D1372468

# CONGRATULATIONS

## You now have access to Mosby's "Get Smart" Bonus Package!

### Here's what's included to help you "Get Smart"

**sign on at:**

**http://www.mosby.com/MERLIN/medsurg_phipps**

A Web site just for you as you learn maternity nursing with the new 6th edition of Medical-Surgical Nursing

**what you will receive:**

Whether you're a student, an instructor, or a clinician, you'll find information just for you. Things like:

- Content Updates
- Links to Related Products
- Author Information . . . and more

**plus:**

LIFT HERE

PASSCODE INSIDE

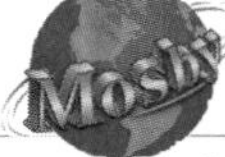


**WebLinks**

An exciting new program that allows you to directly access hundreds of active web sites keyed specifically to the content of this book. The WebLinks are continually updated, with new ones added as they develop. **Simply peel off the sticker on this page and register with the listed passcode.**

If passcode sticker is removed, this textbook cannot be returned to Mosby, Inc.

## Free CD-ROM Companion

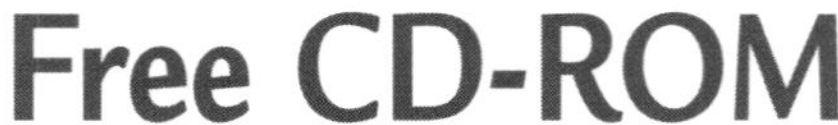

with every copy of Medical-Surgical Nursing, 6th Edition

With Strong Emphasis on Clinical and Functional Relevance this valuable CD-ROM Features:

**Critical Thinking Case Studies**
**Fill-in-the-Blank Questions**
**NCLEX Style Review Questions**
**Vocabulary Review with Sound Pronunciations**

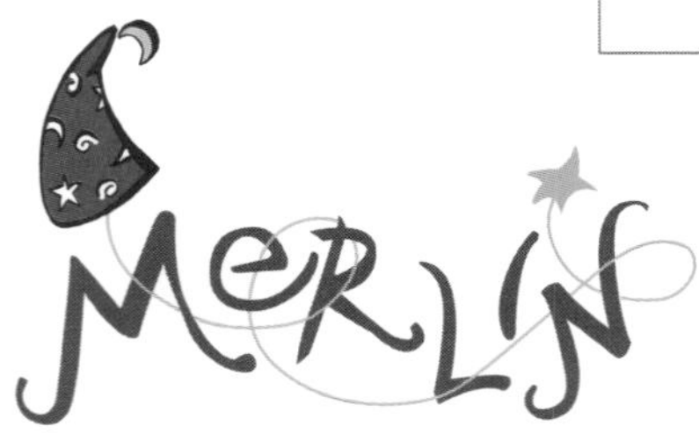


Mosby's Electronic Resource Links & Information Network

Mosby

SIXTH EDITION

# MEDICAL-SURGICAL NURSING

## Concepts & Clinical Practice

**Wilma J. Phipps, PhD, RN, FAAN**
*Professor Emeritus of Medical-Surgical Nursing*
*Frances Payne Bolton School of Nursing*
*Case Western Reserve University*
*Cleveland, Ohio*

**Judith K. Sands, EdD, RN**
*Associate Professor and Director of Undergraduate Studies*
*University of Virginia School of Nursing*
*Charlottesville, Virginia*

**Jane F. Marek, MSN, RN, CS**
*Adult Nurse Practitioner*
*Instructor*
*Frances Payne Bolton School of Nursing*
*Case Western Reserve University*
*Cleveland, Ohio*

*With 906 illustrations*

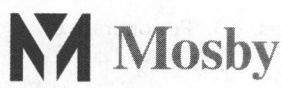


*A Harcourt Health Sciences Company*
St. Louis London Philadelphia Sydney Toronto

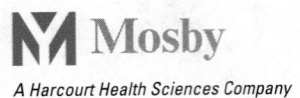

***Publisher*** Sally Schrefer
***Editor*** Michael S. Ledbetter
***Developmental Editors*** Laurie K. Muench and Nancy L. O'Brien
***Project Manager*** Dana Peick
***Project Specialist*** Catherine Albright
***Manufacturing Manager*** Linda Ierardi
***Designer*** Amy Buxton

SIXTH EDITION


A NOTE TO THE READER:
The authors and publisher have made every attempt to check dosages and nursing content for accuracy. Because the science of pharmacology is continually advancing, our knowledge base continues to expand. Therefore we recommend that the reader always check product information for changes in dosage or administration before administering any medication. This is particularly important with new or rarely used drugs.



Printed in the United States of America

Mosby, Inc.
11830 Westline Industrial Drive
St. Louis, Missouri 63146

Medical-surgical nursing : concepts and clinical practice / [edited by] Wilma J. Phipps, Judith K. Sands, Jane F. Marek. — 6th ed.
p. cm.
Includes bibliographical references and index.
ISBN 0-323-00310-9 (alk. paper)
1. Nursing. 2. Surgical nursing. I. Phipps, Wilma J., 1925– . II. Sands, Judith K. III. Marek, Jane F.
[DNLM: 1. Nursing Care. 2. Nursing Process. 3. Perioperative Nursing. WY 150M4894 1999]
RT41.M49 1999
610.73—dc21
DNLM/DLC 98-30558

# Contributors

**Kimberly Adams-Davis, ND, RNC, WHNP, FAAN**
*Assistant Professor*
*Frances Payne Bolton School of Nursing*
*Case Western Reserve University*
*Cleveland, Ohio*

**Martha L. Allen, MSN, RN**
*Chief Operating Officer and Vice President of Nursing*
*University Hospitals Health Systems Bedford Medical Center*
*Cleveland, Ohio*

**Marion Allen, PhD, RN**
*Professor*
*University of Alberta*
*Edmonton, Alberta, Canada*

**Barbara J. Astle, MN, RN**
*Nurse Educator, Faculty of Nursing*
*University of Calgary*
*Calgary, Alberta, Canada*

**Kathryn Ballenger, RN, MSN, CCRN, FNP-CS**
*Instructor of Nursing*
*University of Virginia School of Nursing*
*Charlottesville, Virginia*

**Marilyn Rossman Bartucci, MSN, RN, CS, CCTC, CNN**
*Head Nurse Manager, Transplant Center*
*University Hospitals of Cleveland*
*Cleveland, Ohio*

**Kim Bender-Eggleston, RN, MSN, CEN**
*Administrator, Clinical Management Services*
*University of Virginia*
*Charlottesville, Virginia*

**Mary Jo Boehnlein, MSN, RN**
*Director of Perioperative Services*
*MetroHealth Medical Center*
*Cleveland, Ohio*

**Janet M. Briggs, MSN, RN, CNS**
*Clinical Nurse Specialist/Nurse Practitioner, Infectious Disease*
*Department of Veterans Affairs Medical Center*
*Cleveland, Ohio*

**Mary Vorder Bruegge, RN, MS, CCRN, CNRN**
*Clinician IV, Neuroscience Center*
*University of Virginia Health Sciences System*
*Charlottesville, Virginia*

**Alice Hutchens Carpenter, RN, BSN, CCRN**
*Clinician III*
*University of Virginia Hospitals*
*Charlottesville, Virginia*

**Richard Carpenter, RN, BSN, CCRN**
*Clinician IV*
*University of Virginia Hospitals*
*Charlottesville, Virginia*

**Barbara J. Daly, PhD, RN, FAAN**
*Associate Professor/Co-Director Clinical Ethics*
*Case Western Reserve University*
*University Hospitals of Cleveland*
*Cleveland, Ohio*

**Gladys E. Deters, RN, MSN**
*Formerly Assistant Professor*
*University of Virginia School of Nursing*
*Charlottesville, Virginia*

**Carole A. Drabek, MSN, RN, CNS**
*Clinical Nurse Specialist, Cardiology*
*Department of Veterans Affairs Medical Center*
*Cleveland, Ohio*

**Elizabeth Cameron Eckstein, RN, MSN, CIC**
*Infection Control Nurse*
*Cleveland Veterans Affairs Medical Center*
*Cleveland, Ohio*

**Carolyn Eddins, MN, RN, CETN**
*Assistant Professor of Nursing*
*University of Virginia School of Nursing*
*Charlottesville, Virginia*

**Lisa Forsyth, RN, MSN**
*Clinician IV*
*University of Virginia Health System*
*Charlottesville, Virginia*

**Diane Broadbent Friedman, MSN, RN-C**
*Research Nurse*
*Pennsylvania State University College of Medicine*
*Hershey, Pennsylvania*

**Diane E. Fritsch, MSN, RN, CCRN, CS**
*Clinical Nurse Specialist*
*Trauma Critical Care Nursing*
*MetroHealth Medical Center*
*Cleveland, Ohio*

**Carol J. Green, RN, PhD**
*Nursing Professor*
*Johnson County Community College*
*Overland Park, Kansas*

**Kathy Henley Haugh, MSN, RN**
*Assistant Professor of Nursing*
*University of Virginia School of Nursing*
*Charlottesville, Virginia*

**Shelley Yerger Huffstutler, DSN, RN, CFNP**
*Assistant Professor & Family Nurse Practitioner*
*University of Virginia School of Nursing*
*Charlottesville, Virginia*

**Arlene Keeling, PhD, RN**
*Associate Professor*
*University of Virginia School of Nursing*
*Charlottesville, Virginia*

**Molly Loney, RN, MSN, OCN**
*Clinical Care Coordinator*
*Judson Park*
*Cleveland, Ohio*

**Marilyn S. Lottman, RN, MSN, NP-C**
*Nurse Educator*
*Lake Hospital System, Inc.*
*Willoughby, Ohio*

**Deborah K. Marantides, MSN, RN, CS**
*Adult Nurse Practitioner*
*University Primary Care Practices*
*North Royalton, Ohio*

**Carol Lynn Maxwell-Thompson, RN, MSN, CCRN**
*Faculty*
*University of Virginia School of Nursing*
*Charlottesville, Virginia*

**Jacqueline A. Morgan, MSN, RN, CCRN**
*Clinical Nurse Specialist/Surgery*
*MetroHealth Medical Center*
*Cleveland, Ohio*

**Diana Lynn Morris, RN, FAAN, PhD**
*Associate Professor of Nursing*
*Frances Payne Bolton School of Nursing*
*Case Western Reserve University*
*Cleveland, Ohio*

**Lynn Randolph Noland, RN, PhD, NP**
*Assistant Professor*
*University of Virginia School of Nursing*
*Nurse Practitioner*
*University of Virginia Kidney Center*
*Charlottesville, Virginia*

**Sally J. Reel, PhD, RN, CS, FNP**
*Assistant Professor of Nursing*
*University of Virginia*
*School of Nursing*
*Charlottesville, Virginia*

**Marti Reiser, RN, MSN, CCRN, CNS, NP-C**
*Adult Nurse Practitioner*
*Patricio Aycinena, MD, Inc.*
*Lorain, Ohio*

**Dora A. Rice, MSN, RN, CIC**
*Infection Control Nurse*
*Cleveland Veterans Affairs Medical Center*
*Cleveland, Ohio*

**June Hart Romeo, PhD, RN, NP-C**
*Nurse Practitioner/Researcher*
*Department of Veterans Affairs Medical Center*
*Cleveland, Ohio*

**Helen Schaag, MSN, MA, RN**
*Health Care Consultant*
*Human and System Development*
*Kansas City, Missouri*

**Elizabeth Schenk, MSN, RN, MDiv**
*Pastoral Care*
*Glenbeigh Hospital*
*Rock Creek, Ohio*

**Linda Schuring, MSN, RN**
*Clinical Nurse Specialist*
*Nurse Director, Hearing and Balance Center*
*Mount Sinai Integrated Medical Center*
*Cleveland, Ohio*

**Joan Shettig, FNP, MSN, RN**
*Assistant Professor of Nursing*
*University of Virginia School of Nursing*
*Charlottesville, Virginia*

**Carol E. Smith, RN, PhD**
*Professor*
*University of Kansas School of Nursing*
*Kansas City, Kansas*

**Rachel E. Spector, PhD, RN, CTN, FAAN**
*Associate Professor*
*Boston College School of Nursing*
*Chestnut Hill, Massachusetts*

**Susan B. Stillwell, MSN, RN**
*Clinical Associate Professor*
*Arizona State University*
*Tempe, Arizona*

**Debera Jane Thomas, DNS, ARNP, ANP**
*Associate Professor*
*Florida Atlantic University College of Nursing*
*Boca Raton, Florida*

**Margaret M. Ulchaker, MSN, RN, CDE, NP-C**
*Adult Nurse Practitioner*
*Director of Patient Education/Research Coordinator*
*North Coast Institute of Diabetes and Endocrinology, Inc.*
*Westlake, Ohio*

**Judy Watt-Watson, RN, PhD**
*Associate Professor*
*University of Toronto*
*Toronto, Ontario, Canada*

**Vickie Weaver, RN, MSN, CETN**
*Clinical Monitor: Wound & Skin Care*
*ConvaTec (A Bristol Myers-Squibb Company)*
*Skillman, New Jersey*

**Angela Wilson, MSN, RN, C**
*Instructor*
*Christopher Newport University*
*Newport News, Virginia*

**Arlene Yuan, RN, MSN, FNP-C**
*Assistant Professor*
*University of Virginia School of Nursing*
*Charlottesville, Virginia*

**Lynne C. Yurko, RN, BSN**
*Unit Manager, Burn Center*
*MetroHealth Medical Center*
*Cleveland, Ohio*

**Kathleen M. Zupan, MSN, RN, C**
*Adult Nurse Practitioner*
*VA Medical Center*
*Cleveland, Ohio*

# Reviewers

**Elaine J. Beaupre, RN, BSN, MEd, MSN**
*Instructor*
*Quincy College*
*Quincy, Massachusetts*

**Nancy M. Becker, MS, RN, CS**
*Dean of Allied Health/Director of Nursing*
*Lehigh Carbon Community College*
*Schnecksville, Pennsylvania*

**Carol Boswell, RN, EdD**
*Chairman of Career Ladder Nursing Program*
*Odessa College*
*Odessa, Texas*

**Sylvia E. Bradshaw, MSN, RN**
*Assistant Professor*
*Lenoir-Rhyne College*
*Hickory, North Carolina*

**Anna M. Brock, PhD, RN**
*Professor*
*University of Southern Mississippi*
*Hattiesburg, Mississippi*

**Teresa S. Burckhalter, MSN, RN, C**
*Nursing Faculty*
*Technical College of the Lowcountry*
*Beaufort, South Carolina*

**Joyce B. Campbell, MSN, CCRN, C-FNP**
*Associate Professor*
*Chattanooga State Community College*
*Chattanooga, Tennessee*

**David S. Castelan, RN, BS, CCRN**
*Nursing Instructor, East Los Angeles College*
*Monterey Park, California*
*Charge Nurse Critical Care Unit, Alhambra Hospital*
*Alhambra, California*

**Janet Barkley Coyne, MS, RN**
*Instructor/First Year Coordinator*
*Crouse Hospital School of Nursing*
*Syracuse, New York*

**Hilda Crane-Smith, RN, BSN, MS**
*Assistant Professor*
*Oklahoma State University*
*Oklahoma City, Oklahoma*

**Ruby M. Degener, RN, BSN, MS**
*Assistant Professor of Nursing*
*Catonsville Community College*
*Baltimore, Maryland*

**Rosario T. DeGracia, MS, RN, C**
*Associate Professor*
*Seattle University School of Nursing*
*Seattle, Washington*

**Janet Engstrom, RN, CNM, PhD**
*Associate Professor*
*University of Illinois at Chicago*
*Chicago, Illinois*

**Susan Fowler-Kerry, RN, BA, BSN, MN, PhD**
*Professor*
*University of Saskatchewan*
*Saskatoon, Saskatchewan, Canada*

**Florencetta Hayes Gibson, RN, MEd, MSN, CNS**
*Associate Professor*
*Northeast Louisiana University School of Nursing*
*Monroe, Louisiana*

**Susan K. Giulianetti, MSN, RN, C**
*Family Nurse Practitioner*
*Cleveland Veterans Administration Medical Center*
*Cleveland, Ohio*

**Sister Janet Goetz, CRNP**
*Instructor*
*St. Vincent Health Center School of Nursing*
*Erie, Pennsylvania*

**Susan Stabler Haas, MSN, RN, CS**
*Faculty*
*West Chester University*
*West Chester, Pennsylvania*

**Thelma L. Halberstadt, RN, BSN, MSN, EdD**
*Professor of Nursing*
*Northern Essex Community College*
*Lawrence, Massachusetts*

**Diane Bronkema Hamilton, PhD, RN**
*Associate Professor*
*Western Michigan University*
*Kalamazoo, Michigan*

**Mary E. Hanson-Zalot, RN, MSN, OCN**
*Level IV Coordinator*
*Northeastern Hospital School of Nursing*
*Philadelphia, Pennsylvania*

**Peggy Jenkins, RN, CCRN, BS, MS**
*Associate Professor*
*Hartwick College*
*Oneonta, New York*

**Jennifer Johnson, RNC, BSN, MSN**
*Assistant Professor of Nursing*
*Kent State University*
*New Philadelphia, Ohio*

**Jo Ann Johnson, RN, MSN**
*Director, Sisters of Charity*
*St. Joseph Hospital*
*Southeast Texas Home Care & Hospice*
*Houston, Texas*

**Grace Labaj, RN, BSN, MSN, PhD**
*Associate Dean, School of Nursing*
*University of Mary Hardin Baylor*
*Belton, Texas*

**Nancy L. Lacey, RN, MSN, CAGS**
*Professor (Retired)*
*Massasoit Community College*
*Brockton, Massachusetts*

**Holly Evans Madison, RN, MS**
*Nursing Faculty*
*Southern Vermont College*
*Bennington, Vermont*

**Deborah Marantides, RN, MSN, CS**
*Adult Nurse Practitioner, University Primary Care Practices*
*Cleveland, Ohio*
*Clinical Faculty, Case Western Reserve University*
*Cleveland, Ohio*

**Edwina A. McConnell, RN, PhD, FRCNA**
*Consultant*
*Madison, Wisconsin*

**Louise M. McGee, RN, MS**
*Professor*
*Tompkins-Cortland Community College*
*Dryden, New York*

**Maria E. Nowicki, PhD, RN**
*Director of Nursing Program*
*Mercy College of Northwest Ohio*
*Toledo, Ohio*

**Sandra O'Sullivan, MS, RN, CCRN**
*Instructor*
*Pennsylvania State University School of Nursing*
*University Park, Pennsylvania*

**Mary Russo-Moldenhauer, MSN, RNC**
*Nursing Faculty*
*Maui Community College*
*Kahului, Hawaii*

**Bruce Austin Scott, RN, CS, MSN**
*Nursing Instructor, San Joaquin Delta College*
*Stockton, California*
*Staff Nurse, St. Joseph's Medical Center*
*Stockton, California*

**Ann Coghlan Stowe, RN, MSN**
*Chairperson/Assistant Professor*
*West Chester University*
*West Chester, Pennsylvania*

**Sylvia Tatman, MSN, RN, CS**
*Associate Professor*
*Palomar College*
*San Marcos, California*

**Cesarina Thompson, RN, PhD**
*Chairperson/Associate Professor*
*Department of Nursing*
*Southern Connecticut State University*
*New Haven, Connecticut*

**Janice Topp, RN, MSN, CNS**
*Assistant Professor*
*Purdue University North Central*
*Westville, Indiana*

**Georgianna M. Trofimuk-Thomas, EdD, RN**
*Associate Professor*
*Concordia University*
*Oak Park, Illinois*

**Ann H. White, RN, MSN, MBA**
*Assistant Professor of Nursing*
*University of Southern Indiana*
*Evansville, Indiana*

**Pamela G. Yancy, MSN, RN, CNS**
*Assistant Professor*
*Spalding University School of Nursing and Health Sciences*
*Louisville, Kentucky*

**Marilyn Zierath, ARNP, MS, CETN**
*Medical Surgical Clinical Nurse Specialist*
*Certified Therapy Nurse in Enterostomal*
*Coordinator/Instructor*
*Licensed Practical Nurse Program*
*Clover Park Technical College*
*Tacoma, Washington*

We dedicate this book:

*To Charlie*

**WJP**

*To Mom and Dad for a lifetime of love and support, and to Eric and David who make it all worthwhile*

**JKS**

*To my son, Ian, and in memory of my parents, James F. and Helen Marek*

**JFM**

## MEMORIAM

*Virginia L. Cassmeyer, PhD, RN, ARNP, who served as an editor of the fourth and fifth editions of this textbook, died suddenly at the age of 51 on October 29, 1997. Dr. Cassmeyer began contributing chapters to this textbook with the first edition.*

*Dr. Cassmeyer was an Associate Professor of Nursing at the University of Kansas Medical Center at the time of her death. Her PhD was in physiology, and her major research interest was management and control of diabetes.*

*As an editor she brought knowledge, dedication, and creativity to planning for this textbook. She was actively involved in teaching undergraduate nursing students and was interested in developing a textbook that would inspire and challenge students to become the best practitioners possible.*

*Dr. Cassmeyer was recognized as an outstanding teacher and received two teaching awards while an Assistant Professor at the Frances Payne Bolton School of Nursing at Case Western Reserve University, where she taught after completing her MSN there. She moved to Kansas in 1980 to enter the PhD program in physiology at the University of Kansas. While an Associate Professor in the School of Nursing at the University of Kansas Medical Center, she received the Jayhawker RN Teaching Award three times. She was also the recipient of the Chancellor's Distinguished Teaching Award in 1990 and 1998, the last awarded posthumously in May, 1998.*

*Dr. Cassmeyer's other honors include the Award for Excellence from the Frances Payne Bolton School of Nursing Alumni Associate and Graduate Student Research Presentation Award from the University of Kansas. She was a member of Sigma Theta Tau and Sigma Xi.*

*Her contributions to nursing were many, and she is missed by her former students and many colleagues who are better for knowing her. We will remember Virginia always as a kind, sensitive woman who was devoted to the nursing profession and who willingly shared her knowledge, skills, and expertise with others. We are grateful for her contributions to this textbook.*

# Preface

As the year 2000 approaches, health care delivery in the United States continues to evolve from a primarily hospital-based system to a more diverse delivery system. We have attempted to reflect the changes in the delivery of health care and, thus, in nursing management of care to patients in this revision. Our aim has been to make the content of this revision relevant to the care of the person with a medical-surgical problem, regardless of the setting in which care is being given. We believe that the changes in health care present exciting challenges to nurses, and it is our goal to provide a textbook that assists nurses to meet these challenges. To achieve this, we have sought out clinical experts to write or consult on each of the chapters. Some of our contributors are new to this revision, other contributors have been involved in several editions.

As in previous editions, we refer to the recipients of the services of nurses as *patients* rather than *clients*. Although the word *client* is widely used in the nursing community, we have been interested in the distinction between the two terms. The article, "Complexities and clarity in nurse-client and nurse-patient relationships," by L. Nowakowski, published in the July-August 1985 issue of the *Journal of Professional Nursing*, addresses the distinctions in the two terms. Using her framework, we believe the use of *patient* in this textbook is appropriate. We found her article to be thought-provoking, and we recommend the article to our readers.

## ORGANIZATION

The sixth edition is organized into two parts: Part One, Perspectives for Nursing Practice with Ill Adults; and Part Two, Alterations In Human Functioning. Part One is divided into five units: Perspectives for Health and Illness covers content on managed care and nursing practice in a managed care environment, cultural care, health promotion and prevention, nursing practice with elders, and ethical decision making; Common Concepts for Care of Ill Adults focuses on stress, chronic illness and rehabilitation, and loss, grief, and dying; Common Problems Encountered in the Care of Ill Adults discusses inflammation and infection, cancer, pain, sleep disorders, substance abuse, fluid and electrolyte imbalance, acid-base imbalance, and shock; Perioperative Nursing includes pre-, intra, and postoperative content; and Special Environments of Care focuses on emergency care, critical care, and home care.

Part Two, Alterations in Human Functioning, contains six units focusing on care of persons with specific alterations in body systems. Each system begins with an assessment chapter followed by one or more chapters on the management of persons with disorders of that system. All chapters have been revised to reflect current knowledge in these fields.

## FEATURES

Every chapter offers a consistent format presentation to enhance learning including:

- **Chapter Objectives** at the beginning of each chapter help the student focus.
- **Critical Thinking Questions** at the end of each chapter are designed to test the student's critical thinking and problem-solving skills.
- **Chapter Summaries** at the end of each chapter provide a brief overview of the content from the chapter.

**Assessment Chapters** provide a clear, logical format including:

- Detailed discussions of Anatomy and Physiology, Subjective and Objective Data, and Diagnostic Tests.
- **New**, each chapter includes **Gerontological Assessment** boxes to highlight unique elements to consider in the care of older adults.

**Management Chapters** have been revised to reflect today's approach to care of patients with specific conditions and include:

- **Comprehensive disorders format** presentation includes Etiology, Epidemiology, Pathophysiology, **new** Collaborative Care Management, Nursing Management, Gerontological Considerations, Special Environments of Care, and Complications.
- **New Collaborative Care Management** sections reflect the blurring of traditional lines in health care today. The interventions of health professionals are discussed as collaborative care management without artificial distinctions as to which professional plays which role with the patient. This care is frequently delivered in the community setting.
- **Nursing Management** sections utilize the five-step nursing process format—Assessment, Nursing Diagnoses, Expected Patient Outcomes, Interventions, and Evaluation—and are designed to reinforce the thought process of the nurse during the care planning process. The importance of education for self-care is reflected in a **new** subsection of Interventions entitled Patient/Family Education, a role typically fulfilled by the professional nurse. This helps the student teach patients and families about the care of conditions. Concluding each section of Evaluation are special sections on Gerontological Considerations, Special Environments of Care including **new** Critical Care Management and Home Care Management, and Complications all to provide an understanding of these considerations in the care of conditions.

- **Nursing Care Plans** include clinical situations and use nursing diagnoses and expected outcomes to guide the student in selecting interventions.
- **Clinical Pathways** (eighteen actual examples) are included in select Management chapters to provide students with samples of this collaborative clinical tool.
- **Research** boxes are integrated throughout to provide applications to today's nursing practice.

## NEW FEATURES

- **Full Color Design and Illustration** program enhances the visual appeal to engage the student in the content.
- **Interactive CD-ROM** included with the book provides the student with an exciting tool to complete critical thinking case studies, study and review questions. The CD will also include a key term review with sound pronunciations for students to practice pronouncing words correctly.
- **Patient/Family Teaching** boxes provide students with key information to teach patients and their families about care of conditions.
- **Health Promotion and Prevention** is integrated throughout as a special subsection to Patient/Family Education and in boxed summaries of *Healthy People 2000* goals to highlight important information related to promoting healthy lifestyles and preventing disease.
- **Guidelines for Care** boxes provide step by step instructions for the nurse to follow in caring for specific conditions.
- **Common Medications** tables highlight drugs commonly used in the treatment of specific conditions.
- **Clinical Manifestations** boxes summarize important indications related to certain conditions.
- **Risk Factors** boxes alert the student to important considerations in the care of specific conditions.

## ANCILLARIES

- **Instructor's Resource Manual and Test Bank** includes chapter overviews and teaching suggestions for classroom and practice applications. The test bank has been updated to include 1500 questions in N-CLEX format.
- **Study Guide** has been revised to include more activities, questions, and case studies designed to enhance student learning and stimulate critical thinking.
- **Computerized Test Bank CD-ROM** is the printed test bank from the Instructor's Resource Manual available in hybrid format for Windows or Macintosh users.
- **Mosby's Electronic Resource Links and Information Network (MERLIN)** allows the instructor and student to directly access numerous active web sites keyed specifically to the content of *Medical-Surgical Nursing: Concepts & Clinical Practice, 6th Edition.* Sign on at http://www.mosby.com/MERLIN/medsurg_phipps.
- **Mosby's Electronic Image Collection CD-ROM** provides the instructor with over 100 full color images from the text to enhance their lectures. Images may be imported to presentation software programs or printed out to create transparencies.
- **Mosby's Medical-Surgical Nursing Video Series** includes 12 videos covering major disorders or disease states.


## ACKNOWLEDGMENTS

We welcome Jane F. Marek as a new editor. Jane, who was a contributor to the fifth edition, has an extensive background in operating room and orthopedic nursing. She teaches medical-surgical nursing and is a certified adult nurse practitioner and certified clinical specialist.

We note with sadness the death of Dr. Virginia L. Cassmeyer, who was an editor of the fourth and fifth editions and a chapter contributor since the first edition of this textbook. Dr. Cassmeyer died unexpectedly in October 1997 (see the Memoriam).

Many experts have contributed to the preparation of this sixth edition. For some of them this is their first contribution to this text while others have been involved in more than one edition. We have attempted to make this edition as up-to-date as possible, and we are indebted to all the contributors for sharing their knowledge and expertise with our readers.

We also wish to acknowledge the comments and suggestions of the reviewers who read each chapter. We found their comments to be very helpful, and we trust that they will be pleased with the changes made in response to their suggestions. We would like to acknowledge in particular the extensive review and editing efforts throughout the entire book of Dr. Edwina McConnell of Madison, Wisconsin.

We wish to thank the illustration and composition team at Graphic World who revised the illustrations to reflect the full-color style for this edition. We hope our readers will find the new full-color format and many new illustrations both visually appealing and educational.

We are grateful to Michael Ledbetter, Nancy O'Brien, Laurie Muench, Dana Peick, Catherine Albright, and Amy Buxton for their support and assistance during the preparation of this sixth edition.



**Wilma J. Phipps**
**Judith K. Sands**
**Jane F. Marek**

# Contents

# MEDICAL-SURGICAL NURSING

Concepts & Clinical Practice

chapter 1

# Issues Affecting Adult Health Care

HELEN A. SCHAAG and WILMA J. PHIPPS

## objectives *After studying this chapter, the learner should be able to:*

1. Identify changing characteristics of American society and their implications for nursing.
2. Identify factors that have affected the evolution of the health care system in the United States.
3. Discuss the evolution of health care insurances, including prepaid types, preferred provider organizations, health maintenance organizations, and governmental plans, and their effect on health care facilities, physician practice, and nursing practice.
4. Explain the reasons for the proliferation of ambulatory care centers, home health care services, and long-term care facilities.
5. Discuss the differences between total patient care, team and functional nursing, primary nursing, and case management nursing care.
6. Identify characteristics of potential nursing students and factors that will influence their choice of nursing as a profession.
7. Describe characteristics of nursing schools and nursing practitioners in the twenty-first century.
8. Identify three reasons why total quality management and continuous quality improvement are important aspects of the practice of nursing.
9. Describe six standards of clinical nursing practice developed by the American Nurses Association.
10. Describe how patient outcome variances are used to improve quality of care.
11. Discuss the reasons why interdisciplinary relationships have replaced autonomy of professionals in managed care settings.

Rapid changes in society during the past decade have had profound effects on the health care industry in the United States. Access to care, quality of care, and cost of health care are the most complex and debated issues in the country. These issues have significant implications for the role of nurses and how nursing is practiced now and in the future. This chapter focuses on several major factors that affect these issues and discusses anticipated trends and changes.

## CHANGES IN AMERICAN SOCIETY

### GROWTH OF THE ELDERLY POPULATION AND ITS CARE

Elderly persons, those individuals 65 years of age and older, are the fastest growing segment of our population, and persons 85 years of age and older are the fastest growing portion of the elderly population. By the year 2000, the "old-old" population—those 85 years of age and older—will increase by 30% to a total of 4.6 million. At that time, 35 million people, or 13% of the population, will be 65 years of age or older. By the year 2020, it is expected this number could increase to 51 million. From 1946 to 1964, the most recent baby-boom period, there were 76 million births.[59] This baby-boom generation will be entering the elderly age range beginning in the year 2011. By the year 2030, there will be only three active workers for each retired person, compared with five workers for every retired person today.

The increase in longevity and a simultaneous decline in the birth rate are being experienced by all Western societies. Because of these societal changes some lawmakers have suggested that the eligibility age for retirement under Social Security and access to Medicare coverage be raised from 65 to 67 or 70 years of age. If this suggestion should become law, it would have profound effects on our culture, health care needs, the composition of the workforce, and the work environment itself.

For the aging who live in their own homes, it is evident that additional facilities for their care and well-being, including health care, must be provided. In addition to home health care services, a comparatively new development—the day care center for the chronically ill and the elderly adult—shows evidence of becoming an important part of the health care scene. Such centers would be welcomed by adult working children who care for elderly parents and find it difficult to provide a supervised and structured environment for them. At present, there is minimal third-party reimbursement for this type of service. Medicare does not usually provide reimbursement even though it would be more cost-effective to pay for this type of care than to pay for care in the person's home or in a nursing home.

## GROWTH OF MULTICULTURALISM

The rapid growth of multiculturalism in the United States is another change dramatically affecting the health care industry. The challenge for the health care industry is twofold: as employers of multicultural staff members and as providers of care to multicultural patients. In addition to the expected communication problems, cultural diversity creates the potential for significant problems when there is conflict between the values, beliefs, and attitudes toward treatment and health-promotion practices.[25] Currently, 71% of the United States population is white, 12% is African American, 9% is Hispanic, 7% is of Asian–Pacific Islands origin, and less than 1% is Native American and Inuit.[56] By the year 2000 there will be a decrease to 62% for the white population, with increases to 10% for the Hispanic and 9% for the Asian–Pacific Islands groups.[57] Not only will the workforce be older; it will be more racially and ethnically diverse.[50]

## NEWER HEALTH CARE PROBLEMS

Besides the pressure for health care reform, several patient care challenges have had and will continue to have a profound effect on nursing and the health care industry in the United States. Four of the most significant challenges are care of human immunodeficiency virus (HIV)-positive and acquired immunodeficiency syndrome (AIDS) patients, ethical dilemmas in health care, violence and abuse, and the poor and homeless.

### HIV Infection and AIDS

Although AIDS emerged in 1981 as an unidentified killer of young men, there is still neither a cure for the disease nor a preventive vaccine. The HIV was identified in 1981 as the virus that caused AIDS. The diseases associated with HIV-positive status and AIDS are pandemic (worldwide). At this time 14 million persons worldwide are HIV positive and, of these, more than 3 million are women of childbearing years. Worldwide, 2.5 million people have AIDS.[47] At the end of 1995, more than half a million cases of AIDS had been reported in the United States with a 62% death rate. Approximately 45,000 Americans died of AIDS in 1995.

At present, the largest proportionate increase in reported cases of AIDS is among women, and it is the fourth leading cause of death among women 25 to 44 years of age in the United States. Heterosexual contacts account for the largest proportionate increase in reported cases of AIDS, whereas the incidence of AIDS among homosexual and bisexual persons has decreased. Although homosexual/bisexual men and injecting-drug users still constitute the largest populations in the United States who are HIV positive or have AIDS, the heterosexual population is the most rapidly growing group to become infected. Among men aged 25 to 44 years of age, HIV infection was the leading cause of death in 1997.

In light of the already existing crisis in health care in the United States, the cost associated with providing the necessary care for persons with HIV infection or AIDS is significant. (See Chapter 67 for a detailed discussion of HIV infection and AIDS.)

### Ethical Dilemmas

The administrators and board of directors of each health care facility must identify the basic culture and operating values of the institution to provide the basis for the overall direction and values of the organization. This includes beliefs about how personnel will be managed and valued and how the organization and its personnel will value and treat patients. Patient care outcomes that are unmet or ethical issues that occur can be identified through continuous quality improvement (CQI) activity, which is discussed in more detail later in this chapter.

There are several reasons to focus ethical decision making on CQI activity. First, the rapidly increasing advances in health care will provide more options for patients and providers. Heart transplantation for one patient, for example, means that a family must agree that the heart of a comatose patient who is on a ventilator can be sacrificed. Balancing of individual rights with social good will become more frequent and more difficult in the future. Second, as resources continue to diminish, problems of distributive justice will arise. It is quite possible that in the future some type of health care rationing will exist. For example, who should receive what services? How much? Who should pay? As public policymakers attempt to reduce all care choices to cost-benefit analysis, the nurse must be able to see beyond these calculations and the inability of them to account for human pain and suffering.

Third, nurses, as well as other health care professionals, must participate in ethical decision making or risk losing their unique influence. For example, in cases of the comatose, terminally ill patient, peer review would focus not only on the clinical aspects of death but also on the human dimension. Did the health care provider keep the patient or family members, or both, totally informed? Were the providers guided by the wishes of the patient and family? Did the provider seek competent, objective, and relevant third-party opinions? None of these decisions can be made irrespective of federal or state laws, but questions of quality lie within the realm of CQI activity.

The *Patient Self-Determination Act of 1990* provides persons 18 years of age and older the right to make decisions about their health care, including the right to accept or refuse treatments and the right to formulate advance directives.[45,48] This law strengthens the patient's legal right to make treatment decisions. Advance directives are documents completed in advance of serious illness that indicate an individual's treatment choices during illness or that name someone to make these choices if one becomes incapacitated. Advance directives, such as living wills and durable powers of attorney for health care decisions, provide legal directives for the kind of life-prolonging medical care when one becomes terminally ill and unable to make decisions. Most states have their own living-will laws and forms, and these laws vary somewhat from state to state. Although the Patient Self-Determination Act became effective in December 1991, many individuals have not completed the formal paperwork that is now asked for upon admission to a health care facility. The law requires hospital staff members to ask all persons admitted to a hospital or other health care facility with the capacity to understand the question if they have completed an advance directive; if they have not, they are asked if they would like to do so. If patients have their advance directive form, they are asked if the directives are still current and a copy of the form is placed in their medical record. If a person wants to complete advance directives during admission, representatives will assist the patient to do so. A patient may change his or her mind about specific requests in the directives at any time the person has the capacity to make changes.

Ethical decision making is discussed more fully in Chapter 5.

### Violence and Abuse

The United States is rapidly becoming a more violent society. Public health officials describe a virtual epidemic of youth violence, spreading from the inner cities to the suburbs. Handgun violence is the second leading cause of death in the teen population in the United States. Death from handgun violence also is the leading cause of death in men aged 18 to 24 years. Each year for the past several years approximately 50,000 people were murdered in the United States, and a woman is physically abused every 18 seconds. The incidence of rape also was increasing at an alarming rate. However, in 1995 FBI figures indicated that the rate of rape and other violent crimes decreased for the first time in several years and have decreased each year since. Almost all these victims of violence go to emergency centers for treatment, and, typically, many of the victims of violence do not have any health insurance coverage.

### The Poor and the Homeless

A population that has always been of concern to nurses is the poor. Since the 1980s a population that is of equal concern and that overlaps the poor population is the homeless. Most of the poor and homeless are women and children. There is a greater distance now than in the past between the "haves" and the "have nots" of our society. The number of persons able to pay for increasingly expensive health care insurance is decreasing. Among the more than 40 million Americans who do not have health care insurance are those who have lost their jobs or those who work at low-paying jobs or who can find only part-time work (without health care insurance). The number of uninsured Americans is projected to increase to nearly 46 million by 2002 because fewer workers will be covered by employer health plans.

Many people are homeless, often as a result of job loss or discharge from a mental institution or from another custodial living arrangement without proper follow-up care. Nurses have been and continue to be concerned with these problems. One result of such concern is a clinic established in Atlanta by three nurses, two of them nurse practitioners, for care of the homeless of that city.[55] (For examples of other such clinics see references 17 and 53.)

Nurses may be confronted by any of the issues just mentioned. However, many nurses need support in clarifying their own values, especially when they may differ from those of the persons for whom they are caring. Inservice education programs for nurses related to these topics are helpful. Knowledge about the details of pertinent laws is essential. Ability to use an ethical decision-making model and apply ethical principles in practice is also necessary (see Chapter 5).

## TECHNOLOGICAL ADVANCES

Technological advances have changed health care in the United States in many significant ways. Technology has saved the lives of patients with conditions that only a few years ago would have proved fatal. Diagnostic advancements (1) in the laboratory with new diagnostic screens, (2) in medical imaging with expanded computed tomographic and magnetic resonance imaging scans and ultrasonic equipment, and (3) in pharmaceutical agents have contributed to the rapid growth in the health care industry. Perhaps the technology that has had the most dramatic impact on health care in the past few years is in the field of fiberoptic scoping, especially laparoscopic procedures for exploratory surgeries, cholecystectomies, hysterectomies, and some cardiothoracic and orthoscopic procedures. This technology has significantly reduced the number of inpatient days and decreased the number of days lost from work. It is estimated that by 2030, 80% of all surgery will be fiberoptic. The expense of all these technological advances has "driven up" health care costs dramatically. Increasingly, questions are being raised about how health care monies should be allocated.

Many of the questions have ethical implications and will require hard decisions. For example, will money be allocated to treat chronic illnesses? Will money be used to treat illnesses associated with lifestyles such as abuse of tobacco, illegal drugs, and alcohol? Will the United States decide on allocation of resources as has been done in Great Britain or Canada, where age is an important variable that determines eligibility for certain procedures?

Another issue related to technology includes the ability to prolong life. At present, billions of dollars are spent annually on neonatal intensive care units that keep extremely small, underdeveloped babies alive. If these babies survive, many have lifetime physical problems that require long-term medical care. At the other end of the life span, prolongation of life—especially for those persons who have not communicated their preference about continuing life by artificial means—continues to be a problem. Approximately 28% of Medicare dollars is spent on persons in their last year of life.

Other technological advances such as joint replacements and organ transplantation are widely discussed issues related to health care. Both of these advances are costly. In addition, organ transplantation raises questions about who will receive an organ when the demand for organs always exceeds the supply. Although a law became effective in the late 1980s requiring hospital staff members to ask family members before a patient's death about organ donation for transplantation, the supply of organs remains significantly below the demand.

Will better informed consumers of health care continue to demand the latest in health care technology, despite cost? Evidence indicates that the demand for new technology will continue to increase because many Americans equate technology with increased quality of life. This demand, in turn, will continue to drive up medical costs. For this reason and others the federal government and other third-party payers have begun to exert controls to prevent further escalation of health care costs.

## COST OF HEALTH CARE

In 1992 the cost to the U.S. government of health care exceeded $830 billion, or about 14% of the gross national product (GNP). By the year 2000, at the projected rate with no changes in the health care system, annual health care costs would be $1.6 trillion, or about 16.5% of the GNP.[57] If this projection becomes a reality, nearly one sixth of the total GNP will be spent on health care, compared with one sixteenth of the total GNP in 1965. The growing concern about cost is coupled with a growing uneasiness that the United States has the most expensive health care system in the world, but its population is not more healthy than people in other developed countries.

At present, those 65 years of age and older account for one third of the health care consumption in the United States. It is estimated that people older than 65 years of age comprise almost half of all hospital admissions. The average length of stay (LOS) for this age group is 8.3 days, approximately 3 days more than for persons younger than 65 years of age.[24] As just mentioned, about one fourth of Medicare dollars are spent in the person's last year of life.[31] "Old-old" persons use more than 10 times the health care resources used by persons younger than 85 years of age, and more than 22% of these persons require institutionalization of some kind.

The nursing home population rose by 24% in the 1980s with most of the growth being from those in the old-old group.[41] In the 1990s most of the 1.8 million people in nursing homes were women, outnumbering men by a ratio of almost 3 to 1. Also, the old-old population occupied 42% of all nursing home beds, an increase of 34% from 1980. Of persons 95 years of age and older, 47% are in nursing homes. About half the population in nursing homes suffer from dementia. Estimates indicate that by 2001, between 14 and 27 million older adults in the United States will need some type of nursing home care.

Long-term care costs have been projected to triple from $42 billion to $120 billion between 1988 and 2018. Data indicate that millions of elderly persons are living at home, usually alone rather than with family members. As a result, they often require some type of assisted-living arrangements. The amount and type of assistance required range from meals on wheels for persons in their own homes, to apartments with special services for elders, to group living homes, to skilled caregivers or home aide assistance in the patient's home.

Many elderly persons could not survive without Social Security. The Social Security system (including Medicare and Medicaid) continues to be viewed by some legislators as consuming too much of the GNP, and these legislators are looking for ways to reduce benefits or to freeze increases. The Social Security Act of 1935 was amended in 1965 to include Medicare health care insurance for those 65 years of age and older and for the permanently disabled. The expanded legislation also established Medicaid, a state and federal cost-sharing program to provide medical services for those meeting certain eligibility criteria linked to income as determined by the individual states. Recently many states such as Oregon have received federal permission to control Medicaid within their states.

Medicare reimbursement has been frozen or reduced several times, and the deductible cost (amount not reimbursed by Medicare) has increased almost yearly since the Medicare program began in 1965. Medicare has two parts: Part A and Part B.

For Part A of Medicare (which covers inpatient care and skilled nursing care) the individual currently is required to pay an annual deductible amount of $736 for each episode of illness. From days 61 to 90 of hospitalization, the patient pays $174 per day as coinsurance. Skilled nursing care coverage (for persons who medically qualify for it) extends for 20 days. If additional care is needed, the individual must pay $88 per day as coinsurance for days 21 to 100. Beyond 100 days of skilled nursing care the patient pays all costs.[34] Most persons carry coinsurance such as a medigap policy, which usually pays for all of the amount not paid by Medicare.

Part B of Medicare (which covers outpatient expenses, physician office fees, home health care, and other defined services) provides reimbursement of 80% of Medicare's schedule for cost after the individual pays an annual deductible amount of $100.[34] Currently, the monthly premium for Medicare Part B insurance is $42.50. Coinsurance usually pays for the 20% not paid by Medicare.

The rates for Part A and Part B usually increase every year. Persons 65 years and older are urged to carry private health insurance, referred to as *medigap* or *tie-in* insurance. Those who cannot afford to purchase medigap insurance may be able to receive Medicaid assistance. The financial implications of a growing society of elders, advances in health care technology, and a declining workforce to finance the cost raise questions about how health care for elders will be financed in the future.

Welfare reform passed by Congress in 1996 has had a profound effect on those who were receiving assistance from the federal and state governments. A major concern is that many infants and children previously covered by Medicaid have no health insurance. As this is being written it is too early to determine what the exact effects will be. The individual states will have to determine how they will provide medical services or whether they will provide medical services to this population when they are no longer eligible for Medicaid.

Another significant factor that increased the cost of health care is the practice of "defensive medicine," in which providers order many expensive diagnostic tests and perhaps unnecessary medications to protect themselves from malpractice law suits. An American Medical Association report shows that 8 of 10 fee-for-service physicians (80%) routinely practice defensive medicine.

## HEALTH CARE IN THE UNITED STATES

The tremendous diversity in this country is reflected in the beliefs, expectations, and sociocultural traditions related to health and health care. The words *health, wellness,* and *illness* mean different things to different people. On a health-illness continuum, a person's own concept often defines his or her state of wellness. The term *health,* as used in health care and health insurance, in reality usually means *illness* in our society.

### HISTORICAL PERSPECTIVE

Because social systems exist for the protection and well-being of their members, it would seem that planning for and providing health care would be of great importance. However, the Constitution of the United States makes no provision for the health care of its citizens. In the eighteenth century, health and illness were considered to be individual concerns and were taken care of within the family or community. For many years, waves of immigrants brought with them their own ways of maintaining health and coping with illness, much of which was outside of organized medical care.

Over time, government at several levels became involved in health care. In the early years the federal government established a hospital for merchant seamen, which became the nucleus of the United States Public Health Service. Individual states have been semiautonomous from the beginning of the nation, and they soon found it essential to establish rules and regulations to protect public health in such areas as safe drinking water and food and the threat of communicable diseases. Some cities, especially those on the eastern seaboard, established hospitals to care for homeless immigrants and others who became public charges because of communicable diseases or mental or other illnesses. For example, New York City developed a complex hospital system that was publicly supported from its beginnings.

Today the Social Security Administration, which has overall responsibility for Medicare and Medicaid, is within the Department of Health and Human Services. The Department of Veterans Affairs, which operates one of the largest hospital and ambulatory care services in the world, became a cabinet-level agency in 1991. The legal responsibility for all of these services lies within the domain of the United States Congress.

Another factor in the evolution of health care in the United States is the philosophy of individual initiative and private enterprise. Except for those conditions that threaten the health of large segments of the population and thus come under the aegis of public health, the delivery of health care traditionally has been on a fee-for-service basis.

Every industrialized country in the world today, except the United States, has some kind of national health system that guarantees a basic level of care to all its citizens. In developing countries, the provision of basic health care is usually one of their early goals. National health systems begin with the premises that (1) there should be a minimum of health care services for all citizens, (2) whatever health care is available should be equally available to all, and (3) resources above the minimum should be distributed according to need—with any deviation permitted only if those worse off would be made better off.

### APPROACHES TO HEALTH CARE

In the United States a large aggregate of illness care systems, often poorly articulated with each other, continue to exist. There have been many attempts to establish some kind of an organized system, at least to the extent that everyone would be entitled to basic care. In 1965 Medicare, a form of health insurance for persons 65 years of age and older was established under Title XVIII of the Social Security Act. Medicaid, a health insurance plan for welfare recipients that is administered by individual states, was established under Title XIX of the same act. These entitlements still left large segments of the population without any assurance that they would receive essential care when ill or in need.

During the 1970s some form of national health insurance for U.S. citizens seemed inevitable, even though it was not determined how soon or how broad such a plan would be.[3,28] However, countervailing forces—most of them economic concerns of physicians, hospitals, and other providers—prevailed, and no national plan was agreed on. During the 1970s and 1980s health care cost increased dramatically for a variety of reasons, including inflation, cost shifting of hospital expenses to private payers, and the introduction of more sophisticated technology. In response to these increased health care costs, some employers reduced health care benefits, others increased copayments for employees, and some canceled all health care benefits. At the same time, as new technology became available, everyone expected to benefit from it no matter what the cost.

By the early 1990s legislators and taxpayers acknowledged that not only are the health care systems in the United States out of control relative to cost, but approximately 40 million Americans have no health insurance and another 35 million are believed to be underinsured. The reality of these data can be seen in the number of persons who use emergency departments (the most expensive place to receive health care) as their only access to health care. A survey in four metropolitan areas in the United States indicated that one third to one half of all emergency room patients were seeking help for primary care needs.[42] Health-wellness data in the United States reveal that infant mortality is almost as bad as that of developing countries, and many illnesses that previously were not problematic are now becoming public health crises.

### ILLNESS CARE

Historically, most health care in the United States was really illness care provided by physicians in solo or group practices, operating on a fee-for-service basis. Today, more and more physicians are being employed by hospitals, health maintenance organizations (HMOs), private insurance companies, public health services (federal, state, and local), the Veterans Administration, and the military services. All physicians must be licensed by the state in which they practice, and they continue to be the "gate-keepers" for illness care in the existing health care systems.

Most hospitals in the United States were built during the first decades of the twentieth century when scientific medicine was developing rapidly, and physicians and surgeons needed a workplace for their activities. Even the smallest communities believed they needed a hospital, and they worked hard to obtain one. Fund drives, private philanthropy, and taxes were used to build, maintain, and add to hospitals to meet community needs. The Hill-Burton Act of 1946 provided more than $3 billion of federal tax money to communities over a 25-year span to build or to improve hospitals throughout the country. As a result of this Act, great medical complexes were developed—sometimes more than one in a large city. Medical care became more and more concentrated in large cities while rural areas were underserved. Within these large medical complexes (often associated with schools of medicine), research and technology were producing the miracles of modern medical science.

In the 1960s and 1970s health care insurance began to assume more and more importance as health care costs, both in and out of hospitals, rose sharply. Initially, health insurance was purchased by employers for their employees or by individuals for themselves and their families. Then it was purchased by groups to share cost and spread liability.

The late 1980s saw a dramatic shift of more patient care activity to outpatient areas. Although hospital admission traditionally has been through the patient's personal physician, the number of hospital admissions from hospital emergency departments has increased dramatically. During the 1970s alternative, nontraditional access to health care developed, such as storefront clinics, shopping mall clinics, and mobile screening vans.[35]

## HEALTH CARE INSURANCE

Since the mid 1980s major changes have occurred in the health care insurance options for subscribers and employers. As the cost of health care benefits for employees began to escalate, employers sought ways to reduce these expenditures. Some asked their employees to share some of the costs and introduced the "80-20" plans, which required employees to pay 20% of the cost of their health insurance. Other employers contracted with HMOs or preferred provider organizations (PPOs) to provide health care services to their employees. By 1992 only 4% of workers in public or private settings with more than 200 employees selected a "traditional" type of health care insurance that used no form of precertification or managed care.[19]

### Prepaid Health Care Insurance

The traditional type of health care insurance, such as that offered by Blue Cross and other insurance companies, played a large role in the interplay of health and illness care in the United States. At one time prepaid health insurance represented a small segment of the insurance industry. Blue Cross first offered the prepaid health care insurance plan in 1929. Rapid growth in health insurance coverage, however, did not occur until after World War II. Originally, Blue Cross paid the hospital for all service charges, and Blue Shield paid physicians an agreed amount. With this type of coverage, the subscriber usually had to pay no additional cost, and no questions were asked about the necessity for treatment or surgery. Although this type of coverage is still available, fewer people use it because of its higher premiums.

Health care insurance plans paid for all health care expenses submitted by hospitals with no questions asked. Health care insurance companies continued to raise their premiums to cover their expenses. Eventually, some businesses could no longer afford health care coverage as a benefit for employees and dropped the benefit; thus employees were left with no coverage unless they paid for their own health insurance. Although traditional health insurance is still available, the number of subscribers has declined to about 25% in 1996,[44] as other options became more cost-efficient for the employer and employee.

### Prospective Payment System and Diagnosis-Related Groups

From 1965 to 1983 hospitals were paid for the full costs they incurred in caring for Medicare patients. Whatever the cost, Medicare paid the full hospital bill without question. In 1983 Medicare changed the reimbursement system for hospitals from a retrospective payment system to a prospective payment system (PPS). As part of the PPS, hospitals were notified how much they would be reimbursed for Medicare patients based on patient diagnoses. The diagnoses were grouped into diagnosis-related groups (DRGs), and a specific payment and length of stay (LOS) were predetermined for each DRG. If hospitals are able to provide treatment and care for patients for the specified reimbursement, they will break even financially. If hospitals are able to treat and discharge patients earlier than the predetermined LOS, they are still paid the specified amount for the DRG and can make money that they keep. However, if hospitals cannot discharge patients within the specified LOS, they lose money because they are not reimbursed for the additional days of care. Originally there were 467 DRGs. Because some of the DRGs did not reflect the care needs of all patients in that group, additional DRGs were added. Currently there are 492 DRGs with reimbursement rates determined by Medicare.

The DRG and PPS arrangement has been in existence for about 15 years. In examining the success of hospitals in reducing costs, it becomes clear that some of them are becoming more and more competitive as they seek to attract the patient on whom they can make money (such as patients undergoing cardiac catheterization) and avoid admitting those patients on whom they will lose money. As hospitals learned to operate within the DRG system, some hospitals would transfer patients on whom they would lose money to other hospitals under the pretext that the patient required more sophisticated care than they could provide. This practice is known as "dumping." Many such patients were transferred from community hospitals to teaching hospitals in large medical centers. Dumping became such a large problem that in 1986 Congress enacted Public Law 99-272 to prevent this practice. This law, referred to as the "anti-dumping" law, mandates that heavy fines be levied against an agency that violates the law.

Despite the changes made to control health care costs, it is evident that there is a health care crisis. As mentioned earlier, it is estimated that at least 40 million Americans have no health care insurance. Some are uninsured because of major layoffs, which terminated their health care coverage. Others have been dropped by their insurer because they have conditions that require expensive care, such as that required by patients with malignancies, HIV and AIDS, or chronic conditions such as diabetes. These persons are then unable to obtain insurance from another carrier because of their preexisting conditions.

The need for health care reform has been identified by many Americans, and it was a major factor in determining the outcome of the 1992 presidential election. President Clinton proposed a national plan that would provide health care insurance for all Americans. There were two major provisions of the plan. The first was that the insurance was to be portable and no one who was laid off or changed employment would lose this coverage. The second provision of the plan was that no one could be denied insurance because of a preexisting condition. To make insurance of patients who require large amounts of expensive care more equitable, all insurance carriers would be required to insure some of these patients so that the risk is spread among insurers.

The president's plan was not approved by Congress, and emphasis shifted to a balanced budget and welfare reform. Simultaneously one of the options to reduce hospital costs, managed care, was gaining momentum.

## Managed Care Options

Managed care, which has been evolving for many years, refers to a system of insured health care delivery that offers health care coverage but limits the enrollees' choice of providers and self-referrals. In return, employers and enrollees save money on premiums and copayments.

Most health care insurance companies now offer managed care options along with traditional health care insurance plans. The focus of managed care is to provide cost-effective, outcome-oriented care. Through the use of existing patient outcome data, managed care promotes the identification of expected outcomes, time frames for accomplishing these outcomes and processes, and resources required to achieve the expected outcomes before the patient enters the health care system. Thus the provider and the enrollee know in advance the expected and reasonable outcomes. As with all types of managed care and with Medicare and Medicaid, criteria for patient admission, intensity of service, and severity of illness must be stated before approval for admission is granted. This process is referred to as precertification approval. An insurance company can negotiate with selected physicians and hospitals to provide health care to a large number of enrollees at reduced charges. This approach guarantees physicians and hospitals a volume of potential patients.

Today there are two major types of managed care plans: HMOs and PPOs, which are discussed next.[60]

### Health maintenance organizations

The HMO philosophy is to promote wellness and prevent illness in the enrollees and to provide incentives to the health care provider to minimize the use of expensive inpatient care. Enrollees have access to all services but have a limited choice of physicians, self-referrals, and hospitals. Providers usually are paid on a per capita basis. Enrollees pay a set fee for regular preventive and screening services, as well as for illness care. Fees are prepaid, usually on a monthly or yearly basis similar to other insurance plans. Although HMOs have been in existence for more than 50 years, their rapid growth began only about 20 years ago. The HMO model has been adopted by many third-party insurers and by some private medical practice groups, many of which use advanced nurse practitioners as providers.[22] HMOs fare best financially when enrollees are helped to stay well and kept out of the hospital. There are more than 650 HMOs across the country with approximately 70 million enrollees, which is about 25% of the total U.S. population.[44]

### Preferred provider organizations

The rapid growth of PPOs is directly attributable to several factors. These include (1) the response of fee-for-service physicians to the competition from HMOs and (2) actions by third-party health insurance providers to offer PPO services at a reduced rate to their subscribers. In return, the contracted physicians and hospitals are guaranteed that a large number of patients will use their health care services. PPOs provide members with a greater range of choice in selecting "preferred" physicians, hospitals, and providers than do HMOs. Also, enrollees can use a provider or facility not on the preferred list by paying additional money for the services. This variation of a PPO is referred to as the point-of-service (POS) option. In this variation, members have the option of seeking care outside the plan at an additional fee.[20]

### Variations of HMOs and PPOs

Many hybrids and mixed models are emerging from HMOs and PPOs. Thus the names and initials are constantly evolving to reflect a new incentive or plan.

A variation of the HMO is the independent practice association (IPA) option. Within an IPA, physicians provide care out of their own offices instead of a central site.[20] Concerns with the IPA are that it may not be as efficient as an HMO and patient records may become decentralized rather than kept in one location.

Another variation of managed care that seems to be gaining popularity is the Physician-Hospital Organization (PHO). The PHO is still a fairly new phenomenon and the majority of PHOs are owned by their physicians and hospitals.

By 1996, more than two thirds of U.S. households were enrolled in managed care plans.[26] The success and profitability associated with managed care options have led to the development of many more of these organizations. HMOs have experienced a 10% annual increase in enrollment.[26] However, the greatest percentage of increase has been in PPOs. Currently, more than 28% of all U.S. households are enrolled in a

PPO. This is a 16.5% increase since 1994.[26] Continuous quality improvement (CQI) is an important issue with HMOs and PPOs because of a perceived or actual decrease in quality in an attempt to reduce costs and increase profits. A recent survey indicated that consumer satisfaction with Medicare under managed care options has decreased since 1994.[26]

To ensure quality, The Health Care Finance Administration (HCFA) will require managed care plans contracting with Medicare to complete a quality report. Beginning in 1997, the plans were required to use the *Health Plan Employer Data and Information Set* (3.0 version), commonly referred to as HEDIS.[64] This objective tool has more than 60 quality indicators that describe the managed care organization's structure and care delivery processes, such as quality of care, member access and satisfaction; membership and utilization, finance, and health care plan management activities. The National Committee for Quality Assurance (NCQA), which accredits HMOs, supported the development and use of this tool.[23]

#### Managed competition

Managed competition is a phrase commonly used. The organizing principles of managed care are directed at improving quality, managing costs, promoting competition among health care plans, and increasing cost-consciousness on the part of consumers. Many hospitals in large cities are currently practicing many of the principles of managed competition through partnerships, affiliations, and so forth. Experience in countries with universal health coverage has shown that costs can be reduced by focusing on health promotion and prevention of illness.

## HEALTH CARE DELIVERY SYSTEMS

All hospitals or health care delivery systems can be classified into one of two types of ownerships: private and government (public). On the private side, ownership can be grouped into not-for-profit and for-profit organizations. On the government side, ownership can be grouped into federal, state, or local.

### Not-for-Profit and for-Profit Hospitals

The two categories of private hospitals are not-for-profit and for-profit. All hospitals or health care delivery systems seek to make a profit, that is, an excess of income over expenses. How the profits are used is what differentiates the two types. Not-for-profit hospitals use profits to enhance the content or quality of their health services or to control costs. In the United States, more hospitals are not-for-profit than are for-profit.

The goal of for-profit hospitals is to make a profit that is paid to owners/investors. Most often these are large corporations that own several hospitals in a region and/or across the country. In 1997, Columbia/HC HealthCare Corp. was the largest for-profit chain of hospitals in this country. Although some for-profit hospitals have existed for about 40 years, they have proliferated since the 1980s and have become an important segment of the competitive scene in the health care industry. Typically they have concentrated on providing medical and surgical services to those patients who are able to finance their own care, either because they are well insured or because they are financially able to pay for their care. Generally these corporations provide minimal or no care to the medically indigent. They have attracted well-qualified physicians by providing them with the latest technology and equipment, office space attached to their hospitals, an office support system at a reasonable cost, and joint stock-ventures. They also have the resources to build modern, up-to-date hospitals with amenities that are aimed at attracting the paying consumer. Because of their ability to buy supplies and equipment in volume and because of their centralized accounting and billing services, these corporations have been able to control costs and provide a profit for their investors. It appears that they will continue to proliferate and prosper, often at the expense of those hospitals that provide care to all segments of society, regardless of the patients' ability to pay for their care.

It is projected that by the year 2016 at least one third of all hospitals across the nation will be for profit and almost everyone in the United States will be covered by some form of managed care plan.[44]

### Vertical and Horizontal Integration

Hospitals continue to grow larger and more complex each year. To remain competitive they have had to review their methods of offering services. Since the early 1980s, two major changes have occurred in how hospitals organize their delivery of services: vertical and horizontal integration.

Vertical integration of the delivery of care within one hospital involves providing "full-service" delivery of care, including all inpatient care services, skilled nursing care, outpatient care, long-term care, and home health care services. Horizontal integration involves the consolidation of several hospitals into multihospital complexes, which allows for sharing of technology, facilities, and expertise, resulting in economies of scale and increased influence in the health care market.

### Ambulatory Care and Home Health Care Sevices/Long-term Care

The areas of health care delivery that have experienced the most rapid growth (as a result of DRGs, managed care plans, and other cost control measures) are ambulatory care and home health care services. (See Chapter 23 for a detailed discussion of home health care of the ill adult.)

Until the early decades of the twentieth century and before the great boom in hospital construction and use, nearly all illness care was managed in the physician's office or in the patient's home. People were born and died at home. Several agencies for the care of ill people at home developed from the early days of this nation. Many visiting nurse associations were founded to offer help to persons who were ill at home. Many tax-supported public health agencies also provided some care for the ill in their homes, although their first mission was controlling and preventing communicable disease and protecting the health of the public. The term *community health agency* is an overall designation, with the added *home health agency* used to indicate that many expanded services—such as physical therapy and home-maker care—also are available. Many of these agencies began or expanded their services because Medicare paid for the delivery of certain kinds of home health care to the homebound. (See Chapter 7 for a discussion of these services for the chronically ill.)

## NURSING IN THE UNITED STATES

### HISTORICAL PERSPECTIVE

Professional nursing in the United States is about 100 years old, and it has assumed an indispensable role in every aspect of health care delivery. It is the largest professional group involved in health care. Nurses are employed in acute and chronic care hospitals clinics, physician offices, long-term care facilities, home health care services, HMOs, and health care insurance companies. Some are entrepreneurs in private business. The greatest number of professional nurses continue to work in acute care facilities, where the salaries tend to be higher.

### NURSING CARE DELIVERY SYSTEMS

After World War II the hospital and health care industry began its tremendous growth as more and more patients who had health insurance for the first time in their lives entered hospitals for care. As nursing services in hospitals matured, different types of nursing care delivery systems were developed.

The objectives of nursing care delivery systems include assessing the patient, identifying patient needs, providing the necessary nursing care, and evaluating the effectiveness of the nursing care. The patient care goals are short, usually extending only through hospitalization and are based on nursing diagnosis. From the 1940s to the 1990s some remarkable trends, evolutions, and repackaging of nursing care delivery systems have occurred. There have been many attempts to find the ideal way of providing nursing care to groups of persons designated as ill or in need of care. It is likely that all of these models of nursing care delivery systems are used in one form or another, even coexisting within the same organization.

However, today as budget constraints continue to be a major consideration for chief nurse executives (CNEs), the blend of professional to nonprofessional staff continues to change. The use of nursing assistants or unlicensed assistant personnel continues to increase while the number of licensed personnel (RNs and LPNs) decreases. This means that the RN is responsible for supervising the care administered by a mainly unlicensed staff. As this goes to press some hospitals have begun to increase the number of professional nurses in response to dissatisfaction with the quality of nursing care expressed by patients, nurses, and physicians.

#### Total Patient Care

Before World War II total patient care was the usual type of nursing care delivery system. Registered nurses worked almost exclusively in hospitals, and RNs and nursing students gave complete care to patients. At present, total patient care is the typical nursing care delivery system used in intensive care units. This seems appropriate because intensive care patients are critically ill, have an unstable health status, and thus require the expertise and knowledge provided by RNs.

#### Functional and Team Nursing

During World War II many nurses were in the military, and civilian women volunteered to work in hospitals under the sponsorship of the Red Cross. These women were known as "gray ladies" because of their gray uniforms. Many of these volunteers were socially prominent women who had the time to volunteer as their part of the war effort. They were taught basic tasks, such as bathing patients, making beds, and transferring and repositioning patients. After the war, when these women left hospitals, aides were trained on the job to do these tasks, inasmuch as the gray ladies had demonstrated that lay persons could be taught to do these tasks. At this point there was no secretarial help on the nursing unit, and RNs were responsible for transcribing orders and charting on all patients.

After the war, the supply of nurses did not meet the demand for nurses to care for an increased number of hospitalized patients, and a nursing shortage was declared. As the nursing shortage continued, team nursing was introduced as a method to deliver patient care and to make the best use of the limited number of RNs. In team nursing, RNs served as team leaders. They were responsible for assessing all the patients on their team and deciding which ones needed their professional expertise and which ones could be assigned to nursing aides, nursing students, or in some hospitals, practical nurses. The team leader was responsible for developing a nursing care plan for each patient assigned to her team. The nursing care plan was written to provide guidance to non-RN caregivers. The RN administered all medications and treatments for these patients. She or he also gave direct patient care to patients who were judged to have the most complex needs—not always in terms of physical care but often those with the greatest emotional, teaching, and rehabilitation needs. The team held daily nursing conferences to discuss the needs of individual patients. All persons involved with a particular patient attended the conference, reviewed the nursing care plan, and evaluated the care given. The RN team leader revised the patient's plan of care using new data supplied by direct caregivers. A characteristic of functional nursing that differentiates this model from team nursing is the practice of having specific patient care tasks completed for some or all patients by different direct caregivers.

In reality, team nursing usually did not work as conceptualized. The main problems were fragmented care for patients, the lack of time needed by the team leader for effective team planning, and the difficulty of team leaders in finding time to supervise and coordinate the care provided by their team members. Although team and functional nursing continued for many years and even to the present, both models generally are considered by health care providers and by patients to be unsatisfactory because of the fragmentary nature of care.

#### Primary Nursing

In the late 1970s and in the 1980s primary nursing evolved as the method to best care for the increased number of acutely ill patients in hospitals. Primary nursing must be distinguished from primary care, which is discussed later. In the *primary nursing* model, a professional nurse is completely responsible for assessing, planning, implementing, delivering, and evaluating the nursing care given to a relatively small number of patients during their total hospitalization. The essence of primary nursing is to establish a therapeutic relationship between the nurse and the patient to help the patient achieve his or her goals. The primary nurse assumes 24-hour responsibility for all aspects of the patient's care, from admission to discharge on that unit. The designated primary care nurse cares for the same patient throughout the stay on the unit and is accountable for the outcomes of care that result from nursing interventions.

To those who were active in nursing before World War II primary nursing does not appear to be a new method but a coming to full circle. The model was demonstrated early at the Loeb Center for Nursing and Rehabilitation in New York City, where for many years nurses had been providing care through the primary nursing model.[10] Many agencies have since moved to primary nursing because studies indicate that primary nursing is more satisfying both to patients and nurses, and it is more cost-effective than team nursing. It also makes the RNs accountable for the care the patient receives, and this is most important with the emphasis on quality assurance. In the nursing care delivery systems previously mentioned, accountability is hard to determine and sometimes it appears as if "everyone who cares for the patient is equally accountable; thus no one is really accountable." It is generally accepted that primary nursing is a way of organizing work and staff members in a common-sense system based on professional principles. Studies have clearly demonstrated that in addition to the satisfaction of patients and nurses, physicians and other health care providers also are more satisfied with primary nursing, because they know with whom they should communicate their questions and suggestions about the patient.

Primary nursing markedly changed the role of the head nurse, who in the past in some institutions was the only person who gave and received all communications regarding patients. With the complexity of patient care, especially in larger hospitals and medical centers, it is clearly impossible for the head nurse to know all that is necessary to know about 30 or more patients.

Although many positive aspects about primary nursing make it a desirable model as a nursing care delivery system, several problems emerge. Ideally, only RNs should be primary nurses and associate nurses. The fiscal restraints on nursing services under managed care make it almost impossible to employ a sufficient number of RNs to be primary and associate nurses. In addition, the supply of RNs in some areas of the country is not adequate to meet the demand. Thus many hospitals substituted LPNs for RNs as primary nurses or associate nurses. In some facilities, primary nursing was delivered during the day shift when RNs functioned as the primary nurse, and another type of nursing care delivery system was employed on the other shifts. With these alterations, the objectives of primary nursing were soon lost.

The second problem encountered with the primary nursing model was the impact of 12-hour shifts and the increasing number of RNs who work part-time. Twelve-hour shifts are popular because they allow nurses the flexibility of full-time status while working only 3 days a week, with 4 days off to meet personal and family needs. The reality of a primary nurse working 3 days a week means, at best, that the RN will care for a patient only 3 of the 5 days of an average length of stay. The same problem exists when RNs work part-time because these nurses are available only during a part of the average hospital stay. Thus it was impossible for a nurse who works only 1 to 3 days per week to be responsible for patients 24 hours a day, from admission to discharge unless their stay in the hospital is very brief or unusually long.

### Case Management

Case management is the process of identifying, coordinating, and monitoring the implementation of services needed to achieve desired patient care outcomes within a specified period. Managed care health insurance plans are effective in controlling the cost of health care because of their ability to regulate the amount and type of health care provided and to control its cost. Contracted physicians agree on the reimbursement rate for services such as office visits, hospital visits, and surgeries. Contracted hospitals agree on cost-per-day rates for hospital stays, for costs of inpatient and outpatient tests, and so on. Multiple mandatory preapproval processes are involved for many medical interventions, including most diagnostic procedures, second opinions before surgeries, admission to hospitals, and many therapeutic interventions. Most of these controlling activities occur before a patient is admitted to a hospital. After the patient is admitted, managed care plans expect physicians and hospital services to provide quality care that is effective and efficient. If physicians and hospitals meet this expectation, their contracts most likely will be renewed. If physicians and hospital services do not provide quality care that is effective and efficient, it is more than likely that their contracts will not be renewed. Many hospitals have established case management programs to ensure that effective, efficient, and high-quality care is given throughout the patient's hospitalization. The essence of achieving case management goals lies within the nursing case management delivery system. Managed care and case management have the capacity to improve patient care by using nurses throughout the health care delivery system.[15]

#### Nursing case management

Nursing case management is the latest nursing care delivery system, and it is rapidly gaining in popularity. This system complements the expectations of managed care programs: cost-efficiency, effective interventions, and assured quality.[29] On a unit level, nursing case management is a patient care delivery system that combines some of the best qualities from the previously mentioned delivery systems. Nursing case management acknowledges fiscal limitations with staffing dollars and utilizes all levels of nursing personnel. Nurse case managers who are RNs are the key team members. They coordinate, communicate, collaborate, and facilitate all the care given to their caseload of patients.

Nursing case management organizes patient care by case type or major diagnosis and focuses on achievement of predetermined outcomes within specific time frames and resources. The major components of nursing case management are (1) collaboration of care with all health care team members, (2) integration of anticipated patient outcomes with time frames to evaluate clinical practice (use of critical pathways), (3) utilization of principles of CQI and variance analysis, and (4) promotion of professional practice.[36] Some nurses, physicians, patients, and hospital administrators have been highly satisfied with this new delivery system, while others are very dissatisfied with it.

Nursing case management is based on predetermined practice patterns for specified types of patients. The results of care tend to reduce the length of stay for patients, reduce unnecessary diagnostic procedures, and ensure continuous quality of care to patients. These predetermined practice patterns are put into written form in a tool generically referred to as a *critical pathway* (several chapters in Part II of this book give examples of critical pathways). Critical pathways are developed by the appropriate members of the health care team, including physicians, in a collaborative manner for patients with a specified medical condition. Priority for the development of critical pathways is given to patients with medical diagnoses that represent a high volume of admissions, patients with medical conditions that frequently result in complications and increased lengths of stay, and patients with conditions that cause the hospital to lose money.

It is generally accepted that nurse case managers (NCMs) are the key to the success of this nursing care delivery system. It is highly recommended that NCMs be clinical nurse specialists or master's-prepared nurses who can function as collaborators, problem solvers, communicators, facilitators, and enhancers of patient care.[49,58,60] The NCM is usually responsible for a caseload of 10 to 15 patients from admission to discharge as they move from unit to unit throughout the hospital. NCMs work 8-hour shifts and collaborate with all health team members, including physicians, to ensure that practice patterns reflect the predetermined interventions agreed on in the critical pathways.

The activities of NCMs, the implementation of the system, and the follow-up of any variances from the critical pathways are coordinated by a case management coordinator. The NCM has a team that includes RNs, LPNs, and NAs or other unlicensed assistant personnel to provide direct care to patients. The NCM reviews the critical pathway and the patient's response to interventions, with the person providing care to ensure that all desired outcomes are achieved on time and, if not, to determine what factors prevent them from being achieved. The NCM also solves any system, provider, or patient problems that are hindering the achievement of the desired patient outcomes stated in the critical pathway. If the problem is a patient problem—for example, if the patient develops a complication such as a cerebrovascular accident—the NCM documents the problem and in a collaborative manner modifies the critical pathway to match the patient status. Problems affecting the achievement of the patient outcomes as identified on the critical pathway (system, provider, or patient) are handled as *variances,* and these variances are followed up with total quality management/continuous quality improvement (TQM/CQI) activities through the case management committee, which is led by the case management coordinator. Although NCMs are the key to the success of the nursing case management program, the visible support and the involvement of the chief executive officer (CEO), the chief nurse executive (CNE), the chief financial officer (CFO), and the chief of staff (CS) are paramount to the overall success of the case management program (Figure 1-1).

## ADVANCED PRACTICE NURSES

The four categories of advanced practice nurses (APNs) are the clinical nurse specialist (CNS), the nurse practitioner (NP), the certified nurse midwife (CNM), and the certified registered nurse anesthetist (CRNA).[36] Advanced practice nurses involved in the nursing care of medical-surgical patients are the NP and CNS. A discussion of these two roles follows.

In the late 1980s and 1990s changes in the federal laws governing reimbursement of health care providers in federally operated programs enabled advanced practice nurses to be directly reimbursed for services.[36] Direct reimbursement for APNs is still limited to these federally operated programs. Significant barriers to their practice remain, however, in the areas of legal scope of practice, reimbursement, and prescriptive authority.[36,39] Direct reimbursement gives APNs, as primary care

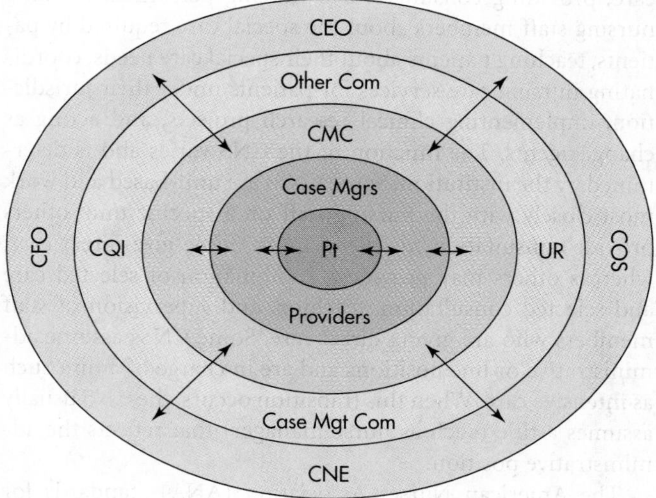


**fig. 1-1** Case management model demonstrating the central role of the patient *(Pt).* The key role of nurse case managers *(Case Mgrs)* and care providers *(Providers)* is emphasized by the central placement of these persons and the arrows showing the continuous interaction. Providers include physicians, nurses, pharmacists, dietitians, respiratory therapists, social service workers, and others.

providers, recognition, credibility, and visibility. An estimated $6.4 billion and $8.75 billion could be saved in the United States annually if APNs were used to their fullest potential as primary health care providers.[46] It is believed to be only a question of time before third-party payment for health care services provided by APNs becomes widely accepted, because research data indicate positive public acceptance, quality care, and cost-effectiveness of their practice.[43]

Primary health care describes the kind of care that most of the people need most of the time. It generally denotes a person's first contact with the health care system. Primary health care may be preventive, including identification of health problems at an early stage, or through a regular screening activity (e.g., mammogram or chest x-ray), or it may be care of patients with minor, noncritical, and chronic illnesses. Results of a 1996 study indicated that certified nurse midwives provided a quality of care that is equivalent to the quality of care provided by obstetricians. Additionally, women cared for by nurse midwives had fewer cesarean sections. Patients were more satisfied with the care provided by nurse midwives than the care provided by physicians relative to the amount of information conveyed, the reduction of professional mystique, and the cost of care.

### Clinical Nurse Specialists

The clinical nurse specialist is a registered nurse who has completed a master's degree program in a clinical specialty—usually with a specified population of patients, such as medical-surgical, maternity, geriatric, or psychiatric patients, or with a population of patients with specific problems, such as renal, cardiovascular, or diabetic patients. Typically, the CNS is in a nonadministrative or a staff position within a hospital or other agency. Duties may include giving direct patient care, providing consultation to nursing personnel, teaching nursing staff members about the special care required by patients, teaching patients about their special care needs, coordinating nursing care services for patients under their jurisdiction, implementing clinical research projects, and acting as change agents. The function of the CNS varies and is determined by the institution. Some CNSs are unit-based and work most closely with the nursing staff on a specific unit; others provide consultation to several units. Some give direct care, whereas others may provide a combination of selected care and selected consultation, teaching, and supervision of staff members who are giving direct care. Some CNSs assume administrative or line positions and are in charge of a unit such as intensive care. When this transition occurs, the CNS usually assumes a title (such as nurse manager) that reflects the administrative position.

The American Nurses Association (ANA) standards for CNS state that the title of *clinical nurse specialist* is limited to nurses with a Master of Science degree in nursing.[3] Further, a nurse must hold this degree to be eligible to sit for the CNS certification examination. However, some hospitals and other agencies employ nurses as clinical nurse specialists, even though they do not have a Master's degree.

### Nurse Practitioners

The title of *nurse practitioner* was first used in 1965 when pediatric nurse practitioners were prepared to provide health care to children in rural areas of Colorado seriously underserved by physicians. Although in the past NPs have been educated in a variety of ways—from very short certificate-awarding programs to master's degree programs—the trend now is toward the latter, because of the broad background of knowledge needed by the practitioner. There are different clinical specialty areas for NPs. The most common ones are pediatric NP, women's health NP, family NP, adult NP, and gerontology NP.[37] Nurse practitioners typically work in primary care settings, providing direct care to prevent illnesses and to treat patients with noncritical, nonacute, minor, or stable chronic illnesses. NPs often manage the medical treatment of patients, using protocols established with physician colleagues.

Until recently, mainly because of the fee-for-service problem, it was more common to find the nurse practitioner in a group practice with physicians and other professional health care providers. However, this is changing, and many NPs are practicing alone or in groups with other NPs. Many are employed by HMOs, mental health centers, schools, and nursing homes. Their practice is in a collegial relationship with other health care providers within the work setting: the NP is a team member in terms of professional expertise in practice, consultation, referral, and planning.

The issues of responsibility and accountability for one's own professional actions are vital in this type of practice. Practice is governed by individual state laws regarding medical and nursing practice, although most state laws allow nurses to practice *nursing* independently.

Although the distinctions between the CNS and the NP may sound fairly clear, it is not always so. Many CNSs practice in facilities other than acute care settings and work in a more generalist role. On the other hand, many NPs work in acute care settings with a specialty group, for example, the neonatal NP. Some authorities believe that there will be a merging of the two titles (NP and CNS) over time.[13,25]

## NATIONAL CERTIFICATION

Many nursing specialty organizations offer certification examinations for nurses practicing in their specialty. Each of these organizations sets its own criteria; many require a certain level of education to sit for the certification examination in a particular area. In many instances the educational requirement is becoming stricter. This is particularly true for nurse practitioner certification and for all certification examinations administered by the ANA. At present the ANA has 29 areas in which a nurse can receive national certification, including certification examinations for clinical nurse specialists.[7] It is important to understand that not all certification leads to advanced practice nursing. See p. 11 for a discussion of the requirements for advanced practice. However, it is predicted that in the future the increasing sophistication of nursing and health care will demand higher educational preparation for nurses sitting for any certification examination.

## CHALLENGES AND OPPORTUNITIES FOR NURSES AND NURSING

Nurses and the nursing profession must be alert to ways in which nurses can have the greatest impact on the changing health care delivery system. Nurses will have to be risk takers in identifying areas where nursing input can affect the health care delivery system. This includes entrepreneurship and incorporation by groups of nurses to provide a variety of services in a wide variety of settings. It will be helpful to nurses and the profession to understand the changes that have occurred in health care delivery, which two experts have called *transformations.*[24a] There transformations are a change from (1) the person as customer to the population as customers, (2) illness care to wellness care, (3) revenue management to cost management, (4) autonomy of professionals to the interdependence of professionals, (5) patient as a nonconsumer of cost and quality to patient as consumer of cost and quality, and (6) continuity of provider to continuity of information.

### RELATIONSHIPS BETWEEN NURSES AND PHYSICIANS

The relationship between nurses and physicians has a significant impact on patient care outcomes.[1,18,52] This relationship is receiving more and more attention as health care organizations look at systems and models to deliver effective and efficient quality care. Health care organizations are realizing that the relationship between nurses and physicians significantly affects the provision of effective and efficient care.

One hallmark of professionalism is autonomy. With the change to managed care the autonomy of professionals is being replaced by interdependence of professionals and other workers.[34] Today physicians, nurses, and managers must involve key stakeholders, including the patient and the population being served, in decision making. It has been difficult for many professionals, especially physicians, to practice in an environment that prescribes what care a patient may receive.

In the past, professionals dominated patient care organizations. Now interdependence has supplanted professional autonomy to achieve both patient care and financial goals. This means that decisions must be reached by consensus and requires a negotiated agreement among health professionals and the customer (patient) about what needs to be done and how it will be done.[24a] The interdependence among physicians, nurses, and administrators calls for an interdisciplinary relationship. The ability to work together involves trust and respect not only of each other but also of the work and perspectives each contributes to the care of patients. Interdisciplinary relationships between nurses and physicians improve patient outcomes and, in many situations, reduce patient costs. Working together is essential to effectively evaluate patient care outcomes, analyze variances in outcomes, and modify necessary practice patterns, resulting in improved quality of patient care.

Many health professionals and patients are concerned about the changes in health care. One evidence of this concern is the book, *Abandonment of the Patient: the Impact of the Profit-Driven Health Care on the Public.*[9] The book has chapters by those who have experienced the changes in hospital care including a patient, a nurse, a physician, a nursing administrator, and a hospital administrator.[9] The nursing administrator comments on her concerns in the following:

> What is badly misunderstood in the work-redesign paradigm is that if the nurse and patient cannot have a sufficient and continuous relationship there can be no care . . . . Our tendency is to measure what the nurse does rather than whether the patient's needs are met. Tasks and procedures are then misconstrued for practice. While there is a place in care-delivery models for persons who assist the nurse, assistive personnel cannot simply be substituted for nurses if care is to be given and received. . . . Resisting change or trying to preserve the status quo will serve no one well, least of all the persons who need care. But the central question is what to change?[9]

The last chapter of the book, "Conclusion: What Can We Do to Protect Quality Care?" presents strategies for those concerned about the present health care crisis. These are publicity, political action, and coalition building, each of which is discussed in detail.[9]

### COLLABORATION BETWEEN NURSING PRACTICE AND NURSING EDUCATION

The many changes in the health care delivery system and pressures on educational institutions are forcing the issue of increased collaboration between education and practice. There has been some movement toward such collaboration for at least 30 years, but today's pressures are causing both nursing service directors and nurse educators to examine the issue even more seriously.

There are several good reasons for collaboration including (1) both groups of nurses have the patient as their focus, (2) nursing education requires a practice laboratory for students, and (3) health care agencies must rely on nursing schools to produce practitioners to work in their agencies. Also, nurses engaged in practice may not have the preparation or time to carry out their own nursing research. However, they can work closely with nursing faculty engaged in research to identify problems that should be systematically studied.

An increasing number of nurses are earning PhD degrees in nursing. This is accelerating the amount of research in areas important to nursing practice. In this regard the National League for Nursing (NLN) recommended in 1993 that the emphasis for nursing research shift to an increase in the number of studies concerned with health promotion and disease prevention at the group and community levels.[40] The findings of nursing research will form a knowledge base for the science of nursing. Nursing scholars are examining the results of this research, identifying theories, and organizing the knowledge derived from research. These results will be incorporated into nursing education and practice as nursing moves toward the future. At present, nurses are examining the use of conceptual frameworks for nursing practice and will be expected to use a conceptual framework to guide their practice. Classification systems and nursing diagnoses will be used to help describe the nursing care delivered to patients. This is essential if the impact of nursing care on a patient's recovery is to be delineated and documented.

## ISSUES IN NURSING EDUCATION

### Nursing Schools in the Twenty-First Century

All the changes discussed have affected and will continue to affect nursing education. In 1993 the NLN[40] and the American Association of Colleges of Nursing (AACN)[2] issued proposals for preparing nurses for the twenty-first century. Both proposals reflect recommendations made in *Nursing Agenda for Health Care Reform,*[4] published by the ANA, and in the Surgeon General's report, *Healthy People 2000.*[62]

With increasing emphasis on health promotion and prevention of illness, the focus of nursing education is changing from the hospital to the community. Students will continue to have experience in acute care and increased experience in community-based, community-focused health care settings. Several schools of nursing have developed community nursing centers, and others are moving to do so. These "nurse-managed care agencies" provide cost-effective, easily accessible, quality primary care with focus on disease prevention and "wellness" care. By the end of 1993 (the latest available figures) revealed that more than 66 nursing schools had established community nursing centers[38] (Figure 1-2). These centers serve as practice sites where students learn from advanced practice preceptors how to function in a community-based, community-focused health care system. An estimated 250 centers are needed to meet the diverse requirements of individuals and communities.[38]

Other possible community practice sites are patients' homes, schools, workplaces, ambulatory settings, long-term care facilities, and shelters for the homeless. The sites used should reflect the community in which they are based and ideally will offer experiences with culturally diverse populations. Because not all university faculty are certified as advanced practice nurses, clinical preceptors for students often are certified APNs in the community agencies in which the students practice. Increasingly, junior faculty are pursuing formal courses to prepare them to sit for an APN certifying examination.

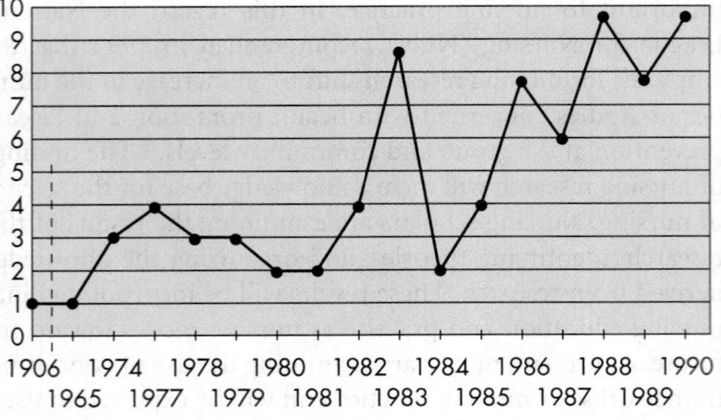


**fig. 1-2** The increase in the number of nursing centers founded per year, based on the NLN/Metropolitan Life Sample.

Skills that students will need to develop are critical thinking, collaboration, shared decision making, a socioepidemiologic viewpoint, and the ability to analyze the effectiveness of interventions in terms of outcomes for individuals, groups, and the community. They also will need to learn how to delegate and work through others to achieve desired outcomes.

To be prepared to function in a new health care delivery system, nurses with baccalaureate degrees desiring to serve as APNs will require advanced degrees.[12]

Because of changes in information processing, all nursing students and practicing nurses must be computer literate. Much of the basic information that nurses need to know will be transmitted by computer-assisted instruction (CAI) and less by textbooks, lectures, and so on. Currently, many nursing programs use CAI materials, and new materials continue to be developed. This knowledge will help nursing students to acquire the vast amount of knowledge they must master to use in their practice. There is no doubt that all nursing programs will need to address the question of how nurses can assist those they serve to *attain, maintain,* or *regain* the highest level of health possible. Although nursing students will gain experience working with patients of all ages in a variety of settings, emphasis needs to be placed on the health care of the rapidly increasing number of elderly persons and on what nurses can do to assist them.

In addition, there is a movement within the profession to move preparation of nursing to the postbaccalaureate level.[54] Case Western Reserve University established the first doctorate of nursing (ND) program in 1979,[32] the second program was instituted at Rush University in 1989, and a third program was founded at the University of Colorado in 1990. In addition, several other schools are considering instituting ND degrees. Continued interest in promoting ND programs was evidenced by a conference on ND education sponsored by the University of Colorado in the spring of 1994. At present some universities (Yale, Pace) offer a generic master's degree.

### The Nursing Doctorate and Generic Master's Degree Programs

The basis for these degrees is the belief that preservice preparation for nursing should be built on a strong undergraduate base as is true in other professions such as medicine, dentistry, pharmacy, or law.[54] In this respect, the establishment of the ND degree is an evolutionary process similar to that which has occurred in comparable professions.

For example, a remarkable increase in the last 25 years has occurred in the number of programs leading to the PharmD degree. Although some universities continue to offer both the bachelor's degree and the doctorate in pharmacy, others have phased out their undergraduate program.

The following reasons support the prediction that the number of ND and generic master's programs will increase in the future.

1. The recognition that current nursing education is too vocational and narrow as it tries to encompass both liberal and professional education in one program[51]
2. The move to have nursing recognized as an autonomous health profession

3. The need to prepare nurses who will be able to function at a higher level and compete for positions in a much more competitive health care system
4. The need to provide nurses with more parity with other health professionals, especially physicians; symbols such as degrees are becoming even more important in today's society
5. The fact that persons making a midlife career change to nursing who already hold a baccalaureate or higher degree in another field are drawn to a degree different from a second baccalaureate degree

## Characteristics of Nursing Students

The population of nursing students is more heterogeneous today than it was 30 years ago, and this heterogeneity will continue. Thus the need to recruit more culturally diverse students and faculty is ongoing. An increasing number of men are entering nursing schools, as well as are women and men who are selecting nursing as a midlife career change. Future students will be more concerned with what the nursing profession has to offer them. Some of the factors that will determine whether potential students will be interested in nursing as a profession are listed in Box 1-1.

## Nursing Supply and Demand

### Staff nurses

Although some experts believe that a nursing shortage persists (ranging from 8% to 12%), in some areas of the country new graduates are having difficulty finding jobs in acute care hospitals. At the same time there is a demand for nurses in home care nursing because of the increased use of sophisticated technology in the home care setting. When possible, agencies providing home care nursing give priority in hiring to nurses with acute care experience who are comfortable with this sophisticated technology.

The decrease in hospital RN positions is the result of several factors. First, the decreased length of stay (LOS) of hospitalized patients has reduced the demand for acute care beds. Second, the number of acute care hospitals throughout the country continues to decrease as more patients are treated in subacute and ambulatory care settings. Third, the number of acute care beds in hospitals continues to be reduced as hospitals "downsize" their operations. Most troubling to nursing, however, is the substitution of less well-prepared workers for RNs.[8] In some institutions whose nursing staff comprised almost 100% RNs, the new goal is a 60% RN and 40% LPN/NA mix.

The rationale for this change is the need to reduce hospital costs, which is achieved primarily by reducing salary costs. Among the troubling issues related to this trend is the threat to quality of care. If RNs are to monitor and supervise staff members who are not registered nurses, they will spend more time in nonpatient care activities and less time providing direct care to patients. In addition, shorter LOSs and more intensely ill patients in hospitals will make it more difficult for fewer RNs to effectively assess, analyze, coordinate, and collaborate in care for more patients during shorter LOSs and yet maintain quality of care. To measure quality of care the entire organization must be committed to TQM and support an effective CQI program. As organizations consider changing the RN staffing mix, an objective means to measure quality of patient care is imperative.

Because of the concern about the quality of care in acute care settings the ANA Board of Directors launched several activities directed toward the safety and quality of patient care and the measurement of outcomes of care.[6] One result of their efforts resulted in Nursing Quality Indicators for Acute Care Settings. The seven quality indicators are listed in Box 1-2.

Because nursing personnel provide the majority of care given in hospitals, nursing leaders need to have a central role in designing new models of patient care. As health care expands to the community, nurses are in an ideal position to develop models of care that improve coordination of care from one health care setting to another.

With the shift of health care from hospitals to the community, some experts predict that acute care hospitals will soon consist only of intensive care beds. Presently experienced critical care nurses are in demand, and this demand can be expected to continue because less well-prepared workers are not able to function effectively in these units.

### Nurses with additional preparation

By the year 2005 the shortage of nurses is estimated to be 600,000: 400,000 at the baccalaureate level and 200,000 at the master's and doctorate levels.[56] The need for more nurse gerontologists is obvious in view of the growing number of

**box 1-1 Factors Influencing Choice of Nursing as a Profession**

1. Status and image of nursing
2. Remuneration when compared with other professions
3. Autonomy of own practice
4. Opportunities for practice

**box 1-2 Nursing Quality Indicator for Acute Care Settings**

1. Nosocomial infection rate (based on urinary infection rate per 1000 patient acute care days)
2. Patient injury rate (based on number of patient falls that result in injury per 1000 patient days)
3. Patient satisfaction with nursing care
   a. Satisfaction with pain management
   b. Satisfaction with educational materials
   c. Satisfaction with care
4. Skin integrity rate per 1000 patient days (number of patients hospitalized 72 hours or more who develop pressure ulcers divided by total number of patient days)
5. Nurse staff satisfaction
6. Mix of RNs, LPNs, and unlicensed staff caring for patients in acute care settings
7. Total nursing care hours provided per patient day

elders. At least 50% of all adult patients in acute care facilities are 65 years of age or older. Further, the intensity of nursing care required in acute care facilities continues to increase as length of stay decreases. Nurses must be able to think critically and solve a diversity of problems. Nurses in long-term facilities must provide not only "high-touch" care but also "high-tech" care and have the appropriate knowledge base to direct and manage the complex health care needs of their patients.

There also is a need for additional advanced practice nurses because the United States does not have enough primary care providers. It is estimated that about 250,000 primary care providers will be needed to manage the goals of any health care reform plan. In the late 1990s there were only 55,000 to 60,000 primary care physicians in the United States. At present more than 100,000 APNs are already providing primary care as NPs, CNMs, CRNAs, and CNSs. An additional 400,000 RNs either are delivering primary care or could be trained to do so in 18 months or less.[37] Thus the nursing profession is at a pivotal point in assuming a major role in providing primary health care as health care reform continues to evolve.

It is crucial that nursing education be equipped to prepare more nurses to function as nurse practitioners. Failure to do so will open the door to other groups such as physician assistants, who will be happy to assume the role of primary care providers if nurses do not meet this need.

Beginning in 1993, several nursing programs began offering special courses in primary nursing care for nurses already holding the Master of Science in Nursing (MSN) degree. These programs are two to four semesters in length depending on the background of the individual student. In addition, nursing programs have reoriented their master's programs to include more emphasis on primary care and preparation of the graduates to function as nurse practitioners.

The nursing profession needs to continue supporting the evolution of differentiated nursing practice.[12] Differentiated practice legitimizes and rewards the expert who is practicing nursing at an advanced level of competency and responsibility. Advanced education at the MSN and doctoral levels is highly specialized and prepares nurses for a variety of increasingly complex roles, responsibilities, and broadened career choices. Education at the advanced level incorporates the primary components of theory, special clinical practice, consultation experiences, education principles, and research expertise. The expectation is that nurses with master's degrees and those with doctorates have the ability not only to apply these theories and principles in their practice but also to refine and generate new theories and principles.[21] They also serve as excellent patient care role models.

Conway-Welch, the Dean of Nursing at Vanderbilt University, points out that nursing education is inextricably linked to the structural changes brought about by health care reform, managed care, and managed care organizations (MCOs). She believes that the survival of nursing is linked to nursing responsiveness to these needs.[12] In this new health care environment she believes that nurses must have the skills listed in Box 1-3 to survive.[12]

## EVALUATING THE OUTCOMES OF PATIENT CARE

### HEALTH CARE REGULATORS

The individual states, as part of their powers (the power to protect the health, safety, and welfare of the public), have enacted legislation to license certain types of health care facilities such as hospitals, nursing homes, and ambulatory care centers. It is essential that health care facilities be licensed by federal, state, and/or local authorities. However, states cannot regulate the activities of federal health facilities within their state because of a stipulation in the Constitution that separates these two levels of government. On the federal level the Health Care Financing Administration (HCFA), a component of the Department of Health and Human Services (HHS), is responsible for administering Medicare and Medicaid programs. The need for safe quality care resulted in the development of review organizations and accreditation agencies.

### PROFESSIONAL REVIEW ORGANIZATION

Since the Medicare program began in 1965, the federal government has made several efforts to ensure appropriate use of Medicare funds and to contain costs while maintaining quality. In 1972 Congress created the Professional Standards Review Organization (PSRO), a program designed to review the medical necessity of services provided to Medicare patients. This program proved to be unsuccessful. Subsequently, a state-level agency, the Professional Review Organization (PRO), was cre-

**box 1-3** *Skills Required for Nurses to Function in Managed Care*

1. Move patients across the continuum of care and use transition (or "handoff") points as grounds for outcomes-based research.
2. Use process technology and demonstrate expertise in continuous improvement techniques.
3. Design patient approaches that are satisfactory from the viewpoints of patients, families, and MCOs.
4. Be enthusiastic about infrastructure change.
5. Understand care as a system of product lines, teams, and relays.
6. Question every example of waste and repetition in resource allocation and management.
7. Direct interdisciplinary teams and redefine the concept of team members (e.g., include the office nurse who is miles from the integrated health care delivery system).
8. Develop, collect, and analyze data to define, refine, and continuously improve the value of their care.
9. Use data to benchmark and improve clinical outcomes.
10. Be highly skilled in information systems technology.

ated by the Social Security Act Amendments of 1983. It is responsible for monitoring quality assurance and cost containment. The purpose of the PRO, like its predecessors, is to determine whether hospitals will receive payment for care given to Medicare patients. PRO staff members randomly select medical records of patients receiving Medicare to determine whether they meet certain criteria (Box 1-4). If the PRO review panel finds that the criteria were not met, the hospital is informed in writing of the discrepancies. If the hospital is unable to provide an acceptable explanation for the discrepancies or cannot supply data acceptable to the panel, the PRO will either deny payment for all or part of the hospital days and/or levy penalty points against the hospital. If a hospital accumulates a specified number of points in a defined period of time, the percentage of Medicare records reviewed at random is increased. If similar discrepancies are found at the next review, additional punitive measures are levied against the hospital.

In 1990 the Institute of Medicine completed a congressionally mandated study that recommended a new approach for ensuring quality of care, referred to as the health care quality improvement initiative (HCQII). Under this plan, Medicare's PRO is committed to quality improvement with a focus on improving patient care outcomes and creating a cooperative, rather than confrontational, exchange among the HCQII reviewer, hospitals, and physicians. The new format devotes fewer resources to case-level review, using instead statistical analyses of the overall patterns of outcomes. If standards of care are not met, the PRO will continue to deny payment for care.

## Accreditation of Health Care Organizations

Without a doubt, no other voluntary organization has had as much impact on the health care industry as has the Joint Commission on Accreditation of Healthcare Organizations (JCAHO), formerly known as the Joint Commission on Accreditation of Hospitals (JCAH). In 1918 the American College of Surgeons established a standardization program to improve the hospital-based practice of medicine. In 1952 JCAH was formed.

The American Osteopathic Hospital Association has a similar national accrediting process for osteopathic hospitals. Its review organization is the American Osteopathic Association (AOA).

The importance of JCAH or AOA accreditation took on special significance with the passage of the Medicare Act in 1965. Congress mandated that hospitals would have to be accredited by either JCAH or AOA to receive Medicare reimbursement. Although seeking JCAH or AOA accreditation is voluntary and not the same as licensure or certification by the state or local authorities, the congressional action made it appear that accreditation was mandatory. In the late 1980s, the Joint Commission's name change reflected the total spectrum of health care organizations accredited by them. Accreditation has come to be recognized as a benchmark of quality and is used by some regulatory agencies as one criterion for licensure or certification and by some insurance agencies as a condition for reimbursement. Acknowledging the importance of accreditation by the Joint Commission, many AOA-accredited hospitals also are accredited by the Joint Commission.

In 1987 the Joint Commission initiated its *Agenda for Change,* which refocused its standards for accreditation toward patient outcomes instead of how care is given to patients. Since 1987 the Joint Commission has been collecting patient care data from several hundred of its accredited hospitals around the country. The data will be used to establish baseline parameters for outcomes of care for a variety of patient care areas, including infection control, obstetrics, anesthesia, cardiovascular care, home infusion therapy, and medication use. Some consider the development of the Joint Commission's indicator monitoring system the most significant quality assessment tool within the Agenda for Change era.

By 1994 any hospital accredited by the Joint Commission could voluntarily submit its outcomes of patient care within specified care areas to the commission. By 1996 participation in the indicator monitoring system was mandatory for accreditation. The expectation is that the requested data will be submitted on a quarterly basis. A hospital will then receive information on how its outcomes of patient care compare with those of other hospitals in its region and to all hospitals in the nation. Thus hospitals will receive continuous feedback on their performance. When a hospital has negative outcome indicators, a meeting between the Joint Commission and the hospital will address the problems, clarifying them, and, if necessary, outlining the process to correct the problems. Another change in the commission's standards is the transition from a quality assurance system to a CQI system. The change of focus from reviewing the process of care to reviewing the outcomes of care complements the Agenda for Change model.

In 1993, for the first time in the Joint Commission's history, a registered nurse was appointed to the board of directors for a 3-year term.[61]

**box 1-4** *Questions Addressed in a PRO Review*

1. Did the patient meet predetermined parameters for hospital admission?
2. Was the patient medically ready for discharge?
3. Was the care delivered to the patient appropriate?
4. Did the care delivered meet professionally accepted standards of quality?

## Professional Standards for Nursing

In 1991 the ANA released a revised *Standards of Clinical Nursing Practice* for the purpose of ensuring the public of quality nursing care (Box 1-5).[5] The primary responsibility for implementing these standards, however, rests with the individual nurse, who bears the responsibility for ensuring that these criteria are met in his or her own practice setting. To fulfill this responsibility, professional nurses must be familiar with both the generic (general) and the specific standards pertinent to

**box 1-5** *ANA's Standards of Clinical Nursing Practice*

**Standard I.** ***Assessment:*** The nurse collects client health data.

**Standard II.** ***Diagnosis:*** The nurse analyzes the assessment data in determining diagnosis.

**Standard III.** ***Outcome identification:*** The nurse identifies expected outcomes individualized to the client.

**Standard IV.** ***Planning:*** The nurse develops a plan of care that prescribes interventions to attain expected outcomes.

**Standard V.** ***Implementation:*** The nurse implements the interventions identified in the plan of care.

**Standard VI.** ***Evaluation:*** The nurse evaluates the client's progress toward attainment of outcomes.

From American Nurses Association: *Standards of clinical nursing practice,* Washington, DC, 1991, The Association.

**box 1-6** *Joint Commission on Accreditation of Healthcare Organization's Review Sections*

1. Patients rights and organization ethics
   a. Assessment of patients
   b. Care of patients
   c. Education (of patients and family)
   d. Continuum of care
2. Improving organization performance
   a. Leadership
   b. Management of the environment of care
   c. Management of human resources
   d. Management of information
   e. Surveillance, prevention, and control of infection
3. Governance
   a. Management
   b. Medical staff
   c. Nursing

From Joint Commission on Accreditation of Healthcare Organizations: *Comprehensive accreditation manual for hospitals,* Chicago, 1996, The Commission.

the care of the patient population for which they are responsible. These standards identify the elements of nursing care that must be met to ensure quality care. They also provide a baseline for measuring that quality.

Three other sets of professional standards also must be considered: nurse practice acts, medical practice acts, and the standards set by the JCAHO. At present, all states have nurse practice and medical practice acts; both constitute sources on which to base standards for nursing practice. Taken together they define and delineate the content and scope of practice of medicine and nursing from a legal standpoint.

*Nurse practice acts* define the scope of nursing practice. *Medical practice acts* further delineate nursing practice by outlining those areas that constitute the exclusive province of the physician. Such exclusions restrict the activities in which nurses may engage. Neither act sets actual standards for practice; rather the acts designate general areas of activity for both professions, and they establish the legal relationship of the nurse to society and to other health care professions.

The Joint Commission is a highly influential external source of nursing standards. Beginning in 1976 the Joint Commission added a section on quality of professional services to its *Accreditation Manual for Hospitals,* which is revised yearly. The overall focus of the review performed by the JCAHO is presented in Box 1-6. Consequently, the hospital's major goal should be to help each employee improve the processes in which he or she is involved—at the same time fulfilling its responsibility to address serious problems involving deficits in knowledge or skill of staff members.

## QUALITY ASSURANCE, TOTAL QUALITY MANAGEMENT/CONTINUOUS QUALITY IMPROVEMENT

Quality assurance (QA) is defined as a process that involves evaluating the degree of excellence of the observable and measurable characteristics of delivered nursing care. Quality assurance can be described on two levels. In its strictest sense it is described as a set of techniques for assuring the maintenance and improvement of standards and the efficiency and effectiveness of nursing care. More broadly, it is an effort to control nursing practice. As such, it involves relationships between nurses and consumers and between nurses and governmental bodies.

For many reasons the transition in health care motivated hospital administrators, providers, and insurance companies to focus on outcomes of patient care as a measurement of quality. The Joint Commission, too, changed its focus for measuring quality. The primary focus had been on reviewing the process of care, such as staff members' consistency in using appropriate policies and procedures for providing care. Thus the QA program of many hospitals focused on how well certain standards for care were met. The Joint Commission's Agenda for Change requires a continuous quality improvement program that focuses on patient outcomes, that is, why patient outcomes were not achieved. Thus TQM/CQI is a commitment by the organization to provide quality care to achieve expected and predetermined patient outcomes (see Table 1-1 for a comparison of QA and TQM/CQI).

An example that will help differentiate the two systems is a review of patient falls. The QA approach would examine "why" the patient fell, and the manager would focus on altering the causes for these patient falls. The cause might be

**table 1-1** *Comparisons Between Quality Assurance and Total Quality Management/Continuous Quality Improvement*

| QA | TQM/CQI |
|---|---|
| **FOCUS** | |
| Problem | Patient |
| Provider/employee | System |
| Single issue | Multiple issues |
| Solve problem | Improve process/outcome |
| Management control | Provider/employee control |
| Inspection driven | Process driven |
| **TIMING** | |
| Retrospective | Prospective |
| Reactive | Proactive |
| Episodic based on problems | Continuous goal to maintain quality |
| **INVOLVEMENT** | |
| Limited staff involved | Many staff involved |
| Top-down directed | Bottom-up directed |
| External-to-problem | Internal-to-problem |
| **QUALITY** | |
| Not assured when problem solved | Integrated in process |

Developed by Helen A. Schaag.

poor lighting (especially at night), beds not lowered to their lowest position, patients' mobility problems, or inadequate staff to supervise patients at risk for falls. The TQM/CQI focus is on "why" the patient fell and allowing the staff members caring for patients to determine how they will reduce patient falls. TQM/CQI focuses on the system and all issues involved with falls, such as staff-patient ratio, environment, types of patients, situations preceding the fall, and ways to avoid or reduce the frequency of these falls. TQM/CQI looks at falls and other problems in general and not at one situation.

See Figure 1-3 for a CQI flowchart that focuses on analyses of falls. TQM/CQI is carried out by all staff members and is not management-directed. TQM/CQI builds in checks to assess whether problems are solved. QA activity, on the other hand, usually focused only on the employee or employees involved with the problem, and the manager would work to change the deficient behavior or procedures; other staff members were not involved in analyzing and resolving the problem. Naturally, the interaction between the manager and the staff member causing the problem occurred some time after the incident. Although the responsible person might not cause this problem again, there was no assurance that falls would not recur. As it evolves, TQM/CQI seems to be less threatening to staff and a more effective problem-solving approach than QA.

QA activity was used during the 1970s and 1980s and achieved the goals it was designed to meet. It served a valuable function in that it was the first organized system to review and document patient care problems.

Three major concerns prompted the health care industry to make the transition from QA to TQM/CQI: (1) the Joint Commission's new requirements to adopt some form of CQI activity (see preceding details), (2) the demand by health insurance programs and employers paying high premiums to ensure quality coverage for the money being spent, and (3) consumer demand for improved quality of health care. Consumerism was the spark that began the patients' rights movement in hospitals, acknowledging the right of patients to participate in their care and to make their own health care decisions. This movement has resulted in an increased knowledge base that has made consumers better informed about the business of health care and about treatment and diagnostic options. More knowledgeable consumers have become more confident in asking physicians about the care they are receiving or would like to have. In addition, data banks that contain information on the performance of physicians and hospitals are beginning to be released to the public—for example, data comparing hospitals in geographic areas as to the number of deaths from open heart surgery, providing the name of the cardiac surgeon, the number of patient deaths in general by hospital, the costs for specific diagnostic tests, and the number of cesarean sections performed. These data are used by some businesses to determine which hospitals and physicians will be covered in their health insurance plans.

An important reason to adopt the TQM/CQI system is an estimate that 94% of all errors made in the hospital are because of "system" problems versus provider or employee problems.[16] The main focus of TQM/CQI is on patient outcomes and the systems that support attaining these outcomes.

## Definition of TQM/CQI

*TQM* is the philosophy of an organization, it is customer driven, and the focus is on every aspect of an organization. TQM, which uses the scientific method, continuously strives to exceed customer expectations.

*CQI* complements the philosophy of TQM. The focus of CQI is on the need for an organization such as a hospital to continually seek opportunities to enhance the quality of its services by use of statistical analyses of these services. The overall expectations are that both quality and efficiency of care will be enhanced with the adoption of TQM and CQI because they force the organization to systematically examine its practices.

To be successful in using TQM and CQI, people in organizations must undergo a shift in the way they think about quality improvement. The mind set of "If it ain't broken, don't fix it" must be changed to "If it ain't broken, that's the best time to make it better."[30] TQM provides a

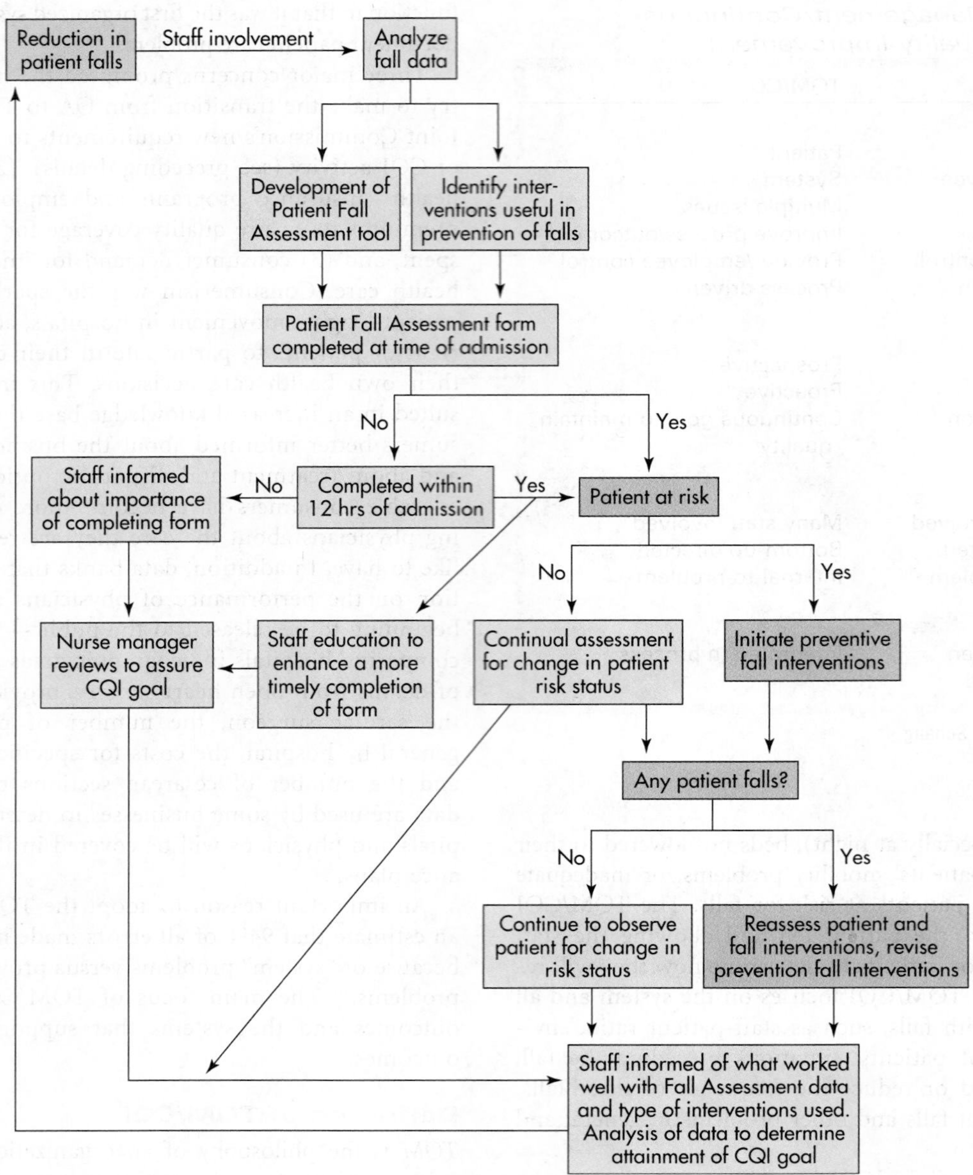


**fig. 1-3** Flowchart for continuous quality improvement (CQI) focused on reduction of patient falls. Note that CQI starts with a goal. Also note the continual reassessment and "grass roots" level of nursing staff involvement.

mechanism for organizations to be proactive; that is, its ongoing review of all systems prevents crises from developing. With CQI, quality meets or exceeds the patient's or customer's needs.

After World War II, a then unknown engineer named W. Edwards Deming was unsuccessful in his attempts to introduce to the leaders of this country's largest industries a new method for ensuring quality control. Businesses and industries were booming, and no one in the United States was interested. At the same time Japan was struggling with its postwar problems, including the worldwide perception that Japanese products were of inferior quality. The Japanese believed they could not compete with American-made products. Deming accepted an invitation to help Japanese business leaders improve the quality of their products. Today "everyone" in the United States is studying and adopting Deming's management model,[16,33,63] and it has been recognized as the single most important factor responsible for transforming large American companies into global competitors. An estimated 80% of all manufacturing companies in the United States incorporate some form of quality improvement in their businesses.

### Continuous quality improvement

The goal of CQI is to identify variations in patient care outcome and to reduce or eliminate as many specific variations as possible. The case management process uses *critical pathways* to identify variances in patient care outcomes. The health care professionals on the case management committee differentiate between random, nonspecific variations and nonrandom, specific variations. There needs to be ongoing documentation of the continuous improvement activities used to correct the nonrandom, specific variations.

When an interdisciplinary team begins to develop a clinical pathway for a particular group of patients or a specific diagnosis, members of the team use their own "expert" interventions and/or "community standards" as the target performance level. There are some individuals who believe that perhaps there could be a "better way" of achieving the desired patient outcomes than the usual way. *Benchmarking* is a process used to seek out the very best, compare the results or outcomes with previous results, pick out the best features, and then incorporate the new steps into the process.[14]

Benchmarking has the potential of truly giving an interdisciplinary team the very best interventions or process that may result in more positive outcomes than the previous "community standard." Use of benchmarking with the CQI activity provides a better focus when resolving a problem or determining if there is a problem.

The Shewhart cycle is a CQI or TQM technique used to test innovations.[14] The process is referred to as the *P-D-C-A cycle,* an ongoing interaction using four steps: *P,* plan what to do; *D,* do it; *C,* check effect of action; and *A,* act. The Shewhart cycle is a helpful tool to keep the focus on outcomes and on the process. That is, it initiates actions that had positive results or revises actions that had unwanted results, and then the P-D-C-A cycle activity is resumed.

## UTILIZATION REVIEW

The utilization review (UR) program for hospitals was first mandated by JCAH in 1978. It has as its primary goal the appropriate allocation of a hospital's resources and patient LOS. In most acute care facilities the activities of UR have merged with the case management program's activities.

## INFECTION CONTROL

All employees who have direct contact with patients are involved in programs to monitor and control infection rates. An infection control report provides monthly data on the number and types of nosocomial infections on a given hospital unit. Questions can then be raised about procedures or practices used not only by nursing personnel but also by physicians, respiratory therapists, phlebotomists, and so on. Variances from patient care outcomes (identified through critical pathways) that deal with nosocomial infections are analyzed, and appropriate CQI activity is initiated. (See Chapter 10 for more information about infection control.)

## RISK MANAGEMENT

The focus of risk management (RM) is on decreasing the probability of incurring an adverse outcome and thus reducing the organization's exposure to risk of a lawsuit. The goals of RM, which closely parallel the goals of CQI, focus on increasing the probability of achieving desired (patient care) outcomes. Although lawsuits will never be totally eliminated, everyone in the organization has a role in identifying and reporting risk incidence and in designing CQI activities to reduce or eliminate risks that could result in the hospital or physicians being sued.

## CONFIDENTIALITY

Confidentiality of all data is an issue usually associated with risk management. The availability and use of evaluative data about a patient or groups of patients have always been of concern to health professionals. The increasing use of computerized data has generated enormous concern for the potential threats to the privacy of sensitive information. Most quality review activities and case management analysis can be conducted without recording patients' names and are reported in terms of aggregate data. Review of care provided to a particular patient requires constant vigilance to ensure the protection of the patient's identity, as well as protection of the identity of the health care team members. Confidentiality of employee data is another sensitive issue that needs to be protected. *Maintaining confidentiality should be a constant goal of everyone in health care.*

# FUTURE CONCERNS

Changes in the delivery of health care and the allocation of monies undoubtedly will receive the attention of most persons in the United States over the next few years. Increasingly the public is expressing concern that the quality of health care is taking second place to the cost of that care. Properly designed and executed TQM programs and CQI activities are vital feedback mechanisms that can help assure the "customers" of health care—patients, health care insurance plans, physicians, nurses, and others—that an acceptable quality of health care is maintained.

As this book goes to press, both political parties are proposing a Patient's Bill of Rights in response to the public's dissatisfaction with HMOs and the control of medical decisions by insurance companies rather than the patient's physician. It is clear that the quality and adequacy of medical care is a predominant concern of the American public and will demand political attention in the coming years.

### critical thinking QUESTIONS

1 What are the reasons for the increased utilization of alternative health care facilities?

2 What are the responsibilities associated with attaining the status of advanced nurse practitioner?

3 Why is differentiated practice necessary?
4 What are the major differences between the goals of quality assurance (QA) and the goals of continuous quality improvement (TQM/CQI)?
5 How could the variances identified by the continuous quality improvement process be used in research?
6 What are the major values and dilemmas that have led to the current health care crisis?
7 How do you believe money should be allocated for health care in the United States?

## chapter SUMMARY

### CHANGES IN AMERICAN SOCIETY

- American society is aging, and the greatest increase is in persons older than 85 years of age, called the "old-old."
- Questions are being raised about the ability of a proportionately smaller working population to support Social Security for elders.
- Technological advances have dramatically changed medical care and driven up costs.
- Ethical problems arise in the use of technological advances such as organ transplantation and life-sustaining interventions.

### COST OF HEALTH CARE

- There has been no decision in the United States concerning how health care reform is to be financed.

### HEALTH CARE IN THE UNITED STATES

- The United States is the only industrial society that does not have some form of national health insurance.
- The many changes in health care insurance coverage include the health maintenance organization (HMO) and the preferred provider organization (PPO). Clinical nurse specialist and nurse practitioner are types of advanced practice positions in nursing.
- Patients are being discharged sooner from the hospital as the result of diagnosis-related groups (DRGs) and other cost-containment measures, resulting in an increased need for ambulatory care, home care services, and skilled nursing units.

### NURSING IN THE UNITED STATES

- Several methods have been used to deliver nursing care in the hospital, including team nursing, total patient care, primary nursing, and case management.
- Primary nursing, which clearly defines accountability for the care of each primary patient to the assigned primary nurse, requires a greater proportion of RNs to total nursing staff.
- Alternate health care settings such as home care are rapidly growing in the United States.
- Health promotion is becoming a major focus of nursing care, with individuals expected to assume more responsibility for their own health.
- A major concern to nurses is that the United States is rapidly moving toward a two-tier health care system—one for the "haves" and another for the "have nots."

### CHALLENGES TO NURSES AND NURSING

- Collaboration, viewed as a positive move, is increasing between nursing practice and nursing education.
- The increase in "high tech" in hospitals demands an increase in "high touch." Nurses are being challenged to provide high-touch care to patients who are attached to highly complex equipment.
- The demand for nurses continues to increase even though more nurses are employed now than ever before.
- Nursing schools are changing to reflect the changes in society, for example, the need for all students to be computer literate.
- Some nursing schools are advancing the preparation of nurses to the postbaccalaureate level, which is what other professions (such as pharmacy) have chosen to do.
- Nursing's commitment to professional excellence includes monitoring the quality of care given.
- Four factors that have influenced quality of practice in nursing are (1) health care legislation, (2) changes in third-party reimbursement, (3) economic factors, and (4) professional standards.
- The American Nurses Association's Standards of Clinical Nursing Practice includes six standards to be followed by all nurses who provide nursing care.

### EVALUATION OF THE OUTCOMES OF PATIENT CARE

- The Joint-Commission on the Accreditation of Healthcare Organizations is a voluntary organization that accredits hospitals and other health care organizations. It publishes an annual accreditation manual that includes a standard for quality of professional services. This standard provides the basis for evaluating patient care.
- The Joint Commission has replaced quality assessment (QA) with continuous quality improvement (CQI) as the system to ensure that quality of care is continuously improved by focusing on patient care outcomes.
- The main goals of CQI are to improve patient care by focusing on patient care outcome variances and by reducing or eliminating specific, nonrandom variances.
- Case management is a patient care delivery system that organizes patient care by specific case types and that focuses on achievement of outcomes within specific time frames and resources.
- The main goals of case management are to increase quality of care, nurse/patient/family satisfaction, and collaborative care and to decrease length of stay and use of resources.
- Critical pathways are patient outcome-focused tools that require an interdisciplinary approach to identify usual interventions for high-volume or high-risk patient diagnostic groups. The tool is designed to provide specific interventions with specific patient outcomes and specific time frames throughout the hospital stay.

## References


1. Alpert HB et al: 7 Gryzmish: toward an understanding of collaboration, *Nurs Clin North Am* 27(1):47-59, 1992.
2. American Association of Colleges of Nursing: *Position statement: nursing education's agenda for the 21st century,* Washington, DC, 1993, The Association.
3. American Nurses Association: *The role of the clinical nurse specialist,* Washington, DC, 1986, The Association.
4. American Nurses Association: *Nursing's agenda for health care reform,* Washington, DC, 1991, The Association.
5. American Nurses Association: *Standards of clinical nursing practice,* Washington, DC, 1991, The Association.
6. American Nurses Association: *Nursing quality indications for acute care settings and ANA's safety and quality initiative,* 1996, Washington, DC, The Association.
7. American Nurses Credentialing Center: *Am Nurse,* p 29, Sept-Oct 1996.
8. Anderson CA: From the editor: making the invisible visible, *Nurs Outlook* 41(6):246-247, 1993.
9. Baer ED, Fagin CM, Gordon S, editors: *Abandonment of the patient: the impact of the profit-driven health care on the public,* New York, 1996, Springer Publishing.
10. Bower-Ferres S: Loeb Center and its philosophy of nursing, *Am J Nurs* 75:810-815, 1975.
11. Cejka S: The changing healthcare workforce: a call for managing diversity, *Healthcare Exec,* pp 20-23, Mar-Apr 1993.
12. Conway-Welch C: Who is tomorrow's nurse and where will tomorrow's nurse be educated? *N&HC: Perspect Community* 17(6):286-290, 1996.
13. Cook S: Breaking with tradition, *Academic Nurs,* pp 19-21, summer 1993.
14. Corbett MW: Flo chart to benchmark, *Best Pract Benchmarking Healthcare,* 1(3):161-166, 1996.
15. delBueno DL: Paradigm shifts—what's good and not so good for health care, *Nurs Health Care* 14:100-101, 1993.
16. Deming WE: *Out of crisis,* Cambridge, Mass, 1986, Center for Advanced Engineering Study, Massachusetts Institute of Technology.
17. Dunkle RM: Parish nurses help patients—body and soul, *RN,* pp 55-57, May 1996.
18. Fagin CM: Collaboration between nurses and physicians: no longer a choice, *Nurs Health Care* 13:354-363, 1992.
19. Friedman E: Managed care: where will your hospital fit in? *Hospitals* 67(7):18-23, 1993.
20. Fries JF et al: Reducing health care costs by reducing the need and demand for medical services, *N Engl J Med* 329:321-325, 1993.
21. Frik SM, Pollock SE: Preparation for advanced nursing practice, *Nurs Health Care* 14:190-195, 1993.
22. Griffith H: Who will become the preferred provider? *Am J Nurs* 85:539-542, 1985.
23. Grimaldi PL: Monitoring managed care's quality, *Nurs Manage Special Suppl* 27(10):18-20, 1996.
24. Hull K: Outpatient acceleration: 1992 survey traces continued ambulatory care growth, *Hospitals* 67(9):40-41, 1993.

24a. Issel LM, Anderson RA: Take charge: managing six transformations in health care delivery, *Nurs Econom* 14(2):78-85, March/April 1996.

25. Jackson LE: Looking toward an NP/CNS merger by the year 2000, *Nurs Pract* 18(4):15-19, 1993.
26. Jenson J: HMO satisfaction slipping: consumers, *Mod Healthcare* 26(41):86-88, 1996.
27. Joint Commission on Accreditation of Healthcare Organizations: Quality assessment and improvement. In *Accreditation manual for hospitals,* Chicago, 1998, The Commission.
28. Kennedy EM: Congress and the national health policy (Rosenhause lecture), *Am J Public Health* 68:241-244, 1978.
29. Ling K: Initiation and evolution of managed care at the Johns Hopkins Hospital, *Nurs Adm Q* 17(3):54-58, 1993.
30. Lopresti J, Whetstone WR: Total quality management: doing things right, *Nurs Manage* 24:34-36, 1993.
31. Lubitz LD, Riley GF: Trends in Medicare payments in the last year of life, *N Engl J Med* 328:1092-1096, 1993.
32. Lutz EM, Scholtfeldt RM: Pioneering a new approach to professional education, *Nurs Outlook* 33:139-143, 1985.
33. McCabe WJ: Total quality management in a hospital, *QRB Qual Rev Bull* 18:134-140, 1992.
34. *Medicare: 1996 highlights,* Baltimore, 1996, US Department of Health and Human Services.
35. Milio N: *The store front that didn't burn,* Ann Arbor, 1970, University of Michigan Press.
36. Mittelstadt PC: Federal reimbursement of advanced practice nurses' services empowers the profession, *Nurs Pract* 18(1):43-49, 1993.
37. Morgan WA: Using state board of nursing data to estimate the number of nurse practitioners in the United States, *Nurs Pract* 18(2):65-74, 1993.
38. National League for Nursing: Nursing centers enter policy arena, *PRISM—the NLN Res Policy Q* 1(1):1-2, 1993.
39. National League for Nursing: A promising trend in the American care system, *PRISM—the NLN Res Policy Q* 1(1):3-5, 1993.
40. National League for Nursing: *A vision for nursing education,* New York, 1993, The League.
41. Nursing homes' population up, *Kansas City Star,* p 6A, June 28, 1993.
42. One in 3 ED patients is seeking primary care, *Am J Nurs* 93(8):9, 1993.
43. Packard NJ: The price of choice managed care in America, *Nurs Adm Q* 17(3):8-15, 1993.
44. Pallarito K: The future: for-profits, managed care to grow, *Mod Healthcare* 26(35):92, 1996.
45. Patient self-determination act, *Omnibus Reconciliation Act of 1990,* Washington, DC, 1990.
46. Pearson IJ: 1992-93 update: how each state stands on legislative issues affecting advanced nursing practice, *Nurs Pract* 18(1):23-26, 1993.
47. Projections of the number of persons diagnosed with AIDS and the number of immunosuppressed HIV-infected persons—United States, 1992-1994, *MMWR* 41(RR-18):1-29, 1992.
48. American Hospital Association: *Put it in writing: questions and answers on advance directives,* Chicago, March 1991, The Association.
49. Robinson JA, Robinson KJ, Lewis DJ: Balancing quality of care and cost-effectiveness through case management, *Am Nephrol Nurs Assoc J* 19(2):182-188, 1992.
50. Sabatino F: Culture shock: are U.S. hospitals ready? *Hospitals* 67(10):23-28, 1993.
51. Sakalys JA, Watson J: Professional education: post-baccalaureate education for professional nursing, *J Prof Nurs* 2:91-97, 1986.
52. Sandrick K: Collaboration: a prerequisite to effective reform, *Health Care Exec* 8:17-19, 1993.
53. Scheller-Janquist F: Walk-in health clinic for the homeless, *N&HC: Perspect Community* 17(3):119-123, 1996.

54. Schlotfeldt RM: The professional doctorate: rationale and characteristics, *Nurs Outlook* 26:302-311, 1978.
55. Selby T: Nurses establish clinic for the homeless, *Am Nurse* 17:1,20, 1985.
56. Sherer JL: Nursing education: addressing post-reform needs, *Hospitals* 67(10):25, 1993.
57. Should health care cost concern you? *AIDE Magazine,* pp 6-9, Apr 1993.
58. Simmons FM: Developing the trauma nurse case manager role, *Dimen Crit Care Nurs* 11(3):164-170, 1992.
59. Suzman R, Riley NW: Introducing the oldest old: health and society, *Milbank Q* 63:177-186, 1985.
60. Trinidad EA: Case management: a model of CNS practice, *Clin Nurse Spec* 7(4):221-223, 1993.
61. Update: nurse chosen to fill Joint Commission Board seat, *J Nurs Adm* 22(12):9, 1992.
62. US Department of Health and Human Services, Public Health Service: *Healthy people 2000: national health promotion and disease prevention objectives,* Washington, DC, 1990, US Government Printing Office.
63. Wakefield DS, Wakefield BJ: Overcoming the barriers to implementation of TQM/CQI in hospitals: myths and realities, *QRB* 19:83-88, 1993.
64. Weissenstein E: HCFA to require HMO quality data, *Mod Healthcare* 26(42):26, 1996.

# chapter 2 CulturalCare Nursing

RACHEL E. SPECTOR

## objectives

*After studying this chapter, the learner should be able to:*

1. Identify the sociocultural issues that make the study of CulturalCare imperative.
2. Contrast allopathic and homeopathic philosophies and health care cultures.
3. Analyze the factors inherent in heritage consistency.
4. Discuss the importance of cultural phenomena—time orientation, spatial orientation, communication, biological variations, and environmental control—to CulturalCare.
5. Describe the HEALTH traditions model.
6. Compare the HEALTH traditions among Americans of Asian origin, African origin, Hispanic origin, North American Indian origin, and European origin.
7. Synthesize CulturalCare and the nursing process.

> *"When there is a very dense cultural barrier, you do the best you can, and if something happens despite that, you have to be satisfied with little success instead of total successes. You have to give up total control."*
> *Anne Fadiman*

As we enter the twenty-first century we are perched on the edge of enormous demographic, social, and cultural change. These changes are destined to play a profound role in the delivery of nursing care in general and adult health nursing care in particular. These changes can be analyzed from countless perspectives; several are presented in this chapter.

Nurses commonly come from different ethnic, cultural, and religious backgrounds than their patients. In institutional settings, where the *patient* may be viewed as the "guest," the nurse, to a greater or lesser degree, is the caretaker and "decision facilitator." However, rapid changes in health care are moving increasing amounts of care into the community and home environment. In these settings the *nurse* is the guest and the patient and family make their own health care–related choices and decisions. In many of these situations, there are "cultural collisions" with peoples from different ethnocultural backgrounds. The term *cultural collision* refers to the contentious phenomena, stemming from cultural miscommunication, that may occur when a person who lives by the health traditions of his or her ethnocultural heritage does not accept the recommendations and care modalities of present-day health care. Nurses must understand that patients may have differing world views and interpretations concerning health and illness that are based on their unique sociocultural and religious beliefs. When nurses are aware of and sensitive to the patient's unique health and illness beliefs and practices, good rapport can be established and culturally effective nursing care can be delivered.

CulturalCare nursing is culturally sensitive, culturally appropriate, and culturally competent. The term *CulturalCare* refers to the provision of nursing care across cultural boundaries that takes into account the context in which the patient lives, as well as the situations in which the patient's health problems arise. An awareness of the importance of cultural diversity in health care arose in the 1990s. CulturalCare is critical to meet the complex nursing care needs of individuals and families as health care approaches a new millennium. The nurse is considered to be culturally competent if he or she demonstrates understanding of the total context of the patient's situation in planning nursing interventions. Cultural competence involves a complex combination of knowledge, attitudes, and skills. Basic knowledge of and constructive attitudes toward the health traditions observed by the diverse cultural groups found in the practice setting enable the nurse to be culturally sensitive. The care is culturally appropriate when the nurse applies this basic cultural knowledge to provide a given patient with the best possible health care. The nurse who becomes skillful in CulturalCare can appreciate the total diversity of our society and strive to meet the needs of all patients.

This chapter presents an overview of the following:

1. The sociocultural issues relevant to CulturalCare (e.g., population changes, barriers to health care, and the sociological phenomenon of "-isms").
2. The profound philosophical and cultural differences between allopathic and homeopathic health beliefs and practices.
3. The HEALTH traditions of people from several different sociocultural backgrounds. *Note:* The term HEALTH is used in this context to designate a state of balance among the person's body, mind, and spirit.
4. An overview of cultural phenomena affecting HEALTH as identified by Giger and Davidhizar.[15]

The nursing process can be effectively used to deliver CulturalCare. Nursing assessment is expanded in this chapter to include "heritage assessment," an exploration of the patient and family from an ethnocultural perspective. A heritage assessment determines the degree to which a given person or the members of a family relate to the traditions of their ethno-religio-cultural heritage, and how strongly they identify with this heritage. Heritage assessment is discussed together with guidelines for implementation and interpretation. Assessment also includes a HEALTH traditions assessment, which is a universal method for describing health traditions related to the maintenance, protection, and restoration of physical, mental, and spiritual health in a nine-dimensional interrelated fabric.

## SOCIOCULTURAL ISSUES

Countless factors determine the sociocultural settings in which CulturalCare is delivered. This discussion focuses on issues of population changes, selected barriers to health care, and the influence of "-isms."

### POPULATION CHANGES

Two major population factors contribute to the increasing need to practice CulturalCare. One factor is the profound shift in population demographics; the other is the outcome of the enormous wave of immigration that has occurred since 1970.

#### Demographic Factors

"Demography is destiny." The percentage of people of European origin in the United States was 80.3% in 1990 but is expected to be only 54% by the year 2000. Low birth rates among the European majority and high birth rates among Asian Americans, African Americans, and Native Americans are combining to shift the population in America toward an "emerging majority" of people of color. Figure 2-1 compares the United States population in 1980 and 1990.

On January 1, 1995, the population of the United States was 261,638,000. This figure represented a 1.0% increase from 1994 and a 5.2% increase since the 1990 census. The number of elderly continues to increase. The number of Americans 65 years old and over increased by 7.3% in 1995 from the 1990 census. The number of people in the oldest segment, that is, over 85 years of age, increased 18.5% since the 1990 census. This differential increase in the population 85 years old and over is the result of improvements in the life expectancy at advanced ages, continued high levels of births during the first decades of the century, and a high rate of European immigration during the early part of the century. "Baby boomers" (those persons born from 1946 to 1964) currently constitute 30.3% of the total population and will begin to add their numbers to the swelling pool of elders early in the twenty-first century.

#### Immigration Factors

Since 1970 more than 30 million foreign citizens and their descendants have been added to the population of this country. In fact, since 1990, nearly 1,000,000 people per year have immigrated to the United States. These numbers represent a massive, legal demographic change. Social outcomes related to this rapid increase in new residents include increased poverty, lowered wages, the inability of large numbers of residents to communicate in English, and the unhealthy and unsafe return of sweatshop work environments. This population change is stressing the health care system in general and nursing practice in particular.

### BARRIERS TO HEALTH CARE

Innumerable barriers restrict people's access to and utilization of the health care system; the major obstacle is poverty. Closely related problems include transportation, language barriers, and the occurrence of "-isms." These problems are common among but not exclusive to the poor.

#### Poverty

There are countless ways to answer the question "What is poverty?" Poverty is partially defined by the receipt of government programs or subsidies such as public housing, Medicaid, Aid to Families with Dependent Children (AFDC), or food stamps. The federal government established a "poverty threshold" in 1965 that is based on pretax income and excludes income from capital gains and noncash benefits such as food stamps or Medicaid. The poverty threshold for an average family of four was $13,547 in 1992. The U.S. Bureau of Labor Statistics counts the poor and describes them by age, educa-

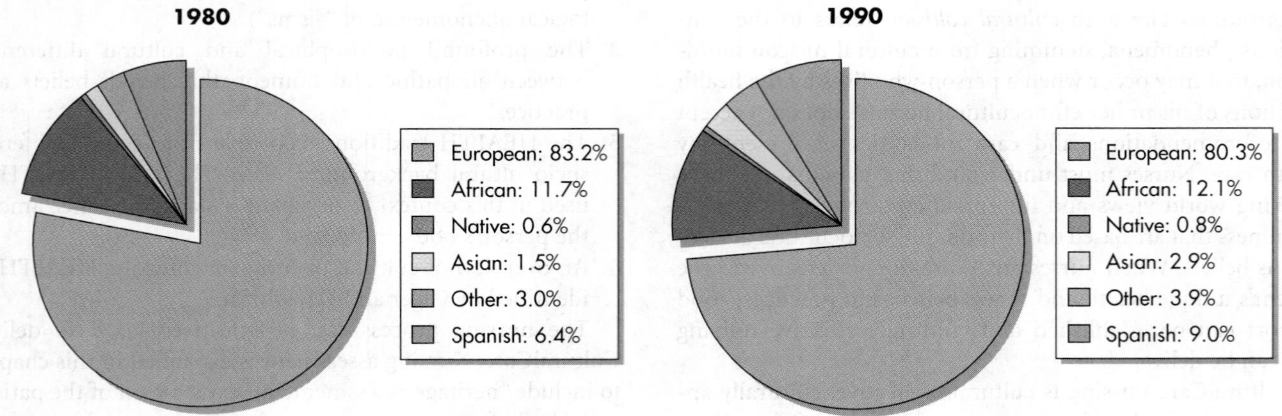


**fig. 2-1** United States population comparison: 1980-1990 census.

tion, location, race, family composition, and employment status. Facts about poverty in America include the following:

1. Forty-seven percent of students in high-poverty schools have low achievement scores, compared with 11.9% in low-poverty schools, regardless of their individual poverty status.
2. One in four African American high school graduates and almost one in eight white graduates are unlikely to earn more than a poverty-level income.
3. Whites make up only 17% of urban poor but 55% of rural poor. African Americans represent 49% of the urban poor and 32% of the rural poor, and Hispanics make up 29% of the urban poor and 8% of the rural poor.
4. Every 30 seconds a child is born into poverty.
5. One in five American children, a total of 14.6 million, is poor.
6. One out of 10 Americans makes use of food pantries, soup kitchens, and other food distribution programs.
7. Poverty cuts off phone access for 1 in 20 U.S. households. Almost one fifth (18.5%) of households nationwide living in poverty are without phone service.
8. Only 27% of the families with incomes below $14,000 are covered by Medicaid; 35% have private insurance, and 37% have no coverage at all.[18]

### Access

Several factors can limit a family's access to the health care delivery system, including the availability and location of health care facilities, transportation to these facilities, and the availability of affordable health insurance. Lack of insurance, whether public (Medicaid) or private, is a rapidly increasing problem.

### Transportation

The issue of transportation is a never-ending and ever-changing one. All too frequently patients and their families are unable to get to health care services because of geographic distance and must depend on other family members or friends for transportation. In many settings, the hospital designated to provide free care is not in the same location as the families needing this care. Public transportation is commonly expensive and, in some locations, nonexistent.

### Language

Many "new Americans" retain their native language, as do many "old Americans," who may have immigrated a generation ago. More and more immigrants arrive in the United States every year, increasing the need for adequate language services. All too often these services are not available. Accurate patient-professional communication is clearly a major necessity in health care delivery systems.

### "-Isms"

Several powerful "-isms" further complicate the issues of poverty access and transportation. These include the following:

*Ethnocentrism* is the belief that one's own cultural, ethnic, or professional group is superior to that of others. One judges others by a personal "yardstick" and is unable or unwilling to see the positive aspects of other groups.

*Xenophobia* is the morbid fear of strangers.[24]

The "-isms" must constantly be addressed, redressed, and monitored to create a safe and caring environment in health care. The sociocultural realities of population change, barriers to health care, and "-isms" set the stage on which nurses practice. They influence the scope of nursing practice and often determine the patient's access to health care resources.

## HEALTH CARE

Recovery from illness is one of life's most incredible phenomena. In today's society, the physician is most often viewed as the "healer," with other professional members of the health care team all playing significant roles in the prevention, detection, and treatment of disease. Yet human beings have existed for more than 2 million years, and for most of human history people recovered from illness without the intervention of high-technology scientific medicine. It is evident that numerous forms of healing existed long before the advent of modern technology.

In the natural course of any illness a person becomes ill, either acutely with pain, fever, nausea, or bleeding or insidiously with a gradual progression and worsening of symptoms. If the illness is mild, the symptoms may disappear with self-treatment or even no treatment. If the illness is more severe or of longer duration, the person may seek expert help from a "healer," usually but not always a physician or nurse practitioner. Other choices for help exist, and these choices are affected by economic, social, and cultural factors. Homeopathic HEALTH care encompasses a wide range of alternative/complementary and ethnocultural/traditional options that people may elect to use, often moving easily between health care options. Figure 2-2 demonstrates the range of options available to patients seeking care and healing.

The ill person recovers or expects to recover. Recovery is by and large a natural biological phenomenon that

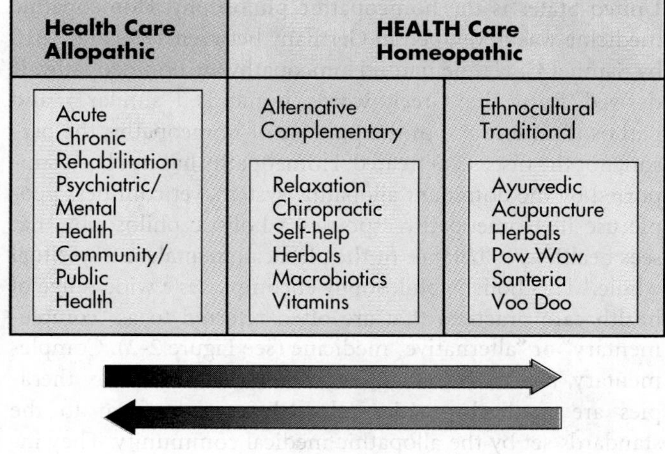


**fig. 2-2** Health and HEALTH care options continuum.

occurs regardless of the nature and extent of treatment provided. This fascinating process of recovery defies full understanding and has been documented throughout human history. It also has given rise to the development of numerous forms of healing that all attempt to explain or augment this natural phenomenon. Over the generations natural healing has been attributed to all sorts of rituals, including cupping, magic, leeching, and bleeding. From medicine man to sorcerer, the art of healing has been passed through succeeding generations.

## THE ALLOPATHIC PHILOSOPHY

The dominant health care system in the United States is "allopathic." It is predicated on a dualistic philosophy that sees the person as "body and mind." Allopathic practices are derived from scientific models of inquiry and involve the extensive use of technology. Interestingly, the word *allopathy* has two quite divergent origins. One origin is Greek from a root meaning "other than disease," reflecting the use of drugs that have no consistent or logical relationship to the patient's symptoms. The second origin of allopathy is from German roots that mean "all therapies." In this context allopathy is a "system of medicine that embraces all methods of proven value in the treatment of diseases." The American Medical Association adopted the second definition of allopathy in 1855 and has subsequently exclusively determined who can practice medicine in the United States. For example, in the 1860s the American Medical Association refused to admit women doctors to medical societies, practiced segregation, and demanded the purging of homeopaths from the practice of medicine. Today, allopathic physicians continue to show little tolerance or respect for other providers of health care, such as homeopaths, osteopaths, and chiropractors, and for such traditional healers as lay midwives, herbalists, and medicine men. The foundation of contemporary nursing education also rests within the domain of the allopathic philosophy.

## THE HOMEOPATHIC PHILOSOPHY

Another health care philosophy that is operational in the United States is the homeopathic philosophy. Homeopathic medicine was developed in Germany between 1790 and 1810 by Samuel C. Hahnemann. Homeopathy, or homoeopathy, is derived from the Greek words homoios ("similar") and pathos ("suffering"). In the practice of homeopathy, the person, not the disease, is treated. Homeopathy has not been supported by the dominant allopathic system, yet countless people use it. Homeopathy espouses a holistic philosophy that sees health as a "balance of the physical, mental, and spiritual whole." This holistic philosophy encompasses a wide range of health care practices that are often referred to as "complementary" or "alternative" medicine (see Figure 2-2). Complementary, alternative, unconventional, or unorthodox therapies are medical practices that do not conform to the standards set by the allopathic medical community. They include such therapies as acupuncture, massage therapy, and chiropractic medicine. These therapies are not taught widely as part of medical and nursing education and are not generally available in the allopathic health care system. Box 2-1 describes a few of the common forms of alternative/complementary therapies.

**box 2-1** *Common Forms of Alternative/ Complementary Therapy*

*Aromatherapy.* An ancient science, presently popular, that uses essential plant oils to produce strong physical and emotional effects in the body.

*Biofeedback.* The use of an electronic machine to measure skin temperatures. The patient learns to control responses that are usually involuntary.

*Hypnotherapy.* The use of hypnosis to stimulate emotions and involuntary responses such as blood pressure.

*Macrobiotics.* A diet and lifestyle from the Far East and adapted for the United States by Michio Kushif. The principles of this vegetarian diet consist of balancing yin and yang energies of food.

*Massage therapy.* Use of manipulative techniques to relieve pain and return energy to the body, now popular among many groups both modern and traditional.

*Overheating therapy (hyperthermia).* Used since the time of the Ancient Greeks, the natural immune system is stimulated with heat to kill pathogens.

*Reflexology.* The natural science dealing with the reflex points in the hands and feet that correspond to every organ in the body. The goal is to clear the energy pathways and the flow of energy through the body.

There are two types of care in the homeopathic system. One is classified as complementary or alternative, and the other is traditional or culture bound. Alternative therapies refer to therapies that are not a part of an individual's ethnocultural or religious heritage; traditional therapies are derived from an individual's traditional cultural heritage. For example, a European American electing acupuncture as a method of treatment is seeking alternative treatment; a Chinese American using this treatment is using traditional medicine. Terms used in traditional therapies are defined in Box 2-2.

The use of alternative therapies is growing rapidly, and they are currently used by patients with cancer, arthritis, chronic back or other pain, stress-related problems, acquired immunodeficiency syndrome (AIDS), gastrointestinal problems, and anxiety. In 1993 a national survey of 1539 subjects reported that approximately one third of all American adults use some form of unconventional medical treatment. The most common users are educated, upper-income white Americans in the 25- to 49-year-old age group who live on the West Coast. The total 1990 projected out-of-pocket expenditure for alternative therapy was $10.3 billion. Alternative therapies used included relaxation techniques; chiropractic; imagery; commercial weight-loss programs; lifestyle diets such as macrobiotics; megavitamin therapy; self-help groups; biofeedback; and hypnosis.[11] The use of traditional healers and therapies by members of the emerging majority was not included in the study.

**box 2-2** *Selected Terms Related to Traditional Health Care*

*Acupuncture.* The traditional Chinese medical way of restoring the balance of yin and yang that is based on the therapeutic value of cold. It is used in a disease in which there is an excess of yang.

*Amulet.* An object with magical powers, such as a charm, worn on a string or chain around the neck, wrist, or waist to protect the wearer from both physical and psychic illness, harm, and misfortune.

*Ayurvedic.* This 4000-year-old method of healing originated in India and is the most ancient existing medical system that uses diet, natural therapies, and herbs. Its chief aim is longevity and quality of life.

*Charm.* Objects that combine the functions of both amulets and talismans but consist only of written words or symbols.

*Chinese doctor.* The physician educated in China who uses traditional herbs and other therapeutic modalities in the delivery of health care.

*Natural folk medicine.* Use of the natural environment and use of herbs, plants, minerals, and animal substances to prevent and treat illness.

*Occult folk medicine.* The use of charms, holy words, and holy actions to prevent and cure illness.

*Santeria.* A syncretic religion that comprises both African and Catholic beliefs.

*Soul loss.* The belief that a person's soul can leave his or her body and wander and then return.

*Spirit possession.* The belief that a spirit can enter a person, possess that person, and control what he or she says and does.

*Susto (soul loss).* The traditional Hispanic belief that the soul is able to leave a person's body.

*Taboo.* A culture-bound ban that excludes something from common use.

*Talisman.* Consecrated religious objects that confer power of various kinds and protect people who wear, carry, or own them from harm and evil.

*Voodoo.* A religion that is a combination of Christianity and African Yoruba religious beliefs.

*Witched.* An example of a traditional Native American belief that a person is harmed by witches.

*Yang.* Male, positive energy that produces light, warmth, and fullness.

*Yin.* Female, negative energy—the force of darkness, cold, and emptiness.

## HEALTH CARE CULTURES

Allopathic and homeopathic "cultures" differ in countless ways. Table 2-1 lists selected differences between the systems. What causes a given person to choose to use one or both of these systems? The answer to this question is complex and is predicated on choice, preference, and need.

Thus far, in this chapter, the sociocultural factors impinging on the health care consumer and available health care options have been discussed. Cultural issues related to individuals and families—heritage, cultural phenomena, and HEALTH traditions—are explored next.

## HERITAGE CONSISTENCY

Belief systems can be analyzed from different perspectives. It is possible to assess health beliefs by determining a person's ties to traditional beliefs and his or her stage of acculturation. The "melting pot" theory views people as acculturated and assimilated into the dominant culture through school, television, radio, and motion pictures.[23] Heritage consistency theory looks at acculturation as a continuum. With this perspective the nurse would not only analyze the degree to which a person identifies with the dominant culture but also the degree to which he or she identifies with a traditional culture.

The heritage consistency theory was developed in 1980 by Estes and Zitzow[12] to assess and counsel Native American alcoholics within a cultural context. It describes the degree to which one's lifestyle reflects his or her tribal culture. The theory has now been expanded to attempt to study the degree to which any person's lifestyle reflects his or her traditional culture, whether it is European, Asian, African, or Hispanic. Some aspects of an individual's lifestyle may reflect cultural heritage, but other aspects are inconsistent with that heritage because the person has undergone acculturation. Factors related to heritage consistency and inconsistency are described in Table 2-2. An individual's degree of heritage consistency is evaluated by determining the importance of culture, ethnicity, and religion in his or her daily life. It is often difficult to evaluate the specific influence of these factors in shaping a person's worldview. Figure 2-3 illustrates the way these variables intertwine in socialization.

### CULTURE

Culture is the socially inherited characteristics of a human group that are transmitted from one generation to the next. These characteristics include worldview, values, beliefs, and patterns of social conduct. Culture is a learned series of symbols that serve as the framework of our individuality, our personhood, and our social relationships. Culture influences both a person's cognitive and behavioral development and shapes a person's way of experiencing health and illness. These symbols become an integral part of the individual's life.

### ETHNICITY

Ethnicity is a cultural group's sense of identification with its common social and cultural heritage. It includes the characteristics a group may have in common. These characteristics encompass nationality, race, language, religious faith, food preferences, and folklore, as well as many traits relevant to physical appearance. There are more than 106 ethnic groups and 500 Native American tribes in North America.[28]

### RELIGION

Religion is the belief in divine or superhuman powers to be obeyed and worshipped as the creators and rulers of the

**table 2-1** *Comparison: Allopathic and Homeopathic Cultural Characteristics*

| Cultural Characteristic | Allopathic Culture | Homeopathic Culture |
|---|---|---|
| Beliefs | Standard allopathic definitions of health and illness that view health and illness as a mind-body balance or imbalance<br>The omnipotence of technology—with a strong emphasis placed on knowledge of the use of the most recent scientific discoveries and equipment | Holistic homeopathic definitions of health and illness see health and illness as a balance or imbalance of physical, mental, and spiritual elements<br>Respect for tradition and traditional beliefs such as the "evil eye" that relate traditional aspects of one's heritage to health and illness care and healing |
| Practices | Maintenance and protection of health through such mechanisms as the avoidance of stress and the use of immunizations, health education, and behavioral change<br>Annual physical examinations and diagnostic procedures, such as Pap smears | Maintenance and protection of health through such mechanisms as the use of substances and objects that are hung in the home, worn, or carried<br>Use of "spiritual" resources to maintain, protect, and restore HEALTH |
| Habits | Charting<br>Use of jargon | Indirect conversation<br>Use of familiar language |
| Likes | Scientific methodology<br>Promptness<br>Neatness and organization<br>Compliance with regimens | Intuitive knowledge<br>Floating concept of time<br>Adaptation to circumstances<br>Use of familiar diagnostic methods and remedies |
| Dislikes | Tardiness<br>Disorderliness and disorganization | Compulsive procedures<br>Strict adherence to regimens |
| Customs | Hand washing<br>Scrubbing<br>Gloves used to touch people | Cleanliness observed<br>Human contact and touch practiced with permission of traditional cultureAreas of body taboo to touch of others |
| Rituals | Men examine women<br>Physical examination<br>Surgical procedures<br>Limiting visitors and visiting hours | Entire family may desire to be with patient all the time |

Source: Spector RE: *Cultural diversity in health and illness,* ed 4, Stamford, Conn, 1996, Appleton & Lange.

**table 2-2** *Factors Related to Heritage Consistency or Inconsistency*

| Heritage Consistency Factors | Heritage Inconsistency Factors |
|---|---|
| Childhood development occurred in the individual's country of origin or in a U.S. neighborhood of like ethnic group. | Childhood development did not occur in the individual's country of origin or in an immigrant neighborhood of like ethnic group. |
| Extended family members encouraged participation in traditional religious or cultural activities. | Extended family members did not encourage participation in traditional religious or cultural activities. |
| Individual engaged in frequent visits to the country of origin or to the "old neighborhood" in the United States. | Individual does not engage in visits to the country of origin or the "old neighborhood" in the United States. |
| Family homes are within the ethnic community. | Family home was not in the ethnic community. |
| Individual participates in ethnic cultural events such as religious festivals, "national holidays," singing, dancing, and costumes. | Individual does not participate in ethnic cultural events. |
| Individual was raised in an extended family setting. | Individual was not raised in an extended family setting. |
| Individual maintains regular contact with the extended family. | Individual does not maintain contact with the extended family. |
| Individual's name has not been Americanized. | Individual's name has been Americanized. |
| Individual was educated in a parochial (nonpublic) school with a religious or ethnic philosophy similar to personal background. | Individual was educated in public schools. |
| Individual engages in social activities primarily with others of the same ethnic background. | Individual does not engage primarily in social activities with others of the same ethnic background. |
| Individual has knowledge about the ethnic culture and language. | Individual does not have knowledge about ethnic culture and language. |
| Individual possesses elements of personal pride about the national and ethnic origin. | Individual does not possess elements of personal pride about the national and ethnic origin. |
| Individual incorporates elements of historical beliefs and practices into personal philosophies. | Individual does not incorporate elements of historical beliefs and practices into personal philosophies. |

Modified from Spector RE: *Cultural diversity in health and illness,* ed 4, Norwalk, Conn, 1996, Appleton & Lange.

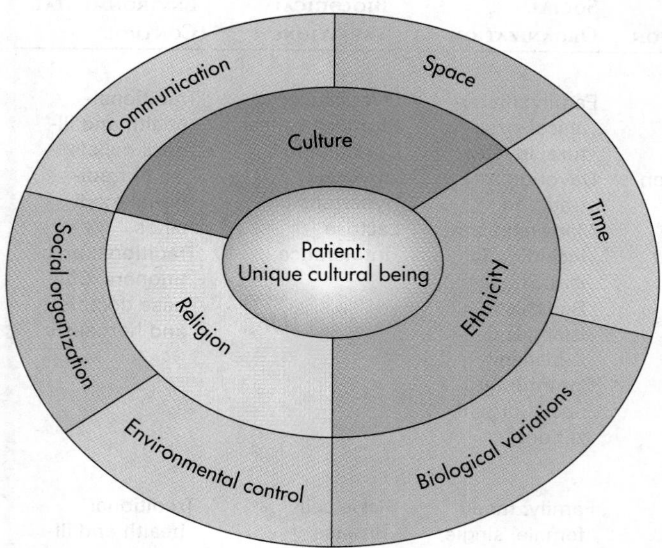


**fig. 2-3** Model of the patient within a culturally unique heritage and the cultural phenomena that have an impact on nursing care.

universe. Religious and ethical values, a system of beliefs and practices, further clarify ethnicity by providing a frame of reference within which to organize information.[1] The major religions in North America are Protestant, Catholic, Jewish, Eastern Orthodox, Muslim, Hindu, Baha'i, and Buddhist.[10] There are countless religious beliefs and practices that relate to health and illness.

### SOCIALIZATION

Socialization is the process of learning a culture. Initially, young children are socialized into the culture of their families. Later they attend schools, where a great deal of socialization into the dominant culture takes place. The adult person is socialized into adult and occupation roles.

Heritage consistency occurs on an ever-changing continuum. The concept does not stereotype or diagnose, but assists the nurse to understand a patient's or family's sociocultural background and how this background influences the way the patient views and interprets life events. The patient and family may interpret events through a traditional or modern viewpoint.

## CULTURAL PHENOMENA AFFECTING HEALTH

Six major phenomena have been identified by Giger and Davidhizar[15] as affecting health; their manifestations vary both within and between cultural groups.

### TIME ORIENTATION

Time may be viewed in the present, past, or future. Future-oriented people have long-range goals; this is the orientation of the dominant American culture. Other people are more present oriented and are less concerned about planning ahead or being on time. Present-oriented people do not plan their daily activities by a clock or calendar (e.g., dinner at 6:30 PM). They respond to needs as they arise (e.g., eating when hungry, going someplace when able).

Time orientation varies among cultural groups, and these differences may become important in long-term health care planning or explanations about when medications should be taken. Table 2-3 provides examples of time orientation found among people from several nations of origin.

### SPATIAL ORIENTATION

Personal space involves a person's set of attitudes and behaviors toward the space around the self. Territoriality is a defensive attitude or emotional reaction that is triggered when someone encroaches on a space or territory claimed by an individual or group. The phenomena of personal space and territoriality are strongly influenced by culture, and groups have varying norms related to the use of space. The modesty practiced by members of some groups may prevent them from seeking health care. For example, women who are prohibited from being touched by men may be reluctant to be examined by a male physician or nurse. In some cultures men are not permitted to be touched by women. Table 2-3 provides examples of spatial orientation found among people from several nations of origin.

### COMMUNICATION

Communication is an integral part of culture, because one definition of culture is that of a metacommunication system. Communication, like culture, influences and reflects how feelings are expressed and what verbal and nonverbal languages mean. Table 2-3 provides examples of spoken languages found among people from several nations of origin.

When the patient and family come from a traditional culture and neither understand nor choose to use allopathic ways, a "cultural collision" occurs that can have highly charged and fatal results.

A capable interpreter may be needed to communicate with the patient, especially to understand the more subtle aspects of verbal and nonverbal communication. All too often modes of communication are used in ways that can be misconstrued, such as shouting, focusing on the task instead of the patient, or doing things to the patient without speaking. Body language is also important. Standing with the arms folded across the chest conveys anger and hostility to many patients.

### SOCIAL ORGANIZATION

This phenomenon includes aspects of the family unit (nuclear, single parent, extended family, blended family, paternal or maternal orientation, etc.) and social-group organizations (religious or ethnic) with which cultural identification takes place. The family, and the support of family members, is often most important to the patient.

Family visits and presence often play an essential role in the patient's care, especially in the strange hospital setting. Family members also play a vital role in discharge planning because they often provide the necessary follow-up care. Numerous

**table 2-3** *Cross-Cultural Examples of Cultural Phenomena Affecting Nursing Care*

| Nations of Origin | Time Orientation | Spatial Orientation | Communication | Social Organization | Biological Variations* | Environmental Control |
|---|---|---|---|---|---|---|
| **ASIA** | | | | | | |
| China<br>Hawaii<br>Philippines<br>Korea<br>Japan<br>Southeast Asia (Laos, Cambodia, Vietnam) | Present | Noncontact people | National language preference<br>Dialects, written characters<br>Use of silence<br>Nonverbal and contextual cuing | Family: hierarchical structure, loyalty<br>Devotion to tradition<br>Many religions, including Taoism, Shintoism, Buddhism, Islam, and Christianity<br>Community social organizations | Liver cancer<br>Stomach cancer<br>Coccidioidomycosis<br>Hypertension<br>Lactose intolerance | Traditional health and illness beliefs<br>Use of traditional medicines<br>Traditional practitioners: Chinese doctors and herbalists |
| **AFRICA** | | | | | | |
| West Coast (as slaves)<br>Many African countries<br>West Indian Islands<br>Dominican Republic<br>Haiti<br>Jamaica | Present or future | Close personal space | National languages<br>Dialect: Pidgen, Creole, Spanish, and French | Family: many female, single parent<br>Large, extended family networks<br>Strong church affiliation within community<br>Community social organizations | Sickle cell disease<br>Hypertension<br>Cancer of the esophagus<br>Stomach cancer<br>Coccidioidomycosis<br>Lactose intolerance | Traditional health and illness beliefs<br>Folk medicine tradition<br>Traditional healer: root worker |
| **EUROPE** | | | | | | |
| Germany<br>England<br>Italy<br>Ireland<br>Other European countries | Future or present | Noncontact people<br>Aloof<br>Distant<br>Southern countries: closer contact and touch | National languages<br>Many learn English immediately | Nuclear families<br>Extended families<br>Judeo-Christian religions<br>Community social organizations | Breast cancer<br>Heart disease<br>Diabetes mellitus<br>Thalassemia | Primary reliance on modern health care system<br>Traditional health and illness beliefs<br>Some remaining folk medicine tradition |
| **NATIVE AMERICAN** | | | | | | |
| 170 Native American tribes<br>Aleuts<br>Eskimos | Present | Space very important and has no boundaries | Tribal languages<br>Use of silence and body language | Extremely family oriented<br>Biological and extended families<br>Children taught to respect traditions<br>Community social organizations | Accidents<br>Heart disease<br>Cirrhosis of the liver<br>Diabetes mellitus | Traditional health and illness beliefs<br>Folk medicine tradition<br>Traditional healer: medicine man |
| **HISPANIC COUNTRIES** | | | | | | |
| Spain<br>Cuba<br>Mexico<br>Central and South America | Present | Tactile relationships<br>Touch<br>Handshakes<br>Embracing<br>Value physical presence | Spanish or Portuguese primary language | Nuclear family<br>Extended families<br>*Compadrazzo:* godparents<br>Community social organizations | Diabetes mellitus<br>Parasites<br>Coccidioidomycosis<br>Lactose intolerance | Traditional health and illness beliefs<br>Folk medicine tradition<br>Traditional healers: *Curandero, Espiritista, Partera, Señora* |

Modified from Giger JN, Davidhizar RE: *Transcultural nursing assessment and intervention,* ed 2, St Louis, 1995, Mosby.
*Indicates a high morbidity incidence.

social organizations, of both a religious and an ethnic nature, may play influential roles in the lives of the patient and family, and these organizations can also be an important source of care and assistance. Table 2-3 provides examples of family structures and community organizations that traditionally influence various ethnic groups.

## BIOLOGICAL VARIATIONS

Many biological variations or physiological differences exist among ethnic groups regarding susceptibility to disease, dermatological conditions, and food and eating habits.

### Susceptibility to Disease

Because of genetic or lifestyle differences, some ethnic groups exhibit an increased susceptibility to certain diseases and conditions. In general, groups with lower socioeconomic status are more susceptible to acquired diseases and conditions such as malnutrition and infections. Refer to Table 2-3 for selected variations in disease susceptibility associated with various ethnic groups.

### Dermatological Conditions

Skin color is an important factor in physiological assessment. Because individuals within a race vary widely in skin color, skin color assessment depends more on the individual than on racial or genetic factors. Color changes in dark-skinned patients must be determined differently from those in whites. For instance, in a dark-skinned person, pallor is the absence of the underlying red tones that normally give brown and black skin its glow. Pallor causes black skin to appear ashen gray and brown skin to appear yellow brown.[15] Keloid formation, an exaggerated skin healing process after trauma, is more common among blacks, as are conditions that cause hypopigmentation and hyperpigmentation.

### Food Preferences

Food and eating customs vary widely among cultural groups, and these customs usually carry emotional and social significance. Therefore it helps to have a general understanding of a patient's food habits. In many cases, family members can bring special foods to hospitalized patients who are unhappy with hospital food.

### Reactions to Pain

Reactions to pain are highly individual, but these reactions are also influenced by cultural background. Pain expression varies widely among ethnic groups. It is essential to understand an individual's pattern of pain expression to be able to collaboratively evaluate a patient's pain response. (See Chapter 12.)

## ENVIRONMENTAL CONTROL

Environmental control is the perceived ability of members of a particular cultural group to control natural events. Environmental control includes complex systems of traditional health and illness beliefs, the practices of folk medicine, and the use of traditional healers. These beliefs and practices shape the response of a person/family/community to the health care system. They also form a link to heritage assessment and the health traditions model. Table 2-3 offers several examples of environmental control beliefs and practices.

## HEALTH TRADITIONS MODEL

The HEALTH traditions model defines HEALTH as a state of balance between the person's body, mind, and spirit. The HEALTH traditions model aids in the understanding, assessment, and analysis of the beliefs and practices the person or family may follow to maintain, protect, and restore physical, mental, and spiritual health. This model is used to analyze the needs of individuals who may practice their HEALTH care within their ethnocultural heritage. The model also describes the HEALTH traditions the individual uses to maintain, protect, and restore physical, mental, and spiritual HEALTH in a nine-dimensional interrelated grid, as illustrated in Figure 2-4. Examples include:

- **Maintain** (e.g., daily health practices such as diet, activities, clothing, and so forth)
- **Protect** (e.g., food taboos; seasonal activities; protective items worn, carried, or hung in the home)
- **Restore** (e.g., diet changes; rest; special clothing, substances, or objects)

## HEALTH MAINTENANCE

A person's HEALTH maintenance beliefs are the *daily* or *frequent* activities that the person carries out to maintain HEALTH on an ongoing basis. An infinite number of substances or objects can be used daily to maintain health. Thus HEALTH maintenance beliefs may include the following:

- **Diet** (e.g., dietary restrictions such as the kosher diet and diets balancing yin and yang, or hot and cold)
- **Exercise** (e.g., specific exercises such as tai chi)
- **Rest** (e.g., observing a specific day of rest, such as the Sabbath)

**HEALTH Traditions Model**

| | Physical | Mental | Spiritual |
|---|---|---|---|
| Maintain health | Proper clothing<br>Proper diet<br>Exercise<br>Rest | Concentration<br>Social and family support systems<br>Hobbies | Frequent religious worship<br>Prayer<br>Meditation |
| Protect health | Special diets<br>Symbolic clothing | Avoid certain people who can cause illness and harm<br>Family activities | Religious customs<br>Superstitions<br>Amulets<br>Talisman |
| Restore health | Homeopathic remedies<br>Liniments<br>Herbal teas<br>Special foods<br>Massage | Relaxation<br>Exorcism<br>Curanderos and other traditional healers<br>Nerve teas | Religious rituals<br>Special prayers<br>Meditation<br>Traditional healings<br>Exorcism |

fig. 2-4 The HEALTH traditions model.

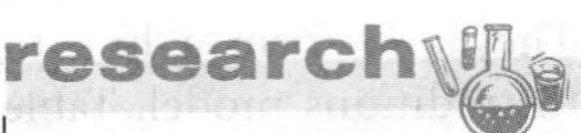

Reference: Smith CA: The lived experience of staying healthy in rural African American families, *Nurs Sci Q* 8(1): 17, 1995.

Research has indicated that persons of low socioeconomic status engage in fewer health-promoting activities than persons with higher incomes and underutilize all types of health care services. African Americans are known to have a higher incidence of diseases that are considered to be responsive to prevention and protection strategies. This qualitative study explored the experience of staying healthy with 21 adults from 10 participant families with children enrolled in a Head Start program in a rural southern community. Participants were interviewed in their homes about the beliefs and practices they used to stay healthy. Traditional qualitative analysis methods were used on the data.

Central themes that emerged included the following: (1) taking care of yourself as a way to maintain God's blessing and protection; (2) learning to care effectively for the self and family creates both physical and emotional strength to meet life's challenges; and (3) being healthy means being happy and not worrying about things. Each family reported consulting trusted sources about health-related issues, but in no circumstance did a trusted source include a health care professional. Family, religious, and community supports were used. The researcher concludes that health care professionals must incorporate health values, beliefs, and practices into their patient care and not seek to change the established patterns of others.

**Clothing** (e.g., dressing modestly, with women covering most of their bodies)

See the accompanying Research Box above.

## HEALTH PROTECTION

A person's HEALTH protection beliefs include the use of specific methods to protect the self from external harm. An infinite number of substances or objects can be used daily to protect health. Objects of a magical nature are worn, carried, or hung in the home for protection from "evil spirits."

Protection of HEALTH rests in the ability of the person to understand the cause of a given illness or set of symptoms. People who hold traditional health and illness beliefs usually regard illness causation differently from allopathic models of etiology. In "traditional epidemiology," illness is often attributed to the "evil eye." The evil eye is a belief that someone can project harm by gazing or staring at another's property or person. Belief in the evil eye is probably the oldest and most widespread of all superstitions, and it exists in many parts of the world, such as Southern Europe, the Middle East, and North Africa. Various evil eye beliefs were carried to the United States by immigrant populations and may be strong among newer immigrants and heritage-consistent peoples. The nature of the evil eye is defined differently by different populations. Variables include how it is cast, who can cast it, who receives it, and the degree of power that it possesses. In the Philippines, the evil is cast through the eye or mouth; in the Mediterranean, it is the avenging power of God; in Italy, it is a malevolent force such as a plague and is prevented by wearing amulets.[21] Table 2-4 lists additional evil eye beliefs.

**table 2-4** *Practices to Prevent the "Evil Eye"*

| Origin | Practices |
|---|---|
| Scotland | Red thread knotted into clothing<br>Fragment of Bible worn on body |
| South Asia | Knotted hair or fragment of Koran worn on body |
| Eastern European Jews | Red ribbon woven into clothes or attached to crib |
| Sephardic Jews | Wearing a blue ribbon or blue bead |
| Italians | Wearing a red ribbon or the corno |
| Greek | Blue "eye" bead, crucifix, charms<br>*Phylact*—a baptismal charm placed on baby<br>Cloves of garlic pinned to shirt |
| Tunisia | Amulets pinned on clothing consisting of tiny figures or writings from the Koran<br>Charms of the fish symbol—widely used to ward off evil |
| Iran | Cover child with amulets—agate, blue beads<br>Children often may be left filthy and never washed to protect them from the "evil eye" |
| India/Pakistan | Hindus—copper plates with magic drawings rolled in them<br>Muslims—slips of paper with verses from the Koran<br>Black or red string around the baby's wrist |
| Guatemala | Small red bag containing herbs placed on baby or crib |
| Mexico | Amulet with red yarn |
| Philippines | Wearing of charms, amulets, medals |
| Puerto Rico | *Mano negro* |

Modified from Spector RE: *Cultural diversity in health and illness*, ed 4, Stamford, Conn, 1996, Appleton & Lange, p 143.

Other agents of disease include "soul loss," "spirit possession," "spells," and "hexes." Rituals are used to protect oneself and one's children from these agents. Other examples of HEALTH protection practices include the following:

**Prayer** (e.g., use of prayer or meditation)
**Diet** (e.g., food taboos)
**Exercise** (e.g., special, seasonal activities)
**Clothing** (e.g., protective items of clothing that are worn at certain times of the day or year)
**Association** (e.g., avoidance of people who may cause the person unknown harm)

## HEALTH RESTORATION

A vast number of substances or objects of a magical nature are used to restore HEALTH. Religion strongly affects the way that people choose to restore HEALTH and to face death when it is imminent.

Many people believe that illness can be both prevented and treated by strictly adhering to religious codes, morals, and practices. They may view illness as a punishment for breaking a religious code. Belief in religious healing is strong, and traditional healers are actively used. Countless rituals guide the dying process, including the Catholic ritual of "anointing the sick" that is used when a person is extremely ill or at the moment of death. Numerous other religious practices must be performed at the moment of or just before death that require the active participation of family members. In some ethnocultural groups, ritual washing and anointing of the body is necessary. Other groups, such as Gypsies, believe that the person should die close to the earth and request that the patient be placed on the floor to die.

When an illness is attributed to the forces of evil, various methods of restoring HEALTH may be used. The sick person may be isolated from the rest of the family and community. Special prayers and incantations may be chanted on the sick person's behalf. The healer may chant in a language foreign to the ears of the general population ("speaking in tongues") and use practices that seem strange to the observers. Sacrifices and dances may also be performed in an effort to cure the ills.

### Religious Beliefs and Healing

Religious beliefs and practices related to healing are found in most religions, and a full description of these practices is beyond the scope of this chapter. A discussion of religious healing beliefs from the Judeo-Christian tradition is included by way of example. The Old Testament does not focus on healing to the extent the New Testament does. God is seen to have total power over life and death and is the healer of all human woes. God is the giver of all good things and of all misfortune, including sickness. Sickness represents a break between God and humans.

The healing practices of the Roman Catholic tradition include a variety of practices, of both a preventive and healing nature. For example, Saint Blaise, an Armenian bishop who died in AD 316 as a martyr, is revered as the preventor of sore throats. The blessing of the throats on his feast day (February 3) derives from the tradition that he miraculously saved the life of a boy by removing a fishbone that he swallowed. Some of the saints concerned with various aspects of illness are listed in Table 2-5. Many more saints could be included.[24]

**table 2-5** *Roman Catholic Saints Concerned with Illness*

| Saint | Problem |
|---|---|
| Our Lady of Lourdes | Bodily ills |
| St. Peregrine | Cancer |
| St. Francis de Sales | Deafness |
| St. Joseph | Dying |
| St. Vitus | Epilepsy |
| St. Lucy | Eye disease |
| St. Teresa of Avila | Headache |
| St. John of God | Heart disease |
| St. Roch | Being bedridden |

People make pilgrimages to a number of shrines in the United States in search of special favors and petitions. These shrines include but are not limited to the following:

- The OHEL (burial place) of the Rebbe Menachem Mendel Schneerson, in Queens, New York. This Jewish shrine was founded when the Rebbe died in 1992. It is visited by thousands of people who ask for the blessings of health and good fortune. Countless letters and petitions are left at the shrine each day. They are collected and burnt, and the ashes are buried behind the OHEL.
- Our Lady of San Juan in San Juan, Texas. This shrine houses a statue of the Virgin that was brought to Mexico by the Spanish missionaries in 1623. The statue caused a miracle, and devotion to La Virgen de San Juan spread. The statue was brought to Texas in the 1940s after a woman claimed to have seen an image of the Virgin in the countryside around San Juan. The statue is currently housed in a beautiful new church, and pilgrims arrive daily to ask for healing and other favors. Countless letters are on display attesting to the healing powers of the statue.[24]
- St. Peregrine for Cancer Sufferers, in the Old Mission San Juan Capistrano in California. This statue is housed in a small grotto in the shrine. St. Peregrine was born in Italy in 1265 and died in 1345. He was believed to have miraculous powers against sickness and could cure cancer. This won for him the title "official patron for cancer victims." Many years ago a woman was afflicted with cancer and an acquaintance gave her a prayer to St. Peregrine. The woman prayed diligently for 6 months, and her cancer was arrested. In gratitude, the woman had a statue of the saint placed in the mission. Today, belief in this saint has spread, and countless documents attesting to his healing powers are on display in the mission.[24]
- Shrine of the Blessed Virgin Mary in the Christ of the Hills Russian Orthodox Monastery in New Sarov, Blanco, Texas. Here, in this shrine, is an icon painted in 1983. The icon is said to have begun to weep tears of myrrh in 1985 and has been a place for healing pilgrimages since then. Hundreds of thousands of pilgrims have come to this icon seeking healing. Many documents attesting to its healing powers are on display in the church. Table 2-6 summarizes the beliefs of people from several religious backgrounds with respect to health, healing, and other events related to nursing and health care delivery.

*Text continued on p. 39*

**table 2-6** *Selected Religions' Responses to Health Events*

**BAHA'I**
**"ALL HEALING COMES FROM GOD."**

| | |
|---|---|
| Abortion | Forbidden |
| Artificial insemination | No specific rule |
| Autopsy | Acceptable with medical or legal need |
| Birth control | Can choose family planning method |
| Blood and blood products | No restrictions for use |
| Diet | Alcohol and drugs forbidden |
| Euthanasia | No destruction of life |
| Healing beliefs | Harmony between religion and science |
| Healing practices | Prayer |
| Medications | Narcotics with prescription<br>No restriction for vaccines |
| Organ donations | Permitted |
| Right-to-die issues | Life is unique and precious—do not destroy |
| Surgical procedures | No restrictions |
| Visitors | Community members assist and support |

**BUDDHIST CHURCHES OF AMERICA**
**"TO KEEP THE BODY IN GOOD HEALTH IS A DUTY—OTHERWISE WE SHALL NOT BE ABLE TO KEEP OUR MINDS STRONG AND CLEAR."**

| | |
|---|---|
| Abortion | Patient's condition determines |
| Artificial insemination | Acceptable |
| Autopsy | Matter of individual practice |
| Birth control | Acceptable |
| Blood and blood products | No restrictions |
| Diet | Restricted food combinations<br>Extremes must be avoided |
| Euthanasia | May permit |
| Healing beliefs | Do not believe in healing through faith |
| Healing practices | No restrictions |
| Medications | No restrictions |
| Organ donations | Considered act of mercy; if hope for recovery, all means may be taken |
| Right-to-die issues | With hope, all means encouraged |
| Surgical procedures | Permitted, with extremes avoided |
| Visitors | Family, community |

**ROMAN CATHOLICISM**
**"THE PRAYER OF FAITH SHALL HEAL THE SICK, AND THE LORD SHALL RAISE HIM UP."**

| | |
|---|---|
| Abortion | Prohibited |
| Artificial insemination | Illicit, even between husband and wife |
| Autopsy | Permissible |
| Birth control | Natural means only |
| Blood and blood products | Permissible |
| Diet | Use foods in moderation |
| Euthanasia | Direct life-ending procedures forbidden |
| Healing beliefs | Many within religious belief system |
| Healing practices | Sacrament of sick, candles, laying on of hands |
| Medications | May be taken if benefits outweigh risks |
| Organ donations | Justifiable |
| Right-to-die issues | Obligated to take ordinary, not extraordinary, means to prolong life |
| Surgical procedures | Most are permissible except abortion and sterilization |
| Visitors | Family, friends, priest<br>Many outreach programs through Church to reach sick |

**CHRISTIAN SCIENCE**

| | |
|---|---|
| Abortion | Incompatible with faith |
| Artificial insemination | Unusual |
| Autopsy | Not usual; individual or family decide |
| Birth control | Individual judgment |
| Blood and blood products | Ordinarily not used by members |
| Diet | No restrictions<br>Abstain from alcohol and tobacco, some from tea and coffee |
| Euthanasia | Contrary to teachings |
| Healing beliefs | Accepts physical and moral healing |
| Healing practices | Full-time healing ministers<br>Spiritual healing practiced |
| Medications | None<br>Immunizations/vaccines to comply with law |
| Organ donations | Individual decides |
| Right-to-die issues | Unlikely to seek medical help to prolong life |
| Surgical procedures | No medical ones practiced |
| Visitors | Family, friends, and members of the Christian Science community and healers, Christian Science nurses |

Adapted with permission from Andrews MM, Hanson PA: Religion, culture, and nursing. In Boyle JS, Andrews MM, editors: *Transcultural concepts in nursing care,* ed 2, Philadelphia, 1995, JB Lippincott, pp 371-406; and Spector RE: *Cultural diversity in health and illness,* ed 4, Stamford, Conn, 1996, Appleton & Lange, pp 153-157.

*Continued*

**table 2-6** *Selected Religions' Responses to Health Events—cont'd*

**CHURCH OF JESUS CHRIST OF LATTER-DAY SAINTS**

| | |
|---|---|
| Abortion | Forbidden |
| Artificial insemination | Acceptable between husband and wife |
| Autopsy | Permitted with consent of next of kin |
| Birth control | Contrary to Mormon belief |
| Blood and blood products | No restrictions |
| Diet | Alcohol, tea (except herbal teas), coffee, and tobacco are forbidden<br>Fasting (24 hours without food and drink) is required once a month |
| Euthanasia | Humans must not interfere in God's plan |
| Healing beliefs | Power of God can bring healing |
| Healing practices | Anointing with oil, sealing, prayer, laying on of hands |
| Medications | No restrictions; may use herbal folk remedies |
| Organ donations | Permitted |
| Right-to-die issues | If death inevitable, promote a peaceful and dignified death |
| Surgical procedures | Matter of individual choice |
| Visitors | Church members (Elder and Sister) family and friends<br>Relief Society helps members |

**HINDUISM**
**"ENRICHER, HEALER OF DISEASE, BE A GOOD FRIEND TO US."**

| | |
|---|---|
| Abortion | No policy exists |
| Artificial insemination | No restrictions exist but not often practiced |
| Autopsy | Acceptable |
| Birth control | All types acceptable |
| Blood and blood products | Acceptable |
| Diet | Eating of meat is forbidden |
| Euthanasia | Not practiced |
| Healing beliefs | Some believe in faith healing |
| Healing practices | Traditional faith-healing system |
| Medications | Acceptable |
| Organ donations | Acceptable |
| Right-to-die issues | No restrictions<br>Death seen as "one more step to nirvana" |
| Surgical procedures | With an amputation, the loss of limb seen as due to "sins in a previous life" |
| Visitors | Members of family, community, and priest support |

**ISLAM**
**"THE LORD OF THE WORLD CREATED ME—AND WHEN I AM SICK, HE HEALETH ME."**

| | |
|---|---|
| Abortion | Accepted |
| Artificial insemination | Permitted between husband and wife |
| Autopsy | Permitted for medical and legal purposes |
| Birth control | Acceptable |
| Blood and blood products | No restrictions |
| Diet | Pork and alcohol prohibited |
| Euthanasia | Not acceptable |
| Healing beliefs | Faith healing generally not acceptable |
| Healing practices | Some use of herbal remedies and faith healing |
| Medications | No restrictions |
| Organ donations | Acceptable |
| Right-to-die issues | Attempts to shorten life prohibited |
| Surgical procedures | Most permitted |
| Visitors | Family and friends provide support |

**JEHOVAH'S WITNESSES**

| | |
|---|---|
| Abortion | Forbidden |
| Artificial insemination | Forbidden |
| Autopsy | Acceptable if required by law |
| Birth control | Sterilization forbidden<br>Other methods individual choice |
| Blood and blood products | Forbidden |
| Diet | Abstain from tobacco, moderate use of alcohol |
| Euthanasia | Forbidden |
| Healing beliefs | Faith healing forbidden |
| Healing practices | Reading scriptures can comfort the individual and lead to mental and spiritual healing |
| Medications | Accepted unless derived from blood products |
| Organ donations | Forbidden |
| Right-to-die issues | Use of extraordinary means an individual's choice |
| Surgical procedures | Not opposed, but administration of blood during surgery is strictly prohibited |
| Visitors | Members of congregation and elders pray for the sick person |

*Continued*

**table 2-6** *Selected Religions' Responses to Health Events—cont'd*

| JUDAISM<br>"O LORD, MY GOD, I CRIED TO THEE FOR HELP AND THOU HAS HEALED ME." | |
|---|---|
| Abortion | Therapeutic permitted; some groups accept abortion on demand |
| Artificial insemination | Permitted |
| Autopsy | Permitted under certain circumstances<br>All body parts must be buried together |
| Birth control | Permissible, except with orthodox Jews |
| Blood and blood products | Acceptable |
| Diet | Strict dietary laws followed by many Jews—milk and meat not mixed; predatory fowl, shellfish, and pork products forbidden; kosher products only may be requested |
| Euthanasia | Prohibited |
| Healing beliefs | Medical care expected |
| Healing practices | Prayers for the sick |
| Medications | No restrictions |
| Organ donations | Complex issue; some practiced |
| Right-to-die issues | Right to die with dignity<br>If death is inevitable, no new procedures need to be undertaken, but those ongoing must continue |
| Surgical procedures | Most allowed |
| Visitors | Family, friends, rabbi, many community services |

| MENNONITE | |
|---|---|
| Abortion | Therapeutic acceptable |
| Artificial insemination | Individual conscience; husband to wife |
| Autopsy | Acceptable |
| Birth control | Acceptable |
| Blood and blood products | Acceptable |
| Diet | No specific restrictions |
| Euthanasia | Not condoned |
| Healing beliefs | Part of God's work |
| Healing practices | Prayer and anointing with oil |
| Medications | No restrictions |
| Organ donations | Acceptable |
| Right-to-die issues | Do not believe life must be continued at all cost |
| Surgical procedures | No restrictions |
| Visitors | Family, community |

| SEVENTH-DAY ADVENTISTS | |
|---|---|
| Abortion | Therapeutic acceptable |
| Artificial insemination | Acceptable between husband and wife |
| Autopsy | Acceptable |
| Birth control | Individual choice |
| Blood and blood products | No restrictions |
| Diet | Encourage vegetarian diet |
| Euthanasia | Not practiced |
| Healing beliefs | Divine healing |
| Healing practices | Anointing with oil and prayer |
| Medications | No restrictions<br>Vaccines acceptable |
| Organ donations | Acceptable |
| Right-to-die issues | Follow the ethic of prolonging life |
| Surgical procedures | No restrictions<br>Oppose use of hypnotism |
| Visitors | Pastor and elders pray and anoint sick person<br>Worldwide health system includes hospitals and clinics |

| UNITARIAN/UNIVERSALIST CHURCH | |
|---|---|
| Abortion | Acceptable, therapeutic and on demand |
| Artificial insemination | Acceptable |
| Autopsy | Recommended |
| Birth control | All types acceptable |
| Blood and blood products | No restrictions |
| Diet | No restrictions |
| Euthanasia | Favor nonaction<br>May withdraw therapies if death imminent |
| Healing beliefs | Faith healing seen as "superstitious" |
| Healing practices | Use of science to facilitate healing |
| Medications | No restrictions |
| Organ donations | Acceptable |
| Right-to-die issues | Favor the right to die with dignity |
| Surgical procedures | No restrictions |
| Visitors | Family, friends, church members |

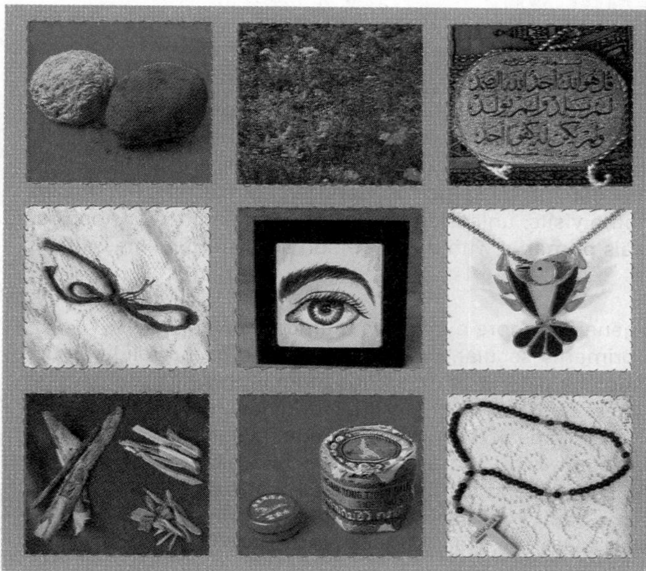

fig. 2-5 HEALTH traditions quilt.

The "quilt" (Figure 2-5) contains the following symbolic illustrations of substances or objects used within selected, representative traditions to maintain HEALTH, protect HEALTH, and restore HEALTH. The illustrations correspond with the categories of the HEALTH traditions model.

- Maintain HEALTH
  *Thousand-year eggs* (China) represent traditional foods that may be eaten daily.
  *Nature*—the enjoyment of nature may be a universal way of maintaining mental health.
  *Islamic prayer*—East Jerusalem prayer may be a way of maintaining spiritual health.
- Protect HEALTH
  *Red string* (tomb of Rachel in Bethlehem, Israel) may be worn, especially on new babies and women, to protect physical health.
  *Eye* (Cuba) may be hung in the home to protect the mental health of the household members.
  *Thunderbird* (Hopi Nation) may be worn for spiritual protection.
- Restore HEALTH
  *Herbal remedy* (Africa) represents herbs that may be used in a wide variety of preparations.
  *Tiger balm* (Singapore)—massage may be a way of restoring mental HEALTH.
  *Rosary beads* (Italy)—prayer and meditation may be used in the spiritual restoration of HEALTH.

### Traditional Healers

In the traditional context, healing is the restoration of the person to a state of HEALTH. Within a traditional community, specific healers have the power to heal. The healer (man or woman) is most often a person thought to have received the gift of healing from a divine source. Healers commonly receive their gift in a vision and are unable to explain how they know what to do. Other healers learned their skills from parents or teachers.

A person who is heritage consistent may consult a traditional healer. The healer may be seen before, instead of, or concurrently with a Western health care provider. The relationship between the person and healer is often much closer than that of the person and the health care professional. The healer understands the problem within the cultural context, speaks the same language, and shares a similar worldview. The following are examples of traditional healers:

1. *Medicine man*—the traditional healer of the Native Americans
2. *Señora*—a Puerto Rican woman knowledgeable in the treatment of illness
3. *Esperitista*—a person who possesses more sophisticated skills than the Señora
4. *Curandero*—a person with a god-given ability to heal using a religious approach
5. *Partera*—a Mexican American midwife
6. *Root worker*—an African American who is able to determine the cause of an illness and the treatment[26]

HEALTH beliefs, HEALTH practices, and the use of traditional healers have been a part of human cultures throughout their existence. The methods used to maintain, protect, and restore HEALTH have been developed over generations by trial and error, with religious beliefs and social circumstances contributing to their development. The effective methods have been preserved and adapted to meet changing needs and circumstances. The traditional healer and nurse are compared in Table 2-7 and in the accompanying Research Box.

## CROSS-CULTURAL HEALTH TRADITIONS

The following CulturalCare capsules provide a general overview of Asian American, African American, Hispanic American, Native American, and European American cultures. Each capsule includes a synopsis of the group's demographic background, traditional HEALTH beliefs, and selected examples of traditional HEALTH practices. These capsules illustrate both the similarities and differences between groups of people. However, it is important to remember that the beliefs of a cultural group are not necessarily shared by each individual in that group, and this information simply provides a foundation for increasing cultural awareness and sensitivity.

### ASIAN AMERICANS

Asian Americans originated in China, Pacific Islands, the Philippines, Korea, Japan, Laos, Cambodia, and Vietnam. Many Asian Americans have lived in the United States for several generations; others arrived more recently, and still others are currently in the process of entering the country. Asian Americans are the second largest ethnic group in the U.S. population. During 1994 the Asian and Pacific Islander population grew by 3.8% and was the only population group whose net international migration added more people than natural increases.[30]

**table 2-7** *Comparison: Healer and Nurse*

| HEALER | NURSE |
|---|---|
| Maintains an informal, friendly, affective relationship with the entire family | Is business-like and formal, dealing primarily with the patient |
| Comes to the house day or night | Stays in a "professional" institution, office or clinic where the patient must go for services; rarely, if ever, makes home visits, unless community health practice or hospice |
| For diagnosis, consults with head of house, creates a mood of awe, talks to all family members, is not authoritarian, has social rapport, builds expectation of cure | Deals primarily with the ill person and specific illness |
| Is generally less expensive than a physician | Is generally more expensive than the healer |
| Has ties to the "world of the sacred," has rapport with the symbolic, spiritual, creative, or holy force | Is primarily secular, pays little attention to the religious beliefs of a patient or meanings of an illness |
| Shares the worldview of the patient (i.e., speaks the same language, lives in the same neighborhood or in the same similar socioeconomic conditions, may know the same people, understands the lifestyle of the patient) | Generally does not share the worldview of the patient (i.e., may not speak the same language, live in the same neighborhood or in the same socioeconomic conditions, may not understand the lifestyle of the patient) |

Modified from Spector RE: *Cultural diversity in health and illness,* ed 4, Norwalk, Conn, 1996, Appleton & Lange. Source: Adapted from Potter PA, Perry AG: *Fundamentals of nursing: concepts, process, and practice,* ed 4, St Louis, 1997, Mosby, p 361.

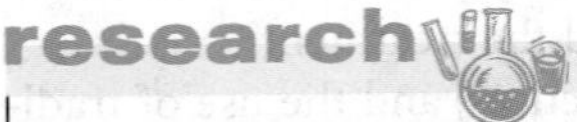

Reference: Engebretson J: Comparison of nurses and alternative healers, *Image J Nurs Sch* 28(2):95, 1996.

Both nurses and alternative healers subscribe to a holistic framework with a focus on health and well-being. This study compared the models of healing and health as described by nurses and alternative healers. The sample was composed of 18 nurse faculty and 23 alternative healers. The nurses were women between 30 and 65 years of age with master's or doctoral preparation in nursing. The alternative healers were primarily women between 25 and 80 years of age, and most had attended at least some college.

Participants were asked to list all the things that one could do to be healed or stay healthy. The items were analyzed and condensed into a final list of 20 to 30 items for each domain, which were then sorted according to similarity and differences. Participants were also asked to discuss the reasons for their choices. Domains included physical, mental, attitudinal, relational, spiritual, self-caring, and help-seeking activities.

There were many overlapping responses between the two groups, but the nurses did not identify any activities related to self-caring under healing despite a rich variety of activities related to staying healthy. Other differences were primarily related to practice setting. Healers usually practice independently in the community, whereas nurses practice in medical settings. Nurses and healers share many beliefs about healing and can benefit by sharing openly with each other. Nurses can work as bridges between patients, providers, and healers in the overall plan of care for the patient.

## Community Overview

The following is a brief sketch of the population:

- The median age of this population in 1990 was 29.8 years.[29]
- 73.6% of the members over age 25 have completed a high school education.[31]
- Personal earnings for people working full time in 1989 averaged $31,979.[30]
- 11% of people over 25 years of age in this group were below the poverty level in 1991.[16]

The family consists of a hierarchical structure, and loyalty among members is valued. There is a devotion to tradition, and many religions, including Taoism, Buddhism, Islam, and Christianity, are practiced.

## HEALTH Beliefs

Within the Asian community, Chinese medicine provides an overall framework for Asian cultures. HEALTH beliefs include the belief that HEALTH is a state of spiritual and physical harmony among body, mind, and spirit in harmony with nature. In addition, the forces of *yin* (female, negative energy) and *yang* (male, positive energy) must be in balance. The body is viewed as a gift from parents and ancestors. It is not the person's personal property and must be cared for and maintained. The primary role of the physician in ancient China was to help safeguard the body and to prevent illness. If a person became ill despite preventive measures, it was not necessary to pay the physician for treatment.

Illness may be caused by an upset in the balance of yin and yang. The weather, overexertion, and prolonged sitting may also cause illness. Illness may be prevented by adhering to a proper diet to maintain the body's balance, exercising, avoiding temperature changes, and taking certain remedies.

## HEALTH Practices

HEALTH is maintained by adhering to dietary rules; protected by wearing amulets, such as jade; and restored with the use of countless herbal remedies, acupuncture, and moxibustion. *Moxibustion* is the practice of applying heat to the designated location on the body to restore the balance of yin and yang.

The following traditional remedies are used to maintain, protect, or restore HEALTH in the Asian tradition:

- *Chi Chung Shui.* A pleasant-tasting liquid diet supplement added to soups to maintain HEALTH.
- *Essential Balm.* A soothing, pleasant-smelling balm that is massaged on the body to relax muscles in an effort to maintain HEALTH.
- *Daishi (Omanori).* An amulet from Japan that is hung in the car and believed to protect the person and ensure safe driving. It may also be hung in the home or in one's place of business for protection.
- *Jen Shen Lu Jung Wan.* A brown-colored, gummy substance encased in white wax. It is indicated in the treatment of general debility, anemia, lack of well-being, mental overstrain, and loss of appetite, and it may be taken before elective surgery.
- *Ginseng root.* A substance that has universal medicinal usage in "building the blood," especially after childbirth. Ginseng root is the most famous Chinese medicine. Chinese legend states that the more the root looks like a human being, the more effective it is. Ginseng is native to the United States and is used in this country as a restorative tonic.
- *Acupuncture.* A method of treating disease by puncturing the skin with thin metal needles at specific points on the body; moxibustion can also be applied to these same points.[24]

## AFRICAN AMERICANS

Most African Americans have ancestors who were brought to the United States as slaves between 1619 and 1860 from the western coast of Africa. Today, many black people have also immigrated to the United States from countries such as the West Indies, the Dominican Republic, Haiti, and Jamaica. The 1990 population of African (black) Americans was 29,986,000 people, or 11.7% of the total population of the United States. This population grew by 1.5% in 1994.

### Community Overview

The following is a brief sketch of the population:

- The median age of the population in 1990 was 28.1 years.[29]
- 59.8% of the members over age 25 have completed a high school education.[31]
- Personal earnings for people working full time in 1989 averaged $22,525.[30]
- 25% of people over age 25 in this group were below the poverty level in 1991.[29]

The family often consists of a matriarchal structure, and there are many single-parent households headed by females; there are strong and large extended family networks. There is a continuation of tradition and a strong religious affiliation within the community. Many African Americans use traditional medicines and healers when these resources are available.

### HEALTH Beliefs

The traditional definition of health stems from African beliefs about life and the nature of being. Life is viewed as a process rather than a state, and the nature of a person is viewed in terms of energy rather than matter. When healthy, a person is in harmony with nature. Illness is seen as a disharmony of the mind, body, and spirit or as a disharmony between humanity and nature. Researchers and epidemiologists have noted chronic illness patterns that are associated with African American culture. A correlation between psychological stress and hypertension was found in African Americans.[3] Illness (disharmony) is often attributed to demons and evil spirits. Several methods are used as protection from these forces, including the ancient practice of voodoo. Voodoo is believed to cause, as well as prevent, the action of malevolent forces. "White" magic protects against malevolent forces and "black" magic directs their energy to a specific person or body area. The extent of belief in voodoo is unknown.

### HEALTH Practices

HEALTH protection may focus on avoiding people believed to carry evil spirits. Prayer and a well-balanced diet are also considered helpful methods of protection.

The following traditional remedies are used to maintain, protect, or restore HEALTH among African Americans:

- *Egg with mating couple.* A ceramic egg from Ethiopia represents the linkage of art forms to symbolic beliefs related to HEALTH maintenance. The couple is depicted mating within the egg (representing fertility), and the shell is decorated with a tree of life.
- *Bangles.* Silver bracelets worn by people originating from the West Indies. They overlap but are open to let out evil and closed to prevent evil from entering the body. They are worn from infancy and are replaced as the person grows. These bracelets tarnish and leave a black ring on the skin when a person is becoming ill. The black ring serves as a signal to rest, improve the diet, and take any other needed precautions. Some people wear many bangles, believing that their sound frightens away evil spirits. Some people believe that they are extremely vulnerable to evil, even to death, when the bangles are removed, so removal of these bracelets can cause a great deal of anxiety.
- *Talismans.* Objects worn on a string around the waist or carried in a pocket or purse. They protect the HEALTH of the wearer from sickness.
- *Asafoetida.* A foul-smelling, gummy, protective substance worn to ward off colds and evil. It is known as the incense of the devil.
- *Voodoo candles.* Candles having a particular spiritualistic character and used for sacred rituals and rites to restore HEALTH. Colors also have significance. For example, pink means love, white means peace, and blue means success and protection from harm.[24]

## HISPANIC AMERICANS

Members of the Hispanic community originated in Iberia (Spain and Portugal) and Cuba, Mexico, Puerto Rico, and other Spanish- or Portuguese-speaking countries of Central and South America. With a 1990 population of 22,354,059 (9% of the U.S. population), Hispanic Americans are the most rapidly growing ethnic group in the United States. In 1994 the growth in the Hispanic population was larger than the growth in the white, non-Hispanic population.

### Community Overview

The following is a brief sketch of the population:

- The median age in 1990 was 25.5 years.[29]
- 47.1% of the members over age 25 have completed a high school education.[31]
- Personal earnings for people working full time in 1989 averaged $22,383.[30]
- 21.3% of people over age 25 in this group were below the poverty level in 1991.[31]

The family often consists of a nuclear family, with large, strong, extended family networks, and *compadrazzo*—godparents. There is a continuation of tradition and a strong church affiliation within the community. Many, but not all, Hispanics are Catholic.

### HEALTH Beliefs

Health is often believed to be the result of good luck or a reward from God for good behavior. Health represents a state of equilibrium within the universe in which the forces of hot, cold, wet, and dry are balanced. Blood is hot and wet, and yellow bile is hot and dry; phlegm is cold and wet, and black bile is cold and dry. The concept originated with the early Hippocratic theory of the four humors. Health exists when the four humors are in a balanced state. Health is maintained by diet and other practices that keep the humors balanced.

Illness is viewed as misfortune or bad luck, punishment from God for evil thoughts or actions, or the imbalance of hot and cold. Several factors cause illness. A hot-cold imbalance, for example, is primarily caused by improper diet. Food substances are classified as hot or cold without regard to their actual temperature. The classification can vary from person to person, but certain foods are known to be hot, and others are known to be cold. Examples of cold foods are chicken, honey, avocados, bananas, and lima beans. Examples of hot foods are chocolate, coffee, corn meal, garlic, kidney beans, onions, and peas. Illness can occur if these foods are eaten in improper combinations or amounts. For example, *frialdad del estómago* (cold stomach) is caused by eating too many cold foods. Adherence to this hot-cold system is particularly important during conditions such as menstruation and pregnancy. A pregnant woman avoids hot foods. During menstruation and after childbirth she avoids cold foods. An infant who requires formula that contains a hot food such as evaporated milk may also be fed a cold food such as whole milk.

Other factors believed to cause illness are the "dislocation of body parts" (such as fallen fontanel) and magic or supernatural causes such as *mal ojo* (bad eye). Diagnostic techniques include divination, observation, and exorcism. *Envidia* (envy) is also a cause of both illness and bad luck, and many means are used to prevent it. Many Hispanic people believe that to succeed is to fail—that is, when a person's success provokes the envy of friends and neighbors, misfortune or illness may follow.

### HEALTH Practices

HEALTH is protected by following a proper diet, avoiding "harmful" people, wearing amulets for protection, and using candles and prayer. Hispanic people may be treated by traditional healers, such as Curanderos, Santeros, or Señoras, and commonly use herbs to restore HEALTH.

The following remedies are used among Hispanic people to protect or restore HEALTH:

- *Mano negro (black hand).* A Puerto Rican amulet may be placed on a baby at birth and is believed to protect the infant from the evil eye.
- *Jabón de la Mano Milagrosa (soap of the miraculous hand).* A soap used to cleanse and protect a person.
- *Amulet.* A medium-sized bottle from Peru that is carried in the pocket for protection. The bottle contains holy oil, a picture of the Mano Milagrosa, feathers, ribbon, worms, seeds, beans, shells, chain with beads, cloth, string, or staples.
- *Manzanilla.* An herb made into tea and used to treat stomach and intestinal pain, uterine cramps, anxiety, and insomnia.
- *Anis.* Star-shaped seeds used to treat painful gases, upset stomach, colic, and anorexia and to increase production of breast milk.[24]

## NATIVE AMERICANS

There are over 200 American Indian Nations and 500 tribes in the United States. They are predominantly located in the Western states. Each nation has its own unique cultural heritage and traditional HEALTH beliefs and practices. Although many Native Americans remain on reservations, many live in the larger society. With a 1990 population of 1.9 million, or 0.7% of the total population of the United States, Native Americans are the smallest ethnic group in the American population.

### Community Overview

The following is a brief sketch of the population:

- The median age of the population in 1990 was 26.2 years.[29]
- 60.5% of the members over age 25 have completed a high school education.[31]
- Personal earnings for people working full time in 1989 averaged $23,121.[30]
- 23.7% of people over age 25 in this group were below the poverty level in 1991.[16]

The family often consists of a nuclear family, with strong biological ties and large extended family networks. Children are taught to respect traditions. Community organizations provide a growing number of social and cultural services to the population.

### HEALTH Beliefs

Health reflects the ability to live in total harmony with nature and to survive under extremely difficult circumstances. People are believed to have an intimate spiritual relationship with nature; to stay healthy, a person must maintain a positive, balanced relationship with the natural world. The earth is considered to be a living organism, the body of a higher individual, with a will and a desire to experience health. Both the body and the earth must be treated with respect. Because the earth provides humans with food, shelter, and medicine, it must be protected. "The land belongs to life, life belongs to the land, and the land belongs to itself."

Traditional Native Americans view the body as divided into two halves, and in every whole there are two energy poles, a positive and a negative. People have the power to control their body's energy through spiritual power. HEALTH is described as the harmony or balance between the two halves or the two energy poles. Illness is disharmony of the body, mind, and spirit.

Sources of illness vary from nation to nation and tribe to tribe. Hopi Indians associate illness with evil spirits and therefore strive to avoid or ward off these spirits. Navajos view illness as the result of displeasing the holy people, annoying the elements, disturbing animal and plant life, neglecting the celestial bodies, misusing a sacred Indian ceremony, or tampering with witches or witchcraft. Hawk Littlejohn,[20] an Eastern Band Cherokee medicine man, describes illness as an imbalance of the body, mind, or spirit caused by an excess in one domain and the neglect of the other two. For example, a student who spends too much time studying—developing the mind—may neglect the body and spirit and be vulnerable to disharmony and illness. The main principle for illness prevention is the maintenance of harmony with the body, mind, and spirit and the avoidance of factors that cause disharmony.

### HEALTH Practices

Many Native Americans use traditional medicines and healers and are knowledgeable about these resources. They may be treated by a traditional medicine man, and the sweat lodge and herbs are commonly used to treat mental symptoms. Diagnostic techniques include the use of divination, conjuring, and stargazing.

The following examples are remedies used by Native Americans to prevent or treat illness:

- *Corn-husk mask.* A mask worn to hide the self from the devil or evil spirits.
- *Sweet grass.* The medicine man burns the grass as a rite of purification to protect HEALTH.
- *Sand painting.* A creation of the Navaho medicine man while diagnosing an ailment. The painting is created in an elaborate diagnostic ceremony of motion of the hand. When the hand moves in a certain way, the medicine man knows that it indicates a specific illness, and he is able to prescribe the correct treatment.
- *Thunderbird.* An amulet worn for good luck and protection.
- *Medicine bag.* A small leather drawstring bag with medicinal herbs carried by the traditional medicine man.[24]

## EUROPEAN AMERICANS

Members of most European American communities originated in Europe and have been migrating to this country since 1620. This population is a diverse mixture of people from many countries, speaking numerous languages and observing a wide variety of health beliefs and practices.

### Community Overview

The 1980 census was the first to attempt to break down the European American population by country of origin. The largest groups were found to be from Germany, England, Ireland, and France. During 1994 the population grew by 0.8%. The following is a brief sketch of the population:

- The median age in 1990 was 34.4 years.[29]
- 74.6% of the members over age 25 have completed a high school education.[31]
- Personal earnings for people working full time in 1989 averaged $31,419.[30]
- 8.8% of people over age 25 in this group were below the poverty level in 1991.[29]

### HEALTH Beliefs

Health and illness are defined in many ways by European Americans. Definitions of health include the ability to perform activities of daily living; a state of physical and emotional well-being; and a state free of illness. Illness is defined as the inability to perform activities of daily living, the presence of disease symptoms and pain, and the malformation of body organs.

To European Americans, traditional beliefs about the causes of illness are many and varied. Beliefs include breaking religious rules, punishment from God, climate changes, exposure to causative factors (e.g., drafts), and the abuse of the body. A wide variety of methods for preventing illness are found among European Americans, including diet, exercise, religious rituals, and the wearing of shawls or amulets.

### HEALTH Practices

The following are a few examples of remedies reported among European Americans:

- *Malocchio.* An Italian horn worn to protect the wearer by preventing the evil eye. The hunchbacked man *Gobo* worn on a horn offers extra protection; he holds a horseshoe for luck in his left hand and points the index and baby finger of his right hand to ward off the evil spirit.
- *Syrup of Black Draught.* An over-the-counter laxative used to maintain HEALTH by keeping the body clean.
- *Father John's Medicine.* A family medicine that has been used to restore HEALTH by treating colds and coughs since 1855.
- *Swamp root.* An over-the-counter liquid used as a diuretic to restore HEALTH.
- *Sloan's Liniment.* A product that restores HEALTH through the temporary relief of minor pains resulting from arthritis and other ailments.

This brief overview is designed to introduce the student to the richness of HEALTH traditions that are part of nursing practice with a diverse population. This introduction can increase the nurse's cultural awareness and sensitivity and serve as a first step toward cultural competence in nursing practice.

## CulturalCare AND THE NURSING PROCESS

The provision of CulturalCare mandates an awareness of and sensitivity to the patient's unique sociocultural background and HEALTH traditions. The nursing process can be effectively adapted to assess a patient's health and illness beliefs and practices and determine the impact of their cultural, ethnic, or religious values on the proposed plan of care. Health beliefs and

**table 2-8** *CulturalCare Nursing Process*

| Process | Action |
|---|---|
| **ASSESSMENT** | |
| Heritage consistency | Perform heritage-consistency assessment (see Box 2-3) on self and patient. |
| HEALTH traditions | Ask the patient what is done to maintain, protect, or restore HEALTH. |
| Environmental control | Ask about the patient's beliefs of the nature of the health problem and actions being taken at home or in the community to treat and resolve it.<br>Ask about other health care resources being used. |
| Biological variations | Ask about nutritional preferences.<br>Observe body structure, skin tone, and color.<br>Be aware of health problems that may be more common in patient's background. |
| Social organizations | Conduct community activities. |
| Communication skills | Determine the needs of the patient who does not speak the nurse's language and provide competent interpreters. |
| Space | Be aware of territoriality; seek permission before intruding in the patient's territory.<br>Be aware of touch and eye-contact expectations. |
| Time | Understand the differences in time orientation. |
| **NURSING DIAGNOSIS** | |
| Development of problem list | Ask about the patient's interpretation of the problem and possible effective interventions. |
| **PLANNING/GOAL SETTING** | Include patient, family, and community in plans as needed. |
| **IMPLEMENTATION** | Alter usual ways of interacting to adjust to patient's social interaction and etiquette.<br>Incorporate interventions agreeing with patient's cultural heritage, educational level, and language skills. |
| **EVALUATION** | With patient, determine whether nursing care has met expectations and needs. |

Modified from Potter PA, Perry AG: *Fundamentals of nursing: concepts, process, and practice,* ed 4, St Louis, 1997, Mosby, p 366.

practices must be recognized and respected, and not challenged. With this level of cultural competence the nurse can prevent cultural collisions between the modern health care world and the patient's traditional world. Blending these divergent viewpoints is challenging, but not impossible. The systematic thinking process inherent in the steps of the nursing process facilitates the provision of individualized CulturalCare nursing. Table 2-8 identifies the components of the CulturalCare nursing process.

Nurses can increase their sensitivity and appreciation for a given ethnoreligious community by visiting the community and witnessing its daily life. Box 2-2 lists various social factors to explore to increase cultural sensitivity and awareness. The "answers" can generally be found in libraries or through interviews with people from the community. Answers can also be acquired by walking through the community and viewing the churches, social organizations, and health-related services that are available. A visit to a community health care provider or clinic, a church or community center that serves the target group, and grocery stores and pharmacies in the area allows the nurse to increase his or her cultural knowledge base concerning the people in the target community.

## CulturalCare ASSESSMENT

A variety of tools are available to assist the nurse to assess the patient and family from a CulturalCare perspective. It is equally important, however, for the nurse to carefully assess his or her own sociocultural heritage and health and illness beliefs. We are each the product of our own unique heritage and upbringing, and nurses are affected by this process as strongly as patients. The nurse cannot expect to enter any situation value free, but it is reasonable to expect the nurse to have a clear view of his or her own belief system and how it may affect a patient's care. Nurses are also representatives of the dominant allopathic health care philosophy and will need to work carefully to communicate an openness to alternative/complementary and traditional practices of health and healing.

In addition to the general assessment, the nurse assesses:

- *The patient's and family's English language skills.* When the patient and family members do not speak or understand English, it is imperative that competent interpreters, who are neither family members nor children, are available 24 hours a day. The interpreters not only translate the spoken words, but also help interpret the nonverbal subtleties of the culture.
- *The patient's and family's cultural heritage.* The Heritage Assessment Tool found in Box 2-3 aids in this process. If a patient scores high in terms of heritage consistency, there is a high probability that this person adheres to traditional HEALTH beliefs. Additional assessment is then undertaken to fully understand the patient's circumstances.
- *The patient's and family's ethnocultural and social organizations.* The assessment tool in Box 2-4 can be used to enhance the nurse's understanding of the patient's community. Other resources, human and literature, that may be used to help the nurse understand the patient's cultural worldview are listed in Box 2-5.

**box 2-3** *Heritage Assessment Tool*

1. Where was your mother born? ______
2. Where was your father born? ______
3. Where were your grandparents born?:
   a. Your mother's mother? ______
   b. Your mother's father? ______
   c. Your father's mother? ______
   d. Your father's father? ______
4. How many brothers ______ and sisters ______ do you have?
5. What setting did you grow up in? Urban ______ Rural ______ Suburban ______
6. What country did your parents grow up in?
   Father ______ Mother ______
7. How old were you when you came to the United States? ______
8. How old were your parents when they came to the United States?
   Mother ______ Father ______
9. When you were growing up, who lived with you?
   Nuclear ______ or Extended ______ Family
10. Have you maintained contact with:
    a. Aunts, uncles, cousins? (1) Yes ______ (2) No ______
    b. Brothers and sisters? (1) Yes ______ (2) No ______
    c. Parents? (1) Yes ______ (2) No ______
    d. Your own children? (1) Yes ______ (2) No ______
11. Did most of your aunts, uncles, cousins live near to your home?
    (1) Yes ______ (2) No ______
12. Approximately how often did you visit your family members who lived outside of your home?
    (1) Daily ______ (2) Weekly ______ (3) Monthly ______ (4) Once a year or less ______ (5) Never ______
13. Was your original family name changed?
    (1) Yes ______ (2) No ______
14. What is your religious preference?
    (1) Catholic ______ (2) Jewish ______
    (3) Protestant ______ Denomination ______ (4) Other ______ (5) None ______
15. Is your spouse the same religion as you?
    (1) Yes ______ (2) No ______
16. Is your spouse the same ethnic background as you?
    (1) Yes ______ (2) No ______
17. What kind of school did you go to?
    (1) Public ______ (2) Private ______ (3) Parochial ______
18. As an adult, do you live in a neighborhood where the neighbors are the same religious and ethnic background as yourself?
    (1) Yes ______ (2) No ______
19. Do you belong to a religious institution?
    (1) Yes ______ (2) No ______
20. Would you describe yourself as an active member?
    (1) Yes ______ (2) No ______
21. How often do you attend your religious institution?
    (1) More than once a week ______ (2) Weekly ______ (3) Monthly ______
    (4) Special holidays only ______ (5) Never ______
22. Do you practice your religion in your home?
    (1) Yes ______ (2) No ______ (if yes, please specify)
    (3) Praying ______ (4) Bible reading ______ (5) Diet ______ (6) Celebrating religious holidays ______
23. Do you prepare foods of your ethnic background?
    (1) Yes ______ (2) No ______
24. Do you participate in ethnic activities?
    (1) Yes ______ (2) No ______ (if yes, please specify)
    (3) Singing ______ (4) Holiday celebrations ______ (5) Dancing ______
    (6) Festivals ______ (7) Costumes ______ (8) Other ______
25. Are your friends from the same religious background as you?
    (1) Yes ______ (2) No ______
26. Are your friends from the same ethnic background as you?
    (1) Yes ______ (2) No ______
27. What is your native language? ______
28. Do you speak this language?
    (1) Prefer ______ (2) Occasionally ______ (3) Rarely ______
29. Do you read your native language?
    (1) Yes ______ (2) No ______

The greater the number of *yes* answers, the more likely the patient is to strongly identify with a traditional heritage. (The one *no* answer that indicates heritage identity is "Was your name changed?")

From Spector RE: *Cultural diversity in health and illness,* ed 4, Norwalk, Conn, 1996, Appleton & Lange.

**box 2-4** *Ethnocultural Social Organization Assessment Tool*

- Demographic data that include
  - Total population size of city or town
  - Breakdown by areas: residential concentrations of target group
  - Breakdown by ages
  - Education
  - Occupations
  - Income
- Traditional health and illness beliefs found within target group
- Traditional health and illness practices within target group
- Use and sources of home remedies
- Identity of traditional healers

Source: Potter PA, Perry AG: *Fundamentals of nursing: concepts, process, and practice,* ed 4, St Louis, 1997, Mosby, p. 367.

The patient or family members are asked about the cause of the illness or problem in a manner that suggests a familiarity with traditional HEALTH beliefs. The patient and family may not believe in the epidemiological or medical model of disease causation. Therefore they may not understand the rationale for modern treatment modalities and may not follow the recommended treatment regimen. When HEALTH beliefs are expressed, the impending cultural collision can be prevented. A compromise solution that recognizes the values of both sides may be possible.

It is also vital to determine whether the patient is using traditional resources, such as a healer, or taking any remedies to treat the symptoms. If the patient is being treated by a traditional healer, it is important to understand the scope of the treatment. Patients commonly move between the two treatment worlds and take the remedies that have the fewest side effects. Traditional remedies can be synergistic or antagonistic to prescribed drugs, and this interaction can create a risk to the patient.

### CulturalCare NURSING DIAGNOSES

The diagnoses recognized as problems in CulturalCare are derived from the assessment and commonly address areas of potential conflict between the allopathic and homeopathic or traditional health care systems. The preceding assessment allows the nurse to cluster relevant cultural data and develop actual or potential nursing diagnoses related to the cultural, religious, or ethnic needs of the patient. Noncompliance is a diagnosis that should be considered a "red flag" for the possibility of cultural collision. The patient's behavior may seem inappropriate to the nurse while being completely consistent with the patient's cultural heritage. The identification of problem etiologies further individualizes the nurse's plan of care and guides the selection of appropriate interventions. At times, the etiologies may be too subtle to accurately describe, but even with an "unknown etiology" a targeted nursing diagnosis can be addressed in a beginning way. Novices may need to enlist the support of nurse experts who practice CultureCare nursing to assist in the diagnostic reasoning process.

**box 2-5** *CulturalCare Selected Resources*

The following resources are suggested:

Fadiman A: *The spirit catches you and you fall down,* New York, 1997, Farrar, Straus, Giroux.

This book *must* be read by all nurses who are involved in CulturalCare. It is the story of a Hmong child who has epilepsy, believed by her parents to be caused by spirits; her American doctors, who had a medical etiology for her illness; and the collision of two cultures. There was limited communication between the cultures, and the outcomes of the illness trajectory, tragic in their own right, were further complicated by the lack of CulturalCare.

Dresser N: *Multicultural manners,* New York, 1997, Wiley.

There are new rules of etiquette for our rapidly changing society, and this book delineates them. The book includes do's and dont's for cross-cultural interaction and communication, tips on avoiding embarrassment in work, and the meaning of different customs.

The 1998 Calendar of Multicultural Celebrations and Foods and the 1998 Multi Cultural Resource Calendar for Health Practitioners. These invaluable calendars are extremely pragmatic in the scope of information they cover relevant to daily living. They will be annual publications and can be ordered from CULTURALINKS—Amherst Educational Publishing and in Amherst, Massachusetts, by calling 1-800-865-5549.

Spector RE: *CulturalCare: maternal child perspectives,* Baltimore, 1997, Williams & Wilkins (videotape).

This videotape depicts the role that culture plays in traditional HEALTH practices and illustrates daily life in several ethnocultural communities. It can be ordered from

Williams & Wilkins<br>351 West Camden Street<br>Baltimore, MD 21201<br>1-800-572-3344

The Transcultural Nursing Society, a professional nursing organization devoted to meeting the cultural needs of people, publishes the *Journal of Transcultural Nursing* twice a year. Membership is open to students. The Society can be reached at Madonna University, College of Nursing and Health, 366000 Schoolcraft, Livonia, MI 48150. The phone number is 1-888-432-5470.

The Center for the Study of Multiculturalism and Health, Inc. This center, located at P.O. Box 889, Chautauqua Institution, Chautauqua, NY 14722, publishes *The Journal of Multicultural Nursing and Health* twice a year.

### CulturalCare PLANNING AND EXPECTED OUTCOMES

The nurse considers cultural variables related to the patient and family as care outcomes are established. It is always important to collaborate with the patient and family in goal setting, but in CulturalCare it is absolutely essential. When health care professionals do not approach this process collaboratively, the planning process is destined to fail before it begins. The nurse synthesizes the cultural data from the assessment process to establish the parameters for what the patient and family find to be acceptable and to determine how to effectively combine allopathic and homeopathic approaches. Including the extended family in this process communicates respect for the family's beliefs and traditions.

HEALTH beliefs and practices, such as the use of special prayers and amulets, special foods, and traditional remedies, are integrated into the plan of care if possible. It is especially important to consider the patient's heritage, educational level, and language skills when planning patient education. The nurse asks the patient to rephrase, summarize, or provide return demonstrations to avoid confusion, misunderstanding, or cultural conflict. The assistance of a qualified interpreter may be appropriate. When patients are not comfortable in English it is also important to plan additional time to orient the patient to the routines and equipment in use in the hospital setting. The nurse should anticipate that the patient will be unfamiliar with most of the hospital environment, which can easily become overwhelming when language barriers make it difficult to ask needed questions.

## CulturalCare NURSING INTERVENTIONS

Specific nursing interventions will be directed toward the unique problems of each patient. A few broad areas of intervention apply to many situations and would be used by any nurse seeking to practice in a culturally competent way. Perhaps the most important intervention is for the nurse to show respect for the patient's unique heritage and to honestly attempt to blend that heritage with the essential aspects of the patient's allopathic medical plan of care. The nurse may need to alter customary ways of interacting to avoid offending or alienating a patient who has different attitudes toward social interaction and etiquette. For example, a patient who is modest and self-conscious about the body may need psychological preparation before some procedures and tests that are usually viewed as routine, such as obtaining a chest x-ray or electrocardiogram. When necessary, arrangements can be made to ensure that women are examined by women and men by men.

Visiting is another broad area where the nurse can demonstrate respect for the patient's unique needs. The nuclear or extended family may provide crucial support to the patient during hospitalization. The nurse makes every effort to support open visiting, as long as the rights and privacy of other patients are not violated. When medical necessity truly dictates restriction in visitation, the nurse attempts to honestly explain these needs to the family. Visitation may also include alternative healers, and the worth and contribution of these practitioners is supported if possible.

Food is another important area. Food has special meaning to many cultural groups, and the nurse attempts to integrate unique cultural food items into the patient's overall plan of care. This is one area where a natural collaboration exists between the nurse and the family. The nurse makes an effort to learn and understand the unique dietary needs and choices of the cultural group so unnecessary confrontation can be avoided.

Dying rituals are another broad area of CulturalCare intervention. The death of a loved one is traumatic and should not be made more difficult by confrontation over pre-death or dying rituals. In this crucial area the nurse allows the family to take the lead and acts as a facilitator as needed with rule-bound administrators. When the nurse can demonstrate an understanding of the death-related rituals that are essential to a particular ethnic or religious group, the first step in respecting differences is achieved.

## CulturalCare EVALUATION

The evaluation of the outcomes of nursing care is done by determining the extent to which the individualized goals of care have been met. The outcomes of CulturalCare are evaluated in the same way. Evaluation is ongoing throughout the CulturalCare nursing process and includes feedback from both the patient and family.

Self-evaluation, of both a personal and professional nature, is another crucial aspect of caring for and interacting with patients from diverse backgrounds. Some nurses believe that they should treat all patients the same. This attitude conveys a sense of equality, but it fails to acknowledge that real cultural differences exist between people. It is not possible to act in exactly the same manner with all patients and still hope to deliver effective, individualized, holistic care. On the other hand nurses can become so self-conscious about cultural differences, and so afraid of making a mistake, that they fail to ask needed questions about areas of difference and again fail to deliver individualized care. The process of ongoing self-evaluation can help the nurse become more comfortable providing care to patients from diverse backgrounds. Nurses who are attempting to increase their cultural competence can monitor their own activities through the use of some simple self-assessment questions.

## critical thinking QUESTIONS

1 Begin your quest for *CulturalCare* knowledge by determining the HEALTH traditions practiced in your family.

2 What is your ethnocultural heritage?

3 How deeply do you identify with your religion and ethnic background?

4 Interview a senior member of your family and ask what his or her mother, grandmother, or grandfather did to maintain, protect, and restore HEALTH.

5 Explore the community where you practice nursing and locate the traditional resources that may be available to your patients.

6 Read several books written by authors from the ethnocultural heritages of the patients you are caring for.

7 Monitor the sociopolitical situations that have an impact on your patients, such as changes in the immigration laws and welfare reform. Write letters to the press and legislators and take other action as warranted when you observe situations wherein HEALTH is compromised by social policies.

## chapter SUMMARY

### CulturalCare

- The term *CulturalCare nursing* refers to the provision of effective nursing care across cultural boundaries. It incorporates cultural sensitivity, cultural appropriateness, and cultural competence.
- Sociocultural issues that are relevant to CulturalCare include population changes, barriers to health care, and the sociological phenomenon of "-isms."

- Varying birth rates, aging, and immigration are combining to create an emerging majority of people of color in the United States.
- Poverty is an important contributing factor that affects access to health care.

### HEALTH CARE

- The natural process of recovery from illness remains a complex mystery. Cultures have developed a myriad of explanations for both illness and healing to explain what is essentially unexplainable.
- The two major health care philosophies are allopathic and homeopathic. Allopathic medicine is the scientific medical approach. Homeopathy incorporates alternative, complementary, and traditional healing therapies.
- Allopathic physicians have traditionally been antagonistic toward all forms of homeopathy.

### CULTURAL PHENOMENA AFFECTING HEALTH

- Heritage consistency reflects the degree to which individuals practice and adhere to the traditions of their culture. It reflects ethnicity, religion, and socialization into the dominant culture.
- Time orientation, spatial orientation, communication, social organization, biological variations, and environmental control are the six phenomena included in the Giger and Davidhizar[15] cultural model.
- The HEALTH traditions model can be used to analyze the beliefs and practices of an individual in regard to HEALTH. It weaves together nine dimensions related to health maintenance, protection, and restoration.
- African American, Asian American, Hispanic American, European American, and Native American are the major ethnic groups that need to be understood in nursing practice in the United States.

### CulturalCare AND THE NURSING PROCESS

- The nursing process can be easily adapted to meet the needs of cultural assessment and CulturalCare.
- The Heritage Assessment tool can provide valuable information about a patient's adherence to traditional health care beliefs and practices.
- Communication, open visiting, inclusion of the family, providing traditional food, and supporting dying rituals are important ways that the nurse can practice CulturalCare.
- Evaluation of the effectiveness of nursing interventions looks directly at patient outcomes but also asks the nurse to engage in an ongoing process of self-assessment concerning his or her own attitudes and responses to cultural practices that differ from those supported by allopathic medicine.

## References


1. Abramson HJ: Religion. In Thermstrom S, editor: *The Harvard encyclopedia of American ethnic groups*, Cambridge, Mass, 1980, Harvard University Press.
2. Beck R: *The case against immigration*, New York, 1996, WW Norton.
3. Berg J, Berg BL: Compliance, diet, and cultural factors among black Americans with end-stage renal disease, *J Natl Black Nurses Assoc* 3(2):18, 1989.
4. Bohannan P: *We, the alien*, Prospects Heights, Ill, 1992, Waveland Press.
5. Boyle JS: The practice of transcultural nursing, *Transcultural Nursing Society Newsletter* 7:2, 1987.
6. Budge EAW: *Amulets and superstitions*, New York, 1978, Dover Publications. (Originally published in London, 1930, by Oxford University Press.)
7. Buehler J: Traditional Crow Indian health beliefs and practices, *Journal of Holistic Nursing* 10(1):18, 1992.
8. Deardorff K, Montgomery P: *National population trends*, Washington, DC, 1997, US Census Bureau.
9. DeSantis L, Thomas J: The immigrant Haitian mother: transcultural nursing perspective on preventive health care for children, *J Transcult Nurs* 2:2, 1990.
10. Eck D: *World Religions in Boston*, Cambridge, 1995, Harvard University Press.
11. Eisenberg DM, Kessler RC, Foster C, et al: Unconventional medicine in the United States: prevalence, costs, and patterns of use, *N Engl J Med* 328:251, 1993.
12. Estes G, Zitzow D: Heritage consistency as a consideration in counseling Native Americans. Paper presented at the convention of the National Indian Education Association, Dallas, 1980.
13. Fadiman A: *The spirit catches you and you fall down*, New York, 1997, Farrar, Straus, Giroux.
14. Fejos P: Man, magic, and medicine. In Goldstone I, editor: *Medicine and anthropology*, New York, 1959, International Universities Press.
15. Giger JN, Davidhizar RE: *Transcultural nursing assessment and intervention*, ed 2, St Louis, 1995, Mosby.
16. Go GV: Changing populations and health. In Edelman CL, Mandle C, editors: *Health promotion throughout the lifespan*, ed 3, St Louis, 1994, Mosby.
17. Hodgkinson H: The changing demographics of minority populations and their effects on American higher education: trends, projections, and larger implications. Address delivered at the Conference on Developing Multi-Cultural Leadership for the Twenty-First Century, Boston, Mass, June 15, 1988, Boston College.
18. Lavelle R: *America's new war on poverty: a reader for action*, San Francisco, 1995, KQED Books.
19. Lipson J: Culturally competent nursing care. In Lipson J, Dibble S, Minarik P, editors: *Culture and nursing care: a pocket guide*, San Francisco, 1996, University of San Francisco Press.
20. Littlejohn H: Interview, Boston, 1979.
21. Maloney C, ed: *The evil eye*, New York, 1976, Columbia University Press.
22. McGee P: Culturally sensitive and culturally comprehensive care, *Br J Nurs* 3(15):789, 1996.
23. McLemore S: *Racial and ethnic relations in America*, Newton, Mass, 1980, Allyn & Bacon.
24. Spector R: *Cultural diversity in health and illness*, ed 4, Norwalk, Conn, 1996, Appleton & Lange.
25. Spector R: Culture, ethnicity, and nursing. In Potter PA, Perry AG: *Fundamentals of nursing: concepts, process, and practice*, ed 4, St Louis, 1997, Mosby.
26. Spector R: *Guide to heritage assessment and health traditions*, Norwalk, Conn, 1996, Appleton & Lange.
27. Starr P: *The social transformation of American medicine*, New York, Basic Books, 1982.
28. Thernstrom S, editor: *The Harvard encyclopedia of American ethnic groups*, Cambridge, Mass, 1980, Harvard University Press.
29. US Bureau of the Census: *Current population reports, 1990 census of population and housing, summary population and housing characteristics, United States*, Washington, DC, 1991, US Government Printing Office.
30. US Bureau of the Census: *1990 census of the population, general population characteristics, United States*, Washington, DC, 1992, US Government Printing Office.
31. US Bureau of the Census: *1990 census of the population, education in the United States*, Washington, DC, 1994, US Government Printing Office.
32. Weil A: *Health and healing*, Boston, 1983, Houghton Mifflin.

chapter 3

# Promoting Healthy Lifestyles

JUDITH K. SANDS and ANGELA WILSON

## objectives

*After studying this chapter, the learner should be able to:*

1. Discuss the development of an agenda for health promotion in the United States.
2. Define health promotion.
3. Compare primary, secondary, and tertiary prevention.
4. Explain the role of nutrition, exercise, rest and sleep, self-responsibility, and regimen adherence in healthy lifestyles.
5. Describe common tools that can be used to assess the elements of a healthy lifestyle.
6. Identify the components of a healthy diet.
7. Create a safe exercise plan for a middle-aged or elderly adult.
8. Develop strategies to assist individuals to adhere to a health-promoting lifestyle.

Healthy lifestyles are increasingly recognized as a key component of optimal wellness in young adults, an essential tool for minimizing the incidence and severity of chronic illnesses and their complications, and an effective strategy for gaining control of the steadily rising costs of health care. Healthy lifestyles are the vehicle by which most of the goals of health promotion and prevention are implemented. Professional nursing has a natural connection with the promotion of healthy lifestyles. Nursing has been a strong voice for health promotion and prevention since Florence Nightingale first utilized the principles of hygiene and environmental management in care of the sick and wounded during the Crimean War. Until recently, however, health promotion has received little support within a care system dominated almost exclusively by attention to disease and illness management. Today, after years of minimal attention in our society, health promotion has become fashionable. People are living longer, and the desire to maximize that increasing life span is strong. Our knowledge about the etiology of major causes of morbidity and mortality continues to unfold, and many of these diseases are at least partially related to lifestyle choices in the areas of nutrition, exercise, and alcohol and tobacco use. Nurses today have an unprecedented opportunity to make a significant impact on individual lives and positively affect the health of society by assisting people to make informed and healthful lifestyle choices.

Public health initiatives in the twentieth century began with an emphasis on halting the spread of infectious disease. Sanitation, immunization, and the development of antibiotics all combined to achieve tremendous successes. Diseases such as typhoid and smallpox have been virtually eliminated; most childhood diseases have been brought under control with routine immunization, and epidemics such as polio have been almost totally eradicated. Equally impressive gains have been made through the development of sophisticated technology that can be used for mass population screening (e.g., mammography and Pap smears). A seemingly endless array of pharmacological agents and high-tech interventions perpetuated the widely held belief that all diseases and conditions would eventually be effectively controlled or eliminated.

The goal of disease eradication may still lie in the future, but now we are to some degree victims of our partial successes. Life spans continue to increase, and the elderly represent a steadily increasing proportion of the population. Chronic diseases are now the major challenges in health care, and the twofold goals of prevention and control have replaced cure. Aging is accompanied by a steadily increasing incidence of chronic illnesses, and an estimated 85% of persons over 65 years of age have at least one chronic condition.[4] The challenge is to postpone or prevent these diseases as long as possible. The relationship between lifestyle choices and the incidence and severity of chronic illnesses is clear and indisputable. Genetics continues to play a crucial role in selected situations, but it is apparent that an individual's health status is, to at least some degree, a reflection of his or her style of living. This chapter addresses the major components of healthy lifestyles and nursing interventions to assist individuals to make health-promoting choices.

## A NATIONAL AGENDA FOR HEALTH PROMOTION

The field of health promotion evolved together with the holism and wellness movement of the 1970s. Dunn's concept of "high-level wellness" epitomized this movement with its focus on a continual process of physical and psychoemotional self-actualization. When health promotion finally emerged on the national scene, however, its focus was much broader and had been expanded to incorporate the fields of disease prevention and the maximization of health within the context of chronic illness. The first public health agenda for the United States was released from the office of the Surgeon General in 1979.[16] In 1980 the major themes of this agenda were translated into a list of goals for the decade called "1990 Health Objectives." This 1980 document specifically targeted areas of needed improvement for the nation in several areas: health status, increasing public awareness, decreasing risks, increasing services, and providing environmental protective measures.[17] For the first time the Surgeon General's office addressed the importance of the environment in influencing health and outlined the importance of government intervention and oversight to ensure these health objectives. The importance of clean air and water, food safety, and occupational safety were all included. Smoking was targeted as a national health hazard.

The *Healthy People 2000* report was the next articulation of national health goals.[15] This document was produced as part of the contribution of the United States to the World Health Organization's (WHO) international project of "health for all by the year 2000." It was also a response to evaluation data indicating that many of the health objectives articulated for 1990 were not being met.

*Healthy People 2000* includes objectives related to the major areas outlined in Box 3-1. Health promotion activities, protection services, prevention services, surveillance, and data systems about the nation's health are discussed. The expressed purposes of the project were to decrease morbidity, prevent disability, guide and facilitate the early detection of asymptomatic disorders, and target specific vulnerable populations. *Healthy People 2000* objectives related to lifestyles and health promotion are presented in this chapter, and objectives related to specific diseases and conditions are included in the chapters throughout this text. A thoughtful midpoint review was conducted in 1995, and a 1995 publication contains minor modifications in the original expressed objectives.[14]

**box 3-1** *Year 2000 National Health Objectives: Priority Areas*

**HEALTH PROMOTION**
- Physical activity and fitness
- Nutrition
- Tobacco
- Alcohol and other drugs
- Family planning
- Mental health and mental disorders
- Violent and abusive behavior
- Educational and community-based programs

**HEALTH PROTECTION**
- Unintentional injuries
- Occupational safety and health
- Environmental health
- Food and drug safety
- Oral health

**PREVENTIVE SERVICES**
- Maternal and infant health
- Heart disease and stroke
- Cancer
- Diabetes and chronic disabling conditions
- HIV infection
- Sexually transmitted diseases
- Immunization and infectious diseases
- Clinical preventive services

**SURVEILLANCE AND DATA SYSTEMS**

From US Department of Health and Human Services, Public Health Service: *Healthy people 2000: national health promotion and disease prevention objectives,* Washington, DC, 1990, US Government Printing Office.

## ROLE OF PROFESSIONAL NURSING

The central role of professional nursing in the new commitment to health promotion and prevention is readily apparent. Nursing concepts and theories have focused on self-care, efficacy, and adaptation for decades. Nurses are acknowledged experts in health education and patient teaching and are well prepared to assume a leadership role in this area. In 1992 the American Nurses' Association (ANA) published *Nursing's Agenda for Health Care Reform,* which boldly called for a shift in the health care system from the predominant focus on illness and cure to a focus on wellness and care.[1] Nurses employed in school health, industry, and community agencies have found themselves suddenly on the cutting edge of the future in health care as potent social and economic forces have joined to catapult health promotion into national prominence. The cost of chronic illness management continues to drive the cost of health care steadily upward, and predictions for the future indicate more of the same. Effective self-care management within the context of a health-promoting lifestyle has been shown to decrease the need for office visits and hospitalization and therefore the cost to insurers.[4] Insurers, primarily in health maintenance organizations (HMOs), are acknowledging that it is cost-effective to invest in health promotion and prevention activities for their subscribers to delay or minimize disease management expenditures in the future. Nurses are quickly selected as the best-prepared health professionals to design and implement these activities.

Business and industry increasingly recognize that a healthy workforce decreases lost days from absenteeism and limits expenditures in copayments for health care. Screening services, diet teaching, and exercise facilities are now common benefits in the workplace as companies attempt to positively influence the health of their workers and minimize costs. Incentives for healthy lifestyles are provided in the form of discounts on insurance for nonsmokers or nondrinkers and for maintaining a healthy body weight. Occupational health nurses are at the center of these efforts and programs.

Education for effective self-care is a cornerstone of management in the acute care setting as well and is again the primary domain of nursing. It is ironic that the importance of patient teaching is finally fully acknowledged when downsizing and restructuring activities in acute care facilities have made it extremely difficult for nurses to continue to effectively fulfill this vital role. Nurses must remain deeply committed to this critical independent function and claim it as an integral part of their practice in every setting. Professional nurses must also utilize opportunities to heighten the public's awareness of this important nursing function.

## AN OVERVIEW OF PREVENTION AND HEALTH PROMOTION

Prevention and health promotion are broadly overlapping concepts, and healthy lifestyles play an essential role in both. Prevention is the broadest in scope. The activities included under this umbrella are classified into three general groupings.

### PRIMARY PREVENTION

Most of the activities considered to be components of health promotion can be included within the parameters of primary prevention. Health promotion involves activities that help individuals achieve their maximal health potential. Activities include those designed to prevent the actual occurrence of specific diseases. For example, immunizations and chemoprophylaxis with drugs and other agents are administered to asymptomatic persons in the attempt to decrease their risk of developing disease. Healthy diet and exercise are also partially directed at prevention of diseases such as hypertension, cancer, and coronary artery disease. Societal initiatives as diverse as water fluoridation, nutrient enrichment in foods, clean air and water, the use of seat belts, and the elimination of domestic violence are all strategies for primary prevention. The scope of primary prevention is nearly limitless and is directly influenced by the economic and political climate of the society.

### SECONDARY PREVENTION

Secondary prevention focuses on the early detection of diseases and their prompt and effective treatment, thereby limiting their seriousness and associated disability. Secondary prevention has expanded extensively over the last 25 years and includes many societal interventions. Examples include mammography; blood pressure, cholesterol, glaucoma, and tuberculosis screening; and more recently the development of fecal occult blood and prostate-specific antigen testing. Major screening guidelines developed by eminent research and service groups such as the American Heart Association and American Cancer Society are presented throughout the text in conjunction with their associated disease processes. Treatment modalities are included in the area of secondary prevention and have traditionally received the lion's share of the health care dollar. *Healthy People 2000* goals related to screening and prevention are summarized in Box 3-2.

### TERTIARY PREVENTION

Tertiary prevention is directed toward rehabilitation of the individual after an episode of disease or trauma. Tertiary prevention has gradually become the most significant target of health promotion activities. People rarely die today when diagnosed with diabetes, chronic obstructive pulmonary disease, coronary artery disease, hypertension, arthritis, or human immunodeficiency virus. Instead, they can be expected to live for many years, facing the challenges of optimal and effective disease management and pursuing wellness within the context of chronic disease. Chronic illness management is estimated to consume 75% of annual health care expenditures.[4] The diagnosis or exacerbation of a chronic disease often creates a readiness point for the individual to be open to education concerning risk reduction and healthier living. Individuals who have never seriously considered changing their behavior and lifestyle may be prompted by the implications of their illness experience to make significant adjustments in their lifestyle. These readiness points are fertile areas for intervention by professional nurses engaged in illness care and management. The nurse's interventions are focused not only on the disease but on ways in which the patient can limit the seriousness and progression of the disease process and simultaneously improve quality of life.

### HEALTH PROMOTION

There is no one universally accepted definition of health promotion. It can be broadly defined as a process of fostering awareness, influencing attitudes, and identifying alternatives so that an individual can make informed lifestyle choices that help the person achieve or maintain optimal levels of physical,

**box 3-2** Healthy People 2000 *Goals Related to Health Promotion, Screening, and Preventive Services*

- Increase years of healthy life to at least 65 years.
- Increase to at least 95% the proportion of people who have a specific source of ongoing primary care for coordination of their preventive and episodic health care.
- Increase the proportion of people who have received selected clinical preventive screening and immunization services and at least one of the counseling services appropriate for their age and gender as recommended by the U.S. Preventive Services Task Force.
- Ensure that at least 90% of people for whom primary care services are provided directly by publicly funded programs are offered, at a minimum, the screening, counseling, and immunization services recommended by the U.S. Preventive Services Task Force.
- Increase to at least 50% the proportion of primary care providers who provide their patients with the screening, counseling, and immunization services recommended by the U.S. Preventive Services Task Force.
- Increase to at least 40% the proportion of people aged 50 and older visiting a primary care provider in the preceding year who have received oral, skin, and digital rectal examinations during one such visit.
- Increase to at least 75% the proportion of primary care providers who routinely counsel patients about the following: tobacco use cessation, diet modification, and cancer screening recommendations, which includes providing information on the potential benefit or harm attributed to the various screening modalities and discussion of risk factors associated with breast, prostate, cervical, colorectal, and lung cancers.
- Improve financing and delivery of clinical preventive services so that virtually no American has a financial barrier to receiving, at a minimum, the screening, counseling, and immunization services recommended by the U.S. Preventive Services Task Force.

From US Department of Health and Human Services: *Healthy people 2000: national health promotion and disease prevention objectives,* Washington, DC, 1990, US Government Printing Office.

mental, and emotional well-being. Health promotion targets personal habits, lifestyle patterns, and the environment to reduce risks and enhance health and well-being, thus strengthening the person's capacity to withstand physical and emotional stress. The concept of health promotion has expanded steadily over the last several decades. Originally directed primarily at young healthy adults seeking optimal wellness, health promotion is now acknowledged as an important goal for people of all ages and health status.

### HEALTHY LIFESTYLES

A healthy lifestyle is one in which the person engages in a pattern of positive activities on a daily basis. These activities act in a cumulative fashion to increase the person's level of health and well-being. A healthy lifestyle is the result of literally hundreds of choices that a person makes over the course of a lifetime.[11] Lifestyles and health behaviors have their foundation within the family unit and reflect the family's unique cultural, ethnic, religious, and socioeconomic heritage and beliefs. These behaviors are powerfully reinforced each day as a child is growing up.

Healthy lifestyles are practiced without the supervision of a health care provider, but they can be powerfully influenced by the attitudes and interventions of health professionals. Routine screenings, prenatal and well child visits, school health education, and public information campaigns all provide opportunities to positively influence lifestyle choices. The patient contacts that occur during the treatment of episodic illnesses are also potential windows of opportunity for primary health promotion and prevention education by health professionals. It is particularly important for health professionals to use episodic illness contacts for health promotion education with young adults who visit a health professional infrequently and are usually in the process of establishing the lifestyle patterns that will carry them through their working years.

## A FRAMEWORK FOR STUDYING HEALTHY LIFESTYLES

A discussion of healthy lifestyles can include a diverse range of topics. Research suggests, however, that six relatively straightforward personal behaviors are associated with a significant decrease in individual morbidity and mortality: (1) avoiding smoking, (2) engaging in regular exercise, (3) limiting the use of alcohol, (4) maintaining a desirable body weight, (5) eating a nutritious diet, and (6) getting 7 to 8 hours of restful sleep each night.[11] The effects of these behaviors may also be additive in nature. These six behaviors also line up fairly well with the major categories of risk factors for the primary causes of morbidity and mortality in the United States. Major categories of risk factors usually include age; hereditary factors; lifestyle factors (e.g., diet, exercise, stress, smoking, alcohol use); environmental factors (e.g., pollution, occupational exposure, poverty); and miscellaneous personal choice elements such as unprotected sex, failure to use seat belts, and drunk driving. The discussion in this chapter is grouped into four major categories: (1) diet and nutrition; (2) exercise; (3) stress, sleep, and rest; and (4) self-responsibility. Risk factors and lifestyle choices associated with specific diseases and disorders are discussed throughout the text.

### DIET AND NUTRITION

The relationship between diet, overall health, and the development of a wide variety of disease processes receives constant attention in both the professional and popular literature today. New studies are reported daily that show a relationship between a dietary element and a disease process. Researchers suggest that dietary practices may be the single most important "choice" factor in determining health and longevity. New information is released daily. However, many of the reports are of preliminary work involving limited samples and draw conclusions from studies with less than rigorous designs. Quality diet research is difficult to perform and requires longitudinal approaches to yield data meaningful in affecting long-term health and well-being. Many of the study results appear to be contradictory and do not provide sufficient guidance to make lifestyle choices. Health care professionals need to remain current and informed about the scope of diet research to help consumers appropriately interpret and apply what they read and hear.

Major changes have clearly taken place in the last 50 years in the way we as a society think about diet and nutrition. Nutritional programs that were developed during and after World War II had clear goals directed at eliminating nutrient deficiencies, especially in children and childbearing women. The crucial roles of the basic nutrients—vitamins, minerals, and amino acids—were just beginning to be delineated. Recommended dietary allowances were established and initiatives were launched that resulted in supplementation of iodine in salt, enrichment of grains and bread products with essential nutrients, fortification of milk, and fluoridation of community water supplies. Daily vitamin supplementation became routine in many families. The "four basic food groups" were promoted as the foundation for a healthy diet, and the eradication of hunger and malnutrition was considered a feasible goal.

By the 1970s ongoing research indicated a direct correlation between what we eat and general health. Diet was found to have profound potential effects on the prevention or control of many chronic diseases.[10] Diet was also found to directly affect the development of major disease processes. Media attention escalated as diet practices were clearly linked to the development of heart disease, diabetes, and selected cancers. Research exploded as the contributions and effects of specific elements were identified and described. Vitamins A, C, and E; beta carotene, fiber, cholesterol, and saturated fats; nitrates and nitrites; food additives and chemicals; and even water have all been spotlighted.

In 1992, the United States Department of Agriculture (USDA) released and publicized a new nutritional pyramid that serves as the broad outline for information and teaching about nutrition in America[5] (Figure 3-1). The pyramid contains five food groups instead of four and is based on extensive research, which indicates that a decreased daily fat intake combined with five daily servings of fruits and vegetables significantly decreases the risk of coronary artery disease, diabetes, and cancer. Americans are increasingly aware of the importance of diet choices but have not been able to make significant changes in daily diet patterns. The "average" American diet still contains about 35% fat and is heavily skewed toward convenience and prepared foods.[9] *Healthy People 2000* goals related to nutrition are summarized in Box 3-3.

## Current Issues in Diet and Nutrition

Nutrient research has become increasingly sophisticated, and the next decade will contribute much to our understanding of the effects of specific nutrients on such factors as immune system functioning, aging, and the development of chronic diseases. Additional broad social issues remain important in the area of diet and nutrition as well.

### Obesity

Obesity is found in every age group and has gradually become a national health problem of significant proportions. Obesity affects about 50 million persons in the United States. This represents one in four European American adults and one in three African American and Hispanic adults. The links between obesity and numerous chronic diseases have been well established. Obesity is a major risk factor in coronary artery disease, hypertension, cerebrovascular accident, diabetes, arthritis, and some cancers. Some authorities consider obesity the second leading cause of preventable death in the United States after cigarette smoking. The social toll of obesity is also enormous. Despite its pervasiveness obesity is strongly stigmatized in American society and is clearly associated with numerous adverse social consequences related to employment, marriage and divorce, and life satisfaction.[9] Despite extensive research both the medical community and the public are quick to classify obesity as a simple failure of will. This stereotyping ignores the clear evidence that complex behavioral, genetic, and environmental factors result in obesity.

Obesity is a chronic disease requiring long-term management, and at present our knowledge base does not contain many effective treatment options. Persons of the same gender and body composition have similar basal energy requirements that can be predicted from their proportion of muscle tissue and body fat. However, these data represent only a beginning understanding of how various bodies metabolize nutrients and respond to increased and decreased demands. The futility of most standard treatment approaches reinforces these principles and has been amply demonstrated. However, weight control remains an important goal because even small percentages of weight loss are associated with significant declines in risks. *Healthy People 2000* goals related to weight management are summarized in Box 3-4.

### Malnutrition

Malnutrition is still a problem in the United States despite a variety of social policy safety nets and interventions. The culture of poverty continues to steadily expand, and poor children are extremely unlikely to eat a diet that contains rich amounts

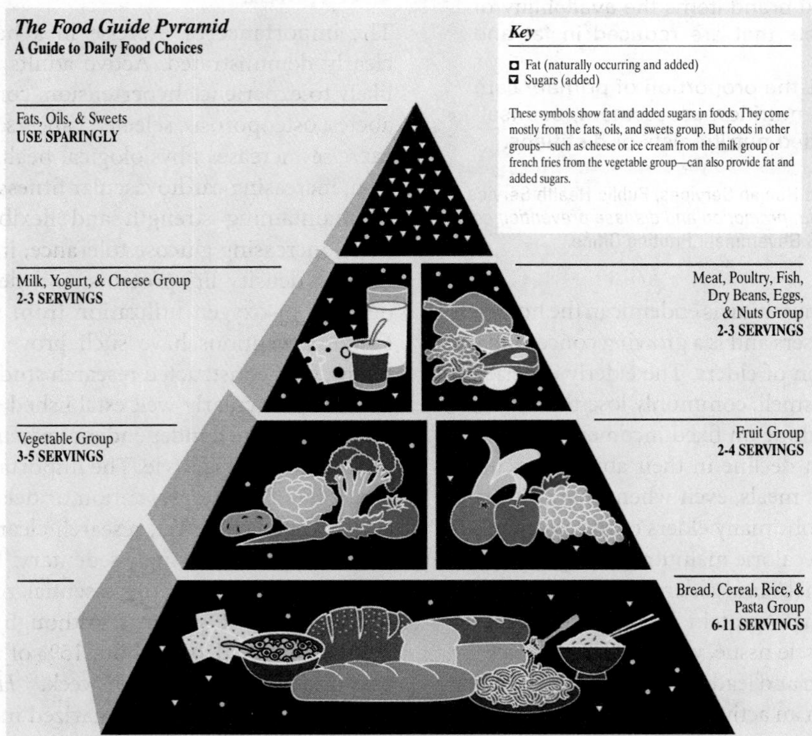


**fig. 3-1** Food guide pyramid: a guide to daily food choices and numbers of servings.

**box 3-3** Healthy People 2000 *Goals Related to Nutrition*

- Increase complex carbohydrate and fiber-containing foods in the diets of people aged 2 and older to an average of five or more daily servings for vegetables (including legumes) and fruits and to an average of six or more daily servings for grain products.
- Reduce dietary fat intake to an average of 30% of calories or less and average saturated fat intake to less than 10% of calories among people aged 2 and older.
- Decrease salt and sodium intake so at least 65% of home meal preparers prepare foods without adding salt, at least 80% of people avoid using salt at the table, and at least 40% of adults regularly purchase foods modified or lower in sodium.
- Increase calcium intake so at least 50% of people aged 11 to 24 and 50% of pregnant and lactating women consume an average of three or more daily servings of foods rich in calcium and at least 75% of children aged 2 to 10 and 50% of people aged 25 and older consume an average of two or more servings daily.
- Achieve useful and informative nutrition labeling for virtually all processed foods and at least 40% of ready-to-eat carry-away foods. Achieve compliance by at least 90% of retailers with the voluntary labeling of fresh meats, poultry, seafood, fruits, and vegetables.
- Increase to at least 85% the proportion of people aged 18 and older who use food labels to make nutritious food selections.
- Increase to at least 90% the proportion of restaurants and institutional food service operations that offer identifiable low-fat, low-calorie food choices, consistent with the *Dietary Guidelines for Americans.*
- Increase to at least 5000 brand items the availability of processed food products that are reduced in fat and saturated fat.
- Increase to at least 75% the proportion of primary care providers who provide nutrition assessment, counseling, or referral to qualified nutritionists or dietitians.

From US Department of Health and Human Services, Public Health Service: *Healthy people 2000: national health promotion and disease prevention objectives,* Washington, DC, 1990, US Government Printing Office.

**box 3-4** Healthy People 2000 *Goals Related to Weight Management*

- Reduce overweight to a prevalence of no more than 20% among people aged 20 and older and no more than 15% among adolescents aged 12 to 19.
- Increase to at least 50% the proportion of overweight people aged 12 and older who have adopted sound dietary practices combined with regular physical activity to attain an appropriate body weight.
- Increase to at least 50% the proportion of work sites with 50 or more employees that offer nutrition education or weight management programs for employees.

From US Department of Health and Human Services: *Healthy people 2000: national health promotion and disease prevention objectives,* Washington, DC, 1990, US Government Printing Office.

of fruits and vegetables. Malnutrition is endemic in the homeless and in alcohol and drug abusers and is a growing concern in the rapidly increasing population of elders. The elderly experience steady declines in taste and smell, commonly lose their natural teeth, and increasingly live alone on fixed incomes. The elderly may experience a significant decline in their ability to acquire food and prepare nutritious meals, even when money is not a concern.[6] Being alone also robs many elders of the essential social aspects of meals. Protein calorie malnutrition is present in a significant minority of homebound elders and those in long-term care facilities. Inadequate protein intake is theorized to contribute to the loss of muscle tissue, which both increases the risk of falls in this population and leads to a steady decline in the ability to pursue or maintain an active, independent lifestyle.

### Osteoporosis

Over 25 million older persons have osteoporosis, and that number will continue to increase as the population ages and female life span increases. Osteoporosis is directly linked to the majority of cases of hip fracture and spinal compression fractures, with their profound direct and indirect costs to the health care system. The toll of pain and suffering from lost independence and admission to long-term care facilities cannot be calculated.

The management of osteoporosis is presented in Chapter 61, but the link between calcium content in the diet and the development or prevention of osteoporosis warrants inclusion among the issues related to nutrition and healthy lifestyles. The current recommended daily calcium intake of 1000 to 1500 mg requires either extremely careful diet planning or appropriate supplementation.

## EXERCISE

The importance of exercise in a healthy lifestyle has been clearly demonstrated. Active adults live longer and are less likely to experience hypertension, coronary artery disease, diabetes, osteoporosis, selected cancers, and depression. Regular exercise increases physiological health by improving circulation, increasing cardiovascular fitness and stamina, increasing or maintaining strength and flexibility, maintaining bone mass, increasing glucose tolerance, increasing the proportion of high-density lipoproteins, and decreasing the age-related declines in oxygen utilization from 9% to 5% per decade.[12] Few interventions have such proven benefits supported by major, well-constructed research studies. The benefits of exercise are particularly well established for elders, who typically achieve sustained independence when they integrate active exercise into their lifestyle. The importance of exercise in weight control and in the prevention or delay of osteoporosis is also clearly established. Yet, research clearly indicates that American society is increasingly sedentary. This apparent dichotomy serves to underscore the essential role that personal choice plays in lifestyle patterns. Although health clubs and gyms have proliferated, only about 15% of adults engage in 20 minutes of active exercise each week.[12] *Healthy People 2000* goals related to exercise are summarized in Box 3-5.

Exercise is generally classified as either aerobic or anaerobic. Aerobic exercise is characterized by activities that involve the large muscle groups and that are performed in a rhythmic and continuous nature, usually for at least 15 minutes at a

**box 3-5** Healthy People 2000 *Goals Related to Exercise*

- Increase to at least 30% the proportion of people aged 6 and older who engage regularly, preferably daily, in light to moderate physical activity for at least 30 minutes per day.
- Increase to at least 20% the proportion of people aged 18 and older and to at least 75% the proportion of children and adolescents aged 6 to 17 who engage in vigorous physical activity that promotes the development and maintenance of cardiorespiratory fitness three or more days per week for 20 or more minutes per occasion.
- Reduce to no more than 15% the proportion of people aged 6 and older who engage in no leisure-time physical activity.
- Increase to at least 40% the proportion of people aged 6 and older who regularly perform physical activities that enhance and maintain muscular strength, muscular endurance, and flexibility.
- Increase to at least 50% the proportion of primary care providers who routinely assess and counsel their patients regarding the frequency, duration, type, and intensity of each patient's physical activity practices.
- Increase community availability and accessibility of physical activity and fitness facilities.
- Increase the proportion of work sites offering employer-sponsored physical activity and fitness programs.

From US Department of Health and Human Services: *Healthy people 2000: national health promotion and disease prevention objectives,* Washington, DC, 1990, US Government Printing Office.

time. Examples include walking, bicycling, swimming, and dancing. Anaerobic exercise is characterized by bursts of energy expended in short time intervals. Activities include weight lifting, baseball, and wrestling. Although aerobic exercise contributes more directly to the development of cardiovascular fitness and endurance, moderate strength training also plays an important role in supporting muscle mass and strength, particularly for women and elders.

## STRESS, SLEEP, AND REST

The effects of stress have been extensively studied from both physiological and psychological perspectives, and the negative effects of chronic and excessive stress are well delineated. (See Chapter 6.) Chronic stress negatively affects health and is associated with an increased incidence of injury and vulnerability to infection. Over half of the adult population consistently reports that they have experienced at least moderate stress in the previous 2 weeks. The incidence of chronic stress rises sharply among well-educated and highly paid individuals. Role stress in particular has received a lot of attention in the last 20 years. Modern lifestyles force many women to experience career versus family conflicts and challenge increasing numbers of women and men to address the multiple demands of single parenthood. The effects of stress are difficult to predict for any individual, but the hectic pace of many contemporary lifestyles significantly reduces the time available for restorative rest and sleep. The number of adults who report that they are "not getting enough sleep" continues to rise.

Despite all of the research conducted on sleep, its precise function remains unknown. The conservation of energy theory suggests that the energy spent during the day is balanced by the low energy demands of deep sleep. More generally accepted is the theory that sleep is a period of recuperation or restoration. Two of the five major sleep stages clearly serve this purpose. Catabolism is decreased and anabolism is increased during stage 4 deep sleep as protein synthesis and adenosine triphosphate (ATP) concentrations increase. Growth hormones are also primarily released at night during deep sleep. Rapid eye movement (REM) or stage 5 sleep appears to be primarily associated with restoring cognitive functioning, processing information and experience, and consolidating memory. Both slow-wave, deep sleep and REM sleep are essential to health, and normal sleep cycles contain both types. See Chapter 13 for a more detailed discussion of sleep.

The amount of sleep an individual requires varies significantly throughout the life cycle, as does the relative percentage of deep and REM sleep. Young and middle-aged adults generally require between 7 and 9 hours of sleep per day; elders tend to sleep less at night but nap more frequently during the day. Sleep patterns vary widely among individuals, but most people are clearly aware of the sleep pattern that best contributes to a feeling of daily well-being. Drugs, alcohol, and stress can all adversely affect an individual's normal sleep patterns.

Sleep and rest are commonly grouped together and share many purposes, but whereas sleep is well researched, our understanding of the more subjective area of rest is extremely limited. Physical rest plays an important role in healthy functioning. Adenosine triphosphate, which is necessary for all types of activities, is not actively stored by the body and must be continuously produced. Physical activity decreases the available pool of ATP, and rest is needed to replenish the supply. Rest also contributes to mental health through effective stress management. The activities that contribute to mental rest and relaxation vary tremendously among individuals and incorporate such diverse strategies as sports, reading, listening to music, and meditation. Strategies for stress management are discussed in more detail in Chapter 6.

## SELF-RESPONSIBILITY

Healthy lifestyles do not just happen. They are the result of conscious and unconscious choices and of commitments to specific, daily behaviors. Therefore the area of self-responsibility is the fourth major and perhaps the single most important element of a healthy lifestyle. Any professional involved in health promotion must understand and respect the complex personal, social, political, and economic factors that shape individual lives. It is a fact of the human experience that most people make the easiest choices that are available to them. The list of self-responsibility issues is almost endless. Most of our current social ills are tied at least in part to individual choices that reflect neither a pattern of health promotion nor self-responsibility. The effects of diet and exercise choices have already been discussed. Other pressing personal choice problems include tobacco use, excess or irresponsible alcohol use, unprotected sex, seat belt use, and domestic violence. Health care professionals must be aware that they cannot make anyone choose a healthy lifestyle, and adhering to a healthy lifestyle regimen can be a devastatingly complex challenge.[11] Many personal choice problems are beyond the scope of this chapter. Others are discussed in other portions of the text, such as alcohol and drug abuse (Chapter 14), sexually transmitted diseases (Chapter 50), and human immunodeficiency virus (Chapter 67). This discussion will focus on the problem of tobacco use and on the broad area of adherence to a therapeutic regimen.

### Tobacco Use

Smoking has been a front-page story for many years now as the Surgeon General's office and numerous citizen's advocacy groups have battled the powerful tobacco industry over the addictive qualities and health risks associated with the use of tobacco. The health risks of smoking have been clearly and specifically identified over the last 20 years, but progress related to smoking cessation has been slow and tobacco use remains a major social concern. In 1995 a reported 50 million Americans still smoked, a staggering total considering the time and money that have been expended to deliver the message of smoking cessation to the public.

The health consequences of tobacco use continue to be impressive. The National Cancer Institute reports that 434,000 people die each year of smoking-related illnesses. Secondhand smoke accounts for approximately 3000 deaths from lung cancer each year and has multiple adverse effects on the developing fetus. From 20% to 30% of low-birth-weight infants can be attributed to maternal smoking during pregnancy, and 10% of the infant mortality rate is also attributed to maternal smoking. Although most Americans are aware that smoking is directly associated with the incidence and mortality of lung cancer and chronic obstructive pulmonary disease, many are unaware of its contribution to cancers of the bladder, kidney, pancreas, and female reproductive organs. Smoking, combined with heavy alcohol use, dramatically increases the incidence of many gastrointestinal tract cancers. Smoking also contributes to the incidence of coronary artery disease, hypertension, peripheral vascular disease, and cerebrovascular disease.

As nicotine is inhaled into the lungs it is absorbed into the bloodstream. Approximately 15% of the nicotine travels to the brain, where it is absorbed within 7 seconds of inhalation. Nicotine stimulates the release of catecholamines, particularly epinephrine. This release of epinephrine causes tachycardia, constricts the peripheral vessels, raises the blood pressure, and produces a feeling of euphoria. The effects of the nicotine on the blood vessels persist well after the cigarette has been smoked. Over time many smokers are able to regulate their intake of nicotine to produce and sustain the feeling of euphoria without the negative side effects of either overdosage or withdrawal. Nicotine is also one of the most powerful known addictions, which is why efforts directed at *preventing* smoking are so essential.

Cigarette smoke also contains carbon monoxide, which binds to the hemoglobin in the blood and has a binding capacity 200 times stronger than that of oxygen. The oxygen-carrying capacity of the red blood cells is significantly decreased. In high-risk individuals a decreased oxygen-carrying capacity results in hypoxia, impairs vision and thinking, and increases the incidence of atherosclerosis. Cigarette smoking is not the only problem. Tobacco may also be chewed (snuff) or smoked in cigars and pipes. Many individuals believe that these methods are "safe" because the nicotine and tar contaminants are not inhaled, but these forms of tobacco use cause their own health-related problems. Smoking cigars and pipes and chewing tobacco are among the leading causes of cancers of the lips, tongue, mouth, larynx, and esophagus.

Eliminating a smoking habit is extremely difficult and requires a significant commitment. But its importance to any discussion of healthy lifestyles is readily apparent. The prevention of smoking is included in Chapter 31. *Healthy People 2000* goals related to smoking cessation are summarized in Box 3-6.

### Regimen Adherence

Regimen adherence is one of the most complex and frustrating phenomena facing health care professionals involved in health promotion and patient teaching. Multiple studies have validated the fact that up to 50% of study populations do not adhere to professional recommendations concerning either disease management or health promotion activities. This fact is reflected in the slow progress and steady resistance associated with even "simple" regimens such as seat belt use, regular daily flossing, and weekly exercise. Dietary changes have proven to be particularly resistant to change because they involve choices that must be made several times each and every day. People cannot simply abstain from food as they can from tobacco or alcohol use. Professionals commonly behave as if "telling" people were enough.[11] Education and awareness are, of course, important elements of lifestyle choices, but they are not the sole factors. People can commonly state the rationale for lifestyle changes and practices but may still be unable to implement this knowledge in their everyday lives, a fact that is clearly demonstrated in smoking cessation.

Pender's model of health promotion continues to be an effective way to illustrate the forces involved in influencing behavior and lifestyle change (Figure 3-2). Pender identified factors that affect the person's perceptions of the problem, factors that modify behaviors, and factors that influence the likelihood

**box 3-6** Healthy People 2000 *Goals Related to Smoking Cessation*

- Reduce cigarette smoking to a prevalence of no more than 15% among people aged 18 and older.
- Reduce smokeless tobacco use by males aged 12 to 24 to a prevalence of no more than 4%.
- Increase to at least 50% the proportion of cigarette smokers aged 18 and older who stopped smoking cigarettes for at least 1 day during the preceding year.
- Increase to 100% the proportion of work sites with a formal smoking policy that prohibits or severely restricts smoking at the workplace.
- Enact in 50 states and the District of Columbia comprehensive laws on clean indoor air that prohibit smoking or limit it to separately ventilated areas in the workplace and enclosed public places.

From US Department of Health and Human Services: *Healthy people 2000: national health promotion and disease prevention objectives,* Washington, DC, 1990, US Government Printing Office.

of health-promoting actions. Motivation to participate in health-promoting behaviors is influenced by the individual's perceptions about health in general and perceptions of self, including self-concept and perceived control of the environment. Persons who do not value health, who do not see a need to improve their health status, or who are not self-motivated are less likely to engage in health-promoting activities. The person's age, sex, and ethnicity are among the many potential modifying factors that may be active in any given situation. Identifying an individual's unique and specific modifying factors requires careful and sensitive assessment. The influence of family and friends can also be powerful factors. Research indicates that family support for health-promoting activities enhances a person's successful adaptation to a health promotion regimen.

Perceived barriers to health promotion and regimen adherence include concrete factors such as cost and availability, as well as highly personal and unique factors such as the reactions of significant others. Major factors that have been identified as barriers to regimen adherence are summarized in Box 3-7. The complexity of the regimen appears to be particularly important. Simpler lifestyle changes are typically easier to make. The degree of behavior change required and the duration of need for the regimen are also critical variables. Changes that must be implemented "for life" are particularly difficult for individuals to sustain over time.

# NURSING MANAGEMENT

## ASSESSMENT

Assessment is perhaps the most critical phase of the nursing process when working with individuals and families to promote healthy lifestyles. A great deal of time and money have been expended in this country on public information campaigns and education materials designed to positively affect lifestyle choices. The public education approach is grounded in the belief that when people understand the importance of making recommended lifestyle changes, they will be able to incorporate those changes into their daily lives. The fallacies of this approach are apparent in our own lives. Most of us can clearly state the health advantages of selected lifestyle changes, but few of us are able to easily make those changes. Most of us want "easy" answers to difficult issues with minimum disruption of our daily habits. Broad-based educational approaches commonly fail to adequately consider individual value systems and are insensitive to differences in various cultural groups.

The assessment challenge of the professional nurse is to understand the lived experience of the patient and family—their values, priorities, life circumstances, interests, intellect, situational constraints, and support network. Valid and reliable assessment tools can gather pieces of information, but an in-depth understanding of the person's life

**box 3-7** *Major Factors Affecting Regimen Adherence*

- Amount of time the regimen requires
- Visibility of the regimen to others
- Amount of energy required to complete the regimen
- Difficulty of the regimen
- Amount of discomfort associated with the regimen
- Frequency of action required
- Expense of the regimen
- Duration of need for the regimen
- Amount of disruption to "normal" activities
- Perceived effectiveness of regimen in controlling or preventing the disease or condition

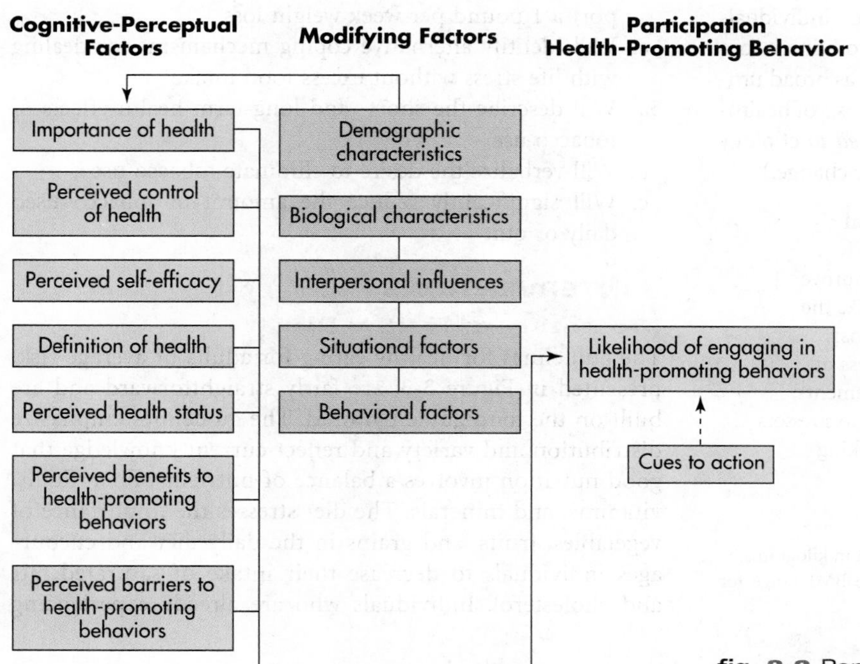


**fig. 3-2** Pender's health promotion model.

circumstances emerges from skilled interviewing. This assessment and interviewing process can also be used to establish a working relationship or partnership with the person and family.

A wide variety of assessment and screening tools exist for evaluating components of the healthy lifestyle. A full presentation of the range of tools is beyond the scope of this chapter. A well-developed functional health pattern assessment tool will provide preliminary data concerning areas such as health beliefs and values, sleep and rest, and exercise. A basic tool can be used to reveal the areas needing in-depth assessment. A sampling of the types of tools or questions that can be used in the initial assessment of the components of the healthy lifestyle are displayed in Boxes 3-8 through 3-11.

Objective assessment is also included in the data gathering process related to healthy lifestyles. The components vary substantially according to the setting and purpose of the nurse's interactions. Common objective areas for assessment include:

General appearance
Height and weight compared with standard reference tools
Body mass index*
Skinfold measurements
Range of motion of joints
Treadmill exercise tolerance assessment
Laboratory tests (e.g., cholesterol, lipids, hemoglobin, and hematocrit)
Vital signs (respirations, pulse, blood pressure)

## NURSING DIAGNOSES

A wide variety of nursing diagnoses may be applicable in any specific patient situation. Promotion of healthy lifestyles will be a goal in working with adults of all ages, regardless of their baseline health status. Efforts can be directed at improving the health status of individuals who are basically healthy; decreasing risk factors in individuals who are asymptomatic but at risk for particular disease processes; and improving the health of individuals already experiencing chronic diseases who need to adhere to a health regimen. The following diagnoses can serve as broad umbrellas for these unique situations. (*Note:* The diagnosis of health-seeking behaviors does not use the standard *related to* etiology and simply states the desired area for knowledge or change.)

| Diagnostic Title | Possible Etiological Factors |
|---|---|
| Health-seeking behaviors | Exercise plan to improve fitness and minimize the effects of osteoporosis |
| Altered health maintenance | Oral intake in excess of metabolic requirements; eating in response to stressors |
| Potential for enhanced management of therapeutic regimen, individual | Desire to quit smoking |

*Body mass index (BMI) is calculated by dividing the weight in kilograms by the height in meters squared. For health maintenance the BMI range for adults is 20 to 25 kg/m$^2$.

**box 3-8 Sample Assessment Questions for Health Beliefs**

**HEALTH PERCEPTION—HEALTH MANAGEMENT PATTERN**

1. How has general health been?
2. Any colds in the past year? If appropriate, absences from work/school?
3. What are the most important things done to keep healthy? Think these things make a difference to health? (Include family, folk remedies, if appropriate.) Breast self-examination?
4. Accidents (home, work, driving)?
5. In past, has it been easy to find ways to follow suggestions of doctors or nurses?
6. If appropriate: What do you think caused this illness? Action taken when symptoms perceived? Results of action?
7. If appropriate: What is important to you while you are here? How can we be most helpful?
8. Use of tobacco?
   Pack year history
   Attempts to quit
9. Use of alcohol? When was last drink?
10. Other drugs?

## EXPECTED PATIENT OUTCOMES

The appropriate outcomes will vary greatly, reflecting the unique personal and etiological factors of the diagnosis. Sample outcomes for the situations reflected in the diagnoses identified above might include:

1. Will participate in a regular physical exercise program that includes weight-bearing exercise of at least 20 minutes' duration a minimum of 3 or 4 times per week

2a. Will verbalize an intent to modify the diet in ways that conform to the recommended food pyramid
b. Will balance food intake and energy expenditure to support a 1 pound per week weight loss
c. Will identify alternative coping mechanisms for dealing with life stress without excess food intake

3a. Will describe the short- and long-term health effects of tobacco use
b. Will verbalize the desire to eliminate tobacco use
c. Will significantly reduce the amount of tobacco used daily or quit

## INTERVENTIONS

### Promoting a Healthy Diet

The guidelines for healthy eating for adults of average risk, presented in Figure 3-3, are fairly straightforward and are built on the food guide pyramid. The guidelines emphasize distribution and variety and reflect current knowledge that good nutrition involves a balance of nutrients, fiber, fluids, vitamins, and minerals. The diet stresses the importance of vegetables, fruits, and grains in the daily diet and encourages individuals to decrease their intake of saturated fats and cholesterol. Individuals who are already experiencing

**box 3-9** *Sample Nutritional History Form*

Patient name ________
Age ________
Gender ________

Marital status ________
Family or significant others ________

Primary medical diagnosis ________

Height ________
Weight ________

Recent weight change (note amount, time period, and cause) ________

Frame (small, medium, large) ________

Allergies (food or drug) ________

Smoking (packs per day) ________

Medications ________

Describe dosage schedule for medications, that is, are they taken with meals or on an empty stomach? ________

Food preferences ________

Food intolerances or restrictions ________

Therapeutic diet or nutritional support prescription ________

What do the patient or family find to be the easiest and most difficult parts of the therapeutic diet or nutritional support plan? ________

What, if anything, would the patient or family like to change about the therapeutic diet or nutritional support plan? ________

Usual daily dietary intake (including fluids) ________

Availability of foodstuffs:
- Who does the shopping? ________
- Where do you shop? ________
- Do you have transportation problems with regard to shopping? ________
- Are you limited by seasonal availability of foods? (Explain) ________

Financial concerns regarding diet ________
Cultural/religious concerns ________

What is the meaning of food to this family (e.g., social or sustenance only)? ________

Food storage:
- Refrigeration: ________
- Hygiene: ________

Food preparation:
- Electricity, gas: ________
- Functioning stove, oven: ________
- Sufficient utensils: ________
- Who prepares the food? ________
- Who makes food decisions? ________

Health problems (describe in terms of onset, chronology, quality, associated factors, aggravating factors, alleviating factors, how the problem is managed, whether the intervention is effective) ________

- Indigestion (preprandial or postprandial) ________
- Dysphagia ________
- Difficulty chewing ________
- Diabetes ________
- Cardiovascular disease ________
- Hypertension ________
- Condition of teeth/gums ________
- Dentures (full, partial) ________

From: Stanhope M, Knollmueller RN: *Handbook of community and home health nursing,* ed 2, 1996, St Louis, Mosby.

chronic illnesses or who are assessed as being at higher risk may need more specific guidelines concerning the balance and distribution of foods. A more detailed description of the principles of healthy eating is provided in the Patient/Family Teaching Box on p. 61.

The nurse assists the person to use the food guide pyramid for effective daily meal planning. Initial assessment reveals the areas of needed dietary changes. The next step is to translate the recommendations into servings and portions that are understandable and that accurately reflect the individual's optimal daily caloric intake.[9] Most sedentary women and older adults need about 1600 total calories per day; this represents the lower end of the serving range on the pyramid. Men usually need about 2200 calories per day, which reflects the upper end of the serving range. Box 3-12 gives examples of standard servings for meal planning purposes. Individuals need to pay particular attention to the serving size for meat because 2 to 3 ounces is a much smaller amount than most people would usually regard as a serving. The individual can use a blank pyramid as shown in Figure 3-4 to adapt the general guidelines to his or her own unique food likes and dislikes. The blank pyramid also facilitates incorporation of cultural or religious food practices into the meal planning process.

The average American diet is at least 10% to 15% higher in total fats than is recommended, and reducing the intake of fats and cholesterol is a major purpose of the pyramid.[10] This purpose becomes even more important for persons who have multiple risk factors or who already have heart or vascular disease. This emphasis on reducing dietary fat is reflected in the *Healthy People 2000* nutrition goals. (See Box 3-4.)

**box 3-10** *Sample Food Habits Assessment Form*

Please answer the following questions and indicate the number of servings of each type of food that you eat in an average day. A partially completed Sample Survey is shown at right.

**Sample Survey**

The food survey at right contains information about Joe's intake of breads and cereals/vegetables and fruits during a typical day.

He typically eats a large bowl of cereal, which is recorded as 2 under "small bowls." He eats a sandwich at lunch and usually a piece of toast at breakfast, which he recorded as "2-3 slices of bread."

**Breads and Cereals**

2-3 slice of bread
__ tortilla
1 small roll, biscuit, or muffin
__ ½ bun, English muffin, or bagel
__ small helping of cooked cereal, rice or pasta
2 small bowl of cold cereal

**Vegetables and Fruits**

2 scoop-sized helping of vegetables
1 small vegetable salad
__ medium-sized potato
1 piece of fruit (an apple, orange, banana, slice of melon, etc.)
__ ½ cup cooked or canned fruit or berries
1-2 small glass of fruit juice

**Name:** ______________

**Date:** ______________

Who purchases food at your home? ______________

Who cooks?

What kind of red meat do you usually buy? ☐ regular ☐ lean

How do you usually cook meat?
☐ fry ☐ bake ☐ broil
☐ stew/slow cook

How many snacks do you eat each day? ______________

How many meals? ______________

How many times each week do you eat away from home? ______________

What restaurant do you go to most often? ______________

Do you take any vitamin or mineral tablets? ☐ Yes ☐ No
If yes, please list the kinds and the amounts: ______________

Do you eat any special foods for health, religious, or personal choice reasons? ☐ Yes ☐ No
If yes, please list the kinds and amounts: ______________

Do you add salt to your food at the table?
☐ Yes ☐ No

Do you add salt to foods when you cook?
☐ Yes ☐ No

**Breads and Cereals**

__ slice of bread
__ tortilla
__ small roll, biscuit, or muffin
__ ½ bun, English muffin, or bagel
__ small helping of cooked cereal, rice, or pasta (large serving equals 2)
__ small bowl of cold cereal (large serving equals 2)

**Vegetables and Fruits**

__ scoop-sized helping of vegetables
__ small vegetable salad
__ medium-sized potato
__ piece of fruit (an apple, orange, banana, slice of melon, etc.)
__ ½ cup cooked or canned fruit or berries
__ small glass of fruit juice

**Milk Group**

__ glass of whole milk
__ glass of 2% milk
__ glass of 1% or skim milk
__ slice of cheese
__ helping of yogurt or cottage cheese
__ small scoop of ice cream

**Meat Group**

__ small piece of meat, fish, or poultry (about 2-3 oz large serving equals 2)
__ 2 eggs
__ 1 cup of dried beans or peas
__ 4 tablespoons of peanut butter

**Mixed Foods**

__ small square of lasagna
__ small serving of spaghetti with meat sauce
__ small serving of macaroni and cheese
__ taco
__ burrito
__ slice of pizza

**Beverages**

__ cups of regular coffee
__ cups of decaf coffee
__ cups of regular tea
__ cups of decaf tea
__ 12 ounce soft drinks
__ 12 ounce diet drinks
__ glass of Kool-aid or fruit punch
__ glass of water

**Sweets and Fats**

__ sweet roll or donut
__ slice of pie or cake
__ 3 small cookies
__ candy bar
__ 10 chips or french fries
__ rounded teaspoonful of margarine or butter
__ tablespoonful of salad dressing

**Alcohol**

__ 12 ounce beer
__ 4 ounces of wine (small glass)
__ shot of liquor

Source: *Physicians' guide to outpatient nutrition,* Arlington, Va, National Dairy Promotion and Research Board.

**box 3-11** *Components of a Sleep History*

1. How easily do you fall asleep?
2. Do you fall asleep and have difficulty staying asleep? How many times do you awaken?
3. Do you awaken early from sleep?
4. What time do you awaken for good? What causes you to awaken early?
5. What do you do to prepare for sleep? To improve your sleep?
6. What do you think about as you try to fall asleep?
7. How often do you have trouble sleeping?
8. Are you tired during the day?
9. Describe your bedtime routine and sleep environment.
10. Do you use any over-the-counter or prescription sleep aids?
11. What foods or drink, if any, affect your sleep pattern?

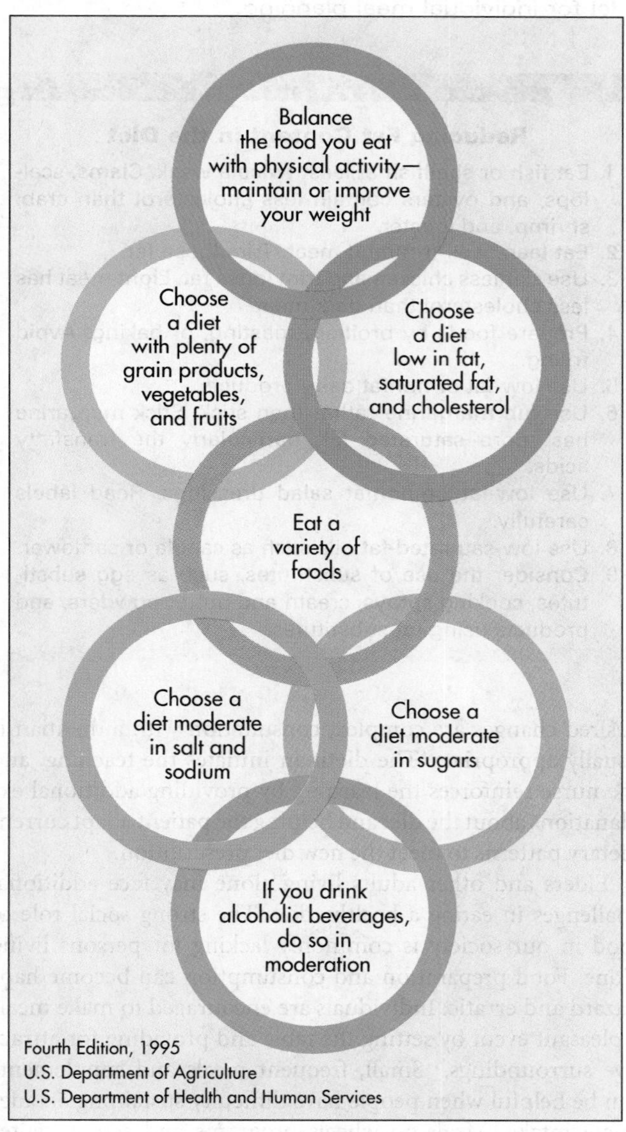


**fig. 3-3** Dietary guidelines for Americans.

**patient/family teaching**

**Guidelines for Healthy Eating**

1. Reduce your daily fat intake to no more than 30% of your total calories (no more than 10% should be from saturated fats).
2. Reduce your cholesterol intake to less than 300 mg per day.
3. Eat five or more servings of vegetables and fruits daily. Be sure to include green and yellow vegetables and citrus fruits.
4. Increase your intake of complex carbohydrates by eating six or more servings of breads, cereals, and legumes.
5. Maintain a reasonable protein intake within the stated fat restriction.
6. Increase the fiber in your diet to 20 to 30 g daily. Add small amounts of fiber daily, and be sure to maintain a liberal intake of water.
7. Drink five to eight 8-ounce glasses of water each day.
8. Drink skim milk daily. It is an excellent source of calcium.
9. Limit the amount of salt you consume each day to 6 g (slightly more than 1 tsp). Limit its use in cooking and avoid adding salt at the table. Eat salty foods such as salt-preserved and salt-pickled foods sparingly.
10. Avoid taking dietary supplements in excess of the recommended daily allowance for any element. Consult with your health care provider before adding supplements to your diet.
11. Alcohol intake is not recommended. If you do drink, limit your intake to no more than 12 ounces of beer, 4 ounces of wine, or 2 to 3 ounces of liquor a day.
12. Balance the amount of food you eat each day with the correct amount of active exercise to maintain a stable body weight.

Adapted from National Academy of Sciences: *Eat for life,* Washington, DC, 1992, National Academy Press.

The nurse encourages individuals to have their baseline cholesterol level determined and provides some simple strategies for reducing dietary fat and cholesterol. Some basic strategies are summarized in the accompanying Patient/Family Teaching Box. Reducing fat and cholesterol is often an extremely difficult change because it targets foods popular in American culture such as high fat cheeses, red meat, and cold cuts. The nurse may also need to teach about the major sources of fat and cholesterol in the average diet.

Permanent diet changes are difficult to sustain and are more likely to be successful when modifications are made gradually. For example, the change to skim milk can be made gradually by first switching to 2% milk and then decreasing the milk fat content again several weeks later. Changing the entire diet is rarely successful, so the nurse encourages the person to select one or two important principles on which to focus his or her efforts. These changes can then be supported through printed materials, written or pictorial, prepared at a reading level that is appropriate and acceptable to the person. Whenever possible diet discussion and teaching should incorporate the whole family or social unit. Success is rarely possible when the family

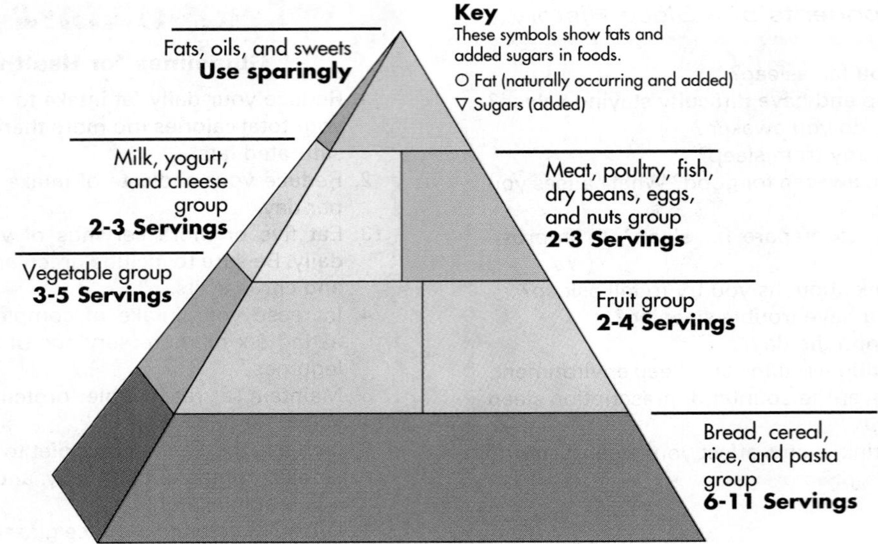


**fig. 3-4** The food guide pyramid—a model for individual meal planning.

**box 3-12** *The Food Guide Pyramid: Standard Foods—What Counts as 1 Serving?*

**BREAD GROUP**
1 slice of bread
½ English muffin or bagel
1 cup ready-to-eat cereal
½ cup cooked cereal or pasta

**FRUIT GROUP**
1 medium apple, banana, or orange
½ cup cooked or canned fruit
¾ cup fruit juice

**VEGETABLE GROUP**
1 cup raw leafy vegetables
½ cup cooked or chopped raw vegetables
¾ cup vegetable juice

**MEAT GROUP**
2-3 ounces* cooked meat, fish, or poultry
1 cup cooked dry beans or peas
2 eggs or 4 tbsp peanut butter

**MILK GROUP**
1 cup milk, yogurt, or ice cream
1-2 ounces cheese
½ cup cottage cheese

*1 ounce of meat or cheese is the size of a matchbox; 3 ounces are the size of a deck of cards; 8 ounces are the size of a paperback book.

Source: US Department of Agriculture and the US Department of Health and Human Services.

does not endorse the needed changes. This is especially true when the patient is not the primary food preparer. The messages given to the patient must be practical and consider financial resources and other environmental constraints such as access to food and equipment for food preparation. When the desired changes are complex, consultation with a dietitian is usually appropriate. The dietitian initiates the teaching, and the nurse reinforces the learning by providing additional explanations about the diet and helping the patient adapt current dietary patterns to meet the new diet prescription.

Elders and other adults living alone may face additional challenges in eating a healthy diet. The strong social role of food in our society is commonly lacking for persons living alone. Food preparation and consumption can become haphazard and erratic. Individuals are encouraged to make meals a pleasant event by setting the table and providing for attractive surroundings.[6] Small, frequent meals and supplements can be helpful when people have difficulty sustaining an adequate intake. Meals-on-wheels programs and senior center services can be viable alternatives for homebound elders or those with limited mobility.

**patient/family teaching**

**Reducing Fat Content in the Diet**

1. Eat fish or shellfish at least twice a week. Clams, scallops, and oysters contain less cholesterol than crab, shrimp, and lobster.
2. Eat lean, well-trimmed meat. Trim loose fat.
3. Use skinless chicken and trim loose fat. Light meat has less cholesterol than dark meat.
4. Prepare foods by broiling, roasting, or baking. Avoid frying.
5. Use low-fat or nonfat dairy products.
6. Use tub margarine rather than stick. Stick margarine has more saturated fat, particularly the transfatty acids.
7. Use low-fat or nonfat salad dressings. Read labels carefully.
8. Use low-saturated-fat oils such as canola or safflower.
9. Consider the use of substitutes, such as egg substitutes, cooking sprays, cream and butter powders, and products using fat substitutes.

### Food labels

Food labels can be an important source of information, and the nurse teaches the individual to interpret labels accurately. The Nutrition Labeling and Education Act, which requires consistent food labeling on nearly all food packages, was passed in 1990. The legislation attempts to facilitate consumer decision making about foods by standardizing serving sizes and clarifying the meaning of terms such as *low, reduced,* and *lean.*[2] The nurse ensures that individuals understand and use the information that is provided on labels to make appropriate diet choices.

### Supplements

The nurse also determines the person's current use of vitamins, minerals, and other supplements. Although more than one third of the adult population is estimated to routinely use supplements, the need for routine, broad-spectrum supplementation is established after carefully assessing the person's daily intake.

Specific supplementation of vitamins A, B, C, or E may be used as chemoprophylaxis to reduce the risk of certain cancers or to bolster immune function. The need for calcium supplementation is explored with women and all elders. If an individual does not consume dairy products, the average diet provides only about 300 mg of calcium per day, which is far below the recommended level of 1200 mg. Each milk product serving provides another 300 mg. A combined calcium and vitamin D supplement is recommended for adults who are not routinely meeting their daily calcium needs through food.

### Promoting an optimal body weight

The complexity of weight loss has been addressed earlier in the chapter. All weight management approaches focus on establishing a lifelong balance between food intake and energy expenditure that supports gradual weight loss if needed. Diet has always received the most attention in weight loss efforts and diet changes remain appropriate, but most exotic and highly restrictive plans have proven to be ineffective for long-term weight control.

Diets are individualized with the caloric intake planned at a level below the person's maintenance needs. A graph of healthy weight ranges is shown in Figure 3-5. The loss of one pound of fat per week requires a calorie deficit of 500 calories per day. The basic food guide pyramid can once again serve as the foundation for diet planning with its primary emphasis on limited use of sugars and fats.[5] Weight loss for some persons may be achieved by eating three average balanced meals a day. Other persons are more successful with frequent small meals. When caloric intake is severely reduced there is often a large initial weight loss through water loss. A plateau is then reached, which lasts 7 to 10 days and may be very discouraging to the dieter. Weight loss then continues at a slower rate as the body adapts to the decreased caloric intake by decreasing the metabolic rate.

Adhering to a diet is often extremely difficult, and the person tends to become preoccupied with food. The use of appetite suppressants is controversial because of long-term inefficiency and associated health risks. Most over-the-counter diet aids contain phenylpropanolamine and bulk-producing agents. Phenylpropanolamine is a sympathomimetic with mild anorectic action but no adverse central nervous system effects. Its effectiveness as a weight loss drug in humans remains questionable. Bulk-producing agents such as methylcellulose expand the stomach and provide a sense of fullness, but the same effect can be achieved by drinking two or three glasses of water before each meal.

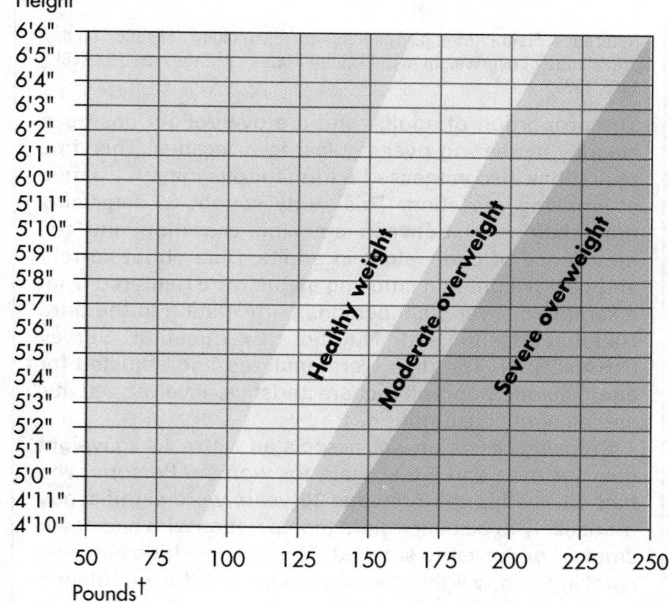


*Without shoes.

†Without clothes. The higher weights apply to people with more muscle and bone, such as many men.

**fig. 3-5** Healthy weights for Americans.

The approval of fenfluramine (Redux) and phentermine for appetite suppression in severe obesity was heralded as the beginning of a new era in obesity management. The initial results were very promising and the drugs have been used successfully in Europe for almost a decade, but a surprising incidence of heart valve problems and cases of pulmonary hypertension have resulted in the abrupt withdrawal of these drugs from the American market.[8] The future of pharmacological support for weight loss therefore remains unclear. The surgical management of severe obesity is discussed in Chapter 40.

Support from others appears to be critical. Positive results are often obtained in the context of weight loss groups such as Weight Watchers.

The role of exercise in long-term weight management continues to expand. Exercise promotes the loss of fat rather than lean body tissue and positively affects serum insulin and lipid levels. Regular exercise also improves general health and well-being and allows the individual increased flexibility in daily meal planning. The following Research Box presents findings of a study that explored the relationship between smoking cessation and weight gain.

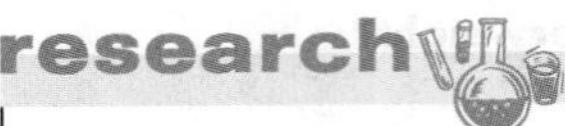

Reference: Flegel KM et al: The influence of smoking cessation on the prevalence of overweight in the United States, *N Engl J Med* 333(18): 1165, 1995.

The proportion of adults who are overweight has been steadily increasing over the last few decades. This time period has also witnessed a tremendous initiative aimed at smoking cessation. This study sought to determine the relationship between smoking cessation and the prevalence of overweight in adults. Data about current and past weight and smoking status were gathered from a sample of over 5000 persons participating in the third National Health and Nutrition Examination Survey (NHANES III). The data were analyzed and adjusted for age, sociodemographic characteristics, level of activity, and alcohol consumption.

Smoking cessation was associated with a 4.4 kg weight gain for men and 5.0 kg gain for women. Persons who had quit within the previous 10 years were significantly more likely to be overweight than persons who had never smoked or currently smoked. The relationships between smoking and weight gain were clear, but this population accounted for less than 10% of the overall increase in overweight prevalence within the general population.

#### Limiting alcohol use

Alcohol use must be included in any discussion of a healthy diet. Alcohol use is pervasive in American society, and the potential for abuse and addiction is tremendous. These problems are discussed in Chapter 14. Although high in calories, alcohol has no nutrient benefits and contributes to a wide variety of medical disorders, including alcoholic cirrhosis. The nurse carefully explores the individual's use of alcohol and its meaning in his or her life. If a person does not currently use alcohol there is no reason to begin. However, if alcohol use is important the individual can safely and appropriately incorporate it into the lifestyle. Some modest health benefits have even been attributed to the occasional use of alcohol in the form of red wine. Daily alcohol intake should be limited to no more than two cans of beer, two small glasses of wine, or two drinks containing no more than 1½ ounces of alcohol each.

### Promoting Exercise

The nurse attempts to assist the person to establish and maintain a program of regular moderate exercise to enhance physical and emotional health. A variety of exercise plans can be used to achieve this goal, but any exercise program should have moderate weight-bearing exercise as its foundation. The recommendations for amount, intensity, and duration of exercise have varied somewhat over the last decade, but it is generally agreed that active aerobic exercise that involves the large muscles and takes place at least three times per week for 20 minutes can achieve all basic health goals.[3] Higher levels of frequency, intensity, and duration can be established for individuals as appropriate. Regular exercise increases the person's energy and feeling of well-being; the individual should feel replenished, not depleted. Moderate-intensity exercise, with brisk walking as the classic example, carries a very low risk of injury and is achievable for adults of all ages. The importance of exercise in a largely sedentary society is reflected in the *Healthy People 2000* goals. (See Box 3-5.)

Consensus is lacking about who needs a physical examination or cardiac screening before beginning an exercise plan. Adults under 45 years of age who do not have significant cardiac risk factors can usually safely begin an exercise program without preliminary screening.[12] The nurse encourages these individuals to begin slowly, increase intensity progressively, and report the occurrence of any unusual or unexplainable symptom promptly. Adults over age 45 should consult with their physician before beginning an exercise program.

Exercise testing can accurately establish the person's maximum oxygen consumption and thereby set definitive maximal and target (70% to 85% of maximal) heart rates for exercise. When testing is not performed the person estimates his or her target and maximal heart rates based on age and a standard formula.[3] A 40-year-old person would have a target heart rate for exercise of 126 to 153 beats per minute. This is established by subtracting 40 from 220 and then taking 70% to 85% of the resultant 180.

An exercise prescription specifically delineates the type, frequency, intensity, and duration of exercise. Intensity and duration can steadily increase as the person's conditioning improves. In addition to this basic aerobic plan the individual may also be counseled to include some strength training. Strength training has proven to be very effective for women seeking to minimize the progression of osteoporosis and for elders who need to maintain muscle mass, strength, balance, and flexibility.

The nurse instructs the person about the importance of both range of motion and stretching exercises before the aerobic phase of exercise, and the importance of a slow cooldown period at the conclusion of exercise so the heart rate can gradually return to its resting level. These precautions help protect the muscles and joints from injury and prevent the incidence of postexercise hypotension and syncope.

Exercise is also commonly prescribed as part of tertiary prevention for persons with chronic illnesses. Exercise has been shown to increase tolerance for activities of daily living (ADL), increase appetite, decrease anxiety and depression, and promote adjustment. The exercise program is specifically tailored to the person's unique needs and abilities. Exercise is begun at a low intensity, and both frequency and duration are modified as needed. Walking, cycling, and swimming are often well tolerated. When specific exercise prescriptions are indicated (e.g., after myocardial infarction or with chronic obstructive pulmonary disease), an exercise physiologist will typically perform the assessment and set the program parameters.

The nurse again uses in-depth assessment to determine the patient's perceived barriers and supports for exercise. Getting started is typically the biggest barrier to the establishment of a regular exercise plan. Both home-based and workplace programs are effective for various groups of people. The nurse reminds the individual that expensive equipment and health club memberships are not necessary for a successful exercise plan. A partner to share the exercise is a strongly positive motivator for most people. Walking remains an ideal choice for many people because the risk of injury is low, the intensity and duration are easily controlled, and the exercise requires no special training.

**patient/family teaching**

**Strategies for Establishing a Successful Exercise Plan**

1. Exercise should be fun or at least pleasurable. Find an activity that you can enjoy.
2. Establish specific time periods for exercise and plan them into your week. You are more likely to exercise if it is a scheduled event.
3. Start in small increments and progress slowly. Monitor your body's response to increases in intensity or duration.
4. Set small, attainable goals and reward yourself as you achieve each goal.
5. Wear proper clothing and use exercise equipment correctly.
6. Be sure to warm up and cool down thoroughly before and after exercise.
7. Avoid exercising in extremes of heat, cold, or humidity.
8. Avoid exercising for about 2 hours after a heavy meal. Do not eat for about 1 hour after active exercise.
9. Share the activity with a friend, or consider joining a structured exercise class. Many community agencies sponsor exercise groups such as swimming, low-impact aerobics, and mall walking.

Adherence to the plan remains a challenge, however, and an exercise plan can easily fall into disuse. Some strategies that can be used to foster adherence to an exercise regimen are included in the Patient/Family Teaching Box above.

### Promoting Rest and Sleep

The nurse will help the person plan for adequate daily rest and sleep. It is easy to allow lifestyle issues to interfere with sleep patterns. Most people experience sleep difficulties at some time, but these problems are usually amenable to correction by simple measures such as those outlined in the Patient/Family Teaching Box, above right.

Exercise can also be used to increase well-being and promote sleep, and the nurse encourages the patient to engage in regular exercise for its multiple positive health benefits. People experiencing actual sleep disorders face more complex challenges. The management of sleep disorders is discussed in Chapter 13.

Stress also negatively affects the individual's ability to achieve adequate rest and sleep. The nurse helps patients improve their overall coping abilities. Relaxation strategies for stress management are discussed in Chapter 6.

### Promoting Adherence to a Healthy Lifestyle

The many benefits of healthy lifestyles are well documented. Most of the components of a healthy lifestyle are low tech, low cost, and seemingly simple. Yet the vast majority of adults do not integrate these components into their daily lives. Nurses have sadly learned that simply educating people about health risks and benefits does not significantly change behavior. The big picture can be discouraging and calls into question the cost-effectiveness of the time and money expended on outreach education for the public. (See the Research Boxes, right and on the next page.)

**patient/family teaching**

**Measures to Promote Restful Sleep**

1. Follow a consistent schedule for getting up and going to bed to promote regular circadian rhythms.
2. Exercise daily but avoid strenuous exercise near bedtime.
3. Engage in some relaxing activity, such as watching TV or reading, before attempting to sleep. Avoid activities that are stimulating or anxiety producing.
4. Avoid eating a heavy meal before sleep; however, a bedtime snack helps many people relax for sleep. Try drinking a glass of warm or cold milk at bedtime. It contains L-tryptophan, a sleep inducer.
5. Avoid drinking caffeine-containing beverages after the evening meal.
6. Make the environment conducive for sleep. Pay attention to temperature, light, and noise.
7. Reserve the bed for sleep and sexual activity. Reading, watching TV, paying bills, and talking on the phone in bed can make it difficult to make the transition to sleep.
8. Avoid late day naps if you are experiencing difficulty falling asleep. Morning naps rarely interfere with sleep patterns.
9. Engage in a pleasant relaxation exercise as you prepare to sleep.
10. Do not lie in bed for more than 20 to 30 minutes "trying" to sleep. Get up and engage in a low-stimulation activity for 15 to 30 minutes and then return to bed.

**research**

Reference: Pruitt RH: Effectiveness and cost efficiency of interventions in health promotion, *J Adv Nurs* 17:926, 1992.

The purpose of this study was to determine the overall effectiveness and cost efficiency of a stress management program incorporating psychological and physiological parameters. The sample was a group of 60 adults drawn from a pool of civilian and military employees at the Pentagon who were invited to participate in a "Fit to Win" program when they were identified as having hypertension or high-normal blood pressure. Participants were randomly distributed between two groups. Both groups participated in the standard offerings of the Fit to Win program, including exercise. One group also took part in a stress management program. The outcomes measured included perceived anxiety, stress-related physical symptoms, blood pressure, and cost estimates.

Both groups experienced an improvement in blood pressure and had less perceived anxiety. These improvements were attributed to the exercise component of the program. In addition, the experimental group also experienced a significant decrease in stress-related symptoms. This change was attributed to the stress management program. The stress management program was evaluated as cost-effective, but the authors note that employers must value employee health and be willing to provide release time for participation in health promotion programs.

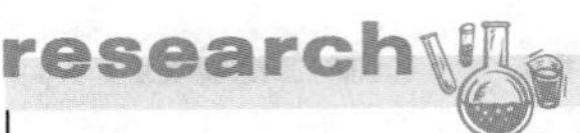


Reference: Frauman A, Nettles-Carlson B: Predictors of a health promoting lifestyle among well adult clients in a nursing practice, *J Am Acad Nurse Pract* 3(4):174-179, 1991.

The purpose of this study was to determine whether selected health-related characteristics or combinations of characteristics would predict the likelihood of persons actually engaging in a health-promoting lifestyle. The sample of slightly more than 300 persons was drawn from a pool of well adults, clients of a nurse practitioner practice that focused on health promotion and maintenance. Pender's health promotion model was used as the conceptual framework for the study. Survey research methods were used to gather data about perceptual and demographic factors and self-reported health-promoting behaviors. The effects of age, gender, marital status, race, education, income, rural/ urban residence, definition of health, importance of health, and health locus of control were all analyzed to determine their effect on health-promoting behavior. Only two variables were found to have a predictive effect. Patients with higher educational levels who embraced a definition of health as exuberant well-being rather than a functional status or simple absence of disease were more likely to engage in healthy lifestyle practices.

The challenges related to regimen adherence are very real and frustrating for health care professionals. The difficulties inherent in making lifestyle changes need to be acknowledged in interactions with patients and families. Regimen adherence is a classic example of personal choice and personal control. The nurse needs to be aware of and respect the person's right to make personal choices that conflict with recommended behaviors. The nurse must also realize that professionals are limited in their ability to "force" positive changes. This does not mean, however, that intervention and teaching are either inappropriate or a waste of time. Successful health promotion outreach acknowledges that the individual retains control over his or her own life choices, but nurses commonly encounter people at moments of readiness when life events have conspired to make health status improvement a priority in the person's life.[11] These opportunities to effect positive change must not be squandered.

The nurse begins by assisting the individual to identify supports and barriers to change and to differentiate between actual and perceived barriers. Teaching and health education remain important parts of the overall intervention plan, but the nurse recognizes that they represent the beginning of intervention and not the end. The nurse is responsible for providing the patient with adequate information to make choices; the nurse is not responsible for the choices that are made. Successful change reflects the person's inner drives and goals. Values clarification can help the person recognize and articulate his or her values related to health and personal responsibility. The nurse directly addresses the issue of self-responsibility and personal choice and helps the person recognize how his or her lifestyle behavior is either congruent or incongruent with the person's core values. The nurse then assists the person to address areas of values conflict. This may provide sufficient impetus for the person to initiate needed behavior change.

The person is next assisted to set goals for health promotion and lifestyle change. The nurse needs to be positive and supportive of the patient's goals. Even seemingly minor changes are positive steps and can reduce health risks and improve overall health. The critical starting point is the person's commitment to take responsibility for his or her health.

The nurse then assists the individual to develop and implement a plan that addresses the targeted lifestyle changes. Appropriate family and community resources and supports are identified. The nurse helps the person explore acceptable alternatives for overcoming actual barriers to adherence. The person must believe that the problem is solvable and that he or she is competent to solve it. The nurse needs to be enthusiastic about the person's ability to make needed changes and provide the individual with positive reinforcement for his or her efforts and accomplishments. Behavior modification principles state that positive reinforcement of desired behaviors increases the likelihood that the behavior will be repeated.

Numerous other practical strategies can be effective in promoting adherence to a health promotion regimen. These include keeping the regimen as simple as possible and allowing the person to adapt it as needed to his or her lifestyle. Formal contracting can occasionally be a powerful tool and underscores the importance of working collaboratively with the patient and family. The family plays a critical role in determining successful outcomes. The nurse needs to be thoroughly familiar with the community resources that are available to help the person integrate the regimen into his or her lifestyle. Printed materials, phone calls, and direct referrals to community support groups can help the person take that important first step. Other strategies that can be effective in promoting adherence to a health promotion regimen are summarized in the following Guidelines for Care Box.

### Promoting Smoking Cessation

The hazards of smoking are well known and widely accepted in American society, but over 46 million persons continue to smoke. Nicotine has been identified as the primary addictive component of cigarettes, and the power of nicotine addiction is now well recognized. Becoming nicotine free is an enormous challenge that has a high risk of failure. The American Cancer Society estimates that over 70% of smokers would like to quit smoking but have either failed in their efforts to quit or fear making the attempt. This number is expected to rise as society continues to make it more difficult and unacceptable to smoke in public settings. The discouraging success rates of smoking cessation efforts reinforce the fears and hesitancies of current smokers. Almost 17 million smokers attempt to quit smoking each year, but only 1 million actually succeed in becoming and remaining smoke free.

There are clearly no magic programs that can create successful nonsmokers. A variety of approaches exist to assist

**guidelines for care**

**Strategies to Increase Patient Adherence to a Therapeutic Regimen**

1. Plan collaboratively with the patient. Remember, the regimen belongs to the individual and not to the nurse.
2. Include the family in all planning and teaching if this involvement is acceptable to the patient.
3. Support the person's overall coping abilities.
4. Simplify the needed regimen as much as possible.
5. Assist the person to incorporate the regimen into his or her preferred pattern of daily activities as much as possible. Encourage the person to tailor the regimen as needed to make it "fit."
6. Be sure that the patient and family understand the rationale for all activities. Provide appropriately written materials for them to keep as references.
7. Explore the idea of contracting with the person for needed behavior change.
8. Provide lots of positive feedback for efforts.
9. Initiate the process of referral to appropriate community self-help and support groups as appropriate. Provide the person with contact phone numbers and addresses and written materials about services. Make the initial telephone contact, if appropriate.

smokers in their efforts to quit, and each has had some degree of success. Hypnosis, acupuncture, aversion therapy, 12-step support programs, psychotherapy, and various forms of nicotine replacement in gums, patches, nasal sprays, and pills are all in use. The programs with the greatest success appear to be those that combine a behavior modification approach with some form of nicotine pharmacological support. It is important to remember, however, that a significant portion of successful "quitters" use no formal program and simply decide to quit "cold turkey." Each smoker clearly has unique needs for support through this process. The American Cancer Society and the American Lung Association are excellent sources of information about specific smoking cessation resources that are available in any local community.

The nurse must remain aware that no one can make someone else quit smoking, no matter how important this action may be from a health perspective. Ultimately, the motivation and effort must come from the individual. However, every health care professional needs to use every opportunity to reinforce education about the hazards of smoking and provide encouragement to persons who are interested in or willing to try smoking cessation. Patients commonly report that no health care professional has ever directly addressed the need for them to stop smoking or encouraged them to try. Approaching patients about the need to quit is clearly the most significant nursing intervention. Nurses commonly interact with patients at times when life and health circumstances have combined to create a readiness point for life changes, and these opportunities need to be promptly and enthusiastically utilized.

**guidelines for care**

**Assisting a Person to Stop Smoking**

1. Assist individual to set a firm "quit" date.
2. Inform individual about available choices for nicotine replacement (e.g., gum, patches of varying concentrations, nasal sprays, pills). Teach about safe and correct use.
3. Explore the advantages of a smoking cessation contract.
4. Encourage the person to use a buddy system or designate a support person to call when he or she experiences cravings.
5. Explore effectiveness of regular gum, hard candy, and so on for use during cravings.
6. Avoid social activities and situations where people smoke during the first weeks of abstinence.
7. Restrict the intake of caffeine if restlessness and anxiety are pronounced symptoms.
8. Incorporate daily exercise into the cessation plan.
9. Use relaxation strategies and imagery to control cravings. Help the person to construct an image of himself or herself as a nonsmoker.
10. Provide regular and enthusiastic support and encouragement for efforts. Openly express confidence that the person can be successful in quitting.
11. Encourage the person to set aside his or her "cigarette money" and spend it on another form of reward for nonsmoking.
12. Encourage involvement with community supports for quitting as available. Remind the family to be enthusiastic and supportive of the person's efforts.

A basic approach to smoking cessation that can be used with any smoker includes the four *A*'s: ask, advise, assist, and arrange. The nurse *asks* the patient about the nature of the patient's smoking habit and *advises* smoking cessation. If acceptable to the patient the nurse *assists* the patient to develop a specific plan for smoking cessation and then *arranges* appropriate follow-up and support. Self-help materials such as brochures, pamphlets, and tapes may prove helpful and should be available in any health care setting. Family involvement and support are critical and can be a defining variable for long-term success. Some type of planned social support during the transition process is helpful for most people. This may involve the family or finding a "buddy" to make smoking cessation a joint effort. Other general behavioral strategies to support smoking cessation are outlined in the Guidelines for Care Box above.

Nicotine replacement preparations were developed to minimize withdrawal symptoms while the smoker learns to live without his or her accustomed smoking-related habits. The power of these habits is reflected in the common yearning for a cigarette after meals, or the expression of not knowing what to do with one's hands without a cigarette. Nicotine gum was first released on the market in the mid-1980s. Nicotine patches were developed next and offered first by prescription and then for over-the-counter purchase. Nicotine is now also available in nasal sprays and pills. The principle of each product is to slowly release sufficient nicotine into the bloodstream to minimize cravings. These products are helpful for many people but are no panacea for withdrawal control. Only 20% of those using the products are able to successfully quit smoking within 6 weeks, and only 10% successfully remain smoke free. They can, however, be a useful adjunct to a more holistic plan to stop smoking.

Nicotine gum must be used correctly to be effective. It is not a traditional gum and cannot be used in that way appropriately. Principles of safe use are summarized in the Guidelines for Care Box below.

The patches release nicotine through the skin, and skin irritation is the most common side effect. Patients are strongly cautioned not to smoke while using the patch because the risk of nicotine overdose exists, particularly for patients with preexisting cardiac disease. Overdose symptoms include headache, abdominal pain, nausea, and vomiting and can progress to severe hypotension and prostration. Patients should also be aware of the predictable symptoms associated with nicotine withdrawal. These symptoms range in severity and duration for any individual but can be extremely severe at times of intense cravings. Classic withdrawal symptoms include irritability, anger, anxiety, restlessness, hunger, decreased concentration, and cravings. See the Research Box on p. 64 for an exploration of smoking cessation and weight gain.

## EVALUATION

Evaluation is specifically targeted to the outcomes that were developed to address the person's unique situation. The range of potential evaluation activities is broad. Successful achievement of the sample outcomes related to a healthy lifestyle would be indicated by the following:

1. Participates consistently in a program of aerobic and strength-building exercise for 30 minutes three times each week
2. a. Plans meals that incorporate the recommendations from the food pyramid
   b. Maintains target goal weight
   c. Uses exercise and progressive relaxation to deal effectively with stress
3. a. Correctly describes the adverse health consequences of smoking
   b. Expresses desire to remain a nonsmoker
   c. Has not smoked cigarettes for 6 months and no longer uses patches or nicotine gum

### guidelines for care

**Safe Use of Nicotine Gum**

- Remember that nicotine gum is not standard gum.
- Take a piece of nicotine gum and chew it a few times to break it down. Chewing will release a "peppery" taste. When this occurs, the gum is parked between the gum and cheek. Do not continue to chew it.
- The nicotine takes several minutes to reach the brain, so the effects are less intense than those achieved with smoke inhalation.
- Repeat at intervals, continuing the chew-and-park strategy for about 30 total minutes.
- Excessive chewing can release the nicotine too quickly. The nicotine mixes with the saliva and may cause dizziness, nausea, and soreness in the mouth and throat. It is not effectively absorbed into the bloodstream and does not reduce cravings.
- Do not smoke while chewing the nicotine gum.

### critical thinking QUESTIONS

1 Nancy is a 38-year-old single mother with four children between the ages of 8 and 16. She works full time and finds it difficult to find time to exercise. She has been slowly gaining weight and is dissatisfied with both her appearance and fitness. Her father died in his forties of a heart attack, and she expresses concern that she is following in his footsteps.

Nancy has actual barriers to establishing an exercise program. She has minimal disposable income, the children get home from school at different times and are all involved in school or community activities, and she is the only driver in the family. She states that she is always tired.

- What approach would you take to help Nancy achieve her stated goal of improving her fitness, considering the constraints of her lifestyle?

2 Mr. Walker is a successful executive who is recovering from a mild heart attack. He is about 35 pounds overweight and admits to an erratic meal pattern. He skips meals, eats a lot of junk food, travels a great deal, and eats heavily when he is entertaining clients. His wife is of Italian background and is an excellent cook. He acknowledges that he needs to make some changes in his diet to decrease the risk of another heart attack and says that he is willing to listen as long as you do not start advocating "the nuts and berries stuff."

- Establish your priorities. What areas will you target and how will you begin to assist Mr. Walker in making changes in his diet?

3 Mrs. Newcomb is 55 years old. She has a history of heart disease and takes medication for hypertension, arthritis, and insulin-dependent diabetes. She has smoked cigarettes for over 30 years and admits to daily alcohol use. She is disabled from her job, lives alone, and is a recent widow. She is quite overweight but states that "all the women in my family are fat and we all live to be 80." Mrs. Newcomb needs to make numerous changes in her lifestyle. The physician wants her to lose weight, bring down her lipid and cholesterol levels, begin exercising, and gain better control of her diabetes. Mrs. Newcomb has confided in you that she thinks it is all "much ado over nothing,"

and she is satisfied with things as they are. "After all," she says, "I'm not in the market for another husband."

- The goal for Mrs. Newcomb is clearly to establish a healthier lifestyle. Where will you begin? Establish goals and priorities and explain your rationale.

## chapter SUMMARY

### EVOLUTION OF A NATIONAL AGENDA FOR HEALTH

- Health promotion has always been a priority concern for nursing but has only recently become recognized as a national health care priority.
- The ANA's *Nursing's Agenda for Health Care Reform* called for a shift in the U.S. health care system from a focus on illness and cure to a focus on wellness and care.
- As the population ages the incidence of chronic illnesses increases. Many of these chronic illnesses are at least partially the result of lifestyle choices.
- The United States did not have an articulated public health agenda until 1980. *Healthy People 2000,* released in 1990, delineated specific goals and objectives concerning the nation's health.
- Managed care insurers and HMOs are increasingly recognizing that promoting healthy lifestyles is one of the most effective methods of controlling health care costs.

### HEALTH PROMOTION AND PREVENTION

- Health promotion and prevention are overlapping concepts.
- Primary prevention involves activities that promote maximum health potential.
- Secondary prevention focuses on the early detection and prompt treatment of disease.
- Tertiary prevention is directed toward rehabilitation after disease is present.
- Health promotion helps individuals make informed lifestyle choices to achieve optimal well-being. It incorporates both primary prevention and rehabilitation through tertiary prevention.

### COMPONENTS OF HEALTHY LIFESTYLES

- The major components of healthy lifestyles include nutrition, exercise, weight control, rest and sleep, and avoiding excess alcohol use and smoking.
- Diet choices play a major role in promoting health and contribute to a wide variety of diseases.
- The nutritional guidelines for health promotion reflect the food pyramid released by the USDA in 1992 and contain five major food groups.
- Obesity is a complex disorder that is steadily becoming a significant national health problem. The links between obesity and the major causes of morbidity are well established.
- Malnutrition and osteoporosis are other major health-related nutritional concerns in the United States.
- The benefits of regular exercise for health have been proven, but the majority of the population does not engage in any regular physical exercise.
- Adequate sleep and rest are essential for health, but many adults report inadequate amounts of daily rest and sleep.
- Self-responsibility and personal choice play a major role in achieving healthy lifestyles. The problem of tobacco use is the clearest example.
- A healthy lifestyle is a form of therapeutic regimen, and long-term adherence to regimens is difficult to sustain.

### NURSING MANAGEMENT

- Assessment is a key role for nursing. Assessment involves both objective measures and attempts to understand the patient's values, motivation, and life experience.
- The two primary nursing diagnoses related to healthy lifestyles are health-seeking behaviors and altered health maintenance.
- Nurses intervene to teach patients how to use the food pyramid, how to reduce the level of fat in the diet, and how to read labels effectively and become informed consumers. Strategies for weight management are provided if the patient exhibits readiness.
- Weight loss focuses on a balanced healthy diet of limited calories combined with daily aerobic exercise.
- Patients are encouraged to slowly begin an exercise plan of active aerobic exercise of at least 20 minutes' duration three times per week. Strength training is also encouraged for elders.
- Several options are available today to assist patients to successfully quit smoking. These include patches of varying concentrations, acupuncture, nasal sprays, and behavior modification. All can be effective with certain persons.
- Nurses assist patients to find ways to increase their adherence to healthy regimens. Basic principles of success include personal goal setting, values clarification, simplifying the regimen, and tailoring the regimen to fit the person's preferred lifestyle, if possible. Involvement of family and friends can be extremely helpful.

## References


1. American Nurses' Association: *Nursing's agenda for health care reform,* Kansas City, Mo, 1992, American Nurses' Association.
2. American Dietetic Association: *Understanding food labels,* Chicago, 1993, The Association.
3. Anonymous: Physical activity: counseling adults and older adults, *Nurse Pract* 22(4):159, 1997.
4. Hoffman C, Rice D, Sung HY: Persons with chronic conditions, their prevalence and cost, *JAMA* 276(18):1473, 1996.
5. Keithley JK, Keller A, Vazquez MG: Promoting good nutrition: Using the food guide pyramid in clinical practice, *Medsurg Nurs* 5(6):397, 1996.
6. Koplan JP, Livengood JR: The influence of changing demographic patterns on our health promotion priorities, *Am J Prev Med* 10(3 suppl):42, 1994.
7. Landis BJ, Brykczynski KA: Employing prevention in practice, *Am J Nurs* 97(8):40, 1997.
8. Manson JE, Faich GA: Pharmacotherapy for obesity—do the benefits outweigh the risks? *N Engl J Med* 335(9):659, 1996.
9. Moore SA: Educating the family and the patient about nutrition, *Prim Care* 21(1):69, 1994.
10. Navia JM: A new perspective for nutrition: the health connection, *Am J Clin Nutr* 61(suppl):407S, 1995.
11. Nichols J: Changing public behavior for better health: is education enough? *Am J Prev Med* 10(3 suppl):19, 1994.

12. Shephard RJ: Exercise and relaxation in health promotion, *Sports Med* 23(4):211, 1997.
13. Turjanica MA: Prevention: what is the cost? *Medsurg Nurs* 4(6):474, 1995.
14. US Department of Health and Human Services: *Healthy people 2000: 1995 review and midcourse corrections*, Washington, DC, 1995, US Government Printing Office.
15. US Department of Health and Human Services, Public Health Service: *Healthy people 2000: national health promotion and disease prevention objectives*, Pub No PHS 91-50212, Washington, DC, 1990, US Government Printing Office.
16. US Surgeon General: *Healthy people: the Surgeon General's report on health promotion and disease prevention*, Washington, DC, 1979, Department of Health, Education and Welfare.
17. US Surgeon General: *Health promotion/disease prevention: objectives for the nation*, Washington, DC, 1980, Department of Health and Human Services.

# chapter 4 Nursing Practice with Elders

DIANA L. MORRIS

## objectives *After studying this chapter, the learner should be able to:*

**1** Discuss the focus of assessment in elderly patients.
**2** Distinguish between primary and secondary changes of aging.
**3** Describe unique patterns of illness in elderly adults.
**4** Explain domains of functional assessment to be addressed in all elderly patients.

## HISTORICAL PERSPECTIVES

Human beings have the longest life span of any animal species, with the potential to live 125 years. For centuries mystery and myth have surrounded the phenomenon of aging. The ancient Greeks believed that life force heat was gradually used up in the normal process of aging. They observed then, as has been confirmed today, that old people are subject to a host of health problems, including dyspnea, joint pains, dizzy spells, insomnia, and visual and hearing losses. The teachings of Sir Francis Bacon (1561 to 1626) marked the beginning of the scientific approach to aging. Bacon believed that the effects of aging accounted for the physical decline of joints and vision. According to Bacon, factors slowing or accelerating the effects of aging included physical stature, temperament, environment, diet, and heredity. These factors remain important correlates that affect health even today. Metchnikoff (1845 to 1916) regarded aging as a natural physiological process beginning at the moment of conception, and Nasher (1863 to 1944) argued that age-related diseases were distinct from aging as a normal process. Today, we continue to emphasize the need to distinguish between normal aging changes and secondary aging changes (diseases). In 1909 Nasher used the word *geriatrics* to refer to diseases of old age. In 1927 Rybrikov, a Russian psychologist, referred to the aging process as the study of *gerontology.* Over time, the following five basic characteristic patterns of aging have been identified:

1. Increased mortality with age
2. Changes in the chemical composition of the body, including a decrease in lean body mass, an increase in fats and lipofuscins, and cross-linking of collagen tissues
3. Progressive deteriorative changes
4. Reduced ability to adapt to environmental changes
5. Increased vulnerability to multiple disease

Nurses have cared for elders and their family members throughout history. In 1904 the American Journal of Nursing published an article on old age and disease. The American Nurses Association (ANA), guided by an understanding of normal aging, the unique needs of elders, and a commitment to scientific care, established a division of geriatric nursing in 1966 to develop standards of nursing care for elders. In 1981 the ANA published standards of care to guide generalist and advanced practice nurses caring for elders. These standards, which serve as a model for practice, apply to all settings and can be used to evaluate care (Box 4-1). Three groups constitute those collectively referred to as elders: the young-old (ages 64 to 74 years); the middle-old (ages 75 to 84 years); and the old-old (ages 85 and older).

### DEMOGRAPHIC TRENDS

America is a nation of aging people. In colonial times, half the population was younger than 16 years of age. In 1900 life expectancy at birth was 49 years. From 1980 to 1990, a period described as "the graying of America," the American population of old-old—those 85 years and older—increased by 38%, whereas the numbers of persons aged 65 to 84 years increased only 20% and those younger than 65 years of age increased by only 8%. By 1990 the so-called "baby boomers" constituted one third of the population of the United States and the number of elders reached 30 million. It is predicted that by 2010 the number of elders will reach 39 million and by 2030, 66 million. This age-group, which comprised 4% of the population in 1900, will increase 23% by the year 2030, with the largest growth occurring among those older than 85 years. Americans indeed reflect an aging population, with four- and five-generational families becoming common as more and more American live into their 100s.

Other dramatic demographic trends include the lower rates of life expectancy for nonwhite persons compared with white persons and the higher number of elderly women than men. In 1991 life expectancy was 72.5 years for African American women and 79.3 years for white women. In 1986 African

**box 4-1** *Standards of Geriatric Nursing Practice*

1. All gerontological nursing services are planned, organized, and directed by a nurse executive. The nurse executive has a baccalaureate or master's preparation and has experience in gerontological nursing and administration.
2. The nurse participates in the generation and testing of theory as a basis for clinical decisions. The nurse uses theoretical concepts to guide the effective practice of gerontological nursing.
3. The health status of the older person is regularly assessed in a comprehensive, accurate, and systematic manner. Information obtained in the health assessment is shared with appropriate members of the interdisciplinary health care team including the older person and family.
4. The nurse uses health assessment data to determine nursing diagnosis.
5. The nurse develops the plan of care in conjunction with the older person, mutually setting goals to address preventive, restorative, and rehabilitative needs of the older person. The plan of care helps the older person attain and maintain the highest level of health, well-being, and quality of life achievable, as well as a peaceful death. The plan of care facilitates continuity of care over time as the client moves to various settings.
6. The nurse intervenes to provide care to restore the older person's functional capabilities and to prevent complications and excessive disability.
7. The nurse continually evaluates the client's and family's response to interventions, to determine attainment of goals and needed revisions.
8. The nurse collaborates regularly with the health care team.
9. The nurse participates in research to generate knowledge development and dissemination of findings into practice settings.
10. The nurse is guided by the ANA code of ethics.
11. The nurse assumes responsibility for professional development, including peer review.

American men had a life expectancy of 66 years compared with 72.6 years for white men. Although the proportions of both men and women in the older than 65 age groups will increase over the next decade, the population of women older than age 65 outnumbers that of men by about 6.1 million. It is projected that in the year 2000, 59% of those older than 65 years of age will be women. The fastest growing group of minority elders are those 85 years of age and older (Figure 4-1).

These demographic trends have had a significant impact not only on families and the labor force but also on the health care system. More and more elders are living longer with chronic illnesses and functional disability and surviving catastrophic acute illnesses. The health care needs of these persons will continue to increase. Those caring for this aging population will need increased knowledge and skills to help this group maintain health and function and avoid complications—all of which will affect the quality and cost of care for elders.

Improving the quality of life, rather than searching for means to increase longevity, is of utmost importance. According to *Healthy People 2000,* the major goal for the 1990s is to increase the span of healthy life for all Americans. For elderly Americans in particular, the focus is on maintaining functional health and preventing disability.

### SIGNIFICANCE FOR NURSING

The U.S. Public Health Service report *Healthy People 2000* is a guide for health professionals and the citizen-consumer. The document provides guidelines for nurses in their daily practice as they provide care to patients. Nurses can anticipate that this report will be used to provide direction for national health policies and future health care priorities and reimbursement. The publication provides a common ground for collaboration with other health care professionals and health service agencies.

The strength of *Healthy People 2000* is that it focuses on health promotion and disease prevention, which traditionally have been emphasized in nursing. All nurses can use this document to support the care and education of patients in all types of settings, no matter what disease process is being treated. The report also provides information about the health promotion and disease prevention needs of specific groups according to characteristics such as age, race and ethnicity, and economic status.

## ASSESSMENT OF ELDERS

### GENERAL ISSUES

Skillful, knowledge-based assessment is the foundation for providing quality nursing care to older adults. In gerontological and geriatric care, the focus of assessment is the older adult's level of function. A basic premise is that function is multidimensional and includes physical, mental, and social function. Further, the position taken in this chapter is that an elder's functional health is influenced by spiritual well-being.

There is a great deal of heterogeneity in the way that people age. Health concerns for aging persons are multidimensional, requiring critical evaluation of what is normative and what is the result of disease. In ethnic minority groups, secondary aging changes and chronic illnesses may present in the late middle years, resulting in earlier functional decline and disability. In addition (as addressed later in this section), illnesses in older adults can present differently than in younger persons. Thus nurses may need to use geriatric assessment guidelines with middle-aged adults.

Elders who are hospitalized are at increased risk for institutionalization. Often such institutionalization is a result of the loss of the ability to carry out activities of daily living (ADL) and instrumental activities of daily living (IADL). Thus time spent on a thorough baseline assessment of an elder's health status with emphasis on functional abilities and periodic follow-up assessment can potentially prevent disability and additional health care cost.

In the 1990s, geriatric research has focused on failure to thrive in elders, a phenomenon first addressed in children that can be catastrophic for elders.[23,66] Failure to thrive in older persons leads to catastrophic disability and preventable deaths.

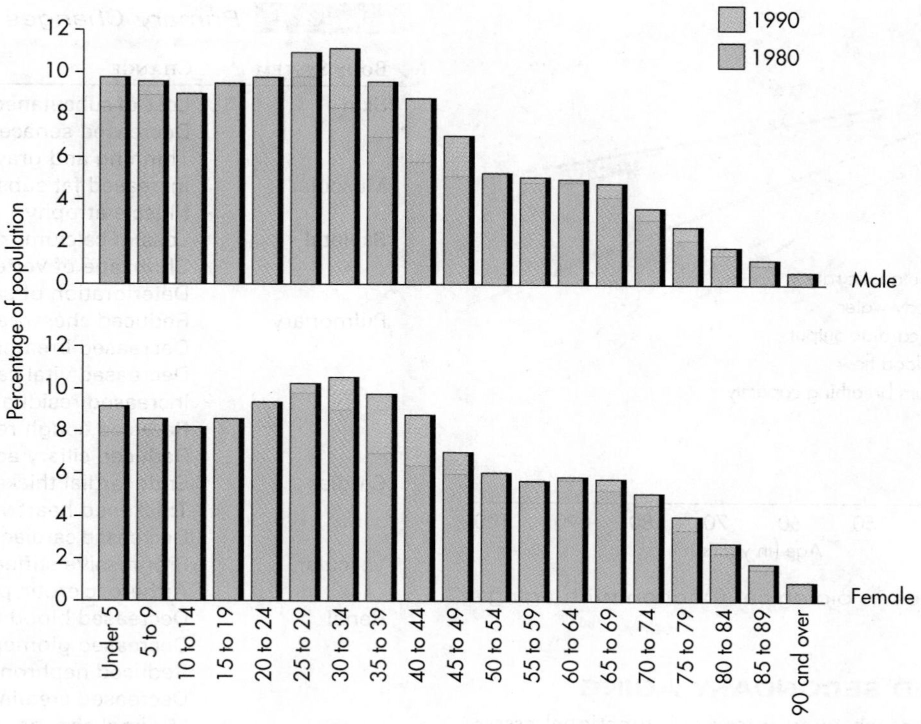


**fig. 4-1** Graphs showing that 1 in 8 Americans is elderly. *Top,* Male population by age in 1980 and 1990. *Bottom,* Female population by age in 1980 and 1990.

This syndrome can be observed in hospitalized elders and could be seen on admission or be noted for the first time during hospitalization. Failure to thrive in elders may be multifaceted and result from factors other than disease processes, such as poor nutrition, depression, losses, medications, alcohol use, and social isolation. Nurses in acute and long-term care settings, therefore, can prevent and assess for failure to thrive in elders.

Institutionalization and failure to thrive are extreme examples of negative health outcomes for hospitalized elders. However, any loss of functional abilities can dramatically affect the quality of life and well-being of older adults.[4,16] A holistic nursing assessment is the necessary foundation for the care of each older adult patient and collaboration with other health care providers. The focus of geriatric assessment is function, and the goal is to enhance or maintain function while preventing loss of function and subsequent disability. As noted in *Healthy People 2000* (Box 4-2), health care providers should assist persons to maintain functional health for as long as possible. This goal will continue to be emphasized as we enter the next century and work toward decreasing the disability curve for aging persons. Nurses will play a key role in meeting this challenge through health assessment that directs primary, secondary, and tertiary intervention. Elders and their family members will be our focus in this endeavor.

The following sections will present critical areas of nursing assessment that should be addressed when caring for older adults no matter what the clinical setting or the acute and chronic diseases being treated. Topics include primary and secondary aging changes, differences in illness presentation, ADL/IADL, falls, spirituality, sexuality, family, nutrition, cognition and sensory perception, depression and suicide, alcohol and medication use, and sleep. The order of presentation of these topics is not meant to imply a hierarchical structure. Although the concepts are presented separately, the elder's functional health status is often affected by the interaction of factors in the physical, mental, social, and spiritual domains. For example, if one has decreased physical function, one can become depressed; if one is depressed, there is a decrease in physical function.

**box 4-2** Healthy People 2000

Health goals and health risks for Americans of all ages were addressed by the Public Health Service in the 1990 report *Healthy People 2000: National Health Promotion and Disease Prevention.*[65] *Healthy People 2000* provides a vision of quality of life and well-being for all citizens as we approach the twenty-first century. The report takes into consideration anticipated changes in the population of the United States. The population is expected to increase by 7% to 270 million people with only about one half of the households having traditional husband-wife partnerships. The median age will be 36 years, with the age of older adults continuing to increase, particularly among those 85 years of age and older. The racial and ethnic composition of the United States will continue to change, with an increase in the number of Hispanic and African American persons, as well as increases in other minority groups. In the next century, those entering the work force are more likely to be women from all racial and ethnic groups and persons from what we currently identify as minority groups.

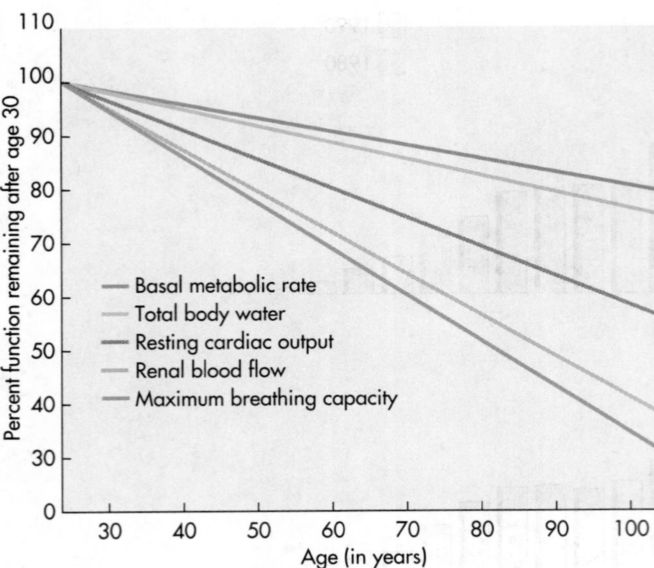


**fig. 4-2** Changes in biological function with aging.

## PRIMARY AND SECONDARY AGING

Critical to any approach to an integrated, functional assessment of elders is understanding of and the ability to differentiate between primary (normative) aging changes and secondary changes (disease related). Normal aging changes are called *primary changes.* Such effects of aging—for example, thinning hair and decreased pulmonary capacity—have been demonstrated through research to occur universally. Increasing knowledge provides evidence that many changes once thought to be associated with aging, such as arthritis and dementia, are actually *secondary changes* and do not occur universally as a part of aging. For example, the muscle atrophy and weakened joints seen in many elders have been discovered to be more related to a sedentary lifestyle than to a primary change of aging. Primary changes of aging are summarized in Table 4-1 and Figure 4-2.

In addition to the primary changes of aging listed in Table 4-1 and Figure 4-2, some other variations in organ function bear mentioning. First, the variation in organ function among individuals is much greater in elders than in younger persons.

Second, the rate of decline from one function to another varies. Basal metabolic rate and total body water of elders decrease only minimally to about 80% of that of young adults.[15] On the other hand, renal blood flow and maximum breathing capacity show a significant decline in most elderly persons.

A third major change related to the aging process occurs in response to stress. Although an aged person may have adequate cardiac output at rest, stress in the form of an infection, exertion, or emotional shock will decrease cardiac output, and it will take much longer for it to return to the person's baseline level. In addition, there is a loss of reserve capacity related to a decline in coordination of brain interactions. This decline causes a slowing of reaction time and a greater susceptibility to infection and accidents.

**table 4-1** *Primary Changes of Aging*

| Body System | Change |
|---|---|
| Skin | Loss of subcutaneous supportive tissue |
| | Decreased sebaceous secretions |
| | Thinning and graying hair |
| Muscular | Increased fat substitution for muscle |
| | Muscle atrophy |
| Skeletal | Loss of calcium from bones |
| | Shrinkage of vertebral disks |
| | Deterioration of cartilage |
| Pulmonary | Reduced chest wall compliance |
| | Decreased breathing capacity |
| | Decreased vital capacity |
| | Increased residual volume |
| | Reduced cough reflex |
| | Reduced ciliary activity |
| Cardiac | Endocardial thickening |
| | Thickened heart valves |
| | Decreased cardiac output (under stress) |
| Vascular | Progressive stiffening of arteries |
| | Artherosclerotic plaques |
| Renal | Decreased blood flow |
| | Decreased glomerular filtration rate |
| | Reduced nephrons |
| | Decreased creatinine clearance |
| Liver | Minimal change |
| Bowel | Minimal change |
| Gastrointestinal | Minimal loss of digestive enzymes |
| | Decreased absorption |
| Endocrine | Decreased utilization of insulin |
| | Cessation of progesterone |
| | Decline, then plateau of estrogen |
| | Gradual decline in testosterone |
| Vision | Deterioration in ability of lens to focus |
| | Loss of color sensitivity |
| | Decreased dark adaptation |
| | Decreased peripheral vision |
| | Decreased sensitivity to glare |
| Hearing | Increased threshold for high frequencies |
| | Difficulty in speech discrimination |
| | Degeneration of cochlea and auditory pathways |
| Sexual | Minimal change in amount of sexual response |
| | Increase in time for full sexual response |
| | Decreased vaginal lubrication |
| | Increased refractory period for men |

From Rossman I: *Clinical geriatrics,* ed 3, Philadelphia, 1986, JB Lippincott.

## UNIQUE PATTERNS OF ILLNESS AMONG ELDERS

A hallmark of gerontology is that disease may have atypical presentations in elders (Table 4-2). Often acute illnesses are superimposed on several chronic illnesses complicated by the effects of primary aging. A careful history, as well as knowledge about the unique clinical presentation in elders, aids the nurse in assessment, establishing nursing diagnoses,

**table 4-2** *How Illness Changes with Age*

| PROBLEM | CLASSIC PRESENTATION IN YOUNG PATIENT | PRESENTATION IN ELDERLY |
|---|---|---|
| Urinary tract infection | Dysuria, frequency, urgency, nocturia | Dysuria is often absent; frequency, urgency, nocturia are sometimes present. Incontinence, confusion, anorexia are other signs. |
| Myocardial infarction | Severe substernal chest pain, diaphoresis, nausea, shortness of breath | Sometimes no chest pain or atypical pain location such as in jaw, neck, shoulder may be present. Shortness of breath may be present. Other signs are tachypnea, arrhythmia, hypotension, restlessness, syncope. |
| Pneumonia (bacterial) | Cough producing purulent sputum, chills and fever, pleuritic chest pain, elevated white blood cell count | Cough may be productive, dry, or absent; chills and fever and/or elevated white count also may be absent. Tachypnea, slight cyanosis, confusion, anorexia, nausea and vomiting, tachycardia may be present. |
| Congestive heart failure | Increased dyspnea (orthopnea, paroxysmal nocturnal dyspnea), fatigue, weight gain, pedal edema, night cough and nocturia, bilateral basilar rales | All of the manifestations of young adult and/or anorexia are seen: restlessness, confusion, cyanosis, falls. |
| Hyperthyroidism | Heat intolerance, fast pace, exophthalmos, increased pulse, hyperreflexia, tremor | Slowing down (apathetic hyperthyroidism), lethargy, weakness, depression, atrial fibrillation, and congestive heart failure may be seen. |
| Depression | Sad mood and thoughts, withdrawal, crying, weight loss, constipation, insomnia | Any of classic signs, plus memory and concentration problems, weight gain, increased sleep may be present. |

Modified from Henderson ML: *Am J Nurs* 85(10):110, 1985.

and intervening effectively. In assessing the health and illness of elders, some general patterns must be recognized. First, an age-related decline in immune function results in a less rapid and less effective response to infections and in an increased incidence of autoimmune and malignant disease.[26] Second, stress situations (either physiological or psychosocial) may produce more pronounced reactions in elderly persons and may require a longer time for readjustment. Third, complex functions that require multisystem coordination show the most obvious decline and require the greatest compensation and support. Fourth, elders frequently have atypical manifestations of an illness. Confusion, restlessness, or other altered mentation is a common occurrence in the presence of illness, including psychiatric disorders such as depression. Obscure or unexplained deterioration of health or function should not be accepted as normal aging and must be evaluated carefully. Multiplicity and chronicity of disease are common among elders, and many patients have several chronic ailments.

## FUNCTIONAL ASSESSMENT OF ELDERS—COMMON CONCERNS

### ADL AND IADL

Assessment is a critical step in effective nursing care for elders. The global aspects of health in elders can be separated into three major concepts: absence of disease, performance of basic self-care activities, termed *activities of daily living (ADL)*, and performance of more complex activities, called *instrumental activities of daily living (IADL)*.

As early as the late 1800s, information on functional health as an estimate of morbidity was obtained in Europe and the United States. During the 1940s, classifications of disability included self-care activities of dressing, toileting, and ambulation. Since that time, three self-maintenance components have consistently been identified: basic activities of daily living (bathing, eating, and toileting), more complex social activities of living (shopping, managing finances, cooking, housekeeping, transportation, and managing medications), and the ability to use a telephone and cope with other aspects of one's environment—that is, instrumental activities of daily living.

Functional disability has been demonstrated to correlate with physical illness, self-care ability, complications during hospitalization, rehabilitation potential, and even mortality. Therefore the concept of functional ability in elders has become a valuable health indicator. Measures of functional status that examine the ability to function independently despite disease are the most useful clinical and research indicators of elders with multiple chronic and acute illnesses.

In addition to assessing the respiratory, cardiovascular, digestive, neurological, and other body systems of the elderly patient, the nurse must carefully assess the elder's functional self-care ability. Subtle changes in appetite or ambulation or even the onset of urinary incontinence may be the initial and only clinical indicator of infections such as pneumonia, urinary tract infections, or even myocardial infarctions. Several functional assessment tools and scales have been widely used in a variety of clinical settings, including the Katz ADL scale and the Barthel index.

## RISK OF FALLS

A major health concern that threatens the function of older adults is the risk of falls that can result in injury and disability.[45] Even falls that do not result in serious injury may affect an elder's function and quality of life. Concern about the risk of falls is heightened when an older adult is admitted to a hospital or long-term care facility. Fortunately, assessment tools (Box 4-3) and protocols are now available to assist clinicians in identifying older patients who are at risk.[40,46] All elderly patients should be assessed upon admission for risk of falling, and then a protocol to prevent a fall from occurring should be instituted.

**box 4-3** *Risk of Falls Assessment Tool*

**FALL ASSESSMENT SCORING SYSTEM** — **POINTS**

**I. AGE**
- 65-79 Years 1
- 80 & Above 2

I. ☐

**II. MENTAL STATUS**
- A. Oriented at all times or comatose 0
  - Confusion at all times 2
  - Intermittent confusion 4

II.A ☐

- B. Agitated/uncooperative/anxious–moderate 2
  - Agitated/uncooperative/anxious–severe 4

II.B ☐

**III. ELIMINATION**
- Independent and continent 0
- Catheter and/or ostomy 1
- Elimination with assistance 3
- Ambulatory with urge incontinency or episodes of incontinence 5

III. ☐

**IV. HISTORY OF FALLING WITHIN SIX MONTHS**
- No history 0
- Has fallen one or two times 2
- Multiple history of falling 5

IV. ☐

**V. SENSORY IMPAIRMENT**
- Sensory impairment 1
  (Blind, deaf, cataracts, not using corrective device)

V. ☐

**VI. ACTIVITY**
- Ambulation / transfer without assistance 0
- Ambulation / transfer with assist of one or assistive device 2
- Ambulation / transfer with assist of two 1

VI. ☐

**VII. MEDICATIONS**

☐ Narcotics ☐ Tranquilizers ☐ Sleeping aids
☐ Diuretics ☐ Chemotherapy ☐ Antiseizure / antiepileptic

For the above medications, check how many the patient is taking currently at home or that the patient will be taking in the hospital.

- No medications 0
- 1 medication 1
- 2 or more medications 2

Add one more point if there has been a change in these medications or dosages in the past 5 days.

VII. ☐

A score of 10 or more indicates a high risk for falling. TOTAL ☐

Indicate high risk and care plan. SCORE ☐

If the patient does not meet a score of 10, but in the nurse's judgement is at risk to fall, initiate the high-risk fall protocol.

From MacAvoy S, Skinner T, Hines M: Clinical methods: fall risk assessment tool, *Appl Nurs Res* 9(4):213, 218, 1996.

## SPIRITUAL WELL-BEING

Spirituality focuses on the meanings one attaches to life, particularly one's own life experience. For some individuals, spirituality includes a connection with and commitment to a particular religious orientation and religious institution. However, belief in specific religious dogma or belonging to a church may not be part of a person's spirituality. Bianchi[5] describes aging as a "spiritual journey" that synthesizes a person's inner contemplative experience and external human concerns. Spirituality is represented by the meaning one attaches to life experiences at any age and represents a holistic integration of physical, social, psychological, cultural, sexual, and theological experiences. The spiritual journey of aging may be grounded in childhood and family experiences. The meaning of life is understood in connection with other human beings and the broader society as one ages and moves toward death. The loss of functional abilities and disability can affect one's spirituality. The opposite is also true. Spiritual distress can result in a loss of physical, mental, and social function.[6,27]

Spirituality is of particular concern for persons who experience illness (see the Research Box below). The experience of physical illness and life crises can precipitate a transforming spiritual change or cause a person to become more introspective and contemplative. The nurse can help a patient explore the meaning of a particular physical or life crisis. This process helps patients find meaning in their lives through definitions of self and personhood that go beyond physical abilities.

The nurse can be instrumental in helping patients express themselves and find meaning in the illness experience. The nurse can provide nonjudgmental support and advocacy for patients and their families as they seek meaning within the illness experience.

To support elders' spiritual well-being, nurses need to include an assessment of elders' spirituality that goes beyond questions about religious affiliation. Older adults should still be asked basic questions about religious practices that comfort them, help them cope, and provide a sense of security. However, spiritual well-being has dimensions beyond religious practices that represent only one aspect of elders' self-care. The JAREL Spiritual Well-Being Scale has been developed for use with older adults.[28] The JAREL scale includes 21 questions for the older patient to answer that the nurse then scores to identify areas of spiritual concern (Box 4-4). Also, a clinical assessment and intervention protocol has been developed for spiritual well-being that can be used to assess a person's spiritual experience during an illness episode.[35]

**research**

Reference: Fehring RJ, Miller JF, Shaw C: Spiritual well-being, religiosity, hope, depression, and other mood states in elderly people coping with cancer, *Oncol Nurs Forum* 24(4):663-671, 1997.

One hundred elderly patients whose average age was 73 years from two acute care units were interviewed. There were 33 men and 67 women with lung, breast, or colon cancer. A positive relationship was found between intrinsic religiosity, hope, and positive mood states. Thus older adults with higher religiosity and hope scores had less depression. Elderly patients with lower levels of intrinsic religiosity and hope were more likely to be depressed and have negative mood states. The implications are that nurses need to assess the religiosity and spiritual well-being of older cancer patients. Further nurses can implement care plans with older patients that support the elder's search for a sense of meaning and hope as a means of coping with illness.

## SEXUALITY

Both men and women maintain interest in sexual activity into the late adulthood years. More women cease having sexual activity after age 65 than do men. The primary reasons for the cessation are lack of an acceptable sexual partner for widows or an ailing husband for married women (rather than lack of interest).[49]

Cultural attitudes toward the elderly influence both genders. Older men and women frequently are thought of as sexually unattractive and lacking in ability to engage in sex. However, Masters and Johnson[42] found that although sexual responses are slower, elders still have the same phases of excitement, plateau, orgasm, and resolution as younger persons.

Sexual problems, however, occur more frequently for elders. Women may have dyspareunia as a result of vaginal thinning and decreased lubrication. These factors are caused by postmenopausal steroid starvation. Men tend to be affected by secondary impotence related to performance anxiety and low self-esteem. Diabetes, alcohol, and medications for hypertension are other prominent causes of impotence.

Masters and Johnson report a condition known as "widowers' syndrome."[42] After an extended period of sexual inactivity, a man cannot achieve or maintain an erection. An equivalent condition occurs in women: the vagina constricts and undergoes atrophic changes. The conclusion is that those who do not engage in sexual activity lose the ability to do so.

Sexuality is more than the physical act of intercourse. Elderly persons continue to need human companionship and love and affection. Nurses need to be aware of components of sexuality and how elders may be affected by chronic illness, loss of a partner, and the need for touch. Being sensitive to family dynamics is just as important for a newly married couple in their seventies as for a young couple. Through counseling the nurse can explain aging changes and suggest vaginal lubrication for women and extra physical stimulation for men. Changes in sexual position and styles of love making are appropriate for those with disabling disease. Nurses have a vital role in enabling elderly persons to express their needs for love and affection. A model for sexual arousal and aging is present in Figure 4-3.[55]

Elders are susceptible to sexually transmitted disease, although not in the same numbers as younger adults.[36] Acquired immunodeficiency syndrome (AIDS) is becoming increasingly prevalent in elders as the epidemic spreads among all age groups. The "at risk" categories differ for elders (e.g., not as many are intravenous drug abusers).[56] However, other risk factors are present, e.g., the decline in the ability of the immune system to ward off infections makes elders more susceptible to organisms of sexually transmitted diseases. Women in

**box 4-4** *JAREL Spiritual Well-Being Scale*

Directions: Please circle the choice that **best** describes how much you agree with each statement. Circle only **one** answer for each statement. There is no right or wrong answer.

| | Strongly Agree | Moderately Agree | Agree | Disagree | Moderately Disagree | Strongly Disagree |
|---|---|---|---|---|---|---|
| 1. Prayer is an important part of my life. | SA | MA | A | D | MD | SD |
| 2. I believe I have spiritual well-being. | SA | MA | A | D | MD | SD |
| 3. As I grow older, I find myself more tolerant of others' beliefs. | SA | MA | A | D | MD | SD |
| 4. I find meaning and purpose in my life. | SA | MA | A | D | MD | SD |
| 5. I feel there is a close relationship between my spiritual beliefs and what I do. | SA | MA | A | D | MD | SD |
| 6. I believe in an afterlife. | SA | MA | A | D | MD | SD |
| 7. When I am sick I have less spiritual well-being. | SA | MA | A | D | MD | SD |
| 8. I believe in a supreme power. | SA | MA | A | D | MD | SD |
| 9. I am able to receive and give love to others. | SA | MA | A | D | MD | SD |
| 10. I am satisfied with my life. | SA | MA | A | D | MD | SD |
| 11. I set goals for myself. | SA | MA | A | D | MD | SD |
| 12. God has little meaning in my life. | SA | MA | A | D | MD | SD |
| 13. I am satisfied with the way I am using my abilities. | SA | MA | A | D | MD | SD |
| 14. Prayer does not help me in making decisions. | SA | MA | A | D | MD | SD |
| 15. I am able to appreciate differences in others. | SA | MA | A | D | MD | SD |
| 16. I am pretty well put together. | SA | MA | A | D | MD | SD |
| 17. I prefer that others make decisions for me. | SA | MA | A | D | MD | SD |
| 18. I find it hard to forgive others. | SA | MA | A | D | MD | SD |
| 19. I accept my life situations. | SA | MA | A | D | MD | SD |
| 20. Belief in a supreme being has no part in my life. | SA | MA | A | D | MD | SD |
| 21. I cannot accept change in my life. | SA | MA | A | D | MD | SD |

JAREL Spiritual Well-Being Scale. Copyright 1987 by J. Hungelmann, E. Kenkel-Rossi, L. Klassen, R. Stollenwerk, Marquette University College of Nursing, Milwaukee, WI 53201. From Hungelmann J et al: Focus on spiritual well-being: harmonious interconnectness of mind-body-spirit—use of the JAREL spiritual well-being scale, *Geriatr Nurs* 17(6):262-266, 1996.

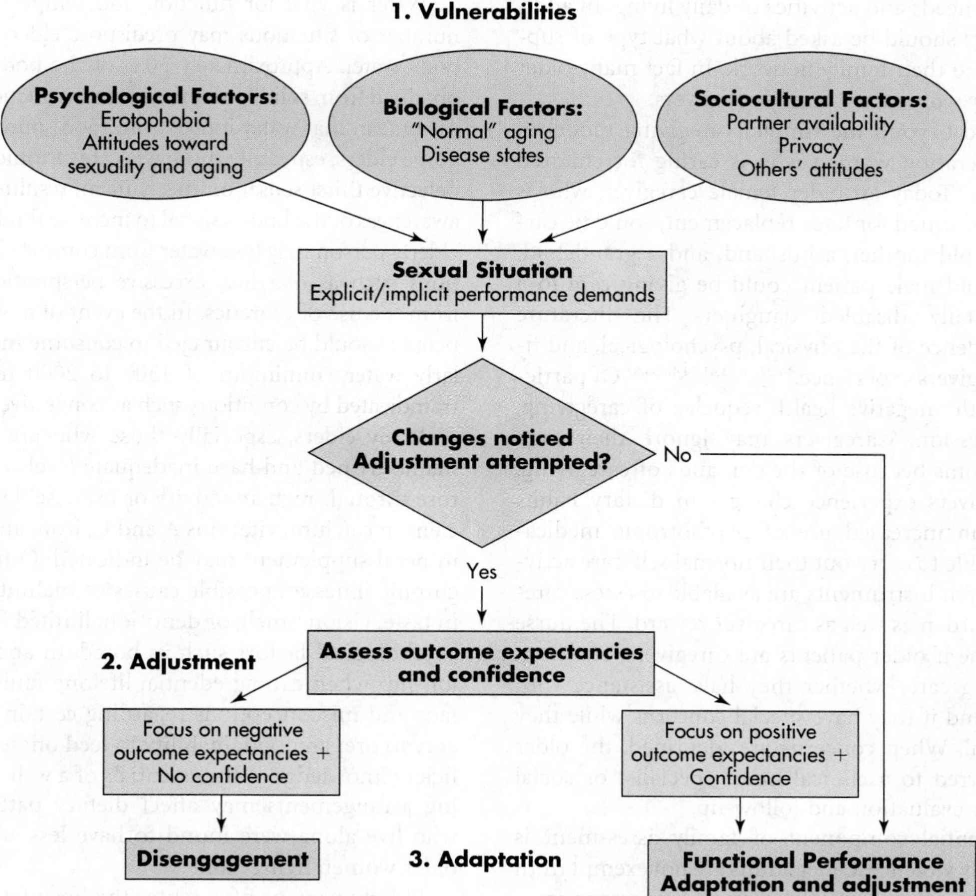


**fig. 4-3** Sexual arousal and aging.

particular are more vulnerable because of the friable vaginal lining that occurs with aging. A final, and often difficult issue for the nurse, is the need to determine if elders are or have been the victims of sexual abuse and violence. Sexual violence against older women is believed to be a growing problem[12] and should be determined as a component of geriatric assessment.

## FAMILY

Although the institutions of marriage and the family are still viewed as the most acceptable in the media and much of society, there is increasing tolerance for diversity in living patterns. Alternatives to traditional family life that are increasingly common include cohabiting with members of the same or opposite sex, living alone, becoming a single parent, remaining a childless couple, and living communally. Other alternative family structures include homosexual couples who make a lifelong commitment and choose to raise a family. Divorce, a common occurrence today, is a highly stressful event that often creates a crisis. Most adults who are divorced, however, go on to marry again. In fact, in more than 45% of all marriages, one or both partners were married previously, with either or both spouses having children from previous marriages, resulting in what is called a *blended family*.[7] Families of older adults also reflect this diversity in family structure. Family, however defined, provides intimacy, affection, and instrumental support to older adults. Also, older adults may be part of multigenerational families and households. Sometimes four or five generations live together and share resources and family tasks. For some older adults, family intimacy and support take place in unrelated (by blood) groups who may or may not live in the same household.

We often think about issues of divorce and alternative lifestyles as only applying to the younger generation. However, older adults are part of diverse family configurations and partnerships. These diverse families play a key role in providing older persons with social support.[61] Thus assessment of the older adult's family as a means of social support is essential, particularly in supporting the functional health and well-being of the older adult. The nurse also needs to assess the role of the elderly patient in providing support to the family. Questions can easily be asked about who older adults get help from when they need it for specific activities; in whom they confide; whether the support is adequate; and most importantly who would they call first that they could count on if they really needed something. Many instruments that measure what support is needed are lengthy,[15,24,28] but a short form[60] is available. The Caregiver Well-Being Scale developed by Tebb[60] includes 45 questions about caregivers' satisfaction with basic human needs and activities of daily living. In addition, older patients should be asked about what type of support they provide to their family network. In fact many older adults, particularly women, are family caregivers.

We have moved beyond the simpler caregiving model of the sandwich-generation woman who is caring for children and aging parents. Today an older female caregiver, who is 70 years old and admitted for knee replacement, could be caring for a 90-year-old mother, a husband, and a grandchild. Another 66-year-old male patient could be giving care to a 44-year-old mentally disabled daughter. The literature abounds with evidence of the physical, psychological, and financial stress caregivers experience.[14,22,30,31,41,44,48,58,67] Of particular concern are the negative health sequelae of caregiving, particularly depression. Caregivers may ignore their own health and symptoms because of the demands of caregiving. Also, many caregivers experience changes in dietary habits and sleep, have an increased use of psychotropic medications, and are unable to carry out their normal self-care activities. Several research instruments are available to assess caregiver stress and burden as well as caregiver reward. The nurse needs to determine if older patients are caregivers, to whom they are providing care, whether they have assistance with their caregiving, and if they have special concerns while they are in the hospital. When concerns are identified, the older adult can be referred to a clinical nurse specialist or social worker for further evaluation and follow-up.

Finally an essential component of family assessment is screening for family violence. Older adults are not exempt from being victims or perpetrators.[20,22] For some older persons, family violence has been an established family pattern. Fulmer and O'Malley also address assessment of elder neglect that results in impaired function.[20] There may be an increased risk for elders being cared for by a family caregiver due to the stress of caregiving. The risk for violence by a family caregiver is greater when there are decreases in the care recipient's function and a lack of adequate formal and informal support for the caregiver. Thus nurses who care for older adults need to determine if older patients are being exposed to violence and neglect in the home. The nurse needs to be aware that in some states mandatory reporting of elder abuse and neglect is required.

## NUTRITION

Nutritional requirements of elders are essentially the same as for other adults, except that calorie needs diminish because of a decrease in lean body mass relative to fat (which burns fewer calories).[15] Fiber (i.e., fruits, vegetables, whole-grain bread, and cereals), although undigestible, is an important constituent in the diet. Fiber holds water in the fecal mass, which softens the stools and enhances regular evacuation. The incidence of diverticulitis, colon cancer, or gallstones is thought to be influenced by diets chronically low in fiber. Persons at or near age 65 may still have a life expectancy of 15 or more years during which dietary fiber deficiencies might play a role in development of colon cancer, diverticulitis, or gallstones. Because the latter disorders and constipation are common problems in elders, moderate amounts of fiber become regularly included in the diet.[15]

Water is vital for function and temperature regulation. A number of situations may predispose elders to a deficiency in body water. Approximately 50% of the body's water supply is obtained from solid foods; therefore a reduction in calorie intake may mean that water intake from food sources is not adequate. Some elders, especially those who are chronically ill, may have a defective thirst sensation mechanism, resulting in a diminished awareness of the body's signal to increase fluid intake. Finally, the elderly person may lose water from commonly occurring conditions such as diarrhea, excessive perspiration, or polyuria or from the use of diuretics. In the event of a water deficit, elderly people should be encouraged to consume more fluids, particularly water (minimum of 1500 to 2000 ml/day unless contraindicated by conditions such as congestive heart failure).

Many elders, especially those who are ill, frequently are malnourished and have inadequate levels of energy expenditure through regular activity or exercise. Diets often are deficient in calcium, vitamins A and C, iron, and zinc. A vitamin-mineral supplement may be indicated. Other than acute and chronic illnesses, possible causes of malnutrition are changes in taste, vision, smell, or dentition; limited financial resources; psychological factors such as boredom and lack of companionship when eating; edentia; lifelong faulty eating patterns; fads and misconceptions regarding certain foods; lack of energy to prepare food; inability to feed oneself; and lack of sufficient knowledge of the essentials of a well-balanced diet. Living arrangements may affect dietary patterns; elderly men who live alone were found to have less adequate diets than older women living alone.[11]

Elderly persons often enter the hospital in a poorly nourished state because of chronic illness or other factors previously described. Trauma, surgery, or sepsis may increase nutritional demands and cause further nutritional deficiencies, particularly in protein and calories, to develop rapidly. Often, a poor state of nutrition upon admission, increased nutritional needs, and decreased appetite coexist in hospitalized elders. A nutritional assessment, including a record of food intake over several days and weight on admission with regular weight checks thereafter, should be a priority in nursing to detect deficiencies early.

It has been suggested that nutritional status be considered a "vital sign."[9] This is particularly true for older adults in acute care. Poor nutrition can lead to functional losses, and functional losses can lead to poor nutrition. For example, in a study of elderly nuns, a 3% weight loss over 1 year increased the risk of an individual becoming dependent in ADL.[62] Other researchers have reported that protein-energy undernourishment in older middle-aged patients (55 to 64 years) and elderly patients is a strong risk factor for mortality 1 year after discharge from a hospital. Therefore one dimension of a geriatric assessment should be nutritional screening.[29,53] Guidelines for clinical assessment are available and can be used by nurses and other health care members.[3] The Mini Nutritional Assessment (MNA) is a relatively simple screening instrument that can be used with older adults in acute care settings (Box 4-5).[24] Some of the areas included in the MNA are dietary habits, medication use, and functional items such as ADL,

**box 4-5** *The Mini Nutritional Assessment Tool*

Last Name: First Name: ____________ M.I. ________ Sex: ________ Date: ____________

Age: Weight, kg: Height, cm: ____________ Knee Height, cm: ____________

Complete the form by writing the numbers in the boxes. Add the numbers in the boxes and compare the total assessment to the Malnutrition Indicator Score.

**ANTHROPOMETRIC ASSESSMENT**

| | Points |
|---|---|
| 1. Body mass index (BMI) (weight in kg)/(height in m)$^2$<br>a. BMI < 19 = 0 points<br>b. BMI 19 to < 21 = 1 point<br>c. BMI 21 to < 23 = 2 points<br>d. BMI ≥ 23 = 3 points | ❑ |
| 2. Mid-arm circumference (MAC) in cm<br>a. MAC < 21 = 0.0 points<br>b. MAC 21 ≤ 22 = 0.5 points<br>c. MAC > 22 = 1.0 points | ❑ ❑ |
| 3. Calf circumference (CC) in cm<br>a. CC < 31 = 0 points b. CC ≥ 31 = 1 point | ❑ |
| 4. Weight loss during last 3 months<br>a. weight loss greater than 3kg (6.6 lbs) = 0 points<br>b. does not know = 1 point<br>c. weight loss between 1 and 3 kg (2.2 and 6.6 lbs) = 2 points<br>d. no weight loss = 3 points | ❑ |

**GENERAL ASSESSMENT**

| | |
|---|---|
| 5. Lives independently (not in a nursing home or hospital)<br>a. no = 0 points b. yes = 1 point | ❑ |
| 6. Takes makes more than 3 prescription drugs per day<br>a. yes = 0 points b. no = 1 point | ❑ |
| 7. Has suffered psychological stress or acute disease in the past 3 months<br>a. yes = 0 points b. no = 2 points | ❑ |
| 8. Mobility<br>a. bed or chair bound = 0 points<br>b. able to get out of bed/chair but does not go out = 1 point<br>c. goes out = 2 points | ❑ |
| 9. Neuropsychological problems<br>a. severe dementia or depression = 0 points<br>b. mild dementia = 1 point<br>c. no psychological problems = 2 points | ❑ |
| 10 Pressure sores or skin ulcers<br>a. yes = 0 points b. no = 1 point | ❑ |

**DIETARY ASSESSMENT**

| | |
|---|---|
| 11. How many full meals does the patient eat daily?<br>a. 1 meal = 0 points<br>b. 2 meals = 1 point<br>c. 3 meals = 2 points | ❑ |

| | Points |
|---|---|
| 12. Selected consumption markers for protein intake<br>• At least one serving of dairy products (milk, cheese, yogurt) per day? yes ❑ no ❑<br>• Two or more servings of legumes or eggs per week? yes ❑ no ❑<br>• Meat, fish or poultry every day? yes ❑ no ❑<br>a. if 0 or 1 yes = 0.0 points<br>b. if 2 yes = 0.5 points<br>c. if 3 yes = 1.0 points | ❑ ❑ |
| 13. Consumes two or more servings of fruits or vegetables per day?<br>a. no = 0 points b. yes = 1 point | ❑ |
| 14. Has food intake declined over the past 3 months due to loss of appetite, digestive problems, chewing or swallowing difficulties?<br>a. severe loss of appetite = 0 points<br>b. moderate loss of appetite = 1 point<br>c. no loss of appetite = 2 points | ❑ |
| 15. How much fluid (water, juice, coffee, tea, milk, . . .) is consumed per day? (1 cup = 8 oz.)<br>a. less than 3 cups = 0.0 points<br>b. 3 to 5 cups = 0.5 points<br>c. more than 5 cups = 1.0 points | ❑ ❑ |
| 16. Mode of feeding<br>a. Unable to eat without assistance = 0 points<br>b. self-fed with some difficulty = 1 point<br>c. self-fed without any problem = 2 points | ❑ |

**SELF-ASSESSMENT**

| | |
|---|---|
| 17. Do they view themselves as having nutritional problems?<br>a. major malnutrition = 0 points<br>b. does not know or moderate malnutrition = 1 point<br>c. no nutritional problem = 2 points | ❑ |
| 18. In comparison with other people of the same age, how do they consider their health status?<br>a. not as good = 0.0 points<br>b. does not know = 0.5 points<br>c. as good = 1.0 points<br>d. better = 2.0 points | ❑ ❑ |

**ASSESSMENT TOTAL** (max. 30 points) ❑❑❑

**MALNUTRITION INDICATOR SCORE**

| | | |
|---|---|---|
| ≥ 24 points | well-nourished | ❑ |
| 17 to 23.5 points | at risk of malnutrition | ❑ |
| <17 points | malnourished | ❑ |



From Guigoz Y, Vellas B, Garry PJ: Assessing the nutritional status of the elderly: the Mini Nutritional Assessment as part of geriatric assessment, *Nutr Rev* 54(1):S59-S65, 1996.

dental health, and depression. A simple method to monitor nutritional status used in long-term care is monthly weighing of all older adults.

## COGNITION AND SENSORY PERCEPTION

Elders differ from their younger counterparts in several aspects of cognitive and perceptual function. Changes occur in the central nervous system, but the peripheral motor neurons and the autonomic nervous system remain relatively constant throughout the life span.

### Cognitive Function

Cross-sectional studies have shown that the highest overall intelligence test performance occurs at some time between the late teens and late twenties. People in their thirties, forties, and fifties tend to score somewhat lower. Longitudinal evidence has shown, however, that general intelligence either remains the same or increases slightly during the adult years. Certain factors, such as education and other sociocultural advantages, may influence intellectual development and performance.

The measure of one's intelligence is more than a score on a standardized examination. Intelligence can include a person's capacity for creativity and understanding of how systems work. Creativity and productivity are possible in old age. Elders do not lose the capacity for creativity as they age. Some, for the first time, have the time to pursue artistic talents that had not been fully developed because of work and family obligations. Active use of mental capacity throughout life contributes to mental productivity in old age.

Aging changes listed in Box 4-6 affect complex processes such as learning, memory, language, and mentation. Although loss of memory is not considered a primary aging change, many older persons have progressively increasing problems with short-term memory. Older persons may need more time to take in information and can experience some problems with retrieval of stored information (memory). Although persons of advancing age perform less well on neuropsychological tests, this performance is not necessarily associated with impaired function.[10] Therefore, any change in cognitive function in the older adult must be taken seriously, and the etiology of the change explored. A change in cognitive function is often the first indication that an elder's health status has changed. Elders with cognitive changes may be misdiagnosed with irreversible organic brain disease (e.g., Alzheimer's). This results in an increased risk of institutionalization. The cause of the cognitive changes may be an undiagnosed medical condition that is reversible with treatment. Reversible cognitive changes may actually be symptoms of disease, depression, delirium due to toxic effects of drugs, dehydration, fecal impaction, infection, and overstimulation to name only a few causes. Changes in cognitive function should then trigger aggressive global assessment of the elder's health status starting with evaluation of the presence of disease or adverse drug effects.

**box 4-6** *Aging Changes Affecting Cognition and Perception*

- Decreased brain weight
- Diminished enzyme activity
- Slowed reflexes
- Decreased sensory receptors for temperature, pain, and tactile discrimination
- Weakening of interneuron connections
- Increased response time
- Chronic hypoxia

The following is an example of what can happen to an older adult who experiences cognitive changes, and the underlying cause is misdiagnosed.

> Mrs. P, a 72-year-old woman, is being discharged from the hospital after a heart attack while on her way to another town to visit her ill husband. While Mrs. P. is in the hospital, her husband dies unexpectedly after elective surgery. She was too ill to attend the funeral and continues to have complications. The physician has asked Mrs. P's daughter to meet him to discuss the need to place her mother in a nursing home. The physician says this is necessary because Mrs. P can no longer care for herself and is unable to remember things, and she is becoming senile. The family places Mrs. P, who does not seem to be the person they once knew, in a nursing home. However, they do seek another opinion to be sure the physician was right. Severe depression is subsequently diagnosed, and Mrs. P is treated. Mrs. P is back living in her own home, driving her car, participating actively in church, and traveling to visit the grandchildren.

The focus of assessment for the nurse then is the level of cognitive function in elderly patients, and cognitive screening is done first. If impairment is present, then information about the person's level of function before hospitalization is obtained from a family member. For those who have impaired function on admission, cognitive screening should continue throughout the hospital stay. A variety of cognitive screening instruments is available. The two most commonly used are the Short Portable Mental Status Questionnaire (SPMSQ), which is quick and easy to administer (see Chapter 9); and the Mini-Mental Status Examination (MMSE),[19] which includes questions that require some level of reading and writing literacy and motor function (see Chapter 9). The SPMSQ and MMSE should be used as screening tools only. If a patient's score is indicative of cognitive impairment, the nurse should refer the elder for further evaluation.

During hospitalization, there needs to be ongoing assessment of the elderly patient's cognitive function. This is necessary because older patients are at risk for developing acute confusional states. Researchers have found that nurses are able to clinically assess marked cognitive impairment but may miss some of the subtle signs of cognitive changes that put the patient at risk for decreased function (see the Research Box on p. 85, left). The NEECHAM Confusion Scale provides nurses with an instrument for systematic, clinical evaluation of acute confusion (Box 4-7).[43,48]

### Sensory-Perceptual Function

Pain, temperature, taste, and touch are all dulled to some extent as one ages. Hearing and vision become less acute as the elder experiences presbyopia and presbyacusis (see Chapter 56). Long-distance vision is less acute, as is night vision,

**box 4-7** *NEECHAM Confusion Scale*

NAME/ID: ______________________ DATE: __________ TIME: __________
SCORED BY: ______________

**LEVEL 1: PROCESSING**

**Processing—Attention: (Attention-Alertness-Responsiveness)**

_4 *Full attentiveness/alertness*: responds immediately and appropriately to calling of name or touch—eyes, head turn; fully aware of surroundings, attends to environmental events appropriately

_3 *Short or hyper attention/alertness*: either shortened attention to calling, touch, or environmental events or hyperalert, overattentive to cues/objects in environment

_2 *Attention/alertness inconsistent or inappropriate*: slow in responding, repeated calling or touch required to elicit/maintain eye contact/attention; able to recognize objects/stimuli, although may drop into sleep between stimuli

_1 *Attention/alertness disturbed*: eyes open to sound or touch; may appear fearful, unable to attend/recognize contact, or may show withdrawal/combative behavior

_0 *Arousal/responsiveness depressed*: eyes may/may not open; only minimal arousal possible with repeated stimuli; unable to recognize contact

**Processing—Command: (Recognition-Interpretation-Action)**

_5 *Able to follow a complex command*: "Turn on nurse's call light" (must search for object, recognize object, perform command)

_4 *Slowed complex command response*: requires prompting or repeated directions to follow/complete a complex command; performs complex command in "slow"/overattending manner

_3 *Able to follow a simple command*: "Lift your hand or foot Mr. ______" (only use 1 objective)

_2 *Unable to follow direct command*: follows command prompted by touch or visual cue—drinks from glass placed near mouth; responds with calming affect to nursing contact and reassurance or hand holding

_1 *Unable to follow visually guided command*: responds with dazed or frightened facial features, and/or withdrawal-resistive response to stimuli, hyper/hypoactive behavior; does not respond to nurse gripping hand lightly

_0 *Hypoactive, lethargic*: minimal motor/responses to environmental stimuli

**Processing—Orientation: (Orientation, Short-Term Memory, Thought/Speech Content)**

_5 *Oriented to time, place, and person*: thought processes, content of conversation or questions appropriate; short-term memory intact

_4 *Oriented to person and place*: minimal memory/recall disturbance, content and response to questions generally appropriate; may be repetitive, requires prompting to continue contact; generally cooperates with requests

_3 *Orientation inconsistent*: oriented to self, recognizes family but time and place orientation fluctuates; uses visual cues to orient; thought/memory disturbance common, may have hallucinations or illusions; passive cooperation with requests (cooperative cognitive protecting behaviors)

_2 *Disoriented and memory/recall disturbed*: oriented to self/recognizes family; may question actions of nurse or refuse requests, procedures (resistive cognitive protecting behaviors); conversation content/thought disturbed; illusions and/or hallucinations common

_1 *Disoriented, disturbed recognition*: inconsistently recognizes familiar people, family, objects; inappropriate speech/sounds

_0 *Processing of stimuli depressed*: minimal response to verbal stimuli

**LEVEL 2: BEHAVIOR**

**Behavior—Appearance:**

_2 *Controls posture, maintains appearance, hygiene:* appropriately gowned or dressed, personally tidy, clean; posture in bed/chair normal

_1 *Either posture or appearance disturbed:* some disarray of clothing/bed or personal appearance or some loss of control of posture, position

_0 *Both posture and appearance abnormal:* disarrayed, poor hygiene, unable to maintain posture in bed

**Behavior—Motor:**

_4 *Normal motor behavior:* appropriate movement, coordination and activity, able to rest quietly in bed; normal hand movement

_3 *Motor behavior slowed or hyperactive:* overly quiet or little spontaneous movement (hands/arms across chest or at sides) or hyperactive (up/down, "jumpy"); may show hand tremor

_2 *Motor movement disturbed:* restless or quick movements; hand movements appear abnormal—picking at bed objects or bed covers, etc; may require assistance with purposeful movements

_1 *Inappropriate, disruptive movements:* pulling at tubes, trying to climb over rails, frequent purposeless actions

_0 *Motor movement depressed:* limited movement unless stimulated; resistive movements

 From Miller J et al: The assessment of acute confusion as part of nursing care, *Appl Nurs Res* 10(3):143-151, 1997.

*Continued*

**box 4-7** *NEECHAM Confusion Scale—cont'd*

NAME/ID: ______________ DATE: ______ TIME: ______

SCORED BY: ______________

**LEVEL 2: BEHAVIOR—cont'd**

**Behavior—Verbal:**

_4 *Initiates speech appropriately:* able to converse, can initiate and maintain conversation; normal speech for diagnostic condition, normal tone

_3 *Limited speech initiation:* responses to verbal stimuli are brief and uncomplex; speech clear for diagnostic condition, tone may be abnormal, rate may be slow

_2 *Inappropriate speech:* may talk to self or not make sense; speech not clear for diagnostic condition

_1 *Speech/sound disturbed:* altered sound/tone; mumbles, yells, swears or is inappropriately silent

_0 *Abnormal sounds:* groaning or other disturbed sounds; no clear speech

**LEVEL 3: PHYSIOLOGICAL CONTROL**

**Physiological Measurements:**

| *Recorded Values:* | *Normal Values:* |
|---|---|
| Temperature | (36-37°) |
| Systolic blood pressure (BP) | (100-160) |
| Diastolic BP | (50-90) |
| Heart rate (HR): regular/irregular | (60-100) (circle one) |
| Respirations | (14-22) (count for 1 full minute) |
| $O_2$ saturation | (93 or above) |

______ Periods of apnea/hypopnea present? 1 = yes, 0 = no

______ Oxygen therapy prescribed? 0 = no, 1 = yes, but not on, 2 = yes, on now.

**Vital Function Stability: (Count abnormal systolic BP and/or diastolic BP as one value; count abnormal and/or irregular HR as one; count apnea and/or abnormal respirations as one; and abnormal temperature as one.)**

_2 BP, HR, temperature, respiration within normal range with regular pulse

_1 Any one of the above in abnormal range

_0 Two or more in abnormal range

**Oxygen Saturation Stability:**

_2 $O_2$ saturation in normal range (93 or above)

_1 $O_2$ saturation 90 to 92 or is *receiving oxygen*

_0 $O_2$ saturation below 90

**Urinary Continence Control:**

_2 Maintains bladder control

_1 Incontinent of urine in last 24 hours or has condom catheter

_0 Incontinent now or has indwelling or intermittent catheter or is anuric

| | | *Total Score of:* | *Indicates:* |
|---|---|---|---|
| ______ | Level 1 Score: Processing (0-14 points) | 0-19 | Moderate to severe confusion |
| ______ | Level 2 Score: Behavior (0-10 points) | 20-24 | Mild or early development of confusion |
| ______ | Level 3 Score: Integrative Physiological Control (0-6 points) | 25-26 | "Not confused," but at high risk for confusion |
| ______ | Total NEECHAM (0-30 points) | 27-30 | "Not confused," or normal function |

and tolerance for glare decreases. The older person has more difficulty hearing high tones and discriminating speech in noisy situations. Of particular concern in geriatric assessment are changes in hearing and vision. Both senses affect an older adult's physical, mental, social, and spiritual function. Losses in either sense, and especially a hearing impairment, affect an older person's ability to communicate with significant others and the outside world. Elders' ability to receive information can become compromised.[33] For example, what appears to be recent memory loss may actually be the result of being unable to take written or spoken information. Specifically, hearing impairment can result in social isolation and depression in the older adult. Approximately one fourth of people older than 65 years of age and one half of those older than 80 years of age have some hearing impairment. Visual impairment is reported in 15% of those 65 years old, and in one third of persons 80 years of age and older.[39] Assessment of hearing and vision should begin by asking the patients to describe (1) what

research

Reference: Pompei P et al: Delirium in hospitalized older persons: outcomes and predictors, *J Am Geriatr Soc* 42:809-815, 1994.

This study examined the rate of delirium in hospitalized elders, compared clinical outcomes in patients with and without delirium, and examined clinical predictors of delirium. There was a 15% rate of delirium in patients during their stay. Elders who experienced delirium had longer lengths of stay and increased risk of death while hospitalized. Predictors of delirium included cognitive impairment, level of comorbidity, depression, and alcoholism. The findings support the critical need for a multidimensional geriatric assessment to be completed by the nurse for all older adult patients. If this is done, at-risk elderly patients can be identified during the initial contact with the nurse. The nurse can then develop a plan of care in collaboration with other health care team members to implement supportive treatment (e.g., for depression or malnutrition) and reduce negative outcomes during hospitalization.

research

Reference: Moore SL: A phenomenological study of the meaning of life in suicidal older adults, *Arch Psychiatr Nurs* 11(1):29-36, 1997.

Eleven older adults aged 64 to 92 were interviewed about their suicidal feelings. The main theme that described the older adults' experience was one of alienation. Suicidal elders talked about broken connections with significant people and a loss of meaningful activities. Respondents spoke of despair, pain, and suffering (Psychache); the feeling that family and others no longer cared about them (No One Cares); and feeling loss of control, loss of independence, and disappointed (Powerlessness). The implications are that assessment should be focused not only on feelings of hopelessness, but also on older persons' sense of connectedness to family, friends, and meaningful activities. Further, the nurse can help the older adult develop a self-care plan that includes continued involvement with people and life-enhancing activities.

problems they may be having, (2) when they were first aware of the problems, (3) whether there have been recent changes, and (4) what are they doing to accommodate losses, including assistive devices. Ebersole and Hess[15] describe basic, clinical observations of the elderly patient's behavior that can be performed by the nurse to assess hearing. They include, but are not limited to, speech quality and loudness, turning head toward speaker, asking that things be repeated, not being able to follow clear directions, not responding to environmental sounds, and thinking that people are talking about him or her. The nurse should also assess the patient for inappropriate anger or irritation when spoken to by staff. In addition, anytime an older adult (or the family) complains of hearing difficulties, visual inspection of the inner ear should be done to assess for cerumen impaction. Assessment of vision can easily be performed using a pocket size Snellen Chart (see Chapter 55).

## DEPRESSION AND SUICIDE

Depression remains the major mental health problem in older adults.[34,51] However, this treatable disorder goes largely unrecognized, undiagnosed, or misdiagnosed, and therefore untreated. Acute and primary health care providers are in the best position to assess the presence of depression in older patients. Depression is present in 12% to 16% of medically ill and long-term care patients; and 20% to 30% of older patients have some depressive symptoms.[51] It has been suggested that late-life depression is a geriatric syndrome with multiple etiologies and requires a multidimensional geriatric assessment.[32] Depression in older adults results in decreased functional health in multiple domains and can lead to suicide (see the Research Box above right). Evidence continues to show that people become more suicidal as they age and at greatest risk are white men older than 85 years of age.[13] Suicidal behaviors may be aggressive and highly lethal or may be more covert such as refusal to eat and not taking necessary medication. Some elderly men who commit suicide commit homicide first by killing their spouses. Even if the older adult is not clinically depressed, the person may be experiencing a level of depressive symptoms that result in functional impairment and poor health. The good news is that depression is treatable in older adults, and timely, appropriate care can prevent suicidal behaviors.

Depression presents differently in older adults than in younger persons. Older persons may find it less acceptable to acknowledge depression. Therefore, structured instruments are helpful in screening. The nurse can easily screen for depression using the Center of Epidemiological Studies Depression Scale (CES-D) or Geriatric Depression Scale (GDS) (Box 4-8).[37] These instruments can be included in the nursing assessment form or used as an addition to it. The questions can be asked of the older patient or read by the older patient and easily scored by the nurse. The CES-D and GDS measure the presence of depressive symptoms but are not used for differential diagnosis of major depression. Standard questions for suicide assessment can be used to assess whether suicidal thoughts are present. If depressive symptoms and suicidal ideas or behaviors are observed, the older person should be referred for more complete psychiatric evaluation.

## ALCOHOL AND MEDICATION USE AND MISUSE

Assessment of alcohol and medication use is an essential component of geriatric assessment for several reasons. This includes the use of illicit drugs although data about illicit use in older adults is minimal, and the types and amount of actual use are uncertain. As middle and younger adults age, assessment of illicit drug use may become more important given younger cohorts' patterns of multiple substance use. First, one needs to screen for potential misuse and abuse of alcohol and drugs in elderly patients. Misuse, abuse, and addiction can result in a variety of functional deficits and have negative effects on body systems.[57] Secondly, nonproblematic use of alcohol in young and middle adulthood may result in functional losses and organ damage because of normal aging changes. Thirdly,

**box 4-8** *Geriatric Depression Scale (Short Form)*

Choose the best answer for how you felt over the past week.

Please circle

| | | |
|---|---|---|
| 1. Are you basically satisfied with your life? | yes | no |
| 2. Have you dropped many of your activities and interests? | yes | no |
| 3. Do you feel that your life is empty? | yes | no |
| 4. Do you often get bored? | yes | no |
| 5. Are you in good spirits most of the time? | yes | no |
| 6. Are you afraid that something bad is going to happen to you? | yes | no |
| 7. Do you feel happy most of the time? | yes | no |
| 8. Do you often feel helpless? | yes | no |
| 9. Do you prefer to stay at home, rather than going out and doing new things? | yes | no |
| 10. Do you feel you have more problems with memory than most? | yes | no |
| 11. Do you think it is wonderful to be alive now? | yes | no |
| 12. Do you feel pretty worthless the way you are now? | yes | no |
| 13. Do you feel full of energy? | yes | no |
| 14. Do you feel that your situation is hopeless? | yes | no |
| 15. Do you think that most people are better off than you are? | yes | no |

The following answers count as one point. Scores >5 indicate probable depression.

| | | |
|---|---|---|
| 1. No | 6. Yes | 11. No |
| 2. Yes | 7. No | 12. Yes |
| 3. Yes | 8. Yes | 13. No |
| 4. Yes | 9. Yes | 14. Yes |
| 5. No | 10. Yes | 15. Yes |

alcohol and medications can have a variety of interactive effects that are detrimental and even life threatening. Finally, the clinical presentation of substance (alcohol, prescribed, and over-the-counter medications) interaction, misuse, and abuse is frequently mistaken by clinicians for irreversible dementia.[25]

## Alcohol and the Elderly

Although alcohol use and misuse decrease with age, 4% of elders abuse or are dependent on alcohol, and 10% are considered problem drinkers.[1] Two patterns of alcoholism have been identified in older adults.[38] Some older alcoholics began drinking at an early age and have survived into their elder years. Other elders are late-onset drinkers who began abusing alcohol in their later years. The abuse often begins in the fifth decade, but alcoholism and related health problems may not be detected until the sixth decade. Of course the abuse of alcohol can occur at any time during the aging process and may actually be a symptom of other functional health problems such as depression and social isolation or may be a self-care behavior to manage insomnia or pain.

**box 4-9** *The CAGE Assessment: Four Questions About Drinking*

C Have you ever felt you should **c**ut down on your drinking?

A Have people **a**nnoyed you by criticizing your drinking?

G Have you ever felt bad or **g**uilty about your drinking?

E Have you ever taken a drink first thing in the morning (**e**ye opener) to steady your nerves or get rid of a hangover?

Positive answers to two or more questions suggest that you may have a problem with drinking.

One or more responses from an elder is significant and deserves follow-up.

Because of the social stigma and cultural values related to alcohol use, it is important that nurses be aware of their personal beliefs about alcohol and experiences with those that use or abuse it. An additional area to address is the attitudes of professionals toward elders who drink, including differences in attitudes related to the gender of the elder. The beliefs, values, and attitudes of professionals can be barriers to accurate assessment. Nurses also need to recognize that older adults may present barriers to assessment because of their own beliefs and attitudes about alcohol use and abuse. Several screening instruments are now available and are easily integrated into multidimensional geriatric assessment such as the CAGE Assessment (Box 4-9) and the Elderly Alcohol Screening Test (EAST) (Box 4-10).[18] One does not have to be an expert in substance abuse to effectively use alcohol-screening instruments. The role of the clinical nurse is to assess an older adult's pattern of alcohol use and screen for abuse so that appropriate referral and management can be implemented. Screening can identify the potential for problems with drug and alcohol interactions and identify those at risk for symptoms of alcohol withdrawal. (See Chapter 14.)

## Medication and the Elderly

The use of both prescribed and nonprescribed medications increases with age. Elders consume disproportionately more of all kinds of drugs than do middle adults, partly because older adults experience more chronic illness. Medications provide tremendous benefits to older adults, but they also can create problems for the patient, family, and health care provider. The medication regimen may be complex and troublesome for the patient or family to administer, and as a result drug misuse can easily occur. Misuse is defined as overmed-

**box 4-10** *Elderly Alcohol Screening Test (EAST)*

Directions: If a statement says something true about you, put a check in the "Yes" box. If a statement says something not true about you, put a check in the "No" box. Please answer all questions.

1. Have you ever drank alcohol? ❑ Yes ❑ No
2. Do you feel that you are a normal drinker? ❑ Yes ❑ No
3. Have you ever awakened the morning after drinking the night before and found that you could not remember a part of the evening? ❑ Yes ❑ No
4. Does your spouse, the people you live with, or your children ever worry or complain about your drinking? ❑ Yes ❑ No
5. Can you stop drinking without a struggle after 1 or 2 drinks? ❑ Yes ❑ No
6. Do you ever feel bad about your drinking? ❑ Yes ❑ No
7. Do friends, your children, or other relatives think you are a normal drinker? ❑ Yes ❑ No
8. Have you ever used alcohol instead of prescribed medications from your doctor to treat your health problems? ❑ Yes ❑ No
9. Do you try to limit your drinking to certain prescribed times of the day or to certain places? ❑ Yes ❑ No
10. Are you always able to stop drinking when you want to? ❑ Yes ❑ No
11. Have you ever been evicted, asked to move, or been denied access to any elderly living accommodations or recreational facilities because of your drinking? ❑ Yes ❑ No
12. Have you ever attended a meeting of Alcoholics Anonymous (AA)? ❑ Yes ❑ No
13. Have you gotten physically or verbally aggressive when drinking? ❑ Yes ❑ No
14. Has drinking ever created problems between you and your spouse, your children, or other family members? ❑ Yes ❑ No
15. Have your children ever avoided contact with you, or not allowed you to see or visit your grandchildren because of your drinking? ❑ Yes ❑ No
16. Has your spouse (or any other family member) ever gone to anyone for help about your drinking? ❑ Yes ❑ No
17. Have you ever lost any friends or had disagreements with neighbors because of your drinking? ❑ Yes ❑ No
18. Have you ever neglected eating, your own daily health maintenance, or your family for 2 or more days in a row because of your drinking? ❑ Yes ❑ No
19. Have you ever drank to relieve the pain and sorrow due to the loss of or death of your spouse or other loved ones? ❑ Yes ❑ No
20. Do you drink before noon? ❑ Yes ❑ No
21. Have you ever been told by your doctor that you have liver trouble? ❑ Yes ❑ No
22. Have you ever had severe shakes, heard voices, or seen things that were not there after heavy drinking? ❑ Yes ❑ No
23. Have you ever gone to anyone for help about your drinking? ❑ Yes ❑ No
24. Have you ever been hospitalized because of your drinking? ❑ Yes ❑ No
25. Have you ever been a patient in a psychiatric hospital or on a psychiatric ward of a general hospital where drinking was part of the problem? ❑ Yes ❑ No
26. Have you ever been at a psychiatric or mental health clinic or gone to a doctor, a social worker, clergyman, or counselor for help with an emotional problem in which drinking played a part? ❑ Yes ❑ No

**ELDERLY ALCOHOL SCREENING TEST SCORING**

| | Yes | No | | Yes | No | | Yes | No | | Yes | No |
|---|---|---|---|---|---|---|---|---|---|---|---|
| 1. | 0 | 0 | 8. | 2 | 0 | 15. | 2 | 0 | 22. | 5 | 0 |
| 2. | 0 | 2 | 9. | 0 | 0 | 16. | 2 | 0 | 23. | 5 | 0 |
| 3. | 1 | 0 | 10. | 0 | 2 | 17. | 3 | 0 | 24. | 5 | 0 |
| 4. | 1 | 0 | 11. | 2 | 0 | 18. | 3 | 0 | 25. | 5 | 0 |
| 5. | 0 | 2 | 12. | 2 | 0 | 19. | 1 | 0 | 26. | 5 | 0 |
| 6. | 1 | 0 | 13. | 2 | 0 | 20. | 1 | 0 | | | |
| 7. | 0 | 2 | 14. | 2 | 0 | 21. | 2 | 0 | | | |

Total possible score: 50
0-3 points: Probably not alcoholic
4-9 points: 80% diagnostic of alcoholism
10 points: Virtually 100% diagnostic of alcoholism

ication, undermedication, inappropriate prescription by the professional, or errors in amount and in administration. Some misuse can result in drug dependency. Medications may be difficult to tolerate and can cause unpleasant side effects, and negative interactions with foods may occur. Other medications may cause adverse reactions and interactions or unpredictable responses in elders. Misuse, dependency, and drug interactions often result in loss of physical, mental, and social function.[17]

### Drug absorption

Numerous age-related physical changes in older adults affect the response to medications. The absorption of drugs may be influenced by the presence or absence of nutrients or by the decrease of hydrochloric acid that normally occurs with aging; drugs that depend on an acid medium may be absorbed less efficiently. Absorption also may be altered because the rate of transit through the gastrointestinal system tends to slow with age.

### Drug distribution

The distribution of drugs within the body affects the loss of lean body mass and the increased proportion of body fat. Fat-soluble drugs tend to be stored in fat, thereby decreasing the intensity of the reaction while increasing the duration. Within the bloodstream the distribution of drugs is affected by the amount of serum protein, specifically albumin, available as binding sites for drugs. In aging persons, the serum albumin levels tend to be lower, resulting in altered concentrations of bound (inactive) and unbound (active) drugs. Unbound drugs in the circulation are active in producing the effects of the drug. The unbound drug can be excreted by the kidneys or metabolized by the liver. A principal mechanism of drug interaction seems to be the displacement of one drug by another from these protein-binding sites. For example, warfarin may be displaced by aspirin, indomethacin, and other drugs, causing increased anticoagulation activity.

### Drug metabolism

The metabolism of drugs in elders may be altered by lower levels of enzyme activity in the liver. The result of prolonged or incomplete metabolism is an increase in the half-life of some drugs that allows the drug to exert its effect over a longer period of time.

### Drug excretion

The kidney is the primary route of excretion of drugs. Changes with aging such as decreased renal plasma flow to the kidney, decreased glomerular filtration rate, and decreased number of functional tubules combine to result in inefficient excretion of active drug. This increases the risk of accumulation of drugs to potentially toxic levels because of decreased renal clearance. The decreased rate of excretion and the changes in binding sites in the blood unite to prolong the elevated blood level and activity of many drugs. Digoxin has a narrow margin of safety and is an example of a drug that is critically affected by the change in renal excretion.

Medications have a definite place in the therapeutic regimen for the older adult, but they must be handled carefully. One general principle in medication therapy is that the drug level should be built up gradually, and the lowest dose and the fewest possible number of drugs should be used. Nurses should check for untoward reactions to medications and report them to the health care provider. The basis for ongoing assessment of an older adult's response to medication is a thorough medication history (Box 4-11). Information from the nutritional assessment of the elder can be used to identify possible food interactions.

**box 4-11** *Patient Medication History**

**GENERAL CONSIDERATIONS:** What is the client/patient's:

1. Cognitive level ________
2. Visual acuity and ability to read labels ________
3. Hand/muscle coordination (to pour, uncap/cap bottle)
4. Ability to swallow without difficulty ________
5. Level of ADL: independent [ ] needs help [ ] ________
6. Lifestyle patterns (alcohol, smoking, activity) ________
7. Beliefs and attitudes toward:
   Self ________
   Illness ________
   Treatments ________
   Prescribing physician or nurse ________
8. Living conditions: alone [ ], with others [ ] ________
   Relationship with others ________
9. Ability to afford cost of medication ________

**SPECIFIC MEDICATION HISTORY:**

10. Medications currently taking (ALL prescribed by ALL physicians and nurses providing care):
    Prescribed: ________
    Over-the-counter
    for pain ________
    constipation ________
    sleep ________
    vitamins ________
    health food products ________
11. Knowledge (reason for taking drug): ________
    Times and frequency of self-medication: ________
12. Are medications shared with: family [ ], friends [ ]
    If so who ________
13. ADR (adverse drug reaction(s)):
    Has experienced ADR(s): yes [ ] no [ ]
    If yes, how was it handled ________
14. Incidence of overuse or underuse of medication:
    yes [ ] no [ ] Describe ________
15. Storage:
    How is medication stored ________
    Where stored ________
    Reason kept that way ________
16. Disposition of old drugs (how handled): ________

From Ebersole P, Hess P: *Toward healthy aging: human needs and nursing response,* ed 5, St Louis, 1998, Mosby.
*If medications administered by spouse or other, the assessment should be done to ascertain caregiver's ability.

**box 4-12** *University Hospitals Nursing Assessment Tool**

Date: ____________ Patient: ____________ ID:
Informant: ____________ Relationship: ____________
Presenting problem: ____________

**MENTAL STATUS**
Appearance: ____________
Mood, affect (including check for depression, orientation): ____________
Cognitive function (examples): ____________
Communication: ____________

**SLEEPING**
Does patient sleep well? ____________ Feel well rested? ____________
If not, explain: ____________
Ease of falling asleep: ____________ Nap pattern: ____________
Hours per night/times up during the night: ____________
Concerns of patient/family: ____________

**SENSES**
Sight:
Hearing: ____________
Taste: ____________ Smell: ____________
Touch: ____________

**ACTIVITIES OF DAILY LIVING**

| | Independent | Dependent | Circle dependent activities |
|---|---|---|---|
| Bathing | | | Initiation of bath<br>Type of bathing (tub, shower, sponge)<br>Bath preparation<br>Get in/out of tub<br>Ability to wash self<br>Hair washing |
| Dressing | | | Clothing selection<br>Putting on garments<br>Doing up buttons, etc.<br>Appropriateness of attire<br>Undressing<br>Laundry |
| Transfer | | | From bed to chair<br>From chair to standing |
| Toileting | | | Able to find bathroom<br>Able to use toilet appropriately<br>Hygiene |
| Bowel continence | | | Frequency and control<br>Constipation |
| Feeding | | | |

*Courtesy University Hospitals of Cleveland, Cleveland, Ohio.

Continued

**box 4-12** *University Hospitals Nursing Assessment Tool—cont'd*

**INSTRUMENTAL ACTIVITIES OF DAILY LIVING**

| | Alone | Assist | Never (N/A) | No longer | |
|---|---|---|---|---|---|
| Telephone | | | | | Look up number<br>Dial |
| Medication | | | | | Preparation<br>Taking |
| Outside of home | | | | | Organization<br>Getting lost |
| Driving | | | | | |
| Housework | | | | | Organization<br>Doing (List what able to do.) |
| Food preparation | | | | | Planning<br>Shopping<br>Preparing |
| Finances | | | | | Banking<br>Paying bills<br>Balancing checkbook |

**URINARY CONTINENCE**

Does patient have "accidents"? (If "yes," when?) ____________________
Patient's knowledge of accidents: ____________________ Frequency: ____________________
Urgency: ____________________ Can patient get to bathroom in time? ____________________
Does patient wet when coughing or sneezing or at other times? ____________________
Where is center of concern about wetting (patient, family, both)? ____________________
Other concerns: ____________________

**MOBILITY**

Walking ability (use of assistive devices): ____________________
Distance able to walk (and frequency): ____________________
Gait, posture:
Stiffness (morning, after inactivity, evening, where?): ____________________

What does patient do to maximize mobility? ____________________
Hand dexterity and function: ____________________
Problems with feet and shoes: ____________________
Other concerns of patient/family: ____________________

**NUTRITION**

No. of meals per day: ____________________ No. of glasses of fluid: ____________________
Indigestion, nausea/vomiting, change in bowels: ____________________
Dentition: ____________________
Appetite: ____________________ Weight stability: ____________________
Concerns of family (need for referral to nutritionist): ____________________

## SLEEP-WAKE PATTERNS

Sleep is a basic requirement for all human beings. Sufficient sleep is needed to maintain energy levels, physical appearance, and well-being. Certain changes in sleep and sleep patterns seem to occur as part of normal aging. These include a prolonged sleep latency (time it takes to fall asleep), an increase in the number of awakenings during the sleep period, a decrease in slow-wave sleep (thought to be associated with physical restoration), and a decrease in rapid eye movement (REM) sleep that occurs in advanced old age (thought to be associated with mental restoration). These changes often result in more fragmented sleep than that experienced in earlier years. Al-

**box 4-12** *University Hospitals Nursing Assessment Tool—cont'd*

**MEDICATIONS**

List medications as prescribed and how they are taken in ( ? ). (Note how long patient has been on medication.)

Patient's knowledge of medications (reason for, side effects, precautions)

Nonprescription medications:

Allergies (medications): (other):

Person responsible for medication administration:

Alcohol intake (past/present): Smoking history:

**SAFETY**

Is patient alone at any time? Gets lost?

Kitchen safety:

Household safety (rugs, cords, railings, stairs):

Other concerns:

**CAREGIVER**

Name of formal caregiver: Relationship:

Informal caregiving system:

Caregiver's role/function:

Impact of caregiving on caregiver/family:

Assessment of stability/security provided in present care environment:

**SUMMARY**

Completed by:

though many elders adapt to these normal sleep changes, others experience acute or chronic insomnia. Physical problems that cause pain, shortness of breath, frequency of urination, incontinence, impairment of mobility, or confusion may disrupt sleep. Other contributing factors include certain drugs (e.g., some antihypersensitive drugs) and environmental factors such as temperature, light, noise, and type of bed and location.

Because quality of sleep can have far-reaching effects on the individual's general well-being, an essential component of the nurse's health assessment of elders must include an evaluation of sleep. A sleep problem that is identified should be analyzed to determine its onset, subjective complaint (how the problem is described by the patient), previous treatments and effectiveness, and sleep patterns before the onset of the problem. Sleep problems are of particular concern during hospitalization when the normal daily routines of older adults are disrupted, and they are exposed to new environmental stimuli. (See Chapter 13.)

Promotion of adequate sleep in elders is based on assessment of an individual's sleep-wake pattern on admission. The nurse's assessment includes a description of the elder's sleep patterns and activities during waking periods, including periods of rest, exercise, and "naps." The elder should be asked about usual bedtime routines as well as what factors disturb and enhance sleep. Some older adults are still working, some are retired from evening or night jobs, or some are caregivers and may have a sleep-wake pattern that is very different from the hospital routine. These data are then used to accommodate the older adult's normal sleep-wake cycle as closely as possible (Box 4-12).

## critical thinking QUESTIONS

1. You are chairing a committee to revise the preadmission assessment for day surgery patients. Sixty percent of the patients admitted are 65 years of age and older. What specific assessment items will you suggest be included for all older adult patients?
2. Mr. J, age 69, is recovering from surgery for a knee replacement. He is refusing to take part in therapy. Mr. J. complains of unspecified, generalized pain. He is suspicious about what his wife is doing while he is in the hospital. At times he is confused and does not remember what he has been told from shift to shift. What areas of function do you need to assess to determine what is affecting Mr. J's status?
3. Mrs. K, age 82, has been hospitalized for 10 days after complications following a myocardial infarction. Three days ago, it seemed that she would be discharged soon. However, Mrs. K has become lethargic and has been sleeping frequently throughout the day. What information from the chart may be helpful in determining what has caused the changes in Mrs. K's condition?

## chapter SUMMARY

### HISTORICAL PERSPECTIVES

- As people lived longer scientists began to study the normal aging process, gerontology, and diseases of aging, geriatrics.
- The fastest growing segments of the American population are persons 65 years of age and minority elders who are 85 years of age and older.
- The largest proportion of persons older than 65 years of age are women.
- Three cohorts constitute the older adult population: young old (ages 65 to 74 years), middle old (ages 75 to 84 years), and old old (ages 85 years and older).

### ASSESSMENT OF ELDERS: GENERAL ISSUES

- Gerontological assessment is multidimensional and includes physical, mental, social, and spiritual function.
- There is a great deal of diversity found in the older adult population.
- Hospitalized older adults are at greater risk for institutionalization as a result of loss of function and disability.
- It is important to distinguish between primary (normal) and secondary (disease) aging changes.
- Non-white persons may exhibit secondary aging changes with loss of function and disability in the late-middle adult years.
- Disease and illness present differently in older adults than in younger patients.

### FUNCTIONAL ASSESSMENT OF ELDERS: COMMON CONCERNS

- Basic self-care activities, called activities of daily living, and the abilities to perform more complex activities, termed instrumental activities of daily living, are basic aspects of gerontological assessment.
- Older adults are at increased risk for falls and must be assessed for risk factors on admission.
- Spiritual well-being focuses on the meaning an older person attaches to life experiences and can affect or be affected by an elder's health status.
- Sexuality continues to be an important issue for persons as they age.
- Older persons are not immune from acquiring sexually transmitted diseases or from sexual violence.
- Family continues to provide a place for intimacy, affection, support, and resources as one ages.
- Older adults are members of diverse types of families.
- Older persons may be family caregivers or may be recipients of family caregiving.
- Elders may be victims or perpetrators of neglect, maltreatment, and abuse within the family or care setting.
- Nutrition should be considered a vital sign of older adults' health status.
- Cognitive changes in older adults are often the first indication of disease and illness.
- Immediate assessment of cognitive changes is critical to determine whether the changes are reversible or irreversible so that appropriate care and treatment can be initiated.
- Sensory perceptual changes, especially hearing and vision, affect an older person's function, particularly mental health and communication.
- Depression is the major mental health problem found in older adults and often goes misdiagnosed or undiagnosed.
- There is an increased risk of suicide as one ages, particularly in older white men.
- Both depression and suicide are treatable in older adults, no matter what the age of the person, once they are diagnosed.
- Early-onset and late-onset alcoholism may go undiagnosed in older adults, resulting in lack of treatment and medical complications.
- Older adults use more prescribed and over-the-counter drugs than younger persons.
- Alcohol and drugs have different effects on the physical and mental function of older persons because of normal aging changes.
- Older adults with health problems that are the result of interactions between alcohol, medication, foods, and disease may be seen in primary, acute, and long-term care facilities.
- Although sleep-wake patterns change with normal aging, sleep continues to be a restorative process that promotes functional health.

## References

1. Adams WL, Cox NS: Epidemiology of problem drinking among the elderly, *Int J Addict* 30(13):1469-1492, 1995.
2. Andelin LC, Alessi CA, Aronow HU: Reliability of screening for sensory impairment in depressed and versus nondepressed older adults, *J Am Geriatr Soc* 43:684-687, 1995.

3. Barrocas A et al: Nutrition assessment practical approaches, *Clin Geriatr Med* 11(4):675-713, 1995.
4. Beck JC, Freedman ML, Warshaw GA: Geriatric assessment: focus on function, *Patient Care* 28(4):10-22, 25, 28, 31-32, 1994.
5. Blanchi EC: *Aging as a spiritual journey,* New York, 1990, Crossroad.
6. Blazer D: Spirituality and aging well, *Generations* 28(4):61-65, 1991.
7. Carter B, McGoldrick M, editors: *The changing family life cycle,* Boston, 1989, Allyn & Bacon.
8. Clipp EC, George LK: Psychotropic drug use among caregivers of patients with dementia, *J Am Geriatr Soc* 38:227-235, 1990.
9. Cope KA: Nutritional status: a basic "vital sign," *Home Health Nurs* 12(2):29-34, 1994.
10. Corey-Bloom J et al: Cognitive and functional status of the oldest old, *J Am Geriatr Soc* 44:671-674, 1996.
11. Davis MA et al: Living arrangements and dietary patterns of older adults, *J Gerontol* 40(4):434-442, 1985.
12. DeLorey C, Wolf KA: Sexual violence and older women, *AWHONN Clin Issues* 4(2):173-179, 1993.
13. Devon CAJ: Suicide in the elderly: how to identify and treat patients at risk, *Geriatrics,* 51(3):67-73, 1996.
14. Dowdell EB: Caregiver burden: grandmothers and their high risk grandchildren, *J Psychosoc Nurs* 33(3):27-30, 1995.
15. Ebersole P, Hess P: *Toward healthy aging: human needs and nursing response,* ed 5, St Louis, 1998, Mosby.
16. Fillit H, Capello C: Making geriatric assessment an asset to your primary care practice, *Geriatrics* 49(1):27-35, 1994.
17. Finlayson RE: Misuse of prescription drugs in the elderly, *Int J Addict* 30(13):1647-1677, 1995.
18. Fioritto P, editor: *Alcoholism and aging: a matter of substance,* ed 2, Cleveland, 1997, School of Medicine, Case Western Reserve University.
19. Folstein MF, Folstein SE, McHugh PR: Mini-mental state: a practical method for grading the cognitive state of patients for the clinician, *J Psychiatr Res* 12:189-198, 1975.
20. Fulmer TT, O'Malley TA: *Inadequate care of the elderly: a health care perspective on abuse and neglect,* New York, 1987, Springer.
21. George LK, Gwyther LP: Caregiver well-being: a multidimensional examination of family caregivers of demented adults, *Gerontologist* 26:253, 1986.
22. Greenberg EM: Violence and the older adult: the role of the acute care nurse practitioner, *Crit Care Nurs Q* 19(2):76-84, 1996.
23. Groom DD: Elder care: a diagnostic model for failure to thrive, *J Gerontol Nurs* 19(6):12-16, 1993.
24. Guigoz Y, Vellas B, Garry PJ: Assessing the nutritional status of the elderly: the Mini Nutritional Assessment as part of geriatric evaluation, *Nutr Rev* 54(1):S59-S65, 1996.
25. Gurnack AM, editor: Introduction: special issue on drugs and the elderly, *Int J Addict* 30(13):1461-1463, 1995.
26. Hazzard W et al: *Principles of geriatric medicine,* ed 3, New York, 1994, McGraw-Hill.
27. Herriot CS: Spirituality and aging, *Holis Nurs Pract* 21(8):60-70, 1996.
28. Hungelmann J et al: Focus on spiritual well-being: harmonious interconnectedness of mind-body–spirit—use of the JAREL spiritual well-being scale, *Geriatr Nurs* 17(6):262-266, 1996.
29. Incalzi RA et al: Nutritional assessment: a primary component of multidimensional geriatric assessment in acute care, *J Am Geriatr Soc* 44:166-174, 1996.
30. Kahana E, Biegel DE, Wykle ML, editors: *Family caregiving across the lifespan,* Thousand Oaks, Calif, 1994, SAGE.
31. Kelley SJ: Caregiver stress in grandparents raising grandchildren, *IMAGE* 25(4):331-337, 1993.
32. Kennedy GJ: The geriatric syndrome of late life depression, *Psychiatr Services* 46(1) 43-48, 1995.
33. Larsen PD, Hazen SE, Martin JLH: Assessment and management of sensory loss in elderly patients, *AORN J* 65(2):432-437, 1996.
34. Lebowitz BD et al: Diagnosis and treatment of depression in late life: consensus update, *JAMA* 278:1186-1190, 1997.
35. Leetun MC: Wellness spirituality in the older adult: assessment and intervention protocol, *Nurs Pract* 21(8):60-70, 1996.
36. Letvak S, Schoder D: Sexually transmitted diseases in the elderly: what you need to know, *Geriatr Nurs* 17(4)156-160, 1996.
37. Lewis CB, Lindsay T, Scott C: Functional assessment in the psychosocial realm, *Top Geriatr Rehabil* 11(4):64-83, 1996.
38. Liberto JG, Oslin DW: Early versus late onset of alcoholism in the elderly, *Int J Addict* 30(13):1575-1594, 1995.
39. Lichtenstein MJ: Hearing and visual impairments, *Clin Geriatr Med* 8:173-182, 1992.
40. MacAvoy S, Skinner T, Hines M: Clinical methods: fall risk assessment tool, *Appl Nurs Res* 9(4):213-218, 1996.
41. Marchi-Jones S, Murphy JF, Rousseau P: Caring for caregivers, *J Gerontol Nurs* 22(8):7-14, 1996.
42. Masters W, Johnson V: *Human sexual response,* Boston, 1966, Little, Brown & Co.
43. Miller J et al: The assessment of acute confusion as part of nursing care, *Appl Nurs Res* 10(3):143-151, 1997.
44. Minkler M, Roe KM, Price M: The physical and emotional health of grandmothers raising grandchildren in the crack cocaine epidemic, *Gerontologist* 32(6):752-761, 1992.
45. Mitchell A, Jones N: Striving to prevent falls in an acute care setting-action to enhance quality, *J Clin Nurs* 5(3):213-210, 1996.
46. Moore TM, Martin J, Stonehouse J: Predicting falls: risk assessment tool versus clinical judgement, *Perspectives* 20(1):8-11, 1996.
47. Mui AC: Perceived health and functional status among spouse caregivers of frail older persons, *J Aging Health* 7(2):283-300, 1995.
48. Neelon VJ et al: The NEECHAM confusion scale: construction, validation, and clinical teaching, *Nurs Res* 45(6):324-330, 1996.
49. Pastorino C, Dickey T: Health promotion for the elderly, *Orthop Nurs* 9(60):36, 1990.
50. Pfeiffer E: A short portable mental status questionnaire for the assessment of organic brain deficit in elderly patients, *J Am Geriatr Soc* 23:433-441, 1975.
51. Proffitt C, Ausgspurger P, Byrne M: Geriatric depression: a survey of nurses' knowledge and assessment practices, *Issues Ment Health Nurs* 17:123-130, 1996.
52. Rossini R et al: Physical performance test and activities of daily living scales in the assessment of health status in elderly people, *J Am Geriatr Soc* 43:1109-1113, 1993.
53. Rueben DB, Greendale GA, Harrison GG: Nutrition screening in older persons, *J Am Geriatr Soc* 43:415-425, 1995.
54. Rueben DB, Valle LA et al: Measuring physical function in community-dwelling older persons: a comparison of self-administered, interviewer-administered, and performance-based measures, *J Am Geriatr Soc* 43:17-23, 1995.
55. Sbrocco T, Weisberg R, Barlow DH: Sexual dysfunction in the older adult: assessment of psychosocial factors, *Sexuality Disabil* 13(3): 201-218.
56. Scura K, Whipple B: Older adult as an HIV positive risk group, *J Gerontol Nurs* 16(1):6-10, 1990.
57. Smith JW: Medical manifestations of alcoholism in the elderly, *Int J Addict* 30(13):1525-1574, 1995.
58. Stull DE, Kosloski K, Kercher K: Caregiver burden and generic well-being: opposite sides of the same coin? *Gerontologist* 34(1):88-94, 1994.
59. Sullivan DH, Walls RC, Bopp MM: Protein-energy undernutrition and the risk of mortality within one year of hospital discharge: a follow-up study, *J Am Geriatr Soc* 43:507-512, 1995.
60. Tebb S: An aid to empowerment: a caregiver well-being scale, *Health Soc Work* 20(2):87-92, 1995.
61. Trenethick MJ: Thriving, not just surviving: the importance of social support among the elderly, *J Psychosoc Nurs* 35(9):27-42, 1997.

62. Tully CL, Snowdon DA: Weight change and physical function in older women: findings from the nun study, *J Am Geriatr Soc* 43:1394-1397, 1995.
63. US Bureau of the Census: *Statistical abstracts of the United States, 1988*, annual ed 108, Washington, DC, 1988, US Government Printing Office.
64. US Bureau of the Census: *1990 Population of census and housing*, Washington, DC, 1991, US Government Printing Office.
65. US Department of Health and Human Services, Public Health Services: *Healthy people 2000: national health promotion and disease prevention objectives*, Washington, DC, 1990, US Government Printing Office.
66. Verdery RB: Failure to thrive in the elderly, *Clin Geriatr Med* 11(4): 653-659, 1995.
67. Wallsten SM: Comparing patterns of stress in daily experiences of elderly caregivers and noncaregivers, *Int J Aging Hum Dev* 37(1):55-68, 1993.

chapter 5

# Ethical Decision Making in Nursing

BARBARA J. DALY

## objectives

After studying this chapter, the learner should be able to:

1. Explain how laws, policies, professional codes, and personal values may contribute to moral judgments in specific circumstances.
2. Apply the concepts of autonomy, beneficence, and justice in examining specific ethical dilemmas.
3. Use a five-step process in analyzing ethical dilemmas.
4. Compare and contrast the living will with the durable power of attorney for health care.
5. Describe nursing responsibilities in caring for a patient with treatment-limitation orders.
6. Identify potential resources to assist the nurse in addressing ethical issues in the workplace.

*Ethics* is the study of the reasoned process of making moral decisions. When we ask ethical questions, we are asking about the morally correct action in a specific situation or about how we ought to behave to live a good or worthy life. Although some make a distinction between the terms *ethical* and *moral*, these words are used interchangeably in this chapter to refer to actions and beliefs that express normative judgments about right and wrong, goodness and evil.

*Ethical dilemmas* are situations in which there seems to be no right answer. Typically these cases involve conflicts between two mutually exclusive rules or principles, such as might occur when a nurse tries to protect a patient's right to make his or her own choices about care and yet feels an obligation to prevent the harm that might occur from an unwise choice.

We encounter ethical questions in our everyday lives. Debates regarding the morality of capital punishment or abortion, justification for civil disobedience, and instances of racial discrimination are examples of ethical issues that affect us all. In addition to our involvement in these issues, health care professionals are likely to face further situations that call for reasoned ethical analysis. Technological advances have made it possible to intervene in health and illness in ways that raise new questions about right courses of action. For example, our ability to prolong life through the use of sophisticated technology sometimes raises doubts about the quality of the life prolonged; discoveries in the field of genetic mapping have created new questions about how to properly use information concerning an individual's genetic predispositions; and improvement in organ transplantation techniques has led to questions about the acceptability of methods to encourage donation.

The current interest in addressing ethical questions also reflects the public's growing awareness of and interest in becoming active participants in these debates. The consumer movement of the 1960s and 1970s, in addition to creating a gradual disillusionment with medicine and science in general, contributed to changing societal norms regarding health care. The recognition and acceptance of patients' rights have fostered new beliefs about the importance of involving patients in decisions about their care, informing them of all options in treatment approaches, and joining with them in mutual attempts to meet their health care needs.

Anyone who attempts to understand an ethical issue and reach a thoughtful decision about the morally correct course of action is acting as a *moral agent.* The purpose of this chapter is to review some of the common principles used by moral agents in ethical reasoning and to consider practical features of health care environments that influence the nurse's ability to make ethical decisions. Situations commonly encountered are discussed.

## MORAL AGENCY

Although moral decisions ultimately must stem from the individual's own decision making, two external sources of direction are relevant to any consideration of how we should resolve an ethical dilemma: the law and the professional code. Although these formal rules should never take the place of individual decision making, they must be considered as part of the process.

Many ethical dilemmas involve questions that have legal aspects. For example, when a nurse considers a patient's request that life support be discontinued, it is appropriate and even necessary to take into account the current laws regarding treatment discontinuation. Laws represent formalized societal norms regarding specific actions, and nurses, like all citizens, are obligated to respect the laws of our country. Knowledge of the law, however, does not always answer moral questions. In many instances laws are too general to be of assistance. In other instances the law is merely silent on the question of what should be done in a specific situation. For example, we generally believe that the nurse has an obligation to be truthful when speaking to the patient; yet there is no actual law forbidding deception.

In many ways the nurse should use an understanding of the law in the same way that he or she uses knowledge of hospital policy in decision making. These external rules tell the nurse what society (in the case of laws) or the hospital (in the case of policies) expects in terms of standards of behavior. These laws and policies describe obligations of the nurse as citizen and employee and in some instances may constrain the options available to the nurse. It is essential, however, that the nurse recognize from the outset that laws and policies, like any kind of general rule, may be unwise, outdated, or just not applicable in a given situation. For this reason the nurse, as moral agent, must know what the laws and policies are but cannot rely on them for complete justification for action. An immoral action performed in accordance with an unreasonable policy is still immoral.

Professional codes of ethics are formal statements made by professional organizations for several purposes. They inform society of what it may expect from a profession, provide guidance to the members of the profession in decision making, and provide standards that the profession can use in judging and regulating members. Rather than providing an explicit set of rules, the American Nurses' Association (ANA) Code for Nurses, developed by the Committee on Ethics of the ANA,[2] expresses the values, goals, and moral commitments of the profession.[3] The values reflected in the Code for Nurses are consistent with those expressed in *Nursing's Social Policy Statement*, the profession's explicit description of nursing's obligations to society.[4] The broad statements and principles contained in the code are intended to serve as a framework within which individual decision making can take place. For example, the code states in the preamble that the most fundamental principle to be used in making clinical judgments is respect for persons. General responsibilities are then described, including confidentiality, public safety, competence, accountability, and collaboration. In addition, the American Nurses' Association issues position statements as further guidance in specific areas such as treatment withdrawal and reporting unethical conduct. The nurse must be aware of the profession's code and should use it for guidance in solving ethical problems (Box 5-1).

**box 5-1** *ANA Code for Nurses*

1. The nurse provides services with respect for human dignity and the uniqueness of the client, unrestricted by considerations of social or economic status, personal attributes, or the nature of health problems.
2. The nurse safeguards the client's right to privacy by judiciously protecting information of a confidential nature.
3. The nurse acts to safeguard the client and the public when health care and safety are affected by the incompetent, unethical, or illegal practice of any person.
4. The nurse assumes responsibility and accountability for individual nursing judgments and actions.
5. The nurse maintains competence in nursing.
6. The nurse exercises informed judgment and uses individual competence and qualifications as criteria in seeking consultation, accepting responsibilities, and delegating nursing activities to others.
7. The nurse participates in activities that contribute to the ongoing development of the profession's body of knowledge.
8. The nurse participates in the profession's efforts to implement and improve standards of nursing.
9. The nurse participates in the profession's efforts to establish and maintain conditions of employment conducive to high quality nursing care.
10. The nurse participates in the profession's effort to protect the public from misinformation and misrepresentation and to maintain the integrity of nursing.
11. The nurse collaborates with members of the health professions and other citizens in promoting community and national efforts to meet the health needs of the public.

Courtesy Committee on Ethics, American Nurses' Association, Washington, DC, 1985.
NOTE: The Code for Nurses is currently under revision; the version printed here is expected to be replaced by 1999.

In addition to appreciating the role of laws, policies, and professional codes in ethical decision making, it is essential that the nurse understand the difference between value judgments and moral decisions. *Values* are expressions of individual preferences and beliefs about things that are important or worthwhile. One's values may include material goods, such as a nice home, or more abstract goods, such as meaningful personal relationships. Values are important determinants of behavior because we tend to act in a way that will help us achieve or obtain the things we think are important in life.

Students are routinely assisted in clarifying their own values and cautioned to avoid imposing their values on others. *Values clarification* is important in helping us understand our own behavior, and it is necessary before we can begin to resolve both intrapersonal conflicts among our own values and interpersonal conflicts between our values and the values of others. By avoiding the imposition of our values on others we avoid interfering in others' pursuit of what they believe a good or worthwhile life to be. This is required because most of us do not ordinarily examine every value we hold; rather, we simply accept that everyone has ideas that are important to them without asking if some of these values are based on false beliefs or are imprudent or more justifiable than others.

In moral issues, however, we must move beyond the level of simply recognizing personal preferences. The entire history of morality is founded on the conviction that there is meaning to the basic concepts of "right" and "wrong," "good" and "evil." This belief entails the recognition that some actions, although they stem from sincerely held values, are morally wrong and should not be performed and that other actions, even if not ordinarily preferred, are morally obligatory. For example, discriminating against others on the basis of belief that people of different races or religions are in some way inferior is morally wrong, even though the discriminatory action stems from strongly held values. Similarly, stopping at the scene of an accident to offer aid is rarely a pleasant or preferred action, yet in some situations may be obligatory.

Bandman and Bandman[6] discuss the need to move beyond values clarification and begin to seek justification for values as one attempts to resolve moral problems. Recognizing that a nurse, physician, or patient holds a certain value does not mean that the value or preference should be acted on. The value in question may not be justified. For example, many people in our country still value segregation between races. They believe that there are differences among people of different races, and they value institutions and practices that promote discrimination. If we examine this value and find, after careful reflection, that it is not justified, that it is based on mistaken beliefs, and that acting on it involves violating important moral principles, we should not respect or even allow those actions to be taken. This does not mean that we cease to respect the person or that we judge the person to be evil; it does mean that we make a judgment that certain actions are morally wrong regardless of the values of the person performing the action.

The caution regarding imposing our own values on others is most important when we interact with others who hold values very different from our own. For example, it could be the case that the nurse may value a lifestyle quite different from that valued by the gay patient with acquired immunodeficiency syndrome (AIDS). The nurse may believe strongly that traditional heterosexual relationships are more valuable and may have difficulty understanding why someone might adopt other patterns of behavior. In this case the nurse must be cautious to avoid interacting with the patient in such a way as to convey condemnation of the patient's chosen lifestyle or the message that this patient is less deserving of care than other patients because of his or her values. Although the nurse sincerely disagrees with the patient's values, this difference is a matter of personal belief and should have no impact on the caring relationship. However, to be alert to inappropriate ways in which our values may affect our behavior, we must first understand what values we hold.

As can be seen, the process of examining values for justification and making decisions about what actions are morally correct is quite complicated. To make these judgments the individual must use both an understanding of basic moral theories and principles and insight into personally held values and beliefs. Because nurses also must fulfill obligations to their patients and sometimes to the other professionals with whom they work, nurses must be knowledgeable about practical steps that can be effective in obtaining the desired outcome of ethical dilemmas. Each of these issues is discussed further in the remainder of this chapter.

## ETHICAL THEORIES AND PRINCIPLES

Ethical theories, like all theories, provide a framework for understanding the phenomena existing within a certain domain. Theories provide us with definitions of the relevant concepts and explain the relationship between concepts. In the study of ethics we are seeking answers to questions such as "What types of acts are right?" "Which traits are praiseworthy?" "What makes certain values justified?" "Which rules should I use to guide my behavior?"[24] Ethical theories offer us a way to answer these general questions by directing the method or approach to use in addressing any ethical issue.

Many specific theories exist, and theories vary widely among different cultures and even within a culture. In Western countries, two types of theories have been particularly influential. One of these is termed *consequentialist* because these ideas instruct us to evaluate the consequences of actions to judge the rightness or wrongness of the action. The other group of theories is referred to as *nonconsequentialist* because the beliefs are based on concepts of fundamental rights and duties, rather than consequences, in choosing the right course of action.

Of all of the consequentialist theories, *utilitarianism* is the most prominent today. Contemporary versions of utilitarianism define right action as any action that promotes human well-being or welfare. When we are confronted with a choice between two actions, we are to assess the expected utility of each action (hence the name utilitarianism) and choose that action which is most likely to produce the largest benefit, or least harm, for the greatest number of people. Everyone's welfare, including the person choosing, counts equally.

Nonconsequentialist theories, also referred to as *deontological*, argue that consequences are not the standard by which we should judge actions. Rather, there are fundamental duties and rights that stem from our nature as rational beings, or, in some theories, as beings subject to the rules of God or a divine power. The morality of any action can be judged according to the dictates of these rights and duties.

All moral theories make use of principles and rules. Although the justification for the principles differs among theories and the strength or rigidity with which we are to follow the rules varies, there is considerable agreement about the importance of several broad principles as guides to action. These principles are general statements about ideals that should be valued, such as honesty and kindness, and they serve as the basis for more specific rules, such as "Always tell the truth." In actual practice it is these principles and rules to which we turn in addressing ethical problems rather than to the more abstract theories that underlie them. Although many different principles are components of each theory, the three that are most common and relevant to nursing practice are autonomy, beneficence, and justice.

### AUTONOMY

*Autonomy* is a term that is derived from the Greek words *autos,* meaning self, and *nomos,* meaning rule or law. The central notion of autonomy is that of self-rule or liberty to follow one's own will.[41] The principle of autonomy is crucial to the study of ethics for three reasons. First, without some sense of persons as autonomous or free, rational decision makers, we have no basis for assigning responsibility for actions. Without this sense that we are responsible for our choices, behaviors, and consequences of actions there is no point to ethical inquiry. Our understanding of human beings as entities at least potentially capable of autonomous decisions and actions underlies all of ethics.

Second, recognition of the principle of autonomy imposes some very important duties on us. If it is the case that people have a right to make autonomous choices, we have a duty not to interfere with these choices. We can interfere with free choice by simply not permitting someone to make a choice, but we also can limit the ability to choose by such acts as withholding necessary information. All of these forms of interference violate the principle of autonomy and will be discussed in more detail.

The third reason autonomy is a significant concept in ethics is that it provides a way of classifying actions that has important implications for other duties. Even if we accept the general rule that we should respect a person's free, rational decisions, what are we to do when someone makes a decision that is clearly not rational? For example, if we believe that someone is acting under the influence of drugs, we generally do not perceive an obligation to facilitate or respect these choices. In fact, in many cases we believe we should actually protect the person from acting on these unwise decisions. Thus we need to be able to differentiate autonomous choices from nonautonomous choices as part of our determination of our own responsibilities toward others.

When we think about autonomy, a tendency exists to confuse the notion of an autonomous person with autonomous choices and autonomous actions. Although it makes sense to ask if someone is ordinarily capable of autonomy, we know that even normally rational adults may at times lose their capacity for autonomy because of an injury, period of emotional disturbance, or ingestion of mind-altering substances. It makes no difference if someone ordinarily is capable of autonomous choices if the particular decision at hand is made while the person is impaired in some way. Consequently it is more helpful to concentrate our discussion on autonomous decisions and autonomous actions rather than autonomous persons.

An autonomous decision is one that (1) is based on the decision maker's values, (2) utilizes adequate information and understanding, (3) is free from coercion or restraint, and (4) is based on reason and deliberation.[43] *Autonomous actions* are those that stem from autonomous decisions, rather than from the person being forced to act or restrained from acting in a certain way. When we think about why anyone, even ourselves, makes certain choices or behaves in a certain way, we realize that we are all under varying amounts of influence from many sources. At any one time we may have other people asking us to do something or telling us we must behave in a certain way. In addition, practical limits always affect the choices available because of factors such as time, access to opportunities, or sometimes the monetary costs associated with certain choices. If we thought that one had to be completely free to make absolutely any choice one wished, we would have to say that none of us has ever made completely autonomous decisions. This would make the concept of autonomy meaningless. Therefore we are interested in determining whether the individual in a given situation was making a decision or taking an action that was "substantially autonomous."[7] That is, we want to ensure that the individual was aware of the right to make a choice; was physically, emotionally, and mentally able to make some evaluation of the options; and had the information necessary to do so.

Both consequentialist and nonconsequentialist thinkers place great importance on autonomy. Consequentialists argue that, in general, each individual is the best judge of what will make his or her life go well, of what choices will contribute most to well-being. As a rule of thumb, then, we should refrain from interfering in the choices of others, even if these choices seem unwise or imprudent to us, up to the point where actions begin to harm or threaten the well-being of others. Nonconsequentialists believe that the respect we owe to each person entails respecting their choices of lifestyles and life projects. By interfering in the decisions others make or forcing them to act in ways not freely chosen, we are expressing disrespect for the person.

The broad principle of autonomy yields many specific rules for health care providers. The best known is the rule of informed consent, which specifies that we must obtain permission from the patient before we do anything to him or her. Although we generally are most conscious of obtaining explicit consent in the form of a written document before invasive or risky procedures, the principle of autonomy actually means that we cannot do anything, even ordinary treatments and procedures, without the patient's agreement. For example, when patients refuse medication or diagnostic tests, we are morally obligated to respect that decision and to refrain from coercing or in any way forcing the patient to take the medicine or accept the test.

Autonomy also can serve as the basis for duties of truth telling. One way in which we can interfere with a person's right to make free choices is by withholding important information or by deceiving the person in some way. To make decisions that will promote our well-being, as conceived by each of us, we have to have accurate information. In making treatment decisions in particular we need to know something about the disease or health problem itself, the range of options for intervention, and the likely benefits and risks associated with each option. If we withhold some of this information, we are interfering in the patient's ability to make a rational decision that is in line with his or her values and preferences, and we are thus violating the principle of autonomy.

As the phrase implies, informed consent has two parts, an informational component and a volitional or consensual component.[15,19] If we are to feel confident that a patient has given truly informed consent, we must be confident that the requirements of both components have been met. An individual, to be "informed," not only must have been provided with all the relevant information about a proposed action or decision but also must have a certain level of understanding or comprehension. For example, if we were to provide a patient with information about a proposed drug regimen by reading the package insert regarding actions and side effects, we would certainly have given some factual information. However, by providing it in a form that is incomprehensible to most laypersons, we would have no reason to think that the patient had any level of comprehension. Thus, even if the patient consented to take the drug, we could not say that this consent was informed.

The volitional component of informed consent is met by ensuring that the patient's agreement is free of coercion or duress. This means that the individual must be able to agree or disagree without fear of reprisal or punishment. Someone could be literally forced to sign a consent form by holding a gun to the person's head or threatening harm if he or she did not consent; clearly the person's signature on a consent form in these cases would not mean that consent had been given freely. For patients, coercion or duress may take the form of fear that health care providers will abandon them or give up on them for not agreeing to the treatment the physicians and nurses think is best. Another common violation of this part of informed consent occurs when patients feel threatened to make decisions quickly, without the opportunity to think things over. When the patient inadvertently is led to believe that a decision has to be made immediately or the opportunity to receive that treatment will be lost or the health problem will become much worse, a subtle form of coercion may be present.

As can be seen, it is the process of obtaining consent to treatment that is morally important, not the simple act of obtaining a signature on a form. Rules about informed consent, based on the principle of autonomy, are so important in our society that they have been formalized in law. Because the concept of informed consent is not a simple one, however, disputes and even lawsuits have arisen regarding the question of whether informed consent was properly obtained before treatment was begun. Although these cases have usually involved physicians and consent for surgical interventions, the nurse is subject to the same requirement to obtain informed consent before initiating nursing actions. Consequently nurses also need to be certain that patients agree to receive the care offered and that this agreement is based on accurate and meaningful information.

This requirement, of course, raises the question of how we are to determine how much information is necessary and how complete the patient's understanding must be before we can feel confident that informed consent has been given. This question has been much debated, and no very specific answer will be correct for all circumstances.[7,19,28] It is unreasonable to expect that absolutely every fact that is known about a proposed intervention be provided to the patient. This is not only a practical impossibility but, as mentioned in the earlier example, probably would be ineffective in that it is likely to confuse most people who do not have the background necessary to understand complex pharmacology or pathophysiology. The ideal might be to try to provide exactly as much information as the individual patient needs in a particular instance to understand the proposed treatment and make a reasoned decision. Although this approach seems right, we have no way of determining in advance exactly how much information and which pieces of information would represent the ideal for every individual. Instead, we need a general guideline that will be appropriate for most cases, recognizing that we will need to tailor this general rule for situations that fall outside the norm.

The guideline that is currently used to judge whether informed consent has been given is termed the reasonable person standard.[7] According to this standard, our obligation in obtaining informed consent is to provide the information that a hypothetical "reasonable person" would wish to have to make a decision about a proposed treatment. Most people, for example, probably would want to know about the expected benefits and the more common risks and complications of a given surgical treatment, as well as all other options with their attendant benefits and risks. In approaching patients to seek permission for interventions, then, we are to provide them with the amount and kind of information that we would expect the average person in this situation to need to know.

Two common issues that arise related to informed consent are the suggestion that, because patients have come to us seeking care, they have already given their consent to treatment, and the worry that we should refrain from giving advice or our opinion about which treatment is best for fear of unduly influencing patients' choices. Regarding the first concern, it seems valid to assume that patients come to the hospital or health care facility because they wish to have some kind of treatment or assistance. However, that tells us nothing about their wishes regarding specific interventions. Patients may come to the hospital for nursing care, for pain relief, or for aggressive, invasive therapies aimed at cure. Until we talk with them, we have no basis for presuming consent. This does not mean that we have to ask explicitly for consent before we do anything, even common interventions such as turning a patient in bed or bathing. It does mean that the nurse must be cognizant of two particular rules. First, as interventions become more invasive, risky, or burdensome, we must begin to *explicitly ask patients* if they consent to the intervention to be certain that we have given them the opportunity to refuse. Second, whenever the competent patient does refuse an intervention, *we must heed his or her refusal and stop what we are doing.*

The second concern—that we may inadvertently pressure patients into making the decisions we want if we tell them what we think they should do—can be addressed by again thinking about what a reasonable person would want to know. Given the fact that the health care provider is more knowledgeable about health, illness, and possible treatments, most people would want to know what the provider thinks about each option, how the provider evaluates each, and what courses of action the provider believes to be best, all things considered. This can be done in such a way as to avoid coercing the patient by being careful to be open about our reasons for recommending a particular intervention and by offering clear reassurance that we will continue to care for the patient regardless of which option is chosen.

The requirements of informed consent are particularly important in conducting clinical research. Nurses may be involved in the research process in many ways, including administering investigational drugs, collecting laboratory specimens, or acting as the principal investigator. Regardless of the specific role, the nurse must be aware of the research procedures and the risks and benefits to the patient of participation, and must ensure that the patient has given informed consent before implementing any part of the protocol.

The discussion of autonomy and the rules of informed consent hinges on the belief that the patient is competent to make an informed, autonomous decision. *Competency* is a legal term and refers to a court's judgment that an individual is capable of exercising the right of self-determination.[14] The most important component of this judgment is the assessment of decision-making capacity and the absence of seriously impaired mental status. This determination is often made by psychiatrists, although each of us informally makes this assessment when we decide to accept or reject a patient's decision.

The question of an individual's capacity to make autonomous decisions is crucial because it determines whether we have a strict obligation to refrain from interfering in the patient's choices. Although patients often make choices that we would not—choices that we believe are not in their best interests—we may not act contrary to these choices as long as the person understands his or her condition, knows the consequences of the decision, and has reasons that make some sense to us.[14]

## BENEFICENCE

In situations in which we believe an individual cannot make an autonomous decision, we rely on the principle of beneficence to direct our actions. *Beneficence* is the duty to do good, to prevent harm, or to reduce harm where it is present. Some include within beneficence the principle of nonmaleficence, or the duty to refrain from doing harm, whereas others treat nonmaleficence as a separate and even more important principle. Although beneficence and nonmaleficence are duties of some importance for everyone, they are especially significant for health care professionals. Part of the core meaning of "professional" is the commitment to act for the good of society in general and individual clients or patients in particular.[39] Nurses feel a particular responsibility to protect patients and to act in their best interests.

For nurses, the notion of *advocacy* is prominent today as an avenue for both supporting patient autonomy and fulfilling duties of beneficence. An *advocate* is one who speaks for the patient as part of a broader effort to protect the patient's rights. As a description of a particular role or activity, "advocacy" is a somewhat vague term, lacking precise definition.[42] It does capture an important function of nurses—that of acting as an interface between the patient and the complex health care bureaucracy. There is no question that nurses are particularly suited, as Winslow[42] notes, to serve as patient confidante, to assist patients in making their wishes known, and to ensure, through education, that patients are properly informed. However, the current emphasis on advocacy does not provide much direction to the nurse who perceives a conflict between the duty to foster patient autonomy and the need to prevent harm and produce benefit.

When patients make choices that clearly will lead to physical dangers to their health, all care providers face a dilemma. For example, patients often object to being restrained or having their side rails up, even after the nurse has carefully explained the danger of falling out of bed. To ignore the patient's wishes seems to be a clear violation of the patient's autonomy. Yet to follow the patient's wishes seems to fail to protect the patient from harm. Dilemmas such as this involve the possibility of paternalistic action.

*Paternalism* consists of actions that, to benefit or protect a person, override that person's wishes, usually with the justification that one "knows better" what is in the patient's best interest.[7] Benjamin and Curtis[8] use the term *parentalism* to reflect the origins of this kind of action in the parent-child model of relationships. The question of when, if ever, we are justified in overriding an autonomous patient's wishes regarding treatment is a major issue in health care.

This is one reason why determination of decision-making capacity is so important. If the patient lacks the capacity to make informed decisions, regardless of whether this is a permanent or temporary impairment, the principle of autonomy is an inadequate guide for us in determining what to do. It is fortunate if friends or family members can speak on the patient's behalf. If not, we are obligated to act according to the principle of beneficence. This moral guideline, as can be seen, does not tell us exactly what to do or how to judge what would be in the best interest of the patient, but it does serve as the basis for our duty to help those who cannot speak for themselves.

When the dictates of autonomy and beneficence appear to conflict, rights of autonomy generally take precedence. The right of patients to accept or reject care has been repeatedly reaffirmed by the courts, and all care providers are both morally and legally obligated to respect the wishes of competent patients regarding their treatment. It may be helpful to the nurse who experiences the conflict to recall that the principle of beneficence directs us to promote good, but it does not specify what that good is. There are many ways in which something might be judged to be "good." For example, a treatment that contributed to physiological stability is a certain kind of good, and production of happiness or relief of suffering is another type of good. Each of these is a rather limited or narrow conception of "good." Most of us, if asked, could identify a higher or more important good. For some this might be ensuring that our family is well cared for, whereas for others it might be retaining a sense of dignity, living in accordance with God's laws, or simply being in control of what happens. In situations in which the nurse finds it impossible to follow the patient's wishes without seeming to act in a way that does not contribute to physiological good, it can be helpful to remember that there are many kinds of goods. Autonomy simply directs us to let the patient's conception of the highest good be most important in our decision making. Thus, when we act to support the patient's choice, thereby helping the individual achieve his or her personal conception of "good," we are acting in accord with both autonomy and beneficence.

## JUSTICE

The third principle relevant to health care is justice. Justice is a very broad principle with many implications. In the most basic sense, justice means treating equals equally and unequals unequally.[30] That is, justice demands that we have equal respect and concern for the rights of others and that differences in how we treat people be in proportion to morally relevant differences. This requirement has important implications for how we treat people generally and particularly for how we distribute scarce resources.

Anytime we are faced with a shortage of valuable resources, we are dealing with a justice problem. For example, the nurse who must decide how to divide a limited amount of time among several patients must decide the fair or just way to apportion this time. The nurse could simply divide the 8-hour shift equally, with each of four patients having 2 hours. This makes no sense, however, because we believe that differences in amount of care needed are morally relevant. Instead, it seems fair to divide the time according to how much care is needed, with the patients who have the greater needs receiving more time and the patients who need less receiving less time. Although the nurse is treating people differently, the difference is in proportion to a morally relevant property—need for care. On the other hand, if the nurse divided his or her time according to something we think is morally irrelevant, such as the race or age of the patient, we would say that this is unfair or unjust. *Morally relevant differences* are those factors or characteristics of individuals that have some logical relation to the resources that are to be distributed or to the treatment in question. In the example just given, a person's race has nothing to do with why he or she became ill, the reason he or she came to the hospital, the burdens of illness, or the benefits of treatment. Race is thus a *morally irrelevant factor* to consider in distributing health care resources.

Although justice problems can occur even at the bedside, the most serious issue for justice today is the national health care distribution system.[13] Health care in our country is currently distributed in a highly uneven fashion. Although some care is provided through social welfare programs (Medicaid and Medicare), many Americans do not qualify for these programs. For those who do not, health care is distributed as a market good. This means that access to care is determined by ability to pay, just as access to cars, houses, and clothing is determined by one's ability to purchase the goods in a free market. The current estimate is that about 40 million Americans do not qualify for either Medicare or Medicaid but also cannot afford to purchase private health insurance.[16]

The question of how our health care system should be reformed to make it more just is a complex one that involves moral issues such as the establishment of a right to care, economic questions about the best way to pay for this care, and practical concerns about how to structure a universal access program. Consideration of these issues would take us beyond the scope of this chapter, but several points are important.

First, as shown by the earlier example, the principle of justice has implications for the individual. Whenever we are faced with deciding how to apportion a scarce resource, such as our time, the last bed in the intensive care unit, or the last open time on the operating room schedule, we must be aware of the patient characteristics we are using in our decision. We should ask ourselves if the criteria for our decisions are fair and if we would be willing to say that resources always should be distributed according to these criteria. Regarding the larger issue of health reform, the nurse must be informed about proposed legislation and be prepared to contribute to these changes at least through knowledgeable use of voting power.

## RESOLVING ETHICAL DILEMMAS

Understanding the moral principles does not in itself provide answers to dilemmas. Rather, the theories, principles, and rules provide us with tools to use in the process of reaching a decision. There are many suggested approaches to ethical decision making, usually involving a series of steps much like the nursing process.[15,27,28] An organized process to guide one's thinking is particularly helpful when the nurse is unfamiliar with ethical analysis. Although there is some variation among models of decision making, most use the five steps discussed in Box 5-2.

### REVIEWING THE FACTS

As with any reasoned problem-solving process, the first step is to collect data and be certain of the facts. Applying ethical theories correctly requires that we know all the relevant facts about a situation, including such factors as data about the patient's condition, patient and family preferences, patient competence, and relevant hospital policies and laws. Formally reviewing the facts with everyone involved in the ethical dilemma is essential for two reasons.

First, we want to be sure that we are proceeding on a full and correct knowledge base. In particular, we need to know something about why the individuals involved hold the views they do. Simply knowing that a patient wants to leave the hospital against medical advice (AMA), for example, is not enough. Does the patient want to leave because he or she believes that care is not being effective, because a problem at home needs to be addressed, because there is concern over the cost of care, because there has been a disagreement with the nurse or physician, or because the patient has consciously and competently decided that the benefits of treatment are not worth the burdens? The answer to this question would have important implications for action.

Second, it often happens that different individuals in the situation have different pieces of information. What initially may be thought to be an ethical disagreement may turn out to be different beliefs about the facts or unjustified assumptions. For example, one nurse may believe that chemotherapy should be stopped because it is not working and is causing the patient unnecessary suffering. Another nurse may have had a

**box 5-2** *Steps in Ethical Decision Making*

1. *Review the facts.* Summarize morally relevant data (medical, social, psychological); differentiate facts from assumptions
2. *Define the problem.* State the specific moral dilemma or question to be answered in this particular case
3. *List the choices.* List all possible options, both immediate and long range, including options that might initially seem unwarranted
4. *Decide on action.* Apply known facts and moral reasoning to choose from available options
5. *Evaluate the choice.* Evaluate the decision for consistency and coherence

discussion with the oncologist about the latest bone marrow biopsy results that showed a reduction in leukemic cells, suggesting that the therapy was in fact beginning to work. If these two nurses did not review the facts together, each might come to a different conclusion about what was in the patient's best interest. This would be a disagreement stemming from different knowledge bases, not a disagreement over moral principles.

## DEFINING THE PROBLEM

Defining the problem consists of making a concise statement specifying the central issues or questions. This might take the form of statements and questions such as the following: "This competent patient wishes to stop life-supporting treatment. Are we obligated to respect this wish and remove the ventilator?" or "The family members of this incompetent patient disagree about what is in the patient's best interest. How should we resolve this question, and what are the implications of this for treatment of the patient?"

Explicit statement of the problem serves several purposes. It focuses discussion on the exact situation, which may help caregivers concentrate on the case at hand rather than becoming distracted by a debate of the more abstract general issues, such as whether autonomy, overall, is more important than beneficence. The theoretical issues are important, but it is neither possible nor necessary to reach complete agreement on these to resolve individual patient problems.

Defining the issue also clarifies that the problem is a moral one and starts to narrow the field of inquiry to the relevant moral questions. For example, the aforementioned problems suggest situations that involve questions about patients' rights to refuse life-supporting treatment in the one case and questions about who should speak for incompetent patients in the second case. Other moral principles, such as duties related to justice, truth telling, and confidentiality, are not involved. Thus describing the problem in one or two sentences helps everyone focus on the central issue of the particular situation at hand.

## LISTING THE CHOICES

When we confront difficult decision-making situations, particularly those in which disagreement among the participants is obvious from the outset, views often become polarized. For example, in the situation in which a patient is requesting the removal of the life-supporting ventilator, members of the health care team might find themselves initially divided into two camps—those who think the patient's wishes should be followed and those who think the patient's wishes should not be followed. If we are not careful first to consider what all of the options might be, we may miss consideration of some actions that actually are better solutions. In our example the complete range of options might include removing the ventilator today, removing it for a short trial period and then allowing the patient to reconsider his or her decision, asking the patient to allow the caregivers a defined period of time to continue selected interventions before making the decision to stop ventilation, or offering the option of going home on the ventilator.

Listing the choices also reminds us that ethical dilemmas always involve choices among several actions. We cannot solve actual problems by choosing values or principles alone. Each of the possible resolutions to a dilemma involves a decision about which course of action is morally justified.

## DECIDING ON THE ACTION

In reaching a decision, the nurse uses the tools of ethical theories and principles discussed earlier. To decide which of all the available options is the morally justified one, the nurse must be able to refer to fundamental principles and rules that direct action, usually specifying duties and rights. To make a choice between supporting a patient's decision to cease treatment or overriding that decision, the nurse must have access to an articulated moral system that specifies the principle, such as autonomy, that takes priority in situations of conflict.

In making a choice, the nurse also will be making use of the facts identified in the first step of the process. We began with outlining all of the relevant data because we need to have these data readily available as part of our justification for action. Even the strongest-held principles and the most important rules have reasonable exceptions. To examine whether an exception is justified in a specific case, we usually appeal to facts about the situation. We might, for example, believe that patients have a right to full information about their condition, and yet choose to put off telling a particular patient the results of his diagnostic tests if we know that in a few days his closest relative will be arriving in town and will be able to support him as he hears disappointing news.

## EVALUATING THE CHOICES

As with any decision-making process, the last step is to evaluate the choice made. In ethical decision making, the nurse examines the choice for its consistency and coherence with other moral decisions. Decisions that are consistent are said to be *universalizable* in that the same decision should be made in any situation that is similar in morally relevant ways. Thus the nurse who chooses to respect a patient's wishes in one situation, believing that autonomy is the most important principle, should expect to make the same decision in all situations involving similar conflicts.

*Coherence* refers to the degree to which the specific decision fits within a fully developed moral system. For example, the moral system of the nurse who chooses to respect the patient's wish to have life-supporting treatment discontinued could not logically support a view in which life itself is thought to be the ultimate value.

These evaluative steps are helpful in two ways. Moral dilemmas take place in complicated real-life situations in which the nurse is subject to many influences, including external constraints of law and policy, the opinion of peers and supervisors, and the nurse's own personal preferences and needs. These influences can make it difficult at times to be sure that the decisions reached are truly the result of thoughtful deliberation rather than the pressure to conform or to choose the option that creates the least controversy.

Taking the step of conscious evaluation also assists the nurse in learning more about his or her own moral values and encourages the process of seeking justification for these values. By asking ourselves if we are being consistent in how we choose to solve problems, if we are willing to commit ourselves to this same answer in all situations similar to this one, and if this answer "fits" with our other values, we can begin to develop a comprehensive moral system that can direct action in a variety of situations.

## COMMON ETHICAL ISSUES IN ACUTE CARE

Although the preceding steps are intended to be used in any situation, two issues are so common in acute care that review of their current status will be helpful to the student. These are the issues of advance directives and treatment limitation.

### ADVANCE DIRECTIVES

*Advance directive* refers to any document that is enacted by an individual before becoming ill, specifying one's wishes regarding treatment should one be unable to express them later on.[5,23] Although one could make an advance directive simply by writing down one's treatment preferences, the two forms of advance directives formally recognized by law in most states are the living will and the durable power of attorney for health care.[17,33]

Living wills generally take effect only when the patient is terminally ill and is unable to voice his or her wishes. Under these two conditions, the living will directs that no life-sustaining treatment is to be administered. In addition, some living will forms include more specific directions regarding the individual's wishes for withholding food and fluid or other specific treatment modalities.

Regardless of the specific form, living wills are not applicable unless the patient is unable to speak for himself or herself. In some states, the living will has an automatic expiration date and must be periodically renewed (e.g., every 5 years or every 7 years).

The presence of a living will can be extremely helpful to caregivers who are faced with treatment decisions for patients who can no longer speak for themselves, but they do not take the place of timely communication. One of the shortcomings of living wills is that, unless we have the opportunity to discuss the document with the patient while the patient is still able to communicate, we cannot be certain of precisely what the patient's wishes were in conditions other than terminal illness. For example, some persons who have experienced a significant neurological insult, such as a massive cerebrovascular accident (CVA), might wish that life-sustaining treatment not be carried out. However, because a CVA does not generally produce a "terminal" condition, the living will is not applicable.

Similarly, the presence of a living will does not imply that a patient would refuse resuscitation in all situations. In addition, research indicates that relatively few patients (15% to 25%) use advance directives. There are probably many reasons for the low use of advance directives, including lack of understanding, reluctance to think about death and dying, and mistrust of health care professionals. Thus we can determine specific treatment preferences only through early and frequent discussions.[17,37]

A second type of advance directive, the durable power of attorney for health care (DPAHC), is more broad and flexible than a living will, and many people choose to have both instruments. The DPAHC transfers all rights that the individual normally has regarding health care decisions—such as accepting and refusing treatment, inspecting the medical record, and accepting or changing physicians—to another person called the "agent" or "attorney in fact."[1] Like a living will, the DPAHC goes into effect only when the individual has lost decision-making capacity. This, however, is the only criterion for activation. Thus, even if the individual is unconscious only for a short time, the DPAHC is in effect during that period; it is not limited to conditions of terminal illness. In addition, because the agent has all decision-making powers, the DPAHC is helpful in seeking any decision about care, including not only life-supporting treatments but also questions related to blood transfusions, antibiotic therapy, and surgical procedures.

Although the DPAHC is applicable in many more situations than is a living will, it does have the disadvantage of leaving all decision making in the hands of the agent. For this reason many people prefer to have both forms of advance directives. A living will is completed to indicate the patient's own wishes and relieve others of the burden of decision making in cases of terminal illness, and the DPAHC is completed to designate someone to make all other decisions.

The Patient Self-Determination Act (PSDA), part of the Omnibus Budget Reconciliation Act of 1991, is a federal law that makes it essential for all nurses to be familiar with the living will and DPAHC laws in their state. The PSDA requires three things of all hospitals, nursing homes, hospices, and home health care agencies. First, these facilities must inform all patients on admission to the facility of their rights under state law to use advance directives. Second, they must tell the patient about hospital policy regarding these directives. Third, they must ask if the patient has any advance directives in effect.[21,23,26] The response must be documented in the medical record. Hospitals have chosen several ways to comply with this law. In some facilities admissions clerks or social workers ask patients about advance directives, whereas in others the nurse who admits the patient to the hospital has this responsibility. Regardless of who raises this subject with the patient initially, the nurse caring for the patient must be prepared to discuss the topic with the patient, answer questions, or obtain other resources to assist patients. Both living wills and DPAHC forms should be available for patients to complete while hospitalized, if they so desire.

### TREATMENT LIMITATIONS

Decisions to limit treatment in some way are always associated with potential ethical concerns. The legal, moral, and practical aspects to these decisions often become intertwined. The fundamental principles involved in situations of limitation of treatment are clear. Patients have an almost absolute legal and moral right to make decisions to limit treatment in any way, regardless of whether that treatment is a life-sustaining one.[10,24,40] The only exception to this position occurs with pregnant women; in these cases courts have sometimes ruled that the concern for the welfare of the fetus justifies overriding the wishes of the mother regarding treatment.

It is important for the student to be aware of attempts that have been made in the past to differentiate acceptable forms of treatment limitation from unacceptable. At various times some have suggested that extraordinary treatments were not obligatory, whereas it was mandatory to administer "ordinary" treatments; that treatments could be withheld but not withdrawn; and that complex technological interventions could be withheld but that hydration and nutrition must always be provided.[29] The arguments involving each of these distinctions are complex, and the reader is referred to texts on bioethics for further discussion.[11] It is important, however, to understand that all these distinctions currently are viewed as unimportant and that any intervention to which a competent patient does not consent must be withheld or withdrawn if already being administered.

Although there is relatively complete consensus regarding the moral acceptability of limiting treatments that the patient wishes to stop or that are ineffective,[22] no such agreement exists regarding acts of active euthanasia. Intervening with the primary intention to cause death, with patient consent, and motivated by the wish to end suffering, is considered to be a form of active euthanasia. Similarly, acts of physicians that provide the patient with the means to end his or her own life are termed *aid-in-dying* or *physician-assisted suicide.* Opponents of such acts argue that in these cases, unlike situations in which medical treatment is withheld or withdrawn, the cause of death is not the illness itself but the person who intervenes. Deliberately causing death in this way is prohibited by law in some states and by all professional codes. Opponents argue that there is no morally relevant difference between withdrawing a treatment such as a mechanical ventilator, with the certain knowledge that death will occur, and administering a drug that will lead to a painless death.[12,29]

Public and professional concern about people who suffer prolonged, painful deaths has resulted in legislative attempts both to eliminate laws prohibiting physician-assisted suicide and to establish legal protection for physicians and others who assist a terminally ill patient in ending his or her life. Oregon is the first state to gain voter approval of such legislation, although this has been challenged in court. The United States Supreme Court has also been requested to review the constitutionality of laws prohibiting assisted suicide. Because the legal status of such acts differs from state to state, the nurse must be knowledgeable about the laws in the state in which he or she practices.[32,38]

Most important, the nurse must become knowledgeable about the moral issues involved and decide on a personal position on the question. Although it is more common for patients to request assistance with ending their life from physicians, nurses often are involved in these discussions with patients and families as they confront terminal illness. Consequently the nurse should be prepared to answer patients' questions about aid-in-dying and discuss the patient's concerns and fears about it.

When a situation occurs in which treatment limitation becomes an issue, inadequate communication leads to confusion. Any decision to limit treatment in any way must be documented in the physician's orders. The most common form of such treatment limitation orders is the do not resuscitate (DNR) order. This order reflects a decision to withhold cardiopulmonary resuscitation in the event of an arrest. Unless additional treatment restriction orders are written, a DNR order does not limit other forms of aggressive treatment, and patients with a DNR order should continue to receive close monitoring and any therapy necessary to prevent an arrest. This may include transfer to an intensive care unit, mechanical ventilation, or use of intravenous vasopressors. One of the most important responsibilities of the professional nurse in caring for the patient with a DNR order is to be certain that the exact intention of the DNR order is understood. Vague phrases such as "no heroics" should not be used because it is unclear to what specific interventions the word *heroics* refers.

The role of the nurse also includes being an active participant in discussions with patients and families regarding their wishes for treatment. It is essential that these discussions be documented and communicated to all persons involved in the patient's care.[21] It is not uncommon for the patient or the patient's family to first mention their thoughts about limiting or withdrawing treatment to the nurse, and the nurse can be instrumental in assisting the patient and family members in raising this issue with the patient's physician. Because issues such as patient requests for treatment termination often are complicated by differing views and uncertainty about the moral principles involved, it is helpful for the nurse to be aware of resources available.

## GENETIC TECHNOLOGY

The National Center for Human Genome Research was established in 1990 as part of the Human Genome Project, an international research effort. The specific aims of genetic research include identification of all human genes, determination of which genes or gene mutations result in abnormal conditions, and discovery of ways to predict, prevent, and treat genetic disorders such as cystic fibrosis, sickle cell disease, and muscular dystrophy.[21]

Knowledge of an individual's genetic predisposition and the potential for altering genetic structure can result in many ethical questions for professionals and persons undergoing genetic testing and therapy. (The most obvious of these are questions concerning confidentiality and privacy.) Information about an individual's genetic makeup may reveal a predisposition for certain diseases, such as breast cancer or Huntington's disease; in such situations, questions arise about who should have access to the data beyond the individual. Should the spouse, children, or insurance company be informed? Because our understanding of the link between specific genetic mutations and the eventual appearance of actual disease is not complete, there is also ongoing debate about the obligation and even the appropriateness of providing such information to persons themselves. Finally, the recently announced ability to clone "perfect" mammals, such as sheep and monkeys, has triggered deep moral concerns about misuse of human genetic technology to support racial prejudices and discriminatory attitudes toward people with less than "perfect" physical attributes.

Because genetic advances raise so many complex ethical issues, the National Institutes of Health established an Ethical, Legal, and Social Implications Branch of the Human Genome Project to analyze and make recommendations about social policy in the United States. In addition, the ANA conducted a study of the implications of genetic advances for nurses. The reader is referred to Scanlon and Fibison[31] for additional guidance when caring for individuals undergoing genetic testing.

## RESOURCES

### ETHICS COMMITTEES

Today many hospitals have ethics committees. These committees are multidisciplinary, and their purpose is to provide consultation to clinicians regarding specific ethical problems. They usually include physicians, nurses, hospital lawyers and administrators, social workers, and clergy. The conclusions of the committee generally are expressed as recommendations, and clinicans are not obligated to follow their advice.[9] Typically, anyone can request that the ethics committee consider a case. These committees are helpful in providing an objective review of the situation by personnel who are familiar with ethics and are knowledgeable about ethical analysis.[18]

In addition to formal committees, some hospitals have ethics consultation services. These services consist of several persons who have expertise in addressing ethical dilemmas and in helping others to resolve them. Consultation services are somewhat more flexible than committees in that the consultant usually can go to the patient care area on rather short notice to meet with the patient and family, perform an independent assessment of the situation, and meet immediately with the caregivers to offer advice.[35]

Even in hospitals in which the nurse does not have access to these formal resources, several general guidelines are available to the nurse who recognizes an ethical dilemma. It is almost always helpful for the nurse to discuss the ethical issue with at least one other person. This action helps ensure that all the data have been considered and that all options have been reviewed. Because ethical dilemmas often involve disagreements and controversy, it is beneficial for the nurse to have the support of peers.

In addition to colleagues, nurses must feel free to express ethical concerns to supervisors and others in the administrative hierarchy. Although most cases can be resolved through thoughtful reflection and clear, planned communication, some issues require administrative action. Policies such as those related to DNR orders, treatment withdrawal, refusal to care for certain patient groups, and concerns about appropriate staffing levels are examples of issues that cannot be resolved by individuals acting alone.

Most important, nurses must continue to develop their understanding of ethical principles and become comfortable with analyzing ethical dilemmas. This process involves gaining knowledge of specific theories, gaining insight into their own moral beliefs, and being willing to examine these beliefs for justification.

## critical thinking QUESTIONS

1 Why is knowledge and application of hospital policy alone inadequate for analyzing moral dilemmas?

2 How can you, as a nurse, assist patients in making decisions about their future health care?

## chapter SUMMARY

- Ethics is the study of the reasoned process of making moral decisions.
- Ethical dilemmas are situations in which there is a conflict between mutually exclusive rules or principles that appears to lack a correct or "right" answer.

### MORAL AGENCY

- Acting as a moral agent involves thoughtful consideration of principled reasons for actions, understanding of relevant laws and policies, and knowledge of the professional code of ethics.
- Unlike value judgments, moral judgments reflect evaluation of values and a search for justification. Judgments that involve the concepts of right and wrong, good and evil, go beyond personal preference and are impersonal.

### ETHICAL THEORIES AND PRINCIPLES

- Ethical theories provide a method for answering questions about right courses of action. The two major categories of ethical theories are consequentialist and nonconsequentialist.
- Virtually all theories emphasize the importance of three principles (autonomy, beneficence, and justice), although the justification for these principles differs.
- Autonomy refers to the right of self-determination. It depends on the possession of decision-making capacity and underlies specific rules of informed consent.
- Beneficence is a duty to benefit or do good. The obligation to help others is particularly important for professionals and directs us to promote the welfare of others when they cannot make autonomous choices. Acting in such a way as to benefit others while overriding or violating their right to make their own decisions constitutes paternalistic action.
- Justice is generally understood as the obligation to treat equals equally through equal concern and respect for their rights. The most important application of principles of justice today is the need for reform of the health care distribution system.

### RESOLVING ETHICAL DILEMMAS

- A five-step process for resolving ethical dilemmas is recommended. These steps are (1) reviewing the facts, (2) defining the problem, (3) listing the choices, (4) deciding on the action, and (5) evaluating the choice.

## COMMON ETHICAL ISSUES IN ACUTE CARE

- Advance directives are written instructions from the patient regarding his or her future health care. Examples of advance directives are the living will and durable power of attorney for health care.
- Do not resuscitate orders reflect the decision to withhold resuscitation should a cardiopulmonary arrest occur. They do not have implications for withholding or withdrawing other treatments, although additional interventions also may be limited by specific orders.
- There is currently much controversy regarding the moral status of patient requests for aid-in-dying, also called active euthanasia or assisted suicide. Professional codes and some state laws currently do not support involvement of nurses or physicians in active euthanasia.
- In caring for any patient for whom treatment limitation is being considered, the nurse should be an active participant in discussions and can play an important role in assisting patients and families in decision making.
- Ethics committees and ethics consultation services can be helpful resources to nurses and others in dealing with ethical problems.
- Documentation, communication, and gaining the support of peers and supervisory personnel are important steps in the process of seeking resolution.

## References


1. Abrams FR: Advance directives: when the patient cannot communicate. In Monagle JF, Thomasma DC, editors: *Medical ethics,* Rockville, Md, 1988, Aspen.
2. American Nurses' Association: *Code for Nurses,* Washington, DC, 1985, The Association.
3. American Nurses' Association: *Ethics in nursing,* Washington, DC, 1988, The Association.
4. American Nurses' Association: *Nursing's social policy statement,* Washington, DC, 1995, The Association.
5. Badzek LA: What you need to know about advance directives, *Nursing* 92(6):58, 1992.
6. Bandman EL, Bandman B: *Nursing ethics through the life span,* ed 2, Norwalk, Conn, 1992, Appleton & Lange.
7. Beauchamp TL, Childress JF: *Principles of biomedical ethics,* ed 3, New York, 1989, Oxford University Press.
8. Benjamin M, Curtis J: *Ethics in nursing,* ed 3, New York, 1992, Oxford University Press.
9. Blake DC: The hospital ethics committee, *Hastings Cent Rep* 22(1):6, 1992.
10. Bosek MSD: Doing good: an ethical quandary, *Medsurg Nurs* 4(2):154, 1995.
11. Brock D: Death and dying. In Veatch RM, editor: *Medical ethics,* Boston, 1989, Jones & Bartlett.
12. Brock D: Voluntary active euthanasia, *Hastings Cent Rep* 22(2):10, 1992.
13. Chafey K: Caring is not enough, *Nurs Health Care* 17(1):10, 1996.
14. Chell B: Competency: what it is and what it isn't. In Monagle JF, Thomasma DC, editors: *Medical ethics,* Rockville, Md, 1988, Aspen.
15. Cisar NS, Bell SK: Informed consent: an ethical dilemma, *Nurs Forum* 30(3):20, 1995.
16. Committee on Ways and Means, US House of Representatives: *Health care resources book,* Washington, DC, 1991, US Government Printing Office.
17. Emanuel L: Advance directives: what have we learned so far? *J Clin Ethics* 4(1):8, 1993.
18. Fletcher JC, Hoffman, DE: Ethics committees: time to experiment with standards, *Ann Intern Med* 120:335, 1994.
19. Gorovitz S: Informed consent and patient autonomy. In Callahan JC, editor: *Ethical issues in professional life,* New York, 1988, Oxford University Press.
20. Greipp ME: A survey of ethical decision making models in nursing, *J Nurs Sci* 1(1-2):51, 1995.
21. Idemoto B et al: Implementing the Patient Self-Determination Act, *Am J Nurs* 93(1):21, 1993.
22. Laffey J, Sr.: Bioethical principles and care-based ethics in medical futility, *Cancer Pract* 4(1):41, 1996.
23. Lo B: The clinical use of advance directives. In Monagle JF, Thomasma DC, editors: *Medical ethics,* Rockville, Md, 1988, Aspen.
24. Meisel A: The legal consensus about foregoing life-sustaining treatment: its status and prospects, *Kennedy Inst Ethics J* 2(4):309, 1992.
25. Meyer C: End-of-life care: patients' choices, nurses' challenges, *Am J Nurs* 93(2):40, 1993.
26. Mezey M, Latimer B: The Patient Self-Determination Act, *Hastings Cent Rep* 23(1):16, 1993.
27. Novak J: An ethical decision-making model for the neonatal intensive care unit, *J Perinat Nurs* 1(3):57, 1988.
28. Purtillo R: *Ethical dimensions in the health professions,* ed 2, Philadelphia, 1993, WB Saunders.
29. Rachels J: Euthanasia. In Regan T, editor: *Matters of life and death,* New York, 1986, Random House.
30. Rakowski E: *Equal justice,* Oxford, 1991, Clarendon Press.
31. Scanlon C, Fibison W: *Managing genetic information: implications for nursing practice,* Washington, DC, 1995, The Association.
32. Scanlon C, Rushton CH: Assisted suicide: clinical realities and ethical challenges, *Am J Crit Care* 5:397, 1996.
33. Schwarz JK: Living wills and health care proxies, *Nurs Health Care* 13(2):92, 1992.
34. Silva MC: The American Nurses' Association's Code for Nurses: purposes, content, and enforceability, *Health Matrix* 11(2):55, 1989.
35. Simpson KH: The development of a clinical ethics consultation service in a community hospital, *J Clin Ethics* 3(2):124, 1992.
36. SUPPORT Investigators: A controlled trial to improve care for seriously ill hospitalized patients: the Study to Understand Prognoses and Preferences for Outcomes and Risks of Treatment (SUPPORT), *JAMA* 274:1591, 1995.
37. Teno JM, Lynn J, Phillips RS, et al: Do formal advance directives affect resuscitation decisions and the use of resources for seriously ill patients? *J Clin Ethics* 5(1):23, 1994.
38. Tilden VP, Tolle SW, Lee MA, Nelson CA: Oregon's physician assisted suicide vote: its effect on palliative care, *Nurs Outlook* 44:80, 1996.
39. Veatch RM: Models for ethical medicine in a revolutionary age, *Hastings Cent Rep* 2(3):5, 1972.
40. Veatch RM: Foregoing life-sustaining treatment: limits to the consensus, *Kennedy Inst Ethics J* 3(1):1, 1993.
41. Wiens AG: Patient autonomy in care: a theoretical framework for nursing, *J Prof Nurs* 9(2):95, 1993.
42. Winslow GR: From loyalty to advocacy: a new metaphor for nursing, *Hastings Cent Rep* 14(3):32, 1984.
43. Wright RA: *Human values in health care,* New York, 1987, McGraw-Hill.

# chapter 6 Stress, Stressors, and Stress Management

DEBORAH K. MARANTIDES and VIRGINIA L. CASSMEYER

## objectives

*After studying this chapter, the learner should be able to:*

1. Describe the process of sensory reception and perception.
2. Compare and contrast stressors and stress response.
3. Correlate the relationship of dealing with stressors to optimal functioning and growth.
4. Describe the neuroendocrine response to stressors.
5. Describe behavioral responses to stressors.
6. Describe types of coping strategies.
7. Identify assessment parameters of anxiety.
8. Develop nursing interventions for persons with anxiety.
9. Evaluate different approaches to crisis intervention.
10. Implement methods of stress management.

*Stress, adaptation,* and *coping* are words commonly used in both lay and professional literature to refer to problematic biophysical-chemical or psychosocial-cultural situations. These words also are used to describe the body's response to or ways of dealing with problematic situations. These terms are entrenched in nursing literature to the extent that it is now understood that a major function of nursing is to help people cope with stressors and adapt to stressful situations.

Yet, when attempting to define these terms to study and understand them better, we find that there is no scientific consensus as to their meanings. Thus how can these terms be used professionally to understand the nature of human problem-solving behavior? Why have they come to such prominence in the helping professions? Is there a set of related phenomena that these terms describe, or should they be abandoned as jargon?

These terms are in the literature to stay, and they describe phenomena regarding the ways human beings deal with life's changing events. Each term provides a general reference point to approach common experiences of persons interacting with their environments even though precise definitions acceptable to most investigators have been elusive. At best, one may recognize common themes that emerge from the multiple perspectives of those who have tried to define these terms precisely.

*Stress* is a general term describing patterns of psychological and physiological responses to a variety of emotional and physical stimuli. Stress responses occur when the ordinary capacity to adapt to life's demands is taxed. Stress can thus be seen as a subset of the concept *adaptation*—or the processes of maintaining psychobiological equilibrium during interaction with the environment. *Coping* comprises those strategies by which adaptation to ordinary or extraordinary environmental demands is accomplished. In this chapter the common themes that have emerged from the scientific study of stressors, stress, adaptation, and coping are presented. These themes are then applied as a framework for management.

Richard A. Ade, RT, BSPA, RN, MPH, assisted in the revision of this chapter.

## STRESS

### HISTORICAL PERSPECTIVE

The term *stress* has been used colloquially for centuries to refer to mental and emotional strain or pressure. In physics, stress has a precise mechanical meaning—the force put on an object. The resulting deformation or response is designated as *strain.* Selye[29] was the first to use the term *stress* in a biological context—the nonspecific response of the body to a variety of noxious stimuli. He termed the stimulus the *stressor.* Initially, Selye[27] avoided the term *stress* because of its common use in connoting emotional turmoil. However, as he came to see that many strong stimuli were capable of provoking the general adaptation syndrome, he postulated that emotional stimuli were equivalent to physical stressors (e.g., heat, cold, or trauma) in evoking the response, and he began to use stress as synonymous with the general adaptation syndrome.[29]

The notion of a general integrated and mutually interacting biological and psychological response to a variety of environmental stimuli was not unique to Selye. In fact, his work was preceded by the philosophic writings of James,[13] who proposed that the perception of visceral responses to emotional events *was* the emotion; by the experiments of Cannon,[7] who observed the similarity of physiological responses of the sympathetic nervous system or the "fight or flight response" during a variety of emotional states; and by Jacobsen,[12] who documented responses of the sympathetic nervous system and skeletal muscles to emotional states. Wihelm Raab subsequently demonstrated the risk effects of excess adrenaline and cortisol.

### STRESSORS

Many different studies have shown that stressors can be biological, physical, chemical, social, developmental, cultural, or psychological stimuli.[32,35] Stressors can vary from an alarm clock that does not go off on time, to an approaching deadline, to the onset of the common cold in a relatively healthy person, to major burns covering more than 50% of the body. The stressors that nurses deal with vary depending on the patient population. Nurses in outpatient settings, in home health care, or in discharge planning may focus more on patients' daily irritations and primary health care problems. Nurses working with patients during the acute or critical stages of illness may deal with more severe physiological stressors.

Box 6-1 lists some common stimuli affecting hospitalized adults that may be perceived as stressors. Although this list is not exhaustive, it contains stressors that might be more universally found in acute and critical care settings. The list can be used during assessment to identify potential stressors. One of the first steps in providing quality care to manage stressors is to be able to identify potential stressors.

**box 6-1** *Common Stimuli Affecting Hospitalized Adults That May Be Perceived as Stressors*

**BIOPHYSICAL-CHEMICAL**

| | |
|---|---|
| Hypoxia | Trauma |
| Hypercapnia | Pain |
| Hypoglycemia | Illness |
| Hypovolemia | Surgery |
| Hypotension | Immobilization |
| Alcohol | Restraints |
| Caffeine | Constant light |
| Drugs | Noise |
| X-ray contrast media | Sleep deprivation |
| Anesthesia | Discomfort |
| Blood transfusions | Fatigue |
| Weakness | Burns |
| Infections | |

**PSYCHOSOCIOCULTURAL**

| | |
|---|---|
| Anger | Uncertainty |
| Fear | Dependency |
| Loss | Invasion of privacy |
| Isolation | Sensory deprivation |
| Sensory overload | Financial burdens |
| Role changes | Language barriers |
| Guilt | Exposure of body |
| Loss of control | Unpleasant sights and sounds |
| Stigma of diagnosis | Change in body image |
| Unfamiliar sounds | Loss of function |
| Anxiety | |

## STRESS RESPONSE

The stress response includes intellectual, behavioral, and emotional components, such as decision-making activities, withdrawal, and anger, as well as physiological components. The physiological components involved in the stress response include the central nervous system, the hypothalamus, the sympathetic nervous system, the anterior and posterior pituitary glands, the adrenal medulla, and the adrenal cortex. The physiological components and their secretions (hormones and catecholamines) are responsible for the neuroendocrine response to stressors. Not all of these components will necessarily be involved in the response to every stressor; however, to provide holistic nursing care, the nurse must know the effects of stimulation of each of these components of the neuroendocrine response to stressors. Understanding the response is critical to (1) identify persons at high risk for impaired ability to deal with stressors, (2) understand how prolonged or repeated stressors can result in disease, and (3) understand how the neuroendocrine component of the stress response eventually can become a threat to health.

The physiological components of the neuroendocrine stress response are diagrammed in Figure 6-1. Stressors—perceived either at the level of the central nervous system or on an unconscious level by baroreceptors, chemoreceptors, or glucoreceptors, which transfer information to the medulla oblongata—serve as the afferent input. This information eventually is forwarded to the hypothalamus, which coordinates the response. The hypothalamus activates the sympathetic nervous system and the anterior and posterior pituitary glands. The adrenal medulla is an extension of the sympathetic nervous system and thus is activated when the sympathetic nervous system is stimulated.

The hypothalamus stimulates the anterior pituitary gland by releasing hormones such as corticotropin-releasing hormone (CRH), growth hormone-releasing hormone (GHRH), and prolactin-releasing hormone (PRH). Some anterior pituitary hormones will be released when the hypothalamus diminishes its secretion of inhibiting hormones. For example, dopamine acts as a prolactin-inhibiting hormone (PIH), and thus prolactin secretion is increased when dopamine secretion is decreased.

Adrenocorticotropic hormone (ACTH), which is released from the anterior pituitary gland, stimulates the release of cortisol from the adrenal cortex. The adrenal cortex also releases the hormone aldosterone in response to ACTH secretion. However, the major control of aldosterone secretion is the renin-angiotensin-system, which is shown in Figure 6-2.

The last endocrine gland activated by the hypothalamus is the posterior pituitary gland. The posterior pituitary gland is also activated by the hypothalamus. When stimulated, the posterior pituitary releases antidiuretic hormone or vasopressin. The effects of stimulation of the sympathetic nervous system, anterior and posterior pituitary glands, adrenal medulla, and adrenal cortex are mediated by the catecholamines and hormones released by the nervous system or the glands.

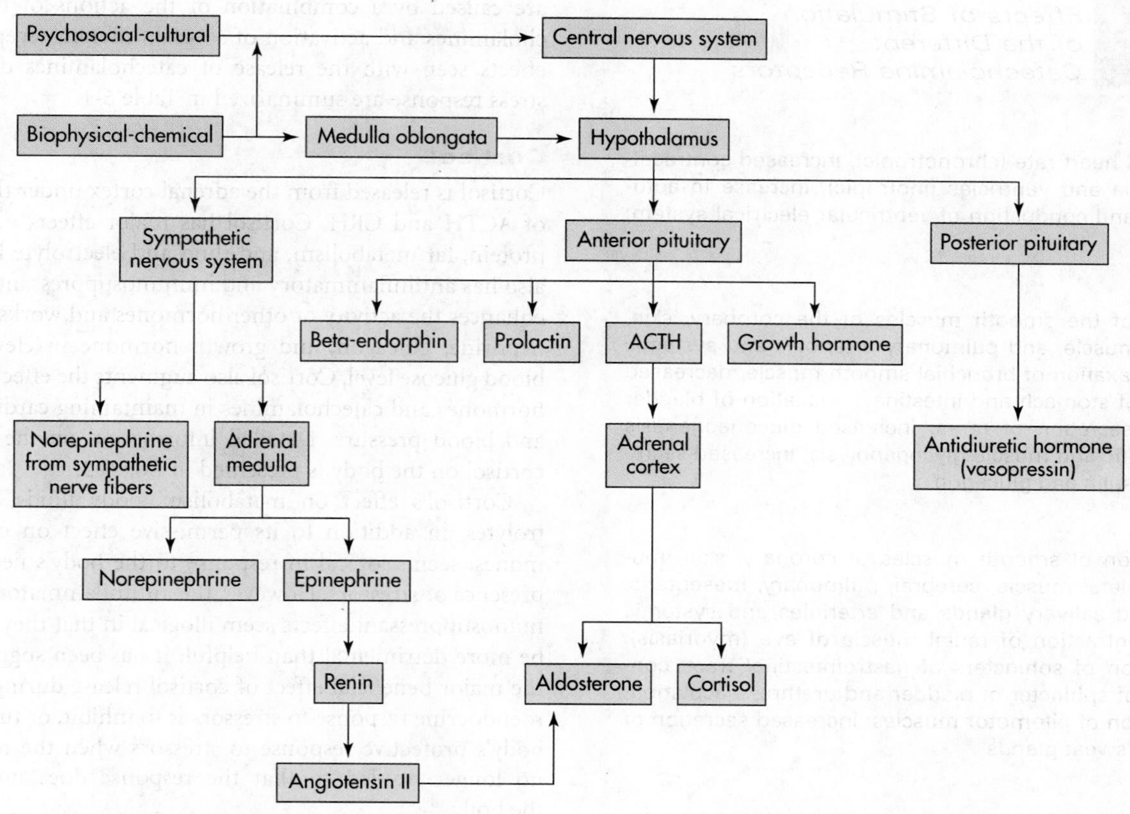


**fig. 6-1** Physiological components involved in the neuroendocrine response to stressors.

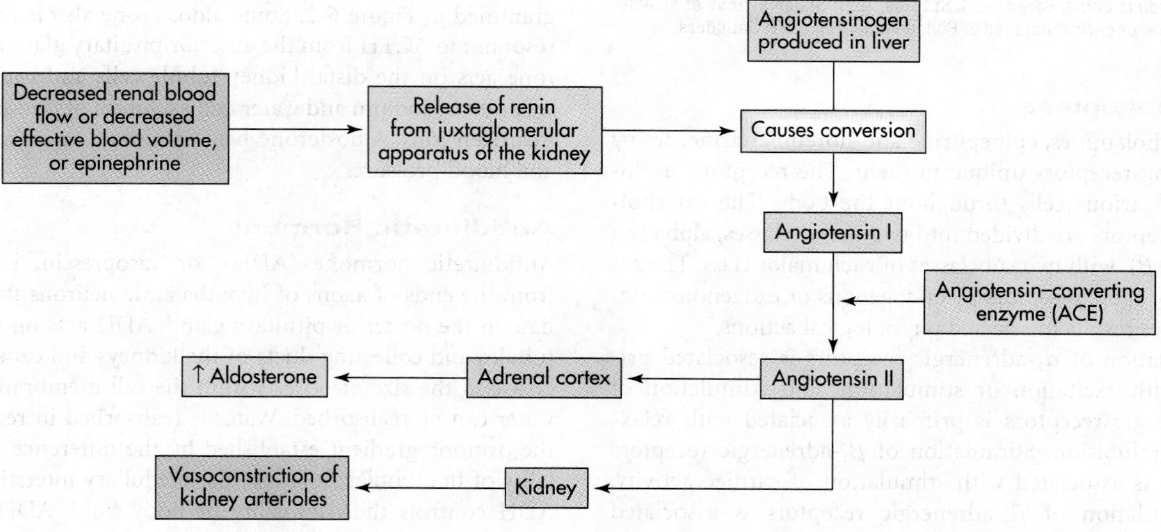


**fig. 6-2** Renin-angiotensin-aldosterone system.

**box 6-2** *Summary of the Physiological Effects of Stimulation of the Different Catecholamine Receptors*

$\beta_1$

Increased heart rate (chronotropic), increased contractility of atria and ventricles (inotropic), increase in automaticity and conduction of ventricular electrical system; lipolysis

$\beta_2$

Dilation of the smooth muscles of the coronary, skin, skeletal muscle, and pulmonary arterioles and systemic veins; relaxation of bronchial smooth muscle; decreased motility of stomach and intestines; relaxation of bladder muscle; secretion of renin; increased gluconeogenesis and hepatic and muscle glycogenolysis; increased secretion of insulin and glucagon

$\alpha_1$

Contraction of smooth muscles of coronary, skin, mucosa, skeletal muscle, cerebral, pulmonary, mesenteric, renal, and salivary glands and arterioles and systemic veins; contraction of radial muscle of eye (mydriasis); contraction of sphincters of gastrointestinal tract; contraction of sphincter of bladder and urethra; ejaculation; contraction of pilomotor muscles; increased secretion of localized sweat glands

$\alpha_2$

Decreased motility of gastrointestinal tract; decreased insulin secretion; platelet aggregation; possibly decreased secretion of intestinal tract

Data from McCance KL, Huether SE: *Pathophysiology: the biologic basis for disease in adults and children,* ed 3, St Louis, 1997; Shoemaker W et al, editors: *Textbook of critical care,* ed 2, Philadelphia, 1995, WB Saunders.

### Catecholamines

The catecholamines, epinephrine and norepinephrine, act by stimulating receptors unique to them. The receptors are located on various cells throughout the body. The catecholamine receptors are divided into two major classes, alpha ($\alpha$) and beta ($\beta$), with two subclasses of each major class. The activation of these receptors by endogenous or exogenous catecholamines results in selected physiological actions.

Stimulation of $\alpha_1$-adrenergic receptors is associated primarily with excitation or stimulation, and stimulation of $\alpha_2$-adrenergic receptors is primarily associated with relaxation or inhibition. Stimulation of $\beta_1$-adrenergic receptors primarily is associated with stimulation of cardiac activity, and stimulation of $\beta_1$-adrenergic receptors is associated with all other effects related to $\beta$ receptors, such as bronchial dilation. (See Box 6-2 for a more detailed description of functions associated with stimulation of specific receptor types.)

During the neuroendocrine response to stressors, both norepinephrine and epinephrine are released. Norepinephrine binds primarily to $\alpha$-adrenergic receptors, whereas epinephrine activates both $\alpha$-adrenergic and $\beta$-adrenergic receptors. The effects of catecholamines during the stress response are caused by a combination of the actions of both catecholamines and activation of several different receptors. The effects seen with the release of catecholamines during the stress response are summarized in Table 6-1.

### Cortisol

Cortisol is released from the adrenal cortex under the control of ACTH and CRH. Cortisol has major effects on glucose, protein, fat metabolism, and fluid and electrolyte balance; it also has antiinflammatory and immunosuppressant effects. It enhances the activity of other hormones and works with epinephrine, glucagon, and growth hormone in elevating the blood glucose level. Cortisol also augments the effects of other hormones and catecholamines in maintaining cardiac output and blood pressure. Detailed information on the effects of cortisol on the body is presented in Box 6-3.

Cortisol's effect on metabolism, body fluids, and electrolytes, in addition to its permissive effect on other hormones, seems logical in response to the body's needs in the presence of stressors. However, the antiinflammatory and immunosuppressant effects seem illogical in that they appear to be more detrimental than helpful. It has been suggested that the major beneficial effect of cortisol release during the neuroendocrine response to stressors is to inhibit, or turn off, the body's protective response to stressors when the response is no longer needed so that the response does not damage the body.[10]

### Aldosterone

Aldosterone is released primarily from the adrenal cortex in response to activation of the renin-angiotensin system as diagrammed in Figure 6-2. Some aldosterone also is released in response to ACTH from the anterior pituitary gland. Aldosterone acts on the distal kidney tubule cells and causes reabsorption of sodium and water and excretion of potassium and hydrogen ions. Aldosterone helps maintain vascular volume and blood pressure.

### Antidiuretic Hormone

Antidiuretic hormone (ADH), or vasopressin, is released from the ends of axons of hypothalamic neurons that terminate in the posterior pituitary gland. ADH acts on the distal tubules and collecting ducts of the kidneys and causes an increase in the size of pores within the cell membrane so that water can be reabsorbed. Water is reabsorbed in response to the osmotic gradient established by the difference in osmolality of the tubular fluid and the medullary interstitial fluid. ADH controls the osmolality of body fluid. ADH in high concentrations can result in arteriole vasoconstriction and can help to increase blood pressure. Vasopressin also stimulates the release of ACTH and thus influences the pituitary-adrenocortical response to stressors.

### Other Pituitary Hormones

Endogenous opiates ($\beta$-endorphins) are released as part of the neuroendocrine response to stressors. These endogenous

**table 6-1** *Systemic Effects of Epinephrine and Norepinephrine Released During the Neuroendocrine Response to Stressors*

| Organ | Physiological Effects | Assessment Findings |
|---|---|---|
| Brain | Blood vessels dilated; blood flow increased; metabolism increased | Patient more alert or restless |
| Eyes | Dilation of pupils | Pupils dilated; patient appears startled |
| Heart | Coronary blood vessels dilated; increased heart rate; increased contractility; cardiac output and stroke volume increased | Tachycardia, increased cardiac output |
| Vascular system | Constriction of arterioles to skin, mucosa, kidneys, and abdominal viscera; increased constriction of veins; ischemia with result of tissue death may occur | Skin pale, cool; urine output decreased; toe temperature decreased; with ischemia of kidneys, fluid retention, increased blood urea nitrogen, and increased serum creatinine level; with ischemia of gastrointestinal (GI) tract decreased bowel sounds |
| Lungs | Dilation of pulmonary vascular bed; bronchodilation; increased rate and depth of respiration; increased $O_2$ uptake and increased $CO_2$ excretion | Tachypnea; hyperventilation; respiratory alkalosis (decreased $Pco_2$ and increased pH) |
| Gastrointestinal tract | Decreased motility and secretion; decreased production of mucus; decreased blood flow to GI tract | Blood in GI secretions (nasogastric or stool) |
| Exocrine pancreas | Decreased enzyme, fluid, and electrolyte secretions | Elevated blood glucose |
| Endocrine pancreas | Decreased insulin secretion | Elevated blood glucose |
| Liver | Increased gluconeogenesis and glycogenolysis; decreased glycogen synthesis; decreased glucose uptake | |
| Adipose tissue | Increased lipolysis and fatty acid production | Increased serum triglycerides and lipoproteins |
| Skeletal muscle | Increased muscle glycogenolysis; decreased glucose uptake; increased contractility | Generalized muscle tension |
| Skin, sweat glands | Decreased blood flow; increased localized secretion of sweat; piloerection | Skin cool, pale, moist; goosebumps present |

**box 6-3** *Systemic Effects of Cortisol Release During the Neuroendocrine Response to Stressors*

**METABOLIC EFFECTS**

1. Maintains blood glucose by increasing gluconeogenesis and decreasing glucose uptake by many body cells, particularly muscle
2. Increases protein catabolism, which provides substrate for glucose formation
3. Promotes lipolysis to provide alternative nutrient sources

**FLUID AND ELECTROLYTE EFFECTS**

1. Promotes sodium and water retention
2. Promotes potassium excretion

**ANTIINFLAMMATORY/IMMUNOSUPPRESSIVE EFFECTS**

1. Decreases eosinophils, basophils, monocytes, and lymphocytes in the circulation
2. Increases neutrophils (polymorphonuclear leukocytes) by movement from bone marrow and circulatory pools
3. Decreases leukocyte accumulation at inflammatory sites
4. Inhibits release of inflammatory substances (kinins, prostaglandins, leukotrienes)
5. Degrades collagen
6. Decreases scar tissue formation
7. Decreases lymphoid tissue mass, participation of T lymphocytes in cellular-mediated immunity, and production of interleukins

**MISCELLANEOUS EFFECTS**

1. Maintains emotional stability
2. Increases red blood cell formation
3. Possibly increases platelet formation
4. Increases gastric acid and pepsin production
5. Is permissive for other hormones and catecholamines (i.e., cortisol is necessary for the full functioning of some hormones and catecholamines), particularly in relation to effects of epinephrine and norepinephrine on blood pressure control, cardiac output, and metabolism

opiates may be involved in the pituitary-adrenocortical response to stressors, and they are known to increase tolerance to painful stimuli. Release of endogenous opiates in stressful situations may account for the analgesic effect present in persons who experience major traumas.

Growth hormone is released from the anterior pituitary during the neuroendocrine response to stressors. Hypoglycemia and strenuous exercise are two stressors associated with an increase in growth hormone. Growth hormone helps to provide nutrients for the energy needs of various cells and tissues during the stress response. Growth hormone decreases glucose use and is an insulin antagonist; thus it helps to maintain the blood glucose level, which provides glucose for the nervous tissue. Growth hormone increases lipolysis, free fatty acid levels, and ketone formation, which furnish nutrients for various tissues, such as skeletal and cardiac muscles.

Prolactin[20] also is released in the presence of certain stressors. The function of prolactin in relation to dealing with stressors is unknown.

## Effects of Stress Response

The catecholamines, ACTH, cortisol, ADH, endogenous opiates, and growth hormone released during the neuroendocrine response to stressors provide a total body response that allows the individual to cope with or to withdraw from the stressors. The total body response includes:

1. Increase in blood levels of substrates necessary for energy—glucose for nervous tissue and fatty acid substrates for other tissues
2. Increase in oxygen uptake to provide oxygen for metabolic processes
3. Maintenance of vascular volume and increase in cardiac function for transport of nutrients and oxygen to tissues and for removal of waste products
4. Increase in respiratory activity for the elimination of excessive carbon dioxide that will be produced while the person is coping with the stressor and for the delivery of more oxygen
5. Increase in muscle activity and alertness that might allow for flight from the stressor
6. Increase in blood flow to brain that might allow for critical decision making, activation of psychological defense mechanisms, or problem solving

The intensity of the stress response depends on a combination of (1) intensity of stimulus, (2) duration of stimulus, and (3) perception of control over the stimulus.

### Intensity of stimulus

Intense physical and psychological stimuli such as trauma, forceful immobilization, and strong fear lead to stress responses in most human beings. Animal research has revealed a graduated multisystem response to graduated increases in intensity of the trauma.[10] A similar graded response is at least partially evident in human response to various traumas and surgical procedures. For example, the metabolic response to burns covering more than 40% of the body area is considerably greater than that to a hernia repair. The psychological component (threat, fear, inescapability, and lack of control) also is greater for the patient with a burn than for the person undergoing elective surgery.

### Duration of stimulus

Some investigators have suggested that although most organisms may have similar emergency responses to acute and intense stimuli, ongoing stimuli may elicit different individual responses. The adaptive response of one organism to ongoing stimuli may either resemble or differ from the response of another organism. The works with colonies of mice by Henry and Ely is the most extensive long-term investigation of the physiological responses of animals to their ordinary social interactions.[11] As these animals established their social dominance hierarchy, those who became the dominant animals exhibited primarily sympathetic-adrenal medullary activation, characterized biochemically by elevated catecholamine levels, behaviorally by muscular activity, and symptomatically by hypertension. In contrast, the animals at the bottom of the social hierarchy showed primarily a pituitary-adrenocortical response: elevated corticosteroid levels, withdrawn behavior, and ultimately enlarged adrenal glands and stomach ulcers. The animals who challenged the dominant animals had profiles midway between the two groups. Although this study is not intended to suggest that socially dominant persons will become hypertensive, it does support the notion that in ordinary daily living, living beings tend to respond in a characteristic mode. This mode depends partially on genetic factors, social position, and learned modes of coping with or responding to everyday events.

### Perception of control

Perception of control over a situation and relevant feedback regarding the effect of one's behavior on the stimulus appear to be potent factors regulating the multihormonal stress response. When a dominant animal from Henry's mouse colony was put into a colony in which dominance had already been established, the previously dominant mouse became submissive, and its behavior and physiological response became that of the submissive mice. One could argue that the mouse perceived itself as no longer being in control. Parachutists in training in Norway exhibited all the characteristic neuroendocrine stress responses before their first jump but rapidly returned to baseline values with subsequent jumps. Their subjective fear decreased as their sense of mastery and control over the task increased.[16] Additional animal studies demonstrated that control over aversive stimuli (shock) and relevant feedback regarding one's efforts reduced and even prevented pathological physiological stress responses in a variety of situations.[10]

The concepts of hardiness and resilience in human beings have been shown to be important factors in maintaining health in stressful situations.[16] Perception of control over life situations is a key component of these concepts. Stress has been linked both in the popular press and in scientific literature with disease, presumably caused by prolonged or excessive physiological responses to a variety of situations. It should be evident from the foregoing that it is not the situations by themselves that create the stress response, but rather the combination of psychological appraisal and sense of control.[25] These concepts lead logically to the notion of coping with change: the perception and appraisal of some relevant but challenging situation and the psychobiological responses emanating from that perception.[25,33]

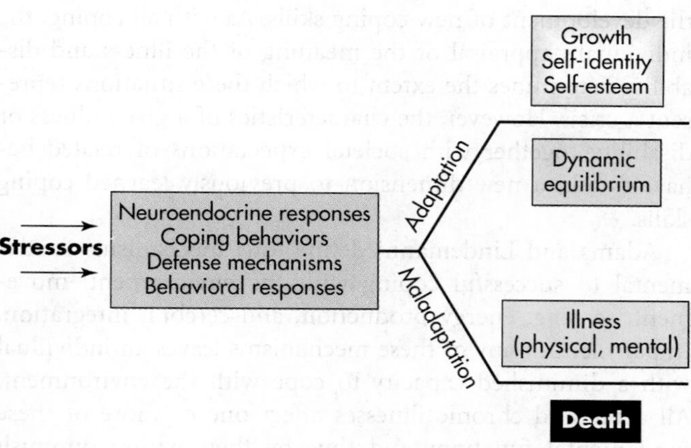


**fig. 6-3** Responses to stressors may lead to adaptation or maladaptation.

## ADAPTATION

Human beings can be conceptualized as open systems that respond to stimuli from the internal and external environments. This process of interaction can be termed *adaptation*. In this context, adaptation has neither positive nor negative values. However, many prefer to use the term in a positive sense to mean the process of interaction with the environment that promotes homeostasis or dynamic equilibrium and growth. The process that leads to inadequate functioning is then termed *maladaptation* or ineffective adaptation. Within the nursing field, the concept of adaptation is most closely associated with Roy.[26]

Human beings adapt biologically, psychologically, emotionally, and socially. The goal of biological adaptation is survival or stability of internal processes. When the ability to maintain this equilibrium is lost, pathophysiological disorders result. Psychological and emotional adaptation is directed toward preservation of self-identity and self-esteem. The person adapting in these modes is mentally healthy, whereas maladaptation leads to mental illness. Social adaptation depends on the sociocultural expectations of the society of which the person is a member. A maladaptive or socially deviant behavior in one society may be acceptable in another.

Although any changing environmental stimuli can initiate the need for adaptation, stressors create major adaptive demands for humans. As shown in Figure 6-3 the neuroendocrine responses, coping behaviors, defense mechanisms, and behavioral responses are major strategies available for meeting adaptive demands associated with stressors. Nurses help patients adapt at many levels by helping patients to:

1. Identify and remove stressors that require adaptive demands
2. Support healthy strategies that meet the adaptive demands of stressors
3. Deal with the psychological responses to stressors
4. Develop alternative coping behaviors or behavioral responses to stressors
5. Deal with the illnesses that result if adaptation is not effective

### General Adaptation Syndrome

Selye's work led him to label the nonspecific response to various agents as the *general adaptation syndrome (GAS)*.[29-31] GAS became known as the *stress syndrome* and was viewed by Selye as having three stages:

1. *The alarm reaction,* during which protective resources are mobilized
2. *The stage of resistance* that occurs when the full syndrome is in place and the stressor is being controlled
3. *The stage of exhaustion* that occurs when the body is not able to control the stressor

Selye[30,31] also proposed that the hormones produced during the GAS were responsible for the "diseases of adaptation." The stress response or GAS involves the sympathetic branch of the autonomic nervous system and the pituitary and adrenal glands. Selye also described the *local adaptation syndrome (LAS),* which is the response to a locally applied stimulus. The inflammatory process is an example of the LAS.

Some major criticisms of Selye's work should be noted. First, in his early work Selye did not acknowledge that psychological events could serve as stressors, although his later writings included this acknowledgment.[30] The work of various persons as early as the 1950s[19] revealed that the GAS could be elicited in response to psychological stimuli.

Another criticism of Selye's work was the idea that stimuli that serve as stressors were stressors for everyone. The work of Lazarus[15] pointed out that a stimulus must be perceived as a stressor before the GAS response is elicited. Important in this perception process is the analysis of the stimulus in terms of the person's resources and the perception of the stimulus as controllable or uncontrollable.

Another important factor in relation to psychological and emotional influences on physiological stressors is that in some experiments[17-20] in which physical stressors were induced while the discomfort, suddenness, or unpleasantness of the stimuli was controlled or minimized, the GAS was not elicited. This may mean that all stressor stimuli must have a psychosocial-cultural component.

One last criticism of Selye's work relates to his description of the stress response as nonspecific. This characteristic means that the same response will occur regardless of the stressor. It has been shown that different hormonal and neurochemical responses occur in response to different stressors.[10] Despite these criticisms, Selye's work provides the basis of the physiological response that can be elicited by stressors and an appreciation of the various stimuli that may serve as stressors in many persons.

## COPING

The definitions of coping are as many and varied as those for adaptation and stress. White[38] considers coping the strategies of adaptation—the means by which adaptation takes place. Coping is often defined as involving problem-solving efforts in situations that are perceived as being highly relevant to the individual and that tax adaptive resources. Although many persons explicitly or implicitly consider coping to be primarily a cognitive process, some authors recognize the interrelationship between physiological and cognitive responses to adverse circumstances. Levine, Weinberg, and Ursin[16] define the ultimate goal of coping processes to be reduction of physiological activation, whereas Murphy[22] divides coping processes into coping I, the capacity to deal with the changing environment (action and cognition), and coping II, the capacity to maintain the internal environment.

In general, then, coping refers to processes or skills that individuals use to deal with events, circumstances, or situations that are out of the ordinary. Coping is an integrated psychobiological process. The stimuli that elicit coping may arise in the external environment in the form of physical stimuli, interpersonal relationships, or community and international events. Similarly, stimuli may arise in the internal environment in terms of thoughts, feelings, and physical illness.

## GENERAL THEMES IN COPING

Coping processes enable us to learn from new situations strategies that may be useful in the future. These strategies emerge from what has been learned from past experience. Coping processes may thus be considered the major means for growth in the continual process of adaptation. When various perspectives in coping are evaluated, recurrent themes are evident: (1) coping stems from appraisal of relevant situations; (2) there is motivation to change; (3) information must be sought and used; (4) either action is practiced and tried or attitudes are changed; (5) there must be relevant feedback regarding coping efforts; and (6) coping takes place in a social context that defines appropriate and inappropriate behaviors. Over time people tend to develop coping styles, by using strategies that have served them well in the past to reduce physiological arousal and to meet the developmental challenges of maturation.

Coping strategies have been categorized as those involving direct action on oneself or on the environment or those involving intrapsychic processes. With direct action one may change the environment or oneself or in some way directly confront or avoid the situation from which the need to cope arises. Intrapsychic processes are largely cognitive ways of changing the meaning of the situation or of dealing with the emotions that arise from the situation. Many investigators have found that those who are judged as coping most successfully with a variety of situations are flexible in using strategies from both categories rather than rigidly repeating the same strategies in each new situation.[33]

## COPING IN ILLNESS AND DISABILITY

Illness often represents a crisis that challenges comfortable coping styles. Chronic illness and physical disability demand the development of new coping skills. As with all coping, the individual's appraisal of the meaning of the illness and disability determines the extent to which these situations represent a crisis. However, the characteristics of a given illness or disability together with societal expectations of related behaviors add a new dimension to previously learned coping skills.

Adams and Lindemann[1] define four mechanisms fundamental to successful coping with the environment: movement, sensing, energy production, and cerebral integration. Impairment of any of these mechanisms leaves an individual with a diminished capacity to cope with the environment. All acute and chronic illnesses affect one or more of these fundamental functions and thus by their nature diminish the available capacity for coping. When experiencing acute or chronic illness, people have two sets of adaptive tasks, as defined by Moos[21]: general tasks, as in any life crisis, and illness-related tasks. The general tasks defined by many authors include maintaining a sense of personal worth or self-esteem, maintaining a reasonable emotional balance, maintaining or restoring relationships with significant persons, and preparing for an uncertain future. Illness-related tasks include dealing with pain and incapacitation, enhancing the recovery of body functions, dealing with the hospital environment, and developing adequate relationships with hospital personnel.

Chronic illness or disability imposes additional adaptive tasks.[34] These tasks include preventing medical crises, controlling ongoing systems, carrying out treatment regimens, adjusting to changes in the disease course, maintaining self-esteem, obtaining funding for survival and ongoing treatment, adapting to or preventing social isolation, normalizing relationships with others, and confronting psychological, marital, and familial problems (see Chapter 7).

A number of coping skills are as relevant to dealing with illness and disability as they are to general crisis situations. They relate to both action (problem-focused) or intrapsychic (emotion-focused) strategies.

Action-focused strategies include seeking relevant information about the illness or disability, learning procedures or tasks specifically related to it, setting concrete and realistic goals, and rehearsing alternative outcomes.[21] For example, a person faced with hemodialysis for renal failure may cope with this major change in lifestyle by learning everything possible about home dialysis, and the procedures that must be mastered to safely accomplish this task. Information regarding expected energy levels, time required for dialysis, and duration between treatments may help the person set realistic goals for employment or education. Rehearsal of alternative outcomes is a strategy by which possible outcomes are thought about and discussed and possible options are considered (e.g., kidney transplantation or death). Rehearsal is one strategy by which all of us "practice" behaviors for anticipated circumstances.

Intrapsychic strategies include reframing the problem or finding some meaning or general purpose in it. If the event is explicable in the context of some larger purpose or understanding of life, distressing emotions may become more manageable and energy can be freed to focus on the problem itself. Simultaneously, one may be requesting reassurance and emotional support from others in the environment. Such support helps reaffirm a sense of personal worth in the face of major change.

There is no one specific or best way to cope with any given situation. What is useful to one individual may be inappropriate for another. The nature of the particular illness, the person's state of development, the social and cultural environment, and the physical and interpersonal resources available influence the style and effectiveness of coping strategies. In nursing, it is most useful to assist a person to cope in ways that are congruent with previously established styles. Weisman[36] suggests seven simple questions that can provide a great deal of information about coping strategies:

1. What problems, if any, do you see this illness creating?
2. How do you plan to deal with them?
3. When faced with a problem you must do something about, what do you do?
4. How does it usually work out?
5. To whom do you turn when you need help?
6. What has happened in the past when you have asked for help?
7. What kinds of problems usually tend to get you upset or down?

These questions establish perception of the current situation, usual style of dealing with problems, sources of help and response to help, and recurrent trouble areas.

## DEFENSE MECHANISMS

Coping strategies are not entirely rational. Emotional responses to crises are dominant and interact with action responses at all points. Emotional strategies that serve to protect us, consciously or unconsciously, from severe distress or anxiety are often called *defense mechanisms*. Defense mechanisms are processes that evolve during personality development and serve to protect the personality, satisfy emotional needs, maintain harmony between conflicting tendencies, and reduce tension or anxiety by modifying reality to make it more acceptable. Defense mechanisms are compromise solutions (see the accompanying Research Box).

There are two levels of defense mechanisms: those that are considered more primitive and those that are of a higher level (Box 6-4). Defense mechanisms are used by all persons. Defense mechanisms become pathological when they are overused. A person may have difficulty making rational decisions, working productively, or engaging in healthy relationships when overused. The alcoholic frequently overuses denial, rationalization, and projection.

A defense mechanism is effective when it succeeds in easing intrapsychic tensions. When lower level defense mechanisms fail, a more pathological process evolves, and the person exhibits psychiatric symptoms. All defense mechanisms are unconscious with the exception of suppression. The hospitalized patient frequently manifests two defense mechanisms, denial and repression.

## SPECIFIC BEHAVIORAL RESPONSES

Stressors and the stress response lead to behaviors that are either adaptive or maladaptive. Persons who display adaptive behavior are those who make appropriate use of their coping mechanisms and do not exhibit symptoms of psychological disturbance. Those with maladaptive behavior are at the other end of the spectrum (Figure 6-4); their psychiatric symptoms are a way of dealing with the increased stress. (For further information on maladaptive behavior consult a psychiatric-mental health text.) Anxiety and other common behaviors resulting from the stress of illness are discussed in the following section.

### Anxiety

Anxiety is a psychological response to stressors that has both physiological and psychological components. Anxiety is a feeling of dread or uneasiness from an unrecognized source. It differs from fear, which is a feeling of dread focused on a recognized source. Anxiety results when a person perceives a threat to the self either physically or psychologically (such as to self-esteem, body image, or identity). Anxiety manifests in different levels, ranging from mild to severe.[24] Box 6-5 presents the behavioral changes that are commonly associated with the different levels of anxiety. Awareness, which is heightened with mild anxiety, begins to decrease until the panic stage, in which perceptions of the environment become distorted. Persons can vacillate among the levels of anxiety. The

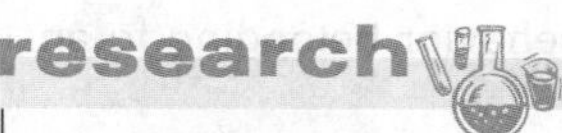

Reference: Leary J, et al: Stress and coping strategies in community psychiatric nurses: a Q-methodological study, *J Advan Nurse* 21:230-237, 1995.

The changing health environment has led to a decrease in inpatient psychotherapy, which in turn has led to a need for more community psychiatric nurses. This study explores the evolving role of the community psychiatric nurse (CPN) in relation to occupational stress, coping strategies, and how these nurses define their stressors. The study evaluated 21 CPNs using semistructured, open-ended interviews. Stressors identified included isolation, communications problems, lack of training, supervision of students, inappropriate referrals, potential violence from patients, unfair expectations, and lack of cooperation. The coping strategies used were organization, planning, decreasing work load, peer support, acceptance of stress, communication, advice seeking, outside interests, independence, and autonomy. The results of this study identified professional isolation as the dominant stressor. Time management practices emerged as the leading method of coping with stress. Further research was suggested to identify the relationship between different areas of stress and coping strategies that are effective in different situations.

**box 6-4** *Defense Mechanisms*

**HIGHER LEVEL: LESS PRIMITIVE MECHANISMS**

**Repression**
Ideas painful to consciousness are forced into the unconscious.

**Suppression**
Thoughts or desires are consciously inhibited.

**Sublimation**
Energy of repressed tendencies is transformed and directed to socially acceptable goals.

**Identification**
Person assumes the personal qualities or elements of the personality of another.

**Compensation**
Person makes up, covers up, or disguises real or fancied inadequacies in another area.

**Displacement**
An emotion is transferred or displaced from its original object to a more acceptable substitute that is less threatening.

**Rationalization**
Plausible explanations are given to account for a belief or behavior motivated from unconscious sources.

**LOWER LEVEL: MORE PRIMITIVE MECHANISMS**

**Denial**
Intolerable thoughts, feelings, or wishes are disavowed; person refutes external elements of reality that are unpleasant or painful.

**Regression**
Person reverts to a pattern of behavior belonging to an earlier stage of development.

**Conversion**
Painful emotional experience is repressed and later is expressed in the form of a physical symptom.

**Projection**
That which is emotionally unacceptable within the self is rejected and attributed to others.

**Introjection**
Person absorbs the emotional attitudes, wishes, ideals, or personality of others into self; the aspirations and self-restraints of others are incorporated into the personality.

**Reaction Formation**
Person adopts attitudes and behavior that are opposites of the impulses to which he or she is reacting.

level of anxiety engendered and its manifestations depend on the individual's maturity, understanding of need, level of self-esteem, and coping mechanisms.

Anxiety is a psychological response that cannot be seen; it is only implied by actions. The state of anxiousness manifested by behavioral changes is communicated interpersonally. Highly anxious persons can transmit the sense of anxiousness to others; for example, very anxious patients can heighten family members' anxieties and vice versa.

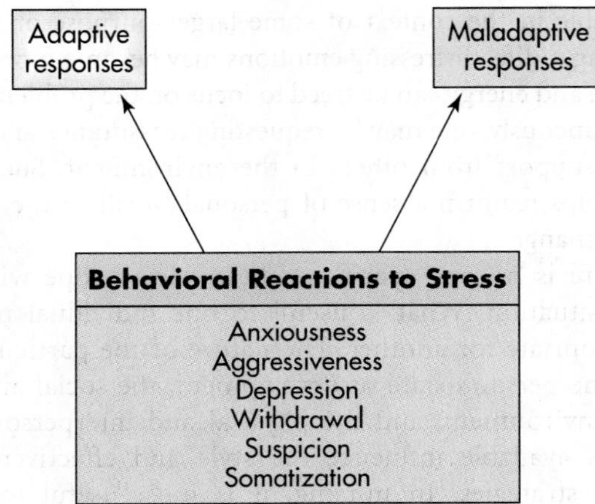


**fig. 6-4** Behavioral response of persons experiencing anxiety from stress, such as illness, range from adaptive to maladaptive behavior.

**box 6-5** *Levels of Anxiety*

**MILD ANXIETY**
Increased alertness
Quick eye movements
Increased hearing ability
Increased awareness

**MODERATE ANXIETY**
Decreased awareness of environmental details
Focus on selected aspects of self (or illness)

**SEVERE ANXIETY**
Disturbances in thought patterns
Incongruency of thoughts, feelings, and actions
Perceptual field greatly decreased

**PANIC**
Distorted perceptions of environment
Inability to see or understand situation
Unpredictable responses
Random motor activity

Although the ego attempts to deal with anxiety through the use of defense mechanisms, certain degrees of anxiety are reflected in behaviors resulting from a discharge of energy necessary to restore equilibrium. These responses range from behavior that is adaptive to behavior that is considered, by societal standards, maladaptive (Figure 6-5). The types of behavioral reactions that occur are influenced by psychosocial-cultural factors, basic personality development, past experiences, values, and economic status. The conclusion that a person is demonstrating anxious behavior can be drawn when several signs of anxiety are present. With mild

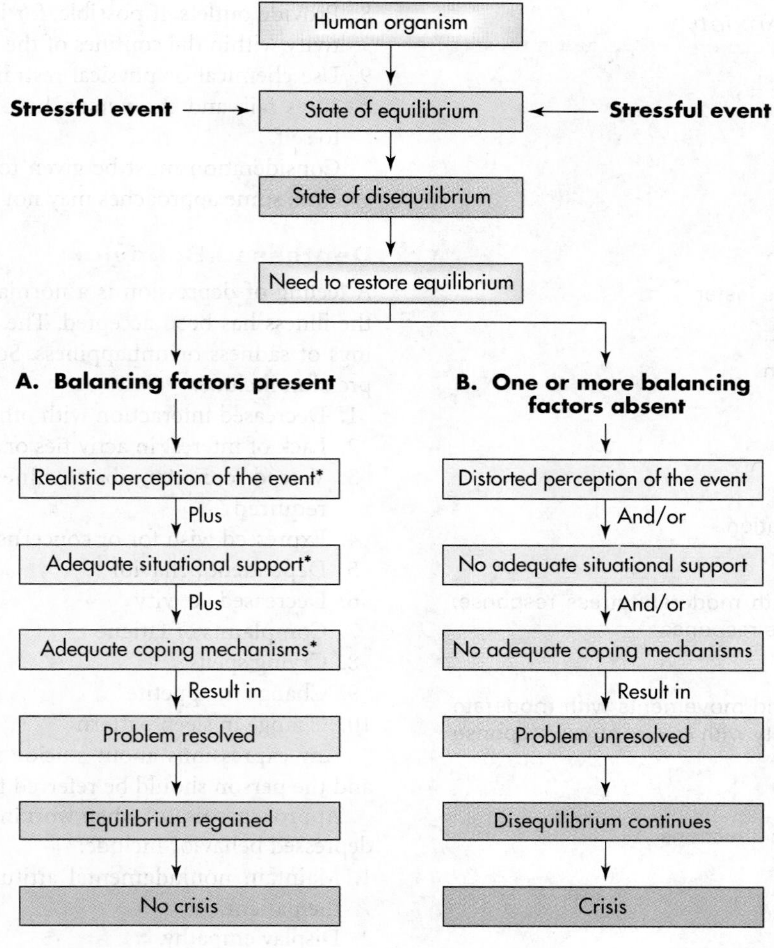


**fig. 6-5** Paradigm: effect of balancing factors in a stressful event.

anxiety the signs are fewer and less prominent. Signs of anxiety are more overt in persons who are experiencing severe anxiety or panic.

Subjective data to be collected to determine the patient's anxiety level include:

1. Statements of feeling apprehensive, uncertain, fearful, out of control, helpless, or anxious
2. Statements of fears of unspecific consequences
3. Statements of feeling overexcited, rattled, distressed, or jittery
4. Statements of feeling tired and having difficulty sleeping

Data from the initial nursing history and the situation (such as proposed surgery, diagnostic tests) may provide clues to possible causes of anxiety.

Objective data related to anxiety are listed in Box 6-6; observations are made about the behavior in addition to the physiological signs. The physiological signs result from the stimulation of the sympathetic nervous system and the adrenal medulla. Restlessness and an increased awareness of the environment are early signs of anxiety. Persons focus more on the self as anxiety increases. Physiological signs usually begin with moderate anxiety and are more prevalent and intense during severe anxiety and panic.

Approaches that prove to be useful in working with persons exhibiting anxious behaviors include:

1. Decrease stimuli.
2. Maintain a calm approach.
3. Provide structure.
4. Explain situation simply and concisely.
5. Help patients use coping mechanisms to bring the anxiety level down to a controllable level.
6. Promote exploration of feelings.
7. Avoid asking patients to make choices.

## Aggressive Behavior

The person whose self-concept is threatened may respond with aggression, which is a way to feel less helpless and more powerful. Aggression involves acting in a hostile manner or launching an attack. Aggression is one way of handling

**box 6-6** *Signs of Anxiety*

**PHYSIOLOGICAL RESPONSE**

**Skin**
Pale or ashen, moist

**Pupils**
Dilated

**Respirations**
Deeper; may or may not be faster

**Pulse**
Increased rate and strength

**Body temperature**
Slightly increased

**Gastrointestinal tract**
Anorexia, nausea, constipation

**Urinary Tract**
Frequency of urination with moderate stress response; oliguria with severe stress response

**Motor System**
Restlessness, frequent hand movements with moderate stress response; immobility with severe stress response

**BEHAVIOR**
Decreased attention span
Decreased ability to follow directions
Increased acting out
Increased somatization

**INTERACTION**
Increased number of questions
Constant seeking of reassurance
Frequent shifting of topics of conversation
Avoidance of focusing on feelings
Focus on equipment or procedures

anxiety. People are often angry at the loss of health status and question what is happening to them. They become irritable and uncooperative and may project their anger on others and become demanding. Expression of anger in socially acceptable ways prevents anger from being turned inward, causing depression.

Approaches that are useful in working with a person who exhibits aggressive behavior include:

1. Provide opportunities for the person to express feelings and the reasons for the feelings.
2. Accept expressions of hostility without retaliation or making the person feel guilty.
3. Anticipate the demands of the patient.
4. Maintain eye contact with the patient.
5. Approach the patient in calm, direct manner without any signs of aggression.
6. Decrease environmental stimuli.
7. Set limits.
8. Provide outlets, if possible, for increased psychomotor activity within the confines of the hospital unit.
9. Use chemical or physical restraints only if all other measures fail, and the person becomes harmful to others or to self.

Consideration must be given to a patient's cultural background; some approaches may not be appropriate.

### Depressed Behavior

A feeling of depression is a normal response to illness, once the illness has been accepted. The person may describe feelings of sadness or unhappiness. Some common signs of depression include:

1. Decreased interaction with others
2. Lack of interest in activities or environment
3. Voiced concern about illness and amount of care required
4. Expressed wish for or concerns about dying
5. Dependent behavior
6. Decreased activity
7. Complaints of fatigue
8. Crying spells
9. Change in appetite
10. Change in sleep pattern

Any expressions about suicide should be taken seriously, and the person should be referred for immediate counseling.

Approaches useful when working with a person exhibiting depressed behavior include:

1. Maintain nonjudgmental attitude when interacting with the patient.
2. Display empathy.
3. Help the person express feelings.
4. Convey acceptance of the right to feel sad.
5. Listen to the person so that the anger can be turned outward.

### Withdrawn Behavior

Withdrawal is commonly noted during illness. Withdrawal permits the person to conserve the mental and physical energy needed to deal with stressors and to promote repair and restoration. Withdrawn patients usually do not pose many problems and are apt to be labeled "good" patients. They demand little from others and thus may be overlooked. Withdrawn patients regress more easily to earlier levels of behavior at which they can accept the patient role. They may have feelings of low self-worth.

Approaches that may be useful in working with the withdrawn person include:

1. Spend time with the patient to increase the person's self-worth—even if you are both silent.
2. Provide gentle encouragement to talk, express feelings, and relate to others.
3. Express acceptance of the withdrawn person.

### Suspicious Behavior

A sense of powerlessness or lack of control as a result of stressors and the stress response and anxiety may lead to behavior that reflects the patient's suspiciousness. Suspicious patients have difficulty with trust and may have had experiences in which they learned to distrust others. They often are suspicious of health care staff members, health care routines, medicines, and procedures. Overheard conversations may reinforce the person's suspicion that others are talking about him or her.

Approaches that may be useful in working with a patient exhibiting suspiciousness may include:

1. Let the person talk about concerns, but do not insist.
2. To promote trust, keep promises made to the person.
3. Avoid an overzealous approach, which may make the person more suspicious.
4. Provide explanations of procedures and routines so that the person knows what to expect.
5. Avoid whispering or talking softly within the person's hearing.

### Somatic Behavior

A familiar reaction to illness is called *flight into illness.* Patients somatize their concerns; that is, they have learned to express anxiety through complaints about a variety of physical symptoms. They may be preoccupied with body functions and feelings of pain. Vague complaints of backache, headache, or fatigue are expressed to legitimize the attention needed. Staff members often become angry at patients who use somatic behavior because of the frequent vague complaints. Staff members feel "caught" if they minimize the symptoms, because there is always the possibility that the complaints are truly connected with an illness. Staff guilt persists for some time if a physical illness is diagnosed in a complaining patient who was ignored.

Approaches that may be useful for the person exhibiting somatic behavior may include:

1. Accept all symptoms and report them.
2. Spend time with the person and listen to physical complaints with some limit setting.
3. Encourage discussion of feelings.

## STRESS-RELATED DISORDERS

In addition to specific behaviors associated with stress and anxiety, many physical illnesses and symptoms are associated with or exacerbated by physiological and psychological stress. Excessive or poorly managed stress affects every body system (Box 6-7).

**box 6-7 Illnesses Exacerbated by Stress**

**NEUROPSYCHOLOGICAL**
Migraines/tension headaches
Panic disorder
Post-traumatic stress disorder

**CARDIOVASCULAR**
Chest pain/angina
Palpitations
Hypertension
Cerebral vascular accident
Atherosclerosis
Peripheral vascular disease

**PULMONARY**
Asthma
Emphysema

**GASTROINTESTINAL**
Inflammatory bowel disease
Irritable bowel syndrome
Peptic ulcer disease
Gastritis
Gastroesophageal reflux disease

**IMMUNE**
Connective tissue diseases

**MUSCULOSKELETAL**
Back pain
Arthritis
Temporomandibular joint dysfunction

**INTEGUMENTARY**
Hives
Allergies
Atopic dermatitis

**ENDOCRINE**
Cushing's syndrome
Addison's disease
Hyperthyroidism
Hypothyroidism
Diabetes mellitus
Premenstrual syndrome

**GENERAL**
Anorexia nervosa
Bulimia
Fatigue
Hyperlipidemia
Sexual dysfunction
Obesity

### Posttraumatic Stress Disorder

Posttraumatic stress disorder (PTSD) is a syndrome seen in persons who have experienced severe physical or emotional trauma.[6] The event generally involves actual or threatened death, injury, or a threat to one's personal integrity. The individual's response involves intense fear, helplessness, or horror.[3]

PTSD was brought to attention of the health community by the Vietnam veterans who had witnessed or been involved in combat. The syndrome has also been identified with victims of rape and other violent crimes. Symptoms include sleep disturbances, irritability, difficulty concentrating and making decisions, hypervigilance, and an exaggerated startle response. Symptoms can last from months to years. Treatment involves psychotherapy, antidepressants, and antianxiety agents.[3,8]

## NURSING MANAGEMENT

### ■ ASSESSMENT

#### Subjective Data

Data to be collected include:

Reports of anxiety: Feelings of apprehension, sleep disorder, decreased concentration, change in appetite, irritability, lethargy, inability to make decisions.

History of traumatic event: Violence or abuse, military service, family stability, support mechanisms.

Somatic complaints: Headache, muscular or skeletal pain, palpitations, chest pain, abdominal pain and burning, nausea, vomiting, history of substance abuse.

#### Objective Data

Data to be collected include:

Increased blood pressure
Increased respirations
Tachycardia
Pallor
Decreased attentiveness
Guarding
Flat or blunted affect

### ■ NURSING DIAGNOSES

Nursing diagnoses are determined from analysis or patient data. Nursing diagnoses for the patient with stress include:

| Diagnostic Title | Possible Etiological Factors |
|---|---|
| Ineffective coping, individual | Personal vulnerability, inadequate support, multiple stressors, multiple life changes |
| Anxiety | Threat to self, change in environment, helplessness, illness, uncertainty, threat to health status |
| Fatigue | Anxiety, change of routine |

### ■ EXPECTED PATIENT OUTCOMES

Expected patient outcomes for the patient experiencing stress may include, but are not limited to:

1a. Verbalizes understanding of problems and stressors, explores feelings, and problem solves.
 b. Identifies stressors and effective methods to manage stress.
2a. Participates in therapeutic programs.
 b. Meets psychological needs by verbalization or expression of feelings, identifying problem-solving techniques, and use of appropriate methods and resources to meet needs.
3. Reports increased energy levels.

### ■ INTERVENTIONS

Many strategies have been developed for stress management. These strategies use physiological, cognitive, or behavioral techniques to diminish the effects of stress. Stress management as a therapeutic process has proliferated in the past 2 decades. Many of its techniques have been scrutinized carefully, and research documents the efficacy of these procedures in the management of stress.

The traditional mode of care in nursing has focused on providing direct care to patients. The direct care mode focuses on the nurse's knowledge and ability to identify and intervene to promote patient health. Patient health in this mode reflects the action and ability of the nurse to monitor, direct, and control the change process.

Effective stress reduction is a function of everyday living and is under the control of the individual person. Intervention by direct care is inadequate for stress reduction except for brief time-limited problems, such as control of anticipatory vomiting in cancer patients. For stress management to be effective in health maintenance and promotion, another mode of care must be implemented.

Stress management embraces a self-management orientation, emphasizing individual responsibility and participation in treatment.[14] The nurse's treatment goal is to provide the behavioral, cognitive, and psychophysiological skills necessary for individuals to manage their own stress responses. In contrast to the traditional relationship between the patient and the nurse, which focuses on "compliance," patients who learn stress management strategies are active change agents. The nurse is cognizant of the limitations of his or her own therapeutic role. Ideally, the nurse is a proficient therapist who acts as an instigator, facilitator, and model to assist the patient to apply relaxation and related stress management skills. The nurse assumes the responsibility for designing with the patient a structured, realistic program of change, but it is the patient's responsibility to implement and maintain the program. Table 6-2 compares the use of direct care and self-management.

#### General Intervention Strategies

General interventions for persons experiencing stressors include various activities, which are described here.

##### *Supporting protective mechanisms*

Rest is essential to maintain energy supply for metabolic functions when a person experiences stressors and stress responses. The patient is kept comfortably warm; overheating causes vasodilation and counteracts the arteriolar constriction necessary to ensure an adequate blood supply to vital organs.

Even minor stress responses can cause annoying discomforts such as backaches, generalized muscle tension, and headaches. These discomforts can act as additional stressors, and comfort measures such as back rubs, position changes, and back supports to relax muscles are indicated. Pain should be alleviated as much as possible, and noise and disturbance should be kept to a minimum. During severe stress responses, food and fluids taken orally may need to be withheld until nausea subsides and gastrointestinal tract activity returns to normal.

##### *Providing structure*

Structure decreases anxiety and is helpful for persons experiencing mild or moderate anxiety. Explanations are one method of providing structure. New experiences should be

**table 6-2** *Contrast of Direct Care and Self-Management According to Care Characteristics*

| | Direct Care | Self-Management |
|---|---|---|
| Locus of control | Professional dominance | Predominantly patient, but nurse takes responsibility for imparting knowledge, skills, and feedback |
| Problem awareness and assessment | Usually depends on clinical observations and judgment of nurse | Self-awareness and self-assessment, with guidance from nurse |
| Goal setting | Most care based on end goal determined by nurse | Negotiation of goals of both patient and nurse |
| Change agent | Action by nurse is medium by which changes are generated | Predominantly patient action or skills to achieve changes |
| Knowledge | Predominantly nurse; knowledge is premise for care | Knowledge is transmitted to patient to use for developing skills to generate care |
| Feedback | Not central for effectiveness of care | Crucial for effectiveness of care and promoting change |

From Kogan H, Betrus P: Self-management in nursing mode of therapeutic influence, *Adv Nurs Sci* 6(4):55-73, 1984.

explained and, if possible, related to other familiar experiences. The higher the level of anxiety, the more simple the explanations need to be.

If patients are to have treatments or tests, they need to be given some ideas of what will be done, necessary preparations, expected sensory perceptions, and the reasons procedures are necessary. To remove water pitchers and inform patients that they cannot have any more water until after x-ray examinations can generate many anxious thoughts: "What x-ray examination?" "I wonder when it is." "What will it be like?" "How will it feel?" "It must be something special if I can't have any water." Anxiety caused by lack of knowledge reflects lack of consideration for patients' rights.

If possible, the patient's anxiety should be at a manageable level to enhance comprehension and retention of information. Explanations should be given in terms understood by patients and at appropriate times and should be repeated as necessary. If patients are very anxious, repeated explanations are necessary because extreme anxiety reduces intellectual function, including memory. Until the problem is resolved, it is not useful to give explanations to patients who are severely anxious or sedated or to those who have high temperatures or severe pain. Repetition often is required for older persons and children because of shorter attention spans or poor recent memory.

Time spent in giving explanations to relatives is not wasted. Not only does it relieve anxieties, which may be transmitted to patients, but it also saves having to untangle misinformation. Often family members are helpful in interpreting necessary instructions to patients in a manner that patients understand and accept.

### Promoting exploration of feelings

In most instances a large part of the nurse's work is to encourage patients to express anxieties, to help them identify the fears in their situations, to help them seek outlets for their fears and tensions, and to allay negative feelings whenever possible. Nurses provide opportunities for patients to talk, but they should not probe. There is a difference between prying into patients' thoughts and beliefs and eliciting information that aids in the understanding of behavior and in planning for care. Without seeming unduly curious, one usually can find topics of interest to patients that provide openings. A picture on the bedside table may be such an example. Nurses who listen with sincere interest and without making judgments may begin to gain insight into patients as persons. More important, patients may begin to speak about personal fears.

As soon as a patient begins to talk about feelings, nurses should encourage conversations, taking cues from what the patient offers. Nurses who feel inadequate or anxious may cut off conversations. For instance, if a patient says, "You know, I don't think I'll ever get to see my little boy again," a common response is, "Oh, don't say that, certainly you will; you're going to be all right" when the patient very well may not be all right. A better response is, "What makes you feel this way?" Such a response allows exploration of subjects and leaves opportunities for the patient to examine concerns. Nurses willing to listen to patients, to be guided by their reactions, and to work with them rather than to make decisions for them will provide needed emotional support. Solving patients' problems, even if it were possible, is not the aim of nursing. Indeed, it would make patients less healthy psychologically.

The art of meaningful communication involves more than just listening; it includes moving conversations so that the patient's attempt to communicate is assisted. Observing patients for facial changes and general body movements provides opportunities for the nurse to discover the full meaning of a situation. For example, consider the patient who sucks in air while talking. The mouth becomes drier and drier, and the tongue seems to stick in the mouth. This patient is not at ease, and even innocuous words may belie anxiety. A simple statement and question such as, "Your mouth seems very dry. Would a glass of water help?" allow the nurse to clarify observations. Such an approach provides an opportunity to tell what the patient is feeling and to gain understanding by talking about it.

The nurse helps patients examine those problems that they are able to bring into awareness. Underlying problems should be handled by professionals trained in psychotherapy. A nurse needs to recognize normal anxiety reactions and to report exaggerated reactions that may indicate the need for psychiatric referral.

When anxiety increases to a high level, the nurse may need to sit with the patient. The nurse's presence is often reassuring. If possible, the patient is helped to recognize the anxiety by the nurse's asking, "Are you uncomfortable?" or "What are you feeling?" In severe anxiety and panic, being there is most important, and touch may be used as a means of reassurance. Some severely anxious persons, however, view touching as an intrusion of their personal boundary, and the nurse needs to keep this in mind. When the patient is able to talk, the nurse helps the patient describe what is happening, what has happened, and what is expected to happen.

### *Facilitating problem solving*

Some persons solve problems in a haphazard manner, whereas others have a highly structured approach. Problem solving can be a means for coping with stressors and the stress response and is more effective if the problem-solving steps are consciously followed. The steps include:

1. Gathering data
2. Identifying the problem (or effect of stressor)
3. Identifying the factors affecting the problem or stressor
4. Determining goals
5. Exploring alternative ways to achieve the goals
6. Implementing actions
7. Evaluating effectiveness of actions

If the stressor has been identified, the nurse first assists the patient in exploring feelings and reactions associated with the stressor. Often persons are not consciously aware of what they are feeling and therefore may select inappropriate actions. Persons vary in their ability to identify problems and in their desire to discuss personal feelings, although it is widely accepted that talking does help. If the patient is urged indiscriminately to talk about problems, the relationship becomes superficial and mechanical. The identification of the consequences of actions often is omitted, but it is an important component if problem solving is to be effective.

Problem solving reduces ambiguity and feelings of loss of control. Persons who do not generally use conscious problem solving as a means of coping with stressors may benefit from learning about problem solving as a strategy for coping with stress.

### *Promoting wellness and reduction in fatigue*

Relaxation exercises are developed from the concept that the stress response of anxiety does not and cannot exist when the muscles of the body are relaxed. Relaxation exercises do not "cure" the stressors or the stress response but do help to minimize effects of the stress response and give the

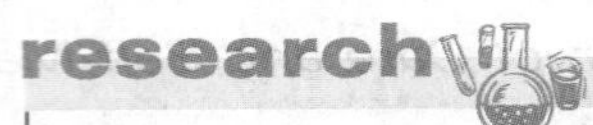


Reference: Collins JA, Hill-Rice V: Effects of relaxation intervention in phase II cardiac rehabilitation: replication and extension, *Heart Lung* 26(1):31-44, 1997.

Cardiac disease is the leading cause of death in the United States. After either a myocardial infarction or coronary artery bypass graft, cardiac rehabilitation programs are available to provide supervised exercise programs, education, risk factor modification, peer support, and counseling. Phase II of cardiac rehabilitation involves a supervised 4 to 6 month outpatient program. The purpose of this study was to determine if progressive muscle relaxation and guided imagery would decrease stress and anxiety and decrease resting pulse and blood pressure for patients participating in cardiac rehabilitation. The behavioral response to stress was documented by self-report on the presence or absence of somatization, anxiety, depression, interpersonal sensitivity, hostility, obsessive-compulsiveness, phobic anxiety, paranoid ideation, and psychoticism. Physiological measurements were recorded by the investigators. The results of the study did not support the hypothesis of lowered subjective anxiety and depression. However, a decreased heart rate and willingness to participate suggests that this intervention may be helpful to cardiac rehabilitation patients.

person a sense of control. A daily program of relaxation exercises has an effect on physiological responses to stressors (e.g., lowering of elevated blood pressure or elevated blood glucose), as well as psychological responses to stressors (e.g., decreased level of anxiety) (see the Research Box). These exercises also are helpful on a short-term basis when anxiety occurs.

There are four basic components of relaxation techniques:

1. *Quiet environment:* eliminating all possible noise and distractions
2. *Comfortable position:* sitting with no undue muscle tension
3. *Passive attitude:* emptying the conscious mind of all thoughts
4. *Mental device:* focusing on a sound, word, phrase, mental image, object, or breathing pattern to shift the mind from logical, externally oriented thoughts

The important factor is that the person empties his or her mind of all thoughts and concentrates on the mental device. It is natural for the mind to wander. When this occurs, a person simply redirects thoughts back to the mental device. Each relaxation session should take approximately 20 minutes.

There are several approaches to performing relaxation exercises. Two approaches are progressive relaxation and Benson's relaxation response.

**Progressive relaxation.** Progressive relaxation consists of tensing and relaxing muscle groups and focusing on the feelings of relaxation (Box 6-8). This technique is similar to guided imagery (see Chapter 20). The systematic application of progressive relaxation has three major effects:[25]

1. Muscle groups are relaxed more and more with each practice.

**box 6-8** *Progressive Relaxation*

1. Assume a comfortable position in a quiet room.
2. Begin by focusing on easy breathing.
3. Tense specific muscle groups (see step 5) for 5 to 7 seconds, then relax quickly.
4. Concentrate for 10 seconds on the sensations of the relaxed muscles.
5. Follow a sequence, repeating each muscle group, tensing two or three times
   a. Hand and arm: clench fist, pull elbow tightly, pull arms tightly into body
   b. Face: wrinkle forehead, close eyes tightly, wrinkle nose, purse lips, smile with teeth tightly clenched
   c. Neck: pull chin to chest
   d. Trunk: pull shoulder blades together, tighten stomach and buttocks
   e. Leg and foot: push down with leg, point toes upward (dorsiflexion) dominant leg first
6. Repeat process in any areas in which increased tension has been identified.

2. Each of the major muscle groups is relaxed one after the other. As a new muscle group is added, the previously relaxed portions also relax.
3. More total body relaxation is experienced as the person moves into the relaxation phase. The relaxed state is maintained beyond the relaxation period.

**Benson's relaxation response.** Benson's relaxation response omits the muscle tensing and is particularly helpful for muscle relaxation in patients who are experiencing pain or discomfort. The nurse should remain with the patient to coach and encourage relaxation,[4] as follows:

1. Assume a comfortable sitting position in a quiet room.
2. Close eyes.
3. Relax body muscles (i.e., "let go").
4. Concentrate on breathing; repeat a word or sound such as "one" or "um-m" after each exhalation.
5. Continue for about 20 minutes.
6. Open eyes.
7. Take time to adjust to surroundings before moving.

For some acute stressors, such as those experienced by hospitalized adults, the nurse may use abridged forms of relaxation techniques that can be implemented more rapidly. Effective abridged relaxation techniques include deep breathing or squeezing and relaxing the hands.

### Implementing music therapy

Music therapy is an intervention that can help patients achieve relaxation and promote coping with stressors and the stress response. Music therapy has been used successfully in various environments, including intensive care units, dentists' offices, and surgery units. Music therapy has been used with patients who have acute and chronic health problems.

When music therapy is used, the patient's preference must be considered, because the type of music that is relaxing and pleasant for one person may be irritating and unpleasant for another. Instrumental music is better than vocal music because words often evoke various emotional responses. In addition, the use of headphones is advocated to help decrease other stimuli. The patient should be able to control the volume.

Music therapy is easily accessible. Only a source of music (tapes or CDs) and a machine are required. Cassette tapes and players are used most frequently because they are least expensive, most portable, and easily available in a variety of clinical settings. Because of the large selection in tapes, individual preferences are easy to accommodate. Frequently music with nature sounds has a relaxing effect, especially the sound of running water. The use of video allows the added dimension of sight and sound to enhance the relaxation. Unlike other relaxation interventions, neither nurses nor patients need special skills to use music therapy. All that is needed is an enjoyment of music.

### Providing antianxiety medications

In some instances, an antianxiety medication may be prescribed to reduce anxiety symptoms. Antianxiety agents may be divided into two groups: the benzodiazepines and the nonbenzodiazepines (Table 6-3). Note that the dosage of benzodiazepines is less for elderly persons, who metabolize the drugs slowly, which can result in a prolonged depressant effect. Dosage also should be reduced for persons with impaired liver or kidney function.

The benzodiazepines are the most frequently prescribed antianxiety agents. These drugs act by inhibiting transmission of stimuli from the limbic system of the brain (septum, amygdala, and hippocampus). Side effects include drowsiness, dizziness, and weakness.

Antianxiety agents produce muscle relaxation and a sense of well-being. The drugs are prescribed for short-term relief of anxiety but not for anxiety from daily stressors. Long-term therapy leads to increased tolerance and dependence; larger doses are then needed to produce the desired effects and drug abuse may ensue.

Persons taking antianxiety agents are cautioned not to drink alcohol or take other central nervous system (CNS) depressants during therapy because of serious complications, even death, as a result of synergistic effects. They also need to be cautious when driving or working around heavy machinery because of possible dizziness.

## Crisis Intervention

Awareness of what occurs during a crisis helps the nurse understand the accompanying behavior. When the ego is met with overwhelming anxiety created by biological, psychological, or social threats to the self, a crisis ensues. The ego is not able to cope successfully with the sudden disequilibrium, and the person needs assistance to use the situation as a growth experience.

**table 6-3** *Common Medications for* ***Anxiety***

| Drug | Action | Nursing Intervention |
|---|---|---|
| **BENZODIAZEPINES** | | |
| Alprazolam (Xanax)<br>Chlordiazepoxide (Librium, Libritabs)<br>Clorazepate (Tranxene)<br>Diazepam (Valium)<br>Halazepam (Paxipam)<br>Lorazepam (Ativan)<br>Oxazepam (Serax)<br>Prazepam (Centrax)<br>Clonazepam (Klonopin) | Exact mechanism of action unknown<br>Acts on limbic, thalamic, and hypothalmic level of CNS; CNS depressant<br>Antidepressant and anxiolytic properties | CNS depressant, avoid use with alcohol, other CNS depressants, potentiates action<br>Caution with renal or hepatic impairment<br>Do not abruptly discontinue drug, taper dose to avoid withdrawal symptoms; abrupt withdrawal may precipitate status epilepticus |
| **NONBENZODIAZEPINES** | | |
| Hydroxyzine HCl (Atarax) | CNS depressant, tranquilizing effect by depressing hypothalamus and brain-stem reticular formation | Cautions<br>Avoid use with other CNS depressants, Causes dry mouth—instruct patient to increase fluids, rinse mouth frequently with water |
| **AZASPIRODECANEDIONE DERIVATIVE** | | |
| Buspirone HCl (BuSpar) | Exact mechanism unknown<br>Decreases serotonin neuronal activity<br>Presynaptic dopamine antagonist<br>Increases norepinephrine metabolism | Cautious use in patients with renal or liver impairment<br>Optimal effect in 3-4 weeks<br>CNS depressant<br>Tardive dyskinesia with long-term use<br>Caution in patients with history of drug abuse<br>Avoid use with MAO inhibitors |

A crisis occurs when a person faces for a time what seems to be an insurmountable obstacle to an important life goal and is unable to use customary methods of coping. A period of disorganization ensues—a period of upset during which many abortive attempts at solutions are made.

Several phases or stages occur during crisis. These stages are similar to the stages of death and dying described by Kübler-Ross.

1. *Initial impact.* During this phase the person experiences shock and depersonalization as reality is clearly perceived. Functioning is organized and automatic, with individual centering and docility.
2. *Realization.* In the second phase the existing self-structure collapses. Reality seems overwhelming, and the person experiences high anxiety, panic, and helplessness. There is inability to plan, reason, or understand the situation.
3. *Defensive retreat.* The third phase is one of regression in which an attempt is made to establish previous identity—to return to better times. Reality is avoided, and denial and wishful thinking may help to relieve the anxiety. When challenged, the ego reacts with anger and the person may experience rage and disorientation. Thinking is situation-bound, and change is resisted.
4. *Acknowledgment.* This is the "yes" stage: "It has happened to me." The individual experiences depression and self-depreciation. Reality imposes itself again and looms large in relating the event to one's life. Without intervention the person may become more disorganized, depressed, and suicidal.
5. *Adaptation.* This is the stage in which change occurs if help is adequate. New identity appears along with hope and renewed sense of personal worth. Anxiety is subsequently decreased and satisfaction is increased as a result of the stabilization and reorganization. Functional improvement is noted without actual change in disability status.

The model offered is a useful approach for explaining what a person experiences during an illness crisis, even though reactions to crisis are individual. People are not equally vulnerable to all categories of stressors, but there is thought to be some commonality in the reactions. Knowledge about the commonalities can facilitate plans for nursing intervention.

The essential element of crisis intervention is the intensive nature of support required to help the ego maintain its integrity and its ability to use coping mechanisms. Crisis is self-limiting. Early intervention can prevent maladaptive behavior, and the individual can emerge a stronger person. Acute or catastrophic illness often precipitates a crisis reaction. The outcome of a crisis is governed by the kind of interaction that takes place between the individual and key figures in the environment during the time of crisis.

Often because of changes in society, previous guidelines for behavior in stressful situations render the individual helpless. In crisis the individual is helped to find ways to facilitate efforts to learn from the experience. A state of disequilibrium produces a felt need to reduce anxiety. The following balancing factors[2] have been identified as being necessary to resolve the problem and avert a crisis:

1. A realistic perception of the event
2. Adequate situational support (staff and family)
3. Adequate coping mechanisms.

When one or more of these balancing factors are absent, the result is an increase in anxiety, with immobilization and an inability to avert the crisis (see Figure 6-5).

In crisis, help should be immediate. Staying with the person, talking through the situation, and encouraging catharsis facilitate recognition and expression of feelings and subsequent relief of guilt. Strengthening coping mechanisms is crucial in preventing the development of symptoms. Personal growth is facilitated by using problem-solving skills.

## Specific Support Approaches

Persons who are having difficulty coping because of severe or multiple stressors may be referred for individual or group counseling. Some may need assistance and support from the nurse in seeking out and initiating counseling.

Therapeutic groups consist of persons who are experiencing common stressors. Peer support is given because the participants share the common experience. Persons often are able to express their feelings more easily when they know that the group members understand what they are experiencing. Sharing approaches is helpful in solving problems common to the group. Therapeutic groups may be self-help groups or be directed by health professionals. Examples of therapeutic groups are Al-Anon (for family member of alcohol-dependent persons), Parents Without Partners, Reach to Recovery (postmastectomy), "ostomy" groups, bereavement groups, and the American Cancer Society's "I Can Cope" program.

## Additional Stress Management Therapies

In dealing with some stressors, particularly chronic stressors or diseases associated with stressors and the stress response, the nurse may use some stress management therapies that require special training or equipment. These are implemented over a long-term basis and usually in outpatient settings. Stress management therapists help patients design and implement structured programs of change to enable them to control and deal more effectively with stressors and the stress response. Some of the therapies include biofeedback, meditation, attitudinal restructuring, autogenic training, behavioral change programs, and systematic desensitization.

### Biofeedback

Biofeedback is a system of learning voluntary control over autonomically regulated body functions so that an individual is able to monitor the physiological stress response and replace it with a nonstressful response. For example, if after a stressful day you notice soreness and muscle tension in your shoulders, you can sit quietly and concentrate on relaxing the shoulder muscles to feel the tension slip away.

With biofeedback, machinery is used to "train" the person to monitor certain parameters. For example, muscle activity can be monitored with an electromyograph, and the stimuli can be converted into a visual or auditory signal. Using this biofeedback, the person can learn how to replace muscle tension with muscle relaxation. Machines also can be used to measure skin temperature or sweat activity, and a similar feedback approach is used. The person is then weaned from the machine to produce the desired effects without machinery. A comprehensive biofeedback program includes feedback from multiple systems and sites.

### Meditation

For centuries the art of meditation has been practiced in the East. Proponents of meditation techniques claim that meditators can control physiological processes, some as dramatic as voluntarily stopping heartbeats.[4] There are many different types of meditation, with differing goals and foci, including Zen Buddhism, yoga, and transcendental meditation (TM). Research has focused on TM because it is one of the most practiced forms of meditation in the West.

TM is not a complicated process. One is given a word, a *mantra*, which is to be repeated silently while one sits in a comfortable position and focuses attention on breathing and repeating the mantra. The purpose of the mantra is to enhance a passive attitude and prevent distracting thoughts. Meditators are instructed to practice twice daily for at least 20 minutes. The physiological relaxation that is produced during meditation is carried over into everyday life as a protection against the effects of the stress response.

### Attitudinal restructuring

The basic premise of rational-emotive therapy, developed by Ellis,[9] is that much if not all emotional suffering (stress response) is due to the irrational ways people perceive the world. The assumptions that people make lead to self-defeating internal dialogues or negative self-talk. The goal of therapy is to replace negative self-statements with positive self-statements. Changing self-talk involves three steps: identifying self-talk, evaluating it, and replacing it with more appropriate self-talk.

Detection of self-talk may be difficult at first because it is "inaudible." Detection of self-talk usually involves keeping a daily log to identify specific thoughts and feelings.

Self-talk often causes a person to distort reality or arrive at false conclusions. The following five questions are useful in examining self-talk and the situations that are antecedent to it:

1. Have I disregarded an important aspect of the situation?
2. Have I exaggerated the meaning of an event?
3. Are my perceptions of the situation overly simplified or rigid?
4. Have I drawn conclusions where evidence is lacking or where evidence supports a contrary conclusion?

5. Have I overgeneralized or generated a false conclusion?

The answers to the five questions should reveal when self-talk is inappropriate and how to restructure it. Negative internal dialogues probably are a major source of stress to many persons.[5]

### Autogenic training

Autogenic training teaches cognitive and physiological behavioral change through passive concentration to decrease sympathetic nervous system activity. The person repeats a statement verbally with the physiological state that is being practiced. The physiological states are heaviness and warmth of extremities, calm and regular heartbeat and breathing, abdominal warmth, and cooling of forehead. The methods are similar to that of TM.

### Behavioral change programs

Some specific stress-related behaviors, such as smoking or overeating, may be eliminated by behavioral conditioning. The programs consist of:

1. Self-monitoring to identify characteristics and situations associated with the behaviors
2. Identifying outcome criteria in precise behavioral terms
3. Developing a formal contract with the therapist, stating short-term goals with rewards and frequency of evaluation

The overall goal is a change in behavior. Behavioral change programs are most effective with highly motivated persons who sincerely *want* to change behavior.

### Systematic desensitization

Systematic desensitization provides specific stressors (such as those related to phobias) in increasing doses while the individual practices relaxation skills. The person is first taught effective relaxation skills. Stimuli eliciting anxieties are then presented in increasing intensity, starting at a minimal level while relaxation techniques are used. Then the person is instructed to relax while imagining the situation in more threatening circumstances. The principle of systematic desensitization is to train the person to behave (relax) in a manner opposite to anxiety behavior (tension). A low initial stimulus that increases in intensity gives the person a sense of control in coping with the undesirable stimulus, thus decreasing the anxiety.

## ■ EVALUATION

To evaluate the effectiveness of nursing interventions, compare patient behaviors with those stated in the expected patient outcomes. Successful achievement of patient outcomes for the patient experiencing stress include:

1a. Identifies stressors, verbalizes feelings, and uses problem-solving techniques.

b. Develops a plan to cope with stressors and identifies effective coping strategies.

2. Participates in a relaxation or stress management program.
3. Reports decreased fatigue and improved sleep patterns.

## critical thinking QUESTIONS

1 Pam, 32 years old with 3 children, is trying to work part-time and care for her children without using child care. Her husband works overtime to make ends meet. She often finds herself easily distracted, and she has difficulty concentrating and sleeping. Paul, 40 years old, travels every week and spends only short periods each weekend with his 8-month-old son and 2-year-old daughter. His wife frequently confronts him about his travel and leaving her to care for the children. Paul's boss confronted him last week about some recent paperwork mistakes. He wakes up early every morning, unable to sleep. Based on these two situations, can any generalizations be made about individuals experiencing stress?

2 Jim, 22 years old, was recently diagnosed with testicular cancer. On admission assessment the nurse notes that Jim is quite defensive. When asked to explain why he was being hospitalized, Jim angrily responds, "I just want to go back to college with my friends and get on with my life." After her interview, the nurse concludes that Jim is experiencing an illness crisis. Analyze this situation, and offer suggestions on how best to handle it.

3 Harry, 58 years old, is a manager of a discount department store. He has been working long hours in preparation for inventory. Many new employees have been added and Harry is responsible for their training. He is complaining of insomnia for one month. When asked why he came to the clinic, he states "My wife thinks I need help. I know I will be fine if only I can sleep at night. I just have too many things going through my head at night." Harry refers to his sleep problem repeatedly, while avoiding eye contact. In which of Selye's adaptation stages would you place Harry? What coping strategies are being used? Are these coping strategies adaptive or maladaptive? Which approaches would work best with this patient?

## chapter SUMMARY

### STRESS

- Responses to stressors include neuroendocrine response, coping behaviors, defense mechanisms, and specific behavioral responses.
- Response to stressors is influenced by the type of stimuli, the intensity and duration of stressors, the meaning of the stressor, perception of stressor, sense of control, coping resources, and health status.
- The general adaptation syndrome consists of three stages: alarm reaction, resistance, and exhaustion. The first two stages occur frequently throughout life; death may ensue from exhaustion.

### STRESS RESPONSE

- The physiological stress response consists of stimulation of the sympathetic nervous system, adrenal medulla, anterior and posterior pituitary glands, and the adrenal cortex.
- The neuroendocrine stress response is integrated by the hypothalamus.

- During the stress response, norepinephrine is released and causes vasoconstriction of blood vessels to skin, mucous membranes, and the organs of the abdomen and pelvis.
- The blood shifted from the vasoconstricted vessels flows to the dilated blood vessels of the heart, lung, and brain.
- In addition to dilating selected blood vessels, epinephrine increases cardiac function, dilates bronchial smooth muscles, and alters metabolism to provide substrates for energy needs.
- Cortisol, acting in concert with catecholamines, growth hormone, and glucagon, helps to mobilize substrates for energy.
- Cortisol may serve a major function by its antiinflammatory and immunosuppressive actions, thus dampening the stress response to prevent over-activity.
- Water and sodium balance, osmolality, and blood volume are protected by the action of aldosterone and ADH, which are released during the neuroendocrine response to stressors.

### ADAPTATION

- Adaptation is a process of interaction with the environment that promotes homeostasis and growth. Maladaptation leads to inadequate functioning.

### COPING

- Types of coping strategies include action, cognitive, intrapsychic, interpersonal, and emotional strategies.

### DEFENSE MECHANISMS

- Defense mechanisms are unconscious mechanisms human beings use to adjust to life stressors. Mentally healthy persons occasionally use defense mechanisms, avoiding more primitive mechanisms.

### SPECIFIC BEHAVIORAL RESPONSES

- Some specific behavioral responses to stressors include anxiety, aggressive behavior, depressed behavior, withdrawn behavior, suspicious behavior, and somatic behavior.
- Anxiety results when a person perceives a threat to the self, either physically or psychologically.
- Anxiety may be mild, moderate, severe, or a state of panic. When anxiety increases, awareness of the environment decreases and physiological signs increase.

### STRESS MANAGEMENT THERAPEUTICS

- Rest and relief of discomfort conserve energy for coping with stressors and the stress response; providing explanations provides structure, which helps to decrease anxiety. Exploration of feelings helps to relieve tension associated with the stress response, and problem solving reduces feelings of loss of control associated with the stress response.
- Relaxation is the opposite of the tension associated with the stress response; it also gives the person a sense of control. Basic components of relaxation techniques are quiet environment, comfortable position, passive attitude, and a mental device to remove externally oriented thoughts.
- Music therapy is an easy-to-apply intervention to decrease stress.
- The most frequently prescribed antianxiety agents are the benzodiazepines. Alcohol or other CNS depressants should be avoided when one takes antianxiety agents.
- Crisis occurs when anxiety overwhelms the self and the person is unable to use coping mechanisms. Crisis is self-limiting. Balancing factors necessary to resolve crises include a realistic perception of the event, adequate situational support, and adequate coping mechanisms.
- Other stress management therapies requiring special expertise include meditation, attitudinal restructuring, biofeedback, autogenic training, behavioral change programs, and systematic desensitization.

## References


1. Adams J, Lindemann E: Coping with long-term disability. In Coehlo GV, Hamburg DA, Adams JE, editors: *Coping and adaptation*, New York, 1974, Basic Books.
2. Aguilera DC: *Crisis intervention: theory and methodology*, ed 7, St Louis, 1994, Mosby.
3. Barker LR, Schmidt CW: Evaluation of psychosocial problems. In Barker LR, Burton JR, Zieve PD, editors: *Principles of ambulatory medicine*, ed 4, Baltimore, 1995, Williams & Wilkins.
4. Benson H: *The relaxation response*, New York, 1975, William Morrow.
5. Betrus P, Kogan H: Stressors in nursing: causes, results and interventions. In *Stressors in nursing: responses and resolutions*, Seattle, 1981, University of Washington Press.
6. Blair D, Ramones VA: Understanding vicarious trauma, *J Psychosoc Nurs* 34(11):24-30, 1996.
7. Cannon WB: *The wisdom of the body*, New York, 1939, WW Norton.
8. Dole PJ: Centering: reducing rape trauma syndrome anxiety during a gynecologic examination, *J Psychosoc Nurs* 34(10):32-37, 1996.
9. Ellis A: *Reason and emotion in psychotherapy*, New York, 1962, Lyle Stuart.
10. Guyton AC, Hall JE: *Textbook of medical physiology*, Philadelphia, 1996, WB Saunders.
11. Henry JP, Ely DL: Physiology of emotional stress: specific responses, *J SC Med Assoc* 75:501-508, 1979.
12. Jacobsen E: *Progressive relaxation*, Chicago, 1938, University of Chicago Press.
13. James W: What is emotion? *Mind* 9:188-205, 1884.
14. Kanfer F, Goldstein A: *Helping people change*, New York, 1975, Pergamon Press.
15. Lazarus RS: *Psychological stress and the coping process*, New York, 1966, McGraw Hill.
16. Levine S, Weinberg J, Ursin H: Definition of the coping process and statement of the problem. In Ursin H, Baade E, Levine S, editors: *Psychobiology of stress: a study of coping men*, New York, 1978, Academic Press.
17. Mason JW: A re-evaluation of the concept of nonspecificity in stress theory, *J Psychiatr Res* 8:323-333, 1971.
18. Mason JW: Specificity in the organization of neuroendocrine response profiles. In Seeman P, Brown GM, editors: *Frontiers in neurology and neuroscience research* (First International Symposium of the Neuroscience Institute), Toronto, 1974, University of Toronto.
19. Mason JW: A historical view of the stress field, *J Human Stress* 1(l):6-12; 1(2):22-36, 1975.
20. McCance KL, Huether SE: *Pathophysiology: the biologic basis for disease in adults and children*, ed 2, St Louis, 1994, Mosby.
21. Moos R. *Coping with physical illness*, ed 2, New York, 1985, Plenum.
22. Murphy LP: Coping, vulnerability and resilience in childhood. In Coehlo GV, Hamburg DA, Adams JE, editors: *Coping and adaptation*, New York, 1974, Basic Books.
23. Murray RB, Zentner JP: *Health assessment and promotion strategies through the life span*, ed 6, Stamford, Conn, 1990, Appleton and Lange.
24. Peplau H: A working definition of anxiety. In Burd S, Marshall M, editors: *Some clinical approaches to psychiatric nursing*, New York, 1963, Macmillan.

25. Roth B, Creaser T: Mindfulness meditation-based stress reduction: experience with a bilingual inner city program, *Nurs Pract* 22(3):150-176, 1997.
26. Roy C, Roberts SL: *Theory construction in nursing: an adaptation model,* Englewood Cliffs, NJ, 1981, Prentice-Hall.
27. Selye H: A syndrome produced by diverse nocuous agents, *Nature* 138:32-35, 1936.
28. Selye H: The general adaptation syndrome and the diseases of adaptation, *J Clin Endocrinol* 6:117-230, 1946.
29. Selye H: *The stress of life,* New York, 1956, McGraw-Hill.
30. Selye H: The stress syndrome, *Am J Nurs* 65:97-99, 1965.
31. Selye H: *Stress in health and disease,* Boston, 1976, Butterworth.
32. Sharp S: Understanding stress in the ICU setting, *Br J Nurs* 5(6):369-373, 1996.
33. Steele RG, Fitch MI: Coping strategies of family caregivers of home hospice patients with cancer, *Oncol Nurs Forum* 23(6):955-960, 1996.
34. Strauss A et al: *Chronic illness and the quality of life,* ed 2, St Louis, 1984, Mosby.
35. Sutterley DC: Stress and health: a survey of self-regulation modalities, *Top Clin Nurs* 1(1):1-29, 1979.
36. Weisman A: *Coping with cancer,* New York, 1979, McGraw-Hill.
37. Weiss JM: Psychological factors in stress and disease, *Sci Am* 226(6):104-113, 1972.
38. White RD: Strategies of adaptation: an attempt at systematic description. In Coehlo GV, Hamburg DA, Adams JE, editors: *Coping and adaptation,* New York, 1974, Basic Books.

# chapter 7 Chronic Illness and Rehabilitation

WILMA J. PHIPPS

## objectives *After studying this chapter, the learner should be able to:*

1. Differentiate between acute and chronic illness.
2. Describe factors that influence chronic illness.
3. Identify areas of assessment for the chronically ill person.
4. Describe psychosocial interventions for the person with a chronic illness.
5. Define rehabilitation and the roles of the patient and team members (especially the nurse).
6. Describe the different types of facilities for continuing care.
7. Describe provisions of the Americans with Disabilities Act.
8. Identify major health goals related to chronic health problems to be achieved by the year 2000.

## IMPACT OF CHRONIC ILLNESS ON SOCIETY

Prevention and control of chronic disease constitute a major aspect of the health problems in the United States today. In the past the impact of chronic diseases on individuals, families, and communities has been overlooked. There is increasing awareness in the United States of great pockets of unmet needs among persons with long-term health problems. These individuals have needs that extend beyond the strictly medical. Their problems demand the use of multiple sources of help and care. In many cases the coping abilities of chronically ill persons are reduced because of advancing age, serious functional impairment and disability, and limited personal, social, and financial resources.

*Chronic disease* is not an entity in itself but an umbrella term that encompasses long-lasting diseases, which often are associated with some degree of disability. Each chronic illness is unique and has a different impact on the individual, family, and community. Nevertheless, common problems and complications that accompany the various chronic health problems can be studied in general to help the nurse understand and care for persons with specific long-term illnesses.

The incidence and prevalence of chronic diseases have increased since the beginning of the twentieth century. *Incidence* refers to the number of cases of illness that had their onset during a specified period of time. Health statistics commonly report the number of new cases for a calendar year. *Prevalence* refers to the total number of cases at a given point in time. Thus prevalence rates are higher than incidence rates because they include all persons (cases) with a specified condition (old cases) and those who acquired the condition during a specified period of time (new cases).

The reason that both the incidence and prevalence are increased for chronic diseases is because fewer persons are dying from acute diseases. There is decreased mortality from infectious diseases such as whooping cough and chickenpox in children and pneumonia in persons of all ages. Improved sanitation, the introduction of effective vaccines and mass immunizations, and the discovery of antibiotics have all contributed to this decrease in deaths from infectious diseases. Unfortunately, immunization rates in some areas of the country have declined, and young children are still dying as a consequence. Most of these deaths are in children living under the poverty level with limited access to medical care. In some states free immunization of these children has become a priority, along with education of the public about the continued need for childhood immunization.

The latest available figures from the U.S. Bureau of the Census show that the number of persons with some limitation in activity has been increasing each year. Another finding of interest is that the number of persons with limited activity decreased as family income increased (Table 7-1). This last finding seems to indicate that persons from higher income levels may be better educated about preventive health measures and that they are able to afford better diet, better housing, and better medical care.

*Disability* refers to any long- or short-term reduction of activity as the result of an acute or a chronic condition. *Limitation of activity* is used to describe a long-term reduction in a person's ability to perform the kind or amount of activity associated with a particular age-group. *Restriction of activity* is generally used to refer to a relatively short-term reduction in a person's activity below his or her normal capacity.

Death rates from heart disease decreased so dramatically in persons 45 to 64 years of age from 1970 until the present that heart disease is no longer the leading cause of death in persons in that age-group. Cancer has replaced it as the leading cause of death in persons between 25 and 65 years of age.[2]

While deaths from heart disease in some age groups were decreasing, death rates from other conditions were increasing. The death rate from HIV infection, which had increased

**table 7-1** *Persons with Activity Limitation by Selected Chronic Conditions and Income, United States, 1985 and 1994 (Figures in Millions of Persons Affected)*

| | 1985 | 1994 | Family Income for 1994 Only: Under $20,000 | $20,000-$34,999 | $35,000 and Over |
|---|---|---|---|---|---|
| **Age (years)** | | | | | |
| All ages | 32.7 | 39.1 | 14.4 | 8.0 | 9.4 |
| 18-44 | 11.6 | 11.1 | | | |
| 45-64 | 10.4 | 11.4 | | | |
| 65 years and over | 10.7 | 11.8 | | | |
| **Sex** | | | | | |
| Male | 15.3 | 18.2 | | | |
| Female | 17.4 | 20.9 | | | |

From US Department of Health and Human Services, Public Health Service, Centers for Disease Control and Prevention/National Center for Health Statistics: *Vital and health statistics: Current estimates from the National Health Interview Survey, 1994,* Hyattsville, Md, 1995.

**table 7-2** *Age-Adjusted Death Rates for 1993 and Percentage Changes in Age-Adjusted Death Rates for the 10 Leading Causes of Death from 1992 to 1993 and from 1979 to 1993: United States*

| Rank | Cause of Death | 1993 Age-Adjusted Death Rate | % Change: 1992 to 1993 | % Change: 1979 to 1993 |
|---|---|---|---|---|
| 1 | Heart disease | 145.3 | 0.7 | −27.2 |
| 2 | Cancer | 132.6 | −0.4 | 1.4 |
| 3 | Stroke | 26.5 | 1.1 | −36.3 |
| 4 | Chronic lung disease | 21.4 | 7.5 | 46.6 |
| 5 | Accidents | 30.3 | 3.1 | −29.4 |
| 6 | Pneumonia and influenza | 13.5 | 6.3 | 20.5 |
| 7 | Diabetes mellitus | 12.4 | 4.2 | 26.5 |
| 8 | HIV/AIDS | 13.8 | 9.5 | — |
| 9 | Suicide | 11.3 | 1.8 | −3.4 |
| 10 | Homicide | 10.7 | 1.9 | 4.9 |

From Centers for Disease Control and Prevention: Mortality patterns—United States, 1993, *MMWR* 45(8):161-164, 1996.

12.7% from 1989 to 1990, increased another 9.5% from 1992 to 1993, the latest year for which figures are available (Table 7-2).

As in the past, death rates for African Americans were higher than for whites for 8 of the 10 leading causes of death. Race-specific ratios were greatest for homicide (6.8) and HIV infection (4.0). The two conditions for which death rates were lower were chronic obstructive pulmonary disease and suicide (Table 7-2). Deaths rates were higher for males than for females for all 10 leading causes of death.

Several factors may have contributed to the increase in homicide: increases in substance abuse, access to handguns, poverty, urbanization and crowding, and family disruption and disorganization.[7] Death rates from homicides were highest among young black men from 15 to 24 years of age. The homicide rate among young black men is attributed to the factors listed above.

For the first time the National Health Survey of 1982 identified major disparities in the health of African Americans and other minorities in the United States compared with the white population. As a result of these findings, the secretary of the U.S. Department of Health and Human Services (DHHS) established a task force on black and minority health.[46] The findings of the task force are discussed on p. 133.

All the leading causes of death have risk factors associated with lifestyle, and many could be prevented by effective control of smoking, blood pressure, diet, and alcohol consumption.

## DEFINITION OF ACUTE AND CHRONIC ILLNESS

An *acute illness* is one caused by a disease that produces symptoms and signs soon after exposure to the cause, that runs a short course, and from which there is usually a full recovery or an abrupt termination in death. An acute illness may become chronic. For example, a common cold may develop into chronic sinusitis. A *chronic illness* is one caused by disease that produces symptoms and signs within a variable period of time, that runs a long course, and from which there is only partial recovery. The National Health Survey defines chronic conditions as follows: (1) the conditions were first noticed 3 months or more before the date of the interview or (2) they belong to a group of conditions (including heart disease, diabetes, and others) that are considered chronic regardless of when they began.[48] This follows the pattern of the

**box 7-1** *Problems Faced by Persons with Chronic Illness*

1. Preventing and managing medical crises
2. Controlling symptoms
3. Following prescribed regimen
4. Maintaining normal interactions with others
5. Adjusting to recurrent patterns in the course of the disease
6. Arranging payment for treatment

From Strauss AL: *Chronic illness and the quality of life*, ed 2, St Louis, 1984, Mosby.

Commission on Chronic Illness, which in 1949 defined *chronic illness as any impairment or deviation from normal that has one or more of the following characteristics:*

1. The illness or impairment is permanent.
2. The illness or impairment leaves residual disability.
3. The illness or impairment is caused by nonreversible pathological alteration.
4. The illness or impairment requires a long period of supervision, observation, or care.

This definition is still in use nearly 50 years later.

The symptoms and general reactions caused by chronic disease may subside with proper treatment and care. The period during which the disease is controlled and symptoms are not obvious is known as *remission*. However, at a future time the disease may become active again with recurrence of pronounced symptoms. This is known as an *exacerbation* of the disease.

Exacerbations of chronic disease often cause the patient to seek medical attention and may lead to hospitalization. The needs of a patient who has an acute illness may be very different from those of the patient with an acute exacerbation of a chronic disease. For example, a young person may enter the hospital with complaints of fever, chest pain, shortness of breath, fatigue, and a productive cough. If the diagnosis is pneumonia, the patient usually can be assured of recovery after a period of rest and a course of antibiotic treatment. If, however, the diagnosis is rheumatic heart disease and the patient is being admitted to the hospital for the third, fourth, or fifth time, the desired reassurance will not be so definite, clear-cut, or easy to give. In such a case it is necessary to begin planning care that will extend beyond the period of hospitalization, taking into consideration many aspects of the patient's total life situation. The concerns of the patient who has repeated attacks of illness will be very different from the concerns of the one who has a short-term illness.

Further, the needs of patients who are admitted to the hospital with an acute illness but who also have an underlying chronic condition must not be overlooked. For example, elderly patients who enter the hospital with pneumonia may receive treatment for the pneumonia and recover from their illness. However, they may still be hampered by the arteriosclerotic heart disease and arthritis that they have had for years. Also, these two chronic conditions may have been aggravated by the acute infection, or the return to former activity may be hindered by joint stiffness resulting from bedrest

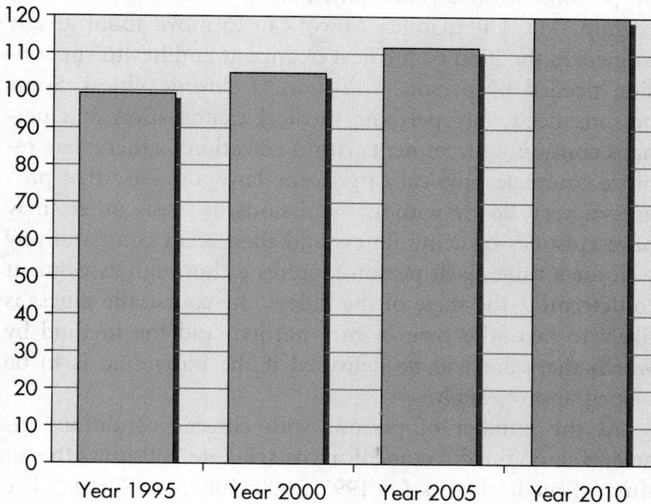


**fig. 7-1** Estimated number of people with chronic conditions (in millions).

and inactivity. Consideration of a patient's multiple diagnoses can help in preventing new problems associated with the chronic illness.

Strauss,[42] a well-known medical sociologist, described some problems experienced by persons with chronic illnesses (Box 7-1).

According to recent surveys an estimated 99 million Americans have one or more chronic conditions, and the number is expected to increase yearly. By the year 2010, 120 million persons will be affected (Figure 7-1). The *National Health Survey* classifies chronic physical conditions into the following categories: (1) selected skin and musculoskeletal conditions, (2) impairments (visual, hearing, speech, paralysis, deformity, or orthopedic impairment), (3) selected digestive conditions, (4) selected conditions of the genitourinary, nervous, endocrine, metabolic, and blood and blood-forming systems, (5) selected circulatory conditions, and (6) selected respiratory conditions.[48]

Many of these conditions cause a limitation of activity, which affects the lifestyle of those who are chronically ill. One of the trends that has been documented is that the impact of acute illness has diminished, whereas the burden of chronic health problems and related disability has increased. Limitation of activity is a measure of long-term disability resulting from chronic health problems or impairment and is defined as the inability to carry on the major activity for one's age-group, such as cooking, keeping house, going to school, or going to work.

Approximately 14% of the population experience some activity limitations, whereas almost half of the persons over 65 years of age are limited in their activities by one or more chronic conditions. Some activity limitations are associated with mental disabilities, but most are the result of physical handicaps caused by heart conditions and arthritis. Because chronic disability increases in direct proportion to age, persons older than 65 years of age are most prone to severe chronic disability.

As the population of the United States ages, the number of persons with chronic illness will continue to increase (Figure 7-1). The inability to work or to move about greatly influences the kind of medical treatment and health supervision needed by persons who have a chronic illness. Some persons need only periodic medical examination and perhaps continuing treatment with medications; others may require complete physical care. Some have a disease that progresses very slowly without remissions, whereas others may have episodes of acute illness and then seem comparatively well for a time. Each person requires a thorough assessment to determine the stage of the illness, the course the illness is likely to take, the type of care needed, and the method by which that care will be delivered if the individual is to be helped appropriately.

As the number of persons with chronic conditions increases so do the direct medical costs. Figure 7-2 shows the estimated medical costs for 1995, 2000, 2005, and 2010.[20] The cost of the care of persons with chronic conditions is spent on hospital care, physician care, other costs, and nursing home care. The 1990 allocation of these costs is shown in Figure 7-3. The "other" category includes the cost of prescriptions, dental care, nonphysician practitioners, home health care, medical equipment for use in the home, and emergency care.[20] Because there is no organized system in the United States for the care of those with chronic conditions, individual states are looking at models for delivering cost-effective care to this population. The Robert Wood Johnson Foundation has a national program, "Building Health Systems for People with Chronic Illness," that is looking at various ways to organize and pay for care for this population.[44a] Some of the approaches being considered by individual states are managed care models and a teamwork approach being studied by the Wisconsin Department of Health and Human Services. In the Wisconsin model the patient can choose a physician, and then community-based organizations put together a care-giving team that works with the physician to develop a comprehensive care plan. The plan is developed with the participant in his or her own home, if possible. This approach helps to identify the individual's strengths, disabilities, and lifestyle preferences and the capabilities of his or her informal support network. In the Wisconsin plan the patients are called "participants" to indicate that they are part of the planning process.

The goal in most programs for persons with chronic conditions is to keep them at home, if possible, because it is less costly, and most persons prefer to stay in their own homes as long as necessary services are available to them. The other issue that is receiving more attention is long-term care insurance. Although long-term insurance is available in most states, sales have been slow. The "Program to Promote Long-Term Care Insurance for the Elderly" is another program sponsored by the Robert Wood Johnson Foundation. There is particular concern because of the number of "baby boomers" who will be retiring in the next 15 to 20 years. More of these persons will need to have private insurance because public financing mechanisms will be inadequate to cover their needs. Because it is almost impossible for persons with chronic conditions to obtain private insurance, it is important that they obtain insurance before they become chronically ill. Figure 7-4 shows the difference in insurance coverage between those who are privately and publically insured.

## FACTORS THAT INFLUENCE CHRONIC ILLNESS

### Age

Different age-groups have different kinds of experiences with acute and chronic diseases. The young are more likely to experience short, intense, acute conditions that are quickly over. Elderly persons are more likely to have long, drawn-out chronic diseases; nevertheless, it is true that anyone can have

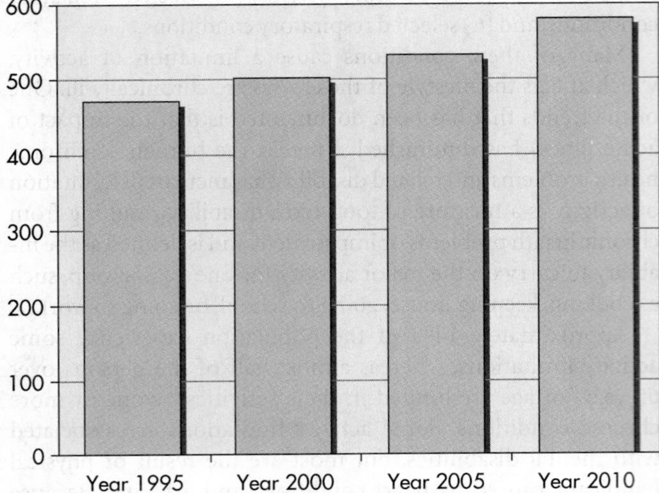

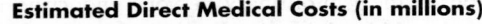

fig. 7-2 Estimated direct medical costs (in millions).

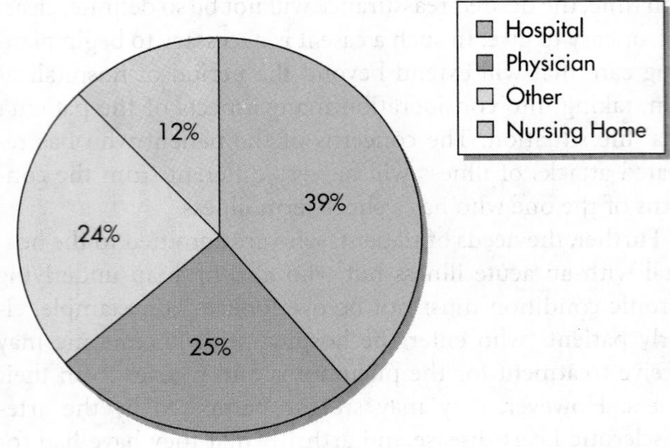


fig. 7-3 Direct medical costs for persons with chronic conditions.

either an acute or a chronic disease at any age. Chronic illness and disability may date from birth (e.g., spina bifida with neurological damage), or they may originate in childhood, adolescence, or early adult life (e.g., multiple sclerosis or rheumatoid arthritis). The major chronic illnesses among those 65 years and older identified in the *National Health Survey* were arthritis, diabetes, heart disease, and hypertension.[48]

Because of strides made in pediatric medicine, children who 30 years ago would have died of diseases such as cystic fibrosis are living longer. The reduction in death rates among the younger age-groups has allowed a higher percentage of the population to reach the age of greatest risk from chronic diseases. Cancer develops far more frequently in older than in younger persons. Because the average age of our population continues to rise, about 30% of persons now alive will eventually develop cancer.[2]

Much remains to be learned about interactions of the normal, pathological, and physiological changes of aging with various diseases. A common question that is asked is "When does aging end and illness begin?" Differences found in age-groups or changes found in individuals as they age represent normal aging—that is, a universal, intrinsic process of growth and development that is inevitable, irreversible, unpreventable, but ultimately detrimental. Even though aging, a normal process, is distinct from chronic disease, a pathological process, chronic illness often accompanies aging. The problems of aging and chronic disease are influenced in major ways by each other; for example, the social problems confronting elders are strongly influenced by the presence and severity of chronic disabilities. Remissions and exacerbations are possibilities with chronic illness; they are not with aging.

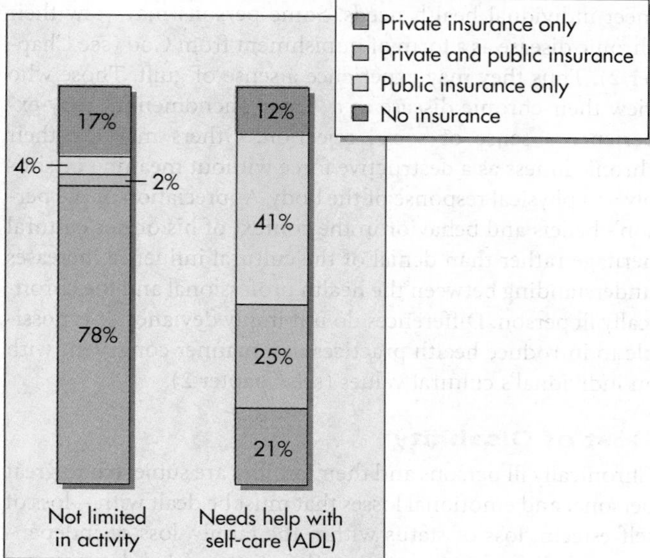


**fig. 7-4** Chronic conditions limit access to private insurance and force reliance on public insurance.

*Healthy People 2000*[47] made the following observations about age and chronicity. Persons in the United States who reach the age of 65 years can now expect to live into their 80s. However, it is not likely that all those years will be active and independent ones. Thus, improving the functional independence and not just the length of later life is an important element in promoting the health of this age-group.

One measure of health that considers quality as well as the length of life is the years of healthy life. Whereas people aged 65 years and older have 16.4 years of life remaining on average, they have an estimated 12 years of healthy life remaining. Thus quality of life is determined by the individual's ability to perform activities of daily living so that he or she can be independent.

## Race and Ethnicity

Race or ethnic group membership is a factor that influences chronic health problems. Race-specific rates measure the association between disease occurrence and race. Data on specific conditions indicate not only that some problems are more prevalent among nonwhites (African Americans, Native Americans, and Asians) but also that many nonwhites fail to receive necessary care.[7] For example, nonwhites are more than three times more likely to die of hypertension than whites of the same age-group. The findings of the Task Force on Black and Minority Health, which were released late in 1985, found that 60,000 excess deaths occur each year in minority populations.[46]

The excess number of preventable deaths is derived by calculating the difference between the number of deaths in the African American population and the number that would have been expected to occur by applying the average annual age-specific rates of the U.S. white population to the U.S. midperiod black population. This means that there would be no excess black deaths if the mortality rates of black and white persons were the same.

Seven causes of death were identified that together account for more than 80% of the excess mortality. The following health problems related to excess deaths are listed in alphabetic order.[12]

- Cancer—16% of excess mortality among African American men younger than 70 years of age.
- Cardiovascular disease and stroke—24% of excess mortality among African American men and 41% among African American women. Most of these deaths were caused by hypertensive heart disease.
- Chemical dependency (measured by deaths resulting from cirrhosis of the liver, associated with excessive use of alcohol)—13% of excess mortality among Native American men and 22% among Native American women younger than 70 years of age.
- Diabetes—38% of excess deaths among Mexican-born Hispanic women.
- Homicides and accidents (unintentioned injuries)—60% of excess mortality among Hispanics younger than 65 years of age.

**table 7-3** *Number of Selected Reported Chronic Conditions per 1000 Persons by Race and Age: United States, 1994*

| Chronic Conditions | White 65-74 | White 75 Years and Over | Black 65-74 | Black 75 Years and Over |
|---|---|---|---|---|
| Arthritis | 481.8 | 529.4 | 486.8 | 651.9 |
| Diabetes | 97.1 | 91.1 | 155.8 | 168.9 |
| Heart disease | 301.5 | 392.0 | 118.5 | 332.6 |
| Hypertension | 338.7 | 376.9 | 439.2 | 543.8 |

From US Department of Health and Human Services, Public Health Service, Centers for Disease Control and Prevention/National Center for Health Statistics: *Vital and health statistics: Current estimates from the National Health Interview Survey, 1994,* Hyattsville, Md, 1995.

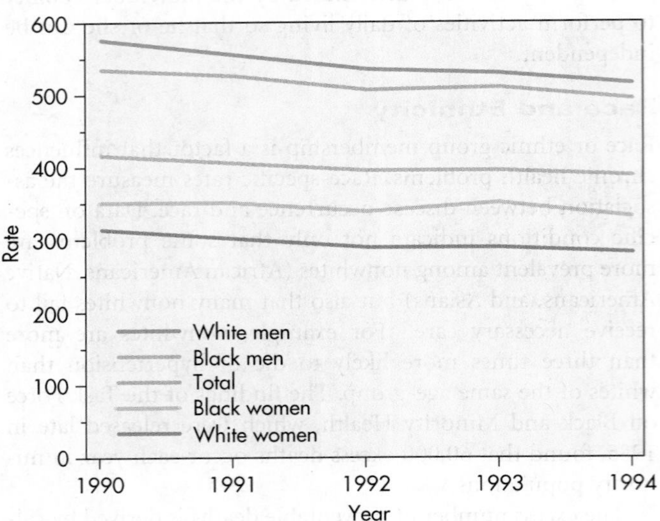


**fig. 7-5** Age-adjusted death rate of ischemic heart disease for adults aged 35 years, by race and sex, United States, 1990-1994.

- Infant mortality—of excess deaths among African American females up to age 45 years, death in the first year of life accounts for 35%.
- Unintentional injuries—44% of excess deaths among male and 30% among female Native Americans. Homicides and unintentional injuries account for 19% of excess mortality among African American men younger than 70 years of age and 38% among those younger than age 45. The figures for African American women are 6% and 14%, respectively. A substantial portion of excess deaths in this category may be associated with excessive use of alcohol and other drugs.

Table 7-3 compares the rates of four major chronic illnesses for whites and African Americans.

Trends in deaths from ischemic heart disease (IHD) from 1990 to 1994 are depicted in Figure 7-5, which compares the rates by race and sex. Death rates are decreasing for both men and women and whites and blacks. The rate of decrease was slower than the decline in the death rate that occurred in the 1980s. Factors contributing to the differential levels and rates of decline by race, sex, and state may include (1) trends in socioeconomic and behavioral risk factors for ischemic heart disease, (2) access to quality health care, and (3) geographic and temporal variation in the medical certification of ischemic heart disease.[49] Other studies have identified that deaths from IHD death rates vary inversely with social, economic, and medical resources. Communities where low-fat and high-fiber foods are available, where persons engage in leisure-time physical activity, and where persons quit smoking and receive medical care for risk factors such as hypertension, hypercholesterolemia, and diabetes show a decline in deaths from ischemic heart disease.[49]

## Cultural Values

Western culture tends to be cure-oriented; therefore, health care for acute conditions is often more valued than is health care for the chronically ill. In contrast with the exciting aspects of sophisticated and mechanical technology, caring for chronically ill persons is often considered boring. The continual struggle to cope with day-to-day living soon becomes tedious for chronically ill persons, their families, and health professionals. The rewards of treating chronic illness cannot be measured by a cure but by the prevention of complications and by helping persons function at their optimal level.

The cultural context has many symbolic meanings, beliefs, and values that health professionals need to understand to meet individual health needs. Some persons may view their chronic disease as a form of punishment from God (see Chapter 2). Thus they may experience a sense of guilt. Those who view their chronic disease as a "leper phenomenon" may experience a sense of social rejection. Others may see their chronic illness as a destructive force without meaning or simply as a physical response of the body. Appreciation of the person's beliefs and behavior in the context of his or her cultural heritage rather than denial of the cultural influence increases understanding between the health professional and the chronically ill person. Differences do not imply deviance. It is possible to introduce health practices in a manner congruent with an individual's cultural values (see Chapter 2).

## Cost of Disability

Chronically ill persons and their families are subjected to great personal and emotional losses that must be dealt with—loss of self-esteem, loss of status within the family, loss of independence, feelings of rejection, and feelings of helplessness are only a few. These can be more devastating than economic deprivation, which is a constant problem for many.

The economic cost to the patient and family is considerable. The cost of hospitalization rises yearly. Frequent or extended hospitalization and medical expenses can be ruinous if patients are inadequately insured or if they cannot afford medical insurance or have been dropped by an insurance company because of the chronicity of their condition. In 1998 it is estimated that more than 40 million Americans had no medical insurance.

Many are forced to seek public assistance merely to survive. Placement in quality nursing homes, which typically costs $3000 or more a month, is financially impossible for most patients or their families to manage. The cost of medications to control or maintain a patient's health status may require a major portion of the family budget. Additional expenses may include special diets and equipment, home modifications (e.g., ramps or widening of doors for wheelchairs), transportation, and support services provided by homemakers, day or live-in attendants, or nurses.

The ability of the individual family to pay its own way is determined in part by which member of the family becomes disabled. Older studies showed that the family suffered less economic deprivation if the wife was disabled. In those studies, three fourths of the chronically ill persons unable to carry out their jobs were men. Today, however, more and more households are headed by women who are single parents and are the only wage earners for the family. Women who head households will need additional help and support, and nurses should be sensitive to their needs.

Some financial assistance is provided by Medicare. This federally administered program provides hospital and medical insurance protection for persons 65 years of age and older, as well as for those younger than 65 years who are disabled and eligible for Social Security benefits. Persons under age 65 who are medically indigent because of health problems may be eligible for assistance through the Medicaid program.

Medicare primarily pays for acute care services. According to the Health Care Finance Agency (HCFA), 58% of Medicare costs covers payments to hospitals, 24% covers physician costs, 14% covers "other" services, and only 5% goes to nursing homes.

Recent changes in federal funding have altered Medicare and Medicaid programs. Persons aged 65 years and older receiving Social Security benefits have a higher fee deducted from their monthly payments to pay for their Medicare premiums. Medicare Part A pays for hospitalization; Medicare Part B covers medical expenses and physician care. Since Jan. 1, 1998, Medicare Part A pays all but $764 for the first 60 days of hospitalization and Medicare Part B covers physician bills, physical therapy treatments, rental of wheelchairs, and other equipment.

Each beneficiary pays a monthly premium of $43.80 for Part B coverage. The premium is deducted from the beneficiary's social security check. Those persons not receiving social security are billed for the monthly premiums quarterly. The monthly premium usually increases yearly. Part B does not cover the cost of medicines, eyeglasses, hearing aids, or dentures. Medicare reimbursement is commonly 80% of the amount billed. Most persons covered by Medicare purchase supplemental health insurance (co-insurance or "gap" insurance) to cover the expenses not reimbursed by Medicare.

There have been severe cutbacks in Medicaid, which is administered by state governments. For example, persons seeking Medicaid assistance in Ohio are not eligible if they have assets of more than $1500. Until recently a person was allowed to keep his or her home if a spouse was living in it. However, some persons who were financially well-off were advised by lawyers to "spend down their assets" to become eligible for Medicaid. That is, they were advised to transfer their assets to children or other relatives so that it appeared they were unable to pay for nursing home care. Because Medicaid was intended to be a program for the indigent, several governors have proposed more stringent eligibility standards and some states have passed laws that make it impossible for well-to-do persons to receive Medicaid after they have "spent down their assets." In Ohio a person is allowed to keep his or her home if a spouse is still living in it; however, the house will be sold by the state after the death of the spouse to recover the amount of Medicaid assistance received by one or both spouses. Because of large state budget deficits beginning in the 1990s, several governors are proposing even more stringent eligibility standards for Medicaid.

Thus persons with chronic illnesses may have considerable difficulty paying for prescribed therapy. For example, antiinflammatory agents used to treat arthritis are very expensive. Many of these medications cost between $0.75 and $1.35 each, and the usual dose is three times daily. Persons with other chronic conditions such as Parkinson's disease may be taking even more expensive drugs (costing as much as $1200/month). It is not uncommon for persons with limited resources to have to decide whether to purchase medications or food because there is not enough money for both.

## EPIDEMIOLOGY

Epidemiology examines the distribution of chronic disease, as well as the measurement of health status in the general population. It is both a body of knowledge and a method for obtaining knowledge. As a methodology, epidemiology can be used to assist in explaining the multifactorial causal patterns of chronic diseases.

### PROBLEMS IN DETERMINING CAUSALITY OF CHRONIC DISEASES

Some of the factors that contribute to the difficulty of studying the cause of chronic disease are:

1. *Multifactorial nature of etiological factors.* The operation of multiple factors is particularly important in chronic diseases. The interaction of factors may be purely additive or synergistic; that is, the combined potential for harm of many risk factors is more than the sum of the individual factors. They interact, reinforce, and even multiply each other. Asbestos workers, for example, have increased lung cancer risk. Asbestos workers who smoke have 30 times more risk than co-workers who do not smoke and

90 times more risk than persons who neither smoke nor work with asbestos.

2. *Absence of a known agent.* Because no specific diagnostic test exists for many chronic diseases, the distinction between persons with a disease and those free of disease may be more difficult to establish than with most infectious diseases.
3. *Long latent period.* Many chronic diseases have a long latent period, which is the equivalent of the incubation period in infectious disease except that it is generally longer. Because of the extended latency, it is often difficult to link antecedent events with outcomes. However, increasing evidence shows that onset of ill health is strongly linked to influences of physical, social, economic, and family environments. It is easy to identify the common exposure to chickenpox in a school setting, but it is much more difficult to identify the impact of drastic alterations in family circumstances caused by mental disorders or slow-onset physical illnesses.
4. *Indefinite onset.* The problem of pinpointing the initial occurrence of the disease exists with many chronic conditions, such as degenerative diseases and mental illnesses. The vague onset of chronic illnesses makes it is difficult to collect statistics on the number of new cases in any given year.
5. *Differential effect of factors on incidence and course of disease.* Factors in the socioeconomic environment that affect health include income level, housing, employment status, culture, and lifestyle. For example, Mormons who abstain from smoking and alcohol have lower cancer rates than the general population as a whole.
6. *Disease-specific mortality rates.* These rates are difficult to determine with chronic illness because the cause of death may result from factors other than the chronic disease itself.

One approach for studying chronic illness from an epidemiological viewpoint is to emphasize that interrelated factors determine illness; that is, disease is a process that results from the breakdown of many factors: biological, cultural, economic, emotional, and social. The multiple interactions involving the host, the environment, and the agent sometimes are described as the "web of causation." With this approach an attempt is made to identify the multiple related factors that lead to the disease process. Until a disease can be understood as a web of causation, it is difficult to make rational decisions regarding therapeutic interventions, and it is even more difficult to identify early preventive actions. To develop a chain of causation, one must identify first the natural history of disease by systematic studies of groups of people.

## NATURAL HISTORY OF DISEASE

All diseases have a natural history. For example, chronic diseases extend over time and develop through a sequence of stages. When people speak of the epidemiology of a disease, they are referring to its natural history. That is, the outcomes of a particular disease are observed over time, and the numbers of the affected persons developing each outcome are measured. This information is used to predict an individual's possible future health. Knowledge of the natural history of disease allows us to intervene to prevent or limit the effects of diseases. The stages involved in the natural history include:

1. *Stage of susceptibility.* The disease has not yet developed, but the groundwork has been laid by the presence of factors that favor its occurrence. These may be referred to as *risk factors.* The need to identify risk factors is becoming more apparent because chronic diseases are a greater health challenge than ever before. Some major risk factors are environmental and behavioral and therefore are amenable to change; for example, smokers can be persuaded to give up smoking.
2. *Stage of presymptomatic disease.* No manifestation of disease is present, but pathological changes have begun. An example of presymptomatic disease is atherosclerotic changes in coronary vessels before any overt signs or symptoms of illness appear.
3. *Stage of clinical disease.* By this stage sufficient anatomic or functional changes have occurred so that recognizable signs of disease exist. At present the natural history of many diseases is not completely understood. For example, it is not known why some individuals with several risk factors do not develop clinical disease, whereas others with fewer risk factors do.
4. *Stage of disability.* Disability, which can result from an acute or a chronic condition, reduces a person's activity. The extent of protracted disability resulting from chronic disease is very significant to the person and society because of the person's reduced income, the impact on his or her psychosocial roles, and the burden on community resources.

The subtlety of the natural history of chronic diseases often leaves the person unaware of a disease process for an extended period. Recently, predisposing characteristics or habits that help identify the person at risk to develop a particular chronic disease have been studied extensively. By altering habits of eating, rest, activity, or smoking, the course of certain chronic illnesses such as emphysema, hypertension, diabetes, or heart disease may be changed. Unfortunately, many chronic conditions begin without the individual's awareness of significant physiological changes. An important step in prevention is early detection of these changes.

## PREVENTION

Because chronic disease evolves over time and pathological changes may become irreversible, the goal is to detect risk factors as early as possible. Although these diseases differ from their infectious disease predecessors, it is now clear that many are preventable.

Generally, prevention means inhibiting the development of a disease before it occurs. More specifically, the term includes several levels of prevention to interrupt or slow the progression of disease: (1) primary prevention, (2) secondary prevention, and (3) tertiary prevention.

*Primary prevention,* appropriate in the stage of susceptibility, is concerned with health promotion and specific protection against diseases. *Secondary prevention,* applied in presymptomatic and clinical disease, includes early detection and prompt intervention to halt the progression of the disease. *Tertiary prevention,* appropriate in the stage of disability, uses rehabilitation activities to prevent further complications and to restore optimal functioning as much as possible.

Another way of looking at prevention has been identified by Albee.[1] He has developed a "prevention equation" for preventing dysfunction:

$$\text{Incidence of dysfunction} = \frac{\text{Stress} + \text{Constitutional vulnerabilities}}{\text{Social supports} + \text{Coping skills} + \text{Competence}}$$

The two major strategies for preventing dysfunction are decreasing the values in the numerator (i.e., decreasing stress or constitutional vulnerabilities) and increasing the values in the denominator (i.e., increasing social supports, coping skills, and competence). It is more difficult to have an impact on the numerator of the prevention equation because stress in our lives cannot always be controlled; however, creative ways to decrease individual and societal stress must continually be sought. It is easier to affect the denominator by strengthening social supports, coping skills, and competence. (For more information on stress see Chapter 6.)

One valuable tool that has been developed to assist persons to identify their own risk factors and change their lifestyles is the health hazard appraisal (HHA).[31] The HHA is a screening process that includes a comprehensive questionnaire and the taking of certain physical measurements. On the basis of probability tables, a risk assessment is then calculated from each person's profile along with goals that would result in risk reduction. Counseling and follow-up are provided to reinforce the data.

## CHRONICALLY ILL PERSONS AND THEIR FAMILIES

The effects of chronic illness on the affected person and family members are numerous and varied. The first impact of the disability may nearly immobilize them. Time must be provided for them to talk through their concerns and fears before they can be expected to begin coping with their new situation.

Marked changes are often required in family living as a result of chronic illness. Some families may find themselves drawn closer together. Other families may drift apart, the individual members being incapable of helping one another. At times, chronic illness may threaten a person's basic emotional stability, and the whole situation may be unbearable to others. Sometimes the person's emotional needs may not have been apparent to family members early in the illness, but when such needs grow obvious, relatives feel inadequate to cope with the situation. The length of illness, periodic hospitalizations, and increased financial, emotional, and social burdens are stressors that threaten the family's integrity.

Many persons struggle on their own to assume the full financial burden of the illness and consequently expose other members of the family to lower standards of nutrition, housing, and care. Many times relatives move in with one another, arguments develop, and family ties are strained or broken. Public assistance may be acceptable to some families, whereas others find it impossible to accept.

Chronic illness imposes additional problems of learning how to cope with restrictions on activities of daily living, how to prevent or identify medical crises that occur, and how to carry out treatment regimens as delineated by the health care provider. Family members also need to learn about the restrictions, not only to be of assistance to the chronically ill person but also to adjust to resultant disruptions in their own activity patterns.

Because chronic illness may have periods of exacerbation when symptoms become more acute and medical crises may occur, patients and family members need to know which symptoms must be reported to the health care provider as well as the time interval for reporting these symptoms. They also need to know how to contact the provider and what measures to take if a medical crisis occurs. For example, if a person has a history of myocardial infarction, family members must know what to do if the person experiences severe chest pain. Should they call 911 or should the person be taken immediately to a hospital emergency room or should the physician be contacted first? Patient and family members should plan in advance the sequence of actions to take during a medical crisis, depending on the nature and extent of the presenting symptoms.

## FAMILY INFLUENCES ON ILLNESS

### DEFINITION OF FAMILY

The definition of *family* has changed over time. In the past the concept of family as extended family was considered the societal norm. With the advent of urbanization, the norm became the nuclear family (mother, father, and children). Today the concept of family includes the single-parent family, the reconstituted family, and the gay or lesbian couple, among others. Family may be defined according to geographic proximity, as in shared households or residential retirement homes. Family also may be defined by shared emotional bonds between individuals or by one's support network. For this reason, in this discussion family is regarded as those people whom the ill individual or spokesperson identifies as family. A flexible definition of the family is especially important among ethnic families such as African Americans and Mexican Americans. African American elders often consider blood, marriage, or friendship relationships as equivalent, and caregivers treat personal care aides of the same cultural background as kin.[23] These nonblood relationships are referred to as *fictive kin.*[8] In addition, Mexican Americans use a "compadre" system or coparent who assumes the parenting role should anything happen to the natural parents.[17]

## MODELS OF FAMILY FUNCTIONING

Models of family functioning provide ways of thinking about the family that allow one to understand and predict behavior. Models are useful because they suggest ways that families may be helped. The two models described here are useful to nurses when they think about how families cope with illness. When selecting a theoretic framework of family functioning to address an ethnically diverse population, the nurse needs to determine if the definition of the family addresses changes in today's family compositions.[17] For example, family systems theory assumes that family members must be together to have relationships. However, family members who live at a distance may be just as intimate as those who live together. Anthropological and developmental perspectives suggest that family must be legally sanctioned or that all families go through the same stages at the same time. Because these two perspectives fail to address nonblood relationships or the earlier ages at which many minority families go through some of the developmental stages, they provide less guidance to the nurse for planning interventions. Despite the limitations of family systems theory, it is still one of the most frequently used family theories because of its focus on the interaction of the family members with the external environment.[28]

### Family Systems Theory

The family systems perspectives is derived from general systems theory (GST), as described in the work of Ludwig von Bertalanffy.[51] Family systems theory conceptualizes the family as an open system that functions within the broader context of the environment. The more open the family system, the greater is the exchange of information with the environment. Within the boundary of the family, dynamic interactions between the members or subsystems (such as the subsystem of parents or children) are governed by the family's organization. The organization of the family system is characterized by roles, relationships, expectations, and rules.

The terms *roles, relationships, expectations,* and *rules* are used to define organization in the family systems literature. Family members occupy and function in roles in relationship to one another. They seem to function in these roles according to the expectations of the whole family. Thus one family member may take on the role of breadwinner, whereas another may take on the role of homemaker. One family member may be the decision maker, another may be the primary caregiver for the small children, and another may be the caregiver for the chronically ill adult.

The term *rules* applies to the family expectations about how each person in his or her role relates to other family members; this becomes a standard for behavior over time. Whether spoken or implicit, these rules result in patterns of relating that characterize the family's interpersonal relationships and their attempts to maintain equilibrium.

The dynamic interactions that take place within the family are governed by the family's organization. According to family systems theory, the interactions are directed toward achieving and maintaining equilibrium within the system. *Homeostasis* reflects the family's striving to maintain equilibrium in the face of internal or external changes. Other family theorists refined the thinking on homeostasis with development of the concepts of morphogenesis and morphostasis.[22,41] *Morphostasis* describes maintenance of the status quo within the family system, and *morphogenesis* reflects the ability of the family to change its basic structure and organization to survive and remain viable. Morphogenesis and morphostasis describe the family system as existing in a dynamic balance between change and stability in response to the environment.

Certain principles describe the characteristics of a system. The principle of circular causality describes family as a group of individuals who are interrelated such that changes in one member evoke changes in another, which in turn affect the first individual. That is to say, individuals living in a family do not exist in a vacuum. They are constantly affected by the behavior of others in the family, which in turn affects their own behavior.

The principle of nonsummativity holds that the family as a whole is more than the sum of the individuals who make up that family. A family cannot be described by the characteristics of its individuals alone because this does not allow for the interaction among them. Thus one cannot look at each member of a family individually and have an appreciation of the characteristics of the family as a whole.

Understood within the framework of family systems theory is the idea that the organism of the family is constantly moving toward goals. The principle of equifinality states that different outcomes may have the same beginnings and that the same beginnings may lead to different outcomes. Because families are open systems, they are constantly exchanging information with the larger environment. Thus the outcome of the system is affected by more than just its initial conditions.

The family systems framework suggests several key assessment areas for the nurse (Box 7-2).

### Family Stress Theory

Family stress theory stems from the work of Hill,[18,19] who described families' responses to dealing with the loss of the father-husband after he was drafted into the armed services. Hill's ABC = X conceptualization of the family's response to stress serves as the foundation for investigation and theory building in the area of family stress research. Although researchers have made some modifications over the years to provide clarity and empiric support to the framework, it has

**box 7-2** *Family Systems Theory—Key Assessment Areas*

1. What are the family rules related to the patient, caregiver, and all other identified family member roles?
2. How flexible is each family member in creating and adapting roles to accommodate changes in the patient's health?
3. What are the patient and family goals related to the illness?
4. What environmental sources of information and support are known and unknown to the family?

remained essentially unchanged. This family crisis framework can be stated as follows:

A (the event) + Interacting with B
(the family's crisis-meeting resources) +
Interacting with C (how the family defines the event) =
X (the crisis)

The A factor represents the stressor event, which can be either external or internal to the family. It can result from normative changes or catastrophic events. In the case of an illness, and in this chapter the chronic illness itself is the stressor event to the family.

The B factor represents family resources, which may be of two types. Resources may be (1) those already available to the family or (2) coping resources strengthened or developed in response to the crisis event. Resources already available to the family might include a family member who is a health care professional or who has had previous experience in caring for an ill person.

The C factor represents the family's perception of the crisis. This is related to the family's view of the event's seriousness as well as what the event means to the family. If a family has experienced the death of a member from a stroke, the family might view a stroke in a second family member more seriously than would another family.

The X factor represents the crisis as experienced by the family. It is the outcome of the stressor event for the family after it is interacted on by family resources and perceptions.

The family's resources, the B factor, represent the area of the family stress framework that has received the most attention by researchers. Family resources may include the family member's personal resources and the family system's internal resources, social support, and coping skills. Two of the most important internal resources are the adaptability and cohesion of the family unit.

### Adaptability and cohesion

*Family adaptability* is the family's ability to reorganize and change roles, rules, and patterns of interaction in response to either situational or developmental stress. Adaptability refers to how flexible family members are in changing roles to accommodate changes in the family. To the extent that family members can be flexible in their roles, rules, and patterns of interaction, the family can successfully manage changes brought about by having a chronically ill member. Families who cannot make the necessary changes in their role structure and who have difficulty changing family rules are described as being rigid. Families at the opposite end of the adaptability continuum are described as being chaotic; they experience such dramatic role shifts and dramatic changes in rules that family members often do not know what rules apply.[32,33]

*Family cohesion* describes the extent to which family members feel bonded to each other and concerned and committed to the family. Cohesion is conceptualized as being on a continuum. Extreme cases of cohesion are (1) enmeshment, an overinvolvement of family members in each other's lives and, at the other end, (2) disengagement, in which family members are detached from the family and have little commitment to it. Healthy families lie somewhere between these two extremes. A sense of commitment in family members is vital if the ill member is to be cared for and the family is to continue.

### Characteristics of families

Particular qualities either increase the family's resources or add to the "pileup," a term used to describe the family experience of having additional stressors at the time of a stressor event. The nurse's awareness of a family's characteristics can give insight into the amount of burden families experience and the resources families have in caring for an ill member. These characteristics include but are not limited to the ones discussed in the following paragraphs.

**Familial relation to the patient.** Spouses and adult children experience caregiving in different ways. Spouses are more concerned about their health and see their physicians more often, rate their own health poorer, report more stress symptoms, and use more psychotropic medications than do adult children. The negative effects on the spouse caregiver's health may be related to the spouse's hesitancy to make use of respite services. Respite services are designed to give a few hours to several days of relief from caregiving activities. Thus the nurse must assess the caregiver's awareness of services and the cultural acceptability of these services and encourage the use or creation of respite by the caregiver. To minimize potential guilt feelings, the nurse should stress the importance of respite for the caregiver's health and continued quality of patient care.

In contrast, adult children are more concerned about family, time, and emotional conflicts. Consequently, adult children often express more burden[24] and place their parents in nursing homes more readily than do spouse caregivers. The fact that adult children perceive more burden may be related to the infrequent visits of family and friends and time spent relaxing.[16] Nevertheless, adult children use respite services more readily and report more benefits than do spouses. Finally, wives are more bothered by their cognitively impaired husband's frequent dangerous behaviors and embarrassing acts, and adult children are more stressed by a parent's inability to bathe himself or herself or stay alone.

**Gender.** Just as differences exist between spouses and adult children, so do differences exist between the genders. Wives tend to be more distressed/burdened during the initial stages of their caregiving role than are husbands,[13,57] and some women throughout the experience describe the situation as more confining and oppressive than do men.[40] Nevertheless, with the passage of time, some wives perceive less burden and reflect attitudes comparable with those of husband caregivers.[58]

Sons perform and experience the caregiving role differently and do not sense any major caregiving problems.[21] This low perception of problems probably is related to the fact that sons often delegate the physically intimate caregiving activities to their wives (i.e., the daughter-in-law) and focus on managing their parents' financial concerns. Daughters usually do not have the opportunity to delegate these activities. Therefore daughters may sense more caregiving problems.

The family life cycle also affects family responses. The family may have the additional burden of caring for both young children and elderly parents, although sometimes older children or young adults can share in the caregiving. Middle-aged daughters are more likely than older wives to have parental, employment, and marital obligations competing with caregiving. As the patient's level of impairment increases and need for the daughter's assistance increases, so does the daughter's sense of burden[16] and rewards.[27,56] Older husbands are more likely than sons to experience burden as caregivers because older men are likely to be full-time caregivers and sons are more likely to be part-time caregivers. Determining where the family is in its life cycle can assist the nurse in identifying potential areas of needed support.

**Ethnicity.** When focusing on diseases such as Alzheimer's, the nurse needs to consider the patient and family's ethnic heritage.[50] The patient's ethnic heritage may produce different human responses to the same phenomenon. Individual responses to catastrophic illness are filtered through differing belief systems and practices.[34] Consequently nurses need to consider the influence of family culture on the selection of coping strategies. White caregivers are more burdened when the patient has dementia and is unable to perform[30] daily living tasks such as preparing meals, laundering clothes, shopping, and paying one's bills. In contrast, African American caregivers are less burdened by the amount of supervision needed by Alzheimer's patients than are white caregivers.[38] Instead, African American caregivers are more burdened by a variety of physical disabilities that require more physical labor. The higher level of burden from physical disabilities among African American caregivers may reflect their overall poorer health status compared with that of white caregivers. Nevertheless, white caregivers are more likely to institutionalize persons with a dementia than are African American caregivers.

Family composition also affects the family response. The family may be large, with several persons who can share in the caregiving, or it may be a single-parent household already pressed to care for its members. The nurse must assess not only the actual participation of household members in caregiving activities but also the caregiver's perceived helpfulness of these acts of caregiver support. A large household does not always mean shared caregiving, and a small household does not always mean more limited support.

**Socioeconomic status.** This determines whether a family can afford to hire extra help to compensate for the activities usually performed by the patient and whether the cost of the illness places an added financial strain on the family.

**Employment status.** The employment situation of the caregiver is also important. The female caregiver may have been forced to quit her job or decrease her hours of work because of caregiving demands. Women who continue to work experience absences, work interruptions, loss of pay, decreased energy to do their jobs well, limited job choices, and a desire to not work.[5] Often women who are forced to quit their jobs score the lowest on mental health measures, which suggests that work may provide some respite for caregivers. Obviously, as the caregiving family's income decreases, the ability to purchase services to support the caregiver will decrease. A nurse referral of the family to a social worker may be helpful to the family at this point.

**Problem solving.** This is another important aspect to consider. Family members may or may not have the knowledge and ability to do the problem solving required to care for an ill member and also meet the family's demands. The perceived caregiver costs and rewards and the helpfulness of available social support are majors factors in the ability to cope.[23,35]

**Family health.** Family health is also important. The caregiver may have a chronic illness as well, which often occurs in a family of elderly persons. African American caregivers often have as many as four chronic illnesses.[25]

**Support network.** A support network composed of persons external to the family who can help the members carry out their tasks and give them emotional support is important for coping. African American elders living in the South have larger, more diverse support networks composed of family, relatives, friends, and fictive kin than do African American elders living in the North.[9,10] Fictive kin or "para-kin" are unrelated individuals with whom interpersonal relationships are so close that they [the fictive kin] are viewed as family members.[15] In addition, fictive kin have the same familial obligations as "blood" relatives.[8] Living in the South tends to increase the actual frequency of support. Not only does region of the country affect the family's caregiver activity, it also affects the type of services used. African American urban elders use more health services than do rural African American elders.[6,54] Rural elders turn first to their families in the case of illness, but urban elders turn to the hospital. The generally higher incomes of urban elders make services more affordable for them than for rural elders. Furthermore, African Americans, Native Americans, poor white persons, and others living in small towns and rural areas are far more dependent on unpaid family members and friends than on public and private service agencies for meeting their everyday needs in life. Also, there are fewer of these services in their area.[52]

**Social support.** It is important to determine whether the family is receiving help with the care needs of the patient, with the family's emotional needs, and with activities outside of the household. Can the family identify persons who visit them, call them, provide respite to them, and/or assist them with decision making? The caregiver's perception of social support decreases the feelings of burden and social isolation.[8,9,37,43,44,57]

**Religion.** The nurse should never overlook the role of the patient's and family's religion during a hospitalization. Religion can affect the patient's practices, acceptable treatments, and attire.[14] Prayer is especially important in the lives of African Americans and Muslims. For many African Americans, frequent prayer demonstrates their belief in the power of God to cure any disease in a faithful person. If the person is not cured, then the person failed to demonstrate sufficient faith. Similarly, devout Muslims must pray to Allah, their supreme being, five times a day. The Muslim patient may be found kneeling on a prayer rug facing Mecca, the Holy Land, during these times. It is important for nursing staff members to assess and arrange for the times the patient will need privacy for prayer. Failure to integrate prayer times into the patient's treatment plan may result in tension between the family and health care professionals. Sometimes the patient's faith that God will provide a cure may interfere with the patient's ability to realize that God sends cure through the hands of health care professionals. Health care professionals may need to employ the assistance of a local religious leader to stress this point.

At other times a patient's religion may forbid the acceptance of a treatment. For example, Jehovah's Witnesses refuse blood transfusions and Orthodox Jews refuse the use of anything electrical on the Sabbath. For Jehovah's Witnesses, to accept a blood transfusion means choosing to give up eternity with Jehovah. Although the health care professional may disagree with the Jehovah's Witness patient's beliefs, he or she must still respect and support the patient. For the Orthodox Jew, the Sabbath begins at sundown Friday and ends at sundown Saturday. During the Sabbath, work of any kind is prohibited, including driving, using the telephone, handling money, and even pushing an elevator button. While caring for one Orthodox Jewish woman with renal failure, the nurses on her medical floor rearranged the time of her hemodialysis on Friday afternoon to the morning hours. Consequently, when the Sabbath began, this patient already had returned to her room and was not in need of the electric elevator for transportation. Furthermore, the patient used battery-powered candles so that she did not have to operate the electric lights. Finally, when the patient needed the head of her bed raised, although she was capable of operating the bedside switches, the nurse brought the patient a bedside bell so that she could use the bell rather than the push-button call bell.

Observance of the Sabbath has ramifications for discharge planning also. Because of the prohibition against operation of a vehicle on the Sabbath, it is important to plan discharge of the Orthodox Jewish patient before or after the Sabbath. Otherwise the patient's family has to find a non-Orthodox Jew to pick up the patient from the hospital. The only exception to strict adherence to these practices is in a situation of life or death. For example, a young Jewish boy was severely injured one Saturday afternoon while playing football. He needed to go to the hospital immediately. The only person available to take him was his Orthodox Jewish grandfather, who drove him the 25 miles to the hospital. Once the boy was safely admitted, his grandfather walked home.[14]

Sometimes patients wear religious symbols, which the nurse must treat respectfully. These religious symbols include rosaries for Catholics, sacred threads around necks or arms of Hindus, medicine bundles for Native Americans, red ribbons for Mexican children, and mustard seeds, which are worn by some Mediterranean people to ward off the evil eye. When a medical procedure needs to be performed, removal of these religious symbols may be a problem. After explaining the rationale for removing the symbol in a calm, soothing tone, the nurse should gently place the symbol in close contact with the patient or at least within eyesight of the patient.

These are just a few cultural characteristics of families that can affect the family's experience as caregivers for a chronically ill member. As positive attributes, they can be indicators of family resources. As negative attributes, they may be predictors of deficits in family coping.

The family stress theory suggests several key assessment areas for the nurse (Box 7-3).

## COMPLIANCE AND NONCOMPLIANCE

Persons with chronic illness often are labeled as "compliant" or "noncompliant" in carrying out regimens prescribed for them. There are many factors that influence the person's ability or motivation to carry out the prescribed regimen. If the person does not carry out the regimen (noncompliant), it does not necessarily mean that the individual is refusing to do so deliberately, although this may sometimes occur.

Before the nursing diagnosis of noncompliance is made, the nurse needs to assess the situation to determine the reasons that the patient is not complying with therapeutic recommendations. The etiology of noncompliance includes the patient's value system (health beliefs, cultural influence, spiritual values).[26] The following are some possible reasons for nonadherence to a prescribed therapy[29]:

1. Failure to understand or internalize the reason for the recommendations
2. Procedures that are difficult to learn and carry out
3. Time required to carry out therapy
4. Inability to pay for prescribed therapy
5. Side effects of therapy (e.g., medications or exercises)
6. Embarrassment about carrying out the regimen in front of others
7. Social isolation and lack of support and positive reinforcement

Conflicts occur within the family structure when one family member recognizes the importance of carrying out the prescribed regimen but another does not. For example, a wife may see the need for continuing check-ups and medication for her husband's hypertension, whereas he may perceive this as a needless expense because he feels well and has no symptoms.

**box 7-3** *Family Stress Theory—Key Assessment Areas*

1. What does the illness mean to the family? Are there different meanings among family members?
2. What family characteristics serve as indicators of possible coping resources?
3. What family characteristics suggest possible deficits in family coping?
4. Has the illness increased or decreased the family's cohesion?
5. Which religious beliefs and practices must be integrated into the plan of care?

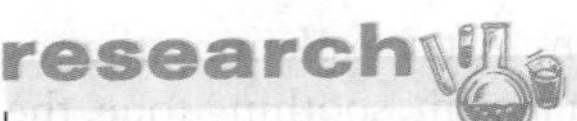

Reference: Burckardt CS et al: Quality of life of adults with chronic illness: a psychometric study, *Res Nurs Health* 12(6):347-354, 1989.

This study was designed to look at the quality of life of middle-aged to older adults with one of four chronic conditions: diabetes mellitus, ostomy secondary to colon cancer or colitis, osteoarthritis (OA), or rheumatoid arthritis. Four instruments, including the quality of life scale, and open-ended questions were used to collect data. All four groups of subjects identified the areas that were important to their quality of life. The major areas identified were independence, being physically active, being able to care for self, being healthy, having a sense of security, and maintaining positive interactions and relationships with others. Persons with OA also emphasized freedom from pain whereas those with diabetes emphasized being in control. These findings suggest that nurses need to be aware of the importance that the persons they are caring for attach to the factors identified in this study.

Persons vary from time to time in the extent of compliance. Those who are not hospitalized are their own health care agents, and they (or their significant others) determine the actions that are taken.

*Coping mechanisms that have been developed should not be tampered with unless, based on a thorough understanding of the situation, viable and more appropriate alternatives can be proposed.* If the goal of maintaining the chronically ill person in the optimal state of health is being interfered with by the individual's or the family's attitudes or capacities, a change in those attitudes or capacities is necessary, but it must be a change that is mutually acceptable. In preparation for giving the highest level of care to persons with a chronic illness, the nurse may find it helpful to review research in this area.[29,36,39,55]

### QUALITY OF LIFE

Nurses and other health care professionals have expressed concern about the quality of life (QOL) of persons with chronic conditions. The accompanying Research Box discusses the results of a study of QOL of middle-aged to older adults. Another report of a study of QOL in patients with heart disease can be found in reference 31a.

## ASSESSMENT OF THE PERSON WITH A CHRONIC ILLNESS

Before a plan of care can be devised for the chronically ill person, a thorough assessment of needs and capabilities must be carried out. Included in such an assessment are the individual's physical, psychological, social, and financial status.

### PHYSICAL STATUS

Because medical diagnoses do not accurately reflect the physical status and functioning of the chronically ill person, the use of a profile system or assessment tool may be instituted as a guide for those working with the patient. One such tool[31] provides a guide for grading the patient in six different categories: (1) physical condition, including cardiovascular, pulmonary, gastrointestinal, genitourinary, endocrine, and cerebrovascular disorders; (2) upper extremities—structure and function—including the shoulder girdle and cervical and upper dorsal spine; (3) lower extremities—structure and function—including the pelvis and lower dorsal and lumbar sacral spine; (4) sensory components relating to speech, vision, and hearing; (5) excretory function, including the bowels and bladder; and (6) mental and emotional status. The ability of the person to carry out activities of daily living (e.g., dressing, feeding, bathing, brushing teeth, combing hair, using the toilet, and moving from place to place) specifically needs to be assessed. The completed assessment should indicate in what areas the patient has difficulty and the extent of that difficulty. Such a guide can be used in planning goals for care, both immediate and long term, and will be useful in assisting the individual and the family to make realistic plans for care. Because a chronic condition is not static, reassessment should be carried out at regular intervals to establish improvement or regression. The assessment tool on p. 150 covers the areas just mentioned.

The impact of chronic illness on the person's desire for or ability to participate in sexual activities should be assessed. Changes in body appearance, shortness of breath, and musculoskeletal or neurological impairments cause some persons to think that they can no longer be sexually active. In addition, the side effects of certain medications tend to decrease sexual desire or cause impotence. The nurse should determine if concern about sexual ability is a problem for the person, and if it is, appropriate action including referral can be taken. (See Chapter 46 for more information about sexuality in health and illness.)

### PSYCHOLOGICAL STATUS

Assessment of the person's psychological needs and capabilities includes determining attitudes and stage of adaptation to the illness, feelings concerning how illness affects the family or significant others, and the person's own goals in regard to living with an illness. For example, those who are almost totally helpless as a result of a long-term chronic condition may seem to have no interest in learning ways to help themselves. Family members may react in the same manner and be of little help to them. Both the affected person and family need interest and support from nurses and other professionals as they learn to cope with the change in their life situations.

Feelings of anxiety, frustration, irritability, bitterness, and guilt may be expressed by some chronically ill persons who face unending pain and loss of economic and social security. Some persons become obsessed with their health problems and spend much of each day thinking about what will happen and what to do. Guilt may result from being unable to work and support oneself or from the belief, as a result of a search for some purpose or reason for the affliction, that one must deserve the suffering. *Depression* is common among chronically ill persons, especially those who feel powerless. *Powerlessness* can be the result of feeling unable to control or overcome what has happened to one.[36] Patients who are depressed may be suicidal, and the nurse should be alert to cues that the patient may be contemplating suicide.

Coping skills may be challenged by persistent, ongoing problems such as chronic pain, recurring medical expenses, or continuing difficulties in carrying out activities of daily living. Usual coping methods may become impossible; for example, a person who usually copes by expending energy in physical activity may become unable to do so. The person who usually copes by discussing problems with family members will need to find an alternative method if family communication patterns break down. The person can be helped to identify usual coping methods and to explore alternative approaches when necessary.

It is important to recognize that chronically ill persons or their families may suffer from unresolved sadness known as *chronic grief.* Chronic grief may be defined as accumulated or prolonged grief. It extends over long periods, with permanent characteristics developing in many persons, and carries with it a potential for decreased functioning. The causes are varied, and new waves of grief are constantly triggered. One example is grief caused by the losses associated with aging: youth, dreams, jobs, hair, friends, family, health, visual acuity, social role, money, body parts, and mobility. Each loss is accompanied by grief, which builds on previous grief, just as individual bricks create a wall. In chronic grief the person may be faced with repeated acute episodes. These episodes may coincide with exacerbation of the condition, facing a new limitation, or meeting new indignities. Each new episode requires a renewed struggle back and forth through the various stages of grief.[36]

The nurse can assist by listening and helping the person explore feelings and the content related to these feelings. Because the grief is ongoing, family members also can be helped to identify their feelings and strengthen the communication patterns within the family structure for normal support of its members.

## SOCIAL AND FINANCIAL STATUS

Social and financial status must be considered because both relate specifically to the kind of support and resources available to meet the person's goals. It would be unrealistic, for example, to plan for a hydraulic bathtub chair if the patient could not afford it, if family members were unavailable to help operate it, or if the patient's apartment manager would not permit it to be installed. Alternative methods of helping the patient to take a tub bath would have to be explored.

The social assessment includes living arrangements, family roles, support of significant others, cultural and social group memberships, education, and vocational and avocational activities. The data collected through the performance of this kind of thorough assessment should make it possible to devise a plan of care directed toward the accomplishment of attainable goals that are mutually acceptable to the patient, the family, and the caregivers.

## ROLE OF THE NURSE IN CHRONIC ILLNESS

### Clarifying Nurse-Patient Values

Before nurses can work effectively with chronically ill persons they need to be able to distinguish between their own values, standards, and goals and those of the patient. In day-to-day contact with individuals who are making little or no progress, it is tempting to make plans for their future because of a sincere interest in helping them. This is particularly true when the patient's age is similar to one's own. There may be a feeling that something must be done to speed progress. One may become frustrated by the feeling of wanting to do something or wanting to see some marked change. However, the nurse must recognize that management of the care of the chronically ill person requires a slow-moving, persistent pace with possibly little or no change for a long time. The person's physical and mental condition must be maintained at its present level or improved, and efforts must be made to progress and encourage the family's adaptation to the patient's condition. Eagerness and readiness to progress will be determining factors for the future. The "doing" in the care of the chronically ill person is not always a physical action with the hands. Often the maintenance of a positive approach and attitude and a demonstration of real interest are the greatest help to the patient. Teaching patients to perform activities related to their own care independently rather than performing those activities for them also may lead to progress.

### Promoting Self-care

Asking the person to identify what is meaningful is a primary step toward helping develop self-care. Physical needs are of paramount importance for chronically ill persons. Meeting these physical needs provides a way to convey to such individuals an interest in their progress and welfare. Chronically ill persons who are hospitalized should be allowed to perform as much of their own care as possible. Persons who have been independent in self-care before hospitalization should not be allowed to regress in these abilities if at all possible. Helping them to take their own baths or showers, attend to toilet needs, and groom themselves can give some sense of accomplishment and help them maintain their self-respect. Helping them to be dressed appropriately promotes a sense of wellness. Success in performing portions of their own self-care may be stimulating enough to strengthen ill persons' motivation; they and their families then may make amazing strides in thinking through and working out future problems themselves. For their planning to be realistic and ultimately functional, all health care personnel must teach chronically ill persons the total physiological ramifications of their disability, as well as methods of coping with those ramifications.

Persons who are in their homes or in substitute homes should be encouraged to dress in regular, comfortable street clothing rather than pajamas or gowns. Visitors to the home and family members who constantly see such individuals dressed in bedclothes think of them as sick and are reminded of their illness. Seeing them dressed as usual helps to maintain normal attitudes, relationships, and expectations.

### Promoting Self-esteem

The care of chronically ill persons requires alertness in feeling, seeing, and hearing. Continued warmth and interest are necessary to the self-esteem of any chronically ill person. Very often a relationship based on an understanding of these requirements promotes self-esteem and helps the individual to become highly motivated. It may be taxing to listen to the same questions and say the same things day after day, but the nature of chronic illness may require this attention, and the manner in which responses are given will convey warmth and interest. The world of chronically ill persons, whether they are in the hospital or elsewhere, becomes narrowed and circumscribed. They treasure and are interested in those things and those people who are close to them. Their conversations may be largely about themselves, their immediate environment, a few close objects, and the persons who are close to them. Although they may be confined to bed and to their room, others can keep them up-to-date on outside news. Depending on their level of adaptation to their illness, they may welcome hearing about outside events, or they may not be able to think beyond themselves. When they reach the stage of being able to look beyond themselves, newspapers, magazines, radio, or television or creating something with their own hands may help to keep up their interest in others and in outside events.

### Supporting the Person with a Progressive Disability

Health care personnel must be prepared to provide care for patients whose disease will follow a course of progressive disability, as with multiple sclerosis, rheumatoid arthritis, or Alzheimer's disease. In these instances, goals of care must be modified to retard the downhill progression of disability rather than to achieve maintenance or improvement of physical status. Helping the patient and family cope with progressive deterioration and in some cases eventual death is a demanding task.

### Providing Community Resources

There has been increasing interest in providing programs for chronically ill persons and in assisting them and disabled persons to assume a more active role in their communities. Volunteer workers may act as readers both in hospitals and in homes or may assist with other diversional activities. Institutions receiving federal funds are required to make aids such as ramps available to persons who are unable to climb stairs or who are in wheelchairs. (See p. 157 for a discussion of the Americans with Disabilities Act.) With the development of structural changes that facilitate mobility, some persons with physical limitations are more involved in local activities and associations. Nurses can assist by supporting the further development of these structural changes in all community buildings and by encouraging the participation of chronically ill persons in community activities of interest. Various information sources may be obtained from national organizations involved with chronic illness and disability. Many of these agencies have services available in the community (Box 7-4). Programs, facilities, and legislation of this nature reflect the public's increasing awareness of the difficulties faced by chronically ill and disabled persons.

## REHABILITATION

Rehabilitation is the process of assisting the individual with a handicap to realize his or her particular goals, physically, mentally, socially, and economically. As such, rehabilitation is an active concept and must be clearly differentiated from the concept of maintenance care. After a thorough assessment of patients' disabilities and capabilities, assumptions can be made regarding the potential for improving their conditions. If improvement can be made, patients are candidates for rehabilitation. If improvement cannot be made, care is directed toward maintaining the current condition, that is, preventing further disability. The process of rehabilitation can be viewed more appropriately as *patient education* rather than *patient care.* One must remember, however, that the rehabilitation of every patient will reach an end point, that is, a point at which no further progress is possible. At that time the focus of care reverts to that of maintenance.

The purpose or extent of rehabilitation ranges from employment or reemployment for the handicapped person to the more limited achievement of developing self-care abilities. This latter accomplishment can be just as important to the individual as earning money and may represent that person's greatest life achievement. This might be true, for example, for a person who was born with a severe physical handicap such as cerebral palsy.

Success in learning to adjust to living with a disability depends on the person's premorbid personality, total life experience, and premorbid family relationships, as well as the person's current behavior and motivation. Certainly, some rehabilitation can occur in any health agency; nevertheless, the greater the number of rehabilitation disciplines made available as needed to individuals, the greater is their chance of achieving their highest potential. The rehabilitation process, as with any form of education, is involved as deeply in the motives and purposes of the teacher as in those of the learner.

Persons with disabilities, whether obvious to others or unrecognizable, should not be viewed from the standpoint of their disability alone. Usually the greatest need is for comprehensive health services and continuing care. Comprehensive care is that which is provided to patients according to their needs in an appropriate, continuous, and dynamic pattern. Accommodating the plan of care to the needs and goals of individual patients rather than to those of the providers of care is the essence of comprehensive care.

## INTERDISCIPLINARY APPROACH

The number of professional persons required to assist the patient and family with rehabilitation will vary. Most often the patient, the family, the physician, and the nurse can work out a practical plan. If a patient's problems are complex, other members may be added to the team. Typically, such a team consists of a physician, nurse, discharge coordinator, medical social worker, vocational counselor, psychologist, speech pathologist, occupational and physical therapists, and a caseworker from the patient's social agency. Figure 7-6 shows members of an interdisciplinary team planning care for a patient. Teamwork requires that members of the team be able to use their special knowledge and skill and understand the value of their contribution to the patient's care. In addition, team members need some understanding of each other's professional functions and contributions. One of the cooperative efforts of the involved team members is to meet regularly to

**box 7-4** *Community Resources Involved in Chronic Health Problems*

Various types of information may be obtained by contacting these national organizations. In addition, services of the various agencies usually are available at the local level.

**GENERAL**

Alzheimer's Disease and Related Disorders Association
4709 Golf Rd.
Skokie, IL 60076
(847) 933-1000

American Association of Diabetes Educators
444 N. Michigan Ave., Suite 1240
Chicago, IL 60611-3901
800-338-DMED

American Association of Retired Persons
601 East St. NW
Washington, DC 20049
(202) 434-2277
e-mail: www.aarp.org

American Cancer Society
1599 Clifton Rd., N.E.
Atlanta, GA 30329
(404) 320-3333
800-ACS-2345
e-mail: www.cancer.org

American Diabetes Association
National Center
P.O. Box 25757
1660 Duke St.
Alexandria, VA 22314
(703) 549-1500
800-ADA-DISC
e-mail: www.diabetes.org

American Heart Association
7272 Greenville Ave.
Dallas, TX 75231-4596
(214) 373-6300
800-242-1793
e-mail: www.amhrt.com

American Lung Association
1740 Broadway
New York, NY 10019
(212) 315-8700
e-mail: www.lung.usa.org

American Parkinson Disease Association
1250 Hylan Blvd., Suite 4B
Staten Island, NY 10305
(718) 981-8001
800-223-2732
e-mail: www.the-health-pages.com

Arthritis Foundation
1330 W. Peachtree St.
Atlanta, GA 30309
(404) 872-7100
800-283-7800
e-mail: www.arthritis.org

Association of Retarded Citizens (ARC-U.S.)
800 E. Border St., Suite 300
Arlington, TX 76010
(817) 261-6003

Brain Injury Association (NHIF)
1776 Massachusetts Ave. NW, Suite 100
Washington, DC 20036-1904
(202) 296-6443
800-444-6443

Cystic Fibrosis Foundation
6931 Arlington Rd., No. 200
Bethesda, MD 20814
(301) 951-4422
800-344-4823

Epilepsy Foundation of America (EFA)
4351 Garden City Dr.
Landover, MD 20785
(301) 459-3700
800-EFA-1000

International Life Sciences Institute–North America (ILSINA)
1126 16th St. NW, No. 300
Washington, DC 20036
(202) 659-0074

Juvenile Diabetes Foundation
120 Wall St.
New York, NY 10005-3904
(212) 785-9500
800-JDF-CURE
e-mail: www.jdfcure.com

Leukemia Society of America, Inc.
600 3rd Ave.
New York, NY 10016
(212) 573-8484
800-955-4LSA
e-mail: www.leukemia.org

March of Dimes Birth Defects Foundation (MDBDF)
1275 Mamaroneck Ave.
White Plains, NY 10605
(914) 428-7100

Mental Health Materials Center
P.O. Box 304
Bronxville, NY 10708
(914) 337-6596

Muscular Dystrophy Association, Inc.
3300 E. Sunrise Dr.
Tucson, AZ 85718
(520) 529-2000
e-mail: www.mdausa.org

National Association for Down's Syndrome
P.O. Box 4542
Oak Brook, IL 60522
(630) 325-9112

National Association for Visually Handicapped
22 W. 21st St.
New York, NY 10010
(212) 889-3141
e-mail: www.staff@navh.org

National Council on the Aging
409 3rd St. SW, Suite 200
Washington, DC 20024
(202) 479-1200
e-mail: www.ncoa.org

National Easter Seal Society (NESS)
230 W. Monroe
Chicago, IL 60606
(312) 726-6200
800-221-6827
e-mail: www.sealsnepa.com

*Continued*

**box 7-4** *Community Resources Involved in Chronic Health Problems—cont'd*

National Hemophilia Foundation
110 Greene St., Suite 303
New York, NY 10012
(212) 219-8180
e-mail: www.hemophilia.com

National Jewish Center for Immunology & Respiratory Medicine
1400 Jackson St.
Denver, CO 80206
(303) 388-4461

National Kidney Foundation
1250 Broadway
New York, NY 10001
(212) 629-9770
e-mail: www.kidney.com

National Mental Health Association
1021 Prince St.
Alexandria, VA 22314-2971
(703) 684-7722
800-969-NMHA

National Multiple Sclerosis Society
733 3rd Ave.
New York, NY 10017
(212) 986-3240
800-FIGHT-MS
e-mail: www.nmss.org

Parents of Children with Down Syndrome
c/o The Arc of Montgomery County
11600 Nebel St.
Rockville, MD 20852
(301) 984-5777

Shriners Hospital for Crippled Children
2900 Rocky Point Dr.
Tampa, FL 33607
(813) 281-0300
800-237-5055
e-mail: www.shriners.com

Sickle Cell Disease Association of America (SCDAA)
200 Corporate Point, Suite 495
Culver City, CA 90230-7633
(310) 216-6363
800-421-8453

Stroke Clubs, International (SCI)
805 12th St.
Galveston, TX 77550
(409) 762-1022

United Cerebral Palsy Associations
1660 L St. NW, Suite 700
Washington, DC 20036
(202) 776-0406
800-USA-5UCP
e-mail: www.ucpok.org

United Ostomy Association
36 Executive Park, Suite 120
Irvine, CA 92714
(714) 660-8624
800-826-0826

**REHABILITATION**

Architectural and Transportation Barriers Compliance Board
330 F St. NW
Washington, DC 20004
(202) 272-5434

Mainstream
3 Bethesda Metro Center, Suite 830
Bethesda, MD 20814
(301) 654-2400
800-661-8239
e-mail: www.mainstrm@aol.com

National Information Center for Children and Youth with Disabilities (NICHCY)
Box 1492
Washington, DC 20013
(202) 884-8200
800-695-0285
e-mail: nichey@aed.org

National Spinal Cord Injury Association (NSCIA)
545 Corcord Ave., No. 29
Cambridge, MA 02138-1122
800-962-9629

Paralyzed Veterans of America
801 18th St. NW
Washington, DC 20006
(202) 872-1300

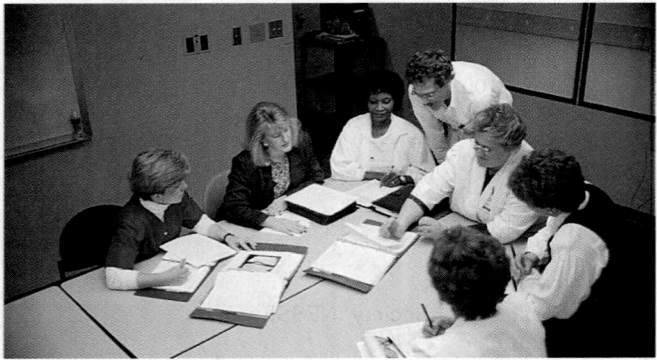

**fig. 7-6** The team approach to rehabilitation is essential.

evaluate patients and their abilities thoroughly. On the basis of this assessment, each patient and the team devise a plan to foster readjustment, compensation, and the learning of new ways to manage self-care and living.

## REHABILITATION CENTERS

Persons with very complex problems of rehabilitation may need to receive care at specialized centers for rehabilitation, or they may receive care at home combined with visits to day rehabilitation centers. The variety of specialized centers includes teaching and research centers (centers located in and operated by hospitals and medical schools), community centers with facilities for inpatients, community outpatient centers, insurance centers, skilled nursing homes with an active rehabilitation service and staff including physical and occupational therapists, and vocational rehabilitation centers. In addition to centers that provide multiple services for the physically disabled, specialized centers provide rehabilitation for blind, deaf, mentally ill, and mentally retarded persons. Most centers offer a wide range of services that usually fall into the following three areas:

**Physical area**
Physical, nursing, and medical evaluation
Physical therapy
Occupational therapy
Speech therapy
Medical and nursing supervision of appropriate activities

**Psychosocial area**
Evaluation
Personal counseling
Social service
Psychometric testing
Psychiatric service
Recreational therapy

**Vocational area**
Work evaluation
Vocational counseling
Prevocational experience
Industrial fitness of programs
Trial employment in sheltered workshops
Vocational training
Terminal employment in sheltered workshops
Job placement

Several advantages exist for patients participating in organized programs for rehabilitation. They have an opportunity to see and be with others who have similar or more extensive disabilities. Often they progress more rapidly when they realize that others have similar difficulties and are overcoming them. Group therapy often arouses a competitive spirit, and a formerly reluctant person may become willing and diligent. On the other hand, all personnel need to be alert to those patients who have the opposite reaction. Patients who see others advance in activity while they either do not improve or progress very slowly may become so discouraged that they give up trying. In some cases the person becomes very depressed and may be suicidal. The nurse should be aware of changes in the person's behavior and be sensitive to any expression of suicidal ideas.

On a rehabilitation unit activities are scaled so that individuals can see their own progress in comparison with their beginning abilities. Patients may take an active interest in keeping their own scores. After a program of therapy has been planned and is scheduled as to time of day, patients can help to keep themselves on the schedule by having a copy of it at the bedside. Patients can then be assisted to gradually assume more responsibility for readying themselves for scheduled activities. In addition, a master plan of activities for all patients on the unit can be a useful device for nurses, physicians, and therapists. The plan can be kept in a central place on the unit and should list name, activity, and time of activity for each patient. This type of plan is also helpful when a patient's progress is to be reevaluated.

A public program for vocational rehabilitation has been serving the United States since 1920. The program involves a partnership between the state and the federal governments. Services for disabled persons are provided by state divisions of vocational rehabilitation. The federal government, through the Social and Rehabilitation Service (SRS), administers grants-in-aid and provides technical assistance and national leadership for the program. Opportunities and services are available in all 50 states, the District of Columbia, and Puerto Rico. All persons of working age with a substantial job handicap resulting from either physical or mental impairment are eligible for help or assistance. The purpose of this service is to *preserve, develop,* or *restore* the ability of disabled persons to earn their own livings. The individual services offered are medical care, counseling and guidance, training, and job finding. All 50 states have separate rehabilitation programs for blind persons. Application for such services can be made to the SRS or to the agency in the state for serving the blind.

## SUBACUTE REHABILITATION FACILITIES

As part of the changes in medical care delivery, patients are being kept in acute rehabilitation units a shorter period of time. Because these patients still require close medical monitoring, intensive rehabilitation nursing, and comprehensive care provided by a multidisciplinary health care team, subacute rehabilitation units have been developed in skilled nursing facilities in nursing homes and step-down units in the hospitals.[4] More community based rehabilitation services as well as home care services are now available. Physiatrists (specialists in physical medicine and rehabilitation) are becoming more involved in community based health maintenance organizations where they work with primary care physicians who may not understand the knowledge that the physiatrist can contribute to patient care. There is also concern that the emphasis on cost cutting may prevent patients from receiving care they need to achieve positive functional outcomes. Measurement of functional change in subacute rehabilitation has recently been started on a systematic basis. Comparison of patient outcomes in different settings is beginning to appear in the rehabilitation literature.[4]

## ROLE OF THE PATIENT

The most important contributions to patients' rehabilitation are made by the patients themselves. The patient, his or her family, the nurse, the physician, the social worker, the occupational therapist, and sometimes others planning together can arrive at the best plans for the future, but the patient's attitudes, acceptance, and motivation are the most important considerations. If the patient cannot adjust to the disability, whatever it is and however extensive, attempts at rehabilitation usually are hindered. Patients must make the decisions, and they change at their own pace. If they are agreeable to suggestions but make little or no effort to try them, one should question if they really have accepted them.

The importance of motivation in rehabilitation was demonstrated by Dennis Byrd, a professional football player for the New York Jets, who was injured in a collision with another player during a game in November 1992. The seriousness of his injury was impressed on those watching the game by the extreme caution with which he was positioned on a backboard while his head was held in midline.

His prognosis was grave, and there was doubt that he would walk again. Yet, less than a year later he was able to walk unaided into the stadium on opening day of the 1993 football season, where he greeted his teammates and fans. From the beginning he believed that he would walk again and he worked hard to achieve this goal. In his book about his rehabilitation, *Rise and Walk,* he discusses the superb support he received from his wife, young daughter, and others and the role that his religious faith played in his recovery. His first-hand report gives the reader an insight into the role his motivation played in his recovery.

Self-care is encouraged within existing limitations. The patient's behavior from day to day can be the first indication of the direction of positive motivation. For example, if the patient makes every effort to resume normal daily activities such as feeding, bathing, and dressing, one can be certain that the person has a sincere desire to be independent. As patients become ready for more advanced activities, such as ambulation and work in the occupational therapy shop, they need continuing genuine interest and support (Figures 7-7 and 7-8). As obstacles arise, patients may be able to accept and eventually overcome them. Patients who are truly motivated to help themselves never seem to give up, finding ways of accomplishing activities that professional personnel might believe impossible. Each person working with the chronically ill patient has seen that many times life has meaning for the individual even though it may not be readily apparent to others. Some patients, however, when faced with an added burden, cannot accept it and give up trying. Guidance and support for the families of such patients become tremendously important. Health care personnel who understand these attitudes and behaviors can help make life satisfying for the chronically ill person and can positively influence the behaviors of the family, professional co-workers, and the public.

## ROLE OF THE NURSE

The concepts of comprehensive nursing care and rehabilitation can be considered synonymous. Helping the patient and family members to help themselves is an integral part of nursing care. Nurses who work with patients who have disabilities have two major responsibilities: (1) to ensure that disability from disease or disuse is limited as much as possible and (2) to see that a rehabilitation program is planned and implemented. Details of the nurse's role and responsibilities are listed in Box 7-5.

### Limiting Disability

Limitation of disability is the nurse's first responsibility and requires attention to the prevention of complications, to the early recognition of symptoms of exacerbations or complications, and to the prevention of deformity. For patients with chronic illnesses, the onset of exacerbations or complications is frequently subtle, marked by minute changes in functional ability or general performance or attitude. Nurses, working closely with such patients and understanding the pathophysiology of their diseases, are frequently the first to recognize initial signs of difficulty and make provision for appropriate intervention.

### Planning and Implementing a Rehabilitation Program

The second responsibility, planning and implementing a program of rehabilitation in accordance with the patient's goals, is a process with which nurses are immediately involved. The

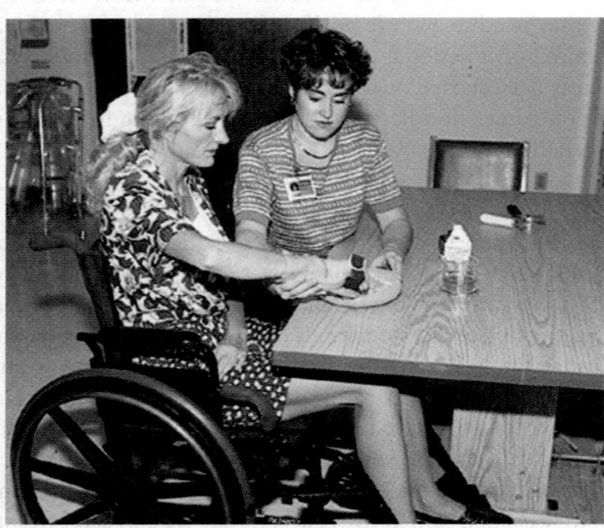

**fig. 7-7** A patient participating in occupational therapy using mobile arm supports and upper-extremity orthotics.

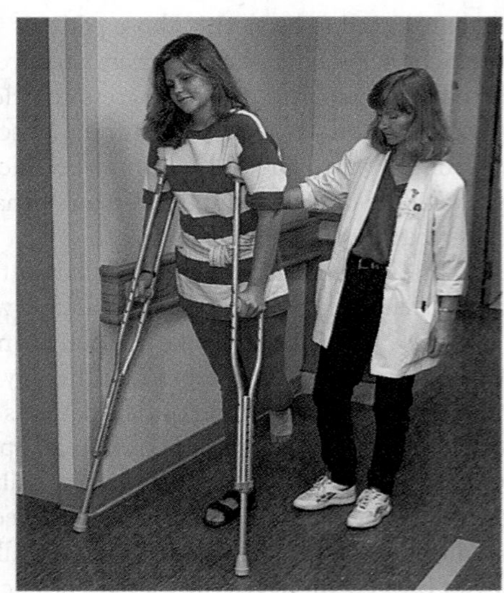

**fig. 7-8** A physical therapist begins a patient's ambulation training by teaching her to walk with crutches.

first step in planning is to take a careful health history in four categories: physical/functional, psychosocial, economic/vocational, and spiritual. A tool for gathering these data can be found in Figure 7-9. Nursing personnel are likely to be in contact with a patient and the family for a longer period each day than are members of any other discipline on the rehabilitation team. Both in the hospital and in the home, nurses are in an excellent position to assist the patient in planning a reasonable care program, as well as to teach the patient, the family, and, if necessary, the employer, about the patient's limitations and rehabilitative expectations.

Much of the nursing activity in the rehabilitation process is no different from basic nursing care. Measures such as appropriate bowel and bladder programs, providing proper diet and fluid requirements, implementing new methods of bathing, and maintaining skin integrity fall within the domain of nursing concern and knowledge. Initially, nursing personnel may assume almost total responsibility for performing these activities for the patient. After assessing patient abilities in these areas, nurses formulate, implement, and evaluate a teaching plan in much the same way as do therapists from other disciplines. The assistance nurses can give the patient and family depends on nurses' ability to understand themselves, personal feelings, and personal behavior as well as the behavior of the patient, family, and other professional team members.

One of the most important aspects of giving continuing care to a patient with a disability is the nurse's own attitude, perseverance, and expectations. Improvement may be slow, and patients may reach a plateau in their progress. Such a time can be critical for patients because they may become discouraged and not wish to continue with their program of care. Realistic encouragement can often sustain patients so that they will not regress before some improvement is noted.

Patients in a rehabilitation program must often learn and practice special physical techniques to strengthen muscles and to improve mobility. Measures such as physical exercise to improve walking, activities to improve self-care abilities, and the use of prostheses require the special knowledge and skills of physical and occupational therapists. To be effective in the rehabilitation process, nurses must have an understanding of the techniques used by the various therapists so that they can plan and work cooperatively with them in caring for the patient. This knowledge is also used to help the patient employ appropriate techniques in carrying out activities of daily living.

## CONTINUING CARE

Traditionally, health care professionals have assumed responsibility for the patient's well-being within the hospital and little to no responsibility for the patient and family in the home setting. This dichotomy between health care in the home and hospital facility made little sense. With chronically ill persons the dichotomy interferes with a smooth transition from hospital to home. The major portion of health care for some persons with chronic illnesses occurs in the home; thus ongoing communications must exist between the patient and health professionals.

*Text continued on p. 155*

**box 7-5** *The Nurse's Role and Responsibilities in Rehabilitation*

I. Limit disability from disease as much as possible.
   A. Prevent complications.
      1. Ensure early recognition of symptoms including patient's condition worsening.
         a. Review signs and symptoms and pathological course of the chronic illness to recognize changes.
         b. Review signs and symptoms of complications frequently associated with the chronic illness, such as infection.
      2. Prevent deformities.
         a. Maintain proper body alignment.
         b. Position limbs to prevent contractures.
         c. Turn patient frequently; keep skin clean and dry to prevent skin breakdown.
         d. Provide adequate nutrition.
         e. Provide adequate fluid intake to maintain bladder and bowel program.
         f. Take precautions to prevent infection.

II. Plan and implement rehabilitation program appropriate to patient.
   A. Determine patient's own goals for rehabilitation.
   B. Plan appropriate nursing interventions based on mutually agreed-on goals.

   Early in rehabilitation the nursing staff may have to assume total responsibility for assisting with activities of daily living (ADL): bathing, dressing, intake of food and fluids, bowel and bladder programs, maintaining skin integrity, turning patient, and so on.
   C. Plan nursing interventions that encourage patient to assume responsibility for own ADL as soon as possible.
      1. Set short-term goals with patient.
      2. Be sure that goals are realistic and attainable.
      3. Reinforce patient's progress (no matter how small) with positive feedback.
      4. Work with other members of the rehabilitation team in providing a consistent, coordinated rehabilitation plan.
      5. Keep patient's significant others informed of patient's progress so they can give positive feedback to patient.
      6. Reassess goals periodically and set new goals as appropriate.
      7. Teach patient, family, and, if necessary, employer about patient's limitations and rehabilitative expectations.

## GUIDELINES FOR RECORDING HEALTH HISTORY

Patient's name ________ Date of birth ________ Age ________
ID number ________ Race/ethnic origin ________
Date of admission ________ Date of initial assessment ________
Medical diagnosis: Primary ________ Secondary ________
Attending physician ________ Primary nurse ________
Rehabilitation team members ________
Informant: Patient: ________ Family member ________
Reliability of historian: Good ________ Fair ________ Poor ________

### PHYSICAL/FUNCTIONAL HISTORY

1. How would you describe your general health? Excellent ________ Very good ________ Good ________ Fair ________ Poor ________
2. Breathing
   a. Have you had any difficulty breathing before or with this admission? No ________ Yes ________
   If yes, describe the difficulty ________
   b. What can be done during your rehabilitation to make breathing easier for you? ________
   c. Do you expect any difficulties in breathing when you return home? ________
3. Nutrition
   a. How would you describe your nutrition? Excellent ________ Very good ________ Good ________ Fair ________ Poor ________
   b. Describe a typical day's food intake ________
   c. What is your weight? ________
   d. What foods do you like the best? ________
   e. What foods do you like the least? ________
   f. Are you now or have you ever been on a special diet? No ________ Yes ________
   If yes, what was the diet? ________
   g. At what times do you usually eat? ________
   h. Have you needed any assistance to eat? No ________ Yes ________
   If yes, what types of assistance? ________
   i. What is the condition of your mouth? Good ________ Cavities ________ Gum disease ________ Other ________ Specify other ________
   j. Do you wear dentures? No ________ Yes ________ Upper ________ Lower ________ Partial ________
4. Elimination
   a. Bladder
   (1) Have you had any difficulty passing urine? No ________ Yes ________
   If yes, what was the problem? ________
   what did you do about it? ________
   what treatment, if any, did you receive? ________
   (2) Do you frequently experience any of the following symptoms?
   Incontinence ________ Foul-smelling urine ________
   Urgency ________ Cloudy urine ________
   Frequency ________ Burning on urination ________
   Pain on urination ________ Bloody urine ________
   If yes, to any of the above problems, what was done about it? ________
   (3) Do you need any assistance with bladder elimination? No ________ Yes ________
   If yes, what type of assistance do you need? ________

*Continued*

**fig. 7-9** Guidelines for recording health history, *cont'd.*

**PHYSICAL/FUNCTIONAL HISTORY — cont'd**

b. Bowel
   (1) How would you describe your bowel habits? Regular _______ Irregular _______
   (2) How often do you usually have a bowel movement? Every day _______ Every other day _______
   Twice a week _______ Once a week _______ Other _______
   (3) What time of day do you usually have a bowel movement? Morning _______ Afternoon _______
   Evening _______
   (4) Tell me if you do any of the following things to assist you in having a bowel movement:
   Eat certain foods _______ Specify _______
   Drink certain fluids _______ Specify _______
   Take medications _______ Specify _______
   Insert suppositories _______ Specify _______
   Perform digital stimulation _______ Perform Valsalva maneuver _______
   Specify other _______
   (5) Do you frequently experience any of the following problems?
   Diarrhea _______ Impaction _______
   Constipation _______ Incontinence _______
   Specify other _______
   If yes to any of the above, what did you do about the problem? _______
   What treatment, if any, did you receive? _______
   (6) Do you need any assistance in getting to the bathroom? No _______ Yes _______
   If yes, what type of assistance? _______

5. Skin integrity
   a. How would you describe the condition of your skin? Excellent _______ Very good _______
   Good _______ Fair _______ Poor _______
   b. Do you bruise easily? No _______ Yes _______
   c. Have you ever had open sores or ulcers that are slow to heal? No _______ Yes _______
   d. Have you ever had rashes? No _______ Yes _______
   e. Have you ever had moles that have grown? No _______ Yes _______
   f. Do you sweat easily? No _______ Yes _______
   g. Have you ever had itchy skin? No _______ Yes _______
   h. If yes to any of the above problems, describe the circumstances and what you did about the problem?
   _______

6. Rest/comfort
   a. Rest
   (1) How would you describe the amount of rest you get? Always enough _______ Enough _______
   Sometimes enough _______ Never enough _______
   (2) What time do you usually go to bed? _______ Get up in the morning? _______
   (3) Do you have any difficulty going to sleep at night? Always _______ Usually _______
   Sometimes _______ Never _______
   (4) Do you awaken during the night? Always _______ Usually _______ Sometimes _______
   Never _______
   (5) Do you take naps? No _______ Yes _______ If yes, when? _______
   (6) What aids, if any, do you use to go to sleep at night?
   Drink warm liquids _______ Read _______
   Take an alcoholic beverage _______ Turn night light on in room _______
   Watch television _______ Take sleeping pills _______

*Continued*

**fig. 7-9** Guidelines for recording health history, *cont'd.*

**PHYSICAL/FUNCTIONAL HISTORY — cont'd**

b. Comfort
   (1) How would you describe your physical comfort? Always very comfortable ______
   Usually comfortable ______ Sometimes comfortable ______ Never comfortable ______
   (2) Have you experienced discomfort in the past? No ______ Yes ______
   If yes, describe ______
   ______
   What did you do about it? ______
   Did it help? No ______ Yes ______ Partially ______
   (3) If you have discomfort during your rehabilitation program, what would you like the nurse or therapists to do about it? ______

7. Personal hygiene/grooming
   a. Have you needed the help of another person with:
   Bathing ______ Shaving ______
   Brushing/combing your hair ______ Applying makeup ______
   Brushing your teeth ______ Feminine hygiene ______
   Applying deodorant ______ Dressing: Uppers ______ Lowers ______ Both ______
   b. Have you used any adaptive aids to assist with any personal hygiene or grooming activities?
   No ______ Yes ______
   If yes, specify ______
   ______

8. Communication
   a. Vision
   (1) How would you describe your vision? Excellent ______ Very good ______ Good ______
   Fair ______ Poor ______
   (2) Do you wear glasses? All the time ______ For reading ______ Never ______
   (3) Do you wear contact lenses? All the time ______ While awake ______ Sometimes ______
   Never ______
   b. Hearing
   (1) How would you describe your hearing?
   Right ear: Excellent ______ Very good ______ Good ______ Fair ______ Poor ______
   Left ear: Excellent ______ Very good ______ Good ______ Fair ______ Poor ______
   (2) Have you ever had pain in either ear? No ______ Yes ______
   (3) Have you ever had ringing in your ears? No ______ Yes ______
   (4) Have you ever had a discharge from either ear? No ______ Yes ______
   (5) If yes to any of these problems, describe ______
   What did you do about it? ______
   What treatment, if any, did you receive? ______
   ______
   c. Sensation/perception
   (1) Do you have any difficulties with feeling pain? No ______ Yes ______
   With feeling temperature? No ______ Yes ______
   (2) Do you have any intolerance to temperature? No ______ Yes ______
   (3) If yes to 1 or 2, describe ______
   What do you do about the problem? ______
   d. Speech/language
   (1) How would you describe your ability to express yourself? Excellent ______ Very good ______
   Good ______ Fair ______ Poor ______
   (2) How would you describe your ability to understand others? Excellent ______ Very good ______
   Good ______ Fair ______ Poor ______

*Continued*

**fig. 7-9** Guidelines for recording health history, *cont'd.*

**PHYSICAL/FUNCTIONAL HISTORY — cont'd**

(3) Have you ever had difficulty expressing yourself? No ________ Yes ________
If yes, describe the circumstances ________
(4) Have you ever had difficulty understanding others? No ________ Yes ________
If yes, describe the circumstances ________

9. Mobility (ask questions appropriate to client's mobility status)
   a. How would you describe your ability to get out of or into a bed or chair? Excellent ________ Very good ________
   Good ________ Fair ________ Poor ________
   b. How would you describe your ability to get into the bathtub? Excellent ________ Very good ________
   Good ________ Fair ________ Poor ________
   c. How would you describe your ability to walk/navigate a wheelchair? Excellent ________ Very good ________
   Good ________ Fair ________ Poor ________
   d. Have you ever had difficulty moving about? No ________ Yes ________
   If yes, describe the difficulty ________
   How did you manage? ________
   e. Do you expect to have any difficulty getting around when you leave the rehabilitation unit?
   No ________ Yes ________
   If yes, what do you expect to do about it? ________
10. Sexuality (ask questions according to patient's marital status)
   a. How would you describe your sex life? Very satisfactory ________ Satisfactory ________
   Not very satisfactory ________
   b. Has there been or do you expect differences in your ability to be a:
   Husband No ________ Yes ________
   Father No ________ Yes ________
   Wife No ________ Yes ________
   Mother No ________ Yes ________
   Significant other No ________ Yes ________
   If yes, describe what you expect the differences to be ________
   ________
   c. Do you expect your sexual functioning to be changed in any way after your rehabilitation?
   No ________ Yes ________
   If yes, describe expected changes ________
   ________
   d. Do you want the nurse to obtain more information about sexual function for you?
   No ________ Yes ________
   If yes, specify interests ________
   Refer you to a sex counselor? No ________ Yes ________

**PSYCHOSOCIAL HISTORY**

1. What is your marital status? Married ________ Divorced ________ Separated ________
   Widowed ________ Never married ________
2. Do you have any children? No ________ Yes ________
   If yes, how many? ________ What are their ages? ________
3. What type of housing do you live in? Upper apartment ________ Lower apartment ________ Ranch ________
   Two or more story dwelling ________
4. How many people live in your home? ________
5. Where do you sleep? ________
6. Where is the bathroom located? ________
7. How would you describe your relationships with others living in your home? Excellent ________ Very good ________
   Good ________ Fair ________ Poor ________
   If fair or poor, would you like to tell me anything about these relationships? ________
   ________
8. Do you have any interests or hobbies? No ________ Yes ________
   If yes, describe ________

*Continued*

**fig. 7-9** Guidelines for recording health history, *cont'd.*

**PSYCHOSOCIAL HISTORY — cont'd**

9. How far did you go in school?
Grammar school ______ College graduate ______
Some high school ______ Some graduate school ______
High school graduate ______ Graduate school degree ______
Some college ______

10. What are your habits?
Smoking ______ How long? ______ How many packs/day? ______
Drinking ______ How long? ______ How much? ______
Drugs ______ How long? ______ How much? ______
Coffee ______ How many cups/day? ______
Exercise ______ Type ______ How often? ______ How long? ______

11. Coping
a. How would you describe your coping abilities? Excellent ______ Very good ______ Good ______
Fair ______ Poor ______
b. What do you do when you are upset? ______
c. Does it help? No ______ Yes ______

12. Relationships
a. Who is the most important person to you? ______
b. How many close friends do you have? ______
c. What effect has your disability had on your family and friends? ______
d. Do you expect your family and friends to visit during your rehabilitation program? ______
e. Who of your friends or family would you most like to assist with your rehabilitation program? ______
f. Who should be notified in case of an emergency? ______
Telephone number ______ Address ______

**ECONOMIC/VOCATIONAL HISTORY**

1. What is your occupation? Present ______ Past ______
Unemployed ______ If unemployed, are you retired? No ______ Yes ______
2. How would you describe your financial resources? Excellent ______ Very Good ______ Good ______
Fair ______ Poor ______
3. How will you pay for your rehabilitation program?
Self, family ______ Vocational rehabilitation agency ______
Insurance plan ______ Medicaid ______
Worker's compensation ______ Medicare ______
Specify other ______

**SPIRITUAL HISTORY**

1. Do you practice a religion? No ______ Yes ______
If yes, what denomination? Catholic ______ Protestant ______ Jewish ______ Muslim ______
Specify other ______
a. Do you attend a place of worship regularly? No ______ Yes ______
b. Do you have any dietary restrictions as part of your religious practices? No ______ Yes ______
c. Would you like to see a chaplain while you are here? No ______ Yes ______
2. Do you feel your spiritual needs are met? Yes ______ No ______
If no, is there anything the nurse can do to assist you in meeting your spiritual needs? ______

**OTHER**

1. What do you know about your current health concerns? ______
2. Do you have any questions right now about your current health concerns? ______

Thank you for answering all my questions. I will be back later to see if we agree on your major health concerns and sit down to establish goals with you for your rehabilitation program.

**fig. 7-9** Guidelines for recording health history, *cont'd.*

Because all persons with long-term care needs cannot be cared for in their own homes, other settings, especially nursing homes, have become centers for these patients. The role of nursing homes in long-term care has become postacute or subacute care. Some hospitals with excess acute care beds have converted them to subacute beds for patients who are expected to recuperate or die. These settings provide convalescent and rehabilitative services formerly provided in acute care hospitals. Most of this type of care is covered by Medicare and Medicaid. In an attempt to limit costs, many states are looking to managed care to reduce Medicaid costs.

At the same time, concern is being raised about the quality of care given under managed care. To monitor the quality of care, there are several ongoing studies designed to compare actual patient outcomes with expected patient outcomes for specific groups of patients. The results of these studies will be used to assess the performance of the managed care program in delivering the level of care necessary to produce expected patient outcomes.

## SELF-HELP GROUPS

Self-help groups are associated with self-care. These groups may or may not include the guidance of health care providers. They provide social support to their members through the creation of a caring community, and they increase members' coping skills through the sharing of information, experiences, and problem solutions. Examples of self-help groups include those for women who have had mastectomies and those for persons who have colostomies, diabetes, or obesity. There are now self-help groups or clubs for patients with a variety of conditions. Nurses should learn what groups are available to patients in their community. A telephone call to a health agency such as the American Cancer Society, American Heart Association, or American Lung Association can elicit information about services available to patients who have the specific condition served by the agency.

In some hospitals and nursing homes nurses have been instrumental in setting up support groups for families of patients with chronic health problems such as Alzheimer's disease. It can be expected that more support groups, both those for patients and those for families, will be developing in the future. Some of the impetus for these groups can be traced to changes in health care.

Both patients with acute and chronic illnesses have shorter hospital stays, and thus their needs for continuing care are greater. It is difficult to predict at this time the changes in Medicare and Medicaid that will occur as the federal and state governments attempt to control costs in these two entitlement programs.

## FACILITIES FOR CONTINUING CARE

It is impossible to include here all the facilities that provide continuing care. Each of the programs mentioned has its own criteria for acceptance of patients for the services it renders. Before application for service is made and before the program is discussed with the patient and family, the individual patient's eligibility for that service should be determined by the health care professional.

### Ambulatory Care

The term *ambulatory care* is used interchangeably with outpatient care and refers to first-contact health care services as well as to continuing contact services in settings that do not require overnight stays. The use of ambulatory care facilities has expanded because of the increase in chronic illness and the increase in cost of inpatient services. A good ambulatory care service constitutes one of the most important elements of the hospital's contribution to community health. There is a trend toward development of ambulatory care facilities in neighborhood health centers to assist disabled, aged, or disadvantaged persons to obtain needed health care. An ambulatory care center usually provides the long-term follow-up care needed by the person with a chronic illness, in addition to preventive health care, diagnostic work-ups, and treatment of acute illnesses for which hospitalization is unnecessary.

### Home Care

Before World War II the home was the place where medical treatment was given. Well-to-do persons rarely went to a hospital; instead, they received the services of a private physician in their own home, and the family or nurses employed by the family were responsible for the day-to-day care. Poor families were among the first persons to use hospitals. The philosophy of home care can be traced as far back as 1796, when the Boston Dispensary provided medical care to the sick poor in their homes.

One of the most obvious reasons for the development of home care programs was to provide care to patients with long-term illnesses who did not need the around-the-clock services of an institution and yet who were too ill to go to an outpatient center. Caring for patients at home is often desired by the individual and family, and it also releases hospital beds for use by acutely ill patients. (See Chapter 23 for more information about home care of the adult.)

Today *home care* is being provided for acutely ill patients discharged from the hospital while they still need skilled nursing care. As a result, many hospitals have set up home care programs to supply nursing care and other services to their patients after discharge. Hospitals that have not set up their own programs are contracting with the Visiting Nurse Association and other nursing agencies to supply nursing care for their patients after discharge.

Frequently the issue arises as to who should pay for home health services and who should be reimbursed for health care provided. The American Nurses Association's position is that reimbursement systems should foster care of individuals in their homes on the basis of the following premises.[3]

1. Home health care is humane and respectful of the individual's dignity and integrity.
2. Home care or care within the community can be less costly than institutional care.
3. Nursing care is the primary element in home care.
4. Payment systems for home care should recognize nurses as the major providers of home care, and nurses should be reimbursed on their own authority.

Home care may not be possible for all patients. For those living in smaller dwellings, adequate space for the patient, necessary equipment such as oxygen, intravenous fluids, and ventilators, and for other members of the family may be at a premium. The choice of home care, independent living center, or institutional care depends not only on the desires of the patient and the family but also on the ability to finance the care.

Some states are testing pilot programs to keep selected elders in their own homes instead of sending them to a nursing home. Carefully selected patients whose needs can be met at home—as long as nursing and other services are available to them—are enrolled in these programs, which are financed by Medicaid funds. The premise for these projects is that keeping patients in their own homes would make it possible to contain Medicaid costs and reduce the number of expensive nursing home beds.

Despite many inconveniences, some families wish to have the patient with them. The family members' understanding of the patient and their ability to assist one another will make a great difference in whether they choose home care or other living arrangements for the patient. Not only may space be inadequate, but many times it is impossible to have a family member at home with the patient during the day. Family members who work cannot afford to sacrifice jobs to stay with the patient. However, many families find it easier financially to have the patient at home and are able to make satisfactory arrangements for his or her care even though their facilities are limited.

Many communities provide portable meals (meals on wheels) for homebound persons. Most programs provide one hot meal daily and food that does not need to be heated for at least one other meal. The cost differs widely and depends on the services offered, such as special diets, and on the sponsorship of the plan. Volunteer groups frequently deliver the meals. This service alone often makes it possible for a chronically ill or aged person to remain at home.

#### Home health aide services

Home health aide services were increased when Medicare came into existence. The greater number of persons eligible for such services under Medicare spurred their growth. The early discharge of patients from hospitals has increased the need for these services even more. Home health aides provide physical care to the patient after a registered nurse evaluates the home situation and the patient's need for physical personal care. They are also responsible for keeping the patient's environment clean and for preparing the patient's meals. Ongoing supervision of the home health aide is the responsibility of the registered nurse assigned by the agency providing the home care.

#### Homemaker services

Homemaker services also have developed with the increased use of home care. These services are increasingly in demand in many communities and may be sponsored by a public or voluntary health or welfare agency or by a private agency that bills the family. Homemakers provide service to families with children and to the person who is convalescing, aged, or acutely or chronically ill. Homemakers are trained to assist in homes where the responsible family manager is temporarily unable to perform his or her usual responsibilities because of illness or absence.

#### Day-care centers

In many communities some senior centers and nursing homes are expanding their facilities and services to include day-care centers. Many chronically ill persons are able to live with their families but require 24-hour attendance. Often the caretaker in the family has to work. Homemaker or home health care aides services are generally not available for the time the caregiver is at work. Day-care centers provide a place where the chronically ill person can be looked after on a daily basis. Nursing services, physical and occupational therapy, recreational therapy, meals, and, in some instances, transportation to and from the center are provided. This form of service may allow a person to remain at home with the family rather than having to resort to institutional care.

#### Respite care services

Some nursing homes and some community hospitals maintain a specified number of beds for respite care. As the name implies, these beds are available on a short-term basis to provide respite for families who have a chronically ill person at home. The day-to-day care of the patient, often 24 hours a day, is a very trying experience for any family and "caregiver fatigue" needs to be addressed. To provide the family or primary caregiver with a period free of this responsibility, respite care may be the answer. Usually the cost of respite care is not reimbursable; however, it may be the only alternative if the primary caregiver cannot continue to care for the family member without a break.

Community health agencies, such as the Visiting Nurse Association, are providing respite services in some cities. They supply respite care in the person's own home for part of a day, for 24 hours, or for extended periods depending on need. As mentioned, the cost of this service is usually not covered by health insurance.

### Independent and Assisted Living Centers

Some persons with chronic illnesses may be unable to cope with the demands of maintaining a home but wish to live as independently as possible. Various options are available in some communities; these range from living units, where persons cook their meals but have the unit maintained, to assisted living units, where persons can have their own physical living area but where one or more meals a day and assistance with activities of daily living is provided. Living units are designed with such features as handrails for support in ambulation, wide doors to facilitate passage of wheelchairs, and emergency call systems. (For more information see reference 11.)

### Foster Homes

Care in foster homes is a service that is now being widely used in many communities. Carefully selected families volunteer to take chronically ill persons into their own homes and provide the nonprofessional care needed. The family is paid either by the patient or the patient's family, from public funds, or by some social agency. The plan is primarily for those patients who have no family and cannot live alone but who neither desire nor need institutional care.

### Institutional Care

Institutional care may be necessary when alternatives are not available, or the type of care needed by the patient requires close professional supervision. This includes chronic disease hospitals, skilled care facilities, convalescent homes, rest homes, homes for the aged, and nursing homes. Veterans Administration hospitals provide services for men and women who have served in one of the U.S. armed forces. The patient's potential for rehabilitation, the need for maintenance care, or the level of physical disability are factors that determine eligibility for placement in any of these facilities. A large or limited selection of outside facilities may be available, depending on the community.

## ROLE OF THE NURSE IN CONTINUING HEALTH CARE

A nurse may be involved in continuing health care in several ways: (1) as an independent nurse practitioner or clinical nurse specialist assisting the person with chronic illness to cope with problems incurred by the illness, (2) as a community health nurse or visiting nurse involved in a primary rehabilitative program in the home, (3) as a supervisor of home health aides, or (4) as a nurse in a hospital concerned about the care patients will be receiving after they leave the hospital, particularly when the patient's rehabilitation program is not completed before discharge or when rehabilitation is not possible. Any of these nurses also may be involved in research pertaining to chronic illness. Some concepts that need further study in the area of chronic disease include social stigmatization, effects of isolation, and effects of chronic illness on the family, marriage, and domestic and occupational roles. Research can make a major contribution to clarification of these general concepts by identifying their relationship to chronic health problems.

Nurses must know the community resources available to patients to inform them and their families about what resources they might obtain, the types of service from which they may benefit, and what referrals they need for obtaining those services (see Box 7-4 for a list of community resources). The hospital nurse should clearly communicate to the continuing care agency the data pertinent to the patient's care so that continuity is ensured. Teamwork and continuity are the keys to successful rehabilitation and management services for patients, and they must be practiced at all stages of care if patients are to realize their fullest potential.

# OTHER FACTORS INFLUENCING CHRONIC ILLNESS AND REHABILITATION NURSING

## AMERICANS WITH DISABILITIES ACT

In 1990 Congress passed the Americans with Disabilities Act (ADA), which some call the Civil Rights Act for the disabled. This law provides protection to the estimated 48 million Americans with disabilities. Its four main components, which address employment, public services, public accommodations and services operated by private entities, and telecommunication services. The provisions under each of the components are listed in Box 7-6.

### Implications for Nursing

It is important for nurses to know about the provisions of the American with Disabilities Act so that they can inform the disabled about their rights under the law.

Nurses working in the rehabilitation settings will be able to employ nursing interventions that will assist the disabled person to function at his or her highest possible level. The role of the nurse in rehabilitation is discussed earlier in this chapter (see p. 148).

All nurses as citizens can be advocates for the disabled and help articulate their needs to the general public. Nurses can be active in their own communities to ensure that the public accommodations and public service provisions are carried out.[53]

A copy of the Americans with Disabilities Act, Public Law 101-239, may be obtained free from the U.S. Government Documents Office in Washington, DC, or from one's congressional representative.

## CENTER FOR MEDICAL REHABILITATION RESEARCH

Another event that is having a favorable impact on persons with disabilities is the establishment of the Center for Medical Rehabilitation Research. The Center, which is within the National Institute of Child Health and Development, is involved in basic, clinical, and applied rehabilitation research. It is expected to have a significant impact on the development of medical rehabilitation therapies and services.

## HEALTH CARE GOALS FOR THE YEARS 1990 AND 2000

In 1979 the surgeon general's report established five goals concerned with reducing death rates in the United States by 1990. Table 7-4 shows the progress made by 1990 and the goals set for 2000. A mid-course review of the 2000 objectives is listed under 1995 status.[49a] The last column indicates whether progress toward the year 2000 goals is in a negative or positive direction.

As follow-up to the 1990 goals, work was begun in 1987 on developing health care goals for the year 2000, which were published in *Healthy People 2000: National Health Promotion and Disease Prevention Objectives.*[47]

The development of the year 2000 goals was a national effort that involved health professionals, citizens, private organizations, and public agencies from every part of the United States. Nearly 300 national membership organizations and health departments from the 50 states were involved, with nurses represented by the American Nurses Association, the National League for Nursing, and several specialty organizations.

Before discussing the goals for the year 2000, it is important to describe the changes in the U.S. population that are expected to occur by 2000.

**box 7-6** *Provisions of Americans with Disabilities Act*

1. Employers may not discriminate against a qualified person with a disability in hiring or promotion.
2. Employers can ask about the person's ability to perform a job but may not ask if someone has a disability or use tests that tend to screen out persons with disabilities.
3. Employers need to provide "reasonable accommodation" to individuals with disabilities, including job restructuring and modification of equipment.
4. Employers do not need to provide accommodations that impose an "undue hardship" on business operations.
5. Employers with 25 or more employees were to comply by July 1992.
6. Employers with 15 to 24 employees were to comply by July 1994.

TRANSPORTATION

1. New public transit buses must be accessible to persons with disabilities.
2. Transit authorities must provide comparable paratransit or other special transportation services to persons with disabilities who cannot use fixed route bus service, unless an undue burden would result.
3. Existing rail systems were required to have an accessible car per train by July 1995.
4. New rail cars must be accessible.
5. New bus and train stations must be accessible.
6. Key stations in rapid, light, and commuter rail systems had to be made accessible by July 1993, with extensions up to 20 years for commuter rail (30 years for rapid and light rail).
7. All existing Amtrak stations must be accessible by July 2010.

PUBLIC ACCOMMODATIONS

1. Restaurants, hotels, and retail stores may not discriminate against persons with disabilities.
2. Auxiliary aids and services must be provided to persons with hearing or vision impairments or other persons with disabilities, unless an undue burden would result.
3. Physical barriers in existing facilities must be removed, if removal is readily achievable. If not, alternative methods of providing the service must be offered, if they are readily achievable.
4. All new construction and alterations of facilities must be accessible.

TELECOMMUNICATIONS

Companies offering telephone service must offer telephone relay services to persons who use telecommunication devices for the deaf (TTDs) or similar devices.

STATE AND LOCAL GOVERNMENTS

State and local governments may not discriminate against qualified persons with disabilities.

**table 7-4** *Progress in Meeting Life-Stage Objectives 1995*

| | Year 1990 Targets* | | Year 2000 Targets* | | |
|---|---|---|---|---|---|
| Age-Group | 1990 Target | 1990 Final | 2000 Target | 1995 Status | Direction |
| Infants (aged <1) | 900 | 908 | 700 | 852 | Negative |
| Children (aged 1-14) | 34 | 30.1 | 28 | 28.8 | Positive |
| Young People (aged 15-24) | 93 | 104.1 | 85 | 95.6 | Negative |
| Adults (aged 25-64) | 400 | 400.4 | 340 | 394.7 | Negative |

From US Department of Health and Human Services: *Healthy people 2000: midcourse review and 1995 revisions,* Washington, DC, 1995, US Government Printing Office.
*Death rates per 100,000 population.

### Profile of Americans in the Year 2000

*Healthy People 2000* describes the demographic changes that will occur between 1990 and 2000.

1. By the year 2000 the population of the United States will have grown about 7% to approximately 270 million people. The slowest growth rate in the history of the country is projected to occur between 1995 and 2000. Average household size is expected to decline from 2.69 in 1985 to 2.48 in 2000, with husband-wife households decreasing from 58% to 53% of all households.
2. By the year 2000 the American population will be older, with a median age of more than 36 years, compared with 29 years in 1975. The number of children younger than 5 years of age will decline from more than 18 million to fewer than 17 million between 1990 and 2000.
3. By the year 2000, 35 million persons older than 65 years of age will represent 13% of the population compared with 8% in 1950. The "oldest old"—those older than age 85—will increase to 30% to a total of 4.6 million by 2000.
4. By the year 2000, the racial and ethnic composition of the American population will change. The number of white persons will decline from 76% to 72% of the population. The forecast is that the number of Hispanic persons will increase from 8% to 11.3%, that is, to more than 31 million by the year 2000. The number of African Americans will increase from 12.4% to 13.1%. Other racial groups, including Native Americans, Native Alaskans, and persons of Asian and Pacific Islands extraction will increase from 3.5% to 4.3% of the total population.
5. By the year 2000, the working population will reflect changes in racial and ethnic populations, and more non-

**box 7-7** *Three Broad Goals for the Year 2000*

1. Increase the span of healthy life for all Americans.
2. Reduce health disparities among Americans.
3. Achieve access to preventive services for all Americans.

From US Department of Health and Human Services, Public Health Service: *Healthy people 2000: national health promotion and disease prevention objectives,* Washington, DC, 1990, US Government Printing Office.

white than white groups will enter the work force. Women of all racial and ethnic groups will be the major source of new entrants into the labor force. The women in the work force will comprise 47% of the total working population compared with 45% in 1988. White men will make up only 25% of the net growth of the labor force.

6. Occupations most likely to grow include service, professional, technical, sales, and executive and management positions.
7. By the year 2000 the American population may increase through immigration by as much as 6 million people. This immigration will be to certain states and cities, with the greatest number settling on the east and west coasts.

The purpose of the *Healthy People 2000* report was to commit the nation to the attainment of three broad goals that will bring us as a nation to our full potential (Box 7-7).

The goals to be achieved by the year 2000 are divided into 22 priority areas. The first 21 of these goals are grouped into three broad categories: *health promotion, health protection,* and *preventive services.* It seems clear that the achievement of the three broad goals would reduce the number of people in the United States with chronic health problems. These goals and the three approaches to them require that individuals take more responsibility *for their own health and for preventing chronic illnesses.* At the same time, health professionals are called on not only to treat disease but to help prevent disease and conditions that result in premature death and chronic disability.

The challenge spelled out in *Healthy People 2000* is for communities to translate these national objectives into state and local action.

Not all the goals for 2000 can be discussed in this chapter. Only those objectives related to chronic conditions are presented. Other goals related to persons with specific health problems are discussed in the appropriate chapters of this text.

## Health Status Objectives Related to Chronic Disabling Conditions

Health status objectives related to chronic disabling conditions include:

1. Increase years of healthy life to at least 65 years from an estimated baseline of 62 years in 1980. Special target populations are listed in Table 7-5.
2. Reduce to no more than 8% (from a baseline of 9.4% in 1988) the proportion of persons who experience a limitation in major activity because of a chronic condition. Special target populations for this objective are presented in Table 7-6.

**table 7-5** *Target Populations—Years of Healthy Life by Year 2000*

| POPULATIONS | 1980 BASELINE | 2000 TARGET |
|---|---|---|
| African Americans | 56 | 60 |
| Hispanics | 62 | 65 |
| People 65 and older—years of healthy life remaining | 12 | 14 |

From US Department of Health and Human Services, Public Health Service: *Healthy people 2000: national health promotion and disease prevention objectives,* Washington, DC, 1990, US Government Printing Office.

**table 7-6** *Prevalence of Disability in Special Population Targets*

| PREVALENCE OF DISABILITY | 1989 BASELINE (%) | 2000 TARGET (%) |
|---|---|---|
| Low-income persons (annual family income: $10,000 in 1988) | 18.9 | 15 |
| Native Americans/ Alaskan natives | 13.4 | 11 |
| African Americans | 11.2 | 9 |

From US Department of Health and Human Services, Public Health Service: *Healthy people 2000: national health promotion and disease prevention objectives,* Washington, DC, 1990, US Government Printing Office.

3. Reduce to no more than 90 per 1000 people the proportion of persons aged 65 and older who have difficulty in performing two or more personal care activities (bathing, dressing, using the toilet, getting in and out of bed) thereby preserving independence. The baseline was 111 per 1000 population in 1984 to 1985. The special target population for this objective is people aged 85 years and older.
4. Reduce to no more than 10% the proportion of persons with asthma who experience activity limitation compared with a baseline of 19.4% in 1986 to 1988.
5. Reduce activity limitation resulting from chronic back conditions to a prevalence of no more than 19 per 1000 by the year 2000 compared with a baseline of 21.9 per 1000 in 1986 to 1988.
6. Reduce significant hearing impairment to a prevalence of no more than 82 per 1000 persons by the year 2000, from a baseline of 88.9 per 1000 persons during 1986-1988. The special target population is persons 45 years and older in whom a prevalence of hearing impairment would be no more than 180 per 1000 compared with a baseline of 203 per 1000 in 1986 to 1988.
7. Reduce significant visual impairment to a prevalence of no more than 30 per 1000 persons by the year 2000, from a baseline average of 34.5 per 1000 during 1986 to 1988. Special target population is people aged 65 and older in whom a prevalence of visual impairment would be 70 per 1000 as compared to 87.7 in 1986 to 1988.

8. There are several objectives related to diabetes. These are presented in Chapter 36.

### Services and Protection Objectives

Services and protection objectives related to the health status objectives[47] include:

1. Increase to at least 60% the proportion of providers of primary care for older adults who routinely evaluate people aged 65 and older for urinary incontinence; impairments of vision, hearing, and cognition; and functional status. Baseline data were not available.
2. Increase to at least 90% the proportion of premenopausal women who have been counseled about the benefits and risks of estrogen replacement therapy (combined with progestin, when appropriate) for prevention of osteoporosis. Baseline data were not available.
3. Increase to at least 75% the proportion of work sites with 50 or more employees that have a voluntarily established policy or program for hiring persons with disabilities. The baseline was 37% of medium and large companies in 1986. This objective reflects the intentions of the Americans with Disabilities Act (see p. 157).
4. Increase to 50 the number of states that have service systems for children at risk of chronic conditions, as required by Public Law 101-239 (Americans with Disabilities Act).

All nurses need to be aware of the goals spelled out in *Healthy People 2000* and the plans developed in the state in which they are residing for bringing these goals to fruition. The goals, if met, should assist all persons in the United States to have as healthy a life as possible.

## critical thinking QUESTIONS

**1** You are caring for two patients, both of whom have advanced, progressive multiple sclerosis. One family adapts well to the debilitated state of their family member while the other family members drift and are unable to offer their support to the patient. Offer an explanation for this difference in family reaction.

**2** How may the care of one person with a chronic illness be generalized to the care of other persons with chronic illnesses?

**3** On admission to the hospital of a patient with a chronic illness, the nurse performs a thorough physical assessment but makes no mention of psychological assessment of the patient. Should this oversight be called to her attention or is the physiological assessment more important?

**4** What resources are available in your community for the care of the chronically ill? Are the facilities adequate for the number of persons needing care? How are these facilities supported financially?

**5** From what you have learned in anatomy, outline in detail the physical movements necessary to rise from a sitting position in a chair to a standing position. Describe how you would assist a patient to stand while allowing him or her to be as independent as possible.

## chapter SUMMARY

### IMPACT OF CHRONIC ILLNESS ON SOCIETY

- Chronic health problems constitute a major area of health problems in the United States.
- The incidence and prevalence of chronic diseases have increased in this century and can be expected to increase even more as the population ages.
- The Bureau of the Census estimates that approximately 110 million persons in the United States have one or more chronic illnesses.
- There are major disparities in the health of African Americans and other minorities in the United States when compared with the white population.
- The characteristics of chronic illnesses include one or more of the following: (1) illness or impairment that is permanent, (2) residual disability, and (3) nonreversible pathological alteration, which requires a long period of care.
- Chronic illnesses may be present from birth or can develop during childhood, adolescence, early adult life, or old age.
- Today some children with chronic illnesses such as cystic fibrosis live into early adulthood because of more effective treatment.
- Major chronic illnesses of adults include arthritis, diabetes, heart disease, and hypertension. The rates for arthritis and hypertension are higher in black than in white persons.
- Cultural values determine how both nurses and patients view chronic illness.
- The economic costs of chronic illness are considerable, and many persons will require some type of financial assistance.

### PREVENTION

- It is important that nurses be involved in prevention of chronic illness.
- There are three levels of prevention: primary, secondary, and tertiary, and the nurse has an important role to play at each level.
- Primary prevention involves health promotion and specific protection against disease (such as immunization against childhood diseases).
- Secondary prevention includes early detection of disease and prompt intervention to halt progression of disease.
- Tertiary prevention includes rehabilitation appropriate to the stage of disability, prevention of further disability, and restoration of functioning to the highest possible level.

### FAMILY INFLUENCES ON ILLNESS

- Family systems theory and family stress theory provide a basis for understanding the effect of a family member's illness on family functioning.
- Selection of the appropriate model of family functioning depends on the model's definition of family that most closely matches the culture of the family.
- Models of family functioning provide ways of thinking about the family that allow the nurse to understand and predict behavior and plan interventions.
- Family systems theory describes the family as an open system that exchanges information with the larger environment.
- Interactions among the family members are governed by roles, relationships, expectations, and rules.
- The key assessment areas for nurses include a determination of the family rules, roles, expectations, and relationships that have been affected by the patient's illness. As

a result, the nurse can determine what environmental sources of information and support are needed by the family.

- Family stress theory proposes that family reactions to an illness are based on characteristics of the illness, the family's resources for meeting the crisis created by the illness, and the meaning of the illness to the family.
- Two important family resources are adaptability, which is the family's ability to reorganize and change roles, rules, and patterns of interaction in response to a stress; and cohesion, which is the extent the family members feel bonded to each other and concerned and committed to family.
- Family characteristics can affect a family's degree of adaptability and cohesion. These include familial relation to the patient, gender, family-life cycle, ethnicity, family composition, socioeconomic status, employment status of the family members, problem-solving ability, family health, support network, social support, and religion.

## CHRONICALLY ILL PERSONS

- Failure to understand or internalize the reason for therapeutic recommendations, procedures that are difficult to learn and carry out, time necessary to carry out therapy, side effects of therapy, inability to pay for prescribed therapy, and social isolation and lack of support and positive reinforcement are possible reasons why a person may be noncompliant with therapeutic recommendations.

## ASSESSMENT OF THE PERSON WITH A CHRONIC ILLNESS

- Depression is common among chronically ill persons, especially those who feel powerless about controlling or overcoming what has happened to them.

## REHABILITATION

- Rehabilitation is best carried out in a setting in which an interdisciplinary team of nurses, physicians, physical and occupational therapists, social workers, and, if necessary, speech therapists are available to work together in planning the therapeutic regimen for the patient and in assisting and supporting the patient with the prescribed therapy.
- The two major roles of the nurse working with persons with disabilities are (1) to limit disability from disease as much as possible and (2) to see that the rehabilitation program is planned and implemented.
- The nurse should be familiar with community facilities for continuing care and the eligibility requirements for each facility.

## OTHER FACTORS INFLUENCING CHRONIC ILLNESS AND REHABILITATION NURSING

- The Americans with Disabilities Act passed by Congress in 1990 provides protection for the disabled in terms of employment, public services, public accommodations, services operated by private entities, and telecommunications services.
- *Healthy People 2000* is a publication prepared for the surgeon general of the United States. It presents more than 300 objectives to improve the health of U.S. citizens by the year 2000.
- Nurses need to be aware of the progress of the state in which they reside in meeting the goals for the year 2000 and beyond.

## References


1. Albee G: In Curtis N, editor: *Self Help Reporter* 3(4), 1977.
2. American Cancer Society: *1998 cancer facts and figures.* Atlanta, 1998, The Society.
3. American Nurses Association: *A national policy for health care: principle and positions,* Kansas City, Mo, 1977, The Association.
4. Branstater ME, Brown SE: Physical medicine and rehabilitation, *JAMA* 275(23):1843-1844, 1996.
5. Brody E et al: Work status and parent care: a comparison of four groups of women, *Gerontologist* 27(2):201-208, 1987.
6. Capitman JA: *Long-term care use by minority elderly: an eldercare information packet,* Waltham, Mass, 1992, Brandeis University.
7. Centers for Disease Control and Prevention (CDC): Years of potential life lost before age 65: United States, 1990 and 1991, *MMWR* 42(13):252-253, 1993.
8. Chatters L, Taylor R, Jackson J: Size and composition of the informal helper networks of elderly blacks, *J Gerontol* 40(5):605-614, 1985.
9. Chatters L, Taylor R, Jackson J: Aged blacks: choices for an informal helper network, *J Gerontol* 41(1):94-100, 1986.
10. Croog S, Lipson A, Levine S: Help patterns in severe illness: the roles of kin network, nonfamily resources and institutions, *J Marriage Fam* 34(1):32-41, 1972.
11. Dardick G: In search of personal power, *Arthritis Today*, Mar-Apr 1994.
12. Desencios JC, Hahn RA: Years of potential life lost before age 65, by race, Hispanic origin and sex—United States, 1986-1988, *MMWR* 4(SS 6):13-23, 1992.
13. Fitting M et al: Caregivers for dementia patients: a comparison of husbands and wives, *Gerontologist* 26(3):248-252, 1986.
14. Galenti GA: *Caring for patients from different cultures,* Philadelphia, 1991, University of Pennsylvania Press.
15. George L: Social participation in later life: black-white differences. In Jackson JS, editor: *The black American elderly: research on physical and psychosocial health,* New York, 1988, Springer.
16. George L, Gwyther I: Caregiver well-being: a multidimensional examination of family caregivers of demented adults, *Gerontologist* 26(3):253-259, 1986.
17. Giger J, Davidhizar R: *Transcultural nursing: assessment and intervention,* St Louis, 1991, Mosby.
18. Hill R: *Families under stress,* New York, 1949, Harper and Brothers.
19. Hill R: Generic features of families under stress, *Soc Casework,* pp 139-150, 1958.
20. Hoffman C, Rice D, Sung H: Persons with chronic conditions: their prevalence and costs, *JAMA* 276(18):1473-1479, 1996.
21. Horowitz A: Sons and daughters as caregivers to older parent: differences in role performance and consequences, *Gerontologist* 25(6): 612-617, 1985.
22. Jackson D: The question of homeostasis, *Psychiatr Q Suppl* 31:79-90, 1954.
23. Jackson D: The study of the family, *Fam Process* 4:1-20, 1965.
24. Johnson C, Catalano D: A longitudinal study of family supports to impaired elderly, *Gerontologist* 23(6):612-615, 1983.
25. Kauffman C et al: *Characteristics and needs of black caregivers and their elderly clients in personal care homes,* Washington, DC, 1987, American Red Cross.
26. Kim MJ, McFarland GK, McLane AM: *Pocket guide to nursing diagnoses,* ed 5, St Louis, 1995, Mosby.
27. Kinney J, Stephens M: Hassles and uplifts of giving care to a family member with dementia, *Psychol Aging* 4(4):402-408, 1989.
28. L'Abate L, Ganahi G, Hansen J: *Methods of family therapy,* Englewood Cliffs, NJ, 1986, Prentice-Hall.
29. Leidy NK: A structural model of stress, psychosocial resources, and symptomatic experiences in chronic physical illness, *Nurs Outlook* 34(4):230-236, 1990.
30. Morycz R et al: Racial differences in family burden: clinical implications for social work, *J Gerontol Soc Work* 10(1/2):133-154, 1987.

31. Moskowitz R, McCann CB: Classification of disability in the chronically ill and aging, *J Chronic Dis* 5:342-346, 1957.

31a. Motzer SU, Stewart BJ: Sense of coherence as a predictor of quality of life in persons with coronary heart disease surviving cardiac arrest, *Res Nurs Health* 19:287-298, 1996.

32. Olsen D, McCubbin H: Circumplex model of martial and family systems. V. Application to family stress and crisis intervention, In McCubbin H, Cauble A, Patterson J, editors: *Family stress, coping and social support,* Springfield, Ill, 1982, Charles C Thomas.

33. Olsen D, Sprenkle D, Russell C: Circumplex model of marital and family systems. I. Cohesion and adaptability dimensions, family types and clinical applications, *Fam Process* 18(7):3-28, 1979.

34. Olsen E: The impact of serious illness on the family system, *Postgrad Med* 47(2):169-174, 1970.

35. Picot S: The relationship between the rewards, costs and coping strategies of black family caregivers, *Disser Abstr Ins* 52(11):5760B, 1992.

36. Pollock SE: Human response to chronic illness: physiologic and psychosocial adaptation, *Nurs Res* 35-90-95, 1986.

37. Pratt C et al: Burden and coping strategies of caregivers to Alzheimer's patients, *Fam Relations* 34(5):27-33, 1985.

38. Pratt C, Wright S, Schnall V: Burden, coping and health status: a comparison of family caregivers to community dwelling and institutionalized Alzheimer's patients, *Gerontol Soc Work* 10(1/2):99-1112, 1987.

39. Raleigh EDH: Sources of hope in chronic illness, *Oncol Nurs Forum* 19(3):443-448, 1992.

40. Robinson B, Thuenher M: Taking care of aged parents: a family life cycle transition, *Gerontologist* 19(6):586-593, 1979.

41. Speer D: Family systems: morphostasis and morphogenesis, or "Is homeostasis enough?" *Fam Process* 9(3):259-278, 1970;.

42. Strauss AL et al: *Chronic illness and the quality of life,* ed 2, St Louis 1984, Mosby.

43. Taylor R: The extended family as a source of support to elderly blacks, *Gerontologist* 25(5):488-495, 1985.

44. Taylor R: Receipt of support from family among black Americans: demographic and familial differences, *J Marriage Fam* 48(1)67-77, 1986.

44a. The Robert Wood Johnson Foundation: Chronic care in Americas: the system that isn't, *Advances* Issue 4:1, 9-10, Princeton, NJ, 1996, The Foundation.

45. US Department of Health, Education and Welfare: *Healthy people: surgeon general's report on health promotion and disease intervention,* Washington, DC, 1979, US Government Printing Office.

46. US Department of Health and Human Services: *Secretary's task force on black and minority health,* Washington, DC, 1985, US Government Printing Office.

47. US Department of Health and Human Services, Public Health Service: *Healthy people 2000: national health promotion and disease prevention objectives,* Washington DC, 1990, US Government Printing Office.

48. US Department of Health and Human Services: *Vital and health statistics: current estimates from the National Health Interview Survey,* 1990, Washington, DC, 1991, US Government Printing Office.

49. US Department of Health and Human Services, Public Health Service, Centers for Disease Control and Prevention National Center for Health Statistics: *Vital and health statistics: current estimates from the National Health Interview Survey 1994,* Hyattsville, Md, 1995, US Government Printing Office.

49a. US Department of Health and Human Services, Public Health Service, Centers for Disease Control and Prevention: *Healthy people 2000: midcourse review and 1995 revisions,* Washington, DC, 1995, US Government Printing Office.

50. Valle R: Cultural and ethnic issues in Alzheimer's disease family research. In Light E, Lebowitz B, editors: *Alzheimer's disease treatment and family stress directions for research,* Rockville, Md, 1989, National Institute of Mental Health.

51. von Bertalanffy L: General systems theory and psychiatry. In Ariti S, editor: *American handbook of psychiatry,* ed 2, New York, 1974, Basic Books.

52. Watson W: *Strengthening family caregivers and the delivery of social services to older blacks in the south: final report,* Award No 90ATO131/01, Washington DC, 1987, Administration of Aging, Office of Human Development Services.

53. Watson PG: The Americans with Disabilities Act: more rights for people with disabilities, *Rehabil Nurs* 156:325-328, 1990.

54. Wood J: Coping with the absence of perceived control: ethnic and cultural issues in family caregiving for patients with Alzheimer's disease, doctoral dissertation, Richmond, Va, 1987, Virginia Commonwealth University.

55. Woog, P, editor: *The chronic illness trajectory framework—the Corbin and Strauss nursing model,* New York, 1992, Springer.

56. Young R, Kahana E: Specifying caregiver burden outcomes: gender and relationship aspects of caregiver strain, *Gerontologist* 29(5):660-666, 1989.

57. Zarit S, Reever K, Bah-Peterson J: Relatives of the impaired elderly: correlates of feelings of burden, *Gerontologist* 20(6):649-655, 1980.

58. Zarit S, Todd P, Zarit J: Subjective burden of husbands and wives as caregivers: a longitudinal study, *Gerontologist* 26(3):260-266, 1986.

chapter 8

# Loss, Grief, and Dying

MOLLY LONEY

## objectives

*After studying this chapter, the learner should be able to:*

1. Recognize how loss affects the individual, family, and community during life changes and the dying process.
2. Identify death as a significant loss and transition in human development.
3. Describe the process of normal grieving and the range of its manifestations.
4. Compare bereavement theories in terms of key tasks for the individual and the family in their grief work.
5. Identify behaviors that place the dying person and family at risk for poor bereavement outcomes.
6. Identify current societal attitudes that influence how nurses, patients, and families respond to situations in which someone is dying or has died.
7. Describe nursing strategies useful in assessing the dying individual and grieving family and in providing palliative care.
8. Discuss factors that affect quality of life for the individual and family during the dying process.
9. Describe self-care strategies for nurses in managing the demands of caring for a dying patient and a grieving family.

> When we think of loss, we think of the loss through death of people we love. But loss is a far more encompassing theme in our lives. For we lose not only through death, but also by leaving and letting go and moving on. And our losses include not only our separations and departures from those we love, but our conscious and unconscious losses of romantic dreams, impossible expectations, illusions of freedom and power, illusions of safety—and the loss of our own younger self. . . the self that thought it always would be unwrinkled and invulnerable and immortal.
>
> These losses are a part of life—universal, unavoidable, inexorable. And these losses are necessary because we grow by losing and leaving and letting go.*

## INTRODUCTION

Throughout time, society has been preoccupied with questions regarding living and dying, while searching for immortality. Despite modern technology and increasing efforts to control the inevitable, death remains a part of life.

Facing the end of life is one of the most difficult losses humans may experience.[7] Although loss and grief are common to any developmental stage or transition, death in all cultures is finite. Losses surrounding dying can be overwhelming and deplete coping resources, as well as the integrity of the individual, family, and community.

The thoughts people have about death affect their lives in many ways. Some are peaceful and inspiring, while others generate anxiety and fear. Living in the shadow of death can motivate further growth[38] and allow the dying to transcend suffering, or it can create a crisis for the dying individual and his or her family.[4] In any culture, how people respond to dying is dependent on the meaning death has in the life cycle of the dying person, the family, and the community.[34,36,57,76] Koestenbaum summarized the many ways that death can positively affect our view of life:[17]

- Death helps one savor life.
- It provides an opposing standard against which to judge being alive.
- It gives a sense of individual existence.
- It helps give life meaning.
- It allows one to evaluate personal achievements.
- It allows retrospective analysis of one's life.
- It gives one strength to express convictions.
- It reveals the importance of intimacy.

Reactions of family and the community can provide needed support or lead to isolation for the dying person.[77,82] Reactions of health care professionals can either enhance or disrupt the quality of care they offer the dying person.[35,41,55] In learning ways to enhance quality of life and guide the patient and family through the dying process, it becomes important for nurses to understand their own experience with loss, grief, and dying.

This chapter offers an understanding of loss, the experience of grief in anticipating or surviving death, factors influencing grieving, societal and ethical issues surrounding death and dying, and nursing strategies for meeting the changing needs of the dying person, family, and self. Perhaps the most beneficial way to learn to effectively care for dying persons and

*Viorst J: *Necessary losses*, New York, 1986, Simon & Schuster.

their families is to understand our own perspectives and those of others on loss, grief, and death.

## THE LOSS EXPERIENCE

Loss is a natural part of human existence. A universal experience that is interwoven into daily life, loss is a pattern that is repeated as one faces change or developmental challenge.[19] As a child learns to become progressively independent in terms of feeding, going to school, making friends, surviving puberty, driving, and wage-earning, a loss occurs for both parents and the child.

Loss is an important force in a person's life because it implies the removal of someone or something that had meaning to an individual.[35] It has been defined as any change that reduces the probability of reaching some desired goal or that deprives a person suddenly of a valued possession or relationship.[7] Although it can be caused by a negative change or a positive developmental event, loss always represents some form of deprivation.[61] According to Viorst,[80] persons grow by having to give up some deep attachment or cherished part of themselves to gain a new level of autonomy and mastery.

Bowlby[7] views loss within a framework of early childhood attachment. During periods of high vulnerability and uncertainty, as in childhood, persons develop strong bonds of affection with significant others who meet their basic needs. These significant others offer safety and security beyond simply meeting physical needs for food and shelter. If attachment bonds are threatened or broken, as with death of a mother, separation anxiety ensues.[35] The ways in which the person learns to cope with this loss of attachment and need gratification in childhood can be a predictor of later coping with adult loss.[88]

Whether a person faces separation or some other significant life changes, experience with loss can result in a crisis. A crisis occurs whenever a person is unable to manage stress and meet basic needs in the usual way. If past coping skills become ineffective or the stress becomes overwhelming, the individual perceives a threat to self-integrity and a loss of control. Feelings of vulnerability and anxiety trigger an adaptive response, and the person tries to resolve the stress by avoidance, finding support, or becoming immobilized.[4] The tension and uncertainty that accompany crisis and loss can motivate regression or growth, depending on the presence of key balancing factors.[48] Mastery involves balancing the stressors with realistic perceptions, using available supports, and regaining some control by tapping constructive coping skills.[4] Growth results when a person develops more resilience in managing life changes in the face of the loss.[31,38]

### TYPES OF LOSS

As a component of crisis, loss can be categorized as developmental or situational (Box 8-1). Developmental loss involves any predictable change in status, role, relationships, or bodily function that normally occurs in life. Although developmental losses require adaptation, we are socially and culturally prepared for making social and biological transitions in reaching a new level of growth and maturity.[4] Situational loss involves an unanticipated change in roles, relationships, or function. The person lacks preparation or role modeling in terms of effective adaptation, except through experience with previous situational losses.[31] Natural disasters, accidents, unemployment, and illnesses are situations that challenge the person's usual adaptive response and may precipitate life crises.[74] Any illness represents several losses occurring simultaneously in all areas of one's life. Situational losses can overwhelm the individual, with each component involving a "small death" and bringing the inevitable reality of one's own mortality into closer focus.[19]

Loss can also be conceptualized as simple, symbolic, or compound. A *simple* loss involves the loss of familiar object, such as misplacing a favorite pair of earrings. The loss carries little attachment value and can easily be replaced. If, however, the earrings were a gift from a grandmother, the loss becomes symbolic and carries with it special meaning. *Symbolic* losses are secondary losses to simple loss and signify cherished roles, relationships, or identities.[62] *Compound* loss involves several symbolic losses occurring together. If the earrings were the gift of a deceased grandmother with whom the person had a special relationship, then the loss becomes compound.[88] Examples of compound loss in this situation include loss of history, support, friendship, maternal figure, self-image, and childhood innocence. Although initially difficult to identify, symbolic losses are important to recognize because they offer insight into possible meanings behind a loss.[65]

Loss can be experienced even when it is not observed. Depending on the degree of threat to self or others, anticipation of loss can trigger an adaptive response similar to an actual loss.[27] Anticipatory loss experienced during a progressive and terminal illness can be as challenging and painful as the death of a loved one as the dying and family confront uncertainty over an inevitably tragic future.[76] Although uncertainty can serve as a motivating force, it also can overwhelm and deplete the adaptive reservoir for coping with loss.[68]

### LOSS WITHIN THE FAMILY

Loss does not occur in a vacuum.[36] An individual's perception of loss is often magnified as each family member and the family as a whole struggle to make sense out of the experience.[16] Because a family is an interactive and functional network of significant relationships,[31] any change in one member affects others. Callanan and Kelley[11] described the family as a mobile, whose balance and structure are disrupted by loss.

**box 8-1** *Types of Losses*

| DEVELOPMENTAL LOSS | SITUATIONAL LOSS |
|---|---|
| Predictable change | Unanticipated change |
| Part of life process | Part of life events |
| Social and cultural preparation | Trial-and-error preparation |
| Potential for crisis | Potential for crisis |
| Observable or anticipated | Observable |

Families try to adapt to change or loss by holding onto the way things were to preserve the family's integrity and identity as a unit. Family members of the dying face unyielding demands in not only meeting the needs of the dying but also meeting the daily needs of all the family members.[35,77,84] Uncertainty and confusion can develop over roles, relationships, rules, and responsibilities.

A teenage son may assume head-of-the-household responsibilities to support his mother and younger siblings when his father is given a prognosis of 3 months or less for end-stage cancer. Although the son may be seeking independence, his added responsibilities prevent him from playing on the basketball team, excelling in school, and getting together with his friends. He is faced with loss of a father figure, normalcy, social support, sources of recognition/achievement, and a somewhat predictable future.

Conflicts may arise between the older son and siblings, who do not recognize his authority. The son and his mother may also be challenged to maintain their parent-child relationship; despite the mother's need for love and intimacy from a male figure. The father may experience loss of self-esteem in feeling inadequate to maintain his role as father and head of the household. The family faces tremendous losses: loss of normalcy, loss of an authority figure and role model, loss of predictability, security, and rules, and loss of relationships with the father.

## FACTORS INFLUENCING LOSS

Individuals differ in their perceptions of loss and their abilities to adapt to loss in growth-producing ways. When the loss represents a major life change, adaptation is challenged. The meaning and extent of loss are interpreted by each person on the basis of many factors, such as personality, cultural and religious background, and coping resources. The extent to which a loss is intensified depends on the importance of the attachment, the possibility of replacing the object or relationship, the person's age and developmental stage, the amount of personal and social disruption caused by the loss, and the availability of a supportive environment (Box 8-2).[19,35,61,88] The more cumulative and meaningful a loss is, the greater its threat and its intensity. Aging, terminal illness, and death represent multiple and often overwhelming losses for any person or family, regardless of adaptive resources.[20,68]

In addition to intensity and meaning, timing is an important factor in determining how loss is perceived. If a person is preoccupied with mastering a developmental task, such as accepting retirement; his or her ability to deal with other life changes may be reduced (Table 8-1). If the same person is also confronted with the sudden death of a spouse, he or she may experience greater difficulty in adaptation. Each loss requires time and effective coping skills for successful integration. Loss cannot be viewed globally. Each person and family will define loss differently. The loss experience is analogous to an onion with multiple interfacing layers. To understand the experience, each layer needs to be peeled away and examined from an inside view, even if the process is painful.

Each loss in life is experienced uniquely in terms of the involved person's or family's developmental stage (Table 8-1) as well as the experience's meaning, relationship to other losses,

**box 8-2** *Factors Influencing Loss*

| INDIVIDUAL | FAMILY |
|---|---|
| Age | Individual factors *plus* |
| Personality | Family's stage of development |
| Developmental level | Family rules and roles |
| Past experience | Belief system and culture |
| Role modeling | Patterns of communication |
| Perception of intensity of loss | Perception of threat to family integrity |
| Meaning of attachment | Flexibility in roles |
| Types of loss | Repertoire of coping skills |
| Replaceability | Relationship to community |
| Timing of experience | Use of community supports |
| Disruption from loss | |
| Threat to self and significant other(s) | |
| Coping skills | |
| Availability of supports | |

**table 8-1** *Developmental Impact of Loss and Death*

| AGE | CONCEPT OF DEATH | POTENTIAL IMPACT |
|---|---|---|
| Younger than 2 yr | Self-centered | Death = need deprivation |
| 2-5 yr | Temporary and concrete | Death = separation, with no distress or fear |
| 5-9 yr | Concrete and logical; unable to link cause/effect; magical thinking | Death = punishment, with anxiety or fear of bodily harm |
| 9-12 yr | Realistic; able to see as inevitable and finite | Death = separation, with fear in leaving home and family; may have daydreams and poor grades |
| 12-18 yr | Abstract and realistic; able to anticipate and predict | Death = threat to independence, with fear of being different from peers; may act out with drugs, alcohol, anger, or aggression |
| 18-25 yr | Abstract and realistic | Death = disruption of lifestyle and separation from peers |
| 25-45 yr | Abstract and realistic | Death = disruption of family unit/roles and threat to history/future |
| 45-65 yr | Abstract and realistic | Death = disruption in productivity in family/work |
| 65-death | Philosophical | Death = series of chronological losses, with separation from support networks |

Adapted from Silverman PR, Nickman SL, Worden IW: Detachment revisited: the child's reconstruction of a dead parent. *Am J Orthopsychiatry* 62(4):494-503, 1992; Griefzu S: Grieving families need your help, *RN* Sept:22-27, 1996.

intensity, and timing.[61,65,88] Individuals also vary in the length of time needed to adapt to or recover from the loss experience. Although a year has been used in the past as a time frame for measuring recovery from a significant loss, current research suggests that true recovery may take years, depending on influencing factors.[86,87]

## DEATH AND LOSS

Although death can be defined as a normal life crisis and a fact of life,[4] it is the most significant loss experienced by an individual or family in today's society.[86] It represents not only separation from an important relationship but also an inevitability that we all face. Despite awareness of our own mortality, death in our culture usually is perceived as untimely and incongruent with laws of nature, especially when caused by an illness or an accident.[19] Death challenges individuals and families to search for "reasons why" in their belief systems and lifestyles. Because of such searching, death always implies several interfacing losses that serve only to remind the survivor(s) of the loved one's death.[51] Concomitant losses of role relationships, normalcy, shared future, identity as a unit (as with a couple or family), sense of control over life events, intimacy, social support, role model, and social approval can all be symbolic of a loved one's death.[61] As a point of transition and potential for growth, death's intensity and complexity challenge the individual's and the family's coping skills. Supportive nursing interventions often are needed to promote the transition from crisis to growth.[4,68]

How successful a family is in adapting to loss depends on the family's developmental stage, rules, belief system, cultural ties, communication patterns, role flexibility, perceptions of threat from the loss, coping skills, and social supports (see Box 8-2).[35,77] When a family faces a loss due to death during a period of high stress or major transition, adaptation is difficult and the family is at risk for ongoing crisis.[4,16,20]

## LOSS WITHIN THE COMMUNITY

Loss also has an impact on the community and its members, especially when finite as with death. All cultures and religions acknowledge death openly or indirectly as a significant loss, both to the family and the community as a whole.[8,34,36] What dying and death mean to the individual and family, as well as how they try adapting to the loss, comes from their culture. It is critical to recognize that[8,35,77]:

1. Culture is not stagnant and can change daily.
2. Members of the same family or community may interpret and practice their identified cultural beliefs differently.
3. Each person and family facing death can experience compounded loss if their cultural patterns of responding to loss are not acknowledged or respected.
4. The dying and their families have much to teach health care professionals about their preferences in how they face a major loss, such as death.

## LOSS AND THE NURSE

Occupational stress involving loss is part of the daily experience of nurses, especially those who work with patients facing terminal illnesses and death.[24,66] By remaining caring and empathic, nurses become vulnerable to identifying with their patients' and families' losses.[40] The observable loss of a patient's independence after learning that cancer has caused irreversible spinal cord compression can symbolize personal losses in the nurse's own family history, as well as professional helplessness.[41,66] A conflict may arise if a nurse perceives his or her role as primarily curing. With the current emphasis in medical care on using technology for cure, nurses are at risk for loss of control, fear of failure, and loss of professional satisfaction when their patients are beyond cure.[24]

Because loss is a universal phenomenon that is experienced by patients, their families and communities, and the nurses who support them, it becomes important to understand the process of adaptation.

## GRIEF: AN ADAPTIVE RESPONSE TO LOSS

Grief and bereavement are companions of adulthood as loss is faced with increasing frequency in the life cycle. Each loss affects the individual and the family by prompting an adaptive response.[4,7,35] Figure 8-1 is an illustrative diagram of adapta-

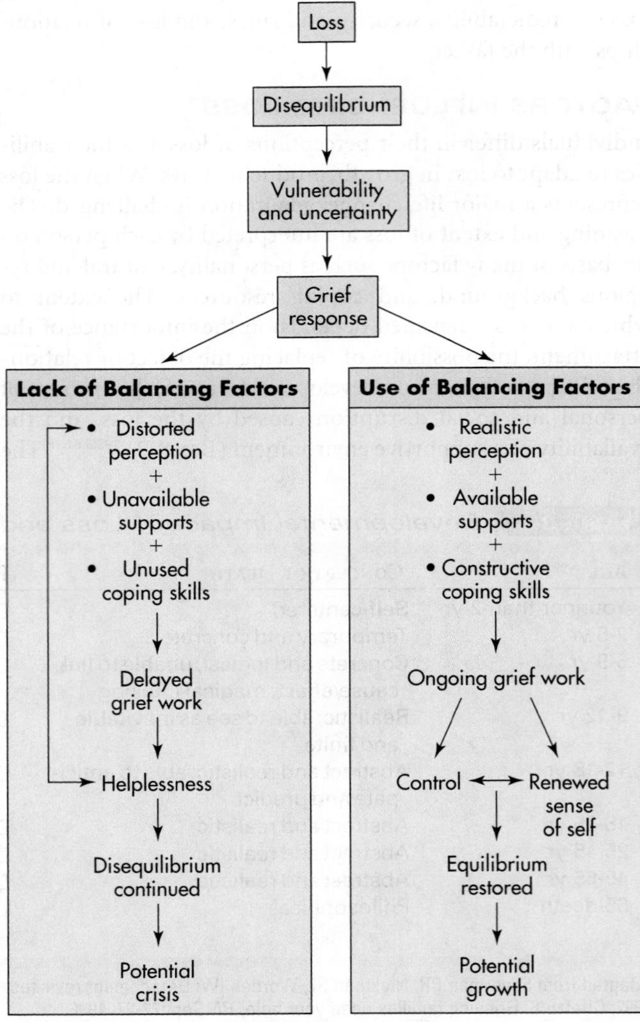


fig. 8-1 Adaptation to the loss experience.

tion to the loss experience. Separation from something or someone of value triggers certain instinctive behaviors through which the person tries to hold onto the loss object. Such behaviors are the basis for grieving.[7,77,88,89]

## DEFINITIONS

*Grief* is the subjective state of anticipating or suffering the loss of a person or object with whom a significant relationship existed. Although used interchangeably with *bereavement*, grief is the normal, expected process of adapting to any loss. It is the total response to the separation caused by the loss which involves psychological, spiritual, cognitive, social, and somatic dimensions.[54,56,77,89]

What makes grief difficult to conceptualize is its universal nature and individual expression. Grief is a lived experience. It depends on each person's or family's perceptions of what is lost and what the loss means at a given point in time.[58] Not only can grief manifest differently from one individual to another, but also individual's and family's expressions of grief can change over time. Because loss is a component of human development, grieving can help a person to adapt to a loss, as well as grow from the experience.[19,31,38]

*Mourning* is the cultural and social response to loss, which includes any manifestation of grief. It is learned through role modeling and socialization during childhood. Mourning is an important term because it often implies how grief is expressed by the individual and family within their cultural norms.[8,65,88]

## HISTORICAL PERSPECTIVE: THE GRIEF PROCESS

In 1915 Freud[26] described grief as a process of gradual withdrawal of the energy that ties the bereaved person to the lost object or person who died.[16,30,34] Freud[26] also described grief as a reaction to loss that caused ego defenses to reduce anxiety and discomfort. The reaction involved a gradual withdrawal of the energy that tied the grieving person to the person who died. In studying victims of fire and war, Lindemann[43] expanded on the definition by identifying both psychological and physical responses to acute loss. Engel[21] legitimized grief as a discrete syndrome with common causative factors and universal manifestations.

Several later theorists have attempted to aid our understanding of grief by defining specific behaviors associated with grief and the sequence in which they occur (Table 8-2). Most agree that grief is an ongoing process of adaptation involving movement through stages or phases of (1) shock and disbelief, (2) awareness and acceptance of the reality of the loss, (3) intense experience of pain over the loss, with disorganization, and (4) recovery or reestablishment of homeostasis.

In working to identify the unique needs of dying patients, Kübler-Ross[37] described five sequential stages of grief, from an initial period of shock and emotional numbness through eventual acceptance of the impending or past loss. Although her conceptualization offered an intimate view of grieving, her stages have been misinterpreted as a series of steps that occur in a neat, chronological order. This misinterpretation, which implies that grief is unidimensional, does not account for individual differences in mourning or adaptation.

Bowlby[7] offered a similar stepwise model of the grief process as a developmental stage in itself for coping with separation from a significant love object or source of need fulfillment. Worden[88] helped redefine grief from a holistic perspective. He identified four tasks of grieving in the Harvard Bereavement Study of elderly widows. A key component is the need to experience the pain of loss in all its dimensions, including physical, cognitive, psychological, social, and spiritual distress (Box 8-3).

Worden[87] offered further insight into the complex grief process including:

1. Grief does not follow any order or sequence.
2. Grief is an individual process through which individuals and families progress at their own rate and in their own ways.
3. Although painful, grief is the only way to adapt to loss.
4. Grief may be so painful for some that the process is denied or delayed, leading to physical complaints and psychological illness.
5. Losses such as death require grief work to reconcile the loss. With each new developmental stage and anniversary of the loss, individuals and families try to make sense of past losses in light of their current situation, roles, and relationships.
6. Unresolved grief may resurface and compound current losses.
7. Even with support, some people never work through their grief.

Rando[62] described grief experienced in times of overwhelming stress or severe trauma as "complicated mourning," defined as abnormal or unresolved grief that persists over time, disrupts one's lifestyle, and interferes with a six-phase process of mourning. Clark[12] elaborated on the definition of *post-traumatic stress* as exposure to a traumatic event that

**table 8-2** *Comparison of Grief Theories*

| STAGE | LINDEMANN | KÜBLER-ROSS | BOWLBY | WORDEN | RANDO |
|---|---|---|---|---|---|
| Initial | Shock and disbelief | Shock and denial | Numbing | Accepting reality | Recognize loss |
| Acute grief | Acute mourning | Anger | Yearning and searching | Experiencing the pain | React to separation |
| | | Bargaining | Disorganization | Withdrawing | Recollect and re-experience |
| | | Depression | | | |
| Recovery | Resolution | Acceptance | Reorganization | Reinvesting | Relinquish old bonds |
| | | | | | Readjust |
| | | | | | Reinvest |

**box 8-3** *Common Manifestations of Grief*

| PHYSICAL | COGNITIVE | PSYCHOLOGICAL | SOCIAL | SPIRITUAL |
|---|---|---|---|---|
| Headache, dizziness | Lack of concentration | Numbness, dulled senses | Withdrawal, isolation | Doubting past beliefs, faith |
| Tightness in throat or chest | Foggy thoughts | Anxiety | Dependency | Hopelessness |
| SOB, deep sighing | Preoccupation with loss | Preoccupation with fears | Helplessness | Searching for meaning of loss |
| Changes in eating, elimination, and sleeping | Hallucinations (auditory and visual) | Denial | Busy with tasks, chores | Changes in religious practices |
| Feeling empty, exhausted | Bargaining | Guilt | Takes on traits of dying person | |
| Restlessness | Searching for reason for loss | Anger | Holds onto possessions of dying person | |
| Malaise | | Hostility, resentfulness | Performance difficulties in work and family roles | |
| Sexual arousal changes | | Ambivalence | Loneliness | |
| | | Crying | | |
| | | Sadness, depression | | |

leads to the survivor's re-experiencing the event in repeated intrusive images that impair the survivor's daily functioning. Although initially associated with war and disasters, such an extreme reaction can result from suffering multiple losses during the dying process, as well as bearing witness to the suffering of others.[3] (See also Chapter 6.)

Solari-Twadell and others added a dynamic, multidimensional structure to the grief process by describing grief as a "pinwheel."[7] "Winds of loss" within the context of an individual's or family's history drive the ongoing cycle of grieving, until emotional surrender and acceptance occur.

Grieving has been described as a three-dimensional rollercoaster with unpredictable ups and downs. The person and family experiencing grief feel "off balance" with no idea of what to expect or of how to return to what used to be a normal course. Ups and downs occur without warning as one emotion comes after another, with forward and backward movement. The difficulty lies in regaining some sense of control and realizing that finding a way back to a pregrief lifestyle may mean having to ride the rollercoaster's entire course.

## DEATH AND GRIEF

Grief is a period of adjustment that requires making a transition in the way one thinks and interacts with the world.[68] Working through grief over dying involves changes in roles, relationships, and identities. As a turning point, death can be a time of immobilization and crisis or potential for growth. Successfully negotiating and making the transition between living and dying can build communication and coping skills in a family, as well as strengthen the family members' ability to face future losses in life.[4,13,16,31,38,68,87]

### Responses by Survivors

Understanding the grieving process and recognizing the behavioral manifestations that usually occur can assist the nurse to prepare survivors for what they can expect or to help them make sense of their feelings and somatic symptoms. Timing of the sharing of information, as well as the type and amount of information given at any one session, is important. Understanding the various processes and behaviors, both anticipated and unexpected, of bereaved persons may help to avert misunderstandings and help to strengthen the survivors and enable them to grow during the period of grieving. Grieving persons are helped by sharing their experiences. Recognizing the "normal" nature of the experiences, even those that seem somewhat bizarre, opens the way for sharing. Nurse researchers are beginning to develop sensitive assessment tools that are consistent with nursing theory (see the following Research Box).

### Shock and Disbelief

The initial response may begin when a terminal prognosis is made and usually lasts for several weeks beyond the funeral.[35,65,86,88] Regardless of whether the death was anticipated or not, the immediate response is shock, numbness, and disbelief. The survivors may feel a sense of unreality, and as a consequence, they may appear to be "taking the death well." After the funeral this feeling of unreality or numbness changes to feelings of pain and separation. Survivors may experience some somatic symptoms, including muscular weakness, tremors, and tightness of the throat. They may experience diaphoresis, sigh deeply, have cold or clammy sensations, become anorexic, or feel exhausted. Bereaved persons exhibit extremes of behavior. They may become sedentary and do little or nothing except nap. On the other hand, they may be so hyperactive that they are unable to sit quietly or to sleep. They may experience extremes of mood such as profound sadness, anger, depression, or guilt or find themselves laughing without an explanation. They may have difficulty concentrating. Coupled with these extremes in mood and behavior may be a continuance of disbelief; although the death is comprehended intellectually. "Searching behaviors" are common. These include dreams in which the deceased is alive and experiences of "seeing" the deceased or "feeling" the deceased's touch. During this phase, offers of comfort are often rejected because the bereaved is focusing on the deceased.

### Yearning and Protest

For several weeks the bereaved have feelings of yearning and protest. They may feel anger toward the deceased for leaving them, toward God for allowing the death to occur, or toward the caregivers for not returning the deceased to health. They may be jealous of others who still have their loved ones. The

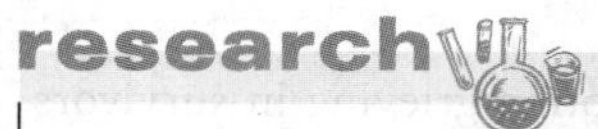

Reference: Lev E, Munro B, McCorkle R: A shortened version of an instrument measuring bereavement, *Int J Nurs Stud* 30(3):213-226, 1993.

The authors developed a tool useful for measuring the grief experience by revising a more complex questionnaire, the Grief Experience Inventory. Parkes' bereavement research was used as a theoretic framework; 418 subjects who had been primary caregivers for significant others before their death completed the revised grief experience questionnaire. Results demonstrated the tool's sensitivity as a concise, valid, and reliable measurement of the highly individual experience of grief.

survivors may wish they had been the ones to die. During this period they may find it difficult to share their feelings or thoughts because they question their own sanity. Knowing that others have had similar thoughts and feelings sometimes is helpful to normalize the experience.

### Anguish, Disorganization, and Despair

As the bereaved begin to focus more on themselves, and as the numbness and rage begin to fade, they begin to recognize the reality and finality of the loss. New feelings and accompanying behaviors emerge. The bereaved may experience a sense of confusion, aimlessness, inability to make decisions, apathy, or a loss of confidence. During this period they may also experience loneliness and depression.

The bereaved experience mood extremes and intense feelings, which are often frightening to them. They fear they will lose emotional control and as a defense become centered on themselves. Family members and friends may interpret this behavior as selfish and either reprimand them or withdraw. Neither behavior is helpful to the bereaved.[46,65,71,86,88]

The experience of anguish leads to a new awareness of the preciousness of life. Life appears fragile. The bereaved may display intense fears of their being hurt or worry over the welfare of family members. At the same time they may smoke or resort to alcohol or chemical abuse. Other health-risking behaviors, such as lack of rest, may occur.

The wish and need to cry fulfill an important function in acknowledging the loss and in receiving support from others. Memories and mental images of the deceased are void of negative characteristics. Feelings of guilt, remorse, fear, and regret may surface. Opportunities to reminisce and to share feelings with others are helpful.[47,63,86,88]

### Identification

The bereaved may adopt the behavior, admired qualities, and mannerisms of their lost beloved ones. Some may take on the symptoms of the last illness of the lost loved one. Care must be taken to distinguish symptoms associated with physical illness from those associated with loss. Symptoms associated with loss will abate as the loss is resolved.[29,77]

### Reorganization and Restitution

The feelings and symptoms of grieving gradually subside; they do not suddenly disappear. Bereaved persons tell us they have periods of depression, as well as periods of well-being as life begins to make sense once again. Reorganization and restitution generally begin approximately 6 months after the loss and last for a few years. The process may be considerably longer or shorter and still be within normal range. Contrary to old popular beliefs, although life stabilizes, the pain of loss may remain for a lifetime. Reactions to loss recur around circumstances that are poignant reminders of the deceased—birthdays, anniversaries, and holidays.[47,77,86,88]

## FACTORS AFFECTING GRIEF RESPONSE

Many factors combine to affect the degree of stress and the particular response of survivors to a death. The major factors include (1) the type of relationship lost, (2) the nature of the death, (3) the characteristics of the survivor, (4) the cultural background, and (5) the nature and use of the support network.

### Type of Relationship and Roles

Feelings of helplessness and emptiness are results of the death of someone such as a parent, spouse, or significant other, upon whom one has been dependent. Perhaps more significant is the intense void that accompanies the loss of the survivor's role as a caring family member when the loved one dies. This sense of loss is intensified in proportion to the survivor's reliance on the deceased for self-validation, identity, and linkage to social and friendship networks.[27,75,77]

Identities and roles are related. A survivor—widow, widower, daughter, or son—is left with incomplete skills because the usual division of labor in everyday life is lost. Loss of children creates its own special problems. The normal course of life events is disrupted when the young die before the old. Feelings of guilt and self-blame may be more pronounced.[86,88]

### Nature of the Death

The nature of the death and the circumstances after a death affect the grieving process. The closer the circumstances are to what the survivors perceive as a "good" death, the more comforting it will be. If survivors' perceptions of the death include intense suffering, confusion over treatment goals, or untimely death (either premature or prolonged), the death may become more difficult to reconcile.[25]

Anticipatory grieving or grieving that began before loss may ease the transition once a loss is complete. However, excessive anticipation and repeated cycles of anticipatory grief may deplete a survivor's energy to complete the grieving process when the death finally occurs.[41,55,75]

### Survivor Characteristics

Individual and family factors that affect adaptation to loss will also influence survivors' grieving (see the above Research Box and Table 8-2).

### Social and Cultural Background

One's cultural background has a profound influence over how illness and death are experienced, as well as how health care professionals are viewed.[36] Cultures all over the world recognize grief and death, but each culture is unique in how it defines what are acceptable expressions of grief.[34,35] Although it is difficult to categorize grief responses from all cultures, some general guidelines can be a useful frame of reference (Table 8-3). Encouraging feedback and validating cultural patterns with survivors in dealing with death can acknowledge and honor their beliefs and promote grieving without compounding loss.[8]

### Social Support

Social support is critical to promoting grieving in survivors. Grieving means expressing the multidimensional pain of the loss with others who both listen and acknowledge what has happened. Such acknowledgment gives survivors opportunities to[41,73,79]:

1. Release feelings.
2. Begin to find some meaning out of the dying experience.
3. Share unresolved concerns.

**table 8-3** *Views of Death Among Major Cultures*

| Cultural Group | Meaning | Life After Death | Grief Expression | Values |
|---|---|---|---|---|
| African American | Natural process<br>Associated with hospitalization | Part of God's plans<br>Eternal life = heaven or oneness with God | Very open in sharing mourning in funeral rituals and church<br>Physical and emotional | Respect aged<br>Large extended family and community support<br>Appearance/dress brings social recognition<br>Food = social bond |
| American Indian | Natural and celebrated process<br>Harmony with nature and gods | Cycle of rebirth in different life forms<br>Spirit lives in oneness with nature/gods | Composed and stoic<br>Search for chance to meet death | Honor aging<br>Actively prepare for death with rituals<br>Multigenerational family (including ancestors) over individual<br>Food and herbs = healing |
| Asian | Natural process<br>Expect to suffer | Cycle of rebirth until reach eternal freedom of spirit | Stoic<br>Somatic complaints | Honor aging and dying<br>Maintain status quo and save face<br>Family over individual<br>Formal relationships |
| East African | Natural and celebrated process<br>Never random event | Transition time between life and death when dead are present<br>Cause = honor or punishment | Very open in sharing mourning with music and dance | Honor aging and dying<br>Multigenerational family and community over individual |
| Hispanic | Natural process<br>Dying = suffering | Life created by death of the gods<br>Reach spiritual state based on how died and family | Men are stoic; women are vocal<br>Somatic complaints | Do not see consequences for health behaviors<br>Extended family and community over individual<br>Open with affection<br>Food = healing |
| Islam | Natural process<br>At peace with Allah and man | Phases of afterlife depending on faith/loyalty (believers find beauty; nonbelievers find ugliness)<br>Day of judgment expected | Stoic with outsiders, especially women<br>Open crying after funeral | Honor men and aging<br>Family and Koran rule<br>Standards for social conduct<br>Relative obliged to stay with dying to pray for atonement<br>After-death care and funeral rituals to prepare for judgment |
| Judaism | Expected but feared process<br>Dying = suffering | Through memories of loved ones and Israeli heritage<br>Hope for new world with coming of the prophets | Open in sharing suffering and loss with times of mourning (first week/month, anniversary) | Respect aged in maintaining history<br>Dying are never left alone until burial<br>After-death and funeral rituals<br>Religious community over individual |
| Western | Natural process in Europe<br>Feared process to be controlled in U.S. | Purgatory as transition until released by prayer for Catholicism<br>Heaven as eternal life for faithful versus hell | Open mourning in Europe<br>Denial and time-limited mourning in U.S. | Respect aging in Europe<br>Deny and fear aging in U.S.<br>Individual autonomy in U.S.<br>Family and church support during funeral ritual |

Modified from Irish D, Lundquist K, Nelsen K: *Ethnic variations in death, dying, and grief,* Washington, DC, 1993, Taylor and Francis; Kemp C: *Terminal illness: a guide to nursing care,* Philadelphia, 1995, JB Lippincott.

4. Validate information about what happened.
5. Remember involvement in trying to support the dying person.
6. Find some beginning closure.

Supportive networks are available but may not used by survivors in an effort to remain composed or protective. Survivors may need to look outside their immediate circle of support, when all are involved in sharing the grieving. The shared experience of grieving may prevent members of the family or network from supporting the most immediate family member(s).[79]

Because inadequate social support for grieving is associated with intense emotions and delayed grief, it becomes important to help survivors share their perceptions of available supports they can use.[3,20,72,79]

## GRIEF RESOLUTION

Debate continues over whether one can ever recover from the experience of loss.[61,86] Lindemann[43] suggested that grief resolution could occur within a few weeks of the loss. Other findings recognize that grief is more appropriately measured in years.[86]

Because grieving is such an individual process, with a wide range of possible manifestations, how can we assess if and when an individual has successfully completed grief work? Engel[22] defined successful mourning as the ability to remember comfortably and realistically both the pleasures and disappointments of the lost relationship. Graininger identified a change in perspective as the key to grief recovery.[29,62] This change in perspective occurs when the person can rise above the emotions of the loss and view the situation more objectively, while finding some meaning in the loss experience.

Silverman and Worden[70] further clarified what is meant by grief recovery. *Recovery* is not simply letting go of the lost object or person. Instead, it is the negotiating and renegotiating of the meaning of the loss over time. Their view reinforces the thought that loss may be permanent and unchanging, but, like development, the grief process is ongoing.

Wolfelt[86] offered *reconciliation* as the term that best describes how acute grief is processed or worked through. Reconciliation means moving on with life even without the presence of the loss object. In reconciliation, there is a renewed energy and a sense of confidence, an ability to fully acknowledge the loss, and a capacity to become reinvolved in normal activities of daily living. Reconciliation involves acknowledging that loss is a difficult yet necessary or growth-facilitating part of life. Wolfelt's view focuses on *reconciliation as a process, not as an event or outcome.* As human beings, we never get over grief; rather we become reconciled to it.

A person's success in grieving at a given point in time will affect future experiences of loss and adaptation. With any loss comes the reliving or resurfacing of old issues involving separation and helplessness. If these issues are not acknowledged in some way and their associated feelings worked through, the griever may carry the pain of the experience into the future.[9,61,65,86,88] Cumulative, unresolved loss has been identified as a significant risk factor for morbidity after bereavement.[56,59,74,86,88] It not only can change perception, but also can confront the person with overwhelming feelings of grief at some future time. When needs for grief work are ignored or denied, even a minor change in the person's routine can serve as a catalyst to resurrect the intensity and burden of past losses.[89] Unresolved loss or grief that is ignored becomes a crisis for the affected individual and family and causes impairment of the usual activities of daily living (Box 8-4).

## NURSING MANAGEMENT

Worden and Cooley state that the role of the caregiver is to assist the griever in releasing emotional ties to the deceased despite the discomfort and sorrow it causes and in subsequently replacing the type of interaction lost.[13,89] The griever must be persuaded to participate in grief work that entails accepting the pain of facing and experiencing the loss. A number of strategies are available to assist grievers. Worden groups these in broad phases that roughly correspond to the process of grief—from shock to reintegration.[88] These activities are useful to health professionals in helping the bereaved.

### ■ ASSESSMENT

Planning interventions for helping grieving persons help themselves must be preceded by accurate assessment of where persons are in their grief, as well as what factors are influencing their grief.[44] Encouraging the grieving individual and family to tell their own stories and describe their lived experiences can provide insight into their grieving as well as help promote

**box 8-4** *Signs of Poor Bereavement Outcomes*

- Overactivity without a sense of loss
- Taking on symptoms belonging to the deceased
- Development of psychosomatic illness
- Withdrawal from relationships with close friends and family members
- Hostility and rage against persons associated with the death or loss
- Wooden and formal conduct that masks rage and hostility
- Lasting loss of social interaction skills
- Destructive behavior (e.g., giving away one's belongings, substance abuse)
- Prolonged and agitated depression, with risk of suicide
- Feelings of worthlessness, self-blame, and need for punishment
- Intense feeling that death or loss occurred yesterday
- Inability to talk about the deceased without emotional distress a year after the loss
- Intense grief triggered by a relatively minor event
- False euphoria after the loss
- Overidentification with the deceased
- Phobias about illness or death
- History of prolonged grieving
- Inability to carry out usual activities of daily living

From Kübler-Ross E: *On death and dying,* New York, 1969, Macmillan; Worden W: *Grief counseling and grief therapy,* ed 3, New York, 1995, Springer; Rando T: *Treatment of complicated mourning,* Champaign, Ill, 1993, Research Press.

grief expression. Assessment cues indicating active grieving are detailed below.

### Subjective Data

Data to be collected include:
- Perception of loss(es) shared in conversation
- Preoccupation with fears (suffering, abandonment, loss of control, or helplessness)
- Asking "Why me?" and "Why us?" questions
- Preoccupation with or avoidance of discussing loss(es)
- Feelings verbalized of "going crazy," "being numb," "loneliness," or "life is empty"
- Reviewing what did or didn't do to help dying or family (i.e., comments with theme of guilt or blame)
- Somatic complaints
- Talking about suicide
- Verbalizing doubts in past religious belief/faith and fairness in the world

### Objective Data

Data to be collected include:
- Deep sighing, breathing changes
- Restlessness, agitation
- Difficulty concentrating
- Hallucinations
- Inability to express feelings without intense emotions (i.e., crying, anxiety, sadness, or anger)
- Lack of emotional expression when talking about loss(es)
- Changes in eating, sleeping, and/or elimination
- Dependent behavior on others
- Withdrawal from family and friends
- Keeping very busy with chores
- Changes in performing daily roles in family and at work
- Taking on behaviors characteristic of dying person

Trying to interpret the importance of any of these cues without having a perception of loss can make assessment difficult. Any assessment needs to be validated and updated on an ongoing basis. Fluctuations in the experiences of the bereaved are to be expected. Interventions that are appropriate for one person are not useful or may even be harmful to another person. Reassessment may address such major topics as:
- Acceptance of the reality of the loss
- Evaluation for need for medical attention and treatment
- Identification of unresolved grief
- Detection of illogical thoughts

Instruments have been developed to identify persons at risk for difficulty in the grieving process or to identify the problems of persons who experienced prolonged bereavement-related distress in widowhood. Behaviors suggestive of the inability to resolve grief include:
- Searching
- Yearning
- Preoccupation with the deceased
- Crying
- Disbelief about loss
- Feeling stunned by loss
- Lack of acceptance of loss of spouse

## NURSING DIAGNOSES

Human responses to the loss of a loved one are varied. Although other nursing diagnoses may be applicable, the one most commonly recognized among persons who experience loss is *grieving*. Grieving is an appropriate diagnostic category for those seeking to promote wellness and to facilitate healing associated with significant loss. At the same time, normal grieving may be associated with dysfunctional or distorted behaviors[1] that can be recognized in a variety of secondary diagnoses. Nursing diagnoses are determined from analysis of patient data. Nursing diagnoses for the person experiencing the loss of a loved one may include but are not limited to:

| **Primary Diagnostic Title** | **Possible Etiological Factors** |
|---|---|
| Grieving | Loss of loved one |
| **Secondary Diagnostic Title** | **Possible Etiological Factors** |
| Anxiety | Loneliness, social isolation; self-reproach; fear of the unknown; financial insecurity; fear of own death |
| Self-care deficit | Depression; anxiety; fatigue; social isolation |
| Nutrition, altered | Anxiety; grief; loss of mealtime companion; inertia because of fatigue; feeling of tightness in throat |
| Coping, ineffective | Depression in response to loss |
| Social isolation | Withdrawal; uncontrolled anger; knowledge deficit regarding support resources; housebound state (unemployed, young children); rejection by significant others |
| Spirtual distress | Inability to understand meaning of loss; anger at God; anxiety; depression |
| Hopelessness | Separation from significant other; inability to achieve goals in life associated with loss; loss of belief in God's care |
| Thought processes, impaired | Grief, anxiety, insomnia; guilt; loneliness; substance abuse; hallucinations |
| Self-esteem disturbance | Hallucinations centered on the deceased; anger; anxiety; preoccupation with the deceased; social isolation; substance abuse; fear of loss of control |
| Sleep-pattern disturbance | Anxiety; hyperactivity; agitation; fear of nightmares; substance abuse |

Grieving is the ultimate price of loving, of attachment, and of a meaningful relationship.[7,89] In some instances the person is unable to mourn in a manner that allows for resolution of the grief and reinvestment in life, and this may result in dysfunctional grief.[74]

NANDA recognizes two independent nursing diagnostic categories in relationship to grieving: (1) anticipatory grieving and (2) dysfunctional grieving. *Anticipatory grieving* is defined as "the state in which an individual or group experiences reactions in response to an expected significant loss,"[20,64] and *dysfunctional grieving* is defined as "the state in which an individual or group experiences prolonged unresolved grief and engages in detrimental activities."[22]

| Diagnostic Title | Possible Etiological Factors |
|---|---|
| Grieving, anticipatory | Perceived loss of a significant other, physiopsychosocial well-being, personal possessions |
| Grieving, dysfunctional | Actual or perceived object loss; thwarted grieving response to loss; absence of anticipatory grieving; multiple losses; chronic fatal illness; loss of others; loss of physio/psychosocial well-being; prolonged denial; intense pining and yearning; ambivalent relationship with the deceased; severe self-reproach; multiple crises; lack of support from family; history of ineffective coping |

## EXPECTED PATIENT OUTCOMES

The expected outcomes associated with grief and the work that is entailed in the grieving process include remembering the loved one without emotional pain and reinvesting emotional energy in life so that the capacity to love is not lost. Cantor speaks of the same outcome as "enriched remembrance."[19] To achieve these outcomes, the grieving person needs to:[86,87]

1. Face the pain.
2. Experience the pain in all its dimensions.
3. Withdraw from ties to the deceased.
4. Adjust to an altered environment without the deceased.
5. Renew or form new relationships.
6. Recall memories without intense grief.

## INTERVENTIONS

Understanding the grieving process as a normal part of loving provides the basis for nursing assessments and interventions. Nursing actions in response to the bereaved call for a delicate blending of being present, listening, expressing honest feelings, and inviting the bereaved to share their experiences and emotions.[44,45,60,81]

After the death, the following nursing interventions may be appropriate:

1. Make contact and assess.
   a. Establish a relationship; simply be present.
   b. Assess the bereaved in her or his grief to plan appropriate future interventions.
2. Reach out.
   a. Take the initiative; reach out in a concrete way. Don't say "call me if you need me." Do be specific in how you can assist or get others to assist. For example: "How about if I call your sister to accompany you to select the casket?" "Suppose I arrange for you to attend a widow-to-widow meeting?"
   b. Do not take refusals personally or give up.
   c. Repeat offers of assistance. Grievers initially may be unable to respond to and appreciate offers of help but will benefit over time.
3. Be physically and emotionally present to offer security and support.
   a. Use physical contact, hugging, touching, and handholding, as appropriate. These actions are important early in the process to convey that the griever is not alone. There may be exceptions. Some people do not like to be touched. You can sit nearby if you perceive that that will be more comforting.
   b. Social supports generally are decreased weeks or months after a death, when the bereaved is forced to resume life without the loved one. Encourage family members to be present after all the intensity of the funeral has subsided.
   c. Encourage regular expression of feelings to help minimize the tendency to become overwhelmed and unable to function.
   d. Encourage others to take charge of routine functions and responsibilities of the bereaved, for example, run errands or prepare meals.
   e. Provide for security through direction concerning meals, rest, and priorities of activities for the day or week.
   f. Help family members focus on one problem at a time.
   g. Address problems to which practical solutions can be found before addressing more complicated problems.
4. Give people "permission" to grieve.
   a. Display nonjudgmental attitudes and behaviors. Be neutral.
   b. Communicate compassionate support through verbal and nonverbal behavior; for example, when the griever's voice cracks, facial muscles quiver, and eyes water, and the bereaved turns to the caregiver, lean forward, relax, do not turn away or offer a tissue, but allow the griever to cry. Display your comfort and approval through your body language; your actions will speak louder than yourwords.
5. Do not allow grievers to remain isolated.
   a. Be present and have others present.
   b. Suggest self-help groups and assist grievers to attend.
6. Maintain a family perspective.
   a. Remember that the family is changed.
   b. Help the bereaved reassess.

### Patient/Family Education

Nursing interventions and guidelines for teaching the patient and family facing death are found in the Guidelines for Care Box.

## EVALUATION

Progress in grieving is difficult to measure because of its ongoing nature and wide range of manifestations.[64] Any assessment needs to be continually updated and revised. Fluctuations in the experiences of the bereaved are to be expected. Interventions that are appropriate for one person may not be useful and may even be harmful to another person.

**guidelines for care**

## Grief Support

| Nursing Interventions | Patient/Family Teaching |
|---|---|
| A. Establish therapeutic nurse-patient relationship.<br>B. Encourage patient/family to talk about the loss and express feelings.<br>C. Acknowledge feelings and the stress involved in dealing with the anticipated or actual losses.<br>D. Use of self and caring presence helps the grieving feel connected to someone who cares.[11,18,39]<br>E. Encourage patient/family to discuss what the loss *means* to them.<br>F. Introduce and encourage use of health care supports.<br>G. Encourage patient and family to share their thoughts about impending death and grieving with each other.<br>H. Guide patient/family in problem-solving ways to deal with the loss:<br>1. Examine ways they have dealt positively with past losses.<br>2. Identify changes needed to adjust now within family or work roles, relationships, responsibilities, and expectations.<br>3. Discuss realistic and available resources to use in making needed changes.[44] | A. Review the normal grief process and its nature.<br>B. Reinforce that everyone deals with grief in his/her own way.<br>C. Explain that feelings over loss are natural and necessary for recovery, even if they are uncomfortable.<br>D. Reinforce the importance of expressing feelings, even negative ones, with someone supportive.<br>E. Emphasize the need to maintain positive habits of self-care when grieving (i.e., eating, sleeping, and elimination).<br>F. Reinforce patient's need for normalcy, support, control, and self-esteem when faced with impending death.<br>G. As questions are raised, briefly review with the dying person and family[35]:<br>1. What to expect in the dying process.<br>2. Choices about the quality of life left that the dying person can make.<br>3. Consequences of those choices (i.e., electing no resuscitation does not mean hastening death).<br>4. Measures being taken to offer comfort and some control. |
| ***Specific Grief Behaviors*** | |
| A. Denial<br>1. Encourage patient/family to describe loss and their perception of the experience.<br>2. Avoid confronting.<br>3. Help discuss changes that have occurred in life since the anticipated or actual loss.<br>4. Give opportunities every shift to share feelings.<br>5. Acknowledge patient/family perceptions and feelings.[13,44] | A. Review normalcy of the grief process.<br>B. Briefly explain denial as a protective mechanism, and the need to give time for each person to work through awareness in his/her own way.<br>C. Review ways to support a grieving loved one who is in denial.<br>D. Explain to family how the dying person may continue denial until the moment of death to maintain hope.[23] |
| B. Bargaining<br>1. Encourage patient/family to ask questions as they arise.<br>2. Acknowledge patient/family's wish that everything was "back to normal."<br>3. Encourage patient/family to express underlying feelings.<br>4. Help patient/family identify realistic versus possibly unrealistic hopes.[15] | A. Offer consistent information.<br>B. Encourage everyday communication of questions with patient's physician.<br>C. Anticipate patient/family needs by explaining briefly all tests, procedures, and care.<br>D. Help patient/family discuss changing goals (from aggressive treatment to palliative care).[11,44] |
| C. Guilt<br>1. Encourage patient/family to express negative or ambivalent feelings constructively.<br>2. Help patient/family examine what they do versus do not have direct control over.<br>3. Acknowledge patient/family's wanting to resolve losses.<br>4. Help define what is realistic control (i.e., maintaining independence with activities of daily living [ADLs]). | A. Reinforce normalcy of the grief process.<br>B. Review concrete ways to maintain some sense of control.<br>C. Review with dying patient ways to remain helpful, if desired, to family.<br>D. Review with family specific ways members can help support and care for their dying loved one.<br>E. Reinforce what care they are giving that is helping.<br>F. Help redefine goals of treatment to palliative care.[13,44] |
| D. Anger<br>1. Encourage patient/family to express negative feelings in constructive ways.<br>2. Acknowledge anger as a legitimate feeling in grief.<br>3. Redirect inappropriate expression of anger toward self or others. | A. Reinforce normalcy of the grief process and importance of expressing *all* feelings, even if negative.<br>B. Review available and constructive outlets for expressing anger.<br>C. Review self-care strategies to prevent anger from building up without some release.[18,20,44] |
| E. Depression<br>1. Encourage patient/family to maintain their ADLs and routine as physically able.<br>2. Help patient/family express sadness over loss (i.e., in talking about lifestyle changes in present and future).<br>3. Provide privacy when crying. | A. Reinforce normalcy of the grief process versus prolonged depression.<br>B. Reinforce depression as a protective mechanism and the need to give each person the time to work through this stage. Explain available resources on the health team. |

*Continued*

**guidelines for care**

### Grief Support—cont'd

| Nursing Interventions | Patient/Family Teaching |
|---|---|
| E. Depression—cont'd<br>4. Help patient/family:<br>• find some positive aspect or characteristic of present situation.<br>• find ways to maximize any positive features.<br>• identify specific hope(s) for the future.[60,63]<br>5. Refer to appropriate health care support for suicidal thoughts that include an intent and plan.<br>6. Encourage patient to participate in activities that increase his/her self-esteem.<br>7. Encourage patient/family to still celebrate moments of joy in everyday life, despite facing death. (i.e., sitting in garden for 30 minutes, watching a family video).[60] | C. Reinforce *important* ways to build up the dying person's self-esteem (i.e., reminiscing, telling the loved one how much he or she did in the past for the family, grace in facing death). |

The grief experience can present an overwhelming challenge to the grieving person, family, and nurse. To face the challenge, measurable outcomes need to be preestablished for *each* person on the basis of the individual's sociocultural situation. The outcomes serve as a yardstick of progress. They offer hope that the intensity of grieving does not last forever.

Successful resolution of the grieving process is indicated by the following:

1. Acknowledging the loss and its impact in changing roles and/or relationships
2. Talking about the *reality* of the loss (e.g., son's deceased father will not be taking him to the park to play ball anymore)
3. Beginning to incorporate the reality of the loss (e.g., wife no longer sets place at table for deceased husband)
4. Displaying *some* sign(s) of grieving, (e.g., cognitive, social, physical, and/or psychological)
5. Indicating an absence of
   a. Destructive behavior (e.g., suicidal thoughts, alcohol, or drug abuse)
   b. Signs of poor bereavement outcomes
6. Using some constructive means to express feelings with a significant other or health care professional about the loss
7. Establishing and maintaining activities of daily life routine in meeting own needs (i.e., rest, nutrition, fluids, elimination)
8. Identifying at least one grief support in significant other or health care professional
9. Beginning to set some goals for own future and decreasing preoccupation with the loss

Evaluation methods that can be useful in measuring grief recovery include the following:

1. Perceptions of the grieving person and family about the experience
2. Observations of responses to nursing interventions
3. Comparisons of current grief behavior with baseline behavior
4. Functional status of the grieving person and family in maintaining lifestyle
5. Mutual discussion of goals and ways to work toward goal achievement
6. Perceptions of the nurse about own grief history

When complicated grief is evident, psychiatric intervention may be required. Parkes identified persons exhibiting the following behaviors as requiring psychiatric care:[56,62,74]

1. An extreme depressive reaction manifested by persistent sadness with no shifts to a normal state; an unresponsiveness to warmth; extreme expressions of guilt and identification symptoms
2. Psychotic break with reality (neurotic anxiety; obsessions; phobic, hysteric, or schizophrenic reactions; acting and speaking as though the deceased were still present)
3. Suicidal tendencies (self-punitive acts, often to expiate guilt)
4. Excessive drinking, drug abuse, or promiscuity (as substitutes for the deceased)

Although the discussion in this section focuses primarily on the survivors, all involved are experiencing loss. The dying person, perhaps, is facing the greatest loss of all. Everyone involved is grieving. The principles apply to all from different perspectives. Nursing care of dying persons includes multiple processes.

Dying persons and their families and friends may or may not experience the grieving process in the same way. Dying persons may grieve over the loss of physical function, the loss of past abilities, the ultimate loss of life, and separation from all they know and love. At the same time, significant others may grieve over the potential loss of the loved one, the hurt they feel, and the emptiness they anticipate.[27,52,61,86,88]

## FACING DEATH: THE FINAL LOSS

Despite the amazing advances of science, technology, nursing, and medical knowledge, dying continues to be a part of living. The fact is that at some future time we will cease "to be." In a sense we are dying even as we are living. To conceptualize living and dying as the opposite ends of a continuum creates a false dichotomy. Living and dying are not opposite ends of a continuum: they *are* the continuum. Recent attention to quality of life in dying has focused on advocating for integration of palliative care into the entire course of illness so that death is a natural transition instead of a crisis.[9,11] When we interact with persons who are known to have a life-threatening illness, we are more directly confronted with their dying and our own vulnerability. This confrontation evokes anxiety, and thus we become more aware of the dying component of living. Although we may identify with the suffering and sorrow of persons as they live their dying, we interact with living persons. To appreciate our own and others' responses to loss, dying, and death, we need an understanding of the context in which they occur and of our own views and reactions within varying contexts.[46]

## SOCIETAL, CULTURAL, AND SOCIAL PERSPECTIVES

### Dying and Death: The Differences

Dying is different from death. *Dying,* a part of living, is a process—the process of coming to an end. *Death,* the permanent cessation of all vital functions—the end of human life—is an event and a state. The event is the moment of death; the state is that of being dead.

Both dying and death have unique aspects that evoke fears, anxieties, and uncertainties. Some aspects of dying such as physical and emotional pain, the loss of others, and the inability to function in familiar ways may also occur under other circumstances (e.g., illness, retirement, or relocation) and therefore are not unique to dying. The unique aspect of dying is that it ends in death. People have no prior experiences to help them understand what it means to be dead. Questions surface: Can dead persons think? Do they have feelings? What is it like to be dead? Is there another life? Where will they go?

At the same time that death is a unique event, it is universal. Because it is universal, each society has had to develop its own beliefs, norms, mores, restrictions, and standards related to loss, dying, and after-death practices. Appropriate ways to respond in one societal or cultural group may be inappropriate in another. Each society dictates the standards and practices that it will support. Thus members of a society have a prescribed set of behaviors from which to choose.[54]

In general, the dominant view of dying, death, and loss of members of any one society is a function of how death fits into the teleological view of life. Individual responses reflect the dominant societal view. However, the repertoire of responses of dying persons or the survivors also is determined by personal beliefs and subcultural group (e.g., social, cultural, religious) affiliations. For instance, Americans may view dying similarly, but their responses may be influenced by their religious beliefs, their views of life after death, their social class, and their occupations.

### Prevailing Societal Attitudes

Death denial, death defiance, death acceptance, and desire for death are four prevailing societal attitudes toward death. As these general attitudes are discussed, it is important to remember that they may vary in different situations, depending on whose death is involved.

Recognition of the prevailing attitudes and their differences helps health care professionals to understand the process of dying, guides them when interacting with others, helps them avoid conflicts among themselves, and, most important, enhances their communication abilities and thus their patient care. Quality care for dying persons and family members must remain the constant goal of health care professionals.[53]

No attitude is good or bad; attitudes are merely different. Our behavior reflects our attitudes. If we recognize our own attitudes toward dying and death in a particular situation, as well as those of other persons involved, we may better understand why all of us feel the way we do and why we are acting the way we are. This recognition and understanding may not always lead to agreement, but it can contribute to modifications of behavior and to decreased conflict in decision making. These attitudes are explored briefly in the following sections.

#### Death denial

Western society has been described as a *death-denying* society.[27,74,83] Many people avoid the subject of dying and death. Health care professionals, particularly physicians, have been described as being unwilling to talk with patients about their dying.[19,55] Both health care professionals and family members often justify their stance by expressing the belief that they are "protecting" the dying person.

The question is, whom are they really protecting? In most situations they are protecting themselves; that is, consciously or unconsciously, they weigh the impact on themselves and decide—or choose—not to act because of fear of the reaction or response. The following questions often arise: What will happen to me? Will I lose emotional control? Will the other person shout, cry, or become angry? Will family members become angry? Will the physician become angry? Will I know what to do or say? What if they do not react at all?

In nursing, a death-denying attitude has taken on a negative connotation. But *no attitude in and of itself is good or bad—it just is.* The actions and consequences of an attitude can be evaluated as good or bad. For example, a death-denying attitude may contribute to a lack of open communication about dying, but it also may contribute to continuing to give care in bleak situations. On the other hand, a behavior or action such as continuation of care may reflect more than one attitude; for example, it may reflect both death denial and death defiance.[27]

#### Death defiance

*Death defiance* is a part of the Judeo-Christian heritage. Throughout the ages people have fought for causes or ideologies, even though they knew that they might die in the attempt. This attitude is reflected in hospitals, especially in critical care units or during emergency situations. The cause is saving a life; the battle is with death.

Although staff members do not die in the battle, they are open to loss. If the patient dies, staff members live with the sense of a battle lost. Moreover, they face again the inevitability of death, despite modern technology.[66]

Death defiance is helpful as we fight for life. It is not helpful when we do not also attend to the realities of the situation.

### Death acceptance

*Death acceptance* is viewing death as a normal, natural, and integral part of living. Becker, a prominent philosopher, defined the resignation to and acceptance of our limited existence as the central task for achieving maturity.[27] With this acceptance, death becomes the conclusion of life's plan. It sounds so simple. Intellectually it calms the fears and pains of dying and of facing our own mortality. Like other attitudes toward death, however, this attitude is not a panacea.

For some, death acceptance is the ultimate achievement of maturation, a form of self-actualization. The dying person must achieve this attitude himself or herself; it cannot be forced on him or her by others. The value of the death-acceptance attitude can be judged by actions and behaviors of the dying person.

### Desire for death

The fourth attitude, the *desire for death,* is more common in our society than people generally like to admit. People may desire their own deaths or the death of others.

Many circumstances give rise to the desire to die or for someone else to die. One major reason is the search for relief from suffering. Suffering takes many forms; pain, loneliness, disability, fear, uncertainty, and economic and emotional crises are only a few. If fears and suffering were prevented with compassionate symptom management, physician-assisted suicide would not exist.[9,54]

Other reasons that contribute to the desire to die may be associated with a relief from suffering but are expressed in a different way. Some persons search for reunion with loved ones. Still others look forward to death as a last phase in the fulfillment of life.

Recognition of how people express their desire to die is important. In many instances the expression of the desire to die is the dying person's or family member's way of confirming his or her recognition that death is inevitable within a predictable period of time in the near future.[10,11]

## Meaning of Death

The knowledge that death is imminent within a predicted period of time adds reality to feelings of fear, anxiety, and uncertainty.[41,46,55] As a result, persons facing imminent death experience these emotions differently than do healthy persons who are speculating about what it is like to be dying. Healthy persons speak of death in the abstract; they talk about the death of another or project it into the distant future. Casual comments such as, "We all have to die someday," "We are all dying from the time we are born," or "Everyone has to die of something," reflect what Freud called "unconscious immortality."[26] The fact that people can continue to think about others who have died causes them to unconsciously believe in their own immortality. Hearing of someone else's dying or death, however, forces them to face their own finiteness.

Neither the casual comments nor the unconscious belief in our own immortality are good or bad in themselves. However, they offer little in the way of understanding or support when made to a dying person or to his or her family. The statements usually are in response to the discomfort we feel when someone tells us that death is imminent. A more understanding response might be, "I'm sorry to hear that."[47,63]

Views toward dying and death vary considerably, depending on whether the discussion is about "my death" or "your death" or whether the discussion is about a member of "my family" or "your family" or someone dear to me or to you. Even when we are discussing hypothetical situations, our closeness to dying or to a dying person can influence our views and our responses.[52,54] The same data are seen differently from different perspectives. We can use age as a common factor and consider how our responses may change. For example, my father is 75 years old, and your father is 75 years old. When death appears imminent, our thoughts may vary, depending on the referent of my father or your father. For example, my father is still young; your father has lived a long and a good life.

It is important to identify the referent under discussion whether we are talking in theoretic terms or about practical situations. In other words, from whose perspective are we evaluating the situation: my perspective, your perspective, the patient's perspective, or a family member's perspective? Lack of recognition of different perspectives can lead to poor communication, faulty nursing judgments, and inappropriate nursing interventions.[46]

## Quality of Life

What constitutes *quality of life?* Who can predict what quality of life is or will be during the dying process? Can one person judge the quality of life of another, especially if the other is dying?

Much has been written on what constitutes quality of life from the research perspective, but there is little on what constitutes quality of life for the dying person. In fact, it has been suggested that if the known instruments were used to measure quality of life, most dying persons would receive low scores, because most instruments focus on objective physical, behavioral, psychological, and economic results of disease and treatment and less on measures of a general sense of well-being, happiness, or satisfaction.[25,53] Dying persons may perceive quality of life differently than those who are living with an acute or chronic illness or who are well.[33,35,53] McMillan[53] studied perceptions of quality of life in cancer patients receiving hospice care. The findings reinforce that social and spiritual aspects of quality of life are enhanced with hospice care (see the Research Box on the next page). What constitutes quality of life differs from person to person and for any one person during the various stages of life. What contributes to the

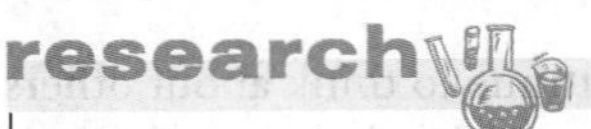

Reference: McMillan S: The quality of life of patients with cancer receiving hospice care, *Oncol Nurs Forum* 23(8):1221-1228, 1996.

This descriptive study evaluated the outcomes of hospice services in having an impact on quality of life for cancer patients and their families. Using the Hospice Quality of Life Index, 118 cancer patients receiving hospice care at home and their primary caregivers were surveyed using a convenience sample. Sampling was done within 48 hours of hospice admission and after 3 weeks of hospice service. Results with factor analysis showed high mean scores of Quality of Life involving social and spiritual issues, with low mean scores involving physical needs and functional issues.

*meaningfulness of life* may be a more cogent question than what constitutes quality of life in considering the dying person.[61] For example, depression can be expected but how much and for how long? A person can live with pain, anxiety, and fear but how much and for how long? How much control does the person have over the situation? Can we increase the control he or she can have in the situation, although the person has lost control over dying? Do the symptoms detract from the meaning of life from the perspective of the dying person? Sometimes trials and tribulations contribute to a person's growth.

Dying persons must have freedom to choose a style of dying and then be assisted in that choice. Patients' preferences are important because they make explicit the values of personal autonomy and self-determination.[5,9,53,67]

*Informed consent,* then, becomes an important factor in supporting meaningfulness of life. It includes giving dying people sufficient information about their diagnoses, prognoses, and possible therapies so that they make informed choices about how they will live or die and about who will help them and in what ways. Informed consent is a person's agreement to allow something to happen on the basis of a full disclosure of facts needed to make an intelligent decision.[19,44] Informed consent reinforces the value of personal autonomy. It assumes that the person has the emotional and mental ability to understand, to process data, to assess benefits and burdens, and to make decisions. This ability is sometimes referred to as competence or *mental capacity.*

Competence and incompetence are used in many ways in everyday life to infer that a person is capable in some way, that is, clinically competent. Actually, the terms *competence* and *incompetence* are best reserved as legal terms. As such they infer reasoning ability and emotional stability sufficient to appreciate the nature and consequences of making decisions regarding such things as wills, contracts, or being a parent. A judge or other proper legal authority makes the judgment of whether or not a person is competent. If a person is judged incompetent, he or she is assigned a guardian. The guardian may be responsible for all decisions for another person, or his or her power may be restricted to *one area* of the dying person's affairs. For example, a person may be deemed incompetent in matters of business but may retain the mental capacity that allows autonomy in decisions about medical treatment.[54]

**box 8-5** *Elements of Quality Care for Patients in the Last Phase of Life*

**PREAMBLE**

In the last phase of life people seek peace and dignity. To help realize this, every person should be able to fairly expect the following elements of care from physicians, health care institutions, and the community.

**ELEMENTS**

1. The opportunity to discuss and plan for end-of-life care.
2. Trustworthy assurance that physical and mental suffering will be carefully attended to and comfort measures intently secured.
3. Trustworthy assurance that preferences for withholding or withdrawing life-sustaining intervention will be honored.
4. Trustworthy assurance that there will be no abandonment by the physician.
5. Trustworthy assurance that dignity will be a priority.
6. Trustworthy assurance that burden to family and others will be minimized.
7. Attention to the personal goals of the dying person.
8. Trustworthy assurance that care providers will assist the bereaved through early stages of mourning and adjustment.

From American Medical Association: *Elements of quality care for patients in the last phase of life,* Chicago, 1997, The Association.

In the health care setting, use of the term *mental capacity* rather than *competence* or *incompetence* offers some clarity. Mental capacity refers to the ability to understand the situation and voluntarily make decisions about it. The mentally capable dying person has the right to refuse or to request treatment. When the request is based on an informed choice, it should be respected, thus reinforcing the value of autonomy. Nurses can enhance the mental capacity of dying patients by educating them about their illnesses and treatments and assisting them to formulate questions for the health care team. They also can provide a safe environment for patients as they deal with uncertainty.

## QUALITY OF DEATH

### Rights of Dying Persons

Some health care consumers are demanding that dying and death no longer be hidden behind closed doors. As a consequence, rights of the dying person have been recognized. Both the American Nurses Association and the American Medical Association have standards for meeting such rights (Box 8-5). One right of dying persons is the right to know that they are seriously ill and that they may die. The assumption is that such information ensures that they will have more control over what happens to them. As a result, they can participate more fully in decisions about their care and will have the opportunity to complete unfinished business.

Another right is the right to die in an atmosphere of hopefulness. Persons have a right to die in peace and dignity, surrounded by loved ones and unencumbered by tubes and machines. They have a right to privacy. Dying persons are entitled to be cared for by sensitive, caring, knowledgeable people who attempt to understand them and their loved ones. They are entitled to die as free from pain or other discomforts as is possible.[67,69] Comfort contributes to dying with a sense of self-esteem and gives meaning to life.[55]

## Advance Directives

Concern that patients be allowed to die in a dignified manner has led to the development of the living will, or *advance directive.* In state statutes it is referred to as the *Natural Death Act.*

The Patient Self-Determination Act was passed by Congress in 1991 to ensure that the rights of the dying were upheld. The law advocates death with dignity when terminal illness precludes treatment. It maintains the right of all patients to make health care decisions and to refuse life-saving treatment, even if they are unable to communicate.

Hospitals, nursing homes, and hospices are required by law to help their patients design an advanced directive for health care. This process involves:

1. Upon admission, advising patients of their rights to:
   a. Accept or refuse medical care in the event they become terminally ill.
   b. Make an advanced directive decision.
2. Documenting the process and the patient's decision.
3. Implementing advanced directive policies.
4. Providing ongoing staff education about advanced directives rights and policies.

Each state has detailed laws that define the types of advanced directives that are legally binding. The state statute should be consulted prior to advising patients regarding the directive.[31] Making an advanced directive decision includes designing a living will and designating a durable power of attorney for health care.[5,35]

Living wills direct decisions for withholding or withdrawing of life-sustaining treatment when the patient is in a terminal condition and death is imminent. Traditionally, life-sustaining treatment has included cardiopulmonary resuscitation and mechanical treatment such as a ventilator. However, with the growing number of court cases, questions have arisen about inclusion of nutrition and hydration.

Living wills are written documents that instruct anyone who may become responsible for the person's health, welfare, or affairs, such as family members, lawyers, physicians, clergy, or representatives of any medical facility in which the person may be. These documents advise them on health care preferences. Living wills include directives to physicians and a durable power of attorney for health care.

Living wills generally request that under conditions in which (1) an individual can no longer take part in decisions about his or her own future and (2) there is no reasonable expectation for recovery, the person be allowed to die and not be kept alive through the use of artificial or extraordinary means. Most living wills also request that the person be kept free of suffering and pain, even though the medications administered for pain relief may hasten the moment of death.

Durable power of attorney for health care is a form of advance directive that enables one to choose an agent to act as decision maker if one becomes too incapacitated to responsibly participate in one's own health care decisions. Included are special directions for life-sustaining treatments and hydration/nutrition issues.[5,19]

Copies of living wills and durable power of attorney documents usually are given to family members, physicians, the person's attorney, and the person's religious advisor. Individuals are advised to sign and date them at least yearly. The wills are likely to be honored if they are written or signed immediately before a person becomes unable to express his or her own wishes about dying care. A sharing with loved ones and primary health care providers of one's philosophy of life and desires related to the process of dying is perhaps the most effective way of ensuring a meaningful death—or what has been referred to as a "good" death.[9,54,78]

## Good Death/Bad Death

Many nurses, and in fact people in general, express concern over dying with dignity or dying a good death. Is there such a thing as a good death? There is no one good death; rather there are many. There is no one right way to die, just as there is no one right way to live. Dying with dignity, or a good death, is really an ideal. The terms offer little in the way of guiding care. There are many views about what constitutes a good death: to die as one lived, to die without pain, or to die in the company of loved ones are all answers.

There are many ways to die well. A good death involves individual perceptions of the living-dying process, as well as shared observations of the death event. *A death is more likely to be labeled as good when dying is viewed as a part of living* and not as a separate phenomenon. A good death also is associated with the way all persons involved interact with each other preceding and during the event—that is, if there is harmony rather than conflict.[9,19,79]

Sometimes nurses refer to deaths as normal or abnormal. Deaths are perceived as *normal* or *good* when most or all persons involved perceive that all was done that could be done and that the wishes of the patient were respected and accepted by most persons involved. In these instances there is a sense of loss, but the loss is accompanied by a sense of fulfillment and closure. Nurses label deaths as *bad* or *abnormal* when there is conflict over the type or length of treatment and when the wishes of the patient are ignored and there are bad feelings about a lack of honesty, especially with family members.

Whether a death is seen as good or bad does not always have to do entirely with the way the person died. Sometimes it has to do with who is present and how they interpret what is happening in the situation. The dying experience can leave a lasting impression on survivors. Family members will retain images of pain, depression, and helplessness.[25,46,53] People's attitudes toward dying and when people should die, as well as the characteristics of the dying person, also influence how they interpret the experience.

### Age and Premature Death

There was a time when people did not make a connection between aging, loss of body function, and general progressive debilitation and dying. For example, primitive people believed that if there were no accidents or magically induced illnesses, no one would die.

The expectations of living have changed as life expectancies have changed. During the Roman period, life expectancy was 20 years; it increased to about 35 years during the Middle Ages. By the late 1800s Americans could anticipate living 50 years; few persons lived past the age of 60 or 70. In contemporary American life, people not only anticipate living more than 70 years; they expect to do so as active, functioning individuals.[54]

Many people believe that any age is too young to die. In contemporary American society death is perceived as premature and clinically unnecessary. The concept of clinical death is well entrenched. Some perceive that people do not die of natural causes or of old age; people die as a result of accidents, homicides, and suicides. They die while receiving treatment for a recognized, diagnosed clinical problem such as heart disease, stroke, disseminated intravascular coagulation, or total body failure. As a consequence, most deaths can be interpreted as avoidable, unnecessary, and premature. If death always is interpreted as avoidable, unnecessary, or premature, it follows that someone must be blamed. Who can be blamed—the physician, the hospital, society? Perhaps it is the fault of the person who died for not seeking help sooner. This interpretation of death as always avoidable contributes to conflict and guilt.[25,27,54]

### Prolonged Dying

Just as there is concern over premature death, there is concern over prolonged dying. Through modern technology and therapy we have become adept at maintaining life in the desperately ill person. Unfortunately, at times the same techniques used to maintain life during temporary crises create dilemmas related to what constitutes life. When are we prolonging dying rather than life? Our ability to prolong dying leads to many moral and ethical issues related to life and death.[41,78]

### Dying: An Achievement or a Failure

Although most dying people express resentment, fear, or sorrow over the major changes that are forced on their lives by their progressive debilitation, some view dying as an achievement.[19] Some persons, especially those with a prolonged course of living with dying, focus on living their dying so as to die well. They speak about their dying to selected persons and at selected times. People who believe that dying well is an achievement sometimes are described by health professionals as denying or defying death. These people recognize their dying but choose therapy or choose to go home and participate in their customary activities. If you listen carefully to what they tell you, you will see that they intend to live their dying the way they wish, and thus from their own perspective they die well. These persons seem to do more than adjust or accommodate. They rise to an unseen challenge and in so doing expand their living rather than extend their dying.[52,53] They transcend what their illness presents as limitations and find strength in facing uncertainty.[14]

A small number of persons may perceive dying as a personal failure or may attribute it to external forces. Some dwell on all they could have accomplished were it not for their illness. They usually exude a sense of powerlessness and futility and express overt anger. Others appear depressed, helpless, and resigned to their situation.[9,46,54]

How people perceive their dying may change throughout the course of their dying. Attitudes, like physical capabilities, do not remain static. Dying encompasses the whole person; it is an emotional, behavioral, and physical process.[35,55]

## FUNERALS AND AFTER-DEATH RITUALS

All societies have funeral practices associated with care and disposal of the body and with the expected behavior of the bereaved. Although the funeral industry has come under scathing attack, funerals and after-death rituals serve many positive functions for the bereaved.[54] They include:

1. Focus on the bereaved by a gathering of friends and family offers sympathy, a recognition of the loss, communication of caring—in short, social support. Wakes, viewings, and visitations are forms of gatherings for family and friends. Nurses and other health care professionals accomplish similar tasks by reviewing together what occurred and sharing past experiences about the person who died or others who have died.
2. Use of ritual, which is often religious in nature, offers some reason or lends some meaning to death.
3. Visual display of the dead body assists survivors with reaching closure or accepting the finality of death.
4. There is opportunity to display grief publicly in a procession that ends at the place of final disposition.
5. Burial, entombment, cremation, or some kind of sanitary disposition of the body reinforces the idea of preservation of life on earth and for some provides a place to return for prayer or reminiscence.
6. Material expenditure for funerals is one way to communicate "the loss of the bereaved to society."

All major changes in life have rituals to help individuals and society adapt to the changed state and cope with the disequilibrium that occurs during the transition from one state to another (e.g., birth, marriage, and death). Funerals serve as a rite of passage[20,68] from life to death. They function to validate the life of the deceased[61] and act as a testimony that a life has been lived.

During the funeral the bereaved begins the process of emancipation from the bondage of the deceased, readjustment to an environment in which the deceased is missing, and incorporation to a new state. The bereaved publicly appears without the living loved one, to be reincorporated into their previous social group in a changed state. The deceased is removed from the social group and admitted to the land of the dead by internment, entombment, or cremation. The relationships are publicly declared changed.[19,61,87]

During the funeral, society bestows rank on the deceased for the last time. The specifics of the ritual (e.g., 21-gun salute), the number of mourners, and the impact of the death on society all reflect the value of the deceased individual.

Funerals meet the needs of mourners and society. They are for the living, not the dead. They offer spiritual, psychological, and social benefits to the survivors and therefore are important.

## THE DYING PROCESS

Thus far we have discussed dying and death in somewhat general terms. Now let us turn more directly to a discussion of dying persons and their characteristics, which will form a basis for nursing support.

### Chronicity of Dying

The nature of dying has changed. Because of modern therapies and technology, patterns of illness have shifted from acute infectious diseases to chronic conditions; as a result, dying has become a chronic process. With the exception of some acute problems such as myocardial infarction, severe infections, fatal accidents, homicides, and suicides, most dying persons experience chronic problems with multiple pathophysiological alterations. These alterations usually are permanent and result in disability, with a need to adjust to loss and to accommodate to change. Multiple series of losses can affect a person's behavioral responses and ability to cope.

Dying takes on many characteristics of chronic illness. Dying persons, just as do other chronically ill persons, express feelings of being socially displaced or isolated. They grieve over the loss of former activities and abilities. They express sorrow over the continued loss of friends, business associates, and acquaintances. They talk of being alive and yet not able to live. They are expected to be present-oriented rather than future-oriented.[20,35]

Whenever the anticipated life span is *perceived* as *shortened,* persons, even though they are healthy, may be viewed as chronically ill or dying and treated accordingly. For example, some elderly persons are perceived and perceive themselves as not having enough time left to make future-oriented plans or decisions. The same perception is associated with some persons with diagnoses of illnesses such as cancer, stroke, and multiple sclerosis. Some people with shortened life spans may perceive themselves or be perceived by others as not deserving of services or not being worthy of the efforts of others because they will not live long; thus they may become displaced, isolated individuals, not allowed to live their living. Furthermore, the chronicity of their dying may force them into experiencing a *social death* while they are functionally and biologically very much alive. Many factors contribute to promoting social dying long before the event of death: these factors are discussed in the next section.[19,35,54]

### The Living-Dying Interval

The theoretic stages and phases of dying are sensitizing schemes to help us remain open to assessing what is "going on" in a situation so that we may understand it better. Our ultimate goal is quality care for dying persons and their families. Understanding, observation, and assessment assist in determining appropriate intervention to better achieve that goal. Another tool to help understand the nature of grief and dying is the patterns of living-dying.[46,47]

The four major patterns and their various combinations are based on the clinical courses of dying patients (Figure 8-2). They describe what has occurred, not what will occur. In other words, they are descriptive, not predictive. They are useful for understanding the variations of behavior among dying persons. They also demonstrate the futility of expecting persons to pass through a series of stages of behavior in any fixed sequence.[46]

#### Peaks and valleys

The *pattern of peaks and valleys* is characterized by periods of greater health (peaks) and periods of crises (valleys). Dying persons refer to the peaks as "hopeful highs" and the valleys as "terrible or depressing lows." Although there are times of greater health, the overall course is downward to the event of death. Many hospitalizations and many moments of increased expectation and dashed hopes are associated with the experience of dying in this pattern. The uncertainties are great; fluctuations in behavior and difficulties in planning and adjustment are to be expected as goals and plans change.[46,47,63]

#### Descending plateaus

The pattern of *descending plateaus* is characterized by an unpredictable number of progressive degenerative steps, with plateaus (periods of stable health) lasting an indeterminate period of time. Again, the overall general course is downward. People do not return to their former level of health or functioning after each crisis. Like the peaks and valleys pattern, the course is fraught with uncertainty and anxiety about whether another crisis will occur and cause more debilitation.

This pattern is associated with expressions of futility and anger. Dying persons and their families grieve over the fact

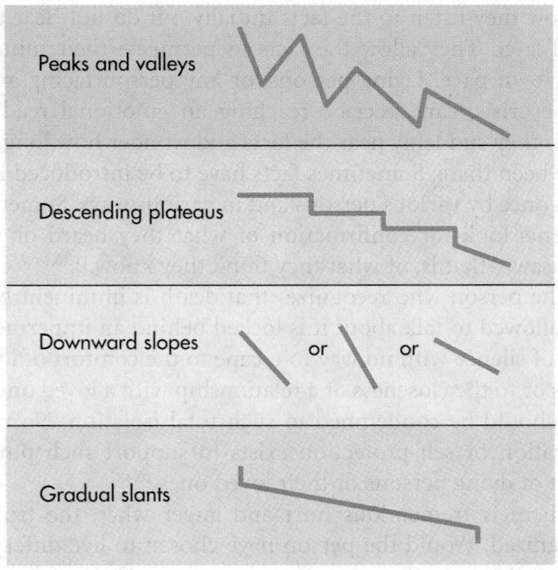


**fig. 8-2** Martocchio's patterns of living-dying.

that functional ability is lost despite concerted rehabilitative efforts to maintain or regain it.[46,47]

#### Downward slopes

The *downward slopes pattern* is characterized by a consistent, persistent, easily discernible downward course. Unlike the other patterns, death is expected within a predictable period of time measured in hours or days. In most instances the dying person loses consciousness, and there is little time to prepare family members for the death of their loved one. These deaths usually occur in critical care units.[46,47]

#### Gradual slants

The fourth pattern of living-dying, *gradual slants,* is characterized by a low ebb of life, gradually and almost imperceptibly culminating in death. Generally these persons experience a debilitating bodily insult from which there is little recovery. In many instances the person is no longer conscious, and life is maintained by life-support systems such as ventilators. This pattern is associated with many of the following questions:
When should life-support systems be discontinued?
Where should these persons be cared for?
Who should be responsible for their care?

In reality, many combinations of the four patterns may occur in one person's experience of living-dying. For example, a person's pattern may change from peaks and valleys to a downward slope or from a downward slope to a gradual slant.[46,47]

### Choice: A Need and a Right

All dying persons eventually learn of their fate. They should be free to choose what role, if any, they will play in the circumstances and manner in which they learn.[9,19,35] Some have recently advocated an individual's choice for also deciding how and when he or she will die.[9,54]

Dying persons describe a system of filtering out or listening only to what they want to know or to realize. They tell us of how they listen to the facts initially but do not hear them until later. They allow the facts to permeate their minds at their own pace. Dying persons, or any person facing an extreme crisis, can describe reaching an emotional readiness when they suddenly hear the facts and wonder how long they have been there. Sometimes facts have to be introduced more than once by various persons and in various ways. Sometimes patients look for confirmation of what they heard or what they saw—that is, of what they think they know.[11,40,89]

The person who recognizes that death is imminent but is not allowed to talk about it is locked behind an impermeable wall of silence with no way to escape to the comfort of loving arms or to the closeness of a relationship with a loved one. No one should be condemned to such total isolation. No rationalization or self-protection exists to support such punishment of dying persons or their loved ones.[10,47]

There is tremendous hurt and anger when the truth is recognized. Would the person have chosen to live differently during the time that can never be returned? What happens to the confidence the person may have had in the nurses, physicians, and health system—the confidence that has been betrayed?

On the other hand, there are patients who sincerely choose not to see or to hear—who choose not to know. If that is their *informed* choice, then it is inappropriate to push them to know that which they do not want to see or hear. To force them to see or hear what they wish to deny is as cruel and inhumane as the conspiracy of silence. The refusal of the patient to know or to discuss the facts creates its own set of problems. The foremost problems, both with lying to patients and with refusal by patients to acknowledge or discuss the facts of dying, are the creation of barriers to comforting and supporting care and communication among interactors and the inability to share feelings and concerns on the basis of the reality of the situation.[6,41,47]

### Role of Confidant

Nurses can introduce the element of choice by fulfilling the patient's need for a *confidant* who will initiate and allow honest talk. The role of confidant is a necessary but difficult role. Talking of dying is not easy, and periods of awkwardness and expressions of fear are inevitable.[11]

Dying persons look to the confidant for honesty and acceptance as they search for understanding of their state. They are not searching for pity, consolation, or sympathy. They are uncomfortable with the helplessness that they see in the eyes of others. The length of time that relationships exist with patients who have long-term chronic illnesses provides both the opportunity and the obligation for nurses to establish *authentic relationships* with dying patients, relationships in which nurses can be viewed as confidants.[13,44,45,84]

The confidant is one to whom patients can voice their deepest fears. They do not voice such fears to business associates; they cannot expect casual friends to understand. They do not reveal their most terrible anxieties to those they love; they protect loved ones from their panic. There are great risks in seeking information about that which they most dread because what they most dread might be confirmed. There is also the superstition that lurks in their minds that what is said aloud might happen or come true; therefore, if they do not talk about it, it will not happen. The result may be fear and silence.

The role of the confidant is primarily to be present, to listen, and to guide as the dying person grapples with the experience of dying. The confidant can help make the period of shifting from living to dying a time for a deepening feeling of closeness, a time for reinforcing family relationships, and a time to do and say what needs to be done and said.[11,47,60,81,89]

Acting as a confidant does not mean that the relationship with the patient is a friendship. A true friendship is characterized by mutuality, with each party having equal rights and equal obligations to be sensitive and concerned for the needs and desires of the other. In contrast, in the nurse/patient relationship, the needs and desires of the patient are the primary concern and provide direction for interaction. Although not a friendship, an atmosphere of emotional closeness is a significant part of the relationship. Within this context, patients can develop and share their agendas for the future, for quality of life, and for what they truly want, without the need to protect the nurse from difficult truths.[10,41,89]

Challenging communication issues confront the nurse confidant and require sensitivity in supporting the patient and family during the dying experience. Callanan and Kelley[11] have described nursing interventions that help operationalize the confidant role (Box 8-6).

Dying persons do not confide in every nurse, nor will the person they select as confidant necessarily be a nurse. Dying persons, just as any other persons, will be selective. Nurses are obligated to offer opportunities to be selected; to demand to serve in the role of confidant is not only inappropriate, but impossible. Nurses who may not be a confidant can support the chosen confidant and learn information that can be useful in guiding care.[13]

## Impact on the Family

Thus far we have focused on the dying person, but the impact of the knowledge that death is imminent extends beyond the dying person to his or her family, social groups, and the society in which he or she lives.

### Cohesive or disruptive force

The experience of dying may serve as a cohesive force in some families and a disruptive force in others. In general, families who have responded to stressors or crises as a unified force in the past will offer each other strength and support. For families who have strained relationships, the dying experience may promote further strain.

Family members generally express remorse over the fact that a family member had to come face-to-face with death before they realized how much they needed each other or cared for each other. But unless this recognition is coupled with assistance in learning how to make the relationship grow, it will not necessarily lead to greater social and emotional solidarity.[15,77]

### Family control

Dying persons at times use their dying to control the behaviors of family members. When dying persons use dying as a means of control for self-gain or as a weapon, the result is anger, resentment, and perhaps retaliation by family members. Retaliation usually takes the form of not visiting, not phoning, or visiting for only short periods. It is an attempt of family members to protect themselves from the control of the dying person even while they wish to be close and loving.

The problem becomes more serious for the family members and the dying person alike if the dying person is being cared for at home. The dying person usually recognizes the antagonism of family members but may interpret it as withdrawal or isolation.[46] More frequently, the dying person may feel rejected and unloved and may not understand that the family loves him or her but not the behavior.

### Dying at home

Although biomedical technological advances continue to encourage that the locus of dying be the hospital, the hospice movement is attempting to deinstitutionalize dying. Hospice nursing is coordinated with the multidisciplinary team to help the terminally ill patient maintain physical, psychosocial, and spiritual well-being in what life is remaining. Symptom management, building family support, and linking the family to community support are central goals.[67,69]

With the increased emphasis on hospice and palliative care and the pressures by Medicare and other insurers to discharge patients as soon as aggressive treatment is discontinued, more persons may choose to die in the privacy of their own homes surrounded by family. *Palliative care,* as defined by the World Health Organization, is the active and total care of people whose disease is not responding to curative treatment. The philosophy of hospice care is based upon palliative care. The goals of palliative care are comfort, control, and quality of living until death.[9,69]

To have those we love die at home, cared for by family, may fulfill the romantic ideas we may have surrounding dying. However, it takes proper, careful, and advanced planning. Two major factors usually are considered: the economic situation and the dying person's wishes. Other important factors to be considered pertain to environmental and caregiver resources. Unless all factors are discussed in advance, family members may be ill-prepared to deal with the most simple tasks. They

**box 8-6** Communicating with the Dying Patient and Family

NURSING INTERVENTIONS

1. Listen to everything the dying patient says for important cues of near-death awareness or messages for family.
   a. Talking about travel, anticipated change, or going home can symbolize approaching death.
2. Help the dying patient describe and share the meaning behind what he or she says, even if it is confusing.
3. Help the family interpret the dying patient's messages and behavior.
   a. Hallucinations can represent the dying patient's sensing the presence of family who have previously died.
   b. Reinforce subtle signs of recognition and comfort when family visit.
   c. Inform the family when the patient shows signs of imminent death.
4. Encourage and guide family communication with the dying patient, whether verbally or through touch.
5. Gently ask about anything not understood.
6. Accept without judgment what the dying patient says.
7. Validate the normalcy of grieving and uniqueness of the patient's own experience.
8. Allow the dying patient to control the conversation. If periods of silence occur, stay with the patient quietly.
9. If silence lasts for more than 10 minutes, acknowledge the patient's efforts in trying to communicate. Let the patient know when leaving the room.
10. Encourage the patient to reminisce when able.
11. Encourage the dying patient and family to put into words any unfinished business.

Adapted from Callanan M, Kelley P: *Final gifts,* New York, 1997, Poseidon Press; Zerwekh J: The truth-tellers: how hospice nurses help patients confront death, *Am J Nurs* (Feb):32-34, 1994.

may not know how to change an occupied bed. They may be concerned about how, what, or even whether to feed the dying person.[81] Family members are suddenly expected to assume nursing responsibilities that they may not desire or feel prepared to do, such as changing dressings, irrigating wounds, and administering medications.

When families are asked to do more than they believe they can accomplish, especially when they do not have readily available assistance, they may feel trapped in an unreasonable situation. Feelings of entrapment can lead to anger, frustration, depression, fear, and despair.[8,61]

Family members who are prepared to care for dying persons in the home need planned times for their own social activities, as well as for grocery shopping and other necessities. Visitors and other family members, as well as the dying person, need help in actively supporting the caretaker. Nurses can help caregivers by helping problem-solve ways to meet their family's and their own needs, while giving them acknowledgment for what they are doing.[15]

## NURSING CARE OF THE DYING PATIENT AND FAMILY

Although each person's experience of dying and grieving is unique and personal, there are similarities. Assessment of the uniqueness of the lived experience coupled with knowledge of some expected common responses can assist nurses in meeting needs of dying people and their families/friends.

### A REALISTIC PERSPECTIVE

To be of most assistance to dying persons and their families, nurses must be realistic about how much they can relieve suffering. Nurses cannot stop the dying process or bring back the dead loved one. Nor can they take away the pain of loss. A realistic perspective helps make the experience better and facilitates grief. Nurses can *reach out* if they objectively accept the fact that fear of pain and suffering is a natural part of facing death.[25]

## NURSING MANAGEMENT

### ■ ASSESSMENT

#### Subjective Data

Nursing assessment is an ongoing process throughout the term of the dying person-family-nurse relationship. It will continue and become the family-nurse relationship at the death of the patient. A thorough initial assessment with subjective input from the dying person and family provides the basis for relationships. Assessment criteria are listed in Box 8-7.

#### Objective Data

The ultimate cause of death depends upon the specific disease process, but certain physiological changes occur to all persons as they approach death. Irreversible failure of the vital organs precedes death. The nurse should recognize the clinical manifestations of death and prepare the family and patient for the impending death. Being present for the death of a loved one may assist the survivors in resolving their loss.

Failure of the respiratory system is characterized by Cheyne-Stokes breathing, which results from alterations in blood $P_{CO_2}$ levels. The hyperpneic and apneic cycles associated with Cheyne-Stokes breathing continue until asphyxia and respiratory failure occur (see Chapter 32). Heart failure may occur as a result of the increased load on the heart and increased ventricular filling during the hyperpneic phase. The results of heart failure include decreased perfusion, ischemia, and eventually cell death. Eventually compensation is no longer effective and myocardial ischemia, liver congestion, and pulmonary congestion result.

Physical manifestations of the failing respiratory and heart systems are manifested as cool skin; skin color changes including pallor, jaundice, or mottling; weak, thready pulse; respiratory stridor (due to accumulated secretions in the larynx or trachea—sometimes termed "death rattle"); decreased urinary output; reduced gastrointestinal motility resulting in impaction; and incontinence as the sphincter muscles relax. As the patient approaches death, the peripheral pulses may not be palpable, and it may be necessary to palpate the carotid or auscultate the apical pulse. The extremities will feel cool and appear cyanotic due to decreased peripheral circulation. The mucous membranes may be dry due to decreased fluid intake. Mouth-breathing will also increase drying of the oral mucosa.

The neurological functioning of the person is decreased due to inadequate cerebral perfusion, usually resulting in confusion, lethargy, and apathy. Severe neurological deterioration is characterized by stupor, absence of reaction to painful stim-

**box 8-7** *Nursing Assessment*

**DYING PERSON AND FAMILY PERCEPTIONS**

**General Perception of Each Individual**

Awareness of clinical diagnosis and prognosis
Philosophy of living while dying and views regarding dying
Perceptions of self and effect on self of the dying process
Expected physiological and behavioral changes
Past experiences with major illnesses or crises
Shared experiences with major illnesses or crises

**Perceived Strengths, Desires, and Hopes**

Personal abilities and coping techniques
Personal support systems
Availability of resources
Beliefs; religious convictions; cultural views of dying, death, and bereavement
Past experiences with death
Expectations about care and dying, use of life supports (present and future)

**INPUT FROM NURSE**

Beliefs, values, attitudes, responses
Support systems: personal and professional
Expertise, including incorporating others in care

uli, and coma. The pupils will react to light sluggishly. As the person experiences neurological failure, the pupils will become unreactive. Not all patients experience neurological deterioration and remain alert to the end. A wide range of emotional responses can be expected from the dying person. Anxiety, fear, restlessness, agitation, or withdrawal are not uncommon. Some persons may exhibit unusual or inappropriate behavior, perhaps due to anxiety. The nurse may observe the dying person speaking to someone when there is no one in the room. Speaking to a deceased loved one in the hours preceding death has been reported around the world and is recognized as part of the dying process.

Objective data indicating that death is imminent include a gradually lowering of the blood pressure, Cheyne-Stokes respirations that become progressively shallow until they cease, fixed and dilated pupils, damp, cool skin, decreased sensorium, and incontinence of bowel and bladder. A weak, irregular pulse indicates the patient is within hours of death.

## NURSING DIAGNOSES

As one reviews the various nursing assessment criteria in caring for dying persons and their significant others, it becomes clear that analyses of the data may lead to identification of nearly all the NANDA nursing diagnoses over the course of the dying process. The complex physiological, psychological, social, and spiritual dynamics that accompany dying help explain the presence of the multiple primary and secondary nursing diagnoses. Perhaps the greatest challenge to nurses is prioritizing—which nursing diagnoses should be addressed and in which order?

Among the most important diagnoses to address are those related to symptom management and anticipatory grief. The physical symptoms that accompany the dying process depend on the particular pathophysiology of the disease responsible for the life-threatening state and the interface with other preexisting emotional and physical health problems. Assessing and understanding the cause of the symptoms is central to determining appropriate interventions. Following is a brief outline of some of the most common nursing diagnoses associated with care of dying persons as they relate to major symptoms/problems. Nursing interventions for these diagnoses are found in the section related to the presenting problem.

| Diagnostic Title | Possible Etiological Factors |
|---|---|
| *Anorexia problems* | |
| Nutrition; altered; less than body requirements | Nausea and vomiting secondary to chemotherapy, medication interactions, obstructions in the gastrointestinal tract, anxiety; altered taste secondary to dysphagia, weakness, depression |
| *Body movement problems* | |
| Activity intolerance, risk for | Depression, shortness of breath |
| Injury (trauma), risk for | Secondary to metastases to bone, confusion, seizures |
| Mobility, impaired physical | Weakness, contractures, pain, infection, semicomatose/comatose state |
| *Bowel elimination problems* | |
| Constipation | Medication reaction, poor fluid-dietary intake, immobility |
| Diarrhea | Impaction, disease process |
| Incontinence, bowel | Secondary to weakened state; semicomatose/comatose state |
| *Fluid balance problems* | |
| Fluid volume deficit | Low fluid intake secondary to weakness, fever, reduced extracellular fluid volume, dysphagia, gastrointestinal fluid losses, oliguria, polyuria |
| Fluid volume excess | Altered cardiac output; effects of medication |
| *Mouth symptoms* | |
| Mucous membrane, altered, oral | Disease secondary to impaired immune system, decreased protein intake; effects of treatment such as chemotherapy, radiation, and continuous oxygen |
| | Decreased fluids, mouth breathing, decreased saliva, medications |
| Pain | Stomatitis secondary to dehydration, continuous mouth breathing and local trauma; dysphagia |
| *Respiratory/ventilation symptoms* | |
| Airway clearance, ineffective | Inability to eliminate secretions |
| Breathing pattern, ineffective | Dyspnea, pain, rales/rhonchi, obstruction, semicomatose/comatose state |
| Gas exchange, impaired | Shortness of breath |
| Tissue perfusion, altered (respiratory) | Respiratory distress syndrome |
| *Skin problems* | |
| Skin integrity, impaired | Edema, immobility, urinary incontinence, sweating, cachexia, fungating tumors |
| | Complications of treatment, reaction to medications |
| | Poor tissue perfusion secondary to infrequent turning/repositioning; circulatory impairment |
| *Sleep and rest problems* | |
| Sleep-pattern disturbance | Fear of dying, uncertainty about the future, pain, shortness of breath, metabolic effects of disease, drug interactions/untoward drug reactions, night sweats, restlessness, depression |
| *Temperature problems* | |
| Temperature, risk for altered body | Medication reaction, decreased fluid intake, altered metabolic rate, sedation; neurological and/or circulatory alterations |
| *Urinary problems* | |
| Urinary elimination, pattern, altered | Reaction to medications, obstruction of the urinary tract, reduced fluid intake, nausea, urinary tract infection |

In addition to the nursing diagnoses associated with physical symptoms, other nursing diagnoses associated with dying persons relate to psychosocial and spiritual dimensions. The following are examples that may be evident:

| Diagnostic Title | Possible Etiological Factors |
|---|---|
| Fear | Death, unknown, loss |
| Coping, compromised (family) | Conflicting perceptions among members, maladaptive coping styles |
| Coping, ineffective (individual) | Pain, effects of medication, lack of family or social support, loss of family, significant other |
| Family processes, altered | Patient's or other family members' inability to fulfill accustomed roles secondary to pain and disability, loss of role |
| Grieving, anticipatory | Association of existence of pain and dysfunction with imminent death |
| Knowledge deficit | Patient's and family's lack of awareness of availability of modern methods of palliation |
| Powerlessness | Dependence on others for care secondary to pain and effects of medication, terminal illness |
| Social isolation | Inability of patient to focus away from symptoms, discomfort of others when confronted with patient's symptoms and dying |
| Spiritual distress | Association of symptoms with punishment, imminence of death, and sense of abandonment by God, loss of significant other |

Because the needs of the dying person and family are complex, it has been suggested that nursing diagnoses and interventions be combined under one heading entitled "terminal care syndrome."[1]

## EXPECTED PATIENT OUTCOMES

Expected patient outcomes for the dying person and his or her family may include but are not limited to:

1. Meets psychological needs and resolves feelings regarding imminent death.
2. Family identifies resources (external and internal) to deal with the patient's eventual death.
3. Accepts imminent death, verbalizes feelings, accepts support from family, friends, and nursing staff.
4. Patient and family express their feelings and acknowledge the impact of the grieving process.
5. Patient and family express hope and express feelings of resolving grief.
6. Family and patient demonstrate effective problem-solving behaviors regarding treatment options.
7. Identifies factors that can be controlled, participates in care and decision making as possible.
8. Identifies friends, family as sources of support.
9. Experiences a dignified death, congruent with his/her personal philosophy and wishes.

## INTERVENTIONS

The nursing needs of dying persons are the nursing needs of living persons. The range of activities is as broad as for any diverse population of patients, family, and significant others. Nursing interventions may occur in a variety of settings, either at home or in various institutional settings.

Direct physical care is a major part of caring for dying persons. Maintenance of comfort, both physical and emotional, is of the essence. Teaching others involved in direct care how to maintain the patient's comfort allows their participation and promotes their feelings of competence and well-being.[15,67]

Nursing interventions may include participation in resuscitative efforts and the maintenance of dying patients on life-support systems. In addition to direct patient care, nurses are responsible for communicating with and supporting family members or for ensuring that someone is providing this service.

In essence, nurses assist patients and families in maintaining control over their individual lives as much as is possible to ensure dignity and self-esteem.[44,64] Expert nursing behaviors have been identified that sensitively address the dying patient's and family's need for control in providing symptom relief, interpreting signs of dying, sharing control, and providing information (Table 8-4).[50]

### Patient/Family Education

The family should be taught in simple terms the physiology of death. Explaining that the gradual slowing of body systems in-

**table 8-4** *Supportive Nursing Behaviors in Terminal Care*

| Key Areas | Positive Behaviors |
|---|---|
| Providing comfort | Reducing physical and psychological pain |
| Responding to family | Meeting family's ongoing need for information |
| | Facilitating transition from focus on cure to palliation |
| | Helping members find something to do and reducing potential for future regret |
| Responding after death | Creating a peaceful scene for survivors |
| | Supporting the realization by family that death has occurred |
| | Demonstrating respect during post-mortem care |
| Responding to anger | Communicating with empathy and respect even when anger is directed at nurse |
| | Offering acknowledgement and redirecting to constructive outlets |
| Responding to colleagues | Providing emotional support and feedback |
| Finding personal growth | Defining a professional and personal commitment in caring for the dying |
| | Reflecting on stories of sharing the dying process with patients and their families |

Adapted from McClement S, Degner L: Expert nursing behaviors in care of the dying adult in the intensive care unit, *Heart Lung* 24(5):408-419, 1995; Steeves R: Loss, grief, and the search for meaning, *Oncol Nurs Forum* 23(6):897-903, 1996.

cludes the gastrointestinal system may help the family accept the patient's refusal of foods or fluids. As death approaches, nausea, vomiting, and pain may result from overloading the gastrointestinal tract.

The patient and family should be reassured that pain will be controlled until death. Dispelling fears of addiction may help the dying person and family. The family should be encouraged to use nonpharmacological methods of pain control, such as reading a favorite story to the patient or bringing in favorite music.

The nurse also serves as a resource for answering difficult questions regarding organ donation, autopsy, and treatment decisions. Informing the patient and family and supporting them during their decision-making process is a vital nursing role.

Nursing responsibilities include being well-informed about organized support systems, agencies, and independent resources within the community and to be prepared to assist patients and their families in contacting and using these resources. Inquiries related to the many alternative modes of care for dying persons, such as hospice and other forms of home care, nursing home care, and other forms of institutional care, should be answered openly and honestly. If the nurse cannot answer the patient's or family's questions, they should be referred to those who can supply the answers.[34]

Health teaching may include measures such as breathing exercises, relaxation techniques, and coping strategies to the dying person and to significant others for use throughout their grieving process.

## EVALUATION

To evaluate the effectiveness of nursing interventions, compare patient behaviors with those stated in the expected patient outcomes. Successful achievement of outcomes for the dying patient and family is indicated by:

1. Verbalizes feelings regarding imminent death.
2. Family verbalizes acceptance of their loss, using coping mechanisms and resources.
3. Patient receives support from family, friends, and nursing staff. Patient verbalizes feelings about own death.
4. Patient and family acknowledge impact of loss on family processes.
5. Patient and family share their grief with one another. Patient and family acknowledge impact of grieving process and begin to look toward future.
6. Patient and family make decisions regarding end-of-life treatments.
7. Acknowledges that some factors are beyond individual control.
8. Receives support from friends and family.
9. Experiences a dignified death according to his or her wishes.

Each nurse is responsible for evaluating his or her own practice as it relates to each patient and family. A sense of control can be an indicator of quality of living and dying. Goals that were mutually set with the dying patient and family will be more achievable. Although accepting losses and death may be encouraged, helping the dying patient and family find some peace in the dying experience is a more realistic outcome.[11,44,86,87]

A nurse will experience loss when a nurse-patient relationship ends with the death of the patient. Evaluation of his or her contribution to the relationship gains importance, especially for each nurse's well-being. Recognition of specific successes and contributions leads to feelings of achievement. Lack of this recognition may lead to perceiving consecutive losses as a sign of failure.

Peer support is beneficial to nurses caring for dying persons. Peer support may be accomplished through formal and informal groups. In addition to groups, one-to-one interactions with a trusted peer or personal significant other may alleviate some of the stress related to working with dying persons.[24,66] More important, such relationships serve as an appropriate avenue for recognizing and reinforcing the inherent rewards of providing nursing care for persons who are living their dying and for those who are sharing the experience.

# SPECIAL ISSUES IN BEREAVEMENT

## ETHICAL PERSPECTIVES

To help a person die well is to support that person's sense of self-respect, dignity, and choice until the last moment of life. Achievement of this goal entails skilled and compassionate nursing care to maximize comfort and minimize suffering. The goal is to provide calm, sensitive, individualized nursing care to each person so that dying, the final human experience, is as free from pain and anxiety as possible.[2]

Historically the profession and activities of nursing have been concerned with life and based on two fundamental principles. These principles are that all people should live (1) as whole persons and (2) long and healthful lives. The expectation has been that nurses and physicians would help to fulfill these principles.[54]

In the past, nurses and physicians fulfilled their obligations by striving to save lives. There were no miracle drugs, life-sustaining machines, transplantation surgeries, or radiation therapies. Intensive and continuous nursing care was the main hope of saving lives. Modalities such as heat, cold, food, fluid, rest, exercise, and maintenance of a sanitary environment were used. Physicians and nurses relied on the natural healing powers of the body. If a body failed to heal despite the efforts of nurses and physicians, the patient died. The power of medicine and nursing simply was no match for the disease that people experienced. Death often was caused by infection and communicable disease. Many people died at young ages.[19,35]

With the advent of miracle drugs and advances in anesthesia, surgical techniques, and life-sustaining technologies, persons who would have succumbed to life-threatening illnesses now seek treatment to restore health and function. The capacity to prolong life and to ease the pain and suffering of seriously ill persons has improved to a great extent. The improvement has been accompanied by some difficult consequences. Increasingly, deaths occur in institutions. In many instances, deaths occur in critical care units to the sound of monitors. More and more often death is caused by someone's decision rather than by the failure of the heart to pump blood or the lungs to breathe.[9]

Death becomes impersonal when the body and the tubes and machines become one and when there is only a deteriorating organ system present. The situation becomes so confusing that those involved have conferences to determine whether life or death is being prolonged.[54]

When a dying person has been termed a "nonperson" and seems neither dead nor alive, all involved persons search for resolution of a situation in which neither grief nor hope is appropriate. Family members long to return to normal living. They search for help in making life and death decisions for loved ones who are no longer able to contribute to decision making. Staff members search for relief from a situation fraught with dilemmas.[9,77]

The dying person does not have to be completely incoherent or comatose for ethical issues to arise. Many ethical issues are inherent in the situation. For example, modern technology has made possible successful treatment of diseases that formerly resulted in fairly immediate death. Now cures for diseases such as cancer are possible. In many instances there are no cures, but there are temporary reprieves; for example, the mechanical ventilator can prolong life. In some situations the result of therapy is ambiguous—for example, therapy that is associated with great discomfort to the patient or the family, such as bone marrow transplantation, or that involves great expense and limited supply, such as organ transplantation.

Discussions of issues such as "quality of life," "right to die," "death with dignity," "living wills," and "informed consent" in lay as well as professional literature demonstrate the extent and awareness of the conflicts associated with modern therapies that extend life but at great cost.[9] Concern over decisions regarding life and death issues has led to the development of organizations that represent differing views. The Hemlock Society, the Society for the Right to Die, and the Americans United for Life[19] are examples of a few of these organizations.[54,69]

The question of who should decide under what circumstances is important. There are other important questions: What is death? What constitutes informed consent? When are therapies ordinary and when are they extraordinary? Should all life be preserved, regardless of quality? Should pain be treated, even though the medication may shorten the life span? What constitutes euthanasia? Is there a distinction between active and passive euthanasia? Is suicide a person's right? All these questions create ethical issues that can make coping with death and dying overwhelming for patients, family members, and the health team.

## ETHICAL ISSUES

Many ethical issues evolve around indications for medical and nursing interventions. These issues arise from questions such as the following: When should medical therapies be started or stopped? When should life supports be discontinued? What constitutes death? Who should decide? (See Chapter 5.)

### Withholding or Withdrawing Treatment

Appropriate consideration of withholding or withdrawing specific therapy occurs when (1) the therapy offers no reasonable expectation of the patient's attaining any human awareness, (2) the therapy is proving medically ineffective and useless after sufficient trial, or (3) therapy is perceived from the expressed point of view of the patient (or the decision-making representative) to be cumulatively a greater burden than a benefit.[67,69]

When decisions are made to withhold or withdraw life-sustaining treatment, the goal of medical and nursing care focuses on keeping the patient comfortable, avoiding suffering and pain, and providing support, comfort, and care on a physical, emotional, and spiritual level. To distinguish those procedures not directed to supportive care becomes more difficult once medical procedures designed to prolong life are withheld or withdrawn. Perhaps the most controversial area is that of determining the proportionate benefit and burden of medical (artificial) nutrition and hydration.[23,35,41] The issue of withdrawing treatment, once it is started, is also present.

### Euthanasia

*Euthanasia* comes from the Greek words meaning "good or pleasant death." It implies that under some circumstances a person may prefer death to life. Euthanasia, or "mercy killing," is a topic surrounded by controversy. At the present time, there is no agreement on whether death is ever preferable to life or on what constitutes euthanasia.[35,78]

The more common distinctions made when discussing euthanasia are those of active and passive and voluntary and involuntary (Box 8-8). *Active euthanasia* refers to an act that directly and intentionally shortens a person's life. It is an act of commission. *Passive euthanasia,* an act of omission, usually refers to letting death occur either by withholding or by withdrawing a treatment that might prolong a person's life.

In looking at questions related to euthanasia, there is a continuum ranging from a strict belief in the sanctity of life (antieuthanasia, treating at all costs) to passive euthanasia (letting die) to active euthanasia (ending life, killing) (Box 8-8).

A persistent moral issue is the question of whether letting death occur is morally equivalent to killing or omission equivalent to commission. Remember, no action is an action. Both active and passive euthanasia are intentional choices. The distinction seems to be that of the intent of the action. The 1986 statement by the AMA Council on Ethical and Judicial Affairs[19,54] holds that the patient and/or immediate family can decide to "discontinue all means of life-prolonging medical

**box 8-8** *Euthanasia*

| DISTINCTIONS | CONTINUUM |
|---|---|
| Active/passive | Antieuthanasia; treating at all costs |
| Commission/omission | Passive euthanasia: letting die |
| Killing/letting die | Active euthanasia: ending life |
| Voluntary/involuntary | |

treatment" even "if death is not imminent but a patient's coma is beyond doubt irreversible." The New Jersey Supreme Court implicitly invoked this distinction when it held that judgments about therapy should be made in terms of the degree of invasiveness of the treatment and its chance of success.[2,78] Ethicists have distinguished ordinary treatment from extraordinary treatment by stating that ordinary treatments offer a reasonable prospect of benefit for the patient without excessive pain, expense, or inconvenience.[41]

In more direct terms, killing is wrong, but letting die in the sense of not instituting extraordinary efforts or by discontinuing extraordinary treatments is morally permissible. In fact, most physicians accept that killing a patient is morally wrong and thus not permissible, but in some circumstances it may become morally required to let a patient die.[54] Nurses generally accept the same view.

## Suicide

Quality of living and quality of dying may be closely associated. A person with terminal illness may assess the situation and decide that living with pain, disability, or despair is not living.[25,53] He or she may ask the question: Is it better to take measures to bring about a peaceful death than to continue in such a state?

Suicide or voluntary euthanasia carried out by the individual on his or her own behalf has been seen as an affirmation of life, a denial of life, and a questioning of life. The traditional religious teaching of the Western world since St. Augustine has condemned all forms of self-destruction. Suicide was and still is considered by some to be a sin and an interference with God's will.[27,34,49] Many assert that human beings do not have the power of disposal of their bodies. They can only treat their bodies as they choose in relation to self-preservation. These views are being challenged in society today as they have been in the past.[22] Some physicians[54] suggest that under some circumstances, when death is imminent, persons who are severely ill should be helped by their physicians to commit suicide. They distinguish this element of the population from the lonely, elderly, and physically handicapped, for whom they do not advocate assisted euthanasia. They point out that, although few laws exist in the United States to cover physician participation, they do exist in Uruguay, Switzerland, Peru, Japan, and Germany. Some cultures, such as the Japanese, and some individuals favor suicide over other negative values such as dishonor.

Individual and societal views regarding suicide run the gamut from opposition to suicide under all conditions and at all costs, to suicide as justifiable under some conditions, to suicide as a person's right. The question of an individual's right to autonomy or self-determination is a basic consideration in discussing suicide. Those who oppose suicide under all conditions usually use some form of the argument that "life is a gift, and no one has the right to take a life." Those at the opposite end of the continuum argue that a person has the right to determine his or her own fate, even if it means destroying his or her own life. Other considerations in arguments opposing suicide include viewing suicide as cowardly, a crime against society, an insult against humanity, and an act that brings great pain to the survivors.[9,78]

Suicide is of particular concern to health care professionals who may be in a position to offer other alternatives and thus prevent it. It is difficult to evaluate what constitutes suicide. Is refusal to eat or to continue with prescribed therapies a form of suicide, or must there be an overt act such as an overdose of medications? Is suicide always a voluntary act, or is a person driven to suicide by rejection of others or by pain that might have been controlled?[9,35,49,78] When is suicide justifiable in the person known to be dying? What do you do when a patient who is dying all too slowly and painfully asks for your assistance in ending it all?

Nurses and physicians, however, are committed to another imperative—that is, to *never abandon care.*[10,11,85] Never to abandon care includes ensuring that a dying person is not alone, that others are aware of his or her dying, and that he or she is free from pain and anxiety. It is not an obligation to assist in ending life. In fact, the ethical basis for suicide prevention is the psychological thesis that a suicide attempt is often a cry for help rather than an unambivalent decision to end one's life. Thus nurses and physicians have a legal and ethical obligation to assess and recognize suicidal risk and depression in patients and to make efforts to assist them in receiving counseling.[31,49] Often suicide is not an act of autonomy but rather is caused by impaired capacity that, in turn, is caused by an underlying emotional conflict or extreme physical discomfort. But what about instances of prolonged dying when it is medically impossible to control pain despite the positive impact of the hospice movement? Life for some dying people does become more of a burden than a gift.

The impact of pain is really a quality of life question that can best be evaluated by the dying individual experiencing the pain.[25,53] If quality of life is determined by the person living the life, is suicide a purely personal decision? It seems that the quality of life of survivors also should be considered. When the survivors have had no prior warning or a part in the decision, and when the suicide is not perceived as an action to achieve comfort, the anguish to the survivors is great. For some the anguish never ends. Their grief is compounded by guilt, shame, and even anger.[62,74] In some instances the survivors become victims of a society that condemns the act as a crime.

Suicide may be a form of control by the dying person, or it may be a form of escape. Some dying people seek an escape from loss of control over the event of dying; others seek an end to suffering. Nurses can be influential in providing dying persons and their families a sense of control by assisting with problems such as pain control, bowel and bladder control, and depression. They can decrease the uncertainty of the situation by explaining what the dying person and family can anticipate over the coming days. In other words, they can assist in promoting quality of life.[11,63]

## Definitions of Death

Much controversy surrounds the question, "What is death?" Is death the irreversible cessation of respiration and circulation, or is death the irreversible cessation of all functions of the entire brain, including the brainstem. In addition, different cultures hold different definitions of death.

The term *brain dead,* in use for some time, still causes much confusion. Originally it referred to a person whose lungs were activated by a ventilator but whose centers in the brainstem were destroyed. Removal from the support system would result in death due to the inability of the person to resume spontaneous breathing. In addition, brain dead means that the person is dead in the sense that a functioning brain is the seat of identity. What decision can be made about persons in a "persistent vegetative state"? They show no evidence of cortical functioning but continue to have sustained capacity for spontaneous breathing and heartbeat.[9,19,54]

Advocates use definitions that reflect their values and provide them with a rationale to act. Each appeal or action has its own consequences. For example, the use of some definitions of brain dead provides more latitude for organ transplantation and experimentation. The rationale for this latitude is that the removal of organs from the person who is brain dead aids the living. A worthy endeavor, but does retrieving organs lead to violation of the dead? What are the constraints? Are the bodies being used with the consent of the donor, or is consent necessary once a person is brain dead?

There are no clear rules that dictate decisions in these matters. Decisions depend on discretion and reflect basic values. They are accompanied by conflict, insecurity, and discomfort. The conflict and emotions that accompany decisions about the life or death of another are entirely appropriate because they are irreversible.[41,78]

The important factor in any ethical issue, regardless of whether it is dealing with euthanasia, suicide, or treatment decisions, is to be aware of the values or forces that lead us to make the decisions we do. An understanding of our own values and perspectives, as well as of formal ethical systems, does not give explicit answers to dilemmas. It does, however, help us be consistent and communicate with others in a way that is understandable. This does not ensure agreement, but it does facilitate discussion and attention to multiple perspectives and to the consequences of actions.

## critical thinking QUESTIONS

**1** Mrs. M, a 60-year-old woman, is admitted for evaluation of progressive back pain, weakness, and weight loss. She is scheduled for magnetic resonance imaging (MRI) to rule out a possible spinal cord tumor. The nurse is preparing Mrs. M for the MRI when the patient remarks, "Why bother? I am going to die like my father no matter what." How should the nurse respond to Mrs. M?

**2** Mr. X is a 45-year-old man with advanced lung cancer and multiple metastases. He is admitted to the hospital with a do not resuscitate (DNR) order. Since requesting DNR status, he has become unresponsive. Mrs. X wants the physician to reverse her husband's DNR order and asks the nurse for help. How should the nurse respond to Mrs. X?

**3** S. G. is a 24-year-old woman who suffered severe head injuries following an motor vehicle accident and is near death. Her family are at the bedside around the clock and ask the nurse caring for S.G. if they can be involved in her physical care. Develop a plan to enable the family to care for their loved one and assist them in the grieving process.

## chapter SUMMARY

### THE LOSS EXPERIENCE

- Coping with loss and dying is an integral part of living.
- Prevailing societal attitudes toward death include death denial, death defiance, death desire, and death acceptance.
- Living wills and advance directives are vehicles used to communicate one's desires related to the process of dying.
- With advances in modern therapies, dying has taken on many characteristics of chronic illness with its accompanying challenges.
- Understanding the stages and phases of grief and dying can aid in assessing the diversity of responses among dying persons and their families, in all cultures.
- Discussions with family members and patients are critical in determining the likelihood of families being able to offer care in the home during the final phases of dying.
- The complex physiological, psychological, social, and spiritual dynamics accompanying dying help explain the presence of the multiple primary and secondary nursing diagnoses and challenge nurses to prioritize them for interventions.

### GRIEF: AN ADAPTIVE RESPONSE TO LOSS

- Grief is the subjective state that occurs as a result of having suffered the loss of a significant person; grief is also the total response (thoughts, feelings, and behaviors) to the emotional suffering caused by a loss.

### DEATH AND GRIEF

- Normal grieving includes a wide range of physical, psychosocial, cognitive, and spiritual manifestations—of shock and disbelief, yearning and protest, anguish, disorganization and despair, identification, reorganization and restitution—that are often frightening and misunderstood by the grieving person.
- Some individual characteristics of survivors are associated with a high risk for problems with the grieving process.
- Nurses can help the dying person and family maintain comfort, communication, and control even in dying.

## References


1. Adams P, Nichols B: An exploration of the nursing diagnosis terminal syndrome, *Nurs Diagn* 7(4):135-140, 1996.
2. American Medical Association: *Elements of quality care for patients in the last phase of life,* Chicago, 1997, The Association.
3. American Psychiatric Association: *Diagnostic and statistical manual of mental disorders: DSM-IV,* ed 4, Washington, DC, 1994, The Association.
4. Aquilera D, Messick J: *Crisis intervention: theory and methodology,* St Louis, 1994, Mosby.
5. Berrio M, Levesque M: Advance directives: most patients don't have one . . . do yours? *Am J Nurs* 96:25-28, 1996.

6. Berry D, Dodd M, Hinds P, Ferrell B: Informed consent and clinical issues, *Oncol Nurs Forum* 23(3):507-512, 1996.
7. Bowlby J: Attachment and loss: retrospect and prospect, *Am J Orthopsychiatry* 52(4):644-677, 1972.
8. Brown-Saltzman K: Multicultural perspectives in palliative care, *Oncol Nurs Forum* 3:41-47, 1994.
9. Byock I: *Dying well: the prospect for growth at the end of life,* Evanston, Ill, 1997, Riverhead.
10. Callanan M: Breaking the silence, *Am J Nurs* 1:22-23, 1994.
11. Callanan M, Kelley P: *Final gifts,* New York, 1997, Bantam.
12. Clark C: Posttraumatic stress disorder: how to support healing, *Am J Nurs* 97(8):27-32, 1997.
13. Cooley M: Bereavement care: a role for nurses, *Cancer Nurs* 15(2): 125-129, 1992.
14. Coward D: Self-transcendence: a resource for healing at the end of life, *Issues Ment Health Nurs* 17(3):275-286, 1996.
15. Czerwiec M: When a loved one is dying: families talk about nursing care, *Am J Nurs* 5:32-36, 1996.
16. Davies B: *Fading away: the experience of transition in families with terminal illness,* Amityville, NY, 1995, Baywood.
17. Dean G: Symptom management for the dying patient, *Qual Life: Nurs Challenge* 3(3):61-66, 1994.
18. de la Fuente E: Counseling dying adults and their significant others. In Lego, S, editor: *Psychiatric nursing: a comprehensive reference,* Philadelphia, 1996, JB Lippincott.
19. DeSpelder L, Strickland A: *The last dance: encountering death and dying,* ed 3, Mountain View, Calif, 1992, Mayfield.
20. Ebersde P: *Toward healthy aging: human needs and nursing response,* ed 5, St Louis, 1998, Mosby.
21. Engel G: Is grief a disease? *Psychosom Med* 3(1):18-22, 1961.
22. Engel G: A life setting conducive to illness: the giving-up given-up complex, *Ann Intern Med* 69:355-365, 1968.
23. Farnslow-Brunjes C: Hope: offering comfort and support for dying patients, *Nursing 97* Mar:54-57, 1997.
24. Feldstein MA, Gemma PB: Oncology nurses and chronic compound grief, *Cancer Nurs* 18(3):228-236, 1995.
25. Ferrell B: *Suffering,* Boston, 1997, Jones & Bartlett.
26. Freud S: *Instincts and their vicissitudes: collected papers,* New York, 1915, Basic Books.
27. Fulton G, Madden C, Minichiello V: The social construction of anticipatory grief, *Soc Sci Med* 43(9):1349-1358, 1996.
28. Glass B: The role of the nurse in advanced practice in bereavement care, *Clin Nurs Spec* 7(2):62-66, 1993.
29. Glick I, Weiss RS, Parkes CM: *The first year of bereavement,* New York, 1974, John Wiley & Sons.
30. Griefzu S: Grieving families need your help, *RN* 9:22-27, 1996.
31. Haber J et al: *Comprehensive psychiatric nursing,* ed 5, St Louis, 1996, Mosby.
32. Haisfield-Wolfe M: End-of-life care: evolution of the nurse's role, *Oncol Nurs Forum* 23(6):931-935, 1996.
33. Highfield M: PLAN: a spiritual care model for every nurse, *Qual Life Nurs Challenge* 2(3):80-84, 1993.
34. Irish D, Lundquist K, Nelsen V: *Ethnic variations in dying, death, and grief: diversity in universality,* Washington, DC, 1996, Taylor and Francis.
35. Kemp C: *Terminal illness: a guide to nursing care,* Philadelphia, 1995, JB Lippincott.
36. Koenig BA, Gates-Williams J: Understanding cultural differences in caring for dying patients. In Caring for patients at the end of life (special issue), *West J Med* 163:244-249, 1997.
37. Kübler-Ross E: *On death and dying,* New York, 1969, Macmillan.
38. Kübler-Ross E: *Death: the final stage of growth,* Englewood Cliffs, NJ, 1975, Prentice-Hall.
39. Laferriere R: Orem's theory of practice: hospice nursing care, *Home Healthcare Nurse* 13(5):50-54, 1995.
40. Larson D: *The helper's journey,* Champaign, Ill, 1993, Research.
41. Lev E: Issues for the nurse caring for dying patients. In Hubbard S et al, editors: *Oncology nursing: patient treatment and support* 1(1): 1-10, 1995.
42. Lev E, Munroe B, McCorkle R: A shortened version of an instrument measuring bereavement, *Int J Nurs Stud* 30(3):213-226, 1993.
43. Lindemann E: Symptomatology and management of acute grief, *Am J Psychiatry* 101:141-148, 1944.
44. Loney M: Death, dying, and grief in the face of cancer. In Burke C, editor: *Psychosocial dimensions of oncology nursing care,* Pittsburgh, 1998, Oncology Nursing Society.
45. Martocchio B: Authenticity, belonging, emotional closeness, and self-representation, *Oncol Nurs Forum* 14(4):23-27, 1985.
46. Martocchio BC: *Living while dying,* Bowie, Md, 1982, Robert J Brady.
47. Martocchio BC: Grief and bereavement: healing through hurt, *Nurs Clin North Am* 20(2):327-341, 1985.
48. Maslow A: *Motivation and personality,* New York, 1954, Harper & Brothers.
49. Massie MJ, Gagnon P, Holland JC: Depression and suicide in patients with cancer, *J Pain Symptom Manage* 9(5):325-338, 1994.
50. McClement S, Degner L: Expert nursing behaviors in care of the dying adult in the intensive care unit, *Heart Lung* 24(5):408-419, 1995.
51. McCue K: *How to help children through a parent's serious illness,* New York, 1994, St Martin's.
52. McIntyre M: Understanding living with dying, *Can Nurse* 93(1): 19-25, 1993.
53. McMillan S: The quality of life of patients with cancer receiving hospice care, *Oncol Nurs Forum* 23(8):1221-1228, 1996.
54. Nuland SB: *How we die: reflections on life's final chapter,* New York, 1994, Random House.
55. Oaks J, Ezell G: *Dying and death: coping, caring, understanding,* Scottsdale, Ariz, 1993, Gorsuch Scarisbrick.
56. Parkes CM, Weiss RS: *Recovery from bereavement,* New York, 1983, Basic Books.
57. Pickett M: Cultural awareness in the context of terminal illness, *Cancer Nurs* 16(2):102-106, 1993.
58. Pilkington F: The lived experience of grieving the loss of an important other, *Nurs Sci Q* 6(3):130-138, 1993.
59. Prigerson H et al: Complicated grief and bereavement-related depression as distinct disorders: preliminary empirical validation in elderly bereaved spouses, *Am J Psychiatry* 152(1):22-30, 1995.
60. Radziewicz R: Go light your world, *Oncol Nurs Forum* 24(10):1689-1997, 1997.
61. Rando TA: *Grief, dying and death,* Champaign, Ill, 1983, Research Press.
62. Rando T: *Treatment of complicated mourning,* Champaign, Ill, 1993, Research Press.
63. Ray C: Seven ways to empower dying patients, *Am J Nurs* (5):56-57, 1996.
64. Reiner A, Brown B, editors: *Manual of patient care standards,* Gaithersburg, Md, 1993, Aspen.
65. Sanders C: *Grief: the mourning after,* New York, 1989, John Wiley & Sons.
66. Saunders J, Valente S: Nurses' grief, *Cancer Nurs* 17(4):318-325, 1994.
67. Schaeffer C, Goldstein P: Palliative care, *Continuing Care* 6:22-24, 1996.
68. Selder F: Life transition theory: the resolution of uncertainty, *Nurs Health Care* 10(8):437-451, 1992.
69. Sheehan D, Foreman W: *Hospice and palliative care: concepts and practice,* Sudbury, Mass, 1996, Jones & Bartlett.
70. Silverman P, Worden W: Detachment revisited: the child's reconstruction of a dead parent, *Am J Orthopsychiatry* 62(4):494-503, 1992.

71. Solari-Twadell P, Bunkers S, Wang C, Snyder D: The pinwheel model of bereavement, *Image* 27(4):323-326, 1995.
72. Spiegel D: *Living beyond limits: new hope and help for facing life-threatening illness,* New York, 1993, Times Books.
73. Spitzer A, Bar-Tal Y, Golander H: Social support: how does it really work? *J Adv Nurs* 22:850-854, 1995.
74. Sprang G: *The many faces of bereavement: the nature and treatment of natural, traumatic, and stigmatized grief,* New York, 1995, Brunner/Mazel.
75. Steele L: The death surround: factors influencing the grief experience of survivors, *Oncol Nurs Forum* 15(5):575-581, 1990.
76. Steeves R: Loss, grief, and the search for meaning, *Oncol Nurs Forum* 23(6):897-903, 1996.
77. Steeves R, Kahn D: Family perspectives: tasks of bereavement, *Qual Life Nurs Challenge* 3(3):48-53, 1994.
78. Sumodi V: Legalization of physician-assisted suicide: point/counterpoint, *Nurs Forum* 30(1):11-17, 1995.
79. Vachon M, Stylianos S: The role of social support in bereavement, *J Soc Issues* 44(3):175-190, 1988.
80. Viorst J: *Necessary losses,* New York, 1986, Simon & Schuster.
81. Watson J: *Human science and human care,* New York, 1988, National League for Nursing.
82. Weatherhill G: Thro' the night: family care when the patient is dying, *Caring* 4:50-53, 1995.
83. Weisman A: *On dying and denying: a psychiatric study of terminality,* New York, 1972, Behavior.
84. Wheeler S: Helping families cope with death and dying, *Nursing 96* 7:25-30, 1996.
85. Wolfelt A: A systems approach to healing the bereaved child, *Bereavement* Jul/Aug: 8-11, 1997.
86. Wolfelt A: *The journey through grief: reflections on healing,* Fort Collins, Colo, 1997, Companion Press.
87. Worden W: Bereavement care, *Semin Oncol* 12(4):472-475, 1995.
88. Worden W: *Grief counseling and grief therapy,* ed 3, New York, 1995, Springer.
89. Zerwekh J: The truth-tellers: how hospice nurses help patients confront death, *Am J Nurs* Feb: 32-34, 1994.

# chapter 9 Impact of Illness on Mentation

JUDITH K. SANDS

## objectives

*After studying this chapter, the learner should be able to:*

1 Describe the process of sensory reception and perception.
2 Compare intensive care unit syndrome with sensory deprivation and sensory overload.
3 Discuss the risk factors for the development of sensory problems in the acute care setting.
4 Differentiate among the terms *confusion, delirium,* and *dementia.*
5 Discuss the major etiologies for acute confusion in hospitalized patients.
6 List the primary laboratory tests used to evaluate acute confusion.
7 Identify the key elements of environmental modification for confused patients.
8 Discuss the parameters for the safe use of physical restraints for the confused patient.

Acute illness and hospitalization commonly result in some negative impact on mentation, and this is particularly true for elderly patients. Changes in mentation can be caused by the underlying disease process, factors in the physical environment, or an adverse response to therapeutic interventions. An estimated 30% to 50% of older patients experience confusion during a hospitalization, and because at least 50% of the patient population in acute care hospitals is over the age of 65, confusion is a significant problem.[13] Additionally, data indicate that patients who develop acute confusion experience increased morbidity and length of stay and are five times more likely to die during the hospitalization than patients who do not experience changes in mental status.[13]

The prevention of altered sensory perception and safe management of confused patients is an essential function of nursing. This chapter lays the foundation for understanding the sensory process and factors that influence sensoristasis (a healthy balance of sensory stimulation and variety). The multiple origins of acute confusion are discussed along with collaborative interventions for effective prevention and management.

## THE SENSORY PROCESS

Human beings depend on an intact sensory processing system to effectively interact with their environment. However, this complex sensory process is largely taken for granted until something disturbs its functioning. The sensory process consists of the ability to receive internal and external stimuli through the sensory receptors and the ability to perceive the data by organizing it in a meaningful way. The process of reception is primarily biological. Sensation originates with a specific stimulus, which activates some of the millions of sensory receptors that are found in the major sense organs, along the entire surface of the body, in the linings of the mucous membranes, and in the viscera, muscles, and joints. The sensory receptors synapse with peripheral nerves and synapse again to join the sensory nerve tracts in the spinal cord. Stimuli then ascend the cord through the reticular activating system (RAS) in the brainstem to the thalamus, and finally to diverse sites in the sensory cortex (Figure 9-1). Chapter 51 provides a more complete review of the structure of the nervous system.

Although reception is primarily biological in nature, the process of reception is largely psychological or cognitive. Through the complex process of perception the brain sorts incoming stimuli into meaningful patterns for interpretation and action. Although the general process of perception is similar in all people, perception represents the unique way that each individual organizes and consciously interprets incoming stimuli.

The RAS plays a major role in both reception and perception. The RAS is a special core of gray matter that is found within the network of neurons known as the reticular formation (RF), which extends from the medulla to the thalamus. The ascending pathways of the RAS control arousal and wakefulness, and they help direct attention to specific stimuli. Without a baseline state of arousal or awareness, stimuli would reach the brainstem, but the cortex would be unable to process them appropriately or take thoughtful action. Both the RAS and RF are believed to play a monitoring or gatekeeping function in perception. Incoming stimuli are collected, combined, and roughly evaluated at this brainstem level of perception. It is theorized that less than 1% of all incoming stimuli are fully processed and interpreted by the cortex. The remaining 99% are blocked or filtered by the RAS and RF to prevent overloading of the cortex. Conscious awareness of sensory stimuli occurs only when the cortex has completed the process of interpretation.

A huge amount of sensory data from the five senses, viscera, muscles, and joints constantly bombards the brain. The brain could never effectively attend to all of these stimuli without being overwhelmed. Grouping stimuli into data sets

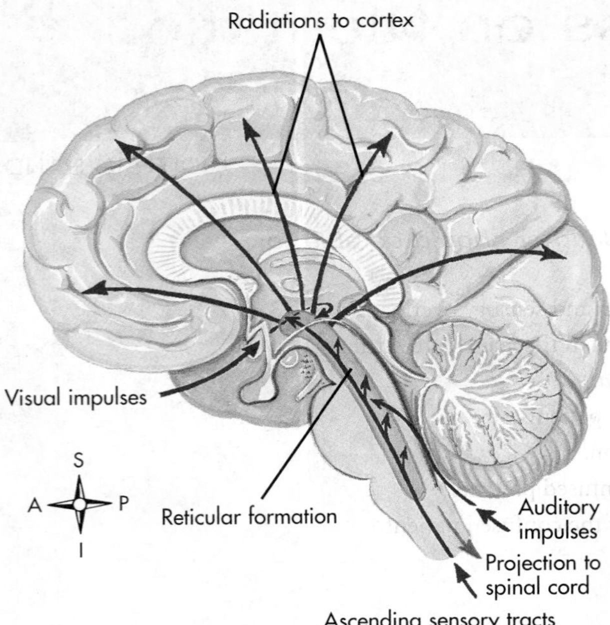


**fig. 9-1** Reticular activating system consists of centers in the brainstem reticular formation plus fibers that conduct to the centers from below and fibers that conduct from the centers to widespread areas of the cerebral cortex. Functioning of the reticular activating system is essential for consciousness.

decreases the number, but many stimuli must simply be filtered out and discarded. Several basic principles govern this process. Intensity influences attention. The larger or stronger the stimulus, the more likely the brain is to perceive it. Stimuli that are repeated frequently also influence attention, but only to a certain limit. Beyond this point a repetitive stimulus begins to be filtered out and ignored. Novelty also influences attention. The brain will generally perceive a change or break in the usual pattern of stimuli. Our acute awareness of sounds in a new environment is a classic example of this process. The meaningfulness of the stimulus also influences attention. This is illustrated by the ease with which parents, even those who describe themselves as heavy sleepers, respond to movement or cries from their infants and children.

## SENSORISTASIS

Sensoristasis describes a state in which a healthy balance of sensory stimulation and variation exists. The amount and type of stimulation required to maintain sensoristasis varies extensively among and between persons and to some extent is a learned process. An individual's culture and family of origin often at least partially determine the amount of stimulation that the individual considers to be "normal." This normal variation manifests itself in a wide variety of lifestyle choices, such as the preference for rural vs. urban lifestyles and the choice of emergency room or critical care nursing vs. primary care or rehabilitation settings. Sensoristasis is generally viewed as the midpoint on a continuum that ranges from sensory deprivation to sensory overload.

**risk factors**

**Sensory Deprivation**

**Receptive Problems**

Eye disease, trauma, surgery
Hearing loss
Loss of taste or smell sensation
Loss of tactile sensation (cerebrovascular accident, spinal cord injury)

**Lack of Meaning in the Environment**

Language barriers
Unfamiliar culture
Multiple care providers, unfamiliar faces
Separation from family and friends

**Lack of Variety**

Bed rest, especially on special air or fluid treatment beds
Isolation
Traction
Paralysis
Monotonous surroundings

**Medication Effects**

Sedatives and narcotics

### Sensory Deprivation

Sensory deprivation has received a great deal of research attention. Interest in this area was stimulated by the "brainwashing" treatment of prisoners during the Korean War and the Vietnam War.[4] Sensory deprivation occurs when there is an absence, blocking, or alteration in reception or perception that reduces sensory input below the level necessary for healthy functioning. The balance of the RAS is disturbed and it is unable to maintain normal stimulation of the cerebral cortex. Sensory deprivation can result from a wide variety of imbalances:

- *Lessened input.* The actual amount of incoming stimuli is reduced. The reduction may be related to a decreased amount of stimuli in the environment or from impairment of receptor organs (e.g., trauma or disease affecting the special senses or the effects of cerebrovascular accident).
- *Decreased meaningfulness.* Stimuli may be strange and lack meaning, or the person may lose the ability to effectively process the stimuli in a purposeful way. This can occur with any condition that affects cognition or from immersion in an environment in which the person does not have the tools to effectively interact (e.g., language barriers).
- *Lack of variety.* Immobility or physical confinement can easily result in a significant drop in the variety of available stimuli. It also results from social isolation and loss of contact with friends and family. The physical environment itself may be bland and monotonous. Patients who are required to lie recumbent have reported the onset of symptoms of mild sensory deprivation in as few as 3 hours.

Risk factors for sensory deprivation are summarized in the box above.

Sensory deprivation can result in a wide variety of symptoms. The changes in thought processing can occur rapidly

**box 9-1** **clinical manifestations**

***Sensory Deprivation***

PSYCHOLOGICAL AND EMOTIONAL

Anxiety, fear
Irritability, restlessness
Boredom
Depression
Labile affect, mood swings

COGNITIVE

Loss of sense of time
Impaired problem solving
Impaired concentration, inability to organize thought
Memory problems
Reduced motor coordination
Vivid sensory images, dreams
Presence of delusions, illusions, or hallucinations
Confusion, disorientation

SLEEP DISTURBANCES, EXCESS SLEEPING
VARIED SOMATIC COMPLAINTS

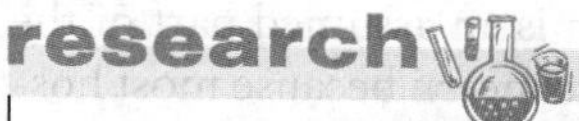

**research**

Reference: Topf M: Effects of personal control over hospital noise on sleep, *Res Nurs Health* 15:19, 1992.

This study explored the relationship between simulated cardiac care unit (CCU) noise, subjective stress levels, and the quality of sleep. One hundred five female volunteers were recruited to spend the night in a simulated hospital environment. They were divided into three groups. Two groups were subjected to an audiotape of CCU nighttime sounds, and the third group had quiet conditions. A sound conditioner was provided to the first two groups, and one group received instruction in how to adjust it to further control the noise level.

The subjects in both groups with background noise had more difficulty falling asleep and staying asleep, awoke frequently during the night, and did not progress effectively through the stages of sleep as documented by polysomnograph and self-report. Less time was also spent in REM sleep than for subjects in quiet environments. Personal control over the sound conditioner appeared to have no positive effects on the quantity or quality of sleep.

under laboratory conditions where the levels of sensory stimulation can be dramatically reduced. Normal, healthy college students develop problems with concentration and decision making in less than 24 hours when they are placed in conditions of severe sensory deprivation.[5] They commonly progress to experiencing perceptual distortions and even hallucinations within a matter of days. It is theorized that the brain's need for stimulation is so great that when it is severely deprived it turns inward in the search for meaning and creates vivid perceptual distortions that severely disturb the individual's ability to perceive reality. The symptoms rarely develop that quickly outside of laboratory conditions, but abrupt, drastic changes in sensory input, such as those that accompany a loss of vision or a loss of tactile sensation through spinal cord injury, can cause significant symptoms of deprivation in a short time.[4] Classic clinical manifestations of sensory deprivation are summarized in Box 9-1.

### Sensory Overload

The concept of sensory overload has not been as widely researched as sensory deprivation, but it is a widely recognized phenomenon. Sensory overload is defined as an increase in the intensity of stimuli to levels beyond normal or the presence of multisensory stimuli. Overload can result from excess stimuli to any of the major senses, but it is best recognized in relation to vision and hearing. In sensory overload the stimuli are too numerous, too intense, too rapid, or too diverse. The effects of sensory overload on hearing are particularly well documented.[15] When an individual is exposed to long-term, high-decibel noise, hearing is gradually impaired. Continuous noise causes anxiety and induces the release of epinephrine and norepinephrine, which elicit the stress response. Excess levels of noise and light are well-documented techniques of torture as reported by prisoners of war. Sensory overload rapidly leads to sleep deprivation and hastens the deterioration of the individual's coping mechanisms. (See the accompanying Research Box.)

Unrelieved pain is another common source of sensory overload in health care situations. There are few clear differences between the symptoms produced by sensory deprivation and sensory overload. Virtually any of the symptoms outlined in Box 9-1 may occur. However, sleep deprivation typically plays an extremely important role in sensory overload, and the person is rarely able to respond to the situation by using sleep as a coping mechanism.

### Intensive Care Unit Syndrome

Sensory overload has been most closely linked in health care with the development and use of intensive care units (ICUs). The unique syndrome associated with ICU placement is referred to as ICU syndrome or ICU psychosis. It was first actively studied in the early 1960s when it was recognized that most patients who underwent open heart surgery developed problems with sensory distortion, confusion, labile emotions, memory loss, and even vivid hallucinations after just 48 hours in the intensive care setting.[3] Incidence rates ran as high as 50% to 80% of cardiac surgery patients. Research into ICU syndrome has served as the impetus for many of the environmental modifications that have taken place in ICUs over the intervening years, including the provision of windows for natural day-night light patterns, separate rooms and carpets to decrease noise levels, the use of clocks and calendars to support orientation to time, and careful attention to supporting natural sleep cycles when possible.

Critical care units clearly possess the potential to cause sensory overload through excessive environmental stimuli. Common stimuli include constant lighting and numerous pieces of equipment, each of which produces its own unique noise pattern. Frequent staff intervention is an assumed part of the environment. Noise is a significant concern because most hospitals have baseline noise levels that are nearly twice the Environmental Protection Association (EPA) recommended levels of no more than 45 dB during the day and 35 dB at night.[16] In addition to its negative effects on sleep, excess noise has been shown to increase requests for pain medication, and it is one of the most common sources of complaint from patients via patient satisfaction surveys.[32,35] Loud voices and staff laughter are reported as being particularly offensive. Sleep deprivation has gradually emerged as one of the most important elements in the ICU syndrome. It is estimated that acute sleep deprivation occurs in ICU patients within 48 hours of admission. Elderly patients are at particular risk because they are more likely to already have fragile baseline sleep patterns and they are easily aroused from sleep by light and noise.

As hospitals continue to increase their acuity level it is clear that the risks of the ICU syndrome apply to most areas of the institution. Stimulus overload can occur anywhere. But the ICU syndrome is believed to incorporate elements of sensory deprivation as well. Stimuli are not just multiple and frequently intrusive to the patient, but they are also usually meaningless. The normal routine sounds of home are absent and are replaced by strange people, strange equipment, frightening alarms, painful procedures, and often overwhelming anxiety. Patients are separated from significant contact with family and friends and may be immobilized. Mechanically ventilated patients are commonly immobilized with paralyzing agents. Elderly patients who live alone and have reduced contact with others in their daily lives are at particular risk when hospitalized. Isolated rural elders are particularly vulnerable. The effects of sedatives and hypnotics diminish the patient's coping resources and ability to interact with the environment in a meaningful way. Intensive care unit placement is usually sudden, and the patient rarely has the opportunity to adequately prepare for the experience. The ICU syndrome presents a significant concern for patient safety because the symptoms can progress rapidly to include terrifying hallucinations, paranoia, and combativeness.

## ACUTE CONFUSION IN HOSPITALIZED PATIENTS

Sensory imbalances are important contributors to the incidence of acute confusion in hospitalized patients, but they are clearly not the only etiological variables. Acute illness and its treatment present multiple challenges to the body's ability to maintain physical homeostasis and psychological equilibrium. Health care professionals must be alert to the possibility of acute confusion in a wide variety of clinical situations and be skillful in identifying potential contributing factors.

*Confusion* is an ambiguous term that refers to a mental state characterized by diffuse cognitive dysfunction that causes problems in comprehension and the loss of short-term memory.[17] Confusion is commonly associated with the presence of delusions and hallucinations. The term *confusion* can be used interchangeably with the term *delirium,* which literally means "off the track."[21] Confusion is seen in people of all ages but it is particularly prevalent in the elderly.[11] Acute confusion has a rapid onset and is generally reversible, which differentiates it from the dementias, which tend to develop slowly and are usually irreversible. Dementia is the most common form of chronic confusion. The demented patient is typically awake and alert but experiences multiple memory problems, a variety of cognitive disturbances (which may include apraxia and agnosia), and impaired social functioning. The cognitive decline is usually progressive and irreversible. Alzheimer's disease is the classic example of a dementia characterized by chronic confusion.

The onset of acute confusion is abrupt—hours to days—and it usually persists for less than 1 week, although it can persist for up to a month.[10] The associated behaviors reflect the severity of the confusion. Mild acute confusion does not always progress to a more severe form. The diagnostic criteria that define delirium and confusion are outlined in Box 9-2.[4]

The incidence of confusion is commonly underestimated because depression often exists as a cofactor, particularly in the elderly. Symptoms such as sleep disturbance and decreased attention span occur in both depression and confusion. Depression typically goes unidentified and untreated, especially in elders, which complicates the management of any episode of altered thought.[29]

### ETIOLOGIES OF ACUTE CONFUSION

Acute confusion is a common clinical manifestation of many neurological and metabolic disorders, and it is often difficult to identify its exact etiology. Acute confusion can be broadly categorized as being related to either use of or withdrawal from alcohol or drugs of abuse, a general medical condition, psychological causes, environmental causes, and treatment effects.[14] Among the most common causes are drug and alcohol effects; the use of prescribed medications with anticholinergic or central nervous system (CNS) effects; systemic infection, particularly urinary tract and respiratory infection in elders; fluid, sodium, and potassium imbalances; and other metabolic disturbances.[14] Box 9-3 lists many of the potential causes of acute confusion.

**box 9-2** *Diagnostic Criteria for Delirium (with Multiple Etiological Factors)*

A. Disturbance of consciousness with reduced ability to focus, sustain, or shift attention
B. Change in cognition (e.g., memory deficit, disorientation) or development of a perceptual disturbance that is not the result of dementia
C. Disturbance that develops over a short period and tends to fluctuate during the course of the day
D. Evidence (from history, physical examination, or diagnostic results) that the delirium has more than one etiological factor, such as several medical conditions or a medical condition and withdrawal from or intoxication with a drug*

Reprinted with permission from the Diagnostic and Statistical Manual of Mental Disorders, ed 4. Copyright 1994, American Psychiatric Association.
*If evidence supports only substance intoxication, the delirium is labeled as *substance intoxication delirium.* If the underlying medical condition is known and is the single etiological factor, the delirium is labeled as *delirium caused by a specific medical condition.*

It is apparent that the potential causes of confusion encompass virtually every condition and treatment with a general systemic effect. Age is the single most important predisposing factor. The severity and duration of the illness and the number of comorbid conditions are also important because most episodes of confusion have multiple causes.[17] The stress of acute illness and sudden hospitalization is a common precipitating event, and the development of confusion in the acute care setting commonly accompanies a major biochemical imbalance, which could be serious or life threatening if not promptly recognized and treated.

### Organic Brain Disorders

Problems that directly involve the brain are common causes of acute confusion. Cerebral thrombosis, "ministrokes," tumors, and degenerative and chronic disorders such as seizures and Parkinson's disease can all precipitate episodes of acute confusion when the individual undergoes the stress of hospitalization or comorbid illness. The person is usually able to successfully adapt to the changes brought on by the primary illness as long as the changes have occurred slowly over time, but the crisis of hospitalization can easily overwhelm the person's fragile coping capacities.

**box 9-3** *Possible Causes of Acute Confusion*

**ALCOHOL AND DRUG USE AND ABUSE**
Intoxication and withdrawal

**CARDIOPULMONARY CAUSES**
Congestive heart failure, myocardial infarction, dysrhythmias
Hypotension
Chronic obstructive pulmonary disease, pneumonia, respiratory failure, pulmonary embolism

**METABOLIC CAUSES**
Liver failure, cirrhosis
Hypothyroidism, hyperthyroidism
Hypoglycemia, diabetic ketoacidosis
Renal failure, uremia, acid-base imbalance

**NEUROLOGICAL CAUSES**
Head trauma, cerebrovascular accident, subarachnoid hemorrhage
Tumors
Infections (meningitis, abscess, encephalitis)
Chronic and degenerative disease (e.g., seizures, Parkinson's disease)

**FLUID AND ELECTROLYTE CAUSES**
Hyponatremia and hypernatremia, hypoosmolality and hyperosmolality (SIADH)
Dehydration

**VITAMIN DEFICIENCIES**
Thiamine, folate, vitamin $B_{12}$, iron, nicotinic acid
Wernicke's encephalopathy

**PHARMACOLOGICAL FACTORS**
Anticholinergics and drugs with central nervous system effects (see Box 9-4)

**ENVIRONMENTAL FACTORS**
Sensory deprivation and overload
Hyperthermia, hypothermia

**PSYCHOSOCIAL FACTORS**
Depression
Loss and grief
Stress and anxiety

### Systemic Conditions

Decreased levels of oxygen or glucose have rapid and dramatic effects on cerebral function. The brain is extremely sensitive to hypoxia. Only a few seconds of anoxia can lead to altered awareness and confusion. Cardiopulmonary conditions that result in a low cardiac output or low blood oxygen levels are common causes. The amount of oxygen available to cells of the cerebral cortex depends on the adequacy of blood flow, blood oxygen tension ($pO_2$), hemoglobin level and saturation, and the arterial pH. Hypoxic encephalopathies result from adverse changes in the cardiopulmonary systems. Problems such as dysrhythmias, congestive heart failure, or chronic obstructive pulmonary disease can readily lead to diminished cerebral oxygenation and acute confusion.[27]

Severe infections frequently result in acute confusion, particularly in the elderly. The urinary tract and respiratory tract are the most common sites of nosocomial infections and can produce subtle behavioral manifestations of acute confusion.[27] Symptoms include difficulty concentrating, restlessness, and disorientation. Metabolic imbalances such as diabetic ketoacidosis can precipitate multiple changes such as inappropriate judgment, decreased alertness, and mental lethargy. Hypoglycemia can be even more dangerous because the brain has no reserve of glucose and depends on a constant blood level. Even brief decreases in serum glucose can result in alterations in alertness and cognition. Depending on the glucose level, the changes can be subtle or abrupt and rapidly life threatening. Fluid and electrolyte imbalances are associated with multiple disorders. Abrupt or severe changes in sodium levels or the osmolality of body fluids can rapidly lead to acute confusion.[27]

### Drug Effects

Drug toxicities can cause confusion in multiple ways. Drugs can reduce cardiac output or decrease blood glucose levels. Drugs can alter the metabolic activity of brain cells, disrupt the activity of neurotransmitters, and alter the brain's oxygen supply. The half-life of many drugs is increased in the elderly, which makes them more vulnerable to adverse effects.[14] Drugs that are classically associated with the development of acute confusion are summarized in Box 9-4.

### Psychological Causes

Depression may mimic the symptoms of acute confusion, and the presence of depression may make acute confusion more difficult to recognize. Anxiety or stress can also cause a person to have difficulty concentrating and become confused. However, the links between depression, stress, anxiety, and confusion are less clear, which makes the assessment more difficult.[29] The nurse needs to use excellent assessment and interviewing skills to recognize the possible correlation between the presence of depression or anxiety and the development of acute confusion.

### Environmental Causes

The effects of altered sensory input have already been discussed. They affect virtually every hospitalized patient. Environmental effects must be explored in every situation that involves the sudden onset of acute confusion. Environmental causes may be primary elements in the development of confusion or may be in the background as contributing causes.

## COLLABORATIVE CARE MANAGEMENT

Acute confusion is an indication of a serious physiological imbalance. The most essential aspect of management is the recognition of the disorder with an immediate search for the causative factors. Subtle confusion and inattention are commonly recognized but ignored by health care professionals, who often assume that elders naturally have a decreased ability to think clearly.[17] Behavior indicative of confusion may be glossed over or assumed to be "baseline" for the patient. The medical specialists who work up the patients in acute care hospitals often have not seen the patient before admission and cannot compare the patient's behavior with his or her preadmission status. This lack of knowledge also makes it more difficult to differentiate between behaviors that are related to confusion and those that are related to depression. Professionals may believe that depression is a normal and inevitable consequence of aging and ignore its potential to mimic the early signs of confusion. The family plays a critical role in clarifying the patient's preadmission mental status.

A diagnostic workup for confusion can include a wide variety of tests, although there are no specific diagnostic tests for confusion. The patient's history can usually provide the necessary indications about potential etiologies to narrow the search. Sample laboratory and diagnostic tests that may be used as part of a workup for acute confusion are displayed in Box 9-5.

Treatment of acute confusion is directed at reversing the underlying problem if possible. Most episodes resolve or at least improve with adequate attention to treating the etiology. Inadequate recognition and treatment could lead to permanent brain damage. Medications play such a common role in the development of acute confusion that it is preferable to discontinue or significantly decrease the doses of all drugs if possible. Polypharmacy is a significant problem with elders, and new drugs tend to be added to the patient's regimen without the removal of old ones. A careful search is initiated to identify contraindications and adverse effects for all drugs in use. Other general measures for managing confusion include addressing nutritional deficiencies, restoring fluid and electrolyte balance, and correcting anemia.

Psychotropic medication may be considered if the episode of confusion is severe and prolonged and the patient does not respond to more conservative measures. Drugs are administered to reduce agitation and support restful sleep. Haloperidol (Haldol) may be prescribed because it is a potent and effective agent but does not produce adverse anticholinergic side effects. It is usually administered intramuscularly. The benzodiazepines may also be used. In extreme situations physical restraints may be necessary to ensure the patient's safety, but their use is not recommended and should always be considered an intervention of last resort. The use of restraints should always be a collaborative decision involving the physician, nurse, and both patient and family if possible. (See the discussion on p. 203.)

**box 9-4 Common Medications That Can Result in Acute Confusion**

**CARDIOVASCULAR DRUGS**
Nitrates, antidysrhythmics
Digoxin, antihypertensives (adrenergic inhibitors, beta blockers, calcium channel blockers)

**GASTROINTESTINAL DRUGS**
Antinauseants (phenothiazines)
Antispasmodics, histamine $H_2$ antagonists

**RESPIRATORY DRUGS**
Antihistamines
Antitussives, decongestants

**NEUROLOGICAL DRUGS**
Anticonvulsants
Antiparkinsonian agents

**MUSCULOSKELETAL DRUGS**
Muscle relaxants
Antiinflammatory agents

**OTHER**
Analgesics, narcotics (particularly meperidine)
Anesthetics
Hypnotics and sedatives (benzodiazepines)
Psychotropics

**box 9-5 Sample Laboratory and Diagnostic Tests for Diagnosing Acute Confusion**

**LABORATORY TESTS**
Serum electrolytes, calcium
Complete blood count
Blood urea nitrogen, creatinine
Blood glucose
Serum $B_{12}$ and folate levels
Arterial blood gases
Blood alcohol, toxicology screen
Serum drug levels
Thyroid and liver function tests
Serum osmolality

**DIAGNOSTIC TESTS**
Computed tomography, magnetic resonance imaging
Lumbar puncture
Electroencephalography
Urine culture

## NURSING MANAGEMENT

### ■ ASSESSMENT

Assessment is a major focus of nursing care for patients experiencing or at risk for acute confusion (see the accompanying Research Box). A thorough admission assessment can provide valuable baseline data for future comparison. The perspective of the family must be included as well to attempt to differentiate between preexisting problems of confusion and new problems that emerge during the hospitalization. The nurse will continuously monitor for changes that may result from specific treatments such as surgery and the effects of any new medications.

#### Subjective Data

##### History

A thorough history is essential in planning care for confused patients. Important data include:

- Onset of confusion
- Past medical history and treatment, with particular attention to the presence and management of cardiovascular, respiratory, renal, and metabolic diseases and disorders
- Changes in personality and self-care abilities
- Presence and severity of sensory deficits and compensatory aids in use
- History and pattern of alcohol and drug use
- Complete record of all prescribed and over-the-counter drugs in use
- Signs of sensory perceptual problem (Box 9-6)
- Presence of illusions, delusions, or hallucinations
- Risk of harm to self or others

##### Environmental assessment

Assessment of the patient's living situation before admission can be important in understanding the risks of acute confusion. This is especially important for the elderly, who are more likely to live alone and have less social contact. When possible, the assessment should include information from the patient about the sensory level that he or she is most accustomed to and tolerates best.[33] The assessment should include the amount and intensity of stimulation currently present in the environment, especially if the person is considered to be at risk for confusion.[36] Environmental stimuli are evaluated for pattern and meaning. The presence and degree of light and noise are particularly important.

#### Objective Data

Although the nurse will establish baseline vital signs and check the patient's most recent laboratory values, ongoing mental status assessment is the key to physical assessment. Frequent observation and reassessment by the same professional nurse will be essential to detect subtle changes in the patient's mental status. The Mini Mental State Exam is widely considered to be the most sensitive tool available for ongoing evaluation of confused patients (Figure 9-2). The Short Portable Mental Status Questionnaire (SPMSQ) is also widely used (Figure 9-3). The Clinical Assessment of Confusion—A (CAC-A) is a behavioral rating scale that emphasizes the nonverbal nature of much confused behavior. All three tools can be administered by nurses at the bedside. The SPMSQ may be superior for use with patients who have physical impairments because it does not require the patient to write. The CAC-A is particularly helpful in focusing the assessment on the patient's behavioral changes.

Mental status tests assess the orientation of the patient to person, place, and time. "Disorientation" is a classic element of confusion. The tools then proceed to evaluate higher-order cognitive functions such as memory, attention, calculation, and use of language.[33] Mental status evaluation can be stressful for the patient, who may become anxious if unable to answer questions appropriately. The nurse needs to be skillful and patient and assist the person to remain as calm as possible. The nurse should also avoid drawing global conclusions from the assessment. The results are documented as specifically and factually as possible.

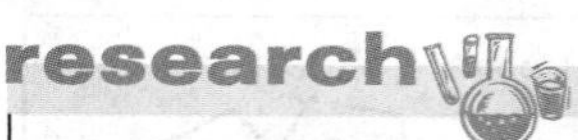


Reference: Yeaw EMJ, Abbate JH: Identification of confusion among the elderly in an acute care setting, *Clin Nurse Spec* 7:192, 1993.

This study examined the rate of delirium in hospitalized elders, compared clinical outcomes in patients with and without delirium, and examined clinical predictors of delirium. There was a 15% rate of delirium in patients during their stay. Elders who experienced delirium had longer lengths of stay and increased risk of death while hospitalized. Predictors of delirium included cognitive impairment, level of comorbidity, depression, and alcoholism. The findings support the critical need for a multidimensional geriatric assessment to be completed by the nurse for all older adult patients. If this is done, at-risk elderly patients can be identified during the initial contact with the nurse. The nurse can then develop a plan of care in collaboration with other health care team members to implement supportive treatment (e.g., for depression or malnutrition) and reduce negative outcomes during hospitalization.

**box 9-6 clinical manifestations**

**Acute Confusion**

- Decreased attention span, distractibility
- Memory impairment
- Disorientation to person, place, or time
- Disorganized thinking
- Fluctuating levels of alertness
- Disturbance of sleep-wake patterns
- Agitation and restlessness, or slowing of movement and speech
- Emotional disturbances (anxiety, fear, apathy, irritability, anger)
- Perceptual disturbances
  - Illusions—misinterpretations of something in the environment
  - Delusions—thoughts or beliefs that have no basis in fact
  - Hallucinations—sensations occurring in the absence of external stimuli (e.g., see, hear, taste, or smell something that is not present)
- Tremor or poor coordination

NOTE: Onset of symptoms is acute or subacute. Changes and fluctuations of symptoms occur with lucid intervals alternating with periods of confusion.

## NURSING DIAGNOSES

A wide range of diagnoses can be applicable to the patient experiencing acute confusion. These include difficulties in performing self-care, maintaining continence, and meeting daily nutritional needs. Complications related to immobility can develop quickly, and the strain of caregiving on the family can create a wide variety of coping-related problems. The following three diagnoses are applicable to the broadest range of patients.

| Diagnostic Title | Possible Etiological Factors |
|---|---|
| Acute confusion | Alcohol, drug abuse; sensory deprivation/overload; biochemical alterations; stress; drug effects |
| Sleep pattern disturbance | Alterations in usual sleep patterns; pain and immobility; excess environmental stimuli; noise |
| Risk for injury | Sensory perceptual alterations; inability to interpret environmental stimuli |

## EXPECTED PATIENT OUTCOMES

Specific outcomes will reflect the unique characteristics of each patient situation. General outcomes may include but are not limited to:

1a. Will receive optimal levels of sensory stimulation
 b. Will demonstrate improving scores on tests of mental status
 c. Will interact appropriately with people and the environment
2a. Will sleep for 4 to 6 uninterrupted hours at night
3a. Will not sustain injury
 b. Will not injure others

## INTERVENTIONS

### Controlling Environmental Stimulation

Acute confusional states are common during hospitalization, particularly for elders. Nurses need to be alert to the significant number of patients who are at risk and actively work to prevent episodes of confusion if possible. Preventing sensory imbalance is far preferable to attempting to reverse it once problems with confusion have developed. The nurse assumes primary responsibility for successfully managing the patient's environment to prevent sensory deprivation, sensory overload, and sleep deprivation to the degree possible within the constraints of the patient's treatment plan. The nurse's most important tool is sensitivity and awareness of the number and variety of stimuli present in the practice environment and the potential adverse effects of these stimuli on the patient's mental status.[23] The patient's family should be involved if possible because studies have demonstrated that only stimuli that are meaningful to the patient are effective in relieving sensory imbalance. Meaningless stimuli are likely to simply increase the patient's agitation. The nurse will also work collaboratively, as discussed on p. 198, to promptly identify confusion when it occurs. This includes monitoring for biochemical imbalances, drug interactions, and changes in oxygenation status.

#### Preventing sensory deprivation

The nurse attempts to add meaningful stimuli to the patient's environment. Human contact is one of the most meaningful forms of stimulation, and the nurse should use a professional presence, as well as visitation by family and friends, to ensure meaningful human contact.[12] This may involve collaborative planning to ease routine constraints on visiting. The nurse will briefly explain all tests and procedures to the patient to help the patient establish some sense of control over the environment.

Most hospitals have become more visually pleasing environments, but the nurse can still place immobilized patients

| Mini Mental State Examination | | |
|---|---|---|
| Maximum score | Patient score | |
| | | **Orientation** |
| 5 | | What is the date (i.e., day of week, day of month, month, year), season? 1 point for each |
| 5 | | Where are we: (hospital) (state) (county) (town) (floor)? 1 point for each. |
| | | **Registration** |
| 3 | | Name three objects, taking 1 s to say each. Then ask the patient to repeat all three. Give 1 point for each correct answer. Then repeat them until patient learns all three. Count trials and record. Number of trials _____ |
| | | **Attention and Calculation** |
| 5 | | Serial 7s. Give 1 point for each correct answer. Stop after five answers. If subject refuses, ask him to spell "world" backwards. |
| | | **Recall** |
| 3 | | Ask the patient to name the three objects cited above. Give 1 point for each correct answer. |
| | | **Language and Praxis** |
| 2 | | Point to a pencil and a watch and ask the patient to name them. (2 points) |
| 1 | | Ask the patient to: Repeat the following: "No ifs, ands, or buts." (1 point) |
| 3 | | Follow a three-stage command: "Take a paper in your right hand, fold it in half, and put it on the floor." (3 points) |
| 1 | | Read and obey the following sign: "Close your eyes." (1 point) |
| 1 | | Write a sentence. (1 point) |
| 1 | | Copy this design. (1 point) |
| 30 | | |
| Maximum score | Patient total | Note: Unimpaired individuals score 25 points or higher. Persons with dementia usually score between 10 to 20 points. |

fig. 9-2 Folstein Mini Mental State Examination (MMSE).

**Short Portable Mental Status Questionnaire (SPMSQ)**
**Eric Pfeiffer, M.D.**

Instructions: Ask questions 1-10 in this list and record all answers. Ask question 4A only if patient does not have a telephone. Record total number of errors based on ten questions.

| + | − | |
|---|---|---|
| | | 1. What is the date today? ____ Month ____ Day ____ Year |
| | | 2. What day of the week is it? ____ |
| | | 3. What is the name of this place? ____ |
| | | 4. What is your telephone number? ____ |
| | | 4A. What is your street address? ____ (Ask only if patient does not have a telephone) |
| | | 5. How old are you? ____ |
| | | 6. When were you born? ____ |
| | | 7. Who is the president of the United States now? ____ |
| | | 8. Who was president just before him? ____ |
| | | 9. What was your mother's maiden name? ____ |
| | | 10. Subtract 3 from 20 and keep subtracting 3 from each new number, all the way down. |

____ Total Number of Errors

To Be Completed by Interviewer

Patient's Name: ____ Date: ____

Sex: 1. Male
2. Female

Race: 1. White
2. Black
3. Other

Years of Education: ____
1. Grade School
2. High School
3. Beyond High School

Interviewer's Name: ____

Scoring:

The data suggest that both education and race influence performance on the mental status questionnaire and they must accordingly be taken into account in evaluating the score attained by an individual.

For purposes of scoring, three educational levels have been established: (1) persons who have had only a grade school education; (2) persons who have had any high school education or who have completed high school; (3) persons who have had any education beyond the high school level, including college, graduate school, or business school.

For white subjects with at least some high school education, but not more than high school education, the following criteria have been established:

| | |
|---|---|
| 0-2 Errors | Intact intellectual functioning |
| 3-4 Errors | Mild intellectual impairment |
| 5-7 Errors | Moderate intellectual impairment |
| 8-10 Errors | Severe intellectual impairment |

Allow one more error if subject has had only a grade school education.
Allow one less error if subject has had education beyond high school.
Allow one more error for black subjects using identical education criteria.

**fig. 9-3** Short Portable Mental Status Questionnaire (SPMSQ).

near windows when possible and use room lighting to reinforce the natural daily patterns of light and dark. Color, incorporated into the room linens, blinds, curtains, rugs, paint, and wallpaper, is helpful. Pictures, calendars, and clocks with large numerals can help keep the patient oriented to time and can be regularly incorporated into orientation activities.[18] The lounge areas can be used to increase the level of stimulation if the patient's condition permits.

The patient should be encouraged and assisted to use any aid to sensory reception such as glasses, hearing aids, and dentures. The use of radio, tapes, or television can help increase sound stimulation, but their use and effectiveness needs to be carefully assessed. The wrong amount or wrong type of music or television can be disturbing to the patient and negate any positive effects. The family is the best source of information about patient preferences in these areas.[12] Patients are encouraged to participate in their own self-care to the degree possible.

A confused patient will usually profit from consistency in the care routine and in care providers.[18] If possible the same staff should care for the patient on a regular basis, and contact with a wide variety of personnel is discouraged. All staff should wear easily read name badges and introduce themselves to the patient each time they enter the room to decrease the sense of isolation and fear. The pace of all activities should be slower and unhurried. It can be helpful to assume that the patient is frightened and use a quiet, reassuring approach. It is important to keep things simple and not to expect the patient to engage in a lot of decision making. The patient may require additional time to respond to questions and interactions because withdrawal is a common coping method for confused persons.[18] Room objects should be kept in the same places and not rearranged, and the patient's attention is regularly drawn to their location and placement. A care routine should be developed and adhered to as much as possible, and the patient should be kept informed whenever circumstances require a break in the established routine.

Reorientation is ongoing every 2 to 4 hours and provides the patient with the security of knowing where they are and why, even if memory impairment does not permit retention of the information. A calm, quiet approach is usually reassuring. There is strong evidence that persons with dementia often do not benefit from reorientation activities and may instead become more agitated, but most patients with acute confusion will profit from it.[12] Reorientation is addressed directly, but constant questioning of the patient should be avoided. The nurse can minimize the potentially demeaning nature of constant questions concerning person, place, and time by routinely incorporating orientation content into interaction—for example, "It's eight o'clock in the morning on Tuesday, January fifth. Breakfast will arrive in about 10 minutes, and Dr. Rogers, your surgeon, is just outside."[11]

The use of touch should be carefully evaluated. It can be a profoundly significant form of contact, communication, comfort, and pleasure, and its importance continues throughout life. It is one of the nurse's simplest and most direct methods of communicating caring to the patient. However, the use and acceptance of touch is bound by cultural and sex role socialization, and it is always important for the nurse to ensure that the use of touch is not interpreted by the patient as intrusive on personal space or unacceptable from another perspective.[26] Back rubs, massage, and range-of-motion exercise are effective ways of incorporating touch stimulation into routine caregiving activities.

**Patient and family education.** The family can play an important role in helping to structure an adequately stimulating environment. The nurse will discuss the importance of visits from loved ones and will work to facilitate family visiting at times when it is convenient within the nurse's broader responsibilities. The nurse will suggest that the family bring clothing and other personal items for the patient from home and use these to provide stimulation and orientation for the patient about his or her place in the world. The family is an excellent source of information about the patient's likes and dislikes concerning music, reading material, television, or other strategies to increase meaningful stimulation. The nurse will teach the family about the cause of the confusion if known, the fact that it will probably resolve within a short time, and the role that the family can play in assisting the patient to maintain or regain reality orientation. Acute confusion is frightening for both the patient and family, and they will need reassurance about the transient nature of most episodes. The importance of loving touch can be reinforced if touch is an accepted part of the family's pattern of functioning.

#### *Preventing sensory overload*

To effectively develop and implement strategies to prevent sensory overload, the nurse must first be sensitive to the risks that are inherent in the acute care setting. Nurses can easily lose sight of the fact that, although the setting is a familiar work environment for the nurse, it is often an overwhelming and frightening environment for patients. Preventing sensory overload requires a commitment to modifying the environment in important but subtle ways. The nurse can thoughtfully plan to reduce the intensity of environmental stimuli and to increase their meaning. The environmental noise level is one area over which the nurse has a significant amount of control. Many of the machines in frequent use have controls that allow the alarm levels to be lowered. This action can be extremely important at night when restful sleep is a priority. Nurses need to be extremely alert to the noise generated by staff conversations and interactions. This is a common area of complaint from patients, and staff laughter is reported on patient satisfaction surveys as being particularly aggravating.[35] This is again particularly important at night. Earplugs and headphones can be used to block noise, but they are no substitute for a staff commitment to reducing noise levels.

Visual stimulation is also commonly excessive, especially in critical care areas. Flashing lights and patterns on monitoring equipment and bright ambient lighting can be excessive, especially for patients who must lie flat in bed, which enhances the effects of room lighting. Dimming lights is both possible and appropriate, and patients can be offered eye shades to block out ambient light for sleep. Dark glasses can be an effective daytime alternative because they mute the light stimulation while still allowing the patient to see and assess the surroundings.[12] Curtains can be partially drawn periodically to decrease the stimulation from constant movement in the area. Control of noxious odors from draining wounds or other sources can also increase the patient's comfort in the environment.

Unrelieved pain is another common source of sensory overload. The nurse can function as a patient advocate to ensure that the medication, route of administration, and dose are adequate and appropriate to control the patient's pain. (See Chapter 12.) The nurse can structure the patient's care, even within the constraints of frequent monitoring, to reduce stimuli and provide periods of uninterrupted rest. A recognizable plan of care can also provide increased meaning for the patient and help with orientation. The nurse acts as the coordinator of the patient's care and collaborates with other providers such as respiratory or physical therapy to minimize the number and frequency of interruptions. Keeping the environment well organized and uncluttered can also be helpful. Patient teaching is ongoing. It is used to help the patient make sense of the sights and sounds of the environment and understand the various treatment interventions. Stimuli that acquire meaning are usually slightly less frightening for the patient.

Providing for consistent caregivers can again be useful in a variety of ways. Consistency not only decreases the number of strangers who have contact with the patient each day but also allows for improved assessment and evaluation of the plan of care.[18] Human contact is clearly an essential intervention, but contact with too many persons can easily overwhelm the patient. The nurse remains calm during all interactions with the patient and speaks in a quiet, clear voice. Patients who are awake should always be addressed by name whenever the nurse or other health care worker enters the room to perform patient assessments and monitor equipment.

Family visiting is usually a positive intervention for the patient, but the nurse may need to intervene to establish limitations on phone calls and visitors if patients become overwhelmed. The nurse can encourage family members to be a quiet presence at the bedside, to reassure and reorient the patient as needed, and to use comforting touch liberally.

### Promoting Sleep

Sleep deprivation is increasingly acknowledged as an important component of acute confusion for many patients. It is of particular concern in intensive care units, where virtually all patients are significantly sleep deprived within 48 hours. Many of the interventions discussed under environmental modification also apply to promoting sleep. Sleep promotion can be successful only when it becomes a priority for the nursing staff, because the structure of most units inherently works against this goal.

Environmental changes to modulate lighting, reduce noise, and group care activities are important strategies. Patients need an average of 70 to 90 minutes to complete a full sleep cycle. (See Chapter 13.) A full 2 hours would be ideal if care demands permit. Early morning napping is another effective strategy. An early morning nap, soon after awakening, allows the patient to easily reenter rapid eye movement (REM) sleep and experience its beneficial effects. Care should be taken to minimize activity and particularly painful interventions during this period. The loss of REM sleep is directly associated with the onset of confusion. Naps taken later in the day do not allow the patient to reach REM sleep levels. Sleeping aids are rarely used with confused patients because sleeping aids alter the sleep cycle and further suppress REM sleep.

The use of structured muscle relaxation exercises and touch through routine back rubs and massage can assist patients to use undisturbed periods effectively for rest and sleep. It is also always important for the nurse to use basic comfort measures such as oral care, fresh linens, and positioning as aids to rest and sleep.

### Preventing Injury

A major focus of care for patients with acute confusion is safety and the prevention of injuries. Patients may put themselves at risk by pulling at tubes, lines, or catheters or climbing out of bed. Patients can also become extremely agitated. Ideally, the confused person is placed in a room near the nurses' station so that frequent monitoring and assessment are possible. The nurse attempts to reassure the patient and make the environment as nonthreatening as possible by explaining the purpose of all tubes and lines, keeping equipment out of the patient's visual field as much as possible, and using touch, if effective, to decrease agitation and promote reality orientation.

The overall goal of care is to achieve patient safety by using the least restrictive device possible. Beds are kept in the low position, but the use of side rails requires careful decision making. Neither side rails nor physical restraints have been shown to reduce injury. If the presence of side rails increases the patient's agitation, their use may not be appropriate. Continuous observation may be a more appropriate strategy. Family members, if willing, may be able to stay with the patient and provide for both safety and the ongoing reassurance of a familiar face and voice. Careful teaching and collaborative planning with the family are essential.

#### *Avoiding restraint use*

The issue of restraint use has presented complex dilemmas for nurses throughout the years. The use of restraints was extremely common in the United States until the early 1990s. Conservative estimates put restraint use at greater than 40% of all residents of nursing homes and about 30% of persons in tertiary care.[8] There is general agreement that staff nurses have traditionally used restraints in a well-intended effort to protect the patient from harm, ensure the continuation of the therapeutic treatment plan, and protect the institution from the threat of legal action related to patient falls and injury[22] (see the Research Box below).

**research**

Reference: Ludwick R, O'Toole AW: The confused patient: nurses' knowledge and interventions, *J Gerontol Nurs* 22(1):44, 1996.

The purpose of this study was to identify nurses' knowledge about confusion and experience with its management. A random sample of 100 acute care nurses from a major medical center were surveyed about their experience with confusion. Most nurses reported regular and recent contact with confused patients, usually within the previous week. They felt knowledgeable about confusion and confident in their ability to identify it. They also overwhelmingly reported a belief in their ability to intervene appropriately in its management. They reported that they had learned confusion management on the job.

The nurses were asked to describe their most recent confused patient. The patient was most likely to be elderly, male, and experiencing a cardiovascular disorder. Eighty-four percent of the nurses reported having used restraints as part of their patient management. Vest restraints were the most common, with extremity restraints also used frequently. Other management strategies included patient reorientation, increased monitoring, and use of side rails.

It is clear that attitudes and practices about restraint use are strongly shaped by the work environment and work relationships because restraint use is virtually nonexistent in health care throughout Europe.[6] Nurses in the United States, however, have traditionally believed that effective alternatives to restraints are extremely limited and not very helpful.[31] Research demonstrates that nurses believe themselves to be knowledgeable about confusion and its management but still use restraints liberally as part of the treatment plan (see the Research Box below).[22,31] Physical restraints are commonly used to prevent falls from the bed or chair, to immobilize agitated patients, to aid in treatment, and to control inappropriate behavior despite the extensive research evidence that they are not very effective in accomplishing these goals.

*Restraints* are broadly defined as devices intended for a medical purpose that limit patient movement. The term includes devices such as safety vests, hand mittens, lap belts, straitjackets, and various forms of anklets or wristlets. They are estimated to still be in use with over 500,000 patients daily despite significant recent declines in their use in long-term care facilities.[34] There is little concrete evidence that restraints succeed in their expressed purpose of protecting the patient from harm. Restraints are directly associated with as many as 200 deaths each year. Death usually results from strangulation by a vest-type restraint as a confused patient attempts to free himself or herself.[20] Restraints are also clearly associated with predictable negative outcomes such as pressure ulcers, incontinence, fecal impaction, aspiration, and other complications of immobility.[20]

The provisions of the Omnibus Budget Reconciliation Act of 1987 (OBRA) combined with guidelines from the Health Care Financing Administration enacted in 1990 have had profound impact on restraint use in long-term care facilities.[25] These regulations have required Medicare and Medicaid skilled nursing facilities to promote and protect patient freedom from physical and chemical restraint. As a result restraint use has decreased 50% nationwide and dropped to less than 5% in model institutions.[20] Positive change has occurred much more slowly in acute care facilities where high-tech interventions are used as a global rationale for extensive patient restraint, particularly in critical care units. Chemical restraint is widely used for intubated patients. The Food and Drug Administration (FDA) now considers restraints to be items requiring physician prescription and also requires that the devices be clearly labeled for correct use.[34] Institutions that use restraints must have a clearly defined policy that delineates all aspects of restraint use, including the following:

- Indications for use
- Alternatives to explore before the use of restraints
- How long restraints can be used (usually no more than 24 hours without renewal of the physician prescription)
- Assessment and monitoring guidelines

Sample care guidelines for patients in restraints are summarized in the Guidelines for Care Box.

The outcomes of decreased restraint use in nursing homes have been clear and positive. There is a higher level of activities of daily living self-care competencies, there are increased rates of continence, and patients have actually sustained fewer injuries.[19] Thoughtful and ongoing confusion assessment is

## research

Reference: Thomas A, Redfern L, Reesa J: Perceptions of acute care nurses in the use of restraints, *J Gerontol Nurs* 21(6):32, 1995.

The purpose of this study was to determine how nursing staff of all levels perceived restraint use and to identify their knowledge of alternatives. The sample included approximately 100 acute care nurses from a large tertiary care facility. Managers, RNs, and LPNs were included. The Strumpf and Evans "Perceptions of Restraint Use Questionnaire" modified for the acute care environment was administered.

The most frequently reported reasons for using restraints were to prevent (1) falls from the bed or chair and (2) pulling out IVs or other tubes. The LPNs attached much greater importance to the use of restraints than RNs and managers. Priority situations for restraint use differed significantly among the various clinical settings. Nurses were also asked to generate a list of alternatives to restraints. Sixty percent of the alternatives were generated by RNs, 30% by managers, and 10% by LPNs. The list included (1) supervision by security staff, (2) sedation, (3) family supervision, (4) close supervision by nursing staff, (5) supervision by volunteers, and (6) diversional activities. Comments added to the questionnaires reflected a high degree of skepticism about the effectiveness of any alternatives to restraints because of low professional staffing levels.

## guidelines for care

### The Patient in Restraints

1. Question why restraints are needed, and explore alternatives first.
2. Use for a strictly defined period (usually no more than 24 hours).
3. A medical prescription is required. Informed consent from the family and the patient if possible should also be obtained.
4. Follow the manufacturer's directions carefully, and keep directions visibly displayed during the period of restraint use. Select the correct type of restraint for the situation, and use the correct size of restraint.
5. Apply the restraint so that it supports comfort and body alignment.
6. Secure the restraint to the bedsprings or frame but never to the mattress or bed rails. The restraint must be able to move as the patient is moved.
7. Assess the patient frequently. Remove the restraints at least every 2 hours to assess the skin and provide for position changes and activities of daily living, particularly toileting.
8. Perform range-of-motion exercises at least every 4 hours while patient is immobilized.
9. Carefully document the need for the restraint—type, alternatives tried, assessments.
10. Consider any restraint a temporary aid, and move as rapidly as possible toward restraint-free care.
11. Reassure and reorient the patient frequently during any period of restraint.

associated with a decreased use of restraints and has enabled professional nurses to recognize patterns in a patient's behavior that reflect unmet needs in areas such as pain, toileting, anxiety, and infection. Attention to these needs has successfully addressed the cause of the confusion rather than dealing only with the results. In addition to professional critical thinking and problem solving, planned reorientation programs have also successfully decreased the incidence of acute confusion.[30] Other strategies that have enabled institutions to decrease their use of restraints have included:

- Multidisciplinary teamwork and a focus on patient rehabilitation rather than custodial care. Involvement of physical therapists and occupational therapists has been important
- Low beds
- Thickly cushioned beds and chairs
- Use of wedge cushions for positioning
- Wheelchair modifications such as footrests and backs with varying positions
- Use of bed alarms for wanderers

Most of these strategies could also be easily transferred to the acute care environment, but little has been done to date. Recent years have seen a sharp decline in the number of professional staff members available on the units, a sharp increase in the number of elderly patients, and a continuing rapid escalation of both the acuity and the technological complexity of care. These factors have combined to place the use of restraints low on the list of issues of concern to nurses and support the ongoing belief among staff nurses that effective alternatives to restraints do not exist. The transition to restraint-free care in the acute care setting may require the establishment of an external accreditation criterion with the weight of the OBRA guidelines.

## EVALUATION

To evaluate the effectiveness of nursing interventions, compare patient behaviors with those stated in the expected patient outcomes. Successful achievement of patient outcomes for patients experiencing an alteration in mentation related to illness or hospitalization is indicated by:

1a. The patient maintains sensoristasis.
 b. The patient is fully oriented as evidenced by tests of mental status.
2. The patient enjoys 4 to 6 uninterrupted hours of sleep each night.
3a. The patient is free of injury and without physical or chemical restraint.
 b. The patient does not injure others.

## critical thinking QUESTIONS

**1** While working on a medical-surgical unit, you are assigned to care for four patients. Mr. Wayne, 69, is being treated for respiratory failure secondary to chronic obstructive pulmonary disease; Mrs. Janes, 53, is being treated for diverticulitis; Mr. Russell, 37, is recovering from a colon resection; and Mrs. Cordera, 79, was admitted for control of her diabetes.

What risks for confusion are present among this group of patients? What additional assessment data do you need to gather to have an appropriate baseline to plan their care? Explain your rationale.

**2** Mr. Gomez is a 45-year-old homeless man admitted for acute tuberculosis. He is in a private room with positive airflow isolation. He was fully oriented on admission but now is acting in an anxious and suspicious manner and appears not to be thinking clearly. On the admission assessment he acknowledged a heavy smoking habit and occasional drug and alcohol use but vigorously denied being an alcoholic. He spoke about his life in positive terms, saying "Don't pity me. I enjoy the freedom of the street. I go where I want and do what I want."

What factors in this situation could be contributing to the development of acute confusion in this patient? What additional assessment data do you need? What will be your initial plan for intervention for his confusion?

**3** You are a float nurse assigned to a busy surgical unit. You are making afternoon rounds and enter the room of an elderly man who underwent major surgery this morning. A patient care assistant (PCA) is in the process of applying a vest and wrist restraints to the patient. When you inquire what the problem is she responds that the patient has become confused and agitated and was trying to get out of bed. When you question the need for restraints she becomes angry and stalks out of the room, saying "On this unit when people are confused we tie them down. That way there's no fall and no lawsuits. You don't like it? Fine—you take care of him." The patient's daughter is at the bedside in tears.

How will you handle this situation? Develop a course of action and explain your rationale.

## chapter SUMMARY

- Acute confusion affects 30% to 50% of hospitalized elders. It is associated with increased morbidity and mortality rates and an increased length of stay.

### SENSORY PROCESS

- The sensory process consists of the ability to receive stimuli from the external environment and the ability to perceive stimuli by organizing them in a meaningful way.
- Reception is primarily biological in nature, whereas perception is primarily psychological and cognitive.
- The RAS and RF are essential to arousal, awareness, and perception. Approximately 99% of incoming stimuli are blocked or filtered at this level.
- Sensoristasis represents a healthy balance in the number and variety of stimuli in the environment. The level varies widely among individuals.
- Sensory deprivation occurs when incoming stimuli are inadequate in number, intensity, or variety to support healthy functioning.
- Sensory overload represents an increase in the number, intensity, or variety of stimuli that overwhelms healthy functioning.
- The ICU syndrome affects patients in ICU settings. It combines elements of both deprivation and overload and is strongly associated with sleep deprivation.

## ACUTE CONFUSION

- *Acute confusion* is a vague term that refers to a state of diffuse cognitive dysfunction. It can be used interchangeably with delirium.
- Acute confusion or delirium has a sudden onset, is transient, and is associated with changes in attention, memory loss, disorientation, impairment in thinking and judgment, sleep-cycle alterations, and altered psychomotor activity.
- Manifestations of acute confusion vary within the same person, throughout the day, among patients, and with different etiological factors.
- Depression may mask confusion because of overlapping behaviors, particularly in the elderly.
- Advanced age is a major predisposing factor for acute or chronic confusion.
- The major causes of acute confusion are drug toxicity, respiratory and urinary tract infections, and electrolyte imbalances.

## COLLABORATIVE CARE MANAGEMENT

- Management of the patient with an alteration in consciousness focuses on identifying the causes, treating the etiological factors, and supporting the patient.

## NURSING MANAGEMENT

- Nursing focuses first on assessment, particularly emphasizing behaviors, presence of systemic diseases, drug and alcohol intake, physical examination, and mental status examination.
- The Mini Mental State Exam and the Short Portable Mental Status Questionnaire are excellent tools for carefully assessing the confused patient's mental status. The Confusion Assessment Scale can be useful when the patient's verbal responses are compromised.
- Modifying the environment to limit sensory deprivation and overload are crucial nursing interventions for both prevention and treatment of acute confusion.
- Measures to promote sleep will help minimize the adverse effects of the noisy hospital environment.
- Although the confused patient may not be aware of the severity of the situation, family members or significant others are aware and need support and education.
- Reorientation and the use of consistent caregivers are important strategies to increase the confused patient's sense of security in his or her environment.
- Preventing injury is an important nursing consideration for confused patients, but the use of restraints should be avoided if possible.
- Restraint use in the United States is high because nurses fear patient falls and subsequent litigation and have little faith in the effectiveness of alternative care strategies.
- Restraint use in long-term care facilities has declined significantly since the passage of the OBRA regulations in the late 1980s, but their use in acute care remains high.

## References


1. Agostinelli B et al: Targeted interventions: use of the mini-mental state exam, *J Gerontol Nurs* 20(8):15, 1994.
2. American Psychiatric Association: *Diagnostic and statistical manual of mental disorders*, ed 4, Washington, DC, 1994, The Association.
3. Baker CF: Discomfort due to environmental noise: heart rate responses of SICU patients, *Crit Care Nurs Q* 15(2):75, 1992.
4. Bolin R: Sensory deprivation: an overview, *Nurs Forum* 13:240, 1974.
5. Chodil J, Williams B: The concept of sensory deprivation, *Nurs Clin North Am* 5:453, 1970.
6. Cutchins C: Blueprint for restraint free care, *Am J Nurs* 91(7):36, 1991.
7. Dellasega C, Morris D: The MMSE to assess the cognitive state of elders, *J Neurosci Nurs* 25(3):147, 1993.
8. FDA Safety Alert: *Potential hazards with restraint devices*, Rockville, Md, July 15, 1992, US Department of Health and Human Services, Public Health Service, Food and Drug Administration, Center for Devices and Radiological Health.
9. Department of Health and Human Services: *Medicare and Medicaid regulations for long-term care facilities*, Federal Register 54:5322, 1989.
10. Francis J, Kapoor W: Delirium in hospitalized elderly, *J Gen Intern Med* 5:65, 1990.
11. Francis J et al: A prospective study of delirium in hospitalized elderly, *JAMA* 263:1097, 1990.
12. Foreman MD, Zane D: Nursing strategies for acute confusion in elders, *Am J Nurs* 96(4):44, 1996.
13. Foreman MD: Adverse psychologic responses of the elderly to critical illness, *AACN J* 3(1):64, 1992.
14. Foreman MD: Complexities of acute confusion, *Geriatr Nurs* 11(3): 136, 1990.
15. Griffin JP: The impact of noise on critically ill people, *Holistic Nurs Pract* 6(4):53, 1992.
16. Grumet GW: Pandemonium in the modern hospital, *N Engl J Med* 328:433, 1993.
17. Hall GR, Wakefield B: Acute confusion in the elderly, *Nursing* 26(7):32, 1996.
18. Holt J: How to help confused patients, *Am J Nurs* 93(8):32, 1993.
19. Janelli LM, Kanski GW, Neary MA: Physical restraints: has OBRA made a difference? *J Gerontol Nurs* 20(6):17, 1994.
20. Leger-Krall S: When restraints become abusive, *Nurs* 24(3):54, 1994.
21. Lipowski ZJ: Delirium. In Hazzard W et al, editors: *Principles of geriatric medicine and gerontology,* ed 3, New York, 1994, McGraw-Hill.
22. Ludwick R, O'Toole AW: The confused patient: nurses' knowledge and interventions, *J Gerontol Nurs* 22(1):44, 1996.
23. Mion LC: Environmental structuring. In Bulechek GM, McCloskey JC, editors: *Nursing interventions: essential nursing treatments,* ed 2, Philadelphia, 1992, WB Saunders.
24. Neufeld R: Alarm devices instead of restraints? *J Am Geriatr Soc* 40(2):191, 1992.
25. Omnibus Budget Reconciliation Act, 4201(C)(1)(A)(II) (Medicare) codified at 42 U.S.C. 1395i-3(C)(1)(A)(II)(supp. 1991), and Public Law 100-203 4211(C)(1)(A)(II) (Medicaid) codified at 42 U.S.C. 1396r-3(C)(1)(A)(II)(supp. 1991), 1987, Health Care Financing Administration, 1987.
26. Pace K: Keeping track of confused patients, *Nursing* 20(6):64, 1990.
27. Schor JD et al: Risk factors for delirium in hospitalized elderly, *JAMA* 267:827, 1992.
28. Shedd PO, Kobokovich KJ, Slattery JJ: Confused patients in the acute care setting: prevalence, intervention, and outcomes, *J Gerontol Nurs* 21(4):5, 1995.
29. Simpson SG, DePaulo JR Jr: Are you recognizing depression in your patients? *Postgrad Med* 94(3):85, 1993.
30. Stolley J: Freeing your patient from restraints, *Am J Nurs* 95(2):27, 1995.
31. Thomas A, Redfern L, Reesa J: Perceptions of acute care nurses in the use of restraints, *J Gerontol Nurs* 21(6):32, 1995.
32. Top SM: Effects of personal control over hospital noise on sleep, *Res Nurs Health* 15:19, 1992.
33. Vermeersch PE: The clinical assessment of confusion, *Appl Nurs Res* 3:128, 1990.
34. Weick MD: Physical restraints: an FDA update, *Am J Nurs* 92(11):74, 1992.
35. Williams M, Murphy JD: Noise in critical care units: a quality assurance approach, *J Nurs Care Qual* 6:53, 1991.
36. Yeaw EM, Abbate JH: Identification of confusion among the elderly in an acute care setting, *Clin Nurse Spec* 7:192, 1993.

chapter 10

# Inflammation and Infection

DORA RICE and ELIZABETH CAMERON ECKSTEIN

## objectives *After studying this chapter, the learner should be able to:*

1 Differentiate between the concepts of self and nonself.
2 Identify the external and internal nonspecific biological defense mechanisms.
3 Describe the mechanism and function of the complement cascade.
4 Describe the steps of the inflammatory process and biological basis of symptoms.
5 Describe the site, structure, and function of each immunoglobulin.
6 Compare the type, genesis, location, and function of the cells involved in the provision of specific immune responses.
7 Compare and contrast the humoral and cell-mediated immune responses and the primary and secondary immune responses.
8 Explain the immunological bases for passive and active immunizations.
9 Describe the chain of infection.
10 Identify high-risk factors for infection.
11 Relate measures to prevent and control nosocomial infections.
12 Describe the major components of the CDC guidelines for Standard and transmission-based Precautions used in hospitals.

## NATURE OF THE PROBLEM

The human body exists in a milieu of antagonistic environmental forces that are constantly attacking and threatening its integrity. In response to these onslaughts, the body exhibits a wide array of adaptations (structures, mechanisms, and responses) designed to provide a defense against these threats and to protect the body from both external and internal deleterious agents. This chapter deals with those anatomical and biological mechanisms that provide protection against environmental factors that physically threaten the patient's body. The implications and applications of the functions of these systems also are discussed. Applications include several aspects of infection control in the hospital and community.

Knowledge of the basic structures and mechanisms that provide this protection helps in the understanding of (1) resistance to infectious disease, (2) diagnosis of disease and physiological state, (3) adaptations in the aging process, (4) immunization against infectious disease, (5) expression of disease of autoimmunity or immunodeficiency, (6) development of allergic reaction, and (7) significance of the localized or systemic inflammatory response. Much of preventive and restorative nursing practice is built on the maintenance or restoration of the cells, systems, and mechanisms that provide defenses against harmful factors in the external and internal environment.

## SELF VERSUS NONSELF

Each human being can be regarded as a genetically and immunologically unique collection of cells and molecules that make up a biological unit of *self.* It is the function of the biological defense mechanisms of the body to protect the integrity of self from encroachment by *nonself* (or foreign) materials. These mechanisms (Figure 10-1) serve to protect the self from both external and internal destructive agents in the following ways:

1. Exclusion of harmful agents from the body
2. Recognition of harmful agents within the body
3. Response designed to dispose of the harmful agents that gain access to the body

The sources of these harmful nonself materials are generally external. These external agents include nonliving materials of the environment such as potentially harmful inorganic chemicals and compounds produced by other living organisms. The most serious external threats to biological integrity, however, come from the living organisms that constantly surround the body. Some of these organisms pose no real threat because the mechanical, biochemical, and metabolic processes of the human body will not support them or offer them shelter. There are myriad living forms, on the other hand, for which the human body is an ideal haven for growth and survival. Most of these organisms, if allowed to penetrate the body, would wreak havoc on its normal functionings. The

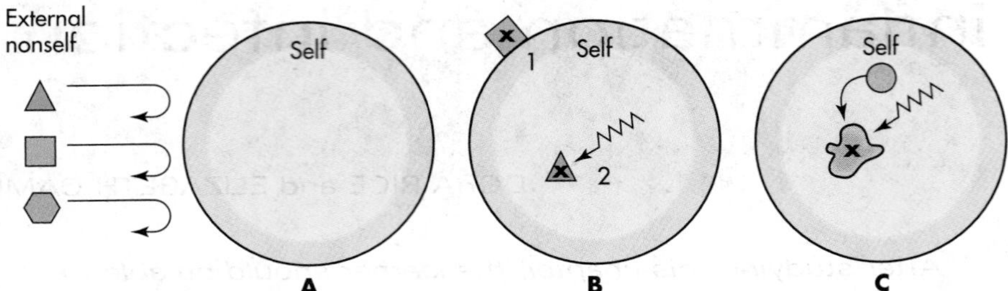


**fig. 10-1** Mechanisms of biological defense in the human body. **A,** Exclusion of external nonself. **B,** Destruction of external nonself by *(1)* nonspecific external mechanisms and *(2)* nonspecific or specific internal mechanisms. **C,** Destruction of altered self. *X* indicates nonspecific mechanisms; → indicates specific mechanisms.

living forms that come to mind in this regard are the organisms classified as *pathogenic* (disease-causing). Although the progress of these organisms in the body can be altered by external agents such as antibiotics, the eradication of the offending organism from the body must be accomplished by the host's own adaptive mechanisms.

In addition to protection against external agents, the defense mechanisms also offer protection against the accumulation of damaged or dysfunctional self material. Without these processes to carry out the systematic, specific removal of damaged or worn-out cellular material, the body would become clogged with debris. Another general function of these systems is recognition of a self's alteration to a potentially dangerous state. When this defense function falters, the tragedy of malignancy (cancer) may result.

## RECOGNITION OF SELF FROM NONSELF

The preceding discussion shows that a critical feature of the protective mechanisms of the human body's immune response system is the ability to discriminate between self and nonself materials. This is accomplished by certain specific protein molecules embedded in the cell membrane of all human body cells, which serve as a cellular fingerprint because the proteins are unique to that individual (Figure 10-2). The recognition process then occurs at the cell membrane surface. Immunoresponsive cells (lymphocytes) have specific protein molecules embedded in their membranes that recognize foreign (nonself) proteins. A person's own immunoresponsive cells recognize nonself proteins on cells that are genetically different, and this triggers a sequence of cellular reactions within the immune response system. This sequence of cellular reactions leads to the elaboration of materials and cells that attack the nonself materials. Contact with self proteins (markers) does not produce an immune attack; that is, there is self-tolerance. This explains why cells from different species or genetically dissimilar members of the same species cannot be transplanted from one host to another without triggering an immunological attack and rejection of the tissue.

In summary, immune system cells have a unique ability to examine the cell surface proteins on any cell or organism with which they come in contact. They interpret these cell surface proteins as either self or nonself and react accordingly.

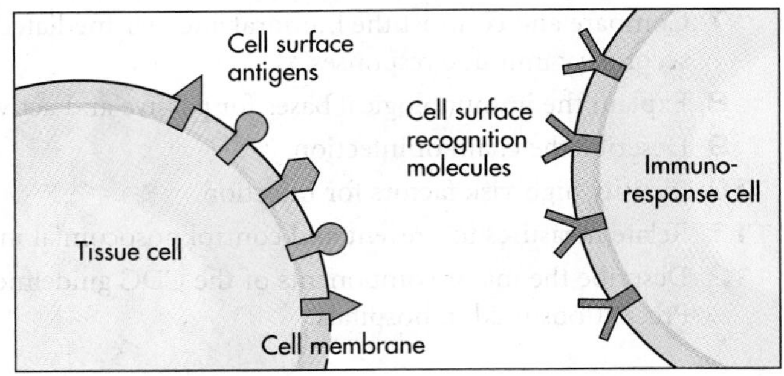


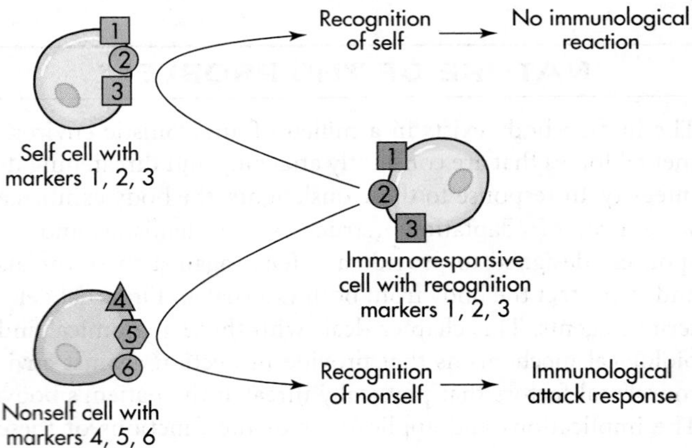


**fig. 10-2** Cell surface markers for recognition of self versus nonself.

## ETIOLOGY: SCOPE OF DEFENSE MECHANISMS

The array of defense mechanisms that have been adapted to protect the normal human body is formidable and complex. For the sake of orderly presentation, they may be divided into nonspecific and specific mechanisms (Table 10-1). The specific and nonspecific mechanisms can be further divided on the basis of where the lines of defense are formed—that is,

**table 10-1** *Biological Defense Mechanisms*

| Nonspecific Mechanisms | Specific Mechanisms |
|---|---|
| **EXTERNAL** | |
| Mechanical exclusion | Immunoglobulin A |
| Physical structures | In mucosal secretions |
| Skin | In mucosal cells |
| Mucous membranes | |
| Specialized structures | |
| Physical actions | |
| Biochemical factors | |
| Body secretions | |
| pH | |
| Lysozyme | |
| Microbial antagonism | |
| **INTERNAL** | |
| Mononuclear phagocytic system | Antigen processing by macrophage |
| Blood | Primary immune response |
| Cellular components | Humoral immune response |
| Fluid components | |
| Complement | Synthesis of circulating immunoglobulins by B cells |
| Acute-phase proteins | |
| Phagocytosis | |
| Inflammatory response | Interaction of immunoglobulins with antigen |
| Interferons | Cell-mediated immune response |
| | Activation of T cell response |
| | Lymphokines |
| | Combined immune response |
| | Secondary immune response |

*external* for the mechanisms of mechanical exclusion, biochemical destruction, and microbial competition and *internal* for the physiological reactions. The nonspecific mechanisms are nonselectively directed against any foreign substance. The specific mechanisms are specifically elicited by unique substances to which the body has acquired the ability to respond.

## EXTERNAL NONSPECIFIC DEFENSE MECHANISMS

### Anatomical Structures and Mechanical Actions

#### Skin and mucous membranes

The first line of defense against penetration by foreign materials, including pathogenic microorganisms, is the skin. When the skin is intact, it serves as an extremely efficient physical barrier to harmful agents and environmental forces such as heat, cold, and trauma. This protection is afforded by the keratinized surface cells, which provide a tough, dense, waterproof covering. Beneath this outermost layer is a dense layer of highly vascularized connective tissue (see Figure 62-1).

Even though some of the fatty acids derived from sebaceous gland secretions have antimicrobial activity, the environment provided by the skin allows the growth of microorganisms on its upper layers and within hair follicles and sweat glands. These resident microorganisms are mainly nonpathogenic; however, when these organisms gain entrance to the tissues of a host exhibiting reduced resistance, they may cause significant problems. Because thorough scrubbing with soap and water removes only the surface organisms, the skin can never be considered sterile.

Any time the physical integrity of the skin is broken—for example, during surgery, with indwelling venous catheterization, or with physical irritation or trauma—there is significant risk of microorganisms gaining entrance to the body. The skin must be kept relatively dry inasmuch as the continued presence of moisture tends to cause maceration of the skin. Further, when essential oils are lost from the skin surfaces, they should be supplemented by lotions to maintain the resilience and unbroken texture of the surface cells. Adequate care of the skin of the hospitalized patient is not just a luxury but a necessity for the provision of an extremely important aspect of biological defense.

Mucous membranes protect the eye and line all body tracts that have external openings. When intact, the mucous membranes, as with the skin, are basically impervious to foreign materials and microorganisms. The surfaces are covered by a viscous secretion that tends to trap and inactivate microorganisms. The mucous membrane of the respiratory tract is further protected by the surface activity of the ciliated epithelial cells, which sweep foreign material out of the tract. The mucous membranes are highly vascularized so that the internal defense mechanisms are readily available to attack any microorganisms that do gain access to the surface of these cells.

Also found in the mucosal secretions and in high concentration within the secretory mucosal cells of the respiratory and intestinal tracts is a specific class of immunoglobulins (antibodies) known as immunoglobulin A (IgA). These specific antibodies are secreted from the mucosal cells and have antibacterial, antiviral, and antitoxic properties. These antibodies serve to prevent microbial adherence and colonization of these tracts by pathogens.

#### Specialized structures and mechanical functions

Other structures and functions of the human body that generally are taken for granted actually serve extremely important roles in defense. The filtration action of the nasal hairs serves to trap particles and microorganisms. The flushing action of saliva and urine prevents the buildup of organisms. The eyes are protected from dirt particles and organisms by the lids and lashes. Foreign material that does gain entrance to the eye tends to be washed out by tears. The constant movement of foods through the stomach and intestines prevents the buildup of organisms and toxic waste products. Even the action of vomiting and the watery stools of diarrhea are active mechanisms of removal of harmful products from the gastrointestinal (GI) tract. Dysfunction or blockage of any of these processes means that special measures must be taken to protect against the establishment of pathogenic organisms and the buildup of toxic materials.

## Biochemical Factors

Many areas of the body are protected not only by mechanical barriers but also by specific antimicrobial chemicals that provide added protection.

### Skin

The acetic acid and salt concentration of perspiration is toxic to many pathogenic microorganisms. Some of the fatty acids released to the skin surface by the sebaceous glands also serve to inhibit the growth of some microorganisms.

### Gastrointestinal tract

In the stomach the acidity (approximately pH 2) of the gastric juice kills many organisms and detoxifies certain potentially toxic substances. For this reason, when gastric pH is increased, special precautions must be taken to avoid introduction of organisms through the nose and mouth. A higher gastric pH is characteristic in neonates; therefore special care should be taken in feeding and handling babies to prevent exposure to pathogens by the oral route. The upper intestine is generally freed of organisms by the action of bile and proteolytic enzymes.

### Vagina

Vaginal secretions allow certain harmless acid-producing bacteria to colonize the vagina and create an acidic environment. This reduces the chance of pathogens colonizing the vagina. When either the amount or the acidity of the vaginal secretions is reduced, a much greater chance exists that a vaginal infection will develop. Because vaginal secretions are not present before puberty and are greatly reduced after menopause, both young girls and older women are more prone to vaginitis. The use of certain types of oral contraceptives may cause a shift in the composition and pH of the vaginal secretions, which increases the possibility of colonization of the vagina, especially by the causative agent of gonorrhea, *Neisseria gonorrhoeae.*

### Lysozyme

The most ubiquitous antimicrobial factor in the body is the bactericidal enzyme lysozyme. It is capable of lysing (splitting) the bacterial cell wall of many gram-positive organisms and causing their destruction. The enzyme is present in mucus, tears, saliva, and skin secretions and is also found in many of the internal fluids and cells of the body. Within the body, lysozyme tends to work in combination with complement and other blood factors to destroy bacteria directly.

## Microbial Antagonism

The skin and mucosal surfaces offer varying nutritional and environmental conditions for the growth and multiplication of certain microbial cells. Although the surfaces of the body are constantly exposed to temporary contamination by organisms from the environment, most of these organisms, known as *transient flora,* do not find conditions suitable for colonization in the body; however, many microorganisms do colonize the skin and mucosal surfaces. These organisms make up what is known as the *normal microbial flora.* Although this normal flora varies from site to site within the body and may vary in response to environmental, hygienic, and physiological changes, it is capable of reestablishment and reflects a fairly predictable pattern. Table 10-2 provides an overview of the body areas normally colonized and shows which organisms most often make up the normal flora of the various areas.

The maintenance of this balanced microbial flora makes it difficult for pathogenic organisms to establish themselves on the body surfaces. Because the normal flora have a selective advantage in their environmental niche, they compete for nutrients and space. Some release antimicrobial substances to retard the growth of transient organisms seeking to occupy the

**table 10-2** *Distribution of Normal Microbial Flora*

| Region of Body | Sterile Areas | Nonsterile Areas | Microorganisms |
|---|---|---|---|
| Skin | None | All skin | *Staphylococcus, Bacillus, Corynebacterium, Mycobacterium, Streptococcus,* transient environmental organisms |
| Respiratory tract | Larynx, trachea, bronchi, bronchioles, alveoli, sinuses | Nose, throat, mouth | *Staphylococcus, Candida, Streptococcus, Neisseria, Pneumococcus,* oral organisms |
| Gastrointestinal tract | Esophagus, stomach, upper small intestine | Esophagus and stomach (transiently), large intestine | Gram-negative rods, *Streptococcus, Bacteroides, Proteus, Clostridium, Lactobacillus* |
| Genitourinary tract | Cervix, uterus, fallopian tubes, ovaries, prostate gland, epididymides, testes, bladder, kidneys | External genitalia, anterior urethra, vagina | Skin organisms, *Lactobacillus, Bacteroides* |
| Body fluids and cavities | Blood, pleural fluid, synovial fluid, spinal fluid, lymph, etc. | None | |

same site. These microbial interferences are known as *microbial antagonism.*

Most of the normal microbial flora are basically nonpathogenic; however, some overtly pathogenic organisms such as *Staphylococcus aureus* and *Streptococcus pyogenes* can be part of the normal flora. The individual who harbors such organisms without demonstrating any symptoms of disease is known as a *carrier.* This carrier state is significant because the carrier may unknowingly be shedding organisms into the environment and infecting others.

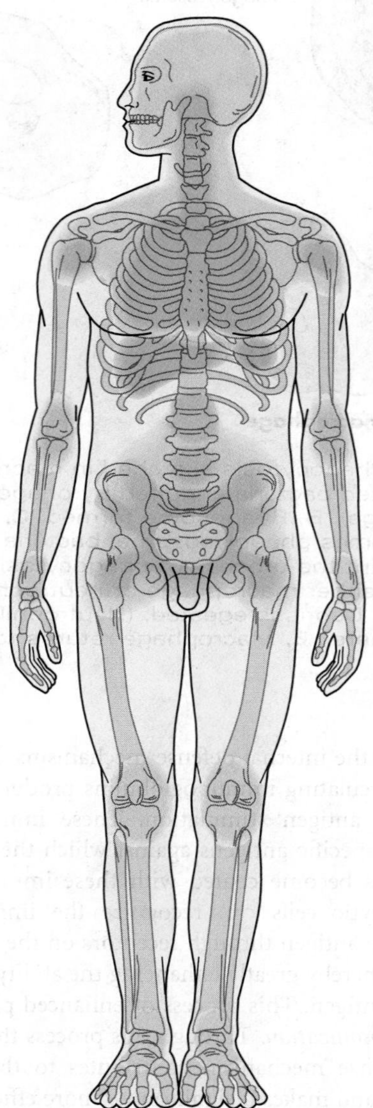

**fig. 10-3** Mononuclear phagocyte system (MPS). Note the anatomical distribution of maximal activity in system, as indicated by shaded areas over the body. To produce such an image, certain radioactive colloidal particles are given to the patient, and radiation detection techniques delineate tissue uptake. Note definition of liver, spleen, and active bone marrow in axial skeleton and proximal parts of long bones.

The protective effects of the normal microbial flora become most apparent when something upsets the microbial balance within the body. The extended use of broad-spectrum antibiotics sometimes creates such an effect. The imbalance may allow a segment of the normal flora to gain ascendence, causing adverse reactions. An example of this phenomenon occurs when certain oral antibiotics induce marked shifts in the normal intestinal flora, allowing organisms generally suppressed by the growth of competitors to thrive to an unusual degree. This imbalance may induce uncomfortable GI tract problems or even allow gastroenteritis to develop.

# PHYSIOLOGY

## INTERNAL NONSPECIFIC DEFENSE MECHANISMS

Once a foreign agent (living or nonliving) penetrates the external resistance barriers, it is met by an even more complex array of defense mechanisms, which provide for the recognition, capture, and disposal of the foreign material. The key to this process is the specific recognition and vigorous action taken against the foreign material and, at the same time, the protection of the host tissues from extensive damage. The physiological reactions that serve to contain and inactivate the foreign agent are carried out through interactions of cells and molecules of the mononuclear phagocyte system, blood, vascular system, and body tissues.

### Mononuclear Phagocyte System

The *mononuclear phagocyte system* (MPS) was formerly known as the reticuloendothelial system. It is a widespread system of *phagocytic cells* (devouring cells) scattered throughout various body tissues (Figure 10-3). The role of these cells is to ingest foreign particulate matter and damaged host tissues. Some of the phagocytic cells are "fixed" in a variety of tissues such as lymphoid tissue, liver, spleen, bone marrow, lungs, and blood vessels. Within the different tissues these anchored cells have been given unique names (Table 10-3). The function of the fixed cells is to capture and destroy foreign materials found in the fluids of their environment.

**table 10-3** *Distribution and Names of Macrophages in Various Tissue Sites*

| TISSUE | NAME |
|---|---|
| Peripheral blood | Monocyte |
| Loose connective tissue | Histiocyte |
| Liver | Kupffer cells |
| Spleen, MPS | Wandering or fixed macrophage |
| Lung | Alveolar macrophage or dust cell |
| Granulomatous tissue | Epithelioid and giant cells |
| Peritoneal cavity, pleural cavity, bone | Macrophages |

Other cells making up the phagocytic network are not stationary and are called *wandering macrophages.* Depending on where they are found, they may be known as *monocytes* (in the bloodstream) or *histiocytes* (in loose connective tissues). The wandering macrophages carry out the important role of final cleanup of a damaged site in preparation for repair. The cells have the capacity to engulf and destroy virtually any type of foreign material or debris within the body. The macrophages also play an important role in the specific response mechanisms discussed later in this chapter.

## Blood

Blood is one of the primary sources of elements designed to provide protection against injurious agents. The blood transports these active factors to the site of an injury or intrusion and through specific vascular changes concentrates these materials at the site. Both the fluid and the cellular constituents of blood contain these factors.

### Cellular components

The important cellular components of blood in this nonspecific response include granulocytes, lymphocytes, monocytes, and thrombocytes (platelets). The granulocytes, also referred to as *polymorphonuclear leukocytes* (PMNs) and the monocytes are the most important because of their phagocytic activity.

One of the key methods of nonspecific defense is the ingestion of microorganisms and other particulate matter by the phagocytic white blood cells (WBCs). The phagocytes carry out the process of phagocytosis in several discrete steps (Figure 10-4). Most infecting microbes are quickly and efficiently destroyed by phagocytosis; however, some pathogens can escape this destruction. Some bacteria, such as strains of streptococci and staphylococci and *Bacillus anthracis* (anthrax), actually produce factors that will kill the phagocyte. Other organisms resist ingestion or digestion. Some organisms may survive within the phagocytes and multiply there. This may lead to the transport of the organism to other sites in the body or may serve as a chronic focus of continued infection.

The granulocytes can be divided on the basis of their structure and function into neutrophils, eosinophils, and basophils. The "granules" found within these cells represent discrete packets of degradative enzymes used to digest the ingested materials. The neutrophils are the most numerous in circulation and are the most efficient and responsive phagocytic cells involved in the inflammatory process. Where there is adequate blood supply to a region, the phagocytes are constantly available to move from the blood vessels to the site of injury or infection. The neutrophils and monocytes are actually attracted to the scene by chemicals released during infection or injury. This cellular response to chemical attractants is known as *chemotaxis,* and the substances released are called *chemotactic substances.*

### Fluid factors

The fluid portion of uncoagulated blood is called *plasma.* Some of the components of plasma provide important con-

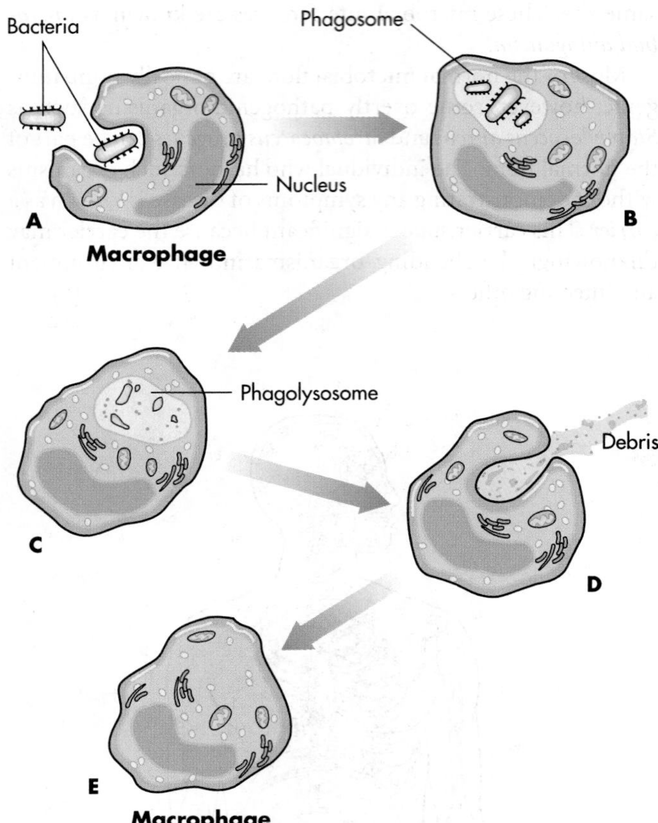


fig. 10-4 Phagocytosis sketched in macrophage. **A,** Opsonized bacteria engulfed by phagocyte (macrophage). **B,** Phagosome formed. **C,** Phagosome becomes phagolysosome; bacteria digested. (To this point the process of phagocytosis is comparable to either macrophage or neutrophil, not shown.) **D,** Debris is egested. (Neutrophil would succumb here.) **E,** Macrophage returns to resting state.

stituents for the internal defense mechanisms. Plasma transports the circulating immunoglobulins produced in specific response to antigen stimulation. These immunoglobulins bind to the specific antigens against which they are formed. The antigens become coated with these immunoglobulins. The phagocytic cells can recognize the immunoglobulin bound to the antigen through receptors on the surface of the phagocyte, thereby greatly enhancing the ability of the cell to engulf the antigen. This process of enhanced phagocytosis is known as *opsonization.* Through this process the specific immune response mechanism contributes to the nonspecific mechanism and makes it significantly more efficient.

Another plasma constituent, fibrin, may create a meshwork around the injured area, sealing it off. Microorganisms may also become trapped within this meshwork, where they are more easily captured by the phagocytic cells.

## Complement

One of the most important constituents of plasma is a complex series of proteins known by the singular name of *complement.* There are as many as 20 different protein components, with

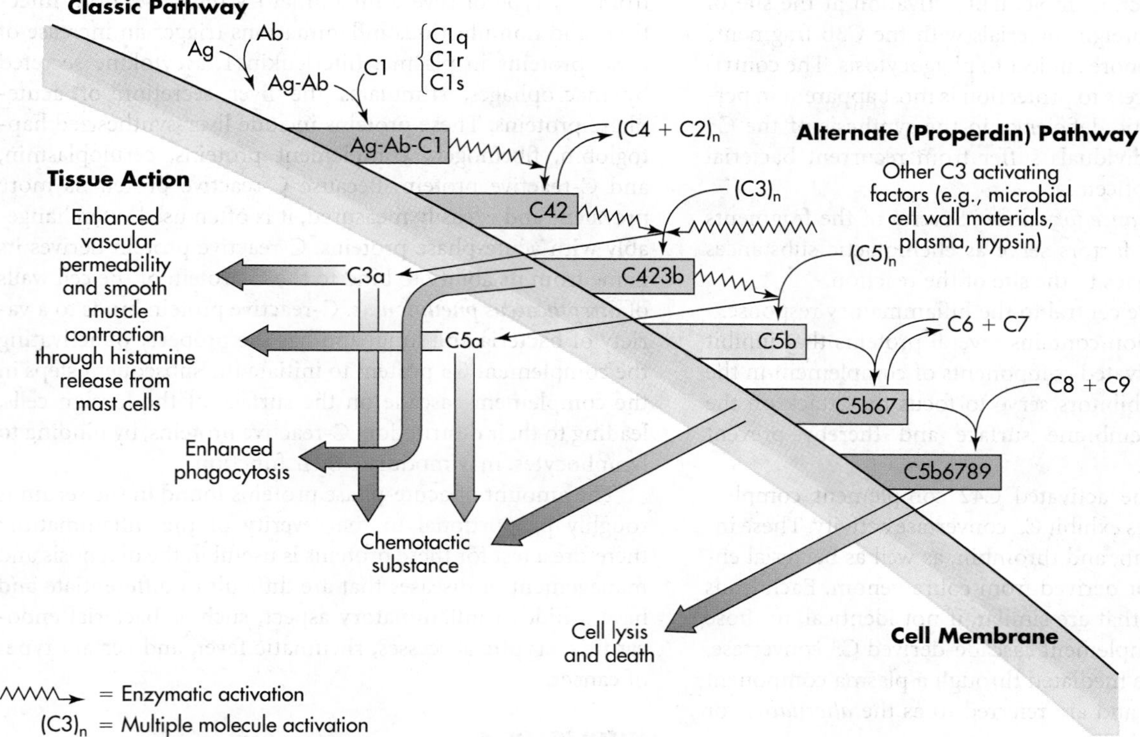


**fig. 10-5** Classic and alternate complement cascade. Sequence of complement activation generates multiple biologically active intermediate molecules, which are active in the inflammatory response.

11 designated as major components in the complement cascade. The liver is the primary site of synthesis of the components of complement. The primary role of complement is to provide specific lysis (rupturing) of cell membranes. The initiation of the *complement cascade* most often is triggered by the binding of the first complement protein to complement-binding immunoglobulins that have already bound to their antigens. Thus complement serves to accentuate or complete the action of an immunoglobulin. The immunoglobulin by itself cannot produce cell lysis, but with the recruitment of complement in the reaction, the cell may be ruptured. However, other nonimmune substances also can activate complement. Complement is considered a nonspecific component of the plasma because it is not increased by immunization. In addition to its cytolytic effects, complement is involved in leukocyte chemotaxis, release of histamines, enhancement of phagocytosis by PMNs, viral neutralization, and bactericidal activity.

The classic activities ascribed to complement depend on the sequential interaction of nine protein subunits (C1 to C9), the first component of which consists of three subfractions termed C1q, C1r, and C1s (thereby accounting for the 11 separate proteins). The C1q, C1r, and C1s components constitute the recognition unit, inasmuch as this unit is capable of recognizing the antibody and fixing to the Fc (for fragment, crystallizable) portion of the antibody. When the first component, C1, is bound by an antigen-immunoglobulin complex on the surface of a cell, it acquires the enzymatic ability to activate many molecules of the next components in the sequence, C4 and C2, to form an active C42 complex (Figure 10-5). (Unfortunately, the numbering system of the complement components reflects their order of discovery and not their sequential additive pattern.) Each of the activated C42 complexes (the activation units) is then able to act on multiple molecules of the next components and so on, producing a cascade effect (a chain reaction) and greatly amplifying the reaction. As each component is added, new enzymatic activity is created to initiate the next step. This cascade effect is similar to that of blood coagulation. The final component, C5b6789, has the ability to create a lesion in the cell membrane and, if enough lesions are created on the membrane, cell death results. This complex is sometimes called the *membrane attack unit.* The intermediate stages in the complement sequence also give rise to complexes and fragments with other significant biological activities. Figure 10-5 depicts the generation of some of these activities, which include the following:

1. *Histamine release.* Histamines cause an extreme increase in vascular permeability and contraction of smooth muscle. A fragment (C3a) split off during the activation of C3 and another fragment (C5a) created by the activation of C5 are released into the surrounding tissues, where they cause the release of histamine from mast cells. The histamines in turn exert their physiological effects on the smooth muscle tissues and vascular system. Because these histamine-mediated reactions are the same as those created during anaphylactic shock (see Chapter 66), these fragments are called *anaphylatoxins.*
2. *Enhanced phagocytosis.* Neutrophils and macrophages have receptors for C3b on their cell surfaces, which add to the

opsonization effect. Complement activation at the site of infection labels foreign materials with the C3b fragments and makes them more subject to phagocytosis. The contribution of the process to protection is most apparent in persons with a genetic deficiency in the synthesis of the C3 protein. Such individuals suffer from recurrent bacterial infections and septicemia.

3. *Chemotactic substance formation.* Several of the fragments and intermediate factors serve as chemotactic substances to attract phagocytes to the site of the reaction.

All these activities are central to the inflammatory response.

The plasma fraction contains several proteins that inhibit the action of the activated components of complement in the fluid phase. Such inhibitors serve to focus the attack on the microorganism's membrane surface and thereby prevent damage to host cells.

In addition to the activated C42 complement complex, several other enzymes exhibit C3 convertase activity. These include trypsin, plasmin, and thrombin, as well as bacterial endotoxins and a factor derived from cobra venom. Each leads to alterations in C3 that are similar, if not identical, to those produced by the complement cascade-derived C3 convertase. These activations are mediated through a plasma component known as *properdin* and are referred to as the *alternative,* or *properdin, pathway.*

The effects of age on the function of the complement system are not clear. There appears to be an increase in the number of complement components or the amount of complement activity from birth to old age, with synthesis beginning as early as the first month of gestation. An increased incidence of conditions whose activities are mediated by complement is seen in elderly persons.

## Acute-Phase Proteins

Acute-phase proteins are serum proteins with concentrations that increase dramatically in the serum of persons suffering from any type of severe inflammatory response. Both infectious and noninfectious inflammations trigger an increase of these proteins in plasma. Interleukin 1, a cytokine secreted by macrophages, stimulates the liver secretion of acute-phase proteins. These proteins include liver-synthesized haptoglobin, fibrinogen, complement proteins, ceruloplasmin, and C-reactive protein. Because C-reactive protein is more prevalent and is easily measured, it is often used interchangeably with acute-phase proteins. C-reactive protein derives its name from its ability to bind to the C protein of the cell walls of *Streptococcus pneumoniae.* C-reactive protein binds to a variety of bacteria and fungi and has the property of activating the complement C3 protein to initiate the subsequent steps in the complement cascade on the surface of the foreign cells, leading to their destruction. C-reactive proteins, by binding to lymphocytes, may modulate their function.

The amount of acute-phase proteins found in the serum is roughly proportional to the severity of the inflammation; therefore a test for these proteins is useful in the diagnosis and management of diseases that are difficult to differentiate and have a hidden inflammatory aspect, such as bacterial endocarditis, cryptic abscesses, rheumatic fever, and certain types of cancer.

## Interferons

Interferons comprise a group of proteins produced by various human cells, usually in response to a viral infection of the cell. When a cell is infected by a virus, the infected cell begins to make interferon almost immediately (Figure 10-6). The interferon is released into its surrounding environment, where it induces uninfected cells to produce alterations that protect those cells from viral multiplication. This antiviral action is exerted before the synthesis of immunoglobulins specific for the virus reach protective levels. The elaboration of interferons from virally infected cells continues for a few hours (up to about 24 hours) after infection, thereby playing a significant

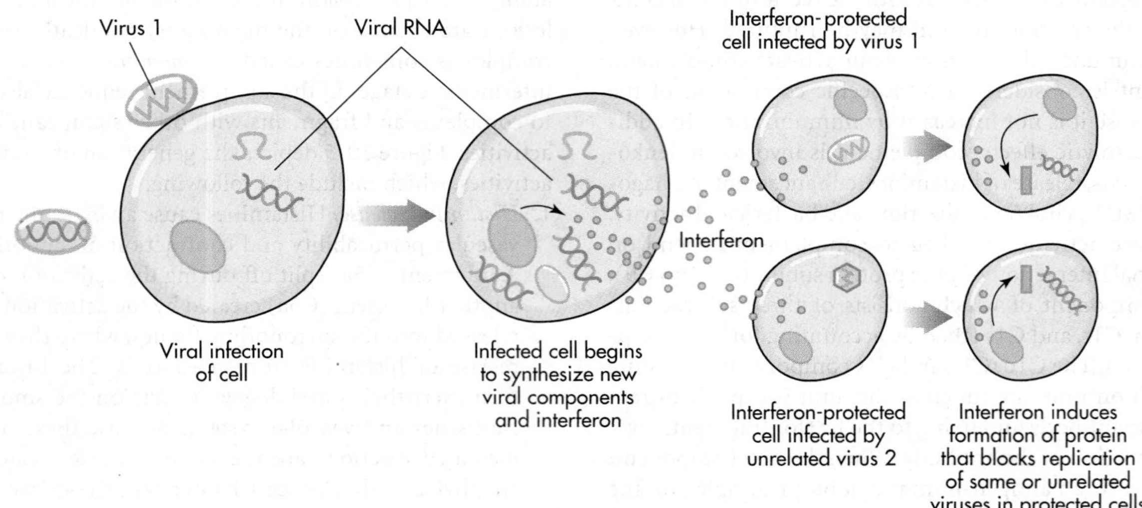


**fig. 10-6** Mechanism of interferon action.

role in isolating the infective foci in many, but not all, viral infections.

Although viruses seem to be the most potent agents for the induction of interferon, production is not restricted to viral infection of cells. Other intracellular parasites such as rickettsia, bacteria, and parasites may also trigger the formation of interferon. Even bacterial and fungal extracts, as well as other materials such as double-stranded ribonucleic acid (RNA), synthetic polymers, and plant extracts, may serve as signals.

Three distinct types of interferons are produced by different cell types in the human body, and each type seems to exert different protective effects. *Alpha-interferon* is produced by lymphocytes and seems to have antiviral activity. *Beta-interferon* is formed by fibroblasts, epithelial cells, and macrophages; it is definitely antiviral. *Gamma-interferon* is produced by T lymphocytes of the specific immune response system and has an immunoregulatory effect. In addition to their antiviral activities, the interferons are capable of inhibiting cell growth; therefore they are being used widely in clinical trials as antitumor agents.

In general, the production of interferon occurs regardless of the viral agent that initiated its formation; thus interferon is said to be *virus-nonspecific* and does not inhibit all viruses equally. Among the viruses that seem to be especially sensitive are the arboviruses, influenza virus, and smallpox virus. Most vertebrate species seemingly are capable of producing interferons; however, each animal species' interferon is protective against viral infection only in that species. This means the bovine interferon has only limited protective value in the human and vice versa. The term *species specificity* is used to describe this quality. This characteristic limited early research into the effects of interferon, because it was difficult to obtain enough human interferon to conduct clinical trials. Through the use of recombinant deoxyribonucleic acid (DNA) technology, the human interferon gene has been introduced into bacterial cells. By growing such bacteria in culture, large amounts of specific types (alpha [$\alpha$], beta [$\beta$], and gamma [$\gamma$]) of interferon can be harvested, purified, and used in clinical studies. The other benefit of this application of genetic engineering is to greatly reduce the cost of the purified interferon.

Interferons slow down cell replication and enhance natural killer cell activity, thereby acting as anticancer agents. Alpha-interferon was approved for the treatment of hairy cell leukemia in 1986 and Kaposi's sarcoma and hepatitis C in 1988.[17]

## SPECIFIC DEFENSE MECHANISMS

### Concepts of an Adaptive Specific Immune System

Specific defense mechanisms within the body provide specific protection against a particular microorganism or molecular entity. This mechanism of protection leads to what is termed *specific immunity.* Depending on the relative levels of protection, the body may be able to defend itself totally or only partially from damage by the agent. The *immune system* is composed of many of the same organs, cells, and molecular entities operating to provide nonspecific defense. It works with the nonspecific mechanisms to focus and amplify the general mechanisms of defense against specifically recognized foreign materials. Refer to Chapter 65 for further discussion of immunity.

The fundamental nature of the specific immune response is characterized by diversity, specificity, recognition, memory, and action. Among the most intriguing aspects of immune response is its diversity of ability to respond *while at the same time responding with specificity of action.* Almost any conceivable organic molecular array on the surface of a molecule has been shown to be able to induce a series of cellular events culminating in the production of antibodies (immunoglobulins).* These antibodies combine with the inducing antigen (immunogen) by virtue of combining sites on the immunoglobulin molecule that exhibit an extremely narrow specificity. The remainder of the immunoglobulin molecule is chemically and structurally similar to all other antibody molecules with distinctly different combining-site specificities.

Recognition and memory are two other aspects of this system that make it unique. The normal organism recognizes its own antigenic make-up and will not produce antibodies against its own antigens. This is known as *recognition of self* or *self-tolerance.* At the same time this intricate system of self-recognition must be able to detect extremely subtle changes in its own cells when incipient tumors that differ only slightly in antigenic constitution are forming. Further, once the immune system has responded to an antigen, subsequent encounters with that antigen produce an even more vigorous and rapid response. This response includes a wide variety of mechanisms designed to take action against the offending agent. Many of these actions are among the most potent biochemical and cellular reactions that the body can produce; yet they are focused so discretely that the foreign agent is rapidly destroyed with a minimum of damage to the host.

### Basic Design of the System

The basic design of the specific immune response system is such that the body provides itself with cells and molecules that can respond to and thwart encroachment of nonself materials rapidly and efficiently. The system has two major interactive divisions: (1) a humorally-mediated system of specifically designed proteins known as *antibodies* or *immunoglobulins* and (2) a cell-mediated system of specifically reactive WBCs known as *activated lymphocytes* or *T cells.* Both arms of the system usually are triggered to respond to encroachment; however, only one of the systems may provide the most protection against certain types of encroachment.

*The terms *antibody* and *immunoglobulin* can be used more or less interchangeably and are used that way throughout this chapter. Specifically, antibody is the original, more general, term describing serum agents that inactivate foreign substances in the body. It was coined in the early part of this century before the specific proteins of the serum had been identified as the globulin proteins of the gamma-globulin fraction. The term *immunoglobulin* more specifically identifies the molecules of the serum that have antibody activity. In the same way, *antigen* is the original, more general, term for foreign materials that elicit the immune response reaction; the newer, more accurate, and interchangeable term for such materials is *immunogen.*

The *humorally-mediated system* provides major immunity against (1) bacteria that produce acute infection (such as *Staphylococcus, Streptococcus,* and *Haemophilus* organisms), (2) bacterial exotoxins (diphtheria, botulinus, and tetanus toxins), (3) viruses that must enter the bloodstream to reach their target tissues (e.g., poliomyelitis and hepatitis virus), and (4) organisms that enter the body from the mucosal tissues (e.g., cold viruses, enteroviruses, and influenza viruses). Even though circulating antibodies may be produced against other organisms (such as tuberculosis, human immunodeficiency virus [HIV], and fungi), these antibodies do not protect the body from infection.

The *cell-mediated system,* on the other hand, offers protection from (1) chronic bacterial infections (e.g., syphillis, tuberculosis, and leprosy), (2) many viral infections (e.g., measles, herpesvirus infections, and chickenpox), (3) fungal infections (e.g., candidiasis, histoplasmosis, and cryptococcis), (4) parasitic infections (e.g., leishmaniasis, toxoplasmosis, and *Pneumocystis carinii*), and (5) transplanted or transformed cells (e.g., tissue transplants and some transformed cells of cancer).

One or both of these systems can be immunodeficient (see Chapter 66). When one system is not functioning properly, the person becomes susceptible to infection or encroachment by the agents against which that system provided primary protection. For example, infection with HIV reduces the protection afforded by the cell-mediated system, making the individual susceptible to fungal infections (candidiasis), protozoan infections (*P. carinii* pneumonia), viral infections (herpesvirus infection), and cancers (Kaposi's sarcoma or lymphoma). Alternatively, the loss of the humorally mediated system that occurs in Bruton's agammaglobulinemia is accompanied by increased incidence of acute bacterial infections, respiratory tract infections, and GI tract problems. If both systems are lost or compromised, the individual is fully susceptible to infectious agents and cannot survive in an unprotected, nonsterile environment.

## Immune Response System

### *Immunogens and immunoglobulins*

**Immunogens (antigens).** An *immunogen* is defined as a substance that, when introduced into an animal, elicits the formation of antibodies, or specifically sensitized cells. The antigen must be recognized as nonself or foreign material within the body. Although most antigens are naturally occurring proteins of at least 10,000 molecular weight, other substances, such as polysaccharides, nucleoproteins, lipoproteins, and glycoproteins, also may serve as antigens. The bulk of the antigen consists of subsurface molecular structures that do not elicit an immune response but do serve as carriers for the multiple antigenic determinants on the surface. Most antigens have many antigenic determinants and are termed *multivalent antigens*; however, some molecules may be monovalent.

Because of their small size, certain molecules cannot induce the synthesis of antibodies; however, when coupled with a high-molecular-weight carrier, they can serve as antigenic determinants. These molecules are incomplete antigens, or hapten. They take on specific significance in the consideration of hypersensitivities, which are allergies to low-molecular-weight compounds such as certain drugs and antibiotics (see Chapter 66).

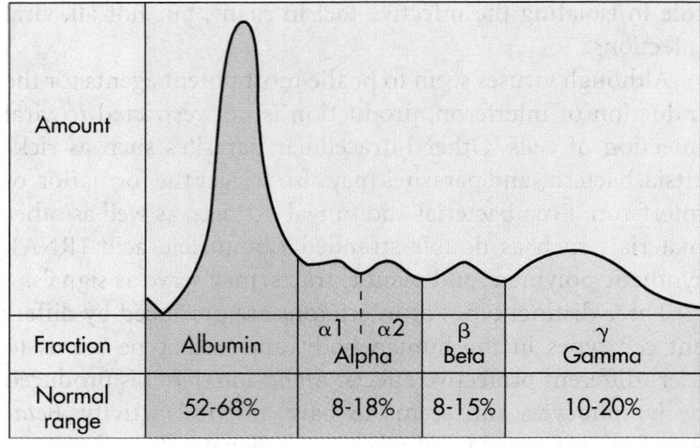


**fig. 10-7** Electrophoretic separation of major serum proteins. Most antibody activity lies within the gamma-globulin fraction. This fraction rises with active synthesis of antibodies in response to antigenic stimulation.

**Immunoglobulins (antibodies).** The body's response to the introduction of an immunogenic substance is the production of a specific, soluble immunoglobulin or a sensitized (antigen-reactive) lymphocyte population. The type of antigen introduced determines the immune response: antibody synthesis or antigen-reactive lymphocyte, or a combination of both.

The circulating antibodies represent modified (e.g., antigen-specific) globulin proteins found in bloodserum. The serum contains several distinct protein fractions, which are separable on the basis of their net electrical charge, molecular size, and molecular conformation into several fractions: albumin, alpha-globulins, beta-globulins, and gamma-globulins (Figure 10-7). The antibody activity of the serum is characteristically associated with the gamma-globulin and beta-globulin fractions. Those gamma-globulins with the ability to bind antigens are called *immunoglobulins.* The immunoglobulins can be further subdivided into different classes on the basis of structure and function of the molecules. The generic symbol for immunoglobulins is Ig, and each of the classes is designated by a letter of the alphabet: IgA, IgD, IgE, IgG, and IgM (Table 10-4).

The basic pattern of structure for all immunoglobulins is based on a four-peptide chain monomeric unit (Figure 10-8). Two of the chains are of higher molecular weight and are termed *heavy* (H) *chains;* two are of lower molecular weight and are called *light* (L) *chains.* Each L chain is linked by disulfide (—ss—) bonds to an H chain, and in turn the H chains are linked to each other by disulfide bonds. When immunoglobulin monomers are visualized by means of electron microscopy, they are seen to have a Y-shaped structure. At the ends of the two arms of the Y are the sites where antigen is bound. Both the H and L chains participate in the forma-

**table 10-4** *Properties of Immunoglobulin Classes*

| PROPERTY | IMMUNOGLOBULIN CLASS IgG | IgM | IgA | IgE | IgD |
|---|---|---|---|---|---|
| Physiochemical | | | | | |
| Percentage of Ig | 75-85 | 7 | 10 | 0.002 | 1 |
| Configuration | Monomer | Pentamer | Monomer, dimer | Monomer | Monomer |
| Half-life in serum (days) | 23 | 5 | 6 | 2 | 3 |
| Functional antigen-binding sites | 2 | 5 | 2 | 2 | 2 |
| Biological | | | | | |
| Principal site found | Internal body fluids | Serum | Serum and exocrine secretions | Tissue bound | Bound to lymphocyte surface |
| Fixed complement | Yes | Yes | No | No | No |
| Crosses placenta | Yes | No | No | No | No |
| Principal functions | Agglutination, detoxification, virus neutralization; enhancement of phagocytosis | Agglutination, cytolysis; enhancement of phagocytosis | Protection of mucosal surfaces | Mediation of immediate type of hypersensitivity | Control of lymphocytic activation and suppression |

tion of these antigen-binding sites. Thus most monomers of immunoglobulin have two antigen-binding sites and are termed *bivalent.* The two arms of the Y are designated the *Fab regions* (for fragment, antigen-binding). The base of the Y is called the *Fc region* (for fragment, crystallizable). The Fc fragment binds to complement and to white blood cells, including macrophages. In the region of the disulfide bond joining the H chains, the molecule seems to be flexible, and this region is known as the "hinge" region.

The predominant class of immunoglobulins in normal adult serum is IgG. It makes up about 75% to 85% of the immunoglobulin fraction. Because of its structure and biological activity, it is also found in the extravascular fluids of the body. IgG is capable of crossing the placenta to provide the newborn with temporary natural passive immunity to those diseases against which the mother has circulating antibodies. It functions primarily in the processes of toxin neutralization and viral and bacterial inactivation and in the formation of antigen-antibody complement immune complexes associated with certain types of hypersensitivity (see Chapter 66). IgG is the immunoglobulin class primarily responsible for the rise in serum antibodies during a secondary (anamnestic, booster) response.

IgM structurally is composed of five monomeric units attached to each other at the Fc region. Thus the star-shaped molecule with the antigen-binding sites pointed outward that results from this macromolecular arrangement is termed a *pentamer.* Sometimes this immunoglobulin class, which constitutes about 7% of the immunoglobulin in serum, is called the *macroglobulin* because of its molecular size. As a result of its size, it is confined primarily to the intravascular fluids. IgM, as with IgG, is capable of binding the C1 component of complement and initiating the complement cascade. In each antigenic stimulation, IgM antibodies are the first to appear, but they neither reach the levels of IgG nor exhibit an

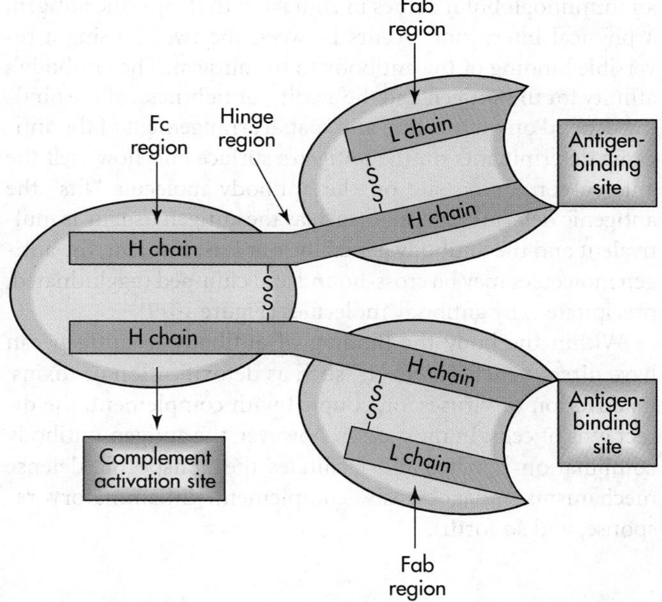


**fig. 10-8** Basic structure of IgG monomer. All immunoglobulin classes are composed of variations of this basic structure with combinations to form dimers (IgA) or pentamers (IgM).

anamnestic response on subsequent antigen contact. They are primarily involved in providing protection against viral and bacterial invaders in the blood. Because of their ability to bind complement, they too are responsible for certain immune complex hypersensitivities and autoimmune diseases, such as rheumatoid arthritis.

IgA constitutes about 10% of the total immunoglobulin in serum. It can be found in a variety of polymeric forms (primarily monomer in serum and dimer in exocrine secretions). IgA is also termed the *secretory immunoglobulin* because it is found in the exocrine secretions of the body (milk, mucin, saliva, and tears). Within these secretions IgA provides specific protection of the mucosal surfaces of the respiratory, digestive, and genital tracts from pathogenic invasion.

IgD makes up only about 1% of the immunoglobulin fraction of serum. Its biological functions are unknown. Most of the IgD is found on the surface of some lymphocytes, where it probably plays a role in the activation and suppression of lymphocyte function. It may also modify the activity of IgM.

IgE is present in the serum in extremely small amounts (0.002%), a sparsity that results from this immunoglobulin's predilection for attachment to the surface of mast cells and basophils. When bound by the Fc region of the monomer to the surface of these cells, which are rich in the potent, physiologically active substances histamine, kinins, and serotonin, IgE serves to mediate the severe and occasionally fatal anaphylactic type of hypersensitivities. These include anaphylactic shock, allergic asthma, and hay fever (see Chapter 66). The protective role of this immunoglobulin is not clear, but it may be effective in providing protection against certain parasitic worms.

**Immunogen-immunoglobulin interactions.** When an immunoglobulin comes in contact with its specific antigen, a physical interaction occurs between the two, causing a reversible binding of the antibody to the antigen. The antibody's affinity for the antigen and the avidity, or tightness, of the binding depend on the location and spatial arrangement of the antigenic determinants on the antigen's surface and how well the antigen-combining site on the antibody molecule "fits" the antigenic determinant. Inasmuch as the antigen usually is multivalent and the antibody generally is at least bivalent, the antigen molecules may be cross-bound and clumped (agglutinated, precipitated) by antibody molecules (Figure 10-9).

Within the body the binding of antibody to antigen can have direct beneficial effects, such as detoxification of toxins, inactivation of viruses, or, coupled with complement, the direct lysis of cells. In most cases, however, the antigen-antibody combination initiates and facilitates the nonspecific defense mechanisms (phagocytosis, complement, inflammatory response, and so forth).

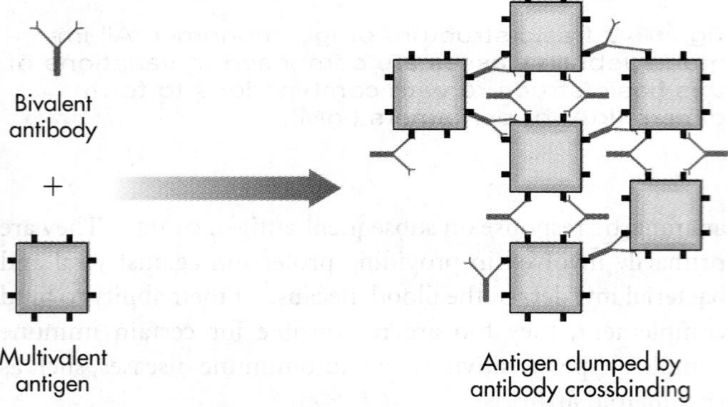


**fig. 10-9** Clumping of multivalent antigen by its specific antibody.

### Cells involved

The cells involved in the specific immune response are all derived from the original undifferentiated stem cells of the bone marrow. The stem cell may develop into any of the blood cells of the body, depending on various signals and influences. The primary cells of the immune response system develop from the lymphocytic cell population (Figure 10-10). One population of lymphocytic cells undergo differentiation under the influence of the thymus gland and become *thymus-dependent lymphocytes,* or *T cells.* These cells become responsible for facilitating the cell-mediated immunity (CMI) response. Another population of lymphocytes mature in a site other than the thymus and are known as *thymus-independent lymphocytes,* or *B cells.* The designation *B cell* comes from the fact that in the chicken, where this process was first detected, a single site exists where this differentiation occurs, that is, the bursa of Fabricius. No such singular lymphoid organ is found in human beings, but it is believed that the process occurs in the bone marrow or possibly the gut-associated lymphoid tissues (tonsils, Peyer's patches of the intestines, and appendix). Because the exact site in humans has not been unequivocably identified, it often is referred to as the *bursa equivalent.* The B cells are responsible for production of the immunoglobulins and provision of the humoral immune response.

The role of the lymphocytes (B or T cells) is to recognize the presence of an antigen and to initiate specific mechanisms of disposal. Just as important, the lymphocyte must recognize a component of host tissues as self and protect that tissue from immunological response reactions.

**table 10-5** *Cytokines Liberated in the Immune Response*

| Cytokine | Function |
|---|---|
| Interferon | Inhibits viral replication<br>Activates macrophages and neutrophils<br>Activates natural killer cells |
| GM-CSF | Stimulates growth and differentiation of myeloid stem cells |
| M-CSF | Stimulates production of monocytes and macrophages |
| G-CSF | Stimulates production of neutrophils |
| Interleukin 1 | Pyrogenic; stimulates helper T cells and B lymphocytes |
| Interleukin 2 | Stimulates production of T lymphocytes |
| Interleukin 3 | Stimulates production of bone marrow stem cells |
| Interleukin 4 | Stimulates growth of B lymphocytes |
| Interleukin 5 | Stimulates growth of eosinophils and function of plasma cells |
| Interleukin 6 | Stimulates growth of B lymphocytes and stem cell production |
| Tumor necrosis factor | Pyrogenic; stimulates secretion of CSFs and some interleukins |

*GM-CSF,* Granulocyte macrophage colony-stimulating factor; *M,* monocyte; *G,* granulocyte.

B and T lymphocytes can be differentiated from each other on the basis of specific markers (membrane-bound proteins) on the surface of the cells. For instance, T cells have a marker that causes the binding of sheep red blood cells (RBCs), whereas B cells are lacking such protein. B cells, on the other hand, usually have immunoglobulins displayed on their cell surface. By the identification of the specific markers on the cell surface, cells can be divided into B or T cell types and even further subdivided into subtypes (see later discussion on helper and suppressor T cells).

A third type of cell directly involved in the immune response, is the *antigen-presenting cell* (APC) (also called *antigen-processing cell*). The macrophage of the bloodstream and lymphoid tissues is the cell type most responsible for antigen processing, although other leukocytes may do this as well.[1] The main role of these cells is to capture antigens introduced into the tissues or draining to regional lymphoid tissues, process the antigen within the cell, concentrate the antigenic determinant, and present the antigen to antigen-sensitive lymphoid cells. The processed antigenic signal is displayed on the surface membrane of the APC. Antigen presented to lymphocytes by cell-to-cell contact triggers the series of events within the lymphocytes that leads to full immunological response.

It is interesting to note that the macrophage is itself activated by activated lymphocytes to its maximal phagocytic efficiency by the release of stimulatory, soluble substances known as *lymphokines,* or cytokines (Table 10-5). In this way the macrophage is stimulated at the site of an immune reaction. Other soluble lymphokines serve to attract the macrophages to the site by chemotaxis. In addition, activated macrophages, sometimes called "angry" macrophages, produce complement components, prostaglandins, and interferon.

Another type of lymphoid cell, called the *null cell,* has characteristics of B lymphocytes, T lymphocytes, and macrophages. Currently it is thought that these cells are not programmed to respond to specific antigens but rather are recruited by immune response reactions to nonspecifically attack and kill tumor cells and virally infected cells. When activated and directed against foreign cells, these are referred to as *natural killer (NK) cells.* After destroying target cells, the NK cell is able to survive unharmed and attack other target cells.

### Organs and tissues involved

The organs and tissues of the specific immune response system include the central organs (bone marrow and thymus) and the peripheral organs (lymph nodes, spleen, and lymphatic vessels). Within the central organs the immune response cells are synthesized and matured, whereas within the peripheral organs the mature cells are concentrated.

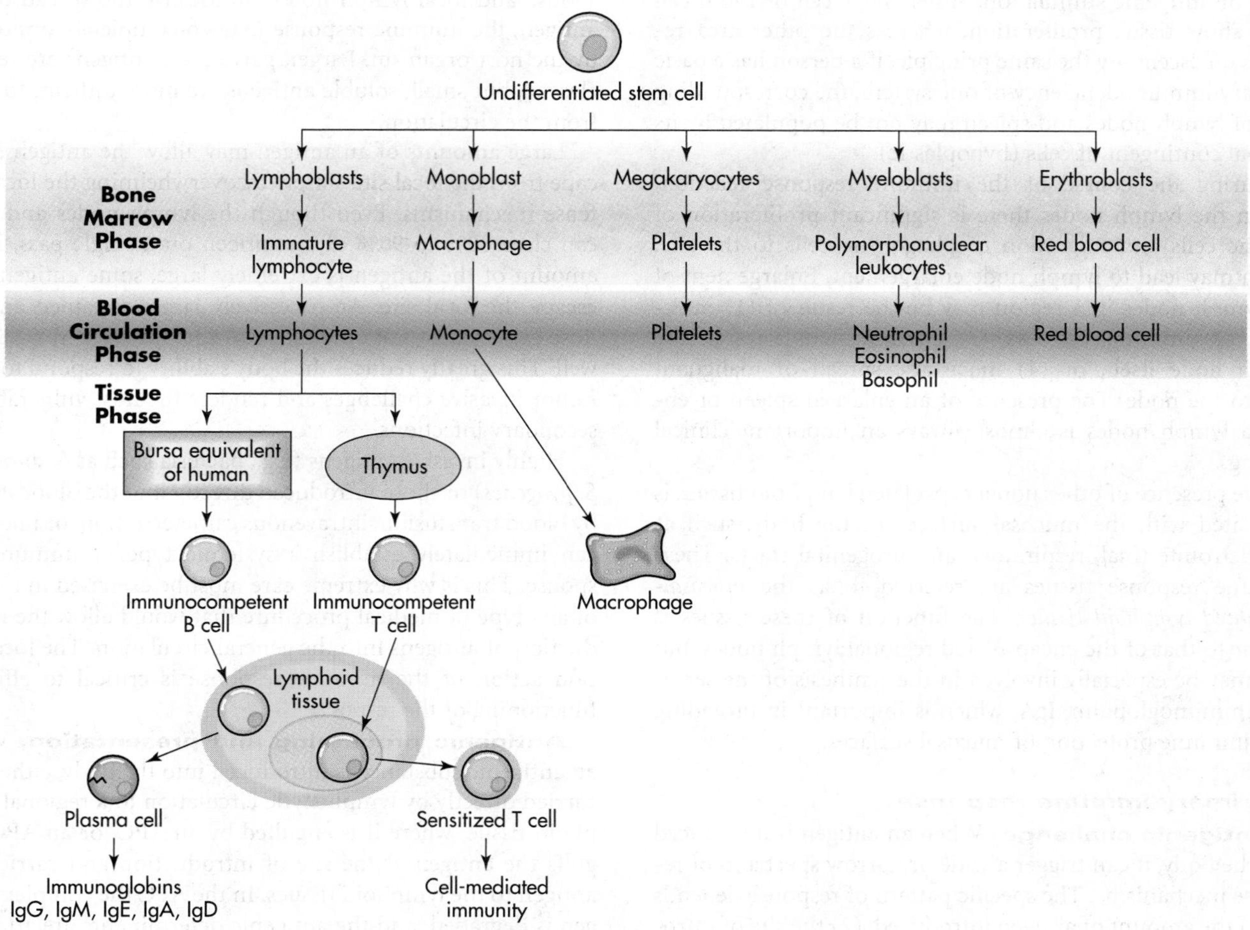


**fig. 10-10** Development of B and T lymphocytes.

The thymus serves as the control organ of the immune system. It is the differentiation site of the T cell lymphocytic populations and, through certain soluble thymic hormones, serves to regulate the overall immune system. The activity of the thymus reaches its peak in childhood, and the organ begins to shrink in size after puberty. If the thymus is removed (thymectomy) very early in an animal's life, a severe state of immunodeficiency is induced and T cell-mediated immunity never develops. The thymectomized animal develops a wasting disease characterized by stunted growth, diarrhea, and death as a result of massive infection by intestinal or respiratory tract normal flora. The B cell function also is reduced, pointing to a cooperative effect between the two basic systems. The loss of the thymus in the adult animal creates less severe reactions, probably because of the establishment of an already functional, long-lived population of T cells.

The lymph nodes and spleen serve as the primary sites of localization of the immune response cells. The lymph node serves to filter the lymph drained from a region of tissue. The structure of the lymph node (Figure 10-11) consists of an inner medullary and paracortical region made up primarily of T cells and an outer cortex composed of clusters, or germinal centers, of B cells known as *follicles.* The spleen is structured on somewhat the same pattern with diffusely packed T cell areas and germinal centers of tightly packed B cells. In certain types of antigenic stimulation, either the T cell or the B cell areas show tissue proliferation, whereas the other area remains quiescent. By the same principle, if a person has a basic primary immunodeficiency of one system, the corresponding area of lymph nodes and spleen may not be populated by its normal contingent of cells (hypoplastic).

During the course of the immune response reaction, within the lymph nodes there is significant proliferation of specific cells and migration of phagocytic cells to the site, which may lead to lymph node enlargement. Enlargement of the lymph nodes in a region may be the result of (1) infections, (2) immune diseases, (3) intrinsic neoplasms of the lymph node itself, or (4) metastatic spread of malignant cells to the node. The presence of an enlarged spleen or enlarged lymph nodes is almost always an important clinical finding.

The presence of other nonencapsulated lymphoid tissues is associated with the mucosal surfaces of the body, such as the gastrointestinal, respiratory, and urogenital tracts. These immune response tissues are referred to as the *mucosal-associated lymphoid tissues.* The function of these tissues is similar to that of the encapsulated regional lymph nodes, but they may be especially involved in the synthesis of the secretory immunoglobulin, IgA, which is important in providing total immune protection of mucosal surfaces.

### *Primary immune response*

**Antigenic challenge.** When an antigen is introduced into the body, it can trigger a wide or narrow spectrum of response mechanisms. The specific pattern of response depends on (1) the amount of antigen introduced, (2) the site of introduction, and (3) the type of antigen introduced.

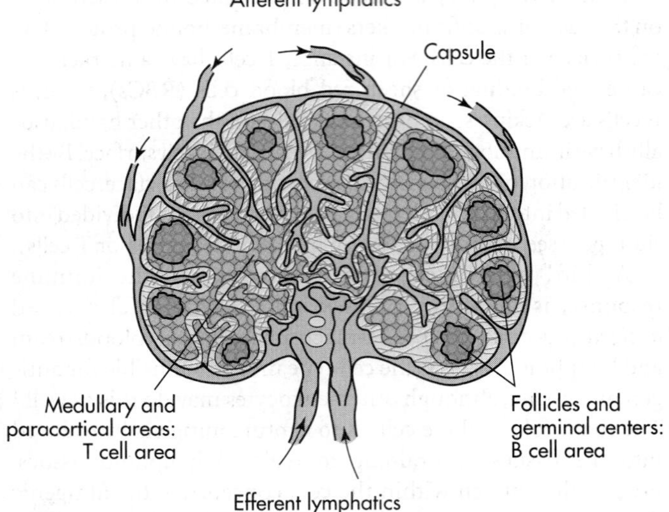


**fig. 10-11** B and T cell areas of lymph node.

Small amounts of a noninvasive, large, particulate antigen introduced at a single body site are quickly and efficiently handled at a local site with little or no systemic involvement beyond the local lymph node. Because the inflammatory response and local lymph node can localize the spread of the antigen, the immune response may go completely unnoticed by the host organism. Larger, particulate antigens are readily cleared, but small, soluble antigens are more difficult to clear from the circulation.

Large amounts of an antigen may allow the antigen to escape from the local site simply by overwhelming the local defense mechanisms. Even though the lymph nodes and MPS can clear 80% to 90% of an antigen on a single pass, if the amount of the antigen is extremely large, some antigen may escape the local site. An excessively large, sustained antigen dose can exhaust not only the local site but the entire MPS as well. This greatly reduces the body's ability to respond to even minor invasive challenges and renders the host vulnerable to secondary infections.

Highly invasive antigens (e.g., bacteria such as *S. aureus* or *S. pyogenes*) or those introduced directly into the bloodstream by blood transfusion, intravenous catheterization, or injection can immediately establish a systemic type of immune response. This is why extreme care must be exercised in the use of any type of medical procedure that would allow the introduction of antigens into the general circulation. The localization action of the immune response is critical to efficient functioning of the response.

**Antigenic processing and presentation.** When an antigenic substance is introduced into the body, either it is carried directly by lymphocytic circulation to a regional lymphoid tissue, where it is engulfed by an APC, or an APC engulfs the antigen at the site of introduction and carries the antigen to the lymphoid tissues. In the APC the complex antigen is degraded, and the antigenic determinants are attached to one of the cell membrane proteins on the APC known as

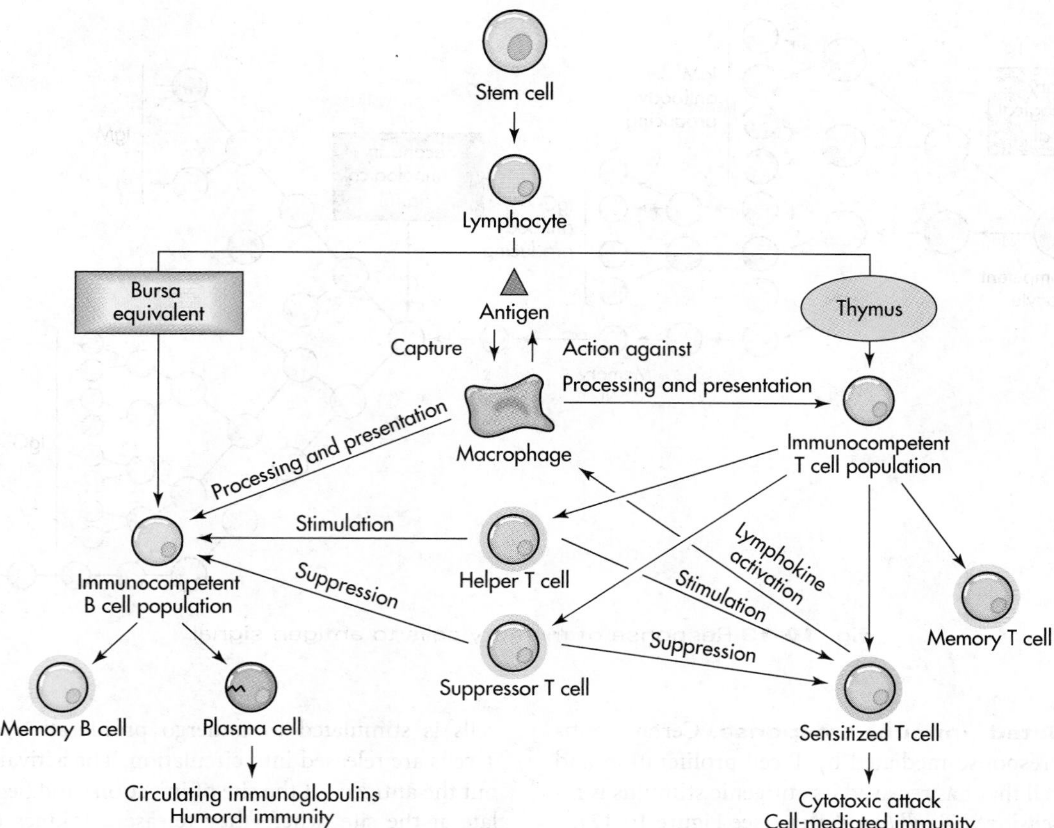


**fig. 10-12** Combined response of B and T cell systems.

a *major histocompatibility complex* (MHC) antigen on its surface. These same MHC antigens are the markers on the surface of the cell that allow recognition of self versus nonself cells (see Figure 10-2). The APC, with the concentrated antigenic determinants, then presents this antigenic signal to specifically reactive B or T cells in the regional lymph node. This is accomplished by a cell-to-cell contact. With this interaction the specific B or T cell is stimulated to undergo proliferation (cell division) and differentiation (change in structure and function). A soluble material known as interleukin 1 (IL-1) released from the APC signals the lymphocyte to divide and differentiate.

**Humoral response.** When the antigen is introduced for the first time, one of three basic mechanisms of response is elicited: (1) the humoral response; a response mediated primarily by B cells, (2) the CMI, a response in which the T cells are primarily involved, or (3) a combined type of response. If the antigen is the type that triggers a humoral response, the first time the body is exposed to the antigen, the B cell system responds with the synthesis of circulating immunoglobulins (Figure 10-12).

Antigen-specific B cells bear receptors to their surface, which allow them to recognize their antigenic stimulant. These receptors are the antigen-specific immunoglobulin molecules that the cell is programmed to produce. They are embedded in the membrane by the Fc region of the monomer with their antigen-binding sites extended out. Seemingly only a few lymphocytes within a lymph node have the ability to respond to the antigen. The stimulated B cell then begins a process of proliferation and differentiation. The progeny of the stimulated cell increases in number within the lymph node, forming *clones* of specifically adapted lymphocytes. With each generation of new cells within the clone, the lymphocytes become more differentiated toward a cell population ideally suited for the synthesis and release of immunoglobulin. These cells are known as *plasma cells.*

With the development of the plasma-cell population in the lymph node (several days after the introduction of the antigen), antibodies can be detected in the lymph node. It is not until about 7 days after the antigenic challenge, however, that detectable levels of specific antibodies appear in the serum. The plasma cell population of the lymph node and the levels of antibody in the blood continue to increase for another 2 to 3 weeks, and then both begin to retreat. Some of the lymphocytes of the activated clone become "memory cells," which are much more responsive, both in time of reaction and efficiency of antibody synthesis, to subsequent contact with the antigen (Figure 10-13).

Humoral immunity responds to antigens and foreign tissue. The humoral response serves to protect the body from such agents as microbial toxins, bacteria within the extravascular spaces in the blood and on mucosal surfaces, and viruses that must pass through the circulatory system to reach their site of infection (e.g., poliomyelitis virus).

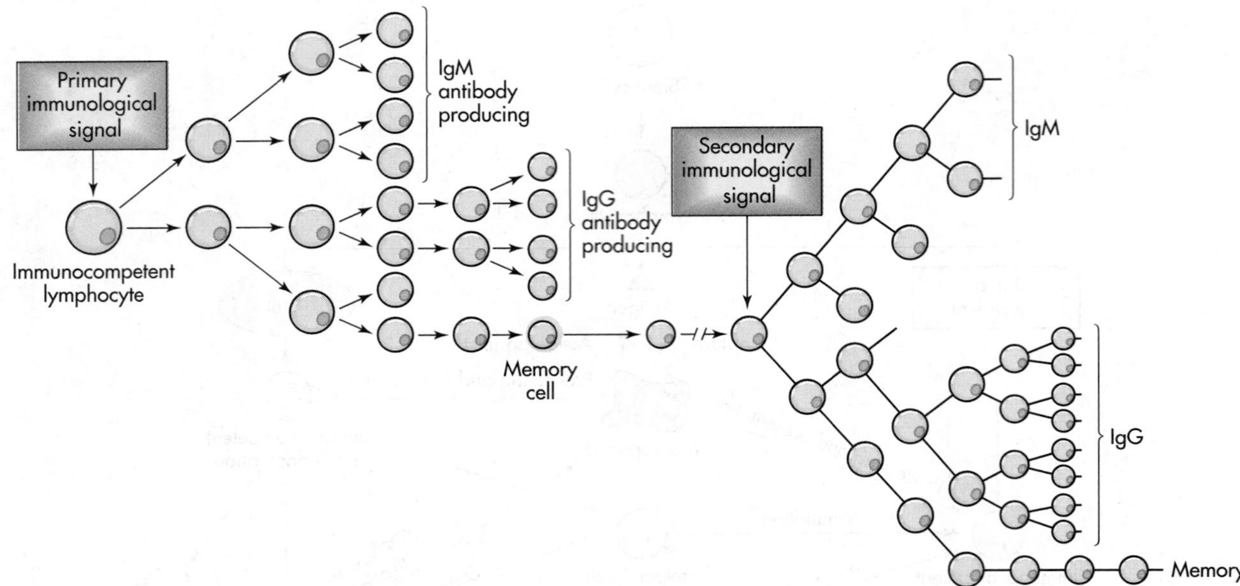


**fig. 10-13** Response of memory cells to antigen signal.

**Cell-mediated immune response.** Certain antigens trigger a response mediated by T cell proliferation and reaction. A T cell that has received its antigenic stimulus is referred to as a *sensitized T cell lymphocyte* (see Figure 10-12).

The initial steps of the CMI response—those involving the antigen processing by the macrophage, or APC—seem to be the same as those in the humoral response. After the presentation of the antigenic stimulus to lymph node T cells, proliferation in the T cell domain occurs. Circulating antibodies are not released; rather, sensitized lymphocytes are released into the circulation. These cells migrate to the site of the antigen's entrance into the body, where the invading agent or residual antigen is found. These activated lymphocytes, along with macrophages, infiltrate the regions of the tissue and begin a direct attack on the antigen or tissue cells labeled with the antigen. The T cells participating in this direct attack are known as *cytotoxic T cells.*

To amplify the site reaction further, the sensitized lymphocytes activate the nonspecific phagocytotic cells (macrophages, PMNs, and null cells) in the region of the antigen. This is accomplished through the release of the soluble cytokines (see Table 10-5), which marshal this additional cellular involvement to attack the antigenic materials.

The observable results of this attack of antigen-labeled tissues are classically illustrated by a positive tuberculin test reaction. In this case the inflammation (erythema, induration) observed at the site of the intradermal injection of a small amount of cell wall extract of *Mycobacterium tuberculosis* represents a T cell attack on the antigen-labeled cells. The positive test result is actually mediated by a secondary immune response (see following discussion) produced by prior exposure to *M. tuberculosis.* With the introduction of the antigen, it is engulfed, processed, and presented by the APC to responsive clones of T cells in the regional lymph node. That clone of cells is stimulated to undergo proliferation, and activated T cells are released into circulation. The activated T cells seek out the antigen (at the site of injection) and begin to accumulate at the site, where they release cytokines (lymphokines) that stimulate null cells and macrophages to attack the tissues at the focal site. The lag time (24 to 48 hours) required for the development of the inflammation at the site is consistent with the time needed to trigger the release of the responsive cells from the regional lymph node and to accumulate at the site of the antigen-labeled tissues.

The CMI response is especially effective in protection against diseases that grow and do their damage intracellularly, where the circulating immunoglobulins cannot reach them. Diseases of this type include viral and rickettsial diseases and those produced by certain chronic types of infective agents, the most outstanding of which are fungal pathogens and tubercle bacillus. One other important function of this system is the provision of cancer cell surveillance.

**Combined immune response.** Most antigens do not cause a purely humoral or purely CMI response; rather, both types of response are evoked. Likewise, our protection against most harmful antigens is the result of both these specific response systems being brought to bear on the antigen involved. In the combined type of response an initial perturbation occurs within the T cell areas of the lymph node. This becomes obvious within about 2 days after the introduction of the antigen. About 3 to 5 days later the B cell areas begin to proliferate.

**Control of immune response.** The production of a full immune response is, of necessity, under control systems. *Cytokines* are soluble protein mediators that induce and regulate various aspects of immunity. They act as hormones and are synthesized by a variety of cells: macrophages, neutrophils, eosinophils, monocytes, and T lymphocytes. These protein mediators have been called by various names as information about them was uncovered. Initially they were termed *lymphokines* when it was recognized that many of them were produced by activated T lymphocytes. When it was generally acknowledged that other cells secreted them as well, they were termed *cytokines*. An even more specific name, *interleukins,* recognizes that the major function of many of the cytokines is communication among various leukocytes. As many as 14 interleukins have been recognized, each with specific functions and structures.

Interleukin 1 is produced by macrophages when they come into contact with bacterial products, the helper T cell, or tumor necrosis factor. Interleukin1 is an endogenous pyrogen; it increases the proliferation of helper T cells, stimulates growth and differentiation of B lymphocytes, and induces the secretion of other interleukins. Interleukin 2 (IL-2) is produced by helper T cells; it increases the growth and differentiation of T lymphocytes and also stimulates increased production of more IL-2 from activated lymphocytes. In addition, it increases nonspecific cytotoxic functions in natural killer cells (lymphokine-activated killer cells). Interleukin 3 (IL-3), produced by helper T cells, stimulates production of immature bone marrow stem cells in the presence of infection. Interleukin 4 (IL-4) and interleukin 5 (IL-5) also are produced by helper T cells; IL-4 stimulates growth and proliferation of B lymphocytes, whereas IL-5 stimulates their differentiation into actively producing antibody cells. Interleukin 6 (IL-6), made by both macrophages and T cells, is thought to have antiviral and possibly antitumor effects. IL-6 stimulates the growth of activated B lymphocytes.

Some of these interleukins are called *colony-stimulating factors (CSFs)* because of their role in stimulating the growth and differentiation of myeloid precursors, including a subset of pluripotent stem cells in the bone marrow. Among the known CSFs are IL-1 (for B lymphocytes), IL-2 (for T lymphocytes), IL-3 (for pluripotent bone marrow cell), IL-4, IL-5, and IL-6 (for B lymphocytes), granulocyte macrophage CSF (for granulocytes and macrophages), granulocyte CSF (for granulocytes), and monocyte macrophage CSF (for mononuclear phagocytes). The potential for important clinical applications of such CSFs is obvious (see Table 10-5 for a summary of the major cytokines).

Another type of control is a nonspecific mechanism known as *antibody feedback,* by which the increasing level of circulating immunoglobulins serves as a negative force on the further synthesis of antibodies. In other words, if circulating immunoglobulin levels are elevated, it is more difficult to stimulate antibody production with further antigenic challenge. This has clinical significance in the case of abnormal antibody production by individuals suffering from gammopathies, such as multiple myeloma or macroglobulinemia (see Chapter 66). These diseases are marked by significant elevation of the gamma-globulin fraction of the blood and a seemingly paradoxic increased susceptibility to infection. The high levels of nonspecific gamma-globulin exert an immunosuppressive effect on further specific antibody synthesis when the host is challenged by a pathogen.

The immune response system also is controlled by the presence of specific regulator T cells. A subset of the T cell population of the body is known as *helper T cells* (designated $T_H$ or $T_4$ cells). The function of these cells is to cooperate with the B cells and T cells to allow the full expression of a B cell or T cell response. If a B cell clone required the aid of a helper T cell clone and the $T_H$ cell clone is missing, the B cell clone will not undergo proliferation and differentiation to form plasma cells that produce the specific immunoglobulin. On the other hand, the presence of *suppressor T cell* clones (designated $T_S$ or $T_8$ cells) prevents or suppresses the full development of the immunoresponsive clones (see Figure 10-12).

If for some reason the normal balance between immunoresponsive T or B cells and $T_S$ and $T_H$ cells is disrupted, control over proper immune response reactions may be lost. The classic example of this problem can be observed in acquired immunodeficiency syndrome (AIDS), in which a disproportionate ratio occurs in the number of $T_S$ ($T_8$) cells compared with $T_H$ ($T_4$) cells in peripheral circulation; this results from destruction of the $T_H$ cells caused by HIV infection. In other conditions, such as some autoimmune diseases, the loss of certain $T_S$ clones may allow the production of antibodies against self antigens.

#### Secondary immune response

As emphasized at the outset of this section, one of the touchstone characteristics of the specific response system is its ability to remember prior contact with an antigen and to provide a more rapid and efficient protective reaction on subsequent contact. The first contact between the immune response system and an antigen leads to the primary response, as just described. When antibody synthesis is measured in a primary response, there is significant lag time to the appearance of antibodies in the circulation (Figure 10-14). Immunoglobulins of the IgM class are the first to appear, but they maintain protective levels for only a short period. Specific IgG antibodies follow and reach protective levels within 12 to 14 days, but they also fall off fairly quickly with only this initial exposure. When the "primed" immune response system encounters the antigen again, a secondary response ensues, which is more rapid, of greater intensity, and longer lasting than the primary response. This secondary response is termed an *anamnestic response.* This "remembered" response is a characteristic of both the B and T cell systems. The prior contact with the antigen is stored in special memory cells of both cell lines. As illustrated in Figure 10-13, the memory cells respond immediately to the antigenic signal, so the lag time between exposure to the antigen and production of protective antibody levels is greatly reduced. This phenomenon provides the basis for active immunization and "booster" doses to maintain the protective levels of immunity. In an immunized person the memory cells elicit the rapid response in time for the immune system to overwhelm the pathogen or toxin before it can produce its damage. These memory cells are long-living lymphocytes, surviving and able to respond for years after their development.

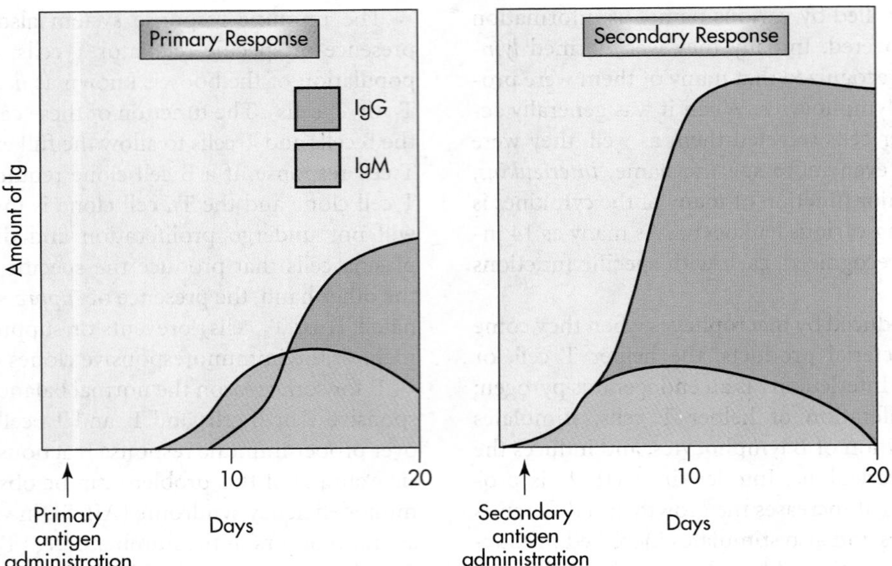


**fig. 10-14** Primary and secondary humoral responses.

## Immune Tolerance

*Immune tolerance* is defined as the state of immunological nonresponsiveness. By some mechanisms the body becomes tolerant to self while maintaining responsiveness to foreign materials. Evidence has established that self-tolerance is acquired primarily during embryonic development; however, the exact mechanisms by which it develops remain an issue. During fetal development the immune system is presented with antigens from the developing tissues. These become identified as self antigens; thus when exposed to these antigens postnatally, the individual is tolerant of them.

One proposed mechanism by which this state could be induced is known as the *clonal selection theory.* This theory states that when potentially responsive clones of B or T cells come into contact with an antigen prenatally, the responsive cell line is killed or controlled, thus eliminating the responsiveness to that antigen from the body. This produces a state of *natural tolerance.* This theory is supported by experimental data showing that, by exposing experimental animals to foreign antigens in utero, a tolerance to that antigen is developed; however, some antigens introduced in this manner are found to be more *tolerogenic* (capable of inducing tolerance) than others. Further, the clonal selection theory does not explain how it is possible to break tolerance in adults, as indicated in certain experimental studies or with certain autoimmune diseases (see Chapter 66). In some cases at least, tolerance is not caused by the total elimination of specifically reactive cells but by the blocking of expression or temporary inactivation of the responsive cells. The action of suppressor T cells or the failure of mobilization by helper T cells has been shown to play a significant role in maintaining the state of self-tolerance.

## Developmental Aspects of Immune Response

Lymphoid cells first appear in the fetus as stem cells in the fetal liver at about the end of the first trimester. The lymphoid tissues of the thymus also develop fairly early in the fetus. At birth, however, the lymph nodes and spleen are still underdeveloped, but T and B cell responsiveness is fully functional. The fetus is capable of some immune response if challenged by an in utero (within the uterus) infection, such as congenital syphilis or rubella. Unless the fetus has been exposed to a congenital infection, at birth the synthesized immunoglobulin levels of the neonate are low (Figure 10-15). The newborn has high levels of transplacentally acquired maternal IgG antibodies. These maternal antibodies have a half-life of about 30 days in the child; this, coupled with the increase in blood volume in the growing infant, leads to a drop in the IgG levels of the blood over the first 3 months. Thereafter the rate of the child's own synthesis of IgG provides for a steady increase in the immunoglobulin concentration within the serum. IgM levels reach adult concentrations by about age 9 months.

Numerous studies in both animals and humans have shown that during the aging process a progressive loss of immunological vigor occurs. The prime immunological age probably is achieved during the late adolescent years, when virtually the full complement of immunities has been developed and the responsiveness of the system peaks. The middle years are characterized by a plateau and slowly falling curve until the later years of life, when a sharp decline becomes evident. This decline is seen in both CMI and humoral response systems. This decrease in immunological sensitivity is associated with an increasingly less effective and more misdirected immune response. There is an increasing frequency of autoimmune disease, susceptibility to pathogenic and opportunistic microorganisms, and incidence of cancer.

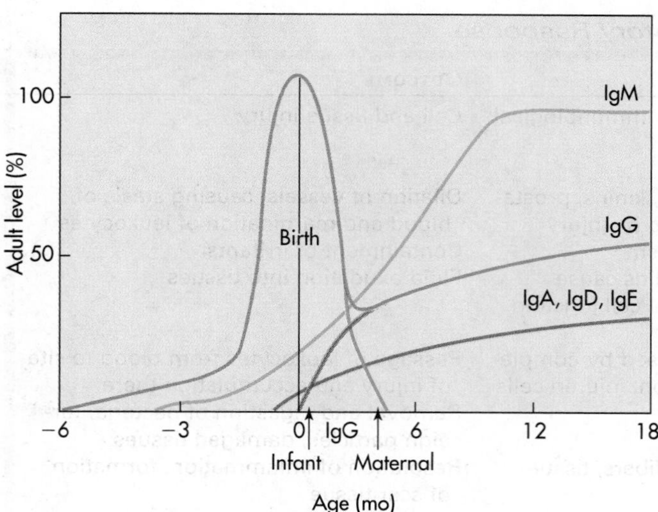


**fig. 10-15** Immunoglobulin levels in fetus and neonate.

### Neuroendocrine Factors Influencing Immune Response

The cells of the immune response system are influenced by and in turn influence the other regulatory communication systems in the body, that is, the endocrine and neural systems. The immune response cells have receptors on their surfaces to receive modifying input from hormones, such as insulin, growth hormone, glucocorticoids, estrogen, and testosterone. Some of these hormone signals (glucocorticosteroids, testosterone, estrogen, and progesterone) have been shown to depress immune function. Other hormones (growth hormone, thyroxine, and insulin) tend to improve immune function. Other neurotransmitters and hormones found in lower doses in the body also influence immune response cell function. The negative effects of the corticosteroids are so great that they are widely used as pharmacological agents to suppress immune function (see Chapters 66 and 68).

The thymus gland functions as an endocrine organ releasing hormones that influence not only immunoresponsive cells and lymphoid tissues but also other body cells that have receptors for these hormones. Interleukin 1 and other cytokines have been shown to stimulate glucococorticosteroid synthesis by influencing the pituitary gland to release adrenocorticotropic hormone. The thymus and lymphoid tissues receive direct innervation from autonomic and sensory neurons that control blood circulation to these organs and also seem to exercise more direct control over the immune response cells themselves.

The physiological control of the neuroendocrine function has long been recognized in the immunosuppressive effects produced by the stress response. Growing evidence suggests that this immunosuppression is also produced indirectly through neural signals to the immunoresponsive tissues.

These interconnections among the three major communication systems of the body has led to the development of the following concept: although many aspects of each system can be considered to stand alone, a broader, more holistic perspective views them as functioning as an interrelated complex. The term *psychoimmunoendocrine system* has been developed to reflect this more inclusive conceptualization. With this perspective in mind, psychotherapeutic methods and cognitive visualization have been increasingly used as adjunctive therapy in immune-related diseases and cancer. However, because most of the connections between these systems are fairly indirect and because our understanding of the control functions of each is still tenuous, these therapies should never be relied on as a primary approach. Also, some potential danger exists in leading patients to believe that they can exercise direct cognitive control over their pathological conditions. When they are not successful, patients may become disillusioned and lose hope, which then removes whatever positive aspects might be derived from the indirect betterment of their overall improved immune state. The emphasis should be on the general and broad improvement of their general immune state.

# PATHOPHYSIOLOGY

## INFLAMMATORY RESPONSE

When injury occurs in the body, all the nonspecific and, to some degree, the specific defense mechanisms are directed toward localizing the effects of the injury, protecting against microbial invasion at the site, and preparing the site for repair. This process is called *inflammation.*

The inflammatory response can be initiated by any type of injury: heat, cold, irradiation, chemicals, trauma, infection, immunological injury, or neoplasia. Whatever the stimulus, the response of the body is the same, but the extent of the involvement of the nonspecific response system's various facets depends on the degree and severity of the injury.

### Steps in the Response

Three major physiological responses occur during the inflammatory process: vascular response, fluid exudation, and cellular exudation (Table 10-6). The *vascular response* consists of a transitory vasoconstriction (stress response) followed immediately by vasodilation. This occurs as a result of chemical substances such as histamine or kinins released at the site of injury or invasion. The amount of blood flow to the area is thus increased (*hyperemia*), causing redness and heat. Blood flow slows as the capillaries dilate. Increased permeability of the capillary walls facilitates fluid and cellular exudation. The extra fluid in the tissues may act to dilute toxins and microorganisms that are in the area.[19]

*Fluid exudation* from the capillaries into the interstitial spaces begins immediately and is most active during the first 24 hours after injury or invasion. Initially the fluid exudate is primarily serous fluid, but as the capillary wall becomes more permeable, protein (albumin) is lost into the interstitial spaces. This increases the colloid osmotic pressure in these spaces, which encourages more fluid exudation. The swelling

**table 10-6** *Summary of the Steps in the Inflammatory Response*

| Steps | Mediators | Outcome |
|---|---|---|
| 1. Injury | Physical, chemical, biological, immunological stimulus | Cell and tissue injury |
| 2. Vascular response | | |
| a. Vascular dilation | Histamine, plasmin, serotonin, kinins, prostaglandins released or activated by injury | Dilation of vessels, causing stasis of blood and margination of leukocytes |
| b. Fibrin clot formation | Activation of clotting mechanism | Containment of irritants |
| 3. Fluid exudation | Histamine, kinins, prostaglandins cause opening of venule-endothelial cell junction | Fluid exudation into tissues |
| 4. Cellular exudation | | |
| a. Leukocyte exudation | Chemotactic substances released by complement activation, clot formation, injured cells | Passage of leukocytes from blood to site of injury and accumulation there |
| b. Attack and engulfment of foreign materials | Neutrophils, macrophages | Removal and digestion of bacteria, foreign particles, damaged tissues |
| 5. Healing | Fibroblasts produce collagen fibers, tissue regeneration | Resolution of inflammation, formation of scar tissue |

of the tissue from the fluid in the interstitial spaces is called *edema.*

*Cellular exudation* refers to the migration of WBCs (leukocytes) through the capillary walls into the affected tissue. An increased number of WBCs are attracted to the vessels in the affected area as a result of chemotactic substances being released from the tissues by cell injury and complement activation. The WBCs adhere to the capillary wall and then pass in ameboid fashion through the widened endothelial junctions of the capillary wall. Neutrophils (PMNs), which make up about 60% of the circulating WBCs, are the first leukocytes to respond, usually within the first few hours. The neutrophils ingest the bacteria and dead tissue cells (phagocytosis); then they die, releasing proteolytic enzymes that liquefy the dead neutrophils, dead bacteria, and other dead cells (pus). Monocytes and lymphocytes appear later. The macrophages continue the phagocytosis, and the lymphocytes play a role in the antigen-antibody response at the site.

## Local Manifestations of Inflammation

The five cardinal symptoms of inflammation were identified many centuries ago. These are redness (*rubor*) and heat (*calor*) caused by the hyperemia, swelling (*tumor*) caused by the fluid exudate, pain (*dolor*) caused by the pressure of the fluid exudate and by chemical (bradykinin and prostaglandins) irritation of the nerve endings, and *loss of function* of the affected part caused by the swelling and pain.

The inflammatory response prepares the tissue for healing and contains the spread of bacterial invasion. To prevent the spread of bacteria, fibroblasts are attracted to the area and secrete fibrin, a threadlike substance that encircles the affected area to wall it off from healthy tissue. If interference occurs with this walling-off process, bacteria can spread into the surrounding tissue. This explains why an abscess should not be incised and drained until it has "come to a head" or until the walling-off process is completed.

## Regional Lymph Node Manifestations

Bacteria may fail to be contained locally and may spread to other parts of the body by means of the lymph system or bloodstream. If picked up by the lymph stream, the bacteria will be carried to the nearest lymph node. These nodes are located along the course of all lymph channels, and bacteria can be ingested and destroyed here as well. If the bacteria are virulent enough to resist the action of the lymph nodes, leukocytes are brought in by the bloodstream to attack and engulf the bacteria in the node. The node then becomes swollen and tender because of the accumulation of phagocytes, bacteria, and destroyed lymphoid tissue. This is known as *lymphadenitis.* Swollen lymph nodes can be palpated primarily in the neck, axilla, and groin.

## Systemic Manifestations

Moderate to severe inflammatory responses can produce generalized systemic manifestations. The three major manifestations are (1) increase in body temperature (fever), (2) increase in WBCs in peripheral circulation (leukocytosis), and (3) increased erythrocyte sedimentation rate (ESR).

Fever is produced by the release of substances known as *endogenous pyrogens* at the inflammatory site. These pyrogens come from injured cells, materials released by WBCs that accumulate at the site, and components of the bacterial cell wall. The pyrogens include prostaglandins, leukotrienes, bacterial endotoxins, and interleukin 1. The substances are carried to the temperature-regulating center in the hypothalamic region of the brain, where they signal a resetting of the body temperature set-point. The body responds by increasing heat production and decreasing heat loss. As long as the pyrogens remain in circulation, the set-point will be elevated. The fever response is designed as part of the defense mechanism and helps increase production of antimicrobial agents such as interferon. It also tends to support increased phagocytic activity of some cells, including fixed and wandering macrophages.

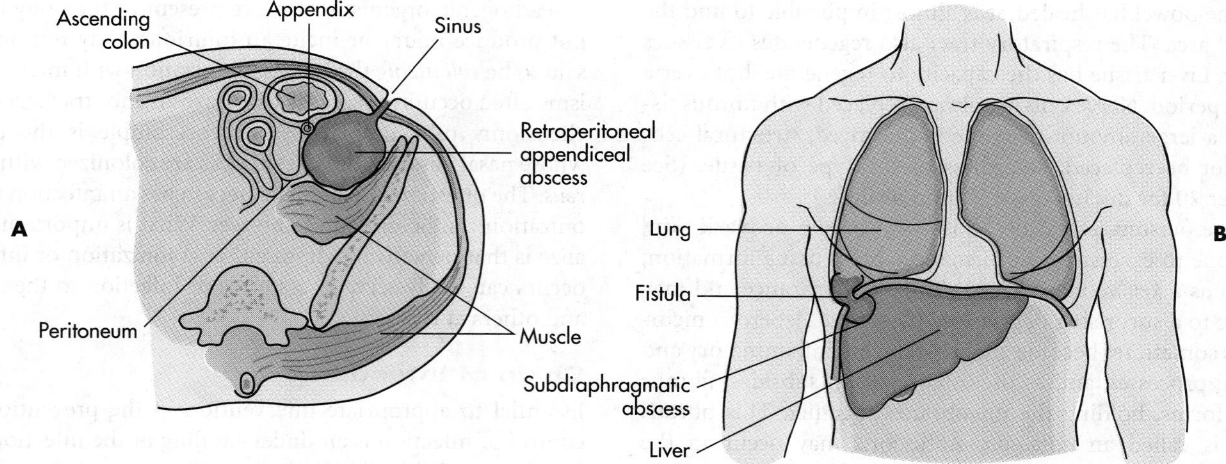


**fig. 10-16 A,** Cross section of torso showing appendiceal abscess with sinus that has developed through abdominal wall. **B,** Subdiaphragmatical abscess that has developed fistula opening into pleural cavity.

Leukocytosis develops when agents released from damaged cells and WBCs accumulating at the inflammatory site are carried by the circulation to the bone marrow, where WBCs are produced. These agents are known as *leukopoietins.* When these agents reach the bone marrow, they signal the release of mature neutrophils held in reserve there. This leads to an immediate rise in the WBC count in the peripheral circulation to greater than 10,000 $mm^3$. The chemotactic agents draw these cells to the inflammatory site. Leukopoietins also increase the production of WBCs in the bone marrow. With prolonged inflammation the bone marrow stores of WBCs are depleted, and the synthesis of mature WBCs may not be able to keep pace with the needs of the inflammatory site; thus the marrow releases more immature neutrophils as the inflammation continues. These less mature cells, known as *bands,* become more prevalent in the peripheral circulation and indicate a significant ongoing inflammation. The condition sometimes is referred to as a "shift to the left." This clinical phrase was derived from the past clinical laboratory method of counting the less mature cells and tabulating them in the left-hand columns of differential count forms.

With inflammation an increased blood sedimentation rate also occurs; that is, when an anticoagulant is added to the blood in the laboratory, the RBCs (erythrocytes) settle to the bottom of a test tube more rapidly than normal. This increase in the erythrocyte sedimentation rate (ESR) is believed to be caused by an increase in fibrinogen, a blood protein essential to the healing process. The ESR is elevated during the acute inflammatory stage of infection, which indicates that the body's defense mechanisms for the repair of damaged tissue are operating.

Inflammations can be classified as acute or chronic. *Acute* inflammations are characterized by a sudden onset and an increase in the fluid exudative response. *Chronic* inflammations have a slower, more insidious onset and are characterized by increased cellular exudation.

Knowledge of the physiological changes that occur during the inflammatory process helps the nurse understand the changes that occur in a variety of diseases. For example, whenever cells die as a result of injury or disease (*necrosis*), such as during a myocardial infarction, the inflammatory process occurs. Fat deposits (*atheromas*) on blood vessel walls cause injury to the lining of the vessel wall and initiate an inflammatory response. Irritation of the peritoneum by trauma or bacterial invasion can cause inflammation of the peritoneum (*peritonitis*).

## Repair and Healing

No healing will occur until inflammation has subsided and pus and dead tissue have been removed. Pus is a local accumulation of dead phagocytes, dead bacteria, and dead tissue. The bacteria most frequently causing this reaction are staphylococci, streptococci, *Neisseria* organisms, and *Pseudomonas aeruginosa* (*Pseudomonas pyocyanea*). A collection of pus that is localized by a zone of inflamed tissue is called an *abscess* (Figure 10-16). An inflammation that involves cellular or connective tissue is called *cellulitis.* When the tissues affected by inflammation produce a fluid that has a low content of cell protein or other solid materials, it is known as a *transudate.* By contrast, an *exudate* is produced when the material produced by the affected tissue contains a high concentration of cell protein or other solid material. An inflammation in which pus collects in a preexisting cavity such as the pleura or gallbladder is called *empyema.* When infection forms an abscess within the body, develops a suppurating channel, and ruptures onto the surface or into a body cavity, it is called a *sinus.* If the infection forms a tubelike passage from an epithelium-lined organ or normal body cavity to the surface or to another organ or cavity, it is called a *fistula.*

After the infected area is clean, new cells are produced to fill in the space left by the injury. They may be the normal structural cells, or they may be fibrotic tissue cells known as *scar tissue.* If they are fibrotic cells, they will not function as the cells functioned formerly but only serve to fill in the injured area. Some body cells readily regenerate; for instance, after the bowel has healed, it is almost impossible to find the injured area. The respiratory tract also regenerates its tissues readily. Liver tissue has the capacity to regenerate, but over a longer period. Nerve cells are always replaced with fibrous tissue. If a large amount of tissue is destroyed, structural cells may not be replaced, regardless of the type of tissue. (See Chapter 20 for discussion of wound healing.)

Some persons, especially those with brown or black skin, are prone to excessive scar formation. Such tissue formation, known as a *keloid,* is hard and shiny in appearance and may enlarge to a surprising degree (see Chapter 62). Serous membranes sometimes become adherent during inflammatory and healing processes, and as the inflammation subsides, fibrous tissue forms, holding the membranes together. This fibrous tissue is called an *adhesion.* Adhesions may occur in the pleura, in the pericardium, about the pelvic organs, and in many other parts of the body. They often occur in and around the intestinal tract, where they may cause an obstruction.

Instead of healing, necrosis (death of the tissue) may occur. Bacteria, both pathogens and nonpathogens, often invade the necrotic tissue and cause decomposition, which is called *gangrene.* The body defenses are useless in preventing or curing gangrene because no blood can get to the area. Gangrenous tissue must be completely removed before healing can occur.

## INFECTIOUS DISEASE PROCESS

A *pathogen* is a microorganism or substance that is capable of producing disease. This discussion is concerned with microorganisms as pathogens. Factors that affect the microorganism's *pathogenicity,* or capacity to infect and produce disease, are listed in Box 10-1. The degree of pathogenicity or a microorganism to invade the host tissue can cause harm is referred to as its *virulence.*

*Infection* is the presence in the body of a pathogen that multiplies and produces effects that are injurious to the host. This injury may result from the presence and spread of the microorganism through the body tissues, known as the pathogen's *invasiveness,* or from the effects on the body of toxins produced by the microorganism, known as its *toxigenicity.* Some organisms, such as pneumococci, are highly invasive and virtually nontoxigenic, whereas others, such as *Clostridium tetani,* present the other extreme of high toxicity but low invasiveness. An infection may be *apparent,* thus causing clinical signs and symptoms, or *inapparent,* in which no perceivable clinical or subclinical signs or symptoms are present (asymptomatic).

**box 10-1** *Factors Affecting Pathogenicity of a Microorganism*

- Ability to live and multiply outside its host
- Virulence
- Host specificity
- Resistance of the host

Pathogenic organisms that are present in the body but do not produce injury or incite an injurious body response are said to be *colonizing* the body. Colonization with microorganisms often occurs in patients who have an endotracheal or tracheostomy tube in place. Another example is the person whose nasal passages or skin surfaces are colonized with *S. aureus.* The question of whether a person has an infection or colonization can be difficult to answer. What is important to realize is that persons in whom either colonization or infection occurs can easily serve as a source of infection to themselves and others at risk.

### Chain of Infection

Essential to appropriate intervention in the prevention and control of infection is an understanding of the infectious disease process. With all infectious diseases, a common sequence of events occurs (Figure 10-17).

First, a causative agent, or pathogen, must exist. This can be a bacterium, virus, fungus, rickettsial organism, protozoa, or helminth (worm). Second, there must be a reservoir where the agent can be found. The reservoir can be animate (human or animal) or inanimate (soil, water, intravenous solutions, equipment, and so on). Human reservoirs can be asymptomatic carriers or persons with an acute clinical infection or colonization. Carriers can (1) be incubating the agent before the onset of signs and symptoms, (2) have a subclinical infection, (3) be in the convalescent stage of an infection, or (4) be chronic carriers of the agent. Viral hepatitis B is an example of an infectious disease that can be transmitted by human carriers in all these stages. Often the reservoir of an agent responsible for an outbreak of an infection is not readily apparent and may never be identified. If the process of infection is well understood, however, appropriate and effective control measures can be instituted, even though the original source of the causative agent is not known.

The agent must have a means of exit from the reservoir. If the reservoir is human, the exit can be (1) the respiratory tract, (2) the GI tract, (3) the genitourinary tract, (4) open lesions on the skin, or (5) across the placenta.

Once the agent has left the reservoir, it needs a mode of transmission to a host. Transmission can be by direct contact, by airborne vehicle, or by vectors. *Contact transmission* includes direct, indirect, or droplet contact. *Direct contact transmission* occurs when there is spread of infection from the source to the host without the presence of an intermediate object. This happens when there is physical contact with or skin shedding onto the host. Gonorrhea is an example of a disease transmitted by direct contact.

*Indirect contact transmission* has an intermediate object between the source and the host. This intermediary can be the contaminated hands of a person who has had contact with an infected source and then touches a susceptible host without washing the hands. An inanimate object that has been contaminated by an infectious source is known as a *fomite.* Bed linen, respiratory therapy equipment, tissues, and silverware are examples of fomites that can be responsible for the indirect transmission of an infectious agent.

*Droplet transmission* occurs when the infectious agent is expelled from the reservoir in the form of droplets, as happens with a sneeze or cough in the direction of a nearby recipient. These droplets do not become airborne but settle on surfaces about 3 to 4 feet from their source. Meningococcal meningitis and influenza are examples of diseases transmitted in this manner.

*Airborne transmission* occurs when the infectious agent expelled from the source remains suspended in the form of droplet nuclei or dust in the air. The agent is then inhaled by a host. These droplet nuclei are 1 to 5 $\mu m$ in size and are smaller than the droplets discussed in droplet transmission, and thus they can be carried by air currents. Chickenpox (varicella zoster) and tuberculosis are diseases that can be spread by this route.

*Common vehicle transmission* occurs when a contaminated inanimate vehicle acts as the intermediary for the infectious agent from the source to multiple hosts. Contaminated water, food, and intravenous fluids are common vehicles. Salmonellosis and hepatitis A are examples of diseases that can be transmitted in this way.

*Vector-borne transmission* occurs when there is an animate intermediary from the source to the recipient. For example, mosquitos are the intermediary in the transmission of malaria, and ticks serve as the intermediary in the spread of Rocky Mountain spotted fever and Lyme disease.

Once the infectious agent has been transmitted to a host, it must gain entry into the host. The portals of entry are similar to the modes of exit from the human reservoir mentioned previously and include the respiratory tract, the GI tract, the genitourinary tract, breaks in the skin or mucous membranes, and across the placenta.

The final step in the process after the inoculation of the host is the maturation and multiplication of the infectious agent. Entry of an infectious agent into a host does not mean that the agent will proliferate and cause infection. Infection depends on the agent's dose, the organism's virulence, and the host's susceptibility. The healthy human body is extremely resistant to infection; however, when the basic biological defense mechanisms of the body are compromised, an organism has a much greater chance of causing an infection. Chapter 65 deals with many biological defense factors exhibited by the host to prevent infection and injury. Some of the factors that affect host susceptibility to infection are (1) age (very young and very old persons being more susceptible), (2) immune status (certain disease states such as HIV infection, diabetes, cancer, or other chronic diseases can impair the immune status), (3) therapeutic treatments such as radiation and certain drugs, especially antibiotics, steroids, and chemotherapeutic agents, (4) surgery, (5) burns, (6) poor nutritional status, and (7) invasive procedures (intravenous catheters, chest tubes, urinary catheters) that break through the normal external defense barriers.

From this discussion of the infectious disease process, it becomes evident that no one factor is responsible for an infection. Rather, variables such as the agent, the environment, and

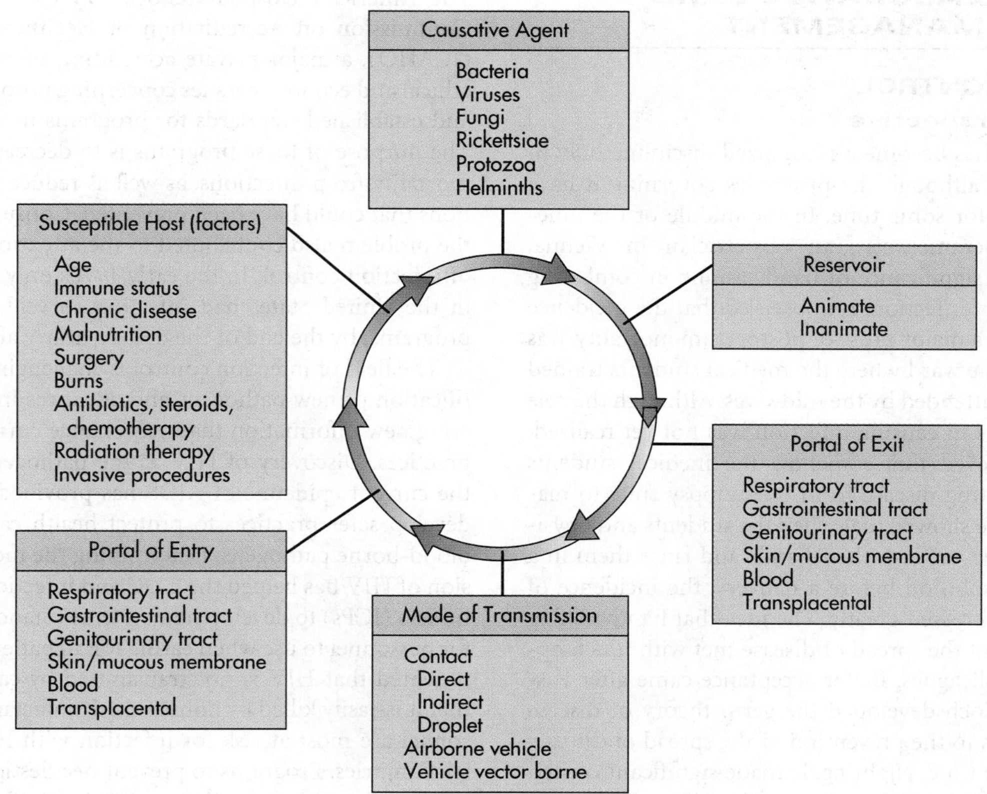


**fig. 10-17** The infectious disease process.

the host determine the outcome. To be able to intervene effectively in the disease process, it is important that all these concepts be understood.

### Clinical Manifestations

Once a pathogen gains access to a susceptible host, a time known as the *incubation period* passes before the clinical symptoms of the disease appear. During this period the organism is establishing itself, spreading to target organs or tissues, and proliferating within various body sites. This incubation period varies depending on the condition of the host but is often predictable and diagnostically significant. The appearance of symptoms depends on the type of injury elicited by the virulent pathogen and the site of the organism within the body. The disease may be described as being *localized* (a focal point of symptoms or injury) or *generalized* (systemic involvement). The course of the disease may be *acute* or *chronic.* An acute disease often incites an immediate violent host response. The outcome of the infection (pathogen over host or host over pathogen) is determined within a relatively short time, as seen in mumps, plague, or smallpox. Conversely, in a chronic infection the pathogen establishes itself more insidiously within the host, does not cause immediate damage, and tends to provoke less of a host response, as in tuberculosis and aspergillosis. Although the terms *acute* and *chronic* are generally useful in describing the relationship between the host and a pathogen, many acute infections become chronic, and vice versa.

## COLLABORATIVE CARE MANAGEMENT

### INFECTION CONTROL

#### Historical Perspective

Infection control has become a recognized discipline only in the past 25 years, although the principles governing it have been in existence for some time. In the middle of the nineteenth century Semmelweiss, an obstetrician in Vienna, demonstrated the significance of handwashing in combating the transmission of infection. He observed that the incidence of puerperal fever, a major cause of postpartum mortality, was much higher on the ward where the medical students trained than on the ward attended by the midwives. Although the role of microorganisms in causing infection was not yet realized. Semmelweiss believed that somehow the medical students could be transmitting disease from the autopsy suite to maternity patients. He showed that when the students and physicians were required to wash their hands and rinse them in a chlorinated lime solution before a delivery, the incidence of puerperal fever decreased greatly. The idea that handwashing alone could prevent the spread of disease met with much opposition by his colleagues. Better acceptance came after Pasteur, Lister, and Koch developed the germ theory of disease and related asepsis to the prevention of the spread of disease. At about the same time, Nightingale made significant contributions to sanitation and isolation practices. From this evolved an era in which medical asepsis was practiced more by ritual than with true understanding of the specific principles on which it was based.

A turning point came during World War II, when the sulfonamides and penicillin were first used successfully to treat infections. As new antibiotics were developed, a false sense of security developed about infection control. It soon became apparent, however, that antibiotics were not the sole answer to infection control. Organisms once well controlled by antibiotics demonstrated the ability to develop resistant strains. In the late 1950s and the 1960s, outbreaks of penicillin-resistant *S. aureus* infections were common, and gram-negative organisms such as *Pseudomonas,* which were previously considered nonpathogenic (incapable of producing disease), were suddenly implicated as the cause of infections acquired in the hospital. Along with drug resistance and the emergence of newly recognized pathogens, the number of persons at risk of secondary infections increased. A longer life expectancy, the use of immunosuppressive agents, and an increase in the use of invasive procedures to diagnose and treat disease increased the risk of infection in certain persons.

The rise in hospital infections made it necessary to examine preventive and control measures, including a reemphasis on aseptic techniques. In 1970 an international conference to address the problem of hospital-acquired *(nosocomial)* infections was held in Atlanta. As a result, the Centers for Disease Control and Prevention (CDC) in Atlanta set forth guidelines for prevention and control of infections in hospitals. The CDC is constantly updating and revising its recommendations based on epidemiological studies and research findings. The American Hospital Association (AHA) and the Joint Commission on Accreditation of Healthcare Organizations (JCAHO), a major private accrediting agency, looked at the ethical and economic issues concerning nosocomial infections and established standards for programs in infection control. The purpose of these programs is to decrease morbidity and mortality from infections, as well as reduce the cost of infections that could have been prevented. Consumer awareness of the problem also contributed to the attention given the issue of infection control. In the early 1970s only 10% of hospitals in the United States had infection surveillance and control programs; by the end of the decade nearly all had them.

The field of infection control is challenging, with the identification of new pathogens and advances in research uncovering new information that may change current thinking and practices. Discovery of HIV as the pathogen responsible for the current epidemic of AIDS has provided the incentive to develop safer practices to protect health caregivers from all blood-borne pathogens. Determining the modes of transmission of HIV has helped the CDC and infection control practitioners (ICPs) to develop new systems (Standard Precautions) for personnel to use when caring for all patients. It is well documented that HIV is not transmitted by casual contact and that it is easily killed by household disinfectants. Hospital personnel are most at risk for infection with HIV from needlestick injuries. Programs to prevent needlestick injuries and to present factual information are essential. (See Chapter 67 for detailed information about HIV infection and AIDS.)

In the late 1980s and early 1990s, antimicrobial-resistant organisms became more prevalent in both the developing world and in hospitals in the United States.[8,17] Examples of such organisms include vancomycin-resistant enterococci and multidrug-resistant tuberculosis. Indiscriminate use of antibiotics and noncompliance with prescribed therapy are largely responsible for this situation. Unfortunately the high cost of drug research has impeded the development of new antibiotics. Nursing implications of the problem include adherence to infection control practices to prevent the spread of resistant organisms from patient to patient.

ICPs serve as a valuable resource as they interact with hospital departments, surveying for infections and teaching prevention and control. When a question or problem about infection control arises, the ICP should be contacted without hesitation. Questions may deal with clinical procedures, products for cleaning and disinfection, waste disposal, isolation systems, or personnel health issues.

All health care facilities should have infection control policies that address the issues of employee health and safety and patient care practices. Incorporated in these policies are Occupational Safety and Health Administration (OSHA) guidelines to protect health caregivers from exposure to bloodborne pathogens such as hepatitis B, hepatitis C, and HIV.[2]

This section presents an overview of the role of the nurse in the prevention and control of infection. For further information regarding a specific infectious disease, the reader should consult the chapter in which the site of the disease is discussed, for example, Chapter 37 for hepatitis or Chapter 32 for tuberculosis.

## INFECTION CONTROL IN THE COMMUNITY

An infectious disease is termed a *communicable disease* when it is highly transmissible to other persons. Smallpox is an example of a communicable disease that, through cooperative efforts worldwide, has been successfully eradicated.[4] The methods used to eradicate smallpox throughout the world can serve as a model of how to eliminate other communicable diseases. The eradication of smallpox also demonstrates the importance of accurate reporting of communicable diseases to the proper authorities so that appropriate prevention and control measures can be instituted.

Efforts are now under way to eliminate rubella and measles (rubeola) in the United States. Rubella vaccine was licensed in 1969, and since then widespread epidemics of rubella and congenital rubella syndrome have been successfully prevented. The continued occurrence of rubella in women of childbearing age has led to recommendations for immunization of both men and women in institutional settings such as hospitals and colleges to prevent outbreaks.

The original vaccine against rubeola licensed in 1963 was successful in reducing the incidence of measles by 99% until 1986. Since 1986 the outbreaks have increased, especially among unvaccinated preschool children and among vaccinated school-aged children and college students. Outbreaks in students vaccinated before 1978 to 1980 are thought to result from instability of the vaccine manufactured before 1980. Current recommendations are for a two-step vaccination for infants in inner-city areas (at 9 and 15 months) and for revaccination of students in outbreaks (if vaccinated before 15 months of age or before 1980). Many schools and colleges now require proof of immunization before enrollment.

On the international level the World Health Organization, a special agency of the United Nations, has as its primary purpose the improvement and standardization of measures to prevent and control disease throughout the world. Its Epidemiological Intelligence Service in Geneva receives immediate notification of large-scale outbreaks of infectious diseases throughout the world and advises the world community of impending epidemics. *The Weekly Epidemiological Record* is an official publication of the agency.

On the national level, the CDC is responsible for programs for the prevention and control of communicable and other preventable disease in the United States. The CDC provides epidemiological and laboratory services to state health facilities on request. It enforces quarantine regulations and conducts foreign quarantine activities; administers international activities for the control of malaria, smallpox, and measles; and provides consultation to other nations in the control of preventable diseases. It also collects, tabulates, and assesses data on reportable diseases from state health departments and publishes the findings in the *Morbidity and Mortality Weekly Report (MMWR)*. Through its continuous surveillance, the CDC is able to detect new cases of diseases and intervene to control disease outbreaks. In addition, the CDC is instrumental in providing guidelines and recommendations for infection control.

The Hospital Infection Control Practices Committee (HICPAC) was established in 1991 to provide guidance to the CDC regarding the practice of hospital infection control, strategic surveillance, and prevention and control of nosocomial infection in U.S. hospitals. HICPAC also advises the CDC regarding updating of guidelines and other policy statements concerning prevention of nosocomial infection.

In the United States the control of infectious diseases is the responsibility of each state. State health officers usually delegate this responsibility to a division of communicable diseases. A staff of physicians, nurses, veterinarians, and sanitary engineers works closely with a state epidemiologist in detection, assessment, and control of specific reportable diseases.

Local public health departments work in conjunction with their state health departments in this effort. The community health nurse plays a vital role in the collection of data, surveillance activities, immunization programs, education, and other control measures. Physicians and health care facilities have a responsibility to report communicable diseases promptly to the health department. Health agencies in the community can use the reported data to determine potential or real problems, identify the causative agent and hopefully its source, and identify the population at risk. A method to control the problem, care for those exposed, and protect the population at risk can then be devised and implemented.

## Prevention and Control Measures

### Environmental

One method of prevention and control of disease in the community involves environmental control measures such as sanitation techniques that ensure a pure water supply and proper disposal of sewage and other potentially infectious materials. These measures have been legislated into building codes, state laws, and federal regulations. Similarly, regulations address health practices in institutions that handle, package, and prepare foods. Another environmental control measure is spraying a designated area to kill mosquitos, which are implicated in the spread of viral encephalitis. Spraying usually is done only after an outbreak has been identified.

Depending on the communicable disease, care of exposed persons and protection of the population at risk for contracting the disease may entail prophylaxis, immunization, or only careful monitoring of new cases. Often, simple adherence to basic principles of hygiene is sufficient. Determination of additional required measures should be made by the local or state health department. Attempts are made to reach those at risk and inform them of the preventive measures. Education of the public is a key component of these efforts.

### Immunization programs

In the United States a marked reduction has occurred in the incidence of infectious diseases that can be prevented by immunization. Because of accessibility and cost, however, there has been a decline in the number of children being immunized. In addition, many persons are concerned that federal monies used to support local immunization efforts have been reduced to such a level that free immunizations are no longer equally available in all 50 states. In 1993 President Clinton requested additional funds for the immunization program. Infections formerly seen only in children are now occurring more frequently in adults because of the failure of the population to develop acquired immunity during early childhood.

Because of air travel, a more recent concern is the elimination of the barriers of time and distance. Thus a person with an infectious disease may be brought from a remote area of the world to a major population center where the disease can be readily spread to a susceptible public.

## Susceptibility and Immunity

The objective of the biological defense mechanisms is to provide the host with protection. The ultimate protection would be total resistance to encroachment or damage by an organism or agent; this usually is termed *absolute immunity.* Absence of such protective barriers is called *susceptibility.* Although these terms generally are applied to immunity from infectious organisms, they can be used to describe the relative susceptibility to encroachment by an external agent. As described earlier, nonspecific immunity, or innate immunity, is provided when the external and internal nonspecific defense mechanisms serve as the barrier excluding or destroying the invading agent. Specific immunity protects against a single, unique agent through the development of specific antibodies or responsive cells in the body. It is acquired from prior contact with the agent (antigen) or through the introduction of specifically protective antibodies or cells into the body.

The acquisition of specific immunity may result from a natural encounter or artificial introduction. Immunity acquired naturally results from natural conditions such as recovery from a disease. Immunity acquired artificially means that the antigen or protective antibodies were purposely introduced into the body by vaccination. The immunity may be active or passive. When an individual is producing the antibodies within the body, the immunity is termed *active.* When an individual receives the protective antibodies from some other source, the immunity is termed *passive.* Thus, when antibodies are transferred from the mother across the placenta, the child is said to have a natural passive immunity. When a vaccine is given so that antibodies are produced within the body, the immunized person is characterized as having an artificial active immunity. Table 10-7 summarizes the different types of acquired specific immunities.

Specific or nonspecific immunity to harmful agents is a relative state. The effects of different dosages of an infectious organism or the toxic products of such organisms in experimental studies clearly demonstrate that administration of sufficiently large numbers of an organism or high dosages of a toxin can overwhelm even the most highly immunized animal. Further, when the normal mechanisms of defense are breached, even in the highly resistant host, disease can result. Thus acquired immunity to infection is not always an absolute condition but depends on many complex variables. These include not only the defense mechanisms of the host but also the dosage, route of contact, and virulence of the harmful agent.

If 90% of the population is protected against organisms that require continued passage through humans to reproduce and live, the disease caused by the organism can be virtually eliminated because there are too few susceptible hosts for organism spread. Smallpox has been eliminated from the world in this way. This type of group protection is called *herd immunity*. It is ineffectual, however, against organisms such as tetanus bacilli that can exist indefinitely (in the soil), and in this instance each person must be immunized to be protected. If the disease is not prevalent in the environment, such as diphtheria in the United States, or is not spread from person to person by direct contact, such as tetanus, the inoculation must be repeated at regular intervals to maintain protection. This inoculation is called a *booster dose*, and usually one tenth of the original inoculating dose is sufficient.

An inoculation often causes a local tissue response. Symptoms of inflammation (redness, tenderness, swelling, and sometimes ulcerations) appear at the site of the injection, and symptoms of widespread tissue involvement (slight febrile reactions, general malaise, and muscle aching) for 1 or 2 days are common. The initial inoculation produces delayed symptoms because the immune response system must become sensitized to the antigen. Usually an accelerated, less severe systemic reaction to subsequent inoculations occurs be-

**table 10-7** *Types of Acquired Specific Immunity*

| Type of Immunity | Acquisition of Immunity | Protection | Examples |
|---|---|---|---|
| **ACTIVE** | | | |
| Antibodies synthesized by body in response to antigenic stimulation | *Natural:* natural contact with antigen through clinical or subclinical case | *Development:* develops slowly; protective levels reached in a few weeks<br>*Duration:* long-term; often lifetime<br>*Spectrum:* specific to antigen contacted | Recovery from childhood diseases (e.g., chickenpox, measles, mumps) |
| | *Artificial:* immunization with antigen | *Development:* develops slowly; protective levels reached in a few weeks<br>*Duration:* several years; extended protection with "booster" doses<br>*Spectrum:* specific to antigen immunized against | Immunization with live or killed vaccines; toxoid immunization |
| **PASSIVE** | | | |
| Antibodies produced in one individual transferred to another | *Natural:* transplacental and colostrum transfer from mother to child | *Development:* immediate<br>*Duration:* temporary; several months<br>*Spectrum:* all antigens that mother has immunity to | Maternal immunoglobulins in neonate |
| | *Artificial:* injection of serum from immune human or animal | *Development:* immediate<br>*Duration:* temporary; several weeks<br>*Spectrum:* all antigens that source has immunity to | Injection of pooled human gamma-globulin; injection of animal hyperimmune sera |

cause the immune response is stimulated at once. The local reaction also is less severe than that after the initial inoculation because the organisms have less opportunity to produce inflammation.

Recommendations concerning current immunization schedules are found in *Morbidity and Mortality Weekly Reports,* which presents recommendations of the U.S. Public Health Service's Advisory Committee on Immunization Practices (ACIP). The reader should refer to this resource when questions arise about proper immunization practices, prophylaxis, interruption in immunization schedules, or adverse reactions and side effects. The ACIP recommends that all children be immunized against diphtheria, pertussis (whooping cough), tetanus, mumps, rubella, poliomyelitis, measles, *Haemophilus influenzae,* and hepatitis B.

### Primary Immunization Schedules

The immunization schedule for diphtheria, pertussis, tetanus (DPT) begins with one dose of combined toxoid and vaccine when an infant is 6 weeks to 2 months old (Table 10-8). The next two doses are given at 4- to 8-week intervals thereafter. The fourth dose is administered 6-12 months after the third dose. This schedule maintains adequate antibody levels until the child enters kindergarten, when a booster immunization is given. Thereafter, booster doses of tetanus and diphtheria are given only every 10 years (Table 10-8).

Oral poliovirus vaccine (OPV), trivalent, is a live vaccine containing all three strains of poliomyelitis virus. OPV is the vaccine recommended for infants and children. Inactivated poliovirus vaccine (IPV) is preferred after age 18 years. IPV is also preferred for immunocompromised persons and their household contacts because it eliminates the theoretical risk to the vaccinee and prevents the spread of vaccine virus to immunocompromised persons. The primary series of OPV consists of three doses. The first usually is given at the same time the DPT series is begun (6 to 12 weeks of age). The next dose is administered 6 to 8 weeks later, and the third dose at any time from 6 to 18 months of age. A fourth dose is given just before entry into school.

A single dose of measles, mumps, rubella (MMR) virus vaccine, live, is given when the child is 12 to 15 months old. A second dose of MMR is given at age 4 to 6 years or 11 to 12 years. As mentioned previously, in urban outbreaks the first dose of monovalent measles vaccine, a live attenuated vaccine, may be given at age 9 months, followed by a dose of MMR at 15 months. Children who have not been vaccinated as infants can be vaccinated at any age.

Mumps vaccine, live attenuated, should not be administered before 12 months of age because of the persistence of maternal antibodies, which may interfere with seroconversion. Mumps vaccine usually is given in a combined vaccine with measles and rubella (MMR) at 15 months of age. All susceptible children, adolescents, and adults should be vaccinated.

As previously discussed, most cases of measles are now seen in young adults, whereas before the vaccine became available in 1969, most cases occurred in school-aged children.

**table 10-8** *Recommended Schedule for Active Immunization of Normal Infants and Children**

| RECOMMENDED AGE | VACCINE | COMMENTS |
|---|---|---|
| Birth | HB vaccine No. 1 | |
| 2 mo | DTP No. 1, OPV No. 1<br>Hib No. 1,<br>HB vaccine No. 2 | Can be given earlier in endemic areas |
| 4 mo | DTP No. 2, OPV No. 2<br>Hib No. 2 | 6-wk to 2-mo interval desired between OPV doses |
| 6 mo | DTP No. 3, Hib No. 3<br>HB vaccine No. 3, OPV No. 3 | OPV No. 3 may be given at 6-18 mo |
| 12-15 mo | MMR, DTP No. 4, Hib booster | Completion of primary series |
| 4-6 yr | DTP No. 5, OPV No. 4, MMR | At or before school entry |
| 11-16 yr | Td† | Repeat every 10 yr throughout life; MMR No. 2 may be given at age 11-12 yr |

Data from *MMWR* 44(RR-5):2, 1995.
*HB,* Hepatitis B vaccine; *DTP,* diphtheria, tetanus, pertussis; *OPV,* oral polio vaccine; *Hib,* vaccine composed of *Haemophilus* b conjugate; *MMR,* measles, mumps, rubella.
*See individual ACIP recommendations for details.
†Tetanus and diphtheria toxoids, adsorbed (for use in persons aged 7 years and older); contains same amount of tetanus toxoid as DTP or DT but a reduced dose of diphtheria toxoid.

Women in childbearing years should be tested for rubella antibodies if they cannot document immunization, because rubella infection in the first trimester of pregnancy is associated with neonatal morbidity and mortality (congenital rubella syndrome). If antibodies are not present, vaccination is recommended. Because of the theoretic risk to the fetus, women of childbearing age are vaccinated only if they are not pregnant, and they are counseled not to become pregnant for 3 months after vaccination.

Administration of *H. influenzae* b (Hib) vaccine conjugate is recommended at 2, 4, and 6 months of age. A booster dose is recommended at 12 to 15 months.

Varicella vaccine was introduced in 1995. It is recommended for susceptible adolescents and adults (especially health care workers), as well as for children between 12 and 18 months of age. The need for boosters and the potential for developing herpes zoster in old age remain unanswered questions.

Routine vaccination against smallpox is no longer recommended by the U.S. Public Health Service because the side effects and complications of the vaccine are greater than the danger of acquiring the disease. The vaccine is indicated only for laboratory workers who are directly involved with smallpox or closely related orthopox viruses. At present, immunization against typhoid fever is recommended only when exposure to a typhoid carrier occurs in the household, when an outbreak of typhoid occurs in a community, or when a person travels to countries where typhoid is endemic (always present). Immunization to protect against other diseases is given on a selective basis; that is, only groups at a high risk are immunized.

### Adult vaccination

Establishing a routine vaccination status assessment at age 50 links vaccination with other established preventive measures. In the United States tetanus is a disease of older adults. Primary or booster administration of tetanus and diphtheria toxoids is recommended at this age.[9]

Because of the prevalence of influenza and its potential for causing death, the ACIP recommends immunization against influenza for all persons at increased risk of adverse consequences from infection of the lower respiratory tract. This includes all persons older than 65 years of age and those more than 6 months of age who because of age or underlying medical conditions are at increased risk for complications of influenza. Health care workers should also be immunized. Protection is obtained by giving an injection of influenza vaccine beginning in October. Infants and children up to 9 years old who are at risk are given a subvirion (split-virus) vaccine in two doses 4 weeks apart. A yearly booster dose is needed to maintain and update immunity. Persons who are allergic to eggs or egg products should not be immunized because of the danger of hypersensitivity reactions.

The current pneumococcal vaccine is a 23-valent polysaccharide vaccine licensed in 1983. It is recommended for adults and children 2 years of age and older with chronic illness who are at increased risk for pneumococcal disease or its complications. It also is recommended for adults older than 65 years of age who are otherwise healthy and for persons of any age with asymptomatic or symptomatic HIV infection. In general, revaccination of persons who received the previous 14-valent vaccine is recommended. Hepatitis A vaccine was introduced in 1995. Vaccination of persons at risk, e.g., drug users, travelers to areas where hepatitis A is endemic, persons with multiple sexual partners or homosexual men, and day care workers, is recommended.

Table 10-9 summarizes various vaccines.

### Passive immunization

Antibodies produced by other persons or by animals such as the horse, cow, and rabbit can be introduced into a person's bloodstream for protection against attack by a pathogen. This

**table 10-9** *Description of Selected Vaccines*

| Vaccine | Description | Comments |
|---|---|---|
| DPT | | |
| Diphtheria | Toxoid<br>Inactivated<br>Diphtheria toxin | Booster dose every 10 years |
| Tetanus | Inactivated<br>Tetanus toxoid | Booster dose every 10 years<br>For contaminated wound management, additional booster given if more than 5 years since last booster dose |
| Pertussis | Killed whole *Bordetella pertussis* | Not recommended for persons older than 7 years of age because risk of pertussis low and reaction possibly severe |
| Measles | Live attenuated virus vaccine | Contraindications: pregnancy, immunocompromised state, history of anaphylactic reaction to eggs |
| Mumps | Live attenuated virus vaccine | Contraindications: pregnancy, immunocompromised state, history of anaphylactic reaction to eggs |
| Rubella | Live attenuated rubella virus grown in human diploid cells | Contraindications: pregnancy, immunocompromised state |
| Polio | | |
| OPV | Live attenuated oral poliovirus vaccine | Contraindications: pregnancy, immunocompromised state |
| IPV | Inactivated poliovirus vaccine | Administered by subcutaneous injection, contraindicated in pregnancy |
| Influenza | Inactivated whole or disrupted (split) influenza viruses | Antigenic content annually changed to reflect influenza A and B virus strains in circulation; administered annually; contraindication: history of anaphylactic hypersensitivity to eggs |
| Pneumococcal | Purified preparation of 23 different types of pneumococcal capsular polysaccharide | Should be given to persons 2 years and older who have chronic illnesses specifically associated with increased risk for pneumococcal disease and to all healthy adults over 65 years |
| Hepatitis A | Killed whole virus grown in human diploid cells | Administered by intramuscular injection with booster in 6 to 12 months |
| Hepatitis B | | |
| Recombinant deoxyribonucleic acid (DNA) | Purified surface antigen of virus produced by recombinant yeast cells | Given in series of three injections, first followed by other two, 1 and 6 months later; indicated for persons who have routine or frequent contact with blood and body fluids; contraindicated for persons allergic to yeast |
| Human serum | Purified, inactivated surface antigen of virus from plasma of human carriers | Administration schedule same as for recombinant DNA form; recommended for hemodialysis patients |
| *Haemophilus influenzae* b (Hib) | Bacterial polysaccharide conjugated to protein | Administration schedule may vary depending on brand of vaccine used |
| Varicella | Live attenuated virus vaccine | Administered by intramuscular injection; transmission of virus to susceptible persons can occur; contraindications: pregnancy, immunocompromised state |

protection is temporary, usually lasting only a few weeks, and stimulates no production of antibodies by the recipient. It is called *artificial passive immunity.* Artificial passive immunization is given to a person who has been exposed to a disease and has no natural or artificial active immunity. It usually is administered before the disease develops but may be given to modify disease symptoms. However, for effectiveness after the disease has developed, it must be administered early, before extensive damage to body tissue.

Passive immunization usually is reserved for persons to whom the disease would be detrimental. For example, it rarely is given to prevent a disease such as chickenpox or mumps in children because they are at an optimal age for the body to respond immunologically with minimal inflammatory response unless the child was immunocompromised. Immunization is given to all age groups exposed to pathogens that cause serious diseases, such as hepatitis A or B, diphtheria, tetanus, or rabies. Antivenins, which are given to persons bitten by poisonous snakes or black widow spiders, are other examples of passive immunological products.

Products used for passive immunization may be specific to the disease. Antitoxins and immune animal and human sera are examples. These materials contain elevated levels of immune globulins, which can specifically detoxify the toxin, neutralize the virus, or inactivate the bacterium. The whole blood of a patient who has recently recovered from a disease against which antibodies are produced also may be used. Antitoxins are available for diphtheria, tetanus, botulism, gas gangrene, and the venom of snakes. Human immune serum is available for measles, tetanus, and rabies.

Immune serum globulin (ISG), or gamma-globulin, is an antibody-rich fraction of pooled plasma from normal donors. The rationale for pooling plasma is that someone among the donors will have had the diseases and will have developed antibodies against them. The globulin fraction of the plasma carries the antibodies, and because it is known not to transmit the hepatitis virus, it is considered safe to use. Because of occasional side effects, it is now recommended that the use of ISG be limited to those disorders in which its efficacy has been definitely established. These are measles prophylaxis or modification, viral hepatitis type A prophylaxis or modification, and immunodeficiency diseases.

Special human ISGs are derived from the sera of persons previously immunized or convalescing from specific diseases. Tetanus immune globulin (human) is of value in prophylaxis and treatment of tetanus in persons who have not received prior immunization. Hepatitis B immune globulin (human) is available for prophylaxis after exposure to hepatitis B. Zoster immune globulin (human) is available for restricted use for prophylaxis against chickenpox.

## NURSING MANAGEMENT IN IMMUNIZATION

Ensuring proper storage and handling of vaccines is basic to an immunization program. A refrigerator with freezer, used only for vaccines and medication with daily monitoring of temperatures, will contribute to vaccine efficacy (Box 10-2).

**box 10-2** *Vaccine Handling and Storage*

Read storage requirements for all vaccines.
Monitor expiration dates monthly.
Date open vials and use within specified time.
Monitor refrigerator and freezer temperatures daily and log.
Store OPV and varicella vaccine frozen (freezer at 7° F [−14° C]).
Refrigerate DPT, diphtheria toxoid, tetanus-diphtheria, IPV, Hib, hepatitis B, pneumococcal, influenza (35-46° F [2-8° C]; do not freeze).
Protect MMR from light and excessive heat at all times.
Use small cooler with ice packs for high-use times.
Dedicate refrigerator for storage of vaccine and medication only.

Probably the greatest responsibility of the nurse in immunization programs is to teach the public the advantages of immunization and encourage widespread participation in programs recommended by the local public health officer.

### PATIENT/FAMILY EDUCATION

In teaching it is advisable to provide the public with the following information: disease protection given, why immunization is desirable, and when booster doses should be obtained. The relative safety of the immunization and the advantages of immunization early in life also should be stressed.

The nurse is responsible for assessing persons before immunization because some contraindications exist to receiving certain immunizing substances. Those that are prepared in chicken or duck embryos may cause an allergic reaction in persons allergic to eggs. Many people are allergic to horse serum, and substances containing horse serum, such as tetanus antitoxin, should never be given unless a small amount of the substance has been injected intradermally (a *sensitivity test*) and no "hive" reaction about the injection site has been produced after 20 minutes. Active immunological products should not be given while a person has a cold or other infection because the inflammatory reaction from the immunization will be greater than usual.

Children with histories of allergy often are *not* given routine immunization against diseases for which there is herd immunity because the danger of severe allergic response to the immunization is greater than the danger of contracting the disease. These children should be immunized against diseases such as tetanus, however, and immunization is achieved by giving the vaccine or toxoid in small doses over several weeks or months. The package inserts accompanying the immunological product should always be read carefully to determine the indications, precautions, and side effects.

Live attenuated virus vaccines should not be given to persons with alterations in the immune status, because virus replication after administration may be unchecked in these

**box 10-3** *Additional Considerations for Vaccine Administration*

In general, inactivated vaccines and live vaccines (except cholera and yellow fever) can be administered simultaneously in separate sites.
Whenever possible, live vaccines should be administered on the same day or at least 30 days apart.
Purified protein derivative (PPD) testing for tuberculosis can be done on the same day as live virus vaccines are given or 4 to 6 weeks later.
Live attenuated vaccines should not be given at the same time as passive immunization because passively acquired antibodies can interfere with the response to live attenuated virus vaccines.
Pregnant women should not receive live attenuated vaccines because of the theoretic risk to the fetus.
If a person has a febrile illness, it is usually best to wait until recovery before vaccination.

individuals. As noted earlier, OPV viruses are excreted by the recipient of the vaccine and are communicable to other persons. Thus individuals who live with an immunocompromised person should receive IPV instead of OPV. Other factors to be considered in the administration of vaccines are listed in Box 10-3.

Before leaving the clinic, the person or family members should be instructed about the expected effects of an inoculation and told to contact the physician or to report to a hospital emergency room if any other symptoms develop. The person is cautioned not to scratch any lesion produced by an inoculation. If a severe local reaction with redness, swelling, and tenderness occurs, the physician may order the application of hot, wet dressings. If the lesion is open, these dressings should be sterile.

When antitoxins, antisera, or antivenins are given, the patient is kept under observation for 20 to 30 minutes. Symptoms of severe allergic response usually will appear within that time. Epinephrine 1:1000 should be available for immediate administration if an allergic response occurs.

## HEALTH CARE WORKERS

Persons employed in health care facilities should be evaluated for immunity against chickenpox, rubella, measles, polio, diphtheria, tetanus, and hepatitis B. Persons at risk for occupational hepatitis B infection or chickenpox should be offered vaccine at the time of employment. Persons with negative tuberculin skin tests should be retested every 6 to 12 months, depending on the prevalence of tuberculosis in the area. Yearly chest roentgenograms are no longer recommended for the routine management of persons with positive tuberculin test reactions. After the initial roentgenogram following a skin test conversion, annual films have not been shown to be of significant clinical value and are not cost-effective in monitoring persons for early disease. If occupational exposure to infectious disease occurs, personnel health should be consulted for prophylaxis and follow up.

## INFECTION CONTROL IN THE HOSPITAL

A *nosocomial* infection is not present or incubating when a person is admitted to the hospital but develops after admission. A *community-acquired* infection is present or incubating at the time of admission to the hospital. The nurse should be aware of the problem of nosocomial infections; their effects on patient morbidity, mortality, and increased hospital costs; and the related legal aspects. The nurse also should be knowledgeable about the types of infections seen most often, the common pathogens and how they are transmitted, factors that predispose a patient to a nosocomial infection, how to recognize persons at risk of infection, and the prevention and control measures necessary to decrease the incidence of nosocomial infections.

At least 2 million persons, or about 5% of all patients admitted to hospitals in the United States each year, develop nosocomial infections. In addition to the considerable morbidity and mortality caused by these infections, their diagnoses and treatment, including additional days of hospitalization, cost more than $4.5 billion per year[4] (Table 10-10). The JCAHO develops and publishes standards for infection control in the *Accreditation Manual for Hospitals.* These standards are designed to help an institution improve its quality of patient care. The JCAHO requires that those institutions seeking accreditation have an effective, hospital-wide program for surveillance, prevention, and control of infection. In addition, infection control indicators (performance measures) are being developed. These indicators would allow the JCAHO to standardize the survey and accreditation process. The CDC and HICPAC have developed guidelines for the prevention and control of infectious diseases for use in patient care centers.

The incidence of nosocomial infections varies with the type of hospital. This can be attributed to differences in the size of hospitals, the severity of illness in the patient population, susceptibility of the patient population, and the number of staff members who have hands-on contact with the

**table 10-10** *Estimated Average Number of Extra Days, Average Amount of Extra Charges per Infection, and Deaths Caused by and Contributed to by Nosocomial Infections—United States, 1992*

| | | | Deaths Directly Caused by Infections | | Deaths to Which Infections Contributed | |
|---|---|---|---|---|---|---|
| Type | Extra Days | Extra Charges* | Total | (%) | Total | (%) |
| Surgical wound infection | 7.3 | $3,152 | 3,251 | (0.6) | 9,726 | (1.9) |
| Lower respiratory tract infection | 5.9 | $5,683 | 7,087 | (3.1) | 22,983 | (10.1) |
| Bloodstream infection | 7.4 | $3,517 | 4,496 | (4.4) | 8,844 | (8.6) |
| Urinary tract infection | 1.0 | $ 680 | 947 | (0.1) | 6,503 | (0.7) |
| Other types | 4.8 | $1,617 | 3,246 | (0.8) | 10,036 | (2.5) |
| All types† | 4.0 | $2,100 | 19,027 | (0.9) | 58,092 | (2.7) |

From Centers for Disease Control and Prevention: Public health focus: surveillance, prevention, and control of nosocomial infections, *MMWR* 41(42):783, 1992.
*1992 dollars.
†Some infections were weighted differently in computing these averages.

patients. The patient with the greatest risk of developing a nosocomial infection has a chronic illness, a prolonged hospital stay, and the most direct contact with various hospital personnel (physicians, students, nurses, therapists, and so on). These factors hold true for variations in infection rates not only from institution to institution but also within an institution. Certain patient care areas are considered to be high-risk areas for the development of nosocomial infections. These areas are where patients who have decreased host defenses or who receive invasive procedures and devices are given care. Areas generally considered to be high risk are (1) intensive care units (including neonatal units), (2) burn units, (3) dialysis units, and (4) oncology units. The infection rate in these areas may well be greater than 20%.[3]

### Persons at Risk

The nurse must recognize patients at the greatest risk of a nosocomial infection. Some of the factors that predispose a person to infection were mentioned previously. Briefly, these include (1) the age of the patient, the very young and the very old being the most susceptible; (2) impairment of normal immune defenses because of an underlying disease process, such as cancer, chronic renal disease, chronic lung disease, diabetes, or AIDS; (3) impairment of the normal immune defenses because of the therapy being given, such as radiation, steroids, or chemotherapy; (4) use of antibiotics, which can eliminate the patient's normal flora, providing opportunity for colonization with pathogenic and drug-resistant organisms that may then cause infection; (5) use of invasive diagnostic and therapeutic procedures and devices, which bypass the patient's normal defense barriers and thus provide a portal of entry into the body (e.g., indwelling urinary catheters, monitoring devices, intravenous catheters, and respiratory assistive devices); (6) surgery; (7) burns; and (8) length of hospitalization. Probably the most important factor that predisposes a patient to acquiring a nosocomial infection is the severity of the patient's underlying disease.

A patient admitted to the hospital with an infection may develop a *superinfection* with another organism during the hospitalization. Often this superinfection is with a more virulent or drug-resistant organism. For example, a patient admitted with a leg ulcer infected with *Staphylococcus aureus* may develop further infection (not colonization) with *Pseudomonas aeruginosa.* Furthermore, if this infection progresses to involve the bloodstream, a secondary bacteremia has occurred. Infection can occur secondary to (1) an existing infection, (2) an underlying disease process, or (3) an anatomical defect that may be causing obstruction. An example of this is the man with benign prostatic hypertrophy (BPH) who develops a urinary tract infection secondary to the obstruction caused by the BPH. These concepts are the most helpful ones when one is trying to determine the cause of a particular infection.

Hospitals participating in the National Nosocomial Infection Study (NNIS) provide the only source of recurring nationwide data on nosocomial infections. In 1986, NNIS revised its surveillance protocols. These now include nosocomial surveillance by service, site of infection, pathogen, device, patient risk factors, and type of hospital.[11]

The most common site for a nosocomial infection is the urinary tract; 75% of these infections are related to instrumentation, including indwelling urinary catheters, catheterizations, and urological procedures. Infected surgical wounds, followed by lower respiratory tract infections, cutaneous infections, and bloodstream infections (some associated with the use of intravascular lines), are the next most frequently encountered types of nosocomial infections. Together these sites account for about 35% of all nosocomial infections.

### Pathogens Causing Nosocomial Infections

The types of pathogens typically responsible for nosocomial infections and their usual reservoirs are listed in Table 10-11. NNIS data from 1986 to 1996 show that the most frequently reported nosocomial pathogens are *Escherichia coli, S. aureus, Enterococcus faecalis, P. aeruginosa,* and coagulase-negative staphylococci.[5]

*E. coli* continues to account for most reported nosocomial urinary tract infections on medical services, and *S. aureus* is the main organism causing nosocomial surgical wound

**table 10-11** *Modes of Transmission of Some Common Pathogens*

| PATHOGEN | COMMON RESERVOIR |
|---|---|
| Gram-positive cocci | |
| *Staphylococcus aureus* | Contaminated objects, hands, and nasal tracts of health care workers, air, self |
| Group A streptococci | Direct contact, air, hands, rarely objects |
| Enterococcus group | Self, hands of health care workers, environmental surfaces |
| Gram-negative rods | |
| *Escherichia, Klebsiella, Enterobacter* | Self, hands of health care workers, contaminated solutions |
| *Proteus, Salmonella, Providencia, Serratia, Citrobacter* | Contaminated food and water, hands of health care workers, self |
| *Pseudomonas* | Contaminated environment, hands, self |
| Anaerobic bacteria | |
| *Clostridium, Bacteroides* | Self, contaminated environment, hands |
| Fungal organisms | |
| Yeasts | Self, hands of health care workers |
| Fungi | Air, contaminated environment |
| Viruses | |
| Varicella | Air, direct contact |
| Herpes | Self, direct contact, air |
| Rubella | Direct contact, air |
| Hepatitis B and C | Contaminated instruments, sharps, direct contact |

infections. *P. aeruginosa* and *S. aureus* are the most common pathogens causing nosocomial pneumonia. Coagulase-negative staphylococci and *S. aureus* are the pathogens most frequently causing nosocomial primary bacteremia.

The reservoirs for *S. aureus* are the respiratory tract and skin. From 10% to 15% of the general population can be persistent carriers of this organism, which is harbored in the anterior nares. Among persons working in hospitals, the carrier rate may be as high as 25% to 30%. Nasal carriers, especially those with respiratory tract infections, are potential sources of environmental and human contact contamination. Methicillin-resistant *S. aureus* (MRSA) especially causes concern among caregivers. Methicillin is one of the penicillins specifically developed to treat *S. aureus* infections. *S. aureus* is a common surgical wound and cutaneous pathogen. Although MRSA is no more virulent than methicillin-sensitive *S. aureus* (MSSA), it is more difficult and expensive to treat. The antibiotic of choice for treating MRSA infection is vancomycin. Institutions have used various strategies in an attempt to eradicate MRSA colonization in their patient populations. These strategies include new cultures on admission, periodic surveillance cultures, isolation, and various antibiotic protocols. All have proved to be largely ineffective.

Enterococci resistant to vancomycin (VRE) have emerged as a significant pathogen within the last 5 years. Enterococci are normally found in the GI tract and in the female genital tract, but can be important nosocomial pathogens. Resistance to vancomycin has developed as a result of indiscriminate use of antibiotics. The limited treatment options and possibility of transfer of resistance to other gram-positive organisms, especially *S. aureus,* are serious concerns with VRE. Consequently, the HICPAC developed recommendations for preventing the spread of vancomycin resistance[10] (see the Research Box at right).

Group A streptococci *(S. pyogenes)* are gram-positive organisms seen in nosocomial infections. Strains of these organisms cause streptococcal sore throat, scarlet fever, and streptococcal skin infections. A particularly virulent strain of this organism is responsible for necrotizing fascitis. Streptococci are found in animate reservoirs, particularly the pharynx and nares, of personnel and patients.

Other organisms involved in nosocomial infections include gram-negative coliform bacteria, *Escherichia, Klebsiella,* and *Enterobacter,* which live in the human intestinal tract. Although these organisms usually are susceptible to antibiotics, they have the capacity to develop antibiotic resistance. The large reservoir of coliform organisms within the general population can be a source for self-infection or for cross-infection from the hands of hospital personnel through the ingestion of foods or through the contamination of other materials. Some strains of these organisms are more likely than others to produce infection. The more pathogenic strains seem to gain ascendency in patients who are receiving antibiotic therapy; immunodeficient patients are particularly susceptible to infection by coliform bacteria.

Although *Salmonella* organisms usually are acquired outside the hospital, the organism is readily transmissible and can be the cause of nosocomial infection. It is transmitted by direct or indirect contact with an infected person or through food (especially raw eggs), dairy products, or water contaminated with the organism. The CDC recommends that no one eat raw eggs. Patients with sickle cell disease, HIV, or malignancies are more vulnerable to infection from these organisms.

*P. aeruginosa,* a gram-negative organism, is present throughout the hospital environment, especially where water is always present (in sinks, irrigating solutions, and nebulizers). It is more frequently found in patients with leukopenia secondary to burns, leukemia, cystic fibrosis, and various immunodeficiency syndromes. It also is known to be a significant cause of infection in patients receiving prolonged courses of antibiotics, immunosuppressive drugs, and inhalation therapy. *P. aeruginosa* can be a threat to patients undergoing instrumentation (tracheostomy and urinary tract catheterization) and receiving renal transplants. Neonates, particularly premature infants, as well as elderly and debilitated persons are the most vulnerable.

*Serratia marcescens* and *Serratia liquefaciens* are gram-negative organisms seen in nosocomial infections. The reservoirs for these organisms are soil and water, and they are found in the hospital similarly to *Pseudomonas.* Previously thought to be nonpathogenic, *S. marcescens* was used because of its red pigmentation to mark air flow and settling patterns of bacteria. It is now recognized as a pathogen that can cause severe infection in a susceptible host. One problem with *Serratia* organisms has been their ability to develop resistance to antibiotics rapidly. This can have devastating consequences in an intensive care or burn unit when an outbreak occurs. Because its mode of transmission is through direct or indirect contact on the hands of personnel or on contaminated articles, good handwashing and aseptic techniques are the most effective measures to prevent outbreaks of infection.

**research**

Reference: Anderson RL et al: Susceptibility of vancomycin-resistant enterococci to environmental disinfectants, *Infect Control Hosp Epidemiol* 18:195-199, 1997.

This study was designed to determine what concentration of commonly used hospital disinfectants would inactivate both vancomycin-sensitive and -resistant enterococci (VSE and VRE). Disinfectants tested included a quaternary ammonium germicidal detergent, a phenolic detergent, and an iodophor detergent germicide. Test strains of *Escherichia faecium* (VRE and VSE) were both inactivated by all the test disinfectants diluted according to manufacturer's instructions. Further dilution of the disinfectants and testing of VRE and VSE showed that strains of enterococci resistant to vancomycin were no more resistant to disinfectants than sensitive strains. The presence of organic material such as stool or blood did affect disinfectant activity. The researchers concluded that any germicidal detergents registered by the Environmental Protection Agency are sufficient for use in all patient rooms, even those where the patient is colonized or infected with VRE.

*Candida albicans* is a yeastlike fungus that can cause infection, especially in immunocompromised patients or those receiving antibiotics. These patients have a decrease in the normal flora, which provides a niche for the *Candida* organisms to settle in and proliferate. Antibiotics suppress bacterial growth but do not affect fungal growth; special antifungal agents are necessary to control these infections unless the normal flora return after discontinuance of the antibiotics.

## Prevention and Control Measures

In the hospital many potential sources of infection exist including patients, personnel, visitors, equipments, linen, and so on. Patients may become infected with organisms either from the external environment *(exogenous)* or as is often seen in the severely immunocompromised host, from their own internal organisms *(endogenous)*. Virtually any microorganism can be a potential pathogen to the immunocompromised patient. Most of the causative organisms are present in the patient's external environment and are introduced into the body through direct contact or contaminated materials. In many instances nosocomial infections could be prevented by strict aseptic technique when giving care and by greater restraint in the use of invasive procedures and antibiotics. Some specific infection control measures follow.

### Control of external environment

Health care providers should be in good health and keep their immunization status up to date. They should report to the employee health service when they feel ill. Visitors also should be in good health, and their number should be limited to prevent overcrowding in the patient's room. Staff members should wear clean clothing and observe good personal hygiene practices, especially thorough handwashing, which decreases transient and resident flora on the hands and thus acts as a deterrent to cross-infection by the hands. Friction and rinsing are the two most important components of good handwashing. Ample handwashing facilities are necessary throughout the hospital and should be used by all personnel before and after patient contact; after contact with excretions, secretions, wound drainage, or any contaminated articles; and before any clean or sterile procedure or contact with clean or sterile equipment. *Handwashing is the most effective method for preventing nosocomial infection*[3,11,16,19] (see the Research Box at right). Dermatological conditions of the hands should be corrected, because dry, cracked skin can more readily become colonized with pathogens, and broken skin is more difficult to rid of transient and resident flora. The person with a skin problem on the hands also tends to avoid proper handwashing, because it can further increase dryness and irritation. The person with active herpes simplex infection of the hand *(herpetic whitlow)* should not give direct patient care until the lesion has healed.

Housekeeping and sanitation practices should be strictly observed to reduce dust and environmental reservoirs of organisms, especially in high-risk areas such as nurseries, operating rooms, and intensive care units. Spills of blood or other body fluids should be cleaned up promptly with an approved hospital disinfectant or a 1:10 dilution of 5.25% sodium hypochlorite (household bleach and water). Linens should be changed with as little contact with the nurse's uniform as possible; linen should not be thrown on the floor or shaken in the air, because this not only will further contaminate the linen but also will stir up dust particles and create air currents that can transmit pathogens. Waste products should be disposed of in the appropriate receptacle. State and federal laws regulate the disposal of infectious waste from health care institutions. Items such as needles and syringes, laboratory cultures and tissue specimens, and other disposable items that are saturated with blood or body substances are considered regulated infectious waste. *Regulated infectious waste must be incinerated or treated (to render it noninfectious) before disposal.* Other waste materials from patient rooms may be disposed of as regular trash. Proper cleaning and sterilization of contaminated reusable articles and equipment are essential. A program should exist to monitor the effectiveness of these practices; however, routine culturing of the environment is not advocated.

Air is generally not considered an important factor in nosocomial cross-infection. However, in the case of *Aspergillus* spores and *M. tuberculosis,* adequate air exchanges are necessary to reduce the number of organisms. Minimal standards for air exchanges in patient care areas are published by the Department of Health and Human Services. Minimal air changes of outdoor air per hour range from 2 in patient rooms to 15 in operating rooms.

### Control of internal environment

Reducing the endogenous sources of infection is more difficult than control of the external environment. Often the source is the patient's own normal flora, and these infections are not directly preventable by the nurse. Preventive measures aim to increase the patient's defense mechanisms and thus decrease the risk of the infection. Teaching the patient about

**research**

Reference: Alvaran MS, Butz A, Larson E: Opinions, knowledge, and self-reported practices related to infection control among nursing personnel in long-term care settings, *Am J Infect Control* 22(6):367-370, 1994.

This study was designed to describe infection control practices of long-term care nursing staff. Participants were asked to self-report practices and opinions to identify factors that predispose nurses to perform appropriate infection control practices such as handwashing. The researchers found no correlation between what nurses knew about infection control and their self-reported handwashing practices. RNs had higher knowledge scores but lower handwashing scores than LPNs or aides. Men had significantly lower handwashing scores than women. The authors concluded that simply improving knowledge would not improve handwashing practices. They suggest that other strategies to encourage and facilitate appropriate handwashing must be developed and enforcement of policies is necessary.

good nutrition and personal hygiene is a practical measure that is part of nursing care. Maintaining the patient's normal flora and preventing colonization with pathogens that can serve as a source of infection are other effective measures. These, however, are not always possible when patients are receiving antibiotics or undergoing chemotherapy, because these measures may disrupt the normal flora and promote colonization. Appropriate use of antibiotics for prophylaxis and treatment helps prevent colonization with pathogens and decreases the incidence of infection with drug-resistant organisms. Good handwashing by all who have contact with the patient decreases the possibility of the patient's inoculation with pathogenic organisms. Staff members should develop the habit of working from clean procedures to dirty procedures when delivering patient care. For example, the nurse should adjust the intravenous infusion rate and check the intravenous site *before* changing the bed of an incontinent patient. A summary of some prevention and control measures is provided in the Guidelines for Care Box.

### *Prevention of urinary tract infections*

As mentioned previously, urinary tract infections (UTIs) are the most common nosocomial infections seen in the hospital. Most of these infections are associated with catheterization and instrumentation of the urinary tract. Urinary catheters should be used only when absolutely necessary. If a catheter must be used, it should be removed as soon as medically feasible, because the longer the catheter is in place, the greater the risk of infection. To prevent transmission of bacteria into the bladder, strict aseptic technique is necessary during insertion of the catheter. Bacteria that are present around the catheter-meatal junction also can be transmitted on the tip of the catheter into the bladder along the thin layer of mucus that surrounds the catheter in the urethra. For this reason the catheter should be securely anchored to prevent it from moving in and out of the urethra. Movement of the catheter can track bacteria into the urethra and up into the bladder along the mucous sheath. Furthermore, the catheter-meatal junction should be kept clean; the patient incontinent of stool can pose a problem in this regard. In some institutions, antiseptic agents are used to cleanse the meatus, and antimicrobial agents are applied

**research**

Reference: Eck EK, Vannier A: The effect of high-efficiency particulate air respirator design on occupational health: a pilot study balancing risks in the real world, *Infect Control Hosp Epidemiol* 18:122-127, 1997.

This descriptive study combined data from seven hospitals to identify factors related to wearing National Institute of Occupational Safety and Health (NIOSH)-approved high-efficiency particulate air (HEPA) respirators, which may increase the likelihood of health care workers (HCW) incurring sharps injury. HCWs who had sustained sharps injuries identified impaired visability, communication, or range of motion as contributory factors for injury. Wearers of selected particulate air (HEPA) respirators were examined at baseline and while wearing each of the respirators. Three contributory factors were rated for each respirator. One of the respirators obstructed part of the visual field of all HCWs examined. Volume and intelligibility of speech were decreased in all but one respirator, and minimal decrease in range of motion was noted with all respirators. The authors conclude that the design of many currently used respirators may contribute to the risk of blood-borne pathogen exposure while they are protecting against airborne pathogens such as tuberculosis. They suggest that a design that sacrifices some efficiency in protection from tuberculosis (the dust-mist-fume particulate respirator) but is less likely to contribute to sharps injuries may be of overall benefit to HCWs.

**guidelines for care**

#### Prevention and Control of Nosocomial Infections

**Control of External Environment (Exogenous Sources of Infection)**

***Health Care Providers***

1. In good health—do not care for patients when ill
2. Keep immunizations current
3. Practice effective handwashing between each patient
   - If skin dry, rough, or broken, seek appropriate attention
   - If active herpes simplex infection of hand (herpetic whitlow), do not give direct patient care until lesion healed
4. Appropriate use of personal protective equipment, based on degree of risk of exposure (e.g., gloves, mask, apron, face shield, shoe covers, air respirator) (see the Research Box at left)

***Housekeeping and Sanitation***

1. Bed linens not shaken in air or thrown on floor
2. Proper disposal of wastes—solid and liquid
3. Proper cleaning and sterilization of contaminated articles
4. Proper ventilation for adequate air exchanges
   - Modern hospitals—patients' room air is under negative pressure
   - Negative pressure keeps air from patients' rooms from moving into hallways
5. Proper mopping and damp dusting to remove dust and other environmental reservoirs of infection

**Control of Internal Environment (Endogenous Sources of Infection)**

1. Preventive measures aimed at increasing patient's defense mechanisms and thus reducing risk of infection
   - Teach patient about good nutrition
   - Teach patient about personal hygiene, especially handwashing
2. Be aware that normal flora of patient can be disrupted when patient is receiving antibiotics or chemotherapy and colonization may occur
   - Give antibiotics on time as scheduled
   - Teach patient about appropriate use of antibiotics and dangers of taking them when not prescribed by physician

around the catheter-meatal junction. Both of these practices are considered controversial. Good handwashing techniques by personnel, cleansing of the patient's meatal area with soap and water, and proper anchoring of the catheter are considered effective ways to reduce the incidence of UTIs in patients with indwelling catheters.

Another portal of entry for bacteria is through the distal catheter-proximal drainage tube junction. Every time the system is disconnected, the risk of introducing bacteria into the system increases, thus a closed drainage system should be maintained. Bladder irrigations should not be a routine practice. If irrigation is necessary, a sterile disposable syringe and sterile solution should be used. If frequent irrigations are necessary, such as in patients who have had a transurethral prostatectomy, in which blood clots are common, a three-way catheter drainage system with continuous bladder irrigation is recommended. In this way a closed system is maintained. Urine specimens should be obtained from the rubber portal on the drainage tubing. The portal should be cleansed with an antiseptic before insertion of the needle into the portal.

Another portal of entry of bacteria into the system is through the collection bag. The bag should be kept below the bladder level at all times to prevent reflux of urine into the bladder. In addition, the bag should be kept off the floor, and the emptying spout should be cleansed with an antiseptic after the urine is emptied. The container used to collect the urine from the bag must be used for only one patient; it should not be shared among patients.

A final control measure in preventing nosocomial UTIs is to place patients with urinary catheters in separate rooms. This is helpful in preventing cross-infection among patients.

#### *Prevention of respiratory tract infections*

Nosocomial pneumonia occurs in approximately 0.6% of hospitalized medical patients (6 cases per 1000 hospital discharges) and is associated with the highest mortality rate of all nosocomial infections.[12] A major risk factor is respiratory intubation because endotracheal, nasotracheal, and tracheostomy tubes bypass the patient's defense mechanisms of the upper respiratory tract. The importance of proper maintenance and decontamination of respiratory therapy equipment in preventing nosocomial pneumonias is well established. Handwashing is essential before and after contact with patients and respiratory assist devices, which contain moisture and are ideal reservoirs for organisms, especially gram-negative species such as *Pseudomonas* and *Serratia.* Suctioning is a sterile procedure necessitating the use of sterile equipment and irrigants (see Chapter 32). Surgical procedures that lead to impaired coughing also are a risk factor. Preoperative patient teaching that stresses the importance and proper technique of coughing and deep breathing is essential to the success of reducing postoperative pulmonary infection. Inappropriate use of antibiotics should be avoided to minimize oropharyngeal colonization with gram-negative bacteria; if aspirated, these may lead to more serious pneumonia. Debilitated patients should be protected from the hazards of aspiration, especially while eating.

#### *Prevention of bacteremias*

Many blood infections (bacteremias) occur secondary to infections at another site; thus prevention may depend greatly on control of the underlying infection. Some bacteremias result from the use of intravascular devices and systems. The sources of infection in these instances are the hands of staff members, the patient's skin, or infusions contaminated either from mishandling by hospital personnel or, less often, at the time of manufacture. Intravenous and intraarterial catheters should be inserted under aseptic conditions, and catheter insertion sites should be cared for aseptically. The insertion site is treated as an open wound and is inspected frequently for any sign of infection, such as redness, swelling, exudate, purulence, or warmth. The patient also may complain of pain at the site.

Central lines should have a sterile dressing to prevent contamination of the insertion site. A controversy exists over the use of transparent dressings rather than gauze dressings. Some studies have shown an increase in site colonization and catheter-related infection with the use of transparent dressings.[6] However, other studies show no increase in the incidence of site infections with the use of transparent dressings.[13]

Peripheral catheters should be changed every 72 hours or more often if a complication such as infiltration or phlebitis occurs. The catheter is secured to prevent in-and-out movement and tracking of bacteria into the cannula site. Aseptic technique should be followed during the mixing and adding of drugs, changing the infusion, or manipulating connections or stopcocks. It is recommended that the tubing also be changed every 72 hours.[13]

Before beginning infusion of a solution, the nurse should check it for turbidity, particulate matter, and leaks in the system. Hyperalimentation solutions require special adherence to these practices because they are composed of nutrients that provide an excellent culture medium for organisms. *Candida* infections occur frequently in patients receiving hyperalimentation, particularly those who are immunocompromised.

### Protection by Isolation

The purpose of isolation is to protect both the caregiver from exposure to infectious agents and the patient from cross-infection. Protective isolation was eliminated from the 1993 CDC guidelines because it had not been shown to reduce the risk of infection in the immunocompromised patient.

Some general principles apply regardless of the type of isolation. Barriers such as gowns, gloves, and masks should be used only once and then discarded in an appropriate receptacle before leaving the patient's room. These barriers should be conveniently available for each patient room. *Hands must be washed before and after each patient contact even when gloves are worn.*

In 1996 the CDC and HICPAC published revised guidelines for isolation precautions in hospitals.[9,14] These new guidelines incorporate the major tenets of both universal precautions (UP) and body substance isolation (BSI). Neither BSI or UP addressed prevention of airborne, droplet, and direct contact modes of transmission. In the early 1990s concern with preventing transmission of tuberculosis including multidrug-resistant tuberculosis required additional precautions. At the same time, the prevalence of multidrug-resistant organisms was increasing, and hospitals needed new ways to deal with this problem. As a result the new CDC/HICPAC guidelines for isolation precautions in hospitals were developed to answer these concerns.

The precautions are described as two tiered. The first tier, *Standard Precautions,* combines UP and BSI techniques and is to be used with all patients regardless of whether the diagnosis is known. These precautions apply to (1) blood, (2) all other body fluids and secretions except sweat, regardless of whether they contain visible blood, (3) nonintact skin, and (4) mucous membranes. Table 10-12 lists the techniques used for Standard Precautions.

The second tier, *Transmission-Based Precautions,* is designed to reduce the risk of airborne, droplet, and contact transmission. It is used when caring for patients with documented or suspected infection with highly transmissible or epidemiologically important pathogens for which Standard Precautions may be insufficient. The three types of transmission-based precautions are (1) Airborne Precautions, (2) Droplet Precautions, and (3) Contact Precautions. Standard Precautions are used in combination with one or more of the Transmission-Based Precautions depending on the disease identified.

*Airborne Precautions* are to be used to prevent airborne transmission of organisms, which are the droplet nuclei of evaporated droplets (5 $\mu$ or less in size) or contained in dust particles. Special air handling, which may include negative pressure, frequent air exchanges, direct-to-the-outside exhaust, HEPA filters, or ultraviolet light, is necessary to prevent airborne transmission. Placing the patient with suspected or diagnosed tuberculosis in a private room with negative pressure room air and 12 air exchanges per hour and having the staff entering the room use HEPA filter respirators is an example of Airborne Precautions. The patient should stay in the room with the door closed until sputum smears indicate that he or she is no longer infectious.

*Droplet Precautions* are used to prevent the contact of the conjunctiva or mucous membrane of the nose or mouth with large-size (larger than 5 $\mu$) particle droplets containing microorganisms generated by cough, sneeze, or talking or by a procedure such as suctioning or bronchoscopy. Generally these droplets are a risk only to persons within a 3-foot radius of the source. They quickly settle onto surfaces and can no longer be inhaled. Placing the patient with suspected *Neisseria meningitidis* pneumonia in a private room and wearing a mask while working within 3 feet of the patient is an example of Droplet Precautions.

*Contact Precautions* are used to interrupt transmission of epidemiologically important organisms by direct (skin to skin) or indirect (skin to contaminated item) contact. Placing the patient with *Clostridium difficile* diarrhea in a private room with single-use or dedicated-to-the-patient equipment and donning a gown and gloves to enter the room to perform any patient care procedure is an example of Contact Precautions.

Because of the special considerations for preventing the spread of VRE, HICPAC developed separate recommendations outlining the additional precautions needed.[10] Contact isolation is used in conjunction with Standard Precautions, with each institution adapting the HICPAC recommendations based on their particular circumstances and endemic rate.

Table 10-13 is a synopsis of types of precautions and patients requiring the precautions. Table 10-14 is a list of clinical syndromes or conditions warranting additional empiric precautions to prevent transmission of epidemiologically important pathogens pending confirmation of diagnosis. Table 10-15 is a list of type and duration of precautions needed for selected infections.

*Text continued on p. 247*

**table 10-12** *Standard Precautions Techniques*

| ITEM | PRECAUTIONS |
|---|---|
| Handwashing | After touching blood, body fluids, secretions, excretions, contaminated items, whether or not gloves are worn |
| Gloves | When touching blood, body fluids, secretions, excretions, and contaminated items and when performing invasive procedures; remove gloves promptly after use and wash hands |
| Mask, eye protection, face shield | To protect mucous membranes of the eyes, nose, and mouth during activities that are likely to generate splashes or sprays of blood, body fluids, secretions, and excretions |
| Private room | Indicated if personal hygiene is poor or if body substances contaminate the environment |
| Needles | Dispose of uncapped and unbent needles at point of use in puncture-resistant container: one-handed or device-assisted recapping if necessary |
| Soiled linen | Placed in leak-proof bags: gown and gloves worn by laundry workers sorting all soiled linen |
| Reusable equipment | Bagged for transport to decontamination area: gowns, gloves, masks, and eye protection worn by decontamination personnel |

Modified from Garner JS and the Hospital Infection Control Practices Advisory Committee: Guidelines for isolation precautions in hospitals. Part II. Recommendations for isolation precautions in hospital, *Am J Infect Control* 22:24-52, 1996.

**table 10-13** *Types of Precautions*

**STANDARD PRECAUTIONS**

Use Standard Precautions for the care of all patients

**AIRBORNE PRECAUTIONS**

In addition to Standard Precautions, use Airborne Precautions for patients known or suspected to have serious illnesses transmitted by airborne droplet nuclei. Examples of such illnesses include:

(1) Measles
(2) Varicella (including disseminated zoster)*
(3) Tuberculosis

**DROPLET PRECAUTIONS**

In addition to Standard Precautions, use Droplet Precautions for patients known or suspected to have serious illnesses transmitted by large particle droplets. Examples of such illnesses include:

(1) Invasive *Haemophilus influenzae* type b disease, including meningitis, pneumonia, epiglottitis, and sepsis
(2) Invasive *Neisseria meningitidis* disease, including meningitis, pneumonia, and sepsis
(3) Other serious bacterial respiratory infections spread by droplet transmission, including:
  (a) Diphtheria (pharyngeal)
  (b) Mycoplasma pneumonia
  (c) Pertussis
  (d) Pneumonic plague
  (e) Streptococcal pharyngitis, pneumonia, or scarlet fever in infants and young children
(4) Serious viral infections spread by droplet transmission, including:
  (a) Adenovirus*
  (b) Influenza
  (c) Mumps
  (d) Parvovirus B19
  (e) Rubella

**CONTACT PRECAUTIONS**

In addition to Standard Precautions, use Contact Precautions for patients known or suspected to have serious illnesses easily transmitted by direct patient contact or by contact with items in the patient's environment. Examples of such illnesses include:

(1) Gastrointestinal, respiratory, skin, or wound infections or colonization with multidrug-resistant bacteria judged by the infection control program, based on current state, regional, or national recommendations, to be of special clinical and epidemiological significance
(2) Enteric infections with a low infectious dose or prolonged environmental survival, including:
  (a) *Clostridium difficile*
  (b) For diapered or incontinent patients: enterohemorrhagic *Escherichia coli* 0157: H7, *Shigella,* hepatitis A, or rotavirus
(3) Respiratory syncytial virus, parainfluenza virus, or enteroviral infections in infants and young children
(4) Skin infections that are highly contagious or that may occur on dry skin, including:
  (a) Diphtheria (cutaneous)
  (b) Herpes simplex virus (neonatal or mucocutaneous)
  (c) Impetigo
  (d) Major (noncontained) abscesses, cellulitis, or decubiti
  (e) Pediculosis
  (f) Scabies
  (g) Staphylococcal furunculosis in infants and young children
  (h) Zoster (disseminated or in the immunocompromised host)*
(5) Viral/hemorrhagic conjunctivitis
(6) Viral hemorrhagic infections (Ebola, Lassa, or Marburg)

From Garner JS and the Hospital Infection Control Practices Advisory Committee: Guidelines for isolation precautions in hospitals. Part II. Recommendations for isolation precautions in hospitals, *Am J Infect Control* 22:24-52, 1996.
*Certain infections require more than one type of precaution.

**table 10-14** *Clinical Syndromes or Conditions Warranting Additional Empiric Precautions to Prevent Transmission of Epidemiologically Important Pathogens Pending Confirmation of Diagnosis*

| Clinical Syndrome or Condition | Potential Pathogens | Empiric Precautions |
|---|---|---|
| Diarrhea | | |
| Acute diarrhea with a likely infectious cause in an incontinent or diapered patient | Enteric pathogens | Contact |
| Diarrhea in an adult with a history of recent antibiotic use | *Clostridium difficile* | Contact |
| Meningitis | *Neisseria meningitidis* | Droplet |
| Rash or exanthems, generalized, cause unknown | | |
| Petechial/ecchymotic with fever | *Neisseria meningitidis* | Droplet |
| Vesicular | Varicella | Airborne and Contact |
| Maculopapular with coryza and fever | Rubeola (measles) | Airborne |
| Respiratory infections | | |
| Cough/fever/upper lobe pulmonary infiltrate in an HIV-seronegative patient and/or a patient at low risk for HIV infection | *Mycobacterium tuberculosis* | Airborne |
| Cough/fever/pulmonary infiltrate in any lung location in an HIV-infected patient and/or a patient at high risk for HIV infection | *Mycobacterium tuberculosis* | Airborne |
| Paroxysmal or severe persistent cough during periods of pertussis activity | *Bordetella pertussis* | Droplet |
| Respiratory infections, particularly bronchiolitis and croup, in infants and young children | Respiratory syncytial or parainfluenza virus | Contact |
| Risk of multidrug-resistant microorganisms | | |
| History of infection or colonization with multidrug-resistant organisms | Resistant bacteria | Contact |
| Skin, wound, or urinary tract infection in a patient with a recent hospital or nursing home stay in a facility where multidrug-resistant organisms are prevalent | Resistant bacteria | Contact |
| Skin or wound infection | | |
| Abscess or draining wound that cannot be covered | *Staphylococcus aureus*, group A streptococcus | Contact |

From Garner JS and the Hospital Infection Control Practices Advisory Committee: Guidelines for isolation precautions in hospitals. Part II. Recommendations for isolation precautions in hospitals, *Am J Infect Control* 22:24-52, 1996.

**table 10-15** *Type and Duration of Precautions Needed for Selected Infections and Conditions*

| Infection/Condition | Precautions: Type* | Precautions: Duration† |
|---|---|---|
| Abscess | | |
| Draining, major | C | DI |
| Draining, minor or limited | S | |
| AIDS | S | |
| Actinomycosis | S | |
| Adenovirus infection, in infants and young children | D, C | DI |
| Amebiasis | S | |
| Anthrax | | |
| Cutaneous | S | |
| Pulmonary | S | |
| Antibiotic-associated colitis (see *C. difficile*) | | |
| Arthropod-borne viral encephalitides (eastern, western, Venezuelan equine encephalomyelitis; St. Louis, California encephalitis) | S | |
| Arthropod-borne viral fevers (dengue, yellow fever, Colorado tick fever) | S | |
| Ascariasis | S | |
| Aspergillosis | S | |
| Babesiosis | S | |

From Garner JS and the Hospital Infection Control Practices Advisory Committee: Guidelines for isolation precautions in hospitals. Part II. Recommendations for isolation precautions in hospitals, *Am J Infect Control* 22:24-52, 1996.

*Type of precautions: *A*, Airborne; *C*, Contact; *D*, Droplet; *S*, Standard; *CN*, until off antibiotic therapy and culture negative; *DI*, duration of illness (with wound lesions, *DI* means until they stop draining); When A, C, and D are specified, also use S.

†Duration of precautions.

*Continued*

**table 10-15** *Type and Duration of Precautions Needed for Selected Infections and Conditions—cont'd*

| Infection/Condition | Precautions | |
|---|---|---|
| | Type* | Duration† |
| Blastomycosis, North American, cutaneous, or pulmonary | S | |
| Botulism | S | |
| Bronchiolitis | | |
| Brucellosis (undulant, Malta, Mediterranean fever) | S | |
| *Campylobacter* gastroenteritis | | |
| Candidiasis, all forms including mucocutaneous | S | |
| Cat-scratch fever (benign inoculation lymphoreticulosis) | S | |
| Cellulitis, uncontrolled drainage | C | DI |
| Chancroid (soft chancre) | S | |
| Chickenpox (varicella) | A, C | |
| *Chlamydia trachomatis* | | |
| Conjunctivitis | S | |
| Genital | S | |
| Respiratory | S | |
| Cholera (see gastroenteritis) | | |
| Closed-cavity infection | | |
| Draining, limited or minor | S | |
| Not draining | S | |
| *Clostridium* spp. | | |
| *C. botulium* | S | |
| *C. difficile* | C | DI |
| *C. pertringens* | | |
| Food poisoning | S | |
| Gas gangrene | S | |
| Coccidiodomycosis (valley fever) | | |
| Draining lesions | S | |
| Pneumonia | S | |
| Colorado tick fever | S | |
| Congenital rubella | C | |
| Conjunctivitis | | |
| Acute bacterial | S | |
| *Chlamydia* | S | |
| Gonococcal | S | |
| Acute viral (acute hemorrhagic) | C | DI |
| Coxsackie virus | | |
| Creutzfeldt-Jakob disease | S | |
| Croup | | |
| Cryptococcosis | S | |
| Cryptosporidiosis (see gastroenteritis) | | |
| Cysticercosis | S | |
| Cytomegalovirus infection neonatal or immunosuppressed | S | |
| Decubitus ulcer infected | | |
| Major | C | DI |
| Minor or limited | S | |
| Dengue | S | |
| Diarrhea acute-infective etiology suspected | | |
| Diphtheria | | |
| Cutaneous | C | CN |
| Pharyngeal | D | CN |
| Ebola viral hemorrhagic fever | C | DI |
| Echinococcosis (hydatidosis) | S | |
| Echovirus | | |
| Encephalitis | | |
| Encephalitis or encephalomyelitis | | |
| Endometritis | S | |
| Enterobiasis (pinworm disease oxyuriasis) | S | |
| Enterococcus species | | |
| Enterocolitis *C. difficile* | C | DI |

*Type of precautions: *A,* Airborne; *C,* Contact; *D,* Droplet; *S,* Standard; *CN,* until off antibiotic therapy and culture negative; *DI,* duration of illness (with wound lesions, *DI* means until they stop draining); When A, C, and D are specified, also use S.
†Duration of precautions.

**box 10-4** *Subjective and Objective Data Suggesting Infection*

**LOCALIZED INFECTION**

| Subjective | Objective |
|---|---|
| Pain | Inflammation |
| Tenderness | Edema |
| Warmth | Redness |
| Swelling | Warmth |
| Itching | Exudate or drainage |
| | Amount |
| | Color |
| | Consistency |
| | Odor |

**RESPIRATORY TRACT INFECTION**

| Subjective | Objective |
|---|---|
| Sore throat | Redness of throat |
| Congestion | Rales |
| Cough | Rhonchi |
| Sputum production | Cough |
| Chest pain | Type |
| Stuffy nose | Frequency |
| Runny nose | Sputum |
| | Amount |
| | Color |
| | Consistency |
| | Odor |

**GASTROINTESTINAL TRACT INFECTION**

| Subjective | Objective |
|---|---|
| Anorexia | Vomitus |
| Nausea | Frequency |
| Vomiting | Amount |
| Diarrhea | Color |
| | Consistency |
| | Odor |
| | Diarrhea |
| | Frequency |
| | Amount |
| | Color |
| | Consistency |
| | Odor |

**GENITOURINARY TRACT INFECTION**

| Subjective | Objective |
|---|---|
| Urgency | Frequency |
| Frequency | Amount |
| Burning or painful urination | Color |
| | Odor |
| Change in color or smell of urine | Purulent, foul discharge |
| | Presence of WBCs and bacteria |
| Flank or pelvic pain | Urinalysis |
| Discharge | Culture |
| Itching | |

**GENERALIZED INFECTION**

| Subjective | Objective |
|---|---|
| Malaise | Fever |
| Muscle aches | Elevated WBC count |
| Headache | Hypotension |
| Weakness | Altered mental status |
| Joint pain | Confusion |
| Anorexia | Convulsions |
| | Shock |
| | Tachycardia |

## NURSING MANAGEMENT

### ASSESSMENT

#### Subjective and Objective Data

The establishment of an infection within the human body leads to several specific and generalized manifestations. The exact signs and symptoms elicited in the host depend on the agent responsible for the infection and the site of the infection. (For details on host response to specific infectious disease, see the particular chapter that discusses the disease site.) Some general subjective, objective, and diagnostic findings can alert the nurse to suspect an infection, even if the causative agent is not known. Recognition of the patient with a suspected infection is a crucial step in initiating early prevention and control measures. Examples of data that would make the nurse suspect the patient may be developing an infection are listed in Box 10-4.

For generalized infections the symptoms may be even more vague. The earliest clinical manifestations of an infection generally are sensed within the host as nondescript, nonspecific reactions such as weakness, headache, lightheadedness, congestion, muscle aches, pain in the joints, decreased appetite, or malaise. These sensations are broadly referred to as *prodromal symptoms* (preceding the infection). As the infection progresses, other manifestations develop. These include fever, increased pulse rate, hypotension, altered mental status, or even jaundice, shock, confusion, and convulsions.

Of all the clinical symptoms mentioned, fever (pyrexia) is one of the most valuable diagnostic indicators of infection, although not all fevers are the result of an infectious process. Most persons with an infectious disease develop fever as a generalized response to the infectious agent.

Another systemic response to infection is the variation in leukocytes (WBCs) in peripheral circulation. The normal WBC count in blood is 5000 to 10,000 WBCs/mm$^3$. With the presence of a serious infection the number of WBCs rises above 10,000/mm$^3$ in response to the infectious inflammation. Leukocyte values between 10,000 and 20,000 are considered slightly elevated; 20,000 to 40,000 moderately elevated, and more than 40,000 greatly elevated. In a few infectious diseases the number of WBCs in circulation actually drops, which is also significant diagnostic data.

Five types of mature WBCs are found in circulation: neutrophils, eosinophils, basophils, lymphocytes, and monocytes. Each type plays a more or less specific role in body defense (see Chapter 65); therefore different diseases produce different reactions among the WBC populations in the blood. These changes in patterns of distribution are detected not only by counting the total number of WBCs in a stained blood smear, but also by classifying them according to morphology and calculating the relative percentage of each cell type present. This type of count is known as a *differential count.* As described earlier, an increase in the number of immature neutrophils is commonly referred to as a "shift to the left" and may indicate an acute infection. The differential count may provide information that can be correlated with other clinical data to help diagnose an infection. Table 10-16 provides some general correlations between leukocyte response and infectious diseases.

None of the signs and symptoms present in localized or generalized infections is diagnostic by itself. Many can be demonstrated by other disease processes. They can, however, serve as helpful clues in the diagnosis of a suspected infectious process.

### Diagnostic Tests

Diagnostic tests are an important adjunct in the diagnosis of an infection. Some of the diagnostic tests used to obtain data include skin tests, radiological tests, gallium and indium scans, ultrasound, computed tomography and magnetic resonance imaging scans, microbiological cultures, serological antibody titers, and complete blood cell (CBC) count. Examples of data obtainable from such tests include the presence of leukocytosis or anemia; an increase in erythrocyte sedimentation rate (ESR); the appearance of C-reactive protein; the presence of proteinemia; positive bacterial, viral, and fungal cultures; and positive radiological findings, all of which may indicate the presence of an infection.

Proper collection and handling of laboratory specimens are essential to ensure accurate laboratory results. Inappropriate collection or handling of specimens may lead to unnecessary delays in test results or inaccurate results, thus affecting the patient's therapy. When an infection is suspected, culture specimens are obtained from the suspected site. In the patient who has a fever and in whom the site of infection is unknown, culture specimens typically are obtained from the blood, urine, sputum, and any other possible sites of infection. This may include spinal fluid cultures, aspirates of body fluid, or intravenous catheter tips. *It is imperative that these cultures be obtained before the initiation of antibiotic therapy because antibiotics can suppress any bacteria present and give inaccurate or false-negative culture results.* Cultures should be obtained in a manner that avoids contamination. Aseptic preparation of the culture site, observance of aseptic technique, and placement of specimens in an appropriate container are crucial factors to be observed in ensuring the best sample. Once obtained, the specimen must be properly stored and transported promptly to the laboratory. Each institution should have guidelines for the proper method for collecting and handling specimens for the laboratory. All specimens must be accompanied by the correct requisition and include the following information: (1) patient's name, (2) date and time of collection, (3) test requested, (4) type of specimen, (5) how specimen was obtained (e.g., clean void or catheter urine, expectorated sputum, or tracheal aspirate), and (6) where the results are to be sent. A record of all tests is kept to avoid unnecessary duplication of tests.

Interpretation of laboratory results is sometimes difficult. Certain body sites have bacteria known as *normal flora*, which reside there in a commensal (intimate) relationship with the host. The skin, upper respiratory tract, vagina, urethra, and bowel are examples of body sites in which normal bacterial flora can be found. The bacteria found vary from site to site, and knowledge of the normal flora is helpful in discerning the significance of laboratory culture results. It must be emphasized that laboratory results alone cannot be used to make diagnostic and therapeutic decisions. Rather, they are used in conjunction with the patient's clinical status to make appropriate diagnostic and therapeutic decisions.

Selection of an antibiotic in response to culture and sensitivities will allow the least disruption of the body's normal

**table 10-16** *White Blood Cell Response to Infections*

| Leukocyte Response | Associated Infectious Process |
|---|---|
| Increase in neutrophils (neutrophilia) | Typical in many acute local and systemic infections caused by bacteria (especially pyogenic bacteria), rickettsia, some viruses, and a few protozoa |
| Decrease in neutrophils (neutropenia) | Frequent in salmonellosis, brucellosis, whooping cough, overwhelming bacterial infections, influenza, infectious mononucleosis, hepatitis A infection, mumps, rubella, rubeola, and some rickettsial and protozoan diseases |
| Increase in eosinophils (eosinophilia) | Frequent in allergic reactions, chronic skin disease, helminthic infections, and scarlet fever |
| Increase in lymphocytes (lymphocytosis) | Frequent in chickenpox, mumps, measles, infectious mononucleosis, influenza, whooping cough, syphilis, tuberculosis, salmonellosis, viral hepatitis, and viral pneumonia; sometimes in convalescent phase of acute bacterial infection |
| Increase in monocytes (monocytosis) | Common in tuberculosis, chickenpox, brucellosis, mumps, syphilis, and certain rickettsial diseases; may occur in certain viral and protozoan diseases and in convalescent phase of acute bacterial infections |
| Decrease in lymphocytes (lymphocytopenia) | HIV |

flora and effective control of the infecting organism. For an immediate response to a serious infection a broad spectrum antibiotic is chosen with activity against types of organisms identified in a Gram stain. Once the culture has grown, the organism has been identified, and sensitivities have been determined, the spectrum of the antibiotic can be safely narrowed.

## ■ NURSING DIAGNOSES

Nursing diagnoses are determined from analysis of patient data. Nursing diagnoses for the patient with an infection include:

| Diagnostic Title | Possible Etiological Factors |
|---|---|
| Hyperthermia | Release of endogenous pyrogens in response to an infectious agent |
| Pain | Inflammation, edema, circulating bacterial toxins |
| Fatigue | Increased metabolic energy production |
| Knowledge deficit related to diagnostic testing, antibiotics, disease process | Lack of exposure |

Other diagnoses are applicable depending on the type and location of infection. Examples include a patient with osteomyelitis who would be at risk for altered mobility or a patient with meningitis who would be at risk for altered cerebral tissue perfusion. The patient is always at risk for developing a systemic infection.

## ■ EXPECTED PATIENT OUTCOMES

Expected patient outcomes for the patient with an infection may include but are not limited to:

1. Returns to normal temperature after defervescence
2. Control of discomforts of malaise, mylagia, and fever
3. Decreased level of fatigue
4. Verbalizes understanding of rationale for diagnosis, e.g., radiological examinations, cultures, and CBC

## ■ INTERVENTIONS

### Promoting Normothermia

Fever is a protective response to pathogens. Treatment is focused on eradicating the causative organism from the body. Nursing interventions include administration of antipyretics and antibiotics to treat the underlying cause of infection. The patient should be monitored for therapeutic and adverse effects of the antibiotic. The nurse should make sure the causative organism is sensitive to the prescribed antibiotic. Superinfection is a side effect of antibiotic therapy and may occur with extended use of certain antibiotics.

Fever causes fluid loss from evaporation of body fluids and increased perspiration. Signs of dehydration include increased thirst, dry mucous membranes, and decreased skin turgor. Encouraging intake of oral fluids and possibly administering intravenous fluids are necessary to support circulating volume and tissue perfusion. Accurate record of intake and output is necessary to assess all sources of fluid loss. The nurse should assess the degree of diaphoresis as the body attempts to increase heat loss by evaporation, conduction, and diffusion. The patient should be bathed and given dry linen after defervescence.

Additional methods of reducing fever include use of hypothermia blankets, ice packs, and tepid water baths. The nurse should be careful not to cool the patient too quickly as this can produce shivering. Shivering causes increased heat production and oxygen consumption. The use of hypothermia blankets should be discontinued when the patient's temperature is within 1° to 3° of the desired temperature.

Vital signs should be monitored including an accurate assessment of core temperature. Seizures and a decreased level of consciousness are potential complications of fever. Dysrhythmias can be caused by dehydration.

### Promoting Comfort

Both pharmacological and nonpharmacological methods of pain relief are indicated (see Chapter 12). Analgesics such as acetaminophen or nonsteroidal antiinflammatory agents (NSAIDs) are effective in reducing discomfort related to fever. NSAIDs will decrease the inflammatory response.

### Promoting Rest

The nurse should encourage adequate rest during the acute phase of infection. The patient should be encouraged to be as independent as possible. Together the nurse and patient should plan for increased levels of activity. Scheduling tests and activities when the patient is fully rested is beneficial.

### Patient/Family Education

The patient and family should be informed of the purpose of treatment modalities. Education regarding medication is essential to prevent recurrence of infection and drug resistance. The importance of completing the entire course of antibiotic therapy should be stressed. Health promotion techniques such as handwashing and avoiding sources of infection should be included in the teaching plan.

Persons with infections frequently are cared for at home. The community health nurse often is asked to teach family members how to care for the patient and how to protect family members, friends, and neighbors. Many of the same principles of infection control apply in the home as in the hospital. Some general principles for home care of persons with an infection are discussed here.

Handwashing is considered the most effective measure in preventing the spread of infection in the home. Hands should be washed before care and after contact with body substances (blood, urine, feces, sputum, vomitus, or wound drainage). Caregivers should wear a smock or coverall to protect their clothes. Gloves should be worn when handling body substances. Soiled dressings, used disposable gloves, and other disposable items that contain body substances should be put in plastic bags before being discarded in the trash. All liquid waste can be flushed down the toilet. Used needles and syringes should be put in a puncture-resistant plastic container or can, which is tightly closed before discarding in the trash. Disposable dishes are not required. Dishes and linen should be washed in hot soapy water. A cup of bleach should be added to the detergent to disin-fect laundry soiled with blood. Blood and body substance spills should be cleaned up using an effective household disinfectant. If gloves are not available, plastic bags can be worn to protect the caregiver's hands. All persons should be taught to cover the nose and mouth when coughing. In general, it is not considered necessary for the caregiver to wear a mask in the home.

### Health Promotion/Prevention: *Healthy People 2000*

Although the last 100 years have seen a reduction in the incidence of infectious diseases, e.g., control of smallpox, diphtheria and polio through the development of vaccines, there exist underimmunized groups. The emergence of newly recognized diseases such as Lyme disease, Legionnaire's disease, and toxic shock and the persistence of diseases such as influenza, bacterial pneumonia, hepatitis B, hepatitis C, tuberculosis, and bacterial meningitis remain as threats to public health. Objectives for the year 2000 include:

- Eliminate measles. Inadequate immunization of low-income preschool children and young adults has resulted in a resurgence of the disease.
- Reduce epidemic-related pneumonia and influenza deaths to no more than 15.9 per 100,000 people aged 65 and older. Pneumococcal pneumonia and influenza immunization of older institutionalized or chronically ill adults must be increased, to at least 80%. Pneumococcal and influenza immunization of noninstitutionalized high-risk populations should be increased to at least 60%.[18]
- Increase childhood immunization levels to at least 90% of 2-year-olds (a 20% increase). Strategies include expanding immunization laws for schools, preschools, and daycare settings and removing financial barriers to immunization.[7]

Other objectives target reducing the incidence of middle ear infections, tuberculosis, surgical wound infections, infectious diarrhea in child care programs, viral hepatitis, rabies, bacterial meningitis, and travel-related typhoid fever and malaria. Strategies include public education programs to reduce infection (see the Patient/Family Teaching Box).

## ■ EVALUATION

To evaluate effectiveness of nursing interventions, compare patient behaviors with those stated in the expected patient outcomes. Successful achievement of patient outcomes for the patient with infection is indicated by:

1. Maintains core temperature within normal range for 24 hours
2. States relief of discomfort
3. Participates in usual levels of activity

4a. Describes rationale for diagnostic examinations

b. Completes course of antibiotics

**patient/family teaching**

**Information to Be Included in Public Education Programs to Reduce Infection**

1. Vaccines that are available to prevent infection; see specific recommendations elsewhere in this chapter
2. Need to report symptoms of generalized infections that persist more than 24 hours (see Box 10-4: Subjective and Objective Data Suggesting Infection)
3. Rationale for completion of entire course of prescribed antibiotics; concept of developing resitance
4. Need to report signs of antibiotic allergy immediately; itching, rash, and respiratory swelling
5. Rationale for reserving antibiotic use for severe infections; avoid disrupting normal body flora

**critical thinking QUESTIONS**

1 Mr. S, a 65-year-old patient with type II diabetes, is admitted for a femoral popliteal bypass graft for impaired circulation to his left lower extremity. Two months before this admission, he was discharged after treatment for an infected left foot ulcer, which grew MRSA and was colonized with VRE. What precautions would you take in planning care for this patient?

2 Ms. P is admitted with a persistent lung lesion in the left upper lobe. Lung cancer is suspected. A bronchoscopy is performed and acid-fast bacillus cultures subsequently grow *Mycobacterium tuberculosis.* The patient had not been in isolation before these results. What action would you take regarding possible exposure of other patients and personnel?

3 Mr. W is admitted for chemotherapy for treatment of acute myelocytic leukemia. He has a right subclavian catheter triple lumen catheter for infusion of his chemotherapy and total parenteral nutrition The site is inspected daily. The nurse tells Mr. W the line must be changed because of induration at the site. Explain why this may have occurred and possible consequences.

## chapter SUMMARY

### EXTERNAL NONSPECIFIC DEFENSE MECHANISMS

- The human body is protected from encroachment by foreign materials and cells by a system of protective structural and biochemical barriers.

### INTERNAL NONSPECIFIC DEFENSE MECHANISMS

- If foreign materials or cells gain access to internal body tissues, they are recognized and attacked by a system of specifically and nonspecifically responding mechanisms.

### SPECIFIC DEFENSE MECHANISMS

- The humorally mediated immune response is mediated by B cell lymphocytes, which produce circulating antibodies that bind antigens.
- The cell-mediated immune response is mediated by T cell lymphocytes, which produce activated T cells that seek out and attack antigen-labeled cells.
- The secondary immune response provides a faster and more efficient response on contact with the specific antigen a second time.

### INFECTION CONTROL: HISTORICAL PERSPECTIVE

- Infection control programs exist to decrease morbidity, mortality, and cost of nosocomial infections.

### THE INFECTIOUS DISEASE PROCESS

- The sequence of events in the chain of infection involves (1) a causative agent, (2) a reservoir, (3) a portal of exit, (4) a mode of transmission, (5) a portal of entry, and (6) a susceptible host.
- Modes of transmission are (1) contact (direct, indirect, or droplet), (2) airborne, (3) vehicle, and (4) vector.
- Fever and a WBC count greater than 10,000/mm$^3$ may indicate a generalized infection.
- When possible, appropriate cultures should be performed before antibiotic therapy is initiated.

### INFECTION CONTROL IN THE COMMUNITY

- In the United States the ACIP recommends that children be immunized against diphtheria, tetanus, pertussis (DTP): measles, mumps, rubella (MMR); poliomyelitis (OPV); *Haemophilus influenzae* (Hib); and hepatitis B.
- Health caregivers who have frequent contact with blood and body fluids should be immunized against hepatitis B virus.
- Passive immunity is temporary, lasting a few weeks without stimulating antibody production in the recipient.
- In general, live attenuated virus vaccines should not be given to persons with alterations in immune status.

### INFECTION CONTROL IN THE HOSPITAL

- A nosocomial infection is one that is not present or incubating when a person is admitted to the hospital but develops after admission.
- Handwashing is the most important measure in preventing cross-infection.
- Urinary catheterization is associated with increased risk for nosocomial urinary tract infection.
- Nosocomial pneumonia occurs in approximately 0.6% of hospitalized medical patients and is associated with the highest mortality rate of all nosocomial infections.
- Aseptic technique is an important factor in preventing nosocomial infection.
- Two tiers of isolation are (1) Standard Precautions and (2) Transmission-Based Precautions.
- Caregivers should direct problems concerning any aspect of infection control to the infection control nurse, the hospital epidemiologist, or the infection control committee in their institution.

### NURSING MANAGEMENT

- Nursing diagnoses related to the care of the person with an infection include hyperthermia, pain, fatigue, and knowledge deficit.
- Nursing interventions include promoting normothermia, promoting comfort and rest, and education regarding infection.
- *Healthy People 2000* goals include increasing the immunization status of adults and the reduction of pneumonia, influenzae, and other infectious diseases.

## References


1. Abbas A, Lichtman A, Pober J: *Cellular and molecular immunology,* Philadelphia, 1994, WB Saunders.
2. American Hospital Association: OSHA's final bloodborne pathogen standard: a special briefing, Chicago, 1992, The Association.
3. Bennett JV, Brachman PS, editors: *Hospital infections,* Boston, 1992, Little, Brown & Co.
4. Centers for Disease Control and Prevention: Recommendations of the ACIP: smallpox vaccine, *MMWR* 34(23):341-342, 1985.
5. Centers for Disease Control and Prevention: National Nosocomial Infections Surveillance (NNIS) Report, data summary from October 1986-April 1996, issued May 1996, *Am J Infect Control* 24:380-388, 1996.
6. Centers for Disease Control and Prevention: Public health focus: surveillance, prevention, and control of nosocomial infections, *MMWR* 41(42):783-787, 1992.
7. Centers for Disease Control and Prevention: Recommended childhood immunization schedule, *MMWR* 44(RR-5):1-9, 1995.
8. Cohen ML: Epidemiology of drug resistance: implications for a post-antimicrobial era, *Science* 257:1050-1055, 1992.
9. Garner JS and Hospital Infection Control Practices Advisory Committee: Guidelines for isolation precautions in hospitals. Part I. Evolution of isolation practices. Part II. Recommendations for isolation precautions in hospitals, *Am J Infect Control* 22:24-52, 1996.
10. Hospital Infection Control Practices Advisory Committee: Recommendations for preventing the spread of vancomycin resistance, *Infect Control Hosp Epidemiol* 16:105-113, 1995.
11. Mayhall CG, editor: *Hospital epidemiology and infection control,* Baltimore, 1996, Williams & Wilkins.
12. Nosocomial infection rates for interhospital comparison: limitations and possible solutions, *Infect Control Hosp Epidemiol* 12:609-621, 1991.
13. Pearson ML, Hospital Infection Control Practices Advisory Committee: Guideline for prevention of intravascular device-related infections, *Infect Control Hosp Epidemiol* 17:438-473, 1996.

14. Pugliese G: Medical news: infection control indicators in 1996, *Infect Control Hosp Epidemiol* 17(1):81-82, 1996.
15. Rumsey KA, Reiger PT, editors: *Biological response modifiers: a self-instruction manual for health professionals,* Chicago, 1992, Precept Press.
16. Soule BM, Larson EL, Preston GA: *Infections and nursing practice: prevention and control,* St Louis, 1995, Mosby.
17. Tenover FC, Hughes JM: The challenges of emerging infectious diseases: development and spread of multiply-resistant bacterial pathogens, *JAMA* 275:300-303, 1996.
18. US Department of Health and Human Services Public Health Service: *Healthy People 2000: midcourse review and 1995 revisions,* Washington, DC, 1995, US Government Printing Office.
19. Wenzel RP, editor: *Prevention and control of nosocomial infections,* Baltimore, 1993, Williams & Wilkins.

# chapter 11 Cancer

GLADYS E. DETERS

## objectives

*After studying this chapter, the learner should be able to:*

1. Describe epidemiological factors related to cancer.
2. Identify the nurse's role in prevention of cancer and in health education.
3. Describe the pathophysiology of cancer, including the characteristics of malignant cells, growth of neoplasms, and nature of metastases.
4. Identify the factors related to carcinogenesis.
5. Relate the pathophysiological changes of cancer to common clinical manifestations.
6. Apply the nursing process to care of the patient in the diagnostic and treatment phases of cancer.
7. Explain the rationale for the four major types of cancer therapy.
8. Discuss the major nursing care concerns for patients undergoing surgery, radiotherapy, chemotherapy, or biotherapy for treatment of cancer.

## NATURE OF THE PROBLEM

Cancer was recognized in ancient times by skilled observers who gave it the name "cancer" (L., *cancri,* crab) because it stretched out in many directions like the legs of a crab. The term *cancer* is an "umbrella" word used to describe a group of more than 270 diseases in which cells multiply without restraint, destroy healthy tissue, and endanger life.

Few diseases cause greater feelings of anxiety and apprehension than cancer. Its physiological and psychological impact on patients and their families results in profound changes in their lifestyles. Cancer may result in death for some and mutilation for others. The legends surrounding malignant disease, often focusing on its incurability, help foster feelings of hopelessness and dread. Yet much progress has been made in prevention, early detection, and treatment of cancer, and research continues in these areas.

Nurses may share the same negative attitudes about cancer that exist in society. For this reason it is extremely important that all nurses examine their own feelings about cancer and try to work through them, both by increasing their knowledge of the disease and its treatment and by discussing feelings openly with members of the health care team. Nurses who have resolved their own feelings are more able to help patients and their familes than are nurses who have not done so.

Cancer nursing has been recognized as a subspecialty in the nursing profession since 1975. Oncology nurses must have a broad base of knowledge in both pathophysiology and the psychosocial arena. They care for patients of all ages, both genders, and in a variety of settings that range from the acute care hospital to health promotion centers, ambulatory care clinics, home care agencies, and hospice care. The oncology nurse fills the role of care provider, manager, researcher, teacher, and consultant. To provide comprehensive care the nurse must have accurate knowledge about the prevention, control, and treatment of cancer. Teaching about cancer is not limited to the practice setting but may take place in industry, at parent-teacher association (PTA) meetings, and at other public forums. In addition to teaching about prevention, the nurse has an active role in treatment and control programs in all settings in which patients are found. Patients and their families look to the nurse for assistance and guidance in all phases of illness, from detection to terminal care.

To be effective as a helping person the nurse must be aware of the emotional impact that the diagnosis of cancer has on the patient and family because this emotional response affects every aspect of nursing care. Cancer nursing challenges the creativity, skill, and commitment of the nurse.

## ETIOLOGY

### MULTISTEP PROCESS OF CARCINOGENESIS

Comprehension of cellular kinetics is necessary to understand the multistep process of cancer development: initiation, promotion, and progression. Initiation begins with exposure of normal cells to carcinogens (substances that can cause cancer). Carcinogens such as radiation, chemicals, drugs, and viruses cause irreversible genetic damage that is referred to as mutation. Promotion, the second step, may last for many years. Promoting factors include cigarette smoking, alcohol abuse, and dietary components that act repeatedly over time on the already transformed cell. Promoters enhance the structural changes within the cell and are thought to facilitate the

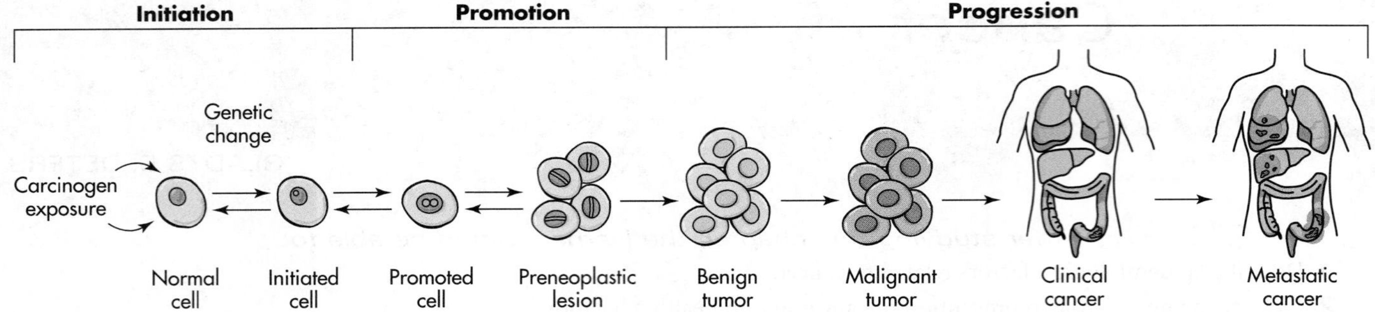


**fig. 11-1** Multistage process of carcinogenesis.

rate of these spontaneous mutations. These mutations produce ever-increasing numbers of abnormal cells.[9] Progression, the final step, is the uncontrolled growth of a malignant tumor capable of metastatic activity.

Carcinogenesis is a dynamic process that is influenced by many independent and poorly defined variables. Etiological agents may act as cocarcinogens. A genetic predisposition for a "weak" immune system along with a viral infection may eventually lead to cancer, or oncogenic viruses may suppress the immune system. Chemical carcinogens may activate latent viral genes or inhibit the immune system's effectiveness in destroying cancer cells. These initiating molecular changes are irreversible. Figure 11-1 illustrates the multistep process of cancer development.

## FACTORS INHIBITING TUMOR GROWTH

Tumor cells compete with normal cells and tissue for blood supply, and tumor growth may be initially impaired by a lack of vascularization. As tumor cells grow, they stimulate vascularization (angiogenesis) with the establishment of new capillary sprouts. Until the capillaries penetrate the tumor, growth is slow and the tumor is termed *avascular.* After capillary penetration, the tumor begins to grow rapidly, is capable of distant metastasis, and is said to be in a *vascular* stage. Carcinoma in situ lesions are in the avascular phase of development, which accounts for their slow and localized growth.

Growth of tumors that arise in tissues regulated by sex hormones may be affected in positive or negative ways. For example, breast cancers that occur during pregnancy often grow rapidly but tend to grow less rapidly after delivery.

Although it is rare, tumors have regressed spontaneously, in some cases as a result of maturation and differentiation of tumor cells. This happens most commonly in neuroblastoma, a tumor of embryonic neuroblasts. The cause and physiological action of spontaneous maturation are not known.

## FACTORS AFFECTING RATE OF TUMOR GROWTH

Knowledge of cell kinetics is important because the sensitivity of the cell to chemotherapy and radiotherapy depends heavily on the proliferative state of the cell at a specific time. In addition, study of cell cycle kinetics helps increase understanding of tumor growth and regulation, laying the foundation for better methods of controlling cancer cells. The rate of growth of a tumor is expressed in terms of volume-doubling time (time required for the tumor mass to double in size). Human tumors generally have a long doubling time, from 1 week to more than 1 year, with a median time of about 60 days. Because tumors contain many different types of cells, the length of the cell cycle (median generation time) varies from 2 to 3 days.

In normal adult tissue, the rate of cell renewal is equal to the rate of cell death. In contrast, cancer cell division continues indefinitely. When the tumor is small and growing rapidly, a relatively high proportion of cells are undergoing division and tumor doubling time is rapid. As the tumor increases in size with a larger cell population, a longer doubling time is needed. This growth pattern is known as gompertzian function (Figure 11-2).

Three factors affect the rate of tumor growth: (1) the rate of the replication of proliferating cells (cell cycle time), (2) the proportion of total cell population that is actively proliferating (growth fraction), and (3) the rate of cell loss from cell death and exfoliation of cells from the tumor surface. Cell cycle time is relatively constant in tumors with similar histology, but it is considerably different from normal tissue. For a given cycle time, a tumor with a high growth fraction will double faster than a tumor with a low growth fraction.

## ROLE OF ONCOGENES

In the early 1970s oncogenes (specific genes that can trigger cancer cell growth) were discovered. One hundred of these cancer genes have now been identified. These oncogenes are similar, if not identical, to genes normally present in the cell, called proto-oncogenes. It seems that these normal genes—when activated by radiation, chemicals, or viruses—are transformed to a malignant state. It is still unclear whether oncogenes are involved in all or just some cancers and how they fit into the overall pattern of carcinogenesis.

The cancer-causing genes and normal genes appear virtually the same, but their functions differ drastically. Although the activation of an oncogene is part of the process of carcinogenesis, it is not in itself usually enough to cause cancerous growth. Tumors may grow from the combined effects of a number of oncogenes, each representing one of the multiple steps of carcinogenesis. The activation of one oncogene may trigger the next oncogene, resulting in a cascade of reactions.

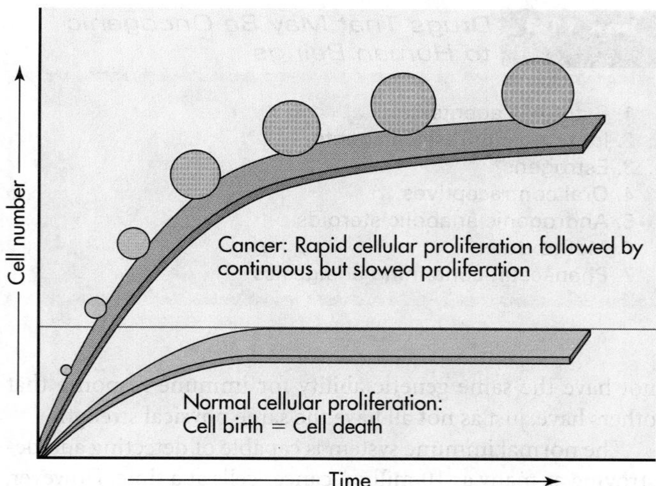


**fig. 11-2** Gompertzian function.

It is hoped that knowledge of oncogenes can eventually be used to treat, cure, or prevent cancer.

## HOST SUSCEPTIBILITY

### Genetic Factors

Research has shown that cancer develops through a multistep process of genetic derangement. Certain conditions and predispositions of the individual seem to contribute to the development of cancer. Studies of genetic factors have examined both specific cancer sites and the disease in general. Deranged genes may be passed to offspring through either autosomal recessive or autosomal dominant transmission. When both parents have the abnormal gene, all future descendents of the transformed cell will be malignant and the strain will be inherited by all future generations (autosomal recessive). Autosomal dominant inheritance is accomplished when a gene from only one parent is abnormal. Thus offspring have a 50% chance of inheriting the deranged cell.[17]

Hereditary cancers have certain general characteristics: (1) an early age of onset, occurring 20 or more years earlier than in the general population; (2) a marked incidence of bilateral cancer in paired organs—for example, breasts, kidneys, and thyroid glands; (3) a greater frequency of the development of the same cancer(s) in multiple primary or multicentered cancers; and (4) appearance in two or more members of one generation.

Leukemia is an example of a malignant condition associated with chromosomal alterations. Chronic myelogenous leukemia (CML) is associated with Philadelphia chromosome 22 translocation, whereas trisomy 21 found in Down's syndrome has been shown to be a risk factor for the development of acute myelogenous leukemia (AML).

It is also possible to inherit a condition that increases a person's risk for eventually developing a certain cancer. Ulcerative colitis can result in cancer the colon even with effective treatment. In familial polyposis, an inherited disease, colon cancer is expected in 100% of all untreated cases. True "cancer families" are rare and differ from other families in whom many cancers seem to develop. Cancer families tend to inherit the same kind of cancer and develop the disease at an early age (Table 11-1).

**table 11-1** *Cancers Associated with Genetic Factors*

| Type of Cancer | Characteristics |
|---|---|
| Wilms' tumor | Purely hereditary |
| Familial polyposis of colon | Precursor of cancer |
| Breast cancer | High incidence in vertical line of descent (mother to daughter) |
| Bronchogenic cancer | Seems to develop from synergistic effect of heredity and cigarette smoking |
| Cancer family syndrome (CFS): adenocarcinoma of colon and endometrium; sometimes of stomach, breast, and ovaries | Autosomal dominant inheritance; transmitted vertically |
| Familial atypical multiple mole–melanoma (FAMMM) syndrome. | Familial disease; genetic factors predispose individuals |
| Xeroderma pigmentosum and disseminated superficial actinic porokeratosis | Autosomal recessive disorders; skin cancer precursors |

### Hormonal Factors

Evidence suggests that hormones may be connected with the development of certain cancers. In addition, some metabolites of cancers may act as antihormones or have new physiological effects. Hormones do not appear to be primary carcinogens but seem to influence carcinogenesis in three ways: (1) by a preparative action on the target tissues, making them susceptible to the carcinogenic agent; (2) by a "permissive" influence on carcinogenesis, allowing the process to progress; and (3) by a conditioning effect on the tumor. Hormones can restrain or enhance tumor growth. Hormone therapy and some surgical therapies (hypophysectomy and oophorectomy) are based on this principle.

There is evidence that tissues that are endocrine responsive (e.g., breasts, endometrium, and prostate) do not develop cancer unless stimulated by their growth-promoting hormones. Estrogens have been associated with adenocarcinomas of the vagina, hepatic tumors, breast tumors, and uterine cancer.

In addition to tissue stimulation by the hormone, carcinogenesis may be determined by the duration of the hormonal effect. The longer the preparative influence of the hormone, the greater the chance of cancer development.

### Precancerous Lesions

Certain benign lesions and tumors have a tendency toward malignant change. The cancers may be preventable if minor precursor conditions are located and treated early. Precancerous lesions belong to a large and heterogeneous group; in some, cancer is inevitable, whereas in others the risk is so low that medical intervention is unnecessary. Precancerous conditions include polyps of the colon and rectum, certain pigmented moles, dysplasias of the cervical epithelium, Paget's disease of the bone, senile keratoses, and leukoplakias of the oral mucous membranes.

### Chronic Irritation

Trauma, chronic irritation, and inflammation are believed to be causative factors in cancer development, but proof has been difficult to obtain. Nevertheless it is prudent to be alert to the possible consequences of trauma or chronic irritation to any part of the body. Efforts are being made to protect workers from the irritation of coal-tar products known to contain carcinogens. Masks and gloves are recommended in some instances, and workers are urged to wash their hands and arms thoroughly to remove all irritating substances at the end of the day's work.

Any kind of chronic skin irritation should be avoided, and moles that are irritated by clothing should be removed. Shoelaces, shoetops, belts, girdles, brassieres, and shirt collars are examples of sources of chronic irritation. Glasses, earrings, dentures, and pipes that are in repeated contact with skin and mucous membranes can also be chronic irritants. Cancer of the mouth sometimes is associated with constant irritation of the oral mucous membrane by rough, jagged teeth. Chewing food thoroughly is recommended to lessen throat and stomach irritation. The habit of drinking scalding hot or freezing cold liquids is also thought to be irritating to the mouth and to the esophagus. Indiscriminate use of laxatives is believed to have carcinogenic effects on the large bowel.

### Immunological Factors

Immunologists have been increasingly aware of the role of the immune system in the natural history of malignant disease. Failure of the normal immune mechanism may predispose a person to certain cancers. Mutated cells are antigenically different and should be recognized as such by the body's immune system. When the immune response is initiated, the malignant cell will be destroyed. The presence of an immune surveillance system is suggested by the following: (1) The two peaks of high incidence of tumors are early childhood and old age—periods when the immune system is weak. (2) Increased tumor development occurs in persons who have immunodeficiency diseases associated with a defect in cellular immunity. (3) Persons who receive immunosuppressive drugs such as cyclosporine or azathioprine used to prevent organ transplant rejection have an increased incidence of neoplasia (e.g., non-Hodgkin's lymphoma).

It is not clear why initial tumor cells progress to clinical cancer if an immune surveillance system exists. Some tumors arise in areas that are poorly served by the immune system, such as the central nervous system or the retrobulbar aspect of the eye. Some tumors do not stimulate antibody formation because they are so similar to normal cells. The normal system that controls the immune response may become overactive and suppress the immune system. And some persons may simply not have the same genetic ability for immune response that others have, just as not all have the same physical strength.

**box 11-1** *Drugs That May Be Oncogenic to Human Beings*

1. Cytotoxic agents
2. Immunosuppressive agents
3. Estrogens
4. Oral contraceptives
5. Androgenic anabolic steroids
6. Methoxsalen
7. Phenacetin-containing analgesics

The normal immune system is capable of detecting and destroying as many as 10 million cancer cells at a time. However, when a tumor mass grows at a rate faster than the normal immunological response can effectively handle, the tumor will continue to grow unchecked. Typically, a tumor mass must be at least 1 cm in size before it can be detected by conventional diagnostic methods. Unfortunately a tumor 1 cm in diameter already contains more than 1 billion malignant cells. Research on the immune system will provide more definitive answers about the interplay of immune function and surveillance and cancer development. (The role of the immune system is discussed further in Chapter 66.)

### Drug Effects

The International Agency for Research on Cancer has identified a number of drugs that are known to have carcinogenic potential in human beings. The list includes some over-the-counter (OTC) drugs easily purchased by consumers, such as mixtures containing phenacetin, as well as a variety of commonly prescribed medications (Box 11-1).

Oral contraceptives, classified as having carcinogenic potential for breast cancer, are now recognized as having a protective effect against ovarian and endometrial cancers.[6] In 1971 a rare form of vaginal cancer in women was linked to the ingestion by their mothers of diethylstilbestrol (DES), which was prescribed to prevent spontaneous abortion.

Cancer therapy itself may increase the risk for other cancers. Intensive alkylating agent therapy is accompanied by significant subsequent risk of acute leukemia. Consequently their use is limited to those cases for which no comparable alternative therapy exists. Further research on disease response to drugs is needed to prevent long-term risks of cancer treatment.

### Environmental Factors

As long ago as 1775 the incidence of prostate cancer was recognized in men employed as chimney sweeps in English homes where coal was burned as fuel. Coal tar, an end product of coal combustion, is now acknowledged as the first recognized occupational chemical carcinogen. The importance of the link between environment and cancer development increases when patterns of incidence and mortality are studied. As people move from place to place throughout the world, the

table 11-2 *Occupations Associated with Exposure to Cancer Risks*

| | |
|---|---|
| **KNOWN HUMAN CARCINOGENS—GROUP 1 RATINGS*** | |
| Aluminum production | Iron and steel founding |
| Auramine, manufacture of | Isopropanol manufacture (strong-acid process) |
| Boot and shoe manufacture and repair | Magenta, manufacture of |
| Coal gasification | Painter (occupational exposure as) |
| Coke production | Rubber industry |
| Furniture and cabinet making | Strong-inorganic-acid mists containing sulfuric acid (occupational exposure to) |
| Hematite mining (underground) with exposure to radon | |
| **PROBABLE HUMAN CARCINOGENS—GROUP 2A RATINGS** | |
| Art glass, glass containers and pressed ware (manufacture of) | Nonarsenical insecticides (occupational exposure in spraying and application of) |
| Hairdresser or barber (occupational exposure as a) | Petroleum refining (occupational exposure in) |
| **POSSIBLE HUMAN CARCINOGENS—GROUP 2B RATINGS** | |
| Carpentry and joinery | Textile manufacturing industry (work in) |

From Stellman JM, Stellman SD: Cancer and the workplace, *CA Cancer J Clin* 46(2):70, 1996.
*Rated by the International Agency for Research on Cancer.

baseline incidence and mortality rates for each type of cancer change. It is theorized that if all the measures already known about cancer prevention were put into practice, up to two thirds of cancers would never occur.[1]

The Occupational Safety and Health Act of 1970 authorized the Occupational Safety and Health Administration to enforce maximal allowable concentrations of exposure to carcinogens (threshold limit values [TLVs]). This task is difficult because the identification of potential human carcinogens in the environment and workplace is a lengthy and time-consuming process. The list of possible carcinogens is ever changing as data accumulate, industrial safety practices are improved, and worker exposure fluctuates. In addition new chemicals are continually being introduced into the occupational setting.[26]

The National Institute for Occupational Safety and Health believes that at present it is not possible to establish precise tolerance levels to chemical carcinogens. It stresses that exposure to any known or suggested carcinogens must be reduced to the least possible level by any means available. Table 11-2 provides a list of occupations that expose workers to cancer risks.

### Ionizing radiation

Radiography and radium may cure cancer, but they also can cause it. Ionizing radiation consists of electromagnetic waves or material particles that have sufficient energy to ionize atoms or molecules (i.e., remove electrons from them) and thereby alter their chemical behavior. In adequate amounts it destroys the cells.

Every living thing is exposed to small amounts of radiation from the sun and from natural elements in the earth, such as uranium, that emit gamma rays ($\gamma$-rays). This is known as natural background radiation. Problems with radiation did not appear until after 1895, when the roentgen-ray (x-ray) machine was developed and became widely used in diagnosis of disease. The development of this machine was followed by the discovery of radium and the use of both radium and radiography for treatment of diseases such as cancer.

Radiologists working with early radiographic equipment showed a higher than normal incidence of skin cancer. Workers employed in painting radium on watch dials had high rates of oral and sinus carcinomas and osteosarcomas. It is well known that survivors of the atomic bombs dropped on the Japanese cities of Hiroshima and Nagasaki during World War II were exposed to high doses of radiation. Within a 10-year period after exposure, a variety of cancers developed in this population at higher than normal incidence rates.

No one really knows how much exposure to radiation is safe for patients having repeated radiographs and the staff members working with them. Relatively small amounts of exposure have produced serious damage in experimental animals, but human beings have not lived through enough generations of relatively high expsure for conclusive evidence to be established. It is reasonable to assume that the less exposure the better.

Radiation exposure results in breakage of either a single or double strand of the DNA helix. The damage is permanent and cumulative following each additional radiation exposure. Exposure of the entire body significantly increases the amount of radiation received. For this reason all of the body except the part being treated is protected from exposure when relatively high doses are given for therapeutic purposes.

The amount of exposure a patient receives from a series of radiographs taken for diagnostic purposes depends on the machine used and the technical skill involved. Usually, the fluoroscopic examination entails more exposure than the use of radiography. The exposure of the average nurse working in a hospital and occasionally assisting a patient while a radiograph is taken is almost negligible.

Systemic reactions to high-dose radiation exposure include leukopenia, leukemia, bone cancer, and sterility or damage to the reproductive cells. Because of the risk, film badges are worn by persons whose daily work exposes them to radiation. The badge, which contains photographic film capable of absorbing radiation, is developed each month. A darkening or blackening of the film indicates excessive exposure. Personnel who are becoming overexposed are removed, at least temporarily, from direct contact with radiation.

Because of the danger to the fetus, particularly between the second and sixth weeks of gestation, pregnant women usually are not employed in radiology departments or in caring for patients receiving radioactive material internally.

**box 11-2** *Chemical Carcinogenic Agents*

Polycylic aromatic hydrocarbons (tar, pitch): skin cancer
Arsenic: skin cancer
Aromatic amines: bladder cancer
Chromium compounds: skin cancer
Asbestos: respiratory and lung cancer
Benzene inhalation: leukemia
Nitrosamines (food additives, nicotine): esophageal cancer
Chloromethyl methyl ether and vinyl chloride (polyvinyl plastics)
Some hair dyes

#### *Effects of the sun*

Our society at times seems sun addicted, and a tanned skin is eagerly sought by many. The carcinogenic effect of sunlight, although not completely understood, appears to be related to ultraviolet B (UVB) radiation. There is speculation that depletion of the ozone may be a factor in the rising rates of skin cancer.[20] Skin cancer occurs most commonly in persons who work in the open air, such as sailors, construction workers, and farmers, and on areas of the body most exposed to sunlight. Light-complexioned individuals are the most cancer susceptible.

#### *Radon and electromagnetic field effects*

Radon exposure in the environment is an increasing concern as a cause of cancer. Radon is an inert gas that emanates from the ground and stone building materials. It results from the decay of uranium, taking the form of radon gas and alpha particles. When the particles are inhaled into the respiratory tract, the resultant alpha irradiation to the bronchial epithelium can result in lung cancer. The radon gas itself is not as important as the alpha particles. The first known association of radon exposure and lung cancer was found among uranium miners.

It is not known whether the same risks apply to indoor exposure, but the possibility is a concern. The leakage of radon is irregular and depends on the condition of both the building structure and the ground beneath. It is believed that the use of central heating and improvements made in building insulation now allow high concentrations of radon to remain indoors instead of escaping into the environment. Radon detection kits are available. Detectors are recommended in several areas of a building, such as the basement and each floor level. Users of home detection kits should seek professional assistance in interpreting results.

The effects of exposure from living or working near electromagnetic fields (EMFs) is another recent environmental concern. Exposure to EMFs can come from household appliances, electrical wiring found in the home, and even from living near electrical power lines and electricity-generating facilities. Electrical transmission lines generate both electric and magnetic fields. Proper grounding blocks penetration of the electric field. However, the magnetic fields can easily pass through body tissue and most materials. The danger from magnetic fields is therefore the focus of most studies.[15] The intensity of the EMF is in proportion to the electrical energy running through the lines. The nearer one is to the source (within 50 m), the greater the exposure. Whether EMFs are carcinogenic remains unclear, but a weak association in leukemia incidence has been shown in children who live near high-voltage electric lines. Occupational exposure has been linked to an increased incidence of leukemia and brain tumors.[15] Cellular telephones are also being studied as a source (and thus a risk) of EMF exposure. At present neither the long-term effects of EMF exposure nor the level of exposure that is detrimental are known.

#### *Air pollution*

The relationship between air pollution and cancer is not completely understood. Two areas of concern are the depletion of the ozone layer as a result of increasing levels of industrial pollutants and the accumulation of gases such as carbon dioxide, nitrous oxide, methane, and chlorofluorocarbons that are known to produce "acid rain." The carcinogenic effects of air pollution are most clearly associated with the risk of lung or skin cancers inasmuch as they are inhaled or have direct contact with exposed skin. The multitude of pollutants in the air we breathe and the complexity of possible interactions make it difficult to identify other organ systems that might be at risk.

#### *Chemical pollutants*

Exposure to chemicals has been blamed for the rising incidence of cancer in the twentieth century. Box 11-2 lists some of the know chemical carcinogens.

Nitrosamines are known to cause a variety of cancers in different species. Nitrates are commonly used as food additives, and nicotine may be a source of amines. A liver carcinogen, aflatoxin 13, has been isolated from a common mold that grows on peanuts, soybeans, fruit, and some meats and cheeses.

Cyclamates, previously used as a sugar substitute, have been banned because they are potentially carcinogenic. Saccharin also has been identified as being carcinogenic in a study of rats, and the Food and Drug Administration (FDA) has recommended that it not be used as an artificial sweetener. Some hair dyes have been implicated in certain cases of cancer.

It is argued that some degree of carcinogenic risk is acceptable; others say that no level is acceptable and that all risks must be eliminated from the environment regardless of the cost. However, regulatory mechanisms and standards have not been established. Agencies such as the Environmental Protection Agency (EPA), Occupational Safety and Health Association (OSHA), and trade unions are aware of the potential health risks and have begun formulating guidelines for prevention and protection of workers and the general public.

## Lifestyle Practices

### Smoking and tobacco use

Cigarette smoking is clearly linked to an increased incidence of lung cancer. In 1997 lung cancer killed approximately 178,100 persons in the United States.[1] Although the incidence of lung cancer in men has been alarming, recent studies have noted a proportionately greater rise in the rate of lung cancer in women. The rise appears to parallel an increase in women smokers, particularly adolescent girls.

Correlation exists between cancer mortality and the number of cigarettes smoked daily, the number of years a person has smoked, and the age at which the person began to smoke. Smokers of two or more packs a day have a lung cancer mortality rate 12 to 25 times greater than that of a nonsmoker. Smoking also has been connected with oral, esophageal, and possibly bladder cancer.[1] If smoking is discontinued even after a habit of 30 or more years, the incidence of lung cancer decreases.

Many smokers have changed to filtered cigarettes, pipe smoking, or the use of smokeless tobacco (plug, leaf, snuff) in the misguided belief that their cancer risk will be lessened or eliminated. Evidence is abundant that there is no "safe" cigarette and that smokeless tobacco is equally unsafe because it places the user at higher risk for head and neck cancers.

The carcinogenic effects of tobacco smoke released into the environment (environmental tobacco smoke [ETS]) have been thoroughly investigated. Results show that ETS contains most of the same carcinogenic compounds that have been identified in mainstream smoke. Consequently nonsmokers inhaling the ambient air near a cigarette smoker are exposed to the same carcinogens as the smoker and their risk for lung cancer, cardiovascular disease, and other respiratory conditions increases.

Since 1971 no cigarette advertising has been permitted on either television or radio. At the same time the warning on cigarette packages was changed from "Caution: cigarette smoking may be hazardous to your health" to either "Warning: the surgeon general has determined that cigarette smoking is dangerous to your health" or a more definitive statement asserting that smoking may cause cancer, heart disease, and emphysema. Although the campaign to convince people to stop smoking has been slow and arduous, changes have been noted in smoking patterns. Two thirds of the population are nonsmokers, and legislation has been enacted to prevent smoking in public places, on domestic flights, and in public buildings. Now with solid scientific evidence of the effects of ETS on nonsmokers, the regulation and restriction of public smoking and the sale of tobacco products are expected to advance on both the local and national levels. Box 11-3 lists strategies that concerned persons can use to eradicate or at least limit smoking.

**box 11-3** *Methods to Control Smoking*

- Encourage young people not to start.
- Educate the public on the hazards of smoking, with the aim of getting the smoker to quit.
- Provide self-help materials.
- Work with the media.
- Recruit ex-smoker volunteers to provide one-to-one help for smokers trying to quit.
- Encourage industries, hospitals, and organizations to conduct their own stop-smoking programs.
- Make available Fresh Start, the American Cancer Society quit-smoking program.
- Support legislation to restrict smoking and the sale of tobacco products in public places.

### Nutrition

The second most significant lifestyle change to reduce cancer risk relates to dietary habits. Nutrition research has increased steadily over the past decade, and a variety of studies indicate a relationship between dietary components and the development of cancer.

The consumption of a diet high in fat and calories has been associated with an increased risk for colon, breast, prostate, pancreatic, and endometrial cancer.[1] These cancers are more prevalent in the United States and Europe and may in part be related to the ability to purchase foods that are high in red meat and fat content. Large-scale, long-term studies of the effect of dietary fat on the incidence of breast and uterine cancer are needed to confirm or rule out the risk.

Diets high in fiber content appear to offer protection against colon cancer. Fiber is believed to reduce cancer risk by diluting colon contents, decreasing colon transit time, and thus limiting contact with carcinogens. Fruits, vegetables, and whole grain foods, which are good sources of vitamins C and D, beta carotene, and selenium, appear to have a cancer-deterrent effect. These vitamins and minerals, known as antioxidants, assist in the repair of cellular damage caused by free radicals. Free radicals damage the genetic makeup of the cell and its natural ability to resist cancer.

A significant association exists between high alcohol intake and cancer of the mouth, pharynx, larynx, and esophagus. However, alcoholism often is also associated with smoking and vitamin and dietary deficiencies. It is speculated that alcohol consumption and nutritional deficiencies may enhance carcinogenesis by increasing the metabolic activity of specific tobacco carcinogens. Tumors of the involved sites occur with greater frequency in men, blacks, elders, and persons from lower socioeconomic groups and urban settings. As a result of nutrition research, dietary recommendations have been established that may reduce or prevent cancer[1] (Box 11-4).

#### Sexual practices

Carcinoma of the uterine cervix is less common in virgins than in sexually active women. The incidence is higher in those who have first coitus at an early age, who have an early first marriage, and who have had multiple sex partners. Teenage women are at greater risk for cervical dysplasia, a precursor stage in the development of cancer of the squamocolumnar junction.

Carcinoma of the penis is virtually unknown among circumcised men. The means by which circumcision provides protection is not clear, but it is probably related to better hygiene. It is no longer believed that coitus with an uncircumcised partner places a woman at risk for cervical cancer.

The correlation between sexual activity and breast cancer is the reverse of that for the uterine cervix. Women in whom breast cancer develops tend to marry and become pregnant later in life. A woman's age at the birth of her first child is also a relevant factor in the subsequent development of breast cancer. Women who give birth to their first child before age 20 have only one third the risk of women older than age 35 who deliver a first child. This fact is not used to advocate for pregnancy at an early age but to help women make informed decisions on when to begin a family. (Box 11-5 summarizes cancer-related factors.)

**box 11-4** *Nutritional Practices to Prevent Cancer*

- *Maintain a desirable weight.* Weight maintenance can be accomplished by reducing intake of total calories and by maintaining a physically active lifestyle.
- *Eat a varied diet.* A varied diet eaten in moderation offers the best hope for lowering the risk of cancer.
- *Include a variety of vegetables and fruits in the daily diet.* Studies have shown that daily consumption of vegetables and fresh fruits is associated with a decreased risk of lung, prostate, bladder, esophagus, colorectal, and stomach cancers.
- *Eat more high-fiber foods such as whole grain cereals, breads, pasta, and vegetables and fruits.* High-fiber diets are a healthy substitute for fatty foods and may reduce the risk of colon cancer.
- *Limit total fat intake.* The American Cancer Society recommends reducing total fat intake to 30% or less of total calorie intake.
- *Limit consumption of alcohol, if you drink at all.* Heavy drinking, when accompanied by cigarette smoking or smokeless tobacco use, increases risk of cancers of the mouth, larynx, throat, esophagus, and liver.
- *Limit consumption of salt-cured, smoked, and nitrite-cured foods.* In areas of the world where salt-cured and smoked foods are eaten frequently, there is a higher incidence of cancer of the esophagus and stomach.

Modified from American Cancer Society: *1996 cancer facts and figures,* New York, 1996, The Society.

### Viruses

Studies in animals have established a viral role in carcinogenesis, but proof that human beings are affected has not been definitely ascertained. Viruses have been isolated and identified as the cause of cancer in mice, rabbits, and frogs.

Cervical cancer may result from a virus introduced into the cervix during sexual intercourse. This virus may be a member of the herpes group, Herpesvirus hominis (HV-II), and is more common in women with dysplasia of the uterine cervix.

Herpes-like viruses have been visualized by use of electron microscopy in Burkitt's tumor and Hodgkin's disease cells. Investigators, however, have been unable to demonstrate human oncogenic viruses in human tumors. The long latency period in humans also makes study of viruses difficult.

### Psychosocial Factors

Stressors such as life changes, loss of a significant other, and personality variables have been suggested as etiological factors in the development of cancer. A "cancer-prone" personality has been suggested, but is unproven. The practical value of such data is also questioned. Little is known about the effect of states of mind on the immune or hormonal systems that may affect the disease, but research with acquired immunodeficiency syndrome (AIDS) patients has indicated a positive effect. Most reports are anecdotal in nature, however, and cannot be subjected to rigorous analysis. Further studies in psychoneuroimmunology may yet reveal the mechanism for these complex interactions.

Social support in the form of institutions, family, and friends also may be an important variable. The person with minimal social support and maximal need may be at a higher risk for developing cancer. In addition, lack of social support may adversely affect coping responses to therapy and to the illness. At

**box 11-5** *Summary of Factors Related to Cancer Causation*

- Genetic predisposition
- Hormonal effects
- Precancerous lesions
- Chronic irritation, trauma, or inflammation
- Immune system function
- Drug therapy
- Environmental factors
  - Ionizing radiation
  - Sun exposure
  - Radon and electromagnetic field effects
  - Chemical pollutants
  - Air pollution
- Lifestyle practices
  - Smoking and tobacco use
  - Nutrition
  - Alcohol consumption
  - Sexual practices
- Viruses
- Psychosocial factors
  - Personality traits and attitudes
  - Social support system

present, however, how one defines the nature of social support and the degree to which it is present or lacking is unclear.

## EPIDEMIOLOGY

The study of epidemiology is essential to identify patterns of cancer occurrence that help determine research, treatment, and financial priorities in cancer care. Cancer affects human beings wherever they live and whatever their race, color, cultural background, or economic status.

Cancer ranks second to heart disease as a cause of death in the United States, but significant progress has been made in prevention and treatment. Success can be attributed to (1) the diagnosis of more cancers in the early localized stage, (2) the treatment of more patients within 4 months of diagnosis, and (3) the development of new diagnostic and treatment modalities, especially chemotherapy.

Despite these advances, an estimated 560,000 persons died of cancer in 1997. According to population figures, approximately 50% of men and 33% of women now alive in the United States will develop some form of cancer in their lifetime. These statistics, however, reflect the growing number of persons who have survived other diseases and who are "available" or at risk for the development of cancer. More than 10 million Americans are alive today who have a diagnosis of cancer, and, of those, 7.4 million are considered cured of their disease.[1] "Cure" refers to those persons who have no evidence of active disease and have a life expectancy comparable to that of a person who has never had cancer. Cancer reflects no differences on the basis of economic or social status, but variations in incidence do exist with regard to gender, site, age, race, and geographic location.

### GENDER AND SITE

Skin cancer is one of the most prevalent and curable types of cancer in both men and women. Other sites with high probabilities for the development of cancer are the lung, colon, and rectum in men. Women are at risk for breast, colorectal, and lung cancer. In both groups the highest incidences are seen for lung cancer and cancer of the colon-rectum (Table 11-3).

Overall survival rates for some people with selected forms of cancer have increased, such as those with cervical cancer, and rates for most other cancers have leveled off in the past 30 years. Increases in survival rates have occurred for cancers of the prostate gland, uterine corpus, thyroid gland, kidney, bladder, larynx, melanoma of the skin, Hodgkin's disease, and chronic leukemia. The survival rates for lung cancer have improved only slightly over a 10-year period; only 13% of these patients live 5 or more years after diagnosis.[1]

The average cancer mortality in developed countries is higher for men than for women. During the past 40 years a decrease in mortality from cancer among American women is a result of a sharp reduction in the number of deaths caused by uterine cancer. It is revealing to note that while the incidence of lung cancer has decreased in men, it has increased in women. In 1987 lung cancer surpassed breast cancer as the number one killer of women. This appears to be related in part to increased cigarette smoking by American women.[1]

**table 11-3** *Reference Chart: Leading Cancer Sites, 1997**

| Site | Estimated New Cases | Estimated Deaths | Warning Signals (if you have one, see your doctor) |
|---|---|---|---|
| Prostate gland | 334,500 | 41,800 | Urinary difficulty, blood in urine, pain in low back, pelvis, or upper thighs |
| Breast | 181,600 | 44,190 | Lump or thickening in breast or unusual discharge from nipple |
| Lung | 178,100 | 160,400 | Persistent cough, sputum streaked with blood, lingering respiratory ailment |
| Colon and rectum | 131,200 | 54,900 | Change in bowel habits, bleeding |
| Kidney and bladder | 83,300 | 23,000 | Urinary difficulty, bleeding, in which case consult physician at once |
| Lymphoma<br>Hodgkin's disease<br>Non-Hodgkin's | 61,100 | 25,280 | Enlarged lymph nodes, itching, fever, night sweats, anemia, weight loss |
| Skin<br>Basal cell<br>Squamous cell | 54,300 | 9,490 | Sore that does not heal or change in wart or mole |
| Melanoma | 40,300 | 7,300 | As above |
| Uterus | 48,400 | 10,800 | Bleeding outside normal menstrual period or after menopause, unusual vaginal discharge |
| Oral (including pharynx) | 30,750 | 8,440 | Sore that does not heal, difficulty swallowing, lump or thickening |
| Leukemia | 28,300 | 21,310 | Fatigue, paleness, weight loss, repeated infections, easy bruising, nosebleeds or other hemorrhages |
| Stomach | 22,400 | 14,000 | Indigestion |
| Larynx | 10,900 | 4,230 | Hoarseness, difficulty in swallowing |

Modified from American Cancer Society: *1997 cancer facts and figures,* New York, 1997, The Society.
*Incidence estimates based on rates from NCI SEER Program (National Cancer Institute Surveillance, Epidemiology, and End Results and population data collected by the US Bureau of the Census, 1979-1993).

The death rate from cancer involving the female genital tract has dropped to one third to one half the rate of 25 years ago. There is ample evidence that the increased use of the Papanicolaou test to detect lesions of the cervix has resulted in early treatment and a higher rate of cure. Figure 11-3 compares cancer incidence and deaths in 1997 by site and gender.

## AGE

Cancer has been called a disease of aging. Some researchers believe that if people live long enough, they will eventually develop a malignancy. Although cancer is the leading cause of death in women 35 to 74 years of age, the three most prevalent malignancies (lung, breast, colorectal) peak between ages 55 and 74 years. In men, this same age span reflects the years in which the most deaths occur from lung, colorectal, and prostate cancer.

### Gerontological Considerations

Today the average life expectancy for women is 78.9 years, and for men it is 72 years. The elderly population has been growing and now makes up about 12% of the population in the United States. In fact, those aged 80 and older are the fastest-growing age group in our society. If predictions hold true, the greatest rise will occur among Hispanics and Asian Americans. This "graying of America" will have immense impact on our present health care system and health care policies. (See Chapter 4.)

Access to health care for many elders is influenced by financial considerations (fixed income, underinsured); transportation (inability to travel to health care facilities); cultural/ethnic/religious practices (lifelong practices not part of mainstream medical care); and language barriers (e.g., among Hispanics and Asians). These factors may account in part for why elderly persons typically are diagnosed with advanced cancer and do not participate in disease-prevention programs to the same degree as younger adults. In addition, elders tend to have more chronic disease states, with signs and symptoms that can mask a malignancy, thereby preventing early detection and treatment while the cancer is still in a localized stage. The ability of elders to withstand the rigors of cancer treatment is compromised by the deterioration of the immune system and their general physical condition. Many elders are poorly nourished. It is estimated that up to 80% of adults over age 65 have chronic conditions that affect their nutritional state. Additionally, 20% have memory loss or confusion, and one in eight are depressed. Thus appetite, digestion, and psychological well-being are affected.[10] It can be readily seen that this group has unique and challenging problems in relation to cancer development and cancer care.

## RACE

The rates of cancer incidence and death for both men and women are higher for African Americans than for white Americans. The overall incidence and mortality rates for the former group are significantly higher in cancers of the lung, stomach, liver, uterine cervix, larynx, prostate, esophagus, and for multiple myeloma. The 5-year survival rate for African Americans diagnosed with cancer is only 44% compared with 59% for white Americans.

Hispanic Americans have lower incidence and mortality rates for cancers than do either African Americans or white Americans. Yet an American Cancer Society survey showed that Hispanic Americans are not adequately aware of cancer

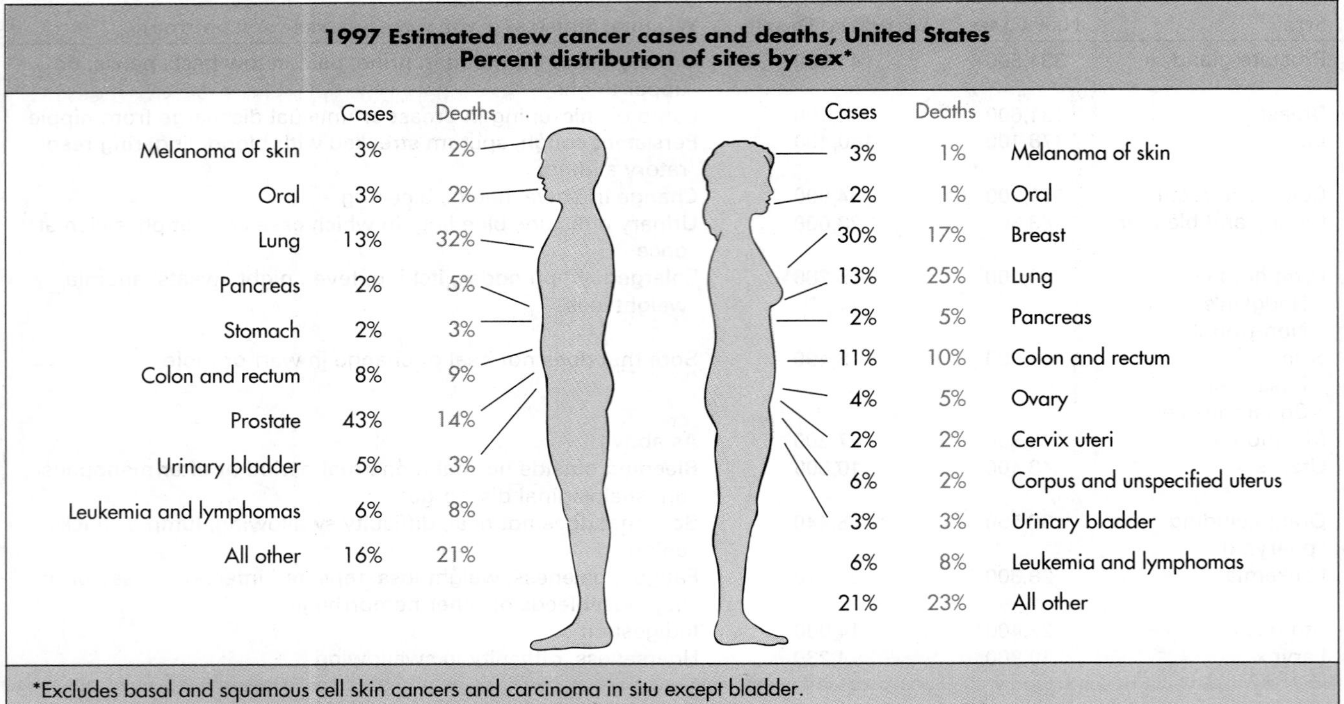

1997 Estimated new cancer cases and deaths, United States
Percent distribution of sites by sex*
Cases Deaths
Melanoma of skin 3% 2%
Oral 3% 2%
Lung 13% 32%
Pancreas 2% 5%
Stomach 2% 3%
Colon and rectum 8% 9%
Prostate 43% 14%
Urinary bladder 5% 3%
Leukemia and lymphomas 6% 8%
All other 16% 21%
Cases Deaths
3% 1% Melanoma of skin
2% 1% Oral
30% 17% Breast
13% 25% Lung
2% 5% Pancreas
11% 10% Colon and rectum
4% 5% Ovary
2% 2% Cervix uteri
6% 2% Corpus and unspecified uterus
3% 3% Urinary bladder
6% 8% Leukemia and lymphomas
21% 23% All other
*Excludes basal and squamous cell skin cancers and carcinoma in situ except bladder.


**fig. 11-3** Comparison of cancer incidence and deaths by site and gender.

warning signals and ways to reduce cancer risk, and they tend not to seek screening or treatment.

Cultural and ethnic behaviors and beliefs, as well as socioeconomic factors such as poverty, play an important role in how quickly a person will seek out health care and treatment. Health care insurance is often unavailable or too expensive for purchase by Hispanic Americans, Native Americans, Asian Americans, and other minority groups.

## GEOGRAPHICAL FACTORS

Differences in the worldwide distribution of cancer exist. For example, primary cancer of the liver is common in Indonesia and parts of Africa and Asia but rare in other regions. Cancer of the breast is more common in the United States and Western Europe than it is in Japan. Ugandans, Nigerians, and South African blacks are at lowest risk for cancer of the lung, stomach, large intestine, uterus, and kidney. Genetic differences among populations may contribute to international variations but are unlikely to explain all variations because migration from one country to another results in major changes in the cancer pattern.

## FACTORS AFFECTING PROGNOSIS

Trends are being evaluated to determine why the incidence of certain cancers has decreased, increased, or remained the same. There is reason to believe that the cure rate and the prognosis of cancer would improve substantially with earlier recognition and more complete reporting of early signs. Patients delay on average 3 months before seeking diagnosis for symptoms suggestive of cancer, thus reducing the chance of cure and long-term survival. Delay is related to the patient's perception of (1) the chance of having cancer, (2) the possibility of early detection and treatment, (3) the inconvenience of examination, (4) the need for relief of symptoms, (5) the need for reassurance, and (6) the ability to pay for health care.

Success in treating many cancers awaits better and more sensitive diagnostic aids to detect lesions in their early stages. In parts of the body that are easily examined, such as the skin and cervix, early recognition and prompt treatment often result in cure.

The prognosis also is affected by the intrinsic characteristics of the tumor, such as histological type and grade, size, and rate of growth. Other important factors are age and the general condition of the patient. The presence of debilitating conditions, such as infection, chronic obstructive pulmonary disease (COPD), or malnutrition, may adversely affect the outcome.

# PHYSIOLOGY

Basic to the understanding of cancer, its development, and subsequent treatment is a knowledge of normal cell kinetics. Much of what is now known about cancer cells is the result of research studies in which normal cells were transformed into malignant cells in a controlled laboratory setting. Cell transformation is recognized as a multistep process originating from a single proliferating cell. The transformed cell then has an altered ability to differentiate and proliferate normally.

## NORMAL CELLULAR PROLIFERATION

### Characteristics of Normal Cells

Normal tissue contains large numbers of mature cells of uniform size and shape, each containing a nucleus of uniform size. Within each nucleus are the chromosomes, and within each chromosome is deoxyribonucleic acid (DNA), the giant molecule whose chemical composition controls the characteristics of ribonucleic acid (RNA), found in the nucleoli and cytoplasm of the cell. The RNA regulates cell growth and function. When the ovum and sperm unite, the DNA and RNA within the chromosomes of each will govern the differentiation and future course of the trillions of cells that finally develop to form the adult organism. In the development of various organs and parts of the body, cells undergo differentiation in size, appearance, and arrangement; thus the histologist or pathologist can look at a piece of prepared tissue through a microscope and know the portion of the body from which it came.

### Mitosis

Mitosis refers to the splitting of one cell into two cells. In the normal cell, multiplication takes place by an orderly process in response to a need such as trauma, surgery, or an inflammatory event. Once the need is met, cell multiplication stops. Normal cells recognize the presence of other cells near them by means of the process of contact inhibition. When cells are in close contact with other cells, they normally adhere closely together. This contact is responsible for inhibiting overlap of cells and disorganized growth. With normal cells these restraints on growth are maintained until need arises because of cell deaths. Some cell turnover rates are rapid, as occurs in the bone marrow, skin, and gastrointestinal tract. The need for cell replacement in these areas is greater than in slower-growing tissue.

### Cell Cycle Time

The concept of cell cycle time is pertinent to understanding normal cell replication and has implications for drug use in cancer therapy. Cell cycle time may be described as the interval from mitosis of a cell to its mitosis into daughter cells. There is a stationary period ($G_0$) of apparent rest after mitosis takes place. The cells are not in the cycle but are viable and capable of undergoing mitosis if necessary. The cell cycle is divided into four phases (Figure 11-4): (1) a quiescent phase consisting of $G_1$ (G denotes a gap) in which RNA and protein synthesis begins; (2) S, a period of DNA synthesis; (3) $G_2$, further RNA and protein synthesis and the development of the mitotic spindle; and (4) mitosis (M).

## NORMAL ALTERATIONS IN CELL GROWTH

Malignant growths represent one form of abnormal cell growth. Other types of cellular growths are benign. Hyperplasia is an increase in cell number, whereas hypertrophy is an increase in cell size but not number. Although many neoplasms are characterized by hyperplasia, normal tissues also may undergo hyperplasia. Wound healing, callus formation, and growth in embryonic tissue are all normal forms of hyperplasia.

Metaplasia is a reversible process in which one adult cell type in an organ is replaced by another adult cell type. The new cell type usually is not one normally seen in the area in which metaplasia occurs. The change of columnar or pseudostratified columnar epithelium of the respiratory tract to squamous epithelium or squamous metaplasia represents the most common type of metaplasia. Dysplasia is an alteration in adult cells characterized by changes in their size, shape, and organization (Table 11-4).

### NORMAL CELL DIFFERENTIATION

All body tissue is derived from stem cells, which are immature cells with no specific cell lineage. These cells have the ability to proliferate rapidly and renew themselves as needed and to develop specialized functions as they grow and mature. The process of cellular differentiation causes the cells to resemble their normal forebears and have fully mature, specialized function and morphology. For example, all kidney cells are similar but are different from muscle cells, and each type has its specialized function.

The method by which differentiation takes place is unknown. One theory is that all cells carry the same genetic material but that selective repression of different genetic characteristics occurs because of buildup of different repressor substances in the cytoplasm. Different cells repress different genetic characteristics. Cell differentiation, once begun, proceeds along a path toward specialized function that cannot then revert to a previous immature state. Figure 11-5 shows the normal cellular differentiation process.

## PATHOPHYSIOLOGY

### CLASSIFYING AND NAMING NEOPLASMS

Tumors derive their names from the types of tissue involved (Table 11-5), but classification of malignant tumors is difficult because many contain several types of cells and may also have benign tissue incorporated within them. In general, the names of benign tumors carry the suffix *-oma* after the name of the parent tissue, for example, neuroma or fibroma; there are some exceptions.

Cancers may be classified according to cell type origin. Two main types are epithelial and mesenchymal (connective tissue). The term *carcinoma* denotes a malignant tumor of epithelial cells, and the term *sarcoma* denotes a malignant tumor of connective tissue cells. When a malignant tumor contains all three types of embryonal tissue, it is termed a *teratoma*.

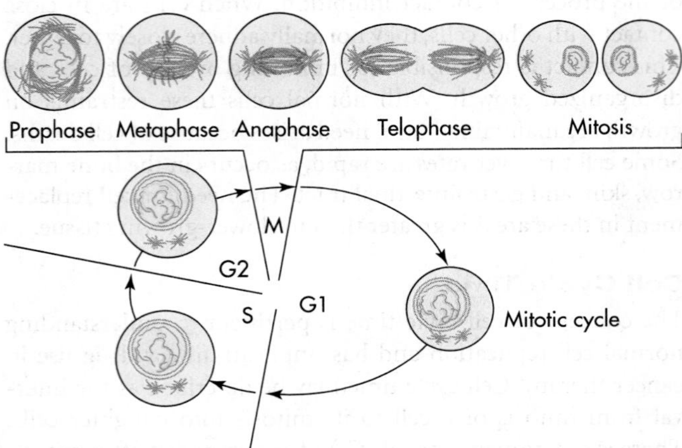


**fig. 11-4** Cell cycle. *GI,* RNA/protein synthesis; *S,* DNA synthesis; *G2,* RNA/protein synthesis and interphase; and *M,* mitosis.

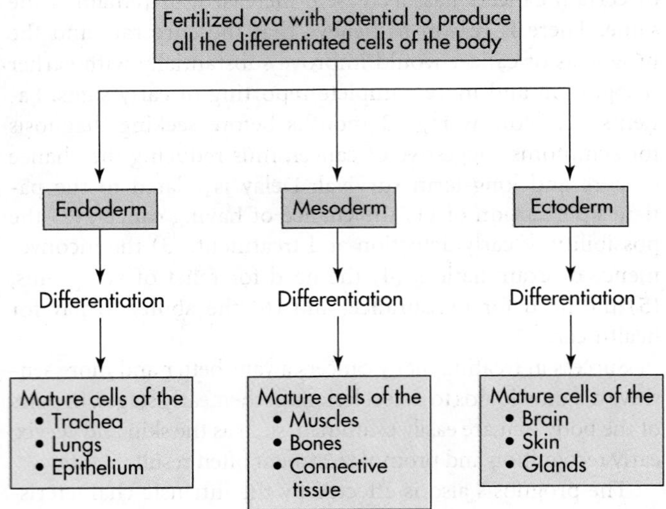


**fig. 11-5** Normal cellular differentiation.

**table 11-4** *Terms Denoting Cellular Changes*

| Type of Cellular Change | Definition | Example |
|---|---|---|
| Mitosis | Formation of new cell by cell division | Normal cell growth |
| Hyperplasia | Increase in cell number | Breast epithelium in pregnancy |
| Hypertrophy | Increase in cell size | Increase in muscle cell size with exercise |
| Atrophy | Decrease in cell size | Decrease in muscle cell size with disuse |
| Metaplasia | Replacement of one adult cell type by a different adult cell type | Replacement of columnar epithelium of respiratory tract by squamous epithelium |
| Dysplasia | Changes in cell size, shape, and organization | Changes in cervical epithelium in long-standing cervicitis |
| Anaplasia | Reverse cellular development to a more primitive cell type | Irreversible change accompanying cancer |
| Neoplasia | Abnormal cellular changes and growth of new tissues | Malignancies |

Tumors also are classified according to cellular maturity. When there is complete loss of identity with the tissue of origin, the tumor is called undifferentiated (anaplastic). Some tumors are known by the names of the scientists who first described them, for example, Hodgkin's disease and Wilms' tumor. Other tumors are named after the organ from which they arise, for example, hepatoma and thymoma.

## METHODS OF CLASSIFYING DEGREE OF MALIGNANCY

The degree of malignancy (grade) is based on microscopic examination of the lesion. Tumors are graded by arabic numerals into four grades; the higher the grade, the worse the prognosis. A grade 1 tumor is the most differentiated (most like the tissue of origin) and therefore the least malignant, whereas a grade 4 is the least differentiated (unlike the tissue

**table 11-5** *Classification of Neoplasms*

| Parent Tissue | Benign Tumor | Malignant Tumor |
|---|---|---|
| **EPITHELIUM** | | |
| Skin and mucous membrane | Papilloma<br>Polyp | Squamous cell carcinoma<br>Basal cell carcinoma<br>Transitional cell carcinoma |
| Glands | Adenoma<br>Cystadenoma | Adenocarcinoma |
| **ENDOTHELIUM** | | |
| Blood vessels | Hemangioma | Hemangiosarcoma<br>Angiosarcoma |
| Lymph vessels | Lymphangioma | Lymphangiosarcoma |
| Bone marrow | | Multiple myeloma<br>Ewing's sarcoma<br>Leukemia<br>Lymphosarcoma<br>Lymphangioendothelioma |
| Lymphoid tissue | | Reticular cell sarcoma (difficult to classify because of cell embryology)<br>Lymphatic leukemia<br>Malignant lymphoma |
| **CONNECTIVE TISSUE** | | |
| Embryonic fibrous tissue | Myxoma | Myxosarcoma |
| Fibrous tissue | Fibroma | Fibrosarcoma |
| Adipose tissue | Lipoma | Liposarcoma |
| Cartilage | Chondroma | Chondrosarcoma |
| Bone | Osteoma | Osteogenic sarcoma |
| Synovial membrane | Synovioma | Synovial sarcoma |
| **MUSCLE TISSUE** | | |
| Smooth muscle | Leiomyoma | Leiomyosarcoma |
| Striated muscle | Rhabdomyoma | Rhabdomyosarcoma |
| **NERVE TISSUE** | | |
| Nerve fibers and sheaths | Neuroma<br>Neurinoma (neurilemoma) | Neurogenic sarcoma<br>Neurofibrosarcoma |
| Ganglion cells | Neurofibroma | Neuroblastoma |
| Glial cells | Ganglioneuroma<br>Glioma | Glioblastoma<br>Spongioblastoma |
| Meninges | Meningioma | |
| **PIGMENTED NEOPLASMS** | | |
| Melanoblasts | Pigmented nevus | Malignant melanoma<br>Melanocarcinoma |
| **MISCELLANEOUS** | | |
| Placenta | Hydatidiform mole<br>Dermoid cyst | Chorion-epithelioma (choriocarcinoma)<br>Embryonal carcinoma<br>Embryonal sarcoma<br>Teratocarcinoma |

of origin) and has a high degree of malignancy. Staging is a form of classification that describes the gross extent of the tumor and its spread (metastasis) rather than its histological appearance. These classifications are useful to the physician in predicting whether the tumor may be expected to respond to treatment (Box 11-6).

Determination of the cancer stage and the site of the original tumor is vital for planning therapy. The International Union Against Cancer has devised the TNM system of classification: *T,* tumor; *N,* regional lymph nodes; *M,* metastases. The TNM system is a uniform system used worldwide for describing the anatomic extent of cancer spread.

Adding a number to the letters (e.g., T1, T2, N1, N2) indicates the extent of the malignancy (Box 11-7). This system provides a type of "shorthand" notation to describe the particular tumor. The purpose of the TNM system is to define categories for all cases and to allow subsequent and more detailed information to be added. Accurate classification is important for treatment, planning, end-results reporting, communication, and clinical trials research.

## TYPES OF NEOPLASMS

### Benign Tumors

Benign (nonmalignant) tumors involve cellular proliferation of adult or mature cells growing slowly in an orderly manner in a capsule. These tumors do not invade surrounding tissue but may cause harm through pressure on vital structures. Benign tumors remain localized, do not metastasize (spread), and do not recur once they are completely removed (Table 11-6).

### Malignant Tumors

A malignant cell is one in which the basic structure and activity have become deranged in a manner not fully understood. It is believed, however, that the basic process involves a disturbance in the regulatory functions of DNA.

The DNA contains information necessary for cell replication: the chemical code for cell growth and development. To convey this information, RNA serves as a messenger. Any small change in DNA (mutation) causes a distortion of biological information, which results in the affected cells running wild. Normal restraints on growth are defective, and the malignant cells lose the specialized function of the normal cell or may take on new characteristics and functions.

**box 11-6** *Classification of Malignant Lesions by Grade and Stage*

| GRADE* | STAGE* |
|---|---|
| **Grade 0**<br>Normal tissue | **Stage 0**<br>Cancer in situ |
| **Grade 1**<br>Well differentiated, with minimal deviation from tissue of origin | **Stage I**<br>Tumor limited to tissue of origin |
| **Grade 2**<br>Moderately well differentiated, with evidence of structural changes from normal tissue of origin | **Stage II**<br>Limited local spread |
| **Grade 3**<br>Poorly differentiated, with extensive structural changes from normal tissue of origin | **Stage III**<br>Extensive local and regional spread |
| **Grade 4**<br>Very anaplastic, with no resemblance to tissue of origin | **Stage IV**<br>Widespread metastasis |

*Not all malignant lesions will have a direct correlation between grade and stage. The pathologist will make the final determination.

**box 11-7** *TNM Staging Classification System*

| | |
|---|---|
| **TUMOR** | |
| T0 | No evidence of primary tumor |
| T1S | Carcinoma in situ |
| T1, T2, T3, T4 | Ascending degrees of tumor size and involvement |
| **NODES** | |
| N0 | No evidence of disease in lymph nodes |
| N1a, N2a | Disease found in regional lymph nodes; metastasis not suspected |
| N1b, N2b, N3 | Disease found in regional lymph nodes; metastasis suspected |
| Nx | Regional nodes cannot be assessed clinically |
| **METASTASIS** | |
| M0 | No evidence of distant metastasis |
| M1, M2, M3 | Ascending degrees of metastatic involvement of the host, including distant nodes |

**table 11-6** *Differences between Benign and Malignant Neoplasms*

| BENIGN | MALIGNANT |
|---|---|
| Limited growth potential | May proliferate rapidly or grow slowly |
| Localized | Spread (metastasize) throughout the body |
| Fibrous capsule | No enclosing capsule |
| Rarely recur after removal | May recur even after treatment |
| Usually regular in shape | Irregular shape with poorly defined border |
| Cells similar to cell of parent tissue (well differentiated) | Cells much different from parent cells (poorly differentiated) |
| Expansive growth | Infiltrative growth |

A characteristic of malignant cells is a loss of differentiation or likeness to the original cell (parent tissue) from which the tumor growth originated. Cancer cells vary in their likeness to the tissue of origin as reflected in the grading system shown in Box 11-6. Generally a cancer with more poorly differentiated cells has a poor prognosis because of a higher degree of malignancy. The loss of differentiation is termed *anaplasia*. Anaplasia is seen only in cancers and does not occur in benign tumors.

The chromosomes that carry genes may also be abnormal. They may be broken apart, have pieces missing or be flipped over, or be shuffled around. The terms *translocation* and *deletion* are used to describe the alteration in position or the absence of parts of chromosomes. Other characteristics of malignant cells include the presence of (1) nuclei of various sizes, many of which contain unusually large amounts of chromatin (hyperchromatic cells), and (2) mitotic figures (cells in the process of division), which denote rapid and disorderly division of cells. (See Table 11-6 for characteristics of malignant cells.)

Tumor cells show less contact inhibition in vitro and therefore "pile up" in cultures, suggesting that surface properties of cancer cells are different from normal cells (Figure 11-6). The proportion of cancer cells actively proliferating in malignant tumors varies from multiplying at a rate equal to normal cells to a very rapid and indiscriminate rate.

Malignant tumors have no enclosing capsules; thus they invade adjacent and surrounding tissue, including lymph and blood vessels. Once these vessels are penetrated, distant spread to other parts of the body is possible.

## CLINICAL MANIFESTATIONS OF CANCER

The clinical manifestations of cancer may be diverse and affect multiple systems, depending on the site and size of the tumor. Nurses need to be aware of these signs and symptoms to aid in early detection of cancer and to monitor the effects of therapy.

### Local Effects

Benign tumors can cause serious problems if they obstruct the lumen of tubular structures such as the ureter, trachea, or intestinal tract. Intraspinal and intracranial tumors cause problems because of the pressure they exert within a closed space. Tumors also may degenerate or cause atrophy and ulceration of overlying epithelium.

Malignant tumors may produce the same problems as benign tumors. In addition, because of their size and ability to infiltrate and destroy surrounding tissue, symptoms of obstruction, hemorrhage, ulceration, and secondary infection may be present.

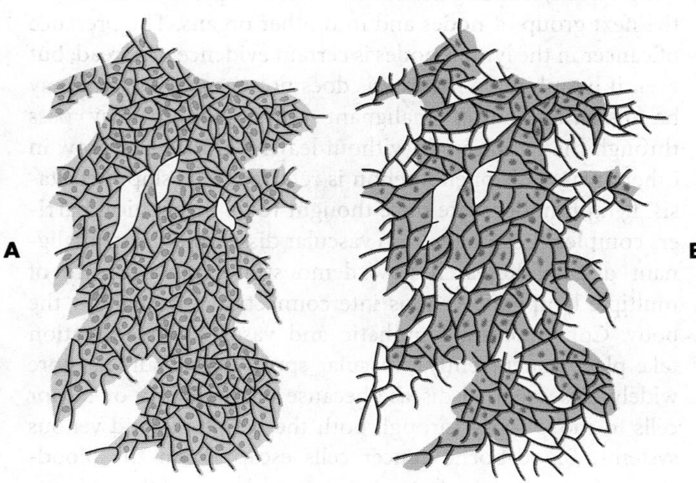


**fig. 11-6 A,** Normal cell appearance. **B,** Abnormal cell appearance.

### Systemic Effects

The term *paraneoplastic syndrome* is used to describe the systemic effects of cancer. These can be divided into the following categories: (1) hematological effects, immunological, and vascular abnormalities; (2) hormonal and endocrinological effects; (3) neuromyopathies; (4) skin and connective tissue disorders; (5) gastrointestinal disorders; and (6) general and metabolic disorders. These effects do not occur in every patient but vary depending on the location and activity of the tumor (Table 11-7).

#### *Cachexia*

Cachexia usually is a sign of advanced cancer. It was once thought to be the result of progressive starvation. Although decreased food intake is a factor, cachexia appears to be a complex derangement of the patient's metabolism. Clinical signs of cachexia include anorexia, early satiety, gradual or rapid weight loss, anemia, and asthenia (Table 11-8). Other factors that may contribute to cachexia include immobilization, drug side effects, reactive depression, insomnia, and a feeling of hopelessness. Any of these factors may contribute to anorexia and cachexia. Therapy for the cachectic state is rarely successful unless the underlying cancer is treated.

#### *Pain*

An estimated 75% of patients with cancer will experience pain sometime during their disease process. Pain is one of the most feared outcomes of cancer. The incidence and severity of the pain depend largely on the site of the cancer, the stage of the disease, and the presence and location of metastasis. The reaction to cancer pain depends on many factors, such as age, pain threshold, and experience with painful events. Cancer pain and its management is discussed in more detail later in the chapter.

#### *Metastasis*

Metastasis refers to the transplantation of tumor cells from one organ or part to another that is separated by distance from the original tumor location. Most deaths from cancer are the result of metastatic disease. A primary tumor or a metastatic site is defined by the presence of a lesion approximately 1 cm in diameter, which contains a billion cells. The process of metastasis no longer is believed to be a random occurrence but a complex sequence of events. An estimated 30% of persons with solid tumors have metastasis at the time of diagnosis.[16]

#### *Types of metastasis*

Cancer spreads in several different ways (Figure 11-7). Cancer cells differ from normal cells in their unique ability

**table 11-7** *Systemic Effects of Cancer*

| Category | Problems | Cause |
|---|---|---|
| Hematological | Anemia, leukopenia, thrombocytopenia | Replacement of bone marrow by cancer cells |
| Immunological | Infection | Deficiency of T and B cells |
| Vascular | Hemorrhage | Blood vessel erosion by tumor, disseminated intravascular coagulation (DIC) |
| Hormonal and endocrinological | Syndromes such as Cushing's, hyperthyroidism | Tumors of endocrine glands cause increased secretions; malignant lung tumors secrete trophic hormones |
| | Cachexia | Hypermetabolism of tumors<br>Increased gluconeogenesis |
| Neuromuscular | Weakness, cerebellar disease, peripheral neuritis | Degenerative changes in central nervous system and peripheral nervous system |
| | Poor pulmonary respiration, stasis of secretions and pneumonia | Destruction of muscle protein, impaired cellular respiration, and failure of abdominal and intercostal muscles |
| | Urinary tract infection and constipation | Failure of smooth muscle in bladder and GI tract |
| Skin and connective tissue | Dermatomyositis | — |
| Gastrointestinal (GI) | Weakness, fatigue, weight loss | Malabsorption, chronic blood loss, impaired digestion |
| General disorders | Ascites | Metastatic implant in abdomen |
| | Pleural effusion | Metastatic implant in pleural cavity |

**table 11-8** *Clinical Signs of Cachexia*

| Signs | Possible Cause |
|---|---|
| Anorexia | Metabolites produced by cancer; food aversions caused by decreased taste and smell and by therapy |
| Early satiety and early filling | Cause unknown—patient is hungry but after a few bites feels full |
| Weight loss | Impaired digestion and absorption, hypermetabolism, negative nitrogen balance |
| Anemia | Decreased red blood cell (RBC) production, increased RBC destruction or loss |
| Asthenia (marked feeling of muscle weakness, easily tired) | Biochemical alterations |

to move without restraint into surrounding tissue. Tumor cells lack adhesiveness (the ability to stay in contact with other cells), so they can easily break away from the tumor mass of which they are a part and directly invade surrounding tissues. This is referred to as local invasion. Local spread may involve hemorrhage, necrosis, ulceration, and fibrous replacement of the involved tissues. This produces the typical local effects of ulcerating, bulky, hemorrhagic masses; or indurative, fibrosing lesions with tissue fixation, distortion of the structure, and the dimpling of the skin that may be seen in some breast cancer.

Infection may accompany the local infiltration. The cancer cells tend to spread along the path of least resistance, such as in tissue clefts, along blood vessels, or along the perineural spaces. The fibrous capsule that covers some organs may limit growth. For example, primary tumors of the kidney, liver, or testes may increase the size of the organ without destroying the capsule. Local spread is not an orderly process but one that occurs unequally and haphazardly. Because of local spread, any cancer excision must include a margin of surrounding tissues to ensure removal of all malignant cells.

Cancer also spreads by lymphatic permeation and embolization. Once cells have invaded the lymph vessels, they then may detach and become emboli, which lodge in the lymph node, forming a metastatic lesion. Spread continues to the next group of nodes and into other organs. The presence of cancer in the lymph nodes is certain evidence of spread, but even if lymph node metastasis does not occur, there still may be dissemination of malignant cells. The cell may pass through the lymph node without leaving a trace and grow in other areas. This phenomenon is referred to as skip metastasis. Lymph nodes were once thought to be mechanical barriers completely separate from vascular dissemination of malignant disease. Research now demonstrates the presence of multiple lymphatic-venous interconnections throughout the body. Consequently, lymphatic and vascular dissemination take place concurrently.[9] Vascular spread can result in more widely disseminated disease because of the ability of tumor cells to move freely through both the lymphatic and venous systems. Blood-borne cancer cells escape from the bloodstream by a process of attachment and invasion through endothelial cells lining the blood vessel (Figure 11-8).

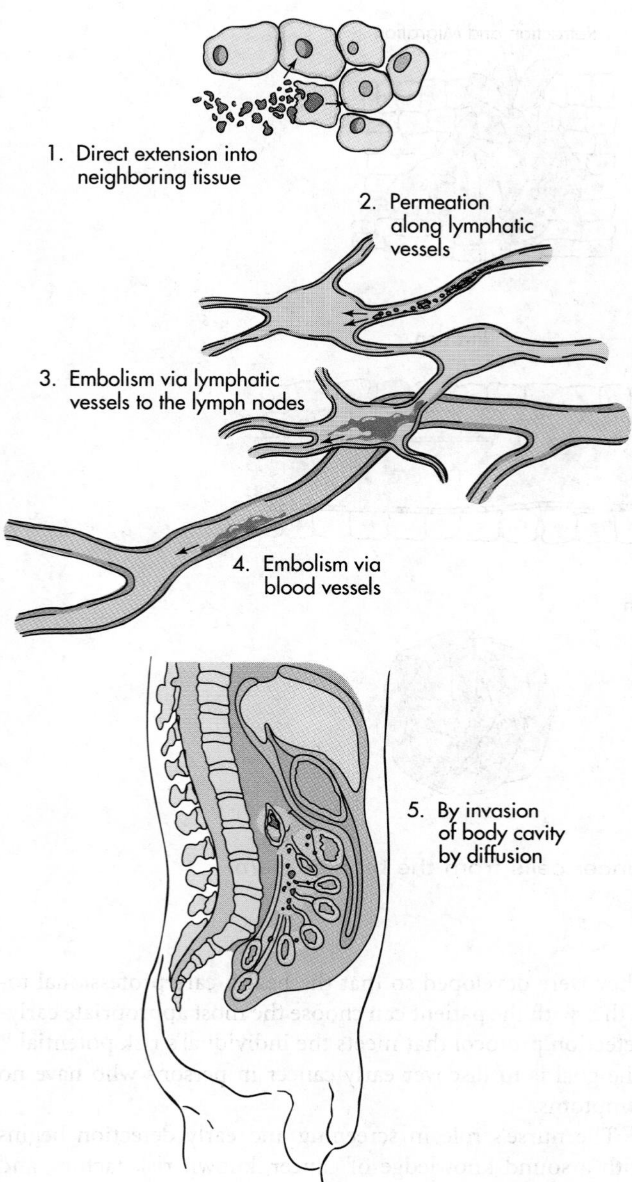


**fig. 11-7** Modes of dissemination of cancer.

Finally, cancer can spread by diffusion, the spread of clumps of cancer cells from the surface of the tumor by mechanical means. This type of spread is particularly prevalent in serous cavities such as the abdominal or pleural cavity. In the peritoneal cavity, cells tend to gravitate to the pelvis. Cancer cells also can be implanted, or "seeded," by the surgeon into the operative area, causing metastatic lesions. Metastasis may regress or disappear without apparent cause and may be dormant for many years, only to resume growth years later.

#### Sites of metastases

The site of metastatic spread depends on the venous or lymphatic drainage of the organ involved, the type of cancer, and the tissue from which the cancer arises. Various body tissues seem to have different attraction for metastases, common sites being, in order, the liver, lungs, bone marrow, brain, and adrenal glands. The spleen, muscle, and skin rarely are involved. Table 11-9 (p. 271) shows the pattern of metastasis of some common primary tumors.

## ONCOLOGICAL EMERGENCIES

Oncological emergencies may occur as a result of the disease process or its treatment. These emergencies include obstructions (increased intracranial pressure, spinal cord compression, superior vena cava syndrome, tracheal or bowel obstruction), metabolic syndromes (hypercalcemia, tumor lysis syndrome, syndrome of inappropriate antidiuretic hormone secretion, hyperviscosity, anaphylaxis, septic shock, disseminated intravascular coagulation), and cardiac toxicities (pericardial tamponade, cardiomyopathy with congestive heart failure) as described in Table 11-10, p. 273. The oncology nurse is the health care professional most often in a position to recognize these emergencies. A careful history and ongoing monitoring for signs and symptoms alert nurses to life-threatening conditions. During these crises the patient may require transfer to an intensive care unit.

## COLLABORATIVE CARE MANAGEMENT

### PREVENTION/HEALTH PROMOTION

Health care professionals have a major responsibility in the prevention of cancer. Because of their knowledge about the disease and their contact with the public in both inpatient and outpatient settings, and in various community activities, they have the opportunity and the obligation to teach about cancer and known risk factors.

A *risk factor* may be defined as something specific to an individual that increases the possibility of developing a malignancy. Risk factors must be identified and reduced if possible. Three types of risk factors for cancer have been identified. *Lifestyle* factors are those over which the person has some control, especially tobacco use, diet, alcohol use, sunlight exposure, and sexual practices. *Environmental* factors include exposure to carcinogens and are at times beyond the individual's control. *Genetic* factors—conditions inherited at conception—are not usually controllable except through genetic counseling services.

#### Primary Prevention

Primary prevention attempts to prevent a person's exposure to any known risk factor that might lead to disease. This is an insurmountable task in cancer prevention, inasmuch as all risk factors are not known or have not been proved as factors in specific cancer development. However, substantial evidence demonstrates a direct link between certain environmental and lifestyle factors and cancer development. Examples include smoking and lung cancer, excessive sun exposure and skin cancer, and low dietary fiber content and colon cancer.

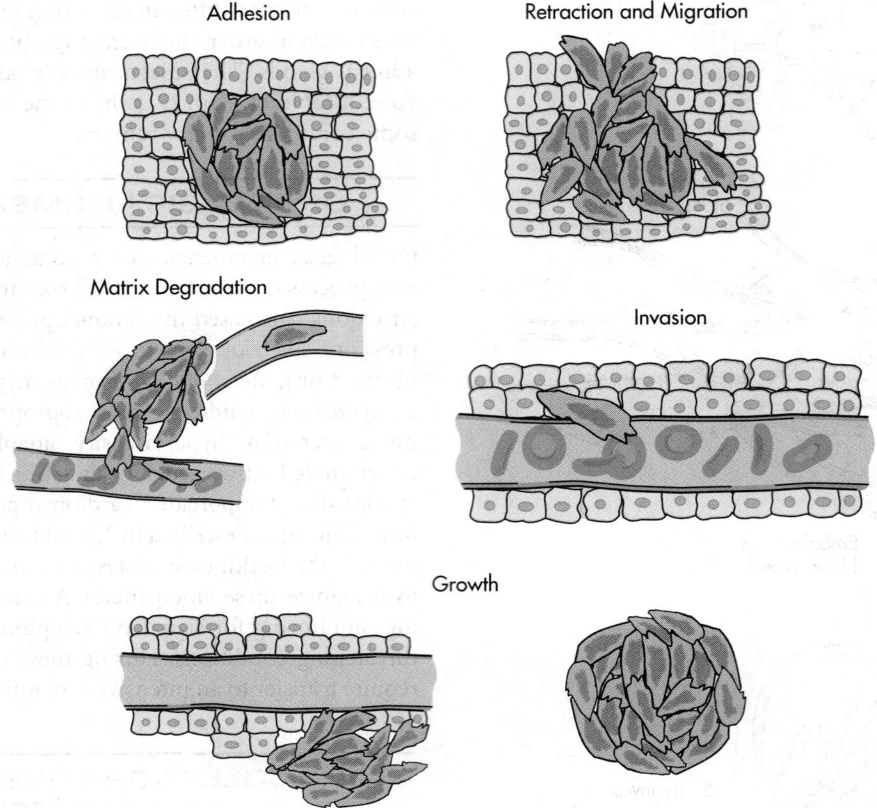


**fig. 11-8** Process of dissemination of cancer cells from the bloodstream.

Nurses who have knowledge of these cancer risk factors must become more active in educating the public. This can be accomplished easily with the hospitalized patient or in the clinic setting, where teaching and counseling are essential components of everyday practice. Participation in community health fairs where educational information and counseling are provided is an area in which all nurses can make meaningful contributions.

### Secondary Prevention

Secondary prevention efforts are aimed at early diagnosis and prompt effective treatment. Once the diagnosis is known, definitive treatment is begun. For successful secondary prevention, there must be a stage in the natural history of the cancer when, if detected, it can be cured. In addition, there must be a means of detecting the cancer at an early stage.

At present, early detection methods through health screening programs are not available for all cancers. The only screening tools that have enabled the detection of early asymptomatic cancers and are known to reduce cancer mortality are mammograms and Pap tests. The use of chest x-ray films to screen for the presence of lung cancer has been largely unsuccessful because metastasis usually has occurred by the time a lesion is large enough to appear on a roentgenogram. The American Cancer Society's guidelines for cancer-related checkups are not recommended for mass screening. They were developed so that the health care professional together with the patient can choose the most appropriate early-detection protocol that meets the individual's risk potential.[18] The goal is to discover early cancer in persons who have no symptoms.

The nurse's role in screening and early detection begins with a sound knowledge of cancer, known risk factors, and the treatment modalities available. Cancer risk assessment must be an integral part of every interaction the nurse has with the public. Data obtained from interviews, the nursing history, physical examinations, social and family histories, health surveys and questionnaires, and employment records help the nurse determine the person's individual cancer risk factors.

Case finding is a responsibility of all health professionals. As an important member of the health care team the nurse must be able to (1) counsel and direct patients to the proper sources of help, (2) have information about those conditions that are known to predispose individuals to the development of the disease, and (3) educate the public about these factors. In addition, the nurse must be sensitive to the needs of patients who may be afraid and embarrassed when confronted with the possibility of cancer. Table 11-11 (p. 275) summarizes the nurse's role in early detection of some common cancers.

Cancer detection is expensive. Education often includes convincing the public that a periodic health examination is

**table 11-9** *Patterns of Metastasis of Common Cancers*

| Primary Tumor | Metastatic Sites | Route of Dissemination | Average Time for Metastasis | Comment |
|---|---|---|---|---|
| Breast | Lymph nodes, lung, liver, bone, brain, soft tissue, skin | Lymphatic, hematogenous, direct extension communication with batson's plexus of paravertebral veins | Variable—50% of recurrences occur in first 2-3 years, but late recurrences can occur | • Systemic disease at onset (experimental studies have shown metastases initiated when primary tumor <0.125 cm) |
| Prostate | Bone, lymph nodes, liver, lung, soft tissue | Direct extension, lymphatic, hematogenous, communication with batson's plexus of paravertebral veins | Long time due to slow growth rate/doubling time (>2 years) | • Bone is primary site of metastases—80% of patients have bone metastasis only<br>• Most frequent bones involved are lumbar vertebrae, pelvis, long bones, and ribs<br>• Natural history of disease (slow but steadily progressive) |
| Lung | Lymph nodes, liver, brain, bone, pleura, adrenals, pericardium, bone marrow, soft tissue | Hematogenous, lymphatic | Early compared with other tumor types—variable based on lung histology (small cell, adenocarcinoma, and large cell metastasize early vs. squamous cell metastasizing later) | • 50% of all lung cancer patients have disseminated disease at the time of diagnosis<br>• Small cell lung cancer, 30-40% of patients have limited disease; 60-70% have extensive disease at time of diagnosis<br>• Brain metastasis accounts for >25% of recurrences in resected NSCLC |
| Colorectal | Liver, lung, brain, bone | Lymphatic, hematogenous, communication with thoracic duct | Most recurrences occur in the first 2 years (70%); almost all within 5 years (90%) | • Predictable course of spread; liver is the primary organ for metastasis (65%); extraabdominal metastasis less common—lung (25%); brain (10%)<br>• Lymph node involvement correlates with depth of invasion and grade of differentiation of primary tumor; low-grade tumor 30% LN+; high-grade tumor 80% LN+<br>• Synchronous liver metastasis occurs in 5-10% of patients. |

Lydon J: Metastasis, *Oncol Nurs* 2(5):9, 1995.

*Continued*

a sound investment. The public attitude toward participation in cancer screening programs is becoming more positive. People are increasingly concerned about living in a more healthy environment and maintaining healthy lifestyles. People also are known to participate in screening programs if they perceive themselves to be at risk for cancer. Some cities have cancer detection centers where a complete physical examination, including chest radiograph, Pap smear, breast examination, proctoscopy, urinalysis, and blood cell count are performed for a moderate fee. Nurses should be aware of resources in their community where persons may be referred.

## Health Teaching

Early detection of cancer can decrease mortality. The nurse must know and be able to explain the significance of the seven warning signs of cancer, stressing that any of these signs should be reported immediately to a physician (Box 11-8). It

**table 11-9** *Patterns of Metastasis of Common Cancers—cont'd*

| Primary Tumor | Metastatic Sites | Route of Dissemination | Average Time for Metastasis | Comment |
|---|---|---|---|---|
| Head and neck | Lymph nodes, lung, liver, brain and bone | Lymphatic, hematogenous | Variable based on site and grade of differentiation<br>Early metastasis occurs in nasopharyngeal, hypopharynx, soft palate, base of tongue, supraglottic larynx; late metastasis occurs in paranasal sinuses, hard palate, lips, buccal mucosa<br>Poorly differentiated tumors metastatize early vs. well-differentiated tumors metastasize late and infrequently | • Advanced head and neck patients have 20-35% metastasis rate<br>• Metastasis above clavicles occurs in 50-80% of patients<br>• Natural history (tends to remain localized and invade adjacent tissues progressively)<br>• Some evidence to suggest control of local regional disease decreases dissemination and metastasis |
| Sarcoma | Lungs, bone | Hematogenous | Variable based on histological type, grade, and stage<br>Early metastasis within 2 years occurs in osteosarcoma, rhabdomyosarcoma in adults, malignant fibrous histiocytoma, lymphangiosarcoma, and angiosarcoma; late metastasis occurs in liposarcoma and embryonal rhabdomyosarcoma | • Approximately 50% of patients have micrometastatic disease at time of diagnosis<br>• Lung is primary site of metastasis<br>• Presence of nodal involvement equivalent to metastasis and overrides grade in determining stage<br>• Resection of recurrent lesions, as well as solitary metastasis, is worthwhile, resulting in some long-term cures<br>• Therapeutic approach requires local control to decrease potential for distant metastasis |
| Ovarian | Intraperitoneal, liver, lung | Surface shedding, lymphatic, hematogenous | Majority of recurrences within 2 years of initial treatment | • 50-70% have advanced disease at time of diagnosis<br>• Relapse and survival rates associated with grade, stage, and amount of residual disease following surgery<br>• At second look 50% will have macroscopic disease, 25% microscopic disease, 25% negative findings<br>• 30-50% of patients relapse after pathological negative findings |

should be emphasized that although these signs should be investigated medically it does not necessarily mean that the person has cancer.

Women should be taught that the breast, lung, gastrointestinal tract, and uterus are the most common sites of cancer. Women should be taught to examine their breasts each month immediately after the menstrual period or, after menopause, on a designated day each month. Even though the value of breast self-examination (BSE) in early detection is questioned (its use has not reduced breast cancer mortality rates), it should still be encouraged until all findings are in. Women of all ages should know the importance of reporting any abnormal vaginal bleeding or other discharge occurring between menstrual periods or after menopause. (See Chapter 47 for details of early symptoms of cancer of the female reproductive system.)

Men should be made aware that their risk is greatest for cancer of the prostate, lung, and gastrointestinal tract. The incidence of testicular cancer overall is small; however, it is most prevalent in young men between the ages of 15 and 40 years.

**table 11-10** *Oncological Emergencies*

| Type | Pathophysiology | Clinical Manifestations |
|---|---|---|
| **OBSTRUCTIVE** | | |
| Increased intracranial pressure | Increased brain mass from tumor, hemorrhage, or edema. Alteration in internal jugular vein flow caused by head/neck tumor or by surgical resection; results in alteration in function. | Change in mental status, vomiting, headache, dizziness, seizures (see Chapter 52) |
| Spinal cord compression | Primary or metastatic lesions causing disruption of reflexes and motor function because of neuron impairment and interruption of motor or sensory nerve fibers. Symptoms depend on location. | Flaccid paralysis, paresthesias, locomotion difficulties, respiratory impairment at C5 level (see Chapter 54) |
| Superior vena cava (SVC) syndrome | Obstruction of the SVC caused by primary (usually lung cancer) or metastatic tumors in the mediastinal or paratracheal nodes. | Dyspnea, facial and neck swelling, chest pain, cough, dysphagia, ruddy edematous face |
| Tracheal obstruction | Reduction in lumen from tracheal stenosis, extrinsic compression, or mass in lumen. | Signs and symptoms of inadequate gas exchange and respiratory function (see Chapter 32) |
| **METABOLIC** | | |
| Hypercalcemia | Bone disease or metastasis increases bone resorption with bone destruction and release of calcium in the extracellular fluid. It is believed the tumor may produce (1) a substance that enables bone resorption of calcium or (2) ectopic parathyroid hormone that increases serum calcium levels. | Nausea and vomiting, constipation, muscle weakness, coma, dysrhythmias, polyuria, nephrolithiasis (see Chapter 15) |
| Tumor lysis syndrome (TLS) | Rapid tumor cell destruction after cytotoxic chemotherapy may result in release of intracellular electrolytes. May occur in cancers characterized by rapid cell growth (leukemia and lymphomas). | Hyperphosphatemia (oliguria, azotemia), hyperkalemia, hyperuricemia (N&V, lethargy, anuria, azotemia), hypocalcemia (see Chapter 15) |
| Syndrome of inappropriate antidiuretic hormone secretion (SIADH) | Increase in ADH seen in cancers such as lung carcinoma (especially oat cell), duodenal and pancreatic carcinoma, thymoma, lymphomas, uterine carcinoma, and central nervous system (CNS) tumors. May also occur with some chemotherapeutic agents (cyclophosphamide, vincristine). | Fluid and electrolyte and neurological changes (see Chapter 52) |

*Continued*

Testicular self-examination (TSE), like BSE in women, has not improved mortality rates but is still stressed for this age group.

Elderly persons, as a group, require more individualized health teaching about cancer risk and detection methods. They are often more reluctant to voice their fears about cancer or to report physical complaints that could be signs of early malignant tumors. Some are reticent about seeking medical intervention because of their tenuous financial state or fears of becoming a burden on their family, or just because they are uncomfortable in discussing their concerns. Still other elderly persons simply are not aware of their increased risk of cancer. All too commonly health care professionals do not encourage elders to participate in health education and screening programs even though it is clear that cancer risk increases with age. The American Cancer Society's guidelines for cancer-related checkups offer a guide related to a broad age range and do not specifically address the needs of persons 65 years and older (see the Guidelines for Care Box, p. 277). Rather, the health care professional must study each guideline for its appropriate application to this population subgroup.

The nurse must take advantage of all opportunities to teach elderly persons. Both the inpatient and clinic settings offer many occasions for assessing the cancer knowledge base of elders and any concerns they may express. In addition, nurses can use health fairs held at churches, nursing homes, and retirement communities to meet the elderly person's cancer education needs.

Two common misconceptions that lead the person to ignore symptoms should be corrected. The first is a belief that a disease as serious as cancer must be accompanied by weight loss. Weight loss usually is a late symptom of cancer. Another

**table 11-10** *Oncological Emergencies—cont'd*

| Type | Pathophysiology | Clinical Manifestations |
|---|---|---|
| Hyperviscosity | Increased blood viscosity from increase in cell number, loss of flexibility of cells, or overproduction of serum proteins. This causes increased resistance to blood flow. | Bleeding from gastrointestinal or urinary tracts or puncture sites; visual disturbance, headache, dizziness, weakness, dyspnea, distended neck veins |
| Anaphylaxis | Hypersensitivity responses (I, II, III, IV) caused by chemotherapeutic agents (asparaginase, cisplatin, neocarzinostatin, VM-26, doxorubicin, daunorubicin, bleomycin, cyclophosphamide, methotrexate, melphalan). | Signs of anaphylactic reactions (see Chapter 66) |
| Septic shock | Increased susceptibility to infection from impaired immune system or effect of immunosuppressive agents, leading to bacterial septicemia. | Signs and symptoms of septic shock (see Chapter 17) |
| Disseminated intravascular coagulation (DIC) | Chronic bleeding consumes all clotting factors; may also result from sepsis. | Thrombocytopenia, bleeding of mucous membranes and tissues (see Chapter 29) |
| **CARDIAC TOXICITIES** | | |
| Cardiac tamponade | Intrapericardial pressure increases from accumulation of fluid from direct tumor invasion, metastatic lesion, or infection or from pericardial thickening after radiation. Results in decreased diastolic ventricular filling, decreased stroke volume and cardiac output. | Dyspnea, cough, chest pain, muffled heart sounds, cyanosis, edema, decreased systolic pressure, decreased central venous pressure (see Chapter 26) |
| Cardiomyopathy with congestive heart failure (CHF) | Chemotherapeutic drugs (such as anthracyclines, mithramycin, mitomycin, and cyclophosphamide) appear to damage cardiac myofibrils, causing sarcoplasmic reticular swelling that leads to destruction of the myofibril; hypertrophy of the heart muscle ensues with decreased function. | Acute: tachycardia, dysrhythmias<br>Chronic: signs of congestive heart failure (see Chapter 26) |

misconception is the belief that the absence of pain means that a problem is minor. It must be repeatedly emphasized that pain is not an early sign of cancer and that cancer often is far advanced before pain occurs.

## Factors That Interfere with Health-Seeking Behaviors

Even though knowledge of cancer is more widespread than before, a more positive attitude toward the disease is essential if persons are to follow good health practices and seek help when warning signs of cancer are noted. Factors that may interfere with health-seeking behaviors include underestimation of the incidence of cancer and negative views about conventional therapies. The poor, minority groups, and the less educated are less likely to have regular physical examinations. It is estimated that direct cancer medical care costs $35 billion annually. Breast, lung, and prostate cancers account for over one half of the direct medical costs. Thus, the uninsured will not seek medical intervention even with obvious symptoms of a disease process.[1]

Unfortunately, anxiety and fear may immobilize the individual. Despite all the public announcements of the past few decades, some people still think cancer must be hidden from others. This attitude stems partly from the fact that cancer in its terminal stages can be a painful and demoralizing disease. Some people fear cancer and shun persons who have the disease because they believe it is contagious. Scientific speculation on the possibility that a virus may be the cause has added to this fear. People must be assured that there is no evidence that cancer can be spread among human beings in a way similar to the spread of infectious diseases.

The positive aspects of cancer care should be emphasized. An estimated one third of persons for whom a cancer diagnosis is made are cured by medical treatment. Another one third could perhaps be cured by medical treatment if the cancer were diagnosed early enough. The remaining third have cancer that occurs in locations in which the disease has advanced beyond medical aid before sufficient signs appeared to warn the patient of trouble. In spite of these facts, some persons still think it is useless to report symptoms early because they

**table 11-11** *Nurse's Role in Early Detection of Common Cancers*

| TYPE OF CANCER | RISK FACTORS | PREVENTION | NURSE'S ROLE |
|---|---|---|---|
| Skin | 1. Light complexion, red hair with freckles<br>2. Frequent exposure to sun or tanning parlors<br>3. Occupational exposure to chemicals, arsenicals, pesticides, coal tar products<br>4. Frequent exposure to ionizing radiation, x-rays, radioisotopes<br>5. Precancerous skin lesions<br>6. Genetic predisposition (xeroderma pigmentosum, albinism)<br>7. Change in mole (color, size, shape) | 1. Limit sun exposure between 10 AM-3 PM; do not exceed 15-30 min/day until tan is established<br>2. Cover exposed skin<br>3. Apply protective sunscreen (factor 15 or more)<br>4. Be aware of medications that increase photosensitivity (e.g., tetracycline)<br>5. Cleanse skin after use of chemical substances<br>6. In industry, wear protective clothing and, if exposed to chemicals, follow guidelines for cleansing skin | 1. Educate public regarding risk factors and behavior/lifestyle modification<br>2. Act as role model |
| Lung | 1. Habitual smoker (cigarettes, pipe, cigars)<br>2. Prolonged inhalation of side-stream smoke<br>3. Exposure to known occupational or environmental carcinogens (asbestos, hydrocarbons, radon)<br>4. Family history of lung cancer | 1. Do not smoke or if a smoker, stop<br>2. Monitor occupational and environmental exposure dosages/risks; wear protective clothing and masks<br>3. Have medical checkup if in high-risk group | 1. Lobby for smoke-free environment and employment setting<br>2. Participate in smoking cessation programs<br>3. Educate youth to risks of smoking<br>4. Conduct research on smoking behavior/attitudes |
| Breast | 1. Family or personal history of breast, endometrial, ovarian cancer<br>2. Never married, no children, or first child after age 30<br>3. Early menarche and late menopause<br>4. History of fibrocystic disease<br>5. Triad of diabetes, obesity, and hypertension<br>6. High-fat diet | 1. Monthly BSE age 18 and older<br>2. Physical examination yearly<br>3. Yearly mammogram >age 40 or as directed by physician*<br>4. Avoid high-fat diet and obesity | 1. Teach BSE<br>2. Educate women on risk factor reduction strategies |
| Colorectal | 1. Black population<br>2. Age >40 years<br>3. Family history of colon cancer<br>4. Personal history of Crohn's disease, Gardner's syndrome, familial polyposis, ulcerative colitis >10 years' duration<br>5. Diet high in fat<br>6. Excess alcohol intake | 1. Diet high in fiber, low in fat (<30% of total calories)<br>2. Avoid salt-cured or nitrite-cured foods<br>3. Avoid obesity<br>4. Annual occult stool examination >age 50 years<br>5. Digital rectal examination >age 50 years<br>6. Sigmoidoscopy every 5-10 years >age 50*<br>7. Total colon examination or double-contrast barium enema every 5-10 years* >age 50 | 1. Educate and counsel blacks and elders on benefits of screening programs and diet modifications<br>2. Participate in cancer prevention/detection programs<br>3. Identify cases of high-risk persons/family |

Modified from White L: *Semin Oncol Nurs* 1(3):184, 1986.
*American Cancer Society Revised Guidelines, June 12, 1997.

*Continued*

**table 11-11** *Nurse's Role in Early Detection of Common Cancers—cont'd*

| Type of Cancer | Risk Factors | Prevention | Nurse's Role |
|---|---|---|---|
| Prostate | 1. Increasing age<br>2. African-American population<br>3. Family history of prostate cancer<br>4. Exposure to cadmium, fertilizers; rubber-industry workers at risk<br>5. Sexual behavior (higher rates in hyperactive or promiscuous)<br>6. Change in bladder habits<br>7. Diet high in fat<br>8. Excess alcohol intake | 1. Annual digital rectal examination >age 40 years<br>2. Test for prostate-specific antigen (PSA) and transrectal ultrasound show promise for early detection | 1. Educate elderly men, especially African-American males, to risk factors<br>2. Promote and participate in screening programs |
| Testicular | 1. Young, white males (15-40)<br>2. History of cryptorchidism<br>3. Testicular atrophy after viral infection (mumps)<br>4. Personal history of testicular cancer<br>5. Trauma<br>6. History of inguinal hernia<br>7. History of maternal ingestion of diethylstilbestrol during pregnancy | 1. Testicular self-examination monthly<br>2. Orchiopexy before age 2 years | 1. Educate and counsel value of self-examination<br>2. Encourage participation in screening program |
| Cervical | 1. Early sexual activity, multiple partners<br>2. Genital infections (herpes viruses)<br>3. Dysplasia<br>4. Multiple pregnancies<br>5. Poor personal hygiene | 1. Barrier protection during coitis<br>2. Lifestyle modification<br>3. Annual pelvic examination and Pap test at age 18 or earlier if sexually active* | 1. Educate to risk factors, especially teenagers; distribute educational materials<br>2. Advocate American Cancer Society (ACS) guidelines<br>3. Participate in screening programs |
| Endometrial | 1. Increasing age<br>2. Triad of diabetes, hypertension, and obesity<br>3. Nulliparity<br>4. Early menarche and late menopause<br>5. History of hormonal therapy | 1. Annual pelvic examination and Pap test<br>2. Endometrial biopsy at menopause | 1. Same as with cervical above |

**box 11-8** *Seven Warning Signs of Cancer*

1. **C**hange in bowel and bladder habits
2. **A** sore that does not heal
3. **U**nusual bleeding or discharge
4. **T**hickening or a lump in the breast or elsewhere
5. **I**ndigestion or difficulty in swallowing
6. **O**bvious change in a wart or mole
7. **N**agging cough or hoarseness

believe that cancer cannot be cured. This attitude can be changed by community-based cancer education programs. The *Healthy People 2000* health status objectives related to cancer are summarized in Box 11-9, p. 278.

## DIAGNOSTIC TESTS

### Laboratory Tests

A complete discussion of the many laboratory tests available and pertinent to the diagnosis of cancer is beyond the scope of this chapter. Many of the same tests can be used to diagnose both benign and malignant conditions. Some of the laboratory tests most often used in cancer detection include a hematology screening profile (complete blood count [CBC]); a serum chemistry profile (sodium, potassium, chloride, carbon dioxide, bicarbonate, glucose, blood urea nitrogen [BUN]); cytology tests; and urinalysis. More specific tests may be employed as indicated by the symptoms exhibited and the organ system involved. For example, a serum prostate-specific antigen (PSA) test may be done if prostate cancer is suspected, or a carcinoembryonic antigen test (CEA) may be performed for suspicious lesions of the gastrointestinal tract. The nurse's role during this phase of care is to prepare the patient for each test and procedure, inform the patient of what to expect, and inform the patient of where and when the test will take place. Table 11-12 (p. 279) covers a number of common malignant conditions with a list of potential laboratory tests and procedures used in their diagnosis.

#### *Cytology*

In 1942 Dr. George Papanicolaou demonstrated that the diagnosis of cancer could be made from the study of cells that have sloughed or exfoliated from a tumor. These cells are

guidelines for care

**Cancer-Related Checkups, 1997***

| TEST OR EXAMINATION | GENDER | AGE (YEARS) | RECOMMENDATION |
|---|---|---|---|
| Breast self-examination | Female | Over 20 | Monthly |
| Breast physical examination | Female | 20-40 | Every 3 years |
| | | Over 40 | Every year |
| Mammography | Female | Over 40 | Every year |
| Papanicolaou test | Female | Over 18; under 18 if sexually active | Every year; after three or more consecutive normal annual exams, the Pap test may be performed less frequently at the discretion of the physician |
| Pelvic examination | Female | Over 18; under 18 if sexually active | Every year |
| Endometrial tissue sample | Female | At menopause or women at high risk | High risk: history of infertility, obesity, failure to ovulate, abnormal uterine bleeding, unopposed estrogen (estrogen alone), or tamoxifen therapy<br>Frequency of tissue sample is at the discretion of the physician |
| Colorectal examination | | | |
| Fecal occult blood test (FOBT) | Male and Female | Over 50 | Yearly |
| FOBT, sigmoidoscopy and digital rectal examination (DRE) | Male and Female | Over 50 or at high risk | Every 5 years |
| OR | | | |
| Colonoscopy and DRE | Male and Female | Over 50 or at high risk | Every 10 years |
| OR | | | |
| Double-contrast barium enema (DCBE) and and DRE | Male and Female | Over 50 or at high risk | Every 5-10 years |
| | | | High risk: personal history of colorectal cancer or adenomatous polyps, family history colorectal cancer or polyps (first-degree relatives < age 60 or two firstdegree relatives of any age), personal history of chronic inflammatory bowel disease, or families with hereditary colorectal cancer syndromes (familial polyposis or nonpolyposis colon cancer) |
| Oral examination | Male and Female | Over 18 | Yearly |
| Skin examination | Male and Female | Over 20 | Every 3 years |
| | | Over 40 | Yearly |
| Prostate examination | | | |
| Digital rectal examination | Male | Over 50 or at high risk | Yearly |
| Prostate-specific antigen (PSA) | Male | Over 50 or at high risk | Yearly |
| | | | High risk: strong familial history (two or more first-degree relatives) or African Americans may begin testing earlier (e.g., age 45) |

*Data from American Cancer Society Revised Guidelines, June 12, 1997.

found in body secretions such as cervical discharges, sputum, gastric washings, pleural fluid, and urinary washings. The secretion is spread on a slide, stained, and examined by a pathologist, who can classify the tissue as benign, dysplastic ("suspicious"), or malignant. The main use of the Pap smear, as it is often called, is to diagnose cancer in a person who has no symptoms and to identify precancerous lesions or noninvasive cancer. If suspect cells are found, a biopsy must be performed to diagnose cancer. The Pap smear is most widely used for examination of cervical washings.

## Radiological Tests

### *X-ray and scanning procedures*

X-ray studies usually are ordered. The use of chest radiography is absolutely necessary if the patient is a smoker. Other tests such as the gastrointestinal series or intravenous pyelogram are used for specific areas where lesions are suspected to be present.

Scanning procedures, which permit mapping of organs, play an important part in the evaluation of the patient with cancer. Some of these procedures are described in Table 11-13, p. 280.

**box 11-9** Healthy People 2000: *Health Status Objectives by Year 2000 as Related to Cancer*

**REDUCTION IN DEATH RATES**

1. Reverse the rise in cancer deaths to achieve a rate of 130/100,000 persons.
2. Slow the rise in lung cancer deaths to a rate of no more than 42/100,000 persons.
3. Reduce breast cancer deaths to no more than 20.6/100,000 women.
4. Reduce deaths from cancer of the uterine cervix to no more than 1.3/100,000 women.
5. Reduce colorectal cancer deaths to no more than 13.2/100,000 persons.

**CANCER RISK REDUCTION**

1. Reduce cigarette smoking to a prevalence of no more than 15% among persons aged 20 or older.
2. Reduce dietary fat intake to an average of 30% of calories or less and average saturated fat intake to less than 10% of calories among persons aged 2 and older.
3. Increase complex carbohydrate and fiber-containing foods in the diets of adults to five or more daily servings for vegetables and fruits and to six or more daily servings for grain products.
4. Increase to 60% of the general population those who limit sun exposure, use sunscreens and protective clothing when exposed to sunlight, and avoid artificial sources of ultraviolet light (sun lamps, tanning booths).

**EARLY DETECTION GOALS**

1. Increase to 75% the proportion of care providers who routinely counsel patients about tobacco cessation, diet modification, and cancer screening recommendations.
2. Increase to 80% the proportion of women aged 40 and older who have received a clinical breast examination and mammogram, and to 60% of those aged 50 and older who have received them within the preceding 1 to 2 years.
3. Increase to 95% the proportion of women aged 18 and older with uterine cervix who have ever had a Pap test, and to 85% the number who had a Pap test within the preceding 1 to 3 years.
4. Increase to 50% the number of persons aged 50 and older who had fecal occult blood testing within the preceding 1 to 2 years and to 40% those who have ever had a proctosigmoidoscopic examination.
5. Increase to 40% the number of persons aged 50 and older visiting a primary care provider in the preceding year who had oral, skin, and digital rectal examinations during one such visit.

**SET SERVICE STANDARDS**

1. Ensure that Pap tests meet quality standards by monitoring and certifying all cytology laboratories.
2. Ensure that mammograms meet quality standards by monitoring and certifying at least 80% of mammography facilities.

From US Department of Health and Human Services, Public Health Service: *Healthy people 2000: summary report.*

#### *Radioisotope studies*

Various procedures that involve the introduction of a radioactive substance into the body are used to detect primary or metastatic cancer. The radioisotope either concentrates in the tumor and shows up as a "hot spot" in the scan or fails to concentrate in the tumor and shows up as a "cold spot" surrounded by normal tissue. Radioisotopes used include the following:

1. Radioactive iodine: oral or by injection; used for diagnosis of thyroid disease
2. Radioactive iodine–tagged albumin: injected intravenously; used for locating brain tumors and to determine blood volume

#### *Ultrasound*

Ultrasound probing, or echography, is performed by means of an electronic instrument that detects and records echoes of sound when they are reflected at the junction of tissue with different densities. The procedure is helpful in differentiating between cystic and solid tumors.

### Biopsy

Biopsy is the only definitive way that cancer can be diagnosed. *Incisional biopsy* is the surgical removal of a section of the neoplasm. If the tumor is small, the entire growth may be removed, a procedure termed *excisional biopsy.* When possible, an *aspiration biopsy* (needle biopsy)—removing a small plug of tumor by use of a needle or syringe—is used to avoid the larger incisional or excisional biopsy. Needle biopsy, although inexpensive and relatively simple to perform in an outpatient setting, has the potential of missing the malignant focus and "seeding" tumor cells along the needle track as it is inserted and withdrawn.

The biopsy specimen is examined under a microscope to obtain a histological diagnosis. In some cases it may be possible to determine the degree of malignancy.

### Endoscopy

Hollow metal tubes equipped with a light are used to illuminate various body cavities, permitting visual inspection of the interior of the cavity being examined. These instruments are commonly referred to as scopes and are named for the organs they visualize. Thus a bronchoscope is used to examine the bronchus, a gastroscope is used to visualize the stomach, and a proctoscope is used to visualize the anus and sigmoid colon. A biopsy specimen of tissue or secretions usually is obtained during these endoscopic procedures.

### Other Diagnostic Methods

The search for a universal cancer marker that would indicate the presence of a malignant process regardless of tissue source con-

**table 11-12** *Common Malignant Conditions and Commonly Used Diagnostic Tests and Procedures**

| Malignancy | Laboratory Tests and Procedures Employed | Malignancy | Laboratory Tests and Procedures Employed |
|---|---|---|---|
| Breast cancer | Breast physical examination | Genitourinary cancers | |
| | Ultrasound | Prostate | Digital rectal examination |
| | Mammography | | Bone scan |
| | Tissue and lymph node biopsy | | Biopsy |
| Lung cancer | Chest x-ray | | Urinalysis |
| | Computed tomography (CT) scan | | Laboratory: prostatic-specific antigen, serum acid phosphatase |
| | Sputum cytology | Bladder | Cytology |
| | Fiberoptic bronchoscopy with biopsy and bronchial washings | | Cystoscopy (internal examination of bladder) |
| | Medastinography (endoscopic examination of mediastinum and nodes) | | Intravenous pyelogram (IVP) examination of calyx, pelvis, and lower part of urinary tract using contrast medium) |
| Gastrointestinal cancers | | | Urinalysis |
| Esophagus | Chest x-ray | Kidney | CT scan |
| | CT scan | | Renal angiogram, sonogram |
| | Magnetic resonance imaging (MRI) | | X-ray studies of kidney, ureters, and bladder |
| | Esophagoscopy and biopsy | | Urinalysis |
| | Barium contrast studies (barium swallow) | | IVP |
| | Sputum cytology | Gynecological cancers | |
| Stomach | As above | Cervix | Colposcopy (examination of the vagina and cervix by means of a magnifying lens) |
| | Gastric secretion analysis | | Biopsy |
| | Carcinoembryonic antigen (CEA) | | Papanicolaou (Pap) test (smear) |
| Colorectal | As above | Ovary | Pelvic physical examination |
| | Stool guaiac | | Pap test |
| | Barium enema | | IVP |
| | Proctosigmoidoscopy and biopsy | | Barium enema |
| Liver | As above | | Urinalysis |
| | Liver biopsy | Uterus | Endometrial biopsy and aspiration |
| | Liver enzyme studies | | |

*The diagnostic tests cited are not a comprehensive list of tests and procedures used to detect specific cancers, but are only a representative sample of diagnostic aids employed.

tinues. However, markers have been determined for some specific cancers. Markers include secreted proteins, cell surface macromolecules, hormones, enzymes and isoenzymes, and components of the cytoplasm. It is now recognized that cancer cells resemble embryonic or fetal cells in appearance and in their ability to produce typically fetal cellular macromolecules. Some of these markers have been clinically useful as a means of monitoring the course of the malignant process and as prognostic factors.[3] Table 11-14 notes some common cancer markers in use today.

## SURGICAL MANAGEMENT

Of the four major modes of cancer therapy (chemotherapy, radiation therapy, biotherapy, and surgery), surgery is the oldest modality and most widely used. Surgery may be used for cancer diagnosis and staging, cure, palliation, adjuvant treatment, oncological emergencies, or pain control.

The initial role of surgery is diagnosis and staging of disease. Most cancers require tissue samples to confirm diagnosis. Surgery is often the best way to obtain these samples. The type of surgical biopsy and its extent depend on the site and characteristics of the tumor.

When surgery is used for cure, the malignant lesion must be small, localized, and amenable to complete surgical removal. Cancer is considered a regional disease rather than a disease confined to one specific organ. Currently it is standard procedure to remove a wide margin of tissue surrounding the involved organ and to dissect the regional lymph node chain at the time of surgery. This technique has greatly reduced the incidence of local recurrence and increased survival rates, especially in tumors that disseminate through the lymphatics.[14] Since the advent of newer and more potent cytotoxic agents and improved radiotherapy techniques, more conservative

**table 11-13** *X-ray and Scanning Procedures Used in Cancer Diagnosis*

| Study | Procedure | Comment |
|---|---|---|
| Lymphangiography | Oil-based blue dye and procaine (Novocain) injected in skin of web between first and second toes or index and second fingers to show lymphatic drainage of extremities | Used in diagnosing lymph and metastatic cancer. Lymphomatous nodes have "foamy" or "lacy" structure. Metastatic nodes have "moth-eaten" appearance. Bluish-green skin discoloration from dye may last 1 week |
| Xeroradiography | X-ray image on plate of selenium-coated metal | Provides picture of soft tissue |
| Tomography | X-ray image with ability to penetrate dense shadows | Provides picture of soft tissue |
| Thermography | Constructs photographic images of surface temperature | Identifies skin temperature elevations over inflammatory or malignant lesions |
| Computed tomography (CT) scan | X-ray beam and use of computer | Produces images of plane sections of body; identifies size and location of tumors |
| Magnetic resonance imaging (MRI) | Magnetic fields | Produces a cross-sectional image of the body; spares patient from x-ray exposure |
| Positron-emission tomography (PET) | Scanners that rotate around patient; image formed by positrons emitted by isotope injected into or inhaled by patient | Allows viewing of brain and body processes in three dimensions; gives a picture of biochemical and metabolic processes |

**table 11-14** *Cancer Markers Used to Detect the Presence of Cancer*

| Marker | Type of Cancer |
|---|---|
| Carcinoembryonic antigen (CEA) | Lung, gastrointestinal, breast, and pancreas |
| Alpha-fetoprotein (AFP) | Stomach, colon, and lung |
| Chorionic gonadotropin | Seminomas and choriocarcinomas |
| Ectopic hormone production | Lung, breast, and pancreas |
| Bence Jones protein | Multiple myeloma |
| Prostate-specific antigen (PSA) | Prostate |
| Genetic markers (chromosome translocation/ rearrangements) | Chronic myelogenous leukemia (CML) |
| CA 125 | Ovary |

surgery is the accepted norm. The patient has a better cosmetic outcome and more normal bodily function.

Surgery as a palliative procedure is now a recognized and useful intervention for cancer patients with more advanced disease. Palliative surgery may be used to reduce the bulk of a growing yet unresectable tumor mass. Surgical removal of hormone-producing organs has been used to curb the growth of tumors that depend on the hormone for growth. An example is removal of the ovaries (oophorectomy) for estrogen-dependent breast cancer. The placement of a jejunostomy tube for nutritional support or a tracheostomy to relieve airway obstruction are common palliative procedures.

Adjuvant surgical intervention is used principally to support other treatment modalities such as radiation and chemotherapy. Surgical placement of vascular access devices provides a means of administering chemotherapeutic agents directly into a tumor, organ system, or limb. Radiation therapy can be enhanced through the use of surgically implanted devices that house the radioactive material and provide concentrated therapy to a localized area.

Surgery plays a prominent role in many oncological emergency situations. Debulking some of a tumor mass can relieve the discomfort of obstructions or nerve pain. The formation of a colostomy to relieve colon obstruction or a laminectomy for spinal cord compression are surgical procedures that increase the patient's quality of life but do not have any effect on the cancer itself.

Last, surgery can be a method of pain control through a variety of surgical blocks. Table 11-15 provides examples of surgical interventions currently used in the treatment of cancer. The operative procedures used to treat various types of cancer are discussed in later chapters under the particular organ systems.

## NURSING MANAGEMENT OF THE PATIENT UNDERGOING CANCER SURGERY

### ■ DIAGNOSTIC PHASE

Although the word *cancer* may not be mentioned, it is usually an overriding fear of the patient and family. Diagnostic tests and procedures can cause anxiety and apprehension even when the rationale for their use is clearly explained. The diagnostic phase is not only emotionally draining, but physically taxing for the patient.

**table 11-15** *Surgical Approaches to Cancer Care*

| INTERVENTION | EXAMPLE |
|---|---|
| Diagnosis | Breast biopsy |
| Staging | Staging laparotomy |
| | Second-look laparotomy |
| Treatment of primary tumor | Curative resection (abdominal perineal resection) |
| Reconstruction, rehabilitation | Breast reconstruction |
| | Continent urostomy or ileostomy |
| Palliative | Endocrine ablation |
| | Pericardial window |
| Adjuvant | Paraaortic node dissection |
| | Hickman line insertion |
| Complications of other methods | Excision of bowel stricture |
| | Excision of radionecrotic tissue |
| Resection of metastases | Partial hepatectomy |
| | Pulmonary resection |
| Cytoreductive | Abdominal soft tissue sarcomas |
| | Ovarian peritoneal carcinoma |
| Emergencies | Obstruction |
| | Hemorrhage |
| Cancer prevention | Colectomy (familial polyposis) |
| | Orchidopexy (testicular tumors) |

From Havard CP, Topping AE: Surgical oncology. In Baird S, McCorkle R, Grant M, editors: *Cancer nursing: a comprehensive textbook,* Philadelphia, 1991, WB Saunders.

**box 11-10** *Karnofsky Performance Scale*

**A subjective assessment tool to assess and compare the patient's activity and performance ability**

| | |
|---|---|
| Normal; no complaints; no evidence of disease | 100 |
| Able to carry on normal activity; minor signs or symptoms of disease | 90 |
| Normal activity with effort; some signs or symptoms of disease | 80 |
| Cares for self; unable to carry on normal activity or to do active work | 70 |
| Requires occasional assistance but is able to care for most needs | 60 |
| Requires considerable assistance and frequent medical care | 50 |
| Disabled; requires special care and assistance | 40 |
| Severely disabled; hospitalization is indicated, although death is not imminent | 30 |
| Hospitalization is necessary; very sick; active supportive treatment necessary | 20 |
| Moribund; fatal processes progressing rapidly | 10 |
| Dead | 0 |

Tests and procedures require the patient to go without usual nourishment, and normal sleep and rest patterns are disrupted. Some tests cause discomfort, beginning with the preparation requirements: being immobilized in uncomfortable positions for lengthy intervals and being alone and isolated from family or familiar nursing staff members. The patient and family alternate between fearing the worst possible outcome—a cancer diagnosis—and hoping for a benign condition.

The nurse plays a pivotal role in the management of the patient's care during the diagnostic phase. Plans should be made to support the patient, as well as the entire family, at this critical time. Hospitalization of a family member and the fear of a cancer diagnosis can lead to changes in family roles that cause some members to assume responsibilities and tasks that are new and frightening to them. Adult children may need to take on the role of decision maker and caretaker and possibly provide needed financial assistance. It is the spouse, however, who has the most significant role adjustment. At one time it was assumed that spouses of cancer patients were more or less passive observers instead of being actively involved in the cancer experience.[21] It is now recognized that spouses have the same needs as the patient: knowledge of the typical course of the disease, symptoms to expect, and the treatment options available.

## PREOPERATIVE PHASE

Preoperatively the health care team will assess the physical and emotional factors that will predict how the patient will withstand cancer surgery and that will affect recovery and rehabilitation. These factors include emotional state, age, nutritional status, and performance status, as well as the presence of any active medical problems and the results of laboratory and diagnostic tests (Box 11-10).

During this phase of care the nurse strives to build a therapeutic relationship with the patient and family. This is best achieved through open and honest communication and assisting the patient to maintain a realistic sense of hope. Explanations of the various tests and test results, as well as the role that surgery will play in their particular situation (cure, palliation, or adjuvant treatment), help both patient and family overcome feelings of helplessness and powerlessness when treatment decisions are made. Table 11-16 summarizes family needs during the course of the patient's illness.

The age and physical state of the patient have considerable impact on acceptance of a cancer diagnosis, as well as on postoperative recovery and rehabilitation. Elderly persons may fear dying or becoming a burden to their families, physically and financially. Patients in early adulthood to middle age may appear to have more physical stamina but may have many emotional concerns. These patients are in their most productive years in relation to career advancement, educational opportunities, and sexual activity. They may fear loss of job security, financial independence, disfigurement, role adjustments within the family and community, and loss of reproductive capacity.

The presence of other physical problems, such as a chronic disease (e.g., diabetes or arthritis), can complicate recovery from surgery. The nurse must assess the patient's knowledge about these conditions and discuss the plan of care as it relates to the management of these physical problems.

The nutritional status of the patient requires careful assessment and intervention before surgery. The signs of bodily

**table 11-16** *Information Needed by Cancer Patients and Spouses Over the Course of Illness*

| Diagnostic Phase | Hospital Phase | Treatment Phase | Adaptation Phase | Recurrent Phase |
|---|---|---|---|---|
| Type and purpose of diagnostic procedures to be performed<br>When test results can be expected<br>The person who is coordinating the care<br>The typical emotions that develop while awaiting diagnosis (e.g., anxiety, uncertainty) | Type of surgery planned<br>When pathology report will be available<br>Expected length of hospitalization<br>Role limitations to anticipate when patient is discharged<br>The effects of illness on other family members | Type and length of treatment planned<br>Anticipated side effects and when they may occur<br>Ways to minimize side effects<br>Likelihood of temporary role changes<br>Availability of cancer education and support groups | When follow-up exams or tests are necessary<br>The typical concerns during this phase (e.g., fear of recurrence)<br>Importance of balancing needs of patient and family members<br>Availability of cancer education and support groups | Type of treatment planned<br>Anticipated side effects and when they may occur<br>The typical feelings during this phase (e.g., uncertainty, sadness, fear)<br>Ways to maintain hope regardless of recurrence<br>Availability of support groups and community resources |

From Northouse LL, Peters-Golden H: Cancer and the family: strategies to assist spouses, *Semin Oncol Nurs* 9(3):77, 1993.

wasting (cancer cachexia) may have been present before medical intervention was sought and before a definitive cancer diagnosis was confirmed. Patients will be nutritionally supported before surgery as necessary. Oral supplements, high in protein and calories, or total parenteral nutrition (TPN) if the patient cannot take and retain oral feedings, play a vital role in preoperative management. The nurse discusses with the patient and family the role of good nutrition in a successful surgical outcome. Sound nutrition helps the patient heal more quickly and have more strength and energy and usually means a shortened recovery time and hospitalization. Blood or blood products will be administered on the basis of laboratory values. The nurse documents the patient's response to these interventions promptly and reports to the physician any difficulties encountered.

The patient's preoperative teaching needs are addressed and any questions answered promptly. Discussion of any special equipment that may be needed during postoperative recovery occurs at this time, such as catheters, monitors, infusion lines, or chest tubes. (See Chapter 18.)

## ■ POSTOPERATIVE PHASE

Meticulous postoperative care is especially important for patients with cancer because many are already physically impaired and immunodeficient before surgery as a consequence of the disease process and the rigors of diagnosis. These patients may not have the physical strength to ward off infectious processes. There are numerous sources of infection in the postoperative period (e.g., drains, indwelling catheters, infusion lines). The nurse must carefully monitor each potential source for the presence of infection, document findings, arrange for culture of any suspicious drainage, and notify the physician immediately. Maintenance of strict asepsis is of utmost importance in the immunocompromised patient. The nurse instructs the patient and other caregivers on the need for strict aseptic technique. Visitors with an infectious process should be advised to refrain from physical contact with the patient during this critical period. Antibiotic therapy to cover a wide range of organisms may be prescribed. (See Chapter 20 for a more detailed discussion of postoperative care and Chapter 10 for information about inflammation and infection control.)

### Promoting Comfort

Comfort measures to alleviate and control pain are concerns for all postoperative patients. The cancer patient will have the same type of analgesic orders as other surgical patients; however, the cancer patient may require larger and more frequent medication to achieve adequate pain control. (See Chapter 12 for an in-depth discussion of pain control.)

Health care professionals are often reluctant to provide the cancer patient with sufficient analgesics because of the fear of drug dependency and addiction. These fears are unfounded. Sufficient pain relief will ensure that ambulation, nutrition, and participation in self-care (bathing, dressing, elimination) can be achieved. Because many cancer patients are elderly and more physically debilitated before surgery, there is an urgent need to increase and restore physical stamina as quickly as possible. The nurse must capitalize on all opportunities to enhance the patient's physical strength by active and passive exercises, use of assistive devices (cane, walker), ensuring safety, and providing privacy. Enlisting the aid of physical and occupational therapists will help achieve this goal.

### Promoting Nutrition

Many factors influence the nutritional status of the postoperative cancer patient. The catabolic state that exists during the perioperative period requires high caloric and protein replacement. The patient may have already been in a malnourished state before surgery, showing moderate to severe weight loss, decreased muscle mass, loss of adipose tissue, and an impaired immune response. The surgical procedure itself may necessitate anatomical alterations that interfere with normal ingestion, digestion, and absorption of nutrients. The nurse and dietitian are challenged to devise a plan for nutritional support that can be accepted and adhered to by the patient. Strategies vary with each individual patient but may include daily weights; keeping daily calorie counts; offering food preferences when possible; providing oral, enteral, or parenteral supplements; and teaching the importance of compliance with the prescribed diet. Good oral hygiene and dentation will help facilitate oral intake. Encouraging ambulation, diversional activities, and family visits during mealtimes may add to the patient's enjoyment and compliance with the nutrition regimen.

### Providing Emotional Support

One of the first questions heard from the patient on awakening from anesthesia after surgery may be "Was it cancer?" or "Did they get it all?" The family may have the same questions. Fear that the tumor was malignant or unresectable is normal. The nurse should anticipate these questions and be prepared to respond appropriately. Dealing honestly with the patient is essential to maintaining therapeutic communication and credibility. The nurse needs to be cognizant of what the surgeon has communicated to the patient so that the information conveyed is clear and consistent. For those patients who desire spiritual comfort, their minister, rabbi, or the hospital chaplain can be enlisted to provide strength and support.

After cancer surgery the patient may face the prospect of changes in lifestyle and disruption of sexuality. Patients who have had a mastectomy or colostomy are especially concerned by body changes that make them feel less attractive and less lovable to their significant other. These reactions may be felt strongly but not verbalized to a caregiver or partner. Depression is a common outcome and may manifest as mood disturbances and sexual dysfunction for many months after surgery. The patient who refuses to look at a mastectomy incision or who lets others care for an ostomy is indicating that a serious problem may be present. It is the responsibility of health care professionals to explore the patient's feelings and concerns about bodily changes. The nurse should encourage the inclusion of the partner in any discussion or information-sharing session related to the patient's sexuality or fears of sexual dysfunction. The patient and the patient's partner need to be aware of the patient's decreased energy level in the postoperative and rehabilitation stage. Sexual desire or the ability to perform sexually may diminish. Alternative methods of sexual expression (e.g., hugging, caressing, alternative positioning) can be suggested and information provided on available corrective measures such as breast reconstructive surgery or penile implants. Patients need to know that grieving a lost body part or function is natural, and the patient should be supported during this time. Support groups are helpful to many people, and the nurse ensures that the patient receives the name and phone number of appropriate groups in the local community.

### Discharge Planning

As with any surgical patient, the goal of discharge planning is to provide continuity of care from the acute care setting to the home environment. Depending on his or her physical and emotional state, the cancer patient may or may not be able or willing to be actively involved in discharge planning. Early participation by the spouse or primary caregiver is essential in this process. (Refer to the discussion of surgical discharge planning in Chapter 20.)

The immunocompromised cancer patient is instructed to avoid persons with infection, crowds, and crowded conditions until advised otherwise. Information about wound care, wound healing, and the signs of infection or complications is provided. If the patient is scheduled to begin another form of cancer therapy, such as chemotherapy or radiation, details related to start date, length of therapy, and site where therapy is to be provided should be given in writing. The nurse reminds the patient to expect fatigue to persist and to carefully balance activity and rest after discharge. The importance of optimal nutrition for recovery is once again stressed.

Before discharge the patient and family should be made aware of the need for referral to community health care agencies, such as home or hospice care. The nurse and social worker can assist the patient and family to make this transition as smooth as possible. The nurse can provide a list of resources and agencies that may be useful once the patient is at home, such as the American Cancer Society (ACS) (supplies—e.g., wigs, dressings, beds) and support groups (Reach to Recovery, ostomy associations). A list of local respite care facilities should be included. Last, the nurse provides the telephone numbers of persons the patient or family can contact for advice, for information, or to report changes in the patient's condition. Many hospitals now routinely make follow-up calls after discharge to assess patient and caregivers' adjustment to the home situation.

## SPECIAL ENVIRONMENTS FOR CARE

### Critical Care Management

Some patients undergoing cancer surgery will require care in an intensive care setting. It is routine for certain surgical patients, such as those having thoracic or neurosurgery, to spend the first 24 to 48 hours in the surgical or neurological intensive care unit for ventilatory support and monitoring. When this situation can be anticipated preoperatively, the patient and family should be informed about the need for this specialized care. They are assured that as soon as the patient is stable he or she will be returned to the general surgical unit. Patients who develop complications during the postoperative period may also need specialized nursing care that can be offered only in a critical care area. The care of the patient in an intensive care area is discussed in Chapter 22.

### Home Care Management

Currently, as a result of changes in reimbursement for health care costs, the postsurgical hospital stay is considerably shorter than ever before. Many patients are discharged home with complex care needs that must be provided by family caregivers or friends. This is especially true with the cancer patient. With earlier diagnosis and treatment, cancer patients are surviving longer, making cancer a chronic disease amenable to management in the home setting. Technical advances now permit the cancer patient to go home with central and peripheral venous access devices, and long-term intravenous therapy (chemotherapy, parenteral nutrition, pain management, antibiotics) is commonplace. Rehospitalization is no longer a necessary requirement for treatment, which often can be provided at home by the family with the assistance of a home health nurse. The benefits of home care outweigh the disadvantages for most patients. However, careful assessment of the home environment and caregiver ability and willingness to be involved is critical. Education about procedures, equipment, and troubleshooting is vital. An understanding of aseptic technique is particularly important when patients are immunosuppressed.

Many patients will have radiation therapy at some time during the course of their illness. This is usually performed on an outpatient basis, and the patient remains in the home. For most cancer patients the home has become the primary location in which care is provided, with occasional visits to the clinic or hospital.

## COMPLICATIONS

It is beyond the scope of this chapter to address the multiple complications that may occur in the postsurgical cancer patient. Most complications are related to the debilitated physical state of the patient and the patient's compromised immune status. Infection, as well as the patient's inability to ward off virulent organisms, is a major complicating factor for optimal recovery and is also a common cause of death. Infections involving the lung, kidney and bladder, skin, mouth, and mucous membranes are common. Changes in fluid and electrolyte balance that result from taste changes, anorexia, nausea, vomiting, and diarrhea can lead to severe metabolic derangements. The reader is referred to chapters that deal with postoperative complications and chapters that present the management of specific types of cancers.

## BIOTHERAPY

### Principles Underlying Biotherapy

The immune system has been scrutinized for many years to establish its relationship to cancer. Studies of cancer in lower animals and in human beings show that when the normal cell becomes malignant, it often undergoes biochemical changes that result in the formation of new cellular antigens that may trigger the immune response. A normally functioning immunosurveillance mechanism can eliminate these cancer cells, thus preventing them from growing and spreading within the body. At present the immune response can handle only a limited number of tumor cells, up to 10 million. After growth reaches 100 million tumor cells the immune response is not capable of preventing further growth.

It has also been noted that (1) some tumors spontaneously regress; (2) cancer incidence increases in persons who are immunosuppressed (posttransplant patients, the elderly); (3) there may be a decrease in metastatic tumor size following surgical removal of the primary tumor; and (4) metastatic disease may become dormant after successful local treatment of a tumor.[11,28] These observations have stimulated continuing research on the role of the immune system and the development of new biological agents.

Immunological treatment of cancer may involve either active immunotherapy, specific or nonspecific, or passive (adoptive) immunotherapy, specific or nonspecific. Table 11-17 reviews immunotherapy and biotherapy agents used in cancer treatment.

Biotherapy is now established as the fourth cancer therapy and is effective alone or in conjunction with surgery, chemotherapy, and radiation therapy. The focus of biotherapy is manipulation of the immune system through the use of naturally occuring biological substances (cells, cell products) or genetically engineered agents and drugs that modify the body's response to cancer or cancer therapy. These substances, which function as regulators and messengers of immune function, are referred to as biological response modifiers (BRMs).[12]

Biotherapy is much broader than immunotherapy. Early research centered on nonspecific immunotherapy agents such as the bacille Calmette-Guérin (BCG), *Corynebacterium parvum,* lavamisole, and specific allogeneic or autologous vaccines. These agents were thought to stimulate the body's immune response to cancer cells. Clinical trials using these agents were disappointing. Today immunotherapy is classified as a subcategory of biotherapy.[21]

### Types of Biological Response Modifiers

Most BRMs are classified as cytokines, proteins that modify immune function. The most common BRMs in use are the interferons (IFNs), interleukins (ILs), and colony-stimulating factors (CSFs). The other class of BRMs is monoclonal antibodies. Monoclonal antibodies are produced by hybridoma

**table 11-17** *Immunotherapy and Biotherapy Agents Used in Cancer Treatment*

| Specificity | Active | Passive |
|---|---|---|
| Specific | Inactivated tumor vaccines (autologous, allogeneic)<br>Human tumor hybrids | Monoclonal antibodies<br>Human heterologous antiserum<br>T lymphocytes<br>Monoclonal lymphocytes<br>Bone marrow transplants |
| Nonspecific | Chemical immunostimulants<br>Biological immunostimulants (such as BCG, *C. parvum*)<br>Cytokines (interferon, IL-2, TNF)<br>Chemotherapy | Lymphokine-activated killer cells (LAKC)<br>Activated macrophages |

From McDonald A. In Dow KH: *Nursing care in radiation oncology,* Philadelphia, 1992, WB Saunders.
*BCG,* Bacille Calmette-Guérin; *C. parvum, Corynebacterium parvum;* *TNF,* tumor necrosis factor.

techniques that permit rapid production of large quantities for commercial application. Table 11-18 presents the common BRMs and their clinical applications.

### Interferons

Interferons comprise a group of glycoproteins (alpha, beta, gamma) produced by leukocytes in response to viral infections or other stimuli. All nucleated cells are capable of interferon production, which can be induced by natural or synthetic agents. Interferons are also produced by recombinant DNA technology by the insertion of genes for an INF of each category into *Escherichia coli.*

Interferons have the ability to alter cellular metabolism in both normal and cancer cells. Interferons produce change in cellular enzymes required for cell growth and proliferation, thereby modifying the immune response. Interferons also can activate natural killer (NK) cells, which are mediators that can identify and destroy some tumor cells. At present INFs

**table 11-18** *Types of Biological Response Modifiers with FDA-Approved Applications*

| Agent | Category | Definition and Biological Actions | Approved Indications |
|---|---|---|---|
| Interferons | Cytokine | Family of glycoprotein hormones with antiviral, immunomodulatory, and antiproliferative effects | |
| Interferon-alfa | | Derived primarily from leukocytes | Hairy cell leukemia<br>Kaposi's sarcoma<br>Condyloma acuminata<br>Chronic hepatitis B<br>Chronic hepatitis C<br>Chronic myelogenous leukemia<br>Adjuvant therapy for melanoma |
| Interferon-beta | | Derived primarily from fibroblasts | Multiple sclerosis |
| Interferon-gamma | | Derived from activated T lymphocytes | Chronic granulomatous disease |
| Interleukins | Cytokine | Molecular messengers between cells of the immune system; they activate cells of the immune system and stimulate the production of other cytokines; 17 interleukins have currently been identified | Renal cell carcinoma (interleukin 2) |
| Monoclonal antibodies | Antibodies | Pure immunoglobulins derived from a single cell (hybridoma); they bind to target antigens on tumor cells and signal other cells of the immune system to destroy the tumor through phagocytosis or by complement-mediated lysis | Detection of colorectal and ovarian cancers |
| GM-CSF | Hematopoietic growth factor | Natural hormone-like protein produced by a variety of immune cells that stimulates the maturation, differentiation, and proliferation of granulocytes and monocytes/macrophages | Autologous bone marrow transplantation in patients with nonmyeloid malignancies |
| G-CSF | Hematopoietic growth factor | Natural hormone-like protein produced by a variety of cells, mainly monocytes and macrophages, as well as endothelial cells, fibroblasts, and stromal cells that stimulates the growth and activation of granulocyte precursor cells | Chronic neutropenia<br>Autologous bone marrow transplantation in patients with nonmyeloid malignancies<br>Decrease the incidence of infection after myelosuppressive therapy in patients with nonmyeloid malignancies |
| Erythropoietin | Hematopoietic growth factor | Natural hormone produced by the kidney that regulates and controls red blood cell production and maturation | Chemotherapy-related anemia<br>Anemia related to chronic renal failure and zidovudine administration in patients with HIV |
| Retinoids | Vitamin A derivatives | Class of agents that perform a significant role in vision, growth, reproduction, epithelial cell differentiation, and immune function | All-*trans*-retinoic acid in the treatment of acute promyelocytic leukemia |

From Ferrell MM: Biotherapy and the oncology nurse, *Semin Oncol Nurs* 12(2):82, 1996.
*GM-CSF,* Granulocyte-macrophage colony-stimulating factor; *G-CSF,* granulocyte colony–stimulating factor; *HIV,* human immunodeficiency virus.

appear to be most effective when used with other agents such as chemotherapeutic agents. Interferon may work synergistically with certain cancer drugs and radiation. Interferons hold the most promise for patients whose immune system has not been weakened by previous treatment with chemotherapy or radiation.

Interferon alfa first received Federal Drug Administration (FDA) approval for the treatment of hairy cell leukemia and has since been approved for the treatment of chronic myelogenous leukemia and Kaposi's sarcoma and as adjuvant therapy for melanoma. It is manufactured under the trade names of Intron-a and Roferon-a. Interferons beta and gamma have demonstrated little effect against cancer cells. Table 11-19 details the most common side effects of biotherapy.

### Interleukins

Interleukins comprise a group of biological factors that are capable of sending messages among cells of the immune system (lymphocytes, macrophages, and hematopoietic cells). They are produced by thymus cells and are involved in cell-mediated immunity. Of the 17 interleukins identified, IL-2 has been most thoroughly studied. The gene for IL-2 is produced by recombinant technology and is available for clinical use in the treatment of renal cell cancer under the name Proleukin.

### Growth factors

Colony-stimulating factors are glycoproteins that are now available for clinical use in the development and activation of several hematopoietic cell lines. Human granulocyte colony–stimulating factor (G-CSF) stimulates the growth and activation of granulocyte precursor cells. No evidence exists that G-CSF can stimulate myeloid and megakaryocyte cell lines. However, continued clinical study may reveal a broader range of activity than is presently known. Granulocyte colony–stimulating factor is approved by the FDA under the name of Neupogen. Granulocyte-macrophage colony–stimulating factor (GM-CSF) stimulates myeloid precursor cells and is approved for use after both autologous and allogeneic bone marrow transplantation under the name Prokine. Both G-CSF and GM-CSF have demonstrated ability to accelerate bone marrow recovery of neutrophil counts after myelosuppression.

Erythropoietin (EPO) is another recombinant growth factor that is approved for the treatment of anemia associated with end-stage renal disease and anemia resulting from chemosuppression of the bone marrow. The approved trade names are Epogen and Procrit.

### Monoclonal antibodies

Monoclonal antibodies are produced by hybridoma techniques that involve immunizing animals (usually mice) with antigen, and then fusing B cells from the mouse's spleen with tumor cells to make hybrid cells. Monoclonal antibodies can be produced to bind with almost any antigen. They are effective in the serological detection of tumors inasmuch as cells that have undergone malignant transformation often express

**table 11-19** *Common Side Effects of Biological Response Modifiers and Their Frequency*

| Side Effect | Interferon | TNF | IL-2 | MoAbs | CSF |
|---|---|---|---|---|---|
| Mental status changes | F | F | F | N | N |
| Anxiety | F | F | F | N | N |
| Headaches | F | F | F | O | F |
| Dysrhythmias | F | F | F | N | N |
| Hypotension | F | F | F | N | O |
| Cardiac dysfunction | O | O | O | N | N |
| Angina | O | O | O | N | N |
| Fatigue | F | F | F | F | F |
| Fever | F | F | F | F | F |
| Chills | F | F | F | O | O |
| Respiratory distress | O | O | O | O | N |
| Weight gain/edema | F | O | F | O | O |
| Renal dysfunction | O | O | F | N | N |
| Hepatic dysfunction | O | F | F | O | O |
| Food/taste aversions | O | O | O | N | N |
| Anorexia | F | F | F | O | O |
| Nausea | F | F | F | O | O |
| Diarrhea | F | O | F | N | N |
| Rash/itching | F | F | F | F | F |
| Allergic symptoms | F | F | F | F | F |
| Anemia | O | O | F | N | N |
| Thrombocytopenia | O | O | O | N | N |
| Eosinophilia | O | O | F | N | N |
| Arthralgias | F | F | F | O | O |
| Myalgias | O | O | F | O | O |
| Bone pain | O | O | O | N | O |

From Shelton B, Belcher A. In Ashwanden P et al: *Oncology nursing: advances, treatments, and trends into the 21st century,* Rockville, Md, 1990, Aspen.
*TNF,* Tumor necrosis factor; *MoAbs,* monoclonal antibodies; *CSF,* colony-stimulating factors; *F,* frequently seen; *O,* occasionally seen; *N,* not seen.

antigens that are not usually found on the surfaces of normal cells. These markers may be sensitive enough to detect early cancer and can be used to monitor the progress of disease in patients undergoing therapy.

Cancer therapy with monoclonal antibodies is in early trials. Some tumor responses have occurred, but monoclonal antibodies alone are not toxic enough to kill tumor cells. Anticancer drugs, radioisotopes, and other BRMs may be attached to monoclonal antibodies and targeted directly to tumor cells, thus bypassing normal cells.

Ongoing research efforts will no doubt provide new applications for BRMs in cancer diagnosis and therapy. The use of biotherapy is expensive because of the advanced technology required to produce these products and the length of clinical trials needed to ascertain their usefulness and effects on human subjects.

## NURSING MANAGEMENT

The role of BRMs in the treatment of cancer is rapidly increasing. As ongoing clinical trials are completed, new BRMs will receive FDA approval for treating primary tumors or as adjuvant therapy. Although clinical trials of BRMs are carried out at large research institutions, patients are now able to receive treatment in small community hospitals, in outpatient departments, and in the home setting. It is the responsibility of nurses working with these patients to be knowledgeable about biotherapy, its role in cancer treatment, and how to provide optimal patient care.

### MANAGEMENT OF SIDE EFFECTS

The BRMs currently in use have a number of side effects. Common side effects are presented in Table 11-19. However, the intensity and duration depend on the BRM used; the dosage, route, and schedule; and any other concurrent therapy in use, such as chemotherapy. Most side effects occur shortly after administration and usually dissipate within several days. Agents given continuously for long periods of time may lead to chronic toxicity. Each symptom can create significant discomfort when experienced alone, but when the patient must deal with the combined effects, care needs are significantly increased. The nursing management of side effects should be comprehensive and coordinated to facilitate transition of the patient from acute care to the home setting.

Although any of the side effects noted in Table 11-19 may occur, flulike symptoms, fatigue, and neurological toxicity are the most disruptive to the patient's daily routine. Flulike symptoms such as fever and discomfort from myalgia, arthralgias, headache, and bone pain can be alleviated by the administration of acetaminophen. Aspirin and aspirin-containing products are avoided. Relaxation and diversional activities is encouraged. Fatigue is a side effect reported by almost all patients receiving BRMs and is a common cause for discontinuing therapy or reducing dosage.[24]

Rest periods in a calm, stress-free environment should be incorporated into each day's activities. Neurological toxicities include somnolence, anxiety, depression, and mental status changes. In most cases the patient will have already been treated with one or a combination of cancer therapies and may become discouraged and question the benefit of further treatment. The nurse must continuously assess patient feelings and response in order to provide sympathetic support and understanding. Family caregivers should be made aware of these potential outcomes of biotherapy and be enlisted to observe and report changes immediately.

### PATIENT EDUCATION

For patients to make an informed decision regarding the need for biotherapy, they must have a basic understanding of their malignant condition, how the immune system functions in relation to cancer, and why biotherapy is being prescribed. Although not all side effects are expected to occur in every case, the patient and caregiver should be made aware of the most common ones. A printed instruction sheet that deals with management of side effects, and side effects to report and to whom, will lend support and help facilitate compliance with therapy. In addition, it is essential that teaching be provided about proper drug preparation and storage, aseptic technique for subcutaneous or intravenous administration, and safe handling and disposal of equipment and drug materials. Most BRMs must be reconstituted or diluted and should be prepared immediately before administration. BRMs are generally unstable at room temperature. Agents prepared in a health care facility for home use should be transported in a cooler to maintain stability. A video that demonstrates proper administration is followed by practice time and redemonstration of techniques to the nurse. This increases the patient's self-confidence and skill levels before the start of therapy.

### HOME CARE MANAGEMENT

Biotherapy is complex and side effects are common, but it can be provided safely in the home setting. Biotherapy requires the availability of dependable and supportive caregivers. Because many cancer patients are elderly, have other chronic conditions, have a caregiver spouse of comparable age and health status, or live alone, it is necessary to know the support network and whether therapy can be successfully handled by the patient outside the acute care setting.

Biotherapy is expensive. The patient and family should be made aware that some private insurers may not reimburse them for agents that are self-administered or administered in the home. Often third-party payers will not pay for what they deem "investigational treatments."[27] These factors will will have an impact on successful home management of biotherapy.

## RADIOTHERAPY

Radiotherapy (RT), the use of radiation in the treatment of disease, has been employed in the treatment of cancer since the discovery of x-rays in 1895 and radium in 1898. The principal radiation agents are (1) x-ray, which consists of electromagnetic radiation produced by waves of electrical energy traveling at an extremely high speed; (2) radium, which is a radioactive isotope occurring freely in nature; and (3) the artificially induced radioactive isotopes produced by bombarding the isotopes of elements with highly energized particles in a cyclotron. The most common sources of radiation for external beam therapy are the linear accelerator, the cobalt-60 teletherapy machines, and the betatron. The advantage of using these high-energy beams lies in their ability to penetrate to a greater depth beneath the skin surface. Skin damage is kept to a minimum because only about 20% of the prescribed radiation dose is delivered to the skin. With high-energy beams, higher doses can be administered with fewer side effects.

Radiation therapy has several recognized advantages over chemotherapy and surgery in cancer treatment. Radiotherapy does not create the many systemic toxicities that are limiting factors in the use of many chemotherapy drugs. In addition, RT is not affected by anatomical restraints that can limit the usefulness of surgery. Thus RT can destroy tumor masses while preserving structure, function, and cosmesis of normal tissues.[23]

### Principles Underlying Radiotherapy

Radiation therapy is prescribed in units called grays (Gy). In the past the dosage was measured by the amount of radiant energy absorbed by tissues and expressed in the unit *rad.* Both terms are used in radiation literature and often are referred to interchangeably (Box 11-11).

Ionizing radiation causes cell death either through direct damage to the double strands of DNA or as a consequence of biochemical changes that interfere with cellular repair and reproduction. Before radiation therapy is prescribed, the radiosensitivity of the tissue targeted must be determined. *Radiosensitivity* is a measure of the potential susceptibility of cells to injury from ionizing radiation and the speed at which damage will occur. All body tissue has a known degree of radiosensitivity. The radiation oncologist must calculate the maximal treatment dosage that can be administered safely without compromising the normal tissues surrounding the tumor. Other considerations include the patient's age, tumor size and stage, degree of spread, and the overall prognosis if radiation is used for treating the tumor. Table 11-20 lists selected organs and their sensitivity to radiation.

Cells that are in the mitosis (M) phase of the cell proliferative cycle are the most sensitive to the effects of radiation. However, damage also may occur during DNA synthesis (S). Tissues that have high proliferative rates, such as bone marrow, skin, and gastrointestinal tract are most effected by radiation. Tumor resistance to radiation is a major problem. Tissue hypoxia is one of the major factors contributing to radioresistance. Hypoxic cells are known to be radioresistant and require about three times as much radiation dosage as a well-oxygenated cell requires to achieve the same degree of cell kill. Cell kill refers to the number of tumor cells that are expected to be destroyed during the most sensitive phases of the cell cycle after a radiation treatment. Tumor cells become hypoxic when, because of tumor growth, they become more distanced from their nearest capillary blood supply. Oxygen is metabolized by and useful only to cells nearest to the capillary. The mechanism of how hypoxia makes a cell radioresistant is not fully understood.

A radiation treatment can range from 1 minute to a few minutes. The exact duration depends on the dose to be delivered, the energy, the type of radiation beam, and the depth of the tumor. Frequency of treatment varies, with some patients being treated daily, five times per week.

In some cases patients may receive a "split course" of therapy, receiving part of the total dose followed by a rest of 1 to 2 weeks until the final cumulative dose is achieved. Split course or fractionation is advantageous for several reasons. Normal cells that received a sublethal dose of radiation have time to repair the damage incurred. Tumor cells that were in a nonsensitive cycle phase may progress to a more radiosensitive phase; therefore a larger cell kill will be attained when treatment is resumed. Probably the most compelling reason to use fractionation is to provide time for reoxygenation of tumor cells, making them more sensitive to radiation effects.

The radiation used medically consists of α-rays, β-rays, and γ-rays (Figure 11-9). The α-rays and β-rays cannot pass through the skin; γ-rays, however, have been found to penetrate several inches of lead, although lead shielding offers a considerable degree of protection. X-rays, which are similar to γ-rays, also require lead protection.

Radiation can be delivered to the patient *externally* by exposure to rays, such as from an x-ray machine or from cobalt 60, or *internally,* either by placing radioactive material such as radium within the tissues or body cavity (sealed internal radiation) or by administering the materials intravenously or

**box 11-11** *Terms Related to Radiation*

| | |
|---|---|
| Roentgen | Amount of radiation exposure in the air |
| Rad | Amount of radiation absorbed per dose (1 rad = 100 ergs/g) |
| Gray (Gy) | International measure: 1 gray = 100 rad |
| Rem | Unit of measure used to express the biological effect of one rad of x-rays |

**table 11-20** *Radiosensitivity of Selected Body Organs*

| Organ | Radiosensitivity |
|---|---|
| Bone marrow | High |
| Ovaries | |
| Testes | |
| Intestine | |
| Skin | Medium high |
| Oral cavity and esophagus | |
| Vagina, cervix | |
| Growing bone and cartilage | Medium |
| Fine vasculature | |
| Mature bone and cartilage | Medium low |
| Kidney | |
| Liver | |
| Thyroid | |
| Muscle | Low |
| Brain and spinal cord | |

orally so that they are distributed throughout the body (unsealed internal radiation).

## Types of Radiotherapy

### External radiotherapy

Before any treatment is initiated, the patient will be thoroughly examined in the radiation oncology department and undergo a simulation phase. During simulation the precise target area is defined and outlined with either ink markings or small permanent tattoo markings called ports. These outlines are essential so that only this small, defined area is within the radiation field.

Different ports may be used on different days, or the position may be changed at intervals during a daily treatment so that only a certain amount of radiation is given through each port. When immobilizing or positioning devices are deemed necessary to help maintain proper positioning during the treatment, they are made specifically for the patient. Pediatric and elderly patients often require casts or molds, special boards, or safety belts. The need for organ-shielding devices also is determined during simulation. The pretreatment phase may require several sessions in the radiation oncology department. A picture of the patient in the exact position, with immobilizing devices and shields, is kept in the patient's treatment file. The photograph helps the technician responsible for administering the treatment to correctly position the patient for each treatment. The technician documents the treatment number, the cumulative dose, patient positioning and immobilizing devices used, and any specific patient concerns or problems encountered.

External radiation may be used alone or in conjunction with surgery. Used alone RT can cure cancer of the skin, oral cavity, larynx, uterine cervix, prostate, pelvis, and Hodgkin's disease stages I, II, and IIIA. When radiation is used in conjunction with surgery, it is used either for cure or palliation of symptoms. Cancers of the head and neck, lung, breast, uterus, bladder, bone, and testes can be cured with combined surgery and radiation. When cure is the anticipated outcome, the radiation may be administered preoperatively or postoperatively. The rationale for preoperative treatment is to decrease the tumor size, increase the potential for removal of all the tumor during surgery, eradicate subclinical disease that might be present beyond the intended surgical field, and eradicate lymph nodes where disease could form or provide a mode for metastasis. The disadvantage of preoperative radiation is the delay in wound healing of normal tissues that were within the treatment field and thus damaged.

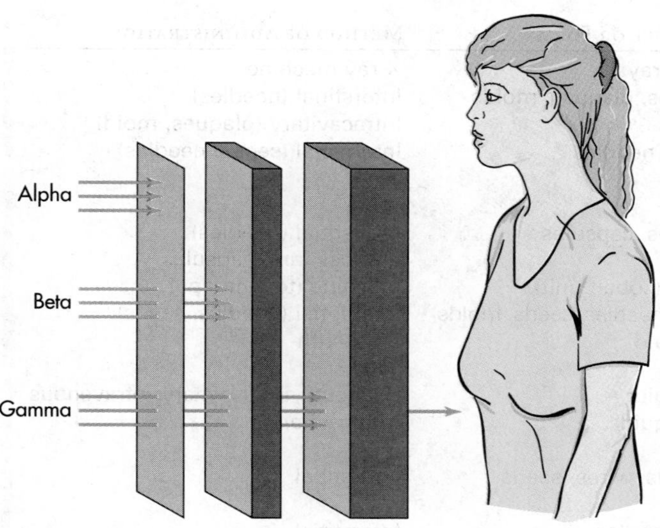


**fig. 11-9** Relative penetrating power of three types of radiation.

Postoperative radiation therapy usually is performed to eradicate any residual tumor and subclinical disease. Higher doses can be administered than could have been used before surgery. The most cited disadvantage of postoperative therapy is the delay in starting treatments until after wound healing is complete. Combination radiation therapy and chemotherapy are discussed in the chemotherapy section.

### Brachytherapy (internal radiation therapy)

*Brachytherapy* is the placement of radioactive sources on or directly into a tumor. Internal radiation may be delivered by sealed or unsealed methods. In either type special precautions may be necessary, depending on the amount of radioactive material used, its location, and the kind of rays being emitted (Table 11-21).

Special precautions are taken if more than a tracer diagnostic dose has been given. Hospitals in which therapeutic doses of radioactive isotopes are administered are required to have a radiation safety officer. Often this person is a physicist. The radiation safety officer determines the precautions to be observed in each situation. Most hospitals have printed instruction sheets stating the precautions to be followed for each substance used. Personnel should be fully acquainted with all precautions and should be supervised in carrying them out. Generally, the patient will be placed in a private room while the radioactive substance is in place. A radiation warning sign is placed on the door to the patient's room, and visitors are restricted.

**Sealed internal radiotherapy.** Sealed internal radiotherapy is used to deliver a concentrated dose of radiation directly to the malignant lesion or tumor area. Usually this involves insertion of radioactive substances within hollow cavities or within tissues. The radioactive isotopes commonly used are $^{60}$CO, $^{198}$Ir, $^{131}$I, $^{32}$P, $^{137}$CS, $^{198}$Au, and $^{226}$Ra (see Table 11-21). These radioactive substances may be used in the form of molds, plaques, needles, wires, special applicators, or ribbons.

Placement of the sealed container may be carried out in the operating room, radiation department, or a treatment room. Exact positioning of the container is essential so that radiation exposure to surrounding tissues and organs is minimized. X-ray films are taken to verify appropriate placement. The patient may then return to a private hospital room where the radioactive substance is inserted. This is called afterloading and is a technique used to prevent unnecessary exposure of staff members in various departments to the radiation source. The length of time the radiation material is left in place depends on the element used and the dose that has been prescribed. Time may range from a few hours to several days. Table 11-22 lists cancers treated with brachytherapy.

**Unsealed internal radiotherapy.** Unsealed internal radiation is delivered to the patient by mouth as an "atomic cocktail" or as a liquid instilled into a body cavity. Persons caring for the patient can be exposed to the radiation from emanations of the substance from the patient (external exposure) or from contact with the patient's discharges that contain the radioactive substance (internal exposure). It may be inhaled, ingested, or absorbed through the skin. The exposure varies with each of the substances used, and safety for the staff members caring for the patient depends on a thorough knowledge of the substance used and its action within the body. Special precautions are not needed with tracer doses used for diagnostic procedures.

Radioisotopes commonly used for unsealed brachytherapy include radioactive iodine ($^{131}I$), phosphorus ($^{32}P$), and gold ($^{198}Au$). These substances may be administered orally or intravenously or by direct instillation into a body cavity. Each isotope can be a source of radiation contamination to health care personnel. The mode of elimination from the body varies with the specific isotope, but generally traces are found in urine, feces, vomitus, sputum, wound drainage, and perspiration. Specific instructions will be provided by radiation oncology personnel to protect staff members working with these patients.

High dose rate (HDR) brachytherapy is now being used for the treatment of inoperable lung cancer and for the palliation of cough, dyspnea, and hemoptysis. Therapy can be performed on an outpatient basis, because treatment time may be as little as a few minutes, repeated at 2-week intervals. The future role of this type of brachytherapy is not yet known.

## Protection of Health Care Professionals from Radiation Hazards

Radiation delivered externally (including x-rays) can harm persons working with the patient only during the time that the patient is being treated. This is true also of the radiation from some radioactive substances used for other methods of treatment. Patients with internal radiation that emits $\gamma$-rays, however, may expose other persons to radiation for varying periods of time, and the length of time that a staff member can be exposed safely to the patient is important in planning care. The time interval required for the radioactive substance to be half dissipated is called its half-life. (See Table 11-21.) This period varies widely, but as the end of the half-life is reached, danger from exposure decreases.

Exposure to radiation can be controlled in three ways: time, distance, and shielding. All emanations are subject to the inverse-square law. For example, a person who stands 2 m away from the source of radiation receives only one fourth as much exposure as when standing only 1 m away. At 4 m only one sixteenth of the exposure will be received. Therefore increasing the distance from the radiation source decreases the exposure (Figure 11-10). Lead-lined gloves and a lead apron, which act as a shield to reduce exposure, should be worn by anyone who attends patients during x-ray treatment or during examination by fluoroscopy.

## Side Effects of Radiation Therapy

When radiation therapy is used, some degree of radiation reaction may occur. The frequency and severity of reaction de-

**table 11-21** *Characteristics of Some Commonly Used Radioactive Agents*

| Radiation Source | Half-Life (Where Applicable) | Rays Emitted | Appearance or Form | Method of Administration |
|---|---|---|---|---|
| X-ray | — | $\gamma$ | Invisible rays | X-ray machine |
| Radium ($^{226}RA$) | 1600 yr | $\alpha$<br>$\beta$ | In needles, plaques, molds | Interstitial (needles)<br>Intracavitary (plaques, mold) |
| Radon | 4 days | $\alpha$<br>$\beta$<br>$\gamma$ (low intensity) | In seeds, needles | Interstitial (seeds, needles) |
| Cesium ($^{137}Cs$) | 33 yr | $\beta$<br>$\gamma$ | In needles, capsules | Interstitial (needles)<br>Intracavitary (capsules) |
| Cobalt ($^{60}Co$) | 5 yr | $\beta$<br>$\gamma$ | External (cobalt unit)<br>Internal (needles, seeds, molds) | Machine (teletherapy)<br>Interstitial (needles, seeds) |
| Iodine ($^{131}I$) | 8 days | $\beta$<br>$\gamma$ (low intensity) | Clear liquid | By mouth |
| Phosphorus ($^{32}P$) | 14 days | $\beta$ | Clear liquid | By mouth, intracavitary, intravenous |
| Gold ($^{198}Au$) | 3 days | $\beta$<br>$\gamma$ | Purple liquid | Intracavitary |
| Iridium ($^{198}Ir$) | 74 days | $\beta$<br>$\gamma$ (low intensity) | In needles, wires, seeds | Interstitial |
| Yttrium ($^{90}Y$) | 3 days | $\beta$ | Beads, needles | Interstitial |

pend on the type of equipment used, the physician's treatment plan, and the patient's compliance with therapy. Early radiation reactions can be observed almost immediately after treatments begin. They generally are mild and last no more than several weeks. The side effects include both local (skin) and systemic sequelae such as fatigue, nausea, diarrhea, and bone marrow suppression. The damage is the result of radiation's effects on actively proliferating cells and the release of catabolic products as cells die. Interventions are of a supportive nature. If these self-limiting reactions become too disabling, their effects can be avoided or lessened by reducing the daily radiation dose.

**table 11-22** Cancers Treated with Brachytherapy

| Cancer | Technique | Radioactive Source |
|---|---|---|
| Endometrial | Intracavitary | Radium, cesium |
| Cervical | Intracavitary | Radium, cesium |
| Prostate | Interstitial | Iodine, gold |
| Breast | Interstitial | Iridium |
| Ocular melanoma | Plaque therapy | Cobalt, iodine |
| Head and neck | Interstitial thermal | Iridium, cesium |
| Rectal | Interstitial | Cesium |
| Esophageal | Intraluminal | Cesium |
| Bronchogenic | Endobronchial | Iridium, iodine |

From Dow KH, Helderley LJ: *Nursing care in radiation oncology,* Philadelphia, 1992, WB Saunders.

Late radiation reactions can occur many months or years after therapy. The late effects are a progression of the earlier self-limiting reactions and are more localized than systemic. There is no consensus at this time on the underlying cause of these late-occurring sequelae.

Radiation therapy, although one of the major cancer treatment modalities, does have carcinogenic potential. The mechanism by which radiation induces cancer is not fully known at this time. It is known that secondary malignant conditions may develop in patients previously treated with radiation therapy. Leukemia or non-Hodgkin's lymphoma may develop in patients receiving irradiation for Hodgkin's disease, and breast cancer may develop in women who undergo multiple fluoroscopies.

Bone marrow suppression is almost always a side effect of radiation therapy. Recovery of the bone marrow depends on the dose used and the tumor volume treated. Full bone marrow recovery is generally expected after chemotherapy, but full recovery may never be achieved after radiation therapy. (Table 11-23 indicates the early and late sequelae of radiation therapy; Table 11-24 presents a toxicity grading system used for evaluating radiation therapy's effects on specific tissues and organ systems.) It is important that patients be provided with information about the immediate and long-term side effects of therapy so that they can make informed decisions related to therapy.

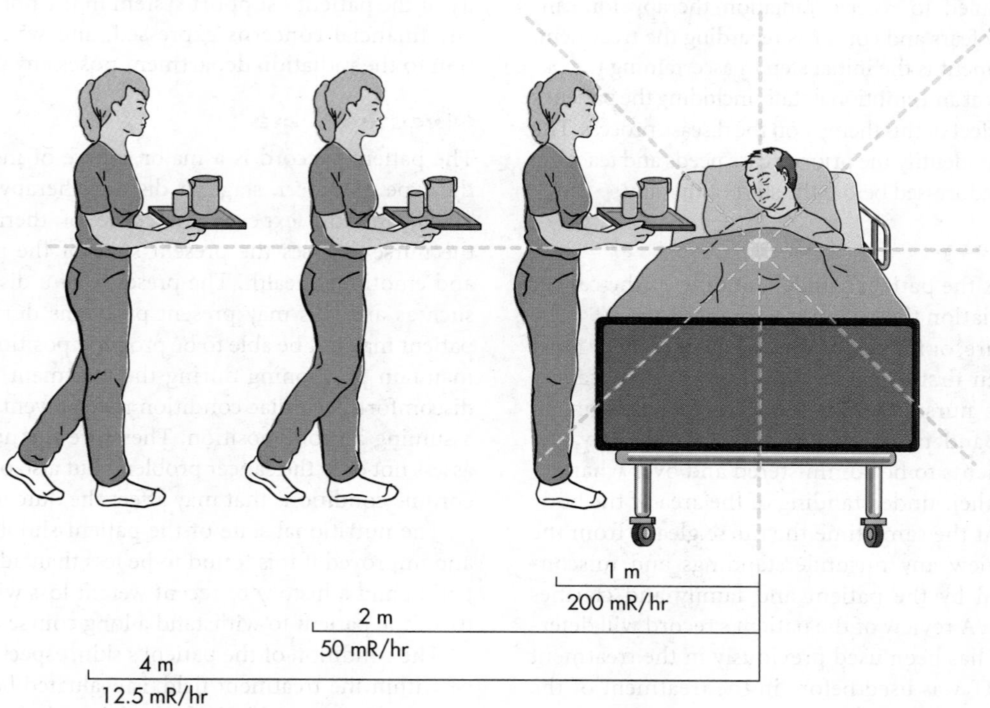


**fig. 11-10** Nurse nearest source of radioactivity (patient) is exposed to more radioactivity.

**table 11-23** *Possible Sequelae of Radiation Therapy*

| Anatomical Site | Acute Sequelae (Early) | Late Sequelae |
|---|---|---|
| Brain | Earache, headache, dizziness, hair loss, erythema | Hearing loss, damage to middle or inner ear, pituitary gland dysfunction, cataracts, and brain necrosis |
| Head and neck | Odynophagia, dysphagia, hoarseness, xerostomia, dysgeusia, weight loss | Subcutaneous fibrosis, skin ulceration, necrosis, thy roid dysfunction, dental decay, osteoradionecrosis of mandible, delayed wound healing, damage to middle and inner ear |
| Lung and mediastinum or esophagus | Odynophagia, dysphagia, cough, hoarseness pneumonitis, carditis | Progressive fibrosis of lung, dyspnea, chronic cough; esophageal stricture<br>Rare: chronic pericarditis, myelopathy |
| Breast or chest wall | Odynophagia, dysphagia, hoarseness, cough; pneumonitis (asymptomatic); carditis; cytopenia | Fibrosis, retraction of breast; lung fibrosis; arm edema; chronic endocarditis, myocardial infarction<br>Rare: osteonecrosis of ribs |
| Abdomen or pelvis | Nausea, vomiting, abdominal pain, diarrhea; urinary frequency, dysuria, nocturia; cytopenia | Proctitis, sigmoiditis; rectal or sigmoid stricture; colonic perforation or obstruction; contracted bladder, urinary incontinence, hematuria, vesicovaginal fistula; rectovaginal fistula; leg edema; scrotal edema, sexual impotency; vaginal retraction or scarring; sterilization<br>Rare: damage to liver or kidneys |
| Extremities | Erythema, dry/moist desquamation | Subcutaneous fibrosis: ankylosis, edema; bone/soft tissue necrosis |

From Perez CA, Brady LW: *Principles and practices of radiation oncology,* ed 2, Philadelphia, 1992, JB Lippincott.

## NURSING MANAGEMENT

### ■ ASSESSMENT

The patient scheduled to receive radiation therapy for cancer may have many fears and concerns regarding the treatment. The nursing assessment is the initial step in ascertaining the patient's overall physical and emotional state, including the patient's perception of the effect of this therapy on the disease process. The assessment will help identify the priority care needs and teaching areas that must be addressed before the start of therapy.

#### Subjective Data

The nurse assesses the patient's understanding of the cancer and the use of radiation therapy in treatment. Is the RT to be used to attempt cure, or for palliation of symptoms? For most patients this is their first encounter with this mode of cancer therapy. Thus the nurse attempts to elicit information on what the patient and family know about the therapy, the number of treatments to be administered and over what period of time, and their understanding of the area of the body to be irradiated. At the same time the nurse gleans from the assessment interview any misunderstandings and misconceptions expressed by the patient and family and clarifies them immediately. A review of the patient's record will determine whether RT has been used previously in the treatment of the cancer. If RT was used before in the treatment of the same cancer, it is important to determine how the patient perceived the therapy and if there were any unpleasant side effects or experiences that might interfere with completing the course of treatments. Generally the first treatment will be administered either just before discharge or at some time after discharge home. The nurse assesses the type and availability of the patient's support system in the home environment, any financial concerns expressed, and whether transportation to the radiation department poses any problems.

#### Objective Data

The patient's record is a major source of information about the type of cancer, stage of disease, therapy previously provided, and the expected outcome of therapy. In addition the nurse assesses the present state of the patient's physical and emotional health. The presence of a disabling condition such as arthritis may present problems during therapy. The patient may not be able to be properly positioned or be able to maintain positioning during the treatment due to pain and discomfort. A cardiac condition may prevent the patient from assuming a prone position. Therefore the nurse will need to assess not only the cancer problem, but also other diseases and chronic conditions that may affect the outcome of therapy.

The nutritional state of the patient should be determined and improved if it is found to be less than adequate. Poor nutrition and a history of recent weight loss will affect the ability of the patient to withstand a long course of treatment.

The condition of the patient's skin, especially skin that will be within the treatment field, is evaluated before the start of therapy. An intact skin is the body's main line of defense. Because skin is always undergoing cellular renewal, it is extremely vulnerable to the effects of radiation beams as they

**table 11-24** *Acute Radiation Toxicity Grading Scale for Specific Tissues and Organ Systems*

| ORGAN/TISSUE | 0 | GRADE 1 | GRADE 2 | GRADE 3 | GRADE 4 |
|---|---|---|---|---|---|
| Skin | No change over baseline | Follicular, faint or dull erythema, epilation, dry desquamation, decreased sweating | Tender erythema, epilation, dry desquamation, moderate edema | Moist desquamation other than skin folds, pitting edema | Ulceration hemorrhage, necrosis |
| Mucous membrane | No change over baseline | May experience mild pain not requiring analgesic | Patchy mucositis; may experience moderate pain requiring analgesic | Fibrinous mucositis; may include severe pain requiring narcotic | Ulceration, hemorrhage, or necrosis |
| Salivary gland | No change over baseline | Mild mouth dryness; slightly thickened saliva; slightly altered taste such as metallic | Moderate to complete dryness; thick, sticky saliva, markedly altered taste | — | Acute salivary gland necrosis |
| Pharynx and esophagus | No change over baseline | Mild dysphagia or odynophagia; may require topical anesthetic or nonnarcotic analgesics, soft diet | Moderate dysphagia or odynophagia; may require narcotic analgesics; puréed or liquid diet | Severe dysphagia or odynophagia with dehydration or weight loss >15% from pretreatment baseline requiring nasogastric (NG) feeding tube, intravenous fluids, or hyperalimentation | Complete obstruction, ulceration, perforation, fistula |
| Upper gastrointestinal (GI) | No change over baseline | Anorexia with <5% weight loss; nausea not requiring antiemetics; abdominal discomfort not requiring analgesics or parasympatholytic drugs | Anorexia with <15% weight loss; nausea or vomiting requiring antiemetics; abdominal pain requiring analgesics | Anorexia with >15% weight loss or requiring NG tube or parenteral support; nausea or vomiting requiring NG tube or parenteral support; abdominal pain (severe); hematemesis or melena; distention | Ileus, obstruction, perforation, GI bleeding; abdominal pain requiring tube decompression or bowel diversion |

Modified from Perez CA, Brady LW: *Principles and practices of radiation oncology,* ed 2, Philadelphia, 1992, JB Lippincott.

*Continued*

pass through each skin layer. Skin that is damaged or broken down from trauma or the effects of a dermatological condition should be noted. The effects of radiation on the body are cumulative. Thus, if an area requires treatment a second time, the overlying skin will be more vulnerable to radiation damage than skin never irradiated.

The age of the patient may also influence the outcome of the therapy. Age is more of a factor if the patient is 65 or older. It is known that immune system function declines with age, and regeneration of the bone marrow takes longer in elderly persons. The effects of fatigue are also more pronounced in the aged. Elderly tissues, especially the skin and mucosa, are less elastic and take longer to repair the damage that may occur with radiation.[23] Consequently, the elderly may not be able to withstand the amount of radiation that would be administered to a younger person with the same cancer. Last, elders may be more frightened and anxious about therapy, especially if they are confused or mentally incompetent. Mild sedation before the treatment may be necessary.

## NURSING DIAGNOSES

Nursing diagnoses are determined from analysis of patient data. Nursing diagnoses for the patient receiving radiation therapy may include but are not limited to:

| Diagnostic Title | Possible Etiological Factors |
|---|---|
| Knowledge deficit | Lack of information on how radiation affects cancer cells and the body; lack of information on expected outcome of therapy on disease process; lack of interest or readiness in learning about radiation therapy |
| Skin integrity, risk for impaired | Radiation effects on skin, nutritional deficits, elderly age group |

**table 11-24** *Acute Radiation Toxicity Grading Scale for Specific Tissues and Organ Systems—cont'd*

| Organ/Tissue | 0 | Grade 1 | Grade 2 | Grade 3 | Grade 4 |
|---|---|---|---|---|---|
| Lower GI including pelvis | No change over baseline | Increased frequency or change in bowel habits not requiring medication; rectal discomfort not requiring analgesics | Diarrhea requiring parasympatholytic drugs; mucous discharge; rectal or abdominal pain requiring analgesics | Diarrhea requiring parenteral support; severe mucous or blood discharge; abdominal distention | Obstruction, fistula or perforation, GI bleeding, abdominal pain or tenesmus requiring tube decompression or bowel diversion |
| Lung | No change over baseline | Mild symptoms—dry cough or dyspnea on exertion | Persistent cough requiring narcotic, antitussive agents; dyspnea with minimal effort but not at rest | Severe cough unresponsive to medications or dyspnea at rest; radiologic evidence of acute pneumonitis; oxygen or steroids required | Severe respiratory insufficiency; continuous oxygen or assisted ventilation |
| Central nervous system | No change over baseline | Fully functional status with minor neurological findings; no medication needed | Neurological findings require home care; nursing assistance may be required; medication including steroids and antiseizure agents required | Neurological findings require hospitalization | Serious neurological impairment and may include paralysis, coma, or seizures; hospitalization required |
| Genitourinary | No change over baseline | Frequency or nocturia twice pretreatment habit; dysuria, urgency not requiring medication | Frequency or nocturia less frequent than every hour; dysuria, urgency, bladder spasm requiring local anesthetic | Frequency and nocturia hourly or more frequently; dysuria, pelvic pain, or bladder spasm requiring regular, frequent narcotic; gross hematuria | Hematuria requiring transfusion; acute bladder obstruction not secondary to clot, ulceration, or necrosis |

## EXPECTED PATIENT OUTCOMES

Expected patient outcomes for the patient receiving radiation therapy for cancer treatment may include but are not limited to:

1. Knowledge of radiotherapy procedure
   a. Describes why radiation therapy will be used to treat the cancer
   b. Correctly describes the treatment plan for the patient's particular disease process
   c. Identifies the most common side effects to expect as a result of radiation treatment
2. Knowledge of effects
   a. Identifies potential skin changes that may occur with radiation therapy
   b. Demonstrates measures to prevent increasing skin impairment while undergoing radiation therapy

## INTERVENTIONS

The word *radiation* is surrounded by a certain mystique of fear and apprehension. Public concern over the consequences of radiation exposure was evident after the nuclear accidents in the United States at Three Mile Island and in Russia at Chernobyl. Therefore, when radiation therapy is prescribed to treat cancer, the patient and family may be anxious and express concerns about its use and safety. A study of the needs of oncology patients who underwent radiation therapy found that receiving correct information about radiation as a treatment method and knowledge of potential side effects were the priority concerns. (See the accompanying Research Box on p. 295.)

### Providing Patient/Family Education

The nurse can play a vital role in dispelling patient and family fears and misconceptions about radiation therapy. The nurse clarifies and reinforces the instruction about the number of treatments planned, the body area to be irradiated, and what will be expected of the patient during preliminary planning and treatment sessions. Treatment planning begins with a consultation with the radiation oncologist who makes the determination if radiation can be used successfully for cure or palliation. In some cases radiation may be considered inappropriate due to the poor radiosensitivity of the tumor. In this event, the nurse anticipates disappointment or anger and is ready to provide understanding and sympathetic support. When radiation is to be used as a treatment, the patient will have one or several simulation sessions, which will pinpoint the exact area to be treated. This target area will be defined with either ink markings or a tattoo. If ink is used, the pa-

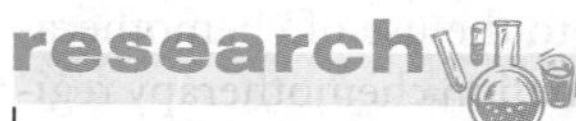

Reference: Hagopian GA: The effects of informational audiotapes on knowledge and self-care behaviors of patients undergoing radiation therapy, *Oncol Nurs Forum* 23(4):697, 1996.

The treatment of cancer is very complex and requires that patients acquire new knowledge and skills at the same time that they are anxious and confused about their disease process. The side effects of radiation therapy (RT) are cumulative and may become debilitating unless properly managed. Understanding of how RT works and self-care strategies to manage side effects will enable patients to more fully participate in their own care and manage their health care problems.

The purpose of this study was to develop and test informational audiotapes about RT and the management of side effects. Audiotapes were used because fatigue from the disease or treatment may cause inability to concentrate. Low literacy skills are also a concern and even the need for new glasses can make reading instructional materials difficult. The study used a posttest format, and patients were randomly assigned to either an experimental or a control group with 27 patients in each group. The control group received standard care (information about the RT department and the nature of radiation therapy, as well as weekly visits with the physician to discuss progress and side effects). The experimental group received the standard care in addition to listening to the audiotapes. Instruments included the Radiation Side Effects Profile (RSEP) used to determine the number and severity of RT side effects, the self-care strategies used by the patient to manage the side effects, and the helpfulness of the self-care measures. Participants also completed a multiple choice knowledge test developed from the content of the audiotapes. Experimental group participants also completed an audiotape survey related to their satisfaction with the use of the tapes.

There were no significant differences between the control and experimental groups in the number of side effects reported or the severity of the side effects. However, the results indicated that those who listened to the audiotapes scored significantly higher on the knowledge test and performed more self-care behaviors in managing their side effects. The study suggests that the use of audiotapes is an effective means of increasing patient knowledge and self-care skills. The audiotapes are inexpensive to produce, easy to use and store, and useful for patients with visual problems or low literacy skills. Audiotapes could easily be prepared for other treatment modalities, such as surgery and chemotherapy. The researcher suggests, however, that other teaching aides, such as videotapes, computer-assisted instruction, and interactive video, might also be useful.

tient is instructed not to wash these markings off when bathing.

Some patients fear that they will be "radioactive" following treatment and a danger to others around them. Still others are anxious that the treatment will be painful. Both are misconceptions. No sensation is felt during treatment. The patient does need to know that he or she will be alone in the treatment room but will be continuously monitored on television and be able to talk to the radiation technician at all times. Immobilizing devices, such as special molds or casts, may be used to maintain proper body position during treatment. Treatments are generally completed in minutes.

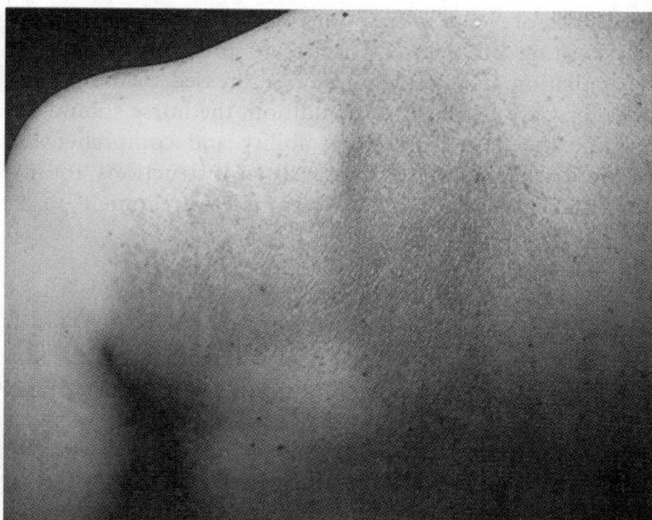

**fig. 11-11** Erythema and dry desquamation of the skin in response to external radiotherapy.

The nurse teaches about common side effects that may be anticipated with radiotherapy. Decreased energy levels and fatigue result from bone marrow depression secondary to treatment. Providing for adequate rest periods throughout the day and 8 hours of sleep at night will help the patient cope with these distressing symptoms. Maintaining good nutrition with a diet high in carbohydrate, protein, and calories will supply the necessary energy for daily activities. Weight is checked weekly to determine if dietary measures are sufficient or if additional supplements are needed. Laboratory studies (blood counts and chemistry evaluations) will be monitored at intervals during treatment to determine the effects of therapy on bone marrow production of essential cellular elements (white blood cell [WBC], red blood cell [RBC], platelet count).

### Promoting Skin Integrity

The skin changes that occur secondary to radiation are addressed before initiating therapy because changes in skin integrity begin with the first treatment. The slight initial erythema may go unrecognized. Initial erythema is the result of radiation effects on capillary blood flow and causes extracapillary cell injury. Vascular vasodilation and congestion occur in phases beginning within minutes of the first treatment, progress to frank erythema in 2 to 3 weeks, and then begin to fade. Figure 11-11 illustrates typical radiotherapy skin reactions, including erythema and dry desquamation. Long-term effects may occur months after irradiation is completed and are attributed to changes in endothelial permeability, edema, and increased skin temperature.[19]

Teaching skin care by demonstration followed by return demonstration and supplementing with verbal and written guidelines prevents unnecessary skin discomfort or alleviates existing problems. Measures to prevent irritation in the radiation treatment field are addressed in the Guidelines for Care Box below. In addition, the nurse should determine the patient's reading ability and comprehension before discharge; appropriate written instructions are important because most patients complete treatment on an outpatient basis.

## EVALUATION

Successful achievement of treatment outcomes for the patient receiving radiotherapy are easily determined. The patient who is able to discuss the rationale for using RT in treating cancer (cure, palliation, or adjunctive to surgery or chemotherapy) is demonstrating retention and comprehension of information on RT's therapeutic use. By stating the exact number of treatments prescribed, the area to be irradiated, and the necessity for completing all treatments, the patient is demonstrating acceptance of the therapeutic plan and responsibility for complying with it. The patient and caregiver confirm their knowledge of skin care measures by answering questions related to strategies employed for hypothetical situations such as cleansing the skin and coping with itch, dryness, or rash. When able to discuss the role of nutrition, adequate rest and sleep, good personal hygiene, and untoward symptoms to report, the patient is ready for self-care.

## CHEMOTHERAPY

Advances in knowledge of cancer growth and chemotherapeutic agents have led to concomitant advances in cancer treatment. Improvement in overall survival and longer disease-free intervals can be directly attributed to the use of chemotherapeutic agents, particularly in combination chemotherapy regimens and as adjuvant therapy.

Chemotherapy may be curative or palliative or have negligible or uncertain effects depending on the type of cancer. Patients and families should be told that "incurable" does not mean untreatable or uncontrollable. Table 11-25 indicates the responsiveness of various neoplastic diseases to chemotherapy.

The expected benefit of chemotherapy (cure, control, or palliation) should be known by the physician, nurse, and patient. This allows for realistic goal setting by the caregivers, patient, and family. Such background also provides a perspective from which to view side effects. The potential for cure, a prolonged disease-free survival, or reduction of symptoms is a benefit that usually outweighs the risk and discomfort of short-term toxic side effects. Conditions in which risk may outweigh benefits include overt or occult infections, bleeding dyscrasias, bone marrow depression, severe metabolic disturbances, renal or liver dysfunction, and pregnancy.

### guidelines for care

**Preventing Skin Irritation During Radiation Therapy**

1. Cleanse radiation field (area within ink markings or inside tattoo outline) daily with mild soap and water. *Do not* erase ink markings if present.
2. Clean and keep dry skin folds that overlap and places where moisture collects (abdominal skin folds, under and between pendulous breasts, between buttocks or perineum).
3. Avoid use of perfumed soaps, lotions, or deodorant on involved skin surface.
4. Guard against irritation from belts, bras, rough clothing on treatment field. Cotton clothing is least irritating.
5. Do not use heating pads, hot water bottles, or ice packs on treated field.
6. Avoid exposure to sunlight. If unavoidable, use sunscreen for protection.
7. Do not swim in salt water or chlorinated swimming pools.
8. Use an electric razor only to shave within treatment area.
9. Do not scratch dry, itchy skin in treatment field.
10. Do not apply any lotions, powders, or ointments to treated area unless advised to do so by radiologist.

**table 11-25** *Neoplastic Disease Response to Chemotherapy*

| Response | Neoplastic Disease |
|---|---|
| Cures in advanced cancer | Gestational trophoblastic tumors<br>Acute lymphoblastic leukemia<br>Acute myeloblastic leukemia<br>Hodgkin's disease<br>Non-Hodgkin's lymphoma (children)<br>Diffuse histiocytic lymphoma<br>Burkitt's lymphoma<br>Testicular tumors |
| Cures with adjuvant chemotherapy | Wilms' tumor<br>Osteogenic sarcoma<br>Rhabdomyosarcoma |
| Minor responses with chemotherapy/adjuvant chemotherapy; no demonstrable prolongation of life | Non–small cell lung carcinoma<br>Head and neck cancer<br>Stomach cancer<br>Pancreatic cancer<br>Cervical cancer<br>Melanoma<br>Cancer of the adrenal cortex<br>Soft tissue sarcoma |
| Complete and partial remissions with uncertain prolongation of survival with chemotherapy/adjuvant chemotherapy | Multiple myeloma<br>Ovarian cancer<br>Endometrial cancer<br>Neuroblastoma<br>Colorectal cancer<br>Liver cancer |
| Complete remissions and increased survival with chemotherapy/adjuvant chemotherapy | Breast cancer<br>Small cell lung carcinoma<br>Acute myeloblastic leukemia<br>Non-Hodgkin's lymphoma, indolent<br>Prostate cancer<br>Chronic granulocytic leukemia<br>Hairy cell leukemia |

Modified from Krakoff IH: *CA Cancer J Clin* 46(3):134, 1996.

Adjuvant chemotherapy refers to chemotherapy administered in conjunction with either surgery or radiation therapy. It is aimed at the destruction of micrometastases believed to be present but too small to be detected by current diagnostic techniques. Left untreated, the micrometastases have a high potential for tumor growth and cancer recurrence. When chemotherapy is used at a time when the malignant cell population is small and likely to be susceptible, complete tumor cell eradication is possible. The goal is cure.

The knowledge that all diagnostic tests are negative for cancer understandably may cause the patient to question the need for adjuvant therapy. This is especially true when side effects are experienced. Sensitivity to these feelings, coupled with the knowledge of the expected benefit of therapy, is the basis for both patient teaching and the support and encouragement often needed to continue therapy.

## Clinical Trials

The general public and, at times, health care professionals view chemotherapy with apprehension. The patient may ask, "Am I a guinea pig?" It is helpful for the nurse to be able to explain that chemotherapeutic drugs are carefully tested before being approved for treatment. Chemotherapeutic drugs reach a phase of clinical trial in human beings according to a drug-screening process established by the National Cancer Institute. This process identifies compounds with antitumor activity, demonstrates the activity in animals, studies and determines all of the pharmacological aspects of the drug (kinetics, absorption, dose, metabolism, and excretion), and defines toxicity. The drugs then go through the four phases of clinical trials outlined in Table 11-26. The effectiveness of the new agent is then compared with standard therapy to determine if the new drug is equal to or better than drugs currently used.

## Principles of Chemotherapy

Normal and malignant cells progress through various phases in the cell cycle as they replicate. (See Figure 11-4.) Cancer chemotherapy is based on the actions of certain drugs that create changes in the cell cycle phases. Figure 11-12 summarizes how some of the commonly used chemotherapeutic agents interrupt cell growth and replication.

**table 11-26** *Phases of Clinical Trials for Chemotherapeutic Drugs*

| Phase | Action |
|---|---|
| I | Identify toxic reactions; determine optimal dose within safe limits and set schedule |
| II | Determine extent of antineoplastic activity |
| III | Compare action of new drug with standard antineoplastic drugs |
| IV | Determine effect on advanced cancer, effect of combined therapy with other antineoplastic drugs, and effect with adjuvant therapy |

Drugs such as antimetabolites and vinca alkaloids that are effective during a particular point of the cell cycle are termed *phase-specific drugs* (Figure 11-13). Drugs that are active throughout the cell cycle (termed *phase-nonspecific drugs*) include the alkylating agents, antibiotics, nitrosoureas, procarbazine, and dacarbazine (DTIC-Dome). Combinations of cycle-specific and cycle-nonspecific drugs have proved useful in treatment regimens. One major factor that influences the response of a cancer to chemotherapy is the fraction of tumor cells in replication at a given time, a percentage that varies among different tumors, among individual patients, and at different times in the same patient.

### Cell population growth

Chemotherapy is more effective when the tumor is small and growing rapidly, a time when a relatively high proportion of cells are undergoing division. At this time, tumor cells are more sensitive to chemotherapeutic agents that are toxic to dividing cells (phase-specific drugs). Larger, slower-growing tumors respond better to drugs that are effective regardless of whether a cell is dividing (phase-nonspecific drugs). Consequently the physician chooses the appropriate drug or combination of drugs, depending on tumor size and rate of growth.

### Combination chemotherapy

Increased knowledge of how specific cytotoxic drugs exert their effect and of the potential for tumor cells to become resistant to a specific therapy, similar to antibiotic resistance, has led to the use of combination chemotherapy. Combination chemotherapy has a therapeutic effect superior to single-agent therapy for many cancers. Drugs considered for combination chemotherapy are those with the following characteristics:

1. Are active when used alone
2. Have different mechanisms of action
3. Have a biochemical basis for possible synergism
4. Do not produce toxicity in the same organs
5. Produce toxicity at different times after administration

Repeated brief courses of drug therapy are given to reduce immunosuppressive effects. Principles of chemotherapy administration are listed in Box 11-12.

### Cell-kill hypothesis

The cell-kill hypothesis explains why patients must often have several or more courses of chemotherapy. Chemotherapy is thought to kill a fixed percentage of the total number of cancer cells. Theoretically, if a drug had a 90% cell-kill rate and 1 million cells were present, the first therapeutic regimen would kill 900,000 cancer cells, leaving 100,000. The second treatment would again destroy 90% of the cells, leaving 10,000. Again, theoretically, after a number of chemotherapy treatments, only one cell would remain and that would be killed by the body's immune system (Figure 11-14).

### Tumor resistance to chemotherapy

Malignant neoplasms can become resistant to the effects of both single and multiple chemotherapeutic agents. The

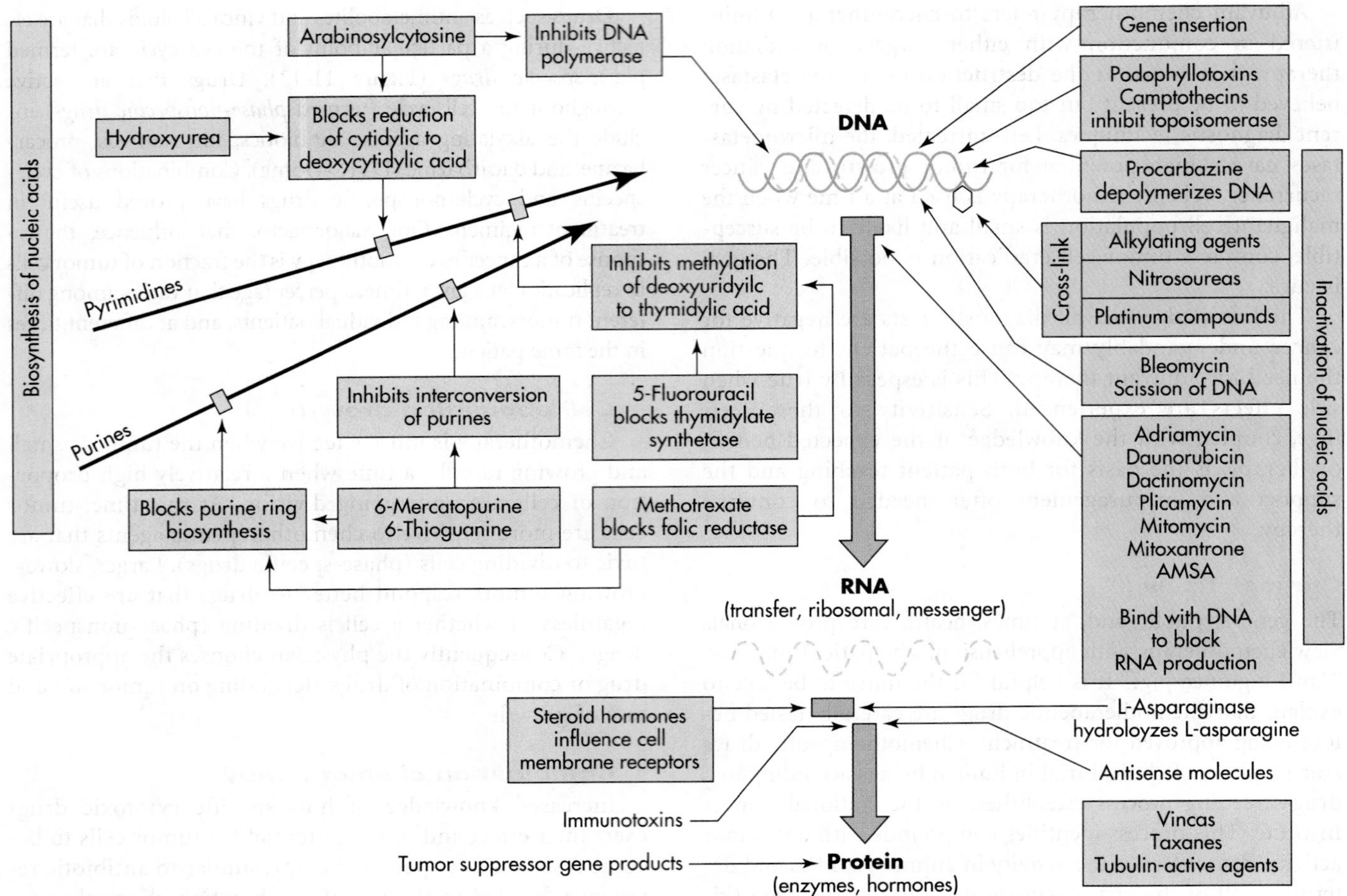


**fig. 11-12** Mechanism of action for chemotherapeutic and biological agents.

resistance is acquired as treatment progresses. The resistance is spontaneous and begins at the individual cell level. As tumor cells are exposed to the chemotherapeutic agent, spontaneous genetic alterations occur, such as mutations, translocations, and deletions, which are then passed on as the cell divides. With each cell division the chance of developing drug resistance becomes greater. This phenomenon can be seen in the treatment of hematological cancers such as acute leukemia and non-Hodgkin's lymphoma. At initial diagnosis 90% of patients with these conditions will respond effectively to a wide range of medications. When the disease relapses, the chemoresponse is less frequent and extends over a shorter period of time. The chance of a cure with use of the same drugs is therefore considerably reduced. As a consequence of this poor response to chemotherapy, the tumor burden (size) increases because cells are no longer sensitive to the chemotherapeutic agent and are not destroyed.

Multiple-drug resistance (MDR) can occur when several agents are used in combination. Multiple-drug resistance is achieved as described for single agents even though their mechanism of action on the cell may occur at different phases of the cell cycle. Acquired MDR is documented in the anthracyclines, vinca alkaloid epipodophyllotoxins, and actinomycin D.[5]

## Protection of Health Care Professionals from Chemotherapy Hazards

Some chemotherapeutic drugs are fetotoxic and carcinogenic. Health care workers who handle antineoplastic drugs can be exposed to low doses of the drug by direct contact, inhalation, and injection. Because the long-term effects of chronic exposure are not completely known, guidelines for safe handling of these agents have been established. The Occupational Safety and Health Administration (OSHA) of the U.S. Department of Labor and other health care institutions have proposed the guidelines summarized in the following Guidelines for Care Box. It is essential that any health care provider working with chemotoxic drugs follow these guidelines to prevent injury to self and to others.

## Chemotherapeutic Agents

Drugs may be classified as alkylating agents, antimetabolites, plant (vinca) alkaloids, antibiotics, and steroids. Table 11-27 (p. 301-304) lists chemotherapeutic agents by classification, action, toxicities, and nursing interventions.

## Common Side Effects of Chemotherapy

There is always some degree of injury to normal cells during treatment with cytotoxic drugs. The bone marrow,

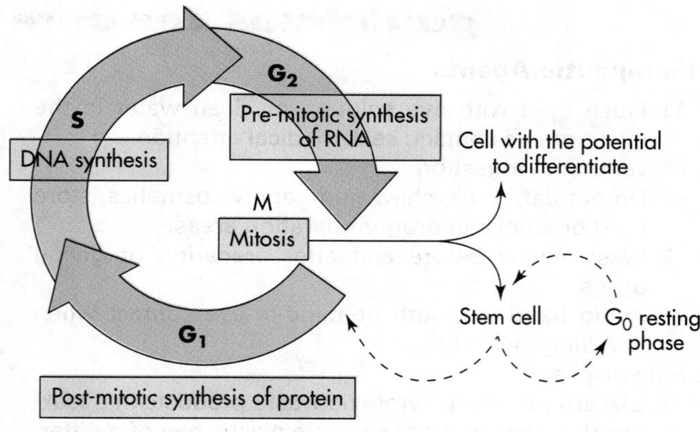


**Cell Cycle Phase-Specific Agents**

**$G_1$ Phase**
Asparaginase
Prednisone

**S Phase**
Antimetabolites
Cytarabine
5-fluorouracil
Hydroxyurea
Methotrexate
Thioguanine

**$G_2$ Phase**
Antibiotic
Bleomycin
Podophyllotoxin
Etoposide

**Mitosis**
Vinca alkaloids
Vinblastine
Vincristine
Vindesine
Paclitaxel

**Cell Cycle Phase-Nonspecific Agents**

**Alkylating Agents**
Busulfan
Carboplatin
Chlorambucil
Cisplatin
Cyclophosphamide
Dacarbazine
Ifosfamide
Mechlorethamine
Melphalan
Thiotepa

**Antibiotics**
Bleomycin
Dactinomycin
Daunorubicin
Doxorubicin
Mitomycin

**Nitrosoureas**
Carmustine (BCNU)
Lomustine (CCNU)
Semustine (MeCCNU)

**Miscellaneous**
Mitoxantrone
Navelbine
Procarbazine

**fig. 11-13** Common cancer chemotherapeutic agents and their activity within the cell cycle.

**box 11-12** *Principles of Chemotherapy Administration*

1. Combination chemotherapy is far superior to single-agent chemotherapy.
2. Complete remission is the minimum requisite for cure and even increased survival.
3. The first round of chemotherapy offers the best chance for significant benefit; therefore the initial therapy should be the type with maximum effectiveness.
4. Maximum doses of drugs are used to attain maximum tumor cell kill. Dose reduction to minimize toxicity has been called "killing patients with kindness."
5. *Neoadjuvant,* or induction chemotherapy, is always recommended for some specific cancers (breast).
6. Chemoprevention shows promise in prevention of some second primary cancers (head and neck).

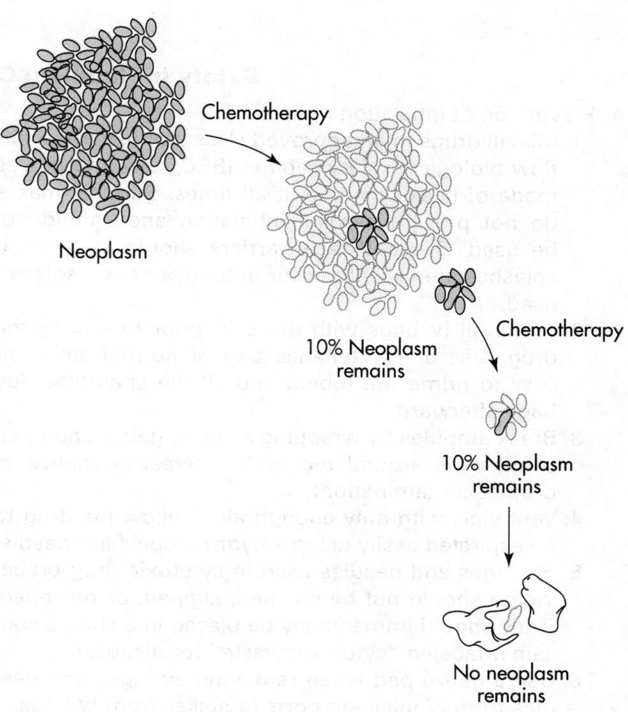


**fig. 11-14** Cell-kill theory. Chemotherapy destroys 90% of neoplasm; repeated chemotherapy repeats process until last neoplastic cell is killed by body's immune response.

gastrointestinal epithelium, and hair follicles are most sensitive to chemotherapy because of their high rate of growth. Other side effects and toxicities include pulmonary effects, cardiac effects (congestive heart failure), genitourinary effects (cystitis, renal damage, sterility), hepatic toxicity, and neurotoxicity (numbness and tingling of the hands and feet, motor weakness). (See Table 11-27.) Toxicities to the bone marrow, gastrointestinal tract, hair follicles, and reproductive system are addressed in the following sections. The Research Box (p. 305) discusses side effects experienced after inpatient chemotherapy.

### Bone marrow effects

Chemotherapy may be toxic to the bone marrow and may produce neutropenia, thrombocytopenia, and anemia. Blood counts are obtained before administration and at regular intervals to identify nadir effect (the time that the blood count is lowest and the patient is most susceptible to infection and hemorrhage). Assessment is also made for signs and symptoms of other organ toxicity (Box 11-13, p. 305).

Infection is a constant threat to the patient receiving chemotherapy. A cold or flu in a person with neutropenia may result in septic shock in a few hours. Intact skin and mucous membranes are first-line defenses against infection; thus care is directed to prevent breaks in skin integrity. Persons receiving chemotherapy are susceptible to middle-ear infections, sinusitis, and pharyngitis. Pneumonia is especially prevalent in patients with leukemia and in elderly persons.

In addition, signs of early infection may be absent and go unrecognized. A rise in body temperature of 1 to 2 degrees

*Text continued on p. 304*

guidelines for care

### Safety in Handling Chemotherapeutic Agents

A. Prevention of inhalation of aerosols
1. Mix all drugs in an approved class II or III vertical air-flow biological safety cabinet (BSC), wearing gloves made of latex or nitrile at all times. Surgical masks do not prevent aerosol inhalation and should not be used. Eye and face barriers should be worn if splashes are likely to occur or sprays or aerosols are used.
2. Prime all IV bags with the BSC prior to adding the drug. Use a maintenance bag of normal saline or $D_5W$ to prime the tubing and all the chemotherapy bags afterward.
3. Break ampules by wrapping a sterile gauze pad or alcohol wipe around the neck (decreases chance of droplet contamination).
4. Vent vials with only enough air to allow the drug to be aspirated easily using a hydrophobic filter needle.
5. Syringes and needles used in cytotoxic drug preparation should not be crushed, clipped, or recapped. They should immediately be placed in a sharps container labeled "cytotoxic waste" for disposal.
6. Use a gauze pad when removing syringes and needles from IV injection ports or spikes from IV bags.

B. Prevention of drug absorption through the skin
1. Wear latex or nitrile gloves and a gown made of nonpermeable fabric with a closed front and cuffed long sleeves.
2. Change gloves every 60 minutes.
3. Remove gloves immediately after spilling drug solution on them or puncturing or tearing them.
4. Wash hands before putting on gloves and after removing them.
5. Cover the work surface with a plastic-backed absorbent pad; change pad when cabinet is cleaned or after a spill.
6. Clean all surfaces or the BSC before and after drug preparation in accordance with manufacturer's instructions. Discard equipment used in a leakproof, puncture-proof, chemical-waste container.
7. Use syringes and IV sets with Luer-Lok fittings.
8. Place an absorbent pad under injection sites to catch accidental spillage.
9. Label all antineoplastic drugs with a chemotherapy warning label.
10. Wash skin areas thoroughly with soap and water as soon as possible in the event of skin contact with drugs.
11. Flush eyes with eye solution or clean water in the event of eye contact; seek medical attention.

C. Prevention of ingestion
1. Do not eat, drink, chew gum, apply cosmetics, store food or smoke in drug preparation areas.
2. Wash hands before and after preparing or giving drugs.
3. Avoid hand-to-mouth or hand-to-eye contact when handling the drugs.

D. Safe disposal
1. Discard nonsharp cytotoxic waste products in a leak-proof, puncture-proof sealable plastic bag of a different color than regular trash bags. Label as "cytotoxic waste."
2. Use a leakproof, puncture-proof container labeled as "cytotoxic waste" for needles and sharp, breakable items.
3. Keep waste containers in labeled, covered waste containers for disposal.
4. Housekeeping personnel should be instructed in safe procedures and should wear latex or nitrile gloves and gowns of nonpermeable fabric.
5. All waste produced by cytotoxic drug administration in the home should be placed in a sealed receptacle and transported in the nonpassenger area of a vehicle to the home agency for disposal.

E. Prevention of contamination by body fluids
1. Wear latex or nitrile gloves and disposable, nonpermeable fabric when handling any body fluids.
2. Empty waste products into the toilet by pouring close to the water to avoid splashing. Close the lid and flush two to three times (in the home).
3. Wear gloves and gown when handling linen soiled with body fluids; place in isolation linen bag for separate laundry.
4. Place soiled linens in separate, washable pillow cases and wash twice, separately from other household linens (in the home).
5. A standard duration of 48 hours is accepted as the time after which most cytotoxic drugs will have been metabolized or excreted. For most cytotoxic agents, urine excretion is complete within 48 hours after administration (range of 1-6 days) and stool excretion is complete within 7 days (range of 5-7 days).

Adapted from Welch J, Silveira JM: *Safe handling of cytotoxic drugs: an independent study module,* Pittsburgh, Penn, 1997, Oncology Nursing Press, Inc.; Gullo SM: Safe handling of cytotoxic agents, *Oncology nursing forum* 15(5):595-601, 1988.

**table 11-27** *Chemotherapy Agents Commonly Used to Treat Cancer*

| DRUG | ACTION | NURSING INTERVENTION |
|---|---|---|
| **ALKYLATING AGENTS*** | | |
| Nitrogen mustard (mechlorethamine)<br>Cyclophosphamide (Cytoxan)<br>Chlorambucil (Leukeran)<br>Busulfan (Myleran)<br>Melphalan (Alkeran)<br>Thiotepa (thiotepa)<br>Ifosfamide (Ifex) | Alkylating agents are cell cycle non-specific and act against already formed nucleic acids by cross-linking DNA strands, thereby preventing DNA replication and transcription of RNA | **Major toxicities**: depend on drugs(s) given<br>• Hematopoietic<br>Anemia<br>Leukopenia<br>Thrombocytopenia<br>• Gastrointestinal<br>Nausea and vomiting<br>Diarrhea<br>• Reproductive<br>Infertility<br>Change in libido<br>• Genitourinary<br>Cystitis and renal toxicity<br>**Nursing interventions**<br>• Hematopoietic<br>Monitor WBC, RBC, platelet count biweekly for pancytopenia<br>Observe for signs and symptoms of infection, bleeding, anemia<br>Provide rest periods and 8 hours sleep per night<br>Teach benefits of good personal hygiene<br>Provide comfort and supportive measures<br>• Gastrointestinal<br>Document N&V times and amount<br>Administer antiemetic drug prn<br>Hydrate to 2000 ml/24 hr if not contraindicated<br>Record intake and output (I&O)<br>Avoid noxious odors<br>Use relaxation techniques or distraction<br>Provide small frequent meals<br>• Reproductive<br>Inform of possibility of temporary or permanent infertility and danger to growing fetus<br>Provide for reproductive counseling as needed<br>• Genitourinary<br>Inform that hemorrhagic cystitis can occur with Cytoxan and ifosfamide therapy<br>Administer mesna (urothelial protection agent) to help prevent cystitis<br>Encourage hydration and complete and frequent emptying of bladder |
| **ANTIMETABOLITES** | | |
| Methotrexate<br>6-Mercaptopurine (6-MP)<br>6-Thioguanine (6-TG)<br>5-Fluorouracil (5-FU)<br>Cytosine arabinoside (ARA-C) (Cytosar-U)<br>Fludarabine phosphate<br>Deoxycoformycin (pentostatin) | Act by interfering with synthesis of chromosomal nucleic acid; antimetabolites are analogs of normal metabolites and block the enzyme necessary for synthesis of essential factors or are incorporated into the DNA or RNA and thus prevent replication; are cycle specific | **Major toxicities**: depend on drug(s) given<br>• Hematopoietic<br>Bone marrow suppression<br>Anemia<br>Leukopenia<br>Thromobcytopenia<br>• Gastrointestinal<br>Mucositis/stomatitis<br>Diarrhea<br>Nausea and vomiting |

*Be aware of potential to develop second malignancy later in life (e.g., leukemia) when on alkylating agents.
*CHF,* Congestive heart failure; *N&V,* nausea and vomiting; *RBC,* red blood cell; *WBC,* white blood cell.

Continued

table 11-27 Chemotherapy Agents Commonly Used to *Treat Cancer*

| Drug | Action | Nursing Intervention |
|---|---|---|
| **ANTIMETABOLITES—cont'd** | | **Nursing interventions**<br>• Hematopoietic<br>(See interventions above)<br>• Gastrointestinal<br>(See interventions above)<br>**Additional nursing interventions**<br>• Mucositis/stomatitis<br>Inspect oral cavity daily for presence of sores, change in taste and sensation<br>Teach oral care and encourage immediately after meals and at bedtime; soft toothbrush and prescribed mouthwash (peroxide and saline, baking soda and water, or others); provide anesthetic agent for mouth sores (e.g., stomatitis cocktail)<br>Report signs and symptoms of oral infection<br>Soft diet with nonirritating foods high in protein, calories; offer high-caloric liquid supplements<br>• Diarrhea<br>Low-residue diet, high protein and calories; maintain hydration<br>Monitor and document number and frequency of stools<br>Administer antidiarrheal medication as needed<br>Provide meticulous skin care in perirectal area<br>Promote good hygiene habits |
| **ANTITUMOR ANTIBIOTICS**<br>Daunorubicin (Cerubidine)<br>Doxorubicin (Adriamycin)<br>Dactinomycin or actinomycin D (Cosmegen)<br>Bleomycin (Blenoxane)<br>Mitomycin (Mutamycin)<br>Plicamycin (mithramycin, mithracin)<br>Idarubicin (Idamycin)<br>Mitoxantrone (Novantrone) | Interfere with synthesis and function of nucleic acids and inhibit RNA and DNA synthesis<br>Agents are cycle nonspecific | **Major toxicities:** depend on drug(s) given<br>• Hematopoietic<br>Bone marrow suppression<br>• Gastrointestinal<br>Mucositis/stomatitis<br>Anorexia, nausea, and vomiting<br>• Integumentary<br>Alopecia<br>Tissue necrosis if extravasation of vesicant drugs<br>• Cardiac and pulmonary toxicity<br>**Nursing interventions**<br>• Hematopoietic<br>(See interventions above)<br>• Gastrointestinal<br>(See previous discussion)<br>• Integumentary<br>Alopecia<br>Warn of potential for hair loss and ways of minimizing loss<br>Extravasation<br>Monitor IV infusion to prevent infiltration; when infiltrated stop immediately and institute agency protocol to prevent tissue necrosis; notify physican immediately; keep extravasation kit available at all times |

*Continued*

table 11-27 Chemotherapy Agents Commonly Used to Treat Cancer

| DRUG | ACTION | NURSING INTERVENTION |
|---|---|---|
| **ANTITUMOR ANTIBIOTICS—cont'd** | | • Cardiac toxicity may occur with daunorubicin and doxorubicin (e.g., CHF, dysrhythmias); should not exceed cumulative lifetime dose of 550 mg/m$^2$<br>Assess for and document cardiac changes<br>• Pulmonary toxicity may occur with bleomycin (pneumonitis and progressive pulmonary fibrosis); should not exceed a lifetime dose of 400 IU<br>Assess respiratory status and document changes |
| **HORMONAL AGENTS** | | |
| Androgens<br>Testosterone propionate<br>Fluoxymesterone (Halotestin)<br>Dromostanolone (Drolban)<br>Testolactone (Teslac)<br>Methyltestosterone | Alter pituitary function and directly affect the maligant cell[4] | **Major toxicities** include fluid retention and masculinization |
| Corticosteroids<br>Cortisone acetate<br>Prednisone (Meticorten)<br>Dexamethasone (Decadron)<br>Methylprednisolone sodium (Solu-Medrol)<br>Hydrocortisone sodium succinate (Solu-Cortef) | Lyse lymphoid malignancies and have indirect effects on malignant cells[4] | **Major toxicities** include fluid retention, hypertension, diabetes, and increased susceptibility to infection |
| Estrogens<br>Diethylstilbestrol (DES)<br>Ethinyl estradiol (Estinyl) | Suppress testosterone production in males and alter the response of breast cancers to prolactin | **Major toxicities** include fluid retention, feminization, and uterine bleeding |
| Progestins<br>Hydroxyprogesterone caproate (Prodrox)<br>Megestrol (Megace)<br>Medroxyprogesterone (Provera)<br>Estramustine (Emcyt) | Promote differentiation of malignant cells[4] | |
| Estrogen antagonists<br>Tamoxifen (Nolvadex)<br>Leuprolide (Lupron) | Compete with estrogens for binding with estrogen receptor sites on malignant cells | Minimal with occasional headache and hot flashes |
| Antiadrenal<br>Aminoglutethimide | Produces the equivalent of a medical adrenalectomy, thereby inhibiting the formation of estrogens and androgenssis and function of nucleic acids and inhibit RNA and DNA synthesis<br>Agents are cycle nonspecific | Adrenal insufficiency<br>**Nursing interventions**<br>• Fluid retention<br>Warn of potential weight gain<br>Weigh bi-weekly; I&O if necessary<br>• Feminization: males<br>Inform about chance of gynecomastia, change in voice, distribution of body fat and hair, and cardiovascular problems<br>Assess fears and concerns and provide psychological support as needed<br>• Virilization: females<br>Discuss risk for facial hair, lowered voice, clitoral enlargement, fluid retention<br>Assess fears and concerns and provide psychological support as needed |

Continued

table 11-27 Chemotherapy Agents Commonly Used to Treat Cancer

| Drug | Action | Nursing Intervention |
|---|---|---|
| **HORMONAL AGENTS—cont'd** | | • Uterine bleeding<br>Prepare postmenopausal women for occurrence<br>Provide support and reassurance<br>• Diabetes<br>Inform patient of potential occurrence<br>Monitor blood sugar for changes<br>Observe for signs and symptoms of diabetes<br>• Adrenal insufficiency<br>Instruct on need to comply with replacement therapy while on medication<br>Reassure that need for therapy will cease when drug discontinued |
| **VINCA ALKALOIDS**<br>Vincristine (Oncovin)<br>Vinblastine (Velban)<br>Vindesine sulfate | Bind to proteins within the cells, causing metaphase arrest thus inhibiting RNA and protein synthesis | **Major toxicities**<br>• Hematopoietic<br>Bone marrow suppression<br>• Integumentary<br>Alopecia |
| **EPIPODOPHYLLOTOXINS**<br>Etoposide (VP-16) | Cause breaks in DNA and DNA-protein cross-links | **Nursing interventions**<br>• Hematopoietic<br>(See previous discussion)<br>• Integumentary<br>(See previous discussion)<br>**Major toxicities**<br>• Neurological<br>Neurotoxicity<br>Muscle weakness, peripheral neuritis, paralytic ileus, loss of deep tendon reflexes<br>**Nursing interventions**<br>• Neurological<br>Gastrointestinal: check for peristalsis frequently; determine usual pattern of bowel elimination; facilitate elimination with laxative regimen<br>Peripheral: observe for numbness, tingling in extremities; institute safety measures (e.g., wearing shoes, use of cane or walker for ambulation); seek assistance for ambulation as needed; teach signs and symptoms to report to physician; provide supportive care and reassurance |

may be the only indication of a potentially dangerous situation. A localized inflammatory response may not occur in patients with severe leukopenia (<1000 cells/mm$^3$). The absence of granulocytes, also referred to as polymorphonuclear leukocytes (PMNs), prevents the formation of pus. Localized tenderness or pain may be the only sign of a skin or wound infection. Reverse isolation or "protective isolation" may be ordered to protect the patient from exposure to infection from caregivers, family members, and friends.

### Gastrointestinal effects

Changes in bowel habits commonly occur but usually do not require intervention. Alertness to the possibility of bleeding or ulceration must be part of the assessment of diarrhea or cramping. Vincristine may cause paralytic ileus; therefore persons receiving this drug are specifically instructed to report constipation. Persons receiving narcotic-based pain medications may develop constipation as a result, and a daily bowel regimen program may be indicated.

### Stomatitis

Stomatitis, an inflammation of the oral mucous membranes, is a common side effect that may range from erythema to mild or severe ulcerations. Nursing strategies for managing stomatitis are summarized in the Guidelines for Care Box (p. 306). Box 11-14 (p. 307) lists some drugs that can cause stomatitis.

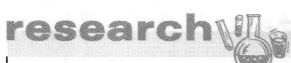

Reference: Foltz AT, Gaines G, Gullotte M: Recalled side effects and self-care actions of patients receiving inpatient chemotherapy, *Oncol Nurs Forum* 23(4):679, 1996.

Chemotherapy is one of the major treatment modalities for cancer. Few data exist on the side effects experienced after discharge from the hospital and the self-care measures used by the patient. The purpose of this retrospective, descriptive study was to identify the most commonly experienced side effects after discharge, determine the intensity of the side effects, and elicit the self-care actions used and their effectiveness. The Nail Self-Care Diary (SCD) was used to gather data.

The sample of convenience consisted of 59 patients with a diagnosis of cancer who received inpatient chemotherapy and could read English. Fifty-seven percent were women, and 43% were men. The majority of patients had been diagnosed with cancer for more than a year and had received multiple cycles of chemotherapy before the study. Breast and lung cancer were the most common cancers.

The study found that the most disturbing side effects in order of incidence and severity were alopecia, fatigue, nausea, taste changes, appetite loss, sleep problems, and constipation. These findings were congruent with prior studies but also identified disruptive symptoms. The SCD showed that self-care actions were used for all of the side effects. Pharmacological interventions were used by many patients, were found to be effective, and were reported as the only action necessary. Nonpharmacological measures included such activities as wearing a wig or hat for alopecia, increasing rest periods or sleep time for fatigue, or increasing fluid or fiber intake to relieve constipation. This study suggests that patients do engage in self-care activities in the home setting to reduce the side effects of chemotherapy. The study also helped identify the most common side effects experienced. Nurses can use these findings to tailor their discharge teaching appropriately.

**box 11-13** *Assessment of Side Effects and Toxicity in the Patient Receiving Chemotherapy*

IDENTIFICATION OF MARROW SUPPRESSION

1. WBC, platelet count, hemoglobin, hematocrit
2. Signs of bleeding (e.g., petechiae, ecchymosis)

IDENTIFICATION OF INFECTION

1. Inspect skin and mucous membranes daily (especially mouth, axillae, and perineum)
2. Auscultate respiratory tract
3. Monitor temperature, pulse, respiration
4. Most important: monitor neutrophil count:
   a. A count of 500/mm³ to 1000/mm³ indicates moderate risk of infection
   b. A count of less than 500/mm³ indicates severe risk of infection

IDENTIFICATION OF OTHER ORGAN TOXICITIES

1. Gastrointestinal toxicity
   a. Inspect mouth for white patches or ulcers
   b. Monitor weight, fluid, and electrolytes
   c. Assess for constipation, decreased bowel sounds
2. Liver toxicity: monitor liver enzymes
3. Cardiac toxicity
   a. Obtain baseline echocardiogram
   b. Check apical pulse for dysrhythmias
   c. Monitor for signs of congestive heart failure
4. Pulmonary toxicity
   a. Auscultate lungs
   b. Monitor for shortness of breath and cough (especially with bleomycin)
5. Urinary toxicity
   a. Monitor urine for blood
   b. Monitor for signs of cystitis (frequency with dysuria)
   c. Evaluate renal function by either serum creatinine or 24-hour urine for creatinine clearance
   d. Keep accurate intake and output
6. Neurotoxicity: assess for paresthesia and motor weakness

### *Nausea and vomiting*

Oncology nurses and patients often identify nausea and vomiting as the most uncomfortable and distressing side effects of chemotherapy. Four emetic syndromes have been identified in patients with cancer: (1) chemotherapy-induced emesis, (2) delayed emesis that occurs 1 to 4 days after treatment, (3) anticipatory emesis that occurs before the next scheduled therapy, and (4) emesis caused by factors other than chemotherapy, such as intestinal obstruction or other drug therapy (e.g., opiates). Depending on the type of emesis, different therapies are indicated. Relaxation techniques can be effective.

For the outpatient, nausea may interfere with the ability to continue work. Persistent vomiting may result in fluid and electrolyte imbalance, general weakness, and weight loss. A decline in nutritional status renders the person more susceptible to infection and perhaps less able to tolerate therapy. Physiological symptoms can accompany or precipitate psychological responses such as depression, withdrawal, and humiliation. The onset and duration of both nausea and vomiting vary greatly from patient to patient and with the drugs given.

### *Alopecia*

Alopecia can occur by two mechanisms. If the hair roots are atrophied, alopecia occurs readily and hair falls out either spontaneously or from combing, often in large clumps. If the hair shaft is constricted because of atrophy or necrosis, the hair will break off near the scalp. The root remains in the scalp, and a patchy, thinning pattern of hair loss occurs.

Alopecia may be one of the most traumatic psychological side effects cancer patients experience. It is a constant reminder of their disease, it makes the illness visible to others, and it may result in a significant change in body image. Strategies to use with patients who experience hair loss are summarized in the following Guidelines for Care Box.

guidelines for care

## The Person Receiving Chemotherapy

1. Teach the patient and significant others:
   a. Signs and symptoms of infection, thrombocytopenia
   b. How to read a thermometer (if appropriate) and when to notify the physician
   c. Good hygiene practices
      (1) Cleanse the perineum from front to back
      (2) Change underwear daily
      (3) Hand washing
   d. Information about prescribed drugs: name, dose, side effects, importance of taking as prescribed
   e. Use of antiemetics
   f. Importance of medical follow-up and blood studies
   g. Available support groups for chemotherapy patients
2. Preventing infection:
   a. Good hygiene, *especially hand washing* (patient, family, health professionals)
   b. Prevent exposure to people with known infection (other patients, staff, family, friends)
   c. Meticulous aseptic technique during intravenous infusions and dressing changes
      (1) Use povidone-iodine for skin preparation (Centers for Disease Control also considers alcohol, tincture of iodine, and chlorhexidine effective)
      (2) Keep one tourniquet for patient's exclusive use
      (3) Use gloves for procedures
   d. Avoid use of aspirin or acetaminophen (to prevent masking fever)
   e. Maintain intact skin and mucous membranes
      (1) Avoid bumping and breaking the skin
      (2) No injections
      (3) Keep fingernails short to prevent small skin breaks (nurse, patient, other caregivers)
      (4) Avoid anal intercourse
      (5) Avoid enemas, rectal medications, rectal thermometers
      (6) Avoid excessive friction and provide vaginal lubrication during sexual intercourse (use water-soluble jelly, if necessary)
   f. Maintain meticulous oral hygiene
      (1) Maintain teeth and gums in good condition; see dentist
      (2) Use mouth wash or oral irrigations (normal saline), mild peroxide solution (1 tablespoon in 240 ml water), sodium bicarbonate (1 teaspoon baking soda in 240 ml water)
      (3) Use Mycostatin tablets or suspension, as necessary
      (4) Relieve dryness: drink water and other fluids
      (5) Use artificial saliva, as needed, in form of spray (Moi-Stir, Salivart, Ora-lub)
      (6) Stimulate saliva with gum, candies, buttermilk, yogurt
      (7) Brush teeth with soft toothbrush (small soft bristles) or use foam stick or swab
      (8) Brush teeth in short horizontal strokes at least 3 to 4 minutes, at least 3 times a day
      (9) Use fluoridated toothpaste or rinse, to prevent caries
      (10) Use Water Pik under low pressure or irrigation, if platelet count is low
   g. Use reverse isolation techniques as needed
   h. Maintain optimal respiratory function: encourage turn, cough, and deep breathe if patient confined to bed
3. Maintaining optimal gastrointestinal function:
   a. Give antidiarrheal medication as needed
   b. Plan daily bowel regimen for constipation, give stool softeners as prescribed
   c. Treat stomatitis
      (1) Oral nystatin (Mycostatin) or other antibiotics as prescribed
      (2) Milk of magnesia or Kaopectate to coat lesions
      (3) Dyclonine hydrochloride (Dyclone), Orabase, lidocaine (Xylocaine) viscous 2%, as local anesthetic before meals and as necessary
      (4) KY jelly, mineral oil, to coat lips and oral mucosa
      (5) Petrolatum (Vaseline) to coat lips (not if neutropenic)
      (6) Diphenhydramine hydrochloride (Benadryl) alone or in combination with Maalox and Kaopectate, as a rinse
      (7) Oral irrigations (see under infection) every 2 hours
      (8) Soft, bland foods, cold liquids tolerated by some persons
   d. Treat nausea and vomiting
      (1) Give antiemetics 30 to 45 min before chemotherapy; use large doses
      (2) Use auditory or diversional stimulation (music, slides, photographs)
      (3) Give antiemetics around the clock for severe nausea and vomiting
      (4) Use relaxation techniques, self-hypnosis, therapeutic touch
      (5) Eat foods that minimize nausea
4. Minimizing or preventing alopecia:
   a. Encourage use of wigs, scarves, eyebrow pencil, false eyelashes
   b. Avoid frequent shampooing, combing, or brushing
   c. Use soft-bristle hair brush
   d. Advise against permanents and hair coloring (increase rate of hair loss)
5. Minimizing or preventing urinary effects—hemorrhagic cystitis, renal toxicity:
   a. Force fluids when taking cyclophosphamide
   b. Take cyclophosphamide early in the day
   c. Check serum creatinine or 24-hr urine for creatinine clearance before giving cisplatin and streptozotocin
6. Minimizing reproductive effects
   a. Provide birth control information and reproductive counseling
   b. Provide information about sperm banking before initiation of therapy for male patients

### Sterility

Cancer chemotherapy has the capacity to affect most body organ systems to some degree. This includes the reproductive organs. Some chemotherapeutic drugs have the potential to cause genetic alterations, which in turn disrupt normal fetal development. In addition, some of the alkylating agents may cause transient or permanent sterility. Persons receiving chemotherapy need to be informed of the known and possible effects on fertility. After completion of chemotherapy, conception and the birth of normal, healthy children are possible. It is customary to recommend that pregnancy be postponed until at least 2 years after completion of treatment. Sperm banking can also be considered.

**box 11-14** *Drugs Causing Stomatitis*

- Bleomycin (Blenoxane)
- Doxorubicin (Adriamycin)
- Cytosine arabinoside (Ara-C)
- Cyclophosphamide (Cytoxan)
- Daunorubicin (Cerubidine)
- Methotrexate
- 5-Fluorouracil (5-FU)

## Methods of Administering Chemotherapeutic Agents

The route of administration is based on the metabolism and absorption of a given drug. The route of choice is that which will deliver the optimal amount of drug to the tumor. Chemotherapeutic agents are given orally, subcutaneously, intravenously, and intramuscularly.

Tumor cells in the central nervous system are difficult to access because many chemotherapeutic agents cannot pass through the blood-brain barrier. Use of the intrathecal route permits the introduction of high drug concentrations directly into the cerebrospinal fluid through a lumbar puncture or through a subcutaneous cerebrospinal reservoir (Ommaya reservoir) (Figure 11-15). Intraarterial and intracavitary routes are also amenable to providing high-dose concentrations of a drug without undue systemic effects. These modes of drug administration may be used when a malignant organ or tissue tumor cannot be treated surgically.

### Long-term drug delivery systems

The use of centrally placed venous access catheters and ports is now a common and accepted part of cancer chemotherapy. The type used depends on the treatment,

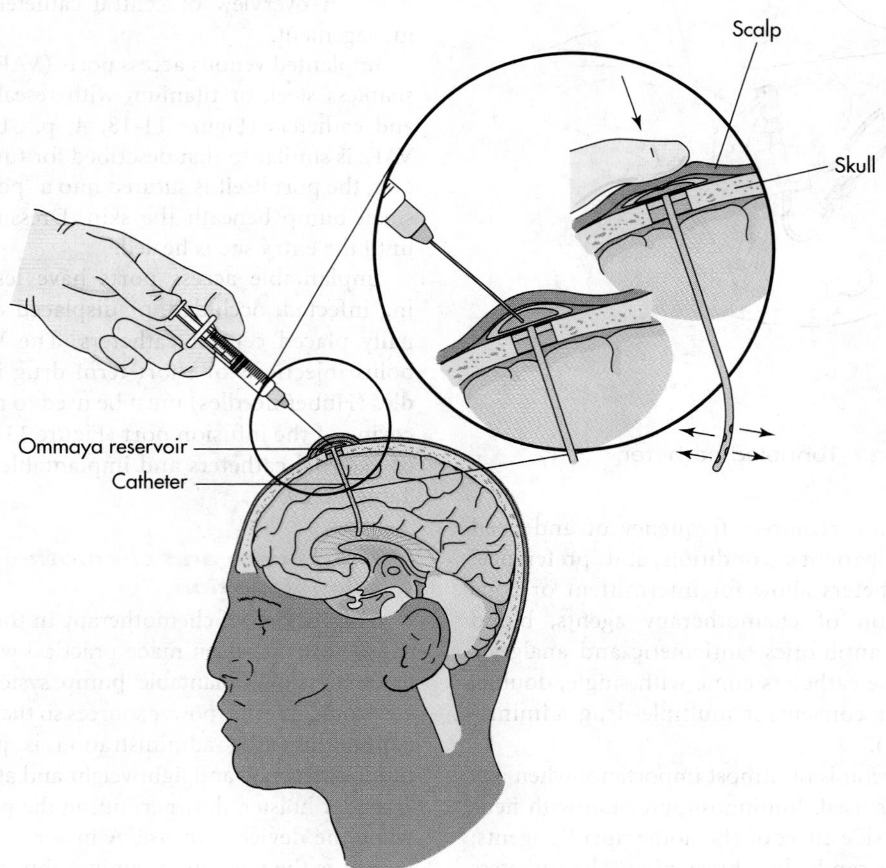


**fig. 11-15** Ommaya reservoir for administration of chemotherapeutic agents directly into the central nervous system. *Note:* Medication is administered into reservoir and moves through a catheter into the lateral ventricle.

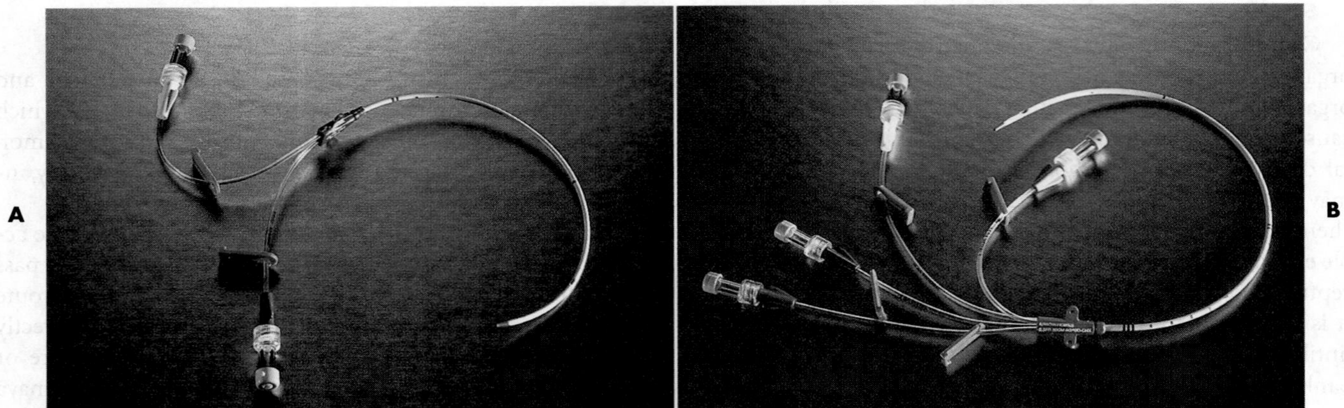


**fig. 11-16** Multilumen subclavian catheters.

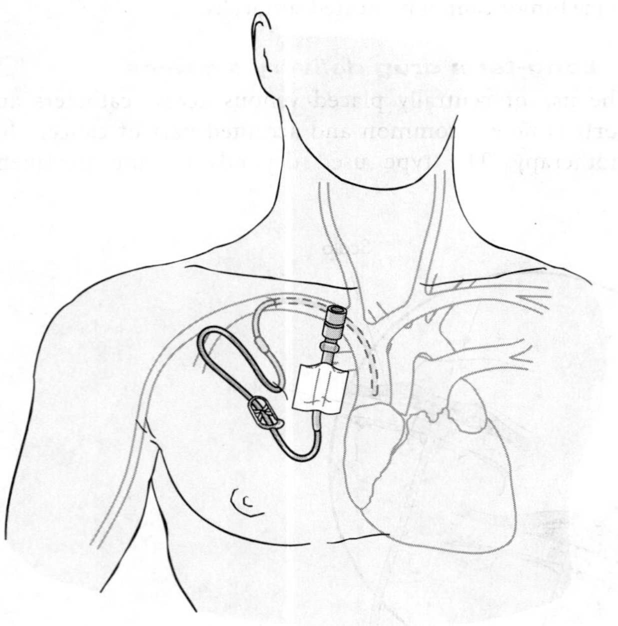

**fig. 11-17** Tunneled catheter.

mode of administration required, frequency of and need for access, and the patient's condition and preference. Centrally located catheters allow for intermittent or continuous administration of chemotherapy agents, blood and blood products, antibiotics, antiemetic and analgesic drugs, and TPN. These catheters come with single, double, and triple lumens for convenient multiple-drug administration (Figure 11-16).

Prevention of infection is of utmost importance when any central access device is used. Immunosuppression with neutropenia is a common side effect of chemotherapeutic agents; therefore any infection can be life threatening. The catheters generally are made of a silicone material and are radiopaque. Their placement can be verified fluoroscopically. The technique of "tunneling" the catheter beneath the skin aids in preventing bacterial entry and growth along the catheter tract. All tunneled catheters have a small "cuff" around which fibroblasts form and help secure the catheter in place. Figure 11-17 shows positioning of a Hickman-Broviac central catheter. The entry and exit sites of central catheters require sterile dressing changes two or three times a week until healing has occurred; then catheter care follows agency protocol. Table 11-28 provides an overview of central catheter infections and their management.

Implanted venous access ports (VAPs) are made of plastic, stainless steel, or titanium with resealable silicone septums and catheters (Figure 11-18, *A*, p. 310). The placement of VAPs is similar to that described for tunneled catheters; however, the port itself is sutured into a "pocket" that appears as a small bump beneath the skin. Dressings may be necessary until the entry site is healed.

Implantable access ports have less danger of becoming infected, occluded, or displaced compared with externally placed central catheters. The VAP can be used for bolus injections or short-term drug infusion. Special needles (Huber needles) must be used to prevent perforation or coring of the infusion port (Figure 11-18, *B*). A comparison of external catheters and implantable ports is presented in Table 11-29.

### Home care and chemotherapy administration

The delivery of chemotherapy in the home or ambulatory care setting has been made practical with the advent of both external and implantable pump systems. The pumps have electronic internal power sources so that either intermittent or continuous drug administration is possible. The external pumps are small and lightweight and attach to either a belt or shoulder holster, thus permitting the patient free ambulation while the device is in use. A major disadvantage of external pumps is the need for a family support person to receive instruction in their care and maintenance because the patient cannot be expected to manage the care alone. An implantable drug-delivery system for ambulatory persons is shown in Figure 11-19, p. 311.

**table 11-28** *Catheter-Related Infections*

| Site of Infection | Signs and Symptoms | Basis for Diagnosis | Management |
|---|---|---|---|
| **LOCAL** | | | |
| Exit/needle | Erythema (>1.0 cm <2.0 cm), tenderness<br>± Fever<br>± Induration or exudate around exit or Huber needle access site (depends on neutrophil count)<br>+ Positive exit/needle site culture | Clinical S&S<br>Exit/needle site culture | Local site care: ↑ frequency of skin care and dressing changes; alternative dressings; antimicrobial ointment<br>Oral antibiotics: nonneutropenic patient, limited inflammation |
| Port pocket | Erythema, swelling, tenderness about port pocket<br>+ Positive exudate culture from port pocket<br>± Fever | Clinical S&S<br>Aspiration and culture port pocket exudate (by physician) | IV antibiotics: neutropenic patient or progressive inflammation<br>IV antibiotics through port if cannulated; through peripheral vein if port not cannulated<br>Consider port removal |
| **TUNNEL** | Erythema, tenderness, and induration along SQ tract >2 cm from exit site<br>± Purulence/inflammation at exit site<br>± Positive culture from exit or insertion site<br>± Fever | Clinical S&S | IV antibiotics<br>Consider catheter removal |
| **SYSTEMIC** (septicemia) | | | |
| Thrombus-related | + S&S of SVC obstruction: neck-arm swelling; discomfort in neck, arm, chest, or back; increased superficial venous pattern<br>Fever and chills | Clinical S&S<br>Radiographic procedures: e.g., venogram, ultrasound<br>Catheter and peripheral blood culture (5-10 times increase in colony forming units catheter vs. peripheral) | IV antibiotics<br>Consider thrombolytic or anticoagulant therapy<br>Consider surgical resection of thrombus and affected vein<br>Consider catheter removal |
| Catheter colonization | Bacteremia or fungemia without catheter tract inflammation<br>Fever and chills | Clinical S&S<br>Catheter and peripheral blood culture (5-10 times increase in colony-forming units catheter vs. peripheral)<br>Positive culture of catheter tip | Bacteremia—IV antibiotics<br>Fungemia—antifungal therapy<br>Consider catheter removal<br>? Antibiotic lock |

From Wickham R, Purl S, Welker D: *Semin Oncol Nurs* 8(2):138, 1992.
*S&S,* Signs and symptoms; ±, presence or absence of a sign or symptom; *SVC,* subclavian vein catheterization.

The implantable pumps are inserted in the manner described for implanted ports. However, because these pumps generally are used for intraarterial chemotherapy for primary and metastatic liver carcinomas, they are situated in a pocket of the abdomen or intraclavicular fossa. The Silastic catheter is then threaded into the hepatic artery, superior vena cava, or subclavian vein. Other uses for implantable pumps now include administration of heparin and morphine. Drugs are added percutaneously through a central inlet septum with a special needle. Drug refills usually are needed every 2 weeks.

The most common complication is development of a seroma over the pump pocket. This is an accumulation of sterile fluid that may be either aspirated by the physician or allowed to be absorbed by the body. Pump pocket infection is rare but may require removal of the pump. Patients are encouraged to resume activities as soon as the incision heals. Written instructions are given to the patient, including telephone numbers of health care professionals who can be consulted.

Patients who use implantable infusion pumps need to be carefully selected. Selection is based on criteria described in Box 11-15, p. 312.

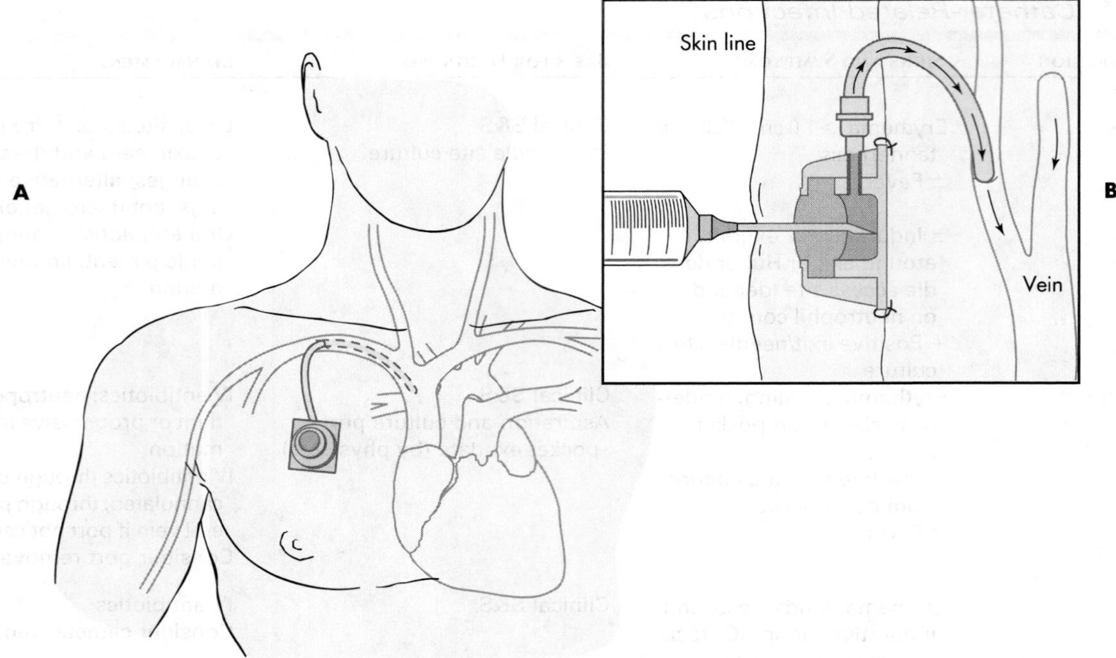


fig. 11-18 **A,** Implantable port. **B,** Cross section of port with needle access.

## NURSING MANAGEMENT OF THE PATIENT RECEIVING CHEMOTHERAPY

### ASSESSMENT

Nurses who care for cancer patients are aware that treatment strategies are complex, and both quality of life and therapeutic outcome vary from patient to patient. This is particularly true when chemotherapy is the primary mode of therapy. Chemotherapy, with its many side effects, can adversely affect the patient immediately or for many months. Thus a thorough assessment of the patient's and family's knowledge base and their expectations related to chemotherapy is completed before the start of treatment.

#### Subjective Data

The nurse first determines the patient's basic understanding of the disease process and whether chemotherapy is to be used for cure, for palliation of symptoms, or as adjuvant therapy. Chemotherapy is the primary treatment for hematological cancer such as leukemia and solid tumors with metastasis. The assessment interview establishes the patient's expectations of therapy and will elicit any fears or anxieties about the treatment. Patients facing chemotherapy for the first time usually know of someone who has been treated with chemotherapy and can recite many of the "negative" aspects associated with it. They may wonder if they will face the same discomforts, such as nausea and vomiting, weight loss, and hair loss. If patients have had chemotherapy previously they may fear resumption of therapy and express doubts regarding the effectiveness of the treatment. They may question whether they wish to subject themselves again to the adverse side effects that go with therapy. It is important to obtain information on what side effects were previously experienced and the measures that were successful in alleviating their severity.

Patients commonly express concern related to the cost of a lengthy course of chemotherapy, especially if they have no health insurance or are inadequately covered. They may fear becoming a financial drain on family resources and may decide to refuse therapy.

#### Objective Data

The nurse can obtain current information from the medical record about the patient's cancer, its stage and extent, and the proposed chemotherapy regimen. Knowledge of the medications included in the chemotherapy protocol will provide the nurse with information about the major side effects to be expected, what organ systems will be affected, and when side effects are likely to occur. This information serves as the basis for developing an individualized patient teaching and care plan.

The nurse assesses the patient's physical state of health. Physical and functional status (from self-care to complete dependency for care) are considered to be more important than chronological age in determining how well the patient will withstand the rigors of therapy. This assessment includes the functional status of the cardiovascular, pulmonary, gastrointestinal, and renal systems, as well as the patient's cognitive state. The side effects of chemotherapeutic drugs affect all age groups but are more pronounced in the person who is over age

**table 11-29** *Comparison of Venous Access Devices*

| External Silastic Catheter | Implantable Ports |
|---|---|
| • May remain in place as long as trouble free | • Silicone septum good for 1000-2000 punctures (varies per product and size needle used) |
| • Technically open system, though catheter closed by injection cap | • Completely closed system |
| • Barrier against infection: Dacron cuff | • Barrier against infection: skin |
| • Surgically inserted and removed | • Surgically inserted and removed |
| • Uses: all intravenous infusions, including transfusions and drawing | • Uses: all intravenous infusions, including blood transfusions and drawing |
| • Features: single, double, and triple lumens available | • Features: single and double lumens available |
| • Maintenance: requires daily heparin flushes, regular dressing, and injection cap changes using aseptic techniques; care is done by the patient or the family; maintenance costs include heparin, syringes, needles, alcohol, dressing supplies, injection caps, etc. | • Maintenance: requires heparin flush every 3-4 weeks; usually done by the nurse; maintenance cost is minimal |
| • Appearance: alteration in body image and physical freedom; changes are considerable with 4-5 inches of external catheter always present | • Appearance: usually minimal alteration because the port is totally under the skin; alteration in body image and physical freedom is limited |
| • Care must be taken with showering, bathing, and swimming | • No disruption in showering or bathing |
| • Access: needle inserted into injection cap at the end of the external catheter; some clothing displacement during infusions | • Access: special needle must puncture the skin to access the port; minimal to significant clothing displacement during infusions depending on site of the port |
| • Placement: can choose exit site for catheter | • Placement: should be placed over bony prominences to assist in stability during access. Potential areas of placement are limited, especially in overweight patients |
| • Complications:<br>1. Catheter-related infections<br>2. Occlusion thrombosis<br>3. Infuses, but cannot draw blood (withdrawal occlusion)<br>4. Catheter damage, leakage, or dislodgement<br>5. Extravasation<br>6. Spontaneous blood backflow | • Complications:<br>1. Port-related infections<br>2. Occlusion thrombosis<br>3. Infuses, but cannot draw blood (withdrawal occlusion)<br>4. Catheter migration<br>5. Extravasation<br>6. Port leakage<br>7. Catheter-needle dislodgement |

From Burke MB et al: *Cancer chemotherapy: a nursing process approach,* Boston, 1991, Jones & Bartlett.

65 or in the individual who has a degree of organ dysfunction. Toxicity is increased when the organ system is actively involved in drug transport, absorption, breakdown, or elimination. Thus comorbid conditions increase the likelihood of more severe side effects. Table 11-30 provides a list of predisposing factors to toxicity of cytotoxic drugs in the elderly.

The nurse records the patient's weight; any signs of recent weight loss or muscle wasting; appetite; ability to eat and retain nourishment; and the presence of nausea, vomiting, diarrhea, or constipation.

The patient's activity and energy level are assessed. Signs of increasing energy loss and fatigue should be known and documented before the start of chemotherapy. Laboratory tests such as the CBC, platelet count, serum electrolytes ($Na^+$, $K^+$, $CO_2$), and BUN provide important data on the patient's current physical state.

When assessing the psychological and emotional state of the patient, the nurse observes for reaction to hospitalization, understanding and acceptance of the cancer diagnosis, and potential for compliance with the treatment plan. Fears and

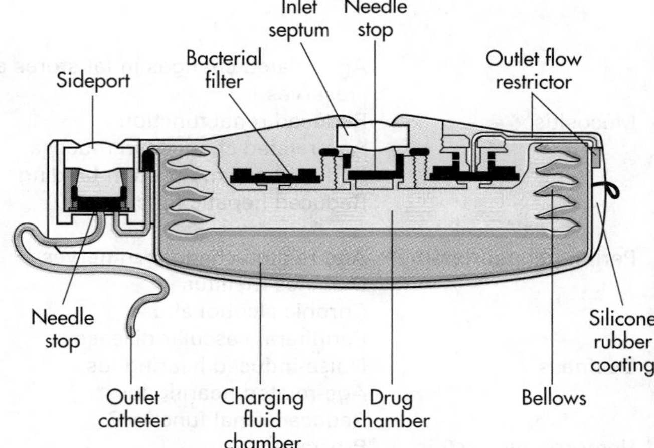


**fig. 11-19** Implantable drug delivery system for ambulatory persons.

misconceptions related to chemotherapy are noted and dispelled as soon as possible. Last, the nurse notes the patient's support network and the degree to which he or she depends on these individuals for physical care, financial assistance, and decision making.

**box 11-15** *Patient Selection Criteria for Implantable Infusion Pumps*

- Clinically stable
- Working access device
- Clean home environment
- No history of severe drug reactions
- Understanding and willingness to participate in self-care responsibilities:
  - Good manual dexterity skills
  - Able to check pump and alarms daily
  - Knowledge of aseptic technique (gloving; safe handling of infusion solutions, tubing, and disposal; dressing care; and protection of pump when bathing)
- Access to emergency medical services

Adapted from Gorski LA, Grothman L: Home infusion therapy, *Semin Oncol Nurs* 12(3):193, 1996.

## NURSING DIAGNOSES

Nursing diagnoses for the cancer patient receiving chemotherapy may include but are not limited to:

| Diagnostic Title | Possible Etiological Factors |
|---|---|
| Infection, risk for | Disease entity, lack of knowledge, decreased nutrition, decreased immune response, chemotherapy effects on bone marrow |
| Fluid volume deficit, risk for | Inadequate fluid intake, side effects of chemotherapy drugs (nausea, vomiting, diarrhea), anticipatory nausea and vomiting |
| Nutrition, altered: less than body requirements | Nausea and vomiting, anorexia, stomatitis, fatigue, weight loss >10% |
| Body image disturbance | Loss of body hair from chemotherapy, cancer cachexia |

## EXPECTED PATIENT OUTCOMES

Expected patient outcomes for the patient receiving chemotherapy for cancer may include but are not limited to:

**table 11-30** *Examples of Predisposing Factors to Toxicity of Cytotoxic Drugs in the Elderly*

| Side Effect | Predisposing Factors | Cytotoxic Drugs Potentially Affected |
|---|---|---|
| Cardiac failure | Reduced cardiac output<br>Ischemic heart disease<br>Cardiac valve disorder<br>Impaired hepatic function | Doxorubicin<br>Daunorubicin<br>Mitoxantrone<br>Epirubicin |
| Pneumonitis | Reduced density of lung<br>Reduced renal function<br>Chronic bronchitis/airways limitation | Bleomycin |
| Myelosuppression | Reduced plasma protein binding<br>Reduced renal function | Methotrexate |
| | Reduced hepatic function | Doxorubicin<br>Epirubicin<br>Mitoxantrone |
| | Age-related changes in fat stores and marrow reserves | Nitrosoureas |
| Mucositis | Reduced renal function<br>Age-related changes in mucosa<br>Reduced plasma protein binding | Methotrexate<br>Fluorouracil |
| | Reduced hepatic function | Doxorubicin<br>Epirubicin |
| Peripheral neuropathy | Age-related changes in nerves<br>Diabetes mellitus<br>Chronic alcohol abuse<br>Peripheral vascular disease | Vinca alkaloids<br>Cisplatin |
| Deafness | Noise-induced hearing loss<br>Age-related hearing loss*<br>Reduced renal function? | Cisplatin |
| Hemorrhagic cystitis | Prostatism | Cyclophosphamide† |
| Constipation | Age-related changes in nerves and bowel function | Vinca alkaloids |

Modified from Rhagavan D et al: In Peckham M et al, editors: *Oxford textbook of oncology,* vol 2, Oxford, 1995, Oxford University Press.
*No obvious increment noted in elderly patients with bladder cancer.
†Theoretical consideration; not observed in a series of 60 cases treated with oral cyclophosphamide.

1a. Understands infection risk during course of chemotherapy
b. Utilizes personal hygiene and good handwashing to prevent infection
2. Uses antiemetics and diet modification to maintain an adequate fluid intake
3. Recognizes why maintaining good nutrition is important while receiving chemotherapy
4. Discusses potential for hair loss and coping mechanisms to deal with change in body appearance

## ■ INTERVENTIONS

The patient who enters treatment with a positive attitude about chemotherapy and who has received both verbal and written information on how the drugs act, expected side effects, and the medications and comfort measures used to alleviate symptoms is much more likely to accept this form of therapy and complete the full course of chemotherapy.

The nurse working with the patient beginning chemotherapy must openly acknowledge the side effects that can and do occur. However, the nurse also provides assurance that the side effects can be managed and that the plan of care will keep the patient as comfortable as possible.

### Preventing Infection

Most chemotherapeutic drugs have some effect on the patient's bone marrow, gastrointestinal tract, and skin. The nurse teaches the patient and family the specific signs and symptoms that can be anticipated for each system. Teaching should include facts on the function of the bone marrow in fighting infection (WBCs, neutrophils), carrying oxygen and nutrients to body tissue (RBCs), and blood clotting (platelets). When a chemotherapeutic drug affects the bone marrow, the body's ability to produce sufficient numbers of each cell type is compromised and cells that are produced may be immature and not function normally. Therefore if insufficient numbers are produced or immature cells result, the patient may be unable to fight infection, may develop bleeding tendencies, and eventually will become anemic. Infection is one of the major causes of mortality in the cancer patient, especially in the leukemic patient.

Both patient and family members require instruction on the need for and purpose of good personal hygiene; the need to avoid family, staff, or visitors who have an infectious process; and how to recognize the signs and symptoms of infection. The patient and caregivers are taught to assess for signs of infection from potential sources, such as wounds, indwelling catheter and tube sites, and areas of skin breakdown. They are instructed on the rationale for frequent monitoring of vital signs, blood cell counts (CBC, hemoglobin, hematocrit, platelets), and blood chemistry tests. If the neutrophil count drops below normal acceptable levels (4000 to 10,000/mm$^3$), the chemotherapy may be discontinued or the dose reduced to protect the person from overwhelming infection. The patient with leukemia is an exception to this strategy. Chemotherapy is continued, and some cancer centers place these highly vulnerable patients in protective isolation. They may even have their food sterilized to prevent exposure to bacterial organisms that may be present. See the Guidelines for Care Box on p. 306 for measures to prevent infection in patients receiving chemotherapy.

### Maintaining Fluid Balance

The gastrointestinal tract is highly sensitive to the effects of chemotherapeutic agents. As a result, patients may lose their appetite (anorexia) and experience nausea and vomiting. Some will have diarrhea as well. The outcome is loss of weight and fluid volume, which may result in dehydration. Nausea and vomiting are some of the more devastating side effects of chemotherapy. When nausea and vomiting are expected, the health care team focuses on either preventing or minimizing the incidence. Prophylaxis and continuous treatment have been successful. Treating nausea and vomiting prophylactically is based on the rationale that once vomiting occurs, it is difficult to stop. It is not easy to control the anxiety and fear that, in some patients, lead to anticipatory nausea and vomiting. If nausea and vomiting are known to occur, the patient usually will be prescribed antiemetic therapy before the chemotoxic drug is administered and then on an around-the-clock schedule. Antiemetic therapy may also be administered on an as-needed basis, but it is not recommended. If the nausea, vomiting, and fluid loss are moderate to severe, the patient will receive rehydration with replacement parenteral fluids. Oral fluids are encouraged as tolerated; normal fluid intake is resumed when side effects decrease. Drug therapy for nausea and vomiting is discussed in Chapter 40.

### Promoting Nutrition

Anorexia can be a direct result of the disease process, as well as an outcome of chemotherapy. It is important that the patient and family be aware that if the patient is able to eat and retain food and fluids, a nourishing diet can help maintain energy level and meet body nutrient and repair needs. The patient needs encouragement to eat even when not hungry. When anorexia is accompanied by nausea and vomiting, an antiemetic is administered 30 minutes before mealtime. The patient is taught to perform mouth care (brush teeth, rinse mouth thoroughly) so that foul taste and odor from vomiting can be eliminated. Resting in bed or in a comfortable chair before meals helps conserve energy needed for eating. Patients often are more agreeable to eating breakfast than other meals, especially when they have had an uninterrupted night of sleep. If the patient must be hospitalized for chemotherapy, family members should be encouraged to join them at mealtimes. It provides a more natural and positive feeling toward food, along with family togetherness. The nurse cautions against "filling up" on fluids such as coffee or tea, which have no caloric value but give a feeling of early satiety. Body weight is monitored frequently so the effectiveness of nutritional interventions can be evaluated. Oral supplements or high-calorie between-meal snacks are commonly ordered. Total parenteral nutrition is used with patients who are more severely malnourished. Anorexia is difficult for both the patient and family. Constant monitoring, encouragement, and creativity are required to ensure that the patient meets nutritional needs.

### Promoting a Positive Body Image

Chemotherapeutic drugs can cause alopecia (loss of body hair), from thinning to total loss. Chemotherapeutic drugs act most efficiently on body cells that have a rapid mitotic cycle. The integumentary cells meet this criterion. Drugs that are most responsible for alopecia are alkylating agents, antimetabolites, and anticancer antibiotics. Box 11-16 lists the drugs most involved in causing hair loss.

Patients scheduled for chemotherapy that causes hair loss should be informed of this likelihood early in the course of therapy so that they can be prepared when hair loss occurs. Some male patients shave their heads or cut their hair very short. Women also may cut their hair to minimize the psychological distress that accompanies hair loss. The use of wigs, head scarves, or caps helps the patient maintain a sense of normalcy, hides the loss, and lessens the visible evidence of the loss. The patient is informed that hair loss will cease when the drug is discontinued. Hair regrows but has been known to change shade and texture with regrowth. Hair loss generally begins within a week or two after the first dose of chemotherapy and reaches its maximal loss in a month or two.

Patients often request the use of scalp tourniquets or hypothermia measures to avoid hair loss. Scalp tourniquets act by constricting blood flow to the scalp hair follicles, and hypothermia (ice packs) produces vasoconstriction of blood vessels in the scalp. These techniques work in theory; however, they are not encouraged. Because chemotherapeutic drugs may not reach some cells of the scalp, the potential exists for cancer cells to find a sanctuary and continue to grow and spread.

Patients are advised to avoid harsh shampoos, vigorous combing or brushing, and the use of hot curling irons or rollers while receiving chemotherapy because these activities will cause increased breakage of the already fragile hair shaft. Although hair loss is one of the most obvious and emotionally painful aspects of chemotherapy, the patient can be well prepared to face the situation when it arises. Reading materials about hair loss and referral to community resources such as the American Cancer Society for wigs can foster effective coping. See the Guidelines for Care Box (p. 306) for a summary of care guidelines.

**box 11-16** *Chemotherapeutic Drugs Most Responsible for Hair Loss*

| | |
|---|---|
| Bleomycin | 5-Fluorouracil |
| Cyclophosphamide | Hydroxyurea |
| Cytosine arabinoside | Methotrexate |
| Dactinomycin | Mitomycin-C |
| Daunorubicin | Mitoxantrone |
| Doxorubicin | Melphalan |
| Etoposide | Vincristine |

## EVALUATION

The nurse evaluates the patient's response to nursing interventions by comparing patient behavior in relation to the expected outcomes. The patient will be able to state that chemotherapy is being used as an adjunctive treatment to follow surgery (e.g., mastectomy, colon resection). The ability to correctly name each drug with its major side effects and the specific measures that will facilitate successful coping indicates a basic understanding of therapy. A knowledge of proper nutrition during chemotherapy may be demonstrated by discussing the need to consume foods high in protein and carbohydrates at each meal. Willingly ingesting high-protein snacks or drinks between meals will show compliance with the nutrition plan. When nauseated the patient will take an antiemetic medication before eating.

Instituting measures to prevent infection can be evaluated by observing the patient washing hands after each trip to the bathroom, taking a complete bath daily, and avoiding contact with anyone with a cold or other infectious process. Describing the signs and symptoms of an infection (redness, swelling, pain, or pus) that must be reported indicates an understanding that infection may become a serious and life-threatening outcome of chemotherapy.

The patient sustaining hair loss from chemotherapy will indicate acceptance of the situation by stating that hair loss is temporary; expressing comfort in the use of a wig or scarf; and being able to identify the drug (or drugs) that caused the hair loss.

## HOME CARE CONSIDERATIONS

Home care management is now an alternative to hospitalization for many cancer patients. Not all chemotherapy administration requires admission to a hospital. Patients are able to receive therapy on an outpatient basis in a designated infusion center or clinic. There are several clear advantages for the patient and family:

1. It is less expensive.
2. Support from family and caregivers is more readily available.
3. The home setting is familiar, comfortable, and less stressful.
4. The risk of infection is decreased.

Another option for the patient is the use of home care infusion services. These agencies have skilled and knowledgable nursing staff capable of providing ongoing therapy, assessment, and education. Additional services that are often available include home health aides and medical social services with 24-hour availability.[13] Many private insurance companies and health maintenance organizations (HMOs) now reimburse for home care. Medicare will cover home care costs for qualified individuals.

## OTHER CANCER TREATMENT MODALITIES

Even with advances in conventional cancer treatment modalities (surgery, radiation therapy, chemotherapy, and biotherapy), cancer remains the second leading cause of death in the United States. Therefore an urgent need exists for the development of new treatment modes or new ways in which existing treatment methods might be used in unique ways. Therapies such as hyperthermia and photodynamic therapy, although not new, are again being studied in clinical trials to determine their value, if any, in cancer treatment.

### Hyperthermia

It has long been known that when normal and malignant cells are exposed to extremely high temperatures (40° to 42° C), they are destroyed. The mechanism by which this cytotoxicity occurs is not completely understood. Because many cancers recur after conventional cancer therapy, it is thought that hyperthermia might be useful as an adjunctive therapy with radiation or chemotherapy. Clinical data seem to indicate a synergistic effect when hyperthermia is used concurrently with chemotherapy or within a few hours of radiation treatment. Rationale for using hyperthermia and radiation therapy together comes from the knowledge that hyperthermia is most cytotoxic in the S phase of the cell cycle, whereas radiation therapy is known to be least effective in this phase. It is believed that hyperthermia may enhance the effectiveness of the cytotoxic drug by increasing its uptake and modifying its pharmacokinetics.

Four methods are used for local or regional hyperthermia: (1) ultrasonic devices, (2) devices using electromagnetic (EM) waves, (3) devices that use alternating electromagnetic fields to heat by induction of electrical currents, and (4) devices using direct coupling of EM currents between needles or plates encompassing the tissue to be heated.

These methods may be either noninvasive (i.e., they do not enter the body) or invasive (e.g., by needle implants, interstitial seeds, and interstitial and intracavitary application of small antennae emitting EM waves). Whole-body hyperthermia has been achieved by immersing the patient in liquid wax or circulating hot water or placing the patient in a heated cabinet.

Information to date on the efficacy of combined hyperthermia and radiation therapy is mixed at best. There is no general consensus on any advantage of combined therapy over radiation therapy alone. Some of the limitations of combined therapy are related to the patient's inability to tolerate the intensity of the treatment and length of time required at each session. Current clinical trials seek to determine the "thermal dose" necessary to destroy specific tumors along with the length of treatment that can be tolerated by the human body.

### Photodynamic Therapy

Photodynamic therapy (PDT) is being studied as a possible treatment for deep-seated tumors. It requires the intravenous administration of a dye (sensitizer)—a specific mixture of hematoporphyrins—that localizes in malignant tissue. When the tissue is subjected to laser light by means of fiberoptic technology, a fluorescent flow can be seen. Once the malignant tissue is identified, it is believed that it can be destroyed by special drugs that are targeted directly at the tumor. As a treatment modality PDT is in the preliminary stage, but it appears to have value as a potential therapy in recurrent breast cancer, in head and neck tumors, and in bronchial, bladder, and early gynecological cancer.[8]

### Bone Marrow Transplantation

Bone marrow transplantation (BMT) is used in patients with a variety of malignant hematological and solid tumors. Conditions treated include acute and chronic leukemias, preleukemic states, lymphoma, multiple myeloma, neuroblastoma, and breast cancer. The patient's bone marrow is treated with high-dose chemotherapy or radiotherapy or a combination of both in preparation for receiving harvested marrow. This intensive therapy eradicates the bone marrow and any malignant cells present and replaces them with harvested marrow from either a human leukocyte antigen (HLA)– matched donor or the patient's own marrow. The goal is to achieve a more normal immune system after transplantation.

There are three types of tissue or bone marrow donors: allogeneic, usually from a sibling who has a close HLA match; syngeneic, from an identical twin; or the most recent type used, autologous bone marrow transplantation (ABMT), in which patients serve as their own donors. This is useful because it is frequently difficult to find a donor with a close HLA match.

Autologous bone marrow "harvest" (the term used for donating the bone marrow) is performed when the patient is in remission or when the tumor burden is small and bone marrow involvement cannot be microscopically identified. The purpose of the harvest is to collect enough stem cells (pluripotent cells) to reconstitute the hematopoietic system after therapy.

The FDA has approved the use of hematopoietic growth factors after BMT. Granulocyte colony–stimulating factor (G-CSF) and granulocyte-macrophage colony–stimulating factor (GM-CSF) are glycoproteins that have the ability to stimulate bone marrow recovery through proliferation and maturation after myelosuppression. They are an important component of therapy for aplastic anemia, myelodysplastic syndrome, acquired immunodeficiency syndrome (AIDS), and bone marrow suppression after chemotherapy for cancer treatment.

Marrow grafting is costly because inpatient hospital stays may run from $50,000 to $120,000. The procedure is extremely stressful for the patient and family. The involvement of staff members and patients is intense in a BMT unit, and nurses may need assistance in coping with the intense physical care that patients require and the emotional challenges of this treatment. Patients and staff swing between the emotional poles of hope and optimism and the devastating reality of a terminal situation. See Chapter 68 for a discussion of bone marrow transplantation.

## UNPROVED CANCER THERAPIES

An unproved therapy is defined as one that is neither based on scientific fact nor demonstrates any effectiveness in the clinical treatment of disease when reviewed by peer experts in the field. The use of unproved, unorthodox, or alternative treatment methods is not a recent phenomenon. Dissatisfaction with the present mode of therapy, fear of uncomfortable side effects of treatment and poor prognostic outcomes, and a perceived lack of responsiveness by health care professionals have prompted many patients to seek unconventional treatment modes. Nowhere is this issue more pronounced than with the cancer patient. An estimated 20% to 50% of those diagnosed with cancer will either try or contemplate trying an unproved therapy.

Unproved therapies most commonly used are metabolic therapy, which consists of special foods, minerals, and vitamins; diet treatment; megavitamins; mental imagery; and spiritual or faith healing. Patients who seek out one of these alternative therapies, even while being treated with conventional therapy, are displaying a lack of faith in conventional medical therapy and expressing a need to try to influence their disease outcome.

Health care professionals have a responsibility to be familiar not only with current conventional treatment methods, but also with the unproven methods available to the public. When approached by the patient or family about "other" therapies, it is important to take time and discuss the potential advantages and disadvantages rather than scoffing at the treatment. Attempting to discern why alternative therapy is being considered may lead to more open communication. Perhaps all that is needed is more time to discuss current treatment and expected outcomes. Encouraging more patient and family involvement in decision making about treatment or listening and acting on patient concerns and fears could make the difference between the patient following accepted and proved therapy versus unproved methods. Often it is possible to incorporate unproved therapies into the current treatment regimen; for example, chemotherapy and relaxation or guided imagery techniques used together may help the patient better handle treatment side effects. Discussion of the use of special, approved dietary supplements while the patient receives radiation might dissuade use of unproved dietary interventions. The patient also can be directed to the American Cancer Society for specific literature that addresses the outcomes of research on unproved therapies.

Not all cancers are curable with available treatment methods. Unorthodox therapies may represent a dying patient's last attempt at cure. It is important for the nurse to accept the patient's needs and continue to support the patient and family with honesty and compassion.

Health care professionals must recognize patients' rights to choose how they want to be treated, and they should be supported in their decision. Should patients wish to return to conventional treatment after attempting an unproved method, they need to know that they will be welcomed back and supported by the health care team.

## CANCER PAIN

Pain is one of the most feared effects of cancer, although contrary to popular belief, it is usually one of the last symptoms to appear. Pain is generally not a problem in the early, localized stage of disease. About 5% to 10% of patients with solid tumors have pain that interferes with activity or mood. As the cancer progresses and metastasizes, upward of 90% of patients will experience pain.

Alleviation of pain is the responsibility and obligation of health care professionals. The Oncology Nursing Society (ONS) developed a position paper on cancer pain in part because pain management is a significant clinical problem faced by the nurse caring for cancer patients and because the assessment and control of cancer pain have been poorly managed. The ONS statement makes the nurse responsible for identifying the problem of inadequate pain management and intervening to achieve optimal pain relief.

### Stages

Three stages of cancer pain have been described: early, intermediate, and late. Early pain usually occurs after initial surgery for diagnosis or treatment and usually subsides after the third day; thus this pain is an acute episode that is short term and temporary.

Intermediate pain results from postoperative contraction of scars and nerve entrapment or from cancer recurrence or metastasis. This pain may subside or be controlled by palliative therapy such as radiation, chemotherapy, neurosurgery, and analgesics. Therapy itself may initiate the pain. The role of primary therapies used in the management of cancer pain is summarized in Table 11-31.

Late pain occurs in terminal cancer when therapy no longer controls the disease. This pain is chronic, may slowly increase in intensity, and at times may be intractable.

### Causes

Malignant neoplasms cause pain by five physiological changes: bone destruction (the most common cause); obstruction of lumina (viscera or vessels); peripheral nerve involvement; pressure of growing tumors that cause ischemia, distention, and inflammation; and infection or necrosis of tissue. The pathophysiology of cancer pain is summarized in Table 11-32. The presence of cancer pain also creates multiple side effects, including fatigue, anorexia, sleeplessness, and decreased movement followed by the complications of immobility, namely muscle weakness, decubiti, contractures, and respiratory dysfunction.

The psychological component of cancer pain is associated with the patient's perception of the threat and stress of cancer and varies from individual to individual. Three categories of stressors have been identified: injury or threat of injury as a result of the cancer; loss or threat of loss (body part or death); and frustration of drives as a result of disabilities from the cancer or from the effect of therapies. Patients may respond with depression, decreased self-esteem, hostility, and irritability.

The sociological effects include decreased interaction and participation in activities of daily living. Decreased productivity is characterized by absence from work, economic problems, and deterioration in family relationships. The spiritual effects of pain are evidenced by loss of hope and trust and an overwhelming feeling of despair, rejection, and sense of isolation.

**table 11-31** *Roles of the Primary Therapies in the Management of Cancer Pain*

| Primary Therapy | Major Pain Indications |
|---|---|
| Radiation therapy | Painful bony metastases<br>Epidural spinal cord compression<br>Cerebral metastases<br>Tumor-related compression or infiltration of peripheral neural structures |
| Chemotherapy | Nociceptive or neuropathic pain syndromes caused by tumors likely to respond to chemotherapy |
| Surgery | Stabilization of pathological fractures<br>Spinal cord decompression<br>Relief of remediable bowel obstructions<br>Drainage of symptomatic ascites |
| Antibiotic therapy | Overt infections (e.g., pelvic abscess or pyonephrosis)<br>Occult infections (e.g., in head and neck tumors or ulcerating tumors) |

Source: Cherny NJ, Portenoy RK: The management of cancer pain, *CA Cancer J Clin* 44(5):272, 1994.

**table 11-32** *Pathophysiology of Cancer Pain*

| Cause | Type of Pain |
|---|---|
| Bone destruction with infraction (fracture without displacement) | Increased sensitivity over area or sharp continuous pain |
| Obstruction of a viscus (gastrointestinal or genitourinary tract) | Severe, colicky, crampy type of pain; may be dull, diffuse, poorly localized |
| Obstruction of an artery, vein, or lymphatic | Dull, diffuse, aching (caused by arterial ischemia, venous engorgement, edema) |
| Infiltration, compression of peripheral nerves or nerve plexus | Continuous, sharp, or stabbing pain; sometimes hyperesthesia or paresthesia |
| Infiltration or distention of integument, fascia, or tissue (e.g., ascites) | Localized, dull aching pain |
| Inflammation, infection, and necrosis of tissue | Varied pain caused by pressure or ischemia |

## Collaborative Management

The ultimate goal of pain management is to provide pain relief that enables the patient to carry on with activities of daily living in as near to normal a manner as possible. Strategies may involve a combination of behavioral techniques, such as relaxation or diversional activities, meditation, hypnosis, or imagery, in addition to the use of conventional management approaches. Interventions that may not be thought of as pain-relief strategies include measures that promote rest and sleep, good body positioning, nutrition, and patient teaching of how to decrease pain perception. Combinations of comfort and behavioral methods are listed in Box 11-17.

At times conventional cancer therapies will themselves be used to achieve pain relief. Surgery may be used (1) to debulk a tumor when it is compressing a nerve or causing obstruction of a vessel and (2) to repair pathological fractures. Surgical procedures also may include nerve blocks to the brachial, sympathetic, intercostal, or epidural nerves. Radiation therapy commonly is used to treat bone pain caused by metastasis and the oncological emergency of superior vena cava obstruction. Chemotherapy and hormonal therapies, although not used as often as radiation therapy and surgery, are believed to have a role in pain relief. See Chapter 12 for a discussion of pain assessment and management.

## Home Care Considerations

Pain often is not effectively managed at home, decreasing the patient's functional ability. Common reasons for not taking medications include misunderstanding dosages, feeling that pain cannot be controlled with the same degree of effectiveness as was achieved in the hospital, and inability to

**box 11-17** *Combination of Comfort Measures and Behavioral Techniques for Pain Relief*

1. Promote comfort
   a. Meticulous hygiene
   b. Clean, dry, bed linen
   c. Control of odors
   d. Good body positioning such as with pillows, bed cradle, foot boards for the bedfast person
2. Maintain nutrition
3. Provide diversionary activities for distraction to decrease pain perception
   a. Physical activities (e.g., working, walking, gardening, swimming)
   b. Mental relaxation activities (e.g., watching TV, reading, crafts, listening to music, comedy cassettes)
   c. Social (e.g., visits from family, friends)
4. Suggest and teach forms of noninvasive pain relief
   a. Guided imagery
   b. Hypnosis
   c. Progressive muscle relaxation
   d. Transcendental meditation
   e. Touch and massage

administer the medication accurately. This is a concern especially if the patient goes home with continuous subcutaneous infusion of an opioid or patient-controlled analgesia (PCA). Patients and families have fears similar to those of health care professionals concerning addiction and dependence on narcotics. It is therefore important that the patient and family be instructed about pain-control measures before discharge. The nurse must stress the need to follow the pain-relief protocol prescribed. If the patient can take medications orally, it is emphasized that omitting doses or taking them on an as-needed basis can lead to breakthrough pain and unnecessary suffering. Subcutaneous infusions or PCAs are most useful for the patient who cannot take oral medications. There are, however, some disadvantages to these methods as the primary means of pain relief. Some patients feel overwhelmed by the technical aspects of these forms of pain management. Some fear the responsibility of self-medication. When the patient or family members indicate anxiety about using PCA, another form of pain relief should be considered. If a family member can take responsibility for assisting with PCA administration, all necessary teaching must be accomplished before the time of discharge. Subcutaneous continuous infusion requires the use of a small portable pump and a pediatric butterfly needle, but these do not appear to interfere with mobility and usually are acceptable to the patient and family. Names and telephone numbers should be provided for contacting persons who can assist in emergency situations or when pain relief cannot be maintained with the protocol in use.

Although complete freedom from pain is not always achieved, the patient can be kept comfortable in most cases. The use of behavioral interventions such as relaxation techniques, self-hypnosis, and meditation should be encouraged in combination with analgesics. In the home setting, surrounded by family members and a familiar environment, these combination strategies may provide a comfort level that cannot be equaled in the hospital setting. Nursing strategies for dealing with the cancer patient's pain are listed in the accompanying Guidelines for Care Box.

**guidelines for care**

**Dealing Effectively with the Cancer Patient's Pain**

- Know the patient and the pattern of pain experienced. Document findings.
- Use an organized pain-assessment method that is easy to use and that provides sufficient data to assist in selecting the most appropriate intervention for relief.
- Understand the pharmacology of the drugs being used, including: classification, probable side effects, route of administration, expected outcomes in terms of when to expect pain relief to occur.
- Understand the difference between addiction, dependence, and tolerance.
- Use appropriate drug combinations.
- Become familiar with equianalgesic doses of common analgesics (see Chapter 12).
- Provide patient and family teaching related to pain control.

## RESOURCES FOR CANCER EDUCATION, DETECTION, AND REHABILITATION

Federal recognition of the need to give intensive assistance to cancer educational programs began in 1926 when Congress proclaimed April of each year as National Cancer Control Month. In 1937 the National Cancer Institute was created within the National Institutes of Health. This institute conducts an extensive program of research in the field of cancer.

Cancer patients may obtain help from both Medicare and Medicaid. The Community Services Administration provides services through state agencies or by direct grants. The Rehabilitation Services Administration arranges and pays for services that help the cancer patient return to productive living. The passage of the National Cancer Act of 1971 provided impetus for the development of cancer clinical research centers. The goal was to translate research results into medical practice so that no one will be denied the most current professional advice and care. These centers combine research capability, patient care, and community outreach programs. Box 11-18 provides a list of organizations that may be used as resources by the cancer patient and family, and Box 11-19 is a listing of cancer-related World Wide Web addresses.

**box 11-18** *National Organizations Providing Cancer Education Materials and Resources*

American Cancer Society
1599 Clifton Road, N.E.
Atlanta, GA 30329

American Academy of Otolaryngology
Head and Neck Surgery, Inc.
1101 Vermont Avenue, N.W.
Suite 302
Washington, D.C. 20005

Breast Cancer Advisory Center
11426 Rockville Pike
Suite 406
Rockville, MD 20857

Leukemia Society of America, Inc.
733 Third Avenue
New York, NY 10017

Make Today Count
514 Tama Bldg.
P.O. Box 303
Burlington, IN 52601

National Cancer Information Clearinghouse
Room 10A18, Building 31
NCI/NIH
Bethesda, MD 20205

National Hospice Organization
1901 North Fort Myer Drive
Suite 307
Arlington, VA 22209

United Ostomy Association, Inc.
2001 West Beverly Blvd.
Los Angeles, CA 90057

**box 11-19** *Selected Cancer-Related World Wide Web Addresses*

| | |
|---|---|
| American Cancer Society | http://www.cancer.org |
| American Medical Association | http://www.ama-assn.org |
| Avon's Breast Cancer Awareness Campaign | http://www.pmedia.com/Avon/avon.html |
| Brain Tumor Clinical Trials | http://www.lanminds.com/local/brain/trial.html |
| Brain Tumor: American BT Assoc. Home Page | http://pubweb.acns.nwu.edu/~lberko/abta_html/abtal.htm |
| CANSearch (NCCS) | http://access.digex.net/~mkragen/cansearch.html |
| CandleLighters | http://cois.com.candle/ |
| FAQ—Cancer | http://www.cancercare.org/faq/cancer_faq.html |
| FAQ—Powerlines/EMF | http://www.cis.ohio-state.edu/text/ |
| Food and Drug Administration | http://www.fda.gov/ |
| ICIC Cancer Information Products | http://wwwicic.nci.nih.gov/icicproducts/html |
| Journal of the National Cancer Institute | http://wwwicic.nci.nih.gov/jnci/jnci_issues.html |
| Kids Home at NCI | http://wwwicic.nci.nih.gov/occdocs/KidsHome.html |
| NCI/ICIC–CancerNet | http://wwwicic.nci.gov |
| National Community of Charitable Aviators | http://www.america.com/~jpringle/acahome.html |
| National Library of Medicine | http://www.nlm.nih.gov/ |
| National Lymphedema Network | http//www.primenet.com/~dean/lymph.html |
| National Cancer Institute Online Publications | http://wwwicic.nci.nih.gov/pubslist.html |
| Office of Cancer Communications Publications | http://wwwicic.nci.nih.gov/occdocs/occpubs.html |
| Oncolink | http://www.oncolink.upenn.edu/ |
| PDQ | http://wwwicic.nci.nih.gov/pdqinci.html |
| PharmWeb: Pharmacy Information Resources | http://www.mcc.ac.uk/pharmacy/ |
| Prostate Cancer Infolink | http://www.comed.com/Prostate |
| Psychosocial and Support Newsgroups | http://brain.psyc.uow.edu.au/usenet.guide.html |
| Self-Breast Exam & Mammography | http://www.net-advisor.com/mammog/ |

Woodworth M, Loochtan A: A road map to cancer resources on the Internet, *Cancer Pract* 4(3):160, 1996.
*NCCS,* National Coalition for Cancer Survivors; *PDQ,* Physicians Data Query.

## critical thinking QUESTIONS

**1** You are speaking to a group of senior citizens at a local retirement home about cancer risk factors. What information about cancer risk would you give them so that they can apply the information to their own chances of developing cancer?

**2** Milton, age 59, is a retired research chemist for a textile manufacturer. Six months after retirement he is diagnosed with acute myelogenous leukemia. What job-related factors might have put him at risk for this malignant condition?

**3** What nursing strategies would you contemplate using to care for a patient who is experiencing side effects from receiving multiple toxic chemotherapeutic drugs?

**4** John is a 66-year-old retired coal miner with metastatic prostate cancer to the bone. He is to begin palliative radiation therapy to help alleviate his bone pain. He tells you that he expects to be completely cured of his cancer by the radiation treatments. How will you address this misunderstanding and yet provide him with a realistic sense of hope?

**5** Larry is a 60-year-old with multiple myeloma. He is in the terminal stages of cancer and is experiencing severe pain. How would you address the problem, and what measures would you use to provide for pain relief?

## chapter SUMMARY

### NATURE OF PROBLEM

- Delay in seeking treatment is the most important factor in a negative prognosis after a cancer diagnosis.
- Underestimation of the incidence of cancer and negative views about the therapy are two of the most important factors that inhibit health-seeking behaviors.

### ETIOLOGY, PHYSIOLOGY, AND PATHOPHYSIOLOGY

- Cancer research focuses on causes of abnormal cell growth (the role of chemicals and other pollutants, genetic factors, and viruses) and therapies for cancer (surgical, drug, radiation, and immune system alteration).
- Changes in cells causing them to become malignant appear to result from disturbance in the regulatory functions of DNA, causing a loss of differentiation and lack of similarity to the original cells.
- Tumor growth may be rapid or slow depending on factors such as immune surveillance, blood supply, hormones, number of cells proliferating, and the length of time in the cell cycle.
- Metastasis may occur through blood vessels, lymph vessels, direct extension, or diffusion.
- Carcinogenesis is a combination of factors that includes carcinogens, host susceptibility, environmental carcinogens, habits, customs, and viruses.
- Cancer has multiple local and systemic effects. Local effects result from obstruction, pressure, and destruction of

surrounding tissue. Systemic effects may involve multiple organ systems and include cachexia, anorexia, pain, and various metabolic disorders.

## EPIDEMIOLOGY

- Cancer occurs most commonly in men and in persons older than 65 years of age.

## COLLABORATIVE MANAGEMENT

- Diagnostic studies for cancer include blood tests; biopsy; and cytological, radiological, and endoscopic examination.
- Nursing care during the diagnostic phase includes assessment of psychological and physiological effects of cancer and interventions to help the patient and family cope.
- Medical management of cancer may include a combination of surgery, chemotherapy, radiation therapy, and biotherapy.
- Nurses teach patients about the expected outcomes of therapy and how to cope with side effects.
- Radiotherapy may be administered externally or internally. Side effects may involve the gastrointestinal system, skin, or other systems.
- A combination of drugs usually is used in chemotherapy because different drugs work in different phases of the cell cycle.
- Chemotherapeutic agents include alkylating agents, antimetabolites, antibiotics, steroids, vinca alkaloids, and various miscellaneous drugs.
- Drugs may be administered orally, subcutaneously, intravenously, intraarterially, intracavitarily, or intrathecally.
- Nursing care during chemotherapy includes assessment, prevention or treatment of infection, gastrointestinal problems, alopecia, and organ toxicities.
- Biotherapy includes use of biological response modifiers such as interferons, interleukins, and monoclonal antibodies.

## ONCOLOGICAL EMERGENCIES

- Oncological emergencies include obstructive, cardiac, and metabolic syndromes.

## CANCER PAIN

- Cancer pain results from physiological and psychological factors and usually can be controlled with a combination of consistently administered drugs and other comfort measures.

## References


1. American Cancer Society: *1997 cancer facts and figures,* New York, 1997, The Society.
2. Anonymous: *Respiratory health effects of passive smoking: lung cancer and other disorders,* Environmental Protection Agency (EPA/600/6-90/006F), Washington, DC, 1990, Office of Health and Environmental Assessment.
3. Bagshawe KD, Gordon J, Rustin JS: Circulating tumour markers. In Peckham M et al, editors: *Oxford textbook of oncology,* vol I, Oxford, 1995, Oxford University Press.
4. Bender C: Implications of antineoplastic therapy for nursing. In Clark JC et al, editors: *Core curriculum in oncology nursing,* ed 2, Philadelphia, 1992, WB Saunders.
5. Borst P, Pinedo HM: Drug resistance. In Peckham M et al, editors: *Oxford textbook of oncology,* vol I, Oxford, 1995, Oxford University Press.
6. Cartmel B et al: Professional and consumer concerns about the environment, life style, and cancer, *Semin Oncol Nurs* 8(1):20, 1992.
7. Coleman CN, Stevenson MA: Biologic bases for radiation oncology, *Oncology* 10(3):399, 1996.
8. Dougherty TJ: Photodynamic therapy: part II, *Semin Surg Oncol* 11:333, 1995.
9. Dudjak LA: Cancer metastasis, *Semin Oncol Nurs* 8(1):40, 1992.
10. Dwyer J: Nutritional problems of elderly minorities, *Nutr Rev* 50(80):S24, 1994.
11. Ferrel MM: Biotherapy and the oncology nurse, *Semin Oncol Nurs* 12(2):82, 1996.
12. Gale D, Charette J: Biologic therapy. In Gale D et al, editors: *Oncology nursing care plans,* El Paso, Tex, 1994, Skidmore-Roth.
13. Gorski LA, Grothman L: Home infusion therapy, *Semin Oncol Nurs* 12(3):193, 1996.
14. Greco M: Achievements and obstacles to progress in cancer surgery. In Peckham M et al, editors: *Oxford textbook of oncology,* Vol I, Oxford, 1995, Oxford University Press.
15. Heath CW: Electromagnetic field exposure and cancer: a review of epidemiologic evidence, *CA Cancer J Clin* 46(1):29, 1996.
16. Lydon J: Metastasis, *Oncol Nurs* 2(5):1, 1995.
17. Mahon SM, Casperson DS: Hereditary cancer syndrome: part I. Clinical and educational issues, *Oncol Nurs Forum* 22(5):763, 1995.
18. Mettlin C: Research in cancer prevention and detection, *Current Issues in Cancer Nursing Updates* 1(4):1, 1992.
19. McDonald A: Altered protective mechanisms. In Dow KH, editor: *Nursing care radiation oncology,* Philadelphia, 1992, WB Saunders.
20. McMillan S: Carcinogenesis, *Semin Oncol Nurs* 8(1):10, 1992.
21. Northouse LL, Peters-Golden H: Cancer and the family: strategies to assist spouses, *Semin Oncol Nurs* 9(3):74, 1993.
22. Oldman RK: Cancer biotherapy: general principles. In Oldham RK, editor: *Principles of cancer biotherapy,* ed 2, New York, 1991, Marcel Dekker.
23. Parker RG, Withers HR: Principles of radiation oncology. In Haskell CM, editor: *Cancer treatment,* ed 4, Philadelphia, 1995, WB Saunders.
24. Sandstrom SK: Nursing management of patients receiving biological therapy, *Semin Oncol Nurs* 12(2):152, 1996.
25. Sporkin E: Patient and family education. In Dow KH, editor: *Nursing care in radiation oncology,* Philadelphia, 1992, WB Saunders.
26. Stellman JM, Stellman SD: Cancer and the workplace, *CA Cancer J Clin* 46(2):70, 1996.
27. Tomaszewski JG, DeLaPena L, Molenda J, et al: Biotherapy module II, overview of biotherapy, *Cancer Nurs* 18(5):397, 1995.
28. Walter D, Quan Y, Mitchell MS: Principles of biologic therapy. In Haskell CM, editor: *Cancer treatment,* ed 4, Philadelphia, 1995, WB Saunders.
29. Wingo PA et al: Cancer statistics for African Americans, *CA Cancer J Clin* 46(2):113, 1996.
30. Yasko JW: Oncogenes and cancer suppression genes, *Semin Oncol Nurs* 8(1):30, 1992.

# chapter 12 Pain and Pain Control

JUDITH H. WATT-WATSON

## objectives

*After studying this chapter, the learner should be able to:*

1. Describe some common misbeliefs about pain management.
2. Describe the physiology of pain and related theories of pain transmission.
3. Compare factors that influence perception and response to pain.
4. Differentiate between acute and chronic pain.
5. Compare pain assessment tools used in clinical practice.
6. Describe pharmacological and nonpharmacological approaches for pain management.
7. Identify five nursing interventions for pain management.
8. Explain the purpose and methods of the team approach for chronic pain management.

## NATURE OF THE PROBLEM

Pain relief is a management problem for many patients, their families, and the health professionals caring for them. Although pain is experienced by everyone to some degree, responses to it are unique for each person. Difficulties in recognizing and understanding someone else's pain are clinically well known. The International Association for the Study of Pain[45] has defined pain as an unpleasant sensory and emotional experience associated with actual or potential tissue damage or described in terms of such damage. Pain therefore is multidimensional and entirely subjective. With verbal children or adults, only the person experiencing the pain can describe or evaluate it. Pain can be evoked by a multiplicity of stimuli, but the reaction to it cannot be measured objectively. Pain is a learned experience that is influenced by the entire life situation of each person.

McCaffery's[38] definition that pain is "whatever and whenever the person says it is," has changed practice by focusing health professionals' attention on the subjectivity of pain. Patients' self-reports about their pain are the key to effective management. However, we now realize that interpreting this definition at the simplest level may cause problems. Patients do not always admit to pain. They do not necessarily know how and when to tell us that they are hurting and/or they "expect to have severe pain so they are not going to complain." Patients may also not differentiate between pain and what the pain means to them, that is, suffering. Therefore, the focus on the individuality of pain in both of these definitions underlines the importance of careful listening and valuing of patient information to understand the patient's pain experience as completely as possible.

Pain accompanies many disorders, as well as some therapies. It is a sensation that is frequently feared by persons undergoing surgery. Although some persons with cancer do *not* experience pain, it is one of the major concerns people have about cancer.

Relief of pain and discomfort is a major nursing objective and one that requires skill in both the art and science of nursing. Knowledge about concepts related to pain, data collection, and useful therapies is essential. Sensitivity and empathy, trying to understand what the person is experiencing, are important components of a systematic approach to the patient in pain. Too often management decisions are made without valid assessment and evaluation, including sufficient input from patients. Consequently, pain management is ineffective.

Recognition of the widespread inadequacy of pain management has prompted recent corrective efforts within multiple health care disciplines, including surgery, anesthesiology, and nursing, as well as in pain management groups. These efforts are reflected in the *Clinical Practice Guideline: Acute Pain Management: Operative or Medical Procedures and Trauma* published by the Agency for Health Care Policy and Research (AHCPR) of the U.S. Department of Health and Human Services.[2] The four major goals for the guideline are the following:

1. Reduce the incidence and severity of patients' acute postoperative or posttraumatic pain.
2. Educate patients about the need to communicate unrelieved pain so that they can receive prompt evaluation and effective treatment.
3. Enhance patient comfort and satisfaction.
4. Contribute to fewer postoperative complications and, in some cases, shorter stays after surgical procedures.

## ETIOLOGY

Pain results from a variety of causes, and its trajectories have different patterns. Some patients may experience both acute and persistent pain depending on the complexity of the problem. Acute pain is usually short-lived with a known cause or pathological process. Trauma, infection, inflammation, diagnostic tests, surgeries, and treatments are common sources of acute pain. Recurrent acute pain can occur in people who experience headaches, dysmenorrhea, arthritis, sickle cell anemia, cancer, or inflammatory bowel disease. Chronic pain is defined as pain that persists beyond the usual time for healing to occur.[45] The term is usually used to describe pain that has been present for more than 6 months. Chronic pain may occur with progressive diseases such as cancer, acquired immunodeficiency syndrome (AIDS), sickle cell anemia, and multiple sclerosis and with neuropathic pain syndromes such as postherpetic neuralgia. Some patients have idiopathic chronic pain for which the cause is not known.

Unnecessary pain can result from incomplete pain assessments or treatments based on assumptions rather than on patient data. Regardless of the etiology of pain, the foundation for effective pain management is to believe that all pain is real and that malingerers (people who deliberately lie about their pain) are rare (fewer than 1%). Patients' self-reports of their pain are critical to the choice of strategies and the evaluation of the effectiveness of interventions. It is important to recognize that patients in pain will not necessarily ask for help until they are in severe pain[50,70] and they may use words such as "pressure" or "soreness" instead of "pain."

Both children and elderly adults frequently experience unrelieved pain because health professionals incorrectly assume that their age minimizes the pain experience.[68] Careful observation, especially of facial expressions at rest and during movement, is particularly important with infants and with cognitively impaired elders.

Unrelieved acute pain has numerous negative consequences. Postoperative pain can cause cardiovascular, pulmonary, and gastrointestinal (GI) complications.[8,15,33,35,49] Atelectasis after surgery has been found to be greater in patients with higher pain intensity.[57] Moreover, early unrelieved postoperative pain for thoracotomy patients was the only factor that significantly predicted pain 18 months later in a major study.[31] The Agency for Health Care Policy and Research[2] has emphasized the importance of effective pain management in order to meet managed care demands for earlier patient mobilization, reduced hospital stays, and reduced costs. Most important of all is research evidence that suggests that early treatment of acute pain before it begins, when possible, may prevent future long-term pain.[7,21,30]

## EPIDEMIOLOGY

Pain is a common reason that people seek help from health care professionals. In the United States alone, 23 million patients have surgery every year and the majority of these experience postoperative pain.[2] Although 90% of cancer pain can be controlled, about 40 to 80% of cancer patients report moderate to severe pain.[3] Unfortunately, people in a variety of settings continue to experience considerable pain in spite of effective treatment options.

For more than 20 years research repeatedly has demonstrated that significant numbers of hospitalized patients experience moderate to severe pain unrelieved by treatment.[11,18,36,37,46,52,65,66,70,71] Inadequate knowledge and problematic attitudes of physicians and nurses have been well documented.[10,12,26-28,61,62] Although health professionals more recently have supported the principle of pain relief, this goal does not appear to have significantly altered practice. Health professionals either have not recognized unrelieved pain or have tolerated poor pain relief as the norm. Many patients have not been asked by health professionals about their pain, or discrepancies have been documented between their pain ratings and those of health professionals.[14,21,27,39,52,70,73] This problematic communication is compounded if patients expect to have pain while hospitalized or are reluctant to ask staff members for help.[11,70] Some commonly held misbeliefs influence our practice and may contribute to this ineffective pain management (Box 12-1).[68] These misbeliefs are crucial to recognize and correct because they influence our approaches to both the assessment and management of pain.

Minimal or no pain should be the goal of pain management. A hospital admission should not automatically mean a pain experience for *any* patient, including elders, children, and infants. Patterns of pain intensity vary, and the diagnosis and/or type of surgery is *not* an effective basis for determining the amount of pain the person is experiencing or the analgesic required. Although not all pain can be eliminated, the use of multiple modalities usually can decrease it to at least the minimal range.

Pain is a complex experience, and multiple strategies rather than only one approach are likely to be more successful in alleviating it. Incorrect beliefs about analgesic administration, particularly opioids, frequently result in the undermedication of patients.[6,70]

It is difficult to understand and recognize another person's pain. Therefore it is crucial to gain as much information about the patient as possible instead of making assumptions about what may be happening.[64] The nurse must be vigilant about personal expectations, biases, and factors that may interfere with the ability to deliver individualized nursing care. One research report discusses the effect of a patient's ethnic group and gender on analgesic administration (see the following Research Box).

## PHYSIOLOGY

### THEORIES OF PAIN

Various theorists through the centuries have tried to explain pain[34,38,44] (Box 12-2). Aristotle's perception of pain as an emotion or "passion of the soul" was rejected by specificity theorists who accepted Descartes' separation of the body from the mind. Specificity theorists believed that pain messages were carried in a specific straight-line transmission from receptors in the periphery to a central pain center; therefore, pain was considered to equal the degree of injury. Pattern theorists questioned this premise, because it was evident that people responded differently to the same stimulus. They proposed that patterns of impulses were more important than specificity in explaining pain. Although these theories contributed to understanding pain mechanisms, they all had major limitations.

### box 12-1 Misbeliefs About Pain

**Misbeliefs are incorrect beliefs that are accepted as truths and frequently used to guide practice.**

**MISBELIEFS ABOUT THE PAIN EXPERIENCE**

1. Patients should expect to have pain in the hospital.
2. Obvious pathological conditions, test results, and, or type of surgery determine the existence and intensity of pain.
3. Patients who are in pain always have observable signs.
4. Chronic pain is not as serious a problem for patients as acute pain.
5. Patients are not the experts about their pain, health professionals are.
6. Patients will tell us when they are in pain and will use the term "pain."

**MISBELIEFS ABOUT PAIN MANAGEMENT**

1. One pain treatment or strategy is all that is needed.
2. Addiction is a major problem with patients taking opioids.
3. The nurse is the best person to administer opioids.
4. Patients must demonstrate pain before receiving analgesic medication.
5. Patients who respond to placebos do not have real pain.
6. Injectable opioids are the most effective.
7. Respiratory depression is a common and severe side effect of opioids in all patients.

**MISBELIEFS ABOUT PAIN AND AGE**

**Children Including Infants**

1. Children do not experience pain.
2. Children cannot accurately describe their pain.
3. Children should not be given opioids for pain.
4. Opioids are best given by the intramuscular route.
5. Children forget painful experiences.
6. Children who are playing or sleeping do not have pain.
7. Parents should not stay with children during painful procedures.

**The Older Person**

1. Pain is a normal part of getting older; pain sensation decreases with age and therefore can never be very intense.
2. Opioids are too potent for elderly patients.
3. Pain cannot be assessed with elderly patients who are cognitively impaired.

From Watt-Watson J: Misbeliefs about pain. In Watt-Watson J, Donovan M, editors: *Pain management: nursing perspective*, pp 36-58, St Louis, 1992, Mosby.

### research

Reference: McDonald D: Gender and ethnic stereotyping and opioid analgesic administration, *Res Nurs Health* 17:45-49, 1994.

Previous studies of gender and ethnic stereotyping in pain management have been inconclusive. In this study, medical records of 180 patients who underwent uncomplicated appendectomies were retrospectively examined (101 male and 79 female patients of whom 40 were from ethnic minorities). White patients were given significantly more opioids overall postoperatively than were ethnic minority patients (Asian, black, or Hispanic). The impact of gender was not as clear. Immediately after surgery, male patients were given significantly larger doses of opioid analgesia than were female patients. However, there was no gender difference in the total dose given postoperatively. As the stereotyping did not persist, women may have taken longer to recover from anesthesia to make their needs known. McDonald suggests that irrelevant cues, such as ethnic differences, may be used in nurses' medication decisions.

### box 12-2 Theories of Pain Transmission

**AFFECT THEORY**

Pain is an emotion and its intensity depends on the meaning of the part involved.
Limitations: Does not include physiological aspects.

**SPECIFIC THEORY**

Specific pain receptors project impulses over neural pain pathways to the brain.
Limitations: Does not account for psychological aspects of pain perception and variability of response.

**PATTERN THEORY**

Pain results from combined effects of stimulus intensity and summations of impules in the dorsal horn of the spinal cord.
Limitations: Does not account for psychological aspects.

**GATE CONTROL THEORY**

Pain impulses can be controlled by a gating mechanism in the substantia gelatinosa of the dorsal horn of the spinal cord to permit or inhibit transmission. Gating factors include effect of impulses transmitted over fast or slow conducting nerve fibers and effects of descending impulses from the brainstem and cortex.

Melzack and Wall built upon the relationships between these theories in proposing their gate control theory (GCT) in 1965. The GCT contributed considerably to our current understanding of the transduction, transmission, modulation, and perception steps of the pain process.[25]

According to the GCT,[43,44] pain is not a simple, sensory experience but a complex integration of sensory, affective, and cognitive dimensions. Pain involves dynamic interactions between ascending and descending neural systems along with ongoing balancing of inhibitory-excitatory mechanisms. Pain perception and responses to pain are not predictable but vary with each person and experience. This variability results from the modulation of noxious (painful) input at several levels of the central nervous system.

Excitatory stimuli, both painful and innocuous, are converted into an action potential that stimulates the primary afferent neurons in the periphery. The message is then transmitted by these neurons to converge onto common second-order neurons in the dorsal horn of the spinal cord. The substantia gelatinosa (SG) in the dorsal horn is the major site where modulation of painful stimuli results from complex excitatory and inhibitory processes acting as a "gate." The GCT postulates that increased activity in the large, non-nociceptive primary afferent neurons (A-beta), such as that produced with massage or transcutaneous electrical nerve stimulation, can reduce pain messages carried by the small, nociceptive afferent neurons (A-delta and C) to cells in the SG. As a result, further transmission of the pain message is inhibited. However, if pain impulses reach a critical level without being blocked, they will be transmitted to second-order neurons in the SG. Pain impulses then are transmitted by nociceptive pathways, which ascend from the second-order neurons to the thalamus and cerebral cortex. These ascending tracts transmit sensory-discriminative data about the quality and intensity of pain, contribute to the motivational-affective dimension about the meaning of pain, and activate descending inhibitory systems. Pain transmission can be blocked by descending inhibition involving neurotransmitters such as enkephalin, serotonin, and norepinephrine.

Impulses sent to the brainstem, the center for motivational-affective and sensory-discriminative actions, can influence cognition or evaluation in the cortex. Impulses are then sent from the cortex back to the SG via corticospinal pathways to inhibit or permit passage of pain impulses. Note in Table 12-1 the various factors that can open or close the gate.

Melzack and Dennis[42] emphasized that noxious stimuli enter an already active nervous system that is a compilation of past experience, culture, anticipation, and emotion. Cognitive processes related to the meaning of the pain act selectively on sensory input and motivation to influence pain transmission via the descending tracts to the dorsal horn. As a result, the amount and quality of pain are determined by individual factors such as previous pain experiences and one's concept of the cause of pain and its consequences. Cultural values can influence how one feels and responds to pain.[44] Therefore, pain is a highly personal experience and more than just a painful stimulus. For example, there is no one standard response to surgery, and the same pain-relieving intervention may not be effective for all patients.

## THE PAIN PROCESS

The process by which a painful stimulus is perceived involves the four steps of transduction, transmission, modulation, and perception.[25] Transduction and transmission involve processing the pain message from the nociceptors to the spinal cord. Modulation in the spinal cord will determine whether the stimuli will be perceived as pain.

### Transduction

Transduction, or receptor activation, involves converting the painful stimulus into an impulse that is carried from the periphery to the central nervous system (CNS). The pain receptors, or nociceptors, are free nerve endings of unmyelinated or lightly myelinated afferent neurons. Nociceptors are located extensively in the skin and mucosa and less frequently in selected deeper structures, such as viscera, joints, arterial walls, and bile ducts. Nociceptors respond to harmful or potentially harmful stimuli that may be chemical, thermal, or mechanical.[25]

The noxious stimulus creates an action potential that activates the nerve fiber to send the impulse to the CNS. Chemical stimuli for pain include histamines, bradykinin, prostaglandins, and acids, some of which are released by damaged tissues. Anoxic tissue also releases chemicals that lead to pain. Tissue swelling may cause pain by creating pressure (mechanical stimulation) on nociceptors in adjoining tissues.

### Transmission

Pain impulses are transmitted to the spinal cord by two types of fibers: thinly myelinated faster-conducting A-delta fibers and slower-conducting unmyelinated C fibers. Pain that may be described as "sharp" or "pricking" and can be easily localized is transmitted by the A-delta fibers. An example of this type of pain is that felt by a needle prick. Pain that may be described as "burning," "dull," or "aching" and that is more diffuse results from impulses transmitted by the C fibers. Impulses transmitted on the larger diameter myelinated A-beta and A-alpha fibers have an inhibitory effect on those transmitted over A-delta and C fibers.

The primary afferent nerve fibers enter the spinal cord through the dorsal root and synapse onto second-order neurons within six interconnected levels or laminae in the dorsal horn (Figure 12-1).

**table 12-1** *Factors Affecting Pain Transmission Based on the Gate Control Theory*

| Site | Close Gate (Block Transimssion) | Open Gate (Permit Transmission) |
|---|---|---|
| Fibers | Impulses transmitted by large, fast, myelinated A-beta and A-alpha fibers | Impulses transmitted by slow, small, A-delta and C fibers |
| | Stimulation of unaffected skin areas (e.g., massage) | Stimulation of affected skin areas (e.g., sunburned skin) |
| Brainstem (descending pathway) | Endorphin effect | No endorphin effect |
| | Sufficient or maximum sensory input (e.g., distraction) | Insufficient sensory input (e.g., monotony) |
| Cortex | Past experiences | Past experiences |
| | Feelings of pain control | Anxiety |

Lamina II comprises an area called the *substantia gelatinosa,* which is the major site for modulation of nociceptive input. Substance P is released at synapses in the SG and is thought to be a major neurotransmitter of pain impulses.[19]

Secondary neurons synapse with projection neurons in the spinal cord. The pain impulses then cross the spinal cord over interneurons and connect with ascending spinal pathways. The most important ascending pathways for nociceptive impulses located in the ventral half of the spinal cord are the spinothalamic tract (STT) and the spinoreticular tract (SRT). The STT is a discriminative system and conveys information about the nature and location of the stimulus to the thalamus and then to the cortex for interpretation. Impulses transmitted over the SRT, which goes to the brainstem and part of the thalamus, activate the autonomic and limbic (motivational-affective) responses. The ultimate perception of pain is dependent on modulation of neuronal impulses in ascending pathways in relation to the activation of descending inhibitory systems.

## Modulation

Discovery of receptors in the brain to which opiate compounds bind led to the discovery of two naturally occurring endogenous morphinelike pentapeptides (5-amino acid compounds), met-enkephalin and leu-enkephalin. These enkephalins are classified as *endorphins* (from the terms *endogenous* and *morphine*). Other endorphins, such as beta-endorphin, also have been identified. The endorphins are thought to suppress pain by (1) acting presynaptically to inhibit release of the neurotransmitter substance P or (2) acting postsynaptically to inhibit conduction of pain impulses.[44] The endorphins are found in high concentration in the basal ganglia of the brain, thalamus, midbrain, and dorsal horn of the spinal cord.

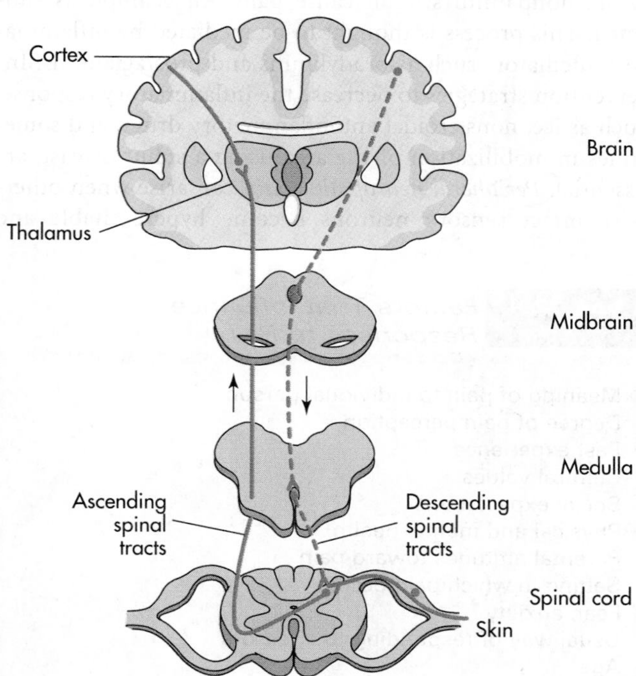


**fig. 12-1** Pathways of pain transmission to and from cortex.

Descending spinal pathways, from the thalamus through the midbrain and medulla to the dorsal horns of the spinal cord, conduct nociceptive inhibitory impulses.[19,44] Serotonin, norepinephrine, and endorphins are released by descending fibers and inhibit the release of neurotransmitters. Therefore, nociceptive stimuli will not be transmitted to second-order neurons. Treatment modalities such as electrical stimulation by means of transcutaneous electrical nerve stimulators can activate opiate analgesia. Acupuncture is also thought to use the opiate pathways.

## Perception

Pain is multidimensional and highly variable.[44] Pain is a subjective, very personal experience that can be influenced by factors such as the meaning of the situation that is unique to each person. Tolerance to pain varies within and between individuals experiencing the same noxious stimulus. Responses to pain are influenced by individuals' interpretation of pain and its meaning to them.

### Pain tolerance

Across cultures there is great uniformity in the minimum level of noxious stimulus that people report as pain.[38] This level is called the *pain detection threshold.* It is primarily biological in nature and is relatively consistent within an individual, relative to the location and type of stimulus. In contrast, pain tolerance involves the cognitive-affective dimension of pain, is very subjective, and varies widely within and between individuals and cultures.

Pain tolerance is the maximum degree of pain intensity a person is willing to experience. It can be increased or decreased by numerous factors (Box 12-3). Tolerance can vary between different individuals in the same situation and in the same individual in differing situations. For example, a woman with a tender breast lump may complain of more pain if her mother died of breast cancer. Individual persons can respond in many ways to any level of pain intensity, and pain tolerance is influenced by the meaning of the pain to the individual. It is important to remember that there is no right or wrong way to experience pain, and the pain experience is subjective and unique to each person.

### The meaning of pain

Pain has different meanings for each person and may differ for the same person at different times. Pain initially has an

**box 12-3** *Factors That Influence Pain Tolerance*

| INCREASE TOLERANCE | DECREASE TOLERANCE |
|---|---|
| Alcohol | Fatigue |
| Drugs | Anger |
| Hypnosis | Boredom |
| Warmth | Anxiety |
| Rubbing | Persistent pain |
| Distraction | Stress |
| Faith | Depression |
| Strong beliefs | |

important protective function of warning the person of impending tissue damage. However, with persistent pain, meanings can change. Some examples of the meanings of pain include the following:

- Harm or damage
- Complication, such as infection
- New illness
- Recurrence of illness
- Fatal disease
- Increasing disability
- Loss of mobility
- Aging
- Healing
- Necessary for cure
- Punishment for sins
- Challenge
- Appreciation for suffering of others
- Something to be tolerated

Numerous factors influence the meaning of pain for an individual, including age, gender, sociocultural background, environment, and past or present experiences. For example, two women may be experiencing pain from a fractured leg. To the 75-year-old woman living alone with few social contacts, pain may be interpreted on the basis of fear of aging and inability to maintain her independent living status. The 28-year-old lawyer might interpret the pain as an expected nuisance, with the realization that healing will occur and she can get back to work soon.

#### *Response to pain*

People respond to pain in different ways, depending on their perception of the pain, including what it means to them. Some may be fearful, apprehensive, and anxious, whereas others are tolerant and optimistic. Some weep, moan, scream, beg for relief or help, threaten to destroy themselves, thrash about in bed, or move about aimlessly when in severe pain; others lie quietly in bed and may only close their eyes, grit their teeth, bite their lips, clench their hands, or perspire profusely when experiencing pain.

On the basis of their cultural beliefs some persons have been taught to endure severe pain without reacting outwardly, whereas others are taught to be very expressive when experiencing any degree of pain. People whose health beliefs and education emphasize prevention tend to accept pain as a warning to seek help. They expect that the cause of pain will be found and cured.

Researchers for many years have attempted to expand Zborowski's[74] qualitative findings that ethnicity influences patients' pain behavior. Research has been inconclusive because of methodology issues as to what differences exist and how they impact pain perception and response.[47] Cleeland[13] examined the relationship between standardized self-report numerical scales of pain intensity and pain interference with cancer patients from several countries. His findings indicated cross-cultural similarity in the self-report ratings. All samples used activity and affect to report how patients reacted to pain. What differed was the focus of interference (e.g., work and activities versus mood and relationships). Therefore, it is important to recognize that ethnic groups may differ in their perception and response to pain, including whether they will approach the caregiver for help. However, there are also many variations *within* groups, and it is important not to stereotype any group.

Numerous factors influence individuals' responses to pain (Box 12-4). One cannot predict how any given person will respond, and value judgments should not be made concerning how a patient responds. It is very important for health professionals to recognize misbeliefs about expected pain responses that prevent effective pain management.

## PATHOPHYSIOLOGY

The pathophysiology of pain includes the processes that are thought to contribute to pathophysiological or persistent pain, i.e., how the nervous system is changed with repeated noxious stimuli. The duration and site of pain determine its clinical manifestations.

### PATHOPHYSIOLOGICAL PAIN

Acute pain results when the sensory endings of primary afferent nerve fibers are activated by strong noxious stimuli, and the brain interprets the input carried by them as painful. This pain is called *nociceptive* as it results from the activity of healthy, intact nociceptive afferent fibers that are aroused only by intense stimuli. Pain that is evoked by repeated or sustained noxious stimuli can sensitize and change the nervous system and is called *pathophysiological* or chronic pain.[16] Three key processes help to explain prolonged or chronic pain problems.[16]

*Peripheral sensitization* occurs when tissue trauma or infection causes sensitization of peripheral nociceptors so that weak, nonpainful stimuli cause pain. An example is sunburn. This process is thought to be mediated by inflammatory mediators such as bradykinins and prostaglandins. Intervention strategies to decrease the inflammatory response, such as ice, nonsteroidal antiinflammatory drugs, and sometimes immobilization of the area using a splint or cast, are essential. *Peripheral neuropathic pain* can arise when otherwise intact sensory neurons become hyperexcitable and

**box 12-4** *Factors That Influence Responses to Pain*

- Meaning of pain to individual person
- Degree of pain perception
- Past experience
- Cultural values
- Social expectations
- Physical and mental health
- Parental attitudes toward pain
- Setting in which pain occurs
- Fear, anxiety
- Usual way of responding to stressors
- Age
- Preparation for pain context
- Health professionals' responses

begin to discharge at abnormal (ectopic) locations along their course. The most important locations of this discharge are at the sites of nerve injury and the associated dorsal root ganglion. Postherpetic neuralgia after shingles is an example. Prevention using early diagnosis of acute herpes zoster, vaccination to prevent chickenpox, and antiviral therapy for acute zoster are being considered. *Central sensitization* involves a progressively increased response to repeated noxious stimuli and hyperexcitability in the dorsal horn (windup). As a result, weak, nonpainful stimuli can cause pain by central amplification (allodynia). For example, surgery can cause central sensitization that increases postoperative pain intensity and the need for analgesia. Administration of opioids before surgery or preemptive analgesia has been shown to reduce windup, resulting in reduced postoperative pain and analgesic requirements.[32,58] Patient-controlled analgesia after surgery helps patients prevent or maintain minimal pain levels and also prevents windup. Central amplification is thought to involve *N*-methyl-D-aspartate (NMDA) receptors and NMDA antagonist drugs such as ketamine and dextromethorphan may help to reduce this.

## LONGEVITY OF PAIN

There are two types of pain syndromes that may occur separately or together: acute and chronic. Unfortunately, many health care professionals do not make this differentiation and provide care for the person experiencing chronic pain as though it were acute pain. There are differences between acute and chronic pain (Table 12-2), and the approaches to pain relief are usually different, although some of the same techniques may be used.

### Acute Pain

Acute pain is essentially a transient episode and informs the person that something is wrong. The onset is usually sudden from a perceived cause, and the painful areas can generally be well identified.

Sudden severe pain activates the autonomic nervous system, which may produce signs of sympathetic overactivity. These signs include tachycardia, increased blood pressure, pupillary dilation, diaphoresis, and stimulation of adrenal medullary secretion. In some situations, such as with severe visceral pain of sudden onset, vasodilation may occur with a subsequent fall in blood pressure and shock. Continuous painful stimulation can also produce a steadily maintained reflex contraction of adjacent or distant muscles, such as abdominal rigidity in persons with intraabdominal pain.

Acute pain is commonly accompanied by increased muscle tension and anxiety, both of which may contribute to increased perception of pain (Figure 12-2). If the pain is moderate or severe, overt physiologic and behavioral signs facilitate assessment of the pain. The person usually seeks pain relief.

### Chronic Pain

Chronic pain persists beyond the usual time for healing and is often present for more than 6 months.[45] Chronic pain may begin as acute pain but then persist (e.g., full-thickness burns), or the onset may be so insidious that the person cannot state specifically when it was first experienced. The source of the pain may be unknown or impossible to determine, such as intractable pain associated with some cancer. The pain sensation can be more diffuse than acute pain so the person is unable to identify a specific pain site. Chronic pain is a major health problem with economic and social implications for both society and the approximately 25% to 30% of the population who suffer from it.[9]

Chronic pain is characterized by irritability (often compounded by insomnia), which leads to decreasing interests and isolation from friends and family.[69] Added to this is the centering of the person's life on the pain experience, with

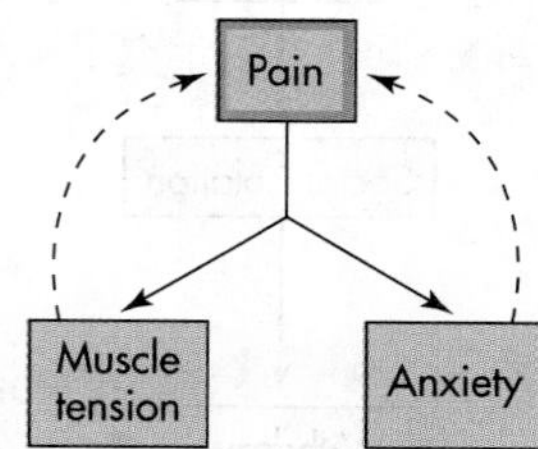


**fig. 12-2** Acute pain.

**table 12-2** *Comparison of Acute and Chronic Pain*

| Characteristic | Acute Pain | Chronic Pain |
|---|---|---|
| Onset | Usually sudden | May be sudden or develop insidiously |
| Duration | Transient (up to 3 months) | Prolonged (months to years) |
| Pain localization | Pain vs. nonpain areas generally well identified | Pain vs. nonpain areas less well identified; intensity becomes more difficult to evaluate (change in sensation) |
| Clinical signs | Signs of sympathetic overactivity (such as increased blood pressure) | Usually no change in vital signs (adaptation) |
| Purpose | Warning that something is wrong | Meaningless; no purpose |
| Pattern | Self-limiting or readily corrected | Continuous or intermittent; intensity may vary or remain constant |
| Prognosis | Likelihood of eventual complete relief | Complete relief usually not possible |

increasing feelings of helplessness and hopelessness as the pain persists. Ultimately the person may withdraw from social interactions (Figure 12-3). Responses to chronic pain can vary, and the unique pattern for each person and family needs to be considered.

The patient's world centers on ways to modify the pain experience. These patients undergo tremendous disruptions in many aspects of their usual activities, including work, family roles, socialization, sleep, and leisure.[62] Some patients go from one physician to another seeking pain relief, which takes time, effort, and money. Even as they seek relief, they often lose faith in the ability of anyone to help them. The lack of continuity of care augments the problem. Physicians often feel helpless when the patient continues to complain of pain. The development of pain clinics and inpatient pain teams has led to successful control of chronic pain for some (but not all) persons. Information about pain centers in the United States and Canada is presented in Box 12-5.

## SPECIFIC TYPES OF PAIN

### Somatic Versus Visceral Pain

Pain may originate in the skin and subcutaneous tissue *(superficial pain)*, in the muscles and bones (deep *somatic pain*), or in the body organs *(visceral pain)*. Somatic and visceral pain differ in their characteristics, particularly in the quality of pain, localization, causes, and accompanying symptoms (Table 12-3).

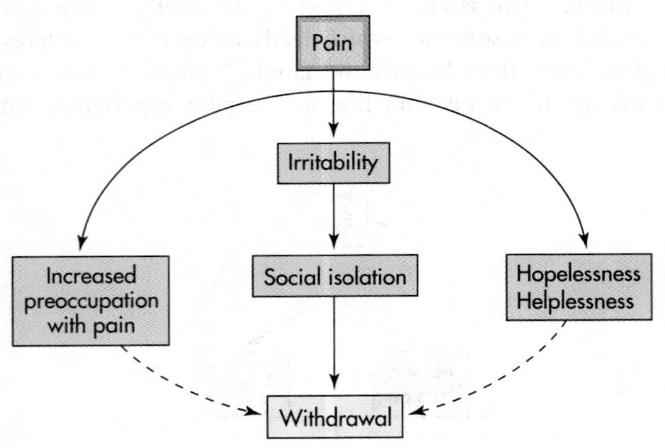


**fig. 12-3** Chronic pain.

### Referred Pain

Referred pain is felt in areas other than those stimulated by injury or disease. For example, the person having a heart attack may complain only of pain radiating down the left arm, when in fact the tissue damage is occurring in the myocardium.

Referred pain occurs most often with damage or injury to the visceral organs, and the pain is referred to cutaneous sur-

**box 12-5** *Organizations Providing Information About Pain-Relief Centers in the United States and Canada*

- American Chronic Pain Association, Box 850, Rockland, CA 95677; (916)632-0922; fax: (916)632-3208; www.members.tripod.com/~widdy/ACPA.html
- National Chronic Pain Outreach Association, 7979 Old Georgetown Rd., Suite 100, Bethesda, MD 20814; (540)997-5004; fax: (540)997-1305; E-mail: ncpoa1@aol.com
- Canadian Pain Society, (416)978-2850; fax: (416)978-8222; www.medicine.dal.ca/gorgs/cps/
- North American Chronic Pain Association of Canada (NAC-PAC), 6 Handel Court, Brampton, Ontario, Canada L6S 14; (905)793-5230; fax: (905)793-8781; E-mail: nacpac@sympatico.ca
- International Association for the Study of Pain, 909 N.E. 43rd St.; Suite 306, Seattle, WA 98105; (206)547-6409; fax (206)547-1703; E-mail: IASP@locke.hs.washington.edu
- American Council for Headache Education, 875 Kings Highway, Suite 200, West Deptford, NJ 08096; (800)255-2243
- The Migraine Association of Canada, Suite 1912, 365 Bloor St., E., Toronto, Ontario M4W 3L4, Canada; (416)920-4916; fax: (416)920-3677; www.migrane.ca; to order information: (800)663-3557; 24-hour information line: (416)920-4917
- Commission for the Accreditation of Rehabilitative Facilities, 101 N. Wilmot Rd., Suite 500, Tucson, AZ 85711; written inquiries preferred

**table 12-3** *Comparison of Superficial, Somatic, and Visceral Pain*

| | Type of Pain | | |
|---|---|---|---|
| | Superficial | Somatic | Visceral |
| Characteristic | Skin and Subcutaneous Tissue | Deep Muscles and Bones | Internal Organs |
| Quality | Sharp, pricking, burning | Sharp or dull and aching | Sharp or dull and aching, cramping |
| Localization | Good | Poor | Poor |
| Referred pain | No | No | Yes |
| Provoking stimuli | Cut, abrasion, excessive heat or cold, chemicals | Cut, pressure, heat, ischemia, displacement (bone) | Distention, ischemia, spasms, chemical irritants (no cutting) |
| Autonomic reactions | No | Yes | Yes |
| Reflex muscle contractions | No | Yes | Yes |

faces (Figure 12-4). The origin of referred pain is complex and not clearly understood and may relate to one or more of the following[44]:

1. Referred pain usually occurs in structures that developed from the same embryonic dermatome.
2. Visceral and somatic nerves enter the nervous system at the same spinal level and share the same spinothalamic tracts.
3. Somatic pain is more common, and the person has "learned" to interpret signals conducted on certain pathways as being somatic in origin.

The cutaneous pattern of various types of referred pain is fairly constant and frequently seen in practice. The nurse should be able to recognize the possibility of visceral organ disease in patients who complain of cutaneous pain.

### Psychogenic Pain

The term *psychogenic pain* has been used to describe pain for which no pathological condition has been found or in which the pain appears to have a greater psychological basis than a physical one.[45] A caution here is that diagnostic tests are not definitive measures and may not be sophisticated enough to detect all pathophysiological changes. Distinguishing between physical and emotional components of pain is difficult, and it is important to remember that *all pain is real.*

### Neuropathic Pain

Neuropathic pain arises from injury to the nervous system and can occur in different forms. Sharp, spasmlike pain can occur along the course of one or more nerves, such as the trigeminal nerve in the face and the sciatic nerve in the lower trunk. Severe burning pain can be associated with injury to a peripheral nerve in the extremities. As a result, the patient may go to great lengths to protect against irritating stimuli, which may be something as simple as the noise of a plane overhead.

*Phantom limb pain* is pain experienced in a surgically removed extremity. This problem is more likely to develop in those who had significant pain before amputation, and it may persist long after healing has occurred. This phenomenon has only recently been successfully prevented in the postoperative period by the administration of effective preemptive analgesia before surgery. Refer to Chapter 27 for a discussion of the management of amputation.

## COLLABORATIVE CARE MANAGEMENT

### PHARMACOLOGIC APPROACHES

### Analgesics

Two groups of analgesics, as well as adjuvant medications, are important components of effective pain management. *Opioid analgesics,* such as morphine, act mainly on the central nervous system to alter the perception of pain. *Nonopioid analgesics,* such as aspirin, block impulses mainly in the periphery and decrease inflammation-related pain by inhibiting the synthesis of prostaglandins. For some types of pain, such as pain with bone cancer, analgesics from both groups are necessary. Adjuvant medications such as diazepam (Valium) relieve pain—for example, muscle spasms—or decrease the side effects associated with some analgesics, particularly opioids.[52]

Standard doses are helpful guidelines for analgesic prescription and administration. However, they need to be evaluated for each individual patient. Although most nurses do not prescribe analgesics, they do make administration choices

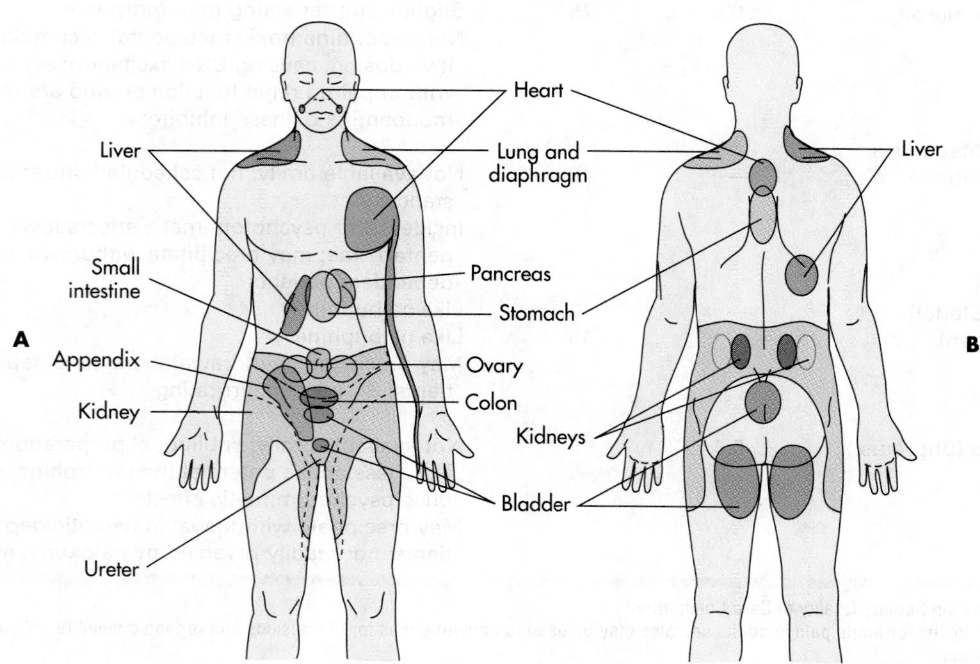


fig. 12-4 Usual sites of referred pain. **A,** Front. **B,** Back.

about the type, dose, and frequency when drug options are given. Nurses are also responsible for evaluating the effectiveness of the medication, including side effects, and for advocating change when needed. It is important to understand the concept of an equianalgesic dose. An equianalgesic dose is the dose of one analgesic that has the same pain-relieving effect as another drug. This concept makes it possible to change one analgesic for another, or to change the route of administration, for example from parenteral to oral opioid doses. It also allows comparisons to be made between weak analgesics such as codeine for mild pain versus stronger analgesics such as morphine for moderate to severe pain. Equianalgesic doses of common opioids are presented in Table 12-4.

### Opioid analgesics

Opioid analgesics can be classified according to the strength of their effect; for example codeine is a weak opioid and morphine is a strong opioid. They are also classified as agonist, antagonist, or mixed agonist-antagonist opioids, depending on their effect at mu, delta, and kappa receptor sites. For example, morphine is an agonist as it binds to and activates the receptors, mainly mu, to produce analgesia. Antagonist opioids, such as naloxone, bind to a receptor without activating it; they also block and displace agonist opioids such as morphine and prevent their analgesic effect. Butorphanol (Stadol) is an example of a mixed agonist-antagonist that acts like naloxone when given to someone who is taking an agonist

**table 12-4** *Equianalgesic Doses of Opioids Commonly Used for Severe Pain*

| Name | Equianalgesic Dose (mg) | | Comments |
|---|---|---|---|
| | Oral | Parenteral* | |
| **Morphinelike agonists** | | | |
| Morphine | 30† | 10 | Standard of comparison for narcotic analgesics; sustained-release preparations (MS Contin, Oramorph-SR) release drug over 8-12 hours |
| Hydromorphone (Dilaudid) | 7.5 | 1.5 | Slightly shorter duration than morphine |
| Oxycodone | 30 | — | |
| Methadone (Dolophine) | 20 | 10 | Good oral potency; long plasma half-life (24-36 hours)<br>Accumulates with repetitive dosing, causing excessive sedation (on days 2-5) |
| Levorphanol (Levo-Dromoran) | 4 | 2 | Long plasma half-life (12-16 hours)<br>Accumulates on days 2-3 |
| Fentanyl | — | 0.1 | Transdermal fentanyl (Duragesic) 25-50 μg/hour roughly equivalent to 30 mg sustained-release morphine q8hr<br>Because of skin reservoir of drug, 12-hour delay in onset and offset of transdermal patch; fever increases dose rate |
| Oxymorphone (Numorphan) | — | 1 | 5 mg rectal suppository = 5 mg morphine IM |
| Meperidine (Demerol) | 300 | 75 | Slightly shorter acting than morphine<br>Normeperidine (toxic metabolite) accumulates with repetitive dosing, causing CNS excitation; avoid in patients with impaired renal function or who are receiving monoamine oxidase inhibitors |
| **Mixed agonist-antagonists** | | | |
| Nalbuphine (Nubain) | — | 10 | Not available orally; not scheduled under Controlled Substances Act<br>Incidence of psychotomimetic effects lower than with pentazocine; may precipitate withdrawal in narcotic-dependent patients |
| Butorphanol (Stadol) | — | 2 | Like nalbuphine |
| Dezocine (Dalgan) | — | 10 | Like nalbuphine<br>May precipitate withdrawal in narcotic-dependent patients; SC injection irritating |
| **Partial agonists** | | | |
| Buprenorphine (Buprenex) | 0.4 | | Not available orally; sublingual preparation not yet in U.S.; less abuse potential than morphine; does not produce psychotomimetic effects<br>May precipitate withdrawal in narcotic-dependent patients; not readily reversed by naloxone; avoid in labor |

Adapted from American Pain Society Quality of Care Committee.[5]

*These are standard IM doses for acute pain in adults and also may be used to convert doses for IV infusions and repeated small IV boluses. For single IV boluses, use half the IM dose.

†Some experts argue that 60 mg of oral morphine is the more accurate equivalent dose and suggest caution in converting patients from high doses of oral morphine to other drugs if the 30-mg equivalent is used.

like morphine on a regular basis. Therefore, people receiving agonist opioids should not be given concurrent agonist-antagonist opioids or a state of withdrawal will result. Confusion, hallucinations, and an analgesic ceiling effect can result from mixed agonist-antagonists such as pentazocine (Talwin), which is no longer a recommended drug.

Opioid analgesics are the most effective analgesics for the relief of moderate to severe pain. They must be given on a regular basis to prevent pain from recurring. Side effects of opioids vary with the physiological state of the patient. Constipation is the most common side effect. Naloxone (Narcan) will reverse any depressive effect.

When opioids are administered, it is important to distinguish between the effects of tolerance, dependence, and addiction as noted here:

Tolerance: Larger doses needed to produce the same analgesic effects

Dependence: Need to continue use of drug to prevent symptoms of withdrawal

Addiction: Behavioral pattern of compulsive drug use; drug used for psychological effect

Drug tolerance occurs with some patients and with some conditions, usually when the patient's pain is first being controlled and/or when the pain increases. This is a physiological response and requires increasing the dose until pain relief is attained. The dose can be steadily increased because there is no ceiling or maximum amount of opioid that can be given. Physical dependence and drug tolerance are involuntary behaviors and are the physiological result of frequent ongoing opioid administration. Although physical dependence and tolerance develop, symptoms of withdrawal rarely occur because, as pain decreases, the dosage is gradually tapered and no symptoms are experienced. Physical dependence and drug tolerance do not represent addiction, and the fear of addiction should not prevent opioid administration, because addiction in hospitalized patients rarely occurs.

### Administration routes

Opioids can be administered by a variety of routes. The oral route is preferred unless the patient is vomiting, is unable or not permitted to swallow, or is in acute pain. Slow-release preparations, such as MS Contin, are given every 8 to 12 hours, allowing less focus on the pain and better control with fewer side effects. In addition to intramuscular and subcutaneous injection, opioids can also be administered rectally, transdermally, sublingually, epidurally, and intravenously.[3,29,52,55] When intravenous access is not possible, sublingual and rectal routes should be considered as alternatives to injections.[2]

Epidural infusions of opioids such as morphine or fentanyl can be administered through a catheter placed in the epidural or intrathecal space by the physician (Figure 12-5). An infusion device attached to the line provides a continuous supply of the opioid. This method relieves pain without diminishing CNS function. Patients with intractable pain can be well managed at home using this route.[41]

Epidural administration is extremely effective, but patients still experience the common related side effects of opioid administration. See the Guidelines for Care Box on p. 342 for a summary of side effect management. In addition patients frequently complain of pruritis (itching), which can be severe. Antihistamines and comfort measures are effective for many patients, but it is occasionally necessary to reduce the opioid dosage or administer low-dose naloxone (Narcan), which generally controls the itching without reversing the analgesic effect.

*Patient-controlled analgesia (PCA)* is a method that allows patients to administer their own opioids whenever they feel it is necessary. PCA may involve oral medications or an infusion system with a pump. With a PCA pump, the patient pushes a button to release a set amount of opioid by bolus intravenously, subcutaneously, or epidurally. A refractory period prevents delivery of another bolus before a preset time interval. The device

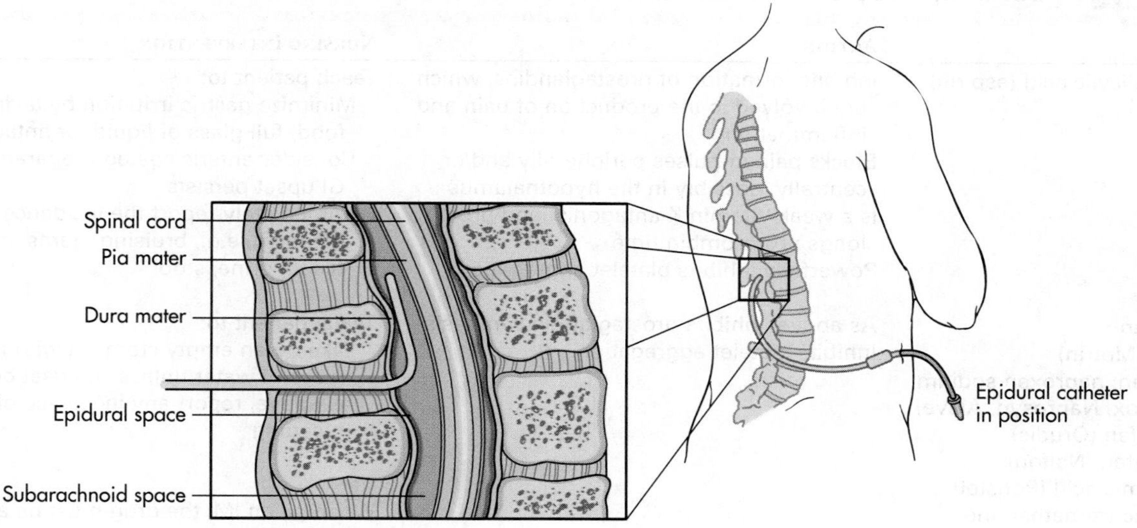


**fig. 12-5** Site of epidural catheter placement.

also records the patient's attempts to receive the opioid in a given time period. A suggested protocol[2] for intravenous PCA includes loading doses such as 3 to 5 mg of morphine, repeated every 5 minutes until the pain is decreased. On-demand doses are usually 0.5 to 1.5 mg of morphine every 6 minutes to a maximum of 10 mg/hr. With shorter hospital stays, patients need to be given oral analgesics as soon as possible and have their pain well managed before discharge. Equianalgesic oral opioids can be started before or when the last PCA dose is given.

People using PCA tend to take less total analgesia than those receiving intramuscular injections.[3,24,52] PCA is used for the management of postoperative pain, other types of acute pain such as sickle cell crisis, and for cancer pain.[24,52]

### *Nonopioid analgesics*

Mild to moderate pain generally can be controlled by nonopioid analgesics, most commonly nonsteroidal antiinflammatory agents such as aspirin, and by acetaminophen.

Acetaminophen (Tylenol, Datril) is comparable to aspirin in analgesic effect, but it does not have any antiinflammatory action. It does not alter the prothrombin level and has fewer side effects, but overdoses can cause severe liver damage. This analgesic is useful for persons who are allergic to aspirin and for whom aspirin is contraindicated, such as persons with peptic ulcers.

The nonsteroidal antiinflammatory drugs (NSAIDs) are the most widely used analgesics because of their general lack of serious side effects and their effectiveness in pain relief.[3,29,52] They act primarily by inhibiting prostaglandin synthesis. Prostaglandins "sensitize" nerve endings and trigger pain. In lower doses these drugs have analgesic properties; in higher doses there is antiinflammatory action in addition to analgesia. NSAIDs are used to control moderate pain of dysmenorrhea, arthritis and other musculoskeletal disorders, postoperative pain, and migraine headaches. They may be used for patients with bone cancer. NSAIDs commonly used for pain management are listed Table 12-5.

NSAIDs and particularly acetylsalicylic acid (aspirin) inhibit platelet aggregation and increase bleeding time. Common side effects include gastrointestinal disturbances, dizziness, tinnitus, and headache. Persons who are hypersensitive to aspirin also may be hypersensitive to other NSAIDs. In addition to blocking prostaglandin synthesis, salicylates also produce analgesia by blocking pain impulses peripherally or centrally, possibly in the hypothalamus. Aspirin is also a weak vitamin K antagonist. It prolongs prothrombin time when given in large doses. Therefore it is contraindicated for persons receiving anticoagulant drugs.

Irritation of the gastric mucosa is a common side effect of NSAIDs, and these drugs should be taken with a full glass of water. If gastric irritation occurs, they should be taken with meals or with a snack such as a glass of milk. Persons with a history of peptic ulcer usually should avoid taking them. Aspirin should be avoided by children and teenagers because of the risk of Reye's syndrome.

### *Adjuvant medications*

Adjuvant drugs may be given *along with* analgesics to augment pain relief.[3,29] They also may be an option for pain relief when other analgesics are not effective.

Sedatives and antianxiety agents sometimes are prescribed for persons with pain. These drugs do not have any analgesic effect but may permit relaxation and decrease anxiety and thus prevent an increase in pain. The drugs may permit the person to sleep and thus be better able to cope with the pain. Phenothiazines such as promethazine (Phenergan) do *not* potentiate the analgesic effect of opioids. However they do increase opioid-related sedation, hypertension, and respiratory depression and should not be used for pain relief.[29] In some

**table 12-5** Common Medications for **Mild to Moderate Pain**

| Drug | Action | Nursing Intervention |
|---|---|---|
| Acetylsalicylic acid (aspirin) | Inhibits formation of prostaglandins, which are involved in the production of pain and inflammation<br>Blocks pain impulses peripherally and/or centrally, possibly in the hypothalamus<br>Is a weak Vitamin K antagonist and prolongs prothrombin time<br>Powerfully inhibits platelet aggregation | Teach patient to:<br>Minimize gastric irritation by taking with food, full glass of liquid, or antacid<br>Consider enteric coated preparations if GI upset persists<br>Immediately report the incidence of any bleeding, e.g., bruising, gums, nose bleed, urine, stool |
| Ibuprofen (Advil, Motrin)<br>Naproxen, naproxen sodium (Anaprox, Naprosyn, Aleve)<br>Ketoprofen (Orudis)<br>Fenoprofen (Nalfon)<br>Mefenamic acid (Ponstel) | As above, inhibits prostaglandin synthesis<br>Inhibits platelet aggregation | Teach patient to:<br>Take on an empty stomach with a full glass of water unless GI upset occurs<br>As above, report any incidence of bleeding |
| Ketoralac tromethamine (Toradol) | | When given IM, the drug must be administered deeply into a large muscle |

persons sedatives and antianxiety agents may lead to disorientation and agitation, which can increase the pain and decrease the person's ability to cope. Treating pain with analgesics is the more effective and preferred method.

Tricyclic antidepressants, such as amitriptyline (Elavil), produce analgesia at doses lower than those used for depression. These drugs are useful in nerve injury pain, such as with postherpetic neuralgia (shingles). They are believed to prevent the uptake of serotonin and norepinephrine in the descending inhibitory modulation in the spinal cord and reduce sensitization mechanisms. Low doses are used for analgesia (average = 70 mg daily).[67]

Anticonvulsants such as phenytoin (Dilantin) and carbamazepine (Tegretol) are used to suppress abnormal (ectopic) nerve discharges that occur in nerve injury pain such as trigeminal neuralgia.[29]

Corticosteroids such as dexamethasone (Decadron) are helpful in relieving pain from increased intracranial pressure, nerve compression, spinal cord compression, and bone metastases. They block the production of arachidonic acid, which is necessary for the synthesis of prostaglandins and other inflammatory chemicals that cause pain.[29] These drugs also stimulate appetite and may elevate mood.

Counterirritants are over-the-counter drugs that relieve local pain by producing counterirritation (stimulation of the large A-beta fibers). Examples of counterirritants include ointments containing methylsalicylate (oil of wintergreen) or ethyl aminobenzoate and oil of cloves (for toothaches).

## NONPHARMACOLOGICAL APPROACHES

Nonpharmacological approaches can be used along with analgesics for effective pain management.[3,22] This type of intervention can alter pain transmission, modify the response to pain, and modify the pain stimulus. Physical strategies that are invasive and/or non-nursing acts will be discussed in this section. Nursing measures will be discussed under Nursing Management.

### Altering pain transmission

#### Electrical stimulators

The purpose of electrical stimulators is to modify the pain stimulus by blocking or changing the painful stimulus with stimulation perceived as less painful. The gate control theory suggests that stimulating large myelinated A-beta fibers closes the "gate" to pain stimuli.[44] Selected forms of electrical stimulation may activate the descending inhibitory system.

Transcutaneous electrical nerve stimulation (TENS) uses a battery-powered stimulator worn externally. This convenient, nonintrusive, nonaddictive type of pain therapy can be learned easily by the patient. Success is variable, and the device is usually used along with other pain therapies.

A number of TENS devices are on the market; all consist of a battery-powered portable pulse generator about the size of a pocket pager. Control knobs on the generator permit adjustment of the impulse. The generator is connected by a pair of cables to electrically conductive tape electrodes placed at appropriate sites on the skin. TENS delivers a balanced biphasic potential in a waveform.

TENS appears to be most useful for postoperative pain, posttraumatic pain, phantom limb pain, peripheral neuralgias, low back pain, and muscle pain. Although it can be effective with mild or moderate pain, it is less effective for severe pain.[65] Nurses are responsible for monitoring the effectiveness of treatments and for patient teaching concerning the safe use of TENS (see the Patient/Family Teaching Box).

TENS electrodes should not be placed over hair, irritated skin, sutures, the carotid sinus (may produce bradycardia), laryngeal or pharyngeal muscles (may trigger spasms), or the uterus of a pregnant woman. A cardiac pacemaker may interfere with TENS effects. Suggested electrode placement may include (1) directly over the painful area, (2) at trigger points along the nerve pathways, or (3) at trigger points in the same dermatome as the pain. Spinal cord stimulators are similar to TENS except that they are intrusive procedures. Instead of electrode placement on the skin, the electrodes are placed on or near the spinal cord. This is achieved either surgically over the ventral surface of the spinal cord or percutaneously through the back into the epidural space. Because the percutaneously inserted spinal cord electrical stimulator can be inserted under local anesthesia, it is preferred over surgical placement of dorsal column stimulator electrodes. Postoperative care after dorsal column stimulator implantation includes the same care that follows laminectomy, with monitoring for infection and leakage of cerebrospinal fluid (see Chapter 61).

#### Nerve block

A nerve block involves the injection of substances such as local anesthetics or neurolytic agents (e.g., alcohol or phenol) close to nerves to block the conduction of impulses. Nerve blocks frequently are used for the symptomatic relief of pain. They are used to treat chronic pain associated with peripheral vascular disease, trigeminal neuralgia, causalgia, and cancer.

#### Acupuncture

Acupuncture is an ancient form of disease treatment that can be used for pain relief. Only recently has the method been used in Western countries. Small needles are skillfully inserted and manipulated at specific body points, depending on the type and location of pain. The gate control theory provides the best explanation for the effectiveness of acupuncture. The

**patient/family teaching**

**The Use of TENS**

Teach patients to:

1. Remove and clean electrodes daily.
2. Wash skin with soap and water.
3. Allow skin to air dry.
4. Wipe skin with a prep pad before reapplying the conductor pad.
5. Check the battery if numbness or tingling is not felt during treatments.
6. Report if sensation is either absent or uncomfortable.

local stimulation of large-diameter fibers by the needles "closes the gate" to pain. It is not known to what extent the psyche and the power of suggestion contribute to the effectiveness of this therapy.

#### Neurosurgical procedures

Neurosurgical procedures do not play a major role in management of chronic pain. Major limitations include short duration of relief, occurrence of dysesthesia (pain induced by gentle touch of the skin), central pain syndrome (burning sensations in skin areas lacking sensation from surgical afferent interruptions), and possible further neurological dysfunction.[38] However, constant, relentless chronic pain cannot be controlled by analgesics *(intractable pain)*; various neurosurgical procedures may be used to reduce or eliminate the pain (Box 12-6).[52] Other forms of pain control usually are attempted before neurosurgical intervention.

**box 12-6** *Neurosurgical Procedures for Pain Control*

NEURECTOMY
Severing of nerve fibers from the cell body

RHIZOTOMY
Resection of posterior nerve root before it enters spinal cord

CORDOTOMY
Severing of ascending anterolateral pain-conducting pathways of spinal cord

SYMPATHECTOMY
Excision or destruction of one or more sympathetic ganglia or nerves

### Modifying Pain Response

A wide range of strategies are available for modifying the pain response. Many of these strategies are within the realm of independent nursing practice and are discussed in the following section. Others may be used by nurses with special training but are frequently interventions used by other members of the collaborative care team.

#### Behavior modification

Behavior modification consists of a planned change in the way a person behaves by means of rewarding desired behavior and ignoring undesirable behavior. Forms of behavior modification are used unconsciously all the time: a young child "throwing a tantrum" may be ignored, but as his behavior becomes more appropriate, his mother may reward him with her time and attention.

Behavior modification may be useful for persons with chronic pain. For example, one protocol for patients with chronic low back pain is to set a limit of 10 minutes daily for discussion of their pain experiences (with the exception of data-gathering interviews). Pain medications are prescribed on a regular schedule to dissociate the feelings of pain with inappropriate use (reward) of analgesics or other unhealthy behaviors.

In using behavioral methods to alter pain-associated behavior or to encourage patient activities, success will occur only with a consistent approach on the part of the health care team. Although patients should always be praised for their efforts to comply or assist with treatment regimens, a true behavior modification program requires careful analysis of patient behavior and the development of a specific and comprehensive treatment plan.

#### Biofeedback and autogenic training

Some persons are able to alter their body functions through mental concentration. In biofeedback training a machine that monitors brain wave activity (electroencephalograph) is used. The individual concentrates on slowing his or her brain wave activity to rates at which pain and distress are unlikely to cause discomfort (i.e., complete relaxation). It may take many months of regular practice to achieve the desired level of control. The nurse should encourage and praise the person's efforts.

In autogenic training the same type of self-regulation is used to alter various autonomic nervous system functions, such as pulse, blood pressure, and muscle tension. The use of transcendental meditation and other methods of concentration and self-control may achieve the same degree of autoregulation without the use of sophisticated physiological monitoring equipment.

#### Hypnosis

Hypnosis may be used in the treatment of various conditions, particularly when these conditions are aggravated by tension and stress. Patients are helped to alter their perception of pain through the acceptance of positive suggestions made to the subconscious. Many persons are able to learn self-hypnosis. Individuals vary widely in their suggestibility and readiness to try this approach. The nurse's most helpful role may be to support the patient's desire to make hypnosis work.

## NURSING MANAGEMENT

### ■ ASSESSMENT

Effective pain management can occur only when systematic and regular assessments take place. It is important for nurses to assess both subjective and objective data at least once a shift and sometimes more frequently when pain is anticipated.[23] Patient input is very important, and it is unfortunate that research has shown that health professionals document patients' pain differently than do patients themselves.[14,18,27,53,70,73] It is crucial to gather as much information from patients as possible to avoid making incorrect assumptions about the pain they are or are not experiencing. A variety of pain assessment tools are available.[17,38]

Although many patients continue to experience postoperative pain, many will not ask for help[70] (see the Research Box).

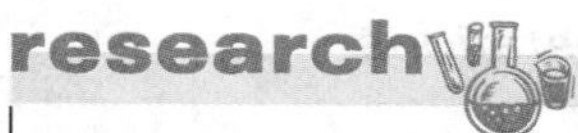

Reference: Ward S, Gordon D: Patient satisfaction and pain severity as outcomes in pain management: a longitudinal view of one setting's experience, *J Pain Symptom Manage* 11:242-251, 1996.

This study explored the reasons why patients were satisfied with their care even when they were in pain. Data were collected from patients during inpatient admission or ambulatory clinic visits (n = 306), telephone interviews of patients after discharge (n = 869), and chart reviews (n = 112). Findings were compared with baseline data obtained 2 years previously before the implementation of pain education programs. Results revealed little change from baseline data. The majority of patients were satisfied with their pain management despite severe pain ratings averaging 7 on a 0 to 10 scale. Almost all orders continued to be written for "as needed" administration. The researchers concluded that patients may have been satisfied with the cyclical pattern of pain relief that occurs with as needed administration. Patients may know they will get relief when the medication is given, although they will not ask until the pain is severe. One needs to be cautious when interpreting satisfaction ratings in isolation from other data. A recommendation of the study is to teach patients about the benefits of scheduled dosing.

For this reason it is best to use a rating scale (e.g., 0 to 10 scale where 0 is no pain and 10 is the worst possible pain) to validate the pain patients are experiencing. The patient's rating of pain intensity is assessed and recorded both before and 1 hour after any analgesic is given. If the pain intensity does not decrease after the analgesic, factors such as the adequacy and timing of the dose and a need for change in dose are assessed.

### Subjective Data

Before pain occurs, it is useful to obtain data concerning the patient's expectation for pain relief. Many persons are unaware that they are expected to speak out when they have pain or discomfort. Some patients think they will be considered "complainers" or "bad patients" if they state that they are in pain.[64]

It is distressing to note that most patients in several studies did not expect to have their pain relieved.[11,36,50] Patients need to be asked on admission about their expectations, knowledge, and concerns about pain. They should then be taught how and when to verbalize their discomfort and the various methods available for pain relief. As already mentioned, the best assessment of pain is the patient's own evaluation.

Data to be collected by the nurse include the location, intensity, quality, timing (onset, duration, frequency, cause), and aggravating and relieving factors. One approach for evaluating these characteristics is the use of the mnemonic PQRST:

**P** provoking factors: what makes the pain worse or relieves it
**Q** quality: dull, sharp, crushing
**R** region or radiation: site and radiation to other areas
**S** severity or intensity
**T** time: onset, duration, frequency, cause

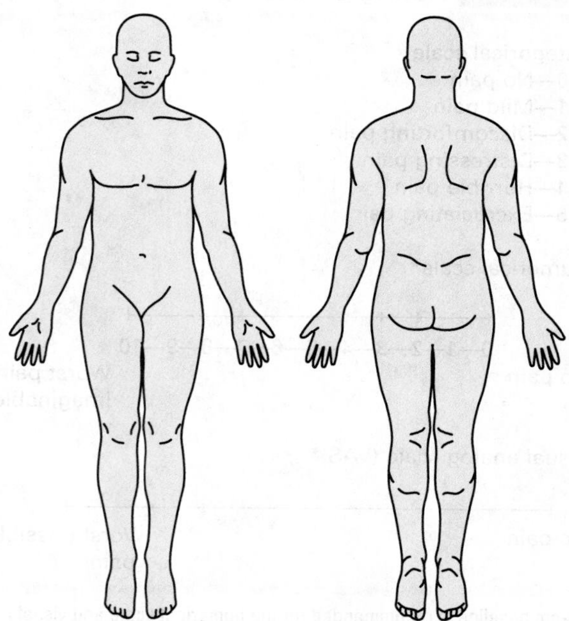

**fig. 12-6** Body diagrams for pointing out sites of pain.

Diagrams of the body can help patients point out the sites of their pain (Figure 12-6). Pain intensity can be assessed using several measures as outlined in Box 12-7. An efficient, reliable, and valid approach is to ask the patient to use a numerical rating to describe the pain or discomfort: 0 (no pain) to 10 (worst pain possible). Ratings need to be documented and intervention options discussed for ratings greater than 3. Ratings can be recorded on a vital sign sheet similar to temperature and blood pressure data. More detailed flow sheets are also helpful to provide ongoing assessment of progression of the pain and the response to various interventions (Figure 12-7). Pain intensity should be assessed at least once a shift or more often if the patient rated his or her pain at 4 or greater (0 to 10) and is receiving interventions for pain (such as analgesics, relaxation exercises, or TENS). When acute pain has subsided, further data can be collected about the meaning of pain for the person. Long-term pain requires a much more in-depth assessment. Hospitals or pain clinics that use a team approach in providing care to the person with chronic pain often develop their own pain history form or questionnaire. This history may be collected by one or more health team members. Types of data collected to assess a patient experiencing chronic pain include:

- Demographic data
- Sociocultural data
- History of the pain pattern from time of onset
- Factors perceived to increase or decrease the pain
- Effects of the pain on the person's lifestyle including work, family responsibilities, sexuality, leisure, sleep, nutrition, and activity.
- Meaning of the pain for the person

**box 12-7** *Examples of Pain Intensity Rating Scales*

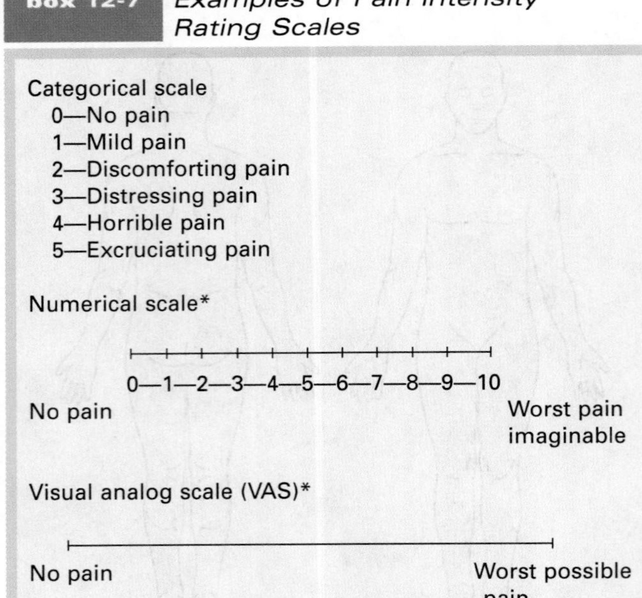

Categorical scale
- 0—No pain
- 1—Mild pain
- 2—Discomforting pain
- 3—Distressing pain
- 4—Horrible pain
- 5—Excruciating pain

Numerical scale*

0—1—2—3—4—5—6—7—8—9—10

No pain — Worst pain imaginable

Visual analog scale (VAS)*

No pain — Worst possible pain

*A 10-cm baseline is recommended for the numerical scale and visual analog scale.

Effects of the patient's pain on other family members or friends

Measures used in the past and present for relief of pain and their effectiveness

### Objective Data

Objective data help the nurse identify possible pain or discomfort in a person who has not reported pain or is unable to do so (Box 12-8). Objective signs of pain are of two types: physiological and behavioral. Physiological signs of pain result from activation of the sympathetic nervous system. With very severe pain, neurogenic shock may result from the stress to the system. The behavioral signs are not specific to pain; therefore, if the observable data suggest that pain may be present, subjective data must be elicited to validate the assumption where possible.

Specific objective data to be collected to assess the patient's pain include:

Appearance (grimacing, gritting teeth, clenching fists, lying rigidly as if afraid to move)
Motor behavior
Affective and verbal responses
Vital signs
Skin moisture and color
Inspection and gentle palpation of painful area; identify trigger points that initiate pain, if present

Sometimes the patient's behavior does not seem to match his or her verbalization of pain. For example, the patient may request an analgesic, a back rub, or other measure to relieve pain, but when the nurse arrives to carry out the request, the patient is found to be asleep. It must be emphasized here that the patient who is sleeping or lying quietly is not necessarily pain free. The patient may be exhausted from the pain, and sleeping is a coping mechanism. Patients may also use distraction such as talking and joking with visitors to manage unrelieved pain. The person's self-report of pain is the key to effective management.

Physiological signs of pain can disappear quickly after only hours for the person with acute pain and are typically not present with chronic pain because of the body's compensatory mechanisms. Although there is adaptation to the pain stimuli, the pain persists. The absence of physiologic signs, therefore, does not indicate absence of pain. Prolonged pain, however, may create changes in the person's appearance over time, perhaps as a result of decreased activity, decreased appetite, lack of sleep, or lack of interest in appearance because of fatigue or depression.

Behavioral responses to chronic pain are varied and unique to the individual person. Here, also, there may be few overt signs to indicate the presence of pain. Changes usually occur in daily patterns related to sleeping, eating, socialization, and libido. If the person is extremely depressed because of the ongoing pain, withdrawal behaviors may be noted.

**box 12-8** *Clinical Manifestations of Acute Pain*

| PHYSIOLOGICAL SIGNS | BEHAVIORAL SIGNS |
|---|---|
| Pulse: increased rate | Rigid body position |
| Respirations: increased depth and frequency | Restlessness |
| | Frowning |
| Blood pressure: increased systolic and diastolic | Clenched teeth |
| | Clenched fists |
| Diaphoresis, pallor | Crying |
| Dilated pupils | Moaning |
| Muscle tension (face, body) | |
| Nausea and vomiting (if pain is severe) | |

## NURSING DIAGNOSES

Nursing diagnoses are determined from analysis of patient data. Nursing diagnoses for the patient with pain include the following direct nursing diagnoses but can also include a wide variety of associated diagnoses that reflect the patient's unique experience and response to the pain.

| Diagnostic Title | Possible Etiological Factors |
|---|---|
| Pain | Tissue pressure, inflammation, trauma or effects of surgery and other treatments |
| Chronic pain | Nervous system sensitization from factors listed for pain; actual etiology unclear |
| Knowledge deficit: pain management strategies | Lack of previous instruction, misunderstanding |

Examples of other pain related diagnoses that may be appropriate after subjective and objective data analysis include:

Activity intolerance
Anxiety

**FLOW SHEET — PAIN**

Patient ______________________________ Date ______________

*Pain rating scale used ______________________________

Purpose: To evaluate the safety and effectiveness of the analgesic(s).

Analgesic(s) ordered: ______________________________

| Time | Pain rating* | Analgesic | R | P | BP | Level of arousal† | Other‡ | Plan and comments |
|---|---|---|---|---|---|---|---|---|
| | | | | | | | | |
| | | | | | | | | |
| | | | | | | | | |
| | | | | | | | | |
| | | | | | | | | |
| | | | | | | | | |
| | | | | | | | | |
| | | | | | | | | |
| | | | | | | | | |
| | | | | | | | | |
| | | | | | | | | |
| | | | | | | | | |
| | | | | | | | | |
| | | | | | | | | |
| | | | | | | | | |
| | | | | | | | | |

* Pain rating: A number of different scales may be used. Indicate which scale is used and use the same one each time. Two common examples:
- 0 to 10 with 0 being no pain and 10 being as bad as it can be.
- Melzack's scale:
 0 = no pain; 1 = mild; 2 = discomforting; 3 = distressing; 4 = horrible; 5 = excruciating

† Possible arousal scale: 1 = wide awake; 2 = drowsy; 3 = sleeping; 4 = difficult to arouse

‡ Possibilities for other columns: bowel function, activities, nausea and vomiting, other pain relief measures. Identify the side effects of greatest concern to patient, family, physician, nurses, etc.

**fig. 12-7** Flow sheet for monitoring patient's response to pain.

Breathing pattern, ineffective
Constipation
Fatigue
Hopelessness
Powerlessness
Self-care deficit
Sexual dysfunction
Sleep-pattern disturbance
Social isolation

## EXPECTED PATIENT OUTCOMES

Expected patient outcomes for the patient experiencing pain may include but are not limited to:

1a. States that pain is decreased to a low rating (e.g., ≤4) on a scale of 0 to 10 (0, no pain; 10, most severe pain imaginable).

b. Demonstrates relaxed facial expression and body position and participates in activities.

c. Discusses concerns about asking for help and taking analgesics.

2. The person with *chronic pain* can
   a. State plans to participate in ongoing therapies.
   b. State plans for increasing independence in activities in daily living.
   c. Identify supports for encouragement and help.

3a. Verbalizes factors that alter the pain and effective control measures.
   b. If future pain is a possibility when patient is discharged, patient or significant other can
      1. Explain how, when, and for how long to apply heat or ice or to exercise to relieve pain.
      2. Explain prescribed medications (actions, dosages, frequency, side effects).
      3. Describe when to seek medical assistance if pain is not relieved as expected.

## INTERVENTIONS

Pain is a complex experience involving sensory, affective, and behavioral components that require a multimodal treatment approach. Pain such as muscle spasms in the lower back may be relieved more effectively by heat and ultrasound than by medications. However, strategies such as breathing exercises, muscle relaxation, imagery, and distraction do not replace analgesics for patients who need pharmacological management, but they can be useful adjuncts in reducing the dose of medication required and in decreasing the pain while the patient waits for pain medication to work. Because pain is multidimensional, encouraging patients to use a broad range of pain relief methods will result in more effective pain management.

### Planning for Pain Management

The nurse's role in planning and monitoring outcomes of care is critical to effective pain management. The initial thorough assessment serves as the foundation on which priorities are established and treatment strategies are devised. The Guidelines for Care Box contains some basic principles of pain management to guide the planning period.[3] The patient's ability and desire to be active or passive in using pain relief measures will need to be considered. Decreased ability results from severe pain, fatigue, sedation, depression, or unconsciousness. Decreased will occurs with some persons with chronic pain who have experienced numerous failures in pain relief. The nurse is able to function independently with many interventions, but careful planning with other members of the health care team is necessary to ensure that all have the same patient outcomes or goals in mind. The patient and family are included in all planning activities if possible.

One aspect of the treatment plan that often is forgotten or omitted is the incorporation of measures the patient thinks may help relieve the pain, even if these measures differ from those usually carried out in that institution. Without encouragement, the patient may hesitate to mention these possible remedies—for example, nonprescription liniments, special applications of heat and cold, unusual positioning, or favorite homemade foods or drinks. If there are no contraindications to the remedy the patient wishes to try, the health care team may consider using it before trying other relief measures.

Current time and staffing constraints can make planning difficult. In addition, patient stays in hospital are shorter or nonexistent. However, planning for the same health care team members to care for the patient regularly would help to ensure a more consistent approach and plan of care. The small group of health care team members and the patient can develop a plan of care in which the patient's decisions are honored, and a daily routine can be developed that will reduce anxiety and frustration about constant changes. The plan should include, if appropriate, items such as specified hours for analgesic administration before uncomfortable procedures, specified blocks of time for rest or napping, and coordination between various departments, such as physical therapy and occupational therapy. For some patients fatigue is a great problem and regular visits to off-unit departments should be interspersed with rest periods; for other patients the most beneficial plan includes ensuring that they go directly from one department to the next so that time is not wasted getting in and out of bed or performing other painful maneuvers.

**guidelines for care**

**ABC Principles of Pain Assessment and Planning**

A Ask about pain regularly.
Assess pain systematically.

B Believe the patient and family in their reports of pain and what relieves it.

C Choose pain control options appropriate for the patient, family, and setting.

D Deliver interventions in a timely, logical, and coordinated fashion.

E Empower patients and their families.
Enable them to control their course to the greatest extent possible.

### Managing Acute Pain

#### *Using physical noninvasive measures*

**Cutaneous (dermal) stimulation.** Cutaneous stimulation is thought to innervate the large A-beta fibers, closing the gate to impulses from the periphery. TENS is a previously

**box 12-9** *Alternatives for Heat Application*

1. Superficial heat
   a. Dry heat: heating pad, hot-water bottle, lamp, sun
   b. Moist heat: whirlpool baths, soaks, hydrocollator packs
2. Deep heat
   a. Short-wave diathermy
   b. Ultrasound vibration
   c. Microwave diathermy (contraindicated if implanted cardiac pacemaker)

discussed example that may be ordered by the physician. Strategies that can be used by nurses include massage, light rubbing of the area involved or of a contralateral site, whirlpool baths, heat, or cold. These interventions are effective, simple, low risk, and not time consuming and do not require expensive equipment. Patients may need to try several to find which ones have the best effects. Box 12-9 lists various alternatives for the application of heat. The Guidelines for Care Box below reviews the basic principles for the safe use of these interventions.

**Positioning.** Patients who are immobilized or who splint (guard) a body part to minimize pain need to be encouraged to perform passive and/or active exercises where possible to prevent complications. Premedication may be necessary to prevent pain or to avoid additional pain when it is already present. For example, when the body or an extremity is moved, supporting the trunk or extremity will prevent an increase in pain by unilateral pulling on muscles, joints, and ligaments. Interventions for nurses and home caregivers to reduce the pain associated with positioning are summarized in the Guidelines for Care Box, at right.

**Modifying the environment.** The patient's physical environment can create sensory overload and potentiate the pain stimuli. If nurses would stand still for 5 minutes in the patient's environment and watch and listen, they might understand that some patients are almost continuously bombarded with noise and visual stimulation. Modifying the environment may be helpful, but not all patients respond positively to the same environment. Some patients may benefit from a quiet room with minimal lighting while others prefer a bright environment with sources of distraction such as television or music. The nurse can explore possible changes with the patient and implement any acceptable suggestions. Potential environmental modifications are listed in the Guidelines for Care Box at the bottom of this page.

### Patient/family education

**Teaching distraction and relaxation strategies.** Patients can be taught to modify their sensory input to control pain by activities that promote distraction or relaxation.[3,22,54] Because anxiety increases pain, measures taken to decrease anxiety may help to decrease pain. (See Chapter 6 for a discussion of stress.)

Distraction interferes with the pain stimulus, thereby modifying the patient's awareness of the pain. Mild or moderate pain can be modified by focusing on activity in the environment. A very quiet environment providing little or no sensory input actually can intensify the pain experience because the person has nothing to focus on but the painful stimulus.

Distraction requires the active participation of the individual in an effort to block out the painful stimulus. This can be enhanced by involving two or more sensory modalities, such as vision, hearing, touch, or movement. The distractors must be powerful enough to involve the person's total interest

#### guidelines for care

**Using Heat and Cold Effectively**

1. Explain the options available and involve the patient in choosing which options to use. Ice is rarely the patient's first choice, but it probably has a better chance than heat of being an effective pain reliever.
2. Apply heat and cold directly to the site of pain, but if this is not possible they can also be used:
   a. around the painful site.
   b. between the pain and the brain.
   c. beyond the pain.
   d. on the opposite side of the body from the pain site.
   e. over acupuncture or trigger point sites.
3. Use heat and cold at a comfortable intensity. They should not cause pain.
4. Apply heat and cold for 20 to 30 minutes at a time. The minimum effective time is about 10 minutes. *Ice should not be applied for longer than 10 minutes to minimize the chance of tissue damage.*
5. Encourage the patient to explore options for frequency of application. Alternating heat and cold can be effective in some situations.
6. Protect the skin with the use of either heat or cold and assess the skin after every application.
7. Use heat and cold before pain becomes severe whenever possible.

Adapted from McCaffery M, Beebe A: *Pain: clinical manual for nursing practice,* St Louis, 1989, Mosby.

#### guidelines for care

**Reducing Pain with Positioning**

1. Give analgesics to prevent or minimize pain before care is given if pain is anticipated.
2. Use a turning sheet for patients with severe neck, back, or general trunk pain.
3. Place a pillow under a painful joint when helping a patient change position.
4. Support limbs at the joints rather than the muscle bellies when handling an extremity.
5. Use special beds (Rotorest, water bed) for patients with severe general or trunk pain.
6. Avoid bumping the bed or moving it suddenly.
7. Use bed cradles to support linens off painful extremities.
8. Assist with range of motion and evaluate joint flexibility.

#### guidelines for care

**Modifying the Environment**

1. Move the patient to a quieter room away from the center of activity.
2. Dim bright lights; pull shades if sunlight is intense.
3. Keep verbal interactions at a minimum when pain is severe.
4. Encourage other patients to use headphones or keep television or radio at a reasonable level.
5. Control the number of persons entering the patient's room according to patient's wishes.
6. Explore the effect of soft music or nature sound tapes.

without resulting in fatigue. Pain of long duration requires a variety of meaningful distractions.

Full relaxation decreases the muscle tension and fatigue that usually accompany pain. It also helps to decrease anxiety, thereby preventing augmentation of the pain stimulus. In addition, relaxation, techniques serve as a form of distraction.

Relaxation exercises may be especially beneficial for persons with chronic pain to help reduce stress that exacerbates the pain and to help the person achieve a sense of control—of being better able to cope with the pain. There are numerous forms of relaxation techniques (see Chapter 6). Success with a relaxation technique requires practice and encouragement.

Examples of common easily used distractors are listed in Box 12-10. Strategies for modifying the environment to reduce anxiety are found in the Guidelines for Care Box below.

**Using guided imagery.** Guided imagery is a term that describes the use of images to improve physiological status, mental state, self-image, or behavior.[3,22,59] Progressive muscle relaxation exercises before the use of this approach facilitate the imaging process. Imagery techniques require practice to be effective and the level of concentration required may be unattainable for patients who are fatigued from acute or chronic pain. Imagery can be used simply to support mental relaxation by visualizing oneself in a favorite setting such as a quiet beach, or it can be a more active part of the pain management plan. Patients can use complex images of their pain such as fire that is gradually extinguished to add a level of conscious control to the pain experience. The technique works best when the patient selects the image and decides how it is to be used.

**Using therapeutic touch.** A less traditional therapy, termed *therapeutic touch,* may be helpful to patients in pain.[59] The rationale for the success of therapeutic touch is not clearly understood and related research is limited. Therapeutic touch is rejected outright by many health care professionals, and it may not be acceptable to the patient, but it has been shown to be helpful for some patients and some types of pain. The nurse would require extensive education and training before attempting to use this technique. The nurse undergoes a brief period of meditation before deliberately moving his or her hands over the patient's body to assess, direct, or modulate body energy patterns. The nurse does not touch the patient's skin.[52] In theory the nurse is focusing his or her

### box 12-10 Common Simple Modes of Distraction

1. Playing games, watching television
2. Talking with someone
3. Listening to favorite music
4. Rhythmic breathing
5. Focusing on an object

### guidelines for care

**Modifying the Environment to Reduce Anxiety**

1. Help the patient explore concerns related to the pain (meaning of pain for the patient).
2. Emphasize the importance of the patients' role in communicating their pain to the nurse (e.g., 0 to 10 pain intensity).
3. Respect the patient's response to pain, even if it differs considerably from what the nurse expects.
4. Teach the family and close friends ways in which they can help the patient, such as massage, encouraging the patient to use distraction or relaxation techniques, or supporting painful parts when moving or changing the patient's position. People often feel helpless when observing a loved one in pain and may need help themselves to cope.
5. Arrange for someone to be with the patient if the person fears being alone.
6. Talk with family or close friends and help them to allay their anxieties so that these are not transmitted to the patient.
7. Use gentle touch in patient interactions if it is acceptable to the patient.

### box 12-11 American Pain Society Guidelines for Managing Acute Pain

1. Recognize and treat pain promptly.
   a. Chart and display patients' self-report of pain.
   b. Commit to continuous improvement of one or several outcome variables.
   c. Document outcomes based on data and provide prompt feedback.
2. Make information about analgesics readily available.
3. Promise patients attentive analgesic care.
4. Define explicit policies for use of advanced analgesic technologies.
5. Examine the process and outcomes of pain management with the goal of continuous improvement.

### research

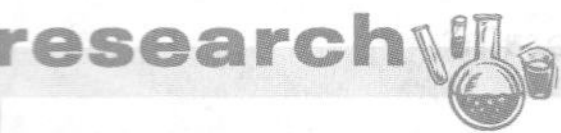

Reference: Ward S et al: Patient-related barriers to management of cancer pain, *Pain* 52:319-324, 1993.

In this study, 207 patients with cancer attending 6 outpatient oncology clinics were asked to identify their concerns about reporting pain and using pain medication. Between 37% and 85% of patients reported concerns, particularly about addiction, side effects, and interpersonal communication issues with health professionals. "Good patients" were thought to avoid talking about pain by 45% of this sample. Women were more concerned about side effects than men. Patients who were older, were less educated, or had lower incomes were more likely to have concerns. Patients with more concerns had higher pain levels and were undermedicated. Health professionals need to assess and address patients' concerns about reporting pain and using analgesics, particularly if they are older and less educated.

own internal energy and then transmitting this healing energy to the patient.

### Administering analgesics

The American Pain Society (APS) quality improvement guidelines[5] identify the two most important components of care for patients with acute pain or cancer pain as being assessment and treatment with analgesic medication. Monitoring outcomes is an important component of their guidelines (Box 12-11). When health professionals are more knowledgeable about pain assessment and management, they are better prepared to clarify patient concerns and help them with management. Patients may have concerns about being a "good" patient or fears about analgesics that interfere with their reporting pain[64] (see the Research Box on p. 340 and Box 12-12). Nurses need to ask patients about these concerns. Nonpharmacological methods are required as well as medications for therapy to be effective.

Concerns about addiction from taking opioids continues to be a concern for both health professionals and patients. Persons receiving opioids for pain relief very rarely develop addiction. The incidence of opioid addiction in hospitalized patients is less than 1%.[56] Patients are taking opioids for pain relief and not for the psychological effect. Patients who are concerned about becoming addicted can be asked, "Would you take this medication if you were not in pain?" Unfortunately, health professionals are also overly concerned about addiction, and opioids are underprescribed by physicians and underadministrated by nurses.[6,70]

Patients can also refuse to take opioid analgesics because of side effects such as constipation and nausea. Laxatives and stool softeners should be given to any patient receiving opioids on a regular basis. Nausea and vomiting are experienced by some; these patients usually respond well to antiemetics. Sedation and drowsiness may occur for the first 48 to 72 hours, but one needs to consider that the patient may be catching up on sleep lost because of the pain. A sedation scale may be used to monitor level of arousal (Box 12-13).

**box 12-12** *Patient Concerns about Reporting Pain and Using Analgesics*

*Addiction:* believe it occurs if they take frequent medication
*Tolerance:* believe they need to "save" medication for later pain
*Side effects:* fear constipation, nausea, mental confusion
*Fatalism:* expect pain to be inevitable and not treatable
*Being a good patient:* means not complaining
*Distract physician:* pain management wastes time that could be spent on treatment
*Progress:* reporting pain means acknowledging disease progression
*Injections:* believe major route is by injection which is not wanted

From Ward S et al: Patient-related barriers to management of cancer pain, *Pain* 52:319-324, 1993.

**box 12-13** *Sample Sedation Scale for Monitoring Opioid Side Effects*

| | |
|---|---|
| S = NORMAL SLEEP | Patient is asleep, but is easily aroused with stimulation |
| 0 = NONE | Alert patient |
| 1 = MILD | Occasionally drowsy patient but easy to arouse |
| 2 = MODERATE | Increased drowsiness but still easy to arouse |
| 3 = SEVERE | Somnolent patient, difficult to arouse |

**guidelines for care**

**Using Opioid Analgesics Effectively**

1. Base all analgesic decisions on thorough and ongoing patient assessment.
2. Administer opioid analgesics on a regular time schedule around the clock for severe pain. Give analgesics to prevent or minimize pain.
   a. Use of PRN administration schedules causes delays in administration and frequently results in inadequate pain control.
   b. Titrate the dose and administration interval to ensure adequate analgesia and minimize side effects. Patients vary greatly in their analgesic dose requirements and responses to opioids. Usual starting doses may be inadequate. Assess and record the effectiveness of each analgesic dose given.
   c. PRN dosing may be utilized late in the postoperative course when continuous pain is no longer present or expected. Ask the patient regularly for pain ratings to ensure adequate control.
3. Intravenous administration is the route of choice after major surgery.
   a. Repeated IM injections are a source of pain and trauma and should be avoided.
   b. Oral administration is convenient and inexpensive, and it is appropriate as soon as a patient can tolerate oral intake. It should be the mainstay of analgesia for the ambulatory population.
4. Morphine is the cornerstone of opioid therapy.
   a. Several types of analgesics may be used together to maximize effects, e.g., adding NSAIDs.
5. Meperidine (Demerol) should be reserved for very brief courses in patients who have allergies or intolerance to morphine and morphine derivatives.
   a. Meperidine is contraindicated in persons with impaired renal function or those receiving monoamine oxidase inhibitors.
   b. Meperidine creates a toxic metabolite, normeperidine, which is a cerebral irritant. Its accumulation can cause irritability, confusion, and mood changes. This is particularly common in elders.
6. Use cognitive/behavioral and nonpharmacological interventions appropriately to augment analgesic pain management.

Adapted from AHCPR: *Acute pain management in adults,* Washington, DC, 1992, US Department of Health and Human Services.

guidelines for care

### Managing Opioid Side Effects

**Opioid Side Effects**

Hypotension (particularly postural hypotension)
Decreased respirations and decreased cough
Dizziness and sedation
Constipation
Nausea

**Preventing Constipation**

Opioids bind to receptor sites in the GI tract and slow GI motility. The resultant constipation is best managed by administering a stool softener or stimulant as soon as the opioid is started. Monitor the patient's bowel pattern carefully and ensure adequate fluids.

**Managing Sedation**

The sedative effects of opioids on the CNS last from 1 to 3 days and then tolerance is built up. Initially it may be beneficial to allow the patient to catch up on needed sleep. If problematic:

- Reduce the opioid dose, add an NSAID if possible, or administer more frequently.
- Change the opioid and evaluate the patient's response.
- Monitor respiratory rate and track the patient's sedation level using a sedation scale.
- Have a reversal agent available for use if needed, e.g., Naloxone (Narcan).

**Managing Nausea**

Nausea is believed to result from stimulation of the chemoreceptor trigger zone in the brain and decreased GI motility. Tolerance to the effects usually develops within a few days. If problematic:

- Administer an antiemetic such as prochlorperazine (Compazine). Administer on a scheduled basis and not PRN.
- Add metoclopramide (Reglan) if antiemetics are initially ineffective.
- Change the opioid if nausea persists.

**Preventing Respiratory Depression**

Effective pain relief allows the patient to be more active in self-care, get out of bed, and ambulate more freely, which counter the effects of respiratory depression. In addition:

- Encourage deep breathing and the use of incentive spirometry.
- Monitor the patient's sedation level. Respiratory depression is usually only a problem when sedation becomes excessive.

**Ensuring Safety**

Orthostatic hypotension and dizziness cause an increased risk for injury. Patients are taught to change positions slowly and should be monitored in their early attempts to be out of bed.

Respiratory depression is rarely a problem with standardized doses and careful titration (slowly increasing the dose). Strategies for managing opioid side effects are summarized in the Guidelines for Care Box above. Nursing activities related to PCA include maintaining the system, recording the number of times the patient activates the system, and monitoring the patient's pain relief. The patient and family members need to know how to monitor the patient's response to the medication and how to care for the line if the patient is at home. Patients need to understand how and when to push the button to get a medication dose. They need to be encouraged to take the next dose when pain increases above mild or above the desired level identified by the patient. In the hospital, the medication button should be clearly differentiated from the call button for help, such as by color or shape.

Whatever the route, patients and families as well as health professionals need to understand how to assess pain and the importance of giving analgesic medication regularly to prevent pain or keep it in the mild range where possible. The importance of preventing or minimizing acute pain needs to be stressed. Ways to help patients do this need to be taught. Patients always have the right to determine their analgesic intake, but it is important to make sure they have adequate knowledge with which to make this decision. The Guidelines for Care Box on p. 341 summarizes basic principles of effective opioid analgesic administration.

The placebo response occurs when people experience pain relief from an intervention that may not be directly related to the applied pain relief method. Health professionals can cause a positive placebo response by the ways they interact with patients. If a person expects relief from pain, anxiety and muscle tension will decrease, and less pain will be experienced. The nurse's empathic approach toward the patient such as listening without judgment, giving ways to express pain and the right to do so, and recognizing the person's unique responses help to facilitate pain relief indirectly. *Medication placebos such as giving saline injections instead of an opioid or giving oral doses of inappropriate drugs such as demerol 50 mg PO are unethical.* Placebo medications can be used in research or in a detoxification setting *after obtaining the patient's consent.*

There are some special considerations for analgesic use with elderly patients. Unrelieved pain in this population has been shown to result in problems after surgery such as confusion. See the Research Box on p. 343.

Opioids usually are well tolerated by elders as long as the person is closely monitored for response to the analgesic prescribed.[29,54] Guidelines to help minimize the risk of side effects from the use of opioids and NSAIDs in the elderly patient are found in the Guidelines for Care Boxes on p. 343.

## Managing Chronic Pain

In recent years knowledge of the nature of chronic pain and the need for coordinated efforts of different health care professionals have resulted in the establishment of pain clinics and inpatient pain teams for control of chronic pain.

Persons with chronic persistent pain sometimes are admitted to a hospital for evaluation or initiation of treatment by a

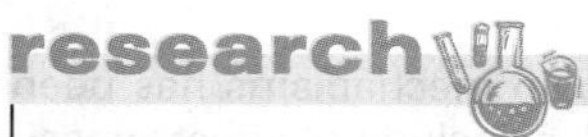

Reference: Duggleby W, Lander J: Cognitive status and postoperative pain: older adults, *J Pain Symptom Management* 9:19-27, 1994.

The purpose of this study was to assess older adults to determine (a) the course of postoperative pain, (b) influences of pain and analgesics on mental status, and (c) relationships among age, mental status, and pain. All 60 patients, aged 50 to 80 years, met the preoperative criteria for mental status and had a total hip replacement. Pain intensity decreased with time after surgery although one third of patients reported moderate to severe pain at the end of their 4th postoperative day. The major predictor of mental status decline was pain and not analgesic intake. Age was not related to pain or mental status. In general, pain was poorly managed for this group of patients. These results suggest an explanation for acute confusion in older patients postoperatively and the need for improved pain management.

**guidelines for care**

**Use of Opioids with Elderly Patients**

1. Height, weight, and body surface are not accurate measures for determining drug dosages in elders.
2. Analgesics usually last longer in elders because their renal and hepatic clearance rates are slower.
3. Age is not significant in determining dose, but it is important in determining frequency of dose.
4. Dose is based on the therapeutic response and undesirable side effects (confusion, untoward CNS effects, respiratory depression).
5. Elders may be hesitant to ask for pain relief. Monitor patients closely for nonverbal signs of pain. The stress of unrelieved pain leads to fatigue, anxiety, and confusion, which are physically and psychologically debilitating.
6. Review other medications the patient is taking to avoid drugs that may interact unfavorably with the analgesic.

**guidelines for care**

**Use of NSAIDs with Elderly Patients**

Precautions to be observed with the use of NSAIDs in elders include:

1. NSAIDs cause more ulcers and bleeding episodes in elders than they do in younger adults.
2. Elders with renal impairment are at increased risk for liver and renal toxicity and need to be monitored closely for signs of toxicity, including serum levels of the NSAID.
3. GI disturbances from decreased prostaglandin production can be reduced by the administration of misoprostol (see Chapter 40). The NSAIDs should also be buffered by food and liquid.

multidisciplinary health care team. One example is a team for evaluation and treatment of chronic back pain or substance abuse. Each team member evaluates the patient separately and shares his or her assessment in a team conference during which a specific treatment plan is developed. Protocols are developed for the approach to be used for control of the chronic pain; all persons providing patient care during the hospitalization need to become familiar with the protocols so that a consistent approach is used.

Nursing responsibilities include patient assessment, documenting observations, carrying out phase-related activities, and patient teaching. The culmination of the hospitalization is a discharge conference with the patient and family members in which future treatment plans and recommendations are presented and discussed.

Most patients with chronic pain profit from an ongoing association with a multidisciplinary pain clinic. Most pain clinics use a team approach that includes physicians (internists, anesthesiologists, surgeons, and psychiatrists), nurses, physical and occupational therapists, social workers, psychologists, vocational rehabilitation counselors, and appropriate others. Each pain clinic is organized differently and emphasizes different aspects of pain relief. Common approaches to the holistic management of chronic pain include:

1. Behavior modification (with patient's approval)
2. Medications: NSAIDs, tricyclic antidepressant, and opioids
3. Exercise and activity prescriptions
4. Hypnosis, acupuncture, or other cognitive/behavioral strategies
5. Family education to support planned goals/activities

The responsibility of the nurse varies depending on the available team members and may include patient assessment, documentation of observations, creating and maintaing a therapeutic milieu, providing emotional support for patient and family, and patient teaching. Nurses who work in pain clinics must be skilled in nurse-patient interactions, be knowledgeable about the mechanisms of pain and the effectiveness of various treatment modalities, and possess patience and understanding as they assist patients in reaching their goals.

## EVALUATION

Successful achievement of patient outcomes for the patient with pain is indicated by:

1a. Assesses pain intensity as being ≤4 on a 0 to 10 scale.
 b. States that does not have pain before the next analgesic dose or that mild pain is acceptable.
 c. Mobilizes and participates in usual activities easily and comfortably.
 d. Is not having side effects such as constipation or nausea.
 e. Asks for help with pain relief when needed.

2a. Participates in holistic chronic pain program.
 b. Is independent in usual activities of daily living, work, family activities, and leisure.
 c. Accurately evaluates the need for additional programs and supports.

3a. Patient and family: Know how to use several nonpharmacological pain relief measures such as heat or cold at home.
  b. Accurately describe action, side effects, dose, and frequency of all medications.
  c. State when and from whom they will seek help if pain is not relieved as expected.

## critical thinking QUESTIONS

1 If you were a scientist who wanted to develop an ideal analgesic, what properties would you borrow from the opioids and the nonsteroidal antiinflammatory drugs if you could select only two properties from each? What side effects would you eliminate if you could eliminate one from each group? Why did you make the choices you made?

2 How does the assessment of acute pain differ from the assessment of chronic pain? Think about two patients for whom you have provided care—one with acute pain and one with chronic pain. In what ways did their responses to pain differ, and how did these responses influence different management approaches?

3 What misbeliefs about pain are most prevalent in your areas of practice, and how have you tried to change them in relation *to your practice* and that of colleagues?

4 Compare the equianalgesic doses and the duration of action for analgesics ordered for patients you are caring for during a 24-hour period.

5 Your 45-year-old male patient says he can be strong and stand his pain which he rates as 8 (0 to10). From your understanding of pain pathophysiology and analgesics how would you respond?

6 Interview three or four patients who are using a nonpharmacological pain intervention. Compare and contrast the method, frequency of use, patient satisfaction, and effectiveness for pain relief. Were several modalities used, and was the combination of approaches successful?

## chapter SUMMARY

### NATURE OF THE PROBLEM

- Pain is a complex universal, yet individualized, experience.

### ETIOLOGY

- Pain results from a variety of causes, and its trajectories have different patterns.
- Unrelieved acute pain has numerous negative consequences such as cardiovascular, pulmonary, and gastrointestinal complications.

### EPIDEMIOLOGY

- Although most acute pain and cancer pain can be controlled, the majority of patients in the hospital report moderate to severe pain.
- Misbeliefs about pain assessment and management are prevalent and prevent effective care.

### PHYSIOLOGY

- Our current understanding of pain mechanisms has been developed from several theories including affect, specificity, and gate control theories.
- The process by which a painful stimulus is perceived involves transduction, transmission, modulation, and perception.
- Nociceptors are pain receptors that respond to chemical, thermal, electrical, or mechanical stimuli through transduction. Chemical stimuli released by damaged tissues include histamines, bradykinins, prostaglandins, and acids.
- Pain impulses are transmitted over A-delta and C fibers to the substantia gelatinosa (SG) of the dorsal horn of the spinal cord. Ascending spinal pathways in the ventral spinal cord carry impulses to the thalamus and cortex.
- Some descending spinal pathways carry pain inhibitory impulses back to the SG. Pain impulses transmitted over A-beta fibers also have a suppressive effect on impulses carried by A-delta and C fibers.
- Substance P is a neurotransmitter of pain impulses. Endorphins and serotonin are neurotransmitters of pain-inhibitory impulses.
- The gate control theory proposes that the SG is a gating mechanism that may modify the pain experience by "opening" or "closing" the gate to pain impulse transmission. The gating mechanism can be closed by impulses from A-beta and A-alpha fibers and from descending pathways from the brainstem and cortex.
- Pain perception is subjective, highly complex, and individual. It is influenced by characteristics of the pain stimuli and transmission and by receptivity and interpretation in the cerebral cortex.
- The pain detection threshold is the intensity of the stimulus necessary for the person to perceive pain.
- Pain tolerance is the maximum degree of pain intensity that the person is willing to endure before seeking relief. Pain tolerance may be enhanced by drugs, warmth, counterirritation, distraction, and strong beliefs; it may be decreased by fatigue, anxiety, boredom, continuous pain, or illness.
- Pain has different meanings for each person and may differ for the same person at different times.
- Pain response is influenced by the degree of pain perception, past experiences, sociocultural values, health status, anxiety, and age.

### PATHOPHYSIOLOGY

- Pain caused by repeated noxious stimuli can sensitize and change the nervous system. Hyperexcitability of the dorsal horn (windup) can result, which is difficult to control. Unrelieved acute pain may become chronic if neural changes become permanent.
- Acute pain is a sudden short-term event, usually with a known source, and is self-limiting or readily corrected. The typical clinical signs are usually present and pain areas generally well identified. Acute pain leads to action to relieve pain, with likelihood of eventual relief. It is characterized by anxiety and muscle tension.
- Chronic pain is a prolonged situation, often with no purpose. Pain areas are less easily defined. Pain may be continuous or intermittent and has few typical clinical signs. It leads to actions to modify the pain experience. Chronic pain is characterized by increased preoccupation with pain, hopelessness, and irritability, all leading to withdrawal.

- Superficial somatic pain is sharp and pricking, well localized, and usually not accompanied by autonomic reactions. Deep somatic and visceral pains are sharp or dull and aching, poorly localized, and usually accompanied by autonomic reactions.
- Referred pain is felt in areas other than those stimulated; it is usually visceral in origin.
- Phantom limb pain is perceived to be occurring in a limb that has been amputated.

## COLLABORATIVE CARE MANAGEMENT

- Opioids provide relief of moderate to severe pain. The oral route is preferred if possible. Constipation is the most serious side effect, and laxatives should be given to patients receiving opioids. Antiemetics to prevent vomiting may also be required, particularly at the beginning of pain control therapy.
- Patient-controlled analgesia is a system of self-administration by means of a pump using an intravenous or subcutaneous set-up, whereby a prescribed preset bolus of opioid may be taken but not repeated until a prescribed refractory time has occurred.
- Acetaminophen and NSAIDs (such as aspirin) provide relief of mild to moderate pain.
- Electrical stimulators include TENS and spinal cord stimulators. TENS is a nonintrusive system, easily learned by the patient, and may be useful for postoperative, posttraumatic, peripheral neuralgia, and muscle and bone pain.
- Approaches to modify the person's pain response include behavior modification, biofeedback and autogenic training, hypnosis, careful explanations, and anxiety reduction.

## NURSING MANAGEMENT

- Subjective data for pain include the location, intensity, quality, timing (onset, duration, frequency, cause), and aggravating or relieving factors.
- Objective data include facial expression, motor behavior, affective and verbal response, vital signs, skin color and moisture, and inspection and palpation of painful areas.
- Pain intensity can be determined by the use of pain scales or visual analog scales, in addition to asking the person to describe the pain.
- General patient/family education for *pain relief* include preparing patients to rate their pain and to communicate when the pain begins to return, varying pain relief measures, trying new approaches, and giving analgesics as effectively as possible.
- Nursing and home caregivers' interventions to *modify the pain* stimulus include preventing pain when possible; modifying the pain stimulus by cutaneous stimulation; positioning and modifying the environment; using therapeutic touch, imagery, distraction, and relaxation exercises; and modifying the pain response by careful explanations and measures to decrease anxiety.

## References


1. Abbott F et al: The prevalence of pain in hospitalized patients and resolution over six months, *Pain* 50:15-28, 1992.
2. Agency for Health Care Policy and Research (AHCPR): *Clinical practice guideline: acute pain management: operative or medical procedures and trauma.* Rockville, Md, 1992, US Department of Health and Human Services.
3. Agency for Health Care Policy and Research (AHCPR): *Management of cancer pain,* Rockville, Md, 1994, US Department of Health and Human Services.
4. American Pain Society (APS): *Principles of analgesic use in the treatment of acute pain and cancer pain,* ed 3, Skokie, Ill, 1992, The Society.
5. American Pain Society (APS) Quality of Care Committee: Quality improvement guidelines for the treatment of acute and cancer pain, *JAMA* 274-1874-1880, 1995.
6. Angell M: The quality of mercy, *N Engl J Med* 306(2):98-99, 1982.
7. Bach S, Noreng M, Tjellden N: Phantom limb pain in amputees during the first 12 months following limb amputation, after preoperative lumbar epidural blockade, *Pain* 33:297-301, 1988.
8. Benedetti C, Bonica J, Belluci G: Pathophysiology and therapy of postoperative pain: a review. In Benedetti C, Chapman C, Moricca G, editors: *Recent advances in the management of pain,* New York, 1984, Raven Press.
9. Bonica I, editor: *The management of pain,* ed 2, Philadelphia, 1990, Lea & Febiger.
10. Brunier G, Carson G, Harrison D: What do nurses know and believe about patients in pain? Results of a hospital survey, *J Pain Symptom Manage* 10:436-445, 1995.
11. Carr E: Postoperative pain: patients' expectations, *J Adv Nurs* 15:89-100, 1990.
12. Clarke E, French B, Bilodeau M, Capasso V, Edwards A, Empoliti J: Pain management knowledge, attitudes and clinical practice: the impact of nurses' characteristics and education, *J Pain Symptom Manage* 11(1):18-31, 1996.
13. Cleeland C: *Culture and pain,* Paper presented at the 8th World Congress on Pain, Vancouver, BC, 1996.
14. Cleeland C, et al: Pain and its treatment in outpatients with metastatic cancer, *N Engl J Med* 330(9):592-596, 1994.
15. Craig D: Postoperative recovery of pulmonary function, *Anesth Analg* 60(1): 46-52, 1981.
16. Devor M: Pain mechanisms and pain syndromes. In Campbell J, editor: *Pain 1996—an updated review, IASP Refresher Course Syllabus,* Seattle, 1996, IASP Press.
17. Donovan MI: A practical approach to pain assessment. In Watt-Watson JH, Donovan MI, editors: *Pain management: nursing perspective,* St Louis, 1992, Mosby.
18. Donovan M, Dillon P, McGuire L: The incidence and characteristics of pain in a sample of medical-surgical inpatients, *Pain* 30(1):69-78, 1987.
19. Dostrovsky J: Pathways of pain: update, *Perspect Pain Manage* 1(1):4-8, 1991.
20. Dunbar P, Chapman R, Buckley P, Gavrin J: Clinical analgesic equivalence for morphine and hydromorphone with prolonged PCA, *Pain* 68:265-270, 1996.
21. Dworkin R: *Acute herpes zoster and postherpetic neuralgia,* Paper presented at the meeting of the 8th World Congress on Pain, Vancouver, BC, 1996.
22. Edgar L, Smith-Hanrahan C: Nonpharmacological pain management. In Watt-Watson JH, Donovan MI, editors: *Pain management nursing perspective,* St Louis, 1992, Mosby.
23. Ferrell B, McCaffery M, Grant M: Clinical decision making and pain, *Cancer Nurs* 14:289-297, 1991.
24. Ferrell B, Nash C, Warfield C: The role of patient-controlled analgesia in the management of cancer pain, *J Pain Symptom Manage* 7:149-154, 1992.
25. Fields H: *Pain,* Toronto, 1987, McGraw-Hill.
26. Fife B, Irick N, Painter J: A comparative study of the attitudes of physicians and nurses toward the management of cancer pain, *J Pain Symptom Manage* 8(3):132-139, 1993.
27. Grossman S et al: Correlation of patient and caregiver ratings of cancer pain, *J Pain Symptom Manage* 6:53-57, 1991.
28. Hamilton J, Edgar L: A survey examining nurses' knowledge of pain control, *J Pain Symptom Manage* 7(1):18-26, 1992.

29. Hardman J, Limbird L: *Goodman and Gilman's the pharmacological basis of therapeutics,* ed 9, New York, 1996, McGraw-Hill.
30. Kalso E: *Prevention of chronicity,* Paper presented at the meeting of the 8th World Congress on Pain, Vancouver, BC, 1996.
31. Katz J, Jackson M, Kavanagh B, Sandler A: Long-term post-thoracotomy pain is predicted by acute post-operative pain. In *Abstracts: 8th World Congress on Pain,* Seattle, 1996, IASP Press.
32. Katz J, et al: Preemptive analgesia: clinical evidence of neuroplasticity contributing to postoperative pain, *Anesthesiology* 77:439-446, 1992.
33. Kehlet H: Pain relief and modification of the stress response. In Cousins M, Phillips G, editors, *Acute pain management,* New York, 1986, Churchill Livingstone.
34. Kim S: Pain: theory, research and nursing practice, *ANS* 2:43-59, 1980.
35. Kollef M: Trapped-lung syndrome after cardiac surgery: a potentially preventable complication of pleural injury, *Heart Lung* 19(6):671-675, 1990.
36. Lavies N et al: Identification of patient, medical and nursing attitudes to postoperative opioid analgesia: stage 1 of a longitudinal study of postoperative analgesia, *Pain* 48:313-319, 1992.
37. Marks RM, Sachar EJ: Undertreatment of medical inpatients with narcotic analgesics, *Ann Intern Med* 78:173-181, 1973.
38. McCaffery M, Beebe A: *Pain: clinical manual for nursing practice,* St Louis, 1989, Mosby.
39. McDonald D: Gender and ethnic stereotyping and narcotic analgesic administration, *Res Nurs Health* 17:45-49, 1994.
40. McGuire D: Comprehensive and multidimensional assessment and measurement of pain, *J Pain Symptom Manage* 7:312-319, 1992.
41. McKenry LM, Salemo E: *Mosby's pharmacology in nursing,* ed 18, St Louis, 1992, Mosby.
42. Melzack R, Dennis S: Neurophysiological foundations of pain. In Steinbach R, editor: *The psychology of pain,* New York, 1978, Raven Press.
43. Melzack R, Wall PD: Pain mechanisms: new theory, *Science* 150:971-979, 1965.
44. Melzack R, Wall PD: *The challenge of pain,* New York, 1996, Penguin Books.
45. Merskey H, Bogduk N: *Classification of chronic pain: descriptions of chronic pain syndromes and definitions of pain terms,* ed 2, Seattle, 1994, IASP Press.
46. Miaskowski C, Nichols R, Brody R, Synold T: Assessment of patient satisfaction utilizing the American Pain Society's quality assurance standards on acute and cancer-related pain, *J Pain Symptom Manage* 9(1):5-11, 1994.
47. Neill K: Ethnic pain styles in acute myocardial infarction, *West J Nurs Res* 15(2):531-547, 1993.
48. Oberle K: Pain, anxiety and analgesics: a comparative study of elderly and younger surgical patients, *Can J Aging* 9(1):13-22, 1990.
49. O'Gara P: The hemodynamic consequences of pain and its management, *J Intensive Care Med* 3:3-5, 1988.
50. Owen H, McMillan V, Rogowski D: Postoperative pain therapy: a survey of patients' expectations and their experiences, *Pain* 41(3): 303-308, 1990.
51. Owen H, Plummer J, Hopkins L, Cushnie J: A comparison of nurse-administered and patient-controlled analgesia. In Bond M, Charlton E, Woolf C, editors, *Proceedings of the VIth World Congress on Pain,* Oxford, 1991, Elsevier Science.
52. Paice J: Pharmacological management. In Watt-Watson JH, Donovan MI, editors: *Pain management: nursing perspective,* St Louis, 1992, Mosby.
53. Paice J, Mahon S, Faut-Callahan M: Factors associated with adequate pain control in hospitalized postsurgical patients diagnosed with cancer, *Cancer Nurs* 14:298-305, 1991.
54. Pasero C, McCaffery M: Postoperative pain management in the elderly. In Ferrell B, Ferrell B, editors: *Pain in the elderly,* Seattle, 1996, IASP Press.
55. Payne R: Transdermal fentanyl: suggested recommendations for clinical use, *J Pain Symptom Manage* 7:540-544, 1992.
56. Porter J, Jick H: Addiction rare in patients treated with narcotics, *N Engl J Med* 303(2):123, 1980.
57. Puntillo K, Weiss S: Pain: its mediators and associated morbidity in critically ill cardiovascular surgical patients, *Nurs Res* 43(1):31-36, 1994.
58. Richmond C, Bromley L, Woolf C: Preoperative morphine preempts postoperative pain, *Lancet* 342:73-75, 1993.
59. Spross J, Burke M: Nonpharmacological management of cancer pain. In McGuire D, Yarbro C, Ferrell B, editors: *Cancer pain management,* Boston, 1995, Jones & Bartlett Publishers.
60. Tasker R: Stereotactic surgery. In Wall P, Melzack R, editors: *Textbook of pain,* London, 1994, Churchill Livingstone.
61. Von Roenn J, et al: Physicians' attitudes and practice in cancer pain management, *Ann Intern Med* 119:121-126, 1993.
62. Vortherms R, Ryan P, Ward S: Knowledge of, attitudes toward, and barriers to pharmacologic management of cancer pain in a statewide random sample of nurses, *Res Nurs Health* 15(12):459-466, 1992.
63. Wall P: Comments after 30 years of the gate control theory, *Pain Forum* (1):12-22, 1996.
64. Ward S et al: Patient-related barriers to management of cancer pain, *Pain* 52:319-324, 1993.
65. Ward S, Gordon D: Application of the American Pain Society quality assurance standards. *Pain* 56:266-306, 1994.
66. Ward S, Gordon D: Patient satisfaction and pain severity as outcomes in pain management: a longitudinal view of one setting's experience, *J Pain Symptom Manage* 11(4):242-251, 1996.
67. Watson CPN, et al: Amitriptyline versus placebo in postherpetic neuralgia, *Neurology* 32:671-673, 1982.
68. Watt-Watson J: Misbeliefs. In Watt-Watson J, Donovan M, editors, *Pain management: nursing perspective,* St Louis, 1992, Mosby-Year Book.
69. Watt-Watson JH, Evans R, Watson CP: Relationships among coping responses and perceptions of pain intensity, depression and family functioning, *Clin J Pain* 4(2):101-106, 1988.
70. Watt-Watson J, et al: Patients' perceptions of their pain experience after coronary bypass graft surgery, In *American Pain Society Book of Abstracts,* abstract 747, 1996.
71. Watt-Watson J, Graydon J: Impact of surgery on head and neck cancer patients and their caregivers, *Nurs Clin North Am* 30:659-671, 1995.
72. Woolf C, Thompson J: Stimulation-induced analgesia: transcutaneous electrical nerve stimulation (TENS) and vibration. In Wall P, Melzack R, editors: *Textbook of pain,* London, 1994, Churchill Livingstone.
73. Zalon M: Nurses' assessment of postoperative patients' pain, *Pain* 54:329-34, 1993.
74. Zborowski M: Cultural components in responses to pain, *J Soc Issues* 15(5):531-543.

# chapter 13 Sleep Disorders

DIANE BROADBENT FRIEDMAN

**objectives** *After studying this chapter, the learner should be able to:*

**1** Take a complete sleep history.

**2** Describe the nature, pathophysiology, therapy, and teaching needs of persons with insomnia, narcolepsy, and sleep apnea.

**3** Describe the relationship of sleep to chronobiology and the implications for nursing research.

We usually divide our lives into two parts: waking and sleeping. We also commonly believe that our important activity occurs while we are awake and that sleep is a passive state initiated by simply closing our eyes. This belief contains the two most basic misunderstandings about sleep: sleep is not active or very important to life, and sleep is something that simply comes "naturally." These misunderstandings contribute to health professionals' and their patients' overlooking sleep problems and the role sleep plays in healing and health maintenance.

## INTRODUCTION TO SLEEP PROBLEMS

### ASPECTS OF NORMAL SLEEP

Sleep is difficult to define because as yet it is incompletely understood by researchers. From the sleeper's point of view, sleep is experienced as (1) being the deliberate initiation of a change or reduction in consciousness lasting an average of 8 hours, (2) commencing about the same time each 24-hour period, and (3) usually resulting in a feeling of restored physical, emotional, and intellectual energy. This definition contains three important concepts about normal sleep: *changes in consciousness, deliberate initiation of sleep, and timing of sleep.*

Although the sleeping person or observers may believe the sleeper is unconscious, the sleeping brain alternates among several active states during sleep, producing a series of predictable 90-minute sleep cycles. Unlike the unconsciousness produced by an anesthetic, the brain maintains all body systems during sleep, some of which are more active in sleep (such as secretion of growth hormone), and allows for restoration of alertness if required. Also, unlike animals, only humans can deliberately postpone the initiation of sleep. The record for sleep postponement is about 10 days.

Sleep commences about the same time each 24-hour period. The study of biological rhythms places the study of sleep into a larger context. The timing for sleep is regulated by many subtle external factors (Box 13-1). Internal hormonal factors and neurological activity maintain internal biological clocks. These factors tend to occur at the same time every 24 hours; therefore they help to "anchor" the onset and termination of sleep. Sleep research at the cellular level indicates that changes in the neuronal cell membrane and in the cell nucleus in several brain areas—including the suprachiasmatic nucleus of the hypothalamus, the pineal gland, and the pontine reticular formation of the brainstem—alter the cell's excitability in different stages of sleep.

### NORMAL SLEEP FUNCTION

Sleep is usually initiated in the late evening about 8 hours before arising for morning work or daily routine. Some people require more or less than 8 hours to feel refreshed. Some people are "larks," falling asleep within moments of lying down and awakening alert and ready to go, whereas others are "owls," taking up to 30 minutes to fall asleep and feeling their most alert in the afternoon or early evening.

Sleep is initiated usually within 30 minutes of lying down. Sleep cycles of 90 minutes occur, initiated by very light stage I/II, followed by deep stage III/IV, and ending with lighter *rapid eye movement (REM)*/dream sleep. If awakened from light stage I sleep, sleepers state that they were not asleep, whereas if awakened from other stages, they state that they were asleep or dreaming. Arousal can occur after each REM cycle. As the night progresses, the amount of time spent in stage III/IV shortens, and the amount of REM lengthens. Thus more dreaming time occurs in the morning hours just before final awakening.

### STATES OF CONSCIOUSNESS

Conscious awareness and sleep may be the most fundamental aspects of life to each of us. They are experienced as states of clear-mindedness, relaxation, and restoration. We take them

**box 13-1** *External Factors Regulating Sleep*

Sunrise, sunset, and length of day
Ambient temperature
Physical activity and rest
Timing and composition of meals
Timing of social/environmental cues, such as increased morning traffic noise

**box 13-2** *Some Systems Thought to Be Involved in Sleep and Arousal*

1. Circadian system: eyes, suprachaismatic nucleus, pineal gland[11]
2. Sleep-promoting areas and areas maintaining consciousness: basal forebrain connections to limbic system, basal ganglia, amygdala, frontal lobe and anterior hypothalamus, and thalamic nuclei[9,19,20]
3. Breathing and REM sleep systems: medial pontine reticular formation and other brainstem nuclei[10]
4. Neurotransmitters and humoral factors such as serotonin, gamma-aminobutyric acid, acetylcholine, melatonin, brain lipids, prolactin, and neurotransmitters made in distant locations such as the gut[6,11]
5. Inflammatory response products: cytokines such as interleukin-1 and tumor necrosis factor[10,18]

for granted and, yet, prize them above all else when they are disturbed.

Each person's level of consciousness fluctuates throughout a 24-hour period, making smooth transitions from drowsiness to deep sleep, dream sleep, arousal, clear-mindedness, relaxation, and fatigue. What makes these states occur and what determines their intensity and duration are not completely understood. Moreover, these states can be upset by an illness, an accident, personal distress, and abnormal waking hours.

The study of sleep disorders not only yields remedies for these disturbances but also may give clues to understanding the mechanisms of normal sleep and consciousness itself. In thinking about sleep and sleep disturbances, it is important to keep in mind that sleep and consciousness are maintained by several discrete brain areas in the cortex and midbrain, several networks of neuronal pathways, combinations of neurotransmitters that initiate, enhance, and inhibit neuronal functions, and humoral factors and inflammatory response products produced by agents at distant locations from the brain (Box 13-2). In other words, while sleep is experienced as a simple release of the day's cares, the underlying mechanisms are very complex. When a person experiences fatigue out of proportion to daily activities, too easy sleepiness, alertness at the wrong time, or unusual behavior during sleep, these are indications that the body is attempting to correct a perturbed system. Not only are these serious problems that risk accident or further decompensation, but they can cause worry, irritability, and frustration.

Sleep disorders are a developing area of research and clinical science. A sleep disorders classification system was revised in 1989 to allow for more precise characterization of sleep phenomena and disorders[1] (Box 13-3). Some theoretical distinctions were removed, such as those that distinguished childhood from adult disorders based only on chronological age. The earlier classification (1979) made distinctions between Disorders of Initiating and Maintaining Sleep (DIMS) and Disorders of Excessive Somnolence (DOES), but could not accommodate syndromes that had features of both. Most interesting for nursing research, the new multiaxial classification system allows for the addition of diagnoses that are relevant to a particular patient's assessment for planning, treatment, and predicting the particular patient's outcome. An example of this is a patient who has psychophysiological insomnia and benign prostatic hypertrophy and hypertension for which furosemide is part of the medical treatment. The timing of the furosemide and accommodation for nocturnal bladder emptying will clearly be part of this patient's plan of care and projected outcomes.

Sleep disorders are now organized under four broad topics. *Dyssomnias* are disorders of insomnia or excessive sleepiness. Dyssomnias are further divided into three subtypes: (1) *intrinsic:* produced by factors within the body; (2) *extrinsic:* produced by factors outside the body (Box 13-3); and (3) *circadian rhythm disorders. Parasomnias* are disorders that intrude into or occur during sleep but do not produce a primary dyssomnia. Additionally, there are sleep disorders associated with medical/psychiatric disorders and other proposed disorders.

Although sleep problems are very common, discussion of all disorders is beyond the scope of this chapter, and only common disorders will be presented. Nurses encounter people with disordered sleep every day. Factors causing disordered sleep, such as pain, worry, or sleeping in unusual surroundings are common in medical settings and can cause unwanted effects in only a few days. Sleep problems in turn affect memory, mood, and thinking that not only works against the patient's learning and coping but also is anxiety-producing in itself. The study of sleep disorders and the study of the effects of other medical disorders on sleep present a vast opportunity for alleviation of suffering as well as for nursing research.

## NATURE OF SLEEP PROBLEMS

It is estimated that more than one half of all adults cite difficulties with sleeping at some time in their lives. These problems result in suffering; risk of accident; worry about loss of emotional, intellectual, or neurological functioning; embarrassment; and exacerbation of other health problems. In 1983 and again in 1990, the National Institutes of Health determined that 35% of a nationally representative sample reported "trouble sleeping" in the previous year and that half of this group reported this as a "serious" problem. This means that approximately one of every three persons a nurse encounters may describe a sleep problem. Sleep problems have been historically overlooked, however, especially in the hospitalized patient when other circumstances appear more compelling.

Nurses can have a primary impact on helping persons with sleep problems and preventing sleep problems. The following instances of sleep problems highlight the need to

**box 13-3** *International Classification of Sleep Disorders*

Classification outline:
1. DYSSOMNIAS
   A. Intrinsic sleep disorders
      1. Psychophysiological insomnia
      2. Sleep state misperception
      3. Idiopathic insomnia
      4. Narcolepsy
      5. Recurrent, idiopathic, or posttraumatic hypersomnia
      6. Obstructive sleep apnea syndrome
      7. Central sleep apnea syndrome
      8. Central alveolar hypoventilation syndrome
      9. Periodic limb movement disorder and restless legs syndrome
   B. Extrinsic sleep disorders
      1. Inadequate sleep hygiene
      2. Environmental sleep disorder
      3. Altitude insomnia
      4. Insufficient sleep syndrome
      5. Sleep-onset association disorder
      6. Nocturnal eating (drinking) disorder
      7. Hypnotic-dependent, stimulant-dependant, and/or alcohol-dependent sleep disorder
      8. Toxin-induced sleep disorder
   C. Circadian rhythm sleep disorders
      1. Time zone change (jet lag) syndrome
      2. Shift work sleep disorder
      3. Irregular sleep-wake pattern
      4. Delayed or advanced sleep-phase syndrome
      5. Non-24-hour sleep-wake disorder
2. PARASOMNIAS
   A. Arousal disorders
      1. Confusional arousals
      2. Sleep walking
      3. Sleep talking
   B. Sleep-wake transition disorders
      1. Rhythmic movement disorder
      2. Sleep starts
      3. Sleep talking
      4. Nocturnal leg cramps
   C. Parasomnias usually associated with REM sleep
      1. Nightmares
      2. Sleep paralysis
      3. Impaired sleep-related penile erections
      4. Sleep-related painful erections
      5. REM sleep-related sinus arrest
      6. REM sleep behavior disorder
   D. Other parasomnias
      1. Sleep bruxism
      2. Sleep enuresis
      3. Sleep-related abnormal swallowing syndrome
      4. Nocturnal paroxysm dystonia
      5. Sudden unexplained nocturnal death syndrome
      6. Primary snoring
      7. Infant sleep apnea
      8. Congenital central hypoventilation syndrome
      9. Sudden infant death syndrome
      10. Benign neonatal sleep myoclonus
3. SLEEP DISORDERS ASSOCIATED WITH MEDICAL/PSYCHIATRIC DISORDERS
   A. Associated with mental disorders, including psychoses, mood disorders, anxiety disorders, panic disorders, and alcoholism
   B. Associated with neurological disorders, including dementia, parkinsonism, fatal familial insomnia, sleep-related epilepsy, and sleep-related headaches
   C. Associated with other medical disorders, including nocturnal cardiac ischemia, chronic obstructive pulmonary disease, sleep-related asthma, sleep-related gastroesophageal reflux, peptic ulcer disease, fibrositis syndrome, and sleeping sickness
4. PROPOSED SLEEP DISORDERS

   These disorders include sleep hyperhydrosis, menstrual- and pregnancy-associated sleep disorder, sleep-related laryngospasm and choking, terrifying hypnagogic hallucinations, and others

Adapted from Diagnostic Classification Steering Committee: *The international classification of sleep disorders: diagnostic and coding manual,* Rochester, Minn, 1990, American Sleep Disorders Association.

detect sleep concerns or to prevent sleep problems from developing:

1. A 50-year-old woman describes a 10-year history of inability to stay asleep beyond 5 AM, dating from death of her husband.
2. A 65-year-old man comes to the emergency room for contusions after a minor traffic accident. He works the night shift, driving a newspaper delivery truck, and then stays awake during the day to care for his chronically ill wife.
3. A downcast boy leaves the examining room after his mother describes how he must pass up summer camp because of bed-wetting.
4. An executive, whose head is immobilized in halo traction after a neck injury, describes sleeplessness at night, distorted conversations with physicians (probably related to medications), being awakened at night for procedures, and being disturbed by noises and vibrations amplified by the tongs.
5. A woman states that her husband falls asleep readily, even while sitting up in a chair and that his skin color becomes bluish as he snorts and breathes irregularly.

Sleep problems can be categorized by the disruption in one or more of the aspects of normal sleep. This chapter discusses only the most common types of sleep disorders:

*Dyssomnias* or intrinsic sleep disorders

*Insomnia*—inability to initiate or maintain sleep

*Narcolepsy*—sleep intrusion into wakefulness

*Sleep apnea*—sleep problems involving other body systems

*Circadian rhythm disorders*—sleep problems associated with time zone changes (jet lag) or shift work

*Parasomnias* or disorders of arousal associated with sleep, sleep stages, or arousal

The last section of this chapter discusses research into sleep and circadian rhythms and their impact on nurses both as researchers and as caregivers who must remain awake and alert at night.

Patients with sleep apnea and narcolepsy may need special advice because many states are passing laws that require persons with either of these conditions to surrender their driver's licenses. Additional information about sleep disorders suitable for professionals, patients, and families may be obtained from the organizations listed below:

1. The National Sleep Foundation, 1367 Connecticut Ave. N.W., #200, Washington, DC 20036; (202)347-3471; www.sleepfoundation.org
2. American Sleep Disorders Association, 1610 14th St. N.W., Suite 300, Rochester, MN 55901; (507)287-6006; www.asda.org
3. National Narcolepsy Network, P.O. Box 42460, Cincinnati, OH 45242; (513)891-3522

## DYSSOMNIAS

Included in this section are discussions of insomnia, narcolepsy, and sleep apnea as well as a general description of circadian rhythm problems.

### INSOMNIA

#### Etiology

Insomnia is the difficulty with initiating or maintaining sleep. Insomnia can be caused by various factors:

1. Transient situations of emotional upset (such as loss of a job) or family needs (such as a child's illness)
2. Adoption of nonfunctional sleep habits
3. Psychiatric disorders, such as depression or psychoses
4. Use of drugs or alcohol
5. Respiratory impairment (see later section on sleep apnea)
6. Medical conditions associated with pain, anemia, fever, changes in nutritional status, or immobility
7. Attempting to sleep in nonconducive environmental conditions

It is important to remember that in many instances persons experience altered sleep patterns when the actual cause of the sleep changes may have been resolved long ago. For example, a woman may describe that she habitually arose at 5 AM to nurse her baby, and now several years later, she still awakens at that time and cannot go back to sleep. Another person may report inability to sleep after great anxiety associated with a job loss that has persisted, although the person has now been happily employed for several years.

#### Epidemiology

Epidemiological studies estimate the number of Americans with insomnia to be in the millions. Insomnia is experienced by adults and children and affects male and female subjects equally.

#### Pathophysiology

Sleep onset can be delayed and arousal prolonged by active thought and worry, physical discomfort, or poor oxygenation. Worry and poor habits, such as sleeping with lights on or a TV or radio on, prolong sleep onset and cause arousals during light stage I sleep. Staying in bed longer than 8 hours at a time or napping during the day fragments sleep. The person sleeps 8 hours, but the total time spent in bed is 10 hours, which makes the person believe that the sleep is "poor."

Normally there is a clear boundary between and regular timing of sleep time and awake time. Meals and social and physical activities occur at predictable times during awake hours, and sleep occurs at night in a dark, quiet, comfortable, secure place. Biological clocks are anchored in time by the regular occurrence of these events. For the person with insomnia, the distinction between waking/sleeping time is blurred by spending a prolonged time in bed, by not initiating the day's activities at a prompt time, or by staying up too late at night. These events cause a distortion in sleep and lead to a continuing cycle of poor sleep at the wrong time. Clinical manifestations of insomnia are discussed below.

The person may describe insomnia in many ways, depending on which aspect of sleeplessness is most troubling. Typical comments include the following: "I cannot go to sleep," "I am awake all night," and "I awaken early and can't go back to sleep." Persons with insomnia often monitor sleep by watching the clock. They may turn on the TV, read, or eat while waiting to feel sleepy. They may try to go to sleep earlier, stay in bed longer, take naps, use sleeping pills or alcohol to initiate sleep, or use caffeine to increase alertness during the day. They may also change their pattern of daily activities to compensate for a distorted sleep pattern by declining or omitting activities from the daily routine, saying, "I'm just too tired." Some persons may not recognize a sleep problem at first because they have adapted to a changed sleep schedule over many years.

#### Collaborative Care Management

If the person has used sleeping pills or alcohol to help with sleep, supervised weaning from these substances is required. A schedule of reducing the dose of sleeping pills over a month or more or a course of chlordiazepoxide hydrochloride (Librium) to assist with alcohol withdrawal may be prescribed.

Routine blood work, such as an SMA 18 and complete blood count (CBC), is done to determine whether any hematological, metabolic, cardiac, or respiratory diseases are contributing to sleeplessness. A thorough assessment, including questions to elicit signs of underlying depression or psychosis, should be done.

A *polysomnogram (PSG)* consists of an all-night sleep study conducted in a certified sleep laboratory. The PSG is performed when the person complains of insomnia, and the physician is unable to make the diagnosis from a history and physical examination.

Sleep technicians monitor the following:

1. Sleep time and quality
2. Brain electroencephalogram (EEG) activity to determine stages of sleep
3. Respiratory activity: intercostal muscle movement, air passage from nose and mouth, and oxygen saturation using an ear lobe oximeter

4. Electrocardiogram (ECG) for monitoring cardiac rate
5. Electromyogram (EMG) monitoring of leg movement to detect abnormal movement of eye and face (to determine onset of REM sleep)
6. Occurrence of nightmares or "restless legs"

The *multiple sleep latency test (MSLT)* is a sleep study done in the sleep laboratory during the day to measure daytime sleepiness. At times the MSLT is needed to distinguish the sleepiness caused by poor nighttime sleep and sleepiness caused by narcolepsy.

## NURSING MANAGEMENT

### ASSESSMENT

A complete nursing assessment of people with sleep disorders is listed in Box 13-4. Never jump to a conclusion about a sleep problem without asking systematic questions about all sleep disorders, because one sleep problem can resemble another superficially. Keep in mind that many times insomnia begins as an understandable response to a stress—such as the loss of a spouse, illness of a family member, or loss of a job—or after a difficult hospitalization or other stressful event. The person may come to terms with the stress or loss, but the new maladaptive sleep habits are now in place. The person may state that the sleep pattern began 5 years ago and that nothing is bothering him or her now to prevent sleep. This makes sense when one views insomnia as a series of decisions that perpetuate a certain sleep pattern, unfortunately a pattern that distresses instead of refreshes. The following data are important to highlight for a person with insomnia.

#### Subjective Data

Data to be collected to assess the patient with insomnia include:

Beliefs about the sleep problems and ability to sleep restfully. Some people believe that they have inherited or developed a permanent mental change or disorder that will prevent regaining normal sleep.

Knowledge about normal sleep.

Sources of pleasure and difficulty in the person's life and how the sleep problem has been affected by these.

Potential resources for life changes. For example, if a retired person has nothing to wake up for, can that person find transport to a senior citizens center, volunteer job, or activity group?

#### Objective Data

Objective data include results from diagnostic tests and reports from a bed partner. A person may be asked to keep a sleep diary, recording times of sleep initiation, arousals, naps, and time of awakening in the morning.

### NURSING DIAGNOSES

Nursing diagnoses are determined from analyses of patient data. Nursing diagnoses for the patient with insomnia may include but are not limited to:

| Diagnostic Title | Possible Etiological Factors |
|---|---|
| Sleep pattern disturbance | Adoption of counterproductive sleep habits |
| Knowledge deficit (about insomnia) | Incorrect self-monitoring and self-assessment of sleep |
| Fatigue | Reduced total sleep time |
| Fear | Personal concern about impossibility of ever sleeping well again |
| Diversional activity deficit | Immobility, depressed feelings, perceived loss of usefulness, or of need for activity |
| Coping, ineffective (individual) | Habit of seeking sleep to avoid facing problems or of reviewing problems at sleep initiation |
| Injury, risk for | Sleepiness during the day |

### EXPECTED PATIENT OUTCOMES

Expected patient outcomes for the patient with insomnia may include but are not limited to:

1. Patient/bed partner/family describe the basic aspects of normal sleep, with emphasis on factors that contribute to the patient's problem.
2. Is able to explain what is causing his or her sleep problem and how to improve sleep.
3. Patient/family carry out measures to reduce the insomnia and improve fatigue.
4. Has realistic expectations about the quality of sleep, and fear is reduced.
5. Identifies impediments to activity and develops and implements a plan for increasing diversional activity.
6. Participates in a plan to problem solve and cope with difficulties; does not think about problems at times of sleep.
7. Does not experience an injury because of sleepiness during normal awake period.

### INTERVENTIONS

#### Facilitating Sleep

Encourage the patient to talk about what interferes with his or her ability to fall asleep. Develop with the patient a plan to improve sleep. Have the patient keep a sleep diary listing activities undertaken before sleep, measures taken to improve sleep, and how successful the changes were in obtaining a good night's rest.

#### Promoting Sleep Hygiene

A person with insomnia will benefit most from a reordering of sleep habits. Develop a plan for sleep hygiene with the patient and inform the physician of the plan, as appropriate. Physician advice may be required if intake patterns of alcohol, other drugs, or caffeine need to be changed. Patients must recognize that they must adhere to the plan faithfully every day, no matter what occurs. They are resetting their sleep-wake cycle, which takes several weeks to a month to accomplish. In developing the plan, choose from the elements listed here that apply to the individual's sleep hygiene problem. Not all elements are appropriate for each person. The plan has three important parts: (1) what the person does during the day (use

**box 13-4** *Sleep Interview*

**GENERAL DATA**

1. Statement of the sleep problem by patient, bed partner, or family: obtain a quantifiable answer about sleep, such as never sleeps, dozes off for an hour several times a night, or has trouble sleeping 5 nights out of 7, every other night, or on weekends only
2. Initiation of sleep problem: when possible, elicit cause
3. Factors that make it worse or better
4. Previous occurrences to patient or to other family member or friend
5. Modifications that need to be made for daytime activities or travel
6. Memories of frightening or upsetting incidences during sleep, such as sudden illness or death of a loved one or damage from storm, fire, or robbery
7. Occurrences of accidents or "near misses" as a result of sleep problems *(very important)*

**INSOMNIA DATA**

(Remember that a complaint of insomnia may be caused by sleep apnea or other difficulties with sleep.)

1. Time person gets into bed and time person falls asleep
2. Number and times of awakenings at night
3. Interval before returning to sleep after each awakening
4. Time of final awakening, time of arising from bed, and what wakes the person up, such as noises, alarm clock, or treatment
5. Daytime naps: number, when, and how long
6. Dozing off briefly (same question as napping, but some persons answer this question differently)
7. Lying down to rest on couch or "resting eyes for a moment" (this counts as napping because person may be falling asleep)
8. Practices used to assist with sleep: type and regularity of use
9. Changes in sleep patterns because of sleep deficit
10. Places where sleep occurs more readily, such as somewhere else in the house or on vacation
11. Concerns that delay getting into bed or falling asleep
12. Amount of and recent changes in caffeine intake (coffee, tea, colas, other caffeinated beverages, caffeinated gum) and alcohol
13. Types of weekly exercise and recreational activities
14. Measures of coping with concerns
15. Recent illness or loss of relatives, friends, or pets
16. Activities of others in house or neighborhood that affect sleep, such as child who returns home late, spouse who leaves home early in morning, noise from a neighbor or dog, and noise from a nearby highway or airport
17. Cigarette use/history

**SLEEP APNEA DATA**

1. Description or reenactment by bed partner of the person's breathing pattern, including sound and volume of snoring, length of time that no air passes, and how the person starts to breathe again
2. Description by bed partner of differences in patient's breathing while on back, each side, and stomach and of changes in patient's skin color while asleep
3. Presence of morning headaches
4. Difficulty in awakening for the day
5. Number of pillows used; preference of sleeping in a certain chair
6. Degree of sleepiness during day; falling asleep at a movie, during a conversation, or while driving

**NARCOLEPSY-RELATED DATA**

1. Presence of sudden irresistible urges to sleep; falling asleep and then awakening a few minutes later feeling refreshed
2. Experiences of a sudden loss of muscle tone, leading to drooping of the head or slumping to the floor, that occur during episodes of strong emotions (surprise, laughter, anger)
3. Experiences on awakening of feeling paralyzed until touched by another
4. Presence of visual, auditory, or tactile hallucinations at time of sleep initiation or awakening
5. Family history of unusual experiences in sleep

**SLEEP SCHEDULE DATA**

1. Working hours
2. Experience of going to bed later each night
3. Daily scheduled activities, flexibility
4. Changes in sleep schedule as a result of changes in life schedule, such as retirement or hospitalization
5. Interruption of sleep because of family activities
6. Practice of sleeping through the day or staying up at night because of a specific purpose, such as fear that a calamity will befall during the night

**OTHER SLEEP-RELATED EVENTS**

1. Uncomfortable feelings in legs when ready to fall asleep: location, type of sensation, duration, actions that make it better or worse, attempted remedies, and effect on sleep
2. Reports from bed partner of patient kicking or moving legs in sleep
3. Bed-wetting: frequency, time of occurrence, actions that make it better or worse, and reports of any nights of dryness
4. Dreams: upsetting recurring dreams, frightening nightmares, or sleep terrors
5. Sleepwalking: initiation, frequency, ability to be awakened easily or guided back to bed, experience of injury while sleepwalking, actions that make it better or worse, and steps taken to keep the person safe
6. Teeth grinding during sleep
7. Dysfunctions associated with sleep, such as chest pain, shortness of breath, heartburn/ulcer pain, morning headache, asthmatic attacks, frequent awakenings to urinate, hot flashes in menopausal woman, coughing, choking and gagging, and arthritic or other neuromuscular pain

of time, naps, eating and drinking, exercise, and diversion), (2) what the person does to prepare for sleep, and (3) how the person interprets his or her sleep experience.

The plan is to be followed faithfully for 1 month. If sleep is improved, adjustments can be made for one element at a time, such as resuming a reduced intake of alcohol or caffeine. Once the sleep pattern is established, however, only one element should be modified at a time. If the sleep pattern is weakened, the person can identify an element to which he or she is sensitive. Check with the person weekly to identify how the new plan is proceeding. Be generous with encouragement. Remember that a new way of sleeping is being taught to a person who is still partly convinced that he or she is one of the few persons in the world who never sleeps.

#### Time spent in bed, sleep, and wake-up hours

The person, in collaboration with the health professional, selects a sleep time and a wake-up time for a total time spent in bed of 7 to 8 hours, depending on how much sleep the patient thinks is needed. Ask what constraints the person has, such as time to get up for work or time arriving home from evening work, and what time the person likes to go to bed, based on time spent with family members or favorite late-night TV shows. The bedtime and wake-up time should be followed faithfully, without alteration, for 1 month, so planning ahead for lifestyle preferences is important. This means the person will follow this schedule even if he or she is out late on Saturday nights or wants to sleep in on Sunday mornings. If the person does not sleep well one night, the schedule must be kept because it is an investment in a better night's sleep the next night.

#### Napping

No naps should be taken. This means not lying down during the day and not closing the eyes while sitting in the chair after dinner. If the person gets sleepy reading the paper, the paper should be read while standing up at the counter. If the person is tired an hour before the agreed-on sleep time, he or she should walk around, engage in an activity, or stand up while watching TV. This gives the body a firm message that all sleep will take place in bed during the nighttime hours only. Taking naps at other times fragments nighttime sleep. If, in following the schedule, the person does not sleep much the night before, taking a nap only hinders the possibility that sleep will come more easily the next night, which perpetuates the problem.

#### Caffeine and alcohol

The best and fastest change in sleep quality comes from the elimination of caffeine and alcohol from the diet during the start of this plan. However, persons who drink a lot of caffeine or even one alcoholic drink each day could experience withdrawal symptoms, so it is best to work with the physician on a safe plan for withdrawal. Also, the strength of this plan is to help the person experience improved sleep without experiencing uncomfortable symptoms that might lead the person to resume the previous, more comfortable patterns.

#### Nutrition

It is important to eat three meals a day composed of balanced nutrition at about the same time each day. On awakening in the morning, the person should wash, dress, and have some breakfast to give the body yet another message that it is time for the day to start. Breakfast may be large or simply toast and juice; the point is to give a regular nutritional time cue.

#### Exercise

Increasing activity gives the body another biological message that the day is here. Even if the person is confined to bed, exercises can be developed to enhance a feeling of well-being. For persons who experience tension, stress, or worry or who face difficult problems, exercise can bring a respite from troubling thoughts or can be a time for thinking through problems instead of at bedtime. Any exercise, from active sports to walking to stationary exercise, is encouraged.

#### Diversional activities

It is important for the person to do something each day that brings enjoyment. It is equally important to have both something in life a person can look forward to and something that requires a person's special participation, creating a feeling of being needed. A person facing a continuing illness often experiences a curtailing of usual outlets for diversion and participation. Remember that what a person does with time during the day influences sleep time as well. An important part of a plan for better sleep is a life-participating activity. Even if the person is confined to bed, a telephone is a link with others who could use the person's support and good will.

#### Sleep environment

Evening routines, such as checking door locks or letting the dog out, should be completed before the predetermined bedtime. By bedtime the person should be in night clothes and ready to get into bed. The bed covers should provide the proper comfort. Lights, TV, and radio should be off. The person should not read or eat in bed. Persons can be advised to turn the clock around so it cannot be checked during the night. The person needs to understand that awakening during the night is normal, and sleep activity does not need to be monitored.

#### Relaxation

The final component of a sleep plan is the relearning of skills of relaxing when the person wants to go to sleep. A person can easily adopt the habit of postponing thoughts about troubling issues until in bed with the lights off. This is a habit and can be replaced by a more useful habit. A person cannot lie in bed "thinking about nothing" because the mind simply searches for something interesting to think about and usually selects some unfinished, compelling issues. Relaxation exercises can help persons regain and strengthen the ability to select something enjoyable to think about. If the person consciously selects something pleasant, the tendency to ruminate over troubles is weakened. Relaxation exercises must be practiced each night. If the person has difficulty mastering this task, a referral to a behavioral therapist may be appropriate.

### Promoting Realistic Expectations of Sleep

Reinforce that it is not realistic for the person to expect every night of sleep to be free of awakenings or disturbing thoughts and to be totally refreshing. The goal of the plan is to increase the number of nights that are restful. When this happens, fatigue and fear will be reduced, injury will be avoided, and the person will have the tools necessary to get back on track if problems with sleep occur in the future.

### Patient/Family Education

Teach aspects of normal sleep to patient and family. Persons typically monitor their own sleep. This can contribute to the sleep problem, because the person may mistake a normal phenomenon for something abnormal or for a sign that the new sleep habits are not working.

#### Health promotion/prevention

Prevention involves teaching persons and families about normal sleep and counseling them to be aware of events and activities that can enhance or detract from sleep. Often persons take steps to remedy a sleep problem, such as taking sleeping pills, taking naps, or drinking alcohol, which only exacerbate sleeping problems. Nurses must also teach persons that it is never too late to begin dealing with a sleep problem.

## ■ EVALUATION

The person will monitor his or her own progress and record this daily. When the interventions just discussed are successful, no further follow-up will be necessary.

## FUTURE RESEARCH ABOUT INSOMNIA

Insomnia may not be one diagnosis. There may be subtypes including limb movement with sleep, sleep hygiene disruption, substance overuse or abuse, and others that could show variable responses to interventions.[8]

Chronic insomnia should be distinguished from short-term sleep disturbance. In an experimental setting normal sleepers were awakened according to the sleep patterns produced by study subjects with chronic insomnia. The normal sleepers displayed sleep symptoms of sleep deprivation, different from those with chronic insomnia[3] (Box 13-5). From this the investigators concluded that poor sleep itself may not be the basis of symptoms in chronic insomnia but rather that poor sleep and these other symptoms may have a common basis, such as increased physiological activation.

The distinction of chronic physiological insomnia from mild sleep deprivation is an important one. Fatigue and tiredness may be on the increase because Americans do not make sleep a priority, choosing to devote fewer hours to rest and more hours to maintaining busy schedules.[2]

Subjective perception of sleep latency time (the time it takes to fall asleep) and time spent asleep or awake during the night is becoming a focus of investigation.[5,12] Research suggests that it may be as important to have the *perception* of having been asleep as having actually *been* asleep.[12]

**box 13-5** *Comparison of Responses of Normal Sleepers and Persons with Chronic Insomnia*

| NORMAL SLEEPERS | PERSONS WITH CHRONIC INSOMNIA |
|---|---|
| Decreased tension | Increased tension |
| Increased vigor | Decreased vigor |
| Approximate estimation of total awake time during sleep period | Overestimation of total awake time during sleep period |
| Decreased body temperature | Increased body temperature |
| Decreased sleep latency time | Increased sleep latency time |

From Bonnet MH, Arand DL: The consequence of a week of insomnia, *Sleep* 19(6):453-461, 1996.

## NARCOLEPSY

Narcolepsy is a neurological condition characterized by short, irresistible episodes of sleep intruding into wakefulness and recurring at frequent intervals. Five abnormal sleep features may be present: (1) irresistible sleep attacks with excessive daytime sleepiness, (2) hypnagogic hallucinations, (3) cataplexy, (4) sleep-onset REM periods, and (5) sleep paralysis. Any combination of the five features can be seen in narcolepsy, but at least two must be present to make a diagnosis.

Occasionally a person with normal sleep patterns may experience any one aspect of narcolepsy. The combination of symptoms, however, experienced consistently, sets narcolepsy apart.

### IRRESISTIBLE SLEEP ATTACKS AND EXCESSIVE DAYTIME SLEEPINESS

The sleep attacks, unpredictable and lasting a few moments to an hour, occur not only during monotonous sedentary activity, but also during mental or physical stimulation. The person may also feel unpleasantly drowsy throughout the day, resulting in poor performance of tasks.

### HYPNAGOGIC HALLUCINATIONS

This is the experience of vivid, troubling hallucinations, usually on awakening. The hypnagogic hallucinations are usually visual but can be auditory or tactile.

### CATAPLEXY

Cataplexy is an abrupt, reversible loss of muscle tone, usually brought on by strong emotions, such as fright, laughter, anger, or sudden increased stress. Cataplexy can be experienced variously from a feeling of slight weakness to a loss of strength in skeletal muscles to a complete loss of posture. Typically, the jaw sags, the head nods, the arms droop, and the legs buckle. Because attacks can be precipitated by listening to a funny joke or reexperiencing in memory a strongly unpleasant experience, persons suffering from cataplexy often try to restrict their emotional response to gain some control. This atonia is similar to the atonia seen during REM sleep.

### SLEEP-ONSET REM PERIODS

The normal sleeper passes through several stages of sleep and experiences REM sleep near the end of the 90-minute sleep cycle. In narcolepsy, when sleep occurs during the day in naps or during sleep attacks, the person goes into REM sleep within 5 minutes of going to sleep.

## SLEEP PARALYSIS

This frightening experience occurs just before falling asleep or on awakening. Sleepers find that, although they are completely awake, they cannot move the extremities, cannot speak, and may not even be able to breathe deeply. Sleep paralysis terminates spontaneously within several minutes but can be interrupted by being touched by someone. (One person plagued by sleep paralysis trained her dog to come and lick her hand each morning.) Often sleep paralysis is accompanied by hypnagogic hallucinations.

## ETIOLOGY

Two new research findings are fueling greater understanding of narcolepsy. First, several researchers have found a genetic link among persons with narcolepsy in which mild forms tend to cluster in some families, whereas more severe forms cluster in other families. Some aspects of narcolepsy (cataplexy and excessive daytime sleepiness) are genetically transmitted in some breeds of dogs. Second, a genetic link has recently been discovered between narcolepsy and a class II antigen of the major histocompatibility complex known as DR2. Scientists theorize that narcolepsy may be a disease that links the involvement of the immune system and its response to severe psychological stress with the development of disease in susceptible individuals.[1,8] This may help to explain the finding that in about one half of persons with narcolepsy, an abrupt change in the sleep-wake schedule and/or major psychological stress precedes the first symptom.

## EPIDEMIOLOGY

Narcolepsy is not a rare condition. Its prevalence has been estimated at 0.05% to 0.06%, which indicates that about one of every 2500 people has this disorder, or 250,000 Americans. Males are somewhat more affected than females. The age of onset varies from childhood to the 50s, with a peak incidence in the second decade of life, usually after puberty. Unrecognized and untreated, these irresistible, unwanted sleep attacks can be totally disabling. They interfere with the concentration required in school or at work and can result in accidents, leading to injury and death.

## PATHOPHYSIOLOGY

### Loss of Ability to Suppress Sleep

Normally the thalamus and cortical gray matter are highly active in wakefulness, resulting in general enhanced excitability of neurons, as well as selective inhibition of input. In drowsiness, reduction of synaptic transmissions occurs in the thalamus, despite an unchanged level of sensory input. Exactly which neurotransmitters and synaptic receptors relate to maintenance of alertness and initiation of sleep is not known. Interestingly, the activity of the gray matter and thalamus in REM sleep closely resembles waking activity.

Also not known is what neuronal changes occur with narcolepsy. Because this condition responds to stimulant drugs such as amphetamine, pemoline, and methylphenidate, however, it is hypothesized that some ratio of adrenergic/cholinergic neuronal activity is disrupted in sleep attacks and restored by these drugs.

### Episodic Atonia

Normally, muscle tone is maintained during wakefulness and during all sleep stages except REM by activity in the cerebellum. In REM sleep, centers in the pons activate, producing active inhibition of muscle tone in all muscle groups except those of the eye and penis and those that control respiration. Usually this atonia is briefly interrupted or overcome by powerful excitatory inputs to muscle groups, resulting in the muscle twitches and jerks seen in REM sleep.

In cataplexy, sudden time-limited atonia is experienced, although no change occurs in consciousness. Because this disorder responds to monoamine oxidase (MAO) inhibitors and other tricyclic antidepressants, it is theorized that cataplectic attacks (as well as sleep paralysis and hypnagogic hallucinations) result from some malfunction of norepinephrine, dopamine, and serotonin neurotransmitters or receptors in the brainstem.

### Aspects of Dreaming Intruding into Wakefulness

Dreaming usually occurs in REM sleep. REM sleep occurs at the end of each 90-minute sleep cycle, and longer periods of REM sleep occur at the end of the night. On awakening, all features of REM sleep (atonia and resulting paralysis of all muscle groups, except those for breathing and sight; dreaming) terminate. Less is known about the mechanisms of dreaming intruding into wakefulness. As just noted, however, because the person with narcolepsy responds to administration of tricyclic antidepressants and MAO inhibitors, a disorder of neurotransmitters or receptors may exist somewhere in the brain.[1]

The clinical manifestations of narcolepsy are discussed below. The person with narcolepsy feels chronically drowsy, exhibits memory lapses and poor work performance, and may experience *microsleeps,* sleep periods of a few seconds that may appear as daydreaming. Night sleep can be frequently interrupted by frightening dreams and awakenings. Cataplexy may develop as long as 20 years after the more common symptom of sleep attacks and excessive daytime drowsiness. The paralysis may last from a few seconds to a few minutes. No known measures can terminate an attack, except to remove the emotional trigger so that another attack will not immediately follow recovery from the first.

## COLLABORATIVE CARE MANAGEMENT

The person who has sleep attacks and excessive daytime sleepiness is given central nervous system (CNS) stimulants, such as amphetamine, pemoline (Cylert), or methylphenidate (Ritalin). Some side effects—such as irritability, tachycardia, and nocturnal sleep disturbances, as well as tolerance and drug dependence—may occur. Persons experiencing cataplexy, sleep paralysis, or hypnagogic hallucinations receive a tricyclic antidepressant, such as imipramine, protriptyline, or clomipramine. Doses are usually adjusted to achieve the best balance between improved daytime alertness and unwanted side effects. An experimental drug, gamma-hydroxybutyrate, shows some promise.

Daytime naps may also be prescribed to assist with daytime alertness. Three 15- to 20-minute naps spaced evenly throughout the day often help restore a feeling of alertness.

The PSG and MSLT (see pp. 350 and 351) are the essential tests to distinguish narcolepsy from daytime sleepiness experienced by someone who simply sleeps poorly at night. The night sleep test (PSG) documents the night aspects of sleep. The MSLT, performed the next day, documents how readily the person falls asleep during a half-hour nap (four naps are observed during the next 8 hours after awakening from the PSG) and how quickly REM sleep occurs with each nap. A "normal" person may have one sleep-onset REM episode of four naps and may not be able to fall asleep for all the nap periods. A "sleepy" person may be able to fall asleep each time but does not have more than one sleep-onset REM period. A "narcoleptic" person falls asleep readily during each nap period and has more than one sleep-onset REM period. The physician may try to record a cataplectic attack if the patient reports a history of this with particular stressors.

# NURSING MANAGEMENT

## ASSESSMENT

### Subjective Data

A complete sleep history (see Box 13-4) is obtained from the person suspected of having narcolepsy. Data of particular importance include:

- Understanding of narcolepsy and factors that increase or decrease symptoms
- Experience with antinarcoleptic drugs and side effects (Are the drugs taken on holidays? Are doses self-adjusted?)
- Safety practices and accident history, especially if the person drives
- Family understanding and support
- Problems and adjustments in employment or school performance

## NURSING DIAGNOSES

Nursing diagnoses are determined from analysis of patient data. Nursing diagnoses for the patient with narcolepsy may include but are not limited to:

| Diagnostic Title | Possible Etiological Factors |
|---|---|
| Knowledge deficit (about narcolepsy) | Lack of information |
| Coping, ineffective | Purposeful emotional restriction and (individual) day-to-day difficulties |
| Fatigue | Excessive daytime sleepiness causing difficulty with treatment regimen and misunderstanding by family and employer or teacher |
| Injury, risk for | Sleep attacks, cataplexy |

## EXPECTED PATIENT OUTCOMES

Expected patient outcomes for the patient with narcolepsy may include but are not limited to:

1. Describes the disorder and medication regimen and reports success with explaining narcolepsy to family or employer (or enlists the assistance of a person knowledgeable about narcolepsy).

2a. Identifies purposeful avoidance of strong emotions as a way to cope with cataplectic attacks.

b. Describes a level of participation that satisfies family and work responsibilities.

3a. Reports feeling less fatigue.

b. Reports improved job or school performance.

4. Demonstrates effective strategies for reducing exposure to risk factors in the environment; avoidable accidents and injuries do not occur.

## INTERVENTIONS

### Promoting Understanding of Narcolepsy

Teach aspects of narcolepsy and rationale for the treatment plan. It is important that the person maintain close contact with the physician and nurse to monitor effectiveness of medications and treatment. Telephone follow-up may be used to maintain contact and support. Encourage the person and family to contact one of the sleep resources listed on p. 350, which can provide information on local support networks. Their newsletters contain up-to-date information on recent research findings and provide forums for sharing ideas.

Assess and support the person's efforts to teach others about narcolepsy. Remind the person that it may take some practice before acquiring ease in teaching others.

### Promoting Safety and Preventing Injury

Teach the patient to consider carefully the risks of injury at home and at school or work. Rather than engage in denial or wishful thinking, the patient should consider problems caused by sleep attacks and cataplectic attacks. Some suggestions include the following:

1. Do not drive unless sleep attacks and cataplectic attacks are completely under control; then drive only for short distances during times of high wakefulness.
2. Do food preparation or self-grooming activities (handling knives, curling or clothes irons; cooking on stove) during quiet times (such as before others in the house awaken) to avoid times of surprise or emotion that can trigger an attack.
3. Learn to use the microwave oven for cooking to avoid burns from the stove.
4. If possible, live in a dwelling that has either no stairs or an enclosed staircase to minimize injury during falls.
5. Ask family members/co-workers to use a gentle aural signal before approaching to prevent triggering a sleep attack.

### Promoting Participation in Family Life and Work

Encourage the person to meet with other persons with narcolepsy for mutual support or with the nurse during times of frustration as well as success. Suggest that family members join a local narcolepsy support group to help deal with their own concerns. Narcolepsy can be a very difficult disorder to live with, but personal isolation and withdrawal only make life more difficult.

### Patient/Family Education

The major nursing strategies for the person with narcolepsy and his or her family are teaching and support with effective ways of coping with the disorder. As control of sleepiness and cataplectic attacks is achieved, fatigue should lessen, job or school performance should improve, and the potential for injury will decrease.

#### *Health promotion/prevention*

As yet, no clear evidence exists concerning the prevention of narcolepsy. More effort is being directed toward the early recognition of the disorder, particularly in relatives of affected family members. If a parent has narcolepsy, there is a 1 in 50 chance that each child will have it.

## EVALUATION

1. Explains narcolepsy to family and employer, including purpose and timing of medications.
2a. States ways to avoid strong emotions in coping with cataleptic attacks.
b. Describes participation in family and work responsibilities.
3a. States feeling less fatigued.
b. Carries out school/work responsibilities at a satisfactory level.
4. Describes way to avoid accidents or injuries by performing activities when medication levels will ensure wakefulness.

# SLEEP APNEA

## ETIOLOGY

Sleep apnea is a sleep problem involving other body systems. A mutual relationship exists between sleep and other body systems; the sleep state affects the functioning of *all* body systems to some extent. In addition, the functioning of *any* body system affects the states of sleep. Many disease processes affect sleep or are affected by sleep, including asthma, gastroesophageal reflux, epilepsy, headache, fibrositis, myocardial instability, and chronic pain. This section focuses on sleep apnea and the mutual relationship between body systems and sleep.

## EPIDEMIOLOGY

The gradual development of sleep apnea and its sequelae is incompletely understood. Although factors such as obesity and oropharyngeal architecture have been associated with this disorder, other neurological and genetic factors may play a role even before any symptoms develop. Some researchers hypothesize that sleep apnea is a progressive illness resulting as a systemic response to years of decreased airway patency, reduced airflow, reduced ventilation,[8] stimulation of autonomic functioning, and disruption of reflexes required to maintain breathing during sleep. This produces a maladaptive response that results in a feedback loop of greater impairment. The cardiovascular consequences of undetected or untreated sleep apnea are significant[22] (Box 13-6). A National Institutes of Health (NIH)-sponsored, multicenter prospective study of cardiovascular events (stroke and myocardial infarction) associated with sleep apnea began in 1996.

Many unanswered questions remain concerning sleep apnea, including the following:

1. How much time does it take for sleep apnea syndrome to develop or for cardiac rhythm changes and hypertension to become severe?
2. How many sleepers who snore quietly and sporadically early in life will subsequently develop sleep apnea?
3. How can one predict who will develop milder or more severe forms of sleep apnea?

## PHYSIOLOGY

While reading the following discussion of normal and abnormal breathing during sleep, remember these major points:

1. The understanding of breathing during sleep centers on the complex interrelationships and feedback loops between the neurological and respiratory systems. These interrelationships have significant impact on the cardiovascular system and on sleep itself.
2. The two primary results of severely impaired breathing during sleep are (a) cardiac dysrhythmia, which can result in increased risk of cardiac fibrillation and death, and (b) excessive daytime sleepiness or reduction of daytime alertness, which can result in increased risk of accident, such as falling asleep while driving.

### Control of Breathing

Breathing is initiated by the respiratory center in the medulla. Breathing responds to body requirements through input from three sources: chemoreceptors in the carotid body, stretch/mechanical receptors located in the lung and chest wall, and input from other brain centers (see Chapter 30). In wakefulness, breathing is modified by conscious effort. In sleep, breathing patterns show clear differences between stage I, deeper, and REM (dreaming) sleep, indicating that brain centers controlling[11] sleep have a direct impact on breathing centers as well. In persons with sleep apnea, chemoreceptor responsiveness is reduced, possibly as a result of years of decreased oxygen saturation and increased carbon dioxide levels during sleep. It is not known if ventilatory compensation for

**box 13-6** *Cardiovascular Consequences of Sleep Apnea*

1. Abrupt hemodynamic changes—increase in heart rate, arterial pressure, and decrease in left ventricular stroke volume
2. Failure to display normal nocturnal decline in arterial pressure of 10% to 15% from waking value
3. Sustained diurnal hypertension

resistive loading (stretch receptor responsiveness) is maintained in sleep. During sleep apnea, when many arousals occur in the night, the person becomes sleepier, leading to decreased arousability and longer apneas. Arousal can be induced by several respiratory conditions. It must occur when a cough is necessary to clear secretions from the airway.

### Open Passageway to Lungs

The pharynx is the only nonrigid structure in the passageway to the lungs. The diameter is maintained by toned muscle in the pharyngeal walls, allowing for closure only during swallowing, regurgitation, and speech. In non-REM sleep, this muscle tone is reduced; in REM sleep, it is greatly reduced. Only intercostal, diaphragmatic, and ocular muscles maintain tone in REM sleep. Some sleep experts theorize that the evidence of diminished upper airway tone with maintenance of diaphragmatic and intercostal muscle tone suggests separate neural control of these respiratory muscle groups. The oropharynx of persons with sleep apnea may be anatomically small or may contain enlarged structures, or it may once have been large enough but now has a reduced diameter because of fat deposition in tissues.

## PATHOPHYSIOLOGY

### Response to Internal/External Stimuli

Breathing also depends on responsiveness to changed internal and external stimuli. In sleep, responsiveness to the following factors is reduced:

1. *Bronchial irritation.* Cough is reduced in REM and non-REM sleep and resumes only on arousal.
2. *Isocapnic hypoxia.* Partial oxygen pressure ($PO_2$) may fall as low as 70% of normal before sleepers are aroused. In REM sleep, arousal threshold is further reduced.
3. *Hypercapnia.* Most sleepers awaken before partial carbon dioxide pressure ($PCO_2$) rises to 15 mm Hg above wakefulness level. In REM sleep, arousal is further reduced.
4. *Alcohol and CNS depressants.* During sleep, these substances suppress upper airway tone, as well as arousal by medulla and higher cortical centers.

Responsiveness to all these factors is depressed further in a person whose sleep has been so fragmented as to lead to further depressed arousal thresholds. Moderate degrees of alcohol intoxication can decrease hypoxic and hypercapnic ventilatory responses to 50% of baseline values. Oxygen saturation of less than 80% of normal is considered severe.

**box 13-7** *Definitions of Apnea/Hypopnea*

| | |
|---|---|
| **Apnea** | Breathing ceases for more than 10 seconds. |
| **Hypopnea** | Breathing is reduced, rather than completely eliminated. |
| **Obstructive apnea** | Breathing effort occurs with diaphragmatic and intercostal muscles, but no air passes through the mouth and nose. The pharynx collapses, producing obstruction. |
| **Central apnea** | No breathing effort is expended by thoracic muscles (message to breathe not received by lungs from medulla). |
| **Mixed apnea** | Begins as an absence of respiratory effort; when effort begins, however, obstruction results. |
| **Sleep apnea syndrome** | More than five apneic events per hour of sleep occur. |

### Apneas/Hypopneas

Different types of apneas occur (see Box 13-7 for definitions). Normal sleepers experience a few apneas/hypopneas each night; the apneas may be obstructive, central, or mixed. These apneas are fewer and shorter in duration than those in sleep apnea syndrome. The normal sleeper has a transient drop in oxygen saturation, transient bradycardia, or tachycardia and a transient rise in blood pressure; all return to normal levels when the apnea episode is over. The person with sleep apnea syndrome has decreased oxygen saturation (less than 80%) through the night that results in (1) maladaptive cardiovascular responses, (2) disrupted sleep, and (3) other difficulties, including morning headache, bedwetting, and changes in mood, alertness, endurance, work performance, and intellectual and sexual functioning. The most serious life-threatening results are hypertension, cardiac dysrhythmias (bradycardia, tachycardia, premature ventricular contractions, second-degree atrioventricular block, prolonged sinus pauses, and atrial fibrillation), and accidents from falling asleep while driving or doing other monotonous tasks.

The clinical manifestations of sleep apnea are described next. When sleep apnea is suspected, a sleeping partner is interviewed, as well as the sleeper. The bed partner may report most or all of the following details:

> He falls asleep very easily in the chair or when he goes to bed for the night. Sometimes he is restless and dozes on and off for a while. He may begin snoring as soon as he falls asleep, or it may not start until later in the night. He used to snore only when he fell asleep on his back, but now he snores in any position. He snores very loudly, and you can hear him from other rooms in the house. Sometimes he stops breathing; after several moments, he snorts loudly, shudders or kicks his legs, then takes a deep breath and goes back to sleep. He may answer me if I speak to him, but he doesn't recall it in the morning. He does this all night long, but I think it happens more often in the early morning. He may get up frequently to urinate in the night, and sometimes he perspires heavily from all the moving around in bed. I hate to admit it, but sometimes I have to sleep in another room because the noise and his restlessness keep me awake. Yet, I am worried that he needs me there to wake him up if he goes too long without breathing. I think *I* am developing a sleep problem.

## COLLABORATIVE CARE MANAGEMENT

Medical management of the person with sleep apnea takes a graded approach to match the severity of the problem. For *mild* sleep apnea syndrome, the patient is advised to sleep on a side and to lose weight if obese.[19] In addition, the patient should avoid all sleeping medications, CNS depressants, and alcohol. If these approaches do not provide improvement, drug therapy may be instituted. Medroxyprogesterone may be prescribed for those who also hypoventilate while awake. A trial of protriptyline is initiated for obese persons. Patients need to be followed closely, because the side effects of the drugs may work against the patient taking them faithfully.

For moderate sleep apnea syndrome, an oral surgeon or ear, nose, and throat (ENT) specialist may suggest removal of tonsils or realignment of the bite, either through jaw surgery or use of an appliance during sleep, if specific upper airway obstruction is found. In the absence of obstruction, a nasal *continuous positive airway pressure (CPAP)* system may be recommended. A CPAP system consists of an air pump connected to a mask worn over the nose during sleep. This air pump (to which supplemental oxygen may be added) delivers air to the oropharynx at a pressure sufficient to prevent collapse of the pharynx during sleep. For the first several nights, the CPAP system is worn while the patient sleeps in the laboratory, where sleep technicians adjust the air pressure in the mask to the amount required. When the CPAP system reduces apneic events, the sleeper will experience deeper and longer periods of sleep for the next several nights; arousal to breathe is unnecessary. Because increased REM sleep also means increased time during which the sleeper does not arouse as easily, the person needs to be observed for any difficulties. Wearing the mask takes some personal adjustment; however, most patients experience quick relief from their problems of daytime sleepiness and nighttime symptoms.

Nasal CPAP is recommended as the initial intervention because it is more effective than oral CPAP. Oral CPAP should be tried next if the patient is unwilling or unable to use nasal CPAP.[17] A significant percentage of patients use CPAP inconsistently because of discomfort of the patient or bedpartner. The apneic symptoms return as soon as CPAP use is discontinued. The person with sleep apnea needs continued support with this lifelong problem. More extreme therapy may be required but only after thorough reevaluation in the sleep laboratory using the CPAP appliance.[16]

When a patient demonstrates pronounced oxygen desaturation or frequent cardiac dysrhythmias (severe sleep apnea syndrome), more extreme therapy is recommended. A *uvulopalatopharyngoplasty* may be performed by an ENT surgeon experienced with the treatment of sleep apnea patients. This procedure removes almost all the soft tissue at the back of the mouth to widen the pharynx. The patient must be cautioned, however, that in some people snoring will disappear, but apnea can still be present. In addition, during the first 3 days postoperatively, regional edema can occlude the airway. A tracheostomy may be required to prevent sudden death. It may take a week to 10 days for the patient to swallow comfortably again. Special attention must be given to the obese person so that the airway will not occlude with supine sleeping postures.

The PSG (see p. 350) is the primary test. It should be performed at night because apneic episodes may be more frequent during REM sleep, and a sleeper may not have any REM sleep during afternoon naps. The test may be repeated after the patient undergoes treatment for sleep apnea to determine the degree of response.

Almost routinely the patient is sent for a consulting examination with an otolaryngologist or maxillofacial specialist to determine the extent to which oropharyngeal architecture impacts on the obstructed airway. Pulmonary function tests may also be ordered to detect any underlying contributing factors. The physician may request that much of the pulmonary testing be done with the patient in a supine position.

## NURSING MANAGEMENT

### ASSESSMENT

#### Subjective Data

Data to be collected to assess the patient with sleep apnea include:

- The patient's and family's understanding of the cause of the sleep apnea and the possible risks to health and life
- Understanding of how the cardiac and respiratory systems work
- Awareness of contributing factors of obesity and alcohol intake
- Sleep history, including use of sleeping pills; use of stimulants; and work, hobby, and accident history
- Understanding of possible courses of action
- Assessment of any emotional, social, or economic factors that may contribute to reluctance of patient and family to take part in treatment

#### Objective Data

Data to be collected to assess the patient with sleep apnea include:

- Blood pressure, respiratory assessment (including breath sounds, chest movement, presence of any thoracic deformities), degree of obesity, oropharyngeal assessment, level of awareness, and skin color
- Results of CBC, pulmonary, cardiac, and sleep studies
- Presence of any other health problems

### NURSING DIAGNOSES

Nursing diagnoses are determined from analysis of patient data. Nursing diagnoses for the patient with sleep apnea may include but are not limited to:

| Diagnostic Title | Possible Etiological Factors |
|---|---|
| Breathing pattern, ineffective | Airway obstruction or episodic loss of neurological stimulus to breathe at night |
| Knowledge deficit (about sleep problem) | Lack of information |
| Fatigue | Altered sleep pattern; oxygen desaturation and frequent arousals at night |
| Injury, risk for | Increased daytime sleepiness, fatigue, reduced vigilance and response time |

## EXPECTED PATIENT OUTCOMES

Expected patient outcomes for the person with sleep apnea may include but are not limited to:

1. Breathes easily at night.
2. Patient/family carry out a plan to remedy sleep apnea and will describe measures to take if sleep apnea does not respond to treatment.
3. Patient/bed partner/family can describe the effects of sleep apnea.
4. Sustains no injuries as a result of daytime sleepiness, fatigue, or decreased awareness.

## INTERVENTIONS

### Facilitating Learning

Nursing interventions consist primarily of patient/family teaching and counseling. As sleep apnea decreases with treatment, fatigue and the potential for injuries also decrease.

The nurse may anticipate that the patient or someone in the family may minimize the seriousness of sleep apnea and may not be totally supportive of the means required to respond to the problem. It takes teaching and support to help a family come to the understanding that "plain old snoring" can indicate a serious health problem. In some sleep laboratories, the sleeper is videotaped throughout a night (with consent). If patients or family members doubt the seriousness of the problem, it can be instructive to let them see parts of the tape or sleep record to illustrate how long breathing does not occur or how often during the night the sleeper arouses.

### Promoting Effective Team Response

Successful treatment involves members of separate disciplines providing several modalities of therapy. A satisfactory therapeutic response from the family's point of view often hinges on one team member, such as the nurse, being willing to handle questions and concerns from family and other team members.

Obese patients need to lose weight. Successful participation in weight loss programs requires knowledgeable referral and supportive follow-up by a member of the treatment team. Surgical treatment requires input from many specialists, and patients and families benefit from someone who can handle questions and respond to concerns. A patient using CPAP will need information for the insurance company, as well as a 24-hour telephone number to call should problems with equipment occur in the middle of the night.

### Patient/Family Education

It is important that both patient and bed partner/family understand normal breathing in sleep, the effects of sleep apnea, measures to take to prevent injury, and treatment regimen. Teaching includes:

1. Relationship between the pulmonary and cardiac systems
2. How sleep affects breathing
3. How uninterrupted sleep contributes to daytime functioning
4. How sleep apnea contributes to cardiac problems and leads to increased risk of accidents
5. Restrictions on operating machinery, including appliances and equipment at home, until risk of fatigue-related accidents subsides
6. Drug therapy regimen, side effects, expected time to determine efficacy, and who to contact if problems occur

#### *Health promotion/prevention*

Because sleep apnea is not yet fully understood, steps to prevent its development are not completely known. In addition to encouraging normal weight and good pulmonary habits, any reported symptoms suggestive of sleep apnea should not be overlooked or dismissed.

## EVALUATION

1. Reports breathing easily at night.
2. Describes what bed partner/family will do if apnea occurs.
3. Discusses effects of sleep apnea.
4. Dos not sustain an injury because of daytime sleepiness, fatigue, or decreased awareness.

# CIRCADIAN RHYTHM DISORDERS

A common difficulty experienced by a large majority of shift workers is sleep disturbance.[4] Many researchers have sought to mitigate the effects of the altered sleep/activity cycle on mood, sleep, appetite, and performance through a variety of means including light treatments, precisely timed meals, rest, exercise, and dietary adjustments to hasten and/or consolidate sleep phase change. Yet research indicates that the realities of daily life, such as the requirement for most workers to go out into the environment to get home from work, thereby exposing the eyes to ambient light, undercuts treatment effects.[4] Some employees using these experimental sleep-wake protocols wear welders' goggles to protect the eyes from light. Bright light may manipulate the circadian rhythm system, but it may not have as strong an effect on behavior and performance as it does on temperature cycles. Moreover, given the tendency for increasing sleep fragility in later decades, middle-aged workers may not be as responsive to such treatments as younger research subjects seem to be.[4]

It would be interesting for further study to determine the effect of sleep interruption on the retention of information taught to patients and to determine the effect of hospital sleep interruption on home sleep patterns. It would be of further interest to determine whether a nursing intervention such as waiting until the person has finished an episode of REM sleep before waking her or him or timing nursing interventions to predicted completion of 90-minute sleep cycles based on the time a particular patient fell asleep would improve sleep parameters, mood, memory, physical stamina, and other factors.

Florence Nightingale is often pictured with a lamp as she watches over wounded and sick soldiers through the night. No more apt picture could illustrate the growing body of knowledge concerning the interrelationships among biological rhythms, especially sleep, as they are challenged in illness, modified because of professional commitment, and highlighted by new nursing contributions to this developing research area.

## PARASOMNIAS

Various types of parasomnias or disorders of arousal may occur, especially in children, who may outgrow the dysfunction (Table 13-1). Additionally, Table 13-2 contains an abbreviated listing of some medical/psychiatric sleep disorders. An example of a proposed disorder is sleep hyperhydrosis, profound sweating during sleep, that can occur in patients with disorders such as lymphoma and human immunodeficiency virus (HIV) infection. Several other parasomnias are discussed next.

### SLEEPWALKING

Sleepwalking (somnambulism) is characterized by sitting up or walking about while asleep. The sleepwalker's eyes are open, but the person appears to be in a daze, has purposeless movements, may speak in short phrases, and remembers nothing about it in the morning. Sleepwalking most commonly occurs in children who usually outgrow it, but it may also be seen in adults. Twenty percent of somnambulists have a parent who sleepwalks, and 5% to 15% of the general population has sleepwalked at some time. Sleepwalking usually occurs in the first third of the night during stage III/IV sleep. Up to 50% of all sleepwalkers either experience injury or narrowly avoid it.

Sleepwalkers should be led back to bed without being awakened. If the sleepwalker must be awakened, do not slap or shake the person or splash cold water on the face, but say the person's name over and over. If the sleepwalker lies down to sleep on the floor, cover the person and he or she can stay there until awakening.

To protect the sleepwalker from injury, place a bell at the bedside that will ring if the bedside is moved, or use an intercom in a child's room to awaken the parent when the child stirs. A protective gate or screen door may be placed across the door to the bedroom, but note that this blocks escape if there is a fire. Lock windows and doors to balconies. Imipramine, a tricyclic antidepressant, is sometimes prescribed for adult sleepwalkers who walk frequently and have been injured.

### SLEEP TERROR

Sleep terror (*pavor nocturnus*) usually occurs in children in the first part of the night during stage III/IV sleep. The child screams, arises from bed, wanders about in panic, and cannot be awakened or consoled. Autonomic changes (rapid pulse and respirations, sweating) can be noted. The child may be amnestic for the event. Sleep terror is often associated with sleepwalking.

Interventions include maintaining a regular sleep schedule and not trying to awaken the child, because this may worsen the confusion. Usually, the child will lie back on the pillow after several minutes, never having awakened. Benzodiazepines are sometimes given to patients with severe episodes, because these suppress stage III/IV sleep.[15]

### FAMILIAL SLEEP PARALYSIS

The person with familial sleep paralysis appears asleep but remains conscious. Occasionally, frighteningly vivid hallucinations may occur. The eyes may be open, and the patient can move them, although he or she is unable to move any other muscles. Although this is part of the tetrad of symptoms of

**table 13-1** *Parasomnias*

| Type of Dysfunction | Comments |
|---|---|
| Nightmare (sleep terror) | Panic attack while asleep |
| Sleep-related enuresis | Bedwetting; event begins in stage III/IV sleep, and enuresis occurs as sleep lightens |
| Sleep-related bruxism | Teeth grinding: dental appliance may be needed to preserve teeth |
| Rhythmic movement disorder | Jactatio capitis nocturna, rhythmic head rocking and banging not uncommon in children younger than 5, occurs in stage I/II sleep |
| Sleep paralysis | Inability to move muscles when first awakening; may have a familial component |
| Impairment in penile erections | Changes in sensation or frequency of erections in REM sleep |

**table 13-2** *Medical/Psychiatric Sleep Disorders*

| Type of Dysfunction | Comments |
|---|---|
| Sleep-related epileptic seizures | Seizures occur more often during sleep; explains why sleep is encouraged during short routine electroencephalograms |
| Sleep-related headache | Associated with REM sleep and postponed morning coffee on weekends, relieved with indomethacin and improved sleep hygiene |
| Sleep-related abnormal swallowing | Inadequate swallowing of saliva during sleep |
| Sleep-related asthma | Early morning increase in bronchoconstriction; 46% of asthmatic attacks occur during last third of night |
| Sleep-related cardiovascular symptoms | Includes paroxysmal nocturnal dyspnea, myocardial infarction (peak incidence 4 AM to 6 AM), nocturnal angina, and premature ventricular contractions, which are more common in REM sleep |
| Sleep-related gastroesophageal reflux | Caused more by posture than sleep |

narcolepsy, many normal people experience this. Intervention includes teaching family members to awaken the person by touch each day or allowing a pet dog or cat to awaken the person through touch.

### PENILE ERECTIONS

Men experience erections during REM sleep, regardless of sexual activity or dream content. If impairment of erections occurs during sleep, an underlying illness may be present, such as diabetes mellitus, or it may result from the effect of medications. Painful erections may occur during sleep, even though erections are not painful or difficult while awake. There may be a problem with the foreskin in uncircumcised men or a problem with the penile blood vessels. The man should be referred to a urologist for evaluation.

## CLINICAL CHRONOBIOLOGY: THE DEVELOPMENT OF A NEW AREA OF SCIENCE

The study of normal sleep and sleep problems falls within the broader area of inquiry known as *chronobiology,* or the study of biological activities as they vary or oscillate predictably over time. Sleep is only one of many biological events that occur at the same time every 24 hours. Other events that have predictable cyclic peaks and troughs every 24 hours include the following:

1. Core body temperature
2. Cell division
3. Production of red blood cells
4. Preferential migration of lymphocytes into spleen from the peripheral circulation
5. Production of hormones, such as cortisol and growth hormone
6. Muscle strength and alertness
7. Mental alertness

Even more interesting, some of these events are apparently controlled by the action of internal pacemakers that are somewhat insulated from the activity of the environment, whereas other biological rhythms depend much more on and are driven by environmental cues. For example, some biological events depend on what the person does such as turning out the lights and lapsing into sleep before they begin. Another compelling finding is that under circumstances of environmental change, such as changing time zones during airplane travel, working the night shift, or postponing sleep, some biological rhythms are affected more than others and some take longer to readjust. Therefore, not only does an individual rhythm lose its pattern transiently but also all rhythms that act on this one rhythm can also become asynchronous.

One focus of current sleep research is to determine how sleep changes as people age. Several researchers hypothesize that the circadian oscillators may lose some of their precise interrelatedness in aging, providing evidence for systematic age-related changes in the output of the circadian pacemakers. Living in an institution with a reduction in exposure to bright outdoor illumination and social zeitgebers (an event that provides the stimulus for setting or resetting the biologic clock) probably undermines the organization of sleep-wake rhythm.

These findings are pertinent at the clinical level because the biological rhythms of both patients and caregivers are affected by the patient's hospitalization. Regarding the patient, the following is only a partial list of factors at work when someone is hospitalized:

1. Pain, fatigue, uncertainty, and anxiety
2. Different bed and bedclothes in an unusual sleeping environment
3. Being awakened for procedures, vital signs, or medications
4. Reduced opportunity for exercise
5. Nutrient timing changes or food withheld
6. Medications depressing or accelerating different biological functions
7. Lights being turned on or off during the sleep time
8. Living in an environmental temperature (too hot or too cold) that is not under patient control

It is not yet known to what degree, if any, a change in environmental conditions affects healing, recovery time, feelings of well-being, or response to treatment. All these environmental factors and more are being studied regarding how they affect sleep, response to treatment, and recovery time. What is most exciting for nursing research is that nurses make clinical decisions about many of these environmental factors (see the accompanying Research Box). Nursing research in the future will contribute to the determination of optimal timing for assessments and treatments and the creation of the chronobiologically most synchronous or most supportive environments for the patient.

**research**

Reference: Gall K, Peterson T, Riesch SK: Night life: nocturnal behavior patterns among hospitalized elderly, *J Gerontol Nurs* 16(10):31-37, 1990.

In an inpatient geriatric unit, 21 elderly people (ages 61 to 91; mean, 75.7 years) were visually observed at 30-minute intervals from 11 PM to 7 AM on the second, third, and fourth nights of hospitalization. These persons were not critically ill and not confused and did not have a preexisting sleep problem.

The investigators found that fewer subjects were sleeping at any given hour on the second night of study compared with the first night, and still fewer were sleeping on any given hour of the third night, compared with the first or second nights. By night 3, less than 50% were asleep at any given hour. Treatments or medications interrupted sleep in three fourths of the subjects. Each time sleep was interrupted, it took at least 30 minutes for the person to fall back asleep. Sleep was particularly disrupted at 3 AM and between the hours of 5 and 6 AM.

| Study Night | 3 AM | 5 AM | 6 AM |
|---|---|---|---|
| 1 | 72% asleep | 80% | 40% |
| 2 | 56% | 55% | 20% |
| 3 | 47% | 40% | 30% |

Nurses must remember that their own biological rhythms are also responding to the environment. Ongoing research has described the risks some workers face when they work and sleep at irregular hours[4] and effects on health and performance during day, evening, and night shifts. Some experts recommend that persons rotating from day shift to night shift make the best adjustment in sleep when the night shift is worked for a longer period. For example, rotating to the night shift for a month or more at a time is easier to adjust to than is rotating shifts every 1 or 2 weeks. Other research is focusing on the resetting of biological clocks by exposure to very bright light at times of day that may exert the most influence on circadian oscillators.

## critical thinking QUESTIONS

**1** You are caring for Sam, a patient suspected of having narcolepsy. One evening he calls you to his room and states that he is confused about information received from his doctor. His doctor explained that Sam's MSLT report was positive, but Sam does not understand the test or its results. How would you explain this finding to Sam? Considering all the interventions possible, which is of the highest priority?

**2** Chuck has been found to have a moderate sleep apnea syndrome. Upon examination he is found to have no specific upper airway obstruction; therefore the doctor orders a CPAP system for Chuck. When it arrives Chuck asks you how and why it works. What is the best explanation regarding this treatment method?

**3** Taking into consideration the 90-minute sleep cycle, how could you best time the waking of a patient at night to take his or her vital signs?

**4** If a man with newly diagnosed sleep attacks caused by narcolepsy calls and states that his medication is not helping at all, what factors would you consider as you assess the situation?

**5** What assessment challenges might you expect as you assess a 70-year-old man whose spouse of 45 years has just mentioned that his snoring is a little louder than before, "but it's probably nothing"?

**6** What steps would you take to coordinate the care of a person having severe obstructive sleep apnea?

## chapter SUMMARY

### NATURE OF THE PROBLEM

- More than a half million adults have difficulty with sleeping at some time in their lives.
- Sleep disorders can be categorized by the type of disruption they cause including the following:
  dyssomnias or intrinsic sleep disorders:
    insomnia—inability to initiate or maintain sleep
    narcolepsy—sleep intrusion into wakefulness
    sleep apnea—sleep problems involving other body systems
    circadian rhythm disorders—sleep problems associated with time zone changes (jet lag) or shift work
  parasomnias or disorders of arousal associated with sleep, sleep stages, or arousal

### INSOMNIA

- Persons with insomnia must be taught not to take naps, sleeping pills, caffeine, or alcohol because these may exacerbate insomnia.
- Nurses need to understand the importance of a sleep schedule in treating sleep disorders.
- Problems of initiating or maintaining sleep may continue over many years, even when the precipitating factor has been resolved.
- Helping a patient master a problem with insomnia requires education about normal sleep and careful initiation of new sleep practices.

### NARCOLEPSY

- Narcolepsy is a neurological condition that has five features, two of which must be present to make a diagnosis. The five features are excessive daytime sleepiness, hypnagogic hallucinations, cataplexy, sleep-onset REM periods, and sleep paralysis.
- Persons with narcolepsy are at risk of injuring themselves or others if they fall asleep while driving or operating machinery. The person with narcolepsy needs to understand the risks and take proper precautions.

### SLEEP APNEA

- Loud snoring and breathing disturbances in sleep are symptoms of sleep apnea.

### GENERAL

- Nurses need to take special care with their own sleep habits, particularly when rotating from day to night shifts, because they may be at greater risk for accidents and slips in performance when deprived of sleep.

## References


1. Bergstrom DL, Keller C: Narcolepsy: pathogenesis and nursing care, *J Neurosci Nurs* 24(3):153-157, 1992.
2. Bliwise DL: Historical change in the report of daytime fatigue, *Sleep* 19(6):453-461, 1996.
3. Bonnet MH, Arand DL: The consequence of a week of insomnia, *Sleep* 19(6):453-461, 1996.
4. Campbell SS, Liu L, Fogg LF: Circadian rhythm adaptation to simulated night shift work: effect of nocturnal bright light duration, *Sleep* 18(6):399-407, 1995.
5. Chervin RD, Guilleminault C: Overestimation of sleep latency by patients with suspected hypersomnolence, *Sleep* 19(2):94-100, 1996.
6. Cravatt BF et al: Chemical characterization of a family of brain lipids that induce sleep, *Science* 268:1506-1509, 1995.
7. Diagnostic Classification Steering Committee: *The international classification of sleep disorders: diagnostic and coding manual,* Rochester, Minn, 1990, American Sleep Disorders Association.
8. Edinger JD et al: The empirical identification of insomnia subtypes: a cluster analytic approach, *Sleep* 19(5):398-411, 1996.
9. Kinney HC et al: Decreased muscarinic receptor binding in the arcuate nucleus in sudden infant death syndrome, *Science* 269:1446-1450, 1995.
10. Krueger JM, Toth LA: Cytokines as regulators of sleep, *Ann NY Acad Sci* 739:299, 1994.
11. Lydic R. Biebuyck JF, editors: *Clinical physiology of sleep,* Bethesda Md, 1988, American Physiological Society.
12. Mendelson WB: Pharmacologic alteration of the perception of being awake or asleep, *Sleep* 16(7):641-646, 1993.
13. Mendelson WB: Long-term follow up of chronic insomnia, *Sleep* 18(8):698-701, 1995.

14. Pakola SJ, Dinges DF, Pack AI: Review of regulations and guidelines for commercial and non-commercial drivers with sleep apnea and narcolepsy, *Sleep* 18(9):787-796, 1995.
15. Schenck CH, Mahowald MW: Long term nightly benzodiazepine treatment of injurious parasomnias and other disorders of disrupted nocturnal sleep in 170 adults, *Am J Med* 334(2):99-104, 1996.
16. Standards and Practices Committee of the American Sleep Disorders Association: Practice parameters for the treatment of obstructive sleep apnea in adults: the efficacy of surgical modifications of the upper airway, *Sleep* 19(2):152-155, 1996.
17. Standards and Practices Committee of the American Sleep Disorders Association: Practice parameters for the treatment of snoring and obstructive sleep apnea with oral appliances, *Sleep* 18(6):511-513, 1996.
18. Strambi-Ferini L et al: Slow wave and cyclic alternating pattern in HIV-infected asymptomatic men, *Sleep* 18(6):446-450, 1995.
19. Strobel RJ, Rosen RC: Obesity and weight loss in obstructive sleep apnea: a critical review, *Sleep* 19(2):104-115, 1996.
20. Szymusiac R: Magnocellular nuclei of the basal forebrain: substrates of sleep and arousal regulation, *Sleep* 18(6):478-500, 1995.
21. Terzano MG et al: Precocious loss of physiological sleep in a case of Creutzfeldt-Jacob disease, *Sleep* 18(10):849-858, 1995.
22. Weiss JW et al: Hemodynamic consequences of obstructive sleep apnea: state of the art review, *Sleep* 19(5):388-397, 1996.

# chapter 14 Substance Abuse

ELIZABETH ANNE SCHENK

## objectives

*After studying this chapter, the learner should be able to:*

1. Compare at least three negative compulsions that are considered addictions.
2. Explain legal and educational efforts to prevent alcoholism and drug abuse.
3. Apply knowledge of physiology to explain at least five physical disorders seen with alcoholism.
4. Discuss alcohol withdrawal and actions to treat the three levels of withdrawal symptoms.
5. Compare the six basic types of illicit drugs, including how they are used, their street names, effects, side effects, and symptoms of overdose.
6. Analyze why nurses are at increased risk for chemical dependency and codependency.
7. Identify the knowledge needed to assess the chemically dependent person.
8. Identify the information needed for the management of detoxification of the chemically dependent person.
9. Explain how the medical-surgical nurse can prepare the patient for entry into a chemical dependency treatment.
10. Analyze the rationale behind self-help groups.

Substance abuse is a subject that has an impact on the practice of every medical-surgical nurse. Patients with addictions are seen in all settings. In addition, treatment centers and outpatient counseling centers have emerged in many localities, and growing numbers of nurses are becoming involved in this specialty. There is a recognition that substance abuse entails a complex set of behaviors that are covered under the term *addiction.* The overriding characteristic of addiction is a preoccupation with obtaining the addictive substance, coupled with the inability to stop the associated behaviors, despite negative consequences. Persons may experience one or more addictions concurrently. An example is the alcoholic who also is a drug addict and a compulsive overeater.

The speciality of chemical dependency is being reshaped by managed health care, the availability of new pharmacological treatment, and the understanding of the neuroscience of addiction. Many inpatient treatment centers have closed in recent years, which has made drug and alcohol treatment less readily available. Detoxification is often the reason that patients come in for treatment.

### DEFINITION OF TERMS

Alcoholism and drug addiction are now commonly brought together under the term *chemical dependency.* This is in recognition of the fact that alcohol is a drug and that the person addicted to alcohol is also at great risk for addiction to other drugs.

Most modern definitions of *dependence* consist of two components—physical and psychological dependence. *Physical dependence* refers to a physiological state in which continuous and prolonged consumption of a drug or alcohol leads to the user's adapting to its presence. *Tolerance* then develops. If use of the drug is interrupted, withdrawal symptoms occur. *Psychological dependence* refers to craving for the drug. See Box 14-1 for a description of terms used to describe responses to drugs and alcohol.

The nurse can do much to encourage the treatment of alcoholism by first recognizing that many patients in the hospital may be alcohol- or drug-addicted, even when this is not listed as a diagnosis.

This chapter deals with four examples of substance abuse: *alcoholism, drug addiction,* and *caffeine* and *tobacco dependency.* In addition, two problems linked closely with substance abuse are discussed: *codependency* and the *impaired nurse.* Both have relevance to the medical-surgical nurse.

## ALCOHOLISM

### NATURE OF THE PROBLEM

Alcoholism is very common and may compound the problems of persons with other health disorders. Excessive alcohol intake may lead to coma or near death from acute alcohol poisoning, or if it occurs over time, it may lead to numerous other health disorders. Alcoholism is recognized today as a treatable disease. Changes in the identification and treatment of alcoholism have had a favorable impact on this major health problem.

**box 14-1** *Terms Used to Describe Responses to Drugs/Alcohol*

**Dependence** (also called *habituation* or *compulsive use*) Psychological and/or physical need for a drug or alcohol
**Psychological dependence** Needing a substance to reach a maximum level of functioning or feeling of well-being
**Physical dependence** Adaptation of the body physiologically to chronic use of substance(s); symptoms of withdrawal occur when the substance is stopped or withdrawn
**Tolerance** Need for higher and higher doses of a substance to achieve the same results
**Cross-tolerance** Development of tolerance to one drug of a class leads to tolerance to drugs of the same class
**Withdrawal (abstinence syndrome)** Appearance of physiological symptoms when use of a substance is stopped
**Drug abuse** Use of mind-altering substances in a way that differs from generally approved medical or social practices
**Metabolic tolerance** Substance is detoxified more quickly than normal
**Pharmacological tolerance** Tissue reaction to substance is diminished

## ETIOLOGY

Alcohol abuse can become a problem over a variable period.[1a] The abuse of alcohol is often so episodic that it is difficult to identify. Some persons can drink large amounts for years without becoming alcoholics, whereas other persons become alcoholics after just a short period of heavy drinking. Some alcoholics drink only on weekends. Many may not drink for months at a time. Some drink only episodically, but when they do, the drinking is in a form of a binge, with the person often drinking to the point of unconsciousness.

In alcoholics, however, there is evidence of progression. Alcohol abusers continue compulsive use despite negative consequences. They focus on obtaining alcohol and often have relapses after treatment. The alcoholic begins to develop increasing physical dependence and tolerance for alcohol.[2] The drinking becomes uncontrollable and secretive. Blackouts (loss of memory from episodes of drinking) may start to occur. Feelings of guilt, shame, and remorse may occur, and the alcoholic drinks more to obliterate these feeling. The alcoholic drinks to live and lives to drink.[2]

Of special concern today is the large number of teenagers who abuse alcohol. They often begin to use alcohol at age 14 or younger. Use of alcohol may be just the beginning of experimentation with many drugs.[6,55] Drinking is widespread even though the legal drinking age is now 21 in all 50 states.[42]

Two distinct types of alcoholism can be identified. Type I occurs after the age of 25 and is usually manifested by binges, followed by long periods of sobriety. Individuals with this type of alcoholism have often been found to have particular personality traits—anxiety, dependence, passivity, caution, shyness, and a desire to please others. Type I alcoholism is often found in relatives of alcoholic women. Type II alcoholics, in contrast, are typified by the inability to stay sober for long intervals and are usually uninhibited, impulsive, and socially detached. Symptoms occur before the age of 25 and include legal and medical problems, including driving under the influence (DUI). Type II alcoholism is found more among male relatives of alcoholic men.[3]

Research has found that young men whose fathers were alcoholic but who themselves had not developed the disease are more sensitive to alcohol compared with a control group of men with nonalcoholic fathers.[3]

## EPIDEMIOLOGY

Alcoholism is said to be the third major health problem in the United States. Conservative estimates are that about 90 million people use alcohol, and at least 9 to 10 million persons are alcoholics or "problem drinkers." In addition, alcoholism adversely affects the mental health or functioning of another 30 million friends and relative of alcoholic abusers.[35]

It has been estimated that 70% of alcoholics are male. The number of female alcoholics, however, is increasing,[24,28] and drinking by pregnant women is a major concern because of fetal alcohol syndrome, which is discussed on p. 369. Research has demonstrated that women are more likely to hide their problem drinking. In addition, women are not as likely as men to be involved in the three major systems that give external motivation for treatment (industrial programs, public intoxication and drunk driving laws, and the criminal justice intervention system).

Among college-aged students, binge drinking poses a serious threat to health and safety. Studies show that alcohol is used widely on college campuses, with men having higher rates of use than women.[75]

Alcohol is involved in nearly half of all deaths caused by motor vehicle accidents[16,20,25,59] and fatal intentional injuries, such as suicides and homicides. It has been found that victims are intoxicated in about one third of all homicides, drownings, and boating deaths. Almost half of all traffic fatalities are alcohol-related, and an estimated 40% of persons in the United States may be involved in an alcohol-related traffic crash sometime in their lives. In 1994, 16,589 persons died, and 297,000 were injured in traffic crashes that involved alcohol.[11] Alcohol is involved in at least one quarter of all admissions to general hospitals.[7]

The costs of alcohol-related problems in the United States have been estimated to exceed $70 billion per year, with an additional $44 billion attributed to problems related to drug use.[25] Included in the costs are medical expenses, lost wages, and fire loss. Also included are use and abuse of sick time, extended hospital stays, and increased medical and surgical complications. The cost of treating substance abuse problems in Medicaid recipients in 1994 was almost $8 billion.[30]

More and more employers are offering their employees assistance programs. These programs are becoming a more prevalent point of access to health care for workers with personal problems such as substance abuse, family problems, or emotional distress.

### Theories of the Cause of Alcoholism

Numerous theories have been advanced to explain the cause of alcoholism.[1a] Research is being done to expand the knowledge base about alcoholism. Thus far, no one theory can completely explain the syndrome.

Current theories can be divided into the following three categories:

1. Physiological theories of the cause
2. Psychological theories of the cause
3. Sociocultural-etiological theories (also known as cultural-etiological theories)

### Physiological theories of etiology

These theories operate on the belief that persons are predisposed to develop alcoholism because of some organic defect. Included are theories that suggest that there is a genetically determined biochemical defect in alcoholics, as well as theories that link alcoholism with a dysfunction of the endocrine system.

The incidence of alcoholism is high in families, and the risk of sons of impaired alcoholic men developing alcoholism over their lifetime is 30% to 50%. Studies of twins who have been adopted have also shown that the identical twins of an alcoholic parent will be alcoholic in 60% of the cases, whereas only 30% of the fraternal twins of an alcoholic will be alcoholic. Studies of children of alcoholic parents who were adopted shortly after birth and reared separately from the natural parents indicate that those who were adopted had a higher rate of alcoholism than did normal control subjects.

### Psychological theories of etiology

These theories are based on the assumption that some element in the personality structure and development leads to the development of alcoholism. Included among these theories are the *oral fixation theory* and the *behavioral learning theory.*

Although there has been a search for the "alcoholic personality," most studies have failed to find any specific personality traits that clearly differentiate alcoholics from normal drinkers. Common personality traits that have been identified as occurring in alcoholics include low stress tolerance, dependency, negative self-image, and feelings of insecurity and depression. Whether these traits precede alcoholism or are a result of it is unclear.

There is evidence that two types of personalities are particularly susceptible to alcohol abuse—the antisocial personality, found chiefly in men, and the borderline personality, found chiefly in women.

### Sociocultural or cultural theories of etiology

These theories postulate a relationship between various groups in society and the incidence of alcohol use. For instance, Jews, Mormons, and Moslems have a very low rate of alcoholism, whereas the French have the highest rate. Individual attitudes toward alcohol and alcoholism to a large extent reflect the attitude of one's culture toward drinking. Another part of these theories is that stress factors in cultures may contribute to alcoholism.

One theory that is no longer recognized as valid is the moral etiological theory. This theory held that alcoholism was either a moral fault or a sin of the alcoholic. Much of the early

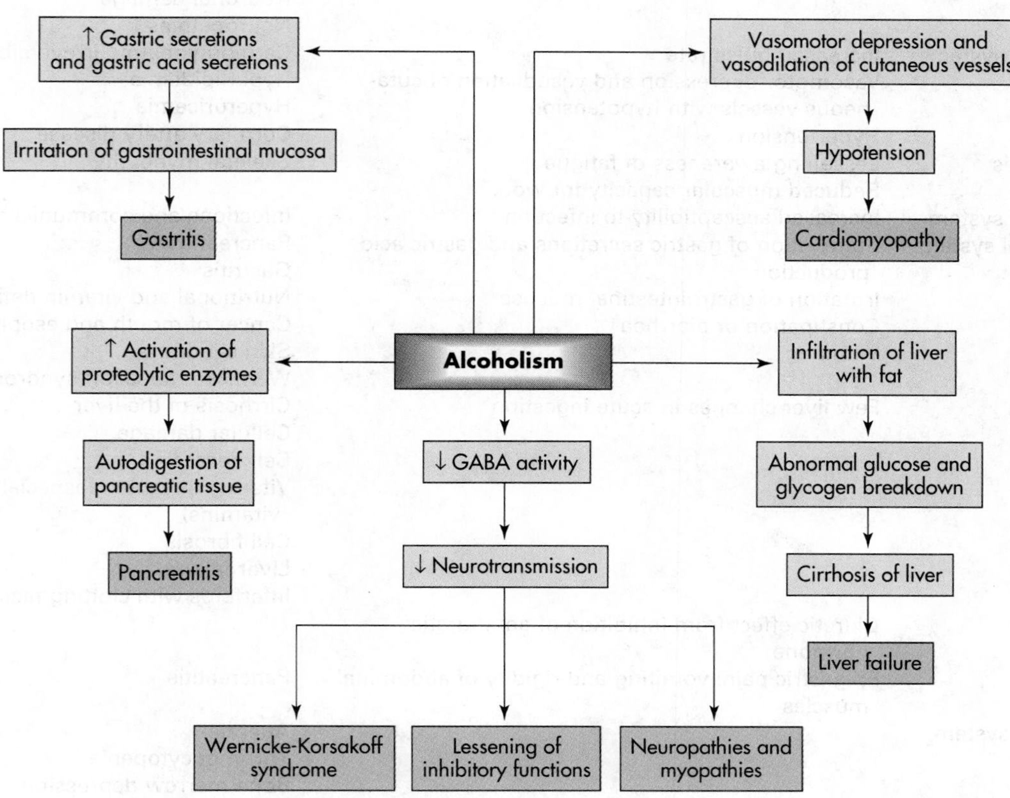


**fig. 14-1** Pathological changes occurring with alcoholism.

treatment of alcoholics was based on this theory, which is still subscribed to by some religious groups.

## PATHOPHYSIOLOGY

Alcohol is a central nervous system (CNS) depressant. It affects the brain by suppressing the activity of the neurotransmitter gamma-aminobutyric acid (GABA). GABA is an inhibitory neurotransmitter. These relationships are diagrammed in Figure 14-1. Thus alcohol inhibits the inhibitor. The so-called stimulating effects of alcohol occur because the first areas affected by the suppression of GABA are the higher centers of the brain governing self-control and judgment, which are inhibitory functions. Slowing the release of GABA to those areas results in a seemingly "stimulating" effect. As alcohol continues to accumulate in the brain, areas of the limbic system and brainstem become inhibited. *Intoxication* occurs and unconsciousness may set in. In fact, the brain may become so overwhelmed by alcohol that it can stop functioning permanently.

### Effects of Alcohol on Organ Systems

Alcohol affects every organ system in the body.[58,60,68] The nurse working in a medical or surgical area is very likely to see an alcoholic patient with various pathological conditions secondary to alcohol abuse. Typical symptoms that may be seen include those listed in Table 14-1. The nurse needs to be aware that alcoholic patients may not admit to drinking excessively or that it is a problem for them. The presence of disease conditions associated with alcoholism should alert the nurse to gather more history about drinking patterns. It is also important for the nurse to assess the intoxicated patient for injuries, such as fractures or lacerations. These often occur when one is intoxicated.[22,33,66]

Cirrhosis of the liver is largely related to heavy alcohol consumption. It is the ninth leading cause of death in the United States. Rates of deaths for nonwhites are almost 70% higher than rates for whites,[8] and the rates for Native American men is triple that of white men.[8] Table 14-2 compares normal function, pathophysiology, and clinical manifestations of alcoholism.

The active ingredient in alcoholic beverages is ethyl alcohol or ethanol (EtOH). Most American beers contain 3% to 6% alcohol, wine contains 2% to 21% alcohol, and hard liquors contain 40% to 50% alcohol. A 12-ounce bottle of beer, a 4-ounce glass of wine, and 1 ounce of hard liquor contain similar amounts of alcohol.

**table 14-1** *Effects of Alcohol on Organ Systems*

| Body System | Effects | Late Effects |
|---|---|---|
| Central nervous system | Depression leading to loss of memory and ability to concentrate<br>Lessening of inhibitory functions<br>Self-control and judgment lessened | Unprovoked seizures<br>Wernicke-Korsakoff syndrome<br>Brain atrophy<br>Sleep disturbances<br>Neuronal damage<br>Neuropathies |
| Cardiovascular system | Increased pulse rate<br>Vasomotor depression and vasodilation of cutaneous vessels with hypotension<br>Hypertension | Cardiomyopathy (irreversible)<br>Hyperlipidemia<br>Hyperuricemia<br>Coronary artery disease |
| Skeletal muscles | Lessening awareness of fatigue<br>Reduced muscular capacity for work | Skeletal myopathy |
| Immunological system | Increased susceptibility to infection | Infections and communicable diseases |
| Gastrointestinal system | Stimulation of gastric secretions and gastric acid production<br>Irritation of gastrointestinal mucosa<br>Constipation or diarrhea<br>Vomiting | Pancreatitis<br>Gastritis<br>Nutritional and vitamin deficiencies<br>Cancer of mouth and esophagus<br>Skin syndrome<br>Wernicke-Korsakoff syndrome |
| Hepatic system | Few liver changes in acute ingestion | Cirrhosis of the liver<br>Cellular damage<br>Cell necrosis<br>Vitamin depletion (especially B complex vitamins)<br>Cell fibrosis<br>Liver failure<br>Interferes with clotting factors |
| Renal system | Diuretic effect from inhibition of antidiuretic hormone | |
| Pancreas | Epigastric pain: vomiting and rigidity of abdominal muscles | Pancreatitis |
| Hematological system | | Anemia<br>Thrombocytopenia<br>Bone marrow depression<br>Prolonged clotting time |

Alcohol does not require digestion and is absorbed in both the stomach and intestine. Absorption is accelerated by increased alcohol concentrations and an empty stomach. After absorption, alcohol is distributed equally throughout body fluids, passing across all mucous membranes. About 2% to 10% is lost through the lungs with respirations and through the kidneys with urination. About 90% of alcohol is disposed of by metabolic processes that occur mainly in the liver (Figure 14-2).

Alcohol has a diuretic effect, partly caused by the increased amounts of fluids ingested. Increased amounts of electrolytes—particularly potassium, magnesium, and zinc—may be excreted in the urine of heavy drinkers. Prolonged use of alcohol has a toxic effect on the intestinal mucosa, which results in decreased absorption of thiamine, folic acid, and vitamin $B_{12}$.

Because alcohol is not converted to glycogen, it cannot be stored, and it provides calories but no minerals or vitamins. One ounce of alcohol provides approximately 200 kcal. Most of the ingested alcohol is metabolized in the liver at a rate of 10 g/hr. The excess remains in the bloodstream, where it acts as a depressant and an anesthetic, which in turn slows down cellular metabolism. The anesthetic action of alcohol can have serious consequences. The margin of safety for the person anesthetized by alcohol is very small.

Blood alcohol levels depend on the amount ingested and the size of the individual. The amount of alcohol that is generally metabolized by the adult is 6 g of pure alcohol in 1 hour (the typical drink). The time from the last drink to maximal blood alcohol concentration is usually 30 to 90 minutes. Most states designate blood alcohol serum levels of 100 mg/100 ml (0.1%) as the legal limit for driving a motor vehicle. Some states such as California have lowered the legal limit for driving to 0.08%. It is illegal to drive with a blood alcohol level above 0.1% in 36 states and above 0.08% in 12 states.[42] Increasing blood alcohol levels have increasingly more serious side effects (Table 14-3).

The main symptom of alcoholism is that the usual drinking behaviors impair the individual's ability to function physically, psychologically, and socially. Usually alcoholism develops slowly, over a period of 10 to 20 years, until the person reaches a point where he "drinks to live and lives to drink."

Several clinical features have been found to occur with alcoholics:

1. Chronicity as a disease or disorder of behavior
2. Undue preoccupation with the intake of ethyl alcohol
3. Loss of control over the drinking pattern itself
4. Use of alcohol in a way that is dangerous to the drinker's physical health, interpersonal relationships, and/or economic functioning
5. Use of alcohol as a universal solution to problems
6. Incorporation of denial and other defense mechanisms as a necessary component of the disease
7. Loss of ability to express feelings; in addition, multiple body systems affected by frequent intoxication

### Fetal alcohol syndrome

Although fetal alcohol syndrome is not a focus of this text, it is mentioned briefly. Medical-surgical nurses may have the chance to educate patients and family members about the risk factors leading to this syndrome.[31] Women who drink during pregnancy have a higher incidence of

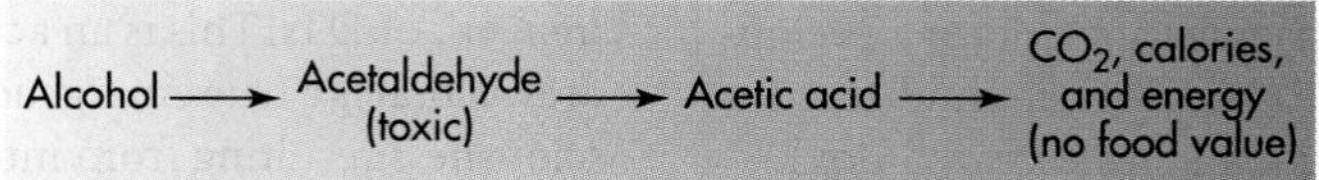


**fig. 14-2** Metabolism of alcohol.

**table 14-2** *Normal Function, Primary Pathophysiology, and Clinical Manifestations in Alcoholism*

| Normal Function | Primary Pathophysiology | Clinical Manifestations |
|---|---|---|
| Gamma-aminobutyric acid (GABA)—(neurotransmitter) | Activity of GABA is inhibited | Lessening of inhibitory functions; self-control and judgment lessened |
| Pancreas—synthesizes protein | Activation of proteolytic enzymes with autodigestion of pancreatic tissue | Epigastric pain; vomiting and rigidity of abdominal muscles |
| Liver—provides glucose during fasting; during carbohydrate ingestion removes glucose and stores it as glycogen | Infiltration of liver parenchymal cells with fat<br>Glucose broken down to acetaldehyde to acetic acid | Jaundice, enlarged liver, increased bleeding time, ascites, possible hepatic coma |
| Stomach and esophagus—normal food ingestion | Increased acid production; irritation of mucosa | Bleeding ulcers, gastritis; cancer of esophagus and mouth |
| Intestine—absorption of vitamins and minerals | Decreased absorption of thiamine, folic acid, and vitamin $B_{12}$ | Malabsorption syndrome, skin conditions, Wernicke-Korsakoff syndrome |
| Immunological system—protection against infection | Increased susceptibility to infection | Infections and illness |
| Neuromuscular system—transmission of impulses | Abnormal transmission of impulses | Neuropathies and myopathies |

**table 14-3** *Effects of Blood Alcohol Levels on Average-Sized Nontolerant Adult*

| Blood Alcohol Levels (per 100 ml of Blood) | Effects |
|---|---|
| 50-75 mg | Pleasant relaxed state, mild sedation, loosening of inhibitions |
| 100-200 mg | Overt signs of intoxication: loosening of tongue, clumsiness, beginning emotional changes |
| 200-400 mg | Severe intoxication: difficulty speaking, stumbling, emotional lability |
| 400-500 mg | Stupor, coma can result in person who is not a chronic alcoholic |
| >500 mg | Usually fatal |

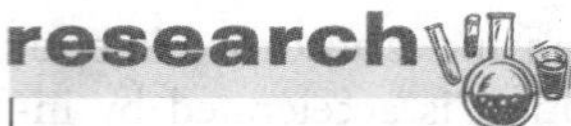

Reference: Larroque B et al: Moderate prenatal alcohol exposure and psychomotor development at preschool age, *Am J Public Health* 85(12):1654-1661, 1995.

Pregnant women were interviewed about their alcohol consumption before pregnancy and during the first trimester. A structured questionnaire measured the amount used. The psychomotor development of 155 children of these women was assessed with the McCarthy scales of children's abilities when the children were about 4½ years old. The results showed that consumption of 1.5 oz of absolute alcohol (about three drinks a day) or more per day was significantly related to a decrease of 7 points in the mean score on the general cognitive index of the McCarthy scales, after other factors were controlled.

children with birth defects. The children of women who drink several times a day throughout pregnancy may be born with fetal alcohol syndrome. The syndrome can include the following:

1. Mental retardation
2. Microcephaly
3. Growth deficiencies
4. Facial abnormalities
5. Malformations of skeletal, urogenital, and cardiac systems

An increase in spontaneous abortions, stillbirths, and infant deaths is also associated with heavy drinking during pregnancy.[80] Even moderate drinking can result in the birth of children with significant lags in mental and motor development.[44,47] The reader is referred to a maternal-child text for further information (see the accompanying Research Box).

### *Alcohol withdrawal*

With continued drinking, a physiological dependency on alcohol and tolerance for increasing amounts of it occur. Alcohol withdrawal affects motor control, mental status, and body functions. Symptoms range from mild tremors to severe agitation and hallucinations when alcohol is withheld. The type and severity of symptoms depend on several factors. Alcoholics at higher risk of experiencing severe withdrawal symptoms are those who are older, who have had previous convulsive seizures or *delirium tremens (DTs)*, and who have coexisting acute illnesses or nutritional deficiencies.

It is important for the medical-surgical nurse to assess the severity of alcohol withdrawal.[36a] Proper medication given early in withdrawal can prevent the development of DTs, as well as possible seizures. The amount and frequency of medication varies, depending on the nature of the alcohol withdrawal. For this reason, the nurse should be familiar with the signs and symptoms of withdrawal.

Mild alcohol withdrawal is characterized by hand tremors, as well as mild restlessness and anxiety. Insomnia or restless sleep is often present. Anorexia and nausea are common. There is usually slight sweating with tachycardia and a normal or slightly elevated systolic blood pressure. The patient remains alert and oriented and generally does not experience seizures or hallucinations.

Moderate alcohol withdrawal is indicated by a worsening of many of the symptoms seen in mild withdrawal. The patient is visibly tremulous with restlessness and anxiety. There is marked insomnia, with nightmares. Vague, transient hallucinations may occur with variable confusion. Marked anorexia is accompanied by nausea and vomiting. Seizures may be present. These seizures are generally not preceded by an aura, but are followed by a postictal stupor. The patient with moderate alcohol withdrawal is diaphoretic. The pulse rate is tachycardic to 100 to 120 beats/min, and the systolic blood pressure is elevated.[20,21]

Severe alcohol withdrawal may also be called *delirium tremens*, or DTs. This is an acute complication of alcohol withdrawal that is a true emergency. It is a pathological state of consciousness resulting from interference with brain metabolism. The onset of DTs usually occurs 3 to 4 days after abstinence but may occur as long as a week after the last drink. DTs that are treated carry a 5% mortality rate, whereas untreated DTs have a 15% mortality rate. The symptoms of this severe withdrawal include uncontrollable shaking, extreme restlessness and agitation, and intense fear and anxiety. This is accompanied by marked confusion and disorientation, with often frightening visual and auditory hallucinations. The patient is wakeful and often refuses all food and fluids. Dry heaves and vomiting may be present. The patient has marked hyperhidrosis (excessive sweating), and seizures are common. The pulse rate is elevated to 120 to 140 beats/min, and there is often marked elevation of the systolic and diastolic blood pressures.[27]

The medical-surgical nurse is responsible for monitoring the patient for symptoms of withdrawal and reporting those symptoms to the physician. A patient who is known to drink may have the initial presenting signs of irritability, a craving for alcohol, and a desire to leave the hospital. Timely and liberal use of PRN medications to prevent withdrawal may avert DTs[61] (see the Research Box on p. 371).

It has been found that a large percentage of trauma patients admitted to hospitals have detectable EtOH concentra-

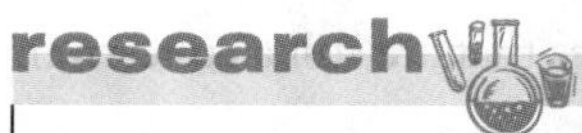

Reference: Saitz R et al: Individualized treatment for alcohol withdrawal: a randomized double-blind controlled trial, *JAMA* 272:519, 1994.

A total of 101 alcoholic patients were randomly assigned either to a fixed-schedule treatment plan (50 patients) or a symptom-triggered plan. Those on a fixed-schedule plan took chlordiazepoxide every 6 hours for 12 doses. Four were 50-mg doses followed by eight 25-mg doses. Those in the symptom-triggered group received between 25 and 100 mg hourly when they were shown to need the medication, according to the Clinical Institute Withdrawal Assessment for Alcohol (CIWA-Ar) withdrawal scale. Those in the fixed-schedule group also received additional medication if their scores on the CIWA-Ar were 8 or greater. The median time of treatment duration was 9 hours in the symptom-triggered group and 68 hours in the fixed-schedule group. The median total amount of chlordiazepoxide administered was 100 mg in the symptom-triggered group and 425 mg in the fixed-schedule group. Thus the patients in the symptom-triggered group received less total medication, and their treatment time was considerably shorter.

tions in their blood. Some studies have found this to be as high as 45%. Unfortunately, withdrawal symptoms in the trauma patient may not be easily detected because of pain and anxiety. Additionally, trauma patients often require analgesics and sedatives, regardless of the use of alcohol. The American College of Surgeons has recommended that level I and level II trauma centers should be capable of determining blood EtOH concentrations 24 hours/day.[27]

Trauma patients with positive blood EtOH concentrations often require larger amounts of benzodiazepines and opioids than patients without detectable concentrations of alcohol. It is also important to administer thiamine to prevent complications related to vitamin B deficiency.[27]

### *Wernicke-Korsakoff syndrome*

One of the consequences of long-term abuse of alcohol is *Wernicke-Korsakoff syndrome.* This can be seen in the medical-surgical areas, especially in elderly patients who may have drank for a long period. The symptoms may also be seen in residents of nursing home facilities. With Wernicke-Korsakoff syndrome, the patient may recover from the initial illness, but amnesia and psychosis may continue. If the residual mental illness is severe, the person may require close supervision and intensive care.

Symptoms of Wernicke-Korsakoff syndrome include ocular disturbances, such as nystagmus and paralysis of the lateral rectus muscle of the eye. Ataxia is usually present, along with symptoms of disturbed mental functioning. The latter can include symptoms of DTs, as well as apathy, listlessness, psychosis, and severe confusion. Memory problems and confusion are commonly seen. At one time this syndrome was believed to be the result of neurological damage from long-term alcohol use. It is now known, however, that nutritional deficiency is the causative factor. The specific nutritional deficiency is thiamine.

**box 14-2** *Protocol for Withdrawal from Alcohol Using Librium*

50 mg q 3 hr prn for the first 24 hr
50 mg q 6 hr prn for the next 24 hr
50 mg q 8 hr prn for the next 24 hr

## Collaborative Care Management

The goal for discharge of patients with alcohol/drug detoxification without rehabilitation as determined by diagnosis-related groups (DRGs) is 4 days. The nurse works collaboratively with the physician for implementation of prescribed medical therapy. Common medical therapy for management of detoxification follows.

Medical management of the alcoholic patient in acute withdrawal focuses on restoration of nutritional and metabolic equilibrium, prevention of seizures, and safe withdrawal from alcohol.[20,21] Medication is used as needed, often in large doses because of the tolerance of the alcoholic for other mood-altering chemicals. These medications are discussed later in this chapter.

## Diagnostic Tests

Routine blood tests often reveal abnormalities that are directly related to alcoholism. These include elevated liver enzyme levels—that is, aspartate aminotransferase (AST/SGOT), alamine aminotransferase (ALT/SGPT), alkaline phosphatase, and bilirubin. Hypoglycemia may also be present if glycogen stores have been depleted. In addition, hypoalbuminemia and hyperglobulinemia are also present in patients with cirrhosis of the liver. Magnesium is often decreased in persons who are alcoholic, usually because of poor dietary intake. It is not uncommon to find anemias and other indicators of poor nutrition in alcoholic patients. Patients who are alcoholics often have an increased mean corpuscle volume (MCV) when the complete blood count (CBC) is done. This and an elevated gamma-glutamyl transferase (GGT) concentration are strong indicators of a possible diagnosis of alcoholism.

Other diagnostic tests demonstrate the concomitant diseases that usually accompany alcoholism. These tests include a urine toxicology screen to determine the use of other drugs. Patients are usually offered an human immunodeficiency virus (HIV) test. This is especially relevant for the patient who is abusing both drugs and alcohol. A urinalysis and urine culture are often done to rule out kidney pathological conditions. A breathalizer test is often used to determine the blood alcohol level on admission.

## Medications

Medications used in the initial detoxification from alcohol include the following:[36a]

1. Chlordiazepoxide (Librium), diazepam (Valium), or similar drugs.
   a. These drugs are used in decreasing doses for their sedating and anticonvulsant effects during detoxification.
   b. See Box 14-2 for an example of a protocol to be used for alcohol withdrawal.
2. Anticonvulsant therapy, such as magnesium sulfate (2 ml of a 50% solution every 8 to 12 hours for several doses).

(This medication is not used as frequently as it once was, but is commonly used in some institutions.)
   a. Phenytoin (Dilantin) may be used for a longer period if the patient has a prior history of seizures or DTs.
3. Multivitamin supplement.
   a. Multivitamin supplements usually are given, at least for the first 3 to 5 days.
   b. Thiamine, 1 g every day is usually given, along with other B complex vitamins because patients may not have been eating a balanced diet for a long period and may have nervous system involvement.
4. Antiemetic agents, such as Tigan or Phenergan, should be used PRN.
5. Antacids should be used for stomach discomfort as needed.
6. Antidiarrheal agents, such as Kaopectate or Lomotil (with serious diarrhea), should be used as needed.

The specific medication used may differ from setting to setting. However, one concept that is important for the nurse to remember is that many alcoholics require medication for safe and effective detoxification. Medication should be given at the first sign of withdrawal symptoms. Detoxification can be dangerous and requires diligent observation by the nurse. Medication should be used freely in the first several days of treatment.

Treatment of DTs consists of the use of tranquilizing drugs, such as chlordiazepoxide or diazepam, and sedatives, such as paraldehyde given rectally, intramuscularly, or orally. High-calorie and high-vitamin diets may have to be given by nasogastric tube. The patient must be protected from physical injury and observed carefully for signs of cardiac failure. If at all possible, restraints should be avoided, because they increase agitation.

## Treatments

### Behavior modification

In the treatment of alcoholism, behavior modification methods may be attempted to discourage drinking behaviors. The best-known aversive agent used is disulfiram (Antabuse), which blocks the enzymatic action necessary to metabolize alcohol. Taken on a regular basis, the drug causes symptoms of nausea, vomiting, palpitations, and general prostration in the person who takes even a small sip of alcohol. The person is then conditioned to avoid alcohol. Disulfiram is usually used as an adjunct to other therapy. Sometimes it is also useful to provide a somewhat forced period of sobriety for an alcoholic who is unable to abstain in any other way. Recently two new drugs, naltrexone[74] and bromocriptine,[48] have been reported to be successful in helping the alcoholic remain abstinent from alcohol.

### Group therapy

Much of the goal of group therapy with the alcoholic is to enable the person to see the relationship between the use of alcohol and the negative consequences that have occurred in his or her life. This in one sense is also a form of behavior modification.

Many alcoholics are socially isolated, and group therapy may assist the person to begin to relate to others in a caring and supportive environment. The group members can help the person look realistically at issues that are still a concern in recovery.

### Self-help groups

Alcoholics Anonymous (AA) is a group of self-acknowledged alcoholics whose aim is to stay sober and to help other alcoholics gain sobriety. There are AA groups that meet regularly in most communities. Meetings are of various types. Open meetings may be attended by anyone, not just the alcoholic. Closed meetings are limited to persons who are alcoholic. There are "lead" meetings, in which a recovering alcoholic tells his or her personal story of alcoholism or meetings in which the members present discuss a topic. There are meetings in most communities for women only, men only, gay persons, young people, and, in larger communities, the deaf. There is no charge for attendance at the meetings—a free-will offering is usually taken.

Local groups are sometimes listed in the telephone directory, and larger communities publish directories of meetings for distribution. A phone call to AA (often the central office) will bring help in the form of telephone conversation, or an AA member will visit the alcoholic desiring help.

In some communities, there is a reluctance on the part of AA members to have persons with other addictions attend meetings. This is partly because of lack of information about the disease of chemical dependence; it is also based partly on fear. With improved methods of diagnosing drug abuse and alcoholism, especially among younger persons, many AA groups are faced with younger people who have not suffered the same number or kind of consequences that the older members may have.

The AA philosophy focuses on the opportunity for the alcoholic to share personal experiences of alcohol abuse and control. Participation in AA may or may not be accompanied by the participation of the patient in other treatment modalities. AA has the highest success rate of any treatment program. The success of AA has led to the formation of other groups that share the same 12-step spiritual approach (Box 14-3). These groups include Al-Anon, Families Anonymous, Narcotics Anonymous, Overeaters Anonymous, Emotions Anonymous, Cocaine Anonymous, and Gamblers Anonymous.[71]

Many communities have alcohol clinics where medical and psychiatric help is available. In addition, many industries have employee assistance programs (EAPs) to aid impaired employees. Treatment centers that offer a variety of inpatient and outpatient programs are also more readily available now than ever before. Information on alcoholism and programs for alcoholics and others are available for interested individuals and groups.

### Promoting rehabilitation

Some persons still believe that it is only when alcoholic patients truly desire and seek help with their alcohol problem that treatment is useful. This is true in some cases, but, often by the time an alcoholic person seeks help, he or she has lost almost everything. Recently, there has been emphasis on the use of a process called *intervention* to assist the alcoholic to receive help.

**box 14-3** *Twelve Steps of Alcoholics Anonymous*

1. We admitted we were powerless over alcohol—that our lives had become unmanageable.
2. Came to believe that a power greater than ourselves could restore us to sanity.
3. Made a decision to turn our will and our lives over to the care of God as we understood Him.
4. Made a searching and fearless moral inventory of ourselves.
5. Admitted to God, to ourselves, and to another human being the exact nature of our wrongs.
6. Were entirely ready to have God remove all these defects of character.
7. Humbly asked Him to remove our shortcomings.
8. Made a list of all persons we had harmed, and became willing to make amends to them all.
9. Made direct amends to such people whenever possible, except when to do so would injure them or others.
10. Continued to take personal inventory and when we were wrong promptly admitted it.
11. Sought through prayer and meditation to improve our conscious contact with God as we understood Him, praying only for knowledge of His will for us and the power to carry that out.
12. Having had a spiritual awakening as a result of these steps, we tried to carry this message to alcoholics, and to practice these principles in all our affairs.

From *Alcoholics Anonymous,* New York, 1976, Alcoholics Anonymous World Sources.

Part of the reason for intervention is that the disease of alcoholism causes delusions or impairs judgment that keeps harmfully dependent persons locked into self-destructive patterns.

Interventions are planned confrontations by individuals who care about the person. It is important to realize that the intervention must be done by a person experienced in organizing and carrying out an intervention. Interventions can be problematic and even dangerous if carried out by someone who is not trained and experienced in this area. Rules for conducting interventions have been summarized as follows:[45]

1. Individuals meaningful to the person must present the facts or data. The most meaningful individual may be the employer or a family member.
2. The data presented should be specific and descriptive of events that have happened or conditions that exist.
3. The tone of the confrontation should not be judgmental.
4. The chief evidence should be tied directly to drinking, whenever possible.
5. The evidence of behavior should be presented in some detail and very explicitly.
6. The goal of the intervention is to have the alcoholic see and accept reality so that the need for help can be accepted.
7. The choices available for treatment should be offered. If possible, immediate treatment should be offered—for example, a bed in a treatment center can be reserved before the intervention, and the employer should stipulate that a condition to the employee's maintaining his or her job is immediate admission to the facility.

### Activity

The alcoholic patient is encouraged to be out of bed as tolerated. In the first several days of withdrawal, stimulation may need to be minimized. It is important for the nurse to be aware of safety concerns with the alcoholic patient. The patient's gait may be ataxic, leading to an increased risk of falls. Because of the risk of falls, side rails should be used while the patient is in bed. As the patient becomes stable, he or she is encouraged to be out of bed most of the day and to take part in unit activities.

### Referrals

Persons experiencing detoxification from drugs and alcohol are commonly referred to a psychologist, chemical dependency counselor, and dietitian. The physician and the nurse working in collaboration may recommend the consultation services of a neurologist and psychiatrist. It is important to consider the importance of transferring the patient to a drug or alcohol treatment program.

## NURSING MANAGEMENT

## ■ ASSESSMENT

Both subjective and objective data are important to assess in the patient with alcoholism. The nurse gains information from interviewing and observing, as well as reviewing information from written sources, laboratory studies, and data from family or significant others. The nurse is reminded that two *cardinal symptoms* of the *untreated alcoholic* are *denial* and *delusion.* Therefore the information gathered from the patient may not always be accurate, and it is helpful to validate it with a family member or friend. It is often helpful for the nurse to mention the dangers of denying or minimizing drug/alcohol use.[5]

The nurse should also be aware of her or his own attitude toward the alcoholic patient and any impact that may have on the interview. Despite a variety of symptoms and the tendency of the alcoholic to be vague about the amount of alcohol used, diagnosis by clinical interview is usually accurate.

### Subjective Data

Data to be collected to assess the patient with alcoholism include:

Normal using or drinking patterns
Date and time of last use or drink
Substances used
Quantity used
Past history of blackouts, tremors, hallucinations, or DTs
Past periods of abstinence/sobriety
Normal dietary pattern
Legal problems
Family problems
Occupational problems
Family history of alcoholism

**box 14-4 Alcoholism Screening Instruments**

Alcohol Use Disorder Identification Test (AUDIT) (10-item self-report measure)
CAGE (4-question screening tool, see Chapter 4)
TWEAK (tolerance, worry, eye-openers, anger, cutting down)
Michigan Alcoholism Screening test (MAST, see Chapter 4)
Short MAST
Self-Administered Alcoholism Screening Test (SAAST)
Short Alcohol Dependence Data Questionnaire (SADD)

Other medications used (mood-altering and over-the-counter)
Use of multiple physicians

These questions are asked of all patients in all settings at the discretion of the nurse.

Several diagnostic instruments can be used to diagnose alcohol dependence (Box 14-4). The reader is referred to Chapter 4 for samples of some of these instruments.

### Objective Data

Data to be collected to assess the patient with alcoholism include:

Abnormal response to preoperative medication, anesthetics, or sedatives
Presence of tremors (usually worse in the morning)
Nausea and/or vomiting, persistent complaints of gastrointestinal distress
Abnormal laboratory findings
Symptoms of vitamin deficiency (pellagra or polyneuropathy)
Body weight in relation to height
Mental functioning
Memory loss
General behavior (e.g., may be argumentative and loud or depressed and withdrawn)
Vital signs
Presence of ascites
Positive blood alcohol or urine alcohol level
Petechiae

## NURSING DIAGNOSES

Nursing diagnoses are determined from analysis of patient data. Nursing diagnoses for the person with alcoholism may include but are not limited to:

| Diagnostic Title | Possible Etiological Factors |
|---|---|
| Airway clearance, ineffective | Fatigue, infection, trauma, decreased consciousness |
| Breathing pattern, ineffective | Neuromuscular impairment |
| Thought processes, impaired | Alcohol- or drug-induced dementia |
| Injury, risk for | Sensory deficits, lack of awareness of environmental hazards |
| Infection, risk for | Decreased nutrition, decreased immune response |
| Fluid volume deficit, actual or risk for | Decreased fluid intake, abnormal fluid loss |
| Sleep pattern disturbance | Pain/discomfort related to withdrawal of substance being abused |
| Anxiety | Change in health status/role functioning |
| Mobility, impaired physical | Decreased strength and endurance, perceptual/cognitive impairment |
| Nutrition, altered; less than body requirements | Anorexia, inability to obtain food |
| Powerlessness | Inability to control alcoholism or drug addiction |
| Self-esteem disturbance | Inability to hold job, do necessary tasks; altered thought processes |
| Hopelessness | Loss of beliefs |
| Denial, ineffective | Unable to admit impact of alcoholism or drug abuse on life pattern |
| Grieving, anticipatory | Loss of use of alcohol or other drugs |
| Coping, ineffective (individual family) | Maturational crises/ situational crises |
| Adjustment, impaired | Disability requiring change in lifestyle |
| Knowledge deficit | Lack of exposure/recall, cognitive limitation |
| Noncompliance | Alcoholic life patterns |
| Spiritual distress | Questioning of personal, spiritual values |
| Social isolation | Unaccepted social behaviors |

## EXPECTED PATIENT OUTCOMES

Expected patient outcomes for the patient with alcoholism may include but are not limited to:

1. Maintains a patent airway.
2. Maintains effective breathing pattern.
3. Improves thought process.
4. Avoids injury.
5. Remains free of infection.
6. Maintains adequate hydration.
7. Maintains normal sleep pattern.
8. Demonstrates decreased anxiety.
9. Achieves optimal mobility.
10. Maintains optimal nutrition.
11. Verbalizes powerlessness over drugs or alcohol.
12. Verbalizes improved self-esteem.
13. Verbalizes a sense of hope.
14. Admits the impact that alcohol or other drug abuse has on life pattern.
15. Verbalizes grief over not being able to drink.
16. Patient and family demonstrate improved and effective coping mechanisms.
17. Patient and family verbalize plan to improve family processes.

18a. Verbalizes knowledge of substances to avoid.

18b. Patient and family verbalize knowledge of disease and treatment.
19. Abstains from alcohol and other drugs.
20. Has decreased spiritual distress.
21. Demonstrates improved social interactions.

## ■ INTERVENTIONS

The patient withdrawing from alcohol is acutely ill and should be placed in an area where he or she can receive intensive nursing care. Discussion of care for these patients follows.

### Acute Care

#### *Maintaining a patent airway*

The patient withdrawing from alcohol is prone to aspiration because of nausea and a decreased mental status and level of consciousness. The head of the bed should be elevated at least 30 degrees, and the patient should be encouraged frequently to cough to clear the airway of secretions. If the patient is unable to clear the airway, suctioning will be necessary. A suction machine should be kept at the bedside or nearby. Fluids should not be offered by mouth until the patient is fully alert.

#### *Maintaining an effective breathing pattern*

Because the effects of alcohol can cause respiratory depression, the patient should be assessed for apnea or other breathing difficulties. Medications that will further compromise respirations, such as morphine, are not given. If narcotic use is suspected, Narcan may be administered. When Valium is used to control DTs, flumazenil (Romazicon) should be available. The patient should also be encouraged to turn, cough, and breathe deeply at frequently intervals to prevent atelectasis.

#### *Improving thought processes*

The person experiencing alcohol withdrawal or DTs may have altered thought processes. This can manifest in symptoms such as disorientation, hallucinations, and paranoia. It is important to reorient the patient as needed and to reassure family members that mentation usually clears as the symptoms of withdrawal end. If this does not occur, the patient needs to be evaluated for Wernicke-Korsakoff syndrome (see p. 371).

The nurse can assist in improving thought processes by medicating the patient liberally with Librium or a similar drug as ordered. The altered thought processes that occur in detoxification indicate the need for aggressive treatment. It may also be helpful to keep the patient from excessive stimulation, which can lead to increased confusion. Visitors are restricted. Lights are kept low, and every effort is made to keep the immediate environment as quiet as possible. Vitamin therapy is given to treat deficiencies, especially of the B vitamins.

#### *Preventing injury*

The alcoholic who has been drinking is at high risk for injury from trauma. Studies have shown that almost one third of all emergency trauma cases involve alcohol. One half of all traffic fatalities and victims of burns have been intoxicated.[66] The cost of treatment of injuries related to the use of alcohol (both to the person, as well as to innocent victims) runs into billions of dollars.

In the initial withdrawal period, the alcoholic may be at risk for seizure activity. Seizure precautions should be taken. Medication is given as ordered to prevent DTs. Side rails should be padded and kept up. The patient is observed closely for signs of impending problems. See Chapter 53 for a more detailed discussion of seizures. The nurse should also realize that patients may have vivid or frightening visual or auditory hallucinations that may cause them to become violent and hurt themselves or others. If the patient becomes so agitated as to pose a risk to self or others, it may be necessary to place him or her in leather restraints. Items that could be harmful or destructive, such as matches and sharp objects, are removed from the patient's area. The patient should be placed in a room adjacent to the nursing station for ease in observation.

#### *Preventing infection*

As alcoholics continue to drink, their health deteriorates. They may suffer from a variety of infections, including tuberculosis. It is important to observe the patient for signs of infection and administer antibiotics as ordered. The patient experiencing detoxification should be encouraged to cough and breathe deeply to prevent atelectasis. The position of the patient who is unable to respond is changed frequently to prevent atelectasis and pressure sores.

Homeless alcohol abusers are at substantially increased risk of contracting tuberculosis. The nurse should monitor the patient for night sweats, late afternoon elevation of temperature, or other symptoms of tuberculosis. Unfortunately, patients with early tuberculosis are usually asymptomatic, and the disease is often well advanced before it is diagnosed (see Chapter 32).

Good nutrition and adequate hydration are essential parts of the treatment of all infections. If skin infections are present, appropriate treatment is begun. The nurse should also be aware that some alcoholics, especially the homeless, may have lice or scabies.

#### *Maintaining adequate hydration*

In the initial period of detoxification, the alcoholic patient may suffer from nausea and vomiting and may require intravenous fluids until nausea and vomiting cease. It may also be helpful to administer an antiemetic agent, such as Tigan. As the amount of alcohol in the body is reduced, the patient will be better able to tolerate fluids. The patient should be educated to drink water and juices, rather than caffeinated beverages or fluid that is high in sugar content, which will cause dehydration secondary to increased urination. Most treatment centers attempt to restrict the use of beverages containing caffeine, because of its stimulating effect.

### Rehabilitative Care

#### *Encouraging normal sleep patterns*

It is very common for the patient going through withdrawal to have insomnia. It may take several months for sleep to return to a normal pattern. Regular physical activity and establishment of a daily routine may help. What is most important is not to use sleeping medication, because the alcoholic is at risk of becoming dependent on the medication. Relaxation tapes and decreasing caffeine use may be helpful in inducing sleep.

#### Decreasing anxiety

Anxiety and depression are common in alcoholics. The patient is encouraged to share concerns and feelings and to learn to deal with anxious feelings. Generally, medications are not used to treat anxiety because of the risk of the person's developing cross-dependence on them. Relaxation exercises and techniques are taught and practiced.

Many persons benefit from a regular exercise program—such as walking, jogging, or swimming, which may help to relieve tension and decrease anxiety. The patient is encouraged to keep a "feeling log" that may be helpful in learning to identify specific feelings and what triggers them. Anxiety usually decreases as long-term sobriety is attained. If not, psychiatric help may be necessary.

#### Promoting mobility

The person entering treatment may be weak because of poor nutrition, as well as because of complications of the alcoholism. As the withdrawal from alcohol occurs, strength improves. Many alcoholics will not have a regular program of physical exercise, and for this reason most inpatient treatment programs include daily periods of physical conditioning. Patients recovering from alcoholism are urged to maintain a regular exercise program after discharge.

As the patient's general condition improves and he or she grows stronger, emphasis can be given to further improving mobility. A physical therapist can assist the patient with appropriate exercises to achieve this goal.

#### Promoting optimal nutrition

Many alcoholics enter treatment with a history of poor nutrition. They may have received as much as a third of their daily intake of calories from alcohol. They often may have been too intoxicated to eat or have had no appetite for normal food. Also, alcohol is the most common cause of *acute gastritis,* which can result in severe vomiting, contributing to poor nutrition. Often addicted persons consume many "empty calories" and are malnourished. Some have chosen to use money for alcohol or drugs, rather than for food.

In the initial detoxification period, the diet is as tolerated, including liberal intake of fluids. As the condition of the alcoholic improves, the appetite usually improves also. Then the emphasis is on three well-balanced meals a day, with free access to snacks. Many patients find that they crave sugar during this initial period, and it is not discouraged because withdrawal from alcohol is the first priority.

Patients usually benefit from assessment by a nutritionist or dietitian. Education about the importance of improved nutrition is essential. If the patient has liver involvement with cirrhosis, dietary restriction of protein is usually necessary. The reader is referred to the section on cirrhosis in Chapter 34 for further information.

#### Accepting powerlessness

The alcoholic person needs to accept that he or she is powerless over alcohol. This is the basis of almost all treatment approaches. It may be a difficult concept for alcoholics to understand—that through becoming powerless they achieve the ability to stay sober. Attendance at Alcoholics Anonymous meetings, group therapy, and discussions with other alcoholics all can help with this. Alcoholics need to understand that taking even one drink of alcohol can start them on the process of active drinking again. Inherent in accepting this powerlessness is the realization that they have no control over alcohol, but that it controls them.

#### Increasing self-esteem

It is important for these patients to build positive self-esteem, enabling them to acknowledge that they are worthwhile. This is important because many alcoholics continue to drink to cover their feelings of inadequacy and lack of self-worth. Positive self-esteem is important for continued recovery.

An important part of treatment of alcoholism leading to positive self-worth is positive reinforcement. This usually occurs in the context of interpersonal relationships with nurses and other staff, as well as with other patients. Caring, emotional support and encouragement are very important. This is demonstrated within the context of honesty and also by pointing out negative behaviors, defense mechanisms, and problems.

#### Decreasing hopelessness

Many alcoholics enter treatment with a great sense of hopelessness. They may have attempted treatment before without success. They may also feel that they will never be able to stop drinking, and that they will never achieve sobriety. In addition, many alcoholics drink to block their feelings of hopelessness, especially about the loss of family and friends and perhaps the loss of a job.

Instilling hope in the alcoholic patient takes time. Often, the most important treatment is the interaction the person has with other recovering alcoholics. Listening to recovering persons "lead" a group meeting will help to instill a beginning sense of hope. Seeing other persons who once were worse off than they are now may help them to see the chance for recovery.

#### Decreasing denial

One of the real challenges in working with the alcoholic patient is facilitating the breaking down of denial. The patient characteristically is not aware of the havoc that his or her alcohol abuse has caused. Group therapy is used to enable the person to see the relationship between the use of alcohol and the negative consequences it has on his or her life.

When the alcoholic becomes sober, many of the problems that have occurred in his or her life can be seen clearly for the first time.

Nurses working with these patients need to assist in pointing out areas of concern and consequences that the person has suffered as a result of alcoholism.

### *Facilitating grieving*

Many alcoholics will actually go through a grieving process for the loss of the alcohol. For the recovering person, the loss and sadness over what has been given up (alcohol) can be quite intense. Practically all persons start drinking or using drugs because it is socially acceptable and fun. No one plans to become addicted and trapped by the compulsion to drink. For some, giving up alcohol may also mean the necessity of giving up their drinking friends. The alcoholic may be angry about the changes required and the realization that drinking is out of the question. Grieving is a natural part of recovery because it implies an emotional response to loss. The nurse can facilitate this grieving by encouraging the patient to talk about feelings and express the grief or anger. Letting the alcoholic know that this grief is normal and expected is helpful.

Depression may occur as the alcoholic recognizes and accepts the illness. Although the decision to stay sober will bring relief and assurance in the long run, alcoholics will have periods when the desire for a drink is so strong that they may become discouraged, even though they are able, with support, to resist the temptation to drink.

Recent studies have shown that a major depression is common in persons with alcohol dependence and that it responds well to treatment with antidepressants. Treatment with these drugs may reduce the rate of relapse.[51]

### *Facilitating coping (individual and family)*

The patient will need assistance in learning to deal with life without the crutch of alcohol or drugs. This includes helping the patient to find a sense of spirituality and perhaps become reconnected with a religious organization or leader. Decision making may be difficult at first, and the person may require support to look at options. Just because the person becomes sober does not mean that all problems will be gone.

Allowing the person to vent emotions and responding with empathy (not sympathy) may assist him or her in letting go of anger or resentment. If indicated, the nurse may suggest professional counseling for the alcoholic.

It is not uncommon for alcoholics to have problems with intimacy and sexuality. They need to learn to trust others and to risk becoming vulnerable with another person. Marriage counseling may be necessary to help a couple regain a healthy marriage, especially if there has been a long history of problems as a result of alcoholism or drug addiction. Family therapy should be discussed and encouraged.

### *Facilitating adjustment*

It is often difficult for the alcoholic person to adjust to the diagnosis of alcoholism, especially if alcoholism is seen as morally wrong. Denial that alcohol is a problem may be part of the difficulty. Denial is discussed earlier in this chapter (see p. 376). The patient is encouraged to focus on one day at a time and to not consider having to stay sober forever. The patient is educated about the disease concept of alcoholism, which usually helps with adjustment. Attendance at daily Alcoholics Anonymous meetings is usually required as a part of both inpatient and outpatient treatment programs. Through daily assignments the person is helped to learn about himself or herself in relation to alcoholism.

Psychotherapy cannot help the patient who continues to drink. It can, however, be helpful as a part of the treatment program. Emotional problems that occur as part of the drinking do not automatically disappear when the person stops drinking. Some patients have problems that are unrelated to their drinking and need to gain insight about them. Therapy directed toward personal insight has been found to be effective only after the patient attains stable sobriety.

### *Improving family processes*

As the alcoholic becomes more involved in the destructive process of the disease, the family also suffers. As a result, when a family of an alcoholic receives help, the family processes are usually in a state of dysfunction. Divorce may have occurred or is being discussed. Spouses, parents, and children have lost respect for and trust in the alcoholic. Other family members may also have become very enabling and codependent.[56]

It is unrealistic to think that family processes can be changed in a short period. Treatment of the family along with the alcoholic is important, not only to help the alcoholic recover, but also to allow the family to work through feelings of fear, distrust, and anger. Adult family members should be referred to Al-Anon, a 12-step support group for persons whose lives are affected by someone who is alcoholic. Children may be referred to Ala-Teen. Adult children of an alcoholic may benefit from referral to an ACOA meeting.

The patient and family often need additional counseling to help them grow together and not apart. In spite of this, the divorce rate among couples where one member is an alcoholic is high, even after the alcoholic achieves sobriety.[56]

### *Increasing compliance*

The object of all treatment for alcoholism is to assist patients in achieving sobriety. When they do stop drinking, they are taught that they can never take one drink without the danger of relapse. In fact, the most complicated and frustrating part of treatment is to prevent relapse.

Some have suggested that alcoholics may be taught to become "social drinkers," but this has not been substantiated. Alcoholics who are currently not drinking are never considered cured, only recovering.

### *Decreasing spiritual distress*

Many alcoholics enter treatment spiritually bankrupt. Generally, they have been cut off from nurturing relationships with others, with self, and with a higher being. The person is forced, because of defense mechanisms, into a grandiose position of becoming a God of sorts. As the disease progresses, values decrease. Many persons may also see God as a punishing force who could never forgive the person for things done while he or she was drinking.

If the patient desires, the service of a chaplain should be offered. The patient should be educated about the difference in the spirituality talked about in AA and religion. As mentioned previously, some persons may have difficulty with the concept of a higher power or God. They can be encouraged to use a power of the group as a higher power until they are able to accept a sense of spirituality.

#### *Decreasing social isolation*

The social isolation experienced by alcoholics can best be handled in a support group. The best-known support group is Alcoholics Anonymous, which is described on p. 372. Participation in AA may or may not be accompanied by participation of the patient in other types of treatment. The chemically dependent person may need to develop a completely different group of friends because associating with persons who drink or use drugs needs to be discouraged. Initially being forced to seek new friends may add to the feeling of isolation, but it is necessary if the patient is to stay sober and straight. As new friends are made, the social isolation usually diminishes.

Initially an alcoholic or drug addict may not feel comfortable in social situations without the substance he or she was using. This, too, improves with time.

### Patient/Family Education

#### *Health promotion/prevention*

Prevention of alcoholism is a complex issue. The goal of primary prevention is to stop involvement with drugs or alcohol before it ever occurs. This is called *primary prevention.* Legally, efforts have been made to restrict the sale of alcohol to minors, as well as to make the consequences of use stringent. Current laws concerning drunk driving focus both on the need of the person to be educated about the disease and on the need to suffer the consequences of the actions caused by the alcoholism. Recent statistics show a decrease in the number of deaths due to alcohol-related accidents.

The key to prevention seems to be grounded in education. This education includes the teaching of fairly young children about the dangers of alcohol use and abuse. Many programs start as early as the first or second grades. In addition, work may be done with children to increase their self-esteem, so that they may better be able to avoid peer pressure to drink as they become older.

Another attempt to educate persons involves the families and employers of alcoholics. They are taught that alcoholism is a disease that needs treatment, but at the same time the person who is alcoholic may need to suffer the consequences of alcohol use so that help may be sought at an earlier time. This has sometimes been called "raising the bottom." Alcoholics are often surrounded by persons who *enable* their use and abuse, for example, the wife who calls in to work for her drunk husband and tells the employer that he is sick with the flu. Without this *enabling behavior,* alcoholics might be forced to seek help earlier.

**table 14-4** *Progress on* Healthy People 2000 *Goals*

| Alcohol and Other Drugs | 1987 Baseline* | Update 1995* | 2000 Target* |
|---|---|---|---|
| Fewer alcohol-related deaths | 9.8 | 6.8 | 5.5 (revised from 8.5) |
| Less alcohol use among youth aged 12 to 17 years | 25.2 | 18.0 | 12.6 |
| Less marijuana use among youth aged 12 to 17 years | 6.4 | 4.9 | 3.2 |

From McGinnis JM, Lee PR: Healthy people 2000, *JAMA* 273(14):1123-1129, 1995.
*Data expressed as rate per 100,000 population.

The importance of prompt diagnosis and treatment is important. This is called *secondary prevention. Tertiary prevention* has as its goal the ending of the compulsive use of alcohol or drugs or the minimization of the negative effects of the use through treatment and rehabilitation. An example of tertiary prevention is the treatment of an alcoholic person in relapse with cirrhosis of the liver in a halfway house.

Complications for the alcoholic patient include those related to the effects of the substance itself and those from nutritional deficits. Complications for persons with drug addictions often occur as a result of diseases acquired from dirty needles or equipment. Many alcoholics and drug addicts continue to drink or use drugs despite the development of life-threatening complications. They will have to deal with these complications long after they have stopped the use of the substance.

The report to the Surgeon General on health goals for the year 2000 contained several recommendations about alcohol and other drugs. These goals are linked with the prevention of alcohol and drug abuse, as well as problems related to these two areas. The reduction of alcohol-related vehicle deaths is very significant. Because of the decrease in the number of deaths, the target goal has been adjusted from 8.5 per 100,000 population to 5.5. See Table 14-4 for an update on progress toward specific *Healthy People 2000* Goals.[52]

#### *Facilitating learning*

Education about the disease of alcoholism is extremely important for the alcoholic and the family or significant others. See the Guidelines for Care Box for important topics that need to be covered. These persons also become sick in the midst of the alcoholic's becoming sicker and need understanding and education to help themselves and the alcoholic to recover.

**guidelines for care**

**Teaching the Alcoholic Patient/Family**

Disease concept of alcoholism
Medical aspects of the disease, including complications
Need for continued abstinence
Importance of expressing feelings to stay sober
Defense mechanisms
Drugs to avoid
Products that contain alcohol (for example, mouthwash and cough medicine)
Importance of being honest with physician and dentist
Signs and symptoms of impending relapse
Importance of aftercare, including AA meetings

Many over-the-counter drugs contain alcohol. Two examples of these are cough medicines and mouthwashes. The alcoholic also needs to know that the use of any mood-altering chemical may lead to relapse.

## EVALUATION

Evaluation of the alcoholic patient involves input from the patient, as well as family members or significant others. To evaluate the effectiveness of nursing interventions, compare patient behaviors with those stated in the expected patient outcomes. Successful achievement of patient outcomes for the patient with alcohol dependency is indicated by:

1. Able to clear own airway of secretions.
2. Has respiratory rate within normal range of 16 to 20/min.
3. Able to think more clearly.
4. Completes detoxification without incurring an injury.
5. Is free of infection.
6. Has good skin turgor, and mucous membranes are moist and pink.
7. Able to sleep between 6 and 8 hours nightly and feels refreshed on awakening.
8. Able to sit or lie quietly without exhibiting nervousness.
9. Has optimal mobility.
10. Eats a well-balanced diet, including foods from all groups in the food guide pyramid.
11. Abstains from alcohol and other drugs.
12. Demonstrates improved self-esteem by speaking positively about self.
13. Able to discuss plans for the future that reflect hopefulness.
14. Able to discuss his or her chemical dependency and plans to remain sober.
15. Able to verbalize grief about no longer being able to drink or use other drugs.
16. Demonstrates improved coping mechanisms, such as becoming less angry and frustrated when things do not go as planned.

17a. Adjusts well to changes in lifestyle.
b. Patient and family verbalize that they were aware of problems in their interactions and are working to improve them.

18. Patient and family discuss chemical dependency and substances to be avoided.
19. Remains sober, attends aftercare meetings, and follows the 12-step program.
20. States that he or she is more comfortable acknowledging dependence on a greater power.
21. Interacts more comfortably with other persons.

## GERONTOLOGICAL CONSIDERATIONS

As many as 3 million Americans aged 60 and older are alcoholics or have some kind of a drinking problem. Physicians often fail to diagnose alcoholism in the elderly. Thus, the elderly constitute a hidden population of alcoholics who may not be identified because of social isolation, despite an increase in diagnosis and treatment of alcoholism among the overall population. (See also Chapter 4.)

The elderly person may have been a "closet drinker" for years, hiding his or her drinking from others. Families and friends are often reluctant to confront the person about the drinking, and thus the person does not receive assistance dealing with the problem. Nurses working with the elderly in hospitals and the community should be alert to the possibility of substance abuse as the cause of confusion, falls, or other injuries. Complications associated with alcohol abuse such as gastric bleeding and cirrhosis of the liver may be more severe than in younger, healthier persons and often result in hospitalization.

The principles of treatment of substance abuse for the elderly person are the same as they are for younger persons. Loneliness has been cited as a prime reason for the use of alcohol and drugs by elderly persons.

# DRUG ABUSE

## NATURE OF THE PROBLEM

Because alcohol is in itself a drug, alcoholism and drug abuse are not mutually exclusive. There is an increasing tendency for persons who abuse substances to mix a variety of drugs and alcohol. Much of the information already covered in the section on alcoholism also pertains to drug abuse.

### Historical Perspectives

The history of nonmedical drug use is thousands of years old. As early as 5000 BC, the Sumerians referred to a "joy plant." This is believed to be a reference to the opium poppy plant. Since then, drugs have played a significant role in almost every culture. Even the results of historic events may have been altered, because the persons involved were under the influence of drugs. Different drugs have assumed importance in different periods of history. For instance, currently use of cocaine is more problematic than ever before. The newest problem drugs are the so-called designer drugs, many of which were unheard of several years ago.[46]

### Definitions

The terms *habituation* and *addiction* have been used to define the nature and extent of drug use. Drug habituation includes repeated use of a drug to a point where there is psychological dependence. Drug addiction involves craving, psychological dependence, and physical dependence. The latter includes development of tolerance for increasing dosages of the drug and the appearance of withdrawal symptoms on cessation of use of the drug. *Drug dependence* is another term that is used. This refers to a psychological or physical dependence on a drug that is taken regularly.

### Types/Classifications of Substances

According to the Controlled Substance Act of 1971, there are five basic classes of drugs:

1. Stimulants
2. Depressants
3. Hallucinogens
4. Narcotics
5. Cannabis

To this list can be added deliriants, such as glue, and paint thinner. Examples of drugs in each of these classifications are presented in Table 14-5. Two drugs (tobacco and caffeine) that are officially classed as stimulants are discussed separately.

Another category of drugs that continue to be abused are the anabolic steroids. They are often used by athletes and body builders to enhance athletic ability and to increase muscle strength. Use of anabolic steroids can be life-threatening and can cause sudden death, usually from cardiac problems.[18,69]

## ETIOLOGY

The cause of drug abuse is unknown. The reader is referred to the Etiology section in the discussion of alcoholism for further insights and information (see p. 366). Some patients with mental illness are also addicted to drugs and alcohol. Drug abuse often exacerbates psychiatric symptoms and leads to violent behavior, homelessness, and poor follow-through in treatment. Cocaine use is a problem especially in the presence of schizophrenia, because cocaine is dopaminergic, and excess dopamine has been associated with the pathophysiology of schizophrenia.[64]

## EPIDEMIOLOGY

In recent years, the incidence of drug abuse has risen sharply. There are no reliable statistics on drug abusers, and experts disagree as to what actually constitutes drug abuse. Some include repeated use of any drug, whereas others limit it to those drugs that, used repeatedly, lead to habituation or addiction.

Use of drugs has increased among adolescents and young adults in the past.[6,15,50] Although efforts to slow this increase seems to be making some headway, drugs are readily available in most elementary and secondary schools and on college campuses. In addition, they are present in many work settings.

The use of injectable drugs is the second most frequently reported risk factor for infection with HIV. Of cases reported to the Centers for Disease Control and Prevention in the past several years, approximately 35% were associated with intravenous drug use.[19,64] Needle-exchange programs have begun in many locations in an effort to reduce the public health concerns associated with intravenous drug abuse.[36] Studies of several needle-exchange programs have found a significant reduction in hepatitis B and hepatitis C among those abusers who participate in needle-exchange.[37,70]

## SPECIFIC DRUGS

### Stimulants

Stimulants are both natural and synthetic drugs that have a strong stimulating effect on the central nervous system. They are accompanied by a feeling of alertness and self-confidence. Drugs included in this category are (1) amphetamines and (2) cocaine.

#### *Amphetamines*

**Physiology.** Amphetamines and amphetamine-like drugs are synthetic psychoactive drugs that are available legally by prescription. They are available in both capsule and tablet forms. A powdered or crystalline-like form of amphet-

**table 14-5** *Effects of Mood-Altering Drugs*

| Drug | Tolerance | Physical Dependence | Psychological Dependence |
|---|---|---|---|
| Narcotics | High | High | High |
| Barbiturates | Moderate | High | High |
| Methaqualone | Moderate | High | High |
| Tranquilizers | High | Moderate | High |
| Amphetamine | High | Low to moderate | High |
| Cocaine | Moderate | Low to moderate | High |
| Lysergic acid diethylamide (LSD) | Moderate | None | Moderate |
| Mescaline | Low | None | Moderate |
| Phencyclidine (PCP) | Low | None | Low |
| Marijuana | Low | None | Moderate |

amine is methamphetamine, which must be injected. It is no longer legally produced in an injectable form.

Methamphetamine (also known as "speed," "crank," "go," and "ice") is the most widely abused type of amphetamine. An estimated 4 million persons in the United States have abused methamphetamine at least once. The number of deaths related to this drug has increased, and related emergency room visits have more then tripled.

Medical uses of amphetamines may include the treatment of narcolepsy, obesity, fatigue, and depression. Methylphenidate (Ritalin), an amphetamine-like drug, is used to treat children who are hyperactive. Common generic and brand names of amphetamines include dextroamphetamine (Dexedrine), methamphetamine (Methedrine), and amphetamine (Benzedrine).

Street names for amphetamines vary, but include the following:

| | | |
|---|---|---|
| Pep pills | Ups | Meth |
| Dexies | Speed | Whites |
| Bennies | Crystal | |

**Pathophysiology.** Amphetamines are CNS stimulants. When swallowed or injected, they speed up the activity of the heart and brain. They dilate the pupil of the eye, increase the pulse rate, and elevate the blood pressure. The use of amphetamines also reduces fatigue, increases concentration, and decreases appetite. However, the feeling of alertness, often coupled with a sense of confidence and well-being, wears off, and the person experiences fatigue and depression, which may be extreme in nature.

Amphetamines have the potential to produce tolerance. The abrupt discontinuation of amphetamines usually does not produce physical withdrawal, although many persons have psychological dependence on these drugs.[36a]

A summary of the clinical manifestations of amphetamine ingestion can be found in Box 14-5.

### Cocaine

**Physiology.** Cocaine is a psychoactive drug that comes from the leaves of the South American coca bush. Medical uses for cocaine include use as an anesthetic of choice for certain procedures and surgery involving the nose, throat, larynx, and lower respiratory passages. It may also be used as an ingredient in Brompton's solution, an oral medication that is used for patients with terminal cancer.

Cocaine is used by sniffing, smoking, inhaling, or injecting. When it is sniffed, or "snorted," the effect of the drug is realized when the cocaine is absorbed through the mucous membranes of the nose. Cocaine may also be freebased, which is the process of heating the drug to separate it from whatever adulterants it may contain. When freebase cocaine is injected, it produces a high that is more intense and more short-lived than when cocaine is smoked. The use of cocaine and heroin together is increasing. The combination of these two drugs is called a "speedball" and is taken intravenously.[9]

Crack is a mixture of cocaine and common baking soda and water. It is smoked, much like free basing, and creates an intoxication more intense than cocaine alone.

Crack is a freebase form of cocaine hydrochloride, so called because the cocaine has been separated from its hydrochloride base. It is called "crack" because of the characteristic crackling sound that is made when the crystals are heated. Cocaine powder is not smoked because heat destroys its effects. Crack is heat resistant and reaches the brain faster and in higher concentrations, producing a more intense euphoria within about 6 seconds. The high is also more intense because crack contains as much as 90% pure cocaine, whereas cocaine hydrochloride may contain only 15% to 25% pure cocaine. The feeling of exhilaration lasts a much shorter time, however—5 to 7 minutes in contrast with 30 minutes after using powdered cocaine. Crack is available in crystal form and is considered to be even more addictive than other forms of cocaine.

Because it is usually less expensive than cocaine, crack has been readily available to less affluent persons. In addition, a recent trend is for heroin to be snorted with crack to prolong the high. The street names for cocaine are listed below:

| | | |
|---|---|---|
| Blow | Flake | Superblow |
| Coke | Nose candy | Toot |
| Crack | Rock | White |
| Dust | Snow | White girl |

**Pathophysiology.** Cocaine acts as a CNS stimulant. It blocks the uptake or reabsorption mechanism of the neurotransmitters, thus prolonging the effects of norepinephrine and dopamine on the brain and peripheral nerves. It also breaks down neurotransmitters. The habitual use of cocaine eventually depletes the brain's supply of dopamine and norepinephrine.[8]

Because of the stimulation of the brain by cocaine, there is a surge in the systolic blood pressure with its use. This surge in blood pressure has been linked with sudden neurological insults, including subarachnoid hemorrhage. Cocaine use in high doses can precipitate fatal ventricular dysrhythmias, often resulting in myocardial infarction or pulmonary edema, as well as seizures.[4,38]

**box 14-5** *clinical manifestations*

**Use of Amphetamines**

1. Restlessness
2. Dizziness
3. Insomnia
4. Lack of appetite, dramatic weight loss
5. Diarrhea or constipation
6. Agitation and anxiety
7. Paranoia, paranoid psychosis
8. Cerebral hemorrhage
9. Myocardial infarction
10. Collapse from exhaustion

*Withdrawal often leads to profound depression and may lead to suicide.*

The use of cocaine during pregnancy causes constriction of the uterine blood vessels, leading to deprivation of oxygen and nutrients to the developing fetus. This increases the risk of spontaneous abortion during the first trimester and can cause premature delivery and premature separation of the placenta. It can also slow fetal growth and cause congenital abnormalities. Use during the first trimester of pregnancy can interfere with the formation of neurological pathways of the brain of the fetus. Cocaine has also been found to lead to in utero brain hemorrhage and stroke.[4,78] Clinical manifestations resulting from the use of cocaine are listed in Box 14-6.

Chronic sniffing of cocaine can destroy the nasal tissues. Smoking it can cause lesions in the lungs.

Concurrent cigarette smoking and cocaine use may also have serious adverse effects on cardiac function.[53] Tolerance and psychological dependence can develop, and an overdose can cause convulsions, respiratory paralysis, and death. A cocaine psychosis that is characterized by a loss of pleasure, loss of orientation, hallucinations, insomnia, concern with minor details, stereotyped behavior, and an increased potential for violence occurs in some persons. Treatment with an antipsychotic medication may be necessary to relieve the symptoms.

Abrupt withdrawal from cocaine can lead to physical symptoms of withdrawal, especially if the cocaine was used on a daily basis. These symptoms include irritability, sleep disturbances, and cravings.[36a]

Currently, there is no effective medication for the treatment of cocaine overdose and addiction. What is known about cocaine is that the dopamine-reuptake transporter is important in the behavioral and biochemical action of cocaine. Cocaine binds strongly to the dopamine-reuptake transporter and blocks reuptake after neuronal activity. Because of this blocking effect, dopamine remains at high concentrations in the synapse and continues to affect adjacent neurons, producing the "high" of cocaine use.[49]

**box 14-6** *clinical manifestations*

***Use of Cocaine***

1. Stimulation of respiration and heart rate
2. Raising of blood pressure and blood sugar levels
3. Suppression of appetite
4. Dilation of the pupils
5. Constriction of certain blood vessels
6. Increase in levels of physical activity
7. Insomnia
8. Trembling
9. Sensations of extreme euphoria
10. Feelings of energy, power, confidence, and talkativeness

*There is a letdown effect of cocaine crash that occurs when the effect of the drug wears off.*

## Depressants

Depressants are synthetic drugs that have a depressant action on the CNS. Drugs included in this category are the following:

1. Sedatives and methaqualone
2. Barbiturates
3. Tranquilizers

### *Sedatives and Methaqualone*

**Physiology.** Methaqualone is a nonbarbiturate sedative-hypnotic. It is the active ingredient in the drugs Quaalude and Mequin. It is available as a prescription drug but has also become a common and popular street drug. It is taken orally. Because of its nonsoluble nature, it cannot be injected.

Common street names for methaqualone are:

| | |
|---|---|
| Ludes | Love drug |
| Soaps, soapers, or sopes | Wallbangers |
| 714s | Lemons |

Methaqualone was first made in the early 1950s as a treatment for malaria in India. In the 1960s it was used as a sedative in Europe; 1965 saw it manufactured in the United States. It was at first thought not to be addicting. Its use as a street drug began in the late 1960s. This drug is no longer available through legitimate channels, but it is available on the street.

**Pathophysiology.** Methaqualone is a CNS depressant that is unrelated to other sedatives or barbiturates. It slows the CNS and impairs coordination, walking, and talking. It also possesses anticonvulsant, anesthetic, and cough-suppressant effects. Its primary effect is drowsiness. If the user resists the sleep-inducing effects of the drug, he or she experiences a relaxed, mellow sense of well-being.

The repeated use of methaqualone produces tolerance, as well as physical and psychological dependence. Withdrawal from the drug produces headache, fatigue, dizziness, nausea, anxiety, skin problems, abdominal cramps, seizures, and vomiting if the withdrawal is not medically supervised.

Overdoses occur when the CNS-depressing effects of the drug slow down the person's rate of breathing to the extent that consciousness is not possible. Most overdoses occur when the drug is combined with other drugs, such as alcohol, that potentiate its action. Symptoms of overdose include delirium, coma, restlessness, convulsions, and vomiting.[36a]

Withdrawal from methaqualone requires the use of medication, which may include diazepam or phenobarbital.

### *Barbiturates*

**Physiology.** Barbiturates are synthetic drugs, arising from barbituric acid, that are classified as "sedative hypnotics." They are used medically to treat epilepsy and insomnia and to sedate patients before and during surgery. Barbiturates are also commonly used street drugs.

Flunitrazepam (Rohypnol) is a hypnotic that is marketed in many countries for insomnia. Its abuse in the United States is increasing. Newspapers and television coverage have focused on its use in date rape.[75]

Barbiturates are taken by mouth (capsule or elixir), used as a suppository, or injected. They were first synthesized in the early 1900s by two German scientists. Currently about 10 derivatives of barbituric acid are in use.

**box 14-7** *clinical manifestations*

***Use of Barbiturates***

1. Feeling of well-being
2. Euphoria
3. Relief from anxiety
4. Side effects, including difficulty in breathing, lethargy, allergic reactions, nausea, and dizziness

There are many common names for barbiturates. The names usually refer to the drug type, the drug effect, the drug name, or the color of the particular capsule. The names are listed below:

| | |
|---|---|
| Yellow jacket (pentobarbital) | Barbs |
| Red devil (secobarbital) | Downs or downers |
| Phennie (phenobarbital) | Rainbows |
| Blue heaven or blue devil (amobarbital) | Blues |
| | Goof balls |

**Pathophysiology.** Barbiturates cause depression of the CNS, including slowing of physical and mental reflexes. The continued use of these drugs can cause physical and psychological dependence, as well as tolerance.

Clinical manifestations of the use of barbiturates are listed in Box 14-7. Alcohol and other CNS depressants tend to potentiate the effects of barbiturates and can be very dangerous when used with them. Accidental overdoses are common. A person who is physically dependent on barbiturates will experience various withdrawal symptoms. Mild withdrawal includes irritability, restlessness, anxiety, and sleep disturbances. An extreme form of barbiturate withdrawal can be life threatening and includes symptoms of convulsions, delirium, and hyperpraxia. Detoxification includes appropriate medication, which may be a long-acting barbiturate given in diminishing dosages.[36a]

### *Tranquilizers*

**Physiology.** Minor tranquilizers are psychoactive drugs that are taken to reduce anxiety. They may also be used as a muscle relaxant. They are the most commonly prescribed drugs in the world today. Tranquilizers are available in prescription form in capsule, tablet, and liquid forms. Illicitly, they are sometimes injected. Common types of tranquilizers are those found in the benzodiazepine family and include the following:

1. Chlordiazepoxide
2. Diazepam (Valium)
3. Prazepam (Antrax or Verstran)
4. Oxazepam (Serax)
5. Lorazepam (Ativan)
6. Clorazepate (Tranxene)
7. Alprazolam (Xanax)

**Pathophysiology.** Minor tranquilizers slow the activities of the CNS. They also have anticonvulsant and muscle-relaxant properties and produce a sense of relaxed well-being. When the effects of the drug wear off, however, users frequently experience an increased level of anxiety. Tranquilizers cause physical and psychological dependence, and tolerance to them can develop. Clinical manifestations of the use of tranquilizers are listed in Box 14-8.

**box 14-8** *clinical manifestations*

***Use of Tranquilizers***

SIDE EFFECTS INCLUDE THE FOLLOWING:

1. Skin rash
2. Headache
3. Nausea
4. Impairment of sexual function
5. Dizziness
6. Light-headedness

SIGNS OF OVERDOSE INCLUDE THE FOLLOWING:

1. Sleepiness
2. Confusion
3. Loss of consciousness
4. Diminished reflexes

Withdrawal symptoms from minor tranquilizers often appear within 12 to 24 hours, especially if the use has been heavy and prolonged. These symptoms include anxiety, sweating, insomnia, vomiting, tremors, delirium, and seizures. The patient must be detoxified with a regimen of medication that is gradually decreased over time.[36a]

### *Hallucinogens*

Hallucinogens are natural and synthetic drugs that affect the mind and produce changes in perception and thinking. Included in this category is phencyclidine (PCP), which is discussed separately from the hallucinogens.

**Physiology.** Hallucinogens include lysergic acid diethylamide (LSD), mescaline, psilocybin, and 3,4-methylenedioxyamphetamine (MDA). They are found on the streets in a wide range of forms, including powder, peyote buttons, mushrooms, capsules, and tablets. LSD may be found as tablets, pellets, blotter paper, chips, and sheets of paper containing tattoos or stamp-like pictures of cartoon figures. Hallucinogens are taken orally, although MDA can be sniffed and injected. They may be put on sugar cubes or mixed in other food.

Common street names for hallucinogens are:

| | |
|---|---|
| LSD | Acid, barrels, blotter, dome, microdots, purple haze, windowpane |
| Mescaline | Buttons, cactus, mesc, mescal buttons |
| MDA | Love drug, mellow drug of America |
| Psilocybin | Magic mushroom, shroom |

Psilocybin and mescaline have been used in religious rites by cultures in the Western hemisphere for centuries. MDA was first synthesized in the 1930s and used as an appetite suppressant. LSD was first synthesized in 1938, and the first "trip" that was documented occurred in 1943 when the drug was accidently absorbed through the skin.

**Pathophysiology.** Most of the effects of hallucinogens are psychological, although nausea and vomiting are not uncommon possible reactions. Clinical manifestations of the use of hallucinogens are listed in Box 14-9. Tolerance to these drugs occurs rather quickly (usually after 3 days of use), and there is cross-tolerance among the four drugs.

Hallucinogens have a profound psychological effect on most people. The effect has been described as a process of amplifications, with the drug being a catalyst. Hallucinogens amplify and distort the users' experience of the environment and put them in touch with thoughts and feelings. In low doses, MDA produces a peaceful euphoria. With higher doses, it mimics LSD experiences without the hallucinations.

The feelings brought on by MDA, mescaline, and psilocybin lasts from 6 to 8 hours, whereas those of LSD usually last 8 to 12 hours. Toward the end of the "trip," the person will gradually reenter reality. A person's attempts to resist the effects of the drug seem to increase the chances of a negative experience, or a "bad trip."

Flashbacks may occur with use of the hallucinogens. In these, the user reexperiences the effects of the drug without having taken it. Bad trips are described as being characterized by tremendous confusion, unpleasant sensory images, and extreme panic. These bad trips often center on a feeling of impending danger or feelings of being threatened. Paranoid behavior is common, as well as psychotic breaks from reality during the bad trip. If the drug has precipitated psychotic breaks, some persons never return to a "normal" or previous state of consciousness.

Care during these situations includes getting the person into a nonstimulating environment and staying with the person until the effects of the trip wear off. Reassurance of the fact that the person is experiencing a drug trip is helpful. Some experts recommend giving niacin (500 mg) as a way to bring the person down from a bad trip.

Although there have been no reports of deaths from LSD, there have been documented instances in which the person died as a result of trying to do something impossible while on a trip. An example is trying to fly—that is, the person actually believes he or she will be able to fly and leaps from a window or rooftop in an attempt to do so.

**box 14-9 clinical manifestations**

***Use of Hallucinogens***

1. Stimulation at first and then depression
2. Anxiety
3. Depressed appetite
4. Increased body temperature
5. Increased heart rate
6. Increased respiration
7. Dilated pupils; with psilocybin, dizziness, numbness of face, and shivering may also occur
8. Altered sensory awareness
9. Senses become more acute
10. Thoughts that colors can be heard and sounds seen
11. Fantasies and illusions
12. Hallucination-like happenings
13. Unawareness that hallucinations are not real
14. Past and present experiences meld together, leading to feeling of oneness, compassion, and love for all things

### *Phencyclidine*

Phencyclidine is a synthetic drug that is generally described as an anesthetic-hallucinogen. However, it is chemically unrelated to hallucinogens such as LSD and mescaline.

**Physiology.** PCP was first synthesized in 1957 and tested as a general anesthetic for humans. Testing stopped in the mid-1960s because of side effects of agitation and delirium. PCP presently is available as an anesthetic agent for use by veterinarians. In the late 1960s and 1970s the drug became available as a street drug. It was banned from legal manufacture for use in humans in 1978 but is still produced illegally.

PCP, produced as a white or yellowish-white powder, has a variety of forms, including tablets and capsules. As "angel dust," it is sprinkled on tobacco or marijuana and smoked. It may also be snorted or injected. Common street names for PCP are listed below:

| | |
|---|---|
| Angel dust | Embalming fluid |
| Animal tranquilizer | KJ killer |
| Crystal | Peace pill |
| Dust | Synthetic marijuana |
| Hog | |

**Pathophysiology.** Different doses of PCP produce different physical effects. These can be found in Box 14-10.

**box 14-10** *Dose-Related Physical Manifestations of the Use of PCP*

| DOSE | EFFECTS |
|---|---|
| 5 mg | Physical sedation<br>Numbness of extremities<br>Loss of muscle coordination<br>Dizziness<br>Constricted pupils, blurred or double vision, and involuntary eye movements<br>Flushing and profuse sweating<br>Nausea and vomiting<br>Increase in blood pressure, heart rate, and respiratory rate (breathing is shallow) |
| 5 to 10 mg | Marked drop in blood pressure, breathing, and heart rates<br>Shivering, increased salivation, and watering of the eyes<br>Loss of balance, dizziness, and rigidity of muscles<br>In some cases, repetitive movements, such as rocking<br>Analgesic and anesthetic properties apparent |
| >10 mg | Extreme agitation, followed by seizures or coma<br>Symptoms similar to mental confusion and delusion of schizophrenia |

From Scott L: *PCP* (pamphlet), Charlotte, NC, 1981, Charlotte Drug Educational Center.

The psychological effects of PCP ingestion last from 1 to 6 hours, with 24 hours needed to return to baseline. These are found in Box 14-11. Research seems to indicate that the bad trip rate of PCP is five times that of other drugs. Chronic users may experience flashbacks. The dose of PCP may indicate the nature of the effects.

Although there is disagreement about whether PCP is physically addicting, there is wide agreement that it is psychologically habit-forming.

PCP overdoses are dangerous, because the person may die as a result of respiratory or cardiac arrest. Symptoms of PCP intoxication are variable and include the following:

1. Violent or combative until nearly unconscious
2. Little or no pain response
3. Inability to speak
4. Elevated blood pressure and pulse rate with slight fever[63]

The person intoxicated by PCP becomes more agitated by noise, bright lights, and talking. PCP use may result in psychosis that lasts from several days to 2 weeks. It is often mistaken for acute schizophrenia. Individuals may be actively suicidal and become depressed when the acute psychosis has passed.[36a]

### Narcotics

Narcotics are drugs that are derived from the opium poppy or produced synthetically. The use of these has been recorded far back in history. Synthetic production of narcotics has occurred in the past 30 to 50 years. In general, narcotics lower the perception of pain.

**Physiology.** Heroin is one narcotic that is abused to a large extent. There has been a shift toward younger addicts and an increase in the percentage of whites using heroin. On the streets, heroin is known as "H," horse, junk, hard stuff, smack, or scag.

There are several different forms of narcotics. See Table 14-6 for a listing of these drugs, their medical use, and route of administration.

**box 14-11** *Dose-Related Psychological Manifestations of the Use of PCP*

| DOSE | EFFECTS |
|---|---|
| Low | Euphoria and sense of alcohol-like intoxication |
| | Changes in body image |
| | Mood swings from ecstacy to panic |
| | Hallucinations and confusion about time and space |
| | In final stage in some cases, a sense of despair and emotional isolation, possibly leading to a feeling of paranoia and a sense of impending death |
| Moderate | Increase in effects felt at low dose |
| | Loss of sense of contact with environment |
| High | Symptoms of mental and emotional confusion similar to schizophrenia |

From Scott L: *PCP* (pamphlet), Charlotte, NC, 1981, Charlotte Drug Educational Center.

**Pathophysiology.** Heroin and morphine are alkaloids of opium that depress the central nervous system. The clinical manifestations of their use and that of other narcotics appear in Box 14-12. A major concern about heroin users is that they commonly inject the drug with contaminated needles, which places them at high risk of acquiring HIV, hepatitis, and other infections, such as septicemia. Narcotic addicts develop both tolerance and physical and psychological addiction. Withdrawal may be painful and should be under medical supervision. Clonidine (Catapres) is often used for purposes of detoxification from narcotics. The heavier the use, the longer detoxification may take. Symptoms of withdrawal may include nausea, cramps, chills, sweating, watery eyes, running nose, and restlessness.[36a]

Using heroin is an expensive habit, and many addicts resort to crime to support it. Heroin is often mixed ("cut") with other substances primarily to increase its weight for retail sale (mannitol and starch) and to add pharmacological effects (dextromethorphan and lidocaine). But at times heroin may

**table 14-6** *Narcotics*

| Name | Medical Use | Route of Administration |
|---|---|---|
| Heroin | None in the United States | By injection or sniffing |
| Morphine | Ease pain | By mouth, smoking, or injection |
| Opium | Ease pain, treat diarrhea, and suppress cough | By mouth or smoking |
| Codeine | Suppress cough and reduce pain | By mouth or injection |
| Meperidine | Relieve pain | By mouth or injection |
| Methadone | Ease pain and to help those dependent on heroin | By mouth or injection |

From O'Brien R, Cohen S, Evans G, Fine J: *The encyclopedia of drug abuse.* Copyright © 1984 by Greenspring, Inc. Copyright © 1992 by Facts On File and Greenspring, Inc. Reprinted by permission of Facts On File, Inc.

**box 14-12** ***clinical manifestations***

***Use of Narcotics***

1. Relief of pain and feeling of well-being
2. Shallow breathing
3. Reduced hunger and thirst
4. Reduced sexual drive
5. Drowsiness
6. Euphoria
7. Lethargy
8. Heaviness of limbs
9. Apathy
10. Loss of ability to concentrate
11. Loss of judgment and self-control
12. Overdoses can cause coma, convulsions, respiratory arrest and death

be contaminated with dangerous substances, such as scopolamine (known as "point on point" or "sting").[14]

**Methadone maintenance.** One approach to the treatment of narcotic addiction is the methadone maintenance program. The drug is given legally as a part of a rehabilitation program. The drug reduces the severity of the heroin withdrawal but must itself be tapered off.

Studies have shown that high-dose methadone maintenance is important in heroin abstinence.[40] There are many controversies surrounding methadone programs, and many professionals discourage its use, recommending instead detoxification leading to abstinence.

Levo-alpha-acetylmethadol is marketed under the name of OrLAA. It is a long-acting opioid that needs to be taken only every other day. It was approved by the Food and Drug Administration (FDA) for maintenance treatment of opioid dependence in 1993. Another drug that is being studied as a maintenance drug for opioid addiction is buprenorphine. However, as of 1997 it has not been approved by the FDA for the treatment of addiction.[74]

### *Cannabis*

**Physiology.** Cannabis, or marijuana, comes from the Indian hemp plant. It can grow wild or is fairly easily cultivated. Marijuana is usually smoked as a cigarette (joint, reefer) or in a pipe. Other paraphernalia may be used, including water-filled pipes known as "bongs." There are many slang terms for marijuana, including the following: dope, grass, herb, joint, pot, reefer, roach, smoke, stuff, and weed.

Marijuana has been used as both a medical and nonmedical drug for more than 3000 years. It has been used since the 1850s in the United States. Its popularity as a street drug began to occur in the twentieth century. It is still one of the most popular and commonly abused drugs, especially among young people.

Hashish, or hash, is a resinous extract of the leaves and flowering part of the marijuana plant. It is more concentrated than marijuana and has more intense effects. Although marijuana use declined for a time, its use by teenagers increased in the 1990s.[54]

A few patients have been able to obtain marijuana legally for therapeutic purposes. Since 1978, legislation permitting patients with certain disorders to obtain marijuana with a physician's approval has been passed in 36 states. Therapeutic uses include to treat nausea and vomiting induced by chemotherapy, to lower intraocular pressure in glaucoma, as an anticonvulsant, as a muscle relaxant, and to stimulate the appetite of persons with acquired immunodeficiency syndrome (AIDS). It also has been advocated to relieve phantom limb pain and other types of chronic pain.[36]

**Pathophysiology.** Marijuana and other forms of cannabis seem to act as CNS depressants. They depress higher brain centers and consequently release lower centers from inhibitory influences. The physical manifestations of marijuana use appear in Box 14-13. Research indicates that marijuana may affect chromosome segregation during cell division. Because marijuana is a fat-soluble molecule, parts of it may be stored in the body for 30 days or more.

In addition to its physical effects, marijuana has important psychological effects, including distortion of time (Box 14-14). A classic description of the time distortion is that "seconds seem like minutes, minutes seem like hours, and hours seem like days."

Psychological addiction develops in users. Crisis situations may occur in the form of an anxiety reaction to the marijuana high. A calming and reassuring approach has been found to be helpful.

### *Deliriants*

**Physiology.** Deliriants are any chemicals that give off fumes or vapors that, when inhaled, produce symptoms similar to intoxication. They may also be called inhalants. Vasodilators—such as amyl nitrate and butyl nitrite, which are used medically—are also considered inhalants.

The fumes or vapors from inhalants are sniffed through the nose, or the vapors are put into a bag or captured in a balloon to increase the concentration of the inhaled fumes.

The history of the use of inhalants is traced back to ancient Greece. Sniffing commercial products and solvents was first documented in the 1950s. No medical use exists for commercially prepared inhalants. Of course, vasodilators and anesthetic agents have a legitimate medical purpose.

Deliriants or inhalants have a psychoactive or mood-altering effect when the vapors are inhaled or sniffed. Most fall into one of three categories:

1. Solvents (glue, gasoline)
2. Aerosol sprays
3. Anesthetics

**box 14-13** *Physical Manifestations of the Use of Marijuana*

1. Drying of the eyes and mouth
2. Increase in appetite and food consumption
3. Can produce glucose intolerance, leading to hyperglycemia, which can be a problem in those with diabetes
4. Reddening of eyes
5. Impairment of short-term memory
6. Increased heart rate and blood pressure
7. Decreased body temperature
8. Impairment of coordination

**box 14-14** *Psychological Manifestations of the Use of Marijuana*

1. Altering of perception (e.g., altering of sight, sound, touch, sense of time, and taste)
2. Feeling of well-being and intoxication, although depression and panic may occur
3. Confusion and distortion of reality may occur

Solvents include commercial products that are not commonly thought of as drugs. These include glue, gasoline, kerosene, lighter fluid, paint products, lacquer thinner, spot remover, and nail polish remover. Products such as hair spray, deodorant, insecticides, and cookware coating sprays are examples of aerosols. Anesthetics that are used recreationally include ether, chloroform, and nitrous oxide.

Typically, persons using solvents and aerosols are among the youngest drug users, with most being teenagers.

**Pathophysiology.** Almost all inhalants are CNS depressants that slow the user's heart rate, brain activity, and breathing. The clinical manifestations of the use of inhalants can be found in Box 14-15.

The prolonged use of inhalants may lead to liver, kidney, blood, and bone marrow damage. The sniffing of toluene, found in gasoline and commercial cleaners, has been demonstrated to cause irreversible brain damage. This may be demonstrated as forgetfulness, inability to think clearly, depression, irritability, hostility, and paranoia.

Deliriants also have an impact on the peripheral nervous system and produce symptoms similar to those of multiple sclerosis. These include poor coordination, inability to walk, poor bladder control, decreased mobility, and decreased ability to perform activities of daily living and to meet basic needs.

Some inhalants cause tolerance. Physical dependency is a possibility. Symptoms of withdrawal include chills, hallucinations, headaches, stomach pains, cramps, and DTs.

The psychological effects of deliriants include a feeling of stimulation and energy. At higher doses, the user may feel intoxicated. The development of psychological dependence is a real possibility.

Use of large amounts of aerosols or solvents can cause death as a result of cardiac arrest after dysrhythmias. Death from inhalants is usually caused by suffocation because of the displacement of oxygen in the lungs. Sniffing inhalants from a bag or balloon increases the risk of suffocation. Misuse of commercial aerosol products used to chill food has been reported to cause death by freezing the lungs of the user.

**box 14-15** *clinical manifestations*

***Use of Inhalants***

1. Slurred speech
2. Blurred vision, bloodshot eyes
3. Inflamed mucous membranes, nosebleeds
4. Bad breath
5. Light-headedness
6. Ringing in the ears
7. Watering eyes
8. Loss of coordination
9. Excessive nasal secretions
10. Loss of consciousness or seizures lasting 20 to 45 minutes with large doses

The CNS effects of inhalants are potentiated by other CNS depressants, thus increasing the chances of overdose.

## OTHER DEPENDENCIES

### CAFFEINE

#### Physiology

Caffeine is the most accepted and used psychoactive substance in the United States. Many beverages and other products contain caffeine. Because of its availability and widespread use, most persons do not view caffeine as a drug.[26]

The use of tea leaves in China dates back at least 4000 years. In the 1200s the Arabians used coffee. Caffeine was first isolated from coffee in 1820. In its pure state, caffeine is a white powder or white needle-shaped crystals. It has been used as an additive in carbonated beverages since the early 1900s.

Medically, caffeine is present in many headache remedies, cold medications, diuretics, diet aids, and other prescriptions. (See Box 14-16 for the amount of caffeine in commonly used beverages.)

#### Pathophysiology

Caffeine stimulates the CNS, as well as the digestive system and the kidneys. The clinical manifestations of this stimulation appear in Box 14-17. Physical dependence occurs with regular intake of 350 mg for an adult. The withdrawal symptoms include severe headaches, irritability, and tiredness.

Caffeine makes most people feel energetic and alert. Too much caffeine can precipitate an anxiety attack. Long-term involvement can lead to depression, persistent anxiety, low-grade fever, nausea, ringing in the ears, and chronic insomnia.

**box 14-16** *Caffeine Content of Products*

| | |
|---|---|
| Coffee | |
| Brewed, per cup | 75 to 155 mg |
| Instant | 60 to 90 mg |
| Decaffeinated | 2 to 4 mg |
| Tea, per cup | 25 to 75 mg |
| Carbonated sodas (all colas [except those labeled caffeine-free], Dr. Pepper, Mountain Dew, Sunkist Orange) | 30 to 70 mg |
| Chocolate | |
| Hot cocoa | 30 to 70 mg |
| Candy (1 oz) | 6 mg |
| Over-the-counter drugs | |
| Anacin, Excedrin, Vanquish, Doan's Pills | 16 to 65 mg |
| No-Doz, Vivarin | 100 to 200 mg |
| APC tablets | 30 to 100 mg |
| Diet aids | |
| AYDS, Dexatrim, Prolamine | 140 to 200 mg |

**box 14-17** *clinical manifestations*

*Use of Caffeine*

1. Increased blood pressure
2. Increased urination
3. Stomach distress (acidity)
4. Tachycardia
5. Headaches
6. Nervousness
7. Insomnia

(4–7: with large doses)

A fatal dose of caffeine is considered to be about 10 g or 10,000 mg.

Research seems to indicate that excessive use of caffeine may contribute to the development of heart disease, as well as to bladder cancer.

## NICOTINE

### Physiology

More than 50 million Americans smoke more than 600 billion cigarettes yearly. From 1965 through 1993, the annual prevalence of cigarette smoking among adults in the United States declined 40%. However, the prevalence of smoking among adolescents has been found to be increasing.[12,15,22,25,57]

Cigarettes are among the most addicting products known. The vast majority of persons who quit smoking relapse within a short time. It has been estimated that only 2% to 3% of smokers become nonsmokers each year. In addition, between one third to one half of those who smoke occasional cigarettes go on to become physically addicted to nicotine. Half of all smokers die prematurely of tobacco-related diseases.[34,65]

### Pathophysiology

Nicotine is a water-soluble and liquid-soluble base. Smokeless tobacco is readily absorbed across the mucosal membranes of the mouth and nose, which explains the rapid absorption associated with it. Cigarette smoke is acidic and must be inhaled to be absorbed by the pulmonary alveoli, where absorption occurs rapidly. From the lung, nicotine is absorbed into alveoli capillary blood and carried to the heart, brain, and other organs.[38]

The effects of nicotine that are associated with dependence include changes in regional blood glucose metabolism, electroencephalographic changes, the release of catecholamines, tolerance, and physiological dependence.[34]

The nicotine in tobacco acts as a stimulant to the CNS. Nicotine is present in the brain within a few seconds of the beginning of smoking. Smokers claim that smoking produces relaxation; however, smoking releases epinephrine, which may create physiological stress. Nicotine acts as an appetite suppressant and some smokers fear gaining weight if they stop smoking. In large doses it produces tremors, decreased urine output, and a rapid respiratory rate.

When nicotine is stopped abruptly, withdrawal symptoms begin within a few hours. They peak within a few days, and last for several weeks.[34] Withdrawal symptoms include the following:

1. Decreased heart rate
2. Weight gain
3. Impairment of psychomotor performance
4. Nervousness and anxiety
5. Headaches
6. Fatigue
7. Insomnia
8. Constipation or diarrhea

The craving for a cigarette often continues for an extended period.

Because those addicted to nicotine find it difficult to give up tobacco, medications containing nicotine are some-time used. These medications replace, at least partially, the nicotine formerly obtained from tobacco. The first of these medications was nicotine polacrilex (nicotine gum). Four transdermal-delivery systems are also available: Habitol, Nicoderm, Nicotrol 16, and Prostep. It is important to educate the person using any of these medications to abstain from tobacco. Smoking or chewing tobacco while using nicotine gum or a patch can lead to relapse and cardiac effects.[41]

Nicotine addiction has implications for the medical-surgical patient. This may include management of respiratory status after surgery or the management of the person who has developed chronic pulmonary disease as the result of years of smoking. It is one of the most physically damaging and addictive habits in which a large number of people engage. Smoking has been linked to heart and blood vessel disease; chronic bronchitis and emphysema, and cancer of the lungs, larynx, mouth, esophagus, bladder, pancreas, and kidneys. It is far easier to become addicted to cigarettes than to alcohol or other drugs.

Tobacco is used by smoking, chewing, or inhaling. Snuff is usually placed between the gums and the cheek.

## NURSING MANAGEMENT

### ■ ASSESSMENT

Most early indications of drug use are covered in the preceding description of individual classes of drugs. The reader is also referred to the assessment section in the discussion on alcoholism on p. 373.

#### Subjective Data

As with those persons who are alcoholic, the subjective data given by the patient may or may not be truthful. It is helpful to collect subjective data from several sources so that the information can be compared. The questions asked under this section in the discussion of alcoholism on p. 373 also apply here.

### Objective Data

Breaks in the skin are an objective sign that must be noted when assessing for drug addiction. If the person has been "mainlining" (that is, injecting the drug directly into the vein), needle marks, scars, or small scabs can be seen on the hands and forearms or instep. Other veins used as points of entry to conceal addiction include the dorsal vein of the penis, the sublingual blood vessels of the tongue, or the conjunctival artery of the eyelid.

A complication that can occur with intravenous drug use is wound botulism. Many cases are caused by subcutaneous injection or "skin popping" of black tar heroin. The number of cases of wound botulism has been steadily increasing.[17]

## ■ NURSING DIAGNOSES

The nursing diagnoses for the patient with drug addiction are the same as for the alcoholic patient. The reader is referred to p. 374.

## ■ EXPECTED PATIENT OUTCOMES

The reader is referred to this section in the discussion on alcoholism (p. 374).

## ■ INTERVENTIONS

The treatment of withdrawal from drug abuse is discussed in each section under the specific drugs. See Table 14-7 for more details on acute intoxication and withdrawal. General rehabilitation follows the guidelines for treatment of the alcoholic. These can be found in the section on alcoholism (p. 375). Today, most treatment centers treat alcoholics and drug addicts side-by-side. In fact, the majority of persons receiving treatment for chemical dependency today have a history of abuse of both alcohol and drugs.

One difference between drugs and alcohol is that in most cases the possession and use of drugs is illegal. In the United States, the addiction to narcotics has been considered a crime since the passage of the Harrison Narcotic Act of 1914. Education is making the public more aware of the primary nature of the disease of drug addiction.

Because of the expense involved, users often sell their belongings, steal, or become prostitutes to obtain money to supply their drug habit. Each day abuse of drugs costs the American economy millions of dollars.

It is important for the nurse caring for the drug-addicted person to examine her or his attitudes about caring for the patient who is addicted. Attitudes that include negativity, moral superiority, anger, indifference, or sympathy are seldom, if ever, helpful. The nurse also should realize that punishment and/or deprivation of the person is also counterproductive. In addition, attempts to control the person are usually counterproductive. Instead, efforts should focus on controlling environmental factors (accessibility to drugs). Finally, the nurse should realize that substances can be and often are brought into the hospital by visitors. The person needs to be observed for signs of recurrent drug use, because many drug- and alcohol-addicted persons are very resourceful in securing substances and in covering up their use.

### Controlling Pain

Medical-surgical nurses often have questions about pain control when dealing with drug-addicted and alcoholic patients. They often undermedicate the patient, fearing that giving prescribed pain medication will increase addiction. It is important to realize that not keeping the patient comfortable may actually predispose the patient to a relapse of the addiction. The patient should receive the pain medication for only as long as he or she requires it, in the view of the nurse or other professional who knows the patient. It is common for the drug-addicted patient, in particular, to require higher doses of pain medication than the average person. It is also important to realize that addiction tends to increase the amount of drug required to produce anesthesia. Thus these persons will require a longer time to recover from the anesthesic.

### Patient/Family Education

The reader is referred to the discussion of this area under alcoholism (p. 378).

## ■ EVALUATION

Evaluation of the patient with drug abuse is the same as that for the person with alcoholism (p. 379).

# OTHER ADDICTIVE BEHAVIOR PATTERNS

## CODEPENDENCE

Another example of addictive behavior that is often encountered by the medical-surgical nurse is codependence. An overview of this problem is included here because the codependent person's approach to the substance abuser can have an effect on the care provided by the nurse. In addition, nurses themselves are often drawn into negative patterns of behavior, which are thought to be a chief cause of "burnout."[39] Nurses who give too much to others without taking care of themselves often become depleted. In addition, they are at high risk for developing alcoholism or drug dependence themselves.

Codependence has often been used to describe a person who is emotionally involved with a chemically-dependent person. The codependent is someone who develops an unhealthy pattern of coping as a reaction to someone else's drug or alcohol use. Recently, however, the definition of codependence has been expanded. It is now seen as a disease entity with a definable onset, a set of physical and psychological symptoms, and a predictable medical course.

Definitions of codependence vary, but there is agreement that these persons manifest dysfunctional responses to life,

**table 14-7** *Clinical Manifestations and Treatment of Acute Intoxication and Withdrawal of Mind-Altering Drugs*

| Drug Group | Acute Intoxication: Clinical Manifestations | Acute Intoxication: Treatment | Clinical Manifestations of Withdrawal |
|---|---|---|---|
| Narcotics | Respiratory depression, bradycardia, hypotension, cold clammy skin, decreased body temperature; deep sleep, stupor, or coma; pin-point pupils | Maintain ventilation, provide oxygen<br>Give narcotic antagonist: naloxone (Narcan) 0.4 mg IV<br>Monitor vital signs every 15-30 min until patient is conscious<br>Treat for shock | (Not life-threatening)<br>Early: restlessness, irritability, drug craving, yawning, lacrimation, diaphoresis, rhinorrhea, followed by "yen" sleep (intense desire to sleep; sleeps restlessly)<br>Later: awakens with more severe symptoms, nausea, vomiting, anorexia, abdominal cramps, bone and muscle pain, tremors, piloerection (goose-flesh) |
| Other CNS depressants | Same as narcotics (above) | Lavage if recent oral ingestion with possible activated charcoal treatment<br>Maintain ventilation, provide oxygen<br>Monitor vital signs every 15-30 min until patient is conscious<br>Position patient side-lying or prone, not supine<br>Treat for shock<br>Hemodialysis for renal shutdown | (May be life-threatening)<br>Insomnia, restlessness, tremors, anorexia, followed by convulsions, and symptoms similar to DTs (confusion, visual and auditory hallucinations), fever, dehydration |
| CNS stimulants | Labile cardiovascular symptoms (flushing or pallor, pulse and blood pressure changes, dysrhythmias), hyperpyrexia, mental disturbances (agitation, paranoia, hallucinations), convulsions, circulatory collapse | Give chlorpromazine, 25-50 mg IM<br>Provide a quiet environment<br>Orient patient to reality<br>Monitor vital signs until stable | (Withdrawal is not severe)<br>Somnolence, apathy, irritability, depression, fatigue |
| Hallucinogens | Physiological toxicity low at doses that produce strong psychological effects<br>Acute panic reaction (bad trip) may lead to suicide<br>"Flashback" episodes<br>Prolonged psychotic disorders (paranoia, depression)<br>Phencyclidine: CNS depression or stimulation may lead to death | Provide quiet, supportive environment and constant attention<br>Give diazepam (Valium), 2-10 mg IM and/or major tranquilizers (thorazine IM) for severe anxiety | No evidence of withdrawal symptoms |
| Cannabis | Adverse reactions infrequent<br>Simple depression, paranoid ideation, confusion, disorientation, hallucinations | Provide support and reassurance<br>Give tranquilizer for agitation | (Withdrawal symptoms rare)<br>Insomnia, anorexia |
| Deliriants | Slowing of heart rate, brain activity, and breathing<br>Slurred speech, blurred vision, inflamed mucous membranes, excessive tearing, and nasal secretions<br>With high doses, loss of consciousness and seizures may occur<br>Brain damage may occur (memory loss, depression, paranoia, hostility)<br>Feeling of stimulation and energy<br>Death may occur from suffocation or cardiac arrest | Maintain airway<br>Maintain respirations<br>Provide quiet environment and provide support<br>Monitor vital signs<br>Orient patient to reality | Chills, hallucinations, headaches, stomach pains, cramps, DTs |

and they derive their self-esteem from their ability to control themselves and others.

Characteristics of codependence include the following:[39,76]

1. Perfectionism
2. Denial
3. Poor communication
4. Caretaking
5. Inability to identify, express, and manage feelings
6. Difficulty forming and maintaining close relationships
7. Feeling responsible for others' behavior or feelings
8. Constantly seeking approval from others
9. Feelings of powerlessness
10. Feeling morally superior
11. Difficulty in setting limits
12. Feeling "super responsible" or "super irresponsible"
13. Martyrdom
14. Need to control
15. Any addictive behavior
16. Stress-related illness

Recovery from codependence starts with the person learning to care for himself or herself. The use of a journal to record feelings may be helpful. Breaking through the denial of the codependent person is often difficult. The person also requires help to learn to set appropriate boundaries, grieve past losses, and acquire the skill of reparenting. Daily affirmations may be used to reinforce the self-worth of the person.

## IMPAIRED NURSES

The issue of the impaired nurse is important to nurses in many different settings. This includes the medical-surgical areas of nursing. It has been estimated that between 6% and 8% of registered nurses will develop an addiction to drugs or alcohol before she or he leaves nursing. A nurse will rarely spend time working in a hospital or other health care setting without having to confront the issue of an impaired nurse.[29,67]

Over the past several years, many states have developed programs to assist the nurse who is impaired by either alcoholism or drug addiction. One of the main reasons for the establishment of these programs is that the rate of chemical dependence in nurses or other health professionals is greater than in the general public, principally because these persons have greater access to mood-altering substances. For instance, nurses may handle narcotics every day and may succumb to the temptation to use them. Before the inception of peer assistance programs (through either the state boards of nursing or state nursing associations), the nurse often was fired and then was free to migrate to another facility, where the cycle might start over again.

In March 1978, nurses from several states attended a meeting held in Manhattan to discuss the problem of the alcoholic nurse. By 1980 two organizations of nurses interested in alcoholism were active in encouraging help. These were the Drug and Alcohol Nursing Association (DANA) and the National Nurses Society on Addiction (NNSA). In 1981 the American Nurses Association (ANA) created a Task Force on Addiction and Psychological Disturbance to formulate guidelines for state nursing associations to develop programs to help the impaired nurse. At their 1982 convention, the ANA adopted a resolution that recognized its responsibility to assist nurses who are impaired.

In 1980 two states, Maryland and Ohio, had peer assistance programs in place. This effort has grown so that almost every state now has a program.

The peer assistance programs have several goals: (1) to assist the nurse who is impaired to receive treatment; (2) to protect the public from the untreated nurse; (3) to help the recovering nurse reenter nursing in a systematic, planned, and safe way; and (4) to assist in monitoring the continued recovery of the nurse for a period of time. The reentry of the nurse may include a restriction from handling controlled drugs for a period of time.

The basis of these programs is one nurse helping another. Many volunteers in these programs are nurses who are themselves recovering or who are working in the field of chemical dependence.

### critical thinking QUESTIONS

**1** Dean, 39, is admitted to the hospital for acute pancreatitis. He is having severe pain, rated as a 12 on a scale of 1 to 10. He is a known abuser of narcotics and is requesting pain medication every 1 to 2 hours. How would you go about problem solving and making a decision regarding the treatment of Dean's pain?

**2** Carrie, 19, is addicted to barbiturates. She frequently takes pentobarbital and secobarbital in combination with alcohol. On any given day Carrie is euphoric and calm. Today she is experiencing difficulty breathing, lethargy, and nausea. What classification of drug do barbiturates represent? Distinguish between the expected clinical manifestations of barbiturates and side effects that Carrie is experiencing.

**3** Mary, 79, is a patient on your medical-surgical unit. She recently was widowed and talks often of how lonely she is. She denied drinking on her admission history, but the emergency room reported that she had a blood alcohol level that indicated intoxication. She has had numerous falls in the past year. She is unkempt and is underweight for her height. When her children and grandchildren are approached with a concern about her drinking, they become angry and vehemently deny it. They want the doctor to find the reason for the falls. What would you do?

**4** David is a nurse on your unit who works evenings. His behavior at work has become erratic at times. You have noticed over the past several weeks that he is moody and that his documentation is not always adequate. He has been going to the bathroom a lot, and you have noted that he seems to spend a lot of time around the narcotic cabinet. Yesterday a patient complained of pain, an hour after the record said she was medicated. When you questioned

David, he became defensive. How would you go about resolving this situation? Who would you consult and what should you document?

## chapter SUMMARY

### INTRODUCTION

- Addictions, including alcoholism and drug addiction, are considered diseases and are commonly referred to as chemical dependence.
- Dependence includes physical and psychological dependence and is defined as the need to continue use of the substance to prevent withdrawal symptoms.
- Tolerance, a decreased susceptibility to the effects of a substance, develops with increased use of alcohol or drugs.
- Enabling behavior by friends or co-workers allows the alcoholic or drug addict to continue the use of the substance.

### ALCOHOLISM

- Alcoholism is the third most common major health problem in the United States and affects more than 10 million persons.
- No one theory has been found to explain alcoholism.
- Alcohol is a central nervous depressant that affects the brain by suppressing the activity of the neurotransmitter gamma-aminobutyric acid (GABA).
- Ninety percent of alcohol is metabolized in the liver.
- The amount of alcohol in the blood at any one time is called the blood alcohol level.
- Delirium tremens (DTs) is an acute complication of alcohol withdrawal that requires aggressive therapy to prevent mortality and morbidity.
- Alcoholics Anonymous (AA) is a group of self-acknowledged alcoholics whose aim is to stay sober and to help other alcoholics gain sobriety. AA also is open to drug abusers and helps them stay off drugs.

### DRUG ABUSE

- Drug habituation is the repeated use of a drug to the point of psychological dependence; while drug addiction includes craving, psychological and physical dependence.
- The basic categories of drugs of abuse include stimulants, depressants, hallucinogens, narcotics, cannabis, and deliriants.
- Caffeine is the most accepted and widely used psychoactive substance in the United States and is found in many beverages and health products.
- It is not unusual for persons with chemical dependence to also experience symptoms of a psychiatric disorder.

### OTHER ADDICTIONS

- A codependent is a person who has let someone else's behavior affect him or her and is obsessed with controlling other people's behavior.
- Nurses and other health professionals are at increased risk for the development of chemical dependency because of their proximity to mind-altering substances.

## References


1. *Alcoholics Anonymous,* New York, Alcoholic World Service, 1976, Classic.

1a. Allen K: Essential concepts of addiction for general nursing practice, *Nurs Clin North Am* 33(1):1, 1998.

2. American Psychiatric Association: *Diagnostic and statistical manual of mental disorders,* ed 4, Washington, DC, 1994, The Association.
3. Antai-Otong D: Helping the alcoholic patient recover, *Am J Nurs* 95(8):22-30, 1995.
4. Blank-Reid C: How to have a stroke at an early age: the effects of crack cocaine and other illicit drugs, *J Neurosci Nurs* 28(1):19-27, 1996.
5. Buchsbaum DG et al: Screening for drinking problems by patient self-report: even "safe" levels may indicate a problem, *Arch Intern Med* 155:104-108, 1995.
6. Bukstein OG, Kaminer Y: Nosology of adolescent substance abuse, *Am J Addict* 3(1):1-13, 1994.
7. Caces FM, Stinson FS and Dufour MC: *Surveillance report #32: trends in alcohol-related morbidity among short-stay community hospital discharges,* United States, 1979-92, Rockville, Md, 1994, National Institutes on Alcohol Abuse and Alcoholism.
8. Cassidy J: On the rocks, *Nurs Times* 91(49):14-15, 1995.
9. Castaglia PT: Smokeless tobacco, *J Pediatr Health Care* 8(6):274-276, 1994.
10. Centers for Disease Control and Prevention (CDC): AIDS associated with injecting-drug-use—United States, 1995, *MMWR* 45(19):382-398, 1996.
11. Centers for Disease Control and Prevention (CDC): Alcohol involvement in fatal motor-vehicle crashes—United States, 1993-1994, *MMWR* 44(47):886-7, 1995.
12. Centers for Disease Control and Prevention (CDC): Cigarette smoking among adults—United States, 1993, *MMWR* 43:925-929, 1993.
13. Centers for Disease Control and Prevention (CDC): Increasing morbidity and mortality associated with abuse of methamphetamine—United States, 1991-1994, *MMWR* 44(47):882-888, 1995.
14. Centers for Disease Control and Prevention (CDC): Scopolamine poisoning among heroin users—New York City, Newark, Philadelphia, and Baltimore, 1995 and 1996, *MMWR* 45(22):457-460, 1996.
15. Centers for Disease Control and Prevention (CDC): Tobacco use and usual source of cigarettes among high school students—United States, 1995, *MMWR* 45(20):413-418, 1996.
16. Centers for Disease Control and Prevention (CDC): Update: alcohol-related traffic crashes and fatalities among youth and young adults—United States, 1982-1994, *MMWR* 44(47):869-874, 1995.
17. Centers for Disease Control and Prevention (CDC): Wound botulism—California, 1995, *MMWR* 44(48):889-892, 1995.
18. Cheever K, House MA: Cardiovascular implications of anabolic steroid use, *J Cardiovasc Nurs* 6(2):19-30, 1992.
19. Chitwood DD et al: Risk factors for HIV-1 seroconversion among injection drug users: a case-control study, *Am J Public Health* 85(11): 1538-1542, 1995.
20. Compton M, Naegle MA, D'Arcangelo JS: *Nursing care in acute intoxication.* In Naegle MA, editor: *Substance abuse education in nursing,* vol 2. NLN Pub 85-2463:347-408, 1992.
21. Compton M, Naegle MA, D'Arcangelo JS: Nursing care in withdrawal. In Naegle MA, editor: *Substance abuse education in nursing,* vol 2, NLN Pub 85-2463:409-462, 1992.
22. Corrigan JD, Rust E, Lamb-Hart GL: The nature and extent of substance abuse problems in persons with traumatic brain injury, *J Head Trauma Rehabil* 10(3):29-46, 1995.

23. Cross GM, Hennessey TG: Principles and practices of detoxification, *Patient Care Clinicians Office Pract* 20(1):81-93, 1993.
24. Dawson DA, Grant BF, Chou P: Gender difference in alcohol intake. In Zakhari C, Hunt W, editors: *Stress, gender and alcohol seeking behavior.* NIAAA Research Monograph 35, 1996.
25. Dufour MC, Ingle KG: Twenty-five years of alcohol epidemiology: trends, techniques, and transitions, *Alcohol Health Res World* 19(2): 77-84, 1995.
26. Elkind AH: Caffeine abuse, *Headache Q Curr Treat Res* 6(4):279, 1995.
27. Erstad BL et al: Recognition and treatment of ethanol abuse in trauma patients, *Heart Lung* 25(4):330-336, 1996.
28. Felbinger D: Substance abuse in women: a growing challenge for nurses, *Med Surg Nurs Q* 1(1):101-109, 1992.
29. Finke LM, Hickman LC, Miller, EL: Personal drug and alcohol use by staff nurses at work, *Addiction Nurs Network* 3(1):25-29, 1993.
30. Fox K et al: Estimating the costs of substance abuse to the Medicaid hospital care program, *Am J Pub Health* 85(1):48-54, 1995.
31. Fuchs CS et al: Alcohol consumption and mortality among women, *N Engl J Med* 332(19):1245-1250, 1995.
32. Garfein RS et al: Viral infections in short-term injection drug users: the prevalence of the hepatitis C, hepatitis B, human immunodeficiency, and human T-lymphotropic viruses, *Am J Public Health* 86(5):655-661, 1996.
33. Gentilello LM et al: Alcohol interventions in trauma centers, *JAMA* 274(13):1043-1048, 1995.
34. Giovino GA et al: Epidemiology of tobacco use and dependence, *Epidemiol Rev* 17(1):48-65, 1995.
35. Grant BF et al: Prevalence of DSM-IV alcohol abuse and dependence: United States, 1992, *Alcohol Health Res World* 18(3):243-248, 1994.
36. Grinspoon L, Bakalar JB: Marijuana as medicine: a plea for reconsideration, *JAMA* 273(23):1875-1876, 1995.
36a. Haack MR: Treating acute withdrawal from alcohol and other drugs, *Nurs Clin North Am* 33(1):75, 1998.
37. Hagan H et al: Reduced risk of hepatitis B and hepatitis C among injection drug users in the Tacoma syringe exchange program, *Am J Public Health* 85(11):1531-1538, 1995.
38. Haim DY et al: The pulmonary complications of crack cocaine: a comprehensive review, *Chest* 107(1):233-240, 1995.
39. Hall S, Wray L: Codependency: nurses who give too much, *Am J Nurs* 89(11):1546, 1989.
40. Hartel DM et al: Heroin use during methadone maintenance treatment: the importance of methadone dose and cocaine use, *Am J Public Health* 85(1):83-88, 1995.
41. Henningfield JE: Nicotine medications for smoking cessation, *N Engl J Med* 333(18):1196-1203, 1995.
42. Hingson R et al: Reducing alcohol-impaired driving in Massachusetts: the saving lives program, *Am J Pub Health* 86(6):791-797, 1996.
43. Hollander JE: Cocaine-associated myocardial infarction: mortality and complications, *Arch Intern Med* 155:1081-1086, 1995.
44. Jacobsen JL, Jacobsen SW: Prenatal alcohol exposure and neurobehavioral development: where is the threshold? *Alcohol Health Res World* 18(1):30-37, 1994.
45. Johnson V: *Intervention,* Minneapolis, 1987, Hazeldon Foundation.
46. Jones C, Dickinson P: Substance abuse: from ecstasy to agony: methylene-dioxymethamphetamine, *Nurs Times* 88(13):27-28, 30, 1992.
47. Larroque B et al: Moderate prenatal alcohol exposure and psychomotor development at preschool age, *Am J Public Health* 85(12): 1654-1661, 1995.
48. Lawford BR: Bromocriptine in the treatment of alcoholics with the D2 dopamine receptor Ai allele, *JAMA* 274:1254, 1995.
49. Leshner AI: Molecular mechanisms of cocaine addiction, *N Engl J Med* 335(2):128-129, 1996.
50. Litt IF: Prevention of substance abuse, *J Adolesc Health* 18(1):10, 1996.
51. Mason BJ et al: A double-blind, placebo-controlled trial of desipramine for primary alcohol dependence stratified on the presence or absence of major depression. *JAMA* 275:761-767, 1996.
52. McGinnis JM, Lee PR: Healthy People 2000, *JAMA* 273:1123-1129, 1995.
53. Mendelson JH, Mello, NK: Management of cocaine abuse and dependence, *N Engl J Med* 334(15):965-972, 1996.
54. Miller CA: Editorial: a contract on America's children, *Am J Public Health* 86(4):473-474, 1995.
55. Muramato ML, Leshar L: Adolescent substance abuse, *Primary Care Clinicians Office Pract* 20(1):141-54, 1993.
56. Navarra T: Enabling behavior: the tender trap, *Am J Nurs* 95(1):50-52, 1995.
57. Nelson DE et al: Trends in cigarette smoking among US adolescents, 1974 through 1991, *Am J Public Health,* 85:35-40, 1995.
58. Parker DR et al: High-density-lipoprotein cholesterol and types of alcohol beverages consumed among men and women, *Am J Pub Health* 86(7):1102-1127, 1996.
59. Perrine M et al: Epidemiological perspectives on drunk driving. In *Surgeon General's workshop of drunk driving: background papers,* Washington, DC, 1989, US Department of Health and Human Services.
60. Randin D et al: Suppression of alcohol-induced hypertension by dexamethasone, *N Engl J Med* 332(26):1733-1737, 1995.
61. Saitz R et al: Individualized treatment for alcohol withdrawal: a randomized double-blind controlled trial, *JAMA* 272(7):519-523, 1994.
62. Seale JP, Muramato ML: Substance abuse among minority populations, *Primary Care Clinicians Office Pract* 20(1):167-180, 1993.
63. Shaird R, Meggs WJ, Lewin NA: PCP Ingestion, *Emer Med Serv* 22(11):32-34; 36; 38-39, 1993.
64. Shaner A et al: Disability income, cocaine use, and repeated hospitalization among schizophrenic cocaine abusers, *N Engl J Med* 333(12): 777-783, 1995.
65. Slade J et al: Nicotine and addiction: the Brown and Williamson documents, *JAMA* 264(3):225-233, 1995.
66. Sommers M: Alcohol intoxication and multiple trauma: a catastrophic combination, *Med Surg Nurs Q* 1(1):110-121, 1992.
67. Stewart C. Research update: part 1: psychological characteristics of substance abusing nurses, *J Addiction Nurs* 7(4):111-116, 1995.
68. Sullivan EV et al: Alcohol and the cerebellum: effects on balance, motor coordination, and cognition, *Alcohol Health Res World* 19:142-147, 1995.
69. Tanner S: Steroids: a breakfast of young champions, *Orthop Nurse* 14(6):26-30, 1995.
70. Toews DW: A community needle/syringe disposal program, *Am J Public Health* 85(10):1447-1448, 1995.
71. Tonigan JS, Shiller-Sturmhofel S: Alcoholics Anonymous: who benefits? *Alcohol Health Res World* 18:308-310, 1994.
72. Torkelson DJ, Anderson RA, McDaniel RR: Interventions in response to chemically dependent nurses: effect of context and interpretation, *Res Nurs Health* 19:153-162, 1996.
73. US Department of Health and Human Services, Public Health Service: *Healthy people 2000: national health promotion and disease prevention objectives,* Washington, DC, 1990, US Government Printing Office.

74. Volpicelli JR et al: Naltrexone and the treatment of alcohol dependence, *Alcohol Health Res World* 18(4):272-278, 1994.
75. Wechsler H et al: Health and behavioral consequences of binge drinking in college, JAMA 272:1672-1677, 1994.
76. Weisner C, Greenfield T, Room R: Trends in the treatment of alcohol problems in the US general population, *Am J Public Health* 85(1):55-60, 1995.
77. Wesson DR, Ling W: Addiction medicine, *JAMA* 275(33):1792-1793, 1996.
78. Yates JG: Are you losing yourself in codependency? *Am J Nurs* 94(4):32-36, 1995.
79. Young ME et al: Alcohol and marijuana use in a community based sample of persons with spinal cord injury, *Arch Phys Med Rehabil* 76(6):525-532, 1995.
80. Zabaleta I et al: Maternal use of cocaine, methadone, heroin, and alcohol: comparison of neonatal effects, *Neonatal Intensive Care* 8(3): 40-43, 1995.

# chapter 15 Fluid and Electrolyte Imbalance

JANET M. BRIGGS and CAROLE A. DRABEK

## objectives

*After studying this chapter, the learner should be able to:*

1. Describe the mechanisms for maintaining fluid and electrolyte balance.
2. Compare the mechanisms and effects of fluid deficit and excess.
3. Discuss the mechanisms and effects of deficits and excesses of sodium, potassium, calcium, and magnesium.
4. Relate data indicating fluid and electrolyte imbalances.
5. Formulate a nursing care plan for a patient with a fluid and electrolyte imbalance.

## INTRODUCTION

Body fluid is divided into two major compartments. The first, cellular fluid, comprises fluid contained within the billions of body cells and accounts for approximately three fourths of total body fluid. The intracellular fluid is encased within the second compartment of fluid, the extracellular fluid. In the nineteenth century, a French physiologist, Claude Bernard, limited though he was by the technology of his time, understood that the human body functioned through a myriad of chemical balances between and among its cells. It was he who first envisioned the two types of body fluid as separate entities. He designated the intracellular fluid as the environment of life, and the extra cellular fluid as the *milieu interieur.*

Through subsequent discoveries it was postulated that human cellular fluid may have had its origins in the simple single-celled creatures of the pre-Cambrian era. The ocean water that surrounded those first microorganisms contained all that was necessary to sustain life. There was a constant exchange of nutrients, salts, and dissolved gasses between the microorganism and its watery environment. The composition of human cellular fluid bears a striking resemblance to the composition of the pre-Cambrian sea. Over the course of millennia, the single-celled organisms joined, forming metazoa. More millennia, and the multicelled creatures developed the ability to encase and circulate the sea water around their cells. Finally, multicelled creatures arose from the sea, having developed the ability to take it within them.[15]

This chapter presents an overview of normal fluid and electrolyte balance. The prevention, causes, assessment, and nursing management of the more commonly encountered fluid and electrolyte imbalances are reviewed. Each imbalance is discussed separately, although in most instances a disturbance in the balance of one is accompanied by a resultant disturbance in one or several of the others. Nursing interventions are listed where applicable throughout the text, but are reviewed in more detail in the Nursing Management section.

Fluid and electrolyte balance are fundamental to the process of life. In the presence of a severe imbalance, the most perfectly conditioned heart cannot beat; neurons either cannot transmit at all or fire uncontrollably; digestion cannot take place; skeletal muscle cannot contract. At the cellular level, operations and exchanges that are primary to the life of the cell cannot take place. In acknowledging the elemental impact fluid and electrolyte balance has on life itself, nurses carry out the following functions:

1. Identify situations likely to cause imbalances, and implement the interventions necessary to prevent or limit them.
2. Recognize signs and symptoms of fluid and electrolyte disturbances, and identify measures necessary to alleviate them.
3. Implement preventive and therapeutic measures prescribed by the physician, and monitor the patient's response to these measures.

## ETIOLOGY

Fluid and electrolyte imbalances are common problems of patients in virtually all clinical settings. Physiological homeostasis is closely related to fluid and electrolyte balance, and alterations in fluid balance usually are accompanied by electrolyte abnormalities. Any disease process can potentially affect the fluid and electrolyte balance. The causes of deficits or excesses are varied and are discussed separately in each section.

## PHYSIOLOGY: MAINTENANCE OF FLUID AND ELECTROLYTE BALANCE

This section briefly reviews basic principles from chemistry and physiology used in homeostasis. Major electrolytes are presented, but the pathophysiological states that result from their imbalance are more thoroughly dealt with in subsequent sections.

## BODY FLUID AND ELECTROLYTE COMPARTMENTS, DISTRIBUTION, AND FUNCTION

Fluid and electrolytes are found within the body either in the cell (intracellular) or outside the cell (extracellular). The *extracellular fluid (ECF)* is contained in two compartments: the *interstitial fluid* (fluid between the cells) and *intravascular fluid* (fluid in the blood vessels). A third type of fluid, *transcellular fluid,* denotes fluid separated by a layer of epithelial cells from other ECF.[13] Transcellular fluid includes digestive juices; water and solutes in the renal tubules and bladder; intraocular fluid; and cerebrospinal fluid. Some authorities consider this to be a part of the extracellular compartment, and others consider it a separate compartment. Transcellular fluid makes up 1% to 3% of body weight. Water is the largest single constituent of the body, representing 45% to 75% of body weight. The volume and distribution of body water vary with age and gender (Figure 15-1). In the newborn, almost three fourths of the body weight is water, with the greatest percentage found in the extracellular compartment. The volume and distribution change over time. In the young adult man, 60% of the body weight is water, with two thirds of this being in the intracellular compartment. In the average young woman, approximately 50% of body weight is water. The difference between men and women is caused by the increased amount of fat in women. Fat is essentially water-free.

Body water has multiple functions. Intracellular fluid (ICF) provides the internal aqueous medium for cellular chemical function. The extracellular water maintains blood volume and serves as the body's transport system to and from cells. Body water cushions and lubricates, helps give the body its structure, hydrolyzes food in the digestive system, and acts as a reactant and medium for the chemical reactions that occur within the cell. Adequate body water balance is necessary for (1) the maintenance of normal body temperature, which is achieved by distributing heat and by cooling the body via evaporation from the skin, (2) the elimination of waste products, and (3) all transportation within the body.

Electrolytes are chemical compounds that develop an ionic charge when dissolved in water. The most prominent of these are the positively charged ions *(cations)*—hydrogen, sodium, potassium, and calcium—and the negatively charged ions *(anions)*—chloride, bicarbonate, sulfate, and phosphate. The precise concentrations of the electrolytes are vital to body functions that require particular ions or pH. Electrolytes also serve to maintain fluid osmolarity and volume within the intra and extracellular compartments.[20] All body fluids contain electrolytes (Table 15-1).

Nurses practicing in acute and critical care areas handle solutions containing multiple electrolytes. These solutions can be as diverse as dialysate and hyperalimentation solution. Although the concentration of these solutions will be calculated by teams of medical, nursing, and pharmacy specialists, it is useful for nurses who are handling these solutions to have a general understanding of the systems of measurements used.

Understanding the millimole (mM) measurement enables one to equate the milliequivalent (mEq) values among the electrolytes. The atomic or molecular weight of the element or compound in milligrams is divided by the *valence* (the numerical measure of the combining power for one atom of a chemical element). Valence also reflects the number of hydrogen atoms that can be held in combination or displaced in a reaction by one atom of an element. If a substance is *univalent* (e.g., chloride) 1 mM equals 1mEq. If a substance is *bivalent* (e.g., calcium), 1 mM equals 2 mEq. Hence, 2 mM (2 mEq) of a univalent substance reacts chemically with only 1 mM of a bivalent substance. Box 15-1 gives the formulas for these conversions.

Transcellular fluids have very distinct patterns of electrolyte concentrations. For example, gastric secretions have a high hydrogen ion concentration, pancreatic secretions have

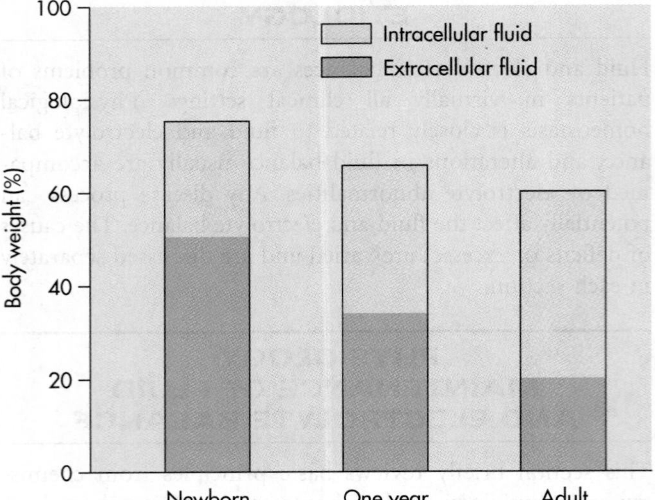


**fig. 15-1** In the newborn infant more than half of total body fluid is extracellular. As the child grows, proportions gradually approximate adult levels.

**table 15-1** *Normal Electrolyte Content of Body Fluids**

| Electrolytes (Anions and Cations) | Extracellular: Intravascular (mEq/L) | Extracellular: Interstitial (mEq/L) | Intracellular (mEq/L) |
|---|---|---|---|
| Sodium ($Na^+$) | 142 | 146 | 15 |
| Potassium ($K^+$) | 5 | 5 | 150 |
| Calcium ($Ca^{++}$) | 5 | 3 | 2 |
| Magnesium ($Mg^{++}$) | 2 | 1 | 27 |
| Chloride ($Cl^-$) | 102 | 114 | 1 |
| Bicarbonate ($HCO_3^-$) | 27 | 30 | 10 |
| Protein ($Prot^-$) | 16 | 1 | 63 |
| Phosphate ($HPO_4^=$) | 2 | 2 | 100 |
| Sulfate ($SO_4^=$) | 1 | 1 | 20 |
| Organic acids | 5 | 8 | 0 |

*Note that the electrolyte level of the intravascular and interstitial fluids (ECFs) is approximately the same and that sodium and chloride contents are markedly higher in these fluids, whereas potassium, phosphate, and protein contents are markedly higher in ICF.

a high bicarbonate concentration, and renal tubular and bladder fluids vary daily. Gastric, pancreatic, and intestinal juices and bile all contain high concentrations of sodium. Although the concentration of electrolytes varies, electrical neutrality is maintained in all fluid compartments; that is, the solution contains equal quantities in terms of chemical activity (milliequivalents per liter) of anions and cations. This concept will assume greater importance later in the chapter when the laboratory measurement of anion gap is discussed.

Each electrolyte has specific functions. The general functions of all electrolytes are to (1) promote neuromuscular irritability, (2) maintain body fluid volume and osmolarity, (3) distribute body water between fluid compartments, and (4) regulate acid-base balance.

In addition to milliequivalent values, the concentration of electrolytes in solution is also taken into consideration. The terms osmolality and osmolarity are used to discuss this concept. Technically, the terms osmolality and osmolarity mean slightly different things. *Osmolality* refers to 1 g mole (or osmole) of solute in 1000 g (or 1 kg) of distilled water. As a result, the total volume will be 1 L of water plus the relatively small volume occupied by the solutes. *Osmolarity* is most accurately used when referring to the concentration of particles in 1000 ml of solution or osmoles per liter of solution. Thus, osmolality is measured in milliosmoles per kilogram of water and osmolarity is measured in milliosmoles per liter.[19] In the clinical setting, the concentrations dealt with are much smaller so osmolality or osmolarity is reported in milliosmoles (thousandth of an osmole) and is written as mOsm/kg of solvent (water, serum, or plasma).[16] The difference in the terms osmolality and osmolarity is of practical interest to a research chemist who may be using electrolytes dissolved in different types of solutions. In clinical practice, the difference in these terms is negligible because of the low solute concentrations in the body fluids, all of which are basically water. Throughout this chapter the term *osmolarity* will be used.

The significance of plasma osmolarity is that it is the main regulator of the release of antidiuretic hormone (ADH). In the state of dehydration osmolarity will rise, stimulating the release of ADH, which signals the kidneys to conserve water and produce concentrated urine.

Measuring plasma and urine osmolarity is useful in several circumstances. Plasma osmolarity averages 290 ± 5 mOsm/kg and is relatively constant from day to day. Symptoms due to increased osmolarity usually occur at levels greater than 350 mOsm. Coma occurs at approximately 400 mOsm or greater. An osmolar gap exists when the measured and calculated (or expected) values differ by more than 15 mOsm/kg. This signifies the presence of substances in the plasma or urine that are not normally found in homeostasis (i.e., toxins or poisons).

**box 15-1** *Formulas for Calculating Milliequivalent Quantity of an Ion and of a Salt from Weight (in Milligrams) and Conversion Between Milliequivalents per Liter and Milligrams per 100 Milliliters*

**CALCULATION OF MILLIEQUIVALENT QUANTITY OF AN ION**

$$\text{mEq} = \frac{\text{Atomic weight of ion}}{\text{Valence}}$$

**CALCULATION OF MILLIEQUIVALENT QUANTITY OF A SALT FROM WEIGHT IN MILLIGRAMS**

$$\text{mEq} = \frac{\text{Weight in milligrams}}{\text{Atomic weight}} \times \text{Valence}$$

Example: 0.5 g of NaCl = 500 mg; molecular weight of NaCl = 23 (atomic weight of $Na^+$) + 35.5 (atomic weight of $Cl^-$) = 58.5; valence = 1

$$\text{Thus } \frac{500}{58.5} \times 1 = 8.5\text{, or 500 mg of NaCl}$$

$$= 8.5 \text{ mEq of NaCl}$$

**CONVERSION OF MILLIEQUIVALENTS PER LITER TO MILLIGRAMS PER 100 ML**

$$\text{mg/100 ml} = \frac{\text{mEq/L} \times \text{Atomic weight}}{10 \times \text{Valence}}$$

**CONVERSION OF MILLIGRAMS PER 100 ML TO MILLIEQUIVALENTS PER LITER**

$$\text{mEq/L} = \frac{\text{mg/100 ml} \times 10 \times \text{Valence}}{\text{Atomic weight}}$$

## NORMAL EXCHANGE OF FLUID AND ELECTROLYTES

In the healthy human being, body fluids (water and electrolytes) are constantly being lost and replaced. The fluid that is lost is not pure water but contains some electrolytes; thus both water and electrolytes must be replaced daily. Knowing the approximate concentrations of fluid and electrolytes in the various compartments enables the nurse to anticipate which imbalance will occur with abnormal losses from any particular site.

In homeostasis body fluids are lost daily from the kidneys, lungs, gastrointestinal tract, and skin. Negligible amounts are also lost in saliva and tears. Two processes demand continual expenditure of water: control of body heat and excretion of metabolic waste products. The volume of fluids used in these processes depends on factors such as external temperature, humidity, metabolic rate, and physical activity. In normal fluid balance, output equals intake. A balanced diet provides excess amounts of electrolytes, which are excreted. The result is that balance is maintained. This balance is regulated primarily by the function of the kidney tubules.

Table 15-2 summarizes the normal routes of gains and losses of fluid in an adult consuming approximately 2500 calories/day. Note that approximately two fifths of the normal fluid intake is obtained from water in food, or "preformed water." Solid foods such as meat and vegetables are 60% to 90% water. The fact that a large quantity of water is obtained from food has important implications if a person's food intake decreases substantially.

**table 15-2** *Normal Fluid Intake and Loss in an Adult Consuming 2500 Calories per Day (Approximate Figures)*

| Intake | | Output | |
|---|---|---|---|
| Route | Amount of Gain (ml) | Route | Amount of Loss (ml) |
| Water in food | 1000 | Skin | 500 |
| Water from oxidation | 300 | Lungs | 350 |
| Water as liquid | 1200 | Feces | 150 |
| | | Kidneys | 1500 |
| TOTAL | 2500 | TOTAL | 2500 |

The insensible route (skin, lungs, and gastrointestinal tract) accounts for approximately two fifths of fluid lost daily. These losses are not perceptible. Insensible loss through the skin refers to invisible perspiration, not visible sweat. When visible perspiration occurs, the loss of water through the skin is greater than the normal 500 ml/day. Fecal loss is proportionately larger in the presence of diarrheal or loose stools. Certain pulmonary conditions cause a loss greater than the normal 350 ml/day from the lungs. It is important to note that increased fluid loss through the insensible routes also results in the loss of electrolytes.

## INTERNAL REGULATION OF BODY WATER AND ELECTROLYTES

The human body uses a number of remarkable operations to closely regulate both the volume and composition of body fluids. Fluid and electrolyte balance depends on an adequate intake and output. This means that the intake must equal the output.

The control of intake and output is regulated by various internal mechanisms. In this section the regulation of body water and major electrolytes is summarized. See standard physiology texts for a more in-depth review.

### Thirst

The major control of fluid intake is thirst. The thirst center is located in the ventromedial nucleus of the hypothalamus. Impulses from this center can stimulate the cerebral cortex, which interprets this stimulation as the perception of thirst. The thirst center itself is stimulated by hypertonic body fluid, isoosmotic contraction, decreased blood pressure, decreased cardiac output, dryness of the mouth, and angiotensin. How these factors generate the stimulus to the thirst center is not fully understood. The dehydration of cells in the thirst center is thought to stimulate the neurons, which transmit an impulse to the cerebral cortex, which in turn translates the sensation to that of thirst. Most of the time thirst is not consciously thought of as a control of water intake. Social and cultural habits exert an important influence on the quantity and type of liquid that human beings drink. This may be an important consideration in some plans of care. Some evidence suggests that human beings also have a salt appetite. This may be important during periods of extreme sodium depletion, such as with prolonged heat exposure and perspiration.

### Sodium

Sodium, the most abundant extracellular cation, influences the degree of water retention and is an important participant in the control of acid-base balance. Deficiency may result in neuromuscular dysfunction. Excess may result in hypertension. Ingestion and excretion control the total volume of plasma sodium, while the degree of its dilution in water determines the concentration, or osmolarity, of plasma sodium. Factors affecting the volume and osmolarity of plasma sodium include (1) ingestion of sodium, (2) excretion of sodium, (3) antidiuretic hormone (ADH), (4) aldosterone-renin-angiotensin system, and (5) atrial natriuretic peptide (ANP).[14]

### Kidney

The major organ controlling extracellular fluid and electrolyte balance is the kidney. In addition to its commonly portrayed function as the organ of excretion of some metabolites and drugs, the kidney plays a powerful role in maintaining a vital balance of substances such as sodium, potassium, bicarbonate, chloride, $H^+$, glucose, and others. When the kidney properly regulates the balance of water and ions, homeostasis is achieved. This is accomplished through filtration, reabsorption, secretion, and synthesis.

Filtration occurs through the glomerular membrane. This membrane contains three layers: the capillary endothelium, the inner wall of Bowman's capsule, and the basement membrane. By design, the outer and inner layers of the glomerular membrane leak. The cells do not adhere to each other and have spaces between them to permit the passage of small molecules. The larger molecules, particularly proteins, are constrained by these small spaces. The large negatively charged molecules have more difficulty passing through the basement membrane due to the ionic charge relationships within the membrane itself.[9]

Glomerular filtration in the kidney is an involved topic (see Chapter 43). Three factors determine glomerular filtration: glomerular capillary blood pressure, the hydrostatic pressure of Bowman's capsule, and plasma protein concentration. Many factors and pathophysiological states can affect these three factors and thus change glomerular filtration. Conditions such as shock and hypertension change glomerular capillary blood pressure. Changes in the pressure of Bowman's capsule can be caused by urinary obstruction. A decrease in plasma protein concentration can occur with increased loss, decreased intake, or decreased production of proteins. Damage to the basement membrane of the capsule, as with glomerular nephritis, will decrease filtration from the glomeruli.

Within the renal lumen, the dynamics of reabsorption and excretion are driven by molecular polarity. Nonpolar molecules are reabsorbed more easily than polar ones and can be affected by introducing drugs that specifically block transport through the tubular epithelium. An example of these is the thiazide diuretics, which block the reabsorption of sodium in the distal tubule. Because the sodium is then excreted, for osmotic

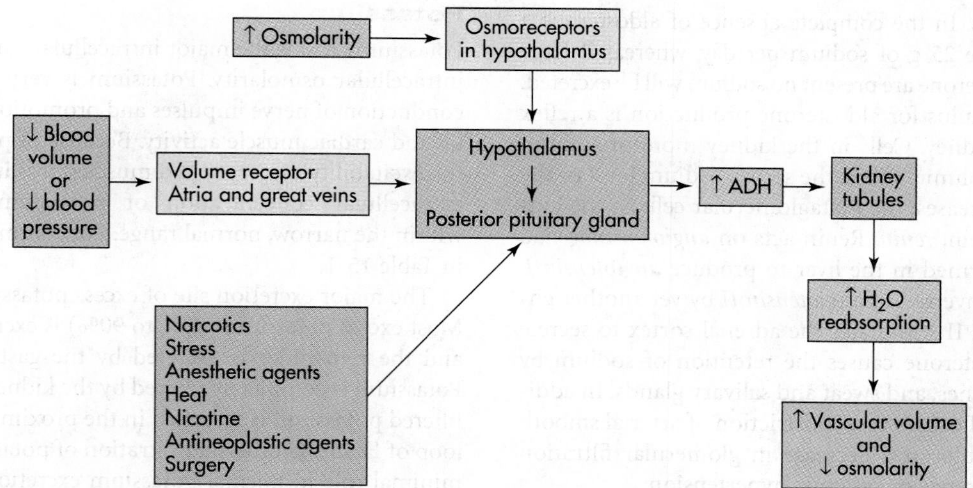


**fig. 15-2** Factors and mechanisms involved in antidiuretic hormone (ADH) production and effect of ADH.

reasons water follows. There is a subsequent volume loss in extracellular fluid. Reabsorption of sodium in the renal tubule involves active transport throughout its length. This is not true of other organic molecules, which depend on carrier proteins that are specific to certain areas of the tubule.

Molecules that do not filter through the glomerulus pass into the efferent renal arteriole to the peritubular capillaries, where they are secreted into the tubular lumen. Some molecules are neither filtered nor secreted significantly (albumin). However, some are both filtered and secreted (potassium). Finally, the kidney synthesizes certain molecules that affect osmolarity and acid-base balance, such as glucose and bicarbonate.[9]

## Antidiuretic Hormone

ADH is a hormone produced by the supraoptic and paraventricular nuclei of the hypothalamus and released from the posterior pituitary gland. The neurons in the hypothalamus receive input from volume receptors in the left atrium and great veins and from osmoreceptors in the hypothalamus. Volume receptors are stimulated by changes in atrial blood volume or blood pressure. Impulses from the volume receptors are transmitted by afferent nerve fibers to the hypothalamus. Increased blood volume or blood pressure augments the firing of the volume receptors, stimulates the hypothalamus, and inhibits ADH production. Conversely, decreased blood volume or blood pressure dampens the firing of the volume receptors and stimulates the production of ADH.

Osmoreceptors are stimulated by changes in cell size. The addition of water to the body fluids increases the size of the cells in the osmoreceptor and leads to the stimulation of ADH production. A loss of water causes the cells to shrink and stimulates the secretion of ADH. Angiotensin, narcotics, stress, heat, nicotine, antineoplastic agents, and anesthetic agents also stimulate the secretion of ADH. Figure 15-2 depicts the factors and mechanisms involved and the results of ADH production.

ADH acts on the kidney cells by stimulating 3′,5′-cyclic adenosine monophosphate (AMP) release, which regulates cellular metabolism. In the kidney, ADH causes increased water reabsorption in the distal convoluted tubules and collecting ducts. Additionally, it stimulates the sodium pump in the loop of Henle and regulates the rate of blood perfusion, both of which lead to water reabsorption. Under the influence of ADH, the kidney can concentrate urine to 1200 mOsm/kg $H_2O$. The conservation of water increases blood volume and pressure and decreases osmolarity. Because ADH can be secreted in response to factors other than a deficit of water (narcotics, anesthetic agents, and stressors), fluid overload can occur.

Inappropriate ADH secretion can be a life-threatening event. This condition is known as the *syndrome of inappropriate secretion of ADH (SIADH)*. The features of this phenomenon are plasma hyponatremia and hypotonicity. Simultaneously, the urine is itself hypertonic and contains appreciable amounts of sodium. In this syndrome there is an absence of hypokalemia and edema. Cardiac, renal, and adrenal functions are normal. Despite the increased urine output there is no evidence of dehydration or hypovolemia. The presence of low serum blood urea nitrogen and uric acid levels assists in confirming the diagnosis. The secretion of ADH is "inappropriate" in that it continues despite the decreased osmolarity of the plasma. The serum sodium concentration and serum osmolarity are the most easily available indices of this process. The treatment consists of restriction of fluid intake and, when applicable, therapy for the underlying disorders (e.g., administration of cortisone for Addison's disease or discontinuation of causative medications). Administration of salt (sodium chloride solutions) is usually of transient benefit, but is useful in patients in whom water intoxication is severe.[14]

## Aldosterone-Renin-Angiotensin System

Aldosterone is a hormone produced by the zona glomerulosa of the adrenal cortex. It increases the kidney's reabsorption of sodium and thus water in the proximal tubules and the distal convoluted tubules. In the complete absence of aldosterone a person may excrete 25 g of sodium per day, whereas if large quantities of aldosterone are present no sodium will be excreted.

The major stimulus for aldosterone production is a reflex initiated by the kidney. Cells in the kidney monitor sodium levels and blood volume. When the serum sodium level or the blood volume decreases, the juxtaglomerular cells in the kidney secrete a protein, *renin.* Renin acts on *angiotensinogen,* a plasma protein formed in the liver to produce *angiotensin I.* This, in turn is converted to *angiotensin II* by yet another enzyme. Angiotensin II stimulates the adrenal cortex to secrete aldosterone. Aldosterone causes the retention of sodium by the kidneys, intestines, and sweat and salivary glands. In addition, angiotensin II causes vasoconstriction of arterial smooth muscle, which results in a decrease in glomerular filtration rate and the occurrence of systemic hypertension.

Some aldosterone may be secreted in response to adrenocorticotropic hormone (ACTH). Sodium and water retention may be precipitated by liver failure because aldosterone is catabolized by a normally functioning liver. Figure 15-3 depicts the factors and mechanisms involved as well as the effects of aldosterone production.

### Atrial Natriuretic Peptide

ANP, also called atrial natriuretic factor, is a hormone produced from specialized cells in the atrial muscle of the heart.[22] This substance is a 28-amino acid peptide released in response to stretching during periods of volume overload, such as congestive heart failure, renal failure, hypertension, and certain dysrhythmias. ANP may also be secreted in direct response to a number of vasopressor substances, including vasopressin and epinephrine.[8] The main effects of ANP are direct arterial vasodilation, increased glomerular filtration rate, and diuresis (due to the increased renal blood flow).[23] It is speculated that ANP may be the primary counteractant of the plasma renin-angiotensin-aldosterone system.[10]

### Potassium

Potassium ($K^+$) is the major intracellular cation and regulates intracellular osmolarity. Potassium is very important in the conduction of nerve impulses and promotion of proper skeletal and cardiac muscle activity. Because of potassium's role in the excitability of nerves and muscles, it is important that the extracellular concentration of potassium be maintained within the narrow, normal range. Potassium values are shown in Table 15-1.

The major excretion site of excess potassium is the kidney. Most excess potassium (80% to 90%) is excreted in the urine, and the remainder is excreted by the gastrointestinal tract. Potassium is completely filtered by the kidney, but most of the filtered potassium is resorbed in the proximal tubules and the loop of Henle. Glomerular filtration of potassium plays only a minimal role in normal potassium excretion. The control of renal excretion of potassium resides in the ability of the distal tubular cells to secrete potassium into tubular fluid. As extracellular potassium levels rise, more potassium moves into all cells, including the distal tubular cells. The higher concentration in the cells facilitates potassium secretion into tubular fluid because of the gradient difference between the distal tubular cells and the fluid in the tubular lumen. Conversely, if potassium intake is low or if more potassium is lost through the gastrointestinal tract, the potassium level in the distal tubules is decreased. This causes a decrease in the gradient, and less potassium is secreted.

Even though glomerular filtration plays only a minimal role in the amount of potassium excreted in the urine, it is an important point to remember. Certain situations interfere with the resorption of the filtered potassium in the proximal tubules, and this can lead to an increased loss of potassium. Osmotic diuretics and disease states that produce osmotic diuresis interfere with the reabsorption of potassium. Tubular diuretics, such as hydrochlorothiazide and furosemide, also enhance the loss of potassium.

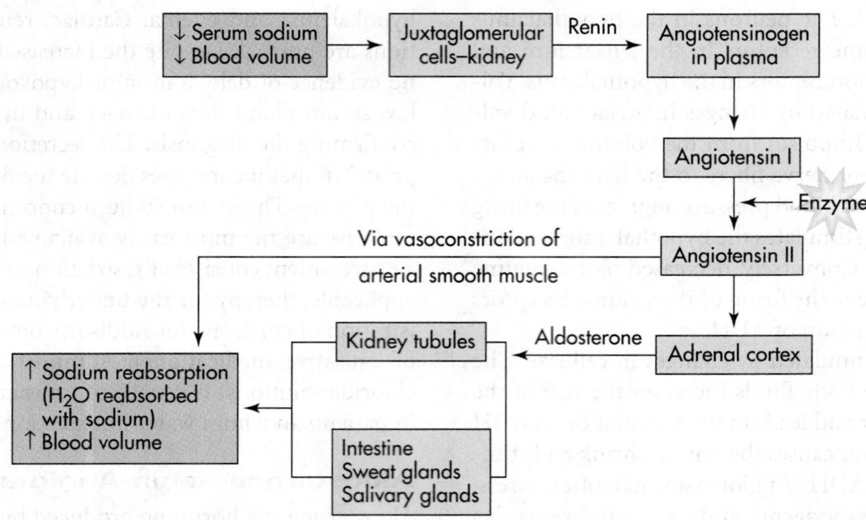


**fig. 15-3** Factors and mechanisms involved in aldosterone production and effects of aldosterone production.

Aldosterone can increase the amount of potassium secreted by the distal tubules. The aldosterone-secreting cells of the adrenal cortex are sensitive to the extracellular concentration of potassium. If the extracellular concentration of potassium increases, aldosterone is secreted and stimulates the distal tubular cells to secrete more potassium. The renin-angiotensin system is not involved in this stimulation of aldosterone.

Electrolyte levels themselves can affect potassium balance. Hydrogen ion concentration is the most common example. The existence of a low hydrogen ion concentration increases potassium excretion and leads to systemic depletion (hypokalemia). Conversely, a high hydrogen concentration (acidosis) decreases potassium excretion and leads to systemic excess (hyperkalemia).

## Calcium

### Factors affecting distribution

Calcium ($Ca^{++}$) plays a major role in the promotion of neuromuscular irritability and muscular contractions. Calcium and phosphorus are found primarily in the bones and teeth (99%), with a very small amount dissolved in the blood (1%). The amounts of dissolved calcium and phosphorus are in inverse relationship. As one increases, the other decreases. This inverse relationship must be maintained; if both are elevated at the same time, they form an insoluble precipitate. The dissolved portion of calcium is carried in the blood in two forms: bound to protein, particularly albumin; and ionized. The serum levels that usually are reported are measures of total dissolved calcium (both bound and ionized). The ionized fraction can be measured separately, but this is a more expensive test and is not routinely performed. Only the ionized fraction is involved in the promotion of neuromuscular activity.

The ionized portion must be maintained within fine limits because a decrease in ionized calcium has profound effects on the body, for example, tetany (see p. 414). In a person with normal serum protein and albumin levels and a normal calcium level, the ionized fraction is usually a little greater than 50% of the total dissolved level. Because part of the dissolved calcium is bound to protein, the concentration of serum calcium varies as the protein level varies. If the total protein and albumin levels fall, the total serum calcium level will fall. Patients with serum calcium levels below normal resulting from a decrease in protein or albumin may exhibit no symptoms of hypocalcemia because, although their total calcium level is low, the ionized fraction may still be within normal limits.

The ratio between the dissolved calcium that is bound and the ionized fraction is affected by acid-base status. Acidosis causes more calcium to be ionized, whereas alkalosis causes more of the ionized fraction to become bound. These changes are probably not detrimental to people with a normal serum calcium level. However, alkalosis in a person who already has a low serum calcium level can lead to tetany. Calcium also binds to other agents such as citrate, which normally is metabolized by the liver. Because citrate is commonly used as an anticoagulant in stored blood, patients receiving a large number of transfusions rapidly should be watched carefully for signs of hypocalcemia. Some authorities recommend that for every 3 to 4 units of blood given rapidly, the patient should receive 10 ml of calcium gluconate.[3]

### Control of calcium levels

The serum level of calcium depends on three hormones: parathyroid hormone, vitamin D, and calcitonin. *Parathyroid hormone* is a hormone produced by the parathyroid gland in response to decreased serum calcium levels. Parathyroid hormone causes increased movement of calcium from the bone, increased absorption of calcium from the gastrointestinal tract, and increased reabsorption of calcium from the renal tubules. These activities result in increased serum calcium levels. Parathyroid hormone also increases the excretion of phosphorus by the kidneys.

*Vitamin D* is a hormone that is formed by the action of sunlight on a provitamin present in the skin and can be obtained in its completed form from dietary sources. The liver and kidney hydroxylate vitamin D to its active form, which is essential for the absorption of calcium from the gastrointestinal tract. Parathyroid hormone cannot increase the absorption of calcium from the gastrointestinal tract unless activated vitamin D is present. In addition, vitamin D significantly increases the effectiveness of parathyroid hormone in bone reabsorption. The major control point for the blood concentration of vitamin D is the hydroxylation step in the kidney, which is stimulated by parathyroid hormone. The feedback mechanism begins with a low calcium level stimulating the secretion of parathyroid hormone, which then activates vitamin D; both then increase the absorption of calcium from the gastrointestinal tract and the reabsorption of calcium from the bone.

*Calcitonin,* a hormone produced by the thyroid gland, decreases calcium levels by preventing bone reabsorption of calcium. It opposes the effects of parathyroid hormone and vitamin D on bones. High calcium levels stimulate the thyroid gland to release calcitonin, which inhibits the release of calcium from the bone, thus lowering serum calcium levels.

# MOVEMENT OF FLUID BETWEEN COMPARTMENTS

The components previously discussed are not static, nor are the different compartments of fluid closed to each other. Instead, there is a constant dynamic process between compartments. Materials are carried to and waste products removed from the cells via the movement of solutes and water.

## Solute and Fluid Transport Between Extracellular and Intracellular Compartments

Fluid and electrolytes flow across cell membranes by passive or active processes. Passive transport across a membrane is called *diffusion.* Solutes move from a more concentrated solution to a less concentrated solution until both are equal. If a higher concentration of a substance exists outside the cell, it will diffuse into the cell if the cell membrane is permeable. Cell membranes are largely lipid; hence lipid-soluble molecules enter easily. Certain water-soluble molecules can diffuse into cells with the assistance of proteins in the cell membrane by the process of *facilitated diffusion.*[20]

Some electrolytes and other solutes flow from lower to greater concentrations or against the concentration gradient. To accomplish this uphill feat requires the help of carrier ions and energy. The energy source is in the form of adenosine triphosphate (ATP). It has been shown that with the expenditure of one high-energy phosphate bond from ATP, three sodium ions move out of the cell, and two potassium ions move into the cell. Active transport uses a large percentage of the energy formed each day, because sodium and potassium are constantly diffusing into and out of the cell. Active transport is required to keep the proper concentrations of the two electrolytes within the cell. Water, like solutes, moves between the extracellular and intracellular compartment. The movement of water is controlled by the osmolarity of the two compartments. Sodium is the main regulator of extracellular osmolarity, while potassium is the main regulator of intracellular osmolarity.

Unaided, water or solutes move in a predictable direction from high concentration to low concentration. This movement or process is called *osmosis* and will continue until the osmolarity between the two compartments is equal. For example, if the water content increases or the solute content decreases in the extracellular compartment, water moves into the cells to equalize osmolarity. Should the reverse conditions prevail and the solute concentration increase extracellularly beyond the intracellular concentration, the flow of water will also reverse until osmolarity is equalized. Solutes also move back and forth between the two compartments, but the cell membrane is more permeable to water than it is to solutes.

The mechanisms controlling water and sodium levels also control osmolarity and thus the movement of fluid between the extracellular and intracellular compartment. Various pathological states including disease and trauma can affect osmolarity and cell membrane permeability. These in turn are the causes of cellular edema or cellular dehydration, the signs and symptoms of which shall be discussed later in the chapter.

## Fluid Transport Between Vascular and Interstitial Spaces

The control of fluid movement between the vascular and interstitial spaces is defined by Starling's law of the capillaries. Two different types of pressure influence the flow of fluid between the vascular space. These are hydrostatic pressure and colloid osmotic pressure (oncotic pressure). *Hydrostatic pressure* is the pressure caused by blood pressing against the walls of the blood vessels. Hydrostatic pressure also exists in the tissue but is minimal (5 torr or less), and some authorities believe that the hydrostatic pressure in the tissue is actually a negative pressure.[4] Hydrostatic pressure effectively pushes fluid out of the vascular bed into the interstitial space.

*Colloid osmotic pressure* is the pressure needed to overcome the pull of proteins (colloids), especially albumin, in the blood. The proteins do not pass freely through the walls of the capillaries because of their size. A few proteins are present in the interstitial space, but a much larger concentration is in the intervascular space. The colloid osmotic pressure within the vascular space serves to *pull* or *absorb* fluid from the interstitial space.

The difference between hydrostatic pressure and colloid osmotic pressure in the vascular space determines the movement of fluid between the vascular and interstitial spaces. For example, in Figure 15-4, the hydrostatic and the colloid osmotic pressures in the tissue would be zero. The hydrostatic pressure at the arteriole end of the capillary (approximately 40 torr) is greater than the hydrostatic pressure at the venule end of the capillary (approximately 10 torr). The colloid osmotic pressure stays approximately the same throughout the vascular bed and equals about 25 torr.

The difference between the hydrostatic pressure and the colloid osmotic pressure at the arteriole end of the capillary is +15 torr (40 torr − 25 torr = 15 torr) and favors the movement of fluid out of the vascular compartment. The difference between the hydrostatic pressure and the colloid osmotic pressure at the venule end of the capillary is −15 torr (10 torr − 25 torr = −15 torr) and favors the movement of fluid into the vascular compartment (Figure 15-4).

Hydrostatic pressure can be conceived of as "push," and colloid osmotic pressure as "pull." These forces are constantly opposing each other in the movement of solutions and substances. The competing forces fall into four categories. (1) *Vascular hydrostatic pressure* is the blood pressure at the capillary level, which is related to the pressure wave each time the heart contracts. (2) *Vascular colloid osmotic pressure* is the pull exerted by the plasma proteins in the blood, which normally remains fairly constant. However, if a large amount of protein leaves the capillary, vascular osmotic pressure drops, further reducing the vascular spaces' ability to retain fluid. (3) *Interstitial fluid hydrostatic pressure* is the push exerted by interstitial fluid against tissues and individual cells, especially those making up the capillary membrane. (4) *Interstitial fluid colloid osmotic pressure* is the pull exerted by the protein in the interstitial fluid.[5]

Overall, this system allows fluids high in nutrients and oxygen to diffuse out of the vascular bed at the arteriole end of the capillary and fluids containing waste products to move back into the vascular bed at the venule end of the capillaries. The system is not perfect, however, and some

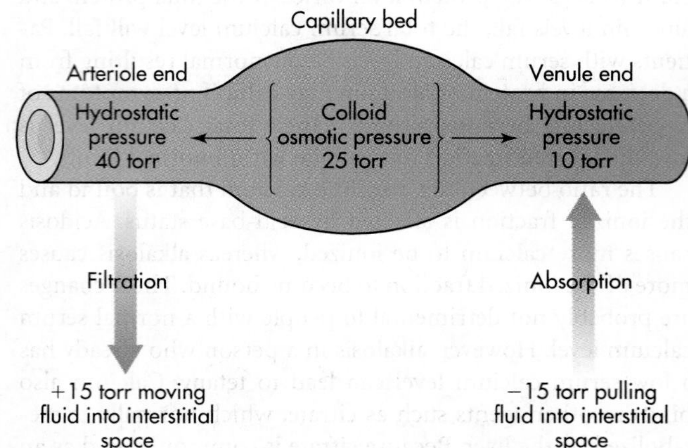


**fig. 15-4** Pressure difference across capillary provides for movement of fluid, nutrients, and waste between interstitial and vascular spaces.

fluid is left in the interstitial space. In addition, some protein may escape from the vascular bed, and if allowed to accumulate, acts as a force to pull even more fluid from the vascular space. The lymphatic system picks up the excess fluid and the escaped proteins and returns them to the vascular space.

Many factors affect hydrostatic pressure. At the arteriole end of the capillary, the hydrostatic pressure depends on the volume and viscosity of blood, force of the heartbeat, and resistance of the blood vessels. Hydrostatic pressure at the venous end depends on the venous pressure. In turn, the venous pressure depends on the structural integrity of the veins, respiration, and skeletal muscle contractions. The colloid osmotic pressure depends on the protein level. The protein level itself is dependent upon dietary intake, the liver's ability to produce proteins, and the body's ability to retain, not lose, protein. Various pathological states can interfere with any of these mechanisms and result in edema.

## FLUID IMBALANCE

Sodium is the most prevalent electrolyte in the extracellular fluid. Therefore, changes in extracellular fluid volume are often associated with alterations in sodium balance and may be described in the context of that abnormality. As a result of fluid and electrolyte imbalance, patients may experience severe, potentially life-threatening pathological changes.

When a change occurs in the sodium : water ratio, a disturbance in osmolarity results; that is, the ECF becomes hypoosmolar or hyperosmolar. When the change in ECF volume occurs with a proportionate change in extracellular solutes (particles dissolved in solution, i.e., electrolytes, urea, or glucose), the ECF remains isotonic. Loss of fluid homeostasis may occur as a result of fluid excess or deficit. The fluid disruption may be associated with hypoosmolarity or hyperosmolarity or the fluid may remain isotonic (Table 15-3).

As with all clinical problems, the same pathophysiological change is not of equal significance to all people. For instance, consider a 24-hour viral syndrome with associated nausea and diarrhea. In one individual, this may result in some extracellular volume depletion, but not significant electrolyte disturbance. On the other hand, the same viral syndrome in someone without the ability to concentrate urine (due to hormonal or renal factors) may cause severe, even life-threatening fluid and electrolyte imbalance. Therefore it is essential to evaluate each episode of real or potential fluid imbalance in the specific physiological context in which it occurs. That is, consider the patient from a holistic perspective.

### Fluid Deficit

An ECF deficit may occur as a result of (1) reduced fluid intake, (2) loss of body fluids, or (3) sequestration (compartmentalizing) of body fluids.

#### Etiology

**Decreased intake.** Anyone without fluids available to drink, who is unable to take fluids independently, or who does not respond to thirst appropriately may develop a fluid deficit. Patients who are unable to ask for fluids, identify their need for fluid, or swallow easily may develop a fluid deficit. Thus someone with a cerebrovascular accident and aphasia may be unable to communicate a desire for fluids or may have difficulty swallowing fluids that are offered. A confused or disoriented patient may be unaware of thirst. Patients who are comatose, weak, or catatonic may develop fluid deficits because of the inability to ask for fluids, swallow, or respond to thirst. People with oropharyngeal discomfort may avoid oral fluid intake in an effort to avoid worsening the pain. In a disaster such as a flood or an earthquake, a supply of potable water or fluids may be unavailable, and people may suffer dehydration as a result.

**Fluid loss.** Excessive fluid loss is very common and occurs for a variety of reasons. Most of the fluid in the gastrointestinal tract is absorbed in the small intestine and proximal colon, leaving only small amounts to be excreted with the feces. In disease states with severe diarrhea, however, liters of fluid can be lost via the gastrointestinal tract resulting in severe volume deficits in a short period of time. Other losses from the gastrointestinal tract, such as vomiting, gastrointestinal suctioning, and bleeding, may also result in significant fluid loss. Table 15-4 shows ECF volumes.

**table 15-3** *Water and Sodium Imbalances*

| Type of Imbalance | Water Imbalance | Sodium Imbalance |
|---|---|---|
| Hyperosmolar | Water ↓ in relation to sodium and other solutes | Sodium or other solutes ↑ in relation to water |
| Hyposmolar | Water ↑ in relation to sodium and other solutes | Sodium ↓ in relation to water |
| Isotonic volume excess | Water ↑ proportionally with sodium | Sodium ↑ proportionally with water |
| Isotonic volume deficit | Water ↓ proportionally with sodium | Sodium ↓ proportionally with water |

**table 15-4** *Extracellular Fluid Volume**

| | Approximate ml of Fluid (Daily) |
|---|---|
| Saliva | 1500 |
| Gastric juice | 2500 |
| Intestinal juice | 2000 |
| Pancreatic juice | 1500 |
| Bile | 500 |
| TOTAL | 8000 ml/24 hr |

*Note that approximately 8 L of fluid are used daily for digestive purposes. Normally, most of this fluid is reabsorbed. Some of each of the ions found in blood plasma is present in each of the fluids listed, but the individual concentration varies with each fluid.

Polyuria can be associated with a fluid deficit. For instance, diabetes insipidus is a clinical syndrome that results in excessive loss of urine. The etiology may be central or nephrogenic, acquired or congenital. Diabetes insipidus may occur as a result of another disease or be provoked by a variety of drugs. It is characterized by polyuria and polydipsia. If a patient with diabetes insipidus is able to maintain adequate intake, severe fluid shifts are avoided. However, anything that interferes with fluid intake quickly results in severe volume depletion.[19]

Fluid loss may be provoked by changes in the osmolarity of ECF. For example, in diabetes mellitus, large amounts of glucose can accumulate in the blood. If diabetic ketoacidosis develops, ketone bodies collect as well. In response to these increased solute levels, a hyperosmolar state occurs, which leads to an osmotic diuresis and concomitant fluid loss.[16]

There are many other problems that may result in significant fluid loss. Hyperventilation, marked perspiration, bleeding, diaphoresis, and excessive tracheostomy secretions are examples of other potential causes of fluid deficit.

**Sequestration of body fluids.** Occasionally extracellular fluid can be sequestered in areas that do not normally contain a large volume of fluid. The pleural, peritoneal, and pericardial cavities are potential spaces that generally contain only a small amount of fluid. Table 15-5 shows fluid collection in potential spaces.

In some clinical problems, one or more of these potential spaces may contain a large volume of fluid that has been lost from the vascular space.[12] This sequestration of body fluids in a potential space is called *third-spacing* and is associated with an intravascular volume deficit. Although not lost from the body, the fluid is unavailable for use. Therefore, symptoms consistent with volume deficit may develop. Eventually, when the fluid begins to return to the vascular space, symptoms of volume overload may be evident. Third-spacing may occur in the context of several clinical problems, e.g., during the postoperative period after major abdominal surgery, with pancreatitis, and with hepatic failure.[16]

### *Pathophysiology*

A fluid volume deficit may occur with sodium loss or sodium excess. When the extracellular sodium content is low, renal absorption of water is diminished in an attempt to restore normal proportions of sodium to water in the ECF. The resulting fluid deficit occurs as a result of the hypoosmolar state. Fluids lost through vomiting, diarrhea, and sweating have a high sodium content, which may precipitate hyponatremia. Diuretics (thiazides, loop, and potassium-conserving) may also contribute to sodium loss.

Fluid deficit may occur in hypernatremia as well. For example, in diabetes insipidus large amounts of urine are excreted, and the sodium content of the ECF may become more concentrated. Hyperosmotic dehydration occurs.

When an extracellular fluid deficit occurs, water moves out of the cells to replace water lost from the extracellular compartment in an attempt to maintain an adequate circulating blood volume. If the water deficit is not corrected, the cells eventually become unable to compensate for extracellular losses and cellular dehydration ensues. When cells are unable to continue providing water to replace the extracellular fluid, signs of circulatory collapse appear. As both intracellular and extracellular fluid volumes decrease, cell function is impaired due to inadequate diffusion of food, oxygen, and waste products. Because brain cells are particularly sensitive to these metabolic alterations, mental changes occur.

Thirst and weight loss are early symptoms of water deficit and become more pronounced as the deficit increases. Note that weight loss is not present with third-spacing phenomena, as fluid has not been lost from the body, just to a nonfunctional compartment. Signs of ECF depletion are listed in Box 15-2.

As a fluid deficit evolves, body temperature begins to rise, and fever may be noted. A dry mouth and throat may cause difficulty with speech. When cells are unable to continue providing water to replace the ECF losses, signs of circulatory collapse ensue: blood pressure drops, tachycardia occurs, and the respiratory rate increases. Table 15-6 shows signs and symptoms of water deficit.

### *Collaborative care management*

Nurses are instrumental in preventing fluid volume deficit. Identification of vulnerable patients is essential. Included are those with (1) a compromised mental state who may not recognize or respond appropriately to thirst; (2) physical limitations that impair the ability to obtain adequate fluids and nutrition; (3) disease states that may alter fluid and electrolyte balance; or

**table 15-5** *Fluid Collection in Potential Fluid Spaces*

| Potential Fluid Space | Location | Fluid |
|---|---|---|
| Intrapleural | Between lung and chest wall | Pleural effusion |
| Pericardial | Between heart and pericardial sac | Pericardial effusion |
| Peritoneal | Between intestines and abdominal wall | Ascites |

**box 15-2** *Signs of Extracellular Fluid Depletion*

Skin: poor turgor
Mouth: dry mucous membranes
Cardiovascular: postural hypotension (early), low blood pressure, tachycardia, increased respiration, decreased vein filling
Weight: loss
Urine: low output, increased specific gravity

(4) limited access to adequate food and fluids due to social, environmental, recreational, or occupational circumstances.

When a patient at risk for fluid and/or electrolyte imbalance is identified, a plan of care is developed. The patient and family members should be educated about the importance of adequate fluid and nutrition intake. Collaboration among the nurse, patient, family members, and other health care providers results in an on-going plan for the continued assessment and treatment of problems. An evaluation of serum electrolytes is essential for the recognition of specific problems. An accurate record of intake and output is maintained. A detailed action plan to replete fluid and restore electrolyte balance is initiated. Factors that may alter fluid and/or electrolyte states, such as certain medications (particularly diuretics), hyperventilation, fever, burns, diarrhea, and diabetes must be noted and appropriate interventions undertaken.

A fluid volume deficit may be mild to severe. People who are mildly dehydrated may notice only symptoms of increased thirst or dry mouth. On the other hand, the fluid deficit may be so profound as to be associated with circulatory collapse and eventually death. Obviously, severe fluid depletion is a clinical emergency requiring rapid but thoughtful fluid repletion, restoration of electrolyte balance, and perhaps circulatory support. While hemodynamic stability is being established, efforts are directed toward identification and treatment of the underlying cause. Once the etiology and precise nature of the deficit are established, interventions specific to the pathophysiological mechanisms can be initiated, and plans to prevent future compromise developed.

Fluid replacement needs are often calculated according to weight. Because 1 L weighs 1 kg, the amount of weight (in

**table 15-6** *Signs and Symptoms of Water Deficit*

| | Moderate Deficit | Severe Deficit |
|---|---|---|
| Skin | Flushed, dry | Cold, clammy |
| Mouth | Dry mucous membranes | Dry, cracked tongue |
| Eyes | — | Soft, sunken eyeballs |
| Cardiovascular system | — | Tachycardia, low blood pressure, rapid respirations |
| Central nervous system | Apprehension, restlessness | Lethargy, coma |
| Blood | — | Hemoconcentration, increase in hematocrit, BUN, electrolytes |
| Urine | High specific gravity, scant amount (except with osmotic diuresis) | Oliguria, concentrated urine |
| Other | Thirst, weight loss | Thirst, weight loss, fever |

kilograms) lost during the period of fluid depletion approximates the volume of water deficit. That is, if 2 kg were lost, the approximate fluid loss is 2 L. Repletion requires intake of the volume lost plus an additional 1.5 L to fulfill the current daily needs.[16] Fluid replacement may require several days of therapy to avoid the complications of rapid volume infusion such as intercompartmental fluid shifts and pulmonary edema.

Oral fluid resuscitation is preferable, but if the patient is unable to tolerate oral fluids, intravenous therapy may be ordered. The type of intravenous solution is based on the patient's fluid and electrolyte status as well as volume needs and is discussed in greater detail later in the chapter.

Vital signs should be assessed regularly. Postural (orthostatic) hypotension is common in persons with a fluid volume deficit. To assess for postural blood pressure changes, the blood pressure is taken with the patient supine. Then the patient is asked to stand, and the blood pressure is taken immediately. The blood pressure is taken again after the patient has remained standing for several minutes. A drop in the systolic blood pressure of greater than 15 mm Hg or a heart rate increase of more than 15 beats/min is consistent with intravascular volume depletion.[16] Observe the patient closely during evaluation for postural hypotension. Marked reductions in standing blood pressure can result in dizziness and, if severe, in syncope. Do not leave the patient unattended. Be prepared to quickly assist the patient to a sitting or supine position should significant symptoms occur. Daily weighing is useful to monitor fluid balance as well. Review laboratory results for serum and urine electrolytes and report abnormalities so appropriate adjustments in therapy can be initiated.

## Fluid Excess

### Etiology

Fluid excess may occur as a result of (1) overhydration, (2) excessive sodium intake, or (3) failure of renal or hormonal regulatory functions.

### Overhydration

Polydipsia may occur in the setting of psychiatric (often psychotic) disorders, SIADH, and certain head injuries involving the hypothalamus. Under normal circumstances, the renal response to increased fluid intake causes the excretion of large volumes of urine to maintain fluid balance. However, when regulatory pathophysiological conditions, such as renal dysfunction exist, intake may substantially exceed output, and extracellular fluid overload may occur.

An iatrogenic fluid excess may occur as a result of intravenous or nasogastric fluid administration. Intravenous fluids such as 0.9% sodium chloride and lactated Ringer's solution contain significant amounts of sodium and may not be tolerated well in large volumes, particularly in compromised patients.

### Excessive sodium intake

Dietary sodium indiscretion may result in hyperosmolarity of the extracellular fluid, which promotes renal conservation of fluid. As the extracellular fluid volume expands to restore normal osmolarity, signs of extracellular volume excess develop.

### Failure of regulatory mechanisms

As mentioned earlier, excess or inappropriate secretion of ADH occurs in response to stressors, drugs, and anesthetics. SIADH may also accompany inflammatory conditions of the lung (tuberculosis, pneumonia, and abscesses) and brain (encephalitis and meningitis), endocrine disturbances, certain infections in the lungs, and some malignancies. ECF volume increases in response to the increased ADH. Other endocrine problems, such as hyperfunction of the adrenal glands and adrenal adenomas, may result in aldosterone excess. Aldosterone promotes sodium retention which, in turn, results in mild volume expansion.

### Pathophysiology

Extracellular fluid excess can be evident in a hypoosmolar or hyperosmolar milieu. Inappropriate secretion of antidiuretic hormone illustrates hypoosmolar overhydration. Initially ADH stimulates the renal tubules to absorb water. As the extracellular volume expands and the sodium remains static, the fluid becomes progressively hyponatremic. When the extracellular fluid is hypoosmolar, fluid moves into the cells to equalize the concentration on both sides of the cell membrane, resulting in cellular swelling. Because brain cells are particularly sensitive to the increase in intracellular water, the most common signs of hypoosmolar overhydration are changes in mental status. Confusion, ataxia, and convulsions may also occur (Box 15-3).

In hypernatremic states, as may occur with increased sodium intake, increased aldosterone secretion, or Cushing's syndrome (see Chapter 34), extra body water is retained in an attempt to restore a normal proportion of extracellular fluid and sodium. The fluid volume excess occurs in response to a hyperosmolar state.

Fluid volume excess is associated with a weight gain that may develop over a short period of time, e.g., several pounds in a 24-hour period. Peripheral edema may occur, particularly in hyperosmolar overhydration. Signs of circulatory overload include neck vein distention, crackles in the lungs, and bounding pulse. If fluid excess is severe or cardiac function is compromised, pulmonary edema and respiratory failure can occur. Assessment techniques are covered in greater detail later in this chapter.

**box 15-3** *Signs of Overhydration*

- Changes in behavior: confusion, incoordination, convulsions
- Hyperventilation
- Sudden weight gain
- Warm, moist skin
- Increased intracranial pressure: slow bounding pulse with an increase in systolic and decrease in diastolic blood pressures
- Peripheral edema, usually not marked

### Collaborative care management

The goals of treatment are to restore normal fluid balance, provide symptomatic care until homeostasis is achieved, and prevent future fluid volume excess. Identification of patients vulnerable to fluid overload is essential. Patients with altered renal, cardiac, hypothalamic, and adrenal function are at risk for fluid imbalance.

Pharmacological therapy includes the administration of diuretics, as long as renal failure is not the cause of the excess fluid. Osmotic diuretics are used initially to prevent electrolyte imbalances. If these are not effective, loop diuretics (furosemide) are prescribed. Accurate monitoring of intake and output, weight, and electrolytes are important nursing responsibilities.

Patients on a low-sodium diet need to know foods to avoid. Education is imperative if sodium restriction is indicated. Long-term dietary modifications may be necessary to control fluid volume. Many processed foods contain large amounts of sodium; patients should be taught to read product labeling so high-sodium foods can be avoided. Patients and family members should be educated about food preparation techniques and seasoning options that minimize sodium use. Assistance with meal planning may be necessary. Sometimes it is necessary to limit fluid intake to avoid overhydration. This may be particularly difficult in the setting of psychogenic polydipsia.

As with fluid deficits, fluid volume excess ranges from mild to severe. Mild volume overload may be associated with transient polyuria. On the other hand, severe volume overload, particularly in persons with compromised renal or cardiac function, may be associated with pulmonary edema, a potentially life-threatening emergency. Once again, if the patient's condition is stable, the primary goal of therapy is identification of the etiology of fluid imbalance and institution of the appropriate therapy.

Excess fluid in the tissues results in poor cellular nutrition as cells are pushed farther apart and away from capillaries. Normal exchange of nutrients and wastes is interrupted. Edematous tissues are therefore poorly nourished, susceptible to trauma and infection, and heal poorly. Caution must be taken to protect edematous parts of the body from prolonged pressure, injury, and temperature extremes. Skin over these parts should be kept well lubricated to prevent dryness. If edematous areas are exposed to extensive moisture from incontinence or perspiration, they should be cleansed and dried frequently to prevent maceration.

## Edema

*Edema* is a collection of excess fluid in body tissue. Usually, edema is extracellular, but it may be intracellular as well. Although edematous states may exist in the setting of overhydration, edema is *not the same* as overhydration. The distinction is important. Do not assume that edema indicates fluid volume overload. Whenever edema is noted, the nurse assesses the patient for potential etiologies such as inflammation, vascular impairment, tissue injury, and volume excess.

### Etiology

**Intracellular edema.** Cellular membrane permeability may be altered when the cell is severely deprived of nutrients or when cell metabolism is so profoundly altered that normal movement of electrolytes across the cell membranes fails. Thus intracellular edema may occur as a result of reduced tissue metabolism and severely impaired cellular nutrition.

When impaired tissue blood flow deprives cells of nutrition, the transmembrane electrolyte movement that maintains intracellular osmotic neutrality becomes dysfunctional. Normally, sodium ions leak into the intracellular space and are removed by active transport mechanisms. In patients with severe cellular malnutrition, ionic pump integrity is compromised, and the sodium cannot be removed from the cell. The relative hypertonicity of the intracellular space results in the osmotic intrusion of water and causes cellular swelling.[12] This usually heralds tissue death and may be seen in severe peripheral vascular disease or hypothermic injury.

Cellular swelling may also develop as a result of the enhanced cellular membrane permeability that occurs in inflammation. Sodium and other ions leak into the cell interior and osmotically attract fluid, resulting in cellular edema. Intracellular edema is part of the complex response to endotoxins seen in septic shock.[12]

**Extracellular edema.** Extracellular edema is much more common than intracellular edema. The two general causes of extracellular fluid accumulation are (1) leakage of plasma fluid across a capillary membrane into an interstitial space (as occurs in pulmonary edema) and (2) collection of fluid in interstitial spaces due to compromised lymphatic function.

### Pathophysiology

Leakage of plasma into an interstitial space may occur as a result of (1) increased capillary fluid pressure, (2) decreased plasma colloid osmotic pressure, and (3) increased capillary (Table 15-7).

**Increased capillary fluid pressure.** An increase in capillary fluid pressure results from vascular compartment overload. The high pressure pushes fluid out of the vessels into the surrounding interstitial tissues. If there is increased hydrostatic pressure in the pulmonary vasculature, fluid will be pushed across the alveolar-capillary membrane into the interstitial spaces of the lung. If the fluid accumulation is sufficient, pulmonary edema will occur.[12]

Increased capillary filtration pressure may be caused by giving too much fluid within a short period of time to a person who, because of advanced age (reduced vessel elasticity) or circulatory or renal disease cannot dispose of the surplus. As the pressure gradient increases, fluid moves into the interstitium.

**table 15-7** *Causes of Edema According to Underlying Physiological Mechanism*

| Fluid Pressure | Oncotic Pressure |
|---|---|
| **INCREASED CAPILLARY FLUID PRESSURE** | **DECREASED CAPILLARY ONCOTIC PRESSURE** |
| **Increased Venous Pressure** | **Loss of Serum Protein** |
| Vein obstruction | Burns, draining wounds, fistulas |
| Varicose veins | Hemorrhage |
| Thrombophlebitis | Nephrotic syndrome |
| Pressure on veins from casts, tight bandages, or clothing | Chronic diarrhea |
| Increased total volume with decreased cardiac output | **Decreased Intake of Protein** |
| Congestive heart failure | Malnutrition |
| Fluid overloading | Kwashiorkor |
| **Sodium and Water Retention, Increased Aldosterone** | **Decreased Production of Albumin** |
| Decreased renal blood flow | Liver disease |
| Congestive heart failure | **INCREASED INTERSTITIAL ONCOTIC PRESSURE** |
| Renal failure | **Increased Capillary Permeability to Protein** |
| Increased production of aldosterone | Burns |
| Cushing's syndrome | Inflammatory reactions |
| Aldosterone added to system | Trauma |
| Corticosteroid therapy | Infections |
| Inability to destroy aldosterone | Allergic reactions (hives) |
| Cirrhosis of liver | **Blocked Lymphatics: Decreased Removal of Tissue Fluid and Protein** |
| | Malignant diseases |
| | Surgical removal of lymph nodes |
| | Elephantiasis |

**Decreased plasma colloid osmotic pressure.** Proteins in the blood (particularly albumin) are necessary to create the oncotic pressure that holds fluids in the vessels. When the colloid osmotic pressure is decreased, fluid moves out of the vascular compartment into the interstitial space. When serum proteins are low because of inadequate intake (severe malnutrition), loss through denuded skin (burns and wounds), renal disease, or decreased production in the liver, edema results.[12]

**Increased capillary permeability.** An increase in capillary permeability may result in extrusion of fluid from the cell into the interstitial space and result in edema.[12] This process is operative in many infectious states, in burns, and with histamine release. Increased capillary permeability contributes to the profound pulmonary compromise in adult respiratory distress syndrome (see Chapter 32).

**Compromised lymphatic function.** Blockage of lymphatic flow can quickly result in significant fluid accumulation. When lymphatic flow is blocked, proteins that have leaked into the interstitial space have no route of escape. As protein accretion occurs, the colloid osmotic pressure rises, and fluid moves into the interstitium.[12] Lymphatic blockage may occur in infections, as a result of an occlusive tumor, or as a result of surgical node excision. (See Chapter 29 for further discussion of lymphedema.)

#### Collaborative care management

Treatment is dependent upon the cause of the edema. Nursing management of persons with edema is discussed in section on Interventions.

## ELECTROLYTE IMBALANCE

As noted earlier, sodium, potassium, calcium, and magnesium are the principal cations in the body. Chloride and bicarbonate are the principal anions. Life cannot be sustained unless body fluids contain exactly the right amount of each in the right concentration within each of the fluid compartments. In addition, no single electrolyte can be out of balance without causing other electrolytes to be out of balance also.

### SODIUM

Sodium is the predominant electrolyte in extracellular fluid. The normal concentration of sodium in the blood is 135 to 145 mEq/L. Its concentration is the major determinant of extracellular fluid volume. Sodium is essential for many physiological activities, including maintenance of acid-base balance, cellular membrane active and passive transport mechanisms, and intracellular metabolism. Disorders of sodium balance are commonly seen in clinical practice and generally occur in association with fluid imbalance.

### Hyponatremia

*Hyponatremia* refers to a serum sodium concentration less than 135 mEq/L.

#### Etiology

Hyponatremia is very common with thiazide diuretic use, but it may be seen with loop and potassium-sparing diuretics as well. While diuretic-provoked hyponatremia is generally mild, it can become severe if confounded by other factors that cause sodium wasting or if sodium intake is markedly restricted, as may be the case in patients with severe congestive heart failure.

Hyponatremia occurs frequently in patients with acquired immunodeficiency syndrome (AIDS), and in patients with midspectrum human immunodeficiency virus (HIV) infection. The etiology may be multifactorial: vomiting and diarrhea, SIADH, adrenal insufficiency, and salt-wasting syndrome.[1]

Postoperative hyponatremia is very common and may be related to several factors, including temporary alteration in hypothalamic function, loss of gastrointestinal fluids by vomiting or suction, or hydration with nonelectrolyte solutions. While equally common in men and women, postoperative hyponatremia is a much more serious complication in premenopausal women. The etiology of this gender/age-related aberrance is unknown. Nevertheless the effects of hyponatremia may clearly be more devastating and potentially fatal in premenopausal women.[16] Judicious monitoring of serum sodium levels and careful assessment for symptoms of hyponatremia are critical for all postoperative patients.

Sodium depletion may also occur as a result of profuse sweating, gastrointestinal or biliary drainage, and draining fistulas. Recall that there are numerous etiologies for SIADH; each also represents a potential cause of hyponatremia.

#### Pathophysiology

Sodium loss from the intravascular compartment causes fluid from the blood to diffuse into the interstitial spaces. As a result, sodium in the interstitial fluid is diluted. In response to this reduction in sodium concentration in the ECF, potassium moves out of the ICF. Therefore the patient with a sodium imbalance is also likely to have a potassium imbalance.

The decreased osmolarity of ECF that exists with sodium loss creates a condition similar to water excess; that is, water moves into the cells by osmosis and leaves the extracellular compartment depleted. This differs from water intoxication because there is not an excess of total body water, but an intercompartmental movement of water that depletes the extracellular compartment.

The laboratory test for plasma sodium does not always give an accurate indication of total body sodium. Some clinical conditions in which the level of serum sodium is not an accurate indicator of total body sodium are listed in Table 15-8. Sodium readily combines with bicarbonate and chloride to help maintain acid-base balance. Signs and symptoms of hyponatremia are listed in Box 15-4.

#### Collaborative care management

Recognition of people at risk for hyponatremia is essential to its prevention. Athletes and persons working in hot environ-

**table 15-8** *Comparison of Serum Sodium Levels with Total Body Sodium**

| Condition | Serum Sodium | Total Body Sodium |
|---|---|---|
| Prolonged sweating | Low (hyponatremia) | Low |
| Diuretics and low-sodium diets | Low | Low |
| Addison's disease | Low | Low |
| Edema (cardiac, renal hepatic disease) | Low or normal | High |
| Excretion of dilute urine, early stages of gastrointestinal sodium loss | Normal | Low |
| Excess oral or IV sodium intake | High (hypernatremia) | High |
| Water and sodium loss with water loss > sodium loss | High | Low |

*Note that a low or high serum level does not necessarily correspond with total body sodium.

ments are encouraged to hydrate with fluid and electrolytes. If salt is not replaced along with water, hyponatremia is aggravated by further dilution. Management includes educating vulnerable people to recognize signs of sodium depletion and maintaining sufficient sodium and water intake to replace skin and insensible fluid loss. Generally, an increased dietary intake of sodium and fluid provides adequate treatment.

People with adrenal insufficiency require special instructions to manage their disease safely. Education about the importance of sodium and fluid balance and the rationale for prescription medications is important. Daily weighing and intake and output monitoring are useful.

The general goal of treatment for hyponatremia is to correct sodium imbalance and restore normal fluid and electrolyte homeostasis. However, specific interventions are guided by the severity of the hyponatremia and the clinical presentation. In the presence of severe hyponatremia and marked symptoms (seizures, coma, and respiratory arrest) aggressive intervention is required. In mild hyponatremia, simply increasing dietary sodium may be sufficient to correct the imbalance.

As sodium replacement is undertaken, continue to monitor serum sodium values to assess the effectiveness of therapy. Evaluate the patient for signs of worsening hyponatremia. Patients receiving vigorous repletion therapy should be monitored for further deterioration of mental status that may occur with too rapid replacement.[16]

If sodium cannot be given orally or by gastric feeding, intravenous fluids are necessary. Generally, 0.9% sodium chloride or lactated Ringer's solution is prescribed. Hypertonic sodium solutions are only given in emergency situations and with very judicious monitoring to avoid dangerous complications.

**box 15-4** *Signs and Symptoms of Hyponatremia*

| | Severe |
|---|---|
| Headache | Mental confusion |
| Muscle weakness | Delirium |
| Fatigue and apathy | Shock |
| Postural hypotension | Coma |
| Anorexia, nausea, and vomiting | |
| Abdominal cramps | |
| Weight loss | |

Too rapid restoration of sodium balance may provoke brain injury due to rapid fluid shifts. The recommended rate of repletion is controversial. It has been suggested that maximum sodium replacement for asymptomatic individuals is 0.5 mEq/L/hr or 12 mEq/L/day. However, 1.5 to 2 mEq/L/hr for 3 to 4 hours is appropriate for severely hyponatremic patients showing significant neurological deficits.[19]

Recall that monitoring of fluid balance is always important when intravenous fluids are given. Patients with compromised cardiac or renal function are particularly vulnerable to fluid overload. Patients should be assessed regularly for the signs of fluid accumulation previously described.

## Hypernatremia

A serum sodium level above 145 mEq/L is termed *hypernatremia.* Hypernatremia may occur as a result of fluid deficit or sodium excess.

### Etiology

Because sodium is inextricably linked to fluid regulation, hypernatremia frequently occurs with fluid imbalance. Hypernatremia develops when an excess of sodium occurs without a proportional increase in body fluid or when water loss occurs without proportional loss of sodium.

Excess dietary or parenteral sodium intake, watery diarrhea, and diabetes insipidus increase the risk of hypernatremia. Thirst is the normal defense mechanism against hypernatremia. People with a preserved thirst mechanism, who have the cognitive ability to process that desire, have unlimited access to fluids, and retain the motor ability to drink those fluids will probably be able to avoid hypernatremia. People most vulnerable to hypernatremia are infants, the elderly, those with physical or mental status compromise, and people with hypothalamic dysfunction.

### Pathophysiology

If sodium becomes concentrated in the ECF, osmolarity rises, water leaves the cell by osmosis and enters the extracellular compartment to dilute fluids there, and the cells are water depleted. The presence of hypernatremia suppresses aldosterone secretion, and sodium is excreted in the urine. Signs and symptoms of hypernatremia are listed in Box 15-5.

**box 15-5** *Signs and Symptoms of Hypernatremia*

Thirst
Dry, sticky mucous membranes
Low urinary output
Firm, rubbery tissue turgor

SEVERE
Manic excitement
Tachycardia
Death

#### *Collaborative care management*

Preventive measures include the recognition of persons at risk for the development of hypernatremia. Bedridden patients should have water readily available. Those who are unable to access water at will should be offered fluids at least every 2 hours. A patient with diabetes insipidus and fluid deprivation requires diligent attention to fluid replacement. An accurate record of intake and output permits quick recognition of a negative fluid balance.

The elderly, the very young, and debilitated patients require careful monitoring to avoid electrolyte imbalance. People with kidney failure, congestive heart failure, or increased aldosterone production may require dietary sodium restriction.

Usually osmolar balance can be restored with oral fluids. If not, the parenteral route may be necessary. Correction of chronic hypernatremia should not exceed a rate of 0.7 mEq/L/hr. In acute, symptomatic states, more rapid correction is indicated: 6 to 8 mEq/L/hr in the first 3 to 4 hours, followed by a rate not to exceed 1 mEq/L/hr.[16]

Recall that fluid resuscitation must be undertaken with particular caution in patients with compromised cardiac or renal function. The nurse should closely monitor the patient's response to fluids, always alert to symptoms of fluid overload.

## POTASSIUM

The normal concentration of potassium in the blood is 3.5 to 5.9 mEq/L. Because most of the potassium in the body is intracellular, the serum potassium level does not necessarily indicate the total body potassium content. Maintenance of serum potassium concentration within the normal range, however, is vital to normal body functions.

Potassium has a direct effect on the excitability of nerves and muscles, contributes most to the intracellular osmotic pressure, and helps maintain acid-base balance and normal kidney function. A potassium deficit is associated with excess alkalinity (alkalosis) of the body fluids, and a potassium excess accompanies an excess of acid (acidosis). These conditions are discussed in Chapter 16.

Potassium is the major cation of the cells. During the formation of new tissues (anabolism) or when glucose is converted to glycogen, potassium enters the cell. With tissue breakdown (catabolism), such as that occurring with trauma, dehydration, or starvation, potassium leaves the cell. The body conserves potassium less effectively then, even when the body needs it. Normally about 5% of the total body potassium is excreted each day.

### Hypokalemia

A low level of serum potassium, less than 3.5 mEq/L, is known as *hypokalemia*.

#### *Etiology*

The patient who has food withheld for several days, is dehydrated, or is given large amounts of parenteral fluids with no replacement of potassium develops potassium depletion. The parenteral administration of 5% dextrose in water without the addition of potassium tends to dilute the potassium in the extracellular fluids. This dilution, in addition to the lack of a balanced diet and to potassium loss caused by catabolism of body proteins, accounts for many instances of electrolyte imbalance in the postoperative patient. People who eat an inadequate diet, who take no food for an extended period of time, or who are losing large amounts of fluid from the gastrointestinal tract through vomiting, diarrhea, or a draining fistula usually are given intravenous solutions that contain potassium.

Severe hypokalemia may be seen in patients with purging eating disorders who induce vomiting or those who abuse laxatives. Chronic hypokalemia may provoke some adaptive response, as even the severely depleted person may not demonstrate symptoms usually seen with marked hypokalemia.[2]

Medications such as diuretics, amphotericin B, some penicillins, and gentamycin may precipitate hypokalemia as a result of renal potassium loss.[16] Aldosterone promotes potassium excretion by the kidneys. Therefore primary or secondary aldosteronism provokes hypokalemia.[19] Figure 15-5 summarizes the causes and effects of hypokalemia.

#### *Pathophysiology*

Movement of sodium (inward) and potassium (outward) across the cell membrane causes depolarization of the membrane and initiates an action potential, which creates nerve and muscle activity. When extracellular potassium concentration is low, the resting membrane potential increases (hyperpolarization), and the cell becomes less excitable. For this reason, the major symptoms of hypokalemia are muscle weakness and atony.

Recall that potassium moves out of the cells when hydrogen ions move into the intracellular compartment in acidosis. Therefore hyperkalemia accompanies acidosis. As the acidosis is treated, potassium moves back into the cells, and hypokalemia may develop. In alkalosis the potassium concentration is lowered because (1) of movement of potassium into cells and (2) potassium excretion by the kidneys as hydrogen ions are being retained.

Whenever sodium is retained in the body through reabsorption by the kidney tubules, potassium is excreted. Thus whenever aldosterone secretion is increased, such as during the stress response, potassium is excreted. Potassium also may be lost in the urine when there is considerable urinary output and as a result of therapy with certain diuretics (the thiazides and furosemide) and the corticosteroids.

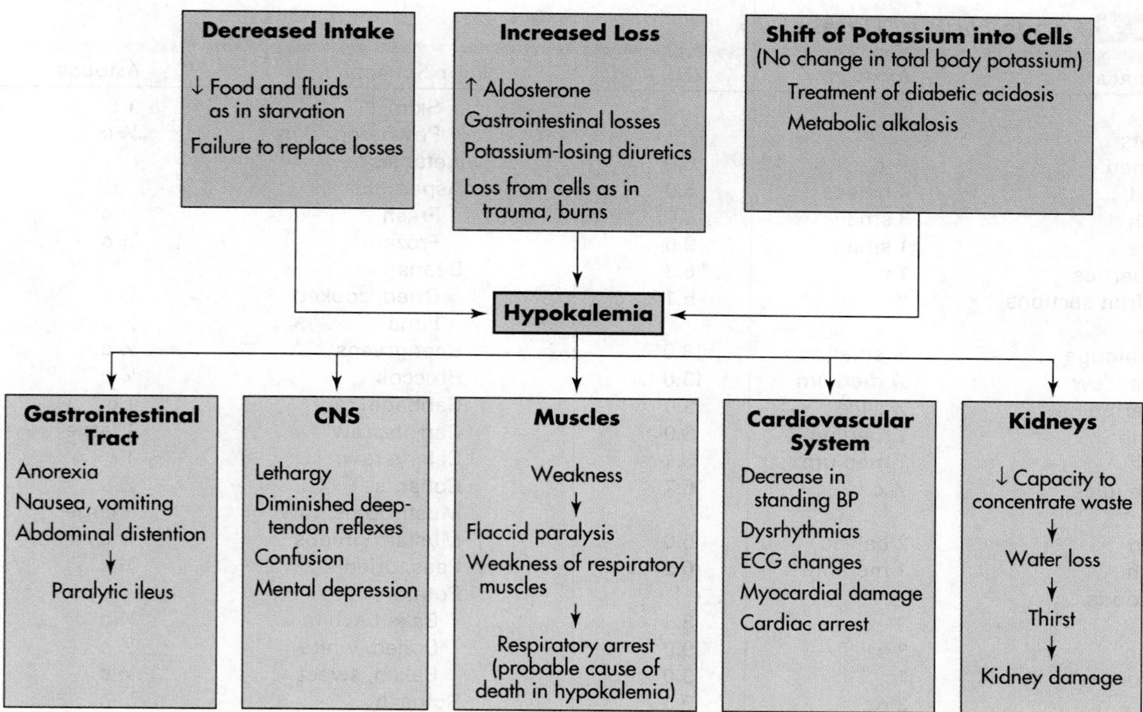


**fig. 15-5** Causes and effects of hypokalemia.

Potassium balance is critical for the maintenance of normal cellular metabolism and excitation. Potentially life-threatening cardiac dysrhythmias may occur in the setting of potassium imbalance. Hypokalemia potentiates the action of digitalis preparations; hence patients receiving these drugs are at particular risk for cardiac rhythm disturbance.

### Collaborative care management

Hypokalemia can be prevented by being alert to the conditions that cause potassium depletion (vomiting, diarrhea, and diuretics) and by monitoring the patient for early warning signs. If there is an order for enemas until results are clear, the nurse should not give more than three enemas to a patient without consulting the physician.

Patients receiving potassium-wasting diuretics should be educated about their effects and taught the importance of adequate dietary intake of potassium. They should be cautioned that in the presence of other problems provoking potassium loss, their health care provider should be contacted.

With severe hypokalemia the patient may die unless potassium is administered promptly. The safest way to administer potassium is orally. When potassium is given intravenously, the rate of flow must be monitored closely to prevent hyperkalemia and a host of cardiac dysrhythmias. Because it is very irritating to the vein, potassium must be diluted before intravenous administration. The usual rate of infusion generally does not exceed 20 mEq/hr. As cardiac dysrhythmias may be provoked by both hypo- and hyperkalemia, cardiac monitoring is useful; it is essential for those with marked disturbance.

In some instances of severe depletion, potassium may be given in a concentrated solution (40 mEq/100 ml) over a 4-hour period. When it is delivered in this concentrated manner, an intravenous infusion pump is essential to safely control the flow rate. If possible, a central line is desirable for the concentrated infusion, due to the irritating nature of the solution.

Persons who are receiving potassium-wasting diuretics should be instructed to include foods high in potassium in their diet (Table 15-9). If low serum potassium levels are shown to result from diuretic therapy, a potassium supplement may be prescribed, usually in the form of potassium chloride (elixir of potassium chloride), or a potassium-sparing diuretic such as triamterene (as found in Dyazide) may be used. People taking diuretics at home should be taught to recognize symptoms of potassium depletion, such as muscle weakness, anorexia, nausea, and vomiting and to report these symptoms to the health care provider. Because potassium supplements are irritating to the gastrointestinal tract, they should be taken with at least one-half glass of water.

## Hyperkalemia

A serum potassium level greater than 5 mEq/L is termed *hyperkalemia.* This condition does not occur as frequently as hypokalemia, especially if renal function is normal.

### Etiology

Hyperkalemia is caused by the movement of potassium out of the cells, increased intake of potassium, and decreased excretion of potassium. Movement of potassium out of the cells occurs with severe tissue damage in sepsis, fever, trauma, or

**table 15-9** *Foods High in Potassium*

| Food Source | Amount | mEq | Food Source | Amount | mEq |
|---|---|---|---|---|---|
| Fruits | | | Skim | 1 c | 8.8 |
| Apricots | | | Powdered, skim | ¼ c | 13.5 |
| Canned | ½ c | 6.0 | Vegetables* | | |
| Dried | 4 halves | 5.0 | Asparagus | | |
| Fresh | 3 small | 8.0 | Fresh | ½ c | 4.7 |
| Banana | 1 small | 9.6 | Frozen | ½ c | 5.5 |
| Strawberries | 1 c | 6.3 | Beans | | |
| Grapefruit sections | ¾ c | 5.1 | Dried, cooked | ½ c | 10.0 |
| Melon | | | Lima | ½ c | 9.5 |
| Cantaloupe | ½ small | 13.0 | Beet greens | ½ c | 8.5 |
| Honeydew | ¼ medium | 13.0 | Broccoli | ½ c | 7.0 |
| Watermelon | ½ slice | 5.0 | Cabbage, raw | 1 c | 6.0 |
| Nectarine | 1 medium | 6.0 | Carrots, raw | 1 large | 8.8 |
| Orange | 1 medium | 5.1 | Celery, raw | 1 c | 9.0 |
| Orange juice | ½ c | 5.7 | Collards | ½ c | 6.0 |
| Peach | | | Mushrooms, raw | 4 large | 10.6 |
| Dried | 2 halves | 5.0 | Mustard greens | ½ c | 5.5 |
| Fresh | 1 medium | 6.2 | Peas, dried | ½ c | 6.8 |
| Protein foods | | | Potato | | |
| Beef | 3 oz | 8.4 | Baked, white | ½ c | 13.0 |
| Chicken | 3 oz | 9.0 | Boiled, white | ½ c | 7.3 |
| Frankfurters | 1 | 3.0 | Baked, sweet | ½ c | 8.0 |
| Liver | 3 oz | 9.6 | Spinach | ½ c | 8.5 |
| Pork | 3 oz | 9.0 | Tomatoes | ½ c | 6.5 |
| Veal | 3 oz | 11.4 | Brussels sprouts | ⅔ c | 7.6 |
| Scallops | 1 large | 6.0 | Squash, winter, baked | ½ c | 12.0 |
| Turkey | 3 oz | 8.4 | Miscellaneous | | |
| Milk | | | Peanut butter | 2 tbsp | 5.0 |
| Whole | 1 c | 8.8 | Nuts, unsalted | 25 | 4.5 |
| Powdered, whole | ¼ c | 10.0 | Beverages that contain large amounts of cocoa, cola drinks, and dry, instant coffee and tea. | | |
| Buttermilk | 1 c | 8.5 | | | |

*Most raw vegetables contain potassium, much of which is lost during cooking.

surgery. This movement also occurs in metabolic acidosis and insulin deficiency/hyperglycemia.

The kidney's efficient excretion of potassium is a safety factor that guards against hyperkalemia. However, people with impaired renal function are at risk for hyperkalemia. This is a particularly important consideration when medications (angiotensin-converting enzyme inhibitors, β-blockers, cyclosporine, nonsteroidal antiinflammatory drugs, lithium, heparin, and others) that also promote potassium retention are prescribed for persons with renal dysfunction.[23] Potassium supplements are generally avoided for people with aldosterone deficiency, as these individuals have a tendency for developing hyperkalemia.

Spurious hyperkalemia may result from drawing a test blood sample from a site proximal to the site of an infusion containing potassium, by using a needle for blood collection that is of so small a bore that cell lysis occurs (21 gauge or smaller), or by drawing the sample after prolonged tourniquet application particularly in combination with isometric hand grip.[16] Spurious potassium elevation must be ruled-out before treatment is instituted, or iatrogenic hypokalemia may be provoked. See Figure 15-6 for causes and effects of hyperkalemia.

### *Pathophysiology*

Time is an important factor in the development of hyperkalemia. A rapid increase in serum potassium of only 1 to 3 mEq/L can be lethal. On the other hand, some persons with renal failure develop severe hyperkalemia slowly and seem to be able to adjust to the potassium excess with few symptoms.

Alterations in the stimulation properties of muscle may result in weakness, even paralysis, in patients with severe hyperkalemia. Generally, these problems do not occur until the serum potassium exceeds 8 mEq/L.[16] Nausea, diarrhea, and intestinal colic may also occur in hyperkalemia. Alterations in cardiac muscle stimulation (depolarization) and relaxation (repolarization) occur as well. These changes in the myocardial action potential result in changes in the surface electrocardiogram, such as wide QRS complexes and tall, peaked T waves. Ventricular dysrhythmias and cardiac arrest may occur.

### *Collaborative care management*

Patients at risk for hyperkalemia should be identified. People with impaired renal function should be cautioned about the possibility of hyperkalemia and advised to avoid over-the-counter medications (such as nonsteroidal antiin-

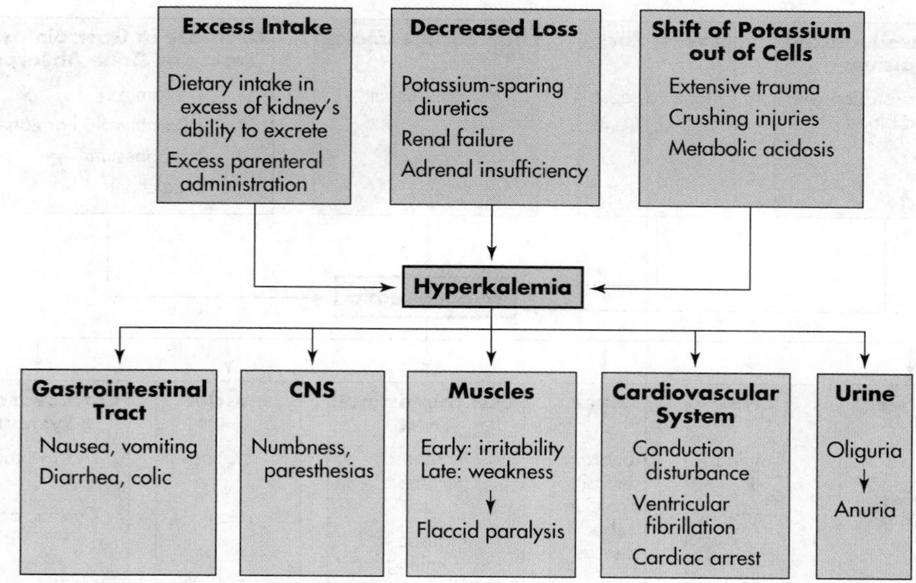


**fig. 15-6** Causes and effects of hyperkalemia.

flammatory drugs) that may provoke hyperkalemia and salt substitutes that are high in potassium. Intravenous potassium repletion should be monitored carefully to avoid iatrogenic hyperkalemia.

The severity of the hyperkalemia guides therapy. Mild hyperkalemia may be relieved by simply withholding the provoking agent (i.e., potassium supplement or medication). With more severe hyperkalemia, a cation-exchange resin, such as polystyrene sulfonate (Kayexalate) may be ordered. Exchange resins act by exchanging the cations in the resin for the potassium in the intestine. The potassium is then excreted in the stool. Bowel function must be maintained if this therapy is to be effective. Potassium-wasting diuretics may be prescribed to promote further loss. If the patient is in acute renal failure, dialysis will be necessary to eliminate the excess potassium.

Severe hyperkalemia (generally greater than 6 mEq/L) is a medical emergency and requires prompt intervention. These patients should be in a unit where continuous cardiac monitoring may be done. Aggressive treatment is indicated if tall, peaked T waves, wide QRS complexes, or ventricular dysrhythmias are present on 12-lead electrocardiogram. Intravenous calcium gluconate may be prescribed to counteract the cardiac effects of hyperkalemia; insulin infusions and intravenous sodium bicarbonate may be used to promote intracellular uptake of potassium.

## CALCIUM

Calcium is necessary for many physiological activities: nerve transmission, cardiac excitability, muscular contraction, blood clotting, and hormone regulation. The normal total serum calcium level is 8.5 to 10 mg/dl. This includes the nonionized (bound to albumin and in combination with citrate or phosphate) and ionized (metabolically active) calcium.[16]

Both vitamin D and parathyroid hormone must be present for calcium to be absorbed from the gastrointestinal tract. As you recall, parathyroid hormone maintains the serum calcium level within normal limits by mobilizing calcium from bone. Calcium is excreted principally through the gastrointestinal tract, with normally only very small amounts being lost in the urine.

### Hypocalcemia

*Hypocalcemia* is defined as a total serum calcium concentration of less than 8.5 mg/dl or an ionized calcium concentration of less than 4.0 mg/dl.

#### *Etiology*

Calcium deficit results from inadequate intake, vitamin D deficiency, hypoparathyroidism, interruption of normal calcium absorption from the gastrointestinal tract, excess loss of calcium through the kidneys, and kidney disease leading to the inability of the kidney to change provitamin D to functional vitamin D. People with pancreatic disease or disease of the small intestine may fail to absorb calcium normally from the gastrointestinal tract and may excrete large amounts of calcium in the feces. Persons with chronic pancreatitis have chronic hypocalcemia related to vitamin D deficiency. Draining intestinal fistulas also cause excess calcium loss.

The hypocalcemia seen with chronic alcoholism is probably multifactorial. Decreased calcium intake, malnutrition, acid-base disturbance, associated pancreatitis, hepatic dysfunction, and gastrointestinal loss are all potential contributors. The causes and effects of hypocalcemia are shown in Figure 15-7.

#### *Pathophysiology*

Calcium ions are thought to line the pores of cell membranes. Because both calcium and sodium ions carry a positive charge, they tend to repel each other. The presence of calcium in the pores of cells (especially neurons) has a blocking effect on permeability to sodium. When serum calcium levels

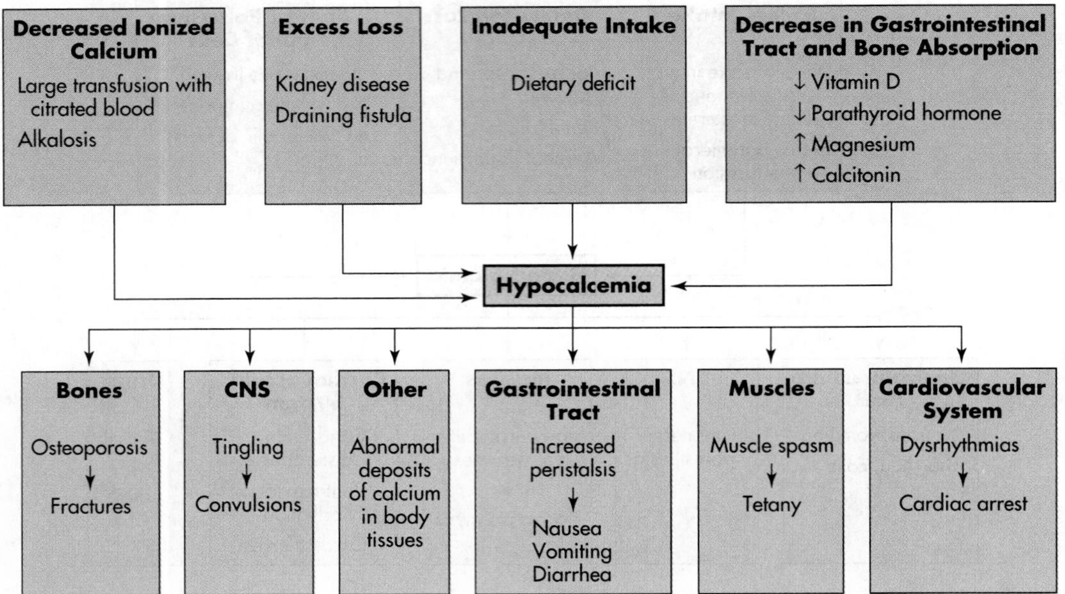


**fig. 15-7** Causes and effects of hypocalcemia.

are low, this blocking effect is minimized, sodium then moves more easily into the cell, and depolarization takes place more readily.[12] This results in increased excitability of the nervous system, leading to muscle spasm, tingling sensations, and if severe, to convulsions and tetany. Skeletal, smooth, and cardiac muscle functions are all affected by overstimulation.

*Tetany* is the most characteristic sign of severe hypocalcemia. The patient who has calcium deficiency usually complains first of numbness and tingling of the nose, ears, fingertips, or toes. If calcium is not given at this time, painful muscular spasms (tetany), especially of the feet and hands (carpopedal spasms), muscle twitching, and convulsions may follow.

Two tests are used to elicit signs of calcium deficiency. *Trousseau's sign* is elicited by grasping the patient's wrist or inflating a blood pressure cuff on the upper arm to constrict the circulation for a few minutes. Palmar flexion, a positive response, may be present in hypocalcemia. *Chvostek's sign* is elicited by tapping the patient's face lightly over the facial nerve (just below the temple). Facial muscle twitching indicates a positive Chvostek's sign. Although positive Trousseau's and Chvostek's signs may be present in hypocalcemia, neither is very sensitive nor specific. That is, a person may have hypocalcemia in the absence of these signs or not have hypocalcemia in the presence of these signs.

Calcium is very important for normal cardiac muscle function as well as normal impulse propagation. Hypocalcemia may be associated with myocardial pump dysfunction, hypotension, and a host of potentially life-threatening cardiac dysrhythmias.

As almost half of the total serum calcium is bound to albumin, the report of serum calcium must be evaluated with consideration of the total albumin. In the presence of a normal serum albumin concentration, ionized calcium constitutes 47% of the total serum calcium. However, in the case of hypoalbuminemia, ionized serum calcium may be easily underestimated. Therefore, in the presence of alkalosis, an ionized serum calcium deficit may be unrecognized. Alkalosis promotes the binding of calcium to protein; hence less calcium is available for physiological activities. Therefore, with alkalosis ($pH > 7.4$), the patient may be hypocalcemic, due to a low level of ionized calcium, despite a normal total serum calcium level.[16]

Hypocalcemia often coexists with hypomagnesemia. Magnesium affects the availability and action of parathyroid hormone. When hypocalcemia occurs as a result of hypomagnesemic hypoparathyroidism, the treatment of choice is magnesium replacement.[16]

### *Collaborative care management*

Inadequate calcium intake, excess calcium loss, and vitamin D deficiency place persons at risk for developing hypocalcemia. Patients who have extremely poor diets or who have calcium-depleting conditions should be monitored for signs of hypocalcemia. Patients should be educated about the importance of adequate calcium and vitamin D intake.

Patients undergoing thyroid, parathyroid, and radical neck surgery are particularly vulnerable to hypocalcemia secondary to parathyroid hormone deficit. Monitoring of serum calcium levels and correction of deficits are very important for these patients.

As discussed earlier, patients receiving transfusions of large amounts of whole blood are at risk for hypocalcemia. Citrate is added to stored blood to prevent coagulation. When the blood is transfused, the citrate binds with circulating calcium. Usually, this does not present a problem, because the citrate is quickly metabolized by the liver. However, if the patient has a preexisting calcium deficit, has a hepatic dysfunction that impairs metabolism, or is receiving large amounts of whole blood very rapidly, hypocalcemia may occur. Vulnerable patients should have serum calcium levels checked during and/or after transfusions.[16]

For persons with acute hypocalcemia, 10 to 20 ml of a 10% intravenous solution of calcium gluconate given slowly may

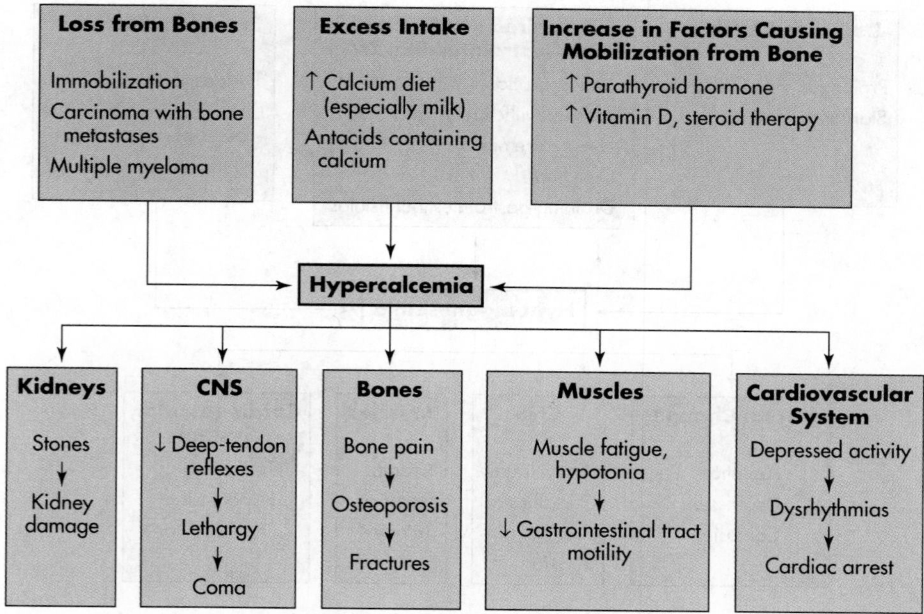


**fig. 15-8** Causes and effects of hypercalcemia.

be prescribed. Although calcium chloride provides more readily available ionized calcium, it is so irritating to the vein that it is generally not used. Patients receiving intravenous calcium replacement should have continuous cardiac monitoring.

For patients with mild hypocalcemia, a high-calcium diet or oral calcium salts may be sufficient. When decreased parathyroid hormone or vitamin D is the causative factor, these substances must be supplied. When the serum phosphorus level rises, the calcium level falls. Hence aluminum hydroxide gel can be given to lower a high serum phosphorus concentration (via phosphorus binding of calcium).

After thyroid, parathyroid, or radical neck surgery, patients must be watched closely for symptoms of calcium deficiency because of the possibility that the parathyroid glands may have been inadvertently removed or are temporarily suppressed by local edema. Intravenous calcium gluconate should always be available for emergency use during the postoperative period.

Bone demineralization may occur with prolonged hypocalcemia. Therefore, while patients should ambulate cautiously, they should be encouraged and assisted to do so to minimize bone resorption.

## Hypercalcemia

*Hypercalcemia* refers to a total serum calcium concentration greater than 10 mg/dl.

### Etiology

Hypercalcemia can result from excessive intake of calcium, especially in milk and absorbable calcium-containing antacids (milk-alkali syndrome), from excessive vitamin D intake, and from conditions that promote release of calcium from the bones into ECF. These causes and their effects are shown in Figure 15-8.

The most common causes of hypercalcemia, however, are malignancy and hyperparathyroidism (see Chapters 11 and 34). An elevated serum calcium level may occur in malignancy as a result of tumor secretion of parathyroid hormone or alteration of bone metabolism.[16]

### Pathophysiology

Hypercalcemia acts like a cellular sedative, depressing nerve and muscle activity. Generalized muscle weakness may be noted. Deep tendon reflexes may be decreased or absent. Myocardial function is altered, and cardiac dysrhythmias may occur. Gastrointestinal motility decreases, and constipation, nausea, and vomiting may occur. Mental status changes (lethargy, confusion, memory loss, and coma) may occur.

When someone is immobilized, calcium leaves the bone and becomes concentrated in the ECF. Normal retention of calcium in the bones is caused by weight-bearing forces on the skeleton. When a large amount of calcium accumulates in the ECF and passes through the kidneys, calcium can precipitate and form stones (calculi), a relatively common complication of immobility.

Calcium precipitates more readily in alkaline solution. This can be a problem in a person with a urinary tract infection, which increases the alkalinity of the urine, because renal calculi are more likely to be formed.

### Collaborative care management

Mild hypercalcemia may be treated with hydration and education about avoiding foods high in calcium or medications that promote calcium elevation. Hypercalcemia as a complication of immobilization may be avoided with ambulation as appropriate when the person is able, and the use of active weight-bearing exercises as appropriate. Appliances such as a trapeze or resistance devices may be applied to a hospital bed to provide opportunities for exercise. When a patient cannot ambulate or do active exercises, a tilt table may be used for weight-bearing exercise.

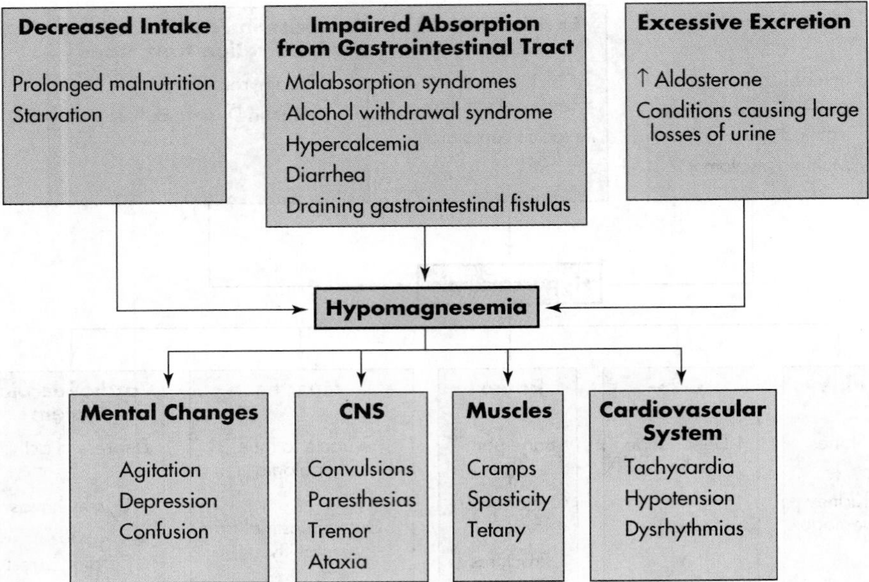


**fig. 15-9** Causes and effects of hypomagnesemia.

People with marked hypercalcemia have often lost calcium from their bones or have malignant involvement of bone, therefore special care should be taken to prevent pathological fractures. Although exercising as able is important to minimize further demineralization, consideration must be given to the danger of fractures, and as usual, an individualized plan of care developed.

Careful attention must be directed to the prevention of renal calculi. Encouraging oral fluids can help prevent concentrated urine. Unless contraindicated, 3000 to 4000 ml of fluid per day is desirable. Acid-ash fruit juices, cranberry juice, and prune juice, are particularly useful as they promote a more acid urine, thus discouraging stone formation.

Severe hypercalcemia is a medical emergency. Continuous cardiac monitoring is necessary and emergency equipment should be readily available. Initial treatment for severe hypercalcemia is hydration. As the hydration regimen may be vigorous (possibly several 100 ml/hr for several hours), cardiac and renal status must be assessed before the fluids are begun and reassessed at least every 2 hours during fluid therapy. Intravenous furosemide may be given to promote diuresis. If additional treatment is required, calcitonin and/or mithramycin may be given to prevent bone resorption. Serum and urinary electrolytes should be checked every 2 hours during treatment of severe hypercalcemia.[23] An example of a Clinical Pathway for the patient with hypercalcemia is found on p. 417.

## MAGNESIUM

The normal serum magnesium level is 1.5 to 2.5 mEq/L. Most is found in bone, 30% to 35% in the intracellular fluid, and only a small amount is found in the extracellular fluid. Therefore serum magnesium levels do not necessarily reflect total body magnesium. Magnesium participates in many enzymatic reactions, especially those involving energy use or production. It is important in the maintenance of normal neural and muscular excitability. Magnesium has a sedative effect on the central nervous system similar to that of calcium.

### Hypomagnesemia

*Hypomagnesemia* is a serum magnesium level of less than 1.5 mEq/L.

#### *Etiology*

Hypomagnesemia is a very common clinical problem. It frequently coexists with hypokalemia and less often with hypocalcemia. Magnesium levels may be decreased as a result of many factors including (1) loss of intestinal fluids through draining fistulas, diarrhea, and gastrointestinal suction; (2) prolonged malnutrition; (3) renal disorders; (4) drug therapy with aminoglycosides and loop diuretics; and (5) endocrine disorders, such as increased secretion of ADH, aldosterone, and thyroid hormone, and diabetes mellitus. The hypomagnesemia often seen in chronic alcoholism is multifactorial and related to decreased dietary intake of magnesium, increased gastrointestinal losses, and intestinal malabsorption.[16] Causes and effects of hypomagnesemia are shown in Figure 15-9.

Cardiac patients may be at particular risk for hypomagnesemia for several reasons. Renal conservation of magnesium occurs at the loop of Henle. Loop diuretics, commonly prescribed for cardiac patients, enhance magnesium loss. Gastrointestinal edema, common in patients with congestive heart failure, diminishes intestinal reabsorption of magnesium and provokes gastrointestinal symptoms that promote magnesium

## clinical pathway *The Patient with Hypercalcemia*

**Directions:**
1. Review coordinated care track (CCT) approximately every 8°.
2. Appropriate and completed interventions need no additional documentation.
3. Cross through any interventions that are not applicable.
4. Circle any intervention not completed.
5. The plan of care—nursing interventions and outcome evaluation statements—may be added to the CCT as necessary.

DRG 239 Expected LOS 5 days
Physician(s) ______

Admit Date ______
Discharge Date ______
Primary Diagnosis ______

Date of last Chemo ______
Date of last Radiation ______

Comorbid Conditions:
☐ CHF ☐ COPD
☐ IDDM
☐ Angina
☐ Dehydration
☐ Malnutrition

Imprint/Label

Complications during this admission:
☐ Pulmonary embolus ☐
☐ Deep vein thrombosis ☐
☐ ☐
☐ ☐

Risk Factors:
☐ Obesity ☐ ETOH/Substance Abuse ☐ Smoking ☐

| DATE | PROBLEM LIST | DISCHARGE CRITERIA | DATE INITIALLY MET | MET ON DISCHARGE YES | MET ON DISCHARGE NO |
|---|---|---|---|---|---|
| | 1. Confusion<br>2. Safety<br>3. Constipation<br>4. Dehydration<br>5. Renal failure | 1. Normal calcium level<br>2. Patient/caregiver has knowledge, resources, and ability to provide care outside of the hospital environment.<br>3. Able to consume 1000 cc fluid/day.<br>4. Renal function returns to prehypercalcemic level. | | | |
| | | Explain any discharge criteria not met: | | | |

Courtesy The Cleveland Clinic Foundation, Department of Advanced Practice Nursing, Cleveland, Ohio, 1996.
*ADL*, activities of daily living; *CHF*, congestive heart failure; *COPD*, chronic obstructive pulmonary disorder; *IDDM*, insulin-dependent diabetes mellitus (type 2).

Continued

## The Patient with Hypercalcemia—cont'd

| TIME FRAME LOCATION | HOSPITAL DAY 1 DATE UNIT | HOSPITAL DAY 2 DATE UNIT | HOSPITAL DAY 3 DATE UNIT | HOSPITAL DAY 4 DATE UNIT | HOSPITAL DAY 5 DATE UNIT |
|---|---|---|---|---|---|
| PATIENT SATISFACTION | "HOW CAN WE ENHANCE YOUR STAY AT THE CCF?" | "HOW CAN WE ENHANCE YOUR STAY AT THE CCF?" | "HOW CAN WE ENHANCE YOUR STAY AT THE CCF?" | "HOW CAN WE ENHANCE YOUR STAY AT THE CCF?" | "HOW CAN WE ENHANCE YOUR STAY AT THE CCF?" |
| DISCHARGE PLANNING PATIENT EDUCATION | Identify primary caregiver ________<br>Identify learning needs | Team conference<br>Consult Social Worker, Chaplain<br>Teach signs/symptoms of hypercalcemia<br>Teach aspiration precautions | Team & family conference<br>Consult Hospice<br>Consult ASC<br>Evaluate need for SQ injection teaching if pt. to be discharged on calcitonin | Confirm discharge disposition<br>SQ injection teaching if pt. to be discharged on calcitonin | Give RTC appts. |
| TESTS/ PROCEDURES/ CONSULTS | CBC, SMA 17<br>Weigh patient<br>Monitor I & O<br>IV hydration and diuresis | Calcium level<br>Weigh patient<br>Monitor I & O<br>IV hydration and diuresis | Calcium level<br>Weigh patient<br>Monitor I & O<br>Decrease IV hydration | Calcium level<br>Weigh patient<br>Monitor I & O<br>Consider discontinuing the IV hydration | Calcium level<br>Weigh patient<br>Monitor I & O |
| ALLIED HEALTH | Nutrition Services ☐<br>Palliative Care Consult ☐ | | | | |
| NURSING INTERVENTIONS | Initiate calcitonin per doctor's order<br>Establish usual bowel pattern ________<br>Institute bowel regimen for constipation (i.e., stool softeners, laxatives, enemas)<br>Aspiration precautions<br>Assess swallowing before giving fluids/food<br>Review meds pt taking prior to admission<br>Exclude meds contributing to confusion or hypercalcemia (i.e., Vit D, antacids, etc.) | Continue calcitonin per doctor's order<br>Continue bowel regimen for constipation (i.e., stool softeners, laxatives, enemas)<br>Assess for bowel movement<br>Aspiration precautions<br>Assist patient with ADL | Evaluate need for further calcitonin<br>Continue bowel regimen for constipation (i.e., stool softeners, laxatives, enemas)<br>Assess for bowel movement<br>Aspiration precautions<br>Assist patient with ADL | Evaluate need for further calcitonin<br>Continue bowel regimen for constipation (i.e., stool softeners, laxatives, enemas)<br>Aspiration precautions<br>Assist patient with ADL | Aspiration precautions<br>Assist patient with ADL<br>Continue bowel regimen for constipation (i.e., stool softeners, laxatives, enemas) |
| OUTCOME CRITERIA | Vital signs stable<br>Weight stable or ↓ from admission<br>Drug therapy initiated<br>Patient satisfaction addressed | Free from injury<br>No aspiration<br>Calcium level decreased from admission<br>Patient satisfaction addressed | Calcium level decreased from previous day<br>Patient satisfaction addressed<br>Free from injury<br>No aspiration | Free from injury<br>No aspiration<br>Calcium level decreased from admission<br>Patient satisfaction addressed | Able to verbalize s/s of high calcium<br>Free from injury<br>No aspiration<br>Normal calcium level<br>Patient satisfaction addressed |

loss. The effects of digitalis preparations are potentiated by a low magnesium level. Therefore when hypomagnesemia occurs, the patient is at risk for digitalis toxicity. In some cases, hypomagnesemia may contribute to the development of atherosclerosis, coronary artery spasm, and cardiomyopathy. Magnesium deficit may precipitate life-threatening cardiac dysrhythmias.[6]

#### Pathophysiology

A low serum magnesium level leads to increased neuromuscular irritability by increasing acetylcholine release, increasing the sensitivity of the myoneural junction to acetylcholine, diminishing the threshold of excitation of the motor nerve, and enhancing the force of myofibril contraction.[19] Magnesium is excreted by the gastrointestinal tract when a large amount of calcium is present, as the calcium is preferentially absorbed. The kidneys effectively conserve magnesium when intake is low. Hypomagnesemia is suspected when hypocalcemia and hypokalemia are refractory to treatment.

Metabolically, magnesium is closely interrelated with both calcium and potassium. Magnesium inhibits transport of parathyroid hormone from the glands, causing a decrease in the amount of calcium being released from bone that results in a calcium deficit. Hypomagnesemia usually manifests with behavioral and neurological symptoms such as confusion, increased reflexes, tremors, muscle spasms, arrhythmias, and paresthesias.[16]

#### Collaborative care management

Recognition of patients at risk for hypomagnesemia is important. People taking loop diuretics and digoxin should be encouraged to consume foods rich in magnesium, such as fruits, vegetables, cereals, and milk.[7] As magnesium is primarily an intracellular electrolyte, serum magnesium levels may be normal, despite total body magnesium depletion. Recognition of signs and symptoms of magnesium deficiency should not be ignored. Magnesium is essential for potassium reabsorption, so if hypokalemia does not respond to potassium replacement, hypomagnesemia should be suspected.[16]

Treatment of the underlying cause is the first consideration in hypomagnesemia. If the deficit is severe, parenteral magnesium replacement is indicated. When intravenous administration of magnesium is necessary, continuous cardiac monitoring is advisable. The infusion should be given via an infusion pump so that accurate dosing is assured. Patients experiencing mental status changes as a result of the hypomagnesemia require special attention be given to safety measures.

### Hypermagnesemia

*Hypermagnesemia* is a serum magnesium level greater than 2.5 mEq/L.

#### Etiology

Hypermagnesemia seldom develops in the presence of normal renal function. However, magnesium excess may inadvertently occur as a result of magnesium replacement or when magnesium sulfate is administered to prevent seizures resulting from eclampsia. Therefore, careful assessment of patients receiving magnesium therapy is essential.

#### Pathophysiology

Magnesium has what might be loosely described as a sedative effect: as the magnesium level rises, the patient becomes drowsy and lethargic and reflexes diminish. Respirations may become so severely depressed that respiratory arrest occurs. Because a loss of deep tendon reflexes occurs before severe respiratory problems occur, periodic assessment of reflexes during magnesium administration is essential. Cardiac effects of hypermagnesemia include slow heart rate and atrioventricular conduction block. As peripheral vasodilation occurs, hypotension, flushing, and increased skin warmth may be noted.[16]

#### Collaborative care management

Patients with impaired renal function are at risk of hypermagnesemia and should be cautioned to avoid over-the-counter medications that contain magnesium (i.e., Milk of Magnesia and Mylanta). Any patient receiving parenteral magnesium therapy should be assessed frequently for signs of hypermagnesemia.

Withholding magnesium-containing medications may correct mild hypermagnesemia. For renal failure, dialysis may be required for adequate treatment. Severe hypermagnesemia may require treatment with intravenous calcium gluconate (10 to 20 ml of 10% calcium gluconate administered over 10 minutes). If cardiorespiratory collapse is imminent, the patient may require temporary pacemaker and ventilator support.[16]

## NURSING MANAGEMENT

Nursing management of persons with alterations in fluid and electrolyte imbalances is discussed in the following section.

### ■ ASSESSMENT

#### Subjective Data

Imbalances in fluid and electrolytes are likely to account for many of the symptoms in various clinical conditions, or they can be caused by the therapy itself. The nurse needs to recognize the symptoms of fluid and electrolyte imbalance and make ongoing physical assessments (Table 15-10). Subjective data such as the presence of headache, thirst, nausea, dyspnea, and time of onset, extent, and aggravating and relieving factors are obtained.

#### Objective Data

Objective data should be compared with baseline assessments. In addition to assessing physical structures, the process of intake and losses by any route needs to be monitored.

Data of particular importance in assessing fluid and electrolyte imbalance are the comparison of intake to output and changes in the patient's weight. These are nursing measures that can be instituted independent of doctors' orders. If patients and families are given explanations, they can participate

**table 15-10** *Assessment of Fluid and Electrolyte Imbalance*

| PARAMETER | FLUID EXCESS | FLUID LOSS/ELECTROLYTE IMBALANCE |
|---|---|---|
| Behavior | Tires easily; change in behavior, confusion, apathy | Change in behavior, confusion, apathy |
| Head, neck | Facial edema, distended neck veins | Headache, thirst, dry mucous membranes |
| Upper gastrointestinal tract | Anorexia, nausea, vomiting | Anorexia, nausea, vomiting |
| Skin | Warm, moist, taut, cool feeling where edematous | Dry, decreased turgor |
| Respiration | Dyspnea, orthopnea, productive cough, moist breath sounds | Changes in rate and depth of breathing |
| Circulation | Loss of sensation in edematous areas, pallor,* bounding pulse, ↑ blood pressure | Pulse rate changes, dysrhythmias, postural hypotension |
| Abdomen | Increased girth, fluid wave | Distention, abdominal cramps |
| Elimination | Constipation | Diarrhea, constipation |
| Extremities | Dependent edema, "pitting," discomfort from weight of bedclothes | Muscle weakness, tingling, tetany |

*Pallor: edema decreases the intensity of skin color by increasing the distance between the skin surface and the pigmented or vascular areas. In the dark-skinned person, pallor is observed by absence of underlying red tones that give brown and black skin "glow." The brown skin appears more yellow-brown, and the black skin appears more ashen gray.

in measuring and recording intake and output. The intake and output are totaled at intervals that are determined by the severity of the patient's condition. A patient in a critical care unit may have hourly measurements, whereas a patient in a stepdown unit or on a medical floor may have them totaled once per shift.

Because symptoms of fluid and electrolyte imbalance are frequently not specific, a good rule is to be alert for changes in behavior, level of consciousness, vital signs, skin, turgor, muscle strength, and condition of mucous membranes. Baseline observations made during the first encounter with a patient are essential for comparison with subsequent observations to detect changes.

Careful observation contributes significantly to determining fluid and electrolyte balance. The following summarizes useful bedside observations.

- Body temperature can alternately indicate fluid and electrolyte imbalance or can cause the imbalance. Dehydration (with resultant increased serum sodium) causes temperature elevations. Fluid volume excess unrelated to infection can cause a decrease in body temperature. A profound decrease in circulating blood volume results in extremities that are cool to the touch. With fever, because of increases in metabolism and respiration, fluid loss is increased.
- Pulse rate is affected by imbalances in potassium, sodium, and magnesium, volume depletion, and plasma to interstitial space shift. Pulse volume is affected by circulating blood volume. Dysrhythmias can indicate imbalances in potassium and magnesium.[12]
- Respiration is a sensitive indicator of body pH. An example of this is the respiratory pattern in metabolic alkalosis, which is evidenced by decreased rate and depth and periods of apnea. Slow, shallow respirations favor carbon dioxide retention and hence carbonic acid and hydrogen ions. The changes caused by the alkalotic state of the arterial blood gases depress the respiratory centers to compensate for the alkalosis. Hypoventilation also occurs in potassium and calcium imbalances due to muscle weakness. Metabolic acidosis increases both the rate and depth of respirations as the lungs attempt to blow off the carbon dioxide. During periods of abnormalities, respirations should be counted for a full 2 minutes.
- Blood pressure variations are useful in evaluating fluid disturbances. In circulatory volume loss, the systolic pressure falls faster than the diastolic, resulting in diminished pulse pressure.
- Jugular neck veins provide a built-in manometer for central venous pressure, providing the patient is not in congestive heart failure. Flat neck veins in a supine patient indicate decreased plasma volume. Normal jugular vein distention (JVD) at a 45° angle is no higher than 2 cm above the sternal angle. Jugular neck veins distended from the manubrium to the angle of the jaw indicate high venous pressure.[14]
- Hand veins are another useful measure of plasma volume. Normally, hand veins empty in 3 to 5 seconds when elevated. Conversely, they fill in 3 to 5 seconds when placed in a dependent position. Decreased plasma volume causes the hand veins not to show or to fill more slowly. Increased plasma volume causes the hand veins to empty more slowly.
- Assessments of skin turgor and mucous membranes are commonly used in detection of fluid volume. In normal skin turgor, gently pinched skin should fall back to its normal position when released. Because of decreased elasticity, evaluating skin turgor is not useful in the elderly. Mucous membranes in mouth breathers can be dry from evaporative processes rather than a fluid volume deficit. However, the area where the cheek and gum meet should be moist even in mouth breathers as long as they have no fluid volume deficit.
- The type of edema that represents excess interstitial fluid (pitting edema, dependent edema, or refractory edema) is an obvious indication of increased total body sodium. As has been previously demonstrated, edema is not produced by retention of water alone. In assessing the patient, it is important to differentiate between pitting edema and lymphedema. Pitting edema is an excessive accumulation of interstitial fluid and is either generalized or localized.

When the amount of generalized edema is great, it is termed *anasarca.* To demonstrate the presence of edema the thumb is pressed into the skin against a bony surface. When the thumb is withdrawn, an indentation persists for a short period of time. The depth of the indentation should be estimated and recorded in millimeters. Terms such as "3+" are meaningless, and should not be used. The distribution should also be noted. Obstruction of lymphatic channels produces *lymphedema.* Lymphedema is differentiated by its woody or brawny feel, as opposed to the more pliant feel of interstitial edema (see Chapter 29).

- Episodes of muscular weakness, fatiguability, and decreased activity tolerance may be descriptive of potassium deficit.
- Severe ECF deficit produces sunken eyes, while excess ECF produces periorbital edema.
- Behavior, while not diagnostic, can augment other observations. Sharp decreases in plasma pH cause disorientation and finally coma. With alkalosis, one of the symptoms is overexcitability, such as unexplained anxiety or nervousness. The extreme of this spectrum can be convulsions.[14]

### Laboratory Values

Laboratory determinations of serum levels of the specific electrolytes help in making decisions concerning electrolyte excesses or deficits. When there is water excess, hemodilution occurs and the hematocrit, hemoglobin, blood urea nitrogen (BUN), and electrolyte levels are decreased. With excessive fluid loss hemoconcentration occurs, and the hematocrit, hemoglobin, BUN, and electrolyte levels are increased. Urine specific gravity and anion gap, both of which will be explained in greater detail in the Interventions section, are also useful measurements of fluid and electrolyte balance.

## ■ NURSING DIAGNOSES

Nursing diagnoses are determined from analysis of patient data. Nursing diagnoses for the patient experiencing fluid and electrolyte imbalances include, but are not limited to:

| Diagnostic Title | Possible Etiological Factors |
|---|---|
| Fluid volume deficit | Active fluid volume loss (hemorrhage, diarrhea, gastric intubation, wounds, diaphoresis), inadequate fluid intake, failure of regulatory mechanisms, sequestration of body fluids |
| Fluid volume excess | Excess fluid intake, excess sodium intake, compromised regulatory mechanisms |
| Alteration in comfort | Thirst, nausea, vomiting, xerostoma, dsyphagia, edema, dry skin |

## ■ EXPECTED PATIENT OUTCOMES

Expected outcomes for patients with fluid and electrolyte imbalances may include, but are not limited to:

1. Maintains functional fluid volume as evidenced by adequate urinary output, stable weight, normal vital signs, normal urine specific gravity, moist mucous membranes, balanced intake and output, elastic skin turgor, prompt capillary refill, and absence of edema.
2. Verbalizes understanding of treatment plan and causative factors that led to the imbalance.
3. Reports relief of symptoms (thirst, dry oral mucous membranes, nausea, vomiting, dry skin, and weakness).

## ■ INTERVENTIONS

### Evaluation of Degree of Deficit or Excess

In this section, some interventions that were listed in the Collaborative Management and Assessment sections will be dealt with in more detail.

#### *Intake and output monitoring*

The intake record should show the type and amount of all fluids the patient has received and the route by which they were administered. This includes fluids taken orally, parenterally, rectally, or by tubes (percutaneous esophageal gastrostomy [PEG], nasogastric, etc.). A record of solid food intake is sometimes necessary, especially with very young children. Foods that are eaten in a semisolid state but which are basically water based such as gelatin or popsicles are recorded as fluids. In a strict sense, milk-based fluids are considered solids and as such are not totaled in with fluids. Ice chips are recorded by dividing the amount of chips by one half (60 ml of chips would equal 30 ml of water). Patients may receive a considerable amount of fluid intake through the frequent sucking of ice chips.

The output record is equally important. Vomitus, gastrointestinal drainage, and liquid stools are measured as accurately as possible and are described by color, content, and odor. Gastric secretions are normally watery and pale yellow-green; they usually have a sour odor. However, if the acid-base balance has been upset, gastric secretions may have a fruity odor because of the presence of ketone bodies (acetone). Bile is somewhat thicker than gastric juice and may vary from dark green to brown in color. It has an acrid odor, and patients may report a bitter taste if vomiting bile. Intestinal contents vary from dark green to brown, are likely to be quite thick, and have a fecal odor. The amount of fluid used in irrigating nasogastric tubes is added to "intake" and needs to be subtracted from total drainage before it is recorded. It is difficult to determine accurately the amount of water lost in the stools, but a record of the consistency, color, and number of stools and the approximate amount of each gives a reasonable estimate.

Disease states that cause increased vascular hydrostatic pressure and/or interstitial fluid colloid osmotic pressure result in fluid loss to the interstitial spaces, or third-spacing. Examples of this are pleural or peritoneal effusions and ascites from hepatic or renal disease. Drainage of peritoneal or pleural fluid during the active disease state can exacerbate intravascular losses caused by continued shifts from the vascular compartment. Peritoneal or pleural fluid drainage is also noted as output, with the amount and color (clarity) recorded. Body weights are used to track fluid shifts and retention such as is found in third spacing. Body weight is discussed in more detail later in this chapter.

Noting the character and volume of urine is essential to evaluating fluid and electrolyte status. Urinary output is documented by recording the time and amount of each voiding. If renal function is a major concern, as in a severely burned patient, an indwelling catheter is inserted to measure the amount of urinary output hourly. The fluid intake is then regulated with respect to the output. Obviously, accuracy is critical. A frequent complaint is that nothing is more difficult to obtain in a modern hospital than an accurate record of urinary output. The patient and family should be instructed to save all urine. Measuring devices can be placed under the toilet seat to collect urine. Signs posted on the patient's chart and in the utility room and bathroom help to prevent discarding urine before it is measured.

Another parameter of importance in evaluating fluid and electrolyte status is the specific gravity of the urine. Specific gravity indicates the kidney's ability to dilute or concentrate urine. It is the weight of a specified amount of urine compared with the weight of an equal amount of distilled water. The specific gravity of water is 1.000. The specific gravity of urine in healthy persons ranges from 1.003 to 1.030. A highly concentrated specimen implies a state of dehydration; a dilute sample in a person with healthy kidneys indicates adequate hydration or possibly overhydration. As a matter of interest, a more accurate way of ascertaining renal concentrating ability is the simultaneous measurement of serum and urine osmolarity. Recall that normal serum osmolarity is $290 \pm 5$ mOsm/kg. The range of urine osmolarity is 40 to 1600 mOsm/L.[16]

As mentioned previously, to maintain chemical neutrality the total concentration of cations and anions must be equivalent in all body fluids in terms of milliequivalents per liter. However, because there are a number of anions and cations present in the blood that are not routinely measured, a "gap" exists between the total concentration of anions and cations and the concentration normally measured in the serum. This gap is composed primarily of unmeasured anions and is calculated by the formula $Na - (Cl + HCO_3^-)$. The mean is approximately 12 mEq/L (range 8 to 16 mEq/L). The anion gap has important diagnostic significance in acid-base disorders, particularly metabolic acidosis. An increased anion gap may indicate endogenous metabolic acidosis, anion ingestion (ethylene, methanol, paraldehyde, and salicylates), acidosis secondary to therapeutic agents (paraldehyde, penicillin, and carbenicillin), and increased plasma proteins. A decreased anion gap may indicate increased unmeasured cations (hypercalcemia, hyperkalemia, and hypermagnesemia) or increased globulins (found in myeloma or lithium toxicity). Four commonly occurring clinical conditions associated with a high anion gap include: (1) renal failure, (2) ketoacidosis, (3) reactions to drugs or toxins, and (4) lactic acidosis. In the absence of renal failure or intoxication with drugs and toxins, an increase in anion gap is assumed to be due to ketoacids or lactate accumulation.

All drainage from body orifices or artificial openings should be measured. This would include drainage from an ileostomy or a T tube after exploration of the common bile duct or from any catheter draining a surgical area. If there is excessive drainage from a wound, it may be necessary to weigh the dressings. Fluid loss is the difference between the wet dressings and the dry weight of the dressing.

Fluid aspirated from any body cavity such as the abdomen (paracentesis) or pleural space (thoracentesis) must be measured. The fluid contains not only electrolytes and water but also proteins. Blood loss from any part of the body is measured carefully. Diaphoresis is difficult to measure without special laboratory equipment. In some patients, however, it may be important to estimate the loss of fluid by this route. A careful note of excessive perspiration and its duration is made. If the clothing and bed linen become saturated, wet and dry weights may be taken. Accurate recording of body temperature helps the physician determine how much fluid should be replaced. Fluid loss through the skin and lungs increases as the body temperature rises. A patient who has a high fever and is breathing rapidly can lose as much as 2500 ml of fluid per day through the lungs.

#### Daily weight

Trends in weight are often the best way to determine the onset of dehydration or the accumulation of fluid, either as generalized edema or as "hidden" fluid in body cavities. An increase of 1 kg in weight is equal to the retention of 1 L (1000 ml) of fluid in the edematous patient. If the weight record is to be accurate, the patient must be weighed on the same scale at the same hour each day and be wearing the same amount of clothing. Circumstances that may affect the weight should be kept as nearly identical as possible from day to day. Usually weights are taken early in the morning after the patient had voided for the first time, but before he or she has eaten or defecated. When precise weights are needed, all clothing and even wound dressings are removed. A person maintained on intravenous fluids other than those specifically designed for parenteral nutrition can be expected to lose approximately 0.2 to 0.5 kg/day.

### Replacement of Fluid and Electrolytes

#### General principles

To review, replacement of fluid and electrolyte losses are accomplished by one of the following: (1) oral intake, (2) tube feeding (gavage), (3) intravenous infusion, and/or (4) total parenteral nutrition. The healthiest method of fluid and electrolyte replacement is by oral intake because it is believed to maintain motility and integrity of the gastrointestinal system.

When fluids can be metabolized by the gastrointestinal system but cannot be swallowed, methods are used to bypass the esophagus such as nasogastric tubes, PEG tubes, and G-tubes (see Chapter 40). Normal saline solution and plain water should also be given by slow drip to replace daily fluid loss. When it is not possible for a patient to take food or fluid through the alimentary tract, the most common method of replacement is by intravenous infusion. Usually a vein in an extremity is used; however, when these are unavailable, a vein in the neck or groin is used. The intravenous infusion may be given by threading a needle or an intracatheter into a vein and securing it by taping it in place at the insertion site. An alternate method of access is to make an incision (cutdown) and thread a polyethylene catheter (intracatheter) into the vein. A peripheral inserted central catheter (PICC) is such an intravenous device. The insertion site is usually the brachial vein, and the catheter tip lies in the superior vena cava, providing a peripheral access to the central circulatory system. This access device permits use of more concentrated and/or irritating solutions than can be safely or comfortably administered with peripheral access devices. PICC lines also allow long-term administration of antibiotics, chemotherapeutic agents, parenteral nutrition, or hydrating fluids. RNs certified in the procedure may insert PICC lines. See Chapter 40 for further discussion of PICC lines and central venous access devices.

Fluids administered by any route are most effective when apportioned over a 24-hour period, which helps maintain normal body fluid levels and provides better regulation of the electrolyte balance. This in turn prevents end metabolic products from being excreted in concentrated form, which reduces the potential of formation of calculi and renal damage. In addition, fluid-spacing prevents circulatory overload, which may result in fluid and electrolyte shifts. Side effects from rapid fluid and electrolyte shifts include diarrhea and pulmonary edema. Side effects such as these can precipitate significant morbidity, and in some cases can contribute to mortality in severely ill patients.

Concentrated solutions of sodium, glucose, or protein should always be given slowly because they require body fluids for dilution. Hypertonic solutions cause fluid to diffuse from the tissues to equalize concentrations in the vascular compartment. The rapid dilution by the volume of blood in the superior vena cava makes it the preferred site for infusions of hypertonic solutions. An example of a hypertonic solution is the solution used for total parenteral nutrition (see Chapter 41).

Administering large amounts of a hypertonic solution into the alimentary tract causes a rapid shift of fluid from the vascular compartment into the intestinal lumen with a resultant decrease of blood volume. This process can lead to shock. "Dumping syndrome," which sometimes occurs after a gastric resection, is caused by this abnormal shift of fluid (see Chapter 40). In older therapies to reduce cerebral edema an attempt would be made to shift the edema through administration of hypertonic solutions. Newer pharmacological therapies for cerebral edema are more precise and safer. It is important to remember that unless in the tightly controlled situation of a "fluid challenge," administration of a large amount of fluid is potentially dangerous, even in an apparently healthy person. Under most circumstances, fluids of any kind should be replaced at the speed with which they are lost.

The size of the patient is another important consideration in fluid administration. The small adult has less fluid in each compartment, especially in the intravascular system. Hence, a small person becomes seriously dehydrated more quickly than a larger adult. Consequently small persons need fluid replacement at a lesser volume than a larger person. In addition, persons with small or inelastic vasculature become overhydrated easily.

### *Promoting oral intake*

Adults who have no circulatory or renal malfunction usually are given between 2500 and 3000 ml of fluids per day. Precautions should be taken so that the overzealous patient does not drink too much fluid in a day or does not take in too much (3 to 4 glasses) at one time. Excessive water intake may cause water intoxication.

When ill, many people find it difficult to eat or drink despite the need to do so. Nurses have a responsibility to encourage adequate food and fluids, thereby avoiding the need for parenteral hydration or nutrition. Water-based fluids such as fruit drinks, lemonade, punch, and noncarbonated beverages may be considered within the water requirement. Juicy fruits and popsicles are yet another way of offering fluids. Despite being water-based, coffee, tea, and some colas have a diuretic effect; caution should be exercised when using them to meet a fluid requirement. Carbonated beverages also have a high sodium content. In a strict sense, milk, eggnog, ice cream, frozen yogurt, cocoa, and nutritional supplements such as Ensure or Sustacal are actually considered solids because they are either protein-, lipid-, or milk-based. Soup and bouillon can provide both fluid and electrolytes. Sport drinks that are high in electrolytes are another way of replacing fluid and electrolytes. It is important to remember the bolus concept discussed earlier in the Intervention section when using sport drinks for replacement. Sometimes it is necessary to dilute the sport drink with water to avoid diarrhea. Be sure that the replacement modality is permitted in the patient's diet. For example, regular soda or sport drinks would be poor choices for fluid replacement in the diet of a person with diabetes because both contain large amounts of glucose.

The methods used in presenting food and fluid to patients may influence their consumption; often a small amount of either offered at frequent intervals is more useful than a large amount presented less often. Serving foods the patient is familiar with and likes helps to stimulate appetite. For example, familiar carbonated beverages are helpful to a nauseated patient. Consideration should always be given to the cultural and aesthetic aspects of eating.

Mouth care should be given to a dehydrated patient before and after meals and before bedtime. Dry oral mucous membranes (xerostomia) may lead to disruptions in the tissues of the oral cavity. Care should be taken to avoid irritating foods (spicy foods or those with high acidic content or fluids with temperature extremes). Stimulation of saliva may be aided by hard candy or chewing gum. Alternatively, an order for carboxymethylcellulose (artificial saliva) may be obtained. Lips should be kept moist and well-lubricated.

Vomiting and diarrhea are common symptoms of many illnesses, and most people suffer from them from time to time. Sodium and potassium are lost in vomiting and diarrhea, whereas chloride is lost only in vomitus. Replacement fluids include salty broth (for sodium replacement) and tea (for potassium replacement). Sport drinks are another electrolyte replacement option discussed earlier. Orange juice is an old standard for replacing potassium. Soda crackers are a sodium replacement option if fluids are not well tolerated.

A patient with a draining fistula from any portion of the gastrointestinal tract loses sodium, calcium, and potassium. Dietary supplementation is necessary. Milk will replace all the losses, and the patient who is lactose tolerant should be instructed to increase milk intake over normal levels. Medications are available for those with lactose intolerance. Lactase enzyme preparations, available over the counter, enhance the digestion of milk in those who are unable to do so. Consultation with a knowledgeable dietitian will yield a wealth of information concerning milk substitutes used for specific replacement needs. Patients with a permanent fistula or ostomy need to be especially careful to supplement sodium and potassium if vomiting, diarrhea, or fever occurs, which adds to their high electrolyte loss.

It is helpful to know the relative amount of various essential nutrients contained in the most commonly used foods (see Chapter 3). When losses must be restored, the patient needs to consume more than the usual daily requirement. Bananas, citrus fruits, all fruit juices, some fresh vegetables, coffee, and tea are relatively high in potassium and low in sodium. Salty broth and tomato juice provide extra sodium in addition to potassium. Milk, meat, eggs, and nuts are high in protein, sodium, and potassium. Current nutrition literature and the dietitian or nutritionist should be consulted liberally.

The nurse may encounter an order to "force" or "encourage" fluids. The amount required depends on the size of the patient, the amount of fluid loss, and the patient's circulatory and renal status. Taking these factors into account, the nurse is required to make an informed judgment to determine the amount. This information is then relayed to the rest of the nursing care team, including involved family members, or other caretakers.

If an elderly person living at home complains of pronounced weakness without apparent cause, the nurse should ask if cathartics or enemas have been used. If so, stopping this practice, replacing the sodium and potassium loss, and increasing fluid may reverse this symptom. Then the nurse may address the issue of proper bowel care.

Any patient with renal or circulatory impairment (shock, cardiac decompensation, or constriction of blood vessels due to disease) may develop electrolyte imbalances. Sodium and water may be held in the tissues, the potassium level of the blood may increase, acidosis may develop from inadequate tissue oxygenation, or the kidneys may be unable to excrete waste products properly. Patients with cardiac and renal impairments are instructed to avoid foods containing high levels of sodium, potassium, or bicarbonate.

### Gavage (tube feeding)

Either water, a physiological solution of sodium chloride, high protein liquids, or a regular diet can be blended, diluted, and given by gavage (see Chapter 40). As previously mentioned, high-protein tube feeding can cause water deficit through osmotic diuresis. The water content in the tube feeding needs to be increased when (1) the patient complains of thirst; (2) the protein or electrolyte content of the tube feeding is high; (3) the patient has a fever or a disease causing an increased metabolic rate, (4) the urinary output is concentrated, or (5) signs of water deficit develop.

### Parenteral fluids

**Types of solutions.** The nurse needs to be familiar with the commonly used parenteral solutions (Table 15-11). The physician's order will include the type and amount of solution and the rate of administration. A hypotonic solution of 5% dextrose in distilled water is often used to maintain fluid intake or reestablish water volume. Ascorbic acid and vitamin B (Solu-B) are frequently added for patients receiving IV fluids for several days. Dextrose 5% in saline solution may be given depending upon the serum levels of sodium and vascular volume; potassium chloride is frequently added to meet normal intake needs and replace losses. A physiological solution of sodium chloride is given primarily when sodium chlo-

**table 15-11** *Solutions for Intravenous Use*

| | Contents of Solutions | | | | | | | | |
|---|---|---|---|---|---|---|---|---|---|
| | Cations (mEq/L) | | | | Anions (mEq/L) | | | | |
| Type of Solution | $Na^+$ | $K^+$ | $Ca^{++}$ | $Mg^{++}$ | $NH_4^-$ | $Cl^-$ | $HCO_3^-$ Lactate | $PO_4^-$ | Glucose (g/L) |
| 5% dextrose in water | | | | | | | | | 50 |
| 10% dextrose in water | | | | | | | | | 100 |
| Normal saline (0.9%) | 154 | | | | | 154 | | | |
| 3% saline | 513 | | | | | 513 | | | |
| Ringer's solution | 147 | 4 | 4 | | | 155 | | | |
| 5% dextrose in Ringer's lactate | 130 | 4 | 3 | | | 109 | 28 | | 50 |
| Ringer's lactate | 130 | 4 | 3 | | | 109 | 28 | | |
| Ammonium chloride (0.9%) | | | | | 170 | 170 | | | |
| Sodium lactate ⅙ molar | 167 | | | | | | 167 | | |
| 5% dextrose in 0.2% saline | 34 | | | | | 34 | | | 50 |
| 5% dextrose in 0.45% saline | 77 | | | | | 77 | | | 50 |

ride has been lost in large amounts. Sodium and chloride deficit occurs with loss of gastrointestinal fluids, with burns, and with vascular volume deficits. A one-sixth molar lactate solution may be ordered when sodium but not chloride needs replacement; an ammonium chloride solution may be used to replace chlorides when added sodium is undesirable. Balanced solutions that contain several electrolytes may be used to replace fluid loss in surgical patients. Ringer's solution and lactated Ringer's solution are examples.

Body needs for carbohydrates may be partially met by giving fructose or 10% to 20% glucose in distilled water. These solutions are hypertonic, and therefore require additional water for excretion.

Amino acid preparations (Aminosol) are generally given into the central vasculature rather than peripherally. Whole blood or packed red cells are used to replace blood loss, but plasma, 25% salt-poor albumin, or plasma expanders can be given to substitute for blood protein loss and are used to reestablish normal volume and prevent shock. Dextran, the most commonly used plasma volume expander, increases the oncotic pressure of the blood, thus increasing the resorption of fluid from interstitial spaces and increasing plasma volume. Low-molecular-weight dextran decreases the blood viscosity and allows greater flow of blood through the capillaries. Thus it is useful in treating cardiogenic, hemorrhagic, or septic shock (see Chapter 17). Dextran may cause a prolonged bleeding time and is contraindicated in patients with renal failure, severe bleeding disorders, and severe congestive heart failure.[16]

**Administration.** The speed at which intravenous solutions containing electrolytes are infused should be regulated according to the patient's condition and electrolyte concentration. The patient is watched carefully for untoward signs, which would include those of excess fluids or electrolytes. Hyperkalemia can be particularly dangerous because it may cause cardiac arrest. When solutions containing electrolytes are administered, the nurse monitors the urinary output carefully. Marked decreases are reported immediately to the physician. Because the kidneys select the ions needed and excrete the surplus, a normal output is essential. If the nurse is planning the sequence of intravenous fluids, hydrating fluids such as one-half strength physiological solution of sodium chloride or glucose in water should be given first for the patient with a primary water deficit. Renal failure and untreated adrenal insufficiency are contraindications for the use of potassium. If these conditions are known or suspected, the nurse should verify orders for potassium administration. Physicians usually write the daily intravenous fluid orders after reviewing the most recent blood chemistry results.

The rate of administration of fluids is ordered by the physician and depends on the patient's illness, the fluids to be administered, and the patient's basic state of health. An infusion is rarely run at a rate faster than 4 ml/min. If the infusion is given continuously, or is given in the presence of impaired cardiac or renal function, the rate of administration is rarely faster than 2 ml/min. The usual rate for fluid loss replacement is 3 ml/min. This rate allows time for the fluid to diffuse into ECF compartments and avoids circulatory overload or increases in the blood volume to the point of producing a diuretic effect. It is important to note that when administering an IV infusion by gravity, different brands of administration equipment vary in drops per milliliter. To determine the rate of delivery, the nurse must check the packaging of the equipment used. The most important factor in determining the rate of delivery is the millimeters per minute, not drops per minute. Drops per minute are dependent on millimeters per minute.

For reasons cited earlier in the text, nurses should question the practice of increasing the rate of flow of intravenous solutions to complete the infusion at a specified time. The rate of flow should never be increased when administering parenteral nutrition. Nurses should recognize the signs of pulmonary edema (bounding pulse, engorged peripheral veins, hoarseness, dyspnea, cough, and rales) and monitor patients for signs of fluid overload (see Chapter 32). Persons at risk include those receiving concentrated solutions or rapid infusions, and those whose age or physical condition places them at special risk. At the first sign of increased blood volume, the rate of flow should be reduced to "keep vein open" rate (20 to 30 ml/hr depending on institution policy), and the physician should be notified. Particular care needs to be taken when delivering fluids to infants, elderly patients with circulatory or renal impairments, patients with cardiac disease, those who have had plasma shifts such as burn patients, and those with extensive tissue trauma from other causes. Patients whose plasma has shifted need to be watched carefully because the shift reverses itself after a few days, flowing from the interstitial spaces to the vascular space. This may potentiate an increase in blood volume with resulting pulmonary edema.

It is imperative that the nurse check the labels of fluid containers carefully for correct content and accurately record the fluids given. Expiration dates are also an important feature of the container label. A current text discussing the fundamentals of nursing provides useful information about contemporary equipment and practices used in parenteral fluid administration.

Patients receiving fluids intravenously are monitored for symptoms of hypervolemia or hypovolemia so that rates can be adjusted accordingly (Table 15-12). The insertion site is checked regularly, several times per shift, for signs of infiltration or inflammation. If infiltration occurs, the infusion should be stopped immediately and relocated. Peripheral IV sites are generally rotated every 72 hours. Dressing changes over peripheral IV sites are also changed every 3 days; institutional policy may vary. Electrolyte solutions that contain potassium are very irritating. Extravasation of these solutions may cause tissue necrosis. Infiltration of these solutions require a physician's attention. When dextran and other plasma expanders or other protein solutions are being given, the patient is observed for anaphylactic reaction (apprehension,

**table 15-12** *Complications of Intravenous Fluid Therapy*

| Observations | Nursing Actions |
|---|---|
| **CIRCULATORY OVERLOAD** | |
| Bounding pulse, venous distention, hoarseness, dyspnea, cough, pulmonary rales, restlessness | Notify physician<br>Reduce flow to "keep open" rate<br>Raise head of bed to facilitate breathing |
| **LOCAL INFILTRATION** | |
| Decreased rate or cessation of fluid flow<br>Tissue around needle or catheter site cold, pale, swollen, hard<br>Complaint of local pain | Stop infusion<br>Arrange to restart infusion at another site<br>Apply moist heat<br>Elevate lower arm |
| **THROMBOPHLEBITIS** | |
| Pain, redness, warmth, edema along vein | Same as for local infiltration<br>Cold compresses may be applied initially |
| **PYROGENIC REACTION** | |
| Fever, chills, general malaise, nausea, and vomiting 30 min after infusion started<br>Hypotension (if severe) | Switch to another infusion solution and run at "keep open" rate<br>Notify physician<br>Monitor vital signs<br>Save infusion fluid for culture |
| **ANAPHYLACTIC REACTION (WITH PROTEINS)** | |
| Apprehension, dyspnea, wheezing, tightness of chest, itching, hypotension | Switch infusion to nonprotein solution and run at "keep open" rate<br>Notify physician<br>Monitor vital signs |

dyspnea, wheezing, tightness of chest, angioedema, itching, hives, and hypotension) (see Chapter 66).

### Promoting comfort

People with fluid and electrolyte imbalance often have extreme thirst, nausea, and vomiting. These symptoms are distressing. This section discusses symptom management with comfort as the goal.

**Relieving thirst.** Thirst, the first and most insistent sign of dehydration, can cause a patient more misery than major treatments or the disease itself. Thirst may develop when fluids have been withheld for even a few hours. If fluids are being withheld intentionally, thirst may be made more bearable by explaining to the patient the reasons for withholding fluids, and when intake will be resumed. Mouth care will allay some of the discomfort of thirst. This care includes cleaning the tongue, teeth, and mucous membranes lining the oral cavity. A soft-bristled toothbrush or sponge designed for this purpose should be used. A mixture of half-strength peroxide and saline may be used for rinsing. It may be necessary to repeat this procedure every hour. Solutions that contain glycerin or alcohol should be avoided because of their drying effects.

When fluids are not permitted, the water pitcher at the bedside is removed. If it is questionable whether the patient will follow instructions, special provisions may be necessary. These may include involving the patient in activities that will distract him or her from thirst, such as reading, watching TV, conversation, or other activities. Thirst may compel some patients to obtain water in any way possible. The family should be involved to assist the patient in complying with restrictions.

Pronounced and continued thirst despite the administration of fluids is not normal and should be reported to the physician. In the immediate postoperative period, this kind of thirst suggests internal hemorrhage, temperature elevation, or some other untoward development. In the chronically ill patient, thirst may indicate the onset of a disease such as diabetes mellitus in which extra water is used by the kidneys to eliminate glucose. Thirst is also a symptom of hypercalcemia.

**Relieving nausea and vomiting.** Fluid and electrolyte imbalances may cause nausea and vomiting. Vomiting in turn leads to further fluid and electrolyte imbalances as a result of the loss of gastric secretions. A pathological cycle may be set up. Treatment for severe nausea and vomiting consists of replacing fluids and electrolytes by parenteral methods and the administration of antiemetic medications. The care of the person experiencing nausea and vomiting is discussed in greater detail in Chapter 40.

### Patient/family education

Education of the patient and family is important in the prevention and early detection of future fluid and electrolyte imbalances. Many of the principles discussed in the Interventions section have relevance as home-going instructions. Patients at particular risk for developing imbalances include those with chronic diseases, especially renal insufficiency, congestive heart failure, diabetes, and cancer. The teaching plan should include the signs and symptoms of deficit or excess, causative factors, and measures to prevent alterations in homeostasis. If drug therapy is included in the treatment plan, the patient and family should be instructed regarding the correct method of administrating the medication, correct dose, and therapeutic and adverse effects.

Depending upon the type of deficit or excess, certain food or fluids may be encouraged or restricted. The patient and family should be provided with a list of foods that are permissible, as well as those to be avoided. The nurse should instruct the patient to discriminate between fresh and prepared foods and read the package labels to determine the nutritional content of prepared foods. For example, the patient needing restrictions in potassium should be instructed to avoid organ meats, fresh and dried fruits, and salt substitutes. The patient should also be provided with a list of foods and their fluid content. Obviously it is important to include the caretaker in the teaching. The patient and caretaker should be informed of the need for periodic reassessment. Teaching should also include measures to prevent complications such as alterations in skin integrity or oral mucosa and infection. Skin assessment and care are important points to include in teaching. Persons with fluid excess and deficits are at risk for breaks in skin integrity. Caregivers should be taught positioning techniques for patients with mobility restrictions. Bony prominences and edematous skin are prone to breakdown. Healing is especially difficult in persons with edema.

## EVALUATION

To evaluate the effectiveness of the nursing interventions, compare patient behaviors with those stated in the expected patient outcomes. Successful achievement of patient outcomes for the patient with disturbances in fluid and electrolyte imbalance is indicated by:

1. Maintains functional fluid volume level; has adequate urinary output, vital signs within patient's normal limits, specific gravity of urine within 1.003 and 1.035, moist mucous membranes, stable weight, intake equal to output, elastic skin turgor, and no edema.
2. Patient and caregiver understand the treatment plan by stating possible causes of imbalance and verbalize plan to prevent recurrence of imbalances.
3. Reports a decrease or absence of symptoms causing discomfort.

## critical thinking QUESTIONS

**1** M.G. is a patient on your unit with a diagnosis of dehydration. The physician has ordered "force fluids." You must make a judgment as to type and amount since these were not specified in the order. Identify the additional patient data needed to make an appropriate nursing decision.

**2** A.J. has advanced cancer of the lung. He has been nauseated for several weeks after chemotherapy and has become malnourished. A serum chemistry profile indicates a serum albumin level of 2.2 mg/dl. Identify the data relevant for assessing calcium balance/imbalance and data needed to confirm your conclusions about the patient's electrolyte status.

**3** S.B. has end-stage AIDS and an opportunistic infection of the small intestine, which at this stage of his HIV infection can be treated but not cured. The opportunistic infection gives him copious amounts of diarrheal stools. Identify the foods and fluids and the information needed to approximate amounts needed to maintain fluid and electrolyte balance.

**4** E.L., an 83-year-old with cardiomegaly and periodic episodes of atrial fibrillation, insists on taking laxatives several times per week. Evaluate the risk this situation presents to E.L.'s fluid and electrolyte balance, and list the possible consequences. Describe a detailed teaching plan to correct this.

**5** C.L., a well-toned 30-year-old engineer, has volunteered to ride his bicycle in a 150-mile ride for charity that will take place over 2 days. This event is planned for early August, when the ambient temperature averages 85° to 90°F. As the nursing consultant helping to plan this event, list the fluid and electrolyte considerations for riders such as C.L.

## chapter SUMMARY

- Body fluid is divided into two major compartments; intracellular and extracellular, and has multiple functions. Electrolytes are chemical compounds that develop an ionic charge when dissolved in body fluids. The positively charged ions are cations and the negatively charged ions are anions. The precise concentrations of electrolytes in body fluids are vital to body function.
- In homeostasis, fluids and electrolytes are constantly being lost and replaced. In health, output equals intake. This balance is regulated primarily by the kidneys, but is assisted by the mechanism of thirst, by ADH, by the aldosterone-renin-angiotensin system, and by ANP.
- There is a constant dynamic process between fluid compartments. Diffusion across a cell membrane is accomplished by osmosis, or by expenditure of ATP. Fluid transport between vascular and interstitial spaces is controlled by hydrostatic pressure and colloid osmotic pressure.
- Each of the electrolytes exerts a particular effect on body function and has a specified range of concentration in the body fluids. Amounts of electrolytes over or below the specified normal range result in various disease states.
- Assessment of fluid and electrolyte balance includes monitoring of laboratory values, fluid intake and losses, frequent body weights, vital signs, skin turgor, muscle strength, condition of mucous membranes, presence of edema, level of consciousness, and changes in behavior.
- Management of fluid and electrolyte imbalances include intravenous and oral replacement, as well as management of the underlying cause of the imbalance. Collaborative management is the key to successful outcomes. In addition to physicians, dietitians and pharmacists are strong resources to consult in the plan of care.

## References


1. Bevilacquq J: Hyponatremia in AIDS, *Bailliere's Clin Endocrinol Metab* 8(4):837-844, 1994.
2. Bonne O et al: Adaptation to severe chronic hypokalemia in anorexia nervosa: a plea for conservative management, *Int J Eating Disord* 13 (1):125-128, 1993.
3. Brensilver J, Goldberger E: *A primer of water, electrolyte and acid-base syndromes,* ed 8, Philadelphia, 1995, FA Davis Co.
4. Brocklehurst JC, Allen S: *Geriatric medicine for students,* ed 3, New York, 1987, Churchill Livingstone.
5. Cirolia B: Understanding edema, *Nursing 96* 26(2):68-70, 1996.
6. Douban S et al: Significance of magnesium in congestive heart failure, *Am Heart J* 132:664-671, 1994.
7. Ferrin M: Magnesium, *RN* 59:31-34, 1996.
8. Giles T et al: Prolonged hemodynamic benefits from a high-dose bolus injection of human atrial natriuretic factor in congestive heart failure, *Clin Pharmacol Ther* 50:557, 1991.

9. Goldberg S: *Clinical physiology made ridiculously simple,* Miami, 1995, MedMaster Inc.
10. Gottlieb SS et al: Prognostic importance of atrial natriuretic peptide in patients with chronic heart failure, *Am Coll Cardiol* 13:1534-1537, 1989.
11. Groer MW, Shekleton ME: *Basic pathophysiology: a holistic approach,* ed 3, St Louis, 1989, Mosby.
12. Guyton AC, Hall JE: *Textbook of medical physiology,* ed 9, Philadelphia, 1996, WB Saunders.
13. Horne M, Heitz UE, Swearingen PL: *Pocket guide to fluid, electrolyte, and acid-base balance,* ed 3, St Louis, 1996, Mosby.
14. Hudak Cet al: *Critical care nursing: a critical approach,* ed 6, Philadelphia, 1994, JB Lippincott.
15. Margulis L, Sagan D: *Microcosmos: four billion years of microbial evolution,* New York, 1986, Summit Books.
16. Metheny NM: *Fluid and electrolyte balance nursing considerations,* ed 3, Philadelphia, 1996, Lippincott.
17. Miller M: Hormonal aspects of fluid and sodium balance in the elderly, *Endocrinol Metab Clin North Am* 24(2):233-248, 1995.
18. O'Donnell M: Assessing fluid and electrolyte balance in elders, *Am J Nurs* 11:41-45, 1995.
19. Rose BD: *Clinical physiology of acid-base and electrolyte disorders,* ed 4, New York, 1994, McGraw-Hill Inc.
20. Sims J: Making sense of tonicity and IV therapy, *Nurs Times* 92:42-43, 1996.
21. Symposium on fluid, electrolytes, and acid-base balance, *Nurs Clin North Am* 22(4):749-872, 1987.
22. Tan A et al: Atrial natriuretic peptide: an overview of clinical pharmacology and pharmacokinetics, *Clin Pharmacokinet* 24(1):28-45, 1993.
23. Young L, Koda-Kimble M: *Applied therapeutics: the clinical use of drugs,* ed 6, Vancouver, Wash, 1995, Applied Therapeutics Inc.

chapter 16

# Acid-Base Imbalance

MARTI REISER

## objectives

*After studying this chapter, the learner should be able to:*

1. Describe the mechanisms that maintain acid-base balance.
2. Differentiate between metabolic and respiratory acidosis and alkalosis.
3. Apply the pathophysiological principles of acid-base balance to interpretation of arterial blood gas (ABG) measurements.
4. Analyze components of ABGs to identify the type of acid-base disturbance.
5. Describe the causes and effects of each type of acid-base imbalance.
6. Utilize ABG findings in formulating the care of the patient with an acid-base imbalance.
7. Describe the management of patients with acid-base imbalance.

## NATURE OF THE PROBLEM

The human body functions optimally in a state of homeostasis. The maintenance of acid-base balance, which is one part of homeostasis, is evidenced by an arterial plasma pH value of 7.35 to 7.45. Many mechanisms in the body work together to achieve and maintain this delicate narrow range of pH that is essential for normal cellular function. This chapter presents these mechanisms along with the etiology, physiology, and pathophysiology of acid-base imbalances. The management of patients with acid-base imbalances is also discussed. The primary acid-base imbalances presented are metabolic and respiratory acidosis and metabolic and respiratory alkalosis.

Although the prescription of medical therapy to prevent and treat imbalances is the responsibility of the physician, nurses have the following responsibilities:

1. Recognizing situations likely to cause imbalances
2. Intervening to prevent imbalances
3. Carrying out preventive and therapeutic measures prescribed by the physician and monitoring patients' responses to these measures
4. Recognizing signs and symptoms of acid-base disturbances
5. Monitoring patients to prevent and recognize imbalances related to their specific conditions or treatments
6. Alleviating the effects of disturbances on the comfort and safety of patients.

## ETIOLOGY

Before discussing the etiologies of acid-base disturbances, it is essential to review the normal values of the acid-base system. An arterial blood gas (ABG) measurement will give the information needed to determine if the primary disturbance of acid-base balance is respiratory or metabolic in nature. It is necessary, therefore, to know the normal parameters for ABGs. Analysis of the patient's arterial blood gases requires an arterial puncture, but is highly accurate[1] (see the Research Box on the next page).

Arterial blood gases give information about a patient's oxygenation and ventilation in addition to acid-base balance. See Table 16-1 for the parameters, normal values, definitions, and implications. It is important to note the patient's temperature on the requisition when the blood sample is drawn since the ABGs must be corrected for temperature, especially fever, which increases oxygen consumption and the metabolic rate.[8]

The information ABG measurements provide reflects the functional status of alveolar and capillary diffusion, alveolar ventilation, pulmonary circulation, and pulmonary gas exchange. They are useful in identifying the cause and extent of the acid-base disturbance and in guiding and monitoring treatment.[5] The partial pressure of oxygen in arterial blood ($PaO_2$) is a measurement of the pressure oxygen exerts in its free form when dissolved in the plasma.[5] Normal $PaO_2$ values range from 80 to 100 mm Hg. The partial pressure of carbon dioxide in arterial blood ($PaCO_2$) reflects the measurement of the pressure of $CO_2$ dissolved in the plasma.[7] Normal $PaCO_2$ values are 35 to 45 mm Hg. The level of the buffer bicarbonate is measured by the $HCO_3$, which reflects the renal component of the ABGs; the kidneys compensate for changes in pH.[5] The normal value is 22 to 26 mEq/L. Base excess is a measurement of the total buffer base in the body. The base excess value is not essential for interpretation of acid-base disturbances.[6] Base excess normal ranges are 0 (+2 to −2 mEq/L). The anion gap reflects the difference between the unmeasured cations ($K^+$, $Mg^{++}$, and $Ca^{++}$) and unmeasured anions (albumin, organic anions, $HPO_4^-$, and $SO_4^-$) and is useful in identifying types of metabolic acidosis. For example, an anion gap of 16 to 20 indicates acidosis caused by retention of organic acids as in diabetic ketoacidosis. A normal range for anion gap is 12(±4) mEq/L.[4]

**table 16-1** *Arterial Blood Parameters Used for the Analysis of Acid-Base Status*

| PARAMETER | NORMAL VALUE | DEFINITION AND IMPLICATIONS |
|---|---|---|
| $Pa_{O_2}$ | 80-100 mm Hg | Partial pressure of oxygen in arterial blood (decreases with age)<br>In adults <60 years:<br>60-80 mm Hg = mild hypoxemia<br>40-60 mm Hg = moderate hypoxemia<br><40 mm Hg = severe hypoxemia |
| pH | 7.40 (±0.05 [2 SD])<br>7.40 (±0.02 [1 SD]) | Identifies whether there is acidemia or alkalemia; the value using 2 standard deviations (SD) from the mean is the common clinical value.<br>pH <7.35 = acidosis; pH >7.45 = alkalosis |
| $[H^+]$ | 40 (±2) nmol/L or nEq/L | The hydrogen ion concentration may be used instead of the pH |
| $Pa_{CO_2}$ | 40 (±5.0) mm Hg | Partial pressure of $CO_2$ in the arterial blood<br>$P_{CO_2}$ <35 mm Hg = respiratory alkalosis<br>$P_{CO_2}$ >45 mm Hg = respiratory acidosis |
| $CO_2$ content | 25.5 (±4.5) mEq/L | Classic method of estimating $[HCO_3^-]$; measures $HCO_3^-$ + dissolved $CO_2$ (latter is generally quite small except in respiratory acidosis) |
| Standard $HCO_3^-$ | 24 (±2) mEq/L | Estimated $HCO_3^-$ concentration after fully oxygenated arterial blood has been equilibrated with $CO_2$ at a $P_{CO_2}$ of 40 mm Hg at 38° C; eliminates the influence of respiration on the plasma $HCO_3^-$ concentration. |
| Base excess | 0 (±2) mEq/L | Reflects pure metabolic component<br>Base excess = 1.2 × deviation from 0<br>Negative in metabolic acidosis<br>Positive in metabolic alkalosis<br>Misleading in respiratory and mixed acid-base disturbances<br>Not essential for interpretation of acid-base disturbances |
| Anion gap | 12 (±4) mEq/L | Anion gap (or delta) reflects the difference between the unmeasured cations ($K^+$, $Mg^{++}$, $Ca^{++}$) and unmeasured anions (albumin, organic anions, $HPO_4^=$, $SO_4^=$); useful in identifying types of metabolic acidosis; value >16-20 indicates acidosis is caused by retention of organic acids (for example, diabetic ketoacidosis) |

**USEFUL FORMULAS**

Plasma anion gap = $[Na^+] - ([HCO_3^-] + [Cl^-])$

Calculation of third acid-base parameter when two are known:

$$[H^+] = 24 \times \frac{Pa_{CO_2}}{[HCO_3^-]}$$

Conversion of pH into $[H^+]$ (use formulas below):

pH of 7.4 = $[H^+]$ of 40 mEq/L

For every 0.1 increase in pH above 7.4, multiply 40 × 0.8

For every 0.1 decrease in pH below 7.4, multiply 40 × 1.25

For example, pH of 7.60 = 40 × 0.8 × 0.8 = $[H^+]$ of 26 mEq/L

From Price SA, Wilson LM: *Pathophysiology: clinical concepts of disease processes*, ed 5, St Louis, 1997, Mosby.

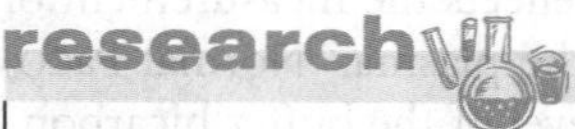


Reference: Christensen MA et al: Comparing arterial and end tidal carbon dioxide values in hyperventilated neurosurgical patients, *Am J Crit Care* 4(2):116-121, 1995.

In this nursing study, 19 adult patients who required hyperventilation to reduce increased intracranial pressure after head injury or neurosurgery were enrolled. The objective of the study was to compare the accuracy of end-tidal $CO_2$ values (a noninvasive, cost-effective method) versus the $CO_2$ measured by an ABG, which is known to be accurate, but a more expensive and invasive method. Researchers found that in this patient sample end-tidal $CO_2$ values did not accurately reflect changes in arterial $CO_2$ levels in the critical care setting. Recommendations were that further technological advances may lead to a more cost-effective, noninvasive method of $CO_2$ monitoring.

## PHYSIOLOGY: REGULATION OF ACID-BASE BALANCE

### ACIDS, BASES, AND pH

Acids are substances having one or more hydrogen ions ($[H^+]$) that can be liberated into a solution. Bases are substances that can accept or bind $H^+$ ions in a solution. Acid-base balance is actually homeostasis of the hydrogen ion concentration in body fluids.[4] The body produces large amounts of acids from normal metabolism everyday, yet despite this large addition of acids to the body fluids, the $H^+$ ion concentration remains low.

Hydrogen ion concentration is represented by the pH. This pH scale was devised by chemists to express the small quantity of $H^+$ ions in blood or body fluids.[4] The scale consists of

**table 16-2** *Mechanisms Regulating Acid-Base Balance*

| Action Time | Effect |
|---|---|
| **CHEMICAL BUFFERS IN CELLS AND ECF** | |
| Instantaneous | Combine with acids or bases added to the system to prevent marked changes in pH |
| **RESPIRATORY SYSTEM** | |
| Minutes to hours | Controls $CO_2$ concentration in ECF by changes in rate and depth of respiration |
| **KIDNEYS** | |
| Hours to days | Increases or decreases quantity of $NaHCO_3$ in ECF<br>Combines $HCO_3^-$ or $H^+$ with other substances and excretes them in urine |

14 points with water having a pH of 7. Water is considered to be neutral, i.e., acids and bases are in balance. The pH is the negative logarithm of the concentration of $H^+$ ions; therefore, as $H^+$ ion concentration increases, the pH decreases and vice versa. A low pH, therefore, indicates an acidic solution, while a high pH indicates a basic or alkaline solution.[2-4] A change in pH by 1 unit results in a 10-fold change in $H^+$ concentration.[2] Even minute changes, e.g., a change from 7.4 to 7.3, mean a major increase in $H^+$ ion concentration in the solution.

Normal arterial blood pH is 7.35 to 7.45. When the pH is in this range, the ratio of base ions to acid ions is 20:1. If there is an increase of $H^+$ ions, the pH decreases (<7.35), and the patient is said to have acidemia. The process of becoming acidemic is called *acidosis.* Alternately, if the ratio of bases to acids is increased, i.e., if there is an excess of bases, the pH will increase (>7.45), and the patient is said to have *alkalemia.* The process of becoming alkalemic is called *alkalosis.*

Even though this normal $H^+$ ion level is minute, a stable level needs to be maintained for normal cellular functions to occur. Minor changes in $H^+$ ion levels have major effects on enzymatic activities.[4] Hormone and enzyme shape and activity may be altered so much that their function is impaired; electrolyte concentrations or balance may be altered, which may cause decreased or increased responses in excitable membranes.

Hydrogen ions circulate throughout the body fluids in two forms: the volatile hydrogen of carbonic acid and the nonvolatile form of hydrogen in organic acids, such as sulfuric, pyruvic, phosphoric, and lactic acids. In a day's time, many acids are produced as the end products of metabolism. In the normal person, the lungs excrete 13,000 to 30,000 mEq/day of the volatile hydrogen in carbonic acid ($H_2CO_3$) as $CO_2$, and the kidneys excrete approximately 50mEq/day of nonvolatile acids. Mechanisms that regulate acid-base balance include chemical buffer systems, the respiratory system, and the kidneys (Table 16-2).

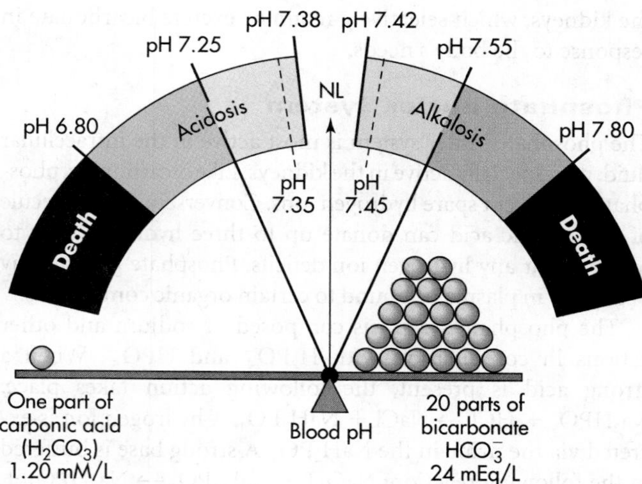


**fig. 16-1** Note that the relationship of 1 part carbonic acid to 20 parts bicarbonate maintains hydrogen ion concentration (pH) within normal limits. Increase in $H_2CO_3$ or decrease in $HCO_3^-$ causes alkalosis.

## CHEMICAL BUFFER SYSTEMS

The body cells are very sensitive to changes in pH, which the buffer systems in the body keep relatively constant. A buffer is a substance that can act as a chemical sponge, by either soaking up or releasing hydrogen ions so that the pH value remains stable.

The main buffer systems of the body are the carbonic acid–bicarbonate system, the phosphate system, and protein buffer system. The carbonic acid–bicarbonate buffer system is the system that is monitored clinically. If this buffer system is stable, the other buffer systems are stable.[4]

### Carbonic Acid–Bicarbonate Buffer System

The carbonic acid–bicarbonate system is present in extracellular fluid (ECF). Carbonic acid is formed by the combination of carbon dioxide and water: $CO_2 + H_2O \leftrightarrows H_2CO_3$. When a strong base is added to the body fluids, it is buffered by carbonic acid to a bicarbonate salt and water: $H_2CO_3 + NaOH \rightarrow NaHCO_3 + H_2O$. When a strong acid is added to the system, the bicarbonate buffer changes it to a salt and carbonic acid: $HCl + NaHCO_3 \rightarrow NaCl + H_2CO_3$. This carbonic acid then dissociates into carbon dioxide and water and can be excreted by the lungs and kidneys.

The ability to maintain a stable pH depends essentially on maintenance of the normal ratio of 20 parts bicarbonate to 1 part carbonic acid. The normal serum bicarbonate level is 22 to 26 mEq/L. The carbonic acid level is determined by taking the $PCO_2$ level (normally 40 mm Hg) and multiplying it by the constant 0.03, the dissolvability factor of $CO_2$. This computation gives an approximate value of 1.2. From these figures it can be seen that the normal bicarbonate-carbonic acid ratio is 20:1 (Figure 16-1).

This ratio of 20:1 is maintained by the lungs and the kidneys. The carbonic acid concentration is controlled by the amount of carbon dioxide excreted by the lungs. The depth and rate of respiration change in response to changes in carbon dioxide. The bicarbonate concentration is controlled by the kidneys, which selectively retain or excrete bicarbonate in response to the body's needs.

### Phosphate Buffer System

The phosphate buffer system is most active in the intracellular fluid; it is especially active in the kidneys. Like bicarbonate, phosphate can accept spare hydrogen ions. Conversely, one molecule of phosphoric acid can donate up to three hydrogen ions to make up for any hydrogen ion deficits. Phosphate groups may occur free in plasma or bound to certain organic compounds.

The phosphate system is composed of sodium and other cations in combination with $H_2PO_4^-$ and $HPO_4^-$. When a strong acid is present, the following action takes place: $Na_2HPO_4 + HCl \rightarrow NaCl + NaH_2PO_4$. A hydrogen ion is excreted via the urine in the $NaH_2PO_4$. A strong base is buffered in the following reaction: $NaOH + NaH_2PO_4 \rightarrow Na_2HPO_4 + H_2O$. $Na_2HPO_4$ is a weak base and minimizes the pH change.[4]

### Protein Buffer System

The protein buffer system is located in the plasma and inside cells; the protein hemoglobin in red blood cells is one of the proteins involved. Although most protein buffers are intracellular, they assist in buffering ECF. Some of the amino acids in proteins contain free acid radicals, —COOH, which can dissociate into $CO_2$ + H, thus adding a hydrogen ion. Other proteins have basic radicals, —$NH_3OH$, which can dissociate into $NH_3^+$ and $OH^-$; the $OH^-$ combines with a hydrogen ion to form water, thus removing one hydrogen ion from body fluid. The protein buffer system is the most plentiful chemical buffer system in the body.[4]

## RESPIRATORY CONTROL OF pH

The respiratory control center in the brain responds to increases of carbon dioxide and hydrogen ions in body fluids. Rate and depth of respiration are in turn controlled by the respiratory control of pH as follows: (1) when the pH value decreases (more acidic), respiratory rate and depth are increased, and there is greater excretion of carbon dioxide through the lungs; thus less carbon dioxide is present to produce carbonic acid by the reaction, $CO_2 + H_2O \leftrightarrows H_2CO_3$, and the pH increases toward alkalinity; and (2) when the pH value rises above the normal range (more alkaline), the respiratory center is depressed, rate and depth of respiration decrease, carbon dioxide is retained, and more carbonic acid is formed, moving the pH toward acidity. The respiratory system is extremely efficient and reacts quickly to changes in acid-base balance.

Because carbon dioxide is constantly being formed as a product of metabolism, the concentration of carbon dioxide in ECFs must be continuously balanced between the rate of metabolism and the rate of pulmonary excretion. The buffering capacity of the respiratory system is more than double that of all the chemical buffers combined.

## RENAL REGULATION OF pH

Both chemical buffers and respiratory regulation have limited ability to make complete adjustments in the pH level, and the kidneys make permanent adjustments in the pH level of body fluids. The renal regulation of the pH level is affected by control of the retention or excretion of bicarbonate and hydrogen ions. The kidneys usually excrete an acid urine because of the excess of acid metabolic products (nonvolatile acids), which must be eliminated by the renal route. Normally, almost all of the bicarbonate formed by the kidneys is retained.

Hydrogen ions secreted by kidney tubule cells and bicarbonate filtered into the glomerular filtrate combine in the kidney tubules to form carbon dioxide and water, which is excreted through exhalation ($CO_2$) and in urine ($H_2O$). In acidosis, excess hydrogen ions are secreted into the kidney tubules, where they combine with buffers and are excreted in the urine. In alkalosis, bicarbonate ions enter the tubules, which lack hydrogen ions that they normally combine with to form carbonic acid; the bicarbonate ions combine instead with sodium or other cations and are excreted in the urine. Hydrogen ions can be exchanged for sodium and potassium ions in the kidney tubules; therefore excretion or conservation of hydrogen ions can result in imbalances of sodium and potassium.

# PATHOPHYSIOLOGY

## COMPENSATORY MECHANISMS

The kidneys and lungs serve a compensatory function to maintain acid-base balance. In a disease state that leads to an acid-base imbalance, the normal bicarbonate–carbonic acid ratio of 20 : 1 is lost. In compensation, the kidneys attempt to compensate for changes in blood $CO_2$ by making a corresponding change in blood bicarbonate, and the lungs attempt to compensate for abnormal changes in blood bicarbonate by making corresponding changes in blood $CO_2$ (Box 16-1).

**box 16-1** *Expected Directional Changes with Acid-Base Imbalances*

| | pH | $HCO_3$ | $PCO_2$ |
|---|---|---|---|
| **Respiratory Acidosis** | | | |
| Uncompensated | ↓ | Normal | ↑ |
| Partly compensated | ↓ | ↑ | ↑ |
| Compensated | Normal | ↑ | ↑ |
| **Respiratory Alkalosis** | | | |
| Uncompensated | ↑ | Normal | ↓ |
| Partly compensated | ↑ | ↓ | ↓ |
| Compensated | Normal | ↓ | ↓ |
| **Metabolic Acidosis** | | | |
| Uncompensated | ↓ | ↓ | Normal |
| Partly compensated | ↓ | ↓ | ↓ |
| Compensated | Normal | ↓ | ↓ |
| **Metabolic Alkalosis** | | | |
| Uncompensated | ↑ | ↑ | Normal |
| Partly compensated | ↑ | ↑ | ↑ |
| Compensated | Normal | ↑ | ↑ |

From Sands JK, Dennison PE: *Clinical manual of medical-surgical nursing concepts and clinical practice,* ed 3, St Louis, 1995, Mosby.

Compensation is an effort to maintain the normal 20 : 1 ratio. Figure 16-2 illustrates the events in metabolic acidosis and the compensatory mechanisms for acid-base imbalance. See Table 16-3 for types of acid-base imbalances and the expected compensatory responses.

Another compensatory mechanism that can be used by the body in the presence of acid-base problems is shifting of hydrogen ions from the extracellular to the intracellular compartment or vice versa. With an increased level of hydrogen ions (metabolic acidosis), these ions can be shifted into the intracellular compartment in exchange for potassium. This shift alone increases the pH level of the blood. In addition, because the hydrogen ion concentration is now higher in the renal tubule cells, hydrogen is excreted in exchange for the

**table 16-3** *Types of Acid-Base Disturbances and Compensatory Mechanisms*

| Physiological Causes | Expected Response | Method of Compensation |
|---|---|---|
| **RESPIRATORY ACIDOSIS** | | |
| Carbonic acid excess: lungs not removing sufficient $CO_2$ (hypoventilation) | Acute: For every 10 mm Hg increase in $Paco_2$, 1 mEq/L increase in $HCO_3^-$<br>Chronic: For every 10 mm Hg increase in $Paco_2$, 3.5 mEq/L increase in $HCO_3^-$ | Bicarbonate production by kidneys increased; bicarbonate retained and chloride excreted instead by kidneys; secretion and excretion of hydrogen ions in urine increased |
| **RESPIRATORY ALKALOSIS** | | |
| Carbonic acid deficit: lungs removing too much $CO_2$ (hyperventilation) | Acute: For every 10 mm Hg decrease in $Paco_2$, 2 mEq/L increase in $HCO_3^-$<br>Chronic: For every 10 mm Hg decrease in $Paco_2$, 5 mEq/L increase in $HCO_3^-$ | Kidneys increase excretion of bicarbonate ions |
| **METABOLIC ACIDOSIS** | | |
| Bicarbonate deficit: retention of acid metabolites, diabetic ketoacidosis, excess acid intake (salicylate poisoning), hyperkalemia, or loss of bicarbonate | For every 1 mEq decrease in $HCO_3^-$, 1.2 mm Hg decrease in $Paco_2$ | Increased rate and depth of respiration cause increased excretion of $CO_2$ by lungs; formation of bicarbonate ions in the kidneys increased |
| **METABOLIC ALKALOSIS** | | |
| Bicarbonate excess: excess intake (sodium bicarbonate, carbonated drinks) or retention of bicarbonate, potassium depletion, loss of acid | For every 1 mEq increase in $HCO_3^-$, 0.7 mm Hg increase in $Paco_2$ | Rate and depth of respiration decreased; lungs retain more $CO_2$; kidneys excrete bicarbonate |

Adapted from Price SA, Wilson LM: *Pathophysiology: clinical concepts of disease processes,* ed 5, St Louis, 1997, Mosby.

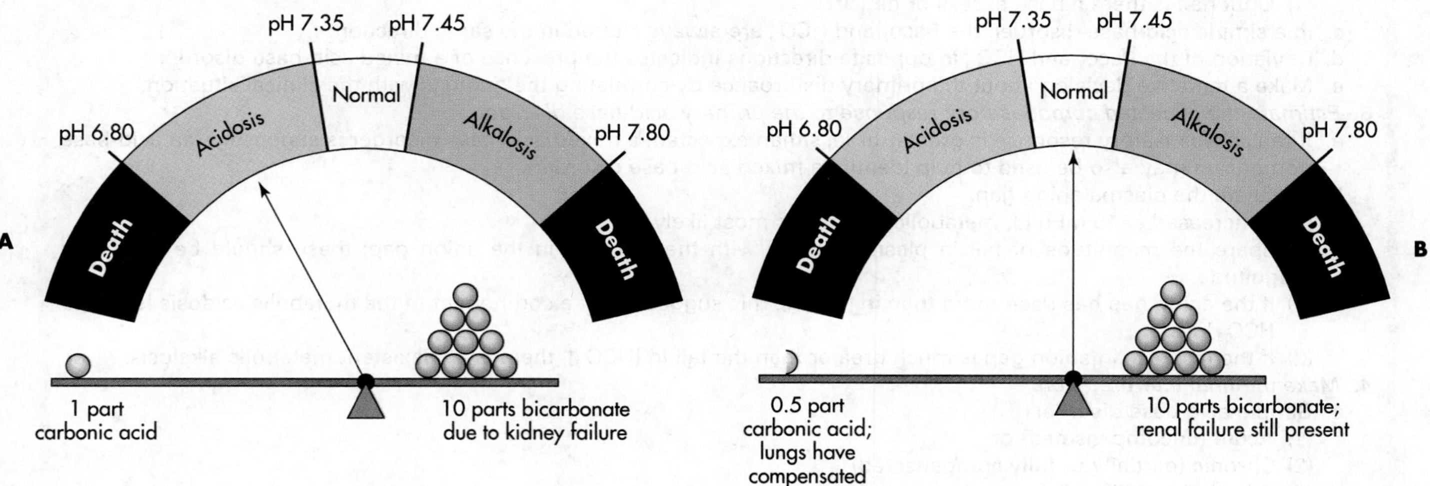


**fig. 16-2** **A,** Example of metabolic acidosis. Bicarbonate is decreased because of renal failure. Carbonic acid to bicarbonate ratio is 10:1; acid is present. **B,** Example of compensation. Note that acid is also decreased. Ratio returned to 20:1; pH level is normal.

reabsorbed sodium. In metabolic alkalosis, hydrogen ions are pulled from the intracellular compartment, and potassium ions are shifted into the intracellular compartment. Again, this shift alone helps to lower the pH level. Also, because potassium ion concentration is now higher in the renal tubule cells, potassium is excreted for the conserved sodium, and hydrogen ions are also conserved. These compensatory mechanisms can lead to hyperkalemia when acidosis is present and hypokalemia when alkalosis is present.

It must be remembered that the buffer systems and the compensatory mechanisms provide for only temporary adjustment, and the underlying cause of the disturbance must be identified and corrected. However, the kidneys can make permanent adjustments, as seen in persons who have respiratory acidosis as a result of chronic obstructive pulmonary disease (see Chapter 32).

## TYPES OF ACID-BASE DISTURBANCES

The two types of acidosis and alkalosis are respiratory and metabolic. The major effect of acidosis is depression of the central nervous system, as evidenced by disorientation followed by coma. Alkalosis is characterized by overexcitability of

### box 16-2 A Systematic Approach to the Assessment of Acid-Base Disturbances

**BEGIN WITH A HIGH DEGREE OF CLINICAL SUSPICION**

1. Examine the *clinical history* for disease processes that may lead to simple acid-base disorders.
   a. This requires knowledge of the pathogenesis of the various acid-base disorders.
   b. For example, one might expect a person with advanced chronic obstructive pulmonary disease to develop respiratory acidosis.
2. Note *clinical signs and symptoms* that suggest an acid-base disorder.
   a. Unfortunately, many of the signs and symptoms of an acid-base disorder are subtle or nonspecific.
   b. For example, Kussmaul respirations in a diabetic patient may represent respiratory compensation for metabolic acidosis.
3. *Examine laboratory reports of the electrolytes and other data* that suggest disease processes associated with acid-base disorders.
   a. For example, hypokalemia is often associated with metabolic alkalosis.
   b. For example, an elevated serum creatinine level indicates renal insufficiency, and renal insufficiency and failure are usually associated with metabolic acidosis.

**EVALUATE ACID-BASE VARIABLES TO IDENTIFY THE TYPE OF DISORDER**

1. First, *examine the arterial blood pH* to determine the direction and magnitude of the acid-base disturbance.
   a. If decreased, the patient has acidemia with two potential causes: metabolic acidosis or respiratory acidosis.
   b. If increased, the patient has alkalemia with two potential causes: metabolic alkalosis or respiratory alkalosis.
   c. It is helpful to note that the renal and respiratory compensations rarely return the pH to normal so that a normal pH in the presence of changes in the $Paco_2$ and $HCO_3^-$ suggests a mixed disorder; for example, a person with a combined respiratory acidosis and metabolic alkalosis might have a normal pH.
2. *Examine the respiratory ($Paco_2$) and metabolic ($HCO_3^-$) variables in relation to the pH* to tentatively characterize the primary disturbance as a respiratory, metabolic, or mixed disorder.
   a. Is the $Paco_2$ normal (40 mm Hg), increased, or decreased?
   b. Is the $HCO_3^-$ normal (24 mEq/L), increased, or decreased?
      (1) Optional: Is there a base excess or deficit?
   c. In a simple acid-base disorder, the $Paco_2$ and $HCO_3^-$ are always altered in the same direction.
   d. Deviation of the $Paco_2$ and $HCO_3^-$ in opposite directions indicates the presence of a mixed acid-base disorder.
   e. Make a tentative decision about the primary disturbance by correlating the findings with the clinical situation.
3. *Estimate the expected compensatory response to the primary acid-base disorder.*
   a. If the compensatory response is greater or less than expected, a mixed acid-base disorder is suggested (an acid-base nomogram may also be used to help identify a mixed acid-base disorder).
   b. Calculate the plasma anion gap.
      (1) If increased (>16 mEq/L), metabolic acidosis is most likely.
   c. Compare the magnitude of fall in plasma [$HCO_3^-$] with the increase in the anion gap; these should be similar in magnitude.
      (1) If the anion gap has risen more than in [$HCO_3^-$], this suggests that a component of the metabolic acidosis is due to $HCO_3^-$ loss.
      (2) If the increase in anion gap is much greater than the fall in [$HCO_3^-$], there is a coexistent metabolic alkalosis.
4. *Make the final interpretation.*
   a. Simple acid-base disorder
      (1) Acute (uncompensated) or
      (2) Chronic (partially or fully compensated)
   b. Mixed acid-base disorder
   c. Normal or wide anion gap: metabolic acidosis

From Price SA, Wilson LM: *Pathophysiology: clinical concepts of disease processes,* ed 5, St Louis, 1997, Mosby.

the nervous system, and the muscles may go into a state of tetany and convulsions. Acid-base imbalance always produces an imbalance of the body's other cations as well; therefore symptoms of these imbalances can also occur. Therefore using a systematic approach to assessment of acid-base disturbances is imperative (Box 16-2).

## Respiratory Acidosis: Carbonic Acid Excess

Any factor that decreases the rate of pulmonary ventilation increases the concentration of dissolved carbon dioxide, carbonic acid, and hydrogen ions and results in *respiratory acidosis.* An excess of carbon dioxide (hypercapnia) can cause carbon dioxide narcosis. In this condition, carbon dioxide levels are so high that they no longer stimulate respirations but depress them. Associated with the decreased respiratory rate are lack of oxygen and hypoxia. During respiratory acidosis, potassium moves out of the cells, producing hyperkalemia. Ventricular fibrillation may occur if the blood potassium level is greatly increased.

Respiratory acidosis can result from a number of pathological conditions that cause hypoventilation and $CO_2$ retention: (1) damage to the respiratory center in the medulla; (2) obstruction of respiratory passages, for example, pneumonia or chronic bronchitis; (3) loss of lung surface for ventilation, for example, atelectasis, pneumothorax, emphysema, or pulmonary fibrosis; (4) weakness of respiratory muscles, for example, poliomyelitis or hypokalemia; and (5) severe depression of respirations, for example, as a result of an overdose of respiratory depressant drugs. Chronic obstructive pulmonary disease (COPD) is the most common cause of chronic respiratory acidosis. Causes of respiratory acidosis are summarized in Box 16-3.

## Respiratory Alkalosis: Carbonic Acid Deficit

Excessive pulmonary ventilation decreases hydrogen ion concentration and thus causes respiratory alkalosis. A common cause of respiratory alkalosis is hyperventilation. A person who hyperventilates blows off large amounts of carbon dioxide. Hyperventilation may be caused by anxiety, pain, hypoxia, or lesions affecting the respiratory center in the medulla (brain tumor or encephalitis). Other causes of respiratory alkalosis are conditions that greatly increase metabolism (hyperthyroidism) and the overventilation of patients with mechanical ventilators. Causes of respiratory alkalosis are summarized in Box 16-4.

### box 16-3 *Causes of Respiratory Acidosis*

- Damage to respiratory center in medulla (head injury)[8]
- Depression of respiratory center by drugs (narcotics, ethanol, barbiturates, anesthetics)
- Obstruction of respiratory passages: pneumonia, chronic bronchitis
- Loss of lung surface for ventilation
  - Atelectasis
  - Pneumothorax
  - Emphysema
  - Pulmonary fibrosis
- Weakness of respiratory muscles
  - Poliomyelitis
  - Hypokalemia
  - Guillain-Barré syndrome
  - Amyotrophic lateral sclerosis (ALS)
  - Increased carbohydrate intake from tube feedings in patients being mechanically ventilated

## Metabolic Acidosis: Bicarbonate Deficit

When excess organic acids are added to the body fluids or when bicarbonate is lost, a metabolic acidosis or nonrespiratory acidosis results.

In conditions such as uncontrolled diabetes mellitus or starvation, glucose either cannot be used or is unavailable for oxidation. The body compensates for this by using body fat for energy, producing abnormal amounts of ketone bodies in the process. In an effort to neutralize the ketones and maintain the acid-base balance of the body, plasma bicarbonate is exhausted. The resultant acid-base imbalance is called metabolic acidosis, or *ketoacidosis.* This condition can develop in anyone who does not eat an adequate diet and whose body fat must be burned for energy. The reason that nutrition experts criticize extremely low-carbohydrate or high-protein–no carbohydrate reduction diets is the resulting ketoacidosis.

Metabolic acidosis can also develop whenever excessive amounts of lactic acid are produced, such as in prolonged strenuous muscle exercise or when oxidation takes place in cells without adequate oxygen, which may occur in heart failure or shock. Loss of large amounts of alkaline intestinal secretions, such as in severe diarrhea or through fistulas, can also create a bicarbonate deficit.

The normal functioning kidney excretes an excess of hydrogen ions in conditions of acidosis and, in so doing, retains potassium so that hyperkalemia, as well as acidosis, is present. In kidney failure, metabolic acids accumulate in the bloodstream. Causes of metabolic acidosis are listed in Box 16-5.

## Metabolic Alkalosis: Bicarbonate Excess

When excessive amounts of acid substance and hydrogen ions are lost from the body or when large amounts of bicarbonate

### box 16-4 *Causes of Respiratory Alkalosis*

- Hyperventilation syndrome (caused by anxiety, hysteria)
- Hyperventilation caused by the following:
  - Fever
  - Hypoxia
- Pulmonary disorders (pulmonary emboli, asthma, pneumonia)
- Lesions affecting the respiratory center in the medulla
  - Brain tumor
  - Encephalitis
- Excess assisted ventilation
- Hyperthyroidism

**box 16-5** *Causes of Metabolic Acidosis*

Increased acid production
- Ketoacidosis (uncontrolled diabetes mellitus, starvation)
- Uremic acidosis (renal failure)
- Lactic acidosis (shock, respiratory or cardiac arrest)

Increased acid ingestion
- Salicylates, ethanol, ethylene glycol

Loss of bicarbonate
- Severe diarrhea
- Intestinal fistulas

Adrenal insufficiency

**box 16-6** *Causes of Metabolic Alkalosis*

Loss of stomach acid
- Gastric suctioning
- Persistent vomiting

Excess alkali intake, e.g., overuse of antacids, Milk of Magnesia, or $NaHCO_3^-$; citrate in blood transfusions
Intestinal fistulas
Hypokalemia
Cushing's syndrome or aldosteronism
Potassium-depleting diuretic therapy

or lactate are added orally or intravenously, the result is an imbalance in which there is an excess of base elements. This imbalance, called *metabolic alkalosis,* does not occur as often as metabolic acidosis. In alkalosis, potassium enters the cells and hypokalemia results. A potassium loss causes a metabolic alkalosis, whereas an alkalosis causes hypokalemia.[4] An excess of bicarbonate in distal tubular fluid causes obligatory potassium loss.

Metabolic alkalosis can occur in the following conditions: (1) loss of hydrochloric acid from the stomach caused by vomiting or gastric drainage from a nasogastric tube (loss of chloride leaves more sodium to combine with and retain bicarbonate in the kidneys), (2) loss of potassium ions through intestinal fistulas, diarrhea, or in the urine, (3) ingestion of large amounts of sodium bicarbonate or other systemic antacids to treat indigestion or ulcers, (4) infusion of excessive amounts of bicarbonate or lactate intravenously, (5) diuretic therapy, and (6) excessive mineralocorticoids. Causes of metabolic alkalosis are listed in Box 16-6.

In metabolic alkalosis, breathing becomes depressed in an effort to conserve carbon dioxide for combination with water in the blood to raise the blood level of carbonic acid.

## COLLABORATIVE CARE MANAGEMENT

### RESPIRATORY ACIDOSIS

Treatment is aimed at increasing the alveolar ventilation rate to improve the exchange of carbon dioxide and oxygen. This objective is accomplished by identifying and treating the cause of the inadequate ventilation. Bronchodilators may be used to reduce bronchial spasm. Respiratory infections may be treated with antibiotics. Postural drainage and chest clapping are necessary for persons with obstructions of respiratory passages. Adequate hydration is also important to assist in removal of secretions. Supplemental oxygen may be used as necessary.

Because the respiratory center is narcotized by the increased amounts of carbon dioxide, the lowered oxygen tension of the blood is the stimulus for respiration. If a patient whose respiratory drive is dependent on a low $Po_2$ level is given large amounts of oxygen, the stimulus for breathing is removed, and respirations will cease. For this reason, uncontrolled oxygen delivery is never used with patients with carbon dioxide narcosis.

Low-flow oxygen (1 to 3 L/min) is given to a patient with COPD who maintains a chronically high $Pco_2$ level. Respiratory treatments are usually given using compressed air or room air instead of oxygen in these situations. If signs of ventilatory failure are present, the $Pco_2$ level is greater than 50 to 60 mm Hg, and the $Po_2$ level is less than 50 mm Hg, the patient may require intubation and mechanical ventilation.[5]

The major nursing responsibility is to recognize patients who have the potential for developing respiratory acidosis because of conditions that interfere with normal respiratory gas exchange. A patient whose airway is compromised by the presence of secretions must be encouraged to cough frequently or may need to undergo nasopharyngeal or tracheal suctioning. Pulmonary hygiene measures may be used to promote removal of secretions.

### RESPIRATORY ALKALOSIS

Treating the underlying condition usually resolves the respiratory alkalosis. Respiratory alkalosis becomes especially dangerous when it leads to cardiac dysrhythmias caused partly by a decreased serum potassium level. If a patient who is receiving assisted ventilation complains of dizziness or shows any signs of muscle irritability, it is likely that the depth of respiration is too great, and the respiratory rate of the machine should be decreased. If tetany is present, calcium gluconate is given intravenously (see Chapter 15). Renal function must be maintained to promote renal compensation of the disturbance.

### METABOLIC ACIDOSIS

Treatment of acidosis is directed toward the underlying cause and restoration of electrolyte balance. If the acidosis is severe, intravenous sodium bicarbonate is sometimes given. Bicarbonate preparations must be administered with caution, because they can induce a metabolic alkalosis and lead to tetany and convulsions. When acidosis is caused by renal failure, renal dialysis is necessary.

As the acidosis is corrected, potassium moves back into cells, and hypokalemia develops. If a patient being treated for acidosis needs to receive potassium, it is given after the acidosis has been partially corrected and as the pH level is returning to normal. It is important to bear in mind that even

**table 16-4** *Major Signs and Symptoms and Therapy for Acid-Base Imbalances*

| Signs and Symptoms | Therapy |
|---|---|
| **RESPIRATORY ACIDOSIS** | |
| Hyperpnea | Bronchodilators |
| Visual disturbances | Postural drainage |
| Headache | Chest clapping |
| Late: confusion, drowsiness, coma | Mechanical ventilation |
| Potassium excess | |
| **RESPIRATORY ALKALOSIS** | |
| Lightheadedness | Treatment of underlying condition |
| Numbness or tingling of fingers or toes | |
| Late: tetany, convulsions | |
| Potassium deficit | |
| **METABOLIC ACIDOSIS** | |
| Headache and mental dullness | Treatment of underlying condition |
| Kussmaul's respirations | Sodium bicarbonate (IV) |
| Late: disorientation, coma | Fluid and electrolyte replacement |
| Potassium excess | |
| **METABOLIC ALKALOSIS** | |
| Confusion, dizziness | Treatment of underlying condition |
| Numbness or tingling of fingers or toes | Diuretic: acetazolamide (Diamox) |
| Late: tetany, convulsions | |
| Potassium deficit | Fluid and electrolyte replacement |

**research** 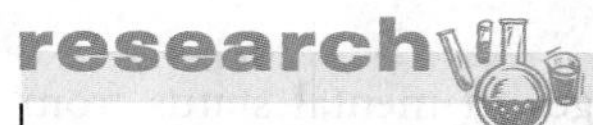

Reference: Szaflarski NL: Emerging technology in critical care: continuous intra-arterial blood gas monitoring, *Am J Crit Care* 5(1):55-65, 1996.

Ongoing research has sought ways to conserve blood in the critically ill patients. One way to conserve blood is to decrease the number of times a patient's blood is drawn for ABG measurements. Blood conservation may be critical in the adult as well as in the pediatric population. This article is a literature review on continuous intra-arterial blood gas monitoring. This type of continuous ABG monitoring conserves blood and provides up-to-the-minute information on the patient's acid-base balance allowing for quicker therapeutic interventions. Every 20 to 30 seconds the $Pao_2$, $Paco_2$, and pH are displayed on the monitor along with the derived values of oxygen saturation, bicarbonate, base excess, and total $CO_2$ content. Other benefits include: decreased risk of blood exposure to hospital personnel; increased efficiency of nursing care due to decreased time spent obtaining, processing, and retrieving ABGs results; and a potential decrease in nosocomial infection rate due to decreased entry into the intra-arterial system.

Problems that occur with the continuous intra-arterial blood gas sensor include aberrant blood gas values due to patient movement and blood gas sensors inadvertently touching the wall of the inner lumen of the artery. Other sensor difficulties were formation of microthrombi on the sensor. Sensors are only calibrated before insertion and are unable to be recalibrated once in the artery in contrast to ABG analyzers that are frequently recalibrated to allow for accurate ABG results. The author suggests further research to weigh patient satisfaction and morbidity associated with this system as well as cost savings due to decreased length of stay.

though acidosis is accompanied by hyperkalemia, the patient may be potassium depleted. The potassium leaves the cells in exchange for the hydrogen ions, and much of it is excreted.

Maintenance of adequate respiratory function in a patient with metabolic acidosis facilitates the excretion of carbon dioxide. If the kidneys are functioning well, they can help correct the acidosis by producing more bicarbonate. Because some conditions that lead to metabolic acidosis cause a hyperosmolar state as well, osmotic diuresis will take place, and the patient will need fluid replacement along with careful monitoring of intake and output. If changes in the sensorium have resulted, safety precautions are instituted.

## METABOLIC ALKALOSIS

Treatment is aimed at correcting the cause of the metabolic alkalosis. Sodium chloride or ammonium chloride may be given orally or intravenously. If the condition is associated with loss of sodium chloride, potassium, given as potassium chloride, must be restored because it is lost with the sodium. A diuretic that acts as a carbonic anhydrase inhibitor (Diamox) may help relieve the alkalosis by increasing excretion of bicarbonate by the kidneys.

The nurse assists in maintenance of optimal respiratory function so that compensation can take place through this mechanism. Careful monitoring of the patient for adequate renal function and safety precautions are important in the nursing care of patients with metabolic alkalosis. Because convulsions may occur, precautions are taken for the patient's protection.

It is important to treat the underlying cause of the acid-base imbalance (Table 16-4). In mixed acid-base imbalances, signs and symptoms as well as management vary. Frequent analysis of arterial blood gas measurements is necessary to monitor effectiveness of treatments (see the Research Box).

## NURSING MANAGEMENT OF PATIENTS WITH RESPIRATORY ACIDOSIS

### ■ ASSESSMENT

#### Subjective Data

Data to be collected include complaints of headache, confusion, lethargy, nausea, irritability, anxiety, and blurred vision.[6]

### Objective Data

Objective data may include changes in mental status from confusion to lethargy, to stupor, and then to coma. Tachycardia and hypertension may be present as well as cardiac dysrhythmias. Respirations may be slow and shallow secondary to respiratory center depression.[8] Hyperkalemia results from movement of potassium out of cells as the hydrogen ions move in.

## NURSING DIAGNOSES

Nursing diagnosis are determined from analysis of patient data. Nursing diagnosis for the patient with respiratory acidosis may include but are not limited to:

| Diagnostic Title | Possible Etiological Factors |
|---|---|
| Gas exchange, impaired | Hypoventilation |
| Thought processes, altered | Central nervous system (CNS) depression |
| Anxiety | Hypoxia, hospitalization |
| Ineffective family coping, risk for | Illness of family member |

## EXPECTED PATIENT OUTCOMES

Expected patient outcomes for a patient with respiratory acidosis include but are not limited to:

1. Maintains patent airway and adequate breathing rate and rhythm with return of ABGs to patient's normal.
2. Is alert and oriented to person, place, and time or to his or her normal baseline level of consciousness (LOC).
3. Copes with anxiety.
4. Patient/family are aware of effective support systems with effective coping exhibited.

## INTERVENTIONS

### Promoting Oxygenation and Comfort

The patient with respiratory acidosis requires thorough and frequent assessment of breath sounds, respiratory rate and rhythm, and maintenance of a patent airway. The nurse needs to be prepared for the potential of using artificial airways. Providing a position of comfort for the patient allows for ease of respirations. Obtaining and monitoring ABG results and vital signs and reporting changes in the patient's condition are crucial to patient care. The nurse provides and monitors supplemental oxygen as ordered. Turning the patient every 2 hours and as needed (prn), providing pulmonary hygiene as ordered and prn, providing comfort measures such as mouth care, and assisting with activities of daily living are all part of nursing care for this patient. The patient should be instructed regarding coughing and deep breathing techniques.

### Promoting Tissue Perfusion

The patient with respiratory acidosis requires frequent neurological assessment. The person's baseline LOC should be documented and monitored frequently. Reorientation to reality is done as necessary by providing calendars, clocks, familiar objects,[8] and frequent family visits.

### Relieving Anxiety

Assess the patient for visible signs of anxiety. Provide a calm, relaxed environment. Give clear, concise explanations of treatment plans. Encourage the patient to express feelings. Provide comfort measures. In addition to orienting the patient to reality frequently, providing support and information to the patient and family helps allay anxiety and fears. Relaxation techniques may be useful in reducing anxiety. As pain and anxiety are closely related, ensure that the patient's pain is under control. However, the patient must be monitored for signs of respiratory depression, which is an adverse effect of narcotic analgesics. Assist the patient to identify coping mechanisms to deal with anxiety and stress.

### Enhancing Coping Mechanisms

Patients in respiratory acidosis are frequently confused and anxious. The patient's family often feels anxious and has difficulty coping. The nurse provides support and information to family members about the patient's ongoing condition. The nurse encourages questions and open communication with entire staff and facilitates family and physician communication.

### Patient/Family Education

The nurse develops an individualized teaching plan based on patient and family learning needs. Diet and medications as well as signs and symptoms of respiratory acidosis are some potential learning needs. Patients with chronic obstructive pulmonary disease are at high risk for this acid-base disorder and may require further pulmonary rehabilitation.[8]

## EVALUATION

To evaluate the effectiveness of the nursing interventions, compare patient behaviors with those stated in the expected outcomes. Successful achievement of expected outcomes for the patient with respiratory acidosis is indicated by:

1a. Demonstrates improved ventilation and oxygenation.
 b. Vital signs, ABGs, and cardiac rhythm are within patient's normal range.
2. Returns to the patient's normal LOC.
3. Reports reduced anxiety.
4. Family utilizes adequate coping mechanisms.

# NURSING MANAGEMENT OF PATIENTS WITH RESPIRATORY ALKALOSIS

## ASSESSMENT

### Subjective Data

Subjective data may include anxiety (most common cause of hyperventilation), shortness of breath, muscle cramps or weakness, perioral tingling, palpitations, panic, and dyspnea.[6]

### Objective Data

Light-headedness and confusion occur as a result of cerebral hypoxia. The person with respiratory alkalosis may exhibit hyperventilation, tachycardia, muscle weakness, and a positive Chvostek's sign or Trousseau's sign indicating a low ionized serum calcium level secondary to hyperventilation and alkalosis.[3,8] Deep tendon reflexes may be hyperactive, the patient's gait may be unsteady, and muscle spasms or tetany may be present.[8] The patient may be agitated, irrational, belligerent, or psychotic. Seizures may occur in extreme cases. Serum potassium levels will be decreased.

## NURSING DIAGNOSES

Nursing diagnoses are determined from analysis of patient data. Nursing diagnoses for the patient with respiratory alkalosis may include but are not limited to:

| Diagnostic Title | Possible Etiological Factors |
|---|---|
| Anxiety | Stress, fear |
| Breathing pattern, ineffective | Hyperventilation |
| Thought processes, impaired | CNS excitability, irritability |
| Injury, risk for | Change in LOC and potential for seizures |

## EXPECTED PATIENT OUTCOMES

Ascertaining and treating the cause or causes of the patient's anxiety and hyperventilation are the goal. Expected outcomes for the patient with respiratory alkalosis may include but are not limited to:

1. Reports decreased anxiety; verbalizes methods to cope with anxiety.
2. Returns to normal respiratory rate and rhythm or at least decreased hyperventilation, with return to baseline ABGs.
3. Exhibits reorientation to person, place, and time as per patient's baseline.
4. Is free from injury.

## INTERVENTIONS

### Allaying Anxiety

The patient with respiratory alkalosis usually hyperventilates because of anxiety. The nurse helps to allay the anxiety and gives antianxiety medications as ordered. Sometimes the intervention may be having the patient breathe into a paper bag. This will trap $CO_2$, allowing the patient to rebreathe and thus increase the $CO_2$ level and slow the respiratory rate. Relaxation techniques may be useful adjuncts to allay anxiety (see Chapter 6).

### Promoting Oxygenation

A thorough frequent assessment of respiratory rate and rhythm is essential, in addition to encouraging the patient to slow his or her respiratory rate. Maintain a calm, comforting attitude when dealing with the patient and family. Position the patient to promote maximal ease of inspiration. Assist the patient with relaxation techniques.

### Promoting Tissue Perfusion

The patient may need frequent reorientation. If possible, ask the family to bring in familiar objects from home, such as calendars, clocks, or photographs. Encourage the family to assist in reorientation. Reading the paper aloud or watching the news may be helpful to review current events. When giving instructions, use simple direct statements and allow the patient adequate time to respond.

### Preventing Injuries

The patient should be frequently assessed for potential injuries. A neurological assessment should be performed and documented. Any changes in neurological functioning should be reported. Utilize the agency's fall prevention program and/or family members to prevent falls or injuries. Institute seizure precautions as needed. Assess the environment for potential hazards. Assess the patient's muscle strength in addition to gross and fine motor coordination.

### Patient/Family Education

The nurse develops an individualized teaching plan based on the etiology of the patient's respiratory alkalosis; for example, a stress reduction class to learn other strategies to decrease stress as a cause of hyperventilation. The patient and family should be taught how to prevent, recognize, and treat hyperventilation. The patient and family should be taught safety precautions for medications, especially those containing aspirin.

### Health Promotion and Prevention

Referrals for psychiatric counseling may be necessary to relieve the patient's anxieties. Other strategies may include teaching the patient muscle relaxation techniques, controlled therapeutic breathing, and visualization techniques.

## EVALUATION

To evaluate the effectiveness of nursing interventions for the patient experiencing respiratory alkalosis, compare the patient's condition with the stated expected outcomes. Successful achievement of expected outcomes for the patient with respiratory alkalosis is indicated by:

1. Reports reduction in anxiety levels.

2a. Demonstrates effective normal breathing pattern.

b. Has ABG results within patient's normal baseline.

3. Returns to normal LOC and orientation level.
4. Remains free from injury. No seizure activity.

# NURSING MANAGEMENT OF PATIENTS WITH METABOLIC ACIDOSIS

## ASSESSMENT

### Subjective Data

Subjective data may include complaints of anorexia, nausea, vomiting, abdominal pain, headache, and thirst if the patient is dehydrated.

### Objective Data

Objective data indicative of metabolic acidosis include confusion; hyperventilation; warm, flushed skin; bradycardia; and other dysrhythmias, decreasing LOC[4]; nausea and vomiting; Kussmaul respirations, especially if acidosis is due to ketoacidosis; and acetone on the breath if due to ketoacidosis. Symptoms may progress to coma if untreated.

## ■ NURSING DIAGNOSES

Nursing diagnoses are determined from analysis of patient data. Nursing diagnoses for the patient with metabolic acidosis include but are not limited to:

| Diagnostic Title | Possible Etiological Factors |
|---|---|
| Thought processes, altered | Secondary to CNS depression |
| Cardiac output, decreased | Dysrhythmias |
| Injury, risk for | Secondary to altered mental state |

## ■ EXPECTED PATIENT OUTCOMES

Once the underlying cause is detected and treated, expected outcomes for the patient with metabolic acidosis include but are not limited to:

1. Returns to usual baseline LOC.
2. Returns to normal baseline parameters for vital signs with improved cardiac output and decreased or resolved dysrhythmias.
3. Remains in a safe, secure environment without injury.

## ■ INTERVENTIONS

### Promoting Tissue Perfusion and Oxygenation

The nurse monitors the patient's LOC frequently and reorients as necessary. Other interventions include monitoring vital signs, especially respiratory rate and rhythm; blood pressure to assess cardiac output, temperature to assess for fever, and ABGs to assess the effects of treatment. Cardiac monitoring may be indicated to detect any dysrhythmias.

### Promoting Safety

The nurse provides a safe, secure, monitored environment for the patient. Safety precautions are especially important for a confused patient.

### Patient/Family Education

An individualized teaching plan is formulated by the nurse to meet the patient and family needs. If ketoacidosis is the cause, teaching about diabetes may be instituted to prevent recurrence of symptoms.

### Evaluation

To evaluate effectiveness of nursing interventions, compare patient behaviors with those stated in the expected patient outcomes. Successful achievement of patient outcomes for the patient with metabolic acidosis are indicated by:

1. Exhibits baseline-level of consciousness and orientation.
2. Returns to normal baseline parameters for vital signs and cardiac output with cardiac dysrhythmias resolved.
3. Remains free from injury.

# NURSING MANAGEMENT OF PATIENTS WITH METABOLIC ALKALOSIS

## ■ ASSESSMENT

### Subjective Data

These data may include reports of prolonged vomiting or nasogastric suctioning; frequent self-induced vomiting; muscle weakness; lightheadedness; ingestion of large amounts of licorice; muscle cramping, twitching, or tingling; and circumoral tingling.[6]

### Objective Data

The patient may exhibit mental confusion, dizziness, and changes in LOC. Other data may include hyperreflexia, tetany, dysrhythmias, seizures, respiratory failure; a positive Chvostek's or Trousseau's sign if the patient has a low ionized serum calcium level, decreased hand grasps secondary to muscle weakness, and generalized muscle weakness. A decreased calcium and/or potassium level may be present. There may be impaired concentration and potentially seizures. Electrocardiographic changes consistent with hypokalemia may be present.

## ■ NURSING DIAGNOSES

Nursing diagnoses are determined from analysis of patient data. Nursing diagnoses for the patient with metabolic alkalosis include but are not limited to:

| Diagnostic Title | Possible Etiological Factors |
|---|---|
| Thought processes, altered | CNS excitation |
| Cardiac output, decreased | Dysrhythmias and electrolyte imbalances |
| Injury, risk for | Muscle weakness, tetany, confusion and possible seizures |

## ■ EXPECTED PATIENT OUTCOMES

Expected outcomes for the patient with metabolic alkalosis may include but are not limited to:

1. Is oriented to time, place, and person as per baseline status.
2. Returns to normal baseline range for cardiac output with resolution of electrolyte imbalances and cardiac dysrhythmias.
3. Maintains a safe, secure environment.

## ■ INTERVENTIONS

### Promoting Tissue Perfusion and Oxygenation

The nurse monitors the patient's LOC and reorients the patient frequently. The use of familiar objects with frequent visits of significant others aids in reorienting the patient.

### Promoting Return of Electrolyte Balance

The nurse monitors serum electrolytes and ABGs and administers replacement therapy such as potassium and chloride as ordered. The nurse observes the patient for any signs or symptoms of electrolyte deficiencies. Antiemetics may be administered to relieve vomiting. An accurate record of intake and output should be kept (see Chapter 15).

### Promoting Safety

The nurse maintains a safe, secure environment for the patient. The nurse institutes seizure precautions and falls prevention as necessary.

### Patient/Family Education

The type of teaching depends on the etiology of the alkalosis. The goal of patient and family education is to prevent recurrence of the imbalance. The patient and family should also be taught signs and symptoms of metabolic alkalosis to detect the onset of any recurrence. If the cause of alkalosis was related to diuretic therapy, reinforcement regarding correct medication use is warranted. Information should be given regarding excessive use of antacids. Teaching the patient how to manage persistent vomiting may prevent future episodes of metabolic alkalosis. If an eating disorder is suspected, a referral to a psychologist is indicated.

## ■ EVALUATION

To evaluate the effectiveness of nursing interventions, compare patient behaviors with those stated in the expected patient outcomes. Successful achievement of expected outcomes for patients with metabolic alkalosis is indicated by:

1. Mental status has returned to baseline.
2. Cardiac dysrhythmias are resolved.
3. Remains free from injury.

## GERONTOLOGICAL CONSIDERATIONS

The elderly, particularly those with COPD, are at risk of developing acid-base disorders that can lead to respiratory depression. Older patients are also at risk of developing any acid-base imbalance as a result of susceptibility to pH disturbances caused by normal physiological aging. In addition, several medications may alter the activity of normal pH compensating mechanisms. Preexisting or underlying conditions such as renal, cardiac, pulmonary, and endocrine disorders increase the risk of an elderly person developing an acid-base disturbance. Once an acid-base disorder develops, the elderly patient is less able to compensate for imbalances because of age-related changes in the kidneys.

## critical thinking QUESTIONS

**1** A 32-year-old administrative assistant comes to the urgent care center with a 72-hour history of vomiting secondary to influenza. She is lethargic and states, "My muscles are twitching." Her respirations are 18/min and heart rate is 110/min, and she has a fever of 100.4° F (orally). Her blood pressure is 110/68 which she states "is about normal for me." Her ABG values are as follows:

| | |
|---|---|
| pH | 7.57 |
| $Pa_{O_2}$ | 92 |
| $Pa_{CO_2}$ | 41 |
| $HCO_3$ | 36 |

Describe her acid-base status, probable cause for the imbalance, and treatment.

**2** A 55-year-old man, whose wife died unexpectedly last week, is found by his daughter to be unconscious on the sofa. On the coffee table is an empty bottle labeled Seconal. He is rushed to the emergency room. Objective data include the following:

| ABGs | | Vital Signs | |
|---|---|---|---|
| pH | 7.13 | BP | 104/68 |
| $Pa_{O_2}$ | 53 | Respirations | 7/min and shallow |
| $Pa_{CO_2}$ | 70 | Heart rate | 82/min |
| $HCO_3$ | 23 | Temperature | 99.6° F (rectally) |

What is your analysis of the situation? What treatment is indicated?

## chapter SUMMARY

### REGULATION OF ACID-BASE BALANCE

- Mechanisms that regulate acid-base balance include chemical buffer systems, the respiratory system, and the kidneys.
- The respiratory control center in the brain responds to increases of carbon dioxide and hydrogen ions in body fluids by changing the rate and depth of respiration.
- The renal regulation of the pH level is effected by control of the retention or excretion of bicarbonate and hydrogen ions.

### TYPES OF ACID-BASE DISTURBANCES

- The major effect of acidosis is depression of the central nervous system, as evidenced by disorientation followed by coma.
- Alkalosis is characterized by overexcitability of the nervous system, and the muscles may go into a state of tetany and convulsions.
- Any factor that decreases the rate of pulmonary ventilation increases the concentration of dissolved carbon dioxide, carbonic acid, and hydrogen ions in the blood and results in respiratory acidosis.
- Excess pulmonary ventilation decreases hydrogen ion concentration and thus causes respiratory alkalosis.
- When excess organic acids are added to the body fluids or when bicarbonate is lost, metabolic acidosis results.
- When excessive amounts of organic acid substance and hydrogen ions are lost from the body or when large amounts of bicarbonate or lactate are added, the result is an imbalance in which there is an excess of base elements, or metabolic alkalosis.

## References


1. Christensen MA, Bloom J, Sutton KR: Comparing arterial and end-tidal carbon dioxide values in hyperventilated neurosurgical patients, *Am J Crit Care* 4(2):116-121, 1995.

2. Gould BE: *Pathophysiology for the health-related professions,* Philadelphia, 1997, WB Saunders.
3. Methany NM: *Fluid and electrolyte balance,* ed 3, Philadelphia, 1996, JB Lippincott.
4. Price SA, Wilson LM: *Pathophysiology: clinical concepts of disease processes,* ed 5, St Louis, 1997, Mosby.
5. Sands JK, Dennison PE: *Clinical manual of medical-surgical nursing concepts and clinical practice,* ed 3, St Louis, 1995, Mosby.
6. Sommers MS, Johnson SA: *Davis's manual of nursing therapeutics for diseases and disorders,* Philadelphia, 1997, FA Davis.
7. Szaflarski NL: Emerging technology in critical care: continuous intraarterial blood gas monitoring, *Am J Crit Care* 5(1):55-65, 1996.
8. Tasota FJ, Wesmiller SW: Assessing ABGs: maintaining the delicate balance, *Nursing* 24(5):34-44, 1994.

# chapter 17 Shock

MARTHA L. ALLEN

## objectives *After studying this chapter, the learner should be able to:*

1. Contrast three major types of shock.
2. Explain early and late pathophysiological changes that occur with shock.
3. Describe organ compromise that may occur with shock.
4. Relate methods of monitoring for shock.
5. Describe methods of fluid replacement during shock.
6. Correlate effects of pharmacological agents used to treat shock and nursing measures for patients receiving drug therapy.
7. Describe therapeutic measures for shock other than fluids and drug therapy.

## NATURE OF THE PROBLEM

Shock is a syndrome characterized by hypoperfusion of body tissues that results in a lack of oxygen to cells and cellular hypoxia. Any condition that prevents cells from receiving adequate blood and oxygen can interfere with cellular metabolism and produce shock.

Blood flow depends on pressure changes within the vascular compartment. Blood flows from areas of greater pressure to areas of lesser pressure. In the systemic circulation, the mean pressure is highest in the aorta, where the blood leaves the left ventricle, and lowest in the right atrium. For the necessary pressure gradients to exist so that blood can flow, the following factors are required:

1. Adequate circulating blood volume
2. The ability of the heart to pump blood in adequate amounts to meet the body's oxygen and metabolic needs
3. Blood vessels with good tone, able to constrict and dilate to maintain normal pressure

Shock results from the disruption of one or more of these factors.

## ETIOLOGY

Shock may be classified as hypovolemic, cardiogenic, or distributive (Box 17-1).

### HYPOVOLEMIC SHOCK

Hypovolemic shock is the most common type of shock. Any condition that reduces the volume within the vascular compartment by 15% to 25% can result in hypovolemic shock. The signs and symptoms of hypovolemic shock progress in direct proportion to the percentage of blood loss from the intravascular spaces (Table 17-1). Common causes of hypovolemic shock are:

1. Excessive blood loss: trauma (most common cause), gastrointestinal (GI) bleeding, coagulation disorders, and surgery
2. Loss of body fluids other than blood: excessive diuresis (diabetic ketoacidosis or other hyperosmolar states), plasma loss from excessive vomiting or diarrhea
3. Abnormal shifting of fluid from the vascular compartment to a body compartment that does not usually contain a large amount of fluid, such as the gastrointestinal tract, peritoneal cavity, or the interstitial space. An example of this abnormal shifting is the movement of 5 to 10 L of fluid from the intravascular space into the bowel during a bowel obstruction. Peritonitis may result in the accumulation of 4 to 6 L of fluid in the peritoneal cavity within 24 hours. The collection of an excess amount of fluid in a body compartment other than the vessels or the cells is referred to as *third spacing of fluid.*

### CARDIOGENIC SHOCK

Cardiogenic shock results from the inability of the heart to pump sufficient blood to perfuse the cells of the body. Because cardiac output is the product of stroke volume and heart rate, the body compensates for decreased stroke volume by increasing heart rate. Initially this will maintain cardiac output. Tachycardia, however, can further compromise heart function and decrease cardiac output. Oxygen consumption is increased, and because the coronary arteries fill during diastole, the filling time is decreased. The heart thus needs more oxygen and receives less.

Although cardiogenic shock may be caused by various cardiac conditions including cardiac tamponade, restrictive

**table 17-1** *Clinical Manifestations of Hypovolemic Shock*

| Parameter (for a 70-kg male) | Class I: Early | Class II: Moderate | Class III: Major or Progressive | Class IV: Severe or Profound |
|---|---|---|---|---|
| Approximate blood volume loss (ml) | Up to 750 | 750-1500 | 1500-2000 | 2000 or more |
| % of blood volume | Up to 15% | 15-30% | 30-40% | 40% or more |
| Neurological/ behavioral status | Slightly anxious | Mildly anxious, restless; muscle fatigue and weakness evident | Agitated, confused; progressive decrease in activity; progressive thirst evident | Stuporous, lethargic, unconscious; dilated pupils may be evident |
| Heart rate | <100 | >100 Mild tachycardia | >120 Tachycardia | 140 or higher Irregular pulse, decreased pulse amplitude |
| Blood pressure | Normal | Normal | Decreased | Severe hypotension |
| Pulse pressure (mm Hg) | Normal or increased | Decreased | Decreased | Decreased |
| Respirations | 14-20, normal | 20-30, normal | 30-40, hyperpnea | >35, shallow, irregular |
| Urine output (ml/hr) | 30 or more | 20-30 | 5-15 | Negligible |
| Capillary blanch test | Normal | Slight delay | Defined delay | No refilling observed |
| Skin | Pale flushed, slightly cool | Slightly cold, pale | Cold and moist | Cold and cyanotic, mottled |

From McQuillian KA, Wiles CE: Initial management of traumatic shock. In Cardona DV et al: *Trauma nursing from resuscitation through rehabilitation,* Philadelphia, 1988, WB Saunders.

**box 17-1** *Types of Shock*

| | |
|---|---|
| HYPOVOLEMIC | Shock from loss of fluid from vascular system (through blood loss or fluid loss) |
| CARDIOGENIC | Shock from inability of heart to pump blood to tissues (decreased cardiac output) |
| DISTRIBUTIVE | Shock from massive vasodilation (from interference with sympathetic nervous system or effects of histamine or toxins) |

pericarditis, pulmonary embolism, severe valvular disease, or dysrhythmias, the most common cause is myocardial infarction. Studies have shown that in most patients who die from cardiogenic shock, at least 40% of the left ventricle was damaged by a recent infarction or by a recent infarction plus a previous scar. Despite improvements in managing cardiogenic shock, the mortality still remains greater than 80%.

## DISTRIBUTIVE SHOCK

Distributive shock is caused by a massive abnormal dilation of the blood vessels, resulting in a disproportion between the size of the vascular space and the amount of circulating blood. As vessels dilate, blood pressure falls and blood pools in dilated vessels, resulting in a decrease in venous return to the heart and a fall in cardiac output.

Types of distributive shock include neurogenic, anaphylactic, and septic. It may also occur with vasodilator drugs or acute renal insufficiency. *Neurogenic shock* results from interference with the sympathetic nervous system, which helps maintain vasomotor tone. Spinal cord injury, spinal anesthesia, and rarely brain damage are among the causes. *Anaphylactic shock,* which is a type of allergic reaction (see Chapter 66), may occur when a sensitized person has contact with an antigen to which he or she is sensitive. This hypersensitive reaction leads to the release of vasoactive substances including histamines, kinins, and prostaglandins. The body's response is massive vasodilation. The endothelial cells that line the capillaries separate and expose the basement membrane, which is permeable to fluid and plasma proteins. Large quantities of fluid may leak out of the capillaries, causing severe hypovolemia.[16]

### Septic Shock

*Septic shock* is a form of distributive shock that may result from infection, including those caused by gram-positive and gram-negative bacteria, viruses, and fungi. Gram-negative bacteria—including *Escherichia coli, Klebsiella-Enterobacter-Serratia (KES), Pseudomonas,* and *Proteus*—are the most frequent causative organisms in septic shock. Infections anywhere in the body can result in septic shock. The most common sites of infections leading to septic shock are the urinary tract, the respiratory tract, and blood. Some gram-negative organisms that may cause sepsis and septic shock are normal flora of the intestinal tract. As long as they remain in the intestinal tract, they do no harm and are even beneficial. However, if these organisms enter the bloodstream, they are lysed by leukocytes and release an endotoxin, which causes cellular injury and the cardiovascular changes associated with septic shock.

The release of the endotoxins from gram-negative organisms into the bloodstream causes the release of numerous vasoactive substances within the body, including histamine, prostaglandins, serotonin, bradykinin, and endorphins. Some of these cause massive vasodilation, others cause selective vasoconstriction, and some cause an increase in capillary permeability. The result is major maldistribution of blood within the body. The massive vasodilation results in hypotension despite the presence of very high cardiac output in the early stage of septic shock. The high cardiac output (hyperdynamic state) is thought to cause the skin's warm, flushed appearance in this stage of septic shock. Septic shock can be viewed as part of the continuum from infection to sepsis to septic shock to *multiple organ dysfunction syndrome (MODS)*.[2]

Conditions that predispose to septic shock include:

1. Extremes of age (very young or very old)
2. Immunosuppressive and steroid therapy
3. Chronic illness affecting the immune system (e.g., acquired immunodeficiency syndrome)
4. Surgery, especially urological and gastrointestinal
5. Malnutrition
6. Invasive instrumentation (e.g., intravenous lines and indwelling catheters)

Men with benign prostatic hypertrophy (BPH) are particularly susceptible to septic shock. A high incidence of urinary tract infections and multiple invasive urological procedures are common in persons with BPH and may contribute to the development of septic shock.

The mechanism by which septic shock occurs is not completely understood. Current thinking is that massive alterations in the microcirculation, including fluid leak from the vascular system, result in hypoperfusion of organ tissues, which in conjunction with the toxic effects of attacking, infecting organisms causes cellular and organ destruction.[17] Another prevailing view is that a cascade of inflammatory events occurs with septic shock and results in the release of biochemical mediators. These mediators cause a faulty cellular metabolism, which leads to multiple organ dysfunction and hypoperfusion of cells.[11]

Research indicates that hypoxemia may alter cell functioning in a way that can stimulate cellular processes. It is suggested that cellular changes include the production of tumor necrosis factor, interleukin 1, and interleukin 8; which affect the cells' "signaling system" and thus normal cellular activity.[43] As septic shock progresses, cardiac output falls, and the clinical picture resembles that of other types of shock.

Septic shock is of particular importance, because it has a high mortality rate and is likely to have resulted from a hospital-acquired infection. It is the 13th leading cause of death in hospitals and the most common cause of death in intensive care units. Septic shock, or *systemic inflammatory response syndrome (SIRS)*, will develop in 40% of all patients with sepsis and of those who develop septic shock, 50% to 60% will die.[30] When septic shock involves at least four bodily systems (MODS), the mortality climbs to 100%.[1, 44]

# PHYSIOLOGY

## MAINTENANCE OF NORMAL BLOOD FLOW

As previously noted, shock results from a catastrophic disruption in one or more components of the cardiovascular system. As long as the functional integrity of this system remains intact and the demand for oxygen and nutrients keeps pace with supply, cells and tissues function normally.

To assess normal functioning, oxygen use must be determined. This is done by assessing two key parameters—oxygen delivery ($DO_2$) and oxygen consumption ($SvO_2$). $DO_2$ is the product of cardiac output multiplied by oxygen saturation and hemoglobin level. $SvO_2$ is the product of cardiac output multiplied by hemoglobin level and the difference in arterial and venous saturation.[34a]

Oxygen use is directly affected by the adequacy of the blood supply, the pumping effectiveness of the heart, and the functional integrity of the vascular system. These three essential components of the cardiovascular system sustain the balance between the blood added to the arterial system with each heartbeat and the blood flowing through arteries to the vascular beds through precapillary arterioles.

Functional control of the cardiovascular system is designed to maintain effective arterial pressure and to sustain adequate blood flow to vital organs. This is done this by regulating control of both blood pressure and blood volume. The neural hormonal responses of the autonomic nervous system regulate this control by four mechanisms: neural regulators, circulating mediators, autoregulation, and local mediation.[39]

*Neural regulation* of arteriolar muscles is accomplished by the sympathetic component of the autonomic system. Stimulation of $\alpha$-adrenergic receptors causes vasoconstriction, and stimulation of $\beta$-adrenergic receptors causes vasodilation. *Circulating mediators* are the blood-borne hormones, such as glucocorticoids, that can be activated in times of stress. These hormones increase the sensitivity of muscle cells to catecholamines, which directly affect vasomotor tone.

*Autoregulation* is accomplished by myogenic reflexes that allow regulation of the vascular bed blood flow by automatically altering vascular resistance with changes in arterial pressure. This maintains pressure and volume in individual organ systems, especially the brain. *Local mediators* (e.g., lactic acid, carbon dioxide, and potassium), which are products of metabolism generated by tissues adjacent to arterioles, affect arterial pressure by vasodilation. During periods of high metabolic demand, this mechanism significantly increases blood flow to local areas of need.[38]

When shock occurs, these same mechanisms play key roles in survival of cells and vital organ systems. When they fail or are overwhelmed by the extent of the stress, there may be a drop in blood pressure and maldistribution of blood flow, which is directly related to hypoxia, oxygen debt, shock, and shock-related organ failure.[35]

## PATHOPHYSIOLOGY

### EARLY STAGE

In the early stage of shock, the body responds to hypoperfusion as it would to any other stressor. Many changes that occur are mediated through the sympathetic nervous system. Stimulation of the sympathetic nervous system results in secretion of norepinephrine from the sympathetic fibers and epinephrine and norepinephrine by the adrenal medulla. Both α- and β-adrenergic receptors are stimulated throughout the body. α-Receptors respond by causing vasoconstriction; β-receptors respond by causing vasodilation ($\beta_1$) and increasing rate (chronotropic) and strength of contraction (inotropic) of the heart ($\beta_2$). Other organs with $\beta_2$-receptors are also stimulated (respiratory system). The skin and the abdominal organs, which are rich in α-receptors, receive a decreased blood supply because of vasoconstriction. The heart and skeletal muscles, which are rich in β-receptors, receive an increased blood supply because of vasodilation. The heart beats faster and harder, and the respiratory rate increases in response to β-stimulation, thereby increasing oxygen delivery to the tissues. All the compensatory responses mediated through the sympathetic nervous system occur rapidly.

The overall effect of the sympathetic nervous system response in hypovolemic and cardiogenic shock is an increase in *systemic vascular resistance (SVR)*, the resistance in the vascular system against which the heart must eject blood. The widespread vasodilation characteristic of septic shock negates the effect of norepinephrine, resulting in decreased SVR.

Another compensatory response, mediated through the renin-angiotensin system, occurs more slowly. As cardiac output falls, the blood flow to the kidneys decreases. The juxtaglomerular cells of the kidneys convert plasma protein to angiotensin I. Angiotensin I circulates to the lungs where the angiotensin-converting enzyme stimulates its conversion to angiotensin II, a potent vasoconstrictor. Increased secretion of aldosterone by the adrenal cortex also occurs. Aldosterone causes the kidneys to retain sodium and water and secrete potassium, resulting in an increased blood volume. The secretion of potassium may result in *hypokalemia* during this stage of shock. In addition, decreased cardiac output results in decreased hydrostatic pressure in the capillaries, causing fluid to shift from the interstitial space into the capillaries. This also improves blood volume.

For a short period the compensatory mechanisms have a beneficial effect. The most vital organs, the heart and the brain, receive an adequate blood supply at the expense of the less vital organs, such as the kidneys and other abdominal organs. This allows time for the underlying cause of shock to be corrected. However, if the underlying problem is not or cannot be corrected, the compensatory mechanisms will not be able to continue to perfuse vital organs sufficiently, and the mechanisms themselves will have a deleterious effect on the body. Shock will then progress to a later stage.

There are few signs of shock in the early stage; the patient may be restless, and the pulse and respiratory rates may be increased. In distributive shock, the extremities are warm and flushed because of vasodilation; this is often referred to as "warm shock." Signs in the later stage of any type of shock include cool, clammy skin; decreased blood pressure; and lethargy or unconsciousness; this is referred to as "cold shock" or late shock. Table 17-2 summarizes the pathophysiological changes in early and late shock. The signs and symptoms of shock are reviewed in Table 17-3.

### LATE STAGE

As shock progresses, blood flow to all body tissues becomes impaired. Cells in vasoconstricted organs receive insufficient oxygen, and aerobic metabolism is replaced by anaerobic metabolism. Energy in the form of adenosine triphosphate (ATP) is produced very inefficiently. Only 2 mol of ATP are produced for each mol of glucose metabolized, in contrast to 38 mol in aerobic metabolism. In addition, lactic acid is formed and cannot be further metabolized in the absence of oxygen. Acidosis and energy deficiency result. Without enough energy, the sodium-potassium pump fails. Potassium leaves the cells, and sodium and water enter, damaging various organelles. Lysosomes, which have an important role in phagocytosis, contain digestive enzymes that are ordinarily contained within a wall. When the lysosome is damaged, the digestive enzymes spill into the rest of the cell and destroy it. As these enzymes come in contact with adjacent cells, these cells also are destroyed and release their digestive enzymes. Cellular death results in organ death.

Acid metabolites cause dilation at the arteriole end of the capillaries (precapillary sphincter) and constriction at the venule end (postcapillary sphincter). Increased hydrostatic pressure within the capillary results and causes fluid to shift from the capillary into the interstitial space; the blood volume is decreased even further. In addition to the increase in pressure within the capillaries, increased capillary permeability may occur. This is most likely to occur in septic shock because of the release of large amounts of histamine and serotonin in response to the presence of gram-negative toxins. Proteins are able to leak through the capillary walls, increasing the osmotic pressure in the interstitium. This causes a further shift of fluid out of the capillaries. Long-standing hypoxemia of the capillaries also can result in increased capillary permeability, so that in the late stages of cardiogenic and hypovolemic shock, this type of fluid shift also may occur. Decreased blood supply to the kidneys results in oliguria or anuria. The serum creatinine and the blood urea nitrogen (BUN) levels increase. The kidneys are unable to excrete the increasing amounts of potassium that are accumulating in the blood as a result of cellular damage, and hyperkalemia results, which is worsened by the acidosis. *Hyperkalemia* depresses the conduction and contractility of the heart.

Vasoconstriction of the splanchnic vessels in response to sympathetic stimulation causes ischemia of the abdominal organs. Of particular importance is the pancreas. In response to hypoxemia, the pancreas forms and secretes a substance called *myocardial depressant factor (MDF)*, which depresses the contractility of the heart. As this enzyme is initially released in the bloodstream, it alters the overall efficiency of cardiac muscle

**table 17-2** *Major Pathophysiological Changes in Shock*

| Change | Effect |
|---|---|
| **EARLY STAGE (COMPENSATORY/NONPROGRESSIVE)**[11] | |
| Increased epinephrine and norepinephrine | |
| Alpha- and beta-adrenergic-receptors stimulated | Increased cardiac output to increase blood flow to tissues |
| Alpha effects: skin and most viscera | Vasoconstriction and decreased blood supply |
| Beta effects: heart and skeletal muscles | Vasodilation and increased blood supply and heart rate |
| Renin-angiotensin response | Vasoconstriction and secretion of aldosterone; sodium and water retention, which supports intravascular volume; potassium loss |
| Increased glucocorticoids and mineralocorticoids | Sodium and water retention to increase intravascular volume; potassium loss |
| Hypoxemia | Hyperventilation and bronchodilation; provides more oxygen to tissues; may cause respiratory alkalosis |
| Decreased hydrostatic fluid pressure | Fluid shifts from interstitial space to intravascular space to increase vascular volume |
| **LATE STAGE (NONCOMPENSATORY/PROGRESSIVE)**[11] | |
| Decreased blood flow to heart | Impaired cardiac pumping ability (decreased cardiac output); blood pressure decreases |
| Anaerobic metabolism | Acidosis; decreased adenosine triphosphate; failure of cellular sodium-potassium pump (potassium leaves cell; sodium and water enter cell); cellular damage |
| Arteriolar dilation and venule constriction | Fluid shift from intravascular to interstitial space, reducing blood pressure |
| Decreased blood flow to kidneys with acute tubular necrosis | Decreased kidney function (oliguria or anuria, retention of nitrogenous waste products and potassium) |
| Decreased blood flow to pancreas | Production of myocardial depressant factor (MDF) |

**table 17-3** *Comparison of Signs and Symptoms in Early and Late Shock by Body System*

| | Early Shock | Late Shock |
|---|---|---|
| Respiratory system | Hyperventilation; ↑ minute volume; ↓ $Paco_2$;* normal $Pao_2$; bronchodilation | Respirations shallow; breath sounds may suggest congestion; ↑ $Paco_2$; ↓ $Pao_2$; pulmonary edema; ↓ pulse oximetry |
| Cardiovascular system | Blood pressure normal to slightly lowered; ↑ diastolic pressure; ↓ pulse pressure; tachycardia; cardiac output normal in hypovolemic shock, slightly decreased in cardiogenic shock, and increased in septic shock; mild vasoconstriction in hypovolemic and cardiogenic shock; vasodilation in septic shock | ↓ Blood pressure; ↓ cardiac output; tachycardia continues; vasoconstriction worsens in hypovolemic, cardiogenic, and septic shock |
| Renal system | Decreased urine output; ↑ urine osmolality; ↓ urine sodium concentration; hypokelemia | Oliguria or complete renal shutdown; hyperkalemia; buildup of waste products |
| Acid-base balance | Respiratory alkalosis | Metabolic acidosis; respiratory acidosis |
| Vascular compartment | Fluid shift from interstitial space to intravascular compartment; thirst | Fluid shift from intravascular to interstitial and intracellular spaces, causing edema |
| Skin | Minimal to no changes in hypovolemic and cardiogenic shock; warm, flushed skin in septic shock | Cool, clammy skin in hypovolemic, cardiogenic, and septic shock; cool, mottled skin in neurogenic and vasogenic shock |
| Hematological system | Release of red blood cells (RBCs) from bone marrow to increase vascular volume; platelet aggregation | Disseminated intravascular coagulation (DIC); ↓ hematopoiesis leading to ↓ white blood cells, ↓ hemoglobin, ↓ hematocrit, ↓ platelets |
| Mental-neurological system | Restless; alert; confused | Lethargy; unconsciousness |
| GI-hepatic system | No obvious changes | Perfusion decreases; bowel sounds possibly diminished; gastric distention; nausea, vomiting |

*$Paco_2$, Arterial carbon dioxide pressure; $Pao_2$, arterial oxygen pressure.

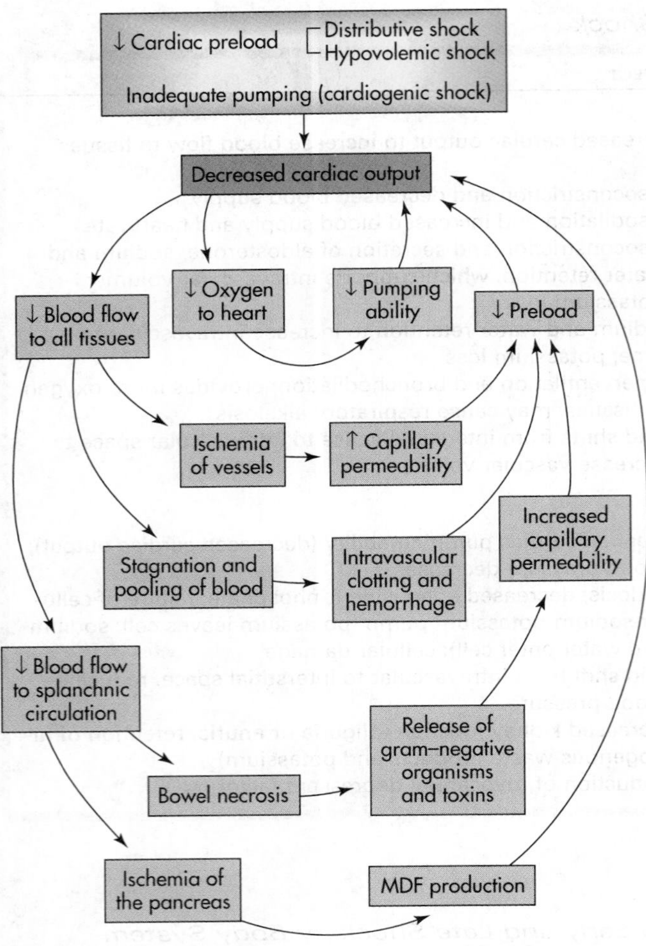


**fig. 17-1** Shock causes shock.

function. Although cardiac function may be sustained initially by the compensating tachycardia that occurs, a lowered stroke volume reflective of left ventricular failure occurs. Eventually cardiac output falls and the heart itself, despite the compensatory mechanisms, receives an inadequate blood supply. This further impairs its electrical and mechanical activity. Finally, cardiac output becomes so inadequate that effective oxygenation delivery and end organ perfusion are impossible.[15]

Shock is a dynamic process, with shock itself causing shock[29] (Figure 17-1). At some point a cycle begins that cannot be interrupted, and an irreversible stage of shock develops. Even if the primary problem is corrected and good supportive care is given, the patient will die. However, the exact point at which shock becomes irreversible is not known. Regardless of the symptoms, all efforts should be made to reverse the progression of shock to prevent damage to vital organs.

## ORGAN COMPROMISE

### Brain

Blood flow to the brain is under the control of local influences rather than the autonomic nervous system. In response to decreased blood flow, the vessels dilate so that the brain, as with the heart, is preferentially perfused. As shock progresses, the local control mechanisms are inadequate, and decreased perfusion of the brain occurs. Cerebral hypoxia results in lethargy and eventually coma. The accumulation of toxic substances and acidosis may compound the signs of hypoxia.

### Heart

Although deterioration of cardiac function is a primary problem only in cardiogenic shock, the heart eventually is affected in all types of shock. As stated previously, in the early stage of most types of shock, the heart is unimpaired. As shock worsens, the pumping ability of the heart is affected and cardiac output decreases. As the heart muscle becomes increasingly hypoxic, it begins to show disturbances of electrical activity. Dysrhythmias have a detrimental effect on cardiac output, and some may be fatal. In the later stages of shock, deterioration of myocardial function is probably the most important factor in the further progression of shock.[8] A factor called the "shock index" (the ratio of heart rate to systolic blood pressure) can be used as a method to assess the degree of this deterioration in the left ventricle of the heart in shock states.[29]

### Lungs

The effect of shock on the lungs has been determined only recently. During the Vietnam War, many victims of shock after trauma survived the early complications because of the use of massive blood transfusions and renal dialysis. The effect of shock on the lungs surfaced as a later complication. The pulmonary condition that results from hypoperfusion of the lungs has been known by various names, including shock lung, white lung, Da Na lung, and more recently adult respiratory distress syndrome. It is now generally known as acute respiratory distress syndrome (ARDS) (see Chapter 32).

ARDS can result from any condition that causes hypoperfusion of the lungs but is seen most often as a consequence of hemorrhagic, traumatic, anaphylactic, or septic shock. Characterized by permeability defects including a diffuse nonuniform injury to the epithelium and the pulmonary capillaries that increases permeability to proteins and water, ARDS is manifested as noncardiac pulmonary edema. There are also changes in airway diameter, injury to the pulmonary circuit, and disruptions in the systemic oxygen transport and utilization mechanisms.[40]

Type 2 pneumocytes are destroyed, impairing the production of surfactant that normally prevents collapse of the alveoli. Alveoli either become filled with fluid, causing pulmonary edema and/or collapse, causing the lungs to become stiff and significantly reducing lung capacity.

In the early stages, hypoxemia results from impaired gas exchange, and hyperventilation occurs, resulting in hypocapnia and respiratory alkalosis. Platelet aggregation in the pulmonary capillaries further damages the lungs. Hypoxemia persists despite administration of increasing amounts of oxygen. As shock progresses, ventilation is impaired, and carbon dioxide is retained, resulting in respiratory acidosis. As hypoxemia increases, platelet aggregation increases, and a destructive cycle is initiated.

### Gastrointestinal Tract

Sympathetic stimulation, which occurs early in shock, causes redistribution of blood flow to vital organs. This results in decreased blood flow to the GI tract. Bowel function decreases, and paralytic ileus may result. If the blood supply is severely impaired for a time, necrosis of the intestinal mucosa may occur. Microorganisms that are normally found in the bowel lyse and release endotoxins when they are attacked by the leukocytes in the blood. Shock, from whatever cause, will now also have a septic component. The gastric mucosa commonly ulcerates when it becomes ischemic, which may result in occult bleeding or massive hemorrhage.

### Kidneys

The kidneys contain about 2.4 million nephrons, each capable of forming urine. Each nephron is composed of a glomerulus that is made up of capillaries and collecting tubules (see Chapter 43). Under normal conditions the pressure within the glomerulus is sufficiently high to force fluid out of the capillaries into the collecting chamber. When the systolic pressure falls below 70 mm Hg, glomerular filtration ceases, and the body is unable to rid itself of fluid and nitrogenous wastes. Normal electrolyte balance is altered. Urinary output is decreased in both the early and the late stages of shock. In the early stage, low output is caused by sympathetic stimulation of the $\alpha$-receptors in the kidneys, resulting in vasoconstriction and a fall in pressure within the glomeruli. Decreased pressure causes a drop in the glomerular filtration rate, diminishing urine production and output. Also, the secretion of aldosterone and antidiuretic hormone causes sodium and water reabsorption.

As shock progresses, the tubules—which are perfused by the peritubular capillaries—begin to suffer from a lack of oxygen and nutrients, and *acute tubular necrosis* develops. The tubular epithelial cells slough and block the tubules, causing loss of nephron function.

### Liver

Sympathetic stimulation causes vasoconstriction in the liver. In the early stages of shock, this can be beneficial. Normally the liver is capable of storing large amounts of blood in its veins. With vasoconstriction it can release up to 350 ml of blood into the general circulation, resulting in improved cardiac output. With continued sympathetic stimulation and decreased blood flow, liver tissue is affected. In septic shock there is an increase in oxygen uptake and a decrease in energy production in the liver.

All types of shock affect liver functioning including its synthesizing, detoxifying, and immunological (reticuloendothelial) functions. Metabolic functions are impaired, leading to a decreased ability to metabolize and synthesize nutrients and a decreased ability to metabolize and eliminate bodily wastes.

The sinusoids of the liver are lined with Kupffer cells, which are part of the mononuclear phagocyte system (MPS). These cells are very powerful phagocytes and destroy the many bacteria from the colon that reach the liver by way of the portal system. Normally, only a very few bacteria get past the MPS. With the destruction of the MPS, bacteria enter the general circulation and produce toxins, which under normal circumstances would be detoxified by the liver. The liver can no longer perform this function, and overwhelming infection and toxicity result.

Alterations in all functional elements of the liver contribute to problems with other organ systems. Low levels of albumin and clotting factors are evidence of the liver's altered capacity to synthesize proteins. The decreases in circulating albumin and clotting factors in turn contribute to the instability of the blood coagulation system, making shock patients at great risk for bleeding and hemorrhage.

### Blood

Disseminated intravascular coagulation (DIC) (see Chapter 29) can cause or result from shock. Characterized by intravascular clotting, DIC results in the formation of microthrombi in the capillaries. Clotting factors in the blood may be activated by acidosis, stagnation, and procoagulation substances. Acidosis and stagnation are common in all forms of shock. Therefore DIC may occur with all types of shock. In septic shock, however, the bacterial toxins and the prostaglandins that are released enhance coagulation and make DIC even more likely.[37] Clotting in the capillaries causes a depletion of clotting factors in the rest of the body. Hemorrhage may then occur from surgical incisions, injection sites, intravenous insertion sites, or the GI tract. Intravascular clotting results in a further decrease in tissue perfusion and acidosis, and a vicious cycle ensues. The hemorrhage caused by DIC decreases the cardiac output even further and worsens tissue perfusion. The mortality in patients with DIC in association with infection and shock is very high.[17]

## COLLABORATIVE CARE MANAGEMENT

Medical and nursing management is determined by the stage of shock and the patient's signs and symptoms. The details of treatment are included under the intervention section later in this chapter.

## NURSING MANAGEMENT

### ■ ASSESSMENT

#### Subjective Data

The nurse collects a complete history from the patient or family, focusing on risk and causative factors that may explain signs/symptoms of evolving shock. Questions should relate to recent illnesses, infections, trauma, surgery, and medication use. While obtaining subjective data, the nurse is observing the manner in which the patient responds to the questions, his or her attention span, and the patient's general mood and behavior. Some of the early manifestations of shock may include an inability to retain focus on the question being asked; expressions of a sense of restlessness, and changes in mood, mental status, or behavior. If possible, the nurse should

**box 17-2** *Parameters for Assessing Status of the Patient in Shock*

**HEMODYNAMIC MONITORING**
- Blood pressure (cuff and/or intra-arterial)
- Heart rate
- Central venous pressure
- Pulmonary artery pressure
- Pulmonary capillary wedge pressure
- Cardiac output
- Electrocardiogram
- Pulse pressure
- Systemic vascular resistance
- Capillary refill

**RESPIRATORY MONITORING**
- Respiratory rate, depth
- Breath sounds
- Blood gas levels
  - pH
  - $Pa_{O_2}$
  - $Pa_{CO_2}$
- Percent $O_2$ saturation
- Mixed venous return ($Sv_{O_2}$)
- Lung capacity

**FLUID AND ELECTROLYTE MONITORING**
- Serum electrolyte levels
- Blood lactate and pyruvate levels
- Intake
  - By mouth
  - Intravenous
  - Nasogastric
  - Irrigation solutions
  - Solution in medications
- Output
  - Urinary
  - GI tract
  - Sweating
  - Dressings
- Weight
- Serum creatinine level
- BUN level
- Serum and urine osmolality
- Urine specific gravity

**NEUROLOGICAL MONITORING**
- Alertness
- Orientation
- Confusion
- Pupil response
- Responsiveness to stimulation

**HEMATOLOGICAL MONITORING**
- Erythrocytes
- Hematocrit and hemoglobin levels
- Leukocytes
- Platelets
- Prothrombin and partial thromboplastin times
- Clotting time
- Fibrin degradation factor

**OTHER MONITORING**
- Bowel sounds
- Skin temperature and color

validate suspected mood or behavior changes with family members or the patient's significant other.

### Objective Data

There are few obvious signs in evolving, early shock. The patient may be restless and complain of feeling weak. There may be subtle but persistent increases in both the patient's pulse and respiratory rates. The patient's skin will appear diaphoretic, pale (unless the patient has early septic shock), and cool to the touch. As these symptoms become more pronounced, the blood pressure will persistently decrease, and lethargy or unconsciousness will evolve as shock advances into the late phase. Monitoring of certain key parameters is critical to early identification and treatment of shock. The various methods for monitoring shock and the parameters used in assessing shock appear in Box 17-2 and are discussed in more detail below.

#### *Hemodynamic assessment*

Hemodynamic alterations are often the first sign of the onset of shock. The patient's hemodynamic status can be assessed at various levels (Figure 17-2).[34a]

**Vital signs.** Vital signs are assessed frequently. In the early stages of shock, the pulse is usually increased. As shock progresses, the pulse becomes quite weak and easily obliterated. Irregularities in the pulse may develop as cardiac dysrhythmias occur.

Early in shock the blood pressure may be normal, slightly decreased, or even elevated because of compensatory vasoconstriction. Blood pressure can be heard without difficulty at this stage. As shock progresses, the blood pressure may be difficult to auscultate, and it may be possible to obtain the systolic pressure only by palpation or by electronic device. If

| Level | Parameters |
|---|---|
| VIII. | Stroke volume index* |
| VII. | Vascular resistance |
| VI. | Cardiac output + Stroke volume |
| V. | Pulmonary artery pressure |
| IV. | Central venous pressure, Blood gases + Electrolytes |
| III. | Urinary output + Electrocardiogram |
| II. | Heart rate + Blood pressure + Venous pulses |
| I. | Mentation, Skin color + Temperature |

**fig. 17-2** Levels of hemodynamic monitoring. *As shock progresses, sophistication of hemodynamic monitoring increases.

intraarterial pressure monitoring is not instituted, Doppler ultrasound may be helpful in obtaining the blood pressure.

Venous pulsation in the neck is noted. Both the external and the internal jugular veins should be examined. Generally the external jugular vein is easier to see, but the internal jugular is more reliable as a sign of elevated right-atrial pressure. Normally, venous pulsations are visible when the patient is lying flat, but not when the head is elevated to 45°. Neck veins that are not visible when the patient is in the horizontal position may indicate an abnormally low intravascular volume. This may be seen in both hypovolemic and distributive shock. In cardiogenic shock the neck veins are often distended, even when the head of the patient's bed is elevated more than 45°, indicating excessive fluid volume (Figure 17-3).

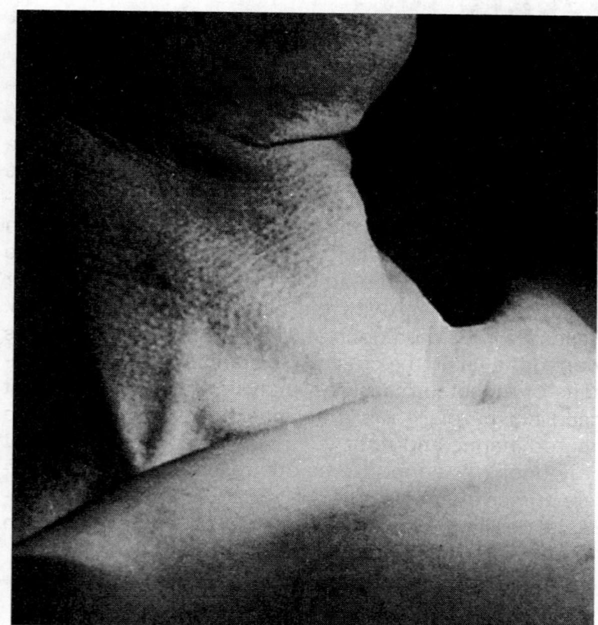

fig. 17-3 Distended external jugular neck vein of the patient with failure of the right side of the heart.

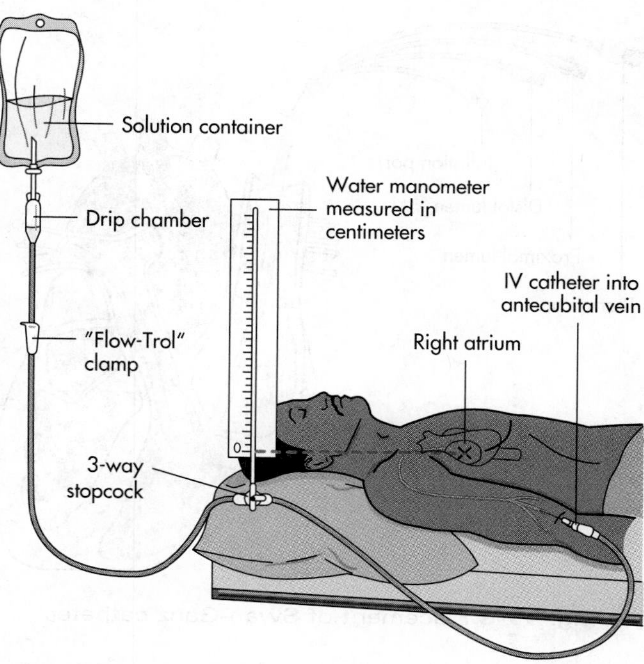


fig. 17-4 Measurement of central venous pressure (CVP) using water manometer. Zero point on manometer is at level of midright atrium, and CVP reading is 7 cm $H_2O$.

**Central venous pressure.** Central venous pressure (CVP) is a more accurate means than general clinical assessment for determining the fluid status of a patient in shock. CVP measures right-ventricular filling pressure, circulating blood volume, and the degree of peripheral vasoconstriction. As a result, CVP is altered by changes in circulating blood volume returning to the right side of the heart and by pressure in the great veins. Thus it is particularly useful in assessing volume status in patients with absolute or relative hypovolemia, including those with distributive, neurogenic, and hypovolemic shock.

To obtain an accurate CVP reading,[23,28,29] one inserts a catheter into a major vein and threads it through the superior vena cava into the right atrium. The catheter is attached by a three-way stopcock to an intravenous infusion and a water manometer (Figure 17-4) or to a pressure transducer. The intravenous solution (usually 5% dextrose in water) is allowed to drip slowly into the vein to keep the intravenous access open. When a reading is to be taken using the water manometer, the stopcock is opened to the manometer, and the manometer is filled with the intravenous solution. The stopcock is then turned to the venous opening of the patient. The fluid level in the manometer should fluctuate with each respiration. The fluid is allowed to stabilize before a reading is taken, and the highest level of the fluid fluctuating in the column is used for the CVP reading. As soon as the reading is taken, the stopcock is returned to the solution position, and the infusion is continued.

For the CVP reading to be accurate, the patient must be relaxed, and the zero point of the manometer must always be at the level of the right atrium, which in most people is level with the midaxillary line at the fourth intercostal space. If the patient cannot lie flat in bed, the zero point on the manometer is adjusted to the level of the right atrium with the patient in a sitting position. Any change in the patient's position requires that the zero point be recalibrated. The initial CVP reading and the position that the patient was in when it was taken should be recorded, because these will serve as a baseline for comparison with subsequent readings. The patient should be placed in the same position for each reading because even a slight change in position alters the CVP.

A range of 5 to 15 cm $H_2O$ is usually considered normal. In hypovolemic shock the CVP is usually very low because the blood volume is decreased. In distributive shock the CVP will also be low, because the blood has pooled in the expanded vascular space and fluid has been lost into the interstitium as a result of increased capillary permeability. In cardiogenic shock the CVP is likely to be high because of the excess intravascular fluid. It is important to note that a change in the trend of the CVP is more important than a numeric reading.

When the catheter is attached to a pressure transducer, a routine practice in intensive care settings, monitoring techniques change. The electronic transducer converts fluid pressure transmitted through the catheter to an electrical signal. The electrical signal is displayed as a waveform on a monitor, thus allowing the pressure to be measured continuously.[34]

Central venous catheters can also be used to obtain blood samples, to assess venous oxygen saturation determinations, and to administer fluids and medications. The catheter

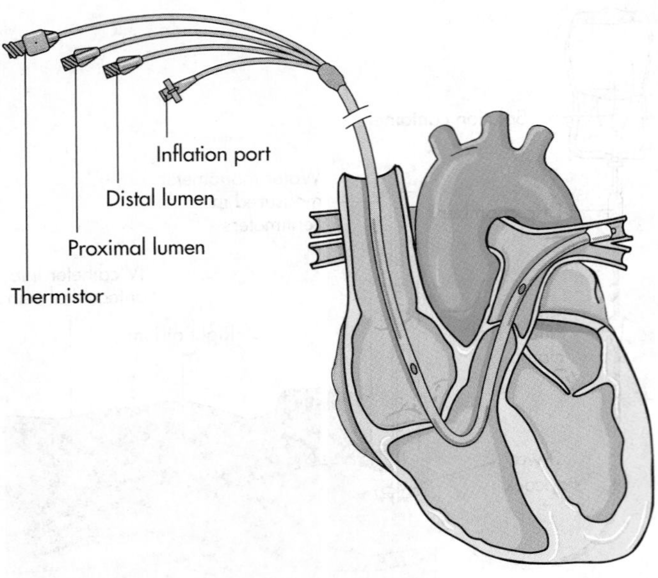


**fig. 17-5** Placement of Swan-Ganz catheter.

**research**

Reference: Wilson AE et al: Effect of backrest position on hemodynamic and right ventricular measurements in critically ill adults, *Am J Crit Care* 5(4):264-270, 1996.

In this study, pulmonary artery measurements were done on 39 subjects, 55% of whom were men and 45% women. Backrest elevation was measured using a draftsman's professional protractor. The degree of elevation was measured by placing the protractor level with the horizontal plane of the adjustable arm of the protractor at 30° or 45°, level with the elevated head of the bed. Readings were then done at 0°, 30°, or 45°. All measures were done using the critical ICU standard of practice. Results of repeated measures analysis show that a patient need not be placed in a flat position to obtain reliable hemodynamic and right ventricular measurements. Not only does this support previous research, but it also offers nurses alternative, accurate options for obtaining reliable hemodynamic readings while maintaining both the patient's comfort and treatment schedules.

insertion site should be kept scrupulously clean to minimize the possibility of phlebitis. Patient movement is not restricted as long as the catheter and tubing are secured adequately and intravenous flow is maintained.

**Pulmonary artery pressures.** The status of the left side of the heart can best be evaluated by the measurement of *pulmonary artery pressure (PAP)* and *pulmonary capillary wedge pressure (PCWP)*. A mean PAP of less than 10 mm Hg may indicate decreased blood volume, resulting in decreased preload in the left ventricle. A mean PAP of more than 20 mm Hg may indicate poor myocardial contractility and left-ventricular overload (see Chapter 24 for assessment of the cardiovascular system).

These pressures are measured with a special balloon-tipped (Swan-Ganz) catheter (Figure 17-5). The catheter is inserted into a vein, usually the subclavian, and advanced to the atrium. The balloon is inflated and carried by the blood flow into the right ventricle and then to the pulmonary artery. The balloon is then deflated, and the tip of the catheter is left floating in the pulmonary artery. The other end of the catheter is connected to low-compliance tubing, which in turn is connected to a transducer. The transducer converts the pressure that it senses through the catheter to an electrical signal, which is displayed on a monitor. Thus the pressure in the pulmonary artery can be monitored continuously. A continuous flush system infusing through a specially designated small-bore, rigid intravenous tube usually is used to maintain patency of the catheter and quality of the waveform.

Traditionally, hemodynamic measurements using a pulmonary artery catheter have been done with the patient in the supine position. Although it is easy to perform the readings with the patient in this position, the discomfort for the patient and the disruption in essential care routines have made doing the procedure in this manner problematic.[45] Current research findings indicate that accurate readings can be obtained as long as the patient's backrest position elevation is placed anywhere from 0° to 45° (see the Research Box).

In individuals without lung or pulmonary vascular disease, PAP is a good indicator of how well the left side of the heart is functioning. Pressure changes in the left ventricle are reflected in the left atrium and back to the pulmonary artery. However, if any disease exists in the lungs, as frequently occurs in shock, the PAP does not accurately reflect left-ventricular pressure. In this case the PCWP should be obtained. By inflating the balloon, which is near the tip of the catheter, the pulmonary artery is temporarily obstructed. This blocks communication between the pulmonary artery and the lumen of the catheter, allowing for pressure that is ahead of the occluded artery to be transmitted through the catheter. The PCWP is identical to the left atrial pressure.

The nurse caring for the patient with PAP monitoring must be aware of the common complications that can occur with this type of invasive monitoring (Table 17-4). The appearance of either a right ventricular or PCWP waveform on the monitor can have serious consequences for the patient. Dislodgement of the tip of the catheter from the pulmonary artery into the right ventricle can result in the occurrence of premature ventricular beats (PVBs) or even ventricular tachycardia. Progression of the catheter into a small vessel in the pulmonary vasculature can occlude the vessel and result in pulmonary infarction. Prolonged inflation of the balloon can have the same effect. The nurse must be able to distinguish the normal PAP waveform from both right-ventricular and PCWP waveforms (Figure 17-6). It is essential that sterile technique be maintained during insertion of the PAP catheter and during dressing changes.

**Intraarterial monitoring.** Intraarterial monitoring is usually instituted along with PAP monitoring. A catheter is inserted into a radial, brachial, or femoral artery and attached to a transducer in much the same way as the pulmonary artery catheter (Figure 17-7).

**table 17-4** *Complications of Pulmonary Artery Pressure Monitoring*

| COMPLICATIONS | MANIFESTATIONS | INTERVENTIONS |
|---|---|---|
| Infection | Chills<br>Headache<br>Malaise<br>Generalized aching<br>Flushed face<br>Warm skin<br>Elevated temperature | 1. Notify physician immediately.<br>2. Prepare for removal of catheter.<br>3. Administer antibiotics as prescribed.<br>4. Provide symptomatic relief. |
| Ventricular dysrhythmias: premature beats (PVBs), or short runs of ventricular fibrillation | Irregular pulse<br>PVBs noted on cardiac monitor | 1. Notify physician immediately.<br>2. Prepare for repositioning of catheter.<br>3. Administer antidysrhythmic drugs if problem persists after repositioning. |
| Sustained ventricular tachycardia or ventricular fibrillation | Light headedness, progressing to loss of consciousness<br>Pulselessness<br>Dysrhythmia noted on cardiac monitor<br>Respiratory arrest | 1. Notify physician immediately.<br>2. Prepare for repositioning of catheter.<br>3. Defibrillate and institute advanced cardiac life support (ACLS). |
| Pulmonary infarction | Chest pain<br>Hemoptysis<br>Fever<br>Friction rub<br>Elevated lactate dehydrogenase<br>Areas of opacity on chest roentgenogram<br>Subnormal $PaO_2$ | 1. Notify physician immediately.<br>2. Administer oxygen.<br>3. Prepare for repositioning of catheter.<br>4. Provide symptomatic relief. |
| Pulmonary artery rupture | Lightheadness progressing to loss of consciousness<br>Acute chest pain<br>Hemoptysis<br>Loss of blood pressure<br>Rapidly decreasing $PaO_2$ | 1. Page physician as an emergency.<br>2. Apply oxygen and prepare to intubate with double lumen endotracheal tube to isolate nonhemorrhaging lung.<br>3. Prepare for insertion of intravenous line with large bore access.<br>4. Prepare for emergency thoracotomy.<br>5. Type and cross-match for transfusion. |

From American Society of Anesthesiologists: Practice guidelines for pulmonary artery catheterization, *Anesthesiology* 78:380-394, 1993.

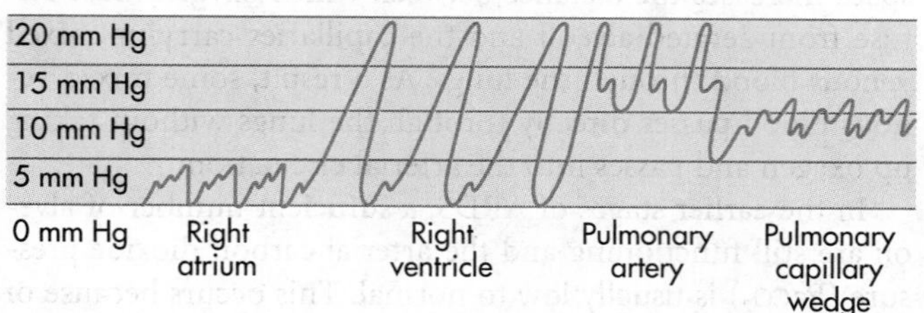


**fig. 17-6** Characteristic waveforms of pulmonary artery pressure (PAP) monitoring.

As was the case with the pulmonary artery catheter, a continuous flush system infusing through a small-bore, rigid intravenous tube maintains the patency of the catheter and the quality of the waveform. Because hemorrhage is a possible complication, the insertion and connections in the system must be monitored frequently. The extremity distal to the insertion site must be monitored for signs of arterial occlusion (color, temperature, movement, presence or absence of pulses, or pain) (Table 17-5). It is essential that sterile technique be maintained during insertion of the catheter and during dressing changes. A patient who is ill enough to require hemodynamic monitoring has little reserve to fight infection.

**Cardiac output and cardiac index monitoring.** Pulmonary artery catheters allow for cardiac output and cardiac index to be monitored at the bedside. Such catheters have a port through which fluid can be injected into the right atrium. A *thermistor* (sensor to measure temperature) is located at the tip of the catheter and is attached to a wire that runs through the catheter to a cardiac output computer. Iced or room-temperature saline solution is injected into the right atrium. The solution travels with the blood into the pulmonary artery. The thermistor senses the extent of temperature change, and from these data the computer is able to calculate cardiac output. Although iced injectate solution improves the accuracy and precision of the cardiac output measurement, room temperature injectate is most often used to gain steady-state results. This solution does not cause the acute, transient changes in heart rate (e.g., bradycardia) that can alter cardiac output. For this reason, room temperature injectate is preferable when cardiac output is measured by the thermodilution technique.[23,46] In addition to its use in determining cardiac output and cardiac index, the thermistor can be used to monitor core body temperature. The data from the pulmonary artery catheters can be used to measure systemic vascular resistance (SVR). There is an inverse relationship

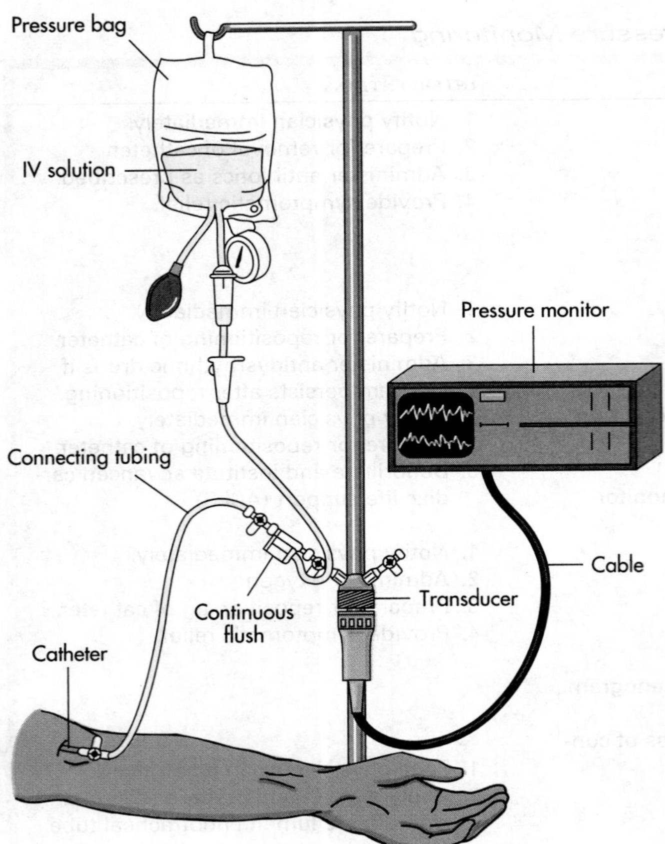


**fig. 17-7** Connections between intraarterial catheter, transducer, monitor, and fluid.

between cardiac output and SVR. As SVR increases, cardiac output falls.

**Oxygen utilization monitoring.** In all types of shock a discrepancy exists between the amount of oxygen delivered to the cells and the amount required. Oxygen delivery is affected by cardiac output, serum hemoglobin concentration, and the amount of oxygen in the blood (measured by arterial oxygen pressure [$Pa{O_2}$]). If any of these decreases, the cells normally compensate by extracting more oxygen than normal from the blood. Blood in the veins then has a lower-than-normal oxygen content. By sampling blood that is a mixture of venous blood from the entire body, oxygen utilization by the body can be determined. Blood in the pulmonary artery is used for this purpose. The difference between the oxygen saturation of arterial blood ($Sa{O_2}$) and the oxygen saturation of the mixed venous blood ($Sv{O_2}$) reflects cellular utilization of oxygen. In both hypovolemic shock and cardiogenic shock, the fall in cardiac output causes the cells to extract more oxygen, with a resultant decrease in $Sv{O_2}$. In septic shock, however, especially in the early stages, this is not the case. The $Sv{O_2}$ may be abnormally high, despite the cells apparently not receiving enough oxygen. This may be a result of the high cardiac output seen in early shock. Other possible reasons include the inability of the cells to extract oxygen because of the effects of endotoxins and the passage of blood through some organs, with little gas exchange occurring because of clogged capillaries.

The $Sv{O_2}$ can be measured by withdrawing blood from a pulmonary artery catheter. However, the preferred way is to monitor the $Sv{O_2}$ by use of a fiberoptic pulmonary artery catheter, which will display a continuous value on a monitor. Table 17-6 lists the hemodynamic parameters found in various types of changes in shock.

### *Respiratory assessment*

As discussed earlier, hypoperfusion of the lungs, which frequently occurs in shock, may result in ARDS. This may be suspected very early in the course of the disease from changes in the patient's mentation as a result of cerebral hypoxemia. The patient is observed for cough and dyspnea, which develop as ARDS progresses. Changes in respiratory rate and in the color of the mucous membranes and skin are important indicators of pulmonary status. Breath sounds are auscultated. Early in the course of the disease the lungs may be clear, but as ARDS progresses, crackles and gurgles may be heard.

If the patient is receiving mechanical ventilation, the amount of pressure required to deliver a specific tidal volume is noted. As the lungs become increasingly stiff, the pressure required to deliver the volume increases. With ARDS, the PAP may rise from pulmonary capillary congestion, although the PCWP remains normal.[40]

Arterial blood gas levels may provide valuable information and are monitored as indicated, depending on the patient's condition. Characteristically with ARDS, the $Pa{O_2}$ level falls despite ventilation with increasing amounts of oxygen because of physiological shunting of blood through the lungs to the left side of the heart.

Physiological *shunting* occurs because many alveoli are either collapsed or filled with fluid and diffusion cannot occur. Collapsed and/or fluid-filled alveoli create airless spaces (sometimes referred to as "dead space") in the lung. Dead space increases the distance between which oxygen must diffuse from aerated alveoli and the capillaries carrying mixed venous blood through the lungs. As a result, some mixed venous blood passes directly through the lungs without taking up oxygen and passes into the arterial circulation.

In the earlier stages of ARDS, a sufficient number of alveoli are still functioning and the arterial carbon dioxide pressure ($Pa{CO_2}$) is usually low to normal. This occurs because of the rapid diffusion of carbon dioxide and the hyperventilation that results from hypoxia.

However, as ARDS progresses and the lungs become increasingly stiff, an acute restrictive condition occurs, and ventilation and diffusion are impaired. In this stage, $Pa{CO_2}$ and $Pa{O_2}$ are affected. The $Pa{CO_2}$, which was decreasing as a result of hyperventilation, begins to increase as a result of hypoventilation.

Arterial blood gas determinations are also used to assess the acid-base balance of the patient. In the early stages of shock, mild respiratory alkalosis typically occurs from the hyperventilation that is part of the stress response. As shock progresses and tissue becomes progressively hypoxemic, anaerobic metabolism takes place and metabolic acidosis occurs.

Because oxygen uptake is an essential component in the supply-demand relationship that is so critical in the body's ability to respond to shock, any phenomenon that affects oxy-

**table 17-5** *Complications of Intraarterial Pressure Monitoring*

| COMPLICATIONS | MANIFESTATIONS | INTERVENTIONS |
|---|---|---|
| Hemorrhage | Obvious excessive bleeding<br>Tachycardia<br>Hypotension<br>Pallor<br>Diaphoresis<br>Tachypnea<br>Restlessness<br>Dizziness<br>Headache | 1. Control bleeding<br>a. If bleeding occurs at the puncture site, apply pressure.<br>b. If part of the system has become disconnected, immediately turn the stopcocks to stop bleeding.<br>2. Attach a syringe containing sterile saline until contaminated parts of the system are replaced with sterile parts.<br>3. Notify the physician if a large amount of blood has been lost.<br>4. Prepare the patient for blood replacement if significant loss. |
| Thrombus or embolus | Pallor, loss of pulse, and coolness of skin distal to the site of the thrombus<br>Pain | 1. Notify the physician immediately.<br>2. Instruct patient to lie quietly.<br>3. Prepare to administer $O_2$. |
| Infection of catheter site | Redness and warmth at the site<br>Possible fever | 1. Notify the physician.<br>2. Prepare for removal of the catheter.<br>3. Send the catheter tip for culture. |
| Bacteremia | High fever<br>Chills | 1. Notify the physician.<br>2. Prepare for removal of the catheter. |

Modified from Asheervath J, Blevins D: *Handbook of clinical nursing practice,* Norwalk, Conn, 1986, Appleton-Century-Crofts.

gen uptake affects physiological functioning in this state. Anaerobic metabolism and the associated metabolic acidosis compound the cellular problems with the oxygen supply. Severely acidotic states cause the affinity of hemoglobin for oxygen to diminish and thus reduce the oxygen-carrying capacity of blood. This in turn worsens the anaerobic state and can facilitate the rapid clinical deterioration of a patient in shock. In the advanced stages of shock, as respiratory compensation decreases and ARDS becomes progressively worse, respiratory acidosis and respiratory failure become pronounced.

### Fluid and electrolyte assessment

The urinary output and the CVP most accurately reflect fluid status. An indwelling urinary catheter is usually inserted, and the urine output is measured hourly. Other output—such as GI drainage, wound exudate, or perspiration—is measured or estimated as accurately as possible. Body weight often gives a more accurate assessment of fluid changes than does the measurement of intake and output; however, this can be an inaccurate determinant of intravascular volume when third spacing of fluid occurs. Noting the presence of edema, auscultating the chest for the presence of fluid, and measuring the abdominal girth for the development of ascites are means of assessing fluid collection in the third space.

In the early stages of shock, the serum potassium concentration may be abnormally low as a result of increased levels of aldosterone in response to stress. However, as shock progresses, the serum potassium level may become abnormally high as damaged cells release potassium. As urinary output falls, the body is unable to eliminate the excess amounts of potassium accumulating in the serum. If potassium is administered in the early stage of shock, it is extremely important that the urinary output and serum electrolytes be monitored frequently.

**table 17-6** *Hemodynamic Parameters in Various Types of Shock*

| | HYPO-VOLEMIC | CARDIO-GENIC | DISTRIBUTIVE* |
|---|---|---|---|
| Cardiac output | Low | Low | High |
| PCWP | Low | High | Low |
| $SvO_2$ | Low | Low | High |
| SVR | High | High | Low |

*In the late stage of septic shock, severely depressed cardiac function results in a clinical picture similar to that of cardiogenic shock.

The concentrations of other serum electrolytes may be abnormal as a result of acid-base abnormalities, altered renal function, or fluid therapy. Serum enzyme levels may be elevated because of ischemia and damage to the heart, liver, and pancreas.

### Neurological assessment

In shock the brain may be adversely affected by hypoxia, acid-base imbalance, or toxins. Often, subtle changes in mentation are the earliest signs of cerebral hypoxia. The patient is observed for increasing restlessness. Sedation should not be given until the patient's status has been assessed further, and it has been determined that the restlessness does not have an organic cause. In the late stages, when perfusion of the brain is severely impaired, loss of consciousness occurs. Vital signs and arterial blood gas determinations can aid in assessing the cause of subtle neurological changes.

### Hematological assessment

The hemoglobin and hematocrit levels are valuable tools for assessing blood loss in hypovolemic shock secondary to hemorrhage. It must be remembered, however, that the hemoglobin and hematocrit levels do not drop immediately with loss of an excessive amount of blood, because plasma is lost along with the blood cells. The blood that remains in the intravascular compartment initially will have a normal concentration of red blood cells (RBCs). Within a few hours after a blood loss, the hemoglobin and hematocrit levels begin to decrease as the kidneys retain water and electrolytes in response to low perfusion.

An increase in hemoglobin and hematocrit levels may be seen in some types of shock. Increased capillary permeability, which occurs primarily in septic and anaphylactic shock, permits water and electrolytes to move out of the capillaries, leaving behind blood with a high concentration of cells. Hematocrit levels also are relative to fluid volume and may be decreased by hemodilution due to fluid replacement.

Patients in shock are assessed for the development of DIC. The nurse may be the first to observe that the patient is bleeding for an excessively long time after a venipuncture or that blood is oozing from an incision. If DIC is suspected, laboratory studies are initiated; clotting factors (including fibrinogen and platelet counts) are decreased, prothrombin time (PT) and partial thromboplastin time (PTT) are prolonged, and fibrin degradation products are increased.

### *Abdominal assessment*

Decreased blood flow to the intestines may result in decreased peristalsis or paralytic ileus (see Chapter 41). Abnormal fluid shifts and occasionally abdominal hemorrhage occur, causing increased abdominal girth. Decreased or absent bowel sounds are noted. Assessment of gastric drainage and stools for occult blood is necessary because of the high incidence of GI tract bleeding with shock.

## NURSING DIAGNOSES

Nursing diagnoses are determined from analysis of patient data. Nursing diagnoses for the person with shock may include but are not limited to:

| Diagnostic Title | Possible Etiological Factors |
|---|---|
| Airway clearance, ineffective | Decreased energy, endotracheal intubation |
| Gas exchange, impaired | Decreased lung complaince, interstitial edema |
| Breathing pattern | Inadequate perfusion, respiratory muscles ineffective |
| Cardiac output, decreased | Myocardial hypoxia, myocardial depressant factor |
| Tissue perfusion, altered (cardiopulmonary) | Hypovolemia, decreased cardiac output |
| Fluid volume deficit | Blood loss, increased capillary permeability, vasodilation |
| Injury, risk for | Confusion from hypovolemia |
| Infection, risk for | Invasive monitoring, indwelling catheter, decreased immune response |
| Anxiety | Threat of death |
| Activity intolerance | Imbalance between oxygen supply and demand |

## EXPECTED PATIENT OUTCOMES

Expected patient outcomes for the person with shock may include but are not limited to:

1. Airway remains free from secretions.
2. Blood gas levels ($PaCO_2$ and $PaO_2$) are within patient's normal limits.
3. Respiratory rate and tidal volume are within patient's normal limits.
4. Intravascular volume, as noted by hemoglobin and hematocrit levels and hemodynamic values, returns to normal limits.
5. Demonstrates increased cardiopulmonary perfusion.
6. Urinary output and hemodynamic values are within normal limits.
7. Mental status improves and the patient is free from injury.
8. Free from signs of infection, invasive lines' sites free from erythema, drainage.
9. Offers statements of feeling relaxed and comfortable and shows no physical signs of anxiety.
10. Tolerates activity and care without an increase in pulse rate of more than 20 per minute.

## INTERVENTIONS

Treatment of shock varies to some extent, depending on the cause of the shock, the organ systems affected, and the preexisting condition of the patient. In the early, acute phase of shock, the major role of the nurse is continuous assessment of the patient's clinical status and assisting with administration of therapies necessary to stabilize the patient's condition.

Fundamentally, the same priorities that exist for treating any life-threatening emergency hold true for shock. The priorities for shock management are:

1. *Airway:* A patent airway must be maintained to maximize oxygen uptake and carbon dioxide removal. To accomplish this, a nasal or oral airway may be inserted. When respiratory failure is a high potential, the patient's airway is secured with an endotracheal tube.
2. *Breathing:* Oxygen is administered immediately at the level ordered. This may include preparations to ventilate the patient by mechanical ventilation. These measures support breathing and enhance ventilation and gas exchange between the airway and the circulation.
3. *Circulation:* The pump (the heart) is supported by the administration of fluids—including blood—to increase blood volume, improve cardiac output, and maximize oxygen transport to the cells. Vasoactive and cardiogenic drugs may also be prescribed to enhance cardiovascular functioning and oxygen transport to the cells.
4. *Diagnosis:* Shock can be treated most effectively if the underlying cause can be determined and treated. For example, if the cause of shock is hypovolemia secondary to massive bleeding, efforts will be made to find the site of the bleeding and stop it, if possible. Administration of blood and fluids will be used to improve intravascular volume and cardiac output, thus improving exchange of oxygen and carbon dioxide at the cellular level. If the cause of

shock is sepsis, antibiotics, antiviral agents, or antifungal agents is administered intravenously, and if the cause is anaphylaxis, epinephrine is given.

### Assisting with Respiratory Support

Most patients in shock have some degree of hypoxemia. Oxygen is usually administered because tissues are already suffering from oxygen deprivation caused by decreased blood flow or anemia. Because the energy system of the body is impaired, the muscles used in ventilation may not function adequately, and breathing may have to be assisted. If symptoms of ARDS develop, positive end-expiratory pressure (PEEP) may have to be used. Positive pressure at the end of expiration prevents surfactant-deficient alveoli from collapsing, resulting in atelectasis. Coughing and deep breathing are important. If the patient is too weak to cough or if an endotracheal tube is in place, suctioning is necessary to keep the airway free of excessive secretions.

Because ARDS is a common sequelae of shock and often requires endotracheal intubation to prevent complete respiratory failure, management of the patient's respiratory system is critical to the patient's care. Maintaining oxygen saturation is an essential element of sustaining the patient's respiratory system and can be compromised if effective endotracheal suctioning is not done. Current research indicates that consistency in the methods of tracheal suctioning (oxygenation, hyperinflation before and after suctioning, and number of passes of the suction catheter) can affect either positively or negatively both ventilation and cardiovascular functioning (see the Research Box).[22]

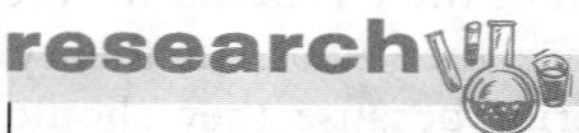


Reference: Mancinelli-Van Atta J, Beck SL: Preventing hypoxemia and hemodynamic compromise related to endotracheal suctioning, *Am J Crit Care* 1(3):62-79, 1996.

This study offers a bridge between research and practice to clinicians to determine ways to reduce the negative effects of endotracheal suctioning. It summarizes the research done between 1984 and 1991 related to oxygenation techniques before, during, and after endotracheal suctioning. While the review points out issues related to research methodologies used in previous studies and offers recommendations for better controlled studies in the future, it also offers recommendations for current practice.

Recommendations include:

- Standardize procedural variables that contribute to oxygen desaturation and hemodynamic instability.
- Hyperoxygenate ($FIO_2$ at 100%) or hyperinflation combined with greater than baseline oxygenation before and after endotracheal suctioning (ETS)
- Evaluate the patient's response to ETS. If the risk of decreased Sao is greater than the risk of increasing mean arterial blood pressure, continue hyperinflation and hyperoxygenation. If not, discontinue hyperinflation, minimize frequency of passes of the suction catheter, and continue 100% oxygenation before and after each ETS pass.

Meticulous mouth care is necessary while the endotracheal tube is in place, because the mouth remains open and swallowing may be difficult. The patient with an endotracheal tube in place is unable to talk; therefore a nonverbal form of communication, such as a magic slate, is necessary.

### Assisting with Cardiac Support

When the left ventricle becomes severely impaired, as in cardiogenic shock or in the late stages of any type of shock, its function may be augmented by the use of the intraaortic balloon pump[33] (see Chapter 26). A balloon-tipped catheter is inserted into the aorta by way of the femoral artery. The catheter is attached to a machine that inflates and deflates the balloon in synchrony with the patient's cardiac cycle. During systole the balloon is deflated as the heart pumps blood into the aorta. During diastole the balloon inflates, enhancing blood flow to the heart (particularly the coronary arteries), which is perfused during diastole, and to the rest of the body. During the next period of systole the balloon deflates again, leaving a space in the aorta that must be filled. This causes a reduction in resistance, which allows the heart to eject a larger quantity of blood with less effort than would normally be required. The balloon counterpulsation is then timed (either by conventional or real timing) to correspond to the cardiac cycle to support effective circulation while resting the impaired heart muscle.[8]

Complications may occur with use of the balloon pump, the most common being vascular insufficiency of the extremity distal to the insertion site. Frequent assessments are made of the pulses, color, temperature, movement, and sensation of the extremity, and any abnormality is reported immediately. Infection may occur with this procedure, as with any invasive procedure; therefore the patient's temperature is also monitored.

The use of the intraaortic balloon pump is a temporary measure intended to enhance cardiac output only until the heart is able to function adequately on its own.

Other devices now exist for emergency cardiopulmonary support for patients who have experienced hemodynamic collapse. These devices often provide a bridge to more long-term therapy such as a heart transplant and have proved successful in improving survival.[26] One such device is the "Hemopump" or *left ventricular assist device (LVAD).* The LVAD, while very useful in the treatment of postcardiotomy shock, acute myocardial infarction, and cardiogenic shock, is not practical for long-term use. Studies are in progress to determine the effects of long-term use of these devices on patients' quality of life. The size and experimental nature of this device make it an unrealistic option for supporting the long-term survival of patients with critically failing hearts.[42]

### Promoting Fluid Balance and Cardiac Output

#### Fluid replacement

The need to administer fluids to the patient with hypovolemic shock is obvious. At times, fluid replacement is the only therapy needed in this type of shock. Distributive and septic shock are accompanied by hypovolemia because fluid is leaking out of the capillaries and because the vascular space has increased with the vasodilation. Fluids are always part of the treatment. However, patients with cardiogenic shock also *may* require fluid therapy, although many may require fluid restriction or removal of fluid. Before fluid therapy is instituted for cardiogenic shock, a pulmonary artery catheter is inserted, and the pulmonary end-diastolic pressure is measured. If the pressure is less than 18 mm Hg and the cardiac index is less than 2.2 L per minute, volume replacement should be given.[32,33]

Current therapies for cardiogenic shock focus on improving tissue perfusion by enhancing oxygen delivery to vital organs during shock. Two means of accomplishing this are by increasing hemoglobin levels and/or by increasing cardiac output. Hemoglobin levels and the oxygen-carrying capacity of blood can be improved by infusing packed RBCs. Cardiac output from the left side of the heart can be impaired because of low circulating volume in some instances. *Fluid challenges,* limited controlled intravenous infusions of crystolloids or colloids, can be given to improve circulation and thus oxygen delivery. Such fluid challenges tend to be no greater than 200 ml and rarely are given without exact continuous monitoring of cardiac function using the pulmonary artery catheter.[5,31,34]

Various fluids may be given to the patient in shock. It is generally agreed that the patient who has sustained a large blood loss will require whole blood replacement. Much disagreement surrounds what other types of fluids should be used to treat shock. Both advantages and disadvantages exist to all types of resuscitative fluids, including blood.

Table 17-7 lists fluids used for replacement therapy in shock.

**Whole blood.** The administration of whole blood for shock is not risk free especially when massive transfusions are required, such as in *class IV* hemorrhage (loss of more than 40% of total blood volume). This condition is life threatening and is characterized by marked tachycardia and hypotension, very narrow pulse pressure, low urine output, and an obvious depression in mental status.[4]

Administration of whole blood has the advantage of increasing the oxygen-carrying capacity of the blood. It also has many disadvantages (transmission of diseases, transfusion reactions, and cost). If massive transfusions are given, additional problems may result. Because blood for transfusion contains an anticoagulant to prevent it from clotting while it is being stored, the patient who receives large amounts of blood may develop clotting defects. Stored blood is also deficient in platelets and other clotting factors. Massive transfusions of cold blood can result in hypothermia, which can cause cardiac dysrhythmias.

Stored blood also contains some debris resulting from the aggregation of platelets, leukocytes, and fibrin. It is believed that some of this debris is able to pass through standard blood filters and is eventually filtered out of the blood by the pulmonary capillaries. This probably causes little difficulty in the patient who receives only a few units of blood, but it is likely to cause a problem for the patient who receives massive transfusions. It is recommended by some that microfilters be used when large quantities of blood (e.g., massive transfusions of 10 units of whole blood or packed cells in less than 24 hours) are transfused.[23,41]

The pH value of stored blood is lower than that of normal blood. The added anticoagulant makes the blood more acidic. Also, because blood is stored in an airtight bag, the metabolism that continues is anaerobic, and the end products are lactic and pyruvic acid. Despite all the disadvantages, until a blood substitute is available for general use, blood must be given to maintain relatively normal hemoglobin and hematocrit levels. Blood also increases preload, which improves cardiac output and facilitates the oxygen-carrying capacity in the circulation.[5]

Some patients who are losing large amounts of blood may be given transfusions with their own blood, which has been collected from the bleeding site with special equipment. *Autotransfusion* has been used in patients bleeding massively from an uncontaminated wound, as well as in patients who bleed excessively during surgery (see Chapter 19). Although autotransfusion eliminates transfusion reactions, human immunodeficiency virus (HIV) infection, and viral hepatitis, it is not without risks. The most common complication of autotransfusion is hemolysis resulting in renal failure, coagulopathy, embolization of debris, and sepsis.[3,13] Its main use is in patients who are bleeding so rapidly that the supply of stored blood is becoming depleted.

**Other types of fluid therapy.** Fluids generally are classified as either crystalloid or colloid solutions (see Table 17-7). Controversy over which of these is better for the patient in shock has existed since the 1960s. In theory, colloids would seem to be superior because they should have the ability to hold fluid within the vascular compartment. However, when shock results in increased capillary permeability, the colloidal particle may leak into the interstitium and be followed by water. Another important consideration is cost. Colloids are generally much more expensive than crystalloids and therefore should be used only if their effect can be shown to be clearly superior to that of crystalloids.[10,36]

Regardless of the type of fluid that the patient receives, the nurse must carefully monitor the rate of administration. The patient is assessed frequently for signs of hypovolemia, fluid overload, or adverse reactions to the type of fluid being administered (see Chapter 15). Neck veins are observed for distention, and lungs are auscultated for signs of fluid (crackles, gurgles) and signs of reaction (e.g., rash or swelling).

### *Fluid redistribution*

Another way in which fluid resuscitation may be accomplished is by the use of *military antishock trousers (MAST).* This suit consists of three inflatable parts, one for each leg and one for the abdomen (Figure 17-8). When they are inflated, the trousers autotransfuse the upper circulation with up to

*Text continued on p. 463.*

**table 17-7** *Fluids Used for Replacement Therapy in Shock*

| Type | Uses/Indications | Advantages | Disadvantages | Special Considerations |
|---|---|---|---|---|
| **BLOOD AND BLOOD PRODUCTS** | | | | |
| Whole blood | Replaces blood volume and maintains hemoglobin (Hb) level at 12-14 g/100 ml<br>RBC concentration pulls fluid into intravascular space | Provides intravascular volume<br>Increases oxygen-carrying capacity of blood | Potential associated risks of hepatitis, HIV infection, and allergic reactions<br>Delayed administration because of necessary typing and cross-matching<br>Possibility of type and cross-match errors<br>Prolonged storage carries the risk of coagulopathy because whole blood is devoid of functional platelets after 24-48 hr | Whole blood should be stored at 1°-6°C (32°-50°F), but warmed at least 20-30 min before administration (*never* infuse cold blood).<br>Use *fresh* whole blood whenever possible to avoid adverse metabolic changes related to stored blood.<br>Administer via Y-connector tubing with normal saline to increase infusion flow rate. |
| RBCs (packed, concentrate)<br>Fresh, frozen (also called leukocyte-poor) | Increase hematocrit to minimum level of 30%<br>Corrects RBC deficiency and improve oxygen-carrying capacity of blood<br>Useful for patients with history of febrile nonhemolytic transfusion reactions | Concentrated form helps prevent excess fluid administration in patients with cardiogenic shock (increases oxygen-carrying capacity with less volume loading)<br>Associated with fewer risks of metabolic complications when compared with stored whole blood (decreased amount of transfused antibodies, electrolytes, and so on)<br>Provides economic use of blood as a resource; frees other blood components, such as platelets and clotting factors to be concentrated and stored | Same as above for whole blood<br>Slow infusion rate because of increased viscosity<br>Decreased content of plasma proteins and coagulation factors when compared with whole blood<br>Inadequate (alone) for volume replacement and correction of hypovolemia<br>Altered blood clotting with administration of more than 20 units; for every 4 units of RBCs over 20, 1 unit of fresh frozen plasma should be administered to replenish clotting factors<br>High cost of frozen (thawed) RBCs | Washed RBCs (resuspended in saline) can be given to persons in shock to decrease red cell adhesiveness (washing decreases cell's fibrinogen coating). |
| Human plasma (fresh, frozen, or dried) (FFP) | Increases oncotic pressure, thus improving circulating volume<br>Restores plasma volume in hypovolemic shock without increasing the hematocrit level<br>Restores clotting factors (except platelets)<br>Provides coagulation factors in selected patients with liver disease | Effective for rapid volume replacement<br>Contains clotting factors | Expensive<br>Deficient of RBCs<br>Should not be used as plasma expander if colloids/crystalloids can be used | Human plasma carries risk of hepatitis, HIV infection, and allergic reactions.<br>Administer fresh frozen plasma promptly after thawing to prevent deterioration of clotting factors V and VIII. |

From Alverdy JC, Levine E, Gould SA: Principles of blood replacement. In Sivak DE et al, editors: *The high risk patient: management of the critically ill,* Baltimore, 1995, Williams & Wilkins; and Fluids used for replacement therapy in shock. From American Society of Anesthesiologists: Practice guidelines for blood component therapy, *Anesthesiology* 84:732-746, 1996.

*Continued*

**table 17-7** *Fluids Used for Replacement Therapy in Shock—cont'd*

| Type | Uses/Indications | Advantages | Disadvantages | Special Considerations |
|---|---|---|---|---|
| **COLLOID SOLUTIONS** | | | | |
| Plasma protein fraction (Plasmanate, Plasma-Plex) | Expands plasma volume in hypovolemic shock (while cross-matching being completed)<br>Increases the serum colloid osmotic pressure | Can be used interchangeably with 5% human serum albumin<br>Osmotically equivalent to plasma<br>Associated with low risk of hepatitis | Expensive<br>Deficient of clotting factors<br>Associated with larger number of side effects, such as hypotension and hypersensitivity, than those reported with 5% albumin (because of presence of globulins)<br>Hypotension induced by rapid intravenous administration (greater than 10 ml/min)<br>Associated with risk of HIV infection | Plasma protein fraction is prepared from pooled plasma heated to 60°C (140°F) for 10 hr.<br>This procedure reduces risk of transmission of hepatitis viruses.<br>Rapid administration of large dosages can alter blood coagulation.<br>This solution should be used cautiously in patients with congestive heart failure (caused by added fluid and rapid plasma volume expansion) and in patients with renal failure (caused by added proteins). |
| Albumin<br>5%<br>25% (salt poor) | Increases plasma colloid osmotic pressure<br>Rapidly expands plasma volume | Rare allergic reactions (less than 0.01% in all albumin solutions combined)<br>Rare transmission of hepatitis virus<br>An important transport protein for drugs (e.g., antibiotics) and ions (e.g., calcium and magnesium) | Potential leakage from capillaries in shock states associated with increased capillary permeability<br>Possible precipitation of congestive heart failure after rapid infusion in patients with circulatory overload and compromised cardiovascular function | Albumin does not contain preservatives; therefore each opened bottle should be used at once.<br>Rate of administration of 5% albumin should not exceed 2-4 ml/min.<br>Rate of administration of 25% albumin should not exceed 1 ml/min.<br>25% albumin is reserved for use in patients with pulmonary or peripheral edema and hypoproteinemia.<br>Administer with a diuretic to ensure diuresis. |
| **PLASMA EXPANDERS** | | | | |
| Dextran<br>Low-molecular-weight dextran (LMWD) (dextran 40, Rheomacrodex, Gentran 40) | Rapidly expands plasma volume | All dextrans: associated with low incidence of anaphylactic reactions; less expensive than protein solutions<br>LMWD: associated with fewer allergic | LMWD: 70% excreted unchanged in urine, so urine osmolality and specific gravity are altered; potential osmotic nephrosis and renal tubular shutdown; possible bleeding from raw | Avoid use of dextran in patients with active hemorrhage, hemorrhagic shock, coagulation disorders, and thrombocytopenia. |

*Continued*

**table 17-7** *Fluids Used for Replacement Therapy in Shock—cont'd*

| Type | Uses/Indications | Advantages | Disadvantages | Special Considerations |
|---|---|---|---|---|
| Dextran—cont'd<br>High-molecular-weight dextran (HMWD) (dextran 70, Gentran 70 and 75, Macrodex) | | reactions than HMWD; facilitates blood flow by decreasing RBC adhesiveness<br>HMWD: leaks from the capillaries less readily than LMWD; can effectively increase plasma volume for up to 24 hr | surfaces caused by decreased platelet adhesiveness; side effects include decreased levels of hemoglobin, hematocrit, fibrinogen, and clotting factors V, VIII, and IX<br>HMWD: 50% excreted unchanged in the urine, so urine osmolality and specific gravity altered; higher incidence of allergic reactions when compared with LMWD; increases blood viscosity and platelet adhesiveness | Bleeding times can be prolonged when the correct dose of dextran 70 (1.2 g/kg/day) or dextran 40 (2 g/kg/day) is exceeded.<br>Administer dextran in dextrose solutions to patients with sodium restriction. |
| Hetastarch (Hespan, Volex) | Expands plasma volume | Same volume expansion characteristics of 5% albumin but with a longer duration of action (up to 36 hr)<br>Has longer serum half-life than albumin with 50% of osmotic effects persisting after 24 hours<br>Associated with low risk of allergic and anaphylactic reactions (0.085%)<br>Cost of hetastarch is about one half that of plasma protein fraction and albumin<br>Nonantigenic<br>No danger of transmission of hepatitis virus | Potential dilution of plasma proteins and decreased plasma colloid osmotic pressure<br>Potential dilution of clotting factors with resultant coagulation changes<br>Potential circulatory overload in patients with severe congestive heart failure and compromised renal function<br>Increased serum amylase level (>200 mg/100 ml), peaking within 1 hr of intravenous administration of hetastarch and persisting for 3-4 days (caused by action of amylase in hetastarch degradation) | Do not use if solution is cloudy or deep brown or if it contains crystals.<br>Monitor clotting studies and platelet counts, observing for prolonged PT and PTT and thrombocytopenia.<br>Safety and compatibility of additives with hetastarch have not been established; manufacturer recommends infusing hetastarch through separate line, when possible, or piggy-backing second drug.<br>Maximum infusion rate in acute hemorrhagic shock is 20 ml/kg/hr.<br>Monitor serum albumin level; if it falls below 2 g/100 ml, consider substituting albumin for hetastarch. |
| Mannitol (Osmitrol) | Raises intravascular volume<br>Reduces interstitial and intracellular edema<br>Promotes osmotic diuresis | Reduces intracellular swelling<br>Increases urinary output | Potential circulatory overload in patients with congestive heart failure, pulmonary congestion, and renal dysfunction | |

*Continued*

table 17-7 *Fluids Used for Replacement Therapy in Shock—cont'd*

| Type | Uses/Indications | Advantages | Disadvantages | Special Considerations |
|---|---|---|---|---|
| **CRYSTALLOID SOLUTIONS (ISOTONIC)** | | | | |
| Normal saline | Raises plasma volume when RBC mass is adequate<br>Replaces body fluid | Considered by some to be most important salt for maintaining and replacing extracellular fluid<br>Increases plasma volume without altering normal sodium concentration or serum osmolality | Potential fluid retention and circulatory overload caused by sodium content<br>Tends to be rapidly excreted because does not improve oncotic pressure | |
| Lactated Ringer's solution (Hartmann's solution) | Replaces body fluid<br>Buffers acidosis | Lactate converted to bicarbonate in liver, which buffers acidosis<br>Lactate replaces bicarbonate, preventing precipitation of calcium bicarbonate and calcium carbonate<br>Lactate more stable than bicarbonate and more compatible with ions present in solution | Increased lactic acidosis in shock caused by lactate<br>Fluid retention and circulatory overload caused by sodium content<br>Added $K^+$ possible problem in patients with renal failure or adrenal insufficiency<br>Added $Ca^{2+}$ risky in patients because $Ca^{2+}$ promotes the "no-flow" phenomenon after resuscitation from hemorrhagic shock | Lactate conversion requires aerobic metabolism; therefore it should be used cautiously in shock and other hypoperfusion states. |
| Ringer's solution | Replaces body fluid<br>Provides additional potassium and calcium | Does not contain lactate, so can be given to patients with hypoperfusion | Potential hyperchloremic metabolic acidosis caused by high chloride concentration<br>Potential fluid retention and circulatory overload caused by sodium content | |
| **CRYSTALLOID SOLUTIONS (HYPOTONIC)** | | | | |
| One-half normal saline | Raises total body fluid volume | | Potential interstitial and intracellular edema caused by rapid movement of this fluid from vascular space<br>Dilution of plasma proteins and electrolytes | |
| 5% dextrose in water (D5W) | Raises total body fluid volume<br>Provides calories for energy (200/1000 ml) | Distributed evenly in every body compartment (acts as free water)<br>Reverses dehydration<br>Prevents hyperosmolar state<br>Maintains adequate renal tubular flow (facilitates water excretion) | Dilution of plasma proteins and electrolytes caused by rapid metabolism of glucose and resultant free water | |

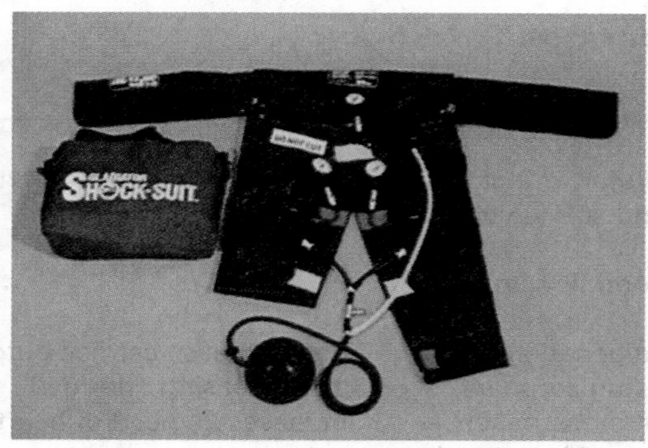


**fig. 17-8** Military antishock trousers (also called pneumatic antishock garment) can be effective in managing shock patients.

2 L of blood from the lower extremities, redirecting blood to the heart, lungs, and brain.[19,24] The trousers also increase peripheral resistance, which helps compensate for decreased blood volume. If bleeding in the lower extremities is present, the suit helps to control bleeding by tamponade (counterpressure). The suit is used as a temporary measure until adequate fluid can be administered. When the suit is to be removed, it must be deflated gradually to prevent a sudden fall in peripheral resistance and a return of shock.

**Positioning.** One position that should be avoided if possible in shock states is the Trendelenburg position. Although this position facilitates venous return, it has a negative effect in shock states. This head-down position causes fluid to rapidly shift to the upper thorax, activating the baroreceptors in the aortic arch and carotid arteries. Activation of these receptors sends incorrect signals that blood pressure is elevated, shutting off the body's sympathetic nervous system response to the shock state.

Fluid resuscitation may be facilitated by positioning the patient in a way that enhances fluid redistribution toward the upper body. If possible, the patient should be placed in the supine position with the legs elevated. This will promote venous return from the legs to the heart, thus improving cardiac output and organ reperfusion. In some instances the patient's clinical deterioration may be such that this type of positioning impairs the patient's ventilation. In such situations, elevation of the patient's head 30° to 45° should aid breathing.

### Medications

If fluid therapy alone is not sufficient to reverse the shock state, vasoactive drugs may be given. Most vasoactive drugs are catecholamines, which stimulate $\alpha$- or $\beta$-adrenergic receptors in the body. Generally, stimulation of $\alpha$-adrenergic-receptors causes vasoconstriction, and stimulation of $\beta$-adrenergic receptors causes vasodilation. Stimulation of $\beta$-adrenergic-receptors also causes the heart to increase its rate *(chronotropic effect)* and strength of contraction *(inotropic effect)*. The abdominal viscera, skin, and muscles respond primarily to the $\alpha$ effects of the catecholamines. (See Chapter 6 for review of effects of stimulation of adrenergic receptors.)

Mixed $\alpha$- and $\beta$-adrenergic drugs are used most often (Table 17-8). In the very early stage of shock, particularly shock characterized by vasodilation, the patient may benefit from drug therapy that results in vasoconstriction. This would enhance the body's normal compensatory mechanisms and increase the blood supply to the brain and the heart, allowing time for the primary problem to be corrected. However, if the primary problem is not or cannot be corrected, compensatory vasoconstriction itself can harm the body. Vasoconstrictive drugs, if used after the early stages of shock, may harm the kidneys and result in renal failure. They may also cause ischemia of the bowel, resulting in bowel necrosis and sepsis and ischemia of the pancreas, resulting in the release of MDF.

Vasodilatory drugs may be effective in counteracting the adverse effects of the body's compensatory mechanisms. They also decrease the pressure against which the failing heart has to pump, thereby decreasing the oxygen needs of the heart. However, they are not without danger. They may cause a fall in an already low arterial pressure, reducing coronary artery filling and making the heart even more hypoxic. Fluid therapy must be given with vasodilator drugs to maintain cardiac output. *Dopamine*, the most frequently used drug in the treatment of shock, has a variable effect depending on the dose administered. In certain dosage ranges it increases cardiac output by an inotropic effect on the heart and at the same time selectively dilates the renal and mesenteric vessels, increasing perfusion of the kidneys and the abdominal viscera. Selecting the proper drug depends to some extent on the cause of shock and how far it has progressed.

A combination of drugs may be given. Dopamine and nitroprusside may be given together to increase cardiac output by combining the inotropic effect of dopamine with the decreased peripheral resistance effected by nitroprusside. Low-dose dopamine may be given for its effect on renal and mesenteric perfusion along with dobutamine for its inotropic effect.

Patients receiving vasoactive drugs require very careful monitoring. Ideally, intraarterial and pulmonary pressure monitoring should be instituted. If the blood pressure is being measured by both cuff and intraarterial line, the two readings may vary. It is imperative that everyone working with the patient use the same measurements in adjusting the rate of drug infusion.

Steroids are often administered to patients in shock; however, their use is controversial. Many benefits from their use have been suggested, the most important being stabilization of lysosomal membranes, thereby preventing the leak of destructive enzymes.[20] There is a significant debate among physicians, however, about whether steroids enhance survival chances from shock. Studies have consistently failed to show any increase in patient survival after use of steroids in the treatment of shock, such as septic shock.[12,31]

**table 17-8** *Common Medications for* ***Vasoactive Treatment of Shock***

| | Effect | Advantages | Disadvantages |
|---|---|---|---|
| **MIXED α- AND β-ADRENERGIC DRUGS** | | | |
| Norepinephrine (levarterenol) | $\beta_1$: Pronounced effect in low doses<br>Positive inotropic and chronotropic effects | May improve cardiac output by increasing rate and stroke volume | Increases $O_2$ need of heart |
| | $\beta_2$: Weak effect<br>Dilation of coronary arteries | May improve blood flow to heart | |
| | α: Pronounced effect, especially in higher doses<br>Vasoconstriction | May improve oxygenation of heart by increasing coronary artery perfusion pressure, especially in presence of hypotension | May decrease cardiac output by increasing afterload<br>Increases $O_2$ need of heart |
| Epinephrine | $\beta_1$: Pronounced effect<br>Positive inotropic and chronotropic effect | May improve cardiac output by increasing stroke volume and rate | Increases $O_2$ need of heart |
| | $\beta_2$: Pronounced effect, especially in lower doses<br>Dilates coronary arteries and vessels in skeletal muscles | May increase blood supply to heart | May shunt blood away from vital organs because of dilation of vessels in skeletal muscles |
| | α: Pronounced effect in higher doses | May improve oxygenation of heart by increasing coronary perfusion pressure | May decrease cardiac output by increasing afterload<br>Increases $O_2$ need of heart |
| Dopamine | Dopaminergic receptors: pronounced effect in low (2-5 μg/kg/min) and moderate doses (5-10 μg/kg/min); α effect in high doses (>10 μg/kg/min) | Improves perfusion of kidneys and abdominal viscera | |
| | $\beta_1$: Pronounced effect in moderate dose range<br>Positive inotropic and chronotropic effect | Improves cardiac output | Increases $O_2$ need of heart |
| | $\beta_2$: Moderate effect<br>Dilates coronary arteries | Increases blood supply to heart | |
| | α: Pronounced in high doses<br>Offsets dopaminergic and β effects<br>Vasoconstriction | May improve oxygenation of heart by increasing coronary perfusion pressure | May decrease cardiac output by increasing afterload<br>Increases $O_2$ need of heart<br>Increases $O_2$ need of heart |

*Continued*

Many drugs are being used experimentally in the treatment of shock, particularly in septic shock. These include the use of α- and β-adrenergic agonists as well as dopaminergic receptors that may modulate severe immune responses seen in sepsis: prostaglandin inhibitors, nonsteroidal antiinflammatory drugs, endotoxin antibodies, and other agents.[9,14,15,18,25] Care of patients receiving vasoactive drugs is summarized in the Guidelines for Care Box.

### Preventing Injury and Infection

In the early stages of shock the patient may exhibit restlessness, which may then progress to confusion. During this time, injury is likely to occur if preventive measures are not taken. If the patient attempts to remove or disconnect life-saving equipment, soft restraints may have to be applied.

Infections occur often in patients with shock because of the many invasive procedures that are performed and the depres-

**guidelines for care**

**Patients Receiving Vasoactive Drugs**

- Monitor blood pressure every 5 to 15 minutes at the beginning of the infusion and every 15 minutes thereafter to maintain a *mean* blood pressure at prescribed level, usually 80 mm Hg.
- Drug must be diluted in a compatible solution and administered slowly by intravenous pump (for control).
- Observe peripheral site of infusion (if used) frequently for signs of infiltration; necrosis and sloughing of tissues may occur with infiltration.
- If infiltration occurs, infiltrate area around site with norepinephrine blockers (phentolamine [Regitine]) as prescribed.
- Monitor urinary output.
- When discontinuing drug infusion, taper infusion slowly while continuing to monitor blood pressure every 15 minutes.

**table 17-8 Common Medications for Vasoactive Treatment of Shock—cont'd**

| | EFFECT | ADVANTAGES | DISADVANTAGES |
|---|---|---|---|
| Dobutamine | $\beta_1$: Pronounced effect<br>Positive inotropic effect<br>Minimal chronotropic effect | Improves cardiac output by increasing stroke volume<br>Lack of rate increase allows more coronary filling time than other inotropic drugs | May decrease cardiac output by increasing afterload<br>Increases $O_2$ need of heart<br>Increases $O_2$ need of heart |
| | $\beta_2$: Weak effect<br>Some dilation of coronary arteries<br>$\alpha$: Minimal effect | May improve coronary artery blood flow | |
| **β-ADRENERGIC DRUGS** | | | |
| Isoproterenol | $\beta_1$: Very pronounced effect<br>Strong positive inotropic and chronotropic effects | Increases cardiac output by increasing stroke volume and rate | Pronounced increase in $O_2$ need of heart<br>Cardiac dysrhythmias |
| | $\beta_2$: Very pronounced effect<br>Dilates coronary arteries and vessels in skeletal muscles<br>Lowers peripheral resistance | May increase blood supply to heart<br>May improve cardiac output by decreasing afterload | Decreased blood pressure may decrease coronary artery perfusion pressure |
| **NONCATECHOLAMINE AGENT** | | | |
| Amrinone | Acts directly on cardiac cells | Increases myocardial contractility<br>Increases cardiac output | Decreases blood pressure by vasodilation |
| **VASODILATORS** | | | |
| Nitroprusside | Acts directly on smooth muscle, dilating both veins and arterioles | Decreases $O_2$ need of heart by decreasing both preload and afterload<br>Decreases pulmonary congestion by decreasing preload<br>Increases cardiac output by decreasing afterload | Decreases in peripheral resistance can decrease coronary artery perfusion pressure |
| Nitroglycerine | Acts directly on smooth muscle<br>Effect on veins—pronounced<br>Effect on arterioles—weak | Decreases $O_2$ need of heart by decreasing both preload and, to a lesser extent, afterload | Decrease in preload can decrease cardiac output and coronary artery perfusion pressure |

sion of the immune system associated with the stress response and ischemia that leads to cellular and tissue death. Some potential sources of infection are indwelling catheters, arterial lines, pulmonary artery catheters, intravenous lines, endotracheal tubes, surgical incisions, and traumatic wounds. Meticulous sterile technique must be used with endotracheal suctioning, dressing changes, tubing changes, and urinary catheter care. Patients who are receiving steroids or who have experienced excessive blood loss are at even greater risk of developing infection.

Complications of immobility must be prevented. The patient in shock may remain in one position for an extended period because of hypotension from loss of intravascular fluid, the limitation of movement from invasive technologies, and the constant activity occurring at the bedside. Such immobility can predispose the patient to complications, such as thrombi, pneumonia, and pressure ulcers.

Daily, detailed skin assessment is essential. Frequent turning (when clinically possible) and maintenance of clean, intact skin aid in prevention of ischemic skin and pressure ulcers. If immobility is prolonged or hypoperfusion severe, the use of therapeutic (low-pressure or pressure-minimizing) mattresses and beds should be considered.

## Promoting Comfort and Rest

The patient should be kept as comfortable as possible. Patients in shock should remain flat, with the legs elevated approximately 45° if necessary. If a patient in shock has difficulty breathing, a small pillow may be used to elevate the head slightly.

Rest is important. All nonessential activities should be eliminated because activity increases the body's need for oxygen and nutrients, substances already deficient in the cells of the patient in shock.

Ambient temperature should be kept at a comfortable level. Excessive warmth increases the metabolic rate of the tissues, thereby increasing their oxygen need. Excessive coolness may cause the blood to flow even more sluggishly through the microcirculation, enhancing the formation of microthrombi. Patients with an endotracheal tube in place or who are very lethargic may not be able to express how they feel. Covers should be used according to the room temperature.

Both the conscious patient and the family will probably experience considerable anxiety. The nurse should remain calm and explain all interventions whenever possible. It may be necessary to repeat explanations frequently to both patient and family, because anxiety can interfere with their ability to comprehend and to remember.

### Facilitating Learning

Patients who are in shock usually require close monitoring to supportive therapies such as oxygen and intravenous drug therapies, and testing and monitoring requiring the use of sophisticated electronic equipment. Such an environment and the uncertainty of the situation can cause significant stress and anxiety for patients and their families.

Educating the patient and family about the equipment and therapies can greatly reduce their anxiety and help diminish stress. Clear, simple explanations about what functions equipment and therapies perform provide them with information about the illness and the indicators that the professional staff are looking for as signs of clinical improvement in the patient's condition (see the Guidelines for Care Box).

## ■ EVALUATION

To evaluate the effectiveness of nursing interventions, compare patient behaviors with those stated in the expected patient outcomes. Successful achievement of patient outcomes for the patient in shock is indicated by:

1. Airway is clear of secretions.
2. Arterial blood gas levels are within normal limits (pH of 7.35 to 7.45; $Paco_2$ of 35 to 45 mm Hg; and $Pao_2$ of 80 to 100 mm Hg).
3. Respiratory rate is 16 to 20/min, with a normal tidal volume.
4. Intravascular volume is normal, as evidenced by hematocrit level of 42% to 52% for men and 37% to 47% for women (levels above 32% may be acceptable); hemoglobin level of 14 to 18 g/dl for men and 12 to 16 g/dl for women; CVP, PAP, PCWP, etc. measurements are within normal limits.
5. Cardiopulmonary perfusion is adequate, as evidenced by warm, dry skin; strong, palpable, symmetrical peripheral pulses; vital signs within patient's normal range; and absence of edema.
6. Urinary output is at least 50 ml/hr.
7. Experiences no injuries.
8. Is free from signs and symptoms of infection.
9. Offers statements of feeling relaxed; demonstrates no physical signs of anxiety; makes needs known.
10. Tolerates activity without an increase in pulse rate of more than 20 beats/min.

### guidelines for care

#### Instructing Patients/Families About Equipment Use in Management of the Patient in Shock

**Equipment Alarms and Use**

- Equipment often makes noise. Most noises are designed into the equipment to aid nurses/physicians in the monitoring of the patient.
- Almost all monitoring equipment has built-in alarms that have light and sound devices that alert the nurses and physicians something has changed.
- Alarms that go off do not always mean the patient is becoming more ill. Alarms mean the caregiver needs to check the patient and check the equipment.
- Understanding what equipment does to help you or your family member is important. Any time you see anything you do not understand, please ask the caregivers to explain its use and the alarms to you.

### critical thinking QUESTIONS

1 During report the nurse from the previous shift tells you that she suspects that Mr. C.'s myocardial contractility is compromised. When you ask about Mr. C.'s data that may suggest decreased myocardial function, the nurse replies that his mean PAP is above 10 mm Hg. How would you respond when given this information?

2 While assessing the 48-hour IV flow rates on a patient receiving a vasoactive drug, you note that each shift has been infusing the drug at a different rate. What are some of the possible explanations for a variation in flow rate?

3 Compare and contrast the assessment findings of a patient in cardiogenic shock and a patient in hypovolemic shock.

### chapter SUMMARY

**NATURE OF PROBLEM**

■ Shock is a syndrome characterized by hypoperfusion of body tissues and tissue hypoxia.

**ETIOLOGY**

■ The major classifications of shock are hypovolemic, cardiogenic, and distributive.

**PHYSIOLOGY**

■ Shock results in a derangement of cellular metabolism; if shock advances, it can affect all body systems.

## PATHOPHYSIOLOGY

- The early stage of shock is characterized by a stress response.
- At some point in the progress of untreated shock, the process becomes irreversible and results in death.

## NURSING MANAGEMENT

- The management of shock includes the following:
  a. Fluid therapy—blood and blood products, plasma expanders, colloids, crystalloids
  b. Drug therapy—vasodilators, vasoconstrictors, inotropes
  c. Supportive care—cardiac support, respiratory support, prevention of injuries and infections, and promotion of comfort

## References


1. Abello PA, Buchman TG, Bukley GB: Shock and multiple organ failure. In Armstrong P, editor: *Free radicals in diagnostic medicine,* New York, 1994, Plenum Press.
2. Ackerman MH: The systematic inflammatory response, sepsis and multiple organ disfunction: new definitions for an old problem, *Crit Care Nurs Clin North Am* 6(2):243-250, 1994.
3. Alverdy JC, Levine ES: Principles of blood replacement. In Sivak DE et al, editors: *The high risk patient: management of the critically ill,* Baltimore, 1995, Williams & Wilkins.
4. American Society of Anesthesiologists, Inc: Practice guidelines for blood component therapy: a report by the American Society of Anesthesiologists Task Force on Blood Component Therapy, *Anesthesiology* 84:732-747, 1996.

4a. American Society of Anesthesiologist, Inc: Practice guidelines for pulmonary artery catheterization: a report by the American Society of Anesthesiologists Task Force on pulmonary artery catheterization. *Anesthesiology* 78:380-394, 1993.

5. Baron BJ, Scalea TM: Acute blood loss, *Emerg Med Clin North Am* 14(1):35-55, 1996.
6. Barone JE: Treatment strategies in shock: use of oxygen transport measurements, *Heart Lung* 20(1):81-86, 1991.
7. Bone RC: A critical evaluation of new agents for the treatment of sepsis, *JAMA* 266(12):1686-1691, 1991.
8. Cadwell AC: Intra-aortic balloon counterpulsation timing, *Am J Crit Care* 5(4):254-261, 1966.
9. Calandra T et al: Treatment of gram-negative septic shock with human IgG antibody to *Escherichia coli j5*: a prospective double blind, randomized trial, *J Infect Dis* 158(2):312-319, 1988.
10. Cone A: The use of colloids in clinical practice, *Br J Hosp Med* S4(4):156-159, 1995.
11. Crowley SR: The pathogenesis of septic shock, *Heart Lung* 25(2):124-134, 1996.
12. Cronin L et al: Corticosteroids treatment for sepsis: a critical appraisal and meta-analysis of the literature, *Crit Care Med* 23(8):1430-1439, 1995.
13. Gannon DM et al: An evaluation of the efficacy of postoperative blood salvage after total joint arthroplasty. *J Arthroplasty* 1(2):109-114, 1991.
14. Gorelick K et al: Randomized placebo-controlled study of *E5* monoclonal antitoxin antibody. In Larrick J, Borrebaeck C, editors: *Therapeutic monoclonical antibodies,* New York, 1990, Stockton Press.
15. Hazinski MF: Mediator-specific therapies for the systemic inflammatory response syndrome, sepsis, severe sepsis and septic shock: present and future approaches, *Crit Care Nurs Clin North Am* 6(2): 309-319, 1994.
16. Higgins TL, Chernow B: Receptor physiology and pharmacology in circulatory shock. In Silvak E et al, Editors: *The high risk patient: management of the critically ill,* Baltimore, 1995, Williams & Wilkins.
17. Hinshaw LB: Sepsis/septic shock: participation of the microcirculation, *Crit Care Med* 24(6):1072-1078, 1996.
18. Huston MC: Pathophysiology of shock, *Crit Care Clin North Am* 2(2):143-149, 1990.
19. Krausz MM: Controversies in shock research: hypertonic resuscitation: pros and cons, *Shock* 3(1):69-72, 1995.
20. Lefering R, Neugebauer EAM: Steroid controversy in sepsis and septic shock: a meta-analysis, *Crit Care Med* 23(7):1294-1303, 1995.
21. Littleton MT: Prostaglandins and leukotrienes as mediators of shock and trauma, *Crit Care Nurs Q* 11(2):11-20, 1988.
22. Mancinelli-Van Atta J, Beck SL: Preventing hypoxemia and hemodynamic compromise related to endotracheal suctioning, *Am J Crit Care* 1(3):62-79, 1996.
23. Marino PA: *The ICU book,* Philadelphia, 1991, Lea and Febiger.
24. McSwain NE: Pneumatic anti-shock garment: state of the art 1988. *Ann Emerg Med* 17(5):506-526, 1988.
25. McCarthy S et al: Cytokine production and its manipulation by vasoactive drugs, *New Horizons* 4(2):252-264, 1966.
26. Overlie PA: Emergency cardiopulmonary support with circulatory support devises, *Cardiology* 84:231-237, 1994.
27. Owings JT and Holcraft JW: Fluid resuscitation of the critically ill patient. In Sivak DE et al: *The high risk patient: management of the critically ill,* Baltimore, 1995, Williams & Wilkins.
28. Phipps WJ: The patient with pulmonary problems. In Long BC, Phipps WJ, Cassmeyer, VL, Editors: *Medical surgical nursing: a nursing approach,* 3rd ed, St. Louis, Mosby, 1993.
29. Rady MY: Triage of critically ill patients, *Emerg Med Clin North Am* 14(1):13-33, 1996.
30. Ramamoorthy S: Current understanding and treatment of sepsis, *Infect Med* 12(6):261-268, 274, 1995.
31. Rice V: Shock: a clinical syndrome: an update. I. An overview of shock, *Crit Care Nurs* 11(4):20-27, 1991.
32. Rice V: Shock, a clinical syndrome: an update. III. Therapeutic management, *Crit Care Nurs* 11(6):41-43, 1991.
33. Rogers GR: Cardiovascular shock, *Med Clin North Am* 13(4):794-809, 1995.
34. Shoemaker WC: Monitoring and management of acute circulatory problems: the expanded role of the physiologically oriented critical care nurse, *Am J Crit Care* 1(1):38-53, 1992.

34a. Shoemaker WC: Pathophysiology, monitoring and therapy of acute circulatory problems, *Crit Care Nurs North Am* 6(2):295-307, 1994.

35. Shoemaker WC et al: Hemodynamic and oxygen transport monitoring to titrate therapy in shock, *New Horizons* 1(1):145-157, 1993.
36. Shoemaker WC et al: Resuscitation from severe hemorrhage, *Crit Care Med* 24(2):s12-s23, 1966.
37. Shelton BK: Disorders of hemostasis in sepsis, *Crit Care Nurs Clin North Am* 6(2):373-388, 1994.
38. Suhl J: Patients with septic shock. In Clochlsey J et al, editors: *Critical care nursing,* Philadelphia, 1993, WB Saunders.
39. Tortora JG, Grabowski SR: The cardiovascular system: blood vessels and hemodynamics. In Tortora JG, Grabowski SR, editors: *Principals of anatomy and physiology,* New York, 1993, Harper Collins College Press.
40. Vollman KM: Adult respiratory distress syndrome: mediators on the run, *Crit Care Nurs Clin North Am* 6(2):341-358, 1994.
41. Von Ruden KT: Sequelae of massive fluid resuscitation in trauma patients, *Crit Care Nurs Clin North Am* 6(3):463-472, 1994.

42. Wampler RK: Baker BA, Wright WM: Circulatory support of cardiac interventional procedures with the Hemopump™ cardiac assist system, *Cardiology,* 84:194-201, 1994.
43. West MA, Wilson W: Hypoxia alterations in cellular signal transduction in shock and sepsis, *New Horizons* 4(2):168-178, 1996.
44. Wiessner WH et al: Treatment of sepsis and septic shock, *Heart Lung* 24(5):380-392, 1995.
45. Wilson EW et al: Effects of backrest position on hemodynamic and right ventricular measurements in critically ill adults, *Am J Crit Care* 5(4):264-270, 1996.
46. Yared JP: Pitfalls in hemodynamic and respiratory monitoring. In Sivak DE et al: *The high risk patient: management of the critically ill,* Baltimore, 1995, Williams & Wilkins.

# chapter 18 Preoperative Nursing

JANE F. MAREK and MARY JO BOEHNLEIN

## objectives

*After studying this chapter, the learner should be able to:*

1 Identify the major influences on the emergence of operating room nursing.
2 Describe the preoperative phase as a component of the surgical experience.
3 Identify different classifications of surgeries.
4 Identify the biopsychosocial responses of patients to surgery.
5 Discuss the components of the preoperative patient assessment.
6 Relate the potential for postoperative complications.
7 Identify nursing diagnoses for the preoperative patient.
8 Discuss expected patient outcomes for the preoperative phase.
9 Discuss nursing interventions in the preoperative phase.
10 Discuss final preparations for the preoperative patient.

## HISTORICAL PERSPECTIVE

### HISTORY OF SURGERY

Surgery is defined as "the medical diagnosis and treatment of injury, deformity, and disease by manual and instrumental operations."[8] The word *surgery* comes from the Greek *kheirurgos,* which means working by hand. Hippocrates, the father of surgery, reportedly used wine or boiled water for wound irrigations as early as 450 BC. Surgery became a specific medical discipline approximately AD 130 to 200, at the time of the Greek physician Galen, who was said to have boiled his instruments before use. A variety of surgical techniques were practiced throughout the following years. During the 1500s ligatures were used to control bleeding. Morton's use of ether at Massachusetts General Hospital in 1846 heralded the advent of anesthesia as an adjunct to surgery. Use of the anesthetic permitted the physician to perform slower, more careful, and pain-free procedures. Despite these advances the incidence of wound infection and mortality rates were high. The mortality rate for patients undergoing amputation reportedly was as high as 40%.[10]

Not until the middle of the nineteenth century did surgery emerge as a true medical specialty. Ignaz Semmelweiss's work in 1847 demonstrated the importance of hand washing between procedures and patients in decreasing the incidence of puerperal fever following childbirth (see Chapter 10). In 1867 Joseph Lister published his work on antisepsis in which he advocated the use of antiseptics such as carbolic acid sprays during surgery to kill microorganisms. Neither Semmelweiss's nor Lister's methods were generally adopted until the 1880s and were followed by the introduction of the principles of aseptic technique. The late 1890s brought forth improvements in diagnostics tools, including the discovery of x-rays in 1895 and advancements in the development of surgical instrumentation. At the turn of the century most surgical procedures were limited to the abdomen. William and Charles Mayo, who had performed only 54 abdominal surgeries between 1889 and 1892, published an article in 1904 describing the results of 1000 abdominal procedures.[10] Surgical techniques continued to develop as thoracic, neurological, and cardiovascular procedures were developed. Throughout the twentieth century advances in anesthesia, surgical environment, and technology have allowed more predictable and safer outcomes for patients.

### PERIOPERATIVE NURSING: PAST AND PRESENT

In the early 1900s many surgical procedures were performed in the patient's home. Nursing's role focused on preparing the environment and supporting the patient. Increasingly complex procedures and greater demands on the physician's time made performing surgery in the home inconvenient for the surgeon, patient, and family. To accommodate these needs, physicians began performing surgery in private medical boarding houses, which provided both hotel and nursing services.[10] By the 1920s and 1930s most physicians were affiliated with hospitals. Nurses provided technical assistance to the surgeon.

Perioperative nursing, as it is known today, is an outgrowth of operating room (OR) nursing as it was practiced in its early years. Unlike the earlier focus, however, contemporary perioperative nursing practice is patient centered rather than task oriented.

The role of the registered nurse in the operating room has been expanded, refined, and standardized through the efforts of the members of the operating room nurses' professional organization, the Association of Operating Room Nurses (AORN).

The AORN defines the perioperative nurse as follows:

> The registered nurse who, using the nursing process, designs, coordinates, and delivers care to meet the identified needs of patients whose protective reflexes or self-care abilities are potentially compromised because they are having operative or other invasive procedures. Perioperative nurses possess and apply knowledge of the procedure and the patient's intraoperative experience throughout the patient's care continuum. The perioperative nurse assesses, diagnoses, plans, intervenes, and evaluates the outcome of interventions based on criteria that support a standard of care targeted toward this specific population. The perioperative nurse addresses the physiological, psychological, socio-cultural, and spiritual responses of the individual that have been caused by the prosect or performance of the invasive procedure.[2]

Using the American Nurses' Association (ANA) Code for Nurses with Interpretive Statements, AORN developed perioperative nursing explications of the Code for Nurses. The explications provide perioperative nurses with a framework to relate the ANA code to their own practice.

The *preoperative phase* begins when the decision for surgical intervention is made. The scope of nursing activities includes but is not limited to preoperative assessment of the patient's physical, psychological, and social states; the planning of nursing care that is required to prepare the patient for surgery; and the implementation of nursing interventions. This phase ends when the patient is safely transported to the OR and transferred to the OR nurse for care.

Movement of the patient onto the OR bed begins the *intraoperative phase;* this period lasts until the patient is admitted to the postanesthesia care unit (PACU). During this phase nursing responsibilities focus on the continuing assessment of the patient's physiological and psychological status and the planning and implementation of effective nursing interventions to promote safety and privacy and to prevent wound infection and promote healing. Specific nursing activities include providing emotional support to the patient during induction of anesthesia and throughout the procedure, establishing and maintaining functional positioning, maintaining asepsis, protecting the patient from electrical hazards, assisting in fluid balance, ensuring accurate sponge and instrument counts, assisting the surgeon, and communicating with both the patient's family and other health care team members.

The *postoperative phase* begins with admission to the PACU and ends with the final follow-up evaluation of the patient in the home or in a clinical setting. Nursing activities include ongoing assessment of changes in the physical and psychological status of the patient, along with appropriate planning and implementation of care. Activities include frequent monitoring of airway patency, vital signs, and neurological status, as well as providing intravenous fluids and blood, accurately assessing output from all drains, and providing a thorough summary report of the patient's status to the nurse receiving the patient on the unit and to the patient's family or friends.

**box 18-1** *Common Surgical Suffixes*

*-ectomy:* removal of an organ or gland
*-rrhaphy:* repairing
*-ostomy:* providing an opening (stoma)
*-otomy:* cutting into
*-plasty:* formation or plastic repair
*-scopy:* looking into

## SURGICAL PROCEDURES

### TYPES OF SURGERY

Most surgical procedures are given names that describe the site of the surgery and the type of surgery performed. For example, appendectomy refers to removal (-ectomy) of the appendix. Common surgical suffixes are listed in Box 18-1. Some surgeries carry the name of the surgeon who developed the technique, such as the Billroth procedures (partial gastrectomies). Surgeries may be classified according to the degree of risk, extent, purpose, anatomical site, timing, or physical setting.

### DEGREE OF RISK

The degree of risk involved in the surgical procedure is classified as either minor or major. *Minor surgery* is simple surgery that presents little risk to life. Many minor surgeries are performed with the use of local anesthesia, although general anesthesia may be used. (See Chapter 19.) Although the operation is termed *minor,* it is rarely viewed as a minor episode by the patient and may evoke fears and concerns. *Major surgery* presents a greater risk to the patient and is generally more extensive than minor surgery. It may involve risk to life. Major surgery usually is performed with use of general or regional anesthesia.

### EXTENT

The extent of the surgical procedure can be classified as minimal access, open, simple, or radical. *Minimal access procedures* are performed with the use of fiberoptic endoscopes and do not require traditional or extensive incisions. Endoscopes may be introduced through natural openings in the body or through porthole incisions, which also permit passage of surgical instruments. Endoscopic procedures have both diagnostic and therapeutic purposes. Endoscopic procedures can be performed on a variety of anatomical sites and have gained widespread use. Examples of endoscopic procedures may be found in Table 18-1. Advantages of minimal access surgery include ambulatory status or decreased length of hospital stay, reduced postoperative pain, and earlier resumption of normal activities.

*Open procedures* involve the traditional opening of the body cavity or body part in order to perform the surgery. Because of the more extensive surgical approach, the patient may experience more postoperative pain and a longer recovery period. The extent of the procedure may also influence postoperative infection rates. Infection rate increases with the length of procedure. It is estimated that the infection rate doubles for every hour the surgical procedure continues.[9]

**table 18-1** *Types of Endoscopic Surgical Procedures*

| Surgical Specialty | Possible Procedures Performed |
|---|---|
| General | Cholecystectomy |
| | Appendectomy |
| | Herniorrhaphy |
| | Modified Whipple procedure |
| | Nissen fundoplication |
| Orthopedic | Anterior cruciate ligament repair |
| | Carpal tunnel release |
| | Acromioplasty |
| | Diskectomy |
| Gynecological | Tubal ligation |
| | Laparoscopic assisted vaginal hysterectomy |
| | Hysteroscopy |
| Ear, nose, throat | Temporal mandibular joint repair |
| | Nasal polypectomy |
| | Ethmoidectomy |
| | Frontal antrostomy |
| Urology | Prostatectomy |
| | Bladder neck suspension |
| Thoracic | Mediastinoscopy |
| | Lymph node dissection |

*Simple procedures* are generally limited to a defined anatomical location and do not require extensive exposure and dissection of adjacent tissue. In contrast, *radical procedures,* which are usually associated with malignancies, involve dissection of tissue and structures beyond the immediate operative site. Adjacent lymph nodes, muscle, and fascia that have been invaded by tumor are excised.

## PURPOSE

Surgical procedures may be classified according to the reasons for which they are performed. Breast biopsy is an example of a *diagnostic* procedure performed to determine the cause of symptoms or origin of the problem. The goal of *curative* surgery, for example an appendectomy, is to resolve a health problem or disease state by removing the involved tissue. *Restorative* or *reconstructive* surgical procedures are performed to correct deformity, repair injury, or improve the functional status of the individual. Procedures done to relieve symptoms without the intent to cure are termed *palliative. Ablative* surgery is performed to excise tissue that may contribute to or worsen the patient's existing medical condition (e.g., an orchiectomy performed for a patient with prostatic cancer). *Cosmetic* surgery is preformed to improve personal appearance.

## ANATOMICAL SITE

Surgery may be classified by location of body parts or systems, such as cardiovascular surgery, chest surgery, intestinal surgery, or neurological surgery. Information specific to these types of surgery can be found in appropriate chapters elsewhere in the text.

## TIMING OR PHYSICAL SETTING

The timing of surgical intervention may be classified as *elective, urgent,* or *emergent.* Planned, nonessential surgical procedures are classified as elective. Urgent procedures are unplanned and require timely intervention but do not pose an immediate threat to life. Emergent procedures must be performed immediately to preserve life and limb. The same principles related to preoperative care apply to all types of surgery, although modifications must be made for emergent surgical intervention because of the limited preoperative time.

*Ambulatory surgery* does not require overnight hospitalization and may be performed under general, local, or regional anesthesia. The patient is admitted to the ambulatory facility on the day of surgery, remains for postoperative care, and is discharged within 23 hours. Origins of ambulatory surgery can be traced to Egypt as early as 3000 BC. Rapid-acting anesthetic agents, minimal-access surgical techniques, technological advances, and changes in reimbursement policies by the federal government and third-party payers all contributed to the emergence of ambulatory surgery as a safe and cost-effective method to provide surgical services. Ambulatory surgical care facilities include hospital-based centers, hospital-affiliated satellite centers, freestanding facilities, and physicians' offices.

In the past all patients were admitted to the hospital for preparation 1 or more days before surgery. The most recent trend, in response to the national mandate to reduce health care cost, is same-day surgery. The patient is admitted to the hospital on the day of the planned procedure and remains hospitalized postoperatively. Patient assessment and preoperative teaching are conducted on an outpatient basis before admission.

# SPECIAL CONSIDERATIONS FOR THE PATIENT IN THE SURGICAL SETTING

Surgery is a unique experience for each patient, depending on the underlying psychosocial and physiological factors present. Although some operations are considered minor procedures by hospital personnel, surgery is always a major experience for the patient and family. Surgery is a stressor that produces both physiological stress reactions (neuroendocrine responses) and psychological stress reactions (anxiety, fear). Surgery is also a social stressor, requiring family adaptation to temporary or lasting role changes.

## NEUROENDOCRINE RESPONSE TO SURGERY

Impending surgery evokes the physiological stress response. The body's response to impending stress is coordinated by the central nervous system. The central nervous system activates the hypothalamus, the sympathetic nervous system, the anterior and posterior pituitary glands, the adrenal medulla, and the cortex. This activation results in the release of catecholamines and hormones, which are responsible for the physiological events that occur in response to stress.

Systemic effects of the neuroendocrine response are manifested by many complex changes in the body. Some of these changes include increased heart rate and blood pressure, increased blood flow to the brain and vital organs, decreased motility and blood flow to the gastrointestinal tract, increased gastric acid production, elevated blood glucose, increased respiratory rate, increased perspiration and piloerection, dilation of pupils, and platelet aggregation. The perioperative nurse must be aware of the physiological impact that impending surgery may have on the patient. For further discussion of stress refer to Chapter 6.

## THE PSYCHOLOGICAL RESPONSE

Anxiety is a normal adaptive response to the stress of surgery. Anxiety occurs in the preoperative phase as the patient anticipates the surgery or during postoperative experiences such as pain and discomfort, changes in body image or function, increased dependency, loss of control, family concerns, or potential changes in lifestyle. Anxiety may be decreased if the patient perceives the surgery as having positive results, such as curing disease, relieving discomfort, or creating a more attractive physical appearance. On the other hand, anxiety usually is increased when the underlying pathological condition is, or is believed to be, malignant or life threatening (e.g., open heart surgery).

Previous surgical experiences may positively or negatively affect the patient's level of anxiety. Anxiety is a well-documented motivating force for many types of behavior. However, extended or excessive periods of anxiety can lead to increased protein breakdown, decreased wound healing, altered immune response, increased risk of infection, and fluid and electrolyte imbalance.[6]

Fear is another emotional response that can result from a perceived impending threat such as surgery. Fear of the unknown and loss of control are the most common responses. Other fears are more specific and related to the type, extent, and purpose of surgery (Box 18-2). Fears concerning pain, disfigurement, or permanent disability may be realistic or may be influenced by lack of information or the personal experiences of others.

**box 18-2** *Fears Related to Surgery*

**GENERAL**

Fear of unknown
Loss of control
Loss of love from significant others
Threat to sexuality

**SPECIFIC**

Diagnosis of malignancy
Anesthesia
Dying
Pain
Disfigurement
Permanent limitations

## INFORMED CONSENT

A patient's right to self-determination regarding surgical intervention is protected by the informed consent process.[3] Before surgery the patient is asked to a sign a statement consenting to the operative procedure. The consent implies that the patient has been given the information necessary to understand the nature of the procedure, as well as the known and possible consequences. The physician is responsible for providing the patient with sufficient information to weigh the risks and benefits of the proposed surgery (disclosure duty). The information usually includes the nature of the surgery with its benefits and risks and prognosis if treatment is withheld. Risks include bodily harm or death, but not the more typical potential postoperative complications such as infection. Legal responsibility for obtaining informed consent from the patient resides with the physician.

The necessary components of the consent document include patient's full legal name; surgeon's name; specific procedure(s) to be performed; signature of the patient, next of kin, or legal guardian; witness(es); and date. Witnessing the informed consent does not ensure that the patient has a complete understanding of the surgical procedure and its consequences. By signing the consent form, the witness validates *only* identification of the patient or legal substitute, mental status of the patient at time of signature (not under the effects of mind-altering substances and alert and competent), and voluntary signature.

Signing of the official consent form primarily provides evidence that the consent process has occurred and that the patient is aware of the concept of informed consent. The role of the nurse in this process is one of patient advocate. The nurse should verify that the patient has discussed with the physician the risks and benefits of the surgery and the alternatives. If this discussion has not taken place, the nurse should consult with the physician. Also the nurse should assess the patient's understanding of what is to occur during and after surgery to clarify any misconceptions and to facilitate the decision-making process. Patients may decide to refuse surgery, and it is their right to do so. Nurses have the responsibility to see that the decision is an informed one. It is imperative that this process occur before the patient receives any sedation. If an adult is incapable of giving informed consent, consent must be obtained from the next of kin. The order of kin relationship for an adult, as determined from legal interstate succession, is usually spouse, adult child, parent, and sibling. A parent or legal guardian usually provides consent for a minor child. "Emancipated minors," that is, minors who are married or earning their own livelihood and retaining the earnings, can sign their own permits. The signature of the husband or wife of a married minor is also acceptable. In an emergency, the surgeon may operate without written permission of the patient or family, although every effort is made to contact a family member or guardian if time permits. Consent in the form of a telephone call is permissible in this situation. The call must be witnessed by two persons. If no family member or legal guardian is able to be contacted, the decision for surgical intervention may be made by two physicians who are not associated with the procedure. In this circumstance a relative must sign an operative consent as soon as possible. Patients who are illiterate must understand the verbal explanation of the consent process and may sign the form with an *X*. This process must be witnessed by two persons. Translators must be provided for patients with language barriers. The consent form for mentally incompetent persons may be signed by the legal guardian; in the guardian's absence, a court of competent jurisdiction may legalize the procedure.

## DO-NOT-RESUSCITATE ORDERS

The patient, or the individual with durable power of attorney for health care, has the right to determine treatment options regarding end-of-life decisions. The decision not to initiate cardiopulmonary resuscitation is written as a specific directive by a physician, which is termed a *do-not-resuscitate (DNR) order.* Perioperative nurses may encounter patients with DNR orders who are undergoing surgical procedures to improve the quality of life or for palliative care. Do-not-resuscitate orders are not automatically suspended when the patient enters the operating room. The AORN's position statement on perioperative care of patients with DNR orders is supported by the Patient Self-Determination Act, the Joint Commission on Accreditation of Healthcare Organizations (JCAHO), the American Nurses' Association Code for Nurses, and "A Patient's Bill of Rights."[3] The AORN position statement asserts the following: "Required reconsideration of DNR decisions with patients is an integral component of the care of patients undergoing surgery."[2] Reviewing the DNR status ensures that the risks and benefits of anesthesia and surgery are discussed with the patient or family before surgery. Discussion should include goals of surgical treatment, potential for and nature of resuscitative measures, and possible outcomes with and without resuscitative efforts. The patient or the individual with durable power of attorney will decide whether to maintain, suspend, or modify the DNR orders during anesthesia and surgery. If the DNR order is suspended during the intraoperative period there must be documentation indicating when it is to be reinstated. The perioperative nurse has the obligation to support the patient's decisions regarding end-of-life treatment choices.

## THE SOCIOLOGICAL RESPONSE

The usual role of a person hospitalized—even for one day—is disrupted. This disruption inevitably causes role adaptation on the part of other family members and friends as they help with transportation of the patient to and from the hospital, psychological support of the patient, child care, and other family responsibilities. Inability to work also may be a problem to both the patient and the family. Job security may be threatened, and financial stress may result.

Literature reveals that family members often experience more anxiety than the patient because of their own feelings of helplessness concerning the surgery.[9] Family members and friends may be anxious for a variety of reasons. They may be concerned about the final outcome of the surgery and resultant changes in lifestyle or routines. They may also experience the stress of providing emotional support for the patient at a time when they themselves are stressed. Family members and friends may also have their own memories and unpleasant associations with surgery, which may result in increased stress and anxiety.

# NURSING MANAGEMENT

## ■ ASSESSMENT

Assessment of the patient during the preoperative phase begins with the initial contact between patient and nurse and is ongoing throughout the period. Assessment should be holistic, reflecting the physiological, psychological, spiritual, and social needs of the patient and the family or significant others.

Patient assessment occurs in a variety of settings. The nurse's initial contact with the patient may be in the physician's office, preadmission testing area, inpatient hospital unit, ambulatory surgery facility, or it may be over the telephone. A complete history is compiled to identify factors that may increase surgical risk or the development of postoperative complications (Box 18-3). Some operative and postoperative complications can be prevented or ameliorated if patients at high risk of developing complications are identified early and preventive measures implemented.

### Subjective Data

#### Age

Age affects surgical and postoperative outcomes. Between the ages of 30 and 40 the functional capacity of each organ system decreases by approximately 1% annually.[9] The age of the surgical patient identifies those individuals at increased risk for surgical and postoperative complications. Refer to the section on gerontological considerations for further discussion.

**box 18-3** *Preoperative Subjective Data Collection*

- Age
- Allergies
  - Iodine
  - Medications
  - Latex
  - Cleansing solutions
  - Adhesive tape
- Medications and substance use
  - Prescription drugs
  - Over-the-counter drugs
  - Smoking
  - Alcohol
  - Recreational drugs
- Review of systems
- Current and previous surgical experience
- Cultural and religious background
- Psychosocial

### Allergies

The patient should be assessed for allergies to iodine, medications, latex, cleansing solutions, and adhesive tape. This information is needed because many of these products are used throughout the surgical procedure. Povidone-iodine is commonly used intraoperatively for cleansing the patient's skin. If the patient is unsure whether he or she has an allergy to iodine, the nurse should question the patient regarding allergies to shellfish. It is necessary to elicit information regarding allergies to shellfish because of the high iodine content. Iodine is also a component of many contrast media that may be used intraoperatively. Latex allergy is discussed in Chapter 20.

### Medications and substance use

Data regarding history of smoking, substance abuse, and prescribed and over-the-counter medications are collected. These data are important because of the potential adverse effects of these substances with some anesthetic agents and increased risk for intraoperative and postoperative complications. Smoking causes pathological changes in the respiratory tract that can increase the risk of intraoperative and postoperative complications. Drug and alcohol use can alter the effects of anesthetic and analgesic agents. Aspirin and nonsteroidal antiinflammatory drugs (NSAIDs) affect platelet function and may increase risks for intraoperative and postoperative hemorrhage. Many types of prescription medications may affect reactions to anesthetics or surgery (Table 18-2).

### Medical history

A thorough review of systems is taken to assess the patient's immunological, endocrine, cardiovascular, respiratory, renal, gastrointestinal, neurological, musculoskeletal, and dermatological status. The nurse questions the patient regarding the presence of systemic or chronic illness. Certain chronic or systemic illnesses increase the potential for intraoperative and postoperative complications.

The immunosuppressed surgical patient may be at an increased risk for infection and impaired wound healing. Conditions that result in immunosuppression include the normal aging process, cancer, diabetes mellitus, chemotherapy, radiation therapy, and long-term steroid use.

Patients with diabetes mellitus are at risk for delayed wound healing and infection. The presence of obesity, advanced age, and complications resulting from diabetes place the patient at additional risk. Stress, nothing-by-mouth (NPO) status, anesthesia, tissue trauma, and reduced postoperative activity are all factors that affect regulation of blood glucose levels.

Assessment of a patient's cardiovascular status is essential because of the prevalence of cardiovascular disease in the general population. The presence of cardiovascular disease may put the surgical patient at risk for anesthetic complications, intraoperative myocardial infarction, thrombophlebitis, cerebrovascular accident, and heart failure. A patient with a questionable or positive history of cardiac disease may need a cardiac consultation before undergoing elective surgery.

A chronic pulmonary condition causes physiological pulmonary changes that impede airflow and can cause problems both intraoperatively and postoperatively. Common complications include atelectasis, pneumonia, respiratory insufficiency, and respiratory acidosis. The increased lung compliance, increased airway resistance, and chronic mucus hypersecretion found in chronic obstructive pulmonary disease (COPD) may lead to inadequate ventilation, severe hypoxemia, dysrhythmias, and respiratory failure. Smoking causes blood vessel constriction and increased secretions. The carbon monoxide in smoke binds with hemoglobin, decreasing tissue oxygenation.

The patient is assessed for the presence of renal disease. Decreased renal function can alter the body's ability to excrete waste products, medications, and anesthetic agents. Patients with history of renal disease are at high risk for the development of problems with fluid and electrolyte balance.

### Current and previous surgical experiences

The patient's level of understanding of the proposed surgical procedure and postoperative routine is determined. The

**table 18-2** *Commonly Prescribed Medications and Their Effects on Anesthesia or Surgery*

| Medication | Effect | Nursing Implications |
|---|---|---|
| Anticoagulants<br>Aspirin<br>Heparin<br>Warfarin | Inhibit platelet aggregation<br>Inhibit action of antithrombin<br>Interfere with coagulation factors | Aspirin should be discontinued 7 days before surgery<br>Monitor for signs and symptoms of hemorrhage<br>Monitor coagulation studies, prothrombin time, partial thromboplastin time |
| Nonsteroidal antiinflammatory drugs | Inhibit platelet aggregation, prolong bleeding time | Monitor for sign and symptoms of bleeding |
| Steroids | Decrease neuroendocrine response, antiinflammatory effect, delayed wound healing | Maintain drug therapy perioperatively, may be given IV intraoperatively, monitor closely for signs and symptoms of infection |
| Antihypertensives | Possible hypotensive crisis intraoperatively | Continuous monitoring of blood pressure, pulse during perioperative period |
| Antidepressants SSRIs (Prozac) | Long half-life | Monitor renal and hepatic functioning |

nurse explores the patient's understanding and expectations of treatment. The nurse also assesses the patient's previous experiences with surgery or anesthesia. These data provide the surgical team with information regarding any reactions or complications to surgical procedures or anesthetics, such as malignant hyperthermia (see Chapter 19). A positive family history of malignant hyperthermia is significant, because it is an autosomal dominant inherited syndrome.

### Cultural and religious background

Cultural background influences responses to health, illness, surgery, and death. An awareness of cultural differences may enhance the nurse's knowledge of how the surgical experience may be experienced by the patient and the family. In addition, responses to pain may be influenced by cultural and ethnic background.

Like cultural beliefs, religious beliefs also influence individual and family responses to health, illness, pain, surgery, and death. Religion can be a source of support and comfort for the patient. Some religions allow for little individual control over the environment and therefore may dictate the degree or level of medical interventions a patient chooses. Awareness of a patient's individual religious beliefs enables the nurse to appropriately support the patient's individual decision regarding care throughout the perioperative period. For example, the nurse would be supportive of a Jehovah's Witness's refusal to receive blood transfusions.

### Psychosocial

Preoperative psychological assessment includes the collection of both subjective and objective data. Much of the data concerning knowledge and perceptions of the coming event will be obtained directly from the patient (Box 18-4). Knowing the level of the patient's understanding of the surgical event is required before any teaching can take place. It is important to find out exactly how the surgery is perceived because persons respond on the basis of their perceptions. Patients may not be able to identify specific concerns, and further exploration may be indicated. If the nurse has identified cues on which conclusions are drawn, these conclusions should be validated with the patient.

Signs of anxiety in the presurgical patient are no different from those in other persons. Signs vary from person to person and can be observed in a number of ways. Highly anxious persons may talk rapidly, ask many questions without waiting for answers, repeat the same questions, or change topics frequently during the interaction. They may deny that they have any worries or fears, but their actions are contrary to this denial. Some patients will not talk about the forthcoming surgery, responding only in monosyllables, whereas others cry and display anger; both behaviors are overt signs of anxiety.

Physical signs include increased pulse and respiratory rate, moist palms, constant hand movements, and restlessness. Anxiety results in elevated levels of cortisol and adrenaline, which are normal physiological responses to stress. Prolonged anxiety may lead to increased protein breakdown, decreased wound healing, increased risk of infection, altered immune response, and fluid and electrolyte imbalances.[6] Changes in sleep patterns also provide clues about increased anxiety. Major causes of insomnia are worry, fear, and concerns about the future.

The effect of family members or significant others on the patient's level of anxiety needs to be determined. Some significant others increase the patient's anxiety by transmission of their own anxiety by hovering over the patient, displaying anxious behaviors, or offering false reassurances. Others are calm, and it is observed that the patient's anxiety is reduced when they are present.

Assessing the social situation of the patient and family is particularly important if the nurse is incorporating the family as client in the preoperative period. The financial situation of the patient may have considerable implications for both the immediate surgical intervention and the follow-up care. The social support network for the patient and family also should be assessed during the preoperative phase. The primary source of psychological support for the patient is usually the family or significant others. Knowledge of their coping mechanisms will enable the nurse to assist the patient to cope with the impending events. Preoperatively, family members are often more anxious than the patient, perhaps because of feelings of powerlessness and helplessness.[9]

**box 18-4** *Assessment of Preoperative Anxiety*

**SUBJECTIVE DATA**

1. Understanding of proposed surgery
   - Site
   - Type of surgery to be done
   - Information from surgeon regarding extent of hospitalization, postoperative limitations
   - Preoperative routines
   - Postoperative routines
   - Tests
2. Previous surgical experiences
   - Type, nature
   - Time interval
3. Any specific concerns or feelings about present surgery
4. Religion, meaning for patient
5. Significant others
   - Geographical distance
   - Perception as source of support
6. Changes in sleep patterns

**OBJECTIVE DATA**

1. Speech patterns
   - Repetition of themes
   - Change of topic
   - Avoidance of topics related to feelings
2. Degree of interaction with others
3. Physical
   - Increased pulse and respiratory rates
   - Increased hand movements and perspiration
   - Increased activity level
   - Increased voiding frequency

## Objective Data

### Physical assessment

The nurse performs a complete head-to-toe physical assessment. Objective data are collected in the preoperative phase for two reasons: (1) to obtain baseline data for comparison during the intraoperative and postoperative phases and (2) to identify potential problems that may require preventive nursing interventions before surgery. If the patient has been hospitalized, the admission history and physical assessment should contain much of the pertinent data that can serve as baseline data before surgery. Recording of the data is important for comparison when changes occur during the perioperative period and for planning nursing care. Any abnormalities in the patient's physical assessment are documented and reported to the attending surgeon and anesthesiologist for further evaluation. The surgical procedure may be canceled based on the severity of the abnormal findings. Refer to individual assessment chapters for in-depth discussion of each particular system.

A complete preoperative assessment of the patient's respiratory status is necessary. Interference with ventilation as a result of anesthetics, pooled respiratory secretions, or both is a common postoperative occurrence that may lead to the complications of atelectasis and pneumonia. A preoperative baseline assessment of the person's ventilatory status is important for early identification of whether the patient is at high risk for the development of postoperative respiratory complications.

Patients at high risk include (1) those scheduled for upper abdominal or thoracic surgery, (2) those who will receive inhalant anesthesia, (3) the obese, (4) smokers, (5) patients suffering from chronic lung disease, and (6) elderly persons. Table 18-3 summarizes the major risk factors for postoperative pulmonary complications.

Preoperative assessment of the patient's cardiovascular status is essential for the identification of signs of heart disease that need correction before surgery. A 12-lead electrocardiogram (ECG) to detect signs of cardiac dysrhythmias or heart damage is usually ordered for persons older than 40 years of age.

**table 18-3** *Risk Factors for the Development of Postoperative Pulmonary Complications*

| Condition | Effect |
|---|---|
| **INCREASED RESPIRATORY SECRETIONS** | |
| **Risk Factors** | |
| Smoking | Irritation of lining of bronchial passages |
| Chronic lung disease | Decreased ciliary action to remove secretions |
| Respiratory infection | Secretions will block bronchial passages or alveoli |
| **DECREASED THORAX EXPANSION** | |
| **Risk Factors** | |
| Obesity<br>Age (elderly)<br>Skeletal deformities (e.g., scoliosis) | Lung does not expand fully, resulting in hypoventilation |

Vital signs are obtained. The nurse screens the patient for undiagnosed hypertension. Heart sounds are auscultated, paying particular attention to the presence of extra sounds, irregularities, or murmurs. The nurse evaluates the extremities for the presence and quality of peripheral pulses, capillary refill, warmth, color, and edema.

Adequate renal function is necessary to maintain fluid and electrolyte balance during the perioperative period. The nurse observes the patient's urine for color clarity, quality, amount, and odor. Urinary tract infection, if present, is treated with antibiotics before surgery.

The patient's musculoskeletal status is assessed for abnormalities in joint structure and function. Limitation in range of motion or arthritis may interfere with intraoperative patient positioning. Persons with alterations in musculoskeletal function may be predisposed to postoperative complications associated with immobility.

An evaluation of the patient's neurological status, including level of consciousness, orientation, and motor and sensory function, is performed. This information is necessary to detect any abnormalities from baseline functioning that may occur during the perioperative period. The patient is also evaluated for sensory deficits such as problems with vision or hearing.

The patient's integumentary system is assessed. Alteration in skin integrity may affect intraoperative patient positioning and placement of monitoring devices, skin preparation, drapes, and other surgical equipment.

The nutritional status of the patient affects postoperative outcomes. An estimated 50% of hospitalized patients have some degree of malnutrition.[3] As a result of malnutrition the patient may experience negative nitrogen balance, failure of blood clotting mechanisms, alterations in wound healing, increased risk of infection, electrolyte imbalance, and increased risk of morbidity and mortality. The obese patient is often malnourished from lack of appropriate nutrient intake.

An assessment of the hydration status of the patient is important because of potential alterations in fluid volume balance resulting from NPO status, administration of intravenous fluids, intraoperative and postoperative hemorrhage, and excessive wound drainage. Physical examination findings that suggest alterations in nutrition and hydration status may include weight outside of ideal range, decreased muscle tone, lack of subcutaneous tissue, dry and flaky skin, brittle nails, poor skin turgor, dry mucous membranes, or edema.

### Diagnostics

Laboratory and diagnostic testing are performed before the patient is cleared for surgery. The extent of laboratory testing is determined by patient age and physical condition, type of procedure and anesthetic, and institutional requirements. Laboratory and diagnostic testing may take place in a variety of facilities and may occur up to 30 days before the planned surgical procedure depending on institutional protocol. Admission panel testing protocols are based on age. Patients over 40 years of age generally require ECG, complete blood count

(CBC), electrolyte panel, and urinalysis. Other tests may be indicated according to the patient's medical history, risk factors, and the proposed surgical procedure. Refer to Table 18-4 for examples of common tests that may be performed.

If surgical blood loss is anticipated, a blood sample is sent for type and crossmatching so that packed red blood cells can be available for transfusion intraoperatively and postoperatively. In the case of elective surgery, the patient may choose to do autologous donation. Use of patient's blood eliminates the risk of contracting hepatitis B virus or human immunodeficiency virus (HIV) from blood transfusions. According to the guidelines of the American Association of Blood Banks, the patient's hematocrit must be at least 34% and the white blood cell count must be below 12,000/mm$^3$ for the patient to be allowed to donate. Donations must be completed at least 72 hours before surgery, and the blood is good for 36 days after donation. The patient may be advised to take an iron supplement after donation, depending on the number of units donated and baseline hematocrit. The patient should be informed about autologous donation at the time the decision is made for surgical intervention, to allow sufficient time for donation.

## Surgical Risk

Every person responds to the surgical experience in a unique way. A number of variables influence psychological and physiological responses throughout the entire surgical experience. Some of these include age, the presence of chronic disease or disabilities, impaired nutritional status, and type of surgical procedure performed. Medication use can also affect the patient's reaction to anesthetics and other agents used intraoperatively.

### *Gerontological considerations*

An estimated 11% to 13% of the population are aged 65 years and older, and 50% of the elderly will undergo at least one surgical procedure before death.[4] The ability of the elderly patient to tolerate surgery depends on the extent of the physiological changes that have occurred with the aging process, the duration of the surgical procedure, and the presence of one or more chronic illnesses. In general, the patient over 65 is a greater surgical risk than a younger individual. The mortality rate is less than 1% in individuals younger than 65 years of age, 5% to 10% in those 65 to 80 years of age, and 10% in individuals over 80 years of age. Surgical procedures that present an increased risk for elderly patients include abdominal, thoracic, neurosurgical, and emergency procedures.[7] Increased incidences of mortality and postoperative complications are associated with cardiac disease, pulmonary complications, sepsis, and renal failure.

The normal aging process produces a general decline in organ function, alterations in pharmokinetics, and alterations in thermoregulatory ability. The nurse's knowledge of the normal aging process is essential for planning perioperative interventions for the geriatric patient. A summary of physiological changes associated with aging is presented in Table 18-5.

Assessment of the elderly patient's visual and auditory capacity, nutritional status, and psychological status is necessary. Hearing and visual impairment are common in the elderly. Hearing loss has been identified in 33% to 50% of persons 65 years of age and older.[11] Common causes of visual impairment in older adults include presbyopia, cataracts, age-related macular degeneration, and glaucoma. Nutritional status may be affected by the presence of loose teeth, ill-fitting dentures, or poor dentition.

In addition to the physiological alterations in the geriatric patient, the nurse also needs to be aware that physiological and psychological stressors may cause confusion. It is important to determine the reason for confusion. Common causes of confusion include hypoxia, electrolyte imbalance, cerebral hemorrhage, diabetes, infection, dehydration, medications, Alzheimer's disease, and unfamiliar surroundings.

Depression and alcohol abuse are common in the elderly and are often undiagnosed. Both can effect postoperative

**table 18-4** *Common Preoperative Diagnostic Tests*

| System | Test | Possible Findings |
|---|---|---|
| Cardiovascular | 12-lead ECG | Dysrhythmias, ischemia, infarct |
| | Complete blood count (CBC) with differential | Blood dyscrasias, anemia, blood loss, infection, congestive heart failure |
| | Electrolytes | Electrolyte imbalance |
| | Prothrombin time<br>Partial thromboplastin time | Liver disease, coagulation disorders, anticoagulation use |
| | Blood type and screen or crossmatch | Determine compatibility for transfusion |
| | Chest x-ray | Heart size, congestive heart failure |
| Respiratory | Chest x-ray | Pneumonia, chronic obstructive pulmonary disease, tumors, structural abnormalities |
| | Pulmonary function test | Obstructive or restrictive lung disease |
| | Arterial blood gas | Acid-base imbalances |
| Renal | Urinalysis | Urinary tract infection, kidney disease |
| | Blood urea nitrogen | Hydration status, renal functioning |
| | Serum creatinine | Impaired renal function |
| | Electrolytes | Electrolyte imbalances |
| | CBC | Anemia associated with renal failure |
| Endocrine | Serum glucose | Diabetes mellitus, hypoglycemia, hyperglycemia |

**table 18-5** *Physiological Changes Related to the Aging Process*

| Physiological Changes | Effects | Potential Perioperative Complications |
|---|---|---|
| **CARDIOVASCULAR** | | |
| ↓ Elasticity of blood vessels<br>↓ Cardiac output<br>↓ Peripheral circulation | ↓ Circulation to vital organs<br>Slower blood flow<br>↑ Blood pressure | Shock (hypotension), thrombosis with pulmonary emboli, delayed wound healing, postoperative confusion, hypervolemia, decreased response to stress |
| **RESPIRATORY** | | |
| ↓ Elasticity of lungs<br>Chest wall rigidity<br>↑ Residual lung volume<br>↓ Forced expiratory volume<br>↓ Ciliary action<br>Thoracic kyphosis<br>Arthritic changes of cervical spine<br>Costochondral calcification<br>Tenacious sputum | ↓ Vital capacity<br>↓ Alveolar volume<br>↓ Gas exchange<br>↓ Cough reflex<br>↓ Hyperextension of neck | Aspiration, atelectasis, pneumonia, postoperative confusion<br>Difficulty maintaining airway<br>Difficult intubation |
| **URINARY** | | |
| ↓ Glomerular filtration rate<br>↓ Bladder muscle tone<br>↓ Bladder capacity<br>Benign prostatic hypertrophy (BPH) | ↓ Kidney function<br>Loss of urinary control<br>Stasis of urine in bladder | Prolonged response to anesthesia and drugs, overhydration with IV fluids, hyperkalemia, urinary tract infection, urinary incontinence<br>Incomplete bladder emptying, urinary retention, urinary frequency |
| **MUSCULOSKELETAL** | | |
| ↓ Muscle mass<br>Loss of bone mass<br>Osteoporosis<br>Arthritis | ↓ Activity<br>Skeletal instability<br>Hip and vertebral fractures<br>↓ Range of motion | Deep vein thrombosis, atelectasis, pulmonary embolism, pneumonia<br>Positioning difficulty<br>Immobility |
| **GASTROINTESTINAL** | | |
| ↓ Intestinal motility | Delayed gastric emptying<br>Retention of feces | Aspiration, ileus<br>Constipation or fecal impaction |
| **IMMUNE SYSTEM** | | |
| Fewer killer T cells<br>↓ Response to foreign antigens | ↓ Ability to protect against invasion by pathogenic microorganisms | Delayed wound healing, wound infection, wound dehiscence, pneumonia, urinary tract infection |
| **NEUROLOGICAL** | | |
| Cerebral atherosclerosis<br>Benign hypothermia (temperature < 98.6° F)<br>↓ Basal metabolic rate<br>Impaired thermoregulatory ability | ↓ Cerebral blood flow<br>↓ Thermoregulatory ability<br>↓ Vasoconstriction, lower core temperature<br>↑ Cardiac workload, hypoxia | Cerebrovascular accident<br>Intraoperative and postoperative hypothermia<br>Delayed shivering, delayed recovery from anesthetics |
| **INTEGUMENTARY** | | |
| ↓ Elasticity<br>Small vessel fragility<br>↓ Lean body mass, ↑ in overall body fat<br>↓ Subcutaneous tissue | ↓ Protective function<br>Dehydration<br>Impaired vascular circulation<br>↓ Tissue nutrition<br>↑ Sensitivity to cold environments | Pressure ulcers, bruising<br>Hypothermia<br>Delayed wound healing<br>Delayed recovery from anesthetics because of storage in adipose tissue |
| **METABOLIC** | | |
| Electrolyte imbalances<br>↓ Gamma globulin level<br>↓ Plasma proteins | Hyperkalemia and hypokalemia<br>↓ Inflammatory response | Confusion, dysrhythmias<br>Delayed wound healing, wound dehiscence or evisceration |

**table 18-6** *Physical (P) Status Classification of the American Society of Anesthesiologists*

| Status*† | Definition | Description and Examples |
|---|---|---|
| P1 | A normal healthy patient | No physiological, psychological, biochemical, or organic disturbance |
| P2 | A patient with a mild systemic disease | Cardiovascular disease with minimal restriction on activity; hypertension, asthma, chronic bronchitis, obesity, or diabetes mellitus |
| P3 | A patient with a severe systemic disease that limits activity, but is not incapacitating | Cardiovascular or pulmonary disease that limits activity; severe diabetes with systemic complications; history of myocardial infarction, angina pectoris, or poorly controlled hypertension |
| P4 | A patient with severe systemic disease that is a constant threat to life | Severe cardiac, pulmonary, renal, hepatic, or endocrine dysfunction |
| P5 | A moribund patient who is not expected to survive 24 hours with or without the operation | Surgery done as last recourse or resuscitative effort; major multisystem or cerebral trauma, ruptured aneurysm, or large pulmonary embolus |
| P6 | A patient declared brain dead whose organs are being removed for donor purposes | |

Modified from the American Society of Anesthesiologists, ASA, 520 N. Northwest Highway, Park Ridge, IL 60068. Reprinted with permission.
*In status P2, P3, and P4, the systemic disease may or may not be related to the cause for surgery.
†For any patient (P1 through P5) requiring emergency surgery, an E is added to the physical status, for example, P1E, P2E. ASA 1 through ASA 6 is often used for physical status.

outcomes for the patient and therefore need to be assessed in the preoperative period.

Elderly persons vary in the extent to which physiological changes occur. The greater the number of physiological changes increases the potential for the patient to develop complications.

### ASA status

Surgical risk can be assessed by different methods. An objective method of determining the degree of risk for a particular patient has been developed by the American Society of Anesthesiologists (ASA). The scale is based on the number and severity of preexisting medical conditions. Higher ASA scores indicate a greater risk of perioperative complications and death. Patient assessment and classification are performed by the anesthesiologist or anesthetist preoperatively. Table 18-6 contains the classification status.

Patients with chronic diseases are also at high risk for developing complications in surgery from the surgery itself or from the anesthesia. The existence of one or more chronic diseases does not necessarily increase surgical risk. The nature and extent of the disease or diseases and the degree to which they are under control are the important variables. Nursing assessment and documentation of these conditions are critical in the preoperative period.

### Nutritional status

Patients with impaired nutritional status are at high risk for developing complications from surgery or anesthesia. Patients most likely to have nutritional deficiencies are the elderly and those who are chronically ill, particularly persons with gastrointestinal tract conditions or malignant tumors. The person who is emaciated or cachectic or who has lost weight below an acceptable level usually has a prolonged postoperative recovery.

The malnourished person already has diminished reserves of carbohydrates and fats. Body proteins will be used to provide the necessary energy requirement to maintain metabolic functioning of cells. Nitrogen imbalances will be greater than normal, and less protein will be available for healing. Collagen, the connective tissue that is the substance of scar tissue, is a protein. Wound healing therefore becomes considerably delayed, and wound separation and infection may occur.

If the surgery is not emergent and can be delayed for several weeks, the malnourished patient is placed on a high-protein, high-carbohydrate diet preoperatively. In the preoperative or postoperative period total parenteral nutrition (TPN) may be given until the patient is able to tolerate a high-protein, high-carbohydrate diet by mouth. High protein intake will not result in increased body protein unless there is sufficient carbohydrate to provide the necessary energy. Activity or exercise also is required for protein synthesis.

Nutritionally depleted patients usually have a deficiency of vitamins. Vitamins $B_1$, C, and K are necessary for wound healing and clot formation, and supplemental vitamins may be prescribed. Box 18-5 summarizes the common causes of both preoperative and postoperative malnutrition.

Patients who are 10% over their ideal weight are considered obese and are at risk for increased morbity and mortality from concomitant systemic disease. The obese patient presents several risk factors for surgery, including enlarged organs such as heart, kidneys, and liver. During surgery, fluctuations of vital signs are more common in the obese person, resulting from the excessive demands on the cardiovascular system. The surgeon incising through layers of fatty tissue has to exert more traction on the tissues to expose the surgical site; this increases trauma to the tissues. Incisional hernias may occur at a later date. During the immediate postoperative

**box 18-5** *Persons at High Risk for Delayed Postoperative Recovery Resulting from Malnutrition*

**PREOPERATIVE MALNUTRITION**
Chronic infection
Inflammatory bowel disorders
Chronic pancreatitis
Carcinoma of stomach or colon
Liver disease
Renal disease
Congestive heart failure
Weight loss (10% of body weight in 3 months before surgery)

**POSTOPERATIVE MALNUTRITION**
Abdominal trauma
Severe multiple trauma (especially pelvic, hip, and leg fracture)
Major burns
Wound sepsis
Acute pancreatitis
Small bowel fistulas
Severe peritonitis

period these patients often require more assistance with turning, coughing, and deep breathing. Excess fat deposits often limit movement of the diaphragm, thereby decreasing ventilation. It is also more difficult for obese persons to move about, and they may require additional assistance. Both decreased activity and decreased diaphragm expansion are contributing factors to development of postoperative pulmonary complications. Decreased activity also causes predisposition to thrombophlebitis. Although weight reduction usually cannot be accomplished preoperatively, it is important for the nurse to identify obesity as a risk factor and make appropriate plans for postoperative management.

## NURSING DIAGNOSES

Nursing diagnoses are determined from analysis of patient data. Nursing diagnoses for the preoperative patient may include but are not limited to:

| Diagnostic Title | Possible Etiological Factors |
|---|---|
| Knowledge deficit | Lack of familiarity with perioperative routines |
| Anxiety | Fear of the unknown<br>Cost of care, lack of insurance<br>Body image changes<br>Change in health status |
| Risk for ineffective airway clearance | Anesthesia, sedation, pooled secretions, surgical procedure |
| Risk for altered peripheral tissue perfusion: deep vein thrombosis | Venous stasis, increased coagulability of blood |
| Risk for infection | Inadequate skin preparation, site for organism invasion<br>Contaminated wound |
| Sleep pattern disturbance | Anxiety, environment |

## EXPECTED PATIENT OUTCOMES

Expected patient outcomes for the patient during the preoperative phase may include but are not limited to:

1. Will verbalize an understanding of perioperative routines
2. Will relate an increase in psychological and physiological comfort
3. Will demonstrate effective coughing, adequate air exchange, and patent airway
4. Will have no evidence of deep vein thrombosis
5. Will be free from postoperative wound infection
6. Will report optimal rest

## INTERVENTIONS

Having identified the patient's specific needs and formulated nursing diagnoses, the nurse must collaborate with other health care professionals to implement the plan for treatments, teaching, and emotional support for the patient. A major focus of nursing intervention during the preoperative period is teaching and psychological preparation of the patient and family.

### Patient/Family Education

#### *Preoperative patient education*

The purpose of preoperative teaching is to provide information that addresses individual learning needs, promotes safety, promotes psychological comfort, promotes patient and family involvement in care, and promotes compliance with instructions. Traditionally preoperative teaching was completed 1 to 2 days before surgery. Recent changes in health care have challenged the perioperative nurse to implement preoperative patient education programs in shortened time frames and in alternative settings. Research indicates that effective preoperative teaching has been associated with reduced anxiety levels, earlier ambulation, and increased involvement in postdischarge self-care activities.[12] The preoperative information helpful to most patients relates to preoperative tests and activities, events related to the surgery, and expectations about what will happen postoperatively. Most patients are less anxious and participate more effectively if they know the reasons for tests and preoperative activities. There is inconclusive evidence supporting the most effective time frame for implementing preoperative teaching. The teaching can be done in the physician's office or in a preadmission testing area before the scheduled surgery date. The nurse should select the most effective method of patient instruction. The following Research Box summarizes the current status of preoperative education methods.

Before initiating a teaching protocol it is necessary for the nurse to assess the learning readiness and capability of the patient. It is important to remember that approximately 20% of adults in the United States are functionally illiterate and would not benefit from printed materials with reading levels above the fourth- or fifth-grade level. The average reading level of patient teaching materials has been found to be above the eighth-grade level, with some reported as high as the four-

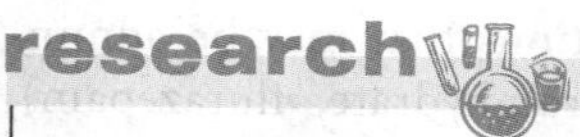

Reference: Cipperly J et al: Research utilization: the development of a preoperative teaching protocol, *Medsurg Nurs* 4(3):199, 1995.

The authors conducted an extensive literature review of preoperative instruction. A summary of their findings follows. Interventions that focused on providing psychological support, health-related information, and patient education resulted in reduced length of stay with resultant reduced cost, increased psychological well-being, decreased postoperative pain, and increased patient satisfaction. These findings were supported by a meta-analysis by Hathaway, who concluded that with low levels of patient fear and anxiety, teaching should be focused on procedural content. Psychological content should be stressed when patients exhibit high levels of fear and anxiety. Many studies focused on the effects of sensory information. Information regarding physical sensations also resulted in decreased length of stay. Structured preoperative teaching has been found to be more effective than unstructured methods. As early as 1976 the effectiveness of preadmission teaching programs in reducing the need for postoperative pain medication, associated increased levels of physical comfort, and improved functional status had been reported. Preadmission instructional booklets also enhanced the effectiveness of preoperative teaching. Patients who received preoperative instruction brochures in the mail required less teaching time, demonstrated increased family involvement and independent learning, and showed increased compliance, increased satisfaction, and more learned behaviors than those who did not.

After reviewing the literature the authors developed a model for preoperative teaching. After an assessment of the patient's fear and anxiety level, one of three uniform systematic teaching protocols was chosen, which included psychological, sensory, and procedural content. This approach allowed the preoperative nurse to address the specific needs of each individual patient. Teaching was initiated 24 to 48 hours before surgery. Teaching protocols were reinforced by means of a take-home instruction booklet and documented by means of a checklist. On admission, all participants in the study were reassessed by the nurse. Anxiety level, knowledge base, and ability to perform coughing, deep breathing, and leg exercises were measured and recorded. Results indicated reduced levels of fear and anxiety and increased involvement in postoperative routines, and all patients reported that sensory and procedural information was helpful. There was only one respiratory complication and no circulatory complications in the sample.

teenth.[5] With this information in mind, the nurse needs to assess the appropriateness of printed materials when using them for patient education. For an in-depth discussion of the principles of teaching and learning refer to a fundamentals of nursing textbook.

Preoperative teaching focuses on information that will increase patients' familiarity with procedural events, thus decreasing anxiety; information regarding activities to enhance physiological healing; and information on prevention of postoperative complications. Content should include information about events that will occur during the surgical experience (procedural), what the patient may experience during the perioperative period (sensory), and what actions may help decrease anxiety (behavioral) (Box 18-6).

**box 18-6** *Preoperative Teaching Content*

**PROCEDURAL**

- Informed consent
- Preoperative screening (laboratory, diagnostic tests, history, physical assessment)
- Preoperative routines (shower, skin prep, vital signs, clothing, personal belongings)
- NPO status
- Preoperative medication
- Transfer to surgical suite (timing, holding area, surgical waiting room, visiting hours, duration of procedure)
- Postanesthesia care unit routines
- Presence of IVs, surgical drains, surgical incision, catheters
- Pain control methods
- Postoperative routines (coughing and deep breathing exercises, leg exercises, antiembolism stockings, pneumatic compression devices, ambulation, diet advancement, expected discharge date, home care needs)

**SENSORY**

- Needle insertion
- Medication effects (drowsiness, dry mouth, amnesia)
- Operating room environment (cold, monochromatic, surgical attire, warm blankets, hard narrow bed, bright lights, noise, face mask for gaseous inhalation)
- Pain (incisional, muscular, sore throat)
- Dizziness when standing or ambulating for the first time
- Sensations associated with invasive devices (Foley, nasogastric tube, etc.) postoperative equipment (pneumatic compression devices, antiembolism hose, etc.)

**BEHAVIORAL**

- Demonstration and explanation of exercise routines (coughing, deep breathing, incentive spirometry, leg exercises)
- Transfer techniques, splinting of incision, progressive ambulation

## Promoting Psychological Comfort

Impending surgery causes anxiety because it is associated with fear of the unknown, pain, body image changes, treatments, altered functioning, loss of control, and death. The JCAHO states that the registered nurse is responsible for assisting the patient and his or her family and significant others in identifying the sources of anxiety and effective coping mechanisms.

The level of the patient's anxiety affects the receptiveness and ability to comprehend preoperative instructions. Mild anxiety enhances learning. However, moderate levels of anxiety are characterized by selective inattention, and severe levels of anxiety may completely impede the individual's ability to comprehend information, and learning may be impossible. When the level of anxiety has decreased sufficiently for learning to take place, the nurse should assist the patient in methods to facilitate learning and enhance problem solving. The nurse can help the patient recall effective coping mechanisms or explore alternative methods of coping with the current situation. Giving someone information does not necessarily mean that the person perceived correctly or understood the information.

Empowering patients by increasing their sense of control before surgery is essential for decreasing patient anxiety. Loss of control is one of the fears associated with surgery. Allowing patients to participate in decision making concerning care helps meet the need for the patient to maintain some control over events. Patients also may be taught activities that help decrease anxiety and gain a sense of control. The most common approaches are deep breathing, relaxation exercises, music therapy, and guided imagery. (See the accompanying Research Box.)

The nurse must consider the patient's family and friends when planning psychological support preoperatively. The patient's family members or close friends are usually as anxious as the patient. This anxiety can be transmitted to patients, increasing their anxiety levels. The same principles described in exploring concerns and giving information to the patient hold true for significant others. Family involvement in preoperative education decreases the anxiety of both the patient and family with resultant increased satisfaction with care and increased patient cooperation with routines.[9]

### Use of Medications

The anxious preoperative patient may require medication to relieve anxiety. Among those drugs most commonly used are midazolam (Versed), lorazepam (Ativan), and diazepam (Valium). Other medications that may be administered include hypnotics (chloral hydrate, flurazepam), narcotics, anticholinergics, and histamine-receptor antagonists (cimetidine, ranitidine). The nurse should be aware that any of these medications may be needed and should not hesitate to ensure that the patient is made comfortable during this stressful time. Table 18-7 lists the dosages and routes of administration for commonly used antianxiety agents.

### Minimizing the Potential for Respiratory Complications

Teaching the patient about the necessity of deep breathing and coughing after surgery is a common component of preoperative education. Deep breathing facilitates oxygenation and removal of residual inhalant anesthetics and also prevents alveolar collapse that leads to atelectasis. Coughing removes secretions that may block the airways. All patients potentially at risk for postoperative pulmonary complications are taught deep breathing and coughing exercises before surgery. Waiting to do so until the patient is awakening from anesthesia decreases the possibility that these exercises will be carried out effectively, because anesthesia and postoperative pain decrease the ability to retain information.

All patients need to know how to perform correct diaphragmatic breathing because it increases lung expansion by permitting the diaphragm to descend fully. Many men normally breathe diaphragmatically, while few women do. With diaphragmatic breathing, the abdomen rises with inspiration and falls with expiration. The nurse assesses the patient's normal breathing pattern by placing a hand lightly on the patient's abdomen and asking the patient to take a deep breath. If diaphragmatic breathing does not occur naturally, the patient can be taught to inspire deeply while pushing the abdomen up against the hand.

Deep breathing and coughing exercises are performed with the patient in a sitting position. The nurse instructs the patient to take a breath through the nose and exhale through the mouth. The patient is then instructed to take a deep breath through the nose and mouth, hold the breath for 3 to 5 seconds, and then exhale completely through the mouth. Deep breathing exercises are repeated three times; the patient is then instructed to cough (Box 18-7).

It is important for the patient to hold the breath for 3 seconds to promote alveolar expansion. If there is diffi-

**research**

Reference: Augustin P: Effect of music on ambulatory surgery patients' preoperative anxiety, *AORN J* 63(4):750, 1996.

This study investigated music as a method to reduce ambulatory surgery patients' preoperative anxiety. Forty-two patients were assigned to either an experimental or a control group. Anxiety levels were measured using the State-Trait Anxiety Inventory, vital signs, and self-report of anxiety. Members of the experimental group were able to listen to their choice of music before surgery in addition to receiving preoperative instruction. The control group received only preoperative instruction. The experimental group had significantly lower heart rates and blood pressure, and respiratory differences were significant. These findings indicate that offering music may enhance preoperative instruction as an alternative method to decrease anxiety in ambulatory surgery patients.

**table 18-7** *Common Anxiolytics*

| MEDICATION | DOSAGE (mg) | ROUTE |
|---|---|---|
| Midazolam (Versed) | 1-4 | IM, IV |
| Lorazepam (Ativan) | 0.5-2 | PO, IM |
| Diazepam (Valium) | 5-15 | PO, IM, IV |

culty with a deep cough, encourage the patient to do a "huff" cough. Repeated huff coughs often stimulate a deep cough. The patient also is shown how to splint an incision with a pillow, a towel, or his or her hands to help decrease pain while coughing.

An additional method of promoting lung expansion is with the use of an incentive spirometry device. Various models are commercially available. The patient is taught to seal the lips around the mouthpiece and inhale. Once maximal inhalation is achieved, the patient should hold his or her breath for 3 seconds and then exhale slowly. The patient should not exceed 10 to 12 breaths per minute. The device can be set to a predetermined volume to achieve maximum lung expansion (Figure 18-1).

### Minimizing the Potential for Deep Vein Thrombosis

A variety of nursing interventions are directed toward promoting adequate peripheral circulation. Measures used to decrease venous stasis include antiembolism hose, pneumatic compression devices, leg exercises, early ambulation, adequate hydration, and deep breathing. Venous stasis in the postoperative period may lead to deep vein thrombosis (DVT), thrombophlebitis, and the potential formation of pulmonary embolus. Risk factors for the development of DVT include age over 40 years, prior history of DVT, decreased mobility, pelvic or cardiovascular surgery, total hip and total knee surgery, fracture or trauma, history of smoking, use of estrogen, and obesity. Refer to Chapter 27 for a full discussion of DVT.

Antiembolism stockings, alone or in combination with intermittent pulsatile compression (IPC) devices or pneumatic compression devices (sequential compression devices or SCD), are often used perioperatively to enhance venous return in the lower extremities. The pneumatic compression device provides intermittent periods of compression starting from the ankle and progressing proximally to promote venous return. The nurse must measure the patient's lower extremities to obtain the appropriate size of sleeves and stockings. These devices are applied in the operating room and are continued until the patient is ambulatory (Figure 18-2).

Leg exercises help prevent venous congestion. The nurse teaches the patient leg exercises preoperatively and has the patient give a return demonstration of proper technique. Refer to Figure 18-3 for an example of teaching material pertaining to postoperative leg exercises.

Additional interventions to decrease venous stasis include early ambulation, frequent turning, and active or passive range-of-motion exercises. Early mobilization prevents pulmonary and circulatory complications, prevents pressure ulcers, stimulates intestinal motility, and decreases pain.

Preoperatively, or during the postoperative period, patients can be taught how to use the side rails effectively for turning and how to sit up on the side of the bed with the least amount of pull on the incision. To turn to right side:

1. Slide hips to left side of bed.
2. Support incision with right hand.

**box 18-7** *Deep Breathing and Coughing Exercises*

**DEEP BREATHING**

1. Lie in semi-Fowler's or high Fowler's position with knees flexed to relax abdomen and allow full chest expansion.
2. Place a hand lightly on the abdomen.
3. Breathe in slowly through nose, letting chest expand and feeling abdomen rise against hand.
4. Hold breath for 3 seconds.
5. Exhale slowly through pursed lips (abdomen contracts).
6. Repeat deep breathing three times, then cough (see below).

**COUGHING**

1. Breathe in as described above.
2. Count to 3.
3. On "3," cough *deeply* three times.
4. If unable to cough deeply, do repeated "huff" coughs (forced expiration with glottis open).

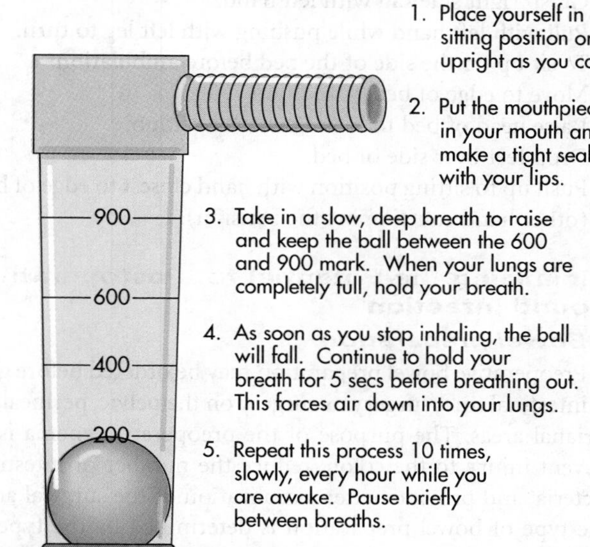

Respirex® 2
To prevent problems with breathing after surgery, it is important to inflate your lungs and keep them clear of secretions. Respirex 2 will help you do this.
To use your Respirex, follow these steps:
1. Place yourself in a sitting position or as upright as you can.
2. Put the mouthpiece in your mouth and make a tight seal with your lips.
3. Take in a slow, deep breath to raise and keep the ball between the 600 and 900 mark. When your lungs are completely full, hold your breath.
4. As soon as you stop inhaling, the ball will fall. Continue to hold your breath for 5 secs before breathing out. This forces air down into your lungs.
5. Repeat this process 10 times, slowly, every hour while you are awake. Pause briefly between breaths.
900
600
400
200


**fig. 18-1** Patient instructions for using incentive spirometer.

**Intermittent Pulsatile Compression Device (IPC)**

The intermittent pulsatile compression device (IPC) gives a regular, gentle massage (or compression) to both legs. This action helps you avoid complications brought about by being less active after surgery.

The IPC is a pair of plastic wrap-around stockings or sleeves. They are put on both legs before surgery. Each sleeve is connected to a small compressor which inflates the sleeves and applies pressure to the calves of your legs. You will feel the pressure as a "milking" action or gentle massage. The pressure lasts for about 10 seconds of each minute. The sleeves then deflate and the process is repeated in a minute.

The sleeves will be removed once you are more active and recovering from surgery. Your nurses will help you with this device and answer any questions you may have after surgery.

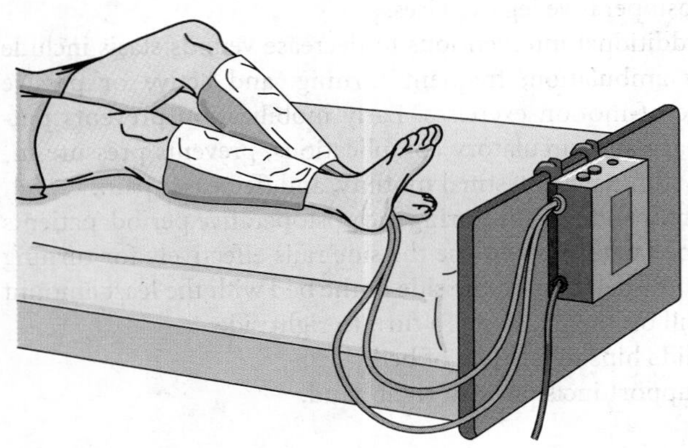

**fig. 18-2** Patient instructions for intermittent pulsatile compression device (IPC).

3. Flex left knee.
4. Grasp right side rail with left hand.
5. Pull with left hand while pushing with left leg to turn.

To sit up on the side of the bed before ambulation:

1. Move to edge of bed.
2. Raise head of bed to high Fowler's position.
3. Drop feet over side of bed.
4. Push up to sitting position with hand closest to edge of bed (other hand can support the incision).

## Minimizing the Potential for Postoperative Wound Infection

### Bowel preparation

Preoperative bowel preparation may be ordered before gastrointestinal tract surgery or surgery on the pelvic, perineal, or perianal areas. The purpose of the preoperative enema is to prevent injury to the colon, reduce the number of intestinal bacteria, and provide better visualization of the surgical area. The type of bowel preparation is determined by the type of surgical procedure and surgeon preference. Common bowel preparations include oral laxatives, clear liquid diets, enemas, and oral antibiotics. Adverse effects and complications depend on the type of preparations used and include abdominal cramping, dehydration, electrolyte imbalance, vagal stimulation, local irritation of bowel and rectal mucosa, fatigue, and anxiety.

Cleansing the bowel by means of enemas is not a routine procedure. Surgeon preference, surgical site, and type of procedure are all determinants of which method of bowel preparation is used. Enemas should be given if a patient has had x-ray studies involving barium immediately before surgery, because barium remaining in the intestinal tract may cause postoperative fecal impactions.

If enemas are to be given until the returns are clear, it is important to remember that fluid excess and potassium deficits can occur with repeated enemas. It is common practice to check with the physician if returns are not clear after the third enema. One method is to give up to three enemas the evening before surgery and then, if the returns are still not clear, to repeat the enemas the following morning. Repeated enemas are tiring to the patient and may irritate rectal and bowel mucosa.

Controversy exists regarding the benefit of antibiotic enemas because of the disturbance of the bowel flora. If antibiotic enemas are ordered, synthesis of vitamin K by intestinal bacteria may be inhibited; supplementary vitamin K may therefore be given to prevent increased bleeding after surgery.

### Skin preparation

The recommended practices developed by AORN provide a guideline for preoperative skin preparation of the operative site. The goal of skin preparation is to reduce the risk of postoperative wound infection by (1) removing soil and transient microbes from the skin, (2) reducing the resident microbial count to subpathogenic amounts in a short period of time and with the least amount of tissue irritation, and (3) inhibiting rapid rebound growth of microbes.

The recommended practices and interpretive statements for skin preparation effective January 1997 include the following:

*Recommended practice I:* The surgical site and surrounding areas should be clean. *Interpretive statements:* Cleansing of the skin can be accomplished by patients showering and by washing the operative site either on the patient unit or immediately before applying the antimicrobial agent in the practice setting.

*Recommended practice II:* The surgical site should be assessed before skin preparation. *Interpretive statements:* Inadvertent removal of lesions traumatizes the skin at the surgical site and provides an opportunity for wound colonization by microorganisms. Hair should remain at the surgical site unless it interferes with the surgical procedure. Hair removal should be performed as close to the time of surgery as possible and in an area outside the room where the procedure will be performed. Use of a depilatory cream or an electric clipper is preferable to shaving with a razor.

*Recommended practice III:* When indicated, the surgical site and surrounding area should be prepared with an antimicrobial agent. *Interpretive statement:* The antimicrobial agent should have a broad range of germicidal action and be nontoxic.[1]

**Postoperative Leg Exercises**

After surgery you will need to do some leg exercises. These exercises will help the blood circulation in your legs and keep your muscles in shape for walking. Before surgery, your nurse will help you practice the exercises you need to know. Your nurse will check or mark the exercises below that you need to practice.

☐ **Ankle Pumps**
*(See Figure 1)*

- Move both ankles by pointing toes up, then down, then in circles to stimulate circulation.
- Repeat at least 10 times every hour.
- You may do this while lying on your back or when sitting and dangling your feet over the side of your bed.

☐ **Quad Sets**
*(See Figure 2)*

- Lying on your back with both legs straight, tighten your thigh muscles so that the backs of your knees press down into the bed.
- Hold your muscles tight for 5 seconds.
- Exhale slowly while holding your muscles tight. Relax.
- Repeat at least 5 times every hour.

**Figure 1: Ankle Pumps**

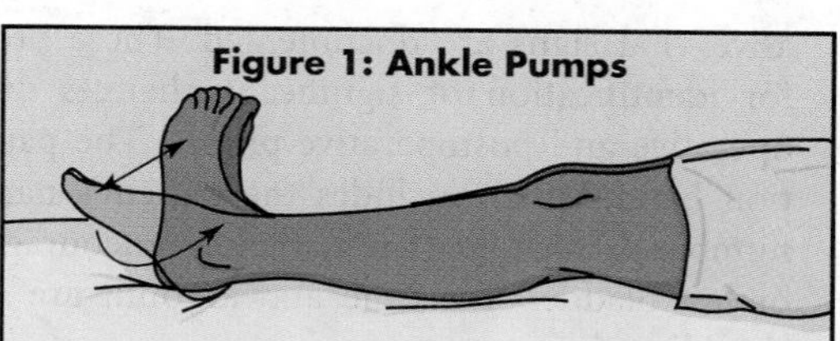

**Figure 2: Quad Sets**

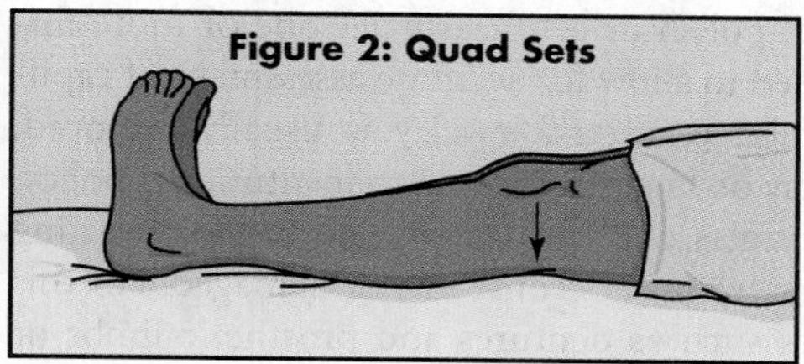

☐ **Gluteal Tightenings**
*(See Figure 3)*

- Lying on your back, tense your buttocks muscles tightly as if holding back a bowel movement.
- Hold these muscles tight for 5 seconds.
- Exhale slowly while holding your buttocks tight. Relax.
- Repeat at least 5 times every hour.

☐ **Straight Leg Raises***
*(See Figure 4)*

- Lying on your back, bend your right hip and knee so your foot rests flat on the bed. This helps to take the strain off your lower back.
- Keeping your left knee straight, point your toes toward the ceiling and lift the leg a few inches off the bed. Exhale slowly while lifting your leg.
- Slowly lower your leg to the bed. Rest.
- Repeat at least 5 times. Then do the same exercise 5 times with your right leg. Do straight leg raises 4 times a day.

** DO NOT do this exercise if you are having abdominal surgery, or if you have back problems.*

**Figure 3: Gluteal Tightenings**

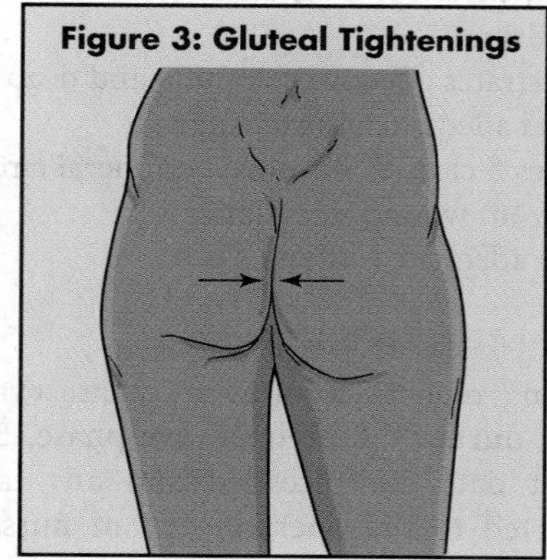

**Figure 4: Straight Leg Raises**

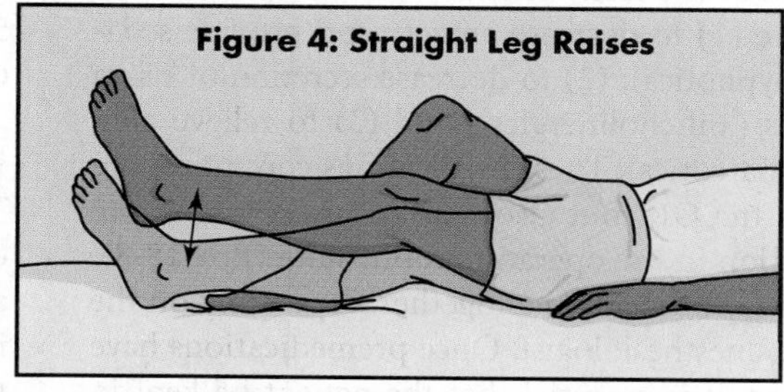

**fig. 18-3** Patient instructions for postoperative leg exercises.

### Promoting Rest and Sleep

Anticipation of surgery can produce stress and anxiety that may interfere with sleep patterns. If the patient is admitted to the hospital before surgery, a sedative may be given in the evening. However, many patients are admitted the day of surgery or have surgery on an ambulatory basis. When the nurse is assessing the patient on a preoperative basis, it may be helpful to explore the patient's methods of relaxation and sleeping patterns to help ensure a restful night before surgery.

### Final Preparations for Surgery

In the final phase of preoperative nursing care the nurse is responsible for ensuring that the patient is ready to be safely transferred to the surgical suite. All of the patient's personal belongings are identified and secured. The patient dons a hospital gown and removes all personal clothing. If the patient is wearing fingernail polish or artificial nails, one or more fingernails are exposed to allow for accurate assessment of capillary refill and pulse oximetry. Jewelry is usually removed; however, rings may be taped according to institutional policy. Objects such as eyeglasses or prostheses sent to the operating room with the patient may become lost or damaged. For this reason, prostheses such as dentures and prosthetic limbs or eyes are usually removed, labeled, and placed in safekeeping. Dentures are removed, labeled, and placed in a denture cup. If dentures are not removed the patient's airway may be compromised with induction of anesthesia. The presence of caps is documented, and this information is also relayed to the anesthesiologist. Patients are usually allowed to wear hearing aids to the surgical suite. This allows the patient to communicate with the surgical team throughout the perioperative period. The presence of the hearing aid must be documented to prevent loss or damage. Patients who want to take religious items or jewelry to the operating room are usually permitted to do so. To prevent loss of the item, a paper emblem obtained from a religious representative is sometimes substituted.

#### *Premedication*

Before any premedication is given, it is imperative that a check is made to ascertain that a consent form has been completed and placed at the front of the chart. The purposes of premedication are (1) to decrease anxiety and provide sedation (sedatives, hypnotics); (2) to decrease secretion of saliva and gastric juices (anticholinergics); and (3) to relieve pain and discomfort (narcotics). These medications commonly are given "on call to the OR" but also may be given just before anesthesia induction in the operating room suite (Box 18-8). Premedications may be omitted altogether, depending on the preference of the anesthesiologist. Once premedications have been administered, it is essential that the patient be kept in bed with the side rails up to ensure safety.

### Preoperative Checklist

A preoperative checklist is a method of summarizing the final patient preparations for surgery (Figure 18-4). Preoperative vital signs are documented. These provide a baseline for identification of significant changes during the intraoperative and postoperative phases. The patient's identification band, which includes the patient's name and hospital number, is secured. The patient is encouraged to empty his or her bladder; the time and amount are recorded on the checklist.

The patient is transferred to a stretcher and transported to the operating room. The patient's chart and archival records, if any, accompany the patient.

**box 18-8** *Common Premedications*

Antianxiety agents
- Midazolam (Versed)
- Diazepam (Valium)
- Lorazepam (Ativan)

Narcotics
- Meperidine (Demerol)
- Morphine
- Fentanyl

Anticholinergics
- Atropine
- Glycopyrrolate (Robinul)

## ■ EVALUATION

To evaluate the effectiveness of nursing interventions, compare patient behaviors with those stated in the expected patient outcomes. Successful achievement of patient outcomes for the patient undergoing surgical intervention is indicated by:

1. Participates in and complies with perioperative instructions and routines; verbalizes an understanding of rationales for care
2. Relates an increase in psychological and physiological comfort; describes own anxiety and uses effective coping mechanisms
3. Demonstrates effective coughing and deep breathing exercises and adequate air exchange
4. Identifies factors to improve peripheral circulation
5. Is free from wound infection
6. Reports adequate rest and sleep.

## ■ DOCUMENTATION

The nursing report serves as a concise evaluation of the care given during the preoperative phase. Biopsychosocial assessment data are recorded and any important findings reported to the operating room nurse. Preoperative teaching and the patient's response should be recorded. In addition, any relevant social factors that need to be considered while the patient is in surgery should be reported. Preoperative medications and laboratory and diagnostic results should be recorded on the patient's medical record.

Items 1-11 and diagnostic results to be reviewed for completion by the RN prior to surgery

Front side to be completed by the RN on the evening prior to surgery

**Preoperative Checklist**

1. Surgical Procedure(s) Verified: Consent _____ Schedule _____ Patient/Family _____
Comments: ____________________

2. Surgical Consent: Signed _____ Dated _____ Witnessed _____
Comments: ____________________

3. Special Consent(s): Signed _____ Dated _____ Witnessed _____ N/A _____
Comments: ____________________

4. History: Physical: Completed _____
Comments: ____________________

5 Pertinent Medical History (circle): Diabetes Hypertension Cardiac
Seizures Pulmonary Disease Liver Kidney Other: ____________________
Comments: ____________________

6. Tentative Anesthesia (circle): G MAC L SP Consult
Comments: ____________________

7. Allergies (List in Red): ____________________
Confirmed with Patient _____ Allergy Band (Location) _____ Labeled on Chart _____

8. ID Band (Location): ____________________

9. Airborne Infection Present: Yes _____ No _____

10. ROM or Physical Limitations (specify): ____________________

11. Major Sensory Deprivations: Hearing Loss: Ear R _____ L _____ Hearing Aid _____
Blindness: Eye R _____ L _____ Prosthesis _____
Language Barrier: ____________________

Criteria:
ECG—Must not be more than 14 days old if normal or unchanged
Labwork—Must not be more than 14 days old if normal
Chest x-ray—Required at discretion of surgeon or anesthesiologist

**Basic Tests Required:**
- General Anesthesia
- Monitored Anesthesia Care
- Regional Blocks

} CBC, Glucose, Potassium, BUN, SGOT, U/A

Local Anesthesia—At the discretion of surgeon or anesthesiologist
Pediatric Patients—CBC, Dipstick Urinalysis, Sickle Prep (Black Patients)

********* A (✔) Is to Be Placed in the Appropriate Box in Each Column *********

Diagnostic Results

**Part A**

| | (✔) Current Results on Chart | (✔) N/A | Abnormal—Physician Notified | Nurse Initial | Not Obtained or Abnormal M.D. Comment | Indicate Person/M.D. Notified |
|---|---|---|---|---|---|---|
| U/A | | | | | | |
| CBC | | | | | | |
| K | | | | | | |
| BUN | | | | | | |
| SGOT | | | | | | |
| Chest | | | | | | |
| ECG | | | | | | |
| Other | | | | | | |
| T+C/T+S | | | | | | |
| Gluc | | | | | | |
| Units Avail. | | | | | | |

**Part B**

Additional Preop Bloodwork (✔) Lab Results

| | |
|---|---|
| GLUC | PT |
| NA | PTT |
| CL | WBC |
| $CO_2$ | HGB |
| | HCT |
| | PLAT CT |
| REPORT NOT ON CHART | |

**Abnormal Test Results Are to Be Reported to the Physician**

Signature of RN: ____________________ Date: _____ Time: _____

*Continued*

**fig. 18-4** Preoperative checklist.

*Items 12-23 to be completed by the RN the morning of or prior to surgery*

12. Items 1-11 Reviewed/Completed ________________ Comments ________________
13. Patient's Vital Signs: T _____ P _____ R _____ BP _____ Time Taken _____
    Height __________ Weight __________
    Vital Sign Criteria: The Department of Anesthesiology requires admission vital signs (T, P, R, BP) and vital signs ×2 within the last 12 hours preop.
14. NPO After Midnight: Yes _____ No _____ If no, time of last meal/intake __________
15. I & O and Vital Sign Flowsheet on Chart: Yes _____ No _____
16. Parenteral Fluids Running: Heparin Lock (Location): ________________
    IV ________________ Rate ________________
    IV ________________ Rate ________________
    IV ________________ Rate ________________
    TPN ________________ Rate ________________
    Lipids ________________ Rate ________________
    Other ________________ Rate ________________
17. Voided or Catheterized Preop: _____
18. Prep Completed: _____ (Bowel, Scrub, Shower, etc.)
19. Valuables:

| Circle if applicable: | Disposition: | Circle if applicable: | Disposition: |
|---|---|---|---|
| Dentures/Partial Plates | | Jewelry | |
| Wigs/Hairpins/Hairpieces | | Glasses/Contact Lenses | |
| Nailpolish Removed | | Prosthesis | |
| Other | | Other | |

20. Preop Medications Given: Yes _____ Recorded and Signed on Med Record _____
    No _____ Consent Form Not Signed _____
    Other: ________________
21. Other medications given day of surgery: Yes _____ No _____
22. Patient on ASA: Yes _____ Amount _____ How Long _____
23. Special Remarks: ________________
    Addressograph Plate on Chart: Yes _____ No _____
    Signature of RN Caring for Patient: ________________ Date: _____ Time: _____

*Items 24-28 to be completed by holding room nurse*

24. Time Control Desk Notified: ________________ Review of Preop Checklist: ________________
25. Local Anesthesia Patient Vital Signs: T _____ P _____ R _____ BP _____
26. Patient Accompanied by: ________________ Location: ________________
27. Comments: ________________

Signature of Holding Room Nurse: ________________ Date: _____ Time: _____

28. Review of Preop Checklist by Operating Room Nurse: ________________
    Date: ________________ Time: ________________

**fig. 18-4, cont'd.** Preoperative checklist.

## critical thinking QUESTIONS

1 Mrs. C, 80, is scheduled for a bowel resection in the morning. A tumor is causing a partial obstruction, but it is not known whether the tumor is malignant. Mrs. C is very concerned about the outcome of her surgery. What data do you need to assess her physiological and psychological status? What postoperative complications pose a potential risk for the patient? What teaching would you include in your plan of care?

2 Mr. D, 45 years of age, has a history of peptic ulcer disease. He has been admitted through the emergency department with a 2-day history of acute abdominal pain and bloody vomitus. He is admitted to your unit, awaiting exploratory laparotomy later in the day. Mr. D speaks Spanish and very little English. He is accompanied by his wife, children, and parents.

How would you ensure that the process of informed consent has been completed?

What laboratory and diagnostic data would be necessary for Mr. D?

What cultural considerations might influence your care?

How would you include his family in his plan of care?

## chapter SUMMARY

### INTRODUCTION

- AORN has developed a framework to guide perioperative nursing practice. Perioperative nursing practice is defined as the activities performed by the professional nurse during the preoperative, intraoperative, and postoperative phases of the patient's surgical experience.

### SPECIAL CONSIDERATIONS FOR PATIENTS IN THE SURGICAL SETTING

- Informed consent includes the nature of surgery with its risks and benefits and prognosis if surgery is withheld.
- Cultural and religious background influences responses to health, illness, surgery, and death.
- Fear and anxiety are common responses to surgery.
- The patient's ASA status is one determinant of surgical risk.
- Surgery is a unique experience for each patient. Surgery is a stressor that produces both physiological stress reactions and psychological reactions. It is also a social stressor, requiring family adaptation to temporary or lasting role changes.

### NURSING MANAGEMENT

Nursing management of the preoperative patient includes physiological, psychological, and family assessment.

- Populations at high risk for surgical anesthetic complications include elderly patients, patients with chronic diseases, and patients with impaired nutritional status.
- Nursing diagnoses for the preoperative patient include knowledge deficit, anxiety, risk for ineffective airway clearance, risk for altered peripheral tissue perfusion, risk for infection, and sleep pattern disturbance.
- Expected outcomes in the preoperative phase include the following: the patient (1) will verbalize an understanding of perioperative routines; (2) relate an increase in psychological and physiological comfort; (3) complications of atelectasis or pneumonia will be minimized; (4) the complications of deep vein thrombosis and postoperative wound infection will be minimized; and (5) the patient will have adequate rest in the preoperative period.
- Nursing interventions to decrease anxiety and increase knowledge include preoperative teaching, emotional support, relaxation, diversion, and medications.
- Preoperative teaching about coughing and deep breathing is essential.
- Preoperative teaching about the importance of mobility in the postoperative phase is essential.
- Final preparations for surgery include documenting care and assessments on the preoperative checklist and transporting the patient to the operating room.

## References


1. AORN recommended practices for skin preparation of patients, *AORN J* 64(5):813, 1996.
2. Association of Operating Room Nurses, Inc.: *1996 Standards and recommended practices,* Denver, Colo, 1996, AORN Publications.
3. Atkinson LJ, Fortunato N: *Berry and Kohn's operating room technique,* ed 8, St Louis, 1996, Mosby.
4. Corey-Plett P: Special considerations of the elderly patient requiring anesthesia, *Can Oper Room Nurs* 13(1):20, 1995.
5. Girdano BP: Ensuring the readability of patient education materials is one way to demonstrate perioperative nurses' value, *AORN J* 63(4): 699, 1996.
6. Martin D: Pre-operative visits to reduce patient anxiety: a study, *Nurs Stand* 10(23):699, 1996.
7. Meeker MH, Rothrock JC: *Alexander's care of the patient in surgery,* ed 10, St Louis, 1995, Mosby.
8. Morris W, editor: *The American heritage dictionary of the English language,* Boston, 1978, Houghton Mifflin.
9. Planchock NY, Wiggins MV: Preoperative assessment and teachings: physiological and psychological preparation, *Seminars in Perioperative Nursing* 3(2):61, 1994.
10. Star P: *The social transformation of American medicine,* New York, 1982, Basic Books.
11. United States Preventive Services Task Force: *Guide to clinical preventative services,* ed 2, Baltimore, 1996, Williams & Williams.
12. Young R, DeGuzman CP, Matis M, McClure K: Effect of preadmission brochures on surgical patients' behavioral outcomes, *AORN J* 60(6): 232, 1994.

chapter

# 19 Intraoperative Nursing

MARY JO BOEHNLEIN and JANE F. MAREK

## objectives

*After studying this chapter, the learner should be able to:*

1. Describe the intraoperative phase as a component of the surgical experience.
2. Identify the subspecialties in surgery.
3. Describe the roles of each member of the surgical health care team.
4. Discuss the significance of aseptic technique maintenance.
5. Explain the purpose of appropriate attire for wear in the surgical suite.
6. Compare and contrast the different types of anesthesia.
7. Describe the physiological stress responses to anesthesia and surgery.
8. Describe the components of the intraoperative patient assessment.
9. Formulate appropriate nursing diagnoses for the intraoperative patient.
10. Relate the potential for the development of intraoperative complications.
11. Identify desired patient outcomes for the intraoperative phase.
12. Discuss nursing interventions to minimize intraoperative risks.
13. Discuss the importance of evaluation of nursing care interventions.

## INTRAOPERATIVE PHASE

The intraoperative phase begins with the transfer of the patient onto the operating room (OR) bed and continues until the patient is admitted to the postanesthesia care unit (PACU). Assessment of the patient's physiological and psychosocial needs provides the nurse with information to determine the nursing diagnoses that are congruent with intraoperative nursing interventions. The intraoperative nursing care plan is developed from assessment data, nursing diagnoses, and identification of expected patient outcomes. The plan is designed to address individual patient needs and safely facilitate the surgical procedure. Throughout the entire intraoperative period, the nurse functions as an active team member who is able to quickly alter the plan in response to changes in the patient's condition.

## SURGICAL SPECIALTIES

Surgery emerged as a true medical specialty in the mid-nineteenth century. The works of Ignaz Semmelweiss, Louis Pasteur, and Joseph Lister became the basis for the current aseptic practices used in the OR.

General surgery is the basis for all surgical specialties. Surgical specialties emerged as a result of understanding the etiology of various disease processes and using specific treatments for various parts of the body.[8] Each specialty involves surgical procedures performed on a specific system or anatomical region (Box 19-1).

## INTRAOPERATIVE PATIENT CARE TEAM

The coordinated efforts of the surgical team are required to deliver safe and effective intraoperative patient care. To accomplish this goal, team members must work as a coordinated unit. Each member of the surgical team must be familiar with the specific surgical procedure, adhere to policies and procedures, and be able to adjust quickly to alterations in the surgical procedure.

The OR team is divided into categories based on the responsibilities of its members. Members of the scrubbed sterile team scrub their hands and arms, don sterile gowns and gloves, and work in the sterile field. Members of this team consist of the primary or operating surgeon, assistants to the surgeon, and the scrub nurse.

Members of the nonscrubbed nonsterile surgical team function outside the sterile field. The team members are responsible for maintaining sterile technique, handling nonsterile supplies and equipment, and providing items for the sterile team. Members of the nonsterile team include the circulating nurse, anesthesiologist and anesthetists, and other allied personnel.

### PRIMARY SURGEON AND ASSISTANTS

The primary or operating surgeon has the knowledge, skill, and expertise to successfully perform the identified surgical procedure. The surgeon is responsible for determining the preoperative diagnosis, the choice and execution of the surgical procedure, the explanation of the risks and benefits of the surgical procedure to the patient, obtaining patient

**box 19-1** *Procedures of Surgical Subspecialties*

**GENERAL SURGERY**
Digestive system structures, abdominal wall, thyroid, and breast—e.g., mastectomy, bowel resection, ventral herniorrhaphy

**GYNECOLOGY AND OBSTETRICS**
Female reproductive system—e.g., hysterectomy, cesarean section

**GENITOURINARY SURGERY**
Male reproductive system, male and female renal system—e.g., prostatectomy, cystoscopy

**ORTHOPEDIC SURGERY**
Musculoskeletal system—e.g., knee reconstruction, fracture repair, spinal fusion, total joint arthroplasty

**NEUROSURGERY**
Brain, spinal cord, and nerves—e.g., cerebral aneurysm clipping, laminectomy

**THORACIC AND CARDIOVASCULAR SURGERY**
Pulmonary structures, heart, great vessels, and peripheral vascular system—e.g., lung resection, femoral-popliteal vein bypass graft, mitral or aortic valve repair

**OPHTHALMIC SURGERY**
Eye structures—e.g., corneal transplantation, vitrectomy, cataract removal

**OTORHINOLARYNGOLOGY, HEAD, AND NECK SURGERY**
Ear, nose, throat, trachea, and esophagus—e.g., stapedectomy, laryngectomy, tracheostomy

**PLASTIC AND RECONSTRUCTIVE SURGERY**
Congenital or trauma-induced abnormalities or disfigurement, cosmetic corrections—e.g., skin grafting, cleft palate repair, face lift

consent for the surgical procedure, and the postoperative management of the patient's care.

Under the direction of the operating surgeon, the surgeon's assistant is responsible for exposing the surgical site, providing hemostasis to prevent blood from obscuring the anatomy, and assisting with suturing throughout the operative procedure. The first assistant may be a surgeon, resident, physician's assistant, or registered nurse (RN).

The Association of Operating Room Nurses (AORN) acknowledged the role of the RN as a first assistant to the surgeon and adopted an official statement recognizing the RN First Assistant (RNFA) in 1984. The association defined the scope of practice, requirements, education, and clinical privileges that are required for the RNFA. Based on the AORN statement, many state boards of nursing have accepted the AORN statement and have incorporated RNFA functions into the scope of nursing practice.[7]

## SCRUB NURSE

The scrub nurse is the nursing team member of the sterile surgical team. This role may be performed by an RN or an OR scrub technologist. The scrub nurse must have an understanding of the specific surgical procedure in addition to knowledge of the basic anatomy and physiology involved in the procedure. Some of the scrub nurse's responsibilities include the preparation of supplies and equipment on the sterile field; maintenance of the safety and integrity of the sterile field; observation of the scrubbed team members for breaks in sterile technique; provision of appropriate sterile instrumentation, sutures, and supplies to the operating surgeon; and adherence to established policies and procedures for sponge, instrument, and sharps counts.

To perform this role effectively, the scrub nurse must possess manual skills and dexterity and strictly adhere to the principles of aseptic technique. All duties need to be consistently performed with precision and accuracy to ensure the patient's safety throughout the surgical procedure.

## CIRCULATING NURSE

The circulating nurse is an RN whose responsibility is to serve as the patient advocate while coordinating events before, during, and after the surgical procedure. The circulating nurse is responsible for creating a safe environment for the patient, managing the activities outside the sterile field, and providing nursing care to the patient.

Before and during administration of the anesthetic, the circulating nurse provides emotional support to the patient and assists the anesthesia team during the induction period. Throughout the surgical procedure, the circulating nurse obtains supplies and equipment for the sterile team members, enforces policies and procedures, and implements measures to ensure patient safety. The circulating nurse is also responsible for documenting intraoperative nursing care and ensuring that surgical specimens are identified and placed in the appropriate medium. Some of the other responsibilities of the circulating nurse include enforcing the principles of aseptic technique; recognizing and implementing actions to resolve possible environmental hazards that involve the patient or surgical team members; ensuring that sponge, instrument, and sharps counts are completed and appropriately documented; and communicating relevant information to individuals outside of the OR, such as family members and other health care workers.

## ANESTHESIOLOGIST AND ANESTHETIST

An anesthesiologist is a physician who specializes in the administration of anesthetic agents and monitoring the patient's response to the agents. An anesthetist is an individual who administers anesthetics under the direct supervision of an anesthesiologist or surgeon. Advanced practice nurses who administer anesthetics are required to pass the certification examination from the Council on Certification of Nurse Anesthetists in order to become certified RN anesthetists (CRNA).[8]

In the preoperative period, the anesthesiologist and anesthetist evaluate the patient and determine the appropriate anesthetic to be administered. Intraoperative responsibilities include anesthetizing the patient, providing appropriate levels of pain relief for the patient, monitoring the patient's physiological status, and providing the best operative conditions for the surgeon. In the immediate postoperative period, the anesthesiologist assumes medical responsibility for the patient.

### OTHER PERSONNEL

A number of allied personnel also contribute to meeting the needs of the surgical patient. Pathologists, radiologists, radiology technicians, perfusionists, environmental services personnel, and clerical staff are a few of the many individuals whose skills and expertise are necessary to provide assistance to the surgical team and ultimately to the patient.

## THE SURGICAL ENVIRONMENT

### DESIGN OF THE SURGICAL SUITE

A surgical suite is designed to provide a safe therapeutic environment for the patient. The design of the suite addresses issues of traffic patterns, infection control, safety, and efficiency.

### TRAFFIC CONTROL

Traffic in and out of the operating suite is kept to a minimum. Only essential personnel are allowed inside the operating room. As the number of persons increases, potential contamination from bacterial shedding and air turbulence increases.

Traffic control patterns are designed to address activity and movement into and out of the surgical suite, as well as within the suite. The floor plan of a surgical suite is divided into three zones. The three-zone concept was developed to define the areas within the surgical suite by the types of activities that occur within each area. The three zones are known as the *unrestricted area,* the *semirestricted area,* and the *restricted area.*

The unrestricted area provides an entrance to and exit from the surgical suite. The holding area, PACU, lounges, dressing rooms, and offices are located in the unrestricted area. In this area street clothes may be worn and traffic is not restricted. The semirestricted area provides access to restricted zones and peripheral support areas within the surgical suite. Peripheral support areas consist of storage for clean and sterile supplies, work areas for processing supplies and equipment, and corridors to the individual ORs. Scrub attire and hair covering must be worn in the semirestricted area. The restricted area includes the individual operating rooms, scrub rooms, substerile rooms, and clean core areas. In this area scrub attire, hair covering, and masks must be worn.

### INFECTION CONTROL

The design of the OR and the materials used within it are chosen to address issues of infection control and safety. Materials used in the interior of the OR address issues of environmental control.

Ceiling and walls are constructed of nonporous, smooth, fire-resistant materials that are easy to clean with microbial agents. Tile wall covering is not advocated because of the potential for microorganisms to grow in porous grout lines.

Materials used for floor coverings have the same specifications as the walls and ceiling. The floors need to be highly wear resistant with slip-proof surfaces to prevent personnel injury.

Sliding doors are used to prevent air turbulence in the OR. Fire regulations dictate that doors should be able to swing open if needed.

### ENVIRONMENTAL CONDITIONS

Temperature and humidity are environmental conditions that need to be controlled to reduce the incidence of infection. Temperature within an OR is maintained between 20° and 22° C (68° and 75° F). Most pathogenic bacteria metabolize and reproduce at or near normal body temperature. Bacterial growth may be inhibited by keeping room temperature below body temperature. The lower room temperature also helps decrease the surgical patient's metabolic demands. The relative humidity in the OR is maintained within the range of 40% to 60%.[19] This level of humidity diminishes bacterial growth and restricts static electricity.

Many ORs have high-efficiency particulate air (HEPA) filters in the air systems to assist with infection control. Inlet air is dispersed from vents in the ceiling and exhausted through vents at the floor level. Slightly less air is exhausted than is introduced, creating a positive pressure gradient within the room. The positive pressure prevents potentially contaminated air from entering the room. This is why all doors to individual ORs remain closed except for patient and team members' entry and exit. There should be at least 15 room air exchanges per hour in each operating room. Three of the exchanges should be fresh air exchanges.[20]

### COMMUNICATION SYSTEM

A reliable communication system is essential in the surgical suite so that OR personnel can call for assistance and communicate with other members of the health care team. Telephones and intradepartmental and interdepartmental intercom systems are used for instant consultation with various departments, such as the blood bank, radiology department, pathology department, and PACU. In addition to intercom systems, a call light system can be used to summon emergent or routine assistance. Some states require the presence of a "code blue" notification system in every OR. The code station should be located close to the work areas of both the circulating nurse and anesthesia staff with the primary indicators located in a central area within the surgical suite.[19]

## INFECTION CONTROL

Surgical wound infections account for 24% of nosocomial infections. They rank as the second most common nosocomial infection for hospitalized patients. An estimated 500,000 infections occur annually with a cost of $10 billion per year. Surgical wound infections are the most common cause of morbidity and mortality for the surgical patient.[19]

*Asepsis* is defined as the absence of microorganisms that cause disease. *Surgical asepsis* promotes tissue healing by deterring pathogens from coming into contact with the surgical wound. Practices that suppress, reduce, and inhibit infectious processes are known as *aseptic technique.*

Infection control policies and procedures guide the practice of aseptic technique in the operating room. The policies and procedures are based on principles of microbiology and bacteriology. Infection control policies are guided by AORN recommended practices for perioperative nursing. The AORN has developed recommended practices for aseptic technique, surgical attire, environmental services activities, sterilization of supplies and equipment, surgical hand scrub, and cleansing of skin.

All members of the OR team are responsible for strict adherence to aseptic technique. It is essential that OR nurses acquire a surgical conscience. *Surgical conscience* is defined as vigilant adherence to aseptic technique throughout the entire perioperative period. This involves constant examination and observation of the patient, OR environment, and personnel. A surgical conscience is completely developed when the nurse automatically attends to sterile technique. To develop a surgical conscience the nurse must understand the principles of asepsis and sterile technique, acquire self-discipline in managing nursing practice, and develop good communication and assertiveness skills to identify patient needs and communicate breaks in sterile technique.

## BASIC RULES OF SURGICAL ASEPSIS

Strict adherence to aseptic technique minimizes the potential for contamination of the sterile field and wound infection. Protocols for creating and maintaining a sterile field have been developed from the seven AORN recommended practices for maintaining a sterile field. Six of the practices address practice issues and will be briefly discussed. The seventh practice addresses the administrative function of establishing and reviewing policies and procedures related to the practice of aseptic technique.

Recommended practice I states that "scrubbed persons function within a sterile field."[4] Scrubbed personnel wear sterile gowns and gloves at the surgical field. Gowns and gloves provide a barrier to restrict the transfer of microorganisms from the scrubbed person's hands and clothing to the surgical wound. The gown of a scrubbed team member is considered sterile in front from the chest to the level of the sterile field, and the sleeves are sterile from 2 inches above the elbow to the stockinette cuff. The stockinette cuff portion of the gown is unsterile and needs to be completely covered by a sterile glove. The unsterile areas of the surgical gown include the neckline, shoulder, axillary region, and back. Articles dropped below the waist or table level are considered contaminated.

The second recommended practice states that sterile drapes are used to create a sterile field.[4] Surgical drapes provide a barrier that impedes the movement of microorganisms from a nonsterile area to a sterile area. Sterile drapes are placed on the patient, equipment, and furniture used within the sterile field. Draped tables are sterile only at the table level; items extending over the table edge are contaminated. Handling of drapes should be kept to a minimum. When placing sterile drapes, gloved hands are protected by a cuff of the drape (Figure 19-1).

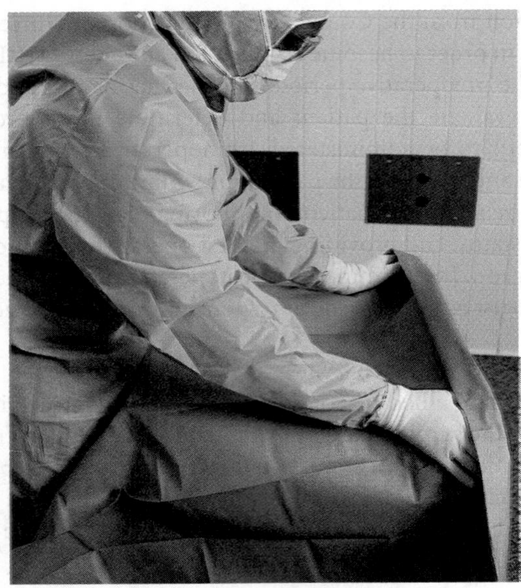

**fig. 19-1** Scrub nurse protects gloves with cuff of drape when opening inner wrapper of pack, which will serve as sterile table cover.

Practice III states that all items used in the sterile field are sterile.[4] If there is a question about the sterility of an item, it must be considered unsterile. Packaging materials must guarantee that items will remain sterile until removed. Before opening a sterile package it must be inspected for seal integrity, tears, pinholes, the presence of a sterilization indicator, and the expiration date as indicated.

The fourth practice addresses the introduction of supplies into the sterile field. Supplies that are introduced into the sterile field are to be delivered in a manner that ensures the sterility of the item and maintains the integrity of the sterile field.[4] A sterile package is opened from the far side first and the near side last; wrapper tails are held when the item is presented to the sterile field (Figure 19-2). Solutions are poured to prevent splashing of liquids onto the field. Once a bottle of sterile solution is opened the entire contents must be presented to the sterile field or discarded. The edges of a bottle cap are considered nonsterile once the cap is removed. If the cap is replaced, the sterility of the bottle contents cannot be ensured; therefore the remaining contents must be discarded.

Recommended practice V addresses the maintenance and monitoring of the sterile field. The possibility for contamination increases with time; therefore the sterile field should be established as close to the time of use as possible. Unattended sterile fields are considered contaminated.[4]

Movement within or around the sterile field by personnel is addressed in recommended practice VI.[4] The integrity of

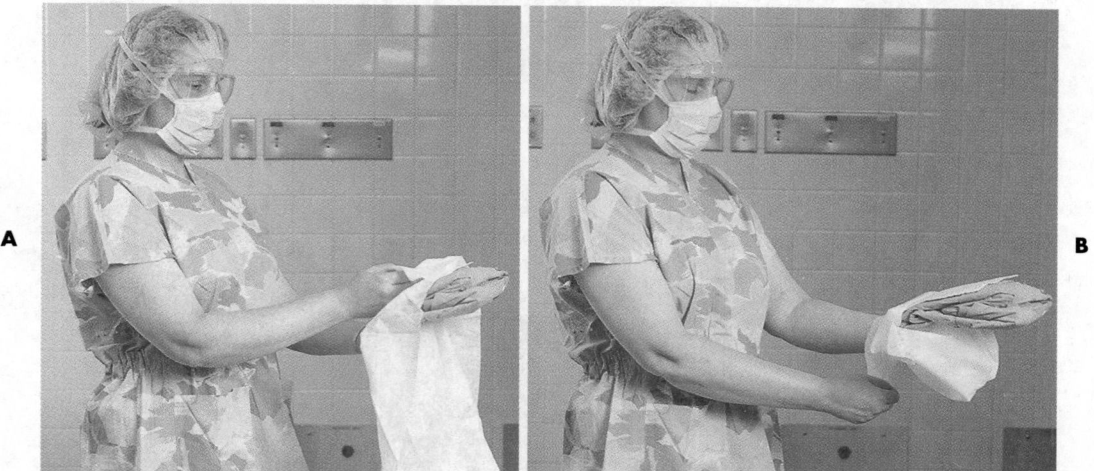


fig. 19-2 **A,** When opening sterile package, circulating nurse opens corner nearest body last to avoid potential contamination of inner pack. **B,** To prevent unsterile corners of outer wrapper from touching scrub nurse or sterile field, circulating nurse draws back corners of opened wrapper when presenting inner package.

the sterile field must be maintained by individuals moving within or around the sterile field. Only scrubbed personnel touch and reach over sterile areas. Sterile persons remain close to the sterile field and never turn their backs to the field. Sterile individuals change positions by passing back to back or face to face. Unscrubbed personnel only touch and reach over non sterile areas. Unscrubbed team members must not walk between sterile fields and must approach sterile fields by facing them.

## INFECTION CONTROL PRACTICES FOR OPERATING ROOM PERSONNEL

All individuals working in the operating room serve as a major source of microbial contamination to the environment because of the large quantities of bacteria that are present in the respiratory tract and on the skin, hair, and attire of all persons. To reduce the risks of OR personnel serving as sources of infection for the patient, it is necessary for everyone to wear surgical attire in the semirestricted and restricted areas of the OR. Surgical attire also provides personnel protection from exposure to infectious microorganisms and hazardous substances.[7] Surgical attire includes a scrub suit, hat or hood, and face mask or shield.

## SURGICAL ATTIRE

Dressing in OR attire proceeds from head to toe. The surgical hat is put on first to prevent contamination of the scrub clothes with hair or dandruff. The hat must be clean, be free of lint, and completely cover all head and facial hair. If the hat does not provide sufficient coverage of facial hair a hood should be worn.

Scrub suits are put on after the hair is covered. The suits, which are laundered daily, should be made of materials that meet the requirements of the National Fire Protection Agency and should be closely woven to minimize bacterial shedding. Scrub shirts are either tied at the waist or tucked into the scrub pants. This is done to decrease bacterial shedding and to prevent contamination of the sterile field by a loose shirt. Unscrubbed personnel should wear long-sleeved warm-up jackets to prevent possible shedding of microorganisms from bare arms. The long-sleeved attire is also described in the Occupational Safety and Health Administration's (OSHA) directive for utilization of personal protective equipment[7] (Figure 19-3).

Footwear should be comfortable. In the interest of safety, clogs, open-toe, and cloth athletic shoes are not recommended. Clogs can be a hazard when a person tries to move quickly, and if sharp objects are accidentally dropped, sandals and canvas shoes provide little protection. Literature suggests that the use of shoe covers in the OR does not affect the incidence of postoperative wound infection.[7] Shoe covers are a part of personal protective equipment and are to be worn whenever it is expected that splashes or spills will happen. If worn, they should be changed when torn, soiled, or wet and removed when leaving the surgical suite.

Masks are necessary to prevent contamination of the surgical environment by respiratory droplets. A mask is to be worn where sterile supplies are open and in areas where scrubbed persons are present. The mask must totally cover the nose and mouth and must be secured to prevent ventilation from the sides of the face. It is either on or off; it should not be saved by being hung around the neck, placed on the forehead, or placed in a pocket. When removing a mask, care should be taken to prevent contamination of the hands. The filter portion of the mask should not be touched. The mask should be removed

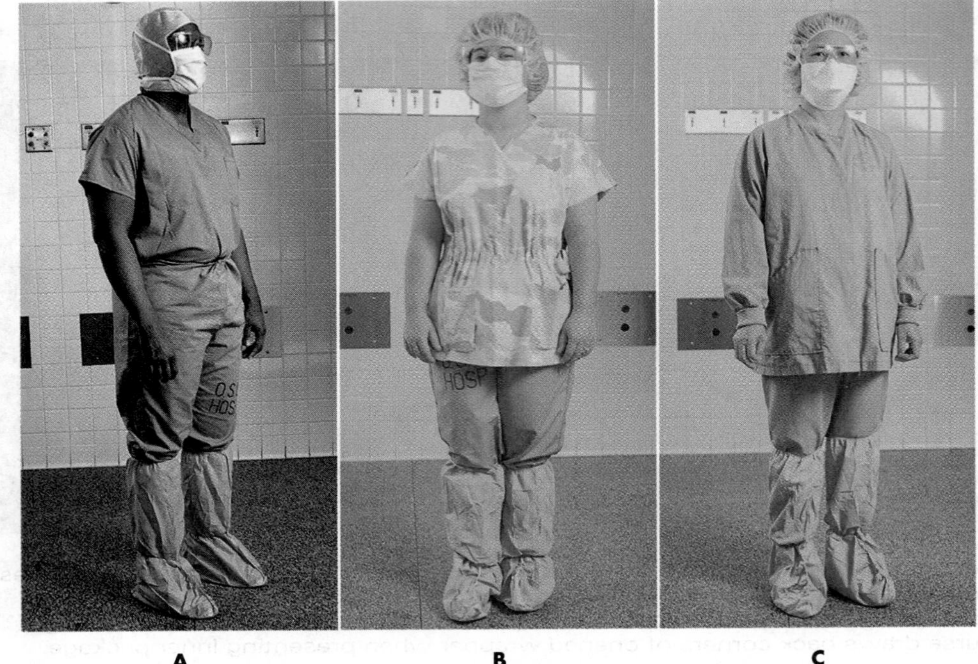

**fig. 19-3** Proper surgical attire consists of a two-piece or a one-piece coverall suit. Shoe covers may be worn; they should be changed whenever they become wet, torn, or soiled. All head and facial hair should be covered in the semirestricted and restricted areas. In the restricted area, all personnel should wear masks. Jewelry should be removed or totally confined. Nail polish or artificial nails should not be worn. When a two-piece scrub suit is worn, loose fitting scrub tops should be tucked into pants **(A)**, or tunic tops that fit close to the body may be worn outside of pants **(B)**. **C,** Nonscrubbed personnel should wear long-sleeved jackets that are buttoned or snapped closed.

only by touching its strings; once removed, it should be immediately discarded (Figure 19-4).

Face shields and protective eyewear are also part of surgical attire. These items are protective barriers used to decrease the risk of splash or spraying of fluids into the mucous membranes of the mouth, nose, and eyes. All personnel who are in close proximity to the operative site should wear protective eyewear.

If jewelry is worn in the OR, it must be completely confined within scrub clothes or cap. Complete confinement of jewelry decreases the possibility of it falling into the surgical wound.

Lead aprons and thyroid shields are protective attire worn to protect OR personnel from radiological exposure. These items are worn when personnel must be present during fluoroscopic procedures or when x-rays are used intraoperatively.

Ideally, OR attire should never be worn outside of the surgical suite because this creates a two-way hazard. Any contaminants that come in contact with the OR team members can become airborne and find susceptible hosts outside of the surgical suite. Conversely, bacteria present outside the suite may be carried back to the surgical suite. If changing scrub attire is not feasible, head and shoe coverings are removed and the scrub clothes are covered. The preferred method is to use a clean cover gown that closes in the back. If a lab coat is worn, it must be completely buttoned to protect the front of the scrub suit. On return to the department, clean scrub attire should be put on because cover gowns and lab coats are ineffective barriers to potential external contaminants.

## STANDARD PRECAUTIONS

A discussion of aseptic technique maintenance is not complete without mention of Standard Precautions. Uncontained blood and body fluids—an inevitable part of surgery—present a great hazard to operating room personnel. Because routine medical history and examination cannot identify all patients with human immunodeficiency virus (HIV), hepatitis, or other blood-borne pathogens, Standard Precautions are used for all patients. The Centers for Disease Control and Prevention (CDC) has outlined these precautions, and OSHA has adopted these standard procedures as part of the requirements for maintenance of a safe working environment. The Standard Precautions are summarized in Box 19-2.

Based on recent epidemiological literature, in 1996 the CDC revised guidelines for infection control in hospitals. The new guidelines have two tiers of precautions. Standard Precautions have replaced Body Substance Isolation Precautions and Universal Precautions. These guidelines are intended for the care of all patients regardless of diagnosis. The second tier of precautions, Transmission-Based Precautions, is to be im-

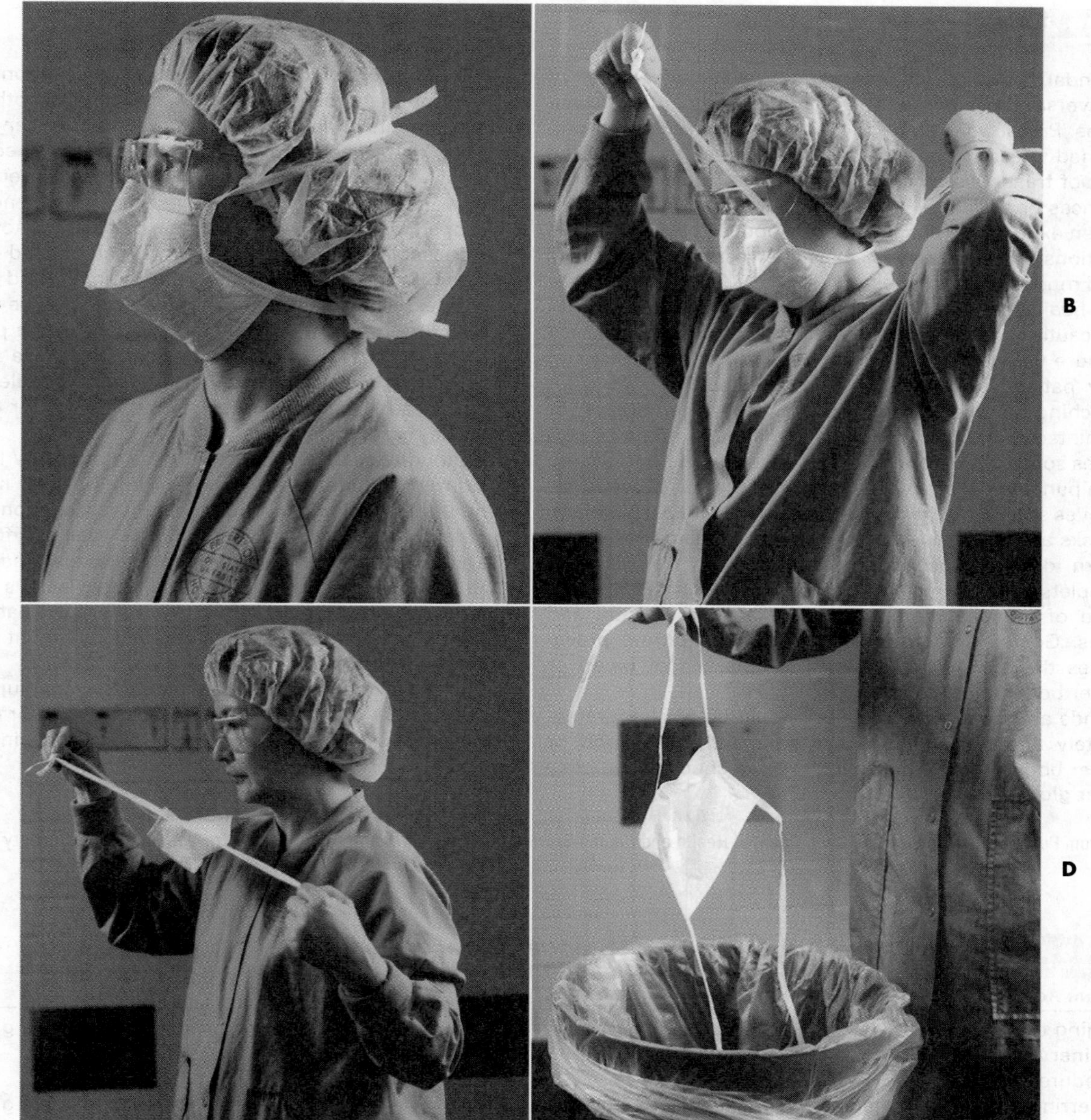

fig. 19-4 Proper handling of mask. **A,** Edges of properly worn mask conform to facial contours when mask is applied and tied correctly. **B** and **C,** Personnel should avoid touching filter portion of mask when removing it. **D,** Masks should be discarded upon removal.

plemented for the care of patients with known or suspected infection by epidemiologically important pathogens spread by airborne, droplet, or contact routes of transmission. (See Chapter 10.)

The proper handling and disposition of needles, knife blades, and sharp instruments, along with strict compliance with the CDC practices of Standard Precautions, protects OR personnel. Adherence to these practices, along with strict adherence to aseptic technique, minimizes the chance of cross-contamination of pathogens between patients and personnel. Table 19-1 provides some examples of how OR nurses can apply the principles of Standard Precautions.

## STERILIZATION OF SUPPLIES

Microorganisms that do not normally invade healthy tissue are capable of causing infection if introduced directly into the body. For this reason all supplies and instruments used for the surgical procedure must be adequately sterilized. Sterilization renders items safe for contact with tissue without transmission of infection as long as their sterility is maintained. The sterilization of products for use in the surgical suite must be performed according to guidelines established by the regulatory agencies that conduct research and set guidelines for the methods, products, and equipment used in sterilization processes. These agencies include the CDC, OSHA, AORN,

**box 19-2** *Standard Precautions*

1. Standard Precautions incorporate the major features of Universal Precautions, or Blood and Body Fluid Precautions. Precautions apply to all patients regardless of presumed infection status. They are designed to reduce the risk of transmission of pathogens from moist body substances or surfaces. Precautions should be implemented when exposure is anticipated to blood; all body fluids, secretions, and excretions, except sweat; nonintact skin; and mucous membranes.
2. All health care workers should use appropriate barrier precautions to prevent skin and mucous membrane exposure when contact with blood or other body fluids of any patient is anticipated. Gloves should be worn for touching blood and body fluids, mucous membranes, or nonintact skin of all patients, for handling items or surfaces soiled with blood or body fluids, and for performing venipuncture and other vascular access procedures. Gloves should be changed after contact with each patient. Masks and protective eye wear or face shields should be worn during procedures that are likely to generate droplets of blood or other body fluids to prevent exposure of mucous membranes of the nose, mouth, and eyes. Gowns or aprons should be worn during procedures that are likely to generate splashes of blood or other body fluids.
3. Hands and other skin surfaces should be washed immediately and thoroughly if contaminated with blood or other body fluids. Hands should be washed immediately after gloves are removed.
4. All health care workers should take precautions to prevent injuries caused by needles, scalpels, and other sharp instruments or devices during procedures; when cleaning used instruments; during disposal of used needles; and when handling sharp instruments after procedures. To prevent needle-stick injuries, needles should not be recapped, purposely bent or broken by hand, removed from disposable syringes, or otherwise manipulated by hand. After they are used, disposable syringes and needles, scalpel blades, and other sharp items should be placed in puncture-resistant containers for disposal; the puncture-resistant containers should be located as close as practical to the use area. Large-bore reusable needles should be placed in a puncture-resistant container for transport to the reprocessing area.
5. Although saliva has not been implicated in HIV transmission to minimize the need for emergency mouth-to-mouth resuscitation, mouthpieces, resuscitation bags, or other ventilation devices should be available for use in areas in which the need for resuscitation is predictable.
6. Health care workers who have exudative lesions or weeping dermatitis should refrain from all direct patient care and room handling of patient-care equipment until the condition resolves.
7. Spills of blood or body fluids should be wiped up as soon as possible with a fresh 10% bleach solution or other antimicrobial solution known to be effective against bloodborne pathogens, such as Staphene.

Adapted from Public Health Service, US Department of Health and Human Services, Centers for Disease Control and Prevention, Atlanta, January 1996.

**table 19-1** *Intraoperative Applications of Standard Precautions*

| Nursing Action | Potential Contaminant | Precautions |
|---|---|---|
| Changing the blood-filled suction liner at the end of the procedure | Blood splashing out of suction liner | Goggles or face shield, nonsterile gloves |
| Transferring an actively bleeding trauma patient to the OR bed | Direct contact with blood | Goggles or face shield, nonsterile gloves, fluid-resistant apron or gown |
| Organizing blood-filled sponges for the sponge count | Direct contact with blood-contaminated items | Goggles or face shield, nonsterile gloves |
| Removing or changing the surgical knife blade | Cuts and direct contact with blood | Instrument or surgical clamp to disassemble knife blade and handle |

Food and Drug Administration (FDA), and American Association for Medical Instrumentation (AAMI). Table 19-2 summarizes methods of sterilization.

## SURGICAL SCRUB

The purpose of a surgical scrub is to remove dirt and microorganisms from the hands, fingernails, and forearms; decrease the resident microbial count to minimum levels; and retard the regrowth of microorganisms. This is accomplished by a mechanical washing of the fingernails, hands, and arms with an antimicrobial soap.

The microbial flora of the skin are classified as transient and resident bacteria. *Transient flora* are acquired by contact and loosely adhere to the skin. The majority of transient microorganisms are removed by chemical and mechanical methods.

*Resident flora* are found deep in the skin in hair follicles and sebaceous glands. These microorganisms are shed from the body with the movement of old cells from the dermal to the epidermal layer of the skin with perspiration and other skin secretions. Because of these actions, resident flora are potential sources of contamination. Resident bacteria are decreased but are not completely removed during the surgical scrub.

**table 19-2** *Major Methods of Sterilization*

| Method | Manner of Sterilization | Advantages | Disadvantages |
|---|---|---|---|
| Steam sterilization | Steam under pressure infiltrates permeable materials with moist heat, causing the denaturation and coagulation of the cellular protein system → death of microbe or spore. | Safe<br>Easy<br>Fast<br>Economic<br>Permeates porous substances<br>Leaves no film on items | Items cannot be sensitive to heat<br>Steam and moisture may corrode items |
| Chemical sterilization (ethylene oxide gas) | Chemical disrupts cellular protein metabolism and reproduction → death of microbe or spore. | Effective for heat-sensitive items<br>Effective against all microorganisms<br>Noncorrosive<br>Permeates dry substances<br>Leaves no film on items | Time consuming<br>Expensive<br>Toxic by-products can formulate |
| Plasma sterilization | Low-temperature hydrogen peroxide creates a gas plasma. The gas plasma consists of ions, electrons, and neutral atomic particles. Free radicals in gas interact with cellular membranes, enzymes, or nucleic acids → death of microbe or spore.[8] | Faster than ethylene oxide gas<br>Dry nontoxic method<br>By-products (water and oxygen) are environmentally safe<br>No aeration<br>Safe for heat-sensitive items<br>Noncorrosive to metal[8] | Incompatible with cotton-woven fabrics and paper[8]<br>Ineffective on small-diameter cannulae |

The skin cannot be sterilized; however, it can be made surgically clean. Obtaining surgically clean skin involves a mechanical process that removes transient flora with friction along with a chemical process that decreases the number of flora on the dermis with the use of an antimicrobial detergent.

Various antimicrobial detergents meet the criteria for effectiveness. The effective agent must be a broad-spectrum antimicrobial, fast-acting in decreasing the microbial count, able to leave a residue on the skin to reduce regrowth of bacteria, and nonirritating and nonsensitizing. The most commonly used agents are povidone-iodine and hexaclorophene.

The procedure and types of material used for the surgical scrub vary from one institution to another. Regardless of the procedure, certain criteria must be met by all personnel before beginning the surgical scrub.

Only individuals who are free of skin problems and upper respiratory infections should scrub. Skin cuts and abrasions can discharge serum, which can provide an environment for microbial growth and therefore increase the potential for infection. Fingernails must be kept short to prevent tearing of surgical gloves and clean to prevent harboring of microorganisms. Nail polish that is chipped or worn for more than 4 days appears to foster larger amounts of bacteria. It is recommended that if nail polish is worn it should be freshly applied and free of chips (see the Research Box).

There are two accepted methods for performing a surgical hand scrub: the timed scrub procedure and the brush-stroke procedure. Both are effective and follow an anatomical pattern of scrub, beginning at the fingertips and ending with the elbows.

The timed scrub takes a minimum of 5 minutes to complete. A 10-minute scrub versus a 5-minute scrub provides no appreciable reduction of microorganisms.[19] In the timed scrub each anatomical area of the hands and forearms is scrubbed for an identified length of time with special attention given to the fingers and hands. At the conclusion of the timed scrub, the hands and arms are rinsed.

The brush-stroke scrub also takes approximately 5 minutes to perform. This method differs from the timed scrub method only in that there is a defined number of brush strokes used

**research** 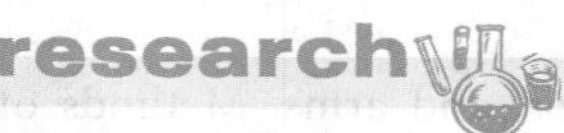

Reference: Wynd CA, Samstag DE, Lapp AM: Bacterial carriage on the fingernails of OR nurses, *AORN J* 60(5):797, 1994.

This study was designed to examine the effects of manicured polished fingernails on bacterial carriage on fingernails of OR nurses. Fingernail lengths, freshly polished fingernails, fingernails with chipped polish, and polish-free nails were examined. The number of bacterial colonies on the nurses' fingernails was measured before and after a surgical scrub.

The 102 OR nurses who participated in the study were randomly assigned into one of three groups: freshly polished fingernails, fingernails with chipped polish, or natural fingernails. Participants in the study scrubbed on a daily basis for a minimum of 2 weeks before joining the study.

Results of data analysis demonstrated that fresh fingernail polish on healthy nails does not increase bacterial count, chipped fingernail polish or polish that has been worn for more than 4 days harbors greater numbers of bacteria, and there is no significant relationship between fingernail length and the number of bacterial colonies in any of the subjects studied.

**table 19-3** *Surgical Scrub Guidelines*

| Action | Comments |
|---|---|
| 1. Don surgical attire making sure all hair and jewelry are covered and mask is properly secured. | Surgical attire decreases possible contamination from the operating room to the patient. |
| 2. Remove all jewelry from hands and arms. | Jewelry harbors microorganisms that may not be removed during hand washing. |
| 3. Moisten hands and arms and wash to 2 inches above the elbows with an antiseptic agent. | A prescrub loosens surface debris. |
| 4. Clean nails and subungual areas with nail cleaner under running water. | Improperly cleaned fingernails and subungual areas can harbor microorganisms. |
| 5. Rinse hands and arms. Allow water to flow from fingertips to elbows, taking care not to splash surgical attire. | Elevating hands higher than the elbows facilitates water flowing from the cleanest area down the arm. Moisture on scrub attire contaminates the sterile gown. |
| 6. Moisten scrub brush, create a lather, and begin the surgical scrub at the fingertips, progressing to the digits, palm, and the back of the hand. | The scrubbing is done vigorously with the scrub brush held perpendicularly to the digit. All sides of the digit and web spaces are scrubbed. Depending on institutional policy, this step initiates either the timed scrub or the scrub-count process. |
| 7. Scrub forearms to 2 inches above the elbow. | Each side of the arm is scrubbed in a circular motion to 2 inches above the elbow. |
| 8. Discard the scrub brush into the appropriate container. Rinse hands and arms thoroughly. Keep hands elevated and proceed into the operating room. | Same comments as for no. 5. |

for each area of the fingers, hands, and arms. Methods of rinsing and entering the operating room are the same as for the timed scrub process. See Table 19-3 for surgical scrub guidelines.

## PATIENT SKIN PREPARATION

The purpose of skin preparation, known as the prep, is to make the surgical incision site as free as possible from transient and resident microorganisms. It is an essential process for the prevention of a surgical wound infection.

Skin preparation can be performed before the induction of anesthesia. If the prep is done when the patient is awake, the circulating nurse needs to explain the purpose of the procedure, attend to the patient's privacy by avoiding unnecessary exposure, and provide for the patient's comfort and safety.

Removal of hair from the surgical site is done only when necessary. Methods for hair removal include wet shaving, use of clippers, and use of a depilatory. There is a greater incidence of wound infection in patients who are shaved preoperatively than for patients who have not had a shave prep, who have a smaller amount of hair clipped, or on whom a depilatory is used.[5]

Data also support the fact that the amount of time between the shave and the operation is related to the wound infection rate.[19] If a wet shave is ordered by the physician it should be performed immediately before surgery in a well-lit area that provides patient privacy. The shave should be performed by an individual who has demonstrated skill in the shave procedure. When performing a shave prep, care should be taken to prevent nicks, scratches, or cuts because any breaks in the skin surface provide a medium for the growth of microorganisms and a resultant infection.

The choice of cleansing agents depends on the surgeon's preference and institution policy. Considerations that are used in the selection of the appropriate agent are patient sensitivity and skin condition; spectrum of activity (the agent must have a broad spectrum of antimicrobial action); toxicity of the agent (some agents can be absorbed from the skin and cause neurotoxicity); and the length of antimicrobial action.[7]

The prep begins with a mechanical scrubbing at the incision site and is extended in a circular fashion away from the site to the periphery. At the periphery the prep sponge is considered contaminated and is discarded. The soiled sponge is never brought back over the area previously scrubbed. Each time the area is scrubbed a new sponge is used. The area of skin that is prepped needs to be large enough to avoid wound contamination by movement of the surgical drapes to accommodate any necessary extensions of the incision and to include all drain sites.

When it is necessary to prep an area that includes an open draining wound or a body orifice, the practice of cleansing from the incision site to the periphery is modified. The alterations of the prep are based on the principle that the cleaning proceeds from clean to dirty areas. The most contaminated area is scrubbed last, even if it is the site of the surgical incision.

# ANESTHESIA

The field of anesthesiology is acknowledged as a major contributor to medicine and has enabled the growth and scientific development of modern surgery. The term *anesthesia* is derived from the Greek word *anaisthesis* meaning "no sensation."[20]

**table 19-4** *Comparison of Types of Anesthesia*

| Type of Anesthesia | Expected Results | Method of Administration | Risks |
|---|---|---|---|
| General anesthesia | Unconsciousness<br>Possible endotracheal tube placement | Anesthetic agent injected into circulatory system<br>Inhalation of anesthetic agents | Sore throat<br>Injury to mouth or teeth<br>Aspiration<br>Pneumonia |
| Spinal or epidural anesthesia | Temporary ↓ or loss of feeling or movement in lower part of body | Anesthetic injected through a needle or catheter into spinal canal or immediately outside the spinal canal | Headache<br>Backache<br>Convulsions<br>Persistent numbness<br>Residual pain |
| Nerve block | Temporary loss of sensation or movement of limb | Anesthetic agent injected near nerves resulting in loss of sensation to the surgical area | Infection<br>Weakness<br>Persistent numbness<br>Residual pain |
| Intravenous regional anesthesia | Temporary loss of sensation or movement of limb | Anesthetic agent injected into veins of arm or leg while using a tourniquet | Infection<br>Weakness<br>Persistent numbness<br>Residual pain |
| Monitored anesthesia care with sedation | ↓ Anxiety<br>↓ Pain<br>Partial or total amnesia | Medication injected into circulatory system<br>Inhalation of anesthetic agents | Unconsciousness<br>Depressed respiration |
| Monitored anesthesia care without sedation | Monitoring of vital signs<br>Immediate presence of anesthesia provider for intervention as needed | None | Increased awareness<br>Anxiety<br>Discomfort |

In the early nineteenth century alcohol or opium was given to patients for pain relief or for muscle relaxation during surgical procedures. Surgeons had to work rapidly to complete the surgical procedure because these drugs were unable to provide sufficient pain relief or relaxation. In 1842 the surgeon Crawford Long began using ether as an anesthetic for surgical patients, but he did not publish his work until 1849. In 1846 dentists Horace Wells and William Morgan used nitrous oxide for dental extractions. Later that year William Morgan demonstrated the use of ether as an effective method for rendering a surgical patient unconscious. Morgan's work provided the foundation for the modern practice of anesthesia.[8]

Anesthesia is the limited or total loss of feeling with or without loss of consciousness. The two broad classifications of anesthesia are general and local. *General* anesthesia produces unconsciousness; *local* anesthesia creates a loss of sensation in a particular area. The method of administering the anesthesia and the choice of anesthetic agent for a particular patient are determined by the anesthesiologist (Table 19-4). Factors that influence the decision include the patient's preference; the patient's age, physical status, and emotional status; the presence of coexisting disease; the type and length of the surgical procedure; the patient's position during the surgical procedure; the postoperative recovery from specific anesthetic agents; and any requirements of the surgeon. The American Society of Anesthesiologists developed a classification system to identify risk factors based on the patient's health status. (See Chapter 18.) As part of the preoperative evaluation the anesthesiologist classifies the patient according to the physical status.

Operating room nurses do not administer anesthetic agents, but they must have an understanding of the various anesthetics used in surgery, the methods of administration, and the potential side effects and complications (Table 19-5). This knowledge enables the nurse to plan intraoperative nursing care and to assist the anesthesia team.

## PREOPERATIVE MEDICATIONS

Preoperative medications may be given to reduce preoperative anxiety (sedatives, hypnotics), to minimize secretions in the respiratory tract and mouth (anticholinergics), to relieve pain (narcotics), and to decrease metabolism so that less anesthetic agent is necessary. Medications are selected on the basis of the preoperative assessment findings and the demands of the intended surgical procedure.

Preoperative medication may be given in the unit before transport to the OR suite or in the holding area after arrival in the OR suite. Patients are observed closely for signs of untoward reactions, which include vomiting, hypotension, and cardiac and sensory changes. It should be noted that the use of preoperative medications has decreased in some settings.

## GENERAL ANESTHESIA

General anesthesia is the depression of the central nervous system with the administration of drugs or inhalation agents. The exact methods by which general anesthetic agents produce unconsciousness, analgesia, and muscle relaxation are unknown. It is thought that each anesthetic affects the central nervous and musculoskeletal systems in unique ways and works with various sites and areas to create these effects.[20]

**table 19-5** *Commonly Used Anesthetic Agents*

| Agent | Indication | Advantages | Disadvantages |
|---|---|---|---|
| **INHALATION AGENTS** | | | |
| Nitrous oxide ($N_2O$) | Maintenance; sometimes for induction | Rapid induction and emergence; additive effects to other anesthetics | Poor muscle relaxation; can depress myocardium |
| Halothane (Fluothane) | Maintenance; sometimes for induction | Rapid induction and emergence; pleasant, nonirritating odor | Sensitizes myocardium to epinephrine; ↓ heart rate and arterial blood pressure; poor muscle relaxation |
| Enflurane (Ethrane) | Maintenance; sometimes for induction | Good relaxation; permits larger amounts of epinephrine to be used than with halothane | Can cause ↑ heart rate and ↓ blood pressure; slightly irritating odor |
| Isoflurane (Forane) | Maintenance; sometimes for induction | Good relaxation; smooth, rapid induction and emergence | ↑ Heart rate; slightly irritating odor |
| **INTRAVENOUS ANESTHETICS** | | | |
| Thiopental sodium (Pentothal) | Induction | Fast, smooth induction and emergence | Large doses may cause respiratory and cardiovascular depression |
| Propofol (Diprivan) | Induction; maintenance; used as part of balanced anesthesia | Rapid onset; minimal excitation during induction | Twitching, bucking, pain at injection site |
| Ketamine (Ketalar) | Induction; occasional maintenance (IV or IM) | Short acting; patient maintains airway | Large doses may cause emergent delirium and respiratory depression |
| Diazepam (Valium) | Amnesia; hypnotic; used for IV conscious sedation | Good sedation | Prolonged duration |
| Midazolam (Versed) | Hypnotic, used for IV conscious sedation | Excellent amnesia; water soluble (no pain with IV injection); short acting | Slower induction than thiopental; concern regarding loss of memory |
| **DEPOLARIZING MUSCLE RELAXANTS** | | | |
| Succinylcholine (Anectine) | Intubation; short procedures | Rapid onset; short duration | May cause muscle fasciculation, postoperative dysrhythmias |
| **NONDEPOLARIZING MUSCLE RELAXANTS (LONGER ONSET AND DURATION)** | | | |
| D-Tubocurarine chloride (Curare) | Maintenance | No effect on intellectual functions or consciousness | Possible interaction with some drugs (antibiotics) causing prolonged relaxation, respiratory depression, apnea<br>• ↓ BP<br>• circulatory collapse<br>• malignant hyperthermia<br>May cause histamine release<br>No anesthetic properties |
| Pancuronimum (Pavulon) | Maintenance | Rapid action | May cause ↑ heart rate and ↑ blood pressure, respiratory depression |
| **LOCAL ANESTHETICS** | | | |
| Bupivacaine (Marcaine, Sensorcaine) | Epidural, spinal, or local infiltration | Good relaxation; long acting | Overdose can cause cardiac arrest |
| Chloroprocaine (Nesacaine) | Epidural anesthesia | Extremely short acting; good relaxation | Can lead to neurotoxicity if injected directly into cerebrospinal fluid |
| Lidocaine (Xylocaine) | Epidural, spinal, peripheral, IV blocks, and local infiltration | Short acting; good relaxation; low toxicity | Overdose can lead to convulsions |
| Tetracaine (Pontocaine) | Spinal anesthesia | Long acting; good relaxation | Possible anaphylaxis |

**box 19-3** *Stages of Anesthesia*

**Stage I** begins with the administration of anesthetic agents and ends with the loss of consciousness. This is also known as the *relaxation* stage.

**Stage II** begins with the loss of consciousness and ends with the onset of regular breathing and loss of eyelid reflexes. This stage is referred to as the *excitement* or *delirium* phase because it is often accompanied by involuntary motor activity. The patient must not receive any auditory or physical stimulation during this period.

**Stage III** begins with the onset of regular breathing and ends with the cessation of respirations. This stage is known as the *operative* or *surgical* phase.

**Stage IV** begins with the cessation of respiration and leads to death.

For anesthesia to be safe, the anesthesiologist must monitor its depth or level. Guidelines to estimate the depth or level of anesthesia used to be based on clearly delineated physiological changes and reflex responses that were seen with the administration of ether (Box 19-3). Because of the variety of anesthetic agents and anesthetic techniques used today, there are no consistent physiological responses to estimate the exact depth of anesthesia. Determination of the level of anesthesia is achieved by monitoring physiological changes in the patient's heart rate, blood pressure, temperature, respiratory rate, oxygen saturation, and airway $CO_2$ tension.

## Phases of General Anesthesia

The three phases of general anesthesia are the induction phase, maintenance phase, and emergence phase. *Induction* begins with the administration of intravenous agents or with the inhalation of a combination of anesthetic gases and oxygen. Endotracheal intubation is performed during this phase. This phase is completed when the patient is ready for positioning, skin preparation, or the incision.

Once it is safe for any of these activities to commence the patient has entered the *maintenance* phase of anesthesia. During this phase the anesthesiologist maintains the appropriate levels of anesthesia with inhalation agents and intravenous medications. The anesthesiologist pays close attention to the surgical field and anticipates the surgeon's actions in order to alter the depth of anesthesia whenever necessary.

The *emergence* period begins when the anesthesiologist decreases the anesthetic agents and the patient begins to awaken. Extubation occurs during this period. Potential complications during this period include laryngospasm, vomiting, slow spontaneous respirations, and uncontrolled reflex movement.

## Inhalation Anesthesia

Inhalation anesthesia is produced by administering a mixture of anesthetic gases and oxygen directly to the lungs. The gases are passed into pulmonary circulation, delivered to the brain and other body tissues, and are readily eliminated through the respiratory system. These agents are administered to the patient by a face mask or directly into the lungs through an endotracheal tube (Figure 19-5).

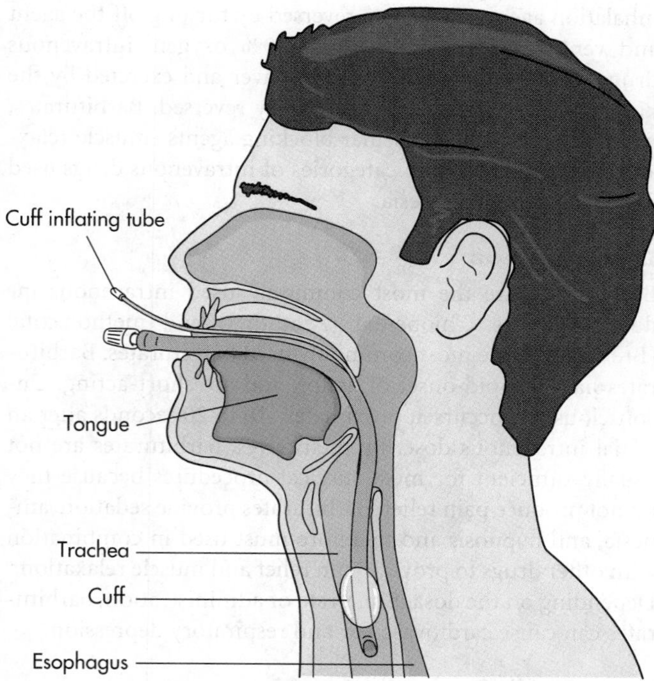


**fig. 19-5** Endotracheal tube in position.

The endotracheal tube may have a balloon that is inflated after insertion; the balloon fills the tracheal space, lessening the chance of aspiration of gastric contents. Regardless of the skill of the anesthesiologist, an endotracheal tube may cause some irritation to the trachea and subsequent edema. It is not uncommon for the patient to complain postoperatively of a sore, irritated throat. Some of the more common inhalation anesthetics in use are described in Table 19-5.

Several measures are used during inhalation anesthesia to promote the safety of both patient and health care workers. Oxygen is administered throughout the procedure, and a method of continuous analysis of the percentage of oxygen in the patient's bloodstream is used. A pulse oximeter is the recommended standard equipment to provide this analysis. A scavenging method for waste anesthetics (carbon dioxide absorber) must be used to avoid unnecessary exposure to health care personnel. In addition, breathing circuits, masks, endotracheal tubes, and reservoir bags are all disposable, providing a clean circuit for each patient, thus avoiding potential cross-contamination.

# INTRAVENOUS ANESTHETIC AGENTS

Intravenous drugs are also used to achieve a safe, reversible state of anesthesia. Patients usually prefer an intravenous anesthesia induction because it is rapid and generally pleasant. Because of patient satisfaction it has become a routine practice to induce general anesthesia with intravenous agents regardless of the agent used for maintenance.

Drugs used for intravenous anesthesia can be used alone as anesthetics or as supplements to inhalation agents. Unlike inhalation agents, which are reversed by turning off the agent and ventilating the lungs with 100% oxygen, intravenous drugs must be metabolized by the liver and excreted by the kidneys. These agents are not quickly reversed. Barbiturates, narcotics, and neuromuscular blocking agents (muscle relaxants) are the three main categories of intravenous drugs used for intravenous anesthesia.

### Barbiturates

Barbiturates are the most commonly used intravenous induction agents. Thiopental (Pentothal) and methohexital (Brevital) are the most commonly used barbiturates. Barbiturates have a rapid onset of action and are short-acting. Unconsciousness occurs approximately 10 to 20 seconds after an initial intravenous dose. By themselves, barbiturates are not usually sufficient for most surgical procedures because they do not produce pain relief. Barbiturates provide sedation, amnesia, and hypnosis and therefore must used in combination with other drugs to provide pain relief and muscle relaxation.[8] Depending on the dosage and rate of administration, barbiturates can cause cardiovascular and respiratory depression.

### Phencyclidine

Ketamine, a phencyclidine derivative, is used to produce a state of dissociative anesthesia. Dissociative anesthesia produces unconsciousness, analgesia, and amnesia. Patients who receive ketamine appear to be awake because the eyes remain open and move, but patients lack awareness and are anesthetized to pain. In the immediate postoperative period patients have been known to experience unpleasant dreams and hallucinations, a condition termed *emergence delirium.* Valium or droperidol can be given to minimize these effects. Having the patient recover in an area of minimum sensory stimulation may also help minimize these effects.

Ketamine can be used as the sole agent for minor surgical procedures that do not require muscle relaxation, or it can be used as an induction agent. Ketamine increases the heart rate and blood pressure and therefore is contraindicated in patients with coronary artery disease or angina.

### Narcotics

Narcotics provide analgesia and sedation and can be used in high doses to provide anesthesia for short surgical procedures. Fentanyl (Sublimaze), meperidine (Demerol), and morphine sulfate are the narcotics commonly used for general anesthesia. The drugs are administered either in bolus doses or by continuous intravenous infusion. The narcotics do not produce muscle relaxation; in fact they may cause an increase in muscle tone. Neuromuscular blocking agents are used intraoperatively to counteract this action.[8]

Postoperatively, patients who receive high-dose narcotic anesthesia are susceptible to respiratory depression. Patients may hypoventilate and become hypoxic; therefore careful monitoring of vital signs is necessary in the postoperative period. Narcotic-induced respiratory depression can be reversed with the administration of a narcotic antagonist such as naloxone (Narcan).

### Neuromuscular Blocking Agents

Neuromuscular blocking agents are used as adjuncts to anesthetic agents. The major action of the neuromuscular blocking agents is the relaxation of voluntary muscles. These agents are used to facilitate the passage of endotracheal tubes, prevent laryngospasm, control muscle tone throughout the surgical procedure, and decrease the amount of general anesthesia used. Neuromuscular blocking agents interfere with the transfer of impulses from the motor nerves to the voluntary muscle cells.

The two categories of neuromuscular blocking agents are depolarizing and nondepolarizing agents. Depolarizing agents react with receptors at the end plate region of the muscle and begin depolarization of the muscle membrane, which causes muscle contraction.[8] The muscle contraction is uncoordinated and is referred to as muscle fasciculation. Postoperatively patients may complain of muscle stiffness and soreness resulting from muscle fasciculation. Succinylcholine is a depolarizing agent. This drug causes muscle relaxation within 1 minute of intravenous administration and is most commonly used for endotracheal intubation.

Nondepolarizing agents cause paralysis of the voluntary muscles, are slower acting, and have a longer duration than depolarizing agents. These agents can interact with other drugs such as antibiotics and lead to a prolonged muscle relaxation. This reaction occurs more commonly with the intravenous administration of antibiotics. (See Table 19-5.)

## BALANCED ANESTHESIA

Balanced anesthesia is one of the most commonly used methods of anesthesia administration. Balanced anesthesia is the practice of combining various agents to produce hypnosis, analgesia, and muscle relaxation with a minimum of physiological disturbances. Each agent is administered for a specific purpose. Intravenous barbiturates are used for induction, regional anesthetics are used for muscle relaxation and analgesia, and inhalation agents are used for maintenance. Variations of this technique are used depending on the patient's physical status and the requirements of the surgical procedure.

## REGIONAL ANESTHESIA

Regional anesthesia causes a temporary loss of sensation in a particular portion of the body from the action of local anesthetics. Local anesthetics temporarily prevent generation and conduction of nerve impulses and may or may not affect motor functions. Local anesthetics do not cause unconsciousness.

Regional anesthetics are used with patients in whom general anesthesia is contraindicated. The advantages and disadvantages of its use are outlined in Table 19-6. The types of regional anesthesia are spinal anesthesia, epidural anesthesia, nerve blocks, and intravenous regional anesthesia.

### Spinal Anesthesia

Spinal anesthesia is usually administered for surgical procedures performed on the lower abdomen, inguinal region, perineum, or lower extremities. With the patient lying on one

**table 19-6** *Advantages and Disadvantages of Regional Anesthesia*

| ADVANTAGES | DISADVANTAGES |
| --- | --- |
| Simplicity<br>Reasonable cost<br>Easily induced<br>Minimum equipment required<br>↓ Postoperative care requirements<br>Fewer systemic effects on body functions | Lack of patient acceptance—patient's fear of being awake during the surgical procedure |
| Avoidance of adverse effects of general anesthesia<br>↓ nausea and vomiting | Impracticality of anesthetizing certain areas of the body |
| Can be used for a variety of patients in circumstances where general anesthesia is contraindicated | Insufficient duration of anesthesia—patient's fear anesthetic will wear off prematurely |
| | Rapid absorption of agent into circulation can lead to cardiac arrest |

side curled into a fetal position or in a sitting position, a local anesthetic agent is injected into the cerebrospinal fluid in the subarachnoid space (Figure 19-6). After the injection of the local anesthetic there is an almost immediate onset of anesthesia at the site.

The duration and level of spinal anesthesia are determined by the site and speed of injection, body height or length of the vertebral column, specific gravity of the anesthetic agent, intraabdominal pressure, and position of the patient immediately following injection.[8] Patient position is extremely important when using hyperbaric agents (agents with a specific gravity heavier than that of the spinal fluid), because gravity moves the anesthetic agents to the lowest point of the vertebral column. Altering the position of the patient causes the hyperbaric agent to be directed up, down, or to a particular side of the spinal cord.[20]

One of the most common postoperative complaints of patients who have spinal anesthesia is headache. The headache occurs because cerebrospinal fluid leaks out of the dura from the opening made by the spinal needle. This leads to a decreased pressure within the spinal cord, which causes the headache when the patient assumes an upright position. Treatment modalities include strict bedrest for 24 to 48 hours, hydration, and application of an abdominal binder to increase pressure.

Recently anesthesiologists have begun using spinal needles that have a sharp point that resembles a sharpened pencil with a hole in the side instead of blunt-bevel spinal needles. Use of this type of needle appears to decrease the occurrence and severity of postspinal headaches. It is postulated that the needle separates the dural fibers instead of cutting them with the blunt-bevel needle.[20]

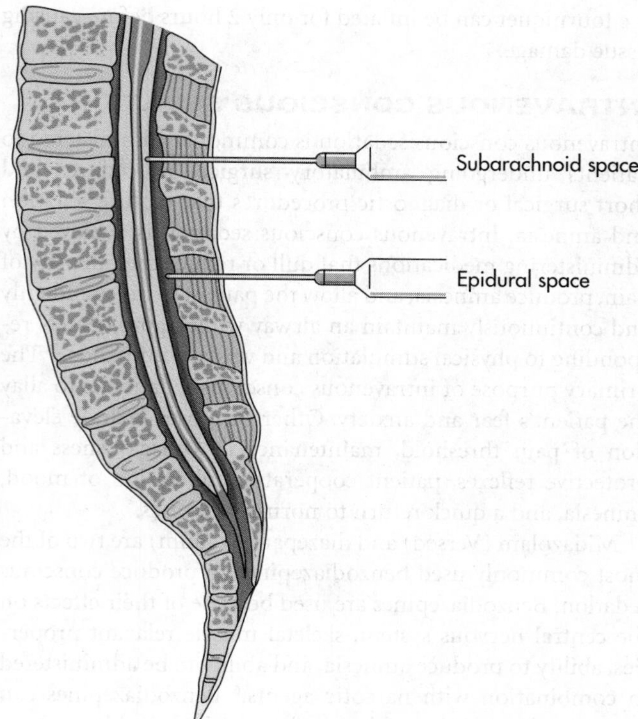


**fig. 19-6** Agent is injected into subarachnoidd space for spinal anesthesia or into epidural space for epidural anesthesia.

### Epidural Anesthesia

Epidural anesthesia is achieved when a local anesthetic agent is injected through the intervertebral space into the space surrounding the dura mater in the spinal column. This type of anesthesia is used in abdominal procedures and orthopedic procedures. In comparison with spinal anesthesia, epidural anesthesia requires greater doses of local anesthetics, has a slower onset of anesthesia, and is not dependent on the patient's position for the level of anesthesia.[20] A distinct advantage of epidural over spinal anesthesia is the absence of postoperative headaches.

### Nerve Block

A nerve block is achieved with the injection of a local anesthetic into or around a nerve or group of nerves that innervates the operative site. Nerve blocks are used to interfere with sensory, motor, or sympathetic transmissions. Onset and length of the block depend on the amount and concentration of the anesthetic. Besides intraoperative use, nerve blocks are also used to relieve chronic pain.

### Intravenous Regional Anesthesia

Intravenous regional anesthesia is achieved by administering local anesthetic agents into the venous system of an exsanguinated extremity. A tourniquet is used to prevent the agent from entering the systemic circulation. Advantages of this technique are a quick onset of anesthesia and a short recovery time. The major disadvantage of this technique is that the tourniquet can be inflated for only 2 hours before causing tissue damage.

## INTRAVENOUS CONSCIOUS SEDATION

Intravenous conscious sedation is commonly administered to patients undergoing ambulatory surgical procedures and short surgical or diagnostic procedures that require sedation and amnesia. Intravenous conscious sedation is achieved by administering medications that dull or reduce the intensity of pain, produce amnesia, and allow the patient to independently and continuously maintain an airway while appropriately responding to physical stimulation and verbal commands.[25] The primary purpose of intravenous conscious sedation is to allay the patient's fear and anxiety. Other purposes include elevation of pain threshold, maintenance of consciousness and protective reflexes, patient cooperation, alteration of mood, amnesia, and a quick return to normal activities.[6]

Midazolam (Versed) and diazepam (Valium) are two of the most commonly used benzodiazepines to produce conscious sedation. Benzodiazepines are used because of their effects on the central nervous system, skeletal muscle relaxant properties, ability to produce amnesia, and ability to be administered in combination with narcotic agents.[6] Benzodiazepines can cause respiratory depression and alterations in blood pressure, heart rate, and heart rhythm. Monitoring parameters for patients receiving intravenous conscious sedation include respiratory rate, oxygen saturation, blood pressure, heart rate and rhythm, level of consciousness, and skin condition.

Narcotics such as fentanyl, meperidine, and morphine are also used for analgesia, sedation, and pain relief. These agents are commonly used in combination with benzodiazepines to achieve intravenous conscious sedation. When narcotics and benzodiazepines are used together, the doses of each agent are decreased to control sedation and respiratory depression.[32]

## MONITORED ANESTHESIA CARE

Some patients undergoing surgical procedures are not ideal candidates for general anesthesia. The surgical procedure can be performed under local anesthesia with a member of the anesthesia team present to monitor the patient's vital signs, respiratory status, and cardiac status and administer oxygen as needed. This type of anesthesia is known as *monitored anesthesia care (MAC)*. Besides monitoring the patient's physical status, the anesthesia provider can administer intravenous analgesics, sedatives, or amnestic agents as necessary for patient comfort. Monitored anesthesia care with conscious sedation has become a popular method of providing anesthesia for patients undergoing minor surgical procedures that do not require muscle relaxation.

## OTHER TYPES OF ANESTHESIA

*Induced hypothermia* may be used as an adjunct to other anesthetic agents. Hypothermia refers to the reduction of body temperature below normal to reduce oxygen and metabolic requirements. Extracorporeal cooling, a method of bloodstream cooling, consists of removing the blood from a major vessel, circulating it through coils immersed in a refrigerant, and returning it to the body through another vessel. Bloodstream cooling is the fastest method for producing hypothermia and is used primarily for patients undergoing open-heart surgery and brain surgery.

## MONITORING THE PATIENT

During any surgical procedure the patient is subjected to many stresses. Potent anesthetic agents, tissue trauma, blood loss, and positioning are all stressors that can interfere with and alter the patient's respiratory and cardiovascular status. Continuous monitoring and assessment are necessary to detect changes in the patient's physiological status and to initiate necessary treatment in a timely manner.

Basic intraoperative monitoring standards have been developed by the American Society of Anesthesiologists to be followed by anesthesia personnel. The Association of Operating Room Nurses has also developed recommended practices to provide guidelines for nurses who monitor patients receiving local anesthetics or intravenous conscious sedation. Both organizations have determined that the basic standards include performing electrocardiograms (ECGs); monitoring blood pressure, heart rate, and temperature; and continuous monitoring of ventilation, circulation, and level of consciousness. Both invasive and noninvasive methods are used for monitoring the patient. Automatic devices are also used to assist in the monitoring processes (Table 19-7). It is imperative that the anesthesiologist and nurse be familiar with the functions and uses of the specialized equipment and ensure that it is in proper working order. Even with the availability of automatic monitoring equipment it is necessary for the anesthesiologist or nurse to remain in close contact with the patient to immediately observe any significant physiological changes.

## ANESTHESIA COMPLICATIONS

The anesthetic-related operative mortality rate is relatively low. For a healthy person the risk is about 0.01%. Some of the more common complications of anesthesia are related to untoward reactions to the anesthetic agent. The major complication is cardiac arrest. Laryngospasm and inhalation of gastric contents are serious potential complications that may occur during the emergence or induction phase of general anesthesia. The perioperative nurse's role is to remain at the patient's side during the induction and emergence phase of anesthesia. In addition to providing emotional support to the patient, the nurse is able to assist the anesthesia team during these critical phases of anesthesia.

During the procedure, monitoring of the anesthetized patient's vital functions is primarily the responsibility of the anesthesiologist. Throughout the surgical procedure the circulating nurse assists in patient monitoring by estimating and reporting blood loss, measuring urine output, and assessing the patient's overall status. In emergent situations, the circulating nurse provides assistance to the anesthesia team. Some less critical complications may occur, such as shivering during the reversal stage in the OR, and extra warmth is provided before the patient is transferred to the PACU. Common postoperative complications and interventions used to prevent or treat them are discussed in Chapter 20.

Both general and regional anesthesia cause a dilation of peripheral blood vessels and a drop in blood pressure. Venous

**table 19-7** *Patient Monitoring Methods during Anesthesia*

| PARAMETER | METHODS |
|---|---|
| Arterial blood pressure | Auscultation method using blood pressure cuff and stethoscope<br>Direct measurement with arterial cannulation and connection to pressure transducer (arterial line)<br>Automatic device that measures systolic, diastolic, and mean blood pressure and heart rate |
| Heart rate | Palpation of superficial artery<br>Auscultation of the heart with a precordial or esophageal stethoscope<br>Doppler monitoring probe applied to radial pulse<br>Electrocardiogram with continual display |
| Respiratory status | Direct observation of chest movements<br>Auscultation of the chest with a stethoscope or esophageal stethoscope |
| Body temperature | Skin surface probes or strips applied to body to monitor surface temperature<br>Core temperature probe inserted into nasophyarynx, esophagus, bladder, or rectum* |
| Urinary output | Indwelling urinary catheter |
| Pulse oximetry | Noninvasive measurement of arterial oxyhemoglobin saturation ($SaO_2$) |
| Capnography—end-tidal carbon dioxide ($E_TCO_2$) | Noninvasive measurement of end-tidal concentration of carbon dioxide<br>Detects changes in respiratory, circulatory, or metabolic status<br>Useful to detect onset of inadvertent hypothermia, malignant hyperthermia, and anesthesia equipment problems |

*Note that core temperature is best measured via esophageal or pulmonary artery probes. Bladder and rectal temperatures are not universally accepted as a true measurement of core temperature.

blood pools in dependent areas, reducing blood return to the heart and lungs for oxygenation and redistribution. General anesthesia depresses the medulla, which maintains cardiac output and peripheral vascular constriction. Muscle relaxants reduce the milking action of normal muscles that assists in venous return. Spinal or epidural anesthesia blocks autonomic output, causing vasodilation and venous pooling. Peripheral vascular injury can occur with occlusion of the vessels. The anesthesiologist constantly monitors the patient and is prepared to compensate for complications of these changes when they occur. The perioperative nurse, knowledgeable about anesthesia methods, patient risk factors, complications, and preventive interventions, is able to provide efficient and appropriate assistance to the anesthesiology team members.

## MALIGNANT HYPERTHERMIA

Malignant hyperthermia (MH), first identified in the 1960s, is a serious and potentially fatal complication of general anesthesia. Even though MH occurs most commonly during induction or during the surgical procedure, it can occur in the PACU or on the nursing unit 24 to 72 hours postoperatively. Malignant hyperthermia can also recur 24 to 72 hours postoperatively.

Malignant hyperthermia is a genetic autosomal dominant defect of the musculoskeletal system that is caused by a disorder of muscle metabolism. It is triggered by certain anesthetic agents (Box 19-4) and extreme physiological and emotional stress. A genetic defect in the muscle cell membrane permits anesthetic agents to trigger a sudden increase of calcium ions within the muscle cells. The rapid increase of calcium starts a series of biochemical reactions that elevate the metabolic rate, causing hyperthermia (with temperatures rising to 43° C), muscle rigidity, respiratory and metabolic acidosis, and cell breakdown.[22]

**box 19-4** *Anesthetic Agents Triggering Malignant Hyperthermia*

**INHALATION AGENTS**
Halothane
Enflurane
Isoflurane
Desflurane

**NEUROMUSCULAR BLOCKING AGENT**
Succinylcholine

**NONDEPOLARIZING MUSCLE RELAXANT**
Tubocurarine chloride

Diagnostic findings include hypercalcemia, metabolic and respiratory acidosis, hyperkalemia, hypermagnesemia, and elevated serum creatine phosphokinase (CPK).

Jaw spasms or fasciculations following the administration of succinylcholine during induction should alert the anesthesiologist to the potential for an MH episode. The earliest and most consistent clinical sign of MH is unexplained ventricular dysrhythmia, specifically tachycardia or premature ventricular contractions, which is associated with an increase in end-tidal carbon dioxide. Other clinical symptoms include tachypnea, cyanosis, dysrhythmias, skin mottling, unstable blood pressure, elevated levels of CPK, and elevated levels of myoglobin.[11] As a result of desaturation, blood at the surgical field may appear dark. Because it occurs in the late stages, an elevated temperature is not a reliable indicator of MH. Other late clinical manifestations of MH include hyperkalemia, acute renal failure, left-sided heart failure, disseminated intravascular coagulation (DIC), pulmonary embolus, and neurological deficits.[8]

Treatment of the patient experiencing MH includes immediate cessation of the inhalation agent or muscle relaxant, administration of 100% oxygen, cooling with ice packs or cooling blankets, lavaging body cavities with iced saline, restoration of acid-base balance, and rapid intravenous infusion of dantrolene. Dantrolene is the only known treatment able to stop an MH crisis. Dantrolene provides skeletal muscle relaxation and retards the biochemical actions that cause muscle contractions. The initial dosage is 2.5 mg/kg of body weight; 10 mg/kg is the recommended maximum dose.[22]

Identification of patients at risk is the primary method for prevention of MH. The preoperative history should include an assessment of the patient's previous experience with surgery, unexplained complications or death of family members who had anesthesia, or known muscular abnormalities. The CPK level may also be elevated, but this is not specific to MH because elevations may also occur as a result of alcoholism or muscle disease. A history of heatstroke in the patient or family is also significant. The key assessment finding in identifying those at risk for MH is unexplained death under general anesthesia. Diagnosis is confirmed by preoperative muscle biopsy. Patients identified at risk for developing MH may be given dantrolene preoperatively as prophylaxis. Anesthetic agents known to trigger MH should not be administered. Family members of individuals with known MH should undergo diagnostic testing as a prophylactic measure.

### INADVERTENT HYPOTHERMIA

Inadvertent hypothermia, a drop in core temperature to 35° C (96° F), is classified as mild, moderate, or severe. Below 20° C (68° F) brain activity ceases. Inadvertent hypothermia occurs in 40% to 70% of surgical patients and is associated with such adverse effects as shivering, decreased drug metabolism, coagulopathy, increased catecholamine production, and postoperative myocardial infarction.[15] Because ischemic cardiac mortality is the number one cause of perioperative death, it is critical to prevent hypothermia and hence cold-induced myocardial ischemia.[15] Anesthesia inhibits the reflexes that generate heat and decreases the thermoregulatory center in the hypothalamus, decreases the basal metabolic rate, and increases vasodilation. In the OR the body may lose core heat by exposure to a cool environment, by skin preparation with cool solutions, and via the surgical incision. Preoperative sedation, the length of the procedure, and blood and fluid losses add to the heat loss. Inadvertent hypothermia may result in cardiac dysrhythmias, metabolic acidosis, hyperglycemia, and coma. Symptoms may not be evident until the postoperative period and include shivering, speech impairment, cyanosis, decreased blood pressure, weak pulse, and dilated pupils. Shivering occurs as result of some anesthetic agents and as a hypothalamic response to a drop in core temperature. Untreated shivering can lead to increased $O_2$ consumption (as much as 400%), increased cardiac workload, and hypoxia. Inadvertent hypothermia should not be confused with induced hypothermia, a special anesthetic technique used during cardiac, neurosurgical, and transplant surgery.

## PHYSIOLOGICAL STRESS RESPONSES TO SURGERY AND ANESTHESIA

Surgery and anesthesia affect all body systems. The organ systems are interdependent, and when one system is affected, to a certain extent all the systems are affected. A thorough understanding of how the various organ systems can be affected by anesthesia and surgery is essential to establish a scientific basis for intraoperative caregiving by the health care team.

### NEUROENDOCRINE RESPONSES

Neuroendocrine responses play a major role in the reaction of a patient to the stress of surgery. The responses include stimulation of the autonomic nervous system (primarily the sympathetic nervous system) and stimulation of selected hormones (primarily aldosterone and glucocorticoid hormones from the adrenal cortex and antidiuretic hormone from the posterior pituitary). Table 19-8 summarizes the effects of endocrine changes on the patient.

Stimulation of the sympathetic nervous system serves to protect the body from further damage. Vasoconstriction of peripheral blood vessels enables the body to compensate for blood loss and redirect blood flow to critical areas such as the heart and brain. Increased cardiac output also helps maintain blood flow. Severe trauma or excessive blood loss, however, will overwhelm the compensatory mechanisms, and blood pressure will fall. Certain types of anesthetics or high spinal anesthesia also may interfere with the compensatory vasoconstriction, producing hypotension.

One aspect of the sympathetic response that may produce undesirable effects is the decrease in gastrointestinal activity. Psychological stress in the preoperative period may lead to anorexia and constipation. After the trauma of surgery, the patient may experience anorexia, gas pains, and constipation from diminished peristalsis in the gastrointestinal tract. Peristalsis may cease completely after abdominal surgery involving manipulation of abdominal organs.

Adrenocortical activity is increased in response to the trauma of surgery, producing greater amounts of aldosterone and cortisol. Aldosterone enhances sodium reabsorption by the kidney. This serves to retain fluid to compensate for fluid lost through blood loss, diaphoresis, and respirations. When sodium is reabsorbed by the kidneys, potassium is excreted; thus after surgery there is a loss of potassium.

In addition to the increase in aldosterone secretion, there is also an increase in antidiuretic hormone (ADH) by the posterior pituitary gland during the first 24 to 48 hours after surgery. Water is reabsorbed by the kidney, and renal output is decreased. After surgery the increased production of aldosterone and ADH is evidenced by a decreased urinary output as compared with fluid intake. Spontaneous diuresis occurs as the amount of ADH is decreased, usually in about 24 to 48 hours.

The increase in the amount of glucocorticoid from the adrenal cortex is thought to mobilize cellular stores of fats and amino acids for energy and protein synthesis. Healing tissues

**table 19-8** *Effects of Endocrine Changes Associated with Surgery*

| PHYSIOLOGICAL CHANGES | RESULTS | OBSERVED EFFECT |
|---|---|---|
| ↑ Norepinephrine secretion | Peripheral vasoconstriction | Helps maintain blood pressure when circulating volume is decreased |
| | ↓ Gastrointestinal activity | May lead to anorexia or constipation |
| ↑ Aldosterone secretion | Sodium retention | Maintains circulating blood volume<br>Increases susceptibility to fluid overload<br>Decreases urinary output |
| ↑ Glucocorticoid secretion | Gluconeogenesis | Provides energy to meet stress of surgery |
| | ↑ Protein catabolism | Provides an additional energy source |
| | Ketogenic effect | Provides amino acids for cell synthesis after tissue destruction |
| | Antiinflammatory effect | Provides fat as an energy source |
| | ↑ Platelet production | Increases susceptibility to infection<br>Promotes clotting to prevent bleeding<br>Contributes to development of thrombophlebitis |
| ↑ Antidiuretic hormone (ADH) secretion | Water reabsorption in the kidney tubules | Maintains circulating blood volume<br>Increases susceptibility to fluid overload<br>Decreases urinary output |

require protein. Glucose is released for energy, with resultant hyperglycemia and glycosuria. Patients who have diabetes must be carefully monitored for signs of ketosis.

## METABOLIC RESPONSES

After surgery the patient is in a relative state of starvation; metabolism is increased, and nutrient intake is decreased. Carbohydrate metabolism increases as a result of the increased production of glucocorticoid hormones. With major surgery, there are periods when the patient is not permitted to eat and receives only intravenous fluids. Commonly used fluids such as lactated Ringer's solution, dextrose, and normal saline are not adequate to meet the body's energy needs. Anorexia also may occur as part of the stress response, thus adding to the problem of inadequate carbohydrate intake even if food is permitted by mouth. The body must supply its glucose needs by the breakdown of stored liver glycogen or by the synthesis of glucose from noncarbohydrate sources.

Fat metabolism increases to allow the mobilization of fat from the cells so that it is available as an energy source. With the decreased intake of carbohydrates and fats after surgery, body fats are metabolized for energy and the patient loses weight.

Protein metabolism is increased after surgery to supply essential amino acids necessary for tissue healing. Body proteins consist of combinations of amino acids, of which nitrogen is an essential component. When tissues break down during catabolism after surgery, some of the nitrogen is lost. As new tissue is formed, essential amino acids are needed. If none of these amino acids is taken in, the body will continue to break down existing tissue proteins to obtain the amino acids that it needs for healing. The "leftover" amino acids not used at that time are broken down to nitrogen end products such as urea and are excreted. A negative nitrogen balance results; nitrogen loss exceeds nitrogen intake.

**box 19-5** *Examples of Medical Supplies Containing Latex*

- Adhesive tape
- Airways
  - Nasal
  - Oral
- Breathing bags
- Breathing circuits
- Bulb syringes
- Catheters
  - Foley
  - Straight
  - Central venous
  - Pulmonary artery
- Elastic bandages
- Electrode pads
- Fluid warming blankets
- Gloves
- IV ports
- Rubber stoppers on multidose vials
- Stethoscope tubing
- Ventilator bags
- Syringe plungers
- Wound drains

## OTHER CONSIDERATIONS

### LATEX ALLERGY

There has been increasing interest among health care workers about the effects of using medical products that contain latex (Box 19-5). The number of individuals who have developed sensitivities to latex has increased during the 1990s.[9] Among health care workers the incidence of latex allergy is 7% to 10% compared with the general population with an estimated incidence of 1%.[21]

Surgical gloves and many of the supplies used in the perioperative area contain latex, which can cause an allergic response in latex-sensitive individuals. The allergic response can be life threatening; therefore it is essential for perioperative nurses to be able to deal with patients and other health care workers who develop sensitivity to latex.

### Natural Rubber Latex

Natural rubber latex originates from the white milky sap of the *hevea brasilinesis* plant, more commonly known as the rubber tree. During the refinement process many accelerators, antioxidants, emulsifiers, stabilizers, extenders, colorants, retardants, ultraviolet light absorbers, and fragrances are added to the sap. The resulting product contains 2% to 3% latex protein.[28]

### Reactions to Latex

There are two types of reactions to latex products. Type I sensitivity produces an immediate reaction and is the most serious form of hypersensitivity. Type IV sensitivity produces a delayed response and is the most common form of hypersensitivity (Table 19-9).

Type I reactions are systemic in nature. Immunoglobulin E (IgE) antibodies are produced in response to the latex allergen. The IgE binds onto receptors on mast cells and basophils. Subsequent exposure to the latex protein causes mast cell proliferation, the release of basophil histamine, and subsequent anaphylaxis. The reactions occur suddenly and range from a skin flare response to wheezing and bronchospasm.[26]

In contrast, there is no antibody formation with a type IV reaction. Macrophages and T lymphocytes are activated in response to the allergen. Activation of the T lymphocytes and macrophages causes tissue inflammation and contact dermatitis. The onset of the reaction is slow and usually requires hours of contact before the appearance of symptoms. The reaction is localized to the area of contact. Type IV reactions are responses to substances used in the manufacturing process and are associated with wearing latex gloves and are therefore not considered latex allergies.[26]

**table 19-9** *Reactions to Latex Products*

| Type I Reactions | Type IV Reactions |
|---|---|
| IgE activated (antibody formation) | T cell activated (no antibody formation) |
| Systemic responses<br>Cutaneous → flushing, diaphoresis, pruritus<br>Gastrointestinal → nausea, vomiting, cramping, diarrhea<br>Cardiovascular → hypotension, tachycardia, dysrhythmias<br>Respiratory → dyspnea, bronchospasm, laryngeal edema | Localized responses<br>Symptoms resolve in 72 to 96 hours<br>Individual remains sensitized and will react with every contact |
| Rapid onset of reactions<br>Immediate response | Delayed onset of reactions<br>Primary reaction occurs within 18 to 24 hours<br>Subsequent reactions can develop sooner |
| Can be life threatening | Causes discomfort but is not life threatening |

### Routes of Exposure

Five routes of exposure to the latex protein can cause severe reactions in latex-sensitized individuals. *Cutaneous* exposure to medical supplies such as anesthesia masks, tourniquets, ECG electrodes, adhesive tape, fluid warming blankets, and elastic bandages can trigger reactions in susceptible patients.

Many of the severe reactions to exposure to latex have occurred as a result of the latex protein coming in contact with the *mucous membranes* of the mouth, vagina, urethra, or rectum. Oral mucosal reactions have occurred in response to the products used in dentistry, as well as to other medical products such as nasogastric tubes. Serious reactions have also been reported as a result of latex exposure to the vaginal mucosa during examinations, sexual intercourse, deliveries, and abortions. Although contact of rectal mucosa with examination gloves, enema kits, and rectal pressure catheters has precipitated reactions, the most severe mucous membrane reactions have occurred as a result of latex exposure to the rectal mucosa with catheters used with barium enemas.[26]

*Inhalation* of the latex proteins also causes severe reactions. Inhalation reactions have been most commonly associated with anesthesia equipment and endotracheal tubes; however, exposure to the latex protein through the aerosolization of glove powder has also been reported. In this circumstance the latex protein binds to the powder used in the gloves. When the gloves are removed from the box or from the hands, the powder is aerosolized and the particles dissipate onto surgical drapes and sponges. The aerosolization increases the risk of exposure for all sensitized individuals.[21]

During the surgical procedure *internal tissue* absorbs the latex protein. A reaction is triggered when internal organs come in contact with surgical gloves and other products such as irrigation syringes, instruments, and catheters used throughout the surgical procedure.

The *intravascular* administration of latex proteins is not well understood. It is postulated that reactions occur from the use of disposable syringes, medications stored in vials with latex plugs, and intravenous tubing that has latex ports.[26]

### Individuals at Risk for Developing Latex Allergy

A number of groups of individuals are at risk for developing a latex allergy (see the Research Box). Individuals at greatest risk are those with neural tube defects. This patient population undergoes multiple surgeries, uses rubber catheters for urinary or bowel programs, and has multiple exposures to latex

**research**

Reference: Steelman VM: Latex allergy precautions: a research-based protocol, *Nurs Clin North Am* 30(3):475, 1995.

A thorough review of research was conducted to determine if significant research was available to develop perioperative practice protocols for patients at risk for a latex reaction. A review of several case reports was also completed to provide information on latex reactions that occurred in clinical settings. Based on the literature and case reviews the determination was made to develop perioperative protocols for latex allergy precautions. A multidisciplinary protocol was developed to direct changes in practice.

The protocol defines patients in high-risk groups for developing latex reactions. These groups are defined as individuals with neural tube defects, congenital urological conditions, positive latex allergy testing, or a history of systemic reactions to latex. The protocol states that during the preoperative assessment each patient is questioned about responses to latex. If any of these conditions is present, latex allergy precautions are started.

The author reports positive patient outcomes as a result of the protocol and supports utilization of research for the development of future patient care protocols.

gloves in daily care. Other at-risk populations include individuals who have urinary conditions requiring continuous or intermittent catheterization; a history of allergies and asthma; a history of reactions to latex products; a history of multiple surgical procedures, especially bowel procedures; food allergies to bananas, avocados, tropical fruits, kiwis, potatoes, and chestnuts (possible cross reaction between the food and the latex allergens); and daily exposure to latex products (individuals working in the medical and dental profession).[21,28]

### Intraoperative Patient Management

A thorough history must be obtained preoperatively to provide safe intraoperative patient care for individuals who are identified as at high risk for a systemic reaction to latex. Once the patient has been identified as having a latex allergy, the information must be documented and relayed to all other health care workers who provide care. The patient and the patient's family should be assured that the team is aware of the latex allergy. The perioperative plan of care that addresses protective measures needs to be explained to the patient and the patient's family members.

Intraoperatively, the circulating nurse ensures that latex-free products are substituted for routine medical equipment. Only latex-free surgical gloves are used. The anesthesia team ensures that the breathing circuit, face mask, and ventilator bag are latex free. Rubber stoppers are removed from vials, and medications are drawn directly from multidose vials. Glass syringes are used to draw medications. Medications are injected through three-way stopcocks instead of through rubber ports. Latex-free tape is used when applying the dressing.

**box 19-6 Perioperative Gerontological Considerations**

- Chronic medical conditions negatively influence morbidity and mortality rates in the elderly population.
- Medication history is especially important because of possible drug interactions and difficulties in anesthetic management.
- Cardiac, vascular, intrathoracic, and intraabdominal procedures pose the most risk for patients over age 80 years with concomitant systemic illness who undergo emergent surgical intervention.
- Elderly patients with a history of hypertension, diabetes, and tobacco use should be monitored for silent myocardial ischemia.
- Geriatric patients are more prone to problems with fluid volume deficit or excess and hypoxia that is due to age-related changes in homeostatic mechanisms.
- Age-related changes in baroreceptor functioning, which are essential for homeostasis, are important factors to consider when the patient is under anesthesia. The elderly surgical patient may not be able to react sufficiently to changes such as hypovolemia, hypoxia, hypercarbia, and hypotension.
- Age-related changes in the kidney and liver result in decreased drug clearance. Dosage of anesthetic agents should be adjusted accordingly.

Adapted from Kelly M: Surgery, anesthesia, and the geriatric patient, *Geriatr Nurs* 16(5):213, 1995.

## GERONTOLOGICAL CONSIDERATIONS

By the year 2020, an estimated one in six Americans will be classified as elderly.[17] The increase in life expectancy necessitates a greater need for health care services and treatment alternatives for the geriatric patient.

Geriatric patients may have multiple chronic health problems that affect recovery from surgical intervention. Morbidity associated with geriatric surgical patients is due to preexisting medical problems. The mortality rate for patients 65 years of age and over undergoing elective surgical procedures is estimated to be 2% to 10%.[14] Geriatric patients generally experience a decline in organ functions and altered reactions to pain, temperature, and medications. The perioperative nurse needs to understand the effects of aging and chronic disease on the outcome of surgery for the geriatric patient. This knowledge allows the nurse to use the nursing process to ensure safe patient care throughout the perioperative experience.

### Intraoperative Considerations

To meet the special care needs of the geriatric patient the circulating nurse takes into account the patient's risk for inadvertent hypothermia during the intraoperative period, the potential complications related to intraoperative positioning, the risk for thrombus formation, and the need for strict monitoring of vital signs. See Box 19-6 for perioperative gerontological considerations.

### Hypothermia

Body temperature is regulated in the anterior hypothalamus. Cutaneous thermoreceptors detect alterations in ambient temperatures and signal the anterior hypothalamus. The sensors in the anterior hypothalamus monitor the temperature of cerebral blood flow. The difference between those temperatures and a set point determined by the hypothalamus triggers the heat-generating response. This response is influenced by age, exercise, medications, and anesthetics.[29]

In the geriatric patient, the shivering response to cold is less sensitive than that of the younger patient. A slower metabolic rate, decreased cardiovascular reserve, thinning of skin, loss of subcutaneous tissue, and diminished muscle mass affect the geriatric patient's ability to produce and conserve body heat. The stress of surgery and anesthesia also suppresses the heat-producing responses in elderly patients. Intraoperative routines, environmental factors, and anesthesia-related factors can also affect perioperative thermoregulation in the geriatric patient (Box 19-7).

The patient is assessed for the risk for developing hypothermia, including assessment of his or her physiological status and body size. Knowledge of the extent of the surgical procedure along with the type of anesthesia planned assists the circulating nurse to formulate a plan of patient care that will decrease intraoperative body heat loss. Increasing the temperature in the OR; covering the patient with warm blankets; warming anesthetic gases, intravenous fluids, and irrigation solutions; warming skin preparation fluids; covering the patient's head; and limiting exposure of body surface are measures that can be taken to prevent inadvertent hypothermia in the elderly patient.

### Positioning

The potential for postoperative skin problems presents a significant risk for the geriatric patient. Decrease of adipose tissue, poor skin turgor, decreased peripheral circulation, and tissue fragility can cause postoperative skin problems. Arthritis, deceased range of motion, and skin fragility make patient positioning one of the most important aspects of intraoperative patient care. Besides causing skin problems, improper positioning can also cause joint pain unrelated to the surgical procedure.

Patients should be lifted into position rather than pulled or slid to avoid skin damage. The patient's limbs should be placed in neutral position to prevent joint strain or fracture. The circulating nurse uses padding and support devices to protect pressure points and bony prominences and to compensate for musculoskeletal deformities of the spine, neck, or extremities. If possible, the circulating nurse modifies the patient's position to improve tissue perfusion to pressure areas.

**box 19-7** *Factors Affecting Perioperative Thermoregulation in Geriatric Patients*

**SURGICAL PROCEDURE RELATED**

Intravenous infusion of cool solutions
Irrigation of incision sites with cool solutions
Lengthy surgical procedures
Surgical procedures involving large body surfaces or open cavities

**INTRAOPERATIVE ENVIRONMENT RELATED**

Cool air temperature in the operating room
Air currents related to air exchanges within the operating room

**ANESTHESIA RELATED**

Inhalation of cool nonhumidified gaseous agents

### Antiembolic measures

Geriatric patients experience cardiovascular changes, increased resistance to peripheral blood flow, and decreased cardiac output.[29] Slowed circulation predisposes the geriatric patient to thrombus and embolus formation. Measures to decrease this risk include use of antiembolic stockings and sequential compression devices.

### Monitoring

Geriatric patients can experience a decrease in renal function, which affects fluid and electrolyte balance and the excretion of medications. Fluid loss is not tolerated well; hypovolemia progresses rapidly in geriatric patients. Fluid loss and urinary output must be closely monitored intraoperatively. Measures to maintain fluid balance are implemented as appropriate. Utilization of invasive monitoring is determined by the patient's physical status and the type of surgical procedure. Pulse oximetry is used to determine oxygenation in peripheral circulation. However, severe vascular disease or hypothermia may obliterate the signal in geriatric patients. End-tidal capnometry is also used to monitor patient oxygenation. Temperature is closely monitored to prevent problems with thermoregulation. Reactions to anesthetic agents are monitored by the anesthesia provider. Alterations in heart rate and rhythm are immediately addressed to prevent cardiac crisis.

## Anesthesia Considerations

Geriatric patients require special consideration when undergoing anesthesia. The normal aging process causes a variety of physiological changes that affect the geriatric patient's response to anesthesia. The patient's response to anesthesia may be unpredictable and significant. Extensive perioperative anesthesia management is essential to monitor the geriatric patient to produce successful outcomes.

The geriatric patient is more susceptible to the action of medications. Decreased liver and kidney function and reduced cardiac output affect the metabolism and excretion of drugs from the body. Therefore geriatric patients require lower doses of anesthetic agents and take longer to eliminate them.

The choice of anesthetic is determined by the patient's preexisting medical conditions, the type and length of the surgical procedure to be performed, and the preference of the anesthesia care provider. Geriatric patients are candidates for general anesthesia, regional anesthesia, intravenous sedation, or local anesthesia. Evidence suggests that geriatric patients undergoing local anesthesia have a better prognosis than those undergoing general or regional anesthesia.[1] Anecdotes relating alterations in cognitive functions following general anesthesia have led to a belief that there is a greater risk of postoperative mental dysfunction in geriatric patients who undergo general anesthesia. Research has been conducted to analyze the effects of general versus epidural anesthesia on the frequency of long-term cognitive dysfunction and cardiac complications on elderly patients following total knee surgery. Results of the study indicate that the type of anesthesia has no effect on the extent or pattern of cognitive dysfunction or the occurrence of significant cardiovascular complications in the group of geriatric patients undergoing total knee replacement surgery.[24] Other studies have also shown that general anesthesia poses no more risks than regional anesthesia to the long-term cognitive function in geriatric patients.[31]

Respiratory problems are found in 10% to 40% of geriatric patients.[14] The presence of pulmonary disease or pulmonary insufficiency causes ventilatory difficulties. The anesthesia care provider relies not only on a physical assessment of the patient's respiratory system but also on the preoperative chest x-ray to plan appropriate perioperative ventilatory support for the geriatric patient.

Alterations in the airway of elderly patients also cause ventilatory difficulties. Loss of teeth and alterations in jaw contours can cause an inadequate fit of the anesthesia mask. Decreased range of motion in the jaw, head, and neck presents difficulties for intubation.

Surgical mortality is greater in the geriatric patient population than the general population. Mortality rates for elderly trauma patients are considerably higher than those of younger patients with similar injuries.[16] Diminished physiological reserves, preexisting medical conditions, and the physical stress caused by anesthesia and surgical intervention pose increased risk. Thorough preoperative assessment and planning along with careful anesthesia management can decrease the rate of morbidity in the geriatric patient.

# NURSING MANAGEMENT

The unique nature of the intraoperative environment creates an inevitable focus on the many technical activities required to facilitate the surgical procedure and maintain patient safety. However, the perioperative nurse is also responsible for meeting the patient's psychosocial needs.

Several factors have an impact when considering the nurse-patient relationship during the operative phase. The operative phase of the perioperative experience is short, and the patient may be sedated or unconscious most of the time. The nurse has a great deal of impact on the patient in a short period of time. The experience is almost universally stressful for all patients. Using Orlando's theory, the perioperative nurse would focus on the patient's needs.[23] The nurse can clarify the patient's concerns and, together with the patient, formulate a plan of care. This approach may be well suited to the operative environment, given the brevity of the relationship. Allowing patients to participate as much as possible in their perioperative care may improve the quality of care. Patients generally view the surgical experience as anxiety producing. Interventions perceived as "good" by patients include human-oriented actions, such as touch, presence, the use of humor, comfort, support, empathy, and respect for human dignity. Patients deserve humane, kind, and professional actions from the perioperative staff.[13] Explanations of procedures and events are critical, because patients may not know what questions to ask. These types of interventions may allow a sense of security and effective coping, thereby making the operative experience a positive one.

Nursing practice in the operating room includes assessment, as well as planning, implementing, and evaluating nursing activities to meet individual needs of patients who require a surgical intervention.

## ASSESSMENT

When patients are admitted to the OR suite, the perioperative nurse must assess the patient's physical and emotional status, paying particular attention to any factors that would increase surgical risk. A preoperative interview should take place on the patient's arrival to the OR admission suite. Astute interviewing skills and communication of a caring attitude are important for a thorough assessment of both physical and emotional status of the patient.

### Subjective and Objective Data

Preoperative data should include an assessment of the physiological and psychosocial health status. Psychosocial assessment should include the patient's family or significant other.

The patient is typically brought to the holding area by transport personnel. The circulating nurse will meet the patient in the holding area and review the chart and preoperative checklist. The perioperative nurse assesses and verifies the patient's physical and psychological readiness for surgery (Table 19-10).

A thorough preoperative assessment will reveal risk factors for fluid volume deficit in patients, which include trauma, preexisting bleeding disorders, the presence of fluid deficit, recent intake of anticoagulant medications, impaired renal function, and age (the very young and elderly persons are subject to fluid imbalances more readily because of immature or impaired body functions). A deficit in fluid volume occurs more commonly in patients who are receiving nothing by mouth, who have intraoperative blood and body fluid losses, who have age-associated decreases in total body water and plasma volumes, or who experience neuroendocrine responses to surgery and anesthesia. Hypovolemia usually occurs when intraoperative bleeding is not controlled and can result in hypovolemic shock.

Risk factors for fluid volume excess include a rapid intake of fluid or sodium, the presence of chronic renal failure or congestive heart failure, neuroendocrine responses to surgery and anesthesia, and corticosteroid therapy (results in sodium retention). Excess intake of intravenous fluid causes hypervolemia and can result in congestive heart failure and edema.

**table 19-10** *Perioperative Assessment Data*

| Assessment | Examples |
|---|---|
| Identify patient | Patient statement<br>Identification bracelet |
| Verify procedure, site, surgeon | Patient statement<br>Consent form<br>Surgeon statement |
| Assess vital signs | Temperature, pulse, respiration, blood pressure, pulse oximetry |
| Review allergy and medication history | Medication, food, topical allergies<br>Possible medication interactions with anesthesia, anticoagulant use aspirin, nonsteroidal antiinflammatory, steroid use |
| Mobility, functional status | Range of motion, loss of body parts, contractures, deformities |
| Skin integrity | Rashes, previous incisions, pressure ulcers, lesions, bruising |
| Sensory status | Hearing, vision, speech, tactile deficits |
| Presence of prostheses, implants | Dentures, pacemakers, joints, lens implants |
| Nutritional status | Nothing-by-mouth status, height, weight, skin turgor |
| Cardiovascular status | Electrocardiogram report, apical pulse, patient history |
| Renal status | Urinalysis, intake and output, creatinine, blood urea nitrogen |
| Respiratory status | Color, lung sounds, respiratory rate |
| Review laboratory findings | Abnormalities in complete blood count, electrolytes, chest x-ray, special diagnostics<br>Blood availability autologous or banked |
| Mental status | Orientation, anxiety, support system available, coping methods |
| Religious, philosophical beliefs | Religious preferences, wish for chaplain, do-not-resuscitate status, advance directives<br>Blood transfusions, treatments |
| Cultural beliefs | Family members present, dominant language, alternative therapies |
| Outcome of treatment | Patient's perception of outcomes |

During the immediate preoperative interview, the nurse is able to identify patients at risk for potential problems due to positioning. Influencing factors that may potentiate complications from positioning include preexisting conditions such as arthritis, diabetes, thin body build, immunosuppressed status, preexisting pressure ulcers, obesity, nerve dysfunction, age (very young or elderly persons), decreased muscle tone, compromised cardiopulmonary status, and malnutrition.

After a review of the information accumulated during the immediate preoperative assessment, the nurse formulates nursing diagnoses, expected patient outcomes, and an intraoperative plan of care. Assessment continues during the patient's transfer to the OR, positioning on the OR table, and induction of anesthesia, and during and immediately after the surgical procedure.

## NURSING DIAGNOSES

Nursing diagnoses provide guides for the nursing activities of the perioperative nurse immediately before, during, and after surgical procedures. The nursing diagnoses discussed in this chapter focus on high-incidence problem areas for patients during a surgical intervention.

Nursing diagnoses for the patient in the intraoperative phase of surgery may include but are not limited to:

| Diagnostic Title | Possible Etiological Factors |
|---|---|
| Anxiety, risk for elevated | Unfamiliar environment, fear of impending surgery/anesthesia, intraoperative diagnosis |
| Perioperative positioning Injury, risk for | Immobility, improper positioning, obesity or emaciation, elderly, edema |
| Injury (trauma), risk for | Misidentification, neuromuscular damage, burns from chemical or electrical hazards, physical hazards, retention of foreign objects |
| Infection, risk for postoperative wound | Excessive body cavity exposure, decreased body defense mechanisms, break in aseptic technique, preoperative health status of patient |
| Thermoregulation, ineffective (risk for alteration in normothermia) | Cool operative environment, of anesthetics, prolonged exposure, cool solutions, elderly |
| Fluid volume deficit, risk for | Rapid loss of blood/body fluid during the surgical procedure, stress of surgical intervention, anticoagulant therapy, trauma, preexisting disorders (e.g., bleeding disorders), elderly |
| Fluid volume excess, risk for | Rapid intake of excessive fluid or sodium, stress of surgical intervention, corticosteroid therapy, preexisting conditions (e.g., Cushing's syndrome, congestive heart failure), elderly |

## EXPECTED PATIENT OUTCOMES

Expected patient outcomes for the patient in the intraoperative phase of surgery may include but are not limited to:

1. Shows little or moderate subjective or objective evidence of anxiety
2. Remains free of signs of skin and tissue injury beyond 24 to 48 hours after the procedure
3. Remains free from injury or trauma related to electrical, chemical, and physical factors

4. Remains free of postoperative wound infection
5. Is at or near normothermia at the end of the immediate postoperative period[2]
6, 7. Maintains adequate fluid volume

## INTERVENTIONS

Having identified the patient's specific needs and formulated nursing diagnoses, the nurse must collaborate with other members of the health care team to implement the plan for patient care during the intraoperative phase of the surgical experience. As discussed previously, anesthesia and all the components of the surgical experience place great stress on the body and may result in postoperative complications for the patient. The major focus of nursing intervention during this period is maintenance of patient safety and prevention of postoperative complications.

### Patient/Family Education

The patient and family should be instructed about perioperative routines on arrival in the OR suite. Although this information was covered in a teaching session (location will vary depending on circumstances), reinforcement is beneficial, because of the anxiety the patient may be experiencing. Anticipating both the patient's and family's questions will help allay their concerns. The family should be told where to wait and the anticipated length of events. During the procedure and recovery period, phone reports of the patient's progress can be given to the family.

### Minimizing Anxiety

Most patients experience some anxiety when facing a surgical intervention. As discussed in Chapter 18, an important part of preoperative nursing intervention is helping the patient cope with anxiety. Anxiety may be due to preconceived ideas and fears related to the surgical experience, illness, and hospitalization. Perioperative events such as the disclosure of possible complications, anesthesia, intraoperative diagnosis, or postoperative pain may trigger an increase in anxiety level immediately before surgery.

The perioperative nurse usually can identify anticipatory anxiety in the patient on admission to the operative suite because the patient is likely to exhibit signs of anxiety when the surgery is imminent. Interventions at this time focus on providing support by gentle physical contact, maintenance of personal dignity, a quiet and unhurried surgical environment, attentiveness to the needs of the patient, and provision of comfort accessories such as a warm blanket or pillow. In addition, providing information about the environment and what to expect before performing a nursing action decreases the patient's fear of the unfamiliar environment. Soothing words and an empathic attitude help promote a nurturing atmosphere in the OR's high-technology environment. Despite the tremendous technological advances made in surgery and nursing, patient needs for personal contact, help to cope with anxiety, and explanations of procedures remain constant.[12] Patient-centered care remains the focus of the perioperative nurse. By communicating an overall attitude of caring and providing physiological and emotional support, nurses can make a noticeable difference in a patient's preoperative emotional state. The successful use of methods to reduce anxiety can significantly enhance the effectiveness of preoperative medications, permit a reduction in dosage, or even eliminate the need for them. During the induction phase of anesthesia, provision of physical security, maintenance of personal dignity, and close, constant attendance by the perioperative nurse are necessary activities that help minimize the patient's fears and thereby facilitate the induction of anesthesia.

### Minimizing Risks for Injury to Skin and Tissues

A breakdown in skin integrity may occur from improper positioning. Prolonged pressure on the bony prominences, pressure on the peripheral nervous or vascular systems, or shearing force of sheets and drapes during patient movement may be responsible for areas of skin breakdown. Irritation or burning from solutions used in skin preparations, as well as burning from misuse of electrical equipment, also can result in postoperative skin breakdown.

#### *Patient positioning*

The patient may be placed in a variety of positions for the surgical procedure. Each has its own unique risks for the patient. Figure 19-7 illustrates common surgical positions and indicates the associated pressure points. The perioperative nurse must understand the basic components of safe positioning and participate in the teamwork necessary to assess, plan, implement, and evaluate the care necessary to keep the patient free from injury and trauma resulting from complications of positioning. A thorough knowledge of the physiological consequences of positioning, patient limitations, positioning equipment, and procedures is necessary to facilitate coordination among all members of the health care team.

Anesthetic agents increase the risks associated with positioning because of their effects on body systems. Physiological changes during positioning affect the respiratory, circulatory, nervous, skeletal, and integumentary systems. Coupled with the effects of anesthesia and surgery on body systems, positioning can become a potential great danger for all surgical patients.

The respiratory system is influenced greatly by positioning. The respiratory system is most vulnerable in the prone and the lithotomy positions. The thoracic cage normally expands in all directions except posteriorly. In these positions there is mechanical restriction of lung expansion at the ribs or sternum and the reduced ability of the diaphragm to push down against abdominal muscles. Respiratory function is impaired because of interference with normal movements. Lung tissue compliance is decreased, thereby reducing the volume of air that can be inspired for rapid exchange. In addition, a change in position alters the pulmonary capillary blood flow volume, thereby affecting the amount of blood available for oxygenation.

Several changes in the cardiovascular system that occur with positioning also may result in complications. Pressure or

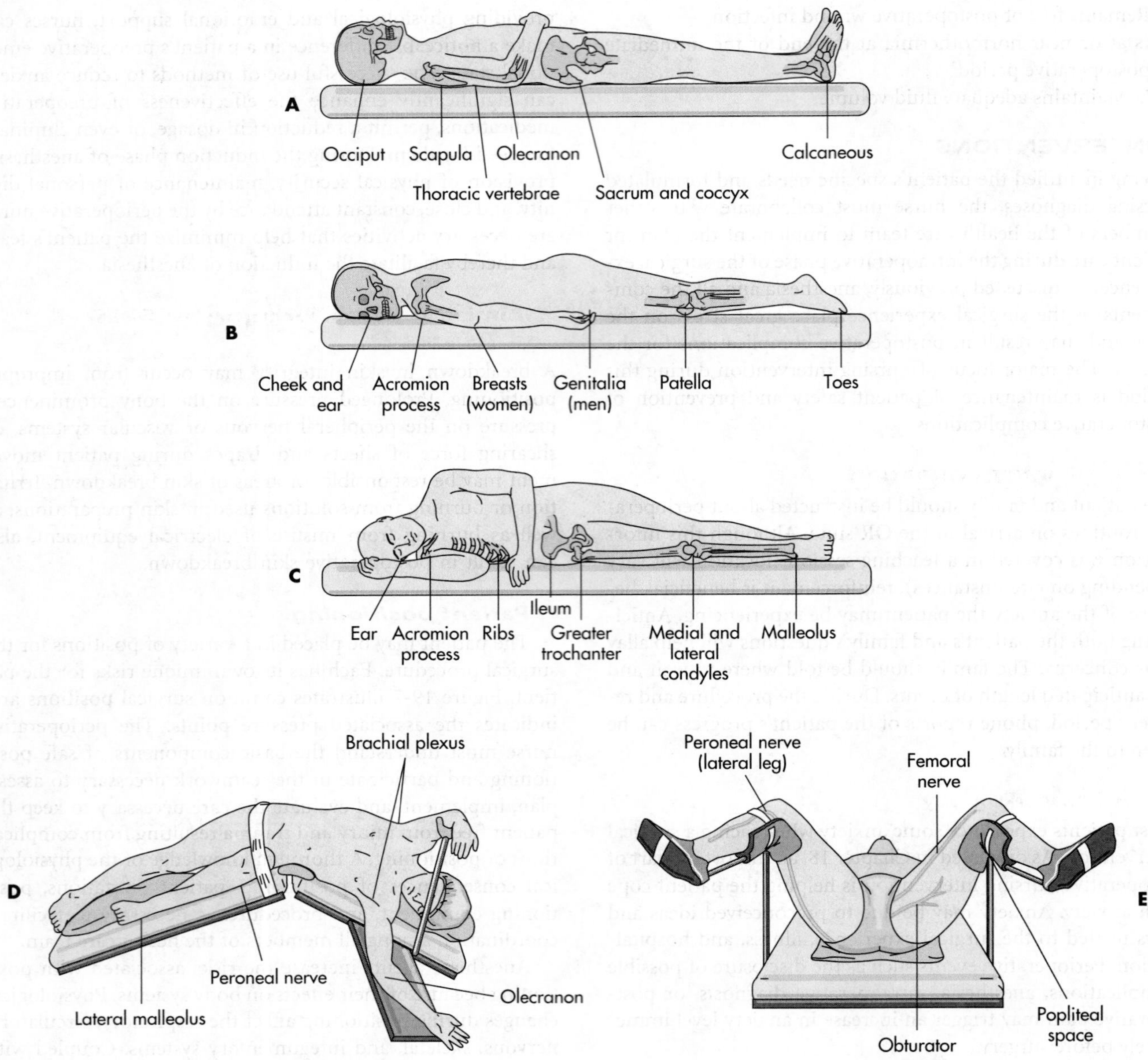


**fig. 19-7** Examples of common surgical positions and their associated potential pressure points. **A,** Supine (dorsal recumbent) position. **B,** Prone postion. **C,** Lateral position. **D,** Lateral (kidney) position. **E,** Lithotomy position.

obstruction of a vessel, or both, causes the greatest amount of damage to the cardiovascular system. A tight restraint, crossed legs, or limb hyperextension can compromise blood flow by compression of a vessel against a bony structure. The volume of blood returned to the heart and lungs can be reduced, affecting oxygenation and distribution of oxygenated blood. Rapid movements during changes in positioning may cause sudden hypotension. An example of this occurs when legs are lowered quickly from the lithotomy position. The lithotomy position also may lead to circulatory pooling in the lumbar region and compression of abdominal contents on the inferior vena cava and abdominal aorta. In both situations, there is a decrease in venous return, which affects cardiac output.

Most of the problems associated with the neurological system are not discovered until recovery from anesthesia is complete. Postoperative sedation may mask symptoms of peripheral nerve damage for days. Most postoperative neuropathies result from an inappropriate position on the operating table. Damage to peripheral nerves usually is the result of direct mechanical pressure. Ischemia and insufficient blood supply caused by stretching or compression are chief factors in nerve injuries. The lithotomy position is especially likely to cause injury to the saphenous and common peroneal nerves. These in-

**table 19-11** *Commonly Used Operative Patient Positions*

| Description | Comments |
|---|---|
| **SUPINE** | |
| Flat on back with arms at side, palms down, legs straight with feet slightly separated | Most commonly used position; venous pooling in the legs may result from a reduction of venous pressure |
| **PRONE** | |
| Patient lies on abdomen with face turned to one side, arms at sides with palms pronated, elbows slightly flexed; feet elevated on pillow to prevent plantar flexion | Patient is anesthetized in supine position and then placed prone; respiratory excursion is decreased; risk for injury to facial nerve, genitalia, and breasts |
| **TRENDELENBURG** | |
| Patient supine; head and body are lowered into a head-down position; knees are flexed by "breaking" table | Respiratory excursion is decreased from upward movement of abdominal viscera; cerebral edema or venous thrombosis may occur because of congestion of the cerebral vessels |
| **LITHOTOMY** | |
| Patient lies on back with buttocks to edge of table; thighs and legs are placed in stirrups simultaneously to prevent muscle injury; head and arms are secured to prevent injury | Elastic wraps or antiembolic stockings may be used on legs to prevent thrombus formation; risk for vein compression in legs, increased intraabdominal pressure, injury to obturator and femoral nerves because of flexion of thighs; injury to common peroneal nerve caused by fibular neck resting against stirrups; risk for acute hypotension when legs are lowered |
| **LATERAL** | |
| Patient lies on side; table may be bent in middle | Risk for injury to dependent brachial plexus and dependent common peroneal nerve, pressure sore development over the dependent greater trochanter of femur; potential interference with cardiac action because of possible shift in heart position |

juries result from either misplaced stirrups or acute flexion of the thighs. In all positions in which the arms are extended on armboards, hyperextension of the arms may cause damage to the brachial plexus.

Positioning injuries may be temporary and resolve within 48 hours or develop into stage IV pressure ulcers. Preserving the integumentary system is a major nursing responsibility in the operating room. Poor positioning can result in the development of pressure ulcers. Tissue perfusion is a critical factor in the prevention of pressure sores. Compression of vessels, external pressure, uneven body weight distribution, and constant pressure on bony prominences can result in pressure sores.

Gravity, which forces patients against the hard surface of the OR bed, compresses skin, muscle, and bone and increases capillary interface pressures. Normal capillary interface pressure is 23 to 32 mm Hg. Pressures in excess of normal can alter tissue perfusion and cause ischemia.[18] Persons with peripheral vascular disease or paralysis may be affected by pressures lower than normal. Pressure injuries commonly occur over bony prominences, such as the occiput, spine, scapulae, coccyx, sacrum, or calcaneous, or in deep tissues. Commonly used operative patient positions are described in Table 19-11.

Many interventions can be initiated to minimize the complications in patient positioning. Distribution of body weight should be as even as possible, and the patient should be maintained in correct alignment.

Positioning devices come in a wide variety of shapes, styles, and materials. Some examples include foam pads and mattresses, face guards, sand bags, bean bags, air mattresses, gel pads, frames, and rolls. The perioperative nurse selects the appropriate device based on the procedure and individual patient. The device chosen should maintain the desired intraoperative position and minimize the potential for injury by redistributing pressure and preventing excessive stretching.[18] To reduce pressure, the device must have the documented ability to reduce capillary interface pressure to 32 mm Hg or less.[18] Ideally, the device should be durable, nonallergenic, radiolucent, easily stored, resistant to moisture and microorganisms, able to be disinfected or disposed, and cost-effective.[18]

Positioning of extremities must not exceed a 90-degree angle to the body. Bony prominences such as heels, elbows, and sacrum are vulnerable pressure points and should be well padded. The safety strap should be applied 2 inches above the knees to avoid pressure on the popliteal nerve. Compression of the popliteal nerve from stirrups or knee braces also should be avoided. Surgical equipment, such as pneumatic saws and drills and retractors, placed directly on the patient may lead to pressure injuries. The circulating nurse monitors members of the team at the field to ensure that they do not lean on the patient during the procedure. Antiembolic stockings or intermittent pneumatic compression devices should be used to decrease venous pooling in the lower extremities. Changing positions gradually is important to prevent drastic shifts in blood volume from one area of the body to another. Foam-filled cushions can be used to maintain adequate respiratory excursion and to prevent pressure on the chest, breasts, genitalia, and abdominal structures. Guidelines related to patient positioning are summarized in the Guidelines for Care Box.

A detailed procedure for each surgical position should be written and available for OR personnel who are responsible for or assist with positioning of patients. Detailed documentation by the perioperative nurse should include the type of position, any changes in positioning made intraoperatively, placement of extremities, type and placement of positioning aids and supplemental padding, and the site of placement of the electrosurgical conduction pad.

### *Electrical, chemical, and physical hazards*

Many perioperative nursing activities are focused on the protection of the patient from electrical, chemical, and physical hazards. The use of electricity introduces hazards of electric shock, power failure, and fire to patients. Faulty wiring, inadequately maintained equipment, and a lack of regard for precautionary measures can cause a spark, resulting in a fire. If a voltage exists between any two electrical conductors touching the patient, the flow of current can result in electric shock or electrocution. If the voltage is high enough, ventricular fibrillation and sudden death may result. The OR is an area containing many potentially life-threatening and mechanically injurious situations related to electrical shock, burn, fire, and explosions. It is imperative that all members of the surgical health care team have current knowledge of the equipment and supplies most often involved in such incidents. The most significant hazards are inadequately trained personnel, malfunctioning equipment as a result of improper maintenance, inappropriate design of OR suites, and inappropriate surveillance by team members.

Federal regulations govern the marketing and safety standards of electronic devices used in ORs, and the Joint Commission on Accreditation of Healthcare Organizations also has standards that must be met. When electrical equipment is in use, hazards can be minimized or prevented by the following perioperative nursing interventions:

**guidelines for care**

**Preventing Complications of Surgical Positioning**

Maintain patient in correct alignment, and distribute body weight equally.

Pad all bony prominences well with foam-filled cushions, gel pads, or full-length flotation mattresses as needed.

Use antiembolic hose and intermittent pneumatic compression devices to decrease venous pooling.

Change patient positions gradually to avoid drastic shifts in blood volume.

Avoid local compression from safety straps, knee braces, stirrups, equipment, or personnel.

Position extremities at no more than a 90-degree angle to the body.

- Use only electrical equipment designed for OR use.
- Use cords of adequate length.
- Ground the patient correctly.
- Test equipment before use.
- Establish and follow sound clinical engineering testing and maintenance programs.
- Participate in inservice sessions for new equipment, and maintain an adequate knowledge base for correct use of all electrical equipment.
- Verify that correct attachments for a piece of equipment are being used.
- Report faulty equipment immediately.
- Maintain humidity levels at 50% or higher to minimize static electricity.
- Prevent the pooling of fluids under the patient.

Laser technology is an effective treatment modality; however, it presents hazards for patients and members of the surgical team. *Laser* is an acronym for light amplification by stimulated emission of radiation. When the high-powered beams of light are directed into tissue, the resultant intense heat vaporizes the tissue and causes a rapid coagulation of blood vessels.

When lasers are used, special equipment is necessary to protect both the patient and surgical team members. Eye protection specific to the type of laser (argon, carbon dioxide, etc.) is used to prevent retinal damage from misdirected beams of light. If aberrant light beams land on surgical drapes, they can cause fire. Improperly functioning surgical instruments can deflect light to other tissue. Measures such as the use of coated instruments, wet towels on the field, smoke evacuation methods, and warning signs on the door of the operative suite are routinely taken to protect the patient and OR team members.

Chemical hazards in the operating room include exposure to solutions used for cleaning, cementing bone, gas sterilization of instruments, and skin preparation. Iodine and iodophors are bactericidal agents used commonly in skin preparations. These are two of the most effective solutions for preoperative skin scrubbing but are irritants to the skin if the concentration is too high. In addition, alcohol, which sometimes is used in incision site preparation, is flammable. Precautions necessary for prevention of injury from any hazardous chemicals are many. As patient advocates, the nursing personnel must ensure proper labeling to comply with the National Fire Protection Association standards. Safe storage for hazardous chemicals away from immediate patient areas must be provided for and maintained. All personnel must be aware of and follow safe chemical usage recommendations set by the hospital's safety department and the manufacturing company. It is imperative that the perioperative nurse determine or verify any patient allergies that may increase risk of injury from certain solutions intended for use during the surgical procedure. To prevent skin irritation and electrical shock or burn, solutions used for skin preparation should not be allowed to pool under the patient.

It is the responsibility of the perioperative nurse to protect the patient from injury from physical hazards. Prevention of injury includes careful movement during positioning, the use of appropriate positioning methods, and the use of protective devices such as side rails and safety straps. Safe transfer of the patient to or from the operating room bed is accomplished with lift devices or a minimum of four people. Safety can be promoted by ensuring that sufficient support help is obtained for the transfer, that all tubes are visible and protected from inadvertent removal, and that the movement is coordinated among all team members.

To ensure that injury does not occur from misidentification of the patient or the correct operative site, it is mandatory that the perioperative nurse verify the patient's identity and operative site. This should be done verbally (unless not possible), by patient identification band, and by chart documentation. Absolutely no discrepancy should exist between operative consent information and what the patient states. The perioperative nurse must bring any discrepancy or concerns to the attention of the surgeon, anesthesiologist, patient, and when necessary, the hospital administrator. Surgery should not begin until all issues have been resolved.

### Prevention of foreign object retention

Because of the high level of risk to the patient related to foreign object retention in the surgical wound, counting materials used during a surgical procedure is an important intraoperative nursing intervention. Sponges, sharps, and instruments are counted before the procedure, as additional items are added, at initial closure, and finally at skin closure. An additional count is necessary when either the scrub or circulating nurse leaves the case. Policies and procedures must be written with specific guidelines to be followed for the counting of items during each surgical procedure. The surgical count should be performed by both the circulating and scrub nurse.

The AORN recommended practices state that sharps should be counted on all procedures. Sponges and instruments should be counted on procedures in which there is a possibility that such items could be retained.[3] For example, procedures in which a major body cavity is opened or a deep incision is made would necessitate both a sponge and an instrument count.

Sponges and other products have radiopaque markings in the event of an incorrect count, and arrangements are made for an x-ray film to be obtained to confirm the presence or absence of the missing item in the patient. All counts performed are documented and placed in the patient's record. Any corrective action taken in the event of a discrepancy and the resultant outcome are also recorded.

## Minimizing Risks for Postoperative Wound Infection

All patients who undergo surgery have the potential to acquire an infection. Surgical intervention breaks down some of the body's primary defenses against infection. Infection can have a negative effect on the outcome of surgery and can even endanger the life of a patient. Protecting the patient from infection is a major goal of intraoperative nursing interventions. The goal of nursing interventions is to control the number and types of microorganisms present during surgery. Many of the activities that are directed toward achieving this goal are related to monitoring and controlling the environment. The most important measure in preventing postoperative wound infection is adherence to meticulous aseptic technique principles and to the CDC's two-tiered system. The entire surgical team has a responsibility to uphold principles of aseptic technique and follow the policies and procedures established to ensure that the surgical suite is protected from unnecessary risks resulting from increases in microbial population.

Creating and maintaining the sterile field is the responsibility of the perioperative nurse. The standards and recommended practices for perioperative nursing provide guidelines in areas related to the maintenance of a sterile field. These areas include basic aseptic technique, traffic patterns in the surgical suite, environmental controls, OR attire, sterilization, barrier materials, surgical hand scrub, and preoperative skin preparation of patients. Throughout the surgical procedure, the perioperative nurse monitors adherence to aseptic technique principles by all surgical team members and ensures that breaks in technique are corrected.

The CDC recommends the classification of surgical wounds to predict the probability of postoperative infection. The circulating nurse is responsible for assigning and documenting the classification. Wounds are classified as clean, clean contaminated, contaminated, or dirty (Table 19-12). Documentation of the appropriate wound classification will

**table 19-12 CDC Surgical Wound Classification**

| Classification | Definition | Examples |
|---|---|---|
| Clean wound | Uninfected, primary closure<br>Closed wound drainage system<br>No inflammation present | Total knee arthroplasty<br>Mitral valve replacement<br>Breast biopsy |
| Clean contaminated wound | Respiratory, alimentary, or genitourinary tract entered without spillage<br>No sign of infection, minor break in sterile technique | Total abdominal hysterectomy<br>Radical prostatectomy<br>Pneumonectomy |
| Contaminated wound | Major break in aseptic technique<br>Signs of infection<br>Contamination from gastrointestinal tract<br>Open fresh traumatic wound | Appendectomy for ruptured appendix<br>Laparotomy for perforated bowel |
| Dirty wound | Old trauma with necrotic tissue<br>Preexisting infection<br>Perforated viscera<br>Acute inflammation | Incision and drainage of abscess |

assist the infection control nurse with follow-up planning and nosocomial wound infection reporting.

Because wound infection is a common postoperative complication, much research has been directed toward determining the most effective method of administering prophylactic intravenous antibiotic therapy. Research has shown that despite strict aseptic technique, *Staphylococcus aureus* has been found at surgical sites.[10] These findings support the practice of prophylactic antibiotic therapy as a valuable adjunct to controlling bacterial growth at surgical sites. Antibiotics are chosen based on which microorganisms are most likely to be found at the surgical site. The surgical wound classification described earlier can be helpful in estimating postoperative infection rates and the need for antibiotic therapy. Research regarding the timing of prophylactic antibiotics indicates that they should be administered to patients within 2 hours or at least 30 minutes before incision time to ensure adequate tissue concentration at the surgical site.[10] Antibiotics are most effective when they are present in tissues before bacteria enter the surgical site. Usually, a single dose of antibiotics is necessary for most surgical procedures. However, more research is needed to determine the needs of patients undergoing lengthy surgical procedures. Nursing responsibilities include assessing the patient for drug allergies, administration of the correct drug at the correct time, and monitoring the patient for therapeutic and adverse effects of the drug. Maintaining sterile technique during the venipuncture and fluid administration is also essential to prevent any further sources of infection.

Etiological factors in wound infection and in wound healing are many and may be environmental, host, or pathogenic. (Wound healing is discussed in Chapter 20.) Appropriate closure and drainage of dead space facilitates wound healing. Closure of an incision with minimal trauma is facilitated by placing sutures in close approximation to achieve an anatomically secure wound. Wound edges will not heal readily if not in close contact. A dead space may occur from separation of wound edges or from air trapped between layers of tissue. Serum, blood, or other fluid may accumulate in a dead space and prevent healing.

### Drains

If it is anticipated that fluid may collect in a body area near the wound after surgery, the surgeon usually inserts a tube or drain to permit the fluid to escape. One end of the tube or drain is placed in or near the organ or cavity to be drained, and the other end is passed through the body wall, usually through a separate small incision near the operative site. Drains are usually made of latex or silicone. In some cases, drainage is by gravity through a tube, such as a T tube (Figure 19-8) or Penrose drain. In most cases a self-contained closed suction system is used for wound drainage. Suction drains create a negative pressure in a reservoir. The negative pressure gently suctions fluid from the wound into the attached reservoir. The Hemovac and Jackson-Pratt drains (Figures 19-9 and 19-10) are examples of closed-suction drainage systems. Closed drains also may be attached to wall or portable suction devices for a greater range of suction capacity. The level of suction is based on the amount and area to be evacuated.

Nursing interventions related to drains focus on the preparation of the drainage system components, assessment of patency and drainage, and accurate documentation for postoperative nurses. After the tubing is placed by the surgeon, the sterile connection is attached to the evacuator or suction source using universal adapters and strict aseptic technique. Assessment of the patency of the system and the amount, type, color, and consistency of the drainage is performed. The type and location of drainage and the drainage assessment are thoroughly recorded and included in verbal reporting to the nurse in the postoperative receiving unit.

### Dressings

Protection of incision sites from contamination is a means of minimizing risk for postoperative wound infection. After surgery is completed, a sterile dressing is applied to the

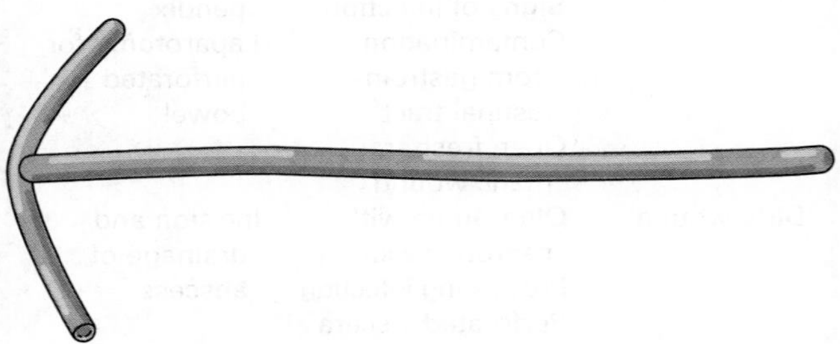

fig. 19-8 T tube drain.

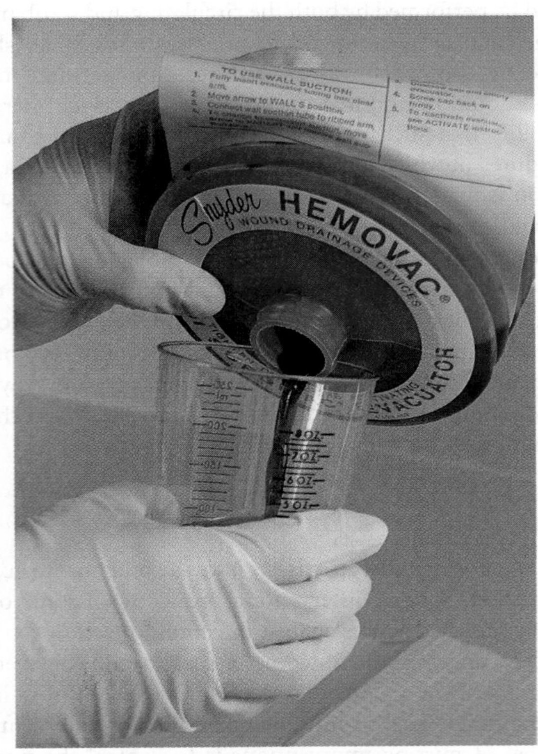


fig. 19-9 Hemovac drain.

wound and secured. Dressings also serve to absorb drainage, protect the incision from trauma, and give support to the incision and surrounding skin. The perioperative nurse is responsible for ensuring dressing security and documenting the condition of the dressing before transfer of the patient to the postoperative unit.

## Minimizing Risk for Alteration in Normothermia

### Hypothermia

Factors that put patients at risk for alterations in body temperature are trauma (because of exposure), advanced age, malnutrition (causes a decrease in metabolism), prolonged preoperative inactivity, and sedation. The greatest heat loss occurs in the first hour of surgery; therefore heat conservation methods should be initiated early by the perioperative nurse.

Prevention is the best treatment of hypothermia. An intervention that can be initiated immediately after admission to the OR is the application of warm blankets. Before surgery begins, the patient should remain covered as much as possible. This necessitates that an ample supply of blankets be available in warming cabinets at all times. Blankets should be warmed to 105° F (40.5° C) and changed every 15 minutes.[8] Another intervention that is used successfully during preoperative preparations is a radiant lamp. The application of thermal coverings, especially a covering for the head, is recommended to reduce radiant heat loss. A plastic head covering will retain the most heat. During surgery the use of an automatic thermal blanket under the patient is a common intervention.

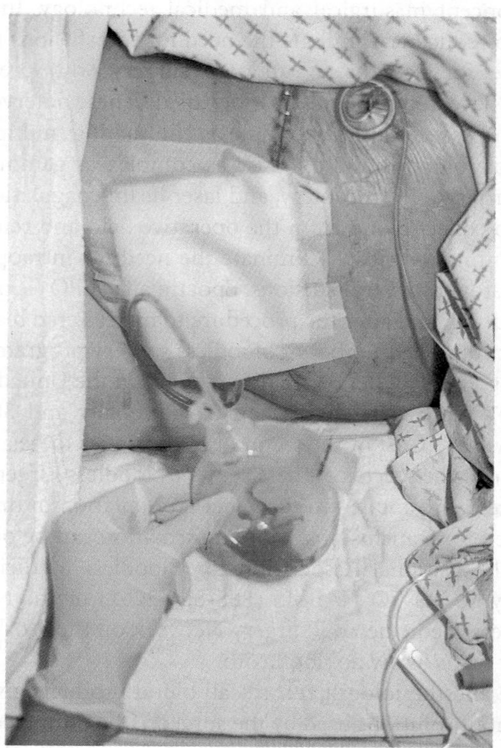

fig. 19-10 Jackson-Pratt drain.

The temperature and humidity of the room should be controlled. The nurse should ensure that the patient's skin is exposed as little as possible during positioning, prepping, and draping. Skin prep solutions can be warmed before use. The nurse should check that the sheets and drapes on and under the patient are dry, both to prevent heat loss and skin irritation and to maintain asepsis. A forced-air warming device (Bair Hugger) is commonly used intraoperatively to conserve body temperature (see the Research Box).

Core body temperature should be monitored throughout the procedure. Sites for measurement of body temperature are chosen based on accessibility, comfort, and safety. Tympanic membrane measurement is considered to be the gold standard for measuring core temperature.[15] Body temperature can also be measured by probes inserted into the esophagus, rectum, or urinary bladder. If the patient is intubated, an esophageal probe may be inserted for continuous temperature monitoring. Temperature probes placed in the distal third of the esophagus are closely correlated with core temperature.[15] Temperatures measured in the mid or proximal esophagus are affected by inhaled gases and are not reliable. Bladder temperature readings are a less reliable indicator of core temperature than esophageal readings but are more reliable than rectal or skin readings. Rectal temperature is a measurement of peripheral temperature and may not accurately reflect the degree of hypothermia present.

During most surgical procedures a large amount of fluid is administered intravenously for replacement and topically for wound irrigation before closure. The perioperative nurse

**research**

Reference: Krenzischek DA et al: Forced-air warming versus routine thermal care and core temperature measurement sites, *J Post Anesth Nurs* 10(2):69, 1995.

This study compared the effectiveness of forced-air warming with conventional methods such as warmed cotton blankets as a means of maintaining core temperature during the intraoperative and postoperative periods. Twenty-nine patients were assigned to two treatment groups: routine thermal care $n = 14$, or forced-air warming $n = 15$. All patients were less than 60 years of age and were undergoing elective vascular, thoracic, or abdominal surgical procedures.

Traditional methods of treating hypothermia consisted of application of warmed cotton blankets. Forced-air convective warming has been shown to increase skin temperature, improve thermal comfort, warm patients rapidly, and reduce the incidence of shivering.

The investigators found that patients treated with forced-air warming experienced less shivering, which resulted in greater patient thermal comfort. Although the sample was small, these findings indicate that it is important to maintain normothermia intraoperatively, which may decrease potential complications and increase patient comfort.

ensures that all fluids presented to the anesthesiologist or added to the surgical field are warm. In the immediate postoperative period, warm blankets are applied as soon as surgical patient drapes are removed. Clonidine may be given to decrease shivering.[8]

### Hyperthermia

Hyperthermia may occur in the surgical patient. Risk factors include dehydration, illness resulting in fever, vasoconstriction from medication, endocrine disorders such as thyroid disease, intracranial infection or injury to the hypothalamus, and a history of malignant hyperthermia.

During surgery, nursing interventions for cooling include removing excessive drapes, applying alcohol or cool water to the patient's skin, assisting with the monitoring of vital signs, use of an automatic cooling blanket, and assisting with the preparation and administration of cool intravenous fluids and emergency medications. A baseline temperature for all patients should be recorded preoperatively. Core body temperature should be monitored throughout the procedure.

As with all nursing interventions, thorough documentation should include all measures taken, equipment used (including serial numbers and temperature settings), and patient responses to treatment. Communication with the postoperative receiving unit is imperative for the continuity of patient care. This is especially important in cases in which an alteration in normothermia resulted in an emergent situation.

## Minimizing Risk for Fluid Volume Deficit or Excess

Intraoperative monitoring of fluid loss and adequate replacement is a responsibility of high priority throughout the procedure for both anesthesiologist and perioperative nurse. The perioperative nurse assists the anesthesiologist in monitoring the patient during surgery. During procedures in which intravenous conscious sedation is used, the perioperative nurse assumes total responsibility for monitoring duties.

The nurse must understand fluid and electrolyte balance, as well as expected patient responses to the parenteral fluids administered. The patient must be monitored for both hypovolemia and hypervolemia. Hypovolemia can result in hypovolemic shock. Excess intake of intravenous fluid causes hypervolemia and can result in congestive heart failure and edema.

The perioperative nurse assists with the preparation and administration of intravenous fluids, ensuring an adequate supply at all times. In addition, the nurse facilitates the preparation and sending of blood specimens to the laboratory. Indwelling urethral catheters are inserted before the start of surgery if the patient is at risk for alteration in normal fluid volume balances, if the surgery is expected to be lengthy, or if the anticipated blood loss may be great. Urine output is recorded hourly. Blood loss is monitored by keeping an accurate record of the fluids administered into the wound, the amount of fluid suctioned from the operative site, and the amount of saturation of all sponges (sponges may be weighed for a thorough estimation). Assessment of the available blood and ordering of additional blood must be performed continuously to remain ahead of anticipated needs.

Blood replacement may be necessary if blood loss exceeds 1200 ml or the hematocrit drops below 30%. Blood or blood products may be transfused to compensate for the loss or to prevent shock. Transfusions may be homologous or autologous. Blood products include fresh frozen plasma, platelets, serum albumin, and blood substitutes. Intraoperatively, blood may be recovered from the field for autotransfusion. Blood can be suctioned from the wound, body cavity, or drapes and sponges. All blood recovery devices must be approved by the Food and Drug Administration. If a microfibrillar collagen has been used for hemostasis, blood may not be salvaged, because of the risk of DIC or adult respiratory distress syndrome (ARDS). Persons with known systemic infections or open trauma are not candidates for autotransfusion.

Three basic systems available for autotransfusions are cell salvage processors, canister collection systems, and salvage collection bags.[8] Operating room personnel must be trained to use these autotransfusion devices. All components of the system must be sterile and disposable. If not used intraoperatively, the blood collected may be processed and bagged for transfusion postoperatively. Alternative methods include salvaging blood from a drainage tube placed in the surgical wound. The blood is anticoagulated and may be collected for a maximum of 6 hours. The red cells are reinfused intravenously.

An alternative exists for patients with objections to receiving blood and blood products. *Bloodless surgery* is a relatively new concept in surgical and medical technology. Interventions to reduce or eliminate the need for transfusions make it possible for patients to undergo surgery who previously would have refused and possibly died. These interventions range from techniques as simple as eliminating multiple preoperative blood draws to those as complex as gamma-knife radiosurgery, electrocautery, and laser beam coagulation. Devices to collect blood from the operative field and reinfuse it in a continuous circuit eliminate the need for intraoperative and postoperative transfusions. Epoetin alfa (EPO) is used before, during, and after the procedure to increase red blood cell production. The number of bloodless surgery programs is increasing. In 1990 there were three centers in the United States; by 1997 there were more than 70 nationally and 30 more worldwide.[30] Cost of the techniques continues to be an issue. Because of the success of these centers, bloodless surgery practices are being applied to the general population to minimize the need for transfusions. More information can be obtained from the National Association for Bloodless Medicine and Surgery at 888-TO-NABMS (888-866-2267) or the National Bloodless Medicine and Surgery Network on the World Wide Web at http://www.noblood.com.

The anesthesiologist records all blood products given, the amount of solutions used by the surgeon, the estimated blood loss, and all intraoperative events concerning fluid imbalances. The perioperative nurse records this information during local procedures when an anesthesiologist is not present. The anesthesiologist and perioperative nurse communicate to the caregiver on the receiving unit collaboratively.

## EVALUATION

Evaluation of perioperative patient care is achieved by comparing the patient's responses to interventions with the expected outcomes. Successful achievement of patient outcomes for the perioperative patient is indicated by:

1. Shows little subjective or objective evidence of anxiety
2. Exhibits intact skin with no discolorations, sensation at preoperative levels
3. Shows no signs of injury or trauma from physical, chemical, or electrical trauma
4. Exhibits no swelling or redness at the incision site
5. Is at or near normothermia

6, 7. Maintains stable vital signs without evidence of hypovolemia or cardiac overload

It is necessary for the perioperative nurse to be astute in assessment techniques to pick up subtle condition changes, as well as obvious ones.

Feedback about postoperative findings from nursing peers on patient care units can supply valuable information for evaluation and should be encouraged. In ambulatory surgery settings, a follow-up telephone call to the patient at home should be made by nursing personnel. This can be useful in obtaining feedback about the nursing care received during the surgical intervention.

## critical thinking QUESTIONS

1 Mrs. G. is an 80-year-old woman scheduled for a hemiarthroplasty for a fractured left hip. On arrival in the holding room Mrs. G.'s oral temperature is 36.1° C. She is oriented to person only. Her past history includes congestive heart failure, chronic obstructive pulmonary disease, and rheumatoid arthritis. What elements of her history will influence her intraoperative management? What nursing interventions should be included in her plan of care to prevent complications?

2 Mr. B. is 17 years old and is scheduled for a right knee arthroscopy and possible anterior cruciate ligament reconstruction. During the immediate preoperative interview, the circulating nurse notes that the patient's perception of the procedure is not congruent with the scheduled surgical procedure and informed consent. What actions by the circulating nurse are appropriate?

3 Ms. K. is scheduled to undergo a diagnostic laparoscopy. She has a documented history of type I allergic response to latex. Devise an intraoperative plan of care for Ms. K.

## chapter SUMMARY

- The intraoperative phase of the surgical experience begins with the patient's arrival in the OR suite and continues until the patient is transferred to the postanesthesia unit.

### TYPES OF SURGERY

- Subspecialties of surgery involve procedures performed in a specific body system or anatomic region.

### THE SURGICAL HEALTH CARE TEAM

- Members of the surgical health care team include the surgeon, surgical assistants, the anesthesiologist or nurse anesthetist, the circulating nurse, the scrub nurse, the RNFA, and other allied support personnel.

### ASEPTIC TECHNIQUE MAINTENANCE

- Postoperative wound infection is a potentially fatal complication. Maintenance of an aseptic environment is a major focus of nursing care during the intraoperative phase.
- Wearing the correct OR attire (scrubs, hair covering, masks) is essential for decreasing the risk of personnel serving as a source of infection.

### ANESTHESIA

- Anesthesia may be general, regional, or local. It is administered by inhalation or by intravenous injection or is localized by regional block or spinal, epidural, or infiltrative means.

### PHYSIOLOGICAL STRESS RESPONSES TO SURGERY AND ANESTHESIA

- An understanding of how the body systems are affected by anesthesia and surgery is essential to establish a scientific basis for intraoperative caregiving by the health care team.

### NURSING MANAGEMENT

- Nursing practice in the OR includes assessment, planning, implementation, and evaluation of nursing activities to meet individual needs of patients requiring a surgical intervention.
- Nursing diagnoses for the intraoperative patient include risk for anxiety, injury resulting from improper positioning, impairment of skin integrity, injury or trauma, postoperative wound infection, alteration in normothermia, and fluid volume deficit or excess.
- Desired patient outcomes include the following: the patient (1) will show little evidence of anxiety, (2) will be free of signs of skin breakdown, (3) will be free from injury and trauma, (4) will be free from signs of postoperative wound infection, (5) will be normothermic, and (6) will maintain adequate fluid volume.
- The perioperative nurse can be instrumental in reducing patient anxiety by providing physiological and emotional support and communicating an overall attitude of caring.
- A major focus of nursing interventions during the intraoperative phase is maintenance of patient safety and prevention of postoperative complications.

## References


1. Alves SL, Deisering LF: Cardiovascular changes associated with aging: the anesthetic implications, *CRNA* 7(1):2, 1996.
2. AORN patient outcomes: standards of patient care, *AORN J* 65(2):408, 1997.
3. AORN recommended practices for sponge, sharp, and instrument counts, *AORN J* 64(4): 616, 1996.
4. AORN recommended practices for maintaining a sterile field, *AORN J* 64(5):817, 1996.
5. AORN recommended practices for skin preparation of patients, *AORN J* 64(5):813, 1996.
6. AORN recommended practices for managing the patient receiving conscious sedation/analgesia, *AORN J* 65(1):129, 1997.

7. Association of Operating Room Nurses, Inc.: *1996 standards and recommended practices,* Denver, Colo, 1996, AORN Publications.
8. Atkinson LJ, Fortunato N: *Berry and Kohn's operating room technique,* ed 8, St Louis, 1996, Mosby.
9. Booth B: Latex allergy: a growing problem in health care, *Prof Nurse* 11(5):316, 1996.
10. Butts JD, Wolford ET: Timing of perioperative antibiotic administration, *AORN J* 65(1):109, 1997.
11. Donnelly AJ: Malignant hyperthermia: epidemiology, pathophysiology, treatment, *AORN J* 59(2):393, 1994.
12. Gillette VA: Applying nursing theory to perioperative nursing practice, *AORN J* 64(2):261, 1996.
13. Hankela S, Kiikkala I: Intraoperative nursing care as experienced by surgical patients, *AORN J* 63(2):435, 1996.
14. Kelly M: Surgery, anesthesia, and the geriatric patient, *Geriatr Nurs* 16(5):213, 1995.
15. Krenzischek DA, Frank SM, Kelly S: Forced-air warming versus routine thermal care and core temperature measurement sites, *J Post Anesth Nurs* 10(2):69, 1995.
16. Letizia M: Perioperative care of elderly trauma patients, *AORN J* 63(5):932, 1996.
17. Lusis SA: The challenges of nursing elderly surgical patients, *AORN J* 64(6):954, 1996.
18. McEwen DR: Intraoperative positioning of surgical patients, *AORN J* 63(6):1059, 1996.
19. Malangoni M: *Critical issues in operating room management,* Philadelphia-New York, 1997, Lippincott-Raven.
20. Meeker MH, Rothrock JC: *Alexander's care of the patient in surgery,* ed 10, St Louis, 1995, Mosby.
21. Redmond MC: Latex allergy: recognition and perioperative management, *J Post Anesth Nurs* 11(1):6, 1996.
22. Riveria PH, Worley C: This looks like malignant hyperthermia! *J Post Anesth Nurs* 10(5):265, 1995.
23. Rosenthal BC: An interactionist's approach to perioperative nursing, *AORN J* 64(2):254, 1996.
24. Russo W, Sharrock NE, Mattis S, et al: Cognitive effects after epidural vs general anesthesia in older adults, *JAMA* 274(1):44, 1995.
25. Shaw C, Weaver CS, Schneider L: Conscious sedation: a multidisciplinary approach, *J Post Anesth Nurs* 11(1):13, 1996.
26. Steelman VM: Latex allergy precautions: a research-based protocol, *Nurs Clin North Am* 30(3):475, 1995.
27. Struebing VL: Differential diagnosis of malignant hyperthermia: a case report, *J Am Assoc Nurse Anesthetists* 63(5):455, 1995.
28. Strzyzewski N: Latex allergy: everyone is at risk, *Plast Surg Nurs* 15(4):204, 1995.
29. Tappen RM, Andre SP: Inadvertent hypothermia in elderly surgical patients, *AORN J* 63(3):639, 1996.
30. Vernon S, Pfeifer GM: Are you ready for bloodless surgery? *Am J Nurs* 97(9):40, 1997.
31. Winslow EH: Research for practice, *Am J Nurs* 96(5):51, 1996.
32. Woodin LM: Resting easy: how to care for patients receiving IV conscious sedation, *Nursing* 26(6):33, 1996.
33. Wynd CA, Samstag DE, Lapp AM: Bacterial carriage on the fingernails of OR nurses, *AORN J* 60(5):796, 1994.

chapter

# 20 Postoperative Nursing

MARY JO BOEHNLEIN and JANE F. MAREK

## objectives *After studying this chapter, the learner should be able to:*

1. Describe the postoperative phase as a component of the surgical experience.
2. Identify postoperative complications that may compromise a patient's safety and stability after anesthesia and surgical intervention.
3. Discuss the patient's risk factors for potential postoperative complication.
4. Discuss postoperative patient assessment.
5. Formulate relevant postoperative nursing diagnoses.
6. Identify desired patient outcomes for the postoperative phase.
7. Describe nursing interventions to prevent or treat postoperative complications.
8. Relate the interventions to minimize anxiety in patients and their families during the postoperative course.
9. Discuss the relevance of evaluation and documentation of nursing care interventions.
10. Identify the benefits of follow-up communication and referrals for the patient's later postoperative recovery.

The postoperative phase begins with the transfer of the patient from the operating room to the appropriate postoperative unit and ends with the discharge of the patient from the surgical facility or the hospital. The focus of nursing care in the postoperative phase is the patient's return, as quickly as possible, to an optimal level of functioning.

The primary focus of this chapter is the nursing care of the patient in the postanesthesia care unit (PACU). The postoperative nursing care on the patient care unit is reviewed in lesser detail. The nursing diagnoses and interventions address the postoperative patient care needs in both the PACU and also the patient care unit.

The immediate postanesthesia phase presents multifaceted challenges in patient care. Anesthesia and surgical interventions place great stress on all body systems (see Chapter 19). The postanesthesia nurse must understand the patient's risks for postoperative complications in body system functioning, alterations in comfort and skin integrity, and the biopsychosocial responses that may occur. Special clinical expertise is required to deliver maximal patient care when complications, often of an emergent nature, arise. In addition, expertise is needed to ensure the patient's return to a state of physiological homeostasis that is the same or improved over the preoperative state.

To meet the criteria for transfer from the PACU to the clinical unit or to the home, the patient must be stable and free from symptoms of complications. The potential for the development of postoperative complications, however, continues beyond the immediate postoperative phase. Ongoing, thorough nursing assessment is essential to providing care after the patient is transferred to a specific clinical unit. Nursing interventions focus on minimizing the potential for postoperative complications and promoting partnership with the patient in planning and implementing recovery. Effective preoperative patient teaching (see Chapter 18) prepares the patient for a role in facilitating the recovery course. In the postoperative phase, the nurse reinforces this information. In addition, the nurse continues planning for the patient's discharge.

In the present era of health care reform, more and more patients are being discharged the same day of surgery or the following day. In addition to economic incentives, improvements in surgical techniques and new anesthesia techniques have made ambulatory and short-stay surgery both safe and efficient. The time that the patient remains at the health care facility has been greatly reduced. As a result, increased responsibility has been placed on the patient and significant others to follow through with observations and treatments after they return home. For this reason, assessing the patient's needs and providing assessment-based informational support before discharge are crucial responsibilities for nurses who care for these patients in the early postoperative period.

## HISTORICAL BACKGROUND

General anesthesia has been used since the late 1890s, and surgical procedures date back to the Egyptian age. However, a specially designated area for the recovery of postsurgical patients is comparatively new. The concept was first conceptualized by Florence Nightingale in 1863. She described the use of a small room adjacent to the operating theater where the patient remained until he or she recovered from the immediate effects of the operation.[2] Even though Nightingale described this concept in the nineteenth century, it was World War II that had the greatest impact on the development of the modern-day PACU. Because of the shortage of nurses there was a need to centralize patients and equipment to efficiently deliver care.

Many PACUs opened in the 1940s after it was discovered that the specialized unit decreased patient morbidity and mortality and shortened length of stay.[12] Postoperative mortality within the first 24 hours after administration of anesthesia and surgical intervention was caused by obstruction of airway, laryngospasm, hemorrhage, cardiac arrest, and medication error. Other factors that contributed to mortality included lack of standardized patient care and absence of medical and nursing supervision.[2] As a result of these findings, many hospitals opened these units staffed with specially trained nurses for the care of patients recovering from anesthesia. Today, most patients recovering from general or regional anesthesia are transferred from the operating room (OR) to the PACU before discharge or transfer to a nursing division. Critically ill patients may be directly transferred from the OR to an intensive care unit (ICU).

## IMMEDIATE POSTANESTHESIA CARE

The PACU is usually located adjacent to the operating rooms. The basic design consists of a large open room divided into individual patient care spaces. The number of spaces depends on the number of individual operating rooms in the surgical suite. In general, there is 1 to 1.5 PACU patient care spaces per OR. Each individual patient care space is supplied with a cardiac monitor, blood pressure monitoring device, pulse oximeter, airway management equipment, suction, and oxygen. Emergency medications and equipment are centrally located. Isolation rooms are available if needed. The PACU length of stay is generally less than 24 hours.

### PERSONNEL

Registered nurses in the PACU are specially educated and have an in-depth knowledge of anesthetic agents and patient responses to these agents, pain management techniques, and surgical procedures and potential complications. The PACU nurse demonstrates competence in physical assessment and managing emergency situations. A collaborative relationship with anesthesiologists and surgeons is essential.

In 1986 the American Society of Post Anesthesia Nurses (ASPAN) devised specialty certification for RNs working in the PACU. Certification in ambulatory postanesthesia (CAPA) is available for nurses working in ambulatory surgical settings.[2] Other staff assisting the nurse in the PACU include licensed practical nurses and unlicensed assistive personnel.

### PHASES OF POSTANESTHESIA CARE

The ASPAN has identified three distinct phases of care: the preanesthesia phase, postanesthesia phase I, and postanesthesia phase II. The focus of the *preanesthesia phase* is the patient's emotional and physical preparation before surgery.[2] *Postanesthesia phase I* is characterized by the care of the patient emerging from anesthesia until the patient is physiologically stable and does not require one-to-one care. During this phase the PACU nurse makes a preliminary assessment of breath sounds, respiratory effort, oxygen saturation, blood pressure, cardiac rhythm, level of consciousness, and muscle strength. *Postanesthesia phase II* begins when the patient's level of consciousness returns to baseline; the patient has a patent airway and intact upper airway reflexes; the patient has manageable pain; and the patient has stable cardiac, pulmonary, and renal functioning. During this phase the patient is transferred to the nursing division or short-stay unit.[9]

### TRANSFER TO THE POSTANESTHESIA CARE UNIT

The circulating nurse informs the PACU of the patient's estimated time of arrival in the unit and also of any special care needs or equipment required. A detailed report is given when the patient is admitted to the unit.

**box 20-1** *Patient Status Report on Admission to the Postanesthesia Care Unit*

- Patient demographics
- Need for life support equipment
- Pertinent medical history
- Baseline vital signs
- Allergies
- Surgical procedure performed
- Presence of implants
- Type and length of anesthetic
- Time and type of reversal agents given
- Medications administered
- Estimated blood loss
- Intravenous and invasive lines
- Amount of fluid replacement intraoperatively
- Vital signs
- Intraoperative complications
- Intraoperative positioning
- Patient skin condition
- Drainage tubes and locations
- Dressings
- Orders to be initiated in PACU
- Preoperative patient anxiety
- Presence of family in waiting area

The nurse-patient ratio on admission to the PACU is 1:1. While connecting the monitoring equipment, applying oxygen, and making an immediate physiological assessment, the PACU nurse receives reports from the anesthesiologist, surgeon, and circulating nurse. The verbal report includes data regarding the surgical procedure and intraoperative patient responses. Data in the report are based on recommendations made by the ASPAN in 1992 (Box 20-1).[12] The anesthesiologist is in attendance until the PACU nurse accepts responsibility for the patient. The anesthesiologist's presence is mandated by the American Society of Anesthesiologists Standards for Postanesthesia Care 1991.[12]

After the verbal reports and immediate assessment of the patient's airway, respiratory, and circulatory status, the PACU nurse performs a more thorough patient assessment. The ASPAN has also made recommendations for the components of the initial PACU assessment (Box 20-2). Nursing units differ in the method of organizing patient assessment data. Some use a head-to-toe approach; others use a major body systems approach (Figure 20-1).

Nursing care in the immediate postoperative phase focuses on maintaining ventilation and circulation, monitoring oxygenation, preventing shock, and managing pain. Assessments of respiratory, circulatory, and neurological functions are performed and documented at frequent intervals. Many institutions use clinical pathways to deliver safe, efficient, cost-effective patient care. An example of a Clinical Pathway (coordinated care track) for use in the PACU can be found on p. 529.

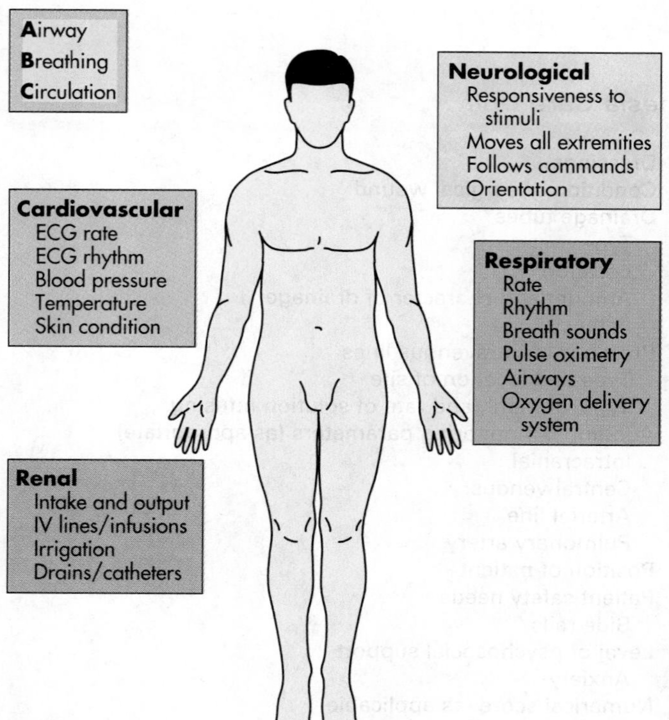


**fig. 20-1** Body system approach to assessment.

## NURSING MANAGEMENT

## ASSESSMENT

### Nursing Care Considerations in the Postanesthesia Care Unit

The PACU nurse cares for a diverse patient population ranging from the ambulatory surgical patient to the individual requiring continuous invasive monitoring and mechanical ventilation. The diversity of operative procedures and anesthetic techniques presents a challenge to PACU nurses.

#### *Respiratory status*

Assessing respiratory status is of primary importance during the immediate postoperative period. Both a patent airway and adequate respiratory function should be ascertained. Immediate respiratory complications that may occur include airway obstruction, hypoxemia, hypoventilation, aspiration, and laryngospasm.

**Respiratory complications.** Respiratory complications are the leading cause of morbidity and mortality in the immediate postoperative period.[1,2] Although respiratory complications are more common in patients with known respiratory disease or other risk factors, the potential for complications exists for all patients. Identified risk factors include age over 60, obesity, male gender, emergent surgical procedures, length of surgery in excess of 4 hours, abdominal and thoracic procedures, and choice of anesthetic agents and techniques (Box 20-3).[1,2]

***Airway obstruction.*** Airway obstruction is commonly thought to occur as a result of movement of the tongue (relaxed from anesthesia) into the posterior pharynx (Figure 20-2). However, research indicates that airway obstruction may be due to anesthetic-induced changes in pharyngeal and laryngeal muscle tone and structural alterations in the airway, with obstruction from the epiglottis.[1] Secretions or other fluid collecting in the pharynx, bronchial tree, or trachea may also cause airway obstruction. Airway obstruction may occur following intubation because of laryngeal or subglottic edema; however, this is seen most commonly in pediatric patients. Clinical manifestations include gurgling, wheezing, stridor, sternal and intercostal retractions, hypoxemia, and hypercarbia. Initial treatment consists of administration of 100% oxygen, physical maneuvers to maintain airway (jaw-thrust maneuver), suctioning of secretions, and insertion of an oral or nasal airway. Insertion of an oral airway must be accompanied by the jaw-thrust maneuver. If these interventions are unsuccessful, endotracheal intubation, cricothyroidotomy, or tracheostomy may be necessary.

***Hypoxemia.*** Hypoxemia is a common complication and occurs in up to 40% of all postsurgical patients.[1] Hypoxemia may occur as a result of hypoventilation, which diminishes the exchange of oxygen between the alveoli and the atmosphere.

Tissue hypoxemia is the result of decreased oxygen delivery. The following factors can place the patient at high risk for inadequate respiratory function:

- Narcotics (respiratory center depression)
- Insufficient reversal of neuromuscular blocking drugs (residual muscle paralysis)

- Increased tissue resistance (emphysema, infections)
  - Decreased lung and chest wall compliance (pneumonia, restrictive diseases)
  - Obesity; gastric and abdominal distention
  - Constrictive dressings
  - Incision site close to the diaphragm
  - General rather than regional anesthesia
  - Postoperative pain

***Aspiration.*** Aspiration is the inhalation of gastric contents or blood into the tracheobronchial system. Aspiration usually is caused by regurgitation; however, aspiration of blood may result from trauma or surgical manipulation (e.g., after tonsillectomy). Aspiration of gastric contents can cause chemical irritation, pneumonitis, destruction of tracheobronchial mucosa, and an increased risk of secondary infection.

Risk factors for aspiration include decreased level of consciousness, dysphagia, delayed gastric emptying, head and neck surgery, history of hiatal hernia, and emergent intubation of a patient with a full stomach.

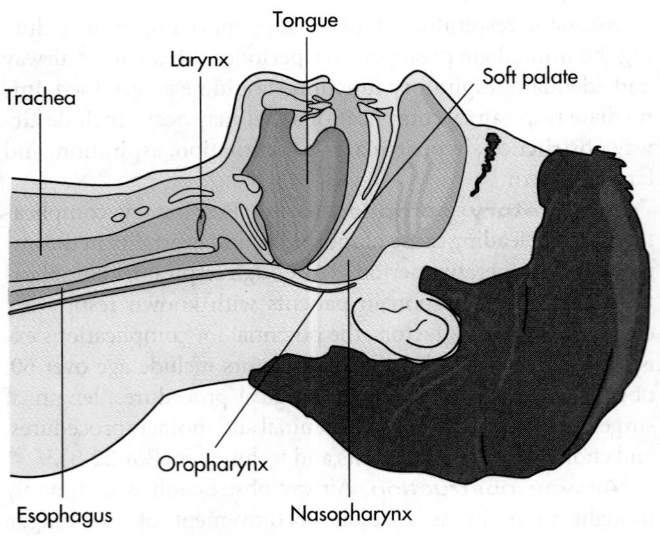


**fig. 20-2** Obstruction of airway by tongue blocking oropharynx in unconscious person lying supine.

**box 20-3** *Factors Contributing to Respiratory Complications*

- History of respiratory disease
- Advanced age
- Morbid obesity
- Diseases of respiratory muscles (myasthenia gravis)
- Anesthetic techniques and agents
  - Inhalation agents
  - Barbiturates
  - Sedatives
  - Hypnotics
  - Opioids
- Emergency operative procedures
- Abdominal and thoracic surgical procedures
- Head and neck surgical procedures

**box 20-2** *Nursing Assessment in the Postanesthesia Care Unit*

- Vital signs
  - Presence of artificial airway
  - Ventilator settings as needed
  - Oxygen saturations
  - Respiratory assessment
  - Blood pressure (cuff or arterial line)
  - Pulse (apical, peripheral)
  - Monitored cardiac rhythm
  - Temperature (include method of measurement)
- Level of consciousness
  - Ability to follow commands
- Pupillary response
- Urinary output
- Skin integrity
- Neurovascular assessment of extremities (as appropriate)
- Motor assessment
- Pain
  - Location
  - Presence
  - Severity
  - Character
  - Pain scale rating
  - Patient-controlled analgesia
- Dressings
- Condition of surgical wound
- Drainage tubes
  - Type
  - Location
  - Amount and character of drainage
  - Patency
- Presence of intravenous lines
  - Type and location of site
  - Type, amount, and rate of solution infusing
- Additional monitoring parameters (as appropriate)
  - Intracranial
  - Central venous
  - Arterial line
  - Pulmonary artery
- Position of patient
- Patient safety needs
  - Side rails
- Level of psychosocial support
  - Anxiety
- Numerical score (as applicable)

Adapted from Meeker MH, Rothrock JC: *Alexander's care of the patient in surgery,* ed 10, St Louis, 1995, Mosby.

**clinical pathway** *Postanesthesia Care Unit Coordinated Care Track*

| *Patient Classification: III*<br>DATE: | PATIENT IMPRINT |
|---|---|

| TIME FRAME | TIME OF ADMISSION: 0-30 MIN | 30-90 MIN | 90-180 MIN | TIME OF TRANSFER: 3-6 HR |
|---|---|---|---|---|
| **Patient Satisfaction** | Pediatric support person at bedside | | What can we do to enhance your stay with us? | |
| **Discharge Planning** | Identify risk factors for prolonged recovery | | Plan for bed availability | Discharge to Regular Nursing Floor (RNF) or extended recovery/ICU |
| **Airway Management** | Airway Assessment<br>Ventilator settings as ordered/$O_2$ as ordered<br>Monitor $O_2$ Saturation<br>Vital signs per protocol | Assess for readiness to wean | Wean ventilatory support/$O_2$ per protocol | Wean to room air<br>Incentive spirometry q2h after extubation |
| **Hemodynamic Management** | Hemodynamic monitoring<br>Hemodynamic support as necessary | Monitor need for hemodynamic support | Wean from hemodynamic support as tolerated | |
| **Nursing and Medical Interventions** | Identify patient by name and arm band<br>Identify allergies<br>Level of consciousness assessment<br>Dressing assessment<br>Systems assessment<br>Dermatome assessment<br>Report from anesthesia<br>Initiate surgical-specific protocols<br>Pain management—provide pharmacological therapies<br>Rewarming initiated<br>IV and arterial line management<br>Initiate stir-up regimen<br>Place necessary consults<br>Admission documentation | Review chart for patient information<br>Pain management—provide pharmacological and nonpharmacological therapies<br>Review orders<br>Implement physician orders<br>Continue stir-up regimen<br>Emotional support<br>Treat nausea/vomiting if necessary<br>Monitor for potential surgical complications | Labs, x-rays complete<br>Consults complete<br>Wean from rewarming devices<br>Patient repositioned<br>Mouth care given<br>Monitor for potential surgical complications<br>Assess need for extended observation | Monitor for potential surgical complications<br>Assess need for extended observation or ICU care |
| **Patient Education** | Family notified patient in PACU<br>Orient to person, place, and time<br>Explain activities of care while providing care | Answer patient questions<br>Reinforce pain scale | Family called for update on patient's condition<br>Orient to expectations of PACU discharge | Family visit for 15 minutes<br>Instruct on postop pain management<br>Instruct on importance of coughing, deep breathing, and exercising limbs |
| **Outcome Criteria** | Vital signs within normal parameters<br>Oxygenation within normal range<br>Dressing and drains intact | Vital signs within normal parameters<br>Dressing and drains intact<br>No excessive bleeding<br>Pain minimized | Oriented to person and place/returned to baseline mentation<br>Hemodynamically stable | Postanesthesia Score >8<br>Temp 35.5°-38.4° C<br>Coughing and deep breathing<br>Pain < 4<br>Minimal nausea/vomiting<br>No evidence of surgical complications<br>All appropriate physician orders initiated |

Courtesy Cleveland Clinic Foundation, Department of Advanced Practice Nursing, Cleveland, Ohio.

***Laryngospasm.*** Laryngospasm is a spasm of laryngeal muscle tissue and may manifest as complete or partial closure of the vocal cords and result in obstruction of the respiratory tract. Untreated, laryngospasm can cause hypoxia, cerebral damage, and death. Therefore laryngospasm is a potential emergency in the immediate postoperative period. Patients at risk for laryngospasm are those who have been exposed to airway irritation. Irritation can be caused by certain anesthetic agents, laryngoscope blades used in intubation, endotracheal tube placement, or surgical stimulation (e.g., bronchoscope passage). In the PACU, repeated suctioning and irritation by the endotracheal tube or artificial airway can cause laryngospasm after extubation. Dyspnea, crowing sounds, hypoxemia, and hypercapnia are symptoms of laryngospasm.

### Cardiovascular status

Assessing the patient's postoperative cardiovascular status is a priority for nursing care. Surgery and anesthetic agents predispose patients to complications of the cardiovascular system. Hypotension, hypertension, and cardiac dysrhythmias occurring as a result of the influence of anesthetic agents on the central nervous system (CNS), myocardium, and peripheral vascular system are the most commonly encountered cardiovascular complications in the immediate postanesthesia period.

#### Cardiovascular complications

***Hypotension.*** Hypotension is defined as a 30% decrease from the patient's baseline measurement.[1] The most common cause of hypotension is a decreased preload secondary to hypovolemia.[12] Hypovolemia is caused by hemorrhage, inadequate fluid replacement, pneumothorax, vasodilation caused by drugs or anesthetic agents, or pulmonary embolus. Postoperative hypotension is often caused by blood loss or inadequate fluid replacement. Other causes of hypotension include shock, ischemia, hypoxia, myocardial infarction, dysrhythmias, third-space fluid loss, and congestive heart failure. Clinical manifestations of hypotension and hypovolemia include increased heart rate, decreased urinary output, pallor of extremities, confusion, and restlessness.

***Hypertension.*** Common causes of hypertension include pain, hypoxia, hypercarbia, preexisting hypertension, hypovolemia, sympathetic stimulation, bladder distention, and anxiety. Of the patients who experience postoperative hypertension, approximately 50% have a preoperative history of hypertension.[1] Treatment of hypertension depends on the etiology. Untreated hypertension may lead to cardiac dysrhythmias, myocardial ischemia and infarction, left ventricular failure, pulmonary edema, and cerebrovascular accident.

***Cardiac dysrhythmias.*** Common dysrhythmias occurring in the immediate postoperative period include sinus tachycardia, sinus bradycardia, and supraventricular and ventricular dysrhythmias. Determination of etiology is essential before initiating treatment. Initial treatment includes assessment of airway patency, adequate ventilation, medications, and supplemental oxygen. Causes include preexisting cardiac disease, hypoxia, hypercarbia, respiratory acidosis, fluid and electrolyte imbalance, hypothermia, and pain.

### Thermoregulation

Premedications, anesthesia, and the stress of surgery interact in a complex fashion to disrupt normal thermoregulation (see Chapter 19). Both hypothermia and hyperthermia are associated with physiological alterations that may interfere with recovery. Patients at the age extremes and those who are extremely debilitated are at even greater risk for the development of postoperative temperature abnormalities.

**Hypothermia.** Prevention of abnormalities in thermoregulatory responses begins preoperatively with the nursing admission history (see Chapter 18). Postoperatively, hypothermia can extend recovery and increases postoperative morbidity. An estimated 60% of patients in the PACU experience hypothermia.[12] Shivering is a potential response to anesthetic agents. It is an involuntary skeletal muscular activity initiated by the hypothalamus to produce heat. Muscle tone is increased and heat is produced. Shivering increases oxygen demands by 300% to 400%, simultaneously increasing the metabolic rate 50% to 100%, resulting in increased myocardial workload. It may cause airway obstruction and increased somnolence.[12] For the patient without cardiac disease there are usually no significant sequelae; however, the patient with coronary artery disease or cardiac myopathy may decompensate.

Temperature of the postanesthesia patient affects recovery time—the lower the core temperature, the longer the recovery time from anesthesia. There is a prolonged elimination of muscle relaxants in hypothermic patients.[12]

Hypothermia also affects coagulation. Fibrinolysis increases and platelet activity decreases as the body temperature drops, increasing chances for bleeding.

Vasoconstriction occurs as a result of hypothermia. Vasoconstriction probably causes a fluid shift from the extracellular space, resulting in intravascular volume loss. Vasodilation occurs as the patient rewarms and approaches normothermia. To avoid hypovolemia during rewarming, the patient may require large amounts of intravenous fluids.

Rewarming is essential in the immediate care for the patient in the PACU (see the Research Box). Patients report feelings of discomfort associated with hypothermia. Unrecognized or untreated periods of hypothermia can pose a significant risk for patients in the immediate postoperative period.

**Hyperthermia.** Hyperthermia is defined as core temperature above 39° C. In the early postoperative period hyperthermia may be caused by an infectious process, sepsis, or malignant hyperthermia. Although malignant hyperthermia is most often associated with the intraoperative period, it may occur or recur 24 to 72 hours postoperatively. If unrecognized or untreated malignant hyperthermia will result in death. (See Chapter 19.)

### Fluid and electrolyte imbalances

Fluids are lost during surgery through blood loss and increased insensible fluid loss (by hyperventilation and exposed skin surfaces). Because of fluid retention at the surgical site, fluids also may be "lost" to the circulation after major surgery in which tissue dissection was extensive.

Excessive blood volume lost during surgery requires replacement therapy intraoperatively and postoperatively. Blood,

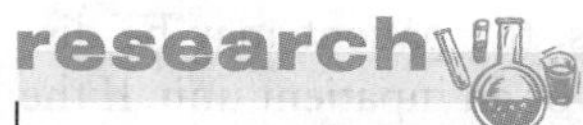

Reference: Hershey J, Valenciano C, Bookbinder M: Comparison of three rewarming methods in a postanesthesia care unit, *AORN J* 65(3): 597, 1997.

This study was designed to compare the effectiveness of three PACU nursing interventions to rewarm postoperative patients. The study was conducted in a 565-bed center with a 17-bed operating room and 23-bed PACU. The sample consisted of 140 adult patients between the ages of 20 and 60 years who had undergone a laparotomy under general anesthesia, were in stable condition, and were admitted to the PACU with temperatures lower than 36° C. The study was limited to these patients in an effort to control the effects of body surface exposure during the procedure.

Patients were divided randomly into three groups to determine the time differences among each of the rewarming methods. The methods consisted of covering the patients with two warmed thermal blankets and a hospital bedspread (standard PACU protocol); two warmed thermal blankets, a hospital bedspread and a reflective blanket; and two warmed thermal blankets, a reflective head covering, a hospital bedspread, and a reflective blanket.

Results indicated no significant differences among the three methods and patients' duration of hypothermia. However, patients receiving the second method (standard PACU protocol plus reflective blanket) reached normothermia 8 minutes faster than those in the other groups. Findings indicate that the standard PACU protocol plus a reflective blanket is a safe, efficient, cost-effective method of reaching normothermia and increasing patient comfort.

blood products, colloids, and crystalloids may need to be replaced. In addition, volume may be replaced with intravenous fluids such as normal saline or lactated Ringer's solutions. Postoperative parenteral fluid requirements vary with the patient's preoperative status and the surgical procedure.

The normal body response to the stress of surgery is renal retention of water and sodium. For at least 24 to 48 hours after surgery, fluids are retained by the body because of the stimulation of antidiuretic hormone (ADH) as part of the stress response to trauma and the effect of anesthesia. During surgery renal vasoconstriction and increased aldosterone activity also occur, leading to increased sodium retention with subsequent water retention. Overhydration can occur with vigorous fluid replacement, especially in the small elderly patient. Both water intoxication and pulmonary edema can occur, depending on the type and amount of fluids given.

Electrolyte disturbances also may be seen in the postoperative period. Although these disturbances are more common in patients with diabetes and renal failure, they also may occur in the young, the elderly, and the debilitated patient. Such electrolyte disturbances should be treated promptly. See Chapter 15.

**Monitoring fluids.** The patient receiving fluids intravenously is monitored for signs of pulmonary edema (dyspnea, cough) or water intoxication (change in behavior, confusion, warm moist skin, sodium deficit). The patient also is monitored for fluid and electrolyte imbalances. Extra potassium may be necessary to replace losses by gastric secretion.

If hydration is adequate, a patient usually voids within 6 to 8 hours after surgery. Fluid intake will exceed fluid output during the first 24 to 48 hours. Although 2000 to 3000 ml of intravenous fluid usually are given on the operative day, the first voiding may not be more than 200 ml, and the total urinary output for the operative day may be less than 1500 ml. As body functions stabilize, fluid and electrolyte balance returns to normal within 48 hours.

### Gastrointestinal disturbances

Nausea and vomiting are common postoperative problems affecting many patients in the PACU. These disturbing occurrences are often associated with general anesthesia, obesity (due to decreased elimination of anesthetic agents), abdominal surgery, the use of opiate analgesics, history of motion sickness, and psychological factors. Preoperative measures are often taken to decrease postoperative nausea and vomiting. Postoperative vomiting can lead to fluid and electrolyte imbalance, dehydration, stress on abdominal incisions, aspiration, and increased intracranial pressure. Vomiting, diarrhea, and prolonged nasogastric intubation may result in the loss of gastrointestinal secretions high in sodium and potassium. See Chapter 15.

### Pain

Pain is a common occurrence after nearly all types of surgical procedures. Incisional pain is the most common; however, pain may also result from positioning or pressure areas during surgery. Pain results from cutting, pulling, and manipulating tissues and organs. Postoperative pain is most severe after intrathoracic, intraabdominal, and major orthopedic surgeries. Pain may result from stimulation of nerve endings by chemical substances released at the time of surgery or from tissue ischemia caused by interference of blood supply to tissue. Reduced blood supply may be caused by pressure, muscle spasm, or edema. Trauma to the nerve fibers in the skin produces sharp, localized pain. Extensive dissection and prolonged retraction of muscle and fascia produce deep, long-lasting pain. Pain originating in the visceral organ may be referred to a distant portion of the body surface or deep within a different area and is usually characterized as a deep, aching pain. A hollow, visceral organ such as the ureter or bile duct can develop muscle spasms characterized as cramping pain.

After surgery, other factors can add to the pain sensation: pressure from tissue edema, distended bladder, gas used during endoscopic procedure, infections, distention, muscle spasms surrounding the incisional area, tight dressings or casts, the pain threshold of the patient, and response to pain. The presence of pain can prolong convalescence because it can interfere with return to activity.

When the patient complains of pain in the postoperative period, it should not be assumed that the pain is incisional in nature. It is important to ascertain the possible cause of the pain. Remember that pain is a subjective experience and occurs when the patient says it does. See Chapter 12 for a complete discussion of pain.

### Neurological status

Immediately after surgery, the patient's level of consciousness can vary from unconscious to wakeful, depending on the type of anesthetic agent used during the surgery. Generally patients are able to breathe without the assistance of an Ambu (breathing) bag or mechanical ventilation. Most patients return to an oriented state in approximately 1 hour, with a tendency to fall asleep when left alone. However, these patients are arousable by either verbal or tactile stimulation.

Neurological status is ascertained by observing the patient's level of consciousness. Response to verbal or noxious stimuli is noted. Pupils are assessed for responsiveness to light and equality. Equality and strength of hand grip also are assessed. A hand grip sustained for 5 seconds is an indication that neuromuscular function is returning. The ability to move all extremities also is assessed and noted.

**Complications of general anesthesia.** Prolonged somnolence and muscle weakness are major nervous system complications that may occur immediately after general anesthesia. Failure to awaken promptly or completely is usually the result of the anesthetic's residual effect. Other causes of stupor include severe hypoxia, hypothermia, metabolic imbalances, hyponatremia, hyperglycemia, and severe hypercapnia. Muscle weakness usually results from prolonged effects of muscle relaxants. Renal failure and electrolyte imbalances can delay recovery from muscle relaxants. Emergence delirium is another alteration in level of consciousness that may occur during the immediate postanesthesia phase. In this short-lived state the patient exhibits increased motor activity, disorientation, and vocalizations.

**Complications of regional anesthesia.** Complications, although rare, can occur if a patient has received spinal anesthesia. These complications are the result of neurological injury caused by local anesthetic toxicity, needle trauma, or cord ischemia. Symptoms can include hypoxia, agitation, hypotension, nausea, and motor or sensory loss.

Spinal anesthesia interferes with innervation of the bladder. The abdomen is palpated to assess for bladder distention.

### Discharge from the postanesthesia care unit

The PACU nurse documents all assessments and interventions for the duration of the patient's stay in the unit. Patients usually remain in the PACU for a minimum of 1 hour or until they are capable of reasonable self-care and their vital signs are stable. Discharge from the PACU is determined by physician order or a numerical scoring system (postanesthesia recovery [PAR] score) approved by the department of anesthesia. The Aldrete score is the most common tool in use. The Aldrete score measures such criteria as respiration, activity, circulation, consciousness, and oxygen saturation. Each criterion is scored from 0 to 2, with a total score of 9 or 10 warranting discharge from the PACU. See Figure 20-3 for PAR score.

Depending on admission status, the patient may be discharged to a short-stay unit, home, or an inpatient unit. If the patient remains hospitalized, the PACU nurse telephones the report to a nurse on the inpatient unit who will assume responsibility for care. The report includes information regarding the patient's preoperative history, surgical procedure and recovery, type of anesthetic and medications administered, and physician orders.

## GERONTOLOGICAL CONSIDERATIONS

Because of the changes associated with the aging process, the prevalence of chronic diseases, the alteration in fluid and nutrition status, and the increased use of medications, the geriatric patient has special care requirements in the postoperative period. Geriatric patients commonly have a slower recovery from anesthesia. Their decreased metabolic rate affects their ability to quickly eliminate sedatives and anesthetic agents.

### Respiratory considerations

The geriatric patient population is at a higher risk for regurgitation, aspiration, and postoperative atelectasis because of diminished airway reflexes, less efficient coughing, and a higher incidence of hiatal hernia.[11] The physiological changes in the pulmonary system alter lung function, which causes a reduced partial pressure of arterial oxygen tension ($PaO_2$).[8] The physiological changes in conjunction with the effects of narcotics, muscle relaxants, and the presence of residual anesthetic agents increase geriatric patients' risks for developing hypoxia. Hypoxia in geriatric patients may be exhibited as combativeness or restlessness. Assessment and maintenance of the airway and adequate ventilation are essential. Pulse oximetry to monitor oxygen saturation is necessary to assist in determining the need for supplemental oxygen. Administration of humidified oxygen enhances ventilation and perfusion and prevents drying of mucous membranes.

### Cardiovascular considerations

Hypertension is a common postoperative complication for elderly patients. Pain stimulates release of sympathomimetic amines, which increases oxygen demand of the myocardium, thereby increasing the potential for the development of myocardial ischemia.[10] Congestive heart failure can occur as a result of fluid overload, which can be an initial sign of myocardial infarction.[11] Diligent monitoring of vital signs, IV fluid administration, and urine output is essential to detect cardiovascular changes and institute timely interventions.

### Hypothermia

Geriatric patients are susceptible to inadvertent hypothermia. Metabolic changes, decrease of subcutaneous fat, reduced muscle mass, intraoperative factors, and anesthesia-related factors alter the elderly patient's ability to produce and conserve body heat. (See Chapter 19.) Postoperative shivering increases oxygen consumption; it can increase tissue oxygen requirements by 200% to 500% in geriatric patients.[10] Postanesthesia care unit nursing interventions to maintain nor-

*Text continued on p. 536*

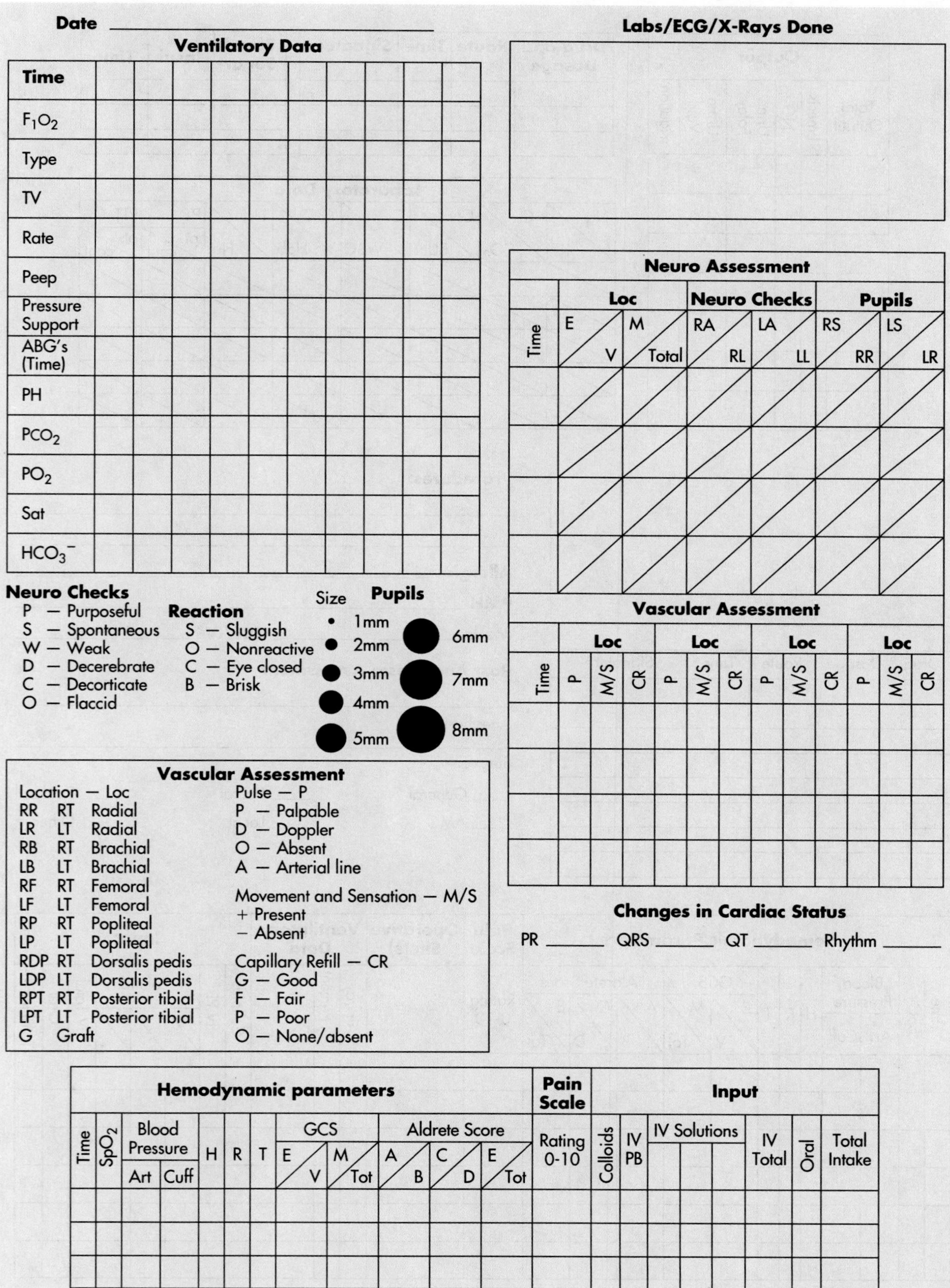

Date ______________________

**Ventilatory Data**

| Time | | | | | | | | | | |
|---|---|---|---|---|---|---|---|---|---|---|
| $F_1O_2$ | | | | | | | | | | |
| Type | | | | | | | | | | |
| TV | | | | | | | | | | |
| Rate | | | | | | | | | | |
| Peep | | | | | | | | | | |
| Pressure Support | | | | | | | | | | |
| ABG's (Time) | | | | | | | | | | |
| PH | | | | | | | | | | |
| $PCO_2$ | | | | | | | | | | |
| $PO_2$ | | | | | | | | | | |
| Sat | | | | | | | | | | |
| $HCO_3^-$ | | | | | | | | | | |

**Neuro Checks**
P — Purposeful
S — Spontaneous
W — Weak
D — Decerebrate
C — Decorticate
O — Flaccid

**Reaction**
S — Sluggish
O — Nonreactive
C — Eye closed
B — Brisk

Size **Pupils**
1mm
2mm
3mm
4mm
5mm
6mm
7mm
8mm

**Vascular Assessment**

Location — Loc
RR RT Radial
LR LT Radial
RB RT Brachial
LB LT Brachial
RF RT Femoral
LF LT Femoral
RP RT Popliteal
LP LT Popliteal
RDP RT Dorsalis pedis
LDP LT Dorsalis pedis
RPT RT Posterior tibial
LPT LT Posterior tibial
G Graft

Pulse — P
P — Palpable
D — Doppler
O — Absent
A — Arterial line

Movement and Sensation — M/S
+ Present
− Absent

Capillary Refill — CR
G — Good
F — Fair
P — Poor
O — None/absent

**Labs/ECG/X-Rays Done**

**Neuro Assessment**

| Time | Loc | | | Neuro Checks | | | | Pupils | | | |
|---|---|---|---|---|---|---|---|---|---|---|---|
| | E / V | M / Total | | RA / RL | | LA / LL | | RS / RR | | LS / LR | |
| | | | | | | | | | | | |
| | | | | | | | | | | | |
| | | | | | | | | | | | |
| | | | | | | | | | | | |

**Vascular Assessment**

| Time | Loc | | | Loc | | | Loc | | | Loc | | |
|---|---|---|---|---|---|---|---|---|---|---|---|---|
| | P | M/S | CR | P | M/S | CR | P | M/S | CR | P | M/S | CR |
| | | | | | | | | | | | | |
| | | | | | | | | | | | | |
| | | | | | | | | | | | | |
| | | | | | | | | | | | | |

**Changes in Cardiac Status**

PR ______ QRS ______ QT ______ Rhythm ______

| Hemodynamic parameters | | | | | | | | | | | | | | | | Pain Scale | Input | | | | | | | |
|---|---|---|---|---|---|---|---|---|---|---|---|---|---|---|---|---|---|---|---|---|---|---|---|---|
| Time | $SpO_2$ | Blood Pressure | | H | R | T | GCS | | | Aldrete Score | | | | | | Rating 0-10 | Colloids | IV PB | IV Solutions | | | IV Total | Oral | Total Intake |
| | | Art | Cuff | | | | E / V | M / Tot | | A / B | C / D | E / Tot | | | | | | | | | | | | |
| | | | | | | | | | | | | | | | | | | | | | | | | |
| | | | | | | | | | | | | | | | | | | | | | | | | |
| | | | | | | | | | | | | | | | | | | | | | | | | |

Continued

**fig. 20-3** Postanesthesia care unit record.

| Output | | | | | |
|---|---|---|---|---|---|
| Total Output | Emesis | NG | Urine Foley | Urine Void | Irrigation |
| | | | | | |
| | | | | | |
| | | | | | |
| | | | | | |
| | | | | | |
| | | | | | |
| | | | | | |

| Drug and Dosage | Route | Time | Signature |
|---|---|---|---|
| | | | |
| | | | |
| | | | |

| Blood Sugar | Insul | Time |
|---|---|---|
| | | |
| | | |
| | | |

| Laboratory Data | | | | | | | |
|---|---|---|---|---|---|---|---|
| Na / K | Cl / $CO_2$ | Glu / BUN | Cr / WBC | RBC / Hgb | Hct / Plat | PT / pt. / cont. | PTT / pt. / cont. |
| | | | | | | | |
| | | | | | | | |
| | | | | | | | |
| | | | | | | | |
| | | | | | | | |
| | | | | | | | |

**Procedures:** ________________

**Allergies** ________________

**PMH** ________________

**Meds** __________ **EBL/IVF** __________

**Post Anesthesia Assessment**

Anesthesiologist ________________

Surgeon ________________

____ General ____ Spinal ____ Epidural

____ AMC ____ Local ____ Other

| Drug & Dosage | Route | Time | Signature |
|---|---|---|---|
| | | | |
| | | | |
| | | | |
| | | | |
| | | | |
| | | | |
| | | | |
| | | | |

| Hemodynamic Parameters | | | | | | | | | | | | | | Pain Scale | Operative Site(s) | Ventilatory Data | | Input | | | | | | | | |
|---|---|---|---|---|---|---|---|---|---|---|---|---|---|---|---|---|---|---|---|---|---|---|---|---|---|---|
| Time | $SpO_2$ | Blood Pressure | | H | R | T | GCS | | | Aldrete Score | | | | Rating 0-10 | | Airway | $O_2$ Percent | Colloids | IV PB | IV Solutions | | | IV Total | Oral | Total Intake |
| | | Art | Cuff | | | | E / V | M / Tot | | A / B | C / D | E / Tot | | | | | | | | | | | | | |
| | | | | | | | | | | | | | | | | | | | | | | | | | |
| | | | | | | | | | | | | | | | | | | | | | | | | | |
| | | | | | | | | | | | | | | | | | | | | | | | | | |
| | | | | | | | | | | | | | | | | | | | | | | | | | |
| | | | | | | | | | | | | | | | | | | | | | | | | | |
| | | | | | | | | | | | | | | | | | | | | | | | | | |

*Continued*

**fig. 20-3, cont'd** Postanesthesia care unit record.

**Glasgow Coma Scale (GCS)**

| | ≥ 2 yrs. | ≤ 2 yrs. |
|---|---|---|
| E — Eyes | | |
| 4 — | Open spontaneously | Open spontaneously |
| 3 — | Open to speech | Open to speech |
| 2 — | Opens to pain | Opens to pain |
| 1 — | No response | No response |
| V — Verbal | | |
| 5 — | Oriented | Coos and babbles |
| 4 — | Confused | Irritable cry |
| 3 — | Inappropriate words | Cries to pain |
| 2 — | Incomprehensible words | Moans to pain |
| 1 — | No response | No response |
| T — | Intubated or TRACH | |
| M — Motor | | |
| 6 — | Obeys commands | Spontaneous movements |
| 5 — | Localizes pain | Withdraws to touch |
| 4 — | Withdraws to pain | Withdraws to pain |
| 3 — | Flexion | Flexion (decorticate) |
| 2 — | Extension | Extension (decerebrate) |
| 1 — | No response | No response |

Activity (A)
2 — Able to move 4 extremities voluntarily
1 — Able to move 2 extremities voluntarily
0 — Unable to move any extremities

Respiration (B)
2 — Able to breathe and cough freely
1 — Dyspnea or limited or shallow breathing
0 — Apneic or assisted ventilation

Circulation (C)
2 — BP = 10-20 of preanesthetic level
1 — BP = 20-50 of preanesthetic level
0 — BP = 50 of preanesthetic level

Color (D)
2 — Pink or normal
1 — Pale or dusky, mottled, or flushed
0 — Cyanotic

Consciousness (E)
2 — Fully awake
1 — Arousable on calling
0 — Not responding

Discharge summary  Time
Level of consciousness ______
BP: ___ P: ___ R: ___ T: ___
Breath sounds: ______
Bowel sounds: ______
Dressings: ______

Neurovascular checks: ______

Pt. belongings:
PO intake ______ Urine: ______
IV intake: ______ Emesis/NG ______
Other: ______ Drains: ______
Total in: ______ Total out: ______
Discharge IV and site:
Other:

**Plan of Care**

**Standard Care Statement Initiated:**

____ Post/Anesthesia Patient ____ Other ______

**Additional Protocols Initiated**

Evaluation of Goals: By discharge patient will:

| Met | Not Met | N/A | |
|---|---|---|---|
| ____ | ____ | ____ | 1. Achieve/Maintain pre-anesthetic and optimal level of respiratory function. |
| ____ | ____ | ____ | 2. Achieve (pre-anesthetic) normal fluid and electrolyte balance. |
| ____ | ____ | ____ | 3. Express a decrease or improvement in discomfort as evidence by verbal/non-verbal communication. |
| ____ | ____ | ____ | 4. Acknowledge understanding of recovery procedures. |

| Output | | | | | | Progress Notes |
|---|---|---|---|---|---|---|
| | | | | | | **Admission Assessment** |
| Total Output | Emesis | NG | Urine Foley | Urine Void | Irrigation | IV Site ______ Drains ______ Breath Sounds ______ Bowel Sounds ______ |
| | | | | | | |
| | | | | | | |

The patient has met the criteria for discharge:

Anesthesiologist signature: ______

Recovery RN ______ Transferred to: ______

Transported by: ______ Report given to: ______

Written discharge instruction given
Title

**fig. 20-3, cont'd** Postanesthesia care unit record.

mothermia are essential to prevent complications in geriatric patients. See the Research Box earlier in this chapter for a discussion of rewarming interventions.

### Pain management

Pain perception does not diminish or decrease with age. Postoperative pain may be more intense and last longer in elderly patients than in younger patients.[14] Geriatric patients may be less likely to complain of pain because they may be less able to differentiate different degrees of pain.[11] In the immediate postoperative period, pain may restrict breathing, increase blood pressure, stimulate dysrhythmias, and aggravate confusion. Acute confusion, which involves disturbances in consciousness, thought, memory, orientation, performance, and attention, can significantly impede the geriatric patient's ability to communicate needs to caregivers.[13] See the Research Box for a discussion of discomfort and confusion in elderly patients. Confusion is a significant problem among elderly surgical patients. It is estimated that 15% to 40% of the elderly population is affected by acute confusion.[13] Delirium or acute confusion affects 10% to 15% of all elderly patients postoperatively.[11]

Geriatric patients may be more sensitive to pain medications and their potential side effects because of slower metabolism. To adequately manage postoperative pain, the PACU nurse needs to administer opioids as quickly as possible. The effects of opioids are stronger and last longer in geriatric patients. The goal of postoperative pain management in elderly patients is to administer the lowest possible dose of an opioid to produce effective relief and minimize the potential side effects of sedation, respiratory depression, and urinary retention.

It is recommended that the initial dose of an opioid be 25% to 50% of the suggested adult dosage and slowly increased to achieve satisfactory pain control.[14] Until geriatric patients are warmed, the intravenous route of opioid administration is the quickest method to get severe pain under control. Absorption is delayed when there is intramuscular injection of an opioid into a cold muscle. Because of the decreased absorption, adequate pain relief may not be achieved; therefore more opioids may be administered. When the patient begins to warm, the blood vessels dilate and absorption is increased, which can lead to an overdose.[11]

On the nursing unit, pain medications should be administered in decreased doses that have been titrated to obtain relief. Lower dosage of pain medications administered on a routine basis instead of on an as-needed basis provides more effective pain control for elderly patients.[11] Nonnarcotic agents that effectively manage pain should be administered as soon as possible. Nonsteroidal antiinflammatory drugs (NSAIDs) are effective in managing moderate levels of pain. However, because of a greater degree of renal insufficiency present in geriatric patients, these medications must be used with caution.

## Ongoing Postoperative Care

### Admission to the surgical unit

If the patient is to remain hospitalized, he or she is transferred from the PACU to the surgical division. The patient is moved onto the bed with assistance as necessary. The patient is oriented to the room, call light is within reach, and side rails are up until the patient is completely oriented. The nurse on the surgical division completes a head-to-toe patient assessment and reviews all perioperative documentation.

**research**

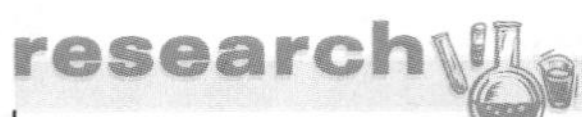

Reference: Miller J et al: A study of discomfort and confusion among elderly surgical patients, *Orthop Nurs* 15(6):27, 1996.

The purpose of this study was to explore the assessment of discomfort among elderly confused surgical patients in an effort to reduce discomfort among hospitalized elders. A convenience sample of 47 patients over 71 years of age (range 75 to 96, average age 83) was screened for confusion within 72 hours of admission. The Neecham Confusion Scale was used to determine the presence and severity of acute confusion in older adults. Thirty-six patients were identified as acutely confused or at high risk for developing confusion. The researchers examined cognitive status, discomfort, and nursing actions to manage discomfort.

The investigators found that patients experienced a notable amount of discomfort during postoperative nursing activities. Sixty-two percent rated discomfort greater than 5 (scale 0 to 10), although 41% were unable to rate their discomfort. Subjects who were observed to have more discomfort were also more confused. With increased levels of confusion, patients were less able to report the discomfort to nursing staff. The researchers reviewed medication records to evaluate analgesia use before nursing actions associated with discomfort.

Further research is indicated to develop methods of assessing discomfort in elderly surgical patients. Nurses should develop methods of assessing and preventing discomfort in elderly confused surgical patients and incorporate such interventions into practice.

### Cardiovascular status

Immediate complications of hypotension and dysrhythmias were previously discussed. Later complications include venous thrombosis and pulmonary embolism. Early recognition and management of cardiovascular complications before they become serious are critical.

**Venous thrombosis.** The formation of clots (deep vein thrombosis [DVT]) in the veins of the pelvis and the lower extremities, which impairs circulation, is a potentially serious postoperative complication. Blood clots develop because of a roughness in the vessel wall such as occurs from trauma, venous stasis (slowing of blood flow), and hypercoagulability (Virchow's Triad). Platelets adhere to the vessel wall, and the resulting inflammatory response stimulates blood coagulation and fibrin development, resulting in a blood clot on the vessel wall (thrombophlebitis). Postoperative clots often form in a vein of the foot, calf, thigh, or pelvis. The clot grows, usually in the direction of the slow-moving blood. Clots can occur in either a deep or superficial vein (Figure 20-4).

Venous stasis occurs postoperatively for a number of reasons. A major contribution to venous stasis is inactivity of the

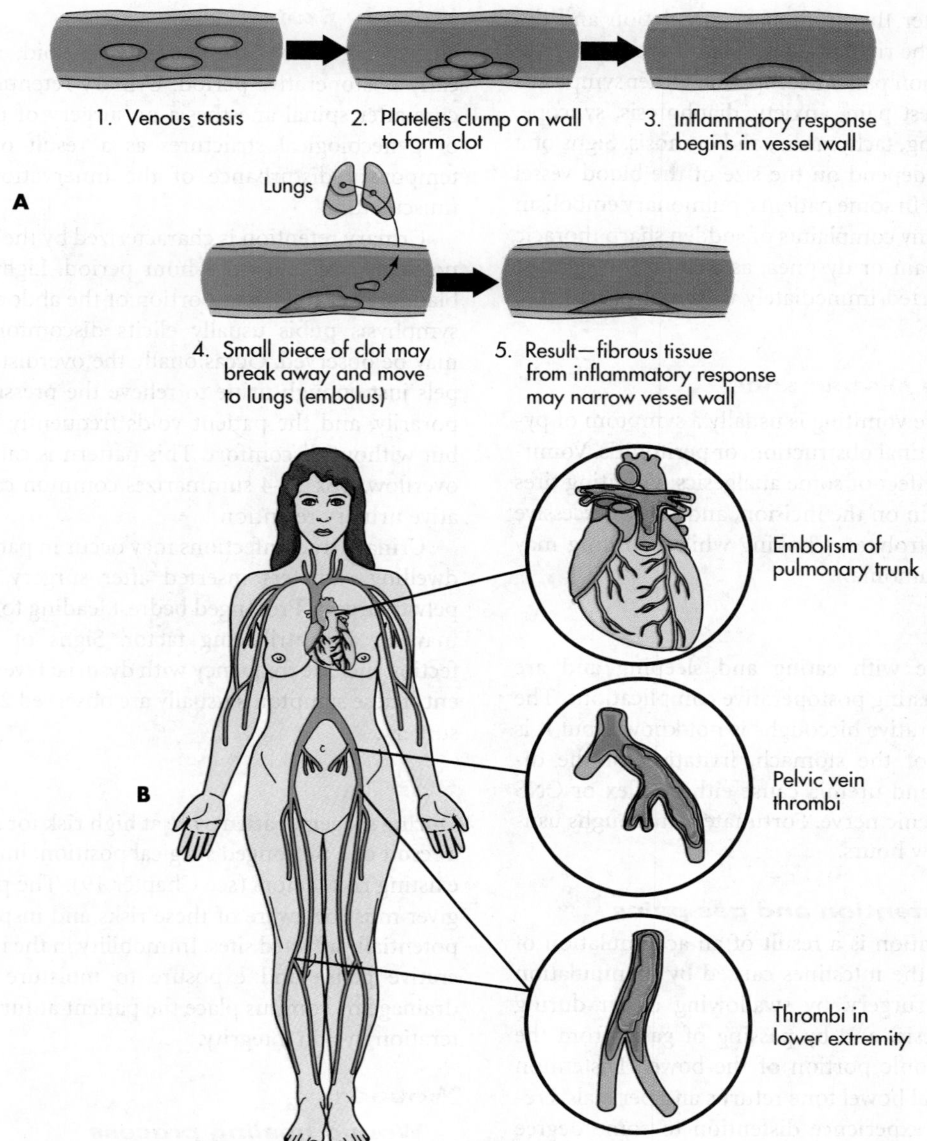
1. Venous stasis
2. Platelets clump on wall to form clot
3. Inflammatory response begins in vessel wall
A
Lungs
4. Small piece of clot may break away and move to lungs (embolus)
5. Result—fibrous tissue from inflammatory response may narrow vessel wall
Embolism of pulmonary trunk
B
Pelvic vein thrombi
Thrombi in lower extremity

**fig. 20-4 A,** Formation of thrombus on wall of vein after venous stasis, resulting in narrowing of blood vessel. **B,** Common locations of venous thrombi.

legs. Every time the leg is moved, the muscle compresses the vein, pushing the blood toward the heart (venous pump); valves prevent the blood from moving backward. Exercise therefore promotes return of venous blood to the heart and prevention of venous stasis.

The development of postoperative venous thrombosis may be attributed to several risk factors. Intrinsic factors include older age, obesity, malnutrition, and contraceptive use. Pathological conditions that increase risk are malignant conditions, congestive heart failure, history of previous DVT, and polycythemia. Patients who undergo pelvic, abdominal, thoracic, or total hip or total knee replacement surgery or who have had fracture of the hip or lower extremities are at greater risk. In addition, prolonged sitting with the legs dependent, decreased mobility, intestinal distention, pressure on the popliteal area, anesthetic effects, and tight dressings or casts on lower extremities also contribute to the potential for the development of venous thrombosis. A venous blood clot may develop without any local symptoms (phlebothrombosis). Homans' sign (pain on dorsiflexion of the foot) indicates a phlebothrombosis, but this sign may not always be present. Pain and local tenderness in the leg are signs of thrombophlebitis. The first indication of difficulty may be a pulmonary embolism. See Chapter 27 for further discussion of DVT.

**Pulmonary embolism.** A clot or portion of a clot may break away and flow through the heart into the pulmonary circulation until it occludes a pulmonary vessel (pulmonary embolism). Emboli alter the pulmonary circulation and decrease the function of the right and left sides of the heart. Dyspnea is the most common patient complaint. Other symptoms include tachypnea, chest pain, anxiety, diaphoresis, syncope, rales in the affected lung, tachycardia, and cyanosis. Signs of a pulmonary embolism depend on the size of the blood vessel that has been occluded. In some patients, pulmonary embolism causes sudden death. Any complaints of sudden sharp thoracic or upper abdominal pain or dyspnea, as well as any signs of shock, should be reported immediately to the physician (see Chapter 32).

### Gastrointestinal Disturbance

Persistent postoperative vomiting is usually a symptom of pyloric obstruction, intestinal obstruction, or peritonitis. Vomiting is also an adverse effect of some analgesics. Vomiting tires the patient, puts a strain on the incision, and causes excessive loss of fluids and electrolytes. Choking while vomiting may lead to aspiration pneumonia.

#### *Hiccoughs*

Hiccoughs interfere with eating and sleeping and are among the most exhausting postoperative complications. The exact cause of postoperative hiccoughs is not known, but it is known that dilation of the stomach, irritation of the diaphragm, peritonitis, and uremia cause either reflex or CNS stimulation of the phrenic nerve. Fortunately, hiccoughs usually resolve within a few hours.

#### *Abdominal distention and gas pains*

Postoperative distention is a result of an accumulation of nonabsorbable gas in the intestines caused by manipulation of the bowel during surgery, by swallowing of air during recovery from anesthesia, and by passing of gases from the bloodstream to the atonic portion of the bowel. Distention will persist until normal bowel tone returns and peristalsis resumes. Most patients experience distention to some degree after abdominal and renal surgery.

Patients with abdominal distention complain of diffuse abdominal pain. Distention may cause dyspnea by pressure on the diaphragm and may lead to atelectasis. Abdominal girth is increased because of the collection of gas; this can be measured with a tape measure to determine progress. Percussion produces a drumlike (tympanic) sound as compared with a dull sound occurring with ascites or obesity. Acute gastric dilation may produce signs of shock (restlessness; rapid, weak thready pulse; hypotension) and overflow vomiting. Gas pains in the intestinal tract, which usually occur as peristalsis returns, can be extremely painful. The return of peristalsis may not occur for 24 hours or more.

A decrease or absence of bowel sounds that occurs after surgery is known as *paralytic ileus.* This condition is characterized by diffuse abdominal discomfort, few or absent bowel sounds, distention, vomiting, and lack of flatus. Fever, decreased urine output, and respiratory distress may accompany this condition. (See Chapter 41.)

### Urinary Status

Urinary retention, the inability to void, may occur in the early postoperative period. Urinary retention commonly occurs after spinal anesthesia or surgery of the rectum, colon, or gynecological structures as a result of local edema or temporary disturbance of the innervation of the bladder musculature.

Urinary retention is characterized by the voiding of little or no urine over a 6- to 8-hour period. Light palpation of the bladder over the lower portion of the abdomen just above the symphysis pubis usually elicits discomfort, and distention may be observed. Occasionally the overdistended bladder expels just enough urine to relieve the pressure within it temporarily, and the patient voids frequently in small amounts but without discomfort. This pattern is called retention with overflow. Box 20-4 summarizes common causes of postoperative urinary retention.

Urinary tract infections may occur in patients who have indwelling catheters inserted after surgery, particularly after pelvic surgery. Prolonged bedrest leading to urinary stasis also may be a contributing factor. Signs of urinary tract infection include frequency with dysuria; fever also may be present. These symptoms usually are observed 24 to 48 hours after surgery.

### Skin Integrity

During surgery, patients are at high risk for skin breakdown as a result of a prolonged surgical position, immobility, and preexisting risk factors (see Chapter 19). The postoperative caregiver must be aware of these risks and inspect for affected or potentially affected sites. Immobility in the immediate postoperative phase and exposure to moisture from body fluid drainage or vomitus place the patient at further risk for an alteration in skin integrity.

### Wounds

#### *Wound healing process*

Tissues may heal by one of three ways: primary, secondary, or tertiary intention. Wound healing by *primary intention* occurs in most surgical incisions. The incision is a clean straight line with all layers of the wound (muscle, subcutaneous tissue, and epithelial tissue) well approximated by suturing. If these wounds remain free of infection and do not separate, healing is quick with minimal scarring (Figure 20-5).

**box 20-4** *Causes of Urinary Retention*

- Recumbent position
- Effects of anesthetics that interfere with bladder sensation and the ability to void
- Pain caused by movement
- Pain at the surgical site after bladder or urethral surgery
- Prolonged immobility

Wound healing by *secondary intention* is seen in wounds such as ulcers with edges that cannot be approximated. It is characterized by tissue loss and an inability to approximate wound edges; tissues heal from the inside out. Healing occurs by a filling in of the wound by granulation tissue over a larger area. Scar tissue formation is extensive. Healing is longer than by primary intention. These wounds have a greater possibility for infection.

Wound healing by *tertiary intention* occurs when there is a delay of 3 to 5 days or more between injury and suturing. The time period permits more microorganisms to penetrate the wound; therefore there will be a greater inflammatory reaction.

**Influencing factors.** Major factors that can delay wound healing are age, nutrition (lack of sufficient vitamin C or protein), circulation (provides blood components and nutrients at the site), corticosteroids (suppress inflammation), presence of foreign bodies, infection, dead space, and irradiation (affects fibroblastic activity). Enzymatic activity in wounds is highest during the early stages of wound healing; therefore new wounds are more sensitive to factors that delay healing.

Wounds in children normally heal more rapidly than those in adults because of increased metabolism and good circulation. Wounds in elderly persons often heal more slowly because of decreased fibroblastic activity and impaired circulation.

Obese persons have excessive subcutaneous tissue that is poorly supplied with blood vessels, and therefore wounds may heal more slowly. Persons with peripheral vascular disease have impaired circulation to the legs, which can cause delayed healing of leg ulcers.

*Keloids,* excessive connective tissue or scar formation, often occur in patients with darker skin. If their appearance is bothersome to the patient, keloids can be surgically excised.

### Hemorrhage

Hemorrhage is most likely to occur within 48 hours after surgery. Hemorrhage may be caused by the slipping of a ligature (suture) or the dislodging of a clot. During surgery small vessels may go unnoticed because of decreased blood pressure or use of a tourniquet. Hemorrhage may occur with the reestablishment of blood flow. Careful assessment of wound dressings and drainage systems is required.

### Wound infection

After surgery the patient remains at risk for wound infection. Excessive body cavity exposure and decreased body defense mechanisms are among the contributing factors to postoperative wound infection. Wound infection is a major type of nosocomial infection. A wound may become infected as a result of factors intrinsic to the patient, factors that can delay healing, and the effectiveness of aseptic technique used by health care personnel.

Objective signs of infection include fever, swelling, erythema, purulent discharge, and increased white blood cell count. These signs usually occur after the immediate postoperative period, but prevention begins preoperatively and continues throughout the perioperative experience. Understanding the principles of standard precautions, isolation, wound healing, and wound care is imperative when caring for the surgical patient.

### Wound dehiscence and evisceration

Wound disruption, or *dehiscence,* is a partial to complete separation of the wound edges. Wound *evisceration* is protrusion of an internal organ through the incision and onto the skin. This typically occurs in the abdomen (Figure 20-6). Wound separation that occurs during the first 3 days usually is related to technical factors, such as the suturing. After the early postoperative period, dehiscence usually is associated with postoperative complications such as distention, vomiting, excessive coughing, dehydration, or infection. Many of these complications can be prevented by careful assessment and continued monitoring, as well as the institution of vigorous preventive measures (ventilatory exercises, ambulation, adequate fluid intake, aseptic technique) on the part of the nurse. Factors such as cachexia, hypoproteinemia, avitaminosis, increased age, decreased resistance to infection, malignant tumor, multiple trauma, chronic steroid use, and hypothermia also can cause wound separation.

On a subjective level, the patient may report a "giving" sensation at the incision or a feeling of wetness. If evisceration has occurred and if a loop of bowel is obstructed, the patient will complain of severe localized pain at the incision. The dressing

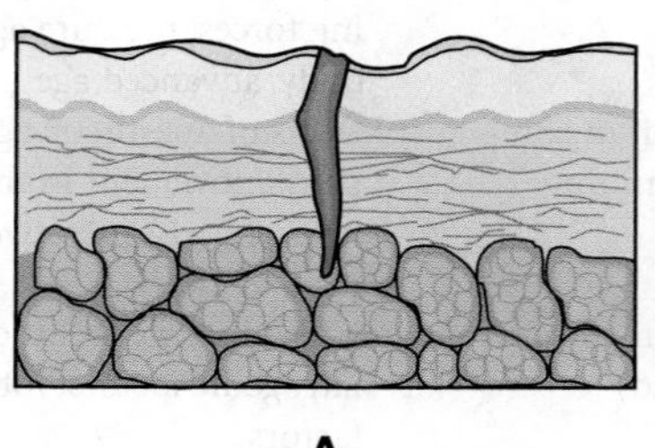


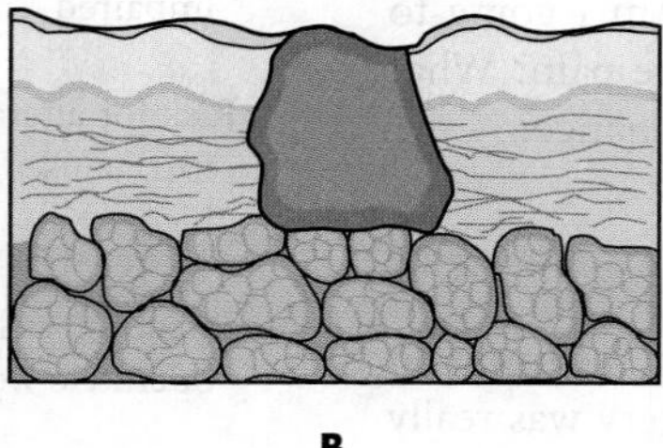


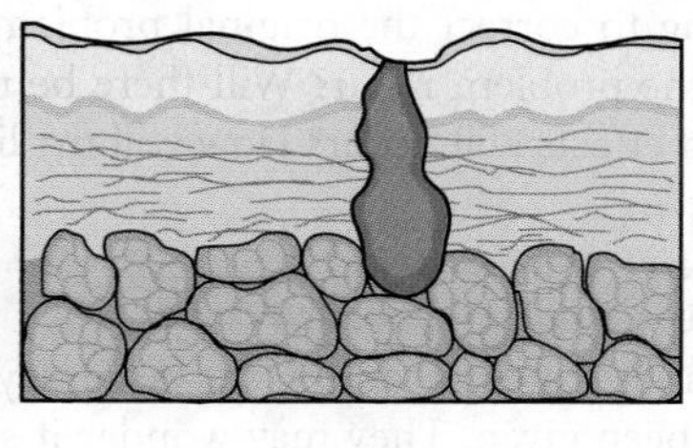


**fig. 20-5** Types of wound healing. **A,** Primary, **B,** Secondary, **C,** Tertiary.

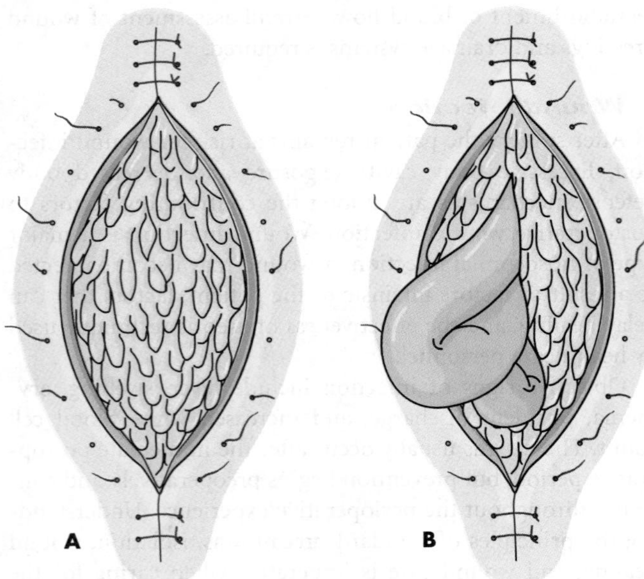


fig. 20-6 A, Wound dehiscence. B, Wound evisceration.

will be saturated with clear pink drainage. The wound edges may be partially or entirely separated, and loops of intestine may be lying on the abdominal wall. Signs of shock may occur.

## Psychosocial Aspects

The immediate postanesthesia period is often a frightening time for the patient. Psychological support is imperative for physical and emotional well-being. Immediately after surgery, most patients are somnolent. As the patient awakens, anxiety is often a major concern.

### Anxiety

Some of the concerns that were present in the preoperative period (see Chapter 18) may continue into the postoperative period. These concerns generally focus on the performed surgery, the results of the surgery, and the temporary or permanent effects that may change a patient's lifestyle.

Anxieties are expressed in many different ways. It must be remembered that expressions such as anger, resentfulness, crying, excessive joking, inappropriate laughter, or withdrawal may all be signs of anxiety and often are seen in the postoperative period.

Fears commonly exist relating to prognosis. Is the surgery really going to correct the original problem? Am I going to die? Will the problem recur? Will there be more pain? What permanent effects will occur? How will my life change?

### Concerns specific to the surgery performed

Sometimes patients doubt the accuracy of information they have been given. They may wonder if surgery was really needed. They may still worry that they have cancer but that nobody is telling them. If they do have cancer, they may think that it is more extensive than they have been told.

### Alterations in body image

Many surgeries involve removal of tissue. If an organ such as the uterus or part of the colon is removed or if part of a limb, breast, or face is removed, patients are faced with a change in self-image. They may experience grief over the lost part. For complete recovery the patient needs to identify feelings and cope with the perceived changes.

### Concerns about the future

The patient may have concerns about changes in roles, return to work, lifestyle, emotional status, economic implications of the surgery, or prognosis. An overriding concern may actually be the patient's inability to predict and control the future. Dealing with uncertainty becomes a major theme.

## NURSING DIAGNOSES

Nursing diagnoses are determined from postoperative analysis of patient assessment data. Nursing diagnoses for the postanesthesia patient may include but are not limited to:

| Diagnostic Title | Possible Etiological Factors |
|---|---|
| Airway clearance, ineffective | Secretions from anesthesia, airway obstruction, improper positioning |
| Gas exchange, impaired | Drug effects, incisional pain, constrictive dressings |
| Aspiration, risk for | Decreased consciousness, suppressed protective reflexes |
| Cardiac output, decreased | Hypotension, preexisting cardiac problems |
| Injury (trauma), risk for | Sensorimotor deficits, residual anesthesia effects, disorientation, venous stasis |
| Fluid volume excess/deficit, risk for | Excess/insufficient intravenous fluids, stress on renal/endocrine systems |
| Thermoregulation, ineffective | Cold environment, prolonged exposure during surgery, anesthetic agents, excessive warming methods, infection, malignant hyperthermia, increased age |
| Pain, acute | Surgical incision, positioning |
| Urinary retention | Surgery, anesthesia, and drug effects |
| Skin integrity, risk for impaired | Improper positioning, shearing forces, pressure against body, advanced age |
| Risk for alteration in comfort: nausea, vomiting, hiccoughs | Effects of anesthetic agents pain, movement in the immediate postoperative period, anxiety |
| Infection, risk for (in postoperative wound) | Break in sterile technique, iatrogenic factors, intrinsic factors |
| Anxiety, risk for | Pain, strange environment, possible change in health status |

## EXPECTED PATIENT OUTCOMES

Expected patient outcomes for the postanesthesia patient may include but are not limited to:

1. Will maintain a patent airway with lungs clear to auscultation
2. Will maintain normal baseline arterial blood gas values and have oxygen saturation level at 96% or above
3. Will successfully eliminate blood, mucus, or vomitus through the mouth and not aspirate
4. Will display pulse and blood pressure at or near preoperative baseline
5. Injury
   a. Will not experience injury related to falls, pressure, or improper positioning
   b. Will return to a state of wakefulness or demonstrate the ability to move all extremities
   c. Will experience adequate venous return and absence of deep vein thrombosis and pulmonary embolism
6. Will maintain a stabilized fluid volume and avoid signs and symptoms of dehydration or overhydration
7. Will maintain a body temperature within normal range
8. Will not show signs of severe pain (facial grimacing, guarding, diaphoresis); pain at 4 or less on a scale of 1 to 10
9. Will successfully empty the bladder within 8 to 10 hours after surgery
10. Will maintain skin integrity
11. Will not have uncontrolled nausea and vomiting or hiccoughs
12. Will display timely healing of surgical wound without signs of infection
13. Will demonstrate the ability to cope with fears, frustrations, and concerns over surgical events

## INTERVENTIONS

### Patient/Family Education

Patient and family education in the postoperative period is primarily a continuation of what was taught in the preoperative period (see Chapter 18). The information might need to be reinforced and clarified. If procedures are being taught, demonstrations of techniques may clarify any misconceptions the patient may have. Explanations regarding rationales for treatment may increase patient cooperation and compliance with postoperative routines. Planning for discharge will require additional teaching. The nurse will have to instruct the patient regarding postoperative medications (dose, frequency, administration techniques, adverse effects), wound care, signs and symptoms of complications, activity restrictions, and the plan for follow-up care. A family member or significant other should be included in the teaching, especially if the patient will require assistance at home.

### Promoting Optimal Respiratory Function

The goal of respiratory care for the postanesthesia patient is to maintain pulmonary ventilation that is adequate to prevent hypoxemia and hypercapnia. Nursing management plays a critical role in the prevention of respiratory complications. In the immediate postanesthesia period, two of the most common causes of inadequate pulmonary exchange are airway obstruction (ineffective airway clearance) and hypoventilation (impaired gas exchange).

#### *Maintaining airway patency*

Excessive secretions from the nasopharynx or tracheobronchial mucosa can lead to partial or complete airway obstruction (Figure 20-7). When secretions pool in the lower airway as a result of shallow breathing and immobility after surgery, pulmonary infection may occur. Removal of these secretions in the early postoperative period can prevent obstruction and the occurrence of infection. Unless the patient can manage these secretions by coughing them up and expectorating them, they must be removed by suctioning. Pharyngeal suctioning often is all that is required. If endotracheal suctioning is necessary, the patient should receive hyperventilation with 100% oxygen before and after each introduction of the catheter into the trachea. When thick secretions are a problem, humidification is increased to keep secretions as thin as possible and to prevent dry air from further irritating the respiratory passages. Blockages can be prevented by keeping secretions moist, taking deep breaths, and coughing up the secretions.

The patient may arrive in the PACU with an oral, nasal, or pharyngeal airway or an endotracheal tube. The airway or endotracheal tube will remain in place until the patient is able to breathe independently and maintain his or her own airway.

If airway obstruction occurs, it may be necessary to intubate the patient or insert an airway. The insertion of an oral airway alone may be insufficient to relieve airway obstruction caused by anesthetic-induced changes in the pharynx and larynx.[1] Insertion of an oral airway should be accompanied by the jaw-thrust maneuver and positive pressure ventilation if necessary.[1] The presence of a nasal airway may cause epistaxis, which will increase airway obstruction.

The pharyngeal airway is most commonly used (Figure 20-8). It keeps the air passage open and the tongue forward until the pharyngeal reflexes have returned. It is removed as soon as the patient begins to awaken and has regained cough and swallowing reflexes. After this time the presence of an airway can be irritating and can stimulate gagging, vomiting, or laryngospasm.

The endotracheal airway not only prevents the tongue from falling back but also prevents airway obstruction resulting from laryngospasm. The endotracheal tube is removed when the patient is awake and able to maintain the airway, as evidenced by the patient's ability to raise the head and grip a hand, as well as by normal blood gas levels.

The endotracheal tube also allows mechanical ventilation. The tube should be left in place until spontaneous and adequate respirations are ensured.

#### *Promoting gas exchange*

Gas exchange is promoted by the delivery of oxygen; by encouraging deep breathing, yawning, and coughing; by proper positioning; and by administering medications to reverse the

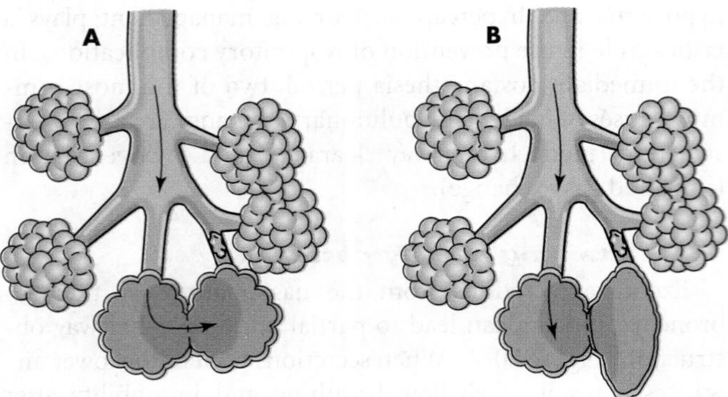


**fig. 20-7** Mucous plug blocking alveolar duct in obstructive atelectasis. **A,** Aeration of blocked alveolus through intraalveolar duct with deep inspiration. **B,** Collapse of blocked alveolus with shallow inspiration.

effects of anesthetic agents. Oxygen is given postoperatively to almost all patients because anesthesia decreases pulmonary expansion and leads to areas of atelectasis. The net result can be hypoxemia. Ventilation is promoted in the postanesthesia phase by oxygen therapy, breathing exercises, and respiratory treatments. Oxygen is administered by nasal prongs or disposable face mask or through the endotracheal or tracheostomy tube.

The duration of postoperative oxygen therapy depends on the individual patient. As a general rule, all patients should receive oxygen at least until they are conscious and able to take deep breaths on command. Prolonged use of oxygen therapy is guided by oxygen saturations and/or arterial blood gas determinations. Patients with thoracic or upper abdominal incisions or preexisting pulmonary disease may be given oxygen for several hours, perhaps until the next day. Special care must be taken in administering oxygen to patients with chronic obstructive pulmonary disease so that hypoxemia, which is the stimulus to breathe, is not entirely corrected. Any patient experiencing shivering, which dramatically increases oxygen consumption, should receive oxygen therapy until the shivering ceases.

Continuous monitoring of oxygen saturation ($SaO_2$) level is a necessary postoperative intervention and can be easily accomplished by use of a pulse oximeter. Portable $SaO_2$ monitoring or pulse oximetry measures the amount of oxygenated hemoglobin in arterial blood. Pulse oximetry is a less expensive, noninvasive method of monitoring arterial oxygen saturation without the risks associated with arterial blood gas measurement or continuous arterial catheters.

All patients need to be instructed and encouraged to perform deep breathing exercises at frequent intervals. Taking deep breaths or yawning also can prevent atelectasis.

### Positioning to support ventilation and prevent aspiration

The most desirable position to ensure maintenance of a patent airway depends on the size and condition of the patient, the anesthesia used, the surgery performed, and the

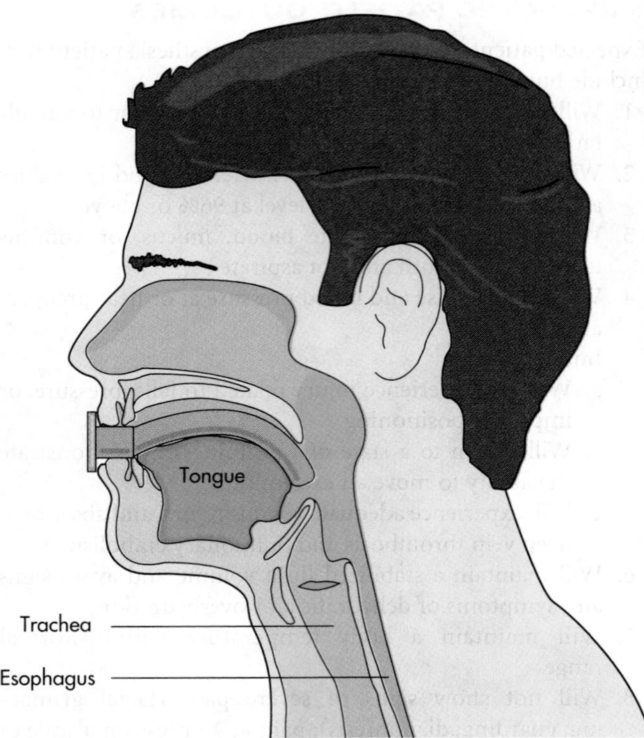


**fig. 20-8** Pharyngeal airway in place to prevent tongue from blocking oropharynx.

amount of experienced nursing care available. Ideally the patient should be in a position to breathe normally with full expansion of all portions of the lungs. Positioning also attempts to facilitate drainage and removal of blood, secretions, or vomitus and to prevent aspiration.

Until protective reflexes have returned, the best position for most patients is side lying or semiprone, with the head tilted back and the jaw supported forward. Aspiration can occur unless the whole body is turned. Turning the patient's head when the chest and shoulders remain in the back-lying position is useless. The disadvantages related to diminished chest expansion in the side-lying position can be reduced by turning the patient frequently and by raising the flexed upper arm and placing it on a pillow.

The supine position with head hyperextended permits full expansion of the lungs, but this is potentially dangerous in the immediate postanesthesia period because of the potential for aspiration. If the supine position must be used, suctioning equipment must be available at the bedside and the patient should be monitored frequently.

### Facilitating drug reversal

The effects of neuromuscular blocking agents used in general anesthesia to facilitate endotracheal intubation and relaxation during the surgical procedure may need to be reversed. Anesthesia may paralyze the natural physiological response for proper ventilation. Barbiturates, narcotics, muscle relaxants, and inhalation anesthetic agents depress respirations. The anesthesiologist will determine if it is necessary to administer drugs to reverse these effects. Naloxone (Narcan) may be used for reversal of narcotics. Nondepolarizing muscle relaxants may be reversed with antagonists, such as anticholinesterases (neostigmine methyl-sulfate [Prostigmin], edrophonium [Tensilon]). Atropine sulfate may be given to minimize such side effects as bradycardia and excessive secretions.

#### *Promoting coughing*

All of the ventilatory measures used to ensure adequate postsurgical ventilation are followed by deep coughing to remove loosened secretions. Coughing may be contraindicated in a few instances, such as after brain, spinal, or eye surgery, because of the increased intracranial or intraocular pressure that can result.

A shallow cough is ineffective in mobilizing secretions and produces fatigue; therefore the patient is encouraged to cough deeply. Patients with abdominal and thoracic incisions are told that it will be painful to cough but that assistance will be given. Narcotics given before ventilation exercises may facilitate patient cooperation; however, narcotics decrease the cough reflex and depress respirations, so exercises must be performed thoroughly and frequently.

Mechanical assistance may be provided by the nurse to promote coughing. Measures include splinting the incision, positioning and turning, increasing activity, and use of an incentive spirometer. Incentive spirometry should be performed every hour.

A simple but helpful nursing intervention is splinting the incision with a drawsheet, towel, small pillow, or placement of the hands firmly on either side of the incision with exertion of slight pressure. Such splinting prevents excessive muscular strain around the incision and reduces acute pain. Family members should be included in the demonstration and teaching. They can be instructed to remind the patient to perform breathing exercises and coughing at regular intervals.

The lungs are auscultated before and after ventilatory measures to determine effectiveness. If the patient has noisy breathing but is unable to cough up secretions, respiratory tract suctioning may be required. Postoperative nursing interventions to facilitate adequate ventilation are continued throughout the postoperative course as necessary inasmuch as the effects of anesthesia may persist for days, particularly in elderly and obese patients.

### Maintaining Circulation

Adequate circulation is important in the postoperative period to provide adequate oxygenation to all tissues, especially to the traumatized tissue to aid in wound healing. Pallor in light-skinned patients and a dullness or decrease in red tones in dark-skinned patients indicates decreased circulation to the skin. Pallor in dark-skinned patients may be more easily assessed by examining the mucous membranes of the mouth. Vasoconstriction may result from cold temperatures or a decrease in the amount of circulating blood as a result of blood loss or from the neuroendocrine response to stress. The nail beds are assessed for prompt capillary return.

Significant changes from baseline data in pulse, blood pressure, or bleeding status are reported to the physician. A weak, thready pulse with a significant drop in blood pressure may indicate hemorrhage or circulatory failure. The surgeon, anesthesiologist, or both are notified at once if any of these signs occur, especially if the skin becomes cold, moist, pale, or cyanotic or if the patient suddenly becomes restless or apprehensive. Oxygen therapy is initiated to increase the oxygen saturation of the circulating blood. Treatment for shock may be necessary (see Chapter 17).

In addition, a dressing that appears constrictive should be loosened, if permissible, or the condition should be reported at once to the physician. Positioning should not constrict circulation.

To avoid the multisystemic complications of immobility, patients are ambulated as soon as permitted by the surgeon. Most patients will be dangled the evening of surgery or the following day. After the patient demonstrates the ability to assume the upright position without orthostatic changes or syncope, activity is advanced as tolerated. Preoperatively the patient should have been instructed regarding the proper technique of leg exercises. See Chapter 18. Until the patient is fully ambulatory these exercises should be performed at least every 2 hours. In some instances these exercises may be contraindicated, such as with femoral popliteal bypass grafts. If the surgical procedure involves one or both of the lower extremities, check with the surgeon before initiating leg exercises.

Before getting out of bed for the first time, the patient is dangled. Dangling is done to assess the patient's activity tolerance and ability to withstand progressive ambulation. Dangling, as a nursing intervention, was described in the literature over 25 years ago.[16] When a patient stands, approximately 500 to 700 ml of blood shifts from the thorax to the pelvis and lower extremities because of the effects of gravity. This redistribution of blood, which is almost complete within 2 to 3 minutes, reduces cardiac output by approximately 20%, with a resultant drop in arterial pressure.[16] This drop in pressure activates compensatory mechanisms to maintain blood pressure.

To avoid orthostatic changes in blood pressure when dangling, patients should be taught leg exercises to prevent muscle deconditioning. The use of antiembolic hose is advisable, especially for patients with varicosities. Patients should be taught to take slow, deep breaths to promote venous return and to prevent vagal stimulation. To maintain spatial orientation, remind patients to keep their eyes open and look ahead. To maintain venous flow while standing, instruct patients to wiggle their feet and contract the leg muscles. By contracting the muscles of the lower extremities a 90 mm Hg force is generated, propelling blood back to the heart. The nurse should assist the patient to change positions gradually and avoid passive standing for more than 3 minutes to avoid pooling of blood in the lower extremities. Continuous assessment of the patient's heart rate, blood pressure, color, and level of consciousness is essential throughout the procedure.

To increase patient cooperation in postoperative ambulation, the nurse should ensure that the patient's pain is under control before ambulation. Literature suggests that 36% of patients do not receive analgesia before ambulating.[5] Uncontrolled pain can limit transfer ability and tolerance of ambulation. Jaw relaxation has been studied as a relaxation method to control postoperative pain. It has been shown to be an effective method to reduce the sensation and distress of pain associated with postoperative mobility in certain postoperative populations.[6] Pain can also cause rapid, shallow breathing and a hesitancy to cough, which may lead to stasis of pulmonary secretions, atelectasis, and pneumonia. Encouraging early activity and mobility in the postoperative period can reduce the risk and severity of cardiovascular, pulmonary, gastrointestinal, and urinary complications.

### Preventing Injury

The nurse who provides postanesthesia care must place great emphasis on patient safety until the patient is fully awake or has complete return of sensations after regional blocks. The unconscious patient must be protected from falling and injury as a result of improper positioning. Side rails should be maintained in the upright position. The patient should be turned frequently and placed in proper body alignment to prevent nerve damage from pressure and to prevent muscle and joint strain caused by lying in one position for a long time.

If emergence delirium should occur, the muscle activity and increased movement may result in injury to the patient. Preventive measures such as use of padded side rails should be taken.

Unconscious patients and patients who have had spinal or epidural anesthesia have a loss of sensation and thus are unresponsive to sensory stimuli. Warming blankets, heat lamps, or cast driers must be used with great care to prevent burns. In addition, pressure to anesthetized extremities must be avoided and care must be taken during positioning of extremities.

#### *Facilitating venous return*

Antiembolic stockings may be applied preoperatively to facilitate blood return from the lower extremities to the heart. These remain in place until the patient is ambulatory.

Postoperative thrombophlebitis often can be prevented by nursing management. No pressure should be permitted on the popliteal area. If legs are supported on pillows, pressure should be equally distributed along the entire leg. Because of the danger of dislodging a clot, the muscle portion of a patient's leg should *not* be massaged postoperatively. A patient who is observed rubbing a leg should be questioned about discomfort. The patients' family should also be instructed not to massage the leg. Nursing interventions to recognize and prevent deep vein thrombosis may also prevent pulmonary embolism from occurring.

An intermittent external pneumatic compression device may be used, either alone or in combination with antiembolic hose on the lower extremities. They should also remain in place continuously until the patient is ambulatory (see Chapter 18).

### Maintaining Fluid and Electrolyte Balance

Fluid volume deficits require fluid replacement after major surgery. Most patients receive intravenous fluids to maintain fluid and electrolyte balance. The exact amount and type of fluid administered depend on the surgical procedure, as well as the patient's age, weight, body surface area, preoperative status, intraoperative course, and individual response to stress. A solution of 5% dextrose in 0.9% sodium chloride commonly is given. Lactated Ringer's solution may be given for prolonged periods to supply the necessary electrolytes. Potassium may be added to an intravenous solution after the first 24 postoperative hours to prevent hypokalemia. Careful monitoring of the patient's intravenous fluid administration is essential to ensure adequacy of replacement and prevention of fluid overload. Output must be measured and monitored, especially urinary output. A preoperative and intraoperative high-volume infusion of isotonic electrolyte solutions (Plasma-Lyte) has been effective in reducing postoperative complications such as nausea, vomiting, drowsiness, headache, and hypotension.[17]

The intravenous site should be checked to ensure that the needle or cannula remains in the vein and that no extravasation has occurred. The arm should be positioned to facilitate the flow of intravenous fluids. The tubing should be checked for patency. The flow rate should be monitored at least hourly. Infusion rates vary, but the average for an adult patient in the PACU ranges from 80 to 120 ml per hour.[9]

Oral administration of fluids is begun as soon as bowel sounds are positive and the cough and gag reflexes are present. Sips of water are offered first. Some persons cannot tolerate iced fluids but are able to suck on ice chips.

### Maintaining Normothermia

Body temperature is monitored frequently during the postoperative period. The patient may have mild hypothermia on arrival in the clinical unit. Rewarming interventions can protect the patient from the development of cardiac dysrhythmias and further complications. Fever (indicated by temperature over 38.5° C) should be reported promptly to the surgeon. Slight elevations in temperature are common on the night of surgery and usually respond promptly to improved pulmonary ventilation and an increased fluid intake.

Body temperature is obtained on admission to the PACU and monitored continually. Axillary, rectal, and oral temperature measures indicate shell (skin) temperature. Tympanic and esophageal temperatures are accurate measures of core temperature.

#### *Treating hypothermia*

Various methods are commonly used to assist the patient in returning to normothermia. Interventions for hypothermia include constant body temperature monitoring, administration of warm intravenous solutions, and the use of warm blankets, hydrothermia mattresses, forced warm air devices, and warming lights (radiant heat). In addition, the nurse may increase room temperature or apply head or body coverings on the patient.

Factors influencing the amount of time required for rewarming include the patient's age, procedure performed, length of procedure and anesthesia, starting temperature, and the temperature and amount of fluids administered.[3] The time required for rewarming varies with the methods used, and different methods have shown different results. A study of cardiac surgical patients indicated that patients rewarmed with circulating-water blankets had a significantly higher rate of core and skin temperature increase than patients rewarmed with convective-air devices.[3]

### *Treating malignant hyperthermia*

Malignant hyperthermic reaction occurs most commonly during the general anesthesia period. However, malignant hyperthermia may occur or recur during the recovery period up to 48 to 72 hours postoperatively. Nurses should be familiar with the condition and be able to respond quickly and appropriately if necessary.

## Promoting Comfort

The literature states that the most commonly used nursing diagnosis is pain.[4] This is understandable, especially in the postoperative period. Pain is a complex process that involves sensory stimuli, neural processes, individual experiences, cultural background, and anxiety.

Racial background also influences individual perceptions of pain. Research indicates that whites have the highest tolerance to pain, blacks second, and Asians the lowest tolerance.[4]

Pain results in the stress response with accompanying changes in the cardiovascular system, hormonal release, anxiety, tension, and muscle contraction. From the patient's point of view the distress of postoperative pain is probably the most significant postoperative problem. Adequate and prompt pain relief is a critical nursing intervention. Effective management of pain begins with a trusting nurse-patient relationship. Involving patients in their pain management program is beneficial. The offer of support, objectivity, and reassurance assists in pain relief and increases the patient's ability to relax.

The amount of perceived control over pain influences the perception of the pain experience.[4] Active participation and empowerment can increase the effectiveness of a pain management program. In the immediate postanesthesia period, narcotic analgesics are given for pain when warranted, with the realization that pronounced depression of the respiratory, circulatory, or central nervous system may follow. Because the patient generally has not completely recovered from the effects of anesthesia, the first postoperative dose of a narcotic usually is reduced to about one half the dose to be received after full recovery from anesthesia. The goal is to keep the patient comfortable without overmedication. The nurse should adjust the dose and interval of medication until satisfactory pain relief is achieved. It is usually necessary to administer narcotics during the first 12 hours after major surgery. If severe pain is expected, medication should be offered to the patient at regular intervals around the clock to maintain effective blood levels.

Analgesics have greater effect if they are administered before pain becomes severe. One method to determine the severity of pain that a patient is experiencing is to use a pain-rating scale in which the patient rates pain level on a scale of 0 to 10.

Analgesics may be given by several methods. The intramuscular route may be used for patients with stable circulatory functions. If circulation is decreased, as with shock, medication given intramuscularly may remain in the tissue and then be absorbed suddenly when circulation is restored, leading to overdosage. The intravenous route is safer and faster and often is preferred.

One intravenous method that is widely used is the administration of narcotics by patient-controlled analgesia (PCA). The infusion control device can be set to administer a basal rate of medication, or the patient can receive a predetermined bolus of narcotic intravenously by activating a hand control when pain relief is desired. The effective use of PCA is based on the assumption that patients can best evaluate and manage their own pain. The mechanism is set to prevent repeated dosage at too-frequent intervals. Assessing and documenting the patient's response to the PCA therapy are nursing responsibilities.

Another method of administering analgesia is the delivery of the drugs directly into the epidural or subarachnoid space. Patient-controlled analgesia may also be administered via the epidural route. The catheter is inserted by an anesthesiologist. Epidural analgesia blocks pain transmission at the spinal cord level. Evidence is accumulating that epidural analgesia is the treatment of choice for controlling many types of pain, including postoperative pain. Epidural narcotics produce analgesia for 15 to 16 hours without significant respiratory depression or sympathetic, motor, or sensory disturbances. Epidural analgesia is highly effective for major orthopedic surgery of the lower extremities. Epidural catheters should be well secured with tape. To prevent dislodgment of the epidural catheter, great care must be taken in moving patients.

The amount of analgesic medication required by patients varies according to age and type of surgery. Numerous individual variables relate to pain perception and reaction. In general, after the first 48 to 72 hours following surgery, pain usually decreases in severity and may be controlled by a less potent analgesic. Physicians commonly write "prn" orders for different analgesics and doses, thus permitting the nurse to select the combination that best meets the patient's immediate needs.

Morphine sulfate and meperidine are commonly used narcotics. An alternative to narcotic analgesics is the use of NSAIDs to relieve postoperative pain. These drugs have the advantage over narcotics of not suppressing the cough center. In addition, NSAIDs do not affect the rate or depth of respirations. They may however, cause GI ulceration and bleeding.

Pain is often accompanied by anxiety. Nonpharmacological methods for managing pain and anxiety are helpful adjuncts to traditional methods of pain management. In 1992 the Agency for Health Care Policy and Research (AHCPR) published guidelines for managing pain using a holistic and interdisciplinary approach. The most effective method of pain control involves both pharmacological and nonpharmacological interventions (Research Box).[7] Inadequate pain management can lead to prolonged healing time, increased length of stay, and patient dissatisfaction.[7]

### Promoting Urinary Elimination

Urinary output is closely monitored after surgery until normal urinary function is reestablished. A urinary output of at least 30 ml per hour is required to maintain adequate kidney function, but 50 ml per hour is desirable. Urinary output typically is less than fluid intake during the first 24 hours because of the fluid shifts that occur in response to the stress of surgery. In addition, the specific gravity of the urine will be high. The bladder is palpated for distention when output is low to identify possible urinary retention.

Initial postoperative voiding may be facilitated by measures such as offering fluids, getting the patient up to the bathroom or commode as permitted, running water in the bathroom, pouring water over the perineum, and ensuring the patient time and privacy. If these measures are not effective, urinary catheterization may be required. An indwelling catheter may be necessary if the inability to void persists. Indwelling catheters are inserted intraoperatively before certain procedures, such as pelvic surgery, that commonly are complicated by pelvic edema and urinary retention. Meticulous catheter care is imperative. Fluids by mouth are encouraged as soon as they can be tolerated. Increasing the patient's fluid volume aids in "flushing" the bladder.

**research**

Reference: Heiser RM et al: The use of music during the immediate postoperative recovery, *AORN J* 65(4):777, 1997.

The purpose of this study was to determine the differences between patients who listened to music intraoperatively during the last 30 minutes of the procedure and postoperatively during the first hour of the PACU stay and patients who did not listen to music during their surgical experience. Patients selected for the study were scheduled for elective lumbar microdiskectomy.

Researchers tested the following hypothesis: patients who listen to music will have lower pain and anxiety visual analog scores than the control group. The experimental group will experience greater satisfaction with their anesthetic experience and will request the use of music during future surgical procedures. The researchers also investigated the amount and type of analgesia used in the first 24 hours after surgery and differences in heart rate, blood pressure, and respiratory rates between the two groups.

Most patients in the experimental group stated that the music added relaxation, decreased anxiety, and functioned as a distracter. Many described the music as familiar and relaxing. Music therapy should be considered as an effective intervention to decrease pain and anxiety in the perioperative period.

### Maintaining Skin Integrity

Maintaining skin integrity is another nursing responsibility in the postoperative period. Interventions focus on the treatment of any reddened or affected areas reported by the perioperative nurse, as well as the prevention of unnecessary pressure on vulnerable points of the body.

Suspicious or reddened areas must be monitored and treated. Positioning the body in proper alignment, padding bony prominences, and avoiding weight or pressure on extremities are effective interventions. Turning a patient frequently in the early postoperative period until the person is able to turn independently also is important.

Linens should be changed as often as necessary to avoid the problem of having skin exposed to moisture for prolonged periods. Skin exposed to moisture from blood or body fluid drainage should be cleansed and dried as quickly as possible. Dressings should be reinforced to contain drainage.

Special attention should be given to the elderly patient, who is extremely vulnerable to skin breakdown as a result of loss of skin elasticity and diminished subcutaneous fat. Pressure against or weight on any area of the body and shearing forces against the skin during movement should be avoided.

### Relieving Nausea and Vomiting

To prevent possible aspiration, the patient who is vomiting should be positioned in a side-lying position. Frequent oral care is provided. When vomiting has subsided, and unless contraindicated, sucking on ice chips, sipping clear liquids, or eating small amounts of dry solid food may relieve the patient's nausea. Antiemetics such as ondansetron (Zofran), trimethobenzamide hydrochloride (Tigan), or prochlorperazine dimaleate (Compazine) may be administered by injection. If vomiting is caused by gastric distention, a nasogastric tube may be passed to drain stomach contents. Because vomiting can be a sign of drug idiosyncrasy, the presence of other side effects should be carefully assessed and the pattern of vomiting in relation to the administration of drugs noted. Accurate recording of intake and output of fluids and electrolyte balance is important.

#### *Relieving hiccoughs*

Hiccoughs may be relieved by having the patient rebreathe carbon dioxide at 5-minute intervals by inhaling and exhaling into a paper bag held tightly over the nose and mouth. Aspiration of stomach contents will stop hiccoughs caused by gastric dilation. Chlorpromazine hydrochloride (Thorazine) is used to treat mild cases of hiccoughs and is theorized to reduce hypersensitivity of the phrenic nerve.

#### *Relieving abdominal distention*

Ambulation is one of the most effective means for stimulating peristalsis and expelling flatus. Ambulation usually is begun and encouraged as early as permissible. Dilation of the stomach can be relieved by aspiration of fluid or gas with a nasogastric tube. Hot or cold liquids tend to cause gas buildup and thus should be avoided when peristalsis is sluggish; ice chips do not have the same effect because the water warms before it reaches the stomach.

## Preventing Wound Infection

Adherence to standard precautions and meticulous wound care are major components of nursing interventions to prevent infection. Interventions to prevent wound infection are necessary throughout the postoperative course. An expected outcome is that wounds will remain clean, dry, and intact. Frequent assessment of dressings and accurate recording of findings are vital in the immediate postoperative period. The surgeon must be notified immediately if signs of complications are noted.

### Caring for the wound

Meticulous care of the surgical incision is an important nursing measure that facilitates wound healing. When a surgical wound site is redressed or treated, strict aseptic technique must be scrupulously followed.

There is a closed connection between drains and drainage bags or suction ports. The primary purpose of catheters, tubes, and drains is to permit the escape of body fluids that may be harmful to a patient if allowed to accumulate within a body cavity. Fluids are removed by either gravity or mechanical means. All drains should be observed frequently in the early postoperative period. Accurate recording regarding the amount and character of output from drains is critical. Excessive or abnormal drainage should be reported to the surgeon immediately. (Commonly used drains are discussed in Chapter 19.)

Antibiotics commonly are ordered as prophylaxis against infection. Administration of antibiotics must take place at the scheduled times to maintain adequate blood levels.

Hemorrhage can interfere with wound healing. The best intervention for hemorrhage is early detection. When bleeding is noted on a dressing, the amount can be outlined with a pen and rechecked at 10- to 15-minute intervals for signs of change. If bleeding is profuse, measures to control it are instituted. For example, a pressure dressing can be applied over an existing dressing. In addition, constant monitoring of vital signs is required. A patient who is bleeding internally or in profuse amounts usually is returned immediately to surgery, where the incision is opened and the bleeding vessel is ligated.

### Treating wound dehiscence and evisceration

A wound dehiscence or evisceration disrupts healing. If either of these occurs, the surgeon is notified immediately. The patient is placed in a low Fowler's position, kept quiet, instructed not to cough, and provided with emotional support. Protruding viscera are covered, preferably with a warm, sterile saline dressing. Interventions to treat shock are initiated if signs and symptoms of shock are present. (See Chapter 17.) A minor wound dehiscence may be either resutured or allowed to remain open and heal by secondary intention. In the presence of infection or drainage, the wound usually is left open. The treatment for evisceration is immediate closure of the wound under local or general anesthesia.

## Relieving Anxiety

On awakening from anesthesia, the patient needs frequent orientation to place and reassurance of not being alone. The patient also needs to know that the operation is over and that recovery from anesthesia is satisfactory. Reassurance should be offered that family or significant others have been notified of the patient's safe arrival in the recovery room. Careful explanations of procedures should be given even when it appears that the patient is not alert. The need for privacy should be considered at all times. The patient who receives this type of support usually recovers from anesthesia faster, with fewer complications, and with less incisional pain. The patient who has had regional anesthesia needs the same considerations and reassurance that sensation and movement in the extremities will return.

The environment of a postanesthesia unit is sometimes noisy and hectic. Florence Nightingale first noted that unnecessary noise is detrimental to patients.[7] Patient care needs change swiftly and sometimes dramatically. Among the many challenges for the postanesthesia nurse is the incorporation of caring practices into planning. A balance of caring and technological skills provides a safe and supportive approach to patient care. Choosing to share positive information, using nonstressful words and touch, and promoting comfort can help relieve patient anxiety.

Pain and anxiety are often closely related. One method of controlling stress, anxiety, and the muscle tension associated with pain is relaxation techniques. To promote the effectiveness of relaxation techniques, the patient should be in a quiet environment, have an object to contemplate, and assume a comfortable position. Persons who indicate a need to control their pain, display a tense posture, and suffer from muscle spasms may benefit most from relaxation techniques. Postoperatively, questioning the patient regarding the past use of relaxation techniques and demonstration of the technique accompanied by written or visual instruction facilitates positive results with the use of relaxation. Pain management techniques should be initiated before the pain becomes too severe to control. The PACU environment, which is usually very busy and sometimes noisy, may contribute to anxiety and pain. Dimming the lights, providing privacy, soothing music, and involving family when feasible may alleviate some stress associated with the environment. According to research, short relaxation techniques such as deep, slow, rhythmic breathing and jaw relaxation are the most effective techniques for postoperative and elderly patients.[6] Relaxation techniques are effective methods of managing anxiety by decreasing the responsiveness of the sympathetic nervous system. The most effective techniques involve focusing on a repetitive word, phrase, or action; disregarding other thoughts; and relaxing muscles.[5,15] In addition to relieving anxiety, relaxation techniques have decreased postoperative pain, decreased the amount of analgesics required and thus lessened serious side effects, decreased length of stay, and increased patients' coping methods (see the Research Box).[15]

### *Supporting exploration of concerns*

Later in the recovery period, taking the time to sit down with the surgical patient and discuss the person's concerns is just as important a nursing action in many instances as any of the interventions for physical care. Time must be allotted for this practice. With the trend toward ambulatory surgery, early hospital discharge, and downsizing, place and time constraints exist for opportunities for effective nurse-patient interaction in addressing some issues. Finding innovative methods to effectively meet patients' psychosocial needs in today's health care environment is a challenge to the perioperative nurse. Follow-up phone calls may help address the need.

### *Including the family*

Family needs also must be considered. The family is kept informed of the patient's postoperative progress. Information that can be shared with family members helps lessen their anxiety.

The level of anxiety can be reduced in postoperative adult patients by allowing family visitation. Family visitation early in the postoperative period can alleviate fears, enhance communication between health care personnel and family members, and prepare family members regarding discharge or transfer. Policies regarding visitors need to be flexible to accommodate persons of diverse cultures.

**research**

Reference: Tusek D et al: A significant advance in the care of patients undergoing elective colorectal surgery, *Dis Colon Rectum* 40(2):172, 1997.

The study explored the effects of guided imagery used during the perioperative period on patients undergoing colorectal surgical procedures. The sample included 130 patients between the ages of 18 and 75 years (average age 40). Exclusion criteria included a history of substance abuse, chronic pain, morphine intolerance, psychiatric history, and inability to use a PCA pump. The control group received routine postoperative care consisting of intravenous PCA. The experimental group received routine postoperative care in addition to listening to guided imagery tapes for 3 days preoperatively.

Results indicated that analgesic requirements were significantly lower in the control group, as was length of time to the first bowel movement. Patients who used guided imagery techniques reported less pain and anxiety each day. They also reported that the tapes helped them during the perioperative period. Other responses included beliefs that the tapes improved the quality of sleep and enhanced recovery.

Guided imagery is one method of empowering surgical patients during an otherwise seemingly powerless experience. It is a simple and inexpensive intervention to add to perioperative protocols.

Most surgeons discuss the results of the operation with the family immediately after the surgery and also visit the patient, briefly telling what was found and providing reassurance. Family members commonly are highly anxious about the patient's condition and may not perceive or understand all that the surgeon tells them. Patients often experience periods of amnesia during the hours when they first regain consciousness and may not remember what they have been told. To provide satisfactory answers to the patient's and family members' questions, the nurse needs to know what information was given. The family also needs to know what to expect when the patient returns to the unit and when the patient is ready for discharge.

## Discharge Needs and Home Care Considerations

It is important for the nurse to recognize that the patient who is discharged directly to home after surgery may be unable to absorb a great deal of information. Therefore a follow-up telephone call should be made by nursing personnel to complete both the education and evaluation. The nurse should also consider any cultural influences that may interfere with routine postoperative instructions. During this call the nurse can provide information and reinforce predischarge teaching. The nurse also can provide emotional support and referral if necessary. Usually an appointment is made for a follow-up examination in the surgeon's office or clinic within 1 to 2 weeks after discharge. Referrals to home health nurses, rehabilitation programs, support groups, and other health professionals also should be made on the basis of individual patient needs.

## EVALUATION

To evaluate the effectiveness of nursing interventions, compare patient behaviors with those stated in the expected patient outcomes. Successful achievement of patient outcomes for the surgical patient in the postoperative phase is indicated by:

1. Maintains patent airway, with lungs clear to auscultation
2. Maintains blood gases within normal limits and oxygen saturation 96% or above
3. Demonstrates effective cough without aspiration
4. Maintains regular pulse and stable blood pressure at preoperative levels
5. Injury
   a. Has no injuries or falls
   b. Is oriented to time, place, and person
   c. Is able to move all extremities
6. Has urine output greater than 30 ml per hour and no observable swelling or edema
7. Maintains normal body temperature
8. States that pain level is acceptable and shows no evidence of facial grimacing or guarding
9. Voids spontaneously within 8 to 10 hours after surgery
10. Displays intact skin
11. Has no nausea or vomiting and tolerates oral fluids
12. Shows wound healing without evidence of dehiscence or infection

13. States that anxiety is relieved and indicates that patient and caregivers are confident and capable of providing needed care after discharge.

Many institutions have developed surveys that ask patients to evaluate the care and attention they received while they were hospitalized. These postoperative surveys can be a valuable quality improvement tool. Feedback obtained from the surveys has been used to modify standards of patient care.

The postanesthesia patient care record is a legal document and should be clear and concise. Standards of care or clinical pathways for care should be written and implemented. A written care plan reflecting the nursing process ensures that the attainment of outcomes and goals for patient care can be determined by the nursing team. Implementations or variations from the standard of care should be thoroughly recorded. Complete documentation portrays accountability for the care delivered to the patient.

Written information about the patient from one health care worker to another helps maintain continuity of care. Records can be used to identify what actually happened during a patient's surgical experience if a question arises at a later time. In addition, records may be used by researchers to collect retrospective data for a study. For these reasons, accurate documentation is extremely important.

## critical thinking QUESTIONS

1 An 81-year-old woman has been transferred to your unit from the PACU. She has undergone an exploratory laparotomy for bowel obstruction. She received general anesthesia and 1 U of packed cells intraoperatively. She has a history of congestive heart failure, hypertension, asthma, and rheumatoid arthritis. She has a Jackson-Pratt drain to self-suction and a nasogastric tube to continuous suction. Five percent dextrose in 0.45% saline is infusing via a central venous catheter at 100 ml per hour. Medication history includes digoxin 0.125 mg PO qd, Lasix 40 mg PO qd, Slo-Bid 60 mg PO bid, prednisone 20 mg PO qd, and lisinopril 20 mg PO qd. Describe the assessments you would make in priority order and the rationale for each. What laboratory tests would you expect to be ordered for the next few days? Provide the rationale for each. What complications is this patient most at risk of developing and why? Develop a postoperative plan of care for this patient.

2 A 54-year-old male patient is being discharged following a split-thickness skin graft to an ulcer on his foot. He has type I diabetes. He is a sales manager and will have to be off work for at least 2 months. How might his medical condition and prolonged recovery time affect his role performance within his family and job? Describe how normal wound healing might be altered for this patient. What assessments must be made before his discharge? What information would you give him as home-going instructions?

3 Compare and contrast the immediate and ongoing care of the postoperative patient.

## chapter SUMMARY

- The postoperative phase of the surgical experience begins with the patient's arrival in the postanesthesia care unit and continues until the patient returns home.
- The goal of the postoperative phase is the patient's return to physiological homeostasis that is the same as or improved over the preoperative state.
- The postanesthesia care nurse must understand the patient's risks for postoperative complications and be prepared to intervene when they occur.
- To assess, plan, and implement care of the postoperative patient, preoperative information must be ascertained and compared with postoperative data.
- Assessing respiratory status is crucial during the immediate postoperative period. Both a patent airway and adequate respiratory function should be ascertained.
- Continuous monitoring of oxygen saturation level is a necessary postoperative intervention and can be easily achieved by the use of pulse oximetry.
- Prolonged somnolence and muscle weakness are major nervous system complications that may occur in the immediate postoperative period. Prevention of injury is foremost at this time.
- Hypotension and the occurrence of cardiac dysrhythmias are the most commonly encountered cardiovascular complications in the immediate postanesthesia period.
- Excessive blood volume and body fluid loss during surgery requires postoperative intravenous replacement.
- Tympanic temperature measurement is an accurate indication of core body temperature. It is fast and noninvasive and presents little discomfort to the patient.
- Changes associated with the aging process, prevalence of chronic diseases, alterations in fluid and nutrition status, and increased use of pharmacological treatments are factors that influence the care requirements of geriatric patients in the postoperative period. Geriatric patients are at a greater risk for respiratory and cardiovascular complications and are susceptible to inadvertent hypothermia in the postoperative period.
- Meticulous care of the surgical incision is an important nursing intervention that facilitates wound healing.
- Effective management of pain begins with a trusting nurse-patient relationship. Providing adequate postoperative pain relief is essential. Relaxation techniques are effective adjuncts to pain management. Narcotics or NSAIDs may be used.
- Among the many challenges for the postanesthesia nurse is the implementation of caring practices into a busy environment. A balance of caring and technological skills provides a safe and supportive approach to patient care.
- Family needs must be considered. Family members should be kept informed of the patient's postoperative progress.
- Cultural considerations are essential and should be integrated throughout the total postoperative period.

## References

1. Aker J: Immediate care in the postoperative period, *Curr Rev Post Anesth Care Nurses* 16(17):145, 1994.
2. Atkinson LJ, Fortunato N: *Berry and Kohn's operating room technique,* ed 8, St Louis, 1996, Mosby.
3. Clinical news: in postop rewarming, water is faster than air, *Am J Nurs* 97(3):10, 1997.
4. Atsberger DB: Relaxation therapy: its potential as an intervention for acute postoperative pain, *J Post Anesth Nurs* 10(1):2, 1995.

5. Good M: Relaxation techniques for surgical patients, *Am J Nurs* 95(5):39, 1995.
6. Good M: A comparison of the effects of jaw relaxation and music on postoperative pain, *Nurs Res* 44(1):52, 1995.
7. Heiser RM et al: The use of music during the immediate postoperative recovery period, *AORN J* 65(4):777, 1997.
8. Hoot Martin JL, Larsen PD, Hazen SE: Interpreting laboratory values in elderly surgical patients, *AORN J* 65(3): 621, 1997.
9. Kaempfe G, Goral VJ: Monitoring postop patients, *RN* 59(7):31, 1996.
10. Kelly M: Surgery, anesthesia, and the geriatric patient, *Geriatr Nurs* 16(5):213, 1995.
11. Lusis SA: The challenges of nursing elderly surgical patients, *AORN J* 64(6):954, 1996.
12. Meeker MH, Rothrock JC: *Alexander's care of the patient in surgery,* ed 10, St Louis, 1995, Mosby.
13. Miller J, Moore K, Schofield A, Ng'andu N: A study of discomfort and confusion among elderly surgical patients, *Orthop Nurs* 15(6): 27, 1996.
14. Pasero CL: Managing postoperative pain in the elderly, *Am J Nurs* 96(10):39, 1996.
15. Tusek DL et al: Guided imagery: a significant advance in the care of patients undergoing elective colorectal surgery, *Dis Colon Rectum* 40(2):172, 1997.
16. Winslow EH, Lane LD, Woods RJ: A review of relevant physiology, research and practice, *Heart Lung* 24(4):263, 1993.
17. Winslow EH, Jacobson AE: Preop fluid bolus reduces adverse surgical effects, *Am J Nurs* 97(3):62, 1997.

# chapter 21 Emergency Care Environment

KIM BENDER EGGLESTON

## objectives *After studying this chapter, the learner should be able to:*

1. Discuss the unique challenges of nursing practice in an emergency care environment.
2. List nursing interventions that increase patient and staff safety in the emergency department.
3. Identify the components of an initial trauma assessment.
4. Describe the principles of collaborative management of the trauma patient.
5. Discuss the role of the emergency department nurse in caring for a person who was sexually assaulted.
6. Outline the guidelines for care of victims of domestic violence.

Emergency nursing is a diverse and multidimensional specialty area of professional nursing. It crosses all age groups and includes care that ranges from disease management and injury prevention to lifesaving resuscitative measures. Astute decision-making abilities, analytic and scientific inquiry, and critical thinking skills are very much a part of the practice of the emergency department (ED) nurse.

The demands on emergency nursing continue to grow and become more challenging as health care changes. A continued increase in the incidence of violence and the numbers of uninsured, and the advent of managed care provide for a challenging practice arena. Managed care is one of the primary financing mechanisms for health care and is of great importance in current ED practice as insurance programs increasingly dictate who receives care, what care can be provided, and which care settings may be used. The challenge of providing health care to the large numbers of uninsured and underinsured individuals and families falls heavily on departments of emergency services, which are commonly used in lieu of a primary care provider. Combined market forces and legislation seem to indicate that managed care payment mechanisms will continue to be a major force in health care for the foreseeable future.

This chapter on emergency care provides an overview of the unique environment of emergency nursing, triage practice, trauma assessment, and the impact of violence on emergency nursing practice.

## SCOPE OF PRACTICE FOR EMERGENCY NURSING

The Emergency Nursing Scope of Practice was approved by its association in 1988 and uses the same framework as the American Nurses' Association's social policy statement.[7] The scope of emergency nursing practice encompasses assessment, diagnosis, treatment, and evaluation of physical and psychosocial problems that may be episodic, primary, or acute.[8] Treatment of these problems may require minimal care or lifesaving measures, patient and family education, and appropriate referral. The quality of practice depends on the nurse's psychomotor, interpersonal, and decision-making skills. Care is delivered in a variety of settings, including the acute care facility, the prehospital setting, or during air or ground transport. Some of the many characteristics unique to emergency nursing practice are listed in Box 21-1. (See also the accompanying Research Box.)

Emergency nursing activities occur in a sequential arrangement or flow pattern based on the acuity of the person's condition. Emergency nursing includes provision of care to persons whose problems range from nonacute to life threatening. In fact, most persons who request ED service are ambulatory and have nonacute conditions; therefore many EDs have developed a specific care area for these persons. Some hospitals use the terms *fast track* or *urgent care* to identify a designated area in or near the ED for persons with nonacute conditions. These areas may be open only after physicians' offices have closed, or they may provide quick service 12 to 24 hours a day. Fast track or urgent care areas have been developed because these care environments are less expensive treatment areas. Persons treated in these areas require less time with the health care staff because of the nature of their signs and symptoms. Regardless of whether EDs are designed to separate the nonacute from the acutely ill person, and regardless of ability to pay, every person requesting care must be evaluated on arrival.[11]

## TRIAGE

Because the needs of patients seeking care in EDs vary greatly, triage systems have been implemented. This initial triage assessment usually is completed by an ED nurse. *Triage* is a continuous and highly visible process in the ED today. The word *triage* is derived from the French word *trier,* meaning "to pick out or sift."[17] The triage system is used to identify those patients whose condition is most seriously compromised so that they are the first to receive medical intervention. The choosing, sorting out, and placing of priorities on care have been practiced since patient care began and have been used

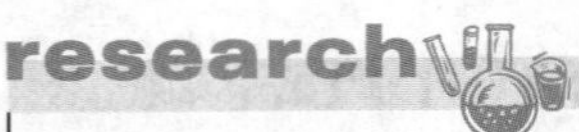

Reference: Kidd P, Sturt P: Developing and evaluating an emergency nursing orientation pathway, *J Emerg Nurs* 21(6):521, 1995.

An orientation pathway was developed to evaluate orientee clinical decision-making skills. The pathway was developed using principles of case management by preceptors who identified critical indicators of role performance in the emergency department. These indicators were organized into categories based on Benner's theory of clinical knowledge development. Four proficiency levels were developed for each category. The progress in orientation of seven new graduates was compared with the expected transitions identified by the expert preceptors. Orientees progressed faster than expected in all categories. It took 8 weeks for an orientee to attain the highest proficiency level in all categories. The fastest progress was made in the category "accurately evaluates patient responses." The slowest progress was made in the category "safety in blood and drug administration."

extensively in disasters and wars. A standardized four-color-coded triage system (used during disasters) quietly communicates to all health care providers the priority of treatment (Box 21-2). However, triage as a systematic method to be used by health care personnel in both prehospital situations and EDs has come into its own.

The most important function of triage is to provide an initial assessment of patients. This assessment is the basis for the assigning of a triage urgency category.

Persons who need to be seen immediately have an emergent or life-threatening situation; persons who need to be seen as soon as possible have an urgent condition that has the potential of becoming a life-threatening situation; and persons who can be seen as time allows have nonurgent conditions, with no life-threatening symptoms at the time of presentation and no symptoms that typically become life threatening. This system of prioritization of patients is used by the Emergency Medical Service (EMS) system. The use of these common terms provides for understanding of the situation and more uniform prehospital and in-hospital communication and care. Fast track or urgent care areas treat patients with urgent or nonurgent conditions. Persons with emergent conditions are seen in the usual ED area.

To increase efficiency and best outcome for patients, many EDs have developed a chest pain center (CPC) within their department. Chest pain centers represent an organized and systematic approach to the evaluation, diagnosis, and treatment of patients with chest pain.[3] The goal of the CPC is the immediate diagnosis and treatment of acute myocardial infarction. Patients are triaged directly into the CPC with a triage category of emergent. Box 21-3 presents a listing of the typical emergent, urgent, and nonurgent complaints of persons seeking care at a level I trauma center over a 24-hour period. Level I trauma centers are usually based in large metropolitan teaching hospitals. (See p. 556 for a description of the levels of trauma care.)

**box 21-1** *Characteristics Unique to Emergency Nursing Practice*

1. Assessment, diagnosis, and treatment of emergent, urgent, and nonurgent individuals of all ages
2. Triage and prioritization
3. Disaster preparedness
4. Stabilization and resuscitation
5. Crisis intervention
6. Provision of care in uncontrolled or unpredictable environments

Modified from Emergency Nurses Association: *Standards of emergency nursing practice*, ed 2, St Louis, 1991, Mosby.

**box 21-2** *Four-Color–Coded Disaster Triage System*

**0—BLACK: DEAD**

**1—RED: CRITICAL OR LIFE-THREATENING**
These victims have a reasonable chance of survival only if they receive immediate treatment. Emergency treatment is initiated immediately and continued during transportation. This category includes victims with respiratory insufficiency, cardiac arrest, hemorrhage, and severe abdominal injury.

**2—YELLOW: SERIOUS**
These victims can wait for transportation after they receive initial emergency treatment. They include victims with immobilized closed fractures, soft-tissue injuries without hemorrhage, and burns on less than 40% of the body.

**3—GREEN: MINIMAL**
Victims in this category are ambulatory, have minor tissue injuries, and may be dazed. They can be treated by nonprofessionals and held for observation if necessary.

### Triage and Managed Care

All ED health care providers must be well informed about the provisions of the Consolidated Omnibus Reconciliation Acts (COBRA) and the Emergency Medical Treatment and Active Labor Act (EMTALA), which outline guidelines for service provision and reimbursement in emergency departments. The EMTALA provisions require that each patient who comes to the ED must receive a screening examination to determine whether an emergency condition exists. Medical screening, often an extension of triage, but a separate process, must be thorough enough to facilitate determination of the patient's condition.[6] Many patients come to the ED without preauthorization from their managed care organization. The responsibility for providing a medical screening examination and securing preauthorization falls on the ED staff.

### Triage and Computerized Tracking

A universal concern in all EDs is patient flow. Tracking of patients provides clinicians with an automated patient locator

**box 21-3** *Presenting Complaints of Persons Seeking Emergent, Urgent, or Nonurgent Care at a University Teaching Hospital Over a 24-Hour Period*

Abdominal pain
Abdominal problem
Alcohol intoxication
Assault
Asthma
Back pain
Behavioral problem
Broken tooth
Cardiopulmonary arrest
Cardiovascular problem (chest pain)
Cough
Depression
Diarrhea
Difficulty breathing
Dizziness
Earache
Electrical shock
Environmental injury (heat stroke)
Eye injury
Eye problem (blurred vision)
Eye problem (infection)
Eye problem (conjunctivitis/pink eye)
Fever
Foreign body removal
Genital problem (sore and discharge)
GI bleeding (black stools)
GI bleeding (bloody stools)
GI bleeding (vomiting blood)
Head injury
Head wound (cut/scrape)
Headache
Head/neck problem (stiff neck)
Hernia
Insect bite
Joint pain
Lower extremity injury (sprain/strain)
Lower extremity problem (swelling, no history of injury)
Lower extremity wound (cut)
Meningitis
Multiple injuries (auto accident)
Multiple problems (achy, dizzy, tired)
Multiple trauma
Multiple wounds (cuts, scrapes from fall)
Nausea/vomiting
Neck injury
Neck wound
Neurological problem (confusion)
Neurological problem (weak one side, unable to walk)
Nosebleed
Overdose
Palpitations (heart racing, skipping beats)
Pregnancy problem (abdominal pain)
Pregnancy problem (bleeding)
Rash
Respiratory problem (drowning)
Seizures
Shortness of breath
Sick (feel bad, tired, irritable)
Trunk injury
Trunk wound
Unresponsive
Upper extremity injury
Upper extremity problem (swelling, inflammation)
Upper extremity wound (cut)
Urinary problem (burning, pain, frequency, blood in urine)
Vaginal bleeding (nonpregnant)
Vomiting
Weakness
Wheezing

board. Patient name, arrival time, chief complaint, and caregiver names are available on the screen. Registration and triage staff are always aware of open beds and the location of patients via the patient tracking systems.

Tracking systems take advantage of abbreviations, symbols, color codes, and icons to note current patient status. Many systems also use color codes to identify which caregivers have already seen a patient, as well as admission or discharge pending information. The tracking system can also be used to improve efficiency in gathering triage information during initial patient assessment and is an excellent tool for research and analysis of department utilization. Computerized tracking also improves communication among department personnel.

## CRITICAL PATHWAYS IN EMERGENCY DEPARTMENTS

Time tracking of patients in the ED is essential for many reasons, such as to ensure quality of care practice, to track and trend workload activity, and to have appropriate staffing to match workload. Many hospitals are using critical (clinical) pathways to achieve these goals. Use of critical pathways in the ED increases the consistency and rapidity of diagnosis and treatment, with earlier initiation being key to effectiveness.[13] For example, a person with an arm injury and signs of a fracture will have an x-ray examination to determine the type of fracture. A critical pathway for this type of patient identifies the x-ray examination as the major diagnostic activity to be accomplished and a time frame for completion, such as 20 minutes after the assessment and evaluation by the ED physician and the ED nurse. Once mutually identified interventions, outcomes, and times are determined for a particular patient population or diagnosis, the nurse can assume that the interventions and outcomes should be completed within the time period. Although critical pathways are tools and guidelines, they provide standardization of care, consistency with interventions, and a means to evaluate effectiveness of care. Thus critical pathways promote quality of care, increase effectiveness of care, increase staff communication, and increase staff and patient satisfaction.

## COMMUNICATION

Maintaining effective communication in any clinical setting is a challenge. However, in the ED the challenge is compounded because of the number of health care personnel involved in the care of the patient and because of the emergent situation. All health care providers should keep in mind that communication is the process through which the patient-clinician relationship develops. The patient may base his or her perception of care provided on the communication and interpersonal skills demonstrated by the nurse, as well as the level of the nurse's competence.

Regardless of the type or location of the emergent incident, one extremely important communication need is the ability to access emergency help. All agencies and communities that provide health care have a code or system that activates a call for help within an extremely short period of time. Most communities in the United States (but not all) have a 911 access number for activating the EMS system. The chain of survival following emergent injuries requires excellent communication skills to access care and initiate appropriate emergency services.

Managing violent situations in the ED also requires the nurse to use excellent communication skills. Nurses need to be able to deescalate a pattern of violent behavior before it is out of control. Appropriate techniques to deescalate such a situation include a calm and interested demeanor, a lowered and controlled voice, and a willingness to avoid interrupting the verbal responses of those involved. If a nurse finds it impossible to apply these communication skills in a particular situation, another nurse may be asked to take over or assist.

Other communication principles to apply in an environment of uncontrolled behavior include the following:[9]

1. Keep communication on the here and now, and make no promises.
2. Keep hands at waist level and open toward the other person to demonstrate nonverbally that you are hiding nothing.
3. Use the rule of five, that is, no more than five words in a sentence with all words less than five letters. For example, "Stand still now."
4. Communicate only requests that are achievable.
5. Avoid commands that include "should not" and "cannot" statements.

Consistent use of these principles can decrease the potential for uncontrolled behavior and improve communication.

## ENVIRONMENT

The nurse working in the emergency arena focuses on controlling environmental factors that can infringe on quality care. Noise is a major environmental factor and a significant stressor in the ED. Nurses must make an effort to work quietly and to identify this approach (quiet work) as a standard for the ED. As new EDs are being constructed, soundproofing is being included whenever possible. However, many other noise-controlling behaviors can be implemented, including the following:

1. Setting all telephones on soft ring
2. Equipping all dispatch radios with telecommunication devices that limit the broadcast to one person (e.g., earphones, telephones)
3. Setting alarms on monitors as low as safely possible
4. Closing doors quietly and as appropriate
5. Use of pagers (on vibrate mode) to locate staff, rather than overhead paging

Implementation of these few activities greatly enhances the quality of the caregiving environment.

**box 21-4 Steps to Increase Security in the Emergency Department**

1. Limited access (should be as few entrances to the ED as possible)
2. Metal detectors
3. Security personnel at entrances
4. Secure triage areas
5. Placement of panic buttons
6. Video cameras
7. Enforce visitor control measures

### Emergency Environment and Violence

Treating critically ill and injured patients is stressful enough without the addition of violent acts. Violence is often triggered by stressors that patients and families are unable to cope with effectively. The two biggest triggers for violence are delays in treatment and frustration with a particular situation. Fear is often a prime motivator for hostility.[2] Other environmental triggers are unpleasant waiting areas, lack of access to refreshments, insufficient and uncomfortable seating, and lack of feedback to patients and significant others about a patient's condition or progress. Attention to these details deescalates the potential for violent behavior and provides a safer working environment.

External violence has also increased in the ED setting in association with the continued increase in street violence, family violence, and drug and alcohol use. Nurses are often called on to manage both the victim and the victimizer in the health care setting. Health care providers always need to be extremely aware of their environment and its potential for violence. Triage nurses and registration staff are at greater risk because they are often situated at the entrance of the ED and in a more isolated spot. Steps to increase security within the ED are reviewed in Box 21-4.

## LEGAL AND FORENSIC CONSIDERATIONS

Nurses must be aware of state and local regulations that require mandatory reporting of cases of suspected child and elder abuse, accidental deaths, and suicides. Each ED has written policies and procedures to assist nurses and other health care providers make appropriate reports.

Physical evidence is real, tangible, or latent matter that can be visualized, measured, or analyzed. Emergency department nurses are often called on to collect evidence, and all hospitals should have policies governing the collection of forensic evidence. It is of utmost importance that chain of custody be followed to ensure the integrity and credibility of the evidence.

The chain of custody is the pathway that evidence follows from the time it is collected until it has served its purpose in the legal investigation of an incident.

## TOPICS OF CONCERN IN EMERGENCY CARE

### TRAUMA

Trauma is the most common cause of death in persons younger than 40 years of age and is the fourth leading cause of death in persons of all age groups. More than 60 million injuries occur annually in the United States. Unintentional injuries are a major source of morbidity and mortality in the United States; therefore accident prevention is a major public health goal.[18] The U.S. Public Health Service and the American Public Health Association actively promote accident prevention. National health care objectives for the year 2000 related to accidents, derived under the direction of the Department of Health and Human Services and the Public Health Service, are listed in Box 21-5. Suggestions for achieving these goals include the following:

1. Enacting laws
   a. Requiring use of vehicle safety belts and motorcycle helmets
   b. Requiring that handguns be designed to minimize the likelihood of accidental discharge, especially by children
   c. Requiring installation of sprinkler systems in residences where fire hazards exist
2. Increasing functional smoke detectors to at least one per floor of every residence
3. Teaching injury prevention and control in all schools
4. Requiring use of effective head, face, eye, and mouth protection for sports that pose risk of injury
5. Improving signs, signals, markings, and lighting of roads for increased visibility

#### Prevention of Trauma

Accidents are the underlying cause of trauma. Although accidents have no single cause, human error is a predominant factor. Onset of illness such as a cerebrovascular accident or myocardial infarction accounts for only a small percentage of accidents. More than one half of all accidents involving motor vehicles are the result of improper driving practices or human error. A much smaller percentage of accidents are caused by vehicle defects or poor road conditions. Alcohol is a factor in approximately 50% to 75% of all fatal motor vehicle crashes. Young drivers are significantly overrepresented in alcohol- and drug-related crashes. Illegal drugs, as well as many legally prescribed medications, can slow reaction time and contribute to the occurrence of accidents.

The home is a dangerous place. Falls account for about one half of the deaths that result from trauma in the home, and they are usually preventable. Falls commonly occur as persons, particularly the elderly, walk from room to room. Some falls are caused by heavily waxed floors, loose rugs, poor lighting, scattered toys, and other preventable conditions (Box 21-6). People fall from roofs, windows, high ladders, and steps, often because they have not used proper equipment or taken appropriate precautions.

**box 21-5 Healthy People 2000 *Objectives Related to Accidents***

1. Reduce deaths caused by unintentional injuries to no more than 29.3 per 100,000 people.
2. Reduce deaths from falls and fall-related injuries to no more than 2.3 per 100,000 people.
3. Reduce residential fire deaths to no more than 1.2 per 100,000 people.
4. Reduce drowning deaths to no more than 1.3 per 100,000 people.
5. Reduce deaths caused by motor vehicle crashes to no more than 1.5 per 100 million vehicle miles traveled (VMT) and 14.2 per 100,000 people.
6. Reduce deaths caused by alcohol-related motor vehicle crashes to no more than 5.5 per 100,000 people.
7. Reduce deaths from work-related injuries to no more than 4 per 100,000 full-time workers.
8. Reduce work-related injuries resulting in medical treatment, lost time from work, or restricted work activity to no more than 6 cases per 100 full-time workers.
9. Increase use of helmets to at least 80% of motorcyclists and at least 50% of bicyclists.
10. Extend to 50 states laws requiring helmets for bicycle riders.
11. Increase use of safety belts and child safety seats to at least 85% of motor vehicle occupants.
12. Extend to 50 states laws requiring safety belt and motorcycle helmet use for all ages.
13. Increase the presence of functional smoke detectors to at least one on each habitable floor of all inhabited residential dwellings.
14. Extend to 20 states the capability to link emergency medical services, trauma systems, and hospital data.

Modified from US Department of Health and Human Services, Public Health Service: *Healthy people 2000: national health promotion and disease prevention objectives*, Washington, DC, 1990, US Government Printing Office.

Burns and other injuries result from improper use of solvents and cleaning agents. The number of electrical appliances used in the home has increased the danger of electrical shock and fire from overloaded circuits. Many persons die in fires caused by cigarette ashes dropped on furniture or rugs or discarded in waste containers, and by cigarettes that are dropped when the smoker falls asleep. Homeowners with older heating systems need to be encouraged to have these systems checked for gas leaks or other unsafe features. Members of a household should hold fire drills and know what to do if a fire occurs. Smoke alarms in kitchens, bedrooms, hallways, and basements should be considered essential.

Children are the victims of most accidental poisonings, although adults also are at risk. All poisonous substances should be kept in original containers, tightly capped, and *never* placed in containers such as soft-drink containers, drinking glasses, or cups. Medications should never be removed from the source bottle and placed in an unmarked bottle. Likewise,

**box 21-6** *Measures to Increase Home Safety*

**FLOORS**
Anchor large rugs and carpets.
Use nonskid backing on small rugs.
Avoid floor wax unless nonskid.

**STAIRS**
Ensure uniform height.
Use nonskid treads.
Mark risers with contrasting color.
Have strong hand rails at appropriate heights.
Have adequate lighting.

**BATHROOM**
Have hand rails in tub or shower and by toilet.
Use skidproof bath mats.
Apply treads in tub or shower floor.
Have shower seat for elderly or unstable persons.

**OTHER**
Have smoke alarms on every level.
Have working fire extinguisher in kitchen.
Have escape ladder if home is more than 1 story.
Secure all medications and cleaning products out of reach of children.

medications should never be taken from unmarked or poorly marked containers.

Each year in the United States 300,000 children are treated in EDs for bicycle injuries. Head injuries cause 67% of bicycle-related deaths, 68% of bicycle-related hospital admissions, and 33% of bicycle-related ED visits. Bicycle helmets are effective in decreasing bicycle-related head injuries. Emergency nurses are in a unique position to teach children proper bicycle safety.

Nurses should also alert the public to the importance of accident prevention. As participants in legislative activities, community committees, and community education, nurses must continually emphasize the role of human error and violence in trauma. Legislative initiatives focus on prevention as the primary method for decreasing the incidence, effects, and related costs of trauma to society.

### Good Samaritan Statute

Nurses may encounter trauma situations as bystanders or because of trauma to family members. When an off-duty nurse happens on an accident, an ethical and moral, if not a legal, duty to stop and render assistance exists. To encourage professionals to help accident victims, the legislatures of all states have passed statutes that grant health care professionals immunity from liability for negligent acts. These statutes, named after the biblical "Good Samaritan," state that a health care professional who stops and aids accident victims without compensation will not be liable for untoward results related to his or her acts.

There is, of course, an exception to the Good Samaritan statute. The law does not exempt a nurse from acts that constitute gross negligence. The statute states that if care was rendered in good faith and an emergency existed, the nurse will be free from liability. If, however, the nurse acts willfully, with gross negligence, a judgment of liability is possible.

### Trauma Centers

Trauma centers are classified according to national designations that are implemented by state rules and regulations. Facilities are classified as level I, level II, or level III trauma centers. Level I–designated facilities are usually tertiary referral centers located in large metropolitan areas and have a strong commitment to manage all types of trauma and emergencies. To offset the cost of the trauma service, as well as to ensure that clinical skills are maintained at a high level, at least 1000 trauma patients per year are treated. A level I trauma center must have clinicians and specialists immediately available 24 hours a day. Level II trauma facilities have similar characteristics, with the exception of in-house availability of specialists. Specialists are on call and must be available within an established time frame, usually 20 to 30 minutes.[4] Level III facilities are most often located in smaller institutions in communities in which a level I or II facility is unavailable. Level III centers have a responsibility to adequately stabilize trauma patients and follow clear and concise protocols for transfer to level I or II facilities. Facilities may also elect to have a nontrauma ED. This designation needs to be clearly communicated to the local community and EMS systems.

## COLLABORATIVE CARE MANAGEMENT OF TRAUMA

Emergency nurses and trauma systems can have an impact on patient outcomes by understanding the trimodal distribution of trauma deaths. The trimodal distribution illustrates the time frame in which the highest incidences of death occur after injury. The first peak occurs within minutes of injury, and death usually results from severe injury to the brain, upper spinal cord, heart, aorta, and other major blood vessels. The second peak occurs within 2 hours of injury and death is related to subdural or epidural hematomas, hemopneumothorax, ruptured spleen, lacerated liver, fractured femurs, or other injuries causing major blood loss. The third peak occurs days to weeks after the injury, and death usually results from complications such as sepsis and multiple organ failure.[15]

In the prehospital care setting nurses and paramedics (e.g., flight crews, rescue squad) can possibly reduce the first death peak with rapid and accurate lifesaving interventions. The second death peak is of importance to all ED nurses because it usually occurs in EDs.

Trauma is a "team sport." All members of the trauma team must work together efficiently and effectively to deliver optimal and comprehensive trauma care. The emergency nurse is an important member of the trauma team, and although he or

**box 21-7** *Nursing Trauma Care Activities*[15]

1. Perform a rapid, initial assessment of the trauma patient to identify injuries.
2. Institute appropriate lifesaving interventions.
3. Monitor patient responses to resuscitative efforts.
4. Communicate with other team members.
5. Perform as a patient advocate.
6. Document care of the trauma patient.

**box 21-8** *Trauma Assessment*

**PRIMARY SURVEY**

**A**irway
**B**reathing
**C**irculation
**D**isability
**E**xpose

**SECONDARY SURVEY**

Rapid head-to-toe assessment to determine all injuries

**box 21-9** *Severe Injuries Often Seen in Multiple Trauma*

Crushing and penetrating chest injuries
Crushing pelvic injuries
Spinal cord injuries
Multiple bone or soft-tissue injuries
Injuries causing hemorrhage with shock
Head injuries with decreasing level of consciousness

she may provide trauma care in a variety of settings, certain nursing functions are common to trauma patient care regardless of the setting (Box 21-7).

## Assessment

In trauma care a systematic process for initial assessment of the trauma patient is crucial for recognizing life-threatening conditions and initiation of appropriate interventions. This process is summarized in Box 21-8 in order of priority.

The initial assessment of all trauma patients (prehospital or ED) is based on specific priorities of care. The initial assessment is divided into primary and secondary surveys and should be completed within minutes unless resuscitative measures are needed. If life-threatening conditions exist, the assessment should not proceed until appropriate interventions are instituted to manage these problems.

The *primary survey* is an assessment of airway, cervical spine stability, breathing, and circulation. Disability (brief neurological assessment) is also part of the primary survey, as is exposing the patient to ensure assessment of all body areas. The *secondary survey* is a systematic head-to-toe assessment, with the objective of recognizing all injuries. If possible, additional information is gathered at this time, such as mechanism of injury, patient information, past medical history, allergies, tetanus status, and current medications. Figure 21-1 presents information on complete primary and secondary surveys.

The primary and secondary surveys begin the initial cycle of trauma care:[4]

1. Cycle I, field stabilization and resuscitation
2. Cycle II, in-house resuscitation and operative phase
3. Cycle III, critical care
4. Cycle IV, intermediate care
5. Cycle V, rehabilitation

Assessment, analysis, and action are ongoing in the trauma situation. Figure 21-2 (p. 560) depicts another portion of a trauma flow record, which reveals ongoing data that are recorded and demonstrates how some of the data from the primary and secondary surveys are combined to identify a trauma score. Other information being collected and recorded includes fluids, medications, blood or blood components administered, and the response of the patient; urine, blood, nasogastric, and other secretion loss; and cardiac rate and rhythm strips.

Analysis of data occurs concurrently with data collection. Some of the major judgments demanded of the nurse caring for the patient who has experienced trauma are presented next.

### *Multiple trauma*

Many trauma patients sustain *multiple trauma,* or injury to two or more body systems (Box 21-9). Motor vehicle crashes and falls, two major causes of trauma, may involve injury to the head or neck, an extremity, or the chest or abdominal area. Penetrating wounds to the chest wall may also affect the abdomen.

Persons with severe injuries require administration of intravenous fluids as soon as possible to prevent or control shock. In the field or ED, two or three large-bore intravenous catheters are placed to administer fluids and drugs. A central line may be inserted. An indwelling bladder catheter is inserted to monitor urinary output, as well as core body temperature.

In multiple trauma, the trauma team first focuses on the highest-priority problem of the particular patient and then moves to the next highest priority problem. Some problems such as penetrating wounds of the heart and aorta require immediate surgery. In other types of injury, if bleeding is controlled, surgery can be delayed while the team focuses on other problems. Although the trauma team has priorities, the needs of the total patient must be kept in focus.

The trauma team must always consider that treatment of one system may add to the problems of another injured system. For example, large amounts of fluid given to prevent or alter renal problems may compromise an inadequate

*Text continued on p. 562*

TRAUMA FLOW SHEET

**University of Virginia Medical Center**
**Emergency Medical Services**
**Trauma Flow Sheet**

**Patient Name Label**

**Date:**
**Arrival time:** __:__ Injury time __:__ Transferred from:
**Arrived by:** Helicopter: Squad: ALS/BLS
**Documentation received:** ER Record X-Rays CT Scan
**Mechanism:** **MVA:** Driver/Passenger Location in vehicle: Carseat Y/N
**Restraint:** Type: Vehicle damage:
**Vehicle speed:** High/Low Rollover Ejected Head-on T-Bone Rear-end
**Pedestrian struck/Fall:** Speed of vehicle/Height of fall:
**GSW/stab:** Caliber/Size of weapon: Distance:
**Other:**
**Past Medical HX:** Cardiac Renal Respiratory HTN Diabetic Other:
**Medications:**
**Allergies:** **Approx. wt:** kg
**Last menses:** **Last tetanus:**
**HPI:**

**Family Notification:** Notified/Enroute Phone consent Y/N Unable to notify Present
Contact person: Phone:

**Prehospital Intervention**
**Airway:** Oral/Nasal Combi Intubated
**$O_2$:** High flow Cannula None BVM
**IV Access:** GA Total fluid
**IV Access:** GA Total fluid
**Immobilized:** Y/N
**CPR:** Y/N Time begun: __:__
**Procedure:**
**Procedure:**

**Response**

| Service | Time | PTA | Name |
|---|---|---|---|
| Trauma res | __:__ | | |
| Trauma chief | __:__ | | |
| Neurosurgery | __:__ | | |
| Anesthesia | __:__ | | |
| Radiology | __:__ | | |
| E.R. Attending | __:__ | | |
| Surg. Attending | __:__ | | |

**Primary Survey**

**Airway:** Patent Obstructed
**Intervention:** Oral/Nasal Airway size MM
Intubated: Oral/Nasal size MM Depth CM
Procedure: Cric size MM Depth CM

**Breathing:** No Distress Distressed <10 >26 Assisted BVM/Vent
Expansion: Symmetrical/Asymmetrical Flail R/L Tracheal Deviation R/L
**Intervention:** $O_2$-high flow Assisted — BVM
Chest tube R/L Size FR Amt out CC
Chest tube R/L Size FR Amt out CC

**Circulation:** Skin — Warm Dry Moist Cool Pink Pale Cyanotic
Cap refill — Brisk Delayed None
Pulses Present: All present Deficit
Obvious Bleeding site
**Intervention:** Bleeding control
IV Access: Cent/Periph site GA NS/LR by
IV Access: Cent/Periph site GA NS/LR by
Procedure: Thoracotomy ACLS Protocol ATLS Protocol
Other:

**Disability:** Awake Responds to verbal Responds to pain Unresponsive

*Continued*

**fig. 21-1** Trauma flow sheet—primary and secondary surveys.

## Secondary Survey

Time: __:__

Date: ____

**Neuro:**
Mental status: A V P U
GCS: E__ V__ M__
Pupils: R __ L __ EOM: Intact Deficit ____
Drainage: Nasal Ears R/L Clear/Bloody None
Motor and sensory: Grossly intact Deficits ____
Other: ____

**Respiratory:**
Trachea: Midline Deviated R/L
Chest expansion: Symmetrical/Asymmetrical Flail R/L
Resp effort: Unlabored 12-18/min Distressed <10 >26 Absent
Breath sounds: R ____ L ____
Other: ____

**Cardiovascular:**
Skin: Warm/Dry Other ____
Cap refill: Normal Delayed
Pulses: All present Deficit ____
Heart sounds: S1, S2 Rub Murmur Other ____
Other: ____

**GI/GU:**
Abd: Soft/Nontender Flat Firm Rigid Distended Tender ____
Pelvis: Stable Unstable
Bowel sounds: Y/N Other ____
Rectal: Heme: +/− Tone: NL Flaccid
Blood at urinary meatus: Y/N
Other: ____
Skeletal: ____

**Interventions**

Time
__:__ Cardiac monitor
__:__ NIPB
__:__ Pulse oximeter
__:__ 12 LD EKG
__:__ Foley size __ Heme +/−
__:__ NG/OG size __ Heme +/−
__:__ ICP bolt
__:__ A-line- Rad R/L Fem R/L
__:__ DPL
__:__ Warming ____

**Radiology**

Time in Time out
__:__ __:__ Portable C-spine, Pelvis, Chest
__:__ __:__ Plain films
__:__ __:__ CT ____
__:__ __:__ A-Gram ____
__:__ __:__ Repeat ____
__:__ __:__ Repeat ____
__:__ C:spine cleared by: ____
__:__ C-collar removed by: ____
__:__ Backboard removed by: ____

Musculoskeletal

A = Abrasion
B = Burn
D = Deformity
E = Ecchymosis
F = Foreign body
H = Hematoma
L = Laceration
M = Amputation
P = Penetrating
T = Tenderness
Av = Avulsion

Rule of Nines

Burns

18 Front
18 Back
9 9
18 18

18
18 Front
18 Back
9 9
14 14

2 3 4 5 6 7 8 9

Pupil Gauge
Diameter by millimeter

**Glasgow Coma Score**

| | | |
|---|---|---|
| Eyes | Open spontaneously | 4 |
| | To verbal command | 3 |
| | To painful stimuli | 2 |
| | No response | 1 |
| Verbal | Oriented and converses | 5 |
| | Disoriented and converses | 4 |
| | Inappropriate words | 3 |
| | Incomprehensible sounds | 2 |
| | No response | 1 |
| Motor | Obeys command | 6 |
| | Localizes pain | 5 |
| | Flexion/Withdrawal | 4 |
| | Flexion/Abnormal | 3 |
| | Extension | 2 |
| | No response | 1 |

**Pediatric Coma Scale**

| | |
|---|---|
| **Eye Opening** | |
| Spontaneous | 4 |
| To verbal command or shout | 3 |
| To pain | 2 |
| No response | 1 |
| **Best Verbal Response** | |
| > 5 years | |
| Oriented and converses | 5 |
| Disoriented and converses | 5 |
| Inappropriate words | 3 |
| Incomprehensible sounds/garbled | 2 |
| No response | 1 |
| 2-5 years | |
| Appropriate words and phrases | 5 |
| Inappropriate words | 4 |
| Cries, screams | 3 |
| Moans, grunts | 2 |
| No response | 1 |
| 0-23 months | |
| Smiles, coos, cries appropriately | 5 |
| Cries | 4 |
| Inappropriate crying, screaming | 3 |
| Moans, grunts | 2 |
| No response | 1 |
| **Best Motor Response** | |
| Obeys commands | 6 |
| Localizes pain | 5 |
| Withdraws (normal flexion) | 4 |
| Abnormal flexion (decorticate) | 3 |
| Extension (decerebrate) | 2 |
| No response | 1 |

**fig. 21-1 cont'd** Trauma flow sheet.

**Intake**

| IV # | Time | Solution | Amt. | Amt. Inf. | PO |
|---|---|---|---|---|---|
| | | | | | |
| | | | | | |
| | | | | | |
| | | | | | |
| | | | | | |
| | | | | | |
| | | | | | |
| | | | | | |
| | | | | | |
| | | | | | |
| | | | | | |
| | | | | | |
| | | | | Total infused | |

**Blood Products**

| Bag # | Time | Product | Amt. | Site | Amt. Inf. |
|---|---|---|---|---|---|
| | | | | | |
| | | | | | |
| | | | | | |
| | | | | | |
| | | | | | |
| | | | | | |
| | | | | | |
| | | | | | |
| | | | | | |
| | | | | | |
| | | | | | |
| | | | | | |
| | | | | | |
| | | | | | |
| | | | | Total infused | |

**Output**

| Time | Urine | NGT | CT-RT | CT LT |
|---|---|---|---|---|
| | | | | |
| | | | | |
| | | | | |
| | | | | |
| Totals | | | | |
| | | | Total output | |

**Arterial Blood Gases**

| Time | PH | PC02 | P02 | HC03 | BE | Fi02 |
|---|---|---|---|---|---|---|
| | | | | | | |
| | | | | | | |
| | | | | | | |

**Labs** **Date:** ______

**Sent** **Time**

Type and cross X____ ____ : ____
Trauma bloods ____ : ____
UA/C&S ____ : ____
Beta HCG ____ : ____
Spun HCT ____ : ____
Repeat HCT: ____________ ____ : ____
Other: ____________ ____ : ____

Urine dip : Heme +/−
DPL : In________ Out________ Heme +/−
Other:____________

**Results**

| | | | | | |
|---|---|---|---|---|---|
| WBC | ____ | GLUC | ____ | CA | ____ |
| HGB | ____ | NA | ____ | MG | ____ |
| HCT | ____ | K | ____ | PHOS | ____ |
| PLT | ____ | CL | ____ | AMY | ____ |
| PT | ____ | C02 | ____ | BILI | ____ |
| PTT | ____ | BUN | ____ | BETA | ____ |
| Lactic acid | ____ | CR | ____ | ETOH | ____ |

**Belongings**

Clothes - Cut off
Shirt/Sweater
Pants
Dress/Skirt
Shoes/Socks
Underwear
Coat/Jacket
Wallet/Purse
Money $ ____________
Watch
Ring
Earring
Bracelet

Necklace
Hearing aid
Glasses
Contacts
Denture
Upper
Lower

Other ____________
Other ____________
Other ____________

**Disposition:** With patient, Police, To family, Morgue

Safe/Security Envelope # ____________

*Continued*

**fig. 21-2** Trauma flow sheet.

| Time | BP | HR | RR | SA 02 | T | GCS E | GCS V | GCS M | | | Meds | Notes | Date: |
|---|---|---|---|---|---|---|---|---|---|---|---|---|---|
| | | | | | | | | | | | | | |

| Time | MD Order | Time | MD Order |
|---|---|---|---|
| | DT .5 ml IM X 1 if >5 years since previous | | |
| | Gastrografen 1/4 oz in 240 cc H20 PO/NG q20′ until CT (or 10cc/kg - Peds) prn / as possible | | |
| | Ancef 1 gram IV now | | |
| | Foley to straight drainage | | |
| | Gastric tube to suction | | |
| | $O_2$ | | |
| | Fentanyl 50-100 mcg IV PRN pain with SBP >100 and RR > 16 | | |
| | Versed 1 - 2 mg IV PRN sedation with SBP > 100 and RR > 16 | | |

Primary RN signature ____________ Procedure RN ____________ Recording RN ____________

Disposition: Unit/Room ____________ Home time: ___ : ___

Report given to: ____________ RN. By: ____________ RN.

UPJ-960798/1074 Revised 12/95

**fig. 21-2 cont'd** Trauma flow sheet.

ventilatory system, leading to failure of both systems. Assessment, analysis, and action in trauma require focusing on these multiple-system problems.

### Airway and breathing

The rate, depth, and character of respirations provide clues to the presence of ventilatory, central nervous system (CNS), or metabolic problems. Most trauma victims breathe a little faster than normal (18 to 24 respirations per minute). In the presence of abnormal respiratory effort (nasal flaring; suprasternal, intercostal, or substernal retractions), the airway may be partially obstructed. The following respiratory findings suggest specific emergency care problems:

1. Rate
   a. Slow (below 10 respirations per minute): ventilatory or CNS problems
   b. Rapid (above 26 respirations per minute): hypoxia, acidosis, shock
2. Depth
   a. Shallow: shock, chest pain, chest injuries
   b. Deep: hypoxia, hypoglycemia, metabolic acidosis
3. Sounds
   a. Inspiratory stridor: upper airway obstruction (above tracheal bifurcation)
   b. Expiratory wheezes or stridor: lower airway obstruction
4. Frothy, blood-tinged sputum: lung injury, pulmonary edema, pulmonary embolus

### Circulation

Pulse quality, locations, and rate are assessed. Skin color and any obvious sources of bleeding are assessed. Life-threatening conditions that may be found when assessing circulation include uncontrolled external bleeding, shock, and pericardial tamponade.

Persons who sustain major trauma or a major stressor to the body usually develop shock (hypovolemic, neurogenic, multisystem failure shock). Signs of shock vary depending on the type and severity of the shock. (See Chapter 17.)

### Disability—neurological assessment

After the primary survey is completed, a neurological assessment is performed. Level of consciousness may be altered in trauma, and such alterations have many causes (Box 21-10). Refer to Chapters 51 and 52 for further information regarding neurological assessment and injury.

**box 21-10** *Possible Causes of Changes in Level of Conciousness*

1. Hypoxia (decreased oxygen to brain)
   a. Respiratory insufficiency
      (1) Airway obstruction from foreign body, secretions
      (2) Pneumothorax
      (3) Spinal cord injury
   b. Shock
      (1) Cardiogenic cardiac arrest
      (2) Hypovolemic hemorrhage
      (3) Multisystem failure shock
2. Metabolic (chemical brain depressants)
   a. Extrinsic
      (1) Drugs: alcohol, narcotics, barbiturates, antihistamines, tranquilizers
      (2) Poisons: carbon monoxide, carbon tetrachloride, hydrocarbons, methane gas
   b. Intrinsic
      (1) Ketones: diabetic ketoacidosis, starvation
      (2) Glucose: hypoglycemia, hyperglycemia
      (3) Ammonia: liver failure
      (4) Urea: kidney failure
      (5) Hormonal hypofunction: hypothyroidism, adrenocortical insufficiency
      (6) Electrolyte imbalance: sodium, potassium, calcium, hydrogen ions
3. Brain pathological conditions
   a. Trauma: concussion, brainstem contusion, intracranial hematoma
   b. Seizures: epilepsy, tumors, idiopathology
   c. Cerebrovascular accident: cerebral hemorrhage, thrombosis
   d. Tumors: benign, malignant
   e. Infections: meningitis, encephalitis

## General Trauma Interventions

Some general principles of management for accidental injuries or sudden illnesses serve as guidelines in giving first aid at a scene.

1. Remain calm and think before acting.
2. Summon assistance or be sure that emergency services has been contacted.
3. Identify yourself as a nurse to victim and bystanders.
4. Do a primary survey for *priority* data (cessation of breathing or heartbeat, interference with breathing, hemorrhage, coma).
5. Carry out measures as indicated by the primary survey. (See Box 21-8.)
6. Do a secondary survey.
7. Keep the victim lying down or in the position in which he or she is found (unless cardiopulmonary resuscitation [CPR] is necessary), protected from dampness or cold. Position the person to support airway management and some degree of comfort.
8. Avoid unnecessary handling or moving of the victim; move the victim only if danger is present.
9. If the victim is conscious, explain what is occurring and provide assurance that help is on the way.
10. Do not give oral fluids if there is a possibility of abdominal injury or if anesthesia will be necessary within a short time.

Lifesaving measures are implemented when the primary survey indicates the presence of breathing or circulatory difficulties. After breathing has been reestablished and excessive bleeding controlled, other interventions are carried out when the secondary survey is completed.

Rescue squad and ED personnel are trained to detect and respond to the patient's physical life-threatening needs. Because these needs assume priority, it is easy to overlook the psychological needs of the victim and significant others. The impact of severe trauma or critical illness can be devastating not only for the patient but for the patient's family and significant others. Care of the emergency patient always extends beyond the patient to the psychosocial care of the patient's family and friends. In times of crisis families need support but may not be able to provide it for each other. Emergency nurses must be there to help provide empathy, support, and direction, as well as act as resource persons. A calm, interested approach that conveys concern for the victim as a person is helpful.

Giving information frequently during all phases of emergency care to both patient and significant others helps them understand what is occurring, thus decreasing some of the anxiety. During resuscitation attempts, it is imperative that contact be made with the family. The family needs clear information regarding their family member's prognosis and condition. The nurse contacts chaplains, social workers, or family friends who can stay with the family. Some hospitals have volunteers who can stay with patients or families during crisis periods. The nurse is honest and does not offer false hope about the patient's condition or expected outcome.

The nurse offers family and friends the option of seeing the patient, even if only for a fleeting moment before the patient is rushed to surgery or an intensive care unit. This contact is crucial for the family. If the patient has injuries or multiple tubes, the nurse prepares the family members for what they will see before taking them into the room.

## SEXUAL ASSAULT: RAPE

Sexual assault is a horrifying, even life-threatening, experience. The number of reported rapes has been steadily increasing, but it is still estimated that two to three times that number of rapes go unreported.

Accurate statistics about rape, rapists, and victims of rape are difficult to compile because of the large number of unreported cases. There are also many misconceptions concerning rape. Some *facts* include the following:

1. Rape occurs among persons of all social classes.
2. Rape occurs mostly between persons of the same race.
3. Most rapes are committed by someone the victim knows.
4. Males, especially young boys, may be rape victims; the attacker usually is heterosexual male.

### Sexual Assault Resource Agencies

Sexual assault resource agencies are available in many cities. The services of these centers differ but usually include one or more of the following:

1. Direct service and counseling to the survivor
2. Service to professional agencies (health, law)
3. Community education

Service to health professionals and community education are efforts to help change the system for the rape victim.

Many victim services agencies are staffed by volunteers who serve as victim advocates throughout the medical examination and police interview. Some form of follow-up service, such as counseling, may be available. Some resource agencies also have attorney volunteers who offer the victim legal advice or representation.

### Rape Trauma Syndrome

Rape is a traumatic event for the victim physically, psychologically, and socially. *Rape trauma syndrome* refers to the emotional state of discomfort and stress resulting from memories of an extraordinarily catastrophic experience. More than 3.8 million adult American women are estimated to have experienced rape-related traumatic stress disorder.[14]

Rape is an act of physical violence, and force often is used. A weapon may be used either to threaten or injure the victim, or the hands or fists may be used to beat or choke the victim. Injury also can occur if the victim struggles or attempts to defend herself. The vagina and perineum may be injured by the force of the sexual attack, and the rectum also may be lacerated if anal sex has been attempted. Sexually transmitted diseases, including human immunodeficiency virus (HIV), may be contracted.

The psychological trauma of rape usually is severe; the rape victim is in a state of crisis. Fear is an overwhelming emotion because the victim perceives the rape as life threatening. Other feelings expressed by victims are depersonalization, shame, degradation, defilement, violation, guilt, humiliation, and anger. The victim not only has been harmed or threatened with harm but also may have been subjected to multiple sexual assaults by one or more persons. Fellatio (oral sex) commonly is demanded, and some rapists will urinate on the victim before leaving. There is also the fear of pregnancy or contracting a sexually transmitted disease.

The person who has been raped goes through the same phases as any person facing a crisis situation. The initial phase is one of shock, disbelief, and disorganization. After the initial acute phase, there is a period of pseudoequilibrium when the victim rationalizes the event or attempts to suppress thoughts concerning the rape. Later, as the survivor tries to reorganize her life, there may be periods of depression, phobic reactions, and nightmares.

The rape victim also experiences sociological crisis. If the victim is married, the marital relationship may be affected. If she is single, she often fears repeated occurrences and may feel the need to relocate, especially if the attack occurred in her home or apartment. The victim needs to make decisions about the incident, because loss of needed support from family and friends may occur. Job security or relationships with co-workers may be threatened. Sociological problems may emerge during the initial emergency period and may take considerable time to resolve. The social importance of rape in the overall context of violence is reflected in its inclusion in the *Healthy People 2000* goals presented in Box 21-11.

**box 21-11** Healthy People 2000 *Objectives Related to Violence*

1. Extend coordinated, comprehensive violence prevention programs to at least 80% of local jurisdictions with populations over 100,000.
2. Reduce rape and attempted rape of women aged 12 and older to no more than 108 per 100,000 women.
3. Reduce physical abuse directed at women by male partners to no more than 27 per 1000 couples.
4. Reduce to less than 10% the proportion of battered women and their children turned away from emergency housing because of lack of space.
5. Reverse to less than 22.6 per 1000 children the rising incidence of maltreatment of children younger than age 18.
6. Increase to at least 30 the number of states in which at least 50% of children identified as neglected or physically or sexually abused receive physical and mental evaluation with appropriate follow-up as a means of breaking the intergenerational cycle of abuse.
7. Extend protocols for routinely identifying, treating, and properly referring suicide attempters, victims of sexual assault, and victims of spouse, elder, and child abuse to at least 90% of hospital emergency departments.
8. Reduce homicides to no more than 7.2 per 100,000 people.
9. Reduce assault injuries among people aged 12 and older to no more than 8.7 per 1000 people.
10. Reduce firearm-related deaths to no more than 11.6 per 100,000 people from major causes.
11. Enact in 50 states laws requiring that new handguns be designed to minimize the likelihood of discharge by children.
12. Enact in 50 states and the District of Columbia laws requiring that firearms be properly stored to minimize access and the likelihood of discharge by minors.
13. Reduce by 20% the proportion of people who possess weapons that are inappropriately stored and therefore dangerously available.

## Prevention

All persons need to know basic rape prevention measures to help prevent rape from occurring (Box 21-12). Some communities include issues of rape and self-defense in secondary school curricula. Classes in self-defense are available in most communities. Sexual assault agencies and police stations may provide information about classes in the local community.

Persons who are raped may seek medical help directly or call the police, who will then take the person to the appropriate facility for medical examination. Some survivors fear reprisal by the rapist or are unwilling to let others know about the rape and therefore do not seek medical attention. Rape survivors need to be encouraged to report the incident.

Most hospitals have developed protocols for care of the rape survivor in the ED, including the following measures:

1. High priority in triage
2. Provision for privacy without leaving the victim alone

**box 21-12** *Rape Prevention Measures*

**PREVENTION OF ATTACK**

Set house lights to go on and off by timer.
Keep light on at all entrances.
Install safety locks on windows and doors.
Have key ready before reaching door of house or car.
Look in car before entering.
Never let a stranger enter the house; insist on identification from all service personnel; check identity with agency if suspicious.
Do not list first name on mailbox or in telephone directory.
Be alert when walking; stay in lighted areas.
Walk down center of street if possible.
Avoid lonely or enclosed areas.

**IF ATTACKED**

Run toward a lighted house; yell "Fire!".
Spit in rapist's face; act bizarre; vomit.
Rip off rapist's glasses.
Step hard on rapist's foot (instep).
Aim at eyes; try to gouge eyes, scrape face.
Hit throat at Adam's apple (larynx).
Use fighting and screaming with caution; this may scare some rapists, encourage others.
Try talking to avoid rape.
Make close observations about rapist, car, location.

3. Provision of a victim advocate (such as a worker from the sexual assault resource agency)
4. Development of sexual assault nurse examiner (SANE) programs
5. Routines to ensure protection and comfort of the victim (if the hospital does not have a SANE program)
    a. Person(s) designated to have primary contact with the victim
    b. Authority of the primary contact person to make the decision about the victim's readiness for medical examination or police interview (if no life-threatening injury is present)
    c. Ensure "chain of evidence" for specimens is maintained (i.e., clear documentation of injuries and collection and storage of specimens according to protocols)

### Sexual Assault Nurse Examiners

Providing care to survivors of sexual assault involves unique challenges. The victim requires skilled and empathetic care to begin the process of emotional recovery, but professional, thorough, and accurate examination is essential to gather the evidence needed for a successful prosecution of the rapist. The sexual assault nurse examiner role was developed to respond to the multiple challenges of caring for survivors of sexual assault. The first SANE program was developed in Memphis, Tennessee, in 1976, and the role has rapidly spread throughout the country. The SANE is able to provide a more time-efficient evidentiary examination process by shortening the time a victim may have to wait for a physician or resident to be available to complete the examination. The forensic quality of the examination is improved as well, because the SANE knows exactly what forensic evidence to collect and how to meet the crisis intervention needs of the survivor.

## NURSING MANAGEMENT OF SURVIVORS OF SEXUAL ASSAULT

### ASSESSMENT

#### Subjective Data

The victim is asked many questions by the SANE to determine the details of the assault and the nature and extent of all injuries. The victim's general demeanor and emotional state are assessed. The victim may express feelings of degradation, shame, guilt, and feeling "dirty" and may express anger toward the assailant or project the anger toward health care personnel. The SANE also collects data related to pain or discomfort (localized, generalized, or diffuse). The victim may complain of a sore throat if choking occurred or if oral sex was forced. Nausea may also be present. Some victims respond emotionally and cry, shake, laugh inappropriately, or are extremely restless. Other victims appear outwardly calm and subdued.

#### Objective Data

The expertise of the SANE is particularly important in the assessment of objective signs of the rape. A head-to-toe assessment is conducted for signs of physical trauma. Any serious physical trauma is treated before collection of evidence. Data regarding the victim's last menstrual period, medical history, history of the assault, and vital signs are obtained.

##### *Evidence collection*

After the SANE explains the procedure to the survivor and obtains her permission, the collection of evidence begins. This process is both time consuming and difficult for the survivor. The SANE collects scrapings from beneath the victim's fingernails, pulls head and pubic hairs, obtains saliva samples, swabs the genitalia and vagina, and conducts a vaginal examination. Some SANE protocols also include colposcopy to obtain photographic evidence of all injuries. A colposcope is a movable microscope that is positioned outside an inserted speculum, and it can provide significant magnification of microtrauma and internal injuries. Used to assess trauma that is difficult to visualize without magnification, the colposcope also has a camera attached to take photographs of the injuries.

A pregnancy test is done, and tests for HIV antibody are performed. Tests for other sexually transmitted diseases are conducted and repeated at appropriate intervals.

### NURSING DIAGNOSES

| Diagnostic Title | Possible Etiological Factors |
|---|---|
| Rape-trauma syndrome: acute phase | (No etiology is necessary with this diagnosis) |

### EXPECTED PATIENT OUTCOMES

Expected patient outcomes for the patient experiencing rape trauma syndrome may include but are not limited to:

1a. Will acknowledge the traumatic effect of the rape
b. Will begin to express feelings and responses to the rape
c. Will identify available rape counseling and support resources in the community
d. Will understand rationale for treatment and evidence collection procedures

### INTERVENTIONS

#### Providing Emotional Support

Most victims need to talk with someone who cares about what is happening to them and who is nonjudgmental. The nurse uses crisis intervention theory to decide how best to help the survivor. Many hospitals have contacts with sexual assault agencies, and the victim is given the choice of having a victim advocate from the center be present during the entire examination period, both medical and legal. Interviews by the police are often done as a team interview with the SANE.

Preparation for the physical examination is carried out in advance. Having a pelvic examination after a sexual assault can be a traumatic experience, especially if the survivor has never had a pelvic examination.

#### Addressing Sexual Concerns

The survivor often has concerns related to sexuality. Time is needed to work through these concerns, and long-term counseling is helpful for many victims.

Concern about possible pregnancy depends on the circumstances—whether the woman is in the childbearing years, whether birth control was used during the assault, and at what point in the menstrual period the rape occurred. If pregnancy is a possibility, postcoital hormone contraceptive therapy usually is initiated immediately.

Concern about sexually transmitted diseases is common. Antibiotic therapy is given after the initial examination as a preventive measure. The victim needs to know that medical follow-up is important and that she should be retested for sexually transmitted diseases and screened for HIV infection at appropriate intervals. In addition, the woman may experience vaginal discharge, itching, and a burning sensation caused by an acute vaginal infection (vaginitis).

#### Planning for Discharge

Clean clothes need to be provided, and no survivor of sexual assault should ever be sent home alone. Every ED should maintain a current list of battered women's shelters. Social workers may be called on to help the victim secure a safe place to stay. The survivor needs to know about the availability of follow-up medical and counseling services. Some medical centers have psychiatrists who are especially expert in counseling rape survivors. The survivor may go to the police station to follow up with the police report after medical care is completed.

**guidelines for care**

**The Sexual Assault Survivor**

1. Assess severity of all injuries and treat accordingly.
2. Obtain consent for evidence collection.
3. Document chief complaint and history of assault.
4. Complete vital signs, history of medications, allergies, and pertinent health history.
5. Observe and document emotional status.
6. Observe and document physical injuries (written, diagrams, and photographs).
7. Observe and document genital injuries (using toluidine blue dye, Wood's light, and colposcopy).
8. Complete evidence collection.
9. Order laboratory studies per protocol.
10. Order additional testing based on the results of the examination.
11. Plan for the patient's discharge, including referrals, prescriptions, and follow-up care.

**research** 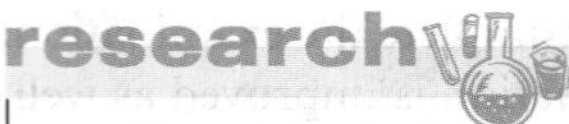

Reference: Varva F, Gesmond S: ED physician house staff response to training on domestic violence, *J Emerg Nurs* 23(1):17, 1997.

Many EDs do not provide any training on domestic violence for physicians and residents. The purpose of this study was to report the response of the ED house staff (residents, interns, and medical students) to a training program on domestic violence against women. This was an exploratory, descriptive study with a three-group pretest and posttest design. The sample consisted of 37 members of the ED house staff. The topics that the house staff rated as most helpful in their day-to-day practice were awareness of the problem, referral as intervention, documentation of abuse, and references and resources. Attitudes and beliefs after training suggested an increased need for the assessment, treatment, and referral of domestic violence for the women who enter the ED for treatment of medical problems or injuries. House staff also showed an increase in belief that help should be given to those who are abused. Before this training, 65% of the house staff had no previous training in domestic violence.

The accompanying Guidelines for Care Box summarizes the care provided to sexual assault survivors.

## ■ EVALUATION

To evaluate effectiveness of nursing interventions, compare patient behaviors with those stated in the expected patient outcomes. Successful achievement of patient outcomes for the survivor of rape experiencing rape trauma syndrome, acute phase, is indicated by:

1a. Expresses the understanding that she is a victim in the assault, and not to blame
b. Expresses her feelings about the rape
c. Identifies community resources available for support and counseling and expresses a commitment to seek follow-up support
d. Describes the rationale for all steps of evidence collection

### DOMESTIC VIOLENCE

Research suggests that 10% to 15% of all women who come to the ED are victims of domestic violence. The link between domestic violence and sexual assault is striking—as many as 33% to 46% of women who have been physically abused by their partner were also sexually assaulted.

For many of the 4 to 8 million women who are abused each year, the ED is their primary source of medical care after abusive episodes. Although the battered woman may come to the ED, opportunities for domestic violence intervention are often lost because health care providers do not ask the right questions. (See the Research Box.) Physicians and nurses should directly ask all injured women if they are in an abusive relationship. Battered women cannot be predicted based on socioeconomic status, race, profession, or educational level. Battering is an equal-opportunity problem.

Emergency department staff follow several principles in caring for patients suspected of sustaining physical abuse. First, nurses incorporate questions and observations into the initial patient assessment. Historical questions and examination techniques may elicit information or evidence about domestic abuse. Victims may not readily share this information if it is not solicited. However, if given the opportunity, the victim often shares the information. Second, nurses must know the resources available for victims of domestic violence. Financial help and "safe housing" are often priority concerns. Victims, once placed in safe environments, can be helped to use the legal system to maintain their safety. Long-term counseling, vocational rehabilitation, and other support are necessary to promote total health. Last, the ED staff must have clear procedures on how to handle victims of domestic violence and must define the process used to notify local authorities.

**critical thinking QUESTIONS**

1 While skating on her new in-line skates, Debi was hit by a bicyclist. You are the first to arrive at the scene of the accident. Debi is sitting up, crying, alert but anxious. What should you do?

2 There has been an increase in violence in your local community. What steps should the ED personnel initiate to ensure a safe work environment?

3 Todd, 28, fell off a roof while working. He has a wrist fracture, several small lacerations, and a swollen ankle. You are the triage nurse in a busy ED. To what category will you assign Todd when presented for care? Provide rationales for your decision.

## chapter SUMMARY

### EMERGENCY NURSING SCOPE OF PRACTICE

- Emergency nursing has grown as a nursing specialty during the past 25 years as indicated by (1) development of a scope of nursing practice, (2) a certification offering, and (3) publication of a professional journal.
- Changes in health care needs of society, caused by the rising incidence of social and domestic violence, the lack of adequate health insurance, and an increase in managed care, have increased the demands on emergency nurses.
- Triage is the process used in the ED to ensure that the patient who most needs the care gets it.
- The use of critical pathways for patient care in the ED provides a system of checks and balances that promote quality and efficiency.
- Excellent communication skills have a key role in emergency nursing.
- Control of the ED environment, particularly decreasing noise and modifying potential violence, is a key nursing goal.

### TRAUMA

- Trauma is the leading cause of death of young people—one of the nation's most valued resources.
- The single most important factor in the cause of accidents is human error.
- Trauma centers, which are designated as level I, II, or III centers by national standards, are governed by specific rules and regulations of the state in which the trauma center is located.
- Primary and secondary surveys are key tools in the assessment of a person who has undergone traumatic injury. These surveys begin cycle I of trauma care.
- Statutes protect off-duty health care personnel who render assistance with good faith and without gross negligence.
- The principles of intervention for use at the scene of an accident or injury are to (1) remove the patient from a hazard only when the risk (e.g., fire) outweighs the danger of moving the patient; (2) call for help; (3) establish an airway, usually by elevating the jaw; (4) initiate cardiopulmonary resuscitation as indicated; (5) control obvious hemorrhage, usually with direct pressure; (6) splint spine and extremity injuries; and (7) transport as soon as possible.
- The person who experiences multiple trauma will need immediate insertion of intravenous lines to allow for fluid and drug administration and management of shock. Management of depressed level of consciousness, respiratory support, and control of pain are also priority concerns.
- Signs of respiratory distress seen in trauma patients are rapid, shallow respirations, abnormal breath sounds, changes in sputum, sinus tachycardia, high or low blood pressure, poor oxygenation, and anxiety or confusion.
- Level of consciousness is altered in trauma for a variety of reasons.
- General trauma interventions at a scene include remaining calm and thinking before acting, identifying oneself as a nurse to the victim and bystanders, conducting a rapid assessment, carrying out lifesaving measures as indicated by the primary survey, performing a secondary survey, and initiating first aid measures.

### SEXUAL ASSAULT: RAPE

- Rape crisis centers have three main functions: victim service, service to professional agencies, and community education.
- A rape survivor suffers psychological, sociological, and physiological trauma.
- Rape survivors require high-priority triage, need to have someone in constant attendance, and need protocols to be followed exactly, especially notifying the local authorities and ensuring the chain of evidence with all specimens.
- Nursing interventions for rape survivors include emotional support; knowledge about sexually transmitted disease testing and care, including testing for HIV infection; knowledge about pregnancy prevention; and knowledge about resources to deal with sexuality-related concerns.
- Rape victims should never be sent home alone.

### DOMESTIC VIOLENCE

- An estimated 10% to 15% of all women who come to the ED are there for reasons of domestic violence.
- The ED must develop clear protocols on how to care for victims of domestic violence Clear guidelines also outline the reporting process to local authorities.

## References


1. American Health Consultants: Domestic violence: how ED's can address the legacy of pain, *ED Management* 7(10):109, 1995.
2. American Health Consultants: Managing violence in the ED crucial to providing top-notch patient care, *ED Management* 8(2):13, 1996.
3. American Health Consultants: CPC: enhancing quality patient care in the ED, *ED Management* 7(6):61, 1995.
4. Cardona V et al: *Trauma nursing from resuscitation through rehabilitation,* Philadelphia, 1995, WB Saunders.
5. Easter C, Muro G: Clinical forensics for perioperative nurses, *AORN J* 50(4):585, 1994.
6. Edelberg C: Coping with COBRA/EMTALA and MCO's, *ED Management* 7:S5-S8, 1996.
7. Emergency Nurses Association: Emergency nursing: scope of practice, *J Emerg Nurs* 5(4):361, 1989.
8. Emergency Nurses Association: *Standards of emergency nursing practice,* ed 2, St Louis, 1991, Mosby.
9. Fazio J: Violence in the emergency department: strategies for survival, Course presented at the Emergency Nurses Association Scientific Assembly, Seattle, 1993.
10. Injury Control Recommendations: Bicycle helmets, *MMWR* 44(RR-1):1, 1995.
11. Laros N: *Assessment and intervention in emergency nursing,* ed 3, Norwalk, Conn, 1992, Appleton & Lange.
12. Ledray L, Simmelink K: Efficacy of SANE evidence collection: a Minnesota study, *J Emerg Nurs* 23(1):75, 1997.
13. Mayer T, Augustine J: Managed care and triage, *Top Emerg Med* 19(2):12, 1997.

14. National Victim Center and Crime Victims Research and Treatment Center: *Rape in America: a report to the nation,* Arlington, Va, 1992.
15. Rea R: *Trauma nursing core course provider manual,* ed 3, Chicago, 1991, Emergency Nurses Association.
16. Skinner C, Forster G: The coexistence of physical and sexual assault, *Am J Obstet Gynecol* 172:1644-1645, 1995 (letter).
17. Somerson SW, Markovchick AB: Development of the triage system. In Salluzo R, Mayer T, Strauss R, Kidd P, editors: *Emergency department management: principles and applications,* St Louis, 1997, Mosby.
18. US Department of Health and Human Services, Public Health Service: *Healthy People 2000: national health promotion and disease prevention objectives,* Washington, DC, 1990, US Government Printing Office.
19. Zimmerman M, Clinton T: Computerized tracking, triage and registration, *Top Emerg Med* 17(4):49, 1995.

# chapter 22 Critical Care Environment

RICHARD CARPENTER and ALICE H. CARPENTER

## objectives *After studying this chapter, the learner should be able to:*

1. Describe the physical and psychological environment of critical care units.
2. Identify the types of data needed for the care of critically ill patients.
3. Develop interventions to alleviate physiological stressors that are specific to the critical care setting.
4. Explain the rationale for interventions to prevent and alleviate psychological stressors for the critically ill patient, the family, and the nurse.

The critical care unit is a unique environment in which the most sophisticated medical, nursing, and technical interventions are integrated to combat life-threatening illness. Since nursing's earliest days the sickest patients have been placed near the nurse's station, underlining the importance of frequent assessment and rapid intervention. From the development of postoperative wards and polio centers to the evolution of the coronary care unit, this concentration of highly specialized caregivers with access to unique technology has remained the guiding principle for the evolution of *critical care environments.* These units are referred to as intensive care units (ICUs), critical care units, coronary care units (CCU), and other names that identify the type and intensity of patient care.

The role of the nurse in the care of the critically ill patient remains the key to the success of the critical care unit. Through the vigilant observation of a patient's ever-changing condition, the critical care nurse is able to monitor the complex treatment regimen, quickly identify problems and initiate appropriate therapies, and intervene to prevent or correct life-threatening situations.

The geographical layout and purpose of the critical care unit vary. Multipurpose ICUs, predominant in small community hospitals, are designed for the care of almost all critically ill patient populations. Specialized ICUs, on the other hand, are uniquely designed to care for specific patient populations and often house "unit-specific" equipment and staff.

In any critical care setting the goal of nursing remains the same: to provide continuous, optimal nursing care to patients in life-threatening situations, remaining alert to the physiological, psychological, and social needs of the patient. This chapter provides an overview of some common aspects of critical care nursing and the critical care environment. Effects of the critical care environment on patient, family, and staff are discussed. Assessment of the critically ill patient is described, followed by selected interventions designed to alleviate physiological, psychological, and social stressors experienced by critically ill patients, families, and the clinicians who staff the units.

## THE CRITICAL CARE UNIT ENVIRONMENT

### PHYSICAL ENVIRONMENT

The critical care unit is designed, equipped, and staffed to meet the anticipated needs of patients in life-threatening situations. The physical layout is frequently a modified circle that allows for direct visualization of all patients at all times. Patients may be separated into individual cubicles or situated in a large open area with curtains for partitions. The advantage of direct nurse-patient visualization is accompanied by the disadvantages of limited privacy and patient exposure to frequent crisis interventions.

Although direct visualization of patients facilitates patient monitoring, maximizes the use of available staff, and may even be required by some hospital accrediting organizations, the cost to the patient in terms of sensory overload and loss of control can be significant. Optimal patient care requires that a careful and sensitive balance be maintained between the needs of patients and those of caregivers.

The central nurse's station contains sophisticated monitoring and even video equipment that enables nurses to continuously monitor vital data for each patient. Supplies and equipment in critical care areas are highly sophisticated and must be readily accessible. Certain technologies are available for constant use at each bedside (e.g., cardiac monitor, oxygen, hemodynamic monitoring equipment, and suction equipment), whereas others must be available within seconds (defibrillator, ventilator, 12-lead electrocardiogram [ECG] machine, emergency medications).

Still other technologies must be available for constant or intermittent use with certain patient populations, e.g., intraaortic balloon pumps, continuous venovenous hemofiltration or hemodialysis, extracorporeal membrane oxygenator, temporary or permanent pacemakers, ventricular assist devices, intermittent conventional hemodialysis, and a variety of pumps for infusion of intravenous fluids or enteral feedings.

The concentration of complex technological equipment also combines to create a unique hazard in the critical care environment—the risk of electrical microshock. The invasive monitoring and therapeutic interventions used with critically ill patients often create a direct pathway to the heart, e.g., central venous pressure lines, pulmonary artery catheters, and temporary pacemakers. Direct contact with stray or leaked current could prove fatal, particularly to critically ill patients whose resistance may be further decreased through other breaks in skin integrity or through electrolyte imbalances. Critical care nurses are responsible for the safe and proper use of electrical equipment, as well as for the implementation of appropriate electrical safety precautions.

In older institutions existing hospital space has often been converted to critical care use, and as the need for more specialized and sophisticated critical care equipment grows, the critical care environment often becomes overcrowded. Even in newer, carefully preplanned units, the critical care environment is so dynamic and new technology develops so rapidly that available space can be quickly overwhelmed with monitoring and other care-delivery equipment. The use of centralized or headwall power columns designed to support the complex power needs for monitoring equipment, oxygen, suction equipment, and electrical outlets; to store equipment; and to provide a workspace at each patient's bedside has become popular in newer or remodeled critical care environments. Ongoing research and development of critical care equipment focuses on how to provide the most service in the smallest available space. Figure 22-1 illustrates a typical high-technology critical care environment.

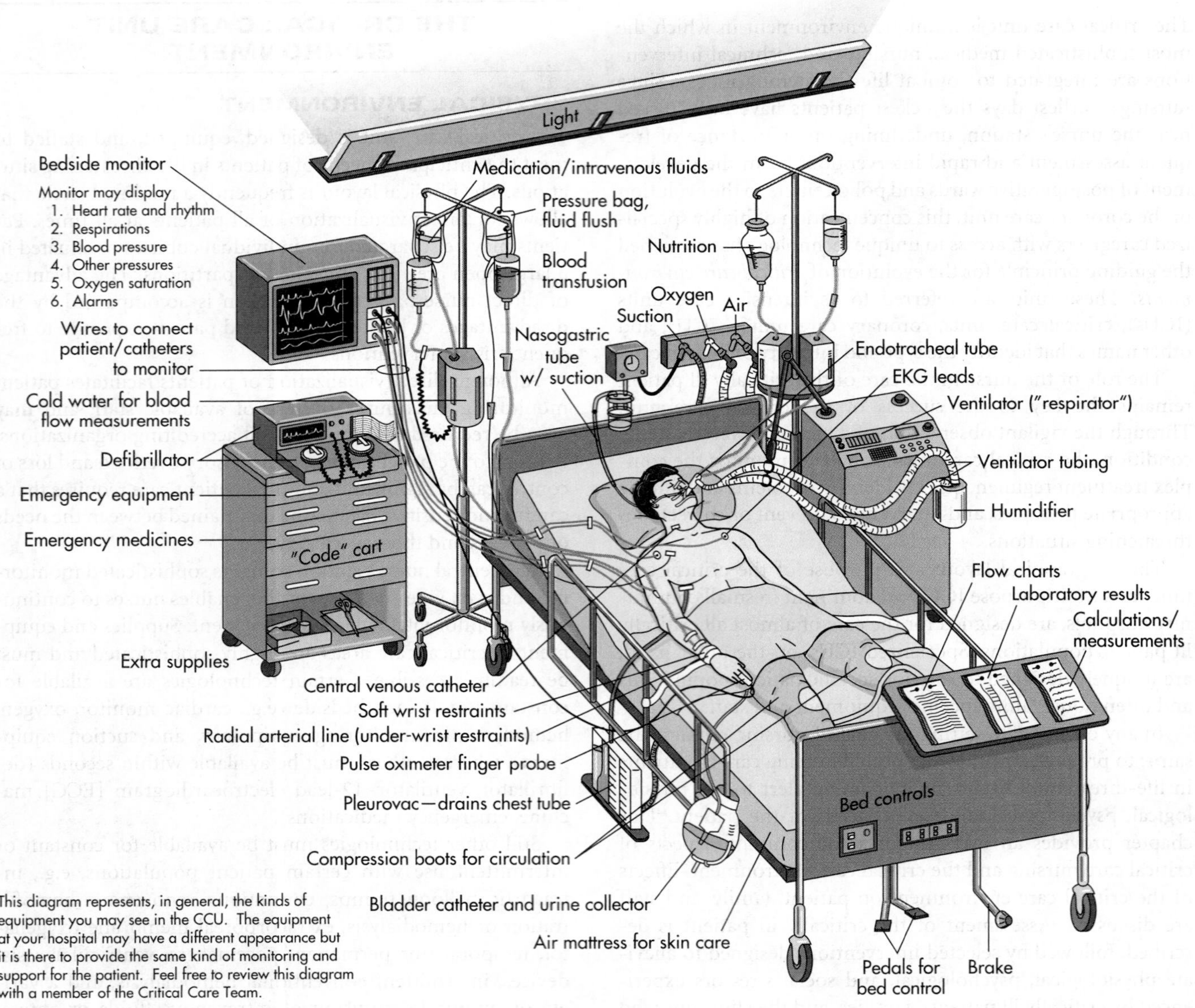


**fig. 22-1** A look at a critical care unit room and equipment.

## PSYCHOLOGICAL ENVIRONMENT

The critical care environment confronts patients with advanced forms of medical and nursing therapies. Although the patient and family are partially aware of the dynamics of critical care, their attention primarily focuses on the appearance of this confusing and frightening environment: flashing lights, buzzing machines; painful procedures; and a noisy, brightly lit, crowded, hyperactive environment. The stressors on the patient and family are immense, heightened by treatment modalities that may prove lifesaving. Some factors that potentiate stress, especially in the ICU environment are sensory input—both deprivation and overload, sleep deprivation, and acute confusion.

### Sensory Deprivation and Overload

The term *sensoristasis* refers to the level and variety of sensory stimulation that allows an individual to interact optimally with the environment. Sensoristasis involves stimulation of all five senses, and the optimal level varies significantly among individuals. Patients in a critical care unit have little or no control over the amount and/or frequency of stimuli that they receive. Too many stimuli can be as undesirable as too few stimuli. ICU environments rarely contain the type of sensory stimuli that are familiar or understandable to patients. Instead, the majority of the sounds, sights, and smells are unique to the critical care unit. Unfamiliar voices, equipment noise, continuous bright lights, and frequent assessment interventions all add to the patient's stress level. This level of stimulation also does not disappear during the night and is in fact minimally diminished.

The stimulation of the critical care environment is continuous, 24 hours per day, 7 days per week. Staff members, who often operate at a much higher level of sensoristasis than their patients, may not realize the impact of this level of stimuli and frequently perpetuate it. Staff, of course, are also able to leave the high-energy critical care environment at the end of their shift while the patient is unable to escape it.

Years of research indicate that sensory overload and deprivation in the critical care environment frequently result in perceptual distortion, hallucinations, and paranoia. (See Chapter 9 for a more complete discussion of sensory deprivation and overload.) The nurse needs to be constantly aware of the type and amount of stimuli directed toward the patient and to help maintain the level of stimulation within tolerable limits. Every effort should be made to reduce noise and other controllable variables and assist the patient to understand this complex environment, thereby reducing the stress of the unknown.

### Sleep Deprivation

An essential part of the 24-hour cycle, sleep accounts for approximately one third of a person's life. An adequate amount of uninterrupted sleep is essential to prevent exhaustion or illness and maintain physiological and psychological well-being. Rapid eye movement (REM) sleep, an important component for mental restoration, occurs primarily in the last cycles of uninterrupted sleep and is the most likely form of sleep to be affected by sleep deprivation in the ICU. (See Chapter 13 for a further discussion of sleep and sleep disturbances.)

Hourly intervention is frequently necessary in the critical care unit to maintain physiological homeostasis. This recurrent disruption in the sleep cycle quickly leads to a lack of REM sleep. Adverse effects of REM sleep deprivation include irritability, anxiety, physical exhaustion, and disruption of metabolic functions. Respiratory distress has also been associated with a lack of REM sleep.

The bedside nurse must assess the patient and determine if adequate periods of uninterrupted time have been provided to promote all stages of sleep. Sleep periods should be included in the plan of care and adhered to as much as possible. Consideration must be given to the importance of interventions versus the necessity of uninterrupted sleep periods. Patients should not be subjected to activity or stressful procedures during the early morning hours unless they are imperative to maintain homeostasis. Visiting times should also be tailored to balance the needs of the patient and family while supporting adequate rest. Recent studies suggest that longer but less frequent visits may be more desirable than the traditional plan of a few minutes each hour.

### Acute Confusion

The risk of developing acute confusion is high in the critical care setting. The high-technology environment is overwhelming and can be very frightening for the patient. The presence of serious or traumatic illness adds additional psychological and physiological stress. Confusion is common among all patients in ICUs but is especially common in the elderly population. It has a rapid onset and is generally reversible but can be very distressing for both patient and family. Symptoms of acute confusion include hallucinations (both visual and auditory), restlessness, memory impairment, and fluctuations in the patient's level of awareness.

The initial patient assessment should include information about the patient's mental status before admission. If the patient was able to adequately perform activities of daily living, it is reasonable to expect that the patient can return to that level of functioning once the acute confusion resolves.

Overwhelming stress is a frequent contributor to acute confusion, and the nurse must make every effort to make the critical care environment therapeutic rather than stressful. In the recent past, patients have been physically restrained to protect them from harm. This type of intervention controls the patient's behavior but frequently increases the patient's confusion and causes a level of struggle or combativeness that may necessitate chemical sedation. Interventions ideally focus on removing stressors, rather than adding to the problem. Current thinking focuses on alternatives to physical restraints. Fostering reality orientation by spending time with the patient and encouraging interaction with family and significant others should be a priority with the confused patient.

Reality orientation is an ongoing, repetitive regimen of providing information to the patient at regular intervals and again as needed. This intervention is initiated immediately after admission to the ICU and is maintained until the patient can repeat the information on request.

## THE CRITICAL CARE CLINICIAN

The critical care environment is also an exceptionally stressful environment for the nursing staff. The stress on the nursing staff stems partially from very high expectations: advanced knowledge of physiology related to all body systems, astute observational and physical assessment skills, ability to quickly prioritize and make decisions regarding patient care, and technical proficiency in operating the highly sophisticated equipment. Nurses are also increasingly faced with complex ethical issues that consume their time and emotional energy. In addition, the constant vigilance and emergency-ready atmosphere may promote an uneasy sense of impending crisis. Critical care nurses must be able to remain calm in stressful circumstances and communicate effectively with the patient and family during crisis situations.

Most critical care nurses select this area of practice at least in part because they feel stimulated by a fast-paced environment where they are expected to effectively integrate a detailed knowledge base, excellent assessment skills, and significant technological proficiency. Manageable stress levels can promote creativity and productivity. However, continuous high-level stress can be as detrimental to the nurse as to the patient. Box 22-1 summarizes some of the multiple stressors that can be present in the critical care environment.

**box 22-1** *Stressors on Patients, Families, and Staff in the Critical Care Environment*

| PATIENT/FAMILY | STAFF |
|---|---|
| Unfamiliar environment, new faces | Expectations of self |
| Noise, light levels | Expectations of peers, clinical supervisors, other health care team members, hospital administrators |
| Sensory deprivation/overload | Intricate machinery and techniques |
| Interruption of sleep/wake cycles | Closed, crowded work area |
| Inaccessibility of family, friends | Constant contact with seriously ill, dying patients |
| Lack of privacy | Continual vigilance over multiple patients |
| Lack of information/understanding of prognosis, care plan | Constant emergency readiness |
| Lack of information/understanding of policies, procedures | Sustained high activity level |
| Anticipation of painful interventions | Limited breaks away from the high-stress unit |
| Confusion/disorientation related to physiological factors | Limited communication with many patients related to intubation or altered level of consciousness |
| Impaired communication related to intubation | Limited opportunity to communicate with some families |
| Observation of crisis intervention in other patients | Isolation from other nurses in the hospital |
| Fear related to diagnosis | Ethical conflicts related to issues of resuscitation and use of life-support equipment |
| Fear of death | Legal issues |
| Conflict between patient/family goals and staff goals | Exposure to infectious diseases |
| Pain | |

Critical care nurses must understand how stressors affect the patient and family but must also be aware of the presence and effects of their own stressors. Critical care nurses must guard their own physical and psychological health and recognize how insufficient or ineffective coping mechanisms can lead to burnout.

All critical care clinicians should be aware of the symptoms of stress and develop strategies for recognizing and decreasing their own stress levels. Most young professionals graduate from nursing school with skill and commitment toward meeting the needs of patients and families. It is essential that these clinicians also develop an ability to understand and respond appropriately to their own needs for support in the daily work environment as well as the needs of their colleagues. Failure to develop self-care strategies may decrease the nurse's ability to respond appropriately to patient needs and ultimately leads to nurse burnout and exit from the health care field.

Long-term involvement with patients in a critical care environment is a relatively new phenomenon and is accompanied by significant new stressors. Technology currently enables medical science to extend the life of some critically ill patients for significant periods of time. Patient populations, such as those awaiting organ transplantation, may have critical care hospitalizations that extend over a period of weeks to months. Consistent nurse caregivers are clearly helpful to the patient and family in coping with the stressors of the critical care environment, and they are more likely to develop a strong therapeutic relationship with the patient and family. They may even be able to more quickly assess and respond to changes in the patient's condition. However, nurses caring for patients on an ongoing basis may also find themselves becoming so close to the circumstances of the patient's illness that their own psychological health suffers. It is important for the clinician to be able to recognize when caring for a patient on an ongoing basis results in undue stress and to develop strategies for protecting their mental health. Some strategies include:

1. Develop support networks among nursing peers.
2. Utilize employee assistance personnel (counselors, social services personnel, and chaplains; critical stress debriefing) to cope with stressful circumstances.
3. Develop interests outside of the critical care environment to help keep personal and professional worlds separate.
4. Carefully self-evaluate the values, beliefs, and feelings associated with the critical care milieu.
5. Utilize a multidisciplinary team approach to nursing care. Multiple resources are available to the critical care clinician to accomplish the work of patient care. The nurse will collaborate with direct caregivers such as physicians; respi-

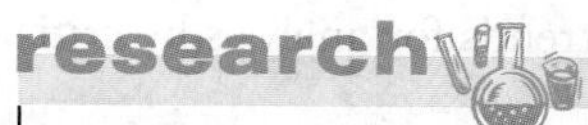

Reference: Porte-Gendron RW et al: Baccalaurete nurse educators' and critical care nurse managers' perceptions of clinical competencies necessary for new graduate baccalaureate critical care nurses, *Am J Crit Care* 6(2):147-158, 1997.

This study sought to determine and compare the perceptions of baccalaureate nurse educators and critical care nurse managers concerning the clinical competencies required of new graduates entering the critical care setting. Former research had indicated wide gaps between the perceptions of these two constituencies. The study used a mailed questionnaire that was sent to a random sample of nurse educators and nurse managers drawn from association listings for each group. A sample of 42 educators and 45 managers was acquired.

The questionnaire included a listing of 105 competencies drawn primarily from an American Association of Critical Care Nurses (AACN) document related to integrating critical care skills into the baccalaureate curriculum. The participants were asked to rate each competency as to its importance for new graduates entering ICU practice ranging from essential to not required. Analysis of results found that there were no significant differences between the two groups on their perception of the relative importance of the various ICU competencies. The current list of competencies showed little overlap with the lists used for similar research a decade ago, but there was strong agreement between both groups of participants that the competency list correctly identified the skills and knowledge that are essential for new graduates to begin practice in this environment.

ratory, speech, and physical therapists; as well as other care providers, such as nutritionists, pharmacists, venipuncture teams, chaplains, social workers, radiology technicians, clerical assistants, and hospital volunteers.

6. Acknowledge the need to occasionally change assignments to provide respite care for the clinician.
7. Set up regular clinical care conferences with the patient, significant others, and other multidisciplinary team members to help the patient feel less dependent on just the nursing staff. The use of conferences allows the patient and family to provide important input into the overall plan of care and feel the tangible involvement of various members of the multidisciplinary team. This approach is particularly important for the long-term critical care patient. Care goals can be reevaluated, modifications agreed upon, or new goals established.

Experience has demonstrated that new graduate nurses can succeed in a critical care environment, but the hiring of novice nurses requires careful attention to both their orientation and mentoring (see the Research Box). Particular emphasis needs to be focused on the need for novices to develop both expertise in clinical skills and the emotional maturity needed for handling the stresses of the critical care environment. The subtle changes in the condition of a critical care patient are more quickly identified by the experienced clinician. If adequate time, support, and supervision are not provided to the new graduate clinician, the presence of a novice simply escalates the stress experienced by other critical care clinicians. Ultimately, patient care suffers.

## NURSING MANAGEMENT OF THE CRITICALLY ILL PATIENT

The nursing process is the same in critical care situations as it is in any other patient setting. Management of critically ill patients requires establishing a database, identifying actual and potential collaborative problems, delineating priorities, defining outcome criteria, executing the planned interventions, and modifying future interventions and plans on the basis of current outcomes. Management of critically ill patients differs from management of other patients because of an ever-changing database; a larger number of complex, interrelated problems; frequent priority reorganization; a greater variety of equipment and methods for measuring changes in patient status; and time limitations imposed by the patient's rapidly changing condition.

### ■ ASSESSMENT

The assessment process for the critically ill patient differs from the assessment of other patients only in terms of the technologies available to assist in data collection. The cardiac monitor, hemodynamic monitoring lines, and laboratory analyses provide data that must be incorporated into the total patient assessment. Technologies are adjuncts to the data the nurse gathers through observation, history taking, and physical examination. Monitored data are useless unless correlated with physical findings and integrated into meaningful analysis by the critical care nurse.

The complete history and physical examination provide the necessary foundation for further ongoing data collection in the critical care setting, and the importance of accurate and thorough initial information cannot be overemphasized. However, the multiple sources of data and the continually fluctuating condition of critically ill patients make constant priority reorganization a necessity. The critical care nurse continually updates the database to reformulate short-term goals and interventions.

Patient assessment must be thorough, yet rapid. The physical and psychological reactions of an entire organism under stress must be taken into account and not be limited by the usual or the expected. Patient assessment also must be organized and repetitive so that small alterations or deviations from previous findings will be apparent. Finally, the assessment must be individualized, with time and attention given to particularly significant aspects.

#### Subjective Data

The critically ill patient may arrive in the critical care unit as (1) a direct admission, usually through the emergency department; (2) a transfer from another patient care division in the same or a different hospital; or (3) a postoperative admission after certain operations. Data from the patient and family, written history, and the transfer report of other nurses are all integrated into the patient's initial treatment plan. Consultation between transferring and receiving nursing unit staffs is essential to accomplish this process effectively. These data sources help ensure continuity of care and communication of all issues important to the patient or family. The nurse carefully explores the patient's and family's response to the need for critical care placement. A full patient profile may be deferred until later in the hospitalization as hemodynamic stabilization is always the first priority of care. The initial contact with the ICU personnel sets the tone for all future interactions and is an invaluable opportunity for the nurse to demonstrate competence and caring and begin to establish that essential foundation of trust.

## Objective Data

The physical assessment of the patient, while augmented by the technology of the ICU, still uses the skills of inspection, palpation, percussion, and auscultation to determine the patient's care needs and evaluate responses to interventions. The critical care nurse combines these physical assessment skills with information received from the patient and appropriate monitoring data to establish an initial plan of care and set priorities. In the critical care setting physical assessment may take place hourly or even more frequently as patient status dictates. All disciplines involved in the patient's care participate in the ongoing assessment process from their own perspective. The ongoing dynamic and collaborative nature of critical care assessment allows for rapid responses to be made to any changes in patient status but may also contribute significantly to the patient's sensory overload. The need to evaluate status changes frequently may leave the patient with little time for rest and privacy. Significant nursing skill is required to balance the need for information gathering with the need for patient rest. It may take years of experience for the nurse to gather and synthesize several pieces of data simultaneously, thoroughly, and rapidly, with the least disruption to the patient.

### *Monitored data*

Nurses in all clinical settings use tools such as stethoscopes, sphygmomanometers, thermometers, and scales to collect patient data. Critical care nurses also have access to tools such as cardiac monitors, hemodynamic pressure lines, intracranial pressure monitoring devices, and airway pressure monitoring devices that are capable of continuous data collection. The explosion in critical care technology since the 1970s provides the critical care nurse with amazing quantities of objective data. Computerized monitoring systems that occupy less space and provide more capabilities than ever before are widely available. The most sophisticated patient data management systems take information from all the monitored parameters (ECG, respirations, intraarterial pressure, pulmonary artery pressure, venous oxygen saturation [$S\bar{v}O_2$], central venous pressure, intracranial pressure, and body temperature), combine it with manually entered data (such as body weight, height, intake and output, and times of drug administration), and produce a wide array of hemodynamic and pulmonary calculations and patient response trends for analysis by critical care practitioners.

In the next century, information systems are expected to integrate data collection and appropriately modify clinical interventions. For example, computerized intravenous medication administration systems now exist that can titrate the dosage of vasoactive drugs by adjusting infusion pump flow rates in response to continuously measured intraarterial pressure. The clinician sets the parameters, but the computer within the pump executes the command. Computers also assist the interdisciplinary team to determine the course of treatment based on input data and treatment paths. As technology assumes an ever increasing role in the treatment of critically ill patients the physical assessment skills of the critical care nurse become an essential backup to ensure the appropriateness of any computer-initiated interventions.

Technological adjuncts to critical care assessment are continuously undergoing change, combining older and well-tested monitoring systems with newer advances. Certain types of monitoring equipment are in use in all critical care environments. Waveforms and other data produced by these devices may be viewed continuously on a video screen or be graphed for a permanent record. Many monitoring systems involve fluid, tubing, and transducing equipment and act as portals of entry for microorganisms. Strict aseptic technique is essential to prevent complications associated with nosocomial infections.

**Cardiac monitoring.** Cardiac monitoring is a noninvasive procedure that poses minimal risk to the patient. It consists of placing conductive electrodes on the patient's chest that recognize the electrical activity of the heart and relay it to a video display screen. Depending upon the sophistication of the monitoring equipment, the clinician may be able to view the patient's ECG and heart rate at the bedside and at remote locations in the critical care unit, monitor changes during activity (with mobile equipment), and set flexible monitoring parameters as changes in cardiac status occur. Parameters may include changes in heart rate and rhythm, respiratory rate and rhythm, analysis of dysrhythmias, and even changes in specific ECG segments, such as the ST segment for ischemia recognition. Alarms notify the clinician when preset limits have been reached. Most monitors default to preset limits if the clinician does not set specific alarm parameters and only allow clinicians to silence the alarms for limited periods of time.

**Hemodynamic monitoring.** Hemodynamic monitoring refers to invasive monitoring of the arterial or venous system. Monitoring is accomplished through catheters that measure changes in air and fluid pressures and can also be used to administer intravenous fluids and obtain arterial or venous blood for laboratory analysis. The air and fluid pressure readings are interpreted by transducers connected to the system and display the results as waveforms on cardiac monitoring equipment (Figure 22-2). The two most commonly used hemodynamic monitoring systems are intraarterial monitoring and pulmonary artery monitoring.

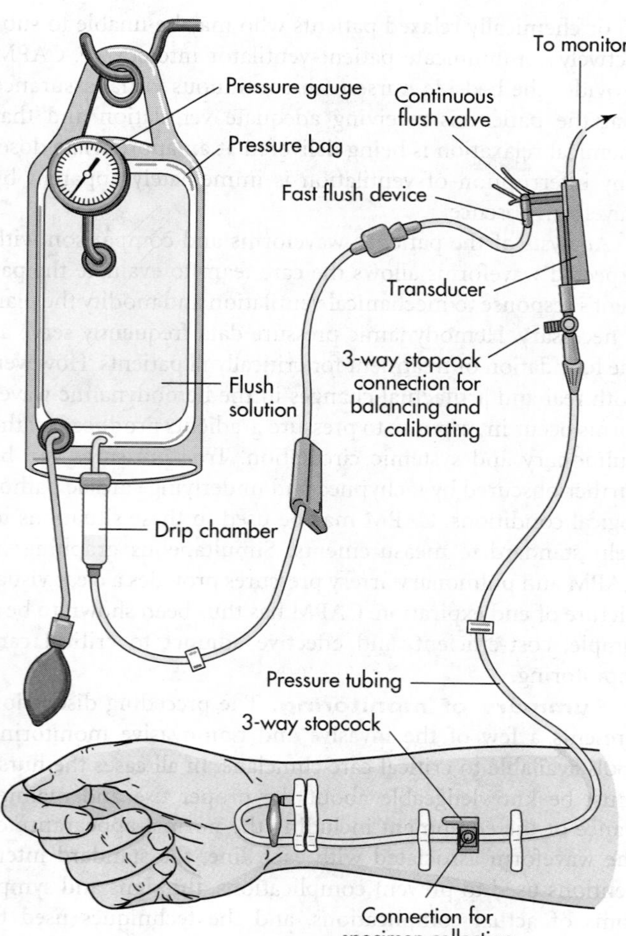


**fig. 22-2** Components of a pressure monitoring system. The cannula, shown entering the radial artery, is connected via pressure tubing to the transducer. The transducer converts the pressure wave into an electronic signal. The transducer is wired to the electronic monitoring system, which amplifies, conditions, displays, and records the signal.

It is important for the nurse to verify the digital display of waveform values with a manual blood pressure cuff, regularly calibrate the transducing equipment with the transducer positioned at specific landmarks on the patient's body, and assess the entire system for patency and accuracy. A thorough knowledge of waveform interpretation is required to appropriately interpret and respond to the values displayed on the screen or on a manual printout. Even minor errors in reading and interpreting values or small problems in the patency of the system, such as a tiny air bubble in the transducing system, can result in inaccurate data and may cause profound complications for the patient. Aseptic technique is critical to maintain these systems with the least possible risk to the patient. Ongoing assessment of the patient's response to the equipment is also critical to avoid dangerous complications such as air emboli, bleeding, malposition of catheters, tissue damage, or hemodynamic compromise as a result of foreign body insertion or malposition. (See Chapter 17 for additional information about hemodynamic monitoring.)

**Intraarterial monitoring.** Intraarterial monitoring involves inserting a catheter into an artery, usually through the radial or femoral artery, and connecting the catheter to a high-pressure flush system filled with either a heparinized or nonheparinized saline solution. The high-pressure flush counterbalances arterial resistance to maintain patency of the system. Intraarterial systems display a continuous reading of the patient's blood pressure and provide ready access to obtain arterial blood gas or other laboratory specimens.

**Pulmonary artery (PA) monitoring.** PA monitoring involves inserting a catheter through the subclavian or internal jugular vein and advancing it into the pulmonary artery, usually under fluoroscopic guidance to ensure accurate placement. These catheters have several lumens encased within a larger lumen, and each opens at a different point along the length of the catheter. Each lumen may be used for fluid administration, and specific lumens may be used to attach monitoring and transducing equipment. The large bore of the lumens and placement of the catheter in large arteries permit the administration of more caustic intravenous solutions that could damage peripheral veins. A balloon at the distal tip of the catheter is filled with approximately 1 ml of air when the natural flow of blood through the patient's heart pulls the balloon into place in the pulmonary artery.

When the catheter is correctly placed, the balloon is deflated. Monitoring and transducing equipment are attached to the catheter. Significant data can be gathered about the patient's hemodynamic and cardiac function as the balloon is inflated and deflated, stopcocks are opened and closed to direct fluid through the transducer, and fluids cooler than body temperature are injected through the catheter and past a thermistor at the catheter tip. Available data include pulmonary artery and central venous pressure recordings and cardiac output measurements. Combining these values with parameters such as blood pressure and body surface area make it possible to calculate additional information that is not directly available from catheter readings. Newer monitoring equipment calculates these values automatically when data are entered into the database, decreasing the chance for error from manual calculation. The pulmonary artery catheter rapidly provides valuable information to evaluate the patient's response to vasoactive drugs by providing data about left and right heart function. It is also a significant tool for managing severe cardiac failure and cardiogenic shock.

A central venous pressure (CVP) catheter may be used in lieu of a pulmonary artery catheter when evaluation of pulmonary artery pressure and left heart function is not required. CVP catheters may be transduced and used to measure right heart pressures and deliver intravenous fluids, but they are more limited in the scope of data they provide than are pulmonary artery catheters. A newer type of central line is called a peripherally inserted central venous catheter (PICC). The external portion of the PICC is assessed and maintained by nurses, and patients and families may be instructed in these techniques for home use. PICC lines are long-dwell catheters that require the same aseptic care as other central lines. They can be used to administer long-term intravenous fluid therapy but at present have no monitoring capabilities. PICC lines are more commonly used for long-term fluid and medication administration.

**Intracranial pressure monitoring (ICP).** ICP monitoring involves placement of a catheter through the skull into either the subarachnoid space or the cerebral ventricle to monitor changes in pressure within the cranial cavity. A transducer and tubing system gather the data that are displayed on the monitoring screens (see Chapter 52). Newer monitoring systems have the capacity to sense changes in intracranial pressure and display pressure readings on a bedside monitor without the use of fluid-filled pressure tubing and transducer systems. Although insertion through the skull into the cranial cavity is still required, these newer systems reduce the risk of contamination by microorganisms. Patients with unstable intracranial pressure may be quite sensitive to routine nursing interventions such as turning, suctioning, and changes in bed position. The continuous display of intracranial pressure readings allows the nurse to constantly evaluate the patient's responses to all interventions and take prompt action if the patient's pressure reaches unsafe levels. The catheter also can be used to aspirate cerebrospinal fluid for analysis or culture and to relieve elevated ICP. The nurse is also responsible for identifying changes in pressure readings, analyzing trends, evaluating patient responses to interventions or therapies, and preventing complications.

**Continuous airway pressure monitoring (CAPM).** CAPM is a relatively recent advance in critical care monitoring systems. CAPM is a simple noninvasive technique that uses a transducer cable, high-pressure tubing (as used for measuring pulmonary and arterial pressures), and a display monitor. The monitoring equipment is connected to a ventilator circuit at the Y connector near the airway. Standard calibration procedures are used, but the monitoring tubing is filled with air, not fluid, and the transducer can be at any level while calibration is performed. The absence of fluid in the transducing system minimizes the risk of infection. The waveforms produced by CAPM may be continuously displayed, graphed, and compared with hemodynamic waveforms. The waveforms produced by the system enable the clinician to continuously monitor the patient's response to various modes of mechanical ventilation or to mechanical ventilation itself, and assess the patient's response to therapeutic interventions.

CAPM is also useful in identifying one of the most common complications of mechanical ventilation—patient-ventilator asynchrony or intolerance. Asynchrony can result from mechanical malfunction, inappropriate ventilator mode selection, inadequate inspiratory flow rate, airway obstruction from excessive secretions, or patient anxiety or agitation. Asynchrony increases the work of breathing and can result in inadequate gas exchange. When a patient experiences asynchrony, the CAPM waveforms deviate from the expected patterns, alerting the nurse to the need for prompt intervention. CAPM can be especially helpful in monitoring sedated, very ill, or chemically relaxed patients who may be unable to subjectively communicate patient-ventilator intolerance. CAPM provides the bedside nurse with continuous visual assurance that the patient is receiving adequate ventilation and that chemical relaxation is being delivered at an appropriate dose. Any interruption of ventilation is immediately apparent by waveform absence.

Analysis of the patient's waveforms and comparison with expected waveforms allows the care team to evaluate the patient's response to mechanical ventilation and modify the plan if necessary. Hemodynamic pressure data frequently serve as the foundation of treatment for critically ill patients. However, both real and artifactual changes in the hemodynamic waveforms occur in response to pressure gradients produced by the pulmonary and systemic circulation. True pressures can be further obscured by tachypnea and underlying cardiac pathological conditions. CAPM may be used in these situations to help standardize measurements. Simultaneous graphing of CAPM and pulmonary artery pressures provides a clear visual picture of end expiration. CAPM has thus been shown to be a simple, cost-efficient, and effective adjunct to critical care monitoring.

**Summary of monitoring.** The preceding discussion presents a few of the invasive and noninvasive monitoring tools available to critical care clinicians. In all cases the nurse must be knowledgeable about the proper use and maintenance of the equipment including the normal appearance of the waveform associated with each line, the standard interventions used to prevent complications, the signs and symptoms of actual complications, and the techniques used to troubleshoot the monitoring systems when problems develop. The patient risk associated with invasive monitoring lines is significantly reduced when the lines are managed by knowledgeable personnel. In addition to the various invasive lines used for monitoring, critical care nurses also must be skillful in using central lines for medication, fluid, and nutrition administration.

As monitoring techniques become increasingly sophisticated, it is tempting to treat the patient solely based on the numbers and waveforms produced by the equipment. It is essential for the clinician to remember that these data must always be combined with data obtained from routine physical assessment that include the patient's general appearance and subjective response to all therapeutic measures. A flat line on a waveform may be the result of a disconnected wire or tubing rather than a change in the patient's condition. The nurse must remain vigilant and keep one eye on the monitor and one eye on the patient to avoid treating the equipment instead of the patient. The nurse must also individualize the use of each monitoring technique to the uniqueness of each patient situation.

## ■ NURSING DIAGNOSES

The range of nursing diagnoses that can be appropriate in any specific critical care patient situation is virtually limitless. The discussion of nursing interventions that follows addresses broad categories of interventions that are applicable in a wide variety of situations. Similarly, commonly encountered nursing diagnoses might include but are certainly not limited to:

| Diagnostic Title | Possible Etiological Factors |
|---|---|
| Decreased cardiac output | Alterations in preload or afterload, disturbances in cardiac rate/rhythm |
| Impaired gas exchange | Altered oxygen supply, changes in the alveolar capillary membrane |
| Altered tissue perfusion (cerebral, cardiopulmonary) | Interruption of blood flow, exchange problems |
| Anxiety | Situational crisis, threat of death or disability |
| Acute confusion | Sensory deprivation/overload, lack of sleep, pain, hypoxia |
| Knowledge deficit: critical care environment and routines | Lack of exposure |
| Altered family processes | Temporary family disorganization and role changes |

## EXPECTED PATIENT OUTCOMES

Expected patient outcomes are tailored to the unique needs of each individual patient. Broad outcomes that might apply to the identified diagnoses include:

1. Maintains systolic blood pressure above 100 mm Hg, urine output greater than 30 ml/hr, and cardiac rate and rhythm within acceptable limits.
2. Demonstrates satisfactory pulmonary function (adequate blood oxygenation, hemoglobin saturation, and forced expiratory volume in 1 second [$FEV_1$]) and exhibits a satisfactory respiratory rate and pattern.
3. Exhibits stable vital signs and intracranial pressure no greater than 15 mm Hg.
4. Reports an increase in psychological comfort and an absence of restlessness or other behavioral manifestations of anxiety.
5. Experiences fewer episodes of confusion.
6. Expresses understanding of routines and environment of the critical care unit.
7. Identifies stresses of critical care admission on family unit and identifies resources available to assist with coping.

## INTERVENTIONS

### Preventing and Alleviating Physiological Stressors

The ultimate goal of nursing intervention for any patient is to promote, sustain, and restore optimal levels of physiological, psychological, and social functioning. However, in a critical care setting, the immediate goal of ensuring a patient's survival determines the priorities for intervention; physiological problems must be addressed first. Once life-threatening stressors have been alleviated, priorities can be reevaluated, and other problems can be addressed.

Physiological priorities are determined by the degree of threat to the person's survival. Certain body systems are more prone to disorders requiring intensive therapeutic interventions and are frequently encountered in the critical care unit. At the most basic level, these priorities can be organized in the same "ABC" framework as basic cardiac life support. Establishment of airway, breathing, and circulation remains the foundation for therapeutic management of the critical care patient. When the ABCs of basic life support are applied, the critical care nurse is able to move from the most pressing to least pressing patient problems. When a critical care nurse determines that a patient's physiological status has begun to deteriorate, actions are immediately taken to reverse the problem. Airway patency is ensured by correct positioning of the endotracheal tube with suctioning as needed to ensure an unobstructed airway. The nurse then assesses the patient's ability to breathe and the effect of physical restraints or physiological conditions such as acute respiratory failure. Circulatory needs are addressed next, such as the establishment of normal cardiac rhythm, intravenous access for administration of medications, and adequate cardiopulmonary perfusion of vital organs. The critical care clinician may continue to use this basic ABC principle in ongoing assessments to ensure that problems are recognized before complications develop.

### Preventing and Alleviating Psychological Stressors

In addition to continuous assessment for physiological derangements, the nurse also must focus attention on recognizing the psychological stressors that confront the patient and family. The emotional discomfort and distress that the patient and family endure not only affect the patient's psychological health but also have a direct impact on physical recovery.

The initial step in preventing or alleviating psychological stress is to identify the patient's and family's perception of the critical event. Their perceptions will be affected by their individual personalities, current psychological health, general understanding of the present situation and its projected outcome, tolerance for ambiguity, and normal patterns of coping. Initial perceptions are often significantly affected by previous exposure to similar events, either positive or negative, and general level of familiarity with medical interventions and the hospital environment. Specific interventions nurses can use in any setting to reduce the psychological stress of illness are detailed in the following discussion.

### Supporting Expression of Feelings

Because the critically ill person is separated from familiar surroundings and is dependent on others to meet the most basic needs, the patient becomes partially or totally isolated from usual support systems. Feelings of helplessness, powerlessness, loneliness, and depersonalization, as well as disturbances in body image, are common. Modes of expressing and therefore relieving the frustration, anger, hostility, fear, and depression generated by these feelings are limited by the physical constraints of the critical care environment. Consistently assigned caregivers can be an effective way to establish a therapeutic relationship with the patient and family.

An atmosphere of openness and acceptance that encourages expression of feelings can help provide patients with a means of coping. The nurse talks openly and honestly with patients and attempts to decrease the patient's feelings of depersonalization, isolation, and alienation. Anger and hostility are often indications of fear and anxiety. Depression and withdrawal may be signs of hopelessness, loneliness, powerlessness, or loss and are normal and expected. The nurse encourages the patient and family to express their feelings and assists the patient to identify the fears and concerns that may be causing unusual or inappropriate behavior. The nurse is nonjudgmental and avoids communicating a message that the patient's behavior is "wrong" or unacceptable.

Nurses or other health care team members who help patients talk about feelings must be ready to accept whatever emotionally laden information might be expressed. Nonjudgmental recognition and acceptance of the patient's feelings help reinforce the patient's right to the feelings.

Intubated patients are unable to express their feelings freely even when alert and oriented and are therefore particularly vulnerable to psychological stressors. It is natural to communicate less with persons who cannot talk easily, and the nurse must guard against this. Strategies such as keeping a letterboard, paper and pencil, or a "magic slate" within the patient's reach and providing assistance when the patient desires it help to reduce the sense of isolation. However, such methods do not allow the patient to truly express feelings and concerns. The nurse carefully assesses the patient for cues concerning his or her emotional state and anticipates common concerns among critically ill patients. The nurse can verbalize the potential concerns, allowing the patient to validate them as appropriate. The direct expression of empathy for the patient and family conveys acceptance and understanding.

### Providing Information

The patient's perception of stressors and not the stressor itself determines the patient's reaction to the illness and the critical care environment. It is essential that the patient and family receive adequate information and simple explanations. Without explanations the critical care environment presents a mysterious and threatening array of noxious stimuli, which may be perceived as extremely unnatural and even magical. The highly sophisticated equipment increases the patient's feelings of vulnerability, and the patient may worry that the cardiac monitor is actually keeping the heart beating, that a blood transfusion indicates hemorrhaging, or that chest physiotherapy signifies pneumonia. A very common misconception of patients after coronary artery bypass surgery is that "open heart" surgery involved cutting the heart wide open and sewing it back together again. Such a perception can lead to a drastic alteration in body image.

The nurse is an important source of information for the patient and family and usually leads the patient education effort. Patient teaching in critical care has a short-term focus. Pain, discomfort, weakness, anxiety, and transient confusion are some of the obstacles to learning what critical care patients experience. The nurse provides simple repetitive explanations of all interventions and their purpose and introduces the patient and family to the overall plan for ongoing care. Patients may not understand or believe what they are told the first time, and anxiety and denial may prevent accurate retention. The nurse may need to reinterpret and reiterate the diagnosis, prognosis, goals of treatment, types of interventions, and expectations of the patient and family during the entire critical care stay. Explanations are ideally provided by the primary caregivers to encourage continuity of care and minimize the confusion of differing approaches and wording. If the patient and family are apprised of the patient's current status, as well as all changes in plans, the situation can be perceived accurately, and they are able to plan realistically for the future and participate fully as members of the health care team.

### Supporting Family Involvement

The essence of crisis intervention is helping persons cope with a major life crisis that a critical illness may precipitate. Critical care nursing is far broader in scope and more future oriented than crisis intervention alone, but specific situations frequently require the immediacy and limited focus of crisis intervention. At that time the nurse assists the patient and family to establish short-term goals and minimizes the number and scope of decisions they must make. As the crisis situation stabilizes, the nurse provides the patient and family with additional information and assists them to accept additional responsibility for decision making and goal setting.

When the patient and family are knowledgeable about the goals of therapy and understand the patient's diagnosis, current status, and prognosis, they can be involved in many aspects of care planning and make decisions consistent with the treatment regimen.

The involvement of significant others decreases the patient's feelings of powerlessness, frustration, and anxiety. The family is likely to be needed in a direct caregiver role at some point in the patient's recovery, and it is important for the multidisciplinary team to begin including them in care planning as soon as possible. The patient is reassured by having a loving advocate represent his or her wishes and concerns. Even when a patient is unconscious, visits by key support figures who talk to and touch the patient may have positive, if unmeasurable, effects on the patient while helping to decrease the family's feelings of helplessness.

The nurse actively involves all alert patients in goal setting and care planning. The nurse seeks to increase the patient's feeling of personal control in structuring the daily schedule of activities. The knowledge that the preferences of the patient are important to the nursing staff and that the patient is viewed as capable of making decisions reinforces the importance of the patient's role in recovery.

The environment of the critical care unit presents multiple stresses to both the patient and family. Narcotics and sedatives, anxiety, hypoxia, sleep deprivation, and multiple metabolic derangements all combine to create acute confusion, disturbed thought processes, and perceptual distortions. The nurse uses reality orientation on an ongoing basis to assist patients to regain their mental stability. Although some environmental factors cannot be altered, the nurse can use a vari-

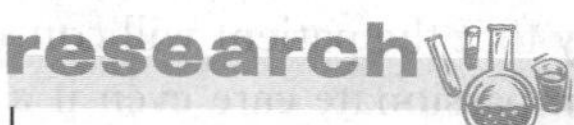

Reference: Simon SK et al: Current practices regarding visitation policies in critical care units, *Am J Crit Care* 6(3):210-217, 1997.

This study explored visiting hour practices in the critical care units of five hospitals in a metropolitan area. Nurses' perceptions about open versus restricted visiting and the effect of those policies on families were also explored.

A mailed questionnaire was sent to a potential pool of 600 ICU nurses. The sample included 200 nurses for a return rate of 33%. Results indicated that 70% of the units had official visitation policies that were restrictive, but 78% of the participants indicated that they were nonrestrictive in their own practice, using their own judgment about the degree of visitation to permit. The nurses overwhelmingly preferred restrictive visitation despite an expressed belief that open visiting had positive effects for both the patient and family. Benefits of restricted visiting were seen to be control over the patient's environment, less noise, and increased rest. At the same time open visiting was assessed as being extremely beneficial to the family and patient. Most participants were more open to "who" could visit than to "when" they could visit and wished to retain control over access even when expressing a belief in the benefits of open visiting to patients.

ety of strategies to control the sensory level of the critical care unit.

Critical care units are increasingly recognizing the importance of visits by the patient's significant others in minimizing the psychological stressors of the environment. The practice of restrictive and minimal visitation is increasingly being replaced by varying degrees of open visitation (see the Research Boxes). Open visitation policies range in scope from longer and more frequent visitation hours to the practice of true open visitation where the patient and family participate fully in care activities and care team rounds. While these policies appear to improve the ability of the patient and family to develop trust and a therapeutic relationship with the care team, the nurse must be careful to avoid overwhelming the family with the daily stress and sensory overload of the critical care unit. With more open visiting in place it is frequently important for the nurse to encourage significant others to meet their own needs for rest, nutrition, psychosocial support, relaxation, and spiritual renewal. Many significant others need to be supported in their decision to leave the critical care environment at regular intervals even when visitation policies would allow them to remain.

## Preventing and Alleviating Social Stressors

In the critical care setting the patient's physiological needs often assume priority over psychological needs, and the patient's needs as a social being may be virtually ignored. Limited visiting hours, the strange technical environment, and the aura of danger in the critical care unit isolate patients from their supportive family and friends and prevent them from participating in their usual social roles. For the most part, staff members view a person who is critically ill primarily in the patient role. The more significant roles of spouse, parent, child, lover, sibling, friend, or provider may go virtually unrecognized unless staff members initiate interventions to provide continuity in these relationships.

Continuity in social roles is fostered through some of the same types of interventions used to reduce psychological stress: increasing visiting between patient and family; including the family in discussions of disease process, prognosis, and plans of care; and reporting by family of events and activities occurring in the other significant spheres of the patient's life. Relaying telephone messages between the patient and distant friends is one way the nurse can help the patient maintain contact with his or her broader external world.

**research**

Reference: Chesla CA, Stannard D: Breakdown in the nursing care of families in the ICU, *Am J Crit Care* 6(1):64-71, 1997.

This study was a subpart of a major ongoing study of socialization and development of expertise by critical care nurses. Its purpose was to describe the broad areas of breakdown in care of families in ICU settings. It used a sample of 130 ICU nurses from eight hospitals who had been selected for inclusion in the larger study. The sample participants were interviewed in small groups a minimum of three times by an experienced interviewer. The interviews were analyzed for content and meaning using standard qualitative methods.

The three primary needs of families in the ICU have been identified as assurance, proximity to the patient, and information. Analysis of the participants' responses showed that nursing care for families broke down when nurses engaged in five groups of behaviors:

1. Making efforts to distance the family physically from the patient. This was manifested as control over visitation and asking the family to leave the room during all care activities or "to support rest." Nurses engaged in numerous power struggles in this area.
2. Distancing themselves from the patient and family. This took the form of not interacting with either patient or family or refusing to answer phone calls or sit down with families.
3. Labeling the family's behavior as pathological. Nurses were quick to consider anxious or questioning behavior on the part of the family as indicative of pathological behavior.
4. Dissipating responsibility for family care. This usually took the form of referring all issues to the nonavailable physician.
5. Taking an elemental rather than a family systems perspective. Nurses rarely exhibited the knowledge or skill to analyze the functioning of the family unit and instead dealt with each person and behavior as it arose.

The researchers were struck by how quickly and thoroughly the nurses were socialized into antagonistic relationships with families when restrictive policies were in use on the unit, regardless of their knowledge of the importance of family roles and supports for patients.

One of the most effective and important ways to prevent disruption in relationships is for the nurse to carefully prepare family or friends for their first visit with the patient in the critical care unit. The patient's physical appearance and the critical care environment are explained thoroughly before the visitor enters. Visitors need to understand the patient's level of consciousness, as well as ability to communicate and comprehend communication. They need to understand the importance of their presence to the patient and the patient's need for their support. When visitors approach the bedside, the nurse remains with them if possible to facilitate their initial interaction with the patient. Family frequently need to be encouraged to touch the patient and offer other physical expressions of their love and support. Fear of hurting the patient or disrupting the multiple monitoring devices can virtually immobilize the family member. The nurse can help family members find safe places to stand and explain the basic purpose of the various lines and tubes. The nurse also encourages the family to speak with the patient, especially unconscious or intubated patients. At each subsequent visit the nurse caring for the patient meets with the family to answer questions and apprise them of the patient's progress.

In addition to supporting the maintenance of the patient's current roles and relationships, the critical care nurse also recognizes the inevitability of actual role change for some patients and families during a critical illness. Roles of provider, decision maker, employer, and employee may be altered, reversed, or eliminated. Family and friends may need to assume some or all of the responsibilities of the patient at this time.

During the critical phase of illness the family members will be trying to cope with significant role changes and may need help in working through problems that arise as family members and friends assume or fail to assume these additional responsibilities. The nurse needs to be sensitive to these challenging problems and provide the family with professional guidance, such as from a social worker, to assist in reorganizing themselves and their resources. The nurse may help the family appoint a temporary family representative, someone who knows and is able to represent the wishes of the family as a whole and who can be contacted in the event of emergency. The nurse also may help the family to plan visiting schedules that meet the patient's needs without preventing family members from fulfilling their own responsibilities. This is a period of great emotional stress for both patient and family.

Emotional stress may climax in the death of the critically ill patient. (See Chapter 8 for a discussion of death and dying). The following suggestions may be helpful in caring for a dying patient:

1. Examine your own feelings about death.
2. Listen attentively to the expressed needs of the patient and family.
3. Remain available to the patient and family both physically and emotionally.
4. Use touch, if culturally acceptable, in caring for the patient and family.
5. Reassure the patient and family that the patient will continue to receive skilled and compassionate care even if a "do not resuscitate" decision has been made.
6. Attempt to remain nonjudgmental about family or hospital issues.
7. Respect the strengths and limitations of the patient-family relationship, which existed long before the patient-hospital relationship.
8. Include the family in care.
9. Provide for patient and family privacy.
10. Provide the opportunity for the family to exercise religious or cultural traditions.

Providing comprehensive care to critically ill patients and their families is a challenging opportunity. The critical care nurse combines the technological sophistication of this unique setting with a personal, individualized care approach to maximize the potential outcomes for the patient.

## Supporting Ethical Decision Making

In many ways, the major technological advances available in hospitals have evolved faster than society's ability to understand and keep pace with the associated ethical dilemmas (see Chapter 5). Life can be prolonged in ways that were previously impossible. Not infrequently, life can be maintained past all known hope of recovery. Tremendous emotional, financial, legal, and social ramifications exist as patients are stabilized into conditions for which long-term health care options are very limited. For example, few families and even fewer skilled care facilities have the resources to care for a patient who requires continuous mechanical ventilation.

With the advent of advance directives, nurses frequently assume responsibility for gathering information about the patients' wishes concerning the extent of their care or treatment. Patients frequently have not prepared advance directives or are incompetent to render such a decision, leaving the family and significant others to determine the type and extent of medical care the patient would or would not want in this situation. Critical care nurses frequently assist families with highly emotional decisions such as foregoing resuscitation or withdrawing life support systems. Assisting families with these decisions is painfully complex.

All health care professionals must examine their own beliefs about life and death, termination of life, organ/tissue donation, and use of limited resources. Education and support for the nurse are available from formal classes, support groups, peers, and hospital ethics committees. Ethics committees are also available to patients, families, and staff members who wish consultation and support in difficult or divisive situations.

Biomedical advances at times seem to challenge the compassionate aspects of caregiving. The critical care nurse is the professional caregiver best qualified to play a pivotal role in identifying and supporting the patient's wishes (see the following Research Box).

## Preparing the Patient/Family for Transfer

Transfer from the critical care unit to another setting can cause significant stress for patients and their families. The crit-

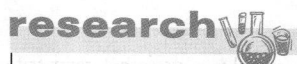

Reference: Stillwell SB et al: The impact of do-not-resuscitate orders on nursing workload in an ICU, *Am J Crit Care* 6(5):400-405, 1997.

This study assessed nursing workload associated with caring for patients with do-not-resuscitate (DNR) orders in several ICUs in a major medical center in the attempt to determine (1) the level of nursing care required by these patients and (2) any differences in nursing care hours required before and after DNR orders were given. The study sample consisted of 60 patients who had been placed on a DNR status during an ICU stay over the study period of 3 months. Nursing workload was measured with the Medicus workload and productivity system and severity of illness was measured using the APACHE prognostic scoring system.

Patients with DNR status were found to require the highest intensity levels of care both before and after DNR orders were given. No differences were found in the level or intensity of care required. Forty of the patients died within 14 hours of DNR status, which influenced the lack of difference in care needs. The remaining 20 were discharged. The proximity of death for most patients stimulated the researchers to conclude that immediate transfer out of the ICU upon DNR status was not in the best interests of either the patients or families, but staffing plans need to incorporate the reality that care needs do not diminish.

ical care area represents security and protection with its sophisticated electronic equipment and attentive, highly skilled staff members. Patients know that transfer means moving to an area where there are fewer nursing personnel per patient, less direct contact with nursing personnel, no automatic or obvious monitoring devices, and no direct observation of the patient from the nurses' station. Greater independence and higher levels of activity will be expected of patients on the transfer unit, and the support of familiar nursing staff members will be lost. Patients may experience ambivalent feelings about the transfer, particularly if they do not feel as well or as independent as anticipated at the time of transfer.

The anxiety precipitated by the transfer can be prevented or reduced if the patient and family are taught to interpret the meaning of particular signs and symptoms and are helped to understand the true purpose of equipment and routines. The nurse continuously points out the signs that indicate patient progress. The nurse begins to include transfer plans in discussions with the family as soon as the patient's condition begins to stabilize. This will help the family to adjust and prepare for the relocation. Along with the projected date of transfer the patient and family need to know what to expect on the new unit and what will be expected of them. Ideally, a nurse from the receiving unit meets the patient and family before transfer. After transfer, visits from the critical care staff are helpful in conveying ongoing concern for the patient's welfare, as well as in providing objective validation of continued progress. With careful planning and execution, transfer from the critical care unit can be a triumphant rather than a traumatic event.

With the increasing trend toward managed care insurance plans and decreased scope of third-party reimbursement for hospitalization patients are increasingly discharged directly from the critical care environment to the home. These patients may require a wide variety of care regimens that their significant others need to manage effectively. Families are also frequently required to perform various nursing therapies. A family member may need to learn to manage sophisticated machinery such as home ventilators or oxygen equipment and understand how to safely troubleshoot routine problems with machinery. Critical care clinicians need to begin working with the patient's family early in the hospitalization to establish a good therapeutic relationship and ensure that home issues are resolved before the day of discharge. Family caregivers must be both technically proficient and confident that they can effectively manage the patient's care. The nurse can instill that confidence in a family caregiver, and confidence is an essential component of successful home management. Planning for respite care for a family caregiver is also important to ensure that the caregiver does not become overwhelmed with the multiple responsibilities of home care. Early referral to community-based home care agencies is also essential to provide the patient and family with the needed physical and psychological resources to manage the transition to home. Discharge is otherwise a lonely and overwhelming experience.

## EVALUATION

To evaluate the effectiveness of nursing interventions the patient's behaviors are compared with those stated in the expected patient outcomes. Successful achievement of the broad outcomes for the critically ill patient is indicated by:

1. Has stable vital signs; all monitoring parameters within accepted limits
2. Demonstrates satisfactory gas exchange and pulmonary function
3. Has pulse oximetry and intracranial pressure levels within accepted limits
4. States an increase in comfort and decreased anxiety in the critical care environment
5. Remains oriented to self and surroundings
6. Understands the nature and scope of critical care monitoring and interventions
7. Family functions successfully with the assistance of personal and community resources

### critical thinking QUESTIONS

1 Compare the priorities and organization of patient care in a critical care environment with those of the acute care unit.

2 What strategies for stress management should the nurse clinician address?

3 How does the utilization of critical care monitoring technology affect the delivery of patient care in the critical care environment?

4 How could the nurse clinician utilize a multidisciplinary approach to optimize patient care planning?

## chapter SUMMARY

### ENVIRONMENT OF THE CRITICAL CARE UNIT

- Numerous types of critical care units exist. They are designed, equipped, and staffed to meet the anticipated needs of patients in life-threatening situations.
- Inherent in the critical care environment are multiple stressors for the patient, the family, and the nurse. Identification and amelioration of these physiological, psychological, and social stressors are the goals of critical care nursing.

### NURSING MANAGEMENT CRITICALLY ILL PATIENT

- Critical care nurses build on clinical knowledge from all specialties. Any organ system dysfunction may result in critical illness, requiring invasive or specialized equipment for assessment and intervention.
- The nursing process is the same in critical care situations as in other patient care settings. The nurse establishes a database, identifies actual and potential nursing diagnoses, defines outcome criteria, and executes the planned interventions based on clinical priorities. Evaluating the results and modifying the plan are ongoing processes.
- The assessment of the patient in a critical care environment incorporates data from cardiac monitoring and hemodynamic monitoring.

### ALLEVIATING AND PREVENTING PSYCHOLOGICAL STRESSORS

- The critical care environment results in separation of patients from their families. Nurses must provide care to the family as well as to the patient.
- The nurse involves the patient and family in all decision-making and goal-setting activities.
- Minimizing sensory overload or sensory deprivation is a major focus of care in critical care settings to decrease psychological stressors.
- Although stressful, the critical care environment provides a feeling of security; patients and families need to be prepared for transfer from the critical care environment.
- The advancement of health care technology has made the prolongation of life possible in ways never before experienced. Careful attention to the ethical, social, and financial implications of critical care technology is necessary to maintain the focus on the patient's quality of life.

## References


1. Abi-Nader JA: Peripherally inserted central venous catheters in critical care patients, *Heart Lung* 22(5):428-434, 1993.
2. Aloi A, Burns S: Continuous airway pressure monitoring in the critical care setting, *Crit Care Nurse* 15(2):66-74, 1995.
3. Atkinson B: The current state of critical care, *Intensive Care Nurs* 7(2):73-79, 1991.
4. Baker C: Discomfort to environment noise: heart rate responses of sick patients, *Crit Care Nurs Q* 15(2):75-90, 1992.
3. Burns S, Hutchens AL: New graduates in critical care: how long do they stay? *Crit Care Nurse* 12(8):74-79, 1992.
4. Carnevale F: High technology and humanity in intensive care: finding a balance, *Intensive Care Nurse* 7(1):23-27, 1991.
5. Chesla CA, Stannard D: Breakdown in the nursing care of families in the ICU, *Am J Crit Care* 6(1):64-71, 1997
6. Henneman B: Building the model ICU, *Crit Care Nurs Q* 15(8):112-114, 1992.
7. Hickey MI, Leske JS: Needs of families of critically ill patients: state of the science and future directions, *Crit Care Clin North Am* 4(4):645-649, 1992.
8. Hudak C, Gallo B: *Critical care nursing, a holistic approach,* ed 6, Philadelphia, 1994, JB Lippincott Co.
9. Jezewski MA et al: Consenting to DNR: critical care nurses' interactions with patients and family members, *Am J Crit Care* 2(4):302-309, 1993.
10. Lazure LLA, Baun MM: Increasing patient control of family visiting in the coronary care unit, *Am J Crit Care* 4(3):157-164, 1995.
11. Lewis DJ, Robinson JA: ICU nurses coping measures and response to work related stressors, *Crit Care Nurse* 12(2):18-26, 1992.
12. McConnell EA: Medical devices and medical futility: when is enough enough? *Nursing* 27(8):32hn1-32hn4, 1997.
13. Porte-Gendron RW et al: Baccalaureate nurse educators' and critical care nurse managers' perceptions of clinical competencies necessary for new graduate baccalaureate critical care nurses, *Am J Crit Care* 6(2):147-158, 1997.
14. Simon SK et al: Current practices regarding visitation policies in critical care units. *A J Crit Care* 6(3):210-217, 1997.
15. Stillwell SB: *Mosby's critical care nursing reference,* St Louis, 1992, Mosby.
16. Stillwell SB et al: The impact of do-not-resuscitate orders on nursing workload in an ICU, *Am J Crit Care* 6(5):400-405, 1997.
17. Swearingen PL, Keen JH: *Manual of critical care: applying nursing diagnoses to adult critical illness,* St. Louis, 1991, Mosby.
18. Taylor C: Medical futility and nursing, *Image* 27(4):3-1-306, 1995.
19. Thelan LA et al: *Critical care nursing diagnosis and management,* ed 2, St Louis, 1994, Mosby.

chapter

# 23 Home Care Environment

CAROL E. SMITH and JUDITH K. SANDS

## objectives

*After studying this chapter, the learner should be able to:*

1 Describe the trends in health care leading to the expansion of home care for medical-surgical patients.
2 Discuss the nursing responsibilities in managing the transition from acute care to home care.
3 Apply the nursing process to plan care for home care patients and their families.
4 Discuss the unique challenges of the home as an environment for providing nursing care.
5 Identify current social and economic issues in home care.

Health care has been provided in the home setting for centuries, but its place and importance steadily eroded in the twentieth century with the rapid rise of hospital-based medical practice. The last decade has witnessed an abrupt reversal in the dominance of hospital-based care as managed care forces have begun to assume control of the health care market. Home care is the fastest-growing segment of the health care system. Its growth reflects the belief that cost control in health care can be most effectively achieved by minimizing hospital stays and transferring as many services to the community and home setting as possible.

Although controversy exists over whether home care is synonymous with or separate from the broader field of community health, it is usually considered to be a subspecialty of that discipline. Home care is a branch of nursing that meets the acute and chronic health care needs of patients and families in the home setting and blends many of the elements of traditional medical-surgical nursing with a community- and family-based focus. The range of possible services provided through home is large, as seen in Box 23-1. It incorporates services to new mothers, the chronically ill, homebound elderly, and dying patients, and it provides high-technology support for patients experiencing a wide variety of pathophysiological conditions. Agencies providing home care services include public agencies supported by tax funds; private, not-for-profit agencies supported primarily by endowments or donations; institution-based agencies, which operate under a larger organization such as a hospital; and private, for-profit agencies owned by individuals or corporations.

This chapter presents an overview of the unique elements of the home care environment. Most medical-surgical conditions involve a significant component of self-management in the home. These elements of nursing management are addressed in the separate problem chapters throughout the text. This chapter focuses on the unique challenges and opportunities associated with providing nursing care in the patient's home.

## TRENDS IN HOME CARE

Economic trends in health care, technological innovations, and population demographics have resulted in increasing numbers of adult patients who require medical-surgical nursing care in the home setting. The growth in home care services is perhaps the most visible outcome of managed care philosophies. Cost-cutting efforts have resulted in dramatically decreased hospital stays nationwide, closure of significant numbers of acute care hospital beds, and a corresponding decline in nursing job opportunities in acute care settings. Health care forecasters predict that the process of institutional consolidation and closure will continue over the next 5 to 10 years. At the same time, the need for and availability of home care services has increased by about 30% a year (Figure 23-1).[18] More than 19,000 agencies currently provide home care services,

**box 23-1 Common Home Care Service Lines**

- Intermittent skilled services
- Hospice services
- Home medical equipment—beds, wheelchairs, ventilators
- Psychiatric program
- Early obstetrics discharge
- Parenteral therapy program—hydration, antibiotics, total parenteral nutrition, chemotherapy
- Respite program
- Rehabilitation program—occupational therapy, physical therapy, speech therapy
- Personal care services—activities of daily living
- Supplies
- Private duty
- Pediatric home care
- Ventilator care
- Newborn home care
- Oncology program
- Prenatal monitoring

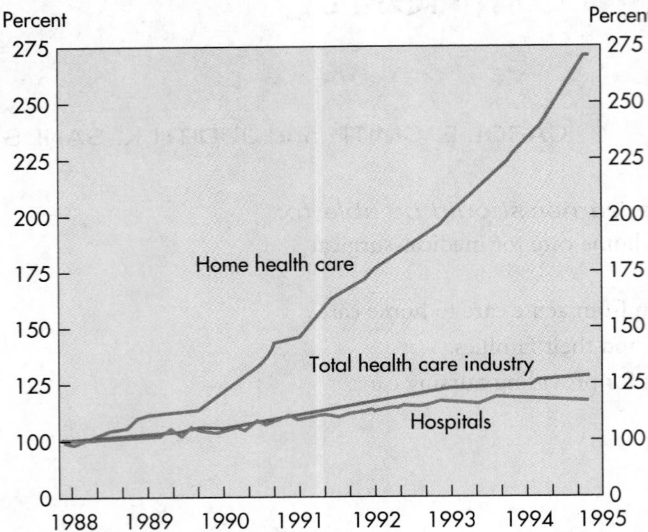


**fig. 23-1** Employment growth as a percent of 1988 levels in selected health agencies.

**table 23-1** *Where Nurses Are Employed*

| Place | Percentage of Nurses |
|---|---|
| Hospitals | 66.3 |
| Community and public health | 10 |
| Ambulatory | 8 |
| Nursing home/extended care facilities | 7 |
| Nurse education | 2 |
| Student health | 2.7 |
| Occupation health | 1 |
| Miscellaneous | 3 |

Reprinted with permission from American Nurses Association, *Nursing facts: today's registered nurses, numbers & demographic,* © 1995 American Nurses Publishing, American Nurses Foundation/American Nurses Association.

**table 23-2** *Number of Home Health Care Workers (1993) and Certified Agency Full-Time Employees (1995)*

| Type of Employee | No. Employees | No. Full-Time Employees |
|---|---|---|
| Registered nurse | 90,950 | 135,694 |
| Licensed practical nurses | 32,240 | 29,545 |
| Physical therapists | 7,600 | 12,470 |
| Home care aides | 215,220 | 120,994 |
| Other | 104,160 | 72,787 |
| **Totals** | **450,170** | **371,490** |

Reproduced by permission of the National Association for Home Care, from *1996 Basic statistics about home care.* Not for further reproduction.

and an estimated 9 to 11 million individuals are in need of services.[18] Job opportunities for experienced nurses in the home care environment have steadily expanded (Tables 23-1 and 23-2). Expenditures for home care in 1996 were in excess of $27 billion. This figure, though impressive, still represents only 3% of the total national expenditure on health care but is expected to continue to rise (Table 23-3).[18]

Home care has been documented as cost-effective in financial analysis studies conducted by insurance companies, health care professionals, pharmaceutical laboratories, and federal regulatory agencies.[5] In-home use of technology costs approximately one third as much as hospital care and even less when skilled services are not needed 24 hours a day. The total daily cost of acute care hospitalization was estimated at $1800 in 1995. This compares with a $300 per day cost in a skilled nursing facility and an $85 fee for a home visit.[18] The economic advantages are clear, and cost considerations are clearly the primary driving forces behind the dramatic growth of home care, but quality and choice also play a role in the broad acceptance of home care by consumers. The privacy and safety of the home environment are clear preferences as the site of care for most patients and families. Other advantages of home care over institutional care include decreased nosocomial infection and improved nutritional status. Home care allows for the resumption of more normal interactions and routines. Care can be more easily personalized to the unique needs of the patient and family, and patients experience a greater sense of control and higher morale when they are cared for in their home environments.

Technological progress has influenced home care greatly. Patients can now be monitored at home through computer linkages to sophisticated diagnostic systems. Technological innovations such as small, easily programmed intravenous infusion pumps have made parenteral home therapies safe and affordable. A variety of respiratory therapies, ranging from oxygen compression tanks to mechanical ventilators, are widely used today with elders or patients with multiple chronic illnesses. Infusion of blood, home defibrillators, and home monitoring of patients at risk for cardiac dysrhythmias are common today. Developing technology will continue to increase the population of patients dependent on such care at home.[3,17,21]

The changing demographics of our population also have influenced the increase in home health care. The number of elders will more than double by the year 2030, whereas the younger generation is decreasing in numbers. Home care is delivered to patients of all ages, but increasing age and functional disability are two major predictors of the need for home care. Elders represent over 50% of the home care population.

Home care is clearly successful in meeting the complex care needs of patients in their preferred setting, but this success comes at a price. Family involvement is integral to the success of home care, and the direct or unspoken message to families is an expectation that they assume this caregiving role regardless of the cost. The interest or willingness of the family is rarely seriously considered. The burden of caregiving can be

**table 23-3** *National Health Care Expenditures, 1995*

| | PERCENTAGE |
|---|---|
| Total personal health care | 100 |
| Hospital care | 40.2 |
| Physicians' services | 21.6 |
| Nursing home care | 9.1 |
| Drugs and other medical nondurables | 9.7 |
| Other professional services | 6.9 |
| Dentists' services | 4.8 |
| Home care | 3.7 |
| Other personal health care | 2.3 |
| Vision products and other medical durables | 1.7 |

Reproduced by permission of the National Association for Home Care, from *1996 Basic statistics about home care.* Not for further reproduction.

**table 23-4** *Medical-Surgical Conditions Commonly Managed in the Home Setting*

| DIAGNOSIS | % CLIENTS RECEIVING HOME OR HOSPICE CARE |
|---|---|
| Neoplasms | 72.3 |
| Circulatory disorders | 38.1 |
| Endocrine, nutritional, metabolic, and immune disorders | 9.8 |
| Musculoskeletal and connective tissue disorders | 9.3 |
| Neurological and sensory disorders | 9.0 |
| Injury and poisoning | 7.3 |
| Respiratory disorders | 6.5 |
| Infection and parasitic diseases | 5.9 |
| Skin and subcutaneous disorders | 4.6 |
| Digestive disorders | 3.5 |
| Diseases of the blood and blood-forming organs | 2.9 |
| Genitourinary disorders | 2.2 |

Reproduced by permission of the National Association for Home Care, from *1996 Basic statistics about home care.* Not for further reproduction.

extensive, yet it is difficult to formally quantify. Not all homes are suitable for caregiving, especially when high-technology care is required, and the demands of monitoring and implementing high-technology care can overwhelm the caregiver.

The needs of home care patients vary significantly and range from patients requiring assistance with personal care and activities of daily living (ADL), to long-term technology-dependent patients, to patients who need short-term skilled interventions following surgery. Patients may require one or two home visits or around-the-clock nursing care. Today, almost any medical-surgical problem dealt with in the hospital setting can also be effectively managed in the home if the patient is stable.[19] Table 23-4 summarizes the major types of disorders that are treated in the home. Cancer clearly creates the greatest need.

The home as the environment for nursing care offers a particular challenge to those involved in home care. Nurses use many standard medical-surgical nursing skills to provide care to their patients, but they also need to develop special skills to work effectively with patients in their homes. Home care administrators have quickly discovered that the home care environment is unique, and skills, even high-technology critical care skills, cannot always be successfully transplanted from one setting to another.[4]

Nurses working in home care may be expected to serve as case managers in a managed care environment. This role can take a variety of forms. Case-managed care is supported by private industries and the federal government as a means of reducing insurance costs and making early hospital discharge to the home safe and less expensive. The nurse can be employed by a home health agency, a hospital, a health maintenance organization (HMO) discharge program, or an insurance company. Some nurse entrepreneurs have established their own companies that provide case-managed services for major insurance carriers or the employees of large corporations. These nurses have become skilled in matching the patients' needs with the most cost-effective resources available.[23]

The nurse case manager may provide direct care to patients or coordinate the efforts of other personnel involved in the patient's care. The role also commonly involves the supervision of unskilled certified nursing assistants (CNAs) and personal care attendants. In either role the case manager conducts a detailed assessment of the patient's needs, discusses options with the patient and family, arranges for selected services to be coordinated with the home care agency staff, and ensures quality care by evaluating patient outcomes on a regular basis. Open communication among the patient, family, and nurse case manager is essential for successful home care.

The home care nurse's caseload routinely includes patients with diverse illnesses such as cardiac disease, respiratory disease, diabetes, cancer, and neurological problems. The home care nurse may provide or direct nursing services to assist with ADL, manage wound care and high-technology interventions, and teach families self-management skills.

## Reimbursement Issues

Medicare is the single largest reimbursement source for home care services, and the number of patients receiving home care through Medicare increased more than twofold between 1991 and 1994. The serious concerns over home care reimbursement are reflected in the fact that patient and family self-pay represents the second-largest source of payment. Medicare's service and reimbursement guidelines are used as models for most other insurers. Home care cannot be initiated without a physician order, and it cannot proceed without a physician-approved plan of care. Box 23-2 summarizes the basic requirements for service and scope of reimbursable services for Medicare and Medicaid.[1]

Home care reimbursement from most insurers covers skilled care provision, assessment and monitoring of unstable conditions, and initial teaching for self-care.[8] Personal care

**box 23-2** *Eligibility Requirements for Medicare and Medicaid Home Care Services*

**MEDICARE**

Covers skilled nursing, physical therapy (PT), occupational therapy (OT), and speech therapy; medical supplies and equipment; and home health aide or social services if delivered in conjunction with skilled service.

Persons covered:

1. 65 years or older and entitled to Social Security benefits
2. Under 65 years if qualifies for Social Security disability benefits
3. End-stage renal disease patients

Requirements:

1. Must be homebound
2. Services must be "medically necessary" and be prescribed in a physician plan of care
3. Must require skilled nursing, PT, or speech/language therapy

*Note:* The skilled provider is authorized to (a) assess an acute process or change in condition, (b) teach about a new or acute situation, and (c) perform a skilled procedure or hands-on service that requires the skill, knowledge, and judgment of an RN.

**MEDICAID**

Must cover intermittent nursing service, a home health aide, and medical supplies and equipment. May cover PT, OT, speech/language therapy, private duty nursing, or personal care services. Persons covered:

1. Recipients of Aid to Families with Dependent Children (AFDC)
2. Recipients of Aid to the Aged, Blind, and Disabled (AABD) with income criteria
3. Others who meet federal or state income guidelines

Requirements:

1. Must be homebound
2. Services must be "medically necessary" and be prescribed by a physician
3. Additional requirements vary by state; participation in case management may be required

from a professional nurse is rarely covered. The treatment plan is used as the basis for reimbursement, and only specifically identified interventions are reimbursed.[1] The components of a plan of care are stipulated as shown in Box 23-3. The continued medical dominance of the health care system and its persistent focus on illness is reflected in the fact that general health maintenance, health promotion, and interventions such as psychoemotional support are not covered services, despite the complexities of most home care situations. Covered services do not consider the full range of nursing practice or the realities of the lives of most patients and caregivers. This often creates dilemmas for the nurse as she (or, less commonly, he) attempts to reconcile the perceived needs of the patient and family with the reality of the limitations of covered services.[2] Figure 23-2 shows a sample home health certification and plan of care form.

**box 23-3** *Medicare's Required Data for the Plan of Care*

1. All pertinent diagnoses
2. A notation of the beneficiary's mental status
3. Types of services, supplies, and equipment ordered
4. Frequency of visits to be made
5. Patient's prognosis
6. Patient's rehabilitation potential
7. Patient's functional limitations
8. Activities permitted
9. Patient's nutritional requirements
10. Patient's medications and treatments
11. Safety measures to protect against injuries
12. Discharge plans
13. Any other items the home health agency or physician wishes to include

## Sociocultural Issues

Effective home care acknowledges and incorporates the patient's cultural background and religious beliefs. The plurality of American society necessitates that the nurse have knowledge of and respect for the patient's unique cultural orientation. (See Chapter 2.) There may be sociocultural or religious conflicts between the family's and the health care professional's approaches to the patient's care, and the nurse may need to incorporate alternative medicines and folk remedies into the total care plan.[11,27] Families may ignore the advice and teaching offered by the health care team and elect not to follow the prescribed regimen. Control over the patient's care is clearly in the hands of the family.

The dynamics of the extended family may also need to be explored and utilized. The promotion of patient and family involvement in care is fundamental as the home care nurse recognizes that self-care may be the only option when insurance and other benefits are depleted.

Families can easily become overwhelmed with the burdens of caregiving. To manage home care, the family members must acquire new knowledge and skills, be motivated to help the patient, and adapt to the changes in role expectations of family members.

The problems typically reported by families who provide home care include the burden of providing daily physical care, steady financial drain, lack of support or resources, and difficulty coping with individual role and schedule disruptions.[22] Other problems include the stress of learning the required nursing care, difficulty accepting help from others, and observing any negative changes in the patient's status such as infection or malnutrition. (See the Research Box on p. 588.)

Long-term caregiving may necessitate developing skills in equipment troubleshooting, require structural remodeling of the home, and result in social isolation for the caregivers. The greatest challenge for the home care nurse is assisting families to find solutions that work within the context of their own unique lifestyle.

The need for custodial or respite care also may be apparent. Care of dying patients in the home has increased significantly

Department of Health and Human Services
Health Care Financing Administration

Form Approved
OMB No. 0638-0357

**Home Health Certification and Plan of Care**

| 1. Patient's HI Claim No. | 2. Start of Care Date | 3. Certification Period From: To: | 4. Medical Record No. | 5. Provider No. |
|---|---|---|---|---|

| 6. Patient's Name and Address | 7. Provider's Name, Address and Telephone Number |
|---|---|
| 8. Date of Birth / 9. Sex ☐ M ☐ F | 10. Medications: Dose/Frequency/Route (N)ew (C)hanged |
| 11. ICD-9-CM / Principal Diagnosis / Date | |
| 12. ICD-9-CM / Surgical Procedure / Date | |
| 13. ICD-9-CM / Other Pertinent Diagnoses / Date | |
| 14. DME and Supplies | 15. Safety Measures: |
| 16. Nutritional Req. | 17. Allergies: |

**18A. Functional Limitations**

1 ☐ Amputation
2 ☐ Bowel/Bladder (incontinence)
3 ☐ Contracture
4 ☐ Hearing
5 ☐ Paralysis
6 ☐ Endurance
7 ☐ Ambulation
8 ☐ Speech
9 ☐ Legally Blind
A ☐ Dyspnea With Minimal Exertion
B ☐ Other (Specify)

**18B. Activities Permitted**

1 ☐ Complete Bedrest
2 ☐ Bedrest BRP
3 ☐ Up As Tolerated
4 ☐ Transfer Bed/Chair
5 ☐ Exercises Prescribed
6 ☐ Partial Weight Bearing
7 ☐ Independent At Home
8 ☐ Crutches
9 ☐ Cane
A ☐ Wheelchair
B ☐ Walker
C ☐ No Restrictions
D ☐ Other (Specify)

19. Mental Status: 1 ☐ Oriented 2 ☐ Comatose 3 ☐ Forgetful 4 ☐ Depressed 5 ☐ Disoriented 6 ☐ Lethargic 7 ☐ Agitated 8 ☐ Other

20. Prognosis: 1 ☐ Poor 2 ☐ Guarded 3 ☐ Fair 4 ☐ Good 5 ☐ Excellent

21. Orders for Discipline and Treatments (Specify Amount/Frequency/Duration)

22. Goals/Rehabilitation Potential/Discharge Plans

| 23. Nurse's Signature and Date of Verbal SOC Where Applicable: | 25. Date HHA Received Signed POT |
|---|---|
| 24. Physician's Name and Address | 26. I certify/recertify that this patient is confined to his/her home and needs intermittent skilled nursing care, physical therapy and/or speech therapy or continues to need occupational therapy. The patient is under my care, and I have authorized the services on this plan of care and will periodically review the plan. |
| 27. Attending Physician's Signature and Date Signed | 28. Anyone who misrepresents, falsifies, or conceals essential information required for payment of Federal funds may be subject to fine, imprisonment, or civil penalty under applicable Federal laws. |

Form HCFA-465 (C-3) (02-94) (Print Aligned)

**PROVIDER**

**fig. 23-2** Sample home health certification and plan of care form.

with the success of the hospice movement. The family's coping skills and a focus on palliative care become issues in long-term terminal care. Home care nurses must be open to discussion of spiritual concerns, life review, and reconciliation.

## THE TRANSITION FROM ACUTE TO HOME CARE: DISCHARGE PLANNING

The process of discharge planning coordinates the transition of the patient from hospital to home and ensures seamless continuity of care. Discharge planning prepares the patient and family for transition from one health care setting to another and includes assessing patient needs at discharge, making arrangements and referrals for follow-up care and assistance, and coordinating the various professional and volunteer services to be used in the patient's care at home.[13] Hospital discharge planning takes a wide variety of forms, from a cursory assessment of needs by an assigned staff nurse on the day of discharge to a multidisciplinary planning process conducted under the guidance of an institution-wide or unit-based discharge planner.[6] This individual is usually a professional nurse, but social workers also fulfill this responsibility in some institutions. Effective discharge planning is by nature a multidisciplinary group

**research**

Reference: Boland DL, Sims SL: Family care giving at home as a solitary journey, *Image J Nurs Sch* 28(1):55, 1996.

Studies have consistently found that home caregiving creates a tremendous burden on the family. This qualitative study explored issues related to home caregiving with 17 families who were caring for patients with a wide range of needs and spanning infancy to 87 years. An interview guide was used to direct discussion.

The central theme of the data was the experience of caregiving as a solitary journey. Related concepts included burden or responsibility, isolation, and sharing of care. The home was valued as a healing place, and its importance shaped the caregiving experience. Burdens consisted of emotional, physical, financial, and psychosocial components. The caregivers commitment to caregiving moderated the very real burden of the experience. In each family there was one primary caregiver, usually a woman, who shouldered most of the burden, and this individual rarely perceived that there were other family members who could or would share the responsibilities. The woman rarely gave up other family responsibilities and managed the tasks of caregiving in addition to her other responsibilities. Caregiving was seen as an intense responsibility without respite. Time orientation was exclusively the present; no future was envisioned. Stress was a constant companion, and all caregivers expressed feelings of isolation and aloneness. Caregivers' commitment to care was their primary coping resource for dealing with all of the burdens of the role of caregiving.

process. Planning complex discharges usually necessitates a team conference in which professionals from a variety of disciplines discuss the patient's discharge needs and plans with the patient, if possible, and the family. However, the luxury of team conferences for discharge planning is not readily available to support the discharge of most patients, and the nurse planner often must work individually with each discipline to determine the full extent of the patient's needs for service and support after discharge. Keeping the patient and family fully involved in the planning process is challenging but essential.

The discharge planning process encompasses assessment of the family's needs for teaching, counseling, and nursing care after discharge from the acute care setting. (See the Research Box, above right.) An important component of discharge planning is determining the resources within and external to the family that will be available when the patient returns home. The nurse accomplishes formal discharge planning by matching the patient's and family's abilities to provide self-care with appropriate and acceptable community and family resources.[13] Resources range from home health nursing care to equipment rental. Discharge planning commonly includes referral to a home care agency. However, if the patient and family are able to meet their own needs after discharge, they may not require any further assistance at home.

The current practice of early hospital discharge ensures that many patients could profit from the short-term involve-

**research**

Reference: Reiley P et al: Discharge planning: comparison of patients' and nurses' perceptions of patients following hospital discharge, *Image J Nurs Sch* 28(2):143, 1996.

The purpose of this study was to determine how well primary nurses predict the functional status of their patients after discharge and to assess whether patients and nurses agree about patients' level of understanding of the home treatment plan. The sample for the study included 97 nurse-patient pairs. The patients were drawn from a pool of English-speaking, cognitively intact adult patients admitted to a major urban teaching hospital with a diagnosis of myocardial infarction or community-acquired pneumonia. Patient interviews and demographic data collection were conducted at admission, 2 weeks after discharge, and 2 months after discharge. Patients were asked about the hospitalization experience, health perceptions, and functional status. The primary nurse for each patient was also interviewed within 48 hours of the patient's discharge.

Comparison of nurse and patient responses showed that the nurses significantly overestimated the predicted functional disability of their patients. Considerable disagreement was found concerning predicted functional status and the patient's reported status 2 months after discharge. Opposite results were found concerning the patient's knowledge of the home treatment plan. Patients understood their medication regimens, but only 57% understood medication side effects and interactions. Nurses believed that greater than 95% of the patients understood both the regimen and drug side effects. Fifty percent of the patients also reported that they did not know when they could resume normal activities, despite the belief of the nurses that 99% of the patients knew this.

ment and supervision of a home care nurse after discharge. Family members often underestimate the difficulties they will face when caregiving is required 24 hours a day.

Assisting families in accepting outside help is a valuable but sometimes difficult task.[21] For some patients a telephone call after discharge can be used to evaluate self-care status and provide continuity of care. The telephone call is organized to ask specifically about the patient's condition and caregiver fatigue so that follow-up care can be instituted as necessary.

The key to the discharge planning process is communication with the patient and family. The nurse coordinates the communication and documents the discharge plan on the health care record. Effective discharge planning begins well before discharge and identifies patients needing home care. Characteristics of patients and various aspects of their medical-surgical treatment that influence their need for home care are listed in Box 23-4.

These criteria reflect common situations that necessitate home care follow-up, but they are not the only variables to consider. Discharge planning truly needs to be initiated at admission and then continued as an ongoing process throughout the hospitalization. Short hospital stays necessitate prompt initiation of the planning process if a serious gap in

**box 23-4** *Characteristics of Patients That Influence the Need for Home Care*

1. Patients who cannot manage nursing care on their own
   a. Comatose or semicomatose patients
   b. Disoriented, confused, or forgetful patients
   c. Frail elderly persons
   d. Patients who live alone
   e. Patients who do not live alone, but persons at home cannot care for patients adequately
   f. Patients who have no home, or those whose present home is no longer adequate
2. Patients who need dressings and wound care
   a. Patients who have complicated dressings
   b. Patients who cannot do the dressing themselves
   c. Patients who will probably not do the dressing unless supervised
3. Patients who need equipment and transportation (function shared with social services)
4. Patients with medication schedules
   a. Patients with complex schedules or infections
   b. Patients who are noncompliant
5. Patients with ostomies (for example, colostomy, ileostomy)
6. Patients with special teaching needs (for example, new diabetic, complex diet, injections)
7. Patients who are terminally ill
8. Patients receiving therapy (occupational, physical, speech)
9. Patients with tubes (Foley, gastrostomy, suprapubic, nasogastric, tracheostomy)
10. Patients being transferred
    a. From another hospital or nursing home
    b. To another hospital or nursing home (e.g., Veterans Administration hospital)

The typical patients who need referrals are those with chronic illness, such as arthritis, cancer, cerebrovascular accident, chronic renal failure, congestive heart failure, diabetes mellitus, emphysema, hypertension, or myocardial infarction, and those who are ventilator dependent.

Modified from Rasmusen L: *Nurs Manage* 15(5):39, 1984.

services is to be successfully avoided. It is not uncommon for patients with complex needs to be discharged and then wait for 24 to 48 hours before they are first contacted by the home care agency. Families are left alone to cope with the patient's needs during the most vulnerable portion of the transition home and may not have the necessary skills, equipment, or support to provide needed care. This service gap can have serious consequences for both the patient's care and the family members' confidence in their ability to successfully manage care at home. The arrival of the home care nurse becomes not support but family rescue. Ideally, a representative of the home care agency meets with the patient and family before discharge to complete the needs assessment and ensure the acquisition of needed supplies and equipment. Unfortunately this first contact is usually viewed more as a luxury than a necessity, and families take patients home with little knowledge of who will be providing needed care and support.

The goal of effective discharge planning is to provide the patient and family with the following: (1) information about what to expect after discharge; (2) instruction in appropriate self-care; (3) identification of family and community resources; (4) awareness of procedures to follow for emergencies; (5) knowledge of follow-up care; (6) family teaching specific to the patient's concerns; and (7) explanation of home care services, telephone numbers, and, when possible, introductions to home care personnel.

Clinical pathways can be extremely useful tools in the discharge planning process as the individual steps of the planning process are directly assigned to specific days of the hospitalization.[24] Used correctly, these pathways establish a manageable and sequential timetable for ensuring that discharge planning takes place in a timely and thoughtful manner.

## Determining Discharge Planning Needs

Discharge planning includes a careful assessment of the patient's home environment. The unique demands of the patient's physical care are compared with the resources available in the home (e.g., running water, refrigeration, and dry storage space). The nurse also assesses the patient's and family's resources and support systems, including the immediate and extended family, neighbors, friends, and religious supports. A basic discharge planning assessment is presented in Box 23-5.

The nurse needs to determine whether the patient and family have adequate coping mechanisms to manage the illness and the common stressors of home care. The patient's attitude toward discharge to home, family members' reactions to the caregiver role, and the family's ability to accept help from the home care team all influence the outcome of care. Before discharge, the patient's and family's attitudes toward home care are determined. The patient's motivation to return home and the family's willingness to provide and accept home care are important determinants of successful home management. The patient's and family's perceptions and concerns about recovery will influence acceptance of home care.

## Financial Assessment

Financial assessment must be undertaken before discharge because home care can be a significant financial burden for families. Home health care can be expensive and is usually not completely reimbursable. Patient and family self-payments are the second-largest source of payments for home care services. Cost analyses indicate that home care expenses vary in relation to the type, intensity, and length of services needed. Medicare, Blue Cross–Blue Shield, and an increasing number of private insurance companies pay for acute, posthospital home care services to reduce the length of hospital stay. For such coverage, however, the care required must be defined as intermittent rather than ongoing. Medicaid and a few insurers will pay for longer-term home care services for those whose condition is chronic. Supplemental coverage can be obtained in some cases from agencies that provide old-age assistance,

**box 23-5** *Discharge Planning Needs Assessment*

**HOME ENVIRONMENT**
Living arrangements
House or apartment
- One floor or multilevel
- Stairs—how many to reach bedrooms, bathrooms, kitchen

Adequacy of heating, cooling, electricity, plumbing, telephone service, etc.

**CARE NEEDS**
Equipment and supplies
Adequacy of storage facilities

**SUPPORT SYSTEMS**
Who is present in the home, family roles?
Extended family, kinship network
Family coping strategies
Knowledge of and willingness to use external supports from community
Friendship, neighborhood, community, and church supports available

**LEARNING NEEDS**
Knowledge base
Skill acquisition
Comfort with caregiver role

**EMOTIONAL RESPONSES**
Feelings about diagnosis, discharge, home care expectations
Potential role conflicts and burdens for caregivers

**FINANCIAL ASSESSMENT**
Family resources
Insurance coverage
Supplemental care expenses

workers' compensation, disability, Medicaid, or other financial aid programs.

Even when care is reimbursable, the family must usually pay deductibles, and only a percentage of the total cost is reimbursable. There may also be extra expenses associated with home care that are not covered by any insurance or government program, and these can become significant out-of-pocket expenses. For example, utility bills may increase because of equipment necessary for care. Special services from a pharmacist or supplies such as enteral feeding products may be costly yet are reimbursable only on a limited basis. Caring for the patient in the home also may have caused a family member to quit work or reduce employment hours, thus reducing income.

Each of the major reimbursement sources varies in the requirements the patient must meet, the length of time benefits are allowed, and the types of equipment or supplies provided. Typically the complete descriptions of the therapies, equipment, and services covered are included in the manuals available from each insurer.

Financial assessment is often difficult for nurses to undertake, and in larger hospitals this aspect of discharge planning is usually the responsibility of a social worker. However, nurses need access to financial data to ensure that patients receive the full benefits for which they are eligible under government or private insurance. Nurses need to understand the services that are reimbursed by different insurers. In today's economic climate, with the high costs of health care, even middle-income families may need assistance because they may be ineligible for governmental programs or other assistance. Box 23-6 lists financial resources that may be available to patients requiring home care. The involvement of a social worker or financial discharge planner who is aware of the current eligibility and reimbursement criteria is essential, especially for elders.

**box 23-6** *Financial Resources Screening Checklist*

1. Check the governmental or private resources available to the patient (benefits vary with each plan):

| | |
|---|---|
| ______ Medicaid | ______ Financial help from family |
| ______ Medicare A (home care services) | ______ Disability payments |
| ______ Medicare B (home care equipment) | ______ Retirement pensions |
| ______ Health insurance including HMOs and PPOs | ______ Welfare programs |
| ______ Employer insurance | ______ Meals-on-wheels |
| ______ Social Security | ______ United Way agencies |
| ______ American Cancer Society (free bandages, equipment) | ______ Private insurance |
| ______ Multiple Sclerosis Society (wheelchair loans) | ______ Savings accounts |
| ______ Volunteer or charitable organization resources | ______ Veterans Administration |
| ______ Old-age assistance | ______ Military retirement |
| ______ Supplemental Security Income | |

2. Do you think that your total income for this year was enough to meet your (the patient and other family members) usual monthly expenses and bills?

   ______ Yes ______ No

3. In the past 6 months, has money been spent on the patient's physician, hospital, nursing home, or medication bills that has not been reimbursed by insurance?

   ______ Yes ______ No

## NURSING MANAGEMENT

The family home is a unique environment for providing care to the adult patient and must be taken into account in the development of the patient's plan of care. The combined influences of the physical and psychological environments of the home continuously affect the outcomes of care provided. The physical environment of the home is evaluated for safety, accessibility, and modifications needed to provide care.[16] The psychological factors affecting home care include motivational factors, patient and family expectations, and social and community attitudes and influences.

Growing numbers of patients and their families successfully manage home care with mechanical ventilators, parenteral nutrition infusions, home hemodialysis, intravenous antibiotics or chemotherapy, and other life-sustaining interventions. Home care, even in the face of technological dependency, allows families to exert control over their lives and maintain their highest level of functioning.

### ASSESSMENT

The home care nurse must be skillful in conducting patient and environmental assessment. Careful assessment of the patient's needs should have been completed as part of the discharge planning process, but the home care nurse needs to promptly and efficiently verify the accuracy of the predischarge assessment and determine any additional or unique needs for equipment, care, or support.

#### Assessment of Expectations

Both the patient's and family's willingness and motivation for home care must be assessed in light of their expectations. The nurse explores the family's expectations concerning the degree of involvement that the nurse will have in the patient's daily care.[9] The roles and responsibilities of the family caregiver(s) versus the nurse or home health aide may need to be clarified. It is important to ensure that family caregivers have thoughtfully considered the changes in their daily lives and schedules that will result from the assumption of the challenges of caregiving.

Cultural values may make it extremely difficult for some families to accept the presence of strangers in their home. The nurse needs to be extremely sensitive to the family's cultural beliefs and respect these in the planning process.[7] Cultural network resources can also be explored as an additional source of potential support for the family. The success of home care depends to a large extent on the ability and willingness of family members or significant others to draw on and use internal and external resources. Internal resources include the family's or individual's positive attitude toward home care, ability to problem solve or seek advice, and willingness to accept help or assistance from external resources. Accepting help from friends, neighbors, and church or community groups often is difficult for families. The home health care nurse can determine the availability of these and other external resources and then assess the family's willingness to accept such help.

Each family member's reactions to the role he or she carries out in relation to home care influences the family's internal resources. The home care nurse may need to periodically assess family members' role responsibilities in home care inasmuch as these change over time. Also, individual reactions to responsibilities and the energy required to carry them out vary with the length of time that caregiving continues. Situational depression in both patients and caregivers is not uncommon. Families also react to changes, whether improvement, decline, or stabilization, in the patient's condition during home care. Interview questions that can be used to assess caregiver roles and reactions are listed in Box 23-7.

When family responses are regularly assessed and evaluated, the nurse may be able to promptly intervene with assistance in obtaining occasional or regular respite care so that the caregivers can spend some worry-free time away from the caregiving situation. The nurse must realize that as home care continues, the resources, motivation, and emotional reactions of the family and patient will change and must be taken into account in revising the home care plan.

#### Assessment of the Home

The home is the physical environment for delivery of nursing care. The criteria used to assess the safety of the home depend to some extent on the patient's abilities and needs. The home of a patient who is discharged with equipment for hemodialysis may require alterations to provide a safe environment for care. Modifications in the home environment for safety also may be based on the patient's disabilities or physical condition, such as the need for high-rise toilet seats, grab bars in the bathroom, or changing a living room into a bedroom.[16]

Guidelines for assessing the physical environment should always include basic information about the home within that community. The location of the residence in relation to

**box 23-7** *Caregiver Role Assessment*

1. How have the responsibilities of the members of the family changed since the patient has been at home?
2. How do you and other family members feel about these changes in responsibility?
3. Has your health changed since you have been caring for the patient at home? If so, describe how.
4. Family members tell us they have emotional reactions to the changes in the person they are caring for. What has your experience been with these emotional reactions?
5. Family members often state that responsibilities of home care can be overwhelming and difficult. Do you find this true or not true?
6. Family members also have found they have gained strengths or a sense that they are successful in caring for the patient at home. Do you find this to be true or not true?
   Tell me the successes you have experienced.
   Tell me about when you have not felt successful.

necessary home care services, durable medical equipment companies, and care sites for emergencies is important. Some rural residents may be willing and motivated to provide home care but are 50 miles away from the closest home health care provider. Even urban dwellers may find out that their metropolitan area does not have an agency that provides necessary equipment, such as mechanical ventilators.

Another factor is the availability of transportation to and from needed resources. Arrangements for trips to the grocery, pharmacy, and clinic are part of the safety of home management. Finding appropriate community resources to ensure safe care is a common challenge for the home care nurse.

The physical environment of the home should always be assessed for basic factors that affect the patient's health and adjustment to home care (Box 23-8). Adequacy of heating, cooling, electrical outlets, plumbing, and refrigeration, as well as access to a telephone, should be determined. Lack of these basic resources does not preclude home care, however, unless they are necessary for safety.

Infestation by insects or rodents can also compromise the safety of the patient and ability to maintain cleanliness for needed care supplies. Plumbing and toilet facilities are also assessed in light of the patient's care needs. The actual physical layout of the home, particularly in relation to the patient's bedroom, also is assessed. The patient may be bedridden, unable to climb stairs, or restricted to one area because of medical equipment. Creative problem solving may be necessary to ensure that family members can use the space in their home in the way they desire and that medical equipment does not cause too much noise or interference. Physical modifications are often necessary to support long-term care provision.

Part of the assessment of the overall safety and preparedness of the home setting is assessment of the family's knowledge of emergency procedures.[16] Each family should know how to use the community's emergency telephone system and how to contact the home health care nurse for less serious situations. Family members can be taught cardiopulmonary resuscitation (CPR). Equipment checks are a specific and important part of home care assessment. Typically, each piece of equipment comes with written materials that outline the safety checks, cleaning procedures, and routine maintenance. The family must understand the manuals and incorporate safety checks into everyday schedules.

**box 23-8** *Sample Home Assessment*

**GENERAL**

1. Is there good lighting available, especially around stairwells?
2. Are there handrails on both sides of the staircases? Are nonskid treads in use?
3. Are the edges of rugs tacked down?
4. Is a telephone present? Are emergency numbers written in large print and kept near the telephone?
5. Are electrical cords, footstools, and other low-lying objects kept out of walkways? Are electrical cords in good condition?
6. Is adequate heating and cooling available?
7. Is furniture designed to accommodate easy transfers on and off?
8. If fireplaces or other heating devices are present, do they have protective screens?
9. Are smoke detectors present?
10. Are there alternative exits from the house?

**KITCHEN**

1. Are spaces for food storage adequate? Are shelves at eye level and easily reachable?
2. Is a sturdy stepstool present for reaching?
3. Are electrical circuits overloaded with too many appliances?
4. Are cleaning fluids, polishes, bleaches, detergents, and all poisons stored separately and clearly marked?

**BATHROOM**

1. Are there grab bars in the bath, in the shower, and around the toilet?
2. Are toilet seats high enough to get on and off of without difficulty?
3. Are bathroom doorways wide enough for easy wheelchair and walker access?
4. Are there nonskid rubber mats in the bath, in the shower, and on the floor?
5. Do medication containers have childproof tops? Are they labeled in large print?
6. Have all outdated medications been discarded?
7. Do you notice any medications (both prescription and over-the-counter) that could cause adverse side effects or drug interactions that the client is unaware of?
8. Can the water temperature be easily regulated?
9. Are electrical cords, outlets, and appliances a safe distance from the tub?

Adapted from Stanhope M, Knollmueller RN: *Handbook of community and home health nursing*, ed 2, St Louis, 1996, Mosby.

## Assessment of the Patient

Assessment of the adult patient in the home environment encompasses many of the same data collection procedures used in the acute care setting, but the patient and family caregivers are the major data collectors. The patient and family caregivers are asked to describe the patient's condition and discuss any concerns. The nurse may never have seen the patient before the initial home visit and may have only the limited data provided on the home care referral form. The nurse depends on the family's observations and monitoring for ongoing specific data.

Assessment proceeds in an orderly fashion. The nurse asks the patient and family members about their concerns and gathers specific data about each identified medical problem, nursing diagnosis, or symptom that the patient is experiencing. Because an interval of several days or more may occur between visits, detailed assessment is necessary to provide a solid basis for comparison on follow-up visits.

Assessment also includes the patient's and primary caregiver's responses to home management. The primary caregiver is the person who provides most of the physical or daily care for the patient. This may be a spouse, parent, sibling, significant other, grown child, or friend. Multiple persons may be involved in the patient's home care. The responsibility of providing care can be both physically and psychologically demanding, and the nurse needs to openly assess the severity of the burden being experienced by the caregivers.

### Assessment of the Treatment Plan

The treatment plan outlines the general care the patient needs and any special skills the patient and family must master. General areas for assessment include basic care needs, medications, nutrition, home environment, emergency procedures, specific patient needs, and equipment checks. General care assessment includes needs for assistance with hygiene, elimination, communication, rest and activity schedules, transportation, socialization, and continued contact with health care professionals.

The treatment plan includes prescriptions for medication, diet, exercise, and physical or psychological care. The nurse discusses with the patient the specific therapy he or she was given and exactly how it is being carried out. In addition, the nurse asks the patient and family about any difficulties with treatments, obtains their opinions about the benefits or drawbacks of the therapy, and discusses these issues with them.

The nurse also identifies all prescription and over-the-counter medications in use and the patient's and caregivers' knowledge of their purpose, desired effects, proper administration, and possible side effects. Careful consideration is given to the possibility of adverse drug interactions among the medications. Written patient education materials about all medications should be available as resources for the patient and family to refer to, and the nurse reviews these carefully with the patient and caregiver to ensure understanding.

Confusion over multiple medications is a common problem. Patients may resume taking medications they took before hospitalization but that no longer are prescribed. The nurse asks about what is taken daily and when it is taken and requests the patient to count the remaining number of pills in the prescription to determine how many were taken. Assessing actual dose taken versus prescribed dose is critical because there may be various reasons why patients and families change the dosage, including finances or forgetfulness.

Drug boxes can be another useful way to assist the family in medication administration and allow the nurse to more accurately monitor the patient's adherence to the medication regimen. Regular assessment of the supply of medications also helps ensure that necessary prescriptions are refilled before they run out.

The nurse also regularly assesses the patient's nutritional status. The ability to follow through on diet prescriptions is affected by food costs, accessibility, and lifelong eating patterns. Objective data about nutritional status obtained through interval measurements of body weight, intake and output, or calorie counts can be useful.

### Assessment of Learning Needs

Patient and family education is an essential responsibility for home care nurses. The nurse must be skillful in assessing readiness to learn, providing information, and evaluating outcomes of teaching. The steps for teaching the family are similar to those for individual patient teaching. Family education, therefore, begins with assessment and diagnosis of learning needs.[12] Assessing the patient's and family's understanding of the illness and its treatment establishes a baseline for teaching. Box 23-9 provides sample interview questions to determine what patients already know about their health care. The nurse can link new knowledge to information the family already has and reinforce behavior change. Any barriers to learning that the patient and family may have, such as reading difficulties or lack of desire to learn, need to be assessed. Learning is influenced by attitudes, beliefs, and values and varies for each person through the various stages of home health care.[9] Patients and families who are in a stage of denial will have difficulty learning.

The nurse also must assess the information that family members desire. In addition to information about the patient's biological condition, family members have personal knowledge and skills needs.

**box 23-9 Sample Interview Questions in Assessing Patients' Knowledge About Their Health Care**

1. Can you tell me what you have learned about your illness?
2. You have had surgery before. Can you tell me what you remember from that experience?
3. When you spoke with your physician/pharmacist, what did he or she tell you was important to know about your medications?
4. Have you heard about your therapy from anyone else who has had your health problem?
5. Have you read or heard reports about the treatments your physician wants you to undergo?

For patients who have physical limitations, careful assessment of their abilities should be done before determining the type of teaching plans and evaluation to use. For instance, some stroke patients' perception and knowledge can be evaluated by using picture boards to assist them to identify frequently used articles.

Modified from Smith CE. *Patient education: nurses in partnership with other health care professionals,* New York, 1987, Grune & Stratton.

## NURSING DIAGNOSES

Nursing diagnoses are based on the assessment data collected in the home and on the data gathered through discharge planning. The nursing diagnoses should reflect each family's actual and potential problems and responses to the condition, treatment plan, and rigors of home care. By diagnosing strengths, the nurse identifies abilities family members can use in dealing with the actual and potential problems they will face. The nurse also analyzes the data to determine the coping skills, external resources, and other family strengths essential for managing the home care alone.

A wide variety of diagnoses may be applicable in any particular situation. These include all of the specific disorder-related diagnoses identified throughout the text. A few diagnoses are more specifically applicable to the uniqueness of the home care situation. The nurse also needs to be aware that patients and family members may experience stress and anxiety when they leave the acute care setting, a problem termed *relocation stress syndrome,* which needs to be acknowledged and planned for before the patient's discharge from the acute care setting. Extensive preparation—through teaching and involvement of the patient and family in coordinating resources that are readily accessible and economically feasible—lessens relocation stress.

Commonly encountered diagnoses in home care include:

| Diagnostic Title | Possible Etiological Factors |
|---|---|
| Risk for impaired home maintenance management | Lack of knowledge of home care and community resources |
| Risk for caregiver role strain | Unrealistic expectations or demands, insufficient opportunities for respite |
| Risk for loneliness | Time demands of caregiving, inability to participate in family and social activities |
| Decisional conflict | Uncertainty about choices for meeting long-term care needs |

## EXPECTED PATIENT OUTCOMES

The ultimate goal of home care is to assist the patient and family to their maximal level of functioning. In some cases this may be the patient's complete recovery and return to work. In other situations, maximal function may be the family's ability to manage the patient's care in the home without professional assistance.

Specific patient outcomes will again reflect the unique aspects of each patient and family situation and their identified needs. The following are broad outcomes that would be applicable for the home care related diagnoses addressed previously.

Patient and caregivers will:

1a. Demonstrate the ability to perform necessary patient care skills
 b. Identify needs for further skills or knowledge to effectively manage the patient's home care regimen
 c. Adapt the home environment successfully to ensure patient safety
2a. Successfully balance caregiving demands with other components of lifestyle
 b. Obtain routine respite services to ensure time away from caregiving
3. Identify ways to increase meaningful social interactions and relationships
4a. Discuss advantages and disadvantages of options for long-term care management
 b. Share fears and concerns regarding choices for long-term care and reactions of others

## INTERVENTIONS

### Gaining Access to the Home

Home care services may be crucial to the patient's successful discharge and home maintenance, but patients and families may still view the process as an invasion of their privacy. Providing nursing care in a person's home cannot be undertaken without developing a successful approach or introduction to home care services. It is hoped that the nurse and other professionals in the acute care setting will initiate discharge planning and that the family members will accept the need for the home care nurse and possibly other professionals in their home.

Ideally the first visit with the patient and family should be conducted in the hospital before discharge, but often the first visit is to the home. Therefore the initial contact with the patient is almost always by telephone. The nurse clearly identifies herself and the home care agency and makes arrangements for the initial home visit, which should take place as soon as possible to confirm the patient's specific care needs. A specific appointment is set up, and the nurse clarifies with the family members how they prefer the nurse to enter the home. An agency contact telephone number is provided to the family for use in making changes in the appointment schedule or to access assistance in case of an abrupt change in the patient's status. This initial phone contact sets the tone for the nurse's working relationship with the patient and family and begins the process of rapport and trust building. When timely and appropriate discharge planning has been performed, the transition to home care can be smooth.

Safety concerns for the nurse working in the community setting are always important, especially on the first home visit. The nurse always needs to be aware of her environment and sensitive to environmental cues that would indicate an unsafe situation. Family members can be approached with questions about safe places to park, walk, and use phones in their neighborhood. Some general precautions that apply to all nurses working in home and community settings are presented in the Guidelines for Care Box.[23]

Families are often unsure of the nurse's exact role in the home and need to clearly understand the scope and boundaries of the nurse's practice. At the first visit the patient's needs are assessed and available home care options are discussed. The nurse confirms her professional role but must always be aware of and sensitive to her status as a "guest" in the patient's home. Control of the home care situation clearly rests with the patient and family, and this fact must be recognized and respected. The nurse is often welcomed to the home in a social manner on the first home visit and may be offered refreshment. The nurse uses this visit to establish trust, rapport, and a warm working relationship with the primary caregiver, and the nurse emphasizes the collaborative nature of their partnership in the patient's care.[23] It is helpful to be clear about the time limits for the visit and to refocus the discussion on issues related to care provision as needed. The nurse explains the steps of the assessment process and the services that will be provided.

Clear information is also provided to the patient and family about the costs of home care services, insurance reimbursement, and other economic details that the family will need. Options to reduce home care expenditures safely, such as family members providing wound dressing changes 3 days a week or the nurse reducing visits to twice weekly, should be explored. The nurse should note that most insurers have restrictions on the lifetime number of visits that the patient can receive. Insurers also have limits on how much they will pay

guidelines for care

### Safety Precautions for Home Visiting

1. Let the agency know your planned schedule in advance and phone numbers of the patients to be visited.
2. Have accurate information about the exact location of the patient's home and parking availability. Always carry a detailed street map.
3. Park in a well-lighted, busy area near the patient's home. If possible, schedule visits only during daylight hours.
4. Reconfirm appointments with the family before arrival.
5. Maintain your car in good working order. Keep the car free of personal belongings. Keep any needed supplies in the trunk, and always keep the car locked.
6. Avoid carrying a purse or wearing jewelry.
7. Be alert at all times. If you do not feel safe, leave the area. Visit high-crime areas only with a second nurse, never alone.
8. If a patient, family member, or visitor is drunk or hostile, leave the home and then reschedule the visit.
9. If a serious argument, fight, or abuse is occurring in or around the home, leave and then report the incident to the proper authorities.
10. Always carry agency identification and emergency phone numbers. A cellular phone provides added security.

for selected patient conditions. Discussing the economics of the health care situation with families can be difficult, but understanding that cost-effective use of their insurance will maintain coverage for them at a later date is essential. The initial visit concludes with mutual understanding and agreement about the patient's care needs, the distribution of care responsibilities between the family and home care agency, and the frequency and nature of future visits.

## Implementing Family Education

The knowledge and skills that the patient and family must have to manage the patient's care safely and effectively are specifically related to the patient's unique diagnosis and treatment plan. Patient/family teaching is directed at (1) understanding the illness and treatment plan, (2) competence in managing the patient's care, and (3) fostering effective coping with the lifestyle implications of home care. Understanding the patient's and family's lifestyle helps the nurse to plan with them about how to make necessary changes with the least disruption. When a care regimen causes minimal disruptions in lifestyle, the patient is more likely to comply with it. Teaching is more effective when it includes not only knowledge of treatment but also assistance in tailoring the needed care regimen to meet the unique lifestyle circumstances and preferences of the family. Flexibility and creative problem solving are essential.

The Guidelines for Care Box (above right) identifies interventions the nurse may use for improving patients' willingness or motivation to learn the necessary home care regimen.[9]

guidelines for care

### Enhancing Willingness or Motivation to Learn

1. Provide counseling to reduce patient or family anxieties.
2. Explore past teaching experiences that created negative attitudes toward learning.
3. Compliment individuals and groups on information already learned.
4. Determine what the person wants to learn and teach this first.
5. Take steps to overcome deficiencies in perceptual skills, such as vision limitations and memory loss.
6. Complete discharge planning so that financial, housing, or other needed assistance can be found to decrease patient's worries.

Modified from Smith CE: *Patient education: nurses in partnership with other health care professionals,* New York, 1987, Grune & Stratton.

Implementation of teaching plans can take many forms in home health care. The use of computer-assisted instruction and videotapes in the home has been successful. Particularly useful is the technique of videotaping the teaching session in the patient's home and leaving the tape there for future viewing. Videotapes illustrating problems that arise in home care, such as contamination of intravenous antibiotic injection ports, slipping of an occlusive dressing, and even signs and symptoms of infection, can be portrayed. Solutions to the problems also are modeled on the videotape for the patient and family members to review. One-to-one demonstration of technical procedures also is effective and can include "walking" a caregiver step by step through a procedure over the telephone.[12] Methods of teaching that incorporate the whole family and emphasize the need to change behavior are most likely to have positive results. Using praise and reinforcement and providing an opportunity to ask questions and to evaluate learning effectiveness are important parts of implementation.

Research on home-based patient/family education indicates that behaviorally oriented programs that emphasize changing the environment in which patients care for themselves are the most successful in improving the clinical course of chronic diseases. An example of environmental modification would include rearranging furniture so that it is in the field of vision of the patient who is rehabilitating from a cerebrovascular accident (CVA) and has residual hemianopsia. Modification of the environment actively enlists the patient in changing behavior to meet desired objectives.

Establishing cues as reminders for new behavior increases adjustment to home care. For example, encouraging patients with many treatments to try to schedule these with meals or other regular activities helps them remember to perform the activities.

The nurse must remember to bring teaching materials for the home visit even if the patient has received handouts before discharge. Duplication of materials and information reinforces previous teaching.

Family members may make statements such as, "We are being taught something different now than what the hospital nurse or doctor instructed." The nurse must coordinate patient teaching and clarify consistency of information for the family.[23] Often it is only the terminology or differences in language that cause confusion. The nurse builds on teaching materials already given to the patient so that it does not appear that only new content is being taught. Also, duplication of teaching efforts must be avoided. For example, the nurse and physical therapist should decide who will be responsible for teaching range-of-motion exercises, thus reducing duplication of effort.

The nurse needs to be skillful in evaluating the cognitive and developmental abilities of patients and families. The nurse should select and use appropriate teaching materials for each specific situation.[12]

Literacy reports suggest that less than 20% of the adult population reads above the fifth-grade level and that in the United States the median literacy is approximately at the tenth-grade level. Many times the educational materials distributed are above the patient's reading level. A mismatch of written material and the patient's reading ability can account for unsuccessful learning.[9]

Not only should the printed word be at an appropriate level for the patient, but also the vocabulary used by the nurse. Results of patient education studies indicate that common "medical words" are not understood by patients. Using the patient's own terms is usually most effective. Even for functionally literate patients, the stress associated with illness may reduce their comprehension of spoken words, written materials, and even visual teaching resources. Teaching and reteaching, with opportunities for patients to ask about terms and ideas they do not understand, are important aspects of treating knowledge deficits.[20]

Instruction is incorporated into patient care activities rather than presented as something that is "in addition to." Documentation of specific teaching activities is also crucial. Although patient education is clearly one of the most essential professional interventions in home care, it remains a struggle to secure reimbursement for education services. Reteaching patients is usually not reimbursable, regardless of learning or need, and may need to be included in other reimbursable care or charged directly to the family. Patients and families often state that carrying out procedures they were taught or observed in the hospital seems more complicated at home. Adaptations in procedures are often necessary in the home, and health care personnel are not immediately available to provide assistance. The caregivers' confidence in their ability to successfully and safely manage care may falter. The complexity of scheduling the total care, including bathing, feeding, and technical treatments, may be difficult. The varied aspects of transferring learning into the home ideally need to be discussed with the family before the patient's discharge. An emphasis on problem solving that incorporates the patient and family environment, including daily routines, will prove helpful. The nurse reassures family members that they can contact the home health agency if they have questions at any time.

Physical problems of the patient and caregiver may make learning the self-care regimen more difficult, especially for elders. Pain, electrolyte imbalances, or the primary disease process can alter the patient's cognitive functioning and prevent the patient from being an active partner in the learning process. The patient may also simply lack sufficient mental or physical energy for learning. Arthritic problems may compromise an elderly caregiver's ability to master psychomotor tasks. The effort to manipulate small objects such as needles and syringes can be frustrating. Nurses must determine any physical changes that might hamper learning and take steps to alleviate these barriers when teaching patients and families.

Another personal factor that can make a difference in the patient's and family's learning is their mental or psychological state. Much has been written about how anxiety affects perceptions and behavior. It generally is accepted that persons who have moderate to severe anxiety may be able to focus only on their immediate concerns. Consequently, the information given during hospitalization, when the patient and family are experiencing moderate to severe anxiety, may be so distorted that the person does not learn what is intended. Nurses may need to employ methods to reduce anxiety so that the patient and family can attend to learning. For some patients, complex equipment may be overwhelming and create increased anxiety. The nurse initially may need to perform the technical care and gradually teach self-care as the patient or family is able to manage it.

Cultural factors can profoundly influence the patient's response to teaching. These factors can include language barriers and cultural beliefs related to health practices. Folkways about health practices also affect home care, and nurses may include these remedies (when safe) in their teaching.[9] It is always good practice to ask patients what they believe will add to their success in home care management and try to incorporate folk remedies, when safe, into the patient's care.[7] Because the patient controls his or her own care, folk remedies are commonly used, and the nurse may be unaware of this.

### Reducing Caregiver Role Strain

Successful home care management usually necessitates changes in the family's daily schedule, routines, and household responsibilities. This shifting of responsibilities may make some family members feel overwhelmed. These changes in lifestyle may be permanent or temporary, depending on the patient's situation and the resources available to the family.[22]

A spouse as the home caregiver may have to drastically change the role previously assumed (e.g., from noncook to cook, yard work only to housekeeper). The designated caregiver may perceive home care as an overwhelming burden. The studies of caregiver burden indicate that it is the *perceived* burden more than the actual physical or financial drain that predicts role performance problems.[1] Home care generally disorganizes a family, at least temporarily. Communication patterns will be altered. The length of home care affects coping within the family. The longer that home care is required, the more the family's coping skills can become depleted. More situational crises arise during prolonged home care, which also challenges the family's coping abilities. Other contributing factors include past experiences and realistic expectations of home care. Families with positive past experiences who can accurately predict the length of home care and who have realistic expectations about the daily schedule are better able to cope with prolonged home care.

Family members' fatigue and stress are problems the home care nurse must address. The nurse can assist family members to predict the disruptions that home care might create and support them in adjusting to these disruptions.[12]

The family may be reluctant to accept help from outside the family. The family may be a closed system that does not desire help from the outside or feels shame when members cannot provide care by themselves.[11] The nurse may need to use values-clarification strategies to assist the family with this issue. Other interventions for caregiver burden include teaching about new responsibilities and social support. Social support in the form of helping with everyday care, contacts with a network of peers, acceptance of caregiving by family members, and provision of emotional concern or praise seems to ease the perception of burden in a caregiver.

The nurse also ensures that the family is aware of and appropriately accessing all support systems available in the community. Volunteer organizations may be available to assist with transportation for physician or clinic appointments, and charitable organizations such as the American Cancer Society can be a source of supplies and equipment that can decrease the costs of care. Local communities typically have a variety of specific social support resources that can be mobilized to assist the family.

Religious denominations, neighborhood associations, community centers, voluntary service groups, and professionally led support groups can all be sources of social support. These groups can be used so that the patient or family caregiver does not become isolated and overburdened with care. Studies have indicated that social and community support also can lessen the depression that the caregiver may experience from the demands and changes brought on by home care.[20]

If the family has an adequate financial resource base, the part-time involvement of a compatible home health aide to assist with daily care demands can release the primary caregiver to devote some time and attention to his or her own needs.

Caring for a family member in the home may alter individual members' everyday activities, interactions, and pattern of social contacts. Participation in religious, leisure, and school activities may be affected. Caregivers may lose familiar and meaningful family interactions such as intimate talks, humorous exchanges, the comfort of physical contact through hugs, and the joy of intimate sexual contact. The caregiver can feel increasingly isolated from normal social contact. The possibility of acute loneliness in both patient and caregiver in the context of overwhelming daily care demands is a very real concern.

Friends may fear that activities are too much of a physical strain for the patient with a chronic illness. Extended family members may believe that visiting the home causes the family more grief over the patient's disability. Many people feel uncomfortable when there are visible changes in the patient and environment and avoid visiting.[22] The nurse can assist the family to explore how home care has changed family function. The family members own descriptions will help clarify the alterations in communications and personal exchanges they are missing. The patient and family need assistance to anticipate these problems and suggestions on how to deal with such reactions. Respite care can be an essential strategy for addressing the problems associated with both caregiver burden and its risk of associated loneliness.

## Assisting with Decision Making

Dealing with the patient's chronic disability and its home care management creates constraints on family members' daily schedules and use of the home for activities. The family must make many decisions each day about the patient's home care. These decisions may result in conflicts between family members. The patient and family members have direct responsibility for managing such conflicts. Patients and families experiencing chronic illness must live with the constraints imposed by the disease and the home care.

Insufficient financial resources are a common problem reported by families at home. Reimbursements from insurance companies or Medicare vary widely and are constantly changing. The home care nurse must be skilled in understanding governmental regulations and advocating for the patient's eligibility for coverage. The nurse may enlist the help of a social worker familiar with home care coverage regulations to ensure that information on the costs of home care covered by insurers is made available to the family. In addition, the nurse (with the assistance of the social worker) needs to identify any voluntary sources of financial support for families.

The nurse also must be concerned about specialty services available to the family. In some instances, the technical support services needed by the patient may be at such a distance that safety is a concern. When this occurs, the nurse must ensure that the family recognizes and can readily manage emergencies such as equipment failure or lack of supplies.

The physical and financial burdens of caregiving may eventually overwhelm the family's coping abilities and necessitate a decision about placement of the patient for long-term care. This is usually an exceedingly stressful decision for everyone concerned. The home care nurse can assist the caregivers to realistically evaluate their situation, explore alternatives, and achieve a degree of comfort related to their ultimate decision. The collaborative involvement of a social worker to explore realistic placement options and associated costs can be helpful.

## EVALUATION

Evaluation consists of making a judgment as to whether home care has been successful. This judgment depends on comparison of the patient's and family's status with the expected outcomes of home care.

If the patient's physical function falls short of the expected outcomes, the nurse must identify factors contributing to this problem. The nurse may see signs that the patient's pathophysiological condition is worsening. Referral to the physician or arrangements for transportation to a medical facility may be necessary. Evaluation might reveal that the expected outcomes have not been achieved. The patient may have misunderstood what he or she was taught, the resources arranged at discharge may not have been obtained, or the family members may have found home care overwhelming. Expected outcomes may have been unrealistic in terms of the allotted time. The nurse reassesses the situation and establishes new outcomes in conjunction with the patient and family.

Evaluation also reveals many instances in which patients have achieved their expected outcomes. The nurse should acknowledge this with the patient and family. When families are given recognition for their achievements, they feel supported in their efforts. All evaluation data, whether indicative of outcome achievement or not, must be documented. Evaluation data may be used for justification for reimbursement of extended home care or for the involvement of other home care resources. For the patient to continue to receive Medicare home health care benefits beyond the 2 to 3 weeks of intermittent care allowable, "exceptional circumstances" must be proved. Patients may qualify for up to 2 months of home care reimbursement when the nurse provides data that document the need for continued home care.

Outcomes assessment data from an individual patient may be blended with data from patients with similar needs to project future trends and needs in home care. These data are used to refine the clinical pathways used for effective case management. Outcome data can also be used to evaluate the quality of nursing care, to determine whether specific nursing interventions were successful, and to determine whether resource allocation was appropriate within the specific situation. The need for predictable, cost-effective nursing interventions is great, and data from home care is an important source of patient data.

## DOCUMENTATION

Documentation plays an essential role in nursing practice in any setting, and home care is no exception. The patient's service record establishes a legal record of the care provided, demonstrates that established standards of care have been met, and serves as the basis for cost reimbursement. Agencies are becoming increasingly dependent on third-party reimbursement, and appropriate documentation is the key to cost recovery. The Medicare and Medicaid reimbursement guidelines dictate the exact and narrow nature of reimbursable services, and these elements must be clearly reflected in the documentation of each home visit.[14] The nurse needs to clearly explain to the patient and family the exact nature, extent, and purpose of any records that will be kept and how the confidentiality of the patient and family are protected.[10] The nurse may use a combination of written notes, tape-recorded notes, or a laptop computer, and the use of these tools should be shared with the family.

As is true with hospital-based care, each agency uses its own unique documentation forms and procedures, but common elements characterize effective documentation. Documentation is completed as soon as possible after care is provided, and time should be scheduled into the visit parameters to allow for this task to be accomplished. Laptop computers enable the nurse to promptly record data and transmit it to the agency in a timely way. Hands-on care, assessments, and health teaching are recorded, as well as all attempted or completed telephone contacts with the patient and family.[10] Box 23-10 contains some tips for accurate and appropriate home care documentation.

Clinical pathways are increasingly being used in the home setting to clearly establish the nature and goals of nursing interventions.[15] They also provide a solid framework from which to construct accurate documentation. A sample Clinical Pathway for use in home care is found on p. 599.

### box 23-10 *Home Care Documentation*

Whatever form the documentation takes, it should clearly indicate the following:

1. Why the service was initiated
2. What skilled interventions are needed and why
3. Where the plan of care is going
4. What plans exist for preparing the patient to manage without home visits

**UNIQUE ELEMENTS IN HOME CARE DOCUMENTATION**

1. The patient's basic homebound state needs to be regularly reaffirmed because this is the primary criterion for care. The limitations that keep the patient homebound need to be reiterated (e.g., fracture, paralysis, shortness of breath, pain).
2. Documentation needs to reflect the patient's ongoing need for care. Entries focus on the patient's limitations rather than strengths and progress.
3. Entries should provide specific factual information about the exact services provided.
4. Each reimbursable service needs to be reflected in the documentation. The need for every visit must be clearly indicated.
5. The entry should clearly indicate in what way the care has been tailored to meet the unique needs of the patient or home situation.

## clinical pathway *Home Care*

**CEREBRAL VASCULAR ACCIDENT (CVA), HPN, DYSPHAGIA, TIA** ICD-9 CODE(S) 436.0, 401.9, 784.5, 435.9

PATIENT NAME ______ PT. ID NO. ______ SOC DATE ______ DISCHARGE DATE ______

| DATE NOTED | EXPECTED OUTCOMES | ACHIEVED | | | VARIANCE CODES | DATE NOTED | NURSING/FUNCTIONAL DIAGNOSES | DATE CLOSED |
|---|---|---|---|---|---|---|---|---|
| | | Y | N | DATE | | | | |
| | 1. Stable cardiovascular status as evidenced by cardiovascular assessment, per protocol, and blood pressure, between *130/90* and *148/98* by visit no. *4*. | | | | | | Caregiver role strain, high risk for<br>Outcome(s) no. *5,6,7,8*: | |
| | 2. Stable neurological status as evidenced by clinical assessment, per protocol and within desired range, by visit no. *8*. | | | | | | Fluid volume, excess<br>Outcome(s) no. *1*: | |
| | 3. Stable functioning of bladder and bowels as evidenced by patient/caregiver understanding of and compliance with home therapeutic regimen by visit no. *4*. | | | | | | Injury, high risk for<br>Outcome(s) no. *2,4*: | |
| | 4. Stable swallowing status, as evidenced by safe swallowing techniques and functional communication by visit no. *5*. | | | | | | Management of therapeutic and medication regimen<br>Outcomes(s) no. *1,2,4, 5,6,7*: | |
| | 5. Personal care and hygiene needs stabilized and transferred to patient/family/caregiver by visit no. *25*. | | | | | | | |
| | 6. Patient/caregiver demonstrates understanding of and compliance with dietary and hydration regimen as evidenced by clinical assessment by visit no. *4*. | | | | | | Skin integrity, impaired<br>Outcome(s) no. *2,3*: | |
| | 7. Patient/caregiver demonstrates compliance with home therapeutic regimen: medication regimen as evidenced by assessment by visit no. *4*. | | | | | | Thought processes, altered<br>Outcome(s) no. *2*: | |
| | 8. Patient/caregiver demonstrates understanding of home safety and exercise program as evidenced by safe ambulation by visit no. *12*. | | | | | | Other:<br>Outcome(s) no. ____: | |
| | 9. Other | | | | | | Other:<br>Outcome(s) no. ____: | |
| | 10. Other | | | | | | Other: Outcome(s) no. ____: | |
| | 11. Other | | | | | | Other: Outcome(s) no. ____: | |

From Marrelli TM, Hilliard LS: *Home care and clinical paths,* St Louis, 1996, Mosby.

*Continued*

## clinical pathway *Home Care—cont'd*

**CEREBRAL VASCULAR ACCIDENT (CVA), HPN, DYSPHAGIA, TIA—cont'd** ICD-9 CODE(S) 436.0, 401.9, 784.5, 435.9

**PATIENT NAME** ______ **PT. ID NO.** ______ **SOC DATE** ______ **DISCHARGE DATE** ______

| ASSESSMENTS/INSTRUCTIONS/INTERVENTIONS | VS No. 1 | VS No. 2 | VS No. 3 | VS No. 4 | VS No. 5 | VS No. 6 | VS No. 7 | VS No. 8 | VS No. 9 | VS No. 10 |
|---|---|---|---|---|---|---|---|---|---|---|
| Explain patient rights and responsibilities. | | | | | | | | | | |
| Assess for home safety management. | | | | | | | | | | |
| Assess vital signs. *(Every visit)* | | | | | | | | | | |
| Assess neurological status. *(Every visit)* | | | | | | | | | | |
| Assess hydration and nutrition status. *(Every visit)* | | | | | | | | | | |
| Assess coping skills of patient/caregiver. *(Every visit)* | | | | | | | | | | |
| Assess patient/caregiver's willingness and ability to provide home therapeutic regimen. *(Every visit)* | | | | | | | | | | |
| Assess patient/caregiver's strengths/weaknesses related to therapeutic regimen. *(Every visit)* | | | | | | | | | | |
| Assess patient's need for personal care assistance and schedule home health aide, as indicated by visit no. 1. | | | | | | | | | | |
| Refer to: Physical/occupational therapist for home exercise and activities of daily living program (specify visit number). *#2* | | *PT* | *OT* | *PT/OT* | *PT/OT* | *PT/OT* | *PT/OT* | *PT* | *PT* | *PT* |
| Refer to: Speech language pathologist for swallowing safety/communication | *SLP* | | | | | | | | | |
| (specify visit number). *#1* | | *RD* | | | | | | | | |
| Refer to: Dietitian for nutritional assessment (especially if receiving tube feedings). | | | | | | | | | | |
| Refer to: Social worker for linkage to appropriate community resources. | | | | | | | | | | |
| Instruct patient/caregiver on home safety. *(Every visit)* | | | | | | | | | | |
| Instruct patient/caregiver on home maintenance program. *(Every visit)* | | | | | | | | | | |
| Instruct patient/caregiver on medication regimen and compliance (especially note symptoms of medication toxicity). | | | | | | | | | | |
| Venipuncture for ordered laboratory tests *PT & PTT* on visit no. *as ordered*. | | | | | | | | | | |
| Other: | | | | | | | | | | |
| Medical Supplies/Home Medical Equipment Needs | | | | | | | | | | |
| 1. Bedside commode | | | | | | | | | | |
| 2. Wheelchair/walker | | | | | | | | | | |
| 3. Other ______ | | | | | | | | | | |
| 4. Other ______ | | | | | | | | | | |

Variance codes
1. Patient related
2. Situation related
3. Systems related

Team member signature ______ Initials ______
Team member signature ______ Initials ______
Team member signature ______ Initials ______

Case manager name ______

Patient signature
(involved in care planning) ______

## critical thinking QUESTIONS

1 Edward Jenkins, 55, has chronic pancreatitis requiring antibiotic therapy every 6 hours and total parenteral nutrition (TPN) therapy at night. His wife works part time, his son Marvin is an auto mechanic and lives nearby, and his daughter Jane is a nurse's aide who works at night and lives 20 minutes away. Mr. Jenkins' care includes administration of the antibiotics and TPN via a multilumen central venous catheter.

Mr. Jenkins remains nauseated and fatigued and is unable to fulfill his responsibilities in the home. Analyze this situation and develop a teaching plan for Mr. Jenkins and his family. Discuss alternatives for who should learn which aspects of care.

2 Brad Jones, 75, has severe coronary artery disease, a history of myocardial infarction, and hypertension. He is on multiple medications and frequently forgets to take them. What strategies would you use to assist Mr. Jones to improve his adherence to the medication regimen?

3 Mrs. Flora Billings, 62, has metastatic breast cancer and is now homebound. Her health insurance was cancelled when she had to quit her job. Mr. Billings is 75 years old and unable to meet her daily care needs. The couple lives on Mr. Billings' social security and on his small pension. What resources will you explore to meet the couple's needs for care and support?

## chapter SUMMARY

### TRENDS IN HOME CARE

- Health care forecasters predict that hospital closings will continue, whereas home care services will increase. Medical-surgical nursing care in the home will be necessary for a wide range of adults.
- Economic limitations on expenses in health care and the demographics of an aging population are the primary forces increasing the need for and use of home care services.
- Medicare is the primary source of reimbursement for home care services. Most other insurers model their guidelines on Medicare. Requirements for home care service are narrow rather than holistic and focus on medical problems rather than the needs of the entire family unit.

### TRANSITION FROM ACUTE CARE TO HOME CARE

- Discharge planning includes resource management, coordination of hospital and community services, and adequate preparation for home care. The nurse may act as the primary planner or coordinate the multidisciplinary team.
- The acuity level of persons who require care in their homes will continue to rise, and the technological aspects of care, including use of mechanical equipment or invasive procedures such as intravenous therapies, will increase in home care.
- The uniqueness of the residence as the environment for care must be taken into account with an adult who requires home care.
- The plurality of U.S. society necessitates that home care nurses be culturally competent in their interactions with patients and families. The nurse is a guest in the home rather than the primary decision maker.
- Many nurses are uncomfortable with financial resource assessment; however, nurses must be skillful at identifying all potential resources for the patient's care. Home care services are rarely completely reimbursable.

### NURSING MANAGEMENT

- Patients may require one or two home visits or around-the-clock nursing care. The nursing management of persons in home care includes expanded assessment of the patient and the home environment, development of nursing diagnoses based on family data, generation of expected outcomes negotiated with the patient and family, implementation of appropriate care, and extensive evaluation of the effectiveness of care for continuous quality improvement.
- The nursing process in home care is an expansion of that used with hospitalized patients. Assessment is broadened to include recognition of environmental, financial, social, and community influences on care. The assessment of the patient's condition, psychological status, and response to treatment is undertaken in light of family analysis.
- Home caregiving can put a tremendous strain on the caregiver. Nurses must carefully assess for caregiver strain and seek out services for providing respite for family caregivers.

### DOCUMENTATION

- Documentation is a unique challenge in home care because it serves as the only basis for service reimbursement. The nurse focuses on documenting the patient's ongoing weaknesses and needs rather than on strengths and progress.

## References


1. Allen SA: Medicare case management, *Home Healthc Nurse* 12(3): 21, 1994.
2. Aroskar MA: Managed care and nursing values: a reflection, *Trends Health Care Law Ethics* 10(1 & 2):83, 1995.
3. Arras JD: The technologic tether: an introduction to ethical and social issues in high-tech home care, *Hastings Cent Rep* 24(5):51, 1994 (special supplement).
4. Benefield LE: Making the transition to home care nursing, *Am J Nurs* 96(10):47, 1996.
5. Brent N: Healthcare reform: implications for home health care nursing and agencies, *Home Healthc Nurse* 12(1):10, 1994.
6. Brooten D, Brown LP, Hazard-Munro B, et al: Early discharge and specialist transitional care, *Image J Nurs Sch* 20:64, 1988.
7. Campinha-Bacote J: The quest for cultural competency in nursing care, *Nurs Forum* 30:19, 1995.
8. Dee-Kelly PA, Heller S, Sibley M: Managed care: an opportunity for home care agencies, *Nurs Clin North Am* 29(3):471, 1994.
9. Dela Cruz EA: Clinical decision making styles of home care nurses, *Image J Nurs Sch* 26:222, 1994.
10. Ellenbecker CA, Shea K: Documenting in home health care practice: evidence of quality care, *Nurs Clin North Am* 29(3):495, 1994.
11. Grossman D: Cultural dimensions in home health nursing, *Am J Nurs* 96(7):33, 1996.
12. Hellwig K: Health teaching: the crux of home care nursing, *Home Healthc Nurse* 8(4):35, 1990.

13. Hester LE: Coordinating a successful discharge plan, *Am J Nurs* 96(6):35, 1996.
14. Magliozzi H: Home care: charting that makes it through the Medicare maze, *RN* 53(6):75, 1990.
15. Marrelli TM, Hilliard LS: *Home care and clinical paths,* St Louis, 1996, Mosby.
16. Mattox DB: Stay safe, *Home Health Focus* 2(1):4, 1995.
17. McNeal GJ: High-tech home care: an expanding critical care frontier, *Crit Care Nurse* 16(5):51, 1996.
18. National Association for Home Care: *Basic statistics about home care,* Washington, DC, 1996, National Association for Home Care.
19. O'Neill ES, Pennington EA: Preparing acute care nurses for community-based care, *Nurs Health Care* 17(2):62, 1996.
20. Smith CE: A model of caregiving effectiveness for technologically dependent adults residing at home, *Adv Nurs Sci* 17(2):27, 1994.
21. Smith CE: Technology and home care, *Annu Rev Nurs Res* 13:137, 1995.
22. Smith CE: Quality of life and caregiving in technological home care, *Annu Rev Nurs Res* 14:95, 1996.
23. Stanhope M, Knollmueller RN: *Handbook of community and home health nursing,* ed 2, St Louis, 1996, Mosby.
24. Wells S: Adding an "at home" path to your discharge plan, *Am J Nurs* 96(10):73, 1996.
25. Williams PD, Williams AR, Griggs C: Children at home on mechanical assistive devices and their families: a retrospective study, *Matern Child Nurs J* 19(4):297, 1990.

# chapter 24 ASSESSMENT OF THE Cardiovascular System

SHELLEY YERGER HUFFSTUTLER

## objectives After studying this chapter, the learner should be able to:

1. Recall subjective and objective data that are significant in a cardiovascular examination.
2. Discuss the basic structure and function of the heart.
3. Explain the conduction system of the heart in relation to the cardiac cycle.
4. Analyze factors that affect cardiac output.
5. Discuss physiological changes that occur in the cardiovascular system with aging.
6. Differentiate common manifestations of altered cardiac functioning.
7. Explain various diagnostic tests used to assess cardiac functioning and the significance of each.
8. Compare nursing care of a patient undergoing cardiac catheterization and electrophysiological study.

Cardiovascular disease, specifically coronary artery disease, continues to be the leading cause of death in the United States. Every year at least 1.7 million years of potential life are lost to cardiovascular disease.[1]

The majority of persons who have a myocardial infarction (MI) are under the age of 60. It is estimated that in the United States 1 man in 5 will have an MI before the age of 60 and that 1 in 10 to 15 men in this age group will die of coronary artery disease. Although onset of coronary artery disease in women is typically 10 years later than in men, women account for at least half of all deaths from MIs each year. In fact, after age 65, the mortality rate from coronary artery disease is 11% higher for women than men.[7]

Therefore, even though the mortality rate from coronary artery disease has declined over 20% in the last 25 years, the aforementioned statistics strongly support the need for continued education of the public about the disease. Continued emphasis must be placed on lifestyle modifications such as diet, exercise, and smoking cessation to further reduce risk factors. More effective medical management, improved surgical techniques, and advances in technology and pharmacotherapy will contribute to the reduction in mortality and morbidity from cardiovascular disease.[11]

This chapter is the first of four chapters that focus on the heart and vascular system. A review of anatomy and physiology of the cardiovascular system, along with assessment (including diagnostic tests), is included.

## ANATOMY AND PHYSIOLOGY OF THE HEART

### BASIC STRUCTURE

The heart is a relatively small organ that weighs 300 g and is approximately the size of a fist. It is located in the middle of the mediastinum, where the lungs partially overlap it. This pulsatile four-chambered pump beats approximately 72 times per minute, pumping more than 5 L of blood each minute, or about 2000 gallons per day. It continually propels oxygenated blood into the arterial system and receives poorly oxygenated blood from the venous system. The heart muscle rests on the diaphragm and is tilted forward and to the left so that the apex of the heart is rotated anteriorly.

The heart is enclosed by the pericardium, which consists of two layers: the inner layer (visceral pericardium) and the outer layer (parietal pericardium). The two pericardial surfaces are separated by a pericardial space that normally contains approximately 10 to 20 ml of thin, clear pericardial fluid. This lubricating fluid moistens the contacting surfaces of the pericardial layers and serves to reduce the friction produced by the pumping action of the heart. The visceral pericardium encases the heart and extends several centimeters onto each of the great vessels. The parietal pericardium is attached anteriorly to the manubrium and xiphoid process of the sternum, posteriorly to the vertebral column, and inferiorly to the diaphragm.

The three layers of cardiac tissue are *epicardium*—the outer layer of the heart, which is the same structure as the visceral pericardium; *myocardium*—the middle layer of the heart, which is composed of striated muscle fibers and is responsible for the heart's contractile force; and *endocardium*—the innermost layer of the heart, which consists of endothelial tissue. The endocardium lines the inside of the heart's chambers and covers the heart valves.

### CHAMBERS

The heart is divided into two halves by a muscular wall (septum) (Figure 24-1). Each half has an upper collecting chamber (atrium) and a lower pumping chamber (ventricle). Oxygen-poor venous blood enters the right atrium, flows from the right atrium to the right ventricle (mainly by gravity) when the tricuspid valve is opened, and is pumped into

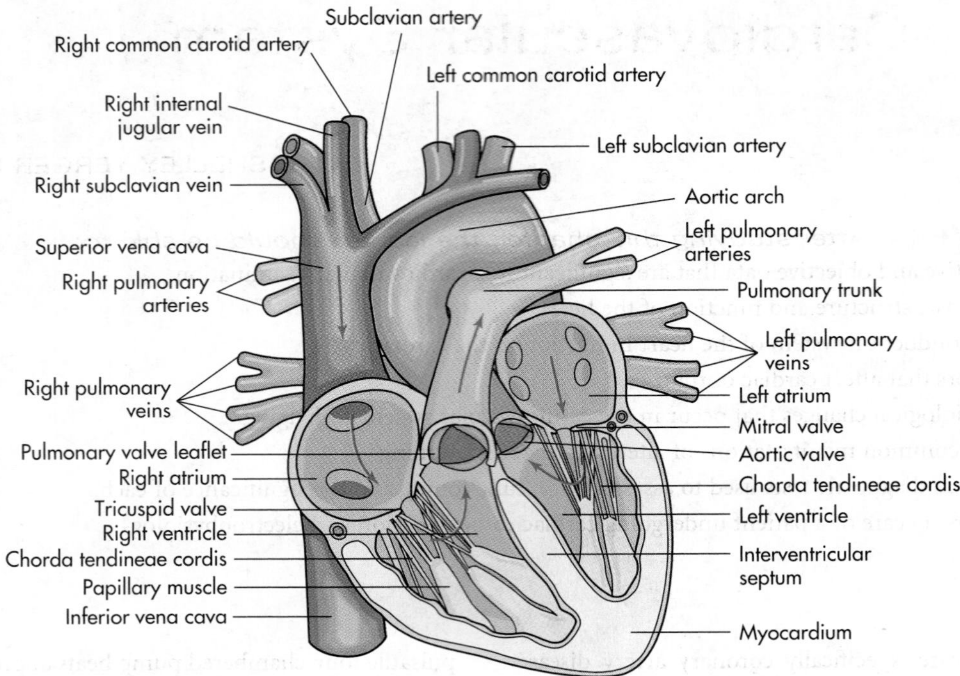


**fig. 24-1** Heart in frontal section; course of blood through the chambers.

the pulmonary artery to the lungs. Oxygen-rich blood returns from the lungs to the left atrium, enters the left ventricle when the mitral valve is opened, and is ejected into the aorta for distribution to the peripheral tissues.

The right atrium is a thin-walled structure that serves as a reservoir for venous blood returning to the heart. Venous blood returns to the heart via the superior and inferior vena cavae and the coronary sinus, which drains venous blood from the heart muscle. Blood is temporarily stored in the right atrium during right ventricular systole (contraction). During ventricular diastole (filling), approximately 80% of the venous return to the right atrium flows by gravity into the ventricle through the tricuspid valve. The remaining 20% of the venous return is delivered to the ventricles during atrial systole. This additional 15% to 20% of the venous return, which is actively propelled into the ventricles, is called the *atrial kick.*

The right ventricle is normally the most anterior structure of the heart and is situated immediately beneath the sternum. The right ventricle receives venous blood from the right atrium during ventricular diastole. During ventricular diastole this blood is propelled through the pulmonic valve into the pulmonary artery and then to the lungs. Because the pulmonary system is a low-pressure system, the overall workload of the right ventricle is much lighter in comparison to the left ventricle. The right ventricle has a crescent-shaped chamber and a thin outer wall that is 4 to 5 mm thick. This thin structure is suitable for right ventricular systole, because the right ventricle contracts against low resistance.

The thin-walled left atrium receives oxygenated blood from the four pulmonary veins and serves as a reservoir during left ventricular systole. Blood flows by gravity from the left atrium into the left ventricle through the opened mitral valve during ventricular diastole. Left atrial contraction then propels the remaining 20% of the venous return and provides a significant increment of blood volume to the left ventricle. This atrial kick serves to stretch the ventricle preparing for ventricular ejection.

The left ventricle receives blood from the left atrium through the opened mitral valve during ventricular diastole. Blood is then ejected through the aortic valve into the systemic arterial circulation during ventricular systole. The left ventricle must contract against a high-pressure systemic circulation to deliver blood flow to the peripheral tissues. Therefore the left ventricular chamber is surrounded by 8 to 15 mm of thick musculature, which is approximately two to three times the thickness of the right ventricle. The thick musculature and ellipsoidal-sphere shape contribute to the powerful expulsive ability of the left ventricular chamber during systole.

## VALVES

The four cardiac valves are flaplike structures that function to maintain unidirectional (forward) blood flow through the heart chambers. These valves open and close in response to pressure and volume changes within the cardiac chambers. The cardiac valves can be classified into two types: the atrioventricular (AV) valves, which separate the atria from the ventricles, and the semilunar valves, which separate the pulmonary artery and the aorta from their respective ventricles.

### Atrioventricular Valves

The AV valves are the tricuspid valve, located between the right atrium and the right ventricle, and the bicuspid (or mi-

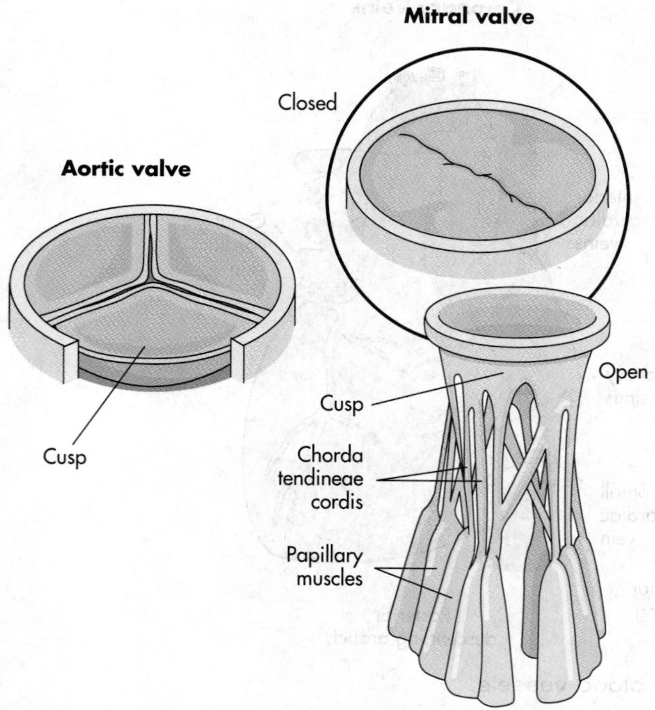


**fig. 24-2** Aortic and mitral (bicuspid) valves.

tral) valve, located between the left atrium and left ventricle. The tricuspid valve contains three leaflets held in place by fibrous cords called the *chorda tendineae cordis,* which in turn are anchored to the ventricular wall by the papillary muscles. The mitral valve on the left side of the heart is a bicuspid valve with two valve cusps or leaflets. It also is attached to chorda tendineae cordis, which extend to the papillary muscles (Figure 24-2). The chorda tendineae cordis are extremely important because they support the AV valves during ventricular systole to prevent valvular prolapse into the atrium. Some leaflet overlapping occurs during closure of the AV valves, which helps prevent the backward flow of blood. Damage to the chorda tendineae cordis or to the papillary muscles allows valvular regurgitation of blood back into the atrium during ventricular systole, resulting in increased pressure and volume. During diastole the AV valves serve as a type of funnel inasmuch as they allow blood to flow from the atria to the ventricles. The diameter of the AV cusps is almost double that of the orifice occluded by the valve. In general, the AV valves are structurally much more complex than the semilunar valves.

### Semilunar Valves

The semilunar valves are the pulmonic and aortic valves. The structural design of the semilunar valves is quite different from the AV valves; each consists of three cuplike cusps. (See Figure 24-2.) The pulmonic valve lies between the right ventricle and the pulmonary artery. The aortic valve lies between the left ventricle and the aorta. These valves are open during ventricular systole (contraction) to permit blood flow into the aorta and the pulmonary artery. They are closed during diastole (relaxation) to prevent retrograde flow from the aorta and the pulmonary artery into the ventricles.

## CORONARY ARTERIES

The coronary arteries arise from the aorta (just behind the cusps of the aortic valve) in an area known as Valsalva's sinus. The function of the coronary artery system is to provide an adequate blood supply to the myocardium.

There are two main coronary arteries, the left and the right (Figure 24-3). The left coronary artery (LCA) divides into two branches: the left anterior descending (LAD) artery and the circumflex coronary artery (CCA). The LAD branch supplies the left ventricular myocardium, the septum, the anterior papillary muscle, and portions of the right ventricle. In addition, the LAD artery usually supplies the anterior apex and some portion of the posterior apex. The CCA typically emerges at a sharp 90-degree angle from the LCA and is then directed toward the lateral left ventricle and apex. The CCA and its branches supply most of the left atrium, the lateral wall of the left ventricle, and part of the posterior wall of the left ventricle. Diagonal branches arise between the LAD artery and the CCA and are distributed along the free wall of the left ventricle.

Two important external landmarks are used in tracing coronary circulation. These anatomical landmarks are sulci, or grooves, and include the following: the atrioventricular groove, which encircles the heart between the atria and the ventricles; and the interventricular groove, which divides the right and left ventricles. The meeting of the two anatomical grooves on the posterior side of the heart is known as the crux of the heart. The location of the crux is significant because this is where the AV node is located. The terms *dominant left circulation* and *dominant right circulation* refer to whether the left or the right coronary artery turns at the crux of the heart and supplies the posterior interventricular groove. Therefore, if the CCA extends as far as the posterior interventricular groove, the circulation is considered to be dominant left. This condition occurs in only 10% to 15% of all persons.

The right main coronary artery (RCA) arises from the right Valsalva's sinus off the aorta and courses around the right AV groove. Its branches supply the right ventricle, a portion of the septum, and in more than 50% of all persons, the sinoatrial (SA) node. In approximately 67% of all persons, the RCA turns at the crux of the heart and descends in the posterior interventricular groove. These hearts are classified as dominant right. The posterior descending branch of the RCA then supplies the posterior aspect of the septum and the posterior left papillary muscle before terminating in several branches to the left ventricular wall.

Great variation exists in the branching pattern of the coronary arteries. In approximately 18% of the population, the CCA reaches the crux of the heart with the RCA; this is the "balanced" coronary artery pattern. In the remaining persons, no true posterior interventricular branch exists; rather, many branches from either main coronary artery supply the posterior septum.

Blood flow to the myocardium occurs almost exclusively during diastole, when coronary vascular resistance is

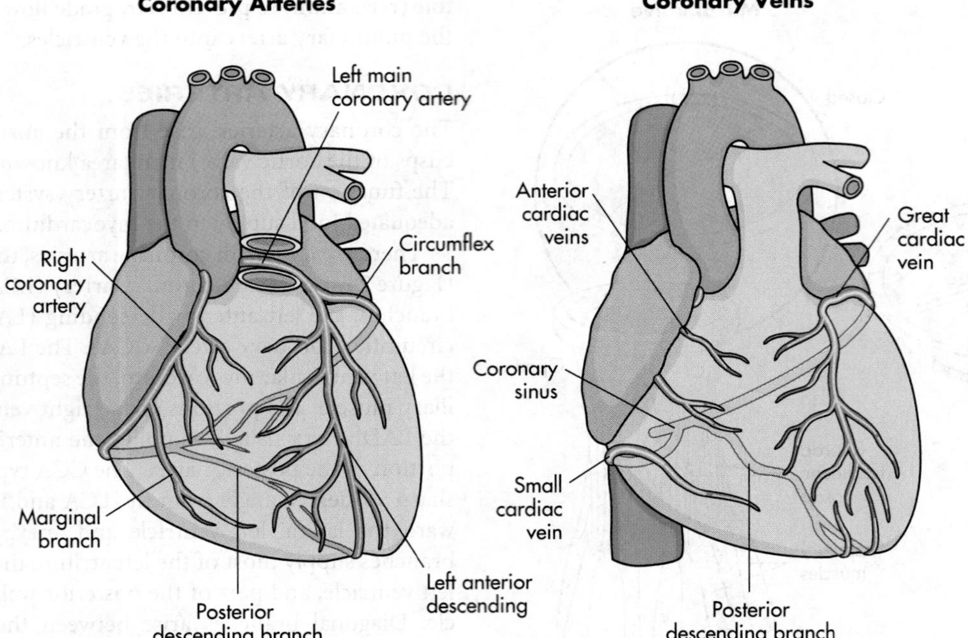


**fig. 24-3** Coronary blood vessels.

diminished. During systole, coronary vascular resistance is increased because of the increased ventricular wall tension produced by ventricular contraction. During diastole, blood enters the coronary arteries at the pressure that exists at the moment in the aortic arch. This is termed *aortic diastolic pressure.*

Coronary venous drainage is accomplished via three subdivisions of the heart's venous system: (1) the thebesian veins drain a portion of the right atrial and right ventricular myocardium; (2) the anterior cardiac veins drain a large portion of the right ventricle; and (3) the coronary sinus and its branches drain the left ventricle and most myocardial venous return.

## CONDUCTION SYSTEM

### Properties of Cardiac Muscle

The mechanical contraction of the heart is the product of a stimulus-response process. The following properties are integral components of the electromechanical events in the heart.

#### Automaticity

The ability of the heart to initiate impulses regularly and spontaneously is known as automaticity, or rhythmicity. Although most cardiac cells have this ability, it is the prominent property of the SA node, making it the dominant pacemaker in the normal heart. Pacemaker cells are known to have lower resting membrane potentials than other myocardial cells and exhibit spontaneous depolarization.

#### Excitability

The ability of cardiac cells to respond to a stimulus by initiating a cardiac impulse is known as excitability. It should be noted that excitatory cells differ from pacemaker cells in that pacemaker cells do not require a stimulus to initiate an impulse.

#### Conductivity

The ability of cardiac cells to respond to a cardiac impulse by transmitting the impulse along cell membranes is referred to as conductivity. Cells that specialize in this function are found in the conduction system. The arrangement of cells outside the conduction system ensures rapid conduction through intercalated disks joining adjacent cells.

#### Contractility

The ability of cardiac cells to respond to an impulse by contracting is known as contractility. Contractile cells compose the largest mass of the myocardium.

### Anatomy of Conduction System

The pacemaking center of the normal heart is the SA, or sinus, node (Figure 24-4). It is composed of a group of highly specialized tissues located in the right atrium adjacent to the superior vena cava. Automatically and at regular intervals, an electrical impulse is emitted from the SA node at a rate of 60 to 100 beats per minute. The atria are then depolarized, and the impulse travels to the AV node via three tracts designated as anterior, middle, and posterior internodal tracts. A fourth tract, called *Bachmann's bundle,* branches off the anterior nodal tract and transmits the impulse to the left atrium.

The three internodal tracts meet at the atrionodal junction. The junctional area refers to the region where atrial and ventricular tissues merge. This junction contains the AV node. The junctional cells above and below the AV node are capable of pacemaking activity under many circumstances (e.g., failure of the SA node to fire).

The AV node itself is located on the right side of the interatrial septum. These cells lack the ability to initiate electrical

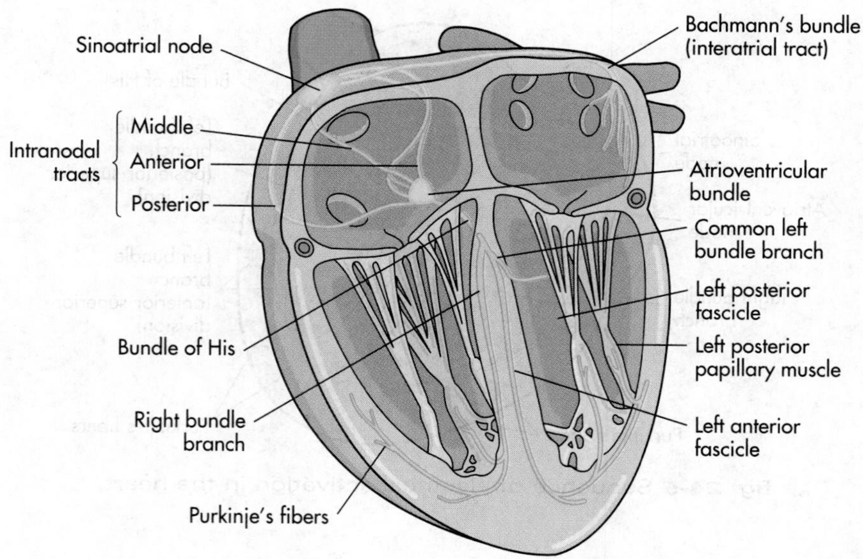


**fig. 24-4** Schematic diagram of heart illustrating the conduction system.

impulses (i.e., automaticity), but they are uniquely responsible for a brief physiological delay in the conduction of the impulse to the ventricles.

The bundle of His begins anatomically at the "tail" of the AV node. It is a short, thick cable of fibers separated by collagen septa that bifurcate into the right bundle branch (RBB) and the left bundle branch (LBB).

The RBB extends down the right side of the interventricular septum and is covered by a connective tissue sheath. It extends to reach the anterior papillary muscle of the right ventricle, where it merges with the Purkinje system. It lies close to the septal surface for much of its length, and therefore its functional ability is vulnerable to right ventricular pressure changes.

The LBB bifurcates into anterior and posterior fascicles. The anterior fascicle extends anteriorly down the left side of the interventricular septum to reach the anterior papillary muscle. The posterior fascicle is shorter and thicker and extends to the posterior papillary muscle of the left ventricle. Both fascicles connect with the Purkinje system and share equally in the spread of the impulse to the left ventricle.

Purkinje's fibers lie as a network on the endocardial surface and penetrate the myocardium of both ventricles. They are responsible for the transmission of the impulse to both ventricular free walls. Purkinje's cells are elongated and contain intercalated disks, which contribute to the superiority of conductivity in myocardial tissue.

Cells outside the conduction system also play a role in the conduction of an impulse. A surface membrane, the sarcolemma, surrounds each cell and acts as a selectively permeable barrier to sodium and potassium ions. Adjacent myocardial cells are connected end to end by a thickened portion of the sarcolemma known as an intercalated disk. These disks act as low-resistance pathways to the transmission of an impulse between cells.

## Sequence of Cardiac Activation

Depolarization (activation of the cardiac muscle) is initiated by an impulse from the SA node. The impulse first spreads through the right atrium and then activates the left atrium. Atrial activation normally is accomplished in 0.11 second or less.

Shortly after the impulse reaches the left atrium, it also activates the junctional region and subsequently the AV node. The AV node delays the impulse about 0.1 second before the impulse enters the bundle of His.

On reaching the bundle of His, the impulse is transmitted along the bundle branches. Within the ventricles, the first structure to be activated is the ventricular septum. The septum is activated by the impulse traveling from the left side to the right side (Figure 24-5).

The impulse then continues down the remaining length of the bundle branches and into the Purkinje network, thus activating the ventricular walls almost simultaneously. Activation of the ventricular muscle then proceeds from the apex back toward the base of the heart to complete the process.

Depolarization of cardiac musculature proceeds from endocardium to epicardium. Repolarization in the atria follows this same pathway. In contrast, repolarization of ventricular musculature proceeds from epicardium to endocardium. Knowledge of the sequence of activation is fundamental to analysis of the electrocardiogram (ECG).

### Action potential

The resting myocardial cell has a membrane potential (i.e., an electrical charge) as a result of the relative distribution of

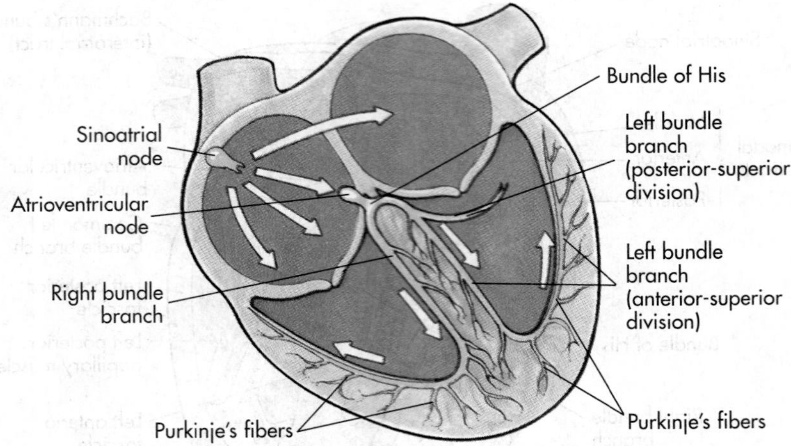


fig. 24-5 Sequence of electrical activation in the heart.

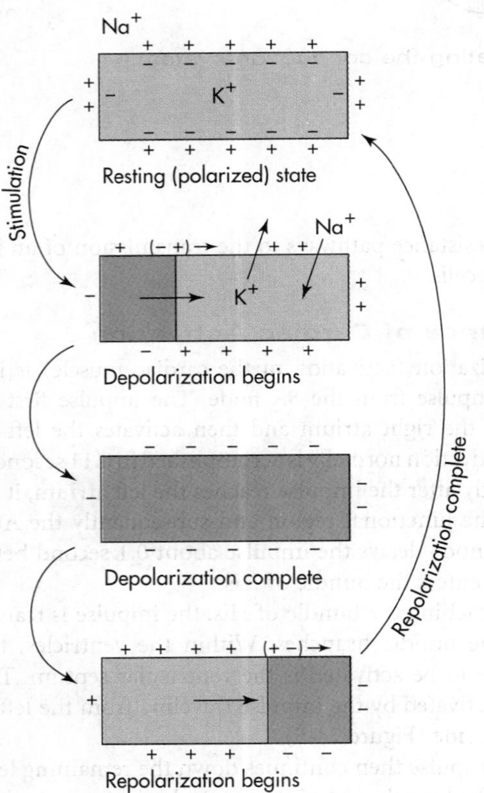


fig. 24-6 Schematic diagram illustrating process of depolarization and repolarization.

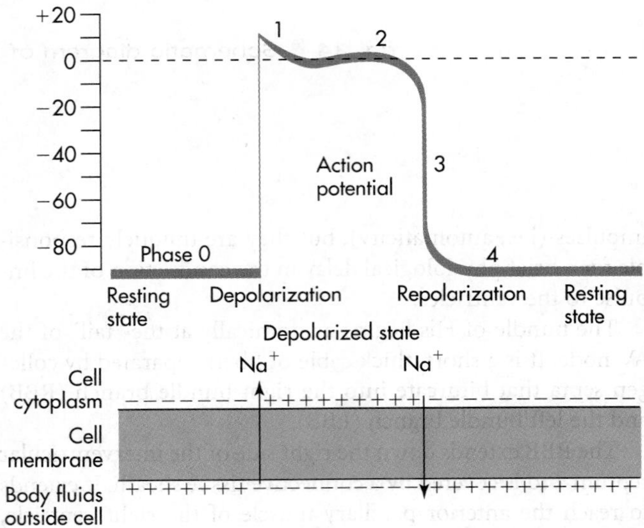


fig. 24-7 Phases of the action potential of cardiac muscle.

sodium and potassium ions extracellularly. Whenever the cell is stimulated, the membrane potential undergoes a change. A graphic record of this change forms the basis for an ECG. The change in electrical potential in response to a stimulus is known as the action potential. The two components of the action potential are depolarization and repolarization.

### Resting membrane potential

In the resting state the inside of the cell is negative with respect to the outside (Figure 24-6). Initiation and conduction of cardiac impulses depend on the cell's ability to maintain an electrical potential gradient when the cell is at rest. The main factor that contributes to the −90 mV resting membrane potential is the cell's permeability to potassium and not to sodium. The sodium-potassium exchange pump is responsible for actively transporting sodium out of the cell and potassium into the cell. The hydrolysis of adenosine triphosphate (ATP) provides the energy for the functioning of this pump. Because more sodium is pumped out of the cell than potassium is moved in, a net outward current of positive ions further enhances the cell's negativity during the resting phase.

### Depolarization

The initiation of a cardiac impulse begins with the process of depolarization. Depolarization indicates the rapid reversal of the resting membrane potential, which results from the following sequence of events: (1) the cell membrane permeability to sodium increases spontaneously (as in pacemaking

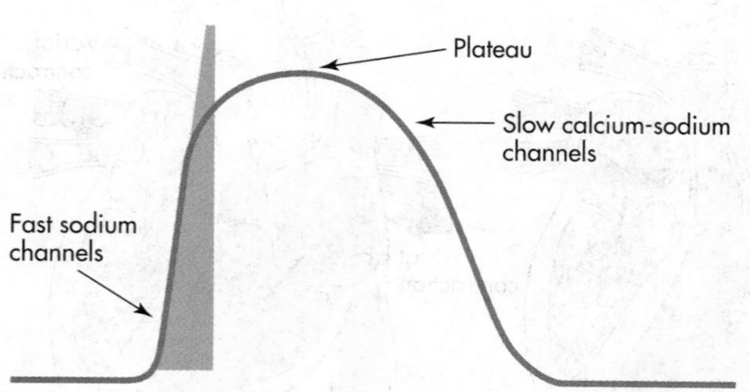


fig. 24-8 The differing effects of the fast sodium channels and the slow calcium-sodium channels on the action potential. The flow of sodium throughout the fast sodium channels initiates the action potential, and then these channels close *(shaded area)*. The flow of current through the slow calcium channels is responsible for the plateau and duration of the action potential.

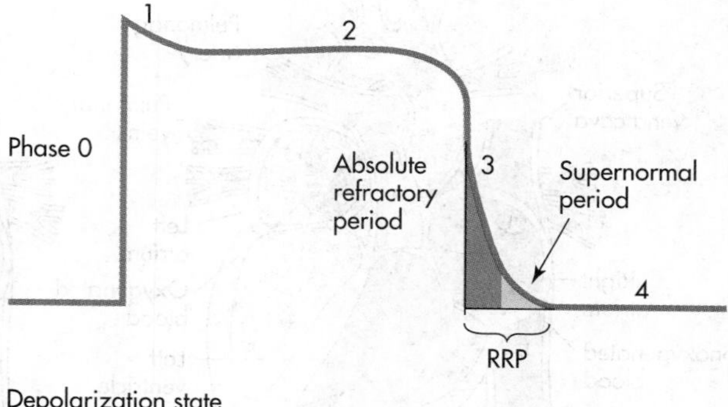


fig. 24-9 Schematic of the action potential showing the absolute and relative refractory period *(RRP)*. A strong stimulus will produce a response in the first part of the RRP and a mild stimulus in the latter *(supernormal period)*.

cells) or in response to a stimulus; (2) a rapid influx of sodium occurs; and (3) potassium moves out of the cell. This movement of ions across the membrane creates an electrical current. When the amount of sodium entering the cell reaches a critical level, an electrical impulse is generated. The impulse may spread as a wave of depolarization to adjacent cells.

#### Repolarization

Repolarization is the process by which the cell is returned to the resting state. The cell membrane permeability to sodium decreases, and sodium leaves the cell. Potassium returns through an active ion transport system.

#### Phases of action potential

**Phase 0.** Phase 0 is the tall upstroke of the action potential that occurs when the cell is stimulated, causing the cell membrane to become permeable to sodium ions. Fast sodium channels open to allow sodium to rush into the cell, creating a positive intracellular membrane potential of 0 to +20 mV (Figure 24-7).

**Phase 1.** Phase 1 represents a brief period of rapid repolarization secondary to an outward positive current carried mainly by potassium ions. Further, sodium influx is abruptly terminated as soon as the cell depolarizes. These two factors cause a slight decline in intracellular positivity.

**Phase 2.** Phase 2 of the action potential is often referred to as the plateau phase. It is sustained by an influx of positive ions, primarily calcium, through the slow calcium channels into the cell (Figure 24-8). This supplies the cell with the calcium needed for contraction. This inward current results in a prolonged refractory period by maintaining the cell in a depolarized state, allowing time for completion of muscular contraction.

**Phase 3.** During phase 3 the sodium pump, along with the increased loss of intracellular potassium, causes a rapid restoration of negativity to the cell.

**Phase 4.** Phase 4 is the return of the cell to the resting membrane potential.

#### Refractoriness

The inability of cardiac cells to respond to successive stimuli is known as refractoriness. During the absolute refractory period, no stimulus will produce a response. This period begins with depolarization and extends through a portion of the repolarization period until the sodium ion carrier sites are again free to transport the sodium ions necessary for depolarization (Figure 24-9).

Refractoriness progressively diminishes in the relative refractory period, which occurs in the final stage of repolarization. During this interval a stimulus of sufficient strength will produce a response. When the resting state is attained, the cell is no longer refractory and a mild stimulus will initiate a cardiac impulse. This is known as the supernormal period.

### Cardiac Cycle

The action potential itself does not cause the myofibrils to contract. The electrical stimulation initiates muscular contraction by stimulating the release of calcium ions in the sarcoplasmic reticulum of the muscle. Calcium ions then catalyze the chemical reaction that promotes the interdigitating and sliding of the actin and myosin filaments along each other, producing muscle contraction. (See Chapter 59.)

The cardiac cycle has two phases, diastole and systole. Relaxation and filling of both atria and then both ventricles take place during diastole. Contraction and emptying of both atria and then both ventricles occur during systole.

#### Diastole

The diastolic phase of the cardiac cycle is subdivided into the following phases: (1) isovolumetric ventricular relaxation, (2) rapid ventricular filling, (3) slow ventricular filling, and (4) atrial systole (Table 24-1 and Figure 24-10, *A*).

Isovolumetric ventricular relaxation begins as soon as the aortic and pulmonic valves close. During this time the myocardial muscle relaxes, and ventricular pressure falls. However, the falling ventricular pressure is still higher than atrial pressure; therefore the AV valves remain closed. Because these

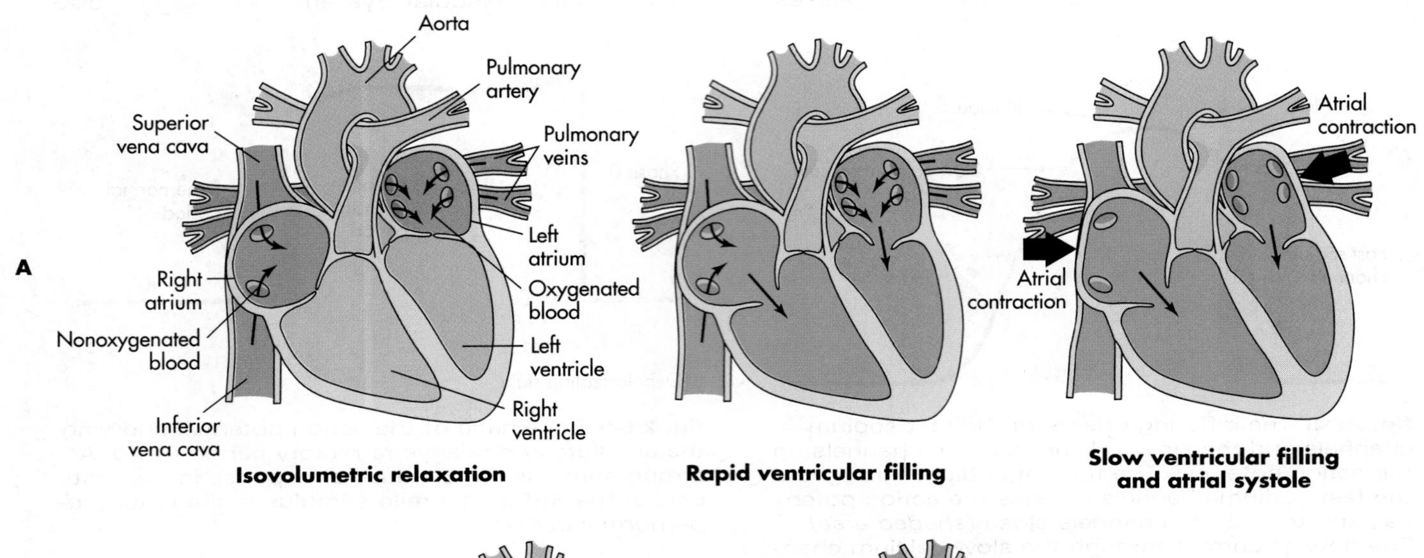


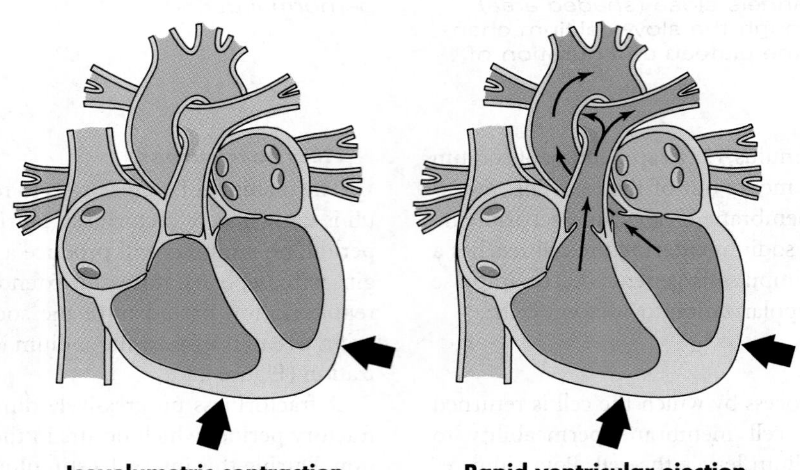


**fig. 24-10** Events during the cardiac cycle. **A,** Diastole. **B,** Systole.

**table 24-1** *Events During the Cardiac Cycle*

| Phase | Valves: Pulmonary and Aortic | Valves: Mitral and Tricuspid | Actions | Pressure (P) Changes |
|---|---|---|---|---|
| **DIASTOLE** | | | | |
| Isovolumetric relaxation | Closed | Closed | Blood collects in atria. | Atrial P increases until greater than ventricular P. |
| Rapid ventricular filling | Closed | Open | Blood flows rapidly into ventricles from pressure differential. | Atrial P decreases; ventricular P increases. |
| Slow ventricular filling | Closed | Open | Blood flows passively into ventricles. | Same as for rapid filling. |
| Atrial systole | Closed | Open, then closed | Atrial contraction pushes additional blood into ventricles. | Ventricular P becomes greater than atrial P. |
| **SYSTOLE** | | | | |
| Isovolumetric contraction | Closed | Closed | Myocardial tension increases. | Ventricular P increases; aortic P decreases until ventricular P greater than aortic P. |
| Maximal ventricular ejection | Open | Closed | Blood is pumped from ventricles into pulmonary artery and aorta. | Ventricular P decreases. |
| Reduced ventricular ejection | Open, then closed | Closed | Some blood ejected. | Ventricular pressure decreases rapidly when ventricles relax. |

valves remain closed, a large amount of blood collects in the atria. As ventricular pressure begins to drop more rapidly to its low diastolic level, the higher pressure in the atria pushes the AV valves open and allows blood to flow rapidly into the ventricular cavity. This second phase of diastole, rapid ventricular filling, lasts for approximately the first third of diastole and causes intraventricular pressures to rise. As ventricular pressure increases, it impedes further rapid filling, and the resultant slowing of ventricular filling marks the third phase of diastole. This phase of slow ventricular filling is referred to as *diastasis.* Both the atrial and the ventricular chambers are relaxed, and blood entering the atria flows passively into the ventricles. During the phase of atrial systole, electrical depolarization spreads through the atria and pauses at the AV node for 0.10 second. The atrial musculature then contracts, propelling an additional 20% to 30% of blood into the ventricle before ventricular contraction.

#### Systole

The ventricular systolic phase of the cardiac cycle is subdivided into phases of isovolumetric ventricular contraction, maximal ventricular ejection, and reduced ventricular ejection. (See Table 24-1 and Figure 24-10, *B.*)

During the isovolumetric ventricular contraction phase, myocardial tension and intraventricular pressure increase, whereas no change occurs in blood volume or muscle fiber length. At this time the aortic valve is closed because pressure in the aortic root exceeds left ventricular pressure. The higher pressure in the aortic root is the result of a previous systole that has just ejected blood into the aorta. As this aortic blood is distributed to the periphery, aortic pressure falls slowly. At the same time, intraventricular pressure and tension are increasing. When intraventricular pressure exceeds aortic root pressure, the aortic valve opens and maximal ventricular ejection begins. Blood from the ventricles is pumped into the pulmonic and systemic circulations. As the ejection rate starts to slow, the phase of reduced ventricular ejection, or protodiastole, begins. The ventricles remain contracted, but little blood is being ejected from the ventricle into the aorta. Ventricular pressure actually falls slightly below aortic root pressure, but some blood is still being ejected simply because of the momentum built up by the contraction. At the end of systole, ventricular relaxation begins suddenly, and a rapid decrease in intraventricular pressure occurs. The higher pressure in the large arteries and in the aortic root immediately pushes blood back toward the ventricles, thus snapping shut the semilunar valves.

### Cardiac Output

The amount of blood ejected from the left ventricle into the aorta per minute is called the cardiac output (CO). Although the right ventricle ejects an equivalent amount of blood into the pulmonary artery, it is not included in the measurement of total CO. Rather, CO is equivalent to stroke volume (SV) (volume of blood ejected from the left ventricle with each contraction) times heart rate (HR) (number of heartbeats per minute):

$$CO = SV \times HR$$

The average CO ranges from 4 to 8 L/min in the adult male. However, during periods of strenuous exercise, the CO may reach 20 to 25 L/min. Because cardiac requirements vary according to individual body size, a more accurate means of assessing tissue perfusion is to compute the cardiac index. The cardiac index is obtained by dividing the CO by the patient's total body surface area:

$$\text{Cardiac index} = \text{CO (L/min)/Body surface area (m}^2\text{)}$$

Therefore the cardiac index represents the CO in terms of liters per minute per square meter of body surface. This corrects an individual's CO to match body size. The normal range for cardiac index is 2.4 to 4.0 L/min. For example, the average 70 kg man has an approximate cardiac index of 3 L/min.

#### Stroke volume

Stroke volume is the amount of blood ejected by the left ventricle into the aorta per beat. At the completion of each filling phase, or diastole, the ventricle contains approximately 120 ml of blood (end-diastolic volume [EDV]) (Figure 24-11). Under normal circumstances, the heart ejects approximately two thirds of the EDV. The blood that is ejected is called the ejection fraction. The volume of residual blood in the ventricle at the end of systole is known as the end-systolic volume (ESV). Therefore stroke volume can be defined as the difference between the volume of blood contained in the ventricle at the end of diastole and the volume of blood remaining at the end of systole:

$$SV = EDV - ESV$$

#### Control of cardiac output

Cardiac output depends on the relationship between two important variables—stroke volume and heart rate. Despite fluctuations in one of these two variables, CO can be maintained at relatively constant levels by compensatory adjustments in the other variable. For example, if the heart rate

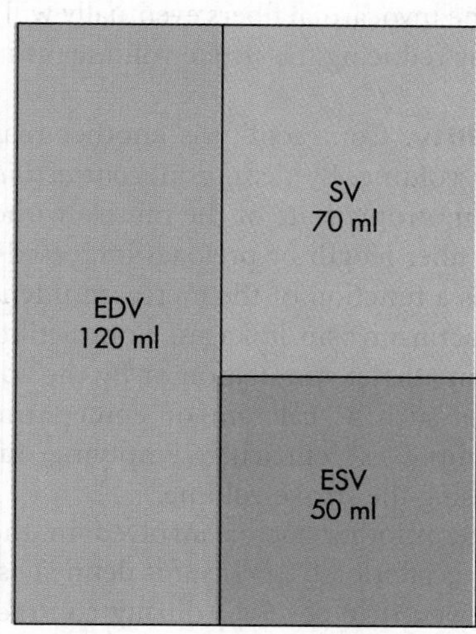


**fig. 24-11** Representation of normal ventricular function, illustrating relationship between end-diastolic volume *(EDV)*, stroke volume *(SV)*, and end-systolic volume *(ESV)*.

slows, the time for ventricular filling (diastole) is lengthened. This lengthened period allows for an increase in preload and a subsequent increase in stroke volume. Conversely, if the stroke volume falls, the heart rate can increase to compensate temporarily and maintain CO. Therefore the actual determinants of CO are the mechanisms regulating stroke volume and heart rate.

#### Control of stroke volume

Three significant factors determine stroke volume and thus CO: preload, contractility, and afterload.

**Preload.** Starling's law of the heart states that myocardial fiber responds with a more forceful contraction when it is stretched. An example of this phenomenon is increasing the stretch of a rubber band to obtain a more forceful recoil when the rubber band is released. Myocardial fibers can be stretched by increasing the volume of blood delivered to the ventricles during diastole. The degree of myocardial stretch before contraction is expressed in terms of preload. *Preload* is defined as the volume of blood distending the ventricles at the end of diastole. Preload is based on the amount of venous return and the ejection fraction, which determines the amount of blood left in the ventricle at the end of systole.

According to Starling's law, increasing venous return and thereby increasing left ventricular end-diastolic volume (preload) facilitates ventricular contraction and promotes increased ventricular function by stretching the myocardial fibers. Stretching of the sarcomeres increases the number of interaction sites for actin-myosin linkages and therefore increases ventricular contraction. Under normal conditions the sarcomere is stretched to 2 mm during ventricular diastole. Maximal ventricular force is developed at a sarcomere length of 2.2 mm. At this length, actin and myosin are able to use the most interaction sites. When myocardial stretching exceeds 2.4 mm, the myofilaments become partially disengaged, and fewer contractile sites are activated. Because Starling's length-tension relationship is functional only within physiological limits, it is important to note that prolonged, excessive stretching of the myocardial fibers eventually will lead to a decrease in CO by reducing the stroke volume (as in ventricular hypertrophy).

**Contractility.** Contractility is another major determinant in stroke volume. By definition, *contractility* refers to a change in the inotropic state of the muscle without a change in myocardial fiber length or preload. Increased contractility (inotropism) is a function of the increased intensity of interaction at the actin-myosin linkages. Contractility can be increased by sympathetic stimulation or by the administration of medications such as calcium or epinephrine. Increased contractility improves ventricular emptying during systole, thereby increasing the stroke volume.

**Afterload.** Another factor involved in the control of stroke volume is afterload. *Afterload* is defined as the amount of tension the ventricle develops during contraction to eject blood from the left ventricle into the aorta. The major impedance against which the left ventricle must pump is peripheral vascular resistance. Increase in pressure resulting from hypertension or vasoconstriction produces an increased resistance to pumping and will necessitate an increase in ventricular tension to eject blood. The afterload on the heart is affected not only by the amount of aortic pressure but also by the size of the heart. This relationship between ventricular tension, arterial pressure, and ventricular size is known as Laplace's law:

$$\text{Ventricular tension} = \text{Arterial pressure} \times \text{Ventricular radius}$$

Both hypertension and dilation of the ventricular chamber increase ventricular tension (increase afterload). Therefore, if arterial pressure increases, the ventricle must pump against higher resistance to empty adequately. Also, if ventricular radius increases, ventricular volume will increase. Thus at the same level of aortic pressure, the afterload against which an enlarged or dilated left ventricle must work is greater than that encountered by a normal-sized ventricle. This would result in an impaired ventricular emptying, thereby reducing stroke volume and CO.

#### Control of heart rate

The autonomic nervous system (ANS) regulates the heart through the sympathetic and the parasympathetic nervous systems.

The sympathetic fibers arise from the thoracic spinal cord and reach the entire atria and ventricles, as well as the SA and the AV nodes. Control of the heart by the ANS is mediated by neurotransmitters. The sympathetic neurotransmitter is norepinephrine. The sympathetic fibers have both positive chronotropic (increase rate) and inotropic (increase force) effects. Therefore with an increase in sympathetic stimulation, the neurotransmitter norepinephrine is released from the nerve endings and increases heart rate, atrial and ventricular contractility, and the speed of electrical conduction through the AV node.

The parasympathetic fibers originate in the medulla and have their innervation primarily in the atrial musculature and the SA and AV nodes; however, parasympathetic stimulation has been shown to reach the ventricles. The parasympathetic fibers have a negative chronotropic effect and may exert a slightly negative inotropic effect; however, in the healthy circulatory system, this negative inotropic effect is compensated for by the increased filling that occurs as a result of a lengthened diastole. Stimulation of the parasympathetic system causes the release of the neurotransmitter acetylcholine at the vagal nerve endings, which has basically the opposite effect of norepinephrine. Parasympathetic stimulation causes a decrease in the rate of discharge of the SA node, a decrease in the rate of conduction from the atria to the ventricles, and a decrease in the force of atrial contraction and probably also of ventricular contraction. The final effect of ANS control of the heart is a balance between these two opposing nervous systems. Normally, the heart is under the control of vagal inhibition and maintains a resting heart rate of 60 to 90 beats per minute.

The effects of the ANS can be greatly influenced by several additional factors, such as the central nervous system (CNS) and pressoreceptor reflexes. Impulses from the cerebral cortex can have a significant effect on heart rate. Pain, fear, anger, and excitement can cause substantial increases in the heart rate. Also, reflex changes caused by stimulation of the pressoreceptors can influence heart rate. The baroreceptor reflex, with afferent branches in the aortic arch, carotid sinus, and other pressoreceptor zones, functions as a negative feedback mechanism to regulate pressure in the arteries and regulate the resistance of vessels in the vasculature. Consequently, an episode of hypotension would cause a sudden drop of blood pressure in the aorta or carotid sinus and would stimulate the pressoreceptors less intensely. Subsequently, stimulation of the cardiac inhibitory center would decrease in frequency resulting in a reflex increase in the heart rate.

Other important factors involved in the control of heart rate include body temperature, medication, catecholamines, arterial blood gas tensions, hormones other than epinephrine, and plasma electrolyte concentrations. However, these are beyond the scope of discussion for this chapter.

## ANATOMY AND PHYSIOLOGY OF THE PERIPHERAL VASCULAR SYSTEM

The vascular system is a closed circuit consisting of the systemic and pulmonary circulations. Blood circulates from the left side of the heart to the tissues and back to the right side of the heart. It then flows through the lungs and back to the left side of the heart. The main components of the vascular system are the arteries, capillaries, and veins.

### ARTERIES

Arteries are thick-walled vessels transporting oxygen and blood via the aorta from the heart to the tissues. Figure 24-12 shows the principal arteries. As the arteries approach the tissues, they branch into smaller vessels called arterioles. Arteries are composed of three tissue layers:

1. Inner layer of endothelium (intima)
2. Middle layer of connective tissue, smooth muscle, or elastic fibers (media)
3. Outer layer of connective tissue (adventitia)

The media forms the major portion of the vessel wall and in larger arteries is composed primarily of elastic and connective tissue. This enables the artery to respond to alterations in blood volume while maintaining a constant flow. In the smaller arteries and arterioles there is much less elastic fiber; the smooth muscle contracts and relaxes by nervous, chemical, and hormonal factors.

### CAPILLARIES

Capillaries, composed of a single layer of cells, are minute, thin-walled vessels located in the tissues. The capillaries connect the arterioles to the smallest veins and venules, allowing for the exchange of essential cellular products. Nutrients, oxygen, and regulatory substances move into the cells; waste products, carbon dioxide, and cellular secretions move from the cells into the blood.

### VEINS

Veins are thin-walled vessels transporting deoxygenated blood from the capillaries back to the right side of the heart. Veins are composed of the same three layers as arteries (intima, media, and adventitia), but in contrast to arterial walls, venous walls have little smooth muscle and connective tissue. This makes the veins distensible, enabling them to accumulate large volumes of blood. The sympathetic nervous system innervates the veins, causing venoconstriction, decreased venous volume, and increased circulating blood volume. Major veins, particularly those in the lower extremities, have one-way valves that promote blood flow against gravity and thereby prevent retrograde flow. Additionally, the squeezing action of skeletal muscle contraction creates an opposing force against gravity. Figure 24-13 shows the major veins in the body.

## PHYSIOLOGICAL CHANGES WITH AGING

The number one cause of death in persons who are 65 years of age or older is cardiovascular disease. Age-related changes take place in the chemical composition, cells, and tissues of the heart and blood vessels and influence many aspects of cardiovascular functioning. However, despite the physiological changes of aging, the heart is able to meet the day-to-day demands and function adequately. Only under unusual circumstances or increased stress is the changing function of the heart apparent. Coronary atherosclerosis is more prevalent in elders, but it commonly manifests as an occult (hidden) disease (see the Gerontological Assessment Box on p. 616).

### Heart

Progressive left ventricular hypertrophy occurs with aging and is accompanied by a rise in systolic blood pressure. Heart weight increases in women but not in men. Ventricular septal thickness and the circumference of all four cardiac valves increase. By age 40 years, the circumference of the aortic valve generally surpasses that of the pulmonic valve. In both genders the leaflet thickness and calcification of the mitral and aortic valves increase progressively and significantly with advancing age. These rigid valves can lead to audible systolic murmurs, usually of an ejection nature.

An increase in average myocyte (muscle cell) size explains the increase in heart mass; however, the simultaneous change in the amount and functional properties of myocardial collagen plays a key role in the development of aging-related cardiovascular abnormalities. The increased connective tissue contributes to myocardial stiffness and decreased cardiac compliance. The amount of subendocardial fat increases, and the endocardium undergoes fibrosis, thickening, and sclerosis.

A decreased peak-systolic left ventricular wall stress occurs with aging. Increasing left ventricular wall thickness and increasing body surface area with age are presumed to be contributing factors. The isovolumetric relaxation period also is prolonged, resulting in incomplete relaxation during early diastolic filling. However, enhanced ventricular filling occurs later in diastole as a result of a compensatory, augmented atrial contribution to ventricular filling.

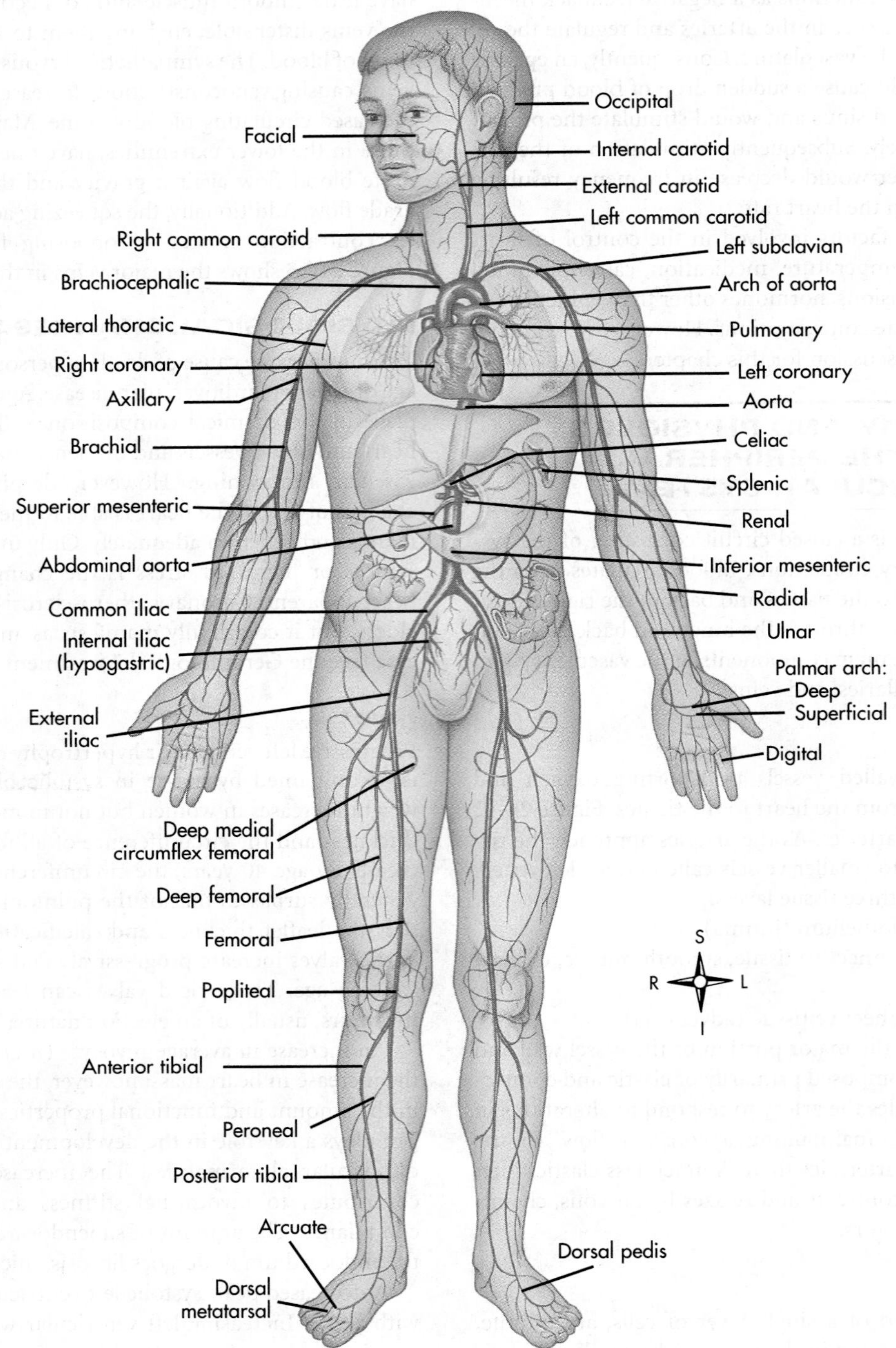


fig. 24-12 Principal arteries of the body.

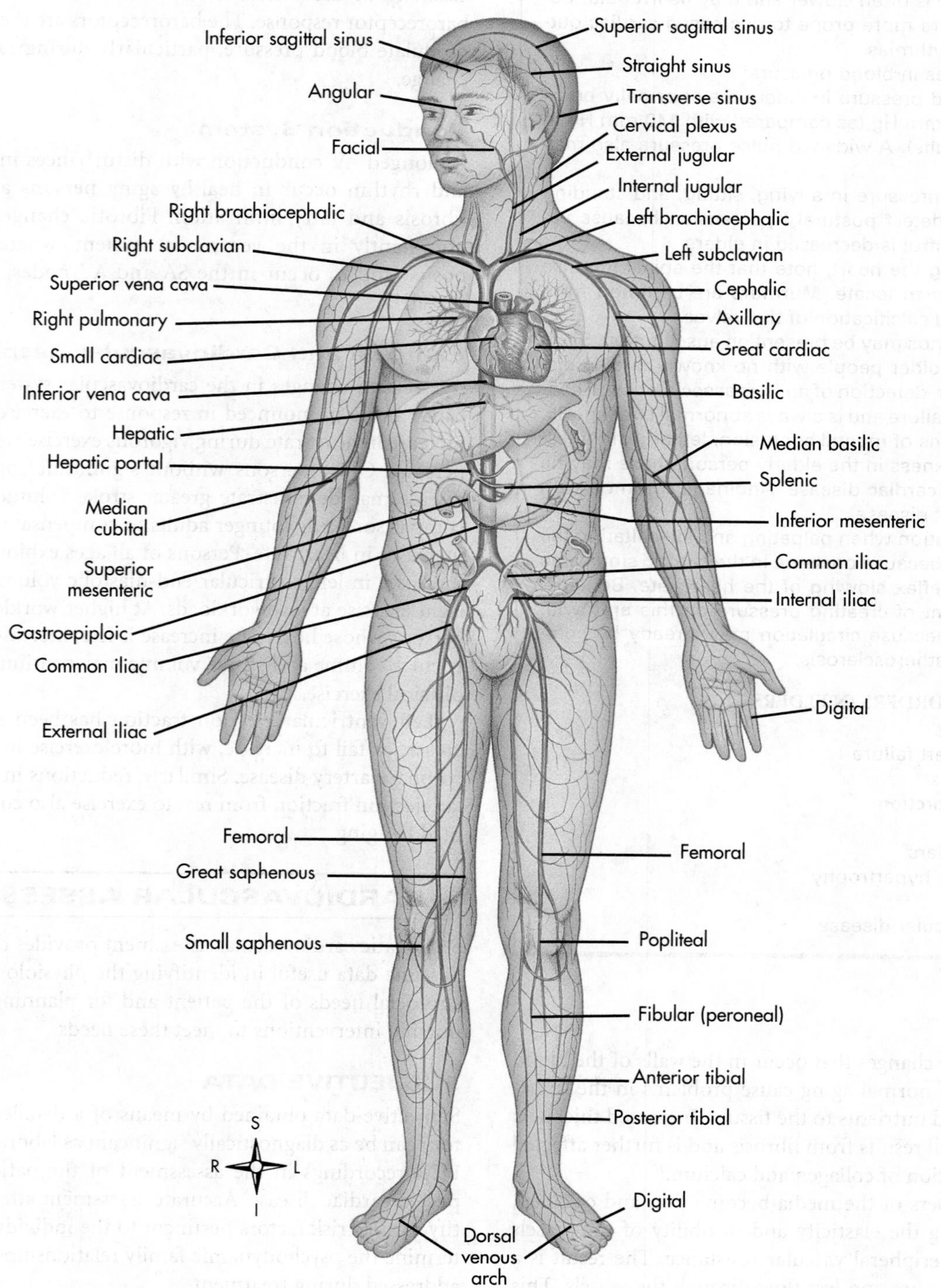

Inferior sagittal sinus
Superior sagittal sinus
Straight sinus
Angular
Transverse sinus
Cervical plexus
Facial
External jugular
Internal jugular
Right brachiocephalic
Left brachiocephalic
Right subclavian
Left subclavian
Superior vena cava
Cephalic
Right pulmonary
Axillary
Great cardiac
Small cardiac
Inferior vena cava
Basilic
Hepatic
Median basilic
Hepatic portal
Splenic
Median cubital
Inferior mesenteric
Superior mesenteric
Common iliac
Internal iliac
Gastroepiploic
Common iliac
External iliac
Digital
Femoral
Femoral
Great saphenous
Small saphenous
Popliteal
Fibular (peroneal)
Anterior tibial
Posterior tibial
S
R
L
I
Digital
Dorsal venous arch

**fig. 24-13** Principal veins of the body.

## gerontological assessment

**ASSESSMENT**

Count the pulse for a full minute at rest and after exertion. The pulse is often slower and may be irregular because elders are more prone to decreased cardiac output and dysrhythmias.

Monitor changes in blood pressure:

- Systolic blood pressure in elders may normally be as high as 160 mm Hg (as compared with 140 mm Hg in younger adults). A widened pulse pressure also may be observed.
- Check blood pressure in a lying, sitting, and standing position to detect postural hypotension because vasomotor control is decreased in elders.

When assessing the heart, note that the apical impulse may be harder to locate. Murmurs are common from thickening and calcification of the valves.

Extra heart sounds may be present on auscultation. $S_4$ often occurs in older people with no known cardiac disease. However, detection of an $S_3$ is associated with congestive heart failure and is always abnormal over age 35.

Monitor for signs of mental confusion, lethargy, indigestion, and weakness in the elderly person; these may be early signs of cardiac disease. Angina is common with ischemic heart disease.

Always use caution when palpating and auscultating the carotid artery because pressure in the carotid sinus area can cause a reflex slowing of the heart rate. Be especially cognizant of creating pressure on this area with older adults because circulation may already be compromised by atherosclerosis.

**COMMON DISORDERS IN ELDERS**

Atherosclerosis
Congestive heart failure
Angina pectoris
Myocardial infarction
Dysrhythmias
Valvular disorders
Left ventricular hypertrophy
Hypertension
Peripheral vascular disease

### Arteries

The degenerative changes that occur in the walls of the blood vessels as part of normal aging cause problems in the transport of blood and nutrients to the tissues. Increased thickness in the intimal wall results from fibrosis and is further affected by the accumulation of collagen and calcium.[10]

The elastic fibers of the media become thin and calcified, greatly decreasing the elasticity and flexibility of the vessels and increasing peripheral vascular resistance. The result is a rise in blood pressure and less flow through the vessels. This results in a decreased supply of oxygen and nutrients to the tissues coupled with an accumulation of cellular secretions, waste products, and carbon dioxide.

Both the aorta and its branches and the large pulmonary arteries and their branches undergo progressive dilation and elongation with age. Because the enlargement is both transverse and longitudinal, the aorta tends to become tortuous. However, the large pulmonary arteries do not dilate longitudinally because the vessels are anatomically shorter and maintain a considerably lower pressure. The generalized loss of elasticity in the arterial system can also lead to a sluggish baroreceptor response. The baroreceptors are then less able to modulate blood pressure, particularly during rapid postural change.

### Conduction System

Prolonged AV conduction with disturbances in cardiac rate and rhythm occur in healthy aging persons as a result of fibrosis and fatty infiltration. Fibrotic changes occur predominantly in the ventricular system, whereas fatty deposits tend to occur in the SA and AV nodes, as well as in the atria.

### Exercise and Cardiovascular Response

Age-related changes in the cardiovascular system are significantly more pronounced in response to exercise. The overall increase in heart rate during vigorous exercise is less in elderly persons. Older persons without significant coronary artery disease may demonstrate greater stroke volume increases in comparison with younger adults to compensate for the lesser increases in heart rate. Persons of all ages exhibit comparable increases in left ventricular end-diastolic volume during upright exercise at low workloads. At higher workloads, in older persons whose heart rate increase is less, increases in left ventricular volume and stroke volume may continue throughout physical exercise.

Left ventricular ejection fraction has been shown to decrease, or fail to increase, with more exercise in persons with coronary artery disease. Similarly, reductions in left ventricular ejection fraction from rest to exercise also could be attributed to aging.

## CARDIOVASCULAR ASSESSMENT

Systematic cardiovascular assessment provides the nurse with baseline data useful in identifying the physiological and psychosocial needs of the patient and for planning appropriate nursing interventions to meet these needs.

### SUBJECTIVE DATA

Subjective data obtained by means of a detailed patient history can be as diagnostically significant as laboratory data and ECG recordings in the assessment of the patient with suspected cardiac disease. Accurate assessment attempts to identify cardiac risk factors pertinent to the individual and to determine the psychodynamic family relationships that must be addressed during treatment.

Classic symptoms of heart disease include dyspnea, chest pain or discomfort, edema, syncope, palpitations, and excessive fatigue. Cardiovascular function, which may be adequate at rest, may be insufficient during exercise or exertion. Therefore careful attention is directed to the effects of activity on the patient's symptoms.

## Dyspnea

Dyspnea, one of the most common and distressing symptoms of cardiopulmonary disease, is described as an abnormally uncomfortable awareness of breathing. The patient complains of shortness of breath. Dyspnea is a subjective experience and is associated with anxiety and a variety of disease processes.

Assessment of dyspnea must include factors that precipitate and relieve dyspnea and data regarding the patient's body position when dyspnea occurs.

Dyspnea on exertion is a common symptom of cardiac dysfunction. In the early stages of heart failure, dyspnea usually is provoked only by effort and is relieved promptly by rest. It is important to identify the amount of exertion necessary to produce dyspnea, because the lower the cardiac reserve (heart's ability to adjust and adapt to increased demands), the less effort is required to precipitate dyspnea.

Orthopnea refers to dyspnea in the recumbent position. It is usually a symptom of more advanced heart failure than is exertional dyspnea. Patients relate that they require two or more pillows to sleep restfully. When the person assumes the recumbent position, gravitational forces redistribute blood from the lower extremities and splanchnic bed, increasing venous return. The augmentation of intrathoracic blood volume elevates pulmonary venous and capillary pressures, resulting in a transient pulmonary congestion. Orthopnea usually is relieved in less than 5 minutes after the patient sits upright.

Paroxysmal nocturnal dyspnea, also known as cardiac asthma, is characterized by severe attacks of shortness of breath that generally occur 2 to 5 hours after the onset of sleep. This condition is commonly associated with sweating and wheezing. Classically, the person awakens from sleep, arises, and quickly opens a window with the perception of needing fresh air. These frightening attacks are precipitated by the same physiological mechanisms that cause orthopnea. The diseased heart is unable to compensate for this increase in blood volume by pumping extra fluid into the circulatory system, and pulmonary congestion results. Paroxysmal nocturnal dyspnea is relieved by the patient sitting on the side of the bed or getting out of bed. However, unlike simple orthopnea, 20 minutes or more may be required for the patient with paroxysmal nocturnal dyspnea to obtain relief.

## Chest Pain

Although pain or discomfort in the chest is one of the cardinal symptoms of cardiac disorders, chest pain can be precipitated by various conditions. For example, chest pain may be caused by anxiety, ischemic heart disease, acute dissection of the aorta, acute pericarditis, pulmonary disorders (e.g., pleurisy and pulmonary embolism), esophageal spasm or reflux, and peptic ulcer disease. To evaluate chest pain accurately the following factors should be addressed during the assessment.

1. *Onset.* When was chest pain first noticed?
2. *Manner of onset.* Did the pain or discomfort start suddenly or gradually?
3. *Duration.* How long did the pain last?
4. *Precipitating factors.* Ask patient to describe possible precipitating factors (e.g., exertion, food, anxiety, emotions).
5. *Location.* Where did the pain originate? Did it radiate? To what area?
6. *Quality.* Ask patient to describe how symptoms feel (e.g., sharp, dull).
7. *Intensity.* Ask patient to describe severity of the pain (e.g., if pain interfered with any activities).
8. *Chronology and frequency.* Has this pain occurred in the past? If so, how often?
9. *Associated symptoms.* Do any other signs or symptoms occur at the same time?
10. *Aggravating factors.* What makes the pain worse?
11. *Relaxing factors.* What makes symptoms less intense?

The same list of factors can also be used to evaluate leg pain. Responses will assist the examiner in establishing a diagnosis of peripheral vascular disease. Furthermore, the analysis will allow for differentiation of arterial versus venous disease.

## Syncope

Syncope is defined as a generalized muscle weakness with an inability to stand upright, accompanied by loss of consciousness. The most common cause of syncope is decreased perfusion to the brain. Any condition that results in a sudden reduction of CO and therefore reduced cerebral blood flow could potentially cause a syncopal episode. In patients with cardiovascular disorders, conditions such as orthostatic hypotension, hypovolemia, or a variety of dysrhythmias (e.g., heart block and severe ventricular dysrhythmias) may precipitate syncope.

## Palpitations

Palpitation is a common subjective phenomenon defined as an unpleasant awareness of the heartbeat. It may be precipitated by a change in cardiac rate or rhythm or by an increase in myocardial contractility. Patients may describe their heartbeat as "pounding," "racing," or "skipping." Palpitations that occur either during or after strenuous activity are considered physiological. Palpitations that occur during mild exertion may suggest the presence of heart failure, anemia, or thyrotoxicosis. Other noncardiac factors that may precipitate palpitations include nervousness, heavy meals, lack of sleep, and a large intake of caffeine-containing beverages, alcohol, or tobacco.

## Fatigue

Fatigue and lassitude have many causes, and therefore these symptoms are not diagnostic of cardiovascular disorders. However, fatigue may be a direct consequence of heart failure. The exact physiological mechanism is not known, but it is probably a consequence of an inadequate CO. Such fatigue can occur during effort or at rest and generally worsens as the day progresses. Fatigue that occurs after mild exertion may indicate a low cardiac reserve if the heart is unable to meet even small increases in metabolic demands.

## OBJECTIVE DATA

Physical examination of the cardiovascular system includes the standard assessment techniques of inspection, palpation, percussion, and auscultation.

### Inspection

#### Skin color

The color of the patient's skin and mucous membranes is noted. A person's "normal" color depends on race, ethnic background, and lifestyle and is an indication of adequate CO and circulation. Pallor may indicate anemia, hypoxia, or peripheral vasoconstriction. Cyanosis, a bluish discoloration of the skin, is most easily observed by examining the earlobes, the oral mucosa at the base of the tongue, the lips, and the nailbeds.

There are two types of cyanosis: central and peripheral. In central cyanosis the tongue is characteristically cyanotic. This form of cyanosis is caused by low arterial oxygen saturation and generally is seen in patients who have congenital heart defects or in those with pulmonary diseases that interfere with ventilation or diffusion.

Peripheral cyanosis results from low CO and generally is accompanied by decreased skin temperature and mottling. In contrast to central cyanosis, no cyanosis of the tongue is present.

Skin color of the extremities is also assessed. It is important to note any erythema or pigmentation changes, as well as the presence of shiny or dry, scaly skin, which may indicate a vascular disorder. Hair distribution, venous pattern, and size of extremities should be assessed.[9]

#### Neck vein distention

A general estimate of venous pressure can be obtained by observation of the neck veins (Figure 24-14). Normally, when a person is supine, the neck veins are distended. However, when the head of the bed is elevated to a 45-degree angle, the neck veins are collapsed. If jugular distention is present, assess the jugular venous pressure by measuring from the highest point of visible distention to the sternal angle. Measurements above 3 cm are considered elevated.

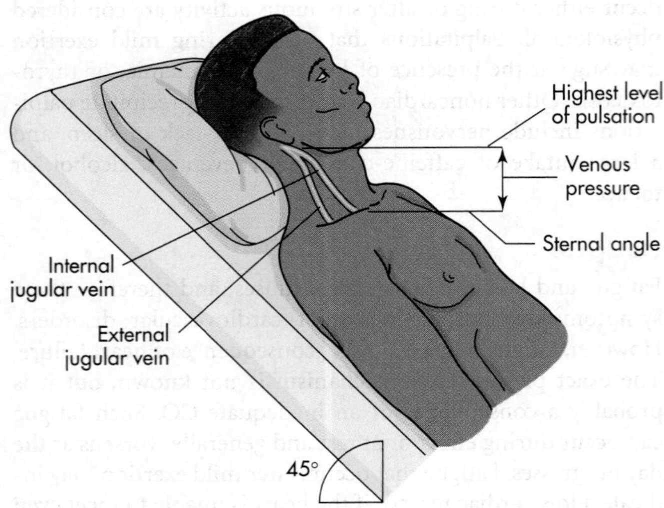


**fig. 24-14** Position of internal and external jugular veins used in measuring venous pressure.

The jugular veins reflect venous tone, blood volume, and right atrial pressure. Therefore distended neck veins suggest increased venous pressure, which may be caused by right-sided heart failure, circulatory volume overload, superior vena caval obstruction, or tricuspid valve regurgitation.

#### Respirations

The rate and character of the patient's respirations are important to assess. Normally, an adult breathes comfortably at a rate of 12 to 20 times per minute. Particular attention is paid to the ease or difficulty in breathing and the patient's general demeanor.

#### Pulsations

Inspection of the anterior chest is best accomplished with the patient lying supine, either flat or with the head slightly elevated. Observe the precordium for the apical impulse, which is a pulsation of the chest wall caused by the forward thrusting of the left ventricle during systole. When visible, the apical impulse occupies the fourth or fifth intercostal space, at or inside the midclavicular line. The apical impulse was formerly known as the point of maximal impulse. The apical impulse is not always visible, but it is palpable in about half of adults.

#### Clubbing and capillary refill

The nails are assessed for clubbing and capillary refill. The exact cause of clubbing is not known; however, clubbing of the fingers is typical in congenital heart defects and pulmonary arteriovenous (A-V) fistulas with right-to-left shunting. Capillary filling, or blanching, is an indicator of peripheral circulation to the fingers and toes and can be tested in all nailbeds. The examiner presses a thumbnail against the edge of a patient's fingernail or toenail and then quickly releases it. The normal response is whitening (blanching) of the area when pressure is applied and brisk return of color when pressure is released. Lack of the blanching response may indicate lack of circulation to the finger or toe because of arterial insufficiency secondary to atherosclerosis or spasm; however, severe vasoconstriction may be the causative factor.

### Palpation

#### Peripheral pulses

One method for evaluating the arterial flow of the vascular system is to palpate the extremities simultaneously to determine skin temperature. A second method is to palpate the peripheral pulses, which are evaluated bilaterally on the basis of their absence or presence, rate, rhythm, amplitude, quality, and equality. Each pulse, except the carotids, should be palpated on the left and right sides simultaneously to evaluate contralateral symmetry (Figure 24-15).

Pulses are rated on a scale of 0 to +4 as follows:

0 = Absent
+ = Palpable, but diminished
++ = Normal, or average
+++ = Full and brisk
++++ = Full and bounding, often visible

Several abnormalities may be detected during palpation of pulses. A hypokinetic (weak) pulse signifies a narrowed pulse pressure, that is, decreased difference between systolic and diastolic pressures. It usually is produced by a low CO and is associated with increased peripheral vascular resistance. This type of pulse is often detected in such conditions as severe left ventricular failure, hypovolemia, or mitral and aortic valve stenosis.

A hyperkinetic (bounding) pulse represents a widened pulse pressure. It usually is associated with an increased left ventricular stroke volume and a decrease in peripheral vascular resistance. This type of pulse is often found in hyperkinetic circulatory states caused by exercise, fever, anemia, or hyperthyroidism.

*Pulsus alternans* is a condition in which the heart beats regularly, but the pulses vary in amplitude. It is caused by an alternating left ventricular contractile force and usually indicates severe depression of myocardial function. Pulsus alternans may be detected by palpation but is more accurately assessed by auscultation of the blood pressure.

*Pulsus paradoxus* signifies a reduction in the amplitude of the arterial pulse during inspiration. Variations in pulse strength can be palpated, but a paradoxical pulse is most readily detected by sphygmomanometry. Pulsus paradoxus is an accentuation of the normal decrease in systolic arterial pressure with inspiration. This is a result of decreased left ventricular stroke volume and the transmission of negative intrathoracic pressure to the aorta. Pulsus paradoxus may occur in conditions such as cardiac tamponade and constrictive pericarditis, but it also may occur in patients with chronic obstructive airway disease who have wide swings of intrapleural pressure during respiration.

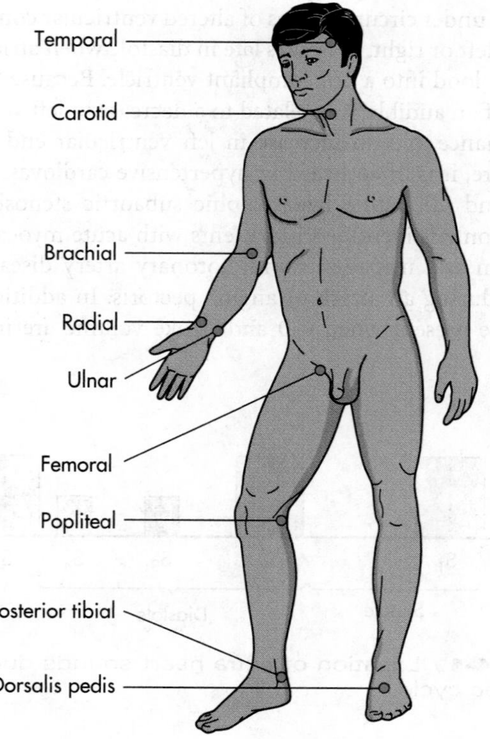


**fig. 24-15** Body sites at which peripheral pulses are most easily palpated.

Normally, the apical impulse is felt as a single, light tap. The presence of anything other than a single, light tap may suggest a myocardial pathological condition and should be reported to the physician. A thrill, or palpable murmur, indicates the presence of significant turbulent blood flow across an intracardiac shunt or a severely stenotic valve. A thrill is often described as a vibration similar to that of a cat's purr and is more readily palpated after the patient exhales forcefully. Having the patient in a left lateral position or leaning forward may accentuate the vibration.

### Edema

Edema is defined as an accumulation of fluid in the interstitial spaces. It maybe localized to one particular body part, organ, or tissue, or there may be a generalized distribution. However, retention of considerable amounts of extracellular fluid may occur without associated edema. In fact, weight gains of up to 7 kg of water can occur before the abnormality is detected. Because early manifestations of edema may be subtle, careful comparison of daily weights is required to determine weight gains resulting from fluid retention. Normally, basal body weight varies little from day to day; therefore subtle weight gains resulting from fluid retention are readily detectable.

An important indicator of cardiovascular function is the presence or absence of peripheral edema, especially in the feet, ankles, legs, and sacrum. This is caused by gravity flow or by interruption of the venous return to the heart as a result of constricting clothing or pressure on the veins of the lower extremities. Edema often disappears on elevation of the body part.

In contrast, pitting edema does not disappear with elevation of the extremity or body part, and it may indicate fluid overload or a pathological condition (e.g., congestive heart failure). Pitting edema is present if an indentation is left in the skin after a thumb or finger has been used to apply gentle pressure (Table 24-2).

### Percussion

The use of percussion for detecting cardiac enlargement generally has been replaced by the chest x-ray, which is much more accurate. Therefore the use of percussion in the

**table 24-2** *Pitting Edema Scale*

| SCALE | DEGREE | RESPONSE |
|---|---|---|
| 1+ Trace | Slight | Rapid |
| 2+ Mild | 0-0.6 cm (0-0.25 in) | 10-15 sec |
| 3+ Moderate | 0.6-1.3 cm (0.25-0.5 in) | 1-2 min |
| 4+ Severe | 1.3-2.5 cm (0.5-1 in) | 2-5 min |

+1 2 mm · +2 4 mm · +3 6 mm · +4 8 mm

From Thompson J, Wilson S: *Health assessment for nursing practice,* St Louis, 1996, Mosby, p 376.

cardiovascular examination is considered to be somewhat limited. Usually only the left border of cardiac dullness can be determined, inasmuch as this is located near the apical impulse, or within the midclavicular line. Cardiac dullness is characteristic of cardiac hypertrophy. Unfortunately, mild to moderate degrees of cardiac hypertrophy are not usually detectable by percussion.

## Auscultation

### Heart sounds

The first heart sound ($S_1$), called lub, generally is thought to be produced by the almost simultaneous closures of the mitral and tricuspid valves. $S_1$ lasts approximately 0.10 second and signals the onset of ventricular systole. $S_1$ is generally loudest at the apex but can be heard over the entire precordium. $S_1$ is longer and lower pitched than the second heart sound ($S_2$), called dub (the first and second heart sounds together are referred to as lub-dub), and $S_1$ corresponds to the beat of the carotid pulse. $S_2$ is caused mainly by the closure of the semilunar valves (aortic and pulmonic). $S_2$ usually is loudest at the base of the heart and is described as shorter, higher pitched, and "snappier" than $S_1$. The sounds of the cardiac cycle are depicted in Figure 24-16.

The diaphragm chest piece of the stethoscope is most useful in listening to high-pitched sounds and murmurs. These include $S_1$, $S_2$, ejection sounds, and clicks. The diaphragm should be placed firmly on the chest wall so that an indentation is present on the patient's skin when the diaphragm is removed. The bell chest piece is most useful in detecting low-pitched sounds and murmurs. These include the third heart sound ($S_3$), the fourth heart sound ($S_4$), and mitral and tricuspid diastolic rumbles. The bell should be placed lightly on the chest wall, barely creating an airtight seal. If the bell is placed firmly on the skin it acts as a diaphragm.

**Splitting of $S_1$ and $S_2$.** The two main components of $S_1$ (closure of the mitral and tricuspid valves) are asynchronous, because left ventricular systole usually occurs slightly ahead of right ventricular systole. The $S_1$ may be split in persons who have RBB block, left-sided mechanical defects (e.g., mitral stenosis), or tricuspid valve dysfunction associated with pulmonary hypertension.

Because left ventricular contraction slightly precedes right ventricular contraction, the aortic valve also normally closes slightly before the pulmonic valve. On inspiration, intrathoracic pressure decreases and facilitates an increase in venous blood return to the right side of the heart. This increased blood return delays the closure of the pulmonic valve and results in a normal physiological split $S_2$. On expiration, closure of the aortic and pulmonic valves occurs almost simultaneously and therefore is heard only as a single sound. In conditions of increased blood flow or increased right ventricular pressure there may be a "fixed" splitting of $S_2$; that is, both components of $S_2$ are heard in both inspiration and expiration. A fixed split is considered abnormal and may occur in RBB block, pulmonary hypertension, and right ventricular failure related to atrial or ventricular septal defects.

**Extra heart sounds.** Extra heart sounds include ejection sounds (systolic clicks), opening snaps, $S_3$, and $S_4$. The two most common extra heart sounds are $S_3$ and $S_4$, or ventricular gallop and atrial gallop, respectively (Figure 24-17).

Ventricular diastolic gallop, or $S_3$, is a faint, low-pitched sound produced by rapid ventricular filling in early diastole. This occurs when the volume of early filling is increased or a decrease occurs in ventricular compliance. Ventricular "gallop" recalls the gallop of a horse, which is mimicked at heart rates greater than 100. When this sound is present in healthy children and young adults, it is almost always a normal condition and is referred to as a physiological $S_3$. An $S_3$ heard in an older person usually is a pathological sign and commonly is one of the first signs of serious heart disease or cardiac decompensation. $S_3$ is typically present in such states as left-to-right shunts, mitral regurgitation, congestive heart failure, and constrictive pericarditis.

Atrial diastolic gallop, or $S_4$, is a low-frequency sound that occurs under circumstances of altered ventricular compliance, either left or right. $S_4$ occurs late in diastole when atrial systole ejects blood into a noncompliant ventricle. Because the presence of an audible $S_4$ is related to a decrease in left ventricular compliance and an increase in left ventricular end-diastolic pressure, it is often heard in hypertensive cardiovascular disease and idiopathic hypertrophic subaortic stenosis. An $S_4$ commonly is identified in patients with acute myocardial infarction and in patients with coronary artery disease, especially during an attack of angina pectoris. In addition, an $S_4$ may be present when CO and stroke volume are increased,

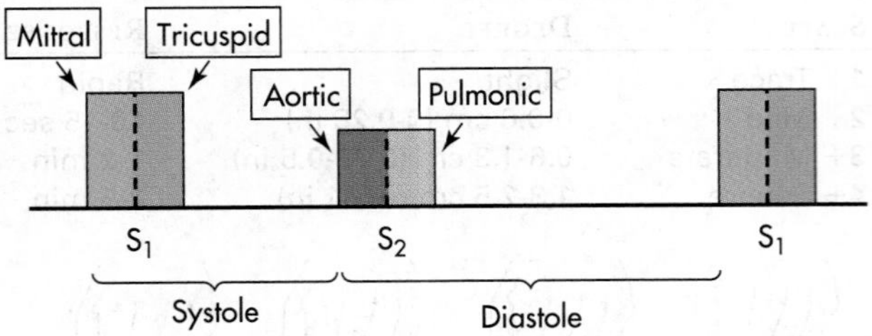

Mitral
Tricuspid
Aortic
Pulmonic
$S_1$
$S_2$
$S_1$
Systole
Diastole

**fig. 24-16** Heart sound $S_1$ is the closure of mitral and tricuspid valves: $S_2$ is the closure of the aortic and pulmonic valves. Systole is the interval between $S_1$ and the start of $S_2$; diastole is $S_2$ to the start of $S_1$. Diastole is longer than systole.

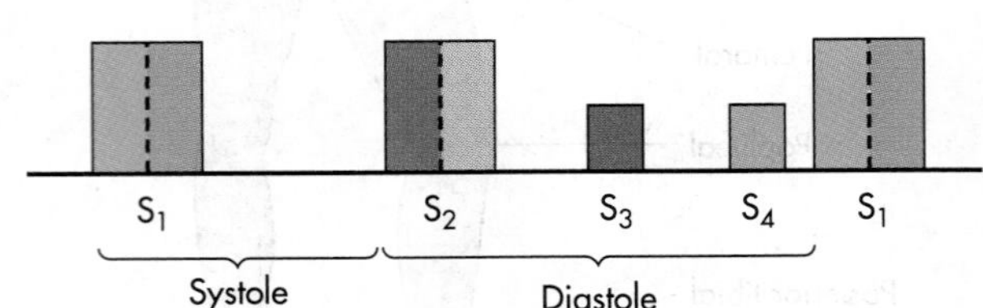


**fig. 24-17** Location of extra heart sounds during cardiac cycle.

such as in severe anemia, thyrotoxicosis, and large A-V fistulas. Although the $S_4$ sound occurs close to $S_1$, it can be easily differentiated because $S_4$ is lower pitched than $S_1$.

**Murmurs.** Murmurs are audible vibrations of the heart and great vessels that occur because of turbulent blood flow. They may be produced by hemodynamic events or by structural alterations occurring in the heart or in the walls of the great vessels. In general, murmurs are heard most distinctly over the area of the valve or altered cardiac structure responsible for the vibrations. The major factors involved in the production of cardiac murmurs include the following: (1) increased velocity of blood flow through normal or abnormal valves; (2) forward flow through a stenotic or irregular valve orifice; (3) backward (regurgitant) blood flow through an incompetent valve, septal defect, or patent ductus arteriosus; and (4) turbulent blood flow produced in a dilated chamber, such as in a ventricular or aortic aneurysm.

Murmurs generally are characterized according to timing (position in the cardiac cycle), intensity, quality, pattern, posture, pitch, location, and direction of radiation. These characteristics provide data concerning the location and nature of the cardiac abnormality.

**Pericardial friction rub.** A pericardial friction rub is an extra heart sound originating from the pericardial sac and is often a sign of inflammation, infection, or infiltration as the heart moves. The sound is high pitched and scratchy, similar to sandpaper being rubbed together. The sound is best heard with the diaphragm of the stethoscope while the patient is in an upright position and leaning forward.

## DIAGNOSTIC TESTS

Cardiovascular diseases usually are diagnosed by reviewing laboratory test results combined with findings from the patient interview and the physical examination. The laboratory tests ordered most commonly in patients with heart disease include blood tests, urinalysis, electrocardiography, invasive hemodynamic monitoring, sonic studies, dynamic studies, radiography, scintigraphic studies, and angiography.[4]

The nurse may be directly or indirectly involved in these tests and procedures. It is essential that the nurse possess an understanding of the various tests or procedures and the importance of the data to an accurate diagnosis. This information enables the nurse to prepare the patient adequately before any diagnostic procedure and to document signs and symptoms while caring for the patient.

### Laboratory Tests

A complete blood cell count (CBC) is ordered for all patients with documented or suspected heart disease. Data concerning red blood cells (RBCs) and white blood cells (WBCs) are helpful in diagnosing infectious heart disease and myocardial infarction (Table 24-3). The RBC count may be elevated as a physiological response to inadequate tissue oxygenation. The erythrocyte sedimentation rate (ESR) is a measurement of the rate at which RBCs "settle out" of anticoagulated blood in 1 hour. The rate of RBC settling is increased if the proportion of globulin to albumin increases or if fibrinogen levels are excessively increased. Nonspecific increases in globulin and fibrinogen levels occur when the body responds to injury or inflammation, as seen with infectious heart disorders and myocardial infarction.

Blood coagulation tests, including prothrombin time (PT), international normalized ratio (INR), and activated partial thromboplastin time (APTT), indicate the rapidity of blood clotting.[8] These tests are useful during anticoagulation therapy. (See Table 24-3.) A blood urea nitrogen (BUN) determination is useful as an indicator of renal function. Decreased CO leading to a low renal blood supply and reduction in glomerular filtration rate will elevate the BUN.

**table 24-3** *Selected Laboratory Tests for Cardiovascular Disorders*

| Test | Normal Values | Significance in Heart Disorders |
|---|---|---|
| Serum red blood cell count | Men: 4.7-6.1 million/mm³<br>Women: 4.2-5.4 million/mm³ | Decreased in subacute endocarditis<br>Increased with inadequate tissue oxygenation<br>Decreased in some congenital heart disease with right-to-left shunt |
| Serum white blood cell count | 5000-10,000/mm³ | Increased in acute and chronic heart inflammations and in acute myocardial infarction |
| Erythrocyte sedimentation rate (ESR) | Men: up to 15 mm/hr<br>Women: up to 20 mm/hr | Increased in acute myocardial infarction and infectious heart disease |
| Prothrombin time (PT) | 11-12.5 sec<br>100% compared to control | Indicates rapidity of blood clotting; used to monitor anticoagulant therapy with warfarin (Coumadin) |
| International normalized ratio (INR) | 2.0-3.0 | Ratio of patient's prothrombin time to the normal standard prothrombin time of the testing laboratory; used to monitor anticoagulant therapy with warfarin (Coumadin) |
| Activated partial thromboplastin time (APTT) | 30-40 sec | More sensitive than PT; used to monitor heparin therapy |
| Blood urea nitrogen (BUN) | 5-20 mg/100 ml | Increased with decreased cardiac output |
| Serum proteins | 6-8 g/100 ml | Levels below 5 g/100 ml seen with edema |

**table 24-4** *Initial Classification of Total, Low-Density Lipoprotein, and High-Density Lipoprotein Cholesterol and Triglycerides*

| Classification | Total Cholesterol | Low-Density Lipoprotein Cholesterol | High-Density Lipoprotein Cholesterol | Triglycerides |
|---|---|---|---|---|
| Desirable/normal | <200 mg/dl | <130 mg/dl | 30-70 mg/dl | <200 mg/dl |
| Borderline-high | 200-239 mg/dl | 130-159 mg/dl | — | 200-400 mg/dl |
| High | ≥240 mg/dl | >160 mg/dl | — | 400-1000 mg/dl |
| Very high | | | — | >1000 mg/dl |

### Blood lipids

The blood (plasma) lipids are composed mainly of cholesterol, triglyceride, phospholipid, and free fatty acids, all of which are insoluble in water and require a "carrier" to transport them. The carriers for plasma lipids are the proteins to which they are bound, thus the name lipoproteins. There are four major classes of lipoproteins: chylomicrons, very-low-density lipoproteins, low-density lipoproteins, and high-density lipoproteins, all of which contain varying levels of cholesterol, triglycerides, and phospholipids.

Chylomicrons are composed mainly of triglycerides and originate in the intestine after the absorption of dietary fat. Chylomicrons should not be found in the plasma after 12 to 14 hours of fasting. Elevated chylomicron levels do not appear to be associated with heart disease.

Very-low-density lipoproteins (VLDLs) are composed primarily of triglycerides and are synthesized in the liver. Sustained elevations of VLDLs sometimes have been associated with atherosclerosis; however, the exact relationship of triglycerides to heart disease is not yet clear.

Low-density lipoproteins (LDLs) are composed of approximately 50% cholesterol and are thought to have the greatest correlation with coronary artery disease. The LDLs are believed to enter the arterial intima and produce arterial endothelial injury. Subsequently, this process can result in progressive atherosclerotic plaque formation and eventually ischemic heart disease. Lipoprotein (a), or Lp(a), is a protein associated with LDL. High plasma levels of Lp(a) have been correlated with an increased risk for atherothrombotic cardiovascular disease. Structurally Lp(a) is similar to plasminogen, which explains its ability to interfere with the processes involved in plasmin generation and clot lysis.

High-density lipoproteins (HDLs) are composed of mostly protein with a modest amount of cholesterol and a considerable amount of phospholipids. This lipoprotein appears to have the lowest atherogenic potential. In fact, studies have demonstrated that HDLs are inversely associated with coronary heart disease. The HDLs may carry cholesterol away from tissues, including atheromatous plaques, and may even provide protection against coronary heart disease.

Lipid assessment includes total cholesterol, LDL, HDL, and triglyceride levels (Table 24-4). Adjustments in target levels are made for individuals with coronary artery disease risk factors such as hypertension, diabetes mellitus, or family history of premature coronary disease.

Evaluation of individual components is important, but the most significant predictor of coronary artery disease is the ratio of total cholesterol to HDL.[7] Before blood lipid tests are performed the patient must fast for 12 hours. No alcoholic beverages or lipid-influencing drugs (e.g., estrogens, oral contraceptives, steroids, salicylates) should be taken. Because lipid levels may fluctuate greatly from day to day, repeated blood samples are obtained before a definitive diagnosis of hyperlipidemia is made.

### Blood cultures

Blood cultures are crucial in the diagnosis of infectious diseases of the heart such as endocarditis. Culture results help identify the organism responsible for the infective process and the organism's sensitivity to various antibiotics.

### Enzyme studies

Enzymes, which are located in all tissues, catalyze the biochemical reactions of the body. When cell membranes are damaged, such as in myocardial infarction, enzymes leak out of the damaged myocardial cell and escape into the serum. The serum enzyme measurements that are used to detect myocardial necrosis are serum aspartate aminotransferase (AST), creatine kinase (CK), troponin I, lactic dehydrogenase (LDH), and hydroxybutyrate dehydrogenase (HBD). Because these enzymes are located in various body tissues, numerous conditions other than myocardial damage may produce enzyme elevations; for example, the brain, pancreas, and liver are all rich sources of AST. If a person were to develop chest pain concurrently with pancreatic or liver disease, an elevated AST level may be mistaken for myocardial necrosis. Fortunately, three of the enzymes, CK, troponin I, and LDH, have isoenzymes that are thought to be present almost exclusively in myocardial muscle.[2]

The CK molecule has two subunits, which have been identified as follows: M, associated with muscle; and B, associated with brain. The brain and gastrointestinal tract contain modest amounts of the BB dimer, and skeletal muscle contains large amounts of the MM form. Heart muscle contains huge quantities of MM, but it also contains the MB hybrid form

**table 24-5** *Time Course of Cardiac Enzymes after Acute Myocardial Infarction*

| Enzyme | Onset | Peak | Return to Normal |
|---|---|---|---|
| Troponin I | <1 hr | 12 hr | 7 days |
| CK | 3-6 hr | 12-24 hr | 3-5 days |
| CK-MB | 2-4 hr | 12-20 hr | 48-72 hr |
| LDH | 24 hr | 48-72 hr | 7-10 days |
| $LDH_1$ | 4 hr | 48 hr | 20 days |
| $LDH_2$ | 4 hr | 48 hr | 10 days |

of CK. Because CK-MB is not found in any other tissue, its presence in the serum is a sensitive indicator of myocardial damage.

Cardiac troponin I is the newest enzyme study. Troponin is normally found in minuscule amounts and is specific to heart muscle. It is immediately released from damaged myocardial cells and is present in the blood for about 1 week after release.

Of the five LDH isoenzymes, $LDH_1$ has been found to be the most sensitive indicator of myocardial damage. Their use in the diagnosis of myocardial infarction has largely been replaced by troponin and CK-MB. See Chapter 25 for a more detailed description of cardiac enzymes in the diagnosis of myocardial infarction.

The different enzymes are released into the blood at varying periods after myocardial infarction. It is crucial to evaluate the enzyme level in relation to the time of the onset of chest discomfort or other symptoms. See Table 24-5 for the time course of cardiac enzymes.

#### Serological tests

Syphilis can play an important role in the development of aortic disorders. The patient may have aortic insufficiency, aortic aneurysms, or disease of the orifices of the coronary arteries. Because of the relationship between syphilis and heart disease, a routine Venereal Disease Research Laboratories (VDRL) test is performed on all cardiac patients.

#### Urinalysis

A routine urinalysis is performed to determine the effects of cardiovascular disease on renal function. Mild to moderate proteinuria (usually albuminuria) may be seen in patients with malignant hypertension and venous congestion of the kidneys secondary to congestive heart failure or constrictive pericarditis. The presence of RBCs in the urine may indicate infective endocarditis or an embolic kidney disease.

The detection of myoglobin in the urine (myoglobinuria) has been useful in the diagnosis of myocardial infarction. Clinical experience with this test remains limited; however, it may prove to be a sensitive indicator of myocardial damage. Destruction of striated muscle by infarction liberates myoglobin, and because of its small size, the molecule can filter through the glomerulus and be excreted in the urine.

**box 24-1** *Diagnostic Uses for the ECG*

The ECG may be used to evaluate the following:
- Tachycardia, bradycardia, or dysrhythmias
- Sudden onset of dyspnea
- Pain occurring in the upper portion of the trunk and in the extremities
- Syncopal episodes
- Shock state or coma
- Preoperative status
- Postoperative hypotension
- Hypertension, murmurs, or cardiomegaly
- Artificial pacemaker function

### Radiological Tests

#### Chest radiography

A radiograph (x-ray film) of the chest may be taken to determine overall size and configuration of the heart, as well as individual cardiac chamber size. Most abnormalities of heart size and calcification in the heart muscle, valves, and great vessels can be detected with a standard posteroanterior and lateral view of the chest.

#### Cardiac fluoroscopy

Cardiac fluoroscopy facilitates observation of the heart from varying views while the heart is in motion. Fluoroscopy can be used to detect ventricular aneurysms, monitor prosthetic valve movement, or assess the position of cardiac calcifications during the cardiac cycle. Because of the radiation risk associated with fluoroscopy, many institutions no longer use this diagnostic technique.

### Special Tests

#### Electrocardiogram

The ECG is a graphic representation of the electrical forces produced within the heart. The ECG is an essential tool for cardiac evaluation, but it must be combined with other data sources for accurate diagnosis. A resting ECG may be normal, even in the presence of heart disease. Conversely, abnormal variances may be seen in the ECG of a normal heart.

An ECG may be used for a wide variety of diagnostic purposes (Box 24-1). The patient should be informed of the step-by-step procedure and assured of its safe, painless nature.

**Standard 12-lead ECG.** The ECG tracing represents the net electrical activity or electrical potential variations of the atria and ventricles as each depolarizes and repolarizes. The electrical currents passing through the heart can be detected by electrodes and measured when they reach the surface.

The conventional 12-lead ECG machine uses several electrode sites to measure the electrical potential differences between a series of locations on the body surface. Each pair of electrodes, consisting of a positive and a negative terminal, constitutes an ECG lead. Representative tracings obtained from the 12 leads are shown in Figure 24-18. The standard lead sites are right arm, left arm, right leg, and left leg. The chest (or precordial) electrodes are placed across the chest wall in six different locations. These 10 sites are combined in

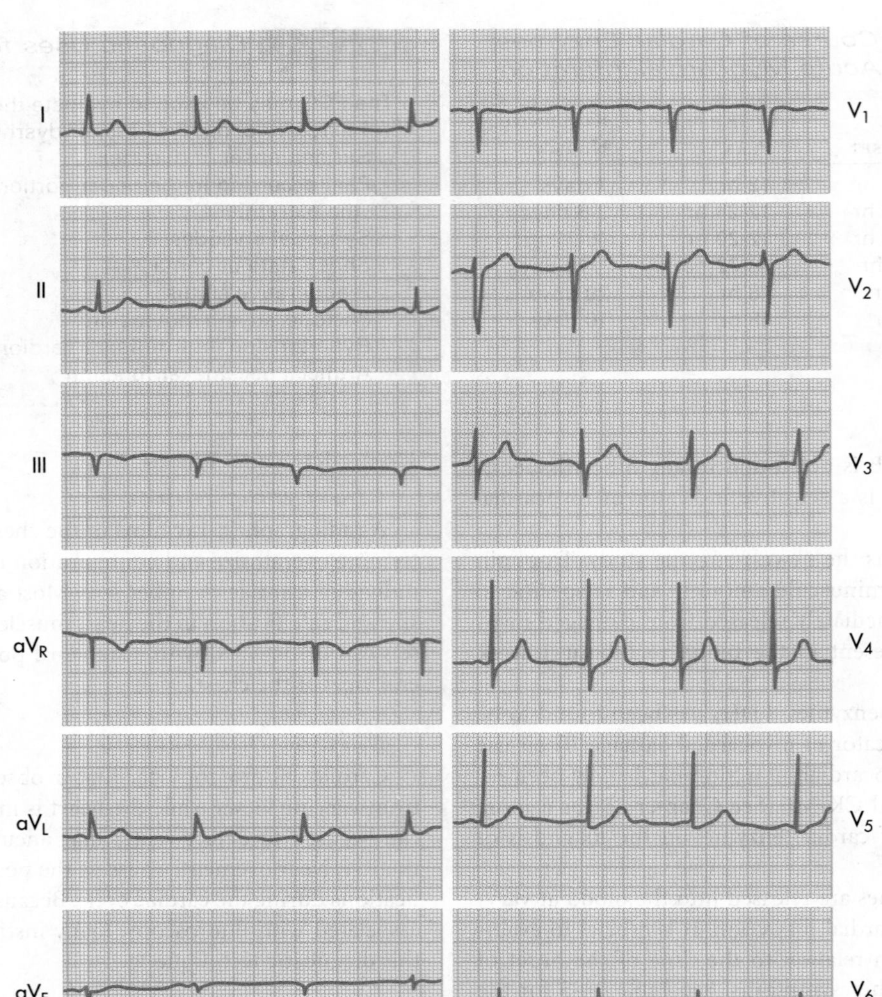


**fig. 24-18** Twelve-lead ECG showing normal sinus rhythm.

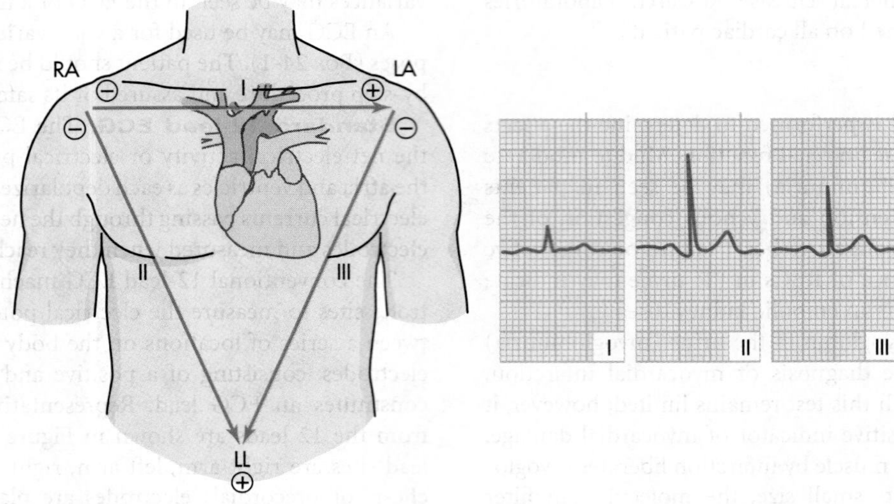


**fig. 24-19** Schematic representation of standard limb lead system.

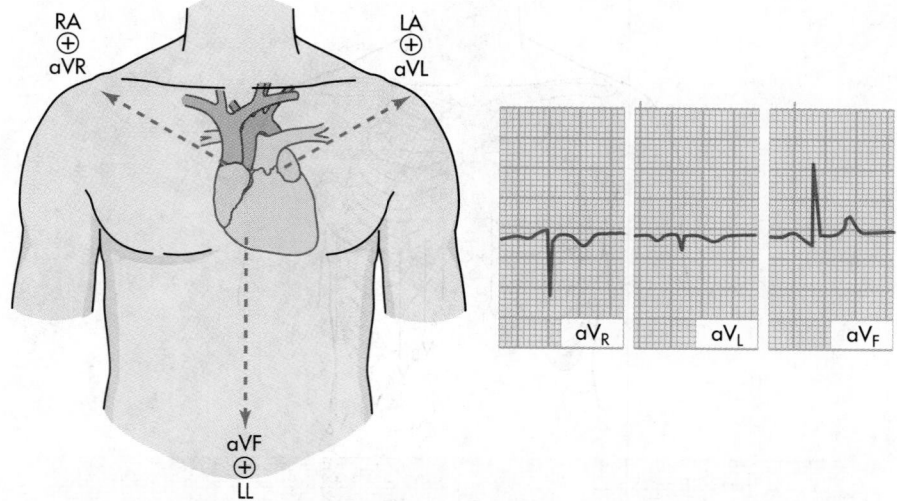

fig. 24-20 Schematic representation of augmented unipolar limb lead system.

pairs through a switching network in the ECG machine. Effective contact between the skin and the electrode is established by the use of electrode jelly, which contains electrolytes and an abrasive capable of penetrating the waterproof layer of the skin.

**Limb leads.** The standard bipolar limb leads, designated by Roman numerals I, II, and III, are created by electrodes applied to the right arm (RA), left arm (LA), and left leg (LL) (Figure 24-19). The right leg (RL) electrode acts as a grounding electrode.

*Lead I* records the difference between the RA and LA potentials.
*Lead II* records the difference between the RA and LL potentials.
*Lead III* records the difference between the LA and LL potentials.

The augmented unipolar limb leads are designated by the abbreviated forms aVR, aVL, and aVF. For these leads the right arm (*R*), left arm (*L*), and left leg (*F*) become the respective positive electrodes (Figure 24-20).

For clinical purposes, the amplitude of the recordings from these electrodes is augmented by approximately 50% to produce a tracing that is easier to interpret. Together, the augmented and standard limb leads provide the six frontal plane leads.

**Precordial leads.** There are six precordial or chest leads designated by the symbols $V_1$ through $V_6$. These leads register the electrical variations of the heart in the horizontal plane (Figure 24-21). The positive electrode is placed on six different sites across the chest as shown in Figure 24-22.

**Monitoring.** To perform continuous cardiac monitoring the conventional ECG leads have been modified to eliminate cumbersome wiring. The most popular leads for continuous dysrhythmia monitoring are lead II and lead $V_1$. The patient wears two, three, or five electrodes, which are attached by small lead wires to a cable connected to a wall-mounted monitor with an oscilloscope screen.

An alternative type of continuous monitoring is known as telemetry. The telemetry system requires no cables that would restrict patient mobility. The electrical impulses are

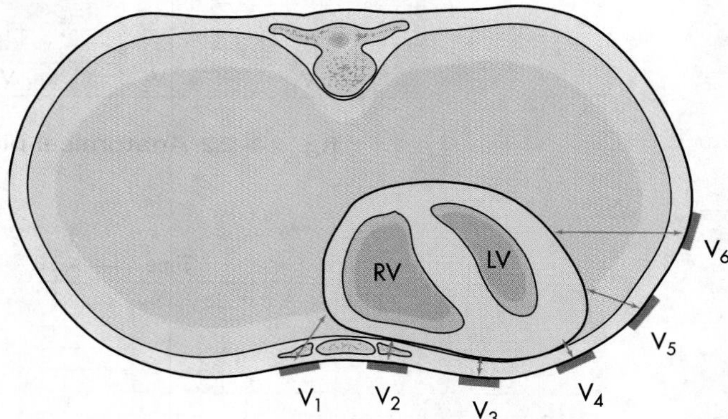


fig. 24-21 Cross section of heart showing precordial leads $V_1$ through $V_6$ in a horizontal plane.

transmitted by antennae to an oscilloscope at another location.

Lead II is produced by placing the negative electrode on the right arm (modified and placed near the right shoulder below the clavicle) and the positive electrode on the left leg (modified and placed on the lower left rib cage eighth intercostal space).

Lead $V_1$ is produced by placing the negative electrode on the left arm (modified and placed near the left shoulder below the clavicle) and the positive electrode at the fourth intercostal space to the right of the sternum. With these modifications, $V_1$ is known as $MCL_1$. The $MCL_1$ lead is the most helpful lead for determining the origin of premature beats and determining the presence of bundle branch blocks.

**Electrocardiographic tracing.** The ECG tracing is recorded on graph paper that is divided into millimeter squares. The millimeter squares are grouped and divided into larger squares by thick lines occurring every fifth square (Figure 24-23).

Horizontally, each millimeter square represents 0.04 second of time elapsed. Each thick line denotes the passage of

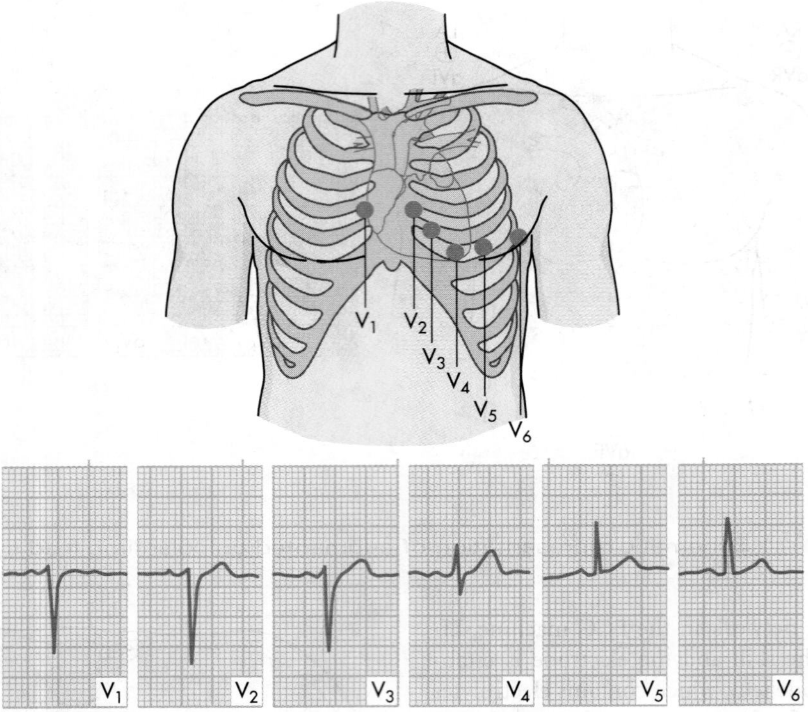


fig. 24-22 Anatomical placement of precordial leads.

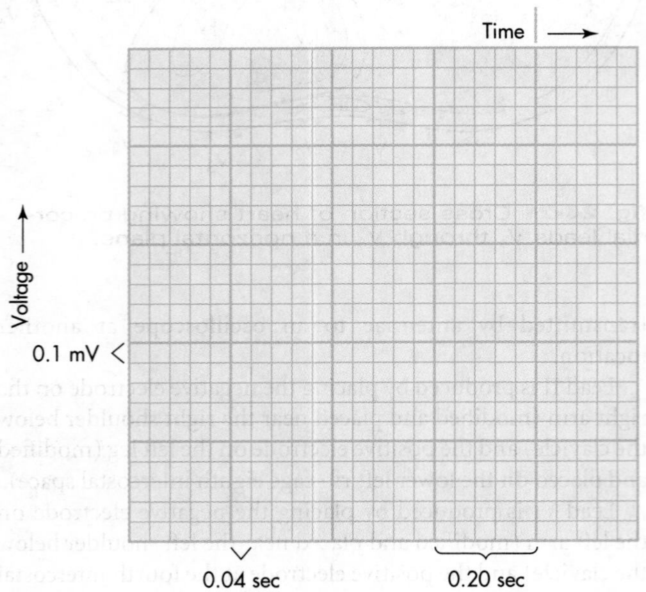


fig. 24-23 Components of ECG paper.

0.20 second. Fifteen hundred (1500) small, or 300 large, squares represent 1 minute. With this information, the duration of any complex or interval on the ECG can be determined by counting the number of small squares and multiplying by 0.04 second. Heart rate may be measured or estimated by various methods (Box 24-2).

Vertically, each small square is 1 mm in height and represents 0.1 mV of voltage. Thus each large square represents 5 mm or 0.5 mV. The voltage or amplitude of a wave or complex in a given lead indirectly indicates the electrical activity of the muscle below the positive electrode. Hypertrophied myocardium produces abnormally high voltage in some leads, whereas infarcted myocardium may produce no voltage or low-voltage waves.

### box 24-2 Three Methods for Estimating Heart Rate from the ECG Tracing

1. Measure the interval between consecutive QRS complexes, determine the number of small squares, and divide 1500 by that number. This method is used only when the heart rhythm is regular.
2. Measure the interval between consecutive QRS complexes, determine the number of large squares, and divide 300 by that number. This method is used only when the heart rhythm is regular.
3. Determine the number of RR intervals within 6 seconds and multiply by 10. The ECG paper is conveniently marked at the top with slashes that represent 3-second intervals. This method can be used when the rhythm is irregular. If the rhythm is extremely irregular an interval of 30 to 60 seconds should be used.

The baseline of the ECG tracing is known as the isoelectric line. Waves are deflections, either above (positive) or below (negative) the isoelectric line. The direction of deflection is determined by (1) the direction in which the electrical impulse flows, (2) the distance between the source of the impulse and the positive electrode, and (3) the site of the electrode. As a rule, when the flow of electrical current is directed toward the positive electrode, the deflection will be positive, and when the flow of current is directed away from the positive electrode, the deflection will be negative (Figure 24-24).

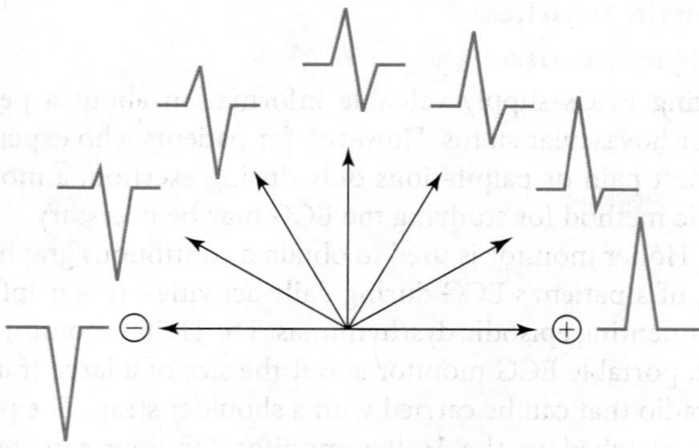

fig. 24-24 Several vectors and their resultant ECG complex. Note: (1) a current perpendicular to the axis produces an equiphasic deflection, and (2) a current parallel to the axis results in the tallest or deepest complex possible.

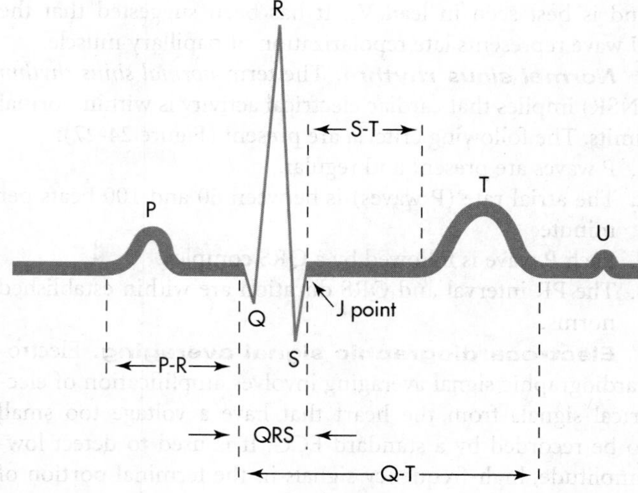


fig. 24-25 Schematic drawing of ECG waves produced by the cardiac cycle.

The waves recorded by the ECG have been arbitrarily designated by the letters P, Q, R, S, T, and U (Figure 24-25). The P wave represents the depolarization of the atria (Table 24-6). Normally the P wave is gently rounded, does not exceed 2 to 3 mm in amplitude, and is 0.11 second or less in duration. It is normally positive in leads I, II, aVF, and $V_4$ to $V_6$. It is negative in lead aVR and variable in all other leads. Repolarization of the atria also produces a wave, but it generally is hidden within the QRS complex.

The PR interval is a measurement of the amount of time taken for the impulse to travel from the SA node to the ventricular musculature. It includes the normal physiological delay of impulse conduction by the AV node. This interval is measured from the beginning of the P wave to the beginning of the QRS complex. Normally the PR interval measures from 0.12 to 0.20 second.

The QRS complex represents depolarization of the ventricles and is often the most significant portion of the ECG. The Q wave is a negative initial deflection from the isoelectric line and may not always be present. A small Q wave of less than 0.04 second duration is a normal finding in leads I, II, III, aVL, aVF, and $V_4$ to $V_6$. The first positive deflection from the isoelectric line is an R wave. The negative deflection following an R wave is an S wave. The full duration of the QRS complex is measured from the first deflection from the isoelectric line (whether it is a Q or an R wave) to the point where the QRS complex ends and the ST segment begins. The normal QRS complex is 0.05 to 0.10 second.

The ST segment represents the plateau (phase 2) of the action potential. It is normally isoelectric because all cells are at zero potential and no current flows. Slight elevation no greater than 1 mm or a subtle depression no greater than 0.5 mm is considered normal. Abnormal elevations or depressions of the ST segment can occur as a result of myocardial muscle injury, conduction disturbances, hypertrophy, and the effect of digitalis.

The T wave represents phase 3 of the action potential, when the ventricles are being rapidly repolarized. It is normally rounded, slightly asymmetrical, and of the same polarity as the QRS complex. The height of the T wave should not exceed 5 mm in a limb lead or 100 mm in a precordial lead. It is normally a positive wave in leads I, II, and $V_3$ to $V_6$. The T wave is a negative deflection in lead aVR and variable in all other leads.

**table 24-6 Electrical Activity of the Heart and Resultant ECG Findings**

| Electrical Activity of Heart | ECG Events |
|---|---|
| SA node fires | Not recorded |
| Wave of depolarization spreads through atria | P wave |
| Slight pause at AV node | Isoelectric baseline between P wave and QRS complex |
| Atrial repolarization | Not recorded; overpowered by electrical activity of ventricles |
| Ventricular depolarization | QRS complex |
| Ventricular repolarization | T wave |

The effective refractory period is present during the beginning of the T wave. At the peak of the T wave, more of the fast sodium channels have recovered and therefore a stronger-than-normal stimulus can produce a successful action potential. However, some fibers are still unresponsive, and electrical chaos and subsequent ventricular fibrillation may occur. The approximate location of this vulnerable period is illustrated in Figure 24-26.

The QT interval is measured from the beginning of the QRS complex to the end of the T wave. It represents the entire duration of ventricular depolarization and repolarization. The normal QT value varies with age, gender, and heart rate but generally should be less than half the preceding RR interval. The termination of the T wave is sometimes difficult to determine, and measuring the QT interval accurately is not always easy.

The U wave is a small wave sometimes seen after the T wave. It usually deflects in the same direction as the T wave and is best seen in lead $V_3$. It has been suggested that the U wave represents late repolarization of papillary muscle.

***Normal sinus rhythm.*** The term *normal sinus rhythm* (NSR) implies that cardiac electrical activity is within normal limits. The following criteria are present (Figure 24-27):

1. P waves are present and regular.
2. The atrial rate (P waves) is between 60 and 100 beats per minute.
3. Each P wave is followed by a QRS complex.
4. The PR interval and QRS duration are within established norms.

**Electrocardiographic signal averaging.** Electrocardiographic signal averaging involves amplification of electrical signals from the heart that have a voltage too small to be recorded by a standard ECG. It is used to detect low-amplitude, high-frequency signals in the terminal portion of the QRS complex to identify patients at risk for ventricular tachycardia. Approximately 200 identical QRS complexes are grouped and averaged, resulting in a waveform that appears smooth and continuous. Signal averaging minimizes the noise that contaminates the ECG signal and thereby exposes signals of a microvolt level normally hidden within the noise.

The rate of postinfarction sudden death precipitated by ventricular tachycardia that degenerates into ventricular fibrillation is approximately 10% to 15%. Thus identification of patients who will need treatment is critical for prevention of this life-threatening complication.

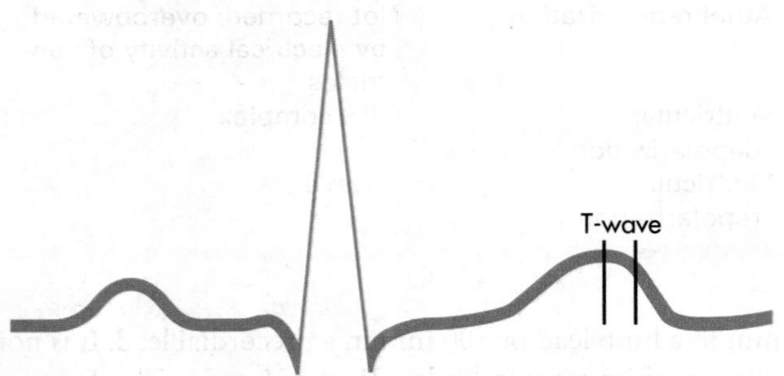


**fig. 24-26** Approximate location of the vulnerable period of ventricular repolarization.

## Dynamic Studies

### *Holter monitor*

Resting ECGs supply valuable information about a person's cardiovascular status. However, for patients who experience chest pain or palpitations only during exertion, a more dynamic method for studying the ECG may be necessary.

The Holter monitor is used to obtain a continuous graphic tracing of a patient's ECG during daily activities. It is helpful in documenting episodic dysrhythmias. The Holter monitor is a small, portable ECG monitor about the size of a large transistor radio that can be carried with a shoulder strap. The patient is attached to the Holter monitor for approximately 24 hours. During this time the patient keeps a log or diary of daily activities. The log includes activities, medications taken, and unusual sensations the person experiences while attached to the monitor. At the end of the monitoring period the physician compares the ECG with the patient's log to determine whether any correlations exist between the ECG and the patient's activities.

### *Stress testing*

Stress testing (ECG during exercise), or exercise testing, is a noninvasive test to evaluate cardiovascular response to a progressively graded workload. Stress testing may be performed for a variety of reasons and is often combined with an echocardiogram to obtain additional information about heart function (Box 24-3).

The exercise test can be performed with a stationary bicycle with adjustable resistance to pedaling or a treadmill. Various protocols are used during the procedure, but the patient's blood pressure and ECG are characteristically monitored closely during and after the stress test. Because the stress test is designed to progressively increase myocardial oxygen demand, some patients may experience untoward effects (e.g., ventricular tachycardia, a significant change in peak systolic blood pressure, premature ventricular contractions, or chest pain) and the test may need to be terminated.

Adequate preparation for stress testing is important. Although the procedure is not painful, it can be fatiguing; patients may become anxious because they will be exercising at a level that might produce symptoms such as dyspnea, palpitations, and chest pain. The nurse reviews the purpose and

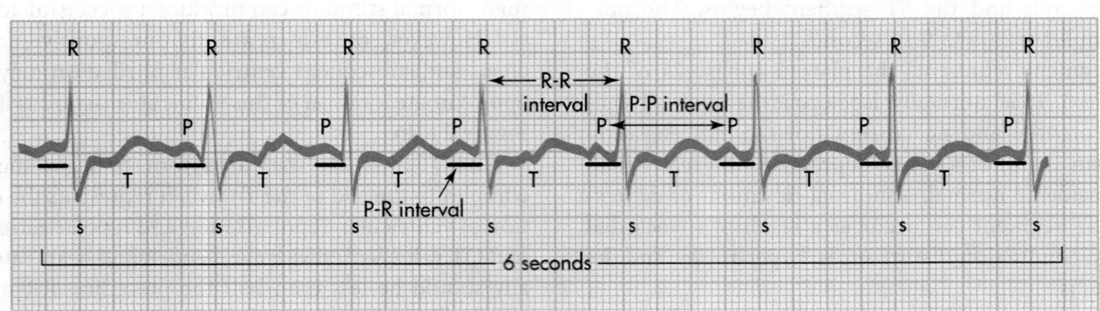


**fig. 24-27** Normal sinus rhythm showing R-R, P-P, and PR intervals.

method of stress testing and encourages the patient to do the following:

1. Avoid coffee, tea, and alcohol the day of the test.
2. Avoid smoking and taking nitroglycerin during the 2 hours immediately before the test.
3. Wear comfortable, loose-fitting clothes. (Women should be advised to wear a brassiere for support.)
4. Wear sturdy, comfortable walking shoes.
5. Consult with the physician about taking any medications before the test.

## Scintigraphic Studies

Various types of myocardial imaging can be used to identify myocardial infarctions, evaluate myocardial perfusion, and assess left ventricular function. In all these examples, myocardial imaging can provide a relatively safe and noninvasive technique for evaluating myocardial function. Techniques of myocardial imaging are occasionally combined with stress testing to improve the depth and accuracy of information about myocardial function.

### Stannous pyrophosphate scan

The pyrophosphate scan, referred to as "hot spot" imaging, typically uses technetium 99m stannous pyrophosphate. A minute dose of the radioisotope is injected into an antecubital vein, and the heart is visualized after about 2 hours. The healthy myocardium shows a homogeneous distribution of the radioisotope, whereas the damaged heart shows an increased uptake of the radioactive material. A gamma scintillator camera is used to identify the area of increased uptake (hot spot). The test is best performed 1 to 3 days after the infarction.

### Thallium imaging

Thallium imaging is referred to as "cold spot" imaging because the uptake of the isotope is greater in healthy myocardial tissue in comparison with the infarction area; thus this area remains a cold spot. A gamma scintillator is used to detect the distribution of the radioisotope. Thallium imaging, which most often is combined with exercise testing, can provide valuable information about the extent and severity of myocardial infarction.

**box 24-3** *Indications for Performing a Stress Test*

- Evaluation of the patient with symptoms suggestive of coronary artery disease
- Determination of the patient's physical work capacity and aerobic capacity
- Determination of the patient's functional capacity after a myocardial infarction and as an aid in planning an exercise rehabilitation program
- Evaluation of exercise-induced dysrhythmias
- Evaluation of the symptom-free person older than 40 years of age who is at risk for coronary artery disease
- Evaluation of pharmacological interventions for dysrhythmias, angina, or ischemia

Thallium scanning can be helpful in quantifying the amount of myocardium at risk during acute infarction by use of two resting scans to localize the affected area. The resting scan is obtained in the very early phase, and a redistribution scan is obtained 3 to 4 hours later. The total area of ischemia and infarction is visible on the initial scan. A smaller cold spot is visible during the redistribution scan as the ischemic tissue has successfully extracted the isotope. This technique is useful in assessing the efficacy of therapeutic interventions, such as thrombolytic therapy, as well as providing direction for further treatment based on the degree of myocardium still in jeopardy. Risk is minimal because the amount of thallium injected is small.

### Pharmacological myocardial perfusion imaging

Dipyridamole is a potent coronary vasodilator. By blocking cellular reuptake of adenosine, dipyridamole acts to increase blood and tissue concentrations of adenosine, which in turn promotes optimal coronary vasodilation. In normal coronary arteries, dipyridamole increases flow to three to four times that of baseline values. In stenosed arteries the increase in flow is less, and with severe stenosis a flow increase may not occur.

Adenosine perfusion imaging has been proposed as an alternative to dipyridamole perfusion imaging primarily because of its significantly shorter half-life (2 to 10 seconds for adenosine vs. several minutes for dipyridamole). Furthermore, adenosine elicits more consistent maximal coronary vasodilation over a shorter period than does dipyridamole. Side effects are common and include headache, dyspnea, chest pain, and facial flushing. Side effects generally disappear within 1 to 2 minutes and rarely require the administration of aminophylline as an antagonist.

### Technetium 99m sestamibi myocardial perfusion SPECT imaging

Technetium 99m sestamibi (Cardiolite) is a nonredistributing radionuclide agent being used in the evaluation of outcomes of thrombolytic and other interventional therapy in the treatment of acute myocardial infarction. Typically technetium 99m sestamibi is administered in the emergency department, followed by thrombolytic or interventional therapy. Once hemodynamic stability has been established, perfusion imaging is performed. Because minimal redistribution occurs with this agent, delayed images still delineate the initially nonperfused myocardial region. Improvements noted in repeat scintigraphy provide an assessment of salvaged myocardium.

### Multiple gated acquisition scanning

Multiple gated acquisition (MUGA) scanning has the ability to demonstrate cardiac wall motion to enable assessment of injury and residual cardiac function. The technique lends itself well to the portable imaging techniques required to scan acutely ill patients.

Gated blood pool imaging is a noninvasive radionuclide technique. The ECG leads are applied, and the ECG is synchronized to a computer and a gamma scintillator camera. A small amount of technetium 99m is injected intravenously.

After the radioactivity reaches a state of equilibrium (approximately 3 to 5 minutes), the patient is placed supine with the gamma scintillator camera positioned over the precordium. The computer then constructs an average cardiac cycle that represents the summation of several hundred heartbeats. Enough data are generated so that an outline of the left side of the heart in all phases of the cardiac cycle can be seen.

Gated blood pool imaging offers several advantages. Because all RBCs are tagged, their counts reflect blood volume. Thus, if the heart can be positioned to isolate the left ventricle on the scan, the left ventricular ejection fraction can be determined. The ejection fraction may provide an early indicator of deteriorating cardiovascular functioning. This information is extremely useful in patients with congestive heart failure or low CO.

Right ventricular ejection fraction also can be determined but is less accurate. The effects of pharmacotherapeutics (e.g., nitroglycerin, vasodilators) on ventricular function can also be evaluated.

Stress-testing ventriculography can be performed to evaluate the ejection fraction during exercise. Some patients with coronary artery disease demonstrate a normal ejection value at rest but experience a decline under the stress of exercise.

#### Positron emission tomography

Positron emission tomography (PET) is a radionuclide-based imaging technique that uses short-lived radionuclides as tracers to report both perfusion and metabolic events. The tracers are administered by intravenous injection or inhalation. Myocardial uptake is proportional to the quantity of tracer delivered by the blood flow. The tracer elements readily pass through the tissues and are detected by counters placed on opposite sides of the body.

Under normal circumstances the well-perfused, aerobically metabolizing myocardium prefers free fatty acids for energy production. When ischemia is present, more glucose and less fatty acid tend to be used. Positron emission tomography is particularly useful in demonstrating this process because the radioisotopes are incorporated into biochemically relevant components. It also provides the basis for medical management of asymptomatic coronary atherosclerosis and is useful in evaluating the effectiveness of interventions such as thrombolysis and percutaneous transluminal coronary angioplasty (PTCA).

### Sonic Studies

#### Echocardiography

Echocardiography uses ultrasound to assess cardiac structure and mobility noninvasively. It is useful in the diagnosis of a variety of cardiac conditions (Box 24-4). A small transducer is placed on the patient's chest at the level of the third or fourth intercostal space near the left lower sternal border. The transducer transmits high-frequency sound waves and then receives these waves back from the patient as they are reflected from different structures. The ultrasonic beam that is reflected back from the patient's heart produces "echoes" that are viewed as lines and spaces on an oscilloscope. These lines and spaces represent bone, cardiac chambers and valves, the septum, and muscle. A copy of the echocardiogram is recorded on paper.

Because echocardiography is a noninvasive procedure, it is safer than cardiac catheterization and is usually performed first. There are virtually no contraindications to the echocardiogram, and it can be performed at the bedside of critically ill patients. No special preparation is necessary for the test; the patient can eat and medications can be administered without interruption. Patient teaching regarding the echocardiogram should include the purpose of the test and the facts that the test is painless and takes approximately 30 to 60 minutes. The patient lies quietly in a supine position during the test with the head elevated 15 to 20 degrees. The patient may resume normal activities as soon as the test is completed.

#### Transesophageal echocardiography

Transesophageal echocardiography (TEE) allows high-resolution ultrasonic imaging of the cardiac structures and great vessels via the esophagus. It permits echocardiography to be used effectively with patients who have chronic pulmonary disease or are mechanically ventilated and poor candidates for ultrasound testing. This technique uses a transducer affixed to the tip of a modified, flexible endoscope that is advanced into the esophagus and manipulated to produce clear posterior images of the heart. The left atrium, the left atrial appendage, and the aortic and mitral valves are easily visualized with TEE. It is, however, unable to visualize the aortic arch and arch vessels. Indications for TEE are summarized in Box 24-5. This procedure can be performed at the bedside without contrast dye.

**box 24-4** *Conditions Detected or Evaluated by Echocardiography*

- Abnormal pericardial fluid
- Valvular disorders, including prosthetic valves
- Ventricular aneurysms
- Cardiac tumors, such as atrial myxomas
- Some forms of congenital heart disease, such as atrial septal defects
- Cardiac chamber size
- Stroke volume and cardiac output
- Some myocardial abnormalities, such as idiopathic hypertrophic subaortic stenosis (IHSS)
- Wall motion abnormalities

**box 24-5** *Clinical Indications for Transesophageal Echocardiography*

- Aortic dissection/aneurysm
- Mitral valve prosthetic dysfunction
- Mitral valve regurgitation
- Infective endocarditis
- Congenital heart disease
- Intracardial thrombi (especially left atrium and left atrial appendage)
- Cardiac tumor
- Intraoperative assessment: left ventricle function, adequacy of valve repair/replacement

The procedure is performed under local anesthesia and sedation. The patient receives nothing by mouth for at least 4 to 6 hours before the test. Preprocedure assessment includes any history of esophageal dysfunction or surgery.

Initially, the patient assumes a chin-to-chest position to facilitate passage of the endoscope through the oropharynx. The scope is advanced 30 to 35 cm to allow posterior visualization of the left atrium by the transducer. To view the left ventricle, the scope is advanced into the stomach and flexed upward for an inferior view. The procedure usually takes about 5 to 20 minutes.

Suction and resuscitation equipment are kept readily available. Cardiac rhythm, vital signs, and oxygen saturation ($SaO_2$) are monitored throughout the procedure. The patient is given a topical anesthetic by spray or gargle to reduce coughing or gagging during probe insertion. Additional sedation, usually diazepam (Valium) or midazolam (Versed), may be given.

The priority for post-test monitoring is the prevention of aspiration. The patient is given nothing by mouth until the gag reflex fully returns. The patient is kept in an upright or side-lying position to support ventilation. Throat lozenges and saline rinses can help alleviate throat discomfort. Other potential complications include esophageal perforation, pharyngeal bleeding, dysrhythmias, and transient hypoxemia.

## Phonocardiography

Phonocardiography involves the use of electrically recorded amplified cardiac sounds. Special microphones attached to the patient's chest pick up cardiac sounds produced by pressure changes in the heart and great vessels. The sounds are graphically recorded on special phonograph paper. Phonocardiography can be helpful in determining the exact timing and characteristics of murmurs and extra heart sounds. Phonocardiograms may be used in conjunction with echocardiograms so that a comparison can be made between sound (phono) and motion (echo). Patient preparation is similar to that described for the echocardiogram.

## Cardiac Catheterization

Cardiac catheterization is an extremely valuable diagnostic tool for obtaining detailed information about the structure and function of the cardiac chambers, valves, and coronary arteries. Cardiac catheterization may include studies of the right side of the heart, the left side of the heart, and the coronary arteries. Indications for cardiac catheterization are summarized in Box 24-6.

### Right-sided heart catheterization

Right-sided heart catheterization is performed to evaluate congenital heart disease and valvular disorders. Blood samples and pressure readings are taken, and cineradiographs of the right chambers of the heart and the pulmonary arterial circulation are made.

To perform a catheterization of the right side of the heart, a catheter is inserted via cutdown or percutaneously into a large vein (e.g., the medial cubital, brachial, or internal jugular). The catheter is then threaded with the use of fluoroscopy into the superior vena cava, the right atrium, the right ventricle, the pulmonary artery, and pulmonary capillaries. As the catheter is passed through the various chambers and vessels, blood samples are taken to determine the oxygen content and saturation. Blood pressure measurements also are recorded (Figure 24-28). The pressure is highest in the left ventricle because of the stronger ventricular contractions. Normally the pulmonary artery pressure (PAP) is approximately 25/10 mm Hg or approximately one fifth of the systemic blood pressure. Elevations in chamber pressures such as an elevated left atrial pressure can indicate valvular problems or possibly left ventricular failure.

### Left-sided heart catheterization

Left-sided heart catheterization is performed to evaluate pressures on the left side of the heart, valvular competency, and

**box 24-6** *Indications for Cardiac Catheterization*

- Confirmation of the presence of suspected heart disease, including congenital heart disease, valvular disease, and myocardial disease
- Determination of the location and severity of the disease process
- Preoperative assessment to determine if cardiac surgery is indicated
- Evaluation of ventricular function after surgical revascularization
- Evaluation of the effect of medical treatment modalities on cardiovascular function
- Performance of specialized cardiac interventions such as internal pacemaker placement

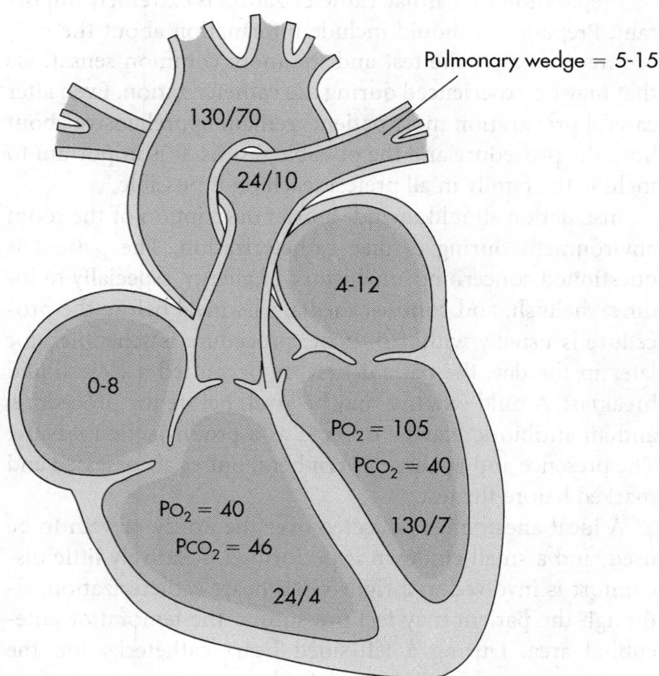


**fig. 24-28** Pressure readings and blood gases in millimeters of mercury (mm Hg) in chambers of heart and major blood vessels.

left ventricular function. A catheter is passed into the aorta from either the brachial or the femoral artery with the use of fluoroscopy. After reaching the aorta, the catheter is manipulated around the aortic arch, down the ascending aorta, and through the aortic valve into the left ventricle. Pressure-gradient measurements are obtained to detect pressure changes across the valves.

Ventricular angiography may be performed during the left-sided heart catheterization. This procedure involves the injection of contrast material into the ventricle while x-rays are taken. Information about contractility, aneurysm formation, valvular disorders, and the ejection fraction can be obtained.

Selective coronary arteriography also may be performed during the left-sided heart catheterization. The catheter is threaded to the aortic roots, and the tip of the catheter is then advanced into the right and left coronary arteries. Contrast medium is injected into each coronary artery, which outlines the entire coronary circulation, and cineangiographic films are taken to monitor the progression of the dye. This outlines the number and severity of stenotic segments and the presence of collateral vessels.

The introduction of the dye may temporarily displace the blood flow in the coronary arteries and may produce transient ischemia and chest pain. Sublingual nitroglycerin may be administered to relieve the discomfort. In addition, medications such as isosorbide (Isordil) may be given to dilate the vessels so that greater visualization may be achieved. Occasionally, the injection of contrast material into the right coronary artery may suppress the SA node, producing bradydysrhythmias, and intravenous atropine may be required.

#### *Patient preparation*

Preparation for cardiac catheterization is extremely important. Preparation should include information about the procedure, care after the test and the more common sensations that may be experienced during the catheterization. Even after careful preparation most patients remain apprehensive about both the procedure and the possible results. It is important to include the family in all pretest teaching if possible.

Instruction should include a brief description of the room environment during cardiac catheterization. The patient is questioned concerning any history of allergy, especially to iodine, shellfish, and contrast media. The meal before the procedure is usually withheld. If the procedure is scheduled for later in the day, the patient may be permitted a clear liquid breakfast. A mild sedative may be given before the procedure, and an antibiotic may be ordered as a prophylactic measure. The presence and quality of peripheral pulses are assessed and marked before the test.

A local anesthetic is injected over the artery or vein to be used, and a small cutdown is performed. Relatively little discomfort is involved in a right-sided heart catheterization, although the patient may feel pressure in the femoral or antecubital area. During a left-sided heart catheterization the patient may experience a warm, flushing sensation as the contrast medium is injected. This flushing sensation lasts for approximately 30 seconds. The patient also may experience nausea and "fluttering" sensations produced by catheter manipulation or from catheter advancement through the heart.

The body's physiological responses to cardiac catheterization are numerous and vary with each person. Therefore it is essential that the patient understand the importance of reporting any unusual sensations that might occur during the catheterization.

#### *Nursing care after catheterization*

The postprocedure nursing care following both types of heart catheterization is similar. These procedures generally last from 1 to 3 hours and can be tiring for the patient. Many patients prefer to rest or sleep after the examination.

The patient's pulse and blood pressure are monitored every 15 minutes for 1 hour and then every 30 minutes for 3 hours. It is essential to check the pulses distal to the catheter insertion site to determine the patency of the cannulated artery. The amplitude of the pulse may be slightly diminished for approximately 24 hours because of arterial spasm or edema at the site. At times thrombus formation may totally obliterate the distal pulse, and surgery may be necessary to correct impaired circulation. The cutdown site is closely monitored for signs of bleeding, inflammation, tenderness, or swelling (hematoma).

If a femoral approach was used, the patient is kept on bed rest for approximately 3 to 4 hours.[6] Various modalities are presently being used to prevent hemorrhage at the insertion site. Historically, sandbags or weights were used; however, these have been replaced by mechanical devices called Fem Stops, which are an external mode of compression.[3] Additionally, invasive devices referred to as hemostatic plugs are becoming increasingly popular. It is essential that the nurse monitor the patient closely after the procedure regardless of the method used. None of these options replaces close bedside monitoring of the insertion site during the initial phase of recovery. The patient should not have the head of the bed elevated more than 30 degrees and should keep the affected leg extended.

If the brachial site is used, the arm is kept straight for several hours, usually with an armboard, but the patient can be up in the room as soon as vital signs are stable. If any bleeding occurs from the cutdown site, firm pressure is applied directly over the site and the physician is notified. Intake and output are monitored in all patients regardless of the approach used. This intervention is important to ensure an adequate intake to flush the dye from the circulation and to monitor the patient's renal status. Hypotension may develop as a result of the diuretic effect of the contrast material used during angiography.

Complications during cardiac catheterization are not common; however, cardiac dysrhythmias such as ventricular fibrillation can occur. The development of tachycardia or any dysrhythmia is reported to the physician immediately.

### Electrophysiological Study

The electrophysiological (EP) study systematically assesses the electrical stability of the heart. This procedure requires electrode placement within the heart to record intracardiac electrical activity. The degree of invasiveness depends on the area of the heart to be studied. More detailed information about the heart's electrical activity can be obtained with the

EP study than with the surface ECG because of the proximity of the catheters to the cardiac conduction system. The test demonstrates the exact sequence of atrial and ventricular activation, localizes areas of conduction disturbances (such as accessory pathways, areas of ischemia and infarction, and dysrhythmia foci), and evaluates the effectiveness of antidysrhythmic management. Although EP studies are used more often than in the past, they are not routinely ordered. Use is currently reserved for persons not responding to treatment.

An EP study is performed under laboratory conditions with fluoroscopy to guide the pacing electrodes into position. The electrodes are typically inserted through the femoral, brachial, and basilic veins. Arterial cannulation is performed only when left ventricular stimulation is necessary.

Before the test antidysrhythmic drugs usually are discontinued for approximately five half-lives to prevent pharmacological interference with the study. Three to six intracardiac pacing catheters are inserted and connected to a multichanneled electrogram. A surface ECG is recorded simultaneously for comparison and evaluation. When indicated, dysrhythmias may be initiated by applying a series of programmed extra stimuli to areas of the heart, and the effects of various antidysrhythmic drugs are evaluated. Pacing also may be used to terminate a tachycardia by inhibiting impulse transmission in conduction pathways.

The EP study usually lasts 2 to 4 hours. At the completion of the test, catheters are removed and pressure is applied at the insertion site, followed by application of a pressure dressing. Patients may be monitored in a telemetry or intensive care unit after the test, where they can be closely observed. Complications of EP studies are similar to those of cardiac catheterization. Patients should be closely monitored for hemorrhage, perforation, hematoma, pulmonary emboli, deep vein thrombus, infection, cerebrovascular accident (stroke), angina, and dysrhythmia.

Nurses play a key role in preparing patients for the EP study. Reinforcing physician information about the indications for the test, the procedure itself, and risks may allay anxiety for the patient and the family. A description of the equipment used and the room's appearance also may be helpful. It is important to inform patients that they will be awake throughout the procedure.

Postprocedural monitoring includes vital signs, peripheral pulses, insertion site, and color, warmth, and sensation of extremities. Initially these observations are performed every 15 minutes and then gradually increased to every 4 hours. The affected extremity is immobilized, and the patient is placed on bed rest for 4 to 6 hours. Documentation of stability or changes in rhythm and frequency of ectopy is essential.

## Invasive Hemodynamic Monitoring

Invasive hemodynamic monitoring is not a typical diagnostic test, but it is used to evaluate the hemodynamic status of the critically ill patient and has greatly increased the database on which health professionals can plan and evaluate therapeutic modalities. Numerous devices are used in hemodynamic monitoring.

### *Central venous pressure*

Central venous pressure (CVP) measurements reflect the pressures in the right atrium and provide information regarding changes in right ventricular pressure. The CVP is used to monitor blood volume and the adequacy of venous return to the heart. The primary factors affecting CVP are the circulating blood volume, right-sided pump function, and the degree of peripheral vasoconstriction. Because the CVP reflects the pressure in the great veins as blood returns to the right side of the heart, a low (or falling) reading may indicate an inadequate blood volume (hypovolemia). A high (or rising) CVP usually is secondary to left-sided pump failure. Unfortunately, the patient's hemodynamic status may be severely altered before representative changes in the CVP are evident.

The normal values for CVP will vary with different equipment; however, a range of 5 to 15 cm $H_2O$ is acceptable. It is important to note that a change or a trend in the CVP is more important than the actual numerical value.

### *Intraarterial blood pressure measurement*

In the critically ill patient, the CO may be decreased to such an extent that standard blood pressure readings may be inaccurate. As the stroke volume falls, Korotkoff's sounds become increasingly more difficult to auscultate. Invasive arterial blood pressure monitoring may be implemented, which will more accurately reflect actual blood pressure.

Arterial catheters may be placed in various arteries; however, the radial, brachial, and axillary arteries are used most often. The arterial catheter is attached to a transducer that converts the mechanical pressure of the pulses to electrical impulses, which can be viewed as waveforms on an oscilloscope.

The patient with an arterial line requires frequent observation. It is essential that the extremity with the arterial line be kept uncovered so that the insertion site is monitored for bleeding and the pulse, color, sensation, and temperature of the extremity distal to the catheter are assessed every 2 hours.

### *Pulmonary artery and pulmonary capillary wedge pressures*

A balloon-tipped catheter (Swan-Ganz catheter) may be introduced into the pulmonary artery to obtain essential information regarding left ventricular function.[5] The pulmonary artery catheter permits the measurement of the pulmonary artery end-diastolic pressure (PAEDP) and the pulmonary capillary wedge pressure (PCWP) (Table 24-7).

The best indicator of left ventricular function is the left ventricular end-diastolic pressure (LVEDP). Elevations in LVEDP result from impaired left ventricular contractility that does not permit adequate emptying of the ventricles.

The PAEDP and the PCWP will be similar in a healthy person. However, in the presence of increased peripheral vascular resistance such as that found in pulmonary embolism, the PAEDP will rise while the PCWP remains normal. Therefore, to evaluate the true LVEDP accurately, the PCWP must be monitored.

Insertion of the pulmonary artery catheter is accomplished using several different approaches. These include a small incision (cutdown) made in an antecubital vein or percutaneously

**table 24-7** *Pulmonary Artery and Capillary Wedge Pressures*

| Type | Common Abbreviation | Normal Values |
|---|---|---|
| Left ventricular end-diastolic pressure | LVEDP | 12-15 mm Hg (elevations result from inadequate emptying of the ventricles) |
| Pulmonary artery end-diastolic pressure | PAEDP | 4-12 mm Hg (elevations result from increased peripheral vascular resistance) |
| Pulmonary capillary wedge pressure | PCWP | 4-12 mm Hg (levels >25 mm Hg indicate imminent pulmonary edema) |

through the internal jugular or subclavian veins. The catheter is threaded through the superior vena cava, through the tricuspid valve, and into the pulmonary artery. One of the lumens of the catheter is attached to a monitor that presents a numerical reading and a display of waveforms that indicate the location (capillary bed, pulmonary artery, or right ventricle) of the catheter. The balloon is then inflated, which causes the catheter to wedge in a distal branch of the pulmonary artery (Figure 24-29). The reading obtained when the balloon is inflated is the PCWP and reflects pressures in the pulmonary capillary bed and left-sided heart function. When the balloon is inflated, it occludes the pressure produced by the right side of the heart; therefore it should never be left inflated for more than a few seconds in order to prevent damage to the pulmonary circulation. The nurse usually obtains measurements of the PCWP every 2 to 4 hours; however, readings should be obtained more frequently if the patient's condition is unstable.

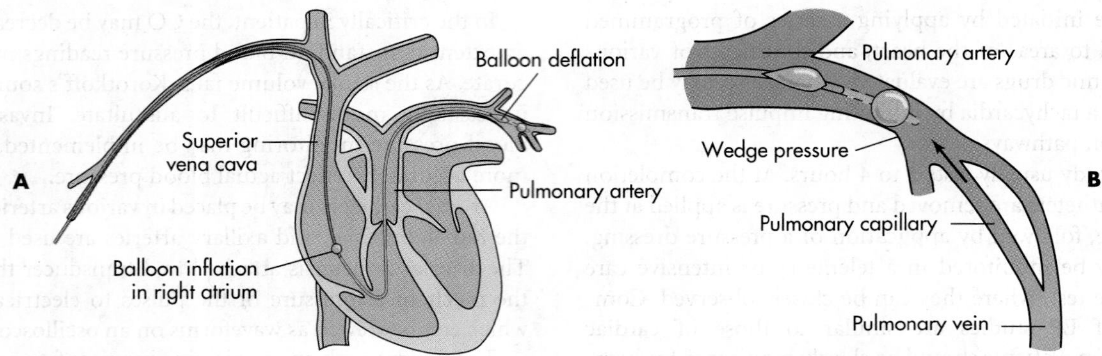


**fig. 24-29** **A,** Flow-directed, balloon-tipped catheter showing inflation of balloon in right atrium and consequent "floating" of catheter through the right ventricle and out to distal pulmonary artery branch. Balloon is deflated, advanced slightly, and reinflated slightly to obtain pulmonary capillary wedge pressure (PCWP). **B,** During the initial positioning of the balloon-tipped catheter in pulmonary artery, balloon is deflated. Catheter is then advanced and balloon is reinflated just long enough to obtain PCWP.

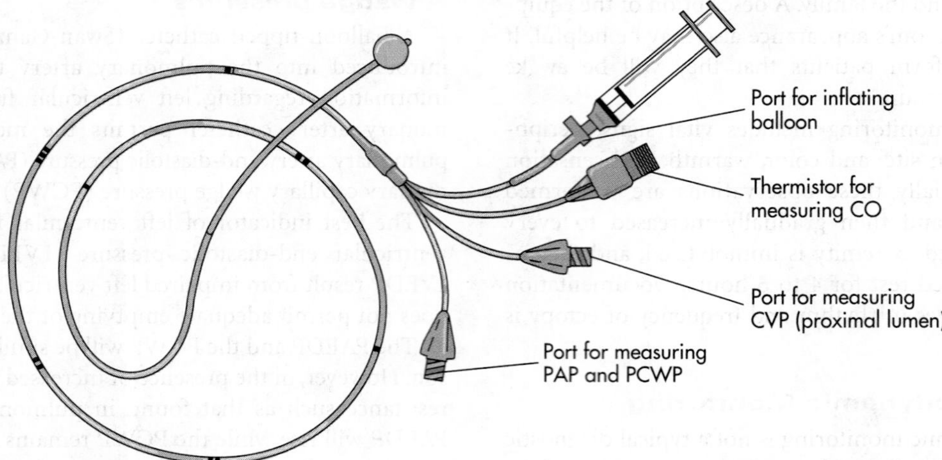


**fig. 24-30** Four-lumen thermodilution pulmonary artery catheter for measuring cardiac output *(CO),* central venous pressure *(CVP),* pulmonary artery pressure *(PAP),* and pulmonary capillary wedge pressure *(PCWP).*

Various types of pulmonary artery catheters may be used that allow measurement of additional hemodynamic parameters. Some catheters have a third lumen that contains a thermistor that is used to determine cardiac output by the thermodilution technique. A fourth lumen that ends at the level of the right atrium can be used to monitor CVP and to obtain blood samples. A four-lumen thermodilution catheter is illustrated in Figure 24-30.

## VASCULAR DIAGNOSTIC STUDIES

Both noninvasive and invasive vascular diagnostic studies are conducted to evaluate vascular blood flow throughout the body. Most vascular studies require active pretest or posttest interventions by the nurse. Others simply require an adequate explanation of the procedure.

### Noninvasive Tests

#### Ankle-brachial index

Ankle-brachial index is the most commonly used parameter for overall evaluation of arterial vascular status in the lower extremity. Blood pressure measurements are obtained over both the dorsalis pedis and posterior tibial arteries using a regular blood pressure cuff. The Doppler probe is placed over the pulse and the cuff is inflated to above systolic pressure. The point at which the pulse returns after cuff deflation is documented as the systolic endpoint number. Typically, the higher of the two pressures is used as the indication of vascular status. This number is divided into the higher of two brachial artery pressures. (For example, an ankle pressure of 70 mm Hg with a brachial pressure of 140 mm Hg gives an index of 0.5.) Normal foot arteries have an index of 1.0 to 1.2. Indexes below 1.0 indicate arterial obstruction.[9]

#### Impedance plethysmography

Venous outflow in the lower extremities is measured by inflation and deflation of pneumatic cuffs around the thighs. The assumption is that because blood is a good conductor of electricity, the electrical resistance will change as blood volume is altered. Electrodes are attached to obtain measurements and determine quality of blood flow. Sharp rises in venous volume suggest venous occlusion, such as blood clots. If a DVT is present in a major vessel, the increase in blood volume during the test is less than expected because the veins are already full. During the procedure, the patient is supine with the leg elevated and knee flexed.

#### Doppler ultrasound

Doppler ultrasound, or ultrasound imaging, aids in the diagnosis of carotid artery disease, peripheral artery disease, venous occlusive disease, valvular insufficiency, and deep vein thrombosis.[10] Ultrasonic waves directed at an artery or vein reflect off red blood cells, producing a waveform or audible sound. Arterial waveforms should be pronounced, with peaks and valleys reflective of the systolic and diastolic pressures; a flattened waveform indicates obstruction. Venous waveforms are in phase with respirations and are of continuous amplitude.

#### Exercise testing

The treadmill test is used to obtain an objective measurement of the severity of intermittent claudication. This test is similar to the test used for coronary patients, except the walking speed is usually 1.5 to 2 miles per hour with a grade elevation of 10% to 20% and a time limit of 5 minutes. Walking times of 5 minutes suggest mild disease, and 1 minute indicates severe disease. Patients should wear loose-fitting clothing and good walking shoes. The exercise will be stopped at the maximal level of exertion or when symptoms become disabling.

#### Magnetic resonance imaging

Magnetic resonance imaging (MRI) capabilities include evaluation of the vascular network, measurement of blood flow velocities, and assessment of stages of vascular disease. Radiofrequency pulses excite the protons, which give a signal creating a three-dimensional image of the vessels. This test does not require ionizing radiation or any injections into the vascular system; therefore it may be preferred to arteriography. However, MRI is expensive and time consuming, which makes it a less likely choice for routine screening and follow-up. The patient should be informed that the noise level during the test may be high and require use of earplugs. Additionally, the confinement to a relatively small area of space is sometimes problematic for patients who have a tendency toward claustrophobia.

### Invasive Tests

#### Contrast angiography and venography

Contrast angiography, or arteriography, is a standard in vascular diagnostic imaging. It is the most invasive test used in evaluation of peripheral disease and has the greatest risk for the patient. Angiography assists in the diagnosis of arterial emboli, arterial trauma, aneurysm, Buerger's disease, and reevaluation of the patency of arteries following grafting. The procedure involves insertion of a radiopaque catheter into the vessel under local anesthesia followed by injection of a contrast medium. X-ray films are obtained that visualize the arterial system.

Venography is performed in a similar manner except that the venous system is examined. It is the definitive test in the diagnosis of deep vein thrombosis; another common use of this test is with patients suspected of having incompetent vein valves. The test takes about an hour and is uncomfortable for the patient.

The procedure and nursing interventions are similar to a cardiac catheterization, but the peripheral system is being examined instead of the coronary vessels (see discussion on p. 631-632). The patient must be assessed for allergies to contrast media before the procedure. Informed consent is obtained, and the patient is told that it is common to experience a flushing or burning sensation after injection of the contrast medium. There is disagreement regarding the need to abstain from food and fluids before the test; some physicians prefer patients to have nothing by mouth for 6 to 8 hours before hand, but others recommend a clear liquid diet to prevent possible dehydration and concomitant hemoconcentration.

A pressure dressing may or may not be placed at the insertion site after the procedure. However, the extremity must be kept straight while the site is closely monitored for hemorrhage, hematoma, and inflammation. Postprocedure protocols vary, but vital signs, distal pulses, skin temperature, and the insertion site are usually monitored every 15 minutes for the first hour, every 30 minutes for the second hour, and hourly for the remaining time. Assessment of motor and sensory function is important. Mild analgesics may be administered for pain at the insertion site. The physician is notified if the patient experiences severe pain.

Potential complications include an allergic reaction to the contrast medium, thrombi, perforation of the vessel, emboli, renal failure, and pseudoaneurysms. Creatinine levels should be monitored to evaluate renal function.

### Digital subtraction angiography

Digital subtraction angiography, or digital vascular imaging, is a computerized fluoroscopic procedure that visualizes the vascular system. It is less expensive and quicker than angiography. Again, contrast medium is injected through a catheter and x-ray films are taken under local anesthesia. A state-of-the-art video system displays the vessels on a television monitor while a computer subtracts images that are not necessary. Separate injections are required for different views of the limb. Patients must be assessed for allergies to contrast media before the procedure. Posttest nursing care is similar to that provided after arteriography.

## chapter SUMMARY

### ANATOMY AND PHYSIOLOGY

- The heart consists of four chambers. The two upper chambers, called atria, are thin-walled reservoirs for holding blood. The two lower chambers are called ventricles and are thick-walled, muscular pumping chambers.
- Electrophysiological properties of the heart include automaticity, excitability, conductivity, and contractility.
- The action potential has two components: depolarization and repolarization. The main ions involved in this process are sodium, potassium, and calcium.
- Phases of the cardiac cycle include diastole (isovolumetric relaxation, rapid and slow ventricular filling, atrial systole) and systole (isovolumetric contraction, maximal and reduced ventricular ejection).
- Determinants of stroke volume include preload, afterload, contractility, and heart rate.

### ASSESSMENT

- Subjective data for cardiovascular assessment includes the presence of dyspnea, chest pain, leg pain, syncope, palpitations, and fatigue.
- Objective data collection is accomplished by a systematic and organized process using the steps of inspection, palpation, percussion, and auscultation.
- Diagnostic tests used to assess cardiovascular functioning include laboratory tests, radiological tests, electrocardiography, sonic studies, dynamic studies, scintigraphic studies, cardiac catheterization, electrophysiological studies, and invasive hemodynamic monitoring.
- Vascular diagnostic studies include both noninvasive tests, such as ankle-brachial index, impedence plethysmography, Doppler ultrasound, exercise testing, and magnetic resonance imaging, and invasive tests, such as contrast angiography, venography, and digital subtraction angiography.

## References


1. American Heart Association: *Heart and stroke facts, 1995 statistical supplement,* Dallas, 1994, The Association.
2. Barker LR et al: *Principles of ambulatory medicine,* ed 4, Baltimore, 1995, Williams & Wilkins.
3. Bogart MA: Time to hemostasis: a comparison of manual vs. mechanical compression of the femoral artery, *Am J Crit Care* 4(2):149, 1995.
4. Cooley DA: *Texas Heart Institute heart owner's handbook,* New York, 1996, Wiley.
5. Darovic GO: *Hemodynamic monitoring: invasive and noninvasive clinical applications,* ed 2, Philadelphia, 1993, WB Saunders.
6. Keeling A et al: Reducing time in bed after cardiac catheterization, *Am J Crit Care* 4(2):277, 1996.
7. Moser DK: Correcting misconceptions about women and heart disease, *Am J Nurs* 97(4):26, 1997.
8. Selig PM: Management of anticoagulation therapy with the international normalized ratio, *J Am Acad Nurse Pract* 8(2):77, 1996.
9. Sieggreen M: Limb and life: principles of leg ulcer management, *Advance for Nurse Practitioners* 5(3):16, 1997.
10. Thibodeau GA, Patton KT: *Anatomy and physiology,* ed 3, St Louis, 1996, Mosby.
11. US Department of Health and Human Services, Public Health Service: *Healthy people 2000: national health promotion and disease prevention objectives,* Washington, DC, 1990, US Government Printing Office.
12. Verderber A et al: Preparation for cardiac catheterization, *J Cardiovasc Nurs* 7(1):75, 1992.

chapter 25

# MANAGEMENT OF PERSONS WITH Coronary Artery Disease and Dysrhythmias

KATHY HENLEY HAUGH and ARLENE KEELING

## objectives

*After studying this chapter, the learner should be able to:*

1 Discuss the role of risk factors in the pathogenesis of coronary artery disease.
2 Recognize the signs and symptoms of coronary artery disease.
3 Explain the collaborative management of angina pectoris, unstable angina, and myocardial infarction.
4 Discuss the nursing role in the care of the patient with coronary artery disease.
5 Recognize common dysrhythmias associated with the cardiac conduction system.
6 Discuss the collaborative care management of patients with cardiac dysrhythmias.
7 Describe the basic components of cardiopulmonary resuscitation.

Patients with coronary artery disease (CAD) often seek health care after experiencing angina or myocardial infarction (MI). Coronary artery disease is directly implicated in other cardiovascular diagnoses such as dysrhythmias, heart failure, and cardiomyopathy. All nurses need to be familiar with the collaborative care management of CAD because of its high prevalence in the industrialized world. This chapter discusses the origins and management of CAD and its progression along the continuum of angina, unstable angina, and MI. It also discusses the recognition and management of common dysrhythmias.

## CORONARY ARTERY DISEASE

### ETIOLOGY

Coronary artery disease is a generic designation for many different conditions that involve obstructed blood flow through the coronary arteries. The two most prevalent etiologies of CAD are atherosclerosis and coronary vasospasm. Atherosclerosis is by far the most common etiology and is the focus of the presentation. A discussion of the unusual nonatherosclerotic forms of CAD is beyond the scope of this chapter.

### EPIDEMIOLOGY

Coronary atherosclerosis is the leading cause of death in the industrialized Western world. Approximately 700,000 persons are hospitalized with the diagnosis of acute MI each year in the United States, and about 400,000 Americans die from CAD or its complications annually.[15] Coronary artery disease remains the number one health problem in the United States today. Some populations have an increased occurrence of CAD because of definable characteristics or risks.

The incidence of CAD varies according to concurrent disease states and behaviors that increase an individual's risk for CAD. Risk factors are classically categorized as noncontrollable and controllable or manageable. Uncontrollable risk factors include age, gender, race, and family history. Controllable risk factors include diabetes, hypertension, the use of tobacco, sedentary lifestyle, obesity, and how a person manages stress. (See the Risk Factors Box.) Table 25-1 links the major risk factors for CAD with their specific physiological effects.

#### Age and Gender

Clinical evidence of CAD rarely occurs before the second and third decades of life. For men, CAD is a leading cause of mortality as early as 35 to 45 years of age. The incidence of death can be as high as 40% for men between the ages of 55 and 64. In women, the incidence of CAD greatly increases after menopause, when the beneficial effects of estrogen in preventing atheroma formation are no longer available. One in three women over age 64 has some form of CAD.[1] The mortality rate from CAD is 11% higher for women than men after the age of 65.[19] Coronary artery disease is the leading cause of death in women, exceeding that of cancer. With increasing longevity in the Western world, the incidence of CAD among both male and female octogenarians and nonagenarians also will increase.

#### Race

Coronary artery disease is nondiscriminatory, affecting all races. The independent role of race as a variable in CAD is unclear. The relationship of race and CAD may be attributed to other risk factors such as hypertension and obesity. Lifestyle, including cultural practices, ethnic traditions, and individual choices, may play the more significant role in the development of CAD.

#### Family History/Heredity

The likelihood that an offspring will have CAD increases if the biological parent manifests CAD before the age of 55. Again, it is difficult to determine the independent role of genetics in the pathogenesis of CAD. Contributing variables include the

**risk factors**

**Coronary Artery Disease**

- Age and gender
- Family history
- Diabetes
- Hypertension
- Tobacco use
- Sedentary lifestyle
- Diet
- How one manages stress

extent to which environmental factors and individual lifestyle choices influence the development of CAD. However, individuals with familial hyperlipidemias have a high rate of CAD.

### Diabetes

The incidence of CAD in individuals with diabetes mellitus is two to three times higher than in nondiabetic individuals.[7] In patients with diabetes, elevated levels of circulating insulin may begin the process of atheroma formation by initiating damage to the arterial intima. Insulin also affects fat metabolism, contributing to lipid deposition in the coronary artery. Control of diabetes with medication and diet can blunt the severity of CAD should it occur.

### Hypertension

Hypertension, defined as a measured elevation in blood pressure above 140/90 on at least three occasions, increases the incidence of CAD twofold to threefold. Hypertension affects the ability of the blood vessel to constrict and dilate. In addition, shearing forces on the intimal lining from hypertension predispose the artery to atherosclerosis.[16] Control of hypertension with medication, diet, or exercise may decrease the incidence of CAD in the hypertensive population.

### Tobacco

The risk of death from CAD is significantly higher in smokers than in nonsmokers, and the risk is proportional to the amount of tobacco used. Cigarette smokers have the highest incidence of CAD; however, pipe and cigar smokers, as well as tobacco chewers, have an increased risk of developing CAD compared with nonusers. The unifying factor promoting CAD in this population is nicotine.

### Sedentary Lifestyle

In 1996, the Surgeon General released a report on physical activity and health. This report noted the incidence of CAD to be higher for individuals who do not participate in regular physical activity compared with those who exercise. Sixty percent of U.S. adults report no pattern of regular activity. (See Chapter 3.) The Surgeon General's report concludes that regular physical activity decreases the risk of coronary heart disease.[24]

### Diet

Research findings consistently report an association between CAD and the dietary intake of cholesterol and fats. Recent findings report that elevated plasma lipoprotein (a) is an independent risk factor for the development of premature CAD in men.[4] An increased nonfasting triglyceride level is also a strong and independent predictor of future risk of MI, especially in combination with a high total cholesterol level.[22] Hyperlipidemia may be either primary (familial) or secondary to some other process.

### Obesity

Although obesity is commonly cited as a significant coronary risk factor, the extent to which it has an independent effect in predisposing a person to CAD is controversial. Obese persons are more prone to diabetes, hypertension, and hyperlipidemias. In addition, obese individuals often demonstrate other behaviors, such as sedentary lifestyles, that are known risk factors for CAD. These known CAD risk factors may be the link between obesity and CAD.

### Stress

Previously, much discussion existed in the literature about the relationship between stress and CAD. It was generally agreed that individuals with type A behavior, described in terms of competitiveness, aggression, hostility, and time urgency, had a higher incidence of CAD than individuals who were more re-

**table 25-1** *Role of Risk Factors in Coronary Artery Disease*

| Risk Factor | Physiological Effect |
|---|---|
| Age and gender | Decrease in elasticity of arteries with age<br>Estrogen in females lowers serum cholesterol |
| Heredity: family history of CAD | Undetermined |
| Diabetes | Damage to intima<br>Insulin modifies lipid metabolism |
| Hypertension | Decreased elasticity of blood vessels<br>Tearing effect on arteries<br>Increased resistance to ejection of ventricular volume |
| Tobacco use (nicotine) | Decreased high-density lipoproteins (HDLs)<br>Displacement of oxygen from hemoglobin<br>Increased catecholamines in response to nicotine, increasing heart rate and blood pressure<br>Increases platelet adhesiveness<br>Accelerates atheroma formation<br>Coronary spasm |
| Sedentary lifestyle | Alters lipid metabolism<br>Decrease in HDLs |
| Diet (hypercholesterolemia, familial hyperlipidemia) | Provide more substrate for lesion formation<br>Increase levels of low-density lipoproteins, increasing atherogenesis |

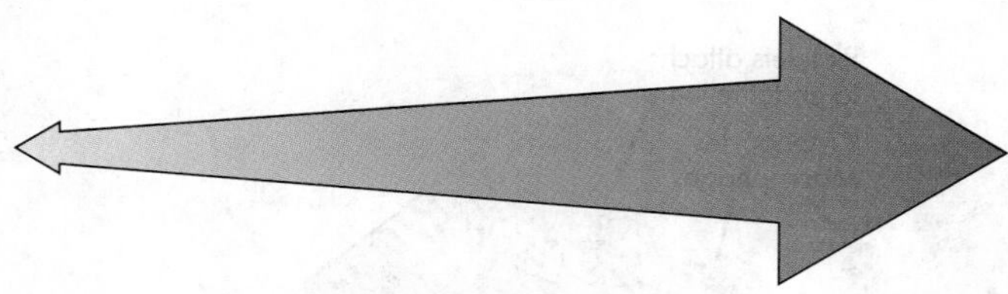


**fig. 25-1** The continuum of CAD. Large arrow depicts the increased severity of the continuum to the right.

laxed, or type B. Today, many professionals question this relationship between personality type and CAD.

Catecholamines, released during the stress response, increase platelet aggregation and may also precipitate vasospasm. However, a complete understanding of the effects of stress on circulation, lipid metabolism, and coagulability requires additional research.

## PATHOPHYSIOLOGY

Coronary artery disease refers to the development and progression of plaque accumulation in the coronary arteries. The continuum in Figure 25-1 illustrates the dynamic nature of CAD. The three stages along the continuum are stable angina, unstable angina, and MI. A patient with CAD may seek treatment at any point along this continuum. After resolution of the initial problem, the patient may move to another point on the continuum. The following sections discuss the pathophysiological evolution of stable angina, unstable angina, and MI.

### Stable Angina

The coronary arteries are small arteries that constrict and dilate on a surface that is constantly moving, the beating heart. (See Figure 24-3 in Chapter 24.) The arteries lie on the epicardial surface and branch often. The small arterial size, constant tension on the arteries, and turbulence created at bifurcations promote the development of atherosclerotic lesions.

Normally, the endothelium of the coronary artery allows for unrestricted blood flow to the myocardium. Any kind of trauma or irritant can disrupt this protective endothelium. The body's response to the injury is a complex interplay of chemical mediators designed to protect the area. Endothelial injury causes the release of thromboxane, which minimizes the extent of injury through local vasoconstriction and by stimulating platelet aggregation (Figure 25-2). The intima releases prostacyclin in response to the effects of thromboxane. Prostacyclin works to restore equilibrium through local vasodilation and by opposing platelet aggregation. With repeated injury, the deteriorated intima cannot produce enough prostacyclin, and platelet aggregation forces predominate.

Platelets and accumulating monocytes release powerful growth factors into the arterial wall. These factors stimulate the proliferation and migration of medial smooth muscle cells into the intima. This structural change causes an increased permeability of the vessel wall to cholesterol. The accumulation of cholesterol produces a fatty streak that protrudes into the lumen of the artery. Smooth muscle cells and fibrous tissue form a fibrous cap over the fatty streak.

The fatty streak continues to grow, invading both the intima and media. Involvement of the media affects the ability of the vessel wall to vasodilate and vasoconstrict. The artery may continue to maintain the supply of oxygen and nutrients to the myocardium as long as the blockage is less than 70% of the arterial lumen. Concomitant conditions such as anemia, smoking (carbon monoxide displaces oxygen in the bloodstream), and hypovolemia further compromise the delivery of oxygen to the myocardium.

The presence of risk factors accelerates atherogenesis, thereby decreasing oxygen supply. Risk factors can also increase the myocardium's demand for oxygen. (See Table 25-1.)

The demand of the myocardium for oxygen can be met only by an adequate blood supply. As long as supply is greater than or equal to demand, aerobic metabolism occurs. When demand is greater than supply, the myocardium must switch to anaerobic metabolism for nourishment. Anaerobic metabolism produces lactic acid, which is believed to be responsible for ischemic anginal pain. This pain is the most common initial symptom of CAD. With stable angina, the patient usually experiences a known threshold beyond which myocardial oxygen demand exceeds supply. Myocardial oxygen demand increases with any condition causing an increase in heart rate, an increase in resistance to ejecting blood volume, and an increase in myocardial size.

### Unstable Angina

Atherosclerosis may remain stable if the blockage in the coronary artery does not progress beyond 70%, if collateral (alternate) vessels develop to maintain nourishment to the myocardium, and if the fibrous cap remains intact. However, pressure within the lesion (plaque) can increase to the point of plaque rupture. Rupture of the fibrous cap exposes the inner plaque to the circulating blood. In an effort to heal, collagen accumulates, smooth muscle cells proliferate, and clotting factors are activated. (See Figure 25-2.) Aggregating platelets activate the coagulation system immediately to seal the rupture (Figure 25-3). With plaque disruption, stable angina becomes unstable. In 1991 alone, 570,000 hospitalizations for unstable angina resulted in 3.1 million hospital days.[5]

Risk factors contribute to this pathophysiology. Nicotine from tobacco use increases platelet adhesion and increases the potential for clotting at the site of disruption. Catecholamines released during the stress response also increase platelet aggregation.

Several scenarios can occur after plaque rupture (Figure 25-4, *A* and *B*). The area can heal over with the platelet plug absorbed into the plaque under a new cap. The larger plaque creates a smaller lumen. The second scenario shows a

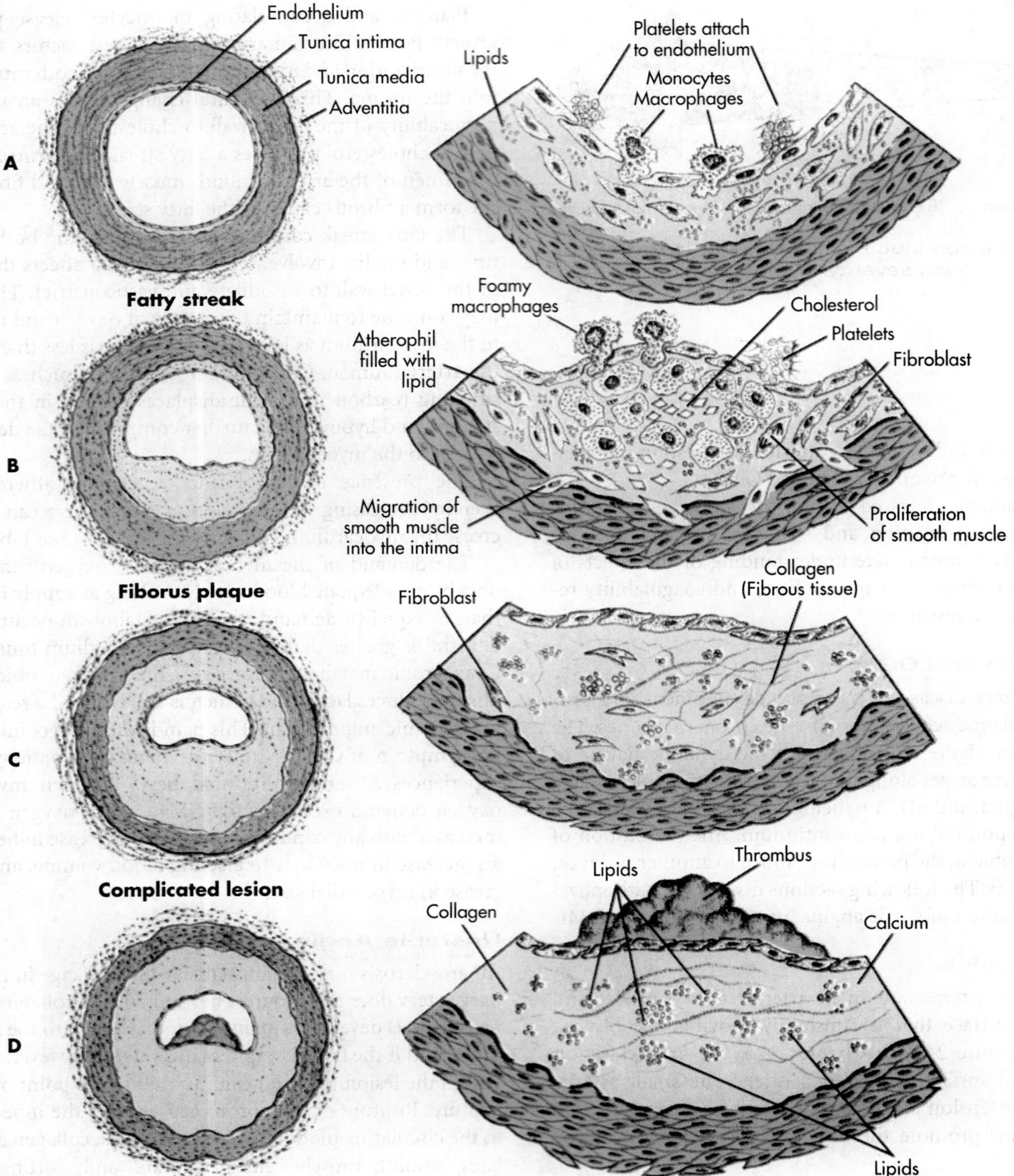


**fig. 25-2** Progression of atherosclerosis. **A**, Thromboxane stimulates platelet aggregation. **B**, Medial smooth muscle migrates into the intima, increasing permeability of the wall to cholesterol. **C**, Fibrous cap seals plaque. **D**, Rupture of the plaque stimulates thrombus formation.

residual fibrous clot extending into the lumen, partially obstructing the artery.

## Myocardial Infarction

A third scenario that can occur is complete obstruction of the coronary artery with the fibrous clot. This is termed *coronary thrombosis* or *coronary occlusion* (Figure 25-4, *C*). Coronary occlusion creates a rapid series of physiological events. The first of these events is immediate myocardial ischemia distal to the occlusion. Ischemia alters the integrity and the permeability of the myocardial cell membrane to vital electrolytes. This instability depresses myocardial contractility and predisposes the patient to sudden death from dysrhythmias (see complications section). Figure 25-5 illustrates the spiraling series of

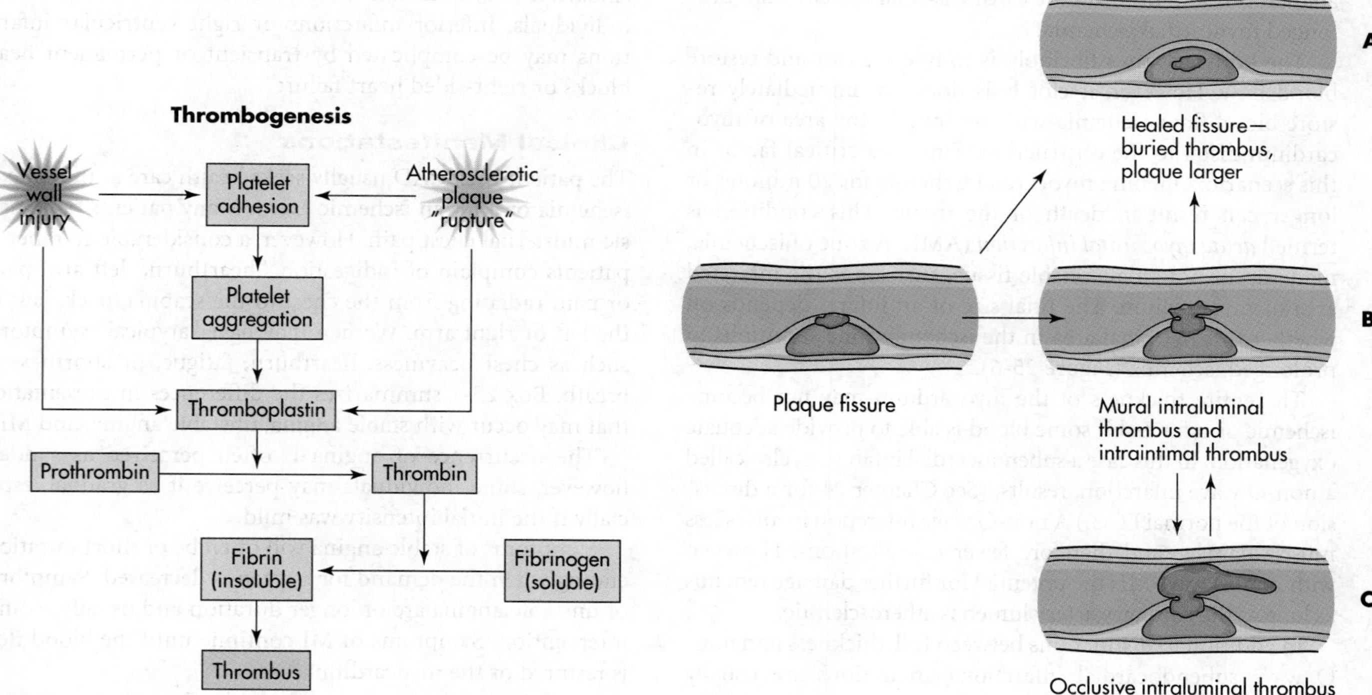


**fig. 25-3** The process of thrombogenesis.

**fig. 25-4** Possible pathophysiological scenarios following plaque fissure. **A**, Clot is resorbed into plaque, healing over area of fissure, but with a smaller lumen resulting. **B**, Clot remains at site of fissure, decreasing lumen diameter. **C**, Clot extends into lumen, completely obstructing lumen (myocardial infarction).

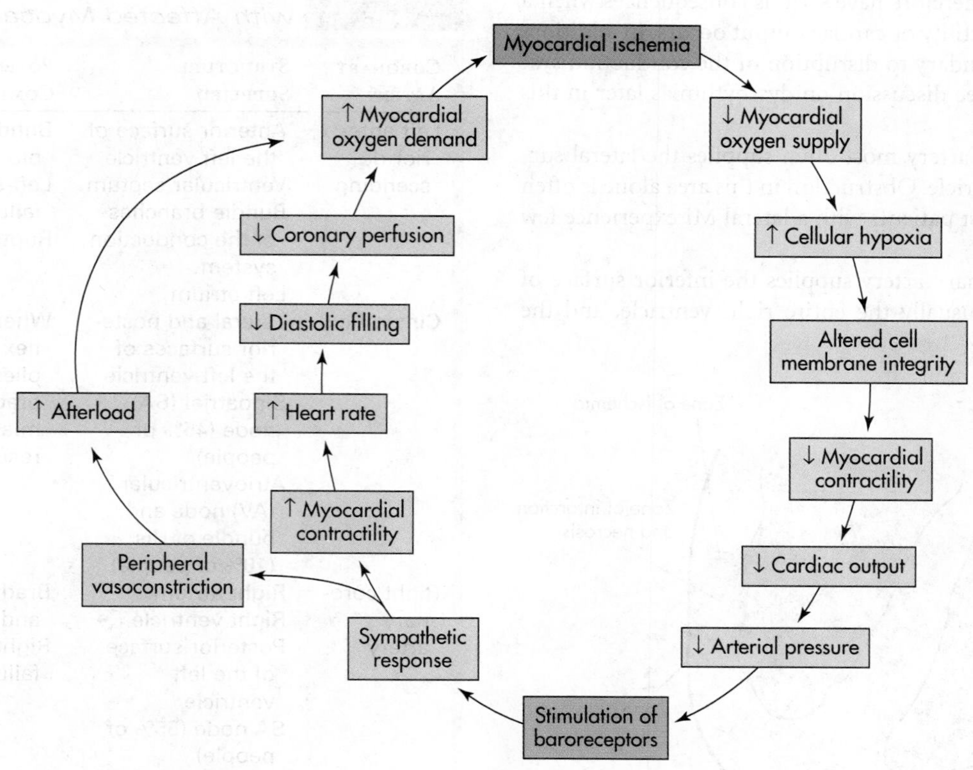


**fig. 25-5** Effects of prolonged myocardial ischemia.

adaptations that occur in the cardiovascular system from prolonged myocardial ischemia.

The body activates fibrinolysis to lyse the clot and restore blood flow. However, if clot lysis does not immediately restore blood flow, ischemia will continue in the area of myocardium distal to the obstruction. Time is a critical factor in this scenario. Ongoing myocardial ischemia for 20 minutes or longer can result in death of the tissue. This condition is termed *acute myocardial infarction* (AMI). A zone of ischemia, made up of potentially viable tissue, surrounds the infarcted area of myocardium. The final size of an infarct depends on whether this marginal area in the ischemic zone succumbs to prolonged ischemia (Figure 25-6).

The entire thickness of the myocardium may not become ischemic or infarcted if some blood is able to provide adequate oxygenation. In this case a subendocardial infarction, also called a non-Q wave infarction, results. (See Chapter 24 for a discussion of the normal ECG.) A non-Q wave infarction involves less muscle damage and therefore fewer complications. However, with non-Q wave MIs the potential for further damage remains as long as the coronary artery lumen is atherosclerotic.

In addition to distinctions between full-thickness and non-Q wave subendocardial infarctions, infarctions are usually classified according to anatomical location (Table 25-2). The left anterior descending (LAD) artery supplies the anterior surface of the left ventricle and the bundle branches of the conduction system. This area of the heart is responsible for most of the contractility generated to eject blood systemically. It requires a substantial source of oxygen to generate the force needed to pump against the aorta's high-pressure system. Lesions in the LAD therefore have serious consequences when a decrease in contractility or cardiac output occurs. In addition, sudden death secondary to disruption of the conduction system may occur. (See discussion on dysrhythmias later in this chapter.)

The circumflex artery most often supplies the lateral surface of the left ventricle. Obstruction in this area alone is often well tolerated. Most patients with a lateral MI experience few complications.

The right coronary artery supplies the inferior surface of the left ventricle, usually the entire right ventricle, and the sinoatrial (SA) node and atrioventricular (AV) node in most individuals. Inferior infarctions or right ventricular infarctions may be complicated by transient or permanent heart blocks or right-sided heart failure.

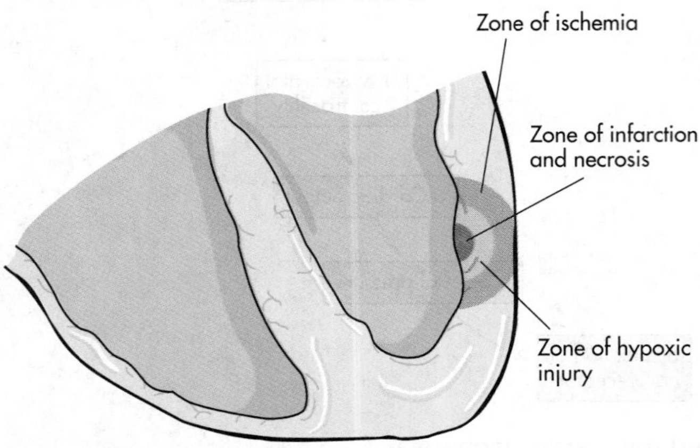


**fig. 25-6** Zones of myocardial ischemia and infarction.

## Clinical Manifestations

The patient with CAD usually seeks health care at the time of ischemia or after an ischemic event. Many patients have classic midsternal chest pain. However, a considerable number of patients complain of indigestion, "heartburn," left arm pain, or pain radiating from the chest to the scapula, neck, jaw, or the left or right arm. Women may have "atypical" symptoms such as chest heaviness, heartburn, fatigue, or shortness of breath. Box 25-1 summarizes the differences in presentation that may occur with stable angina, unstable angina, and MI.

The occurrence of angina is often perceived as sudden; however, some individuals may perceive it as gradual, especially if the initial intensity was mild.

Symptoms of stable angina will often be of short duration, ending when the demand for oxygen is decreased. Symptoms of unstable angina are of longer duration and usually require intervention. Symptoms of MI continue until the blood flow is restored or the myocardium dies.

Precipitating factors for stable angina include any circumstance that increases myocardial oxygen demand, such as exercise, stress, sexual intercourse, and smoking. Precipitating factors for unstable angina and MI can include similar activities, or there may not be an identifiable precipitating event.

**table 25-2** *Correlation of Coronary Artery with Affected Myocardium*

| Coronary Artery | Structure Supplied | Potential Complications |
|---|---|---|
| Left anterior descending | Anterior surface of the left ventricle<br>Ventricular septum<br>Bundle branches of the conduction system<br>Left atrium | Bundle branch blocks<br>Left-sided heart failure<br>Rupture of septum |
| Circumflex | Lateral and posterior surfaces of the left ventricle<br>Sinoatrial (SA) node (45% of people)<br>Atrioventricular (AV) node and bundle of His (10% of people) | When the circumflex artery supplies the SA node, bradydysrhythmias may result |
| Right coronary artery | Right atrium<br>Right ventricle<br>Posterior surface of the left ventricle<br>SA node (55% of people)<br>AV node (90% of people) | Bradydysrhythmias and heart blocks<br>Right-sided heart failure |

The onset of unstable angina and MI often occurs at rest or on awakening when platelets are stimulated.

The classic location of ischemic pain is retrosternal. The pain may radiate down the left arm or both arms, upward to the neck or jaws, or backward to the scapular region. Some patients will not experience pain. This is especially true for elderly patients or patients with diabetes due to alterations in sensory perception. Therefore the quality and intensity of pain may be unreliable indicators of the severity of ischemia. For example, some patients with MI describe the pain as "mild indigestion" or "tightness" while others describe the pain as excruciating and viselike.

In addition to chest pain, patients may complain of dizziness, dyspnea, nausea, vomiting, or anxiety. Patients experiencing an acute MI often report a feeling of doom or feeling as though they are "going to die."

Changes in vital signs may include tachycardia or bradycardia, increased or decreased blood pressure, and shortness of breath. Dysrhythmias may develop from myocardial ischemia. Decreased cardiac output can result in classic "shocky" symptoms such as pale, cool, diaphoretic skin.

## COLLABORATIVE CARE MANAGEMENT

### Diagnostic Tests

When a patient has signs or symptoms of CAD, diagnostic tests help determine whether the patient has stable angina, unstable angina, or MI. (See Figure 25-1.) If MI is ruled out by diagnostic tests, the patient's history often distinguishes between the diagnoses of stable or unstable angina.

**box 25-1** ***clinical manifestations***

***Coronary Artery Disease***

The following may occur with stable angina, unstable angina, or acute myocardial infarction:
- Chest pain or anginal equivalent (jaw pain, left arm pain)
- Nonverbal indicators of pain: clutch, rub, stroke the chest
- Increase or decrease in heart rate
- Dysrhythmias
- Increase or decrease in blood pressure

The following is unique to stable angina:
- Angina that occurs with predictable level of exertion

The following are unique to unstable angina:
- Angina not necessarily associated with activity
- ECG: ST depression

The following are unique to myocardial infarction:
- Angina not relieved by rest or nitroglycerin therapy
- Associated symptoms: dizziness, dyspnea, nausea, vomiting, feeling of impending doom
- Altered neurological status, if decreased cardiac output
- Rales, if decreased contractility creates left ventricular function
- Presence of $S_3$ or $S_4$ gallop
- Diminished pulses
- Pallor
- ECG: ST elevation, Q waves, T wave abnormalities
- Labs: elevated CK-MB, elevated troponin I, elevated glucose, leukocytosis, elevated erythrocyte sedimentation rate

### *Electrocardiography*

The electrocardiogram (ECG) remains a critical tool in diagnosing CAD, but it is most useful when the patient is symptomatic. The ECG interpretation for ischemia focuses on the ST segment of the ECG.

ST segment elevation is the hallmark of acute myocardial ischemia leading to infarction (Figure 25-7). ST elevation resolves with restoration of blood flow or completion of the MI. If the full thickness of the myocardium becomes necrotic, significant Q waves evolve over the next week. Future ECGs will continue to show the significant Q wave, indicating that the patient suffered an MI in the past. When only the subendocardial surface infarcts, Q waves do not develop. A subendocardial infarct is referred to as a non-Q wave MI. T wave abnormalities occur at the time of acute infarction as well. ST depression on the ECG represents ischemia and resolves with improved perfusion.

The 12-lead ECG represents 12 different anatomical views of the myocardium. (See Chapter 24.) ST changes occur in leads specific to the area of myocardium involved. Table 25-3 shows the correlation of leads to the affected area of myocardium. The 12-lead ECG remains one of the most important diagnostic tools in the assessment of chest pain.

#### *Blood tests*

When the patient has unrelenting angina, cardiac isoenzymes are obtained immediately. Injured myocardial cells release the enzyme creatine kinase (CK) during AMI. The CK elevation begins within 4 to 8 hours after an AMI, peaks in 12 to 18 hours, and returns to normal in 3 to 4 days (Table 25-4). Brain tissue and skeletal muscle also release CK with injury. The isoenzyme CK-MB is specific to the myocardium rather than skeletal muscle or brain tissue and is the fraction currently tested.

Another laboratory test for MI is serum troponin (comprised of three proteins: cardiac troponin, troponin I, and troponin T).[12] Cardiac troponin I, a relatively new marker of AMI, was approved by the Food and Drug Administration (FDA) in 1995 and has a high specificity for myocardial injury. Cardiac troponin I rises earlier than CK-MB (within 3 hours) and persists over time (up to 7 days). An elevated cardiac troponin I on admission in a patient with chest pain has been associated with an increase in complications and mortality. Because the serum troponin level in normal individuals is usually undetectable, any elevation of this protein, measured by troponin T or troponin I, indicates myocardial cell damage. Both troponin T and troponin I levels increase in patients with unstable angina. The normal serum level of troponin T is 0.0 to 0.1 ng/ml. The normal range of troponin I is 0.0 to 3.1 ng/ml. Before the use of troponin measurement, lactic dehydrogenase (LDH) was often used as an indicator of late myocardial cell death. Level of LDH rises within 8 to 12 hours after the infarction and persists for 8 to 14 days.

Measurements of serum myoglobin, an oxygen-binding protein found in cardiac and skeletal muscle, may also indicate myocardial cell death. Myoglobin levels increase within 1 hour after MI, reach peak levels in 4 to 6 hours, and return

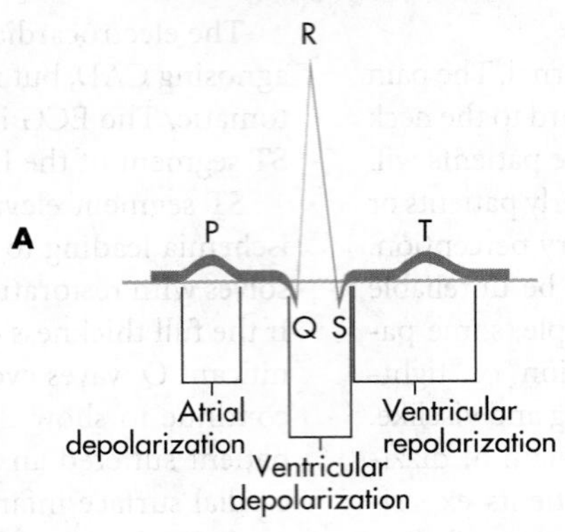


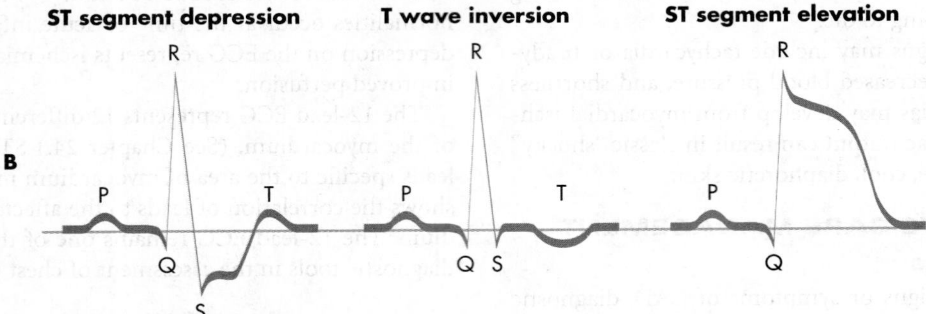


**fig. 25-7** ECG and ischemia. **A**, Normal ECG. **B**, Electrocardiographic alterations associated with ischemia.

**table 25-3** *Correlation of ECG Findings with Cardiac Anatomy*

| Acute Changes in Leads | Anatomical Location of Infarct |
|---|---|
| 2, 3, avF | Inferior |
| 1, avL | Lateral |
| $V_1$-$V_3$ | Anteroseptal |
| $V_4$-$V_6$ | Anterolateral |
| Tall R waves in $V_1$, $V_2$ | Posterior |
| $V_4R$, $V_5R$, $V_6R$ (right precordial lead placement) | Right ventricular |

**table 25-4** *Cardiac Enzyme Serum Levels in Acute Myocardial Infarction*

| Cardiac Enzyme | Elevation (hours) | Peak Elevation (hours) | Duration (days) |
|---|---|---|---|
| Creatinine kinase (CK) | 4-8 | 12-24 | 3-4 |
| Creatinine kinase MB (CK-MB) | 4-8 | 8-16 | 2-3 |
| Troponin T | 3.5 | 2-5 | 7 |
| Troponin I | 4-6 | 2-5 | 7 |
| Lactate dehydrogenase (LDH and $LDH_1$) | 8-12 | 72-144 (3-6 days) | 8-14 |
| Myoglobin | 1 | 4-6 | 1-2 |

to normal within 24 to 36 hours. In some patients, normalization may occur even faster.

Blood chemistry tests and a complete blood count (CBC) are done to determine concurrent disease states and help with differential diagnosis. Patients with AMI may have elevated blood glucose levels secondary to the stress response. The white blood cell (WBC) count may also increase (leukocytosis). Leukocytosis begins within a few hours after the onset of symptoms as an inflammatory response to the injured cardiac tissue. The WBC count can reach 12,000 to 15,000/mm$^3$ and last for approximately 3 to 7 days. The erythrocyte sedimentation rate (ESR) also rises during the first week after infarction and remains elevated for several weeks. Cholesterol levels decrease secondary to altered metabolism during the stress response. Therefore cholesterol screening tests for risk factor modification are deferred for 4 to 6 weeks after an AMI.

### Stress testing

With the introduction of managed care, risk stratification of CAD has taken on increasing importance. Risk stratification refers to the use of diagnostic tests and physical assessment to determine patient management and prognosis. Cardiologists must decide which diagnostic tests to use, and when, to maximize quality patient care and minimize health care costs.

Typically, the patient with stable angina will complete an exercise stress test with or without nuclear imaging. Stress testing, often of modified intensity, may be safely performed with patients after the infarction. An exercise stress test demonstrates the significance of coronary artery blockages relative to the patient's functional status. This noninvasive test indicates areas of the myocardium that do not receive adequate perfusion at peak exercise. The use of nuclear imaging allows comparison of underperfused areas at peak exercise with nuclear images taken at rest. Differences between images indicate infarction (fixed defect) or ischemia (redistribution). Because ECG findings during the exercise component of the test correlate to anatomical locations, these tests can also indicate which coronary arteries might be involved. When a patient cannot exercise due to arthritis, peripheral vascular disease, or general debility, pharmacological agents (e.g., dipyridamole, dobutamine) can be administered intravenously to simulate the exercise response in the coronary arteries.

Echocardiography is another noninvasive test that may be used. Variations include echocardiography with exercise and dobutamine stress echocardiography. This test is being used more often and has merit in given situations and in the hands of skilled technicians.

### Cardiac catheterization

Cardiac catheterization is an invasive cardiac procedure used to assess coronary anatomy, ventricular function, and hemodynamic status. Cardiac catheterization is indicated for patients who have recurrent symptoms after maximal medical management and for patients with one or more recurrent, severe, or prolonged (greater than 20 minutes) ischemic episodes, especially with hemodynamic or ECG changes. Patients who may also benefit from catheterization include those with prior angioplasty, bypass surgery, or MI; those with high-risk clinical findings or noninvasive test findings; and those with significant heart failure or left ventricular dysfunction.

Right-sided heart catheterization provides information on the hemodynamic status of the heart. These findings are especially useful in managing intravenous fluid therapy in complicated MI. Left-sided heart catheterization includes coronary angiography and left ventriculography. Coronary angiography visualizes the coronary arteries using radiopaque dye. Angiography provides an indirect estimate of the percentage of blockage in the coronary arteries and their branches. Blockages of more than 70% are considered significant.

Ventriculography, often done at the same time as arteriography, involves the injection of dye into the left ventricle. Cardiac output can be calculated from the amount of dye ejected from the left ventricle during systole.

Fluoroscopic imaging allows direct visualization of the contractility of the left ventricle. Areas of poor contractility (hypokinesis), overcompensation (hyperkinesis), nonmovement (akinesis), and asynergy (dyskinesis) can be identified with ventriculography. An infarcted area is usually akinetic.

## Medications

Drug therapy plays a major role in the management of CAD. Table 25-5 presents an overview of drugs commonly used.

### Antiplatelet agents

The primary antiplatelet agent used in the treatment and prevention of CAD is acetylsalicylic acid (ASA), commonly known as aspirin. The ASA is given in the emergency department (or in the prehospital setting by emergency medical technicians) to any patient suspected of having an MI. Research has shown that a dose of ASA as low as 81 mg (one baby ASA) once a day effectively maintains an antiplatelet effect. Enteric-coated forms can be prescribed for individuals who cannot tolerate pure ASA. Ticlopidine 250 mg twice a day may be used for patients with a significant allergy to ASA. ReoPro, an antiplatelet drug used to treat the patient undergoing angioplasty, is often used in conjunction with weight-based heparin dose regimens. Given intravenously in the cardiac catheterization laboratory after percutaneous transluminal coronary angioplasty (PTCA), ReoPro acts to inhibit platelet aggregation, thereby preventing reocclusion of the treated coronary artery. Patients receiving ReoPro must be carefully monitored and must be kept on bed rest with the affected leg extended for at least 6 hours. Manual pressure is maintained on the groin insertion site for at least 30 minutes after sheath removal.

### Nitrates

Nitrates are effective in the treatment of both stable and unstable angina, as well as acute MI. Nitrates cause vasodilation, reducing the amount of blood returning to the heart from the venous system, thus decreasing preload. As a result, there is a decrease in workload for the heart and therefore a decrease in the demand of the myocardium for oxygen. Nitrates also dilate the peripheral arteries, decreasing the resistance against which the left ventricle must pump. This decrease in systemic blood pressure contributes to a decreased afterload. Because the left ventricle can pump with less force, there is a decrease in myocardial oxygen demand. In addition, nitrates act specifically to dilate the coronary arteries, especially those that are not atherosclerotic. As a result, collateral flow increases to the parts of the myocardium that are ischemic.

Many preparations of nitrates are available for use. The drug used most commonly for acute episodes of chest pain is sublingual nitroglycerin. The tablets, absorbed within minutes, are highly effective in relieving the acute symptoms of angina by increasing oxygen supply to the myocardium while simultaneously decreasing oxygen demand. Intravenous nitroglycerin is often necessary to manage prolonged chest pain.

Nitrates are also available as topical preparations. Both ointments and patch preparations provide a sustained therapeutic effect. Shorter-acting ointment preparations are preferred within the hospital environment as medications are adjusted. An advantage of the ointment is the ability to quickly remove it from the skin surface if hypotension occurs. Patches and oral preparations, such as isosorbide dinitrate and Imdur, are usually prescribed for long-term management.

### *Beta blockers*

Beta blockers are often prescribed for the treatment of angina. The sympathetic nervous system has two types of beta receptors: beta 1 and beta 2. Older beta blockers blocked both beta 1 and beta 2 receptors, causing the undesired effects of bronchoconstriction and vasoconstriction. Most beta blockers used today are cardioselective, blocking predominantly the beta 1 receptor. Blockade of beta 1 receptors causes a decrease in the force of contraction, a slowing of heart rate, and a slowing of impulse conduction. These three mechanisms of action cause a decrease in myocardial oxygen demand. In addition, by slowing the heart rate, beta blockers indirectly increase the supply of blood to the myocardium by increasing diastole, thus increasing the amount of time for coronary artery perfusion. Beta blockers also decrease blood pressure (thereby decreasing both afterload and myocardial oxygen demand) through their effect on the renin-angiotensin system.

**table 25-5** Common Medications for **Coronary Artery Disease**

| Drug | Action | Nursing Intervention |
|---|---|---|
| Antiplatelet agents (Aspirin, ticlopidine) | Inhibit platelet aggregation | Aspirin should be prescribed unless a true hypersensitivity reaction is present or the patient has a severe risk of bleeding. |
| Nitrates<br>Isosorbide dinitrate<br>Isosorbide mononitrate<br>Nitroglycerin | Decrease myocardial oxygen demand:<br>Venodilate (decrease preload)<br>Peripherally vasodilate (decrease afterload)<br>Increase myocardial oxygen supply<br>Coronary vasodilate | Patients should be lying or sitting with administration of sublingual nitrates.<br>Intravenous nitroglycerin is titrated to relief of symptoms or limiting side effects such as headache or systolic BP $< 90$ mm Hg. IV preparations are usually replaced with oral or topical preparation when the patient has been symptom free for 24 hours.<br>Cautious use with known aortic stenosis.<br>Anticipate headache, administer analgesics as appropriate.<br>Tolerance to nitrates can develop within 24 hours. A nitrate-free interval of 6 to 8 hours may improve responsiveness to therapy.<br>Topical nitrates must be cleaned from the skin surface before applying new dose. Appropriate areas of application include any hair-free area, preferably in noticeable areas when the initial dose is being determined. Application areas should be rotated. Gloves should be worn when applying topical preparations. |
| Beta blockers<br>Atenolol<br>Metoprolol<br>Timolol<br>Nadolol<br>Esmolol<br>Propranolol | Decrease myocardial oxygen demand:<br>Decrease contractility<br>Slow heart rate<br>Slow impulse conduction<br>Decrease BP (through renin interaction)<br>Increase myocardial oxygen supply<br>Slow heart rate, thereby increasing diastolic filling time and coronary perfusion<br>Decrease incidence of morbidity and mortality after acute MI | IV metoprolol is given in 5 mg increments over 1 to 2 minutes. Propranolol, esmolol, and atenolol may be prescribed IV instead of metoprolol. All IV preparations are followed by oral preparations after the patient is stabilized.<br>Monitor for atrioventricular block (including measuring PR interval), symptomatic bradycardia, hypotension, left ventricular failure (rales, decreased cardiac output), and bronchospasm.<br>Beta 1 cardioselective agents are the preferred drugs. Beta 2 agents should be avoided in patients with respiratory or peripheral vascular disease.<br>Target heart rate for beta blockade is 50 to 60 beats per minute. |
| Calcium channel blockers<br>Amiodipine<br>Diltiazem<br>Verapamil<br>Nifedipine | Decrease myocardial oxygen demand or increase myocardial oxygen supply by inhibiting the influx of calcium through the slow calcium channels. Heart rate decreases and conduction through the AV node slows (decrease demand, indirectly increase supply).<br>Inhibition of calcium influx into the arterial cell also promotes vasodilation of peripheral arteries (decrease demand) and coronary arteries (increase supply). | Often prescribed when vasospasm is considered part of the pathology or if significant hypertension exists.<br>Monitor for symptomatic bradycardia, prolonged PR intervals, advanced heart blocks, hypotension, congestive heart failure, peripheral edema. |

*Continued*

Beta blockers are often used alone or in combination with nitrates for the management of stable angina. Beta blockers decrease the incidence of morbidity and mortality when administered within 48 hours of MI and continued for 2 to 3 years after AMI. For this reason, beta blockers are often administered intravenously in the emergency department to individuals with probable MI. After the patient with AMI is stabilized, beta blockers are administered orally. Many beta blocker preparations end with the suffix *-olol* and include metoprolol and atenolol as cardioselective examples.

### Calcium channel blockers

Calcium channel blockers are another class of drugs commonly prescribed for the treatment of CAD. Calcium channel blockers vary greatly within the class in specific physiological effects. These agents inhibit the influx of calcium through the slow calcium channels, which must open and allow calcium to enter the cell before an electrical impulse can occur. Diltiazem is one commonly used calcium channel blocker. By slowing the heart rate, diltiazem decreases the myocardial oxygen demand and indirectly increases myocardial oxygen supply by increasing the time for coronary perfusion during diastole. Diltiazem also blocks calcium used for myocardial contractility, decreasing the force of contraction (and hence oxygen demand).

Another calcium channel blocker, verapamil, also inhibits the influx of calcium into cells, thereby decreasing automaticity of conduction cells and decreasing contractility. For patients with CAD, verapamil's predominant role is blocking

**table 25-5** *Common Medications for* ***Coronary Artery Disease—cont'd***

| Drug | Action | Nursing Intervention |
|---|---|---|
| Heparin (intravenous) | Prevents propagation of an established thrombus by rapidly inhibiting thrombin | Heparin PTTs should be measured 6 hours after any change in dose. Dose is weight based. Therapeutic levels should be maintained between 1.5 and 2.5 times patient control.<br>Hemoglobin, hematocrit, and platelets should be followed for downward trends. Platelets should be followed for heparin-induced thrombocytopenia.<br>Recurrent ischemia, active bleeding, and hypotension may signify subtherapeutic or supratherapeutic dosages and should be evaluated immediately. |
| Thrombolytics<br>Streptokinase<br>Tissue plasminogen activator (tPA) | Given in acute myocardial infarction to activate plasmin for lysis of obstructive clots in the coronary artery (not all agents are clot specific, therefore systemic lysis may occur) | Patients must be carefully screened before administration of thrombolytic agents.<br>The nurse monitors for reperfusion, reocclusion, and bleeding complications with thrombolysis administration.<br>Interventions are directed toward preventing bleeding complications. |
| Morphine sulfate | Blunts the deleterious consequences of sympathetic stimulation with pain<br>Vasodilates, creating decreased preload | Establish baseline vital signs, level of consciousness, and orientation.<br>Monitor for hypotension, respiratory depression, changes in level of consciousness. Doses are usually given in increments of 2 to 5 mg. |
| Oxygen | Increased arterial oxygen saturation | Monitor for adequate arterial oxygenation with finger pulse oximetry. Maintain saturation levels above 90%. |
| Cholesterol-lowering agents<br>Atorvastatin<br>Lovastatin<br>Pravastatin<br>Simvastatin<br>Gemfibrozil<br>Nicotinic acid | Reduce the substrate for lipid deposition in the coronary artery | Side effects vary with drug class. Intolerance to side effects may limit the usefulness of certain medications.<br>Lipid levels should be obtained at regular intervals to monitor for success in effecting changes.<br>Patients must be educated that cholesterol-lowering agents do not substitute for dietary modifications. |
| Angiotensin-converting enzyme inhibitors<br>Captopril<br>Enalapril<br>Benazepril<br>Lisinopril<br>Fosinopril | Decrease afterload and preload, thereby decreasing the workload of the heart. This prevents remodeling of the left ventricle. (Remodeling refers to hypertrophy of the unaffected left ventricle to compensate for the infarcted area.)<br>Long-term consequences of remodeling are increased oxygen demand and heart failure | Monitor for adverse effects: angioneurotic edema, cough, hypotension, hyperkalemia, pruritic rash, renal failure.<br>First doses require BP before and 30 minutes after administration. |

vasoconstriction. As a result, vasodilation predominates, afterload decreases, and myocardial oxygen demand decreases.

A group within the calcium channel blocker class, the dihydropyridines, affects both peripheral and coronary arteries. Vasodilation of the coronary arteries directly increases myocardial oxygen supply while peripheral vasodilation decreases the work of the heart.

Calcium channel blockers can be used alone or in conjunction with beta blockers and nitrates for the management of CAD. In patients with unstable angina, calcium channel blockers increase oxygen supply by dilating the coronary arteries. Calcium channel blockers are not a first-line drug for the treatment of AMI but may be prescribed for long-term management for the beneficial effects on supply and demand.

#### Angiotensin-converting enzyme inhibitors

Angiotensin-converting enzyme (ACE) inhibitors may be used in the management of CAD to decrease afterload and preload. This decreases the overall workload of the heart. Decreasing workload prevents remodeling of the left ventricle. The term *remodeling* refers to the compensatory development of hypertrophy of the unaffected left ventricle. This hypertrophy attempts to compensate for the loss of function in the infarcted area. The long-term consequence of this remodeling process can be a steady increase in myocardial oxygen demand for the enlarged muscle and the development of heart failure.

#### Anticoagulants

Anticoagulants are often prescribed for the patient with unstable angina or AMI. Intravenous heparin prevents clot formation at the site of plaque rupture. Heparin blocks the conversion of prothrombin to thrombin and fibrinogen to fibrin. Heparin administration continues until the person's risk of future myocardial events can be determined through diagnostic testing.

#### Thrombolytics

Thrombolytic agents are the standard of care for patients treated within 6 hours of the onset of AMI. Thrombolytics activate the fibrinolytic processes to lyse the clot that has formed from plaque rupture and is occluding the lumen of the coronary artery. Thrombolytics are administered intravenously when ECG confirms the diagnosis of acute myocardial infarction. The potential for bleeding from the administration of clot dissolution agents necessitates thorough screening of all patients for bleeding risks. Commonly used thrombolytics include tissue plasminogen activator (t-PA) and streptokinase. Streptokinase activates the conversion of plasminogen to plasmin, which degrades fibrin and fibrinogen into fragments. Tissue plasminogen activator also activates plasmin, but preferentially at the site of occlusion. The greatest success in aborting MI or minimizing its complications occurs when thrombolytics are administered within 6 hours after symptom onset. Research supports the benefit of thrombolytics in both men and women.[25] (See the Research Box.)

#### Analgesics

Even though thrombolytics, ASA, and heparin may open the coronary arteries and decrease chest pain, severe chest pain often persists. Pain activates the sympathetic nervous system, increasing heart rate and producing vasoconstriction. These changes decrease myocardial oxygen supply and increase myocardial oxygen demand. The immediate administration of intravenous narcotic analgesics interrupts the deleterious effects of pain. The agent of choice is morphine sulfate. Morphine not only blunts the sensation of pain, its vasodilating effect also decreases preload.

#### Oxygen

Oxygen is administered immediately to the patient experiencing angina, unstable angina, or AMI. This simple but effective intervention is key to increasing myocardial oxygen supply. Oxygen may be administered by nasal cannula or mask. Arterial oxygen saturation levels should be maintained above 90.

#### Cholesterol-lowering agents

Because considerable evidence links hypercholesterolemia to atherosclerosis, drugs that can reduce plasma lipids and lipoproteins are often prescribed in the treatment of patients with CAD. Two fibric acid derivatives, gemfibrozil (Lopid) and clofibrate (Atromid-S), decrease plasma concentrations of triglycerides and cholesterol. Lovastatin (Mevacor) reduces both total cholesterol and low-density lipoprotein (LDL) serum levels. Atorvastatin has been most successful in decreasing total cholesterol and LDL with fewer side effects than the other drugs in this group. The "statin" group of drugs (HMG-CoA reductase inhibitors) predominantly block the production of LDLs. These lipid-lowering agents are espe-

### research

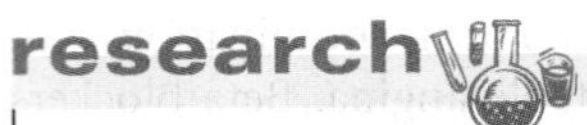

Reference: Weaver WD et al: Comparisons of characteristics and outcomes among women and men with acute myocardial infarction treated with thrombolytic therapy, *JAMA* 275:777, 1996.

Acute myocardial infarction occurs commonly in women, manifests about 10 years later than in men, and is associated with a high rate of mortality. In this study, part of the Global Utilization of Streptokinase and Tissue Plasminogen Activator for Occluded Coronary Arteries (GUSTO-I), a total of 10,315 women and 30,706 men with acute myocardial infarction were followed for 30 days after one of four thrombolytic regimens. The researchers found that women were on average 7 years older than men and delayed 18 minutes longer after symptom onset before coming to the hospital. Women more often had a history of diabetes, hypertension, and smoking than did men. Time to treatment was significantly longer in women (10 to 15 minutes longer after arrival at the emergency department than men), and women had more nonfatal complications after treatment, including shock, heart failure, serious bleeding, and reinfarction. They concluded that although both men and women benefit from thrombolytic therapy after acute myocardial infarction, women who receive thrombolytic therapy for treatment of acute myocardial infarction were at greater risk for both fatal and nonfatal complications than men.

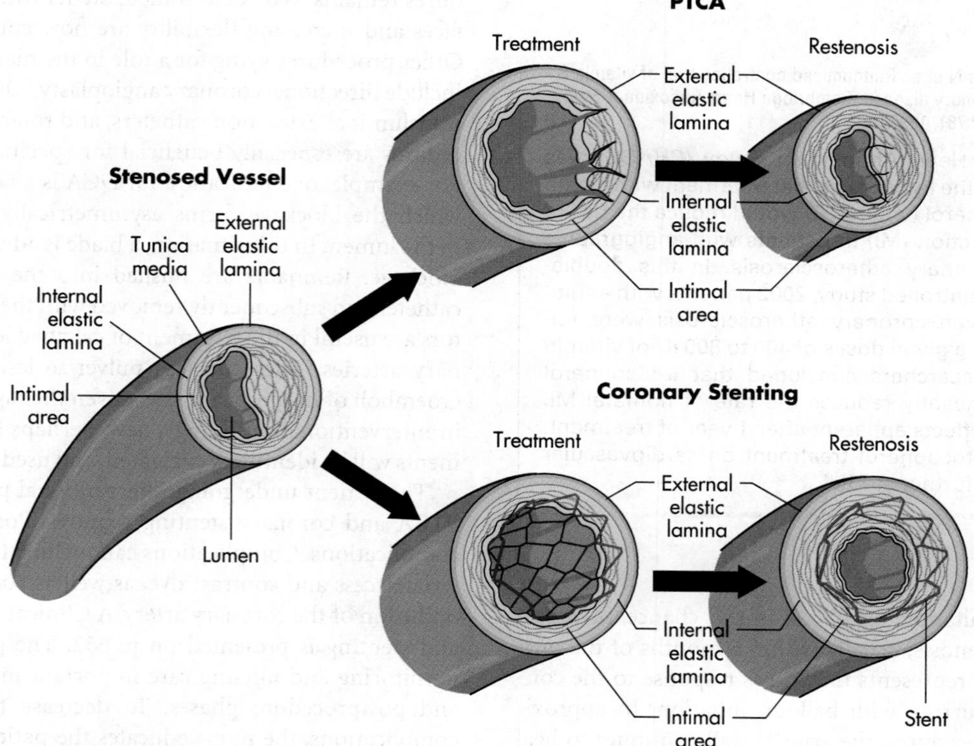


**fig. 25-8** Possible mechanisms of restenosis after PTCA and coronary stenting. Left figure illustrates atherosclerosis. Upper figure illustrates PTCA to the left and restenosis following PTCA on right. Bottom figure illustrates coronary stenting to the left and restenosis of stent to the right.

cially useful as adjuncts to dietary management of patients with familial hypercholesterolemia. (See Table 25-5.)

Vitamin E administration has greatly increased over recent years. Vitamin E and other antioxidants inhibit atherosclerosis by preventing the oxidation of LDLs. Oxidation of LDLs increases the uptake of LDLs by macrophages, thus increasing fatty deposition. Research continues to support the use of vitamin E in patients with CAD.[23] (See the Research Box on p. 650.)

## Treatments

### *Intraaortic balloon pump*

Patients experiencing MI who have symptoms refractory to medical management and those who have symptoms in conjunction with hemodynamic instability may benefit from placement of an intraaortic balloon pump (IABP). The IABP, inserted into the descending thoracic artery, inflates during diastole, thus augmenting early diastolic pressure and coronary artery perfusion. The balloon deflates rapidly at the end of diastole, decreasing afterload, resulting in an increase in cardiac output. A full discussion of intraaortic balloon pumps is included in Chapter 26.

### *Interventional procedures*

**Coronary angioplasty and intracoronary stents.** Percutaneous transluminal coronary angioplasty (PTCA) has been an accepted medical interventional procedure for the treatment of CAD since 1976. The PTCA procedure takes place in the cardiac catheterization or interventional laboratory. It can be performed at the same time as diagnostic cardiac catheterization or as a separate procedure. In both instances, the patient is sedated with combinations of anxiolytics such as diazepam or midazolam, narcotics such as fentanyl, and diphenhydramine. A local anesthetic is injected at the femoral arterial insertion site (alternatively, the brachial or radial artery may be used). After insertion of a sheath in the femoral artery, the catheter is guided through the arteries to the aorta, where radiopaque dye is injected directly into the coronary arteries. The coronary anatomy is viewed and the lesion identified. Technical feasibility of performing PTCA is then determined. A guide wire is advanced across and beyond the lesion. A catheter with a cylindrical balloon is then advanced over the guide wire, and the balloon is positioned centrally in the blockage. The balloon, filled with radiopaque dye and saline, is then inflated at pressures great enough to reconfigure the blockage. This reconfiguration includes the controlled dissection (splitting) of the intima and to a lesser extent vessel dilation (Figure 25-8). The controlled dissection creates passages that allow for an increase in arterial blood flow. At times, the dissection may create enough turbulence to stimulate clot formation or actually interfere with blood flow by obstructing the coronary lumen. In these situations, anticoagulation or additional interventional measures (such as intracoronary stenting) are necessary to prevent occlusion.

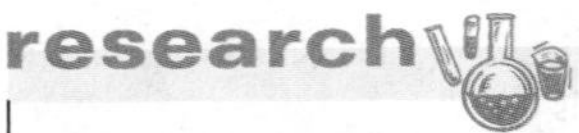

Reference: Stephens N et al: Randomised controlled trial of vitamin E in patients with coronary disease: Cambridge Heart Antioxidant Study (CHAOS), *Lancet* 347:781, 1996.

The Cambridge Heart Antioxidant Study (CHAOS) was designed to test the hypothesis that treatment with a high dose of $\alpha$-tocopherol (vitamin E) would reduce the risk of myocardial infarction (MI) in patients with angiographic evidence of coronary atherosclerosis. In this double-blind, placebo-controlled study, 2002 patients with angiographically proven coronary atherosclerosis were followed, after being given doses of 400 to 800 IU of vitamin E daily. The researchers concluded that $\alpha$-tocopherol treatment significantly reduces the rate of nonfatal MI, with beneficial effects apparent after 1 year of treatment. The effect of $\alpha$-tocopherol treatment on cardiovascular deaths requires further study.

The major limitation of PTCA is the chance of lesion recurrence or restenosis, usually within 6 months of the procedure. Restenosis represents the body's response to the controlled injury occurring with balloon inflation. In approximately 30% of procedures, the arterial wall continues to heal with smooth muscle proliferation into the arterial lumen. Although this is not the same lipid accumulation that caused the original atherosclerotic lesion, it nevertheless compromises myocardial blood flow and results in myocardial ischemia. Indications for PTCA include almost any given anatomical situation, such as small distal branches, multiple lesions in one or more grafts, and long lesions. Primary angioplasty is now considered a first-line treatment for AMI where facilities and personnel are readily available.[10] The decision for PTCA occurs after physician-patient consultation regarding coronary anatomy, symptoms, coexisting disease states, the surgical risks of coronary artery bypass graft surgery, and the patient's feelings regarding open heart surgery. Care of the patient undergoing PTCA is summarized in the accompanying Guidelines for Care Box on p. 651.

**Stents.** Intracoronary stenting, another medical intervention, maintains patency of coronary arteries with a decreased incidence of restenosis (see Figure 25-8). The stent is introduced into the coronary artery on a balloon catheter. With balloon inflation, the stent is deployed and remains in the coronary artery as a scaffold. The delivery balloon catheter is then removed. The stent endothelializes over 3 weeks, decreasing the risk of thrombus formation on the foreign material. Despite these benefits, the potential for restenosis still exists after stent placement. Although stent designs vary among manufacturers, they all serve to increase lumen diameter. The cardiologist decides whether to balloon or stent based on lesion characteristics. The use of intravenous ultrasound may be helpful in the decision process.

**Other procedures.** Besides PTCA and intracoronary stenting, other interventional procedures can be used to treat coronary artery occlusion. The efficacy of some of these procedures remains to be determined. Stents with heparinized surfaces and increasing flexibility are now entering the market. Other procedures vying for a role in the management of CAD include directional coronary angioplasty (DCA), laser therapy, transluminal extraction catheters, and rotablators. These procedures are especially beneficial for specific types of lesions. For example, one indication for DCA is an eccentric lesion in which the blockage forms asymmetrically (not concentric) in the lumen. In this situation, a blade is advanced to shave the blockage. Remnants are pushed into the nose cone of the catheter and subsequently removed with the catheter. Rotablators are useful in the treatment of calcified lesions in the coronary arteries. These devices pulverize lesions, creating microemboli of insignificant size. Given the rapid pace of change in interventional cardiology, new, perhaps less invasive treatments will be identified, evaluated, and used in the near future.

The patient undergoing interventional procedures such as PTCA and coronary stenting requires close monitoring for complications. Complications can include those related to arterial access and contrast dye, as well as complications of reocclusion of the coronary artery. A Clinical Pathway for PTCA and stenting is presented on p. 652. The pathway addresses monitoring and nursing care important in the preprocedure and postprocedure phases. To decrease the occurrence of complications, the nurse educates the patient about the procedure and postcare interventions. When the patient understands the rationale behind bed rest and fluids, for example, the patient can then actively assist the health care team to decrease the chance of complications. (See the Guidelines for Care Box on p. 657 and the Clinical Pathway on p. 652-653.)

### Surgical Management

In coronary artery bypass graft (CABG) surgery the surgeon attaches an artery or vein graft to the coronary artery beyond the areas of blockage. This creates a bypass around the obstruction, thereby reestablishing blood flow (Figure 25-9, p. 654). The decision to proceed with surgery must consider the anatomy of the coronary lesion and the surgical risks and benefits. The decision includes consultation with a thoracic cardiovascular surgeon in collaboration with the patient and family. Although CABG surgery is not curative because the grafts can also occlude, it improves the quality of life for many patients. Chapter 26 presents information related to CABG surgery in detail.

The two most commonly used grafts are the saphenous vein and the internal mammary artery. The internal mammary artery remains patent longer than a saphenous vein graft. Explanations for this include the need for one attachment, the preexisting higher-pressure arterial system, and the more congruent artery-to-artery sizing. Alternative conduits are increasing in use, including the gastroepiploic artery, the brachial artery, and the cephalic vein.

Bypass graft surgery is a major surgical procedure that usually requires an open heart approach. In a limited number of situations, CABG surgery can be performed without the open heart approach. This new procedure, referred to as a mini-CABG, can be used only for selected patients. Chapter 26 dis-

**guidelines for care**

### The Patient Undergoing PTCA

#### General Concepts to Reinforce

Indication for the procedure
Review of rationale for PTCA vs. other interventions
PTCA is not a surgical intervention: no incisions, no general anesthesia
Risk factors associated with procedure, including <1% chance of emergency surgery in noncomplicated PTCAs

#### Preprocedure Preparation

Tests performed before procedure: lab work, ECG
Anxiolytics for anxiety
IV access started to give medications/fluids
NPO after midnight, except medications, clear liquid breakfast if late procedure
If groin access, groin will be shaved and scrubbed
Pedal pulses marked
Cardiac monitor placed

#### Intraprocedure Expectations

Cath lab environment—cool, sterilely draped, staff with masks and gowns, camera close to body
Anxiolytics for anxiety
Cardiac monitor at all times
Local anesthetic to groin or other access site
Back or arm discomfort might occur from positioning—notify staff
Chest pain or anginal equivalent with balloon inflations
Balloon filled with dye and saline so can see it on the fluoroscopy
Need to cough to clear dye and deep breathe to provide a better picture of anatomy
Duration of procedure varies from 30 minutes to 2 hours

#### Postprocedure Expectations

Groin site: need to keep affected leg still until 4 hours after sheath removed
Dressing: clear dressing over entry site
Sheath: cardiologist may continue heparin overnight; if so, sheath must stay in overnight; once heparin is discontinued, sheath can be removed after activated clotting time falls below 180 (usually 3 to 4 hours)
Head of bed (HOB): while sheath is in, HOB should be less than 30 degrees; flexible sheaths allow HOB up to 60 degrees; after sheath is removed, HOB needs to be flat with patient on bed rest for 4 additional hours
Back pain: may logroll with assistance; back rubs, pain medication available
Vital signs and neurovascular assessments every 15 minutes ×4, every 30 minutes ×2, then every hour until stable
ECG: Routine ECG after procedure
Should notify staff if feels warm or wet at puncture site; any pain: anginal, back, leg; inability to void with abdominal fullness
Food: can eat after procedure if sheath remains in overnight; if sheath removed same day, NPO until sheath pulled
Fluids: encouraged, unless contraindicated, to flush dye from system

#### Discharge Expectations

All teaching relevant to angina or MI patient (see Nursing Management), plus the following:
Groin restrictions—no heavy lifting, tub baths for 2 days
PTCA not a cure—should carry nitroglycerin and use as instructed in CAD teaching
Restenosis can occur per no fault of patient; restenosis represents ineffective, inefficient healing at PTCA site; most likely time of occurrence is within 6 months; need to contact cardiologist or primary care provider for symptoms similar to those experienced with balloon inflations
Aspirin must be taken daily; if stent, ticlopidine also taken bid for 30 days

cusses the details of open heart surgery and the associated nursing interventions.

Transmyocardial laser revascularization is a medical or surgical procedure still under clinical investigation. A carbon dioxide laser, under computer guidance, creates holes in the left ventricle. These holes serve as channels for blood flow. The channels seal epicardially but allow blood to enter the endocardium from the left ventricle.

### Diet

The patient being evaluated for acute chest pain is given nothing by mouth (NPO—Latin, *nil per os*) until the diagnosis of AMI is ruled out. Keeping the patient NPO prevents blood from being redirected to the gastrointestinal system at a time when the heart is ischemic and demanding an increased blood flow. Keeping the patient NPO also prevents vomiting, which commonly accompanies chest pain from vagal effects. Patients may also be NPO before cardiac procedures. When not NPO, the diet recommended for patients with cardiac disease is low fat and low cholesterol.

Because of the role of cholesterol and lipids in plaque formation, most patients with a diagnosis of CAD will be offered diet counseling. Counseling begins with careful assessment of the patient's usual daily diet and knowledge of the relationship between diet and CAD. Diet teaching usually includes reducing the fat content of the diet, substituting polyunsaturated fat for saturated fat, and maintaining body weight at normal levels. Patients are encouraged to keep saturated fats at less than 10% of total calories, restrict monounsaturated fats to 10% to 15% of calories, restrict polyunsaturated fats to less than 10% of calories, and restrict cholesterol to less than 300 mg per day. Studies have shown that dietary intake of large amounts of saturated fat raises the serum cholesterol level. When polyunsaturated fats replace saturated fats the blood cholesterol level tends to fall. Sources of polyunsaturated fats include corn, cottonseed, soy, and safflower oils and margarines incorporating these oils in liquid form. Hydrogenated oils contain more saturated fat, as do tropical oils, butterfat, and animal fats. Transfatty acids are created when an oil is hydrogenated. Hydrogenation is a process

*Text continued on p. 654*

## clinical pathway *Percutaneous Transluminal Coronary Angioplasty*

| ADMISSION/CLINIC | IMMEDIATELY PREPROCEDURE | INTRAPROCEDURE | POSTPROCEDURE SHEATH IN | POSTPROCEDURE SHEATH OUT | DISCHARGE |
|---|---|---|---|---|---|
| **Assessment** | | | | | |
| Height/weight<br>History/physical<br>Nursing assessment: baseline data, including medications, allergies, body systems, chronic back pain history; emotional, spiritual, dietary, financial, educational needs | Assessment of systemic perfusion: warmth, peripheral pulses, BP, urine output, exercise tolerance, heart rate and rhythm, level of consciousness, breath sounds<br>Mark peripheral pulses with pen/marker | Assess beneficial effects of anxiolytics<br>Assess for presence and tolerance of anginal or back pain<br>Assess hemodynamic tolerance to procedure, including rhythm disturbances and ST changes<br>Assess for dye reactions | Vital signs, neurovascular, and access site checks q15min ×4, q30min ×2, q1h × 2, and then q2h until sheath removal<br>Cardiac monitor<br>Assess for dye reactions<br>Continue to assess for anxiety and back pain<br>Monitor for reocclusion<br>Monitor for urinary retention<br>With sheath pull, monitor for vasovagal reaction | VS, neurovascular, and access site checks q15min ×4, q30min ×2, q1h ×2<br>Continue to assess for anxiety and back pain<br>Monitor for reocclusion<br>Orthostatic BP and HR before ambulation<br>May discontinue telemetry 6 hours after sheath pull unless contraindicated<br>Assess for bruit after dressing removed | VS every shift<br>Monitor for reocclusion<br>Assess site for signs and symptoms of infection<br>Assess for presence of bruit, pseudoaneurysm, and hematoma |
| **Laboratory/Diagnostic Tests** | | | | | |
| ECG<br>CBC with platelets<br>Chem 7<br>PT<br>PTT | Notify physician of abnormal laboratory results | ACT after heparin bolus to maintain level >300-350 sec<br>For patients receiving Reopro, ACT ≥ 200 sec | ECG postprocedure and prn chest pain or anginal equivalent<br>For overnight sheath, heparin PTT 6 h after procedure and with any change in dose<br>For patients receiving Reopro, CBC with platelets 2 h after bolus and in morning<br>To discontinue sheath: ACT<br>May pull when ACT < 180 sec | BUN and creatinine for renal function<br>CBC and platelets if bleeding concerns | |
| **Medications/IVs** | | | | | |
| Prescribed medications: prednisone 60 mg per orders for known contrast allergy | ASA 325 mg before procedure<br>1000 cc 0.9 NS KVO<br>Diazepam PO, diphenhydramine PO on call, or both<br>60 mg prednisone with diphenhydramine 50 mg PO on call for known contrast allergy | Manage back pain with positioning when possible and the administration of analgesics such as morphine or fentanyl<br>Manage pain with deep breathing, relaxation mechanisms, and calm, competent approach<br>Anxiolytics prn such as fentanyl, diazepam, or midazolam | Resume scheduled medications<br>Anxiolytics and analgesics prn<br>IV fluids appropriate to renal and ventricular dysfunction, heparin to keep PTT 1.5-2.5 control<br>Discontinue heparin 4 h before planned sheath pull<br>ASA 325 mg daily<br>Ticlopidine 250 mg PO bid for stent procedures<br>Before sheath pull: morphine, atropine prn, and local lidocaine | Scheduled meds, including aspirin and ticlopidine<br>Anxiolytics and analgesics prn<br>Discontinue KVO IV after sheath pull and adequate PO intake | Scheduled meds, including aspirin and ticlopidine<br>Discontinue saline lock |

| ADMISSION CLINIC | IMMEDIATELY PREPROCEDURE | INTRAPROCEDURE | POSTPROCEDURE SHEATH IN | POSTPROCEDURE SHEATH OUT | DISCHARGE |
|---|---|---|---|---|---|
| **Medications/IVs—cont'd** | | | | | |
| | Foley catheter or external catheter if needed<br>Void on call to procedure | Set up arterial line flush<br>Foley catheter or external catheter if needed<br>I&O | Foley or external catheter if needed | Remove Foley or external catheter at completion of bed rest<br>Discontinue I&O unless contraindicated | |
| **Dressings** | | | | | |
| | Groin shave and prep on arrival to cath lab | Groin prep/drape<br>Clear dressing over site at completion of procedure | Clear dressing over site | Remove dressing at end of bed rest | |
| **Activity** | | | | | |
| Activity as tolerated | As tolerated | Bed rest | Bed rest with affected limb straight, roll with assist, no chin to chest<br>Head of bed not greater than 30-60 degrees depending on sheath used<br>Back rub prn | Bed rest with affected limb straight 4 h after sheath removal, roll with assist, avoid chin to chest<br>Back rub prn<br>After completion of bed rest, dangle with orthostatic checks; OOB with assist first ambulation | Up ad lib<br>Restrict lifting, tub baths, excessive stairs for 2 days |
| **Diet** | | | | | |
| If morning procedure, NPO except for medications after midnight<br>If evening procedure, clear liquids for breakfast | NPO | NPO | For same day sheath pull: NPO<br>For overnight sheath: heart-healthy diet; on return to unit NPO until sheath removed | Heart-healthy diet<br>Encourage PO fluids unless contraindicated | Heart-healthy diet |
| **Education and Interdisciplinary Involvement** | | | | | |
| Initiate appropriate referrals as per assessment<br>Implement guidelines for patient education<br>Informed consent<br>Advise family where to wait<br>Review pathway with patient/family<br>Address any questions/concerns | Communicate any delays to patient and family<br>Address any concerns or question | Orient to lab<br>Update family<br>Instruct patient to communicate needs/questions | Reinforce immediate postprocedure groin precautions and activity progression | Reinforce immediate postprocedure groin precautions and activity progression | Review S&S of restenosis<br>Review site complications and precautions<br>Reinforce risk factor modification<br>Review protocol for chest pain |

Adapted from University of Virginia Health Sciences Center, Division of Patient Care Services. Used with permission.
*ECG*, Electrocardiogram; *PT*, prothrombin time; *PTT*, partial thromboplastin time; *Chem 7*, sodium, potassium, chloride, bicarbonate, blood urea nitrogen, creatinine, glucose; *ACT*, activated clotting time; *BUN*, blood urea nitrogen; *ASA*, aspirin; *NS*, normal saline; *KVO*, keep vein open; *I&O*, intake and output; *OOB*, out of bed.

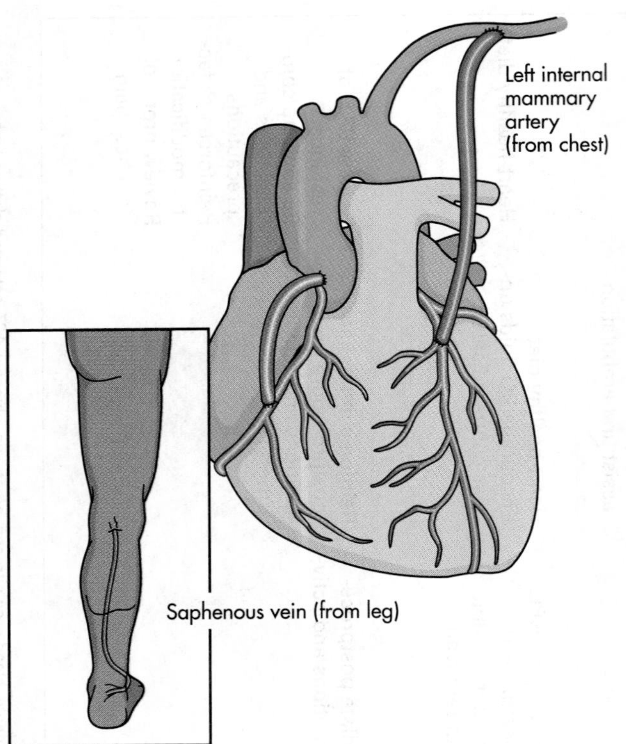


**fig. 25-9** Coronary artery bypass surgery. Common grafts: saphenous vein and internal mammary artery.

**guidelines for care**

### Advancing Activity Levels

**Activity Progression—Admission**

0 to 12 hours: bed rest with bedside commode

12 to 24 hours: orthostatic check; out of bed to chair with meals, ad lib in room

**Activity Progression—Day 2 to Discharge**

Duration: first session, ambulate 1 to 2 minutes; increase duration 1 to 2 minutes per session if patient tolerates (see below)

Frequency: initially 1 to 4 times per day, duration less than 10 minutes

Intensity: maintain heart rate no greater than 20 beats per minute over baseline; patient should be able to converse on ambulation without shortness of breath

**Criteria for Progressing Activity**

Heart rate* within 20 beats per minute of standing baseline heart rate

Systolic blood pressure* within 20 mm Hg of standing baseline blood pressure

Absence of chest pain, pressure, or anginal equivalent; shortness of breath; dysrhythmia; fatigue; light-headedness; diaphoresis

*Blood pressures and heart rate checks are taken in a standing position preambulation and immediately postambulation. Postambulation heart rate should be measured by taking pulse for 10 seconds and multiplying by 6.

that makes an oil more solid at room temperature, extending the shelf life of the product. When an unsaturated fat converts to a transfatty acid, it then acts in the body in much the same way as a saturated fat. Transfatty acids increase LDLs and total cholesterol and may even decrease high-density lipoproteins (HDLs). Patients should avoid transfatty acid products such as stick margarines, shortenings, and foods prepared with these products. The nurse and dietitian work collaboratively with the patient and family to plan realistic changes in the diet.

#### Activity

Initially the patient experiencing chest pain is restricted to complete bed rest. This activity restriction decreases myocardial oxygen demand until enzyme levels peak and a definitive diagnosis of MI can be made. After the patient is hemodynamically stable and free of chest pain, activity can be increased gradually (see the Guidelines for Care Box). Assessment for activity tolerance includes monitoring for orthostatic changes in the blood pressure, dysrhythmias, appropriate changes in blood pressure and heart rate, and the presence of symptoms. The presence of symptoms or hemodynamic changes indicates the potential for ischemia and requires cessation of activity until the patient stabilizes.

Before discharge or soon thereafter, most postinfarction patients undergo stress testing to determine a safe individual exercise level. Ideally, postinfarction patients will enroll in outpatient cardiac rehabilitation programs.[26] These programs direct the progression of activity and offer variety in modes of exercise (bicycle, steps, weights). Unfortunately, not all insurance companies recognize the benefit of structured rehabilitation programs, and financial constraints may prevent enrollment. In these situations standardized home exercise programs are recommended. (See the Patient/Family Teaching Box on the next page.) These activity prescriptions consider the location and extent of myocardial damage, results of stress testing when available, and specific patient needs.

Patients with stable and unstable angina may not require a formal activity progression or program. However, the importance of exercise in preventing disease progression is significant and cannot be overstated. A regular exercise regimen can decrease LDLs, increase HDLs, increase collateral circulation, decrease resting heart rate, and decrease blood pressure (BP). Despite these benefits of exercise, patients with known cardiac disease must take precautions to prevent stressing the already compromised myocardial oxygen supply and demand balance. Therefore the same home walking guidelines can be given to patients with stable and unstable angina. These guidelines promote conditioning and simultaneously prevent overexertion that could further increase myocardial oxygen demand.

#### Referrals

Managing the care of the patient with CAD requires collaboration among members of the cardiac health care team. For the patient newly diagnosed with stable angina, referrals may be made to cardiologists, nutritionists, stress management therapists, and exercise physiologists. For the patient admitted with MI, referrals most often include members of inpatient and outpatient cardiac rehabilitation staffs: RNs, exercise physiologists, nutritionists, and social workers. Other professionals who may be consulted include vocational reha-

**patient/family teaching**

**Home Walking Program**

**Count Pulse**

Take your pulse before, during, and immediately after your walk. Stop and rest if your heart rate is higher than 20 beats over resting heart rate, and then continue at a slower pace.

**Safety**

Carry your nitroglycerin with you and use as directed if symptoms occur.

**Warm-up**

Start with 1 minute of arm/chest exercises followed by 4 or 5 minutes of stationary walking. Purpose: To gradually increase blood flow to the muscles, preventing injury.

**Walk**

Walk at moderate intensity for 5 to 10 minutes. Increase your time by 1 to 2 minutes each time you walk with a goal of a 30- to 45-minute walk. Intensity: stay within a heart rate not higher than 20 beats above your resting heart rate and less than 120 beats per minute initially. If you are taking beta blockers, you must stay within 20 beats of your baseline.

**Cooldown**

Cool down with 5 to 10 minutes of low-intensity walking followed by stretching. Purpose: to gradually decrease effort and prevent a drop in blood pressure causing dizziness.

**General Guidelines**

Preferably walk on a level surface. If you must walk uphill, go more slowly.

Walk at least three times per week.

In the summer, do not walk if the temperature is higher than 85° F or if the humidity is higher than 75%. Wear loose clothing. Drink plenty of water to prevent dehydration.

In the winter, do not walk outside if the temperature is lower than 40° F. Wear a hat and a face scarf.

Avoid exercise for 1 to 2 hours after eating. Diabetic walkers should have a light snack before walking.

Do not use tobacco for 1 hour before exercise.

bilitation workers, chaplains, marriage counselors or sex therapists, and stress reduction therapists. Given the decreased length of hospital stay for patients with MI, much of the care provided occurs after discharge from the hospital.

## NURSING MANAGEMENT

### ASSESSMENT

#### Subjective Data

Chest pain: location, severity, intensity, quality, duration, time of onset; patient may be asymptomatic; classic pattern is retrosternal pain that may radiate down left arm or both arms, upward to neck or jaws, or backward to scapular region; may be described as crushing, or worst pain ever experienced
- Precipitating factors (e.g., exercise, stress, sexual intercourse, smoking)
- Measures attempted to control pain (e.g., nitroglycerin, lying down, eating or drinking, using antacids); effectiveness

Other symptoms (e.g., indigestion, heartburn, dizziness, dyspnea, nausea or vomiting, anxiety and/or feeling of doom)

Risk factors for CAD (e.g., positive family history, lipid profile, tobacco use, history, stress levels, exercise pattern)

Other illnesses (e.g., diabetes, hypertension); current management regimen

Support systems, insurance coverage, financial resources for rehabilitation

#### Objective Data

Posture indicating presence of chest pain (e.g., clutching or rubbing chest, leaning forward)

Changes in vital signs: tachycardia or bradycardia, hypertension or hypotension

Dyspnea or shortness of breath, rales

Presence of $S_3$ or $S_4$

Dysrhythmias

Altered level of consciousness

Vomiting

Declining urine output

Pale, cool, diaphoretic skin

### NURSING DIAGNOSES

Nursing diagnoses are determined from the analysis of patient data. Nursing diagnoses for the patient with CAD may include but are not limited to:

| Diagnostic Title | Possible Etiological Factors |
|---|---|
| Chest pain | Myocardial ischemia, imbalance between myocardial oxygen supply and demand |
| Risk for altered tissue perfusion | Decrease in cardiac output, hypoxemia |
| Risk for injury (bleeding) | Altered clotting factors, pharmaceutical agents (thrombolytics), decrease in platelet adhesiveness (aspirin) |
| Anxiety | Threat of death; threat to or change in health status, socioeconomic status, role functioning, interaction patterns; lack of information about cardiac procedures; general uncertainty |
| Activity intolerance | Deconditioning associated with bed rest, imbalance of myocardial oxygen supply and demand |
| Altered sexuality patterns | Illness, medical treatment, lack of information about safe guidelines for sexual activity, medication side effects, impaired relationship with significant other |

## EXPECTED PATIENT OUTCOMES

Expected patient outcomes for the patient with CAD may include but are not limited to:

1. Will be free of chest pain or pain will be reduced or controlled effectively by medication
2. Will have perfusion to all organs restored to baseline and maintained
3. Will not experience bleeding or bleeding will be effectively controlled and treated if it occurs
4. Will experience only manageable levels of anxiety, permitting patient to seek and process information
5. Will tolerate gradually increasing levels of activity
6. Will verbalize the guidelines for resuming sexual activity, discuss concerns that arise, or seek counseling as needed

## INTERVENTIONS

In managing the care of patients with CAD, the nurse has numerous opportunities to collaborate with other health care professionals in determining appropriate interventions. Some interventions depend on physician's orders, such as the administration of oxygen, thrombolytics, narcotics, and intravenous fluids. Others, such as the provision of psychological support and specific information, may be initiated by the nurse. Interventions should always address the patient's specific needs.

### Controlling Chest Pain

Because ischemic cardiac pain results from an imbalance between myocardial oxygen supply and demand, treatment of pain attempts to increase myocardial oxygen supply while reducing myocardial oxygen demand (see the Guidelines for Care Box below). Immediate collaborative interventions include the administration of oxygen, narcotics, nitrates, and thrombolytics. Before medication administration, the nurse validates the absence of allergies and bleeding risks and establishes baseline vital signs, level of consciousness, and orientation. The nurse observes the patient for deviations from baseline after the administration of nitrates, thrombolytics, and narcotics.

#### Sublingual nitrates

Because of the vasodilatory effects of nitrates, the patient should be lying down before administration. A 12-lead ECG may also be obtained before the first dose of nitroglycerin. When the patient has documented CAD and the treatment strategy has already been determined, nitroglycerin administration is initiated before a diagnostic ECG. This prevents additional delays in treating known CAD.

It is helpful to have the patient rate pain on a scale of 0 to 10, where 0 is no pain and 10 is the worst pain ever. Having this baseline helps evaluate the effectiveness of the immediate interventions of thrombolytics, nitrates, and analgesics. Additional information about the safe and effective use of sublingual nitroglycerin is provided in the Patient/Family Teaching Box.

**guidelines for care**

**The Patient Experiencing Angina**

Stay with patient. Ask for assistance in obtaining needed equipment (e.g., 12-lead ECG and oxygen setup).

Assess the presence of chest pain (or anginal equivalent). Document baseline intensity.

Obtain baseline vital signs. Continue to monitor vital signs every 5 minutes during interventions.

Apply oxygen when available.

Ensure IV access.

Obtain an ECG as soon as possible. For diagnostic purposes, an ECG should be performed before administration of nitroglycerin. If patient has known CAD, nitroglycerin may be administered before ECG. Obtain a repeat ECG.

Administer nitroglycerin and morphine per orders until pain resolves. If pain is not responsive to sublingual nitroglycerin and morphine, anticipate additional interventions such as IV nitroglycerin.

Treat alterations in vital signs with appropriate medications. If ECG indicates acute myocardial infarction, anticipate and prepare for thrombolytic therapy or primary angioplasty.

Assess patient's level of anxiety and offer realistic reassurance. Explain all interventions. Approach patient and family in a calm, confident manner. Minimize environmental stimulation.

**patient/family teaching**

**Use and Storage of Nitroglycerin**

**Use of Sublingual Nitroglycerin**

- Sit or lie down at onset of angina/chest pain.
- Place tablet under the tongue and allow tablet to dissolve; do not chew.
- If pain is not relieved within 5 minutes, take a second tablet. A third tablet can be used after an additional 5 minutes if pain persists. Continuing pain after 3 tablets and 15 minutes indicates a need to receive immediate medical evaluation.
- Tablet will cause a tingling sensation under the tongue.
- Rest for 15 to 20 minutes after taking nitroglycerin to avoid faintness.
- A tablet may, with the physician's permission, be taken 10 minutes before an activity known to trigger an anginal attack.
- Anticipate the occurrence of hypotension, tachycardia, and headache in response to the medication. Headache may persist for 15 to 20 minutes after administration.
- Keep a record of the number of anginal attacks experienced, the number of tablets needed to obtain pain relief, and the precipitating factors if known.

*Note:* Sublingual spray is administered under or onto the tongue following the same guidelines as above.

**Storage of Nitroglycerin**

- Carry tablets for immediate use if necessary. Do not pack in luggage when traveling.
- Keep tablets in tightly closed, original container. Tablets need to be protected from exposure to light and moisture.
- Tablets should be stored in a cool, dry place.
- Check expiration date on prescription. Tablets should be discarded after 6 months once the bottle has been opened. Plan for replacement of supply.

#### Topical nitrates

Topical nitrates, supplied as ointments, creams, and pastes, may also be used for CAD. These preparations must be handled carefully by the nurse administering the medication. Usually this requires the use of clean gloves when applying the topical nitrate. The nurse places the topical nitrate on the chest or upper arm after the hair has been removed by shaving. The site of application is rotated with each dose. An advantage of topical nitrates is their easy removal if untoward effects develop. This advantage proves useful during dose adjustment in the early phases of treatment. However, oral nitrates typically replace topical nitrates for long-term therapy. Nitrate tolerance may develop in some individuals. Nurses should ensure nitrate-free intervals, usually at night, to minimize potential for nitrate tolerance.

#### Intravenous nitroglycerin

Intravenous nitroglycerin may be used to treat severe unstable angina or AMI. During the administration of intravenous nitroglycerin, the nurse monitors the patient's BP frequently. Intravenous nitroglycerin is titrated to keep the patient pain free while maintaining a systolic blood pressure above 90 mm Hg. Because of the vasodilator effects of nitroglycerin on cerebral arteries, many patients receiving nitroglycerin complain of headache requiring analgesic administration.

#### Thrombolytic therapy

Thrombolytics are used emergently to open the coronary artery, increasing blood supply to the myocardium and thus relieving pain. Before thrombolytic administration, all members of the health care team participate in screening the patient for bleeding risks. (See the Guidelines for Care Box.) No question is asked too often in this situation. Thrombolytic therapy must be administered without delay, preferably within 4 to 6 hours of symptom onset. The nurse assisting in the administration of thrombolytics must be knowledgeable of all current thrombolytic treatment protocols to decrease preparation time. The nurse obtains baseline vital signs and completes a physical examination for signs and symptoms of overt or covert bleeding. During the administration of thrombolytics the nurse monitors the patient's pain status and observes the ECG for resolution of ST segment elevation. Should increasing pain or further signs of myocardial injury develop, the nurse anticipates the possibility of emergency interventional cardiac procedures (PTCA, stent placement, atherectomy, bypass surgery) and helps mobilize the cardiac team.

Treatment efforts also address the need to decrease the patient's myocardial oxygen demand. During the acute episode of chest pain myocardial oxygen demand decreases when the patient sits or lies down. The nurse intervenes to modify environmental conditions that may increase myocardial oxygen demand. Examples include restricting visitors who increase anxiety or prevent the patient from getting adequate rest, and modifying environmental heat or cold. In addition, the nurse attempts to decrease the patient's anxiety level. The patient should be approached in a calm and quiet manner (often quite the opposite occurs in the hectic setting of the emergency department or coronary care unit), and explanations should be offered about care and procedures that will affect the patient.

### Monitoring Tissue Perfusion

Patients with AMI may experience alterations in tissue perfusion of the skin, brain, kidneys, and other organs in addition to alterations in myocardial perfusion. These alterations occur from a decrease in cardiac output that results from the impaired myocardial contractility. Monitoring for these alterations is a critical part of nursing management of patients with MI. Frequent measurement of vital signs is necessary.

**guidelines for care**

**The Patient Receiving Thrombolytic Therapy**

**Patient Eligibility**

Within 4 to 6 hours of symptom onset
Symptom duration of at least 30 minutes
ECG pattern strongly suggestive of acute myocardial infarction

**Patient Screening**

Screen for bleeding risks: severe hypertension, active bleeding or known bleeding disorders, current anticoagulation therapy, recent surgery or trauma (including CPR), intracranial neoplasm, aneurysm, AV malformation, history of cerebral hemorrhage
Establish baseline vital signs and physical exam for overt/covert bleeding, such as unexplained hypotension or tachycardia, rigid abdomen, subtle neurological changes

**Monitor for Successful Reperfusion**

Resolution of chest pain
Resolution of ECG ST changes
Presence of reperfusion dysrhythmias, such as accelerated idioventricular rhythm
Early peak of cardiac isoenzymes

**Minimize Risk of Bleeding**

Continue assessment for bleeding, including intracranial, internal, retroperitoneal, and puncture sites
Monitor for frank and occult blood (heme/guaiac)
Monitor laboratory values for therapeutic ranges
Use caution with patient transfers
Limit and coordinate venipunctures; avoid establishing noncompressible IV access sites
Apply pressure to all venous and arterial access sites
Avoid arterial punctures after thrombolysis
Maintain a safe, clean environment

**Monitor for Reocclusion**

Recurrence of chest pain
Return of ST abnormalities
Evidence of hemodynamic compromise

**Support Patient and Family during Crisis**

Approach in a calm, quiet manner
Provide simple explanations of procedures and care
Offer realistic reassurance
Encourage family presence when interventions permit

The nurse performs frequent head-to-toe assessments that include level of consciousness and orientation, breath sounds, heart sounds, dysrhythmias, pulse amplitude, bowel sounds, urine output, and skin turgor and hydration. Abnormal findings require nurse-physician collaboration to prevent further complications.

### Preventing/Monitoring for Bleeding

The patient experiencing an acute MI who receives thrombolytic therapy has an increased risk of bleeding. All health care professionals participate in screening patients before the administration of thrombolytics. The nurse frequently assesses the patient for signs and symptoms of bleeding. Relevant findings include the onset of unexplained hypotension or tachycardia, the presence of a rigid abdomen, subtle neurological changes, frank blood in the urine, and guaiac-positive stools.

In addition to monitoring for bleeding complications, the nurse acts to prevent patient injury. Blood coagulation studies are performed at prescribed intervals, and abnormal values are reported immediately to the physician. The nurse assists in all transfers to ensure minimum abrasion to skin surfaces. The nurse limits the number of venipunctures. After either venipuncture or arterial puncture, direct manual pressure is applied to the site until complete hemostasis is obtained. Arterial punctures are avoided once thrombolytic therapy is begun, especially at sites that cannot easily be compressed to control bleeding.

#### *Monitoring anticoagulation therapy*

Anticoagulation therapy is often used in the treatment of patients with unstable angina and as adjunctive therapy to thrombolytics. Anticoagulation prevents clot formation rather than lysing existing clots as in thrombolytic therapy. Nursing interventions for the patient receiving anticoagulants (e.g., heparin) are the same as those for the patient receiving thrombolytics. These interventions include physical assessment for bleeding, prevention of physical injury, and ensuring hemostasis of puncture sites. During the administration of heparin, the nurse monitors the patient's partial thromboplastin time (PTT) for effectiveness of therapy. Notification of the physician for subsequent dose adjustment is necessary if PTTs are outside the therapeutic range of 1.5 to 2.5 times the control.

**research**

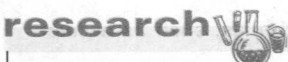

Reference: Crowe J et al: Anxiety and depression after acute myocardial infarction, *Heart Lung* 25:98, 1996.

This study analyzed survey data from 785 hospitalized patients with acute myocardial infarction (AMI), with 1-year follow-up of 201 selected patients from the sample. The purpose of the study was to determine (1) the incidence of symptoms of anxiety and depression in these patients; (2) the association among gender, infarct severity, and history of previous MI and symptoms of anxiety and depression; (3) the incidence of symptoms of anxiety and depression during the first year after AMI; and (4) the association between educational and occupational status and symptoms of anxiety and depression at the time of hospitalization. The Stait-Trait anxiety and the Beck Depression Inventory were used. The researchers found that symptoms of anxiety were prevalent among hospitalized patients who had an AMI, whereas depressive symptoms were rare. During the first 24 weeks, symptoms of moderate to severe depression were reported by 10% of the selected group of patients. No associations were found among anxiety/depression and gender, cardiac enzymes (infarct size), previous AMI, education, or occupational status.

### Relieving Anxiety

Nursing interventions to relieve anxiety are best directed at the etiology. For the MI patient, the threat of death is real. Psychological support, realistic reassurance, brief explanations about care (to the extent desired by the patient), and family visiting should be priorities for patients with MI.

After the patient's condition stabilizes, the nurse makes appropriate referrals for inpatient cardiac rehabilitation and discharge planning. Consultations include social workers, financial advisors, vocational rehabilitation advisors, case managers, chaplains, counselors, acute care nurse practitioners, and advanced nurse clinicians. The experienced staff nurse recognizes when she or he is able to meet the needs of the patient and when it is more appropriate to refer the patient to someone with greater expertise, ability, or time for immediate crisis intervention or long-term follow-up.

Anxiolytics also may be used to decrease patient anxiety. The use of anxiolytic agents is especially important during the acute phase of MI. Severe anxiety is common and increases the patient's myocardial oxygen demand at a time of decreased oxygen supply.[8] (See the Research Box.) Persistent anxiety may be effectively managed with stress reduction techniques, alone or in combination with anxiolytics. Stress reduction techniques include relaxation therapy, guided imagery, music therapy, and exercise. Although all are beneficial, an exercise program may provide the best overall outcomes for the patient with CAD.

### Improving Activity Tolerance

After an MI, the contractility of the infarcted area diminishes, and cardiac output often decreases. As a result, many MI patients experience activity intolerance. Overexertion leads to further damage because the myocardium must contract more forcefully than its weakened state allows. Guidelines for activity progression exist to increase patient conditioning without negatively affecting the balance of myocardial oxygen supply and demand. Bed rest results in deconditioning. Exercise increases collateral blood supply, increases HDLs to remove cholesterol-depositing LDLs, and effectively reduces stress. A structured rehabilitation program is ideal for patients with myocardial infarction or unstable angina. Rehabilitation begins in the acute care setting. The nurse monitors the patient for activity tolerance and makes decisions about advancing the activity level. (See the Guidelines for Care Box on advancing activity levels, p. 654.) Before ambulation, blood pressure and heart rate are checked while the patient stands. Readings are obtained before ambulation, immediately after ambulation, and 5 minutes after ambulation. Heart rate is measured for 10 seconds and then multiplied by 6. This method of heart rate calculation allows the nurse to determine an accurate postambulation heart rate before the heart rate returns to baseline. Additional parameters the nurse monitors include symptoms of pain, dyspnea, fatigue, or lightheadedness; oxygen saturation; and dysrhythmias. The nurse may collaborate with an exercise physiologist in advancing the patient's activity after MI.

After discharge from the acute care setting, patients benefit most from a structured cardiac monitored program. Exercise sessions include warm-up, aerobic exercise, and cool down. The equipment used and the intensity and duration prescribed are individualized for each patient. Once the patient safely exercises in a monitored program without experiencing adverse effects, the patient advances to an unmonitored program. The unmonitored exercise regimen is based on guidelines established for the patient during the monitored program.

Some patients may not be able to enroll in a structured program because of inaccessibility, finances, time constraints, or other reasons. The nurse reviews with these patients the components of exercise and safe programs, the benefits and limitations of exercise, and the dangers of exercise. Stress test results, when available, can be used to individualize the patient's exercise program. In different settings, the nurse, exercise physiologist, or physician may be responsible for establishing such a program. Patients with stable angina are encouraged to begin a home walking program or individualized program.

The nurse includes information about returning to work and sexual activity as part of the overall activity guidelines. A discussion of sexual activity follows for the diagnosis of altered sexuality. Return to work is individualized to the patient's occupation. A patient with a desk job and low stress levels receives different guidelines from the patient with high occupational stress or heavy labor demands.

Medications often improve a patient's tolerance of activity. Nitroglycerin taken before an activity that is known to cause angina may allow the patient to complete the activity without experiencing chest pain. Beta blockers decrease the sympathetic response to exercise, allowing patients to exercise at an increased intensity but with a safer heart rate. Myocardial oxygen demand and efficiency improve with the use of beta blockers.

Fatigue commonly limits the patient's exercise tolerance and can be related to medications. The most often cited medications producing fatigue are the beta blockers. The nurse instructs the patient about potential fatigue and what to do if it occurs. The patient taking beta blockers is cautioned not to discontinue the medication abruptly, because this can result in rebound angina and hypertension. The nurse encourages the patient to discuss concerns with a primary care provider. Interventions for medication-induced fatigue include altering the dose, prescribing another type or class of medication, and offering additional counseling or referral, particularly if the fatigue is associated with depression.

### Facilitating Return to Normal Sexual Patterns

Patients with CAD may have many concerns related to sexuality. They may be concerned about the occurrence of chest pain during sexual intercourse or their ability to perform sexually. In addition, patients may have concerns about aging or concerns related to self-concept. If a therapeutic relationship has been established between the patient and the nurse, it is usually easier for the nurse to address these concerns with the patient. The nurse reassures the patient that concerns about sexuality after MI or with the diagnosis of angina are normal and that it is important to discuss them.

The patient with unstable angina or MI requires additional guidance about resuming sexual activity safely. For the patient with unstable angina, nitroglycerin may be taken before intercourse if intercourse is known to cause angina. For the post-MI patient, guidelines for sexual activity are based on successful progression through home walking or structured outpatient exercise programs.

When the patient tolerates climbing two flights of stairs without symptoms, sexual intercourse can usually be safely

**patient/family teaching**

**Guidelines for Sexual Activity After Myocardial Infarction**

During sex, your heart beats about 117 times a minute.

**Stages of Sexual Response**

Arousal: flushed; breathing and heart rate increase; blood pressure (BP) goes up slightly.

Plateau: increase in respirations, BP, and heart rate.

Orgasm (15 to 20 seconds): pulse may reach 150 beats per minute, BP may reach 160/90.

Resolution: return to resting state within seconds; angina or palpitations are most likely to occur during resolution.

**General Guidelines**

Sexual foreplay at a relaxed pace allows your heart rate and BP to increase more slowly.

Hugging, stroking, and touching are safe ways to get back in touch with your partner.

Talk with your partner. Express your feelings.

Extramarital affairs or sex with new partners may produce more stress.

Avoid positions for sex that require you to support yourself on your arms for a long time.

Have sex in a pleasant, comfortable environment.

Do not take very hot or cold baths or showers before or after sex.

Be rested before sex.

Do not have sex after a heavy meal or drinking alcohol.

If you have any questions about side effects of any drug, do not stop taking the drug, but talk to your health care provider.

Masturbation and manual or oral stimulation are not harmful to your heart. Anal intercourse may lead to an irregular heartbeat. Avoid this choice unless you clear it with your health care professional.

resumed. The patient's spouse or partner may also have fears about the effects of sexual activity on the patient's heart. Therefore he or she should be included in all counseling and educational sessions. See the Patient/Family Teaching Box on p. 659 for additional specific information about the safe resumption of sexual activity after MI.

Beta blockers may cause impotence in some male patients. This is a very real problem and one that must be addressed. The nurse is honest in communicating the side effects of these drugs. The patient who is aware of the possibility of impotence will perhaps be better able to cope with the problem should it occur.

### Patient/Family Education

Educational plans specific to interventional procedures have been discussed earlier. For patients with CAD, the nurse develops an educational plan based on the individual's unique risk factors. An overview of educational guidelines for patients with CAD is presented in the Patient/Family Teaching Box below.

Before the patient's hospital discharge, medications are reviewed with the patient and family. The nurse reviews the purpose of the medication, dose, and possible side effects and establishes a medication schedule suited to the patient's lifestyle. This collaborative effort with the patient promotes adherence to the medical regimen. The nurse reminds patients of the need to discuss drug side effects with their health care providers and not to discontinue any medications without consultation.

The family should be included in discussions of activity progression after MI. Disagreements over activity are a major source of conflict between spouse and patient, adding to the stress of this crisis situation.

The nurse also facilitates discussion regarding the stress of this illness on children of all ages, who commonly exhibit behavior changes, sleep disturbances, and somatic complaints in response to the stress of MI involving a parent.[17]

Low-cholesterol, low-fat diets are reviewed with patients and their families before discharge. The nurse explains the results of the patient's lipid profile. Patients who have sustained an MI should have lipid profiles drawn 6 weeks after the MI to ensure an accurate baseline, because lipid metabolism is altered in the peri-MI period. The nurse teaches the patient about cholesterol-lowering agents, including the potential for unpleasant side effects such as insomnia and myositis (muscle inflammation) commonly associated with these medicines. The nurse emphasizes that lipid-lowering medications do not obliterate the need for the patient to follow recommended dietary guidelines.

#### Health promotion/prevention

Many of the *Healthy People 2000* goals are targeted at the prevention of CAD. Box 25-2 highlights the national health objectives related to coronary artery disease.

**patient/family teaching**

**The Patient with Coronary Artery Disease**

1. Risk factor modification
   a. Provide specific instructions on smoking cessation, daily exercise, and diet modification.
   b. Consider referral to a smoking cessation program or outpatient cardiac rehabilitation program.
   c. Encourage adherence to a diet low in calories, saturated fats, and cholesterol.
   d. Discuss the benefits of stress management techniques in decreasing negative effect on oxygen demand. Refer to individual or group counseling as needed.
2. Resumption of activity
   a. Discuss guidelines for resuming sexual relations (e.g., 2 weeks for low-risk patients to 4 weeks for post-CABG patients).
   b. Provide specific instructions on activities that are permissible and those that should be avoided.
   c. Discuss resumption of driving and return to work.
3. Medications
   a. Ensure understanding of the role of aspirin.
   b. Instruct patient that recurrent symptoms lasting more than 1 to 2 minutes should prompt the patient to stop all activities, sit down, and take a sublingual nitroglycerin tablet. This may be repeated at 5-minute intervals for two additional tablets if needed. If symptoms persist, access emergency medical services (call 911).
   c. Teach correct use and storage of nitroglycerin (see the Patient/Family Teaching Box on p. 656).
   d. Instruct patient in purpose, dose, and major side effects of each medication prescribed.

**box 25-2** *Year 2000 National Health Objectives: Highlights of the Priority Areas Specific to Cardiology*

- Reduce coronary heart disease deaths to no more than 100 per 100,000 people.
- Increase to at least 75% the proportion of adults who have had their blood cholesterol checked within the preceding 5 years.
- Increase to at least 75% the proportion of primary care providers who initiate diet and drug therapy at levels of blood cholesterol consistent with current management guidelines for patients with high blood cholesterol.
- Increase to at least 50% the proportion of work sites that offer blood pressure and cholesterol education.
- Increase to at least 90% the proportion of adults who have had their blood pressure checked within the preceding 2 years.
- Increase to at least 90% the proportion of people with high blood pressure who are taking action to help control their blood pressure.
- Reduce dietary fat intake for the general population to an average of 30% of calories.

From US Department of Health and Human Services Public Health Service: *Healthy People 2000: summary report,* Boston, 1992, Jones & Bartlett.

## EVALUATION

To evaluate the effectiveness of nursing interventions, compare patient behaviors with those stated in the expected patient outcomes. Successful achievement of patient outcomes for the patient with CAD is indicated by:

1. Absence of chest pain or anginal equivalent, or effective control of angina through the use of medications
2. Adequate cardiac output to maintain perfusion to all organs
3. Absence of bleeding or appropriate treatment when bleeding occurs despite precautionary measures
4. Ability to seek and process information
5. Activity progression working toward baseline
6. Ability to discuss concerns, including sexuality issues, and develop a plan to explore resolution of issues.

## GERONTOLOGICAL CONSIDERATIONS

The prevalence of CAD increases with advancing age. In assessing chest pain in the elderly, the nurse is aware that elderly patients may have atypical signs and symptoms and may delay seeking care. Older patients often experience "silent MIs," coming to the emergency department with shortness of breath, heart failure, or pulmonary edema, but without chest pain. Absence of chest pain as a classic symptom often impedes recognition of the fact that the elderly person might be experiencing a heart attack. Elderly patients may therefore delay longer in seeking medical care for the evaluation of their "heart condition," especially when they have a long history of angina. Elderly patients also may delay seeking care because they are reluctant to go to the hospital, do not want to "bother" anyone, or are experiencing loneliness and depression. Diminished cardiac reserve and altered response to inotropic medications place the elderly patient at risk for the development of heart failure or cardiogenic shock.

Elderly patients may be especially sensitive to certain medications. The nurse carefully observes for side effects and drug interactions. The nurse anticipates that the elderly patient may require higher doses of vasoactive agents to achieve desired effects.

**research**

Reference: Keeling A, Dennison P: Telephone follow-up after acute myocardial infarction: a pilot study, *Heart Lung* 24(1):45, 1995.

The purpose of this study was (1) to determine the receptivity of acute myocardial infarction (AMI) patients and spouses to postdischarge follow-up telephone calls from a nurse and (2) to describe the content of nurse-patient/spouse telephone conversations during early convalescence at home. Twenty-one AMI patients and their spouses/significant others were telephoned by an advanced practice nurse 3 times during the first 3 weeks after hospital discharge. All subjects were receptive to telephone follow-up. Five content themes emerged: (1) difficulty accepting the changed health status, (2) reports of attempts at risk factor reduction, (3) concern for financial difficulties, (4) dealing with uncertainty, and (5) an expression of appreciation for the nurse-initiated phone call. The cardiac nurse clinicians provided information and emotional support and made referrals. Developing the nurse-patient/spouse relationship in the hospital and extending it to the home to provide assistance during highly stressful, transitional periods enhances the process of recovery and promotes satisfaction with the health care delivery system.

## SPECIAL ENVIRONMENTS FOR CARE

### Critical Care Management

With the advent of coronary care units (CCUs) in the 1960s attention focused on the early hospitalization of patients with chest pain. During that era, the patient typically spent 5 to 7 days in the CCU and at least 10 to 14 days in a step-down unit. The prolonged hospitalization allowed time for significant patient teaching before discharge. Today, with the use of thrombolytic therapy, PTCA, stents, and atherectomy, as well as the influences of managed care, the average hospital stay after an MI has been significantly decreased. The patient is kept in the CCU for 24 hours or until stabilized. The care provided in the CCU is as outlined in the collaborative care discussion. Patients who are not critically ill are admitted directly to monitored units designed specifically for cardiac patients. The average length of stay is 5 to 7 days after MI and 2 to 3 days for patients undergoing PTCA.

### Home Care Management

Given the trend of earlier hospital discharge, much of the recovery from AMI (or from PTCA, stent, or atherectomy) takes place in the patient's home. Before discharge the patient and family must receive sufficient information about what to expect during this recovery period so that they can adequately manage the patient's care at home. Of particular importance is information about medications, activity progression, what to do for recurrent chest pain, and what to do if bleeding from an arterial catheter insertion site should occur. Many patients and families have questions about their care when they get home that they did not think to ask in the hospital. It is helpful if the nurse telephones patients within 24 hours of hospital discharge to provide additional education and support[18] (see the Research Box).

## COMPLICATIONS

The most common complications of CAD are congestive heart failure, dysrhythmias, and pericarditis. The likelihood of complications increases with severe multivessel CAD and with AMI. Additional complications include cardiogenic shock, ventricular septal defect, free wall rupture, ventricular aneurysms, and ischemic cardiomyopathy.

## HEART FAILURE

Heart failure in CAD occurs in response to a decrease in contractility secondary to an ischemic myocardium. A hypokinetic or akinetic myocardium will not generate the inotropic action needed to sustain an adequate cardiac output. The amount of ischemic or infarcted myocardium determines the onset and severity of heart failure. Heart failure is most often seen in patients having large MIs, particularly MIs involving the anterior surface of the myocardium. Nursing management of the patient with heart failure is presented in Chapter 26.

## DYSRHYTHMIAS

Dysrhythmias often occur secondary to the ischemic processes of CAD. Ischemia alters the stability of the myocardial cell membrane. Ischemia of the specialized conduction pathways (SA node, AV node, and bundle branches) can result in heart blocks. Direct damage to the myocardial cell creates electrolyte imbalances that alter the action potential. Individuals with right coronary artery blockages and inferior MIs may have heart blocks and bradycardia because the right coronary artery most often supplies the SA and AV nodes. Patients with left anterior descending artery blockages may have complete or incomplete bundle branch blocks and ventricular dysrhythmias, because the left anterior descending artery supplies the bundle branch system and a disproportionately large surface of the anterior myocardium. The management of common dysrhythmias is presented later in the chapter.

## PERICARDITIS

After AMI, the pericardial lining of the heart can become inflamed and fluid may accumulate between the parietal and visceral layers. The patient complains of severe precordial chest pain that closely resembles that of AMI. The presence of a characteristic pericardial friction rub is helpful in the differential diagnosis. Pericarditis is usually treated with nonsteroidal antiinflammatory drugs (NSAIDs) or occasionally corticosteroids. Pericarditis is presented in greater detail in Chapter 26.

## DRESSLER'S SYNDROME

Post–myocardial infarction syndrome, or Dressler's syndrome, is a late complication of AMI. Classic signs and symptoms include pericardial chest pain, low-grade fever, a pericardial friction rub, and pericardial and pleural effusions. These signs and symptoms occur 2 to 10 weeks after the MI. The syndrome resembles an autoimmune response, and the patient receives symptomatic treatment.

## ISCHEMIC CARDIOMYOPATHY

As more aggressive interventions for CAD and specifically MI become standard, patients are surviving with hearts that may be severely damaged. Myocardial contractility decreases in the patient with ischemic cardiomyopathy. This decrease in systolic function decreases cardiac output and can result in episodes of heart failure. (See Chapter 26.)

## CARDIOGENIC SHOCK

Cardiogenic shock is caused by myocardial dysfunction that is severe enough to cause end-organ hypoperfusion. This form of shock is characterized by the following: (1) a systolic BP less than 80 mm Hg with normal heart filling pressures (i.e., no hypovolemia); (2) a decrease in urinary output; (3) an altered mental status; (4) compensatory tachycardia; and (5) cold, clammy skin. Cardiogenic shock occurs in 5% to 10% of patients with AMI and has an in-hospital mortality rate of 80% despite aggressive treatment. Survivors are usually young, received early treatment during the evolving MI, and were responsive to pressor agents.

Cardiogenic shock is a medical emergency, and early diagnosis is imperative. Therapy is aimed at correcting factors that contribute to decreased tissue perfusion, such as dysrhythmias, hypoxemia, and decreased cardiac output. Intervention to maintain cardiac output must occur before left ventricular function decreases further from decreased coronary artery perfusion. If untreated, a series of events occur that spiral the patient toward lactic acidosis and death. Pressor agents such as dobutamine and dopamine are often used in combination to support perfusion. An IABP may be inserted to augment coronary artery perfusion during diastole and decrease afterload. The most effective treatment for cardiogenic shock appears to be primary PTCA. Survival rates are significantly improved if the occluded artery can be opened quickly. However, PTCA cannot be used to treat occlusion in the left main coronary artery, and surgical bypass grafting is performed on an emergent basis. See Chapter 17 for a further discussion of shock.

## VENTRICULAR SEPTAL DEFECT

Ventricular septal defect (VSD) is a relatively uncommon early complication of AMI, occurring in 1% to 3% of patients. Ventricular septal defect occurs most often in the female patient who has a history of hypertension and is suffering her first MI as a result of single-vessel occlusion. In these circumstances collateral circulation has usually not been established. The classic manifestation of VSD is the development of a new systolic murmur within the first 3 days after infarction. An echocardiogram confirms the presence of VSD, and surgical repair is required. Ventricular septal defect is associated with a high mortality rate.

## FREE WALL RUPTURE

Free wall rupture refers to the rupture of an area of weakened myocardium that is not supported by the septum. This complication accounts for 5% to 7% of infarct deaths. Women with hypertension and transmural infarction are at high risk for developing this fatal complication.

## VENTRICULAR ANEURYSM

A ventricular aneurysm develops in 12% to 15% of patients experiencing transmural infarcts. The aneurysm is a noncontractile, thinned left ventricular wall that may bulge outward during systole, reducing stroke volume. Blood can collect in the aneurysm, resulting in emboli formation. Most aneurysms occur in the apex of the heart.

The diagnosis is made from the presence of a ventricular gallop, persisent ST elevations after MI, and chest x-ray showing an enlarged left ventricle. A paradoxical expansion of the aneurysmal sac during systole can be seen on fluoroscopy during cardiac catheterization or on echocardiogram.

Ventricular aneurysms can cause heart failure, systemic emboli, and ventricular tachycardia. Treatment is directed toward surgical repair of the aneurysm (aneurysmectomy) and

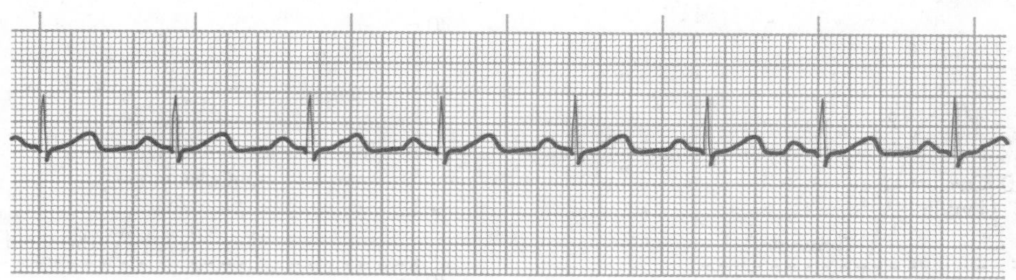

fig. 25-10 Normal sinus rhythm; heart rate, 80.

control of complications. Prognosis depends on the size of the aneurysm, severity of CAD, and the degree of left ventricular impairment.

## CARDIAC DYSRHYTHMIAS

### Etiology/Epidemiology

Normal sinus rhythm begins with the spontaneous depolarization of the SA node. The impulse conducts through the atria to the AV node and then through the bundle of His and bundle branches to the Purkinje fibers. (See Figure 24-5.) A rhythm is classified as "normal" when it meets the following criteria: presence of one upright and consistent-appearing P wave before each QRS complex, all PR intervals between 0.12 and 0.20 seconds, and a consistent-appearing QRS complex of less than 0.12 seconds. The RR interval is consistent, and the heart rate is between 60 and 100 beats per minute (Figure 25-10). Chapter 24 presents the normal heart rhythm in more depth.

Cardiac dysrhythmias are the result of alterations in impulse formation or propagation. Dysrhythmias are often classified by the anatomical site of the dysfunction, for example, sinus dysrhythmias and atrial dysrhythmias. The underlying etiology varies with each specific dysrhythmia. Common etiologies including underlying cardiac disease, sympathetic stimulation, vagal stimulation, electrolyte imbalances, and hypoxia.

Benign dysrhythmias such as sinus bradycardia and occasional premature beats are common in the general population, but dysrhythmias are more prevalent in patients with cardiac disease. In patients with CAD, a benign rhythm may have negative consequences because the myocardium is already impaired. The most common dysrhythmia is atrial fibrillation.

The collaborative management section presents the common dysrhythmias along with the diagnostic criteria and medical and nursing interventions related to each. Unique factors related to the etiology and epidemiology of each dysrhythmia will also be discussed when appropriate.

### Pathophysiology

An understanding of normal cardiac electrophysiology is necessary to grasp the pathophysiology of dysrhythmias. Chapter 24 provides a thorough overview of the heart's normal conduction physiology.

Alterations in impulse formation and propagation arise from one of three pathophysiological processes: altered auto-

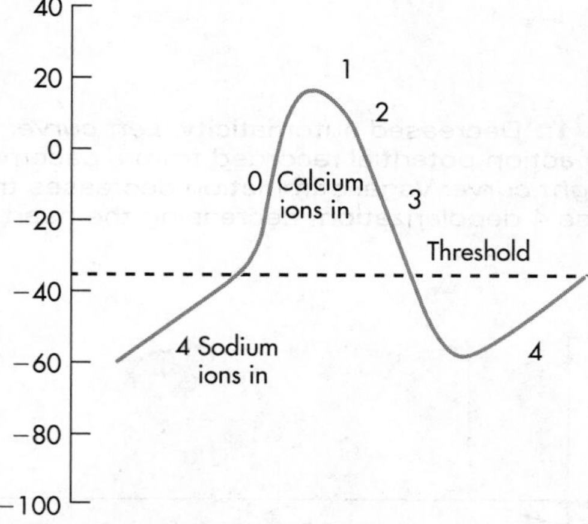


fig. 25-11 The action potential recorded from a pacemaker cell.

maticity, altered conduction resulting in delays or blocks, and reentry mechanisms.

#### Alterations in automaticity

Automaticity, the ability to depolarize spontaneously without external stimulation, is a property that normally is confined to the cells of the SA node. The SA node usually depolarizes at a faster rate than other potential pacemaker cells because of the steep slope of phase 4, allowing sinus cells to reach threshold at a faster rate (Figure 25-11). A variety of conditions can alter the automaticity of the SA node and produce faster or slower than usual heart rates. Vagal stimulation will decrease this slope, resulting in a slower heart rate (Figure 25-12). Sympathetic stimulation and hypoxia will steepen phase 4, resulting in faster heart rates (Figure 25-13).

If the rate of phase 4 depolarization found in the AV node or ventricular conduction system increases, enhanced automaticity is said to exist. The result may be premature beats or tachycardias. Some causes of enhanced automaticity are hypoxia, catecholamines, hypokalemia, hypocalcemia, atropine, heat, trauma, and digitalis toxicity.

Even cells that do not normally have automaticity may develop abnormal automaticity if the resting membrane potential or threshold potential is altered. Increasing the threshold slows the heart rate because it then takes longer to reach threshold (Figure 25-14). If the resting membrane potential is

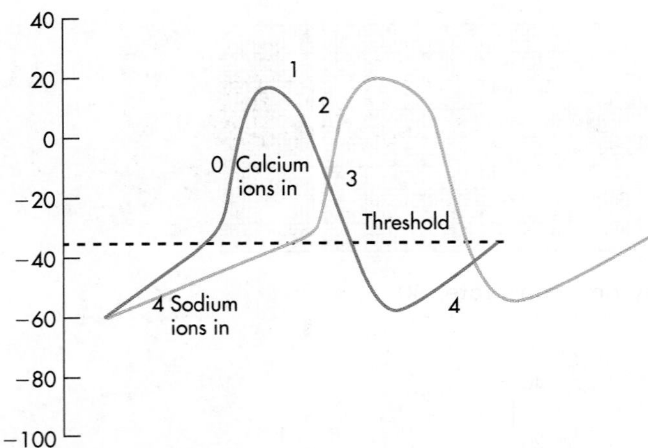


**fig. 25-12** Decreased automaticity. *Left curve:* The normal action potential recorded from a pacemaker cell. *Right curve:* Vagal stimulation decreases the rate of phase 4 depolarization, decreasing the heart rate.

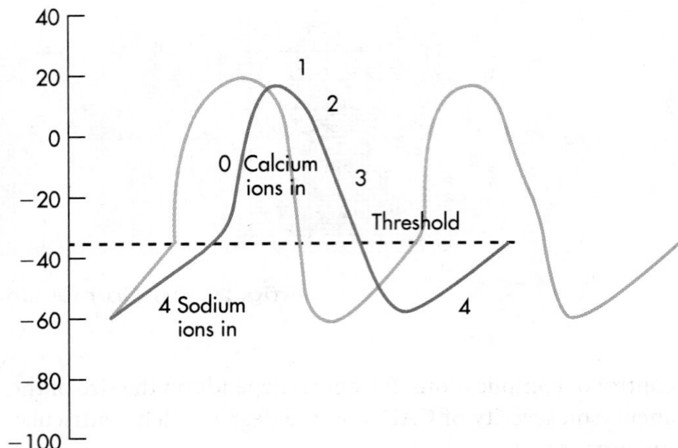


**fig. 25-13** Increased automaticity. *Left curve:* Sympathetic stimulation and hypoxia steepen phase 4 depolarization, increasing the heart rate. *Right curve:* The normal action potential recorded from a pacemaker cell.

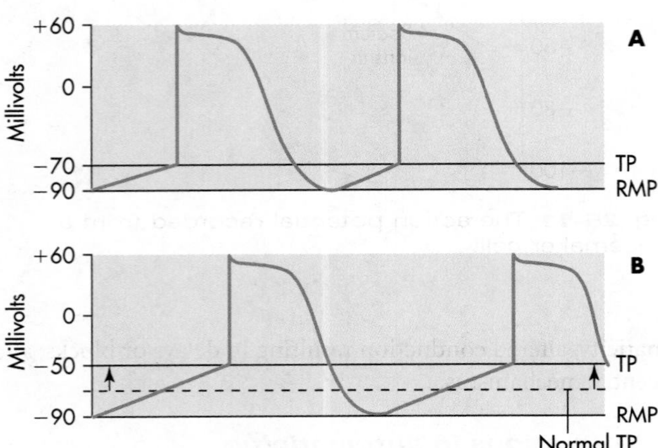


**fig. 25-14** Decreased automaticity. **A,** Normal action potential recorded from a nonpacemaker cell. **B,** Making the threshold potential less negative increases the time needed to reach threshold, decreasing heart rate.

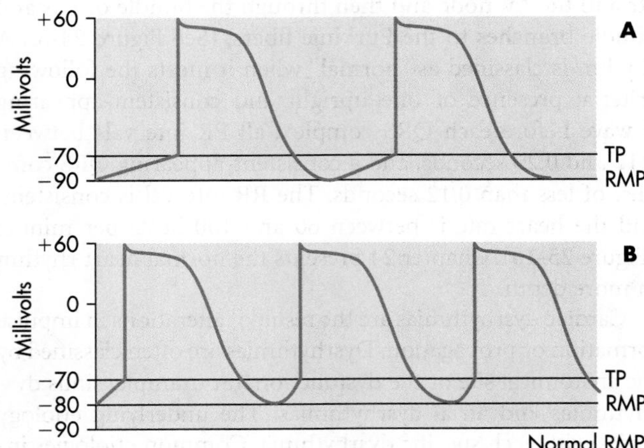


**fig. 25-15** Increased automaticity. **A,** Normal action potential recorded from a nonpacemaker cell. **B,** Making the resting membrane potential less negative makes it easier to reach threshold, increasing heart rate.

made less negative, automaticity will increase because it is easier to reach threshold (Figure 25-15). Altered automaticity may be a consequence of ischemia, infarction, hypokalemia, hypocalcemia, or cardiomyopathy. This abnormal automaticity is not easily suppressed by the activity of faster pacemakers.

### *Alterations in conduction*

When the rate or amplitude of depolarization decreases, conduction also decreases. Electrolyte imbalances affect the rate of depolarization by altering the resting membrane potential. Hyperkalemia causes the resting membrane potential to be more positive, decreasing the rate of depolarization and slowing conduction. Any condition that decreases the amplitude of the action potential, such as ischemia, hypercalcemia, or calcification of the conducting fibers, can cause cardiac conduction disturbances. Abnormalities in conduction occur anywhere in the conduction system, including the SA node, the AV node, and the bundle branches. The severity of impaired conduction ranges from a slight delay to complete cessation or block of impulse transmission.

### *Reentry*

Reentry occurs when an impulse is delayed within a pathway of slow conduction long enough that the impulse is still viable when the remaining myocardium repolarizes. The impulse then reenters surrounding tissue and produces another impulse.

This typically occurs when two different pathways share an initial and final segment. The first impulse travels down the

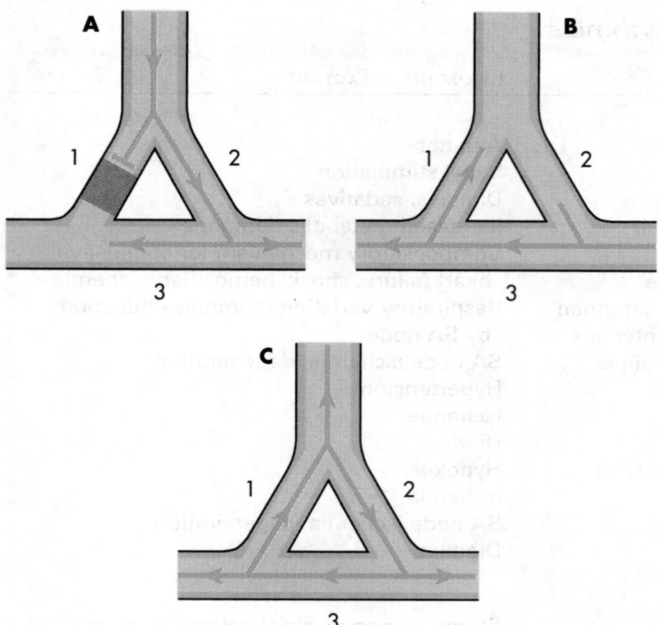


fig. 25-16 Reentry. A, Shaded area shows refractory area after the first impulse passes down path 1. Premature impulse is then blocked from entering path 1 but can travel down path 2. B, Path 1 is no longer refractory to stimulation; therefore, a premature impulse can travel backwards up path 1. C, Reentry down path 2 establishes circuitous pathway.

faster pathway, leaving behind its refractory trail. Should a second, early impulse follow, it will be blocked because that path is refractory. The second impulse then enters the slow pathway and can return retrograde through the fast path, initiating a circuitous pattern (Figure 25-16).

### Clinical manifestations

Many patients with dysrhythmias are asymptomatic as long as cardiac output meets the body's metabolic demands. The clinical manifestations associated with most dysrhythmias directly relate to decreases in cardiac output from slow or fast heart rates. Significant changes in heart rate may not allow adequate time for the ventricles to fill and empty. Clinical manifestations include those listed in Box 25-3. In addition, patients may complain of palpitations (e.g., a "racing heart" or "skipping beats") related to changes in heart rate and stroke volume. These symptoms often create acute anxiety.

## Collaborative Care Management

The diagnosis of dysrhythmias begins with the 12-lead ECG. Each dysrhythmia exhibits characteristic changes in the ECG tracing. A systematic approach to analyzing the ECG rhythm helps distinguish the different dysrhythmias (Box 25-4). Table 25-6 outlines the rhythm criteria that define each common dysrhythmia and its common associated etiologies. Other diagnostic tests used in the evaluation of dysrhythmias include signal-averaged electrocardiography, ambulatory Holter monitoring, and electrophysiology studies (see Chapter 24).

**box 25-3 Clinical Manifestations of Cardiac Dysrhythmias**

**GENERAL**

Palpitations (racing heart, skipped beats)
Anxiety
Fatigue

**ALTERED CARDIAC OUTPUT**

Pallor
Cool, clammy skin
Cyanotic
Shortness of breath
Rales
Decreased blood pressure
Confusion
Dizziness
Weakness
Presyncope
Syncope with loss of consciousness
Chest pain
Atrial thrombi (may dislodge to cause systemic emboli)

**box 25-4 Systematic Interpretation of ECG Tracing**

1. Rate (atrial and ventricular)
2. Rhythm (atrial and ventricular)
3. Presence or absence of P waves
4. PR interval 0.12-0.20 sec
5. QRS complex 0.06-0.12 sec
6. Relationship of QRS to P wave
7. QT interval <0.55 sec
8. Interpretation

*Note:* A normal sinus rhythm has an atrial (P) and ventricular (QRS) rate of 60 to 100 beats per minute, a regular rhythm (constant PP and RR intervals), and a P wave before every QRS.

Medical and nursing management of dysrhythmias focuses on alleviating symptoms from altered cardiac output and eliminating or reversing the etiology. Interventions specific to each dysrhythmia are included in the discussion that follows.

### Sinus bradycardia

Sinus bradycardia is characterized by atrial and ventricular rates of less than 60 beats per minute (Figure 25-17). In all other respects, sinus bradycardia has the normal parameters for sinus rhythm. It may develop gradually or occur suddenly for a brief period.

Bradycardia generally results from increased vagal tone or decreased symphathetic tone. It is commonly seen in athletes and may also be associated with sleep, vomiting, and MI. Carotid sinus stimulation and drugs such as digoxin, morphine sulfate, and sedatives induce sinus bradycardia in many patients.

**table 25-6** *Comparison of Selected Cardiac Dysrhythmias*

| Dysrhythmia | ECG Diagnostic Criteria | Etiological Factors |
|---|---|---|
| **DYSRHYTHMIAS OF SINUS NODE** | | |
| Sinus bradycardia | P waves present followed by QRS<br>Rhythm regular<br>Heart rate <60 | Athletes<br>Vagal stimulation<br>Digitalis, sedatives |
| Sinus tachycardia | P waves present followed by QRS<br>Rhythm regular<br>Heart rate 100-150 beats per minute | Increased metabolic demands<br>Compensatory mechanism for congestive heart failure, shock, hemorrhage, anemia |
| Sinus dysrhythmia | Phasic shortening with inspiration, lengthening with expiration of PP and RR intervals | Respiratory variation in impulse initiation by SA node |
| Sick sinus syndrome | Sinus bradycardia alternating with sinus tachycardia | SA node ischemia, degeneration<br>Hypertension<br>Ischemia<br>Digoxin |
| Sinus exit block/sinus arrest | Isoelectric line (pause) without P or QRS | Hypoxia<br>Ischemia<br>SA node ischemia, degeneration<br>Digoxin |
| **ATRIAL DYSRHYTHMIAS** | | |
| Premature atrial beats | Early P wave<br>QRS may or may not be normal<br>Pause follows QRS | Stress, ischemia, atrial enlargement, caffeine, nicotine |
| Wandering atrial pacemaker | P waves of different appearances or buried in QRS; varying PR intervals | Cardiac disease<br>Drug toxicity |
| Atrial tachycardia | P wave present (may be hidden in previous T wave), QRS usually normal, heart rate usually >150 beats per minute | Sympathetic stimulation, caffeine, nicotine, drug toxicity<br>Pulmonary disease |
| Atrial flutter | Atrial rate 250-350; F waves usually in a ratio to QRS complexes such as 2:1, 3:1; QRS complexes normal | Heart disease<br>Pulmonary disease<br>Valve disease<br>Cardiac surgery |
| Atrial fibrillation | Rapid, indiscernible P waves (>350/min)<br>Ventricular rhythm irregularly irregular<br>Ventricular rate varies | Rheumatic heart disease<br>Atrial ischemia<br>Coronary atherosclerotic disease<br>Hypertension<br>Thyrotoxicosis<br>Cardiac surgery<br>Alcohol |
| **JUNCTIONAL DYSRHYTHMIAS** | | |
| Premature junctional beat | Early beat<br>P before, during, or after QRS<br>P inverted or retrograde<br>PR interval <0.12 if P before QRS<br>QRS normal | Increased metabolism<br>Nicotine<br>Caffeine<br>Ischemia<br>Electrolyte imbalance |
| Junctional rhythm | P before, during, or after QRS<br>P inverted or retrograde<br>PR interval <0.12 if P before QRS<br>QRS normal<br>Rate 40-60, junctional rhythm<br>Rate 60-100, accelerated junctional rhythm<br>Rate >100, junctional tachycardia | Accelerated:<br>Heart disease<br>Caffeine<br>Pain<br>Digoxin |
| **VENTRICULAR DYSRHYTHMIAS** | | |
| Premature ventricular beats (PVBs) | Early, wide, bizarre QRS, not associated with a P wave<br>Rhythm irregular | Stress, acidosis, ventricular enlargement<br>Electrolyte imbalance<br>Myocardial infarction<br>Digitalis toxicity<br>Hypoxemia, hypercapnia |
| Accelerated idioventricular rhythm (AIVR)/ventricular tachycardia (VT) | P not associated with QRS, QRS wide and bizarre<br>VT: ventricular rate >100, usually 140-240<br>AIVR: rate 40-100 | VT: hypoxemia, drug toxicity, electrolyte imbalance, bradycardia, CAD<br>AIVR: reperfusion |

Continued

**table 25-6** *Comparison of Selected Cardiac Dysrhythmias—cont'd*

| Dysrhythmia | ECG Diagnostic Criteria | Etiological Factors |
|---|---|---|
| **VENTRICULAR DYSRHYTHMIAS—cont'd** | | |
| Torsade de Pointes | No associated P waves<br>Wide, bizarre QRSs twist along isoelectric line<br>HR >100 | Medications<br>Electrolyte imbalance<br>Congenital prolonged QT interval |
| Ventricular fibrillation | No recognizable complexes<br>Wavy line of varying amplitude | Myocardial infarction<br>Electrocution<br>Drowning |
| Ventricular asystole | No complexes<br>"Straight line" | Myocardial infarction<br>Chronic diseases of conducting system |
| **IMPULSE CONDUCTION DEFICITS** | | |
| First-degree atrioventricular (AV) block | PR interval prolonged, >0.20 sec | Rheumatic fever<br>Myocardial infarction<br>Cardiac medications |
| Second-degree AV blocks | | |
| Mobitz I | P waves usually occur regularly at rates consistent with SA node initiation.<br>PR interval lengthened before nonconducted P wave; QRS may be widened | Acute myocardial infarction<br>Increased vagal tone<br>Electrolyte imbalance<br>Infection |
| Mobitz II | Constant PR intervals<br>Nonconducted P waves at random or patterned intervals | Coronary artery disease<br>Myocardial infarction<br>Rheumatic heart disease<br>Digoxin |
| Complete third-degree AV block | Atria and ventricles beat independently<br>P waves have no relation to QRS<br>Ventricular rate may be as low as 20-40/min if ventricular; 40-60 if junctional | Digitalis toxicity<br>Coronary artery disease<br>Myocardial infarction |
| Bundle branch block | Same as normal sinus rhythm except QRS duration >0.10 | Hypoxia, acute myocardial infarction, congestive heart failure, coronary atherosclerosis, hypertension |

Generally, sinus bradycardia is a benign rhythm. In association with MI, it may be a beneficial rhythm because it reduces myocardial oxygen demand. If the heart rate is too slow to maintain adequate cardiac output, the patient may be predisposed to syncope and congestive heart failure. Administration of atropine or isoproterenol is usually effective in increasing the heart rate.

### *Sinus tachycardia*

Sinus tachycardia is characterized by an atrial and ventricular rate of 100 beats per minute or more (Figure 25-18). Generally the upper limit of sinus tachycardia is 150 beats per minute. The P waves are sinus in origin, but they may be buried in the T wave with very high heart rates. Intervals and complexes are within normal limits. The onset of sinus tachycardia usually is gradual as the sinus node rate increases in response to higher metabolic needs.

Sinus tachycardia is associated with the ingestion of alcohol, caffeine, and tobacco. It is a normal physiological response to exertion, fever, fear, excitement, acute pain, or any condition that requires a higher basal metabolism. Clinically sinus tachycardia is a short-term compensatory mechanism associated with heart failure, anemia, hypovolemia, and hypotension. Sinus tachycardia is also seen with hyperthyroidism and may be produced by drugs such as atropine and amphetamines.

Generally, sinus tachycardia is a benign rhythm that slows with resolution of the etiology. The patient may complain of palpitations or have no symptoms. In the patient with a compromised myocardium, the tachycardia may cause a decrease in cardiac output with resultant lightheadedness, chest pain, and heart failure. Sinus tachycardia can usually be slowed with digoxin, beta blockers, or diltiazem if necessary.

### *Sinus dysrhythmia*

Sinus dysrhythmia is the most common dysrhythmia. It is typically found in young adults and elderly persons. Sinus dysrhythmia is an irregular rhythm in which PP intervals vary by more than 0.16 second. The P waves have a constant morphology, and the PR interval and QRS duration are within normal limits. Changes in PP intervals are accompanied by changes in RR intervals (Figure 25-19).

The cyclic pattern of changing PP or RR intervals correlates with the patterns of inspiration and expiration. During inspiration the intervals shorten as the heart rate increases. Conversely, the intervals lengthen during expiration.

Sinus dysrhythmia is not treated unless the bradycardia phase is marked, causing symptoms. With slower heart rates,

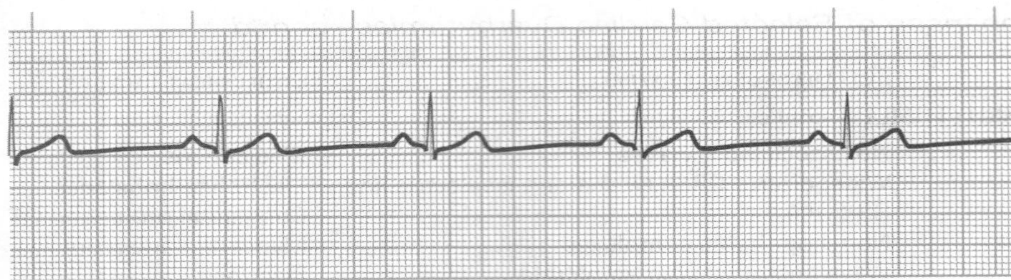

fig. 25-17 Sinus bradycardia; heart rate, 40.

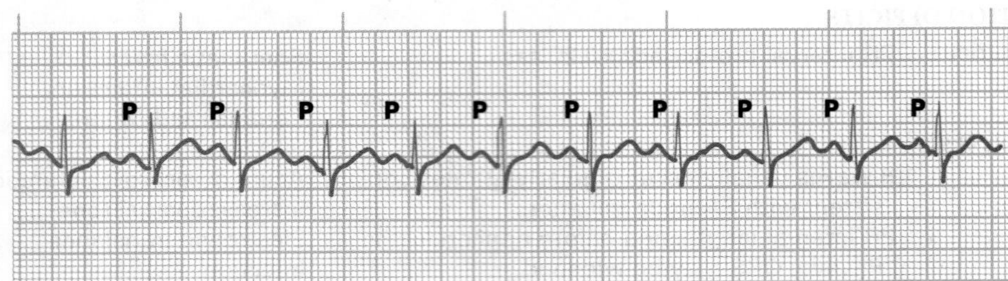


fig. 25-18 Sinus tachycardia; heart rate, 110.

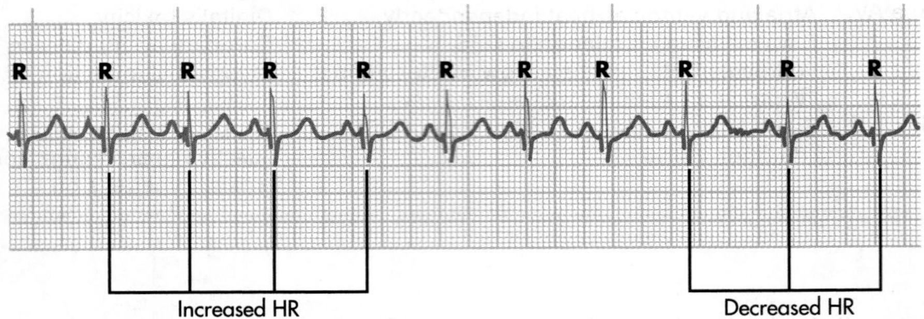


fig. 25-19 Sinus dysrhythmia. Heart rate increases with inspiration and decreases with expiration; overall heart rate, 100.

some patients may experience palpitations or dizziness if the PP intervals are unusually long. Atropine may be effective in treating symptomatic bradycardia.

### Sick sinus syndrome

Tachycardia-bradycardia syndrome is characterized by the presence of bradycardia with intermittent episodes of tachydysrhythmias. The episode of tachydysrhythmia often is followed by a long pause before returning to sinus bradycardia. Sick sinus syndrome (SSS) is one type of tachycardia-bradycardia syndrome. In SSS, the bradycardia and tachycardia are both sinus in origin. Complications of this inefficient rhythm include heart failure and cerebrovascular accident resulting from thromboembolism. In addition, cerebral blood flow may be decreased, producing confusion in the elderly person. Sick sinus syndrome is associated with ischemia or degeneration of the SA node.

Some patients may remain free of symptoms or complain only of palpitations. For the patient with severe symptoms, the heart rhythm is stabilized with a permanent implantable pacemaker for the slow phase and the administration of digoxin or beta blockers to control the ventricular rate of the tachycardia phase.

### Sinus exit block and sinus arrest

Sinus exit block occurs when an impulse originates in the SA node but is blocked immediately (Figure 25-20). No P wave or QRS complex is generated, resulting in a long pause. The next impulse occurs in a time interval representing the normal PP interval. Sinus arrest infers that the SA node never fired; therefore there is no P or QRS complex. The next impulse is asynchronous to the normal PP interval.

Sinus exit block and sinus arrest may occur as a result of medications such as digoxin, hypoxia, myocardial ischemia, and damage or injury to the SA node. The patient is symptomatic from a decrease in cardiac output when the pauses are long or frequent. The patient may feel palpitations from the strong stroke volume that accompanies the next beat after the pause. When the patient is symptomatic, atropine may be adminis-

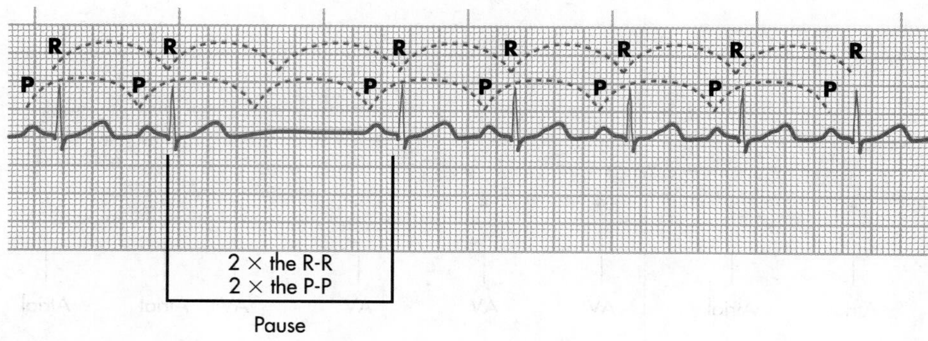


**fig. 25-20** Sinus exit block. Pause equal to two complete cardiac cycles; overall heart rate, 70.

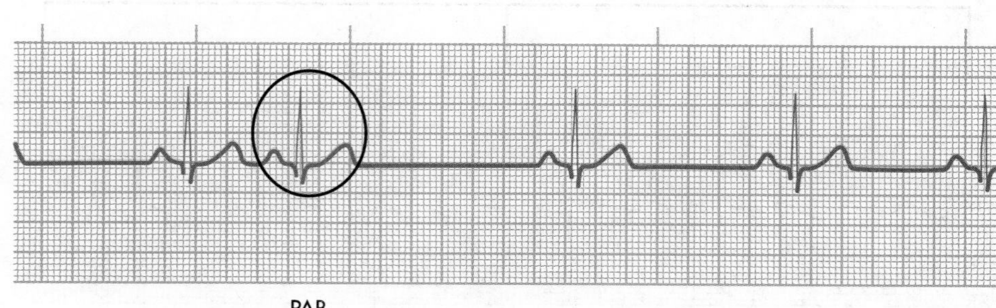


**fig. 25-21** PAB in a sinus bradycardiac rhythm; heart rate, 40.

tered to increase the heart rate and cardiac output. Definitive therapy includes the insertion of a permanent pacemaker.

### Premature atrial beat

A premature atrial beat (PAB) is initiated by an ectopic focus in the atria (Figure 25-21). It is characterized by a premature P wave with a contour different from that of a sinus P wave. The location of the ectopic focus within the atria determines its shape. The QRS complex may or may not be normal. The PAB is often followed by a pause. The atrial impulse may be nonconducted (blocked) because of refractoriness of the AV node at the time the impulse arrives. The nonconducted atrial beat (blocked PAB) is a common cause of irregularity in the heart rhythm.

The PAB may be associated with stress or the use of caffeine or tobacco products. It also is seen in the clinical setting with hypoxia, atrial enlargement, infection, inflammation, and myocardial ischemia. Frequent PABs may warn of impending atrial fibrillation or tachycardia.

In the absence of organic disease, no treatment is required. Often the elimination of caffeine and tobacco will suppress the atrial focus. Premature atrial beats may produce palpitations. Cardiac output is generally not effected unless PABs are frequent or there is a high occurrence of blocked beats.

### Wandering atrial pacemaker

Wandering atrial pacemaker occurs when at least three ectopic sites create the impulse for the cardiac rhythm (Figure 25-22). The ECG shows P waves of different shapes and PR intervals of different lengths. The impulse can originate from the area around the AV node creating inverted P waves from retrograde conduction. Impulses from this lower area may also cause stimulation of the atria at the same time or after the ventricle. The P waves then appear buried in the QRS or occur inverted after the QRS.

Wandering atrial pacemakers usually signify underlying heart disease or drug toxicity. The patient with wandering atrial pacemaker is usually asymptomatic unless the heart rate increases or decreases enough to affect cardiac output. The nurse monitors for changes in the rhythm and in the patient's symptoms.

### Atrial tachycardia

In atrial tachycardia the atrial rate is approximately 150 to 250 beats per minute. P waves are present but may be hidden in the T waves of the preceding beats when the ventricular rate is high. The QRS complex generally is normal, and the ventricular rhythm is regular.

When atrial tachycardia occurs suddenly, it is called paroxysmal atrial tachycardia (PAT) (Figure 25-23). Transient episodes of PAT may occur in children and young adults in the absence of heart disease. When underlying disease is present, it usually is of pulmonary origin or rheumatic heart disease. When the P waves vary in appearance, the rhythm is called multifocal atrial tachycardia (MAT).

The patient may complain of palpitations and experience anxiety during a tachycardic episode. Short, infrequent episodes

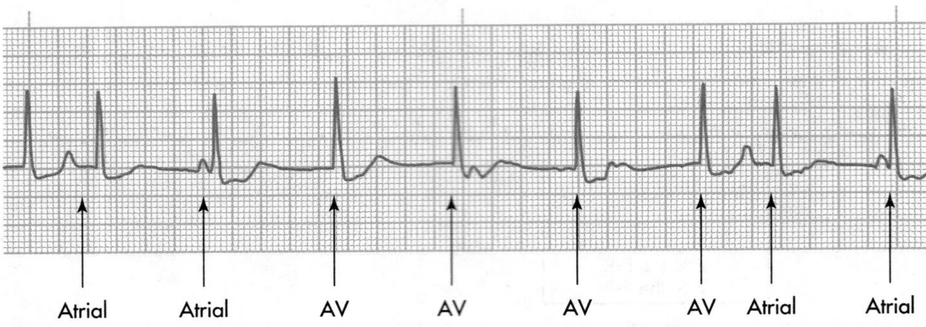


**fig. 25-22** Wandering atrial pacemaker. Sites of origin; heart rate, 90.

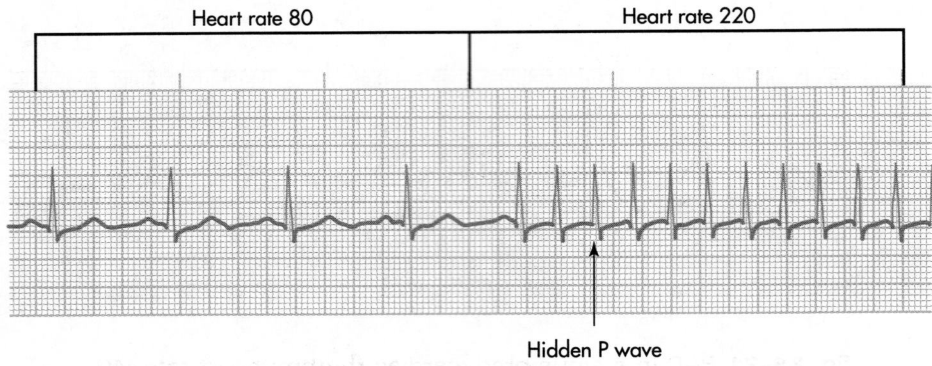


**fig. 25-23** Normal sinus rhythm; heart rate, 80, progressing to PAT; heart rate, 220.

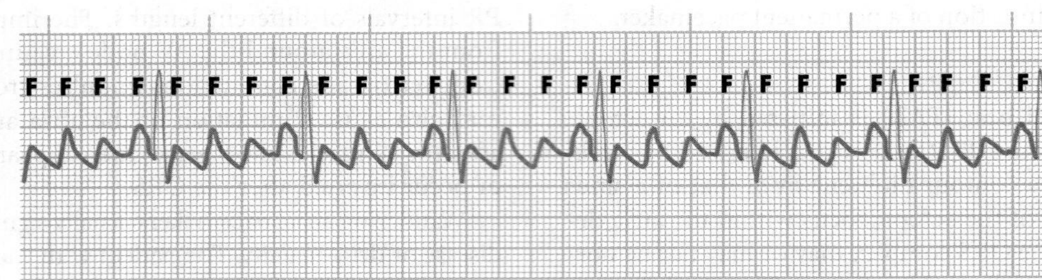


**fig. 25-24** Atrial flutter, 4:1 block. Atrial heart rate, 260; ventricular heart rate, 60.

require no treatment. Generally, hemodynamic changes are not severe unless the episode is persistent, the rate is greater than 200 beats per minute, or underlying disease exists. Lengthy paroxysms may respond to carotid sinus pressure or vagal stimulation. Some patients may benefit from receiving instruction in the performance of Valsalva's maneuver to cause slowing of the rate. Adenosine is the drug of choice to control the ventricular response. If the rate is unresponsive to adenosine, verapamil, digoxin, diltiazem, or beta blockers may be effective.

Atrial tachycardia with block is characterized by the same rapid atrial rate, but some impulses are not conducted into the ventricles (i.e., they are blocked). The AV nodal conduction ratio is usually 2:1, producing a ventricular rate of 75 to 125 beats per minute. This dysrhythmia is associated with organic heart disease. Digitalis toxicity and potassium deficit are two conditions that favor its development. The treatment depends on the clinical picture and often is aimed at correcting the underlying cause. Digitalis antibody may be indicated for hemodynamic compromise secondary to digitalis toxicity.

### Atrial flutter

In atrial flutter the atria depolarize at a rate of 250 to 350 beats per minute. The atrial depolarizations produce flutter (F) waves that give the baseline a sawtooth appearance (Figure 25-24). The QRS configurations are normal. There is no measurable PR interval because it is difficult to determine electrocardiographically which atrial impulse actually is conducted to the ventricles. With rapid atrial rates, the AV node

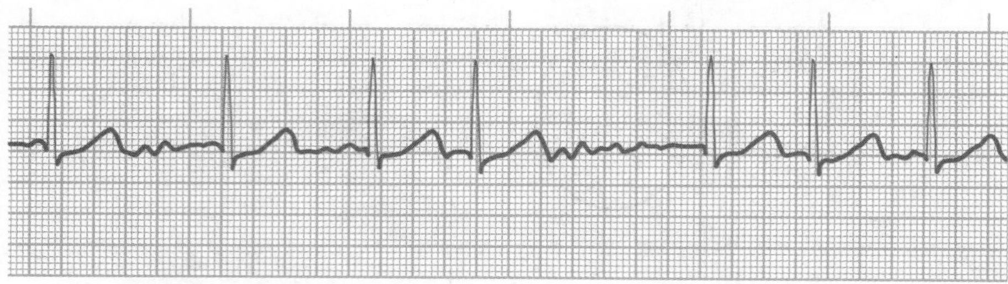

fig. 25-25 Controlled atrial fibrillation. Ventricular heart rate, 70.

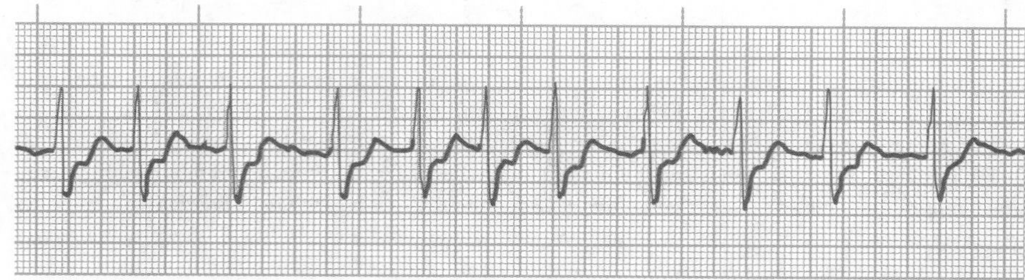

fig. 25-26 Atrial fibrillation with a rapid ventricular response. No distinguishable P waves. Ventricular heart rate, 110.

physiologically prevents conduction of each atrial impulse. The ventricles often respond to the impulses at a regular rate. The number of flutter waves to QRS complexes is expressed as a ratio (e.g., atrial flutter, 3:1 block).

Atrial flutter usually indicates underlying disease. It is associated most commonly with CAD, pulmonary embolism, mitral valve disease, thoracic surgical procedures, and chronic obstructive pulmonary disease (COPD).

The potentially rapid or slow ventricular rate of atrial flutter may result in a decrease in cardiac output. The major goal of treatment is control of the ventricular rate. Diltiazem, digoxin, or beta blockers usually succeed in slowing the ventricular rate. Atropine may be used to augment heart rate when the ventricular response is slow.

Cardioversion is highly successful in converting atrial flutter to sinus rhythm. (See the discussion of cardioversion on p. 679.) Atrial pacing may be used when pharmacological intervention and external cardioversion have been unsuccessful.

### Atrial fibrillation

Atrial fibrillation (AF) is the most rapid atrial dysrhythmia (Figures 25-25 and 25-26). It is generated and perpetuated by one or more rapidly firing ectopic foci. The atria depolarize chaotically at rates of 350 to 600 beats per minute. The baseline is composed of irregular undulations without definable P waves. The QRS complex usually is normal, but the ventricular rhythm is irregularly irregular.

Atrial fibrillation affects more than 1 million Americans, most of whom are 75 years of age or older.[11] Atrial fibrillation may be paroxysmal and transient or chronic. The latter generally indicates underlying heart disease. It is typically associated with pericarditis, thyrotoxicosis, cardiomyopathy, CAD, hypertensive heart disease, rheumatic mitral valve disease, cardiac surgery, heart failure, and excessive alcohol intake ("holiday heart").

Because of ventricular rhythm irregularity and the loss of synchronous atrial contractions (atrial kick), cardiac output is decreased. Symptoms include fatigue, dyspnea, and dizziness. Thrombi may form in the atria and cause emboli, which may lodge in the pulmonary or peripheral blood vessels. The goal of therapy is to prevent complications through control of the ventricular rate and the restoration of normal sinus rhythm (NSR). The risk of emboli may necessitate long-term anticoagulation in certain patients.

Drugs used to control fast ventricular rates include diltiazem, digoxin, and beta blockers. Digoxin is often the drug of choice in heart failure. When reentry occurs through accessory pathways, procainamide is the drug of choice. In atrial fibrillation with a slow ventricular response, atropine may be necessary to increase heart rate and cardiac output. When medications are ineffective in controlling the rate and the patient is symptomatic from an ineffective cardiac output, cardioversion may be successful in restoring a more normal heart rate.

The severity of the patient's symptoms and hemodynamic instability guide treatment decisions. Approximately 50% of patients with new-onset atrial fibrillation convert to NSR without intervention within 48 hours.[20] Several antidysrhythmics may be successful in converting AF to NSR, including procainamide, propafenone, sotalol, and amiodarone. Amiodarone has been effective for refractory AF. Adverse side effects of pulmonary toxicity, thyroid dysfunction, and skin discoloration limit its usefulness for some patients. These drugs can have a prodysrhythmic effect, and patients require careful monitoring.

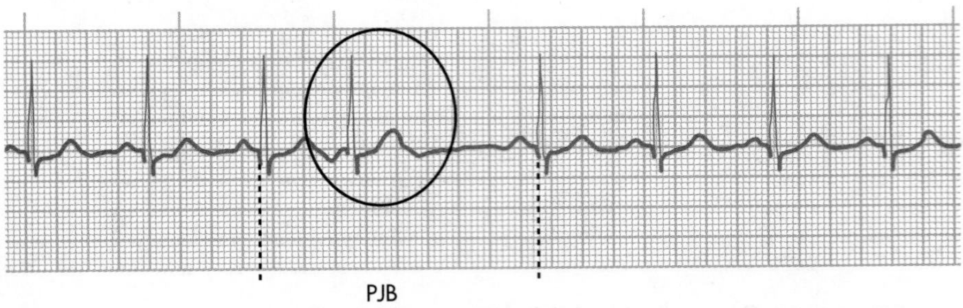


fig. 25-27 Sinus rhythm with a PJB; heart rate, 80.

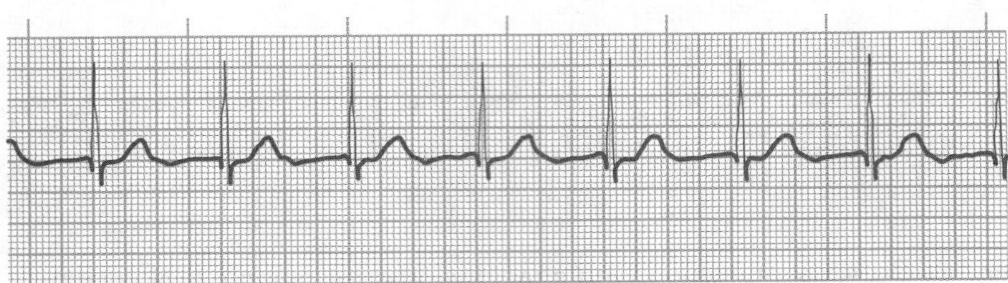

fig. 25-28 Accelerated junctional rhythm with hidden P waves; heart rate, 70.

Cardioversion is the most commonly used nonpharmacological approach for restoring NSR. Internal atrial defibrillation using less than 2 joules of energy is another treatment option. The maze procedure may also be used. In this procedure sinus impulses travel down channels created by multiple atrial incisions to reach the AV node. Endocardial radiofrequency catheter ablation isolates and treats specific areas of atrial activity and has been successful in selected situations. Permanent pacemakers may also have a role.

Conversion to NSR by pharmacological or nonpharmacological approaches can lead to systemic emboli. When AF persists beyond 48 hours, anticoagulation therapy with warfarin is initiated. An international normalized ratio (INR) of 2.0 to 3.0 is maintained for about 3 weeks before pharmacological or electrical cardioversion is attempted. Even after conversion to NSR, thrombi may form until the atria contract effectively and in synchrony. Therefore anticoagulation therapy is continued for 4 weeks after conversion to NSR. If the patient is hemodynamically unstable or has refractory symptoms, the need to electrically cardiovert may be more immediate. Transesophageal echocardiography (TEE) may be helpful in determining the presence of atrial thrombi. If no thrombi are found, heparin may be administered for 2 days, followed by electrical cardioversion and 4 more weeks of warfarin therapy. When conversion to NSR is unsuccessful, the patient receives warfarin to maintain an INR of 2.0 to 3.0. If warfarin cannot be safely administered, 325 mg of aspirin daily is recommended.[20]

### Premature junctional beats

Premature junctional beats (PJBs) arise from an ectopic focus either (1) at the junction of atrial and AV nodal tissue or (2) at the junction of AV nodal tissue and the bundle of His. If the PJBs arise from the first junction, the P wave will be inverted and premature and will precede the QRS complex. In the second case, the P wave is either hidden in the QRS or is inverted and follows the QRS (Figure 25-27). The abnormal timing and the inversion of the P wave are caused by depolarization of the atria in a retrograde fashion. The QRS is normal, but the PR interval is less than 0.12 second.

Premature junctional beats may occur in the normal heart. They also may result from digitalis toxicity, ischemia, hypoxia, pain, fever, anxiety, nicotine, caffeine, or electrolyte imbalance. Treatment, when needed, is directed toward correcting the underlying cause.

### Junctional rhythms

When the SA node fires at a rate less than 40 to 60 beats per minute, the automatic cells in the AV junction may initiate impulses (escape beats) to stabilize the rhythm. A succession of beats from the junction is a junctional escape rhythm.

The P waves may occur before, during, or after the QRS. The QRS is normal, and the ventricular rhythm is regular. Junctional escape rhythm occasionally is found in the well-trained athlete or as a complication of an acute inferior wall MI. Junctional escape rhythm generally is not treated unless the loss of atrial kick produces symptoms of low cardiac output. These patients may require artificial pacing.

When the automaticity of a junctional pacemaker increases to a rate greater than 60 beats per minute, it may usurp the SA node as the pacemaker of the heart. At a rate of 60 to 100 beats per minute, the rhythm is called an *accelerated junctional rhythm* (Figure 25-28). Accelerated junctional rhythm may be due to heart disease, pain, anemia, caffeine, or amphetamines.

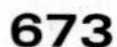

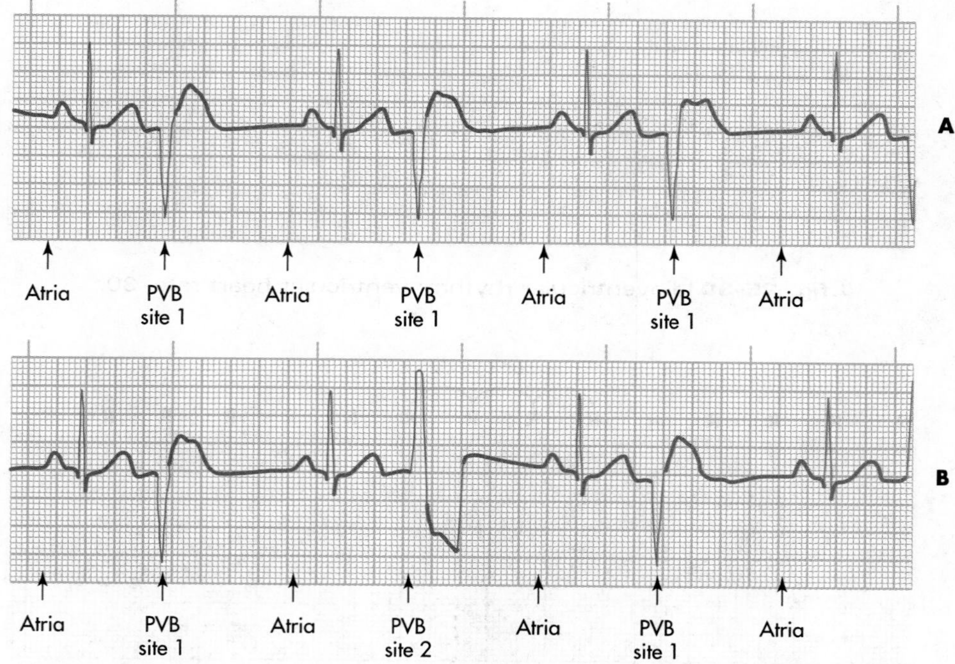


**fig. 25-29** Bigeminy. **A**, Sinus rhythm with unifocal bigeminy PVBs; heart rate, 70. **B**, Sinus rhythm with multifocal bigeminy PVBs; heart rate, 70.

A junctional tachycardia exists when the rate exceeds 100 beats per minute. Junctional tachycardia is associated with digitalis toxicity, acute rheumatic fever, and heart disease. Treatment is aimed at alleviating the underlying cause. If rate control is needed for a symptomatic decrease in cardiac output, vagal maneuvers may be attempted followed by digoxin, beta blockers, or diltiazem administration.

Junctional tachycardia may occur paroxysmally. Because of the rate, it is often difficult to distinguish it from PAT. Both junctional tachycardia and PAT are referred to as supraventricular tachycardia (SVT), indicating that the rhythm originates above the ventricles.

### Premature ventricular beats

A premature ventricular beat (PVB) is an early beat arising from an ectopic focus in the ventricles. The characteristic wide, bizarre QRS (usually greater than 0.12 second) makes the PVB readily identifiable on the ECG tracing (Figure 25-29). There is no associated P wave, and the T wave is in the opposite direction from the main QRS deflection. Most PVBs are followed by a pause until the next normal impulse originates in the SA node.

If PVBs are of different configuration in an ECG tracing, they are said to be multifocal. This indicates the presence of more than one ectopic focus in the ventricles, or one ectopic focus with multiple reentry pathways, thus producing complexes of differing forms. Premature ventricular beats also may have varying degrees of prematurity. The relationship of the PVB to the Q, R, S, and T waves of the preceding beat is important. An electrical impulse of any kind that stimulates the heart near the peak of the T wave (thereby preventing full repolarization of the ventricles) may precipitate a more dangerous or lethal dysrhythmia. The frequency and morphology of PVBs determine their importance. When every other beat is a PVB, the term *bigeminy* is used; every third beat, *trigeminy;* and so forth. Two PVBs together are termed a *couplet.*

Premature ventricular beats occur in the absence of heart disease and increase in number with age. The incidence and frequency of occurrence are higher, however, for the population with heart disease. Clinically, PVBs are associated with heart failure, digitalis toxicity, hypoxia, stimulants, catecholamines, and electrolyte imbalances. In the latter cases treatment of the underlying cause may abolish the dysrhythmia. Pharmacological suppression of PVBs is accomplished with lidocaine or procainamide.

### Ventricular rhythms and tachycardia

If the SA node and AV junction fail to initiate impulses, a ventricular pacemaking cell will automatically begin to initiate impulses at a rate of 20 to 40 beats per minute. This is known as idioventricular rhythm (Figure 25-30). P waves, when seen, are not associated with the ventricular rhythm. The QRS complex is greater than 0.12, wide, and bizarre.

If the rate of the ventricular-initiated rhythm increases to 40 to 100 beats per minute, it is known as an accelerated idioventricular rhythm (AIVR). An AIVR may be seen in hypoxia, in digitalis toxicity, as a complication of an AMI, and as a reperfusion dysrhythmia after thrombolytic therapy. Suppression of the heart's dominant and perhaps only rhythm could be hazardous. Therefore idioventricular rhythms are not treated except to correct underlying abnormalities.

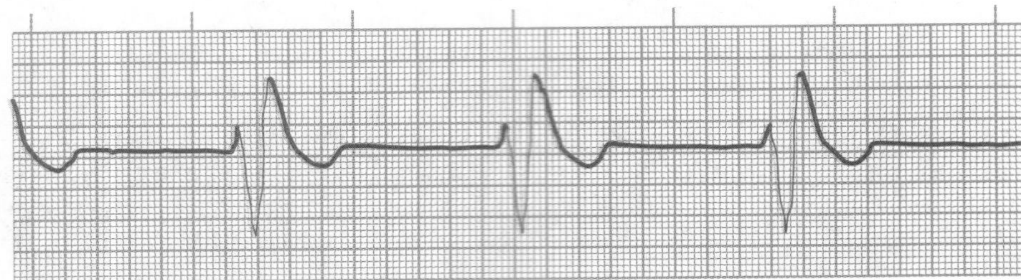

**fig. 25-30** Idioventricular rhythm; ventricular heart rate, 30.

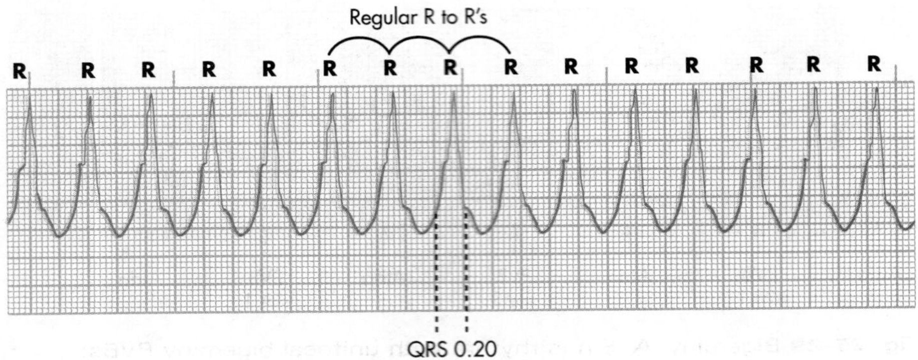


**fig. 25-31** Ventricular tachycardia with regular R to R intervals and QRS greater than 0.12 second; heart rate, 150.

If the cardiac output is low and symptoms of heart failure, syncope, or hypotension develop, the patient may require temporary or permanent artificial pacing. Atropine may be helpful in stimulating the return of SA node activity.

By definition, three or more successive PVBs constitute ventricular tachycardia (VT) (Figure 25-31). The ventricular rate is greater than 100 beats per minute and usually is 140 to 240 beats per minute. The rhythm is regular or slightly irregular. P waves may be present but are not associated with the QRS complexes. Ventricular tachycardia may complicate any form of heart disease and may be a direct result of a PVB striking during the heart's vulnerable period. Conditions that favor its occurrence include hypoxemia, drug toxicity, electrolyte imbalance, and bradycardia. Abnormal automaticity may occur in the postinfarction period as a result of the loss of fast sodium channels, contributing to the development of VT.

Ventricular tachycardia is classified as sustained (lasting more than 30 seconds) or nonsustained. Nonsustained VT may occur in patients with or without cardiac disease and may be associated with palpitations or recurrent syncope. In the presence of severe ventricular dysfunction, nonsustained VT may be a precursor of sustained VT and sudden death. With increasing heart rates, cardiac output decreases as the ventricles do not have time to fill and empty. Symptoms vary depending on the length of the VT and the rate.

Intravenous lidocaine is often the first drug used. Intravenous procainamide is another option because it prolongs the refractory period and slows conduction in the ventricle. If pharmacological measures are unsuccessful, the alternative is cardioversion. Ongoing VT suppression is obtained with oral antidysrhythmic medications such as amiodarone or special procedures such as radiofrequency ablation.

### Torsades de pointes

Torsades de pointes, a variation of VT, can also progress to ventricular fibrillation if not managed appropriately. A long QT interval (over half of the corresponding RR interval) commonly precedes torsades de pointes. P waves, when seen, are dissociated from the QRS complexes. The QRS complexes are greater than 0.12 second and bizarre. The QRS complexes "twist" along the isoelectric baseline, varying in size and direction (Figure 25-32).

The rhythm may result from prolonged repolarization, characterized on the ECG by the prolonged QT interval. Prolongation may occur secondary to various medications or electrolyte abnormalities, or it may be congenital in origin. Cardiac output decreases from inadequate ventricular filling and emptying with the increased heart rate.

Magnesium sulfate is administered first to stabilize the electrical membrane. Lidocaine may be administered, although other agents that do not prolong the QT interval may be tried. Cardioversion is commonly necessary. After resolution, etiological factors are eliminated or corrected, if possible.

### Ventricular fibrillation and asystole

In ventricular fibrillation (VF) the ventricular activity is chaotic, similar to the atria in atrial fibrillation. The ECG tracing consists of unidentifiable waves. The fibrillatory waves may be coarse or fine (Figure 25-33). The most common cause is coronary artery disease. With VF, there is no depolarization and therefore no effective ventricular contraction.

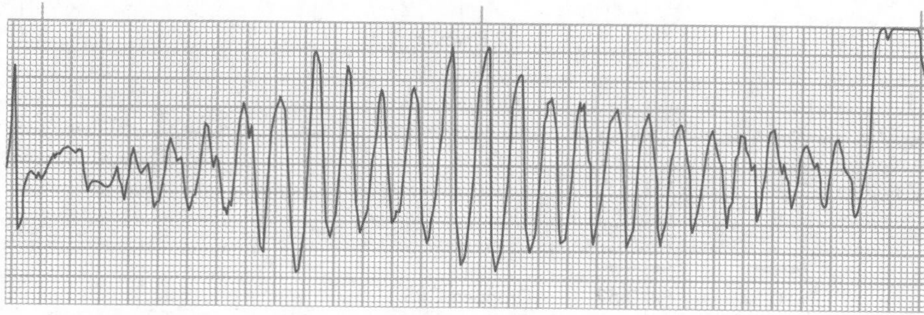

**fig. 25-32** Torsade de pointes; heart rate, 240-250.

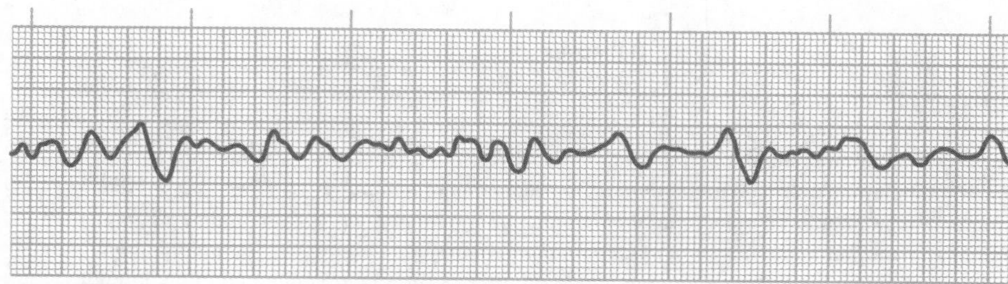

**fig. 25-33** Coarse ventricular fibrillation; heart rate, not measurable.

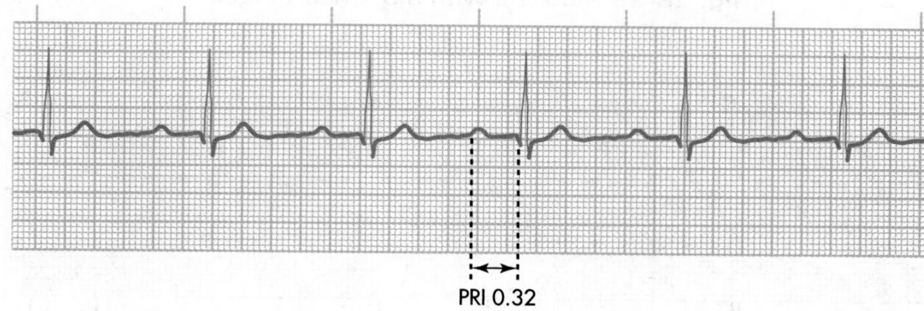


**fig. 25-34** First-degree heart block. PR interval greater than 0.20 second.

Commonly VF is the terminal event in sudden cardiac death. It may occur without warning after reperfusion.

Defibrillation is the only intervention, and it must be performed as soon as possible. The administration of epinephrine may increase the effectiveness of defibrillation.

In asystole, the ECG tracing is a flat line. No electrical activity is noted; all pacemaking cells have failed. The patient has no blood pressure, pulse, or audible heartbeat; respirations quickly cease. Cardiopulmonary resuscitation (CPR) must be instituted immediately. Epinephrine, atropine, and external pacing are all used in the effort to restore cardiac excitability.

### *Atrioventricular block*

A block to conduction of an impulse may occur at any point along the conduction pathways. One common area is the AV junction. The severity of the block is identified by degrees, that is, first-, second-, or third-degree AV block.

First-degree AV block is present when the PR interval is prolonged to greater than 0.20 second, indicating a conduction delay in the AV node (Figure 25-34). It usually is found in association with rheumatic fever, digitalis toxicity, acute inferior MI, and increased vagal tone. When a first-degree AV block occurs in isolation, the patient is usually asymptomatic and no treatment is necessary.

Second-degree AV block may be divided into two categories. Type I (Wenckebach or Mobitz type I) is characterized by a PR interval that progressively lengthens until a P wave is not followed by a QRS complex (Figure 25-35). The pathology is usually within the AV node and produces QRS complexes less than 0.12 second. The nonconducted impulse arrives at the AV node during the refractory period. The ratio of P waves to QRS complexes may be 5:4, 4:3, 3:2, or 2:1 and creates a clustered appearance.

Any drug that slows AV conduction may cause a type I block, but such blocks are most often seen in the patient with an acute inferior wall MI, digitalis toxicity, increased vagal tone, electrolyte imbalance, acute myocarditis, or after cardiac surgery. Type I blocks often are transient and reversible. Generally no treatment is required unless symptoms develop. Atropine may be effective in increasing cardiac output.

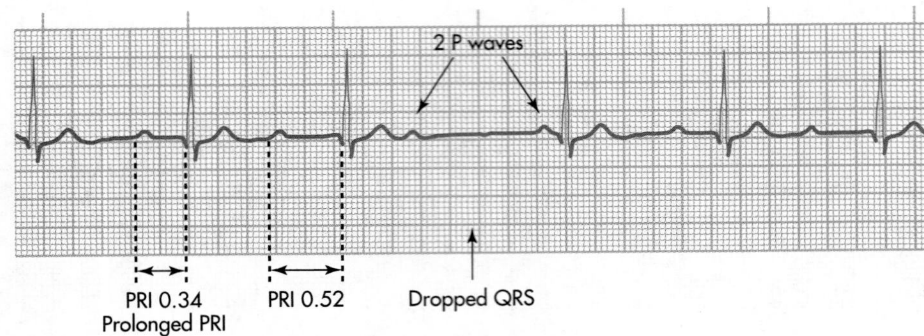


**fig. 25-35** Mobitz I heart block. Atrial heart rate, 60; ventricular heart rate, 50.

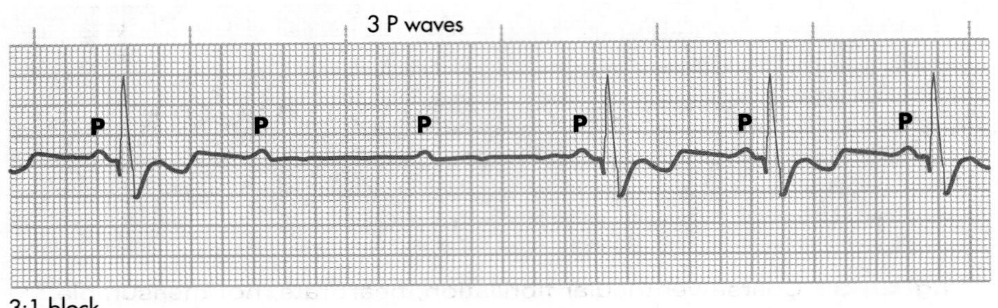


**fig. 25-36** Mobitz II with a 3:1 heart block.

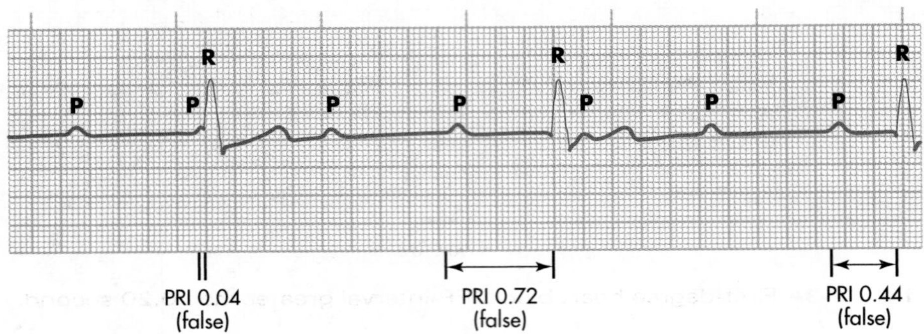


**fig. 25-37** Separate P waves and QRS complexes of third-degree heart block. Atrial heart rate, 70; ventricular heart rate, 30.

Type II (Mobitz type II) second-degree AV block is less common but more serious. A type II block is characterized by nonconducted sinus impulses despite constant PR intervals for the conducted P waves. The nonconducted P waves may occur at random or in patterned ratios (2:1, 3:1, etc.) (Figure 25-36). The QRS complexes are widened unless the block is within the bundle of His.

Type II blocks may occur in CAD, MI, rheumatic heart disease, cardiomyopathy, and chronic fibrotic disease of the conduction system. If cardiac output is decreased, a temporary pacemaker usually is inserted prophylactically until the conduction stabilizes. If the block is persistent, the patient will benefit from a permanent implantable pacemaker. Atropine may be ineffective and may only increase the atrial rate.

In third-degree AV block (complete heart block) all the sinus or atrial impulses are blocked, and the atria and ventricles beat independently. The ventricles are driven by either a junctional or a ventricular pacemaker cell. The usual lesion is in the bundle of His or the bundle branches but may also be at the AV junction. The rate and dependability of the ventricular rhythm are related to the level of the lesion. If a junctional pacemaker drives the ventricles, the ventricular rate will be at least 40 to 60 beats per minute. The QRS complexes are typically narrow. This block may be a transient complication of inferior posterior MI or digitalis toxicity, or it may result from severe heart disease.

If a ventricular pacemaker drives the ventricles, the rate will be 20 to 40 beats per minute, and the patient may experience syncope, heart failure, altered mentation, or angina. The QRS complex is abnormally wide, indicating that the block lies below the AV junction (Figure 25-37). The prognosis is more serious if complete heart block accompanies anterior MI. Generally the patient will require a permanent pacemaker.

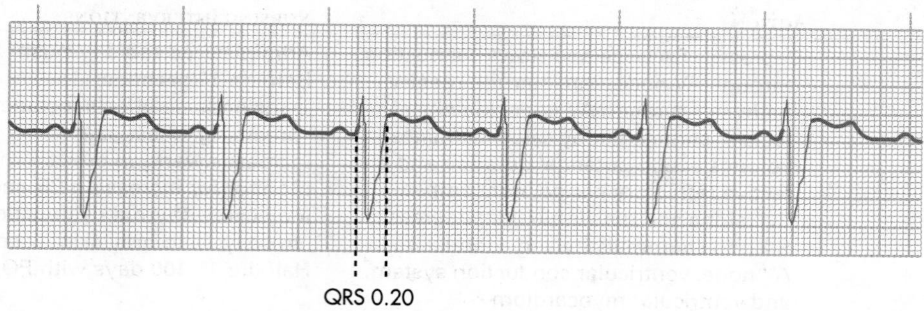


**fig. 25-38** Sinus rhythm with a BBB; heart rate, 60.

Epinephrine or isoproterenol administered intravenously may increase the ventricular rate temporarily until artificial pacing can be instituted.

### Bundle branch block

In bundle branch block (BBB), one or both bundle branch paths of the conduction system are blocked. The impulse must travel a different path to stimulate the ventricle; therefore the QRS is prolonged greater than 0.12 second. Instead of a synchronous QRS complex, each ventricle independently depolarizes, creating characteristic QRS complexes (Figure 25-38).

A BBB occurs as a permanent defect or as a transient block secondary to tachycardia, heart failure, AMI, pulmonary embolus, hypoxia, or metabolic derangements.

The right bundle branch is the more delicate of the two bundles and has a longer refractory period in some persons. In the younger patient right BBB often results from right ventricular hypertrophy, whereas CAD usually is the cause in the older patient. Among the most classic ECG changes is the M-shaped QRS in $V_1$ and $V_2$. In the absence of other conduction defects, no intervention is necessary.

The left bundle branch has a main trunk that bifurcates into the left anterior and left posterior divisions. A block may occur in the main trunk or in either of the divisions. (Blocks of the anterior or posterior division are known as left anterior hemiblock or left posterior hemiblock, respectively.) A block in the main trunk produces a complete left BBB resulting in a QRS greater than 0.12 second, large R waves in $V_5$ and $V_6$, and deep, wide S waves in $V_1$ through $V_3$. Left BBB is associated with severe CAD, valvular disease, hypertensive disease, cardiomegaly, and acute anterior wall MI. It also may occur as a result of degenerative changes in the conduction system. Whenever sufficient blockage is present to leave the heart dependent on one fascicle for conduction to the ventricles, the patient is a candidate for a permanent artificial pacemaker.

### Treatment options for dysrhythmias

Collaborative care for the patient with a dysrhythmia includes diagnosing the specific dysrhythmia and its associated etiology and treating the disorder with medications or interventional procedures. Medications commonly used to manage dysrhythmias are presented in Table 25-7. The nurse must be knowledgeable about the mechanism of action of specific drugs and their associated nursing interventions. Careful attention must be given to potential drug interactions and synergistic effects when combination therapy is used. The metabolism and excretion of medications may be impaired in the elderly and in patients with decreased perfusion to the kidneys and liver. The nurse must be aware of new agents approved for the management of cardiac dysrhythmias and how to monitor their safe use.

Nursing management of the patient experiencing dysrhythmias includes interventions to decrease oxygen demand. The nurse spaces activities and encourages frequent rest periods. While medication therapy is being adjusted, patients are on continuous monitoring (telemetry). Rhythms are documented every 4 to 8 hours and as needed. Skin care is provided to minimize the irritation of the monitoring electrodes.

The nurse must be alert to changes in a patient's rhythm. Assessments for changes in cardiac output are documented. Emergency drugs should be available, and intravenous access should be ensured. Ancillary equipment such as defibrillators, oxygen, suction, and temporary pacemakers should be readily available and in good working condition.

Interventions such as cardioversion, defibrillation, coronary ablation, pacemaker therapy, automatic implantable cardioverter-defibrillators, and cardiopulmonary resuscitation are also part of the collaborative care strategies used for patients with dysrhythmias. An overview of each of these interventions is presented on p. 679-680.

### Patient/family education

The nurse directly addresses the patient's and family's fears and concerns, recognizing that living with a potentially life-threatening dysrhythmia is a huge challenge. Patients and families need to understand the importance of seeking medical attention promptly if symptoms recur. They should also know how to take the patient's pulse and the types of pulse changes that need to be reported. Patients are taught about the specific dysrhythmia and the treatment plan. The nurse reviews the common side effects of the dysrhythmic agents with the patient. The patient is cautioned to discuss the incidence and severity of side effects with a health care professional and not to adjust the dose or discontinue the use of any prescribed medication. Follow-up is essential in monitoring medication therapy and response.

## table 25-7 Common Medications for *Dysrhythmias*

| Drug | Action | Nursing Interventions |
|---|---|---|
| Adenosine | Depresses SA node and slows conduction through AV node; can interrupt reentry pathways through AV node; inhibits effects of stimulation by catecholamines | Administered rapid IV push<br>Half-life 10 seconds<br>Transient side effects include flushing, labored breathing, chest pain |
| Amiodarone | Prolongs action potential duration and effective refractory period, noncompetitive alpha and beta inhibition; depresses SA node automaticity and conduction in AV node, ventricular conduction system, and ventricular myocardium | Increases warfarin effect<br>Monitor for increasing PR and QT intervals<br>May cause thyroid dysfunction, pulmonary toxicity, blue-gray skin discoloration<br>Half-life 15-100 days with PO onset 1-3 weeks |
| Atropine sulfate | Increases heart rate by blocking vagal simulation, increasing automaticity of SA node and conduction in AV node | May be given IV or endotracheally<br>Increases oxygen demand with increased heart rate |
| Beta blockers<br>Atenolol<br>Esmolol<br>Metoprolol<br>Propranolol<br>Sotalol | Interfere with sodium influx; depress automaticity and prolong effective refractory period of AV node | Administered PO or slow IV push<br>Monitor PR interval and BP<br>Patients should be taught not to discontinue abruptly because this may precipitate angina<br>Monitor for CHF in susceptible patients |
| Bretylium tosylate | Inhibits release of norepinephrine by postganglionic nerve endings; prolongs action potential duration and effective refractory periods | Given IV followed by maintenance infusion<br>Monitor for hypotension, nausea, and vomiting |
| Calcium channel blockers<br>Diltiazem hydrochloride<br>Verapamil hydrochloride | Increase effective refractory period in AV node; inhibit calcium ion influx across cell membrane during cardiac depolarization; slow SA and AV node conduction times | Administered PO or slow IV push<br>Avoid in patients with accessory pathways or wide-complex tachycardias<br>May cause hypotension |
| Calcium chloride | Cation needed for cardiac contractility | Give slow IV; extravasation will result in necrosis |
| Digoxin | Decreases conduction velocity through AV node; prolongs effective refractory period | Check apical pulse for 1 minute; if less than 50, notify physician before administration<br>Hypokalemia increases risk of digoxin toxicity<br>Monitor for therapeutic drug levels<br>Administered PO or slow IV push<br>Will increase contractility<br>Benefit of the drug in heart failure must be weighed against the increase in oxygen demand |
| Epinephrine hydrochloride | Beta 1 and beta 2 agonist increasing automaticity | Given IV or endotracheally<br>Increases oxygen demand |
| Isoproterenol hydrochloride | Causes increased contractility and heart rate by acting on beta 1 and 2 receptors in heart | Given IV<br>May be used in diagnostic electrophysiology studies |
| Lidocaine hydrochloride | Inhibits sodium influx during phase 0 depolarization, decreasing automaticity; increases electrical stimulation threshold of ventricle, His-Purkinje system; shortens repolarization and action potential | Given IV push followed by maintenance infusion<br>Toxic effects include confusion, psychosis, decreased hearing, seizures |
| Magnesium sulfate | Reduces SA node impulse formation, prolongs conduction time in myocardium | Monitor magnesium levels |
| Procainamide hydrochloride | Inhibits sodium influx during phase 0 depolarization; prolongs action potential and effective refractory period in atrium, bundle of His, and ventricle | Administered PO or slow IV push followed by maintenance infusion; monitor for hypotension with IV initiation; monitor for increasing PR and QT intervals; avoid use in preexisting long QT syndrome and torsades de pointes; monitor blood levels; may cause systemic lupus symptoms |
| Propafenone | Decreases sodium influx during phase 0 depolarization; slows conduction velocity; reduces membrane responsiveness; inhibits automaticity; increases effective refractory period with little effect on action potential duration; slight beta blocker activity | Significantly decreases inotropic activity; therefore use with caution in depressed left ventricular function |

### Cardioversion and defibrillation

Cardioversion and debrillation use electrical energy to convert a cardiac dysrhythmia to a rhythm that is hemodynamically stable, preferably a sinus rhythm. Electrophysiologically, the electrical countershock produces a simultaneous depolarization of a critical mass of cardiac fibers, thus halting the asynchronous chaos of a fibrillation or the rapid firing of a tachycardia. In some cases, especially in elective cardioversion, the shock will be delivered more than once until the required level of voltage is reached. Once the heart is fully depolarized, the SA node is better able to resume control.

Defibrillation generally applies to unsynchronized electrical countershock during a ventricular fibrillation emergency. The paddles from the defibrillator are placed at the third intercostal space to the right of the sternum and the fifth intercostal space on the left midaxillary line. Conducting gel or saline pads are applied between the paddles and the skin to ensure conductance and to minimize skin burning. The button on each paddle is depressed simultaneously to release 200 to 360 watt-seconds (joules) to the patient. Defibrillation must be performed quickly for ventricular fibrillation and most cases of ventricular tachycardia.

Cardioversion differs from defibrillation in that the electrical discharge is synchronized with the R wave to avoid triggering ventricular fibrillation by accidental discharge during the vulnerable period. Indications for cardioversion include hemodynamically unstable atrial flutter, atrial fibrillation, and paroxysmal atrial tachycardia. To decrease the risk of emboli the patient should be fully anticoagulated for 3 weeks with an INR of 2.0 to 3.0. The anticoagulant of choice is warfarin. If the patient requires cardioversion on a more immediate basis, a transesophageal echocardiogram (TEE) should be performed to rule out intraatrial thrombi before the procedure.

Patients should be prepared psychologically for what to expect and be reassured that they will be sedated. The procedure is best done in a special laboratory and not the patient's room. The patient generally is given diazepam (Valium), midazolam (Versed), or fentanyl intravenously. The defibrillator is synchronized so that when the buttons are pressed, the impulse is not initiated until the next R wave. Because of this precaution, the danger of entering the vulnerable period is eliminated. For most elective procedures, the amount of watt-seconds or joules required for conversion is lower than that required for defibrillation. The patient is monitored after cardioversion until vital signs are stable.

### Radiofrequency catheter ablation

Catheter ablation selectively destroys the site of origin of a dysrhythmia or destroys the pathway necessary for its propagation. Radiofrequency energy is a form of high-frequency electromagnetic waves. The thermal energy produced burns the area selected for ablation. Indications for ablation include the presence of a slower secondary pathway creating reentry rhythm or the presence of specific irritable foci, such as occurs with some atrial fibrillation and ventricular tachycardia rhythms. The amount of damage caused by the catheter is relatively small because of the precision in regulating and focusing the energy delivered. The patient remains in the electrophysiology laboratory for a short interval after the procedure for observation. After this rest period, attempts are made to reinitiate the dysrhythmia. The dysrhythmia recurs if the ablation merely stunned the tissue. Additional ablation bursts are then administered until successful ablation occurs. The reported rate of recurrence is approximately 5%, and most recur within 6 weeks of the procedure.[6]

Complications of the procedure are rare but may include vascular access problems (hematomas, femoral pseudoaneurysms); the formation of catheter-induced thrombi; and myocardial perforation. The procedure takes place in the electrophysiology laboratory under sedation, using femoral arterial and venous site access. Cardiologists advance the catheters endovascularly to the areas of focus while fluoroscopy guides catheter placement. The procedure may last 2 to 3 hours when diagnostic electrophysiology occurs concurrently. Guidelines for care include those used with patients undergoing electrophysiology studies. (See Chapter 24.) A major focus of nursing interventions is patient and family education to alleviate anxiety over the procedure and its potential complications. (See the Patient/Family Teaching Box.)

**patient/family teaching**

**The Patient Undergoing Radiofrequency Catheter Ablation**

**Preprocedure**

Indication for procedure
Potential complications
Withholding of antidysrhythmics per physician orders
Avoid caffeine and alcohol 24 hours before procedure
NPO for 8 hours before the procedure
IV access for fluids, sedation, and cardiac medications
Shaving and scrub of femoral site and right neck
Preprocedure tests: clotting studies, chest x-ray, baseline ECG

**Intraprocedure**

Sedation throughout procedure
Possible discomfort in groin and neck
Cardiac monitor at all times
Sterile drapes to prevent infection at access sites
Medications readily available to test effectiveness of procedure or to treat dysrhythmias should they occur.

**Postprocedure**

Access sheath pulled immediately after procedure
Vital signs and neurovascular checks q15min ×4 then q30min until patient stabilized
Baseline 12-lead ECG obtained

**Discharge**

May be discharged same day
Daily aspirin if ablation performed on left side of heart
Avoid prolonged sitting for first day
Avoid strenuous activity for 72 hours
Avoid driving for 24 hours
Signs and symptoms of infection or complications at access site
Signs and symptoms of dysrhythmia recurrence

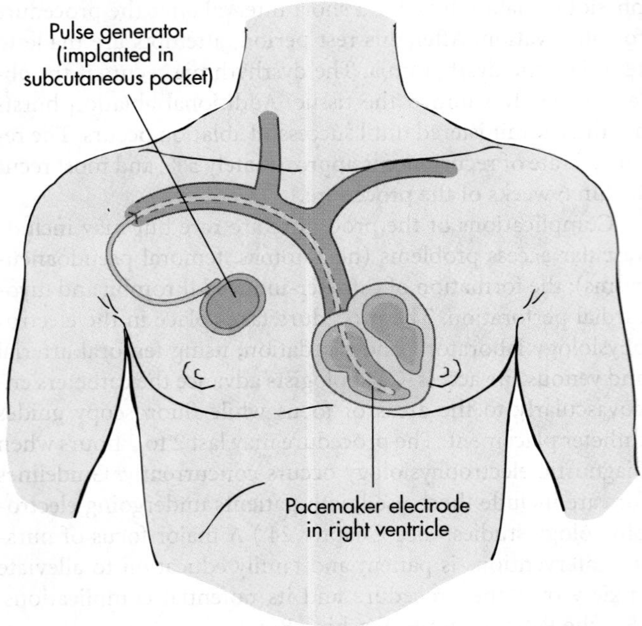


**fig. 25-39** Permanent pacemaker placement.

### Pacemakers

Indications for pacemakers include symptomatic chronic or recurrent dysrhythmias unresponsive to pharmacological therapy. Examples include sick sinus syndrome, higher-level heart blocks, severe bradycardias, tachycardias, and rhythms in which the loss of atrial kick (the blood volume delivered to the left ventricle from coordinated atrial contraction) significantly affects cardiac output. Pacemakers may be permanent, temporary, or external.

Permanent pacemakers use a pulse generator as the "control center" for the pacemaker's functions. The generator attaches to one or two leads positioned in the right ventricle or right atrium (Figure 25-39). These leads are flexible, insulated wires with electrodes for sensing the heart's rhythm and delivering electrical impulses when necessary. The leads are introduced into the myocardium transvenously through the subclavian or jugular vein. A guide wire under fluoroscopy facilitates correct placement of the leads against the atrial or ventricular endocardium. A surgically created subcutaneous pocket encloses the generator, most often supraclavicularly.

The procedure is performed with sedation and local anesthesia. Before insertion of a permanent pacemaker, the patient receives information about the indication for the pacemaker, potential complications, the procedure itself, and pacemaker care. (See the Patient/Family Teaching Box.) Nursing responsibilities before and after permanent pacemaker implantation are summarized in the Guidelines for Care Box on the next page.

A nursing plan of care for the patient with a permanent pacemaker addresses patient concerns over device failure. The pacemakers in use today have many capabilities. A five-letter pacemaker code describes the specific pacemaker's programmable functions (Table 25-8). All pacemakers use the first three letters of the code. Special features of pacemakers are denoted by the last two letters and include antitachycardic pacing and rate-responsive pacing.

When an antitachycardic pacemaker senses a heart rate above its programmed limit, it paces at a heart rate above the patient's tachycardia to take control. The pacemaker then slows the rhythm to an acceptable rate. Rate-responsive pacemakers allow pacing at accelerated heart rates when the pacemaker senses programmed indicators of increased activity such as changes in oxygen saturation, cardiac output, or blood temperature.

Figure 25-40 shows the ECG appearance of pacemaker-stimulated heartbeats. Paced beats are readily identifiable by the sharp spike that precedes a paced ECG complex. The paced QRS complex is wide because initiation of the impulse occurs in the ventricle (as with a PVB).

**patient/family teaching**

**The Patient with a Permanent Pacemaker**

**Permanent Pacemakers—Procedural**

Indication for pacemaker
Potential complications
NPO for 8 hours before the procedure
Pretests, including baseline 12-lead ECG and bleeding function studies
Cardiac monitor at all times during the procedure
IV access for fluids, cardiac medications, and sedation
Prep and shave area where generator will be implanted
Anesthesia of access sites
Sterile field during procedure
Analgesics offered postprocedure
Restricted movement of affected arm for 48 hours
Routine chest x-ray to check placement

**Permanent Pacemaker—Discharge**

Monitor site for infection and bleeding the first week
Avoid immersion of site in water for 3 days (tub bath OK)
Steri-strips will come off in about 1 week
Limit range of motion of affected arm and wear loose covering over incision for 1 week
Avoid contact sports
Contact health care professional with fatigue, palpitations, or recurrence of symptoms (may indicate battery depletion or pacemaker malfunction)
Importance of follow-up via transtelephonic means or office visits
Carry pacemaker information at all times—trigger alarms some airport security
Pacemaker may need to be programmed to fixed mode
Special grounding precautions taken for certain medical procedures (electrocautery, radiation therapy, MRI)
Move away from electrical devices if dizziness experienced
Avoid working over large, running motors
How to take radial pulse—notify health care professional for rates outside those programmed (may indicate pacemaker malfunction or battery depletion)

guidelines for care

## The Patient Undergoing Permanent Pacemaker Insertion

### Preprocedure

Establish assessment baselines: vital signs, 12-lead ECG, peripheral pulses, heart and lung sounds, mental status.
Patient teaching as per patient/family education guidelines
Maintain NPO status for 8 hours
Establish IV access for administration of IV fluids, sedation, and emergency drugs
Assess anxiety level and intervene appropriately with active listening, reassurance, education, and sedation as needed

### Intraprocedure

Shave and scrub access site
Sterile field maintained
Cardiac monitor at all times
Assess patient's anxiety level and intervene appropriately with reassurance and sedation as needed

### Postprocedure

Monitor for complications of insertion such as pneumothorax, hemothorax, perforation, tamponade
Be alert to lead dislodgement, manifested by hiccups if diaphragm being paced or ECG changes
Pain control
Baseline ECG—monitor for loss of sensing, loss of capture, or failure to pace
Assess insertion site for bleeding and infection
Bed rest for 12 hours
Limit range of motion of affected arm for 12 to 24 hours
Apply ice pack to minimize pain and swelling for first 6 hours
Do not administer aspirin or heparin for 48 hours
If defibrillation necessary, anterior-posterior placement is preferable; avoid area surrounding generator site
If patient symptomatic from pacer malfunction: bed rest, safety precautions for syncope potential, frequent vital signs, 12-lead ECG to diagnose malfunction
Continuous telemetry monitoring, IV access (with atropine at bedside), oxygen if needed, chest x-ray to check lead position, pacemaker magnet to convert pacemaker to fixed mode
Discharge teaching

**table 25-8** *Intersociety Commission for Heart Disease (ICHD) Codes for Pacemakers*

| Chamber(s) Paced | Chamber(s) Sensed | Mode of Responses (sensing function) | Programmable Functions | Special Tachydysrhythmia Functions |
|---|---|---|---|---|
| V = Ventricle | V = Ventricle | T = Triggered | P = Programmable | B = Bursts |
| A = Atrium | A = Atrium | I = Inhibited (demand) | M = Multiprogrammable | N = Normal rate competition (dual demand) |
| D = Double (dual) | D = Double (dual) | D = Double (dual function: T and I) | O = None (permanent pacemakers only) | S = Scanning |
| | O = None | O = None (continuous) | | E = External |
| | | R = Reverse | | |

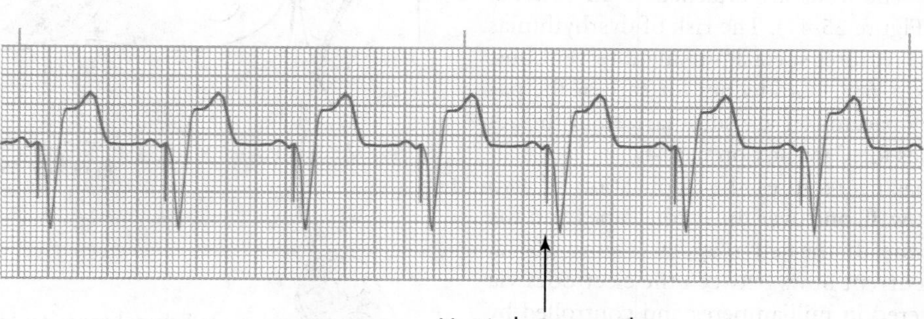


**fig. 25-40** Ventricular pacemaker rhythm with pacer spikes.

**table 25-9** *Troubleshooting Pacemaker Malfunction*

| Problem | Definition | ECG Finding | Physiological Effect | Nursing Action |
|---|---|---|---|---|
| Loss of sensing—oversensing | Pacemaker senses an extraneous signal as an impulse and therefore does not pace | Pause | Decreased cardiac output | Decrease sensitivity of pacemaker<br>Check for electromagnetic interference and proper grounding of equipment (temporary pacemaker) |
| Loss of sensing—undersensing | Pacemaker does not sense heart's own impulse and therefore thinks it has to pace the heart | Inappropriate pacing (extra beats) | Danger of pacing in the vulnerable period causing ventricular tachycardia | Increase sensitivity to heart's rhythm |
| Loss of capture | Pacemaker fires but does not depolarize the ventricle | Spike present but without QRS complex | Decrease in cardiac output | Increase milliamperes (energy delivered); turn to left side (bring lead in better contact with endocardium)<br>Check all connections (temporary pacemaker)<br>Determine etiology of ventricle not responding and correct electrolyte abnormality, ischemia, lead dislodgment |
| Failure to pace | Electrical impulse never initiated | Pause without spikes | Decrease in cardiac output | External/temporary pacemaker at bedside<br>Assess response and treat symptoms until etiology determined and corrected (dislodged lead, battery depletion, malfunctioning pulse generator) |

The patient with pacemaker malfunction usually has recurrence of symptoms. However, the nurse must be able to diagnose the following ECG indicators of pacemaker malfunction: loss of sensing, loss of capture, and failure to pace. Table 25-9 describes common pacemaker problems and interventions to troubleshoot pacemaker malfunction. A Nursing Care Plan for a patient undergoing pacemaker insertion follows.

Temporary pacemakers are indicated for the short-term management of dysthythmias until the patient's rhythm stabilizes or a permanent pacemaker can be inserted. For temporary pacing the pacer wire usually is advanced transvenously to the right ventricle. The leads are attached to an external pulse generator box (Figure 25-41). The risk of dysrhythmias from electrical hazards requires special nursing interventions. (See the Research Box p. 684.) Guidelines for care of the patient with a temporary pacemaker are summarized in the accompanying Guidelines for Care Box on p. 684.

External cardiac pacing requires the application of two electrodes to the chest wall, one over the cardiac apex and the other on the back beneath the left scapula (Figure 25-42, p. 684). An electrical current flows between the electrodes via an output pulse delivered in milliamperes and controlled by the operator. Most external pacing devices function in the demand mode. An oscilloscope allows monitoring of pacer activity. External pacers are primarily used for patients with unstable rhythms in emergency situations.

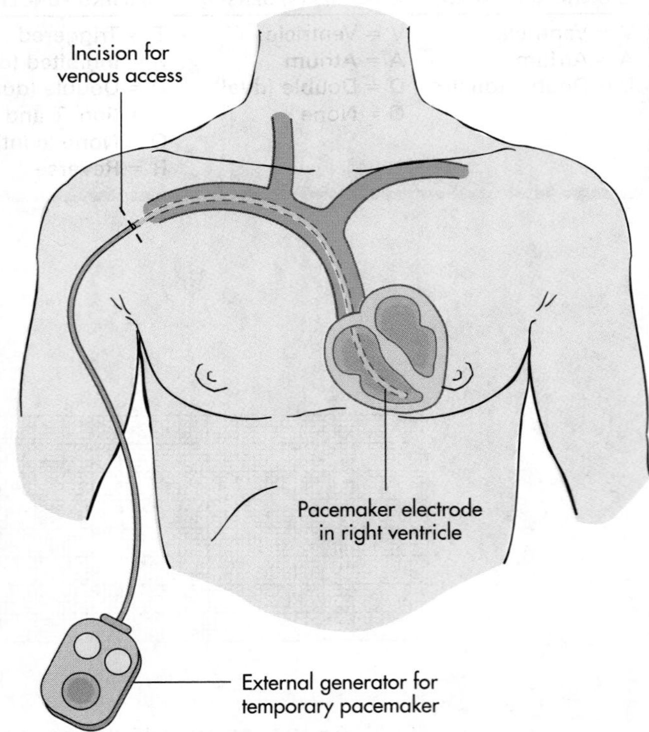


**fig. 25-41** Transvenous temporary pacemaker placement.

## nursing care plan *Patient Receiving Permanent Pacemaker*

**DATA** Ms. P. is a 75-year-old woman who was admitted with shortness of breath, chest pain, and heart failure. Past medical history includes a coronary artery bypass graft of the right coronary artery 10 years ago and an NQMI 2 years ago. Noncardiac history includes hiatal hernia, transient ischemic attacks times two, hypothyroidism, and chronic renal insufficiency. Ms. P.'s admitting diagnosis was unstable angina. Cardiac catheterization revealed native right coronary and left anterior descending coronary artery disease and occlusion of the graft to the right coronary artery. Following the catheterization, Ms. P. experienced symptomatic junctional bradycardia requiring placement of a temporary pacemaker. Because of the potential for heart failure from her bradycardiac rhythm and the ischemic blood supply to her conduction system, the decision was made to proceed with a permanent pacemaker. Ms. P. had a DDD pacemaker placed 6 days after admission. Her postprocedure course was uncomplicated, and the plan is to discharge her to her home tomorrow.

The nursing history also identified the following:

- Ms. P. has no family in the immediate area who can help her at home after discharge.
- Ms. P states she is afraid the pacemaker will fail and she will not know what to do.

Collaborative nursing actions include monitoring for the following:

- Cardiac dysrhythmias
- Pacemaker malfunction (failure to sense, failure to pace, or failure to capture)
- Infection or hematoma at incision
- Procedural complications (pneumothorax, perforation of right ventricle)

**NURSING DIAGNOSIS** *Fear related to knowledge deficit of pacemaker care*

| expected patient outcome | nursing interventions | rationale |
|---|---|---|
| Relates an increase in psychological and physiological comfort | Provide information to reduce distortions. | Misinterpretation can increase fear unnecessarily. |
| Describes effective and ineffective coping patterns | Teach patient how to problem solve. Have patient verbalize signs and symptoms experienced during dysrhythmic event. | Knowing when to worry vs. appropriate expectations helps the patient identify areas requiring follow-up. |
| | Teach skills to enhance control: instruct patient how to self-monitor for signs and symptoms of pacemaker malfunction or incision complications (daily pulse checks, transtelephonic recordings, incision care). | Understanding home care (including incision care and monitoring for pacemaker malfunction) increases confidence in ability to comply with recommendations. |
| | Initiate referral for skilled home health nursing until first follow-up visit with cardiologist (purpose: monitor surgical site, follow-up on knowledge retention and application). | The availability of initial follow-up provides positive reinforcement of the patient's actions for self-care. |
| | Provide written materials that reinforce teaching. | Written information provides a valuable resource for information that may be forgotten or misinterpreted. |
| | Arrange for the patient to meet with another patient who successfully lives at home independently with a permanent pacemaker. | Learning from others can help identify misconceptions and determine areas needing assistance. |

**NURSING DIAGNOSIS** *Impaired physical mobility related to incisional site pain, activity restrictions, and fear of lead displacement*

| expected patient outcome | nursing interventions | rationale |
|---|---|---|
| Performs activities of daily living (ADL) with minimal complaints of discomfort | Provide analgesics before activity while hospitalized. For discharge, encourage the patient to self-administer analgesics before activities requiring arm movement. | Appropriate timing of pain medication allows patient to perform ADL with less pain and more independence. Also decreases risk of immobility complications. |
| Describes resources to assist with ADL until physical mobility improves | Explore with patient community options to help during time of physical immobility—church, neighbors, friends, home health aides. | Encouraging the patient to list activities requiring assistance (meals, lifting, shopping) helps the patient identify appropriate resources. |
| Verbalizes prescribed restrictions | Reinforce the need to limit activities that stress the incision site for 4 weeks (most often includes lifting more than 25 pounds, activities using arms over the head, and recreational activities such as bowling). | Limiting activities that overuse the affected arm will help stabilize the pacemaker by fibrosis around the pacemaker and electrodes (decreases risk of electrode dislodgment). |

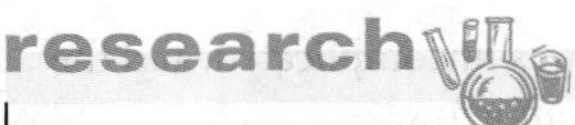

Reference: Baas LS, Beery TA, Hickey CS: Care and safety of pacemaker electrodes in intensive care and telemetry nursing units, *Am J Crit Care* 6(4):302, 1997.

The transmission of microshocks across temporary pacemaker wires can cause lethal dysrhythmias. Current practice guidelines are not consistent and are not validated by research as to their efficacy in preventing this microshock transmission. The authors sought to investigate current practice guidelines to report on existing shortfalls in the care of patients with temporary pacemakers and to identify areas requiring nursing vigilance. A survey that focused on environmental factors triggering static electricity, equipment in use with temporary pacing, and existing nursing practices was mailed to 895 hospitals nationwide with a 43% return reported. Many units reported wearing gloves with temporary pacemaker manipulations even though policy did not mandate gloves. Awareness of environmental hazards for microshock was found to be low. In addition, little attention was given to safeguarding the connection between the external pulse generator and the pacemaker cable. The authors recommend that specific policies and procedures be developed and enforced to reduce electrical hazards. Primary prevention should focus on decreasing the generation of static electricity from carpet, shoes, and humidity. The efficacy of nursing measures currently in use for patients with temporary pacemakers warrants further research.

**guidelines for care**

## The Patient with a Temporary Pacemaker

### Assess Patient's Tolerance of Heart Rhythm

Patient assessment: mental status, blood pressure and rhythm, urine output, skin color and warmth, pulses, heart sounds, and lung sounds

Continuous ECG monitoring

### Check System for Proper Functioning

Check pacing threshold (the minimum amount of milliamperes needed to pace the heart every 8 hours); set milliampere level 2 to 3 times the threshold as a safety margin; adjust as needed and notify physician

May need to replace battery in generator or connecting cable for failure to pace

Adjust sensitivity for undersensing or oversensing; notify physician

Secure all connections; secure generator box to patient or bed

### Maintain Electrical Safety

Maintain insulation cover over uninsulated ends

Wear rubber gloves when handling exposed terminals

Do not touch the patient and electrical equipment at the same time

Prevent liquids from coming in contact with the generator, cables, or insertion site

Keep ungrounded electrical equipment from contact with the patient

### Monitor for Complications at the Insertion Site

Inspect site daily for infection

Change dressing every 48 hours using central line dressing sterile technique

### Assess Patient Safety and Comfort

Explain the purpose of the pacemaker to decrease anxiety

Position patient comfortably, avoiding accidental tension on external wires and generator

When mobility is limited, assist the patient to find diversional activities

#### *Implantable cardioverter defibrillators*

More than half of the deaths from CAD in the United States each year are sudden deaths occurring within 24 hours of the onset of symptoms, and commonly before the patient reaches the hospital. The pathophysiology of sudden cardiac death remains obscure. Only 20% of sudden death events are associated with MI. Many researchers conclude that the cause of sudden cardiac death is not occlusive thrombosis or myocardial damage but a derangement in the heart's electrical stability, most often deteriorating into ventricular fibrillation. The incidence of sudden death is greater in patients with cardiomyopathy, long T intervals, myocarditis, prodysrhythmic medications, and electrolyte imbalance.

The implantable cardioverter-defibrillator (ICD) is indicated for (1) those who have survived one or more episodes of sudden cardiac death resulting from ventricular tachycardia or ventricular fibrillation, not associated with AMI, and (2) those who have experienced recurrent, refractory, life-threatening ventricular dysrhythmias that can induce sustained ventricular tachycardia or fibrillation, or both, despite conventional antidysrhythmic drug therapy.

The ICD consists of a pulse generator and two or three lead systems that continuously monitor heart activity and automatically deliver a countershock to correct a dysrhythmia. Current ICDs have many more applications than those first developed in 1980. The pacemaker-cardioverter-defibrillator models can pace patients out of tachycardiac rhythms and pace bradycardiac rhythms. These devices can override the heart's pacemaker to gain control or cardiovert the heart at different energy outputs if overpacing is ineffective. Retrieval of an event record is another feature that allows evaluation of the events and the appropriateness of ICD therapy.

Implantation of the device uses the subclavian transvenous lead system approach similar to permanent pacemaker insertion. A surgically created subcutaneous pocket is made for the generator subclavicularly or intraabdominally. The nurse protects the patient from situations that may cause malfunction of the ICD, such as magnetic resonance imaging or diathermy. Special precautions are necessary for procedures such as lithotripsy and radiation therapy. Electrical interference may occur with stereo systems, high-powered motors, and arc welders. Patients and family members commonly respond to the device with anxiety, depression, fear, and anger. Teaching guidelines are included in the Patient/Family Teaching Box on p. 685. Research continues concerning the quality of life of patients with ICDs[13] (see the Research Box on p. 686).

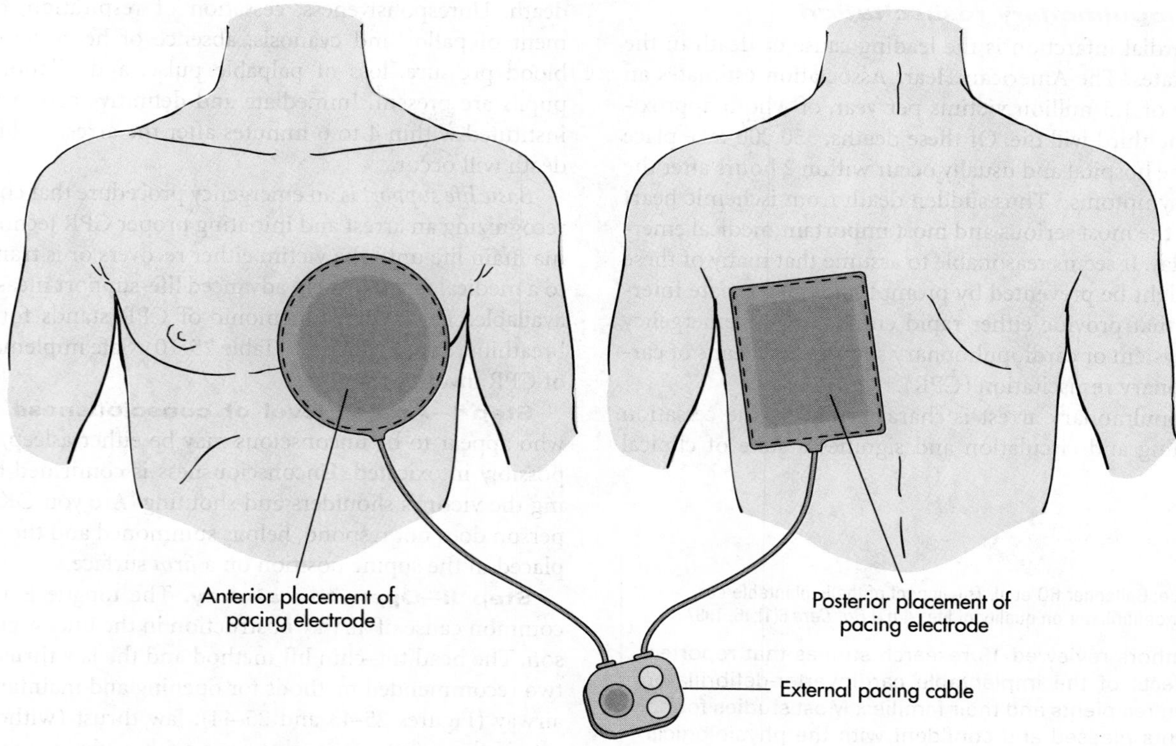


**fig. 25-42** Transcutaneous external pacing.

## patient/family teaching

### The Patient with an Implantable Cardioverter Defibrillator

**Implantable Cardioverter-Defibrillator (ICD)—Procedural**

Indication for ICD device
Potential complications
NPO for 8 hours before the procedure
Pretests, including baseline 12-lead ECG and bleeding function studies
Cardiac monitor at all times during the procedure
IV access for fluids, cardiac medications, and sedation
Prep and shave area where generator will be implanted
Anesthesia of access sites
Sterile field during procedure
Analgesics available postprocedure
Restricted arm movement for 48 hours if implant site is subclavicular
Routine chest x-ray to check placement

**ICD—Discharge**

***Insertion Site***

Monitor site for infection and bleeding the first week
Avoid immersion of site in water for 3 days
Steri-strips will come off in about 1 week
Wear loose covering over incision for 1 week

***Activity***

Avoid contact sports
Increase activity gradually after implantation of device (should be at full preimplant activity level once incision has healed)
Driving restrictions individualized and must be discussed with cardiologist

***Health Care Follow-up***

Importance of follow-up via office visits
If experience signs or symptoms of decreasing cardiac output with dysrhythmia, sit or lie down
Notify health care professional for
  Signs or symptoms of dysrhythmia similar to those before ICD
  Rapid, irregular heart rate
  Chest pain or shortness of breath

***Safety***

Will experience a mild sensation with shock delivery for patient and others in physical contact with patient
Carry ICD information at all times—will alarm some airport security
Consult with cardiologist before undergoing diagnostic or surgical interventions
Move away from devices if dizziness experienced
Avoid working over large, running motors
How to take radial pulse—notify health care professional for rates outside those programmed

### Cardiopulmonary resuscitation

Myocardial infarction is the leading cause of death in the United States. The American Heart Association estimates an incidence of 1.5 million victims per year, of whom approximately one third will die. Of these deaths, 350,000 take place outside the hospital and usually occur within 2 hours after the onset of symptoms.[1] Thus sudden death from ischemic heart disease is the most serious and most important medical emergency today. It seems reasonable to assume that many of these deaths might be prevented by prompt and appropriate interventions that provide either rapid entry into the emergency medical system or cardiopulmonary support by means of cardiopulmonary resuscitation (CPR).

Cardiopulmonary arrest is characterized by the cessation of breathing and circulation and signifies a state of clinical death. Unresponsiveness, cessation of respiration, development of pallor and cyanosis, absence of heart sounds and blood pressure, loss of palpable pulse, and dilation of the pupils are present. Immediate and definitive action must be instituted within 4 to 6 minutes after the arrest or biological death will occur.

*Basic life support* is an emergency procedure that consists of recognizing an arrest and initiating proper CPR techniques to maintain life until the victim either recovers or is transported to a medical facility where advanced life-support measures are available. The "ABC" mnemonic of CPR stands for airway, breathing, and circulation (Table 25-10). Safe implementation of CPR involves five steps.

**Step I—Assess level of consciousness.** Persons who appear to be unconscious may be either asleep, deaf, or possibly intoxicated. Unconsciousness is confirmed by shaking the victim's shoulders and shouting "Are you OK?" If the person does not respond, help is summoned and the victim is placed in the supine position on a *firm* surface.

**Step II—Open the airway.** The tongue is the most common cause of airway obstruction in the unconscious person. The head tilt–chin lift method and the jaw thrust are the two recommended methods for opening and maintaining the airway (Figures 25-43 and 25-44). Jaw thrust (without head tilt) is the safest approach to use with a victim with a suspected neck injury. The head must be carefully supported to avoid turning or tilting it backward. While maintaining an open airway, the rescuer should take 3 to 5 seconds to *look, listen,* and *feel* for spontaneous breathing. The rescuer places an ear over the victim's nose and mouth while looking at the victim's chest. The rescuer looks to see if the chest moves with respiration, listens for air escaping during exhalation, and feels for air movement against the face.

**Step III-Initiate artificial ventilation**

***Mouth-to-mouth ventilation.*** To initiate artificial ventilation give two breaths lasting 1 to 2 seconds each, and observe for adequate ventilation. If the patient does not resume breathing, continue mouth-to-mouth ventilation. One breath is delivered every 5 seconds.

1. Maintain victim in head tilt-chin lift position.
2. Pinch nostrils.

### research

Reference: Gallagher RD et al: The impact of the implantable cardioverter defibrillator on quality of life, *Am J Crit Care* 6(1):16, 1997.

The authors reviewed 18 research studies that reported the effects of the implantable cardioverter-defibrillator (ICD) on recipients and their families. Most studies found recipients pleased and confident with the physiological outcome of maintaining or improving life expectancy. Many patients resumed normal activities, including returning to work whenever possible. Some patients reported altering their normal activities (sleep, recreation, sexual activity, and driving) because of the device. It was reported that 6% of drivers receive shocks while driving, although all pulled over in sufficient time to avoid vehicular accidents. Psychological reactions included fear over the unpredictability of the shock and the fear of pain. Overall, the anxiety level of patients with ICDs was reported to be higher than the general population; however, the degree of anxiety varied considerably. Optimism was the most often reported coping mechanism, followed by self-reliance, confrontation, and seeking social support. Adjustment disorders, major depression, and panic disorders have been reported. The incidence of these disorders was higher where family support was perceived to be inadequate.

**table 25-10** *Sequence of Cardiopulmonary Resuscitation*

| Findings | Action | ABCs of Action | Timing |
|---|---|---|---|
| No response | Activate EMS | | |
| Absence of respirations; cyanosis, dilated pupils | Open airway | A—Open *airway* | 3-5 sec to assess for respiration |
| Respirations still absent | Initiate artificial ventilation | B—Restore *breathing* | Deliver 1 breath every 5 sec 1.5 to 2 sec (12/min), per breath |
| Carotid pulse not palpable | Initiate external cardiac compressions | C—Restore *circulation* | 10 sec to establish pulselessness |
| ECG; ventricular fibrillation | Drug therapy; defibrillation | D—Provide *definitive* treatment | Compression rate of 80-100/min<br>Compression depth 1.5-2 in |

*EMS,* Emergency medical services.

3. Take a deep breath and place mouth around outside of victim's mouth, forming a tight seal. Use a rescue airway if available.
4. Blow into victim's mouth.
5. Adequate ventilation is demonstrated by
   a. Rise and fall of chest
   b. Hearing and feeling air escape as victim passively exhales.
   c. Feeling the resistance of the victim's lungs expanding.

***Mouth-to-nose ventilation.*** Mouth-to-nose ventilation is indicated when the mouth is seriously injured or if a tight seal cannot be established around the mouth. The rescuer places one hand on the forehead to tilt the head back and uses the other hand to lift the lower jaw and close the mouth. After taking a deep breath, the rescuer seals the mouth around the victim's nose and begins blowing until the lungs expand. Occasionally, when mouth-to-nose ventilation is used, it may become necessary to open the victim's mouth or lips to allow air to escape on exhalation because the soft palate may produce nasopharyngeal obstruction.

***Mouth-to-stoma ventilation.*** Direct mouth-to-stoma artificial ventilation is performed for the laryngectomy patient. For the patient with a temporary tracheostomy tube, mouth-to-tube ventilation should be initiated after the cuff is inflated.

***Mouth-to-barrier ventilation.*** An alternative to direct mouth-to-mouth ventilation is use of a barrier device such as a face shield and mask device. Most mask devices have a one-way valve so that exhaled air does not enter the rescuer's mouth; many face shields have no exhalation valves, which cause air leakage around the shield. The barrier device (face

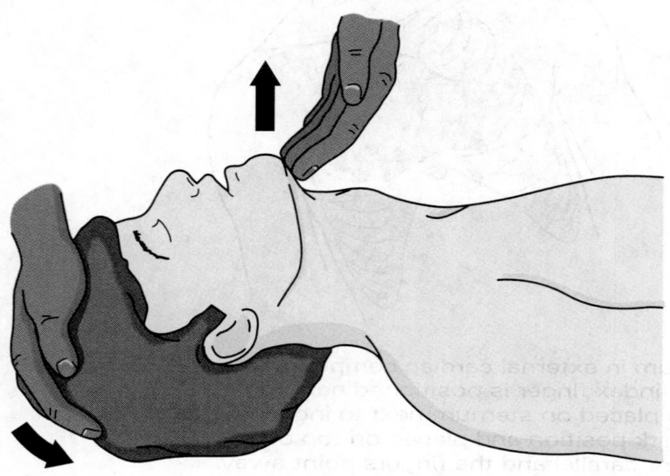

**fig. 25-43** Head tilt-chin lift maneuver for opening airway. Place one hand on forehead and place tips of fingers of other hand under lower jaw near chin. Bring chin forward while pressing forehead down.

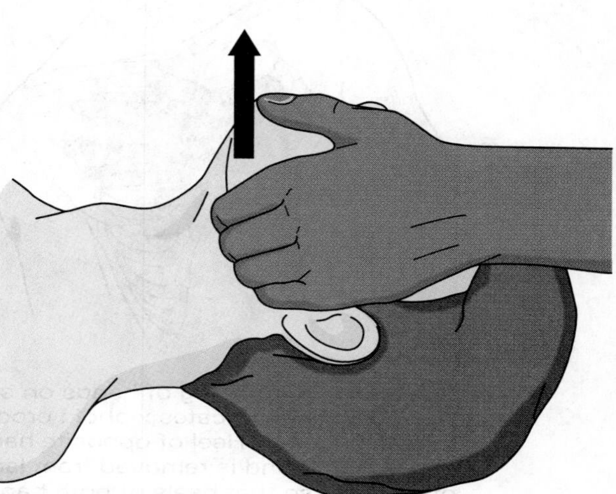

**fig. 25-44** Jaw thrust maneuver for opening airway.

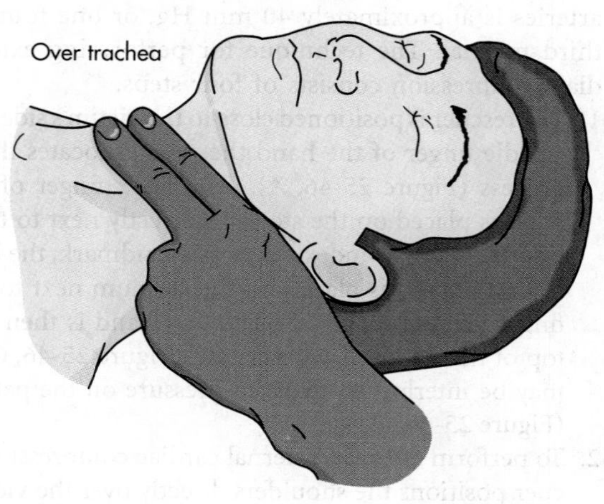


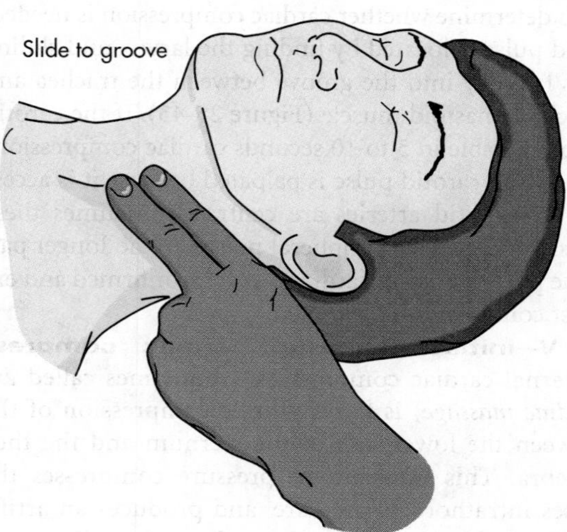


**fig. 25-45** Locating carotid artery.

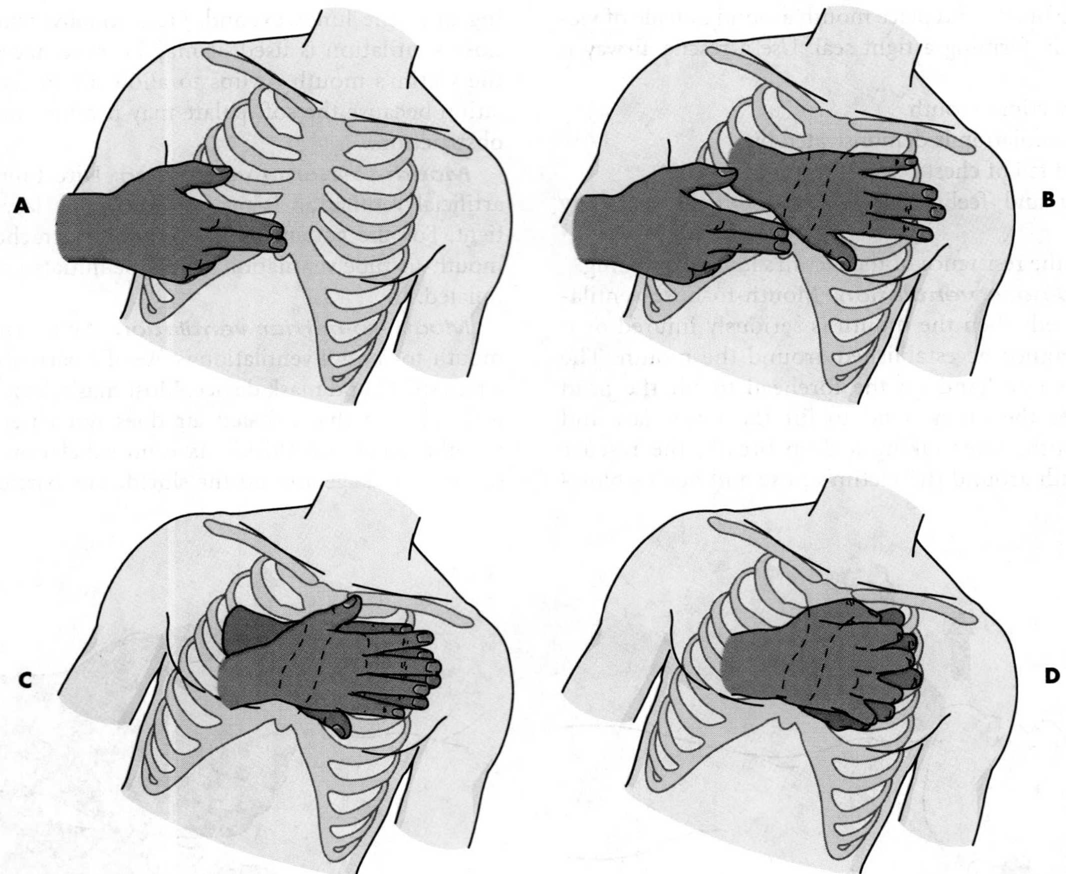


**fig. 25-46** Positioning of hands on sternum in external cardiac compression. **A**, Middle finger locates xiphoid process; index finger is positioned next to middle finger. **B**, Heel of opposite hand is placed on sternum next to index finger. **C**, First hand is removed from landmark position and placed on top of other hand so that heels of both hands are parallel and the fingers point away. **D**, Fingers may be interlocked to avoid pressure on the ribs.

mask or face shield) is positioned over the victim's mouth and nose, ensuring an adequate air seal.

**Step IV—Assess circulation.** The carotid pulse is palpated to determine whether cardiac compression is needed. The carotid pulse is located by finding the larynx and sliding the fingers laterally into the groove between the trachea and the sternocleidomastoid muscle (Figure 25-45). If the carotid pulse is not palpable in 5 to 10 seconds cardiac compressions are initiated. The carotid pulse is palpated because it is accessible and the carotid arteries are central. Sometimes these pulses persist when more peripheral pulses are no longer palpable. If the pulse is absent, cardiac arrest is confirmed and external chest compression is initiated.

**Step V—Initiate external cardiac compression.** External cardiac compression (sometimes called *external cardiac massage*) is the rhythmic compression of the heart between the lower half of the sternum and the thoracic vertebra. This intermittent pressure compresses the heart, raises intrathoracic pressure, and produces an artificial pulsatile circulation. Correctly performed cardiac compressions can produce a peak systolic blood pressure of more than 100 mm Hg. The diastolic pressure is close to zero, however, and the mean blood pressure in the carotid arteries is approximately 40 mm Hg, or one fourth to one third normal. The technique for performing external cardiac compression consists of four steps:

1. The rescuer is positioned close to the victim's side. Using the middle finger of the hand the rescuer locates the xiphoid process (Figure 25-46, *A*). The index finger of the same hand is placed on the sternum directly next to the middle finger. Using the index finger as a landmark, the heel of the opposite hand is placed on the sternum next to the index finger (Figure 25-46, *B*). The first hand is then placed on top of the hand on the sternum (Figure 25-46, *C*). Fingers may be interlocked to avoid pressure on the patient's ribs (Figure 25-46, *D*).
2. To perform effective external cardiac compression, the rescuer positions the shoulders directly over the victim's sternum, keeps the elbows locked in a straight position, and depresses the lower sternum 1½ to 2 inches. The compres-

sions should be regular, smooth, and uninterrupted. After each compression the rescuer must release the pressure completely to allow the heart to refill. A compression rate of 80 to 100 per minute can be achieved with a ratio of compressions to breaths of 15:2. The rescuer delivers 2 full breaths after every 15 compressions (Figure 25-47).

3. When two rescuers are available to administer CPR, one rescuer is positioned at the victim's side and performs external cardiac compression while the second rescuer remains at the victim's head to perform artificial ventilation. If two rescuers are available, the cardiac compression rate remains the same but a 5:1 ratio of cardiac compression to ventilation is established. The rescuer who is ventilating the victim quickly delivers one full breath (1½ to 2 seconds) after every five compressions during a pause in compressions. Two-rescuer CPR is advocated only for skilled providers because of the complexity of coordinating the timing of interventions.
4. After the first minute of CPR, the carotid pulse is palpated to assess the effectiveness of CPR and to check for the return of spontaneous circulation. If two rescuers are performing CPR, the person ventilating the victim also can assess pulses and monitor for the return of spontaneous breathing. Rescuers should continue to perform CPR until one of the following takes place:
   a. Spontaneous circulation and ventilation return.
   b. Another rescuer takes over basic life support.
   c. The victim is transported to an emergency facility.
   d. The victim is pronounced dead by a physician.
   e. The rescuer is exhausted and unable to continue.

For a summary of CPR steps, see the accompanying Guidelines for Care Box.

**guidelines for care**

**Cardiopulmonary Resuscitation for the Adult Victim**

Activate EMS after establishing unresponsiveness

Airway:
- Assess for respirations (3 to 5 seconds)
- Rescue breaths per minute = 1 every 5 seconds (12 per minute)
- Rate of breaths = 1.5 to 2 seconds

Circulation:
- Assess for carotid pulse (up to 10 seconds)
- Determine hand position
- Achieve compression rate of 80 to 100 per minute.
- Compression depth 1.5 to 2 inches
- Ratio compressions to breaths, one-person CPR: 15:2
- Ratio of compressions to breaths, two-person CPR: 5:1

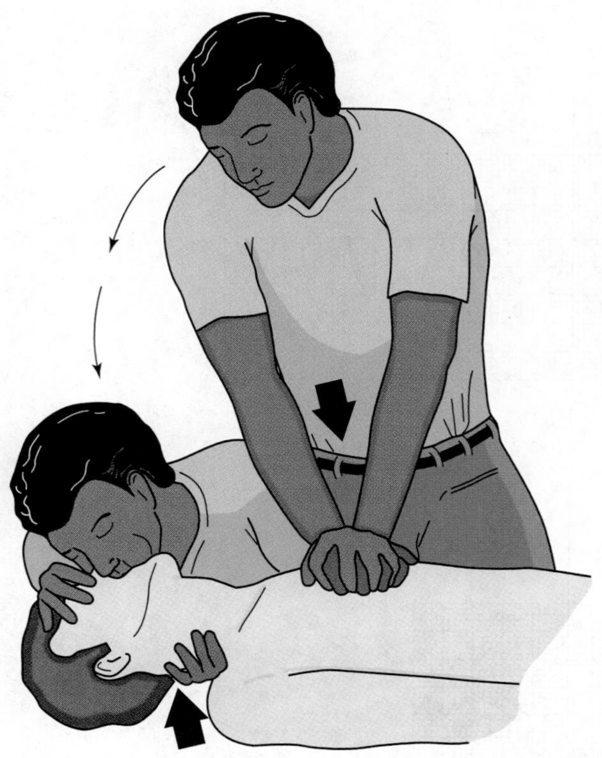

fig. 25-47 One-person rescuer CPR. The person delivers two rapid inflations after every 15 compressions.

### Advanced cardiac life support

Most hospitals have trained teams of personnel, including physicians, nurses, anesthesiologists, and technicians, who can provide immediate care in the event of a cardiac arrest. Equipment needs include an ECG machine, a suction device, oxygen, a defibrillator, a breathing bag, a laryngoscope, a variety of endotracheal tubes, a cutdown set, intravenous fluids, and a tracheostomy set. Medications administered during a cardiac arrest are usually stored on an emergency cart. Algorithms for advanced life support are reviewed and updated regularly by the American Heart Association (AHA). A local AHA office can provide the most current practice guidelines and information about available training sessions.

### Complications of cardiopulmonary resuscitation

The most common complication of external cardiac compression is fracture of the ribs. This may occur even when the technique of external cardiac compression was performed correctly. Other possible complications include fractured sternum, costochondral separation, and lung contusions. Any indication of labored respiration, paradoxical pulse, muffled heart sounds, tachycardia, decreased breath sounds, or drop in blood pressure may indicate pericardial tamponade from the injection of intracardiac medications and must be reported to the physician immediately. Laceration of the liver also may occur as a result of compressions performed over the xiphoid process.

The long-term effects of CPR on cardiac arrest survivors is a topic of current nursing research (see the Research Box on p. 690).

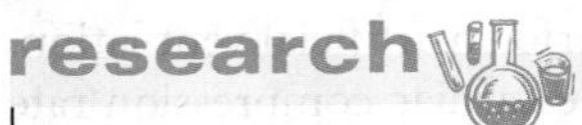

Reference: Sauve MJ et al: Factors associated with cognitive recovery after cardiopulmonary resuscitation, *Am J Crit Care* 5(2):127, 1996.

The probability of sustaining some degree of cognitive impairment after sudden cardiac death is high. Nurses can best help survivors if they know the expected types of impairment and clinical variables that predict cognitive outcomes. This study followed for 6 months the cognitive outcomes of 45 patients who had sustained sudden cardiac death. Independent variables included time to cardiopulmonary resuscitation (CPR), time to defibrillation, duration of CPR, time to awakening, ejection fraction, New York Heart Association class I to IV, tension, anger, and depression. Seven standardized neuropsychological instruments were used to calculate nine cognitive outcomes: orientation, attention, memory (immediate recall, early recall, delayed recall), recognition, reasoning, motor speed, and motor variability. A reported 84% of survivors had mild to severe deficits in one or more cognitive areas while hospitalized; 50% remained impaired in one or more areas at 6 months. Delayed recall was the most frequently occurring impairment. Time to awaken accounted for a unique portion of the variance in orientation and memory outcomes over time. Differences in left ventricular function accounted for recovery with motor speed. The authors concluded that half of the long-term survivors of sudden cardiac death were cognitively intact at 6 months after CPR. They also noted 25% of those patients surviving sudden cardiac arrest will have moderate to severe impairment in memory.

## critical thinking QUESTIONS

**1** A 48-year-old African-American woman with a history of hypertension is admitted to the CCU with her first transmural MI. Within an hour her BP drops from 100/60 to 70/50. She suffers cardiac arrest and dies. Autopsy report shows free wall rupture. Discuss the reasons for this complication in this particular case.

**2** A 58-year-old white male is admitted to the CCU with the diagnosis of acute anterior infarction 13 hours after onset of chest pain. CK > 450. On admission, his monitor shows sinus tachycardia at a rate of 110 with occasional PVBs, BP 110/70. Within 24 hours, his BP is 80/60, HR = 130, respirations = 28. He is lethargic. Urinary output = 15 cc/hr. CVP = 12. Discuss the nursing diagnoses particularly relevant to this patient, and design a plan of care.

**3** The following rhythm strip shows sinus rhythm with conversion to
a. Atrial fibrillation
b. Paroxysmal atrial tachycardia
c. Ventricular tachycardia
Discuss possible causes and treatment.

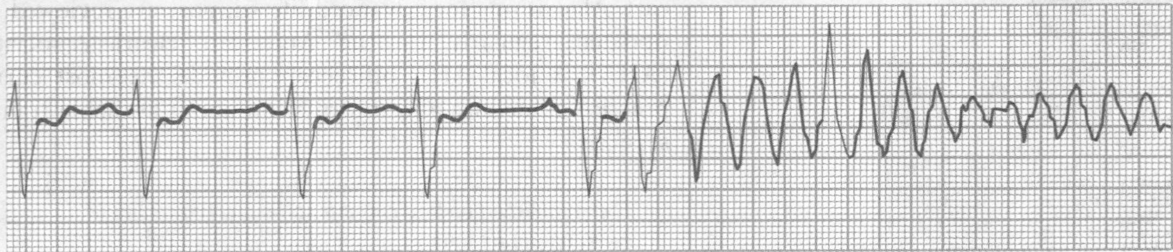

**4** The following rhythm strip shows
a. Sinus tachycardia
b. Atrial tachycardia
c. Ventricular tachycardia
Discuss possible causes and treatment indicated.

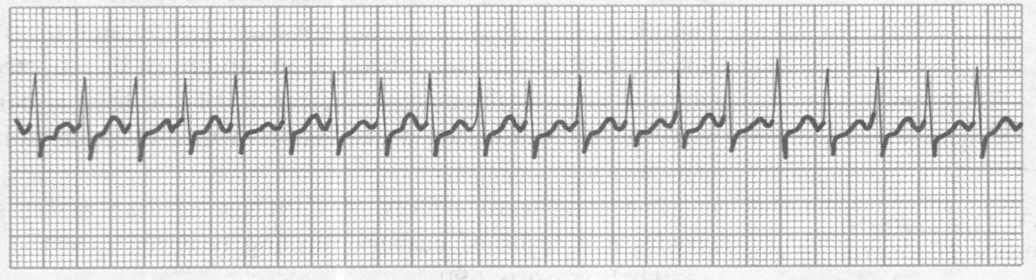

## chapter SUMMARY

### CORONARY ARTERY DISEASE

- Nonmodifiable risk factors for CAD include advancing age, gender (males), race, and a positive family history of CAD.
- Major modifiable risk factors for CAD include hyperlipoproteinemia, hypertension, diabetes mellitus, and cigarette smoking; a diet high in cholesterol and saturated fats contributes to the risk.
- Behavioral and psychosocial influences are associated with the occurrence of CAD.
- Angina pectoris is chest pain caused by reversible myocardial ischemia. Treatment involves increasing myocardial blood and oxygen supply (with medications or surgery) and reducing myocardial oxygen demands. The most commonly used drugs for treating angina pectoris are vasodilators, beta blockers, and calcium channel blockers.
- Myocardial infarction is the result of prolonged myocardial ischemia, which causes irreversible cellular damage. The clinical consequences depend on the location of the coronary artery occlusion and the extent of necrosis.
- Diagnosis of MI is based primarily on the clinical picture, ECG findings, and elevation of serum enzyme levels. Medical interventions include promotion of improved coronary circulation and tissue oxygenation, relief of pain, and prevention of further tissue damage and complications.
- Thrombolytic agents to activate fibrinolytic processes to lyse the clot must be given within 3 to 6 hours of the initial infarction.
- Coronary artery bypass graft consists of circumventing a coronary occlusion using a saphenous vein or internal mammary artery graft.
- An alternative to CABG for selected persons is PTCA. A balloon-tipped catheter is inserted into the coronary artery, and the balloon is inflated to increase lumen diameter by remodeling the plaque.
- Intravascular stenting increases the lumen diameter through a metallic implant that expands to maintain the cylindrical lumen.
- Nursing interventions for CAD include promoting oxygenation, tissue perfusion, adequate cardiac output, comfort, activity, nutrition, and elimination; providing rest; promoting relief of anxiety; and patient teaching.
- Complications of MI include dysrhythmias, cardiogenic shock, congestive heart failure, ventricular aneurysm, post-myocardial infarction syndrome, pericarditis, and embolism.

### CARDIAC DYSRHYTHMIAS

- The mechanisms responsible for the genesis of dysrhythmias include altered automaticity, conduction abnormalities, and reentry.
- Dysrhythmias originating in the SA node include sinus dysrhythmias, sinus tachycardia, sinus bradycardia, sick sinus syndrome, and sinus exit block or sinus arrest.
- Dysrhythmias originating in the atria include premature atrial beat, wandering atrial pacemaker, atrial tachycardia, atrial flutter, and atrial fibrillation.
- Dysrhythmias originating in the AV junction include premature junctional beats and junctional rhythms.
- Dysrhythmias originating in the ventricle include premature ventricular beats, ventricular rhythms and tachycardia, ventricular fibrillation, and asystole.
- Conduction abnormalities include AV block and bundle branch block.
- Treatment for cardiac dysrhythmias involves identification and elimination of the cause (if possible), pharmacological or electrical suppression of ectopic impulse initiation, and modalities to regulate heart rate (drugs, regulation of oxygen demand, artificial pacemakers).
- General nursing interventions for persons with dysrhythmias include promoting adequate cardiac output, activity and rest, tissue perfusion, comfort, relief of anxiety and a feeling of well-being, and patient/family learning.
- Artificial pacing may be accomplished using temporary or permanent pacemakers. Complications include infection, dysrhythmias, and electrical interferences.
- Radiofrequency catheter ablation may be indicated in dysrhythmias refractory to medications. Selected foci or pathways are destroyed to restore stability to the cardiac rhythm.
- Cardioversion and defibrillation are two methods for using electrical energy to convert a cardiac dysrhythmia to one that is more hemodynamically stable. Defibrillation is unsynchronized electrical countershock, whereas cardioversion synchronizes with the R wave to prevent accidental discharge during the ventricular vulnerable period.
- The implantable cardioverter-defibrillator is an implanted device that automatically delivers a countershock on sensing ventricular fibrillation. Models often include antitachycardiac pacemakers as the primary therapy followed by defibrillation if unsuccessful.

### CARDIOPULMONARY RESUSCITATION

- Steps of basic life support include assessment of level of consciousness, opening of airway, initiation of artificial ventilation, assessment of circulation, and initiation of external cardiac compressions.

## References


1. American Heart Association: *Heart facts,* Dallas, 1992, The American Heart Association.
2. Ashton KC: Perceived learning needs of men and women after myocardial infarction, *J Cardiovasc Nurs* 12(1):93, 1997.
3. Baas LS, Beery TA, Hickey CS: Care and safety of pacemaker electrodes in intensive care and telemetry nursing units, *Am J Crit Care* 6(4):302, 1997.
4. Bostom AG et al: Elevated plasma lipoprotein(a) and coronary heart disease in men aged 55 years and younger: a prospective study, *JAMA* 276(7):544, 1996.
5. Braunwald E et al: *Unstable angina: diagnosis and management. Clinical practice guideline number 10 (amended),* AHCPR Pub No 94-0602, Rockville, Md, 1994, Agency for Health Care Policy and Research and the National Heart, Lung, and Blood Institute, Public Health Service, US Department of Health and Human Services.
6. Bubien RS, Knotts SM, Kay GN: Radiofrequency catheter ablation: concepts and nursing implications, *Cardiovasc Nurs* 31(3):17, 1995.
7. Centers for Disease Control and Prevention: *Diabetes surveillance,* Atlanta, 1983, USDHHS, PHS, CDC.
8. Crowe J et al: Anxiety and depression after acute myocardial infarction, *Heart Lung* 25:98, 1996.
9. Cummins RO et al: In-hospital resuscitation: a statement for healthcare professionals from the American Heart Association Emergency Cardiac Care Committee and the Advanced Cardiac Life Support, Basic Life Support, Pediatric Resuscitation, and Program Administration Subcommittees, *Circulation* 95:2211, 1997.
10. Futterman LG, Correa LF, Lemberg L: Thrombolysis or primary angioplasty? An ongoing controversy in the management of acute myocardial infarction, *Am J Crit Care* 5(2):160, 1996.

11. Futterman LG, Lemberg L: Atrial fibrillation: an increasingly common and provocative arrhythmia, *Am J Crit Care* 5(5):379, 1996.
12. Futterman LG, Lemberg L: SGOT, LDH, HBD, CPK, CK-MB, MB1MB2, cTnT, cTnC, cTnI, *Am J Crit Care* 6(4):333, 1997.
13. Gallagher RD et al: The impact of the implantable cardioverter defibrillator on quality of life, *Am J Crit Care* 6(1):16, 1997.
14. Guidelines for cardiopulmonary resuscitation and emergency cardiac care, *JAMA* 268(16):2184, 1992.
15. Hunick MGM et al: The recent decline in mortality from coronary heart disease, 1980-1990: the effect of secular trends in risk factors and treatment, *JAMA* 277(7):535, 1997.
16. Kannel WB: Blood pressure as a cardiovascular risk factor: prevention and treatment, *JAMA* 275(24):1571, 1996.
17. Keeling A: The family experience after acute myocardial infarction, doctoral dissertation, Charlottesville, 1992, University of Virginia.
18. Keeling A, Dennison P: Telephone follow-up after acute myocardial infarction: a pilot study, *Heart Lung* 24(1):45, 1995.
19. Moser DK: Correcting misconceptions about women and heart disease, *Am J Nurs* 97(4):26, 1997.
20. Prystowsky EN et al: Management of patients with atrial fibrillation: a statement for healthcare professionals from the subcommittee on electrocardiography and electrophysiology, American Heart Association, *Circulation* 93(6):1262, 1996.
21. Sauve MJ et al: Factors associated with cognitive recovery after cardiopulmonary resuscitation, *Am J Crit Care* 5(2):127, 1996.
22. Stampfer MJ et al: A prospective study of triglyceride level, low-density lipoprotein particle diameter, and risk of myocardial infarction, *JAMA* 276(11):882, 1996.
23. Stephens N et al: Randomized controlled trial of vitamin E in patients with coronary disease: Cambridge Heart Antioxidant Study (CHAOS), *Lancet* 347:781, 1996.
24. USDHHS: *Physical activity and health: a report of the Surgeon General,* Washington, DC, 1996, USDHHS.
25. Weaver WD et al: Comparisons of characteristics and outcomes among women and men with acute myocardial infarction treated with thrombolytic therapy, *JAMA* 275:777, 1996.
26. Wenger NK et al: *Cardiac rehabilitation as secondary prevention. Clinical practice guideline. Quick reference guide for clinicians,* AHCPR Pub No 96-0673, Washington, DC, 1993, US Department of Health and Human Services, Public Health Services, Agency for Health Care Policy and Research and National Heart, Lung, and Blood Institute.

# chapter 26 MANAGEMENT OF PERSONS WITH Inflammatory Heart Disease, Heart Failure, and Persons Undergoing Cardiac Surgery

KATHY HENLEY HAUGH and KATHERINE BALLENGER

## objectives

*After studying this chapter, the learner should be able to:*

1 Discuss the collaborative care management of patients with pericarditis, endocarditis, and heart failure.

2 Explain the pathophysiology associated with each of the clinical manifestations seen in patients with heart failure.

3 Describe the differences between dilated, hypertrophic, and restrictive cardiomyopathy.

4 Differentiate mitral stenosis, mitral regurgitation, and mitral valve prolapse in terms of etiology, impact on the heart's function, presentation, and treatment.

5 Differentiate aortic stenosis and aortic regurgitation in terms of etiology, impact on the heart's function, presentation, and treatment.

6 Identify at least three important aspects of patient and family education for patients with cardiac valve disorders.

7 Describe six indications for cardiac surgery.

8 Discuss the four major physiological sequelae of cardiopulmonary bypass in the context of post-operative care of the cardiac surgery patient.

9 Discuss the assessment, monitoring, and follow-up of patients receiving anticoagulation after cardiac valve surgery.

Heart disease can be divided into two general groups: congenital and acquired. Congenital heart disease is caused by error in the embryological development of the heart's structures. In acquired heart disease heart damage may occur because of inflammation, infection, chemical agents, or diminished blood supply. Onset may be sudden or gradual. For example, inflammation may cause scarring of heart valves, muscle, or outer coverings that can impair the heart's function. Any changes in the coronary vessels that supply the heart muscle can decrease its efficiency.

Heart disease can be classified according to a specific cause such as rheumatic fever, infective endocarditis, or hypertension. It also is classified according to anatomical changes such as valvular scarring. Progression of any of these diseases can lead to cardiac failure and cardiac dysrhythmias. These complications cause many of the symptoms commonly associated with heart disease, but with early diagnosis and treatment, these problems may be prevented or controlled.

## INFLAMMATORY HEART DISEASE

### PERICARDITIS

#### Etiology/Epidemiology

Pericarditis is an inflammatory process of the visceral or parietal pericardium. It can be acute or chronic and can spread from or to the myocardium. Pericarditis can occur as a result of bacterial, viral, or fungal infection. It also can occur as a complication of a systemic disease process such as rheumatoid arthritis, systemic lupus erhythematosus, scleroderma, uremia, or myocardial infarction or as a result of trauma, including operative procedures.

#### Pathophysiology

In acute pericarditis, the membranes surrounding the heart become inflamed. The inflamed membranes rub against each other and produce the classic pericardial friction rub of pericarditis. The friction rub sounds scratchy and harsh on auscultation and lasts throughout systole and diastole. The patient complains of severe precordial chest pain, which may closely resemble that of acute myocardial infarction. The pain intensifies when the person is lying supine and decreases with sitting. The pain also may intensify when the patient breathes deeply.

Typically temperature elevation occurs and a leukocytosis of 10,000/mm$^3$ to 20,000 mm$^3$ is present. Malaise and tachycardia are common. The electrocardiogram (ECG) shows diffuse nonspecific ST segment abnormalities representative of pericardial inflammation over the entire surface of the heart.

The accumulation of fluid within the pericardial sac is called a pericardial effusion (Figure 26-1). The fluid may be serous, purulent, or hemorrhagic. Serous effusions usually accompany heart failure. Purulent effusions indicate underlying disorders, such as tuberculosis or neoplasms. Hemorrhagic effusions most often occur from trauma, aneurysm rupture, or coagulation abnormalities. An echocardiogram provides the most definitive diagnosis of pericardial effusion. The ECG may show bradycardia with low-voltage QRS complexes. When fluid accumulation is gradual, the patient may not develop symptoms until as much as 1 L of clear or serosanguinous fluid is present.

When fluid accumulates in the pericardial sac, cardiac tamponade (compression of the heart) may occur. The compression decreases venous return to the heart, resulting in a decrease in ventricular filling and therefore a decrease in stroke volume. These events can lead to cardiac failure, shock, and death. Signs of cardiac tamponade include diminished heart sounds, tachycardia, paradoxical pulse (see Chapter 24), a narrowed pulse pressure, and distended neck veins.

Chronic pericarditis can be constrictive or adhesive. Chronic constrictive pericarditis may result from fibrosis of the pericardial sac secondary to surgery, uremia, or radiation. The thick fibrous pericardium tightens around the heart, decreasing cardiac filling and output (Figure 26-2). Patients may complain of dyspnea and fatigue and exhibit symptoms of heart failure as a result of the diminished ability of the heart to pump.

### Collaborative Care Management

Treatment is specific to the underlying cause of the pericarditis, if known. If the pericardial effusion is small, therapy is supportive, with administration of nonsteroidal antiinflammatory agents, including indomethacin. Corticosteroids are prescribed if the inflammation is refractory to nonsteroidal agents. One of the main complications of pericarditis is recurrence after the antiinflammatory drug therapy is completed.

A pericardiocentesis (pericardial tap) may be performed to remove excess fluid from large effusions. A common approach is through a small anterolateral thoracotomy. A pericardial fenestration (pericardial window) is created to allow for continuous drainage of pericardial fluid when necessary. Complications include atelectasis and introduction of infection. Corticosteroids may be administered to reduce inflammation. The nurse monitors for drainage quality and amount and reports increases or changes in drainage character immediately.

In chronic pericarditis, removal of the pericardium (pericardiectomy) may be necessary to restore cardiac function. An open approach through a median sternotomy provides good access to the pericardium, as well as to most cardiac structures in the event of unexpected problems. Postoperative care is similar to that for other cardiac surgery (see p. 735-743). Adjunctive measures similar to those used for heart failure may be prescribed to restore the heart's pumping efficiency.

With both acute and chronic pericarditis, the nurse monitors pulses and heart sounds for changes that suggest cardiac tamponade. Analgesics are used judiciously to control pain and facilitate lung expansion. Pain control is especially important for patients undergoing pericardial windows and pericardiectomy. Antiinflammatories and comfort measures are used to control fever and general malaise. Nursing interventions include encouraging an adequate fluid intake, modifying bed covers and clothing, pacing activities to allow rest periods, and using distraction or other nonpharmacological methods to manage pain.

#### *Patient/family education*

The nurse teaches the patient and significant others about the nature of the disease and the purpose and correct use of all medications. This includes a discussion of all medication side effects. The nurse teaches measures to decrease fatigue and provides information on how to minimize the risks of com-

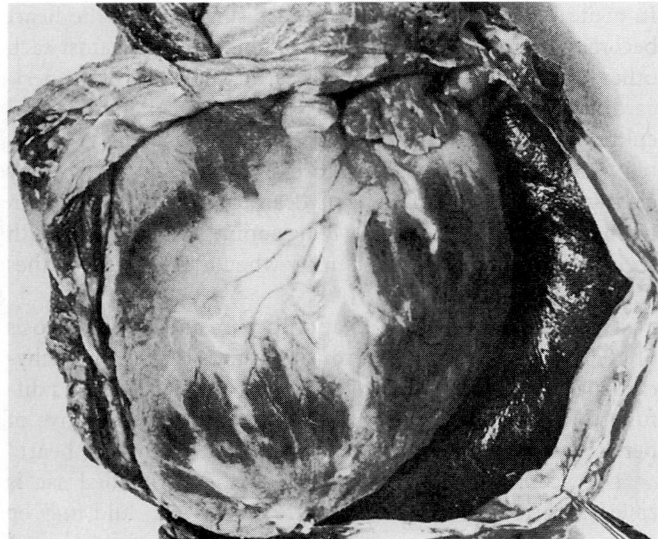

**fig. 26-1** Exudate of blood in the pericardial sac from rupture of aneurysm.

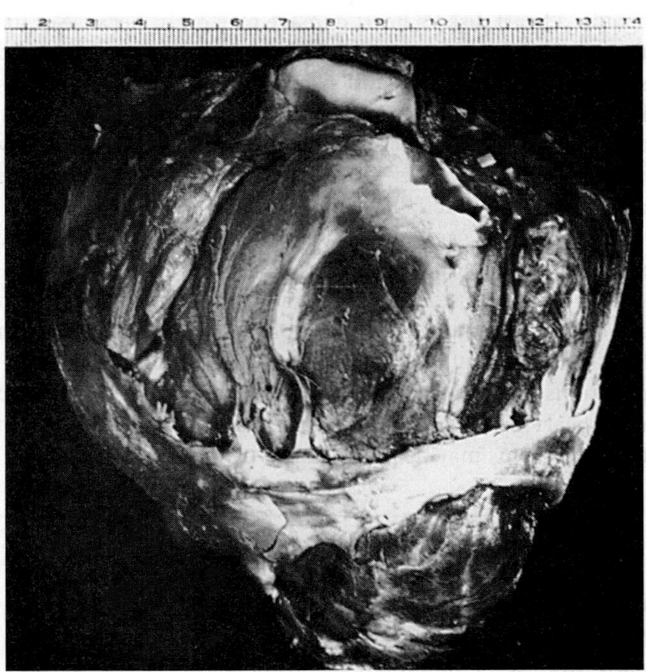

**fig. 26-2** Constrictive pericarditis. Notice band of calcified tissue that constricts heart.

plications. The nurse also provides an overview of the signs and symptoms of recurrent pericarditis that would need to be promptly reported to the health care provider.

## INFECTIVE ENDOCARDITIS

### Etiology/Epidemiology

Infective endocarditis is an infection of the endocardium, most often of the heart valves. Acute endocarditis occurs rapidly, often on normal heart valves, and if untreated may cause death within days to weeks. Subacute bacterial endocarditis (SBE) develops more gradually, usually on previously damaged heart valves, and responds well to treatment.

Infective endocarditis can also be classified based on the causative organism. Hemolytic streptococci are the major causative organisms, especially in the subacute form. Other major infective agents include staphylococci, such as *Staphylococcus aureus* and *Staphylococcus epidermidis,* and enterococci.

Persons at high risk for endocarditis are those with underlying cardiac pathological conditions, including rheumatic valvular disease, congenital heart disease, and degenerative heart disease. Endocarditis develops in 1% to 4% of persons who have artificial heart valve implants. In some cases, endocarditis occurs after intrusive procedures such as dental procedures, minor surgery, gynecological examinations, and insertion of indwelling urinary catheters or renal shunts. Persons who inject "street drugs" directly into the veins are also at high risk because of the possibility of bacteremia from contaminated needles and syringes. Box 26-1 identifies specific patient populations at risk for infective endocarditis.

### Pathophysiology

A damaged cardiac valve or a ventricular septal defect produces turbulent blood flow, which allows bacteria to settle on the low-pressure side of the valve or defect. The hallmark of endocarditis is the platelet-fibrin-bacteria mass on the valve called a vegetation (Figure 26-3). The organisms surround the heart valve, become embedded in the valve matrix, and result in vegetative growths that may scar and perforate the leaflets. Emboli can occur if the vegetative growths break free of the valves and enter the bloodstream. If the vegetative emboli enter organs such as the spleen and kidney, abscesses may form.

The onset of SBE is gradual, and the patient reports malaise and general achiness. Low-grade fever is usually present, although a high fever usually occurs with *S. aureus* infection. Other commonly reported symptoms include headache, arthralgias, arthritis, low back pain, myalgia, tenosynovitis, anorexia, weight loss, chest pain, night sweats, and occasional hemoptysis. Physical examination may reveal splenomegaly, clubbing of the fingers, the presence of Osler's nodes (small, raised, tender, bluish areas) on fingers or toe pads, and small capillary hemorrhages (petechiae) in the conjunctiva, in the mouth, and on the extremities. Auscultation reveals murmurs over the affected cardiac valves. A normocytic normochromic anemia is usually present.

### Collaborative Care Management

Diagnostic tests include blood cultures to guide antibiotic therapy, echocardiography (preferably transesophageal) to demonstrate valvular vegetations, and occasionally cardiac catheterization to evaluate ventricular and valvular function. Deteriorated heart valves are surgically replaced with prostheses when necessary.

Cellular and humoral host defenses are impaired over the affected areas because the colonized bacteria are embedded in the valve matrix, preventing host defenses from reaching the bacteria. The major aim of therapy is to eliminate all

**box 26-1** *Patient Populations at Risk for Infective Endocarditis*

**HIGH RISK**
- Prosthetic heart valves
- Previous history of endocarditis
- Complex congenital cyanotic heart disease
- Surgically constructed systemic pulmonary shunts or conduits

**MODERATE RISK**
- Patent ductus arteriosus
- Ventricular septal defect
- Primum atrial septal defect
- Coarctation of aorta
- Bicuspid aortic valve
- Acquired valvular dysfunction
- Hypertrophic cardiomyopathy
- Some clinical presentations of mitral valve prolapse*

*See complete American Heart Association guidelines in Dajani et al[13] for specific indications.

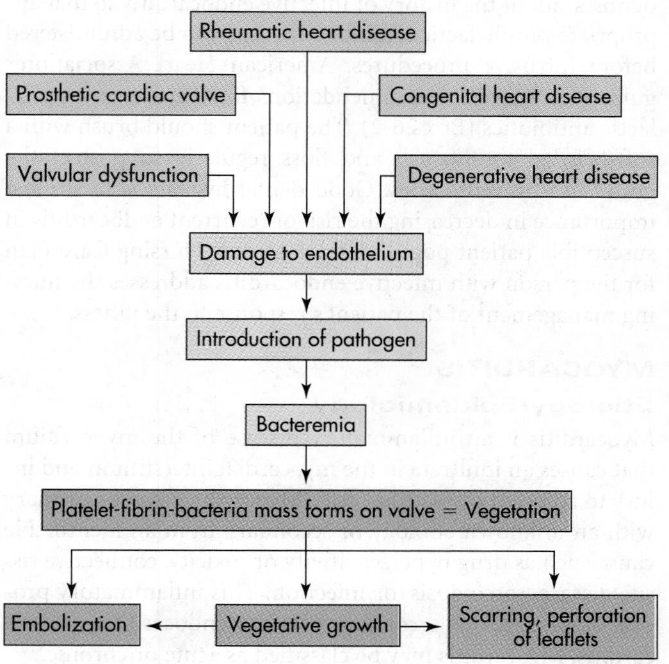


**fig. 26-3** Infective endocarditis. Relationship of endothelial damage, bacteria introduction, and subsequent vegetative growth.

microorganisms from the vegetative growths and prevent complications. If infective endocarditis goes untreated for weeks or months, the incidence of embolic complications and progressive involvement of the heart valves greatly increases. Therefore antibiotic therapy is initiated after three blood cultures are obtained to identify the infecting organism. Antibiotic therapy continues even after symptoms abate, usually for 4 to 6 weeks.

Peak and trough drug levels are evaluated to ensure therapeutic outcomes of antibiotic administration and avoid potential negative patient outcomes. The nephrotoxic effects of many antibiotics necessitate ongoing assessment of renal function through serum blood urea nitrogen (BUN) and creatinine levels.

Health care professionals monitor the patient for the onset of new murmurs or changes in preexisting murmurs. With impaired valve function, the patient is at risk for developing heart failure. Assessing breath sounds and monitoring fluid status alerts the clinician to early signs of heart failure. The risk of decreased tissue perfusion also affects the peripheral vasculature and alters the person's activity tolerance. An assessment of blood pressure and pulse at rest, during activity, and immediately after activity provides information on activity tolerance. When bedrest is necessary, active or passive range-of-motion exercises are performed as tolerated. The nurse encourages rest periods of 30 to 60 minutes between all activities.

#### Patient/family education

The nurse teaches the patient to avoid excessive fatigue and to stop activity immediately if chest pain, dyspnea, lightheadedness, or faintness occurs. Patients should also avoid others with infections. The nurse instructs the patient to inform all primary care providers, including physicians and dentists, about the history of infective endocarditis so that appropriate prophylactic antibiotic therapy can be administered before intrusive procedures. American Heart Association[13] guidelines provide recommendations for the use of prophylactic antibiotics (Box 26-2). The patient should brush with a soft-bristled toothbrush and floss regularly to protect the gums and prevent caries. Good dental hygiene is of utmost importance in decreasing the risk of recurrent endocarditis in susceptible patient populations. A sample Nursing Care Plan for the person with infective endocarditis addresses the nursing management of the patient's response to the illness.

**box 26-2** *American Heart Association Recommendations for Antibiotic Prophylaxis of Infective Endocarditis*

**DENTAL, ORAL, RESPIRATORY TRACT, OR ESOPHAGEAL PROCEDURES**

Pathogen: *Streptococcus viridans*

Antibiotic of choice: amoxicillin 2 g 1 hour before procedure; alternatives if unable to take oral preparation or if allergic to penicillin:

- Ampicillin, intravenous (IV)
- Clindamycin, oral or IV
- First-generation cephalosporins—cefazolin IV
- Azithromycin or clarithromycin

**GENITOURINARY AND NONESOPHAGEAL GASTROINTESTINAL PROCEDURES**

Pathogen: *Enterococcus faecalis*

Antibiotic of choice: parenteral ampicillin or oral amoxicillin

## MYOCARDITIS

### Etiology/Epidemiology

Myocarditis is an inflammatory disease of the myocardium that causes an infiltrate in the myocardial interstitium and injury to adjacent myocardial cells. Myocarditis may be primary with an unknown etiology or secondary from an identifiable cause such as drug hypersensitivity or toxicity, connective tissue disease, sarcoidosis, or infection. This inflammatory process often develops secondary to acute endocarditis or pericarditis. Myocarditis may be classified as acute or chronic.

Viral infection is the most common cause of myocarditis. The most commonly implicated viral agent is picornavirus. Coxsackievirus B accounts for nearly 50% of the cases, and coxsackievirus A, echovirus, and poliovirus account for most of the remainder. Other viruses include influenza A and B, rubella, mumps, rabies, Epstein-Barr, and hepatitis. Myocarditis can be caused by several other infections, by noninfectious agents, or by an autoimmune reaction. Myocarditis has been associated with acquired immunodeficiency syndrome (AIDS); possible mechanisms include opportunistic viral infection or the human immunodeficiency virus (HIV) itself.

### Pathophysiology

During the acute viral phase symptoms are flulike and include fever, lymphadenopathy, pharyngitis, myalgias, and gastrointestinal complaints. Hepatitis, encephalitis, nephritis, and orchitis also can occur. The most common cardiac symptom during the acute phase is pericardial pain, which may be associated with a friction rub because the pericardium is so inflamed. Other cardiac manifestations include signs of congestive heart failure, syncope, pericardial effusion, and ischemia. Electrocardiogram changes include ST segment elevation, T wave flattening or inversion, appearance of Q waves, and QT interval prolongation. Ventricular ectopy can include multiple forms of premature ventricular beats and ventricular tachycardia. Electrocardiogram abnormalities may disappear after recovery or persist for several years.

Preliminary laboratory findings are nonspecific, including elevation of the erythrocyte sedimentation rate, viral titers, and levels of various enzymes (such as lactic dehydrogenase, creatine kinase, and the transaminases). Mild to moderate leukocytosis with atypical lymphocytes may be seen. Chest radiographs may show the heart size to be normal or enlarged. In the acute form of myocarditis, pulmonary rales may be auscultated. Echocardiography shows dilated chambers, depressed systolic function, and a minimum to no pericardial effusion. Although the diagnosis of myocarditis may be suspected clinically, it must be confirmed histologically by endomyocardial biopsy at a time when lymphocytic infiltration

## nursing care plan | Person with Infective Endocarditis

**DATA** Mr. B. is a married, 73-year-old retired naval officer with a history of aortic regurgitation first noted 4 years ago. He also has a history of irritable bowel syndrome with 7 weeks of diarrhea. Six weeks before admission, Mr. B. underwent a colonoscopy revealing polyps, erosive gastritis, and duodenitis. Multiple biopsies were taken. After the colonoscopy, Mrs. B. noticed a decrease in Mr. B.'s normal activity level. He would complain of muscle aches and the need to rest after simple yard work. Thinking of flu symptoms, Mrs. B. monitored his temperature, but it never rose above 100° F. Two nights ago, Mr. B. began experiencing night sweats. He went to his physician, who noticed small, raised, tender, bluish areas on his fingers and multiple petechiae over his extremities. He also noted an increase in intensity from Mr. B.'s baseline aortic murmur. Mr. B. was admitted with the diagnosis of infective endocarditis. A transesophageal echocardiogram confirmed the presence of vegetations on the aortic valve. Blood cultures were quickly obtained and antibiotic therapy initiated. After 1 week of intravenous antibiotics, the patient complained of headaches and vision changes. The next night Mr. B. awoke acutely short of breath. These events were attributed to vegetative embolization and resolved without further complications. Mr. B. will be discharged in another week with plans for ongoing administration of intravenous ampicillin at home.

The nursing history also identified the following:

- Mr. B. recalls being instructed about antibiotic prophylaxis before intrusive procedures but had done so well over the years that he "forgot" to mention his valve history, with all the gastrointestinal discomfort he was having.
- Mrs. B. finds it hard to help Mr. B. in dependent situations because of his need to have all the facts and feel in control of his health.
- Mr. B. is used to being active and on the go. Being confined and resting for any time is hard for him to accept.

Collaborative nursing actions include monitoring for the following:

- Signs and symptoms of heart failure: rales, $S_3$, edema, decreasing blood pressure, tachycardia, breathlessness, decreased activity tolerance
- Signs of embolization: distal pulses, neurological changes, acute shortness of breath, abdominal or peripheral pain

**NURSING DIAGNOSIS** *Activity intolerance related to imbalance between oxygen supply and demand*

| expected patient outcome | nursing interventions | rationale |
|---|---|---|
| • States that fatigue is decreased<br>• Has stable pulse, respiration, and blood pressure with increased activity | • Assess the patient's response to exercise by monitoring vital signs before and after activity. | • Activity tolerance depends on the ability to physiologically adapt to changes in demand. Heart rate and blood pressure should increase with increasing demand but decrease to near baseline within 3 minutes after activity stops. |
| | • Instruct the patient to report dyspnea, chest pain, palpitations, and fatigue during activity. | • Abnormal subjective responses indicate intolerance of activity. |
| | • Instruct the patient to perform activities more slowly. | • Energy conservation minimizes the risk of exceeding the heart's oxygen requirements. |
| | • Assist the patient in sequencing activities to provide rest periods. | • Rest decreases myocardial oxygen consumption, allowing intervals of low energy demand. |
| | • Provide an environment conducive to rest. | • Environmental stimulation inhibits the patient's ability to enter state of relaxation and subsequent rest. |

*Continued*

and myocyte damage are present (within 6 weeks of the acute illness).

### Collaborative Care Management

Patients with myocarditis are treated with bedrest and digitalis to prevent heart failure and cardiogenic shock. Immunosuppression may be beneficial in reducing inflammation and preventing irreversible myocardial damage. Medical therapy also includes treatment of the underlying disease with antibiotics, conventional therapy for congestive heart failure, and management of dysrhythmias. Nursing care includes ongoing monitoring of the patient's physiological status. Patients are commonly anxious about the sudden onset of heart disease and its implications for the future. The nurse provides emotional support and encourages verbalization of feelings.

Postbiopsy nursing care focuses on the potential for injury that can occur, such as hematoma or bleeding at the cannulation site, cardiac tamponade, or pneumothorax. The site is inspected for bleeding, ecchymosis, or swelling. Shortness of breath, changes in breath sounds, dyspnea, and alterations in respiratory rate and pattern of breathing must be reported to a physician. A chest x-ray film may be obtained to rule out pneumothorax. Vital signs are monitored closely to assess for continued hemodynamic stability.

## Person with Infective Endocarditis–cont'd

**NURSING DIAGNOSIS** *Ineffective management of therapeutic regimen, related to complexity of therapeutic regimen, knowledge deficits—cont'd*

| expected patient outcome | nursing interventions | rationale |
|---|---|---|
| • Practices preventive behaviors to minimize future episodes of endocarditis | • Provide verbal and written instructions in the following areas: pathophysiology of endocarditis, treatment plan, medications, and signs and symptoms of endocarditis. | • Teaching reinforces the need to comply with recommended management. Written material provides additional resource for home reference. |
| | • Teach the importance of appropriate antibiotic prophylaxis as recommended by the American Heart Association guidelines. | • Adhering to recommendations helps decrease the risk of recurrence of disease. |
| | • Emphasize good oral care, avoidance of trauma to the gums, and the need for regular dental checkups. | • Proper oral hygiene decreases the risk of pathogen entry. |
| | • Teach the importance of wearing an identification bracelet or necklace to inform health care providers of heart condition. | • Proper identification can decrease the risk of inadvertent exposure to pathogens without appropriate prophylaxis. |
| | • Stress the importance of compliance with follow-up. | • Repetitive explanations may help improve compliance. Proper follow-up is essential. |

**NURSING DIAGNOSIS** *Pain related to arthralgias, myalgias, and embolization*

| expected patient outcome | nursing interventions | rationale |
|---|---|---|
| • Patient will report relief of pain through management strategies | • Administer analgesics to relieve pain as ordered. | • Analgesics may lower pain level to tolerance, working synergistically with other nonmedication strategies. |
| | • Assess and document response to medications. | • The effectiveness of medications needs to be evaluated to minimize risk of side effects and tolerance. Ineffective strategies should be replaced. |
| | • Encourage adequate rest. | • Sleep deprivation lowers the pain threshold. |
| | • Monitor for signs of decreased tissue perfusion from embolization. | • A patient with endocarditis is at an increased risk for embolism. Complete physical assessments should be done every 8 hours to establish baseline. Early detection of problems enables prompt intervention to minimize serious complications. |

Monitoring for heart failure is an important nursing consideration. Measures to decrease cardiac workload include frequent rest periods, provisions for a quiet environment, and the use of semi-Fowler's position.

#### Patient/family education

The nurse emphasizes to the patient and significant others the importance of energy conservation for an extended period. The risk of myocardial damage increases with exercise. The nurse encourages slow progression of activity, with frequent rest periods. The use of nonsteroidal antiinflammatory drugs (NSAIDs) in viral myocarditis also appears to increase myocardial damage. The nurse emphasizes to the patient the need to avoid NSAIDs until medically cleared by the primary care provider. The patient is instructed about a heart-healthy diet and early symptoms of heart failure that need to be reported promptly.

## RHEUMATIC HEART DISEASE

### Etiology/Epidemiology

Rheumatic heart disease is an acute inflammatory reaction. Somewhat fewer than 10% of persons with rheumatic fever develop rheumatic heart disease, and about one half of those with rheumatic heart disease have mitral stenosis. Rheumatic fever and rheumatic heart disease with mild symptoms may go undiagnosed, or the disease may be subclinical with no noticeable symptoms. Thus the discovery of rheumatic heart disease is made years later. Careful recall of childhood illnesses may include a recollection of "growing pains," confirming the likelihood that the patient had rheumatic fever during childhood.

### Pathophysiology

The inflammation of rheumatic heart disease may involve (1) the lining of the heart or endocardium (endocarditis), including the valves, resulting in scarring, distortion, and stenosis of the valves; (2) the heart muscle (myocarditis); or (3) the outer covering of the heart (pericarditis), where it may cause adhesion to surrounding tissues. The development of symptoms of chronic rheumatic heart disease depends on the location and severity of the damage.

### Collaborative Care Management

Prophylactic penicillin is prescribed during acute episodes of rheumatic fever and for several years thereafter. Lifelong antibiotic prophylaxis may be necessary for persons with significant rheumatic heart disease. Corticosteroids may be prescribed during acute rheumatic fever to decrease the cardiac inflammation. If congestive heart failure occurs, bedrest, sodium and fluid restrictions, diuretics, and inotropes usually are prescribed.

#### *Patient/family education*

The nurse emphasizes to the patient and family the importance of rest and adequate nutrition. Additional educational content appropriate to the patient with rheumatic heart disease is included in sections of this chapter on pericarditis, endocarditis, myocarditis, valve disease, and heart failure.

# HEART FAILURE

## ETIOLOGY

Heart failure occurs when the myocardium cannot maintain a sufficient cardiac output to meet the metabolic needs of the body. This condition results from systolic dysfunction or diastolic dysfunction.

Systolic dysfunction results from inadequate pumping of blood from the ventricle. The decrease in pumping power results in a decrease in cardiac output. Any process that alters myocardial contractility can produce systolic dysfunction. Coronary artery disease and hypertension are the most common causes.[26]

Diastolic dysfunction (stiff heart syndrome) occurs when the ventricle does not fill adequately during diastole. Inadequate filling decreases the amount of blood in the ventricle for cardiac output. Systolic function is often normal or augmented. Systemic hypertension and coronary artery disease are again the primary causes of diastolic dysfunction, but it also occurs secondary to fibrosis of aging, infiltrative diseases (such as myocarditis), and constrictive pericarditis (Box 26-3).

The etiologies for both systolic and diastolic dysfunction are similar, but they affect the ventricle in different ways to result in heart failure. Systolic dysfunction is the more common form of heart failure. Diastolic dysfunction is more common in elderly patients. Nearly all patients with systolic dysfunction will develop some degree of diastolic dysfunction over time.

**box 26-3** *Common Etiologies of Heart Failure*

| SYSTOLIC | DIASTOLIC |
|---|---|
| Coronary artery disease | Coronary artery disease |
| Hypertension | Hypertrophy |
| Metabolic disorders | Fibrosis of advanced age |
| Myocarditis | Constrictive pericarditis |
| Alcohol | Myocarditis |
| Cocaine | Hypertension |
| Cardiac valve disease | Aortic stenosis |
| Dilated cardiomyopathy | Ventricular remodeling |
| | Collagen diseases |
| | Cardiomyopathy |

Additional classifications of heart failure include right or left-sided heart failure, biventricular failure, forward or backward failure, high- and low-output failure, and acute or chronic failure (Box 26-4). Such terms are helpful for descriptive purposes, but they do not explain the underlying dysfunction.

## EPIDEMIOLOGY

Approximately 4.7 million Americans have heart failure,[39] with 400,000 new cases diagnosed each year.[2] Fifty percent of all patients with heart failure will die within 5 years of the diagnosis.[26] Heart failure is the only major cardiovascular disorder that is increasing in incidence, prevalence, and mortality rate.[40]

The incidence of heart failure increases with advancing age and coronary artery disease. An increase in the number of survivors of myocardial infarction is in part responsible for the increasing numbers of patients with heart failure. Additional predictors of heart failure include diabetes, cigarette smoking, obesity, an elevated total cholesterol-to-high-density lipoprotein cholesterol ratio, an abnormally high or low hematocrit level, and proteinuria.

A major research study developed from the original Framingham Heart Study recently confirmed the strong association between hypertension and the development of heart failure.[27] The study found that in 91% of the new cases of heart failure, hypertension predated the heart failure diagnosis. The risk for developing heart failure was approximately two times greater in men and three times greater in women compared with normotensive persons. Hypertension causes the left ventricle (LV) to contract more forcefully to eject blood into the aorta. Over time, the muscle fibers thicken (hypertrophy) to sustain an adequate cardiac output. The increase in LV pressure needed for contraction and the increased metabolic needs of a hypertrophied ventricle increase myocardial oxygen consumption. Failure occurs when the heart can no longer meet its demand for oxygen.

Morbidity from heart failure has made this diagnosis the number one reason for hospital admission. Almost 1 million hospitalizations occur each year at an estimated cost of 7 billion dollars.[26] Outpatient expenditures account for an

**box 26-4** *Categories of Heart Failure*

**LEFT-SIDED VS. RIGHT-SIDED HEART FAILURE**

| | |
|---|---|
| Left-sided heart failure | LV cardiac output is less than volume received from the pulmonary circulation; blood accumulates in LV, LA, and pulmonary circulation |
| Right-sided heart failure | RV cardiac output is less than volume received from the peripheral venous circulation; blood accumulates in the RV, RA, and peripheral venous system |

**FORWARD VS. BACKWARD FAILURE**

| | |
|---|---|
| Forward failure | Decreased CO results in inadequate tissue perfusion |
| Backward failure | Blood remains in ventricle after systole, increasing atrial and then venous pressure; rise in venous pressure forces fluid out of capillary membranes into extracellular spaces |

**HIGH-OUTPUT VS. LOW-OUTPUT FAILURE**

| | |
|---|---|
| High-output failure | Occurs in response to conditions that cause the heart to work harder to supply blood; the increased oxygen demand can be met only with an increase in CO; systemic vascular resistance decreases to promote CO |
| Low-output failure | Occurs in response to high blood pressure and hypovolemia; results in impaired peripheral circulation and peripheral vasoconstriction |

**ACUTE VS. CHRONIC FAILURE**

| | |
|---|---|
| Acute failure | Occurs in response to a sudden decrease in CO; results in rapid decrease in tissue perfusion |
| Chronic failure | Body adjusts to decrease in CO through compensatory mechanisms; results in systemic congestion |

*LV,* left ventricle; *LA,* left atrium; *RV,* right ventricle; *RA,* right atrium; *CO,* cardiac output.

additional 3 billion dollars. With the prevalence of heart failure and its associated morbidity, the diagnosis creates multiple socioeconomic dilemmas related to health care costs, death, and dying.

## PATHOPHYSIOLOGY

In most cases, heart failure begins with left ventricular (LV) systolic dysfunction. Three of the more common causes of decreased LV contractility include coronary artery disease, aortic stenosis, and systemic hypertension. Coronary artery disease decreases contractility by diminishing oxygen supply to the mitochondria of the myofibrils. In aortic stenosis the LV must increase pressure to pump its volume through the tight valve. With systemic hypertension, the LV must generate pressures higher than systemic pressures to eject its volume.

The diminished pumping power of the LV results in ejection fractions (EFs) of less than 40%. Blood remains in the LV at the end of systole. Left atrial pressure increases to empty its volume into the LV. When the left atrium (LA) cannot completely empty its volume, blood backs up into the pulmonary circulation. The additional blood volume increases pressure within the pulmonary capillaries. Increased pressure drives fluid out of the smaller pulmonary capillaries into the interstitium and alveoli. High pulmonary pressures then impede the flow of blood from the right ventricle (RV) to the lungs. The RV must generate more force to move blood into the pulmonary system. The remaining blood backs up into the right atrium (RA) and ultimately the peripheral venous circulation.

Right ventricular dysfunction most often results from LV dysfunction. High pulmonary pressures resulting from primary pulmonary hypertension and chronic obstructive pulmonary disease are additional causes of RV dysfunction. The high pulmonary pressures impede the ability of the RV to pump blood to the pulmonary vessels. The RV must generate higher pressures to overcome this resistance. This causes the pressure within the RA to increase, resulting in higher systemic venous pressures.

With left ventricular diastolic dysfunction, the LV is abnormally "stiff" (noncompliant) during diastole and cannot fill at normal low pressures. The reduced LV volume results in a decrease in stroke volume. If atrial pressures increase to fill the LV, pulmonary congestion occurs. The inability of the heart to relax during diastole, myocardial fibrosis, and hypertrophy of the ventricle can all cause ventricular noncompliance.

Elevated calcium concentrations inhibit diastolic relaxation by maintaining ventricular pressure. Calcium concentrations rise when the sarcoplasmic reticulum is unable to remove calcium from the myofibril, as seen in ischemia, hypertrophy, and advanced age. Fibrotic changes prevent the ventricle from expanding. Fibrosis occurs with aging, myocardial infarction, and constrictive pericarditis. Hypertrophy represents an increase in muscle mass. This additional mass of muscle is most often thick, stiff, and noncompliant. The LV is not able to expand effectively to receive additional blood volume, decreasing left ventricular filling. This results in a decrease in stroke volume (the actual volume pumped per beat); the ejection fraction may be normal. The decline in stroke volume produces a cardiac output that is insufficient to meet the body's metabolic demands. Hypertrophy results from hypertension, cardiac valve disease, and ventricular remodeling. In remodeling, myocardium surrounding an area of infarction hypertrophies to compensate for the loss of contractile tissue.

### Compensatory Mechanisms

Arterial and venous pressure changes secondary to systolic or diastolic heart failure affect every organ and tissue. Indeed, all body systems are subject to failure in the presence of heart failure. The body compensates for the decrease in cardiac output through specific responses. These compensatory mechanisms arise from the sympathetic nervous system, the kidneys, and the heart itself (Figure 26-4).

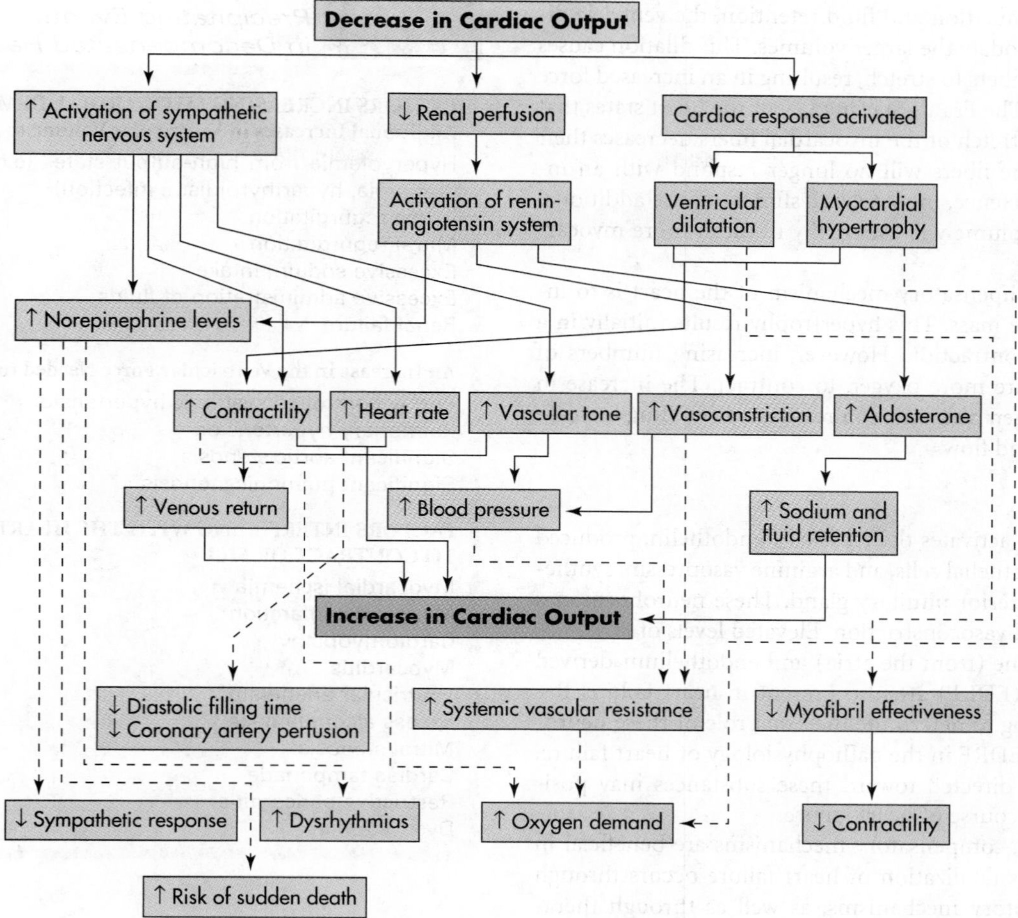


**fig. 26-4** Compensatory mechanisms seen in response to the decreased cardiac output and blood pressure of heart failure. Dotted lines represent the negative effects of sustained compensatory mechanisms.

### *Sympathetic nervous system*

The sympathetic nervous system responds to a drop in cardiac output by working harder. Additional stimulation of beta receptors in the myocardium increases both heart rate and contractility. Systemic vascular tone increases, causing a rise in systemic blood pressure. The rise in venous tone causes an increase in the amount of blood returning to the right side of the heart. The increase in heart rate, contractility, and venous return all work to increase cardiac output. The increase in sympathetic activity also causes a rise in the plasma levels of norepinephrine.

Unfortunately, these mechanisms lose their effectiveness over time. With increasing heart rates, the time for diastole shortens. Less time is available for adequate ventricular filling. Coronary blood flow (and oxygen delivery) also decreases because the coronary arteries are perfused during diastole. An increase in contractility requires more oxygen, and an increase in blood pressure raises the systemic vascular resistance (SVR). The SVR is the pressure the LV must overcome to eject its blood volume. The additional work required of the LV again increases myocardial oxygen demand. High levels of norepinephrine eventually decrease the heart's ability to respond to sympathetic stimulation and may cause cardiac dysrhythmias and sudden death.

### *Renal system*

Insufficient cardiac output decreases renal perfusion. The decrease in renal blood flow activates the renin-angiotensin system to correct a perceived hypovolemia. Increased secretion of renin converts angiotensinogen to angiotensin I. Converting enzymes change angiotensin I to angiotensin II, a potent vasoconstrictor. Angiotensin II also promotes the release of norepinephrine from cardiac nerve endings and raises the blood pressure. The decrease in renal perfusion and rising levels of angiotensin II stimulate an increase in aldosterone secretion that results in sodium and fluid retention.

The increase in fluid volume and blood pressure acutely increase cardiac output. However, in systolic dysfunction, any additional fluid volume increases the amount of fluid the failing ventricle must pump. Vasoconstriction increases SVR, which requires the ventricle to increase its pressure to eject its volume.

### *Ventricular dilation and myocardial hypertrophy*

The heart tries to compensate for its failing performance in two additional ways: ventricular chamber dilation and myocardial hypertrophy. With increasing venous return from sympathetic stimulation and fluid retention, the ventricle dilates to accommodate the larger volumes. This dilation causes the myocardial fibers to stretch, resulting in an increased force of contraction. The Frank-Starling law of the heart states that continued overstretch of the myocardial fibers decreases their effectiveness. The fibers will no longer respond with an increase in force. Hence, in systolic dysfunction, the additional increments in volume will eventually result in more myocardial failure.

A second compensatory mechanism of the heart is to increase its muscle mass. This hypertrophy results initially in a more forceful contraction. However, increasing numbers of myofibrils require more oxygen to contract. The increase in myocardial oxygen demand requires a corresponding increase in coronary blood flow.

### Other

Heart failure activates the release of endothelin, produced by vascular endothelial cells, and arginine vasopressin, synthesized in the posterior pituitary gland. These neurohormones cause additional vasoconstriction. Elevated levels of atrial natriuretic hormone (from the atria) and endothelium-derived relaxing factor (EDRF) are also present in heart failure. Research is ongoing to determine the exact role of these neurohormones and EDRF in the pathophysiology of heart failure. Future therapy directed toward these substances may positively affect the course of heart failure.

As discussed, compensatory mechanisms are beneficial in the short term. Stabilization of heart failure occurs through these compensatory mechanisms, as well as through therapeutic interventions. However, each compensatory mechanism also works against the heart to further increase myocardial oxygen demand (see Figure 26-4). With additional demands on the heart or additional heart damage, rapid decompensation of heart failure may occur (Box 26-5).

**box 26-5** *Precipitating Events in Decompensated Heart Failure*

**FACTORS INCREASING MYOCARDIAL DEMAND**

**Additional Increases in Ventricular Volume to Be Pumped**

- Hypervolemia from high-output states (e.g., pregnancy, anemia, hyperthyroidism, infection)
- Aortic regurgitation
- Mitral regurgitation
- Excessive sodium intake
- Excessive administration of fluids
- Renal failure

**An Increase in the Ventricular Force Needed to Eject Blood**

- Poorly controlled systemic hypertension
- Pulmonary hypertension
- Significant aortic stenosis
- Significant pulmonic stenosis

**FACTORS INTERFERING WITH THE HEART'S ABILITY TO CONTRACT OR FILL**

- Myocardial ischemia
- Myocardial infarction
- Cardiomyopathy
- Myocarditis
- Ventricular aneurysm
- Excess alcohol intake
- Mitral stenosis
- Cardiac tamponade
- Restrictive pericarditis
- Dysrhythmias

## CLINICAL MANIFESTATIONS

Classic symptoms of heart failure include dyspnea with exertion, orthopnea, nocturnal dyspnea, a dry, hacking cough, and unexplained fatigue. When volume overload contributes to the pathology, the following additional symptoms occur: rales, a third heart sound, peripheral edema, unexplained weight gain, jugular venous distention, hepatic engorgement, ascites, and worsening dyspnea. Compensatory mechanisms account for many of the clinical signs and symptoms of heart failure. Box 26-6 lists the more common symptoms as well as symptoms encountered with progressive heart failure. A discussion of each symptom follows.

Dyspnea, an abnormally uncomfortable awareness of breathing, occurs when high pulmonary pressures force fluid out of the pulmonary capillaries into the alveoli. The fluid in the alveoli interferes with effective gas exchange. Dyspnea may occur at rest or may occur only on physical exertion when oxygen requirements increase.

Orthopnea, dyspnea in the recumbent position, may be present in heart failure. In the recumbent position, chest expansion diminishes, resulting in decreased ventilation. In addition, venous return to the right heart increases with elevation of the legs. Patients experiencing orthopnea must often sleep using several pillows or in a semi-Fowler's position.

Although orthopnea may occur immediately after the patient lies down, it often does not occur for 2 to 5 hours. The patient awakes suddenly with severe shortness of breath, often in panic, a condition called paroxysmal nocturnal dyspnea. The severe dyspnea resolves only after being upright for 10 to 30 minutes.

With severe heart failure the patient may experience alternating periods of apnea and hyperpnea (Cheyne-Stokes respiration). Poor gas exchange causes an inadequate delivery of oxygen to the brain, which makes the respiratory center in the brain insensitive to the amounts of carbon dioxide in the arterial blood. Respirations cease until stimulation of the respiratory center occurs from either an increase in the carbon dioxide content in the arterial blood or critically low levels of oxygen. The patient then experiences hyperpnea. The rapid rate of respirations decreases the carbon dioxide content of arterial blood, resulting in apnea.

A persistent hacking cough is a common symptom of heart failure. Coughing results from congestion of trapped fluid, which is irritating to the mucosal lining of the lungs and bronchi. On auscultation, rales (crackles) are heard as a moist popping and crackling sound at the end of inspiration.

Patients with heart failure commonly note fatigue after activities that ordinarily are not tiring. The fatigue results from

**box 26-6** *clinical manifestations*

### *Heart Failure*

**RESPIRATORY**
Dyspnea
Orthopnea
Paroxysmal nocturnal dyspnea
Persistent hacking cough
Alternating periods of apnea and hyperpnea
Rales (crackles)

**CARDIOVASCULAR**
Angina
Jugular venous distention
Tachycardia
Decrease in systolic blood pressure with increase in diastolic blood pressure
$S_3$ or $S_4$ heart sounds

**GASTROINTESTINAL**
Enlargement and tenderness in the right upper quadrant of the abdomen
Ascites
Nausea
Vomiting
Bloating
Anorexia
Epigastric pain

**CEREBRAL**
Altered mental status (confusion, restlessness)

**GENERALIZED**
Fatigue
Decrease in activity tolerance
Edema (peripheral, pitting)
Weight gain

**PSYCHOSOCIAL**
Anxiety

**box 26-7** *New York Heart Association Classification of Heart Failure*

| | |
|---|---|
| Class I | No symptoms, tolerates ordinary physical activity |
| Class II | Comfortable at rest; ordinary physical activity results in symptoms |
| Class III | Comfortable at rest; less than ordinary physical activity results in symptoms |
| Class IV | Symptoms may be present at rest; symptoms with any physical activity |

inadequate tissue perfusion as a result of the decreased cardiac output. The reduction in tissue oxygen decreases the aerobic production of adenosine triphosphate (ATP), the immediate energy source for muscle contraction. Inadequate perfusion also decreases removal of metabolic waste products, further decreasing muscle function. Activity intolerance is common in both systolic and diastolic dysfunction. It is often the initial symptom with diastolic dysfunction because (1) stroke volume cannot increase when the LV prevents an adequate end-diastolic volume and (2) exercise-induced tachycardia decreases the diastolic filling time further. The severity of activity intolerance, while subjective, is often recorded in objective terms. One of the most widely used classification systems for activity intolerance is the New York Heart Association classification shown in Box 26-7. Angina can occur from decreased blood flow to the myocardium, but the pain is most likely to occur in patients with preexisting coronary artery disease.

Engorgement of the low-pressure peripheral venous system results from pressure increases in the right heart. Distention of the internal jugular vein (jugular vein distention [JVD]) is often observed with the patient in a semi-Fowler's position. With sharply elevated venous pressure, pulsations of the earlobes may occur when the patient sits upright.

High venous pressures force fluid into extravascular tissue. The patient often notices this as pitting, nontender edema in dependent areas, usually the lower extremities. As the edema becomes more pronounced, it progresses up the legs into the thighs, external genitalia, and lower portion of the trunk. If the tissue becomes extremely engorged, the skin may crack and fluid may "weep" from the tissues. Increasing fluid volume is most often responsible for the unexplained weight gain experienced by patients in heart failure. Fluid volume increases as urine output diminishes from poor renal perfusion.

The liver also becomes engorged with intravascular fluid, resulting in enlargement and tenderness in the right upper quadrant of the abdomen. Altered hepatic blood flow adversely affects liver function. Among its many functions, the liver metabolizes aldosterone and antidiuretic hormone and many of the medications used to treat heart failure. Adjustments to the patient's medication regimen may be necessary. Pressure within the portal system can increase further, forcing fluid through the blood vessels into the abdominal cavity. The resulting ascites can create nausea, vomiting, bloating, and epigastric pain and can even displace the diaphragm, resulting in severe respiratory distress.

Tachycardia is often present as the sympathetic nervous system attempts to compensate for the low cardiac output. The skin is cool and clammy as the sympathetic nervous system causes vasoconstriction. Additional physical assessment findings include a decrease in systolic blood pressure with an increase in diastolic blood pressure. $S_3$ and $S_4$ heart sounds are often heard over the mitral or right ventricular area. These sounds reflect the resistance to ventricular filling.

The diagnosis and symptoms of heart failure create uncertainty and may trigger persistent anxiety. Confusion and restlessness can occur if cerebral blood flow diminishes.

The clinical presentations of systolic and diastolic dysfunction are often similar. Both pathologies result in a decrease in cardiac output and altered cardiac pressures. Although there are important differences in cardiac pressures between systolic and diastolic dysfunction, these differences are often evident only with diagnostic testing.

## COLLABORATIVE CARE MANAGEMENT

### Diagnostic Tests

#### *Chest radiograph*

When blood backs up into the pulmonary vasculature, congestion appears on the chest film as whitened dense areas. A normal size heart with pulmonary congestion suggests acute new-onset heart failure or diastolic dysfunction. An enlarged heart (cardiomegaly) signals chronic heart failure with hypertrophy or dilation. An additional feature is the appearance of Kerley's B lines, which occur at the bases of the lungs and extend to the pleura. Kerley's B lines represent lymphatic drainage of the overloaded pulmonary vasculature. The presence of liver congestion on x-ray may signify right-sided heart failure.

#### *Laboratory blood tests*

Blood tests can be useful in determining precipitating factors for heart failure. Tests include hematological studies for anemia or thyroid function tests for hyperthyroidism. Heart failure directly alters many laboratory findings as well. Table 26-1 lists common laboratory findings in heart failure with a brief rationale for the abnormal values.

#### *Electrocardiography*

The ECG may be normal in heart failure. However, the ECG of a patient with substantial left ventricular dysfunction is usually abnormal, reflecting the etiology of heart failure, such as ischemia, infarction, tachydysrhythmias, hypertrophy, and tamponade.

#### *Echocardiography*

The aforementioned tests, along with the history and physical, may not be sufficient to differentiate dilated cardiomyopathy, left ventricular diastolic dysfunction, valvular heart disease, or perhaps a noncardiac etiology. Echocardiography provides data about left and right ventricular function, abnormal areas of contractility, and valve function and can clarify the pathology responsible for heart failure. A nondilated, normally contracting LV rules out systolic dysfunction. Left ventricular ejection fraction and cardiac size reflect the severity and progression of the heart failure. An ejection fraction below 45% is often confirmation of left ventricular dysfunction. However, patients with ejection fractions above 40% may still have heart failure from valvular disease or diastolic dysfunction. Doppler echocardiography analyzes blood flow and may reveal a reduction in early filling of the LV.

#### *Cardiac catheterization*

In patients with known coronary artery disease (CAD), cardiac catheterization provides additional information for diagnosis and management of heart failure. With diastolic dysfunction, cardiac catheterization of the right side of the heart demonstrates an elevated end-diastolic pressure at normal or decreased left ventricular volumes. A summary of hemodynamic findings in heart failure is provided in Table 26-2.

#### *Other*

In patients without ECG evidence of CAD, exercise stress testing is sometimes helpful in determining CAD as a factor in heart failure. Radionuclide ventriculography (multiple gated acquisition [MUGA]) uses radioactive dye and radiology to determine ejection fraction. Multiple gated acquisition is superior to echocardiography for obtaining quantitative data and assessing the right ventricle.

**table 26-1** *Common Laboratory Value Abnormalities with Heart Failure*

| Laboratory Value | Alteration | Rationale |
|---|---|---|
| Sodium | Decreased | An increase in total body water dilutes body fluid |
| Chloride | Decreased | Associated with sodium loss |
| Potassium | Increased | Depressed effective renal blood flow and low glomerular filtration rate |
| Blood urea nitrogen | Increased | Decreased renal perfusion |
| Creatinine | Increased | Impaired renal function |
| Red blood cell count | Decreased | Decreased production of erythropoietin with renal involvement |
| Liver function tests | Increased | Hepatic congestion |
| $Pao_2$ | Decreased | Fluid in alveoli limits exchange of oxygen |
| $Paco_2$ | Decreased | Compensatory increase in respiratory rate decreases $CO_2$ |

**table 26-2** *Altered Hemodynamic Findings in Heart Failure*

| Hemodynamic Variable | Finding in Heart Failure | Rationale |
|---|---|---|
| Cardiac output (CO)/ index | Decreased | Systolic or diastolic dysfunction |
| Systemic vascular resistance (SVR) | Increased | Compensate for decreased CO |
| Pulmonary artery wedge pressure (PAWP) | Increased when left side of heart affected | End-diastolic pressure or volume in left ventricle rises due to inadequate emptying or inability to relax during diastole |
| Central venous pressure (CVP) | Increased when right side of heart affected | Reflects increased pressure and volume within right side of heart |

## MEDICATIONS

Pharmacological agents play a central role in the management of heart failure. Prescribed agents include diuretics, vasodilators, angiotensin converting enzyme inhibitors, and inotropes. These medications decrease the volume of blood that the heart must pump (preload), decrease the resistance the heart must overcome to eject its volume (afterload), or increase the force of myocardial contraction (positive inotropic action). Recent research also supports the use of select beta blockers in the management of heart failure. The choice of agents depends on the etiology of the dysfunction and the need for either acute interventions or long-term management. Figure 26-5 is an algorithm for the pharmacological management of heart failure developed by the Agency for Health Care Policy and Research.[26] Table 26-3 lists specific pharmacological agents and the mechanism of action for each. A discussion of each drug group follows; associated nursing interventions are discussed in the section on nursing management.

### Diuretics

Diuretics are administered when clinical signs of volume overload exist. Several classes of diuretics may be used to manage heart failure. Commonly administered diuretics include loop diuretics, thiazides, and potassium-sparing diuretics. Diuretics increase urinary output, resulting in decreased blood volume, preload, and ultimately cardiac workload. A decrease in preload can adversely affect patients with diastolic dysfunction, and their use requires careful monitoring. Diuretics are administered intravenously to stabilize acute events and orally for long-term management of fluid overload.

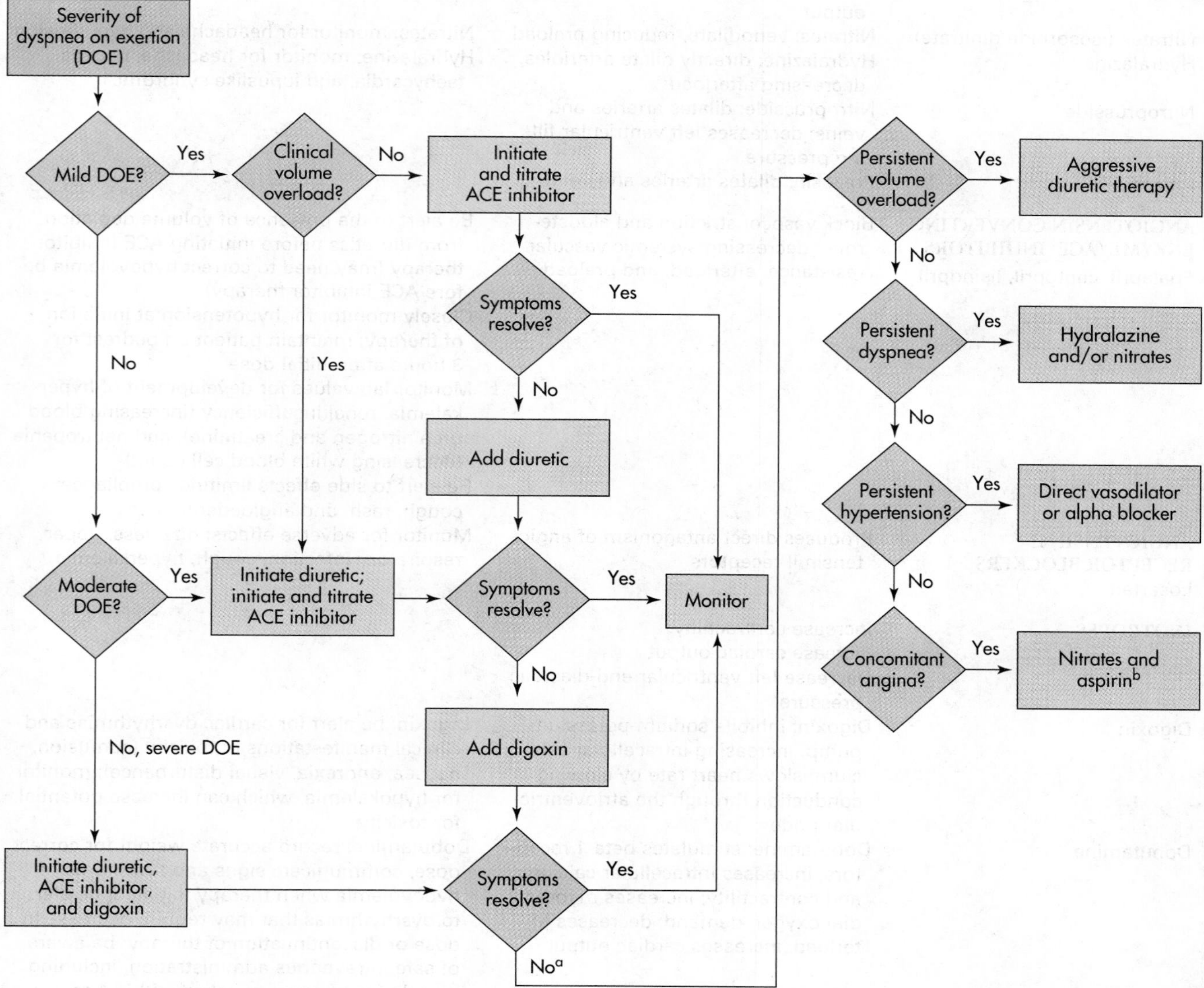


[a] Obtain cardiology consult if not already done.
[b] Beta blockers and calcium-channel blockers may also be effective but should be considered investigational.

**fig. 26-5** Pharmacological management of patients with heart failure.

**table 26-3** Common Medications for ***Heart Failure***

| Drug | Action | Nursing Intervention |
|---|---|---|
| **DIURETICS** | Decrease volume overload<br>Increase urinary output<br>Decrease preload | |
| Loop diuretics (furosemide, bumetanide, torsemide) | Loop diuretics: enhance the excretion of sodium, chloride, potassium, calcium, and magnesium | Loop diuretics, thiazides: monitor labs for hypokalemia, hyperglycemia, hyperuricemia; observe for postural hypotension and rashes |
| Thiazides (hydrochlorothiazide); thiazide-related (metolazone) | Thiazides: block reabsorption of sodium, chloride, water in distal tubule | |
| Potassium sparing (spironolactone, triamterene) | Potassium sparing (spironolactone): inhibits action of aldosterone, interferes with sodium reabsorption in distal tubule | Potassium sparing: monitor for increasing potassium levels, especially when administered with ACE inhibitors |
| **VASODILATORS** | Decrease cardiac workload<br>Improve stroke volume and cardiac output | |
| Nitrates (isosorbide dinitrate) | Nitrates: venodilate, reducing preload | Nitrates: monitor for headache and hypotension |
| Hydralazine | Hydralazine: directly dilate arterioles, decreasing afterload | Hydralazine: monitor for headache, nausea, tachycardia, and lupuslike syndrome |
| Nitroprusside | Nitroprusside: dilates arteries and veins; decreases left ventricular filling pressure | |
| Prazosin | Prazosin: dilates arteries and veins | |
| **ANGIOTENSIN CONVERTING ENZYME (ACE) INHIBITORS**<br>Enalapril, captopril, lisinopril | Block vasoconstriction and aldosterone, decreasing systemic vascular resistance, afterload, and preload | Be alert to the presence of volume depletion from diuretics before initiating ACE inhibitor therapy (may need to correct hypovolemia before ACE inhibitor therapy)<br>Closely monitor for hypotension at initiation of therapy; maintain patient on bedrest for 3 hours after initial dose<br>Monitor lab values for development of hyperkalemia, renal insufficiency (increasing blood urea nitrogen and creatinine), and neutropenia (decreasing white blood cell count)<br>Be alert to side effects limiting compliance: cough, rash, and angioedema |
| **ANGIOTENSIN II RECEPTOR BLOCKERS**<br>Losartan | Produces direct antagonism of angiotensin II receptors | Monitor for adverse effects: dizziness, upper respiratory infection, cough, hyperkalemia |
| **INOTROPES** | Increase contractility<br>Increase cardiac output<br>Decrease left ventricular end-diastolic pressure | |
| Digoxin | Digoxin: inhibits sodium-potassium pump, increasing intracellular calcium; slows heart rate by slowing conduction through the atrioventricular node | Digoxin: be alert for cardiac dysrhythmias and clinical manifestations of toxicity (confusion, nausea, anorexia, visual disturbance); monitor for hypokalemia, which can increase potential for toxicity |
| Dobutamine | Dobutamine: stimulates beta-1 receptors, increases intracellular calcium and contractility; increases myocardial oxygen demand; decreases afterload; increases cardiac output | Dobutamine: record accurate weight for correct dose; communicate signs and symptoms of hypovolemia when therapy initiated; be alert to dysrhythmias that may require decrease in dose or discontinuation of therapy; be aware of safe intravenous administration, including knowledge of onset of action within 1 to 2 minutes, titrating dose to blood pressure and heart rate, tapering drip when discontinuing therapy, monitoring site for infiltration |

Continued

**table 26-3** *Common Medications for* ***Heart Failure—cont'd***

| Drug | Action | Nursing Intervention |
|---|---|---|
| **PHOSPHODIESTERASE INHIBITORS**<br>Amrinone<br>Milrinone | Vasodilate by relaxing vascular smooth muscle, decreasing afterload and preload; increases cardiac output by increasing cyclic adenosine monophosphate levels | Amrinone: carefully monitor for dysrhythmias, thrombocytopenia, hypotension, chest pain; administer loading dose over 3 to 5 minutes; note peak effect within 10 minutes<br>Milrinone: observe for chest pain, hypotension, dysrhythmias, hypotension; administer loading dose over 10 minutes; note onset within 5 to 15 minutes |
| **MORPHINE SULFATE** | Decreases anxiety<br>Promotes venous pooling, decreasing preload and workload | Monitor vital signs before and after administration, with special attention to respiration depression; evaluate effect on anxiety |
| **DOPAMINE** | At low doses: stimulates dopaminergic receptors in renal vessels, increasing renal blood flow, increasing diuresis; increases myocardial contractility; vasodilates peripheral arterioles | Note onset of action within 10 minutes; monitor site for infiltration; if extravasation occurs, prepare for Regitine to infiltrate site; titrate drip to blood pressure and urine output; taper dose when discontinuing infusion |
| **ANTICOAGULANTS** | Patients with a history of systemic or pulmonary embolism or recent atrial fibrillation should be anticoagulated to an INR of 2 to 3 | Communicate bleeding precautions and safety measures to all care providers; teach importance of follow-up coagulation studies, minimizing changes in dietary intake of vitamin K, and need for safety to prevent bleeding occurrences |

Loop diuretics act in the ascending limb of the loop of Henle to enhance the excretion of sodium, chloride, potassium, calcium, and magnesium. The loop diuretics, including furosemide, bumetanide, and torsemide, are powerful and can be administered intravenously or orally. Electrolyte imbalance can be problematic in many patients, predisposing them to dysrhythmias.

Thiazide diuretics block the reabsorption of sodium, potassium, and water in the proximal portion of the distal tubule of the nephron. A combination of a thiazide agent with a loop diuretic often increases diuresis. One often-prescribed combination is metolazone, administered 30 minutes before furosemide.

Potassium-sparing diuretics include spironolactone, amiloride, and triamterene. Spironolactone inhibits aldosterone, causing sodium to be excreted in the distal tubule, but sparing potassium. Amiloride, a weak diuretic, inhibits sodium uptake in the distal tubule and collecting ducts but inhibits the loss of potassium. Triamterene inhibits potassium secretion in the distal tubule and promotes sodium loss.

### Vasodilators

Cardiac workload in heart failure decreases with arterial or venous dilation. Nitrates administered intravenously dilate arteries and veins, whereas nonparenteral nitrates predominantly affect the systemic veins, reducing preload. Hydralazine is a direct arteriolar vasodilator that reduces afterload and therefore workload. The decrease in afterload improves both stroke volume and cardiac output. Hydralazine may be given intravenously with nitrates to stabilize acute episodes of heart failure and orally with nonparenteral nitrates for long-term management.

Nitroprusside dilates both arteries and veins, resulting in an increase in cardiac output and stroke volume and a decrease in left ventricular filling. Nitroprusside is administered intravenously and only for stabilization of acute heart failure. Prazosin, an alpha-adrenergic blocker, also dilates both arteries and veins and can be administered orally.[7]

### Angiotensin Converting Enzyme Inhibitors

Angiotensin converting enzyme (ACE) inhibitors block the enzyme that converts angiotensin I to angiotensin II, thereby blocking vasoconstriction and the stimulation of the adrenal gland's production of aldosterone. The resulting decrease in systemic vascular resistance reduces afterload. Hypotension is usually well tolerated because of the increase in cardiac output. The decrease in aldosterone production causes less sodium and water retention, resulting in a decrease in preload. Renal blood flow increases, promoting natriuresis.

Several major research studies have concluded that ACE inhibitors reduce mortality rates in patients with heart failure, and they are at present the drug of choice for all patients with heart failure.[7,8,10,35] The ACE inhibitors can be administered intravenously and orally. They are prescribed for patients who are asymptomatic with known low ejection fractions and for patients requiring long-term therapy after stabilization of an acute episode.

Angiotensin II production does not occur solely through the renin-angiotensin pathway. Losartan is a direct antagonist of the angiotensin II receptor; therefore it affects the site of action of angiotensin II, not its production. This new drug class may prove to be even more effective than the original ACE inhibitors in managing heart failure.

### Inotropes

Digitalis preparations remain the most commonly prescribed inotropic agent. Digoxin, the most widely prescribed form of digitalis, inhibits the sodium-potassium pump, causing an increase in intracellular sodium. Concentration gradients force sodium out of the cell in exchange for calcium. Higher intracellular calcium levels increase the force of contraction, increasing cardiac output. The improved ejection of blood decreases left ventricular end-diastolic pressure and pulmonary pressures. Digoxin also blocks slow calcium channels of the atrioventricular nodes, which slows heart rate, increasing time for ventricular filling. Digoxin's ability to decrease cardiac burden is now believed to be the key to its effectiveness rather than its ability to increase contractile force. Digoxin may not benefit all patients and can even be deleterious in diastolic dysfunction because the increase in intracellular calcium increases LV stiffness.[18]

Dobutamine, a sympathomimetic agent, acts primarily on beta-1 receptors, stimulating cyclic adenosine monophosphate (cAMP), which increases intracellular calcium and results in a greater contractile force. The increase in cardiac output causes the body's own compensatory sympathetic stimulation to decrease, slightly decreasing afterload. Dobutamine must be administered intravenously and may be prescribed short term until an acute episode of heart failure stabilizes. Dobutamine therapy may be used continuously or intermittently until alternative interventions such as heart transplant become available. Dobutamine therapy has also been adapted for intravenous administration in the home setting.

Amrinone and milrinone block the activity of phosphodiesterase, which breaks down cAMP, resulting in an increase in contractility that improves stroke volume and cardiac output. They also increase vasodilator activity and relax smooth muscle, decreasing afterload and preload. Phosphodiesterase inhibitors act independently of beta receptors and may be effective when sympathomimetic agents lose their effectiveness. These agents are administered intravenously and are usually prescribed short term for refractory heart failure. Additional phosphodiesterase inhibitors, Pimobendan and Vesnarinone, remain under clinical investigation.[15]

### Beta Blockers

Beta blockers may be beneficial for the patient with predominantly diastolic dysfunction. Beta blockers halt the spiraling effect of the sympathetic nervous system on the failing heart. The decrease in heart rate allows more complete emptying of the left atrium, thereby improving left ventricular volume. Myocardial oxygen demand also decreases along with the decrease in heart rate and contractility.

### Calcium Channel Blockers

Newer calcium channel blockers with predominantly vasodilatory action may be safely used in patients with heart failure. Although not first-line drugs, these agents decrease systemic vascular resistance and lower neurohormonal activity to exert a positive effect. Calcium channel blockers also reduce intracellular calcium and LV hypertrophy, which may have positive effects, especially in diastolic dysfunction.

### Adjunctive Pharmacological Agents

Morphine sulfate decreases anxiety and sympathetic stimulation and is used in acute episodes of heart failure. Morphine also decreases venous pooling, resulting in a decrease in preload and cardiac workload. Supplemental oxygenation is appropriate when inadequate oxygenation and gas exchange occur, often evidenced by oxygen saturation levels below 90%. Mechanical ventilation reduces the work of breathing associated with anxiety or labored breathing.

Dopamine hydrochloride in low doses (2 to 5 μg/kg/min) is often used in combination with inotropes, vasodilators, or diuretics. Low-dose dopamine stimulates dopaminergic receptors in renal vessels, resulting in an increased renal blood flow and a more effective diuresis. The net result is an increase in cardiac output. Doses above 10 μg/kg/min stimulate alpha receptors and cause profound vasoconstriction.

Some patients with heart failure have an increased risk of blood clots due to stagnant blood flow. Current recommendations include anticoagulation for heart failure patients with a history of systemic or pulmonary embolism, recent onset of atrial fibrillation, or existing LV thrombi. Long-term anticoagulation with warfarin is prescribed prophylactically to maintain an international normalized ratio (INR) of 2.0 to 3.0.[26]

## TREATMENTS

The goal of management for heart failure is to improve cardiac performance without increasing cardiac workload. This requires interventions that manipulate preload, contractility, and afterload. Medications are the mainstay of such management; however, adjunctive therapies are effective in specific patient populations.

Patients with heart failure and renal impairment may require additional interventions such as ultrafiltration (hemofiltration) or hemodialysis to effectively reduce blood volume. Vascular access is established, and blood flows through a hemofilter within an extracorporeal circuit that supports the removal of fluid and metabolic wastes. The two primary methods of ultrafiltration are continuous arteriovenous hemofiltration (CAVH) and continuous arteriovenous hemofiltration and dialysis (CAVHD). Patients who are hypotensive on maximum inotrope support can seldom tolerate the removal of large fluid volumes through hemodialysis. For these patients, CAVH or CAVHD are appropriate alternatives.[37]

With chronic heart failure, beta receptor responsiveness diminishes, causing the heart's compensatory mechanisms to fail and medications to become ineffective. It then becomes necessary to decrease cardiac workload through nonpharmacological interventions such as intraaortic balloon pump (IABP) counterpulsation and ventricular assist devices. Counterpulsation by the IABP decreases afterload, thus decreasing the workload of the heart (see p. 734). The failing heart also receives an increase in coronary perfusion during diastole when the balloon inflates. Patients in a low-output state or with a structural abnormality may require stabilization with a ventricular assist device (VAD). The VAD withdraws blood from the ventricle or atrium and infuses the blood directly into either the pulmonary or systemic circulation. This rerouting of blood rests the failing ventricle.

## SURGICAL MANAGEMENT

Surgical interventions can reverse the course of heart failure from some etiologies. Corrective surgeries include pericardiectomy, cardiac valve replacements or valvuloplasty, surgical repair of septal defects, and ventricular aneurysmectomies. Revascularization through coronary artery bypass graft surgery may be of benefit for patients with heart failure and severe or limiting angina. Revascularization for patients with heart failure entails significant morbidity and mortality. Current research does not support the use of revascularization for patients with heart failure who do not have angina.

With refractory heart failure, cardiac transplantation may be the only option. Ischemic heart disease and dilated cardiomyopathies account for approximately 90% of cardiac transplant procedures. Survival rates are 80% at 1 year, 65% at 5 years, and 45% at 10 years.[24] Patient evaluation for transplantation is extensive and includes tests of ventricular function and noncardiac tests, such as pulmonary function tests and renal studies. The criteria for heart transplantation continue to change as surgical experience improves. Heart transplant remains an option for only a minority of patients because of the shortage of donor hearts. Transplantation is presented in detail in Chapter 68.

Cardiomyoplasty is another surgical option for end-stage heart failure. The procedure entails surgically wrapping the latissimus dorsi muscle around the heart, limiting additional dilation of the ventricle. Stimulating electrodes are placed in the proximal portion of the latissimus dorsi muscle and connected to a synchronizing cardiomyostimulator placed within an abdominal subcutaneous pocket. The muscle is allowed to recover for approximately 2 to 3 weeks after surgery and develop adhesion to the heart muscle before it is activated. Graded muscle stimulation is then initiated, and the wrapped muscle supports LV contraction. Cardiomyoplasty remains in clinical trials but may be considered an alternative to cardiac transplantation for some patients.[17]

## DIET

A "no added salt" diet is recommended for patients with mild heart failure. This diet eliminates salt in food preparation and avoids obviously salted foods. Sodium-restricted diets of 2 g of sodium daily decrease extracellular water and blood volume. Sodium restrictions of less than 2 g daily are rarely prescribed because the diet is unpalatable and expensive, resulting in poor patient adherence. The use of salt substitutes requires careful attention to potassium content if patients are taking potassium-sparing diuretics.

Fluid restrictions may be necessary for the patient with acute or chronic heart failure. Such restrictions consider weight fluctuations, intake and output ratios, and the electrolyte status of the individual patient. Fluid restrictions are often unnecessary unless the patient is hyponatremic. For patients with diuretic-induced thirst, an upper limit of 64 oz is a valid daily guideline.

Calorie and protein needs often increase as heart failure progresses. Albumin levels may fall as a result of nutritional deficiencies and fluid overload. With decreasing albumin levels, the ability to pull fluid out of the interstitium into the intravascular space diminishes. Serum albumin levels below 3 g/dl require investigation and proper management. Guidelines for alcohol use include abstinence or reduction of alcohol intake to one drink per day. One drink is defined as one glass of beer or wine or a mixed drink containing no more than 1 oz of alcohol. Minimizing caffeine intake is advisable for patients with tachycardic heart rhythms.

## ACTIVITY

Patients experiencing acute heart failure need to be on bedrest to minimize oxygen demands. However, activity should increase as soon as possible after blood pressure, heart rate, and oxygen saturation stabilize. Recent studies report an overall improvement in peak exercise performance when patients with LV dysfunction participate in monitored aerobic exercise programs.[9,23,25] These studies found that patients with ejection fractions as low as 13% could safely exercise without adversely affecting ejection fraction or wall motion or experiencing exercise-related complications. Considering these new findings, heart failure patients without ongoing ischemia should receive exercise prescriptions that include activity frequency, intensity, type, and duration (see Chapter 25). Patients with heart failure need to recognize their individual tolerance levels for physical activity and limit activity until their symptoms resolve. Patients with heart failure and ongoing ischemia are advised to undergo revascularization whenever possible before beginning a conditioning program.

## REFERRALS

Multidisciplinary health care professionals work collaboratively to improve quality of life for patients with heart failure. These individuals include nutritionists, exercise physiologists, nurses, stress management professionals, chaplains, respiratory therapists, social workers, physicians, and psychosocial counselors. Coordination of care is essential to decrease the frequency of hospital admissions, limit length of stay, and increase both the quality of care and patient satisfaction. Even with the best care, heart failure patients may experience exacerbations that require hospitalization.

## NURSING MANAGEMENT

### ASSESSMENT

#### Subjective Data

Members of the health care team collect subjective data as they perform the initial baseline assessment and in all subsequent interactions. The symptoms relate to the clinical manifestations discussed earlier and include:

- Paroxysmal nocturnal dyspnea
- Orthopnea
- New-onset dyspnea on exertion
- Fatigue
- Lower extremity edema
- Persistent cough
- Recent weight gain—documented or perceived

The nurse records a diet and activity history to serve as a baseline and facilitate teaching. Additional areas for assessment include concerns and anxieties of the patient and significant others and the effectiveness of support systems.

#### Objective Data

Physical signs are not unique to heart failure, but must be evaluated with subjective data. Objective data from the physical assessment may include:

- Third heart sound
- Respiratory distress, including increased effort and respiratory rate
- Pulmonary rales
- Elevated jugular venous pressure
- Peripheral edema
- Increase in daily weight without increased intake
- Abdominal distention
- Cool extremities and decreased pulses
- Alterations in level of consciousness
- Decreased urine output

### NURSING DIAGNOSES

Nursing diagnoses are determined from analysis of patient data. Nursing diagnoses for the patient with heart failure may include but are not limited to:

| Diagnostic Title | Possible Etiological Factors |
|---|---|
| Decreased cardiac output | Alteration in preload, afterload, or inotropic changes in heart |
| Impaired gas exchange | Alveolar capillary membrane changes |
| Fluid volume excess | Compromised regulatory mechanism |
| Activity intolerance | Imbalance between oxygen supply and demand |
| Hopelessness | Failing or deteriorating physiological condition |

Additional diagnoses that may be applicable to specific patients with heart failure include sleep pattern disturbance, impaired adjustment, anxiety, ineffective individual/family coping, fatigue, impaired home maintenance management, ineffective management of therapeutic regimen, altered nutrition: less than body requirements, sexual dysfunction, and risk for infection.

### EXPECTED PATIENT OUTCOMES

Expected patient outcomes for the patient with heart failure may include but are not limited to:

1a. Hemodynamic parameters (cardiac output, central venous pressure, pulmonary artery wedge pressure, blood pressure, and heart rate) will improve or remain at patient's baseline
b. Urine output will be greater than 30 ml per hour (exception: renal failure)
c. Peripheral pulses, capillary refill time, and skin temperature will improve or remain at patient's baseline
d. Dysrhythmias will be effectively suppressed or absent
e. Signs of systemic circulatory insufficiency (hepatomegaly, nausea, dependent edema) will be absent or at the patient's baseline
f. Will be alert and oriented ×3 or at patient's baseline
2a. Adventitious breath sounds will resolve or be at the patient's baseline
b. Will not experience respiratory distress
c. Pulse oximetry will be above 90% with activity (exception in patients with chronic obstructive pulmonary disease)
d. Skin and mucous membranes will be pink
3a. Intake and output will balance
b. Weight will stabilize
c. Will adhere to sodium and fluid restrictions
4a. Will tolerate a progressive increase in activity
b. Will accomplish activities of daily living (ADL) with decreased dyspnea
c. Will have increased energy and endurance
d. Will demonstrate acceptable responses in heart rate and blood pressure to exercise
5a. Will express confidence in a desired outcome
b. Will demonstrate initiative and self-direction in decision making and activities

### INTERVENTIONS

The Guidelines for Care Box summarizes the care of the patient with heart failure. A discussion of interventions appropriate to each diagnosis follows.

#### Improving Cardiac Output

The nurse actively works to improve existing alterations in cardiac output by reducing cardiac workload, promoting venous return and minimizing myocardial oxygen requirements. Interventions include positioning the patient in a semi-Fowler's position or position of comfort, avoiding the Valsalva's maneuver, and promoting a calm, quiet, and comfortable environment. Ongoing assessments focus on changes in cardiac output and include vital signs, hemodynamic parameters, telemetry monitoring, heart sounds, level of consciousness, edema, peripheral temperature, capillary refill, urine output, and chemistry values. With acute failure, assessments occur hourly or even more frequently while medications are being adjusted. As stabilization occurs, the frequency of assessments becomes a nursing judgment.

Patients with pitting edema may be at risk for skin breakdown caused by poor nourishment of the skin and cracks in the skin surfaces. The nurse appropriately positions the patient to minimize pressure points and shearing. Positioning is especially important for the patient confined to bedrest and at risk for the development of sacral edema. Skin care includes gentle cleansing and the application of lotion as needed to decrease disruptions in skin integrity. The use of 4-inch foam and other pressure-relieving mattresses is a standard preventive intervention.

Anorexia may occur when venous engorgement affects the gastrointestinal system. The nurse helps the patient select a diet that meets baseline nutrient needs so that catabolism does not occur. Smaller, more frequent meals reduce stress on the gastrointestinal tract.

### Improving Gas Exchange

The less effective oxygenation of the blood as it passes through the congested lungs greatly reduces the oxygen content of the blood. The patient may be more comfortable and better able to rest while receiving oxygen because it helps reduce dyspnea and fatigue. Oxygen is usually administered by nasal cannula at 2 to 6 L/min. Mechanical ventilation is necessary when the work of breathing significantly increases cardiopulmonary demands. The nurse positions the patient in a semi-Fowler's position, encourages the use of the incentive spirometer, and teaches relaxed, controlled breathing to improve gas exchange. The nurse also monitors respiratory rate, depth, and ease; breath sounds; skin color; and pulse oximetry to evaluate improvement or deterioration in gas exchange.

### Restoring Fluid Volume Balance

To decrease excessive fluid volumes, nurses work with the patient to determine how to best manage fluid and sodium restrictions. The physician orders the amount of fluid permitted, and the nurse and patient develop a schedule to divide fluid allowances throughout the day according to patient preferences. Appropriate and safe concentration of intravenous medications minimizes additional fluid intake. Assessments of fluid balance are ongoing. Parameters include edema; intake and output; laboratory values for sodium, potassium, BUN, and creatinine; and observation for a timely diuretic response to administered medications. The nurse records the patient's weight daily in similar clothing, using the same scale, with an empty bladder, and before eating. Weight gain indicates fluid retention: 1 kg of weight gain represents 1 L of retained fluid. Again, the frequency of assessment decreases as the patient's condition stabilizes.

### Improving Activity Tolerance

Patients with heart failure often experience severe fatigue and have little ability to perform even basic ADL. Bedrest reduces myocardial oxygen demand during acute episodes of heart failure while medications are being adjusted and until the severity of symptoms resolves. The nurse organizes the environment to limit myocardial demands by providing a bedside commode, placing toiletry and safety items within reach, and assisting with ADL as needed. Nursing interventions that promote sleep include offering back rubs, providing comfortable bedding, closing doors, turning off phones, decreasing alarm volumes, minimizing bright lights, and promoting quiet conversations. Sedatives may be beneficial in the acute care setting.

As the acute stage resolves, the patient progresses gradually to sitting, ambulating in the room, and finally ambulating in the hall. The nurse helps the patient pace ambulation times and avoids the 1 hour after meals when gastrointestinal perfusion needs are greatest. The ability to tolerate activity is demonstrated by the appropriate response of heart rate and blood pressure to activity and the absence of symptoms. Fatigue and dizziness may occur for some patients receiving aggressive diuretic therapy.

The patient's ability to tolerate activity while hospitalized guides the discharge activity prescription. An explanation of the importance of exercise can help prevent patients from being afraid to perform daily activities. Cardiac rehabilitation programs are especially beneficial for patients who are anxious about exercising on their own. Walking on level surfaces at least four times a week is a reasonable alternative to a structured outpatient exercise program. The nurse teaches the patient to discontinue walking if the heart rate exceeds 120 beats per minute or if the patient experiences chest discomfort, excessive fatigue, severe shortness of breath, or syncope. Pacing activities to decrease myocardial oxygen demand is the principle of management.

**guidelines for care**

**The Person with Heart Failure**

1. Support oxygenation:
   a. Administer oxygen by nasal cannula at 2 to 6 L/min for oxygen saturation greater than 90%.
   b. Give oxygen as needed for dyspnea.
   c. Patient should be well supported in a semi-Fowler's position.
   d. Encourage use of incentive spirometry q4h.
2. Balance rest and activity:
   a. Reinforce importance of conservation of energy and planning for activities that avoid fatigue.
   b. Encourage activity within prescribed restrictions; monitor for intolerance to activity (dyspnea, fatigue, increased pulse rate that does not stabilize).
   c. Assist with ADL as necessary; encourage independence within patient's limitations.
   d. Provide diversional activities that assist in conservation of energy.
   e. Provide a calm, quiet environment.
3. Perform head-to-toe assessment each shift, including assessment of lab values, daily weights, and I&O.
4. Provide skin care, particularly over edematous areas; use prophylactic measures to prevent skin breakdown.
5. Assist in maintaining an adequate nutritional intake while observing prescribed dietary modifications (offer smaller meals with supplements).
6. Monitor for constipation; give prescribed stool softeners.
7. Give prescribed medications and monitor for adverse effects.
8. Provide patient and family opportunities to discuss their concerns and time to learn about the diagnosis and plan of care.

### Supporting the Patient Experiencing Hopelessness

Heart failure is a chronic illness with a poor prognosis. Patients need counseling regarding the effects of heart failure on body image and role performance. Health care professionals need to encourage patients with heart failure to complete advance directives regarding their health care preferences. All individuals involved in the patient's care need updates on these preferences.

Quality of life remains a priority for patients with heart failure. Nurses encourage patients to be active, using energy conservation guidelines to promote optimal functioning. The accompanying Research Box describes the nurse's role in helping patients adapt to their situation of living with heart failure. Patients who undergo successful cardiac transplantation will likely have an improved quality of life. After the transplant, the improvement in function will continue as the once weakened body catches up to the newly transplanted healthy heart.

### Patient/Family Education

The nurse performs an accurate assessment of the patient's knowledge base before implementing an education plan. (See the accompanying Patient/Family Teaching Box and the Research Box on the following page.) An explanation of heart failure and its probable cause is the foundation on which education builds. The nurse teaches the patient signs and symptoms, what to do if symptoms worsen, and the importance of self-monitoring for symptoms (including daily weights). The nurse emphasizes the importance of preventive health measures, including healthy lifestyle modifications, avoiding individuals with infections, and receiving annual influenza vaccinations. Health care professionals involve the patient and family in the management plan and discussion of prognosis. The patient determines what role each individual will have, including both health care team and family members. Additional content areas for patient teaching include advance directives, stress management techniques, relaxation strategies, and the availability of support groups. The nurse encourages the patient to be as active as possible and provides specific guidelines for aerobic exercise and sexual activity. The nurse or dietitian reviews recommended sodium restrictions and fluid restrictions if indicated. This review includes teaching the patient about the importance of abstinence from alcohol or limiting intake to one serving daily. Permitted foods on the sodium-restricted diet receive emphasis. A list of foods to avoid goes home with the patient and family.

The nurse carefully reviews with the patient all medications, including purpose and side effects. The nurse works with the physician and patient to schedule medications to minimize their effect on daily routines. Administering diuretics in the morning minimizes sleep disturbances but may not be conducive to employment demands. Some medications require consideration of food intake (e.g., furosemide, whose absorption decreases significantly with food). Food does not inhibit the absorption of newer loop diuretics, such as torsemide. The

**research**

Reference: Martensson J et al: Male patients with congestive heart failure and their conception of the life situation, *J Adv Nurs* 25:579, 1997.

In this study, 12 male patients with heart failure, between the ages of 48 and 80 years old, were interviewed to determine how they conceived their life situation. The interview consisted of preliminary questions intended to introduce a number of delimited phenomena. The interviews were processed for statements that described conceptions. Six categories emerged that described the patients' conception of how their life situations had been affected by heart failure: feeling a belief in the future, gaining awareness, feeling support from the environment, feeling limitations, feeling a lack of energy, and feeling resignation. The authors conclude that nursing interventions need to focus on helping patients out of the circle of limitation and resignation. Care should be directed toward a focus on self-care and the possibilities that then exist.

**patient/family teaching**

**Heart Failure**

1. Monitor for signs and symptoms of recurring heart failure, and report these signs and symptoms to the primary provider:
   a. Weight gain of 1 to 1.5 kg (2 to 3 lb)
   b. Loss of appetite
   c. Shortness of breath
   d. Orthopnea
   e. Swelling of ankles, feet, or abdomen
   f. Persistent cough
   g. Frequent nighttime urination
2. Avoid fatigue and plan activity to allow for rest periods. Incorporate ADL, occupational activity, and sexual activity into daily routine by pacing activities.
3. Plan and eat meals within prescribed sodium restrictions:
   a. Avoid salty foods.
   b. Avoid drugs with high sodium content (e.g., some laxative and antacids, Alka-Seltzer)—read the labels.
   c. Eat several small meals rather than three large meals per day.
4. Take prescribed medications:
   a. If several medications are prescribed, develop a method to facilitate accurate administration.
   b. Digitalis: check own pulse rate daily; report a rate of less than 50/min to primary provider and signs and symptoms of toxicity.
   c. Diuretics:
      (1) Weigh self daily at same time of day.
      (2) Eat foods high in potassium and low in sodium (such as oranges, bananas) if on potassium-depleting diuretics.
   d. Vasodilators:
      (1) Report signs of hypotension (light-headedness, rapid pulse, syncope) to physician.
      (2) Avoid alcohol when taking vasodilators.
5. Adopt healthy lifestyle choices: daily routine; develop support groups; smoking cessation; alcohol intake limited to no more than one drink per day; minimize risk of infections.
6. Comply with follow-up appointments.

patient on ACE-inhibitor therapy should avoid potassium-containing salt substitutes. The nurse teaches the patient taking digoxin about the signs and symptoms of toxicity. In addition, the nurse cautions all patients to avoid additional over-the-counter and prescription medications without first consulting their primary care provider.

All health care professionals emphasize the importance of follow-up and compliance. Compliance directly affects mortality rate, and lack of compliance is a major cause of hospitalization. The nurse discusses the importance of compliance and assists the patient in removing barriers to compliance (cost, side effects, complexity of protocols). Family support is critical in helping the patient sustain a commitment to heart failure management.[14]

## EVALUATION

On follow-up visits, the nurse asks about the presence of orthopnea, paroxysmal nocturnal dyspnea, edema, and dyspnea on exertion. Patients are likely to experience changes in symptoms before changes are evident on physical examination. Family members may contribute important information about the patient's physical health and compliance. A thorough evaluation includes an evaluation of physical functioning and quality of life. Achievement of patient outcomes for the patient with heart failure includes:

1a. Has hemodynamic parameters (cardiac output, central venous pressure, pulmonary artery wedge pressure, blood pressure, heart rate) at baseline or improved from baseline
b. Has urine output greater than 30 ml per hour (exception: renal failure)
c. Has peripheral pulses, capillary refill time, and skin temperature at baseline or improved from baseline
d. Effectively suppressed dysrhythmias
e. Demonstrates adequate systemic circulation (edema at baseline or improved)
f. Manifests appropriate orientation and level of consciousness
2a. Demonstrates resolution of adventitious breath sounds
b. Denies respiratory distress
c. Manifests pulse oximetry above 90% with activity (except patients with chronic obstructive pulmonary disease)
d. Manifests skin and mucous membranes free of cyanosis or pallor
3a. Has a balanced intake and output
b. Maintains desired weight
c. Eats diet within sodium and fluid restrictions
4a. Tolerates a progressive increase in activity
b. Accomplishes ADL with decreased dyspnea
c. Increases energy and endurance
d. Demonstrates acceptable responses in heart rate and blood pressure to exercise
5a. Expresses confidence in a desired outcome
b. Demonstrates initiative and self-direction in decision making and activities

When necessary, the nurse alters the plan of care to include new diagnoses or new interventions negotiated with the patient and significant others.

### research

Reference: Hagenhoff BD et al: Patient education needs as reported by congestive heart failure patients and their nurses, *J Adv Nurs* 19(4):685, 1994.

A survey of 30 hospitalized patients with heart failure and 26 nurses suggested that patients value the opportunity to be educated about their illness, particularly with respect to medications. The study examined the difference in importance given to educational content from the patients' and the nurses' perspectives. Both groups rated all content areas as important and realistic to learn; however, patients often rated the information as more important than nurses did for the same area. Little difference was found between responses from patients with and without a cardiac history, indicating that both populations perceive the need for thorough counseling about their participation in treatment.

## GERONTOLOGICAL CONSIDERATIONS

Heart failure is the most common cause of hospitalization in patients over 65 years of age. Older patients with heart failure may not have the common clinical manifestations of dyspnea, rales, and edema. Confusion, fatigue, and failure to thrive may be the only clinical manifestations of heart failure.

Primary health care providers adjust medications in consideration of the physiological changes seen in older patients. Nurses should caution the older patient to make position changes slowly while taking diuretics, because they may not be able to adapt as quickly to venous pooling. Elderly patients are especially sensitive to the first-dose hypotensive effect of ACE inhibitors. Decreases in the initial doses still require assessments of the blood pressure response to subsequent dose changes. When even mild renal impairment is present, older adults may develop acute renal insufficiency. The nurse monitors blood urea nitrogen, creatinine, and potassium routinely for older patients taking ACE inhibitors. The routine use of nonsteroidal preparations for arthritis decreases the effectiveness of ACE inhibitors. All health care professionals need to carefully monitor elderly patients taking digoxin for signs and symptoms of toxicity. The elderly population is at an increased risk for toxicity because of a decrease in renal function and reduced lean body mass.

Research indicates that elders are commonly nonadherent to their medication regimen,[30] and readmission rates for heart failure within 90 days have been reported to be as high as 57% for patients over 70 years of age.[26] A multidisciplinary approach for management after discharge can reduce the rate of readmission for this population.

## SPECIAL ENVIRONMENTS FOR CARE

### Critical Care Management

Patients are often admitted to the coronary care unit for initial stabilization of heart failure. Medications are routinely titrated to fluid status and hemodynamic response. The use of adjunctive treatments for refractory heart failure, such as intraaortic balloon pumping, requires careful observation in the intensive care setting. Once stabilized, the cardiology step-down unit becomes the environment best suited for management of patients in heart failure. This transition allows for continued pharmacological intervention with appropriate monitoring and facilitates education and activity interventions. The cardiology step-down unit is the environment of choice for the management of patients with an exacerbation of heart failure.

## HOME CARE MANAGEMENT

Patients should be discharged to the home environment only when their symptoms are controlled; concomitant processes (such as atrial fibrillation, for example) have been treated and are likewise under control; all education outcomes have been met to the satisfaction of the nurse, patient, and significant other; and arrangements are in place for support and follow-up in the community.[26] Plans for return to home begin on admission with an assessment of the patient's home environment.

The nurse emphasizes the importance of consistent follow-up with primary care providers or nurse-managed heart failure clinics. Follow-up includes physical assessment, compliance evaluation, and ongoing education. Elderly patients with heart failure who follow up with nurse practitioner clinics and home health care nurses have significantly fewer exacerbations than patients not managed by these professionals (see the accompanying Research Box). At times, success in home management requires only the use of supportive agencies. This may include individuals to prepare and serve nutritional meals or additional education about the proper use of mobility aids (bedside commodes, shower seats) to decrease cardiac workload.

The increased prevalence and severity of heart disease coupled with societal demands for cost-effective care has also opened the home to the use of technology once limited to critical care. Home health care now includes continued education; implementation of management protocols, such as home inotrope or intravenous diuretic therapy; assessment of the environment for interventions to minimize cardiac workload; provision of support; and evaluation of outcomes. Research data support the efficacious use of left ventricular assist devices in the home setting.[31] With this technology, the home management of patients with end-stage heart failure becomes increasingly challenging.

**research**

Reference: Rich MW et al: A multidisciplinary intervention to prevent the readmission of elderly patients with congestive heart failure, *N Engl J Med* 333(18):1190, 1995.

This study randomized 282 elderly patients with heart failure before discharge to one of two groups: patients in the treatment group received comprehensive education, a prescribed diet, social-service consultation and planning for an early discharge, a review of medication, and intensive follow-up; the control group received standard care. The principal effect of the intervention was in reducing the number of readmissions for heart failure. The readmission rate for heart failure within 90 days of discharge decreased by 56.2% in the treatment group. The study demonstrated that a nurse-directed, multidisciplinary treatment strategy can significantly reduce hospital readmissions for elderly patients with heart failure.

## COMPLICATIONS

### Acute Pulmonary Edema

Acute pulmonary edema is a medical emergency that may develop as a result of severe ventricular failure from prolonged strain on a diseased heart. Any of the events presented in Box 26-5 can cause decompensation of chronic heart failure, resulting in pulmonary edema.

As in left ventricular failure, pulmonary edema arises from left ventricular overload. This volume overload increases left atrial pressure, resulting in increased pulmonary vein and pulmonary capillary pressures. Pulmonary capillary hydrostatic pressure quickly exceeds intravascular oncotic pressure. The high pressure forces fluid and sodium into the interstitium. The high interstitial pressure then forces fluid from the interstitial spaces into the alveoli. The surfactant that keeps the alveoli expanded loses its effectiveness. The fluid-filled alveoli collapse, preventing the exchange of oxygen and carbon dioxide, and unoxygenated blood returns to the left side of the heart. Red blood cells enter the alveoli, producing the characteristic blood-tinged sputum. The fluid rapidly enters the bronchioles and bronchi, creating the acute life-threatening symptoms that characterize this medical emergency: profound dyspnea, pallor, audible wheezing, and cyanosis. Restlessness, anxiety, and tachycardia accompany the rapid gas exchange symptoms.

All members of the health care team must quickly and effectively manage the anxiety that accompanies pulmonary edema. Catecholamine release from anxiety results in tachycardia and other events that increase oxygen demand and confound treatment. The nurse approaches the patient in a calm, reassuring manner to decrease anxiety. Morphine sulfate is the drug of choice because it blunts the sympathetic response and increases venous capacitance, thereby lowering left atrial pressure. The "air hunger" of pulmonary edema is often the impetus for anxiety. Nursing interventions such as raising the head of the bed and positioning the patient in the bed to maximize chest expansion decrease the air hunger.

Arterial blood gas or pulse oximetry results determine the need for supplemental oxygen. Oxygen may be administered at 40% to 70% with face mask delivery to quickly achieve oxygen saturations above 90%. Humidification will aid in the removal of secretions. Intubation will be necessary for patients not responding to conventional measures. Mechanical ventilation ensures the delivery of adequate tidal volumes and oxygen concentrations to decrease the work of breathing. Intubation also facilitates the removal of secretions by suctioning. Aminophylline may be administered to dilate the bronchi, increase urinary output, and increase cardiac output.

Medications prescribed for pulmonary edema include inotropic agents, diuretics, afterload reducers, and supportive adjuncts such as dopamine hydrochloride to increase renal perfusion. The significant diuresis that typically occurs with treatment requires careful monitoring for electrolyte imbalance.

### Dysrhythmias

Atrial fibrillation is a common complication of heart failure. The backup of blood into the atria causes atrial enlargement and ischemia. The ischemia alters the electrical stability needed for impulse initiation and conduction and increases automaticity and irritability of the atrial tissue. Atrial fibrillation can provoke heart failure or cause an exacerbation in a patient who is in compensated heart failure. Deterioration results from the loss of coordinated atrial contraction, which contributes blood volume to the ventricle in late diastole. For management of atrial fibrillation, see Chapter 25.

Ischemia and irritability in the ventricles result in premature ventricular beats, another complication of heart failure. With progression of the disease, premature beats may initiate more lethal dysrhythmias that are difficult to manage due to altered metabolism and decreased renal excretion of medications. Treatment of these ventricular dysrhythmias is controversial because major research studies have indicated that antidysrhythmic therapy may actually increase mortality rates in patients with mild to moderate failure. Prophylactic treatment is not recommended.

### Multisystem Failure

As noted in the pathophysiology section, heart failure affects every organ system and multiple organ system failure can occur. Clinical manifestations and treatment are specific to the organ that is underperfused.

## CARDIOMYOPATHY

### ETIOLOGY/EPIDEMIOLOGY

Cardiomyopathy (CMP) is a myocardial disease causing specific structural changes within the myocardium. There are three major categories of cardiomyopathy: dilated CMP, hypertrophic CMP, and restrictive CMP (Figure 26-6). In dilated CMP the left ventricular chamber dilates but without a proportional increase in contractility. Possible etiologies for dilated CMP include ischemia, damage from inflammatory processes, toxins such as ethanol and chemotherapy, or familial origin. Long-standing hypertension and valve disorders also contribute to the development of dilated CMP. Hypertrophic CMP refers to a dilated, hypertrophied, and hypercontractile ventricle. Hypertrophic CMP may represent a defect of muscle development and therefore may have a hereditary component. Restrictive CMP occurs when the left ventricle is of normal or small size and the muscle mass is normal or increased (Table 26-4). Infiltrative and proliferative disorders are common etiologies for restrictive CMP. Such disorders include amyloidosis and sarcoidosis. Cardiomyopathy is classified as idiopathic when a specific etiology cannot be identified.

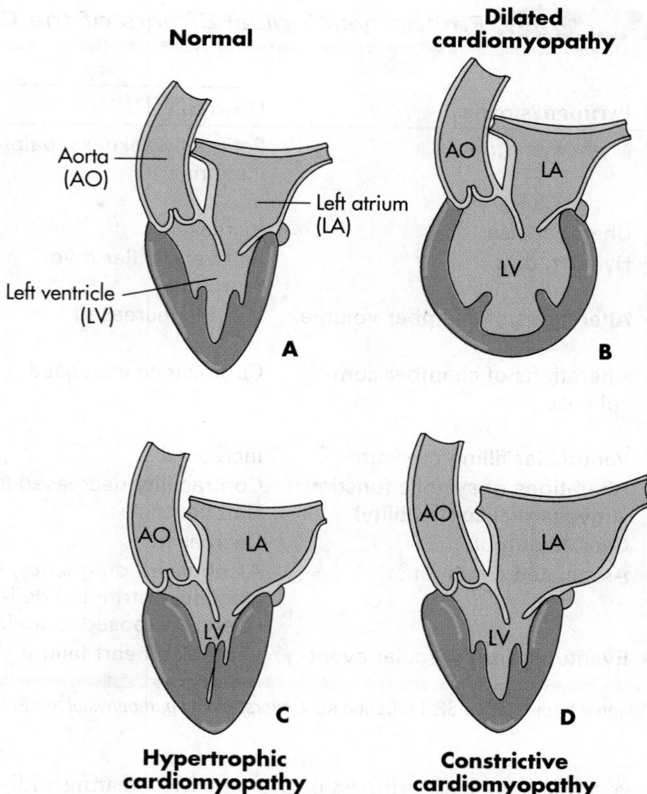


**fig. 26-6** Diagram showing major distinguishing pathophysiological features of the three types of cardiomyopathy. **A,** The normal heart. **B,** In the dilated type of cardiomyopathy, the heart has a globular shape and the largest circumference of the left ventricle is not at its base but midway between apex and base. **C,** In the hypertrophic type, the wall of the left ventricle is greatly thickened; the left ventricular cavity is small but the left atrium may be dilated because of poor diastolic relaxation of the ventricle. **D,** In the restrictive (constrictive) type, the left ventricular cavity is of normal size but, again, the left atrium is dilated because of the reduced diastolic compliance of the ventricle.

### PATHOPHYSIOLOGY

In dilated CMP, the ventricular chamber dilates in response to constant stress. Dilation of the LV increases the capacity for ventricular volume (increased compliance). The stretching of the myocardial fibers, however, displaces the sarcomeres beyond the limits of the Starling curve. As a result, optimum cross-linkages for contractility do not occur, decreasing contractility. Fibrosis from direct toxicity can also inhibit the ability to contract. Therefore, in dilated CMP, there is a larger capacity for ventricular volume but a decrease in contractility. These changes result in a decrease in cardiac output, stroke volume, and ejection fraction. Clinical manifestations reflect this decrease in cardiac output. Major signs and symptoms include fatigue, weakness, and overt manifestations of left-sided heart failure.

In hypertrophic CMP, muscle mass increases but without an increase in LV chamber size. Fibrotic infiltrates of the

**table 26-4** *Pathophysiological Effects of the Cardiomyopathies*

| | Type of Cardiomyopathy | | |
|---|---|---|---|
| Pathophysiology | Dilated | Hypertrophic | Restrictive |
| Major symptoms | Fatigue, weakness, palpitations | Dyspnea, angina pectoris, fatigue, dizziness (syncope), palpitations | Dyspnea, fatigue |
| Chamber size | Increased | Normal or decreased | Decreased or normal |
| Hypertrophy | Left ventricular myocardium | Left ventricular myocardium and interventricular septum | Left ventricular myocardium |
| Alterations of chamber volume | Volume increased | Volume decreased, particularly in left ventricle | Volume normal to decreased |
| Alterations of chamber compliance | Compliance increased | Compliance decreased, particularly in left ventricle | Compliance decreased, particularly in left ventricle |
| Ventricular filling pressure | Increased | Normal or increased | Increased |
| Alterations of systolic function (myocardial contractility) | Contractility decreased in left ventricle | Contractility increased or vigorous | None |
| Cardiac output | Decreased | Normal | Normal or decreased |
| Associated conditions | Alcoholism, pregnancy, infection, nutritional deficiency, exposed to toxins | Possible inherited defect of muscle growth and development | Infiltrative disease |
| Eventual cardiovascular event | Left-sided heart failure | Left-sided heart failure | Heart failure |

Adapted from Huether SE, McCance KL: *Understanding pathophysiology,* St Louis, 1996, Mosby.

myocardium increase stiffness of the ventricle, creating additional hypertrophy. Compliance to LV filling decreases, and the LA dilates in an attempt to increase volume. When the hypertrophied ventricle contracts, it easily ejects the smaller volume of blood from the LV unless a hypertrophied intraventricular septum blocks the flow of blood out of the ventricle. Additional increases in contractility further compromise the patient with hypertrophic CMP. An increase in demand, as would occur with exercise, causes the myocardium to attempt an increase in cardiac output. Such an attempt can result in syncope, serious dysrhythmias, or sudden death. Heart failure is again the eventual outcome as the disease progresses. With hypertrophy, metabolic needs increase and create an imbalance between the high oxygen demand and the reduced cardiac output, thereby precipitating angina. Clinical manifestations include those of dilated CMP plus an increased cardiac impulse, a high ejection fraction in the early stages, and a decreased ejection fraction when heart failure ensues.

In restrictive CMP, the LV is fibrotic and thickened secondary to infiltrates. The ventricle loses its ability to stretch, therefore decreasing compliance. The heart cannot adequately fill, therefore decreasing cardiac output. Heart failure ensues with disease progression. As in hypertrophic CMP, the LA often dilates. The patient may have associated symptoms of infection and amyloid infiltration.

## COLLABORATIVE CARE MANAGEMENT

Diagnostic tests for CMP include chest x-ray, echocardiogram, 12-lead ECG, and physical examination. Complete head-to-toe assessments monitor for subtle changes in systemic perfusion (mental status, heart rhythm, vital signs, peripheral perfusion, oxygenation, fluid status). The nursing assessment seeks to determine how the illness has affected the patient's quality of life.

Management focuses on decreasing the workload of the heart, improving contractile efficiency, and managing symptoms and complications. Medications include all those used in heart failure. Pacing of activities decreases workload; restriction of activities with high metabolic equivalents may be beneficial. Even everyday conversation may create extreme dyspnea, and the nurse cautions the patient to pace this activity to minimize cardiac workload. Proper positioning and supplemental oxygen facilitate breathing. The risk of injury decreases with assessment for orthostatic blood pressure changes and the initiation of appropriate safety measures. Complications may include thromboemboli from stagnant blood flow within the myocardium. Anticoagulation with heparin is prescribed until therapeutic levels of warfarin (Coumadin) are achieved. Chapter 27 discusses nursing interventions for the patient receiving anticoagulant therapy. Dysrhythmias can occur if ischemia creates enhanced automaticity, reentry, or conduction defects. Patients with symptomatic dysrhythmias may benefit from long-term dysrhythmia management. The most commonly occurring dysrhythmias are atrial fibrillation and premature ventricular beats (see Chapter 25 for discussion and management). Altered renal function and electrolyte imbalance occur with decreased renal perfusion and from diuretic therapy. Cardiac transplantation may be an appropriate intervention for the patient refractory to conventional management.

With hypertrophic CMP, medications that increase the obstruction to outflow from the ventricle are avoided. These medications include nitroglycerin, digitalis, and isoproterenol. Beta blockers may be beneficial because they decrease contractility and minimize the obstruction to outflow. Surgery to correct the outflow obstruction with concomitant mitral valve replacement may significantly improve symptoms. Nursing management is similar to that provided for patients with dilated CMP. In addition, the nurse cautions the patient against performing Valsalva's maneuver, which increases outflow obstruction.

With restrictive CMP, management seeks to control heart failure and minimize complications. Nursing management addresses pain from associated diseases (amyloid, sarcoidosis). The nurse also monitors the patient for resolution of the infection.

### Patient/Family Education

To facilitate adherence to the recommended regimens, the nurse provides appropriate explanations of all treatments and interventions. Many of the teaching guidelines appropriate to patients with heart failure are appropriate to the patient with CMP. With hypertrophic CMP, teaching patients to squat or lie down with the legs elevated may relieve symptoms. As noted previously, patients with CMP are at an increased risk of sudden death due to dysrhythmias. Therefore the nurse refers interested family members to an appropriate agency for instruction in cardiopulmonary resuscitation. All health care professionals must emphasize to patients the importance of follow-up care.

**Normal valve**

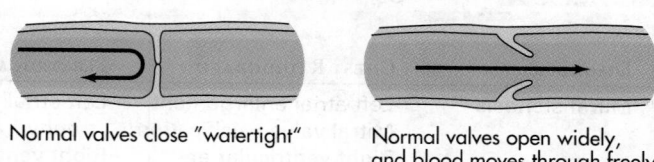

Normal valves close "watertight"

Normal valves open widely, and blood moves through freely.

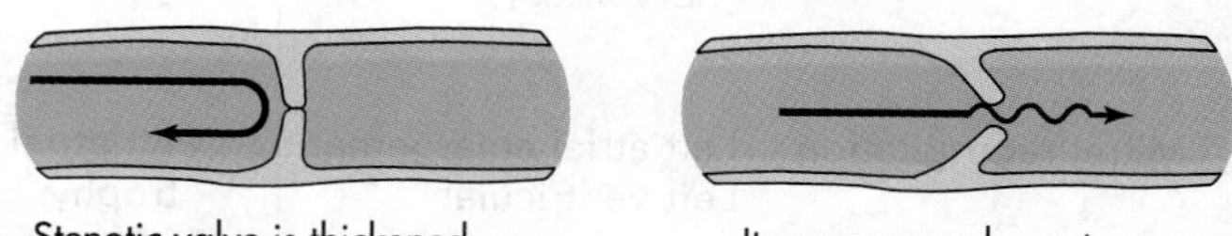


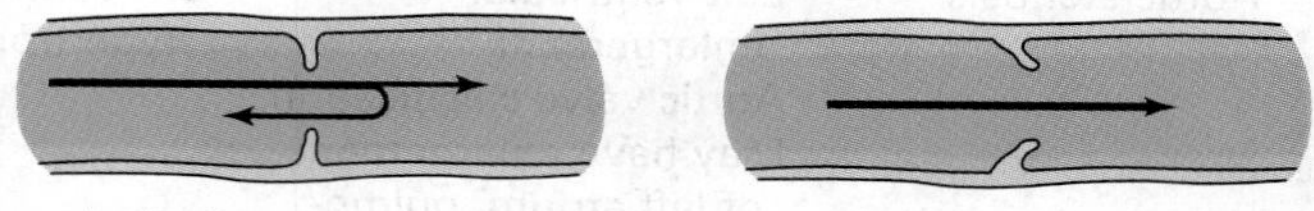

Stenosis or narrowing

It can open only part way.

Regurgitation or leaking
Valve leaflets are puckered and pulled apart by scar tissue—valve cannot close. Blood leaks back into chamber it has just left.


**fig. 26-7** Valvular diseases.

## VALVULAR HEART DISEASE

The cardiac valves are responsible for promoting unidirectional flow of blood through the heart. Cardiac valvular stenosis produces narrowing of the valve lumen, which impedes blood flow through the valve. Valvular insufficiency involves incomplete valve closure, which leads to regurgitation or backward leaking of blood through the valve (Figure 26-7).

The mitral and tricuspid valves (atrioventricular valves) close during ventricular systole to prevent backflow of blood into the atria. During ventricular diastole, pressure changes cause the atrioventricular valves to open, allowing blood to rush into the ventricles. The aortic and pulmonic valves (semilunar valves) prevent blood from flowing back into the ventricles during ventricular diastole. An intact valve structure, including valve leaflets, chordae tendineae, and papillary muscles, is essential to valve competence during all phases of the cardiac cycle.

When a cardiac valve is either stenotic or regurgitant, the heart is able to compensate and maintain function through gradual chamber dilation and myocardial hypertrophy. However, over time the compensatory abilities of the myocardium begin to fail. Excessive myocardial hypertrophy and chamber dilation result in decreased contractility, reduced ejection fraction, and ultimately ventricular failure. Medical therapy supports cardiac function with the use of cardiac glycosides, diuretics, dietary sodium restriction, and antibiotic prophylaxis. Progression of symptoms signifies worsening valvular disease and indicates the need for surgical valve repair or replacement.

The following section reviews the major cardiac valve disorders, including the underlying pathophysiology, clinical manifestations, and related collaborative management. The symptoms and complications of valvular heart disease are primarily related to decreased cardiac output, and the management follows the guidelines presented for patients with heart failure (see p. 694-715). In other words, the various cardiac valve disorders generally result in heart failure, which is the primary focus of medical management. Table 26-5 presents an overview of the specific valvular disorders and the diagnostic findings associated with each. Table 26-6 compares the common clinical manifestations associated with each disorder.

### MITRAL STENOSIS

Mitral stenosis occurs when the blood flow from the left atrium to the left ventricle during ventricular diastole (ventricular filling) is impeded due to thickening or fibrotic changes in the mitral valve.

#### Etiology/Epidemiology

Mitral stenosis is the most common disorder of the mitral valve. The primary etiology is rheumatic fever and carditis, which causes an inflammatory process of the mitral valve's chordae tendineae or commissures (leaflets). Less common causes of mitral stenosis include bacterial vegetation, thrombus formation, calcification of the mitral annulus, and atrial myxoma (tumor).

Forty percent of persons with rheumatic heart disease develop mitral stenosis, and two thirds of all persons with rheumatic mitral stenosis are women. With the decreasing incidence of rheumatic fever in industrialized countries, the incidence of rheumatic mitral stenosis has substantially

**table 26-5** *Findings in Valvular Heart Disorders*

| Disorder | Chest Radiograph | Electrocardiogram | Echocardiogram | Cardiac Catheterization |
|---|---|---|---|---|
| Mitral stenosis | Left atrial enlargement<br>Mitral valve calcification<br>Right ventricular enlargement<br>Prominence of pulmonary artery | Left atrial hypertrophy<br>Right ventricular hypertrophy<br>Atrial fibrillation | Thickened mitral valve<br>Left atrial enlargement | Increased pressure gradient across valve<br>Increased left atrial pressure<br>Increased PCWP<br>Increased right heart pressure<br>Decreased CO |
| Mitral regurgitation | Left atrial enlargement<br>Left ventricular enlargement | Left atrial hypertrophy<br>Left ventricular hypertrophy<br>Atrial fibrillation<br>Sinus tachycardia | Abnormal mitral valve movement<br>Left atrial enlargement | Mitral regurgitation<br>Increased atrial pressure<br>Increased LVEDP<br>Increased PCWP<br>Decreased CO |
| Aortic stenosis | Left ventricular enlargement<br>Aortic valve calcification<br>May have enlargement of left atrium, pulmonary artery, right ventricle, right atrium | Left ventricular hypertrophy | Thickened aortic valve<br>Thickened ventricular wall<br>Abnormal movement of aortic leaflets | Increased pressure gradient across valve<br>Increased LVEDP |
| Aortic regurgitation | Left ventricular enlargement | Left ventricular hypertrophy<br>Tall R waves<br>Sinus tachycardia | Left ventricular enlargement<br>Abnormal mitral valve movement<br>Increased movement of ventricular wall | Aortic regurgitation<br>Increased LVEDP<br>Decreased arterial diastolic pressure |
| Tricuspid stenosis | Right atrial enlargement<br>Prominence of superior vena cava | Right atrial hypertrophy<br>Tall peaked P waves<br>Atrial fibrillation | Abnormal valvular leaflets<br>Right atrial enlargement | Increased pressure gradient across valve<br>Increased right atrial pressure<br>Decreased CO |
| Tricuspid regurgitation | Right atrial enlargement<br>Right ventricular enlargement | Right ventricular hypertrophy<br>Atrial fibrillation | Prolapse of tricuspid valve<br>Right atrial enlargement | Increased atrial pressure<br>Tricuspid regurgitation<br>Decreased CO |

*CO,* Cardiac output; *LVEDP,* left ventricular end-diastolic pressure; *PCWP,* pulmonary capillary wedge pressure.

declined, although it remains a common disorder in developing countries. Refer to the section on inflammatory heart disease for further discussion of rheumatic heart disease and other inflammatory valvular diseases (see p. 693-699).

### Pathophysiology

In mitral stenosis, the mitral valve leaflets become thickened and fibrotic from scar tissue formation and calcification. As the valve leaflets become stiff and fused, the valve lumen progressively narrows and becomes immobile. In addition, the chordae tendineae may shorten and thicken. The mitral valve orifice may decrease in size from its normal 4 to 6 cm to less than 1 cm (Box 26-8).

With progressive mitral stenosis, left atrial pressures elevate as a result of incomplete emptying of the left atrium. Sustained elevated left atrial pressure causes the myocardium to compensate with left atrial dilation and hypertrophy. In addition, high pressures in the left atrium lead to elevated pulmonary venous, capillary, and arterial pressures. Eventually, sustained elevation of left atrial pressure can produce pulmonary hypertension and subsequent right ventricular hypertrophy. With the increased pressure in the pulmonary vasculature, leakage of fluid across the pulmonary capillary membrane into the lung interstitium can occur and produce pulmonary edema (Figure 26-8).

**box 26-8** *Effect of Mitral Orifice Size on Emergence of Symptoms*

| | |
|---|---|
| >2.6 $cm^2$ | No symptoms with exertion |
| 2.1-2.5 $cm^2$ | Symptoms with extreme exertion |
| 1.6-2.0 $cm^2$ | Symptoms with moderate exertion |
| <1.5 $cm^2$ | Symptoms with minimal exertion |

From Hurst JW, editor: *The heart,* ed 7, New York, 1990, McGraw-Hill.

**table 26-6** *Clinical Manifestations of Valvular Stenosis and Regurgitation*

| Manifestation | Aortic Stenosis | Mitral Stenosis | Aortic Regurgitation | Mitral Regurgitation | Tricuspid Regurgitation |
|---|---|---|---|---|---|
| Cardiovascular outcome* | Left ventricular failure | Right ventricular failure | Left-sided heart failure | Left-sided heart failure | Right-sided heart failure |
| General symptoms | Fatigue | Fatigue, weakness | Fatigue, weakness | Fatigue, weakness | Peripheral edema (with heart failure) |
| Respiratory effects | Dyspnea on exertion | Dyspnea on exertion, orthopnea, paroxysmal nocturnal dyspnea, predisposition to respiratory infections, hemoptysis, pulmonary hypertension, and edema | Dyspnea with effort | Dyspnea; occasional hemoptysis | Dyspnea |
| Central nervous system effects | Syncope, especially on exertion | Neural deficits only associated with emboli (e.g., hemiparesis) | Syncope | None | None |
| Gastrointestinal effects | None | Ascites; hepatic angina with hepatomegaly | None | None | Ascites, hepatomegaly (with heart failure) |
| Pain | Angina pectoris | Chest pain | Chest pain (anginal) | None | Palpitations |
| Heart rate, rhythm | Bradycardia, dysrhythmias (with heart failure) | Palpitations (atrial fibrillation) | Palpitations, water-hammer pulse | Palpitations | Atrial fibrillations |
| Heart sounds | Systolic murmur | Diastolic murmur, accentuated first heart sound, opening snap | Diastolic and systolic murmurs | Murmur throughout systole | Murmur throughout systole |
| Most common cause | Congenital, rheumatic fever | Rheumatic fever | Bacterial endocarditis; aortic root disease | Floppy valve; coronary artery disease | Congenital |

Data from Braunwald E, editor: *Heart disease: a textbook of cardiovascular medicine,* ed 4, Philadelphia, 1992, WB Saunders; Hancock EW: Valvular heart disease, *Sci Am Med* 1(I-XI):1, 1992.
*If disease not treated.

Persons with mitral stenosis also have reduced cardiac output. The severity of cardiac output reduction is dependent on the degree of mitral stenosis. Persons with mild to moderate stenosis generally maintain a normal cardiac output at rest but may be unable to tolerate exercise.

Mitral stenosis increases the risk for cardiac dysrhythmias. Atrial fibrillation develops in 50% of persons with mitral stenosis, causing a further decrease in cardiac output. In addition, atrial fibrillation may allow blood to pool and stagnate in the left atrium, resulting in thrombus formation and possible arterial embolization to vital organs.

Many persons with mitral stenosis remain symptom free for approximately 20 years after the initial attack of rheumatic carditis. Symptoms may occur gradually or abruptly depending on the severity of the stenosis (see Table 26-6). When acute symptoms develop, the disease progresses rapidly and death occurs within 5 to 10 years unless surgical correction takes place.

The primary symptom of mitral stenosis is dyspnea, which is largely the result of reduced lung compliance. Dyspnea on exertion (DOE), paroxysmal nocturnal dyspnea (PND), and orthopnea occur as a result of pulmonary hypertension. These symptoms may be precipitated by emotional stress, respiratory infection, sexual intercourse, or atrial fibrillation. Some persons experience a dry cough, dysphagia, or bronchitis because of bronchial irritation from an enlarged left atrium. Pressure exerted on the laryngeal nerve by an enlarged pulmonary artery causes hoarseness. Excessive fatigue and weakness occur as a result of decreased cardiac output. Other symptoms include peripheral and facial cyanosis. Hemoptysis, usually a late sign, occurs from the rupture of a bronchial vein. Eventually right-sided heart failure leads to jugular vein distention, pitting edema, and hepatomegaly.

## Collaborative Care Management

Diagnosis of mitral stenosis is established by the clinical symptoms, such as an opening snap (OS), created by the forceful opening of the mitral valve, followed by a diastolic rumbling or murmur that results from increased velocity of blood flow. The diastolic murmur is absent when the valve is severely calcified. The ECG changes indicate right ventricular

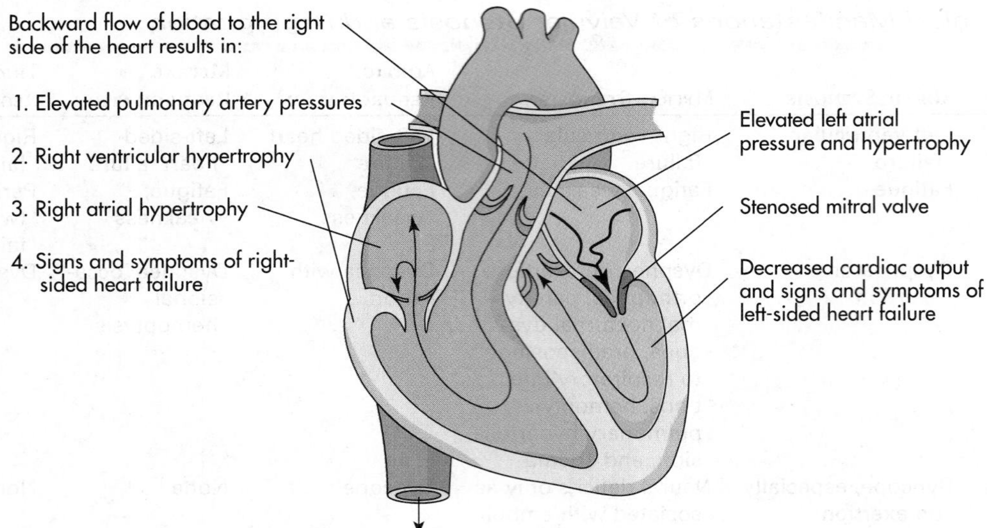
Backward flow of blood to the right side of the heart results in:
1. Elevated pulmonary artery pressures
2. Right ventricular hypertrophy
3. Right atrial hypertrophy
4. Signs and symptoms of right-sided heart failure
Elevated left atrial pressure and hypertrophy
Stenosed mitral valve
Decreased cardiac output and signs and symptoms of left-sided heart failure

**fig. 26-8** Effects of mitral stenosis.

hypertrophy, and chest x-ray films show left atrial enlargement. Mitral stenosis also can be diagnosed with a cardiac catheterization (see Table 26-5). The most sensitive and noninvasive diagnostic test is the echocardiogram, which shows an impedance of flow, fusion of valve leaflets, and poor leaflet separation during diastole.

Mildly symptomatic patients with mitral stenosis are treated with diuretics, and digitalis is used to control heart rate in the event of atrial fibrillation. Anticoagulation therapy with warfarin is used to prevent thrombus formation in patients with moderate to severe mitral stenosis or those with a history of thromboembolism. Medical therapy also includes antibiotic prophylaxis before dental and surgical procedures to reduce the risk of bacterial endocarditis.

Mechanical enlargement of the mitral valve is indicated when the disease causes either loss of exercise capacity or pulmonary hypertension. Percutaneous valvuloplasty using balloon dilation provides a nonsurgical alternative to repair of mitral stenosis. Surgical commissurotomy can also be performed while the valve leaflets remain mobile. Both commissurotomy and valvuloplasty allow patients to retain their natural valve, possibly reducing the need for long-term anticoagulant therapy. Mitral valve replacement using open heart surgery and cardiopulmonary bypass is performed when the valve is severely fibrotic or calcified. In general, patients undergoing mitral valve replacement require permanent anticoagulation therapy.

#### *Patient/family education*

Patients who experience symptoms related to mitral stenosis are prescribed a sodium-restricted diet to help prevent fluid retention and progressive heart failure. Activity is unrestricted for the patient with asymptomatic mitral stenosis. As the patient becomes symptomatic, the activity level is adjusted based on the patient's level of tolerance. Family involvement in activity teaching and planning is encouraged. Patients with moderate to severe stenosis are advised to avoid activities that require sudden increases in cardiac output. Patients receiving anticoagulant therapy must receive instruction in the safe use of the drug and safety measures to follow to prevent bleeding. Important aspects of education for patients receiving anticoagulant therapy are further discussed in Chapter 27.

## MITRAL REGURGITATION

Mitral regurgitation (mitral insufficiency) occurs when the mitral valve fails to completely close during ventricular systole, and consequently some blood flows backward into the left atrium. Mitral regurgitation can be either an acute or a chronic condition.

### Etiology/Epidemiology

As in mitral stenosis, mitral regurgitation can be caused by rheumatic heart disease and is often present in conjunction with mitral stenosis. Other causes of mitral regurgitation include endocarditis, coronary heart disease, dilated cardiomyopathy, a leaky prosthetic mitral valve, mitral valve prolapse, congenital malformation of the mitral valve, and connective tissue disorders such as Marfan syndrome, amyloidosis, and ankylosing spondylitis. A person with idiopathic hypertrophic subaortic stenosis (IHSS) can also develop mitral regurgitation as a result of displacement of the anterior leaflet of the mitral valve during ventricular systole.

Weakness, rupture, or fibrosis of a papillary muscle secondary to ischemic heart disease, ventricular aneurysm, or acute myocardial infarction can cause acute mitral regurgitation. Papillary muscle dysfunction allows the valve leaflets to flop in the direction of the left atrium during systole, and the blood flows backward. In addition, rupture of the chordae tendineae or perforation of a mitral valve cusp can cause acute mitral regurgitation.

Mitral regurgitation occurs more commonly in men than in women and is the most prevalent lesion in patients who ex-

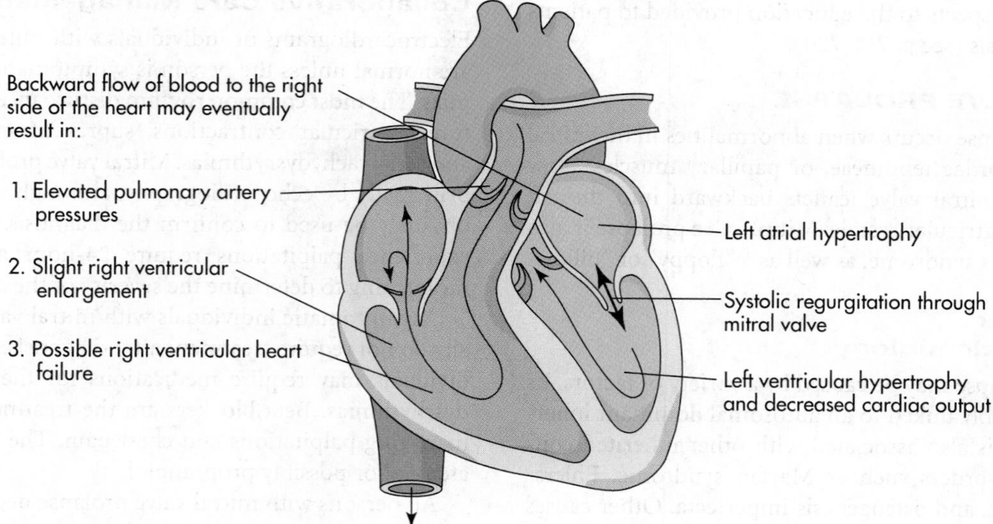
Backward flow of blood to the right side of the heart may eventually result in:
1. Elevated pulmonary artery pressures
2. Slight right ventricular enlargement
3. Possible right ventricular heart failure
Left atrial hypertrophy
Systolic regurgitation through mitral valve
Left ventricular hypertrophy and decreased cardiac output

**fig. 26-9** Effects of mitral regurgitation.

perience heart failure with active rheumatic carditis. With the exception of congenitally malformed mitral valves and connective tissue disorders, mitral regurgitation is primarily a disease of middle-aged and elderly persons.

## Pathophysiology

In chronic mitral insufficiency or regurgitation a variable amount of blood from the left ventricle is shunted back through the mitral valve to the left atrium. This backflow of blood causes both the left atrium and left ventricle to dilate and hypertrophy. In response to increasing preload and left atrial pressure, the pulmonary venous and arteriolar pressures also rise and eventually cause right-sided heart failure (Figure 26-9). As the ventricle hypertrophies, it becomes dysfunctional and cardiac output decreases. Concurrently, the left atrium is often fibrillating, diminishing the cardiac output even further.

Fatigue and weakness related to a decreased cardiac output are the primary symptoms of mitral regurgitation. Right-sided heart failure causes hepatic congestion, edema, ascites, and distended neck veins in severe mitral regurgitation. Some persons experience palpitations or paroxysmal nocturnal dyspnea.

Progressive dyspnea on exertion and pulmonary edema from an elevated left atrial pressure are the primary symptoms of acute regurgitation. The atrial pressure is transmitted immediately to the pulmonary veins, causing the congestive symptoms. Because the ventricle has not yet hypertrophied, the cardiac output remains sufficient and fatigue is not a problem. Although persons with mitral regurgitation commonly develop atrial fibrillation, thrombus formation in the atria is less common than with mitral stenosis because backflow and resultant turbulence of blood limits pooling.

## Collaborative Care Management

The diagnosis of mitral regurgitation is made by the presence of clinical symptoms and auscultation of a blowing, high-pitched systolic murmur and third heart sound. The first heart sound ($S_1$) may not be heard, depending on the severity of regurgitation. A chest x-ray film reveals left atrial enlargement and occasional left ventricular dilation. The ECG tracings show left ventricular hypertrophy and, less commonly, right ventricular hypertrophy (see Table 26-5). The echocardiogram may identify mitral valve cusp prolapse, ruptured chordae tendineae cordis, and enlargement of the left atrium and left ventricle. Definitive diagnosis is made through cardiac catheterization (see Chapter 24), which assesses left ventricular function and the degree of regurgitation.

Patients with mild mitral regurgitation are generally managed medically. For patients with a new onset of acute mitral regurgitation, emergent hospitalization and hemodynamic stabilization are required. Heart failure is managed with diuretics and afterload-reducing agents. Use of a peripheral arteriolar vasodilator facilitates ejection of blood into the aorta. As with other valvular disorders, management of dysrhythmias and control of heart rate with digitalis will promote adequate cardiac output. Antibiotic prophylaxis against bacterial endocarditis is indicated before all dental and surgical procedures.

Patients with mitral regurgitation who develop new-onset atrial fibrillation may need to undergo controlled cardioversion to restore normal sinus rhythm and maximize cardiac output. Patients with long-standing atrial fibrillation or a history of thromboembolism will also receive long-term anticoagulation.

Mitral regurgitation that progresses despite medical therapy necessitates valve repair or prosthetic replacement. Individuals with intact left ventricular function and without other severe noncardiac disease may be referred for open heart surgery and valve replacement.

### *Patient/family education*

Patient/family teaching for patients with mitral regurgitation is directed primarily at symptom management, and is similar in most respects to the education provided to patients with mitral stenosis (see p. 717-720).

## MITRAL VALVE PROLAPSE

Mitral valve prolapse occurs when abnormalities in the mitral valve leaflets, chordae tendineae, or papillary muscles allow prolapse of the mitral valve leaflets backward into the left atrium during ventricular systole. Mitral valve prolapse is also known as Barlow's syndrome, as well as a "floppy" or "billowing" mitral valve.

### Etiology/Epidemiology

Mitral valve prolapse may be caused by a variety of factors. Its incidence is possibly linked to an autosomal dominant inherited trait, and it is also associated with other inherited connective tissue disorders such as Marfan syndrome, Ehlers-Danlos syndrome, and osteogenesis imperfecta. Other causes of mitral valve prolapse include endocarditis, coronary artery disease, myocarditis, cardiomyopathy, cardiac trauma, and hyperthyroidism.

Mitral valve prolapse, the most common valvular disorder in the United States, occurs in approximately 4% to 7% of adults and more commonly in young women. In many patients, mitral valve prolapse is a benign, asymptomatic disorder and may therefore remain undiagnosed.

### Pathophysiology

In mitral valve prolapse, the leaflets of the mitral valve become enlarged or thickened, and the chordae tendineae may become elongated. These changes permit the valve leaflets to billow upward into the left atrium during ventricular systole. Depending on the degree of prolapse and the integrity of the valve leaflets, mitral regurgitation may occur. The subsequent pathophysiology parallels that of mitral regurgitation. In addition, research suggests that individuals with mitral valve prolapse may be associated with some autonomic dysfunction and excessive catecholamine release, leading to a wide array of subjective complaints.

Many cases of mitral valve prolapse are asymptomatic. Individuals who are symptomatic complain of a variety of symptoms. The most common symptom is palpitations, which are secondary to dysrhythmias and tachycardia. Other symptoms may include lightheadedness, syncope, fatigue, lethargy, weakness, dyspnea, and chest tightness. In addition, hyperventilation, anxiety, depression, panic attacks, and atypical chest pain may occur. Many of the symptoms of mitral valve prolapse are vague and puzzling and are not necessarily related to the degree of prolapse.

Although mitral valve prolapse is generally benign, up to 15% of individuals will develop mitral regurgitation and subsequent left ventricular failure. In addition, individuals with mitral valve prolapse are at increased risk for embolic stroke.

On physical examination, most individuals with mitral valve prolapse have a midsystolic click, and if mitral regurgitation is present, a late-systolic murmur is heard. In the absence of auscultatory findings, mitral valve prolapse may be detected on echocardiography.

### Collaborative Care Management

Electrocardiograms of individuals with mitral valve prolapse are normal unless the person is symptomatic from dysrhythmias. The most common rhythm disturbances include premature ventricular contractions, supraventricular tachycardia, and atrial tachydysrythmias. Mitral valve prolapse is diagnosed principally by echocardiography, although cardiac angiography may be used to confirm the diagnosis. Individuals who experience palpitations require 24-hour ambulatory ECG monitoring to determine the severity of the dysrhythmia.

Asymptomatic individuals with mitral valve prolapse usually do not require treatment after diagnosis. Symptomatic individuals may require medications for the management of dysrhythmias. Beta blockers are the treatment of choice for managing palpitations and chest pain. The drug of choice is atenolol or possibly propranolol.

All persons with mitral valve prolapse need regular follow-up and should have an echocardiogram every few years to monitor disease severity and progression. The severity of chronic mitral regurgitation associated with mitral valve prolapse will determine the necessity for surgical intervention.

Antibiotic prophylaxis against endocarditis is indicated before dental and surgical procedures for individuals who have a systolic murmur or echocardiographic evidence of mitral valve leaflet thickening. Asymptomatic individuals do not usually require antibiotic prophylaxis.

#### *Patient/family education*

Individuals with mitral valve prolapse are encouraged to avoid caffeine, which may exacerbate the incidence of tachycardia and atrial dysrhythmias. These episodes can be frightening for the patient and family, who need to thoroughly understand the nature of the problem and how to control or respond to it. No additional dietary restrictions are needed. Activities are also unrestricted, although symptomatic patients may need to adjust their activities in response to the nature and severity of their symptoms.

## AORTIC STENOSIS

Aortic stenosis occurs when the aortic valve leaflets become stiff, fused, or calcified and impede blood flow from the left ventricle into the aorta during ventricular systole.

### Etiology/Epidemiology

Aortic stenosis is caused by congenital malformations of the aortic valve, inflammatory heart disease (endocarditis), or degenerative disease (calcification). Aortic stenosis generally implies impedance to outflow of blood from the left ventricle at the level of the aortic valve, although obstruction to flow can also occur at subvalvular or supravalvular levels. Conditions such as hypertrophic cardiomyopathy may lead to subvalvular aortic stenosis. Coarctation of the aorta is a supravalvular lesion that may mimic aortic stenosis.

The causes of aortic stenosis vary with the age of the patient. In patients less than 30 years of age, aortic stenosis is typically caused by a congenitally stenotic unicuspid aortic valve. Between the ages of 30 and 65, aortic stenosis is more

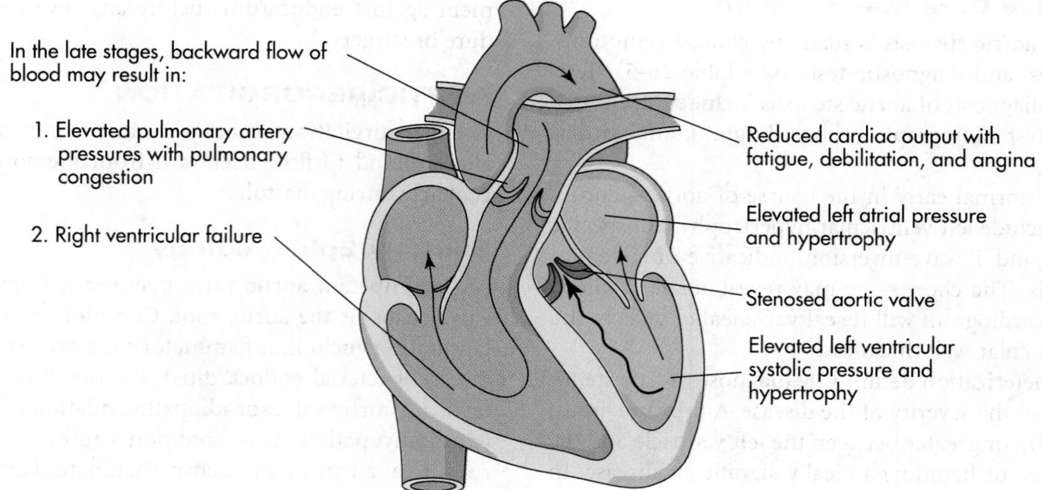


**fig. 26-10** Effects of aortic stenosis.

commonly caused by progressive stenosis of a congenital bicuspid valve, and less commonly by rheumatic heart disease. Although less than 2% of the general population have a congenital bicuspid aortic valve, 50% of these individuals will develop aortic calcification and stenosis by the age of 50. In persons over age 65, aortic stenosis is caused by degeneration and sclerosis of the valve and is equally distributed between men and women. Except in the elderly, men are three to four times more likely to develop isolated aortic stenosis.

### Pathophysiology

Aortic stenosis occurs when the aortic valve narrows and obstructs the flow of blood into the aorta during systole (Figure 26-10). Resistance to blood flow from the left ventricle causes an increase in left ventricular systolic pressure. This pressure increase and the left ventricle's compensatory efforts to increase cardiac output lead to left ventricular hypertrophy. Even though the left ventricle pumps harder to meet the body's needs, the stenotic valve effectively blocks any increase in blood flow from the heart. Hence, in advanced aortic stenosis, cardiac output becomes fixed despite the left ventricle's attempts to increase blood flow.

Worsening left ventricular hypertrophy leads to a constellation of problems late in the course of aortic stenosis, including pulmonary congestion, syncope, and myocardial ischemia. Pulmonary congestion occurs when the combination of aortic stenosis and left ventricular hypertrophy interferes with the forward movement of the blood. Syncope and myocardial ischemia occur because of the fixed-flow condition and inability of the left ventricle to meet the changing needs of the body. The severity of aortic stenosis is determined by the pressure gradient between the left ventricle and the aorta.

Aortic stenosis develops gradually, and symptoms do not appear until late in the course. Life expectancy without medical or surgical intervention is generally less than 4 years after the onset of symptoms. Early symptoms of aortic stenosis include fatigue and dyspnea. The combination of dyspnea, exertional angina, and syncope or near-syncopal episodes indicates severe aortic stenosis. Individuals who demonstrate heart failure survive less than 2 years, whereas patients with either syncope or angina survive longer (5 years and 3 years, respectively). In addition, 15% of those with symptomatic aortic stenosis and 5% of asymptomatic patients suffer sudden cardiac death.

In addition to the symptoms of dyspnea, fatigue, heart failure, angina, and syncope, an array of physical findings is present in individuals with aortic stenosis. The hallmark clinical findings include a grade III/VI or IV/VI systolic ejection murmur over the aortic area radiating upward into the carotid arteries and a pulse pattern that demonstrates a delayed systolic upstroke (Table 26-7). Other clinical findings depend on the degree of heart failure and pulmonary edema.

**table 26-7** *Auscultatory Differences in Valvular Heart Disease*

| Valvular Disorder | General Findings | Murmurs |
|---|---|---|
| Mitral stenosis | $S_1$ snapping, louder<br>Palpable thrill at apex | Soft, low-pitched, rumbling<br>Diastolic |
| Mitral regurgitation | $S_1$ soft or absent<br>$S_3$ present<br>Palpable thrill at apex | High-pitched, blowing<br>Pansystolic |
| Aortic stenosis | $S_2$ soft<br>Left-sided $S_4$<br>Systolic thrill at heart base | Low-pitched, harsh, rasping<br>Midsystolic |
| Aortic regurgitation | $S_3$ present<br>Systolic thrill over aortic area | High-pitched, blowing<br>Diastolic |
| Tricuspid regurgitation | Systolic thrill at lower left sternal border | High-pitched, blowing<br>Pansystolic |

### Collaborative Care Management

A diagnosis of aortic stenosis is made by clinical symptoms, clinical findings, and diagnostic tests (see Table 26-5). Tests that aid in the diagnosis of aortic stenosis include the electrocardiogram, chest radiograph, echocardiogram, and cardiac catheterization.

The ECG is normal early in the course of aortic stenosis. Late changes include left ventricular hypertrophy, nonspecific ST depression, and T wave inversion, indicative of subendocardial ischemia. The chest x-ray may reveal aortic calcification. The echocardiogram will reveal valve leaflet defects and increased ventricular wall thickness.

Cardiac catheterization definitively diagnoses aortic stenosis and quantifies the severity of the disease. A pressure gradient of 50 mm Hg or greater between the left ventricle and the aorta is evidence of hemodynamically significant disease. In addition, the cardiac catheterization evaluates left ventricular function, coronary vessel patency, and the degree of associated aortic and mitral regurgitation before cardiac surgery.

Percutaneous balloon valvuloplasty may be used to alleviate aortic stenosis. This technique involves cardiac catheterization and the introduction of a balloon catheter into the aortic valve orifice. The balloon is repeatedly inflated until the valve lumen is further opened, thus relieving some of the stenosis. Patients receive the same care provided to individuals undergoing cardiac catheterization but may also be monitored in an intensive care unit for 24 to 48 hours after the procedure. Although balloon valvuloplasty improves symptoms for some individuals, the procedure carries a high morbidity and mortality rate and is currently used primarily for individuals who are poor candidates for cardiac surgery and cardiopulmonary bypass.

The definitive therapy for patients with aortic stenosis is valve replacement with a prosthetic aortic valve. Although this surgery carries significant risks, most individuals report substantial improvement in their general health and exercise tolerance.

Although atrial dysrhythmias are uncommon, they are managed aggressively, but the use of beta blockers in patients with aortic stenosis is contraindicated because of their negative effect on left ventricular contractility. Heart failure associated with aortic stenosis is treated with digitalis and diuretic therapy, although caution must be taken to prevent volume depletion and subsequent decrease in cardiac output.

#### *Patient/family education*

The diet for persons with aortic stenosis is unrestricted unless heart failure is present, in which case the nurse instructs patients to restrict their daily intake of sodium and fluid. Activity levels must be carefully monitored because patients are at risk for sudden cardiac death. Patients are cautioned against undue physical exertion or stress, which may precipitate acute heart failure or dysrhythmia. Patients and families need ongoing teaching and support to effectively manage this ongoing challenge in their daily lives. The nurse also reminds patients of the importance of seeking prophylactic antibiotic treatment against endocarditis before any invasive dental procedure or surgery.

## AORTIC REGURGITATION

Aortic regurgitation occurs when an incompetent aortic valve allows blood to flow backward from the aorta into the left ventricle during diastole.

### Etiology/Epidemiology

An incompetent aortic valve may result from disease of the valve cusps or the aortic root. Common causes of aortic regurgitation include inflammatory diseases (rheumatic heart disease, bacterial endocarditis), the presence of a congenital bicuspid aortic valve, or idiopathic dilation of the aortic root (cardiomyopathy). Less common causes include traumatic rupture of an aortic valve cusp, rheumatoid arthritis, ankylosing spondylitis, Reiter's syndrome, connective tissue disorders (Marfan syndrome, Ehlers-Danlos syndrome, osteogenesis imperfecta), and syphilitic aortitis.

Acute aortic regurgitation occurs with sudden dilation of the aortic root and is most commonly associated with an ascending aortic dissecting aneurysm. The most common risk factor for acute aortic dissection is systemic hypertension. Selected connective tissue disorders, especially Marfan syndrome, also pose a risk for acute aortic dissection. Refer to Chapter 27 for further information relating to aortic aneurysms.

The incidence of aortic regurgitation related to rheumatic heart disease has decreased significantly over the past 20 years. Except in cases of rheumatic heart disease, aortic regurgitation is more common in men than in women.

### Pathophysiology

In chronic aortic regurgitation, the backward flow of blood through the incompetent, leaky aortic valve increases the volume of blood in the left ventricle (Figure 26-11). This increased blood volume and subsequent increase in left ventricular end-diastolic pressure serve to increase stroke volume and sustain cardiac output. Over time, however, left ventricular dilation and hypertrophy occur. Ultimately, the left ventricle loses the ability to compensate for the increased pressure and volume, leading to decreased stroke volume and cardiac output and finally left ventricular failure. Progressive aortic regurgitation can also lead to increased left atrial pressures, left atrial chamber dilation, pulmonary congestion, pulmonary hypertension, and possibly right-sided heart failure.

In acute aortic regurgitation as seen with aortic dissection, the left ventricle does not have the ability to compensate for the sudden increase in workload (increased blood volume and increased left ventricular end-diastolic pressure). In such cases, left ventricular decompensation and failure occur rapidly, and these patients require emergent lifesaving care.

Individuals with chronic aortic regurgitation may remain asymptomatic for 20 years or may report mild dyspnea on exertion. With disease progression and left ventricular decompensation, symptoms of heart failure and pulmonary edema develop, including progressively more severe dyspnea, orthop-

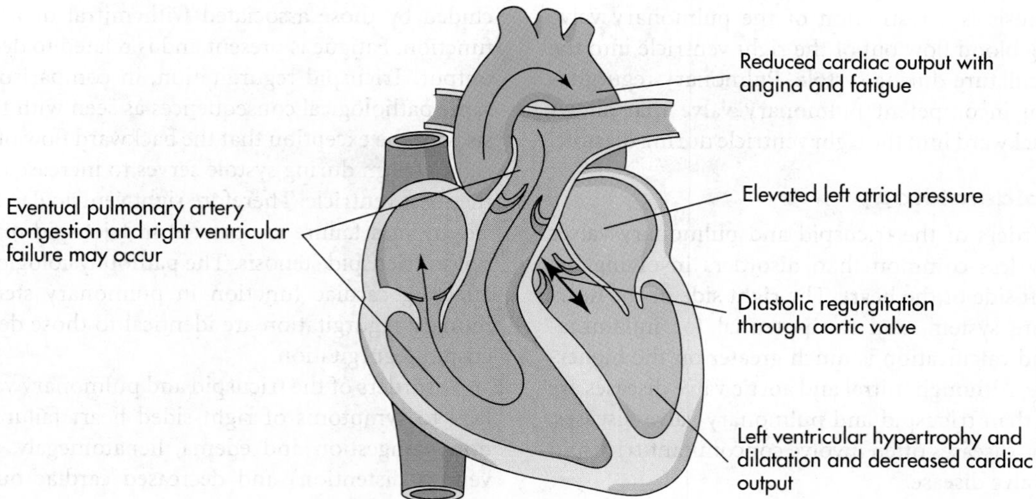


**fig. 26-11** Effects of aortic regurgitation.

nea, paroxysmal nocturnal dyspnea, and angina. The development and progression of these symptoms reflect advanced disease. In the case of acute aortic regurgitation, patients develop fulminant pulmonary edema. Other symptoms in acute aortic regurgitation vary depending on the etiology (e.g., fever with acute endocarditis, severe back pain with aortic dissection).

The hallmark physical finding in individuals with aortic regurgitation is a diastolic murmur that is loudest over the aortic area (see Table 26-7). The duration of the murmur reflects the severity of the regurgitation. Other classic physical findings associated with chronic aortic regurgitation include decreased diastolic pressure, widened pulse pressure, and subsequent water-hammer pulse. Pistol-shot pulse sounds can be auscultated over the femoral arteries, and some persons demonstrate a typical head bobbing with each heartbeat. Individuals with acute aortic regurgitation do not demonstrate the changes in pulse pressure because of the sudden onset of the disease.

### Collaborative Care Management

The diagnosis of aortic regurgitation is made based on the presence of the diastolic murmur and the widened pulse pressure. (See Tables 26-5 and 26-6.) The ECG shows left ventricular hypertrophy in persons with chronic aortic regurgitation but not in persons with acute regurgitation. The ECG in acute aortic regurgitation may show nonspecific ST or T wave changes. The chest x-ray may show cardiomegaly in cases of chronic aortic regurgitation, but again, for individuals with acute aortic regurgitation, the cardiac size may be normal. Echocardiography is useful in assessing left ventricular function, hypertrophy, and aortic root dilation.

Persons with asymptomatic aortic regurgitation do not require any treatment other than yearly follow-up and regular chest x-ray, ECG, and possibly echocardiography. Persons with symptomatic aortic regurgitation are managed medically pending evaluation by a cardiologist and subsequent aortic valve surgery.

Digitalis and diuretic therapy are indicated for individuals who demonstrate heart failure. Afterload-reducing agents may also be used to manage the heart failure.

Because of the high mortality rate associated with symptomatic aortic regurgitation, all symptomatic individuals are evaluated for aortic valve replacement surgery. Aortic valve replacement before the development of left ventricular dysfunction can significantly reduce operative mortality and result in long-term improvement in quality of life.

#### *Patient/family education*

Patients with aortic regurgitation must understand the nature and potential seriousness of their disease and commit to regular medical follow-up and evaluation. Definitive surgical treatment is recommended before the disease process can seriously compromise left ventricular function. Asymptomatic patients do not need to restrict their diet or activity in any way. Symptomatic patients are instructed to reduce their intake of sodium to help control the symptoms of heart failure and to adapt their activity to changes in their tolerance level. Patients need to be knowledgeable about the safe use of any prescribed medications. The nurse reminds patients of the importance of seeking prophylactic antibiotic therapy against endocarditis before any dental or surgical procedure.

## TRICUSPID AND PULMONARY VALVE DISORDERS

Tricuspid stenosis is a restriction of the tricuspid valve orifice that impedes blood flow from the right atrium to the right ventricle during right ventricular diastole (filling). Conversely, tricuspid regurgitation involves an incompetent tricuspid valve that allows blood to flow backward from the right ventricle to the right atrium during ventricular systole.

Pulmonary stenosis is a restriction of the pulmonary valve orifice impeding blood flow out of the right ventricle into the pulmonary vasculature during systole. Pulmonary regurgitation involves an incompetent pulmonary valve that allows blood to flow backward into the right ventricle during diastole.

## Etiology/Epidemiology

In general, disorders of the tricuspid and pulmonary valves are significantly less common than disorders involving the valves on the left side of the heart. The right side of the heart is a low-pressure system, and the potential for inflammatory changes and calcification is much greater on the higher-pressure left side. Although mitral and aortic valve diseases are more common than tricuspid and pulmonary valve diseases, mitral and aortic diseases often involve concomitant tricuspid or pulmonary valve disease.

Disorders of the tricuspid valves are primarily caused by rheumatic fever. Less common causes include endocarditis or congenital malformations of the valve cusps. Tricuspid stenosis is generally seen in women with a history of rheumatic heart disease who suffer from mitral stenosis. Tricuspid regurgitation often accompanies tricuspid stenosis.

Pulmonary valve disorders are rare. Pulmonary regurgitation, like tricuspid valve disease, is caused by endocarditis or rheumatic fever. Congenital malformations and tumors are also causes of pulmonary valve dysfunction.

## Pathophysiology

Tricuspid and pulmonary valve disorders all cause similar consequences to cardiac function. Tricuspid stenosis causes increased pressure in the right atrium and subsequent right atrial enlargement and hypertrophy (Figure 26-12). Over time, systemic venous congestion occurs and causes ascites, hepatomegaly, and edema. Because of reduced flow across the stenotic tricuspid valve, cardiac output is fixed and eventually diminished. Symptoms of tricuspid stenosis are generally precluded by those associated with mitral or aortic valve dysfunction. Fatigue is present and is related to decreased cardiac output. Tricuspid regurgitation, in comparison, involves the same pathological consequences as seen with tricuspid stenosis with the exception that the backward flow of blood into the right atrium during systole serves to increase the workload of the right ventricle. Therefore right ventricular dilation, hypertrophy, and failure are present in tricuspid regurgitation but not in tricuspid stenosis. The pathophysiological mechanisms affecting cardiac function in pulmonary stenosis and pulmonary regurgitation are identical to those described for tricuspid regurgitation.

Disorders of the tricuspid and pulmonary valves ultimately lead to symptoms of right-sided heart failure (systemic venous congestion and edema, hepatomegaly, ascites, jugular venous distention) and decreased cardiac output (fatigue). The ECG will show tall, peaked P waves (atrial hypertrophy) in tricuspid stenosis and tricuspid regurgitation. Right ventricular hypertrophy will also be evident on ECG for tricuspid regurgitation, pulmonary stenosis, and pulmonary regurgitation. Atrial fibrillation may also be present. In tricuspid stenosis, a high-pitched diastolic murmur can be auscultated along the left sternal border. In the other disorders of the tricuspid and pulmonary valves, the murmur is pansystolic and harsh. Radiographic evaluation will show right atrial enlargement, right ventricular enlargement (except in tricuspid stenosis), and a prominent shadow of the superior vena cava. Echocardiogram is used to determine the degree of valve dysfunction.

## Collaborative Care Management

Care for patients with tricuspid and pulmonary valve disorders focuses on the management of right-sided heart failure and decreased cardiac output. The care is similar to that previously outlined for mitral and aortic valve disorders. One exception is that patients do not experience dyspnea and pulmonary consequences with tricuspid and pulmonary valve

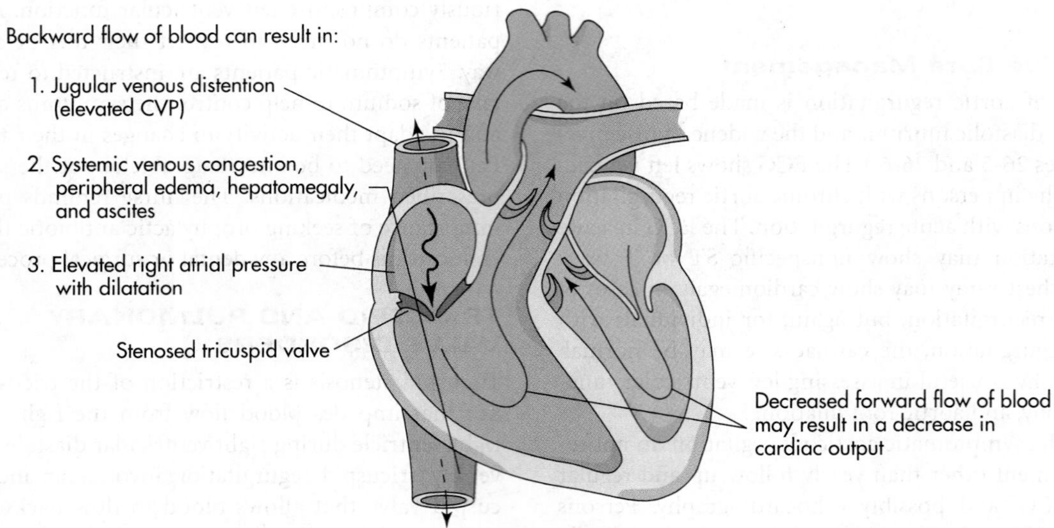
Backward flow of blood can result in:
1. Jugular venous distention (elevated CVP)
2. Systemic venous congestion, peripheral edema, hepatomegaly, and ascites
3. Elevated right atrial pressure with dilatation
Stenosed tricuspid valve
Decreased forward flow of blood may result in a decrease in cardiac output

**fig. 26-12** Effects of tricuspid stenosis.

disease, unless these disorders occur concurrently with aortic and mitral valve disease.

#### Patient/family education

Teaching for patients with tricuspid and pulmonary valve disorders is targeted toward specific symptom management, which may vary substantially from patient to patient based on the severity of the disorder and involvement of valves from the left side of the heart. Patients are encouraged to modify their activities to match their tolerance level and to plan for the presence of chronic fatigue. Congestion within the gastrointestinal tract may lead to chronic anorexia, and the nurse emphasizes the importance of adequate nutrition. Patients are taught to monitor their edema at home and to protect the skin from breakdown. Patients are also instructed in the correct and safe use of all medications and the effective management of expected side effects.

## CARDIAC SURGERY

Although the first attempts to surgically correct cardiac problems date to the 1930s, effective cardiac surgery techniques and favorable outcomes for patients did not develop until the 1950s. In 1954 the development of cardiopulmonary bypass revolutionized cardiac surgery. Since then a variety of cardiac surgical procedures have been developed, and numerous cardiac disorders in both adults and children can now be effectively treated with cardiac surgery.

Numerous diseases and conditions may create the need for cardiac surgery. The most common reason for an adult to undergo cardiac surgery is myocardial revascularization (coronary artery bypass graft). In addition, patients undergo cardiac surgery for valve repair or replacement, repair of structural defects (acquired or congenital), implantation of devices, and cardiac transplantation. Table 26-8 provides a detailed list of indications for cardiac surgery.

Cardiac surgery is classified as either open heart or closed heart, depending on whether the heart is "opened" during the course of the surgery. Cardiac surgery involving the repair of internal structural defects is open heart, whereas myocardial revascularization is a closed heart procedure. Other essential concepts in the care of patients undergoing cardiac surgery include cardioplegia and cardiopulmonary bypass, which are discussed later in the chapter.

**table 26-8** *Indications for Cardiac Surgery and Associated Procedures*

| Problem | Procedure |
|---|---|
| Ischemic heart disease | Coronary artery bypass graft |
| Repair of structural abnormalities | Valve repair<br>Valve replacement<br>Atrial septal defect repair<br>Ventricular septal defect repair<br>Ventricular aneurysm resection<br>Atrial tumor resection<br>Aortic aneurysm (thoracic) repair |
| Implantation of devices | Automatic implantable cardioverter-defibrillator<br>Ventricular assist device<br>Artificial heart chamber |
| Transplantation | Replacement of diseased heart with healthy heart |

## SURGICAL PROCEDURES

### Coronary Artery Bypass Graft

Coronary artery disease is the most common indication for cardiac surgery. When a coronary artery becomes partially or totally obstructed, a coronary artery bypass graft (CABG) may be performed. The graft allows blood to bypass the obstructed portion of the coronary artery and helps provide adequate blood flow to the myocardial tissue distal to the lesion. With improved blood flow to the myocardium, the heart muscle receives increased oxygen. Although coronary artery bypass does not cure the underlying heart disease, the benefits of CABG include a reduction of angina and prevention of myocardial ischemia and infarction.

#### Vein grafts

Patients can undergo a single coronary artery bypass or may simultaneously receive multiple bypass grafts, depending on the nature and severity of the coronary disease. The surgical procedure involves closed heart surgery via a median sternotomy, cold cardioplegia, and extracorporeal circulation with a cardiopulmonary bypass machine. The graft used to bypass the affected coronary artery may be either a vein graft or an artery graft. The most common donor vein used for bypass is a long portion of the saphenous vein, although occasionally a cephalic vein from the forearm is used. After vein harvesting, the donor graft is reversed before insertion because of the presence of directional valves within the vein. The vein graft is anastamosed to the coronary artery distal to the obstructive lesion, and the proximal end is anastamosed to the ascending aorta. Before surgery, Doppler studies of venous flow help pinpoint optimal segments of veins for use as grafts. This enables the surgeon to use minimally invasive vein harvesting in which only the necessary segments, rather than the entire length of the donor graft vein, are removed.

#### Arterial grafts

The artery most commonly used for CABG is an internal mammary artery (right or left), although occasionally a gastroepiploic artery is used. When an artery is used for bypass grafting, only the distal end of the artery is dissected away from the tissues and anastomosed to the coronary artery distal to the obstructive lesion. A more recent trend involves harvesting the radial artery from the forearm and using it as a bypass graft rather than a vein.

Long-term patency rates for internal mammary artery grafts exceed the long-term patency rates for saphenous vein grafts. Studies have shown that 40% to 50% of saphenous vein grafts close within 2 years, whereas 90% of internal mammary artery grafts remain patent 10 years after surgery. However, internal mammary artery grafts are contraindicated for patients with diabetes mellitus (because of the impact of reduced arterial circulation to the chest wall on wound healing), as well as in obese or large-breasted individuals.

The last decade has witnessed dramatic changes in the approach to care of patients undergoing coronary artery bypass surgery, especially during the postoperative recovery phase. Average length of hospital stay for patients undergoing uncomplicated CABG surgery is 4 to 5 days (compared with 2 to 3 weeks in the 1980s). In addition, a new, minimally invasive CABG procedure for disease of the left anterior descending coronary artery allows a single-vessel bypass (using an internal mammary artery) to be performed without median sternotomy, cardioplegia, or cardiopulmonary bypass. In this procedure, access to the internal mammary artery and the left anterior descending artery is gained through a small incision at the left sternal border of the anterior chest wall. Preliminary data show shorter recovery times with an estimated length of hospital stay for this procedure of 2 days (Box 26-9).

**box 26-9** *Minimally Invasive Coronary Artery Bypass Graft*

A new surgical technique allows for coronary artery bypass graft surgery to be performed without the use of a median sternotomy, cardiopulmonary (heart-lung) bypass, or cardioplegia. In this new procedure, a small left chest incision allows the surgeon to directly visualize the heart and complete an internal mammary artery–to–left anterior descending coronary artery bypass. Preliminary data suggest that operative time and postoperative complications are reduced, and hospital stay averages 2 days as opposed to 5 days for traditional heart surgery.

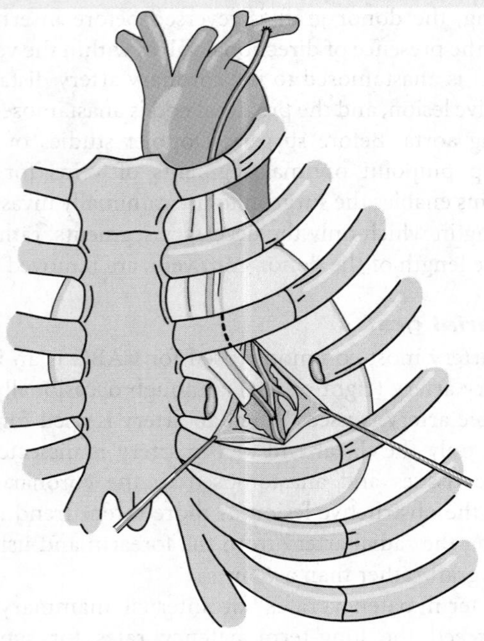

Through a pericardial window anastomosis of the left internal mammary artery to the left anterior descending coronary artery is performed under direct vision.

## Correction of Structural Defects

Another important indication for cardiac surgery is the correction of a structural defect. Cardiac valve dysfunction is the most common structural repair in adults. Options include either a valve repair (annuloplasty, valvuloplasty, or commissurotomy; see Box 26-10) or replacement with a valve prosthesis. Less commonly, adults undergo cardiac surgery to repair structural defects, such as a ventricular aneurysm or atrial or ventricular septal defect; to remove a cardiac tumor; or to repair the heart after trauma.

Surgery involving intracardiac structural defects requires open heart surgery via a median sternotomy, cardioplegia, and cardiopulmonary bypass. Surgery involving extracardiac structures such as repair of a thoracic aortic aneurysm or coarctation of the aorta may include cardiopulmonary bypass and cardioplegia, depending on the location and severity of the lesion. Occasionally during the repair of severe aortic arch defects, total circulatory arrest may be used. This involves deep hypothermia and cessation of cardiopulmonary bypass for a period of time while the aortic defects are undergoing repair. Refer to Chapter 27 for further discussion of aortic aneurysms.

### *Valve repair*

**Annuloplasty.** Annuloplasty is a procedure to reduce an enlarged annulus (fibrous ring surrounding the valve). The procedure involves the use of a prosthetic ring that is sutured into the circumference of the mitral or tricuspid annulus. The stitches are pulled together toward the prosthesis, reducing the size of the valve orifice.

**Valvuloplasty.** Valvuloplasty is direct suture repair of torn leaflets or clefts by open heart surgery. The advantages of operative valve repair over valve replacement include (1) higher survival rates, (2) fewer cardiac complications (especially thromboembolism), (3) lower operative mortality and morbidity, (4) potential improvement in left ventricular function, (5) reduced need for anticoagulation, and (6) lower cost. Mitral valvuloplasty has gained increasing acceptance as the surgery of choice for mitral regurgitation, including cases of rheumatic etiology. A different form of valvuloplasty is per-

**box 26-10** *Types of Valve Repair*

**ANNULOPLASTY**
Repair of ring or annulus of incompetent or diseased valve

**VALVULOPLASTY**
Repair of valve, suturing of torn leaflets

**COMMISSUROTOMY**
Dilation of valve; repair of a leaflet or commissure, fibrous bond or ring

cutaneous aortic balloon valvuloplasty, a nonsurgical procedure for aortic valve repair.

**Commissurotomy.** Mitral commissurotomy is the separation or incision of the stenosed valve leaflets at their borders or commissures. Two techniques are used for a commissurotomy—open or closed. Controversy exists over the two methods, with an open commissurotomy being the procedure of choice.

An open commissurotomy usually is performed through a median sternotomy or a right anterolateral thoracotomy incision. This allows for proper visualization of the mitral valve. Cardiopulmonary bypass is used, and after the incision of the left atrium, the valve is inspected and the atrial thrombus removed.

The commissures are then incised with a scalpel, and new mobilized leaflets are attached to the chordae tendineae cordis. Disadvantages of this approach include those associated with open heart surgery, that is, difficult cannulation during cardiopulmonary bypass and clotting problems. The advantages include fewer thrombotic and embolic complications and fewer atrial tears with resultant hemorrhage. If the valve disease appears to be so advanced that replacement is indicated, the heart is already open.

A closed commissurotomy (without bypass) is performed through a left posterolateral thoracotomy. The fifth rib is removed to prepare for a closed or open operation. Some closed commissurotomies are performed in the fourth and fifth interspace with a transection of a rib, if necessary. After the incision is made, the atrium is palpated to detect any thrombi. If a thrombus is present, the procedure is converted to an open procedure to remove the clot. Otherwise, the surgeon inserts a finger through a small incision, dividing the papillary muscle longitudinally from the apex toward the base as shown in Figure 26-13. The atrium is digitally examined for thrombi, and the valve is examined for calcium particles. Some surgeons may digitally open the fused commissures and use a dilator to open the valve and relieve the stenosis. The advantages of the closed approach include a shorter operating time, greater simplicity, and less blood replacement. Systemic emboli, atrial wall tears, inadequate alleviation of the stenosis, and mitral regurgitation are risks of this method of commissurotomy.

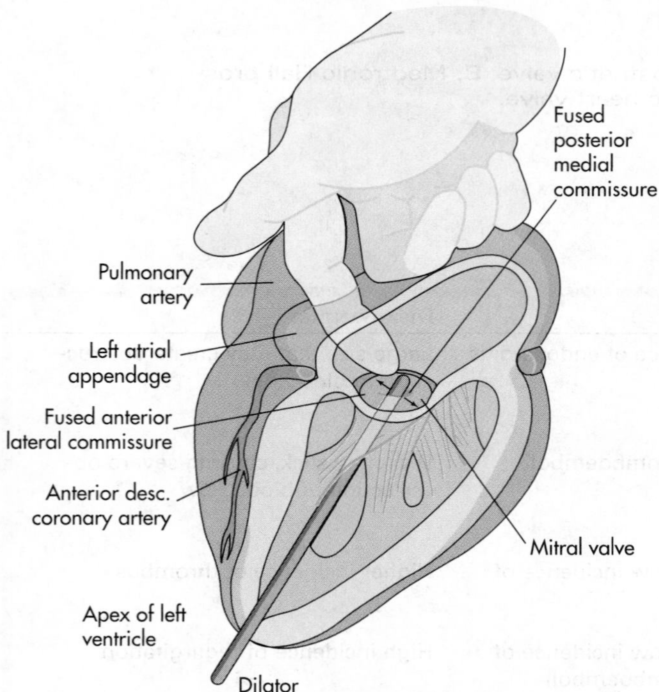


**fig. 26-13** Technique of closed mitral commissurotomy using mitral dilating instrument.

One major advantage of mitral valve repair over a mitral replacement is the mortality rate. The operative mortality rate for a commissurotomy is 1% to 2%, compared with 10% for a mitral valve replacement.

### Valve replacement

Valve replacement is considered when the valve is so stenosed and calcified that repair would not achieve long-term relief of obstruction. Variables that affect the results of the valve replacement include the patient's general clinical condition and level of myocardial functioning before surgery and the type of valve used.

The heart usually is approached by a median sternotomy. Cardiopulmonary bypass is used in an open procedure. The diseased valve leaflets are excised at the annulus, and the remaining annuli are sized with an obturator. The loose chordae are excised to avoid their becoming tangled in the new valve, and the prosthetic valve is sutured into the new annulus. Although the mortality rate with an aortic valve replacement is less than 5%, it is greater for the mitral valve. Risk factors include physiological and chronological age, chronicity, type of valvular lesion, and left ventricular function. Mortality rates of valvular replacement surgery increase in persons older than 70 years of age.[32]

The Ross procedure is an alternative method of aortic valve replacement. It uses the patient's own pulmonary valve, which has all the characteristics of the patient's aortic valve. This procedure is specifically indicated for young patients in whom a long life span is expected. Primary indications include isolated aortic valve disease, severe aortic stenosis, and severe aortic regurgitation with or without dilation of the aortic root. Contraindications include dissection of the aorta, Marfan syndrome, and other diseases that cause significant aortic root enlargement. A routine midline sternotomy is performed, with cannulation of the ascending aorta and right atrium, followed by cardiopulmonary bypass. Extreme care must be taken in removing the pulmonary valve to avoid damage to the left main coronary artery. A homograft valve (human transplant) is carefully inserted into the pulmonary position. The patient's removed pulmonary valve is trimmed of excess fat and muscle and inserted into the aortic root and sutured in place.

### Types of valves

The ideal replacement valve has the following characteristics: durable, hemodynamic accuracy, nonhemolytic, nonthrombogenic, easily inserted, anatomically suitable, and a low incidence of endocarditis. A wide variety of prosthetic

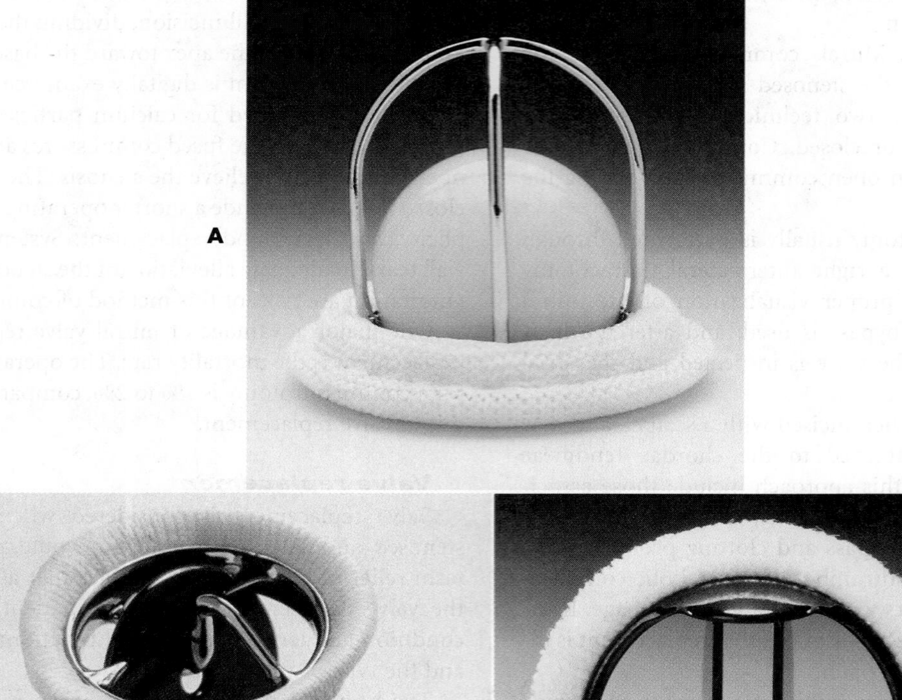

**fig. 26-14** **A**, Starr-Edwards caged ball prosthetic valve. **B**, Medtronic Hall prosthetic valve. **C**, St. Jude Medical tilting disc heart valve.

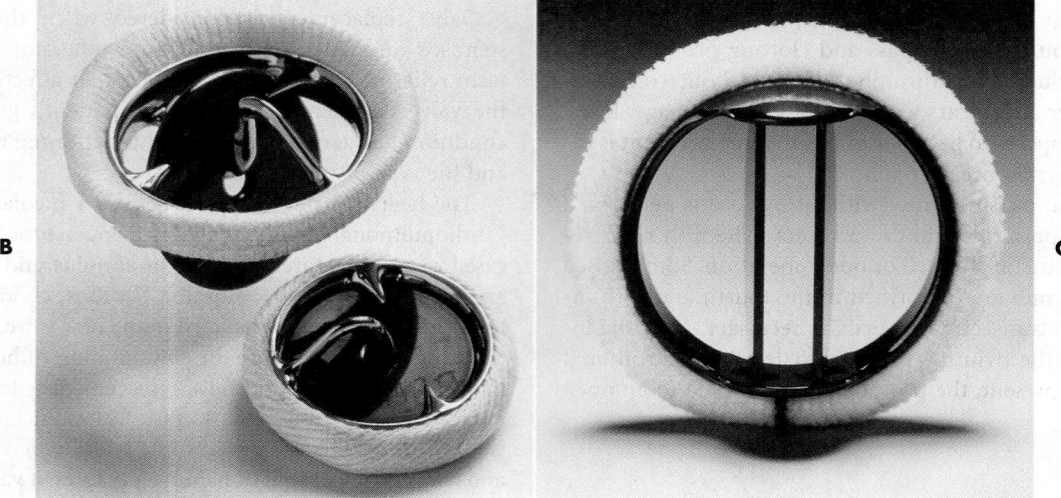

**table 26-9** *Types of Prosthetic Valves*

| Type | Examples | Advantages | Disadvantages |
|---|---|---|---|
| Caged ball | Starr-Edwards<br>Smeloff<br>Braunwald-Cutter<br>McGovern-Cromie | Durable, low incidence of endocarditis | Large size that may create obstruction to blood flow |
| Caged disk | Beall<br>Hufnagel<br>Cross-Jones<br>Kay-Shiley | Low incidence of thromboemboli | Disk may stick, causing severe obstruction of blood flow |
| Tilting disk | Bjork-Shiley<br>Wada-Cutter<br>St. Jude | Central blood flow, low incidence of hemolysis | Higher incidence of thrombus |
| Stenting allograft | Lillehei-Kaste | Central blood flow, low incidence of hemolysis, no thromboemboli | High incidence of regurgitation |
| Xenograft | Porcine | Silent valves, low incidence of thromboembolism or hemolysis | High incidence of calcification over time |

valves are available. The advantages and disadvantages of each valve type are listed in Table 26-9.

Caged-ball prosthetic valves consist of a metal cage with a synthetic, freely moving ball inside; the cage is attached to a sewing ring (Figure 26-14). The ring and struts of the cage are covered by a synthetic cloth. The cloth-covered ring is sutured carefully into the existing valve annulus. Within 2 to 3 months, tissue covers the cloth and the incidence of thromboembolism decreases. Caged-ball valves come in various sizes and slightly varying designs and materials.

Caged-disk prosthetic valves occupy less space in the ventricles than do other valves and require less force to move the occluding disk. This type of valve creates more obstruction to blood flow than do other types of valves. If the disk "sticks" in the cage, causing total obstruction of blood flow, hemodynamics are seriously compromised.

Tilting-disk prosthetic valves have occluders that tilt or pivot within a ring rather than balls or disks that pop back and forth in a cage. This type of valve produces nearly central blood flow through its orifice, providing more normal blood flow. However, the areas under the pivoting points are more susceptible to thrombus formation as a result of the blood stasis.

Stenting allografts are human heart valves that are supported or "stented" by an underlying frame. Allografts provide relatively normal hemodynamic characteristics with central flow, no thromboemboli, and little hemolysis. However, allografts are difficult to procure in quantity.

Xenograft bioprosthetic valves are composed of valves from species other than human, are more readily available than other valves, and can be obtained in all sizes. Porcine xenograft valves are most commonly used. The hemodynamic performance is similar to that of human heart valves. Many patients with this type of valve may not require anticoagulants. Approximately 70% to 80% of patients older than 35 years of age are free of primary tissue failure at 10 years. After 10 to 12 years, calcification of the valve begins to accelerate. Because of the higher incidence of calcification over time, porcine valves are now used less often in young persons.

## Implantation of Devices

Cardiac surgery may involve the implantation of technological devices. An automatic implantable cardioverter-defibrillator (AICD) includes a myocardial sensing electrode and a pulse generator and differs from an artificial pacemaker in purpose and function. The AICD senses the presence of lethal tachydysrhythmias in persons at risk and delivers an electric countershock to restore normal heart rhythm.

Ventricular assist devices (VADs) and artificial heart chambers perform part of the workload of the heart. The primary indication for these devices is the prevention of end-organ damage in a person with a failing heart who is awaiting cardiac transplantation.

## Cardiac Transplantation

Cardiac transplantation is the most effective therapeutic modality to significantly prolong life in patients with end-stage heart disease. Despite the positive outcomes of cardiac transplantation, donor availability and complications from infection, rejection, and immunosuppressive drug therapy continue to be serious problems (see Chapter 68). At least half of all cardiac transplantations are performed for dilated cardiomyopathy and most of the remainder for end-stage heart disease caused by extensive coronary artery disease.[11]

Cardiac transplantation involves excision of the recipient's diseased heart, with subsequent replacement with the donor human heart. Cardiectomy requires transection of the main pulmonary artery and aorta and partial resection of the atria, leaving the posterior walls intact. These portions serve for surgical attachment to the donor heart and also retain their systemic and pulmonary venous connections. The donor heart is trimmed to fit the recipient's atria and great vessels. Anastomoses are made between the recipient left atria, septum, right atria, the aortas, and the pulmonary arteries (Figure 26-15).

Overall condition of the donor heart, ischemic time, myocardial preservation techniques, and pharmacotherapy ultimately

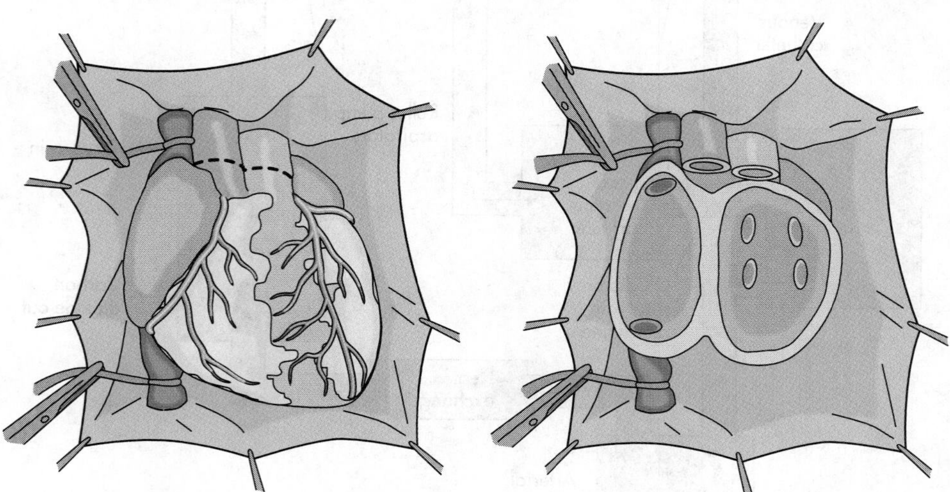

**fig. 26-15** Technique of cardiac transplantation. The diseased heart is removed, leaving the posterior walls of the atria. The new heart is then anastomosed to the atrial walls and great vessels.

influence the integrity of the donor heart's newly independent mechanical and electrical responses. During the immediate postimplantation period, the myocardium must adapt to the absence of autonomic enervation. Commonly it is necessary to augment its inotropic and chronotropic function with intravenous catecholamines, such as dopamine and isoproterenol, until hemodynamic parameters stabilize. See Chapter 68 for additional information on organ transplantation.

## CARDIOPULMONARY BYPASS

Some heart surgery procedures can be performed without artificial ventilation and circulation, but most procedures require either partial or total cardiopulmonary bypass. In partial, or left heart, bypass, blood is drained from the left atrium and ventricle and is passed through a pulsatile or roller pump, which returns the blood to the common femoral artery or the descending aorta. In this type of bypass, the pulmonary circulation is not interrupted.

In total cardiopulmonary bypass, the heart-lung bypass machine is used to provide artificial oxygenation and circulation of the blood during the surgical procedure. Venous blood is removed from the body through large cannulas placed in either the right atrium or the inferior or superior venae cavae (Figure 26-16). The blood passes through the oxygenating mechanism of the bypass machine to become oxygenated. The blood is then pumped back into the arterial circulation of the body through large cannulas placed either in the ascending aorta (most common) or in the femoral artery. A venting tube is usually introduced through the apex of the left ventricle or left atrium and is connected to the pump to aspirate blood from within the heart to maintain decompression of the heart during the surgery. In addition to providing artificial oxygenation and circulation during the surgery, the cardiopulmonary bypass machine also provides a way to administer medications and control body temperature.

Important events during cardiopulmonary bypass include hemodilution, anticoagulation, hypothermia, and cold cardioplegia.

### Hemodilution

The cardiopulmonary bypass machine is primed for use with approximately 2500 ml of crystalloid fluid, mainly lactated Ringer's solution. Although bypass circuits used to be primed with crossmatched type-specific whole blood, advantages of nonblood primer include decreased blood viscosity, limited hemolysis, and no risk of transfusion reaction or disease transmission from the primer solution. With the large and sudden infusion of crystalloid fluid during the initiation of

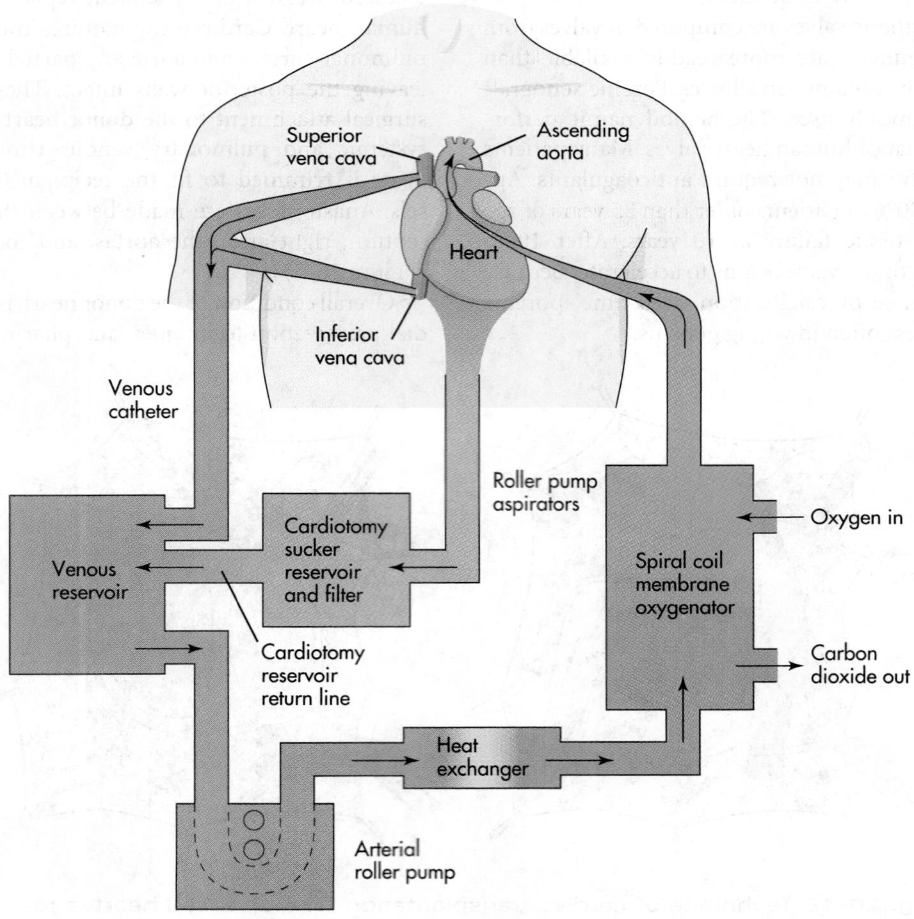


**fig. 26-16** Set-up for cardiopulmonary bypass (CPB).

cardiopulmonary bypass, the patient's hematocrit will fall. To maintain an adequate hematocrit, blood can be transfused through the cardiopulmonary bypass machine. Most commonly, autologous blood (the patient's own blood) is administered. Autologous blood is obtained through preoperative donation or is collected during the surgical procedure by an autotransfusion system.

### Anticoagulation

Systemic anticoagulation with heparin is required to prevent thrombus formation within the cardiopulmonary bypass machine. In addition, anticoagulation prevents the patient from developing a thrombus during periods of reduced blood flow and cardiac output. Anticoagulation is reversed with protamine sulfate on cessation of cardiopulmonary bypass.

### Hypothermia

The cardiopulmonary bypass machine provides systemic hypothermia by cooling the perfusion solution to temperatures that range from mildly (30° to 35° C) to profoundly (15° C) hypothermic. Hypothermia is important because it lowers the metabolic needs of the body's vital organs and tissues by lowering the body's overall oxygen consumption. A reduced need for oxygen helps preserve vital organs and body tissues during the period of aortic cross-clamping, cold cardioplegia, and reduced cardiac output.

### Cold Cardioplegia

Cardioplegia is the intentional arrest of the heart by the surgical team during total cardiopulmonary bypass. The aorta is clamped and a cold cardioplegic solution is infused into the heart and coronary arteries, causing the heart to stop beating. This induced cardiac arrest provides the surgical team with a quiet heart on which to operate. Myocardial tissue preservation is of primary concern during the time in which the myocardium is not perfused. Therefore the cardioplegic solution is cold (to reduce myocardial tissue oxygen demand) and contains an alkaline hyperosmotic solution with potassium, calcium chloride, mannitol, and other substances. The cold cardioplegia solution is infused at the time the aortic clamp is applied, as well as 30 to 45 minutes later or when myocardial temperatures rise above 19° C. A continuous infusion into the pericardium of lactated Ringer's solution at 4° C provides additional external cardiac cooling and protection. Advances in cold cardioplegic techniques have significantly improved myocardial tissue preservation during cardiopulmonary bypass.

### Termination of Cardiopulmonary Bypass

Once the surgical repair is complete, the cardioplegia infusion is terminated. The blood in the cardiopulmonary bypass machine is slowly rewarmed, and the patient's core body temperature is brought back to near normal. The cardioplegic heart is restarted, and the lungs are reexpanded. Once the cardiac rhythm and output become stable, weaning from cardiopulmonary bypass begins. Autologous blood from the bypass machine is collected and returned to the patient. The degree of partial bypass support is systematically decreased and ultimately discontinued. Systemic heparinization is reversed with protamine.

### Side Effects and Potential Complications of Cardiopulmonary Bypass

Although cardiopulmonary bypass has significantly advanced the rapidly growing area of safe and effective cardiac procedures, a number of potentially devastating physiological sequelae exist. Overall, cardiopulmonary bypass creates a shocklike state in which there is a low hematocrit (caused by hemodilution) and decreased systolic blood pressure and perfusion of the body's organs and tissues. If prolonged, this shocklike state can contribute to neurological, myocardial, and renal ischemia and damage. Shearing forces during cardiopulmonary bypass lead to platelet destruction and red blood cell hemolysis, predisposing the patient to coagulation problems postoperatively. Thrombus formation and arterial embolism related to aortic cross-clamping can lead to infarction of vital organs and tissues. Finally, the patient's physiological response to stress causes an increase in circulating catecholamines, leading to hyperglycemia and associated fluid volume deficit postoperatively.

### Cardiogenic Shock and Heart Failure After Cardiopulmonary Bypass

Some patients may experience difficulties in being weaned from extracorporeal circulation. These persons may require circulatory assistance such as the intraaortic balloon pump to temporarily augment their circulatory system.

The various situations in which counterpulsation has been found useful are listed in Box 26-11. In all cases, the timeliness of its application is essential to reduce the workload of the heart and halt the progressive deterioration of the myocardium. Patients have been maintained on IABP assistance for periods of several hours to several months; however, the usual time is 2 to 3 days. The IABP is not indicated for persons whose underlying pathological condition is so severe that eventual weaning from the IABP is considered impossible, unless the individual is being seriously evaluated for heart transplantation.

An alternative approach for patients in ventricular failure is a left ventricular assist device (LVAD) or right ventricular assist device (RVAD). These devices provide rest for the ventricles while artificially replacing systemic pumping. They generally are indicated for profound intraoperative myocardial depression with failure to wean from the cardiopulmonary

**box 26-11** *Intraaortic Balloon Counterpulsation: Indications for Use*

- Cardiogenic shock secondary to acute myocardial infarction
- Other low cardiac output states
- During emergency diagnostic procedures on unstable cardiac patients
- In unstable cardiac patients before and during open heart surgery
- Assistance in removing patients from cardiopulmonary bypass postoperatively
- Drug-resistant, life-threatening dysrhythmias
- Unstable angina pectoris
- Severe acute myocardial infarction

bypass. Patients requiring this type of assistance are critically ill and require care in an intensive care unit.

### Intraaortic balloon pump

A counterpulsation device assists the circulation of blood through the body by pumping when the heart is in ventricular diastole. The hemodynamic result of this action is to augment intraaortic blood pressure during diastole. The physiological effects of counterpulsation are an increase in coronary artery perfusion, a decrease in preload, and a decrease in afterload.

The pump is used to provide temporary assistance to the patient's circulation until the pathophysiological condition is corrected, to afford optimal conditions for repair, or to rest the heart until it can provide adequate circulation unaided.

The intraaortic balloon is inserted percutaneously or by cutdown into the right or left femoral artery. It is advanced into the thoracic aorta and is sutured into place at the insertion site after the balloon tip has been correctly positioned just distal to the left subclavian artery. The end of the balloon catheter is attached to a pump, which alternately inflates and deflates the balloon with helium.

The timing of the inflation-deflation sequence is of the utmost importance in obtaining maximal counterpulsation effect. The ECG is used to trigger the balloon, which is timed to inflate just at the beginning of ventricular diastole, immediately after closure of the aortic valve. The balloon remains inflated during diastole and is then timed to deflate immediately before the next ventricular systolic ejection or just before the aortic valve reopens (Figure 26-17). Improper balloon timing not only defeats the purpose of counterpulsation but also could directly damage the myocardium, particularly if early inflation or late deflation forces the heart to eject blood against a partially inflated balloon.

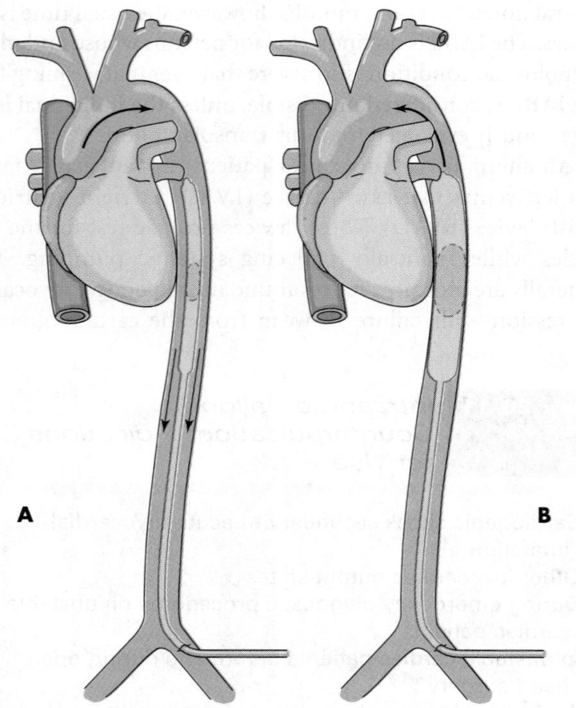


**fig. 26-17** Representation of intraaortic balloon positioned just distal to left subclavian artery. **A,** Balloon is deflated, allowing forward blood flow during systole. **B,** Balloon is inflated to increase coronary perfusion during diastole.

When the balloon is inflated during diastole, it causes an intraaortic pressure rise known as diastolic augmentation. This heightened diastolic pressure forces blood in the aortic arch to flow in a retrograde fashion and provides increased coronary artery filling. This process achieves the goal of improving oxygen delivery to the myocardium.

When the balloon deflates at the end of diastole, it reduces pressure in the aorta, causing blood in the aortic arch to move from an area of higher pressure to one of lower pressure and to fill the space previously occupied by the balloon. This decreases the pressure in the aortic arch, reducing the resistance that the left ventricle must overcome to eject blood during systole; hence afterload is reduced. A sustained reduction in afterload will allow the left ventricle to eject more of its stroke volume during each contraction, thus leaving more space for ventricular filling. This usually results in a secondary decrease in preload as the left ventricle becomes and remains more efficient.

The patient undergoing intraaortic balloon counterpulsation requires intensive nursing observation and care. All vital signs and indexes of cardiac function must be continually observed and recorded. Commonly the patient will be receiving vasopressor and antidysrhythmic drugs, and it is the nurse's responsibility to titrate these for the desired effects. Intubation and ventilatory support may be in place.

Circulation checks of all pulses in both lower extremities are performed before insertion and hourly thereafter until the balloon is removed. No hip flexion is allowed on the catheterized side; well-padded leg restraints must be used if the patient is unable to cooperate. The head of the bed is not elevated more than 30 degrees to prevent balloon migration upward in the aorta. The patient should be tilted and carefully positioned on alternate sides every 2 hours to prevent skin breakdown and other consequences of limited mobility. The dressing on the balloon insertion site must be kept clean and dry and is changed every 24 to 72 hours using sterile technique.

Considerable psychological support is necessary for the patient and family during such critical therapy. The physical size and noise of the pump may be intimidating, and the pump's presence may reinforce everyone's awareness of the frailty of the patient's heart and uncertainty about the future. The nurse provides careful but simple explanations of the pump's action. It is important that patients not get the mistaken idea that the pump is working instead of their heart. Continuous reassurance and repeated simple explanations are essential; some patients may benefit from mild sedation.

## NURSING MANAGEMENT OF THE PATIENT UNDERGOING CARDIAC SURGERY

Care of the person undergoing cardiac surgery involves a multidisciplinary team approach utilizing the skills of a variety of health care professionals, including nurses, physicians, respiratory therapists, physical therapists, social workers, and nutritionists. Clinical pathways guide case managers and help the multidisciplinary team ensure a positive outcome for the patient while using existing resources efficiently. A sample Clinical Pathway to guide collaborative management of a person undergoing cardiac surgery is shown on p. 736.

Cardiac surgery patients are generally admitted to the hospital either the day before or the morning of the planned surgery. After surgery, most patients spend 24 to 36 hours in the intensive care recovery area and are transferred to the floor on the first or second postoperative day. The patient's recovery progresses rapidly so that discharge is achieved on the fourth through sixth postoperative day.

## PREOPERATIVE CARE

The nurse caring for the cardiac surgery patient provides individualized care that is appropriate for the patient's medical condition, health history, and psychosocial history. Important goals for the preoperative period include obtaining an accurate and complete patient history, providing preoperative teaching to the patient and family about the planned surgery, and then preparing the patient physiologically and psychosocially for surgery.

Before surgery, the patient undergoes extensive testing to establish the medical diagnosis and evaluate the severity of the disease process. Preoperative diagnostic tests are usually performed before admission or during previous hospitalizations. Information is obtained from the chest x-ray, cardiac catheterization and coronary angiography, echocardiography, stress testing, and serum blood analyses as appropriate. Particular attention is given to assessing the degree of cardiac impairment and related lifestyle limitations, as well as identification of risk factors that may impede the recovery process.

Risk factors that may contribute to postoperative complications include a history of past cardiovascular disorders such as myocardial infarction, bacterial endocarditis, pulmonary embolism, or coagulation abnormalities. Cigarette smoking, diabetes mellitus, and obesity also increase the risk of complications. Data regarding the patient's psychosocial support systems, coping patterns, and level of understanding help the nurse anticipate the patient's and family's needs related to preoperative teaching, postoperative recovery, and discharge planning.

Many well-established preoperative teaching programs for cardiac surgery patients exist. Although structured, these programs allow the nurse to provide individualized teaching while simultaneously ensuring that all essential information is provided. Refer to the Guidelines for Care Box on p. 739 for the preoperative teaching necessary for the patient undergoing cardiac surgery. Ideally, patients and their families receive preprinted, taped, or video information well before admission for elective cardiac surgery. Before surgery, the nurse provides adjunctive information and verbally reinforces the patient's and family's understanding of the planned procedure. Patients are aware that they are facing a potentially life-threatening situation. The nurse plays a vital role in determining and addressing specific questions, fears, and concerns that the patient and family may express.

A complete baseline database is documented before surgery. Baseline vital signs (including apical and radial heart rates and bilateral arm blood pressures), integrity of all pulses (both proximal and distal), neurological status, height, weight, nutritional status, elimination patterns, and psychological status are assessed and recorded in the immediate preoperative period. Before surgery, patients continue their normal medical and activity routines, with the exception of withholding aspirin 1 to 3 days before the day of surgery. Patients remain NPO after midnight the night before surgery.

## POSTOPERATIVE CARE

After surgery, the goals of care include promoting and maintaining the patient's physical and psychosocial stability, as well as preventing postoperative complications. These goals are initially achieved in an intensive nursing care setting. Refer to the accompanying Guidelines for Care Box on p. 740 for information regarding important aspects of care for patients after cardiac surgery. Ongoing monitoring thorough assessment, careful planning, and knowledgeable intervention may be organized through a systems approach to care.

### Promoting Cardiovascular Function

A major goal of patient care in the immediate postoperative period is to promote cardiovascular function, adequate tissue perfusion, and stabilization of vital signs. Heart rate and invasive arterial blood pressures are monitored continuously and recorded every 15 minutes until stable, then hourly thereafter. Central venous pressure (CVP), pulmonary artery pressure (PAP), pulmonary capillary wedge pressure (PCWP), and cardiac output (CO) measurements are obtained as indicated by the patient's condition. Peripheral pulses are monitored for bilateral strength and symmetry. Apical and radial pulses are compared for evidence of a pulse deficit. Skin color, temperature, and capillary refill are assessed for evidence of adequate tissue perfusion. Urine output, a reliable indicator of cardiac output, is assessed hourly. Chest tube drainage is assessed and recorded hourly to monitor for postsurgical bleeding.

#### *Heart rate and rhythm*

The patient's ECG is monitored continuously postoperatively and compared with the preoperative baseline. Cardiac dysrhythmias are common in the postoperative period and may be caused by operative trauma, anesthesia, extracorporeal circulation, alterations in potassium values, hypotension, hypovolemia, and hypoxia. See Chapter 25 for a discussion of the pharmacological management of dysrhythmias.

Temporary epicardial pacing may be used to manage cardiac dysrhythmias and low cardiac output. Supraventricular tachycardia (SVT) commonly occurs after cardiac surgery because of edema or inflammation of atrial tissue. Atrial flutter, atrial fibrillation, or other supraventricular tachycardias produce decreased left ventricular diastolic filling and subsequent deterioration in cardiac output. Overdrive atrial pacing can effectively restore normal sinus rhythm. Bradydysrhythmias after cardiac surgery are transient and may be associated with low cardiac output. Postoperative temporary pacing may be required to augment cardiac output by increasing heart rate.

Temporary epicardial pacing wires require specialized care and protection, because they are a potential source of lethal

*Text continued on p. 739*

## clinical pathway *Coronary Artery Bypass Graft*

| PREOP VISIT | DAY OF SURGERY | POSTOPERATIVE DAY #1 | POSTOPERATIVE DAY #2 | POSTOPERATIVE DAY #3 | POSTOPERATIVE DAY #4 THROUGH DISCHARGE |
|---|---|---|---|---|---|
| **Interdisciplinary communication** (Consults)<br>Cardiology<br>Chaplain prn | Anesthesia<br>→<br>Respiratory care → | →<br>Respiratory care prn<br>PT consult prn<br>Nutrition consult prn<br>Pharmacy consult prn | Respiratory care smoking cessation consult (prn)<br>→<br>→<br>→<br>→<br>→ | →<br>→<br>→<br>→<br>→ | →<br>→<br>→<br>→<br>→ |
| **Assessments**<br>Adult screening tool (Multidisc.)<br>Ht/Wt (Nsg)<br>H&P (MD)<br>Emotional needs (Nsg)<br>Financial needs (SW)<br>Discharge needs (Nsg, SW) | • Pt systems assessment q1° →<br>• ICU VS Policy →<br>• Wt post-op then q AM<br>• Cardiac monitoring | q 2°-4° in TCVPO<br>Systems assessment q 4-8° →<br>4 W VS Policy →<br>→<br>→ | →<br>→<br>→<br>→ | →<br>→<br>→<br>D/C Cardiac monitoring<br>Assess need for home $O_2$ | →<br>→<br>→ |
| **Diagnostics** (LAB, RADIOL)<br>Cardiac Cath<br>EKG<br>CXR<br>Wt<br>Labs: CBC, u/a, Chem 10, pt/ptt T/X 4u PRBC (8 U if Redo)<br>ABG if Pulmonary Hx | • EKG<br>• CXR<br>• Cardiac indices q 1°-2° and change in status or med adjustment<br>• ACT at bedside<br>• CBC, plats, pt/ptt, chem 6, mg,++<br>• Glucose q2°-4°<br>• ABGs on admission and prn<br>• CBC after PRBC, pt/ptt after FFP | EKG<br>CXR after CT removal<br>Chem 10, CBC with plts q AM until disch. | → | CXR PA + LAT<br>→ | EKG<br>→ |

| PREOP VISIT | DAY OF SURGERY | POSTOPERATIVE DAY #1 | POSTOPERATIVE DAY #2 | POSTOPERATIVE DAY #3 | POSTOPERATIVE DAY #4 THROUGH DISCHARGE |
|---|---|---|---|---|---|
| **Medications** | | | | | |
| D/C as a 48° preop<br>D/C Coumadin 3 days pre-op | • Ancef o.c. to OR → administ. within 1° of incision, then q 8° | D/C IV abx after 3 doses | | | |
| Pre-op cardiac antibiotic orders<br>Continue preop meds | • IV $H_2$ blockers → | D/C $H_2$ blockers when extubated unless pre-op indication | Initiate bowel regimen → | → | → |
| | • ASA supp. within 6° postoperative → | ASA q AM | | | |
| | • Administer/titrate → vasoactive/inotropic infusion per order set | D/C vasoactive/inotropic infusions | → | → | → |
| | • Fluid resuscitation per order<br>• Replace K+/Ca++/Mg++ per orders<br>• Treat glucose per orders | • Restart pre-op meds except antianginals | | | |
| | • IV opiates for pain → | PO pain meds | → | → | → |
| **Dressings tubes/drains** | • Pulmonary artery → | D/C | | | |
| | • A-line → | D/C | | | |
| | • NGT → | D/C 2° after extubation | | | |
| | • Epicardial wires → | D/C ½ hr before MCT removed | | | |
| | • Chest tubes → | D/C (*see activity) | | • Remove CT dressing 48° after CTs D/C'd | |
| | • Foley → | → | D/C Foley | | |
| | • IV/CVP → | → | D/C IV when taking po | → | → |
| | • ETT → D/C when awake and stable | Incision care: → | Incision care BID → | → | → |
| **Interventions/Treatments** | | | | | |
| Antibacterial scrub PM before surgery and AM of surgery | • Mechanical ventilation and weaning | • Initiate $O_2$ via cannula | • Wean $O_2$ per policy → | D/C $O_2$ per policy → | → |
| Incentive spirometer | • $O_2$ therapy | • Incentive spirometry q2° | → | → | → |
| Cardiac skin prep/clip guidelines | • Continuous pulse oximetry | • Deep breath/cough q2° | Deep breath/cough q4° | → | → |
| | • Heat lamps | • Knee-high teds | → | → | → |
| | • Extubation | • Support bra for women | | | |

*This form is a documentation and decision support tool only.



*H&P,* History and physical examination; *TCVPO,* thoracic cardiovascular postoperative unit; *o.c.,* on call; *abx,* antibiotics; *MCT,* mediastinal chest tube.

*Continued*

## Coronary Artery Bypass Graft—cont'd

| PREOP VISIT | DAY OF SURGERY | POSTOPERATIVE DAY #1 | POSTOPERATIVE DAY #2 | POSTOPERATIVE DAY #3 | POSTOPERATIVE DAY #4 THROUGH DISCHARGE |
|---|---|---|---|---|---|
| **Activity**<br>Up ad lib | OR ⟶ TCVPO<br>Bedrest; HOB 30°<br>IF VS within parameters and stable rhythm | TCVPO ⟶ 4W acute<br>Raise HOB for comfort<br>• *Prior to MCT removal; turn patient side to side; or sit patient on side of bed<br>• OOB to chair with assistance | • Ambulate in room and hall with assistance<br>• Physical therapy exercises ⟶ | • Ambulate in room without assistance ⟶<br>⟶ | ⟶<br>⟶ |
| **Nutrition**<br>NPO after MN | NPO except ice | • Advance diet as tolerated to ice chips ⟶<br>Clear liquids ⟶<br>Traditional diet | • Advance from transitional diet ⟶<br>♥ Healthy or<br>♥ Healthy, limited sucrose, if diabetic<br>• Patient should have BM by discharge | ⟶ | ⟶ |
| **Discharge preparation**<br>Identify discharge need via adult screening tool (multi-D) | | • Review D/C plans with patient/S.O.<br>Initiate appropriate support services per D/C planning:<br>• D/C Coordinator<br>• Social work<br>• Dietitian<br>• Nursing<br>• Respiratory care<br>• Physical therapy<br>• Pharmacy<br>• M.D. | • Reinforce need for patient/S.O./family to learn self-care measures<br>⟶<br>Evaluate patient for cardiac rehabilitation | ⟶<br>⟶ | ⟶<br>⟶ |
| **Educational activities**<br>Initiate:<br>• Pre-op teaching<br>• Incentive spirometry<br>• Effective coughing techniques<br>• Introduce teaching folder<br>• Patient pathway | | Initiate discharge patient education plan | Patient/S.O. observe incision care<br>Teach cardiac exercises ⟶ | Patient/S.O. perform incision care<br>Patient/S.O. describe home management | |

guidelines for care

### Preoperative Teaching for the Person Undergoing Cardiac Surgery

1. General information
   a. Places of care during hospitalization
      (1) CCU or ICU after surgery
      (2) Return to general patient care unit in 2 to 3 days
   b. Visiting hours and location of waiting rooms
2. Description of surgery
   a. Simple explanation of anatomy of heart and effect of the patient's cardiovascular disorder (e.g., incompetent valve, obstructed coronary artery)
   b. Explanation of surgical procedure, including planned incision
   c. Definition of any unfamiliar terms: bypass, extracorporeal
   d. Length of time in surgery: 2 to 4 hours
   e. Length of time until able to see family (usually 1½ to 2 hours after surgery)
3. Preparation for surgery
   a. Shower or bath night before surgery with special antimicrobial soap
   b. Surgical shave: shaving of entire chest and abdomen, neck to groin and left midaxillary line to right
   c. Legs shaved if saphenous vein grafts will be used
   d. Preoperative medication
4. Explanation of monitors
   a. Round patches on chest connected to a cardiac monitor that records patient's heartbeats
   b. Monitor makes beeping sound all the time
5. Explanation of lines
   a. Intravenous routes for fluid and medications
   b. Central venous line in neck or chest to monitor fluid status
   c. Pulmonary artery catheter in chest or neck to measure pulmonary pressures and monitor fluid status
   d. Plastic connector line to obtain blood samples without a needle stick
6. Explanation of drainage tubes
   a. Indwelling urinary catheter
   b. Chest tube: bloody drainage is expected
7. Explanation of breathing tube
   a. Tube in windpipe connected to machine called ventilator
   b. Unable to speak with tube in place but can mouth words and communicate in writing
   c. Tube is removed when patient is fully awake and stable
   d. Secretions in lungs or tube removed by nurse using a suction catheter
   e. Food and oral fluids not permitted until breathing tube is removed
8. Explanation and demonstration of activities and exercises
   a. Purpose of activity is to promote circulation, keep lungs clear, and prevent infection
   b. Activity includes:
      (1) Turning from side to side in bed
      (2) Sitting on edge of bed
      (3) Sitting in chair the night of or the morning after surgery
   c. Range-of-motion exercises
   d. Deep breathing using sustained maximal inspiration
   e. Tubes and lines will restrict movement somewhat, but nurse will assist patient
9. Relief of pain
   a. Some pain will be experienced, but it will not be excruciating (different pain than original angina if this was present)
   b. Frequent pain medication will be given to help relieve the pain, but patient should always tell nurse when pain is present

ventricular dysrhythmias if they come in contact with a ground current. These electrodes must be insulated with either a rubber cap or glove when not in use.

#### *Blood pressure*

Maintenance of a stable systemic blood pressure in the postoperative period is critical to the patient's recovery and must be aggressively controlled with the use of pharmacological agents. Postoperative hypertension can lead to complications including excessive postsurgical bleeding, cardiac tamponade, and excessive oxygen demand in the weakened myocardium. Intravenous nitroglycerin or sodium nitroprusside infusions reduce hypertension, reduce systemic vascular resistance, and ease the myocardial workload and oxygen demand. In addition, postoperative hypertension may be caused by the patient awakening from anesthesia and experiencing anxiety and pain. Administration of anxiolytics and adequate analgesia aid in the management of postoperative hypertension.

An unstable low blood pressure in the postoperative period must also be aggressively treated. Causes of postoperative hypotension include hypovolemia and shock. Hypovolemia may be caused by third-space fluid shifts that occur during cardiopulmonary bypass, rewarming from hypothermia, or excessive blood loss. Causes of cardiogenic shock include myocardial depression secondary to anesthesia, trauma from surgery, preexisting heart disease, dysrhythmias associated with an inadequate stroke volume, or cardiac tamponade. Treatment of postoperative hypotension includes fluid resuscitation and gentle rewarming of the patient's core body temperature. Intravenous infusion of inotropic agents such as dobutamine will help stimulate myocardial performance. Dysrhythmias are aggressively managed with antidysrhythmics or temporary cardiac pacing using the surgically implanted epicardial pacing wires. Refer to Chapters 17 and 25 for further discussion of hypovolemic and cardiogenic shock management.

Persistent cardiogenic shock that is unresponsive to these measures may be further treated with the use of a temporary mechanical assist device designed to reduce the myocardial workload. Intraaortic balloon counterpulsation can be used at any point during the preoperative, perioperative, or postoperative period. In addition, the use of a VAD may provide circulatory assistance if the myocardial performance is insufficient to meet the body's needs.

**guidelines for care**

### The Person Who Has Undergone Cardiac Surgery

I. Monitoring
  A Cardiovascular
    1. Blood pressure and pulse (rate, pulse deficit)
    2. Pulmonary artery pressure (PAP), pulmonary capillary wedge pressure (PCWP), cardiac output (CO), central venous pressure (CVP), left atrial pressure (LAP)
    3. ECG for signs of dysrhythmias
    4. Body temperature
    5. Skin color, temperature, capillary filling
    6. Signs of hypovolemic shock (decreased CVP, decreased LAP, decreased PCWP, decreased cardiac output)
    7. Signs of cardiac tamponade (cessation of chest drainage, restlessness, decreased blood pressure, increased CVP, increased PAP, increased LAP)
  B. Respiratory
    1. Respirations: rate, depth, quality
    2. Breath sounds
    3. Chest tubes for patency and drainage
    4. Autotransfuse chest tube drainage
  C. Neurological
    1. Level of consciousness
    2. Pupillary size and reaction
    3. Orientation
    4. Movement and sensation of extremities
  D. Gastrointestinal
    1. Nausea
    2. Anorexia
  E. Urinary
    1. Output (amount)
    2. Color
    3. pH and specific gravity
  F. Fluid and electrolyte balance
    1. Intake/output balance
    2. Daily weights
    3. Serum potassium and calcium levels
  G. Presence of discomfort: pain, fatigue
  H. Ability to sleep
  I. Behavior: depression, fear, disorientation, hallucinations

II. Promoting oxygen/carbon dioxide exchange
  A. Preoxygenation and suction during intubation; suction as necessary after extubation
  B. Position with head only slightly elevated; turn side to side
  C. Encourage breathing exercises; incentive spirometry
  D. Give analgesics before breathing and coughing exercises
  E. Encourage range-of-motion exercises and progressive activity

III. Promoting fluid and electrolyte balance
  A. Record accurate intake and output
  B. Maintain prescribed flow rates of parenteral fluids
  C. Give prescribed supplemental IV potassium chloride

IV. Promoting comfort
  A. Give narcotic analgesics every 3 hours during the first 24 hours, then as needed
  B. Give frequent mouth care
  C. Control environment for comfort
  D. Change bed linens when diaphoresis is present (assure person that this is common)
  E. Plan activities to permit periods of sleep
  F. Provide back rubs for backache
  G. Splint incision during coughing
  H. Encourage patient to share feelings and experiences
  I. Support family visiting

V. Promoting activity
  A. Provide for passive then active range-of-motion exercises
  B. Encourage ambulation when permitted

VI. Teaching
  A. Progressive return to physical activity as recommended by the physician
  B. Rehabilitation exercise program
  C. Sexual activity usually permitted in 3 to 4 weeks
  D. Signs of overexertion include fatigue, dyspnea, pain
  E. Eat a balanced diet with any prescribed modifications (such as no added salt or low cholesterol)
  F. Medications
    1. Name, dosage, schedule, action, and side effects of prescribed medications
    2. Use of prescribed medications as needed
  G. Signs that may persist: dyspnea, pain, night sweats
  H. Signs requiring medical attention (fever, increasing dyspnea, or chest pain with minimal exertion)
  I. Need for ongoing medical care

#### *Maintaining blood volume and chest drainage*

During cardiac surgery, mediastinal chest tubes and possibly pleural chest tubes are placed to drain the surgical area. Refer to Chapter 32 for further information about care of the patient with a chest tube.

Excessive postsurgical bleeding is evidenced by increased drainage of blood from the mediastinal or pleural chest tube. Chest tube drainage should not exceed more than 100 ml per hour during the first 2 postoperative hours and should be approximately 500 ml during the first 24 hours. A sudden increase or cessation in bleeding from the chest tubes may signify a postoperative bleeding problem, and the surgeon must be notified immediately. Postoperative bleeding is aggressively corrected by normalizing clotting studies and possibly reexploring the chest by the surgeon on an emergent basis.

Excessive blood loss through the chest tubes can lead to hemorrhagic shock unless the patient's blood volume is maintained. Fluid volume resuscitation with intravenous crystalloid fluids or blood products is essential to correct the patient's hypovolemic state. Ideally, the chest drainage system allows collection of bloody chest drainage for later autotransfusion in the event of a bleeding complication. In this way, the risks of transfusion reaction and disease transmission from transfusion of homologous (banked) blood are avoided.

A sudden marked decrease or cessation of drainage from the chest tubes indicates clotting of the chest tubes. Clotting

**box 26-12** *Symptoms of Cardiac Tamponade*

Diminished or absent point of maximal impulse
Diminished heart sounds
Tachycardia
Paradoxical pulse
Narrowed pulse pressure
Distended neck veins (increased central venous pressure)

of the chest tubes predisposes the patient to cardiac tamponade, a life-threatening emergency (Box 26-12). Cardiac tamponade leads to cardiogenic shock and is corrected through emergent reexploration of the mediastinum by the surgeon.

#### *Normalizing body temperature*

Although patients are rewarmed before termination of cardiopulmonary bypass, their body temperature remains unstable and low after separation from bypass, leading to postoperative hypothermia. Persistent hypothermia can lead to undesirable shivering, increased myocardial workload, increased carbon dioxide production, and increased lactic acid production. Measures to gently rewarm the patient's body temperature include the use of heat lamps, thermal blankets, perfusion blankets, and vasodilation with intravenous sodium nitroprusside. Once the patient's body temperature has rewarmed, cool or diaphoretic skin may be an indication of shock.

### Promoting a Patent Airway and Effective Gas Exchange

After cardiac surgery, intubation and mechanical ventilation are maintained until the patient is stable and fully recovered from anesthesia. The rate, depth, and quality of respirations are monitored and recorded, and the patient's breath sounds are assessed through chest auscultation. The effectiveness of coughing efforts and sputum production are monitored. Arterial blood gas and oxygen saturation monitoring provide evidence of effective gas exchange. A postoperative chest x-ray verifies proper lung reexpansion and chest tube placement after the surgical procedure. In general, patients are awake and extubated within 4 to 18 hours after cardiac surgery.

The lack of alveolar expansion and ventilation during cardiopulmonary bypass leads to decreased surfactant production and alveolar collapse in the postoperative period. Therefore after extubation the nurse promotes aggressive pulmonary hygiene every 1 to 2 hours while the patient is awake. Administration of adequate pain medication helps the patient cough, deep breathe, and use an incentive spirometer more effectively. Splinting the surgical incision with a small pillow or blanket provides extra support during coughing. Patients unable to clear excessive pulmonary secretions may require nasotracheal suctioning. Frequent position changes while in bed and early ambulation are also critical to preventing pulmonary complications after cardiac surgery.

### Preventing Infection

Cardiac surgery patients receive prophylactic antibiotic therapy to prevent infection from numerous sources during the perioperative period. A broad-spectrum antibiotic is administered intravenously for 2 to 4 days postoperatively. Although an initial postoperative fever is most likely pulmonary in origin, the nurse assesses the patient's skin and all surgical wounds for evidence of infection. Incision care is provided based on the hospital's protocol.

### Monitoring Neurological Status

Patients usually begin to awaken within 1 to 2 hours after surgery. Failure to awaken may be the result of unusually deep anesthesia or of embolization of air, calcium, fat, or thrombotic particles to the brain. A return of consciousness that seems sluggish and in which the patient does not seem to regain full alertness after a day or two may have been caused by poor cerebral perfusion or microembolization during cardiopulmonary bypass.

Pupil size, equality, and reaction to light are checked frequently in the immediate postoperative period. Pupil dilation may be caused by excessive carbon dioxide in the blood or by such cardiac medications as atropine. Constricted pupils may be caused by dopamine. Disorientation and restlessness may be signs of hypoxia or embolization to the brain in addition to being symptoms of pain, fatigue, fear, or sensory overload.

### Monitoring Fluid Balance

Accurate recording of intake and output is essential for the first few postoperative days. Careful observation of hourly urinary output, as well as urine color, pH, and specific gravity, provides essential information about renal function. Adequate urinary output is at least 30 ml per hour. Specific gravity may be elevated because of oliguria or the presence of red blood cells as a result of extracorporeal circulation. Fluids are limited to reduce the chance of fluid overload and increased cardiac workload. Intravenous fluids are carefully titrated by intravenous infusion pumps. Daily weights are obtained, and diuretics are administered if fluid retention occurs.

Renal insufficiency after heart surgery is caused by complications of cardiopulmonary bypass. The destruction of red blood cells can cause sludging in the kidneys. If low-perfusion states occurred during the surgical procedure, the kidneys themselves may have been damaged, resulting in acute tubular necrosis. If the acute tubular necrosis is severe and prolonged, temporary hemodialysis is initiated. Up to 25% of patients may experience some form of renal failure after bypass.

Serum electrolyte levels are checked several times during the first 24 hours and at least daily thereafter. Supplemental potassium may be needed in the immediate postoperative period, particularly if diuretics are in use. The serum glucose may be initially elevated from the stress of surgery and cardiopulmonary bypass, but this is temporary and usually does not require intervention.

Hemoglobin and hematocrit values and prothrombin time are obtained daily to assess the extent of blood loss and the effect of replacement therapy. Plasma and plasma expanders are given to avoid hypovolemia and to maintain a normal osmotic gradient. Crystalloid intravenous solutions are administered to ensure adequate circulating volume.

### Promoting Comfort, Rest, and Sleep

Alleviation of pain is critical in the postoperative period, and patients should be kept as comfortable as possible. This not only adds to a sense of security but also reduces stress on the heart, decreases the need for oxygen, and promotes healing. Other comfort measures are routinely employed, such as positioning, controlling environmental temperature, giving frequent oral hygiene, and supporting visiting from concerned family or friends.

After cardiac surgery the patient is weak and tires easily. Activity periods should be organized so that rest periods are frequent (even if brief) and uninterrupted.

### Supporting Nutrition

Gastrointestinal symptoms, such as anorexia and nausea, may occur after cardiac surgery. Contributing factors include drug therapy, prolonged perfusion time, preexisting gastrointestinal disease, vasopressors, perioperative hypoperfusion or hypotension, systemic hypothermia, stress, and anxiety. Although anorexia occurs more commonly than nausea, the latter is more distressing. Procainamide can affect appetite. Comfort measures to decrease nausea are instituted, and antiemetics are administered if needed. Small amounts of food may be more palatable than a large meal.

### Promoting Activity

Passive arm exercises are started shortly after surgery, followed by active exercises as the person gains strength. The nature and extent of allowed activity depends on the operation and the status of the heart, but most patients are assisted out of bed the first day after surgery.

The nature and duration of activity depend on the patient's progress and condition but progress steadily from dangling at the bedside to sitting in a chair at the bedside. Ambulation begins in the room and if tolerated progresses to walking in the halls.

During ambulation, close supervision is necessary, and activity that causes excessive fatigue, dyspnea, or an increased pulse or respiratory rate is discontinued. If any of these symptoms appear, the patient is returned to bed, and the physician is consulted before further activity is attempted.

### Promoting Psychological Adaptation

The psychological ramifications of heart surgery, sleep deprivation, and sensory overload can be overwhelming. Some persons experience a period of depression or disorientation after surgery, whereas others may become unreasonably fearful or hallucinate. The disorientation may even progress to panic. The nurse should be alert to subtle behavioral changes and reassure the patient and family that these reactions are common and do not mean that the patient is "losing his or her mind." Physiological causes of the behavior must be ruled out.

It is helpful to the patient and family if the nursing staff members attempt to personalize the patient's experience as much as possible. It is easy to lose sight of the person behind the monitoring equipment in an intensive care unit. Calling the patient by his or her preferred name, using frequent physical contact, orienting the patient to time and place, and including the patient in any discussions that are held at the bedside help decrease the sense of isolation.

### Monitoring Anticoagulation

Patients with mechanical or bioprosthetic valves are at high risk for developing systemic emboli. Anticoagulation is necessary to prevent thrombus formation on the surface of the valves. Warfarin (Coumadin) is the most common anticoagulant used with both types of valves, and its use is continued long term. The maintenance dose of warfarin is based on the prothrombin time (PT); a therapeutic PT is 1.2 to 1.5 times the control value. Use of the INR allows for greater standardization in anticoagulant monitoring.

Bleeding is the major risk associated with the use of warfarin. If bleeding occurs, the dose may be lowered or another medication may be substituted. Dipyridamole (Persantine) is another type of antithrombotic agent. It inhibits platelet aggregation while not affecting the PT. Dipyridamole may be used in conjunction with warfarin to prevent embolization. The normal dose to reduce platelet aggregation is 225 to 400 mg per day.

### Patient/Family Discharge Education

In preparation for discharge, the patient is asked to describe normal daily activities. The activities are discussed with the physician to determine their safety and appropriateness. Sexual intercourse usually is permitted within 3 to 4 weeks after surgery. Patients usually are advised to start activities slowly and progress gradually to more energy-consuming tasks. The physician will want the patient to return for frequent medical follow-up examinations, at which time advice will be given regarding additional activities. The person is allowed to do anything that does not cause fatigue or pain but must be advised against attempting too much too soon.

Definite instructions must be provided about climbing stairs. Only two or three steps should be attempted the first time, and the patient is instructed to climb slowly. The patient should rest two or three times while climbing one flight of stairs.

The family is also instructed about the patient's activity guidelines. Because the patient may have been an invalid before surgery, the family may be fearful about an increase in activity. Persons are encouraged to return to work, but the physician needs to give the person specific directions regarding return to work.

The patient and family need to be told that no large improvement will be noticed immediately after the operation—it will be at least 3 to 6 months before the full result of the surgery can be evaluated. Patients are reminded that some dyspnea and pain may still be present postoperatively. Discharge instructions for cardiac surgery patients and a list of symptoms to report are presented in the accompanying Patient/Family Teaching Boxes.

## GERONTOLOGICAL CONSIDERATIONS

As the population ages, the number of very old patients (between 80 and 100 years of age) undergoing cardiac surgery also continues to increase. Advanced age alone is not a contraindication to cardiac surgery, but consideration of the special needs of the elderly cardiac surgery patient is essential to promoting relief of cardiac symptoms and recovery after cardiac surgery.

Cardiovascular age-related changes include decreased cardiac output, decreased vasomotor responsiveness, decreased cardiac conduction tissue, and increased aortic calcification.

These changes can predispose the very old patient to a decreased tolerance to sudden fluctuations in fluid volume status, orthostasis, dysrhythmias, and arterial embolisms, respectively. Age-related changes in renal and hepatic function can lead to altered pharmacokinetics; endocrine and immune system dysfunction can contribute to impaired skin integrity and wound healing. Changes in mobility, functional status, and neuropsychological status can impair postoperative progress and timely recovery. In addition, very old cardiac surgery patients often have significant coexisting medical problems that can complicate recovery from surgery. Elderly cardiac surgery patients require individualized care management that accounts for a potential lower recovery rate and a potential increased risk of postoperative complications (see the Research Box).

## SPECIAL ENVIRONMENTS FOR CARE

### ■ CRITICAL CARE MANAGEMENT

All patients undergoing cardiac surgery are cared for at least temporarily in an intensive care unit (ICU) environment to ensure continuous in-depth physiological monitoring. The care provided in this setting has been discussed in the postoperative care section. With successful surgery this ICU stay may be brief and measured in hours until the patient is successfully stabilized and extubated. Patients requiring intraaortic balloon pump or ventricular assist devices may be extremely unstable and require more long-term management. This is especially true of patients in severe heart failure who may be waiting for a donor heart to become available.

### ■ HOME CARE ENVIRONMENT

Hospital stays after cardiac surgery have been dramatically reduced, and it is expected that a significant portion of the patient's recovery from surgery will take place in the home environment. Careful adherence to clinical pathway elements guides the nurse in evaluating the patient's resources, self-care abilities, and family supports and permits timely referral for home health supervision and monitoring. Basic discharge teaching for the cardiac surgery patient is summarized in the Guidelines for Care Box on p. 740. The nurse ensures that the patient and family are knowledgeable and capable of providing this care. Screening for home care assistance is particularly important for elderly patients, who can expect a longer convalescence and may have limited social supports available to them in the community setting.

## COMPLICATIONS

Many factors can complicate the patient's recovery after cardiac surgery. Pulmonary complications are most common, including atelectasis, pleural effusion, and pneumonia. Cardiovascular complications include hemodynamic instability and cardiac dysrhythmias. Neurological changes, fluid imbalance, fever, immobility, and sleep disturbance are all complications that can impede timely recovery from cardiac surgery. Late complications from cardiac surgery include mediastinitis and postpericardiotomy syndrome.

## MEDIASTINITIS

Mediastinitis after cardiac surgery is an infectious separation of the sternal wound and involves the anterior mediastinal space. The incidence of mediastinitis is 0.5% to 5% of cardiac surgery patients and occurs from 4 to 30 days after the surgery. Signs and symptoms of mediastinitis include pain, erythema, and tenderness of the incisional area; serous or purulent wound drainage; grating of the sternum with coughing; fever; elevated white blood cell count; and positive wound

**patient/family teaching**

**Discharge Instructions After Cardiac Surgery**

**Incision Care**

Clean twice a day
Care of sterile stips, staples, sutures
Incision massage with cocoa butter after 10 days

**Showering**

Wash with soap that is unscented, gentle, bactericidal
No tub baths until incisions completely healed

**Activity**

No lifting greater than 10 pounds
No driving for 6 weeks
No prolonged sitting
Activity as tolerated, cardiac rehabilitation if ordered
May resume sexual activity when comfort level allows

**Nutrition**

Low-sodium, low-fat, heart-healthy diet
Increase protein intake for 4 to 6 weeks

**Medications**

Pain medications: do not drive or operate machinery if taking narcotics

**Miscellaneous**

Women should wear a bra to help support chest
TED stockings
Daily weights—notify physician for gain of 6 pounds in 2 days
Incentive spirometer three times a day
Prevent constipation with fiber, fluids, and stool softeners

**patient/family teaching**

**Symptoms to Report After Discharge**

Incision is red (like a sunburn)
Area around incision feels warm
Incision is swollen
Incision has increased or different drainage (pus)
Fever above 100.5° F
Unusual pain
Return of presurgical symptoms (if angina occurs, rest and take nitroglycerin); seek medical attention for angina unrelieved by three nitroglycerin or for frequent ocurrence of angina
Shortness of breath
Palpitations (skipping of heart beat)
Heart beating too fast or too slow
Severe bruising or bleeding
Worsening fatigue
Flu symptoms (aches, chills, fever, loss of appetite)

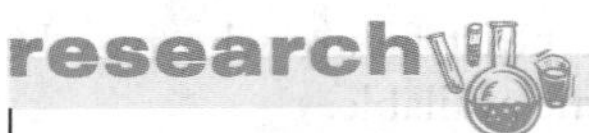

Reference: Finkelmeier B et al: Influence of age on postoperative course in coronary artery bypass patients, *J Cardiovasc Nurs* 7(4):38, 1993.

Patients undergoing elective coronary artery bypass graft (CABG) were divided into two groups according to age: below 65 (group I) or age equal to and above 65 (group II). Comparison of the two groups revealed similarities in preoperative disease, history of myocardial infarctions, number of grafts received, time spent on cardiopulmonary bypass, and operative morbidity and mortality.

Statistical analysis showed that patients in group II required longer overall hospital, intensive care unit, or immediate care unit stays. In addition, patients in group II showed a greater incidence of postoperative disorientation, need for transfusion of exogenous blood, and need for special discharge arrangements. Conclusions reached from this study suggest that CABG patients over the age of 65 have a longer and more complex postoperative course and more special discharge needs than their younger counterparts.

cultures. The most common infecting organisms are normal skin flora such as *S. epidermidis, S. aureus, Candida albicans, Pseudomonas, Klebsiella, Enterobacter,* and *Aspergillus.*

Mediastinitis is prevented through hand washing, meticulous aseptic technique, and antibiotic prophylaxis during the perioperative period. Risk factors for the development of mediastinitis include nutritional deficiency, diabetes, obesity, smoking, and the use of internal mammary artery grafts. Stress to the sternal wound may also predispose the patient to mediastinitis. Such stressors include intense vomiting, coughing, external cardiac massage, and lifting of heavy objects.

Treatment of mediastinitis depends on the depth of the infection and ranges from parenteral antibiotic therapy to surgical debridement of the sternum, mediastinal irrigation, and subsequent sternal dressing changes. Severe cases of mediastinitis may require muscle or omental flaps to revascularize and support the affected area. Muscles commonly used include the pectoralis major, rectus abdominus, and latissimus dorsi.

## POSTPERICARDIOTOMY SYNDROME

Postpericardiotomy syndrome is a form of a post-cardiac injury syndrome that affects between 10% and 40% of patients undergoing cardiac surgery. Symptoms may appear 1 week to several months after the cardiac surgery and include fever, malaise, and pleuropericardial pain. An important physical finding is the presence of a pericardial friction rub on auscultation of the heart. Diagnostic studies may reveal nonspecific ST-T wave changes on ECG, bilateral pleural effusions on chest x-ray, and pericardial effusion on echocadiogram. Laboratory values include an increased eosinophil count, increased white blood cell count, and possibly anemia.

Although the cause of postpericardiotomy syndrome is not completely clear, the most accepted explanation is that it is an immune-mediated reaction. An autoimmune reaction to cardiac injury during surgery leads to the production of anticardiac antibodies. This autoimmune reaction leads to the inflammatory changes seen in the typical patient. Treatment is directed toward reducing the symptoms of fever and pain and consists of administering aspirin, nonsteroidal antiinflammatory agents, or corticosteroids. Postpericardiotomy syndrome generally resolves spontaneously within several days to several weeks.

## critical thinking QUESTIONS

1 Mrs. Hall, 59 years old, was discharged 2 weeks ago with the diagnosis of heart failure after her second myocardial infarction in 18 months. She now comes to the emergency department with acute shortness of breath, chest pain, a positive $S_3$, and significant bilateral rales. Her ECG shows sinus tachycardia at 124 and evidence of her prior anterolateral myocardial infarction. Chemistry shows normal electrolytes with the exception of a potassium level of 3.2. Her complete blood count (CBC) shows a hemoglobin (Hgb) of 7.3 g/dl and hematocrit (Hct) of 25.8%. Her discharge CBC was Hgb 11.2 g/dl and Hct 30.3%.

Discuss the likely precipitating events for Mrs. Hall's exacerbation of her heart failure, including the pathophysiology and collaborative care management.

2 Mr. White has cardiomyopathy and is awaiting a cardiac transplant. When notified that a donor has been found, Mr. White experiences both joy and sorrow about obtaining an organ. Why might Mr. White be having mixed feelings about his transplant?

3 Mr. Panetta is a 49-year-old man with a history of an asymptomatic heart murmur found on physical examination at age 45. While shopping one day with his wife, he suffered an acute cardiac arrest. Bystanders immediately provided basic life support and cardiopulmonary resuscitation. Emergency personnel arrived quickly and provided advanced cardiac life support. Mr. Panetta was successfully resuscitated and transported to a nearby hospital. Diagnostic studies revealed that Mr. Panetta had aortic stenosis with associated left ventricular hypertrophy.

Discuss the following about Mr. Panetta and aortic stenosis:

- Identify the precipitating physiological event that caused his sudden cardiac arrest.
- Discuss the relationship between aortic stenosis, left ventricular hypertrophy, and coronary blood flow.
- Identify the symptoms, physical findings, and diagnostic findings you would most likely expect Mr. Panetta to exhibit.

Mr. Panetta's physician recommends that he undergo aortic valve surgery to correct his aortic stenosis. Mr. Panetta is talking with you, his nurse, about his fears and whether he should proceed with the open heart surgery. How will you respond?

4 Miss Levin is a 27-year-old woman who has been diagnosed by her doctor with symptomatic mitral valve prolapse. She now needs information and education about her condition. Using lay terminology, provide her with the following:

- A description of mitral valve prolapse and the associated changes in heart function
- The relationship between mitral valve prolapse and the symptoms she has experienced or may experience in the future

- Home monitoring actions she will need to take when symptoms occur
- Aspects of lifestyle management that can lessen symptoms of her condition
- Symptoms that require immediate notification of her physician

**5** Mr. B. is a 72-year-old man who has undergone a triple coronary artery bypass graft operation without complications and is preparing to be discharged home tomorrow. Identify essential home assessments you must make as you plan for his discharge.

Discuss home factors that will either impair or facilitate his continued recovery after discharge from the hospital.

## chapter SUMMARY

### CONGESTIVE HEART FAILURE

- Congestive heart failure refers to a syndrome arising from the inability of the heart to effectively maintain a cardiac output sufficient for metabolic needs. Symptoms may involve the pulmonary circulation, the systemic venous circulation, or both.
- Medical therapy for heart failure consists of reducing oxygen requirements through oxygen therapy and rest, optimizing cardiac output with medications (inotropes, diuretics, vasodilators, and ACE inhibitors), and monitoring sodium intake.
- Nursing interventions for heart failure consist of providing oxygenation; promoting rest and activity, nutrition, and elimination; providing skin care and emotional support; promoting tissue perfusion; minimizing fluid volume excess; and patient teaching.
- Pulmonary edema is the most severe form of congestion resulting from left ventricular failure; it requires immediate medical and nursing intervention.

### CARDIOMYOPATHY

- Cardiomyopathy arises from systolic or diastolic dysfunction. Three classifications of dilated, hypertrophic, and restrictive cardiomyopathy distinguish between presence of ventricular dilation and hypertrophy.
- The collaborative care management of cardiomyopathy is aimed at increasing cardiac output and decreasing myocardial oxygen demand, using many of the interventions appropriate to the management of heart failure.

### INFLAMMATORY HEART DISEASE

- All layers of the heart (pericardium, myocardium, and endocardium) may become inflamed. Patients with these conditions have the usual signs of inflammation and also may develop heart failure. Measures to prevent recurrence are important aspects of the treatment regimen.

### VALVULAR HEART DISEASE

- Mitral and aortic valvular disease are more common than pulmonic and tricuspid valvular disease. Rheumatic fever is a common precursor. The two basic problems that compromise normal functioning of the valves are stenosis and regurgitation (insufficiency). Stenosis causes a narrowing of the valvular orifice and impedes the forward flow of blood. Regurgitation causes incomplete closure of the valve and allows blood to flow backward.
- Cardiac murmurs are a common physical finding in patients with valvular heart disease. Depending on the severity of the disease, the patient may develop such clinical symptoms as those associated with heart failure.
- Treatment of valvular disease involves management of clinical symptoms. Surgical repair of the valve or replacement of the valve with an artificial valve may be necessary.

### NURSING MANAGEMENT OF THE PATIENT WITH HEART SURGERY

- Types of heart surgery include repair or replacement of valves, repair of ventricular aneurysms, coronary artery bypass graft, and heart transplantation. Coronary artery bypass graft is the most common procedure.
- Teaching is a major preoperative nursing intervention for cardiovascular surgery and includes information about the intensive care unit, surgery, and preoperative and postoperative procedures.
- In total cardiopulmonary bypass, both the oxygenation and circulation of the blood are bypassed and performed by the bypass machine, thus permitting the heart to be incised and opened for surgery. The machine also permits administration of medications and can provide systemic hypothermia. Side effects of the procedure include hemodilution, decreased platelets, shock, and decreased perfusion to major organs.
- Intraaortic balloon counterpulsation is a method by which a balloon is inserted into the thoracic aorta as temporary assistance for circulation. When inflated, the balloon forces blood retrograde to increase coronary filling; when deflated, it decreases pressure in the aortic arch, thus facilitating afterload.
- Postoperative nursing care after cardiovascular surgery includes monitoring cardiovascular, respiratory, neurological, and urinary systems; monitoring and promoting fluid and electrolyte balance and oxygen-carbon dioxide exchange; promoting patient comfort and activity; and patient teaching.

## References


1. Acuff T et al: Minimally invasive coronary artery bypass grafting, *Ann Thorac Surg* 61:135, 1996.
2. American Heart Association: *Heart and stroke facts: 1995 statistical supplement,* Dallas, Tex, 1994, National Center of the American Heart Association.
3. Braunward E, editor: *Heart disease: a textbook of cardiovascular medicine,* ed 4, Philadelphia, 1992, WB Saunders.
4. Bunzel B, Wollenek G: Heart transplantation: are there psychosocial predictors for clinical success of surgery? *Thorac Cardiovasc Surg* 42:103, 1994.
5. Cardiac Arrhythmia Suppression Trial Investigators: CAST mortality and morbidity: treatment vs. placebo, *N Engl J Med* 324:781, 1991.
6. Cohn JN: The management of chronic heart failure, *N Engl J Med* 335(7):490, 1996.
7. Cohn JN et al: Effect of vasodilator therapy on mortality in chronic congestive heart failure, *N Engl J Med* 314:1547, 1986.
8. Cohn JN et al: A comparison of enalapril with hydralazine-isosorbide dinitrate in the treatment of chronic congestive heart failure, *N Engl J Med* 325:303, 1991.
9. Conn EH, Williams RS, Wallace AG: Exercise responses before and after physical conditioning in patients with severely depressed left ventricular function, *Am J Cardiol* 49:296, 1982.
10. CONSENSUS Trial Study Group: Effects of enalapril on mortality in severe congestive heart failure, *N Engl J Med* 316:1429, 1987.

11. Copeland J et al: Selection of patients for cardiac transplantation, *Circulation* 75:2, 1987.
12. Cox JL: Evolving applications of the maze procedure for atrial fibrillation, *Ann Thorac Surg* 55:578, 1993.
13. Dajani AS et al: Prevention of bacterial endocarditis. Recommendations by the American Heart Association, *JAMA* 277(22):1794, 1997.
14. Dracup K et al: Management of heart failure, II: counseling, education, and lifestyle modification, *JAMA* 272(18): 1442, 1994.
15. Feldman AM et al: Effects of vesnarinone on morbidity and mortality in patients with heart failure, *N Engl J Med* 329:149, 1993.
16. Finkelmeier B et al: Influence of age on postoperative level in coronary artery bypass patients, *J Cardiovasc Nurs* 7(4):38, 1993.
17. Futterman LG, Lemberg L: Cardiomyoplasty: a potential alternative to cardiac transplantation, *Am J Crit Care* 5(1):80, 1996.
18. Garg R, Gonin R, Smith T, Yusaf S (Digitalis Investigation Group): The effect of digoxin on mortality and morbidity in patients with heart failure, *N Engl J Med* 336(8):525, 1997.
19. Glennen S, Metcalf H: Minimally invasive cardiac surgery (MICS), *Nurs Stand* 11(5):54, 1996.
20. Hagenhoff BD et al: Patient education needs as reported by congestive heart failure patients and their nurses, *J Adv Nurs* 19(4):685, 1994.
21. Haque A et al: Hemodynamic effects of supplemental oxygen administration in congestive heart failure, *J Am Coll Cardiol* 27:353, 1996.
22. Hancock EW: Valvular heart disease, *Sci Am Med* 1(1):1-4, 1992.
23. Hoffmann A, Duba J, Lengyels M, Majer K: The effect of training on physical working capacity of MI patients with LV dysfunction, *Eur Heart J* 43, 1987.
24. Hosenpud JD, Novick RJ, Breen TJ, et al: The registry of the international society for heart and lung transplantation: 11th official report-1994, *J Heart Lung Transplant* 13:561, 1994.
25. Kellerman JJ, Ben-Ari E, Fisman E, et al: Physical training in patients with ventricular impairment, *Adv Cardiol* 34:131, 1986.
26. Konstam M et al: *Heart failure: evaluation and care of patients with left-ventricular systolic dysfunction. Clinical practice guideline number 11*, AHCPR Pub No 94-0612, Rockville, Md, 1994, Agency for Health Care Policy and Research, Public Health Service, US Department of Health and Human Services.
27. Levy LG et al: The progression from hypertension to congestive heart failure, *JAMA* 275:1557, 1996.
28. Martensson J, Karlsson JE, Bengt F: Male patients with congestive heart failure and their conception of the life situation, *J Adv Nurs* 25:579, 1997.
29. Mizell J, Maglish B, Matheny R: Minimally invasive direct coronary artery bypass surgery: introduction for critical care nurses, *Crit Care Nurse* 17(3):46, 1997.
30. Monane M, Bohn RL, Gurwitz JH, et al: Noncompliance with congestive heart failure in the elderly, *Arch Intern Med* 154:433, 1994.
31. Moroney DA, Powers K: Outpatient use of left ventricular assist devices: nursing, technical, and educational considerations, *Am J Crit Care* 6(5):355, 1997.
32. Nair CK et al: Ten years' experience with mitral valve in the elderly, *Am Heart J* 124:154, 1992.
33. Packer M et al: The effect of carvedilol on morbidity and mortality in patients with chronic heart failure, *N Engl J Med* 334(21):1349, 1996.
34. Rich MW et al: A multidisciplinary intervention to prevent the readmission of elderly patients with congestive heart failure, *N Engl J Med* 333(18):1190, 1995.
35. SOLVD Investigators: Effect of enalapril on survival in patients with reduced left ventricular ejection fraction and congestive heart failure, *N Engl J Med* 325:293, 1991.
36. Sullivan MJ, Hawthorne MH: Nonpharmacologic interventions in the treatment of heart failure, *J Cardiovasc Nurs* 10(2):47, 1996.
37. Valle BK, Valle GA, Lemberg L: Volume control: a reliable option in the management of "refractory" congestive heart failure, *Am J Crit Care* 4(2):169, 1995.
38. Whitman G: Prosthetic cardiac values, *Progress in Cardiovascular Nursing* 2:116, 1987.
39. Williams JF et al: Guidelines for the evaluation and management of heart failure, *J Am Coll Cardiol* 26(5):1376, 1995.
40. Yamani M, Massie BM: Congestive heart failure: insights from epidemiology, implications for treatment, *Mayo Clin Proc* 68(1):1214, 1993.

chapter 27

# MANAGEMENT OF PERSONS WITH Vascular Problems

CAROL LYNN MAXWELL-THOMPSON and ARLENE YUAN

## objectives *After studying this chapter, the learner should be able to:*

1. Discuss the pathophysiology of arterial and venous disease.
2. Prepare a teaching plan for a person with primary hypertension.
3. Discuss the use of pharmacological agents in the management of vascular diseases.
4. Identify the risk factors associated with the development of vascular disease.
5. Compare the collaborative management of arterial and venous disease.
6. Describe the preoperative and postoperative nursing care for patients undergoing vascular surgery.
7. Develop a plan of care for a patient undergoing amputation related to the complications of vascular disease.

This chapter discusses the management of conditions that interrupt the flow of blood through the arteries and veins except for problems affecting the coronary and cerebral blood vessels. These conditions are presented in Chapters 25 and 53, respectively. The management of hypertension, although not exclusively a vascular problem, is included in this chapter because it is a major risk factor for vascular disease.

## HYPERTENSION

### ETIOLOGY

Hypertension is defined as a consistent elevation of the systolic or diastolic blood pressure above 140/90 mm Hg. The diagnosis of hypertension is not made on the basis of a single elevated value, however, and must be based on at least two elevated blood pressure readings, both sitting and supine, obtained on separate office visits. There are two major types of hypertension: essential (primary) and secondary. Primary hypertension accounts for more than 90% of all cases and has no known cause, although it is theorized that genetic factors, hormonal changes, and alterations in sympathetic tone all may play a role in its development.[1] Secondary hypertension develops as a consequence of a particular underlying disease or condition. Common examples of conditions that can result in secondary hypertension are outlined in Table 27-1. In these situations the treatment plan focuses on correcting or controlling the specific primary disease process. When the underlying disease is successfully managed the secondary hypertension is controlled.

Hypertension can be further classified in stages according to the degree of blood pressure elevation, ranging from stages 1 to 4.[15] This classification system is outlined in Table 27-2. A diastolic blood pressure above 120 to 130 mm Hg is considered to be a hypertensive crisis that requires emergency medical treatment. Crisis occurs in less than 1% of all patients with chronic hypertension.

### EPIDEMIOLOGY

An estimated 64% of the population aged 65 to 74 years have primary hypertension.[29] Hypertension causes no overt symptoms in most cases, and it is impossible to accurately estimate the number of adults who remain undiagnosed and therefore untreated. The importance of hypertension as a health problem in the United States is reflected in several specific *Healthy People 2000* goals, which are summarized in Box 27-1.

Age is the primary risk factor for hypertension because the incidence increases steadily with age.[16] The exception is the rare condition of hypertensive crisis, which occurs more commonly in middle-aged hypertensive patients aged 40 to 50 years. Hypertension is more common among men than women until after menopause, when the incidence in women increases. The incidence of hypertension also varies significantly among different races and cultural groups. Hypertension is twice as prevalent among African Americans as among

**box 27-1 Healthy People 2000 *Goals Related to Hypertension***

- Increase to at least 50% the proportion of persons with high blood pressure whose blood pressure is under control.
- Increase to at least 90% the proportion of persons with high blood pressure who are taking action to help control their blood pressure.
- Increase to at least 60% the proportion of adults with high blood cholesterol who are aware of their condition and are taking action to reduce their blood cholesterol to recommended levels.

From US Department of Health & Human Services, Public Health Service: *Healthy People 2000: summary report,* Boston, 1992, Jones & Bartlett.

**table 27-1** *Causes of Secondary Hypertension*

| DISORDER/CONDITION | MECHANISM |
|---|---|
| **KIDNEY** | |
| Renal parenchymal disease (glomerulonephritis, renal failure) | Most often causes a renin- or sodium-dependent hypertension; physiological changes relate to type of disease and severity of renal insufficiency |
| Renovascular disease | Decrease in renal perfusion from atherosclerotic or fibrotic narrowing of renal arteries; causes marked increase in peripheral vascular resistance and cardiac output |
| **ADRENAL GLAND** | |
| Cushing's syndrome | Increase in blood volume |
| Primary aldosteronism | Increase in aldosterone, causing sodium and water retention that increases blood volume |
| Pheochromocytoma | Excess secretion of catecholamines (norepinephrine increases peripheral vascular resistance) |
| **COARCTATION OF AORTA** | Causes marked elevated blood pressure in upper extremities with decreased perfusion in lower extremities |
| **HEAD TRAUMA OR CRANIAL TUMOR** | Increased intracranial pressure reduces cerebral blood flow; resultant ischemia stimulates medullary vasomotor center to raise blood pressure |
| **PREGNANCY-INDUCED HYPERTENSION** | Cause unknown; generalized vasospasm may be a contributing factor |

**table 27-2** *Classification of Hypertension**

| | CHARACTERISTICS | |
|---|---|---|
| STAGE | SYSTOLIC (MM HG) | DIASTOLIC (MM HG) |
| 1 | 140-159 | 90-99 |
| 2 | 160-179 | 100-109 |
| 3 | 180-209 | 110-119 |
| 4 | ≥210 | ≥120 |

From Report of the Joint National Committee on Detection, Evaluation and Treatment of High Blood Pressure, US Department of Health and Human Services, Public Health Services, NIH Publication, Bethesda, Md, 1992, National Institutes of Health.
*Age 18 or older.

**risk factors**

**Essential Hypertension**

Age: advancing
Sex: male
Race: African American
Family history: hypertension
Obesity: associated with increased intravascular volume
Atherosclerosis: narrowing of arteries increases blood pressure
Smoking: nicotine constricts blood vessels
High-salt diet: sodium causes water retention, increasing blood volume
Alcohol: increases plasma catecholamines
Emotional stress: stimulates sympathetic nervous system

whites and is also usually more severe.[15] The incidence and severity of hypertension are particularly high among African Americans living in the Southeastern United States compared with other areas.[1] The reasons for these variations have not been satisfactorily explained. In addition to age, gender, and race, other risk factors for hypertension include a positive family history, obesity, atherosclerosis, smoking, a high salt intake, excess alcohol use, and emotional stress. Risk factors are summarized in the accompanying Risk Factors Box.

## PATHOPHYSIOLOGY

Blood pressure is the pressure exerted by the blood on the walls of the blood vessels. The regulation of blood pressure is a complex process involving renal control of sodium and water retention and nervous system control of vascular tone. The two primary regulatory factors are blood flow and peripheral vascular resistance. Blood flow is determined by the volume of blood ejected from the left ventricle with each contraction (stroke volume) and the heart rate. Peripheral vascular resistance refers to the size of the peripheral blood vessels. The more constricted the vessel, the greater the resistance to flow; and the more dilated the vessel, the less the resistance. As peripheral vessels become more constricted, the blood pressure becomes more elevated.

Dilation and constriction of the peripheral blood vessels are controlled primarily by the sympathetic nervous system and the renin-angiotension system (Figure 27-1). When the sympathetic nervous system is stimulated, catecholamines such as epinephrine and norepinephrine are released. These chemicals cause increased vasoconstriction, increased cardiac output, and increased strength of ventricular contraction. Likewise, when the renin-angiotension system is activated, angiotension causes vasoconstriction of the blood vessels.

Hypertension is called the "silent killer" because it is a disease that usually occurs without any symptoms. Long-term vasoconstriction of the renal vessels causes permanent renal

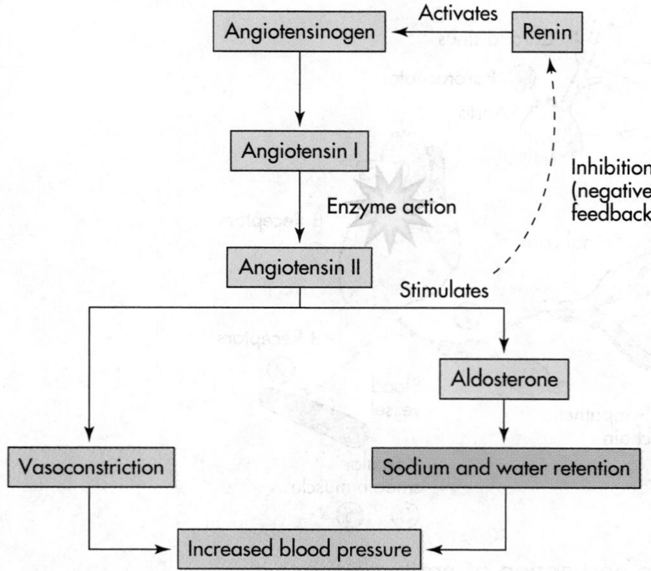


**fig. 27-1** Diagram of the effect of the renin-angiotensin system on blood pressure.

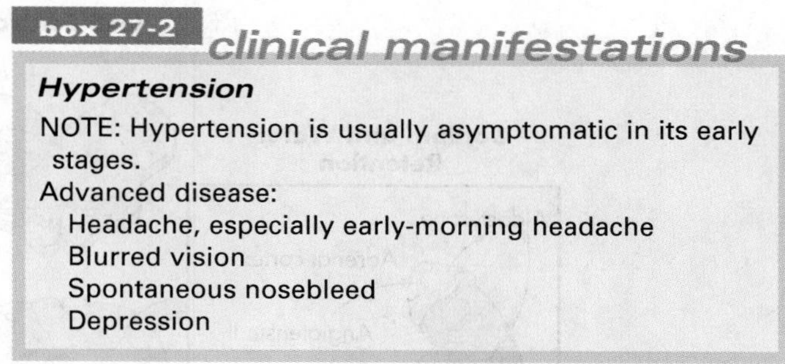

**box 27-2 clinical manifestations**

***Hypertension***

NOTE: Hypertension is usually asymptomatic in its early stages.

Advanced disease:
- Headache, especially early-morning headache
- Blurred vision
- Spontaneous nosebleed
- Depression

damage and may lead to kidney failure. Other important organs such as the brain and heart also suffer long-term damage from untreated hypertension. More advanced disease may produce symptoms such as early morning headache, blurred vision, and spontaneous nosebleed.[15] The clinical manifestations of hypertension are summarized in Box 27-2.

## COLLABORATIVE CARE MANAGEMENT

### Diagnostic Tests

The initial diagnosis of hypertension is made on the basis of two or more elevated blood pressure readings, supine and sitting, obtained on at least two separate occasions. Once the diagnosis is established the health care provider must decide how extensive the hypertension workup needs to be. Specific diagnostic tests will be ordered to rule out an underlying cause or evaluate the extent of organ damage. A comprehensive physical examination is performed, including careful evaluation of the blood vessels of the retina, and is typically supplemented with laboratory tests that will evaluate the neurological, cardiovascular, and renal systems for evidence of target organ damage. These data also serve as a baseline for future comparison. Tests may include the following:

1. Complete blood count (CBC), differential, and serum chemistry
2. Renal function studies (e.g., blood urea nitrogen [BUN], creatinine, urinalysis)
3. Lipid panel to assess for coexisting hyperlipidemia
4. Electrocardiogram (ECG), chest x-ray, and possibly echocardiogram to assess for cardiac enlargement, left ventricular hypertrophy, or aortic calcification

### Medications

Drug therapy is the primary treatment for essential hypertension, and a wide variety of medications are available for use. Figure 27-2 illustrates the sites of blood pressure regulation and the action of major categories of antihypertensive drugs. Table 27-3 (p. 751) summarizes the major drug categories with common examples of each. Drug selection is made on an individual basis with consideration of the patient's age, gender, cultural background, and lifestyle. In general, treatment is started with a low dose of a drug from one drug category that ideally can be administered in a once-a-day format to support patient adherence.[13] Either the frequency of administration or the dose may be increased later based on the patient's therapeutic response. Adjustments are based on a series of blood pressure readings obtained over a period of several weeks.[24] Other classes of drugs may be added or a new drug substituted if the previous medication is unsuccessful in controlling the patient's hypertension after approximately 2 to 3 months of treatment.

It is also important to recognize cultural differences in response to certain classes of blood pressure medications when making treatment decisions.[26] Angiotensin converting enzyme (ACE) inhibitors are most effective in the white young adult population, who tend to have higher levels of renin than African Americans and the elderly.[2] Diuretics, on the other hand, are highly effective in the African American and elderly populations because these groups tend to have higher levels of intracellular sodium.[32]

Adherence is the primary concern with hypertension management. Hypertension is usually completely asymptomatic, and the patient may not understand or accept the importance of adhering to the treatment plan, especially when the medications prescribed represent a substantial financial outlay.[13] (See the Research Box on the next page.) It is therefore desirable to keep the regimen as simple as possible. The goal of treatment is to reduce and maintain the blood pressure at a level that protects the vital organs such as the heart, brain, and kidneys from permanent damage. Adverse side effects of the medications are also minimized when dosage adjustments are made gradually. After 1 year of successful blood pressure control it may be possible to attempt a gradual reduction in the level of antihypertensive therapy.

### Treatments

The management of hypertension does not involve any specific treatments, but management is usually improved when the patient is able to make targeted lifestyle adjustments that support the drug therapy. Two important measures are

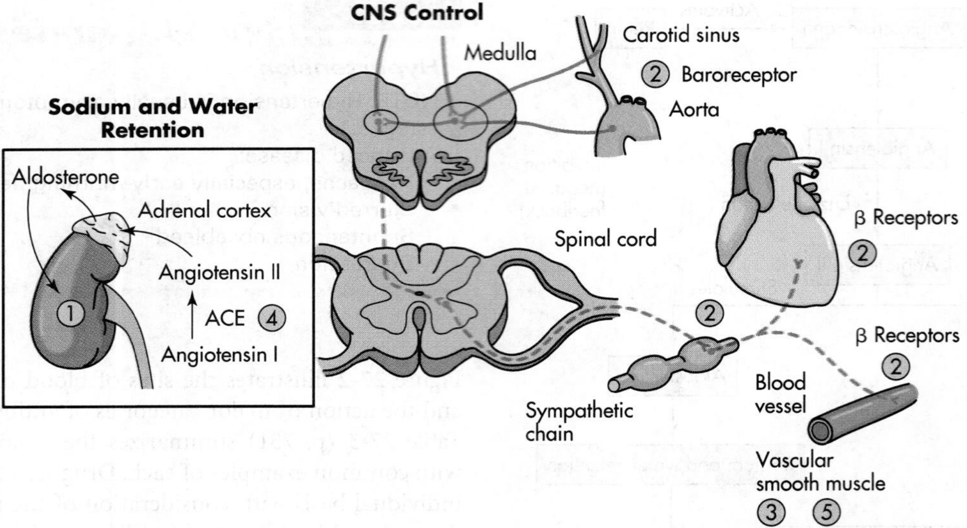


**fig. 27-2** Sites of blood pressure regulation and action of antihypertensive drugs. *1,* Diuretics. *2,* Adrenergic inhibitors. *3,* Vasodilators. *4,* ACE inhibitors. *5,* Calcium antagonist. *ACE,* Angiotensin converting enzyme.

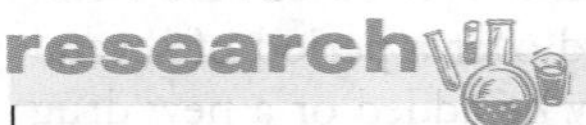


Reference: Wieck KL: Hypertension in an inner-city minority population, *J Cardiovasc Nurs* 11(4):41, 1997.

This study explored the health perception and hypertension awareness of a sample of inner-city minority persons. Nine hundred fifty individuals agreed to participate in a personal interview and blood screening process. The participants completed a health-related questionnaire and had their blood pressure measured.

The responses of a subset of 150 elderly persons were analyzed and compared with the responses of 800 young and middle-aged adults from the total sample. The elders were predictably more likely to have been told that they were hypertensive and to be using medications than were the younger participants. The health perception of both groups was positive, with 64% reporting good to excellent health. No differences were seen in the two groups on other measures of health perception.

There was also a high level of hypertension awareness in both groups, but measured blood pressures were significantly elevated in portions of the sample, particularly among elderly participants. Follow-up interviewing revealed consistent problems related to regimen adherence. Hypertension medication did not assume a top priority among daily living issues. The researchers concluded that current public information efforts are raising awareness of hypertension in all ages, but treatment gaps still exist that are primarily related to adherence to a medication regimen. The problem of nonadherence is particularly important in the elderly.

cessation of smoking and stress reduction or management. Smoking has a direct vasoconstrictive effect on the blood vessels and should be eliminated if at all possible. The role of stress is less clear, but the use of relaxation and stress management strategies is often helpful in blood pressure control.

### Surgical Management

Surgery does not play a role in the treatment of primary hypertension. It would be used in the treatment of secondary causes such as the adrenal tumor, pheochromocytoma, which secretes excessive amounts of catecholamines, or to correct selected renal problems.

### Diet

Diet does not play a major role in the treatment of primary hypertension, but it is another lifestyle modification that may be recommended to the patient. Strict sodium restriction is no longer recommended, but patients are advised to reduce their daily intake of salt, especially in prepared foods, snacks, and at the table. Weight loss can be of significant benefit to some patients, and diet modification plays a major role in this effort. The reduction of saturated fat intake also is recommended to decrease cardiac risk factors. Some patients are able to temporarily eliminate or reduce their need for antihypertensive medication through successful weight loss. Patients are also encouraged to reduce or moderate their intake of alcohol because alcohol has been shown to cause an elevation in blood pressure and has adverse interactions with many of the standard antihypertensive medications.

### Activity

Patients with hypertension are encouraged to develop a pattern of regular aerobic exercise, which may help control their hypertension and also contributes to weight loss and reduces cardiac risk factors. Patients are cautioned to avoid strenuous exercise, particularly activities that involve heavy lifting or the Valsalva maneuver. Weight lifting should be avoided, and sustained moderate exertion is preferable to bursts of effort.

**table 27-3** Common Medications for **Hypertension**

| Drug | Action | Nursing Interventions |
|---|---|---|
| **DIURETICS** | | |
| **Thiazide/Thiazide-Like Diuretics** | | |
| Bendroflumethiazide (Naturetin)<br>Benzthiazide (Aquatag, Exna)<br>Chlorothiazide (Diuril)<br>Chlorthalidone (Hygroton)<br>Cyclothiazide (Fluidil)<br>Hydrochlorothiazide (Esidrix, Hydrodiuril)<br>Hydroflumethiazide (Saluron)<br>Indapamide (Lozol)<br>Methyclothiazide (Enduron)<br>Metolazone (Zaroxolyn)<br>Polythiazide (Renese)<br>Quinethazone (Hydromox)<br>Trichlormethiazide (Diurese, Metahydrin) | Block sodium reabsorption in cortical portion of ascending tubule; water excreted with sodium, producing decreased blood volume.<br>NOTE: Thiazides ineffective in renal failure | Check vital signs before administering in early days of treatment.<br>Monitor lab values of electrolytes, particularly potassium.<br>Monitor patient's weight.<br>Teach patient to<br>• Take drug early in the day<br>• Maintain a liberal fluid intake<br>• Take drug with food if GI upset occurs<br>• Eat a potassium-rich diet (e.g., fruits, legumes, whole grains, cereals, potatoes)<br>• Expect an increased frequency and volume of urination<br>• Report the incidence of muscle weakness, cramping, fatigue, nausea<br>• Change positions slowly |
| **Loop Diuretics** | | |
| Bumetanide (Bumex)<br>Ethacrynic acid (Edecrin)<br>Furosemide (Lasix) | Block sodium and water reabsorption in medullary portion of ascending tubule; cause rapid volume depletion | Same as above, but potassium loss can be severe.<br>Monitor daily weight to assess response to treatment.<br>Monitor lab values for increases in uric acid, glucose, BUN. |
| **Potassium-Sparing Diuretics** | | |
| Amiloride (Midamor)<br>Spironolactone (Aldactone)<br>Triamterene (Dyrenium) | Inhibit aldosterone; sodium excreted in exchange for potassium | Monitor lab values for potassium excess.<br>Weigh patient daily.<br>Teach patient to<br>• Expect an increased volume of urine<br>• Avoid potassium-rich foods<br>• Report incidence of drowsiness or GI side effects |
| **ADRENERGIC INHIBITORS** | | |
| **Beta-Adrenergic Blockers** | | |
| Acebutolol (Sectral)<br>Atenolol (Tenormin)<br>Betaxolol (Kerlone)<br>Carteolol (Cartrol)<br>Metoprolol (Lopressor)<br>Nadolol (Corgard)<br>Penbutolol (Levatol)<br>Pindolol (Visken)<br>Propranolol (Inderal)<br>Timolol (Blocadren) | Block beta-adrenergic receptors of sympathetic nervous system, decreasing heart rate and blood pressure.<br>NOTE: beta blockers should not be used in patients with asthma, COPD, CHF, and heart block; use with caution in diabetes and peripheral vascular disease | Establish baseline vital signs and lab values before treatment.<br>Check blood pressure and pulse before administration.<br>Teach patients to<br>• Change positions slowly<br>• Take drug as prescribed<br>• Avoid abruptly discontinuing use<br>• Report any decline in sexual responsiveness<br>• Report incidence of fatigue, drowsiness, difficulty breathing<br>• Be alert to signs of hypoglycemia if diabetic because drugs mask the symptoms |
| **Centrally Acting Alpha Blockers** | | |
| Clonidine (Catapres)<br>Guanabenz (Wytensin)<br>Guanfacine (Tenex)<br>Methyldopa (Aldomet) | Activate central receptors that suppress vasomotor and cardiac centers, causing a decrease in peripheral resistance. NOTE: rebound hypertension may occur with abrupt discontinuation of drug (except with Aldomet) | Check vital signs before administration.<br>Teach patient to<br>• Change positions slowly<br>• Avoid hot baths, steam rooms, saunas<br>• Use gum or hard candies to counteract dry mouth<br>• Be cautious driving or operating machinery if drowsiness or sedation occur<br>• Report any decline in sexual responsiveness |

*Continued*

**table 27-3** *Common Medications for* ***Hypertension—cont'd***

| Drug | Action | Nursing Interventions |
|---|---|---|
| **Peripheral-Acting Adrenergic Antagonists** | | |
| Guanadrel (Hylorel)<br>Guanethidine (Ismelin)<br>Rauwolfia serpentina (Raudixin)<br>Reserpine (Serpasil) | Deplete catecholamines in peripheral sympathetic postganglionic fibers<br>Block norepinephrine release from adrenergic nerve endings | Check vital signs before administration.<br>Teach patient to<br>• Change positions slowly (dizziness is common)<br>• Avoid hot baths, steam rooms, saunas<br>• Use stool softeners as needed to prevent constipation<br>• Report incidence of edema in hands or feet<br>• Use gum or hard candy to relieve dry mouth<br>• Report any decline in sexual responsiveness |
| **Alpha$_1$-Adrenergic Blockers** | | |
| Doxazosin mesylate (Cardura)<br>Prazosin (Minipress)<br>Terazosin (Vasocard, Hytrin) | Block synaptic receptors that regulate vasomotor tone; reduce peripheral resistance by dilating arterioles and venules | Monitor closely for first-dose syncope occurring 30–90 min after first administration.<br>Give first dose at bedtime.<br>Monitor BP and pulse. Syncope may be preceded by tachycardia.<br>Other interventions as described for other adrenergic blockers. |
| **Combined Alpha- and Beta-Adrenergic Blockers** | | |
| Labetalol (Normodyne, Trandate) | Same as for beta blockers | Interventions are same as for beta blockers. |
| **VASODILATORS** | | |
| Hydralazine (Apresoline)<br>Minoxidil (Loniten) | Dilate peripheral blood vessels by directly relaxing vascular smooth muscle<br>NOTE: usually used in combination with other antihypertensives as they increase sodium and fluid retention and can cause reflex cardiac stimulation | Check BP and pulse before each dose. Palpitations and tachycardia are common during first week of therapy.<br>Teach-patient to<br>• Change positions slowly because dizziness is common<br>• Avoid hot baths, steam rooms, saunas<br>• Take drug with meals<br>• Be prepared for nasal congestion and excess lacrimation<br>• Report incidence of constipation or peripheral edema |
| **ACE INHIBITORS** | | |
| Benazepril (Lotensin)<br>Captopril (Capoten), captropril/HCTZ (Capozide)<br>Enalapril (Vasotec), enalapril/ HCTZ (Vaseretic)<br>Fosinopril (Monopril)<br>Lisinopril (Prinivil, Zestril), lisinopril/HCTZ (Prinzide, Zestoretic)<br>Ramipril (Altace)<br>Quinapril (Accupril) | Inhibit conversion of angiotensin to angiotensin II, thus blocking the release of aldosterone, thereby reducing sodium and water retention | Monitor for first-dose syncope in patients with CHF.<br>Monitor renal function through lab work, potassium levels.<br>Check BP before administering.<br>Teach patient to<br>• Change positions slowly<br>• Report incidence of fatigue, skin rash, impaired taste, chronic cough |
| **ANGIOTENSIN II RECEPTOR ANTAGONIST** | | |
| Losartan (Cozaar) | Selectively blocks the binding of angiotensin II to the angiotensin II receptors found in many tissues and vascular smooth muscle, which blocks its vasoconstrictive and aldosterone-secreting effects | Monitor for first-dose syncope, especially in volume-depleted patients.<br>Check BP before administering.<br>Patient teaching as per ACE inhibitors. |

*Continued*

**table 27-3** *Common Medications for Hypertension—cont'd*

| DRUG | ACTION | NURSING INTERVENTIONS |
|---|---|---|
| **CALCIUM ANTAGONISTS** | | |
| Amlodipine besylate (Norvasc)<br>Diltiazem (Cardiazem, Dilacor XR)<br>Felodipine (Plendil)<br>Isradipine (DynaCirc)<br>Nifedipine (Procardia, Adalat)<br>Nisoldipine (Sular)<br>Verapamil (Calan, Calan SR, Isoptin, Isoptin SR) | Inhibit influx of calcium into muscle cells; act on vascular smooth muscles (primary arteries) to reduce spasms and promote vasodilation | Check vital signs before administering (bradycardia is common).<br>Monitor renal and liver function tests<br>Teach patient to<br>• Take drugs before meals<br>• Change positions slowly<br>• Report incidence of peripheral edema, fatigue and headache |

### Referrals

Patients with hypertension do not require referral to other professional services as part of their primary treatment plan. The disease is self-managed in the home setting. Patients may profit from information concerning community resources that are available to support efforts in smoking cessation, stress management, diet modification, or aerobic exercise. The nurse encourages the patient and family to take advantage of these services as available.

## NURSING MANAGEMENT

### ASSESSMENT

#### Subjective Data

Subjective data to be collected to assess the patient with hypertension include:

Presence of risk factors; family history of heart disease, hypertension, stroke, diabetes, hyperlipidemia
History of hypertension; treatment prescribed; adherence and follow-up care
History or symptoms of cardiovascular, cerebrovascular, or renal disease; diabetes, hyperlipidemia
Smoking history, alcohol use
Usual diet, history of weight gain or loss
Activity and exercise pattern
Occupation, stress level, and stress management
Patient's knowledge of hypertension and its treatment
Social and environmental factors that may influence understanding of and compliance with treatment

#### Objective Data

Objective data to be collected include:

Two or more blood pressure measurements taken in both arms at separate office visits
Height and weight
Funduscopic eye examination; presence of arteriolar narrowing or hemorrhage
Examination of the neck for carotid bruits, distended neck veins, or enlarged thyroid gland
Auscultation of heart for murmurs, $S_3$, $S_4$, increased rate, or evidence of left ventricular hypertrophy
Examination of the abdomen for bruits, aortic pulsations, masses, or organomegaly
Examination of the extremities for warmth, color, edema; palpation of peripheral pulses; auscultation over femoral arteries for bruits
Neurological assessment
Laboratory tests (CBC, chemistries, lipids, BUN, creatinine), ECG, urinalysis

### NURSING DIAGNOSES

Nursing diagnoses are determined from analysis of patient data. Nursing diagnoses for the patient with hypertension may include but are not limited to:

| Diagnostic Title | Possible Etiological Factors |
|---|---|
| Knowledge deficit: hypertension risk factors, medications | Lack of exposure/recall, misinterpretation, unfamiliarity with information sources |
| Ineffective management of therapeutic regimen | Patient value system, treatment side effects, prescription costs |

### EXPECTED PATIENT OUTCOMES

Expected patient outcomes for the patient with hypertension may include but are not limited to:

1. Will be knowledgeable about the disease process and its effective management
   a. Accurately describes hypertension and its effects on vital organs
   b. Identifies lifestyle modifications to reduce risk factors
   c. Accurately describes action of prescribed medications and expected side effects
2. Takes antihypertensive medication consistently as prescribed.

### INTERVENTIONS

#### Patient/Family Education

The goal of treatment for hypertension is to reduce its associated morbidity and mortality. Treatment requires a commitment to lifelong therapy and lifestyle modifications.

Nursing interventions focus on teaching the patient and family about the disease, its associated risk factors, and the importance of adherence to the medical regimen. Although drug therapy plays a central role in hypertension management, effective treatment is also clearly based on lifestyle modification to reduce major risk factors. The nurse focuses patient teaching on the major areas of smoking cessation, diet modification and weight control, exercise, and stress management.

Cigarette smoking is a major risk factor for cardiovascular disease and is an important target of any health promotion effort. Nicotine causes constriction of the blood vessels, which contributes to a chronic elevation in blood pressure and increases peripheral vascular resistance. The nurse needs to explore the issue of smoking cessation directly and openly with the patient and ensure that the patient and family have the information they need about treatment options and community resources available to assist them with this difficult challenge. Smoking cessation is also addressed in Chapter 3.

The primary diet modifications recommended for patients with hypertension mirror those recommended for heart-healthy living in general. The nurse encourages the patient to reduce the intake of dietary fats and use moderate amounts of sodium. Dramatic changes are not necessary. Excess sodium elevates blood pressure because it contributes to fluid retention. Saturated fats have no direct effect on blood pressure and are targeted primarily because of their role in cardiac disease. A patient with both hypertension and hyperlipidemia has an increased risk of major adverse cardiovascular events such as heart attack and stroke. Reduction of saturated fat intake also makes it easier for the patient to achieve personal goals related to weight reduction and the maintenance of a stable body weight. Blood pressure typically drops as the patient loses weight, and less medication may be required. Alcohol use is also discussed as part of the overall plan for diet modification. A moderate alcohol intake can be continued, but alcohol potentiates the effects of certain antihypertensive medications and can increase patient risk.[13] The negative effects of alcohol on major target organs such as the liver and heart are also well documented.

Regular aerobic exercise can help reduce resting blood pressure and improve the response of the heart to exercise and physical exertion.[24] The nurse encourages the patient to begin an exercise plan gradually and slowly work up to a regular program of 30 to 45 minutes of aerobic exercise at least three times per week. The nurse cautions the patient to avoid weight lifting and other forms of exercise that involve bursts of activity or incorporate the Valsalva maneuver. Regular exercise also assists the patient in effective weight control.

The nurse also explores the role of stress in the patient's lifestyle and the patient's interest in or willingness to use stress reduction strategies. Patients may need help in identifying their sources of life stress and recognizing their own unique responses to stress. Simple measures such as relaxation techniques and improved coping mechanisms can be offered to any patient.[32] Patients who are interested in self-management strategies may be encouraged to explore the use of biofeedback as part of their hypertension treatment plan. See Chapter 6 for more discussion of stress and stress management.

Medication teaching is the final major area of regimen education. Lifestyle modifications are a critical component of management, but the vast majority of patients also depend on drugs to control their hypertension, and they need to know how to use these medications safely. Drug therapy is usually lifelong. Patients should know the name, dosage, action, and side effects of each blood pressure medication and should be provided with this information in written form for home reference. The nurse encourages the patient to keep an updated list of all medications on his or her person for easy reference in case of emergency.[26] Family members, especially the spouse or partner, should be included in the medication education process if at all possible. Significant others play an essential role in compliance, particularly for elderly persons. Most antihypertensive medications produce side effects that the patient must manage. The nurse needs to be honest about these side effects and encourage patients to discuss any adverse effects with their health care provider. There are numerous options available in the antihypertensive drug arsenal, and patients can be switched to a different drug if their prescribed agent is unacceptable.

Common side effects of antihypertensive medications include potassium depletion and orthostatic hypotension. Potassium depletion occurs primarily with the use of diuretics and is managed by eating foods high in potassium or taking a potassium supplement. Orthostatic hypotension occurs with the use of many drugs. It is often worse in the morning when blood pressure is normally lower, after alcohol use, and following active exercise. The nurse instructs the patient to change position slowly and sit down immediately if feeling faint. Patients should avoid standing in one position for long periods because this promotes venous pooling. Hot showers, baths, hot tubs, and saunas, which promote vasodilation, should be used with caution.

### Supporting Treatment Adherence

Treatment for hypertension involves a commitment to lifelong therapy. Adherence is a major multidimensional concern that is neither easily understood nor accomplished. The absence of symptoms associated with hypertension makes adherence a greater challenge, especially when financial constraints and troublesome drug side effects are present. The nurse encourages the patient to be involved in the plan of care and all decisions about disease management. Patients are encouraged to take advantage of community opportunities to have their blood pressure regularly checked at sites such as health fairs, grocery stores, walk-in clinics, and so on. A log of blood pressure readings can be kept and brought to the health care provider's office on each visit. These records give the provider more information on the status of the patient's blood pressure control than can be obtained at a single office measurement. The nurse also stresses the importance of keeping regular follow-up visits for ongoing disease management (see the Research Box).

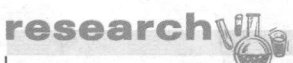

Reference: Pheley AM et al: Evaluation of a nurse based hypertension management program: screening, management and outcomes, *J Cardiovasc Nurs* 9(2):54, 1995.

This study evaluated the effectiveness of a nurse-managed hypertension screening and follow-up program designed to improve hypertension management. The sample of 460 persons included all newly referred patients from a large multispecialty group practice in a suburban midwest region. The hypertension program provided serial blood pressure screening and education about drug therapy, diet, and exercise.

The effectiveness of the managment program was demonstrated first through screening. With careful screening 78% of patients referred because of one elevated blood pressure reading obtained during an office visit were found to be normotensive and not in need of treatment. Significant decreases in both systolic and diastolic blood pressures were found in participants after 12 months of follow-up. Twenty-five percent of the participants were managed nonpharmacologically, 45% were on single-drug therapy, and 30% were on combination therapy. The researchers believe that consistent care and measurement allowed these patients to be successfully managed with the minimum amount of pharmacological intervention.

## ■ EVALUATION

To evaluate the effectiveness of nursing interventions compare patient behaviors with those stated in the expected patient outcomes. Successful achievement of patient outcomes for the person with hypertension is indicated by:

1. Is knowledgeable about the disease process and its effective management
   a. Correctly describes the disease process of hypertension and its effects on vital body organs
   b. Identifies the expected side effects of prescribed drugs and measures to minimize adverse effects
   c. Makes lifestyle adaptations to reduce risk factors
2. Takes antihypertensive medication as prescribed and participates in recommended follow-up care

## GERONTOLOGICAL CONSIDERATIONS

The incidence of hypertension increases with age, making it a problem of particular concern to the elderly. This population is at unique risk related to this disease because elders are increasingly likely to have other chronic health problems for which they are taking medications. Taking multiple medications increases the chance of adverse drug interactions and may significantly increase the monthly cost of medication. Antihypertensive medication can be extremely costly for anyone, but particularly for individuals on fixed incomes. The absence of overt disease symptoms increases the likelihood that hypertension medication will be dropped when cost becomes overwhelming.

Elders are also likely to be more vulnerable to the side effects of hypertension medication, and the development of orthostatic hypertension can pose a significant safety risk for falls. Failing memory may also interfere with medication compliance, and patients may profit from the use of medication boxes that can be filled for the week by family, friends, or visiting nurses. Hypertension is a community-managed problem, and the nurse who manages care for the elderly must plan holistically to meet the patient's needs for safe medication, side effect management, and follow-up care.

## SPECIAL ENVIRONMENTS FOR CARE

### Critical Care Management

Most patients have chronic hypertension, which can be successfully managed on an outpatient basis. Occasionally, blood pressure rises to a critical level above 210 mm Hg and requires immediate emergency treatment. When severe hypertension threatens to cause irreversible organ damage, the patient may be managed in a critical care unit, where drug therapy can be administered intravenously with continuous monitoring. Sodium nitroprusside and nitroglycerine are two of the most commonly used intravenous vasodilators for such emergencies. The goal of therapy is to lower the blood pressure gradually, because too-rapid drops in pressure can lead to organ ischemia and stroke. As the blood pressure begins to respond to these powerful medications, patients are gradually weaned again to oral medication. Once the patient's blood pressure is under control, therapy with oral medication is continued as an outpatient. The patient is instructed to resume the same regimen and lifestyle previously discussed.

### Home Care Management

Hypertension is managed in the home environment with outpatient supervision. The entire discussion of hypertension presented previously therefore addresses the management of the disease in the home. This again underlines the importance of careful and thorough patient education, particularly related to issues of adherence with the drug regimen.

## COMPLICATIONS

Hypertensive crisis and irreversible damage to major body organs are the most serious complications related to hypertension. The end-organ damage can eventually lead to encephalopathy, renal failure, left ventricular failure, and retinal hemorrhage. Untreated hypertensive crisis results in significant morbidity and mortality, as high as 90% within 2 years. When hypertensive crisis is treated successfully, however, the survival rate approaches 94% at 1 year. Appropriate ongoing follow-up appears to be the key variable and is clearly linked to the effectiveness of the patient education provided.

# ARTERIAL DISORDERS

The arteries are thick-walled vessels that transport blood and oxygen from the heart to the tissues. Arterial disease can affect any artery of the body and can manifest itself as an acute or a chronic condition. Disruption of the arterial blood flow can be caused by narrowing or complete obstruction of the wall of

**box 27-3** *Causes of Decreased Arterial Blood Flow*

- Atherosclerotic plaque
- Arterial spasm
- Embolus or thrombus
- Changes in blood pressure
- Increased blood viscosity or hypercoagulability
- Arterial venous fistula
- Trauma
- Heart failure
- Compartment syndrome

the vessel from a variety of causes (Box 27-3). The symptoms associated with arterial disease are primarily related to the severity of interruption in blood flow, which slows the delivery of oxygen and nutrients to the tissues and causes accumulation of waste products and carbon dioxide. If the tissue needs for oxygen and nutrients exceed the blood supply, ischemia (cell damage) and necrosis (cell death) will result.

## CHRONIC ARTERIAL OCCLUSIVE DISEASE

### Etiology

Chronic arterial occlusive disease involves the progressive narrowing, degeneration, and eventual obstruction of the arteries of the extremities. The lower extremities are most commonly involved. Arteriosclerosis obliterans is the most common form of chronic occlusive disease. Atherosclerosis, the buildup of cholesterol and triglyceride plaque within the arteries, combines with the process of diffuse arteriosclerosis or calcification to produce widespread, slowly progressive narrowing of the arteries. The superficial femoral, iliac, and popliteal arteries are the most common sites of involvement.[12] Plaque typically develops at points of arterial branching or bifurcation (Figure 27-3).

### Epidemiology

Chronic occlusive disease is strongly associated with aging, and symptoms usually develop between the ages of 50 and 70.[9] Approximately 10% of adults over the age of 70 are estimated to have symptoms of arterial occlusive disease.[9] The disease is more prevalent in men than in women. Several factors are known to predispose individuals to peripheral vascular disease (PVD). These include smoking, hypertension, diabetes, hyperlipidemia, and a positive family history. The disease is often more aggressive in persons with diabetes and tends to affect the smaller distal vessels below the knee.[12] Advanced vascular disease can be painful, debilitating, disabling, and even life threatening. Lifestyle modification to reduce known risk factors can slow the disease process, but there is no known cure. Risk factors for PVD are listed in the accompanying Risk Factors Box.

### Pathophysiology

The atherosclerotic plaque formation that occurs with arteriosclerosis obliterans causes thickening of the intima and media of the artery, resulting in partial or complete obstruction. The calcification of arteriosclerosis further weakens the arterial wall and increases the chance for both thrombus and aneurysm formation. The disease usually occurs segmentally with lengths of normal vessel interspersed with diseased lengths. The vessel is usually more than 50% occluded before symptoms appear.

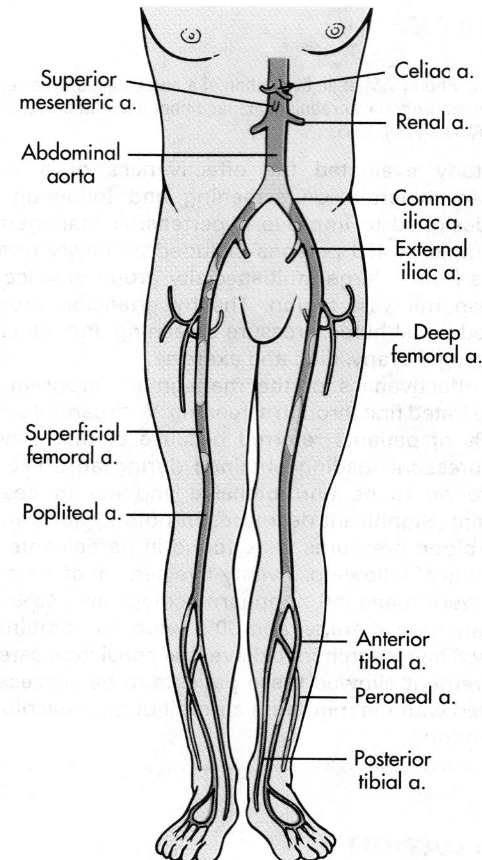


**fig. 27-3** Common sites of atherosclerosis.

Symptoms of arteriosclerosis obliterans gradually appear when the arteries can no longer provide the tissues with sufficient essential nutrients or remove metabolic waste products. Intermittent claudication, an aching pain or cramping sensation in the muscle, is the classic symptom. The term *claudication* means "limp," and claudication occurs when a muscle is exercised without an adequate blood supply.[9] Claudication is an ischemic pain that occurs with exercise and is relieved by rest. The pain is usually distal to the site of obstruction and disappears within 1 to 2 minutes after cessation of exercise. The muscles of the calf are commonly involved as a result of the disease affecting the femoral artery. Muscles of the lower back, buttocks, thigh, and foot are also commonly affected. Symptoms usually occur when a person has walked one half to two blocks and will appear even more rapidly when the person walks uphill. The body attempts to bypass the obstruction by developing collateral circulation with extra vessels in the affected areas. In slowly progressive disease the collateral circulation may reduce the overt symptoms.

Sedentary patients may not develop claudication because they may not ambulate enough to cause ischemia. Pain that

**risk factors**

**Peripheral Vascular Disease**

| | |
|---|---|
| Increasing age | Stress |
| Smoking | Family history of PVD or atherosclerosis |
| Hypertension | Sedentary lifestyle |
| Atherosclerosis | Hyperlipidemia |
| Obesity | |
| Diabetes mellitus | |

occurs at rest, termed *rest ischemia,* indicates severe disease. Rest pain typically occurs at night and is accompanied by coldness, numbness, and tingling of the extremity. Any factor that decreases cardiac output and peripheral arterial blood flow such as elevating the extremities can trigger the pain. The patient may be awakened at night and need to sit up or walk around. Gravity improves perfusion of the tissues and relieves or lessens the pain. In advanced arteriosclerosis obliterans, rest ischemia may lead to necrosis, ulceration, and gangrene, particularly in the toes and distal foot. Ischemic ulcers are pale, round, painful, and crusty in appearance.[11] Either eschar or black necrotic tissue may be present.

Chronic occlusive disease also causes hair loss on the affected extremity; thick, brittle, and slow-growing nails; and impaired motor function. The skin typically appears shiny and taut and is fragile, dry, and scaly.[9] The skin also feels cooler than normal to the touch. The extremity becomes pale when elevated above the level of the heart for 5 minutes and then exhibits reactive hyperemia or redness, which persists for more than 15 seconds when the extremity is lowered. Reddish discoloration or rubor may be present whenever the extremity is in a dependent position. Bruit, or a blowing sound, may be auscultated over the obstructed vessel where the blood flow is turbulent. A Doppler may be necessary to hear either pulses or a bruit in obstructed vessels. Box 27-4 lists the clinical manifestations of chronic arterial occlusive disease.

## Collaborative Care Management

### Diagnostic tests

A variety of tests can be used to diagnose arterial occlusive disorders. Noninvasive tests include ultrasonography, segmental limb pressure, pulse volume recordings, and exercise testing. Arteriography, an invasive procedure, is used to determine the location and extent of the disease process and is an essential part of any plan for surgical intervention. See Chapter 24 for a further description of common vascular tests.

The calculation of the ankle-brachial index (ABI) or the ankle-arm index is an objective measurement of the degree of stenosis present. In a healthy person the pressures in the leg should be the same or slightly higher than the pressures in the arm. As the disease worsens, the blood pressure in the legs drops. To obtain an ABI the patient is placed in a supine position for about 5 minutes and then systolic ankle pressure and systolic brachial blood pressures are obtained with the Doppler. The highest ankle pressure for each foot is divided by the higher of the brachial artery pressures. The ABI in a healthy person would be about 1. Patients with arterial insufficiency have an ABI of 0.5 to 0.95. Patients with ischemic rest pain have an ABI of 0.5 or less. With severe tissue damage and ischemia, the ABI can be 0.25 or lower.

**box 27-4** **clinical manifestations**

**Chronic Arterial Occlusive Disease**

- Intermittent claudication
  - Rest pain in advanced disease
- Diminished hair growth on affected extremities
- Thick, brittle, slow-growing nails
- Shiny, thin, fragile, taut skin
  - Dry and scaly
- Cool temperature
- Diminished or absent pulses
- Pale, blanched appearance with extremity elevation
- Reddish discoloration, rubor with extremity in dependent position
  - Reactive hyperemia
- Decreased motor function
- Ulcer formation with advanced disease
- ABI of 0.5-0.95

### Medications

Pharmacological therapy is used in PVD to improve blood flow and prevent thrombus formation in the affected extremities. Patients with arterial vascular disease commonly are also managing other chronic conditions that affect the blood vessels, such as diabetes, hypertension, and hyperlipidemia. These patients are often prescribed a variety of medications that may have a direct or indirect effect on their occlusive disease process. Patients may be prescribed vasodilators such as hydralazine or minoxidil. Vasodilators directly affect smooth muscle and peripheral resistance and are primarily used for blood pressure control. The calcium channel blockers and dihydropyridines block the entry of calcium into the vascular smooth muscle and also cause vasodilation. They are primarily used in the treatment of hypertension and coronary heart disease but also directly affect the vascular muscle.

Pentoxifylline (Trental) directly treats the peripheral arterial disease. Pentoxifylline increases erythrocyte flexibility and reduces blood viscosity, which directly improves the supply of oxygenated blood to the ischemic tissue.[12] Antiplatelet medications are also commonly used in treatment because arterial thrombi are composed mainly of platelets. Aspirin is the classic drug, but dipyridamole (Persantine) and ticlopidine (Ticlid) are also commonly prescribed. The effectiveness of antiplatelet agents in improving circulation through diseased arteries has not been proven and continues to be studied. Antiplatelet and anticoagulant medications may also be used after bypass surgeries to prevent reocclusion. Drugs commonly used to treat chronic arterial occlusive disease are presented in Table 27-4.

### Treatments

No specific treatments are routinely included in the management of arterial occlusive disease. The patient is assisted to improve the management of other chronic conditions such as

**table 27-4** *Common Medications for* ***Arterial Occlusive Disease***

| Drug | Action | Nursing Interventions |
|---|---|---|
| **ANTIPLATELET MEDICATIONS** | | |
| Aspirin<br>Ticlopidine (Ticlid)<br>Dipyridamole (Persantine) | Inhibit platelet aggregation, prolong bleeding time | Administer with food to reduce GI distress.<br>Monitor coagulation times.<br>Assess for signs of bleeding. |
| **XANTHINE DERIVATIVE** | | |
| Pentoxifylline (Trental) | Increases flexibility of the RBCs, thereby facilitating passage through microcirculation; decreases RBC aggregation; increases fibrinolytic activity | Monitor for side effects—GI upset, tremor.<br>Monitor for effect on claudication and exercise tolerance.<br>Therapeutic effect may take 2-4 weeks. |
| **DIHYDROPYRIDINES** | | |
| Nifedipine (Adalat, Procardia)<br>Isradipine (DynaCirc)<br>Felodipine (Plendil)<br>Nimodipine (Nimotop)<br>Amlodipine besylate (Norvasc) | Selectively block influx of calcium ions across cell membrane of vascular smooth muscle; decreased peripheral resistance increases blood flow; primarily indicated for Raynaud's phenomenon | Monitor blood pressure.<br>Teach patient to change position slowly and report the incidence of edema, fatigue, or headache. |
| **VASODILATORS** | | |
| Hydralazine (Apresoline)<br>Minoxidil (Loniten, Minodyl) | Cause vasodilation and decrease peripheral vascular resistance; useful in PVD only if small vessels can dilate in response to stimulation | Monitor blood pressure and pulse.<br>Teach patient to change positions slowly, take drug with meals, and report the incidence of constipation or peripheral edema. |

hypertension and diabetes. The most significant treatment would be assisting a patient with a smoking history to stop smoking.

A number of interventional radiological procedures may be used in the attempt to manage the disease process. Most are adaptations of procedures used to treat coronary artery disease. Procedures include transluminal angioplasty, laser surgery, atherectomy, and intravascular stent placement. These procedures are used when the patient's condition has deteriorated to the point of being incapacitating. They are discussed in more depth in the section on acute arterial occlusion later in this chapter.

### Surgical management

Various surgical procedures are available for the management of a disabling arterial disease that threatens the patient with the loss of the limb. Surgical options include bypass grafts and endarterectomy, and these options are discussed in more depth in the section on the surgical management of acute arterial occlusion. Amputation unfortunately remains one of the most commonly employed surgical procedures for chronic arterial disease. Amputation is necessary when gangrene is extensive or infection invades the bone.

### Diet

Diet does not play a direct role in the management of chronic arterial occlusive disease, but many patients can profit from interventions that will help them correct obesity and control diabetes. A heart-healthy, low-fat, low-cholesterol diet is recommended to slow the further progression of the disease process.

### Activity

A sedentary lifestyle is a risk factor for atherosclerosis. Increasing daily activity in a carefully planned way can decrease blood lipids, help control hypertension, and improve arterial blood flow by stimulating the development of collateral circulation in the occluded regions. A daily walking program is suggested for patients with arterial occlusive disease. Participation in a structured rehabilitation program is recommended if possible because the patient can receive the professional monitoring and supervision that can ensure safety.

### Referrals

A variety of professionals may be included in the collaborative plan of care for the patient with arterial occlusive disease. Diet counseling is often needed. A nutritionist can provide assistance and guidance in making the needed diet changes to reduce both body weight and overall disease risk factors. Diet teaching is especially important with diabetic patients. Referral for physical or occupational therapy may be appropriate to assist the patient to develop an appropriate exercise plan and regain the strength and endurance to manage activities of daily living independently. Referral to community support groups may also be essential, particularly for patients who are attempting smoking cessation.

## NURSING MANAGEMENT

### ASSESSMENT

#### Subjective Data

Subjective data to be collected to assess the patient with chronic arterial occlusive disease include:

- Presence, severity, and location of intermittent claudication; presence of rest pain, if any
- History of hypertension, diabetes, coronary artery disease (treatment used, adherence to regimen)
- Smoking history, attempts to quit, if any
- Dietary patterns
- Impact of disease on ability to complete activities of daily living (ADL)
- Effect of disease on family, work, social activities
- Effects of disease on sexuality—impotence
- Home living situation and effect on mobility
- Exercise and activity pattern
- Numbness or tingling in extremity

#### Objective Data

Objective data to be collected to assess the patient with arterial occlusive disease include:

- Peripheral pulse assessment by palpation (1 to 4) or Doppler
- Appearance of skin, nails, hair on extremities
  - Signs of skin breakdown
  - Postural color changes, reactive hyperemia
  - Presence of muscle wasting
- Skin temperature
- Ankle-brachial index
- Weight
- Cholesterol and triglyceride levels

### NURSING DIAGNOSES

Nursing diagnoses are determined from analysis of patient data. Nursing diagnoses for the patient with arterial occlusive disease may include but are not limited to:

| Diagnostic Title | Possible Etiological Factors |
|---|---|
| Tissue perfusion, altered (lower extremity) | Decreased arterial blood flow |
| Skin integrity, risk for impaired | Ischemia, immobility |
| Pain | Imbalance between oxygen supply and demand |

### EXPECTED PATIENT OUTCOMES

Expected patient outcomes for the patient with chronic arterial occlusive disease may include but are not limited to:

1. Describes measures to promote tissue perfusion
2. States measures to maintain skin integrity
3. Balances activity and rest to minimize incidence of pain

### INTERVENTIONS

Most of the nursing interventions that are appropriate for patients with chronic arterial occlusive disease fall into the category of patient/family education. The disease is chronic and progressive and is best managed by lifestyle modifications that support peripheral perfusion and prevent injury and complications. The patient needs to assume responsibility for incorporating these measures into her or his home lifestyle in a way that is comfortable and acceptable.

#### Promoting Tissue Perfusion

Patients are encouraged to incorporate a number of lifestyle modifications into their daily activities to improve the delivery of oxygen to the tissues. A warm environmental temperature of about 21° C (70° F) should be maintained. Avoiding exposure to the cold is critical because cold is likely to induce ischemia and pain from vasoconstriction. Socks, layered clothing, and blankets should be used for warmth, and patients are cautioned about the dangers associated with the use of heating pads and hot water bottles. The patient should avoid the use of constrictive or restrictive clothing such as girdles, rolled garters, tight shoes or shoelaces, tight waistbands, and socks with tight banding that could impede circulation.

Positioning is also an important intervention to support perfusion. The legs should be maintained in a position of slight dependency, which uses gravity to enhance tissue perfusion. The legs should not be elevated above the level of the heart because this would impede arterial flow. The patient is encouraged to avoid crossing the legs at the knees, which places pressure on the arteries of the leg, and to avoid sitting in a slumped or slouched posture to prevent acute constriction of the arteries in the pelvis. Both pressure and massage of the extremities should be avoided. The skin is fragile and can break down easily. Vigorous massage can also promote embolus formation.

Eliminating smoking is the other critical lifestyle change to support perfusion. Nicotine causes vasoconstriction and promotes vasospasm, and inhaled carbon dioxide reduces the oxygen carrying capacity of the blood. Smoking cessation is addressed in this text under several discussions of cardiac and respiratory problems, but its importance in PVD cannot be overestimated. The nurse needs to explore the patient's knowledge about the effects of smoking, prior efforts to quit, and interest in quitting. Referral for community support can be initiated after this assessment process is completed.

#### Maintaining Skin Integrity and Preventing Injury and Infection

The skin is at high risk for breakdown because of decreased tissue oxygenation from impaired circulation. The nurse will teach the patient to carefully examine the skin daily for intactness, dryness, redness, and injury. A mirror can be used to inspect areas that are difficult to see such as the heels and the plantar surfaces of the toes. If the patient is hospitalized, the nurse performs a complete assessment at least once each day and equips the bed with antipressure devices to prevent skin breakdown. Daily gentle cleansing of the feet using a mild soap is recommended. The skin is gently dried and moisturizing lotion is applied as necessary to counteract dryness. Cotton socks are recommended and should be changed daily to prevent moisture buildup and irritation. Properly fitted shoes are important, and shoes made out of synthetic materials that do not breathe should be avoided. Soft leather shoes are recommended.

Sensation may be decreased in the feet, which increases the chance for injury. The feet need to be protected from abrasion and irritation as much as possible. The use of direct heat is contraindicated. Toenails should be trimmed straight across using nail clippers. Corns, calluses, and other foot problems should not be self-treated but evaluated by a podiatrist. The health care provider should be contacted immediately if ulceration, infection, or skin breakdown is detected.

#### Reducing Pain and Increasing Exercise Tolerance

Activity improves circulation through muscle contraction and relaxation and also stimulates the formation of collateral circulation that increases blood flow to the ischemic area. The patient needs to be encouraged to exercise or walk to the point of pain because this exercise is the most effective way to decrease the incidence and severity of claudication. The exercise should be slow and progressive. Walking is the preferred exercise, but swimming and use of a stationary bicycle can also be incorporated into the plan. The patient should avoid bedrest as much as possible. The goal is to develop an exercise tolerance of 30 to 45 minutes of walking twice a day. The exercise should be halted immediately when pain occurs. The patient should rest and resume walking only after the pain has completely subsided. Range-of-motion exercises are also recommended.

The Buerger-Allen exercises can also be recommended to patients with advanced disease. These exercises can be used with patients who have minimal exercise tolerance. The patient lies flat with legs elevated above the heart for 2 to 3 minutes and then relaxes with the legs in a slightly dependent position for an additional 2 to 3 minutes. The patient then proceeds to exercise the feet (flexion, extension, inversion, eversion), ankles (rotations and pumps), and knees (flexion, extension) for 30 seconds in each position.

## ■ EVALUATION

To evaluate the effectiveness of nursing interventions, compare patient behaviors with those stated in the expected patient outcomes. Successful achievement of patient outcomes for the patient with arterial occlusive disease is indicated by:

1. Correctly describes measures to promote tissue perfusion
2. Correctly describes measures to maintain skin integrity
3. Is able to engage in daily activities without pain

## GERONTOLOGICAL CONSIDERATIONS

Chronic arterial occlusive disease primarily affects older individuals, particularly those over the age of 70. Therefore all of the management discussion that has been presented applies to this population. The unique needs of elders in terms of learning, making lifestyle changes, and adherence need to be taken into account in planning care. Patients are carefully assessed for the presence of vision or hearing losses that may make it more difficult for them to learn the self-care regimen. Potential obstacles in the home environment also need to be considered and modified if possible.

## SPECIAL ENVIRONMENTS FOR CARE

### Critical Care Management

Critical care management would not be routinely needed in the management of chronic arterial occlusive disease. This is a slowly progressive problem that only rarely causes acute complications. Acute obstruction can occur, however, and may cause an acute limb-threatening emergency. The discussion of care related to acute arterial occlusion is presented on p. 762.

### Home Care Management

Virtually all of the care described for the patient with chronic arterial occlusive disease will take place in the home setting. The patient requires hospitalization only for complications of the disease. All of the teaching that is discussed in the section on nursing interventions is addressed toward successful self-management by the patient at home. Care planning, especially for elders, is based on a thorough assessment of the home setting and the support network available to assist the patient in managing the disease.

## COMPLICATIONS

The major complications of chronic arterial occlusive disease include injury, infection, gangrene, and thrombus or embolus formation. Many of these problems, if not identified and treated promptly, result in the loss of the limb through amputation. Care of the patient undergoing amputation is discussed on p. 770.

Arterial ulcers may also develop as a result of the decreased blood supply. Arterial ulcers are typically located on or between the toes, or on the upper surface of the foot over the metatarsal heads, and are extremely painful.[11] The diabetic patient is particularly vulnerable to the development of ulcers, which may become chronic and nonhealing. Necrotic tissue must be removed before healing can occur. This is accomplished by mechanical debridement, chemical debridement with an enzymatic agent such as Varidase, or autolytic debridement with hydrocolloid and film dressings. Nonrestrictive bandages are used to support circulation and healing. Treatment is difficult, and outcomes are unpredictable. Prevention through the previously discussed strategies is the focus of intervention.

## BUERGER'S DISEASE (THROMBOANGIITIS OBLITERANS)

### Etiology/Epidemiology

Buerger's disease is an obstructive vascular disorder caused by segmental inflammation in the arteries and veins. It typically occurs in men between the ages of 20 and 40 years and is rare in women. Although Buerger's disease occurs worldwide, the incidence is much higher in persons of Indian, Asian, and Jewish heritage. The incidence of Buerger's disease is strongly associated with cigarette smoking—the disease does not occur in nonsmokers. The underlying cause remains unknown. The disease primarily affects the vessels of the lower extremity, and the tibial arteries and the vessels of the foot are the most common sites. Thirty percent of patients with Buerger's disease have upper extremity involvement, primarily affecting the vessels of the forearm and hand.

### Pathophysiology

Buerger's disease causes an inflammatory response in the arteries, veins, and nerves. There is infiltration of white cells and the area becomes fibrotic as healing occurs, which can result in vessel occlusion. The pathology is different from atherosclerotic disease because small and medium-sized arteries and veins are involved. Necrotic lesions form at the tips of the finger and toes, and recurrent superficial thrombophlebitis commonly occurs in both the upper and lower extremities. Symptoms include slowly developing claudication, cyanosis, and coldness, which can progress to necrosis and gangrene. Rest pain is common. The risk of gangrene increases with the presence of collagen disease or atherosclerosis and in response to stress or cold weather.

### Collaborative Care Management

Buerger's disease is difficult to treat, and management is focused on assisting the patient to quit smoking. Neither anticoagulants nor vasodilators are very effective, and the use of calcium channel blockers and antiplatelet drugs has shown mixed results. A sympathectomy may help eliminate vasospasm, but it must be performed early in the disease process. Amputation may ultimately be required.

### Patient/Family Education

The patient must be helped to understand the direct relationship between cigarette smoking and the disease process. Complete abstinence from smoking is essential if the disease is to be successfully controlled. Most patients improve when they stop smoking. In addition to supporting the patient's smoking cessation efforts, the nurse teaches the patient to avoid exposure to the cold and to protect the extremities from injury and trauma.

## RAYNAUD'S DISEASE

### Etiology/Epidemiology

Raynaud's disease is an episodic vasospastic disorder of the small cutaneous arteries, usually involving the fingers and toes. First described by Maurice Raynaud in 1862, it affects an estimated 5% to 10% of the population.[21] Ninety-three percent of those affected are women. More common in winter and in damp cool climates, Raynaud's disease can occur in isolation or in combination with another disease process.[21] When it accompanies another disease it is termed *Raynaud's phenomenon.* Associated disorders include systemic sclerosis, systemic lupus erythematosus, rheumatoid arthritis, hematological disorders, trauma, and arterial obstruction. Other contributing factors include occupation-related trauma and pressure to the fingertips such as that experienced by typists, pianists, and workers who use handheld vibrating equipment. Symptoms are commonly precipitated by exposure to the cold, emotional upset, caffeine ingestion, and tobacco use.

### Pathophysiology

Vasoconstriction is regulated by alpha-2 receptors. Sympathetic stimulation or cold exposure causes the release of noradrenaline, which activates the alpha-2 receptors and causes vasoconstriction and vasospasm. Persons with Raynaud's disease may have an increased number of alpha-2 receptors. They may also have a decrease in beta receptors and calcitonin, which are responsible for vasodilation. The pathological sequence is not completely understood. A positive antinuclear antibody (ANA) is present in 25% of patients with Raynaud's disease.

The symptoms of Raynaud's disease are symmetrical and bilateral. The vasospasm is confined to the digits and does not usually include the thumb. Only the tip of the finger distal to the metacarpophalangeal joint is typically affected. Toes may also be affected in the same pattern.

The classic triphasic color changes of pallor, cyanosis, and rubor of one or more digits of both hands is considered to be diagnostic for Raynaud's disease (Figure 27-4). Pallor is the primary early symptom. The rubor phase occurs as blood flow resumes after the vasospasm relaxes and is acutely painful. The cyanotic phase is not always present. Normal radial and ulnar pulses are usually preserved. Episodes typically last just minutes, but in severe cases they can persist for hours. Lesions and gangrenous ulcers on the fingertips can develop in advanced disease. If unilateral symptoms occur, arterial occlusion should be suspected.

### Collaborative Care Management

Raynaud's disease has no cure and in mild cases does not require treatment because the episodes are self-limiting. It is

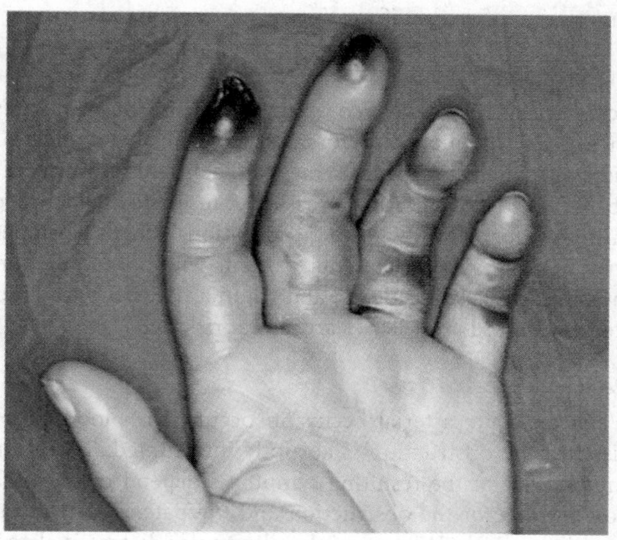

**fig. 27-4** Raynaud's phenomenon.

important to rule out the presence of a treatable secondary condition. Treatment for primary Raynaud's disease focuses on preventing vasospasm. Pharmacological intervention includes the use of calcium channel blockers, vascular smooth muscle relaxants, and vasodilators, although success is variable. A prostacyclin analog, iloprost, has been successfully used to improve circulation and decrease pain in research subjects. Biofeedback techniques to increase skin temperature and prevent spasm have also been used successfully. Sympathectomy may be necessary in severe cases. Persistent uncontrolled spasms can cause gangrene and necessitate surgical intervention (possibly amputation).

#### Patient/family education

Patient education focuses on reassuring the patient that episodes can be effectively managed in most cases. The nurse explores ways that the patient can minimize exposure to the cold through the use of adequate layered clothing. Mittens are encouraged because they do not constrict the fingers and allow the fingers to warm each other. Socks are also important. The patient is cautioned to avoid direct contact with ice and frozen food and to use gloves when handling cold products. Stress management and relaxation techniques can often be effective in decreasing the frequency of vasospastic episodes.

## ACUTE ARTERIAL OCCLUSIVE DISEASE

### Etiology

Acute arterial occlusion can occur in both healthy and diseased arteries. The occlusion can result from an arterial thrombosis that forms in an atherosclerotic artery, an embolism in a healthy artery, or trauma. The occlusion typically occurs suddenly and without warning. An embolus that forms in the heart or an atherosclerotic aneurysm is the most common etiology. The thrombi dislodge and travel to the lungs if they originate in the right side of the heart or to anywhere in the systemic circulation if they originate in the left side of the heart or the peripheral circulation. The occlusion typically occurs at sites of vessel bifurcation or narrowing.

### Epidemiology

Acute arterial occlusion can occur in any patient in the presence of appropriate risk factors. Patients with rheumatic heart disease, artificial heart valves, myocardial infarction, and atrial fibrillation are at particular risk because the incidence of thrombus formation with these conditions is high. Postoperative vascular surgery patients, patients who have undergone invasive arterial procedures, and trauma patients with lacerated or compressed arteries are also at risk.

### Pathophysiology

When an acute arterial occlusion occurs, the blood supply distal to the obstruction is abruptly interrupted. The extent and severity of the resulting symptoms depend on the location and size of the obstruction and the patency of the surrounding vessels. When peripheral vascular disease is already present in the extremity, the symptoms are likely to be much more severe. Acute embolic occlusion usually occurs suddenly, and neither rest nor activity relieves it.[3] The pain of severe occlusion is both severe and unrelenting. The primary symptoms of acute occlusion can be clearly described through the "six *P*'s" of neurovascular assessment. The limb exhibits pain, pallor, pulselessness, paresthesia, paralysis, and poikilothermia (it is most often cool to the touch). The development of paralysis in the affected limb is considered to be a late and ominous sign that usually reflects the ischemic death of nerve cells supplying the extremity.[10] Patients are often unable either to rest or sleep due to the severity of the pain. Limb-threatening ischemia rapidly progresses to necrosis and gangrene and requires limb amputation if successful intervention does not promptly restore perfusion. The window of opportunity for successful treatment can be hours in severe cases. The classic clinical manifestations of acute occlusion are summarized in Box 27-5.

### Collaborative Care Management

#### Diagnostic tests

The diagnosis of acute occlusion is primarily established through physical assessment of the affected limb. Noninvasive tests such as Doppler ultrasonography and ankle-brachial index measurements are commonly employed. Magnetic resonance imaging (MRI) or angiography may be used to map the location and severity of the obstruction before surgical intervention.

#### Medications

Drug therapy may be used as a primary treatment modality or as a follow-up to interventions such as embolectomy. The goal of drug therapy is to dissolve the clot and prevent further clot formation. Anticoagulant therapy with continuous intravenous heparin is usually initiated immediately to prevent further enlargement of the thrombus. Heparin, however, will not dissolve existing clots. Emboli may be treated

**box 27-5** ***clinical manifestations***

**Acute Arterial Occlusion**

NOTE: Symptoms typically occur suddenly and are severe.

*Pain.* When the obstruction is complete, the pain is severe and constant and is not relieved by rest.

*Pallor.* The limb typically appears pale or mottled.

*Pulselessness.* The peripheral pulses are either diminished or completely absent over the path of the affected vessel.

*Paresthesia.* Numbness, tingling, and burning in the extremity are common when ischemia is severe.

*Poikilothermia.* The limb is typically cool, if not frankly cold, to the touch.

*Paralysis.* Mobility of the part is limited. The development of frank paralysis is an ominous sign because it may indicate the ischemic death of nerves in the extremity.

If perfusion is not rapidly restored, the limb will develop signs of necrosis and gangrene, often in a matter of hours.

with thrombolytic agents when the risks associated with ischemia outweigh the risk of bleeding.[14] Thrombolytics also prevent the occurrence of complications associated with the more invasive procedures. Urokinase is used most commonly.[3] Its effectiveness depends on the severity and location of the obstruction.

A percutaneous arterial catheter is inserted into the femoral artery and advanced to the site of obstruction. This allows the drug to be directly administered to the thrombus. The thrombus is dissolved over 24 to 48 hours.[10] The risk of bleeding complications is high; therefore patients need to be carefully selected and screened.

Arterial spasm can also be a problem with an arterial thrombus or embolus. Spasmolytic agents such as papaverine, tolazoline, and calcium channel blockers may be administered to relieve or prevent arterial spasm. Blood pressure control is also important for any patient with an acute arterial condition, especially if surgical intervention is planned. Drug therapy will be used as needed to manage the patient's blood pressure.

Anticoagulant therapy may be used after successful treatment of the thrombus. Any patient considered at risk for future embolization will usually be prescribed long-term anticoagulant therapy with an oral agent such as Coumadin to prevent future acute episodes.

### Treatment

Treatment of an acute arterial occlusion may involve the use of one of the newer endovascular procedures. Endovascular procedures are an evolving specialty in vascular care that allow for treatment within the artery itself to remove blockages.[5] These procedures include balloon angioplasty or percutaneous transluminal angioplasty (PTA), intraluminal ultrasound, laser angioplasty, mechanical atherectomy, and stent placement. Most of these procedures have been adapted from similar procedures developed to treat coronary artery obstruction. Their major advantages include decreased cost, decreased risk, minimally invasive surgery with fewer postoperative complications, and decreased length of hospital stay. Few of the procedures have been used extensively enough to fully evaluate their long-term promise in the management of acute arterial occlusion.

*Percutaneous balloon angioplasty.* This procedure is used for both diagnosis and treatment. A catheter is inserted into a major artery and advanced under fluoroscopic guidance to the site of obstruction. If a red thrombus is visualized, it will be treated with either thrombolytic therapy or by thrombectomy. If a white or yellow-white atherosclerotic plaque is seen, the procedure of choice is usually bypass surgery or recanalization. Balloon angioplasty can also be used to dilate any artery of the body except for the carotids. Angioplasty has been used successfully with coronary, aortic, iliac, femoral, popliteal, tibial, mesenteric, and renal stenoses. Calcified and fibrous lesions cannot be treated in this manner. Patients are typically placed on heparin after the procedure to minimize the risk of restenosis and then are placed on long-term antiplatelet therapy.

*Intravascular ultrasound.* This procedure is used in conjunction with definitive treatment strategies. Ultrasound is employed within the occluded vessel to measure the stenosis. This allows for the safe removal of the atheroma without vessel injury. It may also be used to assist in or evaluate the placement of stents.

*Laser-assisted balloon angioplasty (LABA).* Laser energy is used to reduce the obstructive plaque through vaporization and open an occluded artery so that balloon angioplasty can be effectively performed.[5] The use of the laser is designed to reduce the stenosis and reshape the artery. Papaverine is administered during and after the procedure to prevent vessel spasm.

*Peripheral atherectomy.* This is a percutaneous procedure that directly removes the atheroma or plaque from the diseased artery.

*Intravascular stents.* Restenosis is a common problem after any revascularization procedure. Stents have been developed that can be inserted in the affected artery to provide structure and support vessel patency.

None of the described interventions is without risk. Rethrombosis, embolism, vasospasm, and both local and systemic bleeding are all possible complications of these procedures, especially when patients are also being anticoagulated.

### Surgical management

Surgery may be the treatment option of choice for severe occlusion, or it may be used when more conservative interventions fail to reverse the severe ischemia. Although a variety of surgical procedures are available, the most common and successful operation for arterial ischemia is to bypass the obstruction (Box 27-6). An autologous graft of the patient's own saphenous vein may be used for the bypass. The vein is removed and then reversed so that the valves in the vein allow the blood to flow in the desired direction. These grafts are the preferred option because there is less risk of restenosis and graft failure. Synthetic grafts are also commonly used. Polytetrafluoroethylene (PTFE) grafts, which are also know as Gore-Tex grafts, have been successfully used for many years. Grafts from human umbilical cord veins have also been used successfully.

**box 27-6** Options for Surgical Repair of Acute Arterial Occlusion

*Endarterectomy.* A direct opening is made into the artery to remove the obstruction.

*Embolectomy.* Removal of an embolus from an artery.

*Femoral-femoral bypass.* A graft from one femoral artery to the other.

*Axillofemoral bypass.* A graft from the axillary artery to the femoral artery. It is created subcutaneously on the side of the chest.

*Femoral-Popliteal bypass.* A graft from the femoral artery to the popliteal artery.

*Aortoiliac bypass.* A graft from the aorta to the iliac arteries. The incision is made from the xiphoid process to the pubis.

The aorta and the renal, iliac, femoral, popliteal, and anterior and posterior tibial arteries are common sites of obstruction. The surgeon will determine the optimal graft placement to reestablish patent arterial flow. Grafting from the femoral to the popliteal artery is extremely common (Figure 27-5). Patients with occlusion of the distal aorta may undergo aortoiliac bypass. A femoral-femoral bypass shifts blood from one femoral artery to the other and may be a procedure of last resort for patients who have had prior aortic surgery and are no longer candidates for further surgery on the aorta. Grafts can also be placed subcutaneously from the axillary artery to the femoral artery. Procedures involving the aorta tend to be more extensive and carry a higher risk of complications.

### Diet

Diet does not play a major or direct role in the treatment of acute arterial occlusion. Patients usually receive nothing by mouth (NPO) while the workup is completed and decisions are made about the appropriate intervention. An empty stomach minimizes aspiration risks associated with either the interventional or surgical procedures. The NPO status is extremely important when general anesthesia is used, particularly with abdominal procedures. Patients will be gradually advanced to a normal diet after surgery. Ileus is common after surgery on the aorta, and meticulous abdominal assessment is important. Once a normal oral diet is resumed, attention is again directed toward encouraging the patient to adhere to a heart-healthy diet of low-fat, low-cholesterol foods. Diet is particularly important when diabetes complicates the management of vascular problems.

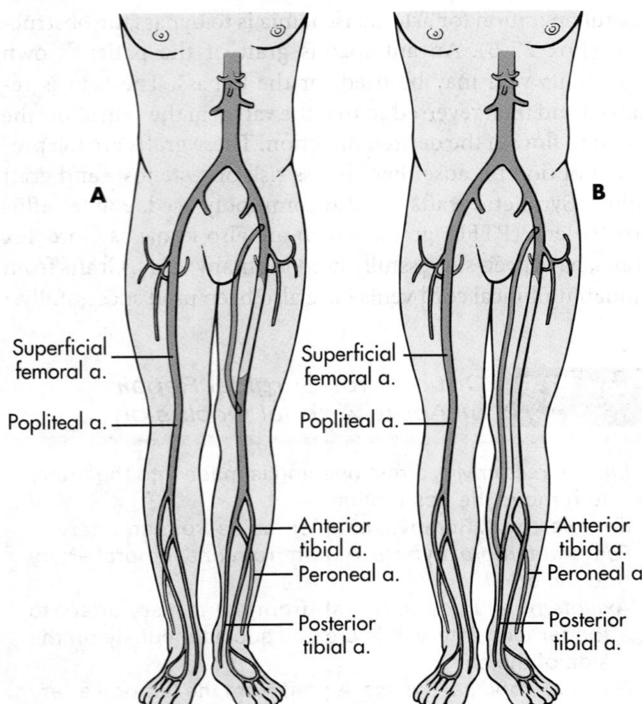


**fig. 27-5** **A,** Femoral-popliteal bypass graft around an occluded superficial femoral artery. **B,** Femoral-posterior tibial bypass graft around occluded superficial femoral, popliteal, and proximal tibial arteries.

### Activity

After interventional procedures patients are kept on bedrest until the invasive arterial lines and thrombolytic agents can be discontinued. Protocols vary based on the nature and extent of the intervention, but bedrest is commonly maintained for 6 to 24 hours. Early ambulation is important after vascular surgery and helps prevent the complications of immobility. Patients are assisted out of bed the first day after surgery as long as they are hemodynamically stable. Activity is then steadily progressed. A daily walking program is usually recommended at discharge. If possible, the patient will be referred to a structured vascular rehabilitation program. Exercise helps support blood flow, improves overall functioning, and increases the patient's general sense of well-being. Heavy lifting is restricted for at least 6 weeks after surgery. Sexual activity may be resumed as soon as the patient's comfort level permits.

### Referrals

A pain service may be used in the preoperative period to help manage the patient's severe ischemic pain. Both patient-controlled analgesia and epidural administration are commonly used. A nutrition referral may be appropriate for diet teaching before discharge. Both physical and occupational therapists are essential collaborative partners in the patient's management. They will assist the patient to develop a manageable exercise plan and adapt daily activities to maintain independence in self-care. Home health referrals may be appropriate for patients who experience complications or for elders who live alone.

## NURSING MANAGEMENT OF THE PATIENT UNDERGOING VASCULAR BYPASS SURGERY

### PREOPERATIVE CARE

Preoperative care focuses on the physical, emotional, and psychosocial preparation of a severely stressed patient. The patient may be undergoing a variety of emergency tests and procedures and will have extensive needs for teaching and support. This is a very anxiety-producing situation for the patient and family. Pain, medication effects, anxiety, and uncertainty all influence the ability of the patient and family to absorb the information being presented. The nurse performs frequent vital signs and neurovascular assessments to assess for any changes in patient status. The nurse is an important liaison between the patient and the rest of the treatment team and attempts to keep the channels of communication open. Guidelines for care of the patient with an acute arterial occlusion are summarized in the accompanying box.

### POSTOPERATIVE CARE

The patient receives meticulous general surgical care. The complications of vascular surgery can affect virtually any organ system. The more invasive the procedure, the greater the risk of complications. Patients with surgery involving the aorta are typically at greatest risk. Potential complications include bleeding, infection at the graft site, cardiac failure, myocardial infarction (MI), dysrhythmias, stroke, renal failure, and injury to adjacent organs and tissues (e.g., ureters, bowel, nerves). The nurse is responsible for meticulous postoperative monitoring of all major body systems. A sample Clinical Pathway for a patient undergoing bypass graft surgery is found on p. 766.

### Supporting Circulation and Perfusion

Patients with vascular disease also commonly have problems with coronary artery disease or hypertension. Cardiac monitoring, vital sign, and peripheral vascular assessments are all critical nursing interventions. The nurse is alert to the development of dysrhythmias or cardiac failure. The nurse assesses and evaluates data from vital signs, pulse oximetry, arterial blood gases, cardiac enzymes, electrolytes, and Swan-Ganz catheter measurements.

Graft patency is a priority concern in the postoperative period because the risk of reocclusion from thrombosis, restenosis, or debris is significant. The nurse monitors the patient's peripheral pulses and limb temperature, as well as the degree of pain, pallor, sensation, and movement.

Anticoagulant therapy increases the risk of bleeding from the suture line and graft anastamoses. The nurse closely monitors appropriate laboratory values such as hemoglobin, hematocrit, and coagulation studies. These values can alert the clinician to potential hemorrhage. Body excretions, particularly nasogastric secretions are tested for blood. The nurse also monitors all incision and arteriogram sites for signs of bleeding. Measuring the patient's abdominal girth and limb circumferences provides an objective means to assess for distention from either internal bleeding or edema.

### Preventing Respiratory Complications

Atelectasis is the most common cause of fever in the first 24 hours after surgery. Atelectasis can progress rapidly to pulmonary infection if aggressive pulmonary toilet measures are not instituted. The nurse encourages the patient to deep breathe and cough to clear the airway as needed and to use an incentive spirometer frequently. Early ambulation is a critical intervention. Patients with abdominal and chest incisions need lots of encouragement plus effective pain management to assist them in complying with essential respiratory and ambulation protocols. Percussion and postural drainage are initiated if needed.

### Supporting Fluid Balance

The kidneys are at particular risk after bypass surgery because many of the procedures involve the aorta or femoral arteries. Hypotension, hypovolemia, and trauma to the kidneys or ureters during surgery can all lead to acute postoperative renal failure. The nurse carefully measures and records the patient's intake and output and daily weight, and monitors laboratory values of BUN, creatinine, and serum electrolytes. The urine is assessed for signs of myoglobinuria.

### Promoting Wound Healing

Wound healing problems and infection are common after vascular surgery, particularly with diabetic and malnourished patients. The incision is cleaned with saline solution at least twice daily, and this technique is taught to the patient or a family member. With the surgeon's approval the patient may shower a few days after surgery. An antibacterial soap without lotions or perfume is suggested. Tub baths are not recommended because of the risk of contamination from standing water. The patient and family are taught the signs and symptoms of wound infection, complications to monitor for after discharge, and the importance of promptly reporting any complications to the surgeon. Infection in the graft is an extremely serious complication with a high mortality rate. Graft infection is usually accompanied by high fevers, prolonged ileus, and a rapidly rising white blood cell count.

### Patient/Family Education

Hospitalization will be brief, and the patient and family need to have adequate education for self-care at home. If the ability of the patient and family to provide adequate care is questioned by either the nurse or the family, a home health referral is promptly initiated. Patients receive standard discharge teaching concerning diet, activity, wound care, and resumption of normal activities. The nurse also provides the patient with information about risk factor reduction to decrease the risk of vascular problems and future complications. A

**guidelines for care**

**The Patient with an Acute Arterial Occlusion**

- Monitor the patient for any change in circulatory status to the affected limb. Monitor temperature, color, sensation, and pain. A change in these parameters may indicate worsening occlusion
- Monitor peripheral pulses bilaterally for presence, strength, quality, and symmetry.
- Keep the extremity warm, but do not apply direct heat or heat lamps.
- Avoid chilling.
- Maintain bed rest unless activity is specifically ordered.
- Keep the extremity flat or in a slightly dependent position to promote perfusion.
- Use an overbed cradle to protect a painful extremity from the pressure of linens.
- Use a sheepskin and 4-inch foam mattress beneath the extremity.
- Do not use the knee gatch on the bed; instruct the patient not to cross the legs at the knee or ankle.
- Do not apply any restraint to the affected limb.
- Keep the head of the bed low to support circulation to the lower extremities.
- Monitor the effects of anticoagulant and thrombolytic therapy. Monitor prothrombin time, partial thromboplastin time, platelets, and other coagulation studies.
- Assess for local and systemic bleeding.

## clinical pathway *Bypass Graft Surgery*

DRG# E-LOS: 6 days ACTUAL LOS

SURGERY: A-GRAM + PVD BYPASS (FEM-POP, FEM-TIB, FEM-PERONEAL)

OTHER MEDICAL DX:

ATTENDING M.D. CASE MGR

| DATE | / / | / / | / / | / / | / / | / / | / / | / / | / / |
|---|---|---|---|---|---|---|---|---|---|
| | **PRE-ADMISSION CLINIC** | **ADMIT DOS** | **POD #1** | **POD #2** | **POD #3** | **POD #4** | **POD #5** | **POD #6** | **POST-DISCHARGE** |
| EDUCATION D/C PLAN | • Pre-op:<br>NPO p MN<br>Incision<br>Pain meds<br>TCDB/IS<br>Activity<br>Surgical consent<br>• Assess:<br>Home support<br>Educational level<br>Functional level | • Pre A-gram<br>• Assess procedure purpose | • Activity—sit less than 1°. Walk to tolerance. | • Activity—progressive walking program →<br>• Incision care (watch) →<br>• S/S of infection<br>→ | • →<br>• — perform →<br>• →<br>• Foot care →<br>Temp of extremity<br>Proper shoes<br>Cleansing<br>• Diet →<br>• Medications → | • →<br>• →<br>• →<br>• →<br>• →<br>• → | • →<br>• →<br>• →<br>• →<br>• →<br>• → | • →<br>• →<br>• →<br>• →<br>• →<br>• → | • Risk factor reduction<br>Smoking<br>Weight<br>Activity<br>• Diabetes F/U<br>• Coumadin teaching<br>• Foot care<br>• Self care<br>• Psycho-social review |
| DIAGNOSTICS | • PVRs<br>• Risk factor evaluation<br>• Labs: CBC, Chem 10, PT/PTT, T/X 4U PRBC, Lipid Profile<br>• ECG<br>• CXR<br>• VS<br>• Weight | • Arteriogram in AM<br>• VS Q4° →<br>(With Doppler pulses)<br>• I/O →<br>• Telemetry Protocol →<br>• Labs: CBC, Chem 7 →<br>• ECG | • →<br>• →<br>• →<br>• PT/PTT<br>• Weight → | • CXR (PA/Lat)<br>• —Q8°→<br>• →<br>• → <br>• → | • →<br>• →<br>• Post-Op PVRs<br>• → | • →<br>• Labs: CBC, Chem 7<br>• → | • →<br>• → | • →<br>• → | • Perfusion assessment<br>• Functional assessment<br>• PVRs<br>• Incision assessment/ wound care<br>• Vital signs<br>• Weight |

| | PRE-ADMISSION CLINIC | ADMIT DOS | POD #1 | POD #2 | POD #3 | POD #4 | POD #5 | POD #6 | POST-DISCHARGE |
|---|---|---|---|---|---|---|---|---|---|
| MEDICATIONS | • DC Coumadin/ ASA 3 days PTA<br>• Continue Cardiac →<br>• Continue AntiHTN<br>• Continue Diabetic | • ? Heparin →<br>• Pain meds IV →<br>• → | • →<br>• ASA/Coumadin<br>• ▲ to PO →<br>• Restart Home Meds →<br>• Lasix/KCL PRN → | • →<br>• →<br>• →<br>• →<br>• →<br>• OBR → | • →<br>• →<br>• →<br>• →<br>• →<br>• → | • →<br>• →<br>• →<br>• →<br>• →<br>• → | • →<br>• →<br>• →<br>• →<br>• →<br>• → | • →<br>• →<br>• →<br>• →<br>• →<br>• → | • Medication review and reinforcement<br>• Assess compliance |
| TREATMENTS | | • OR after A-Gram<br>• Hibiclens scrub<br>• IVF →<br>• Foley →<br>• Cardiac Monitor Protocol → | • Reinforce OR drsg PRN<br>• ▲ to Heparin Lock →<br>• →<br>• →<br>• TC & DB Q2° | • →<br>• →<br>• Incision care BID → | • →<br>• → | • →<br>• → | • →<br>• → | • →<br>• → | • DC staples<br>• Foot Whirlpool<br>• Foot care<br>• Incision care |
| ACTIVITY | • Ad lib | • Bed rest →<br>• Daily weights →<br>• Sheepskin/Foot-cradle →<br>• Geomatt → | • Slouch sit →<br>• →<br>• →<br>• → | • OOB TID →<br>• Ambulate w/assist<br>• →<br>• →<br>• → | • Ambulate in halls w/assist →<br>• →<br>• →<br>• → | • Ambulate in halls →<br>• →<br>• →<br>• → | • Ad lib<br>→<br>• →<br>• →<br>• → | • →<br>• →<br>• →<br>• → | • Ad lib<br>• Activity tolerance assist<br>• Follow up with surgeon 6 wk |
| CONSULT | • Cardiology<br>• Social Work<br>• PT<br>• Diabetic Coordinator<br>• Dietitian | • Anesthesia | | • PT →<br>• OT (PRN) → | • →<br>• → | • →<br>• → | • →<br>• → | • →<br>• → | • Diabetes Coordinator<br>• Dietary consult |
| DIET | • Low cholesterol<br>• NPO p MN PTA | • NPO | • Clears, advance to regular diet, no concentrated sweets | • Reg → | • → | • → | • → | • → | • Assess compliance |

From The University of Virginia Health Sciences Center, Charlottesville Va. Used with permission.
*TCDB/IS,* Turn, cough, deep breathe, incentive spirometer; *PVRs,* postvoid residuals.

summary of discharge instructions for the patient after vascular surgery is presented in the accompanying Guidelines for Care Box.

## GERONTOLOGICAL CONSIDERATIONS

Most individuals with vascular disease are elderly and have multiple health care needs. The presence of diabetes, coronary heart disease, poor nutrition, and other chronic illnesses and conditions may complicate surgical recovery. Other chronic diseases may also impair the patient's ability to ambulate and meet self-care needs. An acute arterial occlusion is an abrupt emergency situation that is likely to upset the patient's and family's normal patterns of support and interaction. The elderly person's sudden need for significant support and physical assistance can have a tremendous impact on all concerned. The nurse needs to use the multidisciplinary care team to coordinate the patient's care and optimize the patient's discharge and recovery. The patient may need home health care or admission to a rehabilitation facility. Discharge planning for elderly patients needs to be immediate and proactive.

## SPECIAL ENVIRONMENTS FOR CARE

### Critical Care Management

Patients with multiple health problems may need close monitoring in an intensive care unit after vascular surgery. This is particularly true after abdominal and aortic procedures. A 1- to 2-day stay is standard to ensure close monitoring, hemodynamic stability, and successful extubation from ventilator support.

### guidelines for care

#### Discharge Teaching After Bypass Graft Surgery

- Shower daily, cleaning the incision gently with a mild or antibacterial soap without lotion or perfume added. Pat dry. Use a shower chair or stool to prevent falling if any instability is present. Avoid tub baths until healing is complete.
- Monitor the incision daily for signs of infection—redness, swelling, increased pain, discharge, or suture or staple separation. Report any of these symptoms to the surgeon promptly.
- Advance activity gradually as tolerated. Initiate a daily walking regimen. Expect to feel fatigued, and plan for rest periods throughout the day. Avoid lifting anything heavier than 10 pounds until approved by surgeon.
- Resume a low-fat, low-cholesterol diet as tolerated. Use supplements as needed to ensure adequate calories, protein, and vitamin C during the healing period. Four to six small meals a day are often better tolerated than three large ones.
- Avoid constipation and straining at stool. Eat a high-fiber diet with plenty of fluids to avoid constipation. Remain active. Take a stool softener daily plus a bulk-forming laxative if constipation cannot be managed through diet and fluids alone.
- Use prescribed pain medications as needed to ensure adequate rest and activity. Take oral medication with food to prevent gastric irritation.

### Home Care Management

The home is the primary site of postoperative care and recovery for all patients as hospital stays continue to shorten. The needs for discharge teaching have been outlined in the Guidelines Box. The unique needs of the older patient have also been addressed. The nurse needs to be alert to the need for temporary or long-term care and support in the home. Referrals to social services are initiated early in the patient's hospital stay so the patient can be discharged with all needed supports in place.

## COMPLICATIONS

Acute arterial occlusions are serious medical emergencies that can be accompanied by a wide variety of complications. Most of the complications have been discussed during the general care presentation. Bypass surgery is complex and associated with multiple potential complications as well. Many patients have associated chronic health problems that can seriously interfere with their recovery from surgery. Infection, reocclusion, and a wide variety of respiratory, circulatory, and renal complications may occur. Finally, whenever acute or chronic arterial occlusion occurs, the possibility exists that treatment will be ineffective. In these situations the ischemia leads to necrosis and gangrene. Therefore amputation must be considered as one of the potential complications of vascular occlusion. The management of the patient undergoing amputation is discussed on p. 770.

## ANEURYSMS

### Etiology/Epidemiology

Aneurysms are points of weakness, dilation, or outpouching of arteries to at least 1.5 times their normal size.[19] The word *aneurysm* comes from the Greek word *aneurysma* meaning widening. Aneurysms occur most commonly in the aorta, but they can occur in any artery of the body. Other common sites include the femoral and popliteal arteries. Aneurysm disease is the thirteenth leading cause of death in the United States. It is more common in men than women and typically occurs between the ages of 50 and 70.[19] Aneurysms are caused by atherosclerotic disease, trauma, syphilis, congenital abnormalities of the vessel, infection, and connective tissue disorders that cause weakness in the wall of the vessel. Cigarette smoking, hypertension, and a genetic predisposition to aneurysm formation are all linked to the development of aneurysms. The steady aging of the population and better diagnostic tools have increased the frequency with which aneurysms are diagnosed. An estimated 50% of all aneurysms larger than 6 cm in diameter will rupture within 1 year.[19]

### Pathophysiology

The abdominal aorta is the most common site for aneurysm formation. Risk factors that weaken the vessel wall act in combination with the forceful turbulent blood flow in this region to gradually dilate the vessel. The three primary types of aneurysms are illustrated in Figure 27-6. A *fusiform* aneurysm involves a circumferential dilation of the vessel wall and is relatively uniform in shape. A *saccular* aneurysm is a localized outpouching that occurs on just one side of the artery. A narrow neck connects the aneurysm sac to the vessel wall. Saccular aneurysms have a higher incidence of rupture. A *dissecting* aneurysm develops from a tear in the intima of the artery that causes an accumulation of blood in the newly formed cavity between the intima and the media. Dissecting aneurysms are further classified by the type of tear and the degree of hematoma or bleeding. Dissecting aneurysms are strongly associated with arterial hypertension and hemodynamic instability and are most common in the thoracic aorta. The growth rate of aneurysms is unpredictable, but in general the larger the aneurysm, the greater the risk of rupture.

Patients with aneurysms are commonly asymptomatic. Abdominal aneurysms may be felt as a palpable mass, and a systolic bruit may be heard. The patient may complain of abdominal or back pain. If the aneurysm leaks or ruptures, the patient will develop severe pain, signs of shock, decreased red blood cell count, and increased white blood cell count. Symptoms of thoracic aneurysms vary and depend on the size and placement of the aneurysm and its effect on the surrounding structures. Most patients are again asymptomatic. Patients may experience anterior chest wall, back, flank, or abdominal pain or may develop signs of shock if the aneurysm leaks. Symptoms such as dyspnea, cough, and wheezing may develop if the aneurysm puts pressure on the trachea or bronchus.

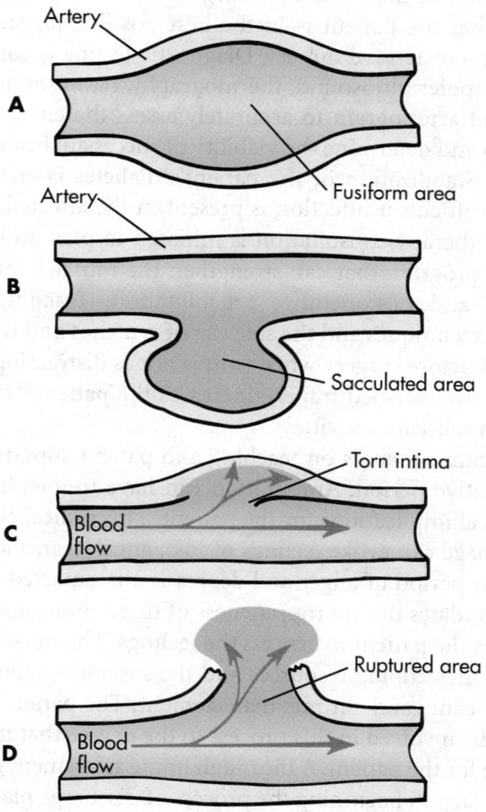

A Artery Fusiform area
B Artery Sacculated area
C Torn intima Blood flow
D Ruptured area Blood flow

**fig. 27-6** Types of aneurysms. **A,** Fusiform. **B,** Saccular. **C,** Dissecting. **D,** Ruptured.

## Collaborative Care Management

Most aneurysms are discovered on routine physical examination or by x-rays. Once the diagnosis is established, the primary therapeutic goal is to prevent aneurysm rupture. The only definitive treatment for an aneurysm is surgical repair, but surgery on the abdominal or thoracic aorta is complex, dangerous, and potentially affects all body systems. The decision to operate is made collaboratively with the patient after a careful workup is completed and all risks and benefits have been discussed. Patients who are symptom free and have small aneurysms may be treated conservatively with careful monitoring. The risk of rupture with aneurysms greater than 6 cm in size outweighs the risks of surgical intervention. Regardless of whether surgery is attempted, maintenance of blood pressure in an optimal range is a high priority of care. Surgical repair involves the use of a synthetic graft to support the weakened area (Figure 27-7). The care of the patient undergoing aneurysm repair surgery is similar to that of patients who undergo vascular bypass surgery as outlined on p. 764.

### *Patient/family education*

The decision regarding whether to undergo surgical repair of the aneurysm is one of the most difficult aspects of patient care. The nurse may play an essential role in helping the patient and family sort through the available data and make an

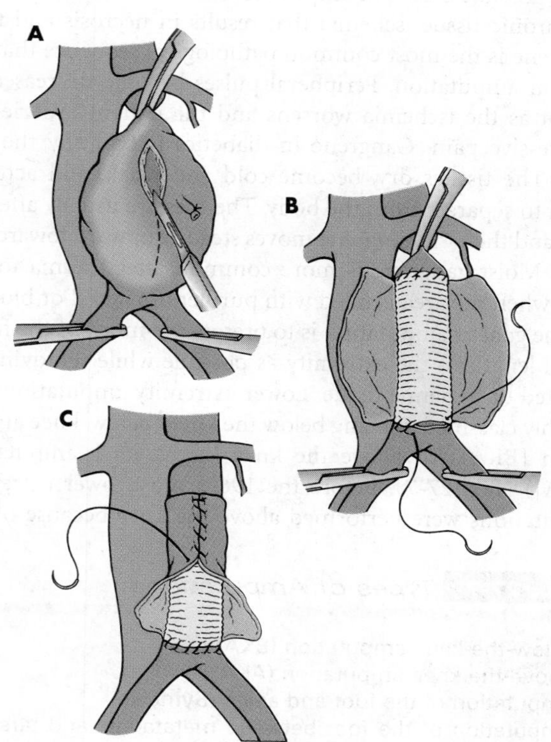


**fig. 27-7** Surgical repair of an abdominal aortic aneurysm. **A,** Incising the aneurysmal sac. **B,** Insertion of synthetic graft. **C,** Suturing native aortic wall over synthetic graft.

informed choice. The nurse helps ensure that the patient's decision is respected and supported. The nurse reinforces the importance of blood pressure control and careful medical follow-up, especially if surgery is not planned. Discharge education for patients undergoing aneurysm repair is similar to that provided to patients after vascular bypass surgery. Teaching highlights are summarized in the Guidelines for Care Box on p. 768.

## NURSING MANAGEMENT OF THE PATIENT UNDERGOING AMPUTATION

Amputation is a surgical intervention commonly used in the treatment of advanced peripheral vascular disease. Amputation is usually considered to be a last resort treatment when other medical and surgical interventions have failed to preserve the limb. Amputation, although radical and traumatic for the patient, can provide relief of chronic pain, the potential to walk again with the use of a prosthesis, and an improved quality of life.

More than 110,000 amputations are performed each year in the United States, and 91.7% of them are lower extremity amputations. Diabetes is the underlying pathology that results in severe peripheral vascular disease in more than 50% of all cases. The rate of amputation is 15 times greater in individuals with diabetes resulting from the effects of coexisting risk factors such as neuropathy and both large and small vessel vascular disease. Birth defects, trauma, and malignancy are other possible causes of amputation.

Chronic tissue ischemia that results in necrosis and then gangrene is the most common pathological sequence that results in amputation. Peripheral pulses become decreased or absent as the ischemia worsens and the patient experiences progressive pain. Gangrene in diabetics is typically the dry type. The tissues dry, become cold and black, and actually begin to separate from the body. The toes are usually affected first, and then the gangrene moves steadily upward toward the knee. Moist gangrene is more common after trauma to the limb when the area is filled with purulent material or blood.[4]

The goal of amputation is to preserve as much of the functional length of the extremity as possible while removing all infected or ischemic tissue. Lower extremity amputations are roughly classified as being below the knee (below-knee amputation [BKA]) or above the knee (above-knee amputation [AKA]) (Box 27-7). Before the 1960s most lower extremity amputations were performed above the knee because of the greater chance for successful wound healing. As diagnostic testing has improved, clinicians are able to more accurately assess the adequacy of perfusion to the extremity. This enables BKAs to be performed more frequently and with greater success.[4] Below-knee amputations preserve the knee joint, which allows the patient an increased range of motion and improves the likelihood of successful prosthesis fitting after surgery. A BKA is usually made at the lower third of the leg, leaving a 12 to 18 cm stump. An AKA can be made at any level, although a longer stump makes it easier to fit a prosthesis.

**box 27-7** *Types of Amputations*

- Below-the-knee amputation (BKA)
- Above-the-knee amputation (AKA)
- Amputation of the foot and ankle (Syme's)
- Amputation of the foot between metatarsus and tarsus (Hey's or Lisfranc's)
- Hip disarticulation—removal of the limb from the hip joint
- Hemicorporectomy—removal of half of the body from the pelvis and lumbar areas

The two major techniques for amputation are closed and open. With the closed method the bone is cut approximately 2 inches shorter than the skin flap. This creates a stump that is suitable for weight bearing with a prosthesis. The incision is closed with sutures in a posterior position so the suture line will not be positioned in a weight-bearing area. This reduces the chances of irritation from the prosthesis. Drains are inserted to prevent excessive swelling and to allow for the drainage of old blood, fluid, and infectious matter.[4] The open amputation is used most commonly when infection is present in the limb. The bone and muscle are cut at the same level, and the wound is left open to allow for drainage. Wound closure is usually achieved at a future point through a second surgical procedure.

### PREOPERATIVE CARE

The preoperative period focuses on the careful evaluation and preparation of the patient for surgery. The medical goal is to ensure that the patient is in the best possible physical state to undergo extensive surgery. Diagnostic testing is completed using Doppler ultrasound, thermography, radioisotope clearance, and arteriogram to accurately assess the circulation to the limb and determine the viability of successful healing after surgery. Stabilization of the patient's diabetes is critical but may be difficult if infection is present in the affected limb. A physical therapy consultation is initiated to plan an effective exercise program that can strengthen the muscles for crutch walking and postoperative rehabilitation. Teaching about transfer techniques and the safe use of crutches and walkers is initiated before surgery when pain is not as distracting for the patient. An over-bed trapeze increases the patient's independence in self-care activities.

The nurse focuses on teaching and patient support in the preoperative period. Amputation can have tremendous psychological implications for the patient. This radical change in body image can evoke feelings of loss, anger, fear, shock, and denial. A period of anger and depression is expected, and the nurse validates the appropriateness of these emotions and encourages the patient to express the feelings. The nurse assesses the patient's coping resources and the support systems available for acute and chronic management. The patient's family should be involved in this process to the degree that it is comfortable for the patient. A thorough home assessment is an important step in beginning the process of discharge planning.

Preoperative teaching emphasizes care that will be delivered in the postoperative period, pain management strategies, plans for prosthesis fitting, and a basic introduction to stump care routines. The patient should be told to anticipate the occurrence of phantom limb sensation, a sensation of aching, tingling, itching, or simple "awareness" of the amputated part. Phantom limb sensation is an expected but still extremely disconcerting aspect of amputation. The sensations typically decrease over time but initially can be quite strong. If chronic pain had been present in the extremity, the patient must also be taught about the possibility of phantom limb pain. Phantom limb pain is similar to the pain experienced before surgery and represents a complex management problem. Phantom sensation occurs in most patients, but fortunately phantom pain is much less common.

## POSTOPERATIVE CARE

### Maintaining Physiological Stability

Monitoring for complications is an important aspect of initial postoperative nursing care. Vital signs and pulse oximetry are closely monitored until the patient stabilizes. The wound dressing and drainage systems are assessed at least every 2 hours to monitor for excessive bleeding because hemorrhage is the primary immediate complication of amputation. A surgical tourniquet may be kept available at the bedside for emergency use. Some serosanguineous drainage is expected, but the appearance of bright red blood should be reported immediately. Tachycardia and hypotension are classic indicators of bleeding. The stump dressing is not usually disturbed for the first 2 to 3 days, but the nurse assesses the operative site as thoroughly as possible. Careful intake and output records are maintained, as well as flow rates for all IVs. Respiratory care and assessment are also critical. The patient is encouraged to begin deep breathing, position changes, and coughing as needed to clear the airway, as soon as he or she is alert. Effective pain management is a critical intervention because severe pain can adversely affect the patient's vital signs, decrease the ability to deep breathe and clear the airway, and compromise the patient's ability to participate in self-care.

### Maintaining Appropriate Stump Positioning

The stump is placed on pillows to reduce postoperative pain and swelling for the first 24 hours. Stump positioning and exercise become critical interventions after this initial period. The stump is supported but not elevated because of the risk of flexion contractures. The flexor muscles in the extremities are stronger than the opposing extensors, and the patient needs to counteract the flexion pull effectively if hip and knee contractures are to be prevented. Position changes are made at least every 2 hours, and the patient is encouraged to lie prone for at least 20 to 30 minutes twice a day to stretch the hip flexor muscles. Positioning is also used to prevent both the abducted and adducted position. Any change in normal hip alignment makes it difficult for the patient to achieve an acceptable prosthesis fit and normal gait. The patient continues to work with the physical therapist to build strength in the muscles needed for ambulation and is encouraged to be out of bed for increasing intervals each day.

### Conditioning the Stump

Stump care is a critical nursing intervention in the early postoperative period, and it remains a major management concern throughout the healing and rehabilitation period. Some surgeons apply an immediate temporary prosthesis after amputation. These devices are composed of a rigid plastic bandage that is applied around the closed stump and attached to a prosthetic pylon with an ankle and foot assembly. The device is applied in the operating room while the patient is still anesthetized. Its main advantages are the potential for early weight bearing and the reduction of edema. The major disadvantage is the inability to directly assess wound healing in the stump. If delayed prosthesis fitting is planned, the stump is initially wrapped snugly in dressings and Ace wraps to provide compression and minimize the accumulation of edema.

Proper stump bandaging supports the shaping of the stump for eventual prosthesis fitting and weight bearing. This compression bandaging is worn at all times, except for needed skin care, and needs to be correctly reapplied whenever it becomes loose or wrinkled. The shrinker bandage is typically reapplied at least daily, and the nurse teaches the patient how to correctly apply the bandage as soon as possible. The bandages need to be washed and changed regularly, and the nurse instructs the patient in the importance of keeping these wrappings clean and intact. Figure 27-8 illustrates the correct method of applying compression or shrinker bandages to above-knee and below-knee amputations.

Daily stump care is also part of the conditioning process. The healing of the incision is closely monitored, and the patient is instructed to carefully assess the stump each day for signs of redness or irritation. The stump should be washed daily after healing is complete and thoroughly air dried before rewrapping. No lotion, oil, or powder should be applied to the stump surface without specific orders from the health care provider or rehabilitation specialist. The goal is to achieve a well-healed and appropriately shaped stump whose surface skin is tough enough to absorb the pressures of weight bearing with a prosthesis.

### Supporting Independence in Self-Care

The physical therapist continues to work with the patient on range of motion, ambulation with an assistive device, and general conditioning. Building upper body strength, particularly triceps strength, is emphasized because these muscles are critical to crutch walking. The therapist teaches the patient the principles of safe transferring, and this skill is practiced on the unit under the nurse's supervision. The loss of the weight of the amputated limb can significantly alter the patient's center of gravity, and the nurse needs to be alert and provide support for the patient while she or he is relearning upright balance. A fall can have serious adverse consequences on wound healing.

### Patient/Family Education

Hospitalizations for all conditions are being continually shortened, and planning for discharge needs to begin before surgery. The nurse needs to create a teaching plan that includes time for the patient to learn stump care, transfer techniques, safe ambulation, prevention of complications and contractures, and the importance of follow-up care from the multidisciplinary care team. Referral to a prosthetist may not occur until after discharge, and achieving a good prosthetic fit can take as much as 2 years because the healing stump

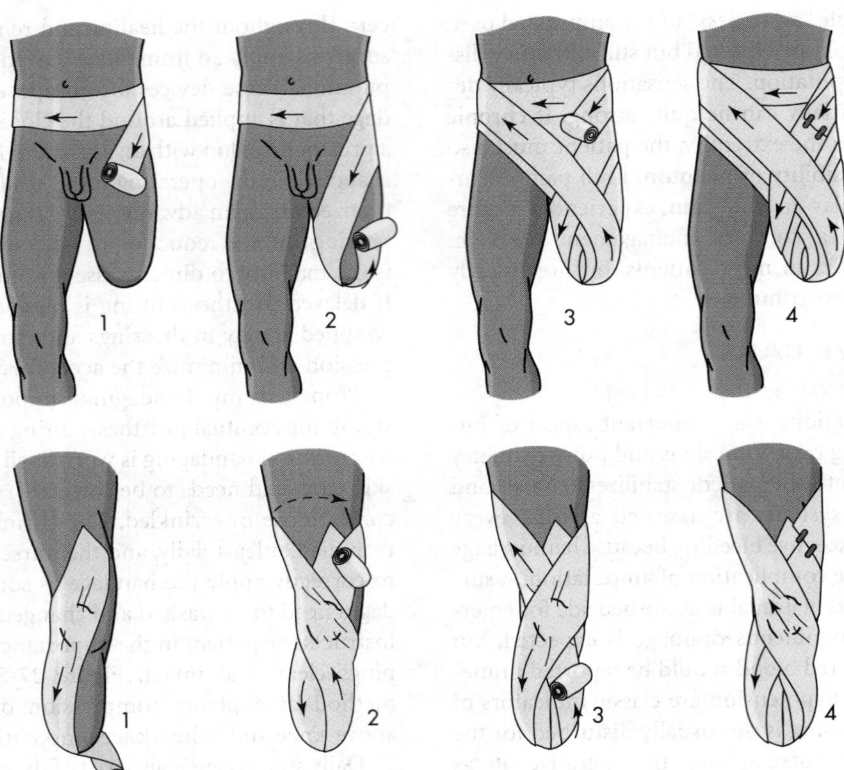

**fig. 27-8** *Top,* Correct method for bandaging midthigh amputation stump. Note that bandage must be anchored around patient's waist. *Bottom,* Correct method for bandaging midcalf amputation stump. Note that bandage need not be anchored around the waist.

**guidelines for care**

**The Person After an Amputation**

- Assess stump and monitor drainage for color and amount; report signs of increased drainage.
- Position patient with no flexion at hip or knee to avoid contractures; encourage prone position.
- Maintain patient in low-Fowler's or flat position after AKA.
- Support stump with pillow for first 24 hours (according to physician preference and avoiding flexion); place rolled bath blanket along outer aspect to prevent external rotation.
- Encourage exercises to prevent thromboembolism:
  - Active ROM of unaffected leg, ankle rotations and pumps
  - Use of overhead trapeze when moving in bed
  - Push-ups from sitting position in bed
  - Quadriceps sets (see Chapter 18)
  - Lifting stump and buttocks off bed while lying flat on back to strengthen abdominal muscles
- Teach care of stump.
  - Inspect for redness, blister, and abrasions.
  - Wash stump with mild soap, rinse with water, and pat dry.
  - Avoid use of alcohol, oils, and creams.
  - Remove stump bandage or stump sock and reapply as needed; use firm smooth figure-of-8 Ace wrapping (Figure 27-8) to reduce swelling and shape stump (if rigid dressing not used).
- Encourage patient to ambulate using correct crutch-walking technique.
  - Keep elbows extended; limit elbow flexion to 30 degrees or less.
  - Avoid pressure on axilla.
  - Bear weight on palms of hands, not on axilla.
  - Maintain upright posture (head up, chest up, abdomen in, pelvis in, foot straight).
- Monitor patient's ability to use a prosthesis.

continues to shrink and alter in shape. The process is slow and often frustrating, and the nurse needs to help the patient and family anticipate the long-term nature of the rehabilitation period. Guidelines for care of the patient after amputation are presented in the accompanying box. A Nursing Care Plan for a patient with a lower extremity amputation is found on p. 773.

## GERONTOLOGICAL CONSIDERATIONS

Lower limb amputations are commonly performed on older patients. The patient's previous ability to ambulate and engage in self-care will profoundly affect the ability to make a successful transition to independence after amputation. Use of a prosthesis for ambulation requires strength and energy. If the elder is already weakened from the presence of other

## nursing care plan Person Undergoing Amputation

**DATA** Mr. Lopez is a 68-year-old Hispanic man who has a long history of non–insulin-dependent diabetes, hypertension, and peripheral vascular disease. He has been experiencing progressively increasing levels of claudication in his right leg over the past 6 months. He is unable to walk across a room without pain and has begun experiencing rest pain at night, which forces him to get out of bed and put his legs in a dependent position. One month ago he developed an ulcer on his great toe that progressed to gangrene despite aggressive treatment. He was admitted yesterday and underwent a right below-the-knee amputation.

Mr. Lopez tolerated surgery well, although both he and his wife indicate that the idea of the amputation is terrifying and he is concerned about becoming disabled and a burden to his family. Mrs. Lopez is particularly distraught but is afraid to let her husband see her concerns. He has Medicare, but no supplemental insurance. Mrs. Lopez is still employed and is concerned that no one will be able to help Mr. Lopez at home after discharge.

His current care routines include the following:

- Out of bed to chair with assistance
- Patient-controlled analgesia with morphine for pain, basal administration plus bolus
- Elevate stump when out of bed; avoid use of pillows under stump when in bed
- Monitor stump for edema, bleeding; evaluate Hemovac drainage every shift
- Accuchecks per routine with sliding-scale insulin coverage as needed
- Physical therapy referral for evaluation for crutchwalking

**NURSING DIAGNOSIS** *Grieving related to loss of limb*

| expected patient outcome | nursing interventions | rationale |
|---|---|---|
| Expresses grief.<br>Verbalizes plan for resocialization. | Assess significance of loss to patient and family.<br>Encourage patient to verbalize feelings.<br>Acknowledge grief and provide support to patient and family.<br>Allow privacy for expression of grief.<br>Consult Clinical Nurse Specialist (CNS) in psychiatry, support group, or rehabilitated amputee for patient counseling. | Effective support and resolution of the grieving process are necessary for the patient to successfully cope with needed lifestyle adjustments and changes. |

**NURSING DIAGNOSIS** *Pain related to tissue trauma and phantom limb sensation*

| expected patient outcome | nursing interventions | rationale |
|---|---|---|
| Verbalizes relief of stump pain.<br>Describes phantom sensations and pain and methods to manage. | Monitor character, intensity, and location of pain.<br>Administer analgesics to maintain comfort.<br>Explain the causes of phantom pain and sensations and methods to treat.<br>Instruct patient on effective use of analgesics and comfort measures. | Pain control is essential to optimal physical therapy training and rehabilitation. |

**NURSING DIAGNOSIS** *Impaired physical mobility related to inadequate crutch walking skill and endurance*

| expected patient outcome | nursing interventions | rationale |
|---|---|---|
| Maintains safe ambulation or mobility with prosthesis or assistive device.<br>Does not develop contractures. | Assess upper extremity strength and cardiopulmonary status and endurance.<br>Assess previous mobility status.<br>Teach ROM and strengthening exercises.<br>Teach positioning and exercises to prevent flexion and abduction contractures.<br>Dangle or up to chair 12-24 hr after surgery.<br>Teach purpose of exercises and interventions. | Upper body strength and optimal conditioning are essential to achieve mobility and perform bed-to-chair transfers.<br>Contractures will prevent proper fitting of a prosthesis and thus limit rehabilitation progress. |

*Continued*

## Person Undergoing Amputation—cont'd

**NURSING DIAGNOSIS** *Impaired skin integrity related to incision and effects of diabetes on wound healing*

| expected patient outcome | nursing interventions | rationale |
|---|---|---|
| Wound heals without infection.<br>Verbalizes and demonstrates actions to maintain integrity of stump. | Assess stump for drainage or bleeding, edema, proximal pulses, and tissue perfusion.<br>Maintain dressing without wrinkles or constriction.<br>Instruct on stump care and hygiene and prosthesis care if indicated.<br>Instruct on signs and symptoms of decreased perfusion to stump.<br>Perform Accuchecks before each meal and at bedtime | Adequate perfusion is necessary for wound healing.<br>Wound healing must be complete for optimal fitting and use of prosthesis.<br>Stress of surgery and infection can result in severe hyperglycemia |

**NURSING DIAGNOSIS** *Self-esteem disturbance related to limb loss and change in functional abilities*

| expected patient outcome | nursing interventions | rationale |
|---|---|---|
| Discusses change in feelings about self.<br>Develops confidence in ability to accomplish goals (physical, social, emotional).<br>Identifies two positive characteristics. | Assess patient's view of self and role relationships.<br>Encourage expression of feelings about self.<br>Assess significant other's view of loss.<br>Clarify misconceptions regarding perception of self:<br>**a.** Encourage open communication between significant other and patient.<br>**b.** Provide information regarding treatment and prognosis<br>**c.** Promote social interaction.<br>**d.** Encourage self-care of stump.<br>Facilitate use of prosthesis as soon as possible.<br>Assist patient to identify personal strengths.<br>Make referrals for counseling and assistance as necessary. | Increased mobility and ability for self-care will foster independence and positive self-esteem. |

debilitating health problems, it may not be possible to fit a prosthesis even if the stump heals adequately. Wheelchair mobility may be a more realistic option. Most elders also require at least short-term admission to a rehabilitation facility after discharge from the hospital to continue with needed therapy.

## SPECIAL ENVIRONMENTS FOR CARE

### Critical Care Management

Patients who undergo lower extremity amputation usually do not require postoperative management in a critical care unit unless serious complications develop. After the initial stabilization and recovery from anesthesia in the postanesthesia care unit, the patient returns to the general surgical floor.

### Home Care Management

Patients are not able to complete their recovery and rehabilitation in the acute care setting. Therefore planning for ongoing management and rehabilitation after discharge is an important consideration that needs to be addressed early in the hospitalization. The degree and duration of support needed by the patient are determined by age, baseline health status, financial and social resources, and living situation. The nurse is responsible for initiating the careful assessment of these variables and then making referrals as indicated through social services, home health agencies, and community physical therapy to ensure that the patient receives all needed support. The family is involved in all planning if possible because significant modifications may need to be considered or implemented in the home environment to accommodate the patient's mobility limitations and establish a safe environment. An occupational therapist can often assist with this needed planning.

## VENOUS DISORDERS

The most common venous disorders result from incompetent valves in the veins and obstructions of venous return to the heart, usually as a result of a thrombus.

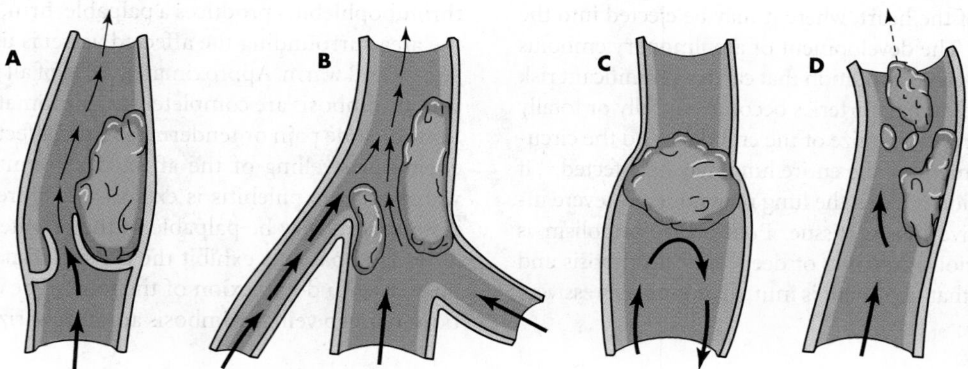


fig. 27-9 Development of deep vein thrombosis with arrows indicating direction of blood flow. A, Thrombus in a valve pocket of a deep vein with blood flowing beside thrombus. B, Thrombi tend to form at bifurcations of deep veins with some slowing of blood flow. C, Complete occlusion of the vein by a thrombus forcing backflow of blood. D, An embolus that has broken off from a thrombus and is floating in the bloodstream could migrate to the lungs and cause pulmonary embolus.

## DEEP VEIN THROMBOSIS

### Etiology

A variety of different terms are used to describe the disorder that results from the formation of a thrombus within a vein (Figure 27-9). The term *phlebothrombosis* refers to the actual process of clot formation. Thrombus formation is commonly accompanied by some degree of vein wall inflammation, and the terms *phlebitis* and *thrombophlebitis* are used to reflect this inflammation.[7] Thrombus formation occurs in either the superficial or deep veins of the body. Superficial thrombophlebitis occurs in the majority of patients receiving IV therapy. Deep vein thrombosis is more serious, often necessitates hospitalization, and carries the risk of potentially fatal embolization.[7]

Venous thrombosis typically results from at least one element of Virchow's triad: venous stasis, damage to the endothelial lining of the vein, and hypercoagulopathy. Venous return to the heart is supported by the action of the vein valves along with the rhythmic contractions of the muscles in the extremities, which compress the veins and help move the blood toward the heart. Any period of relative or partial inactivity or immobility, such as prolonged sitting, surgery, or bedrest, impairs venous return. A decrease in muscle tone and activity in the legs causes pooling and venous distention. The distention causes minor damage to the endothelial lining of the veins and valves, and platelets are attracted to the site.[20] This can result in the development of a thrombus. The presence of IV catheters, central lines, and pacemaker wires and the irritation of drugs and IV solutions can contribute to endothelial damage. Any increase in viscosity or hypercoagulability of the blood increases the likelihood of thrombus formation. Dehydration, pregnancy, clotting disorders, sickle cell anemia, malignancy, polycythemia, systemic lupus erythematosus, and oral contraceptive use can all contribute to the subtle alteration in coagulability that results in thrombus formation. The presence of atherosclerosis and varicosities also increases the risk. Risk factors for deep vein thrombosis are summarized in the accompanying box.

**risk factors**

**Deep Vein Thrombosis**

- Age—the elderly typically have a number of risk factors, which increases the incidence of DVT in this population
- Gender—DVT occurs more often in women
- Positive history of thromboses
- Immobility/stasis
  - Surgery, bed rest, paralysis
  - Prolonged sitting (automobile or air travel)
  - Obesity and pregnancy
- Increased viscosity
  - Dehydration, fever
  - Polycythemia
- Intimal damage
  - Central and peripheral IV catheters, pacemaker wires
  - IV drug abuse
- Associated conditions/disorders
  - Malignancy
  - Varicose veins
  - Inherited coagulation disorders
  - Hemolytic anemias (sickle cell anemia)
- Trauma
  - Fractures, especially involving the pelvis and long bones
  - Burns
- Use of oral contraceptives (risk is primarily related to estrogen content)
- Chronic lung and heart disease

Most thrombi form in the veins of the pelvis and lower extremities, but they can also form in the vessels of the upper extremities and those leading directly to the heart. A venous thrombus that becomes dislodged is called an embolus. An embolus can travel from the site where it formed through the larger veins and into the right side of the heart, where it may be ejected into the pulmonary arteries. The development of a pulmonary embolus is an extremely dangerous condition that carries a significant risk of mortality. The pulmonary arteries become partially or totally obstructed depending on the size of the embolus, and the circulation to a lung segment or the entire lung may be affected.[20] If the area of obstruction is large, the lung may undergo severe infarction with massive loss of tissue. Pulmonary embolism is clearly the most serious outcome of deep vein thrombosis and is the major reason that treatment is immediate and aggressive.

## Epidemiology

Deep vein thrombosis develops in a significant number of people, both in the hospital and the community setting. Deep vein thrombosis is more common in women and the elderly. No racial prevalence has been identified. More than 300,000 persons are admitted for treatment of deep vein thrombosis each year, and many other asymptomatic cases are believed to go undiagnosed.[7] As many as 50% of patients with deep vein thrombosis will develop pulmonary emboli, and approximately 50,000 die from pulmonary emboli each year.[7] The link with deep vein thrombosis is clear because an estimated 90% of pulmonary emboli begin as thrombi in the lower extremities, usually in the popliteal, femoral, and pelvic veins. Few calf thromboses result in emboli.

## Pathophysiology

Thrombi develop from platelets, fibrin, and both red and white blood cells. They typically form in areas where the blood flow is slow or turbulent. The major elements of stasis, increased coagulability, and intimal damage dramatically accelerate the process. Muscle spasm and changes in the intravascular pressure can cause the developing thrombus to dislodge and move toward the heart and lungs. The lungs are rich in heparin and plasmin activators and can effectively dissolve some thrombi. However, if the thrombus is not successfully dissolved, it can lodge in an artery and obstruct perfusion to the lung segment. Pulmonary emboli are further discussed in Chapter 32.[32]

The clinical manifestations of deep vein thrombosis vary substantially according to the size and location of the thrombus and the adequacy of the collateral circulation. Superficial thrombophlebitis produces a palpable, firm, cordlike vein, and the area surrounding the affected vessel is usually tender, reddened, and warm. Approximately 50% of all patients with deep vein thrombosis are completely asymptomatic. Possible symptoms include pain or tenderness in the affected area, unilateral edema or swelling of the affected extremity, and redness or warmth if the phlebitis is extensive (Figure 27-10). A tender venous cord may be palpable in the popliteal fossa. Less than 20% of all patients exhibit the classic Homans' sign (calf tenderness with dorsiflexion of the foot). The clinical manifestations of deep vein thrombosis are summarized in Box 27-8.

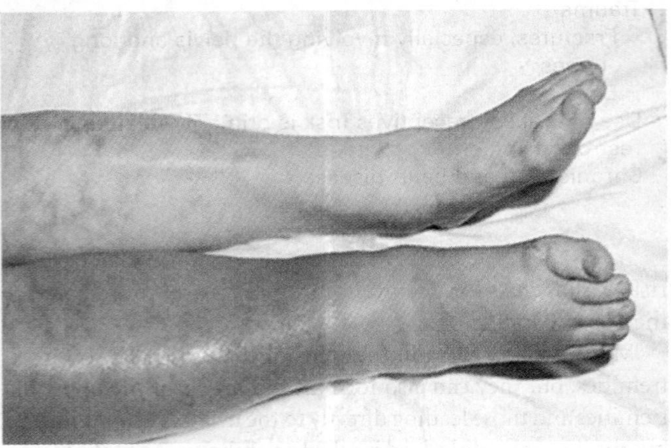

**fig. 27-10** Deep vein thrombosis.

## Collaborative Care Management

### Diagnostic tests

The venogram is the gold standard for the diagnosis of deep vein thrombosis, but even this test is not completely accurate.[9] It may identify filling defects in the vein that can be mistaken for deep vein thrombosis. Venogram is more accurate with peripheral thrombi and is less effective in diagnosing pelvic, renal, or vena caval thrombi. In addition the test is, in itself, irritating to the veins and can trigger phlebitis and thrombus formation. Radiolabeled fibrinogen scans may also be used in diagnosis. The fibrinogen becomes visible at the site of the thrombosis, but there is a lag time of 24 to 36 hours before the fibrinogen reaches the thrombus.

Noninvasive testing with impedance plethysmography and ultrasonography is being increasingly used. Plethysmography measures changes in electrical resistance to blood flow (see Chapter 24), and ultrasonography evaluates the sound of blood flowing through the veins. Duplex scanning combines traditional Doppler scanning with B-mode ultrasonography, which determines the compressibility of the vein.[9] A deep vein thrombosis renders the vein noncompressible. D-dimer testing is also being combined with plethysmography. This newer agglutination assay blood test uses venous blood from a finger stick or venipuncture to assess the degree of agglutination occurring.

### Medications

Drug therapy plays a major role in both the prevention and treatment of deep vein thrombosis. Low-dose heparin is ad-

**box 27-8** *clinical manifestations*

**Deep Vein Thrombosis**

NOTE: Approximately 50% of all patients are asymptomatic.

- Local pain or tenderness
- Unilateral edema or swelling
  - May be bilateral if DVT is located in the vena cava
- Local warmth, redness
- Mild fever
- Tender, palpable venous cord in the popliteal fossa
- Fewer than 20% of all patients with DVT have a positive Homans' sign.

ministered subcutaneously for prevention in doses of about 5000 units every 12 hours. Intravenous dextran may be given to decrease venous stasis and platelet adhesion. Patients at high risk for deep vein thrombosis may also receive low-molecular-weight heparin (LMWH) for both prevention and treatment.[2] Examples of LMWHs are enoxaparin, tinzaparin, and nardroparin. They are administered subcutaneously, do not require blood coagulation monitoring, and can be used as a long-term preventive measure in the home environment.[33] (See the Research Box.)

Heparin is ordered in full anticoagulation doses and administered intravenously once an existing thrombus is identified. The goal of drug therapy is to prevent new clots from forming and prevent the extension or growth of the existing thrombus. Heparin does not dissolve existing thrombi, but it does block the conversion of fibrinogen to fibrin.[28] An initial bolus dose of heparin is administered and then maintained by continuous infusion. Recent studies have indicated that therapeutic levels can be achieved most effectively when the dosage of heparin is calculated by the patient's body weight.[33] A standard protocol calls for the administration of a bolus dose of 75 to 100 U/kg followed by a continuous infusion of 18 U/kg/hr for at least 5 days.[31] Partial thromboplastin times (PTTs) are monitored regularly throughout therapy.

Bleeding is the major adverse consequence of heparin administration, although thrombocytopenia also occurs. The platelet count is therefore monitored throughout therapy. Heparin-induced thrombocytopenia (HITT), or white clot syndrome, is diagnosed when the platelet count falls below 100,000 or falls more than 50% from the onset of therapy. This serious complication of heparin therapy occurs in 5% to 10% of patients receiving heparin and can result in life-threatening thrombosis in either the arteries or the veins.[28] Heparin therapy is discontinued and the effects of the drug are reversed through the administration of protamine sulfate. Plasmapheresis is used to remove the thrombi. The LMWH alternatives appear to have a lower associated incidence of HITT.

Oral anticoagulation with warfarin (Coumadin) is initiated along with the heparin therapy to prevent the recurrence of thrombi. There is little consensus about when Coumadin therapy should be started. Because Coumadin takes several days to reach a therapeutic concentration, some authorities recommend starting it immediately. Others advocate beginning Coumadin administration after 3 days of heparin therapy. A standard beginning dose of 5 to 10 mg is administered and is then gradually adjusted until a therapeutic international normalized ratio (INR) of 2.0 to 3.0 is achieved. Coumadin therapy is usually continued for at least 6 months after an initial episode of thrombosis.

Thrombolytic therapy with streptokinase, urokinase, or tissue plasminogen activator is also used to treat deep vein thrombosis and pulmonary embolus. These agents activate the conversion of plasminogen to plasmin and actively dissolve existing thrombi. Thrombi in the veins of the lower extremities are usually older and larger than those that cause acute arterial occlusions and may not respond as well to the use of thrombolytics.

**research**

Reference: Levine M et al: A comparison of low molecular weight heparin administered primarily at home with unfractionated heparin administered in the hospital for proximal deep vein thrombosis, *N Engl J Med* 334(11): 677, 1996.

This study explored the treatment of deep vein thrombosis in two groups of patients. Approximately 250 persons were assigned to each group. One group received standard DVT treatment, including a 5- to 7-day course of intravenous heparin in a hospital setting, and the other group received treatment with subcutaneous low-molecular-weight heparin (enoxaparin), primarily in the home setting. Both groups underwent baseline plethysmography at the beginning of treatment. Both groups were started on oral Coumadin on day 2 and switched to Coumadin management as soon as their INR ratios were within the therapeutic range, usually after about 5 days.

The study demonstrated that enoxaparin was a safe and effective method of treating patients with DVT in the home setting. The rates of recurrent thromboembolism and major bleeding were the same for both groups. The associated costs for the patients treated in the home setting were obviously much lower.

### Treatments

Many patients are admitted to hospitals for minor procedures or treatments and develop a deep vein thrombosis or pulmonary embolus secondary to immobility. Therefore, several preventive treatment measures are in common use. Preventive treatments include the use of antiembolic stockings, graduated compression stockings (GCS), and external pneumatic compression (EPC) sleeves. The purpose of each of these devices is to increase the venous return from the lower extremities and prevent venous stasis.

Graduated compression stockings apply different degrees of compression to different parts of the legs. The highest degree of compression is applied at the ankle. The pressure is recorded as 100% at the ankle and then decreases to 70% compression at midcalf and 40% at midthigh.[20] Pneumatic compression devices consist of soft plastic sleeves that are applied to the legs. The sleeves are attached to an air pump that regulates the flow of air into the sleeves. This provides gentle intermittent compression by inflating and deflating the sleeves at regular intervals to stimulate venous return (Figure 27-11). Both GCS and EPC devices are contraindicated in patients with arterial disease, severe edema, phlebitis, leg fractures, or skin breakdown. Early ambulation remains the most effective preventive measure.

### Surgical Management

Surgery does not play a major role in the acute management of a deep vein thrombosis, although removal of the thrombus via thrombectomy may be performed when the circulation of the extremity is compromised. Surgical

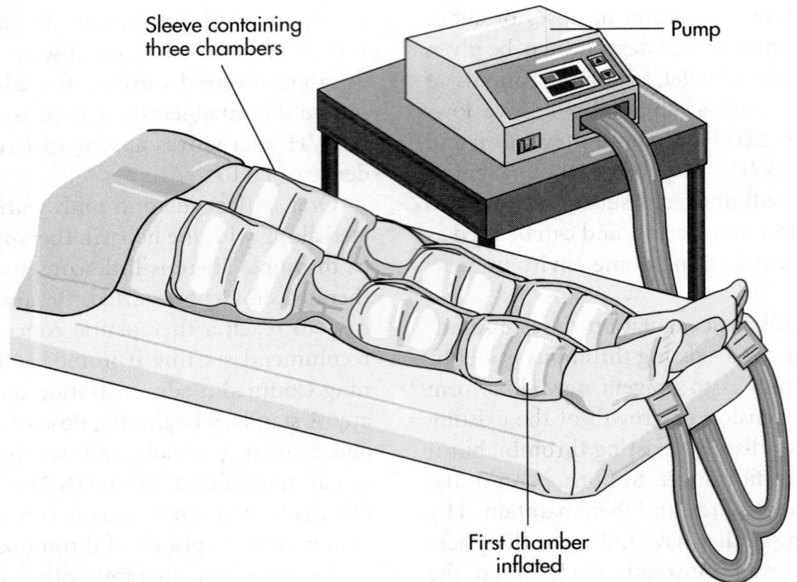


fig. 27-11 Sequential pneumatic compression device. The three-chambered sleeve is connected to a pump that delivers 45 to 60 mm Hg of pressure sequentially to the first, second, and third chambers. The cycle ends with the deflation of all three chambers and begins again.

intervention may be used, however, for patients at risk for recurrent deep vein thrombosis and pulmonary emboli and those who do not respond well to anticoagulant therapy. The primary surgical option is a transvenous filtration device placed in the vena cava to trap emboli before they reach the heart and pulmonary vessels.[27] Two types are currently in use: the Greenfield filter and the bird's nest filter. The Greenfield filter (Figure 27-12) can be inserted surgically or through interventional radiology. The filter is inserted through an incision in the jugular or femoral vein and then advanced to the superior vena cava for placement. The bird's nest filter is a web of stainless steel wires that intercept and trap emboli. It is inserted percutaneously through the femoral vein or occasionally through the subclavian or jugular veins. Both filters are permanently implanted and rarely become dislodged or occluded.[27] Guidelines for care of the patient with a vena cava filter are summarized in the accompanying box.

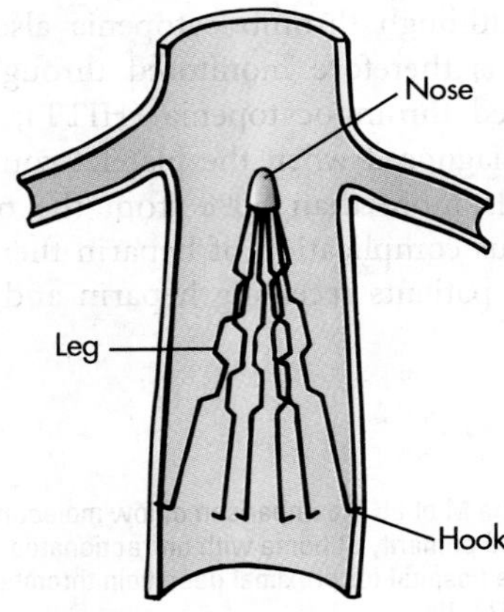


fig. 27-12 Greenfield filter placed in the vena cava.

### Diet

There are no dietary restrictions for a person with a deep vein thrombosis. Patients receiving Coumadin need to restrict their intake of foods high in vitamin K because the vitamin acts as an antidote to the action of Coumadin and can disrupt its therapeutic blood level. Obese patients may also be advised to attempt to achieve a more optimal body weight.

### Activity

Patients with deep vein thrombosis on heparin therapy have traditionally been restricted to bedrest for 5 to 7 days while therapeutic blood levels of heparin were being established. With weight-based heparin dosing, therapeutic levels are achieved within 24 hours and the patient is then permitted to ambulate as tolerated. If severe edema or pain is present in the extremity, the patient is kept on bedrest with the leg elevated.

### Referrals

Patients who will receive long-term oral anticoagulation with Coumadin may need referral to a home health agency for follow-up blood drawing and assessment for complications related to recurrent thrombi, pulmonary emboli, or medication side effects. Home health referral is particularly appropriate for elderly patients, who may have restricted mobility, live alone, suffer visual or other sensory impairments, or be on multiple drug protocols for other chronic health problems. Advanced practice nurses are commonly responsible for managing anticoagulation clinics, and their services and expertise should be consulted as indicated.

**guidelines for care**

**The Patient with a Vena Caval Filter**

- Assess venipuncture site for signs of bleeding or infection. Maintain an adhesive covering over the insertion site.
- Immobilize the extremity after the procedure per institution protocol or physician's order.
- Assess peripheral pulses, temperature, color, and sensation in affected extremity per protocol. Assess for pain and presence of positive Homans' sign.
- Assess respiratory status and monitor pulse oximetry or blood gases as indicated. Position in partial or high Fowler's position.
- Implement bleeding precautions and associated safety measures if systemic anticoagulation is to be continued. Monitor appropriate laboratory test results (e.g., PTT, platelets, Hgb, Hct, INR).
- Teach the patient to monitor for signs of infection at insertion site; signs of systemic bleeding (e.g., blood in urine, stool, gums; nosebleeds; easy bruising); bleeding precautions for home use if anticoagulation is to be continued (e.g., use of soft toothbrush, electric razor, stool softeners); symptoms to report to health care provider (bleeding and infection; DVT, pulmonary embolism—swelling and warmth in extremity; sudden chest pain, dyspnea, tachypnea, restlessness; filter occlusion—localized pain, venous stasis or swelling, unusual symptoms).

## NURSING MANAGEMENT

### ASSESSMENT

#### Subjective Data

Subjective data to be collected to assess the patient with deep vein thrombosis include:

Pain or tenderness in calf or thigh muscle at rest or with exercise
Tenderness over affected area with palpation
Previous history of deep vein thrombosis
Significant risk factors—female, advancing age, prolonged sitting or immobility (see the Risk Factors box on page 775 for complete list)
Sudden onset of chest pain, dyspnea, or tachypnea, which may indicate pulmonary embolus

#### Objective Data

Objective data to be collected to assess the patient with deep vein thrombosis include:

Unilateral or bilateral extremity edema
Increase in circumference over affected area
Warmth or redness over affected area
Abrupt pain on attempted dorsiflexion of the foot
Engorgement of collateral veins in affected area
Positive results from Doppler ultrasonography, venography, or plethysmography

### NURSING DIAGNOSES

Nursing diagnoses are determined from analysis of patient data. Nursing diagnoses for the patient with deep vein thrombosis may include but are not limited to:

| Diagnostic Title | Possible Etiological Factors |
|---|---|
| Tissue perfusion, altered peripheral | Decreased venous blood flow, immobility |
| Pain: leg | Inflammation, edema, venous stasis |
| Knowledge deficit: pharmacotherapy, support stockings, surgery | Lack of exposure/recall, unfamiliarity with information sources |

### EXPECTED PATIENT OUTCOMES

Expected patient outcomes for the patient with deep vein thrombosis may include but are not limited to:

1. Has adequate circulation to lower extremity: palpable distal pulses and warm, pink extremity
2. Shows signs of decreased pain: states feeling more comfortable and has less edema
3. Explains need for medical therapy: understands major action and side effects of anticoagulants and thrombolytics, complies with restriction to bedrest, wears support stocking, avoids prolonged sitting and standing, and identifies signs and symptoms of pulmonary embolism

### INTERVENTIONS

#### Supporting Tissue Perfusion

The nurse monitors the adequacy of perfusion to the affected extremity by regular neurovascular assessment, including pulses distal to the site of the obstruction, the degree of pain, paresthesia if any, temperature changes, and degree of swelling. Calf and thigh circumferences are recorded each shift.[6] When leg circumference is being monitored, the nurse marks the exact site to be used directly on the skin to ensure that the tape measure is placed consistently on the same site.

The patient is initially placed on bedrest with the leg elevated. This activity restriction may be maintained if the patient is experiencing significant pain. Patients receiving LMWH can begin to ambulate after 24 hours. Patients receiving traditional heparin therapy may be kept in bed for 5 to 7 days.[28] Once out of bed the patient is encouraged to ambulate, avoid prolonged standing and sitting, and avoid crossing the legs at the knee or ankle. Compression stockings will be applied to both legs unless contraindicated.

The nurse also carefully monitors the patient for signs of complications related to anticoagulant therapy or pulmonary embolus. The nurse monitors all laboratory results, assesses the patient for signs of bleeding, and tests urine, stool, and any emesis for blood. Bleeding precautions are implemented to protect the patient. These include holding all venipuncture sites for at least 5 minutes, avoiding the use of all IM medications, and checking all body excretions for the presence of blood. The patient's records should be clearly marked to indicate the anticoagulated state to anyone performing venipuncture.

#### Promoting Comfort

Patients with deep vein thrombosis experience both physical and psychological discomfort. Leg pain is managed with mild analgesics as needed, and the nurse assesses the patient's comfort level frequently. Elevating the leg and minimizing activity also help control initial discomfort. Warm soaks may be applied to the leg for comfort if there is active phlebitis in the affected leg. Nonsteroidal antiinflammatory drugs may be used for both their pain relieving and antiinflammatory effects.[6] The patient is also likely to be extremely anxious during the early days of treatment because the risk of pulmonary embolus is very real. The nurse encourages the patient to participate in all care decisions and keeps the patient and family informed about laboratory results and test findings. The nurse encourages the patient to express fears and concerns and offers realistic comfort and reassurance where possible.

### Patient/Family Education

Patients who experience deep vein thrombosis need extensive education because they are likely to need long-term anticoagulation at home. Patients need to be knowledgeable about how to monitor anticoagulant therapy and prevent complications. The nurse instructs the patient about the major action and side effects of the anticoagulants, the rationale for long-term management, and the planned schedule for laboratory monitoring of coagulation levels. The nurse instructs the patient to assess for and report the incidence of any excessive bruising or bleeding. Major elements of patient teaching related to the safe use of anticoagulants are summarized in the Patient/Family Teaching Box.

The patient may also be asked to wear compression stockings after discharge, and the nurse provides instruction about their safe and appropriate use. The patient will need more than one pair of the stockings so that they can be washed regularly. The correct fit of any pair of compression stockings is ensured by careful ankle, calf, and thigh circumference measurement before purchase. The stockings should be smoothly applied before getting out of bed in the morning and worn throughout the day. The skin is carefully inspected for bruising and signs of irritation or breakdown whenever the stockings are removed. Routine cleansing of the legs and feet should be maintained.

#### *Health promotion/prevention*

Preventing the incidence of deep vein thrombosis is a major nursing concern for all hospitalized patients. Early ambulation remains the single best preventive measure available, and the nurse needs to explain the rationale for frequent ambulation to both the patient and family to increase compliance with this measure.[8] High-risk patients are identified and more aggressive preventive measures are implemented, such as low-dose heparin and the use of compression stockings or sequential compression devices. All patients need instruction about the risks associated with prolonged sitting and the importance of taking breaks for ambulation every 1 to 2 hours during long car trips. Ambulating while on airplanes is more difficult but equally important.[30] Patients are also instructed to maintain a high fluid intake to avoid dehydration when traveling, avoid sitting with the ankles or knees crossed, consider the use of compression stockings when traveling, and use ankle and leg exercises every hour if possible.[8] Young women need to be informed about the risks of deep vein thrombosis associated with the use of estrogen-containing oral contraceptives, particularly if they also smoke cigarettes. Not all episodes of deep vein thrombosis can be prevented, but the risks can be decreased with the use of some of these basic measures. Care of the patient with deep vein thrombosis is summarized in the Guidelines for Care Box.

**patient/family teaching**

**Patients Receiving Oral Anticoagulant Therapy**

Teach patient the action, dosage, and side effects of medication.

- Consult with pharmacist about the concurrent use of any other medications because many drugs display strong interactions with anticoagulants (see Table 27-5).

Instruct patient not to take aspirin or any aspirin-containing over-the-counter (OTC) preparation. Aspirin will increase the anticoagulant effect. Teach patient to read all OTC medication labels carefully for aspirin content.

Instruct patient to take the drug at the same time each day and to never discontinue the drug without specific instruction from the health care provider.

Teach the patient to monitor for signs of bleeding and report them to the health care provider (bleeding gums, nosebleeds, blood in the urine or stool, bruising, cuts that do not stop bleeding despite prolonged direct pressure).

Teach patient the importance of follow-up blood tests to monitor anticoagulant levels.

Teach patient to do the following:

- Eat dark green and yellow leafy vegetables moderately because these are rich sources of vitamin K, which can counteract the effect of Coumadin.
- Use alcohol only in moderation because it increases the anticoagulant effect.
- Wear a Medic Alert tag or bracelet that identifies the use of anticoagulants.

**table 27-5** *Drugs Interfering with Oral Anticoagulant Response*

| Drugs Potentiating Response | Drugs Diminishing Response |
|---|---|
| Anabolic steroids (e.g., Dianabol) | Barbiturates (e.g., secobarbital, phenobarbital) |
| Clofibrate (Atromid-S) | Cholestyramine (Cuemid, Questran) |
| Dextrothyroxine (Choloxin) | Ethchlorvynol (Placidyl) |
| Disulfiram (Antabuse) | Glutethimide (Doriden) |
| Metronidazole (Flagyl) | Griseofulvin (Grifulvin) |
| Neomycin | Rifampin (Rifadin, Rimactane) |
| **NONSTEROIDAL ANTIINFLAMMATORY DRUGS** | |
| Oxyphenbutazone (Tandearil) | |
| Phenylbutazone (Butazolidin) | |
| Phenytoin (Dilantin) | |
| Phenyramidol (Analexin) | |
| **SALICYLATES** | |
| **SULFONAMIDES (GANTRISIN)** | |

**guidelines for care**

**The Patient with Deep Vein Thrombosis**

**Bedrest**

The patient on traditional heparin therapy will be on bedrest for 5 to 7 days. Patients on low-molecular-weight heparin (LMWH) can be out of bed after 24 hours if pain level permits.

**Treatments**

Use local heat to extremity when inflammation is acute. Fit the patient carefully for graduated compression stockings and teach correct use.

**Drug Therapy**

Administer bolus of heparin and begin heparin dosing: (a) IV drip with weight-based dosing and traditional heparin; (b) subcutaneous injection of low-molecular-weight heparin with weight-based dosing.

- Monitor APTT to establish desired heparin dosage.
- Monitor antifactor Xa to establish desired LMWH dosage; LMWH does not affect APTT or PT times.

Begin warfarin (Coumadin) treatment on day 2. Monitor INR results to establish desired warfarin dosage. Administer stool softener as needed.

**Patient Teaching**

- Risks and complications of DVT, signs and symptoms of complications
- Risks and complications of heparin administration, signs and symptoms of complications
- Bleeding precautions
- Need for ongoing laboratory follow-up of anticoagulation levels after discharge

## EVALUATION

To evaluate the effectiveness of nursing interventions, compare patient behaviors with those stated in the expected patient outcomes. Successful achievement of patient outcomes for the patient with deep vein thrombosis is indicated by:

1. Has adequate circulation to lower extremity as indicated by palpable distal pulses and warm pink extremity
2. States that pain is decreased and has less edema
3. Correctly explains safe use of all medications, wears support stockings, avoids prolonged sitting and standing, and explains signs and symptoms of complications

## GERONTOLOGICAL CONSIDERATIONS

Deep vein thrombosis is common in the elderly, and preventive measures are particularly important for this group. Early ambulation and avoiding prolonged bedrest are critical measures during any hospitalization and particularly after surgery and interventional procedures. Compression stockings and subcutaneous heparin administration are essential measures to prevent deep vein thrombosis in elders. Elders are more likely to require home health follow-up to monitor for complications when they are discharged on long-term anticoagulation.

## SPECIAL ENVIRONMENTS FOR CARE

### Critical Care Management

Critical care management is not required for the routine management of deep vein thrombosis, but it would become necessary if the patient were to develop a pulmonary embolus. Pulmonary embolus is a potentially life-threatening emergency that necessitates critical care placement for aggressive pulmonary therapy and monitoring. The management of the patient experiencing a pulmonary embolus is discussed in Chapter 32.

### Home Care Management

The initial care for a patient with a deep vein thrombosis is provided in an acute care setting, but the long-term management of the disorder takes place in the home. Patients are likely to be discharged on anticoagulant therapy and require all of the teaching and follow-up care previously outlined. The incidence of deep vein thrombosis also clearly predisposes an individual to a future recurrence of the problem, and patients need to be clearly taught and counseled about the importance of general preventive measures as outlined in the section on patient/family education earlier in this chapter. These preventive measures must be consistently integrated into the patient's daily self-care regimen after discharge.

### Complications

Recurrence of deep vein thrombosis and the development of pulmonary embolus are the two most significant complications associated with deep vein thrombosis. It is not always possible to prevent the development of either of these complications, but the measures outlined in the nursing interventions section earlier in this chapter provide the best available strategies for preventing these complications.

## VARICOSE VEINS

### Etiology/Epidemiology

Varicose veins are prominent, abnormally dilated veins that develop most often in the lower extremities because of the effects of gravity on venous pressure. In 1891 Trendelenburg first noted that varicose veins were caused from vein valve incompetence and abnormal hydrostatic pressure in the lower extremities. Few individuals under the age of 25 develop varicose veins. The exception is young women who have had multiple pregnancies. By 40 years of age 25% of men and more than 50% of women have some varicosities. The incidence rate increases to 50% of men and more than 64% of women by age 50. A hereditary component is theorized in the development of varicose veins, but obesity, prolonged standing, and the effects of chronic diseases such as cirrhosis and congestive heart failure are also well documented.

### Pathophysiology

Blood in the legs flows through the capillaries and then to the superficial veins that lie next to the skin. The blood then moves through the penetrating or communicating veins to the deep veins, which return the venous blood to the heart. Venous blood flow in the lower extremities is constantly working against gravity. The unidirectional intraluminal valves in the veins help move the blood toward the heart in conjunction with the intermittent compression effects of the leg muscles. Over time, the accumulated pressure on the vein valves can cause them to become incompetent. Risk factors such as obesity, prolonged standing, pregnancy, and chronically elevated intraabdominal pressure can significantly increase the pressure within the veins. As the valves fail, the veins will appear progressively swollen and enlarged and may become hard and tortuous (Figure 27-13). The patient may experience no symptoms or may develop swelling and a feeling of heaviness, pressure, or chronic fatigue in the legs, particularly after standing for any length of time.

### Collaborative Care Management

The Trendelenburg test is commonly employed to evaluate valve competence. The patient lies supine and elevates the leg. A tourniquet is applied to the upper thigh and the patient is assisted to a standing position. If the veins fill immediately, varicose veins are present.

Treatment depends on the severity of the disease. Primary interventions include teaching the patient about the importance of regular exercise, leg elevation, and avoidance of prolonged standing. Elastic stockings or another form of external support are usually recommended. Custom-fitted stockings are prescribed to be worn whenever the legs cannot be elevated. The appearance and weight of these stockings have improved over time, but they still may be unacceptable to many women. They are also somewhat difficult to put on, which makes them difficult for elderly patients and those with arthritis.

Sclerotherapy is an option for patients with small localized varicosities. A sclerosing agent, usually 1% to 3% sodium tetradecyl, is injected into the vein. Ligation, stripping, and excision of veins are surgical options that can usually be performed as outpatient surgery if no untoward complications develop.

#### *Patient/family education*

Teaching is an important component of conservative management for varicose veins. The patient needs to understand the relationship between gravity and varicose filling. The nurse assists the patient to find ways to minimize prolonged sitting or standing and to elevate the legs above the level of the heart at intervals throughout the day. The nurse also encourages the patient to maintain an optimal body weight and explore whether symptom improvement can be obtained through weight loss. The nurse also encourages the patient to wear compression stockings. The patient may need to experiment with different types and brands until a style and weight can be found that provides the needed support and is acceptable to the patient for daily use. The nurse reinforces the importance of applying compression stockings before getting out of bed in the morning. Discharge teaching after vein surgery includes monitoring wound healing, assessing for signs of infection, and resting with the legs elevated at intervals throughout the day. Walking is encouraged; prolonged sitting and standing should be avoided.

## VENOUS ULCERS

### Etiology/Epidemiology

Leg ulcers can be caused by many conditions, including venous hypertension, infection, diabetes mellitus, malignancy, connective tissue disorders, rheumatoid arthritis, and damage from deep vein thrombosis or venous stasis. External insults such as trauma, pressure, and insect bites are other possible causes. Although ulcers may be either arterial or venous in nature, more than 85% of all ulcers are venous. One in four Americans over the age of 65 (more than 1.5 million people annually) develop extremity ulcers.[17] Treatment is prolonged and is estimated to cost from $750 million to $1 billion each year. Most ulcers result from a coexisting disease process or trauma, but risk factors for ulcers include a positive family history, pregnancy, obesity, and an occupation that requires prolonged standing.

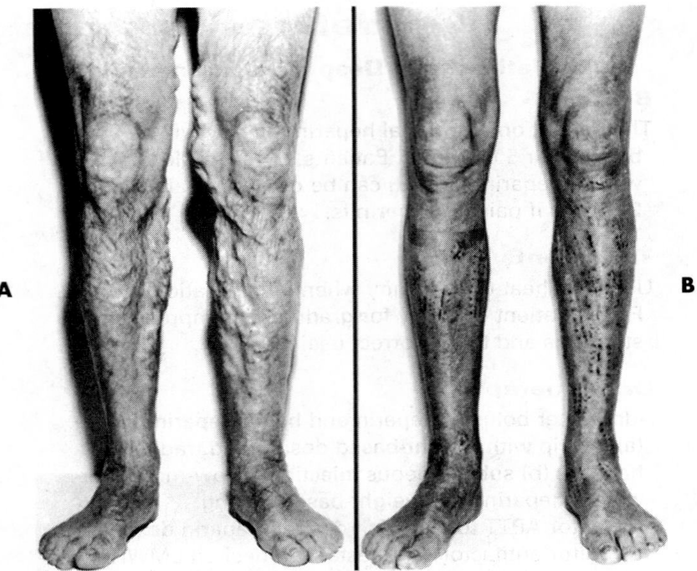


**fig. 27-13** Extensive varicosities (incompetency of the greater saphenous systems). **A,** Appearance preoperatively. **B,** Appearance 2 weeks postoperatively.

### Pathophysiology

Venous ulcers typically develop from a pattern of increased venous tension and valve incompetence that leads to venous stasis, poor venous return, edema, and ultimately ulceration. The pattern is similar in most ways to the pathology of other venous disorders. It is theorized that fibrin cuffs may develop around the dermal capillaries in response to prolonged venous hypertension. These cuffs prevent sufficient oxygen and nutrients from reaching the tissue. The decreased circulation results in ulceration. An alternative theory suggests that capillaries are damaged from prolonged venous stasis and cellular permeability increases due to the release of antiinflammatory substances from the white cells.

Chronic venous hypertension causes varicosities, stasis eczema, and lipodermatosclerosis. The varicosities are the direct result of the incompetent valves, but only 3% of patients with varicosities develop ulcers.[17] Stasis eczema or dermatitis occurs from edema and blistering. Eczema is often the first sign of ulcers. Lipodermatosclerosis occurs when fibrotic tissue develops in response to long-standing extremity edema. The fibrotic tissue replaces the normal tissue and fat in the legs. The leg becomes larger at the calf and smaller at the ankle, and the skin is tough and thick.

The ulcers typically exhibit irregular margins. The wound ranges in appearance from red granulation tissue to fibrinous tissue to necrosis (Figure 27-14). Venous ulcers usually produce copious serous exudate.[18] The ulcers are often located over the medial or lateral malleolus but can develop on other portions of the leg. The skin is brown or brawny in appearance because of the accumulation of waste products from hemolyzed red blood cells. Edema and distention of the veins on the medial aspect of the foot are also typical.

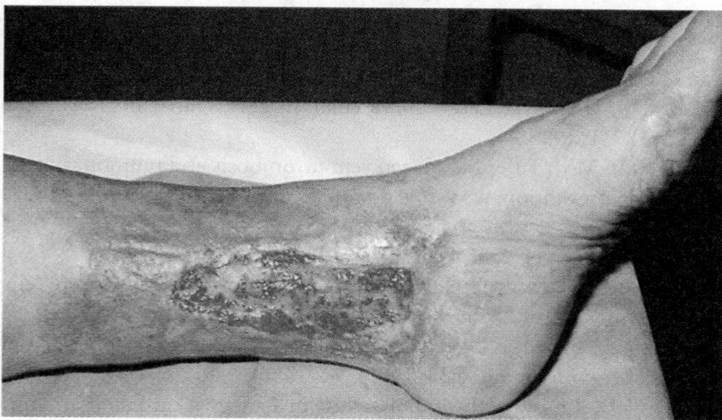

**fig. 27-14** Classic venous ulceration in the malleolar region.

## Collaborative Care Management

Venous ulcers are treated with a combination of compression, elevation, and topical wound care. Compression is directed at improving the blood flow and venous return to the heart. Compression also decreases the edema and therefore assists in the healing process. Two approaches to compression are typically used: the Setopress and Unna's boot. Elastic stockings may also be used as both a treatment and prevention tool. As with other conditions, compression hose are applied before getting out of bed and removed before going to bed. Intermittent compression devices can also be beneficial to patients with venous ulcers.

Unna's boot was developed by Dr. Paul Unna in the late 1800s. It is a continuous compression bandage that contains glycerol and zinc oxide with the option to include diphenhydramine lotion.[22] The extremity is covered by an elastic compression dressing that is wet when applied and requires up to 12 hours to dry. Unna's boot disintegrates in water, so bathing is contraindicated during treatment. Skin and circulatory assessment are essential components of care. Excessive boot pressure can cause arterial compression, so monitoring peripheral pulses and capillary perfusion are important interventions.[22]

Patients with stasis dermatitis may be treated with a topical steroid cream. A hydrocolloid dressing such as Duoderm may be applied over the cream. Any wound needs to be kept clean. Normal saline is an appropriate choice for cleansing noninfected wounds. Infected ulcers may require topical or systemic antibiotics. Infected ulcers need daily wound care. Alginates, hydrocolloids, hydrogels, foams, and transparent films may all be used on the ulcer wounds. Ideally, a wound care specialist develops the overall plan for wound care that is implemented by the patient or other caretakers. A compression wrap is usually applied over the base dressing.

Surgical intervention may be necessary to prevent the recurrence of venous ulcers and promote healing. Thrombosed veins may be surgically removed. Excision of the ulcer followed by split-thickness skin grafting may be needed.

### *Patient/family education*

Venous ulcers are difficult and time consuming to heal. From 70% to 80% of them will recur, so their management becomes a lifelong process. Patients may be admitted to an acute care institution for portions of their care, but most of the wound management will take place in the home. The wound cleansing and dressing routines can be complex and time consuming. Home health assistance may be indicated initially, but most patients will be expected to manage their extended wound care with the help of the family. The nurse plays an essential role in teaching the patient and family about needed wound care techniques and the rationale for all interventions. The patient and family also need to know where to find wound care supplies in their community and how to effectively compare the wide range of wound care products that are available on the market. Compression, elevation, and optimal skin care are the essential components for healing. The nurse will also discuss supportive measures such as weight loss or control, rest, optimal nutrition, and avoiding prolonged standing.

## critical thinking QUESTIONS

1 Maria Lopez, 62 years of age, is recovering from a recent myocardial infarction. She is in atrial fibrillation. She suddenly complains of a severe pain in her left leg. The nurse notes that pulses are absent and the leg is cool to the touch. On further questioning, Mrs. Lopez states that her leg feels somewhat numb. Hypothesize about the possible problem and cause.

2 How would you differentiate between a venous and an arterial disorder?

3 What approaches might you use to assist an elderly patient with hypertension who is noncompliant in taking his prescribed medication?

4 What are the similarities and differences in patient teaching for persons with arterial and venous disorders?

## chapter SUMMARY

### HYPERTENSION

- Hypertension is defined as a consistent elevation of blood pressure above 140/90 mm/Hg. Hypertension is a major cause of coronary artery disease, cardiac failure, strokes, and renal failure.
- Drugs to control hypertension include diuretics (especially thiazides), peripheral- and central-acting adrenergics, beta blockers, vasodilators, ACE inhibitors, and calcium antagonists. Medications are added in steps, as necessary, to control the blood pressure within the desired range.
- Persons with hypertension should take prescribed medications, exercise regularly, avoid excess salt intake, stop smoking, and continue with follow-up care.

### ARTERIAL DISORDERS

- Risk factors for PVD include cigarette smoking, hypertension, hyperlipidemia, obesity, physical inactivity, diabetes mellitus, and a family history of atherosclerosis.
- Arterial disorders develop from any disturbance in the structure of the arteries, causing diminished blood flow and decreased oxygen and nutrients to reach the tissues.
- Clinical manifestations of arterial disorders are caused not by the degree of obstruction but rather by the extent to which the affected tissues are deprived of circulation.
- Medical therapy for patients with arterial occlusive disease includes smoking cessation, a diet low in saturated fats,

weight reduction, regular exercise, and control of associated diseases (diabetes, hypertension).

- Intermittent claudication is a cramplike muscle pain that develops during exercise and ceases 1 to 2 minutes after stopping the exercise. It usually is unilateral, affects primarily the calf muscles, and indicates arterial occlusive disease.
- Positioning a patient with an arterial disorder may include placement of the extremity flat in bed or in a slightly dependent (15-degree) position to promote circulation. Elevation is contraindicated in arterial disorders.
- Thrombolytics such as streptokinase and urokinase dissolve existing thrombi.
- Nursing interventions for the patient undergoing arterial bypass surgery include frequent assessment of peripheral pulses and the graft site, avoidance of flexion in the area of the graft, and position changes to promote circulation.
- A teaching plan for a patient with arterial problems includes measures to prevent infection and injury, maintain skin integrity, and increase peripheral tissue perfusion, as well as methods to alter risk factors.
- An aneurysm is a local or diffuse dilation of an artery. Depending on location and size of the aneurysm, surgical resection may be necessary. A synthetic graft is used to replace the diseased segment.

### VENOUS DISORDERS

- Phlebitis and thrombosis can affect the superficial or deep veins. Deep vein thrombosis can lead to pulmonary embolus.
- Deep vein thrombosis is treated by bedrest and aggressive anticoagulation therapy.
- Anticoagulants such as heparin and warfarin sodium (Coumadin) prolong clotting time, prevent extension of an existing clot, and inhibit further clot formation. Anticoagulants do not dissolve an existing clot.
- A teaching plan for a patient receiving Coumadin must include the prevention of bleeding.
- Protamine sulfate is a heparin antagonist, and vitamin K counteracts the effects of Coumadin.
- Patients with chronic venous disorders such as varicose veins should be taught measures to increase peripheral perfusion. These include avoiding constrictive clothing, never crossing legs at the knee, and avoiding long periods of sitting or standing. Elevating the legs when sitting and wearing compression support stockings are important.
- Leg ulcers can develop secondary to arterial or venous disorders. The primary treatment goal is to promote wound healing and prevent infection.
- Wet-to-dry dressings and debriding chemicals remove necrotic tissue from leg ulcers. A special protective boot (Unna's paste boot) may be applied over ulcers for ambulatory patients. Arterial bypass surgery, endovascular techniques, or an amputation may be necessary for nonhealing chronic ulcers.

## References


1. Alderman M, Elliott W, Oparil S, Wood A: Addressing multiple risks in hypertensive therapy, *Patient Care* 28(14):64, 1994.
2. Anonymous: New drugs. Losartan (Cozaar)—an antihypertensive in a class by itself, *Am J Nurs* 95(12):56, 1995.
3. Apple S: New trends in thrombolytic therapy, *RN* 59(1):30, 1996.
4. Basore C, Lewis ML: Wound healing in lower extremity amputation and a system for amputation prevention, *Semin Periop Nurs* 2(4): 248, 1993.
5. Beal K, Danzig B: Lasers in vascular surgery, *Nurs Clin North Am* 25(3):711, 1990.
6. Blondin MM, Titler MG: Deep vein thrombosis and pulmonary embolism prevention: what role do nurses play? *Medsurg Nurs* 5(3):205, 1996.
7. Bright LD: Deep vein thrombosis, *Am J Nurs* 95(6):48, 1995.
8. Bright LD, Georgi S: How to protect your patient from deep vein thrombosis, *Am J Nurs* 94(12):28, 1994.
9. Bright LD, Georgi S: Peripheral vascular disease. Is it arterial or venous? *Am J Nurs* 92(9):34, 1992.
10. Burns D: Review of thrombolytic use in acute myocardial infarction, pulmonary embolism, and cerebral thrombosis, *Crit Care Nurs Q* 15(4):1, 1993.
11. Cameron J: Arterial leg ulcers, *Nurs Stand* 10(26):51, 1996.
12. Cantwell-Gab K: Identifying chronic peripheral arterial disease, *Am J Nurs* 96(7):40, 1996.
13. Chase S: Antihypertensives, *RN* 59(6):33, 1996.
14. Coen SD, Silverman E: Peripheral intra-arterial thrombolytic therapy for acute arterial occlusion, *Crit Care Nurse* 16(10):23, 1994.
15. Cuddy R: Hypertension: keeping dangerous blood pressure down, *Nursing* 25(8):35, 1995.
16. Haefele L, Dumas MA: Controlling hypertension in the elderly, *Am J Nurs* 96(11):2, 1996.
17. Harris AH, Brown-Etris M, Troyer-Caudle J: Managing vascular leg ulcers—part 2: treatment, *Am J Nurs* 96(2):40, 1996.
18. Harris AH, Brown-Etris M, Troyer-Caudle J: Managing vascular leg ulcers—part 1: assessment, *Am J Nurs* 96(1):38, 1996.
19. Hatswell EM: Abdominal aortic aneurysm surgery, part II: major complications and nursing implications, *Heart Lung* 23(4):337, 1994.
20. Hickey A: Catching deep vein thrombosis in time, *Nursing* 24(10):34, 1994.
21. Hodges H: Raynaud's disease: pathophysiology, diagnosis, and treatment, *J Am Acad Nurse Pract* 7(4):159, 1995.
22. Hull RD, Pineo GF: Low molecular weight heparin treatment of venous thromboembolism, *Prog Cardiovasc Dis* 37(2):71, 1994.
23. Husband LL: The management of the client with a leg ulcer, *J Adv Nurs* 24(3):53, 1996.
24. Johannsen JM: Update: guidelines for treating hypertension, *Am J Nurs* 93(3):42, 1993.
25. Keep NB: Identifying pulmonary embolism, *Am J Nurs* 95(4):42, 1995.
26. Kuncl N, Nelson KM: Antihypertensive drugs, *Nursing* 27(8):46, 1997.
27. Lancaster R, Dinwiddie JR: Filters that trap emboli, *RN* 54(9):56, 1991.
28. Lilly LL, Guanci R: A cautious look at heparin, *Am J Nurs* 96(5):14, 1996.
29. Noel H: Essential hypertension: evaluation and treatment, *J Am Acad Nurse Pract* 6(9):421, 1994.
30. Nunnele JD: Minimize the risk of deep vein thrombosis, *RN* 58(12): 28, 1995.
31. Pearson SD et al: A critical pathway to treat proximal lower-extremity deep vein thrombosis, *Am J Med* 100(3):283, 1996.
32. Solomon J: Hypertension—new drug therapies, *RN* 57(1):26, 1994.
33. Sparks KS: Are you up to date on weight-based heparin dosing? *Am J Nurs* 96(4):33, 1996.
34. White VM: T-PA for pulmonary embolism, *Am J Nurs* 96(9):34, 1996.

# chapter 28 ASSESSMENT OF THE Hematological System

MARILYN S. LOTTMAN and DEBORAH K. MARANTIDES

## objectives *After studying this chapter, the learner should be able to:*

1. Assess persons with suspected hematological disorders.
2. Analyze components of the hematopoietic system.
3. Relate subjective and objective data gathered during a hematological assessment of patients with suspected hematological disorders.
4. Apply diagnostic studies results of the hemoglobin and hematocrit levels, red blood cell indices, and peripheral smear results to the hematological system assessment.
5. Correlate bone marrow examination results to further patients' understanding of a hematological diagnosis.

## ANATOMY AND PHYSIOLOGY

Diseases associated with the reticuloendothelial system (RES) are diverse in their underlying pathological manifestations, disease course, and response to treatment. Most often the accompanying symptoms result from interference with the normal development and function of the blood components: erythrocytes (red blood cells [RBCs]), thrombocytes (platelets), leukocytes (white blood cells [WBCs]), and altered hematopoiesis (blood cell production). Normally, homeostasis is maintained through a balance between the rate of production of normal blood cells and the rate of destruction. Disorders of the blood occur when this balance is lost. Disturbances in the coagulation mechanism also result in blood disorders.

### COMPONENTS OF THE HEMATOPOIETIC SYSTEM

The hematopoietic system includes blood and its components and bone marrow, as well as the RES, which is located throughout the body. The RES function is phagocytizing foreign materials and lysing (breaking down) RBCs.

#### Blood

Blood is an aqueous solution (plasma) that contains water, proteins, electrolytes, and inorganic and organic constituents. Cells make up 7% to 9% of the blood.

The cell components of blood include erythrocytes, leukocytes, and thrombocytes. All normal cells are derived from a single stem cell that can divide into lymphoid and myeloid stem cells. These stem cells can in turn become progenitor cells that divide along a specific single pathway (Figure 28-1). This process is known as hematopoiesis and takes place in the bone marrow of the skull, vertebrae, pelvis, sternum, ribs, and proximal epiphysis of long bones. Production may occur in all the long bones during periods of increased demand, such as with hemorrhage or during cell destruction (hemolysis).

#### *Erythrocytes*

An erythrocyte (RBC) is a nonnucleated biconcave disk that is soft and pliable. These characteristics enable the RBC to change its shape during passage through the microcirculation. The RBC's major component is hemoglobin (Hgb), a protein that transports oxygen and carbon dioxide and maintains normal pH through a series of intracellular buffers (see Chapter 16). The Hgb molecule contains globin (two pairs of polypeptide chains) and four heme groups, each containing an atom of ferrous iron. Thus each Hgb molecule can unite with four oxygen molecules to form oxyhemoglobin (a reversible reaction). Carbon dioxide is carried by the globin portion of the Hgb molecule.

Maturation of RBCs in the bone marrow requires adequate amounts and use of vitamin $B_{12}$, folic acid, proteins, enzymes, and minerals (iron, copper). *Erythropoiesis* (RBC formation) can be greatly stimulated by the secretion of the hormone *erythropoietin* from the kidneys; this occurs when the number of RBCs falls below normal (such as with severe blood loss) or when demand for oxygen increases (tissue hypoxia). The RBCs circulate for 120 days and are then destroyed by the macrophages of the RES. Most of the iron is removed from the heme and can be used to form new heme groups. Small amounts of iron lost daily in urine and feces and through menstrual flow must be replaced by iron ingestion (see Chapter 29). The remainder of the heme is broken down to form bilirubin and is secreted into the bile. Energy in the form of adenosine triphosphate (ATP) is required to maintain cell membrane integrity and the relatively low sodium and high potassium content of the RBC.

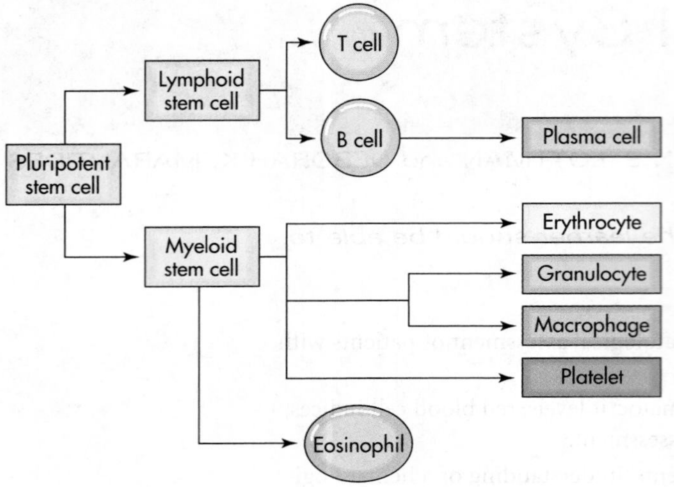


**fig. 28-1** Scheme of stem cell differentiation showing typical progenitor cell for erythrocytes, granulocytes, and platelets.

**box 28-1** *Coagulation Factors*

| | |
|---|---|
| Factor I | Fibrinogen |
| Factor II | Prothrombin |
| Factor III | Thromboplastin, tissue thromboplastin |
| Factor IV | Calcium |
| Factor V | Proaccelerin, labile factor |
| Factor VII | Serum prothrombin conversion accelerator (SPCA) |
| Factor VIII | Antihemophilic globulin (AHG) Antihemophilic factor (AHF) |
| Factor IX | Plasma thromboplastin component (PTC), Christmas factor |
| Factor X | Stuart-Prower factor |
| Factor XI | Plasma thromboplastin antecedent (PTA) |
| Factor XII | Hageman factor, contact factor |
| Factor XIII | Fibrin-stabilizing factor, fibrinase |

### *Leukocytes*

The leukocytes make up the body's mobile defense system against foreign invaders. These cells are formed both in the bone marrow (granulocytes, monocytes, and some lymphocytes) and in the lymphatic tissue (lymphocytes). These cells are classified into two groups: polymorphonuclear granulocytes (neutrophils, basophils, and eosinophils) and nongranular leukocytes (monocytes and lymphocytes). The average life span of a leukocyte is 4 to 5 days, but once activated it lives only 6 to 8 hours in circulation. Monocytes that lodge in tissue become macrophages and can live months to years until they are destroyed in the process of phagocytosis.

Neutrophils make up 50% to 70% of circulating leukocytes. In response to inflammation or infection transient increases in neutrophils will occur *(neutrophilia)*. Neutrophils provide defense in two ways. First, they release the contents of their granules, which contain enzymes to kill and digest bacteria. Second, they are capable of direct phagocytosis of foreign organisms (see Chapter 10).

Eosinophils constitute about 2% of circulating leukocytes. Although not significant in bacterial infections, eosinophils are active in parasitic infections by attaching to the organism and releasing chemicals to aid in destruction of the invader. Eosinophils also participate in the allergic response by preventing local inflammation from spreading throughout the body.

Basophils are less than 1% of circulating leukocytes. The granules of the basophil contain heparin and histamine, as well as small quantities of bradykinin and serotonin. These substances are released during the process of inflammation. In the allergic response, the immunoglobulin E (IgE) antibody attaches to the basophil, causing the release of chemicals and resulting in the localized tissue reaction commonly seen with the allergic response.

Circulating monocytes make up 2% to 8% of the total number of leukocytes. These cells are larger than granulocytes and have a kidney-shaped nucleus. The majority of monocytes are tissue-based and become macrophages as they leave the circulation. The tissue macrophage is the first line of defense against infection. These tissue macrophages participate in phagocytosis of dead and injured cells, cell fragments, and microorganisms.

Lymphocytes make up the remaining 20% to 40% of leukocytes. These cells have a round to oval nucleus. The majority of lymphocytes originate in lymphoid tissue but are also made in the bone marrow. The two types of lymphocytes are circulating T lymphocytes originating from the thymus and noncirculating B lymphocytes. T lymphocytes are long-lived and initiate the cellular immune response, and B lymphocytes are short-lived and initiate the humoral immune response. The function of lymphocytes is discussed in Chapter 10.

### *Thrombocytes*

Thrombocytes (platelets) are not cells but granular, disk-shaped, nonnucleated cell fragments. Approximately two thirds of all platelets are within the circulatory system, and the remaining one third are present in the spleen as a reserve pool. A platelet's life span is approximately 6 to 10 days. Platelets also originate from the stem cells and are essential to hemostasis and coagulation (Figure 28-2). Hemostasis results from the adhesion and aggregation capabilities of platelets to plug small breaks in blood vessels. Platelets also release thromboplastin (factor III), which, in the presence of calcium ions, converts prothrombin into thrombin in the first step of the coagulation cascade (Figure 28-3). In the second step of the coagulation cascade, thrombin promotes the conversion of fibrinogen (a soluble plasma protein) into fibrin (an insoluble strand) (Figure 28-4). Step one requires coagulation factors IV, V, VIII, IX, X, XI, and XII, and step two requires factors IV and XIII (Box 28-1). (For further discussion on hemostasis, see Chapter 29.)

## Reticuloendothelial System

The RES, also called the *mononuclear phagocyte* system or *macrophage* system, includes circulating monocytes and

fig. 28-2 Production, maturation, and function of granulocytes and monocyte-macrophages.

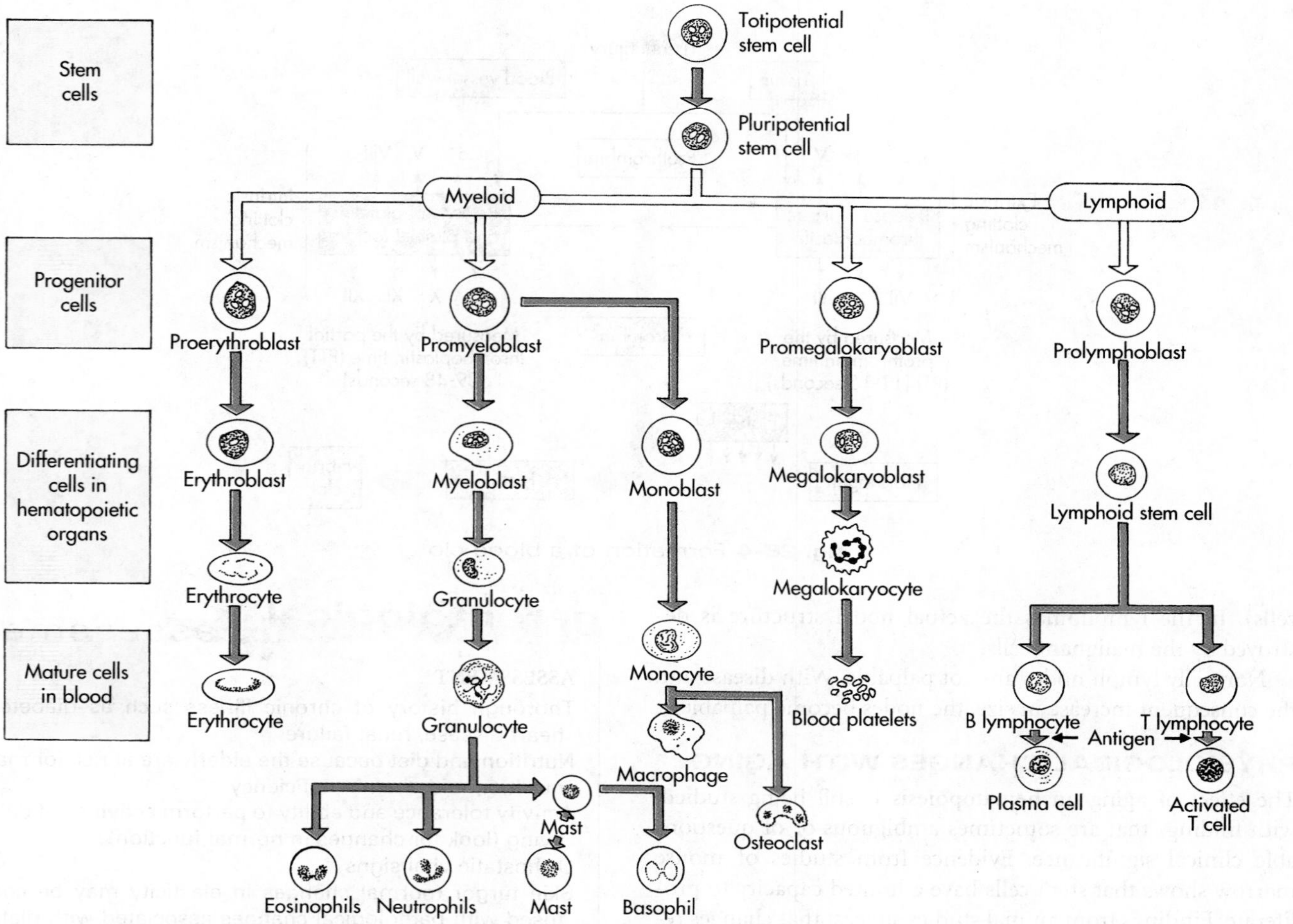

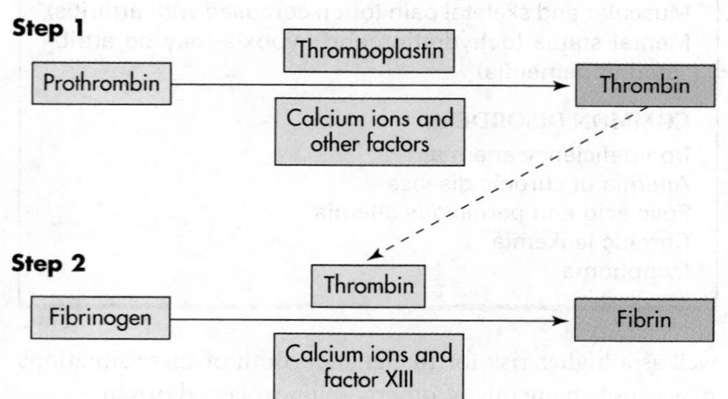


fig. 28-3 Basic steps in the coagulation process.

their precursor cells in the bone marrow. Also included are more or less fixed mononuclear phagocytic cells (also called macrophages) found in blood channels in the spleen and liver (Kupffer's cells), in the lymphatic system, in serosal cavities of the body, in the lungs, in general connective tissue, and in the bone marrow[2,3] (see Chapter 10).

The RES is primarily responsible for *phagocytosis,* the process of engulfing and removing "wasted" white blood cells. In addition to phagocytosis, the RES processes the Hgb of RBCs that have reached the end of their life span, splitting Hgb into an iron-containing substance and bilirubin.

## Lymphatic System

The lymphatic system is an alternative pathway in which fluid can flow between the interstitial spaces and the blood. Its chief function is to remove proteins from the tissue spaces. All tissues of the body contain lymph channels with the exception of the central nervous system, bone, and the superficial skin layers. Lymph fluid circulates throughout the body at a rate of 120 ml/hr. The lymphatic system also plays an important role in the regulation of tissue volume and interstitial fluid pressure.

The normal lymph node consists of connective tissue encapsulating a fine mesh of reticular cells. The reticuloendothelial cells function chiefly in the phagocytosis of cellular debris. The chief function of lymphocytes, which are the main cells constituting the lymph nodes, is to provide an immune response to antigens presented to the node from the structure being drained by the node.

Lymph node enlargement, or *lymphadenopathy,* results from an increase in the number and size of lymphoid follicles with proliferation of lymphocytes and reticuloendothelial cells. Lymphadenopathy also may occur when the node is invaded by cells normally not present (leukemic cells, cancer

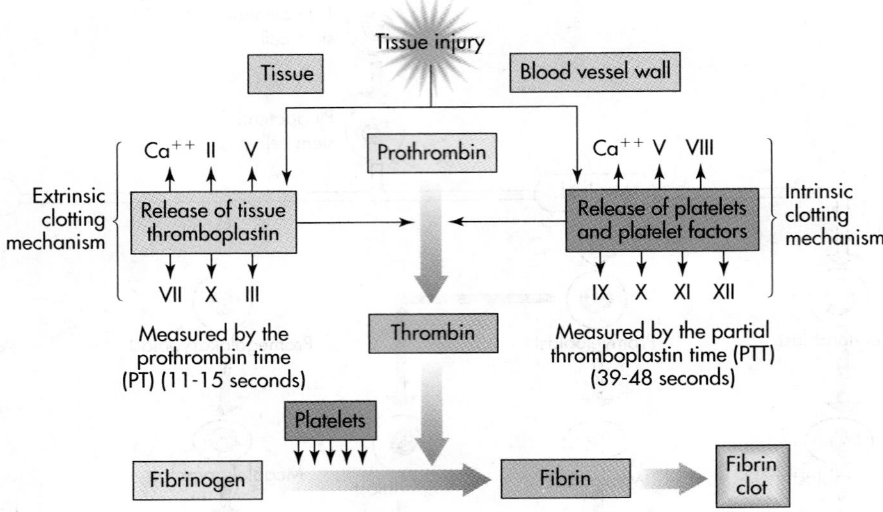


**fig. 28-4** Formation of a blood clot.

cells). In the lymphomas the actual nodal structure is destroyed by the malignant cells.

Normally lymph nodes are not palpable. With disease and the consequent increase in size, the nodes become palpable.

## PHYSIOLOGICAL CHANGES WITH AGING

The effect of aging on hematopoiesis is still being studied, with findings that are sometimes ambiguous or of questionable clinical significance. Evidence from studies of mouse marrow shows that stem cells have a limited capacity to proliferate. Findings from animal studies suggest that changes related to aging do not have clinical significance.[2] The cellularity of human marrow decreases with age, but this may be the result of an increase in fat from osteoporosis rather than a decrease in hematopoietic cells.

In human beings, the total number of leukocytes and differential counts shows no variation through middle age and no gross changes in old age. In general, the leukocyte count does not rise as high in response to infection for the elderly, and studies suggest that elderly persons have a diminished marrow granulocyte reserve.

The Hgb level decreases after middle age, although the decrease in women seems to be relatively less than that in men. Unexplained anemia in elders has been noted, but iron absorption is not impaired; however, use of orally administered iron is reduced because of the side effect of constipation. This anemia does not appear to be related solely to age.[2] Serum iron and iron-binding capacity decrease in elders, and low serum vitamin $B_{12}$ and folic acid levels occur in a significant number of elderly persons—but without anemia. Obvious signs and symptoms of hematological disorders in a younger individual may be mistaken for normal aging in an elderly person. Fatigue, activity intolerance, and pallor may be attributed to advanced age. It is important when assessing an elderly patient to be aware of the normal physiological changes and to discern those from pathological changes related to hematological dysfunction (see the Gerontological Assessment Box). The elderly are also more likely to have a chronic illness, as well as a higher risk for malignancy. Both of these situations may cause an anemia of otherwise unexplained origin.

No age-related changes in platelets have been reported. Some of the plasma coagulation factors have been reported to increase with age (factors I, V, VII, and IX). Partial thromboplastin time (PTT) may be shortened. The RBC sedimentation rate increases significantly, but this rate is of limited value in detecting disease in elders.

### gerontological assessment

**ASSESSMENT**

Thorough history of chronic illness such as diabetes, heart disease, renal failure
Nutrition and diet because the elderly are at risk for malnutrition and vitamin deficiency
Activity tolerance and ability to perform activities of daily living (look for changes in normal function)
Orthostatic vital signs
Skin turgor (normal changes in elasticity may be confused with pathological changes associated with platelet dysfunction)
Vision
Changes in taste and smell
Muscular and skeletal pain (often confused with arthritis)
Mental status (dehydration and hypoxia may be attributed to dementia)

**COMMON DISORDERS**

Iron deficiency anemia
Anemia of chronic disease
Folic acid and pernicious anemia
Chronic leukemia
Lymphoma

## SUBJECTIVE DATA

A variety of disorders affect the hematopoietic system. In addition to primary hematological disorders, secondary effects from disease of another body system may manifest in abnor-

**box 28-2** *Some Drugs Implicated in Hematopoietic Suppression**

Acetophenetidin (1, 3)
Acetylsalicylic acid (aspirin) (1, 2, 3)
Acetyl sulfisoxazole (3)
Aminosalicylic acid (3, 4)
Ammonium thioglycolate (3)
Amodiaquin HCl (3)
Arsenicals (1, 2, 3, 4)
Arsphenamine (1, 2)
Atabrine (1, 2)
γ-Benzene hexachloride (1, 3)
Benzene (1, 2, 3, 4)
Bishydroxycoumarin (3, 4)
Carbamide (2)
Carbon tetrachloride (1)
Carbutamide (Orabetic) (2)
Chloramphenicol (1, 2, 3, 4)
Chlordane (1)
Chlorophenothane (DDT) (1, 2)
Chlorothiazide (3)
Chlorpheniramine maleate (3)
Chlorpromazine (Thorazine) (3)
Chlorpropamide (2)
Chlortetracyline (1, 3)
Cinophen (3)
Coldricine (2, 3)
Cycloheximide (3)
Dextromethorphan HBr (2)
Diethylstilbestrol (2)
Diphenylhydantoin (Dilantin) (4)
Dipyrrone (3)
Ethinamate (2)
Fumagillin (3)
Hair lacquer (3)
Imipramine HCl (3)
Iproniazid (1)
Isoniazid (1, 3, 4)
Lead (1)
Lithium carbonate (1)
Mephenytoin (Mesantoin) (1, 2)
Meprobamate (1, 2, 3)
Methaminodiazepoxide (Librium) (3)
Methapyrilene HCl (4)
Methylpromazine (3)
Mezapine (2)
β-Naphthoxyacetic acid (2)
Nitrofurantoin (4)
Novobiocin (4)
Nystatin (2)
Oxyphenabutazone (2)
Para-aminosalicylic acid (3, 4)
Penicillin (1, 2, 3, 4)
Phenobarbital (1, 2, 3, 4)
Phenylbutazone (Butazolidin) (1, 2, 3)
Pipamazine (1)
Primidone (1)
Prochlorperazine (Compazine) (2, 3)
Pyrimethamine (Daraprim) (1, 2, 3)
Quinidine (2)
Quinine (2, 3)
Reserpine (2)
Stibophen (2)
Streptomycin (1, 2, 3)
Sulfamethoxypyridazine (Kynex) (2, 3, 4)
Tetracycline (3)
Thenalidine tartrate (3)
Thioridazine HCl (3)
Tolazoline HCl (1, 2)
Tolbutamide (1, 2, 3)
Tolbutamide (Orinase) (2)
Trifluoperazine (1, 3)
Trifluoperazine (Stelazine) (3)
Trimethadione (Tridione) (1, 2)

*More than 500 are listed in the latest report of the American Medical Association subcommittee on blood dyscrasias. The drugs listed in this table are those that have produced dyscrasias when given alone. *1,* Pancytopenia; *2,* thrombocytopenia; *3,* leukopenia; *4,* anemia.

mal hematological findings. For example, the anemia associated with renal insufficiency is the consequence of disease outside the hematopoietic system.

The vagueness of symptomatology of disorders of the hematological system makes a thorough assessment essential. Common symptoms include shortness of breath, fatigue, bruising, tarry stool, constipation, lymphadenopathy, flu-like illness, and musculoskeletal pain. Unfortunately, these symptoms occur in a vast number of other common disorders. The cause of any hematological abnormality must be assiduously pursued. The importance of accurate diagnosis, combined with the diverse and usually nonspecific signs and symptoms, makes it likely that the person will become involved in an arduous diagnostic process.

At the time of initial contact with the health care system the patient already is experiencing the stress of sudden onset of illness or the gnawing fear or suspicion that all is not well. The explanations offered and the time allowed for verbalization and questions are means of providing a positive foundation for the long-term care that may follow.

A thorough history includes detailed information about the person's symptoms and a thorough review of systems. In the history taking of a person with suspected hematological disease, other key points to include are family history, drug history, exposure to chemicals, and general nonspecific complaints offered by the patient.

## FAMILY HISTORY

The existence of inherited hematological disorders, such as sickle cell disease and malignant tumors, requires a detailed family history. Questions regarding disease or presence of symptoms among relatives should include reference to parents and siblings (a genogram is an excellent tool to visualize the family's history). More specific disorders, such as hemophilia, may involve questions to grandfathers, uncles, and nephews. For other disorders, female relatives need to be considered. Questions should explore instances of severe or prolonged bleeding after minor trauma, dental extractions, or surgery. The occurrence of jaundice or anemia in relatives also should be ascertained.

## DRUGS AND CHEMICALS

Drugs may induce or potentiate hematological disease (Box 28-2). Most notable are the hematological effects of the cytotoxic drugs used in cancer chemotherapy and the neutropenia associated with chloramphenicol. A thorough history of drugs ingested by a person is a crucial part of assessment. Many persons regularly ingest "something to help me sleep," "something to calm me down," or "just aspirin." Analgesics, tranquilizers, laxatives, and sedatives often are overlooked by persons when asked about drugs. Specific, often rephrased questioning is necessary to obtain a complete drug history. Do not negate the importance of over-the-counter medication.

Certain chemicals may exert a potentially harmful effect on the hematopoietic system. To obtain a history of exposure to chemicals, an occupational history is useful.

## FEVER

Fever is a common manifestation of many hematological disorders and is an important question to be asked during the history. Fever typically occurs in lymphoma, primarily Hodgkin's disease and leukemia. Severe chills may accompany hemolytic disorders. Night sweats commonly are associated with both lymphoma and leukemia.

### FATIGUE AND MALAISE

Fatigue and malaise are difficult symptoms to evaluate because they accompany many physical and emotional disorders. Information regarding the occurrence of these symptoms should be included in the history. When combined with physical and laboratory findings, they are of some diagnostic value. In addition, the person's subjective description of such symptoms lends some insight into perception of the illness, the extent to which the illness is affecting daily living, and the ability of an individual to adapt to changes in homeostasis.

## OBJECTIVE DATA

A thorough physical examination is performed in the assessment of a person with a hematological disorder. It is useful to recognize target organs and alterations that may reflect hematological disease.

### SKIN

Skin manifestations of hematological disease are often readily visible. Petechiae, ecchymoses, and purpura are associated with decreased platelets (thrombocytopenia) and other bleeding disorders. Jaundice may be associated with pernicious anemia, hemolytic disease, or primary liver dysfunction. Pallor is typically associated by the layperson with disorders of the blood. Pallor as a criterion for assessment may be deceptive because many healthy persons have pale complexions, whereas some severely anemic patients may have ruddy complexions. Other skin changes that appear pathological may be normal for a particular patient. It is therefore essential to establish norms for individual patients.

Changes in skin texture also may be observed. Except in severe cases, the patient most likely will not observe such changes. With iron deficiency anemia the patient may notice dry skin, dry hair, and brittle nails. Severe itching, especially on the palms, often is associated with Hodgkin's disease and also may occur with polycythemia vera, especially noted after bathing. In persons with leukemia and lymphoma, infiltrative lesions of the skin may be observed on any portion of the body.

### HEAD AND NECK

The sclerae of the eyes are examined for jaundice and the conjunctivae for pallor. Retinal hemorrhages may occur in persons with severe anemia and thrombocytopenia. Questions also may elicit a history of visual disturbances.

The oral mucosa is observed for pallor, bleeding tendency, and ulceration. The tongue may be very smooth in association with both pernicious anemia and nutritional deficiencies.

The neck is observed primarily for evaluation of lymph nodes. Nodes may be so large as to be visible, but palpation is always used in assessing lymph nodes. A "lump" on the neck often is the reason for seeking medical attention. Enlarged tumors may obstruct breathing or elicit coughing or difficulty in swallowing.

### CHEST

Firm pressure with the fingertips is exerted along the sternum and ribs to elicit any tenderness that may be present. Such tenderness may reflect a leukemic process or multiple myeloma. Lung sounds are assessed for signs of pneumonia, another common occurrence with leukemia or multiple myeloma.

### ABDOMEN

The abdomen is percussed and palpated with special attention to the liver and spleen. Both organs are prone to enlargement in association with hematological disease. Ascites may be a late manifestation of liver failure that could be associated with a hematological disease process.

### BACK AND EXTREMITIES

The skeletal system is evaluated primarily for pain, joint deformity, and arthritis. Bone pain may be associated with malignant conditions of hematological origin. In persons with hemolytic processes and in some hematological malignancies, there is increased uric acid production and a corresponding increase in the incidence of gout. Joint deformities are associated with bleeding disorders, and pathological fractures may be a late sign of a disorder.

### LYMPH NODES

Lymph nodes are widely distributed in the body and are routinely examined by palpation. In the healthy adult, the only palpable nodes are in the inguinal region and less often in the axilla. In a disease process, the cervical and supraclavicular nodes may become palpable. Further evaluation of lymph nodes requires x-ray examination, lymphangiography, and biopsy. It is important to recognize that any enlarged lymph node may reflect a disease process and should be evaluated thoroughly. Enlarged lymph nodes may be painful if they impinge on other organs.

### NERVOUS SYSTEM

Many neurological abnormalities may develop in persons with hematological disorders. These catastrophic complications are caused by bleeding or infection within the central nervous system. Infiltration of malignant leukemic or lymphomatous cells may produce signs and symptoms of a cerebral tumor or stroke. In addition, some of the lymphomas, especially Hodgkin's disease, may produce a dementia as a remote effect. Initial physical examination should therefore include assessment of mental status, cranial nerve function, sensory function (pain, touch, position, vibratory sensation), and motor function (strength, reflexes, plantar response). It is important to know an individual's baseline assessment. Deviations from the baseline should be noted.

## DIAGNOSTIC TESTS

Extensive blood examinations are performed as part of the diagnostic workup of a person suspected of having a hematological disorder (Table 28-1). The most common laboratory tests are Hgb and hematocrit (Hct) levels, red blood cell indices, and peripheral smear, which includes WBC counts and differential. The information obtained from such studies pro-

**table 28-1** *Laboratory Tests for Hematological Assessment*

| Blood Cell | Function | Diagnostic Test |
|---|---|---|
| **ERYTHROCYTES** | To mediate the exchange of oxygen and carbon dioxide between lungs and tissue, the transportation of oxygen, and excretion of carbon dioxide | RBC, hemoglobin (Hgb), hematocrit (Hct), reticulocyte count<br>Blood indices: Hgb, mean corpuscular hemoglobin concentration (MCHC), mean corpuscular hemoglobin (MCH)<br>Red cell fragility<br>Morphological description in stained smear |
| **THROMBOCYTES (PLATELETS)** | To produce platelet plug; to promote thrombin production<br>To provide factor IV to neutralize the action of heparin | Platelet aggregation<br>Platelet count<br>Bleeding time |
| **LEUKOCYTES** | | WBC with differential |
| Granulocytes | | Skin tests for anergy |
| Neutrophils (PMN, SEGs) | To initiate phagocytosis | Immunoelectrophoresis<br>Radial immunodiffusion |
| Eosinophils | To reverse allergic responses, parasitic infestations | |
| Basophils | To mediate hypersensitivity reactions | |
| Lymphocytes | To form immunoglobulins, humoral (B lymphocytes), cellular (T lymphocytes), immune responses | |
| Monocytes | To initiate phagocytosis | |

*PMN,* Polymorphonuclear neutrophils; *SEGs,* segmented neutrophils.

vides important clues as to the pathology of the disorder. In addition to their diagnostic value, blood studies are used to monitor a patient's progress and response to treatment. The confirmation of a hematological disease often depends on an examination of a peripheral blood smear and results of the bone marrow examination. Culture and sensitivity results are important in order to rule out other sources of fever, malaise, or abnormal CBC results.

## HEMOGLOBIN AND HEMATOCRIT

The Hgb test measures the amount of Hgb in circulation. The packed red blood cell volume, or Hct, is the ratio of RBC volume to the whole blood volume (Table 28-2).

## RED BLOOD CELL INDICES

The RBC indices consist of the mean corpuscular volume (MCV), mean corpuscular hemoglobin (MCH), and the mean corpuscular hemoglobin concentration (MCHC). The MCV estimates the average size of the RBC. Both the MCH and the MCHC measure the content of the Hgb in RBCs. The MCHC is considered more accurate than the MCH because it measures the entire blood volume of Hgb rather than just from a single cell. The RBC indices provide a differential diagnosis of the type of anemia. Normal values are indicated in Table 28-2.

## PERIPHERAL BLOOD SMEAR

Each blood cell possesses microscopic features that identify and set the cell apart from other cell types. Examination of the peripheral blood smear provides information concerning the etiology of an anemia. The size and shape of the RBC is observed (Box 28-3). Alteration in the size of the RBC is classified as *anisocytosis;* alteration in shape of the RBC is noted as *poikilocytosis.* The WBC may be examined to provide information about adequate bone marrow production. A decreased platelet count may indicate a tendency for bleeding. Often this information, when combined with data from the history, physical examination, and other laboratory tests, determines the medical diagnosis.

**table 28-2** *Normal Values of Cellular Blood Components*

| Type | Normal Values | |
|---|---|---|
| RBCs | Male: 4.6-6.1 million/mm³<br>Female: 4.0-5.4 million/mm³ | |
| Hematocrit (Hct) | Male: 45-52%<br>Female: 37-48% | |
| Hemoglobin (Hgb) | Male: 13-18 g/100 ml<br>Female: 12-16 g/100 ml | |
| Mean corpuscular volume (MCV) | 80-95 $\mu m^3$ | |
| Mean corpuscular Hgb concentration (MCHC) | 32-36% | |
| WBCs | 5000-10,000/mm³ | |
| Neutrophils | 55-70% | Differential blood cell count—totals 100% |
| Eosinophils | 1-4% | |
| Basophils | 0-1% | |
| Monocytes | 2-6% | |
| Lymphocytes | 25-40% | |
| Platelets | 150,000/mm³ | |

Nurses must have a working knowledge of molecular events involved in the neoplastic transformation process. This knowledge will aid in teaching, supporting, and educating families and patients regarding their disease process.

## BONE MARROW EXAMINATION

An adjunct to the peripheral blood smear is the bone marrow examination. Generally the bone marrow is examined when the diagnosis is not clearly established from the peripheral blood smear or when further information is needed. A bone marrow specimen is obtained by bone marrow aspiration or bone marrow biopsy. Figure 28-5 illustrates sites of active bone marrow.

### Bone Marrow Aspiration

Aspiration is the most common procedure for obtaining a bone marrow sample. The procedure is possible because normal bone marrow is soft and semifluid and can therefore be removed by needle aspiration. Bone marrow aspiration is most likely to be performed in persons with severe anemia, neutropenia (decreased number of WBCs), acute leukemia, and thrombocytopenia (decreased number of platelets).

**box 28-3** *Descriptive Cell Characteristics in Anemia*

| SIZE | HEMOGLOBIN |
|---|---|
| Macrocytic (large) | Normochromic |
| Normocytic | Hypochromic (decreased) |
| Microcytic (small) | |

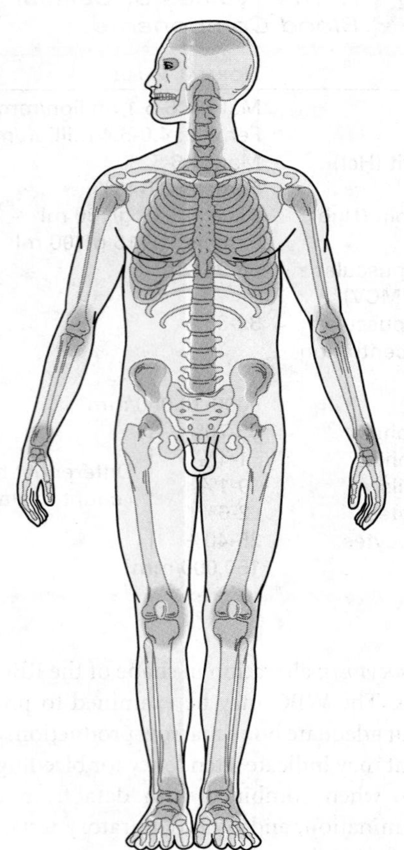

**fig. 28-5** Sites of active bone marrow.

Education, preparation, and emotional support of the patient before bone marrow aspiration can reduce anxiety. Emotional support of the patient and family is necessary because of the potentially life-threatening diagnoses that may result from the examination.

#### Procedure

The skin surrounding the puncture site (Figure 28-6) is shaved (if necessary) and cleansed with an antiseptic such as povidone-iodine complex (Betadine). Sterile towels are placed around the site. The skin and periosteum are anesthetized to decrease pain. First, the most superficial layer of the skin is infiltrated with procaine. After a few seconds, the needle is advanced until it meets bone. Procaine is then injected to anesthetize the periosteum.

The marrow aspiration needle is inserted; when the marrow cavity is entered, the marrow stylet is removed from the needle, and a sterile syringe is attached. The syringe plunger is drawn back until marrow appears in the syringe. As the plunger is drawn back, the person will experience a brief, sharp pain, sometimes described as a burning sensation. The pain is caused by the suction exerted as the plunger is pulled back. At this point the nurse's hands placed gently on the patient's shoulder and a calm reminder to lie still serve well to prevent a sudden jerk or movement.

After the needle is removed, a pressure dressing is applied over the aspiration site to arrest the minimal bleeding that occurs. If the patient has thrombocytopenia, pressure is applied for 15 minutes. The site should be monitored every 15 minutes for 1 hour after the procedure.

Some persons may complain of tenderness at the aspiration site for a few days. Most often, no pain or discomfort is experienced after the procedure.

### Bone Marrow Biopsy

A bone marrow biopsy is indicated when a large sample of bone marrow is needed. Persons most likely to undergo a bone marrow biopsy are those with pancytopenia (a decrease in more than one

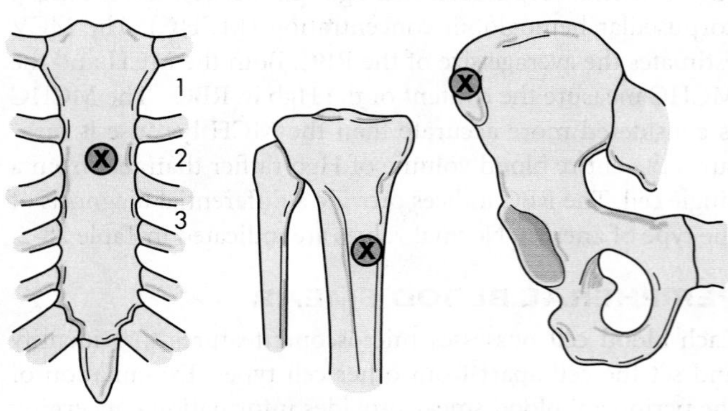


**fig. 28-6** Sites for bone marrow aspiration: sternum, iliac crest (most common), and tibia.

cell type), myelofibrosis, metastatic tumor, lymphoma, and multiple myeloma. The most common site for bone marrow biopsy is the posterior superior iliac spine. The sternum and proximal tibia may also be used. The initial steps in the biopsy procedure are similar to those outlined for bone marrow aspiration. The use of a Jamshidi needle allows for a core of marrow to be collected (Figure 28-7).

After a bone marrow aspirate or biopsy, patients are assessed for bleeding from the site. Other comfort measures, such as assisting the person to freshen up, often are needed to help the person relax and rest comfortably.

From microscopic examination of the bone marrow, iron stores can be determined, as can the morphology of the progenitor cell (see Figure 28-1). Large immature cell changes may be observed; infiltration with leukemic cells and absence of cells, as in aplastic anemia, can be determined.

As mentioned with bone marrow aspiration, emotional support before, during, and after the procedure is indicated. Both the patient and family may be stressed and anxious while awaiting results.

## COAGULATION STUDIES

### Activated Partial Thromboplastin Time and Prothrombin Time

Activated partial thromboplastin time (APTT) (normally 25 to 35 seconds) measures the number of seconds in which a clot forms. It is used to evaluate and identify congenital and acquired deficiencies in the coagulation system, as well as a means to monitor the effectiveness of heparin therapy. The prothrombin time (PT) (normally 10 to 13 seconds or 60% to 140% of normal clotting activity) also measures the time needed to form a clot, but specifically measures factors I, II, V, VII, and X in the coagulation cascade. The PT is used to monitor warfarin therapy and to screen for vitamin K deficiency and disseminated intravascular coagulation (DIC).

The PT may be reported as time in seconds, as a percentage of normal clotting activity, or as an International Normalized Ratio (INR). The INR was developed in the 1980s by the World Health Organization in an effort to standardize results. By the early 1990s most laboratories had begun using the INR.

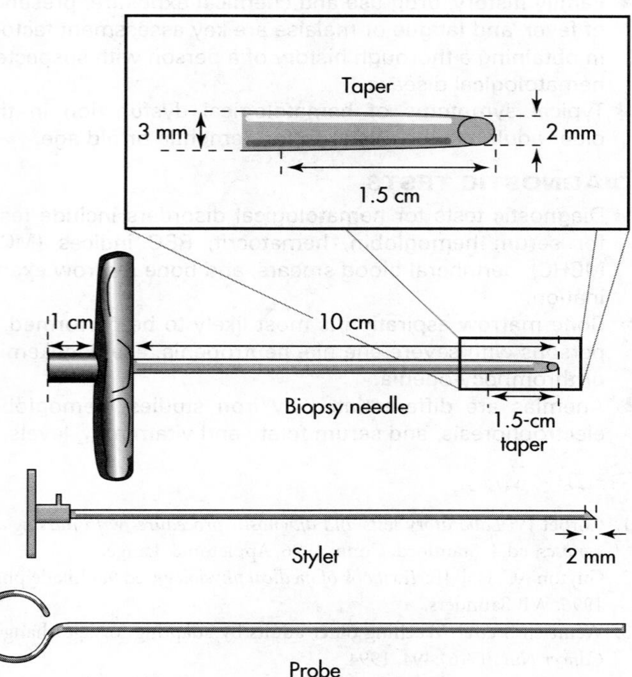


**fig. 28-7** Bone marrow biopsy needle showing shape and size.

### Fibrin Split Products

During the process of fibrinolysis, fibrinogen is broken down into fragments called fibrin split products or fibrin degradation products. Increased levels of these products occur in DIC and are also used to evaluate rejection in transplanted organs.

### Coagulation Factor Assay

To diagnose specific disorders of the coagulation pathway, it is necessary to isolate specific factor level abnormalities. The coagulation factor analysis facilitates identification of specific deficiencies (Box 28-4).

## HEMOGLOBIN ELECTROPHORESIS

Normal hemoglobins found in the adult erythrocyte are types A, $A_2$, and F, with 96% to 98% of hemoglobin being type A. With electrophoresis, abnormal levels of hemoglobin (hemoglobinopathy) and abnormal types of hemoglobin (hemoglobins S and C) can be detected. This test can be used to diagnose sickle cell disease and the thallasemias (Box 28-5).

## IRON STUDIES

Serum iron measures the concentration of iron that is bound to transferrin, which is normally 50 to 150 μg/dl. The total iron binding capacity (TIBC) measures the amount of iron that could still bind to the receptor sites on the transferrin. The serum iron and TIBC should vary conversely and are both used to evaluate microcytic anemia. Serum vitamin $B_{12}$ and serum folate, as well as bilirubin, are also useful in identifying causes and types of anemia (Table 28-3).

**box 28-4** *Coagulation Factor Deficiencies*

Vitamin K deficiency—decreased VII, IX, X
Liver disease—decreased II, V, VII, IX, X
Hemophilia A—decreased VIII
Hemophilia B—decreased IX
Disseminated intravascular coagulation—decreased V, VI

**box 28-5** *Abnormal Hemoglobins*

Hemoglobin A2—>7% beta thalassemia
Hemoglobin S—sickle cell disease
Hemoglobin C—hemolytic anemia
Hemoglobin F—>1% microcytic hypochromic red blood cells

**table 28-3** *Laboratory Values in Anemia*

| | Anemia of Chronic Disease | Iron Deficiency | Vitamin $B_{12}$ Deficiency | Folate Deficiency | Thalassemia |
|---|---|---|---|---|---|
| Mean corpuscular hemoglobin | Normal | Decrease | Increased | Normal | Decreased |
| Iron | Normal | Slight decrease | Elevated | Elevated | Elevated |
| TIBC | Slight decrease | Elevated | Normal | Normal | Normal |
| Bilirubin | Normal | Normal | Elevated | Elevated | Elevated |
| Vitamin $B_{12}$ | Normal | Normal | Decreased | Normal | Normal |
| Folate | Slight decrease | Normal | Normal | Decreased | Slight decrease |

*TIBC,* Total iron-binding capacity.

Other diagnostic tests are discussed throughout the text along with the specific disorders to which they pertain.

## LYMPHANGIOGRAPHY

Lymphangiography is a radiological technique used for visualization of the lymphatic system nodes to detect the presence of disease. This procedure is especially valuable in the assessment of paraaortic nodes that are anatomically too deep in the abdomen to allow for evaluation by palpation. For this procedure a small incision is made between the toes or fingers and dye is instilled. After approximately 30 minutes the lymphatic system is outlined. An iodine-based dye is then injected and radiographs are taken, and then again at intervals of 24 and 48 hours after the procedure. In addition, because the dye remains in the lymph nodes for as long as 6 months after the initial study, disease status and response to therapy can be periodically evaluated with routine abdominal roentgenograms.

Patient preparation includes information regarding the type and length of procedure, associated sensations, and aftercare. The patient may or may not have food and fluids restricted before the procedure. A consent form is necessary. The patient may experience discomfort associated with needle puncture and lying still for the procedure, which may last up to 3 hours. An assessment of the patient's allergy status, particularly to iodine, is necessary because of the contrast media used.

The patient may experience a sensation of warmth and flushing as the iodine-based dye is injected. Local anesthesia is used before the needle insertion.

Postprocedural care includes elevating the affected limb for 24 hours. The nurse should assess the patient for signs of bleeding, infection, or adverse reactions to the dye. The dissection site may require a few sutures, and mild analgesia (acetaminophen or nonsteroidal antiinflammatory) may be indicated.

The affected extremity should be carefully assessed for any changes in sensory-motor function, which suggest possible nerve damage. The nurse should inform the patient that a blue skin discoloration may result from the first dye injected. The stool and urine may also be discolored. Complications include infection and rarely pneumonia if the dye migrates to the lung via the thoracic duct.[1] The patient and family should be instructed to report any respiratory problems to the physician.

Computed tomography (CT) also is used to assess abdominal lymph nodes. The CT scan is used as a monitoring tool to evaluate the patient's disease process, remission during chemotherapy, and response after treatment. Assessment by periodic CT scans (every 6 to 12 months) helps evaluate the remission or detect a relapse. Lymph nodes may also be evaluated by biopsy or endoscopy (mediastinoscopy, laparoscopy). See Chapters 24 and 38.

## chapter SUMMARY

### ANATOMY AND PHYSIOLOGY

- The hematopoietic system is made up of the blood (erythrocytes, leukocytes, platelets) and the reticuloendothelial system (RES).
- The lymphatic system is a ductwork of vessels and nodes controlling protein and fluid levels in the interstitial tissue. The lymph nodes serve as a reservoir for bacteria and protein awaiting destruction by tissue macrophages.

### SUBJECTIVE DATA

- Family history, drug use and chemical exposure, presence of fever, and fatigue or malaise are key assessment factors in obtaining a thorough history of a person with suspected hematological disease.
- Typical symptoms of hematological dysfunction in the older adult may be mistaken for dementia or old age.

### DIAGNOSTIC TESTS

- Diagnostic tests for hematological disorders include tests for serum hemoglobin, hematocrit, RBC indices (MCV, MCHC), peripheral blood smears, and bone marrow examination.
- Bone marrow aspiration is most likely to be performed in persons with severe anemia, neutropenia, acute leukemia, or thrombocytopenia.
- Anemias are differentiated by iron studies, hemoglobin electrophoresis, and serum folate and vitamin $B_{12}$ levels.

## References


1. Corbet JV: *Laboratory tests and diagnostic procedures with nursing diagnoses,* ed 4, Stamford, Conn, 1996, Appleton & Lange.
2. Guyton AC, Hall JE: *Textbook of medical physiology,* ed 9, Philadelphia, 1996, WB Saunders.
3. Weinrich S et al: Teaching older adults by adapting for age changes, *Cancer Nurs* 17(6):494, 1994.
4. Wintrobe MM et al: *Clinical hematology,* ed 9, Philadelphia, 1993, Lea & Febiger.

# chapter 29 MANAGEMENT OF PERSONS WITH Hematological Problems

DEBORAH K. MARANTIDES and MARILYN S. LOTTMAN

## objectives

*After studying this chapter, the learner should be able to:*

1. Correlate different types of anemias in terms of pathophysiology, assessment, and interventions.
2. Relate the genetic factors of sickle cell disease.
3. Describe the nursing care for patients with sickle cell crisis, including teaching strategies.
4. Compare and contrast disorders of hemostasis, platelets, and coagulation (thrombocytopenia, thrombocytosis, hemophilia, vitamin K deficiency, and disseminated intravascular coagulation), including nursing interventions.
5. Analyze nursing interventions and therapeutic modalities in four types of leukemia.
6. Differentiate between Hodgkin's disease and non-Hodgkin's lymphoma and their related interventions.

Management of persons with problems of the hematological system presents challenges to the nurse because of the diversity and vagueness of the presenting symptomatology. Disease processes are as diverse as the components that make up the hematological system. For this reason, the nurse performs a complete and thorough ongoing assessment of the patient to determine the etiology of the patient's health concerns. Interventions should be focused on supporting the patient's return to optimal function and resolution of the hematological alteration. The nurse is responsible for assisting the patient to a better understanding of the hematological system and the complexities therein to obtain an optimal level of health.

## DISORDERS ASSOCIATED WITH ERYTHROCYTES

Common disorders of erythrocytes include underproduction (anemias), overproduction (erythrocytosis), and impaired hemoglobin synthesis (hemoglobinopathies). The term *anemia* refers to a deficiency in the number of circulating red blood cells (RBCs) available for oxygen transport. This condition is determined by an overall decrease in the number of RBCs, the concentration of RBCs (hematocrit [Hct]), and the hemoglobin (Hgb) concentration of the RBC. Anemias can be further subdivided by RBC size (macrocytic or microcytic) or by the concentration of Hgb (hyperchromic or hypochromic). Refer to Table 28-2 for normal values.

Anemias can also be classified by their causative factors. Some causative factors include blood loss, bone marrow dysfunction, nutritional deficits, hemolysis, hemoglobin defects, and chronic disease. The anemias are summarized on Table 29-1.

Jane Stearns, MSN, RN, OCN, CRNH assisted in the revision of this chapter.

### ANEMIA CAUSED BY BLOOD LOSS

#### Etiology/Pathophysiology

##### *Acute blood loss*

The anemia associated with acute blood loss is the direct result of the decrease in circulating RBCs. The adult of average build has a total blood volume of approximately 6000 ml. Usually an adult can lose 500 ml of blood without serious or lasting effects because of the spleen's ability to release stored red cells. If the loss reaches 1000 ml or more, serious acute consequences may result.

Signs and symptoms of acute blood loss include those associated with hypovolemia and hypoxemia (see Table 29-1). Weakness, stupor, irritability, and cool moist skin may be observed. Vital signs indicate hypotension and tachycardia. Decreased Hgb and Hct levels may not be evident until several hours after the blood loss has occurred. The severity of the patient's symptoms correlates with the severity of the blood loss. Acute blood loss is associated with trauma, surgery, platelet dysfunction, and coagulation disorders.

##### *Chronic blood loss*

The body has remarkably adaptive powers and may adjust fairly well to a severe reduction in RBCs and Hgb, provided the condition develops gradually. A person may remain asymptomatic even though the total RBC count may drop to almost half its normal amount. For example, patients with chronic renal failure tolerate hemoglobin levels of less than 8.0 without difficulty. With chronic anemia, determinations of RBC counts, Hgb and Hct levels, mean corpuscular volume (MCV),

**table 29-1** *Types of Anemia and Clinical Manifestations*

| Type | Causes | Clinical Manifestations |
|---|---|---|
| **SECONDARY TO BLOOD LOSS** | | |
| Acute | Hemorrhage | Early: weakness, cool moist skin, tachycardia, hypotension; late: decreased Hgb and Hct |
| Chronic | Gastrointestinal or other malignancy, bleeding ulcers, bleeding hemorrhoids, menorrhagia | Decreased RBCs, Hgb, Hct, MCV, and MCHC; fatigue |
| **SECONDARY TO IMPAIRED PRODUCTION OF RBCs** | | |
| Aplastic anemia | Drugs, chemicals, radiation, chemotherapy, virus, congenital, autoimmune mechanism | Pallor of skin and mucous membranes, fatigue, palpitations, exertional dyspnea, pancytopenia, bleeding tendency, infection |
| Anemia of chronic disease | Chronic illness, renal disease, diabetes | Decreased serum iron concentration, fatigue |
| **HEMOLYTIC ANEMIAS** | | |
| Hereditary spherocytosis | Genetic: inherited as autosomal dominant trait | Spherocytes and increased reticulocytes on peripheral blood smear; fatigue, exertional dyspnea |
| Thalassemia | Genetic: decreased synthesis of one of globin chains of Hgb | Microcytosis, hypochromic RBCs, decreased growth at pubescence, eventual cardiac failure |
| Sickle cell disease | Genetic hemoglobinopathy | Painful episodes; vasoocclusive crises; chronic leg ulcers, chronic renal and ocular problems; sickled cells on peripheral blood smears |
| Enzyme deficiency anemia | Genetic: deficiency of glucose-6-phosphate dehydrogenase (G6PD) | Episodic hemolytic episodes, decreased levels of G6PD |
| Hemolytic anemia | Drug-induced or autoimmune response | Presence of RBC antibody on antiglobin or Coombs' test<br>Splenomegaly, jaundice (may or may not be present depending on cause), pallor |
| **NUTRITIONAL ANEMIAS** | | |
| Iron deficiency anemia | Chronic blood loss, inadequate intake | Fatigue, exertional dyspnea, microcytosis, low serum iron concentration |
| Megaloblastic anemia | Deficiency in vitamin $B_{12}$ or folic acid | Macrocytosis, glossitis and neurological abnormalities with vitamin $B_{12}$ deficiency |

*MCHC,* Mean corpuscular hemoglobin concentration; *MCV,* mean corpuscular volume.

mean corpuscular hemoglobin concentration (MCHC), and reticulocyte count are important diagnostic tests. All indices usually are below normal (see Table 28-2 for normal values).

Chronic blood loss is the most common cause of iron deficiency anemia. When blood loss is continuous and moderate, the bone marrow may be able to keep up with the losses by increasing the production of RBCs. Eventually, if the cause of chronic blood loss is not corrected, the bone marrow will not be able to keep pace with the loss, and symptoms of anemia appear (see Table 29-1).

### Collaborative Care Management

Successful treatment for anemia caused by blood loss requires immediate identification of the source of the loss and institution of appropriate treatment. In addition, transfusion therapy or iron supplements may be needed.

Transfusion therapy is not indicated in the asymptomatic patient with chronic anemia because of the increased risks associated with transfusion therapy. When necessary, the decision to transfuse is based on the severity of the symptoms. General guidelines for symptomatic patients are included in Table 29-2.

Transfusion of whole blood is rarely indicated even in situations of surgical hemorrhage. Instead, packed red blood cells (PRBCs) are used because they reduce the incidence of pulmonary edema and circulatory overload. If colloids and clotting factors are needed, plasma, platelets, and cryoprecipitate may be transfused as separate products.

Patients need to be educated about the risks and benefits of transfusion therapy (see the Research Box). Concerns regarding acquired immunodeficiency syndrome (AIDS) and hepatitis may need to be addressed by the nurse. The nurse also needs to explore the patient's belief system regarding the use of blood products. Certain cultural and religious belief systems (e.g., Jehovah's Witness) prohibit the receiving of blood products. These beliefs need to be respected by the health care team, although this may create some ethical dilemmas for the nurse.

If transfusion therapy is indicated, the nurse must take steps to ensure that the patient is carefully monitored during the process. Transfusion reactions can occur even though lab-

**table 29-2** *Transfusion Guidelines for the Symptomatic Patient*

| Component | Indications | Patient Symptoms |
|---|---|---|
| Red blood cells | Hgb <8 | Shortness of breath, fatigue |
| Platelets | <20,000 | Bleeding, petechiae, bruising |
| Granulocytes | <500 | Sepsis, failure of antibiotic therapy |
| Fresh frozen plasma | Deficiency of coagulation factors | Hemorrhage |
| Cryoprecipitate | Deficiency of factors VII and XIII | Diagnosis of hemophilia, uncontrolled hemorrhage |

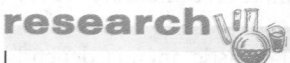

Reference: Higgens V: Leukocyte-blood components: patient benefits in practical applications, *Oncol Nurs Forum* 23(4):659, 1996.

The purpose of this study was to review the types of filters used for RBC and platelet transfusions.

Leukocyte filters are used to decrease the complications of blood and blood component transfusions. Current filters in use are clot filters, microaggregate filters, and leukocyte-removal filters. The incidence of adverse reactions such as hemolytic febrile reactions, alloimmunization, development of refractory reactions to platelets, transmission of cytomegalovirus, and immunomodulation were compared with each filter type. The results of this study demonstrate that the use of leukocyte-reducing filters significantly reduces the incidence of adverse transfusion reactions of all types and provides a cost-effective, convenient method to decrease transfusion-related problems and increase patient safety.

oratory testing was done to verify compatibility of the product (Box 29-1). Because transfusion reactions generally occur within the first 15 to 20 minutes after starting the infusion, it is important for the nurse to observe hospital protocols for administering blood products and to monitor the patient carefully for adverse reactions. The nurse should also teach the patient reportable signs and symptoms.

In addition to transfusion therapy, iron supplementation is used to replace depleted iron stores from increased blood cell production (see section on iron deficiency anemia). Patients experiencing chronic blood loss are also encouraged to eat a well-rounded diet including foods rich in iron and vitamins.

Patients with low hemoglobin may exhibit chronic fatigue and activity intolerance as a result of tissue hypoxia. Activities should be spaced at intervals, allowing the patient frequent rest periods. This optimizes the patient's limited energy reserves.

Routine screening for anemias may be done by occupational health nurses for high-risk populations. Fecal occult

**box 29-1** *Adverse Blood Reactions*

**SIGNS AND SYMPTOMS**

Urticaria
Hematuria
Arthralgias
Rigors
Shortness of breath
Flank pain
Hypotension
Fever

**INTERVENTIONS**

Stop the transfusion
Infuse normal saline
Collect urine and blood samples for evaluation

**MEDICATIONS**

Diphenhydramine
Acetaminophen
Demerol

blood screening is recommended for persons over the age of 50. Most screening takes place during routine physical examinations and includes blood tests.

#### Patient/family education

Nurses in all settings teach about dietary needs for iron and vitamins. Persons with low income can be taught to identify inexpensive food sources of the vitamins and minerals necessary for hematological health. Nurses also can become politically active to ensure adequate governmental funding for low-cost nutritional programs for persons with marginal incomes.

Women who have long-term blood loss because of heavy menstrual bleeding also are at risk for anemias, as are other persons with long-term, slow blood loss. These persons need to know of the risks and the need for continued monitoring of their RBC indices. Patients should also be taught energy-conservation techniques to decrease fatigue.

### Healthy People 2000

*Healthy People 2000* goals highlight improved nutrition not only to decrease fat and obesity but also to improve overall energy levels. Energy levels are improved by increasing intake of fruits, vegetables, and grains rich in vitamins and iron.

## APLASTIC ANEMIA

### Etiology/Epidemiology

Aplastic anemia (anemia as a result of impaired erythrocyte production) affects all age groups and both genders. The incidence is 1:100,000 of the population.[5] In approximately one half of patients with aplastic anemia in the United States, no etiological agent is identifiable. Predictable bone marrow depression occurs with antineoplastic drugs. Aplastic anemia may follow exposure to certain drugs, including chloramphenicol, sulfonamides, phenylbutazone (Butazolidin), and anticonvulsant agents such as mephenytoin (Mesantoin). Insecticides such as DDT and chemicals, particularly benzene, also are thought to cause aplastic anemia. Infections associated with the pathogenesis of aplastic anemia include hepatitis (types B and non-A, non-B), Epstein-Barr virus, cytomegalovirus, and miliary tuberculosis. The defect leading to aplastic anemia is most likely injury or destruction of a common stem cell (see Figure 28-1), which affects all subsequent cell populations. Aplastic anemia also may be congenital.

### Pathophysiology

Aplastic anemia usually is characterized by depression or cessation of activity of all blood-producing elements. There is a decrease in white blood cells (WBCs) *(leukopenia)*, a decrease in platelets *(thrombocytopenia)*, and a decrease in the formation of RBCs, which leads to an anemia (Table 29-3). The process may be chronic or acute depending on the causative factor of the anemia.

Symptoms of aplastic anemia usually develop gradually over weeks or months but in some cases have an abrupt onset. Pallor of the skin and mucous membranes is characteristic, in addition to fatigue, palpitations, and exertional dyspnea. Infections of the skin and mucous membranes occur with severe granulocytopenia; hemorrhagic symptoms (bleeding into the skin and mucous membranes and spontaneous bleeding from the nose, gums, vagina, and rectum) occur with severe thrombocytopenia. Results of a physical examination often are normal. The complete blood count (CBC) characteristically reveals a *pancytopenia* (a marked decrease in the numbers of all cell types). The reticulocyte count is low. Definitive diagnosis is made by bone marrow examination. Attempts at bone marrow aspiration may yield a "dry tap" because of hypocellularity and a decrease in active marrow. Bone marrow biopsy often is necessary for diagnosis of aplastic anemia.

### Collaborative Care Management

The immediate treatment for aplastic anemia is the removal of the causative agent, if known. In the past, treatment for aplastic anemia was aimed mainly at stimulating hematopoiesis through the administration of steroids and androgen therapy. These agents have been shown to be of limited value and can produce toxic side effects. In recent years, bone marrow transplantation (BMT) from a donor with identical human leukocyte antigen (HLA) has emerged as the treatment of choice for persons younger than age 40 years with severe aplastic anemia. The remainder of persons are treated with immunosuppressive therapy. Bone marrow transplantation centers are reporting survival rates of 60% to 80%.[3]

The prognosis for persons with aplastic anemia depends primarily on the severity of the anemia, method of treatment, and general supportive care. In addition, a higher treatment success rate occurs in patients who receive BMT early and have not received blood products, especially from the potential bone marrow donor. Patients who have undergone transfusion have a higher mortality rate from development of graft-versus-host disease. If transfusions are essential, leukocyte-poor RBCs and platelets should be used (see Chapter 66). Patients who are not successfully treated often die

**table 29-3** *Normal Function, Pathophysiology, and Clinical Manifestations in Aplastic Anemia*

| Normal Function | Pathophysiology | Clinical Manifestations |
|---|---|---|
| **RED BLOOD CELLS** | | |
| Major component is Hgb, which provides transportation of oxygen and carbon dioxide to cells | Reduction or depletion of hematopoietic stem cells, with decreased production of erythrocytes, platelets, and leukocytes<br>Decreased tissue oxygenation | Pallor of skin and mucous membranes; fatigue and exertional dyspnea<br>Low Hgb and Hct levels |
| **PLATELETS** | | |
| Adhesion and aggregation capabilities to plug small breaks in small blood vessels<br>Release of thromboplastin, which, in presence of calcium ions, converts prothrombin into thrombin in initial step of coagulation process | Fewer platelets available for blood coagulation | Bleeding tendency, as evidenced by ecchymosis, purpura, and petechiae<br>Bleeding from nose, mouth, vagina, and rectum<br>Low platelet count |
| **WHITE BLOOD CELLS** | | |
| *Neutrophils* serve as primary defense against bacterial infection through phagocytosis<br>*Monocytes* remove dead and injured cells, cell fragments, and microorganisms<br>*Lymphocytes* participate in cellular immune response (T cell) and humoral immune response (B cell) | Fewer WBCs make a person more susceptible to infection (decreased phagocytosis, decreased immune response) | Complaints of many infections, frequent sick days<br>Low WBC count |

of complications associated with repeated hemorrhage and infection.

Nursing care is based on careful assessment and management of the complications of pancytopenia, primarily focused on preventing infection and monitoring for signs of bleeding. To prevent infection in the hospitalized patient who is immunosupressed, the following interventions should be included in the plan of care:

- Private room
- Protective isolation
- Provide and instruct the patient on meticulous hygiene
- Assessment and maintenance of oral care regimens
- Monitor invasive lines for signs of infection
- Avoid bladder catheterization
- Instruct family and visitors on careful hand washing

Nursing interventions aimed at the prevention of bleeding episodes include the following:

- Monitoring invasive line sites
- Testing urine and stool for blood
- Minimizing venipuncture and injections
- Avoiding rectal temperatures, medications, and enemas
- Instructing the patient on use of soft sponges for oral care

Decreased oxygen-carrying capacity of the blood decreases oxygen supply to the tissues, leading to fatigue with activity. Measures to prevent fatigue include providing frequent rest periods, avoiding fatigue-producing activities, and monitoring the patient for signs of excessive fatigue or shortness of breath with activities.

#### Patient/family education

Education of the patient and family members is the cornerstone in the prevention of infection and the avoidance of bleeding episodes in the bone marrow–suppressed patient (see the Guidelines for Care Box). Patients are often hospitalized for several weeks depending on the type of treatment received. The nurse needs to assist the patient in developing coping strategies to deal with the anxiety and isolation of prolonged hospitalization. Music and art therapies are helpful strategies to assist the patient in coping positively with the disease and treatment.

## HEMOLYTIC ANEMIAS

*Hemolytic anemia* is defined as the premature destruction of erythrocytes occurring at such a rate that the bone marrow is unable to compensate for the loss of cells. Hemolysis can occur either extravascularly or intravascularly. In the case of extravascular hemolysis, the spleen removes erythrocytes from circulation at a much more rapid rate, usually because of some perceived problem with the erythrocyte. Examples of this type of hemolytic anemia are the autoimmune anemias and hereditary spherocytosis.

Intravascular hemolysis is secondary to the erythrocyte lysing and spilling the cell contents into the plasma. This occurs as a result of an enzyme deficiency in the erythrocyte membrane or mechanical factors such as dialysis or prosthetic heart valves, which can prematurely weaken the erythrocyte. Hemolytic anemias can also develop as a result of abnormal hemoglobin synthesis, as in thalassemia and sickle cell disease. Regardless of the cause, in each case the spleen identifies the RBC as being "abnormal" and destroys it (Table 29-4).

### Autoimmune Hemolytic Anemia

#### Etiology/epidemiology

Autoimmune hemolytic anemias can be classified as warm-reacting, cold-reacting, and drug-induced. *Warm-reacting* forms are usually idiopathic and are more commonly seen in women. Associated disease entities are systemic lupus erythematosus, rheumatoid arthritis, chronic lymphocytic leukemia, and myeloma. Immunoglobin A has also been identified as an etiological factor in warm hemolytic disease.

*Cold-reacting* disease is less common and affects mostly older adults, with an increased incidence in older females. An example of cold-reacting disease is Raynaud's phenomenon. Cold-reacting disease is associated with mononucleosis, *Mycoplasma pneumoniae,* Epstein-Barr virus, mumps, and legionnaires' disease.

Approximately 15% to 20% of autoimmune hemolytic anemias are *drug-induced.*[7] Drugs causing this type of autoimmune reaction are methyldopa, penicillin, quinine, and quinidine.

**guidelines for care**

**Teaching the Person with Aplastic Anemia**

1. Prevent infection
   a. Use good hand-washing technique.
   b. Avoid contact with those who have infections.
   c. Avoid sharing eating utensils and bath linens.
   d. Take a bath every day (or every other day if skin is dry); keep perineal area clean.
   e. Use good oral hygiene.
   f. Eliminate intake of raw meats, fruits, or vegetables.
   g. Report signs of infection immediately to health care provider.
2. Prevent hemorrhage
   a. Observe for signs such as bloody urine, stool, and petechiae, and report these to physician.
   b. Use a soft toothbrush or swab for mouth care; avoid the use of dental floss.
   c. Keep mouth clean and free of debris.
   d. Avoid enemas or other rectal insertions.
   e. Avoid picking or blowing the nose forcefully.
   f. Avoid trauma, falls, bumps, and cuts; avoid contact sports.
   g. Avoid use of aspirin or aspirin preparations (anticoagulant effect).
   h. Use an electric razor.
   i. Use adequate lubrication and be gentle during sexual intercourse.
3. Prevent fatigue
   a. Take frequent rest periods between ADL and activity.
   b. Avoid excessive workload or heavy lifting, and ask for assistance with strenuous activity.
   c. Increase time necessary for routine care.
   d. Decrease activity if shortness of breath, dizziness, or sensation of heaviness in extremities occurs.
   e. Report signs of increased fatigue with activity to health care provider.

**table 29-4** *Causes of Hemolytic Anemias*

| Type of Hemolytic Disorder | Primary Cause or Associated Disorder | Mechansims of Erythrocyte Destruction |
|---|---|---|
| **ACQUIRED FORMS** | | |
| Immune system–mediated hemolysis | Transfusion reaction<br>Hemolytic disease of the newborn<br>Autoimmune hemolytic anemia | Antibody-mediated erythrocytes by enzymes of the complement system |
| Traumatic hemolysis | Presence of prosthetic heart valves<br>Structural abnormalities of the heart<br>Hemolytic uremic syndrome<br>Disseminated intravascular coagulation<br>Hemodialysis | Physical destruction of erythrocytes by "mechanical" means (trauma) |
| Infectious hemolysis | Bacterial infection (clostridia, cholera, typhoid fever)<br>Protozoal infection (malaria, toxoplasmosis) | Infection of erythrocytes |
| Toxic (chemical) hemolysis | Exposure to toxic chemical agents<br>Hemodialysis or uremia<br>Venoms | Chemical injury of erythrocytes |
| Physical hemolysis | Burns<br>Radiation | Heat or radiation injury |
| Hypophosphatemic hemolysis | Hypophosphatemia (phosphate deficiency in plasma) | Diminished cellular production of substances required for erythrocyte life and function |
| **HEREDITARY FORMS** | | |
| Structural defects | Plasma membrane defects | Fragility of the erythrocyte |
| Enzyme deficiencies | Deficiency of glycolytic enzymes<br>Deficiency of metabolic enzymes (i.e., glucose-6-phosphate dehydrogenase deficiency) | Diminished cellular function |
| Defects of globin synthesis or structure | Sickle cell anemia | Increased membrane fragility and deformation during sickle crises |
| | Thalassemia | Defective hemoglobin structure and function |
| | Miscellaneous hemoglobin defects | Defective hemoglobin structure and function |

From Lee GR et al: *Wintrobe's clinical hematology,* ed 9, Philadelphia, 1993, Lea & Febiger.

### Pathophysiology

In warm-reacting anemias, antibodies (IgG) develop against an individual's own erythrocytes. These antibodies combine more readily at body temperature. Antibody-coated RBCs are destroyed by the reticuloendothelial system, particularly the spleen. Symptoms depend on the onset. In episodes of severe hemolysis, dyspnea, palpitations, and congestive heart failure can occur. Jaundice, pallor, and splenomegaly are common.

In cold-reacting disease, IgM antibodies react with antigens on the erythrocyte, optimally in cold temperatures (below 31° C). Ischemia occurs when red cells clump in the capillary beds, causing cyanosis, pain, and paresthesias. Hemoglobinuria also occurs.

Methyldopa (Aldomet) is associated with production of an autoantibody and a positive Coombs' test result in approximately 20% of patients and a hemolytic anemia indistinguishable from an idiopathic autoimmune hemolytic anemia in 1% of patients. Infrequently, high-dose penicillin produces hemolysis through production of an antibody that requires the presence of penicillin on the RBC membrane for its effects to occur.

### Collaborative care management

Diagnosis is confirmed by demonstrating the presence of the antibody or complement on the RBCs (direct Coombs' test) or in the serum (indirect Coombs' test). Additional laboratory findings will show a decreased hematocrit, increased reticulocytes, and an increased bilirubin. The treatment depends on the cause of the hemolysis.

Mild cases require no treatment. When treatment is indicated, 70% of persons will respond to the administration of corticosteroids or danazol (Danocrine), a gonadotropin inhibiter. Splenectomy is performed for those patients not sufficiently responsive to steroids or danazol and often is successful in controlling or ameliorating the disease. Transfusions may be given cautiously for life-threatening anemia, but this may be difficult and dangerous because of the autoantibody reacting not only with the patient's RBCs, but also with all donor cells. Plasmapheresis may be indicated for critically ill patients.

**Patient/family education.** Nursing management consists of teaching the patient about the drug therapy, preparing the patient for surgery if indicated, and helping the patient and family to cope with the illness. The patient and family need to be instructed regarding precipitating factors associated with autoimmune hemolytic anemia. Teaching should include preventive measures such as avoiding exposure to cold for persons with cold-reacting anemias.

## Hereditary Spherocytosis

### Etiology/epidemiology

Hereditary spherocytosis (HS) is the most common problem of alterations in erythrocyte shape. This anomaly occurs in 1 of every 5000 persons without regard to sex or race.[4] Hereditary spherocytosis, inherited as an autosomal dominant trait, is characterized by a membrane abnormality that leads to osmotic swelling of the RBC and susceptibility to destruction by the spleen. It usually is detected in childhood but may appear initially in adulthood.

### Pathophysiology

In HS there is a defect in the proteins that form the structure of the erythrocyte. This malformation of proteins gives the cells a thick, spherical appearance. This abnormal cell then becomes increasingly permeable to sodium, leading to increased energy demands by the cell. The circulating spherocytes become trapped in the spleen, where the increased energy demands cannot be met and the cells die.[4]

### Collaborative care management

Diagnosis depends on observation of spherocytes on the peripheral blood smear and by laboratory demonstration of increased osmotic fragility of the RBCs. The reticulocyte count usually is elevated, as is the serum bilirubin level. Bilirubin is derived from the breakdown of the hemoglobin released by the destroyed RBCs. Occasionally, red cell survival time will need to be determined. This is accomplished by labeling the cells with radioactive chromium and measuring the rate of decrease of radioactivity for 1 to 2 weeks (chromium survival). Symptoms include those typically associated with anemia (pallor, fatigue, exertional dyspnea), jaundice from the increased serum bilirubin level, and an enlarged spleen from the increased RBC destruction.

The treatment for HS is splenectomy, which will correct the hemolysis, but the underlying spherocytosis will persist. The gallbladder is often also removed because of the increased incidence of gallstones (50%) in patients with HS.

Routine postoperative care is indicated for persons who have undergone splenectomy or cholecystectomy. Nursing management includes careful monitoring for infection and continuing monitoring for signs of anemia.

### Patient/family education

Patient education should include wound management if splenectomy was performed. Genetic counseling is indicated for couples considering childbirth. Energy conservation techniques should be included in the teaching plan.

## Enzyme Deficiency Anemia

### Etiology/epidemiology

Deficiency of enzymes in the pathways that metabolize glucose and generate adenosine triphosphate (ATP) (Embden-Meyerhof and pentose phosphate shunt pathways) commonly leads to premature RBC destruction, known as enzyme deficiency anemia. The most common clinically significant enzyme abnormality is that of *glucose-6-phosphate dehydrogenase (G6PD).* This defect is autosomal recessive and occurs in a mild form among African Americans. A more severe form can occur in certain population groups in the Mediterranean area and may cause chronic hemolytic anemia.

### Pathophysiology

The enzyme G6PD is responsible for the antioxidant reactions in the red blood cell. The lack of this enzyme causes the cell to be susceptible to oxidizing agents. This exposure results in damage to the hemoglobin on the RBC membrane and the subsequent release of hemoglobin into the circulation.

Hemolytic episodes in G6PD deficiency can be caused by viral and bacterial infection or oxidant drugs (antimalarials, antipyretics, sulfonamides, quinidine, vitamin K derivatives, and phenacetin). Hemolytic episodes persist for 7 to 10 days after exposure to oxidating agents. The patient may experience back pain, jaundice, and hemoglobinuria as evidence of the hemolytic process. Diagnosis is established by assay for the enzyme.[4]

### Collaborative care management

Treatment is in the recognition of the disorder and cessation of the offending drugs. During a hemolytic episode, hydration and blood transfusions may be necessary. Prompt treatment of infections is also important in managing these patients.

**Patient/family education.** Nursing care centers on the education of patients and their families on the precipitating factors of the disorder and ways to prevent hemolytic episodes. Teaching should include the rationale for increasing oral fluids during bacterial and viral illnesses and avoiding precipitating drugs.

## Thalassemia

### Etiology/epidemiology

Thalassemia is one of the most common inherited single-gene disorders in the world. This inherited disorder of hemoglobin synthesis primarily affects persons of Mediterranean descent, but it also occurs in Southeast Asians, Chinese persons, and persons of African descent.

### Pathophysiology

Thalassemia is characterized by a decreased synthesis of one of the globin chains of hemoglobin. The beta ($\beta$) chain is most often affected ($\beta$-thalassemia). As a result, there is decreased synthesis of hemoglobin and an accumulation of the alpha globin chain in the erythrocyte. These alterations result in decreased RBC production and a chronic hemolytic anemia.

There are two presentations of thalassemia (Table 29-5). The heterozygous state, *thalassemia minor,* is associated with a mild anemia (usually asymptomatic). No therapy is required. The homozygous condition, thalassemia major, is characterized by a severe anemia. The RBCs are characteristically hypochromic (low MCH) and microcytic (low MCV). Diagnosis is by hemoglobin electrophoresis. Growth failure begins

**table 29-5** *Types of Thalassemia*

| TYPE | STATE | SYMPTOMS | THERAPY |
|---|---|---|---|
| Thalassemia minor | Heterozygous | Mild anemia, usually asymptomatic | None required |
| Thalassemia major | Homozygous | Severe anemia<br>Low MCH<br>Low MCV | Transfusion |

**table 29-6** *Phenotypes for Sickle Cell*

| GENETIC RELATIONSHIP | HEMOGLOBIN ALLELES | SICKLE CELL DISEASE |
|---|---|---|
| Homozygous dominant | Hb A, Hb A | No disease |
| Heterozygous | Hb A, Hb S | Sickle cell trait |
| Homozygous recessive | Hb S, Hb S | Sickle cell anemia |

about ages 10 to 12 years. Eventually, cardiac failure develops, and death usually occurs between ages 17 and 30.[7]

### *Collaborative care management*

At present, the only treatment for thalassemia is transfusion therapy. Bone marrow transplant should be considered in children who are under 5 years of age with thalassemia major.[7] Transfusions may be administered either to alleviate severe symptoms or to maintain the Hgb at a near-normal level to allow for a more normal lifestyle. The latter approach incurs the risk of producing iron overload from frequent transfusions, a problem that can be ameliorated by the use of an iron-chelating agent such as deferoxamine.

The nurse must be familiar with transfusion therapy (see Table 29-2) and sensitive to the emotional needs of patients receiving frequent transfusions. Because the average age at which death occurs is 17 to 30 years, the nurse should be aware of the hopelessness and depression that may occur in this population.

**Patient/family education.** Patients and their families need education about the disease process and rationales for treatment. Couples should be referred for genetic counseling.

## Sickle Cell Disease: A Hemoglobinopathy

Normal Hgb is composed of heme (red) and globin (protein component). The globin portion comprises two pairs of polypeptide chains, $\alpha$ and $\beta$. Each of the polypeptide chains has a specific amino acid sequence and number. Any deviation in the normal number or sequence of essential amino acids results in abnormal Hgb synthesis.

Disorders of hemoglobin synthesis are categorized as *hemoglobinopathies.* They result from abnormalities in one or both of the polypeptide chains ($\alpha$ or $\beta$) or in any one of the more than 500 amino acids. One of the most common hemoglobinopathies is Hb S disease (sickle cell anemia). Abnormalities in Hgb are diagnosed through serum electrophoresis.

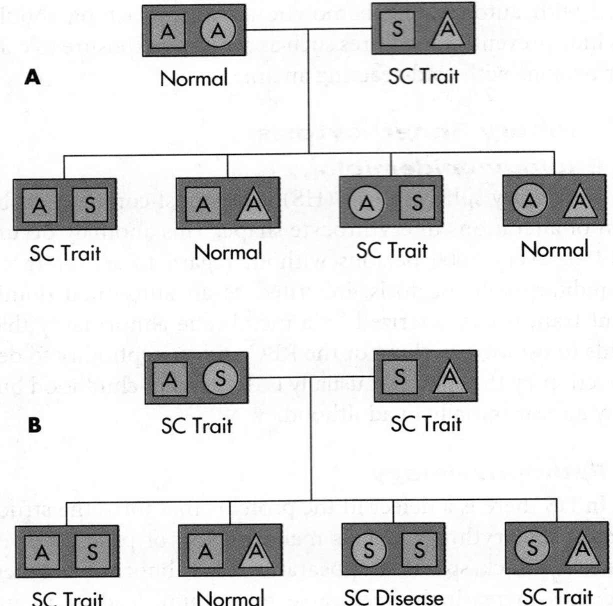


**fig. 29-1** **A,** When one parent has sickle cell trait (Hb SA), a 50% probability (2/4) exists that a child will have sickle cell trait. **B,** When both parents have sickle cell trait, there is a 25% probability (1/4) that a child will have sickle cell disease and a 50% probability of sickle cell trait.

### *Etiology/epidemiology*

Sickle cell anemia is the most common genetic disorder in the United States. Sickle cell disease (Hb SS) is homozygous recessive (Table 29-6 and Figure 29-1) and is characterized by a chronic hemolytic anemia.

Sickle cell anemia occurs predominantly in the black population. An estimated 1 in 12 African Americans is a sickle cell carrier, and 1 in 65 develops sickle cell anemia. To a lesser extent, sickle cell disease also occurs in persons from Asia Minor, India, the Mediterranean area, and the Caribbean area.

### *Pathophysiology*

The basic abnormality lies within the globin fraction of the Hgb, where a single amino acid (valine) is substituted for another (glutamic acid) in the sixth position of the $\beta$ chain. This single amino acid substitution profoundly alters the properties of the Hgb molecule (Table 29-7). Because of the intermolecular rearrangement, Hb S is formed instead of normal Hb A. Hb S has normal oxygen-carrying capacity.

However, when the oxygen tension of RBCs decreases, Hb S polymerizes, causing the Hgb to distort and realign the RBC into a sickle shape (Figure 29-2). The sickle cell in circulation leads to increased blood viscosity, which prolongs circulation time. This decrease in circulation time causes an increase in the hypoxic time of the cell, promoting further sickling. The development of sickle cells leads to plugging of

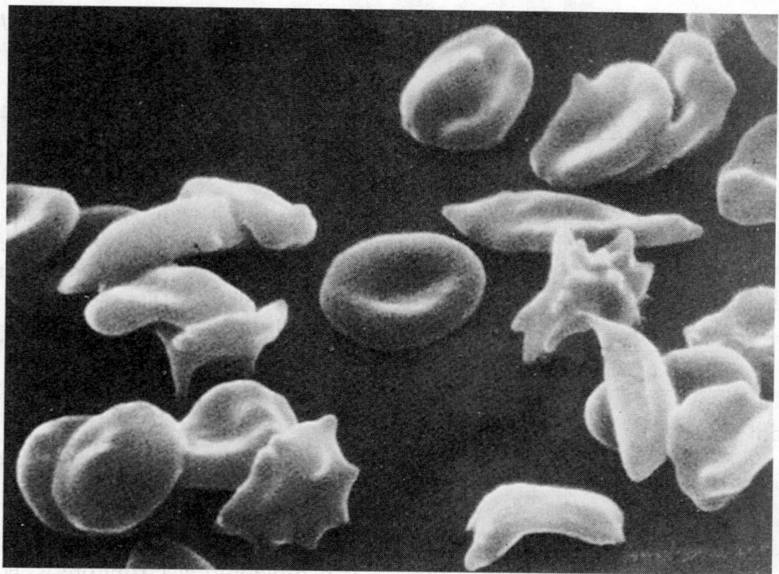

fig. 29-2 Sickled red blood cells.

table 29-7 *Normal Function, Primary Pathophysiology, and Clinical Manifestations in Sickle Cell Disease*

| Normal Function of Hemoglobin | Pathophysiology | Clinical Manifestations |
|---|---|---|
| Hgb A is major Hgb fraction in adults and consists of two $\alpha$- and two $\beta$-chains, which form a smooth, round shape | Inheritance of homozygous Hgb S interferes with function and structural integrity of Hgb molecule | Chronic hemolytic anemia classified as normochromic and normocytic; peripheral blood smears demonstrate sickled RBCs |
| Carries oxygen to tissues and carbon dioxide from tissues to be expelled by lungs | When cellular oxygen tension decreases, RBC distorts itself into sickle shape<br>Sickled cells increase viscosity of the blood, slowing circulation and causing increased cellular hypoxia and plugging of circulation to the organs; infarcts can occur in central nervous system, eyes, lungs, liver, spleen, kidney, joints, and bone | Vasoocclusive or "painful" crisis, cerebrovascular accident (CVA), retinal hemorrhage, pulmonary infarct, hepatomegaly, autosplenectomy, renal failure, enlarged heart, bone and joint abnormalities, leg ulcers |

the small circulation, further decreasing cellular pH and oxygen tension[3] (Figure 29-3). Anaerobic metabolism occurs with resulting tissue ischemia in any organ. This cycle leads to further hypoxia, infarction of organs, and painful crisis. The affected cells have a shortened life span of 7 to 20 days, as compared with the normal 105 to 120 days, after which they are identified as abnormal and destroyed by the spleen.

Different terminologies are used with discussions of sickle cell anemia (Table 29-8). Only the homozygous condition of Hb SS describes the classic form of the disease called sickle cell anemia. The heterozygous state, Hb SA, refers to the often asymptomatic condition called *sickle cell trait.* In addition, a category of sickling disorders, called *sickling syndromes,* is associated with the presence of Hb S.

Sickle cell disease is often diagnosed in early childhood and is fatal by middle age. The gradations of sickling and symptoms vary both in occurrence and intensity. The complexity of this disorder and the problems that can arise from it make sickle cell disease a major health problem.

Anemia usually is severe, chronic, and hemolytic. When hospitalization is necessary, it is usually due to one of many complications inherent in sickle cell disease (Box 29-2).

The painful vasoocclusive episode is the most common event in sickle cell disease. The pain is a manifestation of localized bone marrow necrosis affecting the juxtaarticular areas of the long bones, spine, pelvis, ribs, and sternum. Pain management is a top priority in the care of the patient with sickle cell disease.[15] The frequency of painful episodes varies greatly. Some patients experience one or two episodes per month, whereas others have only one or two per year. The duration of the episode also varies and may last from 1 to 10 days. Physical and probably emotional factors (stress)

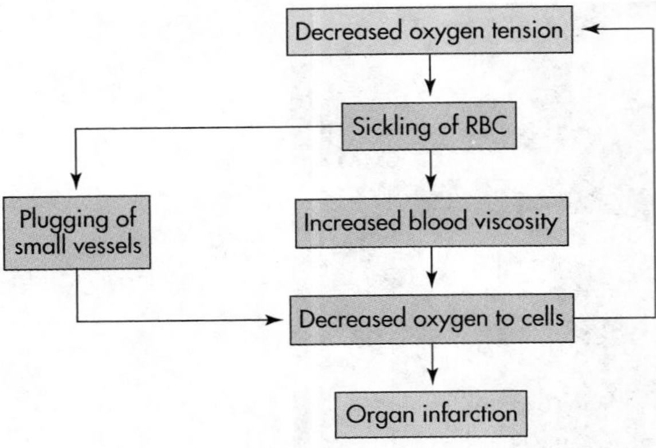


**fig. 29-3** Physiological effects of RBC sickling.

**table 29-8** *Types of Sickle Cell Disorders*

| Term | Characteristic | Hemoglobin Molecule |
|---|---|---|
| Sickle cell trait | Carrier of Hb S<br>Persons are symptom free | Hb SA |
| Sickle cell disease | Presence of sickling with associated symptoms | Hb SS |
| Sickle cell syndromes | Diseases associated with presence of Hb S | Hb SC (sickle cell Hb C)<br>Hb SD (sickle cell Hb D)<br>Hb Sβ (sickle cell thalassemia) |

precipitate a painful episode. Physical factors include events that cause dehydration or change the oxygen tension in the body, such as infection, overexertion, weather changes (cold), high Hgb levels, ingestion of alcohol, and smoking.[15]

Bacterial infection is a major cause of morbidity and mortality in patients with sickle cell disease. Persons with other hemoglobinopathies, such as Hb SC and Hb S, seem to be at lower risk for infection. Persons with sickle cell disease are particularly susceptible, primarily because most experience functional asplenia (no spleen function). Meningitis, sepsis, pneumonia, and urinary tract infections are potential risks for the person with sickle cell disease.

The sudden exacerbation of sickling can bring about a condition known as *sickle cell crisis.* Sickle cell crisis may be thrombotic, aplastic, megaloblastic, or splenic sequestration. *Vasoocclusive* or *thrombotic* crisis is the most common type and is caused by occlusion of blood vessels by the sickled cells. Dehydration, hypoxia, or acidotic conditions can provoke sickling. Fever, infections, anesthesia, exposure to cold or high altitudes, and extreme physical or emotional stress can cause a sickle cell or vasoocclusive crisis. Pain is the primary symptom in thrombotic crisis. *Aplastic crisis* is most often secondary to infection and a temporary decrease in erythropoiesis resulting from the continuous stimulus for production of new RBCs. Because of the shortened RBC survival, the anemia rapidly worsens. Diagnosis may be made by bone marrow examination. *Megaloblastic* crisis appears in some cases to be caused by the depletion of bone marrow stores of folic acid. In such cases the crisis may be treated or prevented by administration of folic acid. *Splenic sequestration* crisis occurs when the spleen suddenly increases in size, leading to pooling of blood in the spleen and subsequent hypovolemia. Signs of shock are present.

### Collaborative care management

**Diagnostic testing.** The diagnosis of sickle cell anemia should be considered with any black patient who has hemolytic anemia. The common screening test for sickle cell is the metabisulfate test or sickle cell solubility test (sickle prep). This test will be positive for both sickle cell trait and sickle cell disease. Examination of the peripheral blood smear will show target cells or sickle cell forms. Also seen are Howell-Jolly bodies and siderocytes. The confirmative test for sickle cell disease is hemoglobin electrophoresis. For the homozygous patient, the usual pattern is 2% to 20% hemoglobin F, 2% to 4% hemoglobin $A_2$, and the remainder hemoglobin S. Routine screening should be performed for all newborns of high-risk populations.

**Medications.** Medication regimens for sickle cell disease are still in the research phase. Hydroxyurea therapy has been shown to increase the hemoglobin F levels and decrease hemolysis. Neutropenia, which results from therapy with hydroxyurea, may contribute to the drug's efficacy.[2] Further research is also being done on the use of butyrate and erythropoietin to stimulate hemoglobin F production.

Current medical management of sickle cell disease is supportive care and also symptomatic management. Supplemental iron, folic acid, and vitamin $B_{12}$ are given to promote RBC production. Antibiotics are used to combat infections early in the course to avoid precipitating a crisis. Analgesia is a challenge for patients during a crisis, as well as chronic pain management. Narcotics are commonly used to control acute pain episodes.

**Treatments.** The cornerstones of treatment continue to be hydration and pain management. Oxygen therapy should be administered during an acute crisis to prevent hypoxemia. Blood transfusions are limited because patients tolerate even severe anemia very well. Exchange transfusions have been done with varying degrees of success during vasoocclusive crisis. Patients are encouraged to eat a well-balanced diet and there are no dietary restrictions. Mobility and activity tolerance can be a problem. Patients are encouraged to maintain regular and consistent exercise patterns.

Patients with sickle cell anemia can be considered for bone marrow transplantation (BMT). A problem is the lack of HLA-identical donors, because of the genetic component of the disease.[7,10] A study of matched-sibling BMT patients found 90% of patients to be free of disease 36 months after BMT (Box 29-3).

Genetic counseling is important in the prevention of sickle cell disease. Parents who both have the sickle cell trait should be informed that the risk of giving birth to an infant with sickle cell disease is one out of four births. Genetic counseling is recommended for persons considering childbirth. Diagno-

**box 29-2** *clinical manifestations*

***Sickle Cell Disease***

**ACUTE EPISODES**

Pain: usually in back, chest, or extremities; may be localized, migratory, or generalized
Fever: low grade, 1 to 2 days after onset of pain
Vasoocclusive crises: occlusion of blood vessels by the sickled cells; may occur in areas such as the brain (CVA), chest, liver, or penis (priapism)
Jaundice: caused by increased RBC destruction and the release of bilirubin

**CHRONIC PROBLEMS**

Leg ulcers: usually of the medial malleolus
Renal problems: renal insufficiency from repeated infarctions
Ocular problems: microinfarctions of the peripheral retina leading to retinal detachment and blindness
Musculoskeletal: necrosis of femoral head

sis of sickle cell disease can be done early in the first trimester of pregnancy.

**Diet.** A diet rich in protein, calcium, vitamins, and adequate fluids should be encouraged. Iced liquids should be avoided, because they may precipitate a crisis.

**Activity.** As mentioned earlier, physical stress or overexertion may precipitate a sickle cell crisis. The patient should be taught to avoid activities such as contact sports that may cause joint injury or swelling. Nonstressful exercise such as walking or swimming is recommended to maintain muscle tone and stimulate circulation. Range-of-motion exercises and regular physical activity are important measures to maintain muscle tone and joint mobility.

**Referrals.** Referrals are indicated for genetic counseling, chronic pain management, and specialty clinics based on manifestations of complications. For example, a referral to an orthopedic surgeon may be indicated in the case of severe joint trauma, hemarthrosis, or avascular necrosis.

## NURSING MANAGEMENT

### ASSESSMENT

#### Subjective Data

Data to be collected concern the person's knowledge and feelings about the disease and factors that appear to precipitate crisis or exacerbate symptoms. Fatigue may be reported when anemia is severe. Data pertaining to pain characteristics are appropriate when pain is present.

#### Objective Data

Objective data to be collected include vital signs, presence of blood in the urine, and overt signs of pain and restlessness.

### NURSING DIAGNOSES

Nursing diagnoses are determined from analysis of patient data. Prioritizing of nursing diagnoses depends on patient status and main concerns. Nursing diagnoses for the patient with sickle cell disease may include but are not limited to:

| Diagnostic Title | Possible Etiological Factors |
|---|---|
| Pain | Imbalance between oxygen supply and demand |
| Fluid volume deficit | Infection, overexertion, weather changes, high Hgb levels, alcohol, smoking |
| Infection, risk for | Decreased immune response |
| Tissue perfusion, altered | Decreased blood flow |
| Gas exchange, impaired | Ventilation/perfusion imbalance |
| Activity intolerance | Imbalance between oxygen supply and demand |
| Coping, ineffective (individual); coping, family: compromised | Crisis, prolonged disability<br>Genetic component of disease |
| Knowledge deficit | Unfamiliarity with information |

**box 29-3** *New Treatments for Sickle Cell Disease*

*Hydroxyurea.* In a study by Charache et al.,[2] hydroxyurea, which stimulates production of fetal hemoglobin, prevented painful sickle cell crisis in adults. Hydroxyurea, however, is not yet approved by the FDA, and the long-term risks of the treatment are unknown.

*Bone marrow transplant.* Walters et al.,[10] studied the effectiveness of allogeneic bone marrow transplants in children less than 16 years old and found that BMT can cure sickle cell anemia. The long-term results, however, have not yet been determined.

The role of new treatments for sickle cell anemia is evolving, and the literature suggests that there is a crucial need for controlled studies to determine the risks and benefits of these new treatments.

### EXPECTED PATIENT OUTCOMES

Expected patient outcomes for the person with sickle cell disease may include but are not limited to:

1. Feels more comfortable and rested
2. Has moist skin and mucous membranes
3. Does not develop infection
4. Has warm skin; reports no tissue pain
5. Breathes easily and regularly
6. Does not complain of fatigue or shortness of breath with activity
7. Makes informed decisions with partner about family planning; demonstrates coping strategies to deal with chronic illness.
8. Describes the basis of the anemia, availability of genetic and regular counseling, measures to prevent infection, and events that may cause crisis

### INTERVENTIONS

#### Promoting Comfort and Oxygenation

The person who experiences weakness and fatigue from the anemia is assisted in planning daily activities to include rest periods. Oxygen is given for dyspnea or excessive fatigue with exertion.

Nursing care for painful episodes involves all the principles of pain management (see Chapter 12). The goal is to relieve the pain but not overmedicate. This usually involves the use of both narcotic and nonnarcotic analgesics. Astute evaluation of the effectiveness of pain medication is most important. Managing pain in sickle cell crisis may include the use of patient-controlled analgesia.

### Promoting Hydration

The vasoocclusive nature of painful episodes requires adequate hydration to decrease blood viscosity. Patients who are supposedly in a steady state of their disease are advised to drink 4 to 6 quarts of water daily; this requirement increases to 6 to 8 quarts of water daily during a painful episode. If intravenous hydration is necessary, careful attention must be given to venous access, with avoidance of multiple punctures and infiltration.

### Preventing Infection

Because patients with sickle cell disease have a high risk for infection, monitoring for early signs is important. Persons with invasive lines and indwelling urinary catheters are at an increased risk for developing infection. Early signs of respiratory infection (cough, abnormal breath sounds) are reported to the health care provider.

### Promoting Tissue Perfusion

The patient is monitored for signs of pain that indicate blood vessel occlusion. Changes in pain or mental status are reported to the physician. To avoid vasoconstriction, the patient should be taught not to smoke. Constrictive clothing should be avoided to enhance circulation and tissue perfusion.

### Promoting Activity Tolerance

Persons who are trying to maintain independence with activities of daily living (ADL) are encouraged to take regular rest periods. Increased time may be needed for daily care because of the patient's fatigue or dyspnea.

### Facilitating Family Planning and Genetic Counseling

Many people are now deciding when or if they want to have children. This is increasingly true for persons with genetic disorders such as sickle cell disease. Some forms of birth control, such as the intrauterine device (IUD), are not as highly recommended as other forms, such as the diaphragm or spermicides, for persons with sickle cell disorders. An IUD has a higher incidence of infection than the diaphragm or spermicides. Tubal ligation, vasectomy, and oral contraceptives are other possible choices for birth control, but they are associated with significant risk. To make a wise decision about contraception, a couple must be provided with accurate information about side effects, risks, and options (see Chapter 47). Such family counseling must be performed by persons who are well versed and knowledgeable about the options.

Family planning for persons with sickle cell disease can be a most difficult issue. The fact that a person carries a gene for the disorder makes it possible that this gene will be carried into the next generation. Although moral and ethical arguments can be made, it is ultimately the personal decision of the involved couple. Information about local services can be obtained from the National Association of Sickle Cell Disease, 3345 Wilshire Blvd., Suite 1106, Los Angeles, CA 90010-1880.

### Facilitating Coping

Sickle cell patients may sometimes be labeled as malingerers because some patients may demonstrate difficult behavior patterns that are influenced by anxiety about their chronic illness. Counseling and the use of support groups are encouraged. Verbalization of fears and anxieties should be encouraged. The patient should be informed that these are normal reactions to chronic illness. The patient and family should be supported while implementing behavior and lifestyle changes necessary to cope with a chronic illness.

### Patient/Family Education

Teaching for the person with sickle cell disease includes:

1. Knowledge of the disease
2. Avoidance of situations that cause crisis (infection, high altitudes, overexertion, emotional stress, alcohol, cigarette smoking); avoidance of trauma
3. Importance of adequate fluid intake
4. Availability of psychological support services and social resources
5. Need for medical follow-up

A Nursing Care Plan for the patient with sickle cell disease is presented on p. 807-808.

## EVALUATION

To evaluate the effectiveness of nursing interventions, compare patient behaviors with those stated in the expected patient outcomes. Successful achievement of patient outcomes for the patient with sickle cell anemia is indicated by:

1. Feels more comfortable and rested
2. Has moist skin and mucous membranes
3. Has no infection
4. Has warm skin and no tissue pain
5. Breathes easily and regularly
6. Has no complaints of fatigue or shortness of breath with activity
7. Has made informed decisions with partner about family planning; implements positive coping strategies to deal with chronic illness
8. Correctly describes the basis of the anemia, availability of genetic and regular counseling, measures to prevent infection, and events that may cause crisis

## COMPLICATIONS

Sickle cell crisis causes occlusion of the microvasculature and hypoxia, which results in further sickling. This sickling process has major effects on many body systems. Infarction and thromboses resulting from anoxia may occur in the brain, kidneys, bone marrow, and spleen. Increased intracranial

## nursing care plan Person with Sickle Cell Crisis

**DATA** Mr. S. is a 24-year-old, married, African-American mail carrier who is the father of one child. He was diagnosed at age 10 years as having sickle cell disease but had been largely symptom-free until 2 years before this admission. When he was admitted with symptoms of sickle cell crisis, he had severe joint pain in upper and lower extremities, moderate fever (38.1° C), and shortness of breath.

**PHYSICAL EXAMINATION** Crackles in both lower lobes, cyanosis of lips and nailbeds, dry scaly skin on both legs, 2+ pitting edema with a small (2 cm) reddened area over each medial malleolus. No hair was visible on toes. His Hgb was 9 g/dl.

**PHYSICIAN ORDERS** Oxygen by nasal cannula, 4 L/min, bedrest with bathroom privileges, morphine sulfate IV via patient-controlled analgesia (PCA). He was given two units of packed cells to be followed by IV fluids. Sickle cell crisis with congestive heart failure was diagnosed.

The nursing history identified the following:

- Mr. S. is very "worried" about the outcome of the hospitalization and his ability to "catch his breath."
- He expresses concern about his ability to support his family and be a "father" to his son and especially to take part in athletic events: "I'm hardly a man." His wife has assumed responsibility for some of the yard work, formerly his responsibility.
- He continues to exercise and jogs several times a week. He smokes one pack of cigarettes per day and states he has never been "a big fluid drinker," although he does have a beer a day. He states that he does not know what brings on the crisis.
- He is concerned about his sexual relationship with his wife because of his general fatigue. They had one child before he was aware of the genetic nature of the disease and expresses concern about having other children who might inherit the disease.

Collaborative nursing actions include those to maintain fluid and electrolyte balance, as well as peripheral and pulmonary oxygen/carbon dioxide balance, and to prevent further vascular occlusion.

Nursing actions include monitoring for:

- Signs of infection: hyperthermia, abnormal fluid, positive blood and sputum cultures, tachycardia, tachypnea
- Signs of increased fluid/electrolyte imbalance, CHF and renal failure: hematocrit, electrolyte levels, intake and output, skin turgor; respiratory status (rate, depth of respiration, presence of crackles or wheezes, skin color, level of consciousness), renal function (creatinine, blood urea nitrogen)

**NURSING DIAGNOSIS** *Anxiety related to threat to self-concept, health status, and role functioning*

| expected patient outcome | nursing interventions | rationale |
|---|---|---|
| Shows decreased signs of anxiety. | Give Mr. S. opportunities to explore concerns about the effects of the disorder. | Making the unknown known may decrease anxiety. |
| | Assess his knowledge of sickle cell anemia and correct misunderstandings. | Relaxation decreases the psychomotor responses to anxiety. |
| | Teach relaxation measures. | |

**NURSING DIAGNOSIS** *Risk for infection related to spleen dysfunction, inadequate primary defense (broken skin), and inadequate secondary defenses (decreased hemoglobin)*

| expected patient outcome | nursing interventions | rationale |
|---|---|---|
| Is free of infection. | Use of standard precautions, medical asepsis. | Aseptic technique decreases patient's contact with pathogenic organisms; infection is predicated on type and number of organisms to which patient is exposed, as well as patient resistance to infection. |
| | Restrict persons (staff members/visitors) with any type of infection. | Restricting persons with infection decreases patient's contact with infectious agents. |

**NURSING DIAGNOSIS** *Pain in joints and chest related to poor pain management techniques, lack of knowledge*

| expected patient outcome | nursing interventions | rationale |
|---|---|---|
| States that he feels comfortable. | Assess effectiveness of PCA at least every four hours. Consult with physician if pain relief is not effective. | Pain of sickle cell crisis is excruciating, and large doses of medication may be required. |
| | Identify measures Mr. S. has found helpful, include these measures in the care. | Patients often have the most accurate information for their pain control. |
| | Support joints gently when assisting patient to do ROM exercises. | Improper support increases stress on joints and increases pain. |
| | Use moist heat or massage, if helpful. | Heat dilates blood vessels and increases circulation to the area. Massage may increase circulation and relax tense muscles. |
| | Use other pain-relieving measures; person with frequent crises may benefit from learning special techniques i.e., biofeedback, self-hypnosis, music therapy. | Biofeedback and self-hypnosis decrease the physiological responses to pain (muscle spasm, increased pulse). |

Continued

## Person with Sickle Cell Crisis–cont'd

**NURSING DIAGNOSIS** *Activity intolerance related to decreased oxygen transport*

| expected patient outcome | nursing interventions | rationale |
|---|---|---|
| Has no dyspnea with activity and feels rested. | Provide prescribed oxygen as needed. | High concentration of $O_2$ in alveoli increases diffusion across membranes. |
| | Limit activities and provide periods of rest. | Decreased activity decreases $O_2$ needs of body. |
| | Administer prescribed transfusion (packed red blood cells). | Packed cells increase the number of RBCs available to carry $O_2$ to tissue cells in the anemic person. |

**NURSING DIAGNOSIS** *Sexual dysfunction related to fatigue, pain, fear of pregnancy*

| expected patient outcome | nursing interventions | rationale |
|---|---|---|
| States that the sexual relationship is satisfying. | Discuss coital positions that require less energy for the person who becomes tired easily. | Coitus requires energy and involves neuromuscular activity; side-lying or male-inferior position is less demanding for male patients. |
| | Suggest coitus at times of day when Mr. S. is less fatigued (morning, afternoon). | Fatigue increases with continued daily activities and demand on cardiovascular system. |
| | Discuss genetic counseling and contraceptive methods. | Knowledge of and use of reliable methods to prevent pregnancy reduce fear that may cause sexual dysfunction. |

**NURSING DIAGNOSIS** *Self-esteem disturbance related to loss of body function, change in lifestyle and masculine role*

| expected patient outcome | nursing interventions | rationale |
|---|---|---|
| States satisfaction with life and self. | Provide opportunities for Mr. S. to discuss feelings about inability to fulfill expected roles. | Verbalization of concerns decreases their impact and assists in problem solving. |
| | Assist Mr. S. to identify personal strengths. | Focusing on strengths and positive factors provides a basis for personal growth. |
| | Assist Mr. S. to explore alternative ways to meet role expectations. | Concern over losses may immobilize patient; providing assistance in exploring alternatives fulfills a nurse's therapeutic role. |
| | Suggest joining a support group or obtaining counseling to minimize dependency behaviors. | Research shows that increased social support from family and groups increases recovery from disease and disability and facilitates rehabilitation. |

**NURSING DIAGNOSIS** *Knowledge deficit related to lack of exposure/recall and unfamiliarity with information sources*

| expected patient outcome | nursing interventions | rationale |
|---|---|---|
| Describes the nature of the disorder and care requirements. | Review with Mr. S. the basis of sickle cell disease and genetic effects. | Knowledge of causes of disease is one factor in ensuring patient compliance with medical regimen and adherence to preventive measures. |
| | Provide resources for family planning and genetic counseling. | Persons and groups with in-depth knowledge of family planning methods help patients identify a family planning method that conforms to the patient's cultural and religious values. |
| | Encourage Mr. S. to avoid situations that cause crises (see the text). | (See the first rationale.) |
| | Teach Mr. S. the importance of drinking 4 to 6 quarts of fluid daily. | Dehydration is a primary cause of RBC sickling. |

pressure may result (see Chapter 52). In younger patients, death may occur from cerebral hemorrhage or shock. There is a high risk of recurrence of thrombotic strokes, especially in persons up to 18 years of age.[7]

Infection is another complication, which usually occurs in tissues damaged from sickling, especially the lungs, urinary tract, and bones. Urinary tract infections may be a chronic problem.

Alterations in skin integrity, such as leg ulcers, are common skin manifestations. Leg ulcers commonly occur on the malleoli and tend to heal poorly.

Bony complications include sickling of the growth plates, which results in uneven bone growth. Avascular necrosis, especially in the shoulders and hips, can lead to arthritis and eventually total joint replacement (see Chapter 61). The vertebrae are also susceptible to bony collapse.

Pulmonary complications include pneumonia, infiltrates, and pulmonary infarction. Fat embolism (arising from the bone marrow) may also occur (see Chapter 60). Long-term pulmonary complications include pulmonary hypertension and cor pulmonale. Multiorgan failure, including pulmonary, renal, neurological, and hepatic involvement, may occur in the person with sickle cell disease.

Cardiovascular complications may result from increased cardiac workload. The patient should be assessed for dysrhythmias and murmurs.

Priapism (prolonged, painful erection) can result from a sickle cell crisis. There is no effective therapy. The best treatment is avoidance of prolonged sexual activity, alcohol, and dehydration.

Although many patients may die during childhood from cerebral hemorrhage or shock, some persons survive into their fifties or older. In the older patient, death usually results from progressive renal damage and uremia (see Chapter 45).

## IRON DEFICIENCY ANEMIA

### Etiology and Pathophysiology

Iron is a fundamental part of the Hgb molecule, and its deficiency leads to production of RBCs with a decreased amount of Hgb and ultimately to fewer RBCs. The average adult body contains approximately 4 g of iron, 3 g of which are in Hgb, 500 mg to 1 g in iron stores in the liver and bone marrow, and the rest in certain tissues and enzyme systems. The body loses approximately 1.5 mg of iron daily; this loss is usually compensated for with daily dietary intake. This tenuous balance may be compromised by chronic blood loss, either physiological, such as menstruation; or pathological, from gastrointestinal (GI) or other bleeding. This compromise results in an iron deficiency anemia.

Gradual development of iron deficiency anemia may permit adaptation with few clinical signs of anemia. Some persons may develop fatigue and exertional dyspnea. Severe iron deficiency anemia causes the nails to become brittle and spoon-shaped (concave) and develop longitudinal ridges (Box 29-4). The papillae of the tongue atrophy, and the tongue has a smooth, shiny, bright-red appearance. The corners of the mouth may be cracked, reddened, and painful (cheilosis). The cells are characteristically hypochromic and microcytic and may be detected by observation of the peripheral blood smear or by blood cell indices. Diagnosis may be confirmed by a low serum iron level and elevated serum iron-binding capacity or by a low serum ferritin level or absent iron stores in the bone marrow.

**box 29-4** ***clinical manifestations***

***Iron Deficiency Anemia***

**MILD**

Fatigue and exertional dyspnea

**SEVERE**

Brittle, spoon-shaped nails with longitudinal ridges
Smooth, shiny tongue
Cheilosis

### Collaborative Care Management

The first step in medical therapy is to determine and correct the cause of the anemia. Repletion of iron stores in the body may then be accomplished by the administration of iron. Oral iron supplement usually is given in the form of ferrous sulfate.

#### *Patient/family education*

Patient teaching is the major nursing intervention, especially with a patient newly diagnosed with iron deficiency anemia. Because ferrous sulfate may be irritating to the GI tract, it should be taken after meals and with orange juice or vitamin C to increase the iron absorption. The person is told that the stools will be black or tarry and that symptoms of diarrhea or nausea should be reported to the health care provider. Constipation is a major side effect of iron supplementation, and a stool softener may be needed. When the patient cannot tolerate oral iron preparations or is unable to absorb iron properly, parenteral iron is administered by Z-track intramuscular injection.

Poor diet is rarely the sole cause of iron deficiency anemia but is usually a contributing factor. An assessment is made of the person's dietary habits and knowledge of principles of nutrition. Persons with insufficient financial means for food, medication, or medical attention may be referred to community resources, including dietitian, social worker, or Meals-on-Wheels.

## MEGALOBLASTIC OR MACROCYTIC ANEMIA

Megaloblastic anemia refers to anemias with characteristic morphological changes caused by defective deoxyribonucleic acid (DNA) synthesis and abnormal RBC maturation. On the peripheral blood smear, macrocytic RBCs and hypersegmented neutrophils (increased number of nuclei) are present. In the bone marrow, erythroid precursors can be found that are two to three times larger than normal, with nuclei that are immature relative to their cytoplasmic development.

## Etiology/Epidemiology

Most megaloblastic anemias are caused by deficiency of either vitamin $B_{12}$ (cobalamin) or folic acid (Table 29-9). Deficiency of vitamin $B_{12}$ can result from dietary deficiency, surgery, malabsorption, or pernicious anemia. *Pernicious anemia* is the most common cause of cobalamin deficiency. Vegetarians can develop cobalamin deficiency as a result of dietary habits. Both are essential in the synthesis of DNA, and their deficiency leads to impaired nuclear development in cells throughout the body. Deficiency of either leads to anemia and often leukopenia and thrombocytopenia. Administration of medication that interferes with DNA metabolism, such as chemotherapeutic agents and anticonvulsants, can also cause megaloblastic anemias.

### *Vitamin $B_{12}$ deficiency*

Vitamin $B_{12}$, obtained from dietary sources, combines with intrinsic factor in the stomach and is carried to the ileum, where it is absorbed and transported by a carrier protein to the tissues of the body. Patients who have had a total gastrectomy or ileal resection will need parenteral cobalamin injections for life. Anemia is caused by the lack of intrinsic factor, which allows absorption of vitamin $B_{12}$.

**table 29-9** *Etiology and Pathophysiology of Megaloblastic or Macrocytic Anemias*

| Anemia | Etiology | Pathophysiology |
|---|---|---|
| Vitamin $B_{12}$ or cobalamin deficiency | Poor dietary intake<br>Malabsorption syndrome<br>Pernicious anemia | Deficiency results in impaired synthesis of DNA, resulting in morphological changes in the blood and marrow. |
| Folic acid deficiency | Poor dietary intake<br>Chronic alcoholism<br>Malnutrition<br>Pregnancy | Folic acid is an essential element required for DNA synthesis and RBC maturation; deficiencies result in morphological changes in blood and marrow. |
| Pernicious anemia | Autoimmune reaction<br>Loss of parietal cells<br>Overgrowth of intestinal organisms<br>Gastrectomy<br>Ileal resection<br>Tapeworms<br>Inflammatory bowel disease<br>Celiac disease | Intrinsic factor produced by the stomach is absent or deficient, resulting in the malabsorption of vitamin $B_{12}$. |

**Pathophysiology.** Diagnosis of $B_{12}$ deficiency is made by demonstration of a low serum vitamin $B_{12}$ level in a patient with macrocytic anemia and megaloblastic bone marrow. In addition to the general symptoms associated with anemia, patients with vitamin $B_{12}$ deficiency may manifest neurological abnormalities; in particular, they may develop a peripheral neuropathy and a loss of balance resulting from an abnormality of the posterior and lateral columns of the spinal cord (subacute combined degeneration).

Loss of proprioception and diminished vibratory sense have been reported in up to 40% of persons with cobalamin deficiency. Other neurological manifestations, including mental status changes, impaired memory, dementia, and depression, are often overlooked or mistaken for Alzheimer's disease in the elderly. Diagnosis of pernicious anemia is confirmed by an abnormal Schilling test result, which demonstrates the inability to absorb vitamin $B_{12}$ unless intrinsic factor also is administered.

**Collaborative care management.** Treatment of vitamin $B_{12}$ deficiency consists of parenteral administration of vitamin $B_{12}$, usually once a month by a nurse in an outpatient setting. The most common cause of relapse in persons with pernicious anemia is their reluctance to continue therapy for life.

***Patient/family education.*** Patient teaching is a focus of nursing care and discharge planning. The patient must be assisted to understand the nature of the illness and the absolute necessity for continued treatment.

### *Folic acid deficiency*

Folic acid deficiency anemia may be caused by dietary deficiency, often in association with chronic alcoholism, overcooking of vegetables, malabsorption syndromes, and medications that inhibit the enzyme involved in normal folate absorption through the intestinal wall.[12] Pregnancy causes an increase in the need for and use of folic acid. Deficiencies during pregnancy may result in neural tube defects.

Signs and symptoms are associated with the underlying disease and anemia in general. Laboratory findings include macrocytic anemia, megaloblastic changes in the bone marrow, and a low serum folate level.

**Collaborative care management.** Most persons respond promptly to oral folic acid and a well-balanced diet. Daily requirements for folic acid are 100 to 200 mg. The body is able to store approximately a 4-month supply of folic acid. Persons with anemia caused by dietary deficiency can be treated with 1 mg of folic acid for a 3-month period. Return visits to nurse clinics and community health nurse home visits will help the person incorporate dietary modifications into daily life. Patients who drink alcohol excessively may be referred to Alcoholics Anonymous. Patients with financial limitations are referred to appropriate community resources.

***Patient/family education.*** Patients should be instructed regarding foods rich in folic acid, including organ meats, eggs, cabbage, broccoli, citrus fruits, and brussels sprouts. Boiling, steaming, and canning of folic acid–rich foods reduces the amount of available vitamin. Persons who consume large amounts of fast foods are susceptible to folic acid deficiency.

## ANEMIA OF CHRONIC DISEASE

### Etiology/Epidemiology

Anemia of chronic disease (ACD) is one of the most common types of anemia, second only to iron deficiency. By definition, ACD is a normochromic, normocytic, hypoproliferative anemia. This anemia commonly accompanies such diseases as chronic inflammatory disorders (systemic lupus erythematosus, rheumatoid arthritis), infections, malignancy, AIDS, and Crohn's disease.[4]

### Pathophysiology

The pathophysiology of ACD is not fully understood but is thought to be related to the failure of erythropoietin (EPO) to stimulate RBC production. Immune activation contributes to the inability of EPO to stimulate the bone marrow. Also contributing to ACD are certain treatments such as chemotherapy, which suppress the marrow's ability to produce RBCs. Symptoms include fatigue, weakness, dyspnea, and anorexia, as well as symptoms of the underlying disease.

### Collaborative Care Management

Diagnosis is made by low serum iron, decreased total iron-binding capacity, and increased serum ferritin. Treatment is supportive and related to appropriate management of the underlying disease process. The anemia is usually mild, but transfusions may be given in more severe cases. EPO therapy has also been shown to improve the anemia associated with chronic disease.

#### *Patient/family education*

Education of the patient and family should center on the relationship of the anemia to the underlying disease process. Patients also need to be taught to maximize periods of high energy and to allow frequent rest periods to avoid fatigue. Risks and benefits of transfusion therapy should also be presented to the patient. Instruction about the self-administration of EPO may also be required.

## ERYTHROCYTOSIS

Erythrocytosis refers to an abnormal increase in erythrocytes. The increase may be secondary to hypoxia (from high altitudes or from pulmonary and cardiac disease), certain erythropoietin-producing tumors, or a primary disorder (polycythemia vera). With hypoxia, RBCs increase as a compensatory mechanism to carry additional oxygen. Principal laboratory tests to determine the nature of erythrocytosis include determination of the arterial oxygen concentration, RBC volume, and plasma volume.

### Polycythemia Vera

#### *Etiology/epidemiology*

Polycythemia vera (PV) is a myeloproliferative disorder of the pluripotent stem cell. The etiology is unknown. Common manifestations are erythrocytosis, thrombocytosis, and leukocytosis. Polycythemia vera typically affects elderly persons at a median age of 60 years. The incidence is approximately 1 to 3 cases per 100,000 annually and appears to be increasing, but this may be attributed to better recognition of the disease.[7] Men over the age of 80 have an increased incidence, as do women between 70 and 79 years of age. The disease is found mainly among Jewish males of European descent. Following diagnosis the mean survival rate is approximately 9 to 14 years.[7] Death is usually a result of thrombosis, leukemia, or hemorrhage. Approximately 7% to 12% of persons with PV will develop acute leukemia.[7]

#### *Pathophysiology*

Polycythemia vera (primary polycythemia) is a bone marrow disorder characterized by erythrocytosis, usually with a simultaneous leukocytosis and thrombocytosis. Hypervolemia, increased blood viscosity from the increased RBC mass, and platelet dysfunction occur.

Symptoms usually are absent in the early stages. As hypervolemia develops, symptoms include headaches, vertigo, tinnitus, and blurred vision. Thromboses with embolization may result from the increased blood viscosity, and the skin may develop a more reddened appearance. Platelet dysfunction may lead to nosebleeds, ecchymoses, and GI bleeding (Box 29-5). Thromboembolic events occur in one third of persons with PV and include deep vein thrombosis, cerebral infarction, myocardial infarction, pulmonary embolism, arterial embolism, and splenic infarction. Thromboembolic events commonly recur and account for the decreased survival rates.

On physical examination, splenomegaly typically is found in persons with polycythemia vera, but it is not common in other types of erythrocytosis. Laboratory tests demonstrate an increased total RBC volume and a plasma volume that is either increased or normal. The Hct at sea level is greater than 53%. Arterial oxygen concentration is usually normal.

#### *Collaborative care management*

The goal of therapy is to decrease the red cell mass. Treatment options are phlebotomy, alkylating agents, radioactive phosphorus, or interferon. Leukemic transformation may be a significant risk in younger persons treated with myelosuppressive therapy.[3] Usual treatment is periodic phlebotomy aimed at maintaining the Hct and Hgb at a normal level.

**Patient/family education.** Teaching for the person with polycythemia vera includes the following:

1. Nature of the disorder
2. Importance of continued medical care, blood tests, and phlebotomy
3. Name, dosage, frequency, desired action, and side effects of prescribed medications

**box 29-5** *clinical manifestations*

***Polycythemia Vera***

EARLY STAGE

No symptoms

MODERATE STAGE

Headaches, vertigo, tinnitus, blurred vision

LATE STAGE

Thromboses, embolization

Nosebleeds, ecchymoses, GI bleeding

4. Signs of thromboembolic events that require immediate medical attention
5. Maintenance of hydration to decrease blood viscosity

## DISORDERS OF HEMOSTASIS, PLATELETS, AND COAGULATION

Normal hemostatic functioning requires vascular integrity, normal numbers and functioning of platelets, and normal clotting factors. Although each of the essential components arises separately and is independently regulated, the balanced interplay among these components is necessary to protect the body from excessive bleeding or excessive thrombi formation.

Primary hemostasis involves the formation of a platelet plug over a damaged area of endothelial cells lining a blood vessel. Primary hemostasis is completed with the formation of the platelet plug. Secondary hemostasis is the formation of a fibrin clot overlying the platelet plug. This process requires the sequential activation in the cascade of clotting factors (Figure 29-4). The major steps are the formation of thrombin from prothrombin leading to the formation of fibrin from fibrinogen. (Coagulation factors are listed in Box 28-1.)

A fibrinolytic mechanism exists to balance clot formation and leads to clot lysis. Two enzymes are involved in clot lysis: plasminogen and plasmin. Plasminogen is the inactive form that circulates in the blood. It is converted to plasmin by the action of active Hageman factor in addition to other factors. Plasmin then degrades and dissolves the clot. Streptokinase is a fibrinolytic enzyme.

Another balance to clot formation are substances called anticoagulants. A naturally occurring anticoagulant is heparin, which acts by interfering with activation of several coagulation factors, including activation of thrombin. Coumarin derivatives interfere with synthesis of coagulation factors II, VII, IX, and X in the liver by interfering with vitamin K. Heparin interferes with the intrinsic mechanism whereas warfarin interferes with the extrinsic mechanism.

Disorders of platelets and coagulation are listed in Box 29-6.

## DISORDERS OF PLATELETS

Disorders of platelet function include both increased and decreased numbers of platelets. *Thrombocytosis* is defined as the presence of an abnormally high number of circulating platelets (Box 29-7). Mild bleeding syndromes may be caused by quantitatively normal but functionally defective platelets. The most common cause of such platelet abnormalities is drugs, particularly aspirin. Aspirin inhibits the release of intrinsic platelet adenosine diphosphate (ADP) and produces a defect in platelet aggregation. The defect remains for the life span of the platelet. A variety of familial and nonfamilial platelet disorders also has been described, and defective platelet function typically occurs in persons with uremia. The abnormality may be detected by a test of bleeding time or, more sensitively, by platelet aggregation tests. Patients with disorders of platelet function have clinical manifestations and patient care needs similar to those of persons with thrombocytopenia, although the bleeding abnormality usually is mild.

### Thrombocytopenia

#### Etiology/epidemiology

*Thrombocytopenia* is defined as a lower than normal number of circulating platelets. Laboratory values for a normal adult platelet count range from 150,000 to 400,000/mm$^3$. The many types of thrombocytopenia may result from (1) decreased platelet production, (2) decreased platelet survival, (3) increased platelet destruction (most common form), or (4) sequestration of blood in the spleen.

The most common cause of increased destruction of platelets is *idiopathic thrombocytopenic purpura (ITP)*; ITP can be divided into acute and chronic forms. Acute ITP is self-limiting, lasts less than 6 months, and generally follows a viral illness. Chronic ITP occurs most often in the second and third decades of life and is caused by production of an autoantibody (IgG) directed against a platelet antigen. It has thus been suggested that this disorder be named autoimmune thrombocytopenic purpura (ATP).[14]

Platelet destruction also may be drug-induced. Approximately 70 drugs (some of which are listed in Box 29-8) have been shown to induce thrombocytopenia.[14] Platelet counts generally return to normal within 1 to 2 weeks after the drug is withdrawn; some drugs such as gold salts may require several months.

Secondary thrombocytopenia may result from aplastic anemia, acute leukemia, and conditions causing splenomegaly (such as cirrhosis or lymphomas) that lead to sequestration of blood in the spleen. Sequestration of blood in the spleen results in splenomegaly.

#### Pathophysiology

The major signs of thrombocytopenia observable by physical examination are petechiae, ecchymoses, and purpura. Petechiae occur only in platelet disorders. The person may give a history of menorrhagia, epistaxis, and gingival bleeding. The patient is questioned about recent viral infections, which may produce a transient thrombocytopenia; drugs in current use; and extent of alcohol ingestion.

**box 29-6 Disorders Associated with Platelets and Coagulation**

| | |
|---|---|
| **PLATELETS** | |
| Thrombocytopenia | Decreased number of platelets |
| Thrombocytosis | Increased number of platelets |
| Bleeding syndromes | Disorders of platelet function |
| **COAGULATION** | |
| **Congenital** | |
| Hemophilia A | Decrease of factor VIII |
| Hemophilia B | Decrease of factor IX |
| von Willebrand's disease | Decrease of factor VIII and defective platelet aggregation |
| **Acquired** | |
| Vitamin K deficiency | Decrease of factors II, VII, IX, and X |
| Disseminated intravascular coagulation | Stimulates first the clotting process, then the fibrinolytic process |

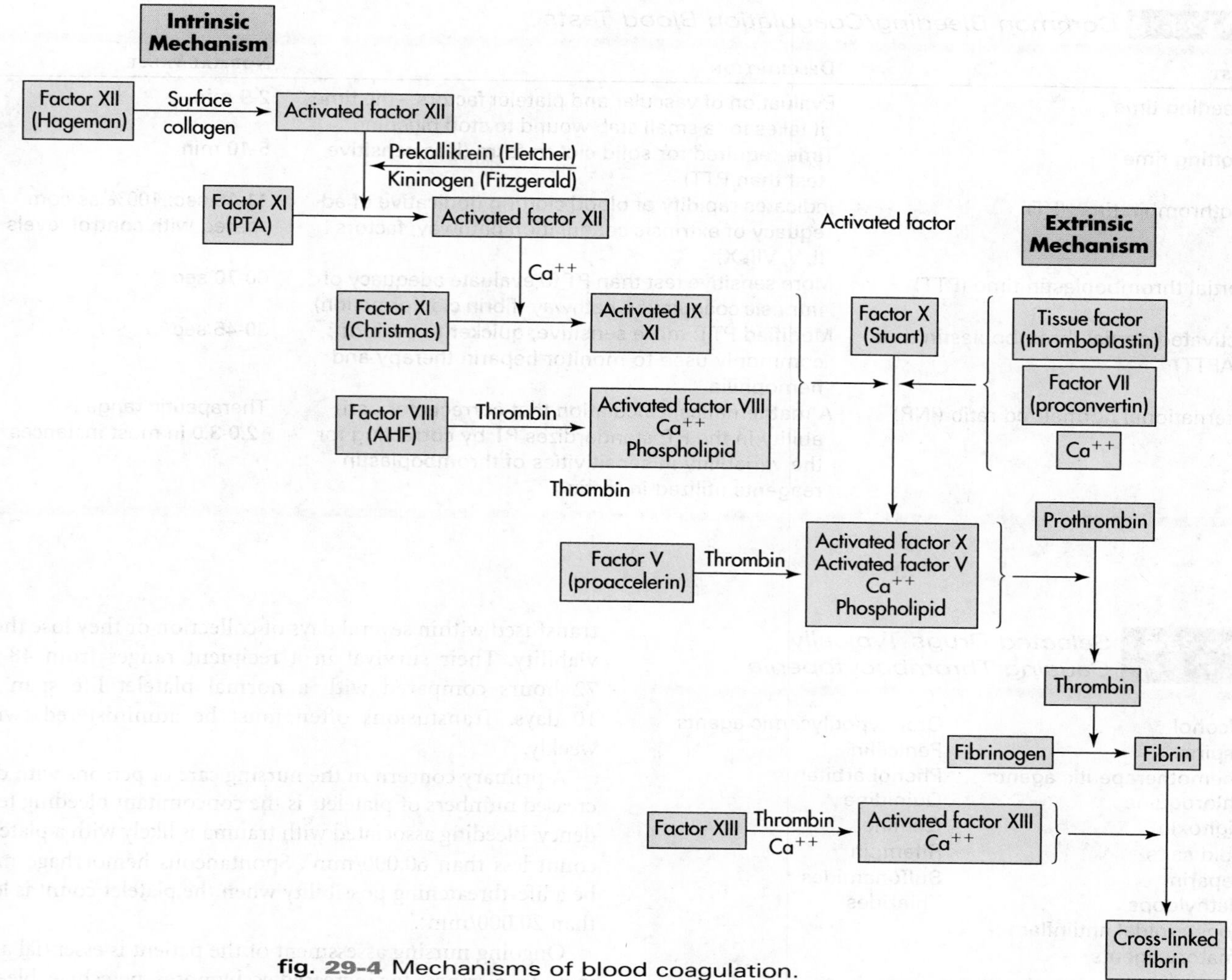


**fig. 29-4** Mechanisms of blood coagulation.

### *Collaborative care management*

Diagnostic tests include complete laboratory studies to ascertain the status of all blood components. The most commonly used tests for assessment of platelets are platelet count, peripheral blood smear, and bleeding time (Table 29-10). In addition, a bone marrow examination is performed to determine the presence of megakaryocytes (precursors of platelets in the bone marrow). Their presence suggests that the thrombocytopenia is caused by peripheral platelet destruction, and their absence or decrease suggests a failure of thrombopoiesis. Examination of the bone marrow also reveals the presence or absence of primary bone marrow abnormalities, such as neoplastic invasion, aplastic anemia, or fibrosis.

The primary treatment modalities for ITP are corticosteroid therapy and splenectomy. Steroids appear to decrease both antibody production and phagocytosis of the antibody-coated platelets. Splenectomy removes the principal organ involved in destruction of the antibody-coated platelets. Other therapeutic modalities include danazol, γ-globulin, or immunosuppressive drugs. Plasma exchange, a form of experimental therapy, may have some efficacy in acute ITP.

**box 29-7** *Thrombocytosis*

Thrombocytosis can be categorized as reactive (hyperactive bone marrow) or essential (myeloproliferative syndrome).

**ASSOCIATED CONDITIONS**

Polycythemia vera
Myelofibrosis
Splenectomy
Iron deficiency anemia
Chronic inflammatory diseases
Hemorrhagic thrombocythemia (thrombocytosis)
Advanced carcinomas

**CLINICAL MANIFESTATIONS**

Thrombosis
Increased bleeding tendencies
Platelet counts >1,000,000/ml

**COLLABORATIVE CARE**

Control of underlying cause
Myelosuppressive drug therapy
Plasmapheresis to reduce circulating number of platelets
Antiplatelet agents (e.g., aspirin, dipyridamole)

**table 29-10** *Common Bleeding/Coagulation Blood Tests*

| TEST | DESCRIPTION | NORMAL VALUE |
|---|---|---|
| Bleeding time | Evaluation of vascular and platelet factors—the time it takes for a small stab wound to stop bleeding | 2-9 min |
| Clotting time | Time required for solid clot to form (less sensitive test than PTT) | 5-10 min |
| Prothrombin time (PT) | Indicates rapidity of blood clotting (indicative of adequacy of extrinsic coagulation pathway; factors I, II, V, VII, X) | 11-16 sec; 100% as compared with control levels |
| Partial thromboplastin time (PTT) | More sensitive test than PT to evaluate adequacy of intrinsic coagulation pathway (fibrin clot formation) | 60-70 sec |
| Activated partial thromboplastin time (APTT) | Modified PTT; more sensitive; quicker to perform; commonly used to monitor heparin therapy and hemophilia | 30-45 sec |
| International normalized ratio (INR) | A mathematical calculation that corrects for variability in the PT; standardizes PT by correcting for the variability in sensitivities of thromboplastin reagents utilized in testing | Therapeutic range is 2.0-3.0 in most instances |

**box 29-8** *Selected Drugs Typically Causing Thrombocytopenia*

Alcohol
Aspirin
Chemotherapeutic agents
Chloroquine
Digitoxin
Gold salts
Heparin
Methyldopa
Nonsteroidal antiinflammatory agents
Oral hypoglycemic agents
Penicillin
Phenobarbital
Quinidine
Quinine
Rifampin
Sulfonamides
Thiazides

**Platelet transfusion.** Transfusion with platelet concentrates may be used in persons with thrombocytopenic bleeding. It is not usually helpful for ITP because the transfused platelets have a short survival time and are rapidly destroyed by the same mechanism as the person's own platelets. In conditions of impaired platelet production, the platelet concentrates increase the platelet count for 1 to 3 days.

Platelets may be obtained from random or HLA-compatible donors. Random donors are logistically easier to obtain and often provide effective platelets for considerable periods, but use of these platelets may eventually lead to decreased efficacy because of antibody production. Because platelets are not always matched for ABO antigens and the infused platelets usually are contaminated with some erythrocytes, antibodies to these antigens may develop. When production of antibody impairs platelet transfusion effectiveness, an attempt should be made to obtain platelets from an HLA-compatible donor. The effectiveness of platelet transfusions may be monitored by performing a platelet count before and 1 hour after transfusion. No increase in the platelet count indicates the transfusion was ineffective. Platelets must be transfused within several days of collection or they lose their viability. Their survival in a recipient ranges from 48 to 72 hours compared with a normal platelet life span of 10 days. Transfusions often must be administered twice weekly.

A primary concern in the nursing care of persons with decreased numbers of platelets is the concomitant bleeding tendency. Bleeding associated with trauma is likely with a platelet count less than $60,000/mm^3$. Spontaneous hemorrhage may be a life-threatening possibility when the platelet count is less than $20,000/mm^3$.

Ongoing nursing assessment of the patient is essential and includes alertness for increased ecchymoses, petechiae, bleeding from other sites, and any change in mental status. The need for avoiding trauma is obvious. Persons with platelet counts below $20,000/mm^3$ should have bleeding precautions instituted. These include the following:

1. Test all urine and stools for blood (guaiac).
2. Do not take temperatures rectally.
3. Do not administer intramuscular injections.
4. Apply pressure to all venipuncture sites for 5 minutes and to all arterial puncture sites for 10 minutes.

**Patient/family education.** Patient teaching is an important component of patient care. Points to be included in the teaching are listed in the accompanying Guidelines for Care Box.

## Thrombotic Thrombocytopenic Purpura

### *Etiology/epidemiology*

*Thrombotic thrombocytopenic purpura (TTP)* is a rare disorder of young adults, occurring more commonly in women than men. In the majority of cases, the etiology is unknown. The increased incidence within families suggests a genetic component. There is also an increased incidence in persons with an immune system disorder (rheumatoid arthritis, systemic lupus erythematosus, and sarcoidosis). Certain drugs

**guidelines for care**

**Teaching the Person with Thrombocytopenia**

1. Nature of the disorder
2. Signs of decreased platelets (petechiae, ecchymoses, gingival bleeding, hematuria, menorrhagia)
3. Name, dosage, frequency, and side effects of prescribed medications (corticosteroids) and importance of not stopping corticosteroid medications abruptly
4. Measures to prevent injury
   a. Use a soft toothbrush or swab for mouth care.
   b. Do not use dental floss.
   c. Keep mouth clean and free of debris.
   d. Avoid intrusions into rectum (e.g., rectal medications, enemas).
   e. Use electric shaver.
   f. Apply direct pressure for 5 to 10 minutes if any bleeding occurs.
   g. Avoid contact sports, elective surgery, and tooth extraction.
   h. Avoid blood thinning drugs, such as aspirin, that decrease sticking ability of platelet.
   i. Increase knowledge of contents of over-the-counter (OTC) medications and effects on platelet functioning. Read labels on OTC medications.
5. Need for follow-up medical care.

have also been associated with TTP. These include iodine, sulfonamides, penicillin, oral contraceptives, and cyclosporine. Lymphoma, pregnancy, and bacterial endocarditis have also been associated with TTP.

#### Pathophysiology

The underlying problem in TTP relates to the depletion of circulating platelets during abnormal clotting processes. The cause of the abnormality in the clotting process is unknown but is thought to be related to vascular injury and the hypercoagulability of circulating platelets. The resulting platelet aggregation results in thrombus formation; the thrombus then lodges in the microvasculature of susceptible organs such as the heart, brain, kidneys, pancreas, and adrenal glands. Symptoms of the disease include fever, anemia, nausea, anorexia, weakness, petechiae, and hematuria. Additional symptoms are related to the organ involved and include renal failure and neurological changes.[8]

#### Collaborative care management

Diagnosis of TTP is made by peripheral blood smear. Findings include low platelets and red cell fragmentation. Other laboratory features include anemia, reticulocytosis, increased serum lactic dehydrogenase (LDH), normal or increased blood urea nitrogen (BUN), and increased fibrin degradation products.

Plasma exchange using fresh frozen plasma is the treatment of choice for TTP. Survival rates are over 80%.[3] Treatment is most effective if initiated as soon as TTP is suspected. Exchanges should be continued until platelet counts and serum LDH levels are near normal. Other therapies include vincristine, cyclosporine, azathioprine, immunoglobulin, and splenectomy. Monitoring the patient's mental status is important, because coma associated with TTP is not uncommon. Monitoring renal and cardiac function is necessary for early treatment of complications. Renal dysfunction occurs in 50% to 75% of patients with TTP.[3]

**Patient/family education.** Patients may require prolonged treatments with plasma exchanges and may require placement of central venous access devices. Patients and families need to be taught correct care in management of these devices (see Chapter 40). Patients should also follow specific guidelines for thrombocytopenia (see the Guidelines for Care Box).

## DISORDERS OF COAGULATION

### Hemophilia

#### Etiology/epidemiology

Hemophilia is a hereditary coagulation disorder. Hemophilia A (factor VIII deficiency), hemophilia B (factor IX deficiency), and hemophilia C (factor XI deficiency) are inherited as sex-linked recessive disorders and are therefore almost exclusively limited to males. An example of the inheritance pattern of hemophilia is shown in Figure 29-5. The incidence of hemophilia A is 1 : 10,000, and for hemophilia B, 1 : 100,000 of the male population. Hemophilia C is rare, with an incidence of 2% to 3% of all hemophilias.

#### Pathophysiology

The diagnosis of hemophilia usually is made in infancy or early childhood. The clinical history is one of lifelong bleeding tendency. A history of excessive bleeding after circumcision or dental extractions commonly is obtained. Persons with hemophilia may give a history of bleeding into any part of the body—spontaneously or after trauma (Box 29-9).

A diagnosis of hemophilia is made by specific assays for factors VIII, IX, and XI. The partial thromboplastin time (PTT), which reflects the intrinsic pathway of coagulation, is prolonged in hemophilia A, hemophilia B, and hemophilia C. The platelet count and prothrombin time (PT) are normal.

Complications associated with hemophilia are the direct result of the bleeding tendency. Commonly the person experiences repeated episodes of spontaneous bleeding into the joints, resulting in joint deformities. Life-threatening bleeding involves retroperitoneal, intracranial, and paratracheal soft tissue hemorrhages.

#### Collaborative care management

Treatment is replacement of the deficient coagulation factor when bleeding episodes do not respond to local treatment (ice bags, manual pressure or dressings, immobilization, elevation, or topical coagulants such as fibrin foam and thrombin). Because the deficient factors are contained in plasma, the treatment used for many years was fresh plasma and blood or fresh frozen plasma. In major hemorrhages, adequate blood levels were difficult to maintain without overloading the person's circulation with large volumes of blood and plasma. The

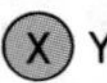


Defective gene is found on X chromosome.

When faulty X chromosome is present in a female,
she will be a carrier of hemophilia.

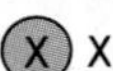


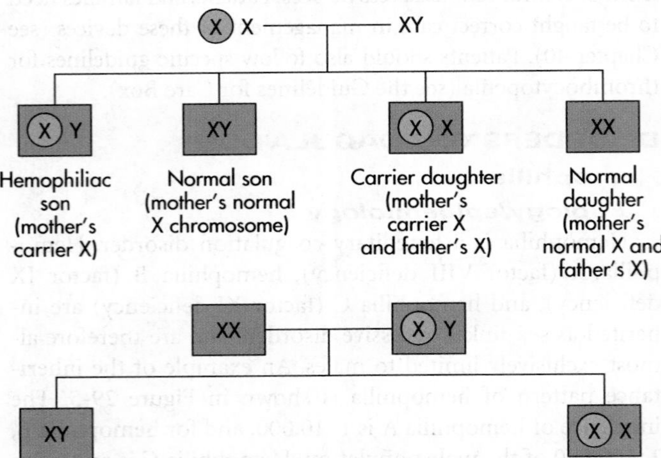


In conception between a normal male and a carrier
female, four possibilities arise:

Hemophiliac son (mother's carrier X)
Normal son (mother's normal X chromosome)
Carrier daughter (mother's carrier X and father's X)
Normal daughter (mother's normal X and father's X)

In conception between a hemophiliac male and a normal
female, son will be normal but daughter will be carrier.

**fig. 29-5** Pattern of inheritance of hemophilia.

discovery of cryoprecipitate in 1964 led the way to the development of commercially prepared concentrated preparations such as fibrinogen, factor VIII, and a concentrate containing the four vitamin K–dependent factors (prothrombin and factors VII, IX, and X). Concentrates avoid the problem of circulatory overload and produce fewer adverse effects (e.g., urticarial or febrile reactions) in some patients. High cost and possible contamination with the virus of serum hepatitis or human immunodeficiency virus (HIV) have been drawbacks to the use of some of the concentrates from pooled blood.

A number of persons with hemophilia A have developed AIDS from transfusions of factor VIII concentrate. This problem has been corrected with the testing of blood donors for evidence of HIV and with heat treatment of the factor VIII concentrates, which kills HIV.

In classic hemophilia the treatment of choice for an acute bleeding episode is infusion of concentrates of the antihemophilic factor (AHF) (factor VIII). One such concentrate is cryoprecipitate. This concentrate is extracted and concentrated by slowly thawing previously frozen plasma at refrigerator temperature. Most of the factor VIII remains as a gel and can be separated from the rest of the plasma by centrifugation. The gel is reconstituted by the addition of saline solution. After the AHF is extracted, the remaining plasma may be used for other purposes. This process results in a concentration of factor VIII as high as 15 to 40 times that of normal plasma. Factor VIII can be produced and stored in any well-equipped

**box 29-9** *clinical manifestations*

***Hemophilia***

- History of lifelong bleeding tendency
- Repeated episodes of spontaneous bleeding into joints
- Excessive bleeding after dental extractions
- Life-threatening hemorrhages: retroperitoneal, intracranial, paratracheal

blood bank at a cost well below that of other concentrates. Treatment with cryoprecipitate is performed in ambulatory care centers. Home infusion of cryoprecipitate controls bleeding episodes effectively, thereby decreasing the need for hospitalization and absence from school or work.

DDAVP (D-amino-8-D-arginine vasopressin) has been demonstrated to increase the factor VIII level in persons with von Willebrand's disease and mild hemophilia A. It is given intravenously and has been associated with few side effects. DDAVP does not carry the risk of transmitting hepatitis, AIDS, or other disorders.

The outlook for the person with hemophilia has been greatly improved by the availability of transfusion therapy. In the past, many persons with factor VIII deficiency died in infancy or in the first 5 years of life. Surgical procedures can now be performed and joint deformity prevented, thus increasing quality of life. Today many persons with moderate or mild hemophilia can live normal, productive lives.

**Patient/family education.** Adults with hemophilia generally are knowledgeable about their disease. They should be aware of the possibility of hemorrhage after dental extraction, injury, or surgery. Persons who have hemophilia should carry a card or wear a Medic-Alert tag that includes their name, blood type, physician's name, and disorder to avoid delay in medical treatment if they should accidentally sustain injury and lose consciousness.

Pain control and the threat of spontaneous bleeding episodes are ongoing stressors the person must confront. Those persons who are able to meet the demands of their illness and adapt their lifestyles accordingly are able to live productive lives. Genetic counseling, aimed at explaining the pattern of inheritance of hemophilia, may be of great value to adults contemplating having children. Such counseling can help potential parents realistically evaluate their ability to raise a child afflicted with hemophilia and to anticipate ways to meet the demands placed on both them and the child.

The National Hemophilia Foundation (110 Greene St., Suite 303, New York, NY 10012; write for information on state and local chapters) is an organization established for persons with hemophilia and their families. The basic function of the national organization is hemophilia research. Other functions include the establishment of standards for chapters, publication of literature, production of films, and promotion of health care legislation in Washington, DC. Local chapter services include special camps for children with hemophilia; parent, child, and adult counseling; group therapy sessions for parents; and a newsletter that reports advances in hemophilic care. A chapter may function as a liaison between hospitals and families with insurmountable bills for blood.

## Vitamin K Deficiency

### Etiology/epidemiology

Vitamin K, a fat-soluble vitamin, is a cofactor in the synthesis of clotting factors II, VII, IX, and X. Approximately 50% of required vitamin K is obtained from a normal diet, and 50% is produced by intestinal bacteria. Vitamin K deficiencies can be anticipated in persons who have a decreased intake and who are given broad-spectrum antibiotics (such as neomycin sulfate) that decrease the growth of intestinal bacteria. Interference with vitamin K absorption occurs with primary intestinal disease (e.g., ulcerative colitis, Crohn's disease), biliary disease, and malabsorption syndromes. Drugs such as coumarin derivatives and large doses of salicylates, quinine, and barbiturates interfere with vitamin K function.

### Pathophysiology

Symptoms are those of hypoprothrombinemia superimposed on the underlying disease. Bleeding is similar to other coagulation disorders—that is, bleeding of the mucous membranes and into the tissues. Postoperative hemorrhage may be observed. In severe cases, GI bleeding may be massive.

### Collaborative care management

Diagnostic features of vitamin K deficiency are prolonged PT and PTT. There is also a decrease in the levels of vitamin K–dependent clotting factors. Treatment consists of therapy for the underlying disorder and cessation of causative drugs. For mild disorders a water-soluble vitamin K preparation (menadione) is given orally or parenterally. In severe disorders a fat-soluble vitamin K preparation (phytonadione) may be given. Fresh frozen plasma will partially correct the disorder immediately, whereas vitamin K therapy takes 6 to 24 hours to be effective and does not have the complications of fresh frozen plasma.

**Patient/family education.** Nursing management includes monitoring of vital signs and patient teaching regarding safety precautions to prevent bruising or bleeding episodes. The patient should be instructed to avoid trauma, use a soft-bristled toothbrush, avoid intramuscular injections, and apply direct pressure immediately on any bleeding sites (see the Guidelines for Care Box on p. 815).

## Disseminated Intravascular Coagulation

Disseminated intravascular coagulation (DIC) is a response of the body's hemostatic mechanisms to a variety of diseases or injury. Disseminated intravascular coagulation is a complicated and potentially fatal process characterized first by clotting and secondarily by hemorrhage. It almost always occurs in response to a primary disease.

### Etiology/epidemiology

Disseminated intravascular coagulation is essentially an imbalance between the processes of coagulation and anticoagulation. Many disease states may alter the normal balance of clotting and fibrinolytic factors, which under normal conditions prevent bleeding while maintaining the fluidity of the blood. Disseminated intravascular coagulation may be directly or indirectly initiated by conditions that trigger at least one of three mechanisms: factor XII formation, activation of factors II and X, and tissue thromboplastin release.[4] A stimulus such as sepsis, anoxia, or a burn most likely causes activation of the intrinsic clotting system by the release of factor XII after endothelial cell wall damage and platelet aggregation. Disseminated intravascular coagulation may be caused by factor VII activation from massive trauma or the release of tissue thromboplastin from an amniotic fluid embolus entering the maternal circulation. Proteolytic enzymes in snake venom can cause direct activation of factors II and X (Box 29-10). Mortality rates vary because of the multiple precipitating factors associated with DIC. Death usually results from uncontrolled bleeding or multiple organ failure.

**box 29-10 Common Precipitating Factors Associated with Disseminated Intravascular Coagulation**

**INFECTIONS**
Hepatitis
Sepsis
Gram-negative infections
Glomerulonephritis

**NEOPLASTIC**
Adenocarcinoma
Acute leukemias
Pheochromocytoma

**OTHER**
Snakebites
Blood transfusion reaction
Surgery
Anaphylaxis
Polycythemia vera
Shock

**OBSTETRIC**
Retained dead fetus
Abruptio placentae
Amniotic fluid embolus
Toxemia
Septic abortion

**VASCULAR**
Aortic aneurysm
Fat embolus
Vasculitis

**TRAUMA**
Crush injury
Brain injury
Burns
Ischemia

### Pathophysiology

The primary disease initiates the clotting process. This response is generalized and occurs throughout the vascular system, creating a state of *hypercoagulability.* The fibrinolytic processes, which normally operate to limit clot extension and dissolve clots, are then stimulated (Figure 29-6). As clotting factors are depleted and fibrinolysis continues, a state of *hypocoagulability* develops.

The most common sequela of DIC is hemorrhage. This paradox is caused by (1) decreased platelets; (2) depletion of clotting factors II, V, VIII, and fibrinogen in the clotting process; and (3) the production of fibrin degradation products (FDP) through fibrinolysis. The FDP act as anticoagulants and increase the hemorrhagic tendency.

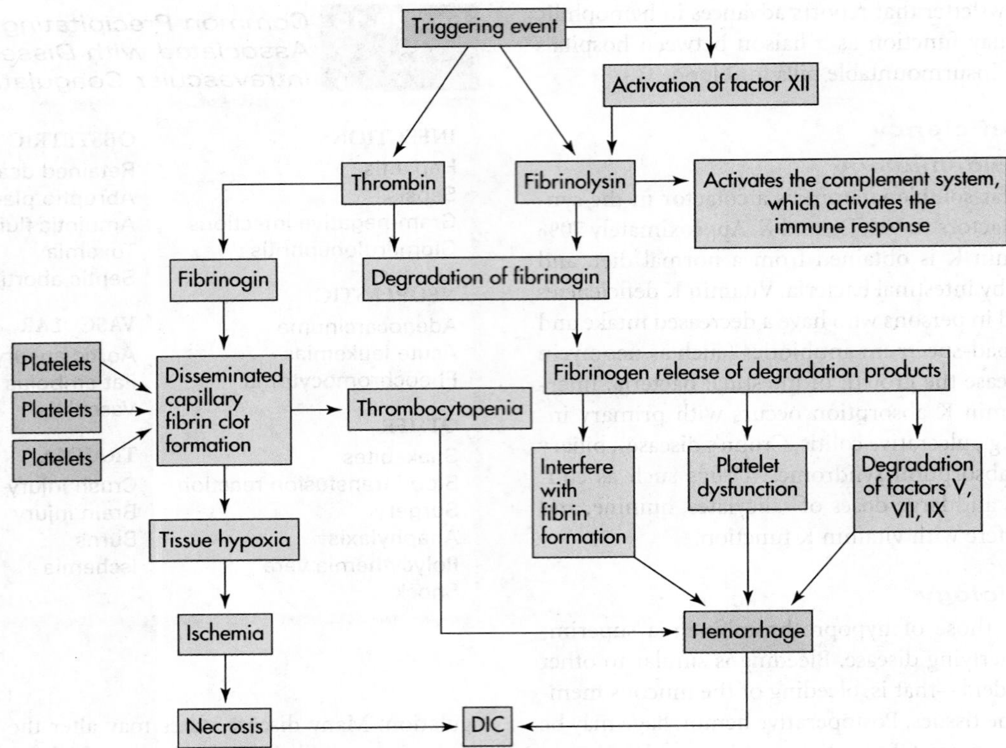


**fig. 29-6** Pathophysiology of disseminated intravascular coagulation.

As the disorder progresses, clinical manifestations may include bleeding of the mucous membranes and tissues (petechiae, ecchymoses). Oral, gastrointestinal, genitourinary, and rectal bleeding and bleeding after injections and venipunctures may occur. Hypoxia, tachypnea, hemoptysis, hypotension, acidosis, and fever may also be present (Box 29-11).

### Collaborative care management

Clinical suspicion of DIC is confirmed by laboratory findings (Table 29-11). Abnormal RBCs may be found on peripheral smear, fibrinolysis reflected in increased fibrin split products, D-dimers, and prolonged thrombin time. The management of DIC always begins with treatment of the primary disease. Once this has been initiated, the goal is to control the bleeding and restore normal levels of clotting factors. Blood products such as fresh frozen plasma, platelet packs, cryoprecipitate, and fresh whole blood may be administered to replace the depleted factors. Heparin has been used to inhibit the underlying thrombotic process; however, it too often promotes rather than decreases bleeding, and its use is controversial.

Nursing management of the patient with DIC is extremely challenging. The person who develops DIC is critically ill and commonly has numerous sites of bleeding. The amount and nature of drainage from chest and nasogastric tubes, oozing from surgical incisions, and progressive discoloration of the skin should be noted and recorded.

Continual observation for new bleeding sites and for an increase or decrease in bleeding is an integral part of the nursing plan, especially if heparin therapy is being used. The susceptibility of these persons to bleeding presents special problems; medications should be given orally or intravenously if at all possible, and small-gauge needles should be used when other injections are necessary. The precautions previously described for patients with thrombocytopenia are applicable to the patient with DIC (see the Guidelines for Care Box on p. 815).

Maintaining fluid balance assumes great importance. Persons with DIC usually lose large quantities of blood and receive frequent transfusions and other fluid replacement. In addition to monitoring blood infusion rates carefully, the nurse must be alert to signs of fluid overload such as slow, bounding pulse and increasing central venous pressure. Hourly urine output is recorded not only as another indication of cardiac function but also because of the possibility of renal thrombi formation and subsequent renal failure.

**Patient/family education.** Commonly the patient is comatose, and the presence of purpura, numerous intravenous lines, and drainage tubes makes the patient's appearance especially upsetting to the family. Most of the primary conditions associated with DIC are of a sudden nature, and the family requires preparation and help in understanding this catastrophic occurrence and support during treatment. Emotional support of the family is paramount because of the

**box 29-11 clinical manifestations**

**Disseminated Intravascular Coagulation**

NEUROLOGICAL
- Confusion
- Irritability
- Headache
- Dizziness
- Seizures
- Fevers
- Increased intracranial pressure
- Vertigo
- Decreased level of consciousness

SENSORY
- Blurred vision/intraocular hemorrhage
- Inner ear bleeding
- Conjunctival hemorrhage
- Epistaxis

CARDIOVASCULAR
- Tachycardia
- Chest pain
- Hypotension
- Absence of peripheral pulses
- Abnormal or increased bleeding from venipuncture or IV insertion sites

RESPIRATORY
- Hemoptysis
- Diffuse infiltrates on x-ray
- Hypoxia
- Dyspnea
- Tachypnea
- Pulmonary embolus
- Pulmonary edema

GENITOURINARY
- Progressive oliguria
- Hematuria
- Renal failure
- Bleeding around indwelling Foley catheters
- Severe bleeding during menstruation
- Vaginal bleeding
- Proteinuria

GASTROINTESTINAL
- Melena
- High-pitched bowel sounds
- Nausea
- Vomiting
- Abdominal distention
- Hematemesis

INTEGUMENTARY
- Cool, moist skin
- Cyanosis
- Petechiae
- Mottling
- Ecchymoses
- Purpura

GENERAL
- Acidosis
- Acral cyanosis

sudden and unexpected onset of DIC. Depending on the etiology and severity of DIC, the family may need support and referrals during the grieving process.

## DISORDERS ASSOCIATED WITH WHITE BLOOD CELLS

The WBC (leukocyte) system is composed of neutrophils, lymphocytes, monocytes, basophils, and eosinophils. All but the lymphocytes are derived from a common stem cell. The primary function of WBCs is to provide for humoral and cellular response to infection. Neutrophils are primarily responsible for phagocytosis and the destruction of bacteria and other infectious organisms. Lymphocytes are the principal cells involved in immunity, which is responsible for the development of delayed hypersensitivity and the production of antibodies (see Chapter 65). Any compromise in the integrity of the WBC system renders a person susceptible to infection.

### NEUTROPENIA

#### Etiology and Pathophysiology

*Neutropenia* is defined as a neutrophil count of less than $2000/mm^3$. Neutropenia may occur as a primary hematological disorder, but more often it is associated with other disorders, including malignant diseases of the bone marrow, aplastic anemia, megaloblastic anemia, use of chemotherapeutic agents, and hypersplenism. The degree of susceptibility to infection is in direct proportion to the degree of neutropenia. Persons with severe neutropenia are at risk of contracting a life-threatening infection.

#### Collaborative Care Management

Severe neutropenia, sometimes referred to as *agranulocytosis,* occurs as a reaction to a variety of drugs and chemicals, including sulfonamides, propylthiouracil, and chloramphenicol. Specific treatment consists of removing the offending agent. Granulocyte transfusion may be used for the patient with severe neutropenia whose condition is life-threatening.

##### *Patient/family education*

A person with a compromised WBC system is highly susceptible to life-threatening infections. Teaching focuses on avoidance of potential sources of infection and recognition of the earliest signs of infection. Family members must be taught to recognize early signs of infection as well. If infection is suspected, the patient should report to the primary health care provider.

Meticulous hand washing by hospital personnel and visitors is mandatory. The environment should be kept scrupulously clean and dustless, and persons with any type of infection should not be allowed contact with the patient. Family members and hospital personnel need frequent reminders of this. Mild colds and respiratory tract infections, taken for granted in daily life, are serious threats to patients with decreased numbers of WBCs.

Patients should be in private rooms with posted neutropenic precautions. When this is not possible, cautious screening of roommates for a potential source of infection is mandatory. The patient should be instructed to wear a mask whenever leaving his or her room. To decrease exposure to bacteria, fresh fruits, vegetables, and flowers are not permitted. Further discussion of nursing care of patients with neutropenia is contained in Chapter 11.

### NEUTROPHILIA

*Neutrophilia* is defined as a neutrophil count greater than $10,000/mm^3$. Such an increase is a normal response to infections, primarily bacterial infections. Prolonged elevation of the neutrophil count, especially in the absence of an apparent cause, demands a diligent search for the underlying cause. Persistent elevated neutrophil counts are associated with leukemia, polycythemia vera, myeloid metaplasia, and various systemic and inflammatory disorders.

**table 29-11** *Laboratory Profile of Disseminated Intravascular Coagulation*

| Diagnostic Test | Normal Value | Expected Value in DIC |
|---|---|---|
| Prothrombin time (PT) | 11-15 sec | Prolonged |
| Partial thromboplastin time (PTT) | 60-70 sec | Usually prolonged |
| Thrombin time | 10-13 sec | Usually prolonged |
| Fibrinogen level | 200-400 mg/100 ml | Decreased |
| Platelet level | 150,000-400,000/mm³ | Normal or decreased |
| Factor assay (II, V, VII, VIII, IX, X, XI, XII) | | Decreased levels of factors V, VIII, and IX |
| Fibrinogin/fibrin degradation products (FDP) | <10 | Increased |
| Protamine sulfate test (soluble fibrin monomer) | Negative | Strongly positive |
| Antithrombin III levels (AT-III) (used to monitor response to therapy) | 89%-120% | Decreased |

Data from Yasko JM: *Guidelines for cancer care: symptom management,* Reston, Va, 1983, Reston.

## LEUKEMIAS

### Etiology/Epidemiology

Leukemia is the fifth leading cause of cancer deaths in men and the sixth leading cause of death in women. It was predicted that 28,000 new cases would be diagnosed for 1997. Leukemia is most common in white males. Five-year survival rates are approximately 38%.[7] Leukemia is a malignant disorder of the hematopoietic system involving the bone marrow and lymph nodes; it is characterized by uncontrolled proliferation of leukocytes and their precursors. With rare exceptions, the bone marrow is involved at the onset, with infrequent manifestations in other hematopoietic organs that lead to organ enlargement (splenomegaly, hepatomegaly). The proliferation of one type of cell often interferes with the normal production of other hematopoietic cells, resulting in the development of immature cells, thrombocytopenia, and anemia. The immaturity of the WBCs leads to decreased immunocompetence and increased susceptibility to infections. The etiology of leukemia is unknown.

Although the causative factors that lead to the development of acute leukemia have not been identified, some predisposing relationships have been discovered. Persons with specific chromosomal aberrations, such as occurs with Down's syndrome, von Recklinghausen's neurofibromatosis, and Fanconi's anemia, have an increased incidence of acute leukemia. Chronic exposure to chemicals such as benzene, drugs that cause aplastic anemia, and radiation exposure has been associated with an increased incidence of the disease. An increased risk for development of acute leukemia has been noted after cytotoxic therapy for Hodgkin's disease, non-Hodgkin's lymphoma, multiple myeloma, polycythemia vera, and breast, lung, and testicular cancers.

The leukemias are classified as acute or chronic and are further subdivided according to cell type or maturity. *Acute* leukemias involve immature cells and are categorized according to the predominant cell in the bone marrow. They are subclassified as acute lymphocytic leukemia (ALL) or acute nonlymphocytic leukemia (ANLL) according to the specific morphology of the leukemic cell. Acute nonlymphocytic leukemia is further classified as acute myelogenous leukemia (AML), promyelocytic leukemia, monocytic leukemia, and other varieties according to cell type. Distinguishing among the various subclassifications of ANLL is difficult, but it is important to do so because newer chemotherapeutic agents appear to have more success against some types and almost none against others. *Chronic* leukemias may be lymphocytic, as in chronic lymphocytic leukemia (CLL), or granulocytic, as in chronic granulocytic or myelogenous leukemia (CML).

Acute leukemias have a rapid onset and a short course ending in death if untreated. The paucity of normal WBCs leads to numerous infections such as pneumonia and septicemia. Early symptoms include fever, lymphadenopathy, pallor and fatigue from anemia, and ecchymoses. The WBC count may be normal, decreased, or increased.

Chronic leukemias have a more insidious onset. Median survival of patients with CML is 3 to 4 years and with CLL 2 to 10 years, depending on the stage at diagnosis. Early signs include fatigue, weakness, anorexia, and weight loss characteristic of a hypermetabolic state. An enlarged spleen and liver usually can be palpated. The WBC count usually is considerably elevated. See Table 29-12 for a synopsis of the four types of leukemia, symptoms, cell type, and commonly used chemotherapeutics.

### Acute lymphocytic leukemia

#### *Etiology/epidemiology*

As mentioned earlier, the etiology of ALL is unknown. Eighty percent of persons affected by ALL are between 2 and 4 years of age. There is a decreased incidence of disease past the age of 10 years.

#### *Pathophysiology*

Acute lymphocytic leukemia is a malignant disorder arising from a single lymphoid stem cell (see Figure 28-1), with impaired maturation and accumulation of the malignant cells in the bone marrow. Diagnosis is confirmed by bone marrow aspiration or biopsy, which typically shows different stages of lymphoid development, from very immature to almost normal cells. The degree of immaturity is a guide to the prognosis: the greater the number of immature cells (increased percentage of lymphocytes and presence of blast cells on a peripheral smear and bone marrow aspiration), the poorer the prognosis.

**table 29-12** *Clinical Manifestations and Common Chemotherapeutic Agents Used in Different Leukemias*

| Leukemia | Peak Age (yr) | Characteristic Symptoms | WBC Level | Bone Marrow Cell Predominance | Common Chemotherapeutic Agents |
|---|---|---|---|---|---|
| Acute lymphocytic leukemia (ALL) | 2-4 | Fever, infections of respiratory tract, anemia, bleeding of mucous membranes, ecchymoses, lymphadenopathy | Decreased, normal, or increased | Lymphoblasts | Regimens with vincristine and prednisone, 6-mercaptopurine, methotrexate |
| Acute myelogenous leukemia (AML) | 12-20, after 55 | Same as ALL except less lymphadenopathy | Normal, decreased, or increased | Myeloblasts | Cytarabine, 6-thioguanine, doxorubicin (Adriamycin), daunomycin |
| Chronic lymphocytic leukemia (CLL) | 50-70 | Weakness, fatigue, lymphadenopathy, pruritic vesicular skin lesions, thrombocytopenia, anemia, splenomegaly | Increased (20,000-100,000) | Lymphocytes | Alkylating agents (e.g., chlorambucil), glucocorticoids |
| Chronic myelogenous leukemia (CML) | 30-50 | Weakness, fatigue, anorexia, weight loss, splenomegaly | Increased (15,000-500,000) | Granulocytes | Busulfan |

Signs and symptoms of ALL include anemia, bleeding, lymphadenopathy, and a predisposition to infection. A blood smear may show immature lymphoblasts. The platelet count and Hct level are reduced in most patients.

### Collaborative care management

Perhaps more dramatically than in any other malignant disorder, chemotherapy has improved the prognosis of children with ALL. Untreated patients have a median survival time (MST) of 4 to 6 months. With current chemotherapy regimens, the MST is close to 5 years, and approximately 50% of children with ALL can be cured.

Complete remissions are obtained in more than 90% of patients treated with chemotherapeutic regimens. Chemotherapeutic protocols for ALL involve three phases: (1) *induction,* often using vincristine and prednisone; (2) *consolidation,* using a modified course of intensive therapy to eradicate any remaining disease; and (3) *maintenance,* usually a combination of drugs, usually including the antimetabolites 6-mercaptopurine and methotrexate. In most chemotherapeutic regimens, vincristine and prednisone are administered intermittently during the maintenance program. Appropriate duration of therapy in patients who remain disease free remains unsettled, but in most centers it is approximately 3 years. The use of "prophylactic" treatment of the central nervous system (e.g., intrathecal administration of methotrexate with or without craniospinal radiation) has greatly diminished recurrences. Because the blood-brain barrier does not allow parenterally infused chemotherapy to reach the leukemic cells, the central nervous system acts as a sanctuary for the leukemia. Intrathecal administration of chemotherapy and/or craniospinal radiation, or both, eradicates the leukemic cells. (See the accompanying Clinical Pathway for acute leukemia.)

**Patient/family education.** Patient and family teaching should include information about the principles of nutrition. The diet should be high in protein, fiber, and fluids. The patient and family should be taught methods to avoid infection (e.g., hand washing, avoiding crowds) and injury. Any signs of bleeding or infection should be reported to the health care provider. Measures to decrease nausea and to promote appetite are important. Oral hygiene and interventions to prevent stomatitis are also important (see p. 827-828). Smoking and spicy and hot foods may alter taste or irritate buccal mucosa. These foods should be avoided.

Teaching should also include the prescribed medication regimen. The patient and family should understand the desired and adverse effects of medications, especially chemotherapeutics. Antibiotics should be taken as prescribed. Pain management is another important intervention. Both pharmacological and nonpharmacological methods should be taught. Finally, the patient and family should be aware of the support services available.

## Acute myelogenous leukemia

### Etiology/epidemiology

Acute myelogenous leukemia is a disease of the pluripotent myeloid stem cell. The cause of the malignant transformation is unknown. Acute myelogenous leukemia can occur at any age but occurs most often at adolescence and after age 55.

*Text continued on p. 825*

## clinical pathway *Acute Leukemia*

*Directions:*
1. Review coordinated care track (CCT) approximately every 8°.
2. Appropriate and completed interventions need no additional documentation.
3. Cross through any interventions which are not applicable.
4. Circle any intervention not completed.
5. The plan of care—nursing interventions and outcome evaluation statements—may be added to the CCT as necessary.

DRG 473 Expected LOS 28.0
Physician(s) ____________

Admit Date ____________
Discharge Date ____________

Surgery/Procedure ____________

Date of Hickman Placement ______
Surgeon ____________

Comorbid Conditions:
❑ CHF ❑ COPD
❑ IDDM
❑ Angina

Leukemia type: ______
Date of Dx: ______
Induction:
1st ____ 2nd ____
Consolidation: ____
Salvage:

Imprint/Label

Complications during this admission:
❑ ICU required ❑
❑ Failure to achieve remission ❑

Last course of chemo: ________

Risk Factors:
❑ Obesity ❑ ETOH/Substance Abuse ❑ Smoking

| DATE | PROBLEM LIST | DISCHARGE CRITERIA | DATE INITIALLY MET | MET ON DISCHARGE YES | MET ON DISCHARGE NO |
|---|---|---|---|---|---|
| | 1. Nausea<br>2. Pancytopenia<br>3. Infection/sepsis<br>4. Pain<br>5. Knowledge deficit | 1. Vital signs stable (afebrile ×24 hr)<br>2. Labs stable (ANC >500)<br>3. Nausea controlled with antiemetics<br>4. Able to tolerate 2 L fluid/day<br>5. Pt has not required platelet transfusions for 48 hr<br>6. Patient/caregiver has knowledge, resources, and ability to safely provide care outside the hospital environment | | | |
| | | Explain any discharge criteria not met: | | | |

## Acute Leukemia—Chemotherapy Phase

**Proceed to Neutropenic Phase when Chemo completed.**

| TIME FRAME<br>LOCATION | HOSPITAL DAY<br>DATE UNIT | HOSPITAL DAY<br>DATE UNIT |
|---|---|---|
| **Patient satisfaction** | "What can we do to enhance your stay with us today?" | "What can we do to enhance your stay with us today?" |
| **Patient Education/ Discharge Planning** | • Initiate PERs:<br>Disease<br>Chemotherapy<br>Labs<br>Restrictions/mouthcare<br>• Assess coping skills (pt/fam) | • Support/resources available to pt/family<br>• Identify primary caregiver<br>________ |
| **Tests/Procedures/ Consults** | • Consult Gen Surg for Hickman cath placement<br>• Consult BMT coordinator for tissue typing<br>• Daily labs as ordered<br>• Weight ________ | WBC ________ K ________<br>Hgb ________ Cr ________<br>Plt ________ Mg ________<br>ANC ________<br>weight ________ |
| **Allied Health Interventions** | • Consult Blood Bank Coord<br>• Consult Nutrition Serv. | |
| **Nursing/Medical Interventions** | • Monitor fluid/electrolytes/replace as ordered<br>• Monitor blood cts/transfuse as ordered<br>• Initiate mouthcare protocol<br>• Hickman dressing change<br>• Initiate neutropenic/thrombocytopenic precautions—<br>Chemo Day 1 ________ | • Monitor fluid/electrolytes/replace as ordered<br>• Monitor blood cts/transfuse as ordered<br>• Continue mouthcare protocol<br>• Hickman dressing change<br>• Guaiac stool, hematest urine<br><br>Chemo Day 2 ________<br>- Chemo Day 10 |
| **Outcome Criteria** | • Chemotherapy begun<br>• Pt/family received info re: disease, treatment, & potential S/E | • Patient satisfaction addressed<br>• Tolerating chemo<br>• Electrolytes stable<br>• No evidence of bleeding |

## Acute Leukemia—Neutropenic Phase

**Proceed to Discharge Phase ANC >100**

| TIME FRAME<br>LOCATION | HOSPITAL DAY<br>DATE UNIT |
|---|---|
| **Patient Satifaction** | "What can we do to enhance your stay with us today?" |
| **Patient Education** | • Teach re:<br>Antibiotics (ATBs)<br>Blood products |
| **Tests/Procedures/ Consults** | WBC ________ K ________<br>Hgb ________ Cr ________<br>Plt ________ Mg ________<br>ANC ________ |
| **Allied Health Interventions** | • Assess for PT/OT |
| **Nursing/Medical Interventions** | • ATBs as ordered<br>• Monitor fluid/electrolytes/replace as ordered<br>• Monitor blood cts/transfuse as ordered<br>• Continue mouthcare protocol<br>• Hickman dressing change |
| **Outcome Criteria** | • Patient satisfaction addressed<br>• Tolerating chemo<br>• Electrolytes stable<br>• No evidence of bleeding |

Courtesy The Cleveland Clinic Foundation, Department of Advanced Clinical Practice Nursing.
*ANC,* Absolute neutrophil count; *PER,* patient education record; *ASC,* alternate site coordinator.

0

## Acute Leukemia—cont'd

### Acute Leukemia—Discharge Phase

| TIME FRAME LOCATION | HOSPITAL DAY DATE UNIT | HOSPITAL DAY DATE UNIT | HOSPITAL DAY DATE UNIT | HOSPITAL DAY DATE UNIT | HOSPITAL DAY DATE UNIT |
|---|---|---|---|---|---|
| **Patient satisfaction** | "What can we do to enhance your stay with us today?" | "What can we do to enhance your stay with us today?" | "What can we do to enhance your stay with us today?" | "What can we do to enhance your stay with us today?" | "What can we do to enhance your stay with us today?" |
| **Discharge/ Planning Patient Education** | • Consult TPN Nurse for Hickman teaching<br>• Assess for home care needs<br>• Consult ASC as needed | • Hickman teaching begun or scheduled | • Discharge teaching re: meds, precautions, dietary needs and Hickman care<br>• Written instructions given | • Review discharge teaching and written Instructions | • Review discharge teaching |
| **Tests/ Procedures/ Consults** | WBC ____ K ____<br>Hgb ____ Cr ____<br>Plt ____ Mg ____<br>ANC ____<br>Weight ____ | WBC ____ K ____<br>Hgb ____ Cr ____<br>Plt ____ Mg ____<br>ANC ____<br>Weight ____ | WBC ____ K ____<br>Hgb ____ Cr ____<br>Plt ____ Mg ____<br>ANC ____<br>Weight ____ | WBC ____ K ____<br>Hgb ____ Cr ____<br>Plt ____ Mg ____<br>ANC ____<br>Weight ____ | WBC ____ K ____<br>Hgb ____ Cr ____<br>Plt ____ Mg ____<br>ANC ____<br>Weight ____ |
| **Allied Health Interventions** | ASC to see & evaluate home needs | | | | |
| **Nursing/ Medical Interventions** | • Monitor fluid/electrolytes/ replace as ordered<br>• Monitor blood cts/transfuse as ordered<br>• Continue mouth care protocol<br>• Hickman dressing change | • Monitor fluid/electrolytes/ replace as ordered<br>• Monitor blood cts/transfuse as ordered<br>• Continue mouth care protocol<br>• Hickman dressing change | • Monitor fluid/electrolytes/ replace as ordered<br>• Monitor blood cts/transfuse as ordered<br>• Continue mouth care protocol<br>• Hickman dressing change | • Monitor fluid/electrolytes/ replace as ordered<br>• Monitor blood cts/transfuse as ordered<br>• Continue mouth care protocol<br>• Hickman dressing change | • Monitor fluid/electrolytes/ replace as ordered<br>• Monitor blood cts/transfuse as ordered<br>• Continue mouth care protocol<br>• Hickman dressing change |
| **Outcome Criteria** | • Patient satisfaction addressed<br>• Afebrile<br>• Nausea & vomiting under control<br>• Electrolytes stable | • Patient satisfaction addressed<br>• Afebrile<br>• Nausea & vomiting under control<br>• Electrolytes stable | • Patient satisfaction addressed<br>• Afebrile<br>• Nausea & vomiting under control<br>• Electrolytes stable<br>• ANC >500<br>• ATBs D/C'd | • Patient satisfaction addressed<br>• Bleeding not present<br>• ANC >500<br>• Afebrile<br>• IV hydations stopped<br>• Able to demonstrate Hickman care | • Patient satisfaction addressed<br>• Afebrile ×48 hr<br>• Pt has not required Plt Tx for 48 hr<br>• D/C criteria met |

Other terms for AML include acute nonlymphocytic, acute granulocytic, and acute myelocytic leukemia.

#### Pathophysiology

Acute myelogenous leukemia arises from a single myeloid stem cell and is characterized by the development of immature myeloblasts in the bone marrow. Clinical manifestations are the same as for ALL (see Table 29-12). The WBC count may be low, normal, or high. Bone marrow aspiration reveals a marked increase in myeloblasts.

#### Collaborative care management

In the untreated patient or the patient who is unresponsive to therapy, the MST is approximately 2 to 3 months. Therapy includes the use of cytarabine, 6-thioguanine, and doxorubicin or daunomycin. Complete remission occurs in 50% to 75% of treated patients, and the MST is approximately 2 to 3 years. Approximately 20% of patients are in complete remission at 5 years and are capable of prolonged disease-free periods (remission). Although patients in remission clearly have an improved quality of life, induction of therapy is arduous, often requiring weeks in the hospital with the need for intensive supportive care (blood component replacement and antibiotic therapy). Bone marrow transplantation with the use of HLA-identical allogeneic bone marrow is being used with increasing frequency. Transplanting the patient's own (autologous) bone marrow obtained after a remission with chemotherapy or radiation therapy is another option (see the Research Box). Several studies have shown the advantages of bone marrow transplantation with the benefits of colony-stimulating factor compared with salvage chemotherapy.[9]

**Patient/family education.** The patient and family should be instructed to avoid sources of potential infection. Signs of potential infection should be recognized and reported to the primary health care provider. Precautions to minimize bleeding should be emphasized (e.g., soft-bristled toothbrush, electric razors). The patient should be instructed to avoid possible injury or tissue trauma (e.g., blow nose gently, avoid constipation). Dietary instructions should include the basics of a nutritionally adequate diet, particularly high-protein and high-fiber foods. Adequate amounts of fluids (2000 to 3000 ml/day) should be encouraged. The patient will also need instruction about medication protocols, side effects, and management of complications (e.g., nausea, vomiting, mouth care). The nurse should inform the patient and family about available support groups and services.

**research**

Reference: Burns JM et al: Critical pathway for administering high-dose chemotherapy followed by peripheral blood stem cell rescue in the outpatient setting, *Oncol Nurs Forum* 22(8):1219, 1995.

The purpose of this descriptive study was to define and explain the rationale for a critical pathway for high-dose outpatient chemotherapy followed by autologous bone marrow transplant with peripheral stem cells. Information was obtained from various published sources. As health care costs skyrocket, safe, cost-effective therapies for advanced cancers need to be developed. It was concluded that a multidisciplinary team is important in the development of complex treatment protocols. Nurses are crucial to the success of coordinated care tracks and should maintain their role as patient advocate while monitoring pathway compliance.

### Chronic Lymphocytic Leukemia

#### Etiology/epidemiology

As with other types of leukemia, the etiology of CLL is unknown. An estimated 8000 new cases occur annually. The incidence of CLL increases with age and is rare under age 35. Chronic lymphocytic leukemia is more common in men than women.

#### Pathophysiology

Chronic lymphocytic leukemia is characterized by a proliferation of small, abnormal, mature B lymphocytes, often leading to decreased synthesis of immunoglobulins and depressed antibody response. The accumulation of abnormal lymphocytes begins in the lymph nodes, then spreads to other lymphatic tissues and the spleen. The number of mature lymphocytes in the peripheral blood smear and bone marrow is greatly increased.

The onset is insidious with weakness, fatigue, and lymphadenopathy. Symptoms include pruritic vesicular skin lesions, anemia, thrombocytopenia, and an enlarged spleen (see Table 29-12). The WBC count is elevated to a level between 20,000 and 100,000; this increases blood viscosity, and a clotting episode may be the first manifestation of disease. Bone marrow biopsy shows infiltration of lymphocytes.

#### Collaborative care management

The MST of persons with CLL is 4.5 to 5.5 years. As a general rule, persons are treated only when symptoms, particularly anemia, thrombocytopenia, or enlarged lymph nodes and spleen appear. Chemotherapeutic agents used in the treatment of CLL are most often one of the alkylating agents, such as chlorambucil and the glucocorticoids. Although no treatment is curative, remissions may be induced by chemotherapeutics or radiation of the thymus, spleen, or entire body.

**Patient/family education.** Patient and family teaching is similar to that described for AML. Education is necessary regarding the course of disease and benefits and possible side effects of treatment. This is especially important because of the age of the affected population and the advantages of conservative therapy. Some persons do well without treatment, especially if asymptomatic.

### Chronic Myelogenous Leukemia

#### Etiology/epidemiology

Chronic myelogenous leukemia accounts for 15% to 20% of all cases of leukemia. The incidence is 1 per 100,000 persons and an estimated 4300 new cases were diagnosed in 1997. The onset of this disease occurs in the fifth and sixth decades of life and is equally distributed between the sexes.[7] The median survival rate is 60 to 65 months.

Although the etiology of CML is unknown, benzene exposure and high doses of radiation have been associated with CML. In 80% to 95% of persons diagnosed with CML, the Philadelphia chromosome (translocation of chromosomes 22 and 9) has been identified.[3] This has led to research regarding a genetic component to this disease, but more studies are needed.

### Pathophysiology

The primary defect in CML is an abnormal stem cell leading to uncontrolled proliferation of the granulocytic cells. As a result of this proliferation, the number of circulating granulocytes increases sharply.

The classic symptoms of chronic types of leukemia also exist in CML. These include fatigue, weakness, anorexia, weight loss, and splenomegaly (Table 29-13). The WBC count ranges from 15,000 to 500,000 depending on the stage of the disease. The peripheral blood smear demonstrates granulocytes in varying degrees of maturity, from blast cells to mature neutrophils, and granulocytic hyperplasia in the bone marrow.

Chronic myelogenous leukemia commonly changes from a chronic indolent phase into an accelerated phase that progresses rapidly into a fulminant neoplastic process sometimes indistinguishable from an acute leukemia. The accelerated phase of the disease (*blastic* phase) is characterized by increasing numbers of granulocytes in the peripheral blood. Often there is a corresponding anemia and thrombocytopenia. Fever and adenopathy also may develop. Of patients with CML, 50% to 60% progress to the blastic phase. Once the CML enters the blastic phase, the chemotherapeutic regimen is similar to that of AML.

The overall survival rate for CML is poor. Only 30% of patients survive 5 years after diagnosis. After the onset of a blast crisis, the life expectancy decreases to 2 to 4 months, and prognosis is grave.[6]

### Collaborative care management

**Diagnostic tests.** The most distinguishing characteristic of CML is the WBC count, which may be greater than 100,000 at the time of diagnosis. The WBC differential count shows a shift to the left. The eosinophil and basophil count will also be elevated. Leukocyte alkaline phosphatase stain, which is low in CML, differentiates this from other types of leukocytosis.

The bone marrow aspirate will be hypercellular with increased myeloid cells. Chronic myelogenous leukemia is confirmed by verifying the presence of the Philadelphia chromosome by genetic karyotyping. In juvenile-onset CML (less than 4 years of age), the Philadelphia chromosome will be missing.

**Medications and treatments.** The goal of treatment for CML is to control the proliferation of WBCs. Two commonly used medications are hydroxyurea and busulfan. Of these two, hydroxyurea is most commonly used because of the high incidence of toxic side effects associated with busulfan. Patients taking hydroxyurea must be instructed about compliance with daily medications and have their blood counts monitored at frequent intervals.

Once CML has converted to the blast phase of the disease, aggressive therapy becomes necessary. Anthracyclines and cytosine arabinoside have been used, but with less than a 20% remission rate. Some success has been seen with the use of the biological response modifier interferon-$\alpha$, and current studies are being done to further evaluate the long-term effects of this medication.[13]

The only potential curative therapy for CML is the bone marrow transplant (see Chapter 68). Transplants with the HLA-matched sibling donors are the most successful if they are done early in the course of the disease in patients who are younger than 50 years of age and who are in good underlying health. Transplant-related complications include graft-versus-host disease, sepsis, and uncontrolled bleeding. These present significant risk to the patient.

**Diet and activity.** Diet and activity are generally unrestricted. Patients who are considered neutropenic (absolute neutrophil count less than 500) should be placed on a low-pathogen diet, which excludes fresh uncooked fruits and vegetables. Patients with platelet counts less than 20,000 should be instructed to avoid activities that may result in injury.

**Referrals.** The patient and family may benefit from referrals to social services and available community resources (see the Patient/Family Teaching Box).

**table 29-13** *Symptomology of the Phases of Chronic Myelogenous Leukemia*

| | Stable | Accelerated | Blast Crisis |
|---|---|---|---|
| Presence of symptoms | None to minimal | Moderate | Pronounced |
| Splenomegaly | Mild | Increased | Marked |
| WBC count | Slight elevation | Erratic | Very high |
| Differential | <1% blasts | Increase immature cells | >25% blasts |

**patient/family teaching**

**Persons with Leukemia**

- Nature of the disease process and its effects
- Prevention of infection
- Drug regimen: name, side effects
- Method of arranging for chemotherapy administration and periodic blood counts
- Symptoms requiring immediate medical attention (fever, bleeding)
- Available community resources (American Cancer Society, Leukemia Society*)
- Need for continual medical follow-up
- Meticulous oral care to prevent stomatitis

*600 Third Ave, New York, NY 10016.

## NURSING MANAGEMENT

### ASSESSMENT

#### Subjective Data

Subjective data to be collected to assess the patient with CML include:

- Presence of fatigue
- History of arthralgia, malaise
- Tenderness in the left upper quadrant (LUQ)
- Abnormal bruising or bleeding
- Weight loss
- Decreased exercise tolerance

#### Objective Data

Objective data to be collected to assess the patient with CML include:

- Vital signs, elevated temperature
- Splenomegaly
- Petechiae
- Presence of bruising
- Lymphadenopathy
- Abdominal tenderness
- Shortness of breath
- Pallor
- Hematuria

### NURSING DIAGNOSES

Nursing diagnoses are determined from analysis of patient data. Nursing diagnoses for the patient with CML include:

| Diagnostic Title | Possible Etiological Factors |
|---|---|
| Infection, risk for | Immunosuppressive therapy, nonfunctioning WBCs |
| Injury, risk for | Decreased platelets, bone marrow suppression |
| Oral mucous membrane, altered | Breakdown of oral mucosa secondary to chemotherapy, neutropenia |
| Fatigue | Anemia, chronicity of disease |
| Knowledge deficit | Treatment options |
| Coping, ineffective | Poor prognosis of disease |

### EXPECTED PATIENT OUTCOMES

Expected outcomes for the patient with CML may include but are not limited to:

1. Maintain normal body temperature and be free from signs of infection
2. Demonstrate measures to minimize the complications of thrombocytopenia
3. Demonstrate measures to restore or maintain the integrity of oral mucosa
4. Maintain level of independence without complaint of fatigue or shortness of breath
5. Participate in support groups and identify effective coping strategies to deal with chronic illness
6. Verbalize understanding of the signs of CML, the signs of conversion to advanced disease, and treatment options available

### INTERVENTIONS

#### Preventing Infection

Patients who are neutropenic from either chemotherapy or leukemia are at an increased risk for infection and sepsis. Interventions aimed at reducing patient risk begin with careful hand washing before patient contact. Instructions must also be given to visitors and patients about the necessity of good hand washing. Proper perineal care after urination and bowel movements will also decrease the risk of infection.

Patients should have private rooms and be placed in protective isolation. A low-pathogen diet eliminating raw fruits and vegetables is appropriate. Foods from outside sources (carryout, fast foods) and fresh plants and flowers should be discouraged.

The skin, oral cavity, phlebotomy sites, and invasive line sites should be carefully monitored for signs of infection. All invasive lines should be maintained aseptically. Patients should be instructed on the signs and symptoms of impending septic shock and to report any related symptoms immediately.

#### Promoting Safety

Bleeding is a constant risk for the patient with CML. Platelet counts are monitored daily during hospitalizations. Platelet transfusions may be indicated for patients whose platelet counts are below 20,000 and who are exhibiting signs of bleeding.

The skin should be assessed daily for the presence of petechiae and ecchymosis. Intravenous lines and all invasive sites should be assessed for bleeding. The nurse should also monitor stool and urine for the presence of blood. Any changes in mental status, severe headache, changes in visual and pupillary response, restlessness, and widening pulse pressure should be reported immediately. All invasive procedures should be avoided. Electric razors should be used to avoid potential trauma, and soft-bristled toothbrushes should be provided to the patient for oral care. Stool softeners should be given to avoid constipation, and the patient should be instructed to avoid straining with bowel movements or blowing the nose forcefully.

#### Providing Oral Hygiene

Stomatitis, mucositis, and esophagitis are serious and painful complications related to depression of the immune system, particularly in patients receiving chemotherapy. Persistent comprehensive oral care should be maintained by the patient (see the Patient/Family Teaching Box). Pain associated with breakdown and infection of the oral cavity can be severe. Narcotics may be administered to relieve the pain.

#### Preventing Fatigue

To minimize fatigue in patients with a chronic disease such as CML, it is important to minimize energy expenditure. Encourage the patient to prioritize activities and maximize energy potential to complete activities that are most valued. Assist the patient in delegating nonessential activities to others, and provide assistance with ADL as needed. The patient's activity level can be increased as tolerated. The day should be structured to allow for frequent rest periods.

Sleep deprivation also contributes to a patient's feelings of fatigue. Limit noise and needless interruptions to the patient's sleep. Perform vital signs and assessments before medicating the patient for sleep, allowing for maximal periods of uninterrupted sleep.

### Promoting Effective Coping

Chronic myelogenous leukemia is a chronic disease with a poor prognosis. Patients and family members must cope with actual and potential losses, as well as the fear of future treatments and possible side effects. Actively listening as patients and families verbalize their concerns while creating a nonjudgmental atmosphere helps facilitate coping. Assisting the patient to establish personal goals will help promote feelings of self-worth despite chronic illness.

Additional strategies to facilitate coping include relaxation, guided imagery, and music therapy. Patients should also be encouraged to seek out support groups. Many organizations provide assistance to persons with cancer, and patients may need assistance locating available help. Sources of assistance include the following:

American Cancer Society ("I Can Cope" programs)
Leukemia Society of America
American Red Cross
National Coalition for Cancer Survivorship

### Patient/Family Education

Patient and family education should initially focus on the disease process and typical course. The patient needs a complete understanding of treatment options to make informed choices.

Knowledge of specific drug therapy and anticipated side effects is also a component of the teaching plan. Of utmost importance in learning is the ability of the person to identify the body's signals that blood abnormalities exist. Petechiae, ecchymoses, and gingival bleeding (indicating infection) are warning signs to seek prompt medical attention. Bone pain, often severe, may signal blastic crisis (acute proliferation of immature cells).

Persons whose illness runs the course of several months to years often become highly knowledgeable about their disease, blood components, related symptoms, and specific chemotherapeutic drugs. These persons sometimes discuss their progress in terms of changes in their blood counts. Many patients are quite knowledgeable about the significance of laboratory results and the effects on the body. For example, they often can predict their count by how they feel. Many such persons respond well to being included in their plan of care during hospitalization and in preparation for discharge.

Establishing a therapeutic relationship with the patient and family allows the patient to vent feelings and fears regarding living with the diagnosis of CML. Allow sufficient time for questions when planning a teaching session. The family should be included whenever possible. See the Patient/Family Teaching Box for the person with leukemia on p. 826.

## EVALUATION

To evaluate effectiveness of nursing interventions, compare patient behaviors with those stated in the expected outcomes. Successful achievement of patient outcomes for the patient with CML is indicated by:

1. Remains free from infection
2. Demonstrates appropriate measures to prevent bleeding episodes
3. Displays intact oral mucosa and demonstrates correct oral hygiene regimen
4. Maintains typical level of function without fatigue or shortness of breath
5. Identifies coping strategies and develops a support group to assist in managing the stress of chronic disease
6. Verbalizes understanding of disease processes and makes informed choices regarding treatment

**patient/family teaching**

**Oral Care for the Patient Undergoing Chemotherapy**

1. Oral care should be done after each meal and at bedtime.
2. Soft brushes or sponges should be used to avoid trauma.
3. Do not use dental floss.
4. Rinses containing alcohol should be avoided because these can cause irritation and increase pain.
5. Tobacco in any form should be avoided.
6. Foods that are extreme in temperature should be avoided.

**Medications Used to Manage Stomatitis**

Nystatin (Mycostatin)—swish and swallow four times a day
Clotrimazole (Mycelex troches)—dissolve in mouth five times a day
BMX (Benadryl, Maalox, Xylocaine)—topical analgesia as needed
Viscous lidocaine as needed
Narcotic analgesics as needed

**gerontological assessment**

**Chronic Myelogenous Leukemia**

| ASSESSMENT FINDINGS IN CML | CHANGES ASSOCIATED WITH AGING |
|---|---|
| Skin changes: petechiae, ecchymoses | Increased fragility and decreased skin turgor |
| Oral cavity: swollen, irritated gums | Ill-fitting dentures |
| Neurological: headache, confusion, decreased nerve response | Alzheimer's disease/ dementia |
| Musculoskeletal: joint pain, inflammation, bone pain | Degenerative joint disease |
| Genitourinary: hematuria, urinary tract infection | Benign prostatic hypertrophy |

## GERONTOLOGICAL CONSIDERATIONS

Chronic myelogenous leukemia is a disease that primarily affects older adults. The typical symptoms of CML may be confused with characteristic changes of aging. Some persons may be asymptomatic; others may report vague symptoms such as malaise, fatigue, headache, and weight loss (see the Gerontological Assessment Box).

## COMPLICATIONS

Complications of CML include those associated with treatment options. Hemorrhage, infection, and mucositis can occur as a result of chemotherapy or the disease process. During the blast phase, lytic bone lesions, soft tissue infiltrates, and epidural tumors causing cord compression may complicate the course of the disease. As stated earlier, prognosis in this phase is grave. Widespread organ damage may occur, caused by large numbers of leukemic cells occluding the vasculature.

The major side effect of hydroxyurea is reversible myelosuppression. Busulfan toxicity includes potentially fatal myelosuppression, organ fibrosis (lung, heart, and bone marrow), and a wasting syndrome similar to Addison's disease.

Toxicity associated with the use of interferon-$\alpha$ manifests as fever, chills, malaise, arthralgia, fatigue, and headache. These symptoms usually resolve after 2 weeks of therapy with interferon-$\alpha$. Late signs of toxicity include hepatitis, proteinuria, hypothyroidism, depression, and psychosis. (See Chapter 68 for complications associated with bone marrow transplant.)

# DISORDERS ASSOCIATED WITH THE LYMPH SYSTEM

## LYMPHEDEMA

### Etiology

*Lymphedema* is an abnormal accumulation of lymph within the tissues caused by an obstruction in flow. Lymphedema can be classified as primary or secondary. Primary lymphedema results from hypoplastic, aplastic, or hyperplastic development of the lymphatic vessels. Symptoms may manifest at birth, during puberty, or in middle age. Secondary or acquired lymphedema most often develops from trauma to the lymph nodes. Common causes include surgical removal of lymph nodes, radiation-induced fibrosis, inflammation, lymphomas, and parasitic infections.

### Epidemiology

Primary lymphedema affects women more commonly than men. Filarial infections, prevalent in tropical climates, are the most common worldwide cause of secondary lymphedema.

### Pathophysiology

The lymphatic vessels carry lymph from the tissues back into the venous circulation. This system is made up of small, thin vessels that are found throughout the body in close proximity to the veins. The lymphatics begin as capillaries that drain the tissues of lymph (a fluid similar to plasma) and tissue fluid that contains cells, cellular debris, and proteins. The lymph flows through oval bodies called lymph nodes, which remove noxious agents such as bacteria and toxins. The flow then drains into the thoracic duct and the right lymphatic duct, which empty into the junction of the internal jugular vein and subclavian vein (see Figure 29-7).

Pathophysiological changes may include (1) roughening of the surface of the lymphatic vessel, (2) dilation of some lymph channels with thickening and edema of the lymphatic tissue, and (3) fibrosis and separation of elastic fibers that may be present in inflammatory states. Recurrent episodes of lymphedema may cause fibrosis and hyperplasia of lymph vessels, leading to a severe enlargement of the extremity, called *elephantiasis.*

Lymphedema of the lower extremities begins with mild swelling at the ankle, which gradually extends to the entire limb. Initially, the edema is soft and pitting, but it then progresses to firm, rubbery, nonpitting edema. Left leg swelling is more common than right leg swelling. This condition is aggravated by prolonged standing, pregnancy, obesity, warm weather, and menstruation.

### Collaborative Care Management

#### *Diagnostic tests*

Diagnostic tests include the use of lymphangiography (see Chapter 28). Radioisotope lymphography involves injection into the foot, with subsequent scanning. A computed tomography (CT) scan may show a honeycomb pattern in the subcutaneous compartment.

#### *Medications*

Diuretics can be prescribed to temporarily decrease the size of the limb. Long-term antibiotic therapy may be indicated to control recurrent cellulitis and infection.

#### *Treatments*

Treatment consists of elevating the foot of the bed on blocks at a height of 8 inches, wearing compression support stockings, and using an intermittent pneumatic compression device. Monitoring the circumference of the extremities can help in determining the effectiveness of treatments.

#### *Surgical management*

Surgery is restricted to severe cases of lymphedema that are unsuccessfully treated by medical management. The most common reason is to reduce the size and bulk of the limb. Surgery also may be used to decrease the incidence of recurrent infections and to improve the cosmetic appearance of the involved limb. The surgical approaches are varied. In general, surgery is directed at restoring lymphatic function or improving the patient's symptoms. Microsurgery involving vein grafting to small lymph vessels has been successful.

#### *Diet*

There is no special diet to treat lymphedema; however, the patient receiving diuretic therapy requires adequate potassium. Salty and spicy foods that predispose to fluid retention and edema should be avoided.

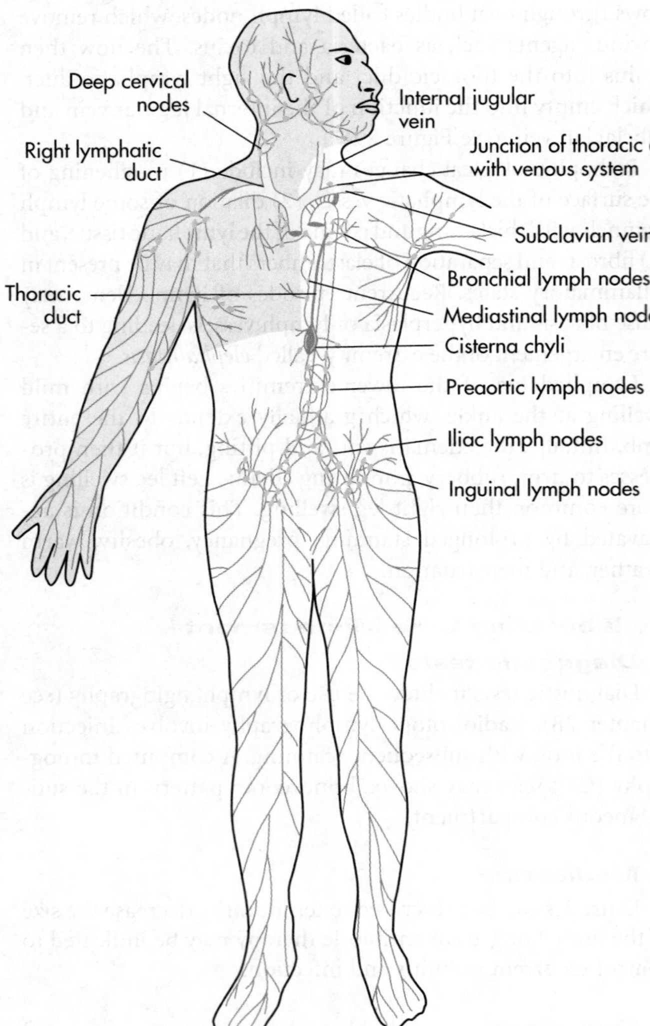


**fig. 29-7** Lymph pathways of the lower limb drain into the subclavian vein.

### *Activity*

Standing still for long periods of time is contraindicated. If infection is present, activity is restricted to bedrest with leg elevation. Otherwise, regular moderate exercise may improve lymph flow.

### *Referrals*

A physical therapy consultation may be appropriate if the patient needs additional assistance with mobility. A wound care specialist may be of help if infection is present.

## NURSING MANAGEMENT

## ■ ASSESSMENT

### Subjective Data

Subjective data to be collected to assess the patient with lymphedema include:

- Onset of swelling in affected limb
- History of surgical removal of lymph nodes, radiation therapy, recurrent inflammation, parasitic infection
- Functional limitation of swelling
- Effectiveness of current therapy to decrease swelling

### Objective Data

Objective data to be collected to assess the patient with lymphedema include:

- Presence of edema—pitting or nonpitting
- Location of edema—more common in left leg
- Comparison in size of extremities
- Texture of skin: firm, rubbery
- Association with prolonged standing, pregnancy, obesity, warm weather, and menstruation

## ■ NURSING DIAGNOSES

Nursing diagnoses are determined from analysis of patient data. Nursing diagnoses for the patient with lymphedema may include but are not limited to:

| Diagnostic Title | Possible Etiological Factors |
|---|---|
| Infection, risk for | Lack of knowledge |
| Body image disturbance | Change in body appearance |
| Knowledge deficit | Lack of exposure/recall |

## ■ EXPECTED PATIENT OUTCOMES

Expected patient outcomes for the person with lymphedema may include but are not limited to:

1. Describes measures to prevent infection
2. Expresses acceptance of body image changes
3. States measures to improve lymph circulation

## ■ INTERVENTIONS

### Preventing Infection

1. Assess skin daily for intactness, swelling, redness, and lesions.
2. Provide meticulous care to skin, especially feet.
3. Complete entire course of prescribed antibiotics.
4. Avoid application of nonprescribed topical ointments and creams.

### Promoting a Positive Body Image

1. Encourage expression of concerns regarding swelling of affected limb.
2. Discuss alteration in clothing and shoes to accommodate swelling.
3. Teach importance of adherence to measures that decrease edema.

### Patient/Family Education

1. Perform passive and active exercise of involved limb.
2. Elevate affected extremity.
3. Avoid standing still for long periods.
4. Wear compression support stockings.
5. Avoid constrictive clothing.
6. Exercise on a regular basis.

7. Elevate foot of bed on 8-inch blocks.
8. Use pneumatic external compression pump as ordered.
9. Take medications as prescribed.
10. Adhere to dietary restrictions as indicated.

## EVALUATION

To evaluate effectiveness of nursing interventions, compare patient behaviors with those stated in the expected patient outcomes. Successful achievement of patient outcomes for the patient with lymphedema is indicated by:

1. Correctly describes measures to prevent infection
2. Expresses acceptance of body image change
3. Correctly describes measures to improve lymph circulation (see Chapter 48 for further discussion of lymphedema associated with breast cancer)

## HODGKIN'S DISEASE

### Etiology/Epidemiology

Hodgkin's disease is a malignant disorder of lymph nodes first described by Thomas Hodgkin in 1832. The etiology is unknown, but there may be a genetic component to the disease. Increased incidence among siblings has been reported. An infectious etiology is under debate. The Epstein-Barr virus has been associated with the development of Hodgkin's disease.[3] The peak incidence of disease occurs in the third decade of life, with a second peak at ages 55 to 75 years.[3] Males are more frequently affected. An estimated 7 persons per 100,000 are diagnosed with Hodgkin's disease in the United States annually.[3]

### Pathophysiology

The presence of the Reed-Sternberg (RS) cell is the pathological hallmark of the disorder, but four histological subtypes of Hodgkin's disease have been recognized: *lymphocyte predominant, nodular sclerosis, mixed cellularity,* and *lymphocyte depletion.* The lymphocyte predominant and nodular sclerosis types have the best prognosis, and lymphocyte depletion has the worst. Nodular sclerosis is the most common type and accounts for 40% to 70% of cases. Nodular sclerosis typically manifests in the supraclavicular and cervical nodes. The origin of the Reed-Sternberg cell is unclear, but it may originate from the B lymphocyte or macrophage. The most important prognostic indicator is the stage of the disease at the time of diagnosis. Accurate staging is crucial to the subsequent treatment regimen. The diagnostic workup is often arduous and difficult, and explanation of the many facets of the complex diagnostic procedures helps provide the emotional support so often needed during this time.

Systemic symptoms that may be associated with Hodgkin's disease include fatigue, weakness, anorexia, unexplained fever, night sweats, and generalized pruritus. Physical examination may show enlargement of lymph nodes, liver, and spleen. Lymphadenopathy is most common in the cervical, axillary, and inguinal nodes. A chest roentgenogram may identify the presence of a mediastinal mass. A bone marrow biopsy is performed to determine if there is marrow involvement. The disease may spread via the lymph system to the liver, spleen, vertebrae, uterus, and bronchi. The liver and spleen are evaluated by radionuclide scanning or by CT scan. Lymphangiography is performed to evaluate the intraabdominal nodes. A *staging laparotomy* is performed in some circumstances to obtain a biopsy specimen of retroperitoneal lymph nodes and both lobes of the liver and to remove the spleen. The rationale for this procedure is the limitations of nonsurgical diagnosis of liver, spleen, and intraabdominal node involvement.

The classification into stages allows for comparison of persons with similar disease involvement and their response to a given treatment regimen. Over time such comparisons have identified the treatment course most appropriate for a described disease. The revised Ann Arbor staging classification for Hodgkin's disease is shown in Box 29-12.

**box 29-12 Ann Arbor Clinical Staging Classification of Hodgkin's Disease**

**STAGE I**

Involvement of a single lymph node region (I) or of a single extralymphatic organ or site ($I_E$)

**STAGE II**

Involvement of two or more lymph node regions on the same side of the diaphragm (II) or localized involvement of an extralymphatic organ or site and of one or more lymph node regions on the same side of the diaphragm ($II_E$)

**STAGE III**

Involvement of lymph node regions on both sides of the diaphragm (III), which also may be accompanied by involvement of the spleen ($III_S$) or by localized involvement of an extralymphatic organ or site ($III_E$) or both ($III_{SE}$)

**STAGE IV**

Diffuse or disseminated involvement of one or more extralymphatic organs or tissues, with or without associated lymph node involvement

The presence or absence of fever, night sweats, or unexplained loss of 10% or more of body weight in the 6 months preceding admission are denoted by the suffix letters B and A, respectively. Biopsy-documented involvement of stage IV sites also is denoted by letter suffixes: M, marrow; L, lung; H, liver; P, pleura; O, bone; D, skin and subcutaneous tissue.

### Collaborative Care Management

Radiation therapy (Figure 29-8) is used for stages IA, IB, IIA, and IIB. This treatment yields a cure rate of approximately 90% for stage I and 80% for stage II. Combination chemotherapy is the treatment of choice for stages IIIB and IV. Therapy of stage IIIA is controversial and involves chemotherapy, radiation, or a combination of these therapies. The most commonly used combination is the MOPP regimen, which consists of mechlorethamine (Nitrogen mustard), Oncovin (vincristine), procarbazine, and

**table 29-14** *Chemotherapeutic Regimens for Treatment of Hodgkin's Disease*

| Name | Drugs | Dosage | Method | Schedule | Cycle |
|---|---|---|---|---|---|
| MOPP | Mechlorethamine (nitrogen mustard) | 6 mg/m$^2$ | IV | Days 1 and 8 | 2 wk with 2 wk rest period |
| | Oncovin (vincristine) | 1.4 mg/m$^2$ | IV | Days 1 and 8 | |
| | Prednisone | 20 mg/m$^2$ | Oral | Days 1-14 | |
| | Procarbazine | 100 mg/m$^2$ | Oral | Days 1-14 | |
| ABVD | Adriamycin (doxorubicin) | 25 mg/m$^2$ | IV | Days 1 and 15 | 2 wk with 2 wk rest period |
| | Bleomycin | 10 mg/m$^2$ | IV | Days 1 and 15 | |
| | Vinblastine (Velban) | 6 mg/m$^2$ | IV | Days 1 and 15 | |
| | Dacarbazine (DTIC-Dome) | 150 mg/m$^2$ | IV | Days 1-5 | |

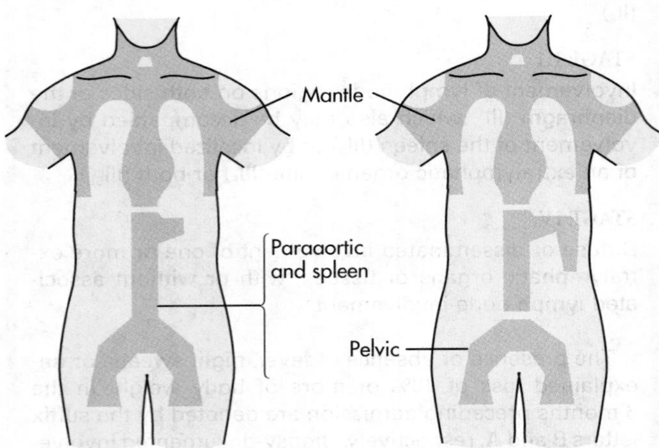


**fig. 29-8** Diagram of mantle and inverted Y fields used in total lymphoid radiotherapy of Hodgkin's disease.

prednisone (Table 29-14). This regimen is administered in a 2-week course each month with prednisone added during the first and fourth courses. The drugs are administered for at least 6 months or for two or three courses after the attainment of complete remission. Complete remissions are achieved in approximately 80% of these patients; long-term, disease-free remissions and probable cures occur in half of this group.[1] Continuing chemotherapy beyond the attainment of complete remission has not been shown to improve survival. Combinations such as ABVD (Table 29-14) are likely to be added to the treatment regimen if relapse occurs, and complete remission can again be attained. Initial use of alternating courses of MOPP and ABVD has increased response rates.

#### *Patient/family education*

Teaching regarding methods to decrease the potential for infection and skin damage is important for the patient with Hodgkin's disease. The patient and family should be knowledgeable regarding the treatment regimen and potential side effects. As with other hematological disorders, the patient should avoid potential injury.

## NON-HODGKIN'S LYMPHOMA

### Etiology/Epidemiology

The non-Hodgkin's lymphomas (NHL) include a broad spectrum of lymphoid malignant diseases with different histopathologies, disease courses, and responses to therapy. The cause is unknown, although viruses have been implicated. An association between the development of non-Hodgkin's lymphoma and immunosuppressed status, particularly persons with AIDS and organ-transplant recipients, has been reported. An increased incidence has also been reported in persons with certain autoimmune disorders such as Sjögren's syndrome.

The incidence of non-Hodgkin's lymphoma has increased over the past 20 years. Men are more commonly affected, with the greatest incidence occurring in persons over 60 years of age. Burkitt's lymphoma, a high-grade tumor, is most common in children and persons with AIDS.

### Pathophysiology

Accurate identification of the histopathology is crucial to the determination of the treatment plan. The classifications are briefly reviewed here so that familiarity with terminology will allow the reader to review charts and treatment plans.

One classification separates the non-Hodgkin's lymphomas into lymphocytic, histiocytic, and mixed cell types, each of which may appear as nodular or diffuse on microscopic examination. These have been subdivided into "favorable" and "unfavorable" histology (Box 29-13). In general, a nodular pattern of cell structures conveys a more favorable prognosis than a diffuse pattern. A lymphocytic cytology is more favorable than a histiocytic one, and a mixed cellularity–histiocytic type is intermediate in its prognosis.

Patients most often have nontender peripheral lymphadenopathy that may appear bulky. The liver and spleen may be moderately enlarged. Other symptoms that may occur include unexplained fever, night sweats, and weight loss.

### Collaborative Care Management

The diagnosis of non-Hodgkin's lymphoma is made by examination of pathological lymph node tissue. Accurate histological classification is of importance, and often slides are sent to major cancer centers for consultation regarding the classification. Once the diagnosis is made, the extent of the disease (staging) must be determined. As with Hodgkin's disease, accurate staging is a crucial factor required to determine the treatment regimen. The staging workup is similar to that for Hodgkin's disease, except that staging laparotomies are less often needed. Explanations of the extensive workup and its

**box 29-13** *Non-Hodgkin's Lymphomas*

**"FAVORABLE" HISTOLOGY**
Nodular poorly differentiated lymphocytic lymphoma (NLPD)
Nodular mixed lymphocytic and histiocytic lymphoma (NML)
Well-differentiated lymphocytic lymphomas of the nodular (NLWD) or diffuse (DLWD) type

**"UNFAVORABLE" HISTOLOGY**
Nodular histiocytic (NHL)
Diffuse poorly differentiated lymphocytic (DPDL)
Diffuse histiocytic lymphoma (DHL)
Diffuse mixed lymphoma (DML)
Diffuse undifferentiated lymphoma (DUL)

importance in determining the treatment plan are an important focus of patient teaching during the diagnostic period.

The complexity of the disease and the array of treatment regimens used encourages nurse-physician discussion of the treatment plan. It is especially important that the goals of therapy be shared, whether curative or only local or systemic palliation.

In general, radiotherapy is the initial treatment when the disease is localized. Local field radiation is used. Total nodal radiation is reserved for patients whose disease is more widespread. Chemotherapy is the mainstay of treatment of non-Hodgkin's lymphomas that are not localized (Table 29-15).

Nodular poorly differentiated lymphocytic lymphoma is the most commonly occurring non-Hodgkin's lymphoma. In some patients, observation is reasonable until the disease shows signs of progression. Treatment with a single alkylating agent, most often chlorambucil, is effective in that it produces a response rate that extends survival. Combination chemotherapy, however, produces higher response rates, including complete remissions, but is not yet shown to be curative. Median survival time is 7 to 10 years.

In diffuse histiocytic lymphoma, which includes most of the cases previously designated as reticulum cell sarcoma, combination chemotherapy has been superior to single-agent therapy. Survival is significantly prolonged in those who demonstrate a complete response, and a significant minority of this group are cured. Chemotherapy regimens produce complete responses in 40% to 60% or more of patients whose MST is well over 3 years.

In nodular histiocytic and nodular mixed histiolymphocytic types, complete responses have been achieved with single agents, and 50% to 70% of those treated with COP, COPP, MOPP, and other combinations have shown an MST of 55 months for those who attained a complete response and 13 months for those in whom only a partial response was attained. See Tables 29-14 and 29-15.

### *Patient/family education*

Hodgkin's and non-Hodgkin's diseases most often affect young adults; therefore special attention needs to be given to minimizing the impact of the illness and its treatment on their lives, not only during the treatment period, but later as well. Before the initiation of treatment, therapy-induced sterility should be discussed. For young women receiving radiation therapy alone, surgical relocation of the ovaries outside the field of radiation may be performed. Sterility commonly occurs in association with chemotherapy. For women, this is often temporary, and the ability to conceive and bear normal children often returns after therapy is completed. For men, sterility is more commonly permanent. For this reason the option of sperm banking should be discussed before beginning either radiation therapy or chemotherapy.

To allow for work and career development, every effort should be made to schedule treatment at those times and days of the week that least interfere with work and other important events in the person's life. The nurse has a crucial role in assisting patients to develop a realistic approach to the illness and to meet successfully the demands and limitations imposed by the illness and its treatment.

Persons with lymphomas have periods of remission and recurrence. Such peaks and valleys are stressful and disruptive. Many patients describe subsequent courses of treatment after a recurrence as more stressful than the initial treatment. Comments include, "Is it worth it? I don't have the same faith." Other patients, realistically encouraged by the initial response to treatment, are able to express an optimistic outlook: "It worked the first time. It will work again." Recognition of the stress involved in therapy requires that support systems be available to the patient. The health care team can provide some of the needed support and guidance as the person learns to incorporate the illness into daily life.

Patient teaching includes:

1. Knowledge of the disorder, its treatment, and prognosis
2. Name, dosage, frequency, and side effects of medications
3. Arrangements for chemotherapy or radiation treatments and for periodic blood cell counts
4. Symptoms requiring immediate medical attention (fever, bleeding)
5. Need for continued medical follow-up
6. Resources available in the community: financial assistance and local support groups (American Cancer Society)

## INFECTIOUS MONONUCLEOSIS

### Etiology/Epidemiology

Infectious mononucleosis is an acute disease caused by a herpes-like virus, the Epstein-Barr virus. It occurs more often in young persons, with the highest incidence occurring between 15 and 30 years of age.

### Pathophysiology

Signs and symptoms of infectious mononucleosis are varied (Box 29-14). It is a benign disease with a favorable prognosis. The onset may be subtle, appearing almost as flu-like symptoms. Malaise is a common early complaint, and it is often accompanied by fever, lymphadenopathy, sore throat, headache, generalized aches and pains resembling those of influenza, and moderate enlargement of the liver and spleen. Pruritis,

**table 29-15** *Chemotherapeutic Regimens for Treatment of Non-Hodgkin's Lymphomas*

| DRUGS | DOSAGE | METHOD | SCHEDULE | CYCLE |
|---|---|---|---|---|
| **COP** | | | | |
| Cyclophosphamide (Cytoxan) | 800-1000 mg/m² | IV | Day 1 | 3 wk |
| Oncovin (vincristine) | 2 mg | IV | Day 1 | |
| Prednisone | 60 mg/m² | Oral | Days 1-5 | |
| **CHOP** | | | | |
| Cyclophosphamide (Cytoxan) | 750 mg/m² | IV | Day 1 | 3 wk |
| Hydroxydaunomycin (doxorubicin, Adriamycin) | 50 mg/m² | IV | Day 1 | |
| Oncovin (vincristine) | 1.4 mg/m² | IV | Day 1 | |
| Prednisone | 100 mg/m² | Oral | Days 1-5 | |
| **CHOP-Bleo** | | | | |
| Cyclophosphamide (Cytoxan) | 750 mg/m² | IV | Day 1 | 3 or 4 wk |
| Hydroxydaunomycin (doxorubicin, Adriamycin) | 50 mg/m² | IV | Day 1 | |
| Oncovin (vincristine) | 2 mg | IV | Days 1 and 5 | |
| Prednisone | 100 mg | Oral | Days 1-5 | |
| Bleomycin | 15 U | IV | Days 1 and 5 | |
| **COPP** | | | | |
| Cyclophosphamide (Cytoxan) | 400-650 mg/m² | IV | Days 1 and 8 | 4 wk |
| Oncovin (vincristine) | 1.4 mg/m² (max, 2 mg) | IV | Days 1 and 8 | |
| Procarbazine | 100 mg/m² | Oral | Days 1-10 | |
| Prednisone | 40 mg/m² | Oral | Days 1-14 | |
| **BACOP** | | | | |
| Bleomycin | 5 U/m² | IV | Days 15 and 22 | 4 wk |
| Adriamycin (doxorubicin) | 25 mg/m² | IV | Days 1 and 8 | |
| Cyclophosphamide (Cytoxan) | 650 mg/m² | IV | Days 1 and 8 | |
| Oncovin (vincristine) | 1.4 mg/m² (max, 2 mg) | IV | Days 1 and 8 | |
| Prednisone | 60 mg/m² | Oral | Days 15-28 | |

*Continued*

**box 29-14** *clinical manifestations*

***Infectious Mononucleosis***

**MILD**
Fever, malaise

**MODERATE**
Enlarged lymph nodes, sore throat, headache, generalized aches, moderate enlargement of liver and spleen

**SEVERE (RARE)**
Rupture of spleen, encephalitis

palatal petechiae, jaundice, and rash may be present. The mode of transmission is via intimate contact with the spread of the virus through the saliva. Rupture of the spleen and encephalitis are rare complications.

## Collaborative Care Management

Diagnosis is established by the heterophil agglutination or monospot blood test. This test is based on a certain substance being present in the blood of a person with infectious mononucleosis that causes clumping, or agglutination, of the washed erythrocytes (antigen) of another animal. The test result is almost always positive after 10 to 14 days of the illness. Other laboratory findings are a great increase in the number of mononuclear leukocytes, which lends the name to the disease, and an increase in atypical lymphocytes. At the height of the disease the WBC count may range between 10,000 and 20,000 cells/mm³.

Infectious mononucleosis is self-limiting, and with rest affected persons usually recover spontaneously within 2 to 3 weeks. Effectiveness of antiviral therapy has not been established. The use of corticosteroids may be indicated in severe cases with tonsillar enlargement and potential airway obstruction. Acetaminophen is effective in relieving fever, sore throat,

**table 29-15** *Chemotherapeutic Regimens for Treatment of Non-Hodgkin's Lymphomas—cont'd*

| Drugs | Dosage | Method | Schedule | Cycle |
|---|---|---|---|---|
| **Pro-MACE** | | | | |
| Prednisone | 60 mg/m² | Oral | Days 1 to 14 | 4 wk |
| Methotrexate | 1.5 g/m² | IV | | |
| Adriamycin (doxorubicin) | 25 mg/m² | IV | Days 1 and 8 | Follow with MOPP regimen (see Table 29-14); then restart Pro-MACE |
| Cyclophosphamide | 650 mg/m² | IV | Days 1 and 8 | |
| Etoposide (VP 16) | 120 mg/m² | IV | Days 1 and 8 | |
| Leucovorin | 50 mg/m² | IV | q6h for 5 days | |
| **M-BACOD** | | | | |
| Methotrexate | 200 mg/m² | IV | Days 8 and 15 | Repeat cycles every 3 wk |
| Bleomycin | 4 U/m² | IV | Days 1 and 21 | |
| Adriamycin (doxorubicin) | 45 mg/m² | IV | Days 1 and 21 | |
| Cyclophosphamide | 600 mg/m² | IV | Days 1 and 21 | |
| Oncovin (vincristine) | 1 mg/m² | IV | Days 1 and 21 | |
| Dexamethasone | 6 mg/m² | Oral | Days 1-5 and 21-25 | |
| Leucovorin rescue | 10 mg/m² | Oral | q6h for 8 doses, beginning 24 hr after each methotrexate dose | |
| **MACOP-B** | | | | |
| Methotrexate | 100 mg/m², then 300 mg/m² | IV<br>IV/4 hr | Wk 2, 6, 10<br>Wk 2, 6, 10 | Cycles may be repeated |
| Leucovorin rescue | 15 mg | Oral | q6h for 6 doses beginning 24 hr after methotrexate | |
| Adriamycin (doxorubicin) | 50 mg/m² | IV | Wk 1, 3, 5, 7, 9, 11 | |
| Cyclophosphamide | 350 mg/m² | IV | Wk 1, 3, 5, 7, 9, 11 | |
| Oncovin (vincristine) | 1.4 mg/m² | IV | Wk 2, 4, 8, 10, 12 | |
| Prednisone | 75 mg | Oral | Daily doses tapered over last 15 days | |
| Bleomycin | 10 U/m² | IV | Wk 4, 8, 12 | |
| NOTE: CNS prophylaxis also given to patients with bone marrow involvement after bone marrow remission | | | | |
| Methotrexate | 12 mg | Intrathecal (IT) | Wk 6-8 | |
| Cytarabine | 30 mg/m² | IT | Wk 6-8 | |

and myalgias. Most persons can return to activities that do not require heavy exertion in 1 to 2 weeks and to normal activities in 4 to 6 weeks. Some persons have persistent fatigue for several months. Nursing management is supportive and focuses on the relief of symptoms and promotion of rest.

### *Patient/family education*

The patient is instructed to avoid heavy lifting or contact sports for at least 1 month or until splenomegaly is resolved. An enlarged spleen is susceptible to rupture. Additional teaching includes the need to increase fluids and to use appropriate hand washing to prevent the spread of disease.

Young adults should be educated regarding the mode of transmission and incubation period of mononucleosis. Persons with mononucleosis should be cautioned against donating blood for at least 6 months after the onset of illness. Reassurance should be given that isolation is not necessary, but that the oral secretions of a person with acute mononucleosis should be considered infectious.

## *critical thinking* QUESTIONS

**1** You are administering a vitamin $B_{12}$ injection to an elderly man in the outpatient clinic. He has recently had a gastrectomy. He asks you why he needs to have these injections and how long he will need them. How do you respond?

**2** A young woman hospitalized with sickle cell crisis asks you why she has to wear oxygen. How do you respond? What other interventions will promote comfort for this patient?

**3** A 63-year-old man recently diagnosed with chronic myelogenous leukemia (CML) is extremely anxious about his diagnosis. He has heard many horror stories about chemotherapy. To relieve his anxiety, what would you explain to him regarding the initial therapy for CML? How does this treatment differ from treatment for acute types of leukemia?

## chapter SUMMARY

- Major health problems of the hematopoietic system include RBC disorders (anemias, erythrocytosis); disorders of hemostasis, platelets, and coagulation; WBC disorders (neutropenia, neutrophilia, leukemia); disorders of the lymph system (lymphomas); and infectious mononucleosis.

### DISORDERS ASSOCIATED WITH ERYTHROCYTES

- Anemias may be caused by blood loss, impaired RBC production, increased RBC destruction, or nutritional deficiencies.
- Weakness and fatigue are major signs of anemia as a result of decreased oxygenation from lack of Hgb and increased energy needs required by increased RBC production.
- Aplastic anemia is anemia that results from impaired RBC production and is characterized by pancytopenia. Treatment is by bone marrow transplantation or immunosuppressive therapy. Nursing interventions include preventing infection and hemorrhage.
- Sickle cell anemia is a hemolytic anemia with a genetic basis. A sickle cell crisis occurs when the RBCs become deoxygenated and sickle shaped, causing plugging of small vessels, leading to organ infarction and necrosis.
- Nursing interventions for sickle cell disease include promoting comfort and hydration, counseling, and teaching.
- Ingestion of iron compounds is part of the therapy for iron deficiency anemia only; it will not help the other types of anemias.
- Megaloblastic anemia is a macrocytic anemia from defective DNA synthesis and abnormal RBC maturation; causes include vitamin $B_{12}$ and folic acid deficiencies and administration of chemotherapeutic and anticonvulsant drugs.
- Erythrocytosis is an abnormal increase in RBCs, as seen with polycythemia vera.

### DISORDERS OF HEMOSTASIS, PLATELETS, AND COAGULATION

- Thrombocytopenia is a decrease in the number of circulating platelets and leads to bleeding; persons with thrombocytopenia need to learn how to prevent injury and hemorrhage.
- Hemophilia is a hereditary coagulation disorder; hemophilia A is a lack of coagulation factor VIII, and hemophilia B is a lack of factor IX; maintenance therapy consists of blood factor replacement therapy and prevention of injury.
- Disseminated intravascular coagulation is a coagulation disorder characterized initially by clotting and secondarily by hemorrhage, resulting from an alteration in the balance between clotting factors and fibrinolytic factors; the person usually is critically ill.

### DISORDERS ASSOCIATED WITH WHITE BLOOD CELLS

- Persons with alteration of WBCs are at a high risk of infection because leukocytes are a major factor in the body's defense against invading microorganisms.
- The leukemias are malignant disorders characterized by uncontrolled proliferation of WBCs and their precursors; the cause is unknown.
- Leukemias may be acute or chronic, lymphocytic or nonlymphocytic (primarily myelogenous). Acute leukemias have a rapid onset and a short course if untreated; chronic leukemias have a more insidious onset and a longer course. The major therapies for leukemias are chemotherapy and bone marrow transplantation.
- Chronic myelogenous leukemia (CML) is diagnosed by the presence of the Philadelphia chromosome and affects persons in the fifth and sixth decades of life.
- Initial treatment for CML consist of oral chemotherapeutic agents. Curative treatment involves bone marrow transplantation.
- Nursing interventions for persons with CML are aimed at prevention of infection and bleeding, education and coping strategies, and prevention of fatigue.

### DISORDERS ASSOCIATED WITH THE LYMPH SYSTEM

- Lymphomas (Hodgkin's disease and non-Hodgkin's lymphomas) are malignant disorders of the lymph system; radiotherapy and chemotherapy are the major medical treatments.
- Lymphedema is a result of an interruption of the flow of fluid through the lymphatics and is commonly seen in breast cancer.
- Treatment for lymphedema includes diuretics, compression devices, and skin and wound management.
- Infectious mononucleosis is a viral illness characterized by fever, lymphadenopathy, and sore throat.
- Treatment for infectious mononucleosis is largely supportive. The mode of transmission is through intimate contact with the saliva of an infected person.

## References


1. Carnevali D, Reiner A: *The cancer experience: nursing diagnosis and management,* Philadelphia, 1990, JB Lippincott.
2. Charache S et al: Effects of hydroxyurea on the frequency of painful crisis in sickle cell anemia, *N Engl J Med* 332(20):1317, 1995.
3. Harmening DM: *Clinical hematology and fundamentals of hemostasis,* ed 2, Philadelphia, 1992, FA Davis.
4. Erickson J: Anemia, *Semin Oncol Nurs* 12(1):2, 1996.
5. Lusher JM et al: Hematology, *JAMA* 275(23):1814, 1996.
6. Parker S et al: Cancer statistics, 1997, *CA Cancer J Clin* 47(1):5, 1997.
7. Rakel RE: *Conn's current therapy,* Philadelphia, 1997, WB Saunders.
8. Shuey K: Platelet-associated bleeding disorders, *Semin Oncol Nurs* 12(1):15, 1996.
9. Stone RM et al: Granulocyte macrophage colony stimulating factor after initial chemotherapy for elderly patients with primary acute myelogenous leukemia, *N Engl J Med* 332(25):1671, 1995.
10. Walters MC et al: Bone marrow transplantation for sickle cell disease, *N Engl J Med* 335(6):363, 1996.
11. Warkentin TE et al: Heparin induced thrombocytopenia in patients treated with low molecular weight heparin or unfractionated heparin, *N Engl J Med* 332(20):1330, 1995.
12. Williams SR: *Nutrition and diet therapy,* ed 7, St Louis, 1993, Mosby.
13. Wujcik D et al: Leukemia management strategies: the next generation, *Oncol Nurs Forum* 23(3):477, 1996.
14. Wyngaarden JB, Smith LH: *Cecil textbook of medicine,* ed 19, Philadelphia, 1992, WB Saunders.
15. Yang Y, Shah K, Watson M, Vipul M: Comparison of cost to the health sector of comprehensive and episodic health care for sickle cell disease patients, *Public Health Rep* 110(1):80, 1995.

# chapter 30 ASSESSMENT OF THE Respiratory System

SUSAN B. STILLWELL

## objectives

*After studying this chapter, the learner should be able to:*

1. Identify the structural components of the respiratory system.
2. Differentiate ventilation from respiration.
3. Describe the respiratory system's primary function of gas exchange.
4. Describe the mechanisms that control ventilation.
5. Describe the defense mechanisms of the lungs.
6. Identify changes in the respiratory system that occur with aging.
7. Identify subjective and objective data to obtain a complete respiratory assessment.
8. Describe diagnostic tests and related nursing care commonly used to evaluate respiratory conditions.

An activity that most of us rarely think about throughout our daily lives is breathing air in and out of our lungs. However, the ease or discomfort with which we breathe has a major impact on the quality of our daily activities. The act of breathing involves two interrelated processes, ventilation and respiration. *Ventilation* is the movement of air into and out of the lungs. *Respiration* refers to the exchange of oxygen and carbon dioxide across cell membranes.

This chapter provides a review of the anatomy and physiology of the respiratory system, identifies subjective and objective data integral to obtaining a health assessment of an individual experiencing a respiratory problem, and describes tests commonly used to diagnose and monitor individuals with respiratory dysfunction.

## ANATOMY AND PHYSIOLOGY

### UPPER AIRWAY

#### Nose and Sinuses

The nose consists of an anterior component known as the vestibule. It extends posteriorly to a point at which its lining changes from skin to mucous membrane and houses the sensory endings of the olfactory nerve. The upper portion of the nose is supported by bone, and the lower portion of the nose is supported by cartilage. The openings to the nose are the nostrils or nares, which are separated by the nasal septum.

Air enters the nares and passes into the nasal cavities. Mucosa-lined curved projections, called *turbinates,* form the lateral walls of the nasal cavities (Figure 30-1) and provide a large surface area for warming, humidifying, and filtering the inspired air. Because the turbinates have a rich blood supply, air that is inhaled is heated to almost body temperature by the time it reaches the posterior nasopharynx. The inspired air is also humidified by the nose and is 100% saturated with water vapor by the time the air reaches the alveoli. This humidification results in an insensible fluid loss of 250 ml/day. Filtration of large particles of dust and other matter is accomplished by trapping of the particulates by the nasal hairs. These irritants can trigger the sneeze reflex to remove the foreign particles. In addition, the mucous membrane of the turbinate bones entraps small particles where they are propelled by cilia (hairlike projections that beat in a wavelike motion) to the pharynx for swallowing or expectoration.

Each turbinate has an opening for draining the nasolacrimal ducts and four sinuses (Figure 30-2) that surround the nasal cavities. These air-filled spaces are lined with mucous membrane that is continuous with that of the nose. The sinuses produce mucus for the nasal cavity and promote vocal resonance and timber.

#### Pharynx

The pharynx, or throat, is divided into the nasopharynx, oropharynx, and laryngopharynx (Figure 30-3). Because it is the only opening between the nose and mouth and the lungs, any obstruction of the pharynx (e.g., tissue swelling, presence of a foreign body, or the tongue falling back into the pharynx) can lead to cessation of ventilation. The nasopharynx is posterior to the nose and above the soft palate and contains the adenoids and openings of the eustachian tubes. The oropharynx is located in the posterior portion of the mouth and contains the tonsils. The adenoids and tonsils are made up of lymphoid tissue that helps to filter bacteria or other foreign matter that enters the nose and throat. The laryngopharynx opens into the larynx and esophagus.

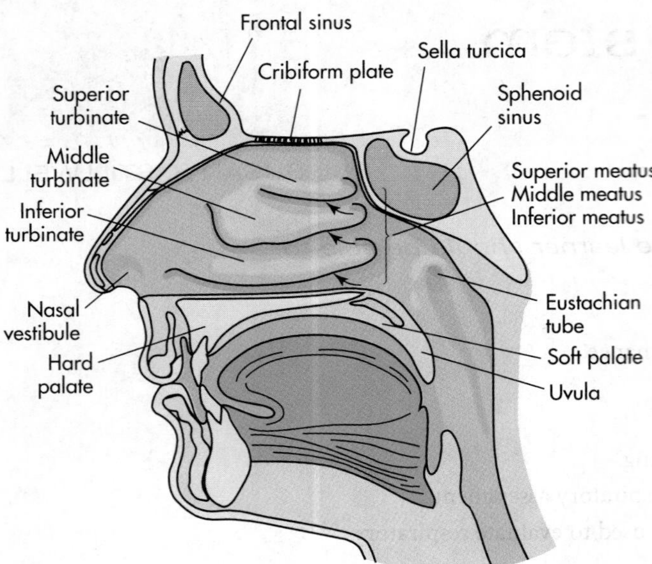


**fig. 30-1** Lateral wall of nose, showing superior, middle, and inferior turbinates.

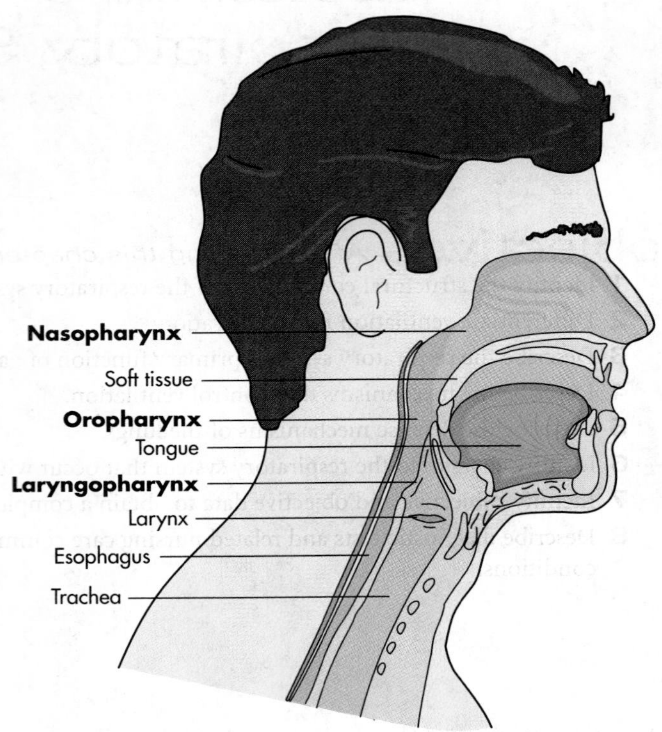


**fig. 30-3** Sagittal section of head showing pharynx and larynx.

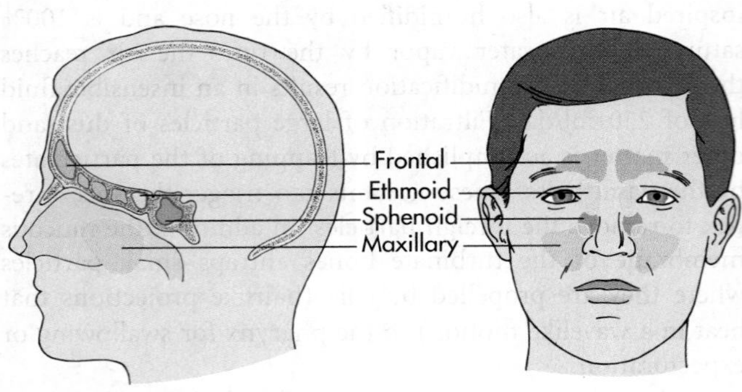


**fig. 30-2** Location of sinuses.

### Larynx

The larynx, also known as the *voicebox*, connects the pharynx to the trachea. It is made up of cartilage, muscle, and ligaments (Figure 30-4) and houses the vocal cords, which form the V-shaped opening of the glottis or entrance to the larynx. Sound is produced as exhaled air is forced through a closed glottis causing the vocal cords to vibrate. The closing of the glottis also allows for an increase in intrathoracic pressure that is needed when a person is coughing or lifting. The entrance to the larynx is protected by a leaf-shaped lid of fibrocartilage, the *epiglottis*, that covers the glottis during swallowing to prevent aspiration of food or fluids into the lungs. The larynx is innervated by the laryngeal nerve, which initiates the cough reflex in response to stimulation by foreign particles, dry mucous membranes, and other irritants. When the muscles of the larynx are paralyzed, foreign materials can enter the lungs.

## LOWER AIRWAY

### Trachea, Bronchi, and Bronchioles

As inhaled air travels through the larynx, it reaches the lower airway consisting of the trachea, bronchi, bronchioles, and terminal respiratory units (Figure 30-5). The *trachea*, commonly known as the windpipe, connects the larynx to the right and left mainstem bronchi. The point at which the trachea bifurcates into the right and left bronchi is called the *carina*. The carina contains cough receptors that can be easily stimulated, for example, by tubes such as suction catheters or endotracheal tubes. The landmark to locate the carina is the manubriosternal junction, also referred to as the angle of Louis.

The trachea and bronchi are supported by incomplete cartilaginous rings that prevent these airways from collapsing when the pressure in the thorax becomes negative. The trachea shares a small muscle with the esophagus at the point where the cartilaginous rings do not meet. This may become a potential site for a tracheoesophageal (T-E) fistula. Cuffed tubes, such as endotracheal or tracheostomy tubes, may lead to T-E fistulas as a result of high pressures within the cuffs.

These conducting airways are lined with goblet cells that trap debris and ciliated epithelium that propel foreign particles toward the pharynx for removal. Mucus and particles are removed from the airway by swallowing, coughing, or sneezing. See Chapter 32 for a complete discussion of pulmonary defense mechanisms.

The bronchi enter the lungs through an opening called the *hilus*. The right bronchus is wider and shorter than the left

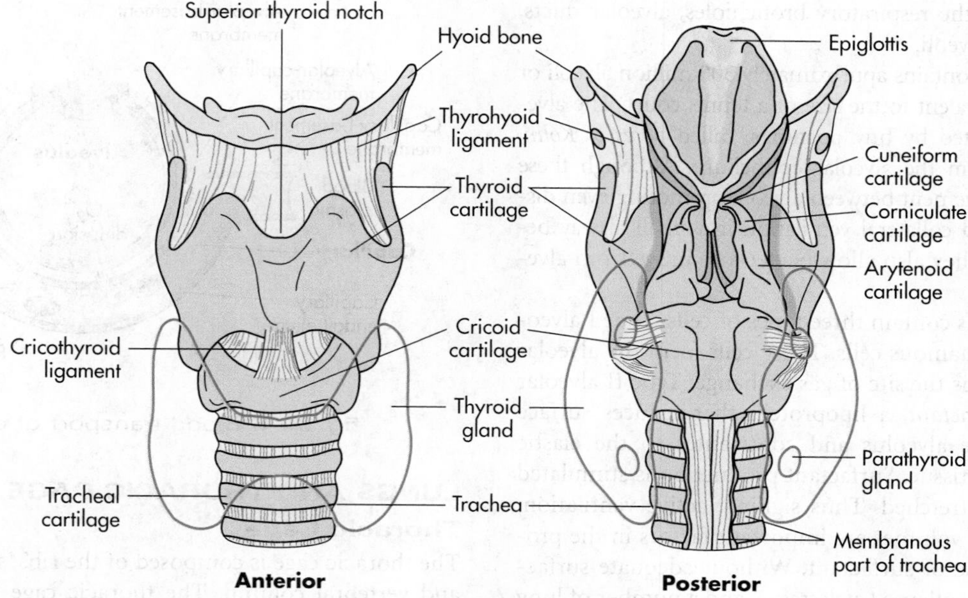


**fig. 30-4** Larynx.

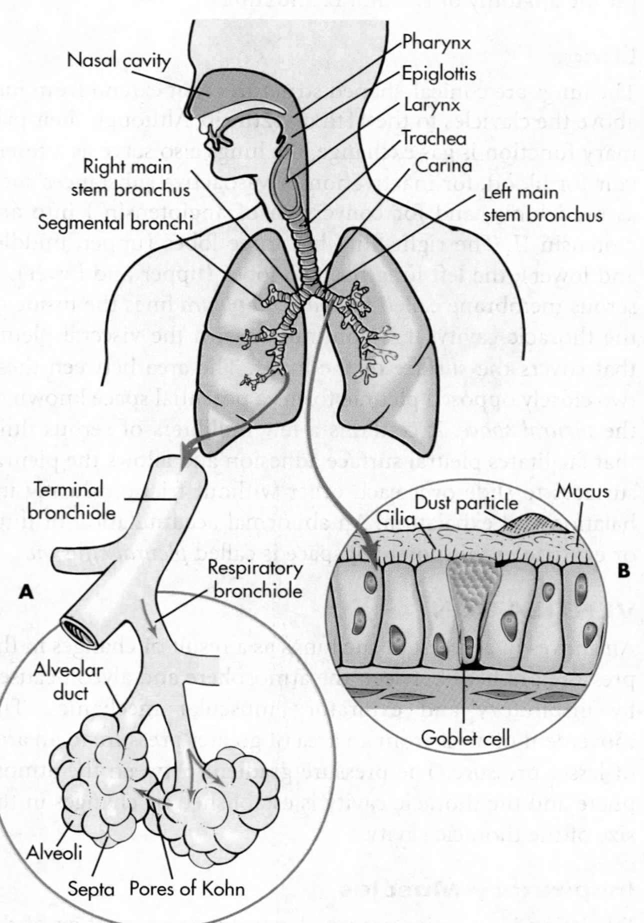


**fig. 30-5** Respiratory system. Inset **A**, Acinus, or pulmonary functional unit. Inset **B**, Ciliated mucous membrane.

bronchus and extends nearly vertically from the trachea. Because of this anatomical feature, the right lung is the more likely site for aspiration or misplaced intubation. Thus, it is important to secure an endotracheal tube so that proper ventilation can be maintained. If the tube is misplaced or slips into the right bronchus, air will not be able to enter the left lung. The left bronchus is narrower and extends at more of an acute angle off the trachea, making it more difficult to pass a catheter into it for removal of secretions from the left lung.

The mainstem bronchi divide into smaller branches: the left bronchus divides into two lobar branches, and the right bronchus divides into three lobar branches. The lobar branches divide into segments that further subdivide into subsegmental bronchi, terminal bronchi, bronchioles, terminal bronchioles, and respiratory bronchioles. Respiratory bronchioles divide further into respiratory terminal bronchioles, alveolar ducts, alveolar sacs, and alveoli.

The bronchioles contain no cartilage for support. Patency of their structure is determined by smooth muscle, which relaxes or contracts, thus affecting the diameter of the bronchioles. The diameter of the airway determines the amount of airway resistance. For example, if the radius of the airway was cut in half, the resistance would increase by 16 times. Mucous plugs, bronchoconstriction, airway edema, and external compression of the airway are conditions that increase airway resistance and impair airflow into the lungs. Cilia and secretory gland cells, which aid in the removal of dust and particles, are absent at the level of the terminal bronchioles.

### Terminal Respiratory Unit

The structures distal to the terminal bronchioles are collectively referred to as acini or terminal respiratory units (Figure 30-5, *A*).

The acini include the respiratory bronchioles, alveolar ducts, alveolar sacs, and alveoli.

The adult lung contains approximately 300 million alveoli or a surface area equivalent to the size of a tennis court. The alveoli are interconnected by tiny openings, called *pores of Kohn,* which are present in the alveolar epithelium. Although these pores allow air movement between alveoli, promoting even distribution of air and collateral ventilation if a small airway becomes obstructed, they also allow bacteria to move from alveolus to alveolus.

The alveolar sacs contain three types of cells. Type I alveolar cells are flat squamous cells. These cells form the alveolar epithelium, which is the site of gas exchange. Type II alveolar cells produce *surfactant,* a lipoprotein that reduces surface tension within the alveolus and contributes to the elastic properties of lung tissue. Surfactant production is stimulated when alveoli are stretched. Thus sighing, active ventilation, and adequate tidal volumes are important factors in the production and release of surfactant. Without adequate surfactant, alveoli would collapse (*atelectasis*), and a number of lung diseases, including acute respiratory distress syndrome, may result. Alveolar macrophages are the third type of cell found in the alveolar sacs. Macrophages are phagocytic cells that are responsible for ingesting and removing bacteria and other foreign particles from the alveolar surface. The macrophages transport the microorganisms to the lymphatics or bronchioles for removal via the mucociliary escalator. The alveolar macrophage is one of the most important defense mechanisms to prevent lung infection.

## LUNG CIRCULATION

### Pulmonary and Bronchial Blood Supply

The lungs receive blood from both pulmonary and bronchial circulation. Bronchial circulation provides nutrients to the tissues of the tracheobronchial tree and warms and moistens inspired air but does not participate in gas exchange.[1] The bronchial arteries originate from the thoracic aorta. The azygos vein returns blood from the bronchial system to the left atrium. Pulmonary circulation is a high-volume, low-pressure circuit made up of the blood received from the right ventricle of the heart that interacts with the airway at the terminal bronchioles. The deoxygenated blood from the right ventricle is transported through the main pulmonary artery that branches into smaller arteries and arterioles and finally to the alveolar capillaries of the acini. Once the blood is oxygenated and carbon dioxide is removed, the blood is returned to the left atrium of the heart via the pulmonary veins. The oxygenated blood then enters the left ventricle where it is pumped out of the aorta to the systemic circulation.

The alveoli are surrounded with a pulmonary capillary network. Each alveolus is separated from the pulmonary capillary by an interstitial space (Figure 30-6), a distance of less than 1 $\mu$m. It is at this site that oxygen travels from the alveolus into the capillary blood where it is returned via the pulmonary veins to the left side of the heart for distribution throughout the body and where carbon dioxide moves from the capillary blood into the alveolus for exhalation.

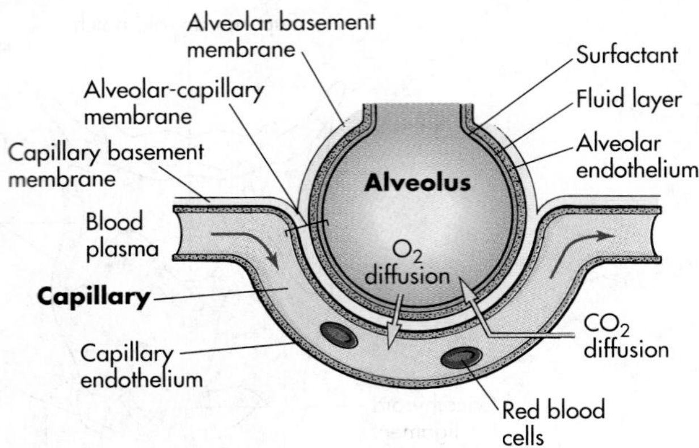


**fig. 30-6** Blood transport of oxygen.

## LUNGS AND THORACIC CAGE

### Thoracic Cage

The thoracic cage is composed of the ribs, sternum, scapulae, and vertebral column. The thoracic cage houses the lungs, heart, great vessels, lymph nodes, thymus gland, and esophagus. Intercostal muscles lie between the ribs, and the diaphragm forms the floor of the thoracic cage. See Figure 30-7 for the anatomy of the thorax and lungs.

### Lungs

The lungs are conical-shaped structures that extend from just above the clavicles to the 11th or 12th rib. Although their primary function is gas exchange, the lungs also serve as a reservoir for blood, for inactivation of vasoactive substances such as bradykinin, and for conversion of angiotensin I into angiotensin II. The right lung has three lobes (upper, middle, and lower); the left lung has two lobes (upper and lower). A serous membrane called the *parietal pleura* lines the inside of the thoracic cavity. It is continuous with the visceral pleura that covers the surface of the lungs. The area between these two closely opposed pleurae forms a potential space known as the *pleural space.* It contains a few milliliters of serous fluid that facilitates pleural surface adhesion and allows the pleural surfaces to slide over each other without friction during inhalation and exhalation. An abnormal accumulation of fluid or exudate in this potential space is called *pleural effusion.*

## VENTILATION

Air moves in and out of the lungs as a result of changes in the pressure gradient between the atmosphere and alveoli caused by inspiratory and expiratory muscular mechanics. The movement of air is from an area of greater pressure to an area of lesser pressure. The pressure gradient between the atmosphere and the thoracic cavity is established by changes in the size of the thoracic cavity.

### Inspiratory Muscles

Inhalation is an active process that requires contraction of the inspiratory muscles, for example, the diaphragm, external intercostal muscles, and scalene muscles. The diaphragm is a large dome-shaped muscle that flattens during contraction, initiating inspiration. It is the primary muscle of breathing and is

fig. 30-7 Anatomy of thorax and lungs.

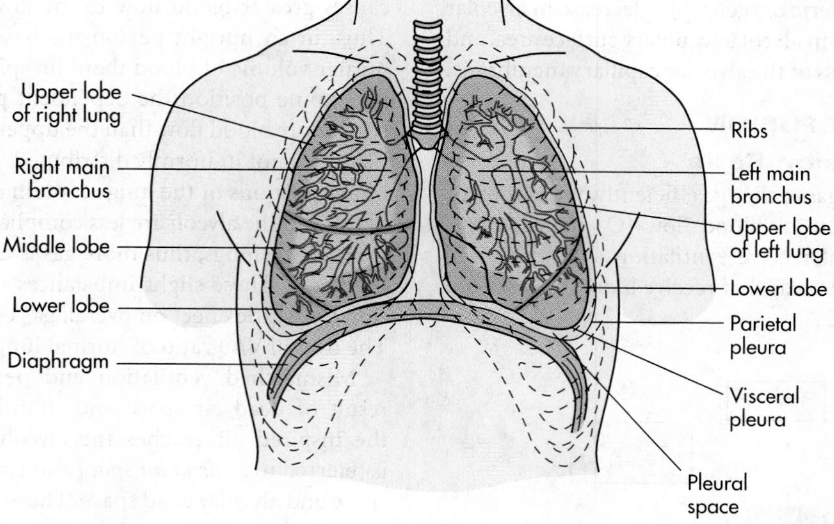

innervated by the right and left phrenic nerves. Injury or damage to the phrenic nerves causes paralysis of the diaphragm, adversely affecting lung movement on the affected side. The chest will move up instead of downward on the side of the paralysis during inspiration. This is known as *paradoxical movement.* Contraction of the external intercostal and scalene muscles causes the anterior portion of the thoracic cage to rise during inspiration, increasing the chest dimensions. During exercise or in diseased states, the sternocleidomastoid muscles, accessory muscles used to assist in inhalation, raise the sternum, increasing the diameter of the thoracic cage. Because of the change in the size of the thorax, the resultant increase in volume causes a change in pressure. The intrapleural pressure as well as the intrapulmonary pressure or airway pressure decreases in relation to atmospheric pressure. This pressure gradient causes air to move into the lungs.

### Expiratory Muscles

Exhalation is normally a passive process produced by elastic recoil of the chest wall and the lungs. Relaxation of the diaphragm and intercostal muscles decreases the size of the thoracic cage. When exhalation is active, for example, as a result of disease, exercise, or coughing, the internal intercostal and abdominal muscles contract. The contraction of these accessory muscles causes the ribs to move upward and the abdominal contents to rise, pushing the diaphragm upward. The resultant decrease in volume leads to an increase in the intrapulmonary and intrapleural pressures. The pressure gradient that is created between the atmosphere and the airways causes the air to flow out of the lungs.

### Compliance and Elasticity

Two properties that permit the lungs to expand and return to their resting state are compliance and elasticity. *Compliance* is a quality of yielding to pressure and represents the ease with which the lungs can be stretched to take in a volume of air. Determinants of compliance include the elastic recoil of the lung and chest wall and the alveolar surface tension. An increase in compliance means that the lungs are abnormally easy to inflate; a decrease in compliance indicates stiffness or difficulty in inflating the lungs.

*Elasticity* of the chest wall is determined by the musculature and bones of the thoracic cage and is reduced in individuals with bony deformities, abdominal distention, and obesity. *Elastic recoil* of the lungs is the tendency of the lungs to return to the resting state. The elasticity of the lungs is determined by the elastic and collagen fibers of the lungs. The fibers are stretched out when the lungs are inflated and contract when the lungs are deflated. Conditions in which lung tissue stiffens, such as pulmonary fibrosis or interstitial lung disease, result in a decrease in compliance.

### Intrathoracic Pressure

The pressure gradient between the atmosphere and thoracic cavity is established by changes in the size of the thoracic cavity. When the diaphragm contracts, the thoracic cage increases in size, expanding the lungs and creating a negative intrathoracic pressure. Because atmospheric pressure (the air pressure at the nose and mouth) is greater than the pressure in the alveoli, air enters the airway and moves through the respiratory passageways into the alveoli. During exhalation, the lungs return to the resting state causing a decrease in thoracic volume. Consequently, intrathoracic pressure increases and moves air out of the lungs.

## GAS EXCHANGE

### Diffusion

Gas movement across the alveolar-capillary membrane occurs by the process of *diffusion.* Once the inspired oxygen reaches the alveoli, it diffuses into the pulmonary capillary because the partial pressure of oxygen of alveolar air is greater than the partial pressure of oxygen in venous blood. Carbon dioxide, on the other hand, diffuses in the opposite direction because the partial pressure of carbon dioxide of venous blood is greater than the partial pressure of carbon dioxide of alveolar air (Figure 30-8). Diffusion of oxygen is decreased by the following: (1) a decrease in atmospheric oxygen, (2) a decrease in alveolar ventilation, (3) a decrease in alveolar-capillary surface area, and (4) an increase in thickness of the alveolar capillary membrane.

## VENTILATION-PERFUSION

### Ventilation-Perfusion Ratio

For the lung to perform gas exchange efficiently, *ventilation* or air flow (V) and *perfusion* or blood flow (Q) must be balanced. That is, areas that receive ventilation should be well perfused with blood, and areas that receive blood flow should be capable of ventilation.

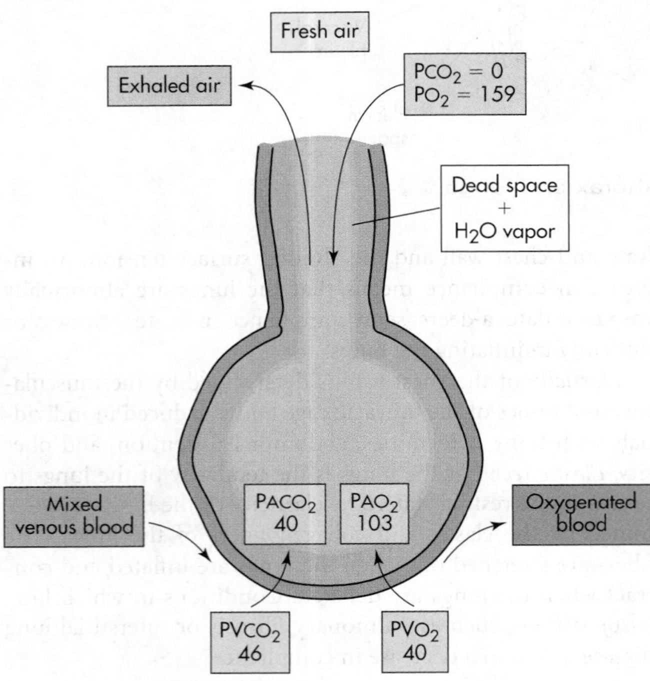


**fig. 30-8** Diffusion of gases across the alveolocapillary membrane. $P_{CO_2}$ and $P_{O_2}$, partial pressure of carbon dioxide and oxygen; $PA_{CO_2}$ and $PA_{O_2}$, alveolar $P_{CO_2}$ and $P_{O_2}$; $PV_{CO_2}$ and $PV_{O_2}$, mixed venous $P_{CO_2}$ and $P_{O_2}$.

In the normal lung, alveolar ventilation is about 4 L/min and pulmonary capillary blood flow is about 5 L/min. Gravity causes greater blood flow to the lower portion of the lungs. Thus, in an upright person the bases of the lungs receive a greater volume of blood than the apices. If an individual is in the supine position the dependent portions of the lungs receive more blood flow than the upper portions. Similarly, ventilation is not uniformly distributed. In an upright person, the upper portions of the lungs contain a greater residual volume of gas and the alveoli are less compliant than in the lower portions of the lungs; thus more gas is distributed to the bases of the lungs. These slight imbalances in ventilation and perfusion have little effect on overall gas exchange in normal lungs. The overall V/Q ratio of normal lungs is 0.8.

Mismatched ventilation and perfusion may occur as a result of dead air space and shunting of blood. Not all of the inspired air reaches the alveoli for gas exchange. This is referred to as *dead air space* and consists of anatomical dead space and alveolar dead space. The air that remains in the conducting airways is termed *anatomical dead space. Alveolar dead space* occurs when there is poor blood flow in relation to the amount of ventilation to the alveoli or if the ventilation is excessive in relation to the amount of blood flow. For example, blood flow (perfusion) to the alveoli may be blocked by a pulmonary embolus, yet the alveoli may be well ventilated. In addition, perfusion may be blocked when gas pressure within the alveolus is greater than within the capillary, causing the capillary to collapse. These are both examples of high V/Q ratios resulting in dead-space ventilation or "wasted" ventilation. Although the air does not participate in gas exchange, it does contribute to the work of breathing.

Low V/Q ratios indicate that the lungs are less ventilated in relation to the amount of blood flow. For example, blood flow to the alveolus may be normal, but fluid in the alveolus, bronchospasm, or mucous plugs increases airway resistance and may prevent adequate ventilation. This V/Q inequality is referred to as *shunting.* The blood perfuses the area of the lung that is not ventilated; thus blood is "shunted" past the area, and no gas exchange occurs. This is known as *wasted perfusion.* Figure 30-9 shows examples of V/Q relationships.

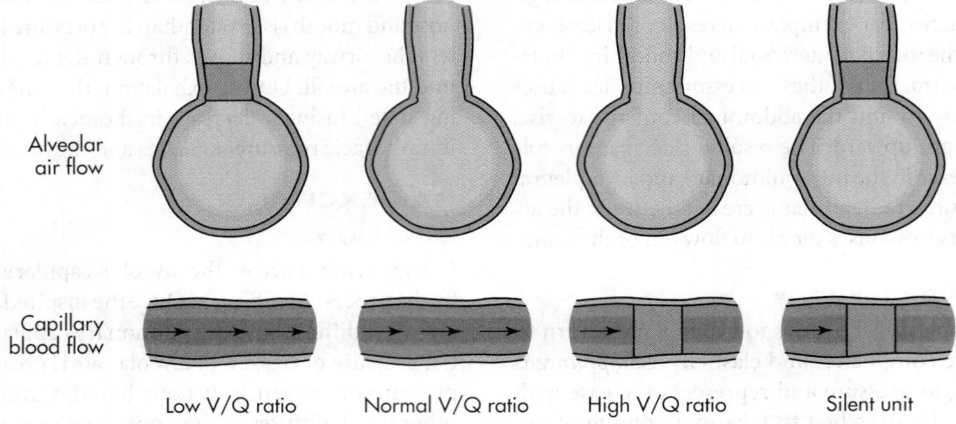


**fig. 30-9** Range of ventilation to perfusion ratios from zero to infinity.

## CONTROL OF RESPIRATION

Breathing can be viewed as an automatic loop process by which sensors (chemoreceptors) continually feed data to a central processor (medulla oblongata and pons) that then directs respiratory muscles to adjust ventilation to meet the needs of the body (Figure 30-10). In addition, an override feature (cerebral cortex) exists, so that ventilation can be consciously altered. The major sensors are the central and peripheral chemoreceptors. Other receptors that affect ventilation include the stretch receptors and J receptors.

### Central Chemoreceptors

Central chemoreceptors, located near the medulla, are sensitive to hydrogen ion concentration (pH) in the spinal fluid. Carbon dioxide readily crosses the blood-brain barrier and combines with water to form carbonic acid, which dissociates into hydrogen ions. A change in arterial carbon dioxide levels affects the pH of the cerebrospinal fluid, which in turn stimulates the chemoreceptors. There is an increase in the depth and rate of ventilation when carbon dioxide levels increase and a decrease in the depth and rate of ventilation when the carbon dioxide levels decrease.

Although ventilation is regulated primarily by the central chemoreceptor response to changes in arterial carbon dioxide levels and its effect on the pH of the cerebrospinal fluid, the central chemoreceptors become less sensitive in individuals with chronically high carbon dioxide levels and thus low oxygen levels. In these individuals, the peripheral chemoreceptors are the primary stimuli for ventilation.

### Peripheral Chemoreceptors

Peripheral chemoreceptors, located in the carotid bodies and aortic arch, primarily respond to low arterial blood oxygen levels ($Pa_{O_2}$ <60 mm Hg) that signal the respiratory center in the medulla. Efferent signals are sent to the respiratory muscles to increase the ventilatory rate. Individuals who rely on their hypoxic drive for breathing (e.g., those with chronic obstructive lung disease [COPD]) depend on the peripheral chemoreceptors for control of ventilation. Administration of an uncontrolled amount of oxygen or not monitoring arterial $Pa_{O_2}$ levels with oxygen administration in these individuals can depress or abolish their hypoxic ventilatory drive, and death may result.

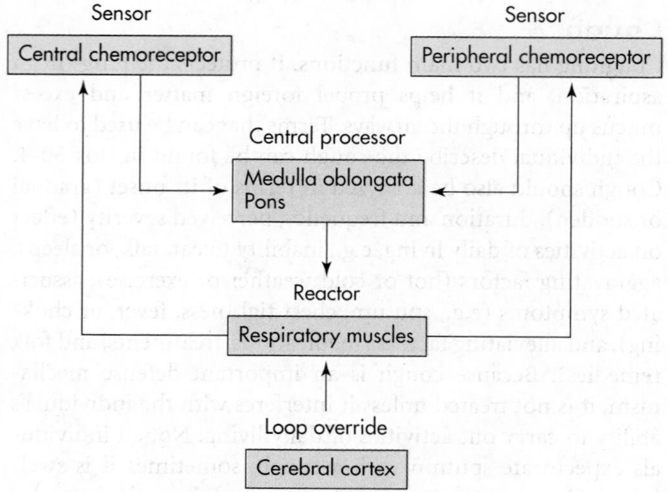


**fig. 30-10** Respiratory control loop.

### Neural Receptors

The *stretch receptors* located in the conducting airways respond to changes in the pressure within the airways. They inhibit inspiration once the lungs are inflated. This is known as the Hering-Breuer inflation reflex and is important to prevent overinflation of the lungs. *J receptors* are located in the alveolar walls and respond with rapid shallow breathing in conditions associated with an increase in interstitial fluid volume, such as pulmonary edema and pneumonia.

## SUBJECTIVE DATA

Respiratory assessment should be tailored to the individual's health status. If the individual exhibits signs of respiratory distress, such as increased restlessness, paradoxical breathing pattern, increased ventilatory rate, complaints of dyspnea and use of accessory muscles, the subjective information should be deferred and an abbreviated physical assessment made. Once the individual is physiologically stable, data collection can resume. Information can also be obtained from a significant other (if available).

## COMMON SYMPTOMS

The most common pulmonary symptoms or reasons a person seeks health care include dyspnea, cough, increased sputum production, hemoptysis, wheezing, or chest pain. Upper airway symptoms may include obstruction of nares, nasal discharge, sinus pain, sore throat, or hoarseness.

### Dyspnea

Dyspnea and breathlessness are frequently used to describe the same symptom. *Dyspnea* is frequently described as the subjective sensation of difficult breathing or "breathlessness." Yet, it is the term often used to describe difficult or labored breathing observable by others. Because of its subjective nature, dyspnea has been difficult to assess. A descriptive study of patient, nurse, and physician views of dyspnea is presented in the Research Box.

Individuals experiencing pulmonary dysfunction, such as breathlessness, tend to perceive their illness in terms of its impact on their ability to carry out activities of daily living (ADL). Dyspnea may cause other problems such as constipation or poor nutrition, as well as psychosocial problems related to poor self-esteem or changes in lifestyle. See Box 30-1 for assessing the effect of breathlessness on ADL.

A quick and easy instrument that can be used to assess how breathless the individual feels is a self-report visual analog scale. Ask the individual to place a mark on the scale consisting of phrases ("no breathlessness" to "extreme breathlessness")

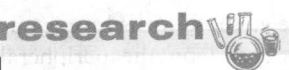

Reference: Hay L, Farncombe M, McKee P: Patient, nurse and physician views of dyspnea, *Can Nurse* 92(10):26-29, 1996.

This study compared dyspnea assessments by a patient or the patient's family with those of the primary nurse and physician. A total of 142 patients completed four scales that measured the degree of breathlessness, and when and how much the dyspnea affected their activities: the Linear Analogue Self Assessment Scale (LASA), the Borg Category Scale (BCS), the Modified Medical Research Council Dyspnea Scale (MMRCDS), and the Oxygen Cost Diagram (OCD). The primary nurses and physicians completed only LASA and BCS because the other scales were entirely subjective. Assessments were completed at similar times by the patient, nurse, and physician. Thirty-two percent of the patients reported some degree of dyspnea as measured by LASA and BCS, 75.6% reported that they had to restrict their activities of daily living secondary to breathlessness as measured by MMRCDS, and 78.5% reported that their dyspnea limited daily activities by as much as 50% as measured by OCD. Primary nurses agreed with the patient assessment of the level of dyspnea in 63 (47%) cases. Nurses overestimated dyspnea in 22% and underestimated dyspnea in 10% of the cases. Physicians agreed in 50% of the cases, overrated dyspnea in 19% of the cases, and underestimated dyspnea in 10% of the cases. Dyspnea is a subjective experience that is oftentimes accompanied by other symptoms. This presents a challenge to health care workers. Both direct and activity-based measures of breathlessness are important to a complete assessment. Awareness of associated symptoms that may mask the need to treat dyspnea is imperative.

**box 30-1** *Assessment of the Effect of Breathlessness on ADL*

How does your breathing difficulty affect your ability to:
- Bathe, dress, and groom yourself
- Walk or exercise
- Prepare meals and eat
- Get about your home or climb stairs
- Sleep
- Perform chores or hobbies
- Get to the bathroom
- Maintain family and social relationships
- Maintain employment
- Perform sexually
- Attend activities away from home

that corresponds with the individual's perception of the severity of the sensation (Box 30-2).

This scale can be used to evaluate the effectiveness of interventions and to monitor the individual's response to therapy. Factors such as stress and anxiety that may contribute to respiratory symptoms should be explored with the individual. In addition, methods that prevent or control breathlessness should also be identified. See Box 30-3 for analysis of dyspnea.

**box 30-2** *Breathlessness Visual Analog Scale*

Extreme breathlessness—shortness of breath is the worst it can be

No breathlessness or shortness of breath

**box 30-3** *Analysis of Dyspnea*

**TIMING**
1. Chronic or acute
2. Episodic or paroxysmal
3. Onset
4. Duration
5. Frequency

**CHARACTERISTICS**
1. Perceived severity
2. Phase of respiratory cycle
   a. Inspiratory
   b. Expiratory
   c. Throughout entire cycle
3. Other symptoms related to dyspnea
4. Associated factors
   a. Time of day
   b. Seasonal or weather changes
   c. Environmental irritants
   d. Anxiety
   e. Body position
      (1) Paroxysmal nocturnal dyspnea (PND): sudden onset while sleeping in recumbent position
      (2) Orthopnea: breathlessness on assuming recumbent position
   f. Activity

Dyspnea is a common cardiopulmonary symptom and is discussed further in Chapter 24.

## Cough

Coughing has two main functions. It protects the lungs from aspiration, and it helps propel foreign matter and excess mucus up through the airways. Terms that can be used to have the individual describe the cough can be found in Box 30-4. Cough should also be analyzed in terms of its onset (gradual or sudden), duration and frequency, perceived severity (effect on activities of daily living, e.g., inability to eat, talk, or sleep), aggravating factors (hot or cold weather or exercise), associated symptoms (e.g., sputum, chest tightness, fever, or choking), and alleviating factors (medications, treatments, and folk remedies). Because cough is an important defense mechanism, it is not treated unless it interferes with the individual's ability to carry out activities of daily living. Not all individuals expectorate sputum with a cough; sometimes it is swallowed. However, the term *productive cough* is used when sputum is produced regardless of the individual's ability to expectorate it.

**box 30-4** *Cough*

**TIMING**
1. Chronic
2. Acute
3. Paroxysmal (periodic forceful episodes that are difficult to control)

**CHARACTERISTICS**
1. Perceived severity
2. Pattern
   a. Occasional
   b. Upon arising
   c. With activity (talking, exercising, eating)
3. Quality
   a. Productive-nonproductive
   b. Dry progressing to productive
   c. Barking
   d. Hoarse
   e. Hacking
4. Other symptoms
   a. Chest tightness
   b. Fever, coryza
   c. Choking

**box 30-5** *Sputum Characteristics*

1. Thick
2. Viscous (gelatinous)
3. Tenacious (sticky)
4. Frothy
5. Mucoid (colorless or clear: noninfectious process)
6. Watery
7. Mucopurulent
   a. Creamy yellow: staphylococcal pneumonia
   b. Green: *Pseudomonas* pneumonia
   c. "Currant jelly": *Klebsiella* pneumonia
   d. Rusty: pneumococcal pneumonia
   e. Pink frothy: pulmonary edema
8. Casts (from bronchioles, rubbery)

**box 30-6** *Bedside Assessment of Hemoptysis and Hematemesis*

| | |
|---|---|
| Hemoptysis | Usually frothy, pH alkaline, bright red |
| Hematemesis | Never frothy, may be mixed with food particles, pH acidic, dark red, or "coffee colored" |

### Sputum Production

As mentioned earlier, a mucous blanket lines the epithelial layer of the tracheobronchial tree and cleanses it of inhaled particles and debris. Mucus is produced by the goblet cells and submucosal glands. The cilia propel the mucus (which contains foreign particles, pus, blood, and debris) upward toward the pharynx where it is coughed up, suctioned, or swallowed. Normal sputum is clear and thin and averages 100 ml/day. However, individuals with pulmonary disease often have sputum associated with their condition making it important to assess baseline sputum characteristics. The characteristics in Box 30-5 can be used to ask the individual to describe the sputum. Have the individual quantify the amount of sputum using teaspoons, tablespoons, or cups as measurements instead of terms such as "scant" or "moderate."

### Hemoptysis

*Hemoptysis* is the coughing up of blood or blood-tinged sputum. The sputum may also contain air bubbles. The source of bleeding may be from anywhere in the upper or lower airways or from the lung parenchyma. Ask the individual to describe the color and appearance of the sputum. Blood that originates in the gastrointestinal tract and is coughed up as dark brown or resembling coffee-grounds in appearance is termed *hematemesis.* Bleeding from the nares (epistaxis) should be assessed as a cause for coughing up blood or vomiting of blood. See Box 30-6 for differences in hemoptysis and hematemesis. Have the individual quantify the hemoptysis in teaspoons, tablespoons, or cups. The coughing up of 400 to 600 ml of blood in a 24-hour period is considered massive.[1]

### Wheezing

Wheezing is a continuous high-pitched, whistling sound produced when air passes through narrowed or obstructed airways. It generally occurs during expiration; however, wheezing can be heard throughout the respiratory cycle. Wheezing is usually heard with a stethoscope; however, wheezing may be audible to the individual or heard by others in close proximity to the individual. Ask the individual if noisy breathing has ever been experienced. An analysis of this symptom should include factors that can cause bronchospasm and produce wheezing, such as asthma, exposure to physiological irritants, stress, or anxiety. Snoring may also be reported by the individual. If airway obstruction is present, "stridor" or loud snoring may be experienced. Individuals who awake frequently due to loud snoring may be experiencing sleep apnea syndrome (see Chapter 13).

### Chest Pain

Chest pain can result from several conditions. A detailed investigation is required to differentiate chest pain of cardiac origin from other causes. Chest pain of cardiac origin is described in Chapter 25. Chest pain of pulmonary origin can originate from the chest wall, parietal pleura, or lung parenchyma. Table 30-1 summarizes the characteristics of pulmonary chest pain.

### Upper Airway Symptoms

Ask the individual if any difficulty breathing through the nose, any nasal discharge or sinus pain, or any vocal changes have been experienced. Changes in voice can be caused by obstruction or congestion of nasal passages as well as inflammation of the vocal cords (hoarseness). Hoarseness may be associated with tumors, laryngeal nerve damage, or laryngitis. Individuals may experience hoarseness after removal of an endotracheal tube.

**table 30-1** *Characteristics of Pulmonary Chest Pain*

| ORIGIN | CHARACTERISTICS | POSSIBLE CAUSE |
|---|---|---|
| Chest wall | Well-localized, constant ache increasing with movement | Trauma, cough, herpes zoster |
| Pleura | Sharp, abrupt onset, increasing with inspiration or with sudden ventilatory effort (cough, sneeze), unilateral | Pleural inflammation (pleurisy)<br>Autoimmune and connective tissue disease |
| Lung parenchyma | Dull, constant ache, poorly localized | Benign pulmonary tumors<br>Carcinoma |
| | Well-localized, sharp, sudden onset | Pneumothorax |
| | Sudden onset, increasing stabbing pain on inspiration, may radiate | Pulmonary embolus and infarction |

## RESPIRATORY HEALTH HISTORY

In addition to a review of the symptom or reason the individual is seeking health care, the individual should be interviewed about risk factors associated with respiratory dysfunction, including smoking, past pulmonary illnesses or exposure to respiratory infections, predisposition to genetic disorders, exposure to environmental irritants, and the psychosocial effects of the respiratory disorder.

### Smoking

Smoking has been implicated as a major cause of lung disease. There is a strong relationship between smoking and the development or exacerbation of chronic bronchitis, emphysema, asthma, lung cancer, and respiratory infections. Passive smoke has also been implicated in increasing the risk for nonsmokers. The individual's current and past history of tobacco use must be assessed. Individuals should be questioned about the type of tobacco (cigars, cigarettes, or pipe) as well as the number of packs and number of years smoked. Pack-years (for cigarette use) can be determined with the following equation: Pack-year = number of years smoked × number of packs smoked per day (e.g., 20 years of 2 packs/day = 40 pack-years). Questions regarding any efforts to quit smoking and smoking by others (in the home or at work) should also be asked. If the individual has quit smoking, pack-years are still determined in addition to the length of time the individual has stopped smoking. The use of cigars, pipes, marijuana, and smokeless tobacco is measured as amount used per day.

### Respiratory Disorders

A history of respiratory illnesses and hospitalizations for lung diseases or disorders should be obtained (e.g., childhood allergies, frequent respiratory infections, influenza, frequent colds, pneumonia, pleurisy, emphysema, asthma, chronic sinusitis, chest surgery or trauma, tuberculosis, and adult-onset allergies). Any exposure to tuberculosis or other respiratory infections or travel to areas with risk for respiratory infections, such as histoplasmosis (Southwest United States) or coccidioidomycosis (Southwest United States, Central America, or Mexico), should also be asked of the individual.

### Family History

Some health problems have a genetic link with respiratory disease. Ask the individual if there is a family history of allergy, asthma, atopic dermatitis, or lung cancer. Also, obtain a family history of documented $\alpha_1$-protease inhibitor deficiency or cystic fibrosis. A strong family history of emphysema or the development of respiratory symptoms at an early age could prove helpful in identifying individuals who are candidates for genetic testing and counseling. Panlobular emphysema is a disease that usually affects young adults and is caused by an $\alpha_1$-protease inhibitor deficiency. Cystic fibrosis is a disease that involves mucus-secreting and eccrine sweat glands. The abnormal secretions affect the lungs by obstructing respiratory passages, impairing oxygenation, and impairing mucociliary clearance.

### Environmental Irritants

Assess the individual's exposure to pollutants and irritants such as dust, fumes, gases, coal dust, and other allergens. Ask about the workplace and type of work the individual does, the home environment and adjacent area for exposure to irritants, and hobbies of the individual to reveal potential pollutant exposure such as pets, glues, and paints. Information about the occupation of the individual's family members may also provide information helpful to assessing the individual's respiratory complaint.

### Psychosocial History

Because dyspnea can affect an individual's functional status, it is important to obtain a history of the individual's perception of the situation as well as coping skills and resources. The quality of life may be perceived as diminished in individuals with respiratory disorders.

Need satisfaction is important to understanding the individual's functional performance. Assess the individual's sense of self, sense of control, satisfaction with family life, safety-security needs, leisure activities, financial resources, and social support. Although symptoms may affect psychosocial functioning, psychosocial effects of a respiratory disorder may also impair cognitive functioning and adaptation to the disorder. This may be manifested as sleeping difficulties, irritability, helplessness-hopelessness, tension-anxiety, depression, and isolation.

An assessment of emotional responses during dyspnea is important to understanding the individual's experiences. Anxiety is frequently experienced during dyspnea as are depression and hostility. Assessing emotional responses to dyspnea such as anxiety, fear, or panic may assist the health care provider to select interventions to prevent or reduce dyspnea. Asking the individual how bothersome or upsetting the shortness of breath is or how nervous or apprehensive he or she becomes helps the health care provider to understand how dyspnea affects the individual.

### Other

Ask the individual about problems with swallowing and ambulating, as well as any history of neurological or muscular disease. Factors that may adversely affect respiratory function include immobility, dysphagia, and diseases affecting muscular strength (e.g., amyotrophic lateral sclerosis, myasthenia gravis, and stroke).

# OBJECTIVE DATA

## RESPIRATORY VITAL SIGNS

### Respiratory Rate and Ventilation

The respiratory rate should be counted, and the depth and rhythm of the breathing pattern assessed. The expansion of the chest should be bilaterally symmetrical. See Figure 30-11 and Table 30-2 for normal and abnormal breathing patterns.

### Pulse Oximetry

Pulse oximetry, referred to as $SpO_2$, is a noninvasive method used to assess oxygenation. The normal $SpO_2$ value is greater than 95%.[3] An arterial blood gas analysis can provide an $SaO_2$ measurement that can be compared with the $SpO_2$ value when pulse oximetry is initiated. See Chapter 20 for further discussion of pulse oximetry.

### Mixed Venous Oxygen Saturation ($SvO_2$)

$SvO_2$ measurement is a valuable tool used to assess oxygenation status in the critically ill person. It can be measured continuously or periodically with a specialized pulmonary artery catheter (see Chapter 24). $SvO_2$ provides information about the amount of oxygen that is supplied to the tissues relative to the oxygen demand at the tissue level. Oxygen demand reflects the amount of oxygen extracted for use at the tissue level. Normal $SvO_2$ is 60% to 80% and indicates adequate tissue perfusion. A decrease in $SvO_2$ ($<60\%$) signifies that the oxygen demand is greater than the supply. An increase in $SvO_2$ ($>80\%$) signifies that the oxygen supply is greater than the oxygen demand. A value of $<60\%$ or a change of $+10\%$ from the individual's baseline is significant.

## UPPER AIRWAY

An examination of the upper airway includes the inspection of the nose and nasal septum for deformities and asymmetry. Some septal deviation is common in adults and is usually asymptomatic (Figure 30-12, p. 849). Each naris is occluded to determine the presence of an obstruction to breathe. The nasal mucosa and turbinates are observed for color, edema, exudate, or polyps. Excessive redness, edema, exudate, or bleeding is an abnormal finding. Red, swollen nasal mucous membranes accompanied by watery to mucopurulent nasal discharge indicates acute rhinitis. Nasal mucosa that is swollen, pale, boggy, and usually gray to dull red indicates allergic rhinitis.

The sinuses are palpated for signs of tenderness of the frontal and maxillary areas. Transillumination can be performed if infection is suspected. Normally, the sinuses will demonstrate differing degrees of a red glow. When disease is present, the light will not penetrate the sinuses, and the red glow will not be seen through the hard palate or above the eyebrow.

The oropharynx is examined with a tongue blade and a mirror. The anterior and posterior tonsillar pillars, the uvula, the tonsils, and the posterior pharynx are inspected for color, symmetry, evidence of exudate, edema, ulcerations, and tonsillar enlargement. Some tonsils are enlarged without being

| Pattern | Description |
|---|---|
| Eupnea | Rhythm is smooth and even with expiration longer than inspiration. |
| Tachypnea | Rapid superficial breathing; regular or irregular rhythm. |
| Bradypnea | Slow respiratory rate; deeper than usual depth; regular rhythm. |
| Apnea | Cessation of breathing. |
| Hyperpnea | Increased depth of respiration with a normal to increased rate and regular rhythm. |
| Cheyne-Stokes respiration | Periodic breathing associated with periods of apnea, alternating regularly with a series of respiratory cycles; the respiratory cycle gradually increases, then decreases in rate and depth. |
| Ataxic breathing | Periods of apnea alternating irregularly with a series of shallow breaths of equal depth. |
| Kussmaul's respiration | Deep regular sighing respirations with an increase in respiratory rate. |
| Apneusis | Long, gasping inspiratory phase followed by a short, inadequate expiratory phase. |
| Obstructed breathing | Long, ineffective expiratory phase with shallow, increased respirations. |

**fig. 30-11** Respiratory patterns.

**table 30-2** *Possible Findings by Inspection in a Pulmonary Examination*

| OBSERVE | NORMAL | ABNORMAL |
|---|---|---|
| General appearance | Quiet respiration<br>Sitting or reclining without difficulty<br>Skin translucent, appears dry<br>Nail beds pink<br>Mucous membranes pink and moist* | Lips puckered when exhaling (pursed-lip breathing)<br>Nasal flaring<br>Audible wheezing<br>Restless and apprehensive<br>Leans forward with hands or elbows on knees (tripod position)<br>Skin: diaphoretic, dull pale, or ruddy<br>Cyanosis: skin or mucous membranes have bluish cast<br>Central cyanosis: results from decreased oxygenation of blood†<br>Peripheral cyanosis: result of local vasoconstriction or decreased cardiac output<br>Digital clubbing: painless enlargement of terminal phalanges related to chronic tissue hypoxia (Figure 30-13) |
| Trachea | Midline in neck | Tracheal deviation; displacement either lateral, anterior, or posterior<br>Jugular venous distension (see Chapter 26)<br>Cough: strong or weak, dry or wet, productive or nonproductive<br>Sputum production: amount, color, odor, and consistency (see p. 845) |
| Rate | Eupnea: 12 to 20 | Tachypnea: rate >20 breaths/min<br>Bradypnea: rate <10 breaths/min |
| Breathing pattern | Minimal effort with inspiration: passive, quiet expiration<br>Inspiration/expiration ratio: 1:2<br>Male: diaphragmatic breathing<br>Female: thoracic breathing | Accessory muscle breathing<br>Paradoxical: portion of chest wall moves in during inhalation and out during exhalation<br>Stridorous: audible, loud, low-pitched sound with inhalation and exhalation |
| Thoracic configuration | Symmetrical appearance<br><br>Anteroposterior (AP) diameter less than transverse diameter<br>Spine straight<br><br>Scapulae on same horizontal plane | Chest expands unevenly<br>Muscular development asymmetrical<br>Barrel chest: AP diameter increased in relation to transverse diameter<br>Kyphosis: increased thoracic curvature<br>Scoliosis: increased lateral curvature<br>Scapular placement asymmetrical |

*Dark-skinned people might have normal bluish-pigmented mucous membranes.
†Central cyanosis is relevant to respiratory status. Observe nail beds, mucous membrane, and lips.

infected. The gag reflex is also tested. Absence of a gag reflex affects the individual's ability to manage the airway.

## CHEST AND LUNGS

### Inspection

Note the individual's thorax for shape and symmetry. Observe the color of the lips, skin, and nail beds. Inspect the fingers for clubbing (Figure 30-13). Table 30-2 indicates possible findings.

### Palpation

The chest and spinal column are palpated for tenderness, bulges, and abnormalities; the trachea is palpated for position; and the chest is palpated for symmetry of expansion. All areas of the chest should be palpated for fremitus. Generally, the individual is asked to repeat a phrase (e.g., "99") while the examiner places the palms of the hands against the individual's chest. Fremitus increases with lung consolidation because vibrations caused by liquid or solid material are transmitted more readily than they are in air-filled spaces. Possible findings are presented in Table 30-3.

### Percussion

Percussion is used to assess lung fields and diaphragmatic excursion (Figure 30-14). Percussion tones (resonance) are produced from vibration created by tapping the chest wall. The degree of percussion note depends on the density of the underlying tissue and the amount of air through which the vibration travels. *Hyperresonant sounds* are produced over areas of trapped gas, such as emphysema. Dull percussion sounds are produced in conditions such as atelectasis or consolidation

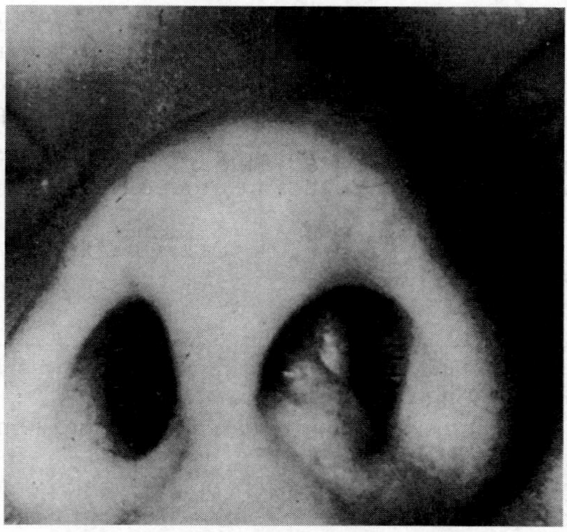

**fig. 30-12** Septal deviation. Anterior end of septal cartilage is dislocated and projects into nasal vestibule.

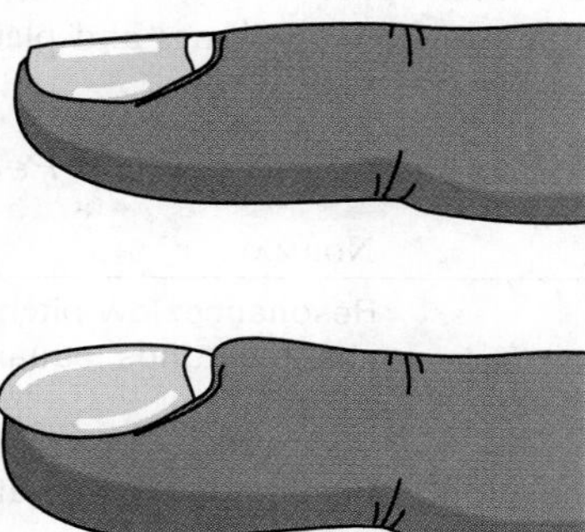

**fig. 30-13** Comparison of normal nail *(top)* and digital clubbing *(bottom)*.

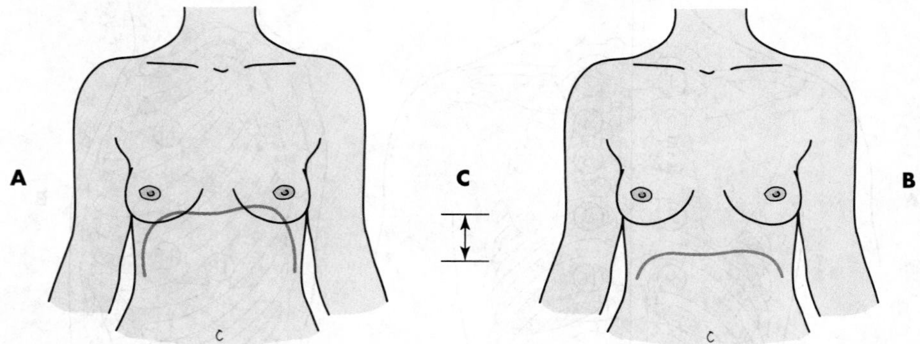


**fig. 30-14** Diaphragmatic excursion. **A,** Position of diaphragm at full-end expiration. **B,** Position of diaphragm at full-end inspiration. **C,** Range of diaphragmatic movement—distance from expiration to inspiration.

**table 30-3** *Possible Findings by Palpation in a Pulmonary Examination*

| Palpate | Normal | Abnormal |
|---|---|---|
| Skin and chest wall | Skin nontender, smooth, warm, and dry | Skin moist or exceedingly dry<br>Crepitation—"crackling" when skin palpated—caused by air leak from lung into subcutaneous tissue |
| | Spine and ribs nontender | Localized tenderness |
| Fremitus* | Symmetrical, mild vibrations felt on chest wall during vocalization | Increased fremitus—a result of vibration through more solid medium, such as lung tumors; pneumonia<br>Decreased fremitus—a result of vibration through increased space (excess air) in the chest, such as pneumothorax or COPD<br>Asymmetric fremitus is always abnormal |
| Lateral chest expansion | Symmetrical 3-8 cm expansion† | Expansion less than 3 cm, painful or asymmetrical† |

*Normal fremitus varies from person to person. An individual's baseline must be established.
†Reduced expansion can result from either an overexpanded chest (barrel chest) or from a restricted chest.

and pleural effusion. Table 30-4 identifies possible findings by percussion.

### Auscultation

Auscultation of breath sounds and voice sounds provides valuable information about the lungs and pleura. The individual should be instructed to take slow, deep breaths through the mouth during the examination. With the diaphragm of the stethoscope, the examiner listens systematically to all lung fields and compares breath sounds of the right and left sides during inspiration and expiration (Figure 30-15). Three normal and distinct breath sounds are produced based upon the

**table 30-4** *Possible Findings by Percussion in a Pulmonary Examination*

| Percussion | Normal | Abnormal |
|---|---|---|
| Lung fields | Resonance: low-pitched, hollow, easily heard sounds; equal quality bilaterally | Hyperresonant: heard with air trapping (emphysema or pneumothorax)<br>Dull or flat: results from decreased air in lungs (tumor, atelectasis, fluid) |
| Diaphragm position and movement | Resting diaphragm at 10th thoracic vertebra<br>Each hemidiaphragm moves 3-6 cm (see Figure 30-14) | High position—stomach distention or phrenic nerve damage<br>Decreased or no movement in either hemidiaphragm* |

*Decreased excursion can result from hyperinflated lungs pushing down on diaphragm, diaphragmatic disorders, or loss of diaphragmatic innervation.

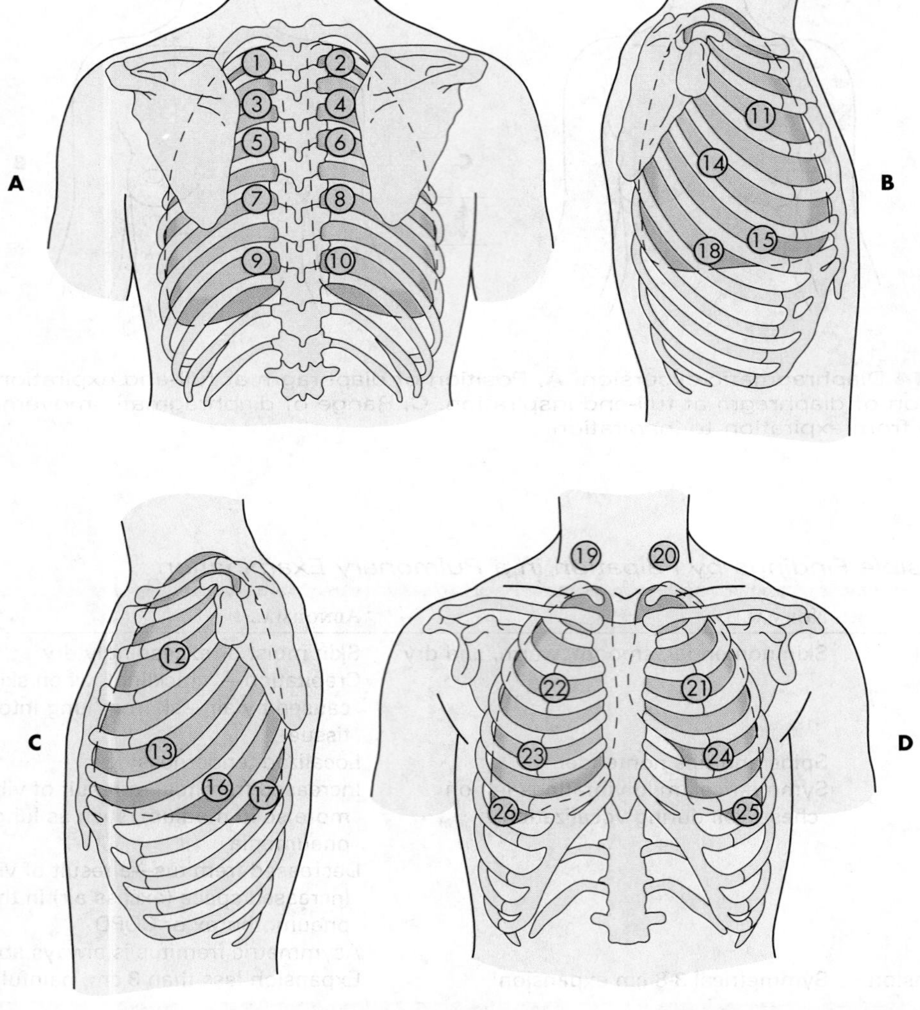


**fig. 30-15** Numbers indicate a recommended sequence for percussion and auscultation during a routine screening examination. **A,** Posterior thorax. **B,** Right lateral thorax. **C,** Left lateral thorax. **D,** Anterior thorax.

specific area of the respiratory tract. Characteristics of breath sounds can be found in Table 30-5.

Adventitious breath sounds (Table 30-6) can be caused by a variety of underlying pathological conditions that cause excess mucus or fluid, tissue inflammation, bronchospasm, or airway obstruction. Bronchial or bronchovesicular sounds auscultated in peripheral lung fields are abnormal. Diminished or absent breath sounds are associated with conditions that lead to alveolar hypoventilation, such as shallow breathing, COPD, pus, or fluid in pleural space. Crackles can be heard more frequently during inspiration and generally do not clear with coughing, rhonchi are more pronounced during expiration and disappear after coughing, and wheezes can be heard during inspiration or expiration.

Normal voice sounds are usually muffled and indistinct. Consolidation in the lung can cause changes in vocal resonance (Table 30-7).

## PHYSIOLOGICAL CHANGES WITH AGING

Changes in respiratory anatomy and physiology that occur with aging can produce variations in clinical findings. The thoracic cage becomes rigid from cartilage calcification, osteoporosis of the ribs, and arthritic changes in the joints of the ribs. *Kyphosis* or the accentuated dorsal curvature of the thoracic spine (hunch back) may also occur with aging. An increase in the anterior-posterior diameter of the chest occurs in the elderly.

Chest wall compliance is reduced because of stiffening of the chest wall and a loss in elastic recoil of the lungs associated with advanced age, resulting in increased work of breathing. Muscle strength decreases with aging, affecting lung volumes and pressures. However, respiratory muscle strength may be enhanced with exercise. Structural changes within the lungs include calcification of bronchial cartilages, increased

**table 30-5** *Characteristics of Breath Sounds*

| Sound | Duration of Inspiration and Expiration | Diagram of Sound | Pitch | Intensity | Normal Location | Abnormal Location |
|---|---|---|---|---|---|---|
| Vesicular | Inspiration > expiration 5:2 | | Low | Soft | Peripheral lung | Not applicable |
| Bronchovesicular | Inspiration = expiration 1:1 | | Medium | Medium | First and second intercostal spaces at the sternal border anteriorly; posteriorly at T4 medial to scapulae | Peripheral lung |
| Bronchial (tubular) | Inspiration < expiration 1:2 | | High | Loud | Over trachea | Lung area |

From Malasanos L et al: *Health assessment,* ed 4, St Louis, 1990, Mosby.

**table 30-6** *Abnormal (Adventitious) Lung Sounds*

| Type | Physiology | Auscultation | Sound | Possible Condition |
|---|---|---|---|---|
| Crackles | Air passing through fluid in small airways, or sudden opening of deflated weakened airways | More commonly heard during inspiration | Fine high-pitched or coarse low-pitched popping sounds that are short and discontinuous | Pneumonia, heart failure, atelectasis, emphysema |
| Rhonchi | Large airway obstructed by fluid | Heard commonly during expiration | Low-pitched continuous snoring sound | COPD, bronchospasm, pneumonia |
| Wheezes | Air passing through narrowed airways | Can be heard throughout inspiration and expiration | High-pitched whistling sound | Airway obstruction, bronchospasm as in asthma, COPD |
| Pleural friction rub | Rubbing of inflamed pleura | May occur throughout respiratory cycle, heard best at base of lung at end of expiration | Scratching, grating, rubbing, creaking | Inflamed pleura, pulmonary infarction |

**table 30-7** *Voice Sounds**

| Type | Instruction to Patient | Normal Sound | Abnormal |
|---|---|---|---|
| Egophony | Say prolonged "e" | Muffled "e" | "a" |
| Whispered pectoriloquy | Whisper "1, 2, 3" | Muffled "1, 2, 3" | Loud, clear "1, 2, 3" |
| Bronchophony | Say "1, 2, 3" | Muffled "1, 2, 3" | Loud, clear "1, 2, 3" |

*Examiner auscultates for characteristic changes when voice sounds are transmitted through chest wall.

anatomical dead space, decreased diameter of noncartilaginous bronchioles, increased size of the pores of Kohn, and enlarged alveolar ducts. Pulmonary diffusion capacity decreases because of a loss in the surface area of the alveolar-capillary membrane and inequalities in the distribution of air or blood. Room air alveolar-arterial oxygen gradient ($PAO_2$-$PaO_2$) increases with aging. Arterial oxygen pressure ($PaO_2$) levels are lower, but carbon dioxide levels and pH are not affected by age. Ventilatory and heart rate responses to brief periods of hypoxia or hypercarbia are also blunted in the older adult. Sleep apnea may be observed in the elderly but has not been reported to be clinically significant.[2] Although total lung capacity is relatively unchanged, the effects of aging on lung volumes and spirometry include an increase in residual volume, a decrease in forced vital capacity, a decrease in forced expiratory volume, a decrease in maximum voluntary ventilation, and a decrease peak expiratory air flow.[4]

Assessment considerations in the elderly are listed in Box 30-7.

**box 30-7** *Considerations in the Elderly*

| Changes Associated with Aging | Effect on Respiratory System |
|---|---|
| Increase in AP chest diameter | Decreased chest expansion |
| Kyphosis | |
| Decreased muscular strength; reduced chest wall compliance | Decreased ability to cough forcefully and breathe deeply<br>Decreased arterial oxygen levels<br>Increased risk for atelectasis |
| Decreased lung defenses | Increased risk for respiratory infections |
| Decreased ability to handle secretions | Increased risk for aspiration<br>Increased risk for infection |
| Decreased chest expansion; decreased ability to deep breathe and cough | Decreased breath sounds, crackles<br>Increased risk for atelectasis<br>Increased risk for respiratory infection<br>Decreased oxygenation<br>Increased risk for hypoventilation |
| Altered pulmonary function | Increased residual volume<br>Decreased forced vital capacity<br>Decreased forced expiratory volume<br>Decreased maximum voluntary ventilation<br>Decreased peak expiratory airflow |

## DIAGNOSTIC TESTS

### LABORATORY TESTS

Nursing care associated with laboratory and noninvasive radiological tests can be found in Table 30-8.

#### $\alpha_1$-Antitrypsin Assay

This blood test is valuable in the identification of individuals with the genetic abnormality that leads to emphysema. $\alpha_1$-Antitrypsin is a globulin that inhibits certain enzymes. Without it, these enzymes destroy the alveolar walls. $\alpha_1$-Antitrypsin deficiencies are inherited, and individuals with this deficiency develop emphysema at a young age.

#### Arterial Blood Gases and Acid-Base Balance

Arterial blood gas analysis provides information about oxygenation, ventilation, and acid-base balance. It is valuable in assessing the efficiency of pulmonary gas exchange and the presence of an acid-base disorder. The arterial blood gas parameters are shown in Table 30-9.

##### *Nursing care*

Explain the purpose of the test and its procedure. There are no food or fluid restrictions. The amount of oxygen should be noted if the individual is receiving supplemental oxygen. The oxygen should not be changed or removed (unless ordered) before the test. In addition, interventions or activities required of the individual should be withheld for 20 minutes before the test. The nurse may be required to obtain a sample or assist in the sample collection and in applying pressure at the arterial puncture site. The site should be observed for bleeding or hematoma formation and any circulatory impairment reported.

##### *Blood sample collection*

The Allen's test should be performed to determine adequacy of collateral blood flow to the radial artery (Figure 30-16). A blood sample is obtained by directly puncturing a radial, brachial, or femoral artery (arterial punctures are contraindicated in individuals receiving thrombolytic agents). A preheparinized syringe is used to collect the sample to prevent blood clotting. Once the 2 ml of blood is obtained, air bubbles are expelled, and the syringe is sealed with an impermeable cap to prevent contact with room air. The blood sample is placed on ice until analyzed. Individuals with blood-clotting abnormali-

**table 30-8** *Diagnostic Tests and Related Nursing Care*

| Test | Nursing Care |
|---|---|
| $\alpha_1$-Antitrypsin assay<br>MM genotype: 2.1-3.8 U/ml<br>MZ phenotype: 1.05-2.1 U/ml<br>ZZ phenotype: 0.5-0.7 U/ml | Explain purpose. No food or fluid restrictions are necessary. No special care is required posttest. |
| Complete blood count | |
| Red blood cells<br>4.2-5.4 million/L (female)<br>4.6-6.2 million/L (male)<br>Hemoglobin<br>12-16 g/dl (female)<br>14-18 g/dl (male)<br>Hematocrit<br>38%-47% (female)<br>40%-54% (male)<br>White blood cells<br>4.5-11.0 × $10^3$/L | Explain purpose. No food or fluid restrictions are necessary. No special care is required posttest. |
| Sputum analysis | Explain purpose. Some tests require specimens collected on consecutive days. Usually 4 ml of sputum is sufficient. Coughing upon awakening is more likely to result in collecting sputum and not saliva. Instruct individual to rinse the mouth with water; demonstrate effective deep breathing and coughing; have individual practice deep breathing and coughing; instruct individual to notify the staff as soon as the specimen is collected. |
| Throat culture | Explain purpose. No special care is required. |
| Chest radiograph | Explain purpose. No food or fluid restrictions are necessary. No special care is required posttest. |
| Computed tomography | Explain purpose. No food or fluid restrictions are required unless contrast medium is used. Check the individual for iodine sensitivity and inform the individual that a warm flushed feeling and salty taste may be experienced. No special care is required posttest. |
| Esophagogram | Explain purpose. Individual is given nothing by mouth until completion of the test. Inform the individual that all metal objects must be removed. Explain that the individual will be required to drink barium contrast medium while films are being taken. The barium may be unpleasant (chalky) tasting. Assess bowel evacuation of barium posttest. |
| Fluoroscopy | Explain purpose. No special care is required; however, if performed with other procedures, pre- and postprocedural care related to that test may be required. |
| Magnetic resonance imaging | Explain purpose. Test takes about an hour. Remove all metal objects before the test. |
| Ventilation/perfusion lung scan | Explain purpose. No food or fluid restrictions are necessary. Assess individual for allergies. Remove all metal objects before the test. Obtain an accurate weight so that the dosage of radioactive agent can be calculated. No special care is required posttest. |

**table 30-9** *Arterial Blood Gases*

| Parameter | Measurement | Value |
|---|---|---|
| Acid-base-balance | pH: hydrogen ion concentration | Normal: 7.35-7.45<br>Alkalemia: ↑ 7.45<br>Acidemia: ↓ 7.35 |
| Oxygenation | $Pa_{O_2}$: partial pressure of dissolved $O_2$ in blood | Normal: 80-100 mm Hg<br>Hyperoxemia: ↑ 100 mm Hg<br>Hypoxemia: ↓ 80 mm Hg |
| | $Sa_{O_2}$: percentage of $O_2$ bound to hemoglobin | 95%-98% |
| Ventilation | $Pa_{CO_2}$: partial pressure of $CO_2$ dissolved in blood | Normal: 35-45 mm Hg<br>Hypercapnia: ↑ 45 mm Hg<br>Hypocapnia: ↓ 35 mm Hg |

ties may require direct pressure over the puncture site for longer than 5 minutes.

An indwelling arterial catheter (see Chapter 22) is commonly used to obtain blood samples in the critically ill; the catheter should be flushed per hospital protocol to prevent clotting. Continuous arterial blood gas monitoring is also available.

### Oxygenation

Both partial pressure of oxygen ($PaO_2$) and oxygen saturation ($SaO_2$) levels are measured to determine the adequacy of arterial blood oxygenation. $PaO_2$ is oxygen dissolved in arterial blood and is influenced by fractional inspired oxygen ($FIO_2$). However, the amount of oxygen carried in the blood in this form is small. The $PaO_2$ can be used to assess the need for oxygen therapy or a change in it. $SaO_2$ measures the percentage of the hemoglobin that is combined with oxygen. About 98% of the oxygen-carrying capacity of blood is accounted for by oxyhemoglobin, with the partial pressure of oxygen acting as the driving force for this chemical combination.

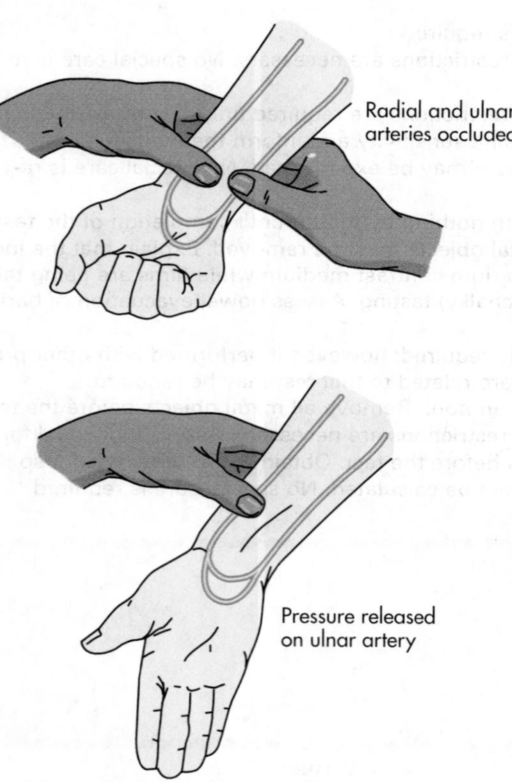


**fig. 30-16** Allen's test. Hold patient's hand with palm up. Have patient clench and unclench hand while occluding the radial and ulnar arteries. The hand will become pale. Lower the hand and have the patient relax the hand. While continuing to hold the radial artery, release pressure on the ulnar artery. Brisk return of color (5 to 7 seconds) demonstrates adequate ulnar blood flow. If pallor persists for more than 15 seconds, ulnar flow is inadequate and radial artery cannulation should not be attempted.

### Oxyhemoglobin dissociation curve

The relationship of $PaO_2$ to $SaO_2$ is demonstrated in the oxyhemoglobin dissociation curve. Although the percentage of hemoglobin that is bound with oxygen increases as the $PaO_2$ increases, this relationship is not directly linear. Many factors affect the affinity of the heme molecule for oxygen. The sigmoid curve represents the saturation percentages that occur at various $PaO_2$ levels (Figure 30-17). In the upper portion of the curve, hemoglobin has an increased affinity for oxygen, so that large changes in $PO_2$ levels can be tolerated without significantly changing the saturation. For example, at a $PO_2$ of 100 mm Hg, hemoglobin saturation is 97%; even if the $PO_2$ level should fall to 70 mm Hg, the saturation would only decrease to 94%. This serves as a protective mechanism that ensures adequate tissue oxygenation despite mild hypoxemia. However, once the $PO_2$ level falls below 60 mm Hg, oxygen saturation drops sharply, thus reducing the ability of the hemoglobin to transport oxygen.

The affinity of hemoglobin for oxygen is influenced by several factors. For example, hypothermia, alkalosis, and hypocapnia are conditions associated with reduced tissue metabolism. These conditions cause the oxyhemoglobin dissociation curve to shift to the left. The result is that there is an increased affinity of hemoglobin for oxygen resulting in less oxygen being released to the tissues. So, an individual who has an alteration in pH (alkalosis) will have more oxygen-bound hemoglobin, e.g., a higher $SaO_2$, than an individual who has the same $PaO_2$ but with a pH in the normal range.

A shift in the oxyhemoglobin dissociation curve to the right means there is decreased affinity of the hemoglobin for

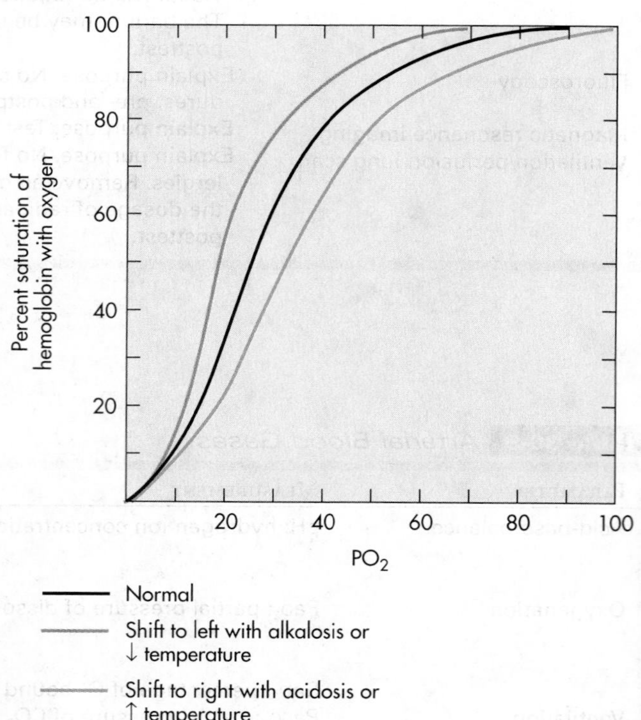


**fig. 30-17** Oxyhemoglobin dissociation curve.

oxygen, and oxygen is easily released from the hemoglobin. Fever, acidosis, and hypercapnia are conditions that shift the curve to the right. These conditions produce an increased need for oxygen because of the associated increase in tissue metabolism. An individual with an altered pH (acidosis) will have a lower $Sa{O_2}$ than an individual who has the same $Pa{O_2}$ with a pH in the normal range. Another condition that causes a shift to the right is an increase in 2,3–diphosphoglycerate.

The amount of oxygen that is delivered to the tissues depends on oxygen saturation, hemoglobin, and cardiac output. $Pa{O_2}$ and $Sa{O_2}$ levels may be normal, yet if the individual is anemic or has inadequate cardiac output, tissue oxygenation may be inadequate. Thus, arterial blood gas results should not be assessed in isolation.

### Ventilation

$Pa{CO_2}$ is the partial pressure of carbon dioxide in the blood and is a parameter that measures the adequacy of ventilation. $Pa{CO_2}$ levels depend on the amount of carbon dioxide produced by the body and the ability of the lungs to eliminate it. A decrease in the ventilatory rate, or *alveolar hypoventilation,* causes the lungs to retain carbon dioxide. This results in an elevated $Pa{CO_2}$ level *(hypercapnia).* An increase in the ventilatory rate, or *alveolar hyperventilation,* causes carbon dioxide to be blown off. This results in a decrease in $Pa{CO_2}$ level *(hypocapnia).* $Pa{CO_2}$ levels are used to assess the need for or change in mechanical ventilatory support.

#### Acid-base balance

Arterial blood pH is a measurement of hydrogen ion concentration and reflects the acidity or alkalinity of the blood. As the hydrogen ion concentration increases, the blood becomes more acidic and the pH value falls. When the hydrogen ion concentration decreases, the blood becomes more alkaline, and the pH value rises. Excess acid can be the result of a respiratory or metabolic disorder or of both a respiratory and metabolic disorder.

Carbon dioxide combines with water to form carbonic acid. Carbonic acid, in turn, dissociates to form hydrogen and bicarbonate ions, as illustrated in this equation:

$$CO_2 + H_2O \leftrightarrow H_2CO_3 \leftrightarrow HCO_3 + H$$

When there is an excess of $CO_2$ in the blood, a result of alveolar hypoventilation, the excess carbonic acid and H ions produce an acidemia. The pH level is $<7.35$, and the individual is said to be in a state of *respiratory acidosis.* When the $Pa{CO_2}$ level decreases as a result of alveolar hyperventilation, too much carbon dioxide is blown off. The decrease in carbonic acid and H ions produces an alkalemia. The pH level is increased ($>7.45$), and the individual is said to be in a state of *respiratory alkalosis.*

In metabolic acidosis an accumulation of metabolic acids causes the increase in hydrogen ion concentration of the blood; and in metabolic alkalosis the excessive loss of acids causes the decrease in hydrogen ion concentration. The respiratory system can rapidly compensate for a metabolic acid-base imbalance by either increasing or decreasing ventilation. If a metabolic acidosis (decrease in bicarbonate level) develops, the lungs respond by increasing ventilation and blowing off excess carbon dioxide *(hypocapnia).* Conversely, if a metabolic alkalosis (increase in bicarbonate level) develops, the lungs respond by decreasing ventilation and retaining carbon dioxide *(hypercapnia).* The kidneys also respond to acid-base imbalances by excreting bicarbonate or reabsorbing bicarbonate ions and secreting hydrogen ions. However, this compensatory mechanism occurs over several days, whereas the respiratory system changes occur within minutes.

An imbalance in acid-base balance may be a result of a respiratory disorder, a metabolic disorder, or a combination of both. Thus, an acid-base assessment requires an evaluation of $Pa{CO_2}$, pH, and bicarbonate levels.

## Complete Blood Count

The complete blood count provides information about red blood cells (RBCs), hemoglobin, hematocrit, and white blood cells (WBCs). The RBC count is valuable in assessing overall oxygen-carrying capacity. Normally there are 4 million (female) to 5 million (male) RBCs in each cubic millimeter of blood, and each RBC contains an estimated 280 million hemoglobin molecules. Oxygen that diffuses into the pulmonary capillary chemically attaches to the hemoglobin for transport to the tissues. An abnormally low hemoglobin level can adversely affect the body's ability to carry oxygen to the cells to meet the metabolic needs of the body. The WBC count provides information to diagnose and monitor infectious states.

## Sputum Analysis

A sputum sample may be ordered for microbiology and cytology testing. Sputum examination may be helpful in evaluating patients in whom tuberculosis, pneumonia, and lung cancer are suspected. Gram stains and cultures are helpful tests to define a causative organism. Sensitivity is a test ordered in conjunction with the culture. It identifies antibiotics to which the organisms present in the sputum are sensitive and thus will not grow. An acid-fast bacilli stain is used to diagnose tuberculosis. Cytological examination identifies cell types to aid in diagnoses, such as in lung cancer. However, an absence of malignant cells in the specimen does not mean cancer is not present. The sputum examination may also reveal the presence of parasites, macrophages, or other cells that may provide information in the evaluation of lung disease.

A bronchodilator or inhalation of a hypertonic solution may be ordered for individuals who have difficulty producing sputum. Individuals who are intubated or who have a tracheostomy will require suctioning via the artificial airway with a catheter and special collection container. Sputum specimens can also be obtained by invasive methods, such as transtracheal aspiration or fiberoptic bronchoscopy.

## Throat Culture

A throat culture is performed to help identify microorganisms so that appropriate treatment can be initiated. To obtain the throat culture, ask the individual to tilt the head back and open the mouth. A tongue depressor is used so that the swab is less likely to come in contact with the normal flora of the mouth. Both tonsillar pillars and the posterior pharynx should be swabbed. The swab is placed in the culture tube, labeled, and transported to the laboratory.

## RADIOLOGICAL EXAMINATION OF THE CHEST

### Chest Roentgenograms

Chest radiographs are obtained to diagnose disorders of the lung, to evaluate effectiveness of treatment, to determine the extent and location of disease, and to assess the progression of lung disease. In addition, chest radiographs can be used to evaluate proper placement of catheters and tubes. Chest radiographs are usually performed in the radiology department when the individual can stand in an upright position with the anterior chest pressed against the film cassette holder. This produces a posteroanterior (PA) radiograph in which the x-ray beam travels through the individual's posterior chest to the x-ray film. However, if the individual is acutely ill, the x-ray can be taken at the bedside with a portable x-ray machine. If the patient can sit up, the radiograph is taken with the x-ray camera positioned toward the individual's anterior chest, and the x-ray beam travels through the anterior chest to the x-ray film that is placed behind the individual's back. This is referred to as an anteroposterior view. A lateral radiograph is generally taken along with a PA radiograph. Generally, the left side of the chest is pressed against the film cassette, and the x-ray beam travels through the side of the body. Figure 30-18 shows PA and lateral chest radiographs. Special views such as the oblique, lordotic, or decubitus may be obtained to visualize specific parts of the chest. Removal of metal objects above the waist is required. The individual will be asked to take a deep breath and hold it. There is no discomfort, although the temperature of the room and film cassette holder may be cool. Personnel may be positioned behind a lead wall or wear lead aprons while the

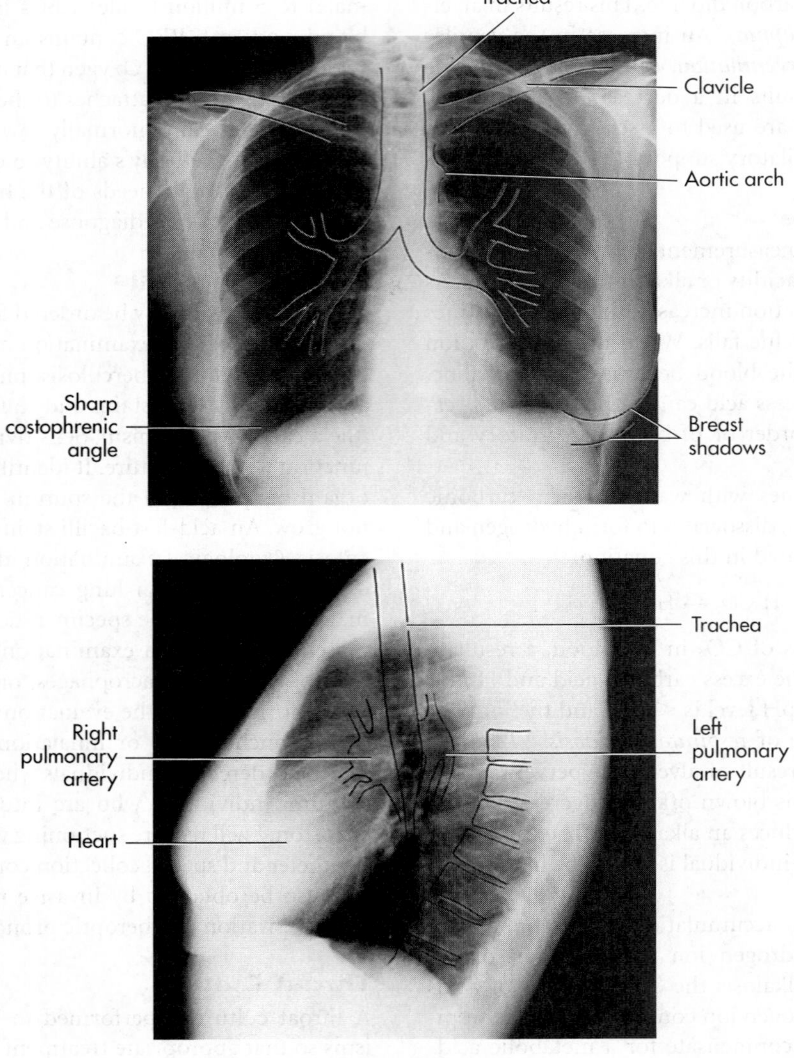


**fig. 30-18** Location of structures on a chest radiograph.

radiograph is taken. Possible radiographical findings are listed in Table 30-10.

## Computed Tomography (CT)

CT scanning, with or without the use of radiopaque contrast media, uses computer programming to permit visualization of multiple cross-sectional "slices" of the lung. Each tomogram represents a specific part of the lung. Lesions that are not clearly visualized on chest radiography can be evaluated more clearly with CT. The individual will be required to remove all metal articles and lie still on an examination table while the x-ray machine rotates to take films.

## Esophagogram

Esophagogram with fluoroscopy visualizes the swallowing of a radiopaque material (barium) to assess patency and contour of the esophagus. The test is used to identify abnormalities of the esophagus and confirm that aspiration is present. There is no pain or discomfort; however, the barium has a chalky taste that some find unpleasant.

## Fluoroscopy

Dynamic information about the chest, such as diaphragmatic movement or lung expansion and contraction can be evaluated with fluoroscopy. Fluoroscopy is a technique used to observe movement in the area being filmed while the specific study is in progress. It can also be used in conjunction with other procedures, such as bronchoscopy, when a biopsy of the lung is obtained. This technique exposes the individual to greater doses of radiation than the standard chest radiograph and is reserved for select patients.

## Magnetic Resonance Imaging (MRI)

MRI is able to produce cross-sectional images of the body that are helpful in detecting subtle lesions. It is superior to CT scanning in detecting lesions of the chest wall and congenital heart disease. However, CT scanning is better for most thoracic abnormalities. An individual who has an object made of ferromagnetic material should not undergo MRI since the device (e.g., prosthetic valve) could shift. The imager may also interfere with the functioning of a cardiac pacemaker.

## Ventilation/Perfusion Lung Scan

Lung scan procedures involve the use of a scanning device that records the pattern of pulmonary radioactivity after the inhalation (ventilation lung scan) or intravenous injection (perfusion lung scan) of gamma ray-emitting radionucleotides. These scans provide the clinician with a visual image of the distribution of ventilation and perfusion in the lungs. Valuable information about ventilation-perfusion patterns can aid in the diagnosis of parenchymal lung disease and vascular disorders, such as pulmonary embolism. The individual will be required to breathe a small amount of radioactive gas through a ventilation system. During the scanning, the individual will be asked to take a breath and hold it. If a perfusion lung scan is to be performed, the individual will receive an injection of a radioactive agent, and a series of images will be taken by the camera.

## Pulmonary Angiography

Pulmonary angiography provides a visualization of the pulmonary vascular system and is used to detect pulmonary emboli and a variety of congenital and acquired lesions of the pulmonary vessels. Additional data obtained with this test include the measurement of pulmonary pressures, cardiac output, and pulmonary vascular resistance. A radiopaque material is injected into a catheter that has been introduced into a peripheral vein and advanced through the right side of the heart to the pulmonary artery. A series of radiographic films

**table 30-10** *Radiographical Findings*

| | |
|---|---|
| Trachea | Midline, translucent, tubelike structure found in the anterior mediastinal cavity |
| Clavicles | Equally distant from the sternum |
| Ribs | Thoracic cavity encasement |
| Mediastinum | Shadowy-appearing space between the lungs that widens at the hilum |
| Heart | Solid-appearing structure with clear edges visible in the left anterior mediastinal cavity; cardiothoracic ratio should be less than half the width of the chest wall on a posteroanterior (PA) film; cardiac shadow appears larger on an anteroposterior (AP) film |
| Carina | Lowest tracheal cartilage at the bifurcation |
| Mainstem bronchus | Translucent, tubelike structure visible approximately 2.5 cm from the hilum |
| Hilum | Small, white, bilateral densities present where the bronchi join the lungs; left bronchus should be 2-3 cm higher than the right |
| Bronchi | Not usually visible |
| Lung fields | Usually not completely visible except for "lung markings" at periphery<br>Blackened area without tissue markings suggests pneumothorax<br>Patchy infiltrates suggest pneumonia, atelectasis |
| Diaphragm | Rounded structures visible at the bottom of the lung fields; right side is 1-2 cm higher than the left; costophrenic angles should be clear and sharp<br>Loss of costophrenic angle sharpness suggests pleural effusion<br>Flattened diaphragm suggests emphysema |

are taken to follow the distribution of the contrast material throughout the pulmonary vascular system. The catheter is removed at the completion of the test and a pressure dressing applied (see the Guidelines for Care Box below).

## ENDOSCOPY

### Bronchoscopy

Bronchoscopy is used to diagnose and treat airway and lung disorders. It can be used to examine vocal cord movement, to obtain specimens by biopsy, bronchial brushing, or bronchoalveolar lavage, and/or to remove foreign bodies or mucous plugs. Specimens can be examined for cytology or bacteriology and cultured for fungi, acid-fast bacilli, *Legionella pneumophila* and *Pneumocystis carinii.* Bronchoscopy can also be used to localize sites of bleeding or tumor.

Fiberoptic bronchoscopy is frequently performed because of the instrument's small size and ability to visualize the segmental and subsegmental bronchi. The fiberoptic scope has two channels to accommodate light, one channel for the clinician to visualize the structures, and one channel to accommodate equipment such as biopsy forceps, suction, cytology brush, or oxygen. A local anesthetic is sprayed or swabbed on the tongue and oropharynx, and the scope is introduced into the nose (the mouth or an endotracheal tube or tracheostomy tube can also be used). The anesthetic is also applied to the scope, and additional anesthetic may be applied through the scope as it advances toward the vocal cords and carina.

Bronchoscopy with the rigid bronchoscope is generally performed in the operating room because general anesthesia is required. It is usually reserved for removing foreign objects, controlling massive hemoptysis, placing airway stents, and dilating tracheobronchial strictures. If bronchoscopy is performed under general anesthesia, the care is similar to that for any individual undergoing general anesthesia (see Chapters 18 and 20). Information to prepare the patient and family for fiberoptic bronchoscopy can be found in the Patient/Family Teaching Box. Postbronchoscopy care can be found in the Guidelines for Care Box below.

### Laryngoscopy

Indirect laryngoscopy involves the placement of a laryngeal mirror into the back of the mouth and rotating it to visualize the larynx. It is used for examination and removal of tissue or foreign objects. Direct laryngoscopy is performed under local or general anesthesia and involves the insertion of a laryngoscope through the mouth into the larynx for examination. Biopsy of a tumor or removal of a foreign object can be accomplished. Postlaryngoscopy care is similar to postbronchoscopy care (see the Patient/Family Teaching Box). Pre-

**guidelines for care**

**Individual Undergoing Pulmonary Angiography**

**Preangiography**

- Explain the purpose of the test and its procedure.
- Give the individual nothing by mouth for 4 to 6 hours before the test.
- Check for the signed consent form.
- Check laboratory data: electrolytes, complete blood count, blood urea nitrogen, creatinine, and clotting studies should be within normal limits.
- Assess the individual for allergies to contrast media and obtain baseline vital signs before the procedure. Inform the individual that the dye may cause flushing, coughing, and a warm sensation.

**Immediately Postangiography**

- Monitor vital signs every 15 minutes.
- Observe dressing and site for bleeding or hematoma development every 15 minutes.
- Assess site for infection or thrombophlebitis (swelling, warmth, redness, or pain).
- Maintain bedrest for 4 to 6 hours.

**patient/family teaching**

**Preparing the Individual for Flexible Bronchoscopy**

- Check for the signed consent form.
- Instruct the individual not to eat or drink for 6 to 8 hours before procedure.
- Reassure the individual and family as necessary. Most individuals are anxious both about the bronchoscopy and about what the results might indicate.
- Explain that a sedative will be given before and during the procedure as needed and that a local anesthetic will be applied to the nose, larynx, and throat.
- Explain that the anesthetic has a bitter taste and that sensations of difficulty swallowing or a thick tongue may be experienced.
- Explain that oxygen will be administered during the procedure and that oxygenation will be monitored with pulse oximetry.

**guidelines for care**

**Individual Undergoing Flexible Bronchoscopy**

- Respiratory rate and pattern are monitored and lungs are auscultated. Observe for changes in breathing pattern and breath sounds.
- Oxygen saturation may be monitored with pulse oximetry.
- Individual is given nothing by mouth until cough and gag reflexes return.
- Individual is positioned in a semi-Fowler's or side-lying position.
- Individual is monitored for bleeding, laryngeal edema, or laryngospasm (stridor) and increasing shortness of breath.
- If a biopsy was performed, explain to the individual that sputum may be blood streaked.
- Manage throat discomfort with warm saline gargles or throat lozenges.

and postprocedural care is similar to that for any individual undergoing general anesthesia (see Chapters 19 and 21).

### Mediastinoscopy

Mediastinoscopy is an operative procedure that allows visualization and biopsy of lymph nodes. The procedure is helpful in diagnosing cancer, tuberculosis, histoplasmosis, and other diseases. A mediastinoscope is an instrument similar to a bronchoscope that is inserted through a small incision in the suprasternal notch. It is advanced into the mediastinum where lymph nodes can be inspected and biopsied. The procedure is generally performed in the operating room with the individual under general anesthesia. A small incision is made to allow entrance of the scope. After the procedure, the incision is sutured, and the individual is taken to the postanesthesia care unit to recover. Pre- and postprocedural care is similar to that for any individual undergoing general anesthesia and surgery (see Chapters 18 and 20). Pneumothorax, hemoptysis, subcutaneous crepitus of neck or face, and laryngeal nerve damage (hoarseness, changes in vocal patterns, and difficulty in swallowing) are potential complications.

### Thoracoscopy

Thoracoscopy is an operative procedure that allows visualization of the contents of the thoracic cavity. It can be used to obtain biopsies, resect tumors, perform esophageal operations, resect pericardium, and perform many other thoracic surgical procedures. A simple fiberoptic mediastinoscope, a rigid bronchoscope, a flexible bronchoscope, or the newer video-assisted laparoscopic instrumentation may be used to perform thoracoscopy. A general or local anesthetic may be administered, depending on the extent of the procedure. Two to four small incisions are made to insert the instrument. The lung on the operative side is allowed to collapse to permit a more panoramic view of the intrathoracic structures and keep the lung immobile while the surgeon performs the desired procedures. A chest tube is inserted and connected to a closed drainage system at the completion of the procedure. Pre- and postprocedure care is similar to that for any individual undergoing general anesthesia and surgery (see Chapters 18 and 19). Care of an individual with a chest tube can be found in Chapter 32.

## PULMONARY FUNCTION TESTS (PFTs)

Pulmonary function testing is a noninvasive method of assessing the functional capacity of the lungs. These tests cannot be used in isolation to diagnose specific disease but are integral to the diagnostic process. PFTs are used to evaluate pulmonary disability, to evaluate pulmonary function in individuals preoperatively, to evaluate the patient's disease progression and response to therapy, and to differentiate obstructive lung disease from restrictive lung disease. The individual is asked to breathe into a mouthpiece that is connected to a spirometer. Noseclips are applied to permit mouth breathing only, and the individual is required to inhale deeply, hold his or her breath, and then quickly and forcefully exhale. Several attempts may be required of the individual. Shortness of breath or lightheadedness may be experienced.

### Nursing Care

Explain the purpose of the test and its procedure. Food and fluids are not restricted; however the test should not be scheduled after a meal since the diaphragm muscle will be exerted during the test. Obtain height and weight measurements before the test. After the test, allow the individual to rest and assess respiratory status.

### Spirometry

Spirometry is the most common pulmonary function test conducted. It is a test in which lung capacities (the sum of two or more lung volumes), lung volumes, and flow rates are determined. The individual breathes through a mouthpiece connected to a spirometer that measures the air moving through the apparatus. A graphic tracing of the lung volumes and capacities is recorded (Figure 30-19).

Tidal volume periodically increases in spontaneously breathing healthy individuals. This is referred to as sighing. Individuals whose breathing pattern is shallow without sighing are at risk for atelectasis and pneumonia. Tidal volume is monitored closely in critically ill individuals who are mechanically ventilated.

Vital capacity (VC) reflects the muscle strength and volume capacity of the lung. It is important to maintain an effective cough, to take a deep breath, and to clear the airways of secretions. In addition to evaluating respiratory function preoperatively, vital capacity is used to monitor and diagnose pulmonary disorders. Vital capacity provides information about airway resistance when measured as forced vital capacity. One of the most meaningful clinical measurements is the forced expiratory volume (FEV). The FEV measures the amount of air in liters that is forcefully expired over a specified amount of time, generally 1, 2, or 3 seconds. When compared with the forced vital capacity (FVC), it can identify the pulmonary impairment as restrictive or obstructive. In obstructive disease,

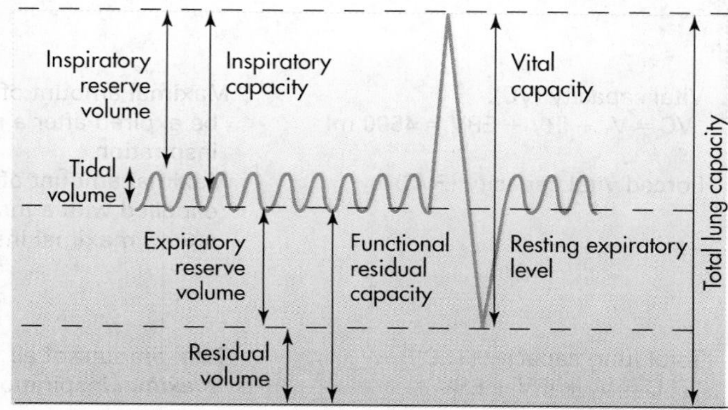


**fig. 30-19** Lung volumes and capacities illustrated by spirography tracing.

blocked airways interfere with expiration more than inspiration. When airway obstruction (resistance) increases, air flow rates decrease. The amount of time necessary to forcefully exhale an amount of air after full inspiration is increased in obstructive disease. The FEV/FVC ratio will be low. In restrictive disease, air can be expelled rapidly and the FEV/FVC ratio is usually high. Most individuals should be able to exhale approximately 75% of their VC in one second.

Functional residual capacity (FRC) reflects the volume of gas remaining in the lungs at the end of a normal passive exhalation and is in continuous contact with pulmonary capillary blood. If FRC is decreased, alveoli collapse and gas exchange is adversely affected.

Lung volumes and capacities are defined, and clinical implications of each measurement are provided in Table 30-11. Normal values for pulmonary function tests are expressed in milliliters, liters, liters per second, or liters per minute or as a percentage of predicted normal depending upon the test performed.

Pulmonary function testing can also be performed during bronchial provocation and while an individual is exercising to identify triggers to bronchospasm, to determine if the obstruction (bronchospasm) is reversible with bronchodilator therapy; and to determine the extent of exercise limitation. Bronchodilators are generally withheld before the bronchial provocation test.

### Flow-Volume Loops

Flow-volume loops aid in determining obstructive versus restrictive lung disorders and intrathoracic from extrathoracic disorders. Inspiratory and expiratory volumes are plotted against flow rates to produce a flow-volume loop. Figure 30-20 presents a comparison of various flow-volume loops. Typically, an individual with obstructive airway disease will have a "scooped out" appearance in the expiratory flow curve. In restrictive disease there is a symmetrical reduction in volume and flow, and it appears as a smaller version of a normal flow-volume loop.

**table 30-11** *Definitions and Implications of Pulmonary Function Tests*

| | Definitions | Implications |
|---|---|---|
| **LUNG VOLUME (Nonoverlapping Measures)** | | |
| Tidal volume ($V_T$) ~500 ml | Volume of gas inspired and expired with a normal breath | Decrease in $V_T$ without an increase in respiratory rate can lead to hypoventilation and respiratory acidosis |
| Inspiratory reserve volume (IRV) ~3000 ml | Maximal volume that can be inspired from the end of a normal inspiration | Not widely used clinically |
| Expiratory reserve volume (ERV) ~1000 ml | Maximal volume that can be exhaled by forced expiration after a normal expiration | Limited use clinically |
| Residual volume (RV) ~1500 ml | Volume of gas left in lung after maximal expiration | Expressed as a ratio<br>>33% of VC suggests presence of COPD<br>Normal in restrictive disease |
| **LUNG CAPACITIES (Combinations of Various Volumes)** | | |
| Inspiratory capacity (IC): $IC = V_T + IRV = 3500$ ml | Maximal amount of air that can be inspired after a normal expiration | Not widely used clinically |
| Functional residual capacity (FRC): $FRC = ERV + RV = 2500$ ml | Amount of air left in lungs after a normal expiration | Reflects expanding forces of chest wall and recoiling forces of lungs<br>When lung tissue is lost, the chest wall forces have less opposition, thus increasing FRC |
| Vital capacity (VC): $VC = V_T + IRV + ERV = 4500$ ml | Maximal amount of air that can be expired after a maximal inspiration | Reflects ability to deep breathe, cough, and clear the airways |
| Forced vital capacity (FVC) | Maximal amount of air that can be expelled with a maximal effort after a maximal inspiration | VC that is forcefully exhaled<br>Important index to evaluate individuals before surgery for postoperative respiratory complications: <20 ml/kg of ideal body weight indicates that the individual is at risk for complications |
| Total lung capacity (TLC): $TLC = V_T + IRV + ERV + RV = 6000$ ml | Total amount of air in lungs after maximal inspiration | Determined by size, age, and sex<br>Increased in obstructive disease and decreased in restrictive disease |

*Continued*

### Pulmonary Diffusion Capacity

The ability of gas to diffuse across the alveolar-capillary membrane is measured by a test called diffusing capacity of the lung for carbon monoxide ($D_{LCO}$). One method involves the individual breathing in a known amount of carbon monoxide and exhaling it after 10 seconds of breath holding (to allow the gas to diffuse across the alveolar-capillary membrane). The carbon monoxide concentration in the blood is estimated by the amount of carbon monoxide exhaled. A normal value is approximately 25 ml/min/mm Hg; however, predicted values are based upon age, height, and gender. The $D_{LCO}$ is decreased in individuals with lung disorders that involve the alveolar-capillary membrane such as emphysema and interstitial lung disease.

## SKIN TESTING

Skin testing is performed to evaluate the body's cell-mediated immune function and to determine the body's sensitivity to infectious agents or allergens. A positive reaction is manifested by induration (thickening or hardening) at the site of the injection within a specified time period. Testing for *Mycobacterium tuberculosis* with tuberculin-purified protein derivative (PPD) is a common type of skin test. A positive reaction indicates that the individual has developed antibodies to the infectious agent, but it does not confirm active disease. A positive skin test reaction must be substantiated with other diagnostic evidence before active disease can be confirmed. Skin controls are sometimes administered to individuals along with the PPD skin test. If the reaction to the control is positive but the reaction is negative for PPD, then it is unlikely that the individual has tuberculosis. If the reaction to the control is negative, then the individual is "anergic" (i.e., has an altered cellular immunity system), and other tests must be performed to make the diagnosis of tuberculosis.

### Nursing Care

Explain the purpose of the test and its procedure. See the Guidelines for Care Box for administration of the Mantoux test.

## THORACENTESIS

Thoracentesis involves the insertion of a needle into the pleural space to remove pleural fluid, instill medications into the pleural space, or biopsy the pleura. The procedure is usually performed at the bedside with the patient under local anesthesia. An abnormal accumulation of fluid in the

**table 30-11** *Definitions and Implications of Pulmonary Function Tests—cont'd*

| | DEFINITIONS | IMPLICATIONS |
|---|---|---|
| **VOLUME/TIME RELATIONSHIPS** | | |
| Minute volume ($\dot{V}E$):<br>$\dot{V}E$ = 4-12 L/min | Volume inspired and expired in 1 min of normal breathing | Index of ventilation<br>Should increase with fever, pain, exercise, and acidosis |
| Forced expiratory volume in 1 sec ($FEV_1$): $FEV_1$/FVC = 75% of VC in 1 sec<br>$FEV_3$/FVC = 95% | Amount of air expelled in the first second of forced vital capacity maneuver | Reflects airflow characteristics; expressed as a percentage of FVC<br>Severe decline in $FEV_1$ results in hypercapnia and respiratory acidosis<br>Forced expiratory flow ($FEF_{25-75}$) is an early indicator of obstructive disorders and reflects degree of airway patency |
| Peak expiratory flow (PEF) | Maximum flow rate achieved during FVC<br>Degree of obstruction:<br>Severe: <100 L/min<br>Moderate: 100-200 L/min<br>Mild: >200 L/min | Correlates with $FEV_1$<br>Useful to assess response to treatment |
| Maximal voluntary ventilation (MVV):<br>MVV = 170 L/min | Amount of air exchanged per minute with maximal rate and depth of respiration | Quick assessment of lungs<br>Reflects compliance, airway resistance, and respiratory muscle status |
| **DIFFUSION/PERFUSION MEASUREMENT** | | |
| Diffusing capacity ($D_{LCO}$) = 25 ml/min/mm Hg | Assesses ability of gas molecules to cross alveolar-capillary membrane | Reported as raw number and percentage of predicted value |
| Nitrogen washout | Determines maldistribution of ventilation | Displayed on a tracing showing a curved pattern<br>If slope of the pattern is uneven, uneven ventilation is suspected |

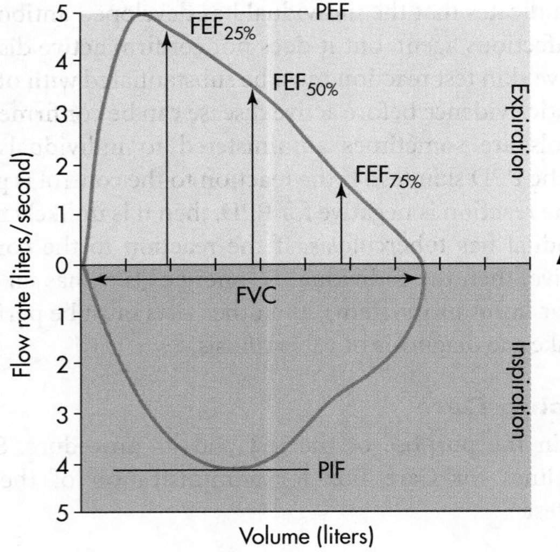


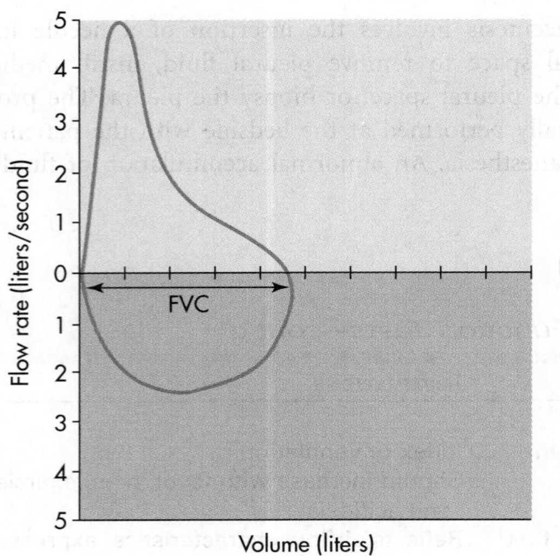


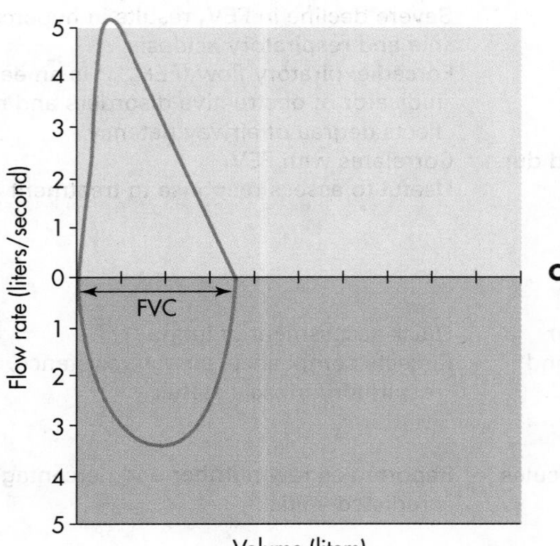


**fig. 30-20** Flow volume loops. **A,** Peak expiratory flow *(PEF);* peak inspiratory flow *(PIF);* forced expiratory flow at X% of FVC *(FEF%),* and forced vital capacity *(FVC);* **B,** Obstructive disorder. **C,** Restrictive disorder.

## guidelines for care

### Administering the Mantoux Test

1. Draw up 0.1 ml (or amount specified by manufacturer) of PPD, using a tuberculin syringe and ½-inch, 25- to 27-gauge needle.
2. Cleanse the site (ventral forearm) with alcohol and let dry.
3. Keeping skin slightly taut, insert the needle (bevel upward) just beneath the skin surface.
4. Inject the solution, creating a 6- to 10-mm bleb. Do not massage the area after withdrawing the needle.
5. Read the test site with a millimeter ruler 48 to 72 hours after injection. The site should be lightly palpated to determine the presence or absence of induration. The largest diameter of induration should be measured and recorded in millimeters. Any erythema at the site should also be noted. Erythema alone does not indicate a positive result.
6. Interpretation of induration:
   a. 10 mm or more = highly significant for past or present infection.
   b. 5 mm through 9 mm = doubtful reaction; however, retesting may be required.
   c. 0 through 4 mm = little or no sensitivity; however, if individual's history indicates exposure, the test should be repeated in 4 to 6 weeks as it may take this long for a tuberculin test to convert from negative to positive.

pleural space can be caused by a number of diseases and can severely impair respiratory function. Thoracentesis is used to obtain fluid for examination, which aids in making a diagnosis, reducing dyspnea, and improving gas exchange. See the Guidelines for Care Box for the care of the individual undergoing thoracentesis.

## chapter SUMMARY

### ANATOMY AND PHYSIOLOGY

- Breathing includes the movement of air in and out of the lungs (ventilation) and exchange of oxygen and carbon dioxide between the pulmonary capillary blood and alveolus (respiration).
- The respiratory system consists of the upper and lower airways, thoracic cage, and pulmonary circulation.
- Gas exchange is dependent upon ventilation of the alveoli, diffusion of the gases across the alveolar-capillary membrane, and perfusion of capillaries.
- Ventilation is involuntary, controlled primarily by chemoreceptors and neuroreceptors.
- Defense mechanisms of the lung protect the lungs from infecting organisms.
- Respiratory changes that occur with aging primarily affect elastic properties of the lungs.

### SUBJECTIVE DATA

- A nursing history of the individual with a pulmonary problem includes information about pulmonary symptoms, functional capacity, risk factors, and current treatment.
- The major pulmonary symptoms are cough, dyspnea, chest pain, sputum production, hemoptysis, and wheezing.

guidelines for care

### Individual Undergoing Thoracentesis

1. The procedure is explained, and a signed consent form is obtained. Emphasize the importance of not moving, breathing quietly, and not coughing during the procedure to avoid damage to the pleura and lung. Explain that the local anesthetic may cause a slight burning sensation and pressure may be felt when the needle is inserted.
2. Assess the individual's respiratory status and vital signs before the procedure. Pulse oximetry may be monitored. Supplemental oxygen should not be discontinued.
3. If possible, the individual should sit on the edge of the bed with the affected side closest to the foot of the bed. Support the individual's feet with a footstool. Raise the bedside table and put pillows on the table so that the individual can lean forward and rest his or her head and crossed arms comfortably on the pillows. If the individual is unable to sit up, place him or her in the position indicated by physician.
4. Reassure the individual and provide physical support, such as holding the individual's hand, as needed.
5. Monitor vital signs, general appearance, and respiratory status throughout the procedure. Up to 1 L of fluid may be removed at one time. If the individual develops pernicious coughing, reexpansion pulmonary edema should be suspected and the procedure terminated. Other signs and symptoms to monitor include hypotension, increased shortness of breath, bloody sputum, tracheal deviation, vasovagal reflex, and hypoxemia.
6. After the needle is withdrawn, a sterile occlusive dressing is applied, and the individual can assume a position of comfort.
7. A postprocedural chest radiograph is taken to check for a possible pneumothorax.
8. Manage postprocedural pain.

- Data collection should be tailored to the individual's respiratory status and may be deferred if the individual exhibits signs of respiratory distress.

## OBJECTIVE DATA

- Objective data collection includes respiratory vital signs and the physical examination.
- The focus and extent of the physical examination is dictated by the degree of respiratory distress. An abbreviated assessment may be a priority.

## DIAGNOSTIC TESTS

- Tests of the respiratory system are performed to diagnose, treat, and monitor respiratory dysfunction.

## References

1. Des Jardins R: *Clinical manifestations and assessment of respiratory disease,* ed 3, St Louis, 1994, Mosby.
2. Peterson DD, Fishman AP: Aging lung. In Fishman AP, editor: *Update: pulmonary diseases and disorders,* New York, 1992, McGraw-Hill.
3. Szaflarski NL: Use of pulse oximetry in critically ill adults, *Heart Lung* 18:444, 1989.
4. Tockman M: Aging of the respiratory system. In Hazzard WR et al, editors: *Principles of geriatric medicine and gerontology,* ed 3, New York, 1994, McGraw-Hill.

chapter 31

# MANAGEMENT OF PERSONS WITH Problems of the Upper Airway

WILMA J. PHIPPS

## objectives

*After studying this chapter, the learner should be able to:*

1. Compare the etiology, pathophysiology, clinical manifestations, and management of the patient with rhinitis and sinusitis.
2. Compare acute pharyngitis with acute follicular tonsillitis and peritonsillar abscess in relation to etiology, clinical manifestations, and management.
3. Describe the nursing care of the patient after nasal surgery.
4. Identify conditions that cause obstructions of the upper airway and their management.
5. Outline the nursing care for the patient who has an endotracheal tube or tracheostomy.
6. Discuss the precautions to be observed when feeding the patient who has an endotracheal tube or tracheostomy tube.
7. Describe clinical manifestations and management of the patient experiencing epistaxis and a malignancy of the upper airway.
8. Contrast the nursing care of the patient after a partial laryngectomy and after a total laryngectomy with radical neck dissection.
9. Differentiate among the three speech methods used by patients after a total laryngectomy.

The upper airway includes the nose and sinuses, upper throat (nasopharynx and oropharynx), and lower throat (laryngopharynx and larynx). Disorders of the upper airway are common, and patients often ask nurses to give them advice about these kinds of disorders.

Disorders that affect the nose or olfactory nerve may lead to *anosmia,* or loss of the sense of smell. Anosmia may result from (1) nasal obstruction, which prevents air currents from reaching the olfactory epithelium; (2) skull fracture across the cribriform plate at the roof of the nose where part of the olfactory nerve enters the nose; (3) viral infections, which affect the olfactory nerve; or (4) some meningiomas, which may form in the olfactory area. A perverted sense of smell, called *parosmia,* may also be present during sinusitis or an upper respiratory tract infection.

## INFECTIONS OF THE NOSE AND SINUSES

The skin around the external nose is easily irritated during acute attacks of rhinitis or sinusitis. Furunculosis (boils) and cellulitis (see Chapter 63) occasionally develop. Infections around the nose are extremely dangerous because the venous blood supply from this area drains directly into the cerebral venous sinuses. Septicemia therefore can occur easily. No pimple or lesion in the area should ever be squeezed or "picked"; hot packs may be used. If any infection in or around the nose persists or shows even a slight tendency to spread or increase in severity, a physician should be consulted.

Mary Lynn Droughton, MSN, RN, assisted in the revision of this chapter.

### RHINITIS

#### Etiology/Epidemiology

Rhinitis refers to inflammation of the mucous membrane of the nose. It may be acute or chronic.

*Acute rhinitis* (coryza, common cold) is an inflammatory condition of the mucous membranes of the nose and accessory sinuses caused by a filterable virus. It affects almost everyone at some time and occurs most often in the winter, with additional high incidences in early fall and spring. Some of the known causes of the common cold are 100 serotypes of rhinoviruses, coronoviruses, adenoviruses, echoviruses, influenza and parainfluenza viruses, and coxsackievirus. The common cold is spread by droplet nuclei from sneezing, and the condition is contagious for the first 2 to 3 days.

Colds also may be spread by the contaminated hands of persons who are frequently sneezing and blowing their noses or by fomites such as a telephone used by these persons. Secondary invasion by bacteria may cause pneumonia, acute bronchitis, sinusitis, and otitis media.

Allergic rhinitis (hay fever) is a type I hypersensitivity reaction (see Chapter 66). Atopic persons can become sensitized to inhaled allergens that have no affect on the rest of the population.[14] More than 35 million Americans have allergic rhinitis.[8] Inhaled allergens are classified as outdoor (seasonal), also called acute, or indoor (perennial), also called chronic. The outdoor (seasonal) allergens are pollens of trees, grasses, or weeds. The indoor allergens are spores of molds, dust mites, and animal danders. Although some persons believe they are allergic to flowers, this is often not so because many flowers, such as roses, are insect pollinated. Only flowers that are pollinated by pollen in the air can cause an allergic reaction. The medications commonly used to treat allergic rhinitis are listed in Table 31-1.

*Chronic rhinitis* is a chronic inflammation of the mucous membrane with increased nasal mucus caused by repeated acute infections, by an allergy, or by vasomotor rhinitis. The cause of vasomotor rhinitis is unclear, but this condition may result from an instability of the autonomic nervous system caused by stress, tension, or some endocrine disorder. Often it is mistaken for nasal allergy, but an allergen cannot be identified. Rhinitis can also be caused by the overuse of nose drops (rhinitis medicamentosa); a rebound phenomenon occurs after the immediate effect of the nose drops with the return to congestion. Discontinuing use of the nose drops usually clears up this condition within 1 to 2 weeks.

## Pathophysiology

All forms of rhinitis cause sneezing, nasal discharge with nasal obstruction, and headache, but the form of these symptoms varies with the different types of rhinitis (Table 31-2). Acute rhinitis also includes signs of acute inflammation (early chilliness followed by "feverishness" and malaise). A painful throat is not always associated with a cold. However, the pharynx may feel sore because of early dryness followed by irritation from postnasal drainage. If uncomplicated, the cold is usually self-limiting and lasts for about 1 week.

In chronic rhinitis, acute symptoms are absent. The chief complaint is nasal obstruction accompanied by a feeling of stuffiness and pressure in the nose. Polyp formation may occur, and vertigo may be present.

## Collaborative Care Management

No specific treatment exists for the common cold. The goals of treatment are to (1) relieve symptoms, (2) inhibit spread of the infection, and (3) reduce the risk of bacterial complications such as sinusitis and otitis media. Studies have indicated that oral antihistamines are not effective in treating viral upper respiratory infections. They are helpful, however, in treating allergic rhinitis. The recommended treatment for relieving nasal congestion and enhancing eustachian tube function is decongestants (sympathomimetic amines). The decongestants are administered as nasal drops or sprays two or three times a day for no more than 3 days[4] (see the Guidelines for Care Box). Decongestants are commonly used to treat symptoms of rhinitis. Topical decongestants include oxymetazoline (Afrin) and phenylephrine nasal sprays (Neo-Synephrine). In persons with severe congestion these med-

**table 31-1** *Common Medications for* ***Allergic Rhinitis***

| Drug | Action | Nursing Intervention |
|---|---|---|
| **NONSEDATING ANTIHISTAMINES** | | |
| Fexofenadine (Allegra)<br>Ceterizine (Zyrtec)<br>Loratidine (Claritin)<br>Astemizole (Hismanal) | Prevents the release of histamine and other substances causing symptoms | Evaluate effectiveness. |
| **LOW-DOSE STEROID NASAL SPRAYS** | | |
| Beclomethasone (Vancenase, Beconase)<br>Flunisolide (Nasalide)<br>Triamcinolone (Nasacort)<br>Budesonide (Rhinocort)<br>Futicasone (Flonase)<br>Dexamethasone (Dexacort) | Depresses inflammatory reactions | Evaluate effectiveness.<br>Ask patient to demonstrate use of nasal spray. |
| **OTHER NASAL SPRAYS** | | |
| Cromolyn sodium (Nasalcrom) | Reduces mucus production and swelling | Evaluate effectiveness. |
| Ipratopium bromide (Atrovent) | Blocks ability of nervous system to stimulate the nasal mucus glands | |

**table 31-2** *Symptoms of Rhinitis*

| Symptom | Acute Rhinitis | Allergic Rhinitis | Chronic Rhinitis |
|---|---|---|---|
| Nasal discharge | Initially watery, then mucoid | Thin, watery | Serous, mucopurulent, or purulent |
| Eyes | Tearing during early phase | Tearing, itching | No tearing |
| Turbinates | Edematous | Pale, edematous, mucoid | Enlarged |
| Nasal polyps | No | Sometimes | Sometimes |
| Headache | Generalized | Generalized | Generalized |

ications facilitate the uptake of other topical drugs such as nasal cromolyn (Nasalcrom) and corticosteroid sprays.

The side effects of sympathomimetic amines include rebound nasal congestion (with chronic use), nervousness, and transient increases in blood pressure. Sympathomimetic amines are contraindicated in patients receiving tricyclic antidepressants or monoamine oxidase (MAO) inhibitors. Room humidifiers are helpful in liquefying nasal secretions.[4]

For allergic rhinitis the treatment consists of maintaining an allergen-free environment (see Chapter 66). Hyposensitization or desensitization (administering the allergen in gradually increasing doses to establish an "immunity") may be helpful. Antihistamines give relief to most persons, but their effectiveness often decreases as the "hay fever season" continues.

For chronic rhinitis a careful medical follow-up is indicated. When nasal obstruction persists, surgery may be necessary to remove polyps (polypectomy) or to remove tissue obstruction (septoplasty) (see p. 871).

If the nasal passages are dry, a nasal spray of normal saline can be purchased over the counter, or it can be made by mixing 1 teaspoon of salt in 1 quart of water. The homemade solution should be made fresh daily. The solution is best administered from a spray bottle with both nostrils open.

#### Patient/family education

Guidelines for teaching the patient and family can be found in the Patient/Family Teaching Box.

## SINUSITIS

### Acute Bacterial Sinusitis

#### Etiology/epidemiology

The sinuses are air-filled cavities lined with mucous membranes. Any inflammation of the mucous membranes of the sinuses is termed *sinusitis.* This is a common disorder, although it has become less common since the advent of antibiotics. Often patients who complain of sinusitis do not have a sinus infection but some other disorder. Of every 100 patients who consult an otolaryngologist because of "sinus trouble," fewer than 10 have sinusitis.[20]

Sinusitis may be acute or chronic. The most common types of acute sinusitis are allergic and viral. It is often difficult to distinguish between these two types, although the patient's history may be helpful. *Allergic sinusitis* is usually seasonal, and redness and itching of the eyes may be present. *Viral sinusitis* is usually accompanied by fever, malaise, and systemic symptoms such as achiness. There may also be a history of recent exposure to an infected person. The common pathogens found in sinusitis are rhinovirus, influenza virus, adenovirus, and parainfluenza virus. The most commonly implicated organisms are listed in Box 31-1. The treatment of rhinosinusitis is nonspecific and includes adequate fluid intake and reporting of any worsening of symptoms.

**guidelines for care**

**Self-Administration of Nose Drops**

1. Wash hands.
2. Assume a position that will facilitate flow of medication:
   a. Sit in chair and tip head well backward, or
   b. Lie down with head extended over edge of bed, or
   c. Lie down with pillow under shoulders and head tipped backward.
3. Turn head to side that will receive the drops.
4. Place no more than 3 drops of solution into each nostril at one time (unless otherwise prescribed).
5. Remain in position with head tilted backward for 3 to 5 minutes to permit solution to reach posterior nares.
6. If marked congestion is still present 10 minutes after nose drop insertion, another drop or two of solution may be administered (nasal constriction from first insertion may facilitate additional drops reaching posterior nares).

**patient/family teaching**

**The Person with Rhinitis**

1. Obtain additional rest.
2. Drink at least 2 to 3 L of fluid daily.
3. Medications: use nasal spray or nose drops two or three times/day as ordered (see the Guidelines for Care Box at left).
4. Prevention of further infection:
   a. Blow nose with both nostrils open to prevent infected matter from being forced into eustachian tube.
   b. Cover mouth with disposable tissues when coughing and sneezing to prevent droplet nuclei from contaminating the air.
   c. Dispose of used tissues carefully.
   d. Avoid exposure when possible (i.e., avoid crowds, people with colds, specific allergens). Elderly persons and those with chronic lung disease are particularly vulnerable and should have a flu shot yearly.
   e. Wash hands frequently and especially after coughing, blowing the nose, sneezing, and so on. Evidence suggests that many colds are transmitted from person to person by hand contact and from touching objects handled by a person with a cold.
   f. Seek medical attention if the following are present:
      (1) High fever, severe chest pain, earache.
      (2) Symptoms lasting longer than 2 weeks.
      (3) Recurrent colds.

**box 31-1** *Microbial Causes of Sinusitis*

| VIRAL | BACTERIAL |
|---|---|
| Rhinovirus | *Streptococcus pneumoniae* |
| Influenza | *Haemophilus influenzae* |
| Parainfluenza | Beta-hemolytic streptococcus |
| Adenovirus | *Klebsiella pneumoniae* |
| | Anaerobic organisms |

### Pathophysiology

The first symptom of acute bacterial sinusitis is usually a stuffy nose followed by slowly developing pressure over the involved sinus. Other signs and symptoms include general malaise and toxicity, persistent cough, postnasal drip, headache, slightly elevated or normal temperature, and mild leukopenia. Symptoms worsen over 48 to 72 hours, culminating in severe localized pain and tenderness over the involved sinus (Table 31-3 and Figures 31-1 and 31-2). The patient often believes that the pain is due to an infected tooth.

In acute frontal and maxillary sinusitis, pain usually does not appear until 1 to 2 hours after awakening. It increases for 3 to 4 hours and then becomes less severe in the afternoon and evening.

**table 31-3** *Location of Pain with Sinusitis*

| Sinus | Pain Location |
|---|---|
| Maxillary | Over cheek and upper teeth (Figure 31-1) |
| Frontal | Above the eyebrow (Figure 31-1) |
| Ethmoid | Medial and deep in the eye (Figure 31-2) |
| Sphenoid | Deep behind the eye, over the occiput, or top of head |

Frontal sinus pain distribution

Ethmoid sinus pain distribution

Maxillary sinus pain distribution

**fig. 31-1** Sinus pain: area of local tenderness and pain referral. Maxillary sinus pain frequently is referred to teeth. Frontal pain is generally localized to supraorbital area. Ethmoid pain is generally deep to eye.

There may be bloody or blood-tinged discharge from the nose in the first 24 to 48 hours. The discharge rapidly becomes thick, green, and copious, blocking the nose. The throat may become inflamed and sore on one side because of the purulent discharge.

On examination, the involved nasal mucosa is hyperemic and edematous, and the turbinates are enlarged. X-ray films show that the involved sinus is clouded, and a fluid level is visible (Figure 31-3).

### Collaborative care management

Diagnostic tests include transillumination of the sinuses, conventional sinus x-rays, computed tomography (CT), and magnetic resonance imaging (MRI). Fiberoptic examination of the nose (rhinoscopy) may also be used. For most patients the diagnosis is made without radiographic studies.[7]

Management of acute bacterial sinusitis centers on relief of pain and shrinkage of the nasal mucosa. Ibuprofen (Advil) and an oral decongestant such as pseudoephedrine (Sudafed) are commonly prescribed. The decongestant is given orally or by nasal spray for 2 to 3 days. In some patients codeine (usually Tylenol No. 3) may be required for pain relief, and it may need to be taken for several days.

The antibiotic of choice is amoxicillin for 10 days. Failure of the infection to respond to amoxicillin is an indication for

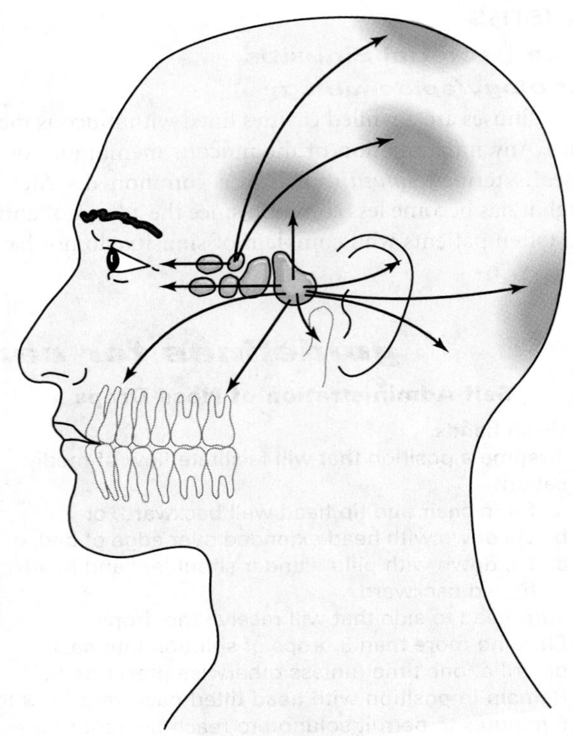

**fig. 31-2** Pain from anterior ethmoid deep to eye. Pain from posterior ethmoid cells and sphenoid refers to the eyes, teeth, ears, or the temporal area of the occiput.

aspiration of the maxillary sinus to obtain a specimen for culture and sensitivity. A list of the antimicrobial agents used to treat acute sinusitis can be found in Box 31-2. If a patient does not improve after 5 days of amoxicillin, a change in antibiotics may be necessary. The antibiotics are usually taken for 10 to 14 days.

Patients may obtain relief from saline nasal sprays, steam from a shower, or a humidifier. Hot wet packs applied to the face over the infected sinus(es) either continuously or for 1 to 2 hours at a time four times a day may provide symptomatic relief. A washcloth wrung out in hot water is a convenient way to provide wet packs.

*Acute frontal sinusitis* with pain, tenderness, and edema of the frontal or sphenoid sinus may require hospitalization because of the risk of intracranial complications or osteomyelitis. High-dose intravenous antibiotics and nasal decongestants orally or by spray are usually ordered. When the infection has subsided the patient is placed on an oral antibiotic and discharged home. In some cases, osteomyelitis of the frontal bone will occur, and *Staphylococcus aureus* is the most common organism responsible. Osteomyelitis is diagnosed by technetium and gallium scans and is treated with a prolonged course of intravenous antistaphylococcal antibiotics.[16]

*Fungal sinusitis* can range from mild infections resembling chronic sinusitis to severe life-threatening invasive infections. Noninvasive fungal sinusitis is often found in patients following other infections or prolonged administration of antibiotics. *Aspergillus* and *Candida* species are commonly found in these situations. Treatment may require surgical drainage of the sinuses.

*Invasive fungal sinusitis* is most likely to occur in transplant patients, patients on chemotherapy, patients with acquired immunodeficiency syndrome (AIDS), or persons with poorly controlled diabetes. *Aspergillus* and *Mucor* are two types of fungi most prone to cause invasive disease. Symptoms include facial fullness, cranial neuropathies, and pain. Proptosis of the eye, facial swelling, and blood-tinged nasal discharge may be present. On examination the nasal mucosa appears gray or black. The diagnosis is confirmed by biopsy of the affected membranes. These patients should be hospitalized. Treatment is with amphotericin B intravenously, aggressive surgical management, and attempts to correct the underlying immunodeficiency. Despite treatment, many patients will not survive.[16]

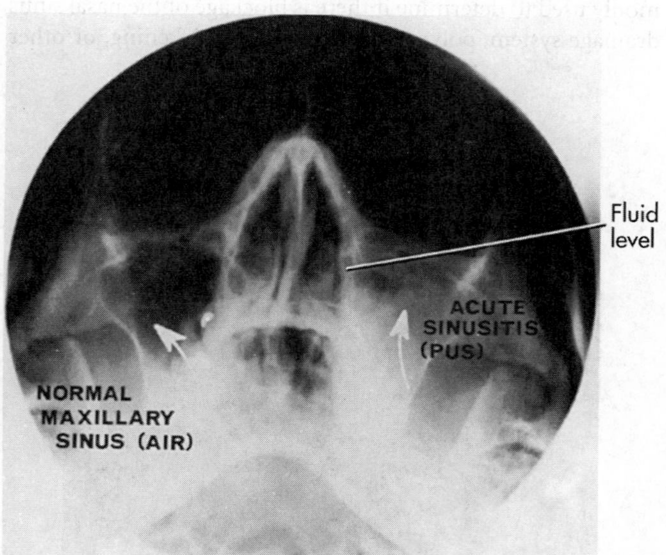


**fig. 31-3** X-ray film of maxillary sinus showing normal sinus on left and acute sinusitis with clouding and visible fluid level on right.

**Patient/family education**

1. Obtain additional rest.
2. Increase fluid intake to 2 to 3 L daily.
3. Medications:
   a. Write out a schedule of times when medications are to be taken.
   b. Take antibiotics as prescribed. If no change in symptoms after 5 days on antibiotic, call health care provider. Your antibiotics may have to be changed.
   c. Take ibuprofen and decongestant as prescribed.
   d. Apply hot wet packs to face using a washcloth wrung out in hot water. Repeat process when washcloth cools off.
   e. Use nasal spray or steam from shower to keep nasal mucosa moist.
   f. Seek medical attention if any of the following are present:
      1) Increase in bloody drainage from nose.
      2) Severe headache or increase in pain in face, teeth, or ears.
      3) Elevation of temperature above 99° F.
      4) Increase in fatigue or general achiness.
      5) Increased nasal stuffiness and inability to clear secretions from nose.

## Subacute Bacterial Sinusitis

### *Etiology/epidemiology*

The measures described previously cure more than 90% of patients with acute bacterial sinusitis. A subacute infection persists in the remaining 10%.[20]

**box 31-2** *Antimicrobial Therapy for Acute Bacterial Sinusitis*

Amoxicillin (Amoxil)
Loracarbef (Lorabid)
Amoxicillin/clavulanate potassium (Augmentin)
Cefaclor (Ceclor)
Cefuroxime axetil (Zihacef IV, Ceftin PO)
Doxycycline (Vibramycin)
Trimethoprim and sulfamethoxazole (Bactrim, Septra)
Clarithromycin (Biaxin)
Azithromycin (Zithromax)
All of the above except azithromycin are prescribed for 10 to 14 days.
Azithromycin is prescribed for 5 days only.

### Pathophysiology

Persistent purulent nasal discharge is the only constant symptom. A sinus x-ray or CT scan determines whether one or more sinus is involved. Because it is uncommon for acute bacterial sinusitis to persist, a persistent infection may be caused by an unusual organism. Special culture techniques may be necessary to identify the organism, especially if it is an anaerobe.[20] Antibiotic sensitivity studies are essential. The most commonly isolated organisms are *Haemophilus influenzae, Haemophilus pneumococcae,* and *Branhamella catarrhalis.* The latter organism is not sensitive to penicillin or amoxicillin, and the following therapy is indicated.

### Collaborative care management

Because *B. catarrhalis* is resistant to penicillin and amoxicillin, systemic sulfonamide therapy or erythromycin with a sulfonamide is indicated. Other organisms are treated with antibiotics to which they are sensitive, usually penicillin or amoxicillin. It is also important to determine whether the patient has an underlying allergy, because persistent sinus infections are common in patients with allergic symptoms.

Other treatment consists of nasal vasoconstriction, moist heat over the sinus(es), and irrigation of the involved sinus. Pain is not severe and requires no medication. Irrigation of the involved sinus may provide some relief. An antral puncture is commonly used when the maxillary sinus is involved and can be repeated several times without causing permanent damage to the nose or the maxillary sinus. Anesthesia is achieved by placing a cotton applicator moistened with 5% cocaine solution high under the inferior turbinate against the lateral wall of the nose. A second applicator is placed under the middle turbinate. After the anesthesia takes effect (in about 5 to 10 minutes), a 16- to 18-gauge needle is inserted under the turbinate until the needle pierces the medial wall of the antrum and enters the sinus cavity (Figure 31-4). A syringe is attached to the needle, and purulent material or air is aspirated from the cavity. The aspirated material is sent to the laboratory for culture and sensitivity testing. Saline solution is instilled to wash out the sinus. Antibiotic solutions may be used, but mechanical cleansing is more important than the solution used (Figure 31-5).

It is impossible to irrigate the ethmoid sinuses directly, and ethmoiditis is treated with systemic antibiotics. The antibiotics should be continued for 10 to 14 days.[20]

Proper treatment of subacute bacterial sinusitis is the best means of preventing chronic bacterial sinusitis, which is discussed next.

## Chronic Bacterial Sinusitis

### Etiology

When suppurative sinusitis is either not treated or inadequately treated during the acute or subacute phase, or when the mucosa is damaged from recurrent attacks, permanent change results. With prolonged infection of soft tissue, pathological change can become irreversible and the patient has chronic sinusitis.[20]

### Epidemiology

The infection is often polymicrobial with anaerobes present in most cases.

### Pathophysiology

The major symptom is nasal congestion with the presence of thick, green, purulent discharge that is present for at least 3 months. Fever or facial pain, or both, may be present. Usually the patient does not have a headache. The most commonly involved organisms are *S. aureus, H. influenzae,* and anaerobes.

### Collaborative care management

**Diagnostic tests.** A CT scan of the sinuses is commonly used to determine if there is blockage of the nasal sinus drainage system, polyps, mucoperiosteal thickening, or other

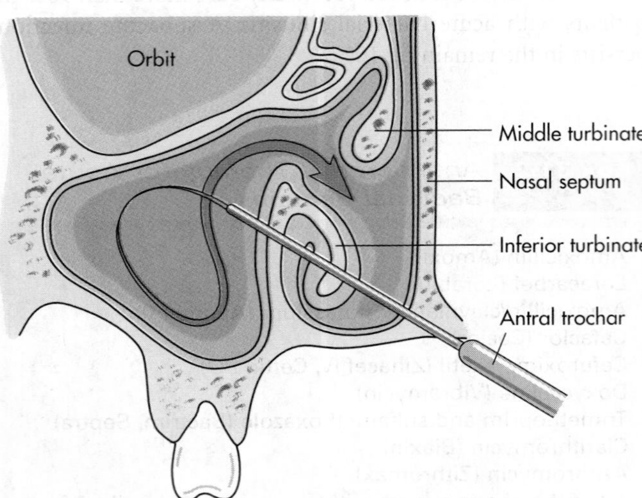


**fig. 31-4** Antral puncture. Trochar inserted under the inferior turbinate (through the medial wall of the antrum). Contents of the sinus are washed into the nose through the natural ostium.

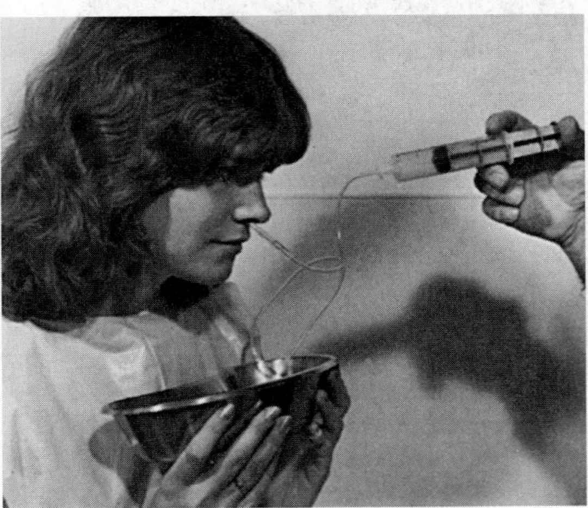

**fig. 31-5** Irrigation of the maxillary sinus. With the head tipped forward, solution returns via the natural ostium and out the anterior portion of the nose for examination and/or culture.

findings that would require endoscopic sinus surgery.[20] The sinuses will be aspirated to obtain organisms for culture and sensitivity. Before endoscopic sinus surgery is used to treat chronic sinusitis, the patient is evaluated with nasal endoscopy and coronal CT scans. The nasal endoscopy reveals subtle changes that cannot be seen in an anterior rhinoscopy using a nasal speculum, and the coronal CT scan determines the underlying cause of sinusitis. The coronal CT scan is best performed after acute inflammation has subsided and medical treatment has been attempted.

**Medications.** Decongestants are usually sufficient treatment. Patients who do not have fever, facial pain, or tenderness are not usually helped by antibiotics. When antibiotics are necessary, the results of the culture and sensitivity will be used to determine the appropriate antibiotic. Antibiotics are prescribed usually for 2 to 3 weeks.

**Treatments.** Nasal saline irrigations and surgery are the major treatments.

**Surgical management.** Treatment of chronic sinusitis involves surgery to remove all diseased soft tissue and bone, to provide adequate postoperative drainage, and to obliterate the sinus cavity when necessary. The goal of surgery is to eradicate infection and leave contiguous structures normal.

Several surgical procedures are used to treat patients with chronic sinusitis (Table 31-4). These procedures are discussed next.

**table 31-4** *Types of Sinus Surgery*

| Procedure | Use |
|---|---|
| **FUNCTIONAL ENDOSCOPIC SINUS SURGERY (FESS)** | |
| Sinus endoscope enters sinus and removes diseased mucosa and opens sinus ostia | Chronic sinusitis<br>Removal of polyps |
| **CALDWELL-LUC (RADICAL ANTRUM OPERATION)** | |
| Clearing out of maxillary sinus through incision under upper lip | Chronic maxillary sinusitis |
| **TRANSNASAL, EXTERNAL, OR TRANSANTRAL ETHMOIDECTOMY** | |
| Various approaches used to excise infected ethmoid or sphenoid cells | Chronic ethmoid or sphenoid sinusitis |
| **FRONTAL SINUSECTOMY** | |
| Complete removal of diseased mucosa of both frontal sinuses; space packed with subcutaneous fat from abdomen | Chronic frontal sinusitis |
| **SPHENOID SINUS SURGERY** | |
| Ethmoid sinus removed and anterior wall of sphenoid sinus opened | Chronic sphenoid sinusitis |

***Functional endoscopic sinus surgery.*** In functional endoscopic sinus surgery (FESS), also known as endoscopic sinus surgery (ESS), a fiberoptic endoscope that illuminates and magnifies is used to enter the sinus. The underlying principle in this type of surgery is to focus on the actual site of the pathology and thus perform a more limited operation.[20] In endoscopic sinus surgery, the surgeon attempts to open normal sinus bone more widely, ensuring adequate drainage from the sinuses and thus alleviating current infection.[20]

Endoscopic sinus surgery has made it possible for patients with sinus disease to be treated without hospitalization and has prevented facial scarring and an extended recovery period.[16] Although the main use of FESS is to treat recurrent or chronic sinus disease, it can be used for other purposes, including (1) the removal of polyps, foreign bodies, or other growths; (2) treatment of recurrent or chronic pain caused by nasal or sinus blockage; and (3) examination with the patient under anesthesia, usually with biopsy.

The purpose of FESS is to reestablish sinus ventilation and mucociliary clearance by removal of tissue from the osteomeatal complex (the area of the anterior ethmoids and middle meatus).

The surgical goals of FESS include removing diseased tissue, promoting sinus drainage, improving sinus ventilation, removing objects or masses, and alleviating pain. The procedure can be performed with the patient under local or general anesthesia. If local anesthesia is used, the procedure is performed in an ambulatory surgery center where the patient is kept for 2 to 3 hours postoperatively and then discharged.

Functional endoscopic sinus surgery is performed as follows: Small nasal endoscopes are used to dissect the diseased tissue. The surgeon uses the CT scan as a guide to nasal anatomy and to locate diseased tissue.[21] In early sinus disease the cells are opened to allow for ventilation and drainage. In advanced disease the cells may need to be removed. A major advantage of fiberoptic endoscopy is that it allows the surgeon to remove all of the diseased tissue while preserving more healthy tissue and thus preserving more of the function of the sinus.[18]

In 1994 powered instruments for use in FESS were introduced. These powered instruments enhance precision and safety in the surgical approach. Other advantages of the use of these instruments are faster recovery time and less time in the postanesthesia unit. For more information about powered instruments see reference 14.

*Diet.* Patients may eat whatever they wish, but the nasal packing and postoperative swelling usually decrease appetite. Protein intake to aid healing is emphasized, and patients may be able to take milk-based drinks. Additional fluids are encouraged.

*Activity.* The patient is encouraged to take it easy and rest more than usual for the first 5 to 7 days to allow the body to heal.

*Referrals.* Usually no referrals are necessary.

***Caldwell-Luc sinus surgery.*** The Caldwell-Luc procedure, also called a radical antrum operation, is the generally accepted operative procedure for *chronic maxillary sinusitis* that cannot be cured with antibiotics and other medical therapy. Local or general anesthesia may be used.

The procedure is performed through an incision under the upper lip (Figure 31-6). Part of the anterior bony wall of the antrum is removed, producing a permanent window (Figure 31-7). All of the diseased mucosa and periosteum is removed through the window. The bone of the lateral wall of the nose in the inferior meatus, which divides the nose from the antrum, is removed.[20] The mucous membrane and periosteum of the lateral wall of the nose are preserved and fashioned into a hinged flap.

The antrum may be packed to prevent bleeding. Packing is removed through the nose 24 to 48 hours postoperatively. As the maxillary sinus heals, the exposed bone is covered by mucosa. Numbness of the upper lip and upper teeth may be present for several months after a Caldwell-Luc operation, because some nerves to these structures pass through the site of the incision.

*Diet.* Because of the oral incision only fluids are given for at least 24 hours and then a soft diet for several days. The need to increase protein intake to aid healing is emphasized.

*Activity.* The patient is encouraged to rest more than usual for the first 5 to 7 days to allow the body to heal.

*Referrals.* Usually no referrals are necessary.

***Ethmoidectomy.*** An ethmoidectomy is performed to remove diseased mucosa, polyps, or mucoceles from the ethmoid sinus. A mucocele is a mucous cyst that is a consequence of repeated infection. Repeated infection causes the sinus ostia from the ethmoid sinus to become blocked by thickened mucosa or scar tissue. Thus mucus cannot drain; it builds up, and a cyst forms. The mucocele continues to enlarge, resulting in pressure necrosis on surrounding bone. It can be seen as a mass at the medial canthus.

Three surgical approaches are used in performing an ethmoidectomy: (1) transnasally, (2) transantrally, or (3) externally. General or local anesthesia with sedation may be used. Ethmoidectomy is commonly used to remove nasal polyps arising in the ethmoid sinus. Ethmoid cells are removed, creating a single large cavity that is packed for 24 to 48 hours. Usually steroids are given intranasally to prevent nasal polyps from recurring.

In the *transnasal approach* the surgery is performed using a headlight and operating microscopes or endoscopes. This approach is technically difficult, and complications to the orbit can cause cerebrospinal fluid rhinorrhea.

In a *transantral ethmoidectomy* a Caldwell-Luc incision is used (see Figures 31-6 and 31-7). The ethmoid cells are removed from below. It is difficult to remove anterior ethmoid cells using this approach, and a combined intranasal and transantral approach may be necessary. Complications of the transantral approach include damage to the infraorbital nerve, causing numbness of the lip or upper teeth.

The *external approach* is preferred for ethmoid surgery because it allows better visualization and reduces the risks of complications such as damage to the optic nerve and cerebrospinal fluid leak. An ethmoidectomy entails removal of ethmoid air cells (see Table 31-4). The incision is made in the inner half to the eyebrow downward along the side of the nose (Figure 31-8). Ethmoidectomy is performed to remove nasal polyps (which commonly originate in the ethmoid cells) and to remove diseased mucosa or mucoceles. A pressure dressing is usually applied over the eye to prevent postoperative edema.

*Diet.* Fluids are given freely for the first 24 hours, progressing to a soft diet. The need to increase protein intake to aid in healing is empathized.

*Activity.* The patient is encouraged to rest more than usual for the first 5 to 7 days to allow the body to heal.

*Referrals.* Usually no referrals are necessary.

***Sphenoid sinus surgery.*** Surgery of the *sphenoid sinus* can be accomplished using an endoscopic technique,

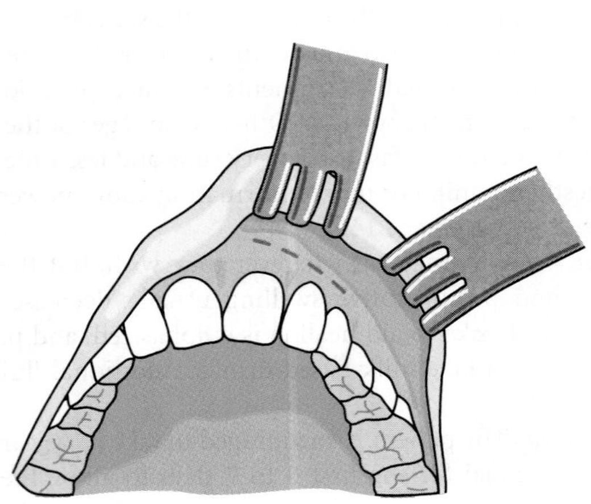

**fig. 31-6** The incision into the maxillary sinus (Caldwell-Luc surgery) is made under the upper lip.

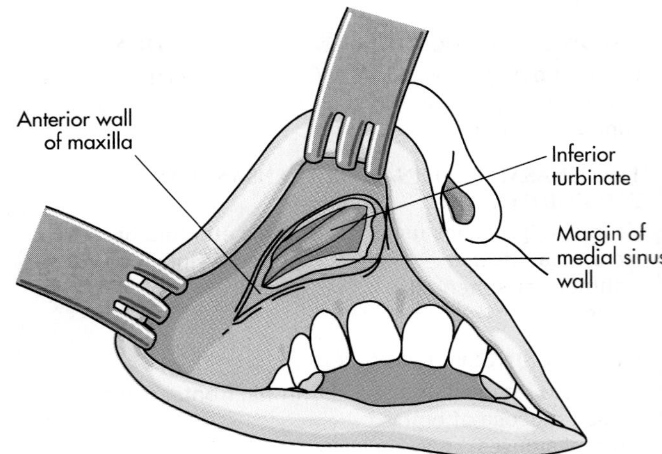


**fig. 31-7** Caldwell-Luc surgery. After removal of the sinus mucosa or polypoid tissue, a window is made into the nose along its floor, allowing dependent drainage from the maxillary sinus. Incision is closed with absorbable sutures.

through an external or transantral ethmoidectomy approach, or through a transseptal approach (see Table 31-4). The ethmoid sinus is usually removed and the anterior wall of the sphenoid sinus opened. Diseased tissue is removed along with the mucous membrane lining the sinus. To facilitate drainage directly into the nasopharynx, the sinus ostium is opened wide.[20]

*Diet.* As for ethmoidectomy, see p. 872.

*Activity.* As for ethmoidectomy, see p. 872.

*Referrals.* As for ethmoidectomy, see p. 872.

***Frontal sinusectomy.*** The advent of the *osteoplastic flap operation* makes frontal sinus surgery different from that performed on the other sinuses. Surgery of the other sinuses basically provides for an open, well-drained cavity, which in the past proved inadequate for the frontal sinuses because recurrence of disease was common. The osteoplastic flap operation allows for complete removal of diseased mucosa of the frontal sinus and for obliteration of the sinus so that it is no longer functional or continuous with the inner nose.

The osteoplastic flap procedure is performed through a "gull-wing" or "crossbow" incision. In men the incision extends along the eyebrows and connects along the bridge of the nose. In women, for whom baldness usually is not a problem in later life, the incision connects both temporal areas a few centimeters posterior to the hairline. Both incisions give excellent postoperative cosmesis and are extended to the periosteum of the bone overlying the frontal sinus.

The skin overlying the sinus is reflected, and a radiograph of the frontal sinus (obtained preoperatively) is used as a template for sawing the lateral and superior borders of the anterior frontal bone. The anterior bone is then reflected inferiorly, thus exposing the entire contents of the frontal sinus. The mucosa is removed under direct vision, and an operating microscope is used to ensure that all fragments of mucosa are removed. An incision is then made in the left lower abdominal quadrant, and subcutaneous fat is obtained for adipose obliteration of the sinus. The bony flap and skin are then repositioned, and a pressure dressing is applied to minimize postoperative swelling.

Postoperatively, pain in the frontal area is not significant after 24 hours. Pain in the abdominal area, however, often lasts several days, and serous drainage from this area is common after the drain is removed. Sutures are removed about the fifth postoperative day. Because nasal packs are not used, special oral hygiene care is not needed. Preoperative and postoperative teaching for patients having sinus surgery can be found in the accompanying Guidelines for Care Boxes.

*Diet.* As for ethmoidectomy, see p. 872.

*Activity.* As for ethmoidectomy, see p. 872.

*Referrals.* As for ethmoidectomy, see p. 872.

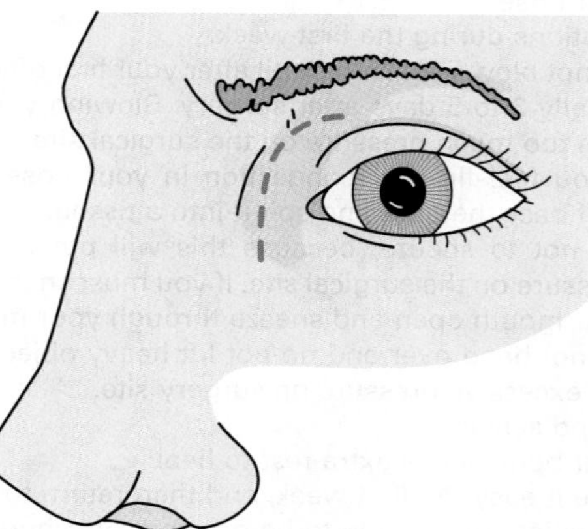

**fig. 31-8** Medial canthal incision for external ethmoidectomy.

## NURSING MANAGEMENT OF THE PATIENT UNDERGOING FUNCTIONAL ENDOSCOPIC SINUS SURGERY

### PREOPERATIVE CARE

Because this is an outpatient procedure, preadmission tests and preoperative teaching are scheduled a few days before surgery. The points to be covered with the patient are outlined in the Guidelines for Care Box below.

### POSTOPERATIVE CARE

The postoperative routine is reviewed with the patient at the time of the preoperative teaching so that the patient can determine in advance of surgery the preparations, if any, that will need to be made at home (see the following Patient/Family Teaching Box). Postoperatively the nurse assesses the patient's progress by a telephone call within 24 hours of discharge.

**guidelines for care**

**Preoperative Teaching for the Person Undergoing Sinus Surgery**

Determine patient understanding about the surgical procedure. Clarify misconceptions and answer patient's and family's questions. Explain that the patient will:

- Have nothing to eat or drink for 6 to 8 hours preoperatively.
- Receive a sedative before surgery.
- Feel pressure, not pain, during surgery.
- Have a nasal pack for 24 to 48 hours postoperatively and may feel like he or she has a "head cold."
- Have a mustache dressing postoperatively (Figure 31-10).
- Have "black eyes" and swelling around the nose and eyes for 1 to 2 weeks postoperatively.
- Have prescription for pain medication as needed.

**guidelines for care**

## Postoperative Care of the Person Undergoing Sinus Surgery

1. After general anesthesia, position patient well onto the side to prevent swelling or aspiration of bloody drainage.
2. Administer cool mist via face tent or collar, or provide humidifier.
3. When the patient is awake, remind him or her to expectorate secretions and not swallow them.
4. Encourage mid-Fowler's position when fully awake to promote drainage and decrease edema.
5. Apply ice compresses over nose (or ice bag over maxillary or frontal sinuses) in the early postoperative period.
6. Monitor the patient for:
   a. Excessive bleeding from nose (may be evidenced by repeated swallowing).
   b. Decreased visual acuity, especially diplopia, indicating damage to optic nerve or muscles of globe of eye.
   c. Complaints of pain over the involved sinus, which may indicate infection or inadequate drainage.
   d. Fever—take temperature rectally.
7. Give frequent mouth care using a soft toothbrush. If there is an oral incision, mouth care is given before meals to improve appetite and after meals to decrease danger of infection.
8. Change nasal pad when it is soiled.
9. Apply ice compresses to ecchymotic areas to constrict blood vessels, decrease oozing and edema, and help relieve pain.
10. Encourage liberal fluid intake. Patient may be very thirsty because of dry mouth from mouth breathing.
11. Teach patient to:
    a. Avoid blowing nose for at least 48 hours after packing is removed to prevent bleeding.
    b. Avoid sneezing; if patient must sneeze, he or she should keep mouth open.
    c. Avoid lifting heavy objects.
    d. Report signs of infection (fever, purulent discharge) to surgeon.
    e. Expect tarry stools from swallowed blood for a few days.
    f. Avoid constipation (Valsalva's maneuver [straining] can cause bleeding).
    g. Expect that ecchymosis of nose and eyes will begin to change color over next 1 to 2 weeks.
    h. Take prophylactic antibiotics as prescribed; do not stop until all medication is taken.

**patient/family teaching**

## Home Care of the Person Undergoing Sinus Surgery

1. Pain.
   a. The discomfort after surgery is more of an ache and pressure from the packing in the nose than actual pain.
   b. The pain may increase during the week after surgery because of swelling and secretions in the sinus.
   c. Most patients obtain relief by taking acetaminophen. If your physician expects you will have more pain, another medication will be prescribed.
   d. Never take aspirin or any product containing aspirin because aspirin can cause bleeding.
2. Drainage.
   a. Drainage will increase after surgery.
   b. A small amount of bright red bleeding is normal and may continue for a week.
   c. Old blood that accumulated during the surgery is reddish brown, and it will drain for a week or more. It is of no concern.
   d. A small dressing (dry pad) will be placed beneath your nose to absorb any drainage.
   e. You may need to change the pad several times each day, depending on the amount of drainage. The drainage pad can be discontinued when the drainage stops.
   f. After drainage stops, a thicker, yellowish green drainage may continue for several weeks.
3. Breathing.
   a. Your head may feel stuffy, and the mucous membranes of your nose may swell. This is normal and expected.
   b. Stuffiness will increase during the first week after surgery and then decrease over the next couple of weeks and breathing through your nose should improve.
   c. Keeping your head elevated and sleeping with an extra pillow will help make you more comfortable. In this position there will be less swelling and better drainage of nasal secretions.
   d. A cool mist humidifier at the bedside will help loosen secretions and prevent crusting of the nose. *Be sure to follow the manufacturer's directions for cleaning the unit so that bacteria will not grow, be dispersed into the air, and infect you or others.*
   e. At your first postoperative visit, the packing will be removed and you will be given instructions for cleaning your nose.
4. Precautions during the first week.
   a. Do not blow your nose until after your first office visit, usually 3 to 5 days after surgery. Blowing your nose puts too much pressure on the surgical site.
   b. If you feel fluid or congestion in your nose, gently sniff back the fluid and spit it into a tissue.
   c. Try not to sneeze, because this will put too much pressure on the surgical site. If you must sneeze, keep your mouth open and sneeze through your mouth.
   d. Do not bend over and do not lift heavy objects; both put excessive pressure on surgery site.
5. Rest and activity.
   a. Your body needs extra rest to heal.
   b. Take it easy the first week, and then return to normal activities. Usual time to be off work or school is 5 to 7 days unless you work in a dusty or dirty environment.
   c. After 1 week you may swim, jog, or do other exercise. If bright red bleeding occurs, stop activity until bleeding stops, and then gradually resume activity.

If inflammation or infection is noted during the surgery, antibiotics will be administered and continued for a total of 10 to 14 days. Some surgeons also order a steroid nasal spray for a few days. To maintain moisture to mucosa all patients will begin normal saline sprays after packing is removed. Saline irrigations may be necessary for those with considerable nasal crusting.

## NURSING MANAGEMENT OF THE PATIENT UNDERGOING CALDWELL-LUC SURGERY

### ■ PREOPERATIVE CARE

Generally the patient is admitted to the hospital the morning of surgery. For the convenience of the patient, preadmission tests and preoperative teaching should be scheduled for the same day. Usually these are scheduled a few days before surgery. Preoperative teaching is summarized in the Guidelines for Care Box on p. 873.

### ■ POSTOPERATIVE CARE

Because general anesthesia is usual, the patient is positioned well onto the side to facilitate removal of secretions and to maintain the airway. This position also prevents swelling of the surgical site and aspiration of bloody drainage. Cool mist is administered by face tent or collar to prevent drying of secretions and to keep mucous membranes moist.

When the patient recovers from anesthesia, the head of the bed is elevated to a mid-Fowler's position to prevent edema and promote drainage. The patient is reminded to sniff secretions to the back of the mouth where they can be expectorated. Ice compresses are applied over the nose or over the maxillary or frontal sinuses for a few hours after surgery. Ice helps reduce swelling in the operative area, constrict blood vessels, reduce bleeding, and relieve pain.

The patient is monitored for the following:

1. Excessive bleeding from the nose (frequent swallowing is a clue).
2. Decreased visual acuity, especially diplopia, which indicates damage to the optic nerve or muscles of the globe of the eye.
3. Pain over the involved sinus, which may indicate an infection or inadequate drainage.
4. Fever. Take temperature rectally or aurally. Temperature cannot be taken orally because of packing in the nose, which causes mouth breathing.

Mouth care using a soft toothbrush is given frequently. If there is an oral incision, mouth care is given before meals to improve appetite and after meals to clean food debris, which could lead to infection if not removed. A liberal fluid intake is urged to prevent drying of secretions. The patient may be very thirsty because of dry mouth from mouth breathing. Postoperative teaching is presented in the Guidelines for Care Box on p. 874.

Patient/family teaching for the person undergoing Caldwell-Luc surgery can be found in the accompanying box.

## NURSING MANAGEMENT OF THE PATIENT UNDERGOING ETHMOIDECTOMY, SPHENOIDECTOMY, OR FRONTAL SINUS SURGERY

### ■ PREOPERATIVE CARE

See the Guidelines for Care Box on p. 873.

### ■ POSTOPERATIVE CARE

See the Guidelines for Care Box on p. 874.

### SPECIAL ENVIRONMENTS FOR CARE

#### Home Care Management

See the Patient/Family Teaching Box on p. 874.

### Complications of Sinusitis

Complications of sinusitis usually are the result of inadequate therapy during the acute stage or a delay in treatment. Signs and symptoms of complications include the following:

1. Generalized persistent headache
2. Vomiting
3. Convulsions
4. Chills or high fever
5. Edema or increasing swelling of the forehead or eyelids
6. Blurring of vision, diplopia, or persistent retroocular pain[19]
7. Signs of increased intracranial pressure
8. Personality changes or dulling of the sensorium
9. Increase in white cell count above 20,000 $mm^3$

Other complications include the following:[19]

1. Orbital or periorbital cellulitis
2. Orbital or periorbital abscess
3. Cavernous sinus thrombosis
4. Bacteremia or septicemia
5. Osteomyelitis

**patient/family teaching**

**The Person Undergoing Caldwell-Luc Surgery**

In addition to general care of the patient following sinus surgery, patient teaching specific to Caldwell-Luc surgery includes the following:

1. Do not chew on affected side until incision heals.
2. Use caution with oral hygiene to avoid injury to the incision.
3. Avoid wearing dentures for about 10 days.
4. Avoid blowing nose for about 2 weeks after packing has been removed.
5. Avoid sneezing; if you must sneeze, keep mouth open.

#### Orbital complications

Most orbital infections (75%) are caused by extension from paranasal sinusitis. Most commonly the ethmoid sinuses are involved. Orbital complications include inflammatory edema, orbital cellulitis, subperiosteal abscess, orbital abscess, and cavernous sinus thrombosis. Complications are treated vigorously with intravenous antibiotics and, in case of abscess, incision and drainage.

#### Cavernous sinus thrombosis

Cavernous sinus thrombosis occurs when there is extension of infection through the venous pathways (usually the angular vein) to the cavernous sinus. The patient is very ill, with chills and a temperature as high as 41° C (106° F). There is pain deep behind the eye, and the patient becomes toxic and may become semicomatose. Cavernous sinus thrombosis is a serious complication of sinusitis that can cause death in 48 to 72 hours if untreated. More than 25% of patients who develop this complication will die even when adequately treated.[20] The primary treatment is with intravenous antibiotics.

**table 31-5** *Types of Pharyngitis, Pathophysiology, and Clinical Manifestations*

| Pathophysiology | Clinical Manifestations |
|---|---|
| **GROUP A BETA-HEMOLYTIC STREPTOCOCCAL (GABHS)** | |
| Uniform infection of pharyngeal walls<br>Purulent exudate, edema of lymphoid tissue of palate, tonsils, uvula | Sore throat, slightly elevated temperature, malaise |
| **GONOCOCCAL OR VIRAL** | |
| Vesicles may be present on pharyngeal walls and tonsils | Minimal discomfort<br>Fever, diffuse sore throat |
| **INFECTIOUS MONONUCLEOSIS (EPSTEIN-BARR VIRUS)** | |
| Exudate on pharyngeal walls and tonsils<br>Spleen may be enlarged | Sore throat, cervical lymphadenopathy, and fever |
| **FUNGAL (ESPECIALLY CANDIDIASIS [THRUSH])** | |
| Develops in patient who is immunosuppressed and on prolonged antibiotics | Pus, dysphagia, white plaques in mouth or on pharyngeal walls |

## INFECTIONS OF THE PHARYNX AND LARYNX

### ACUTE PHARYNGITIS

#### Etiology/Epidemiology

Acute pharyngitis is the most common throat inflammation. It may be caused by hemolytic streptococci, staphylococci, other bacteria, filterable viruses, or fungi. *Group A beta-hemolytic streptococci (GABHS)* are the cause of up to 30% of the cases of acute pharyngitis. The most common cause, however, is viruses, which account for 70% of the cases of acute pharyngitis.[17] There is also increased evidence of gonococcal pharyngitis caused by the gram-negative diplococcus *Neisseria gonorrhoeae.* The disease is increasingly found in both men and women. When gonorrhea is suspected, a throat culture is indicated. A severe form of acute pharyngitis often is termed *strep throat* because of the frequency of streptococci as the causative organism.

#### Pathophysiology

Dryness of the throat is a common complaint. The throat appears red, and soreness may range from slight scratchiness to severe pain with difficulty in swallowing. A hacking cough may be present. Children often develop a very high fever, whereas adults may have only a mild elevation of temperature. Symptoms usually precede or occur simultaneously with the onset of acute rhinitis or acute sinusitis. Pharyngitis is also a common manifestation of infectious mononucleosis (Table 31-5).

#### Collaborative Care Management

Acute pharyngitis usually is relieved by hot saline throat gargles. An ice collar may make the person feel more comfortable. For adults acetylsalicylic acid administered orally as a gargle or in Aspergum may be prescribed. Lozenges containing a mild anesthetic may help relieve local soreness. Moist inhalations may help relieve throat dryness. A liquid diet usually is better tolerated than solid food, and fluids to at least 2.5 L per day are encouraged. Oral hygiene may prevent drying and cracking of the lips and usually refreshes the mouth. If the temperature is elevated, the person should remain in bed and, even if ambulatory and afebrile, should have extra rest.

A throat culture is necessary to identify the offending organism. If beta-hemolytic streptococcus is identified, the drug of choice is penicillin. For the person allergic to penicillin, erythromycin or another antibiotic is prescribed. Persons with a history of bacterial endocarditis or rheumatic fever are usually given penicillin prophylactically.

As with other infections treated with antibiotics, the patient must understand the need to take the prescribed antibiotic until the course is completed. This will vary from 7 to 12 days, depending on the organism and the severity of infection. Patients must understand that they should continue therapy for the prescribed number of days, even if they are symptom free.

#### Patient/family education

The major role of the nurse is patient teaching, which is presented in the accompanying Patient/Family Teaching Box.

**patient/family teaching**

**The Person with Pharyngitis or Tonsillitis**

1. Comfort measures: use warm saline gargles, ice collars, moist inhalations, mouth care
2. Drink at least 2 to 3 L of fluids daily
3. Symptoms of recurrence requiring medical attention: fever, excessive pain, pus, dysphagia
4. Teach rationale for prophylactic antibiotic therapy for pharyngitis in patients with a history of rheumatic fever or infective endocarditis to prevent reinfection

## ACUTE FOLLICULAR TONSILLITIS

### Etiology/Epidemiology

Acute follicular tonsillitis is an acute inflammation of the tonsils and their crypts. It is usually caused by the *Streptococcus* organism. It is more likely to occur when the person's resistance is low, and it is common in children.

### Pathophysiology

The onset is almost always sudden, and symptoms include sore throat, pain on swallowing, fever, chills, general muscle aching, and malaise. These symptoms often last for 2 to 3 days. The pharynx and tonsils appear red, and the peritonsillar tissues are swollen. Sometimes a yellowish exudate drains from crypts in the tonsils. A throat culture usually is taken to identify the offending organism.

### Collaborative Care Management

The patient with acute tonsillitis is encouraged to rest and take generous amounts of fluids orally. Warm saline throat irrigation may be ordered, and antibiotics are given for streptococcal pharyngitis. Acetaminophen (Tylenol) and sometimes codeine sulfate may be ordered for pain and discomfort. An ice collar applied to the neck may relieve discomfort.

#### *Patient/family education*

Because the person with acute tonsillitis is usually cared for at home, the nurse should help in teaching the general public the care that is needed (see the Patient/Family Teaching Box, above). Nurses working in clinics, industry, schools, physician offices, emergency departments, and the community have many opportunities to do this teaching.

### Complications

Complications of untreated tonsillitis include heart and kidney damage, chorea, and pneumonia. Incidence of these complications is decreasing with early diagnosis and the widespread use of penicillin. Most physicians believe that persons who have recurrent attacks of tonsillitis should have a tonsillectomy. This procedure is usually performed from 4 to 6 weeks after an acute attack has subsided (see p. 881).

A peritonsillar abscess is an uncommon local complication of acute follicular tonsillitis in which infection extends from the tonsil to form an abscess in the surrounding tissues. The presence of pus behind the tonsil causes difficulty in swallowing, talking, and opening the mouth; the difficulty in swallowing may be so great that the person is unable to swallow. Pain is severe and may extend to the ear on the affected side.

If antibiotics to which the offending organism is sensitive are administered early, infection subsides. If the peritonsillar abscess is caused by anaerobic organisms, hydrogen peroxide (an oxidizing agent) in the form of a mouthwash may help relieve symptoms. Acute streptococcal or staphylococcal tonsillitis may also cause a peritonsillar abscess to form. If an abscess forms, it will be incised and drained. During the procedure, the patient's head usually is lowered, and suction is applied as soon as the incision is made to prevent the patient from aspirating the purulent drainage. Warm saline irrigations, an ice collar, or narcotics may relieve discomfort. If acute follicular tonsillitis is treated adequately, peritonsillar abscess is not likely to occur.

## ACUTE LARYNGITIS

### Etiology/Epidemiology

Simple acute laryngitis is an inflammation of the mucous membrane lining the larynx accompanied by edema of the vocal cords. It may be caused by a cold, by sudden changes in temperature, or by irritating fumes.

### Pathophysiology

Symptoms vary from a slight huskiness to complete loss of voice. The throat may be painful and feel scratchy, and a cough may be present.

### Collaborative Care Management

Laryngitis in adults usually requires only symptomatic treatment. The person is advised to remain indoors in an even temperature and to avoid talking for several days or weeks, depending on the severity of the inflammation.[11] Steam inhalations may be soothing, and cough syrups or home remedies for coughs provide relief to some patients. Smoking or being near others who are smoking should be avoided. Additional fluids by mouth help prevent dehydration and drying of the throat.[11]

#### *Patient/family education*

The nursing role is mainly patient teaching, which would include the following:

1. Need to take antibiotics as prescribed (not to stop antibiotics when feeling better)
2. Need to increase fluid intake
3. For smoker, need to stop smoking and, for both smokers and nonsmokers, need to avoid smoky environments (secondhand smoke)
4. Referral to a support group for persons wanting to stop smoking
5. Precautions to be observed in using steam inhalations

## CHRONIC LARYNGITIS

Chronic laryngitis occurs in people who use their voices excessively, who smoke a great deal, or who work continuously where there are irritating fumes. Hoarseness usually is worse in the early morning and in the evening. There may be a dry, harsh cough and a persistent need to clear the throat. *All persons with persistent hoarseness should be examined by laryngoscopy to rule out cancer of the larynx.*

Treatment of chronic laryngitis consists of removal of irritants, voice rest, correction of faulty voice habits, steam inhalations, and cough medications. Additional fluids by mouth are encouraged to prevent dehydration and drying of the throat.

# OBSTRUCTIONS OF THE NOSE AND THROAT

## ETIOLOGY/EPIDEMIOLOGY

The upper airway may become partly obstructed, leading to interference with breathing. Obstructions may occur at the base of the tongue (tumor), in the nose (deviated septum, hypertrophied turbinates, or nasal polyps), pharynx (enlarged tonsils and adenoids), or larynx (laryngeal paralysis or edema, cervical esophageal tumor).

## PATHOPHYSIOLOGY

The signs and symptoms of upper airway obstruction include difficulty in breathing through the nose, dry mucosa, postnasal drip, nasal discharge, bleeding from the nose, and loss of sense of smell.

## COLLABORATIVE CARE MANAGEMENT

Management is mainly surgical. The types of surgery are discussed under each of the obstructions.

## NASAL DEFORMITIES

### Reconstruction of the Nose

#### *Etiology/epidemiology*

Deformities of the nose can be present from birth or develop as the result of trauma to the nose from sports injuries, automobile crashes, and the like. Although some deformities may seem to be minor to the casual observor, they may be considered major by the person whose nose size and shape does not please them.

#### *Pathophysiology*

Depending on the deformity, there can be loss of nasal septal cartilage from trauma or infection resulting in marked concavity. This is referred to as a saddle nose. In some persons the nose is considered too long, too wide, or of the wrong shape. In this situation the problem may be entirely anatomical, and the patient's desire for change in the appearance of the nose is for cosmetic reasons. In this case it is important that the plastic surgeon clearly define what results the patient can expect from surgery of the nose.

#### *Collaborative care management*

Cosmetic surgery on the nose is termed *rhinoplasty.* Preparation of the patient is important so that the patient does not have unrealistic expectations about the surgery. Some plastic surgeons have all candidates for cosmetic surgery interviewed by a psychologist to ensure that their expectations are realistic.

Bone and cartilage may be removed from the nose if it is irregular, or they may be inserted if a defect such as a saddle nose is being corrected (Figure 31-9). Most rhinoplasties are performed with the patient under local anesthesia. The incision is usually made at the end of the nose inside the nostril so that it is not conspicuous.

Following a plastic procedure, the nose is usually protected with a plaster of paris splint, adhesive tape dressing, or plastic mold. Firm healing develops on about the tenth day. There will be ecchymosis and swelling around the eyes and nose for 10 to 14 days after surgery. Iced compresses and an ice bag are commonly used to hasten fluid resorption from the surgical site. The patient needs to know that it will

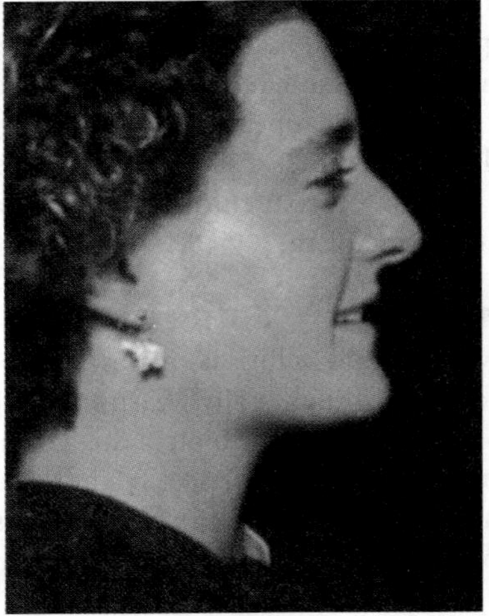


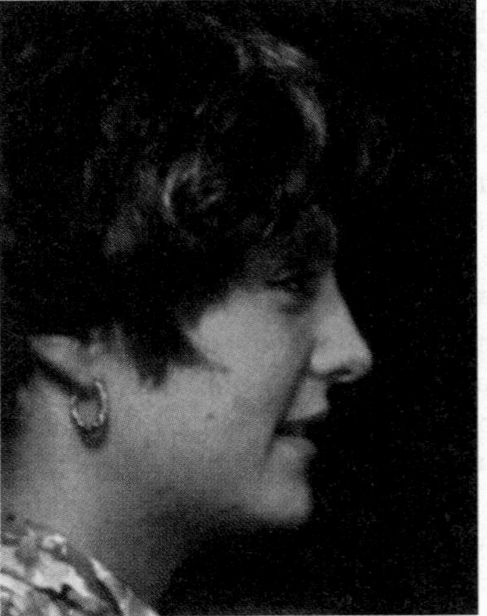


**fig. 31-9** Rhinoplasty. **A,** Preoperative lateral view; **B,** Postoperative lateral view.

be several weeks before the final results of the surgery will be evident.

## Deviated Septum

### Etiology/epidemiology

Normally the septum of the nose is straight and thin. As a person ages, the septum tends to become deviated to one side or the other, and an irregular projection may develop on the septum (see Chapter 30, Figure 30-12).

### Pathophysiology

The nasal septum is made up of cartilage and bone joined by a fibrous attachment. The septum separates the nose into two cavities, provides support, and acts as a shock absorber for the floor of the frontal fossa. Trauma may result in fibrous growth of tissue that fills in the fracture, producing an overgrowth that causes bowing of the septum.

The main symptoms of a deviated septum or nasal fracture are obstruction to breathing through the nose. A deviated septum may also interfere with normal functions of the nose in filtering out foreign substances from the air and in warming and humidifying the air. A deviated septum changes the velocity of air, altering normal functions of the nose. This results in drying of the nasal mucosa, crusting, nasal bleeding, and changes in the lining of the nose.[21]

### Collaborative care management

When a deviated septum is causing the patient problems, a surgical procedure termed a *nasoseptoplasty* may be necessary.

A nasoseptoplasty involves reconstruction of the nasal septum. It is widely used to treat a deviated septum. In this procedure an incision is made through the mucosa at the caudal end of the septal cartilage. The septal mucous membranes are elevated, and the septal cartilage is separated from its bony attachments and straightened. The septal mucous membranes are then approximated to prevent bleeding.

Nasal septal splints made of plastic or Silastic are inserted into the nose to prevent synechiae (a type of scar tissue) and to keep the septum in place. The nose may be packed for 24 to 48 hours to prevent a hematoma from forming between the septal flaps and to hold the septum in place.[20] The patient is usually given antibiotics until the packing is removed. The splints and nasal packing are removed by the surgeon. Reconstruction of the external nose (rhinoplasty) is often combined with septoplasty.

After nasal surgery the patient is placed in mid-Fowler's position to decrease local edema, and cool mist is given via collar or face tent. Iced compresses are usually applied to the nose to lessen the discoloration, bleeding, and discomfort. Patients can usually apply their own iced compresses.

The patient is monitored for signs of hemorrhage (see the Guidelines for Care Box). Some oozing on the dressing below the nose is expected, and this dressing may be changed as necessary (Figure 31-10). If bleeding becomes pronounced, the surgeon is notified and material for repacking the nose is prepared. This material consists of a hemostatic tray containing gauze packing, umbilical tape for posterior packing, a few small gauze sponges, small catheter (used for inserting a postnasal plug), packing forceps, tongue blades, and scissors. The surgeon may require a head mirror, good light, epinephrine 1:1000 or other vasoconstrictor, 4% topical lidocaine (Xylocaine) or 4% cocaine solution, applicators, nasal speculum, and suction.

Because packing blocks the passage of air through the nose, a partial vacuum is created during swallowing, and the person may complain of a sucking action when attempting to drink. Postnasal drainage, the presence of old blood in the mouth, dryness of the mouth from mouth breathing, and loss of the ability to smell often lead to anorexia. Frequent mouth care is important.

**guidelines for care**

**Care of the Person After Nasal Surgery**

1. Assessment.
   a. Monitor for hemorrhage.
      (1) Excessive blood on nasal dressing.
      (2) Bright red vomitus.
      (3) Repeated swallowing (check back of throat with penlight for blood running down throat).
      (4) Rapid pulse.
      (5) Restlessness.
   b. Monitor for infection: fever, elevated white blood cell count (WBC).
2. Discomfort.
   a. Mid-Fowler's position to decrease local edema.
   b. Cool mist via collar or face tent.
   c. Ice compresses over nose for 24 hours prn.
   d. Support and sedation for patient apprehension because of difficulty in breathing caused by blockage of nasal passages.
   e. Use a flashlight or penlight to examine back of throat to ensure that packing has not slipped to back of the throat where it could gag the patient.
   f. Frequent oral care.
   g. Change dressing under nose prn.
3. Nutrition.
   a. Food as tolerated.
   b. Encourage increased fluid intake.
4. Patient/family teaching.
   a. Avoid blowing nose for 48 hours after packing removed.
   b. Avoid constipation (Valsalva's maneuver) and vigorous coughing until healing occurs (can initiate bleeding).
   c. Expect stools to be tarry for several days.
   d. Expect face to be discolored around eyes and nose for several days.
   e. Cosmetic effect from nasal surgery cannot be judged for 6 to 12 months (time for tissue to return to normal and for scar resolution).

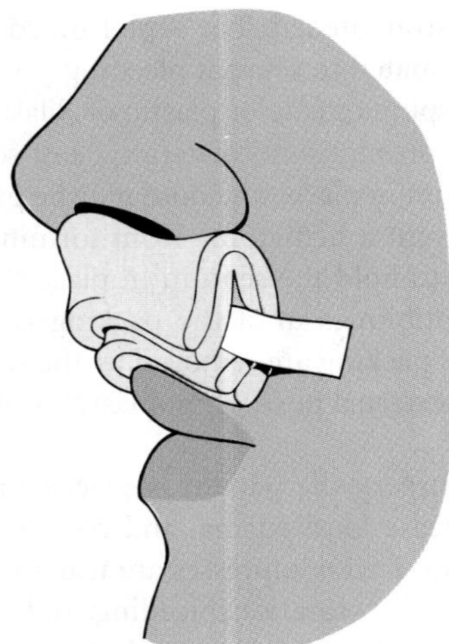

**fig. 31-10** Dressing placed under the nose to catch nasal drainage. Also called a *mustache dressing* or a *drip pad*.

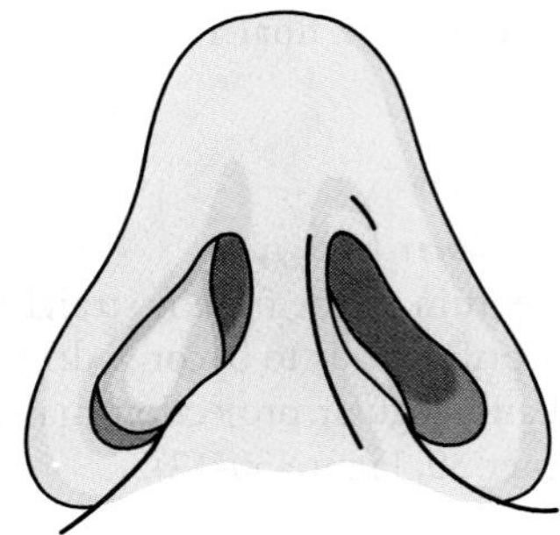

**fig. 31-11** Hypertrophic turbinate.

**Patient/family education.** Patient/family education is described in the Guidelines for Care Box on p. 879.

## Hypertrophied Turbinates

### *Etiology/epidemiology*

Long-standing allergic rhinitis and low-grade inflammation may cause permanent enlargement of the turbinates, especially the inferior turbinate.

### *Pathophysiology*

The turbinates lose most of their normal ability to expand and shrink. This results in continuous nasal obstruction (Figure 31-11).

### *Collaborative care management*

Hypertrophied turbinates may be medically treated by the use of aerosols containing corticosteroids such as beclomethasone dipropionate (Beconase, Vancenase) or dexamethasone (Decadron, Turbinaire). These aerosols are used for their antiinflammatory response and have proven to be effective for allergic and inflammatory nasal conditions, as well as for treatment of nasal polyps.

Although not used as often since the advent of the corticosteroid aerosols, laser surgery on the turbinates may still be used to restore the airway. Debulking (resection) of the hypertrophied mucosa may be necessary.

When surgery is necessary, the care and teaching of the person is the same as for persons having nasal surgery. See the Guidelines for Care Box on p. 879.

## NASAL POLYPS

### Etiology/Epidemiology

Nasal polyps are grapelike growths of the mucous membranes of the sinus mucosa into the cavities of the nose and paranasal sinuses. The exact cause of nasal polyposis is unknown, but some believe it is related to the inflammatory response. Supporting this theory is the fact that persons with chronic viral or bacterial infections have a higher incidence of nasal polyps. Nasal polyps are common and affect men twice as often as women. They are commonly associated with allergies, cystic fibrosis, asthma, disorders of ciliary motility, chronic rhinitis, and chronic sinusitis.

### Pathophysiology

Approximately 8% of patients with nasal polyps also have symptoms of asthma and intolerance to aspirin, indomethacin, and other nonsteroidal antiinflammatory drugs (NSAIDs). The cause of the triad of nasal polyps, asthma, and aspirin sensitivity is unknown, but the patient may have an acute asthmatic attack in response to infection, anesthesia, surgery, or the administration of aspirin. All of the above could be considered stressors for the hyperresponsive airway of the person with asthma.

### Collaborative Care Management

Nasal polyps can be treated with corticosteroid sprays or by local injection of a steroid into the polyp. Steroid sprays are used for long-term reduction of size of polyps, to prevent recurrence, and to reduce the inflammatory response, thus reducing swelling.

Antibiotics such as amoxicillin or erythromycin are prescribed when infection is present. Persistent polyps may require nasal polypectomy to remove the polyps; functional endoscopic sinus surgery, in which polyps are removed (see p. 871); or Caldwell-Luc surgery (see p. 871), in which the maxillary sinus is entered to remove polyps.

### *Patient/family education*

The major role of the nurse is in patient teaching. The points to be emphasized are listed in the accompanying Patient/Family Teaching Box.

# CHRONIC ENLARGEMENT OF TONSILS AND ADENOIDS

## ETIOLOGY/EPIDEMIOLOGY

Tonsils and adenoids are lymphoid structures located in the oropharynx and nasopharynx. They reach full size in childhood and then begin to atrophy during puberty. When adenoids enlarge, usually as a result of chronic infections but sometimes for no known reason, they cause nasal obstruction.

**patient/family teaching**

**The Person with Nasal Polyposis**

1. Elevate head of bed to decrease nasal edema and improve breathing through nose.
2. Increase humidity to thin secretions and reduce dryness of nose. Use central humidifier on furnace or use room humidifier. Increase fluid intake, and use saline nasal spray.
3. Prevent respiratory infections by avoiding persons with upper respiratory infections and avoiding crowds. Notify physician at first sign of infection so appropriate therapy can be started.
4. Seek prompt medical attention if signs of recurrence of polyp(s).
5. Take medications as ordered. Be aware of side effects such as drowsiness if antihistamines are prescribed.

**guidelines for care**

**Care of the Person after Tonsillectomy**

1. Position patient on side until fully awake after general anesthesia or in mid-Fowler's position when awake.
2. Monitor for hemorrhage.
   a. Frequent swallowing (inspect throat).
   b. Bright red vomitus.
   c. Rapid pulse.
   d. Restlessness.
3. Comfort.
   a. Give 30% cool mist via collar.
   b. Apply ice collar to neck (will also reduce bleeding by vasoconstriction).
   c. Use acetaminophen in place of aspirin.
4. Food and fluids.
   a. Give ice-cold fluids and bland foods during initial period (e.g., ice chips, Popsicles, Jello).
   b. Milk is usually not given, because it may increase mucus and cause the patient to clear throat.
   c. Advance to normal diet as soon as possible.
5. Patient/family teaching.
   a. Avoid attempting to clear throat immediately after surgery (may initiate bleeding).
   b. Avoid coughing, sneezing, vigorous nose blowing, and vigorous exercise for 1 to 2 weeks.
   c. Drink fluids (2 to 3 L/day) until mouth odor disappears.
   d. Avoid hard, scratchy foods, such as pretzels, popcorn, or toast, until throat is healed.
   e. Report signs of bleeding to physician immediately.
   f. Expect more throat discomfort between fourth and eighth postoperative days because of membrane separation.
   g. Expect stool to be black or dark for a few days because of swallowed blood.
   h. Resume normal activity immediately, as long as it is not stressful and does not require straining.

The person breathes through the mouth, snores loudly, may have a dull facial expression, and may have reduced appetite, because the blocked nasopharynx can interfere with swallowing. Hypertrophy of the tonsils does not usually block the oropharynx but may affect speech and swallowing and cause mouth breathing.

Approximately 30% of cases of tonsillitis are caused by group A beta-hemolytic streptococci or staphylococci. Other organisms, such as pneumococci, gram-negative organisms, and viruses, may also be the causative agent.

## PATHOPHYSIOLOGY

The tonsils are red and swollen with yellow or white exudate found mainly in the crypts of the tonsils. Signs and symptoms include fever, dry throat, malaise, dysphagia, otalgia, and a feeling of fullness in the throat. Lymph nodes in the upper part of the neck are swollen and palpable.

## COLLABORATIVE CARE MANAGEMENT

The tonsils and adenoids are removed when they become enlarged and cause symptoms of obstruction, when they are chronically infected, when the person has repeated attacks of tonsillitis, or after repeated peritonsillar abscesses. Chronic infections of these structures usually do not respond to antibiotics and may become foci of infection by spreading organisms to other parts of the body, such as the heart and the kidneys.

Tonsillectomy in adults may be performed with either general or local anesthesia. After the tonsils are removed, pressure is applied to stop superficial bleeding. Bleeding vessels are tied off with sutures or by electrocoagulation. The person is monitored carefully for hemorrhage, especially when sleeping, because a large amount of blood may be lost without any external evidence of bleeding. The physician may be able to control minor postoperative bleeding by applying a sponge soaked in a solution of epinephrine to the site. The person who is bleeding excessively often is returned to the operating room for surgical treatment to stop the hemorrhage.

If sutures are used, the person will have more pain and discomfort than that occurring after a simple tonsillectomy and may be unable to take solid foods for several days. Most otolaryngologists prescribe acetaminophen instead of aspirin for pain after tonsillectomy because aspirin increases the tendency for bleeding.

The tough, yellow, fibrous membrane that forms over the operative site begins to break away between the fourth and eighth postoperative days, and hemorrhage may occur. The separation of the membrane accounts for the throat being more painful at this time. Pink granulation tissue soon becomes apparent, and by the end of the third postoperative week the area is covered with normal mucous membrane. Postoperative care, including patient/family teaching, is outlined in the Guidelines for Care Box above.

## LARYNGEAL PARALYSIS

### Etiology/Epidemiology

Laryngeal paralysis may result from disease or injury of either the laryngeal nerves or the vagus nerve. Some causes include aortic aneurysm, mitral stenosis, laryngeal cancer, subglottic or cervical esophageal tumors, bronchial carcinoma, neck injuries, severing or stretching of the recurrent laryngeal nerve during thyroidectomy, and prolonged intubation of patients in intensive care units. The major diagnostic method is laryngoscopy.

### Pathophysiology

Either one or both vocal cords may be paralyzed. If only one cord is affected, the airway is adequate and only the voice may be affected.[20] Efforts to improve the voice in persons with unilateral cord paralysis have been accomplished by injecting a small quantity of Gelfoam or Teflon into the paralyzed cord. This swells the cord and pushes it toward the midline where the other cord can approximate it better during phonation.

Bilateral paralysis causes a poor airway that results in incapacitating dyspnea, stridor on exertion, and a weak voice. A sudden bilateral vocal cord paralysis is uncommon and is usually a result of a massive cerebrovascular accident or blunt trauma, both of which are usually incompatible with life. Treatment of bilateral cord paralysis is aimed at restoring the airway, not at improvement of the voice. Airway management is discussed under Laryngeal Edema.

### Collaborative Care Management

Diagnostic tests and their purposes are listed in Table 31-6. Depending on the patient's symptoms, one or more of the following medications may be prescribed. If the patient is experiencing gastroesophageal reflux, antacids, which neutralize gastric acid, or $H_2$ inhibitors, which reduce the amount of gastric acid produced, may be ordered.

If the patient has signs and symptoms of an infection, appropriate antibiotics will be prescribed. For patients with swelling of the vocal cords, systemic steroids are often ordered, and for those with spastic movements of the cords, botulinum may be injected.

A tracheostomy may be necessary to maintain the airway. Tracheostomy is discussed later in this chapter. Treatment of cord paralysis may involve excision of nodules or polyps, or a thyroplasty, in which a stent is inserted to reapproximate the vocal cords, may be performed.

Other possible procedures include an arytenoidectomy, in which a portion of one of the arytenoid cartilages is resected, thus increasing the diameter of the posterior portion of the glottis sufficiently to improve breathing.[19]

**table 31-6** *Diagnostic Tests and Purposes*

| Test | Purpose |
|---|---|
| Indirect laryngoscopy | To diagnose vocal cord abnormality |
| Videostroboscopy (observe vocal cord vibration during phonation): fiberoptic laryngoscope is attached to a videotape to record actual cord motion | To diagnose abnormal vibrations of cord |
| Electromyography | To determine innervation and thus movement of vocal cord(s) |
| Computed tomography (CT) scan | To determine cause of vocal cord pareses or paralysis such as tumor or aneurysm along course of recurrent laryngeal nerve |

Adapted from Sigler BA, Schuring LT: *Ear, nose and throat disorders,* St Louis, 1993, Mosby.

## LARYNGEAL EDEMA

### Etiology/Epidemiology

*Acute laryngeal edema is a medical emergency.* It may be caused by anaphylaxis, urticaria, acute laryngitis, serious inflammatory disease of the throat, or edema after intubation.

### Pathophysiology

Acute laryngeal edema causes the airway to narrow or close and requires immediate restoration of the airway.

### Collaborative Care Management

Treatment of acute laryngeal edema consists of administering an adrenal corticosteroid or epinephrine. Intubation or a tracheostomy may be necessary (see p. 903). Edema of the larynx caused by irradiation of the larynx or tumors of the neck may be chronic and may require a tracheostomy.

# TRAUMA OF THE UPPER AIRWAY

## FRACTURES OF NASAL BONES AND SEPTUM

Fractures of the nasal bones and septum commonly occur from relatively minor injuries, such as falls, or from more severe injuries, such as automobile accidents or fights. If there is no displacement of the bone, no obstruction to the airway, and no cosmetic deformity, treatment is not needed. When airway obstruction or bone displacement occurs, simple reduction is performed (Figure 31-12). Most simple nasal frac-

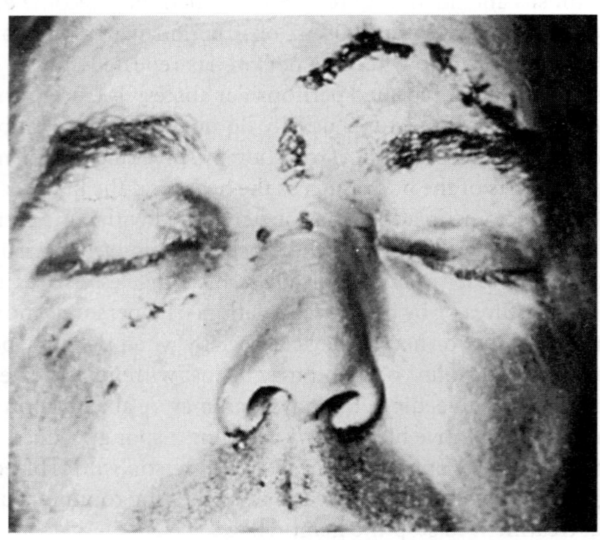

**fig. 31-12** Laterally displaced fracture of nose secondary to trauma. Pressure on convex side will restore alignment.

tures can be reduced by applying firm pressure on the convex side of the nose. Nasal fractures should be reduced within the first 24 hours if at all possible. Local anesthesia is used. After 24 hours the reduction becomes more difficult and may require general anesthesia.

## FRACTURES OF THE MAXILLARY AND ZYGOMATIC BONES

Fractures of the maxillary and zygomatic bones are seen after automobile accidents and fights.[19] These fractures are generally reduced with the patient under anesthesia. Patients may also require wiring of the teeth with all the attendant problems of that procedure.

## EPISTAXIS

### Etiology/Epidemiology

Epistaxis (nosebleed) usually originates from the tiny blood vessels in the anterior part of the septum. Bleeding from the posterior part is more common in elderly persons and is more likely to be severe. In adults, nosebleeds are more common in men than in women.

The most common cause of epistaxis is trauma to the nasal mucosa from damage by a foreign object. Other causes include picking the nose, local irritation of the mucous membrane from lack of humidity in the air, chronic infection, violent sneezing, or blowing the nose. Systemic causes include coagulation defects such as hemophilia, leukemia, and purpura.

### Pathophysiology

Although persons with hypertension do not have more nosebleeds than do normotensive persons, they tend to bleed more profusely when they do have a nosebleed. Nosebleed is usually unilateral, and some persons are more prone to nosebleed than are others. Persons with frequent nosebleeds should have a complete physical examination to determine the cause.

### Collaborative Care Management

Most nosebleeds can be controlled with simple measures (see the Guidelines for Care Box). If these measures are ineffective, medical intervention is necessary. After identifying the site of the bleeding, the physician cauterizes the bleeding point with a silver nitrate stick or electrocautery. If the bleeding point cannot be seen, a postnasal pack may be inserted (Figure 31-13). Because this procedure is extremely painful and may cause complications, patients should be admitted to the hospital. For example, the pressure of the postnasal pack may stimulate the sinopulmonary reflex, causing the patient to stop breathing. In this situation the pack must be removed immediately. If no problems occur, the pack is left in place for 3 to 5 days and then gently removed. Management includes adequate oxygenation, humidification, analgesia, bed rest, blood transfusions, intravenous fluids, systemic antibiotics, and sedation. If the posterior pack fails to control the bleeding, another pack may be placed and the patient may be taken to surgery for ligation of the internal maxillary artery or to the x-ray department for embolization of the bleeding vessels.

Severe epistaxis causes apprehension because of the profuse bleeding from the nose flowing into the throat. The person is kept in mid-Fowler's position and is urged not to swallow blood, because it may cause nausea and vomiting. The position of the postnasal pack must be checked frequently by viewing the posterior oropharynx for bleeding or slippage. Nasal packs may slip out of place and cause airway obstruction. The patient is monitored for signs of complications (confusion, agitation, increased lethargy, and changes in vital signs, especially in respirations and pulse). Nasal packs also make eating and swallowing difficult; a liquid diet is usually better tolerated.

**guidelines for care**

**Initial Care of the Person with Epistaxis**

1. Have person sit up leaning forward with head tipped downward (prevents swallowing or aspiration of blood).
2. Compress soft tissues of nose against septum with finger and maintain pressure for at least 5 minutes.
3. Apply ice or cold compress to nose to constrict blood vessels.
4. If bleeding does not stop with direct pressure, place a cotton ball soaked in a topical vasoconstrictor (e.g., phenylephrine [Neo-Synephrine]) into nose and apply pressure.
5. Instruct person not to blow nose for several hours after a nosebleed.
6. Notify physician.

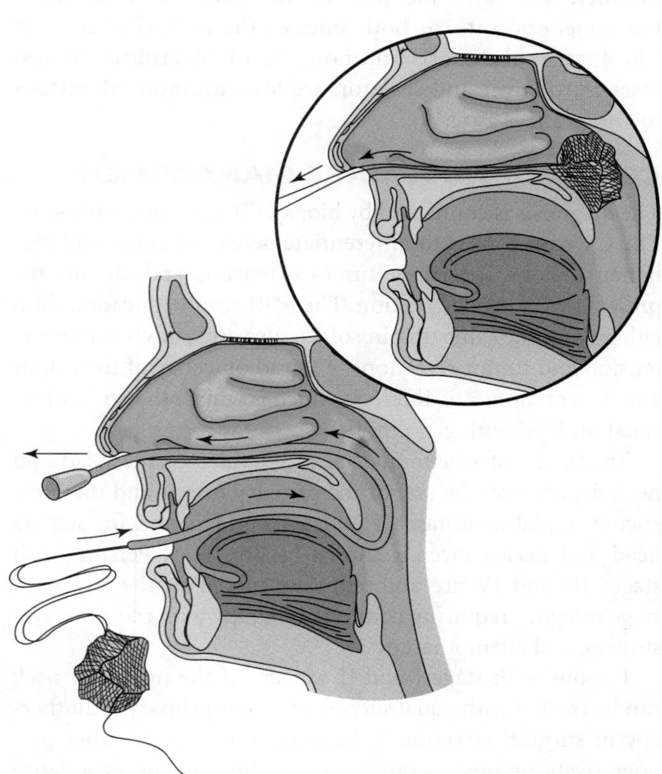

**fig. 31-13** Postnasal packing. Pack is attached to catheter and then pulled through mouth to posterior aspect of nasopharynx.

## MALIGNANCIES OF THE UPPER AIRWAY

Malignancies of the head and neck can occur in several sites, including (1) lip and oral cavity; (2) pharynx: nasopharynx, oropharynx, and laryngopharynx; (3) larynx; (4) paranasal sinuses; (5) salivary gland; and (6) thyroid gland.[15]

### ETIOLOGY/EPIDEMIOLOGY

Ninety percent of cancers of the head and neck are squamous cell carcinoma. The exact mechanism for the development of the malignant phenotype is not understood. Heavy alcohol use and tobacco abuse are considered to be definite etiological factors, with the exception of sinonasal and nasopharyngeal carcinomas.[19] For example, less than 5% of oral cancers are seen in non–tobacco users.[15] The male/female ratio for head and neck cancers varies from 2 : 1 to 8 : 1, depending on the site.

### PATHOPHYSIOLOGY

Squamous cell carcinomas of the head and neck can metastasize to regional lymph nodes. In those areas with rich lymphatic supply, such as the floor of the mouth, tongue, pharyngeal wall, nasopharynx, and supraglottic larynx, metastases occur in 40% to 70% of the patients.[15] There is little correlation between cervical metastases and the size of the primary lesion, because even small lesions may have regional metastases.

The presence of nodal metastases greatly affects patient outcome, and the staging of nodal disease is based on the number, size, and location of the metastases to either the same, opposite, or both sides of the neck (Box 31-3).[19] The lung is the most common site of metastasis. Metastases to the liver and skeleton are less common. Metastasis to the brain is rare.[2]

### COLLABORATIVE CARE MANAGEMENT

The diagnosis is confirmed by biopsy, CT scan, and MRI scan. The CT scan is used to differentiate between benign and malignant lesions, determine tumor extension, and identify the presence of bony destruction. The MRI scan with gadolinium enhances tumor imaging in soft tissues and shows tumor extension and tumor secretions. The radiolucency of the tumor and its secretions are different, which is why both can be identified on MRI with gadolinium.

Treatment of squamous cell carcinomas of the head and neck depends on the size of the primary tumor and the presence of nodal metastasis. The usual TNM system for staging head and neck cancer is shown in Box 31-3. Persons with stages III and IV are automatically placed in the advanced stage category requiring combined therapy with radiotherapy, surgery, and chemotherapy.

Persons with stage I and II cancers of the head and neck can be treated with equal success by either primary radiotherapy or surgical resection.[19] Radiotherapy is given either preoperatively or postoperatively depending on the experience and wishes of the surgeon.

Chemotherapy may also be used, but it is considered experimental. There is no standard chemotherapeutic regimen

**box 31-3** *TNM System for Staging of Head and Neck Cancer**

| | |
|---|---|
| Stage I | $T_1$, $N_0$, $M_0$ |
| Stage II | $T_2$, $N_0$, $M_0$ |
| Stage III | $T_3$, $N_0$, $M_0$; $T_1$, $T_2$, or $T_3$, $N_1$, $M_0$ |
| Stage IV | $T_4$, $N_0$ or $N_1$, $M_0$ |
| | Any T, $N_2$ or $N_3$, $M_0$ |
| | Any T, any N, $M_1$ |

**T,* Primary tumor extent or size; *N,* regional lymph node (number, size, and location); *M,* presence or absence of distant metastases.

used alone or as an adjuvant to radiotherapy and resection for squamous cell carcinoma of the head and neck.[19]

When cervical lymph node metastases are identified at the time of surgery, a neck dissection is performed. In the past a radical neck dissection was performed, in which all affected nodes, lymphatic tissues with the submandibular gland, sternocleidomastoid muscle, internal jugular vein, and spinal accessory nerve were removed. Advances in surgical techniques have led to modified neck dissection, in which an attempt is made to preserve the sternocleidomastoid muscle, internal jugular vein, various chains or sections of lymph nodes, and spinal nerves by themselves or in combination. As mentioned, patients will have radiation treatments before or after neck dissection depending on surgeon preference, the condition of the patient, and the site of the tumor.

## CARCINOMA OF THE NASAL CAVITY AND PARANASAL SINUSES

### ETIOLOGY/EPIDEMIOLOGY

Carcinoma of the nasal cavity has its highest incidence in men between 60 and 70 years of age. Exposure to certain substances has been implicated in some malignancies of the nasal cavity. These substances include wood dust and leather dust (inhaled by furniture workers) and exposure to nickel compounds, chromate compounds, hydrocarbons, nitrosamines, and dioxane. Risk is higher among snuff users, workers in the shoe industry, and textile and asbestos workers.[19]

### PATHOPHYSIOLOGY

When questioned about exposure to the substances just mentioned, the majority of persons give no history of exposure. Most, however, have signs and symptoms of a long-standing chronic sinusitis. Common complaints include a stuffy nose, sinus headache, and facial pain.

Clinical manifestations of malignancies of the nasal cavity and paranasal sinuses are listed in Box 31-4.

### COLLABORATIVE CARE MANAGEMENT

Treatment consists of radiation therapy followed by complete surgical excision of the maxilla. This combination is more effective than either radiation or surgery alone.[19] Some surgeons prefer that radiation be given 8 to 10 weeks before surgery; other surgeons prefer to perform surgery first, followed by

**box 31-4** *clinical manifestations*

### Carcinoma of Nasal Cavity and Paranasal Sinuses

**MAXILLARY SINUS**

Bump on hard palate; nasal obstruction and bleeding as the tumor breaks into the nasal cavity; swelling of cheek with pain; swelling of the gums may cause toothache or result in ill-fitting dentures; if the tumor impinges on the infraorbital nerve there may be numbness of the cheek, increased lacrimation, exophthalmos, and diplopia; more advanced tumors may result in displacement of the eye, extraocular muscle palsy, hyperesthesia of the cheek, and inability to open the mouth.

**FRONTAL SINUS**

Patients commonly have swelling and frontal pain that mimic a sinus headache; pain occurs when the tumor invades bone and causes bony destruction; if tumor invades the ethmoids and orbit, the eye on that side will be displaced, resulting in double vision (diplopia).

**SPHENOID SINUS**

Major complaint is steady, deep-seated temporoparietal headaches; because of its close proximity to the cavernous sinus, a tumor extending into this area causes compression of the third, fourth, and sixth cranial nerves, causing diplopia.

**ETHMOID SINUS**

These tumors cause medial orbital swelling, puffiness of the face, decreased vision, excessive tearing (epiphora), and olfactory complaints; death is caused by direct extension of the tumor into the vital areas of the skull.

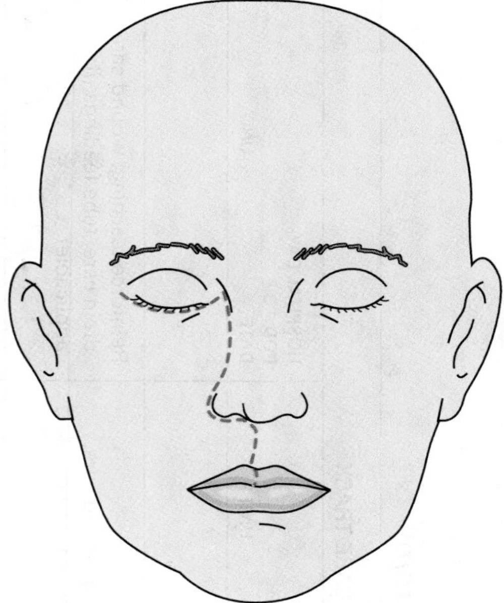

**fig. 31-14** Weber-Fergussonn incision for maxillectomy.

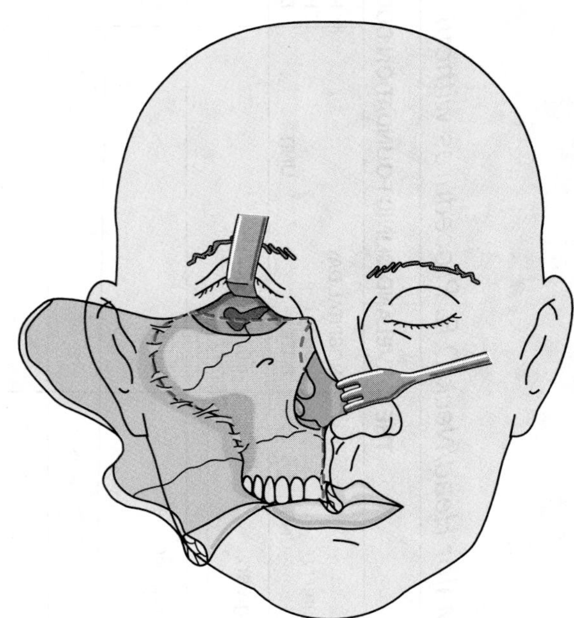

**fig. 31-15** Demonstration of exposure and block removal of maxilla with eye preservation. If the tumor extends through the floor of the orbit, the eye must be removed with the maxilla.

radiation therapy. Chemotherapy in conjunction with surgery and radiation may improve long-term survival, especially in patients with large tumors.[19]

Surgery for maxillary sinus and palate tumors consists of removal of the entire jaw (maxillectomy), removal of the entire palate (hard and soft), and when necessary removal of one eye (orbital exenteration) (Figures 31-14 and 31-15). When possible the eye is preserved. Split-thickness skin grafts are usually applied to the oral defect remaining after surgery. After healing, a dental prosthesis replaces the hard palate and floor of the nose. The patient then has nearly normal speech, swallowing, and appearance. Early diagnosis greatly improves the surgical result.[19]

Radical surgery is required because of the danger of recurrence. Meningitis is a potential postoperative complication, and prophylactic antibiotics are usually prescribed.

Maintenance of an airway postoperatively is critical for these patients, and sometimes a tracheostomy is performed. A Clinical Pathway for a patient who does not require a tracheostomy is shown on p. 886. A nasogastric tube is inserted to ensure adequate liquid and caloric intake, because eating is difficult until the prosthesis is fitted. Several different prostheses are usually needed before a final one fits, because the cavity shrinks as healing progresses. Often they need to be readjusted and sized weekly.

Postoperative care is outlined in the Guidelines for Care Box on p. 888. Persons who undergo radical surgery of this type have a number of emotional adjustments to make. Alteration in their physical appearance is readily visible; the person feels conspicuous and different. In addition to disfigurement, these patients have all the normal fears of surgery and of cancer. Fear, anger, and grief are normal reactions to the situation. Fear is focused on concerns about the future,

*Text continued on p. 888*

## clinical pathway *Major Head/Neck O.R. Procedures without Tracheostomy*

**DRG 49.400 Expected LOS 4 THE CLEVELAND CLINIC FOUNDATION COORDINATED CARE TRACK**

| TIME FRAME<br>LOCATION | HOSPITAL DAY<br>POD Day of surgery<br>DATE UNIT | HOSPITAL DAY<br>POD 1<br>DATE UNIT | HOSPITAL DAY<br>POD 2<br>DATE UNIT | HOSPITAL DAY<br>POD 3<br>DATE UNIT |
|---|---|---|---|---|
| **Discharge Planning** | Identify caregiver: ______ | Screen for ASC | | |
| **Patient Education** | Identify learning needs | | Initiate PERs<br>Begin teaching wound care, drain care, tube feedings (if applicable) | Reinforce teaching: wound care, drain care, tube feedings (if applicable) |
| **Tests/Procedures/ Consults** | | | | |
| **Allied Health Interventions** | | Physical therapy if needed for shoulder ROM<br>Dietician (if on TF) | Physical Therapy | Physical Therapy |
| **Nursing/Medical Interventions** | Monitor vital signs q4 hrs<br>Monitor IV fluids, labs, wound I&O<br>Wound care q shift<br>Drain care/output q shift<br>HOB elevated 45°<br>IV antibiotics<br>NPO vs. clear liquid | Monitor vital signs, I&O, labs, IVF, wound<br>Wound care q shift<br>Drain care/output q shift<br>HOB elevated 45°<br>IV antibiotics<br>Advance diet or start tube feed<br>Decrease IVF<br>Check residuals q4hrs (if applicable)<br>Ambulate with assistance | Monitor vital signs, I&O, labs, wound<br>Wound care q shift<br>Drain care/output q shift<br>HOB elevated 45°<br>IV antibiotics<br>Advance diet/TF's<br>D/C IVF if PO adequate<br>Check residuals q4hrs (if applicable)<br>Ambulate with assistance tid | Monitor vital signs, I&O, labs, wound<br>Wound care q shift<br>Drain care/output q shift<br>HOB elevated 45°<br>IV antibiotics<br>Diet as tolerated/bolus TF<br>Ambulate independently tid |
| **Outcome Criteria** | Vital signs stable<br>Adequate urine output<br>Properly functioning drains/no hematoma<br>No wound complications | Vital signs stable<br>Adequate urinary output<br>Properly functioning drain/no hematoma<br>No wound complications<br>Tolerating PO/TF | Vital signs stable<br>Properly functioning drains/no hematoma<br>No wound complications<br>Increased PO intake vs. advance TF<br>Receptive to teaching | Vital signs stable<br>Properly functioning drain/no hematoma<br>No wound complications<br>Good PO intake vs. tolerating bolus TF<br>Progressing with teaching |

| TIME FRAME<br>LOCATION | HOSPITAL DAY<br>POD 4<br>DATE UNIT | HOSPITAL DAY<br>POD<br>DATE UNIT | HOSPITAL DAY<br>POD<br>DATE UNIT | HOSPITAL DAY<br>POD<br>DATE UNIT |
|---|---|---|---|---|
| **Discharge Planning** | | | | |
| **Patient Education** | Patient/significant other demonstrate care needs | | | |
| **Tests/Procedures/ Consults** | | | | |
| **Allied Health Interventions** | | | | |
| **Nursing/Medical Interventions** | Monitor vital signs, I&O, labs, wound<br>Wound care q shift<br>Drain D/C if <30 ml/24°<br>Diet as tolerated/bolus TF<br>Ambulating tid<br>DC IV antibiotics | | | |
| **Outcome Criteria** | Vital signs stable<br>Ambulating independently<br>Adequate PO vs. TF administration<br>Stable wound<br>D/C home with drain (if applicable)<br>D/C criteria met | | | |

*TF,* Tube feeding; *ASC,* after surgery care-home care program; *PERs,* patient education records; *ROM,* range of motion; *IVF,* intravenous fluids.

**guidelines for care**

**Care of the Person after Paranasal Surgery**

1. Routine tracheostomy care (see p. 908).
2. Nasogastric tube for feeding (see Chapter 40).
3. Monitor patient for signs of meningitis: fever, headache, stiff neck, neck rigidity.
4. Mouth care.
   a. A gentle spray or oral irrigation may be indicated.
   b. Oral irrigating solutions include saline and hydrogen peroxide, weak sodium bicarbonate, or antibiotic solution.
   c. Know where suture line is to prevent damage to it when irrigating mouth.
   d. Because the person may have difficulty in swallowing, it may be necessary to aspirate the irrigating solution from the mouth; care must be taken to prevent trauma to the sutures by the suction. Management of saliva may also be a problem because of the swallowing difficulty.
   e. Patient will have a bolster/bolus dressing or packing in the maxillary sinus cavity. Observe packing to ensure that it is intact and not hanging loose in the back of the throat where it can gag the patient.
5. Adjustment to prosthesis may be a problem because of a poor fit.
   a. Prosthesis causes pressure, leading to pain.
   b. Eating may cause nasal regurgitation and prosthesis may need adjustment.
6. Long-term follow-up after discharge.
   a. Seen weekly for at least 6 weeks.
   b. If receiving radiation therapy postoperatively will be seen for several more weeks.
7. Eye prosthesis.
   a. Have to complete radiotherapy before being fitted for prosthesis.
   b. After radiotherapy, it may take 4 to 6 months for healing to occur and the patient to be ready for the eye prosthesis.

the ability to live normally, and being rejected. Anger and grief are common responses to the loss and the helplessness to control the loss. Oral communication also may be a problem immediately after surgery, and every effort is made to allow the person to express needs and feelings by writing if necessary. Conveying compassion and concern to the person is important.

# CARCINOMA OF THE OROPHARYNX

## ETIOLOGY/EPIDEMIOLOGY

Carcinoma of the oropharynx is second only to laryngeal malignancy in malignancies of the upper respiratory tract. Cancer of the oropharynx is more common in persons between 50 and 70 years of age. The male/female ratio is 5 : 1. The clinical manifestations of malignancies of the oropharynx are listed in Box 31-5.

**box 31-5 clinical manifestations**

***Malignancies of the Oropharynx***

History of prolonged sore throat is the most common symptom.

With a tumor in the palatine arch, ulceration and pain are early symptoms.

Tumors at base of tongue ulcerate later, have fewer nerve fibers, and tend to be discovered later.

Otalgia (deep-seated earache) is a common complaint as pain is referred along the ninth cranial nerve.

Speech difficulties and nasal regurgitation are late symptoms.

Asymptomatic mass in the neck is the first sign of a malignancy in 25% of persons.

## PATHOPHYSIOLOGY

Approximately 90% to 95% of the tumors are squamous cell carcinoma. At the time of diagnosis, nodes are involved in more than 60% of the cases, and in 23% nodal involvement is bilateral. When metastasis occurs it is to the lung, bone, and liver in that order of frequency.

## COLLABORATIVE CARE MANAGEMENT

Radiotherapy and surgery are the treatments for oropharyngeal cancers. Early-stage lesions are managed with excision or radiotherapy alone. Advanced-stage tumors are treated with radiotherapy and extensive resection, requiring reconstruction with skin grafts, local musculocutaneous flaps, distant pedicled musculocutaneous flaps, or microvascular free tissue transfer.

After extensive surgery for oropharyngeal malignancy, the emphasis is on maintaining respiration and nutrition, taking proper care of the graft or flap, and maintaining communication. Edema of the oral cavity or oropharynx can cause airway obstruction, and a tracheostomy is commonly performed. Tracheostomy care is discussed on p. 908. A feeding tube is necessary for nutrition, because the patient cannot swallow properly because of swelling of the mouth, inability to move the tongue and swallow saliva, and weakness. Proper care of the skin flap and the skin graft donor site is essential for a successful patient outcome. Each is discussed next.

### Skin Flap Care

To prevent the formation of a hematoma or serotoma, Jackson-Pratt or Hemovac drains are placed in the incision at the time of surgery. Continuous suction must be maintained postoperatively, and the drains need to be aspirated periodically using sterile technique to remove clots that would interfere with the suction. In some hospitals medicinal leeches are used to reduce venous congestion that threatens flap survival. The patient and family must be psychologically prepared for leech therapy. Adams and Lassen[1] have published an excellent discussion of the nursing role in leech therapy. Pressure on the flap from dressings, tracheostomy ties, and so on is avoided so that circulation to the flap is not compromised.

**patient/family teaching**

**The Person Undergoing Surgery of the Oropharynx**

1. Teach the signs and symptoms of infection (fever, an increase in foul-smelling drainage, change in character of pain) to be reported to surgeon.
2. Teach the patient and family ways to increase protein and calorie intake (milk shakes, eggnogs, dietary supplements such as Ensure, puddings, and ice cream). Keep diary of daily intake.
3. Teach patient and family the need to notify physician about weight loss or change in the ability to swallow.
4. Teach patient and family how to do oral hygiene (use Water Pik or catheter and syringe, and oral swabs to remove debris from flap on graft site).
5. Teach patient and family how to care for skin flap and wound edges and how to eliminate pressure on skin flap so that circulation to flap is not compromised.
6. Teach patient and family how to care for skin graft donor site. (Keep protective dressing on site; avoid pressure on donor site from heavy bed covers and pajama bottoms to help decrease pain. Nurse will make periodic home visits to assess donor site and remove dressings when donor site has dried—usually 7 to 10 days.)
7. Teach patient and family how to care for tracheostomy (see p. 908).

### Skin Flap Donor Site Care

The site is covered with a protective dressing. The outer dressing is removed in 24 hours. There are two types of inner protective dressings: Xeroform gauze and Opsite. Both stay on for 7 to 10 days. The Xeroform gauze is dried with a heat lamp and then soaked in a tub twice daily for 10 minutes. As the edges of the gauze peel, they are trimmed using scissors. Pressure on the donor site by bed covers and pajama bottoms is avoided to decrease discomfort.

Because of the tracheostomy the patient is unable to speak. In the immediate postoperative period the patient may be asked to signify "yes" or "no" to questions by squeezing the nurse's hand, raising a finger, and so on. As the patient recovers, alternative methods, including having the patient write notes, may be used.

### Patient/Family Education

See the Patient/Family Teaching Box above.

# CARCINOMA OF THE LARYNX

## ETIOLOGY

Squamous cell carcinoma of the larynx is increasing in frequency. It is estimated that in the United States over 12,600 new cases and over 3800 deaths associated with carcinoma of the larynx occur every year.[2] Cancer of the larynx limited to the true vocal cords grows slowly because of the limited lymphatic supply. Elsewhere in the larynx (epiglottis, false vocal cords, and pyriform sinuses) lymphatic vessels are abundant, and cancer of these tissues often spreads rapidly and metastasizes early to the deep lymph nodes of the neck.

## EPIDEMIOLOGY

Cancer of the larynx is five times more common in men than in women, and it occurs most often in persons over 60 years of age. There appears to be a relationship between cancer of the larynx and heavy smoking, heavy alcohol intake, chronic laryngitis, vocal abuse, and family predisposition to cancer. Because of an increase in the number of women who are heavy smokers, the incidence of carcinoma of the larynx among this group is increasing. Carcinoma of the larynx may invade deeper structures and cause vocal cord paralysis or metastasis to the neck.

## PATHOPHYSIOLOGY

Squamous cell carcinoma can arise from any part of the laryngeal mucous membrane. It is often preceded by leukoplakia.

The most common presenting symptom of laryngeal cancer is *persistent hoarseness,* often associated with otalgia and dysphagia. Tumors confined to the true vocal cords rarely metastasize to the cervical lymph nodes, whereas tumors of supraglottic and infraglottic portions of the larynx have a 35% to 40% incidence of metastasis to mid- to low-jugular nodes.

*Anyone, but especially any smoker, who becomes progressively hoarse or is hoarse for longer than 2 weeks should be urged to seek medical attention at once.* If treatment is given when hoarseness first appears (caused by the tumor's preventing the complete approximation of the vocal cord), a cure usually is possible. Signs of metastases of cancer to other parts of the larynx include a sensation of a lump in the throat, pain in the Adam's apple that radiates to the ear, dyspnea, dysphagia, enlarged cervical nodes, and cough.

## COLLABORATIVE CARE MANAGEMENT

The expected length of stay for patients having a partial or total laryngectomy is usually 7 to 10 days.

### Diagnostic Tests

Diagnostic tests used to determine the presence of head and neck or laryngeal cancers include direct and indirect fiberoptic laryngoscopy; chest x-ray to determine if there is metastasis to the lung, a second primary tumor, or chronic obstructive pulmonary disease; barium swallow to rule out metastasis to the esophagus, determine extent of tumor, and evaluate swallowing ability; and CT scan to determine if there is metastasis to lymph nodes or adjacent structures. If laryngeal ulceration or mass is found on laryngoscopy, a biopsy is taken for pathological confirmation of the diagnosis.

### Medications

No medications are prescribed after laryngoscopy except medication for pain, if indicated. Preadmission medications such as digitalis preparations or diuretics are continued.

### Treatments

The primary therapy is surgical excision or primary radiotherapy. Patients with early-stage lesions (T1 or T2) that are localized to the glottis have an 85% to 90% cure rate when treated with either of these procedures. Surgery is accomplished with endoscopic laser excision or partial laryngectomy[19] (Table 31-7).

Patients with more extensive tumors (T3 or T4) require a combined approach of surgical resection and preoperative or postoperative radiotherapy. Newer treatment regimens add chemotherapy with cisplatin and 5-fluorouracil along with radiotherapy in an attempt to preserve the larynx. Chemotherapy alone is never curative in these cancers.

If these therapies fail, the tumor recurs, or there are extensive tumors with cartilaginous invasion, a total laryngectomy is required.[19] Some patients will also require a modified neck dissection. A discussion of each of these procedures follows.

#### *Surgical management*

**Hemilaryngectomy.** In hemilaryngectomy, or vertical partial laryngectomy, one half of the larynx is removed (Figure 31-16). This procedure is usually well tolerated; difficulty in swallowing is not a long-term problem, but the patient is not allowed to swallow for 7 to 10 days postoperatively. The quality of the voice is adequate for communication.

Removal of more than one half of the larynx or a portion of the second vocal cord is called a *subtotal laryngectomy.* If more of the second cord is removed, the patient will have more difficulty in swallowing. Thin liquids are the most difficult to swallow, and thickened liquids and soft foods are recommended. Initially, the speech pathologist works with patients on their swallowing postoperatively.[15]

**Supraglottic laryngectomy.** When the supraglottis is invaded by cancer, a supraglottic laryngectomy (horizontal partial laryngectomy) is performed. The procedure usually in-

**table 31-7** *Laryngectomy Surgery for Cancer*

| Type | Description | Voice Result | Swallowing Ability |
|---|---|---|---|
| PARTIAL LARYNGECTOMY | | | |
| Hemilaryngectomy | Opening into larynx through thyroid cartilage with removal of diseased false cord, arytenoid, and one side of thyroid cartilage | Hoarse voice | Initially need swallowing therapy to learn how to swallow without aspirating |
| Supraglottic partial laryngectomy | Horizontal incision passes above true cords (leaving cords intact) with removal of epiglottis and diseased tissue | Normal voice | Same as above |
| TOTAL LARYNGECTOMY | Removal of epiglottis, thyroid cartilage, and 3 or 4 tracheal rings; closure of pharynx with trachea; permanent tracheostomy | No voice | No swallowing problem |

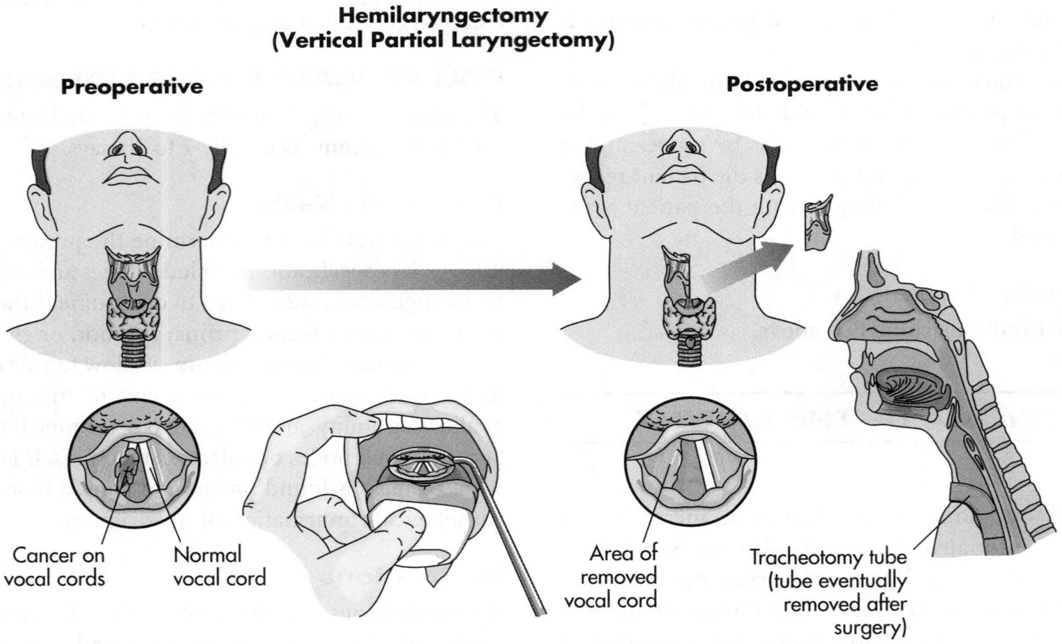

**fig. 31-16** The technique of hemilaryngectomy (vertical partial laryngectomy).

volves the removal of endolaryngeal structures from the tip of the epiglottis down to and including the laryngeal vertical[20] (Figure 31-17). Because the true vocal cords are preserved, the patient's voice quality is excellent. The major postoperative problem is the danger of aspiration because of difficulty in swallowing. Aspiration may occur because the major reflex arc that causes closure of the larynx is initiated by sensory receptors in the supraglottic larynx, which has been removed. These patients will need special swallowing training postoperatively. Patients take variable amounts of time to learn to swallow safely, and it may be 2 to 3 weeks or longer before oral feedings are started.

After partial laryngectomy, a temporary tracheostomy tube is inserted. It is removed when edema in the surrounding tissues subsides. The person is not on absolute voice rest but is advised not to use the voice until the surgeon gives specific approval (usually 3 days postoperatively). In the past whispering was allowed, but it is now believed that whispering can further damage the voice. The person usually adjusts readily to relatively minor limitations of speech. The main problems encountered by persons undergoing partial laryngectomy are those of swallowing and aspiration. Before caring for a patient with a partial laryngectomy, it is important to review the process of swallowing (Table 31-8).

When the risk of aspiration is suspected, methylene blue dye, grape juice, or food coloring is added to drinks and swallowed, and the color is checked for in tracheal secretions. The reader is referred to two recent articles that discuss dysphagia and testing for the ability to swallow safely; both articles help clarify the roles of the speech therapist and the nurse in preventing aspiration in patients with dysphagia.[3,5]

**Total laryngectomy.** When cancer of the larynx is advanced, a total laryngectomy may be performed. This includes

**table 31-8** *The Swallowing Process*

| Phase of Swallowing | Action |
|---|---|
| I. Preparatory | Mastication and release of saliva, with bolus held between the tongue and hard palate. |
| II. Oral | Tongue moves bolus posteriorly, hard palate seals as bolus passes anterior faucial arches, and pharyngeal phase is triggered. |
| III. Pharyngeal | Soft palate elevates and retracts, "blocking" the nasal cavity. Peristalsis of pharynx carries bolus to cricopharyngeal muscle. Larynx closes and elevates to prevent aspiration into respiratory tract; cricopharyngeal muscle relaxes. |
| IV. Esophageal | Bolus passes from cervical esophagus to the cardiac sphincter by peristalsis. |

Modified from Bryce JC: Aspiration: causes, consequences, and prevention, *ORL Head Neck Nurs* 13(2):14, 1995.

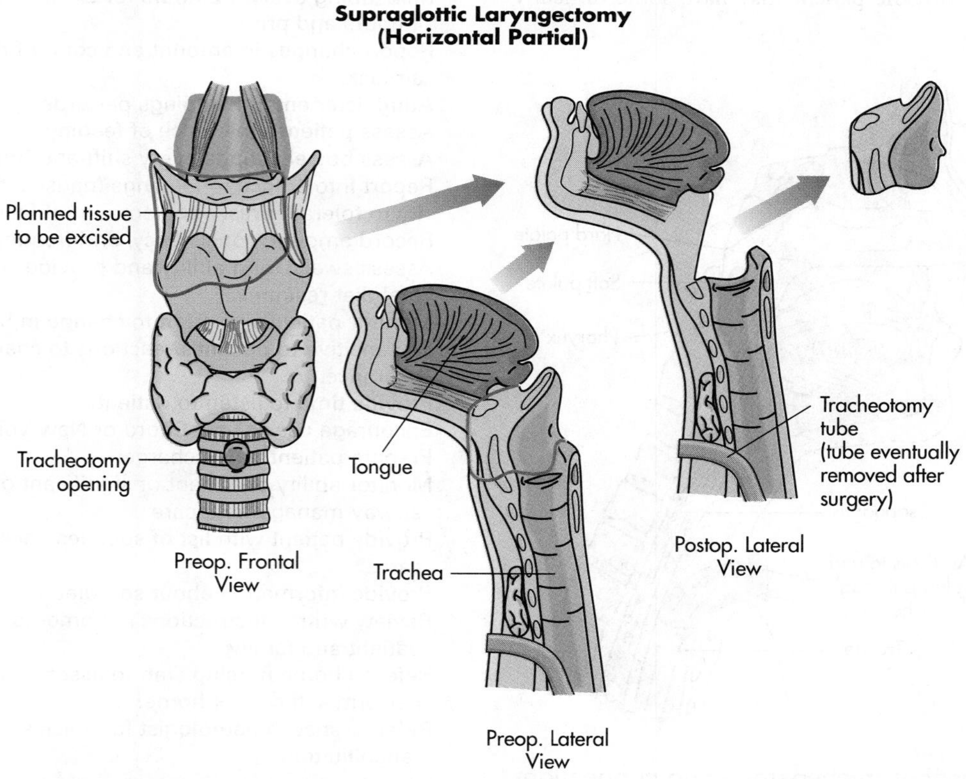

**Supraglottic Laryngectomy (Horizontal Partial)**



**fig. 31-17** The technique of supraglottic laryngectomy. Removal of the endolaryngeal structures from tip of epiglottis down to laryngeal vertical.

removal of epiglottis, thyroid cartilage (larynx), hyoid bone, cricoid cartilage, and three or four rings of the trachea. The pharyngeal opening to the trachea is closed, and the remaining trachea is brought out to the neck wound and sutured to the skin to form a permanent tracheostomy through which the patient breathes (Figure 31-18). The patient loses the sense of smell because breathing through the nose is impossible. Initially, the person has a runny nose because sniffing in and out is not possible. The person has no voice because of loss of the larynx. Nursing care of the patient with a total laryngectomy is outlined in the accompanying Guidelines for Care Box and the Nursing Care Plan.

**Radical neck dissection.** A radical neck dissection may be performed along with the laryngectomy when risk of metastasis to the neck is high. This includes primary tumors whose size and location are known to result in metastasis and palpable cervical lymph nodes found during surgery. In a radical neck dissection the submandibular salivary gland, sternocleidomastoid muscle, internal jugular vein, and spinal accessory nerves are removed to ensure complete removal of node-bearing tissue or to prevent nodal spread.[20] In some patients a modification of a radical neck dissection will be performed. These are referred to as *selective modified, conservative,* or *functional neck dissections* and are used when the nodal metastatic disease is not far advanced. Radical neck dissection causes atrophy of the trapezius muscle, and the shoulder droops on the side of surgery.

Patients can be taught by the physical therapist to do exercises to gradually replace the function of the lost muscles with that of other muscles. Initially, the patient may have some difficulty

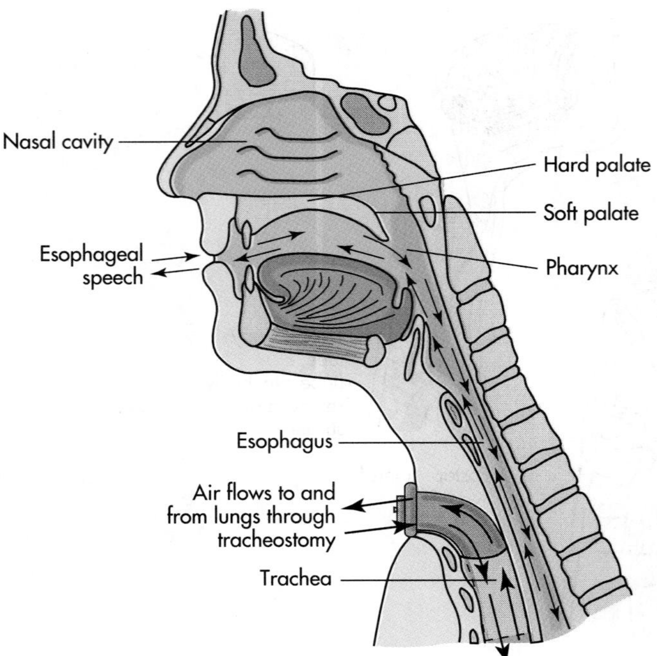


**fig. 31-18** Permanent tracheostomy: no connection exists between trachea and esophagus.

## guidelines for care

### Care of the Person After a Total Laryngectomy

Elevate head of bed 45 degrees.
Encourage coughing, deep breathing every 4 hours.
Maintain oxygen to tracheostomy collar.
Use incentive spirometry if ordered.
Assess airway patency every shift and prn.
Assess vital signs, quality and rate of respiration, and skin color (pallor, cyanosis).
Auscultate lungs every shift and prn.
Monitor hydration and ensure adequate fluid intake to maintain healthy oral mucosa; provide mouth care at least three times daily.
Record intake and output every shift.
Weigh daily at the same time and in same amount of clothing.
Provide stoma and stoma vent care every shift and prn.
Ambulate tid and prn.
Begin teaching laryngectomy care.
Assess anxiety level and provide emotional support.
Assist patient in communicating.
Provide patient with writing materials, picture board.
Use questions that can be answered yes or no.
Reinforce use of artificial speech device and encourage its use.
Assess suture line and stoma site every 4 hours.
Report erythema, purulent drainage, hematoma.
Care for suture line and stoma site as ordered by surgeon.
Monitor drain function and output.
Maintain suction to drain at level ordered.
Milk tubing every 1-2 hours for 24 hours; and then every 4 hours and prn.
Report changes in amount and color of drainage or air leak.
Administer enteral feedings per order.
Assess patient's tolerance of feedings.
Assess bowel sounds every shift and prn.
Report intolerance to feedings (nausea, fullness, inability to tolerate prescribed amount of feedings).
Record amount, consistency, and frequency of stools.
Assess swallowing ability and provide support when oral diet resumes.
Monitor patient's reaction to change in body image.
Be sensitive to patient's reactions to changes in appearance.
Provide time to listen to patient.
Encourage use of Lost Chord or New Voice Club.
Prepare patient for discharge.
Monitor ability of patient or significant other to perform airway management care.
Provide patient with list of supplies necessary for home care.
Provide information about soft diet.
Review written instructions in home-going booklet with patient and family.
Refer to home nursing staff to assess patient's ability to perform self-care at home.
Refer to speech pathologist for voice/speech rehabilitation.

## nursing care plan | Person with Laryngectomy

**DATA** Mr. K., a 68-year-old man, had noted progressive hoarseness for several months. Indirect laryngoscopy and biopsy confirmed cancer of the larynx, and he was admitted for a total laryngectomy. His wife accompanied him to the hospital and planned to be with him as much as possible during his hospitalization. She was attentive and supportive.

The following pertinent data were identified on admission:

- He was visibly apprehensive (pacing the floor, restless, asking repeated questions).
- His major concerns centered on the extent of the cancer and on communication problems postoperatively.
- Height 175 cm (5 ft 10 in), weight 68 kg (150 lb).
- He wears glasses; near vision is poor without glasses.

Before surgery, Mr. K.'s primary nurse spent time with him, encouraging him to explore his concerns and providing information about what to expect in the postoperative period and care that would be provided. After the interaction, Mr. K.'s restlessness decreased and he was observed talking quietly with his wife and watching TV.

During surgery, the larynx was removed; a permanent tracheostomy was performed with insertion of a temporary laryngectomy tube. A nasogastric tube was inserted, to be removed after Mr. K. was swallowing well. During the first postoperative day, Mr. K. again appeared apprehensive (restlessness, pointing frequently to his tracheostomy, pulling on wife's hand, and pointing to the call cord to call the nurse). Breath sounds in the upper lobes were clear but were absent in the lower lobes. Codeine and acetaminophen were prescribed for pain.

**NURSING DIAGNOSIS** *Ineffective airway clearance related to secretions in upper airway and laryngectomy tube*

| expected patient outcomes | nursing interventions | rationale |
|---|---|---|
| Respirations effortless, quiet, and at baseline rate | Place patient in semi-Fowler's position. | Uses gravity to help expand thorax and decrease pressure on lower lobes. |
| Breath sounds clear at all lobes | Suction laryngectomy tube as often as needed as evidenced by noisy respirations, increased pulse and respiratory rate, and restlessness (may only require suctioning every 2-4 hr). | Air blowing through secretions produces noisy respirations; pulse and respirations are increased when oxygen intake is decreased; restlessness may indicate decreased oxygenation. |
| | Provide tracheostomy care. | Keeping tube open will facilitate air exchange. |
| | Provide humidification. | Humidity will help keep secretions liquid for easier removal and prevent mucous plugs. |
| | Encourage deep breathing and coughing. | Deep breathing will help aerate lower lobes; coughing will help expel the secretions. |

**NURSING DIAGNOSIS** *Anxiety related to breathing difficulties and inability to communicate*

| expected patient outcome | nursing interventions | rationale |
|---|---|---|
| Patient rests quietly, does not call frequently for suctioning | Explain to patient and carry out regular suctioning of tracheostomy. | If patients knows tube will be suctioned frequently, fear of possible asphyxiation should decrease. |
| | Develop a means of communication (e.g., cards with needs printed clearly or paper for writing). Be sure patient wears his glasses. | If patient can communicate needs, anxiety should decrease. His glasses are needed for visual communication. |
| | After initial period, and if wife is willing and able, teach her to help with suctioning tracheostomy. | Participating in husband's care may assist wife to feel she is helping, thus decreasing her anxiety (anxiety can be transmitted to patient). |
| | Encourage patient to care for own tracheostomy when feasible. | Self-care enhances feelings of control of situation. |

*Continued*

## Person with Laryngectomy–cont'd

**NURSING DIAGNOSIS** *Pain related to surgery*

| expected patient outcome | nursing interventions | rationale |
|---|---|---|
| Is relaxed and signals feeling comfortable. | Give prescribed analgesic to prevent pain from becoming severe. | Analgesics will decrease transmission and interpretation of pain stimuli. |
| | Encourage other pain-relieving measures such as relaxation exercises or distraction. | Help to minimize pain perception. |
| | Provide nose and mouth care while nasogastric tube is in place. | Tube may irritate nose; mouth becomes dry and uncomfortable from open mouth breathing and decreased lubrication (unable to swallow fluids); also may cause earache. |

**NURSING DIAGNOSIS** *Nutrition, altered: less than body requirements (related to difficulty swallowing)*

| expected patient outcome | nursing interventions | rationale |
|---|---|---|
| Weight is not less than 5 lb from baseline. | Give prescribed tube feedings via nasogastric tube until patient can swallow well. | Tube feedings provide more adequate nutrients than IV fluids; swallowing is impaired initially from postoperative edema of lower pharynx. |
| | When nasogastric tube is removed, give fluids until patient is swallowing well. | Fluids are easier to swallow initially past the edematous area. |
| | Explain anatomical changes to patient (no connection between esophagus and tracheostomy). | This may help decrease patient's concern of choking. |
| | Stay with patient during initial eating of semisolid and solid foods. | He may fear choking and not be willing to swallow initially; encouragement by nurse with assurance of suctioning if necessary may give patient more confidence. |
| | Use measures to encourage eating as necessary (tray for wife so they can eat together, selection of desired foods, etc.). | Return to usual eating patterns may encourage patient to eat. |
| | Encourage him to monitor weight two to three times per week until baseline weight is regained. | Participating in own weight monitoring may motivate him to eat. |

**NURSING DIAGNOSIS** *Impaired verbal communication related to surgery*

| expected patient outcomes | nursing interventions | rationale |
|---|---|---|
| Communicates with others. | Encourage him to communicate via an established system (e.g., electrolarynx, hand signals, writing) during initial period. | With larynx removal, sounds cannot be made by previous method of vibrating vocal cords. |
| Begins speech rehabilitation using electronic larynx. | Support activities of speech therapist:<br>**1.** Encourage practice with device.<br>**2.** Discuss availability of mechanical devices for speech or telephone use.<br>**3.** Discuss TEP as a future goal. Usually occurs 3 months after radiotherapy. | Until he has tracheoesophageal puncture (TEP), electronic larynx will help him communicate. Ability to communicate raises self-confidence. |

*Continued*

## Person with Laryngectomy–cont'd

**NURSING DIAGNOSIS** *Impaired skin integrity related to surgery, malnourished state*

| expected patient outcome | nursing interventions | rationale |
|---|---|---|
| Surgical incision is healing; no evidence of hematoma or dehiscence. | Clean incision using sterile technique. Monitor drainage device for patency. Milk tubing as prescribed and prn. Check appearance of wound and report changes promptly. | Keeping incision clean promotes healing. Keeping drain patent prevents formation of hematoma under tension. Hematoma places pressure on suture line, interfering with approximation of skin edges and possible wound dehiscence, venous congestion, and possible necrosis of flap. |

**NURSING DIAGNOSIS** *Risk for infection related to surgery and poor nutritional status*

| expected patient outcome | nursing interventions | rationale |
|---|---|---|
| Does not develop an infection in suture line. | Clean suture line every 4 hours and prn using sterile technique; monitor negative drainage system for patency. Milk tube as necessary to prevent hematoma. | Keeping suture line clean helps to prevent infection. Preventing hematoma formation reduces opportunity for bacteria to grow in hematoma, which is an excellent culture medium. |

**NURSING DIAGNOSIS** *Knowledge deficit related to lack of exposure/recall*

| expected patient outcome | nursing interventions | rationale |
|---|---|---|
| Describes self-care. | Teach patient:<br>**1.** Description of anatomical changes<br>**2.** Care of stoma, including self-suctioning<br>**3.** Methods to protect stoma<br>**4.** Availability of community resources<br>**5.** Recommended soft diet for 2 weeks after discharge | Providing own care will give him self-confidence; care is needed to keep the tracheostomy open for air exchange.<br>He may be interested in the Lost Chord Club for sharing of experiences.<br>This helps patient develop confidence in eating a variety of foods. |

**NURSING DIAGNOSIS** *Body image disturbance*

| expected patient outcomes | nursing interventions | rationale |
|---|---|---|
| Beginning to accept body change and loss of voice. | Prepare patient and significant other preoperatively for changes in appearance and loss of voice. | Clarify what they perceive surgeon and speech pathologist have told them. Helps determine how realistic their expectations are and allows opportunity to clarify any misconceptions. |
| | Provide time in schedule to sit down with patient and significant other so they can express their feelings. | Allows opportunity for them to ventilate feelings of anger and grief. |
| Willing to attend support group and participate in discussion. | Make referral to other services (speech pathology, social work, etc.) and to support group of patients who have had a laryngectomy. | Supports multidisciplinary approach. Helps patient understand roles of others; allows discussion with other laryngectomees who have had same experiences. |

lifting the head and can lift the head by placing the hands with fingers interlocked behind the head to lift it from the pillow.

The patient can breathe best in a mid-Fowler's position. This position helps reduce facial edema, improve circulation, and reduce or prevent headaches from lymphedema. Pressure dressings are best avoided in radical neck dissection, because they compromise the blood supply to the skin flaps protecting the vital neck structures.[6,15]

Radical neck dissection can be performed without laryngectomy for persons whose primary malignant lesion is in the oral cavity, oropharynx, or parasinuses. Often the procedure accompanies other procedures and is termed a *composite resection.* Composite resections may include either radical neck dissection, in addition to the removal of the mandible; removal of the mandible and resection of the floor of the mouth; or removal of the mandible, the floor

**guidelines for care**

**The Person After Radical Neck Dissection**

Elevate head of bed 30 degrees.
Maintain oxygen mist therapy if ordered.
Encourage coughing, deep breathing, and use of incentive spirometer.
Assess airway for signs and symptoms of increasing airway obstruction (stridor, dyspnea, increased pulse and respiratory rate).
Monitor vital signs every 4 hours.
Maintain venous access with large-bore needle.
If hemorrhage occurs: stat-page physician, apply direct pressure, suction airway, reassure patient.
Care for suture line as ordered.
Maintain drainage function output, color, and consistency.
Maintain suction to drain.
Milk tubing every 1-2 hours for 24 hours; and then q4h prn.
Check for air leak in drain.
Assess for signs and symptoms of infection of suture line (erythema, pus, elevated temperature).
Assess skin flap every shift for signs and symptoms of poor drain patency or infection: swelling, bleeding, oozing of suture line, or dehiscence.
Monitor intake and output and record every shift.
Monitor shoulder droop secondary to loss of nerve supply to trapezius muscle and inability to raise hand over head.
Reinforce need to do shoulder-strengthening exercise 3 times per day.
Consult physical therapist with concerns about patient's exercises.
Monitor patient's ability to ingest optimal caloric intake.
Provide emotional support.
Monitor depression, which is not uncommon after disfiguring surgery.
Identify members of patient support system and involve them and patient in planning and giving care.
Plan for specific time to provide emotional support.
Help patient verbalize feelings about having cancer, changes in body image, and changes in lifestyle.
Monitor for difficulty in swallowing related to postoperative swelling and xerostomia (dry mouth) from radiation therapy preoperatively.
Weigh daily at same time and with same amount of clothing.
Consult with dietitian and physician if desired caloric intake cannot be met.
Teach patient about role of diet in wound healing.
Refer to home care nursing staff to assess patient's ability to care for self at home.
Teach suture line care for home-going. Cleanse site with half-strength hydrogen peroxide followed by antibiotic ointment twice daily to keep incision line free of crusting.
Provide optimal pain management.
Encourage activity.

of the mouth, and the tongue. Patients with a composite resection will usually have a tracheostomy. The nursing care for patients with a radical neck dissection is outlined in the accompanying Guidelines for Care Box. Emotional reactions to this type of radical surgery may be profound. Disfigurement is readily visible, and reactions to the change in body image are marked. In addition to the usual fears of surgery and cancer, the patient having a composite resection may have fears of rejection and fears concerning the future.

Often a Hemovac (Figure 31-19) or another suction device is attached to drains placed in the incision in the operating room. Its purpose is to maintain constant drainage from the neck wound and prevent pressure on the skin flaps. The drain is checked regularly to see that it is working properly and there is no edema, which might indicate that a hematoma is developing. The tubing is milked every 1 to 2 hours for the first 24 hours postoperatively and then every 4 hours and as needed. Changes in the amount or color of drainage should be reported to the surgeon.

### Diet

Diet includes tube feedings postoperatively progressing to soft diet. Protein is encouraged for wound healing.

### Activity

The patient is up in a chair on the first postoperative day and can walk in the hall beginning the second postoperative day.

### Referrals

Common referrals for persons with laryngectomy include social work, speech pathology, respiratory therapy, and physical therapy.

## NURSING MANAGEMENT OF THE PATIENT UNDERGOING LARYNGEAL SURGERY

### PREOPERATIVE CARE

The person who is to have a total laryngectomy is told by the physician that breathing will occur through a permanent opening made in the neck and that normal speech will not be possible. This information is often depressing to the patient, because it may threaten economic status as well as life. The patient will meet with a speech pathologist preoperatively to learn about options for postoperative rehabilitation and speech. In some instances a visit from another person who has made a good recovery from total laryngectomy and who has undergone rehabilitation successfully is helpful. In other instances the visit may depress the patient further. Careful assessment must be made to determine if the person will benefit from such a visit and whether the visit should be made preoperatively, immediately after surgery, or later in the recovery period.

In some medical centers the visit is planned for 5 to 7 days postoperatively. Even though the patient and significant other may be hesitant about the visit, they often indicate that the visit was helpful and improved their outlook about the patient's future.

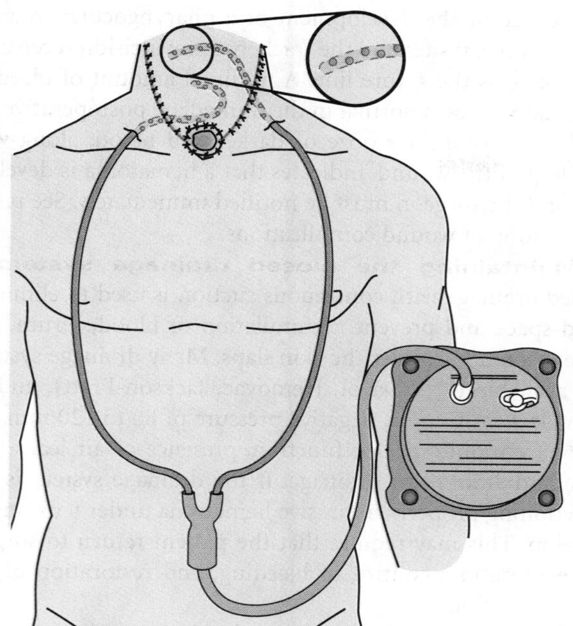

**fig. 31-19** Hemovac apparatus for constant closed suction. In this system of wound drainage, suction is maintained by plastic container with spring inside that tries to force apart lids and thereby produces suction that is transmitted through plastic tubing. Neck skin is pulled down tight, and no external dressing is required. Container serves as both suction source and receptacle for blood. It is emptied as required, and drainage tubes are left in neck for 3 days.

## gerontological assessment

**ASSESSMENT**

Assess nutritional status because many patients with cancer of the larynx have a history of alcohol abuse and may be malnourished.

Assess for signs and symptoms of alcohol withdrawal:
- Tremors: occurs 6-48 hours after alcohol withdrawal
- Seizures: occurs 12-24 hours after last drink; usually are grand mal seizures and not preceded by an aura
- Delirium tremens (DTs): acute complication of alcohol withdrawal; signs and symptoms include restlessness and irritability, paranoia, hallucinations, headache, nausea, insomnia, and nightmares; usually treated with chlordiazepoxide (Librium) or another CNS depressant.

Assess for decrease in hearing and use of hearing aids. Inform all personnel of presence of hearing aid.

Assess for visual changes and use of eyeglasses.

Assess mobility and whether the patient uses an ambulatory assistive device such as a cane.

**INTERVENTIONS**

Work with dietitian to provide a high-calorie, high-protein diet with extra snacks to improve nutritional status.

Encourage physician to order multivitamin, vitamin $B_{12}$, and folic acid daily.

Monitor mental status to determine if patient is exhibiting signs of alcohol withdrawal.

Discuss patient's symptoms of alcohol withdrawal with surgeon to determine if surgery will be postponed.

**COMMON DISORDERS IN ELDERS**

Alcoholism
Malignancies
Pneumonia

Often no one else can give a person reassurance about the return of speech as effectively as can a fellow patient. Many large cities have a Lost Chord Club or a New Voice Club, and the members are willing to visit hospitalized patients. Information regarding these clubs may be obtained by writing to the International Association of Laryngectomees (American Cancer Society, Inc., 1599 Clifton Road NE, Atlanta, GA, 30329. [404]320-3333 or [800]ALS-2345). Local speech rehabilitation centers may supply instructive films and other resources. The local chapter of the American Cancer Society and the local health department also have information. If possible, the family also should learn about the method of esophageal speech that the person will be learning.

## POSTOPERATIVE CARE

Most patients undergoing major head and neck surgery are placed in an intensive care unit or a specialized ear, nose, and throat (ENT) unit because of their needs for intensive nursing care. See under Critical Care Management for a detailed description of the required nursing care.

## GERONTOLOGICAL CONSIDERATIONS

Gerontological considerations can be found in the Gerontological Assessment Box.

## SPECIAL ENVIRONMENTS FOR CARE

### Critical Care Management

#### *Immediate postoperative care*

Most patients undergoing head and neck surgery require care in a specialized unit because of their need for hemodynamic monitoring, airway monitoring, and wound and flap monitoring.[15] The following discussion applies only to patients with a partial laryngectomy. The care of patients with a total laryngectomy is discussed on p. 898.

**Maintaining proper positioning.** To reduce venous and arterial pressure in the neck and decrease the risk of swelling and hemorrhage, the head of the bed is elevated 30 to 45 degrees. The neck is maintained in a slightly flexed position to minimize tension on the suture lines. Some patients will require greater neck flexion or rotation to minimize tension or flexion of the flaps used for reconstruction. The patient is usually up in a chair on the first postoperative day and can walk in the hall with assistance on the second day.[15]

**Maintaining a patent airway.** Some degree of airway obstruction is common in patients with a partial laryngectomy, from either preoperative radiotherapy or swelling from surgery close to the airway.

To prevent emergency airway situations, a tracheostomy is performed at the time of surgery. A cuffed tracheostomy tube is used to (1) allow ventilation postoperatively until the patient wakes from anesthesia, (2) prevent blood from the surgical site from entering the tracheal bronchial tree, (3) prevent pharyngeal and gastric secretions from soiling the bronchial tree, and (4) maintain an adequate airway when edema from surgery or radiation is expected.[15]

The tracheostomy cuff is kept inflated until the morning after surgery or until the patient can manage his or her secretions. When suctioning the cuffed tracheostomy tube, the following steps are followed. To prevent aspiration of secretions accumulated above the cuff, the patient is suctioned orally before the cuff is deflated. The patient is suctioned every 2 to 4 hours to prevent the buildup of secretions in the tracheobronchial tree or in the tracheostomy tube. In some centers 3 to 5 ml of sterile saline may be instilled in the tube to soften and dislodge thickened secretions.

Patients receive cool mist therapy with a T tube or cervical mask. They also receive incentive spirometry and chest physiotherapy (see Chapter 33) and, if necessary, aerosol and systemic bronchodilators.

When a cuffed tracheostomy tube is no longer necessary (not earlier than 3 days postoperatively), an uncuffed tube is inserted. Cuffless tubes are less harmful to the trachea, interfere less with swallowing, and minimize aspiration. Because there is no cuff, secretions cannot accumulate above it. Also, the cuffless tube allows the patient to occlude the tube with a finger and speak, which is a significant psychological boost to the patient. As the patient is able to expectorate secretions and has an adequate airway, the tracheostomy tube is plugged for increasing periods of time (see p. 912). The goal is to remove the tube and allow the opening to close by secondary intention. Some patients' tubes are removed 5 to 7 days postoperatively, when most patients leave the intensive care unit (ICU) and move to a step-down unit. Other patients' tubes remain in for up to 10 days.

**Managing the wound.** In head and neck surgery, complications are always a threat because of extensive undermining of subcutaneous tissues to elevate the skin flaps, contamination at the time of surgery when the upper aerodigestive tract is entered, and the poor quality of tissue in persons who receive preoperative radiotherapy.

Assessment of the operative wound is of crucial importance. The surgical site is closed either with interrupted or running sutures or staples. The site is left exposed (no dressing), which makes it easier to monitor the wound site. The persons caring for the patient need to be familiar with the initial appearance of the wound so that any changes are readily apparent. The viability of the skin flaps is assessed by noting color, temperature, capillary refill, and induration. Slight erythema and induration of the skin flaps are normal in the early postoperative period. The incision should be kept free of crusting and exudates.

The suture line is assessed for signs of approximation, edema, color, and drainage. The incision is cleansed with half-strength hydrogen peroxide solution using clean technique. Cotton swabs are used to remove crusts. Antibiotic ointment is applied to the wound to seal the suture line. Patients who receive radiotherapy preoperatively are more prone to wound dehiscence or the development of a pharyngocutaneous fistula. Drain exit sites and the tracheostomy incision receive the same care as the suture line. A minimal amount of bleeding from skin edges is normal in the immediate postoperative period. A more diffuse ooze of darker, red blood, along with swelling of the wound, indicates that a hematoma is developing, and the surgeon must be notified immediately. See p. 903 for a listing of wound complications.

**Maintaining the closed drainage system.** A closed drainage with continuous suction is used to eliminate dead space and prevent accumulation of blood, serum, and other secretions under the skin flaps. Many drainage systems are available (e.g., Davol, Hemovac, Jackson-Pratt), and all provide a continuous negative pressure of 80 to 120 mm Hg. They are monitored for function, presence of air leaks, and type and amount of drainage. If the drainage system is not functioning properly, a massive hematoma under tension can develop. This may require that the patient return to surgery for exploration, control of bleeding, and restoration of the drainage system.[15]

If air continuously seeps into the drainage system, negative pressure will not be maintained. Air leaks should be corrected immediately. If the air leak is through the suture line, the problem can be solved by adding sutures or applying thick antibiotic ointment to the incision. In some situations a circular dressing is applied to the neck if no reconstruction flap is involved. If the air leak is minimal, the drain can be connected to wall suction. When a massive air leak occurs, the drain may need to be removed. In some situations the patient will return to surgery for closure of the leak and proper drain replacement.[15] When the tubing is milked, the wound is examined to determine if fluid is accumulating under the flaps.

The type and amount of drainage are recorded every 8 hours. The amount of drainage in the first 16 hours can vary from less than 100 ml to as much as 300 ml. Initially the drainage is sanguineous to serosanguineous. The drains are removed when the drainage is less than 30 ml/24 hr. Purulent or granular serous drainage mixed with air (with an odor to it) indicates a probable pharyngocutaneous fistula.[15]

### *Ongoing postoperative care*

Postoperative care of the person with a total laryngectomy is essentially the same as that described for tracheostomy (see p. 908) except that these persons will have a laryngectomy tube in place—a tube that is shorter and wider in diameter than a tracheostomy tube. Some patients may not have a tube in the laryngeal stoma after the operation because the stoma is a permanent one kept open initially by the sutures and because their surgeon believes that there is less tissue reaction and a better laryngeal stoma if no tube is used. If a laryngectomy tube is used, it remains until the wound is healed and a permanent fistula has formed—usually in 3 to 6 months or longer.

A nasogastric tube (inserted during the surgical procedure) is used for the instillation of food and fluids at regular intervals postoperatively (Figure 31-20). The use of a nasogastric tube to give food is thought to minimize contamination of the pharyngeal and esophageal suture lines and to prevent fluid from leaking through the wound into the trachea before healing occurs. The nasogastric tube is removed as soon as the person can swallow safely. The person then needs careful attention in the first attempts to swallow. Aspiration cannot occur because the trachea no longer communicates with the esophagus.[15]

The sense of smell is affected after laryngectomy because breathing through the nose is impossible; therefore the patient does not receive normal olfactory sensations. Some patients report that they are able to smell, and most have drainage from the nose for a period of time. See the Guidelines for Care Boxes earlier in this chapter for a summary of postoperative care of the patient with a total laryngectomy and for postoperative care of the patient with a neck dissection.

Some alteration of appearance is readily visible, which may cause the person to feel somewhat conspicuous. Anger, grief, or denial may be part of the normal response to the change in body image.

**Speech rehabilitation after total laryngectomy.** There are three ways of speaking after a total laryngectomy: (1) artificial larynx, or electrolarynx, which is learned immediately postoperatively; (2) esophageal speech; and (3) tracheoesophageal speech.

Until recently esophageal speech was the primary speech method after laryngectomy. Although this method of speech was successful for many laryngectomees, others could never learn to use it. In addition, the increased use of radiotherapy after total laryngectomy causes fibrous tissue to form, making esophageal speech difficult to master.

***Tracheoesophageal puncture.*** For a number of years, surgeons had been working to develop other forms of speech after total laryngectomy. In 1980 the first successful procedure using surgical-prosthetic voice restoration was introduced. In this procedure a tracheoesophageal puncture (TEP) is made to create a tracheoesophageal (TE) fistula large enough to permit the insertion of a valve prosthesis.

Some surgeons create the TE fistula after the larynx has been resected and a frozen section reveals that all of the carcinoma has been removed. Other surgeons prefer to wait until the patient has completed postoperative radiotherapy. This may be as long as 3 to 6 months after surgery. The reason for deferring TE fistula is that this allows time for edema of the incision to abate. Also, radiotherapy may cause shrinking of the skin around the incision. The TE fistula may require an overnight hospital stay, or it may be performed in an outpatient setting. In this procedure a small fistula is created from the superior wall of the tracheal stoma into the proximal wall of the esophagus.[15] A red rubber catheter is pulled through the fistula into the esophagus at the 12 o'clock position of the laryngostoma and sutured into place (Figure 31-21, *A*). The end of the catheter is occluded with a plug or an umbilical clamp, or a knot is tied in the catheter (Figure 31-21, *A*). The patient is discharged with the catheter in place. The prosthesis is inserted 5 to 7 days later by the speech pathologist or the surgeon. The patient is taught how to speak with the TEP at this time. Figures 31-21, *B*, and 31-22 show placement of the prosthesis.

The prosthesis is a hollow silicone tube with a one-way valve open at the tracheal end and closed with a horizontal slit at the laryngopharyngeal end. When the patient talks, air

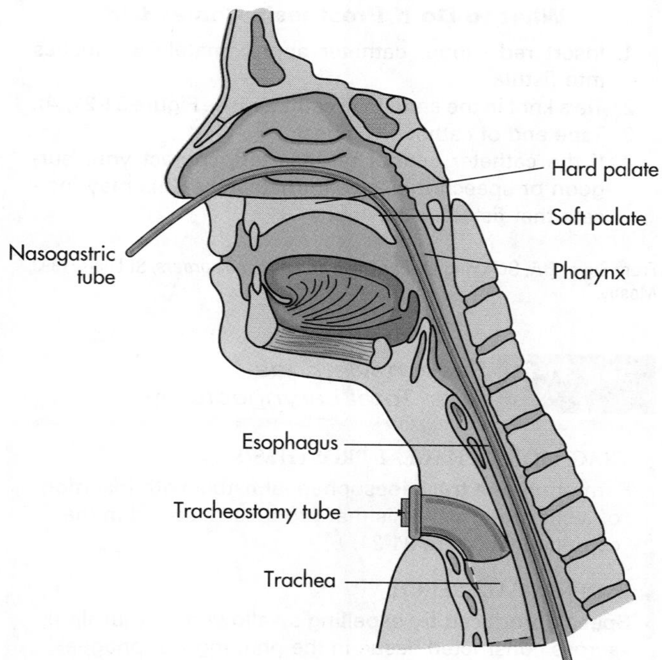


**fig. 31-20** Position of tracheostomy tube and nasogastric tube after total laryngectomy.

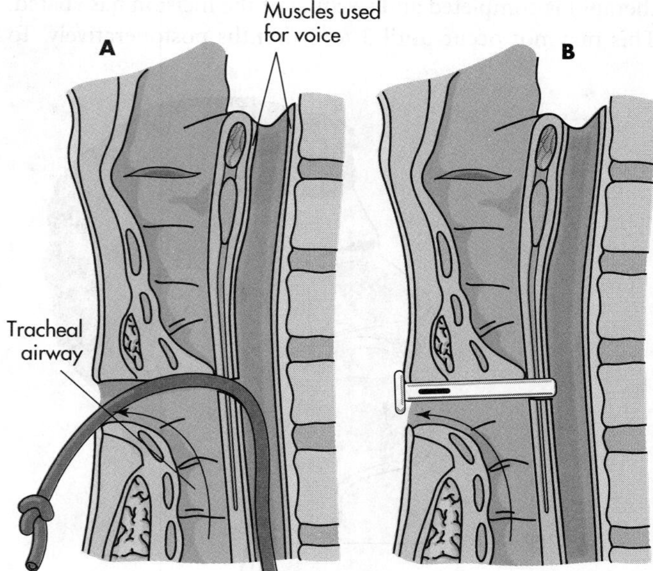


**fig. 31-21** Trachoesophageal puncture (TEP). **A,** Placement of red rubber catheter into TEP. Note knot in end of catheter to prevent passage of stomach contents. **B,** Placement of voice prosthesis into TEP.

pressure opens the closed end, permitting air to enter the laryngopharynx. When the patient stops talking, the laryngopharyngeal end closes, preventing saliva from draining into the trachea. Because air is diverted from the trachea into the esophagus, this form of speech is termed *tracheoesophageal speech.*

The stoma must be occluded during speech, either by placing a finger over the opening of the valve or by using a special tracheostomal valve inserted after the patient has learned to use the prosthesis. The patient or family must be taught to remove, clean, and reinsert the voice prosthesis rapidly so that the fistula does not stenose. Not all patients and families are comfortable with removing and cleaning the prosthesis, and considerable support by the speech pathologist may be necessary. The patient and family need to be taught what to do if the prosthesis comes out (see the Guidelines for Care Box).

Advantages of tracheoesophageal speech include more rapid restoration of voice, speech that is closer to normal in rate and phrasing, and speech that is more pleasing than speech with an electrolarynx. Disadvantages include reliance on a prosthesis and the rapidity with which the tracheoesophageal fistula may stenose.[20] For these reasons, all three methods of speaking are still in use, and none are mutually exclusive. In fact, some patients find it useful to use more than one of the methods (Box 31-6).

Information about devices used to produce electronic speech can be obtained from the American Cancer Society or from the local telephone company. Information about esophageal speech can be obtained from the American Speech and Hearing Association (10801 Rockville Pike, Rockville, MD 20852), the International Association of Laryngectomies, and the American Cancer Society.

The speech pathologist teaches the patient to use esophageal speech after all therapy (including postoperative radiotherapy) is completed and swelling of the incision has abated. This may not occur until 3 to 6 months postoperatively. To learn esophageal speech, the patient must first practice burping. This provides the moving column of air needed for sound, and folds of tissue at the opening of the esophagus act as the vibrating surface. The patient must learn to coordinate articulation with esophageal vocalization made possible by aspirating air into the esophagus. The new voice sounds are natural, although somewhat hoarse. The qualities of speech provided by the use of the nasopharynx are still present. The patient may have digestive difficulty while learning to speak; this is caused by swallowing air during practice, by unusual strain on abdominal muscles, and by nervous tension. Digestive difficulties usually abate with proficiency in speaking.

Most patients learn esophageal speech best at a specialized speech clinic, and some individuals may need to go to a nearby city for this instruction. Motivation and persistent effort are essential in learning this kind of speech. Encouragement from the professional staff and from the patient's significant other is important to the patient's morale. Approximately 75% of all laryngectomees learn some sort of speech, and the average patient can return to work 1 to 2 months after surgery.

One to two days postoperatively the speech pathologist teaches the patient to use an electronic artificial larynx (Figure 31-23). Various mechanical devices are available, and newer ones permit a natural type of speech, providing pitch inflection and volume control. The patient's speech pathologist, the local chapter of the American Cancer Society, or the local telephone company can provide information about purchase of these devices.

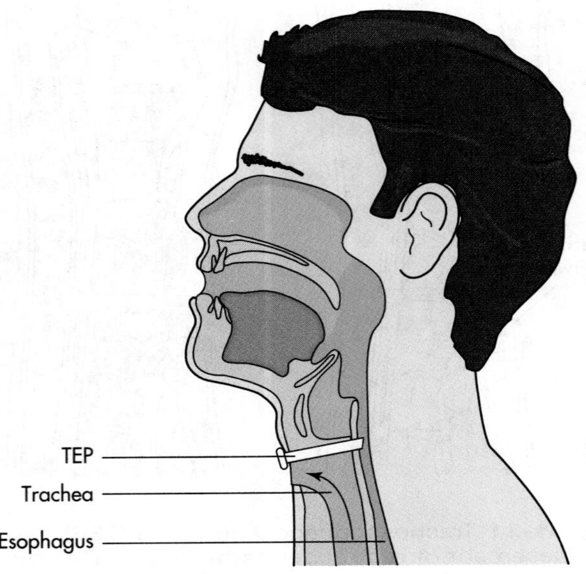


**fig. 31-22** Placement of voice prosthesis in relation to trachea and esophagus.

**guidelines for care**

**What to Do If Prosthesis Comes Out**

1. Insert red rubber catheter approximately 6-8 inches into fistula.
2. Tie a knot in the end of the catheter (see Figure 31-21, *A*).
3. Tape end of catheter to chest.
4. If the catheter cannot be inserted, contact your surgeon or speech therapist immediately. This may indicate that fistula is closing.

From Sigler BA, Schuring LT: *Ear, nose and throat disorders,* St Louis, 1993, Mosby.

**box 31-6** *Speech Methods after Total Laryngectomy*

TRACHEOESOPHAGEAL PROSTHESIS

Formation of a tracheoesophageal fistula with insertion of a silicone prosthesis that produces a sound in the esophagus (Figure 31-21, *B*)

ESOPHAGEAL SPEECH

Speech produced by expelling swallowed air (burping) across constricted tissue in the pharyngoesophageal segment

EXTERNAL SPEECH AIDS

Mechanical devices, such as a vibrator or electronic artificial larynx, used externally (Figure 31-23)

**Reconstructive surgery.** Because of the extensive surgery required to treat malignancies of the head and neck, reconstructive surgery has become common practice. In the past, skin grafts and pedicle or rotation skin flaps were used for reconstruction. Today myocutaneous flaps and free flaps are the major reconstructive flaps used to reconstruct large deficits caused by extensive tumor resection and traumatic defects of the head and neck.[15]

***Myocutaneous flaps.*** Myocutaneous flaps use the axial blood supply that supplies muscle mass, as well as cutaneous and subcutaneous tissue. The inclusion of muscle with its blood supply when transferring the skin allows for a much greater range of rotation of the flap. The pectoralis major, the latissimus dorsi, the trapezius, and the sternocleidomastoid muscles can be used for myocutaneous flaps.

***Free flaps.*** Free flaps consist of harvested tissue separated from the donor site with the vein and artery. The vein and artery are anastomosed to recipient vessels close to the defect (microvascular anastomosis). It is also possible to harvest flaps containing soft tissue and bone to reconstruct the mandible after mandibulectomy.

Close postoperative monitoring of any type of skin flap is essential. Monitoring includes the following:

1. Direct observation, unless the wound is completely covered with a dressing. Some surgeons exteriorize (bring to the outside) a small segment of buried flaps for monitoring purposes.
2. Doppler is used to monitor patency of the anastomoses. The surgeon indicates the area where the Doppler is to be applied. Assessments are hourly for at least the first 24 hours.

To prevent clot formation in the recipient graft, the hematocrit is kept below 30 and sometimes as low as 25 before blood replacement is considered. Some surgeons order low-dose aspirin or even heparin to prevent clot formation. Persons with a below-normal hematocrit fatigue easily because the oxygen-carrying capacity of the blood is reduced.

### Home Care Management

See the Patient/Family Teaching Box on p. 903.

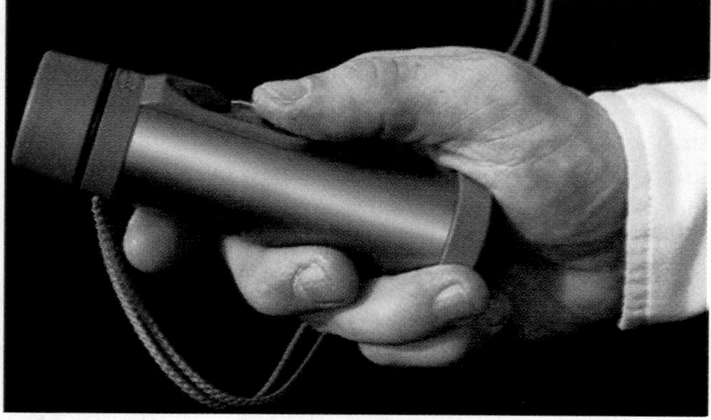

**fig. 31-23** Artificial larynx. Battery-powered electronic artificial larynx for patient who has total laryngectomy.

## COMPLICATIONS

Complications related to the surgical wound include hematoma, wound dehiscence, tissue loss, pharyngocutaneous fistula, and carotid artery rupture. Complications of myocutaneous and free flaps include venous or arterial congestion, flap necrosis, and slough.

## NURSING MANAGEMENT OF THE PATIENT UNDERGOING TOTAL LARYNGECTOMY

### ASSESSMENT

#### Subjective Data

Data to be collected from the patient scheduled to have a total laryngectomy include:

- Complaints of:
  - Pain and difficulty when swallowing
  - Aspiration when swallowing or having a feeling of a foreign body in throat
  - Frequent hoarseness
  - Sore throat on left side of throat and pain in the left ear
  - Shortness of breath (SOB) with exertion
- Number of cigarettes smoked daily and number of years of smoking
- Normal alcohol drinking pattern

#### Objective Data

Data to be collected to assess the patient scheduled for a total laryngectomy include:

- Does the patient appear anxious?
- Body weight in relation to height
- Color of skin, is the patient pale? _____ cyanotic? _____
- Presence of hoarseness
- Noticeable difficulty in swallowing or breathing
- Vital signs: BP _____ T _____ P _____ R _____
- Was patient accompanied by a significant other? _____
  - Relationship to patient _____________

### NURSING DIAGNOSES

Nursing diagnoses are determined from analysis of patient data. Nursing diagnoses for the person undergoing total laryngectomy may include but are not limited to:

| Diagnostic Title | Possible Etiological Factors |
| --- | --- |
| Airway clearance, ineffective | Presence of laryngectomy tube, increased tracheobronchial secretions, crusts, mucus, serosanguineous plugs |
| Anxiety | Threat to self-concept, inability to speak, threat to socioeconomic status, alcohol withdrawal |
| Pain, acute postoperative | Surgery |
| Nutrition, altered: less than body requirements | Swallowing difficulty, malnourished because of alcoholism |
| Communication, impaired verbal | Laryngectomy |
| Skin integrity, impaired | Surgical incision, preoperative radiotherapy, malnourished state |

| | |
|---|---|
| Infection, risk for | Surgical incision, fistula |
| Knowledge deficit | Lack of previous exposure |
| Body image disturbance | Disfiguring surgery |

## ■ EXPECTED PATIENT OUTCOMES

Expected patient outcomes for a person undergoing a total laryngectomy may include but are not limited to:

1. Has a patent airway
2. Exhibits no signs of anxiety (restlessness, increased pulse, respirations, blood pressure)
3. Is comfortable, appears relaxed, and is able to sleep
4. Tolerates tube feedings and does not lose more than 5 lb during hospitalization
5. Communicates effectively
6. Surgical incision healed and free of dehiscence
7. Does not develop an infection in suture line
8. Is able to follow plan of care and asks appropriate questions when reviewing plans for home care
9. Begins to acknowledge feelings about change in body image

## ■ INTERVENTIONS

Nursing interventions can be found in the Nursing Care Plan, earlier in this chapter.

## ■ EVALUATION

To evaluate the effectiveness of nursing interventions, compare patient behavior with those stated in the expected patient outcomes. Successful achievement of patient outcomes for the patient with a total laryngectomy is indicated by the following:

1. Arterial blood gases (ABGs) and pulse oximetry are within normal limits; respirations are quiet and at least 16 per minute; breath sounds are clear. Patient has an effective cough and is not short of breath.
2. Patient appears relaxed, is able to rest at appropriate intervals, and is able to fall asleep without medication.
3. Patient is able to do more of own activities of daily living (ADL) and is able to control discomfort with oral analgesic.
4. Patient is able to swallow, able to eat a soft diet with snacks, and beginning to gain weight.
5. Patient communicates effectively with electronic speech device.
6. Edges of skin wound are clean and approximated well; no drainage from incision; temperature is normal, and white blood cell (WBC) count is not elevated. There is no evidence of a fistula.
7. There is no evidence of infection in surgical incision; suture line has no discharge.
8. Patient demonstrates care of the laryngostoma as it will be done at home.
9. Patient mixes with other patients in a support group, talks about changes in appearance, and appears to be coping well.

## GERONTOLOGICAL CONSIDERATIONS

Special considerations for care of the elderly can be found in the Gerontological Assessment Box, earlier in this chapter.

## SPECIAL ENVIRONMENTS FOR CARE

### Critical Care Management

Critical care management is discussed on p. 892 and in the Nursing Care Plan on p. 893.

### Home Care Considerations

Home care considerations for the person who has had a laryngectomy are presented in the accompanying Patient/Family Teaching Box. In addition, the patient will be seen by a nurse from home care nursing who will visit the patient and evaluate progress. The nurse will also reinforce teaching and assess how well the patient and significant other are coping with the patient's surgery, diagnosis, and change in body image. The patient will have outpatient appointments with a physical therapist for neck exercises and with a speech pathologist for assistance with communicating.

## COMPLICATIONS

Complications are presented on p. 903.

# MANAGEMENT OF THE COMPROMISED AIRWAY

The airway can be partially or completely obstructed by many conditions, several of which are discussed in this chapter. In partial airway obstruction the individual displays respiratory distress and produces sounds such as gurgling, snoring, or stridorous ventilations. When the airway is completely obstructed, the conscious person will have no breath sounds and will display signs of severe respiratory distress progressing to respiratory arrest. Airway obstruction is confirmed in the unconscious person when attempts to ventilate the person do not produce chest movement and no expiratory air passes from the individual's airway.

## AIRWAY MANAGEMENT

The type of intervention used to reestablish and maintain airway patency depends on the individual's level of consciousness, respiratory status, and the cause of airway obstruction. The conscious person with an obstructed airway must be assessed for adequacy of air exchange. If the individual can talk and cough, air exchange is adequate and interventions can be focused on the underlying cause. The conscious person with a completely obstructed airway will be unable to speak or cough and will soon lose consciousness if the obstruction is not relieved. Special maneuvers such as chest or abdominal thrusts and back blows are administered if the obstruction is caused by a foreign object blocking the airway. Organizations such as the American Heart Association and the American Red Cross offer training programs to certify proficiency in these basic lifesaving techniques.

In the unconscious individual the tongue falls back, covering the glottis. Lifting the chin moves the tongue forward, opening the airway. An alternative position to keep the tongue from obstructing the unconscious person's glottis is to place the individual in a side-lying position.

**patient/family teaching**

### Home Care of the Person with a Laryngectomy

The nose normally filters and warms air that we breathe. This function is lost with a tracheostomy or stoma; therefore extra humidity is necessary to moisten the air you breathe. Measures that you can take to increase humidity include the following:

1. Use a cool mist in the room where you spend most of your time. Also use it in your bedroom at night.
2. Cover the stoma during the day with a dampened stoma cover and moisten it when it dries.
3. Wash stoma with a washcloth and warm water and soap daily to remove crusts of mucus that form inside and outside of stoma. Do not use paper tissues to clean around stoma because they may contain lint that may be inhaled into stoma. Crusts that are difficult to remove can be softened with hydrogen peroxide or a few drops of saline solution.
4.* You can use a syringe or eyedropper to instill 3-5 ml of normal saline in your laryngectomy vent or stoma. This will loosen mucous plugs before suctioning. Normal saline can be made by boiling 1 tsp of table salt in 1 qt of tap water for 20 minutes, cooling the solution, and placing it in a clean bottle with a lid. Make new solution every 2 days, because it does not contain a preservative.
5. Keep stoma covered when you go outside to prevent cold air, dust, or pollens from getting in the tube or stoma. Use a scarf, bib, crocheted cover, or shirt that buttons at the neck.
6. If the skin around the stoma becomes irritated, apply a thin coat of plain Vaseline or zinc oxide. Take care not to place it too close to the stoma to avoid inhaling it.

*Other precautions include the following:*

7. You can bathe in a tub or take a shower, being careful to keep soap and water from entering the tube or stoma. A stoma shower guard or a handheld shower can be used.
8. You can shampoo as long as you keep shampoo and water out of the stoma. You may need someone to help you shampoo.
9. Men can shave using an electric or a manual razor. Be sure to cover stoma so that lather and particles do not fall into the opening.
10. You may *not* swim, because water would enter your lungs.
11. Drink at least 8-10 glasses of fluid daily. More fluid is needed during hot weather or when home heating is in use.
12. Avoid persons who have colds or the flu or are not feeling well.
13. Call your physician immediately if you feel like you are getting a cold or other respiratory infection.
14. You can use antihistamines or decongestants, but be aware that they dry secretions; drink extra fluids and increase humidity while taking them.
15. Increasing your activity helps thin secretions and makes them easier to cough or suction up.
16. Wear a medical identification bracelet or carry a card stating that you are a neck breather. Emergency cards stating "I am a total neck breather" can be obtained from your local branch of the American Cancer Society.
17. Persons with a total laryngectomy often have dry mouth and bad breath. Brush with fluoride toothpaste and floss your teeth at least after breakfast and at bedtime. Keep mouth fresh and clean by using baking soda and salt gargle (1 tsp of salt, 1 tsp of baking soda, and 1 qt of water).

**Complications**

Complications related to the surgical wound include hematoma, wound dehiscence, tissue loss, pharyngocutaneous fistula, and carotid artery rupture.

*This step may not be prescribed for all patients. Also see p. 908.

When a person has a mechanical obstruction of the airway and is expected to be unconscious for some time, it may be necessary to use an artificial airway. The methods used to provide an artificial airway are discussed next.

## Artificial Airways

### Oral airways

The simplest type of artificial airway is an *oropharyngeal airway.* The oropharyngeal airway keeps the tongue from falling back over the glottis. This type of airway is never used in a conscious individual, because it may cause vomiting or laryngospasm. An oropharyngeal airway must be inserted correctly to avoid pushing the tongue back against the glottis.

The *esophageal gastric airway* consists of a face mask with two ports. The lower port is for the esophageal tube, which is introduced into the esophagus to prevent gastric contents reflux. The upper port is used for ventilation. The esophageal gastric tube airway is never inserted into a conscious person.

### Endotracheal tubes and tracheostomy

When a person is no longer able to maintain his or her own airway, an endotracheal tube or a tracheostomy is necessary. An endotracheal tube is usually chosen initially as a means of providing the airway; tracheostomy is performed only if airway maintenance is necessary for longer than 10 to 14 days or if trauma to the airway prevents the use of an endotracheal tube. Although the tracheostomy has the disadvantage of a higher risk of infection, it is much more comfortable than an endotracheal tube and allows the person to eat. It is also necessary when a patient requires prolonged mechanical ventilation.

In *endotracheal intubation* a tube is passed through either the nose or mouth into the trachea (Figure 31-24, *A*), whereas in a tracheostomy an artificial opening is made in the trachea into which a tracheostomy tube is inserted (Figure 31-24, *B*). These procedures are used (1) to establish and maintain a patent airway, (2) to prevent aspiration by sealing off the trachea from the digestive tract in the unconscious or paralyzed person, (3) to permit removal of tracheobronchial secretions in the person who cannot cough adequately, and (4) to treat the patient who requires positive pressure mechanical ventilation that cannot be given effectively by mask. Whether an intubation or a tracheostomy is performed initially depends on the facilities available and the wishes of the physician. Most physicians consider it safer to do an emergency endotracheal intubation and then perform a tracheostomy as a nonemergency procedure in the operating room if prolonged support of the airway is needed. The endotracheal tube is not removed until after the tracheostomy opening is made.

A tracheostomy is necessary when an endotracheal tube cannot be inserted or when it is contraindicated, as in severe burns or laryngeal obstruction caused by tumor, infection, or vocal cord paralysis. Once the airway is secured, either by intubation or tracheostomy, secretions are aspirated, and well-humidified oxygen is usually given. If the patient is unable to sustain respiration, a mechanical ventilator is attached to either the endotracheal tube or the tracheostomy tube (see Chapter 32). When mechanical ventilation is required, a cuffed tube is used. Usually an endotracheal tube is not left in place longer than 10 to 14 days. If the patient is unable to maintain a patent airway after this period of time, a tracheostomy is performed.

The endotracheal tube is made of plastic with an inflatable cuff so that a closed system with the ventilator may be maintained (Figure 31-25). The tube is inserted via the mouth or nose through the larynx into the trachea. If an oral endotracheal tube is used, a rubber airway or bite block is often necessary to prevent the patient from biting down on the tube and obstructing the airway.

Two potentially fatal complications can occur in patients with endotracheal tubes: accidental extubation and displacement of the endotracheal tube. Tips of endotracheal tubes have been shown to shift as much as 2 cm in the trachea when patients flex or extend their necks or laterally tip their heads. Usually the endotracheal tube is affixed to the patient's face with waterproof tape above and below the lips and around the endotracheal tube to keep it in place. This method can cause facial skin breakdown, especially in patients with leukemia or who are immunosuppressed. For this reason, commercially available endotracheal tube holders that use no tape are available[13] (Figures 31-26 through 31-28). A research study compared these holders with the tape method known as the Lillihei harness, after the surgeon who designed it (see the Research Box, p. 906).

Tracheostomy tubes are usually made of silicone, pliable plastic, or metal. They may have only a single lumen or may have both an inner and an outer cannula (Figure 31-29).

Most adult-sized plastic tubes have a cuff that is inflated with air to fill the space between the outside of the tube and the trachea when a sealed airway is desired for mechanical ventilation. Usually tracheostomy tubes do not need to be changed more often than every 2 to 3 weeks. Low-pressure cuffs are less likely to cause damage to the trachea. When secretions are thick and copious the tube may have to be changed weekly or more frequently. Some tracheostomy tubes have a single lumen; others have both an inner and an outer cannula. The outer cannula is changed only by the physician or a specially prepared nurse; the inner cannula is removed regularly by the nurse for cleaning. Twill tapes are attached to each side of the tube and tied securely on the side of the neck to prevent the tube from becoming dislodged when the patient coughs or moves. The tapes are

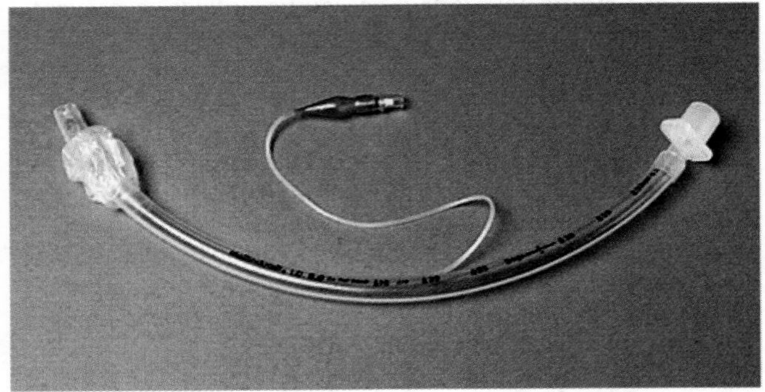

fig. 31-25 Endotracheal tube.

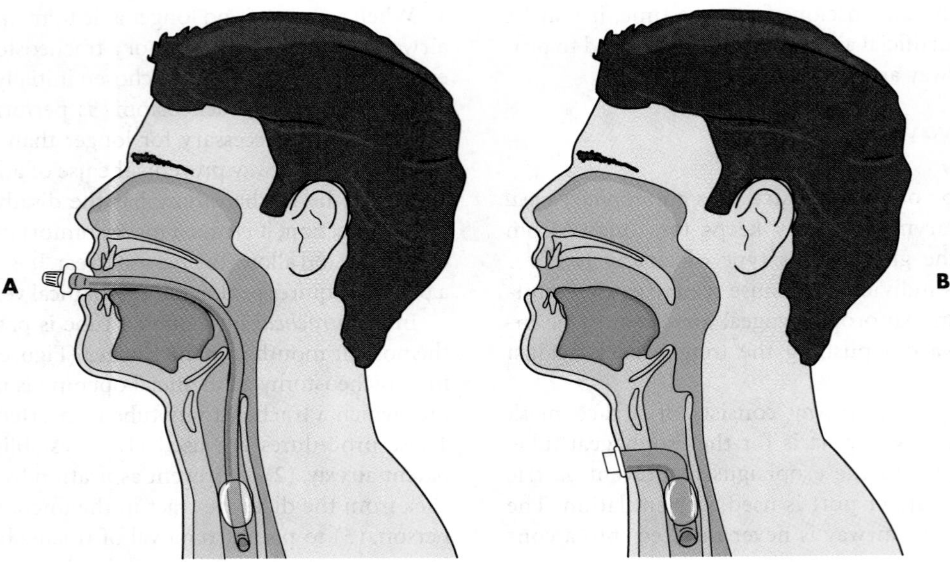


fig. 31-24 A, Position of endotracheal tube. B, Position of tracheostomy tube.

not tied behind the patient's neck because lying on the knot may cause skin irritation and a pressure sore.

Should the tracheostomy tube be coughed out, the opening may close, and the patient will be unable to breathe through it. Therefore a tracheal dilator or curved hemostat is kept at the bedside so that the opening can be held open until the physician arrives to insert a new tracheostomy tube. Some surgeons prefer to place a retention suture on each side of the tracheostomy opening and tape the end of the suture to the skin. If the opening shows signs of closing, tension can be placed on the sutures to widen the opening.

A small dressing may be placed under the tracheostomy tube. Although drainage should be minimal, the wound is inspected frequently for bleeding during the immediate postoperative period. The dressings are changed as they become soiled with mucous drainage.

Depending on the patient's condition, a tracheostomy can be either temporary or permanent; the person who has a total laryngectomy will have a permanent tracheostomy. Any patient who has had a tracheostomy is apprehensive and is often fearful of choking. Thus when feasible, the procedure is thoroughly explained to the patient before surgery. Both patient and family need to understand that the patient will be unable to speak, that the nurses will be able to communicate with the patient, and that constant attendance will be provided until the patient can manage his or her own airway safely.

A fenestrated tracheostomy tube has an opening on the upper surface of the outer cannula that allows air inspired through the nose and mouth to pass through the tube. When the external opening is plugged, air can pass over the vocal cords, allowing the individual to talk. If ventilatory assistance is required, the inner cannula can be inserted so that the patient can be connected to a mechanical ventilator.

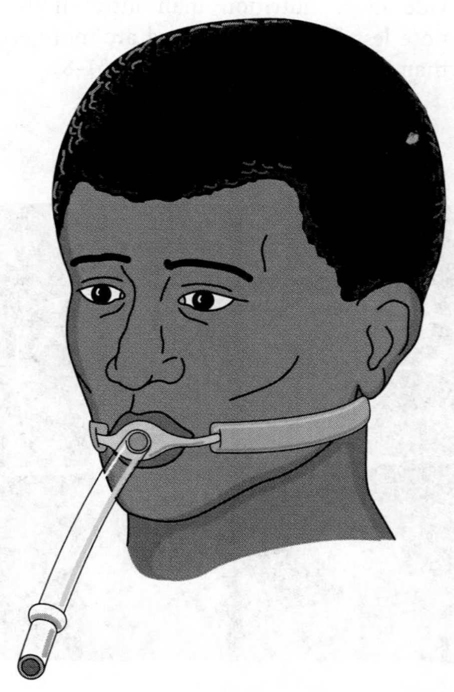

**fig. 31-26** Comfit endotracheal tube holder.

## CRITICAL CARE MANAGEMENT OF THE PERSON WHO HAS AN ENDOTRACHEAL OR A TRACHEOSTOMY TUBE

An endotracheal or tracheostomy tube provides a direct route for introduction of pathogens into the lower airway, increasing the risk of infection. It is essential that the

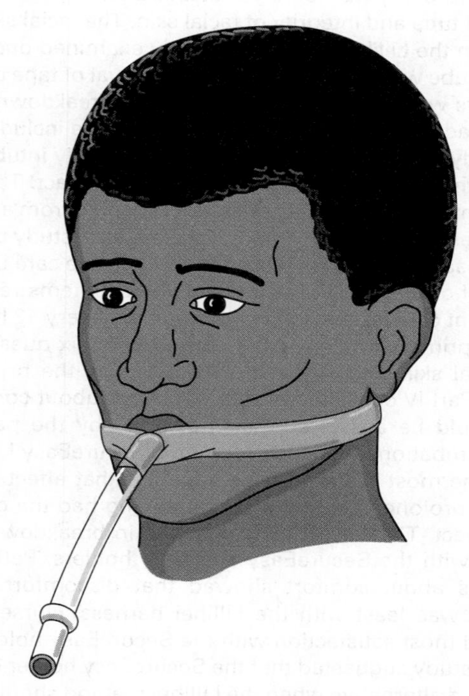

**fig. 31-27** Dale endotracheal tube holder.

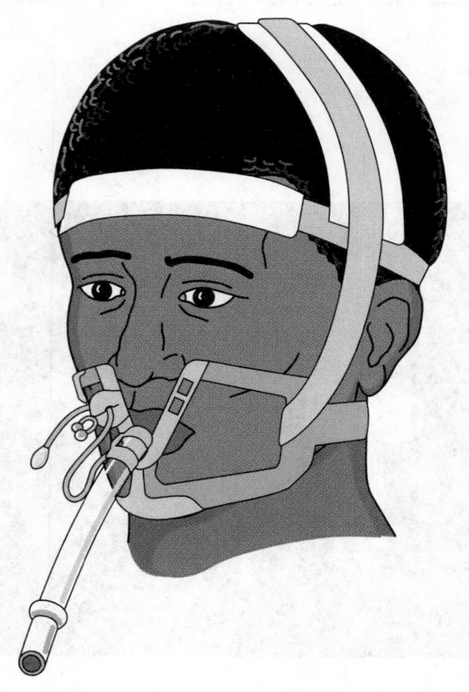

**fig. 31-28** SecureEasy endotracheal tube holder.

## research

Reference: Kaplow R, Bookbinder M: A comparison of four endotracheal tube holders, *Heart Lung* 23(1):59, 1994.

The purpose of this study was to compare four methods (Lillihei harness, Comfit, Dale, and SecureEasy) of securing endotracheal tubes in orally intubated adult patients in one intensive care unit.

The sample consisted of 121 patients. Subjects were evaluated every 12 hours for stabilization of the endotracheal tube and integrity of facial skin. The facial skin of those on the Lillihei method was only examined once after the tube was removed, because removal of tape every 12 hours would increase the risk of skin breakdown. Patients had to meet the following criteria to be included in the study: (1) at least 18 years of age, (2) orally intubated within the last 8 hours, and (3) facial skin intact. The instrument used to collect the data was adapted from a four-part questionnaire developed by Tasota for a study of endotracheal tube holders in a surgical intensive care unit.

Part II of the questionnaire contained 20 items related to patient care issues and was completed every 12 hours by the primary nurse. Part III consisted of six questions on facial skin integrity also completed by the primary nurse. Part IV consisted of four questions about comfort that could be answered "yes" or "no" by the patient after extubation. The study found the SecureEasy holder to be the most secure. Of the variables that affect extubation, prolonged coughing and gagging had the greatest impact. The fewest incidents of skin breakdown occurred with the SecureEasy and Dale holders. Patients' answers about comfort showed that discomfort with turning was least with the Lillihei harness. Nurses expressed most satisfaction with the SecureEasy holder.

This study suggested that the SecureEasy holder is the preferred alternative when the Lillihei method should not be used because of the potential for skin breakdown when tape is used on the face.

following preventive nursing interventions be consistently implemented.

1. Minimize infection risk.
   a. Endotracheal airways irritate the trachea, resulting in increased mucus production. Assess the patient regularly for excess secretions, and suction as often as necessary to maintain a patent airway. See Box 31-7 for sterile suctioning procedure.
   b. Provide constant airway humidification. Endotracheal airways bypass the upper airway, which normally humidifies and warms inspired air. An external source of cool, humidified air must be provided to avoid thickening and crusting of bronchial secretions.
   c. All respiratory therapy equipment should be changed every 24 hours. In addition:
      (1) Replace any equipment that touches the floor.
      (2) Remove water that condenses in equipment tubing. Do not pour condensed water back into humidifier reservoir because it may contain pathogens.
   d. Provide frequent mouth care. Secretions tend to pool in the mouth and in the pharynx, particularly if the cuff of the tube is inflated. An endotracheal tube or oral airway increases the risk of ulceration or abrasion of the lips and oropharynx.
      (1) Gently suction oropharynx as needed.
      (2) Inspect the lips, tongue, and oral cavity regularly.
      (3) Clean the oral cavity with swabs soaked in saline.
      (4) Apply moisturizing agent to cracked lips.
   e. Maintain adequate nutritional levels.
      (1) The person with an endotracheal tube is allowed nothing by mouth. Nourishment will be given parenterally or by gastrointestinal feedings. Gastrointestinal supplemental feedings are preferred because they maintain the function of the gut, provide more nutrition than intravenous feedings, pose less infection risk, and are more economical than intravenous feedings (Box 31-8).

A 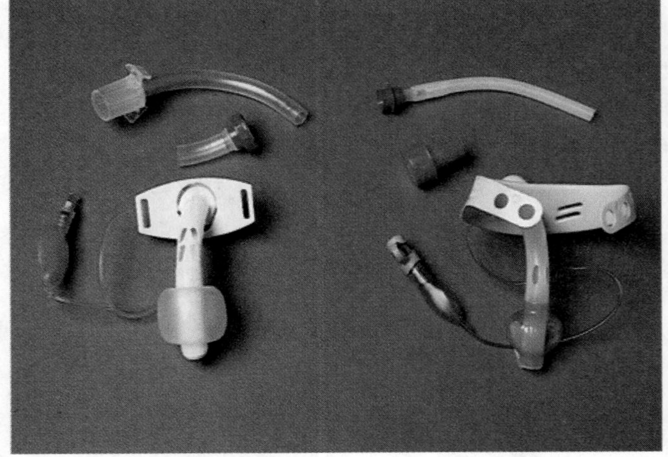

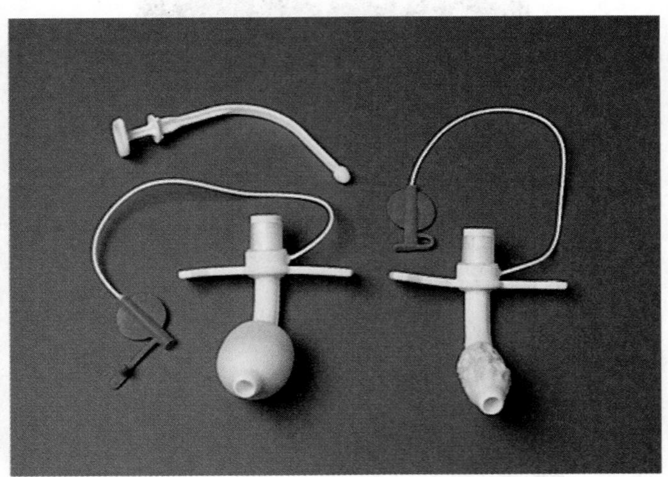 B

**fig. 31-29** Types of tracheostomy tubes. **A,** Shiley and Portex fenestrated tracheostomy tube with cuff, inner cannula, decannulation plug, and pilot balloon. **B,** Bivona (Fome) tracheostomy tube with foam cuff and obturator (cuff is inflated on tube to the left).

**box 31-7** *Performing Endotracheal or Tracheostomy Suctioning*

1. All persons with endotracheal or tracheostomy tubes require suctioning when necessary. The frequency of suctioning is determined by auscultation and observation of the patient. Much of the ability to produce an effective cough is lost, because it is impossible for the person who is intubated to build up the pressure needed to create an explosive cough.
2. The mouth and oropharynx above the cuff are suctioned first. This catheter is discarded and a sterile catheter is used to suction the trachea. It may not be necessary to deflate the cuff each time the patient is suctioned. The nurse may wish to deflate the cuff once per shift to remove pooled secretions above the cuff and ensure that the cuff is properly sealed. When the nurse is ready to suction, the cuff is deflated while the patient is exhaling to prevent aspiration of secretions into the tracheobronchial tree.
3. Suction as deeply as possible. In an adult a catheter can be introduced through an endotracheal tube approximately 45 to 55 cm (18 to 22 in.). The recommended depth through the tracheostomy tube is 20 to 30 cm (8 to 12 in.). The diameter of the suction catheter should be approximately one half the diameter of the tube.
4. A fenestrated catheter with a whistle tip is attached to the suction outlet. The catheter is inserted without suction. When the catheter is in place, suction is applied by placing the thumb over the fenestration in the catheter.
5. Before beginning suctioning the patient is hyperoxygenated with 100% oxygen. The ventilator or an Ambu, anesthesia, or Laerdal bag is used to deliver three breaths of 100% oxygen, one every 5 seconds. Preoxygenation is necessary because oxygen is removed during suctioning.
6. The suction catheter is lubricated with sterile water or a water-soluble lubricant. Suctioning usually stimulates coughing in the patient with a tracheostomy. If the patient coughs, the catheter is removed, because it obstructs the trachea and the patient must exert extra pressure to cough around it. When coughing occurs, the nurse or patient should have tissues ready to receive mucus, which may be forcefully ejected.
7. To prevent hypoxia, the patient is not suctioned longer than 10 seconds at a time and should rest 1 to 2 minutes between aspirations, with 100% oxygen administered between suctioning. The number of aspirations is limited to no more than three (two, if possible).
8. The patient is monitored for signs of hypoxia, such as tachycardia, bradycardia, or ectopic beats.

(2) The patient with a tracheostomy tube is usually able to swallow and have a normal oral intake. Some experts prefer that the cuff on the tracheostomy tube be inflated while the patient is eating to prevent aspiration. Others believe that the inflated cuff bulges into the esophagus and makes swallowing more difficult, and they therefore prefer that the cuff be deflated. Nursing assessment will determine which technique to use. Methylene blue dye can be swallowed before each feeding or mixed with the tube

**box 31-8** *Administering Gastrointestinal Feedings to the Intubated Patient*

1. Assess for bowel sounds and tube placement.
2. Elevate head of bed at least 45 degrees.
3. a. Inflate the tracheostomy tube cuff.
   b. If using a Salem sump nasogastric tube, check the amount of residual feeding. If half the volume of the feeding to be given remains, the tube feeding is withheld.
4. a. Administer the tube feeding over 20-30 minutes.
   b. Keep head of bed elevated for 45-60 minutes after feeding.
5. Assess at regular intervals for aspiration.
6. Regularly assess for tube placement and residual stomach contents.

feeding. If the dye does not appear in tracheal secretions, it is safe to proceed with the meal.

2. Ensure adequate ventilation and oxygenation.
   a. Assess lung sounds regularly. Unless the individual's underlying lung pathology alters lung ventilation, breath sounds should be heard bilaterally, and chest expansion should be symmetrical. If an endotracheal tube is inserted too far it will slip into one of the main-stem bronchi (usually the right) and occlude the opposite bronchus and lung, resulting in atelectasis on the obstructed side. Even if the endotracheal tube is still in the trachea, airway obstruction will result if the end of the tube is located on the carina (area at lower end of trachea at point of bifurcation of main-stem bronchi). This will result in dry secretions that obstruct both bronchi. Although these complications are more common with the use of an endotracheal tube, they can occur with a tracheostomy tube, especially in a small person with a short neck. In either situation the tube is pulled back until it is positioned below the larynx and above the carina. The tube is then fastened securely in place.
   b. Turn and reposition the patient every 2 hours for maximum ventilation and lung perfusion.
   c. Assess respiratory frequency, tidal volume, and vital capacity.
   d. Perform postural drainage, percussion, and vibration as appropriate.
3. Provide safety and comfort.
   a. Most endotracheal and tracheostomy tubes have cuffs for the following reasons:
      (1) To provide a sealed airway for positive pressure mechanical ventilation.
      (2) To prevent aspiration in the unconscious person, during tube feedings.
   b. Assess tube placement at regular intervals.
      (1) The tube is secured around neck with tape or specially designed ties.
      (2) The endotracheal tube is marked to establish a landmark for position comparison and to measure and document the length of tube that extends beyond the patient's lips.
   c. Change tapes or ties whenever soiled to decrease skin irritation.

d. Always keep a spare tube at the bedside.
e. Minimize sensory deprivation.
(1) Patients with endotracheal tubes or tracheostomy tubes with the cuff inflated cannot talk. Therefore an acceptable communication mode must be established.
(a) Organize questions so the patient can use a simple "yes" or "no" response (nodding head, using hand signals, or squeezing the nurse's hand).
(b) The patient may be able to use an erasable board or note pad to communicate.
(c) Always talk to the patient and explain all procedures.
(d) Reorient the patient frequently.
(e) Encourage family and friends to talk to the patient and offer encouragement.
(f) Keep call light (or tap bell) within patient's reach.
(g) Reinforce that the ability to speak will return when the tube is removed.

4. Observe special precautions during the immediate extubation period.
a. Monitor for signs such as increased respiratory distress, increased restlessness, hoarseness, and laryngeal stridor indicating upper airway obstruction secondary to laryngeal edema.
b. Assess for adequacy of cough and gag reflex.
c. After removal of a tracheostomy tube there is a temporary air leak at the incision site. To speak, the patient will have to occlude the opening with a finger.
d. The tracheal stoma can be suctioned. However, frequent use of the stoma for suctioning can delay closure and healing of the tracheostomy incision.

Although the low-pressure cuffs used today reduce the risk of tracheal wall damage, it is important to inflate the cuff with the correct amount of air (Box 31-9).

**box 31-9** *Inflating an Endotracheal or Tracheostomy Cuff*

The cuff should be inflated to a volume that provides adequate occlusion around the tube without increasing the risk of tracheomalacia, tracheal stenosis, tracheoesophageal fistula, or erosion through a major blood vessel. Many experts recommend the "minimal leak technique," which follows.

1. Using a 10 or 20 ml syringe, slowly inject air into cuff.
2. As air is introduced, assess for air leak around tube. This is determined by (1) ability of patient to talk or make sounds, and (2) nurse being able to feel air coming from patient's nose or mouth.
3. When the airway is sealed and no passage of air around the tube can be detected, remove 0.5 ml of air. This creates a "minimal leak" and ensures that the lowest possible pressure is being exerted on the tracheal wall.
4. Auscultate over the trachea while ventilating the patient with either an Ambu bag or a mechanical ventilator. A small amount of air should be heard gurgling past the cuff.
5. If an adequate seal cannot be obtained with 25 ml of air, notify the physician.
6. The exact pressure in the cuff can be measured by connecting the pilot balloon to a handheld meter. To do this, the balloon is inflated with a syringe, in the normal fashion, until a seal is obtained. The syringe is removed and the meter attached. The meter reading, in cm $H_2O$, is then recorded, and the pressure in the cuff is checked each shift to ensure consistency.

## CARE OF THE PERSON WITH A TRACHEOSTOMY

Although nursing care of persons with either endotracheal or tracheostomy tubes is similar, patients with tracheostomies have additional nursing care needs. (See the Clinical Pathway for a simple tracheostomy.) Analgesics and sedatives are given judiciously so as not to depress the respiratory center. The patient is suctioned as often as necessary. Every 1 to 2 hours may be sufficient. The need for suctioning can be determined by the sound of the air coming from the tracheostomy tube, especially after the patient takes a deep breath. When respirations are noisy and pulse and respiratory rates are increased, the patient needs to be suctioned. Patients who are conscious can usually indicate when they need to be suctioned. With any sign of respiratory distress, such as an increase in pulse or respirations, the tube should be suctioned. If mucus is blocking the inner cannula of the tracheostomy tube and cannot be removed by suction, the inner cannula is removed to open the airway. When the mucus is thick, the inner cannula should be cleaned and replaced at once because the outer tube may also become blocked. If, despite these measures, the patient becomes cyanotic, the physician should be summoned at once. A patient who is able to cough up his or her own secretions probably will require suctioning less frequently. The amount of mucus subsides gradually, and the patient eventually may go for several hours without being suctioned. However, even when secretions are minimal, the patient is apprehensive and needs constant attendance.

For about 25 years it has been a common practice to instill normal saline into tracheostomy or endotracheal tubes before suctioning. The reason for this practice was the belief that this would thin secretions and make them easier to remove when suctioning. This practice has been questioned because there is no scientific evidence to support it. At the same time, many nurses who care for patients undergoing head and neck surgery believe that the instillation of a 5 ml bolus of normal saline before suctioning improves airway patency. A recent nursing research study concluded that "using normal saline instillation as part of the suctioning procedure significantly enhanced mobilizing bloody mucus tracheal secretions common in postoperative head and neck cancer patients."[12] They also found that this practice did not cause oxygen desaturation (see the Research Box). On the other hand, a recent study, which sampled patients on mechanical ventilation from surgical, medical, and burn/trauma intensive care units of an academic medical center, found that the instillation of a 5-ml bolus of normal saline before suctioning had an adverse effect on oxygen saturation that worsened over time. The study

*Text continued on p. 912*

## clinical pathway Simple Tracheostomy

**DRG 482 Expected LOS 9.2 THE CLEVELAND CLINIC FOUNDATION COORDINATED CARE TRACK**

| TIME FRAME<br>LOCATION | HOSPITAL DAY<br>POD Day of Surgery<br>DATE UNIT | HOSPITAL DAY<br>POD 1<br>DATE UNIT | HOSPITAL DAY<br>POD 2<br>DATE UNIT |
|---|---|---|---|
| **Patient Satisfaction** | What can we do to enhance your stay with us? | What can we do to enhance your stay with us? | What can we do to enhance your stay with us? |
| **Discharge Planning** | Identify caregiver: ________ | | Screen for ASC (44663)/SW (46552) |
| **Patient Education** | Identify learning needs | Assess knowledge of surgical procedure and postop supports | Initiate patient education record<br>Begin teaching trach/wound care |
| **Tests/Procedures/ Consults** | | | |
| **Allied Health Interventions** | Respiratory therapy | Respiratory therapy | Speech pathology if patient has persistent aspiration<br>Screen for physical therapy |
| **Nursing/Medical Interventions** | Monitor vital signs q4h, I&O, labs, IV fluids<br>Airway: HOB elevated, $O_2$ via cool mist trach collar, I/S, trach care/suction qsh and prn<br>Wound: wound/stoma care qsh, IV ATB<br>Nutrition: NPO vs. C/L<br>Provide emotional support and reassurance regarding trach | Monitor vital signs q4h, I&O, labs, IV fluids<br>Airway: HOB elevated, $O_2$ via cool mist trach collar, I/S, trach care/suction qsh and prn<br>Deflate trach cuff<br>Wound: wound/stoma care qsh, IV ATB<br>Nutrition: clear liquids; advance as tolerated<br>Provide emotional support and reassurance regarding trach<br>Activity: up in chair | Monitor vital signs q4h, I&O, labs, IV fluids<br>Airway: HOB elevated, $O_2$ via cool mist trach collar, I/S, trach care/suction qsh and prn<br>Wound: wound/stoma care qsh, IV ATB<br>Nutrition: advance diet as tolerated; D/C IV with good PO<br>Provide emotional support and reassurance regarding trach<br>Activity: ambulate with assistance |
| **Outcome Criteria** | Vital signs stable<br>Adequate urine output<br>Patent airway<br>No wound complications<br>Patient/family satisfaction addressed | Vital signs stable<br>Voiding without difficulty<br>Patent airway with cuff down<br>No wound complications<br>Tolerating PO without aspirating<br>Patient/family satisfaction addressed | Vital signs stable<br>Voiding<br>Mobilizing secretions effectively<br>No wound complications<br>Increased PO intake without aspirating<br>Receptive to teaching<br>Patient/family satisfaction addressed |

4/1/97 (I:\ccf\pulmonar\simtrach.wpd) SIMPLE TRACHEOSTOMY FOR FACE, MOUTH, AND NECK DIAGNOSES (i.e., UPP With Trach; Trach for Vocal Cord Paralysis, etc.).* The Cleveland Clinic Foundation, 1997.
This is a general guideline to *assist* in the management of patients. This guideline is not designated to replace clinical judgment or individual patient needs.
*I/S,* Incentive spirometry; *ATB,* antibiotics.

*Simple Tracheostomy—cont'd*

**THE CLEVELAND CLINIC FOUNDATION COORDINATED CARE TRACK**

| TIME FRAME<br>LOCATION | HOSPITAL DAY<br>POD 3<br>DATE UNIT | HOSPITAL DAY<br>POD 4<br>DATE UNIT | HOSPITAL DAY<br>POD 5<br>DATE UNIT |
|---|---|---|---|
| **Patient Satisfaction** | What can we do to enhance your stay with us? | What can we do to enhance your stay with us? | What can we do to enhance your stay with us? |
| **Discharge Planning** | | ASC involved with discharge planning | |
| **Patient Education** | Continue teaching | Continue teaching | Continue teaching |
| **Tests/Procedures/ Consults** | | | |
| **Allied Health Interventions** | Respiratory therapy<br>Physical therapy (if needed) | Respiratory therapy<br>Physical therapy (if needed) | Respiratory therapy<br>Physical therapy (if needed) |
| **Nursing/Medical Interventions** | Monitor vital signs, I&O, labs, IV fluids<br>Airway: HOB elevated, $O_2$ via cool mist trach collar, I/S, trach care/suction qsh and prn<br>Wound: wound/stoma care qsh, IV ATB<br>Nutrition: DAT<br>Activity: ambulate independently | Monitor vital signs, I&O, labs<br>Airway: HOB elevated, $O_2$ CMTC, trach care/ suction qsh and prn, change to airlon or button trach<br>Wound: wound/stoma care qsh<br>IV antibiotics<br>Nutrition: DAT<br>Anxiety: emotional support<br>Activity: ambulating | Monitor: vital signs, I&O, labs<br>Airway: HOB elevated, $O_2$ CMTC, trach care/ suction qsh and prn<br>Wound: wound/stoma care qsh<br>D/C antibiotics<br>Nutrition: DAT<br>Anxiety: emotional support<br>Activity: ambulating |
| **Outcome Criteria** | Vital signs stable<br>Voiding<br>Mobilizing secretions effectively<br>Stable wound<br>Adequate PO intake<br>Receptive to teaching<br>Patient/family satisfaction addressed | Vital signs stable<br>Voiding<br>Tolerates trach change<br>Mobilizing secretions effectively<br>Stable wound<br>Adequate PO intake<br>Progressing with teaching<br>Patient/family satisfaction addressed | Vital signs stable<br>Voiding<br>Mobilizing secretions effectively<br>Patent airway<br>Stable wound<br>Good PO intake<br>Progressing with teaching<br>Patient/family satisfaction addressed |

| TIME FRAME<br>LOCATION | HOSPITAL DAY<br>POD 6<br>DATE UNIT | HOSPITAL DAY<br>POD 7<br>DATE UNIT | HOSPITAL DAY<br>POD 8<br>DATE UNIT |
|---|---|---|---|
| **Patient Satisfaction** | What can we do to enhance your stay with us? | What can we do to enhance your stay with us? | What can we do to enhance your stay with us? |
| **Discharge Planning** | | | |
| **Patient Education** | Reinforce teaching | Reinforce teaching | Reinforce teaching |
| **Tests/Procedures/ Consults** | | | |
| **Allied Health Interventions** | Respiratory therapy<br>Physical therapy (if needed) | Respiratory therapy<br>Physical therapy (if needed) | Respiratory therapy |
| **Nursing/Medical Interventions** | Monitor: vital signs, I&O, labs<br>Airway: trach care/suction qsh/prn<br>Wound: wound/stoma care qsh<br>Nutrition: DAT<br>Activity: ambulating | Monitor: vital signs, I&O, labs<br>Airway: trach care/suction qsh/prn<br>Wound: wound/stoma care qsh<br>Nutrition: DAT<br>Activity: ambulating | Monitor: vital signs, I&O, labs<br>Airway: trach care/suction qsh/prn<br>Wound: wound/stoma care qsh<br>Nutrition: DAT<br>Activity: ambulating |
| **Outcome Criteria** | Vital signs stable<br>Voiding<br>Mobilizing secretions effectively<br>Stable wound<br>Good PO intake<br>Progressing with teaching<br>Patient/family satisfaction addressed | Vital signs stable<br>Voiding<br>Mobilizing secretions<br>Stable wound<br>Good PO intake<br>Progressing with teaching<br>Patient/family satisfaction addressed | Vital signs stable<br>Voiding<br>Mobilizing secretions<br>Stable wound<br>Good PO intake<br>Able to do trach/wound care<br>D/C criteria met<br>Patient/family satisfaction addressed |

*DAT,* Diet as tolerated; *CMTC,* cool mist trach collar.

recommended that instillation of normal saline before suctioning should not be used routinely in patients receiving mechanical ventilation who have pulmonary infections.[1a] In an article published in the same journal, nurses and respiratory therapists working in adult ICUs in a large university teaching hospital were surveyed about the practice of instilling saline before suctioning. Of the 187 respondents, 96 (51%) rarely instilled saline before suctioning, whereas 61 (33%) frequently used saline.[20a] Most nurses (64%) *rarely use* saline before suctioning, whereas most respiratory therapists (71%) frequently use saline. Nurses indicated more adverse effects of instillation of saline, specifically oxygen desaturation and the increased risk of pulmonary infections than did respiratory therapists. Respiratory therapists (57%) were more aware than nurses (37%) of the benefit of saline to stimulate a cough. The authors concluded that the results of the survey determined target areas for educational programs for nurses and respiratory therapists, and they are developing a protocol for all who do suctioning. See references 9 and 22 for other information on suctioning.

### Maintaining Air Humidification

Because the insertion of the endotracheal or tracheostomy tube bypasses the upper airway, the patient's ability to humidify and warm inspired air is lost. Therefore, whether the patient is on or off the ventilator, the inspired air should be humidified to prevent mucosal irritation and drying of secretions. Large-bore tubing is needed to provide this mist because water particles condense in small-bore tubing. A noticeable difference in the viscosity of secretions is evident in patients who do not receive mist for even as short a period as 30 minutes. Other important nursing care measures and observations vary with the route of intubation—via the larynx or from below the larynx. The patient who has an endotracheal tube in place usually has an increased volume of oropharyngeal secretions because of irritation from the tube. The patient also has great difficulty in swallowing (especially if an oral tube is used), necessitating frequent oropharyngeal suctioning.

### Providing Nourishment

The patient with an endotracheal tube is allowed nothing by mouth. Nourishment is given intravenously or by nasogastric tube feedings. The patient with a tracheostomy tube in place is usually able to swallow and have a normal oral intake. As mentioned earlier, some experts prefer that the cuff on the tracheostomy tube be inflated while the patient is eating to prevent aspiration.

### Weaning from the Tracheostomy Tube

Patients who have had tracheostomies for a period of time may require progressive weaning before the tracheostomy tube can be safely removed (decannulation). The cuff is deflated to determine the patient's ability to handle secretions without aspiration. If no aspiration occurs, a smaller uncuffed tube is inserted to determine the patient's ability to breathe around the tube and through the nose and mouth. Next, the opening of the tracheostomy tube is occluded for 24 hours to ensure that the patient can breathe through nose and mouth without difficulty. If the patient tolerates this procedure, the tracheostomy tube is removed and decannulation is accomplished. An occlusive dressing is applied to the stoma site to promote healing.

Some patients will have a permanent tracheostomy. A discussion of their home care follows.

## HOME CARE CONSIDERATIONS

### Care of the Tracheostomy Tube

Persons to be discharged with a tube in place are taught to care for and change the tube while in the hospital (Figure 31-30). A mirror will be necessary to perform this procedure, which the patient may begin a few days after surgery.

Patients who go home with the tracheostomy tube in place must be provided with necessary supplies or with instructions as to where to get supplies. The patient will need suction equipment, which can be rented for home use or obtained in many communities through the local chapter of the American Cancer Society.

## research

Reference: Hudak M, Bond-Domb A: Postoperative head and neck cancer patients on artificial airways: the effect of saline lavage on tracheal mucus evacuation and oxygen saturation, *ORL Head Neck Nurs* 14(1):17, 1996.

In this study, 20 postoperative head and neck cancer patients with tracheostomy were studied to evaluate arterial oxygen saturation following suctioning with and without a 5 ml saline bolus. The amount of secretions obtained by these two methods of suctioning was also determined. $Sao_2$ was monitored before suctioning and at 15, 30, and 45 seconds and at 1, 2, 3, and 5 minutes after suctioning. Data were collected from a convenience sample of 20 patients who met the following criteria: all had a tracheostomy performed within the past 12 hours; had a history of smoking (one pack or more per day); had a no. 8 Shiley cuffed nonfenestrated tracheostomy tube; and received continuous oxygen at $Fio_2$ of 40% via a trach collar. The patients served as their own controls. The experimental treatment consisted of a standardized suctioning regimen with pulse oximetry monitoring and instillation of a 5 ml saline bolus before suctioning. The control treatment consisted of a standardized suctioning regimen with pulse oximetry monitoring without a saline bolus before suctioning. The subjects were randomly assigned to receive either the experimental or the control treatment first. Each patient alternated between one experimental and one control treatment. $Sao_2$ levels showed that the saturation level did not drop below 95% in either group. Both the experimental and the control groups had a drop in $Sao_2$ immediately after suctioning, and both groups showed a slight improvement in $Sao_2$ 5 minutes after suctioning. When the $Sao_2$ data were compared, no differences were found between the two groups across time. The mean sputum weight of the suctioned secretions after normal saline installation was greater (7.75) than was the weight without saline instillation (4.53). This study demonstrates that installation of a 5 ml bolus of normal saline before suctioning enhanced removal of tracheal secretions in postoperative head and neck cancer patients and had no harmful effects.

The patient should be given written instructions about how to care for the tracheostomy tube, and the instructions should be reviewed with the patient and significant other before discharge. The patient should practice suctioning the tracheostomy tube before discharge. Points to be included in the written instructions are listed in the Patient/Family Teaching Box.

### Tracheal Buttons

Tracheal buttons are used in some patients with a permanent tracheal stoma. A tracheal button is a hollow Teflon tube with a serrated distal end that is inserted into the tracheal stoma, where the end fits against the anterior tracheal wall (Figure 31-33). When the button is in place, a solid plug is inserted to spread the distal end flanges, which secures the tube in place. The button keeps the stoma tract open and allows the patient to breathe, vocalize, and clear secretions through the upper airway.

If the patient has difficulty breathing, the solid plug can be removed and the patient can be ventilated with an Ambu bag fitted with an adaptor. Routine suctioning through the tracheal button is discouraged, because the suction catheter tends to hit the posterior wall of the trachea, causing ulceration and bleeding. If the tracheostomy tube must be reinserted after several hours or days, it can be easily reinserted because the stoma has been kept open with the button.

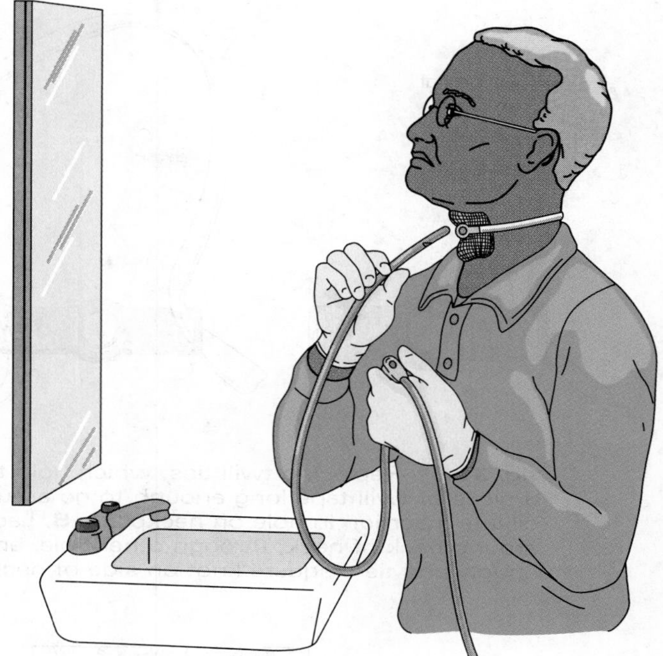

**fig. 31-30** Man using mirror to suction tracheostomy tube. Note that man's left thumb will be placed over the fenestration in catheter, allowing suction to be applied.

## patient/family teaching

### Home Care for the Person with a Permanent Tracheostomy Tube

The nose normally filters and warms the air we breathe. These functions are lost when there is a tracheostomy tube; therefore extra humidity is necessary in the home. To increase humidity, use a cool mist humidifier in the room where you spend most of your time. Also use it in your bedroom when you are napping or sleeping.

Suctioning the tracheostomy tube:

1. Gather the supplies you will need.
   a. Suction machine
   b. Suction catheter (no. 14 French whistle-tip)
   c. Two nonsterile gloves
   d. A clean basin or sink
   e. Hydrogen peroxide
   f. Clean 4 × 4 fine mesh gauze pads
   g. Jar of tap water or normal saline (use distilled water if you have well water)
   h. Clean cotton-tipped swabs
   i. Clean pipe cleaners or small brush
   j. Clean washcloth and towel
   k. Trach tube ties
   l. Clean scissors
   m. Plastic or paper bag for disposal of soiled materials
2. Wash hands thoroughly with soap and water.
3. Sit or stand in front of mirror (can use mirror over sink in bathroom).
4. Put on gloves.
5. Suction the tracheostomy tube (see Figure 31-30).
6. If your tube has an inner cannula, remove it. (If your tube does not have an inner cannula, go to step 12).
7. Clean inner cannula in the basin. Pour hydrogen peroxide over it until it is clean.
8. Clean inner cannula with pipe cleaners or small brush. Discard used pipe cleaners in disposable bag.
9. Rinse the cannula thoroughly with normal saline, tap water, or distilled water.
10. Dry inside and outside of cannula with 4 × 4 fine mesh gauze. Discard used gauze in disposable bag.
11. Reinsert inner cannula and lock in place.
12. Remove soiled gauze dressing from your neck and dispose of it in disposable bag.
13. Inspect skin around stoma for any signs of irritation or infection such as redness, hardness, tenderness, drainage, or foul smell. If any of these are present, call your nurse or physician after you finish your trach tube care.
14. Soak cotton-tipped swabs in hydrogen peroxide. Use swabs to clean the exposed parts of the outer cannula and the skin around it. Discard in disposable bag.
15. Wet the washcloth with tap water, normal saline, or distilled water. Wipe away hydrogen peroxide and clean skin around stoma.
16. Dry area around stoma with the clean towel.
17. Change the trach ties using twill tape recommended to you.
18. Do not completely remove the old tie until you have a new one in place.
19. Cut twill tape as you have been taught (see Figure 31-31).
20. Place fine mesh gauze under the tracheostomy tie and neckplate by folding it or cutting a slit (Figure 31-32).
21. Remove your gloves and discard them in the same bag used for soiled gauze.
22. Wash hands with soap and warm water.
23. Wash basin and small brush with soap and warm water.
24. Put the washcloth and towel in laundry.
25. Wash your hands again.

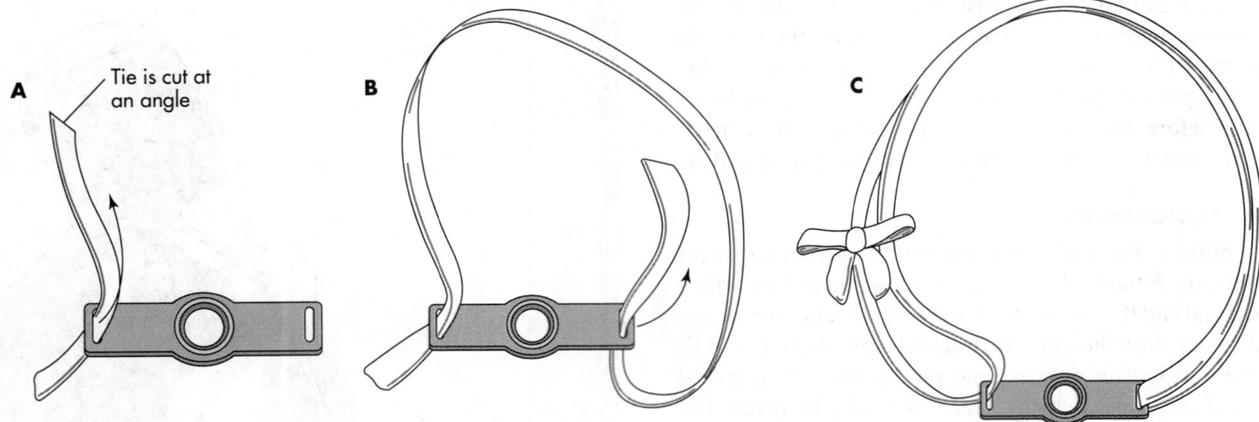


**fig. 31-31** Replacing twill ties, which hold tracheostomy tube in place. Measure and cut a piece of twill tape long enough to go around neck twice. **A,** Cut tape at an angle to facilitate insertion in hole on neckplate. **B,** Lace tape through one hole of the neckplate, around back of neck, through other hole, and around back of neck again. **C,** Pull tie snugly and tie a square knot on side of neck.

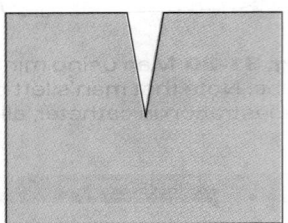


**fig. 31-32** Cut slit in fine mesh gauze so it will go under the tracheostomy tie and neckplate. Alternative is to fold two pieces of fine mesh gauze in triangles and place them under tie and neckplate.

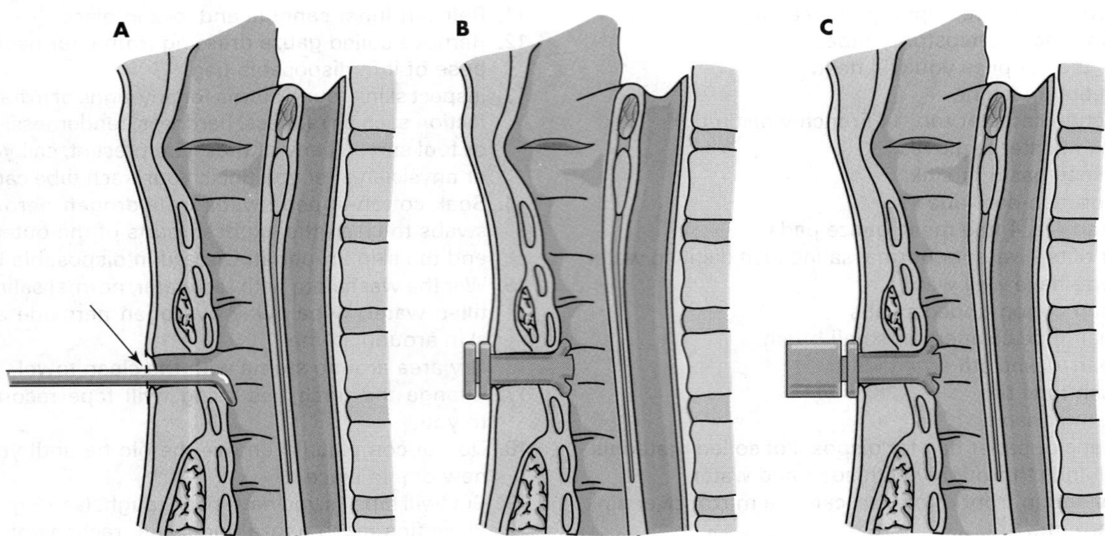


**fig. 31-33** Tracheal button. **A,** Inserting bent pipe cleaner into stoma to measure stoma depth. Pipe cleaner gently pulled back to hook on anterior tracheal wall. Distance from pipe cleaner bend to skin surface determines length of tracheostomy button. As an alternative, several different sizes of tracheal buttons are tried to determine which one is most comfortable for patient. **B,** Solid plug inserted into tracheostomy button prevents button from being coughed out and allows patient to breathe through upper airway and vocalize. **C,** Hollow tube adaptor ("one-way" valve) replaces stoma plug to allow for suctioning and inspiration through button and expiration and vocalization through upper airway.

## critical thinking QUESTIONS

**1** Investigate resources that are available in your community to assist the person who is unable to speak after a total laryngectomy.

**2** Compare the nursing care of a 45-year-old patient who is post–partial laryngectomy with that of a 56-year-old patient who is post–total laryngectomy with radical neck dissection.

**3** Debate the advantages and disadvantages of various vocal restoration methods used for individuals after a total laryngectomy.

**4** What specific behavior might indicate that an individual who has had radical neck surgery or permanent laryngectomy is not adjusting to changes in appearance?

## chapter SUMMARY

### INFECTIONS OF THE NOSE AND SINUSES

- The major infections of the nose and sinuses are rhinitis (common cold), allergic rhinitis (hay fever), chronic rhinitis secondary to repeated infections or allergy, and bacterial or viral sinusitis.
- Persons with allergic rhinitis (hay fever) are usually sensitive to pollen of grasses such as ragweed (see Chapter 66).
- Persons who are allergic need to know which allergens they are allergic to and to avoid these allergens if possible. For this reason they need to know how to prepare an environmentally controlled bedroom (see Chapter 66).
- Persons with acute sinusitis usually have a severe headache and pain over the infected area. Fever is common and is related to the amount of sinus obstruction. If the sinus is abscessed, fever may be as high at 40° C (104° F).
- Subjective assessment of the person with a nose or sinus problem includes a careful history of previous infections, how the infections were treated, and self-treatment by the person, including the use of over-the-counter medications.
- Acetaminophen is recommended instead of aspirin in persons with nasal problems, because aspirin may be associated with nasal polyposis.
- Functional endoscopic sinus surgery (FESS) is being used more often to treat chronic sinusitis. Other procedures include Caldwell-Luc surgery, ethmoidectomy, sphenoid sinus surgery, and frontal sinus surgery.
- Postoperative teaching for persons having sinus surgery includes the following:
  1. Avoid blowing nose for at least 48 hours after packing is removed.
  2. Avoid constipation because Valsalva's maneuver can cause bleeding.
  3. Avoid sneezing or sneeze with mouth open.
  4. Avoid lifting heavy objects or bending over.

### INFECTIONS OF THE PHARYNX AND LARYNX

- The most common throat inflammation is acute pharyngitis. Group A beta-hemolytic streptococci (GABHS), staphylococci, and other bacteria and viruses may be sources of infection. Pharyngitis caused by *Neisseria gonorrhoeae* is being seen more commonly in both men and women.
- A throat culture is taken to obtain material for culture and sensitivity so that appropriate antibiotic therapy can be determined.
- Prophylactic antibiotics are often prescribed for persons with pharyngitis who have a history of rheumatic fever or bacterial endocarditis.

### OBSTRUCTIONS OF THE NOSE AND THROAT

- Obstructions of the nose, such as deviated septum, are treated surgically by nasoseptoplasty.
- Rhinoplasty can be used to correct an anatomical problem or for cosmetic reasons.
- Nasal polyps are common and affect men twice as often as women. They are treated with corticosteroid sprays or injection of steroid into the polyps.
- Tonsils and adenoids are removed surgically when they cause symptoms of obstruction or are chronically infected.
- Laryngeal paralysis is caused by disease or injury of the laryngeal nerves or the vagus nerve. It is diagnosed by laryngoscopy. Laryngeal paralysis may be treated medically but can require surgery.
- Acute laryngeal edema is a medical emergency that is treated with a corticosteroid or epinephrine. If airway obstruction is present, endotracheal intubation or tracheostomy will be necessary.

### MALIGNANCIES OF THE HEAD AND NECK

- Heavy alcohol use and tobacco abuse are etiological factors in persons with head and neck cancers.
- Postoperative care after paranasal surgery includes gentle mouth care with an oral irrigating solution of saline and hydrogen peroxide, weak sodium bicarbonate, or antibiotic solution.
- Oropharyngeal cancers are treated with radiotherapy and surgical excision. With extensive resection, reconstructive surgery with skin grafts or flaps will be necessary. Drains are placed in the incision and attached to a suction device, which requires careful monitoring to ensure that it is draining properly.
- Progressive or persistent hoarseness that lasts longer than 2 weeks requires medical evaluation for cancer of the larynx.
- Carcinoma of the larynx is treated with surgery or radiotherapy.
- Partial laryngectomy may be achieved by hemilaryngectomy or supraglottic partial laryngectomy, after which the person will be able to speak.
- Total laryngectomy is necessary when cancer of the larynx is far advanced. Persons with total laryngectomy are unable to speak normally but will be able to have some form of speech.
- The three major forms of speech following laryngectomy are esophageal, tracheoesophageal, and external speech aid. Tracheoesophageal speech requires the formation of a fistula after all the carcinoma has been removed. This procedure is called a tracheoesophageal puncture (TEP).
- A radical neck dissection is commonly performed along with total laryngectomy because of the risk of metastasis to the neck in some patients.
  1. Postoperatively the person will have a laryngectomy tube and a nasogastric tube in place.
  2. Communication is impaired because of the loss of ability to speak, and the person will require speech rehabilitation.
- Patients undergoing total laryngectomy may benefit from a visit from a member of the Lost Chord Club or New Voice Club who has undergone laryngectomy and is successfully rehabilitated.
- Postoperative care following laryngectomy includes the following:
  1. Proper positioning: head elevated 30 to 45 degrees.
  2. Maintaining patent airway, including proper suctioning of tracheostomy.
  3. Managing the wound by assessing viability of skin flaps (color, temperature, capillary refill, and induration).

4. Suture line assessment (approximation, edema, color, and drainage) and suture line care to remove crusting and keep suture line clean.
5. Monitoring closed drainage system to keep tube patent and avoid a massive hematoma under tension. Monitoring includes milking tubing, recording type and amount of drainage, and checking for air leaks.
6. A nasogastric tube is inserted during surgery and removed as soon as edema subsides, allowing the person to swallow. Many patients are discharged while still on tube feedings and must learn to swallow liquids and eat soft food at home. The assistance of the speech pathologist may be required to assist with swallowing.

- Postoperative care of a patient with a neck dissection is similar to that for a patient with a laryngectomy and includes the following:
  1. Elevating head of bed 30 degrees
  2. Monitoring for airway obstruction
  3. Caring for suture line and assessing skin flaps
  4. Maintaining drainage system
  5. Monitoring shoulder droop and limited range of motion of head, neck, and shoulders
  6. Monitoring ability to ingest optimal calories
  7. Monitoring for depression
- Myocutaneous and free flaps are the major reconstructive flaps used after large tumor resections.

## MANAGEMENT OF THE COMPROMISED AIRWAY

- When a patient cannot maintain his or her own airway, intubation with an endotracheal tube or a tracheostomy may be necessary. Endotracheal tubes are used for short periods of time (10 to 14 days). If longer intubation is required, a tracheostomy performed in the operating room is the treatment of choice.
- General care of the person with an endotracheal tube or a tracheostomy includes measures to minimize infection, including proper suctioning technique, humidification of the airway, proper care of respiratory therapy equipment, frequent mouth care, and adequate nutrition.
- To ensure adequate ventilation and oxygenation, the patient's lung sounds are assessed frequently. Turning and repositioning every 2 hours; assessing respiratory frequency, tidal volume, and vital capacity; and providing chest physiotherapy, including percussion, vibration, and postural drainage, are essential.
- Precautions pertaining to endotracheal tubes or tracheostomies include assessing tube placement at regular intervals, keeping a spare tube on hand for emergencies, minimizing sensory deprivation by developing a method of communication, talking directly to the patient and explaining all procedures, reorienting the patient frequently, encouraging family and friends to talk with the patient, keeping the call light within reach, and reinforcing that the patient will be able to speak after extubation.
- Precautions to be observed after decannulation include frequent monitoring for respiratory distress, adequacy of cough and gag reflex, and care of stoma incision.
- Patients being discharged with an endotracheal tube or a tracheostomy need to be taught how to care for their own tube before discharge. Community sources for equipment and supplies need to be determined before discharge.
- The patient discharged with a tracheostomy tube or laryngostoma is given home-going instructions that include increasing humidity with a cool mist humidifier; covering the stoma with a dampened stoma cover; washing the stoma daily with a washcloth and warm water and soap; suctioning the stoma or tube; keeping the stoma covered when going outside; using precautions when bathing, shampooing, and shaving; and wearing a medical identification bracelet or carrying a card saying, "I am a total neck breather."

## References

1. Adams JF, Lassen LF: Leech therapy for venous congestion following myocutaneous pectoralis flap reconstruction, *ORL Head Neck Nurs* 13(1):12, 1995.

1a. Ackerman MH, Mick DJ: Instillation of normal saline before suctioning in patients with pulmonary infections: a prospective randomized controlled study, *Am J Crit Care* 7(4):261, 1998.

2. American Cancer Society: *Cancer facts and figures 1998,* Atlanta, 1998, The Society.

3. Bryce JC: Aspiration: causes, consequences and prevention, *ORL Head Neck Nurs* 13(2):14, 1995.

4. Corren J, Rachelesky GS: Allergic rhinitis caused by inhalant factors. In Rakel RE, editor: *Conn's current therapy 1996,* Philadelphia, 1996, WB Saunders.

5. deLaminat V, Montravers P, Durell B, Desmonts J: Alteration in swallowing reflex after extubation in intensive care patients, *Crit Care Med* 2:486, 1995.

6. Droughton ML, Krech RI: Head and neck cancer resection and reconstruction from past to present, *Today's OR Nurse* 14(9):25, 1992.

7. Gantz NM: Sinusitis. In Rakel RE, editor: *Conn's current therapy 1996,* Philadelphia, 1996, WB Saunders.

8. Gillyat P: Allergic rhinitis—hay fever is nothing to sneeze at, *Harvard Health Letter* 21(8):6, 1996.

9. Glass CA, Grap MJ: Ten tips for safer suctioning, *Am J Nurs* 95(5):51, 1995.

10. Higgins DM, Maclean JC: Dysphagia in the patient with a tracheostomy: six cases of inappropriate cuff deflation or removal, *Heart Lung* 26(3):215, 1997.

11. Hoffman HT, Karnell MP: Hoarseness and laryngitis. In Rakel RE, editor: *Conn's current therapy 1996,* Philadelphia, 1996, WB Saunders.

12. Hudak M, Domb-Bond A: Postoperative head and neck cancer patients with artificial airways: the effect of saline lavage on tracheal mucus evacuation and oxygen saturation, *ORL Head Neck Nurs* 14(1):17, 1996.

13. Kaplow R, Bookbinder M: A comparison of four endotracheal tube holders, *Heart Lung* 23(1):59, 1994.

14. Krouse HJ, Krouse JH, Christmas DA Jr: Endoscopic sinus surgery in otorhinolaryngology nursing using powered instrumentation, *ORL Head Neck Nurs* 15(2):22, 1997.

15. Lavertu P, Droughton ML: Postoperative management following head and neck surgery. In Sviak E, Higgins D, Scivers A, editors: *The high risk patient: management of the critically ill,* Philadelphia, 1995, Lea & Febiger.

16. Leach JI, Schaeffer S: Sinusitis. In Rakel RE, editor: *Conn's current therapy 1993,* Philadelphia, 1993, WB Saunders.

17. McCarthy JM: Streptococcal pharyngitis. In Rakel RE, editor: *Conn's current therapy 1993,* Philadelphia, 1993, WB Saunders.

18. Miller WF: The role of the outpatient nurse in endoscopic sinus surgery, *ORL Head Neck Nurs* 10(3):20, 1992.

19. Scher RI, Richtsmeier WJ: Otolaryngology: head and neck surgery. In Sabiston DC Jr, Lyerly KH, editors: *Sabiston: essentials of surgery,* ed 2, Philadelphia, 1994, WB Saunders.

20. Schuller DE, Schleunng AJ: *DeWeese and Saunders otolaryngology head and neck surgery,* ed 8, St Louis, 1994, Mosby.

20a. Schwenker D, Ferrin M, Gift AG: A survey of endotracheal suctioning with instillation of normal saline, *Am J Crit Care* 7(4):255, 1998.

21. Sigler BA, Schuring LT: *Ear, nose and throat disorders,* St Louis, 1993, Mosby.

22. Somerson SJ et al: Mastering emergency airway management, *Am J Nurs* 96(1):24, 1996.

chapter 32

# MANAGEMENT OF PERSONS WITH Problems of the Lower Airway

WILMA J. PHIPPS

## objectives

*After studying this chapter, the learner should be able to:*

1. Differentiate between restrictive and obstructive pulmonary disorders.
2. Compare community-acquired and hospital-acquired pneumonias.
3. Describe incidence, preventive measures, and treatment of tuberculosis.
4. Compare fungal infections of the respiratory tract.
5. Explain the pathophysiology of adult respiratory distress syndrome.
6. Describe incidence, prevention, and therapy for lung cancer.
7. Write a teaching plan for the patient who is to have resectional surgery of the lung.
8. List five precautions to be observed in care of chest tubes and a closed drainage system, and give the rationale for each.
9. Differentiate among a closed, an open, and a tension pneumothorax in terms of signs and symptoms, treatment, and nursing management.
10. Explain the pathophysiology of and interventions for chronic bronchitis, pulmonary emphysema, and asthma.
11. Describe how you would teach the patient with chronic obstructive pulmonary disease to use a metered-dose inhaler and an inhaler with a spacer.
12. Discuss the clinical manifestations of cystic fibrosis in adults.
13. Describe the nature of respiratory failure and the care of the patient with an endotracheal tube and mechanical ventilation.
14. Differentiate between a pressure-cycled and a volume-cycled ventilator.
15. Describe the three most common methods used in weaning a patient from a ventilator.

Many diseases, both acute (short term) and chronic (long term), affect the respiratory system. Considerable change in the incidence of diseases affecting the respiratory system has occurred in the past few decades. Although the incidence of some pulmonary diseases such as lung abscess and bronchiectasis has decreased, the incidence of other pulmonary diseases such as chronic bronchitis and emphysema has increased. In addition, the reduction in immunological competence that occurs with cancer chemotherapy, immunosuppressant medications given after organ transplantation, or acquired immunodeficiency syndrome (AIDS) has resulted in an increase in opportunistic lung infections caused by microorganisms that were rarely pathogenic in the past.

The most significant pulmonary diseases are those that are chronic and have increased dramatically in recent years. Current statistics indicate that more than 17 million Americans have emphysema, asthma, or chronic bronchitis. This number can be expected to increase yearly as the number of elderly persons in our society increases. Because most diseases of the respiratory tract are not reportable, the full extent of both acute and chronic illness is difficult to estimate. However, known facts about disability from chronic pulmonary diseases indicate that they are a major health problem and that they cause tremendous losses in productivity in the United States. The Social Security Administration reports that disability payments to persons with chronic pulmonary problems are second only to payments to persons with heart problems. Whereas the mortality rate from tuberculosis has declined, the mortality rate from bronchitis, emphysema, and lung cancer has continued to rise yearly.

Early symptoms of respiratory diseases are probably those most often ignored by the general population. With the exception of acute pulmonary disorders, the major factor preventing early diagnosis and treatment of pulmonary diseases is the insidious nature of their signs and symptoms. Nurses should encourage individuals and families to seek proper medical attention if they have symptoms such as *cough, difficulty breathing, production of sputum, shortness of breath,* and nose and throat irritation that do not subside within 2 weeks. These symptoms suggest respiratory diseases and should be investigated.

Tobacco use is the leading cause of preventable death in the United States. Several organizations, most notably the American Lung Association (ALA), the American Cancer Society (ACS), and the American Heart Association (AHA), along with the federal government, have launched campaigns to

Adele Large, MSN, RN, assisted in the revision of this chapter.

reduce tobacco use in the United States. The stated objective of the U.S. government is to reduce the proportion of smokers in the national population to 15% by 2000. This figure will be difficult to attain because the figures for 1995 showed that 24.7% of adults over age 18 were smokers.[13] These figures show differences in rates by gender, age groups, race, ethnicity, educational level, and socioeconomic status (Table 32-1).

Efforts are underway to decrease smoking among high school students. However, figures released in 1998 indicate that smoking among high school students is increasing rather than decreasing. The Centers for Disease Control and Prevention (CDC) reported that the prevalence of smoking among U.S. high school students increased from 27.5% in 1991 to 36.4% in 1997, with 42.7% of students indicating that they used cigarettes, smokeless tobacco, or cigars during the 30 days preceding the survey.[18]

In a report to the Surgeon General from the Office of Smoking and Health, the committee that worked on the report reached six major conclusions:

1. Nearly all first use of tobacco occurs before high school graduation; this finding suggests that if adolescents can be kept tobacco free, most will never start using tobacco.
2. Most adolescent smokers are addicted to nicotine and report that they want to quit but are unable to do so; they experience relapse rates and withdrawal symptoms similar to those reported by adults.
3. Tobacco is often the first drug used by those young people who use alcohol, marijuana, and other drugs.
4. Adolescents with lower levels of school achievement, with fewer skills to resist pervasive influences to use tobacco, with friends who use tobacco, and with a lower self-image are more likely than their peers to use tobacco.
5. Cigarette advertising appears to increase young people's risk of smoking by affecting their perceptions of the pervasiveness, image, and function of smoking.
6. Community-wide efforts that include tobacco tax increases, enforcement of minors' access laws, youth-oriented mass media campaigns, and school-based tobacco-use prevention programs are successful in reducing adolescent use of tobacco.

**table 32-1** *Percentage of Adults Age 18 and Over Who Were Current Cigarette Smokers by Gender, Age-Group, Racial Ethnicity, Level of Education, and Socioeconomic Status*

| CHARACTERISTIC | 1995 |
|---|---|
| **GENDER** | |
| Men | 24.5 |
| Women | 22.4 |
| **AGE-GROUP** | |
| 18-24 | 24.8 |
| 25-44 | 28.6 |
| 45-65 | 25.5 |
| **RACE/ETHNICITY** | |
| White | 25.6 |
| Black | 25.8 |
| Hispanic | 18.3 |
| Native American/Native Alaskan | 36.2 |
| Asian/Pacific Islander | 16.6 |
| **EDUCATIONAL LEVEL (YEARS)** | |
| 12 | 37.5 |
| 13-15 | 23.6 |
| >16 | 14.0 |
| **SOCIOECONOMIC STATUS** | |
| At/above poverty level | 23.8 |
| Below poverty level | 32.5 |
| Unknown | 23.5 |

From Centers for Disease Control and Prevention: United States National Health Survey, 1995, Cigarette smoking among adults, *MMWR* 46(51):1217, 1997.

In the United States, most daily smokers (82%) began smoking before age 18, and more than 3000 young persons begin smoking each day.[11] Attempting to reduce tobacco use among this group, the CDC published "Guidelines for School Health Programs to Prevent Tobacco Use and Addiction."[12] The guidelines offer recommendations for school health programs for students from kindergarten through twelfth grade. The following seven recommendations summarize strategies that are effective in preventing tobacco use among youth. To ensure the greatest impact, schools should implement all seven recommendations.[12]

1. Develop and enforce a school policy on tobacco use.
2. Provide instruction about the short-term and long-term negative physiological and social consequences of tobacco use, social influences on tobacco use, peer norms regarding tobacco use, and refusal skills.
3. Provide tobacco-use prevention education in kindergarten through twelfth grade; this instruction should be especially intensive in junior high or middle school and should be reinforced in high school.
4. Provide program-specific training for teachers.
5. Involve parents or families in support of school-based programs to prevent tobacco use.
6. Support cessation efforts among students and all school staff who use tobacco.
7. Assess the tobacco-use prevention program at regular intervals.

Although some persons question whether increasing cigarette taxes will decrease cigarette use, a recently published report from the Office on Smoking and Health of the Centers for Disease Control and Prevention indicates that it may be successful in some groups of young people. They reported that the National Health Interview Survey from 1976-1993 indicated that lower-income, minority, and younger populations were more likely to quit smoking in response to a price increase in cigarettes. The greatest decline in smoking (25%) was in Hispanics between 18 and 24 years old; the second greatest decline in smoking (12%) was in non-Hispanic black persons in the 18 to 24 year age group. The least decline was in non-Hispanic whites in the same age group.[15]

Along with the campaign to decrease smoking, there has been increased emphasis on reducing pollution in the environment, which has resulted in legislation such as the Clean

Air Act. Some of the measures taken to reduce pollution are presently threatened, because some persons believe they are too costly for the benefits achieved. This issue will be at the forefront through the 2000s, and nurses, as health professionals and concerned citizens, will need to keep themselves informed about proposed changes and their effects on health.

Several states and the federal government have successfully sued the major tobacco companies for causing increased morbidity and mortality from cigarette use. The companies were accused of lying when they stated in Congressional hearings that cigarette smoking does not cause cancer. They are also being sued for targeting their advertising with cartoonlike figures with special appeal to young children. Some of the companies have agreed to an out-of-court settlement of the claims in the federal suit, and the details of the settlement are being worked out as this is being written. The settlement involves millions of dollars to be paid over several years. Some of the money is earmarked for spending on antismoking education of children. At the state level, the states are trying to recoup money spent by Medicaid to care for patients with tobacco-related diseases. State trials are ongoing, and it may be years before final settlements are made.

The Food and Drug Administration (FDA) has issued regulations aimed at reducing smoking among children. These regulations, which became possible when it was agreed that nicotine is a drug subject to control by the FDA, became effective February 28, 1997. They require that retailers observe the following restrictions when selling cigarettes and other tobacco products:

1. They must not sell cigarettes or smokeless tobacco to anyone under 18 years of age.
2. They must verify that anyone buying cigarettes or smokeless tobacco is at least 18 years old. This involves checking identification that contains the buyer's photo and date of birth.
3. All sales of cigarettes and smokeless tobacco must be a direct face-to-face exchange between seller and buyer.
4. They must not break open any package of cigarettes or smokeless tobacco to sell individual cigarettes.

A copy of these regulations can be obtained from the local branch of the ALA, ACS, or AHA or the local health department.

**table 32-2** *Comparison of Pulmonary Function Test Results in Restrictive and Obstructive Disease*

| Test | Restrictive | Obstructive |
|---|---|---|
| FVC | Decreased | Decreased or normal |
| RV | Decreased | Increased |
| TLC | Decreased | Normal or increased |
| RV/TLC | Normal or increased | Significantly increased |
| $FEV_1$/FVC | Normal or increased | Decreased |
| $FEV_3$/FVC | Normal or increased | Decreased |

*FVC*, Forced vital capacity; *RV*, residual volume; *TLC*, total lung capacity; *FEV*, forced expiratory volume (in 1, 3 seconds).

## CLASSIFICATION OF PULMONARY DISORDERS

The classification of lung diseases used in this chapter differentiates the pulmonary disorders on the basis of how they affect ventilation. This classification divides lung diseases into either *restrictive* or *obstructive ventilatory defects.* A third category of pulmonary disorders consists of those that affect the *pulmonary vascular system* and thus alter the ability of the lung to carry out respiration.

### Restrictive Lung Disease

In restrictive lung disease, there is a limitation to full expansion of the lungs. Static lung volumes are diminished as a result of decreased lung or thoracic compliance (Table 32-2).

Patients with a restrictive disorder may demonstrate respiratory alkalosis caused by a compensatory increase in respiratory frequency (rate) to offset diminished lung volumes. When the increased respiratory rate no longer adequately compensates for the diminished lung volumes, hypoxemia (low arterial blood oxygen) occurs. Clinically, persons with restrictive disorders exhibit some degree of *dyspnea.* Often they will become dyspneic only on exertion. As the restrictive disease progresses, however, persons will become *dyspneic at rest.* Additionally, persons with restrictive disorders often have a *dry, hacking cough.* Table 32-3 lists major disorders that result in primarily restrictive ventilatory defects.

### Obstructive Lung Disease

Obstructive lung disease includes any process that limits airflow on expiration. Both lung compliance (lung expansibility) and airway resistance are increased. These pathophysiological changes alter the ability to move air out of the lungs, which results in characteristic changes in both static and dynamic lung volume measurement (see Table 32-2). Clinically, persons with obstructive lung disease may exhibit a *prolonged expiration time, increased anteroposterior thorax diameter,* and *hyperresonance on percussion.* Persons with pulmonary disorders characterized by the preceding description have been identified as having chronic obstructive pulmonary disease (COPD), which has classically included any mixture of emphysema, chronic bronchitis, and asthma. Discussion of COPD in this chapter includes these three conditions.

**table 32-3** *Restrictive Pulmonary Diseases*

| Alteration | Disease Example |
|---|---|
| Parenchymal inflammation | Pneumonia, adult respiratory distress syndrome |
| Space-occupying lesions | Tumors, malignancies |
| Diffuse pulmonary disease | Silicosis, fibrosis |
| Pleural disease | Pleural effusion |
| Lung collapse | Pneumothorax, atelectasis |
| Resectional surgery | Pneumonectomy |
| Neuromuscular disorders | Poliomyelitis, Guillain-Barré syndrome |
| Central nervous system depression | Narcotics, cerebral edema |

The third category of pulmonary disorders considered in this chapter is those identified as resulting in pulmonary vascular disease. Pulmonary vascular diseases include any process that results in the narrowing or occlusion of pulmonary blood vessels. In pulmonary vascular disease, efficiency of pulmonary respiration is compromised, usually resulting in hypoxemia. Clinically, patients have *dyspnea, increased respiratory frequency, digital clubbing, atelectasis,* and *chest pain.* Pulmonary vascular disease may result from primary pulmonary hypertension or as a result of either circulatory or lung disease. Only pulmonary vascular disease related to pulmonary emboli and pulmonary infarction is discussed here. This chapter presents restrictive diseases first, beginning with the infectious diseases. Obstructive lung diseases and pulmonary vascular diseases are discussed later in the chapter.

**box 32-1** *Lung Defense Mechanisms*

**UPPER AIRWAY DEFENSES AGAINST PULMONARY INFECTION**

**Removing Particulate Matter from Inspired Air**

- Particles greater than 20 μm settle back on surfaces
- Particles 5-10 μm deposited in nose
- Particles 0.1-10 μm remain suspended in air for long periods and are then inhaled
- Particles 1-5 μm deposited in tracheobronchial tree
  - Droplet nuclei 2-4 μm (dried particles from sneezing, coughing, talking)
  - May contain viruses or bacteria
  - Spread organisms from person to person

**Minimizing Microbial Population on Membranes of Upper Respiratory Tract**

- Mucocillary transport
  - Posterior two thirds of nasal cavity, sinuses, and nasopharynx lined by *ciliated epithelium* covered with thin layer of mucus
  - Dense concentration of small blood vessels present beneath ciliated epithelium and mucous layers
  - Mucus and fluid produced = 1000 ml/24 hr in normal persons
  - Mucus and fluid carried at rate of 5-10 mm/min back into hypopharynx by beating action of cilia
  - Substances in secretions inhibit microbial growth and prevent organisms from sticking to mucous membranes
    - Immunoglobulins (secretory IgA)
    - Lysozyme
    - Complement

**Minimizing Possibility of Aspiration**

- Motor function of upper airway
  - Laryngeal mechanism—closes glottis when swallowing to protect larynx
    - Gag reflex also closes glottis
    - Clearing throat/spitting clear upper airway
  - Contamination of lower respiratory tract
    - Impaired clearance of particles in upper airway = spread of bacteria
    - Accumulation of debris and microbes → penetration of tissues = sinusitis, otitis media
    - Accumulation of debris and microbes → aspiration into trachea; lung abscess caused by anaerobic bacteria secondary to severe gingival disease
    - Intoxication or distraction → aspiration
    - Normal sleep → minor aspiration
    - Aspiration of pharyngeal contents → lung → bacterial pneumonia

**LOWER RESPIRATORY TRACT CLEARANCE MECHANISMS**

**Pulmonary Reflex**

- Cough—involuntary reflex elicited by stimulation of irritant receptors in subepithelium of hypopharynx, larynx, and tracheobronchial tree: mediated by vagus nerve
  - Facilitator of mucociliary clearance
  - Aids in dealing with gross contamination from above larynx
- Bronchoconstriction—reflex response to airway irritants
- Decreased size of bronchus and forced expiration and cough propel debris toward mouth
- Excessive bronchoconstriction (asthma) = decreased expiratory airflow, air trapped in lung, difficulty with effective cough

**Mucociliary Clearance**

- Mucus secreted by epithelial goblet cells from submucosal glands; 0.10-100 ml passes up trachea into hypopharynx and is swallowed; amount and nature of mucus secreted are controlled, in part, by parasympathetic nervous system affected by neurohumoral stimulation (adrenergic or cholinergic) and by direct mucosal irritation
- Cilia (200 cilia/each cell surface) beat rhythmically 1200 beats/min mouthward beginning at terminal bronchioles → larynx; beating of cilia → overlying mucous layer → mouthward at rate of 0.5 mm/min in small airways to about 10 mm/min in major bronchi
- Clearance increased by:
  - Bronchodilator drugs
    - Beta-adrenergic agents (ephedrine) stimulate transport of water and salt into mucus = ↓ viscosity of mucus
    - Methylxanthines (aminophylline) = ↑ mucus production and ciliary activity
- Ciliary function depressed by:
  - Chronic exposure to airway irritants—cigarette smoke and other irritants
  - Pharmacological agents—100% $O_2$, anticholinergic agents, alcohol
  - Infection such as viral bronchitis
- Mucus production increased by:
  - Chronic irritation of respiratory tract → increase in number of mucus-secreting goblet cells = ↑ mucus
  - Inflammatory response to irritation = ↑ numbers of phagocytic cells and amount of cellular debris in mucus (especially DNA) = ↑ viscosity of mucus, which is less readily moved along by ciliary action
- Immotile cilia—congenital impairment
  - *Kartagener's syndrome*—sinusitis, recurrent lung infection, and sinus inversus
  - *Cystic fibrosis*—infection, chronic inflammatory increases in respiratory mucus volume and viscosity = impaired lung clearance and progressive lung damage

*Continued*

# RESTRICTIVE LUNG DISEASES

## INFECTIOUS DISEASES OF THE RESPIRATORY TRACT

The respiratory tract is in contact with the environment via inhalation of ambient air. Fortunately, the respiratory tract has a variety of defense mechanisms to prevent contamination of the respiratory tract with infectious agents (Box 32-1).

### Acute Bronchitis

#### Etiology/epidemiology

Bronchitis can be acute or chronic (chronic bronchitis is discussed later in this chapter). Acute bronchitis is an inflammation of the bronchi and usually the trachea (tracheobronchitis).

Although acute bronchitis occurs most often in persons with chronic lung disease, it also occurs as an extension of an upper respiratory infection (URI) in persons without underlying lung disease and is therefore communicable. It also may be caused by physical or chemical agents such as dust, smoke, or volatile fumes. As air pollution increases, the incidence of acute bronchitis increases. Acute bronchitis is typically viral, but bacterial pathogens such as *Streptococcus pneumoniae* and *Haemophilus influenzae* may also cause bronchitis either as a primary or secondary infection (Box 32-2).

#### Pathophysiology

As part of the inflammatory process, there is increased blood flow to the affected area, causing an increase in pulmonary secretions. A painful cough with sputum production, low-grade fever, and malaise are common symptoms. The patient may have pain beneath the sternum caused by inflammation of the tracheal wall. Bronchitis without tracheitis is never seen, and *tracheobronchitis* is a more appropriate term for this condition. Symptoms usually last 1 to 2 weeks but may continue for 3 to 4 weeks. Rhonchi and wheezes are heard on chest examination. If symptoms worsen and there is a high fever, shortness of breath, pleuritic chest pain (pain on inspiration), rapid respirations, and rales or signs of consolidation on physical examination of the chest, pneumonia is suspected.

#### Collaborative care management

Treatment of acute bronchitis is mainly supportive and includes the following:

1. Codeine or dextromethorphan is prescribed for nocturnal cough.

**box 32-1 Lung Defense Mechanisms—cont'd**

**INTRAPULMONARY DETOXIFICATION MECHANISM**

**Phagocytes**

- Alveolar macrophage
  - Phagocytosis of particles—inhaled particulate debris, bacteria, or cell constituents
  - Kills most microbes
- Polymorphonuclear neutrophil present in blood (normally only small number in lung)
  - Avid phagocyte—kills microbes
  - Defends against established infectious processes
  - Infection—products of inflammation attract neutrophils to site of infection (chemotaxis)
- Factors interfering with phagocytosis
  - Inhibition of alveolar macrophage function
    - Cigarette smoke
    - Other inhaled pollutants—ozone, nitrogen dioxide, oxygen
    - Drugs—corticosteroids, antineoplastic and antiinflammatory cytoxic agents, ethanol (alcohol)
    - Metabolic derangements—uremia, hyperglycemia of diabetes mellitus
    - Acquired granulocytopenia—bone marrow depression from cytoxic drugs

**Immunoglobulins**

- IgA and IgG—most important for lung defense; present in secretions of respiratory tract as well as in blood
  - IgA antibodies—specific for viral antigens; neutralize viruses and prevent infection
  - IgG predominates in terminal lung units; antigen-specific IgG contributes to local defense against bacterial infections (important in neutralizing highly pathogenic encapsulated bacteria [especially *Streptococcus pneumoniae* and *Haemophilus influenzae*], which are resistant to phagocytosis)

**Cell-Mediated Immunity (CMI)**

- One half of lymphocytes in and around airways are thymus-derived lymphocytes, or T cells
  - Found in lymphoid aggregates adjacent to bronchi (bronchus-associated lymphoid tissues, or BALT)
  - T cells important in:
    - Resistance to some viral infections
    - Resistance to most fungal infections
    - Infections by organisms that survive and multiply inside host cells: *Mycobacterium tuberculosis, Brucella, Listeria monocytogenes, Pneumocystis carinii*
- Impaired CMI = ↑ susceptibility to infection
  - Deficient T cell function (anergy) associated with:
    - Neoplasms—lymphoma
    - Cytotoxic or corticosteroid therapy
    - Systemic diseases—sarcoidosis, malnutrition
  - Some lung infections occur almost exclusively with severely impaired CMI—pneumonia caused by cytomegalovirus, herpes zoster, *Aspergillus* species, or *Pneumocystis carinii*

**box 32-2** *Infectious Causes of Acute Bronchitis*

**VIRUSES**
Rhinovirus
Adenovirus
Influenza A and B
Parainfluenza virus
Respiratory syncytial virus (RSV)

**BACTERIA**
*Streptococcus pneumoniae*
*Haemophilus influenzae*
*Moraxella catarrhalis*
*Bordetella pertussis*
*Mycoplasma pneumoniae*
*Chlamydia pneumoniae* (TWAR strain)

2. Bronchodilator therapy is prescribed for patients who are wheezing and for those whose peak expiratory flow rate is prolonged.[49] An inhaled $\beta$-agonist such as albuterol (Proventil, Ventolin) or ipratropium (Atrovent) is usually prescribed.
3. Decongestants and antihistamines are used sparingly, if at all, because they tend to dry secretions and make them more difficult to remove.
4. Oral fluid intake of 2 to 3 L per day is encouraged if there is no contraindication to it.
5. Aspirin helps reduce fever and alleviate some of the symptoms of inflammation.
6. Patients who are smokers are urged to quit.
7. Antibiotics are usually *not* prescribed unless there is evidence of bacterial infection. Exceptions include symptoms lasting more than 2 weeks in persons with chronic diseases such as diabetes mellitus, cirrhosis, congestive heart failure, or COPD, as well as elderly persons in general.[49] All of these persons are at a higher risk for pneumonia.
8. Rest is encouraged to give the body a chance to heal.

Nursing care is supportive and is directed toward helping the patient with prescribed therapy and avoiding future infection. Emphasis is on assisting the patient to cough effectively, assisting with comfort, assisting with activities of daily living (ADL), and teaching the patient and family.

The patient must be taught to cough effectively. Receptors for the cough reflex are located in the tracheal and bronchial mucosa, with the largest concentration of them found in the larynx, carina, and bifurcations of the large and medium-sized bronchi. When these receptors are stimulated, impulses are transmitted primarily via the afferent nervous pathways (vagus, phrenic, and spinal motor nerves) to expiratory musculature (larynx, tracheobronchial tree, diaphragm, and abdominal wall).

To produce an effective cough, a deep inspiration must be followed by maximal expiratory effort against a closed glottis. This results in a tremendous increase in intrathoracic pressure. As the glottis opens, mucus and inhaled particles are forced out of the airways at a high velocity.

**table 32-4** *Common Medications for* ***Cough***

| Desired Effect | Medications Prescribed |
|---|---|
| ↑ Secretions | Expectorants<br>Guaifenesin<br>Iodinated glycerol<br>Potassium iodide (saturated solution, SSKI)<br>Terpin hydrate |
| ↓ Secretions | Anticholinergic agents<br>Atropine |
| Thin secretions | Mucolytic agents<br>Acetylcysteine (Mucomyst)<br>Desoxyribonuclease (Dornavac) |
| Depress cough reflex | Antitussives<br>Narcotic<br>Codeine<br>Nonnarcotic agents<br>Benzonatate (Tessalon)<br>Noscapine (Nectadon)<br>Dextromethorpan hydrobromide (Romilar)<br>Carbetapentane citrate (Toclase)<br>Levopropoxyphene napsylate (Novrod)<br>Chlophedianol hydrochloride (Ulo) |

Assist with coughing as necessary by supporting the patient's chest (front and back) with an open palm as the patient coughs. Ask the patient to take a deep breath, force the air out down to residual volume, contract the diaphragm, exhale forcefully, and then cough. Successful airway clearance and an effective breathing pattern should help return vital signs to prebronchitis levels.

Persistent coughing can be annoying and tiring to the patient and those around him or her. Complications of persistent coughing include insomnia, exhaustion, vomiting, urinary incontinence, rib or muscle trauma, pneumothorax, and fainting. If cough persists, give cough medication, if prescribed. Table 32-4 lists commonly used medications and their desired effects.

Additional assistance in achieving therapeutic goals includes the following:
1. Provide for good drainage of tracheobronchial secretions.
2. Give antibiotics on time to maintain therapeutic blood levels.
3. A semi-Fowler's or high Fowler's position usually facilitates breathing.
4. If steam vaporization is prescribed, teach the patient to use the precautions described on p. 927.
5. If a bronchodilator is ordered, teach the patient how to use an inhaler with a spacer (see p. 984).
6. Assist with ADL as necessary.

**Patient/family education.** The patient should be taught to avoid persons with URIs. If URI does occur, the patient should seek medical attention.

**risk factors**

### Hospitalization of Persons with Community-Acquired Pneumonia

Age 50 or older
History of:
- Neoplastic disease
- Congestive heart failure
- Cerebrovascular disease
- Renal disease
- Liver disease

Physical examination findings:
- Altered mental status
- Pulse ≥125/min
- Respiratory rate ≥30/min
- Systolic blood pressure <90 mm Hg
- Temperature <35° C or ≥40° C

Demographic factors:
- Male
- Nursing home resident

Laboratory or radiographical findings:
- Blood urea nitrogen ≥30 mg/dl
- Glucose concentration ≥250 mg/dl
- Hematocrit <30%
- $Po_2$ <60 mm Hg
- pH <7.35
- Pleural effusion

Adapted from Fine MJ et al: A prediction rule to identify low-risk patients with community acquired pneumonia, *N Engl J Med* 336(4):243, 1997.

If the patient smokes cigarettes, he or she should be encouraged to quit smoking. Group programs are helpful to some persons, and the local branches of the ALA, ACS, or AHA can supply the names of local programs to help persons stop smoking.

## Bacterial Infections

### Pneumonia

**Etiology.** Pneumonia is an acute inflammation of lung tissue resulting from inhalation or transport via the bloodstream of infectious agents or noxious fumes or from radiation treatment.

**Epidemiology.** Of all the infectious diseases, pneumonia is the leading cause of death in the United States. More than 4 million cases of pneumonia occur in the United States yearly. Most pneumonias are communicable diseases; the mode of transmission depends on the infecting organism.

There have been significant changes in pathogens causing bacterial pneumonia and dramatic shifts in antimicrobial resistance patterns. Many new antimicrobial agents have been developed in response to pathogen resistance. These include $\beta$-lactamase inhibitors, fluoroquinolones, macrolides, and azalides.

Pneumonia is classified according to whether the infection was acquired in the community or in the hospital. Thus pneumonia is classified as *community-acquired pneumonia (CAP)* or *hospital-acquired pneumonia (HAP)*. Hospital-acquired pneumonia is also called nosocomial pneumonia.

**box 32-3** *Different Clinical Presentations of Community-Acquired Pneumonia*

| PRESENTATION 1 | PRESENTATION 2 | PRESENTATION 3 |
|---|---|---|
| Abrupt onset | Indolent onset | (Mimics influenza) |
| High fever | Low-grade fever developing over days | Nausea |
| Pleuritic chest pain | Malaise | Vomiting |
| Rigors | Fatigue | Headache |
| Purulent sputum | | Myalgias |

**table 32-5** *Causes of Community-Acquired and Hospital-Acquired Pneumonia*

| ORGANISM | COMMUNITY (%) | HOSPITAL (%) |
|---|---|---|
| *Streptococcus pneumoniae* | 33 | 6 |
| *Mycoplasma pneumoniae* | 9 | — |
| *Haemophilus influenzae* | 7 | 5 |
| Virus | 7 | — |
| *Legionella* species | 6 | — |
| *Chlamydia* species | 6 | — |
| *Staphylococcus aureus* | 3 | 8 |
| Aerobic gram-negative bacteria | 5 | 80 |

From Dominguez EA, Rupp ME: Bacterial pneumonia. In Rakel RE, editor: *Conn's current therapy,* Philadelphia, 1996, WB Saunders.

***Community-acquired pneumonia.*** Community-acquired pneumonia is responsible for between 800,000 and 1 million hospitalizations and 50,000 deaths annually in the United States. It may affect healthy individuals, but more than 70% of the cases occur in persons with preexisting diseases (e.g., COPD, coronary artery disease, diabetes mellitus, malignancy, and alcohol abuse) or impaired host defenses (see the Risk Factors Box). The mortality rate for persons with CAP who require hospitalization ranges from 6% to 13%, with even higher rates in elderly and debilitated persons. The economic cost of CAP is estimated to exceed 4 billion dollars yearly. The incidence of specific pathogens varies among patient populations and is dictated by host and environmental factors. *Streptococcus pneumoniae* is the most common cause of CAP in all age groups; it is responsible for about one third of all cases.[24] *Mycoplasma pneumoniae* primarily affects adolescents and young adults, but it can cause severe pneumonia in older and debilitated persons. *Haemophilus influenzae* and aerobic gram-negative bacteria have increased as a cause and are responsible for 12% of cases of CAP. *Legionella pneumoniae* accounts for about 6% of cases of CAP but is associated with a disproportionately high rate of respiratory failure and death.[26] Box 32-3 lists the different clinical presentations of CAP.

***Hospital-acquired pneumonia.*** The pathogens causing pneumonia in hospitalized patients differ from those causing CAP (Table 32-5). From 0.5% to 1% of patients develop pneumonia while hospitalized. However, the mortality

**risk factors**

**Hospital-Acquired Pneumonia**

Residence in an ICU
Mechanical ventilation (those requiring 48 hours or more of ventilation in an ICU have a 10% to 20% chance of developing pneumonia)
Endotracheal intubation or tracheostomy
Recent surgery
Debilitation or malnutrition
Invasive devices
Neuromuscular disease
Depressed level of alertness
Aspiration
Antacid use
Age 60 or older
Prolonged hospital stay
Any serious underlying disease

rate for these patients is 30% to 50% because of coexisting diseases and the high prevalence of gram-negative bacteria that are resistant to many antibiotics. When gram-positive bacteria are involved, the mortality rate decreases to 5% to 20%.[24]

About 80% of cases of HAP are caused by gram-negative bacteria. The remaining cases result from gram-positive bacteria (*Staphylococcus aureus* and *Streptococcus* species). *Pseudomonas aeruginosa* causes 20% to 30% of nosocomial pneumonias and is the most common pathogen found in these patients.

The second most common pathogen responsible for nosocomial pneumonia is *S. aureus,* which occurs when there are impairments in host defenses or other risk factors (e.g., indwelling and central venous catheters, chronic renal failure, residence in a neurosurgical intensive care unit [ICU], coma, recent surgery, arteriovenous shunts or fistulas).[24] *Enterobacter* species are the third most common cause of nosocomial pneumonia. Several factors put hospitalized patients at risk for pneumonia (see the Risk Factors Box above).

Hospital-acquired pneumonia occurs with aspiration of endogenous oropharyngeal bacteria into the lower respiratory tract. Oropharyngeal and tracheal colonization with gram-negative bacteria often occurs when patients have impaired defenses or serious underlying disease. Colonization of the stomach may lead to subsequent colonization of the airway and lower respiratory tract. Agents that increase gastric pH (e.g., antacids, $H_2$ antagonists) have been associated with higher rates of nosocomial pneumonia in critically ill patients being mechanically ventilated.[56]

Environmental factors implicated in the transmission of bacteria are contaminated ventilator tubing and inadequate hand washing by medical staff. Nosocomial pneumonia can also be spread hematogenously to the lung from infections in wounds, soft tissue, or the urinary tract.

**Pathophysiology.** Pneumonia results in inflammation of lung tissue. Depending on the particular pathogen and the host's physical status, the inflammatory process may involve different anatomical areas of the lung parenchyma and the pleurae. Table 32-6 lists the normal function of the respiratory system, primary pathophysiology, and clinical manifestations of pneumonia.

**Collaborative care management.** Not all patients with CAP have to be hospitalized. In general, persons aged 55 years and younger who are in good health and have no serious preexisting condition (e.g., COPD, ethanol abuse, congestive heart failure, renal failure, liver disease, cerebrovascular accident [CVA], malignancy, debilitation) can be treated on an outpatient basis as long as they respond well to oral therapy. Persons who develop systemic toxicity, prostration, respiratory failure, or hypoxemia have to be hospitalized. Parenteral antibiotics for 2 to 3 days often improve the patient's condition sufficiently that oral antibiotics can be substituted and treatment continued on an outpatient basis.

The expected length of stay of patients with pneumonia under managed care is 3 days. Common medical therapy for management of pneumonia is discussed next. Methods used to prevent pneumonia are presented in Table 32-7.

***Diagnostic tests***

1. Chest x-ray film to confirm lung consolidation and distribution and pleural effusion
2. Sputum studies for culture and sensitivity; if unable to obtain specimen by usual means, may use
   a. Transtracheal aspiration
   b. Bronchoscopy with aspiration, biopsy, or bronchial brushing
3. Arterial blood gas (ABG) studies or pulse oximetry
4. Hematology
   a. White blood cell (WBC) count for bacterial pneumonia
   b. Cold agglutinins and complement fixation for viral studies
5. Thoracentesis to obtain pleural fluid specimen if pleural effusion is present

***Medications.*** Unless the clinical findings and Gram's stain are classic for a specific organism, initial treatment of CAP is with a broad-spectrum antimicrobial. Therapy is then modified when more culture data are available.

Hospital-acquired pneumonia, with its high mortality rate, requires aggressive therapy. Therapy is often empirical and uses combinations of broad-spectrum antibiotics. Many experts recommend treatment with a third-generation cephalosporin or an anti-*Pseudomonas* penicillin–$\beta$-lactamase inhibitor combined with an aminoglycoside. Hospital-acquired pneumonia caused by methicillin-resistant *S. aureus* (MRSA) is treated with vancomycin.[26]

***Treatments.*** Oxygen is titrated to maintain $SpO_2$. Turning, coughing, and deep breathing are performed regularly.

***Diet.*** A high-calorie, high-protein diet with frequent small feedings is usually prescribed.

***Activity.*** The patient should be on bedrest but may be out of bed to use the toilet or commode chair.

**table 32-6** *Normal Function of Respiratory System and Primary Pathophysiology and Clinical Manifestations of Pneumonia*

| Normal Function | Pathophysiology | Clinical Manifestations |
|---|---|---|
| **MUCOCILIARY SYSTEM** | | |
| Cleanses inhaled air by trapping particles | Hypertrophy of mucous membrane lining lung, resulting in hypersecretion | Increased sputum production and cough<br>Anaerobic—foul-smelling sputum<br>*Klebsiella*—currant jelly color<br>*Staphylococcus*—creamy yellow<br>*Pseudomonas*—green<br>Viral/mucopurulent |
| | Bronchospasm from increased secretions | Localized or diffuse wheezing, dyspnea |
| **ALVEOLOCAPILLARY MEMBRANE** | | |
| Oxygen–carbon dioxide exchange | Increased capillary permeability resulting in excess fluid in interstitial spaces | Chest x-ray films: consolidation: localized/bacterial; diffuse/viral |
| | Decreased surface area for gas exchange | Hypoxemia |
| **PLEURA** | | |
| Maintains close approximation of lungs and chest wall; minimizes friction during lung expansion and contraction | Inflammation of pleurae | Chest pain, especially on inspiration<br>Pleural effusion<br>Dullness on percussion<br>Decreased breath sounds<br>Decreased vocal fremitus |
| **RESPIRATORY MUSCLE** | | |
| Expands and contracts chest wall and thus pleura and lungs | Hypoventilation | Decreased chest expansion |
| | Respiratory acidosis (in presence of underlying disease) | Hypercapnia and low arterial blood pH |
| **LUNG DEFENSE SYSTEM** | | |
| Protects normally sterile lung from invasion by pathogens | Bacteremia | Elevated white blood cell count: leukocytes (15,000 to 25,000/mm$^3$)<br>Neutrophilia<br>Tachypnea, fever |

**table 32-7** *Methods Used to Prevent Pneumonia*

| Type of Pneumonia | Methods |
|---|---|
| Streptococcal | Pneumonia polysaccharide vaccine for persons 65 years and older and others at high risk, effective 3 to 5 years against multiple strains of pneumococcal polysaccharides |
| Gram negative, gram positive | Frequent hand washing<br>Adequate ventilation<br>Every 24 hours:<br>Changing open container solutions<br>Changing respiratory equipment<br>Tracheostomy and endotracheal airways treated with sterile technique<br>Sterile technique when suctioning<br>Turning and repositioning every 2 hours<br>Necessity of not draining condensation in ventilator equipment back into liquid reservoir |
| Aspiration | Positioning patients with decreased consciousness to facilitate drainage of secretions<br>Inflating endotracheal or tracheostomy cuff before feeding<br>Ensuring proper placement of nasogastric tube before giving tube feeding |
| Viral, *M. pneumoniae* | Prompt treatment of unresolved URI or acute bronchitis<br>Limiting contact with people who have viral infections<br>Maintaining optimal nutrition |

***Referrals.*** Common referrals for the patient with CAP requiring hospitalization include a dietitian, physical therapist, respiratory therapist, and social worker.

## NURSING MANAGEMENT

### ASSESSMENT

#### Subjective Data

Data to be collected to assess the patient with pneumonia include:

History and character of onset and duration of cough, fever, shaking chills, chest pain, sputum production (amount, color, consistency)
Self-care modalities used to treat symptoms
History of exposure to persons with URI or pulmonary irritants

#### Objective Data

Data to be collected to assess the patient with pneumonia include:

Signs of other chronic diseases and general debilitation
Vital signs: elevated temperature (39° C to 40° C [102.2° F to 104° F]) or low-grade temperature elevation; tachycardia/tachypnea
Pulmonary examination
Inspection: accessory muscle retraction, central cyanosis, respiratory grunting on expiration, restricted chest movement
Palpation: decreased expansion on affected side of chest, increased tactile fremitus
Percussion: dullness
Auscultation: bronchial breath sounds, inspiratory crackles (rales), decreased vocal fremitus (pleural effusion), egophony (consolidation)
Laboratory findings
Hematology: WBC—elevated 15,000 to 25,000/mm$^3$; cold agglutinins—complement fixation/viral or *M. pneumoniae*
ABG studies: hypoxemia/respiratory alkalosis; if underlying chronic disease, respiratory acidosis
Chest x-ray: diffuse involvement—atypical pneumonia; lobar involvement—typical pneumonia

### NURSING DIAGNOSES

Nursing diagnoses are determined from analysis of patient data. Nursing diagnoses for the person with pneumonia may include but are not limited to:

| Diagnostic Title | Possible Etiological Factors |
|---|---|
| Airway clearance, ineffective | Decreased energy, fatigue, tracheobronchial inflammation |
| Gas exchange, impaired | Alveolocapillary membrane changes, altered oxygen delivery |
| Pain | Pleural inflammation, coughing paroxysms |
| Infection, risk for | Compromised lung defense system |
| Knowledge deficit: conditions, treatments | Lack of exposure to or unfamiliarity with information |
| Anorexia | Infectious process, sputum production |
| Nutrition, altered: less than body requirements | Increased metabolic needs |

### EXPECTED PATIENT OUTCOMES

Expected patient outcomes for the person with pneumonia may include but are not limited to:

1. Demonstrates effective cough with adequate sputum production. (Both cough and sputum production decreased within 72 hours of treatment initiation. Patient with chronic lung disease returns to prepneumonia status.)
2. Demonstrates improved ventilation and adequate oxygenation of tissues. pH returns within normal limits. Oxygen tension ($PO_2$) during active disease: 60 to 80 mm Hg; after resolution of disease, arterial $PO_2$ ($PaO_2$) is within normal limits.
3. Reports absence of chest pain.
4. Does not develop a superinfection.
5a. States when influenza and pneumonia vaccines should be taken.
 b. Knows the signs and symptoms that should be reported to the physician.
 c. Describes the cause and factors contributing to the occurrence of pneumonia and names common symptoms indicating pneumonia.
6. Has improved appetite.
7. Weight returns to near preillness level.

### INTERVENTIONS

#### Maintaining Effective Airway Clearance

1. Monitor for increased respiratory distress.
2. Assist patient to cough effectively.
3. If unable to clear own airway, suction airway using sterile technique (see Chapter 31).
4. Assist with nebulizer therapy.
5. Administer bronchodilators as ordered. Monitor for side effects and response to therapy.
6. Change position frequently to assist in mobilizing secretions.
7. Ensure fluid intake adequate to thin secretions.

#### Facilitating Breathing

Help the patient breathe deeply and expand the chest to increase ventilation.

1. Place patient in position to facilitate breathing, usually upright or semiupright position (Figure 32-1).
2. A pillow may be placed lengthwise at the patient's back to provide support and thrust thorax slightly forward, allowing freer use of the diaphragm.
3. The patient who must be upright to breathe may find it restful to put head and arms on a pillow placed on an overbed table.
4. For the patient with severe hypoxemia, side rails should be in place. The patient can use them to assist in moving about in bed.

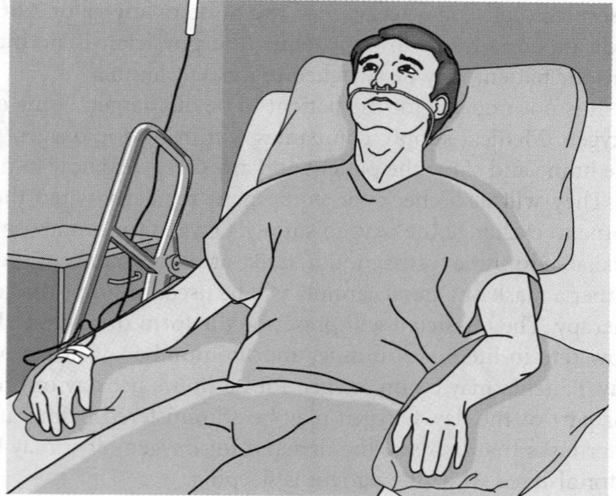

**fig. 32-1** Patient sitting upright with pillow under head and each arm to promote chest expansion and comfort.

5. Some patients may breathe best when sitting up in a large armchair while leaning on a smaller chair placed in front of them. This chair is blocked to prevent it from slipping.
6. Assist with ADL, pacing activities to prevent fatigue and respiratory distress.

#### *Maintaining ventilation, humidity, and comfortable temperature*

1. Most patients are most comfortable if air is cool and not too humid. An air-conditioned room may add to patient comfort.
2. If patient has nose, throat, or bronchial irritation, warm moist air from a humidifier or vaporizer may be helpful.
3. Because of concern about cross-infection from room humidifiers, follow CDC recommendations (Box 32-4).

#### *Vaporizers*

Small electric vaporizers can be purchased at most local drugstores. However, when a patient cannot afford to purchase one, the nurse can assist in improvising equipment for inhalation and proper humidity. An empty coffee can or a shallow pie tin can be filled with distilled water and placed in the person's room to increase humidity.

### Administering Medications and Treatments

1. Before beginning administration of prescribed antibiotic, collect sputum for culture. If blood culture is ordered, also draw blood before therapy is begun.
2. Maintain antibiotic blood levels by giving antibiotics at scheduled times.
3. Give medication prescribed to relieve pain. Codeine may be prescribed because it is less likely to inhibit the cough reflex than more potent narcotics.
4. Begin oxygen therapy.

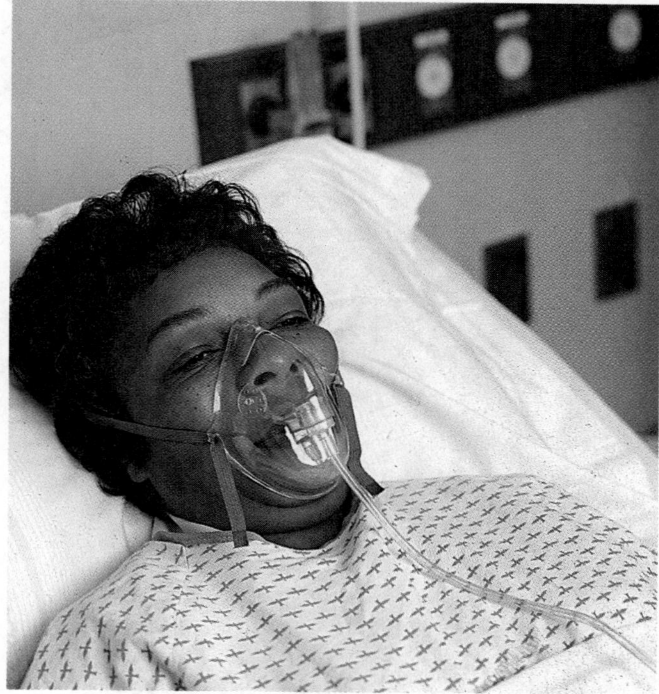

**fig. 32-2** Simple oxygen mask.

**box 32-4** *CDC Recommendations When Using a Humidifier*

1. Use only a direct-heated humidifier or a nebulizer with a bacterial filter. Cold vapor or cool-mist humidifiers are not recommended because they cannot withstand daily sterilization.
2. Use only sterile water in the humidifier, and drain remaining water each time the humidifier is refilled, or at least every 24 hours. Tap water is not safe to use because it may be contaminated with *Pseudomonas, Flavobacterium, Acinetobacter,* or other organisms.
3. Establish a routine maintenance schedule.
4. Set medical guidelines to determine which patients should receive humidification and which should not. It may not be advisable to use humidifiers for immunosuppressed patients.
5. Do not send humidifying unit home with patients because of the concern about transporting highly resistant hospital organisms into the community.

### Administering Oxygen Therapy

Oxygen by mask or cannula (Figures 32-2 and 32-3) is usually ordered when $Po_2$ is less than 60 mm Hg. When supplemental oxygen is necessary, it may be administered by nasal prongs or by mask. The method used depends on the patient's condition and the concentration of oxygen required. The nurse should become familiar with the various devices used to administer oxygen, and when oxygen is in use, the nurse should check the equipment frequently to ensure it is working properly.

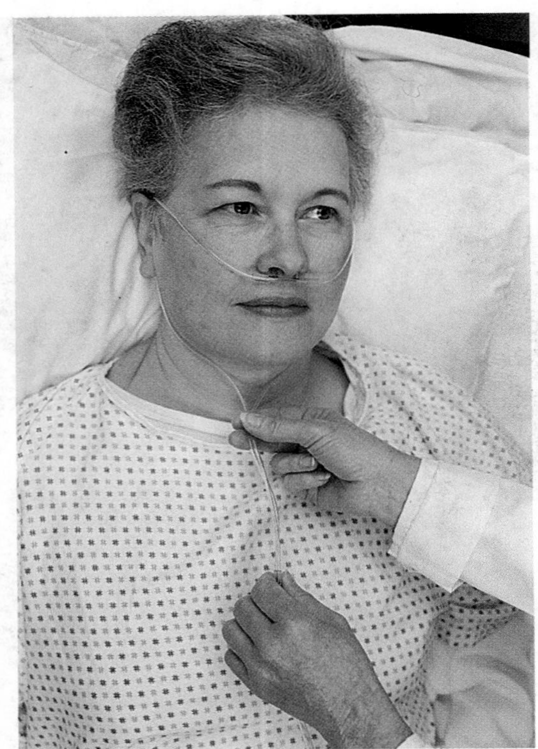

**fig. 32-3** Nasal cannula.

When the patient is having difficulty exchanging oxygen and carbon dioxide, such as occurs in pulmonary edema, oxygen may be given under positive pressure. In some situations, such as COPD, low flow rates of oxygen are indicated. The use of low-flow oxygen is discussed on p. 1016. *In all situations, the nurse should remember that the patient with hypoxemia may not be breathless or cyanotic because cyanosis does not occur until there is 5 g or more of deoxygenated hemoglobin.* In persons with anemia, all the available heme is completely saturated with oxygen, and thus they are never cyanotic even though they may be hypoxemic. For this reason, an increase in the pulse rate or restlessness may be the first indication that the patient is experiencing hypoxemia. Patients receiving oxygen therapy are monitored with ABGs and pulse oximetry. Table 32-8 compares oxygen delivery systems.

Transtracheal oxygen (TTO) therapy may be used to treat patients with hypoxemia who are able to care for themselves. In TTO administration, a small, flexible catheter is inserted into the lower anterior neck. A necklace and a transparent film dressing are used to hold the catheter in place. The catheter is connected to an oxygen hose that is attached to an oxygen source. The oxygen hose is secured to the patient's clothes.[46]

Care of the patient on TTO is the same as that described for other types of oxygen delivery, except for care of the insertion site. The site is cleansed twice daily using a long swab and warm water or hydrogen peroxide. No creams or ointments should be used on the site. The insertion site is monitored for signs of infection. If the patient develops shortness of breath, a severe cough, or wheezing, or the pulse oximetry or ABGs indicate an increase in hypoxemia, the physician is notified and the patient may be switched to a nasal cannula.

It is not unusual for the patient to be discharged home on oxygen. Medical supply companies will bring the oxygen to the home and show the patient and any caregivers how to use it. They will also check the equipment regularly when they come to exchange the oxygen supply. Oxygen for home use is available in three forms: liquid, tank, or oxygen concentrator. Either a mask or a nasal cannula will be used for home oxygen therapy. The physician will prescribe the form of oxygen, the flow rate in liters per minute, and the number of hours per day. Patients may be on oxygen for 24 hours per day or only for part of the day. Oxygen may be administered before and after tasks that increase the demand for oxygen, or it may be administered while the patient is sleeping.

#### *Patient/family education*

1. Be sure that the flow rate is as ordered by the physician.
2. Check the amount of water in the humidifier bottle each time oxygen is used or at least every 6 to 8 hours if used continuously. If the water level is close to the fill line, empty the bottle and refill with sterile or distilled bottled water.
3. Oxygen is drying to the membranes in the nose. Applying a water-soluble lubricant such as K-Y jelly to the inside of the nose may help reduce dryness and cracking. Petroleum jelly (Vaseline) should not be used because it might be inhaled.
4. Always order a new supply of oxygen when the oxygen source reads one-quarter full usually 2 to 3 days before a new tank is needed.
5. Observe safety precautions:
   a. Notify the local fire department that you have oxygen in the house. Most fire departments offer a free safety inspection, along with suggestions for making your home safer while oxygen is in use.
   b. Oxygen is not itself flammable, but it supports combustion. For this reason, no one should smoke in the room where oxygen is being used.
   c. When a patient is using oxygen, he or she should stay away from gas stoves, gas space heaters, or kerosene heaters or lamps.
   d. To prevent leakage of oxygen, always keep the container upright. Make sure the system is turned off when not in use.
   e. Keep an all-purpose fire extinguisher close by.
   f. If fire should occur, turn off oxygen and leave the house immediately. Have a neighbor call the fire department.
6. Notify your physician immediately if any of the following occur:
   a. Your breathing is difficult, irregular, shallow, or slow.
   b. You become restless or anxious.
   c. You are tired or drowsy, or have trouble waking up.
   d. You have a persistent headache.
   e. Your speech becomes slurred, you cannot concentrate, or you feel confused.
   f. Your fingernails or lips are blue.

table 32-8 *Comparing Oxygen Delivery Systems*

| Delivery System | Indications | Concentration | Flow Rate | Considerations |
|---|---|---|---|---|
| **LOW FLOW** | | | | |
| Nasal cannula | Patient with spontaneous respirations and oxygen requirements of less than 50% | 32-36% | 2-6 L/min with no respiratory distress; 5-6 L/min with onset of respiratory distress | Oxygen concentration will increase about 4% for each increase of 1 L/min<br>Questionable efficacy in patients who are mouth breathing |
| Simple face mask | Patient with spontaneous respirations | 35-60% | 6-8 L/min | Liter per minute flow should be *at least* 6 to prevent accumulation and rebreathing of expired $CO_2$<br>May not be well tolerated by claustrophobic patient<br>Effective for patients who are mouth breathing |
| Partial rebreather face mask | Patient with spontaneous respirations and oxygen requirements greater than 50% | 65-75% | 6-10 L/min | Flow rates should be high enough to ensure that reservoir bag remains inflated during inspiration *and* expiration |
| Nonrebreather face mask | Spontaneously breathing patient with profound hypoxia or oxygen requirement | 85-95% | 8-12 L/min | Flow rates should be high enough to ensure that reservoir bag remains inflated during inspiration *and* expiration |
| **HIGH FLOW** | | | | |
| Venturi mask | Patient with spontaneous respirations | 24-50% | Varies (consult manufacturer's directions) | Good for use in patients who require delivery of precise oxygen concentrations<br>Prescribed by concentration, not flow rate |
| **POSITIVE PRESSURE** | | | | |
| One-way valve pocket mask | Patient requiring assistance or control of ventilation | 50-55% (with oxygen supplement) | 10-15 L/min | Prevents direct contact between health care provider and patient<br>Easier to use and obtain adequate tidal volumes than bag-valve mask<br>Should be used with oropharyngeal or nasopharyngeal airway in place to prevent gastric distension |
| Bag-valve mask | Patient requiring assistance or control of ventilation | Approaching 100% with reservoir; 45-50% without reservoir | 10-15 L/min | Prevents direct contact between health care provider and patient<br>Should be used with oropharyngeal or nasopharyngeal airway in place to prevent gastric distension<br>Difficult to use; inexperienced operators may not deliver adequate tidal volumes<br>Short-term device of choice once endotracheal intubation achieved |

From Somerson SJ et al: Mastering emergency airway management, *Am J Nurs* 96(5):25, 1996.

### Promoting Comfort

1. Place in position of comfort; patients are usually most comfortable with head of bed elevated 45 to 90 degrees.
2. Assess for character and location of chest pain.
3. Administer analgesics for chest pain:
   a. Acetylsalicylic acid
   b. Acetaminophen
   c. Codeine
4. Splint chest with hands when patient coughs (see p. 958).
5. Administer frequent mouth care. Protect lips and nares with lubricant.
6. Keep patient warm and dry and avoid chilling.

### Preventing Spread of Infection

1. When Standard Precautions are used, respiratory isolation is unnecessary.
2. Hand washing is the most important way to prevent spread of pneumonia from one patient to another via the hands of hospital personnel.
3. Reducing the likelihood of gram-negative colonization of patients is a primary consideration. For this reason, many hospitals have instituted tighter control policies on the use of antibiotics except in situations where a review panel of physicians approves their use. A reduction in use of antibiotics also reduces the incidence of antibiotic-resistant hospital flora, which are the source of many nosocomial infections (see Chapter 10).

### Facilitating Learning

The major teaching emphasis is on prevention.

1. Assess patient's understanding of pneumonia with questions concerning such information as how pneumonia is transmitted and risk factors.
2. Teach proper handling of secretions. Cover nose and mouth with tissue when coughing or sneezing. Discard tissues in a paper or plastic bag for disposal. Expectorate into specimen container provided.
3. Stress importance of hand washing after coughing, sneezing, and expectorating.
4. Reinforce importance of follow-up care.
5. Reinforce need for immunization.
   a. Two vaccines are now available to prevent respiratory infections: influenza vaccine and pneumococcal vaccine.
   b. Persons at risk for developing complication of influenza (pneumonia) should be immunized unless they are allergic to eggs or egg products or have had a previous reaction to vaccine.[16]
      (1) Influenza vaccine is given yearly.
      (2) Pneumonia polysaccharide vaccine is given only every 3 to 5 years.

### Promoting Adequate Hydration and Nutrition

Dehydration results in thick, tenacious secretions. The best liquefying agent is water, and it is preferable to hydrate the patient adequately rather than attempt to loosen secretions with mist therapy. If the patient does not have cardiovascular disease requiring fluid restriction, a fluid intake of 3 to 4 L per day should be provided.

1. Encourage oral fluids. If patient is receiving intravenous (IV) fluids, monitor rate. Observe for signs of fluid volume deficit or excess.
2. Ask patient what foods he or she would like to eat.
3. Offer small, frequent feedings.
4. Encourage high-carbohydrate and high-protein foods.

#### *Patient/family education*

**Health promotion/prevention.** The major points in patient and family education are discussed under Facilitating Learning. For care of patients who may receive oxygen therapy at home, see the discussion on p. 928.

## EVALUATION

To evaluate the effectiveness of nursing interventions, compare patient behaviors with those stated in the expected patient outcomes. Successful achievement of patient outcomes for the person with pneumonia is indicated by:

1. Cough and sputum are reduced, and lung sounds are clear.
2. $PaO_2$, $PaCO_2$, pH, and pulse oximetry are within normal limits.
3. Patient is free of chest pain.
4. Patient does not develop superinfection.

5a. Patient states the need to receive an influenza shot yearly in September and a pneumonia shot every 3 to 5 years.

b. Patient verbalizes the need for medical attention if cough persists, a fever lasts for more than 48 hours, fatigue is overwhelming, or generalized achiness is present.

c. Patient verbalizes that failure to seek medical attention after a prolonged bout of influenza was the factor that led to pneumonia.

6. Anorexia is improved.
7. Patient has improved appetite, and weight is only 2 pounds less than it was before admission.

## GERONTOLOGICAL CONSIDERATIONS

Nurses working with elderly persons need to be aware of their vulnerability to pneumonia. Interventions are directed toward preventing pneumonia by teaching them to receive a vaccination for influenza yearly and for pneumonia every 3 to 5 years. Also, nurses should emphasize how elderly persons can care for themselves by maintaining activity and good health practices (see the Gerontological Assessment Box).

## SPECIAL ENVIRONMENTS FOR CARE

### Home Care

Persons discharged from the hospital after being admitted with CAP who are otherwise in fairly good health still require 4 to 6 weeks before they feel completely well. Attention to their recuperation includes obtaining extra rest and gradually resuming activities such as returning to work. Many people find it easier to resume work on a part-time basis until they have more energy. An adequate, balanced diet is essential, as are rest periods and adequate sleep at night. As a general rule, the older the person, the longer the period of recovery,

## gerontological assessment

**ASSESSMENT**

Assess lung sounds; diminished lung sounds are common in elderly persons because of thickened alveoli and decreased rib cage expansion (thorax stiffening).

Assess respiratory status with activity; dyspnea with exertion may occur from decreased pulmonary oxygen diffusion.

Monitor effects of drugs that may interfere with breathing, such as narcotics and hypnotics. Elderly persons may have decreased drug clearance from decreased glomerular filtration rate (GFR) and nephron activity or from decreased hepatic function.

Monitor for signs of pneumonia, to which elderly persons are highly susceptible. Elderly patients may have symptoms of mental confusion, tachycardia, or dyspnea rather than the customary signs of cough, fever, and crackles.

**INTERVENTIONS**

Encourage as much activity as the person can tolerate to promote ventilation, such as paced walking.

Suggest patient sit upright for meals and for 20 to 30 minutes after meals to prevent pulmonary aspiration.

Encourage pneumococcal and influenza vaccine prophylaxis.

Teach patient the importance of oral care to clear mouth of pathogens to help prevent pneumonia.

For elderly patient with pneumonia, maintain good hydration (with close monitoring to prevent fluid imbalances), and assist with respiratory therapy and position changes to facilitate removal of secretions.

although many young people recovering from pneumonia remark, "I can't believe how tired I am."

Persons with hospital-acquired pneumonia have an even more protracted period of recovery because their pneumonia was superimposed on a chronic condition such as COPD. They are likely to be even more restricted in their activities because of chronic shortness of breath and resultant fatigue.[24]

Persons living alone should have someone in the home at least part of each day to assist with ADL such as bathing, dressing, and meal preparation. The nurse caring for the patient or a social worker should make a referral to a home health agency before the patient is discharged, unless the patient has a significant other who will assist with these activities. These patients also need to be monitored closely by their health care provider and often need assistance in going to follow-up appointments. For some persons, meals-on-wheels can provide them with a hot meal daily until they are well enough to prepare their own meals. Some persons, however, receive Meals-on-Wheels for several months.

## COMPLICATIONS

With the advent of antibiotics and better diagnostic measures such as x-ray procedures, complications during or after pneumonia are rare in otherwise healthy persons. Atelectasis, delayed resolution, lung abscess, pleural effusion, empyema, pericarditis, meningitis, and relapse are complications that were common in the past. Because pneumonia and influenza rank fifth as a cause of death in the United States, the patient must understand the importance of strict adherence to the prescribed medical treatment. Careful and accurate observation and sufficient time for convalescence also help ensure that the average patient has a smooth recovery. Elderly persons and those with a chronic illness are likely to have a relatively long course of convalescence from pneumonia and are at higher risk for complications. There has been an increase in the incidence of staphylococcal pneumonia subsequent to influenza. Consolidation of lung tissue, pleural effusion, and empyema may occur soon after onset of staphylococcal pneumonia and may cause death.

### *Tuberculosis*

In 1900 tuberculosis (TB) was the leading cause of death in the United States. It remained a major cause of death until the introduction of antituberculosis drug therapy in the late 1940s and early 1950s. The most effective of these agents is isoniazid, which first became available clinically in 1952. The use of isoniazid in combination with two agents introduced earlier, streptomycin and paraaminosalicylic acid, resulted in a striking decrease in TB mortality rates. It also made it possible for patients with TB to be treated on an outpatient basis. However, some patients still have to be hospitalized during their illness, and most nurses will care for a patient with TB at some time in their careers.

**Etiology.** Tuberculosis is an infectious disease caused by the bacillus *Mycobacterium tuberculosis* or the tubercle bacillus, an acid-fast organism.

**Epidemiology.** Although TB is considered a preventable and curable disease, it is a disease that demands constant public health surveillance. In 1993 there was a small decrease in the number of new TB cases, and the case rate has decreased every year since then. In 1997 a total of 19,855 new cases of tuberculosis were reported to the CDC from the 50 states. This was the fifth consecutive year that the number of reported TB cases had decreased (Figure 32-4). The U.S. case rate per 100,000 cases was 7.4. This is the lowest number and case rate of reported TB cases since national reporting began in 1953.[19]

The TB rates per 100,000 population by state ranged from 0.4 in Wyoming to 14.1 in Hawaii. The highest case rate was 20.8 in the District of Columbia. Sixteen states met the interim target rate for the year 2000 of $\leq$3.5 cases per 100,000 population. The number of new cases decreased in both men and women and in all age groups and racial/ethnic groups. The largest decrease was in adults 25 to 44 years of age.[19]

When TB rates among U.S.-born and foreign-born persons are compared, the case rate decreased for U.S.-born persons and increased 6% for foreign-born persons from 1992 to 1997 (Figure 32-5). Seven countries (Haiti, India, Mexico, Philippines, People's Republic of China, Republic of Korea,

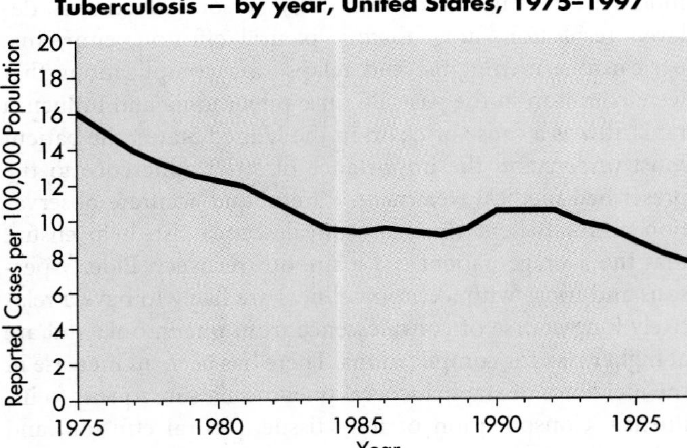


**fig. 32-4** Number of tuberculosis cases per 100,000 population, United States, 1975 through 1997.

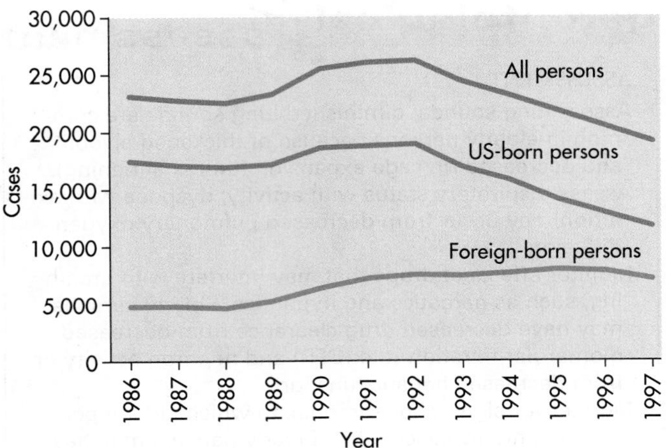


**fig. 32-5** Number of persons with reported cases of tuberculosis, by country of birth—United States, 1986 through 1997.

and Vietnam) accounted for more than two thirds of the cases among foreign-born persons who were infected with TB in their country of origin.

Despite the overall decrease in the number of reported TB cases, some differences bear mentioning. Although the greatest decrease in U.S. cases was in the 25 to 44 age group, this age group still has the greatest number of reported TB cases. It is assumed that this group represents the greatest source of infection for children 14 and under because they probably have the most contact with children.

Cities with the highest number of persons positive for the human immunodeficiency virus (HIV), especially among drug abusers, also have the highest number of TB cases. Usually these cities also are more likely to have many immigrants, many of whom come from countries in which TB is endemic. Another concern is that many persons with HIV are infected with TB organisms resistant to most chemotherapeutic agents used to treat TB. When this is true, infected persons pass their resistant organisms to those they infect, making treatment of newly infected persons particularly difficult.

Because HIV infection is an important risk factor for developing TB among persons who have a positive tuberculin test, the CDC recommends that all HIV-infected persons be screened for active TB and, if infected, receive appropriate therapy. Also, persons with active TB and all tuberculin-positive persons should be evaluated for HIV infection.

**Pathophysiology.** When an individual with no previous exposure to TB (negative tuberculin reactor) inhales a sufficient number of tubercle bacilli into the alveoli, tuberculosis infection occurs. The body's reaction to the tubercle bacilli depends on the susceptibility of the individual, the size of the dose, and the virulence of the organisms. Inflammation occurs within the alveoli (parenchyma) of the lungs, and natural body defenses attempt to counteract the infection.

Macrophages ingest the organisms and present the mycobacterial antigens to the T cells. CD4 cells secrete lymphokines that enhance the capacity of the macrophages to ingest and kill bacteria. Lymph nodes in the hilar region of the lung become enlarged as they filter drainage from the infected site. The inflammatory process and cellular reaction produce a small, firm, white nodule called the *primary tubercle.* The center of the nodule contains tubercle bacilli. Cells gather around the center, and usually the outer portion becomes fibrosed. Thus blood vessels are compressed, nutrition of the tubercle is impaired, and necrosis occurs at the center. The area becomes walled off by fibrotic tissue, and the center gradually becomes soft and cheesy in consistency. This latter process is known as *caseation necrosis.* This material may become calcified (calcium deposits), or it may liquefy (liquefaction necrosis). The liquefied material may be coughed up, leaving a cavity, or hole, in the parenchyma of the lung. The cavity or cavities are visible on chest x-ray films and result in the diagnosis of *cavitary disease.*

Most individuals who are exposed to TB and develop a TB infection (confirmed by a positive tuberculin test) do not develop an active case of TB. The only x-ray evidence of their TB infection is a calcified nodule known as the *Ghon's tubercle.* The evidence on x-ray film of enlarged hilar lymph nodes and a Ghon's tubercle is referred to as the *primary complex.*

Persons who have the primary complex have become sensitized to the tubercle bacillus, and an antigen-antibody reaction results. When the person receives the antigen in the form of a purified protein derivative (PPD) or old tuberculin (OT) in a tuberculin test, the reaction results in a positive tuberculin test. This sensitization, once developed, usually remains throughout life unless something compromises the immune response. Evidence suggests that most persons who have a positive tuberculin reaction and take isoniazid prophylactically for 6 months convert from a positive to a negative tuberculin test. This protection is believed to last for life. A positive tuberculin test does *not* mean that one has TB, however, and nurses should explain this to persons undergoing the test.

Tuberculosis infection is unlike other infections. Usually, other infections disappear completely when overcome by the body's defenses and leave no living organisms and generally no signs of infection. However, persons who have been in-

**table 32-9** *Classification of Tuberculosis*

| Class | Description | Medical Therapy |
|---|---|---|
| 0 | No TB exposure, not infected | None |
| 1 | TB exposure, no evidence of infection | Preventive chemotherapy may be given for persons who have converted their tuberculin test from negative to positive |
| 2 | TB infection, no disease | Isoniazid (INH) for 6 mos (preventive chemotherapy) for *positive reactors* under age 35 |
| 3 | TB: clinically active (persons with completed diagnostic evidence of TB: both a significant reaction to tuberculin skin test and clinical or x-ray evidence of TB) | Antituberculosis drugs: at least 2 of the first-line drugs (INH, ethambutol, rifampin, pyrazinamide, streptomycin) |
| 4 | TB: not clinically active (persons with previous history of TB or with abnormal x-ray films but no significant tuberculin skin test reaction or clinical evidence) | No new therapy (persons may still be receiving chemotherapy) |
| 5 | TB: suspect (diagnosis pending); used during diagnostic testing of suspect persons, for no longer than a 3-month period | Preventive chemotherapy with INH may be instituted |

fected with tubercle bacilli harbor the organism for the remainder of their lives unless they have received prophylactic isoniazid. Tubercle bacilli remain in the lungs in a dormant, walled-off, or so-called resting state. When a person is under physical or emotional stress, these bacilli may become active and begin to multiply. If body defenses are compromised, active TB may develop. Most persons who have active TB developed it in this manner. However, it is generally accepted that only 1 out of 10 persons with a positive tuberculin test will ever develop active TB, and the incidence is expected to be much lower among those who receive preventive therapy with isoniazid.

Tuberculosis that occurs several years after the primary infection is known as *reactivation tuberculosis.* The development of active TB is believed to be caused by defects in T cell function, macrophage function, or both.

Tuberculosis is more likely to occur in persons with HIV infection because in HIV infection, progressive depletion and dysfunction of CD4 cells occur, along with defects in macrophage and monocyte function. Epidemiological evidence suggests that because of these changes, persons with HIV infection and a positive tuberculin test (primary infection) are at risk for reactivation tuberculosis. At the same time, persons with HIV infection who have negative tuberculin tests are at risk of progressing directly from a primary infection to active TB when exposed to someone with TB. Also, extrapulmonary TB is more common among persons with HIV infection, and TB diagnosed in them becomes an AIDS-defining condition. This means that tuberculosis is a more opportunistic infection than is *Pneumocystis carinii* and other infections that indicate that a person has progressed from HIV infection to AIDS.[28]

Two mycobacterial organisms are found in persons with AIDS. In developed countries the *Mycobacterium avium-intracellulare* complex (MAC) is the organism found in middle-class AIDS patients who have no history of intravenous drug use. Pulmonary tuberculosis caused by *M. tuberculosis* is more common in AIDS patients from developing countries and in persons from inner-city minority populations who have a history of intravenous drug use.[14]

***Classification.*** The classification used by states and territories of the United States when reporting TB cases to the CDC of the Public Health Service is outlined in Table 32-9. The six basic classifications cover the total child and adult population, those unexposed to TB, those uninfected even though exposed, those with evidence of infection without disease, those with disease, those with evidence of TB without current disease, and those in whom TB is suspected (diagnosis pending).

***Extrapulmonary tuberculosis.*** Tuberculosis may affect other parts of the body besides the lungs, such as the larynx, gastrointestinal (GI) tract, lymph nodes, skin, skeletal system, nervous system, urinary system, and reproductive system. Tuberculosis is spread to other parts of the body via blood (hematogenously) or lymph (lymphogenously).

Extrapulmonary TB has taken on increased importance because of its extremely high rate of occurrence, usually along with pulmonary tuberculosis, in persons with HIV infection. The lymph nodes are the most common site of extrapulmonary TB in persons with HIV infection. Miliary disease (in which the chest x-ray film looks as though millet seeds are spread throughout both lungs) is also common. Involvement also occurs in bone marrow, the genitourinary tract, and the central nervous system (CNS). Because persons with HIV infection and TB infection usually have bacteremia, blood cultures are recommended when the diagnosis of TB is suspected.

***Mycobacteria other than tubercle bacilli (MOTT).*** These mycobacteria, formerly referred to as atypical acid-fast bacilli, are named *M. kansasii, M. avium-intracellulare* complex, *M. xenopi, M. marinum, M. fortuitum,* and *M. chelonai.* The last two are classified as rapid growers. These organisms are strongly acid-fast but differ from *M. tuberculosis* on culture. They are being isolated with increasing frequency from immunocompromised patients (persons with HIV infection or AIDS, transplant patients, and patients undergoing antineoplastic chemotherapy). MOTT have been found in soil and water and less commonly in foodstuffs and are considered to be opportunistic organisms.

MOTT identified in sputum specimens may mean that the person is colonized and does not have invasive disease. (See Chapter 10 for more information on colonization.) MOTT are often isolated from the sputum of patients with pneumoconiosis, chronic bronchitis, COPD, past history of TB, bronchiectasis, and chronic aspiration from esophageal disease. Table 32-10 summarizes these nontuberculosis organisms.

*Mycobacterium avium-intracellulare* complex is the most common bacterial infection in patients with AIDS. It occurs in 30% to 50% of AIDS patients. Patients with MAC have fever, night sweats, weight loss, diarrhea, lymphadenopathy, and anemia. The diagnosis is usually made from isolator blood cultures, bone marrow, lymph node, or liver biopsy. It is also diagnosed by acid-fast smear of stool in patients with disseminated infection.[47]

***Multidrug-resistant TB (MDR-TB).*** MDR-TB has become a major problem in the United States. In 1997 nearly 8% of TB patients were resistant to isoniazid, rifampin, or both (two of the most effective drugs for treating TB). New York City and California reported the greatest number of cases of MDR-TB.[5]

The emergence of MDR-TB means that increased efforts are required to find every TB patient and to ensure that they are treated with four-drug therapy initially in an effort to prevent further drug resistance. It is also important to protect other patients and health care workers from becoming infected by patients with MDR-TB. The problem is especially great in institutions caring for large numbers of patients with HIV, many of whom also have MDR-TB. Protective methods are discussed in the following sections.

**table 32-10** *MOTT Associated with Human Disease*

| Organism | Sites Typically Involved | Suggested Therapy |
|---|---|---|
| *M. avium* complex (MAC) | Lung, disseminated (AIDS) | Amikacin, clofazimine, (Lamprene), RIF and EMB and clarithromycin |
| *M. kansasii* | Lung | INH, RIF, and EMB for 12-24 months |
| *M. xenopi* | Lung | Amikacin, clofazimine, RIF and EMB (perhaps clarithromycin and quinolone) |
| *M. marinum* | Skin, soft tissue | RIF, trimethoprim-sulfamethoxazole, or minocycline as single agents |
| *M. fortuitum* | Soft tissue<br>Pulmonary<br>Disseminated | Amikacin (parenteral) and cefoxitin or imipenem for 4-6 weeks |
| *M. chelonai* | Soft tissue | Often resistant to INH and PZA; may respond to four or more drugs; surgical excision of localized disease |

**Collaborative care management**

***Diagnostic tests.*** Each of the tests used to diagnose tuberculosis is described in Chapter 30. These tests are (1) tuberculin skin testing, (2) chest x-ray films, and (3) sputum smear and culture. If microscopic study of a slide prepared from the sputum of an individual reveals tubercle bacilli, the individual is said to have positive sputum, which confirms the diagnosis of TB. However, most persons with tuberculosis will not have positive sputum on smear, and a positive sputum culture will be necessary to confirm the diagnosis. Patients who have a positive culture and negative smear are less infectious than are those with both a positive smear and a positive culture.

*Establishing the diagnosis of tuberculosis.* Results of chest x-ray films and sputum examinations will either rule out the possibility or confirm a diagnosis of TB. Bacteriological confirmation of the presence of *M. tuberculosis* is necessary to establish the diagnosis of TB. Because it is impossible to differentiate between typical bacilli and MOTT by a sputum smear, cultures are obtained on all persons. Cultures are also used for antimicrobial susceptibility (sensitivity) studies. Despite the introduction of improved culture media, the *tubercle bacillus grows slowly on artificial media,* and *culture reports are not available for 3 to 6 weeks.* Newer approaches to culturing the bacillus are under development.

Blood-streaked sputum in the absence of pronounced coughing may be the first indication to the person that something is wrong. Pathological changes may have occurred in the lungs, but sputum examination may not show tubercle bacilli. However, if the nodules produced in the parenchyma of the lung become soft in the center and then caseated and liquefied, the liquefied material may break through and empty into the bronchi and be raised as sputum. Cavities in the lung may appear on x-ray film and may be present in more than one lobe of the lung.

***Medications.*** To avoid the emergence of drug-resistant organisms, the Advisory Council for the Elimination of Tuberculosis (ACET) recommends the following beginning therapy for TB:

1. Susceptibility testing.
   a. All persons with TB from whom *M. tuberculosis* is isolated should have drug-susceptibility testing performed on the first isolate.
   b. Drug-susceptibility testing also should be performed on additional isolates from patients whose cultures fail to convert to negative within 3 months of beginning therapy.
2. Initial regimen.
   a. Initial treatment should be with four drugs (Table 32-11). During the first 2 months, the patient should receive isoniazid (INH), rifampin (RIF), pyrazinamide (PZA),

ethambutol (EMB), or streptomycin (SM). When drug susceptibility results are available, the regimen should be altered as appropriate.
b. Health care and correctional facilities that are experiencing outbreaks of TB resistant to INH and RIF or are resuming treatment of a patient who has been treated for TB in the past may need to begin patient treatment with five or six drugs as initial therapy.
c. Patients whose organisms are susceptible to INH and RIF should receive these two drugs for a full 6 months, supplemented with PZA for the first 2 months.

3. Immunosuppressed patients. Patients with HIV infection and other factors that compromise a patient's immune system make them more susceptible to the development of resistant organisms. For this reason, it is recommended that patients with HIV and TB be treated for a total of 9 months and for at least 6 months after their sputum converts to negative. If drug susceptibility results are not available, EMB or SM should be considered for the entire course of therapy because of the rapid progression of TB while the patient is receiving inadequate therapy.
4. Treatment of extrapulmonary TB. The regimen that is used for treating pulmonary disease is also used to treat extrapulmonary disease. Some experts believe that therapy should be for 9 months instead of 6 months for patients with disseminated TB, miliary disease, TB of bone and joints, and TB of the lymph glands.
5. Treatment of TB during pregnancy. Therapy is essential for pregnant women who have TB. SM is not used because it may cause congenital deafness. Routine use of PZA is not recommended because the risk of birth defects in the fetus has not been determined. Nine months of therapy with INH, RIF, and EMB is recommended. Women may breastfeed while receiving TB therapy because the concentration of the drugs in breast milk is so low that drug toxicity does not develop in the newborn.
6. Directly observed therapy (DOT).[14]
   a. A major cause of drug-resistant TB and treatment failure is patient nonadherence to prescribed treatment. Treatment failure and drug-resistant TB can be life threatening and pose other serious public health problems because they lead to prolonged infectiousness of

**table 32-11** *Common Medications for Tuberculosis*

| Drug | Classification | Common Side Effects | Tests | Remarks |
|---|---|---|---|---|
| Isoniazid (INH) | Bactericidal; penetrates all body tissues and fluids, including cerebrospinal fluid (CSF) | Peripheral neuritis, hepatitis, rash, fever | AST (formerly SGOT), ALT (formerly SGPT) (not as routine) | Daily alcohol intake interferes with metabolism of isoniazid and increases risk of hepatitis; antacids containing aluminum interfere with absorption of INH. |
| Rifampin (RIF) | Bactericidal; penetrates all body tissues, including CSF | Hepatitis, febrile reactions, thrombocytopenia (rare), hepatotoxicity increases when given with INH | AST, ALT, platelet count (not as routine) | Urine, sweat, tears may turn orange temporarily; decrease effectiveness of oral contraceptives, anticoagulants, corticosteroids, barbiturates, hypoglycemics, and digitalis. |
| Ethambutol (EMB) | Bacteriostatic; does not penetrate CSF; penetrates other body fluids | Optic neuritis (reversible with discontinuation of drug; very rare at 15 mg/kg skin rash) | Visual acuity; red-green color discrimination; GI irritation | No significant reaction with other drugs. Check vision monthly; give with food. |
| Pyrazinamide (PZA) | Bacteriostatic or bactericidal depending on susceptibility of mycobacterium | Hyperuricemia, hepatitis, arthralgia, GI irritation | Uric acid, AST, ALT | Obtain baseline liver function tests and repeat regularly. Give with food; drink 2 L of fluid daily. |
| Streptomycin (SM) | Bactericidal, aminoglycoside; disrupts protein synthesis; poor penetration into body tissues and CSF | Eighth cranial nerve damage (vestibular or ocular); damage often irreversible; nephrotoxicity | Vestibular function; audiograms; creatinine level determined before therapy started | Monitor kidney function monthly, monitor vestibular function with caloric stimulation test monthly. Monitor hearing with audiograms monthly. Meningitis is treated with intrathecal or subarachnoid instillation of SM. |

the patient and increased transmission of TB in the community. For this reason, direct observation of the patient taking the drugs is recommended.

b. Effective use of DOT requires a setting in which the patient goes to receive drugs either daily, two times a week, or three times a week, depending on the regimen ordered. The setting can be a TB clinic, community health center, homeless shelter, prison or jail, nursing home, school, drug treatment center, or other community settings that can serve as treatment centers.
c. In some situations, a responsible person other than a health care worker may administer DOT. These persons include correctional facility personnel, staff of community-based organizations, clergy, or other community leaders.
d. The use of incentives and enablers may promote patient adherence to a DOT program.
   (1) Providing transportation or taxi/bus fare to the DOT site.[18]
   (2) Use of combined preparations of INH and RIF, which reduce the number of pills the patient has to take.
e. Outreach workers who go into the community to talk with patients are often helpful in stressing to patients the urgency of taking the drugs as prescribed.

***Surgical management.*** Although medical therapy is the primary treatment for tuberculosis, surgery may be used to remove residual pulmonary lesions in some patients.[43] The principle in thoracic surgery for tuberculosis is to preserve as much normal lung tissue as possible. The surgical procedures that are used include wedge resection, in which a wedge-shaped portion is removed from the surface of the lung; segmental resection (segmentectomy), in which one or more segments of the lung are removed; lobectomy, in which a lobe of the lung is removed; and pneumonectomy, in which one lung is removed. Surgery of the lung and care of patients having thoracic surgery are discussed later in this chapter.

***Diet.*** A well-balanced diet containing the essential food groups with a vitamin supplement is recommended. Persons who are homeless or have limited incomes may require food vouchers with which to obtain additional food. Those who are poorly nourished or underweight may benefit from six small feedings of high-calorie, high-protein foods daily rather than three large meals.

***Activity.*** Most patients may be up to use the bathroom, but patients are encouraged to stay in bed as much as possible until their sputum culture converts from positive to negative, indicating that the antituberculosis drugs are effective. Patients who have an elevated temperature and those who appear acutely ill are urged to stay in bed until their temperature returns to normal or they are feeling better. Those whose temperatures are no longer elevated are asked to take morning and afternoon naps in addition to obtaining 8 or more hours of sleep daily. Strenuous exercise is to be avoided.

***Referrals.*** The most common referrals are to social services, nutrition, and community health nursing. Patients who are homeless or have limited incomes are referred to social services for assistance with food and shelter. A social services referral is also recommended for patients who have strained interpersonal relationships related to their diagnosis of TB and the changes it has caused in family relationships.

A nutritionist should meet with the patient and significant others to review the basic food groups and the amount of each nutrient required by the patient. Ways to provide extra calories in small, frequent feedings are also discussed. A community health nurse or another person in the community who will be the clinical supervisor should meet with the patient and significant other to develop a plan for follow-up care.

## NURSING MANAGEMENT

### ASSESSMENT

#### Subjective Data

It is important to determine whether the patient was exposed to a person with TB. *Often the source of the infection is unknown* and may never be determined. However, close contacts of the patient need to be identified so that they may undergo examination to determine whether they are infected and have active disease or a positive tuberculin test. The most common patient complaints are productive cough and night sweats.

#### Objective Data

Data to be collected to assess the patient with TB include:

Productive cough
Afternoon temperature elevation
Tuberculin skin test reaction of 10 mm induration or more (see Chapter 30)
X-ray film showing a pulmonary infiltrate (see Chapter 30)

### NURSING DIAGNOSES

Nursing diagnoses are determined from analysis of patient data. Nursing diagnoses for the person with tuberculosis may include but are not limited to:

| Diagnostic Title | Possible Etiological Factors |
|---|---|
| Knowledge deficit about tuberculosis: spread and treatment | Lack of exposure to information |
| Airway clearance, ineffective | Increased sputum, decreased energy/fatigue |
| Fear | Long-term illness requiring long-term chemotherapy, lifestyle changes until no longer infectious |

### EXPECTED PATIENT OUTCOMES

Expected patient outcomes for the person with tuberculosis may include but are not limited to:

1a. Explains how TB is spread and measures to prevent spread of TB (remain on chemotherapy, cover mouth and nose with tissues when coughing or sneezing)
b. Explains basic food groups and how a nutritionally adequate diet will be achieved
c. States name, dose, actions, and side effects of prescribed medications

d. Explains why two, three, or four chemotherapy agents must be taken together
e. Explains drug-resistant organisms and relates this to the need to take chemotherapy as directed
f. Explains why the health care provider should be notified immediately if for any reason (e.g., side effects) chemotherapy cannot be taken
g. States where to receive new supply of chemotherapy and date it is to be obtained
h. States plans for follow-up care
   (1) Lists signs and symptoms that indicate need for immediate medical care (increased cough, hemoptysis, unexplained weight loss, fever, night sweats)
   (2) States when next sputum test or x-ray film is to be taken and where
   (3) States plans for ongoing follow-up care

2a. Is able to cough effectively and clear airway
b. Amount of sputum is reduced

3a. Appears less fearful
b. Respirations, pulse, and blood pressure are within normal range

## ■ INTERVENTIONS

The major nursing responsibility is to teach the patient about TB and how it is transmitted. Preventing contamination of air with tubercle bacilli is accomplished by treating the patient with antituberculosis drugs and teaching the patient to cover the nose and mouth with tissues when sneezing or coughing.

The most important factor in the transmission of TB is overcrowded living conditions. This is why outbreaks of TB occur in schools, homeless shelters, jails, prisons, and other settings where people are crowded together. To prevent the transmission of TB from person to person it is necessary to prevent contamination of the air with *M. tuberculosis.* This is achieved in two ways:

1. Teach the patient to cover the nose and mouth with a tissue when coughing, sneezing, and laughing so that droplet nuclei are not discharged into the air.
2. Treat the patient with antituberculosis drugs. Most persons who adhere to the prescribed therapy and do not have other mitigating factors such as immunosuppression convert their sputum from positive to negative in a relatively short time (2 to 3 weeks). See the Guidelines for Care Box for a summary of patient teaching about the transmission of tuberculosis.

To improve airway clearance, the patient is taught to sit upright in a chair or in bed. If the patient is confined to bed at home, he or she may find it helpful to sit on the side of the bed with the feet on a chair. The patient is taught to take two or three deep breaths, cover the mouth with tissues, and then cough. Using this method when coughing decreases fatigue because it requires less expenditure of energy than does repeated ineffective coughs.

Many patients can cough most effectively when the mouth is moist, and sips of water or a warm beverage such as tea or coffee can be encouraged before coughing. For patients with thick tenacious sputum, fluid intake is encouraged to thin the secretions and make them easier to expectorate. Water is considered by many experts to be the most effective sputum-liquefying agent.

To reduce fear about the disease and what lifestyle changes it will require, patients are encouraged to ask questions about anything they do not understand or anything that concerns them. The nurse who sits while talking with the patient signals that he or she will take the time to listen to the patient. All questions should be answered as completely as possible, supplying information appropriate to the patient's educational level and ability to comprehend what is being taught. Written materials with diagrams and drawings that reinforce what is being taught are helpful. The materials are given to the patient for use later on. All written materials should be reviewed with the patient and, whenever possible, a family member before they are given to the patient. For patients who do not speak English, a translator and written materials in the patient's language will be necessary. Concerns about interpersonal problems or financial needs indicate the need for a social services referral.

**guidelines for care**

**Preventing the Transmission of Tuberculosis**

Patient must take antituberculosis drugs as prescribed.
- Drugs are always taken as combination of at least four drugs initially.
- Drugs must be taken uninterruptedly.
- Both of the above are necessary to prevent development of resistant strains of *M. tuberculosis.*

Prevent contamination of air with *M. tuberculosis.*
- Cover nose and mouth with disposable tissues when coughing, sneezing, or laughing.
- Place used tissues in paper or plastic bag for disposal.

### Patient/Family Education

#### *Health promotion/prevention*

The decline in the number of TB cases that has occurred yearly in the United States since 1992 reflects improvements in TB prevention and control programs in state and local health departments. These programs received increased federal funding beginning in the 1990s. The increased funding enabled many TB control programs to ensure that each patient completed an adequate course of therapy and that DOT was expanded. Directly observed therapy is discussed on p. 935.

Although the number and rate of reported TB cases in the United States continue to decline, the national goal of TB elimination (an incidence of less than 1 case per 1 million population) by 2010 seems improbable because the 1997 case rate of 7.4 exceeds the goal of 3.5 or fewer cases set for 2000.[19] Because minorities presently account for two thirds of reported cases of TB, special target figures were set for these groups for 2000 (Table 32-12). The rise in TB rates among minorities requires that efforts be redoubled to ensure that those already infected complete therapy so that they will not spread TB to others. The Advisory Council for the Elimination of

**table 32-12** *Special Population Targets for Decrease in the Tuberculosis Case Rate per 100,000 Persons*

| Group | 1988 Baseline | 2000 Target |
|---|---|---|
| Asians/Pacific Islanders | 36.3 | 15 |
| Blacks | 28.3 | 10 |
| Hispanics | 18.3 | 5 |
| Native Americans/ Native Alaskans | 18.1 | 5 |

From US Department of Health and Human Services: *Healthy People 2000: National health promotion and disease prevention objectives.* Washington, DC, 1990, US Government Printing Office.

Tuberculosis (ACET) has issued guidelines for state tuberculosis control programs (Box 32-5).

The major priority of TB prevention and control programs is that all persons with TB be promptly identified and treated with an adequate course of drug therapy. A special effort must be made to identify TB among foreign-born U.S. residents from countries with high TB rates.[20] These high rates reflect the global nature of TB as a public health problem. Tuberculosis control activities aimed at reducing the incidence of TB in other parts of the world need to be strengthened.[14]

Additional resources are needed to implement DOT short course (DOTS) in underdeveloped countries. DOTS is a strategy advocated by the Global Tuberculosis Program of the World Health Organization (WHO) and the International Union Against Tuberculosis and Lung Disease (IUATLD). Their goals are to ensure detection of TB cases with appropriate diagnostic procedures, establish a secure supply of essential anti-TB drugs, and establish a system of record keeping and program assessment. The CDC is collaborating with WHO, IUATLD, and the World Bank to implement and evaluate this strategy. Global efforts to eliminate TB should result in improved TB prevention and control in the United States.

In 1998, the Global Tuberculosis Program members reported on global resistance to antituberculosis drug therapy from 1994-1997. They found resistance to the four first-line antituberculosis drugs in 35 countries. Multidrug resistance was particularly high in the former Soviet Union, Asia, the Dominican Republic, and Argentina. Their findings illustrate that MDR is a potential threat to tuberculosis control programs worldwide because of the ease with which persons travel from one country to another. All of this may make TB prevention and control in the United States more difficult.[44a, 48a]

**Primary and secondary prevention.** To eliminate TB, the organism must be prevented from being transmitted from one person to another. Preventive measures are directed toward the latest ACET recommendations.

Persons over 35 years of age without the risk factors listed here are not given preventive chemotherapy because of the risk of isoniazid-associated hepatitis. Although the risk is small, it is age related and increases from less than 0.2% in those under age 20 to up to 2.3% in those 50 to 64 years of age. If isoniazid-associated hepatitis occurs, the symptoms are mild, nonspecific, and similar to those of any viral illness. (See Chapter 37 for a discussion of viral hepatitis.)

**box 32-5** *Guidelines for State Tuberculosis Control Programs*

States should have systems that incorporate the following guidelines:

- Ensure the mandatory reporting of each confirmed and suspected case of TB, and observe local laws and regulations protecting patient confidentiality.
- Examine persons at high risk for TB infection and disease, prescribe the appropriate preventive or curative treatment for these persons, and monitor their treatment.
- Monitor the treatment of patients, and require that a treatment plan be devised for all hospitalized patients before they are discharged.
- Ensure the rapid laboratory examination of specimens and reporting of results to the appropriate health department and the requesting clinician.
- Ensure that TB-infected patients receive treatment until they are cured.
- Protect the health of the public by isolating and treating persons who have infectious TB and detaining persons who, although not infectious, are unwilling or unable to complete their treatment and are at risk for becoming infectious and for acquiring drug-resistant TB.
- Finance the treatment of indigent patients.

From Centers for Disease Control and Prevention: *MMWR* 41(RR-5):1, 1992.

Contraindications to the use of isoniazid preventive therapy are (1) previous isoniazid-associated liver disease; (2) severe adverse reactions to isoniazid, including fever, chills, rash, and arthritis; and (3) acute liver disease of any etiology.

Persons receiving isoniazid preventive chemotherapy should be seen monthly by a health care provider for the purpose of reinforcing the necessity of taking the chemotherapy regularly and to monitor the patient for any serious side effects. Because most cases of TB in patients with HIV infection occur in those with a history of a positive tuberculin test, all persons with HIV infection should be considered for preventive therapy with isoniazid. Groups that should receive particular attention are IV drug users, prison inmates, and the homeless, since they have an extraordinarily high incidence of HIV and TB infection.

Because of the difficulty in preventing TB among homeless persons, special recommendations have been made for this group.[16]

1. The highest priority should be given to (1) detection, evaluation, and reporting of current symptoms of active TB in homeless persons and (2) completion of an appropriate course of treatment by those diagnosed with active TB.
2. The second priority should be screening and preventive therapy for homeless persons who have, or are suspected of having, HIV infection.
3. The third priority should be the examination and appropriate treatment of persons with recent TB that was inadequately treated.

4. The fourth priority should be screening and appropriate treatment of persons exposed to an infectious (sputum-positive) case of TB. Because contacts are difficult to define in a shelter population, it is usually necessary to screen all residents of a shelter when an infectious case is identified.
5. The fifth priority should be screening and preventive therapy for homeless persons with known medical conditions that increase the risk of TB, for example, diabetes mellitus and other conditions listed in Box 32-6.

Preventive chemotherapy in the United States is isoniazid daily for 6 months. The usual adult dose is 300 mg in a single dose daily. If the person has antibodies to HIV, isoniazid is given daily for 1 year.

In 1989 ACET published *A Strategic Plan for Elimination of Tuberculosis in the United States.* The committee recommended that a goal be established to eliminate TB by the year 2010. To achieve the goal, a case rate of 0.1 per 100,000 persons was set for the year 2010, with an interim goal of a case rate of 3.5 per 100,000 population by the year 2000. As mentioned, this goal may not be achieved, in view of the 1997 case rate of 7.4 per 100,000.

**Vaccination.** Efforts continue in search of a more satisfactory TB vaccine. Presently, bacille Calmette-Guèrin (BCG) vaccine is used worldwide except in the United States and the Netherlands. The vaccine contains attenuated tubercle bacilli that have lost their ability to produce disease. It is administered only to persons who have a negative reaction to the tuberculin test. It is not widely used in the United States because of disagreements as to its safety and effectiveness. Currently, BCG vaccination is recommended only for tuberculin-negative infants and children who have continuing exposure to persons who have isoniazid-resistant and rifampin-resistant active TB. Most persons who have received BCG will have a skin test reaction of less than 10 mm. If a larger reaction occurs to PPD, it can be assumed that the person has a TB infection. The vaccine should be given only by persons who have had careful instruction in the proper technique. A multiple-puncture disk is used to give the vaccine. When there is a positive reaction to skin testing with tuberculin, when acute infectious disease is present, or when there is any skin disease, BCG vaccine is not given. Possible complications of vaccination are local ulcers, which occur in a relatively high percentage of persons vaccinated, and abscesses or suppuration of lymph nodes, which occur in a small percentage.

In countries such as India where living conditions are such that transmission of TB is to be expected, BCG vaccine is given at birth and then repeated after 12 to 15 years. The intradermal method is used to administer the vaccine so that a uniform controlled dose can be given. The BCG vaccine, as mentioned, is not widely used in the United States, although some highly susceptible groups such as migrant workers may be vaccinated.

### Protection of health care workers

Nurses and other health care workers need to know the protective measures they can use when caring for patients who have a positive TB smear or culture. The following measures are indicated.[15]

**box 32-6 Priorities for Preventive Therapy with Isoniazid among TB-Infected Persons**

1. Persons with HIV infection
2. Recent contacts of persons with infectious TB
3. Persons with recent skin test conversions
4. Persons with recent TB disease who have been inadequately treated
5. Persons with negative sputum cultures and stable fibrotic lesions on chest radiographs consistent with inactive TB
6. Persons with medical conditions that increase the risk of TB
   - Leukemia or lymphoma
   - Silicosis
   - Diabetes mellitus
   - Gastrectomy
   - End-stage renal disease
   - Antibodies to HIV

1. The first emphasis should be on preventing *M. tuberculosis* from being expelled into room air by the patient. Most patients will cooperate and cover their nose and mouth with tissues when coughing and sneezing. Those who are too ill to do so or who are confused can have a surgical mask put over their nose and mouth.
2. The patient is placed in a private room, and the door to the hallway is kept closed.
3. If the patient must leave the room for tests or procedures, he or she should wear a mask or particulate respirator with a one-way valve.
4. The air pressure in the room should be negative, which allows air to flow into the room when the door is opened and prevents room air from moving out into the hallway.
5. The air in the room should be exchanged at least six times every hour, with two of the exchanges being with fresh air from the outside. Air from the patient's room should be directly vented to the outside and not recirculated within the hospital.
6. High-energy particulate air (HEPA) filters can be installed in ventilation ducts.
7. Some institutions use ultraviolet lights high on walls or ceilings in patient rooms to disinfect room air. They are placed so that they do not cause a risk to the patients or health care workers.
8. Personnel caring for the patients should wear a disposable particulate respirator. The respirator should fit snugly over the nose and mouth to prevent as much room air as possible from getting in around the edges. The particulate respirator filters out organisms as small as 1 $\mu$; *M. tuberculosis* organisms are 3 to 5 $\mu$.
9. All health care workers should know their tuberculin status. Most younger workers in the United States will be tuberculin negative, and the goal is to keep them that way. All workers who are tuberculin negative should be tested yearly with PPD. Those who have not had a recent test should receive a baseline tuberculin test on

employment and then yearly. Workers who have inadvertently been exposed to a patient with TB (often before the diagnosis of TB is made) should have a tuberculin test 8 to 12 weeks after exposure. It takes this period for a test to convert from negative to positive. The CDC recommends that health care workers involved in the care of patients receiving cough-inducing procedures such as bronchoscopy and tracheal suctioning should be tuberculin tested at least every 6 months.

10. Health care workers who convert from a negative to a positive tuberculin test should have an examination to rule out active TB. Isoniazid preventive therapy is offered to those under age 35 who do not have active TB. Those refusing therapy should have a yearly chest x-ray.
11. Once patients have three negative smears for TB, they are considered noninfectious, and health care workers do not need to wear a mask when caring for them.

## ■ EVALUATION

To evaluate the effectiveness of nursing interventions, compare patient behaviors with those stated in the expected patient outcomes. Successful achievement of patient outcomes for the patient with tuberculosis is indicated by:

1a. Explains rationale for taking four anti-TB drugs without interruption; demonstrates use of empty egg carton to distribute each day's supply of medications divided according to times taken, along with checklist to record each dose as it is taken
 b. States date of next sputum test and date and time of next chest x-ray
 c. States date and time of next appointment with medical provider
 d. States signs and symptoms that indicate need for immediate medical care (e.g., an increase in dyspnea or appearance of hemoptysis)
2. Cough minimal; covers nose and mouth with tissue when coughing or sneezing and disposes of tissues as taught
3. Dyspnea absent; vital signs within normal range

## GERONTOLOGICAL CONSIDERATIONS

Many elderly persons were exposed to tuberculosis when they were children and have a positive tuberculin test, which indicates that they have dormant tubercle bacilli walled off in their lungs. When these persons are subjected to physical or emotional stress, they may develop active tuberculosis. Also, with aging the immune system may be less able to respond effectively to an infection. This includes the ability of the person to react to the tuberculin test. For this reason, it is recommended that the elderly have a yearly chest x-ray. A major concern is that the elderly will develop undiagnosed tuberculosis, which they can spread to their grandchildren and other youngsters with whom they have contact. All residents of nursing homes should have yearly chest x-rays for the same reason. If an active case of tuberculosis is found in a nursing home resident, more frequent x-rays of other residents will be necessary.

Many elderly, especially the frail elderly, have a poor appetite and will need special attention to their nutritional needs. Other elderly persons with limited financial resources will need help in obtaining an adequate diet. Asking the person to keep a daily food diary can help determine whether the person's diet is sufficient to support healing of the tuberculosis.

## SPECIAL ENVIRONMENTS FOR CARE

### Home Care Management

Many persons with active tuberculosis will remain at home and periodically visit a TB clinic or other treatment facility. The community health nurse will assess the home environment and determine whether the patient can be relied on to take all medications as prescribed or whether there is another adult in the home who can be responsible for ensuring that the patient takes all medications as prescribed. If not, other provisions for directly observed therapy will be necessary. The nurse is responsible for teaching the patient about medications, handling secretions, protecting others from infection, and eating an adequate diet. Generally, patients who take their medications as prescribed will convert their sputum from positive to negative within 3 to 4 weeks. Measures to prevent the transmission of tuberculosis are discussed on p. 938. If the patient faithfully covers nose and mouth with tissues when coughing or sneezing, this will prevent contamination of air in the home. Because the incidence of tuberculosis is high among persons who are HIV positive, the patient should be encouraged to have an HIV test.

It is also important that persons who have had sustained contact with someone who has tuberculosis have a tuberculin test and appropriate follow-up care. Contacts (under age 35) who have a positive tuberculin test will be offered prophylactic treatment with isoniazid. They will need follow-up with periodic chest x-rays.

## COMPLICATIONS

The complication of greatest concern is that the patient will develop a resistant strain of tuberculosis that may be extremely difficult to treat and will usually require hospitalization while effective drug therapy is sought. The development of HIV may also occur, and it may not be possible to determine which of the two diseases occurred first. Rigorous treatment of both diseases will be necessary, and hospitalization is often necessary. Complications can also occur after thoracic surgery; these are discussed later in the chapter.

## Lung Abscess

### *Etiology/epidemiology*

A lung abscess is an area of localized suppuration within the lung. It usually is caused by bacteria that reach the lung through aspiration. Some experts suggest that lung abscess might better be called *aspiration lung abscess* because aspiration is the common factor.

### *Pathophysiology*

The infected material lodges in the small bronchi and produces inflammation. Partial obstruction of the bronchus results in retention of secretions beyond the obstruction and the eventual *necrosis of tissue.* The necrotic lung tissue is coughed up, and an air-filled cavity is left in the lung.

Food particles and perigingival debris, which contain both aerobic and anaerobic organisms, are the most commonly aspirated substances. Laboratory cultures of sputum or transtracheal aspirates are necessary to identify the causative organism. When only normal oropharyngeal flora is found, aerobic cultures may demonstrate the presence of fusospirochetal organisms, peptostreptococci, and *Bacteroides* species. All of these organisms are typically found in gingival infections. The most common aerobic bacteria causing lung abscess are *Staphylococcus aureus* and *Klebsiella pneumoniae*. Aerobic gram-negative organisms are found most commonly in persons with nosocomial infections or in persons who are immunosuppressed. Sputum should also be examined for tumor cells and for tuberculosis and fungal organisms. Before the advent of antibiotics and specific chemotherapy, lung abscess was a common complication of pneumonia.

Lung abscess may follow bronchial obstruction caused by a tumor, foreign body, or stenosis of the bronchus. Metastatic spread of cancer cells to the lung parenchyma may also cause an abscess, and occasionally the infection appears to have been borne by the bloodstream. In recent years the incidence of lung abscess caused by infection has decreased, and secondary lung abscess after bronchogenic carcinoma has increased.[42] Bronchoscopy may be used to identify the infected segment and to obtain specimens for culture. Box 32-7 lists clinical manifestations of lung abscess.

### Collaborative care management

The course of lung abscess is influenced by the cause of the abscess and by the type of drainage that can be established. If the purulent material drains easily, the patient may respond well to segmental postural drainage, antibiotic therapy, and good general supportive care. When obstruction interferes with drainage into the bronchi, bronchoscopic procedures are used to improve drainage and to rule out obstructing foreign bodies or neoplasms. Surgical treatment to establish drainage has become increasingly less necessary; however, if after several weeks of medical treatment a cavity persists, a segmentectomy or lobectomy may be performed.[42]

Penicillin G is the drug of choice, and 2 to 3 million units is given intravenously every 4 hours until the fever is relieved and the patient's condition shows marked improvement. Penicillin VK in doses of 500 mg four times daily is then given orally. When the patient has a sensitivity to penicillin, clindamycin (Cleocin), 600 mg every 8 hours, is prescribed. For staphylococcal infections, oxacillin or nafcillin, 6 to 8 g intravenously in divided doses, is often prescribed. Patients with lung abscesses caused by gram-negative organisms are treated with appropriate antibiotics, as determined by in vitro sensitivity tests.

Antibiotic therapy is continued until all signs of the illness have subsided and the chest x-ray films show that the cavity has completely disappeared or has reduced significantly in size. Most cavities close within 6 weeks, but occasionally a cavity may persist for months. Foul-smelling sputum usually disappears within a few days, whereas cough and nonfoul sputum may continue for a longer period. Usually the patient begins to feel better during the first week of therapy, but it may take up to 2 months for the temperature to return to normal.

If the patient does not improve with the therapy just discussed, bronchoscopy is performed to search for a possible obstruction to drainage, such as carcinoma or a foreign body.

Medical treatment cannot cause a walled-off abscess to disappear, and surgery will be necessary. If surgery is necessary, the portion of lung containing the abscess is removed. If the abscess is caused by carcinoma, the surgery may be much more extensive.

The person with a lung abscess is very ill and will be admitted to the hospital. Additionally, patients in the hospital for another condition are at risk of aspiration and lung abscess. The most vulnerable patients are those with suppressed levels of consciousness such as occurs after anesthesia and in head injury, CVA, alcoholism, seizure disorders, drug overdoses, persons with compromised immunological defenses, and elderly persons, especially if immobile.

Nursing responsibilities include:

1. Prevent aspiration in hospitalized patients.
   a. Monitor patients who are at risk of aspiration.
   b. Provide frequent mouth care to persons with diminished levels of consciousness.
   c. Closely monitor persons receiving tube feedings to ensure that tube is in stomach.
   d. If patient is vomiting, place on side in postanesthesia position to reduce aspiration.

**box 32-7 clinical manifestations**

**Acute Lung Abscess**

- High fever: 39° C (102° F)
- Chills and prostration
- Cough and sputum production common
- Night sweats, pleuritic chest pain, anemia, and occasionally hemoptysis
- Putrid sputum in about 50% of patients—foul odor evident in patient's room
- Weight loss in about 40% of patients (foul-smelling and foul-tasting sputum often causes anorexia)
- Mortality rate of primary abscess is 5%
- Up to one third of patients 45 years of age and older have a lung abscess associated with carcinoma
- A diagnostic bronchoscopy should be considered for all high-risk patients, even if they respond well to therapy

**guidelines for care**

**The Person with Lung Abscess**

- Monitor vital signs at least every 4 hours because temperature may spike in afternoon and may persist for as long as 2 weeks.
- Place patient in comfortable position. If patient is conscious, usually is more comfortable with head rest at 45 to 90 degrees.
- Help patient cough up sputum. This helps drain abscess.
- Collect sputum for culture and sensitivity tests to determine organism and antibiotic therapy. This monitors effectiveness of therapy and whether resistant organisms are developing.
- Do postural drainage (see p. 993). This facilitates drainage from the abscess.

e. If patient is unable to expectorate secretions from mouth and oropharynx, oral suctioning may be necessary.
2. Care of patient with a lung abscess is outlined in the Guidelines for Care Box.

## Bronchiectasis

### Etiology/epidemiology

Bronchiectasis is irreversible dilation of the bronchial tree. It has declined greatly since the advent of antibiotics.

### Pathophysiology

When infection attacks the bronchial lining, inflammation occurs, and an exudate forms. The progressive accumulation of secretions obstructs the bronchioles. The obstructed bronchioles then break down, and ciliated columnar epithelium is replaced by nonciliated cuboidal epithelium and sometimes fibrotic tissue, resulting in localized areas of dilation or saccules (Figure 32-6). The expulsive force of the bronchioles is diminished, and they may remain filled with exudate. Only forceful coughing and postural drainage will empty them.

Bronchiectasis may involve any part of the lung parenchyma, but it usually occurs in the dependent portions or lobes, except in TB, when it is usually in the upper lobes. Before the widespread use of antibiotics in treating persons with respiratory tract infections, this disease began to develop in young people, with many showing symptoms in childhood or by age 20. Although the incidence of childhood bronchiectasis is decreasing, it is increasing in individuals with cystic fibrosis, immunodeficiency diseases, or atopic asthma, in which repeated respiratory infections have been successfully treated with antibiotics. These persons now survive the acute episodes of bacterial infection that complicate their underlying disease but sometimes develop bronchiectasis as a sequela.

A contributing factor in bronchiectasis may be a congenital weakness in the structure of the bronchi that results in impairment of elasticity. Bronchiectasis may occur without previous pulmonary disease, but it usually follows such diseases as pneumonia, lung abscesses, TB, cystic fibrosis, or asthma. A computed tomography (CT) scan is used for diagnosis. Box 32-8 lists clinical manifestations.

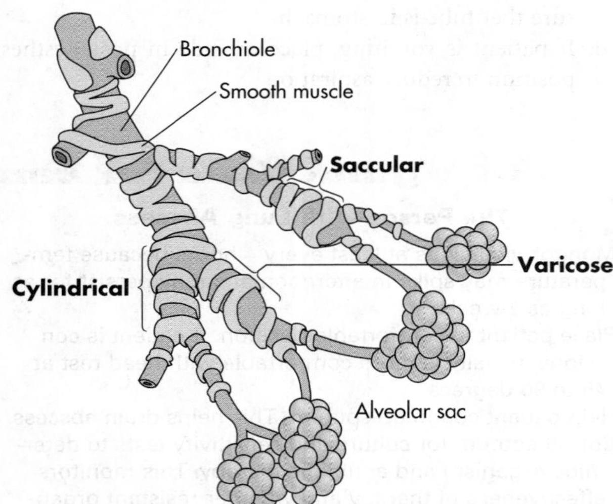


**fig. 32-6** Cylindrical, varicose, and saccular types of bronchiectasis.

### Collaborative care management

Treatment of bronchiectasis includes:
1. Antibiotics
2. Postural drainage to assist in mobilizing secretions to larger airways, where they can be coughed up
3. Bronchoscopy to remove thicker secretions

Surgery is necessary when signs and symptoms of bronchiectasis persist despite medical therapy. The goal in surgery is to preserve as much functional lung as possible. Therefore a segmentectomy or lobectomy is given priority. (See p. 955 for discussion of these procedures.) Some patients have bilateral disease. In this situation, the most involved lung is operated on first to see how much improvement occurs before treating the other side.[28]

Nursing care stresses good general hygiene, which may contribute to relief of symptoms. Adequate diet, rest, exercise, and diversional activity are important; avoiding superimposed infections such as colds should be emphasized. Frequent mouth care is essential, and cleansing the mouth with an aromatic mouthwash before meals often makes food more acceptable.

## Empyema

### Etiology/epidemiology

Empyema is pus within a body cavity, most often the pleural cavity. It usually occurs after pleural effusion secondary to other respiratory diseases such as pneumonia, lung

**box 32-8** *clinical manifestations*

***Bronchiectasis***

Signs and symptoms of bronchiectasis vary with the severity of the condition and may include the following:

**SIGNS**

Cyanosis
Clubbing of fingers
Fine crackles and coarse rhonchi
Dull or flat sounds over areas of mucous plugs
Increased vocal and tactile fremitus over middle and lower lobes
Decreased diaphragmatic excursion
Paroxysms of coughing on arising in morning and when lying down

**SYMPTOMS**

Severe coughing productive of copious amounts of purulent sputum
Hemoptysis
Dyspnea
Fatigue and weakness
Loss of appetite and weight loss

The condition may develop so gradually that the person is unable to tell when the symptoms first began.

abscess, TB, and fungal infections of the lung and also after thoracic surgery or chest trauma. It now occurs fairly often as a complication of staphylococcal pneumonia. Box 32-9 lists clinical manifestations of empyema.

### Collaborative care management

The aim of treatment of empyema is to obliterate the pleural space by draining the empyema cavity completely. The cavity can be drained in the following ways:

1. Initial treatment is often daily thoracentesis with aspiration of the cavity and instillation of antibiotics into the pleural space. Oral or IV antibiotics may also be given. If the cavity cannot be evacuated within a few days or if the lung fails to reexpand to obliterate the space, surgery is necessary.[40]
2. The type of surgery depends on the situation and may include:
   a. *Closed-chest drainage,* in which a trochar is inserted between the ribs at the base of the cavity. A chest catheter is inserted through the trochar, the trochar is removed, and the tube is connected to water-seal drainage (see p. 954). Pus then drains from the cavity into the collection chamber. For closed drainage to be successful, the pus must be thin enough to drain out of the pleural space, and the lung must be able to reexpand to fill the pleural space.
   b. *Rib resection* with open-chest drainage is necessary when empyema is chronic and the lung is incapable of reexpanding to obliterate the pleural space. A portion of one or two ribs is removed, and a large drainage tube is inserted into the empyema cavity. This allows pus to drain into a heavy chest dressing, which will need to be changed once or twice daily. The tube is changed weekly. If the treatment is effective, granulation tissue will form in the space from the inside out, thus obliterating the pleural space.
   c. *Decortication* is necessary in instances of chronic empyema in which a fibrinous peel has formed on the visceral pleura, preventing the lung from reexpanding and filling the space left after the empyema cavity was drained. In decortication, the fibrinous peel is removed from the visceral pleura by blunt dissection, freeing the lung so that it can reexpand and fill the pleural space. Two chest tubes are inserted into the pleural space and connected to water-seal drainage with additional suction. See p. 954 for a discussion of chest drainage.
   d. *Thoracoplasty* (the removal of one or more ribs) may be necessary if none of the preceding procedures are successful in obliterating the pleural space. The removal of ribs alters the shape of the thorax, and the chest wall is brought inward to obliterate the pleural space (see p. 962).

Nursing care depends on the type and effectiveness of the procedure and the patient's symptoms. Some patients require oxygen therapy. Bedrest and coughing and deep breathing exercises may be indicated to improve ventilation. In some cases the patient will go through several treatments before the empyema space is closed. This can be frustrating, and the patient can become very discouraged. A major nursing role is to support the patient and family during the various procedures.

**box 32-9** clinical manifestations

**Empyema**

The patient with a lung infection or chest injury may develop empyema and should be observed closely for the following signs and symptoms of empyema:

- Cough (usually nonproductive)
- Dyspnea
- Tachypnea
- Tachycardia
- Elevation of temperature
- Unilateral chest expansion
- Malaise
- Decreased appetite

The diagnosis can usually be made from the signs and symptoms and the medical history, but it is confirmed by a chest x-ray film that demonstrates the presence of a pleural exudate. A thoracentesis is performed to obtain a sample of the pus for culture and sensitivity studies and to relieve the patient's respiratory symptoms.

From Hill RC: The pleura and empyema. In Sabiston DC Jr, Lyerly LK, editors: *Sabiston essentials of surgery,* ed 2, Philadelphia, 1996, WB Saunders.

## Fungal Infections

There are three major fungal infections of the lungs: *histoplasmosis, coccidioidomycosis,* and *blastomycosis.* They are classified as deep mycoses because there is involvement by the parasite of deeper tissues and internal organs. The etiology, epidemiology, and prevention of these fungal (mycotic) infections are presented in Table 32-13.

### Histoplasmosis

**Etiology/epidemiology.** Inhalation of spores of *Histoplasma capsulatum* causes histoplasmosis (see Table 32-13).

**Pathophysiology.** The inhaled spores are phagocytized by alveolar macrophages within which they germinate. The spores form yeast cells and multiply by budding. In persons previously uninfected, there is a primary or initial infection that resembles the infection in primary TB with involvement of regional lymphatics and early dissemination via lymphatic and blood to other organs. Yeast cells spread hematogenously and are phagocytized by reticuloendothelial cells in the liver, spleen, and bone marrow. The process in the lung is similar to that seen in TB with necrosis and healing by fibrotic encapsulation. Eventually, the original parenchymal foci in the lung and in the hilar lymph nodes show calcification. In immunocompetent individuals, T cell immunity develops in 10 to 14 days, and the initial infection is self-limiting and does not require antifungal chemotherapy. However, some immunocompromised persons may develop a rapidly progressive primary infection that will be fatal without antifungal therapy.

*Reinfection histoplasmosis* and *progressive histoplasmosis* can also occur. Reinfection with *Histoplasma* causes an illness

**table 32-13** *Etiology, Epidemiology, and Prevention of Fungal Lung Infections*

| DISEASE | ETIOLOGY | EPIDEMIOLOGY | PREVENTION |
|---|---|---|---|
| Histoplasmosis | Inhalation of spores of *Histoplasma capsulatum*<br>Soil contaminated with fowl excreta; infected areas they inhabit (caves, bird roosts, chicken coops); can be extremely infectious | Most common systemic mycotic disease in United States; endemic areas in Missouri, Kentucky, Tennessee, Southern Illinois, Indiana, and Ohio; more than 40 million persons in these areas infected | Locate areas where soil is infected with fowl excreta. Teach public to wear a mask to avoid inhalation of dust from infected soil. Infants and elderly persons are especially susceptible. |
| Coccidioidomycosis (Valley fever, San Joaquin Valley fever) | Inhalation of spores of *Coccidioides immitis*<br>Soil contaminated with spores; growth of fungus enhanced by heavy rainfall in desert; inhibited by sunlight; anthrospores which are inhaled, dispersed by liberation of dust in spring | Endemic to well-defined areas in southwestern United States, Mexico, and South America. In United States, endemic in San Joaquin Valley, Southern Arizona, New Mexico, and Southwestern Texas | Encourage wearing of masks by persons working in desert dust such as archeologists and construction workers. |
| Blastomycosis | Believed to be inhalation of *Blastomyces dermatitidis*<br>Soil contaminated with spores that are carried on air currents and inhaled by humans and animals; dogs can acquire the disease; not believed to be spread from animals to man; believed that both humans and animals infected by inhaling spores | Most prevalent in the United States and Canadian valley areas surrounding the Mississippi, Missouri, Ohio, and St. Lawrence rivers; also present in Africa, South America, Mexico, and Asia | Wear a mask to avoid inhalation of spores in soil in areas where cases have been identified. |

resembling the initial infection. Because the initial infection confers some degree of immunity to histoplasmosis, the extent of disease will be modified by the degree of fungal immunity. Heavy inoculation may cause pneumonitis, which is usually self-limiting over days to weeks. The onset is acute with nonproductive cough, fever, malaise, and dyspnea. Some persons who are fully immune may develop a hypersensitivity-like pneumonitis with small, discrete granulomatous foci that may give a miliary appearance on x-ray examination. This means that the infection is spread throughout the lung, giving the appearance of the presence of small millet seeds throughout the lung.

*Progressive histoplasmosis* is usually chronic; chronic pulmonary histoplasmosis is the most common symptomatic form of the disease. It develops almost exclusively in middle-aged white men who have COPD. There are recurrent episodes of necrotizing segmental or lobar granulomatous pneumonitis, which have a tendency to cavity formation, contraction, fibrosis, and compensatory emphysema.

*Progressive disseminated histoplasmosis* occurs in 1 in 2000 exposed individuals with very low resistance to infection (infants, immunocompromised persons). Persons with AIDS who develop disseminated histoplasmosis have a relapse rate of 80% after treatment. For this reason, the goal of therapy is lifelong suppression as opposed to cure, and patients with AIDS receive maintenance therapy with amphotericin B for life.[31] Rarely, disseminated histoplasmosis can occur in adults of both genders and all ages with no known immune disorder. These persons have fever, weakness, weight loss, hepatosplenomegaly, leukopenia, and mucous membrane ulceration involving the oropharynx, tongue, or larynx. Adrenal insufficiency occurs in about 50% of these persons. See Table 32-14 for signs and symptoms and medical therapy.

**Collaborative care management.** See p. 945.

### *Coccidioidomycosis*

**Etiology/epidemiology.** Inhalation of spores of *Coccidioides immitis* causes coccidioidomycosis (see Table 32-13).

**Pathophysiology.** The process after inhalation of spores is believed to be similar to that described under histoplasmosis. The arthrospores reach the alveoli, where they are phagocytized. Disseminated disease is marked by hilar adenopathy, and fungi can be isolated from lymph nodes. A pneumonic disease with necrosis and cavitation may occur after development of delayed hypersensitivity. The disease process is controlled and resolved in most persons as the result of cell immunity to infection. Thus progressive disseminated coccidioidomycosis or progressive pulmonary disease is found only in those persons whose ability to resist infection or develop immunity has been compromised in some way.

Susceptibility to infection is in part genetically determined. Coccidioidomycosis is 50 times more common in Filipino men and 10 times more common in black men than it is in white men. This increased susceptibility to progressive disease in these groups of men parallels their susceptibility to tuberculosis. The increased susceptibility of some races to diseases such as coccidioidomycosis and tuberculosis is believed to be the result of a genetically determined impairment of their capacity to develop cellular immunity to infection.

**table 32-14** *Signs and Symptoms and Medical Therapy for Fungal Lung Infections*

| TYPE OF INFECTION | SIGNS AND SYMPTOMS | MEDICAL THERAPY |
|---|---|---|
| Histoplasmosis | Severe infections; acute onset with fever, chest pain, dyspnea, prostration, weight loss, widespread pulmonary infiltrates, hepatomegaly, and splenomegaly; no symptoms in some persons, benign acute pneumonitis in others | Drug(s) of choice: amphotericin B (Fungizone IV); 75% of patients are cured.<br>Ketoconazole (Nizoral), 400 mg orally daily at bedtime or with meals; without treatment, patient with disseminated disease will die. |
| Coccidioidomycosis (Valley fever, San Joaquin Valley fever) | Asymptomatic upper respiratory tract infection in about 60% of those who inhaled spores: 40% have symptoms ranging from flulike illness to frank pneumonia | Amphotericin B IV.<br>Therapy required for only 10% of those with symptoms; remainder have spontaneous remission.<br>Ketoconazole orally. |
| Blastomycosis | Skin lesions that appear as small papular or pustular lesions on exposed parts of the body such as hands and face<br>Peripheral development of lesions, may become raised but do not itch | Amphotericin B IV; mandatory in immunocompromised patients.<br>Ketoconazole orally.<br>Miconazole (only for patients who cannot tolerate amphotericin or ketoconazole). |

Coccidioidin, 1 : 10 or 1 : 100, is used to test for the disease. The test is read in 48 hours. It takes 3 to 6 weeks after exposure for the test to become positive. In severe disseminated disease the test may be negative, indicating that the patient's immune system is no longer able to respond.

X-ray films of the chest may show pneumonic infiltrate, hilar adenopathy, pleural effusion, or cavitary lesions 2 to 4 cm in size. These cavities usually close spontaneously within 2 years of detection. Approximately 5% of persons with primary pulmonary involvement will have residual lung lesions such as cavities or nodules. Only about 0.5% of infected individuals go on to develop a severe, progressive mycosis.

Extrapulmonary dissemination of coccidioidomycosis can occur. One of the sites of dissemination is the meningeal surfaces of the brain. If there is any indication of CNS involvement, a lumbar puncture is performed. A positive complement fixation titer in the spinal fluid is diagnostic of meningitis.

Dissemination can also occur to skin, soft tissue, liver, and bones; the patient is monitored by physical examination of the skin, gallium scanning of soft tissue, and bone scans. A bone scan should be performed before starting amphotericin B therapy. See Table 32-14 for information about signs, symptoms, and medical therapy.

Surgical intervention for lesions that are localized may involve either excision or drainage to facilitate healing.

**Collaborative care management.** See next column.

### *Blastomycosis*

**Etiology/epidemiology.** Blastomycosis is caused by inhalation of *Blastomyces dermatitidis* (see Table 32-13).

**Pathophysiology.** Although skin lesions may be the first evidence of blastomycosis, the initial site of infection is in the lung. It is assumed that inhaled spores are phagocytized in the alveoli as part of the primary infection. Thus the pathogenesis of blastomycosis is similar to that of TB, histoplasmosis, and coccidioidomycosis.

The infection spreads to other organs by lymph and blood. The skin, bones, and prostate are the most common sites of spread.

*Acute pulmonary blastomycosis* in the form of a self-limiting pneumonia can occur. Otherwise, blastomycosis is a chronic progressive disease with a mortality rate of about 90% when untreated. For this reason, treatment is recommended for every person in whom the diagnosis is established.

The only way to prevent these mycotic infections is to wear a mask to avoid inhaling spores of the organisms. See Table 32-13 for specific details.

**Collaborative care management.** The signs and symptoms and the medical therapy for the three fungal diseases are presented in Table 32-14.

Diagnostic tests include:

1. Direct demonstration of intracellular yeasts in smears of bone marrow and biopsy of lymph nodes, liver, and spleen; cultures of bone marrow, blood, or sputum.
2. Serological tests. Aggulutination, precipitation, and complement-fixation tests are used to help establish the diagnosis of histoplasmosis and coccidioidomycosis. Serology tests become positive about 1 month after the primary infection. Titers of serial tests are used to determine activity of the infection.
3. Skin testing. The skin test for histoplasmosis is used only for screening purposes. In endemic areas, 90% to 95% of young adults have positive test results. The person should be tested with histoplasmin, tuberculin, blastomycin, and coccidioidin because of the likelihood of cross-reaction. The strongest skin reaction indicates the likely cause of the infection.
4. In histoplasmosis and coccidioidomycosis, chest films demonstrate a nodular infiltrate similar in appearance to TB. In blastomycosis, chest films may be nonspecific.
5. The WBC count is usually normal. In acute cases it may increase to 13,000/mm$^2$.
6. Leukopenia and anemia may be present in persons with disseminated disease.

Promoting comfort is important and includes the following:

1. Place patient in position to facilitate breathing.
2. Take measures to reduce fever (if present), such as use of cool sponge baths.
3. Maintain room temperature desired by patient.

Administering and monitoring the effects of medications is the major focus of treatment. The role of the nurse is as follows:

1. Administer medications as prescribed and monitor patient for side effects.
   a. Amphotericin B (Fungizone IV) is the standard therapy for mycotic infection. The dose and length of therapy are determined by the difficulty in eradicating the infection and the likelihood of relapse. The therapy may last 2 to 3 weeks or 2 to 3 months.
   b. Amphotericin B must be given intravenously and has many toxic properties, including local phlebitis, systemic reactions, renal toxicity, hypokalemia, and anemia. In rare instances, anaphylaxis, bone marrow suppression, and cardiovascular and hepatic toxicity develop.
   c. Systemic toxicity (chills, fever, aching, nausea, and vomiting) can be lessened by premedication with acetaminophen along with 25 to 50 mg of diphenhydramine (Benadryl) orally. Heparin and hydrocortisone succinate (Solu-Cortef) are sometimes added to the infusions to minimize phlebitis.
   d. A reversible azotemia occurs when amphotericin B is administered. The level of azotemia is monitored by biweekly blood urea nitrogen (BUN) or serum creatinine determinations. A BUN of greater than 40 or a creatinine nearing 3 indicates a need to reduce the drug or temporarily stop it. Therapy is not continued until the azotemia is improved. Serum potassium levels are checked biweekly, and hypokalemia is treated with oral potassium. Anemia is common, and the hematocrit usually stabilizes at 25% to 35%.
   e. Ketoconazole (Nizoral) is administered orally and is effective in the treatment of systemic mycotic infections. It is given daily for a minimum of 6 months. Toxicity appears to be minimal; pruritus, minor GI intolerance, and liver function abnormalities have been reported.
2. Teach patient about medications and follow-up therapy.

***Patient/family education.*** Persons with mycotic diseases can be seriously ill and may require long-term therapy (as long as 2 to 3 months or more) with IV antifungal agents. Because these diseases are not well understood by the public, the patient and family need to feel comfortable in discussing concerns with the nurse. The nurse is responsible for providing factual information, clarifying misconceptions, and helping the patient and family understand the disease, its therapy, and the required follow-up.

These patients require close medical follow-up for 1 year to prevent relapse. The patient and family must understand the need to avoid infected areas or to wear a protective mask if they have to be in an infected area.

## OCCUPATIONAL LUNG DISEASES

### Etiology/Epidemiology

Many pulmonary diseases are believed to be caused by substances inhaled in the workplace. Occupational lung diseases are more common (1) in blue-collar workers than in white-collar workers, (2) in industrialized areas than in rural areas, and (3) in small and medium-sized businesses than in larger industrial plants.

In some instances it is debatable whether a person's lung disease is clearly occupation specific. This is especially true in cases of bronchitis, asthma, emphysema, or cancer, because all of these conditions can be caused or aggravated by several factors found in many different occupations and by nonoccupational factors such as smoking and air pollution.

Millions of Americans are believed to have job-related diseases. Because these diseases are not reportable, exact statistics do not exist. The U.S. Department of Health and Human Services (HHS) has estimated that 400,000 persons develop job-related diseases each year and that there are 100,000 deaths each year from occupational diseases. The National Heart, Lung, and Blood Institute reports that lung diseases cause more than half of these deaths. More than 5 billion dollars per year is paid out in workers' compensation for job-related illnesses and injuries.

It is well documented that smokers develop occupational lung disease more often than nonsmokers and that smokers' lungs are more vulnerable to the effects of these diseases than are nonsmokers' lungs. The combined effects of cigarette smoke and industrial pollutants are great. The risk of developing chronic bronchitis, emphysema, lung cancer, and heart disease is much increased when the worker smokes. Some of these risks, such as lung cancer in persons who worked with asbestos and who also smoked are becoming more widely known.

Occupational lung diseases can be divided into several categories. The major ones are (1) the pneumoconioses, including silicosis and coal worker's pneumoconiosis (black lung disease); (2) asbestos-related lung disease; and (3) hypersensitivity diseases, including occupational asthma, allergic alveolitis (farmer's lung), and byssinosis (brown lung disease). The etiology, epidemiology, pathophysiology, clinical manifestations, and prevention of the major occupational lung diseases are presented in Table 32-15.

### Pathophysiology

See Table 32-15.

### Collaborative Care Management

Medical therapy of these patients depends on the patient's signs, symptoms, and complications.

The major role of nurses is to be knowledgeable about the cause and prevention of occupational lung diseases so that appropriate information and teaching can be presented to the public.

#### *Patient/family education*

Occupational lung diseases are preventable. However, concerted efforts by the public, governmental agencies, and industry are necessary if these diseases are to be prevented.

Governmental action has been slow and in some instances has occurred only in response to public interest groups that have lobbied for stricter regulation of harmful substances. However, countervailing economic and political pressures have sometimes prevented laws from being passed or have resulted in less strict laws being passed because of the costs

*Text continued on p. 950*

**table 32-15** *Major Occupational Lung Diseases*

| Type | Etiology and Epidemiology | Pathophysiology | Clinical Manifestations and Prevention |
|---|---|---|---|
| **PNEUMOCONIOSES*** | | | |
| Simple (chronic) silicosis | Inhaled silica dust; most common form seen in miners, foundry workers, and others who inhaled relatively low concentrations of dust for 10-20 years | Dust accumulated in tissue → tissue reaction with whorl-shaped nodules throughout lungs | Breathlessness with exercise; 20-30% progress to *confluent silicosis* |
| Complicated silicosis (also called confluent silicosis) | 20-30% of persons with chronic silicosis develop this form | Progressive massive fibrosis (PMF) throughout lungs → ↓ lung function and cor pulmonale | Breathlessness, weakness, chest pain, productive cough with sputum, dies of cor pulmonale and respiratory failure |
| Acute silicoproteinosis | Rapidly progressive disease, leading to severe disability and death within 5 years of diagnosis | Inflammatory reaction within alveoli, diffuse fibrosis<br>Rapid progression to respiratory failure | Prevention: dust control and improved ventilation can reduce dust levels; sandblasters in enclosed spaces can use special suits and breathing apparatuses; some experts believe such protective measures are still inadequate |
| Complicated progressive massive fibrosis (PMF) | 3% of persons with simple silicosis develop PMF; occurs in miners with heavy deposits of coal dust in lungs; *may appear suddenly years after miner has left the mines;* workers who smoke have 5-6 times more lung obstruction than nonsmoking workers; cigarette smoking causes chronic bronchitis and emphysema | Fibrosis develops in some of dust-laden areas; fibrosis spreads and fibrotic areas coalesce; eventually most of lung is stiffened and useless | PMF shortens life span; may die from respiratory failure, cor pulmonale, or superimposed infection; most silicosis-associated deaths are in persons >65 years; National Institute for Occupational Safety and Health (NIOSH) concerned about number of young persons dying from silicosis (Figure 32-7, p. 950); occupations of these young persons include operators of machines used to crush, grind, mix, and blend materials; painters/paint spray operators; construction trades; and laborers<br>More deaths occur in minorities; more women are developing silicosis[17]<br>Prevention: dust control; abrasive blasting with silica sand, to prepare surfaces for painting = exposure to 200 times NIOSH recommendations; workers need to be educated about NIOSH recommendations for avoiding prolonged overexposure to silica dust |
| **ASBESTOS-RELATED LUNG DISEASE** | Asbestos causes lung cancer, malignant mesothelioma of pleura and periosteum, cancer of the larynx, and certain gastrointestinal cancers; also causes asbestosis, a progressive fibrotic lung disease; | Fibrosis caused by asbestos called asbestosis; asbestos fibers accumulate around terminal bronchioles; surrounds fibers with iron-rich tissue, forming asbestos body with characteristic picture on x-ray; | After fibrosis begins, cough, sputum, weight loss, increasing breathlessness; most die within 1-5 years of first symptoms |

*Also known as "dust in the lungs."

*Continued*

**table 32-15** *Major Occupational Lung Diseases—cont'd*

| Type | Etiology and Epidemiology | Pathophysiology | Clinical Manifestations and Prevention |
|---|---|---|---|
| **ASBESTOS-RELATED LUNG DISEASE —*CONT'D*** | risk of these diseases increases with repeated exposure and length of time since first exposure; declared a human carcinogen by the Environmental Protection Agency (EPA) and International Agency for Research on Cancer of the World Health Organization (WHO)[40]<br>Total number of deaths in United States eventually caused by exposure to asbestos is estimated to exceed 200,000; 20-25% of deaths from workers with heavy exposure are from lung cancer; cancer related to degree of exposure and to cigarette smoking, which enhances carcinogenic properties of asbestos; *asbestos workers who smoke are 90 times more likely to develop lung cancer as smokers with no exposure to asbestos*<br>Four commercially important forms of asbestos: chrystolite, crocidolite, amosite, and anthophylline; chrystolite accounts for 95% of current world production; nearly all asbestos used in North America is mined in Quebec, Canada; crocidolite is 2-4 times more potent than chrystolite or amosite in causing mesothelioma; all forms equally potent as cause of lung cancer; new use of asbestos almost completely ended in United States and other developed nations as a result of governmental bans and market pressures; asbestos extensively and aggressively marketed by Canada and other exporting nations in the developing world, where sales remain strong<br>Asbestos Hazard Emergency Response Act (AHERA), passed in 1986, tightened controls on use of asbestos in the United States; mesothelioma accounts for 7-10% of deaths in asbestos workers; inoperable and always fatal; can occur after very little exposure to crocidolite; has been reported in wives of asbestos workers and in persons living near asbestos plants; | more asbestos bodies as more fibers are inhaled; after 20-30 years of exposure, fibrosis begins in lungs; if heavy exposure, appears in 4-5 years<br>Occurs in persons exposed to crocidolite fibers of a certain size; needlelike shape of crocidolite fibers enables them to pass through lung tissue to pleura | Treatment with radical pleurectomy and pneumonectomy; survival only 1-2 years<br>Prevention: enforcement of regulations governing mining, milling, and use of asbestos; a guiding principle of AHERA is that asbestos in a building poses no hazard to health unless fibers become inhaled; removal of asbestos required only when asbestos is visibly deteriorating or when renovation is imminent[40]<br>Protective masks must be used when working with asbestos |

*Continued*

**table 32-15** *Major Occupational Lung Diseases—cont'd*

| TYPE | ETIOLOGY AND EPIDEMIOLOGY | PATHOPHYSIOLOGY | CLINICAL MANIFESTATIONS AND PREVENTION |
|---|---|---|---|
| **ASBESTOS-RELATED LUNG DISEASE—*CONT'D*** | cigarette smoking not a contributing factor in these persons; inhalation of only a few fine, straight crocidolite factors are necessary; swallowing of asbestos-contaminated sputum responsible for cancer of larynx, esophagus, stomach, and intestines | | |
| **HYPERSENSITIVITY DISEASES** | Hypersensitivity diseases fall into occupational category when antigen is found primarily in workplace; lung hypersensitivity can occur in bronchi, bronchioles, or alveoli; coarse dust causes bronchial reactions; fine dust provokes small airway and alveolar reactions | | |
| Occupational asthma | More common in 10% of population who are atopic (genetic tendency to develop an allergy); nonatopic persons can also become sensitized; substances with antigenic properties include detergent enzymes, platinum salts, cereals and grains, certain wood dusts, isocyanate chemicals used in polyurethane paints and other products, agents used in printing, and some pesticides | Hypersensitivity reaction mediated by histamine → bronchoconstriction and ↑ mucus production; repeated attacks if cause unrecognized and asthma is untreated; may lead to permanent obstructive lung disease; asthmatic response that is well established can be provoked by other factors (house dust, cigarette smoke) and by fatigue, breathing cold air, and coughing | Wheezing is major symptom<br>Prevention: total elimination of antigen; desensitization not successful |
| Hypersensitivity pneumonitis (allergic alveolitis [farmer's lung]) | Hypersensitivity disease caused by fine organic dust inhaled into smallest airways; cause of farmer's lung is moldy hay; other dusts can cause allergic alveolitis: these include moldy sugar cane and barley, maple bark, cork, animal hair, bird feathers and droppings, mushroom compost, coffee beans, and paprika; often disease is named for cause (mushroom worker's lung, etc.); fungus spores growing in the apparent antigen are thought in many cases to be real cause of disease | Alveoli are inflamed, inundated by WBCs, sometimes filled with fluid; if exposure infrequent or level of dust low, symptoms are mild, and treatment not sought, chronic form develops over time; eventually, fibrosis occurs, and fibrosis may be so well established that it cannot be arrested | Symptoms begin some hours after exposure to offending dust and include fatigue, shortness of breath, dry cough, fever, and chills; symptoms may be severe enough to require emergency treatment and hospitalization; acute attacks treated with steroids; recovery may take 6 weeks, and patient may have residual lung damage; real cure is permanent separation of patient and antigen<br>Prevention: properly dried and stored farm products (hay, straw, sugar cane) do not cause allergic alveolitis; presumably fungi only grow in moist conditions |

*Continued*

**table 32-15** *Major Occupational Lung Diseases—cont'd*

| Type | Etiology and Epidemiology | Pathophysiology | Clinical Manifestations and Prevention |
|---|---|---|---|
| Byssinosis (brown lung) | Occupational disease occurs in textile workers; mainly in cotton workers but also afflicts workers in flax and hemp industries; cause is found in bales of raw cotton that contain not only cotton fibers but fragments of cotton plant; something in plant matter, rather than pure cotton, is cause | Chronic bronchitis and emphysema develop in time; constriction of bronchioles in response to something in crude cotton; symptoms of asthma and allergy persist as long as there is exposure to cotton antigen | Tightness in chest on returning to work after a weekend away (Monday fever); strong relationship between amount of dust inhaled and symptoms; persistent productive tight chest with chronic bronchitis and emphysema; person leaves industry as respiratory cripple<br>Prevention: dust control measures; pretreating bales of cotton by washing with steam and other agents may inactivate causative agent; try to detect persons who are likely to become sensitized to cotton dust and keep them out of high-risk areas |

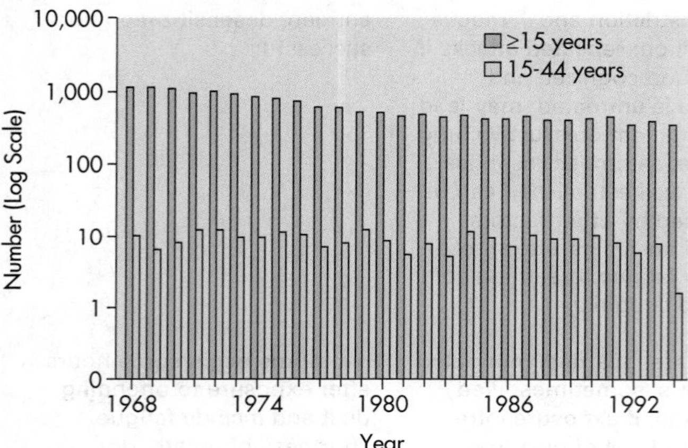


**fig. 32-7** Number of silicosis-associated deaths, by age group and year—United States, 1968 through 1994.

involved in meeting the strict standards required to control certain hazards.

The ALA recommends several measures to reduce the incidence of occupation-related lung diseases: (1) public education about the relationship between polluted air in the workplace and lung diseases; (2) general commitment to reduce, eliminate, or avoid air pollution in the workplace; and (3) elimination of the most prevalent and notorious lung hazard: cigarette smoke.

Education of the public includes not only employers and employees but also engineers and planners who design operations; buyers and purchasers who select ingredients, cleaning agents, and equipment; and physicians and nurses who care for persons with occupation-related diseases. Many times, workers who are instructed about the hazards involved in certain occupations and workplaces are helpful in deciding what preventive measures need to be taken to combat or minimize the effects of hazards. The commitment to reduce, eliminate, or avoid pollution of workplace air requires full consideration of possible health effects whenever operations are planned and improvement of conditions whenever possible.

The year 2000 national health goal for occupational lung disease is to establish in the 50 states exposure standards to prevent the major occupational lung diseases to which their worker populations are exposed (byssinosis, asbestosis, coal worker's pneumoconiosis, silicosis). Because these diseases are not reportable, no baseline data are available. The reader is urged to contact his or her state's department of health to determine what progress has been made in establishing and enforcing exposure standards for these diseases.

## SARCOIDOSIS

### Etiology/Epidemiology

Sarcoidosis is a systemic granulomatous disease of unknown cause. It is worldwide in distribution and is most common in young adults. In the United States, it is more common in black women. Some evidence suggests that the incidence is higher in blacks than whites in other parts of the world, especially if the disease is sought out.

### Pathophysiology

There is evidence of an antigen-antibody reaction manifested by reticuloendothelial response in which both thymus-derived (T) cells and plasma (B) cells participate (see Chapter 65 for more information). It is believed that the antigen is airborne, because bilateral hilar lymphadenopathy is commonly present at the onset and bronchopulmonary macrophages are increased.

The central pathological event involves the growth of noncaseating granulomas and proliferation of lymph tissue. Pulmonary sarcoidosis typically is seen on chest x-ray films as enlarged lymph nodes in the hilar area. The patient with sarcoidosis may initially complain only of vague symptoms of malaise, fever, aching in the joints, or weakness. In addition to mediastinal lymph node enlargement, ocular manifestations, such as uveitis and conjunctivitis, and dermatological changes, such as erythema nodosum, are often found.

Diagnosis of sarcoidosis is based on x-ray film findings, transbronchial lung biopsy, and organ biopsy showing noncaseating granulomas. Organ biopsy yields the most conclusive evidence of sarcoidosis and is most helpful in differentiating it from Hodgkin's disease and TB.

Other diagnostic methods in pulmonary sarcoidosis include gallium scan and bronchoalveolar lavage (BAL) with flexible fiberoptic bronchoscopy. The fluid obtained from BAL is examined to determine the degree of active inflammation in the lung and need for therapy. The patient's symptoms and pulmonary function tests (especially lung volume) are still widely used, however, in deciding whether treatment is required.

### Collaborative Care Management

In many patients, sarcoidosis is a benign, self-limiting process that resolves with no residual damage within 2 years of diagnosis. Other patients will have an acute or chronic form of the disease.

Treatment of acute pulmonary disease is with systemic steroids. Patients are treated with prednisone, 60 mg daily for 2 months, followed by 40 mg of prednisone daily for 2 months. The steroids are then slowly tapered off to a maintenance dose of 15 mg daily. Most patients are treated for 18 to 24 months. The patient is then followed medically for several years for signs of relapse. Relapse usually occurs within 3 to 6 months after the steroids are discontinued, and repeat treatment is necessary.

In chronic forms of pulmonary sarcoidosis, patients are treated with small doses of steroids (5 to 10 mg every other day) for years. About 10% of patients develop the chronic form of sarcoidosis. In this form the disease proceeds to nodular granulomatous depositions in lung tissue and eventual pulmonary fibrosis. In severe cases, pulmonary hypertension and cor pulmonale develop.

Nursing care depends on the severity of the patient's signs and symptoms and medical therapy. Teaching the patient about the precautions and side effects of steroid therapy is a major nursing function.

## CANCER OF THE LUNG

### Etiology

Cancer of the lung may be either metastatic or primary. Metastatic tumors may follow malignancy anywhere in the body. Metastasis from the colon and kidney is common. Metastasis to the lung may be discovered before the primary lesion is known, and sometimes the location of the primary lesion may be found only at autopsy.

### Epidemiology

The past 50 years have seen a startling increase in the incidence of cancer of the lung. The ACS estimates 178,100 new cases in 1997 and 160,400 deaths (29% of all cancer deaths).

**box 32-10** *Effects of Smoking on Lung Cancer Risk*

- Smokers are 10 times more likely to develop lung cancer than those who never smoked.
- Heavy smokers more likely to die of lung cancer than light smokers, suggesting dose-response effect.
- Risk associated with smoking increases with number of years person smokes.
- Risk decreases steadily after person stops smoking.
- Cigarette smokers have higher death rate than pipe smokers.
- Nonsmoking wives of smokers have significantly higher risk of lung cancer than nonsmoking wives married to nonsmokers.

Since 1986 cancer of the lung has surpassed breast cancer to become the number-one cancer killer of women. Thus lung cancer is now the leading cause of death from cancer in both men and women.[1]

The increase in death rates for both men and women is directly related to cigarette smoking. A history of smoking, especially for 20 years or more, is a prime risk factor. Other risk factors include exposure to certain industrial substances such as arsenic, specific organic chemicals, radon, and asbestos, particularly in those who smoke. It is estimated that asbestos workers who smoke have 6 to 10 times more cancer of the lung than the general population. Some evidence also suggests a genetic predisposition to lung cancer.[38]

In the United States the age-adjusted death rate from cancer has been steadily increasing. Most of the increase is directly related to rise in lung cancer death rates. Age-adjusted rates for other cancer sites have been leveling off and in some cases declining. There has been a decline in cancer death rates for all age groups, for males and females, and for blacks and whites, except in people 55 years of age and older, in whom the cancer death rate has increased.[38]

The cause of cancer of the lung is closely related to cigarette smoking. Box 32-10 shows the relationship between lung cancer and smoking. Prevention is the best protection against cancer of the lung because early detection of the disease is difficult. The cancer death rate for male cigarette smokers is more than double that for nonsmokers, and the rate for female smokers is 67% higher than that for nonsmokers.[1]

Because no effective treatment exists for lung cancer, emphasis is on prevention. *Nearly 90% of persons with lung cancer die within 5 years of diagnosis.* This percentage could be reduced with early diagnosis and treatment. Unfortunately, about one third of the persons with lung cancer have inoperable cancer when first seen by a physician. Another one third are found to have inoperable cancer when an exploratory thoracoscopy or thoracotomy is performed.

### Pathophysiology

Because most new growths in the lungs arise from the bronchi, the term *bronchogenic carcinoma* is widely used. A patient's signs and symptoms depend on several factors, including the location of the lesion. Signs and symptoms of lesion in the bronchus and lung include:

1. Approximately 10% of patients are asymptomatic, and cancer is identified on routine chest x-ray film.
2. Approximately 75% have a cough.
3. Approximately 50% have hemoptysis.
4. Shortness of breath and a unilateral wheeze are common.

*Peripheral pulmonary lesions* that perforate into the pleural space cause extrapulmonary intrathoracic signs and symptoms. These include:

1. Pain on inspiration
2. Friction rub
3. Pleural effusion
4. Edema of face and neck when the superior vena cava is involved
5. Fatigue
6. Clubbing of fingers

In the latter stages of the disease, weight loss and debility usually indicate metastases, especially to the liver. Cancer of the lung may metastasize to nearby structures such as the prescalene lymph nodes, the walls of the esophagus, and the pericardium or to distant areas such as the brain, liver, kidneys, adrenal glands, or skeleton.

Histologically, lung cancer is divided into four major subgroups: squamous (epidermoid) cell carcinoma, small cell (oat cell) carcinoma, adenocarcinoma, and large cell carcinoma (Figure 32-8). Table 32-16 shows the type, percentage of cases in the subtypes, and recommended therapy. As with other types of cancer, lung cancer is staged (see Chapter 11 for more details about staging). The International Tumor, Node, Metastasis (TNM) Staging for Lung Cancer is presented in Box 32-11.

Because patients with early lung cancer have no symptoms, they often have inoperable cancer when they seek medical assistance. Some patients with cancers of the lung are diagnosed after a chest x-ray film as part of a routine physical examination. Other patients are not diagnosed until they seek medical treatment for symptoms related to metastases.

Survival rates of patients with non–small cell lung cancer (NSCLC) depend on the size of the tumor, nodal status, and degree of metastases. Table 32-17 gives the 5-year survival rates for patients with NSCLC.

Some patients who undergo surgical resection (pneumonectomy or lobectomy) may also receive radiation therapy or chemotherapy. These adjuvants are given mainly to treat metastases and to relieve some of the patient's symptoms.

## Collaborative Care Management

### *Diagnostic tests*

1. Histological examination of the tumor is necessary to confirm a diagnosis of lung cancer. Four methods are used to collect tissue samples:
   a. Sputum collection: a 3-day pooled sample provides more reliable evidence than a single sample. Sputum is examined for bacteria and cancer cells.

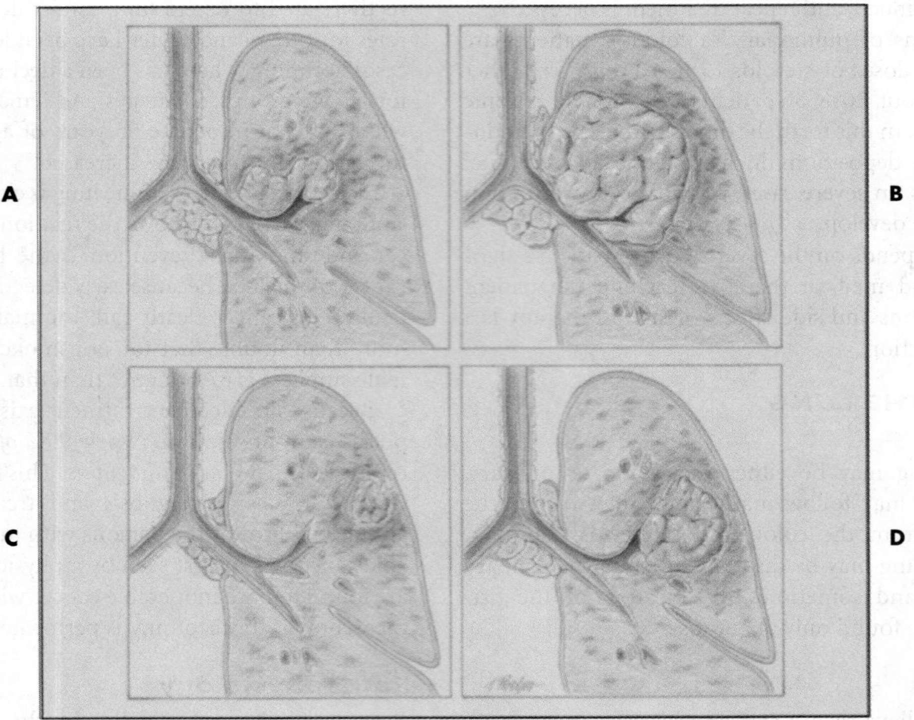


**fig. 32-8** Cancer of the lung. **A,** Squamous (epidermoid) cell carcinoma. **B,** Small cell (oat cell) carcinoma. **C,** Adenocarcinoma. **D,** Large cell carcinoma.

b. Fiberoptic bronchoscopy can be used to remove tissue samples from visible tumors or to perform brushing and washing of peripheral lesions. When hilar or mediastinal lymph nodes are involved, transbronchial needle biopsy (with a bronchoscope) is used to obtain node tissue for examination.

c. Percutaneous transthoracic needle biopsy is used to biopsy lesions visible on fluoroscopy, especially when they are close to the surface of the lung. Analysis of tissue samples can provide a specific diagnosis and sometimes cell type. A small number of patients develop a pneumothorax requiring chest tube drainage.

d. Excision of lesion. A lesion is removed through a small incision. Video-assisted thoracoscopy or thoracotomy is useful for performing small diagnostic wedge excisions; mechanical staplers or lasers are used with these procedures.

**table 32-16** *Histological Subtypes of Lung Cancer and Therapy for Each Type*

| Type | Classification and Percentage of Cases | Therapy |
|---|---|---|
| Small cell carcinoma | Small cell lung cancer (SCLC): 15-25% of cases | Combination chemotherapy such as (1) cyclophosphamide, doxorubicin, and vincristine, or (2) cyclophosphamide, doxorubicin, and etoposide, or (3) cisplatin plus etoposide |
| Adenocarcinoma; most common type: 35-45% of cases<br>Squamous cell carcinoma: 30-40% of cases<br>Large cell carcinoma: about 10% of cases | All three classified as non–small cell lung cancer (NSCLC): 75-85% of cases | Pulmonary resection—only one third are operable; one third inoperable because of advanced lung cancer; one third inoperable because of distant metastases |

**box 32-11** *International TNM Staging System for Lung Cancer*

**TUMOR (T)**

- **TX** Occult carcinoma (malignant cells in sputum or bronchial washings, but tumor not visualized by imaging studies or bronchoscopy)
- **$T_1$** Tumor ≤3 cm in diameter, surrounded by lung or visceral pleura but not proximal to lobar bronchus on bronchoscopy
- **$T_2$** Tumor ≥3 cm in diameter, or with involvement of main bronchus at least 2 cm distal to carina, or with visceral pleural invasion, or with associated atelectasis or obstructive pneumonitis extending to the hilar region but not involving the entire lung
- **$T_3$** Tumor invading chest wall, diaphragm, mediastinal pleura, or parietal pericardium; or tumor in main bronchus within 2 cm of carina but not invading it; or atelectasis or obstructive pneumonitis of entire lung
- **$T_4$** Tumor invading mediastinum, heart, great vessels, trachea, esophagus, vertebral body, or carina; or ipsilateral malignant pleural effusion

**NODES (N)**

- **$N_0$** No regional lymph node metastases
- **$N_1$** Metastases to ipsilateral peribronchial or hilar nodes
- **$N_2$** Metastases to ipsilateral mediastinal or subcarinal nodes
- **$N_3$** Metastases to contralateral mediastinal or hilar nodes or to any scalene or supraclavicular nodes

**DISTANT METASTASES (M)**

- **$M_0$** No distant metastases
- **$M_1$** Distant metastases

**STAGE GROUPINGS**

| | | | |
|---|---|---|---|
| **Occult** | TX | $N_0$ | $M_0$ |
| **Stage I** | $T_{1\text{-}2}$ | $N_0$ | $M_0$ |
| **Stage II** | $T_{1\text{-}2}$ | $N_1$ | $M_0$ |
| **Stage IIIA** | $T_3$ | $N_{0\text{-}1}$ | $M_0$ |
| | $T_{1\text{-}3}$ | $N_2$ | $M_0$ |
| **Stage IIIB** | $T_4$ | $N_{0\text{-}2}$ | $M_0$ |
| | $T_{1\text{-}4}$ | $N_3$ | $M_0$ |
| **Stage IV** | Any T | Any N | $M_1$ |

Modified from American Joint Committee on Cancer.

**table 32-17** *Five-Year Disease-Free Survival Rates for Surgical Resection in Patients with Non–Small Cell Lung Cancer*

| | Stage | 5-Year Disease-Free (%) |
|---|---|---|
| I | $T_1$, $N_0$, $M_0$ | 70-85 |
| | $T_2$, $N_0$, $M_0$ | 55-65 |
| II | $T_1$, $N_1$, $M_0$ | 30-50 |
| | $T_1$, $N_2$, $M_0$ | 25-30 |
| IIIA | $T_3$, $N_0$, $M_0$ | 25-35 |
| | $T_3$, $N_1$, $M_0$ | 15-20 |
| | $T_{1\text{-}2}$, $N_2$, $M_0$ | 9-24 |
| | $T_3$, $N_2$ | 0-5 |

From Jett JR: Primary lung cancer. In Rakel RE, editor: *Conn's current therapy,* Philadelphia, 1996, WB Saunders.

2. Staging techniques:
   a. Imaging techniques: chest x-ray films, CT scans, and magnetic resonance imaging (MRI) are used for clinical staging of lung cancer.
      (1) Lateral chest x-ray film is able to depict tumors, especially those on periphery.
      (2) Contrast-enhanced CT scan or MRI can differentiate an underlying mass from atelectasis or inflammation.
      (3) Chest wall invasion: MRI can be used to differentiate involvement of visceral pleura from involvement of parietal pleura.
      (4) CT scan is also used to reveal malignant pleural effusions, which usually mean inoperability. Malignant cells should be identified in pleural fluid before a decision is made about inoperability.
      (5) Positive emission tomography (PET) has been found to be effective in staging non–small cell lung cancers.
   b. Thoracentesis is routinely performed if there is evidence of pleural effusion clinically or on CT scan. Up to 1000 ml of fluid may be removed.
   c. Thoracoscopy and mediastinoscopy: thoracoscopy is useful for evaluating pleural seeding and for examining mediastinal nodes. Mediastinoscopy is better than CT scan or MRI for assessing mediastinal metastases and effectiveness of preoperative radiation therapy or chemotherapy.

Assessment of surgical risk for pulmonary resection is based on age, pulmonary reserve, cardiovascular disease, and disease so extensive it would require a pneumonectomy. Each is discussed briefly next.

**Age.** Mortality and morbidity related to pulmonary resection increase significantly in persons older than 70 years of age. Some studies suggest higher mortality and morbidity in those 60 to 65 years of age.

**Pulmonary reserve.** Arterial blood gases and pulmonary function tests (PFTs) are used to measure pulmonary reserve. A $PCO_2$ greater than 45 mm Hg indicates inoperability, whereas a $PO_2$ less than 60 mm Hg suggests that pulmonary resection would be risky, unless the low $PO_2$ is caused by complete airway obstruction that results from desaturated blood entering the pulmonary veins from perfused but nonventilated lung (V/Q mismatch). The PFTs are used to evaluate risk of pulmonary resection. A predicted postoperative forced expiratory volume ($FEV_1$) of more than 800 ml is required in most adults. Most patients with a predicted $FEV_1$ less than 30% are usually unable to tolerate pneumonectomy.

**Cardiovascular disease.** Coronary artery disease is present in about 80 of every 1000 patients older than age 65. Previous myocardial infarction, especially when surgery would be necessary less than 6 months after infarction, increases the risk. Left ventricular dysfunction, including signs of congestive heart failure, indicates high risk of death after pulmonary resection. Unstable angina must be controlled before resection. Hypertension has to be under control. Frequent premature ventricular contractions (PVCs) are signs of severe heart disease and are associated with increased perioperative complications and death.

**Pneumonectomy.** Particularly for patients age 70 and over and especially with surgery of right lung (which normally does 60% to 70% of breathing), pneumonectomy is associated with higher risk than lesser procedures.

### *Surgical management*

#### Principles of resectional surgery

1. Endotracheal anesthesia is used for surgery involving the lung in which the pleural space is entered.
2. Endotracheal anesthesia makes it possible to keep the uninvolved ("good") lung expanded and functioning when the chest is opened and atmospheric pressure enters the pleural space.
3. To understand resectional surgery and the purpose of chest tubes and closed drainage system, an understanding of the following is necessary.
   a. Physiology of breathing:
      (1) The pressure in the pleural space (the space between the visceral and parietal pleura) is subatmospheric (less than 760 mm Hg) and is referred to as *negative.*
      (2) The pressure in the pleural space is usually 756 mm Hg and goes down to 751 mm Hg before inspiration. This change in pressure allows air (atmospheric pressure) to enter the lungs.
      (3) When the pleura is entered surgically or with trauma to the chest wall, atmospheric *(positive)* pressure enters the pleural space, and the lung on that side collapses.
   b. Purpose of chest tubes and closed drainage system:
      (1) After resectional surgery of the lung (except pneumonectomy), one or two drainage tubes are inserted into the pleural space. Each tube is connected to a negative-pressure closed drainage system.
      (2) This system allows air and fluid to drain from the pleural space and prevents air or fluid from entering the pleural space.
      (3) In all resectional surgery (except pneumonectomy), the remaining portions of the lung must overexpand and fill the space left by the resected portion.

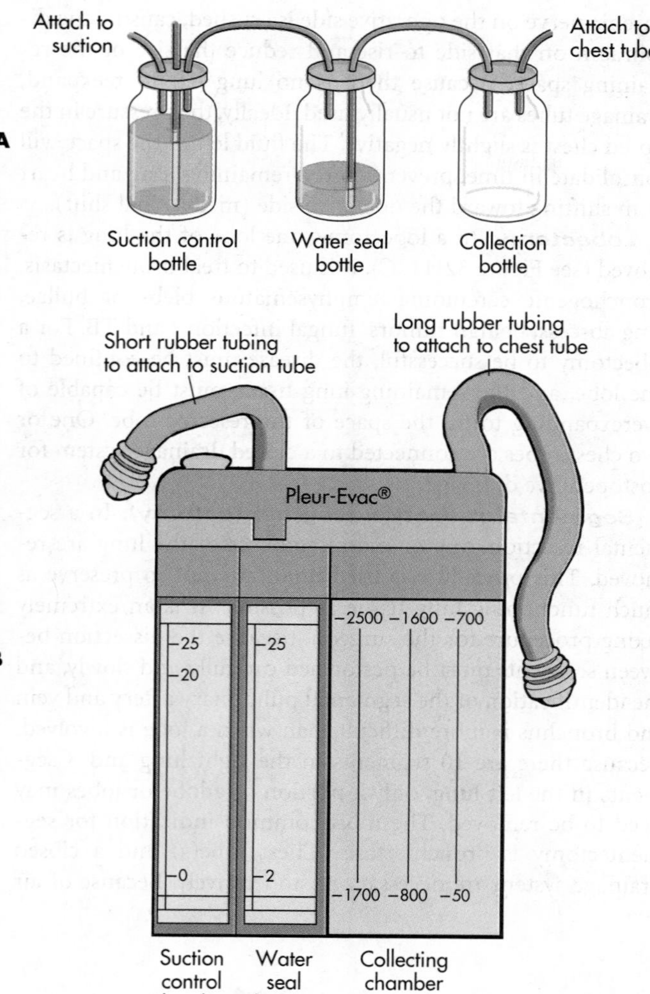


**fig. 32-9** **A,** Water-sealed closed-chest drainage system (original three-bottle design). **B,** Pleur-Evac, one of several brands of disposable chest drainage systems based on the three-bottle design. The unit collects drainage, maintains a seal to prevent air from entering the pleural cavity, and prevents excessive buildup of negative pressure.

(4) The removal of air and fluid from the pleural space accomplishes two basic purposes: (1) to aid in the expansion of the remaining portion of the lung as air (*positive* pressure) and fluid escapes through the drainage tubes, and (2) to reestablish *negative* pressure in the pleural space.

(5) Nursing actions necessary to maintain the integrity of the chest tubes and closed drainage system are discussed under postoperative care.

(6) Older closed-chest drainage systems such as water-sealed bottles may be used (see Figure 32-9, *A*).

**Types of resectional surgery.** Box 32-12 presents the types of resectional surgery and the indications for the use of each type. A brief discussion of each type of resectional surgery follows.

***Exploratory thoracotomy.*** An exploratory thoracotomy is performed to confirm a suspected diagnosis of lung or chest disease. The usual approach is by a posterolateral parascapular incision through the fourth, fifth, sixth, or seventh intercostal space. Occasionally, an anterior approach is used. The ribs are spread to give the best possible exposure of the lung and hemithorax. The pleura is entered and the lung examined; a biopsy usually is taken; and the chest is closed. This procedure may also be used to detect bleeding in the chest or other injury after trauma to the chest. Because the pleural space was entered, a chest tube and closed drainage system are necessary (Figure 32-10).

**box 32-12** *Types of Thoracic Surgery and Indications for Their Use*

**EXPLORATORY THORACOTOMY**
To confirm suspected diagnosis of lung or chest disease, especially carcinoma; to obtain a biopsy; being replaced by noninvasive procedures (thoracoscopy)

**PNEUMONECTOMY**
Removal of a lung; bronchogenic carcinoma when lobectomy will not remove all of lesion; tuberculosis when other surgery will not remove all of diseased lung

**PNEUMOMECTOMY**
*Lung reduction surgery* to reduce lung volume and decrease tension on respiratory muscles in persons with emphysema

**LOBECTOMY**
Removal of one lobe of lung; bronchogenic carcinoma confined to a lobe, bronchiectasis, emphysematous blebs or bullae; lung abscess, fungal infections, benign tumors; tuberculosis

**BILOBECTOMY**
Removal of two lobes from right lung; bronchogenic carcinoma when lobectomy will not remove all of disease

**SLEEVE LOBECTOMY**
Resection of main bronchus or distal trachea with reanastomosis to a distal uninvolved bronchus; bronchogenic carcinoma to preserve functional parenchyma

**SEGMENTAL RESECTION**
Segmentectomy; removal of one or more lung segments; bronchiectasis; lung abscess or cyst; metastatic carcinoma; tuberculosis

**WEDGE RESECTION**
Removal of pie-shaped section from surface of lung; well-circumscribed benign tumors, metastatic tumors, or localized inflammatory disease, including TB

**DECORTICATION**
Removal of a fibrinous peel from visceral pleura; chronic empyema

**THORACOPLASTY**
Removal of ribs; residual air space after resectional surgery; chronic empyema space

***Pneumonectomy.*** A pneumonectomy, the removal of an entire lung, is most often performed to treat bronchogenic carcinoma (Figure 32-11, *B*). It may also be used to treat TB. However, a pneumonectomy is performed only in cases in which a lobectomy or segmental resection will not remove all the diseased tissue. A thoracotomy incision is made in either the posterior or anterior chest using the method described under exploratory thoracotomy. Before the lung can be removed, the pulmonary artery and vein are ligated and then cut. The main-stem bronchus leading to the lung is clamped, divided, and sutured or stapled. To ensure an airtight closure of the bronchus, a pleural flap may be placed over it and sutured into place. This is not necessary if staples are used. The phrenic nerve on the operative side is crushed, causing the diaphragm on that side to rise and reduce the size of the remaining space. Because there is no lung left to reexpand, drainage tubes are not usually used. Ideally, the pressure in the closed chest is slightly negative. The fluid left in the space will consolidate in time, preventing the remaining lung and heart from shifting toward the operative side (mediastinal shift).

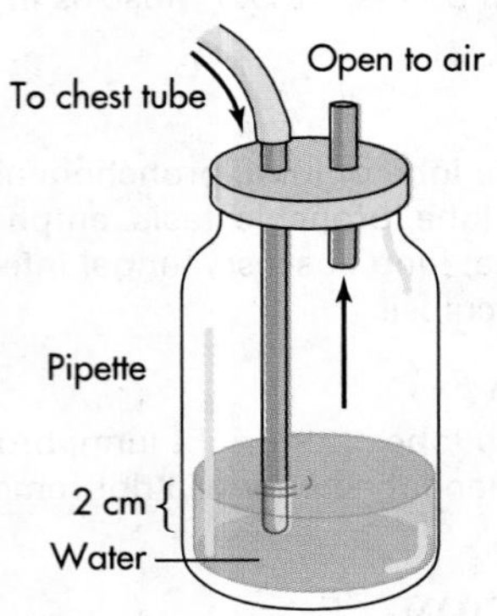


**fig. 32-10** Water-sealed closed-chest drainage showing tip of tube under water.

***Lobectomy.*** In a lobectomy, one lobe of the lung is removed (see Figure 32-11, *C*). It is used to treat bronchiectasis, bronchogenic carcinoma, emphysematous blebs or bullae, lung abscess, benign tumors, fungal infections, and TB. For a lobectomy to be successful, the disease must be confined to one lobe, and the remaining lung tissue must be capable of overexpanding to fill the space of the resected lobe. One or two chest tubes are connected to a closed drainage system for postoperative drainage.

***Segmental resection (segmentectomy).*** In a segmental resection, one or more segments of the lung are removed. This procedure is used in an attempt to preserve as much functioning lung tissue as possible. It is an extremely taxing procedure for the surgeon, because the dissection between segments must be performed carefully and slowly, and the identification of the segmental pulmonary artery and vein and bronchus is more difficult than when a lobe is involved. Because there are 10 segments in the right lung and 8 segments in the left lung, only a portion of a lobe or lobes may need to be removed. The most common indication for segmentectomy is bronchiectasis. Chest tube(s) and a closed drainage system are necessary postoperatively. Because of air

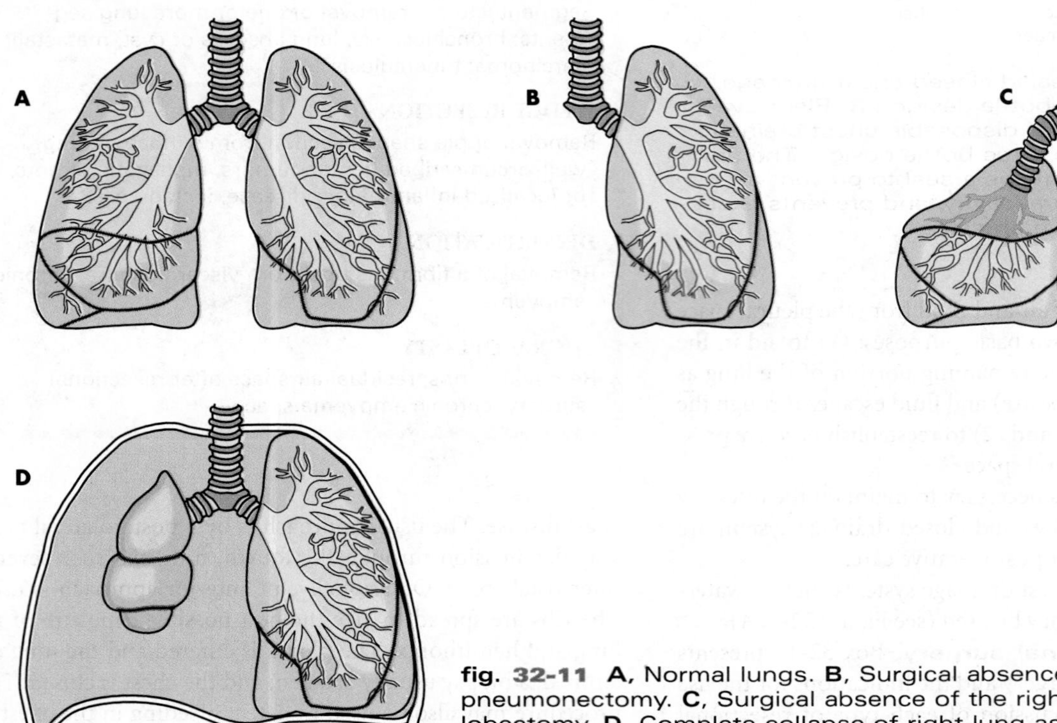


**fig. 32-11** **A,** Normal lungs. **B,** Surgical absence of right lung after a pneumonectomy. **C,** Surgical absence of the right upper lobe after a lobectomy. **D,** Complete collapse of right lung as a result of air in the pleural cavity (pneumothorax).

leaks from the segmental surface, the remaining lung tissue may take longer to reexpand.

***Wedge resection.*** In a wedge resection, a well-circumscribed diseased portion is removed without regard to the segmental planes of the lung. The area to be removed is clamped, dissected, and sutured or stapled. Chest tube(s) and a closed drainage system are used postoperatively.

***Decortication.*** In a decortication, a fibrinous peel is removed from the visceral pleura, allowing the encased lung to reexpand and obliterate the pleural space. This procedure is discussed further under the treatment of empyema (Table 32-18). Chest tube(s) and chest suction are used to facilitate the reexpansion of the lung. If the lung has been encased for a long time, it may be incapable of reexpanding after decorticaton. In this situation, thoracoplasty may be necessary.

***Lung reduction surgery.*** This procedure, which was designed to treat a select group of patients with pulmonary emphysema, has been used only since the early 1990s. The purpose of the surgery is to (1) reduce lung volume; (2) decrease tension on respiratory muscles, thereby decreasing dyspnea; and (3) allow the normal lung, which is being compressed, to expand and improve gas exchange. One approach to this procedure involves "trimming" both lungs to remove distended areas of each lung, thus allowing the compressed lung underneath to expand more fully. Strips of bovine pericardium may be used to help seal the cut surfaces of the lungs and prevent large postoperative air leaks. This procedure has been termed *pneumomectomy* to differentiate it from pneumonectomy. In this approach chest tubes and closed drainage will be required for both lungs. Because the surgery is so new, its long-term effectiveness is still being evaluated.[21]

**Preoperative care and evaluation.** Bronchoscopy and pulmonary function tests are required before thoracic surgery. Both of these procedures are discussed in Chapter 30.

## NURSING MANAGEMENT OF THE PATIENT WITH THORACIC SURGERY

### PREOPERATIVE CARE

The proposed surgery is discussed with both patient and family. The goal of teaching is to prepare the patient for what he or she is expected to do postoperatively. In some hospitals, nurses from the operating room, recovery room, or ICU do the preoperative teaching. Even when this is so, the nurse caring for the patient is responsible for determining what the patient understands about the impending surgery and to be sure that preoperative teaching is completed.

Points to be discussed in teaching include:

1. Patient's knowledge of procedure
2. Explanation of procedure as necessary, including intubation for anesthesia, site of incision, and chest tube(s) and drainage system
3. Oxygen
4. Blood administration and IVs
5. Pain medication, including patient-controlled analgesia (PCA) if used

**table 32-18** *Long-Term Complications of Resectional Surgery*

| COMPLICATIONS | SIGNS AND SYMPTOMS | TREATMENT |
|---|---|---|
| **EMPYEMA** | | |
| Pus in the pleural space is a dreaded complication of thoracic surgery. Pus may drain from chest tube(s) or if chest tubes are already removed, pus can be obtained on thoracentesis (insertion of a needle attached to a syringe with a three-way stopcock used to remove fluid, blood, or pus from pleural space). | Unexplained elevation in temperature<br>Evidence of pleural exudate on x-ray film | Dependent drainage by thoracentesis, intercostal chest tube, or open drainage with rib resection. Chest tube may be connected to a closed drainage system or cut off and allowed to drain into chest dressings. Water seal not necessary if empyema space has a thick wall and there is no danger of lung collapse. Over time as empyema drains out tube, the space becomes smaller and smaller and fills in with granulation tissue. If space persists, a thoracoplasty is necessary. |
| **BRONCHOPLEURAL FISTULA (BPF)** | | |
| Opening in the sutured bronchus that permits communication between bronchus and pleural space. Space usually becomes infected, and empyema develops. Use of an automatic stapling machine to close the bronchus has reduced the incidence of BPF. | Cough (usually nonproductive), fever, leukocytosis, anorexia, expectoration of purulent sputum, and evidence of pleural exudate on x-ray film | Chest tube connected to a water-seal chamber because there is a direct communication between bronchus (positive pressure being inspired) and the pleural space. A persistent bronchopleural fistula is treated by thoracoplasty and a muscle implant to seal off the bronchus. |

6. What patient will be asked to do
   a. Coughing and deep breathing
   b. Arm exercises
   c. Ambulation
7. Where patient will be taken after surgery
   a. To recovery — how long
   b. To ICU—for how long
8. Where family can wait during surgery

## ■ POSTOPERATIVE CARE

The care of the patient after thoracic surgery centers on promoting ventilation and reexpansion of the lung by maintaining a clear airway, maintaining the closed drainage system, promoting arm exercises to maintain full use of the patient's arm on the operative side, promoting nutrition, and monitoring the incision for bleeding and subcutaneous emphysema.

In most hospitals the patient is taken from the recovery room to the ICU. The immediate postoperative nursing care is outlined here.

### Oxygen Therapy

Oxygen is attached to the endotracheal tube in the immediate postoperative period. After extubation, humidified oxygen is given by cannula, usually at 6 L/min. An oxygen mask is not used because of the need to have the patient cough and raise secretions frequently.

### Hemodynamic Monitoring

The patient is usually attached to a cardiac monitor. A Swan-Ganz catheter and central venous pressure line are used for hemodynamic monitoring.

### Position of Patient in Bed

The patient is kept flat in bed or with head elevated slightly (20 degrees) until blood pressure is stabilized to preoperative levels. Once blood pressure is stabilized, the patient can usually breathe best in semi-Fowler's position with a pillow under the head and neck but not under the shoulder and back because of the subscapular incision.

### Monitoring Vital Signs

Vital signs are taken every 15 minutes until the patient is well recovered from anesthesia, every hour until condition has stabilized, and then every 2 to 4 hours. It is not unusual for blood pressure to fluctuate during the first 24 to 36 hours, and close monitoring of the patient is essential. A persistently low blood pressure is reported to the surgeon.

### Initiating Coughing and Deep Breathing Exercises

The patient should be assisted to cough as soon as conscious and extubated. If the blood pressure is stable, the patient is assisted to a sitting position, and the incision is supported anteriorly and posteriorly by the nurse's hands. Firm, even pressure over the incision with the open palm of the hands is a most effective method. The nurse's head should be behind the patient when the patient is coughing (Figure 32-12). The patient is encouraged to breathe deeply, exhale, and then cough. Sips of fluids, especially warm ones such as tea or coffee, often facilitate coughing. Mist therapy may be used to loosen secretions.

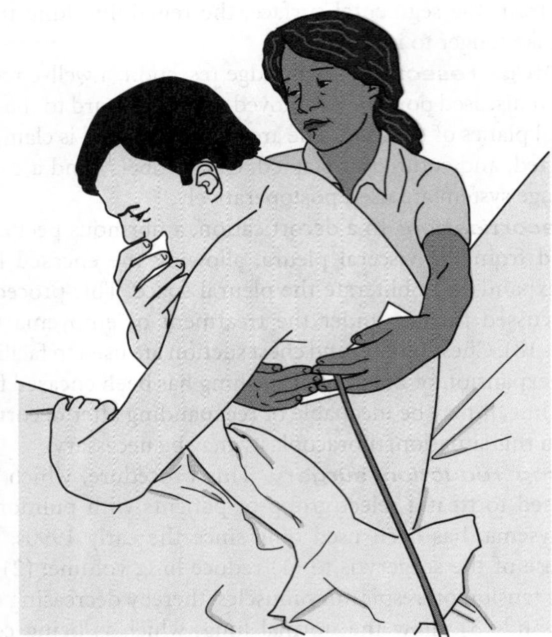

**fig. 32-12** Nurse helps patient cough by splinting incision with firm support from hands. This lessens muscle pull and pain as patient coughs. Note that nurse keeps her head behind patient while he coughs, and patient uses tissue to cover mouth.

Deep breathing and coughing keep the airway patent, prevent atelectasis, and facilitate reexpansion of the lung. The patient should be assisted to cough every hour for the first 24 hours, and then every 2 to 4 hours around the clock. The patient should cough until the chest sounds clear. Otherwise, secretions will accumulate in the tracheobronchial tree. The patient is urged to use incentive spirometry 10 times every hour to help inflate the lungs and mobilize secretions. The patient can cough most effectively 20 to 30 minutes after receiving pain medication, and this should be capitalized on by the nursing staff.

When a patient is unable to cough effectively, tracheobronchial suctioning is performed (see Chapter 31). If suctioning fails to clear the airway, fiberoptic bronchoscopy may be necessary, because it is crucial that the airway is kept clear. In these situations, bronchoscopy is performed at the bedside with a fiberoptic bronchoscope (see Chapter 30).

### Promoting Abdominal Breathing

Abdominal breathing exercises are a valuable adjunct to the care of the patient with chest surgery, because abdominal breathing improves ventilation without increasing pain and assists in coughing more effectively (Figure 32-13). The exercises should be taught preoperatively so that the patient has time to practice them before surgery.

### Promoting Comfort by Pain Relief

Morphine is usually ordered for pain. Medication for pain should be given as needed and may be required as often as

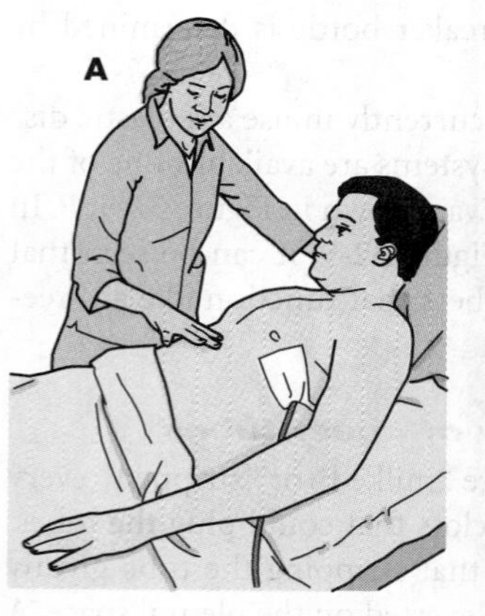


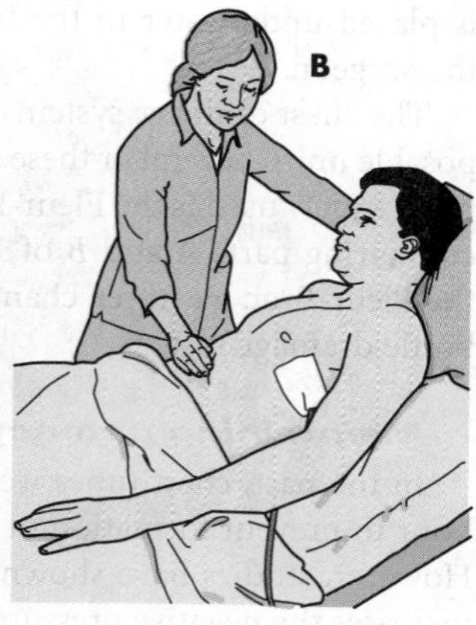


**fig. 32-13** **A,** Physical therapist assists patient in learning augmented abdominal breathing. Patient is instructed to inhale through nose, using abdominal muscles, and to concentrate on moving lower ribs under therapist's hands. This exercise improves ventilation of bases of lungs. **B,** Physical therapist places hand on upper abdomen in assisting patient to exhale fully.

every 3 to 4 hours during the first 48 to 72 hours. The patient is extremely uncomfortable and will be reluctant to cough or turn unless there is relief from pain. The tubes in the chest cause pain, and the patient may attempt rapid, shallow breathing to splint the lower chest and avoid motion of the catheters. This impairs ventilation, makes coughing ineffective, and causes secretions to be retained. It is a nursing responsibility to make the patient comfortable, because this facilitates deep breathing and coughing. Patient-controlled analgesia pumps and epidural catheters are widely used for pain medication management. Pain medication should never be withheld without first consulting with the surgeon, because undermedication is counterproductive. If, despite all efforts, the patient's discomfort is interfering with adequate chest excursion, an intercostal nerve block may be performed.

### Promoting Arm Exercises

Passive arm exercises are usually started the evening of surgery. The purpose of putting the patient's arm through range of motion (ROM) is to prevent restriction of function. Most patients are reluctant to move the arm on the operative side, but with proper pain control, preoperative instruction, and postoperative follow-through, they do so readily. It is important for both the patient and the nurse to understand that the longer the arm is unexercised, the stiffer it will become. The patient should put both arms through active ROM two or three times a day within a few days. The recommended exercises are similar to those used after mastectomy (see Chapter 48). The exercises are best performed when the patient is upright or lying on the abdomen. Exercises such as elevating the scapula and clavicle, "hunching the shoulders," bringing the scapulae as close together as possible, and hyperextending the arm can be performed only in these positions. Because lying on the abdomen may not be possible at first, these exercises are performed with the patient sitting on the edge of the bed or standing.

### Promoting Nutrition

The patient is encouraged to take fluids postoperatively and to progress to a general diet as soon as it is tolerated. Fluids help liquefy secretions and make them easier to expectorate. A diet adequate in protein and vitamins (especially vitamin C) facilitates wound healing.

### Monitoring the Incision for Bleeding or Subcutaneous Emphysema

The dressing is checked periodically for bleeding. *Blood on the dressing is unusual and should be reported to the surgeon at once.* The time and amount of blood are recorded in the patient's record. The surgeon may reinforce the dressing, and in the rare instance when bleeding persists, the patient may be taken back to surgery. The chest wall will be reopened and the source of bleeding located and ligated.

Subcutaneous emphysema is not unusual after chest surgery. In subcutaneous emphysema, air leaks from the pleural space through the thoracotomy incision or around the chest tubes into the soft tissues. The presence of air under the skin is readily detected and has been described as feeling like "tissue paper" or "Rice Krispies" under the skin. Subcutaneous emphysema is most notable in the neck and chest, and if considerable air is leaking, the patient's face and neck will become swollen. Small amounts of air will reabsorb over time and cause no problem. However, if subcutaneous emphysema is worsening, the chest tube may be changed by the surgeon and one with a larger diameter inserted, because air is leaking into the tissues faster than it is being removed by the tube. Additional suction may also be applied to the chest tube(s) in an attempt to remove air more rapidly. Rarely, a patient will need to return to surgery for closure of air leaks.

The patient with a pneumonectomy should have only a small amount of (if any) subcutaneous emphysema. *Progressive subcutaneous emphysema after pneumonectomy is very serious and should be reported to the surgeon immediately because it could indicate a major leak in the bronchial stump.* This is a rare occurrence, requiring immediate return to surgery for reclosure of the bronchial stump.

### Maintaining Chest Tube(s) and Drainage

All patients who have resectional surgery of the lung, except those having a pneumonectomy, will require drainage of the pleural space by one or two chest tubes connected to closed drainage. Usually two tubes are used, although some surgeons may prefer only one tube. At the completion of the surgical resection, each tube is inserted into the pleural space through a stab wound in the chest wall. The tubes are sutured in place. When two tubes are used, one catheter is inserted in the anterior chest wall above the resected area. This *anterior or upper tube* removes air from the pleural space. The second tube is inserted in the posterior chest, and this *posterior or lower tube* is for the drainage of serosanguineous fluid that accumulates as a result of the surgery. The lower tube may be of a larger diameter than the upper tube to prevent it from becoming plugged with clots. Figure 32-14 shows the placement of tubes within the pleural space. When only one chest tube is used, it is usually placed anteriorly above the resected area of the

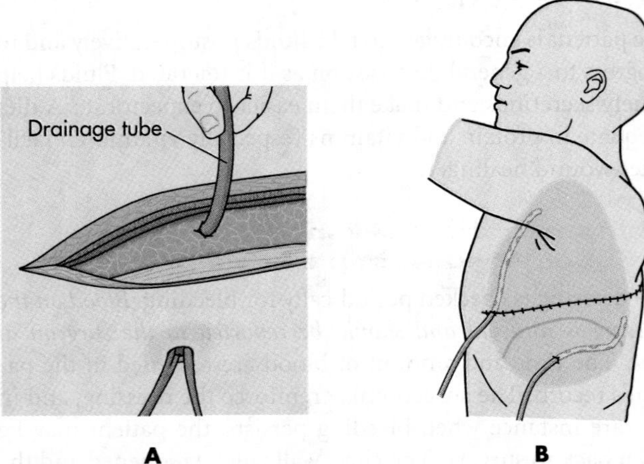


**fig. 32-14** **A**, Drainage tube being inserted into pleural space. **B**, Note that upper and lower tubes are placed well into pleural space.

lung. To initiate chest tube drainage, the chest tubes are connected to a closed-chest drainage system.

#### *Three-bottle water-sealed drainage system*

Although the three-bottle drainage system is used less often today, understanding how it works makes it easier to understand newer plastic disposable drainage systems. In Figure 32-9, *A*, the bottle to the right is connected to the patient's chest tube to drain air and blood from the pleural space. The middle bottle is water-sealed; that is, the tip of the tube is underwater, allowing fluid and air to drain from the pleural space and preventing air from entering the pleural space. The third bottle is a suction control bottle, sometimes called a breaker bottle. The stopper in the control bottle has three openings. One is connected to the water-seal bottle, one is connected to the suction source, and the third contains a glass rod that is underwater and open to the outside. The amount of suction produced is determined by the distance between the surface of the water and the tip of this tube. When the suction source is turned on, the level of water in the open tube will sink in proportion to the amount of negative pressure in the system. Thus if there is 15 cm of water between the surface of the water and the tip of the tube, the amount of negative pressure in the system will be 15 cm of water pressure. Because the water will be at the bottom of the tube when this amount of pressure is reached, any increase in negative pressure will cause air to be drawn in from the outside, *breaking* the suction at this level. Therefore it can be expected that the water in the breaker bottle will bubble almost continuously. If it fails to bubble, the desired level of suction is not being attained, and the tubing should be checked for air leaks. If there are no leaks, the surgeon should be notified at once, because the air leak in the pleural surface may be so great that the amount of negative pressure is not sufficient to overcome it. In this instance, water may be added to the breaker bottle to increase the distance between the surface of the water and the tip of the tube, thereby increasing the amount of negative pressure exerted on the pleural space. The distance the tube is placed underwater in the breaker bottle is determined by the surgeon.

The chest drainage systems currently in use are plastic disposable units. Several of these systems are available; one of the most widely used is the Pleur-Evac shown in Figure 32-9, *B*. In comparing parts *A* and *B* of Figure 32-9, it can be seen that the Pleur-Evac has three chambers that function like a three-bottle drainage system.

#### *Maintaining patency of chest tubes*

In the past, chest tubes were "milked" or "stripped" every hour to prevent formation of clots that could plug the tubes. However, studies have shown that stripping the tube greatly increases the negative pressure exerted on the pleural space. A study by two clinical nurse specialists revealed the following: (1) the pressure generated by stripping was considerably higher than the suction pressures of −15 to −20 cm of water typically applied to chest drainage systems; (2) the amount of pressure was directly related to the length of the tubing stripped; and (3) even stripping only a few centimeters produced pressures near −100 cm of water, and stripping the entire tube produced pressures exceeding −400 cm of water.

Undesirable side effects of increased levels of negative pressure include (1) lung entrapment in the chest tube eyelets and focal tissue infarction and (2) persistent pneumothorax. The persistent pneumothorax occurs when the pleural surface of lung, which normally has air leaks at the close of the procedure, does not seal off. Fibrin will seal the air leaks; however, the presence of an increased amount of negative pressure may prevent the air leaks from sealing and may even increase the size of the air leaks. This is why some thoracic surgeons do not attach suction to the closed drainage system for the first 24 hours or more after surgery. They believe that this amount of time is sufficient in most instances to allow the pleural surface to seal off.

Because the anterior (upper) tube usually evacuates mainly air, there is less reason to believe that this tube will clot off. Posterior tubes, which are inserted lower in the chest, drain more fluid and blood and are more likely to clot off. However, gentle squeezing of the tube is usually sufficient to move the bloody drainage along in the tubing. The nursing measures necessary in maintaining chest tubes and closed drainage are summarized in Box 32-13.

### Removal of Chest Tubes

Chest tubes are removed when there is no tidaling of fluid in the water-sealed chamber and when x-ray films confirm the full reexpansion of the lung. Most patients have their chest tube(s) removed within 48 to 72 hours postoperatively. If there is a persistent air space in the apex of the lung, the upper tube may be left in longer. Surgeons are concerned about leaving tubes in for long periods of time because of the risk of an ascending tube track infection. The patient should receive medication for pain 30 minutes before removal of the tube. Physicians vary in the exact procedure used to remove the tube, but generally a sterile suture set, 4 × 4–inch gauze squares, and 2-inch tape are required. The suture holding the tube in place is cut, the patient is asked to take a deep breath and hold it, and the tube is removed. If a purse-

**box 32-13** *Maintaining Chest Tubes and Closed Chest Drainage*

1. Set up the disposable drainage system following the directions attached to the unit.
2. Connect the tube from the collection chamber to the patient's chest tube. Fasten tubing to bed so that there are no dependent loops between the bed and the drainage system. Dependent loops allow fluid to collect in the tubing, preventing removal of air and fluid from the pleural space (see the Research Box below).
3. Connect the other tubing to the suction source. Follow the directions to set the amount of suction. The desired amount of suction is determined by the surgeon. Suction can be set at −10 to −40 cm $H_2O$. In some drainage systems, water must be added to the suction chamber to the appropriate level. Tape all connections.
4. Turn on the suction source and increase it until the water begins to bubble, indicating that the amount of suction is at the desired level.
5. When the suction level is changed from a higher level to a lower level, the pressure being exerted on the patient's pleural space may remain at the higher level unless the amount of pressure in the closed system is relieved. All systems have some way to reduce the negative pressure in the system (such as a negativity relief valve) that reduces the negative pressure to the desired level.
6. Record the amount of drainage, date, time, and initials on the front of the unit. If there is 200 ml of drainage in 1 hour or bright red drainage, it may mean active bleeding, and the surgeon should be called immediately.
7. Samples of drainage fluid may be withdrawn from self-sealing sample port in the connector tubing. Use an 18-gauge or larger needle attached to a syringe to withdraw samples.
8. To dispose of the chest drainage system, tie off the drainage tubes and wrap the unit tightly in a plastic bag to prevent any leakage. Dispose of according to hospital policy for contaminated materials.

**PRECAUTIONS TO BE OBSERVED WITH ANY TYPE OF CLOSED DRAINAGE SYSTEM**

1. Monitor drainage system for tidaling (fluctuation) in the water-seal chamber. The water level should rise on inspiration and fall on expiration.
2. If the fluid is not tidaling (fluctuating) in the water-seal chamber:
   a. Be sure the patient is not lying on the tubes.
   b. Check connections to be sure the chest tube system is intact.
   c. Ask patient to cough or change position to see if tidaling is restored.
   d. Tidaling will stop when the lung is reexpanded.
3. Never lift the closed drainage system above the level of the patient's chest, because this allows fluid to be pulled into the pleural space.
4. Never clamp chest tubes without a written order from the surgeon, because air (positive pressure) will be trapped in the pleural space, further collapsing the lung.
5. A liter bottle of sterile water is kept at the bedside at all times. If the patient's chest drainage system cracks or breaks:
   a. Insert patient's chest tube into the bottle of sterile water.
   b. Remove the cracked or broken system.
   c. Obtain a new system and connect it to patient chest tube as soon as possible.
6. If the patient's tube is accidentally pulled out of the chest (a rare occurrence):
   a. Apply gloves in accordance with body substance isolation policy.
   b. Pinch skin opening together with fingers.
   c. Apply occlusive dressing.
   d. Cover dressing with overlapping pieces of 2-inch tape. Call surgeon immediately.

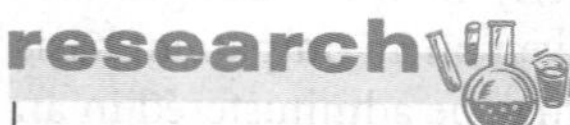

Reference: Gordon PA et al: Positioning of chest tubes: effects on pressure and drainage, *Am J Crit Care* 6(1):33, 1997.

In this controlled laboratory study the position of chest drainage tubes was studied to determine whether keeping the drainage tube free of dependent loops has a beneficial effect on patient outcome. The differences in drainage with tubing in straight, coiled, or dependent-loop (with and without periodic lifting) positions and pressures in each of the four tubing positions were determined. Pressure and drainage were measured for 1 hour with drainage tube in straight, coiled, and dependent-loop positions. When the tube was in the dependent-loop position, it was lifted and drained every 15 minutes. There was no difference in pressure or drainage with the tube in straight or coiled positions. However, with the dependent-loop position, pressure at the "lung" side increased from about −18 cm $H_2O$ to as high as +8 cm $H_2O$. Drainage dropped to 0 in the dependent-loop position until the drainage tube was lifted and drained. The authors concluded that this study supported recommendations to maintain chest tubes in straight or coiled positions. Although frequently lifting and draining a dependent loop will provide the same amount of total drainage as with the tube in straight or coiled position, the pressure within the tube may be altered sufficiently to exceed recommended levels.

string suture was used, it is retied, and a dry sterile dressing is placed over the site. Some physicians cover the site with petroleum gauze or a Telfa dressing instead of gauze squares to ensure an airtight dressing. The dressing is covered securely by three overlapping strips of 2-inch tape.

### Care After Pneumonectomy

The postoperative care discussed previously applies to all patients with resectional surgery except those having a pneumonectomy. The special care required after pneumonectomy is outlined in the Guidelines for Care Box.

**guidelines for care**

**The Person After Pneumonectomy**

1. Chest tubes are not necessary because there is no lung left to reexpand on the operative side.
2. Patient may lie on back or operated side only. Patient is not allowed to lie with operative side uppermost because of fear that the bronchial stump may leak, allowing fluid to drain into the unoperated side and drown the patient.
3. Pressure in the operative side will be checked in the operating room after the chest is closed. A pneumothorax apparatus (which can instill or remove air) will be used to check the pressure in the operative space, and air will be removed or instilled as necessary to bring the pressure to slightly negative (slightly less than 760 mm Hg).
4. The surgeon will palpate the patient's trachea at least daily to determine if it is in midline. Deviation of the trachea toward either the operated or unoperated side is a sign of mediastinal shift. If pressure builds up in the operated side, the trachea will deviate toward the unoperated side. The treatment is to remove air (positive pressure) with a pneumothorax apparatus. Mediastinal shift toward the "good" lung can seriously compromise ventilation and needs to be treated promptly. Deviation of the trachea toward the operated side indicates that more pressure (air) needs to be instilled into the empty space.
5. The patient with a mediastinal shift resembles the patient in congestive heart failure. Neck veins are distended, the trachea is displaced to one side, pulse and respirations are increased, and dyspnea is present.
6. Serous drainage will collect in the operated space and over time will congeal to the consistency of axle grease. This is often sufficient to keep the mediastinum from shifting toward the operative side. Persistent mediastinal shift toward the operative side may have to be treated with thoracoplasty (removal of ribs) to reduce the size of the remaining space and assist in maintaining the mediastinum in midline. Thoracoplasty is described below.
7. The remaining lung needs 2 to 4 days to adjust to the increase in blood flow. For this reason the amount of fluids and blood given intravenously is monitored closely to prevent fluid overload. Central venous pressure monitoring is common. Crackles are often heard over the base of the remaining lung, and vascular markings will be more prominent on x-ray films. Any increase in crackles, in pulse or blood pressure, and in dyspnea may indicate circulatory overload and should be reported immediately. Treatment may include diuretics or digitalization along with discontinuing IV fluids.
8. Deep breathing, coughing, and arm exercises are the same as described earlier (p. 959).
9. Patients who have had a lung removed may have a lowered vital capacity, and exercise and activity should be limited to that which can be performed without dyspnea. Because the body must be given time to adjust to having only one lung, the patient's return to work may be delayed.
10. If the diagnosis is cancer, radiation therapy is usually given, and it may be started before the patient leaves the hospital. (See Chapter 11 for further discussion of nursing care for patients receiving radiation therapy.)
11. The patient who has had a pneumonectomy for cancer is urged to call the physician promptly if hoarseness, dyspnea, pain on swallowing, or localized chest pain develops because these symptoms may be signs of complications.

### Thoracoplasty

A thoracoplasty is an extrapleural procedure involving the removal of ribs to reduce the size of the chest cavity. Before the widespread use of resectional surgery, thoracoplasty was the basic surgical treatment for TB. Today, thoracoplasty is used uncommonly and then only to prevent or treat the complications of resectional surgery. When it is thought that a patient's lung may not be able to expand sufficiently after a resection to fill the space, a thoracoplasty is performed 2 to 3 weeks before the resection. It also may be performed before pneumonectomy, because this will reduce the chance of mediastinal shift after surgery. This type of thoracoplasty is often called a *preresection or tailoring thoracoplasty;* that is, the chest wall is tailored to reduce its size.

If the remaining portions of the lung fail to reexpand sufficiently postoperatively or if another complication such as empyema occurs, a thoracoplasty is performed. In general, it is used when there is a space in the chest that cannot be obliterated by other means. See the accompanying Clinical Pathway.

## GERONTOLOGICAL CONSIDERATIONS

Many elderly persons with lung cancer will not be candidates for thoracic surgery, and some of them will receive radiation as palliative therapy. For those who have surgery, adjunct therapy with radiation or antineoplastic drugs or both may be necessary. The side effects of both radiation and chemotherapy may be more severe in the elderly than in younger persons. Radiation therapy is usually given on an outpatient basis at the hospital, and chemotherapy may be administered in an outpatient clinic or at home. Special emphasis for the elderly is on fluid, dietary, exercise, and sleep requirements, all of which will be affected by the therapy the patient receives.

## SPECIAL ENVIRONMENTS FOR CARE

### Critical Care Management

The care discussed under postoperative care ideally takes place in an intensive care unit. The patient may remain in the ICU until the chest tubes are removed. Chest tubes may have to remain longer than the usual 72 hours in the elderly, because the lung tissue is less distensible than it is in younger persons and it will take longer for the remaining lung to reexpand.

### Home Care Management

Patients with cancer of the lung treated with thoracic surgery will be discharged from the hospital less than a week after surgery. Most will require the presence of a family member or a home health aid to assist them until they regain strength and can care for themselves. Those who must leave their home to receive chemotherapy or radiation therapy will

**clinical pathway** *Major Chest Procedures—4-Day Recovery*

| TIME FRAME LOCATION | 1 TCI → OR → CVICU → RNF | 2 POD #1 | 3 POD #2 | 4 POD #3 | DISCHARGE POD #4 |
|---|---|---|---|---|---|
| **DATE/UNIT** | DATE UNIT | DATE UNIT | DATE UNIT | DATE UNIT | DATE UNIT |
| **Patient Satisfaction** | What can we do to enhance your stay with us? | What can we do to enhance your stay with us? | What can we do to enhance your stay with us? | What can we do to enhance your stay with us? | What can we do to enhance your stay with us? |
| **Discharge Planning** | Patient verbalizes expected LOS and postop activity.<br>PERS initiated.<br>Patient's primary support person identified. | Verbalizes understanding of progress.<br>Patient's needs identified and notify as needed for D/C. | Verbalizes understanding of progress.<br>Patient's needs identified and notify as needed for D/C. | Verify all medications, supplies, services are arranged for discharge. | Discharge instructions given to patient. |
| **Patient Education** | Instruct family to go to surgical waiting room.<br>Orient patient during emergence from anesthesia. | Reinforce IS, C & DB exercises, pain management, and ambulation.<br>Provide patient/family with info R/T discharge needs. | Provide patient/family with information R/T discharge needs/procedures and progress. | Provide patient/family with information R/T discharge needs/procedures and progress. | Discharge instructions R/T medications, activity, diet, treatments, and incisional care. |
| **Tests/ Procedures/ Consults** | CXR, CBC, KP6; ABGs, BPH/ Ventolin q6°; Respiratory therapy; pain management; CHIRP | CXR, oximetry<br>Radiation oncology prn<br>Hemo/oncology prn<br>Home health care prn | CXR, oximetry<br>Respiratory therapy | Oximetry<br>Pulmonary rehab prn | |
| **Allied Health Interventions** | | Respiratory Tx per respiratory consult algorithm. | Respiratory Tx per respiratory consult algorithm. | | |
| **Nursing/ Medical Interventions** | Monitor rhythm; VS routine; I & O; wt qd; $O_2$ N/C; Chest tubes to suction; Foley; wean from vent. | Telemetry; I & O; wt qd; VS routine; IS 10×/hr w.a.; C & DB; D/C 1 CT; Epidural pain control, D/C Foley. | D/C telemetry; D/C I & O; wt qd; VS routine; IS 10×/hr; C & DB; epidural pain control (to be D/C when last CT out); D/C CT; wean $O_2$ to room air; Remove incisional dressings and begin wound care. | Wt qd; VS routine; IS 10×/hr w.a.; pain control with P.O. | VS routine; IS 10×/hr w.a. |
| **Mobility** | BR; turn q2°, HOB ↑ 30°; Up in chair after extub. | OOB with assistance and chair 1 qs. | Chair qs and ambulate hall TID. | UAL | UAL |
| **Nutrition** | NPO; ice chips; clear liquids D5 1/2NS + 20 KCl | Clear liquids → full liquid diet; IV to HL if tolerating liquids. | Advance diet as tolerated. | Preop diet | Preop diet |
| **Outcomes Criteria** | Admission assessment completed.<br>Anesthesia consult documented.<br>Patient assessment completed and WNL.<br>Patient premedicated.<br>Patient/family satisfaction addressed. | Patient with adequate oxygenation per pulse oximetry; hemodynamically stable; alert and oriented ×3.<br>Adequate pain control.<br>Patient/family satisfaction addressed. | Tolerate diet.<br>Has BM normal for patient.<br>Comfort level maintained.<br>Ambulate W/O SOB.<br>Patient/family satisfaction addressed. | Tolerate diet.<br>Has BM normal for patient.<br>Comfort level maintained.<br>Ambulate W/O SOB.<br>Breath sounds and secretions clear.<br>Patient/family satisfaction addressed. | Breath sounds and secretions clear.<br>Ambulates independently W/O SOB.<br>Infection free.<br>Patient/family satisfaction addressed. |

4/1/97 (1:\cct\thoracic\75a-fdr) Thoracic FDR—4 Day Recovery, Courtesy The Cleveland Clinic Foundation, 1997. This is a general guideline to *assist* in the management of patients. This guideline is not designated to replace clinical judgment or individual patient needs.

*CXR,* Chest x-ray; *HOB,* head of bed; *IS,* incentive spirometry; *qs,* quantity sufficient; *CHIRP,* rehab program; *OOB,* out of bed; *D/C,* discharge; *CT,* chest tube; *C & DB,* cough and deep breathe; *R/T,* routine; *UAL,* up ad lib; *W/O,* without, *SOB,* short of breath; *W.A.,* when awake; *HL,* heparin lock.

need someone to drive them to treatments and to care for them after the therapy. Both chemotherapy and radiation therapy can be extremely debilitating, and the patient is often very tired and wants to go to bed as soon as possible after arriving home. Many will be nauseated and will require antiemetics so that they will not become dehydrated.

Despite improvements in the treatment of lung cancer, the 5-year survival rate is only 14%, and only 41% survive for 1 year. For this reason, hospice services should be explained to the patient and family, assuming that hospice care is available in their community. If the patient and family opt to use this service, a hospice nurse will be responsible for managing the care of the patient, and the emphasis will be on keeping the patient as comfortable as possible. Some patients will be able to remain at home with hospice services, others will need to go to the hospital for management of intercurrent problems, and some persons will die in the hospital. Many others will be able to die comfortably at home with the patient and family supported by the hospice staff.

## COMPLICATIONS

In the immediate postoperative period (24 to 48 hours), hypotension, cardiac dysrhythmia, pulmonary edema, and subcutaneous emphysema may occur. Long-term complications include a residual air space, which results from failure of the remaining portions of the lung to reexpand and fill the space. If this space is small, no treatment is indicated. Two major complications of chest surgery tend to occur later in the postoperative period and require treatment: empyema and bronchopleural fistula. The patient may have empyema alone or empyema and a bronchopleural fistula. The signs and symptoms and treatment of these two complications are outlined in Table 32-18.

## ADULT RESPIRATORY DISTRESS SYNDROME

### Etiology

Adult respiratory distress syndrome (ARDS) is a syndrome of acute hypoxemic respiratory failure without hypercapnia. The syndrome was first described in 1967 by Dr. T.J. Petty, who named it *acute respiratory distress syndrome.* In the literature it can be found under both names.

### Epidemiology

Adult respiratory distress syndrome affects 200,000 to 250,000 critical care patients yearly. It is often fatal and is characterized by severe dyspnea, hypoxemia, and diffuse bilateral pulmonary infiltrations after lung injury in previously healthy persons.[45] Several conditions precipitate ARDS (Box 32-14).

### Pathophysiology

The pathophysiological alterations that result in ARDS are typically initiated by a major trauma to the body, often a physical insult to a body system other than the pulmonary system (Figure 32-15). The following physiological alterations result in the clinical syndrome identified as ARDS:

1. As a consequence of the precipitating insult, the complement cascade is activated, which in turn increases capillary wall permeability.

**box 32-14** *Clinical Conditions Associated with ARDS*

1. Shock
   a. Septic
   b. Hemorrhagic
   c. Cardiogenic
   d. Anaphylactic
2. Trauma
   a. Pulmonary contusion
   b. Nonpulmonary, multisystem
   c. Multiple fractures
3. Infection
   a. Pneumonia
4. Fat emboli
5. Aspiration of acid gastric contents
6. Inhaled toxic agents
   a. Smoke
   b. Phosgene
   c. Oxides of nitrogen
7. Severe pancreatitis
8. Oxygen toxicity
9. Alcohol and drug abuse
10. Radiation pneumonitis
11. Hypertransfusion

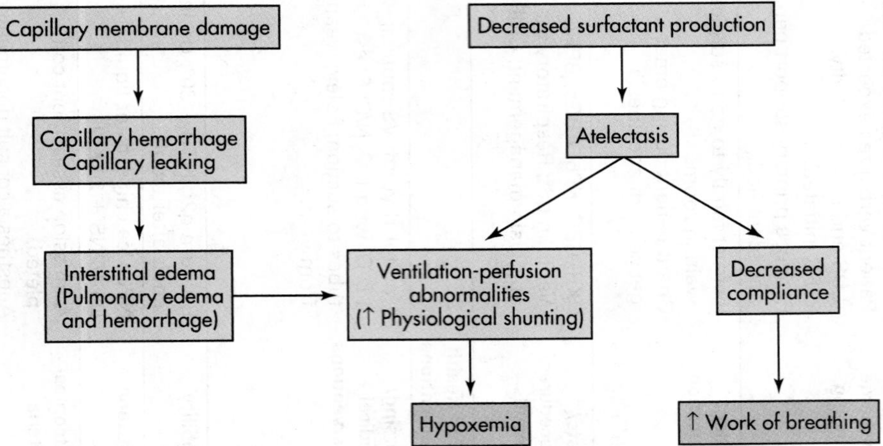


**fig. 32-15** Pathophysiological events in adult respiratory distress syndrome.

2. Fluid, granular leukocytes, red blood cells (RBCs), macrophages, cell debris, and protein leak into the interstitial spaces between the capillaries and alveoli and ultimately into the alveolar spaces.
3. Because of the fluid and debris in the interstitium and alveoli, the surface area for oxygen and carbon dioxide exchange is decreased, resulting in low ventilation/perfusion (V/Q) ratios and hypoxemia.
4. Compensatory hyperventilation of functional alveoli occurs, resulting in hypocapnia and respiratory alkalosis.
5. Cells that normally line the alveoli are destroyed and replaced by cells that do not produce surfactant, thus increasing alveolar surface tension and resulting in atelectasis and increased alveolar opening pressures.

The normal function, pathophysiology, and clinical picture of a person with ARDS are presented in Table 32-19.

Adult respiratory distress syndrome usually occurs in a person who has had a recent physical trauma, although it can appear in persons who appeared to be healthy immediately before onset (e.g., someone with sudden onset of an acute infection). There is usually a latent period of 18 to 24 hours from the time of lung injury to the development of symptoms. The syndrome runs a variable course from a few days to several weeks duration. Patients who appear to be recovering from ARDS may suddenly relapse into acute pulmonary disease from secondary insult such as pneumothorax or overwhelming infection. Box 32-15 lists clinical manifestations of ARDS.

## Collaborative Care Management

### Diagnostic tests

1. Tests of pulmonary function
   a. V/Q— oxygen gradient increased to 300 to 500 mm Hg indicates number of alveolar-capillary units with low V/Q
   b. Shunt factor—may be greater than 15% to 20%; measures degree of intrapulmonary shunting; normal: <6%
   c. Compliance —below normal
   d. Pulmonary capillary wedge pressure (PCWP)—low to normal pressure, <15 mm Hg
2. Arterial blood gases
   a. $PaO_2$ <55 mm Hg; $PaCO_2$ normal to low but may increase
   b. pH elevated at first in response to hyperventilation; as ARDS worsens, pH decreases
3. Lactic acid levels—possibly increased when there is tissue hypoxia; normal: 0.5 to 2.2 mEq/L (venous blood)
4. Chest x-ray films
   a. Early—thickened or blurred margins of bronchi or vessels
   b. Later—diffuse, blurred appearance (heavy wet lungs)

### Medications

There is no specific drug therapy for ARDS. Medications are given as supportive therapy. For example, morphine

**box 32-15 clinical manifestations**

**ARDS**

Signs and symptoms of ARDS include the following:
1. Acute respiratory distress: tachypnea, dyspnea, accessory muscle breathing, and central cyanosis
2. Dry cough and fever that develop over a few hours or days
3. Fine crackles throughout both lung fields
4. Altered sensorium ranging from confusion and agitation to coma

Radiological and laboratory findings include the following:
1. Chest x-ray films: reveal diffuse, bilateral, and usually symmetrical interstitial and alveolar infiltrations
2. ABGs
   Hypoxemia, $PaO_2$ less than 50 mm Hg
   Hypocapnia (early)
   Hypercapnia (late)
   Respiratory alkalosis
   End stage: hypercapnia and respiratory acidosis, death

**table 32-19 Normal Function, Pathophysiology, and Clinical Manifestations of a Person with ARDS**

| Normal Function | Pathophysiology | Clinical Manifestations |
|---|---|---|
| **ALVEOLOCAPILLARY MEMBRANE** | | |
| Oxygen and carbon dioxide exchange between alveolar air and pulmonary capillaries | Increased capillary wall permeability; blood plasma contents infiltrate interstitial and alveolar spaces, resulting in hypoxemia, alveolar hyperventilation, and respiratory alkalosis. | $PaO_2\downarrow$<br>$PaCO_2\downarrow$<br>pH ↑<br>Fine crackles auscultated throughout lungs |
| **LUNG PARENCHYMA** | | |
| Lung tissue that makes up the alveoli | Destruction of normal lung tissue, in particular, alveolar septal walls, normal cells replaced by nonsurfactant producing cells, and presence of edema and debris results in decreased lung compliance (stiff lung). Fibrosis may also develop. | Decreased functional residual capacity and need to use high pressures to ventilate patient<br>Dyspnea at rest |

may be given to a patient on a ventilator who is restless and tachypneic.

### Treatments

1. Oxygen:
   a. Initially may need to administer highest concentration of oxygen available (100%—using nonrebreathing face mask). However, oxygen delivered at levels greater than 50% is associated with oxygen toxicity that worsens already-existing ARDS pathology. Oxygen concentrations can usually be lowered below 50%, by using positive end-expiratory pressure (PEEP) to open closed alveoli for increased ventilation.
   b. Goal is $PaO_2$ of 50 to 60 mm Hg.
   c. Gradually reduce $FIO_2$ while maintaining adequate arterial oxygen levels.
2. Ventilatory support: if oxygen therapy alone is unsuccessful in providing adequate arterial oxygenation, the patient is placed on a mechanical ventilator. The patient may be intubated, or a mask may be applied for noninvasive ventilation with CPAP or BiPAP (see p. 1019).
   a. When the patient is ventilated, a volume-limited ventilator is most commonly used.
   b. Ventilator is set to provide tidal volume equal to 10 to 12 ml/kg body weight, respiratory rate equal to 10 to 14 respirations per minute, and $FIO_2$ of 50%; PEEP is used.
   c. When spontaneous ventilatory pattern interferes with providing adequate ventilation, the patient is sedated or paralyzed. If the individual has high peak airway pressures, high frequency, or an inverse ratio, ventilation techniques may be necessary. See p. 1017 for information on care of the patient on a ventilator.
3. Fluid volume:
   a. A balloon-tipped pulmonary artery catheter is inserted to measure pulmonary capillary pressure.
   b. Diuretics, fluid volume expanders, and hypotensive medications are administered as indicated to maintain optimal fluid volume.
   c. The underlying cause of the patient's ARDS is treated.

Because of the high mortality rate from ARDS, newer therapies are constantly being evaluated. Two of these are *nitrous oxide* and *prone positioning.* Each is discussed below.

Nitrous oxide is a natural local vasodilator. Because it is inhaled, nitrous oxide bypasses nonventilated fluid-filled alveoli and dilates blood vessels in ventilated areas of the lung. This maximizes perfusion in ventilated areas of the lungs and improves oxygenation. Because most patients with ARDS are ventilator-dependent, nitrous oxide is administered by the ventilator during the inspiratory cycle using a ventilator nebulizer modified to deliver nitrous oxide. The nebulizer is connected to a tank containing 400 to 800 parts per million (ppm) of nitrous oxide. The nebulizer's flow meter is set to deliver nitrous oxide in a dose of 5 to 20 ppm.

Nitrous oxide binds with hemoglobin to form methemoglobin, and the nurse is responsible for monitoring methemoglobin levels daily and reporting levels above the normal range of 1.5% to 2.5% of total hemoglobin to the physician. In addition to monitoring methemoglobin levels, pulmonary artery pressure (PAP) is monitored via a pulmonary catheter and oxygenation is assessed by pulse oximetry and ABGs. The effect of nitrous oxide therapy is determined by stopping nitric oxide (challenging) for 30 minutes daily and checking the effect on PAP and oxygenation. Nitrous oxide is discontinued when ABGs and pulse oximetry indicate that the patient can maintain adequate oxygenation without it. The patient is gradually weaned from nitrous oxide over a 24-hour period.[3a] The use of nitrous oxide to treat ARDS is still considered to be experimental pending the results of several on-going studies.

Because infiltrates are not universally distributed throughout the lungs in patients with ARDS, changes in position may improve oxygenation by improving perfusion in ventilated areas of the lungs. In some medical centers the patient is placed in the prone position. The assistance of four to five well-prepared caregivers is required to turn the patient successfully. Because this practice is so labor intensive, it is only being implemented in intensive care units with the resources to do so. When it is not possible to do prone positioning, the *lateral decubitus position* may be used in patients with hypoxemia who are unresponsive to other medical interventions.[39a]

### Diet

The patient is critically ill and usually unable to take anything by mouth. A feeding tube is used when possible; otherwise intravenous feedings are used.

### Activity

The patient is placed on bedrest.

### Referrals

Referrals to a nutritionist and social worker may be appropriate.

## NURSING MANAGEMENT

## ■ ASSESSMENT

Nursing assessment of the patient with ARDS must be tailored to maximize information obtained without increasing respiratory distress.

### Subjective Data

Background information and history of present illness may need to be obtained from family members, because the patient is usually too ill to give details.

### Objective Data

The process of gathering objective data is the same as that described for respiratory failure (see p. 1015).

## NURSING DIAGNOSES

Nursing diagnoses are determined from an analysis of patient data. Nursing diagnoses for the person with ARDS may include but are not limited to:

| Diagnostic Title | Possible Etiological Factors |
|---|---|
| Breathing pattern, ineffective | Decreased lung compliance |
| Gas exchange, impaired | Ventilation/perfusion abnormality |
| Tissue perfusion, altered (cardiopulmonary) | Fluid mobilization to and from third space (interstitium and alveolar space) |
| Fatigue | Increased respiratory effort, hypoxia |
| Anxiety | Threat of death, physical factors (abnormal ABGs, hypoxia) |
| Nutrition, altered: less than body requirements | Unable to eat, increased effort of breathing requires increase in calories |
| Infection, risk for | Invasive procedures, bypass of defense mechanisms |

## EXPECTED PATIENT OUTCOMES

Expected patient outcomes for the person with ARDS may include but are not limited to:

1. Breathing effectively
   a. Respirations regular and between 16 and 20 per minute
2. Improved ventilation and oxygenation
   a. $PaO_2$ maintained at 50 to 60 mm Hg during acute phase of illness
   b. On resolution of ARDS, $PaO_2$, pH, and $PCO_2$ return to acceptable preillness levels
   c. Sensorium returns to preillness level
   d. During acute phase of illness, is able to tolerate mechanical ventilatory assistance
   e. Inspiratory/expiratory ratio: 5 sec/10 sec
   f. Respiratory rate and tidal volume within normal limits
   g. Does not complain of dyspnea
3. Adequate tissue perfusion
   a. Pulmonary capillary wedge pressure (measure of pulmonary capillary pressure) below 18 mm Hg
   b. Urine output at least 30 ml/hr
   c. Peripheral pulses present and extremities warm to touch
4. Fatigue diminished
   a. Able to participate in own care without complaining of being tired or asking to stop to rest
5. Increased physiological and psychological comfort and decreased anxiety
   a. Tolerates ventilator and artificial airway
   b. Acknowledges and expresses fears
   c. Communicates personal needs effectively with staff and family
   d. Cooperates and assists with care
6. Stable body weight within 5 pounds of preillness weight
7. Is free of infection
   a. Vital signs within normal limits; temperature is not elevated
   b. Cultures of pulmonary secretions and urine negative

## INTERVENTIONS

Patients with ARDS are critically ill and are best cared for in an ICU. Their care centers around the following measures.

### Maintaining Adequate Gas Exchange

#### Oxygen

1. Maintain oxygen therapy as ordered.
2. Monitor for signs of hypoxemia.

#### Ventilatory support

1. Maintain a patent airway.
2. If an artificial airway is present (endotracheal tube or tracheostomy), provide necessary care.
   a. Secure tube to avoid movement either in or out of established position.
   b. Position patient for optimal oxygenation; usually head of bed elevated 45 to 90 degrees.
   c. Auscultate lungs hourly to assess placement of endotracheal tube (may slip into right main-stem bronchus).
3. Suction endotracheal tube as needed.
4. Administer bronchodilators as ordered.
5. Check ventilator settings frequently.

### Maintaining Adequate Tissue Perfusion

The maintenance of adequate tissue perfusion is a nursing responsibility.

1. Monitor pulmonary capillary wedge pressure.
   a. Notify physician if pressure is above or below established range.
   b. If pressure is below established range, administer plasma volume expanders or hypotensive medications as ordered.
   c. If pressure is high, administer diuretics or vasodilators as ordered.
2. Assess urine output, vital signs, and extremities hourly.

### Minimizing Fatigue

Space nursing activities to allow for rest periods when possible.

### Decreasing Patient and Family Anxiety

1. Ensure proper ventilator function to deliver adequate tidal volume and oxygen concentration. If patient appears in respiratory distress although ventilator is functioning properly, assess ABG levels.
2. Identify a method for patient to communicate concerns and express feelings (if unable to verbalize because of intubation, try alternative methods of communication).
3. Provide simple explanations about procedures; orient patient to surroundings, and repeat explanations regularly.
4. Offer explanations of care routines and environment to family. Encourage family to approach, talk to, and touch patient, as they desire.

## nursing care plan *The Person on Mechanical Ventilation with PEEP*

**DATA** Mr. R. is a 28-year-old married man admitted to the surgical intensive care unit after a motor vehicle accident. Injuries sustained include a ruptured spleen and liver laceration resulting in hypovolemic shock. Mr. R. was taken to the operating room, where his injuries were repaired and blood losses replaced. His early postoperative course was unremarkable. On Mr. R.'s third postoperative day, he began to experience some respiratory difficulties with a deterioration in his ABGs. Because of severe hypoxemia, Mr. R. was intubated. His chest x-ray film revealed diffuse interstitial and alveolar infiltrates. He had developed ARDS and eventually required PEEP.

Mr. R.'s wife visited her husband daily and often attempted to communicate with him. She would reassure and calm him when he became anxious and resisted the ventilator. Mrs. R. would ask the nurse many questions about her husband's status.

The nursing history identified the following:

- Mr. and Mrs. R. have been married 5 years; they have no children.
- Mr. R. has full hospitalization and medical coverage through insurance at work.
- Mr. and Mrs. R. come from large families that appear supportive.
- Mr. R. is a nonsmoker.

Collaborative nursing actions include those to assist in improving oxygenation through evaluating $FiO_2$ and levels of PEEP, as well as techniques used to wean Mr. R. from the ventilator.

Nursing actions include the following:

- Supporting oxygenation and ventilation to maintain $PaO_2$ over 60 mm Hg and to maximize functional residual capacity
- Weaning from $FiO_2$ and levels of PEEP gradually while monitoring ABGs
- Monitoring patient for signs of hypoxia

**NURSING DIAGNOSIS** *Impaired gas exchange related to ARDS*

| expected patient outcome | nursing interventions | rationale |
|---|---|---|
| Remains adequately oxygenated, as evidence by:<br>**1.** $PaO_2$ on ABG >75 mm Hg<br>**2.** Adequate color<br>**3.** Adequate peripheral circulation | Monitor ABGs to determine $PaO_2$.<br>Suction only when necessary to prevent loss of PEEP secondary to disconnection from ventilator.<br>Monitor required levels of PEEP and $FiO_2$.<br>Assess peripheral circulation for pulses, color of extremities, and warmth.<br>Monitor mixed venous blood oxygen levels. | ARDS is an acute lung injury that results in increased capillary permeability, which permits proteins and fluids to leak out into alveoli and interstitial spaces, thus preventing normal gas exchange to occur. |

**NURSING DIAGNOSIS** *Decreased cardiac output related to decreased venous return*

| expected patient outcome | nursing interventions | rationale |
|---|---|---|
| Does not experience hemodynamic compromise related to PEEP. | Monitor vital signs qh and as needed.<br>Monitor hemodynamic parameters for signs of decreased cardiac output, hypotension, elevated CVP, and oliguria.<br>Monitor intake and output.<br>Check peripheral circulation every 2 to 4 hr and as needed.<br>Elevate foot of bed 10 to 20 degrees to encourage venous return.<br>Perform passive range of motion exercises q4h to q6h to encourage venous return.<br>Administer adrenergic agents as ordered to improve cardiac output.<br>Notify physician of hemodynamic complications. | PEEP may cause decreased cardiac output by increasing intraalveolar pressures, thereby decreasing venous return to the heart. |

*Continued*

## The Person on Mechanical Ventilation with PEEP—cont'd

**NURSING DIAGNOSIS** *Ineffective breathing pattern related to altered lung/thoracic pressure relationship*

| expected patient outcome | nursing interventions | rationale |
|---|---|---|
| Does not experience pulmonary complications secondary to PEEP:<br>**1.** Pneumothorax<br>**2.** Pneumomediastinum<br>**3.** Subcutaneous emphysema | Monitor respirations qh and as needed.<br>Assess breath sounds for adventitious findings.<br>Administer pulmonary toilet q2h and as needed:<br>**1.** Frequent turning<br>**2.** Chest physiotherapy<br>Monitor for signs of pulmonary complications and respiratory distress:<br>**1.** Asymmetrical chest excursion<br>**2.** Sudden sharp pain<br>**3.** Cyanosis<br>**4.** Anxiety<br>Assess for subcutaneous emphysema.<br>Keep chest tube set up at bedside.<br>Monitor ABGs as needed.<br>Notify physician of respiratory complications. | When walls of alveoli cannot withstand the positive pressure from PEEP, perforation may occur.<br>As a result, air leaks into the pleural space, mediastinum, or its subcutaneous space.<br>The result is a pneumothorax, pneumomediastinum, or subcutaneous emphysema, respectively. |

**NURSING DIAGNOSIS** *Altered nutrition less than body requirements related to intubation*

| expected patient outcome | nursing interventions | rationale |
|---|---|---|
| Receives adequate nutritional intake while intubated. | Administer hyperalimentation or enteral feedings as prescribed.<br>Monitor intake and output.<br>Weigh daily.<br>Administer albumin or volume expanders as prescribed.<br>Monitor serum albumin level. | Nutritional status must be maintained to assist in weaning process; protein and volume expanders will increase serum colloidal osmotic pressure, thus maintaining fluid in the intravascular compartment. |

**NURSING DIAGNOSIS** *Anxiety related to ARDS, intubation, and discomfort from PEEP*

| expected patient outcome | nursing interventions | rationale |
|---|---|---|
| Mr. and Mrs. R. exhibit behavioral signs of decreased stress and anxiety. | Assess for signs of anxiety.<br>Explain ARDS to family, including rationale for mechanical ventilation and PEEP.<br>Allow Mr. and Mrs. R. to express concern and fears.<br>Explain procedures before performing them.<br>Provide comfort measures.<br>Provide for a means of communication between Mr. R. and his wife.<br>Attempt to anticipate their needs.<br>Administer light sedation/antianxiety medications if necessary, as ordered. | Intensive care unit, mechanical ventilation, the inability to communicate, and fear of the unknown all contribute to feelings of stress and anxiety for the patient in the ICU, as well as the patient's significant others. |
| | Attempt to calm and reassure Mr. R. if he begins to "buck" or resist the ventilator.<br>Provide Mr. R. and his wife distraction from the ICU environment:<br>• Soft music, TV<br>• Breaks from the ICU for Mrs. R. | Positive-pressure exhalation is often uncomfortable for the patient, who often responds by resisting ventilator. |

### Maintaining Adequate Nutrition

1. Assess fluid and caloric intake hourly to ensure adequate intake.
2. Maintain tube feedings or hyperalimentation in collaboration with physician and nutritionist.
3. Avoid excessive carbohydrate intake, because metabolism of carbohydrates results in the production of carbon dioxide.
4. Monitor for signs of malnutrition resulting from the increased caloric requirements of labored breathing.

### Preventing Infection

1. Wash hands before any contact with patient.
2. Use sterile procedures and equipment.
3. Suction airway only when necessary to avoid trauma to tissue and introduction of bacteria.

#### *Patient/family education*

The patient and family are kept informed about each aspect of treatment, with special attention to intubation and mechanical ventilation when they are necessary.

**Health promotion/prevention.** Prompt treatment of the underlying cause of ARDS is the major focus of preventive care. Additionally, judicious use of the mechanical ventilator and oxygen therapy is required to avoid inducing ARDS as an untoward complication of these treatment modalities.

## ■ EVALUATION

To evaluate the effectiveness of nursing interventions, compare patient behaviors with those stated in the expected patient outcomes. Successful achievement of patient outcomes for the patient with ARDS is indicated by:

1. Breathing effectively at a rate of 16 to 20 breaths/minute.
2. Maintaining own ventilation without mechanical assistance
   a. $PaO_2$: 75 mm Hg
   b. $PaCO_2$: 45 mm Hg
   c. Inspiratory/expiratory ratio: 5 sec/10 sec
   d. Respiratory rate and tidal volume within normal limits
3. Maintaining adequate tissue perfusion
   a. Pulmonary capillary wedge pressure: 17 mm Hg
   b. Urine output 150 to 200 ml at each voiding
   c. Peripheral pulses present and extremities warm to touch
4. Not experiencing fatigue
5. Appears calm and relaxed
   a. Able to sleep at night
   b. Expresses any concerns freely
   c. Appears calm in interactions with family
6. Body weight below preillness level, but appetite improving and patient gaining weight daily
7. Absence of a nosocomial infection

## GERONTOLOGICAL CONSIDERATIONS

Adult respiratory distress syndrome is more severe in the elderly, and the mortality rate is higher than that in younger persons. Although the mortality rate has decreased in persons under 60 years of age, the mortality rate for those 65 years of age and older is above 60%.

## SPECIAL ENVIRONMENTS FOR CARE

### Critical Care Management

Adult respiratory distress syndrome is the most common illness requiring critical care services. According to Petty,[45] the technology exists to save nearly 50% of all patients with ARDS. The care described previously is provided in an intensive care unit.

## COMPLICATIONS

Many complications are possible, including dysrhythmias, pneumonia, GI bleeding, disseminated intravascular coagulation (DIC), renal failure, and respiratory arrest.

## PULMONARY VASCULAR DISEASES

### Pulmonary Emboli and Pulmonary Infarction

#### *Etiology*

Pulmonary embolism (PE) is caused by the lodging of a clot or clots in a pulmonary arterial vessel. Commonly the clot is from a deep vein thrombosis (DVT). Pulmonary emboli can cause massive occlusion of a major portion of the pulmonary circulation (main pulmonary artery embolus). *Pulmonary infarction* results when an embolus is large enough to interfere with the blood supply to a portion of lung tissue, causing necrosis of lung parenchyma. Embolism without infarction occurs when the embolism is not severe enough to cause permanent lung injury. Pulmonary emboli may be chronic or recurrent.[3]

#### *Epidemiology*

Emboli rarely occur without the presence of certain risk factors, although in some cases it may be difficult to identify the cause (see the Risk Factors Box). Pulmonary emboli result from damage to blood vessel walls (surgery, trauma), blood stasis (varicosities), or hypercoaguability of blood (estrogen therapy). They are the most common cause of acute pulmonary disease in hospitalized patients, cause 100,000 deaths yearly, and are thought to contribute to another 100,000 deaths each year. About 50% of the deaths from pulmonary embolization occur within 2 hours of the event and are often undetected.[33]

#### *Pathophysiology*

Emboli travel from their site of origin through the right side of the heart and lodge in the pulmonary vasculature. The size of the pulmonary artery and the number of emboli determine the severity of symptoms.

**risk factors**

**Pulmonary Emboli**

Thrombophlebitis (DVT)
Immobility
Recent surgery (especially orthopedic or gynecological)
Obesity
Congestive heart failure/myocardial infarction
Recent fracture
Estrogen therapy (oral contraceptives)
Pregnancy

Blood flow is obstructed, causing localized tissue hypoxia and ultimately a decrease in the pulmonary vascular bed. Pulmonary vessels vasoconstrict in response to the hypoxia. The resultant V/Q inequality (ventilation greater than perfusion) causes arterial hypoxemia. The normal function, primary pathophysiology, and clinical picture of a patient with PE are presented in Table 32-20.

If the embolus blocks a larger vessel, the person may complain of sudden, sharp upper abdominal or thoracic pain, become dyspneic, cough violently, and have hemoptysis; shock may develop rapidly. If the area of infarction is small, the symptoms are much milder. The patient may have cough, tachypnea, pleuritic chest pain, slight hemoptysis, elevation of temperature, and an increased leukocyte count. An area of dullness or crackles may be detected when checking breath sounds.

### Collaborative care management

**Diagnostic tests.** The diagnosis of PE is not easy to make. Clinical history, changes in blood chemistries, and plain chest x-rays often are not definitive in establishing the diagnosis. The ultimate *standard for diagnosis of PE is pulmonary angiography in which an abrupt cutoff of a vessel or a filling defect indicates the presence of an embolus.* Computed tomography with contrast media and an MRI angiography have been used to diagnose PE. Another test that is helpful in diagnosing PE and is usually used before angiography is a V/Q lung scan. Normal ventilation and decreased perfusion suggest PE.

**Medications.** A major component of medical treatment of PE is anticoagulant therapy. Anticoagulant therapy may either be prophylactic for persons at risk for DVT or curative for persons with an actual pathological event (Box 32-16). When the patient is not responsive to anticoagulant therapy or when it is contraindicated, surgical intervention may be necessary. Therapies available to treat PE are discussed next.

***Anticoagulant therapy.*** The goal of anticoagulant therapy is to limit the growth of the embolized thrombus and prevent reembolization by inhibiting coagulation and preventing deposition of new clots. Heparin is most effective when given as a bolus followed by continuous IV infusion. It

**box 32-16** *Anticoagulant Therapy for Pulmonary Emboli*

1. Prophylactic: often used for high-risk persons
   a. Low-dose heparin: 5000 U subcutaneously every 12 hours preoperatively and every 8 to 12 hours postoperatively until patient is ambulatory
   b. Oral anticoagulants: warfarin, 5-10 mg daily for 3 days, then maintenance on the basis of prothrombin time
2. Curative treatment
   a. Heparin, approximately 5000 U IV bolus, then continuous infusion approximately 1680 U every hour
   b. Long-term treatment (3-6 months) with warfarin, 5-10 mg daily

**table 32-20** *Normal Function, Primary Pathophysiology, and Clinical Manifestations of Pulmonary Embolism*

| Normal Function | Pathophysiology | Clinical Manifestations |
|---|---|---|
| **PULMONARY VASCULATURE** | | |
| To carry venous blood received from right side of heart to alveolocapillary membrane in lung for oxygen–carbon dioxide exchange | Occlusion of pulmonary vessels because of increased vascular resistance, decreased cardiac output (usually occurs only in massive emboli), decreased lung perfusion | Elevated pulmonary artery pressure<br>Dyspnea<br>Hypotension<br>Tachycardia<br>High V/Q ratio as shown on lung scan<br>Hypocapnia and elevated arterial blood pH |
| **AIRWAYS** | | |
| Carry oxygenated air to alveolocapillary membrane for exchange and deoxygenated air out of lung | Airway constriction from lowered alveolar carbon dioxide levels | Underventilated lung areas as shown on lung scan<br>Hypoxemia<br>Tachypnea<br>Cough |
| **ALVEOLI** | | |
| Lung site where gas exchange takes place (alveolocapillary membrane) | Infarction of alveolar tissues caused by complete obstruction, resulting in extravasation of blood cells into alveoli (NOTE: occurs only in more severe cases) | Hemoptysis<br>Radiological opacity |
| **PLEURA** | | |
| Maintain close approximation of lungs and chest wall<br>Minimize friction during lung expansion and contraction | Transudate from damaged vascular structures (pleural effusion) | Pleural friction rub<br>Chest pain during inhalation/exhalation |

can be given subcutaneously to patients with poor venous access. The patient is monitored by partial thromboplastin time (PTT) every 4 to 6 hours. The goal is to achieve a PTT 1.5 to 2 times the control.[33]

Warfarin, 5 to 10 mg daily, is begun once the patient's condition is stable. Warfarin is monitored by prothrombin time (PT). The goal is to achieve a PT of 2 to 3 international normalized ratio (INR). Heparin and warfarin are continued until the PT is at the desired level for 2 consecutive days or warfarin has been given concurrently for 5 days, whichever is longer. Clinical trials of low-molecular-weight heparin (LMWH) are ongoing.

***Thrombolytic therapy.*** This therapy promotes immediate dissolution of the embolus and prompt return of pulmonary function in a patient who is hemodynamically unstable or severely hypoxic.

One of the thrombolytic agents, urokinase, streptokinase, or recombinant tissue-type plasminogen activator (rt-PA), is used. Therapy can be delivered either systemically or directly into the pulmonary artery via selective catheterization, although systemic therapy appears to be superior. The most popular regimen involves the administration of 100 mg of rt-PA as a continuous peripheral infusion over 2 hours. Thus far, the reported results indicate that this strategy is effective in achieving clot dissolution in more than 80% of patients, with bleeding complications occurring in less than 5%. This form of therapy is often not applicable to many postsurgical patients because of the increased risk of bleeding complications at their surgical site.

***Pulmonary embolectomy.*** A small group of patients with PE fail to respond to immediate aggressive medical support, and pulmonary embolectomy, in which PEs are extracted from the pulmonary vasculature, should be considered.[37] This procedure is usually performed with the patient under general anesthesia, although it may be performed with a special IV suction catheter under local anesthesia. The survival rate for this procedure is about 60%.[37]

**Diet.** Diet is as tolerated; the patient is usually started with fluids and progressed to soft foods.

**Activity.** The patient is confined to bed initially.

**Referrals.** The patient may be referred to a vascular surgeon or to social services.

## NURSING MANAGEMENT

### ASSESSMENT

#### Subjective Data

Data to be collected to assess the patient with PE include:

1. Determine the presence of risk factors (see the Risk Factors Box on p. 970).
2. Assess for the recent onset of any of the following symptoms: dyspnea, substernal chest pain, hemoptysis, chest palpitations, pleuritic pain, cough, apprehension: sense of foreboding, or diaphoresis.

#### Objective Data

Data to be collected to assess the patient with PE include:

1. Assess general appearance: patient often appears apprehensive.
2. Assess vital signs for tachypnea, tachycardia, and elevated temperature.
3. Perform pulmonary examination:
   a. Inspection, palpation, and percussion findings are usually normal unless there is an underlying pulmonary disease.
   b. Auscultate, listening for pleural friction rub and localized, decreased breath sounds and crackles.
4. Assess laboratory findings for the following: ABGs, hypoxemia, respiratory alkalosis, chest x-ray film (often normal), lung scan, perfusion scan (positive), ventilation scan (may indicate underventilated areas), and pulmonary angiography (if positive, is definitive for PE). Positive findings indicate vessel filling defect and cutoff (abrupt ending of vessel).

### NURSING DIAGNOSES

Nursing diagnoses are determined from analysis of patient data. Nursing diagnoses for the person with PE may include but are not limited to:

| Diagnostic Title | Possible Etiological Factors |
|---|---|
| Tissue perfusion, altered in pulmonary vascular and lung | Vascular obstruction from emboli resulting in decreased or absent blood flow to region |
| Gas exchange, impaired | High V/Q ratio |
| Pain | Pleural effusion |
| Knowledge deficit: condition and its treatment | Lack of exposure or unfamiliarity with information sources |

### EXPECTED PATIENT OUTCOMES

Expected patient outcomes for the person with PE may include but are not limited to:

1. Demonstrates adequate tissue perfusion
   a. Extremities warm and dry to touch, pulses present
   b. Coagulation studies: PT, PTT within normal limits
   c. IV sites intact and nonreddened
2. Demonstrates adequate ventilation
   a. $PaO_2$: 80 to 100 mm Hg
   b. $PaCO_2$: 40 mm Hg
   c. pH: 7.35 to 7.45
3. States that pain is relieved
4. Patient or significant others are able to
   a. List behaviors that would increase the risk of pulmonary emboli
   b. Identify the signs and symptoms of pulmonary emboli
   c. State the reason for anticoagulant therapy, the prescribed dose and time of administration of medications, any adverse side effects, and need to take medications as prescribed
   d. State plans for follow-up care, including periodic blood coagulation tests

### INTERVENTIONS

#### Promoting Tissue Perfusion

1. Provide antiembolism stockings.
2. Perform hourly active foot dorsiflexion.
3. Elevate lower extremities (do not use Gatch bed).
4. Perform ROM exercises.

5. Assess legs for adequate pulses and measure leg size (do not massage legs).
6. Inspect IV sites regularly.
7. Administer anticoagulants as ordered.
8. Monitor PT and PPT; withhold anticoagulant and notify physician if PT or PTT falls below accepted levels.

#### Promoting Gas Exchange

1. Assist patient to deep-breathe and cough every 4 hours.
2. Administer oxygen therapy as ordered, and monitor with pulse oximetry.
3. Maintain prescribed activity while avoiding overexertion.

#### Promoting Comfort

1. Elevate the head of the bed 30 to 40 degrees.
2. Maintain a quiet, calm environment.
3. Administer pain medications as necessary.

#### Patient/Family Education

Teach the patient about prescribed anticoagulant therapy:

1. Dose, side effects, and time of administration
2. Need to wear Medic Alert bracelet or carry a card stating that patient is taking an anticoagulant
3. Precautions to be observed to prevent bleeding while on anticoagulant therapy, including using a soft toothbrush, not going barefoot, applying pressure to cuts to stop bleeding, and not taking any medication containing aspirin

Teach the patient about signs and symptoms of PE that require immediate medical attention:

1. Dyspnea
2. Substernal chest pain
3. Hemoptysis
4. Chest palpitations
5. Cough
6. Diaphoresis
7. Apprehension

##### *Health promotion/prevention*

Teach the patient about risk factors associated with PE and how to avoid them:

1. Do not wear constrictive clothing such as rolled garters.
2. Avoid standing or sitting for prolonged periods. Be sure to move about at least every 2 hours. Do active dorsiflexion of feet while sitting.
3. Stop smoking. Refer to resource that assists patients to stop smoking.

## ■ EVALUATION

To evaluate the effectiveness of nursing interventions, compare patient behaviors with those stated in the expected patient outcomes. Successful achievement of patient outcomes for the patient with PE is indicated by:

1. Adequate tissue perfusion
   a. Extremities warm and dry, pulses present
   b. Coagulation studies: PT and PTT within normal limits
   c. IV sites intact and give no indication of bleeding from them
2. Adequate ventilation
   a. $PaO_2$: 85 to 100 mm Hg
   b. $PaCO_2$: 40 mm Hg
   c. pH: 7.35 to 7.45
3. Absence of pain
4. Listing behaviors that would decrease the risk of PE
   a. Not sitting in one position for a long time without getting up and moving about
   b. Verbalizing signs and symptoms of PE: dyspnea; sharp pain in chest, especially when taking a deep breath and when exhaling; cough; rapid heartbeat
   c. Taking an anticoagulant to prevent future thrombi and emboli; knowing the dose and time of medications he or she will take after discharge and side effects, such as bruising easily and bleeding gums
   d. Showing card indicating next appointment for blood test; verbalizes the importance of having blood drawn as scheduled; also verbalizes that if for any reason appointment cannot be kept, physician should be called for assistance with alternative plan (sending someone to patient's home to draw blood, assisting patient with transportation, etc.)
   e. Carrying card stating that he or she is on an anticoagulant or wearing a Medic Alert bracelet.

## GERONTOLOGICAL CONSIDERATIONS

Elderly persons are at higher risk for developing DVT and PE because they are more likely to have surgery, such as knee and hip replacements, and they may be less active than younger persons.

## SPECIAL ENVIRONMENTS FOR CARE

### Critical Care Management

Patients with PE are critically ill and will receive the care outlined previously in an intensive care unit until it is believed that it is safe to move them. This period can vary from a few days to a week or more.

## COMPLICATIONS

Complications may include pulmonary infarction, pleural effusion, right ventricular failure, GI bleeding, or bleeding from other sites.

## CHEST TRAUMA

### Etiology/Epidemiology

Chest trauma is a major problem most often seen first in the emergency department. Injury to the chest may affect the bony chest cage, pleurae and lungs, diaphragm, or mediastinal contents.

Injuries to the chest are broadly classified into two groups: *blunt* and *penetrating* (Box 32-17). Blunt, or nonpenetrating, injuries damage the structures within the chest cavity without disrupting chest wall integrity. Penetrating injuries disrupt chest wall integrity and result in alteration in intrathoracic pressures.

The leading cause of *blunt chest injuries* in the United States is motor vehicle steering wheel impact in the person not wearing a seat belt. Blows to the chest with blunt objects or as a result of a fall also cause nonpenetrating chest injury. *Penetrating wounds* usually result from gunshot or stabbing injuries.

### Blunt injuries

#### Rib fractures

***Pathophysiology.*** Rib fractures are the most common blunt injury. Ribs 3 through 10 are most often fractured, because they are less well protected by the chest muscles. The ribs usually fracture at the point of maximum impact, but they may fracture at a site distant from impact. Rib fractures are caused by blows, crushing injuries, or strain caused by severe coughing or sneezing spells. If the rib is splintered or the fracture displaced, sharp fragments may penetrate the pleura and lung, resulting in a *hemothorax* (blood in the pleural space) or *pneumothorax* (air in the pleural space), which are *penetrating injuries.*

Common signs and symptoms of rib fracture include:

1. Pain at the site of injury, increasing on inspiration
2. Localized tenderness and crepitus on palpation
3. Splinting of chest and shallow breathing

Fractures are confirmed by chest x-ray findings.

***Collaborative care management.*** It is important to determine how the patient was injured. If the patient is unable to answer questions, information is obtained from those accompanying the patient. The following questions are asked:

1. How, when, and where did the injury occur?
2. Does the patient complain of pain when taking a breath?
3. Does the patient complain that the chest is tender to the touch?

The patient is observed for splinting of the chest and shallow breathing, which could lead to atelectasis. To improve breathing the patient is placed in a position of comfort; most patients are able to breathe best in Fowler's or semi-Fowler's position. Analgesia is given to relieve pain so that the patient can be encouraged to breathe more deeply. If pain persists despite analgesics, the physician may infiltrate the intercostal spaces above and below the fractured rib(s) with 1% procaine.[27] Most patients with minor rib fractures without penetration of the lung will be sent home with instructions to return in 2 weeks for a chest x-ray.

*Patient/family education*

1. The patient should rest and do nothing strenuous for several days.
2. The patient should take deep breaths every hour.
3. If pain is not relieved by the oral analgesic, call the physician.
4. If shortness of breath, sudden sharp chest pain, or coughing up of blood occurs, return to the emergency department immediately.

### Flail chest

**Etiology/epidemiology.** The etiology/epidemiology of flail chest are the same as those for other blunt injuries discussed in the column at the left.

**Pathophysiology.** When multiple ribs or the sternum is fractured in more than one place, a portion of the chest wall becomes separated from the chest cage, resulting in a flail chest. Thus the chest wall no longer provides the rigid bony support that is necessary to maintain the bellows function required for normal ventilation. This causes *paradoxical breathing,* or paradoxical respiratory movement. During inspiration the dislocated segment is pulled inward by the subatmospheric intrapleural pressure (Figure 32-16, *C*). During expiration the dislocated segment bulges outward as intrapleural pressure becomes less negative (Figure 32-16, *D*).

*Flail chest usually causes localized atelectasis* secondary to decreased ventilation, resulting in hypoxemia. Because of the increased work of breathing, the individual may also develop hypercapnia and respiratory acidosis. Pulmonary contusion is a common occurrence in persons with a flail chest. Box 32-18 lists clinical manifestations of a flail chest.

#### Collaborative care management

*Diagnostic tests*

1. Chest x-ray examination to determine extent of trauma
2. Arterial blood gases to determine $Pa{O_2}$ and $Pa{CO_2}$

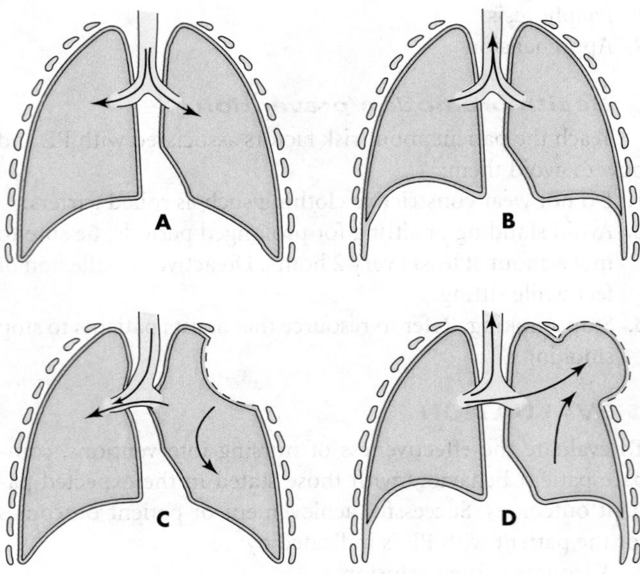


**fig. 32-16** Normal respiration: **A,** inspiration; **B,** expiration. Paradoxical motion: **C,** inspiration, area of lung underlying unstable chest wall sucks in on inspiration; **D,** same area balloons out on expiration. Note movement of mediastinum toward opposite lung on inspiration.

**box 32-17** *Penetrating and Nonpenetrating (Blunt) Chest Injuries*

**PENETRATING**

| | |
|---|---|
| Open pneumothorax (sucking chest wound) | Pulmonary contusion |
| Hemothorax | Diaphragm rupture |
| Tracheobronchial injury | Mediastinal injury |

**BLUNT (NONPENETRATING)**

| | |
|---|---|
| Fractured ribs | Tracheobronchial injury |
| Flail chest | Diaphragm rupture |
| Closed pneumothorax | Mediastinal injury |
| Tension pneumothorax | |

***Treatments.*** Treatment for flail chest includes the following:

1. Stabilizing the flail segment. The individual is usually intubated and placed on a positive pressure ventilator with PEEP. Mechanical ventilation provides internal stabilization of the chest, decreases the work of breathing, and initiates the bellows function normally provided by the intact bony chest cage. If prolonged ventilatory support is required, a tracheostomy is performed.
2. Provide supplemental oxygen; monitor with pulse oximetry.
3. Correct acid-base imbalance. Mechanical ventilation is used to correct respiratory acid-base imbalance.
4. Provide analgesics for pain control.
5. For severe pain, epidural anesthesia may be used.
6. Avoid fluid overload.

***Diet.*** Diet is as tolerated.

***Activity.*** The patient will be confined to bed as long as he or she is on a ventilator.

***Referrals.*** Possible referrals include respiratory therapy, physical therapy, and social services.

## NURSING MANAGEMENT

### ASSESSMENT

#### Subjective Data

Data to be collected include nature of the injury and when it occurred. Often the patient is too badly injured to answer questions, and data are obtained from those accompanying the patient.

#### Objective Data

Data to be collected to assess the patient with flail chest include:

Pain is severe and increases with each respiratory movement.

Mediastinum oscillates, or flutters with each respiration.

There are decreased breath sounds on auscultation.

If there is severe interference with cardiac function, neck veins will be distended.

Vital signs: increased pulse and respiratory rate. Blood pressure will fall if paradoxical motion is not relieved.

**box 32-18** ***clinical manifestations***

***Flail Chest***

Severe chest pain
Paradoxical breathing (asymmetrical chest movement)
Oscillation of mediastinum
Increasing dyspnea
Rapid shallow respirations
Accessory muscle breathing
Restlessness
Decreased breath sounds on auscultation
Cyanosis
Anxiety related to difficult breathing

### NURSING DIAGNOSES

Nursing diagnoses are determined from analysis of patient data. Nursing diagnoses for the person with a flail chest may include but are not limited to:

| Diagnostic Title | Possible Etiological Factors |
|---|---|
| Airway clearance, ineffective | Trauma to chest wall |
| Gas exchange, impaired | V/Q abnormality |
| Pain | Trauma to chest wall |

### EXPECTED PATIENT OUTCOMES

1. Airway clearance is improved.
2. a. $PaO_2$ and $PaCO_2$ are improved.
   b. Patient has normal respiration.
3. Patient is more comfortable.

### INTERVENTIONS

#### Improving Airway Clearance

Because the patient will be placed on a ventilator, care will be provided in an intensive care unit. The patient will be intubated and cannot clear his or her own airway. Shallow breathing and retained secretions can result in a fatal pulmonary infection.

The following nursing actions are indicated:

1. Suction airway as needed to maintain patency.
2. Liquefy pulmonary secretions by providing adequate fluid intake and humidification of the respiratory tract.
3. After extubation, time coughing maneuvers to coincide with peak effect of analgesics.

#### Improving Gas Exchange

Nursing interventions to promote adequate oxygen and carbon dioxide exchange are aimed at stabilizing the flail segment and include:

1. Initially, provide direct support to the flail segment with the hands or sandbags.
2. After spinal injury is ruled out, turn the patient so that he or she is lying on the affected side. This provides stabilization of the flail segment and also encourages lung expansion on the unaffected side until the patient can be intubated and attached to a positive pressure ventilator with PEEP. If the patient has a significant unilateral injury, placing the affected lung down will increase perfusion to that lung and may result in improved gas exchange.

#### Promoting Comfort

Interventions to promote comfort include:

1. Administer analgesics liberally for pain.
2. Splint the flail segment with hands during coughing and deep breathing (see Figure 32-12).

#### Patient/Family Education

The patient and family need to be prepared for intubation and connection to a ventilator. This includes developing a way for the patient and family to communicate. They will be informed that the patient will be weaned from the ventilator as soon as the chest wall is stable, and that once this is accomplished the patient can be extubated and will be able to talk.

#### Health promotion/prevention

The major preventive measure is to ensure that everyone understands the importance of using seat belts when riding in a motor vehicle. Motor vehicle accidents are the source of most serious chest injuries.

## EVALUATION

To evaluate the effectiveness of nursing interventions, compare patient behaviors with those stated in the expected patient outcomes. Successful achievement of patient outcomes for the person with flail chest is indicated by:

1. Has been weaned from the ventilator and is extubated
2a. $Pa{O_2}$: 90 mm Hg; $Pa{CO_2}$: 40 mm Hg; pH: 7.35
 b. Respirations 18 and regular
3. Moves about freely without pain

## GERONTOLOGICAL CONSIDERATIONS

Fractured ribs and a flail chest can be more serious when they occur in an elderly person. However, fewer elderly persons are involved in motor vehicle crashes, because most of these accidents involve teenaged and young adult males.

## SPECIAL ENVIRONMENTS FOR CARE

### Critical Care Management

The care discussed previously will take place in an intensive care unit because the patient is critically ill.

### Home Care Management

The patient with a flail chest is too ill to be cared for at home. However, after recovery and discharge from the hospital, the patient will recuperate at home. The major emphasis will be on regaining strength and improving respiratory capacity.

## COMPLICATIONS

Possible complications include pneumonia, tension pneumothorax, ARDS, and shock secondary to hemothorax.

### Penetrating Injuries

#### Pneumothorax

**Etiology/epidemiology.** In pneumothorax there is air in the pleural space between the lung and the chest wall. Pneumothorax can occur as a result of penetrating or nonpenetrating chest injuries, or it can occur spontaneously.

**Pathophysiology.** A *closed pneumothorax* is caused by fractured ribs that pierce the pleura. It can also occur when there is a sudden compression of the rib cage. Air enters the pleural space, increasing intrapleural pressure and collapsing the lung (Figure 32-17, *B*). A variant of a closed pneumothorax is a *spontaneous pneumothorax* that results from the rupture of an emphysematous bleb on the lung surface. Spontaneous pneumothorax may also follow severe bouts of coughing in persons with a chronic pulmonary disease such as asthma. It commonly occurs as a single or recurrent episode in an otherwise healthy young male. If large enough and left untreated, a closed pneumothorax can become a tension pneumothorax.

A *tension pneumothorax* occurs when air enters the pleural space on inspiration but cannot leave it on expiration. Although usually a result of a closed pneumothorax, a tension pneumothorax can be caused by a penetrating chest injury. The accumulating air builds up positive pressure in the chest cavity, resulting in the following:

1. Lung collapse on the affected side
2. Mediastinal shift toward the unaffected side
3. Compression of mediastinal contents (heart, great vessels) resulting in decreased cardiac output and decreased venous return

An *open pneumothorax* occurs when a penetrating chest wound opens the intrapleural space to atmospheric pressure. Each time the person inspires, air is sucked into the intrapleural space, increasing intrapleural pressure. An open pneumothorax is also called a *sucking chest wound,* because the wound makes a sucking sound on inspiration and expiration. Blood also may leak into the pleural cavity, creating a *hemothorax.*

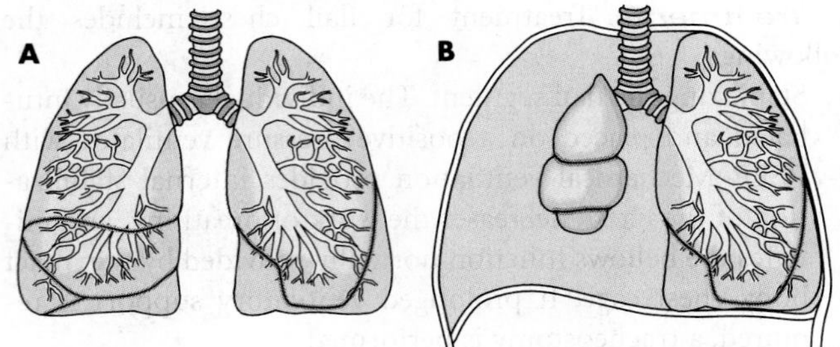


**fig. 32-17** **A,** Normal expanded lungs. **B,** Complete collapse of right lung caused by air in pleural cavity (pneumothorax).

**box 32-19** *clinical manifestations*

**Pulmonary Contusion**

Pulmonary contusion may vary from total absence of symptoms to the full spectrum of symptoms associated with noncardiogenic pulmonary edema. Signs and symptoms (some of which may be delayed) include the following:

- Increasing dyspnea
- Tachypnea
- Increasing restlessness
- Crackles noted on auscultation
- Hemoptysis

**Collaborative care management.** The clinical manifestations and medical management of the various types of pneumothorax are presented in Table 32-21. Nursing interventions associated with the specific types of pneumothorax are presented in Table 32-22.

#### Pulmonary contusion

**Etiology/epidemiology.** A penetrating injury may cause contusion of the lung or pleura. Pulmonary contusion usually results from sudden compression followed by rapid decompression of the thoracic cavity, causing blood to extravasate into the pulmonary tissue.

**Pathophysiology.** The contusion is usually self-limiting because the pulmonary vasculature is a low-pressure system. However, extensive contusion can precipitate pulmonary edema, with resultant hypoxemia, hypercapnia, and respiratory acidosis. Box 32-19 lists the clinical manifestations.

**table 32-21** *Clinical Manifestations and Medical Management of Pneumothorax*

| Pneumothorax | Clinical Manifestations | Medical Management |
|---|---|---|
| Closed (spontaneous) | Small or slowly developing pneumothorax may produce no symptoms.<br>Larger or rapidly developing pneumothorax results in the following:<br>1. Sharp pain on inspiration<br>2. Increasing dyspnea<br>3. Increasing restlessness<br>4. Diaphoresis<br>5. Hypotension<br>6. Tachycardia<br>7. Absence of chest movement on affected side<br>8. Breath sounds absent on affected side<br>9. Hyperresonance on affected side | Observation on outpatient basis<br>Supplemental oxygen<br>Needle aspiration of air from pleural space, if present; insertion of chest catheter connected to a flutter valve or closed drainage system<br>If frequent recurrences, doxycycline or talc instilled into pleural space to cause adhesions between pleurae; if this procedure fails, lung portion with defect resected and parietal pleura abraded |
| Tension | 1. Severe dyspnea<br>2. Agitation<br>3. Trachea deviated from midline toward unaffected lung—mediastinal shift<br>4. Jugular venous distention<br>5. Absence of chest movement on affected side<br>6. Hypotension, tachycardia<br>7. Breath sounds absent on affected side<br>8. Hyperresonance on affected side<br>9. Diminished heart sounds<br>10. Shock<br>11. Subcutaneous emphysema<br>12. Ineffective ventilation | True emergency<br>Defect in chest wall covered with a sterile dressing<br>Insertion of chest tube connected to a flutter valve or closed drainage system |
| Open | 1. Sucking sounds at wound site with respiration<br>2. Tracheal deviation (trachea moves toward unaffected side during inspiration and returns toward midline with expiration) | Occlusion of open wound<br>Same as for closed pneumothorax |

**table 32-22** *Nursing Interventions for Pneumothorax*

| Pneumothorax | Nursing Interventions |
|---|---|
| Closed (spontaneous) | Perform the following:<br>1. Place in semi-Fowler's position.<br>2. Administer oxygen.<br>3. Obtain thoracentesis tray and closed drainage equipment (see p. 959 for care of the patient with chest tubes).<br>For outpatient or for patient after chest tube removal, instruct to:<br>1. Report any increased dyspnea to physician.<br>2. Avoid strenuous exercise or activity that increases rate and depth of breathing.<br>3. Avoid holding breath.<br>4. Follow physician's instructions about resuming normal activity. |
| Tension | Life-threatening event; imperative that interventions be carried out immediately to relieve increased intrapleural pressure; interventions same as those listed for closed pneumothorax<br>Perform the following:<br>1. Monitor vital signs frequently.<br>2. Observe for cardiac dysrhythmias.<br>3. Palpate for subcutaneous emphysema in upper chest and neck.<br>Same discharge instruction as for patient with closed pneumothorax |
| Open | Perform the following:<br>1. Occlude wound with nonporous covering.<br>2. Same interventions as for closed pneumothorax.<br>3. Same discharge instructions as for closed pneumothorax.<br>Same discharge instruction as for closed pneumothorax |

**Collaborative care management.** Medical treatment of pulmonary contusion depends on the severity of the injury. Treatment may vary from outpatient monitoring to intubation and mechanical ventilatory support when pulmonary edema is present.

Nursing care includes the following:

1. Administer analgesia as ordered every 3 hours.
2. Monitor for fluid overload.
   a. Keep accurate record of all intake and output.
   b. Monitor vital signs every 30 minutes. Pulse and respirations can be expected to increase with fluid overload.
   c. Monitor breath sounds every 30 minutes.
3. Monitor ventilatory status every 30 minutes.
   a. Check for signs of respiratory distress:
      (1) Dyspnea
      (2) Increase in respirations
      (3) Change in breath sounds
   b. Check ABG results.
4. Monitor for signs and symptoms of a flail chest, which commonly accompanies pulmonary contusion.
5. Support patient to stay in bed until physical status is stabilized.
   a. Stay with patient. Listen to patient's concerns, and explain what is planned.
   b. Assist with ADL so patient can conserve energy and demands made on the cardiopulmonary system.

***Patient/family education.*** Because pulmonary contusion is the result of an accident, the main emphasis is on preventing injuries by wearing a seat belt. Other education includes teaching the family how to be supportive of the patient.

## OBSTRUCTIVE LUNG DISEASES

### CHRONIC OBSTRUCTIVE PULMONARY DISEASE

*Chronic obstructive pulmonary disease (COPD)* is defined as a disease state characterized by airflow obstruction resulting from chronic bronchitis or emphysema[2] (Figure 32-18). The airflow obstruction is generally progressive, may be accompanied by airway hyperreactivity, and may be partially reversible. In the past, *asthma* was subsumed under COPD. Today asthma is separated out because it is marked by inflammation with participation of complex cellular and chemical mediators. Thus asthma will be discussed separately from chronic bronchitis and emphysema in this chapter.

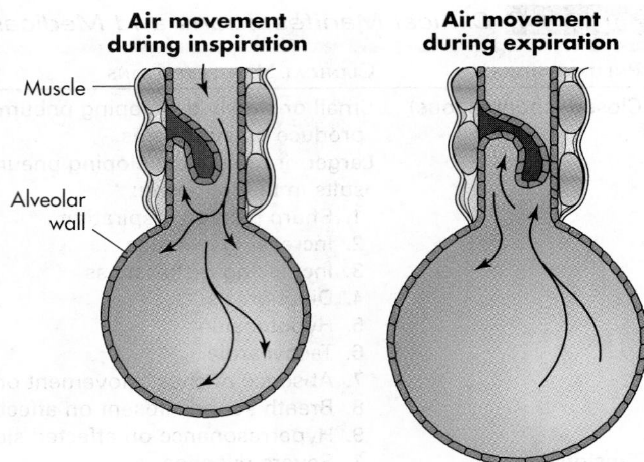


**fig. 32-18** Mechanisms of air trapping in chronic obstructive pulmonary disease (COPD). Mucus plugs and narrowed airways cause air trapping and hyperinflation on expiration. During inspiration the airways enlarge, allowing gas to flow past the obstruction. During expiration the airways narrow and prevent gas flow. This mechanism of air trapping, known as ball valving, occurs in asthma and chronic bronchitis.

#### Epidemiology

More than 14 million persons in the United States have reported that they have chronic bronchitis or emphysema—12.5 million persons with chronic bronchitis and 1.65 million with emphysema. When persons with asthma are included in this statistic, the total number of persons affected by COPD totals 17 million. Persons with chronic bronchitis or emphysema had 169 million days of restricted activity per year, or nearly 2 months of restricted activity yearly for each person. For employed persons with these diseases, frequent absences from work are likely to threaten their jobs.

Both the prevalence of COPD and the death rates attributed to it have reached epidemic proportions. Chronic obstructive pulmonary disease is the fourth-leading cause of death in the United States, after heart disease, cancer, and CVAs. The death rate from COPD increased 32.9% from 1979 to 1991. For this reason, there is little hope of reducing the death rate by the year 2000. The goal set for that year is to slow the rise in deaths from COPD to no more than 25 per 100,000 people. The age-adjusted baseline was 18.7 deaths per 100,000 in 1987. If this trend continues, the CDC estimates that the death rate for COPD will reach 26 to 28 deaths per 100,000 in the year 2000. Given the difference between 18.7 deaths per 100,000 and 26 deaths per 100,000, considerable change will have to occur if the year 2000 goal is to be achieved.

The increase in the death rate from COPD is believed to be related to (1) the growing tendency of physicians to list it as a primary cause of death, (2) the greater use of PFTs to identify persons with COPD, and (3) more emphasis in medical literature on the importance of this syndrome. Despite these facts, it is believed that the mortality rate is even higher than reported, because many persons who were reported to have died from pneumonia, asthma, or congestive heart failure probably had COPD. The major factor in this increase in mortality, in addition to improved reporting and the increased aging of the population, is a history of cigarette smoking. Risk factors for COPD are listed in the accompanying Risk Factors Box.

Although chronic bronchitis and emphysema are classified under the same category, it is clinically important to identify the predominant type of pulmonary disease that is the basis for the individual's COPD. Therefore, in the following presentation, COPD is divided into two major obstructive diseases: chronic

**risk factors**

**Chronic Obstructive Pulmonary Disease**

- Cigarette smoking
- Air pollution
- Occupational factors (cigarette smoke plus hazardous airborne substances)
- Alpha$_1$-antitrypsin deficiency
- Sex—male
- Race—white
- Socioeconomic status—higher incidence in blue-collar than in white-collar workers

From American Thoracic Society: Standards for the diagnosis and care of patients with chronic obstructive pulmonary disease, *Am J Respir Crit Care Med* 152:579, 1995.

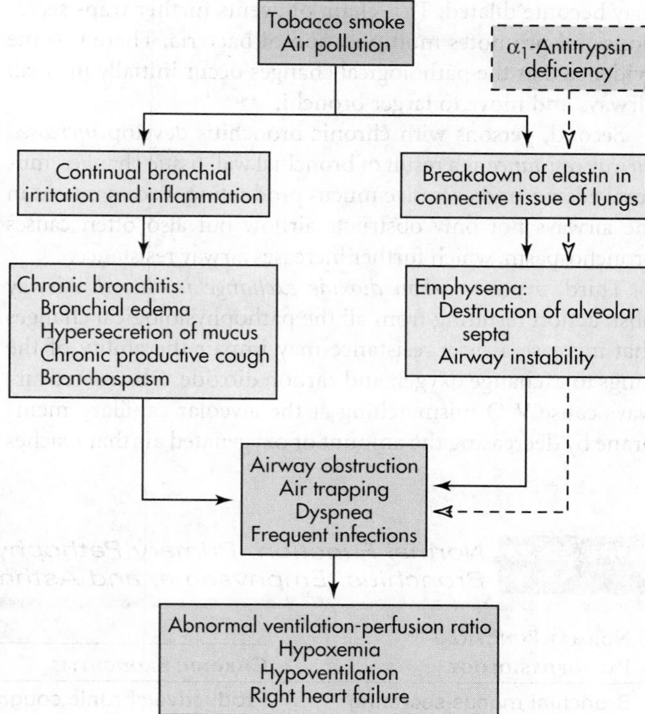


**fig. 32-19** Pathogenesis of chronic bronchitis and emphysema (COPD). (Dashed arrows indicate role of $\alpha_1$-antitrypsin deficiency, if present.)

bronchitis and emphysema. Because the clinical management of chronic bronchitis and emphysema is similar, the care for patients with either of these diseases is presented together.

Appropriate interventions can minimize the progression of COPD. A comprehensive management program will benefit all patients, even those with severe disease. Management programs should be designed to educate patients, retard the progression of airflow limitation, minimize airflow limitation, correct secondary physiological problems, and optimize functional capabilities.

## Chronic Bronchitis

Chronic bronchitis is defined by the presence of a chronic productive cough for a minimum of 3 months per year for at least 2 consecutive years in patients in whom other causes have been excluded. It is characterized physiologically by hypertrophy and hypersecretion of the bronchial mucus glands and structural alterations of the bronchi and bronchioles.

### *Etiology*

Chronic bronchitis is caused by the inhalation of physical or chemical irritants or by viral or bacterial infections. The most common inhaled irritant is cigarette smoke, and heavy cigarette smoking is believed to be the major cause of the disease.

### *Epidemiology*

Occupations in which dust or other irritants are inhaled may cause bronchitis, but the evidence for this is not conclusive. However, in Great Britain it has been recognized for years that the highest incidence of bronchitis occurs in large industrial cities with high levels of air pollution.

### *Pathophysiology*

The two pathological changes that typify chronic bronchitis are hypertrophy of mucus-secreting glands and chronic inflammatory changes in the small airways. First, there is glandular hypertrophy. *Mucous gland hypertrophy* and *hyperplasia* from chronic irritation cause excessive mucus production. The excessive mucus and impaired ciliary movement associated with chronic bronchitis increase susceptibility to infection (Figure 32-19). Bacteria proliferate in the mucous secretions in the lumen of the bronchi. The most common infectious agents are *S. pneumoniae* and *H. influenzae.* As bacteria multiply, they exert a neutrophilic chemotaxis, and pus cells migrate from between bronchial epithelial cells to produce a mucopurulent exudate in the lumen, or the disease may progress to ulceration and destruction of the bronchial wall (Figure 32-20). The presence of granulation tissue and peribronchial fibrosis results in stenosis and airway obstruction. Small airways may be completely obliterated, and others

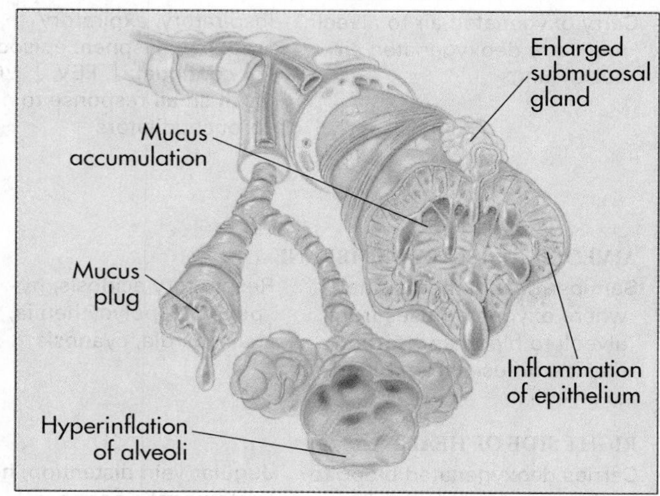


**fig. 32-20** Airway obstruction caused by chronic bronchitis. Inflammation and thickening of mucous membrane with accumulation of mucus and pus leading to obstruction; characterized by cough.

may become dilated. This chain of events further traps secretions and promotes multiplication of bacteria. There is some evidence that the pathological changes occur initially in small airways and move to larger bronchi.

Second, persons with chronic bronchitis develop *increased airway resistance* as a result of bronchial wall tissue changes, mucosal edema, and excessive mucus production. Excess mucus in the airways not only obstructs airflow but also often causes bronchospasm, which further increases airway resistance.

Third, *oxygen–carbon dioxide exchange is altered.* Airway obstruction resulting from all the pathophysiological changes that increase airway resistance may impair the ability of the lungs to exchange oxygen and carbon dioxide. Obstructed airways cause V/Q mismatching at the alveolar capillary membrane by decreasing the amount of oxygenated air that reaches the alveoli. Additionally, the obstructed airways may lead to atelectasis, which further diminishes the surface area available for respiration. The result of these pathophysiological alterations is *hypercapnia, hypoxemia,* and *respiratory acidosis.*

Fourth, right *ventricular decompensation* (cor pulmonale) may result. The hypercapnia and hypoxemia typically associated with chronic bronchitis cause pulmonary vascular vasoconstriction. The increased pulmonary vascular resistance results in pulmonary vessel hypertension that in turn increases vascular pressure in the right ventricle of the heart.

Signs and symptoms of chronic bronchitis are manifestations of the underlying physiological abnormalities that have occurred. Table 32-23 relates the normal function, primary pathophysiology, and clinical picture observed in chronic bronchitis.

**table 32-23** *Normal Function, Primary Pathophysiology, and Clinical Manifestations in Chronic Bronchitis, Emphysema, and Asthma*

| Normal Function/ Pathophysiology | Clinical Manifestations | | |
|---|---|---|---|
| | Chronic Bronchitis | Emphysema | Asthma |
| Bronchial mucus-secreting glands produce mucus to trap foreign particles and transport them out of lungs | Productive chronic cough, grayish white sputum; when infected sputum is yellow, inspiratory; crackles (rales) | | Inflammation, hypersecretion; eosinophils in sputum |
| **BRONCHI AND BRONCHIOLES** | | | |
| Carry oxygenated air to alveoli and carry deoxygenated air out of lungs | Inspiratory, expiratory rhonchi; dyspnea: episodic or continual; ↓ FEV, ↓ VC with small response to bronchodilators | Early onset dyspnea on exertion, which progresses to continuous dyspnea; rhonchi, crackles, accessory muscle breathing; ↓ FEV, ↓ VC with no response to bronchodilators | Episodic dyspnea, accessory muscle breathing; inspiratory/expiratory wheezing; ↓ FEV, ↓ VC with good response to bronchodilators; ↑ work of breathing, pulsus paradoxus |
| **ALVEOLOCAPILLARY MEMBRANE** | | | |
| Semipermeable membrane where oxygen diffuses from alveoli to blood and carbon dioxide diffuses from blood to alveoli | Respiratory acidosis, hypoxemia, polycythemia, tachycardia, cyanosis | Early stage: normal or mild hypoxemia, respiratory alkalosis; late stage: hypoxemia, respiratory acidosis, ↓ diffusing capacity | Respiratory alkalosis with mild hypoxemia; status asthmaticus: respiratory acidosis with hypoxemia |
| **RIGHT SIDE OF HEART** | | | |
| Carries deoxygenated blood to pulmonary vasculature for oxygen/carbon dioxide exchange | Jugular vein distention, hepatomegaly, peripheral edema | Right ventricular decompensation | |
| **LUNG AND CHEST WALL COMPLIANCE** | | | |
| Relationship between lung and chest wall ability to expand and contract during inhalation and exhalation | | ↑ Anteroposterior diameter, ↓ lateral expansion, ↓ diaphragmatic excursion, ↓ breath, heart, and voice sounds, ↑ RV, ↑ FRC, ↑ TLC, hyperresonance, complaint of episgastric fullness | ↓ Fremitus, ↓ lateral expansion, hyperresonance, ↓ breath sounds, ↓ diaphragmatic excursion |

*FEV,* Forced expiratory volume; *VC,* vital capacity; *RV,* residual volume; *FRC,* functional reserve capacity; *TLC,* total lung capacity.

The earliest symptom of chronic bronchitis is a *productive cough,* especially on awakening. This symptom is often ignored by cigarette smokers, who become so accustomed to an early-morning cough that they take it for granted; some of them even refer to it as their "cigarette cough."

Persons with chronic bronchitis often unconsciously reduce their activity level to accommodate their respiratory symptoms in their daily lives. Thus they do not seek medical help until they experience a severe exacerbation of their symptoms, usually precipitated by a respiratory infection.

Pulmonary function tests reveal a limitation to airflow on expiration, as evidenced by a diminished forced expiratory volume. Vital capacity is also reduced, indicating diminished air movement both in and out of the lungs. Lung volumes are usually within normal limits until later in the course of the disease, when the lung volumes may be increased. There usually is no loss of diffusing capacity.

Early in the course of chronic bronchitis, the symptoms tend to be episodic in nature. As the disease progresses in severity, the patient's symptoms are constantly present to some degree. The patient appears increasingly dyspneic, using accessory muscles to breathe. *Chronic hypoxemia* resulting in *polycythemia* causes the patient to appear to be *cyanotic.* Increased pulmonary vascular resistance caused by respiratory acidosis and hypoxemia increases pressure on the right side of the heart, ultimately resulting in right-sided heart failure (cor pulmonale). The person with late-stage chronic bronchitis and cor pulmonale appears stout or overweight from edema, and the skin appears dusky.

Patients with chronic bronchitis complicated by cor pulmonale often have chronic respiratory failure (gradual onset of $Pa{O_2} < 50$ mm Hg and a $Pa{CO_2} > 50$ mm Hg). They are also prone to develop acute respiratory failure (sudden onset of a $Pa{O_2} < 50$ mm Hg and a $Pa{CO_2} > 50$ mm Hg) as a complication of a respiratory infection superimposed on their already diseased lung.

Effective health care management programs for persons who have chronic bronchitis or any of the variant combinations of pulmonary diseases that make up COPD require a multidisciplinary approach. The multidisciplinary approach to the management of COPD is included in the discussion of implementation of care for patients with COPD later in this chapter.

Medical management of chronic bronchitis is included in Table 32-24, which summarizes a typical multidisciplinary program for a person with COPD. Under managed care, the diagnosis-related group (DRG) for chronic bronchitis has been reduced from 6 days to 3 days (see the Clinical Pathway on p. 984).

### *Collaborative care management*

**Diagnostic tests.** The following tests may be used in diagnosing chronic bronchitis:

1. Chest x-ray films. Typical findings in chronic bronchitis are increased bronchovascular markings.
2. Sputum studies for culture and sensitivity. Neutrophils and bronchial epithelial cells usually occur in chronic bronchitis.
3. Arterial blood gas studies (see Chapter 30).
4. Hematology studies (complete blood count).
5. Pulmonary function tests (see Chapter 30).

**Medications**

***Bronchodilators.*** Two categories of bronchodilators—beta-2 agonists (adrenergic agents) and methylxanthines (theophylline)—are used to improve efficiency of breathing. Table 32-25 lists the commonly prescribed adrenergic agents that work at beta-2 sites located in smooth muscles of the airways. Beta-2 agonists have fewer cardiac side effects than Beta-1 agents with receptor sites in the myocardium. For this reason, albuterol, bitolterol, pirbuterol, metaproterenol, salmeterol, and terbutaline may be prescribed for COPD patients.

***Theophylline.*** Theophylline (a methylxanthine) is a weak bronchodilator that improves mucus clearance. Administering long-acting theophylline in the evening has been shown to reduce overnight decline in forced expiratory volume and morning respiratory symptoms. Theophylline may also increase collateral ventilation, respiratory muscle function, mucociliary clearance, and central respiratory drive and may reduce airway inflammation. In severe COPD with cor pulmonale, it can be given intravenously as aminophylline (see the Guidelines for Care Box, p. 984).

***Corticosteroids.*** Some patients benefit from both short-term and long-term administration of steroids, but it is not possible to predict which patients will benefit. Long-term treatment with oral corticosteroids should be prescribed only for patients who have documented improvement in airflow or exercise performance. The lowest possible dose of the steroids is used.[58] Steroid preparations used to treat COPD include methylprednisolone (Solu-Medrol), 0.5 mg/kg intravenously, and prednisone orally.

Patients should have a tuberculin test before beginning long-term steroid therapy. Those with a tuberculin reaction of 10 mm or more are candidates for prophylactic isoniazid therapy (see p. 938).

***Anticholinergic agents.*** Ipratropium (Atrovert) is a bronchodilator that is administered in a metered-dose inhaler (MDI). The usual dose is 2 to 4 puffs three or four times daily. A combination of albuterol and ipratropium in the same MDI is available and may simplify therapy for some patients. A spacer is usually used with the MDI. Ipratropium is well tolerated. Some patients will have a cough and dry mouth, which are side effects of anticholinergic agents.

***Antibiotics.*** During acute exacerbations of COPD, antibiotics may be ordered. Although viruses are the usual organisms contributing to a flare-up of COPD, colonizing organisms such as *S. pneumoniae, H. influenzae,* and *Moraxella catarrhalis* also play a pathological role. The airways of the patient with chronic bronchitis provide a rich culture medium for these organisms.

Recommended antibiotics are ampicillin, 500 mg every 6 hours; tetracycline, 500 mg every 6 hours; trimethoprimsulfamethoxazole, 160 to 1800 mg every 12 hours; or ciprofloxacin, 500 mg every 6 hours for 7 to 10 days.

If the person has frequent flare-ups, some experts recommend that a different antibiotic than the one usually

**table 32-24** *Etiology, Signs and Symptoms, and Medical Therapy for Chronic Bronchitis and Pulmonary Emphysema*

| Bronchitis | Pulmonary Emphysema |
|---|---|
| **ETIOLOGY** | |
| Inhalation of physical or chemical irritants or viral or bacterial infections<br>Most common inhaled irritant—cigarette smoke | Not known; believed that some change in the enzyme-inhibitor balance occurs, allowing proteolytic enzymes to attack lung tissue<br>Not known why some smokers develop bronchitis and others develop emphysema; α-antitrypsin deficiency in some persons who develop severe, disabling emphysema early in life; familial tendency for this type of emphysema |
| **SIGNS AND SYMPTOMS** | |
| **Early Symptoms** | |
| Productive cough on awakening; often ignored by cigarette smokers, who refer to it as their "cigarette cough" | Dyspnea on exertion, may be in acute respiratory distress<br>Using accessory muscles to breathe; ruddy color<br>Thin with a "barrel chest"<br>Usually able to maintain resting $Po_2$<br>Cyanosis uncommon |
| **Later Symptoms** | |
| Significant physical incapacity; breathlessness even when walking on a flat surface, noticeable shortness of breath and use of accessory muscles to breathe; cyanosis common; ankle edema, bloated appearance, distended neck veins | |
| **Late in Disease** | |
| Common complications: cor pulmonale (right ventricular hypertrophy), right-sided heart failure, and respiratory failure | ↑ $Pco_2$<br>Cor pulmonale and respiratory failure possible complications |
| **PULMONARY FUNCTION TEST FINDINGS** | |
| ↓ Expiratory flow rates<br>↓ Vital capacity (VC)<br>↑ Residual volume (RV)<br>Total lung capacity (TLC) usually within normal limits | ↓ Expiratory flow rates, especially forced expiratory volume, and maximal midexpiratory flow<br>↑ TLC<br>↑ RV<br>VC normal or slightly reduced until late stages of disease, $FEV_1/VC$ ratio changed |
| **ARTERIAL BLOOD GAS FINDINGS** | |
| Low resting $Po_2$<br>Elevated $Pco_2$ (if obstruction severe)<br>During exercise $Pco_2$ ↑ and $Po_2$ may also ↑ | $Po_2$ normal or slightly reduced at *rest* but falls during exercise<br>Normal $Pco_2$<br>Late in disease ↑ $Pco_2$ |
| **MEDICAL THERAPY** | |
| Medical therapy for chronic bronchitis and pulmonary emphysema is similar and depends on symptoms, PFT results, and ABG findings. Therapy may include all or some of the modalities outlined here. | |
| **SUPPORTIVE MEASURES** | |
| Education of patient and family about the following:<br>Avoidance of cigarette smoke<br>Avoidance of other inhaled irritants<br>Avoidance of persons with upper respiratory infections<br>Control of environmental temperature and humidity<br>Proper nutrition<br>Adequate hydration | |
| **SPECIFIC THERAPY** | |
| Medications<br>Bronchodilators<br>$\alpha_1$-Antitrypsin replacement for those with ↓ levels<br>Antimicrobials<br>Ampicillin or another broad-spectrum antibiotic usually prescribed to treat respiratory tract infections<br>Corticosteroids<br>May be prescribed to alleviate acute symptoms; prednisone most often prescribed | |

*Continued*

**table 32-24** *Etiology, Signs and Symptoms, and Medical Therapy for Chronic Bronchitis and Pulmonary Emphysema—cont'd*

| Bronchitis | Pulmonary Emphysema |
|---|---|
| **SPECIFIC THERAPY—cont'd** | |
| Digitalis | |
| May be prescribed to treat left ventricular failure if present | |
| **RESPIRATORY THERAPY** | |
| **Aerosol Therapy** | |
| Used to deliver bronchodilators through metered cartridge devices with a spacer | |
| **Oxygen Therapy** | |
| Required for patients who are unable to maintain a $PaO_2$ of 50 mm Hg or more at rest or who cannot carry out ADL without becoming short of breath; 1 to 2 L of $O_2$ given by nasal prongs | |
| **PHYSICAL CONDITIONING** | |
| **Relaxation Exercises** | |
| Progressive relaxation exercises encouraged; best practiced before meals or 2 hours or more after eating because digestion seems to interfere with ability to relax | |
| **MEDITATION** | |
| Meditation becoming more widely used to assist patients to relax | |
| **Breathing Retraining** | |
| Pursed-lip breathing | |
| Leaning forward position for exhalation | |
| Abdominal breathing | |
| Inhalation-exhalation exercises | |
| Exhalation with exertion | |
| **Rehabilitation** | |
| Muscle reconditioning program designed for patient | |

**table 32-25** *$\beta_2$-Agonists and Their Dosages for Metered-Dose Inhalers and Nebulized Solutions*

| Drug | Dose | mg/Puff | Nebulization |
|---|---|---|---|
| Albuterol (Proventil, Ventolin) | 2-3 puffs q4-6h | 0.09 | 0.3-0.5 ml 0.5% solution in 3 ml saline q4-6h |
| Bitolterol (Tornalate) | 2-3 puffs q6-8h | 0.37 | |
| Metaproterenol (Alupent, Metaprel) | 2-3 puffs q4-6h | 0.65 | 0.3 ml 5% solution in 2.5 ml saline q4-6h |
| Pirbuterol (Maxair) | 2-3 puffs q4-6h | 0.20 | |
| Salmeterol (Serevert) | 2 puffs q12h | 0.50 | |
| Terbutaline (Brethaire) | 2-3 puffs q4-6h | 0.20 | |

prescribed be used. Prophylactic administration of antibiotics in persons with COPD is not recommended.

***Mucolytics and expectorants.*** Patients with chronic bronchitis usually have thick, tenacious sputum. The literature suggests that the overall efficacy of mucolytics and expectorants remains unproven. For this reason, they are not ordered as often as previously. Patients who have been using these agents for years and found them to be helpful may want to continue to use them while hospitalized. The patient or the nurse may convey this information to the physician.

***Alpha₁-antitrypsin replacement therapy.*** In patients with alpha₁-antitrypsin (AAT) deficiency, pulmonary function declines more rapidly than in patients with COPD who have normal levels of AAT. A normal AAT level ranges from 180 to 280 mg/dl. A weekly dose of 60 mg/kg of active AAT may be given intravenously. Other experts suggest that taking it every 2 to 4 weeks may be equally effective. The long-term effects of replacement therapy in the AAT-deficient population with emphysema is unknown. However, a national registry has been formed to monitor the effectiveness of AAT therapy.

**Treatments**

***Aerosol therapy.*** Aerosol therapy is one of the most effective ways to deliver bronchodilators, corticosteroids, and cromolyn. The most commonly used methods to deliver an aerosol include a freon-propelled MDI and an intermittent positive-pressure breathing (IPPB) machine. Intermittent positive-pressure breathing is used less commonly and is reserved for persons who cannot inhale repetitively enough to near total lung capacity or who are unable to use an MDI because of lack of coordination or fatigue. Directions for teaching patients to use an inhaler with a spacer are given in the Patient/Family Teaching Box. When bronchodilators are administered as aerosols, the solution should be diluted with either water or saline. Some experts recommend that the diluent be water, because saline solutions already contain a solute (NaCl) in water. All bronchodilator solutions are high-molecular-weight concentrated solutions and have a high solute content. When they are diluted with water, there is a maximal decrease in solute concentration; thus smaller particle size and deeper deposition of the aerosol in the smaller airways result.

**guidelines for care**

### The Person Receiving Methylxanthine Medications

1. Monitor theophylline plasma level results. Therapeutic levels = 10 to 20 μg/ml, although individual response to theophylline levels varies. Notify physician if these levels are exceeded before administering the next dose of medication.
2. Certain types of theophylline formulations must be specifically taken with or without food. Food present in the stomach can either slow or speed up absorption of certain types of theophylline.
3. Cigarette or marijuana smoking significantly increases plasma clearance of theophylline. Patients who quit smoking may experience side effects normally seen with higher levels of methylxanthines. Counsel patients to notify their physician if they quit smoking.
4. Various medications interact with theophylline, altering plasma absorption rates. Counsel patients to inform their physician when they begin any new medication.
5. Liver cirrhosis, hepatitis, cardiac decompensation, cor pulmonale, and viral respiratory infections decrease plasma clearance of theophylline.

Aerosol devices are excellent sites for bacterial growth, and patients using such equipment at home should be advised on how to clean them appropriately.

When a spacer (Figure 32-21), a molded plastic chamber, is fitted on an inhaler, medication can be delivered more safely and effectively for the following reasons: (1) large droplets of the aerosol, which would tend to settle in the mouth and on the vocal cords, land on the walls of the spacer instead; (2) the finer droplets in the aerosol disperse more fully within the spacer and can be carried farther into the airways; (3) it is not necessary to coordinate breathing as carefully as it is with the standard inhaler, and thus patients are medicated more effectively; and (4) spacers can reduce the number and volume of puffs required, thereby reducing the

**patient/family teaching**

### Using an Inhaler with a Spacer

1. Exhale fully.
2. Position nebulizer in mouth *without* sealing lips around it.
3. Take a deep breath while releasing a puff of medication into spacer.
4. Hold breath for 3 to 4 seconds at full inspiration.
5. Exhale slowly through pursed lips.
6. Usually one or two puffs is prescribed.
7. Several breaths may be necessary to receive the entire dose from the spacer.
8. The mouth should be rinsed after completing treatment.
9. The inhaler and spacer should be washed with warm soapy water, rinsed, and dried thoroughly after each use.

**clinical pathway** *Chronic Obstructive Pulmonary Disease without Intubation*

| | DAY 1 | DAY 2 | DAY 3 |
|---|---|---|---|
| **Diagnostic Tests** | CBC, SMA6, ABGs, Sputum C & S, chest x-ray, PFT, theophylline levels (if on theophylline) | | |
| **Medications** | IV@TKO, aerosol Tx: beta agonist + ipratropium. Consider antibiotic. Consider nicotine replacement. | IV saline lock, convert aerosol Rx to MDI. | Discontinue IV saline lock, adjust drugs for home use. |
| **Treatments** | I & O q8h, weight, $O_2$ if indicated. VS with temp. q4h. Assess cardiopulmonary system and LOC q4h, elastic stockings. | I & O q8h, weight, assess need for home $O_2$ unless chronic use, VS q8h, elastic leg stockings. | Weight, discontinue I & O, VS q8h, assess cardiopulmonary systems and LOC q8h, elastic leg stockings. |
| **Diet** | Full liquids, low sodium. Encourage PO fluids, unless contraindicated. | Diet as tolerated, provide six small meals/day, high protein and calorie, low sodium. | |
| **Activity** | Bedrest, head of bed elevated 30 degrees with BRP. | OOB as tolerated. | |
| **Referral/Consultation** | Respiratory therapy, pulmonary medicine, home health | Respiratory rehab, dietary | |

cost of medication because each dose is used more efficiently.

After the medication is in the spacer, the patient can take several breaths, inhaling each time from the spacer, to receive the entire dose. Inhalers with spacers can be used to deliver steroids, $beta_2$-agonists, and cromolyn.

A newer device, a breath-activated MDI, is available. As its name indicates, inhaling triggers the inhaler to release a premeasured dose of bronchodilator. This device offers another way to ensure that patients receive the prescribed bronchodilator in the correct dosage.

**Diet.** See discussion on nutrition on p. 995.

**Activity.** Patients should be up and about as much as possible. Some will have to use portable oxygen while walking or doing other tasks (see p. 997 for further information).

**Referrals.** Common referrals for the patient with chronic bronchitis include respiratory therapy, physical therapy, dietary therapy, and social work.

## NURSING MANAGEMENT

### ASSESSMENT

#### Subjective Data

Data to be collected to assess the patient with chronic bronchitis include:

- History, character, onset, and duration of
  - Cough
  - Sputum production (amount, color, consistency)
  - Dyspnea
  - Pain in right upper quadrant (hepatomegaly)
- Smoking history
- Disease history
  - Influenza
  - Pneumonia
  - Repeated respiratory tract infections
  - Chronic sinusitis
- Past or present exposure to environmental irritants at home or at work
- Self-care used to treat symptoms
- Medications taken and their effectiveness in relieving symptoms

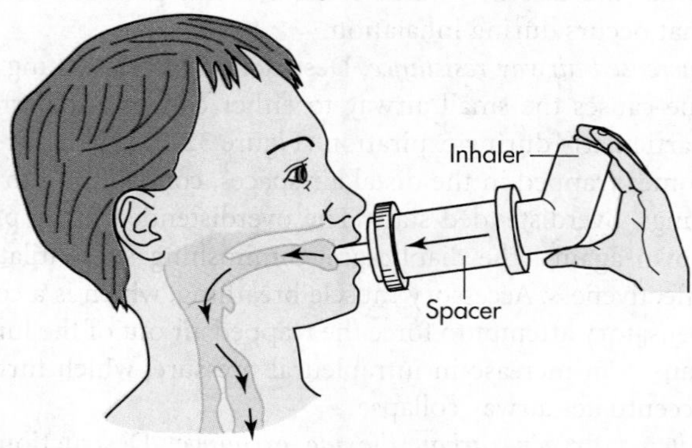


**fig. 32-21** Patient using inhaler with spacer attached to allow for better dispersal of medication.

#### Objective Data

Data to be collected to assess the patient with chronic bronchitis include:

- Assess general appearance.
  - Patient may appear overweight or bloated, and skin is dusky.
  - Check for dependent edema and jugular vein distention.
  - Abdominal assessment may indicate hepatomegaly.
- Assess vital signs.
  - Elevated temperature
  - Tachycardia
  - Tachypnea
- Conduct pulmonary examination
  - Inspection
    - Accessory muscle breathing
    - Forward-leaning posture
    - Central cyanosis
    - Clubbing of fingers
    - Altered sensorium (restlessness or lethargy)
  - Palpation: increased tactile fremitus
  - Percussion: normal
  - Auscultation
    - Inspiratory crackles (rales)
    - Inspiratory and expiratory rhonchi
- Assess laboratory findings.
  - Arterial blood gases
    - Respiratory acidosis
    - Hypoxemia
  - Hematology
    - Elevated hemoglobin and hematocrit
    - Elevated WBC
  - Pulmonary function tests
    - Decreased $FEV_1$
    - Normal diffusing capacity
    - Normal lung volumes (in end-stage chronic bronchitis, lung volumes may appear similar to those found in patients with emphysema)

### NURSING DIAGNOSES

Nursing diagnoses are determined from assessment of patient data. Nursing diagnoses for the person with chronic bronchitis may include but are not limited to:

| Diagnostic Title | Possible Etiological Factors |
|---|---|
| Gas exchange, impaired | Low V/Q ratio |
| Airway clearance, ineffective | Hypersecretion, tracheobronchial infection, decreased energy/fatigue |
| Breathing pattern, ineffective | Decreased energy/fatigue, airway changes |
| Activity intolerance | Imbalance between oxygen demand and requirement |
| Fluid volume excess | Pulmonary hypertension with resultant increased cardiac workload |
| Nutrition, altered: less than body requirements | Dyspnea, anorexia, sputum production, medication side effects, fatigue |
| Infection, risk for | Decreased lung defenses |
| Fear | Long-term illness and disability, change in role functioning |

| Knowledge deficit: condition and its treatment | Lack of exposure/recall, cognitive limitation, unfamiliarity with information source |
|---|---|

Expected outcomes, nursing interventions, evaluation, gerontological considerations, special environments for care, and complications of care for patients with COPD are similar, regardless of the underlying obstructive airway disease. Thus these subjects are included later in this chapter (see the discussion beginning on p. 989).

## Emphysema

Emphysema is defined pathologically by destructive changes in alveolar walls and enlargement of air spaces distal to the terminal nonrespiratory bronchioles. It is characterized physiologically by increased lung compliance, decreased diffusing capacity, and increased airway resistance.

### Etiology

The cause of emphysema is not known; however, evidence suggests that proteases released by polymorphonuclear leukocytes or alveolar macrophages are involved in the destruction of the connective tissue of the lungs. Connective tissue in the lungs is primarily composed of elastin, collagen, and proteoglycan, which can be damaged and destroyed by enzymes such as proteases and elastase. Protease-antiprotease imbalances and cigarette smoke destroy connective tissue. Cigarette smoke directly blocks the inhibitory capacity of AAT and promotes an excess of neutrophils through the attractant effects of alveolar macrophages. The neutrophils release elastases, which are capable of destroying the elastin structure of the lung. Cigarette smoking is also associated with goblet cell metaplasia and bronchiolitis, which contribute to airway obstruction.

Some persons with a deficiency of AAT develop severe, disabling emphysema early in life, usually of the bullous type.

### Epidemiology

Although it is not known when emphysema actually begins, there appear to be many years between the initial pathophysiological changes and the onset of overt symptoms. Symptoms associated with emphysema usually appear in the fourth decade of life, and disability from disease usually occurs in the fifth or sixth decade of life. The typical individual with emphysema is a man of about 55 years of age with a history of smoking tobacco.

Why some smokers develop bronchitis and others develop emphysema is unknown. Differences in susceptibility and the predominant type of disease are believed to be influenced by hereditary or environmental factors or factors in the patient's history. An established familial tendency to AAT deficiency indicates that relatives of persons with this type of emphysema should be screened and provided with counseling, as discussed later.

An estimated 1% of persons with COPD have an AAT deficiency. The mean age for onset of dyspnea related to COPD is 40 to 45 years in persons with AAT deficiency. Their mean life expectancy is 50 to 65 years of age, with smokers dying about 10 years earlier than nonsmokers.

Patients with AAT deficiency can be treated with human $\alpha_1$-proteinase inhibitor (Prolastin), which has been approved by the U.S. Food and Drug Administration (FDA). The cost of Prolastin, which is given intravenously once a week, is estimated to be more than $30,000 a year. Evidence indicates that treating patients with AAT deficiency would be cost-effective because it would decrease complications in those with AAT deficiency and increase their life span. Because AAT deficiency cannot be prevented, it is important that persons who have it not smoke.

### Pathophysiology

The type of emphysema can be determined only by descriptive morphology. The two principal types of emphysema morphologically are centrilobular (centriacinar) emphysema (CLE) and panlobular (panacinar) emphysema (PLE). *Centrilobular emphysema* is characterized by distention and damage of the respiratory bronchioles selectively. Openings develop in the walls of the bronchioles; they become enlarged and confluent and tend to form a single space as the walls enlarge. The disease tends to be unevenly distributed throughout the lung but usually is more severe in the upper portions (Figure 32-22).

*Panlobular emphysema* is characterized by a more uniform enlargement and destruction of the alveoli in the pulmonary acinus. Panlobular emphysema is usually more diffuse and is more severe in the lower lung. It is found in elderly persons who have no evidence of chronic bronchitis or impairment of lung function. It occurs just as often in women as in men, but PLE is less common than CLE. Panlobular emphysema is a characteristic finding in persons with homozygous AAT deficiency.

The clinical diagnosis of emphysema is inferred from the presence of signs and symptoms that are manifestations of known pathophysiological changes associated with the disease. Physiological abnormalities characteristic of emphysema include the following alterations:

1. *Increased lung compliance.* Loss of elastic recoil resulting from destruction of elastin in lung parenchyma causes the lungs to become permanently overdistended. Thus, compared with normal lungs, emphysematous lungs have a larger increase in volume relative to the pressure change that occurs during inhalation.
2. *Increased airway resistance.* Destruction of elastic lung tissue causes the small airway to either collapse or narrow, particularly during expiration (Figure 32-23). Thus air becomes trapped in the distal air spaces, contributing to the lungs' overdistended state. The overdistended lungs press down against the diaphragm, diminishing its ventilatory effectiveness. Accessory muscle breathing, which is a compensatory attempt to force the trapped air out of the lungs, causes an increase in intrapleural pressure, which further accentuates airway collapse.
3. *Altered oxygen–carbon dioxide exchange.* Destruction of alveolar and respiratory bronchiole walls decreases alve-

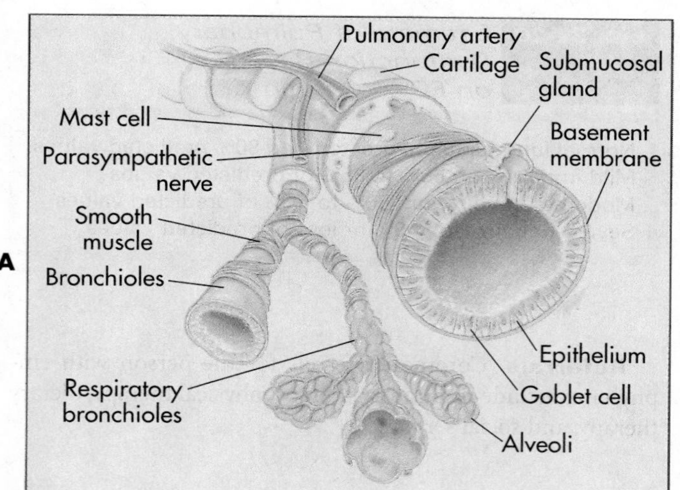


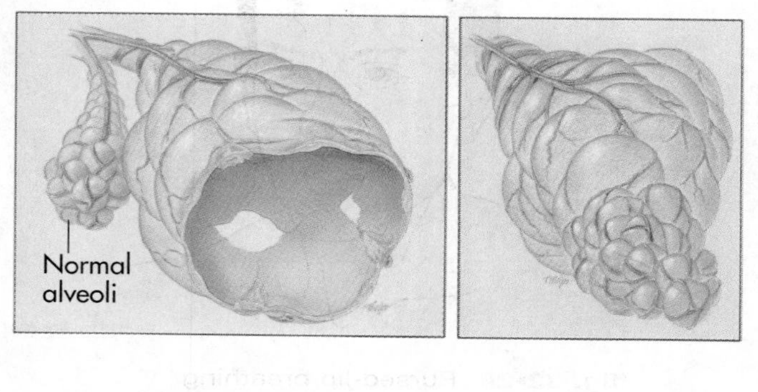


**fig. 32-22** Airway obstruction caused by emphysema. **A,** The normal lung. **B,** Emphysema: enlargement and destruction of alveolar walls with loss of elasticity and trapping of air; *(left)* **panlobular emphysema** showing abnormal weakening and enlargement of all air spaces distal to the terminal bronchioles (normal alveoli shown for comparison only); *(right)* **centrilobular emphysema** showing abnormal weakening and enlargement of the respiratory bronchioles in the proximal portion of the acinus.

olocapillary membrane surface area, which in turn may diminish diffusion of $O_2$ and $CO_2$. Persons with emphysema are able to compensate for these destructive changes by increasing their respiratory rate. Thus ABGs remain relatively normal, although mild hypoxemia may be present. Late in the course of the disease, extensive surface area loss and V/Q inequalities usually cause respiratory acidosis and hypoxemia. Normal function, pathophysiology, and clinical manifestations of emphysema are presented in Table 32-23.

Typically, the first symptom heralding the onset of emphysema is dyspnea on exertion (DOE), which progresses to continual dyspnea. Sputum production tends to be scant or absent. Persons with emphysema usually appear thin and manifest a barrel chest with an increased anteroposterior (AP) diameter from hyperinflation. The characteristic breathing pattern of the emphysematous individual includes accessory muscle breathing, an increased respiratory rate, and a prolonged expiratory phase resulting from airway narrowing or collapse on expiration. These individuals will spontaneously exhibit pursed-lip breathing, which facilitates effective air exhalation (Figure 32-24). (Pursed-lip breathing elevates end-expiratory pressures, which inhibits airway collapse during expiration.)

Pulmonary function studies demonstrate an increased residual volume (RV), functional residual capacity (FRC), and total lung capacity (TLC). Diffusing capacity is significantly reduced because of lung tissue destruction. Diminished respiratory air flow is demonstrated by a decreased forced expiratory volume ($FEV_1$) and maximal midexpiratory flow rate (MMFR). The vital capacity (VC) may be normal or only slightly reduced until late in the disease progression; thus the $FEV_1$/VC ratio is decreased. The degree of respiratory impairment may be estimated on the basis of the ratio of $FEV_1$ to forced vital capacity (FVC) (Box 32-20). A significant finding that differentiates emphysema from the other obstructive airway pathologies is the failure to demonstrate improvement in PFT results in response to the administration of bronchodilators.

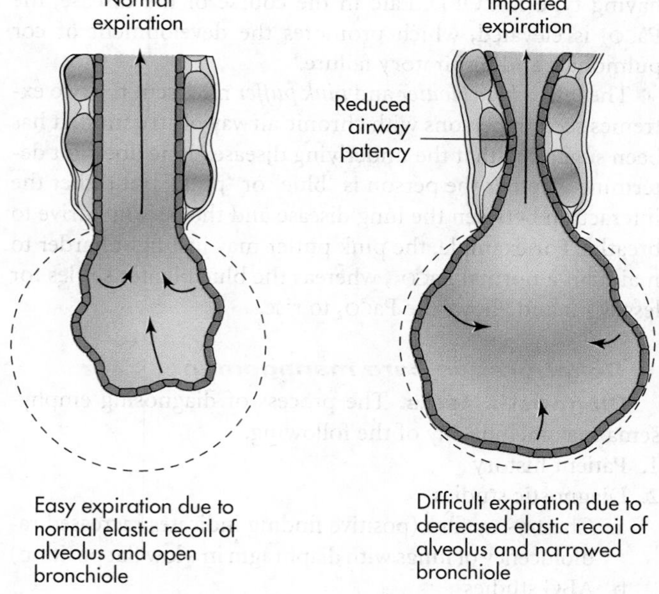


**fig. 32-23** Mechanisms of air trapping in emphysema. Damaged or destroyed alveolar walls no longer support and hold airways open, alveoli lose their elastic recoil. Both of these factors contribute to collapse of alveoli during expiration.

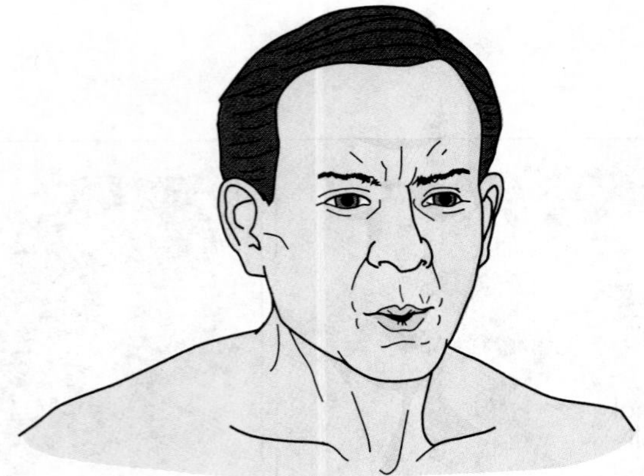

**fig. 32-24** Pursed-lip breathing.

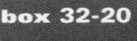

Arterial blood gases are often near normal because of the individual's ability to compensate through increased respiratory rate and tidal volume. Indeed, many people with emphysema overcompensate and develop a mild respiratory alkalosis from hyperventilation. Because resting hypoxemia is absent and ventilation is high, these individuals maintain a normal $Pa_{CO_2}$ despite abnormal gas exchange. A person exhibiting these symptoms of pure emphysema is classified as having type A COPD. Late in the course of the disease, the $Pa_{CO_2}$ is elevated, which promotes the development of cor pulmonale and respiratory failure.

The terms *blue bloater* and *pink puffer* represent the two extremes seen in persons with chronic airway obstruction. It has been suggested that the underlying disease alone does not determine whether the person is "blue" or "pink," but rather the interaction between the lung disease and the person's drive to breathe. For example, the pink puffer may just fight harder to maintain a normal $Pa_{CO_2}$, whereas the blue bloater settles for less work and allows the $Pa_{CO_2}$ to rise.

### *Collaborative care management*

**Diagnostic tests.** The process of diagnosing emphysema may include any of the following:

1. Patient history
2. Diagnostic studies
   a. Chest x-ray film (positive finding indicates increased radiolucency of lungs with diaphragm in a low flat position)
   b. ABG studies
   c. PFTs
   d. Hematology
      (1) AAT assay
      (2) CBC; usually normal
   e. Sputum for culture and sensitivity

Table 32-23 summarizes the components of medical therapy used in the treatment of both chronic bronchitis and emphysema.

**Medications.** See p. 990.

**Treatments.** See p. 991.

**Diet.** See p. 995.

**Activity.** Patients should be up and about as much as possible. They will often have to use portable oxygen when walking and doing other activities.

**box 32-20** *Estimate of Pulmonary Dysfunction Based on FEV/VC Ratio*

Normal lung function: greater than 80% predicted values
Mild impairment: 65% to 85% of predicted values
Moderate impairment: 50% to 64% of predicted values
Severe impairment: 49% or less of predicted values

**Referrals.** Common referrals for the person with emphysema include respiratory therapy, physical therapy, dietary therapy, and social services.

## NURSING MANAGEMENT

### ■ ASSESSMENT

#### Subjective Data

Data to be collected to assess the patient with emphysema include:

- History and onset of the following:
  - Dyspnea: important to investigate if patient correlates the occurrence of dyspnea with any specific illness or other life event; establish how the patient's dyspnea affects ADL.
  - Cough: usually mild or may be absent
  - Sputum production: usually scant white sputum
- Smoking history
- Family history of emphysema
- Past or present exposure to environmental irritants at home or at work
- Self-care modalities
- Medications or other prescribed therapies and their effectiveness in relieving symptoms

#### Objective Data

Data to be collected to assess the patient with emphysema include:

- Assess general appearance: patient usually appears thin with a large chest. (NOTE: this is a normal variant in the elderly; thus it does not always signify pulmonary disease.)
- Assess vital signs for:
  - Tachycardia
  - Tachypnea
- Pulmonary examination
  - Inspection
    - Accessory muscle breathing
    - Forward-leaning posture
    - Pursed-lip breathing
    - Prolonged expiration
    - Barrel chest, increased AP diameter
  - Palpation
    - Decreased lateral expansion
    - Decreased fremitus

Percussion
- Hyperresonance
- Low diaphragm
- Decreased diaphragmatic excursion

Auscultation
- Decreased breath and heart sounds
- Late inspiratory crackles
- Rhonchi (NOTE: adventitious sounds often absent with emphysema)

Laboratory findings assessment
- ABGs
  - Early-stage emphysema—respiratory alkalosis with mild hypoxemia
  - Late-stage emphysema—respiratory acidosis with hypoxemia
- Hematology: positive AAT assay
- Pulmonary function
  - Decreased $FEV_1$, VC, and diffusing capacity
  - Increased TLC, FRC, and RV

## NURSING DIAGNOSES

Nursing diagnoses for patients with COPD are similar regardless of the underlying obstructive airway disease. Nursing diagnoses are determined from analysis of patient data. Nursing diagnoses for the person with COPD may include but are not limited to:

| Diagnostic Title | Possible Etiological Factors |
|---|---|
| Gas exchange, impaired | Low V/Q ratio |
| Breathing pattern, ineffective | Decreased energy/fatigue, airway changes |
| Airway clearance, ineffective | Hypersecretion, tracheobronchial infection, decreased energy/fatigue |
| Nutrition, altered: less than body requirements | Dyspnea, anorexia, sputum production, medication side effects, fatigue |
| Infection, risk for | Decreased lung defenses |
| Fluid volume excess (more common with bronchitis) | Pulmonary hypertension with resultant increased cardiac workload |
| Activity intolerance, risk for | Imbalance between oxygen demand and requirement |
| Sleep pattern disturbance | Dyspnea |
| Fear | Long-term illness and disability, change in role functioning |
| Knowledge deficit: condition and its treatment | Lack of exposure/recall, cognitive limitation, unfamiliarity with information source |

## EXPECTED PATIENT OUTCOMES

The following expected patient outcomes and interventions sections apply to patients with chronic bronchitis, emphysema, or any combination of these two obstructive airway diseases.

1. Demonstrates improved ventilation and oxygenation.
   a. Arterial blood pH and $PCO_2$ returns or stays within acceptable baseline limits.
   b. $PaCO_2$ is at optimal level for individual.
   c. Explains how and when to use oxygen therapy.
2. Demonstrates an effective breathing pattern.
   a. Inspiratory to expiratory ratio is 5 seconds to 10 seconds.
   b. Uses pursed-lip breathing (see Figure 32-24).
   c. Appropriately uses forward-leaning postures (Figure 32-25).
   d. Uses diaphragmatic breathing (abdominal muscle breathing, see Figure 32-26).
   e. Exhales with activity.
   f. Respiratory rate is within near-normal limits, with moderate tidal volume.
3. Demonstrates adequate airway clearance.
   a. Uses effective methods of coughing.
   b. Appropriately uses nebulizers, humidifiers, mistometers, IPPB machine, and medications.
4. Explains dietary changes required after discharge.
   a. Maintains optimal weight for height, age, and gender.
   b. Explains food and fluid requirements and daily plan for achieving them.
   c. Lists specific foods to be avoided.
   d. Explains plan for frequent, small feedings that are soft and that do not require much chewing and the need for increased time required for eating if indicated.
5. Remains infection free.
   a. Temperature remains normal.
   b. Sputum does not change in color, amount, or consistency.
   c. If signs of infection occur, health care provider should be informed.
6. Achieves a normal fluid balance.
   a. Daily weight remains stable.
   b. Electrolyte levels remain within expected levels.
   c. Takes diuretics and digitalis, if prescribed, as ordered.
   d. If signs of edema (weight gain, increase in dyspnea) occur, health care provider is notified.
7. Maintains or works toward an optimal activity level.
   a. Paces activities.
   b. Plans for simplification of activities.
   c. Participates in planned muscle-conditioning program.
8. Uses effective measures to promote sleep.
   a. Determines best position in bed (number of pillows) to minimize dyspnea.
   b. Practices methods that promote sleep (relaxation exercises, meditation, guided imagery, soft music).
9. Demonstrates activities to control stress response to symptoms of fear.
   a. Uses muscle relaxation.
   b. Uses meditation.
   c. Participates in support group.

10-1. Lists common signs and symptoms that require reporting to the health care provider:
   a. Change in sputum color, amount, and consistency.
   b. Increased coughing.
   c. Change in behavior (argumentative, combative).
   d. Increased fatigue.
   e. Increased dyspnea.
   f. Weight gain or loss.
   g. Peripheral edema.
   h. Elevated temperatures.

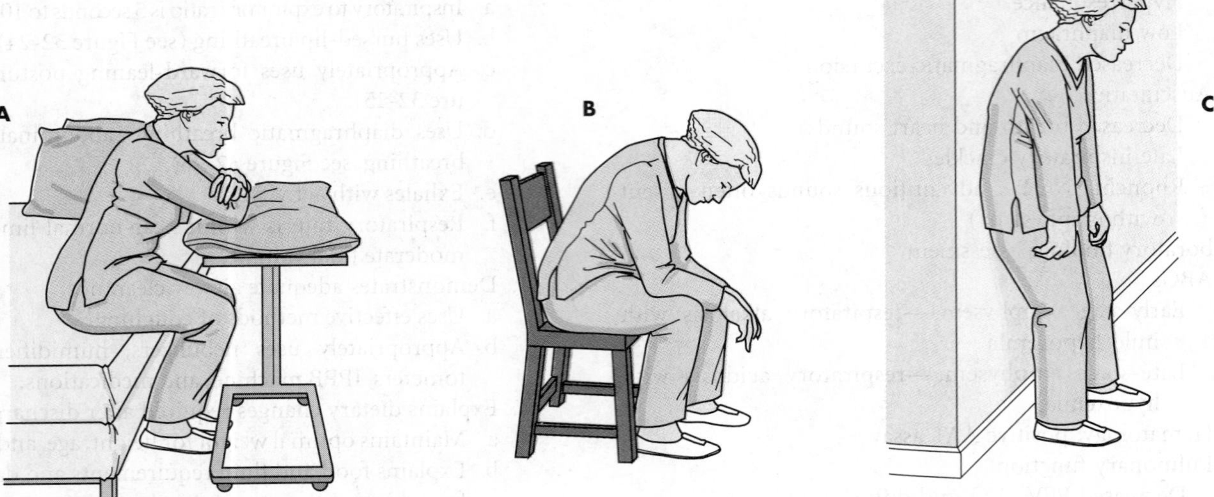


fig. 32-25 Forward-leaning position. A, Patient sits on edge of the bed with arms folded on pillow placed on elevated bedside table. B, Patient in three-point position. Patient sits in chair with feet approximately 1 ft apart and leans forward with elbows on knees. C, Patient leans against wall with feet spread apart, allowing shoulders to sag forward with arms relaxed.

10-2. Demonstrates how to carry out the exercise program to be followed at home, including the following:
   a. Specific exercises to be completed.
   b. Frequency of each exercise.
   c. Criteria for monitoring physical response to exercises, such as heart rate increase or perceived fatigue.

10-3. Demonstrates comprehension of self-care activities.
   a. Explains health maintenance or therapeutic follow-up program.
   b. Describes any home medication or treatment program.
   c. Explains exercise program to be followed at home.
   d. Describes how to obtain professional and community resources necessary to structure a satisfactory home environment.
   e. States plans for ongoing follow-up care.

10-4. Explains the following aspects of home medication or treatment regimens:
   a. Name, dose, action, and side effects of each medication to be used at home.
   b. How and when to use medications ordered on an as-needed basis (e.g., bronchodilators, antibiotics, steroids, antacids).
   c. Techniques necessary for follow-up care (e.g., segmental postural drainage, percussion and vibrating, inhalation therapy treatments).
   d. How to obtain and maintain any needed equipment or supplies (e.g., oxygen, nebulizers, humidifiers, mistometers, IPPB machine, syringes, medications).

10-5. Lists names and telephone numbers of appropriate community support services, such as the Visiting Nurse Association and a home medical equipment supplier.

## INTERVENTIONS

Chronic obstructive pulmonary disease and all of its actual or potential impact on the individual's life are most effectively managed by a multidisciplinary team. Pulmonary health care teams consisting of physicians, nurses, respiratory therapists, occupational therapists, physical therapists, dietitians, social workers, and psychologists or psychiatrists provide a comprehensive approach to assist patients to attain or maintain their optimal level of function within the constraints of their pulmonary disability.

Although it is difficult to measure the physiological effects of these programs, hospitalization of patients who have participated in them is less frequent, and most people state that they feel better. The complex multidisciplinary rehabilitation team is the ideal, but the nurse functioning in a small community hospital or community health agency can provide effective rehabilitation activities for the person with COPD.

Nursing interventions for persons with chronic bronchitis and pulmonary emphysema are the same, and discussion of specific medications and aerosol therapy are discussed in the section on chronic bronchitis. Other medications used less often are discussed next.

### Administering Medications

#### *Digitalis and diuretics*

Digitalis may be prescribed for patients with COPD and left ventricular failure. The patient receiving a digitalis preparation should be carefully monitored for side effects.[25]

Patients with increased dyspnea secondary to pulmonary edema or with right ventricular failure or corticosteroid-induced fluid retention may benefit from diuretics. When diuretics are given, the patient should be carefully monitored for side effects. Those taking thiazide diuretics need to be told to eat foods high in potassium, such as bananas, oranges, prunes, raisins, and potatoes.

#### Psychopharmacological agents

Psychopharmacological agents may need to be prescribed for some patients with severe emotional disturbances. The type of agent and size of dose are individually determined, but in general, the older the patient, the smaller the dose.

### Improving Gas Exchange

Arterial blood gases are monitored for indications of hypoxemia, respiratory acidosis, and respiratory alkalosis. Hypoxemia and hypercapnia often occur simultaneously, and the signs and symptoms of each are similar. These include headache, irritability, confusion, increasing somnolence, asterixis (flapping tremors of extremities), cardiac dysrhythmias, and tachycardia.

If hypocapnia is developing, tachypnea, vertigo, tingling of the extremities, muscular weakness, and spasm are often present. The presence of signs and symptoms associated with altered levels of $PaO_2$ and $PaCO_2$ depend more on the *rate of change than on the degree of change* in the levels. *Rapidly changing signs usually indicate a rapid worsening of the patient's condition.* At the same time, patients with long-standing hypoxemia and hypercapnia may be relatively asymptomatic because they have physiologically accommodated to increased levels of $PaCO_2$ and decreased levels of $PaO_2$.

#### Oxygen therapy

Oxygen therapy is required for patients with COPD who are unable to maintain a $PaO_2$ greater than 55 mm Hg or an oxygen saturation greater than 85% or more at rest and for those who cannot carry out ADL (breathing, eating, dressing, toileting) without becoming very short of breath. In these patients, 1 to 2 L oxygen is usually given via nasal prongs to relieve hypoxemia and decrease pulmonary hypertension, which in turn decreases the load on the right side of the heart. Studies have shown that patients receive the most benefit from oxygen therapy if the oxygen is used continuously. A common misunderstanding expressed by patients requiring ongoing oxygen therapy is that they should use their oxygen only when they are symptomatic (i.e., short of breath) to avoid becoming habituated to the oxygen and thus requiring higher levels of oxygen. The nurse needs to clarify that habituation to $O_2$ will not occur. The nurse also stresses the importance of continual oxygen use in order to receive maximal benefits of the therapy.

Because many patients with COPD have chronic carbon dioxide retention, their stimulus to breathe is their low $PaO_2$ level. Patients must understand that high flow rates of oxygen (greater than 6 L/min) and high concentrations (greater than 40%) may elevate their $PaO_2$ to a level that removes the stimulus by which they breathe, resulting in respiratory failure (see the section on respiratory failure later in this chapter).

### Improving Efficiency of Breathing Pattern

1. Teach patient to slow respiratory rate and to breathe slowly and rhythmically.
2. Discourage patient from taking large gulps of air.
3. Teach patient to increase inspiratory/expiratory ratio so that expiration takes twice as long as inhalation.
   a. Teach patient to count in seconds and to concentrate on increasing time taken to exhale.
   b. Count to 5 on inhalation and to 10 on exhalation.

#### Pursed-lip breathing

Teach pursed-lip breathing if the patient is not already using it (see Figure 32-24). To teach pursed-lip breathing the patient is asked to (1) inhale through the nose for several seconds with the mouth closed and (2) exhale slowly (taking twice as long as inhalation) through pursed lips held in a narrow slit. Pursed-lip breathing maintains patency of collapsible airways during exhalation and helps reduce air trapping. It decreases the respiratory rate, increases tidal volume, decreases $PaCO_2$, and increases $PaO_2$ and $SaO_2$. Some patients use pursed-lip breathing spontaneously with exertion.

#### Forward-leaning position

Teach the forward-leaning position for exhalation. Using a forward-leaning position of 30 to 40 degrees with the head tilted at a 16- to 18-degree angle is an effective way to improve exhalation (see Figure 32-25). As mentioned earlier, patients with emphysema have increased TLC and RV with the diaphragm in a fixed, flattened position. Therefore the diaphragm cannot assist in exhalation as it does normally. Leaning forward allows more air to be removed from the lungs on exhalation. The leaning-forward position can be achieved with the patient in either a sitting or standing position. For example, (1) the patient can sit on the edge of the bed or a chair and lean forward on two or three pillows placed on a table or overbed stand; (2) the patient can sit in a chair with the legs spread apart shoulder width (or wider, if obese) with the elbows on the knees and the arms and hands relaxed; or (3) the patient can stand with the back and hips against the wall with the feet spread apart and about 12 inches (30 cm) from the wall. The patient then relaxes and leans forward. In these positions the patient cannot use the accessory muscles of respiration, and the upward action of the diaphragm is improved.

#### Abdominal breathing and exercises

Teach abdominal breathing, leg-raising exercises, inhalation-exhalation exercises, and muscle-reconditioning exercises.

Abdominal breathing improves the breathing efficiency of persons with COPD because it assists the patient to elevate the diaphragm. Abdominal breathing can be taught in the sitting or lying position. In the sitting position, the patient sits on the side of the bed or in a chair and holds a small pillow or a book against the abdomen. The patient then exhales slowly while leaning forward and pressing the pillow or book against the abdomen. In the lying position, a small pillow or a book is placed on the abdomen and the patient is asked to "puff out" the abdomen and raise the pillow or book as high as possible. The patient then exhales slowly through pursed lips while pulling in on the abdominal muscles. Manual pressure on the upper abdomen during expiration facilitates this maneuver (Figure 32-26). In addition to abdominal breathing, exercises to strengthen the abdominal muscles help patients use their abdominal muscles more effectively in emptying their lungs.

This controlled breathing pattern is to be used while performing various ADL, from sitting, standing, walking, and climbing stairs to more complex activities. As this pattern becomes natural, the patient will use it automatically during periods of increased shortness of breath. Persons who do not know how to use controlled breathing tend to increase their respiratory rate and their work of breathing when they are short of breath. As a result, physiological obstruction increases, oxygen requirements increase, and effective ventilation decreases. Changing a person's respiratory pattern requires much effort by both the individual and those providing care.

This same method of teaching augmented abdominal (diaphragmatic) breathing can be used to teach the patient to cough. The difference is that expiration is forced down to RV. This maneuver often stimulates the cough reflex. If it does not, the person is taught to cough actively at the end of full expiration. Physiologically, forced expiration simulates the effects of a cough and is therefore more effective than telling the patient to take a deep breath and then cough. For more information about raising secretions, see p. 994, 1e.

*Leg-raising exercises,* with each leg being raised alternately as the patient exhales, is one way to strengthen abdominal muscles. Another way is to have the patient raise the head and shoulders from the bed while he or she exhales. With practice and encouragement, the patient can do the exercises 10 times each morning and evening after clearing the lungs as completely as possible of secretions.

*Inhalation-exhalation exercises* emphasize the need to prolong exhalation to at least two times longer than inhalation. Patients who are able to walk can be taught to count in seconds and to concentrate on exhaling slowly and fully. While learning to exhale with exertion, the patient exhales during an activity such as bending over or sitting down.

*Muscle reconditioning* refers to a variety of muscle-toning exercises. For patients who are able to be out of bed, walking, using a treadmill, or riding a stationary bicycle is helpful. The exercise period is started slowly with 10 minutes twice daily three times a week, increasing to 20 minutes twice daily three times a week. The patient needs to be assessed for his or her

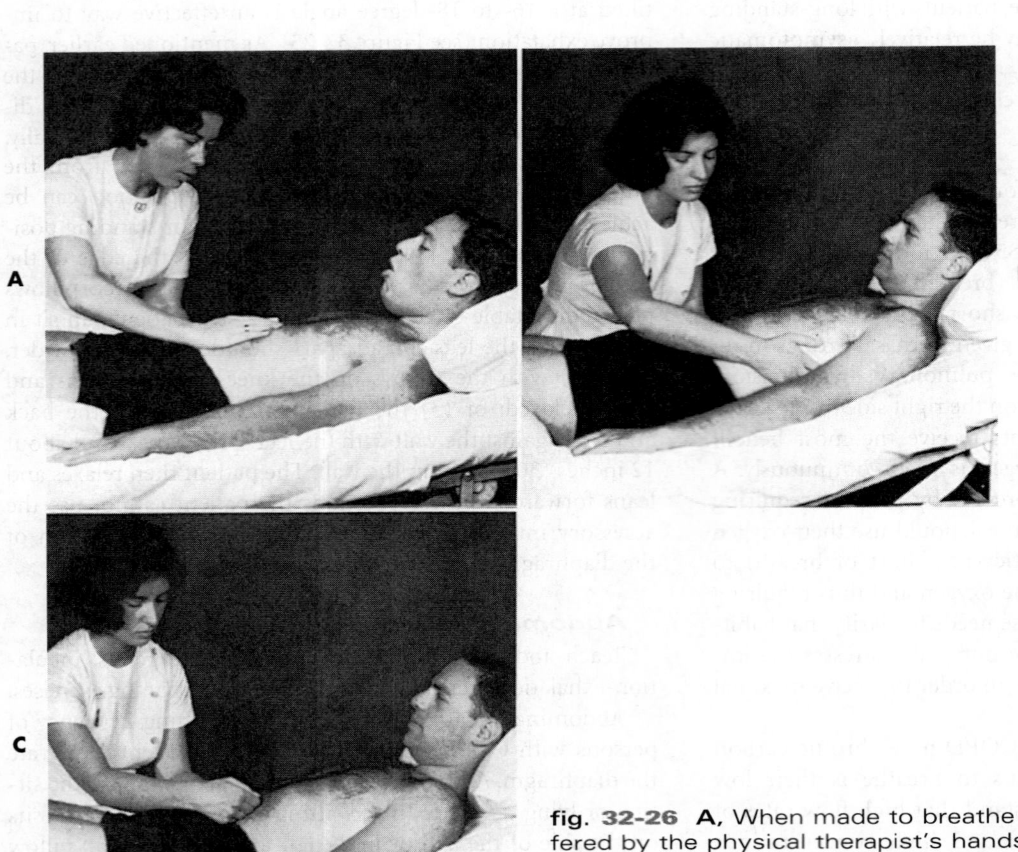

**fig. 32-26** **A,** When made to breathe against the resistance offered by the physical therapist's hands, the patient is made aware of every phase of respiration and use of muscle groups. **B,** The patient learns how to expand fully the lower lobes by breathing against counterpressure applied to the side of the chest during inspiration. **C,** The patient is taught diaphragmatic control by breathing against resistance applied in the costophrenic angle.

ability to carry out such an exercise program, and a staff member should be present during the exercise period.

### Pulmonary physiotherapy

Although pulmonary physiotherapy activities (segmental postural drainage, percussing, and vibrating) may be performed by a physical therapist, they are often part of a nurse's responsibility. Regardless of where the primary responsibility lies, nurses must be familiar with the techniques so that they can demonstrate and reinforce them and ensure that the individual is doing them correctly. Also, the need for pulmonary physiotherapy may occur at a time when the physical therapist is not available to the patient.

### Segmental postural drainage

Segmental postural drainage with percussing and vibration combines the force of gravity with the natural ciliary activity of the small bronchial airways to move secretions upward toward the main bronchi and the trachea. From this point the patient can cough secretions up, or they can be suctioned. In the treatment of COPD, drainage of all segments is usually accomplished by placing patients in various postural drainage positions (Figure 32-27). Treatment may also be directed at draining specific areas of the lung. While the patient is in each position, *percussion* with a cupped hand is performed over the area being drained. This maneuver helps loosen secretions and stimulate coughing (Figure 32-28). After percussing the area for approximately 1 minute, the patient is instructed to breathe deeply. Vibrating (pressure applied with a vibrating movement of the hand on the chest) is performed during the expiratory phase of the deep breath. This assists the patient to exhale more fully. The procedure is repeated as necessary. When the patient cannot tolerate a head-down position, a modified position is used.

Positions that provide gravity drainage of the lungs can be achieved in several ways, and the procedure selected usually depends on the age and general condition of the person, as well as the lobe or lobes of the lungs where secretions have accumulated. A young person usually can tolerate greater lowering of the head than an elderly person whose vascular system adapts more slowly to change of position. A severely debilitated patient may be able to tolerate only slight changes in position.

Postural drainage can be accomplished in several ways. Electric hospital beds can be tilted into a head-down position with little difficulty. If an electric bed is not available (e.g., in the home), blocks can be placed under the casters at the foot of the bed, or a hydraulic lift can be used under the foot of the bed.

The nurse needs to know the part of the lung that is affected and how to position the patient to drain that portion of the lung. For example, if the right middle lobe of the lung is

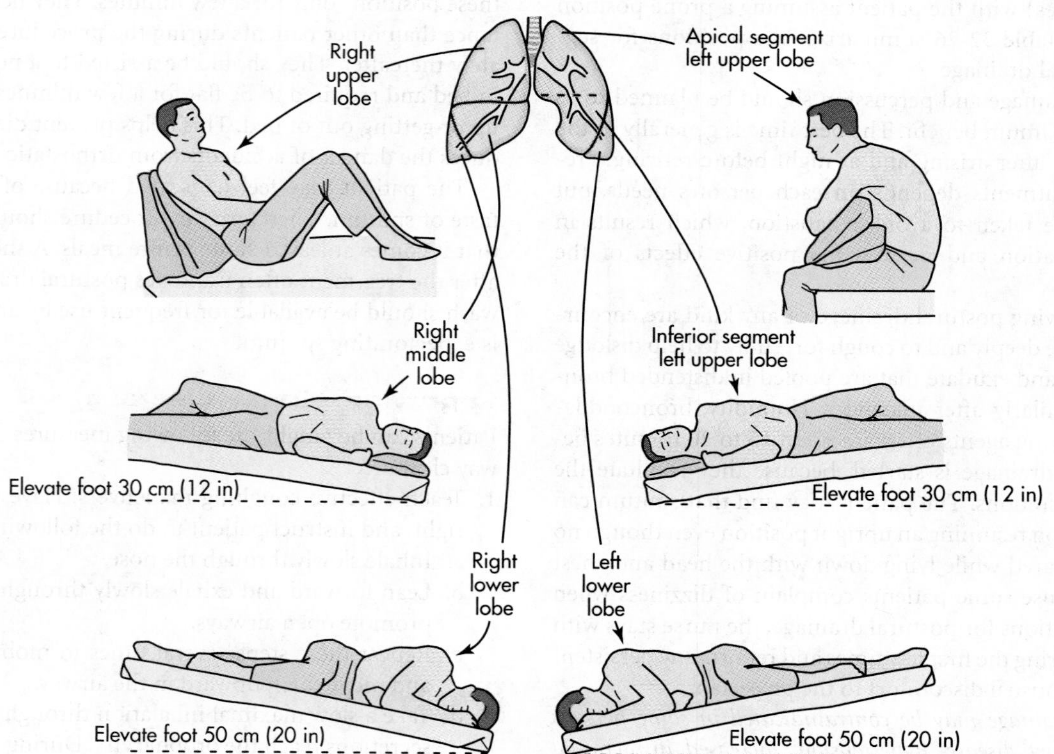


**fig. 32-27** Postural drainage requires that the patient assume various positions to facilitate the flow of secretions from various portions of the lung into the bronchi, trachea, and throat so that secretions can be raised and expectorated more easily. Drawing shows the correct position to drain various portions of the lung.

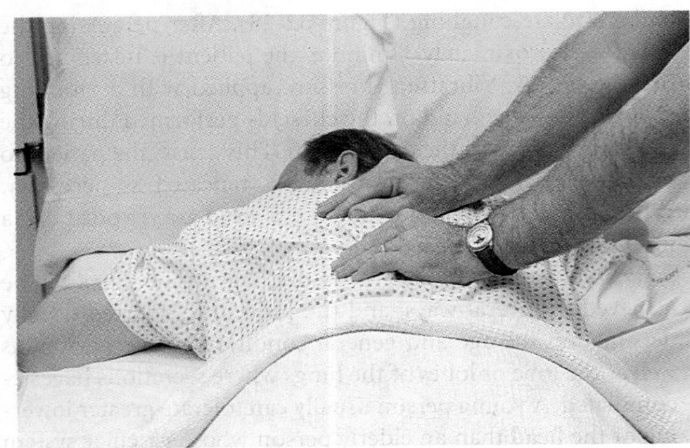

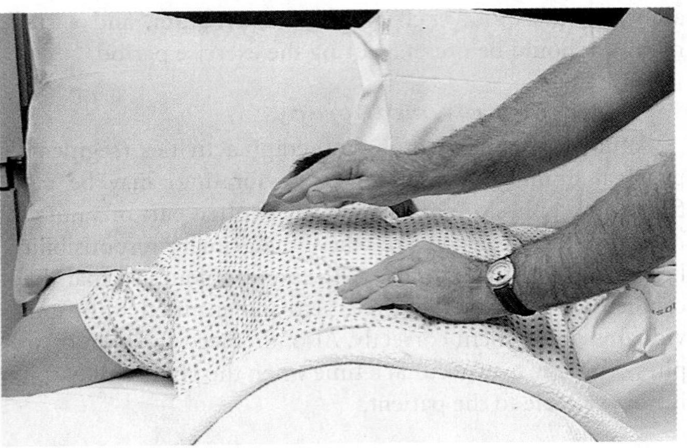

**fig. 32-28** **A**, Hand position for chest wall percussion during physiotherapy. **B**, Chest wall percussion, alternating hand motion against the patient's chest wall.

affected, drainage will be accomplished best by way of the right middle bronchus. The patient should lie supine with the body turned at approximately a 45-degree angle. The angle can be maintained by pillow supports placed under the right side from the shoulders to the hips. The foot of the bed is raised about 30 cm (12 inches). This position can be maintained fairly comfortably by most patients for half an hour at a time. On the other hand, if the lower posterior area of the lung is affected, the foot of the bed can be raised 45 to 50 cm (18 to 20 inches) with the patient assuming a prone position for drainage. Table 32-26 summarizes the positions for segmental postural drainage.

Postural drainage and percussion should be planned so as to achieve maximum benefit. The best time is generally in the morning soon after arising and at night before retiring. Frequency of treatments depends on each person's needs, but care should be taken to avoid exhaustion, which results in shallow ventilation and negates the positive effects of the treatment.

Patients having postural drainage of any kind are encouraged to breathe deeply and to cough forcefully to help dislodge thick sputum and exudate that are pooled in distended bronchioles, particularly after inactivity. Humidity, bronchodilators, or liquefying agents often are given 15 to 20 minutes before postural drainage is started, because they facilitate the removal of secretions. The patient may find that sputum can best be raised on resuming an upright position even though no drainage appeared while lying down with the head and chest lowered. Because some patients complain of dizziness when assuming positions for postural drainage, the nurse stays with the patient during the first few times and reports any persistent dizziness or unusual discomfort to the physician.

*Postural drainage may be contraindicated in some persons because of heart disease, hypertension, increased intracranial pressure, extreme dyspnea, osteoporosis, or advanced age.* However, most people can be taught to assume the positions for postural drainage and can proceed without help after being supervised once or twice.

*Chest percussion is contraindicated* (1) in *patients with pulmonary emboli, hemorrhage, exacerbation of bronchospasms,* or *severe pain* and (2) *over areas of resectable carcinoma.* Often, patients with a chronic pulmonary problem need to be taught to perform postural drainage independently so that they can continue it at home. The position usually is maintained for 10 minutes at first, and the period of time is gradually lengthened to 15 to 30 minutes as the patient becomes accustomed to the position. At first, elderly persons usually are able to tolerate these positions only for a few minutes. They need more assistance than other patients during the procedure and immediately thereafter. They should be assisted to a normal position in bed and required to lie flat for a few minutes before sitting up or getting out of bed. This helps prevent dizziness and reduces the danger of accidents from orthostatic hypotension.

The patient may feel nauseated because of the odor and taste of sputum. Therefore the procedure should be timed so that it comes at least 1 hour before meals. A short rest period after the treatment often improves postural drainage. Mouthwash should be available for frequent use by any patient who is expectorating sputum.

### Improving Airway Clearance

Patients can be taught the following measures to improve airway clearance:

1. Teach effective coughing maneuvers. Have patient sit upright, and instruct patient to do the following:
   a. Inhale slowly through the nose.
   b. Lean forward and exhale slowly through pursed lips to promote open airways.
   c. Repeat these steps several times to mobilize secretions and move them upward in the airway.
   d. Take a slow maximal inhalation through the nose when secretions reach the oropharynx. During exhalation, use short, repeated coughs to minimize bronchospasm.
   e. For patients who have thick tenacious secretions that are difficult to expectorate, a forced expiratory technique known as *huffing* is recommended. In *huffing* the pa-

**table 32-26** *Positions for Segmental Postural Drainage, Percussion, and Vibrating*

| Area of Lung | Position of Patient | Area to be Percussed or Vibrated |
|---|---|---|
| Upper lobe | | |
| Apical bronchus | Semi-Fowler's position, leaning to right, then left, then forward | Over area of shoulder blades with fingers extending over clavicles |
| Posterior bronchus | Upright at 45-degree angle, rolled forward against a pillow at 45 degrees on left and then right side | Over shoulder blade on each side |
| Anterior bronchus | Supine with pillow under knees | Over anterior chest just below clavicles |
| Middle lobe (lateral and medial bronchus) | Trendelenburg's position at 30-degree angle or with foot of bed elevated 35-40 cm (14-16 inches), turned slightly to left | Anterior and lateral right chest from axillary fold to midanterior chest |
| Lingula (superior and inferior bronchus) | Trendelenburg's position at 30-degree angle or with foot of bed elevated 35-40 cm (14-16 inches), turned slightly to right | Left axillary fold to midanterior chest |
| Apical bronchus | Prone with pillow under hips | Lower third of posterior rib cage on both sides |
| Medial bronchus | Trendelenburg's position at 45-degree angle or with foot of bed raised 45-50 cm (18-20 inches) on right side | Lower third of left posterior rib cage |
| Lateral bronchus | Trendelenburg's position at 45-degree angle or with foot of bed raised 45-50 cm (18-20 inches) on left side | Lower third of right posterior rib cage |
| Posterior bronchus | Prone Trendelenburg's position at 45-degree angle with pillow under hips | Lower third of posterior rib cage on both sides |

tient takes a deep breath and while slowly exhaling opens the glottis by saying the word "huff," resulting in a series of coughs that help to clear the airway.

f. Inhale maximally after coughing to reinflate alveoli.

2. To thin secretions, a fluid intake of 3 to 4 L has traditionally been encouraged unless contraindicated. However, evidence suggests that this quantity of fluids may not be needed to keep secretions mobile. Although expectorants are sometimes prescribed, some experts believe they do more harm than good. Water is still considered to be the best expectorant, and adequate hydration without fluid overload should be encouraged.
3. Teach postural drainage, percussion, and vibrating as discussed in Table 32-26.
4. Airway clearance maneuvers may be enhanced by strengthening respiratory muscles.

## Improving Nutrition

Persons with COPD often demonstrate excessive weight loss. The following factors may contribute to weight loss:

1. A feeling of satiety with small amounts of food because the flattened diaphragm compresses abdominal contents
2. Dyspnea interfering with eating
3. Increased dyspnea when eating because the stomach pushes up against the diaphragm
4. Decreased appetite secondary to chronic sputum production
5. Gastric irritation associated with bronchodilators and steroids
6. Increased work of breathing requiring increased caloric intake to maintain weight; makes it imperative that the patient with COPD maintain adequate nutritional levels, because
   a. Diminished total weight is correlated with a dramatic decrease in respiratory muscle (especially the diaphragm) size and strength
   b. Inadequate nutritional status and in particular deficiencies in vitamins A and C decrease resistance to infection
   c. Protein insufficiency decreases colloid osmotic pressure, which increases the risk of pulmonary edema

Nursing actions focused on assisting the patient with COPD to maintain adequate nutrition include:

1. Explore usual dietary habits (collect a 24-hour diet history).
2. Counsel patient to select foods that provide a high-protein, high-calorie diet (Box 32-21) with vitamin supplementation.
3. It is important to counsel the patient to select foods that provide higher calorie levels through higher fat content rather than by high carbohydrate levels. Persons with advanced chronic bronchitis or emphysema are unable to exhale the excess carbon dioxide that is a natural end product of carbohydrate metabolism. Therefore calories obtained from high-carbohydrate foods may elevate $PaCO_2$ levels in persons with COPD.
4. Advise patient that prepackaged food supplements such as milk shakes or snack bars taken between meals provide an excellent source of protein and calories.
5. Teach that smaller, more frequent meals are often tolerated better than three larger meals.
6. Consider financial status and ethnic background when planning meals.

### Preventing Infection

The *most common complication of COPD,* and the cause of most hospital readmissions, is *respiratory infection.* Pulmonary system response to the infectious process includes increased respiratory rate, mucosal irritation, and increased mucus production. Because of these localized responses, patients may have bronchospasm and a change in their pattern of sputum production. If the infection remains untreated, the result is an overall increased work of breathing with eventual respiratory failure. Thus the person with COPD should avoid respiratory infections. The patient should be counseled to take the following steps to *decrease* the chance of contracting a pulmonary infection.

1. Avoid large crowds, especially during known influenza seasons.
   a. Avoid contact with people who have an upper respiratory infection.
   b. Receive influenza and pneumonia immunizations.
2. Contact health care provider if the following common signs and symptoms occur:
   a. Change in sputum color, amount, and consistency
   b. Increased cough
   c. Change in behavior (e.g., more argumentative than usual) that indicates an increase in $PaCO_2$
   d. Increased fatigue
   e. Increased dyspnea
   f. Weight gain
   g. Peripheral edema
   h. Elevated temperature

Antimicrobial agents prescribed to treat respiratory tract infections in persons with COPD are discussed on p. 981.

### Preventing Fluid Volume Excess

Low $PaO_2$ is a potent pulmonary vasoconstrictor, which increases pulmonary arterial pressure and causes pulmonary hypertension. If pulmonary hypertension exists for a prolonged time, the increased workload on the heart's right ventricle will result in right ventricular failure, or *cor pulmonale.* Depending on its severity and duration, patients with cor pulmonale will have neck vein distention, hepatomegaly, dependent peripheral edema, and, as oncotic pressure is exceeded, ascites and pleural effusions. Nursing interventions to prevent fluid volume excess in patients with cor pulmonale are based on the understanding that the disease is treated by intervening with the cause of the pulmonary hypertension. Therefore nursing interventions focus on promoting adequate ventilation for optimal oxygen–carbon dioxide exchange and relieving symptoms that result from the fluid volume excess. Thus a nursing care plan for the person with COPD that promotes optimal ventilation will help prevent fluid volume excess resulting from cor pulmonale. Other interventions focused on the symptoms of fluid volume excess include:

1. Weigh daily in the same amount of clothing and at the same time of day on the same scale.
2. Monitor intake and output accurately. (NOTE: Although it is unknown whether fluid restriction is effective in the actual treatment of cor pulmonale, excess fluid intake may overwhelm an already compromised cardiac system.)
3. Encourage moderate exercise or change patient's position frequently to promote adequate lung perfusion.
4. Measure abdominal girth at regular intervals to assess the possible presence or progression of ascites.
5. Administer diuretics as ordered. When diuretics are given, the patient should be carefully monitored for side effects. Those taking thiazide diuretics will need to be taught about eating foods high in potassium, such as bananas, oranges, prunes, raisins, and potatoes.
6. Administer digitalis as ordered. (NOTE: Digitalis is of questionable usefulness in pure right-sided heart failure.) Persons receiving digitalis should be carefully monitored for side effects.

**box 32-21 Foods to Increase Protein and Caloric Intake**

Offer frequent small feedings of foods high in protein and calories such as the following:
- Milk shakes
- Flavored gelatin or pudding with whipped cream
- Cream soups made with half-and-half
- Peanut butter spread on crackers, bananas, pears, or apples
- Crackers and cheese, nuts, dried fruits, and ice creams readily available for snacks

### Assisting with Breathing and Rest

1. Place patient in position of comfort, usually semi-Fowler's or high-Fowler's.
2. Assist patient with progressive relaxation exercises and meditation (see the Patient/Family Teaching Boxes on the next page).

### Assisting with Control of Environment

Abrupt changes in weather or hot or cold environments can increase sputum production and bronchial obstruction.

### Temperature and Humidity

1. Humidity of 30% to 50% is ideal. This can be achieved by a humidifier as necessary.
2. An air conditioner may reduce dyspnea by controlling temperature and preventing pollutants from outside air from entering. The cost of an air conditioner is a medically deductible expense for persons with COPD.
3. Wearing a scarf over the nose and mouth in cold weather helps warm the air and prevent bronchospasm. Masks for this purpose are also available.
4. Moving to another climate is usually not advised unless there is some other medical indication for doing so. Persons living at high altitudes may be advised to move to a lower altitude or use supplemental oxygen continuously.
5. Travel by airplane is possible. The airline needs to be informed in advance of the need for supplemental oxygen during the flight.

### Avoiding Inhaled Irritants

Air pollution is a common problem in modern civilization and is a serious threat to persons with COPD, who should observe the following:

1. Heed pollution alerts, and avoid being outdoors when an alert is in effect.
2. Use an air conditioner, HEPA filter, or electrostatic filter to remove particulate matter from air.
   a. Keep filters clean.
   b. Follow manufacturer's directions for use.
3. Use an activated charcoal filter if offending odors or gas pollutants are a problem.
4. Avoid secondhand smoke.

### Improving Activity Tolerance

1. Allow ample time for activities; do not rush patient.
2. Provide oxygen as needed before and during activities.
3. Encourage gradual increase in activities such as walking.
4. Provide positive feedback on progress, and encourage new endeavors when patient is ready.

### Assisting with Sleep

Persons with COPD usually sleep only for short periods. Many patients are most comfortable sleeping in an upright position in bed or in a lounge chair with footrest.

1. Assist with relaxation exercises at bedtime.
2. Give backrub at bedtime, and encourage family member to do same at home.
3. Provide relaxing music at bedtime, and encourage same at home.
4. Ascertain preferred position for sleep, usually high Fowler's.
5. Establish regular bedtime to meet patient's usual schedule.
6. Give bedtime snack, if desired.

### Assisting with Fear Reduction

Persons who are short of breath are usually anxious and frightened.

1. Encourage patient to talk about anxiety and fears with nurse and family members.
2. Take measures already discussed to improve airway clearance and breathing.
3. Do not leave patient alone during periods of breathlessness.
4. Explain to family reason for not leaving patient at home alone for long periods; assist them with securing community resources to assist as necessary (e.g., Homemakers, Visiting Nurse Association).

**patient/family teaching**

**Progressive Relaxation Exercises**

1. Contract each muscle to a count of 10 and then relax it.
2. Do exercises in quiet room while sitting or lying in a comfortable position.
3. Do exercises to relaxing music, if desired.
4. Have another person serve as a "coach" by giving command to contract specific muscle, count to 10, and relax muscle.
5. The following are examples of exercises helpful to some persons with COPD.
   a. Raise shoulders, shrug them, and relax for 5 seconds; then relax them completely.
   b. Make a fist of both hands, squeeze them tightly for 5 seconds, and then relax them completely.

### Patient/Family Education

Persons with COPD play a major role in monitoring their own condition and in maintaining their physical and psychological functioning at the maximal possible level (see the Research Box).

For these reasons, it is imperative that the nurse thoroughly assess the patient's knowledge of COPD, including its cause and treatment. Individualized teaching plans based on the patient's knowledge level can then be developed. The Guidelines for Care Box on p. 999 lists areas that may be included in the teaching program.

#### *Health promotion/prevention*

According to the CDC, only 30% of persons at high risk for influenza-related complications, such as persons with COPD, are vaccinated. A year 2000 national health objective is to achieve influenza vaccination levels of at least 60% in noninstitutionalized high-risk persons. Unless more persons who are at high risk can be convinced to receive influenza vaccine, this goal will not be reached by the year 2000.[40]

**patient/family teaching**

**Meditation Exercises**

1. Sit or lie quietly with eyes closed and attempt to relax all muscles, beginning with feet and moving upward.
2. Breathe in through the nose slowly (may help to count slowly to 4 on inhalation) and exhale slowly through pursed lips (mentally count to 6) with a natural rhythm, relaxed and peaceful (this can be coached or performed without assistance).
3. Survey the body for points of tension. Consciously relax the tense areas. The body is peaceful and relaxed.
4. Continue breathing as above, aware of the feeling of well-being throughout your body. This can be continued for 10 to 20 minutes, or after 5 minutes go to step 5.
5. Listen for (or visualize) a special relaxing sound (or image). Listen to it closely (or visualize) all the while breathing as above.
6. At this point, positive suggestion can be used; for example, "I am in control of my body. When I find myself getting tense, I can take a moment to stop and breathe in all the air that I need and let the tension flow away."
7. After mental suggestion, continue breathing easily and slowly come back to normal alert mental state.
8. Meditation can be used at any time to induce a relaxed state of mind (e.g., to promote sleep).

The cornerstone of prevention of emphysema is education. Public education must focus on the pulmonary health risks associated with inhaled irritants, regardless of their source. Increased public awareness of the vital role clean air plays in pulmonary health is essential for the success of any legislative actions promoting air quality standards. Individuals must also be educated to understand the importance of personal responsibility to decrease their own health risk through smoking cessation.

Persons with a family history of emphysema should be screened for AAT deficiency. It is imperative that persons with this enzyme deficiency take active measures to prevent additive lung damage from smoking, air pollution, and infection. Persons identified as being at high risk for emphysema may require vocational counseling if their current work environment is known to have inhaled irritants. These individuals also should be counseled to receive the influenza vaccine yearly and the pneumococcal vaccine every 3 to 5 years.

## research

Reference: Scherer YK, Schmieder LE: The effect of a pulmonary rehabilitation program on self-efficacy, perception of dyspnea, and physical endurance, *Heart Lung* 26(1):15, 1997.

The purpose of this study was to determine the effect of attendance at an outpatient pulmonary rehabilitation (OPR) program on changes in self-efficacy, perception of dyspnea, and exercise endurance in patients with chronic obstructive pulmonary disease (COPD). Sixty patients with the diagnosis of COPD participated in this study. The participants ranged in age from 35 to 82 years with a mean age of 65 years. The subjects were tested with the COPD Self-Efficacy Scale (CSES) and the Dyspnea Scale and the distance walked on the 12-minute walking-distance test (12 MD) before and after the outpatient rehabilitation program. The OPR program consisted of 36 1-hour classes conducted three times per week for 12 weeks by a clinical nurse specialist. Breathing retraining (including pursed-lip breathing and diaphragmatic breathing exercises) were an important part of the education program. Patients were encouraged to incorporate these breathing retraining techniques into the exercise component of the program to make the best use of their ventilatory capabilities. The educational component was followed by exercise training and supervised workout sessions. The subjects' heart rate, blood pressure, and respirations were routinely monitored. Pulse oximetry was used to monitor oxygen saturation. There was a significant difference between preprogram and postprogram scores on the CSES, the Dyspnea Scale, and the 12 MD. These results indicated that higher self-efficacy scores on the CSES were correlated with lowered perceptions of dyspnea and greatest distance walked in 12 minutes. The authors concluded that an OPR can improve self-efficacy or confidence in participants' ability to manage or avoid breathing difficulty. Improvement in self-efficacy also may be a factor in decreased perception of dyspnea and increased exercise endurance. Methods to increase self-efficacy expectations with education and exercise training provide an approach to assist persons with COPD to manage breathing difficulty more effectively.

## EVALUATION

To evaluate the effectiveness of nursing interventions, compare patient behaviors with those stated in the expected patient outcomes. Successful achievement of patient outcomes for the person with COPD is indicated by:

1. Ventilation and oxygenation are improved.
   a. $PaO_2$, $PaCO_2$, and pH are at acceptable levels.
   b. Verbalizes need to use oxygen therapy almost continuously. If not using continuously, use while sleeping and exercising.
2. Breathing pattern is effective.
   a. Takes twice as long to exhale as to inhale (5 : 10 seconds).
   b. Uses pursed-lip breathing when exhaling.
   c. Leans forward on an overstuffed chair to increase ability to exhale.
   d. Concentrates on abdominal breathing when lying in bed and when up and about.
   e. Inhales before beginning an activity and exhales while doing activity.
   f. Has respiratory rate of 24 to 28 respirations per minute and moderate tidal volume.
3. Airway clearance is improving.
   a. Uses inhaler with bronchodilator as necessary to clear secretions.
   b. Is well hydrated.
   c. Inhales deeply and exhales down to RV to empty lungs and initiate cough reflex.
4. Verbalizes dietary changes after discharge.
   a. Prefers to eat several small meals daily because it causes less shortness of breath.
   b. Verbalizes that gas-producing foods such as cabbage, baked beans, and raw green pepper and radishes are to be avoided because they cause discomfort and bloating.
5. Remains infection free.
   a. Temperature is normal.
   b. Sputum is clear.
   c. Knows to call health care provider if sputum color changes to yellow, green, or rusty, or if streaked with bright-red blood.
6. Fluid balance is normal.
   a. Weight remains stable.
   b. Electrolyte levels are within normal range.
   c. Is taking diuretic as prescribed.
   d. Verbalizes need to call health care provider if weight gain, dyspnea, or dependent edema occurs.
7. Maintains or works toward improving activity level.
   a. Does muscle-reconditioning activities daily at home and participates in group reconditioning sessions twice weekly at support group sponsored by local branch of ALA.
   b. Paces activities, using oxygen most of the time.
8. Verbalizes measures used to support sleep.
   a. Uses five pillows to achieve upright position with each arm supported on a pillow.

b. Practices relaxation exercises and meditates to soft music.

9. Is able to control stress response.
   a. Demonstrates muscle relaxation.
   b. Verbalizes how to meditate using taped music to improve relaxation.
   c. Participates in support group at local ALA office.

10-1. Verbalizes signs and symptoms that should be reported to health care provider:
   a. Change in sputum color, amount, and consistency
   b. Increase in cough
   c. Irritability, inability to control temper (both signs of increased $PaCO_2$)
   d. Fatigue, especially when unusual for activity being undertaken
   e. Increase in dyspnea
   f. Weight gain or weight loss
   g. Swollen feet and legs
   h. Elevated temperature

10-2. Demonstrates exercises.

10-3. Demonstrates how to carry out activities with the least expenditure of energy.
   a. Has repositioned several pieces of furniture at home to meet need to have things used frequently nearby.
   b. Knows community resources to call for oxygen equipment and other assistance.
   c. Family member has been taught how to assist with postural drainage. Nurse or physical therapist from home health agency comes in weekly to check progress with activities and exercise.

10-4. Knows names, dose, action, and side effects of all medications.

10-5. Has developed own phone directory of community resources.

## GERONTOLOGICAL CONSIDERATIONS

Many patients with COPD are elderly and may require additional time and support in learning how to take their medications, perform breathing exercises, and use oxygen properly. A multidisciplinary team including social services, nutritional services, and physical therapy may be necessary to assess the patient and assist the nurse with teaching the patient. The patient's significant others need to be involved in each

**guidelines for care**

### Teaching the Person with COPD

The following areas should be addressed in a typical teaching program for persons with chronic bronchitis or emphysema:

I. Patients should be able to explain, in lay terms, the basic function and pathology of their lungs. The ALA offers several excellent booklets for the lay population. (Your local branch of the ALA can provide you with a complete listing of their various publications.)

II. The avoidance of respiratory irritants and maintenance of a proper environment should be emphasized to people with COPD. As discussed earlier, inhaled irritants (especially cigarette smoke) pose a serious threat to these persons. Steps the patient can take to reduce or avoid exposure to these irritants are listed below.
   A. Stop smoking. Many community agencies, including the ALA, AHA, and ACS, offer programs for persons who want to stop smoking. The nurse should be familiar with community programs and give a list of them to the patient.
   B. Ask other persons not to smoke in the immediate environment. Inhalation of secondary smoke can exacerbate symptoms.
   C. Pay heed to announcements on radio and television warning of pollution alerts. Do not go outside during an alert.
   D. Use an air conditioner or HEPA filter or electrostatic filter to remove particulate matter from air.
      1. Keep filters clean.
      2. Follow manufacturer's directions for use.
   E. Use an activated charcoal filter if offending odors or gas pollutants are a problem.
   F. Avoid abrupt environmental temperature or humidity changes because they can increase sputum production and cause bronchospasm.
      1. Use an air conditioner in hot weather.
      2. Use a face mask when going out in cold weather.
      3. Use a dehumidifier or humidifier as appropriate to maintain a humidity of 30% to 50%.
   G. If air travel is required, check with physician about the need for supplemental oxygen.
   H. Avoid large crowds, especially during known influenza seasons.
      1. Avoid contact with people who have an upper respiratory infection.
      2. Receive influenza and pneumonia immunizations.

III. The patient should be able to explain the following aspects of the home medication or treatment regimen.
   A. State name, dose, action, and side effects of each medication.
   B. Explain how and when to use medications ordered on an as needed basis (e.g., bronchodilators, antibiotics, steroids, antacids).
   C. Demonstrate techniques necessary for follow-up care (e.g., postural drainage, percussing and vibrating, aerosol therapy).
   D. Describe how to obtain and maintain any needed equipment or supplies (e.g., oxygen, nebulizers, humidifiers, aerosols, IPPB machines, syringes, medications).

IV. The patient should demonstrate how to carry out the specific home exercise program:
   A. Specific exercises to be completed
   B. Frequency of each exercise
   C. Monitor physical response to exercises, such as heart rate increase, increased respiratory rate, or perceived fatigue

V. The patient should be able to list the names and telephone numbers of appropriate community support services, such as the Visiting Nurse Association and a home medical equipment supplier.

teaching activity so that they will be able to assist the patient as necessary.

## SPECIAL ENVIRONMENTS FOR CARE

### Critical Care Management

If the patient develops respiratory failure, care in an intensive care unit will be required (see discussion later in this chapter).

### Home Care Management

Before the patient goes home, an assessment is made of the home environment (Box 32-22). A home health nurse should meet with the family at home. The nurse will help the family determine whether they can care for the patient without assistance. If the patient is on Medicare, visits by the nurse and physical therapist are covered for a specified number of visits. If the family desires the assistance of a home health aide, the patient will have to pay for this service. Agencies such as the Visiting Nurse Association provide services on a sliding fee scale determined by the patient's financial resources. The main emphasis will be on determining the patient's understanding of his or her treatment plan and how well it is being carried out. It is important that the patient is taking medications as ordered and is able to manage any equipment needed to administer medications, oxygen, and so on. Another major emphasis is determining whether the patient and family know how to protect the patient from infection, because infection is the most common reason for admission to the hospital.

## COMPLICATIONS

Infection and respiratory failure are the major complications.

### Asthma

Asthma is an *inflammatory disease* characterized by *hyperresponsiveness of the airways and periods of bronchospasm, resulting in intermittent airway obstruction.* The onset of asthma is sudden, as opposed to the slow, insidious progression of symptoms seen in chronic bronchitis and emphysema.

**box 32-22** *Assessment of Home Environment*

1. What are the distances between the living areas where the patient spends most of the time (e.g., bedroom, bathroom, kitchen)?
2. Are stairs present, and how often each day must patient climb them?
3. Is the patient's environment safe and free of clutter, to promote ease in ambulation?
4. If the patient is dependent on oxygen, is there room for the equipment, and is equipment portable?
5. Are room temperature and humidity suitable for the patient with COPD?
6. Does the patient require a hospital bed so that the head of the bed can be elevated to assist with effective breathing?

Adapted from Burke MM, Walsh MB: *Gerontologic nursing: holistic care of the older adult,* ed 2, St Louis, 1997, Mosby.

#### Etiology

Asthma is caused by increased responsiveness of the trachea and bronchi to various stimuli that cause narrowing of the airways and difficulty in breathing.

#### Epidemiology

Asthma affects approximately 5% of adults in the United States. Both hospitalizations for the treatment of asthma and deaths from it have been increasing. In 1978, 2000 persons died from asthma. By 1988, the number of deaths from asthma had more than doubled to 4800, and by 1995, the number of deaths had increased to 5000.[6] The reasons for the increase in morbidity and mortality are not well understood. The death rate for blacks is higher than that for whites. Some experts have suggested that the reason for this is that more blacks are among the medically underserved. Women have higher death rates than men, and the highest death rates are among persons 65 years of age and older. Deaths in those over age 65 show increases during December through February, suggesting that a concomitant infection (influenza, pneumonia) contributed to the need for hospitalization and the number of deaths.

#### Pathophysiology

There are two types of asthma: *extrinsic* (atopic) and *intrinsic* (nonatopic). Extrinsic asthma results from an inflammatory response of the airways caused by mast cell activation, eosinophil infiltration, and epithelial sloughing. An *attack* is *triggered by environmental allergens* (dust, pollen, molds, animal danders, and foods). An initial encounter with an allergen stimulates plasma cells to produce antigen-specific IgE antibodies that bind to mast cells in airways. When exposed to the allergen, IgE antigen binding causes mast cell deregulation and release of inflammatory mediators. The result is an intense inflammatory response in the airways.

*Intrinsic asthma* (nonatopic) occurs in adults 35 years of age and older, and the asthma attack is often severe. *Factors that precipitate attacks* include *respiratory tract infection; drugs* (aspirin, *β-adrenergic antagonists); environmental irritants* (occupational chemicals); air *pollution; cold, dry air; exercise;* and *emotional stress.* Chemical mediators interact with the autonomic nervous system, causing inflammation and bronchoconstriction.

An asthmatic attack results from several physiological alterations, including altered immunological response, increased airway resistance, increased lung compliance, impaired mucociliary function, and altered oxygen–carbon dioxide exchange.

**Altered immunological response.** Regardless of the precipitating factors, the basis of extrinsic asthma is genetic or immunological. Extrinsic asthma is the result of an antigen-antibody reaction in which chemical mediators are released. These chemical mediators, which include histamine; bradykinin; leukotrines C, D, E; platelet-activating factor; prostaglandins; thromboxane $A_2$ and chemotactic factors for eosinophils; platelets; neutrophils; and T lymphocytes cause three main reactions: (1) *bronchoconstriction of smooth muscles* of both large and small airways, resulting in bronchospasm; (2) *increased vascular permeability* with mucosal edema and further narrowing of the airways; and (3) *increased mucous gland secretion,* increased mucus production, and impaired mucociliary function. As a result, the person with an asthmatic attack struggles to breathe through a narrowed airway that is in spasm. Because breathing is labored, the person breathes through the mouth, which dries the mucus and further occludes the airway.

Box 32-23 lists common factors triggering an asthmatic attack. Although allergic mechanisms are important in the pathogenesis of asthma, the many nonimmunological precipitating factors indicate that other pathophysiological processes, such as parasympathetic and sympathetic nervous system reactivity, are active in the onset of asthma. *Hypoxemia, hypercapnia,* and *overuse of bronchodilators may lead to an acute asthma attack.*

**Increased airway resistance.** Increased airway resistance results from bronchial smooth muscle spasm, mucosal inflammation, and hypersecretion of mucus. These airway changes cause obstruction to airflow both into and out of the lungs.

**Increased lung compliance.** The lungs become hyperinflated during an acute asthmatic attack as a result of air that becomes trapped in the distal air spaces. During the acute attack, the person with asthma demonstrates the same symptoms of increased lung compliance that are observed in the patient with emphysema.

**Impaired mucociliary function.** Hypertrophy of mucus-secreting glands, thickened mucus, and slowed ciliary movement are common findings in persons with asthma. During an asthma attack, increased mucus production combined with slowed clearance of mucus caused by decreased ciliary movement results in increased water loss from mucus. Thus the mucus becomes increasingly viscous and can ultimately result in the development of mucous plugs, which may block airways (Figure 32-29).

**Altered oxygen–carbon dioxide exchange.** Increased airway resistance and hyperinflation cause the respiratory muscles to work harder, resulting in muscle fatigue and ultimately exhaustion. In mild or short-term asthmatic attacks, the individual compensates with an increased respiratory rate, which results in respiratory alkalosis. Mild hypoxemia from altered V/Q ratios usually accompanies the alkalosis.

In a severe or prolonged attack, if the increased work of breathing cannot be relieved, respiratory muscle exhaustion will result in hypoventilation, which in turn causes respiratory acidosis and severe hypoxemia. If the process cannot be reversed, the person may die.

The signs and symptoms associated with asthma are correlated with normal lung functions and underlying pathophysiological origins (see Tables 32-23 and 32-27). The character of asthmatic attacks can vary on a continuum from

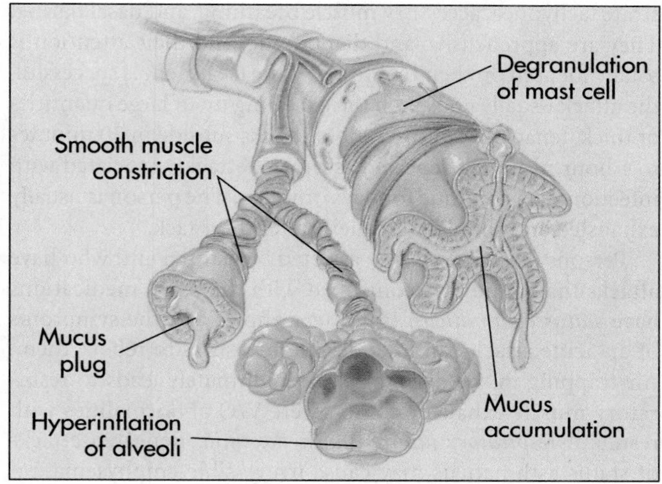


**fig. 32-29** Bronchial asthma; thick mucus, mucosal edema, and smooth muscle spasm cause obstruction of small airways; breathing is labored and expiration is difficult.

### box 32-23 *Common Factors Triggering an Asthmatic Attack*

- Environmental factors
  - Change in temperature, especially cold air
  - Change in humidity: dry air
- Atmospheric pollutants
  - Cigarette and industrial smoke, ozone, sulfur dioxide, formaldehyde
- Strong odors: perfume
- Allergens
  - Feathers, animal dander, dust mites, molds, allergens; foods treated with sulfites (beer, wine, fruit juices, snack foods, salads, potatoes, shellfish, fresh and dried fruits)
- Exercise
- Stress or emotional upset
- Medications
  - Aspirin and nonsteroidal antiinflammatory drugs (NSAIDs), β-blockers (including eyedrops), cholinergic drugs (to promote bladder contraction and as eyedrops for glaucoma)
  - Enzymes, including those in laundry detergents
  - Chemicals: toluene and others used in solvents, paints, rubber, and plastics

### table 32-27 *Asthma Syndromes Classified by Precipitating Factor and Response Pattern*

| Asthma Syndromes | Characteristics |
|---|---|
| Atopic asthma | Childhood onset, allergic rhinitis, allergic dermopathy, identifiable environmental precipitating events |
| Exercise-induced asthma | Airway constriction after exercise |
| Aspirin-hypersensitivity triad | Presence of nasal polyps, urticaria, and asthma after aspirin ingestion |
| Bronchospasm associated with nonbacterial upper respiratory tract infections | As described by patient |
| Industrial asthma | Bronchoconstriction associated with certain industrial precipitating factors |

chronic or acute mild intermittent attacks to life-threatening status asthmaticus.

With chronic mild asthma, symptoms are not noticeable when the person is at rest. However, after exertion (e.g., laughing, singing, vigorous exercise, or emotional excitement) dyspnea and wheezing develop rapidly. These attacks are controlled with medications, and patients usually can continue their mode of living with a few modifications and no serious lung changes. They are not hospitalized, but they sometimes come to outpatient clinics for medical supervision.

Acute asthmatic attacks often occur at night. The person awakens with a sensation of choking caused by the mucosal inflammation and hypersecretion of mucus. Bronchospasm, with resultant increased airway resistance, causes audible expiratory and inspiratory wheezing. During the acute attack, patients appear to be in acute respiratory distress and typically demonstrate tachypnea, accessory muscle breathing, and nasal flaring. They are apprehensive and diaphoretic, and their attention is totally focused on their breathing. If the treatment is successful, the attack usually ends with the coughing up of large quantities of thick, tenacious sputum. Most attacks subside in 30 minutes to 1 hour, although repeated asthmatic attacks associated with infection may continue for days or weeks. The person is usually exhausted and should rest quietly after the attack.

Persons who are severely affected by asthma and who have attacks that cannot be controlled with the usual medications have *status asthmaticus.* In status asthmaticus, the symptoms of an acute attack continue despite measures to relieve them. Air trapping in the distal air spaces ultimately leads to respiratory muscle exhaustion and severe V/Q abnormalities with resultant *respiratory failure and hypoxemia.* Repeated attacks of status asthmaticus may cause irreversible emphysema, resulting in a permanent decrease in total breathing capacity.

Patients with *status asthmaticus* often demonstrate such severe respiratory distress that they are unable to talk. They may be moving minimal amounts of air into and out of the lungs; thus audible wheezing and adventitious lung sounds may *not* be present. During this phase of the attack, *the patient will appear cyanotic and may demonstrate both pulsus paradoxus* and *sensorium changes.* This is a medical emergency, and the patient requires immediate therapy. Most patients arrive in the emergency department, where treatment is begun. Patients remain in the emergency department until their condition is stabilized. Most patients are then admitted to the hospital for ongoing therapy and observation.

Pulmonary function tests characteristic of asthma show reduction in $FEV_1$ to less than 25% of the predicted value. The FEV is usually greatly reduced in proportion to the FVC, although the FVC may also be decreased. Improved flow rates after administration of bronchodilators indicating reversible bronchospasm is a characteristic finding with asthma. The results of ABG studies can vary from respiratory alkalosis with mild hypoxemia to severe respiratory acidosis with profound hypoxemia, depending on the severity and duration of the asthmatic attack.

### *Collaborative care management*

The objectives of medical management of asthma are to promote normal functioning of the individual, prevent recurrent symptoms, prevent severe attacks, and prevent side effects from medication. The chief aim of various medications is to afford the patient immediate, progressive, ongoing bronchial relaxation. One approach to treating an acute asthmatic attack is presented in Table 32-28.

**table 32-28** *Treatment of an Acute Asthmatic Attack*

| THERAPY | EFFECTS AND PRECAUTIONS |
|---|---|
| Inhaled $\beta$-agonist such as albuterol sulfate (Proventil, Ventalin), salmeterol (Serevent), or metaproterenol sulfate (Alupent, Metaprel) in normal saline | Stimulates $\beta_2$-receptors in bronchial smooth muscle resulting in smooth muscle relaxation.<br>Starts to act in 10 minutes; effects last 4-6 hours.<br>Monitor vital signs, lung sounds, and peak expiration flow rate (PEFR) before and after each treatment. |
| *If above is not successful:*<br>Methylprednisolone (Solu-Medrol) IV: loading dose, 2 mg/kg or about 125 mg q 6 hr then 60-125 mg q 6 hr for 48 hours total or until patient stable. | Reduces inflammation and edema of airway and decreases hyperactivity of airway.<br>Benefit seen within 6 hours, full effect in 6-8 hours. |
| When patient is stabilized, change IV to 60 mg prednisone by mouth daily or every other day. | Oral prednisone should be tapered off by 7-10 days. Taper 60 mg over 2 days, 40 mg over 2 days, 30 mg over 2 days, and 10 mg over 2 days. |
| Nebulized atropine sulfate may be tried, or aminophylline may be given IV; a pump is used for better control of infusion. | Relax bronchial smooth muscle. |
| Loading dose of aminophylline: 4 to 6 mg/kg over 15 to 30 minutes and then continuous infusion of 0.45 to 0.70 mg/kg/hr. Patients who have been taking aminophylline at home will be placed on continuous IV therapy. Rate of infusion is determined by theophylline blood level. Desired level is 10 to 20 $\mu$g/ml. | *Too rapid an infusion may cause severe hypotension, premature ventricular contractions, and cardiac arrest.*<br>Monitor heart rate and rhythm closely, and report any changes immediately.<br>Theophylline metabolized by the liver. For persons with liver disease, smaller doses are used. Patients taking cimetidine, erythromycin, or ciprofloxacin require smaller doses. Smokers and those taking phenytoin require larger doses to maintain blood levels. |

**Maintenance therapy.** The *goal of maintenance therapy* is to provide the patient with ongoing therapy that will *keep inflammation in check and prevent an acute asthmatic attack.* The two types of medications used for maintenance are an inhaled corticosteroid to treat airway inflammation and a long-acting bronchodilator such as salmeterol (Serevent). Table 32-29 lists six classes of medications used for maintenance therapy.[9]

Because of concerns that many patients may have been undertreated and that this has contributed to the increase in death rates, *more attention is being given to the role of inflammation in asthma.* The use of an inhaled steroid along with a $\beta_2$-agonist ensures that the medications reach deeper into the lung and do not cause the side effects associated with oral steroids. It is recommended that the inhaled $\beta_2$-agonist be given first to open the airway; the inhaled steroid will then be more effective.

**table 32-29** *Common Medications for Asthma*

| | Administration | Action | Adverse Effects |
|---|---|---|---|
| **MAINTENANCE MEDICATIONS** | | | |
| **Nonsteroidal Antiinflammatory Drugs**<br>Cromolyn (Intal)<br>Nedocromil (Tilade) | Metered-dose inhaler (MDI) or nebulizer | Decrease airway inflammation and irritation | Cough or throat irritation, headaches, bad taste in mouth |
| **Corticosteroids**<br>Beclomethasone (Vanceril, Beclovent)<br>Triamcinolone acetonide (Azmacort)<br>Flunisolide (AeroBid)<br>Fluticasone (Flovent) | MDI | Antiinflammatory | Sore throat, hoarseness, cough, oral thrush |
| **Leukotriene Inhibitors/Receptor Antagonists**<br>Zafirlukast (Accolate)<br>Zilenton (Zyflo)<br>Montelukast sodium (Singulair) | Oral | Antiinflammatory | Headache, nausea, diarrhea, dizziness, myalgia, fever, dyspepsia, elevated alanine aminotransferase level |
| **Theophylline**<br>Theophylline (Theo-Dur, Slo-bid, Uniphyl, Theo-24, Uni-Dur, Slo-Phyllin)<br>Theophylline ethylenediamine (Aminophylline) | Oral, parenteral | Long-acting bronchodilator | Nausea, vomiting, stomach cramps, diarrhea, headache, muscle cramps, tachycardia, irritability, restlessness; serum blood levels should be checked for therapeutic ranges |
| **Anticholinergic**<br>Ipratropium (Atrovent) | MDI, nebulizer, nasal spray | Short-acting bronchodilator | Nervousness, dizziness, headache, palpitations, cough, blurred vision, nausea, gastrointestinal distress, dry mouth |
| **$\beta_2$-Agonist**<br>Salmeterol (Serevent) | MDI | Long-acting bronchodilator | Headache, tremor, tachycardia, palpitations, nasopharyngitis, stomachache, cough, rash |
| **RESCUE MEDICATIONS** | | | |
| **Corticosteroids**<br>Prednisone<br>Methylprednisolone (Medrol)<br>Prednisolone (Prelone)<br>Prednisolone sodium phosphate (Pediapred) | Parenteral, oral | Antiinflammatory | Increased appetite, fluid retention, weight gain, gastrointestinal irritation |
| **β-Agonists**<br>Albuterol (Proventil, Ventolin)<br>Metaproterenol (Alupent, Metaprel)<br>Pirbuterol (Maxair)<br>Bitolterol (Tornalate)<br>Terbutaline (Brethaire)<br>Epinephrine | MDI, nebulizer<br>Albuterol is also available for parenteral administration | Short-acting bronchodilators | Nervousness, tremors, tachycardia, headache, dizziness, vomiting |

**box 32-24 Use of PEFR Measurements in Medical Settings**

1. Assess severity of asthma to make decisions as to admission, discharge, or initiation of oral steroid therapy.
2. Monitor response to therapy during acute exacerbation.
3. Justify patient's therapy.
4. Diagnose exercise-induced asthma.
5. Detect asymptomatic deterioration in lung function in the physician's office to intervene to prevent a more serious episode of asthma.
6. Monitor degree of airflow obstruction during a series of office visits to assess success of therapy.

Modified from US Department of Health and Human Services: *National Asthma Education Program guidelines for the diagnosis and management of asthma,* Washington, DC, 1991, US Government Printing Office.

Some patients are taught to use peak-flow meters and to adjust their medications according to the results. For example, if their peak-expiratory flow rate (PEFR) is below 70% of normal, inhaled medication is increased; below 50%, oral steroids are added; below 30%, emergency measures are called for, and the patient calls the physician and goes to the emergency department for treatment with oxygen and additional drug therapy. It can be anticipated that more and more patients will be taught to use peak-flow meters to monitor response to their treatment and detect changes in airflow—often before symptoms are evident. Peak-flow meters are portable, durable, and inexpensive ($25 to $50) and are not difficult to use.

The National Heart, Lung, and Blood Institute, which is part of the U.S. Department of Health and Human Services, convened an expert panel of physicians to address the increase in asthma morbidity and mortality. This group, the National Asthma Education Program (NAEP), publishes guidelines to help in the diagnosis and management of asthma. This expert panel recommended that PEFR be used in medical settings for the situations listed in Box 32-24.

# NURSING MANAGEMENT

## ASSESSMENT

### Subjective Data

Data to be collected to assess the patient with asthma include:
- History of asthma onset and duration
- Precipitating factors
- Any recent changes in medication regimen
- Medications used to relieve asthma symptoms
- Other medications
- Self-care methods used to relieve symptoms

### Objective Data

Data to be collected to assess the patient with asthma include:
- Assess general appearance
  - Does patient appear apprehensive?
  - Is there any evidence of altered sensorium?
- Assess vital signs
  - Tachycardia
  - Pulsus paradoxus (diminished pulse with inspiration, confirmed by a 6 to 8 mm Hg drop in systolic blood pressure during inspiration)
  - Tachypnea
- Perform pulmonary examination
  - Inspection
    - Accessory muscle breathing
    - Forward-leaning posture
    - Dyspnea
    - Prolonged expiration
    - Cyanosis
  - Palpation
    - Decreased lateral expansion
    - Decreased fremitus
  - Percussion
    - Hyperresonance
    - Decreased diaphragmatic excursion
  - Auscultation (as patient approaches exhaustion from increased work of breathing, breath sounds and adventitious sounds may be absent or faint)
    - Inspiratory and expiratory wheezing
    - Rhonchi
- Assess laboratory findings
  - ABGs
    - Short-term or moderate attack: respiratory alkalosis with mild hypoxemia
    - Prolonged or severe attack: respiratory acidosis with severe hypoxemia
  - Sputum: for eosinophilia
  - PFT: decreased FEV and VC

## NURSING DIAGNOSES

Nursing diagnoses are determined from analysis of patient data. Nursing diagnoses for the person with asthma may include but are not limited to:

| Diagnostic Title | Possible Etiological Factors |
|---|---|
| Airway clearance, ineffective | Ineffective technique, decreased energy/fatigue, impaired mucociliary clearance mechanism, inadequate fluid intake |
| Anxiety | Threat of unknown or death |
| Breathing pattern, ineffective | Bronchoconstriction, underuse of bronchodilator medications |
| Gas exchange, impaired | Mucous plugs, V/Q imbalance |
| Knowledge deficit: predisposing factors, prevention, treatment | Lack of exposure to information, unreceptiveness to information, unfamiliarity with information sources |

## EXPECTED PATIENT OUTCOMES

Expected outcomes for the person with asthma may include but are not limited to:

1. Demonstrates effective airway clearance.
   a. Effective methods of coughing
   b. Appropriate use of medication and equipment

2. Demonstrates activities to control anxiety response to symptoms.
   a. Muscle relaxation
   b. Meditation
   c. Appropriate use of medications
3. Demonstrates effective breathing patterns.
   a. Inspiratory/expiratory ratio of 5 seconds: 10 seconds
   b. Respiratory rate within near-normal limits
4. Demonstrates improved ventilation and oxygenation.
   a. Arterial blood pH and $Pa{CO_2}$ return to or stay within acceptable limits
   b. $Pa{O_2}$ at optimal level for individual
5. a. Patient or significant other states the factors most likely to precipitate an asthmatic attack (e.g., stress, allergens, infections).
   b. Patient or significant other states the importance of keeping a diary of symptoms and medications (time and dose) during an asthmatic attack.
   c. If the cause is allergic, states how to prepare an environmentally controlled bedroom.
   d. Patient or significant other explains any home medication program.
      (1) Gives name, dose, action, and side effects of each medication.
      (2) States conditions under which medications might be increased (e.g., infection: start or increase antibiotics; increased stress or worsening of symptoms: increase corticosteroids).
   e. Patient or significant other demonstrates how to take inhaled medications.
   f. Patient or significant other describes what to do when an acute attack occurs (e.g., take medication and sit quietly).
   g. Patient or significant other states signs and symptoms that indicate need for immediate medical attention (e.g., asthmatic attack unrelieved by usual treatment).
   h. If receiving corticosteroid therapy, shows card to be carried at all times giving data about the drug, dose of drug, and name of physician; alternative is to wear Medic Alert bracelet.
   i. States plans for ongoing follow-up care, including plans for desensitization if appropriate.

## INTERVENTIONS

### Administering Medications

1. Give medications as ordered. Monitor IV rates closely.
2. Monitor patient closely for adverse effects of medications (see Table 32-29).

### Improving Airway Clearance

During an asthmatic attack, secretions tend to become viscous and can plug airways, causing increased airway obstruction. Mobilizing secretions often prevents the need for intubation and artificial ventilation.

1. Ensure adequate systemic fluid intake. (NOTE: Research findings suggest that overhydration may not increase secretion clearance above levels obtained by normal hydration levels.)
2. Provide adequate nutritional levels.
3. Provide extra humidity.
4. Medicate with short-acting bronchodilator and corticosteroid.
5. Teach effective cough maneuvers.
6. If cough is ineffective to produce sputum, administer chest physiotherapy.

### Providing Emotional Support and Preventing Anxiety

1. Never leave patient alone during an asthmatic attack.
2. Encourage relaxation techniques.
3. Guide or assist patient with respiratory maneuvers.
4. Assess for possible medication overuse.

### Improving Breathing Patterns

The nursing role in improving breathing patterns and gas exchange is as follows:

1. Place patient in high Fowler's position.
2. Encourage slow, rhythmic breathing.
3. Encourage patient to breathe through nose and exhale through pursed lips.
4. Administer bronchodilator and antiinflammatory medication as ordered. Monitor patient for both therapeutic response and adverse effects to medications. Table 32-29 lists medications, administration, action, and adverse effects of medications typically used to treat asthma.

### Improving Gas Exchange

Blood gas results should be monitored as follows:

1. If respiratory alkalosis is present, encourage slower breathing.
2. If respiratory acidosis and hypoxemia are present:
   a. Administer oxygen as prescribed.
   b. If oxygen and other therapeutic measures do not relieve the attack, intubation and ventilatory assistance may be required.

### Patient/Family Education

After the patient has recovered from an acute attack, the patient's knowledge about asthma is assessed, and the following points are stressed:

1. Keep a symptom diary to help identify the following:
   a. Possible precipitating factors
   b. Symptom patterns
   c. Efficacy of self-treatment modalities (include time and dose of any self-administered medications)
2. Signs and symptoms
   a. Tightness in chest
   b. Restlessness or vague feeling of uneasiness
   c. Dyspnea
   d. Increased wheezing
   e. Productive cough
3. Self-treatment of signs and symptoms
   a. Take bronchodilator as ordered.
   b. Take inhaled steroid as prescribed by physician.
   c. State conditions under which medication might be increased (e.g., infection: start or increase antibiotics;

increased stress or worsening of symptoms: increase inhaled corticosteroid) (Box 32-25).

d. If another person is not present, call someone so you will not be alone.

e. Try to remain calm and breathe slowly; use relaxation techniques at first sign of attack.

f. If symptoms are not relieved, call physician or go to nearest emergency facility.

4. Know how to use special equipment: MDI (see the accompanying Patient/Family Teaching Box), inhaler with spacer (see the Patient/Family Teaching Box, p. 984), and peak-flow meter if one is prescribed.

## patient/family teaching

### Using a Metered-Dose Inhaler

1. Inhale through nose, then slowly exhale.
2. Place inhaler 1 to 2 inches from mouth.
3. Press down on inhaler while simultaneously inhaling one puff deeply. Breathe in air from around the mouthpiece while inhaling.
4. Hold breath for 5 to 10 seconds to allow medication to reach lung.
5. Repeat second puff if one is ordered.

*Caution:* Some persons with asthma may experience bronchoconstriction after using an MDI. Patients who complain of chest tightness after using an MDI may be reacting to the propellant gases used to deliver the β-agonist.

### Health promotion/prevention

A goal set by *Healthy People 2000* was to reduce to no more than 10% the proportion of people with asthma who experience activity limitation, from a baseline of 19.4%.

Prevention of immunological (atopic) asthma is focused on identifying the allergens to which the person is sensitive. In nonimmunological or mixed asthma, factors precipitating the exacerbation of symptoms may be obscure. However, identification of causative or aggravating factors is still imperative in order to avoid or decrease the incidence of asthma attacks.

There is perhaps no disease in which knowing the patient well is more important than in asthma. Because sensitivity tests can be performed with only a small fraction of the substances with which the patient is in contact, the physician usually makes the diagnosis on the basis of a careful history. Knowing about the person's lifestyle, such as the type of work, leisure-time activities, and even food preferences, may give useful clues as to what precipitates the asthmatic attack (Box 32-26).

*It is imperative to understand that even though psychological factors may precipitate an attack, the response to the attack is physiological and requires the same treatment as that prescribed for an attack precipitated by an allergen or any other factor.*

## ■ EVALUATION

To evaluate the effectiveness of nursing interventions, compare patient behaviors with those stated in the expected pa-

**box 32-25** *Sample Action Plan for the Patient with Asthma*

Assess severity of the episode by rating the severity of symptoms or measuring peak flow.

**MILD EPISODE**

Symptoms: Mild wheeze, cough, chest tightness, shortness of breath occurring with activity but not at rest

Peak flow: 70-90% of baseline (personal best or predicted, as determined by the clinician)

Actions: Take inhaled bronchodilator. If improved, continue medication on regular basis for 24-48 hours. If not improved, take action as indicated for moderate episode.

**MODERATE EPISODE**

Symptoms: Wheeze, cough, chest tightness, and shortness of breath while at rest; symptoms may interfere with daily activity.

Peak flow: 50-70% of baseline

Actions: Repeat inhaled bronchodilator every 20 minutes for 1 hour. If improved, continue medication every 3-4 hours for 24-48 hours. If not improved in 2-6 hours after initial treatment, begin or increase prednisone. Contact your clinician.

**SEVERE EPISODE**

Symptoms: Severe shortness of breath, wheeze (wheeze may disappear with very severe episode), cough, and chest tightness at rest; difficulty walking and talking; perhaps retraction of muscles in chest or neck

Peak flow: Less than 50% of baseline and little response to bronchodilator

Actions: Repeat inhaled bronchodilator, 4-6 puffs, every 10 minutes up to 3 times. Begin or increase prednisone. Contact your clinician if available. **If there is no significant improvement after 20-30 minutes, seek emergency care immediately.**

**Be prepared:**

Have a plan for receiving emergency care quickly in the event of a sudden episode. Keep emergency phone numbers handy. Always carry an inhaler of bronchodilator medication with you.

From US Department of Health and Human Services: *National Asthma Education Program guidelines for the diagnosis and management of asthma,* Washington, DC, 1991, US Government Printing Office.

tient outcomes. Successful achievement of patient outcomes for the patient with asthma is indicated by:

1. Airway clearance is effective.
 a. Taking a deep breath and blowing it out through pursed lips helps initiate cough reflex.
 b. Inhaled medication is effective in dilating bronchioles, as evidenced by a decrease in wheezing.
2. Patient's anxiety is improved.
 a. Demonstrates muscle relaxation while concentrating on breathing pattern.
 b. Practices meditation after acute symptoms subside.
 c. Listens to soft music.
3. Breathing pattern is effective.
 a. Is concentrating on increasing time of exhalation to twice that of inhalation by counting to 5 seconds for inhalation and 10 seconds for exhalation.
 b. Respirations are quieter and slower at 28 per minute.
4. Ventilation and perfusion are improving; $PaO_2$, $PaCO_2$, and pH are returning to patient's baseline levels.

5a. States factors most likely to precipitate an asthmatic attack; for example, attacks are frequently exercise induced and are more likely to occur during times of increased stress.
 b. Has kept a symptom diary for years, and the cues from a review of it have assisted in reducing the frequency of attacks.
 c. Knows name, dose, and adverse effects of prescribed medications.
 d. Has had asthma since childhood. Sleeps in an environmentally controlled room with approved bedding, washable throw rug on hardwood floor, tight-fitting closet doors, and daily damp dusting of furniture and floors. Does not have a dog or cat.
 e. Demonstrates correct use of MDI.
 f. Verbalizes steps to take when an acute attack is beginning. Has peak-flow meter and uses it to determine how much bronchodilator to take and how often.
 g. Verbalizes when physician needs to be called or when a trip to the nearest emergency department is indicated.
 h. Wears a Medic Alert bracelet indicating that he or she takes steroids.
 i. Knows importance of ongoing medical follow-up and has appointment for a complete evaluation in 2 weeks.

**box 32-26** *Identifying Factors Precipitating Asthma*

1. Be alert for casual comments about daily activities the patient might consider insignificant.
2. Encourage patient to keep a symptom diary. Ask patient to perform the following tasks:
   a. Use a small notebook that can be carried at all times.
   b. Record everything that occurred and was present during 24 hours before and during the onset of the attack. When the attack began: What were you doing? Where were you? Who or what else was present? What was the weather like?
   c. Note the time and date that the attack occurred.
3. Write down what you think caused the symptoms to occur, even if it is a guess.
4. Observe patient's interaction with others and reaction to stressors that might aggravate or precipitate an attack.

## GERONTOLOGICAL CONSIDERATIONS

Although the goals of asthma treatment are the same for persons of all ages, they may be more difficult to achieve in the elderly. Some of the problems that may be present in the elderly are: (1) normal lung function may be unattainable or attainable only with high, potentially dangerous, drug doses, (2) elderly persons may have unnecessarily restricted their lifestyle to accommodate their asthma, and (3) they may need additional education to raise their expectations of improvement in their symptoms and restoration and maintenance of an independent, active, and personally satisfying lifestyle. Special problems that may arise include: (1) the need for additional education of the patient, family, and in-home caregivers in the proper use of medications. Elderly persons may have difficulty using metered-dose inhalers because of diminished hand strength and arthritis. They also may be unable to use peak-expiratory flow meters, and PEFR will need to be performed by their home care nurse or the physician. As a substitute to PEFR the elderly person may be encouraged to keep a symptom diary in order to become more sensitive to worsening of their asthma. (2) Medications commonly used to treat asthma may have increased adverse effects in the elderly person. For example, high doses of inhaled steroids cause dermal thinning with potential for bruising. Older women may have dose-dependent bone loss and calcium, and vitamin D supplements may be indicated along with bone density monitoring tests. Systems steroids (oral and parenteral) pose an increased risk because they are cleared from the body more slowly. Additionally, possible adverse effects from long-term use including electrolyte imbalances, hypokalemia, hypertension, hyperglycemia, osteoporosis, worsening of glaucoma because of increased intraocular pressure, aggravation of peptic and gastric ulcer, and depression are more common in elderly patients. Older patients have increased susceptibility to theophylline's adverse side-effects and when theophylline is given to elderly persons with asthma, blood levels of the drug are monitored more closely. Inhaled $beta_2$ agonists also have an increased potential for adverse side-effects, and elderly patients require close monitoring for ECG changes, hypokalemia, tremor, and hypoxemia. Oral long-acting $beta_2$ agonists are usually not given to elderly persons with asthma because of possible tremors, and increased heart rate and blood pressure. Medications used to treat coexisting conditions such as cardiovascular disease, glaucoma, and arthritis may cause problems in persons with asthma, and alternate medications may need to be prescribed. Medications that pose particular problems to persons with asthma include beta adrenergic blocking agents, nonsteroidal antiinflammatory drugs (NSAIDs), diuretics, and angiotensin-converting-enzyme (ACE) inhibitors. A careful medication history is required for every elderly person with asthma, and the patient needs to understand why certain medications may pose a special problem for him or her.

## SPECIAL ENVIRONMENTS FOR CARE

### Critical Care Management

If the person with asthma has an attack that cannot be relieved by the usual therapy, intubation and ventilatory support may be necessary, and the patient will be cared for in an intensive care unit.

### Home Care Management

Most persons with asthma are able to manage their asthma well at home. Patients who adhere to their prescribed therapy and avoid allergens to which they are sensitive may not have an asthmatic attack for years unless they develop a severe respiratory infection.

## COMPLICATIONS

Complications include status asthmaticus and respiratory failure.

### Cystic Fibrosis

#### Etiology

Cystic fibrosis (CF) continues to be the most common fatal genetic disease among whites. It is an autosomal recessive disease, and 1 of every 22 individuals carries the CF gene. When both parents are carriers (heterozygotes), there is a one in four chance with each pregnancy that their child will have CF (Figure 32-30).

There is considerable ongoing research in CF. Table 32-30 summarizes research projects, findings, and future goals. The identification of the CF gene in 1989 was a major breakthrough and has raised hope for future progress in preventing and treating CF.

#### Epidemiology

Approximately 25,000 individuals with CF live in the United States. Of that population, 6500 individuals are adults, according to the Cystic Fibrosis Foundation Patient Care Registry.[23] More important, the number of adults with CF continues to increase steadily because of increased life expectancy and diagnostic advances (Figure 32-31).

Two groups make up this adult CF population: (1) those diagnosed when infants and children and (2) adolescents and adults. Statistics indicate that approximately 20% of the adult CF population is diagnosed after age 15.

Reaching adulthood is now a realistic expectation for infants and children with CF. The average life expectancy in 1997 was 31.5 years with a maximum survival of 35 to 40 years. The major contributing factors to this increased life expectancy include diagnostic advances and improved therapeutic interventions.

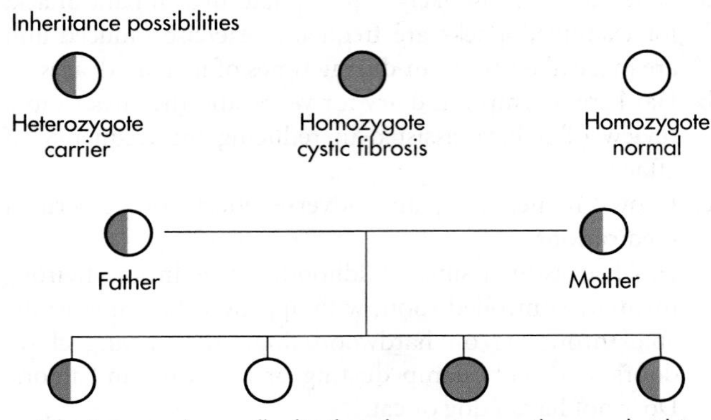


**fig. 32-30** Inheritance of cystic fibrosis (CF) when both mother and father are carriers of the CF gene.

**table 32-30** *Research in the Prevention and Treatment of Cystic Fibrosis*

| Subject | Topic | Findings | Future Goals |
|---|---|---|---|
| Prevention | CF gene | Gene identified in 1989: location, size mutations, and defective protein | To define protein structure and function<br>To treat or alter defective protein<br>To identify and change sodium and chloride ion movement in CF cell<br>To identify causes of CF<br>To develop vaccines to prevent lung infections |
| | Vaccinations | | |
| | Genetic counseling | Phosphatase and pancreatic trypsin for neonatal diagnosis | To identify CF carriers—prenatal and neonatal diagnosis |
| Treatment | Antibiotics | Prophylactic use, early use, aerosolized antibiotics, oral route effectiveness | To treat lung infections effectively<br>To decrease side effects of frequent treatment<br>To decrease hospitalizations |
| | Dornase-alfa | Improve lung function, reduce risk of respiratory infections | Same as for antibiotics |
| | Double lung transplantation | 308 patients received transplants between 1990 and 1994 | To replace damaged lungs<br>To increase number of transplants |

***Pathophysiology***

Cystic fibrosis is an exocrine gland disease involving various systems (pulmonary, pancreatic/hepatic, GI, reproductive). Obstruction of the exocrine gland ducts or passageways occurs in nearly all adult patients with CF. Exocrine gland secretions are known to have a decreased water content, altered electrolyte concentration, and abnormal organic constituents (especially mucous glycoproteins); however, the specific biochemical or physiological defect that leads to obstruction is not known.

The following physiological alterations are found in adults with CF.

1. *Pulmonary damage.* Mucus obstruction, inflammation, edema, and smooth muscle restriction of airways are found in this COPD. Changes in the airways predispose the person to respiratory infection, which can be life threatening. Frequent, recurrent pulmonary infections erode blood vessels, such as bronchial arteries, which branch from the aorta and the lung at high pressures and are most at risk for bleeding *(hemoptysis).*

   Other complications of damage to the airways include *pneumothorax, respiratory insufficiency,* and *cor pulmonale.* These complications account for 95% of the deaths in adults with CF. The normal function, primary pathophysiology, and clinical manifestations in CF are outlined in Table 32-31.
2. *Gastrointestinal and pancreatic involvement.* Intestinal obstruction occurs in 20% of adult patients with CF. Generally, pancreatic insufficiency predisposes to intestinal obstruction. Cramps and abdominal pain in adults with CF should arouse suspicion of intestinal obstruction. Pancreatic insufficiency is reported in 80% to 90% of adults with CF. The pathological lesions in the pancreas decrease pancreatic enzyme production and lead to malabsorption of fat.
3. *Glucose intolerance.* About 40% of adults with CF have glucose intolerance caused by obstruction of islets of Langerhans and pancreatic fibrosis.

Three major clinical symptoms are associated with CF: recurrent respiratory infections, malnutrition, and excessive salt losses. Early identification of CF often rests on the presence of several otherwise unexplained clinical symptoms. In infants, clinical symptoms of CF may include meconium ileus and failure to thrive. Excessive salt losses in infants may first be detected by the infant's mother, who reports that the child tastes salty when kissed. Older children should be suspected of having CF when recurrent respiratory infections and failure to thrive despite large appetites cannot otherwise be explained. Excessive salt losses in older children and young adults with CF may be manifested by heat exhaustion after exercise or exposure to hot weather, or dehydration after fevers. In young adults, the only clinical manifestation of CF may be infertility. Box 32-27 lists the clinical manifestations of CF.

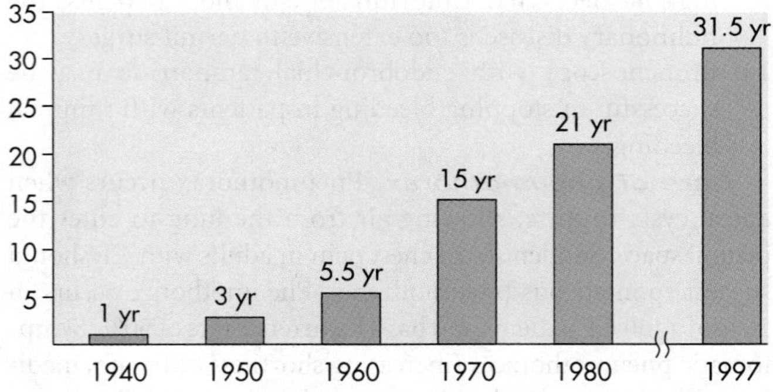


**fig. 32-31** Life expectancy of children born with CF. The number of children surviving to adulthood continues to increase.

**box 32-27** ***clinical manifestations***

***Cystic Fibrosis***

Specific clinical manifestations by system are listed below. Pulmonary signs and symptoms of CF include the following:

1. Chronic productive cough and/or recurrent bronchitis or pneumonia.
2. Crackles and rhonchi, decreased pulmonary compliance, digital clubbing (see Figure 30-13).
3. Shortness of breath and dyspnea on exertion, wheezing, and weight loss occur with respiratory complications and usually indicate need for vigorous therapy.

GI signs and symptoms include the following:

1. Frequent, bulky, greasy stools
2. Weight loss
3. Cramps and abdominal pain—should arouse suspicion of obstruction

Glucose intolerance signs and symptoms include the following:

1. Polyuria, polydipsia, polyphagia
2. Absence of ketoacidosis even with above signs

**table 32-31** *Normal Function, Primary Pathophysiology, and Clinical Manifestations in Cystic Fibrosis*

| NORMAL FUNCTION | PATHOPHYSIOLOGY | CLINICAL MANIFESTATIONS |
|---|---|---|
| Mucus production by goblet cells lubricates airways and entraps foreign particles. | 1. Excessive amounts of mucus production<br>2. Inflammation of small airways, causing hyperinflation of alveoli<br>3. Chronic bacterial infections<br>4. Eroding of a major blood vessel secondary to infection | 1. Increased cough and mucus production<br>2. Fatigue, shortness of breath<br>3. Fever, fatigue, shortness of breath<br>4. Hemoptysis |

### Collaborative care management

**Diagnostic tests.** The diagnosis of CF is confirmed by the presence of *at least two* of the following:

1. A positive sweat test with a chloride level greater than 60 mEq/L
2. COPD demonstrated clinically and on chest x-ray film
3. Exocrine pancreatic insufficiency
4. Positive family history of CF

**Medications.** Dornase-alfa (Pulmozyme), a recombinant form of the naturally occurring human enzyme deoxyribonuclease I (DNase I), which is responsible for the breakdown of extracellular deoxyribonucleic acid (DNA), was released in 1994. It works by reducing the viscoelasticity of CF secretions and is being widely used in the treatment of patients with CF.

The goals of medical management of CF are to minimize bronchial plugging and to inhibit bacterial colonization. Measures to minimize bronchial plugging include:

1. Chest physiotherapy with chest percussion and postural drainage (see Figures 32-27 and 32-28) are performed for 20 minutes two or three times daily and sometimes much more frequently.
2. Administer dornase-alfa, 2.5 mg ampule in compressed air-driven nebulizer.
3. Mucolytic agents may be ordered to thin secretions, although ensuring that the patient is well hydrated may be sufficient to thin secretions.
4. Humidification of air is controversial because it has been associated with bronchospasm and bacterial colonization. It may be helpful for some patients, however, and some physicians may prescribe it.

To minimize bacterial colonization during acute phases of the disease, sputum should be cultured and tested for sensitivity. Antibiotics are prescribed based on the results of these tests. Combination therapy with two or three antibiotics is recommended to prevent bacterial resistance and is usually prescribed for 14 days. Shorter courses of antibiotic therapy are associated with reexacerbation of symptoms. Oral antibiotics may be prescribed long term to inhibit bacterial colonization, although there is little scientific basis for this practice. Inhaled antibiotics are given in very high doses, because only about 10% of the inhaled drug is absorbed.

**Treatments**

***Preventing pulmonary infections.*** Pulmonary infections compromise respiratory status and usually result in the patient being hospitalized for routine pulmonary physiotherapy, or cleanout. This includes the following:

1. Vigorous postural drainage and percussing. Some patients will spend up to 8 hours a day consumed by percussing, vibrating, and postural drainage. Mechanical vibrators may be purchased by the patient with CF when physical therapists, nurses, respiratory therapists, or family members are not able to provide the necessary therapy. Most patients must have postural drainage with percussing every 4 hours. Respiratory personnel and nurses may share the treatments, depending on hospital policy.
2. Room humidification if ordered.
3. Aerosols with a bronchodilator such as Bronkosol R or antibiotics may be administered before postural drainage and percussion.

***Care of hemoptysis.*** Hemoptysis occurs when a blood vessel is eroded as a result of pulmonary disease. The patient may expectorate as much as 300 to 500 ml of blood in 24 hours. When a patient with a pulmonary disease such as CF has an uncontrollable urge to cough, this usually indicates blood in the airways from hemoptysis. The patient will be very anxious and should not be left alone.

Nursing and medical care during hemoptysis include:

1. Elevate head of bed 45 to 90 degrees.
2. Turn patient's head to left side to facilitate expectoration of blood.
3. Have emesis basin and tissues ready for expectoration of blood.
4. Provide clean basin frequently so that patient is not made more anxious by amount of blood.
5. Measure amount of hemoptysis and record time and amount.
6. Postural drainage and percussion are contraindicated when hemoptysis is present. Treatment is withheld during acute episodes of bleeding, usually for at least 24 hours.
7. Vitamin $K_1$ (Mephyton) is sometimes ordered by mouth or subcutaneously to control bleeding.
8. Stay with patient until bleeding has subsided and patient is made comfortable and is feeling less fearful.
9. Hemoptysis usually subsides without surgical intervention. If hemoptysis becomes life threatening, surgical intervention, such as removal of the bronchiectatic lobe, may be necessary. Unfortunately, in most patients, the pulmonary disease is too extensive to permit surgery.
10. Bronchoscopy with endobronchial tamponade may be successful in stopping bleeding in patients with minimal bleeding.

***Care of pneumothorax.*** Pneumothorax occurs when apical cysts rupture, allowing air from the lung to enter the pleural space. Sudden sharp chest pain in adults with CF should suggest spontaneous pneumothorax. Pneumothorax occurs in 20% of adult CF patients and has a recurrence rate of 50%. Symptomatic pneumothoraces (increasing shortness of breath, mediastinal shift) are treated with intercostal drainage as follows:

1. Stab wound is made between ribs, and chest tube is inserted.
2. Chest tube is connected to closed drainage system.
3. After the lung is reexpanded, pleural sclerosis with doxycycline or talc may be used. This procedure causes the visceral pleura to adhere to parietal pleura, obliterating the pleural space.
4. If there is a persistent air leak or pleural sclerosis fails, a partial pleurectomy may be performed. In a partial pleurectomy, the portion of pleura overlying the cysts that ruptured is removed.

***Care of cor pulmonale.*** As the airways become progressively plugged, atelectasis and air trapping occur. The result is a progressive V/Q mismatch, resulting in progressive hypoxemia. Cor pulmonale (right-sided heart failure secondary to pulmonary hypertension) can be expected to develop in patients with cystic fibrosis and advanced lung disease. A resting $Pa{O_2}$ less than 50 mm Hg and a $Pa{CO_2}$ greater than 45 mm Hg usually indicate cor pulmonale. Treatment of cor pulmonale includes the following:

1. Supplemental oxygen to help reverse pulmonary vasoconstriction caused by the hypoxemia and to improve myocardial performance. Oxygen therapy via cannula during sleep is usually prescribed for patients with a daytime resting $Pa{O_2}$ less than 60 mm Hg. Continuous oxygen is prescribed for patients with daytime resting $Pa{O_2}$ less than 50 mm Hg.
2. Long-term diuretic therapy and fluid restriction may be effective therapy. The patient is monitored closely for electrolyte imbalances.
3. Digoxin is of questionable value in patients with right ventricular failure. However, many patients with CF have biventricular failure, and digoxin may be of therapeutic value. Patients are monitored closely for hypoxemia and hypokalemia, which would increase the risk of digitalis toxicity.

**Diet.** Gastrointestinal problems are common and are treated as follows:

1. Supplemental fat-soluble vitamins are used to aid digestion and improve weight.
2. Most patients take multivitamins and vitamin E.
3. Pancreatic enzyme supplement doses are individualized and titrated by patients to control fatty stools to less than three per day.
4. When a patient can take nothing by mouth, minimal doses of pancreatic supplements are necessary.
5. If adequate intake cannot be maintained orally, IV feedings or gastrostomy may be necessary.

**Activity.** The patient is encouraged to be up as tolerated.

**Referrals.** Common referrals include pulmonary physiotherapy, respiratory therapy, social services, and genetic counseling. Most of these patients are readmissions, and they are well known to the services listed.

## NURSING MANAGEMENT

### ASSESSMENT

Assessment data need to be collected to assess the patient with CF in three areas: pulmonary, nutritional/GI, and psychosocial.

#### Pulmonary

##### *Subjective data*

Onset and description of symptoms such as shortness of breath, dyspnea on exertion, fatigue, and wheezing

Patient's understanding of CF pathophysiology and treatment regimens, including postural drainage and percussion; antibiotics; aerosol therapy with dornase-alfa, bronchodilators, and antibiotics; and nutritional supplements such as pancreatic enzymes and vitamins

##### *Objective data*

Auscultation for adventitious breath sounds

Chest pain on inspiration

Cyanotic mucous membrane

Digital clubbing (see Figure 30-13)

Productive cough and color of sputum

Presence of fever, tachypnea

Review ABGs for indications of falling $Pa{O_2}$ or rising $Pa{CO_2}$; review results of pulmonary function tests (decrease in tidal volume, $FEV_1$)

Signs and symptoms of antibiotic toxicity that may cause renal toxicity

Side effects of aerosols (bronchodilators) that may cause tachycardia

#### Nutritional/Gastrointestinal

##### *Subjective data*

Patient's description of color, consistency, and frequency of stools

Patient's description of color, smell, and frequency of urination

Patient's description of appetite and ability to swallow food

Patient's description of daily eating pattern

Medications taken at home and their effectiveness in decreasing stool frequency

Onset and duration of abdominal discomfort

Signs or symptoms of gastric reflux

Weight loss; when began

##### *Objective data*

Color, consistency, and frequency of stools

Appears thin

Presence of polyuria, polydipsia, or polyphagia

Dietary intake

Intensity, frequency, and location of abdominal pain

Absence of bowel sounds

#### Psychosocial

##### *Subjective data*

Description of daily routine as it relates to work or school, pulmonary regimen, medications, and leisure activities

Description of current coping strategies and support network

Concerns about sexuality or fertility

Method of financial support (job, family, other forms of assistance)

Patient's and family's understanding of CF

##### *Objective data*

Identify stage of grieving; symptoms that would infer that patient is grieving: anxiety, sleeplessness, hallucinations.

Identify patient and family strengths.

Identify patient support structure.

Identify normal adult developmental needs.

Identify need for genetic counseling, career counseling, or social services.

## NURSING DIAGNOSES

Nursing diagnoses are determined from analysis of patient data. Nursing diagnoses for the adult with CF may include but are not limited to:

| Diagnostic Title | Possible Etiological Factors |
|---|---|
| Airway clearance, ineffective | Obstruction/thick secretions, tracheobronchial infection, hemoptysis |
| Fatigue | Decreased oxygenation, inadequate nutrition, inadequate rest |
| Gas exchange, impaired | V/Q imbalance |
| Grieving, dysfunctional | Loss of fertility/loss of independence/loss of job or role/loss of control of one's life; unhealthy grief work/withdrawal, preoccupation, sleeplessness |
| Infection, risk for | Increased mucus in airway, decreased nutrition |
| Nutrition, altered: less than body requirements | Pancreatic insufficiency resulting in malabsorption, glucose intolerance/weight loss; shortness of breath makes eating difficult |

## EXPECTED PATIENT OUTCOMES

Expected patient outcomes for the person with CF may include but are not limited to:

1. Improved airway clearance
   a. Decreased mucus production
   b. Clear breath sounds
   c. Decreased fatigue and shortness of breath
   d. Absence of fever
   e. Absence of hemoptysis
2. Reduced fatigue
   a. Oxygenation improved and has less shortness of breath
   b. Is able to sleep better
3. Improved gas exchange
   a. $PaO_2$ 50 mm Hg or above
   b. $PaCO_2$ less than 45 mm Hg
4. Improved grieving skills
   a. Verbalizes actual and potential losses
   b. Identifies own strengths and personal goals
   c. Identifies support person to assist with coping and achievement of goals
5. Decreased risk for infection
   a. Decreased mucus in airway
   b. Environment free of pathogenic bacteria
   c. Nutrition improved
6. Improved nutrition
   a. Maintains weight within 20% of ideal weight
   b. Maintains normal blood glucose
   c. Is able to eat small frequent feedings that permit eating when less fatigued and short of breath

## INTERVENTIONS

Because the adult with CF is most often admitted to the hospital when the airway is compromised, considerable nursing care is necessary. The care of the adult with CF centers around the following measures.

### Improving Airway Clearance

1. Provide with postural drainage percussion every 2 to 4 hours, depending on the severity of the infection.
2. Assist patient to cough effectively.
3. Assess breath sounds before and after each treatment.
4. Encourage patient to increase fluid intake to 3 to 4 L every 24 hours unless contraindicated.
5. Monitor food intake; provide frequent snacks when energy level is improved.
6. Provide quiet environment with frequent monitoring and reassurance.
7. Maintain cool room with temperature below 70° F (21.1° C).

### Monitoring Fatigue

1. Assess fatigue frequently.
2. Provide rest periods between activities.
3. Provide frequent small feedings, which will increase energy stores.

### Improving Gas Exchange

1. Place in high Fowler's position.
2. Encourage slow, rhythmic breathing.
3. Encourage patient to breathe through nose and exhale through pursed lips.
4. Monitor ABG findings and pulse oximetry.

### Helping the Patient Cope with Grief

The nurse can play a major role in helping the patient work through the grieving process.

1. Identify stage of grieving.
2. Allow time for patient to verbalize feelings, hopes, and fears.
3. Support expressions of hope, but avoid false reassurance.
4. Support patient and family through grief work. Recommend CF support group as indicated.
5. Refer as appropriate for genetic counseling, career counseling, or social service.
6. Intervene for pathological symptoms of grief such as anxiety, sleeplessness, and hallucinations.
7. Be aware of your own feelings of grief, and share these with peers or a support group for nurses and other health care providers.

### Monitoring for Infection

Because the adult with CF is extremely vulnerable to infection or superinfection, the nurse needs to be aware of providing an environment that is as free of pathogens as possible.

1. Monitor patient's temperature frequently.
2. Monitor color, volume, and consistency of sputum.
3. Collect sputum specimens correctly, and send for culture and sensitivity as indicated.
4. Give antibiotics as prescribed and on time to maintain adequate blood level.

5. Keep all persons with upper respiratory infections away from patient.
6. Wash own hands frequently, and encourage visitors to wash hands before touching the patient.
7. Provide frequent mouth care, especially after postural drainage.
8. Assist patient to wash hands after coughing.

### Promoting Adequate Nutrition

Because the patient with CF often has difficulty in maintaining nutrition, the nurse may need to be ingenious in promoting nutrition.

1. Perform baseline and periodic assessment of nutrition, including food history, recording of daily intake/output and daily weight.
2. Monitor blood glucose levels so that insulin can be given as prescribed according to blood glucose findings.
3. Provide small, frequent feedings.
4. Work with dietitian and patient to provide feedings that will appeal to patient.
5. Administer pancreatic enzymes and vitamins as ordered.

### Patient/Family Education

Because the adult patient has had CF for several years, teaching is more in the form of review and reinforcement. In addition to the teaching guidelines for patients with COPD (see p. 999), the following areas should be addressed with the patient with CF:

1. Review daily nutrition requirements, vitamins, and the need to check weight daily.
2. Review daily pulmonary exercises and treatments.
   a. Postural drainage and percussion
   b. Aerosol medication before postural drainage
3. Review medications in terms of usual dose, expected effects, and side effects. In some sections of the United States, medications can be obtained at substantial discount through the local Cystic Fibrosis Foundation.
4. Review clinical symptoms that indicate that the health care provider should be notified.
   a. Signs of an acute respiratory infection such as fever, increased fatigue, shortness of breath, increased production of sputum, or change in color of sputum
   b. Hemoptysis
   c. Sudden sharp chest pain
5. Assess patient's knowledge and understanding of fertility, genetic testing, and contraceptive methods.
6. Assess patient's and family's knowledge of community and social resources for assistance with health care reimbursement programs, disability insurance, and finding an appropriate support group.

#### *Health promotion/prevention*

Because CF is a genetically inherited disease, identification of carriers who may pass on the defect and disease to offspring remains the most important preventive strategy. Early identification of carriers combined with genetic counseling minimizes the chance of offspring inheriting this lethal genetic disease. Family histories of possible incidences of CF should be followed up by genetic testing.

## ■ EVALUATION

To evaluate the effectiveness of nursing interventions, compare patient behaviors with those listed in the expected patient outcomes. Successful achievement of patient outcomes for the adult with CF admitted for treatment of a respiratory infection is indicated by:

1. Ability to mobilize secretions and clear own airway
2. Daily schedule that allows ample time for activities so that fatigue is avoided
3. $Pa{O_2}$ of 75 mm Hg and $Pa{CO_2}$ of 40 mm Hg
4. Verbalizing feelings about this latest hospitalization
5. Absence of infection
6. Being 0.5 lb below admission weight

## GERONTOLOGICAL CONSIDERATIONS

Although many persons with CF are living longer, CF is not a condition found in the elderly.

## SPECIAL ENVIRONMENTS FOR CARE

### Critical Care Management

When patients with CF develop respiratory failure, they may be placed in an ICU. However, most of these patients have do-not-resuscitate (DNR) orders and are not moved to an ICU. See following discussion under Complications.

### Home Care Management

The goal in the care of persons with CF is to care for them at home with admission to the hospital being limited to life-threatening conditions that should respond to hospital treatment. The care discussed under Interventions would be given at home by either a family member or a nurse from a home health care agency. The Cystic Fibrosis Association is very helpful to patients and families in terms of supplying names of health care resources and providing support to family members who are caregivers.

## COMPLICATIONS

Patients with CF eventually succumb to progressive respiratory and cardiac failure. Because these patients have a fatal disease, they usually have DNR orders and are not intubated or placed on mechanical ventilation. The patient and family have to be involved in the DNR decision, and nurses play an important role in supporting the patient and family in their decision.

## RESPIRATORY FAILURE

### Etiology

Acute respiratory failure (ARF) is used to describe any rapid change in respiration resulting in hypoxemia, hypercarbia, or both. Acute respiratory failure can be separated into two major categories: *hypoventilation* and *hypoxemia.* They commonly occur together, because an increase in alveolar carbon dioxide tension always results in a decrease in alveolar oxygen tension. However, hypoxemia can occur without hypercarbia in acute parenchymal lung disease. Some experts make a distinction between ARF in a previously healthy person and ARF in persons with COPD, which they call *acute on chronic respiratory failure (AOCRF)*.[22]

### Epidemiology

Many disorders can lead to or are associated with respiratory failure (Table 32-32).

### Pathophysiology

The respiratory system is made up of two basic parts: the gas exchange organ (the lungs) and the pump (the respiratory muscles and the respiratory control mechanisms). Any alteration in the function of the gas exchange unit or the pump can result in respiratory insufficiency or failure.

Regardless of the underlying condition, the resultant events or processes that occur in respiratory failure are the same. With inadequate ventilation, the arterial oxygen falls, and tissue cells become hypoxic. Carbon dioxide accumulates, leading to a fall in pH and respiratory acidosis.

Lung or gas exchange unit respiratory failure is usually seen in persons with underlying primary pulmonary disease such as COPD. In this situation, respiratory failure is a result of pathology directly affecting the respiratory unit.

Pump failure is associated with the extrapulmonary disorders that may precipitate respiratory failure. In this situation the underlying disorder decreases the ability of the lungs to move oxygen and carbon dioxide into and out of the lungs by altering either the central ventilatory control mechanism (e.g., drug overdose), neuromuscular function (e.g., Guillain-Barré syndrome), or chest wall movement (e.g., flail chest).

**table 32-32** *Disorders Associated with Respiratory Failure*

| Pulmonary Disorders | Nonpulmonary Disorders |
|---|---|
| Severe infection | CNS disturbance secondary to drug overdose, anesthesia, head injury |
| Pulmonary edema | Neuromuscular disorders (e.g., Guillain-Barré syndrome, myasthenia gravis, multiple sclerosis, poliomyelitis, muscular dystrophy, spinal cord injury) |
| Pulmonary embolus | Postoperative reduction in ventilation following thoracic and abdominal surgery |
| COPD | Prolonged mechanical ventilation |
| CF | |
| ARDS | |
| Cancer | |
| Chest trauma (flail chest) | |
| Severe atelectasis | |
| Airway compromise secondary to trauma, infection, or surgery | |

**box 32-28** *Physiological Criteria for Acute Respiratory Failure*

Sudden onset of the following:
- $Pa_{O_2}$ 50 mm Hg or less (measured on room air)
- $Pa_{CO_2}$ 50 mm Hg or more
- pH 7.35 or less

Acute respiratory failure is defined by predetermined physiological criteria. Box 32-28 lists physiological parameters that define acute respiratory failure.

Hypercapnia and hypoxemia are present in chronic respiratory failure. In chronic respiratory failure the pH usually stays within the range of 7.35 to 7.40 because of compensation. Patients with chronic respiratory failure develop acute on chronic respiratory failure as a result of a secondary insult to their already compromised pulmonary system, usually in the form of a respiratory infection. The individual can no longer compensate for the altered lung function, and a dramatic decrease in pH (below 7.35), accompanied by severe hypoxemia, occurs. Because carbon dioxide retention (hypercapnia) preexists in these individuals, the $Pa_{CO_2}$ is less relevant than pH and $Pa_{O_2}$ in determining respiratory status. In fact, these patients often display few clinical signs or symptoms, even though they may have major blood gas derangements.

Underlying blood gas alterations are the basis for the clinical signs and symptoms associated with respiratory failure. Box 32-29 lists the common signs associated with hypoxemia, hypercapnia, and respiratory acidosis. The signs and symptoms are presented together because the blood gas derangements causing them usually occur simultaneously.

In acute respiratory failure, VC is markedly decreased. However, PFTs are useful only if the patient is alert and able to cooperate. Vital capacity can be measured at the bedside with a Wright respirometer. It is important for the nurse to recognize that the signs and symptoms associated with hypoxemia and hypercapnia depend more on the rate of change in value than on absolute value. The patient with COPD may show few signs until severe acute respiratory failure occurs. The normal function, pathophysiology, and clinical manifestations of a person with acute respiratory failure are presented in Table 32-33.

### Collaborative Care Management

Collaborative care management of respiratory failure is presented in Box 32-30.

## NURSING MANAGEMENT

### ASSESSMENT

#### Subjective Data

Data to be collected to assess the patient with respiratory insufficiency or failure include:

History of past or present associated disorders (see Table 32-32)

**box 32-29** *Signs and Symptoms Associated with Hypercapnia, Hypoxemia, and Respiratory Acidosis*

| | |
|---|---|
| Headache | Cardiac dysrhythmias |
| Irritability | Tachycardia |
| Confusion | Hypotension |
| Increasing somnolence, coma | Cyanosis |
| Asterixis (flapping tremor) | |

Recent change in respiratory status
- Change in sputum (color, viscosity, odor)
- Increased dyspnea
- Change in mental status
- Complaints of chest tightness or pain

Current medications: any recent changes in medication regimen

Self-care modalities

**box 32-30** *Collaborative Care Management of Respiratory Failure*

1. Medical therapy is based on degree of severity
   a. Severe acute respiratory failure: focus on immediate oxygenation and ventilation
   b. Less severe acute respiratory failure: underlying cause determined and treated concurrently while treating hypoxemia and hypercapnia
2. Clinical evaluation
   a. Diagnostic studies
      (1) ABGs
      (2) Chest x-ray film
      (3) Bedside pulmonary spirometry
      (4) Sputum for culture and sensitivity (C & S)
   b. Treatments
      (1) Oxygen therapy
      (2) Ventilation: may require intubation and mechanical ventilatory support
      (3) Treatment of complications
      (4) Treatment of underlying cause

If available, a family member or friend may be able to provide objective information about changes in the patient.

### Objective Data

Objective data include:

Assess general appearance.

Assess mental status: may vary from agitation to somnolence.

Assess vital signs.
- Tachycardia
- Tachypnea, bradypnea, or apnea (respiratory rates less than 8/min result in alveolar hypoventilation; rates over 35/min cannot be sustained)[22]
- Hypotension

Perform pulmonary examination.
- Select components of pulmonary examination that patient can tolerate. Findings will depend on underlying cause of respiratory failure.

Assess laboratory findings.
- ABGs for blood gas derangements associated with acute respiratory failure
- Sputum culture and sensitivity (C&S): often positive
- Bedside spirometry: VC is less than 15 ml/kg ideal body weight

## NURSING DIAGNOSES

Nursing diagnoses are determined from analysis of patient data. Nursing diagnoses for the person with respiratory failure may include but are not limited to:

**table 32-33** *Normal Function, Primary Pathology, and Clinical Manifestations in Acute Respiratory Failure*

| Normal Function | Pathophysiology | Clinical Manifestations |
|---|---|---|
| **ALVEOLOCAPILLARY MEMBRANE** | | |
| Site of oxygen and carbon dioxide exchange | Interstitial and alveolar edema, airway obstruction from mucus and bronchoconstriction causing inadequate $O_2$ and $CO_2$ transport and exchange, with resultant hypoxemia, hypercapnia, and acidosis | Headache, cardiac dysrhythmias, ↑ $Paco_2$, ↓ $Pao_2$, ↓ pH, irritability, cyanosis, confusion, tachycardia, hypotension, asterixis (flapping tremor), increasing somnolence with eventual coma |
| **RESPIRATORY MUSCLES** | | |
| Expand and contract chest and lungs | Respiratory muscle strength and endurance unable to counterbalance mechanical load placed on muscles | Increased work of breathing, dyspnea, exhaustion, and ↓ vital capacity |
| **CENTRAL AND PERIPHERAL CHEMORECEPTORS** | | |
| Controls rate and depth of ventilation in response to pH and $CO_2$ in CSF (central) or low levels of $Po_2$ (peripheral) | Decreased or absent response to $CO_2$, pH, or $Po_2$ levels | Increasing somnolence progressing to coma if untreated, worsening hypoxemia, hypercapnia, and acidosis |
| **RIGHT-SIDED CARDIAC OUTPUT** | | |
| Right side: receive unoxygenated blood from systemic circulation and carry deoxygenated blood to lungs for reoxygenation | Increased pulmonary vascular resistance from hypoxemia or lung pathology increases pressure on right side of heart, causing increased venous pressure | Peripheral edema, neck vein distention, hepatomegaly |

| Diagnostic Title | Possible Etiological Factors |
|---|---|
| Gas exchange, impaired | V/Q imbalance |
| Airway clearance, ineffective | Fatigue, tracheobronchial infection, airway obstruction |
| Cardiac output, decreased | Increased pulmonary vascular resistance |
| Nutrition, altered: less than body requirements | Unable to maintain intake large enough to balance increased metabolic needs from increased work of breathing |
| Knowledge deficit: prevention and treatment | Lack of exposure or recall, cognitive impairment |

## EXPECTED PATIENT OUTCOMES

Expected patient outcomes for the person with respiratory failure may include but are not limited to:

1. Improved ventilation and oxygenation.
   a. ABG, pH, and $Paco_2$ return to or stay within acceptable baseline limits.
   b. $Pao_2$ at optimal level for individual.
   c. Explaining how and when to use oxygen therapy.
   d. Sensorium returns to or is maintained at pre–respiratory failure level.
   e. Respiratory rate is within or near normal levels, with moderate tidal volume.
   f. Dyspnea is absent or returns to preacute illness level.
2. Effective airway clearance.
   a. Effective coughing maneuvers
   b. Appropriate use of nebulizers, MDI, humidifiers
3. Adequate cardiac output.
   a. Absence of pulsus paradoxus
   b. Blood pressure within acceptable limits
   c. Heart rate and rhythm within acceptable limits
   d. Pulses equal and present in all extremities
   e. Urine output greater than 30 ml/hr
4. Adequate nutritional intake to balance metabolic needs.
   a. Weight stabilizes at preacute illness weight.
   b. If preillness weight is outside acceptable limits for size and age, weight progresses toward an established goal weight.
5. Describing signs and symptoms that should be reported to the physician.

Patients with underlying COPD also meet the outcome criteria for persons with COPD (see p. 989).

## INTERVENTIONS

The level of nursing interventions for acute respiratory failure will depend on the patient's immediate status. The patient's condition may vary from critically ill, requiring immediate life support measures (cardiopulmonary resuscitation), to less urgent, in which aggressive nursing interventions can prevent further deterioration of physical status. Nursing interventions for acute respiratory failure include the following.

### Improving Gas Exchange

Severe hypoxemia is incompatible with life. Thus it is imperative to initiate oxygen therapy rapidly if severe hypoxemia is present. General oxygen therapy is discussed on p. 927.

The effectiveness of oxygen therapy is evaluated with ABG measurements and pulse oximetry. Supplemental oxygen should be provided to maintain a $Pao_2$ of 60 to 90 mm Hg. Persons without underlying pulmonary disease can receive oxygen by either high-flow or low-flow systems. However, hazards are associated with prolonged exposure to high concentrations of oxygen.

*Oxygen toxicity* is the term used to describe the damage to lung tissue that results from prolonged exposure to high oxygen concentrations. Although the exact effects of oxygen in any one individual may depend on the person's underlying pathological condition, exposure to greater than 60% oxygen for more than 36 hours or exposure to 90% oxygen for more than 6 hours may result in atelectasis and alveolar collapse. Breathing very high concentrations of oxygen (80% to 100%) for prolonged periods (24 hours or more) is often associated with the development of ARDS. Thus a firm general principle is to use the lowest amount of oxygen that will achieve an acceptable $Pao_2$.

Special precautions must be taken when administering oxygen to patients with COPD who are carbon dioxide retainers to avoid further elevation of their $Paco_2$ levels, resulting in carbon dioxide narcosis or coma (Box 32-31).

Patients with COPD (who are carbon dioxide retainers) must receive supplemental oxygen via a controlled oxygen therapy system. The Venturi mask provides oxygen at controlled ranges of 24% to 40% (Figure 32-32). When low-flow oxygen is desired, oxygen is given by nasal cannula. However, the actual concentration of oxygen delivered to the lungs by cannula depends on the patient's ventilatory pattern. Regardless of the oxygen delivery system used, the patient's response to oxygen therapy can be accurately assessed only by ABG measurements or pulse oximetry.

Adequate oxygenation is essential for life. Therefore, if adequate oxygenation cannot be maintained without a concurrent rise in $Paco_2$ (hypercapnia), oxygen therapy must still be continued. In this situation, mechanical ventilation is instituted to combat the hypercapnia.

Although *carbon dioxide narcosis* might be precipitated if a chronically hypoxemic person receives high concentrations of oxygen, treatment of the hypoxemia is the first priority in the patient's care. Medical research on the effect of administering high oxygen concentrations to patients with COPD who were in respiratory failure showed little change in their respiratory drive. These findings can be balanced in care of the chronically hypoxemic patient in acute respiratory failure by basing practice on the principle that the first priority for sur-

**box 32-31** *Oxygen Therapy for the Person with Elevated $Paco_2$*

Oxygen therapy resulting in elevated $Pao_2$ levels may decrease the ventilatory drive in patients who retain carbon dioxide and are chronically hypoxemic. Decreased ventilatory drive causes hypoventilation, which causes elevated $Paco_2$ levels, respiratory acidosis, and, ultimately, carbon dioxide narcosis and death.

vival in a person experiencing acute respiratory failure is to receive adequate oxygen. However, patients with COPD are at risk of developing carbon dioxide narcosis; therefore they must be monitored continuously during oxygen therapy in order to intervene if a loss of ventilatory drive should occur.

### Ventilatory Support

Ventilatory support is focused on reversing hypercapnia caused by hypoventilation. Aggressive nursing interventions to improve ventilation can often be effective in preventing the need for intubation and artificial ventilatory support (see interventions to improve airway clearance following the discussion on mechanical ventilation).

### Mechanical Ventilation

If, despite all the measures discussed, the person is unable to maintain ventilation (as indicated by a rising arterial $Paco_2$), mechanical ventilation is necessary. The goal of mechanical ventilation is to deliver a minute ventilation (respiratory rate times tidal volume) with an enriched concentration of oxygen sufficient for adequate tissue oxygenation. The usual tidal volume delivered by a ventilator is in the range of 10 to 15 ml/kg, compared with a spontaneous tidal volume of 5 ml/kg.

Because of the complexity of mechanical ventilation, the ideal place for these patients is in an ICU, where experienced staff can care for them. However, because of the high cost associated with keeping long-term ventilator patients in the ICU, some hospitals have set up special care units for these patients. Other hospitals place long-term ventilator patients on general medical-surgical units. The general principles for care of patients on ventilators follow.

Many different kinds of ventilators are available. In general, there are two types: pressure-cycled and volume-limited ventilators. The Bird and Bennett (PR series) are pressure-limited ventilators used mainly for IPPB treatments. Several volume-cycled ventilators are available (Figures 32-33 and 32-34).

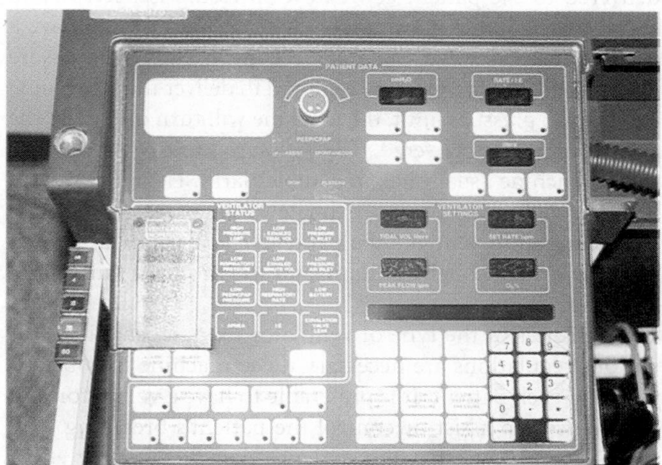

fig. 32-33 Front display panel of a ventilator for monitoring airway pressures and volumes.

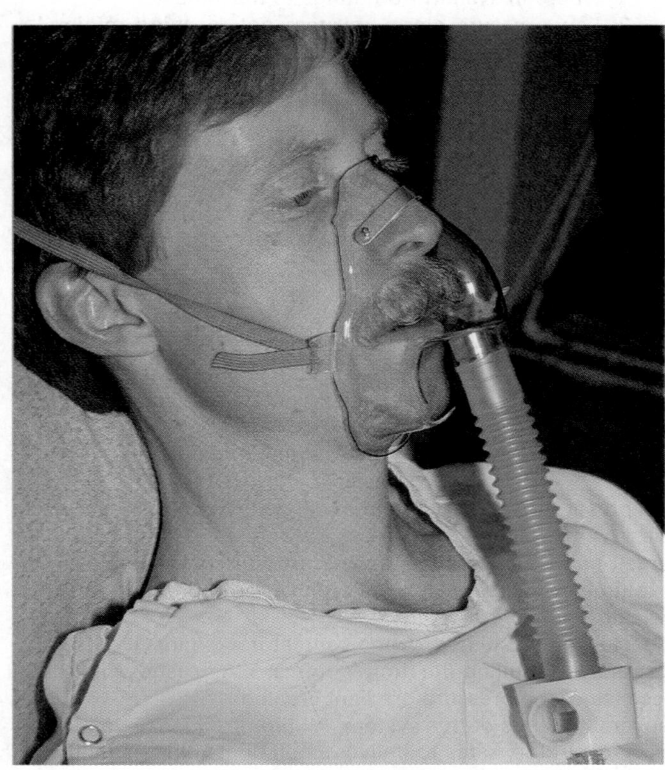

fig. 32-32 Venturi mask.

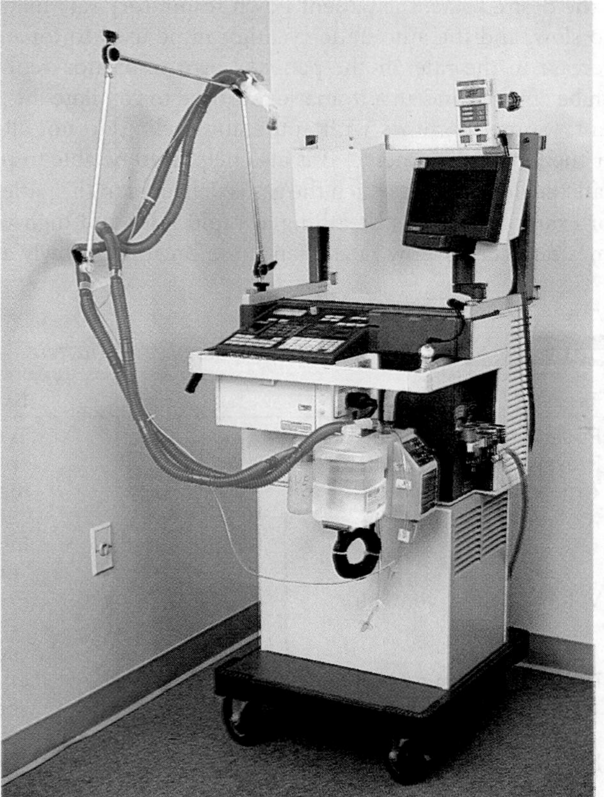

fig. 32-34 A mechanical ventilator.

Table 32-34 lists the types of ventilators and their mode of function.

Volume-cycled ventilators are currently the most often used. They provide a wide range of flexibility to meet individual requirements for adequate oxygen and carbon dioxide exchange. Box 32-32 lists the functions that can be adjusted on the volume-cycled ventilator.

With a volume-cycled machine a *constant volume* of air is delivered with each breath. The volume is preset and is delivered to the patient at whatever pressure is necessary to attain that volume. A volume-cycled machine should have a pressure cut off valve. Such a mechanism allows a pressure limit to be set. If the pressure required to deliver the set volume exceeds the pressure limit, the machine will turn off before the entire volume is delivered. The pressure limit on a volume-cycled machine usually has an audible alarm. The nurse can set the limit slightly above (approximately 5 cm of water) the pressure required to ventilate the patient. The alarm will then go off if the patient coughs, accumulates secretions, or starts to resist the machine.

Regardless of the type of ventilator used, mechanisms for various regulations are necessary if the machine is to be adjusted to each patient. It is preferable to have a ventilator that can be used to assist or control the patient's breathing. The term *assist* means that the patient's own inspiratory effort triggers (turns on) the machine. Most respirators have a sensitivity control knob that can be adjusted to respond to weak inspiratory efforts. The term *control* implies the use of automatic cycling. The patient may be apneic and the machine set at the desired rate; the patient's own respiratory rate may be too slow, and the automatic cycling can be used to force an increase in the rate; or the patient's own respiratory efforts can be ignored and an automatic rate used to ventilate the patient. (Some machines with automatic cycling do not allow for the latter adjustment.) It is also helpful to be able to regulate the flow rates at which the gas is delivered to the patient. For example, patients breathing at rapid rates and high volumes need faster flow rates than those breathing slowly and at moderate volumes. A final necessity is the ability to regulate the inspired concentration of oxygen from 21% (room air) to 100%.

The most common modes of mechanical ventilation are assist/control (AC) and synchronized intermittent mandatory ventilation (SIMV). These two modes can be used alone or with continuous positive airway pressure (CPAP), positive end-expiratory pressure (PEEP), or pressure support ventilation (PSV) (Table 32-35). Regardless of the type of ventilator used, certain parameters must be determined by the physician (Box 32-33).

#### Assist/control

In the AC mode, the ventilator senses each time the patient begins to inspire and delivers a breath. If the patient is unable to trigger the machine, the ventilator delivers the preset number of breaths at the set tidal volume. The AC mode is also called continuous mechanical ventilation (CMV) and gives the patient complete ventilatory support.

**box 32-32** *Functions That Can Be Adjusted with Volume-Cycled Ventilators*

Tidal volume—volume of air in a normal breath

$FiO_2$—oxygenation concentration delivered through the ventilator

Alarm systems—vary from machine to machine; basic alarms usually present:

1. High-pressure alarm—increased resistance somewhere in system from lungs to machine
2. Low-pressure alarm—system not reaching minimal pressure required for ventilation
3. Low-volume alarm—when volume of ventilation does not equal the amount set

Control modes—degree of ventilation that is controlled by the ventilator; can vary from complete ventilator control to almost total patient control

**table 32-34** *Types of Mechanical Ventilators*

| Types | | Basic Function Mode |
|---|---|---|
| Positive-pressure ventilator | Require intubation | Types of positive-pressure ventilators are based on how inspiratory phase is ended. |
| Pressure-cycled ventilator | Require intubation | Inspiration ends at a preset pressure limit; time and volume are variable. |
| Time-cycled ventilator | Require intubation | Inspiration is preset for a given time interval; volume and pressure are variable. |
| Volume-cycled ventilator | Require intubation | Preset volume of air is delivered. Time and pressure are variable. However, volume-cycled ventilators often have pressure- and time-cycled capacities. |
| Negative-pressure ventilator (intubation not required) | | Thorax, at least, is encapsulated. When ventilator expands, it creates negative pressure by pulling the thorax outward. Air rushes into the airways because of the pressure gradient created. |
| High-frequency ventilation (requires intubation) | | There are several variants of this system. All high-frequency ventilators use high respiratory rates to deliver small tidal volumes at low pressures. |

### Synchronized intermittent mandatory ventilation

Synchronized intermittent mandatory ventilation (SIMV) allows the patient to take additional breaths over the set rate of the ventilator. The volume of extra breaths is determined by the patient's ability and effort to breathe spontaneously. In SIMV the number of ventilator breaths can be gradually reduced until the patient is breathing on his or her own.

### Positive end-expiratory pressure

Positive end-expiratory pressure is a ventilator mode that has been shown to increase the effectiveness of mechanical ventilation in certain patients. It involves the maintenance of positive pressure at the end of expiration, rather than allowing airway pressure to return to normal (atmospheric) as usually occurs. By maintaining positive pressure, alveoli that would otherwise collapse on expiration are held open, thus increasing the opportunity for gas exchange across the alveolar capillary membrane. This is accomplished by the increase in FRC. The result is a decrease in physiological shunting and the ability to achieve a higher level of $PaO_2$ with lower concentrations of delivered oxygen ($FiO_2$). Positive end-expiratory pressure has its greatest use in the treatment of ARDS but is also used in treating any patient who would otherwise require unacceptably high concentrations of oxygen.

Positive end-expiratory pressure can be hazardous because of the increase in intrathoracic pressure. Most serious of the dangers related to PEEP is the increased incidence of pneumothorax, particularly in those with friable lung tissue, as seen in persons with emphysema or lung cancer. The sudden disappearance of breath sounds on one side and mediastinal shift, in conjunction with signs of respiratory distress, in the patient being ventilated with PEEP *must be taken as an indication of a pneumothorax.* This can develop into a life-threatening episode if the pneumothorax is large, and the physician must be called immediately. Another serious consequence of PEEP may be a reduction in venous return, caused by the increased intrathoracic pressure and a subsequent fall in cardiac output. This effect seems to be particularly common in patients who are relatively dehydrated and can sometimes be avoided by careful fluid administration.

**box 32-33 Ventilator Settings Prescribed by Physician[22]**

When a patient is placed on a ventilator, the physician prescribes the following:

- Respiratory rate
- Tidal volume
- Inspired oxygen concentration
- Mode
- Positive end-expiratory pressure (PEEP)
- Inspiratory/expiratory ratio

**table 32-35 Ventilator Modes**

| Mode | Description |
|---|---|
| Assist/control (A/C) | Each breath is ventilator assisted. If patient is unable to trigger machine, the ventilator continues to deliver preset number of breaths at the set tidal volume. |
| Bilevel CPAP (BiPAP) | Positive pressure applied to spontaneous breathing allowing inspiratory positive pressure and expiratory positive pressure to be set independently. |
| Continuous positive airway pressure (CPAP) | Positive pressure applied during respiration and maintained throughout entire respiratory cycle. Decreases intrapulmonary shunting. |
| Controlled mandatory ventilation (CMV) | Ventilator delivers a preset volume at a fixed rate regardless of patient's effort to breathe. |
| Independent lung ventilation (ILV) | Each lung is ventilated separately. Used in unilateral lung disease. Requires intubation with double-lumen tube. |
| Intermittent mandatory ventilation (IMV) | Ventilator delivers preset number of breaths. Patient may take unassisted breaths. |
| Positive end-expiratory pressure (PEEP) | Applies positive pressure at end of expiration. Decreases intrapulmonic shunting. |
| Pressure-support ventilation (PSV) | Selected amount of positive pressure applied to airway during patient's spontaneous respiratory efforts. Amount of pressure gradually reduced until patient is receiving no assistance. |
| Synchronized intermittent mandatory ventilation (SIMV) | Intermittent ventilator breaths synchronized with patient's spontaneous breaths. Reduces competition between patient and ventilator. |
| High-frequency ventilation | Special positive-pressure ventilator used in some patients. |
| **HIGH-FREQUENCY VENTILATORS** | |
| High-frequency positive-pressure ventilation (HFPPV) | Extremely short inspiratory times with a total volume equivalent to dead space. Rate 60-100 cycles/min. |
| High-frequency jet ventilation (HFJV) | Small volumes < anatomical dead space are pulsed through jet injector catheter at 100-600 cycles/min. |
| High-frequency oscillation ventilation (HFO) | Small volume of gas is continuously vibrated in airways at rates up to 4000 cycles/min. |

Adapted from Stillwell SB: *Mosby's critical care nursing reference,* ed 2, St Louis, 1996, Mosby.

#### Continuous positive airway pressure

Continuous positive airway pressure is a technique that maintains positive pressure in the lung during spontaneous ventilation. It is used most often with spontaneously breathing patients, although it also can be delivered through the tubing circuits of a volume-controlled ventilator. Continuous positive airway pressure maintains positive pressure continuously. In this way it is similar to PEEP, which is used only for patients being mechanically ventilated. With CPAP, expiration is controlled by a valve in the expiratory circuit that measures airway pressure and stops expiration before airway pressure returns to zero.

One disadvantage of CPAP is that the work of breathing may be increased because of resistance in initiating gas flow. The level of CPAP chosen should be as low as possible to obtain a $Pa{O_2}$ greater than 60 mm Hg with a relatively safe $Fi{O_2}$ of less than 0.6. With CPAP there is lack of backup mandatory ventilation, and careful monitoring of oxygen saturation with oximeters is essential. Respiratory rates, level of agitation, and ABGs must be monitored to prevent unrecognized hypercapnia.

#### Pressure support ventilation

Pressure support ventilation (PSV) relies on patient effort to determine tidal volume and frequency. This mode differs from CPAP in that the patient's inspiratory efforts trigger ventilator airflow until a preset airway pressure is reached. Airflow continues as long as the patient is making sufficient inspiratory effort to keep airway pressure below the preset limit. The advantages of pressure support ventilation may include overcoming the circuit-resistance breathing associated with spontaneous breathing through a ventilator. By decreasing the level of *pressure support* over time, this mode of ventilation can be an effective weaning technique.

#### Biphasic airway pressure

Biphasic airway pressure (BiPAP) delivers PSV for inspiration and CPAP on expiration. It is used primarily to assist breathing during sleep for patients with neuromuscular disorders such as muscular dystrophy and central sleep apnea. To deliver BiPAP, a small mask is fitted over the nose. The use of BiPAP during sleep allows the patient to obtain a restful night's sleep and to awake feeling more refreshed.

#### Suctioning the patient

When the patient on a ventilator needs suctioning, a closed system is preferred. In closed-system endotracheal suctioning, an adaptor is inserted at the endotracheal tube–ventilatory circuitry interface. This allows patients to be suctioned without disconnecting them from the ventilator. The benefits of this form of suctioning are (1) continuation of oxygen supply, (2) the stability of PEEP, and (3) reducing the incidence of ventilator-associated pneumonia.[32,41,42] See Box 32-34, which lists the steps in closed-system suctioning, and also Figure 32-35.

#### General care of the patient on a ventilator

When care is planned for the patient on a mechanical ventilator, knowing the patient's ability to breathe spontaneously in the event of accidental disconnection from the ventilator is imperative. In most facilities, respiratory therapists regularly monitor ventilator function and settings, but the nurse is also responsible for ensuring that the ventilator settings are maintained. Usually a checklist is used to verify the ventilator settings on an hourly basis.

The patient should be assessed on a regular basis and any time a ventilator alarm sounds. The cause of an alarm sounding can be a dysfunction anywhere from the person's lungs to the machine. Troubleshooting should be carried out in a systematic manner, starting with the patient and moving toward the machine. Assessment should include:

1. Patient assessment
   a. Inspection
      (1) Does the person appear to be in respiratory distress?
      (2) Is the person's chest moving with machine-cycled inspiration?
      (3) Is the chest moving bilaterally?
   b. Auscultation
      (1) Are breath sounds present?
      (2) Are adventitious sounds present?
      (3) Are breath sounds coordinated with ventilator inspiration?
2. Assessment of tubing to machine: inspection
   a. Is there an air leak around the endotracheal cuff?
   b. Is there excess condensation in the tubing? (Always remove water from tubing system. Do not empty back into

**box 32-34** *Closed-System Suctioning*[10]

1. Wash hands for 10 seconds as recommended by the CDC.
2. Glove.
3. Select catheter that is one half the diameter of the artificial airway. Catheter has a suction valve at one end, a patient connector at the other end, and is enclosed in a plastic sheath.
4. Attach suction valve to suction source. Select suction pressure between −80 mm Hg and −120 mm Hg. Set the maximum pressure by pinching the suction tubing closed.
5. Attach patient connector to ventilator tubing and the endotracheal tube (ET).
6. Use the ventilator to hyperoxygenate and hyperinflate the patient's lungs before suctioning.
7. Open the access valve and advance catheter through connector into the ET and trachea.
8. Using the suction valve, apply suction for not more than 10 seconds as the catheter is withdrawn. Repeat as necessary.
9. Provide 100% oxygen and deep breaths while suctioning.
10. Withdraw catheter and close access valve.
11. Clean suction tip by attaching a normal saline unit-dose vial or syringe containing normal saline to irrigation port. Squirt the saline on catheter tip and apply suction until catheter is clean and saline is sucked out of catheter.
12. Remove gloves and wash hands for 10 seconds.

humidifier reservoir.) NOTE: Not all ventilators have humidifiers.

c. Check all ventilator settings and readouts.

If the alarm continues to sound and the cause cannot be determined or the patient is in respiratory distress, the patient is disconnected from the machine and manually ventilated with an AMBU bag (or anesthesia bag) with oxygenated air until the problem can be resolved.

### *Weaning from the ventilator*

The decision to wean a person from the ventilator is based on clinical evidence of improved physical status. Weaning is most successful when performed by a nurse who has developed a trust relationship with the patient. The underlying pathology that compromised the patient's respiratory status must be stabilized, or the patient's condition will deteriorate when the ventilator is discontinued. Weaning is initiated when the patient meets certain physiological criteria, including the following:

1. Acceptable ABGs
2. Tidal volume greater than 10 ml/kg
3. VC greater than 15 ml/kg
4. $FiO_2$ less than 0.5
5. Maximal inspiratory pressure greater than −20 cm $H_2O$ (usually prefer −30 to −40 cm $H_2O$)
6. Normal hematocrit

Most patients on long-term ventilator support have hematocrits below 30. They are usually not transfused until their hematocrit falls to about 25. There is general agreement that weaning is most successful when the patient's hematocrit is 30 or higher.

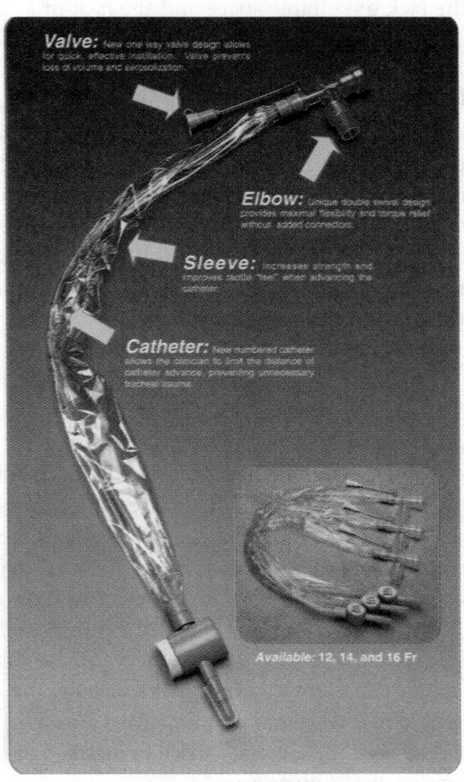


**fig. 32-35** Closed-system suctioning tube.

The weaning process is individualized to meet the patient's needs. The three most common methods of weaning are as follows:

1. T-piece weaning
   a. Place patient in upright position.
   b. Disconnect patient from ventilator.
   c. Connect a T-piece to endotracheal tube cuff to provide oxygenated humidified air.
   d. Observe patient for signs of respiratory distress, and reconnect to ventilator when patient indicates fatigue. Some patients may be able to breathe for only a few minutes on their own; others may do well for 30 minutes.
   e. Time off ventilator is gradually increased.
2. Synchronized intermittent mandatory ventilation (SIMV)
   a. Patient remains connected to the ventilator. The number of synchronized mandatory breaths delivered by machine is gradually reduced, allowing the patient to take an increasing number of breaths independently.
   b. Patient is disconnected from the ventilator when predetermined physiological criteria are maintained.
3. Pressure-support ventilation (PSV)
   a. Patient remains connected to ventilator. The level of preset positive pressure during inspiration is gradually reduced until the patient is receiving no assistance.
   b. This mode helps reduce airflow resistance of artificial airways, making breathing easier.

See the Research Box on the next page for a comparison of four methods of weaning.

Some nurse experts divide the weaning process into three phases: *preweaning, weaning,* and *extubation.* During the preweaning stage, special attention is given to ensuring that the patient will have *normal electrolytes,* including *phosphate, calcium,* and *magnesium.* Malnutrition is to be avoided, but the patient should not be overfed. Overfeeding with carbohydrates and extra calories may result in increased carbon dioxide production and increased ventilatory demand. The recommended 24-hour caloric intake is 1500 to 2500 calories, which should ensure adequate calories for energy expenditure. Protein intake is important, and 1 to 1.5 mg/kg has been suggested. Tube feedings containing these requirements are given to prepare the patient for weaning. Nursing interventions during the weaning process include:

1. Before initiating weaning, prepare the patient. Teach effective breathing techniques. Inform the patient that weaning may take several attempts.
2. Obtain baseline vital signs, tidal volume, and vital capacity.
3. Stay with the patient during the initial weaning process.
4. Coach the patient as needed to breathe slower and deeper with emphasis on increasing the time of exhalation.
5. Suction as needed.
6. Monitor for the clinical signs of hypoxemia and hypercapnia (increased respiratory rate, tachycardia, dysrhythmias, increased blood pressure, agitation, diaphoresis, or increased somnolence).

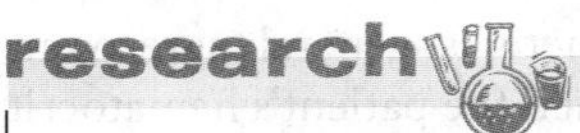

Reference: Esteban A et al: A comparison of four methods of weaning patients from mechanical ventilation, *N Engl J Med* 332(6):345, 1995.

The purpose of this study was to determine which of four methods of weaning patients from mechanical ventilation was the most effective. This study was undertaken because more than 40% of the time a patient spends on mechanical ventilation is spent in weaning, and a large portion of staff time is devoted to weaning. Also, life-threatening complications associated with mechanical ventilation make it important to discontinue ventilator support as early as possible. The study was conducted at 14 teaching hospitals in Spain. The study included 546 patients (378 men and 168 women) with a mean age of 58.2 years. All patients had acute respiratory failure and had been on mechanical ventilation for more than 24 hours with the mean time of 7.5 days of ventilator support. The subjects were randomly assigned to one of four weaning methods (intermittent mandatory ventilation, pressure-support ventilation, intermittent trials of spontaneous breathing, and once-daily trial of spontaneous breathing). A T-tube circuit was used for the intermittent trials of spontaneous breathing and once-daily trial of spontaneous breathing. The median duration of weaning was 5 days for intermittent mandatory ventilation, 4 days for pressure-support ventilation, 3 days for multiple trials of spontaneous breathing, and 3 days for once-daily trial of spontaneous breathing. A once-daily trial of spontaneous breathing led to extubation about three times more quickly than intermittent mandatory ventilation and about twice as quickly as pressure-support ventilation. Intermittent daily trials of spontaneous breathing were equally successful.

7. If patient cannot breathe on own, reconnect to ventilator.
8. Weaning may require several attempts for longer periods of time before the ventilator can be disconnected.

Some experts have suggested that success in weaning is determined more by the ability of the respiratory muscle to cope with an increased respiratory workload than any other factor.[52]

Patients who are able to breathe comfortably after weaning and have satisfactory ABGs are extubated. Some patients may receive supplemental oxygen by face mask for 24 hours. The patient is observed closely for signs of respiratory distress and increased efforts to breathe (e.g., respirations less than 8/min or more than 30/min; increase in respiratory rate of 10 or more from starting rate; increase or decrease in heart rate by 20 beats/min; increase or decrease in blood pressure by 20 mm Hg; decrease in $Pa{O_2}$ or increase in $Pa{CO_2}$; or pH less than 7.35.[50] If a patient develops respiratory distress, the physician is notified, and reintubation may be necessary.

### Failure to wean successfully

There are several reasons why some patients cannot be weaned from a ventilator. These include congestive heart failure, prolonged muscle weakness, diaphragmatic paralysis (occurs when the phrenic nerve is severed unintentionally during cardiac surgery), excessive secretions, small diameter of endotracheal tube, hypophosphatemia, hypomagnesemia, hypothyroidism, and COPD.

Because of the number of patients who require long-term ventilatory support and may be difficult to wean from it, The North American Nursing Diagnosis Association (NANDA) has approved two new nursing diagnoses: dysfunctional ventilatory weaning response and inability to sustain spontaneous ventilation. Dysfunctional ventilatory weaning response is divided into three types: mild, moderate, and severe. Inability to sustain spontaneous ventilation has two categories: major and minor. With either of the diagnoses, related factors are noted. For dysfunctional ventilatory weaning response, the related factors are pathophysiological, such as muscle weakness; situational, such as fear of separation from the ventilator; and treatment errors, such as rushing the weaning process. Related factors for inability to sustain spontaneous ventilation include physiological, such as respiratory muscle fatigue, and psychosocial, such as depression.

### Care of the patient who cannot be weaned

For those patients who are unable to be weaned from the ventilator, three options are available. In a conference with the patient and his or her significant others, each of the options is discussed. These options are (1) being discharged home on the ventilator, (2) being discharged to a nursing home on the ventilator, or (3) being taken off the ventilator and allowed to die (terminal weaning).

Few patients find it possible to go home on a ventilator because of the lack of suitable space and the lack of a significant other who can assume responsibility for the ventilator 24 hours a day for 7 days a week. If the patient is financially well off, he or she may be able to employ nurses to provide 24-hour care at home. If the patient and significant others decide on the patient being discharged home, careful planning is required to ensure that the home can accommodate the patient and the necessary equipment. The assessment of the home is best made by a nurse from a health care agency that will be following the patient and monitoring care at home. (See Chapter 23 for more information on home health nursing care.)

The option of being discharged to a nursing home does not appeal to many patients. Also, few nursing homes can accommodate patients on ventilators, and those that can usually have a limited number of beds for these patients.

The option of being taken off the ventilator and being allowed to die is being chosen by an increasing number of patients. Once the patient indicates that this is his or her choice, the care team meets to discuss how the patient's wishes can best be accommodated. Most patients elect to have a significant others with them when the ventilator is removed. A morphine drip is usually started before the ventilator is disconnected to ease the patient's anxiety. An article by the daughter of a man who chose terminal weaning gives a moving account of the experience.[4] She describes her own struggle with her father's decision and points out:

Finally, Dad confronted the truth: his lungs could never sustain him without the ventilator. He had struggled long and he fought hard, but in the end he knew that if he could not live independently, he did not want to live at all. He made his decision to be disconnected from the ventilator and, as difficult as it was, we all supported him.[4]

### Improving Airway Clearance

Airways clogged with excess mucus are one of the most reversible components precipitating acute respiratory failure. Nursing interventions that promote a patent airway and can prevent deterioration of respiratory status include:

1. Effective cough maneuvers
   a. Have patient sit upright
   b. Inhale slowly through the nose
   c. Lean forward and exhale slowly through pursed lips to promote open airways
   d. Repeat these steps several times to mobilize secretions and move them upward in the airway
   e. Take a slow maximal inhalation through the nose when secretions reach the oropharynx; during exhalation, use short repeated coughs to minimize bronchospasm
   f. Inhale maximally after coughing to reinflate alveoli
2. Sufficient fluid intake to mobilize secretions (3 to 4 L, unless contraindicated, has traditionally been encouraged, but some evidence suggests that this quantity may not be needed)
3. Frequent deep breathing exercises
4. Position changes every 2 hours
5. Elevation of head and chest
6. Nasotracheal suctioning if patient is unable to cough effectively (see Chapter 31)

### Improving Breathing Pattern

Nursing interventions for patients in acute respiratory failure must be implemented in a firm but empathetic manner. The patient may be agitated or nearly exhausted from hypoxemia, hypercapnia, and the increased work of breathing. It is imperative that the patient be gently guided in respiratory maneuvers to improve breathing. The nurse must be alert for signs and symptoms indicating that the patient's condition has changed from acutely ill but adequately ventilating to critically ill with insufficient ventilation to maintain body functions. Nursing interventions include:

1. Encourage forward-leaning postures (see Figure 32-25).
2. Coach patient to a slow, rapid respiratory rate and to avoid gulping large quantities of air.
3. If ordered, assist with IPPB treatments. Although the therapeutic effect of IPPB has been questioned, the treatment, at least for the short term, helps slow respiratory rate and decreases the work of breathing.

### Improving Cardiac Output

Decreased cardiac output may be a complication of acute respiratory failure or may be a precipitating factor related to underlying cor pulmonale. Diminished cardiac output causes tissue hypoxia, which creates a metabolic acidosis in addition to the respiratory acidosis caused by the respiratory failure. Specific aspects of care include:

1. Limiting fluid intake as ordered
2. Monitoring for signs of inadequate tissue perfusion (urine output less than 30 ml/hr, cool extremities with decreased peripheral pulses)
3. Administering medications as ordered

See Chapter 26 for detailed care of the patient with decreased cardiac output.

### Maintaining Adequate Nutrition

Individuals with acute respiratory failure are at increased risk for nutritional deficits because of the increased work of breathing. Nursing interventions are the same as those for the patient with COPD (see p. 995). Additional aspects of care must be considered for patients who require mechanical ventilatory support. The overall focus of nutritional interventions is to prevent or correct malnutrition. Nutritional intake affects ventilatory drive, respiratory muscle function, and the amount of oxygen consumed and carbon dioxide produced from metabolic processes. Persons who have fasted for a few days or have been maintained on 5% dextrose intravenously may have severely depleted glycogen stores necessary for adequate respiratory function. Thus nutritional status can have a major impact on the individual's ability to be successfully weaned from the ventilator. Actions must focus on providing appropriate nutrition to meet their specific metabolic needs while on the ventilator and during and after weaning from it. Nutritional support by either enteral supplementation or parenteral hyperalimentation may be necessary. Whenever feasible, the GI route should be used rather than parenteral therapy because it poses fewer risks and is more economical.

### Health Promotion/Prevention

Prevention of respiratory failure is focused on early identification of persons at high risk for developing ARF. In the inpatient setting, a preventive plan of care should be developed for every person with an increased risk of developing respiratory failure. A preventive plan of care should include but is not limited to the following:

1. Keeping airway clear
   a. Instituting regularly performed deep breathing and coughing maneuvers
   b. Nasotracheal suctioning if necessary
2. Optimal activity level
3. Judicious use of sedatives or analgesics
4. Assessing regularly for signs and symptoms indicating deterioration of respiratory status

Persons with COPD have an increased risk of developing acute on chronic respiratory failure as a complication of their chronic disease. They should be counseled to contact their physician if they experience any change in the following:

1. Sputum production
2. Degree of dyspnea

3. Activity tolerance
4. Changes in ability to think clearly, unexplained irritability, and so on
5. Any change in response to medications

If respiratory failure is a complication of a disease other than COPD, the patient's knowledge needs to be assessed as to causative and contributing factors. Appropriate teaching is then instituted. All patients need to be able to explain homegoing medications and treatments and plans for follow-up care.

## EVALUATION

To evaluate the effectiveness of nursing interventions, compare patient behaviors with those listed in the expected patient outcomes. Successful achievement of patient outcomes for the patient with respiratory failure is indicated by:

1. Improved ventilation and oxygenation.
   a. $PaO_2$, $PaCO_2$, and pH have returned to patient's baseline level.
   b. Is able to maintain $PaO_2$ at optimal level.
   c. Verbalizes how and when to use oxygen therapy (when exercising, when feeling very fatigued).
   d. Is able to think and speak clearly.
   e. Respiratory rate is 16 to 30.
   f. Dyspnea is greatly improved.
2. Effective airway clearance.
   a. Coughs effectively and does not tire self with ineffective coughing.
   b. Uses inhaler correctly.
3. Adequate cardiac output.
   a. Pulsus paradoxus is absent.
   b. Blood pressure is stable.
   c. Heart rate and rhythm are within acceptable limits.
   d. Pulses are equal and present in all extremities.
   e. Urine output is 40 to 50 ml/hr.
4. Adequate nutritional intake to balance metabolic needs; weight is returning to preacute illness level.
5. Describing signs and symptoms to be reported to physician.

## GERONTOLOGICAL CONSIDERATIONS

The elderly person with respiratory failure will need the same care and support discussed for the patient with COPD on p. 1000.

## SPECIAL ENVIRONMENTS FOR CARE

### Critical Care Management

The patient with respiratory failure will require care in an intensive care unit. The care required is discussed above.

### Home Care Management

The patient who requires prolonged ventilator support may be discharged home on ventilator support if a family caregiver is willing to accept the responsibility for the patient's care.[51] Before the patient can be discharged, the designated caregiver will be taught basic skills by the hospital nursing staff. These skills include: (1) clean technique for tracheostomy care and for suctioning, (2) cuff management, (3) tracheostomy tube change, (4) how to recognize breathing problems, (5) medications, and (6) activities of daily living.

The home ventilator company will be contacted as soon as the decision is made to discharge the patient. The home ventilator company will (1) identify the financial obligations of the patient and family for home ventilation care, (2) investigate the patient's insurance coverage, and (3) evaluate the patient's home to determine if a ventilator and other electrical equipment can be operated safely.

The home ventilator company will be asked to deliver a portable ventilator and suction machine to the hospital and coordinate ventilator instruction time with the patient, family, and nurse. The ventilator company will be responsible for the following: (1) instruction on the safe use, setup, maintenance, and troubleshooting of the ventilator, circuits, oxygen, and suction machine; (2) home visits by respiratory therapists for equipment evaluation, cleaning, and maintenance; (3) written reports to the patient's physician about results of home visits; (4) backup equipment service 24 hours a day, 7 days per week; and (5) notification of the fire department, electric company, police, and ambulance service about the patient's arrival home and potential need for their services.

The nurse from the home health agency will evaluate the patient's home nursing requirements and insurance coverage for home nursing visits, home health aides, and physical and occupational therapy.

The DRG for ventilator-dependent patients is 30 days. This amount of time allows for the teaching and supervised practice of the designated caregiver and other family members with the ventilator and suction machine that will go home with the patient. The caregiver must also become CPR certified before the patient can be discharged.

## COMPLICATIONS

Complications of respiratory failure and mechanical ventilation include impaired gas exchange from plugged tube, kinked tube, or cuff herniation; fluid volume excess, electrolyte imbalance; stress ulcer and GI bleeding; infection; increased intercranial pressure secondary to altered cerebral perfusion; tissue hypoxia; and cardiopulmonary arrest.

## critical thinking QUESTIONS

1 What is the quality of air in the community in which you live? If air pollution is a problem, what are the major contributing factors (industries, automobile exhaust, etc.)? Are there community groups working to improve the problem? If so, what activities are they involved in, and how might a nurse be helpful to their efforts?

2 Where is the branch of the American Cancer Society and the American Lung Association nearest your community? What services do they provide for health professionals and for patients?

3 Design a teaching plan or project that you believe would help convince teenagers they should not

smoke. Would you use a different approach for females than for males?

**4** Mrs. Jones has just been admitted to your unit. She has a long-standing history of COPD with chronic respiratory failure. She recently developed a viral bronchitis. She arrives on your unit with ABGs of $Pao_2 = 55$, $Paco_2 = 80$, pH = 7.30. She appears extremely short of breath and is very restless. What information do you need to obtain to assess this patient's current status? What is your immediate plan of care?

**5** Describe the unique developmental needs of young adults with CF.

**6** Considering the trend of increasing life expectancy for patients with CF, what moral and ethical issues may the nurse encounter when caring for these patients?

**7** Develop a nursing care plan for a patient with an artificial airway and mechanical ventilation.

## chapter SUMMARY

### CLASSIFICATION OF PULMONARY DISORDERS

- Pulmonary disorders can be classified by the way ventilation is altered. The three major categories of pulmonary disorders are restrictive, obstructive, and vascular.
- In restrictive diseases, lung volume and lung compliance are reduced.
- Restrictive lung diseases include acute bronchitis, pneumonia, tuberculosis, fungal infections, occupational lung diseases, ARDS, and cancer of the lung.

### INFECTIOUS DISEASES OF THE RESPIRATORY TRACT

- Acute bronchitis may be caused by viruses; bacteria such as *S. pneumoniae, H. influenzae, M. catarrhalis,* and *B. pertussis;* and other organisms (*Mycoplasma pneumoniae, Chlamydia pneumoniae* [Twar strain]). The better term to describe bronchitis would be tracheobronchitis, because bronchitis without tracheitis is never seen.
- Bacterial pneumonia is classified as community-acquired pneumonia (CAP) and hospital-acquired pneumonia (HAP).
- *Streptococcus pneumoniae* causes 33% of cases of CAP in elderly and debilitated persons. Several of the organisms causing CAP are resistant to penicillin and require other antibiotics. Staphylococci (*S. aureus, S. epidermidis*) infections develop in residents of nursing homes or chronic care facilities, patients with Hickman catheters, IV drug abusers, and persons with diabetes or renal failure. *Mycoplasma pneumoniae* primarily occurs in adolescents and young adults.
- Gram-negative bacteria are responsible for the greatest number of cases of hospital-acquired pneumonia. The largest number of cases are caused by *Enterobacteriaceae* and *Pseudomonas aeruginosa.*
- Risk factors for the development of hospital-acquired pneumonia include: being a patient in an ICU, being on mechanical ventilation, having an endotracheal or tracheostomy tube, having recent surgery, being debilitated or malnourished, having invasive devices, having neuromuscular disease or depressed levels of alertness, aspiration, antacid use, age 60 or older, prolonged hospital stay, or any prolonged underlying disease.
- The major nursing responsibility is in preventing spread of pneumonia by careful hand washing between patients.
- Prevention of pneumonia includes pneumonia vaccine for those aged 65 years or older and those who have a chronic disease that makes them more susceptible to pneumonia.
- Regardless of the causative agent, pneumonia results in acute inflammation of lung tissue. Inflamed tissue often involves both the conducting airways and the alveolar tissue; thus both airway clearance and gas exchange may be impaired.
- The number of cases of tuberculosis in the United States has declined, except in persons with HIV and AIDS and immigrants from countries where TB is endemic.
- The mycobacterium responsible for TB in middle-class AIDS patients is the *Mycobacterium avium-intracellulare* complex (MAC). *Mycobacterium tuberculosis* is more common in AIDS patients from developing countries and inner-city minority patients who have a history of IV drug abuse.
- Mycobacteria other than tubercle bacilli (MOTT) are strongly acid-fast bacteria that are being isolated more frequently from immunocompromised patients, persons with HIV and AIDS, and patients on antineoplastic therapy.
- Multidrug-resistant TB (MDR-TB) has become a major problem in the United States, especially in New York City, California, and other areas with many patients with HIV.
- Primary prevention of respiratory infections such as tuberculosis includes prevention of the spread of infection by teaching the infected person to cover nose and mouth when coughing or sneezing so that droplet nuclei are not released into the air and taking antituberculosis drugs consistently as ordered.
- Histoplasmosis, coccidioidomycosis, and blastomycosis are three major fungal infections of the lungs. Amphotericin B is the standard therapy for mycotic infection.
- Lung abscess is usually caused by bacteria that reach the lung from aspiration. It can also follow bronchial obstruction caused by a tumor, foreign body, or stenosis. Up to one third of these patients 45 years of age and older have lung abscess associated with carcinoma.
- Although bronchiectasis is not as common as it once was, it occurs in persons with pneumonia, lung abscesses, TB, cystic fibrosis, immunodeficiency diseases, or asthma who have had repeated respiratory infections.

### OCCUPATIONAL LUNG DISEASES

- Occupational lung diseases are caused by microscopic substances inhaled in the workplace. They can cause severe lung damage, especially in persons who inhale these substances for years. Examples are silicosis, which occurs in foundry workers and spray painters who are exposed to silica dust, and mesothelioma (cancer of the pleura), which occurs in asbestos workers.
- Occupational lung diseases are more common among smokers than nonsmokers, and smokers often have a more severe form of the disease.

### SARCOIDOSIS

- Sarcoidosis is a systemic granulomatous disease of unknown cause. In the United States it is 10 times more common in blacks than whites. It is treated with steroids.

### CANCER OF THE LUNG

- Cancer of the lung is the leading cause of death from cancer in both men and women. Because there is no cure from cancer of the lung, the goal set for the year 2000 in *Healthy People 2000* is to slow increase in the lung cancer deaths because it is impossible to decrease the number of deaths.

- The treatment of choice for lung cancer is surgical removal of the tumor. Unfortunately, one third of persons have inoperable tumors when they first see a surgeon. Another one third are found to have inoperable tumors on exploratory examination, and 90% of the persons who do survive die within 5 years.
- Because there is no cure for cancer of the lung, the emphasis is on prevention, which focuses on keeping persons from starting to smoke and convincing those who smoke to quit, because smokers are 10 times more likely to develop lung cancer than nonsmokers.

## THORACIC SURGERY

- After resectional surgery of the lung (except for pneumonectomy), one or two chest tubes are inserted into the pleural space and connected to a closed drainage system.
- Postoperative nursing care of the patient after thoracic surgery centers on promoting ventilation and reexpansion of the lung by maintaining a patent airway, promoting comfort by pain relief, promoting reexpansion of the lung by coughing and deep breathing exercises, proper maintenance of the closed drainage system, promoting nutrition, and monitoring the incision for bleeding and subcutaneous emphysema.
- Bronchopleural fistula and empyema are long-term complications of resectional surgery of the lung.

## PULMONARY VASCULAR DISEASE

- Therapy for patients with pulmonary embolism includes thrombolytic therapy with urokinase, streptokinase, or recombinant tissue-type plasminogen activator (rt-PA). If this treatment is not successful, a pulmonary embolectomy may be used to extract emboli from the pulmonary vasculature.

## CHEST TRAUMA

- Chest trauma is divided into blunt and penetrating injuries. The most common blunt injury is fractured ribs.
- The major cause of chest trauma is automobile accidents in which the chest hits the steering wheel.
- Chest trauma is managed by stabilization of the fracture site and analgesics to reduce pain.
- When several ribs are fractured or the sternum is fractured in more than one place, the patient may develop a flail chest with paradoxical breathing.
- Management of the person with a flail chest includes stabilizing the fractured ribs, improving gas exchange and airway clearance, and promoting comfort.
- A pneumothorax occurs when air enters the pleural space between the lung and chest wall. There are three main types of pneumothoraces: closed or spontaneous, open, and tension.
- If an open sucking wound of the chest has been sustained, the wound should be covered immediately to prevent air from entering the pleural cavity and causing a pneumothorax.
- Effective breathing patterns can be facilitated by proper positioning and by the use of respiratory assistive devices such as incentive spirometry.

## CHRONIC OBSTRUCTIVE PULMONARY DISEASE

- Obstructive lung diseases result in an obstruction to airflow, predominantly on expiration.
- Chronic obstructive pulmonary disease (COPD) is a chronic limitation of airflow. The most common chronic airflow disorders are emphysema, chronic bronchitis, and asthma.
- Asthma is an inflammatory disease characterized by hyperresponsiveness of trachea and bronchi causing narrowing of airways.
- To facilitate breathing, the nurse teaches the person with COPD abdominal breathing, forward-leaning postures, inhalation-exhalation exercises, muscle-reconditioning exercises, and pursed-lip breathing.
- Persons with COPD who have chronically elevated carbon dioxide and low oxygen levels are considered to have chronic respiratory failure. These chronically ill people are at high risk of developing acute on chronic respiratory failure, in addition to their chronic failure.
- Cystic fibrosis is an inherited disease that causes airway obstruction. It usually develops in childhood.
- Because of more effective treatments, more patients with CF are living into their thirties.

## RESPIRATORY FAILURE

- When the patient is unable to maintain ventilation, $Paco_2$ will increase and $Pao_2$ will decrease, and mechanical ventilation will be necessary.
- Respiratory failure is defined by the physiological criteria of $Pao_2$ = 50 mm Hg or less, $Paco_2$ = 50 mm Hg or greater, and pH = 7.35 or less.
- There are two major types of ventilators: pressure cycled and volume cycled. Currently, volume-cycled ventilators are more commonly used. The patient will be intubated with either an endotracheal or a tracheostomy tube before being attached to a ventilator.
- A volume-cycled ventilator delivers a constant volume of air at a preset pressure with each breath. These ventilators have a cutoff valve, which will stop the cycle if the pressure required to deliver the desired volume exceeds a preset level.
- The patient on a ventilator requires constant attendance and is best managed in an intensive care unit.
- After the patient's underlying pulmonary problem is improved, the patient will be weaned from the ventilator. Weaning is best carried out by a nurse who has developed a trust relationship with the patient.
- There are three major methods of weaning: T-piece, synchronized intermittent mandatory ventilation (SIMV), and pressure support ventilation (PSV). Several attempts for increasing periods of time may be necessary before the ventilator can be discontinued.
- Nursing management to facilitate aeration of alveoli requires interventions that promote optimal airway function, promote effective breathing patterns, and manage pulmonary secretions. Measures to achieve these include hydration, humidification of the airways, nebulizer therapy, segmental postural drainage, and breathing exercises.
- When the patient cannot manage secretions, tracheobronchial suctioning may be necessary. If this is not successful in clearing the airway, fiberoptic bronchoscopy may be used to remove impacted secretions.
- Maintaining transportation of oxygen to body tissues requires several interactive physiological processes. These

include ventilation, perfusion, and diffusion. Also required are sufficient hemoglobin and an adequate cardiac output.

- Several modes are used to deliver oxygen to the patient. These include nasal cannulae and several types of face masks that can deliver various concentrations of oxygen.
- Adult respiratory distress syndrome (ARDS) results in severe hypoxemia without hypercapnia. Patients with ARDS usually require mechanical ventilation with PEEP in order to provide adequate oxygen safely.

## References

1. American Cancer Society: *Cancer facts and figures—1997,* Atlanta, 1997, The Association.
2. American Thoracic Society Statement: Standards for the diagnosis and care of patients with chronic obstructive pulmonary disease, *Respiratory and Critical Medicine Supplement* 152(5):S77, 1995.
3. Andreoli TO, Bennett JC, Carpenter CCJ, Plum F, editors: *Pulmonary vascular disease, Cecil essentials of medicine,* ed 4, Philadelphia, 1997, WB Saunders.

3a. Angelucci P: *A new weapon against ARDS,* RN 59(11):22, 1996.

4. Benner KI: Terminal weaning: a loved one's vigil, *Am J Nurs* 93(5):22, 1993.
5. Bloch KI et al: Nationwide survey of drug-resistant tuberculosis in the United States, *JAMA* 271(9):665, 1994.
6. Borkgren MW, Gronkiewicz CA: Update your asthma care from hospital to home, *Am J Nurs* 95(1):26, 1995.
7. Bradsher RW: Blastomycosis. In Rakel RE, editor: *Conn's current therapy,* Philadelphia, 1996, WB Saunders.
8. Buchanan RJ: Compliance with tuberculosis drug regimens: incentives and enablers offered by public health department, *Am J Public Health* 87(12):2014, 1997.
9. Canales MAP: Asthma management, *Nursing* 97(12):33, 1997.
10. Carrol P: Closing in on safer suctioning, *RN* 61(5):22, 1998.
11. Centers for Disease Control and Prevention: Cigarette smoking among adults—United States, 1992, and changes in the definition of current cigarette smoking, *MMWR* 43(19):342, 1994.
12. Centers for Disease Control and Prevention: Guidelines for school health programs to prevent tobacco use and addiction, *MMWR* 43(RR-2):1, 1994.
13. Centers for Disease Control and Prevention: Cigarette smoking among adults—United States, 1995, *MMWR* 46(51):1217, 1997.
14. Centers for Disease Control and Prevention: Components of a tuberculosis prevention and control program and screening for tuberculosis and tuberculosis infection in high-risk populations, *MMWR* 44(RR-11):1, 1995.
15. Centers for Disease Control and Prevention: *Response to increases in cigarette prices by race/ethnicity, income, and age-groups—United States, 1976-1993,* MMWR 47(29):605, 1998.
16. Centers for Disease Control and Prevention: Supplement to morbidity and mortality reports. Prevention and control of influenza: a recommendation of the Advisory Committee on Immunization Practices (ACIP), *MMWR* 45(RR-4-5), 1996.
17. Centers for Disease Control and Prevention: Silicosis deaths among young adults—United States, 1968–1994, *MMWR* 47(16):331, 1998.
18. Centers for Disease Control and Prevention: Tobacco use among high school students—United States, 1997, *MMWR* 47(12):229, 1998.
19. Centers for Disease Control and Prevention: Tuberculosis morbidity—United States, 1997, *MMWR* 47(13):253, 1998.
20. Centers for Disease Control and Prevention: Characteristics of foreign-born Hispanic patients with tuberculosis—eight U.S. counties bordering Mexico, 1995, *MMWR* 45(47):1032, 1996.
21. Cooper JD et al: Bilateral pneumomectomy (volume reduction) for chronic obstructive pulmonary disease, *J Thorac Cardiovasc Surg* 109:106, 1995.
22. Cottrell JJ, Rogers RM: Acute respiratory failure. In Rakel RE, editor: *Conn's current therapy,* Philadelphia, 1996, WB Saunders.
23. Davis PB, Drumm M, Kontos MW: State of the art: cystic fibrosis, *Am J Respir Care Med* 154:1229, 1996.
24. Dominguez EA, Rupp ME: Bacterial pneumonia. In Rakel RE, editor: *Conn's current therapy,* Philadelphia, 1996, WB Saunders.
25. Esteban A et al: A comparison of four methods of weaning patients from mechanical ventilation, *N Engl J Med* 332(6):345, 1995.
26. Fine MJ et al: A prediction rule to identify low-risk patients with community acquired pneumonia, *N Engl J Med* 336(4):243, 1997.
27. Fink MP: Trauma. In Sabiston DC Jr, Lyerly LK, editors: *Sabiston essentials of surgery,* ed 2, Philadelphia, 1994, WB Saunders.
28. Friedman LN et al: Tuberculosis, AIDS, and death among substance abusers on welfare in New York City, *N Engl J Med* 334(13): 828, 1996.
29. Galgiani JN: Coccidioidomycosis. In Rakel RE, editor: *Conn's current therapy,* Philadelphia, 1996, WB Saunders.
30. Goldhaber SZ et al: A prospective study of risk factors for pulmonary embolism in women, *JAMA* 277(8):642, 1997.
31. Goldman M, Wheat LJ: Histoplasmosis. In Rakel RE, editor: *Conn's current therapy,* Philadelphia, 1996, WB Saunders.
32. Grap MJ, Munro CL: Ventilator-associated pneumonia, *Heart Lung* 26(6):419, 1997.
33. Haire WD: Pulmonary embolism. In Rakel RE, editor: *Conn's current therapy,* Philadelphia, 1996, WB Saunders.
34. Haire WD: Venal cava filters for the prevention of pulmonary embolism, *N Engl J Med* 338(7):463, 1998 (editorial).
35. Hanson MJS: Caring for a patient with COPD, *Nursing* 97(12):39, 1997.
36. Hill RC: The pleura and empyema. In Sabiston DC Jr, Lyerly LK, editors: *Sabiston essentials of surgery,* ed 2, Philadelphia, 1996, WB Saunders.
37. Jaffe MS, Skidmore-Roth L: *Home health nursing,* St Louis, 1997, Mosby.
38. Jett JR: Primary lung cancer. In Rakel RE, editor: *Conn's current therapy,* Philadelphia, 1996, WB Saunders.
39. Jones I, Hannum D: Playing it safe with a particulate respirator, *Nursing* 98(1):50, 1998.

39a. Kollef MH, Schuster DP: *Medical Progress: The acute respiratory distress syndrome,* N Engl J Med 332(1):27, 1995.

40. Landrigan PI: Asbestos—still a carcinogen? *N Engl J Med* 338(12): 618, 1998 (editorial).
41. Mathews PJ: Ventilator associated infections: reducing the risks. Part 1, *Nursing* 97:50, 1997.
42. Mathews PJ: Ventilator associated infections: reducing the risks. Part 2, *Nursing* 97:50, 1997.
43. Metersky ML, Sulavik SB: Primary lung abscess. In Rakel RE, editor: *Conn's current therapy,* Philadelphia, 1966, WB Saunders.

43a. National Institutes of Health, National Heart, Lung, and Blood Institute: *National asthma education program guidelines for diagnosis and management of asthma,* Washington, DC, 1991, National Institutes of Health.

43b. National Institutes of Health, National Heart, and Blood Institute: *NAEPP Working Group Report: Considerations for diagnosing and managing asthma in the elderly,* NIH Publication No. 96-3662, Washington, DC, 1996, National Institutes of Health.

44. Moran JF: Surgical treatment in tuberculosis. In Sabiston DC Jr, Lyerly LK, editors: *Sabiston essentials of surgery,* ed 2, Philadelphia, 1994, WB Saunders.

44a. Pablos-Mendez A et al: *Global surveillance for antituberculosis-drug resistance, 1994-1997,* N Engl J Med 338(23):1641, 1998.

45. Petty TR: Acute respiratory distress syndrome. In *Year book of pulmonary diseases,* St Louis, 1997, Mosby.
46. Rodnick JE: Acute bronchitis. In Rakel RE, editor: *Conn's current therapy,* Philadelphia, 1996, WB Saunders.
47. Schakenbach L: Caring for a patient with TTO, consult STAT, *RN* 60(5):69, 1997.
48. Singh NT, Pesanti EL: Tuberculosis and other mycobacterial diseases. In Rakel RE, editor: *Conn's current therapy,* Philadelphia, 1996, WB Saunders.
48a. Snider DE, Castro KG: The global threat of drug-resistant tuberculosis, *N Engl J Med* 338(23):1689, (editorial), 1998.
49. Somerson SJ et al: Mastering emergency airway management, *Am J Nurs* 96(5):25, 1996.
50. Stilwell SB: *Mosby's critical care nursing reference,* ed 2, St Louis, 1966, Mosby.
51. Thompson KS et al: Building a critical path for ventilator dependency, *Am J Nurs* 91(7):28, 1991.
52. Tobin MJ: Mechanical ventilation, *N Engl J Med* 330:1056, 1994.
53. US Department of Health and Human Services: *Healthy people 2000: national health promotion and disease prevention objectives,* Washington, DC, 1990, US Government Printing Office.
54. US Department of Health and Human Services: National Institutes for Safety and Health: *Protect yourself aganst tuberculosis—a respiratory protection guide for health care workers, pub. 96-102, Cincinnati, 1995,* US Department of Health and Human Services.
55. US Department of Health and Human Services, Public Health Service, National Heart, Lung, and Blood Institute: *Teach your patients about asthma: a clinician's guide,* Bethesda, Md, 1992.
56. US Department of Health and Human Services, Public Health Service: *Tobacco use among US racial/ethnic minority groups—African Americans, American Indians and Alaska Natives, Asian Americans and Pacific Islanders, and Hispanics: a report of the Surgeon General,* Atlanta, 1998, US Department of Health and Human Services, CDC, National Center for Chronic Disease Prevention and Health Promotion, Office of Smoking and Health.
57. Yagan MB: Hospital-acquired pneumonia and its management, *Crit Care Q* 20(3):36, 1997.
58. Ziment I: Chronic obstructive pulmonary disease. In Rakel RE, editor: *Conn's current therapy,* Philadelphia, 1966, WB Saunders.

# chapter 33 ASSESSMENT OF THE Endocrine System

KATHLEEN M. ZUPAN, JUNE HART ROMEO, DOROTHY R. BLEVINS,* and VIRGINIA L. CASSMEYER*

**objectives** *After studying this chapter, the learner should be able to:*

1 Describe the locations of endocrine glands and the mechanisms that control hormone synthesis and release from these glands.

2 Analyze the functions of the hormones secreted by the pituitary, thyroid, parathyroid, adrenal cortex, and adrenal medulla glands and the pancreas.

3 Compare biological effects that occur when there is a deficit or an excess of endocrine hormones.

4 Relate the physiological changes that occur within the endocrine system with aging.

5 Synthesize subjective and objective data of patients with actual or potential health problems of the endocrine system into a nursing care plan.

6 Discuss the common diagnostic tests used to identify endocrine dysfunction and explain the meaning of the results.

The complexity of the human body and the specialization of cells and tissues require an internal communication system that integrates processes in order to function as a unit to meet selected needs. Two systems, the endocrine and nervous systems, function together to enable the body to respond appropriately to changes in the internal and external environments.

The endocrine system consists of the anterior and posterior pituitary, thyroid, parathyroid, adrenal cortex, adrenal medulla, pancreas, gonads, pineal body, and thymus glands. Specialized endocrine cells are also located along the gastrointestinal (GI) tract. The hormones from these endocrine glands are vital to the important life transactions of the organism, including differentiation, reproduction, growth and development, metabolism, adaptation, and senescence.[5] This is the first of three chapters that focus on the role of the anterior and posterior pituitary, thyroid, parathyroid, adrenal cortex, and adrenal medulla glands and endocrine pancreas in these processes. The neuroendocrine response to stressors, which involves the nervous system, the adrenal medulla, and other endocrine glands, is discussed in Chapter 6; the GI hormones are discussed in Chapter 38; and the gonads are discussed in Chapter 46. The thymus, which is critical to development of immunocompetent T lymphocytes, is discussed in Chapters 10 and 65.

## ANATOMY AND PHYSIOLOGY

### GENERAL ENDOCRINE PROCESSES

The endocrine system integrates body functions by the synthesis and release of hormones. Hormones are substances, synthesized and released by the endocrine glands, that act to regulate function of the target cell, tissue, or organ. These substances may influence cells close to the site of origin (*paracrine* action), act within the organ of synthesis (*autocrine* action), or travel via the bloodstream to distant target tissues (*endocrine* action).[3,10] Hormones can be classified by chemical structure into six groups as shown in Table 33-1.

### MECHANISMS OF HORMONE ACTION

The secretion and release of hormones does not occur at a uniform rate. Physiological levels of hormones are determined by the amount of hormone produced, an intact transport system, adequate receptors, feedback systems, and metabolic degradation of the hormone.

#### Hormone Release

Hormone release is influenced by negative feedback systems, intrinsic rhythmicity, and the nervous system. In a negative feedback system the gland responds to a low hormone level by releasing additional hormone. As the level returns to normal, hormone release is inhibited. Calcium regulation is an example of a simple negative feedback system (Figure 33-1). Antidiuretic hormone and insulin release are also regulated through this system.

A more complex feedback mechanism controls the levels of other hormones. The most elaborate feedback mechanism is demonstrated by the interaction of the hypothalamus and the anterior pituitary with the thyroid, adrenal cortex, and gonads. The basic components of this feedback loop are illustrated in Figure 33-2. When the level of hormone produced by the thyroid, adrenal cortex, or gonads is adequate, the release of trophic hormones by the pituitary or releasing hormone by the hypothalamus is inhibited by negative feedback. To control the level of selected hormones, the hypothalamus synthesizes and releases inhibiting hormones (Figure 33-3). The amounts of prolactin and growth hormone released by the anterior pituitary are in part controlled by a prolactin-inhibiting hormone and a growth hormone–inhibiting hormone (GHIH) (somatostatin).

*Deceased.

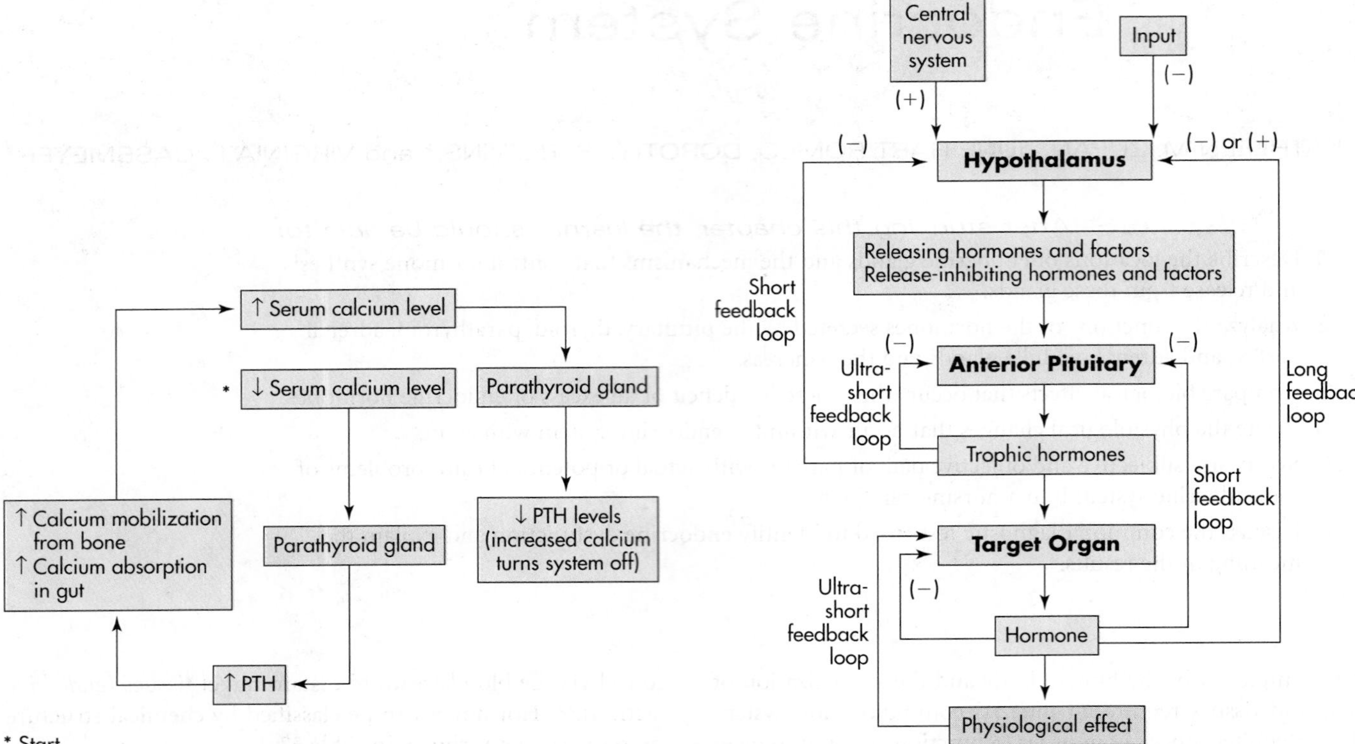


**fig. 33-1** Negative feedback for calcium regulation.

**fig. 33-2** General model for control and feedback to hypothalamic-pituitary target organ systems.

**table 33-1** *Structural Categories of Hormones*

| STRUCTURAL CATEGORY | EXAMPLES | STRUCTURAL CATEGORY | EXAMPLES |
|---|---|---|---|
| Proteins | Growth hormone | Amino acid derivatives | Epinephrine |
| | Prolactin | | Norepinephrine |
| | Insulin | | Thyroxine (both $T_4$ and $T_3$) |
| | Parathyroid hormone | | Melatonin |
| Glycoproteins | Follicle-stimulating hormone | Lipids | |
| | Luteinizing hormone | Steroids (cholesterol is a precursor for all steroids) | Estrogens |
| | Thyroid-stimulating hormone | | Progestins (progesterone) |
| Polypeptides | Thyrotropin-releasing hormone | | Testosterone |
| | Oxytocin | | Mineralocorticoids (aldosterone) |
| | Antidiuretic hormone | | Glucocorticoids (cortisol) |
| | Calcitonin | Fatty acids | Prostaglandins |
| | Glucagon | | Thromboxanes |
| | Adrenocorticotropic hormone | | Prostacyclins |
| | Endorphins | | Leukotrienes |
| | Thymosin | | |
| | Melanocyte-stimulating hormone | | |
| | Hypothalamic hormones | | |
| | Lipotropins | | |
| | Somatostatin | | |

McCance KL, Huether SE: *Pathophysiology: the biologic basis for disease in adults and children,* ed 3, St Louis, 1998, Mosby.

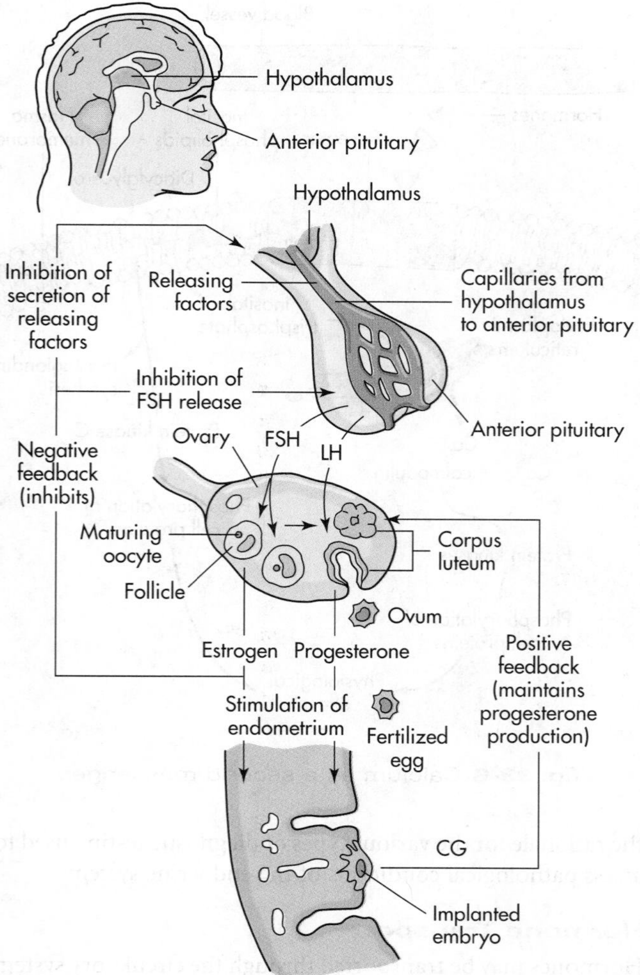


**fig. 33-3** Endocrine feedback loops involving the hypothalamus-pituitary gland and end organs (endocrine regulation).

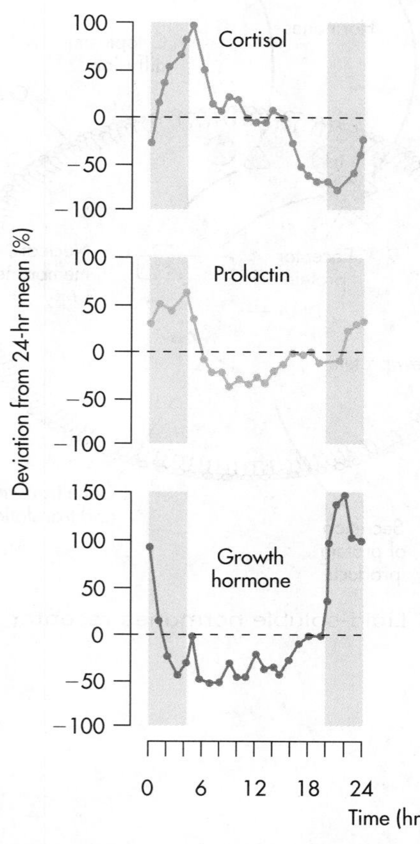


**fig. 33-4** Intrinsic rhythms of cortisol, prolactin, and growth hormone.

Although negative feedback control is a distinguishing feature of the endocrine system, it does not control all hormones.[2] Examples include estrogen in males, testosterone in females, placental hormones, and hormones produced by ectopic tumors. A second factor regulating hormone levels is intrinsic rhythmicity. The intrinsic rhythms can vary over minutes, days, or weeks. For example, prolactin, cortisol, and growth hormone demonstrate daily circadian rhythms (Figure 33-4). These intrinsic rhythms are controlled by various factors.

The environmental factor of sleep-wake patterns influences the circadian rhythms of growth hormone, adrenocorticotropic hormone (ACTH), and cortisol. Age, growth, and development influence the intrinsic rhythmicity of gonadotropins and gonadal steroids. Neurogenic factors influence the intrinsic rhythm of other hormones such as prolactin. In addition to circadian rhythms, hormone secretion may demonstrate pulsatile or cyclic patterns.

Extrinsic factors such as pain, trauma, infection, or other stressors also influence levels of selected hormones. These extrinsic factors can override the normal feedback mechanisms or intrinsic rhythmicity and increase secretion of hormones above normal levels.

The central nervous system (CNS) influences hormone release. The hypothalamus contains neurons and neurosecretory cells. Nerve tracts connect the hypothalamus with the posterior lobe of the pituitary. This neuroregulatory system will be discussed in the section on endocrine structures and hormonal function.

The autonomic nervous system (ANS) is also involved in hormone release. As the ANS responds to a stressor, the adrenal medulla is stimulated to release epinephrine.

Last, the level of hormones is affected by excretion or metabolic inactivation. The liver and the kidneys are primarily responsible for hormonal inactivation and excretion, and diseases of these organs can result in increased hormone levels.

In summary, hormone levels are controlled by multiple mechanisms. Understanding these mechanisms helps clarify

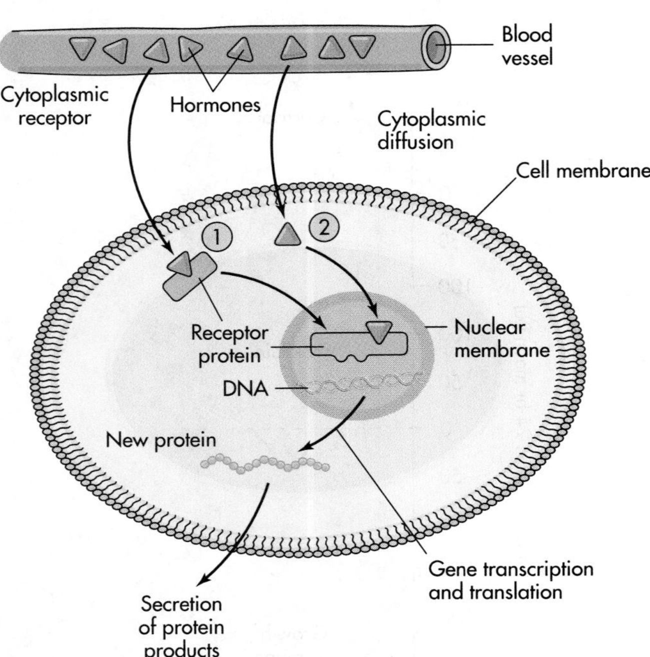


fig. 33-5 Lipid-soluble hormones receptor activity.

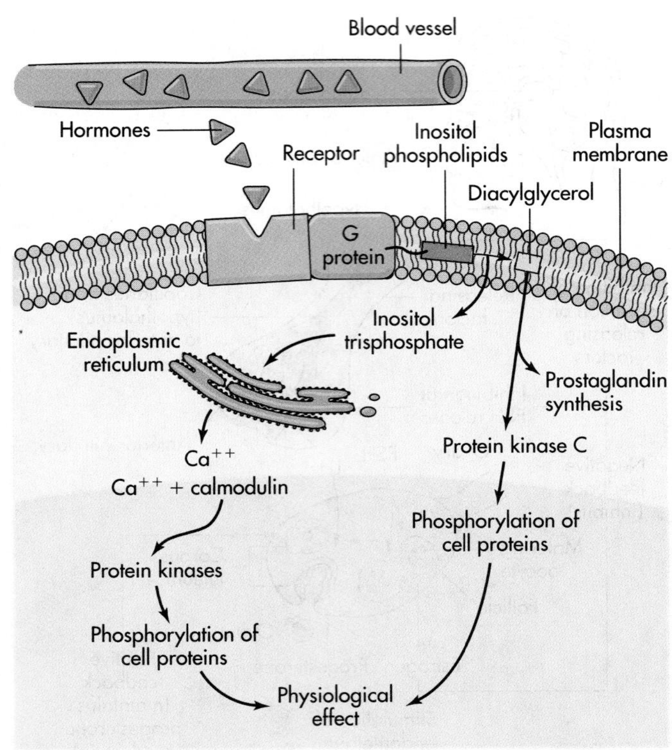


fig. 33-6 Calcium as a second messenger.

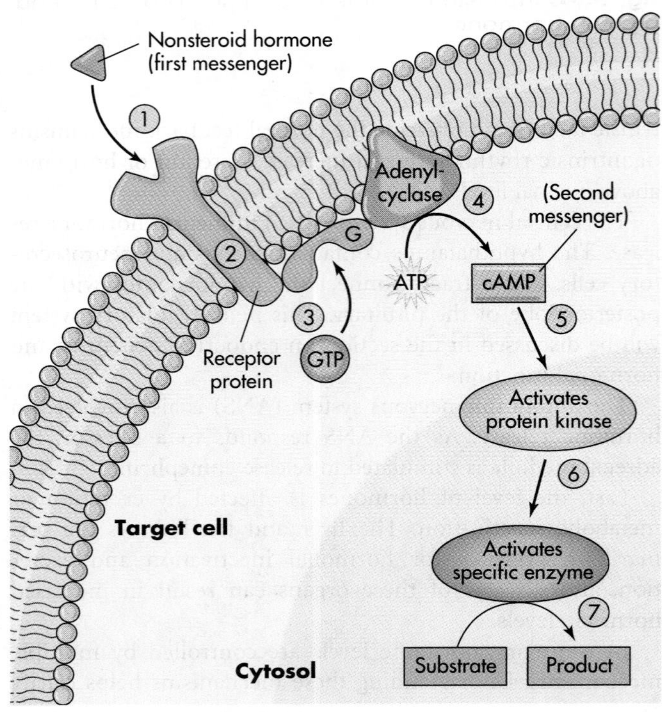


fig. 33-7 Cyclic AMP (cAMP) as a second messenger.

the rationale for the various types of diagnostic testing used to assess pathological conditions of the endocrine system.

### Hormone Transport

Hormones may be transported through the circulatory system in a free state or bound to plasma proteins. Biologically active hormones are transported in the free state. The concentration of free hormones is balanced by the concentration of bound hormones. As the level of free hormones falls, plasma proteins release enough of the bound hormone to reach equilibrium.

### Hormone Action

Hormones stimulate responses by binding either with cell membrane receptors or intracellular receptors. Steroid hormones such as adrenal steroids, gonadal steroids, and active derivatives of vitamin D and thyroid hormone, which are lipid soluble, are believed to use intracellular receptors. These hormones freely cross the plasma membrane and combine with their specific intracellular receptor. The steroid-receptor complex is changed in size and conformation and is translocated to the nucleus, where it combines with acceptor sites located in the nucleus near the deoxyribonucleic acid (DNA) sequences. The binding of the hormone-receptor complex initiates transcription of DNA, translation of ribonucleic acid (RNA), and synthesis of protein. A summary of this model of hormone activation is shown in Figure 33-5.

Water-soluble hormones (hypothalamic-releasing hormones, anterior and posterior pituitary hormones, parathyroid hormone, calcitonin, insulin, glucagon, biogenic amines) are believed to use membrane receptors. The hormone, acting

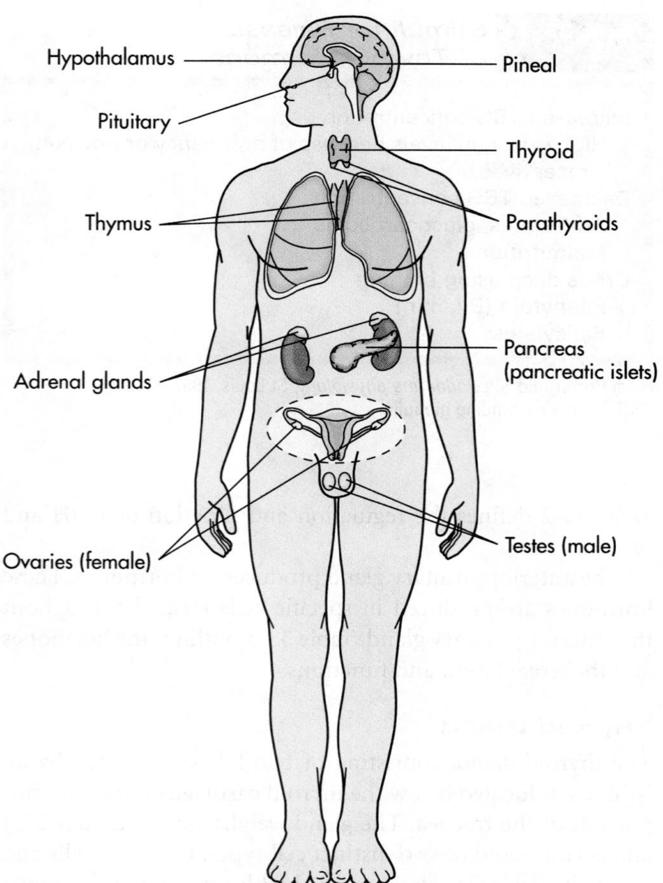


fig. 33-8 The endocrine system.

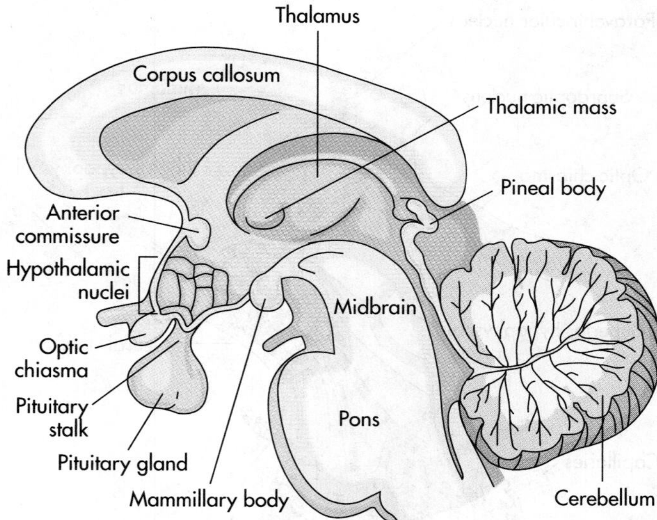


fig. 33-9 Sagittal section through the brain.

as a first messenger, combines with its specific receptor on the plasma membrane, and this hormone-receptor combination activates a second messenger located inside the cell. The second messenger then initiates a sequence of events in the cytoplasm that results in altered cell function. Cyclic adenosine monophosphate (cAMP) has been identified as the second messenger for several hormones. It is hypothesized that the combination of the hormone with the receptor activates adenyl cyclase, which causes the formation of 3′,5′-cAMP from adenosine triphosphate (ATP). The cAMP activates protein kinases. These activated kinases phosphorylate specific proteins in the stimulated cell and result in altered cell function.

Although cAMP has been identified as a second messenger for several hormones, other compounds serve as second messengers. Growth hormone is mediated by insulin-like growth factor 1 (IGF-1), or somatomedin, its second messenger.[7] Calcium ions, calmodulin, adenosine, and prostaglandins are some of the other potential second messengers. A summary of this model of hormone activation is presented in Figures 33-6 and 33-7.

## ENDOCRINE STRUCTURES AND HORMONAL FUNCTION

The endocrine structures are located throughout the body. In addition to the glands depicted in Figure 33-8, there are endocrine cells throughout various parts of the GI tract.

### Hypothalamus and Pituitary Gland

The hypothalamus, a part of the diencephalon, consists of numerous poorly defined nuclei. The hypothalamus forms the lower portion of the lateral walls and the floor of the third ventricle and is bordered anteriorly by the optic chiasma. The hypothalamic sulcus and thalamus lie on the dorsal border; the internal capsule, subthalamic nuclei, and basis pedunculi form the lateral boundaries. On its inferior surface the hypothalamus is continuous with the pituitary stalk. Figure 33-9 shows a sagittal section through the brain. The anterior, dorsal, and inferior boundaries are depicted. Although a very small area of the brain, the hypothalamus receives input directly or indirectly from almost every other part of the brain and is a major controller of the anterior and posterior pituitary gland.

The pituitary gland, which is approximately 1 cm in size and weighs 500 mg, lies in the sella turcica of the sphenoid bone. This gland is composed of two functionally distinguishable components: the adenohypophysis (anterior pituitary) and the neurohypophysis (posterior pituitary). The posterior pituitary is a continuation of the pituitary stalk. The anterior pituitary, which makes up 75% of the total gland, arises embryonically from an outpouching of ectoderm and fuses with the posterior pituitary.

#### *Hypothalamic-pituitary relationship*

The hypothalamus serves as a critical link between the rest of the nervous system and the endocrine system, controlling both the posterior and the anterior pituitary glands. By its control of the anterior pituitary gland, the hypothalamus exerts global control over the entire endocrine system. Figure 33-10 depicts the connections between the hypothalamus and the pituitary gland. The hypothalamus is connected to the posterior pituitary gland by nerve tracts that originate in the paraventricular and supraoptic nucleus of the hypothalamus. Posterior pituitary hormones are actually synthesized in the hypothalamus and transported along

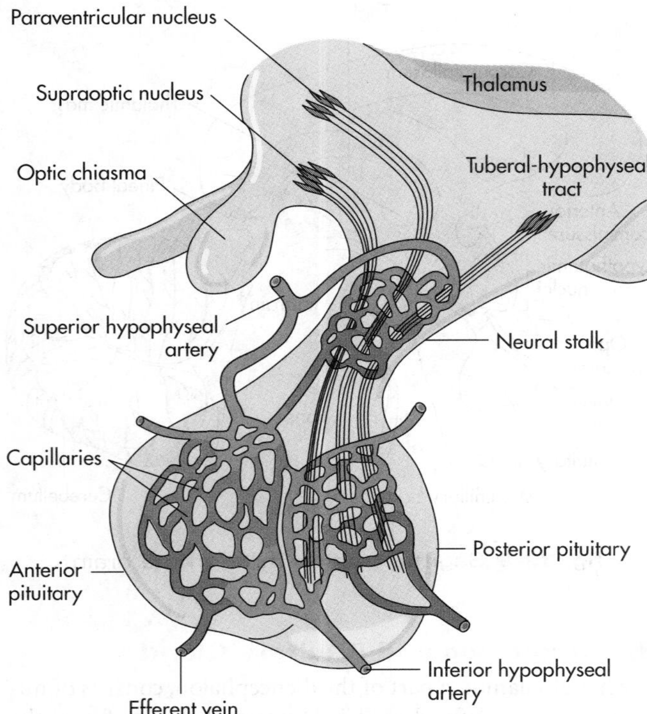


**fig. 33-10** Hypothalamic pituitary connections. Hypothalamus connects to posterior pituitary gland by nerve tracts. Connection between hypothalamus and anterior pituitary gland is vascular.

nerve axons to the posterior pituitary gland, where they are stored.

The hypothalamus and anterior pituitary gland are connected by the hypothalamic-hypophyseal portal blood supply. Blood entering the anterior pituitary gland has first passed through the hypothalamus. The hypothalamus regulates anterior pituitary function by the synthesis and secretion of releasing or inhibiting hormones into the hypothalamic-hypophyseal portal blood supply. These hormones are released in the anterior pituitary gland and stimulate or inhibit the release of appropriate hormones.

The known releasing and inhibiting hormones include the following: growth hormone–releasing hormone (GHRH), growth hormone–inhibiting hormone (GHIH) (somatostatin), thyrotropin-releasing hormone (TRH), corticotropin-releasing hormone (CRH), gonadotropin-releasing hormone (GnRH), prolactin-inhibiting hormone (PIH), and prolactin-releasing factor (PRF). Research is continuing in the area of releasing and inhibiting hormones.

### Pituitary hormones

The posterior pituitary gland stores and releases two hormones: antidiuretic hormone (ADH) or vasopressin, and oxytocin. Both of these hormones are synthesized in the paraventricular and supraoptic nucleus of the hypothalamus. The blood level of these two hormones is controlled by multiple factors that act either as stimulators or inhibitors.

**box 33-1** *Stimuli for Release of Thyroid Hormone*

- Increased TBG concentration
  - High estrogen levels because of pregnancy or oral contraceptives
- Decreased TBG concentration
  - Androgens, glucocorticoids
  - Malnutrition
- Drugs decreasing binding
  - Phenytoin (Dilantin)
  - Salicylates

From Porterfield SP: *Endocrine physiology,* St Louis, 1997, Mosby.
*TBG,* Thyroxine-binding globulin.

Table 33-2 defines the regulation and function of ADH and oxytocin.

The anterior pituitary gland produces six hormones. These hormones are produced in specific cells located throughout the anterior pituitary gland. Table 33-3 outlines the hormones and their regulation and functions.

## Thyroid Gland

The thyroid gland, consisting of two lobes connected by an isthmus, is located below the thyroid cartilage on the superior portion of the trachea. The gland weighs approximately 20 g and is composed of two distinct cell types: follicular cells and parafollicular cells. The gland is highly vascular and receives adrenergic and cholinergic innervation.

Iodine is necessary for the synthesis of thyroid hormone. The thyroid gland has the ability to trap and concentrate iodide. Thyroid hormone is produced in response to one of the following stimuli: low serum iodide levels, factors affecting the binding capacity of thyroxine-binding globulin (TBG), TRH, and TSH (Box 33-1).

The follicular cell is the functional unit of the thyroid. Follicular cells are responsible for thyroxine ($T_4$) and triiodothyronine hormone ($T_3$) production. The follicle consists of a ring of epithelial cells that surround a colloid-filled center. Thyroglobulin is produced by the follicular cells and stored in the colloid. When thyroid hormone is needed, the follicle converts thyroglobulin to $T_3$ and $T_4$, which are secreted into the blood. The amount of $T_3$, the more potent of the two hormones, that is secreted is less than the amount of $T_4$. To become biologically active, $T_4$ must be converted to $T_3$ at the cellular level.[3,4,10]

Thyroid hormone is mainly bound to proteins for transportation. Thyroxine-binding globulin is the protein with the greatest affinity for $T_3$ and $T_4$. Less than 1% of the hormone is free and therefore active. The bound hormone acts as a reservoir to protect the cells against sudden large increases or shortages of thyroid hormone.

The parafollicular cells synthesize and secrete the hormone calcitonin, which is involved in calcium metabolism. The release of calcitonin is influenced by serum calcium levels. As the serum calcium level rises, calcitonin acts to maintain a

**table 33-2** *Posterior Pituitary Hormones: Their Regulation and Function*

| Hormone/Regulation | Function |
|---|---|
| **ANTIDIURETIC HORMONE (ADH, VASOPRESSIN)** | |
| **Stimulators** | Target organ: kidneys |
| ***Primary*** | Major regulator of osmolality and body water volume |
| Increased serum osmolality (as little as 1% increase) via hypothalamic osmoreceptors | Increases permeability of collecting ducts in kidney to water, resulting in increased water reabsorption |
| ***Others*** | May stimulate water intake by stimulating perception of thirst |
| Modest volume depletion via atrial volume receptors | |
| Modest hypotension via baroreceptors | |
| Stressors | |
| Psychological | |
| Pain | |
| Nausea and vomiting | |
| Chemicals | |
| Cholinergic agonist | |
| Beta-adrenergic agonist | |
| Barbiturates | |
| Morphine | |
| Nicotine | |
| **Inhibitors** | |
| ***Primary*** | |
| Decreased serum osmolality (as little as 1%) via osmoreceptors | |
| Modest increased volume and blood pressure via atrial volume receptors and baroreceptors | |
| Chemicals | |
| Alcohol | |
| Alpha-adrenergic agonist | |
| **OXYTOCIN** | |
| **Stimulators** | Target organ: breast tissue and uterus |
| ***Primary*** | Results in milk "let-down" in lactating breast |
| Suckling via neurogenic reflex conducted from afferent fibers in nipple to hypothalamus | Causes increased uterine contraction after labor has begun; role in initiating labor unclear |
| ***Others*** | |
| Uterine contraction via neurogenic reflex from afferent fibers in uterus | |
| **Inhibitors** | |
| Stressors | |
| Psychological | |
| Physical | |
| Alpha-adrenergic stimulation | |

normal level by opposing the action of parathyroid hormone. Table 33-4 outlines the thyroid hormones, their regulation, and their function.

## Parathyroid Gland

The parathyroid glands consist of four minute glands, located on the posterior aspect of the upper and lower poles of each lobe of the thyroid (see Figures 33-8 and 33-11). Occasionally normal extra parathyroid glands are found on the thyroid, on the mediastinum, or behind the esophagus. The parathyroid produces parathyroid hormone (PTH), which regulates calcium levels in the blood. As the serum calcium decreases, PTH secretion increases. This release of PTH is also influenced by serum phosphate and magnesium levels[8,10] (Figure 33-12). Parathyroid hormone acts on bone and kidneys to maintain serum calcium levels. Calcitonin and vitamin D also act to regulate calcium (Table 33-5).

## Adrenal Gland

The adrenal glands cap the upper pole of each kidney. Each gland consists of two glands: the outer gland is the adrenal cortex, and the inner core is the adrenal medulla. The cortex consists of three zones: the zona glomerulosa, zona fasciculata, and zona reticularis.

table 33-3 *Anterior Pituitary Hormones: Their Regulation and Function*

| Hormone/Regulation | Function |
|---|---|
| **GROWTH HORMONE (GH)** | |
| Controlled by GHRH/GHIH<br>GH shows episodic secretion with increases after eating (particularly a high-protein diet) and after onset of deep sleep (usually within 1-2 hours after sleep)<br>Other stimuli that increase GH<br>Exercise (strenuous)<br>Hypoglycemia<br>Stressors<br>Chemicals<br>Arginine infusion<br>L-dopa<br>Clonidine<br>TRH in acromegaly<br>Adrenergic agonists<br>Beta-adrenergic antagonists<br>Hyperglycemia decreases GH | Target organ: whole body<br>Possibly works on most tissue through action of somatomedin(s)<br>Concerned with growth of cells, bones, and soft tissues<br>Increases mitosis<br>Affects carbohydrate, protein, and fat metabolism<br>Increases blood glucose by decreasing glucose utilization; insulin antagonist<br>Increases protein synthesis<br>Increases lipolysis, free fatty acid levels, and ketone formation<br>Increases electrolyte retention and extracellular fluid volume |
| **PROLACTIN (PRL)** | |
| Controlled by PRH and PIH; PRL chronically inhibited by hypothalamus<br>PRL shows episodic secretions occurring during later hours of sleep<br>Other stimulants<br>Stressors<br>Suckling<br>Chemicals<br>Estrogen<br>TRH<br>Dopamine antagonist<br>Chlorpromazine<br>Chemicals that are dopamine agonists (L-dopa, bromocriptine) inhibit PRL | Target organ: breast, gonads<br>Necessary for breast development and lactation<br>Regulator of reproductive function in males and females |
| **THYROID-STIMULATING HORMONE (TSH)** | |
| Controlled by TRH and negative feedback from plasma $T_4$ levels<br>Increase $T_4 \rightarrow$ decrease TSH<br>Decrease $T_4 \rightarrow$ increase TSH | Target organ: thyroid gland<br>Necessary for growth and function of thyroid; controls all functions of thyroid |
| **ADRENOCORTICOTROPIN (ACTH)** | |
| Controlled by CRH and negative feedback by cortisol levels<br>ACTH shows episodic secretion with rhythm that peaks between 6 and 8 AM<br>Circadian pattern (24-hour pattern) related to sleep-wake pattern and caused by increased CRH<br>Physiological and psychological stressors (e.g., hypoglycemia, infections, pain, anxiety) increase ACTH caused by increased CRH (override negative feedback); changes in cortisol influence ACTH<br>Increase cortisol $\rightarrow$ decrease ACTH<br>Decrease cortisol $\rightarrow$ increase ACTH | Target organ: adrenal cortex gland<br>Necessary for growth and maintenance of size of adrenal cortex<br>Controls release of glucocorticoids (cortisol) and adrenal androgens<br>Minor role in release of mineralocorticoids (aldosterone) |
| **GONADOTROPINS**<br>**FOLLICLE-STIMULATING HORMONE (FSH)**<br>**LUTEINIZING HORMONE (LH) (ALSO PREVIOUSLY CALLED INTERSTITIAL CELL–STIMULATING HORMONE [ICSH] IN MALES)** | |
| Secretion controlled by GnRH<br>Amount of FSH secreted is decreased by inhibin in males<br>Amount of LH secreted is decreased by testosterone in males<br>Sex steroids in females exert positive feedback on FSH and LH at certain times in normal menstrual cycle and negative feedback at other times | Target organs: gonads<br>Stimulates gametogenesis and sex steroid production in males and females |

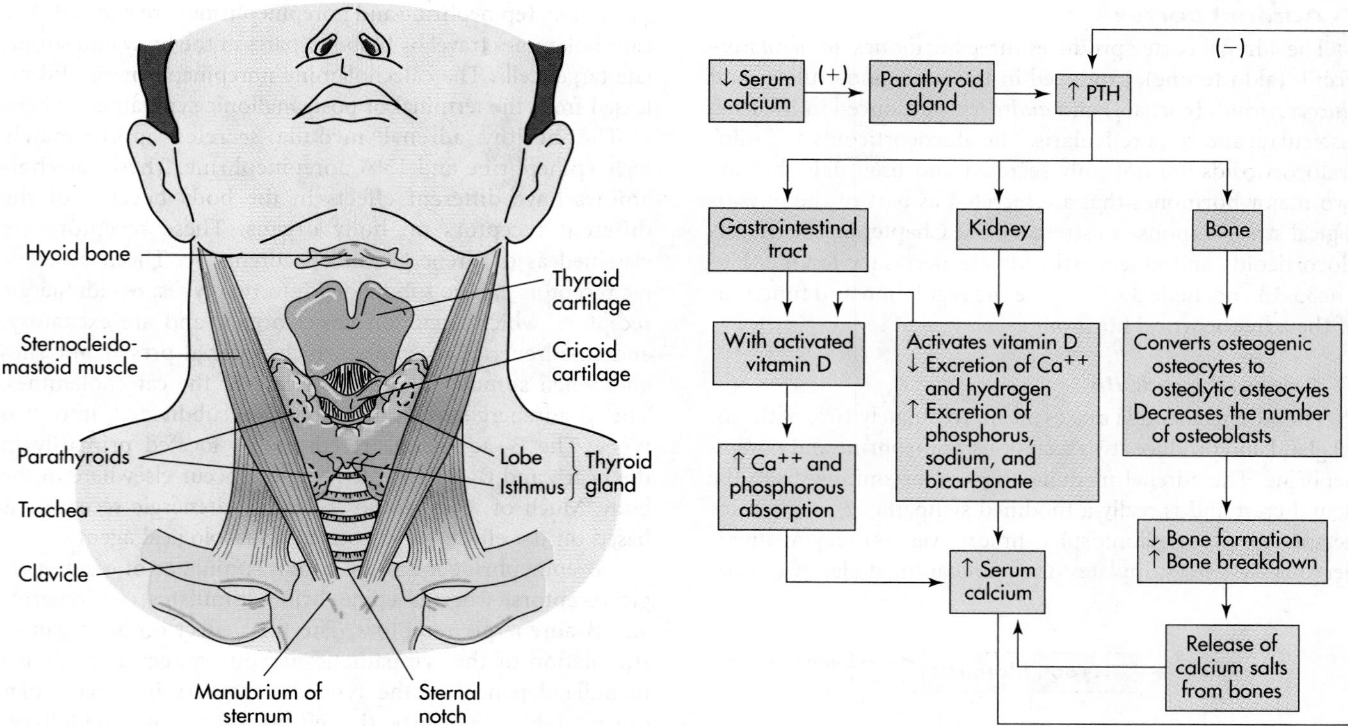


**fig. 33-11** Midline neck structures; note thyroid gland in anterior aspect of neck.

**fig. 33-12** Regulation and function of PTH.

**table 33-4** *Thyroid Gland Hormones: Their Regulation and Function*

| Regulation | Function |
|---|---|
| **THYROXINE ($T_4$) AND TRIIODOTHYRONINE ($T_3$)** | |
| $T_4$ and $T_3$ levels controlled by TSH | Regulates protein, fat, and carbohydrate catabolism in all cells |
| Hormones show diurnal variation with peak during late evening | Regulates metabolic rate of all cells |
| Influences on amount secreted | Regulates body heat production |
| Gender | Acts as insulin antagonist |
| Pregnancy | Maintains growth hormone secretion, skeletal maturation |
| Gonadal steroid and adrenal corticosteroids; increased steroids = ↑ levels of $T_4$ and $T_3$ | Affects central nervous system development |
| Exposure to extreme cold = ↑ levels | Necessary for muscle tone and vigor |
| Nutritional state | Maintains cardiac rate, force, and output |
| Chemicals | Maintains secretions of GI tract |
| GHIH = ↓ levels | Affects respiratory rate and oxygen utilization |
| Dopamine = ↓ levels | Maintains calcium mobilization |
| Catecholamines = ↑ levels | Affects red blood cell production |
| | Stimulates lipid turnover, free fatty acid release, and cholesterol synthesis |
| | Regulates sympathetic nervous system activity |
| **CALCITONIN** | |
| Elevated serum calcium—major stimulant for calcitonin | Lowers serum calcium by opposing bone-resorbing effects of PTH, prostaglandins, and calciferols by inhibiting osteoclastic activity |
| Other stimulants | Also lowers serum phosphate levels |
| Gastrin | May also decrease calcium and phosphorus absorption in GI tract |
| Calcium-rich foods (regardless of serum $Ca^{++}$ levels) | |
| Pregnancy | |
| Lowered serum calcium—suppresses calcitonin release | |

### Adrenal cortex

The adrenal cortex produces three hormones: *mineralocorticoids* (aldosterone), produced in the zona glomerulosa, and *glucocorticoids* (cortisol) and *androgens,* produced in the zona fasciculata and zona reticularis. The glucocorticoids and mineralocorticoids are not only secreted and used daily but are two major hormones that are secreted as part of the physiological stress response to stressors. See Chapter 6. The mineralocorticoids and glucocorticoids are necessary for life. Figure 33-13 and Table 33-6 outline the regulation and functions of the adrenocortical hormones.

### Adrenal medulla

The adrenal medulla makes up approximately 10% of the total gland and produces two secretions: epinephrine and norepinephrine. The adrenal medulla arises embryonically from the neural crest and is really a modified sympathetic ganglion innervated by preganglionic splanchnic nerves. As the sympathetic nervous system stimulates the adrenal medulla, two *catecholamines* (epinephrine and norepinephrine) are released. The catecholamines travel by blood to parts of the body and stimulate target cells. The catecholamine norepinephrine is also released from the terminal of postganglionic sympathetic fibers.

The healthy adrenal medulla secretes approximately 85% epinephrine and 15% norepinephrine. These catecholamines have different effects in the body because of the different receptors on body organs. These receptors are classified as $\alpha$-adrenergic and $\beta$-adrenergic. The $\alpha$-adrenergic receptors can be subdivided into two types: $\alpha_1$-adrenergic receptors, which occur on target organs and are excitatory; and $\alpha_2$-adrenergic receptors, which occur at presynaptic sites and, when stimulated, inhibit release of the catecholamines. The $\beta$-adrenergic receptors are also subdivided into two types. The $\beta_1$-adrenergic receptors are located primarily in the heart, and $\beta_2$-adrenergic receptors occur elsewhere in the body. Much of what is known about adrenergic receptors is based on the effects of various pharmacological agents.

Norepinephrine is a more potent stimulator of $\alpha$-adrenergic receptors, whereas epinephrine stimulates $\alpha$-adrenergic and $\beta$-adrenergic receptors. The final effect on an organ of stimulation of the sympathetic nervous system and adrenal medulla depends on the type of receptors in a particular organ. Table 33-7 lists the effects of adrenal-medullary-sympathetic stimulation on body organs.

A small quantity of catecholamines is released at all times, and this helps maintain homeostasis. In the presence of a major stressor, either physiological or psychological, increased amounts of catecholamines are released in an attempt to overcome the stressor, and all the effects listed in Table 33-7 may be seen. This increased adrenal-medullary-sympathetic stimulation is part of the physiological stress response, which is discussed in more detail in Chapter 6.

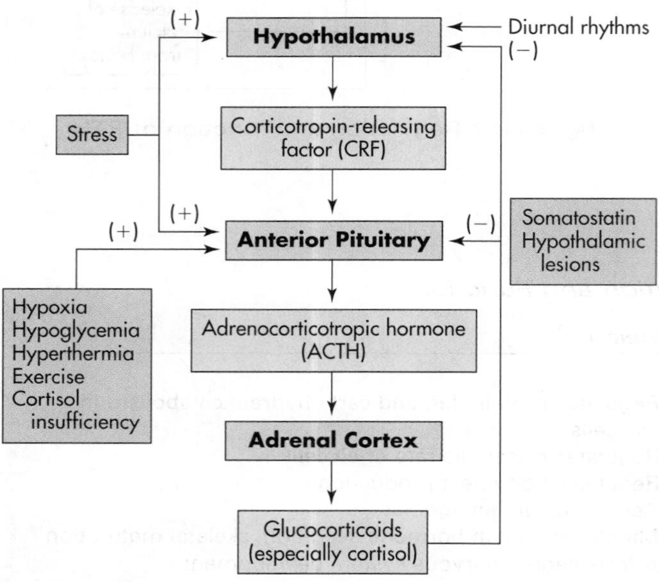


**fig. 33-13** Feedback control of glucocorticoid synthesis and secretion.

## Pancreas

The pancreas is both an exocrine and an endocrine gland. It lies retroperitoneally behind the stomach, with its head and neck in the curve of the duodenum, its body extending horizontally across the posterior abdominal wall and its tail touching the spleen. The cells of the pancreas that serve the endocrine function are the islets of Langerhans. There are over 1 million islet cells spread throughout the total pancreas; these

**table 33-5** *Actions of Calcium Regulatory Hormones*

| | Bone | Kidney | GI Tract |
|---|---|---|---|
| PTH | Increases bone resorption and osteocytic osteolysis | Increases renal calcium reabsorption; lowers Tm for phosphate reabsorption; increases renal conversion of 25-(OH)$D_3$ to 1,25-$(OH)_2D_3$ | No direct action; stimulates activation of vitamin $D_3$, which stimulates calcium and phosphate absorption |
| Calcitonin | Decreases bone resorption | Decreases calcium and phosphate reabsorption | No direct action |
| Vitamin D | Synergizes with PTH on bone; stimulates calcium pump on ECF interface of surface osteoblasts | Minimal renal actions; renal actions appear to increase calcium reabsorption | Increases GI calcium and phosphate absorption |

From Porterfield SP: *Endocrine physiology,* St Louis, 1997, Mosby.
*GI,* Gastrointestinal; *PTH,* parathormone; *Tm,* tubular maximum; *ECF,* extracellular fluid.

cells make up 1% to 2% of the pancreatic mass. The islets of Langerhans consist of four cell types: (1) α-cells, which secrete glucagon; (2) β-cells, which make up 70% of the cells and secrete insulin; (3) delta cells, which secrete somatostatin; and (4) F-cells, which secrete pancreatic polypeptide. Somatostatin inhibits gastric motility and emptying; gallbladder contraction; intestinal absorption of fats, amino acids, glucose, and other nutrients; and insulin and glucagon secretion. Pancreatic polypeptide inhibits pancreatic exocrine secretion and contraction of the gallbladder.

### *Insulin*

Insulin is a protein hormone that is secreted as a prohormone. The removal of a connecting peptide (C-peptide) fragment results in the active hormone. Both insulin and C-peptide are secreted into the blood in equal amounts. Insulin has an unstimulated basal secretion that controls metabolism between meals. Insulin also shows meal-related increases. The major stimulus is glucose, but insulin secretion is also stimulated by the intake of amino acids. Acetylcholine increases insulin secretion, whereas catecholamines acting on α-adrenergic receptors inhibit insulin secretion.

Overall, insulin is an anabolic hormone; it promotes the utilization of ingested food and the storage of nutrients in excess of body needs. Although it can affect every cell in the body, its major effects are seen in liver cells, adipose tissue, and muscles (Table 33-8).

### *Glucagon*

Glucagon, along with epinephrine, growth hormone, and glucocorticoids, functions as a counterregulatory hormone to insulin. Glucagon's overall function is to increase blood glucose. It is stimulated by a decreased blood glucose level and increased amino acid levels. The primary target of glucagon is the liver, where it stimulates *glycogenolysis* (breakdown of glycogen to glucose). When the need for glucose is greater than can be provided by glycogenolysis, glucagon promotes amino acid transport from the muscle and stimulates *gluconeogenesis* (formation of glycogen from fatty acids and proteins rather than carbohydrates). Glucagon also promotes lipolysis and ketone formation. Glucagon works with epinephrine, glucocorticoids, and growth hormone in carrying out the metabolic function designed to maintain blood glucose in times of fasting, starvation, or stress.

**table 33-6** *Adrenal Cortex Hormones: Their Regulation and Function*

| Regulation | Function |
|---|---|
| **GLUCOCORTICOIDS (CORTISOL)** | |
| Level of cortisol is controlled by CRH/ACTH.<br>Cortisol shows episodic secretion with a circadian rhythm that peaks between 6 and 8 AM; this circadian pattern follows the circadian pattern of CRH/ACTH.<br>Physiologic and psychologic stressors (e.g., hypoglycemia, hypoxia, pain, infection, trauma, anxiety) result in increased cortisol via increased CRH and ACTH. This stress response overrides negative feedback cortisol normally exerts on ACTH. | Overall effect: maintain blood glucose level by increasing gluconeogenesis and decreasing rate of glucose utilization by cells<br>Increases protein catabolism<br>Promotes lipolysis<br>Antiinflammatory<br>Degrades collagen<br>Decreases T-lymphocyte participation in cellular-mediated immunity by decreasing circulating level of T lymphocytes<br>Increases neutrophils by increasing release and decreasing destruction<br>Decreases new antibody release<br>Decreases eosinophils, basophils, and monocytes<br>Decreases scar tissue formation<br>Increases red blood cell formation and possibly increases platelet formation<br>Increases gastric acid and pepsin production<br>Promotes sodium and water retention<br>Maintains emotional stability |
| **MINERALOCORTICOIDS (ALDOSTERONE)** | |
| Major regulator is renin-angiotensin system. When vascular volume or sodium is decreased, the renin-angiotensin system is activated (see Chapters 6, 15, and 43), and angiotensin II stimulates release of mineralocorticoids.<br>Other regulators<br>Increased serum potassium ($K^+$) directly stimulates adrenal cortex to release mineralocorticoids.<br>CRH/ACTH system is a weak regulator. | Maintains sodium and volume status<br>Increases sodium reabsorption in distal tubules<br>Increases potassium and hydrogen excretion in distal tubules |
| **ADRENAL ANDROGENS** | |
| Major regulator is CRH/ACTH system. | Responsible for some secondary sex characteristics in females; in males, acts as gonadal steroids |

**table 33-7** *Effects of Adrenal-Medullary-Sympathetic Stimulation on Body Organs*

| Organ | Effect* |
|---|---|
| Heart | Increased conduction velocity, automaticity, contractility, rate, and stroke volume caused by $\beta_1$-stimulation |
| Blood vessels | |
| Coronary vessels, brain, lungs | Dilation caused by $\beta_2$-stimulation and autoregulatory phenomena |
| Skin, mucosa, abdominal viscera, renal and salivary gland vessels | Constriction caused by $\alpha_1$-receptor stimulation; renal vessels also have dopaminergic receptors |
| Veins | Constriction caused by $\alpha_1$-stimulation |
| Bronchial muscles | Relaxation caused by $\beta_2$-stimulation |
| Gastrointestinal tract | Inhibition of production of gastrointestinal secretions; decreased motility and contraction of sphincters |
| Gallbladder | Relaxation |
| Kidney | Increased renin secretion caused by $\beta_2$-stimulation |
| Urinary bladder | Relaxation of detrusor muscle and contraction of sphincter |
| Skin | Pilomotor muscle contraction and localized sweating |
| Liver | Glycogenolysis and gluconeogenesis caused by $\beta_2$-stimulation |
| Pancreas | Decreased secretion of exocrine cells; $\beta_2$-stimulation causes increased secretion of islet $\beta$-cells, but $\alpha$-stimulation causes decreased secretion of islet cells; $\alpha$-effect predominates |
| Fat cells | Lipolysis |
| Brain | Increased alertness, restlessness |
| Eyes | Dilation of pupils and relaxation of ciliary bodies |

*These total effects would be seen in the physiological responses to stressors, as discussed in Chapter 6.

**table 33-8** *Action of Insulin*

| Liver Cells | Adipose Tissue | Muscle |
|---|---|---|
| Increases glycogenesis | Increases fatty acid synthesis | Increases glycogenesis, glycolysis |
| Increases fatty acid synthesis | Increases glycerol synthesis and formation of triglycerides | Increases amino acid uptake and protein synthesis |
| Increases glucose uptake | Decreases lipolysis | Decreases protein catabolism |
| Decreases glycogenolysis, gluconeogenesis, and ketogenesis | Increases glucose uptake | Decreases glycogenolysis |

## PHYSIOLOGICAL CHANGES WITH AGING

Changes in the endocrine system occur with normal aging. Endocrine dysfunction may result from cellular damage caused by aging, wear and tear on the endocrine tissue from long-term use, or genetically programmed cellular changes.[5] Endocrine changes may result in altered synthesis and secretion of hormones, altered metabolism of hormones, altered circulatory levels of hormones, altered biological activity, altered target cell and target tissue responsiveness, or altered intrinsic rhythms.[3] Although findings are not consistent, the following is a summary of the major alterations in endocrine function that are most commonly reported:

1. The most commonly seen change is decreased ovarian functioning, resulting in increased gonadotropins and changes in reproductive and sexual functioning. Although there is no distinct andropause in men, gonadal sensitivity to luteinizing hormone (LH) and androgen production decreases and LH and follicle-stimulating hormone (FSH) levels rise. Sperm production starts to decrease after age 50, and testosterone levels begin to decline.
2. Impaired secretion of hypothalamic hormones or impaired response to feedback may influence endocrine system responsiveness to alterations in the internal environment and thus to stressors. Decreased secretion of GHRH has been reported.[7]
3. The anterior pituitary gland shows morphological changes with increased fibrosis and microadenoma formation, a decrease in basal levels of prolactin in women, and a decrease in growth hormone and somatomedins.
4. Antidiuretic hormone secretion in response to changes in serum osmolality is increased, resulting in increased levels of ADH. However, elderly persons have alterations in renal function that decrease the ability to concentrate urine and can result in hyponatremia. Nocturia is typically present.
5. Various changes in thyroid gland structure, including glandular atrophy, fibrosis, nodularity, and infiltrates, have been found. The following changes in thyroid hormone levels have been reported:
   a. Decreased $T_4$ secretion and metabolism
   b. Decreased plasma $T_3$ levels
   c. Increased basal plasma TSH levels
   d. Decreased responsiveness in TSH secretion to TRH

   Hypothyroidism often occurs in elderly persons. Whether all these changes in thyroid structure, function, or disease can be attributed to the aging process is unclear.

Some of the early clinical manifestations of hypothyroidism, such as skin and hair changes, neurological changes, or GI changes, can be seen in elderly persons for other reasons, leading health care professionals to ignore or potentially misdiagnose the changes.

6. Calcium homeostasis is altered in the older adult. Changes found include decreased intake of calcium, negative calcium balance, bone loss, decreased intestinal adaptation to varied calcium intake, hypercalciuria, and decreased vitamin D levels. Age-related alterations in PTH may explain some of the changes in calcium homeostasis, but more research is needed.
7. The adrenal cortex gland, which is small and contains fibrous tissue, responds to feedback mechanisms and maintains circadian patterns of cortisol secretion in response to circadian patterns of ACTH. However, the amount of cortisol secreted is decreased because of decreased metabolic clearance and decreased usage. Thus increased blood cortisol levels result in decreased secretion. The amount of androgens secreted by the adrenal cortex is decreased, and the renin-aldosterone response to postural changes and volume depletion is depressed.
8. Impaired glucose tolerance in elderly persons is multifactorial. Delayed glucose-induced insulin secretion, altered hepatic handling of glucose, and impaired insulin-mediated glucose uptake are all part of the problem and result in elevated blood glucose levels after glucose loads, such as eating. These changes may result in blood glucose values that are higher than usually considered normal but are not diagnostic for diabetes mellitus.
9. Type 2 diabetes mellitus is one of the more common chronic diseases of elderly persons.

If the changes described in the preceding section are ignored, elderly persons may be misdiagnosed. For example, they may be diagnosed as having diabetes mellitus when further assessment reveals this to be untrue, although diabetes mellitus is more common in elderly individuals than in younger populations. Changes in serum sodium and potassium must be carefully evaluated to differentiate changes related to aging from those that might be caused by drugs such as diuretics, other diseases such as congestive heart failure, or diet. The potential role of changes in PTH in development of metabolic bone disease needs more exploration. It is important to remember that the hypothalamic-pituitary-adrenal axis and the hypothalamic-pituitary-thyroid axis, which are important in daily living and response to stressors, are intact but may be slower to respond.

In addition to the changes just listed, changes in response to actual endocrine pathological conditions have been reported. Some elderly persons with hypothyroidism have subtle signs and symptoms that make diagnosis difficult. Elderly persons tolerate hypothyroidism better, delaying diagnosis and causing a great insufficiency of thyroid hormone when they are first diagnosed. Also, early signs of hypothyroidism may be overlooked because they can occur in normal aging in the absence of a thyroid pathological condition. (See the Gerontological Assessment Box.)

## gerontological assessment

Signs and symptoms of endocrine dysfunction may be subtle, progress slowly, and often mimic normal changes associated with aging.

**NEUROLOGICAL**

Hoarseness, progressive deafness, unsteady gait, and muscle weakness may be caused by hypothyroidism.

Assess for confusion, lethargy, and memory problems. These may be the results of hypothyroidism, hyperthyroidism, hyponatremia, hypernatremia, or hypoglycemia.

Neurological symptoms such as paresthesias, blurred vision, headache, and inability to sense temperature may be attributed to complications from diabetes.

**CARDIOVASCULAR**

Count the pulse for 1 full minute. Assess for angina. Assess for signs and symptoms of congestive heart failure. All may occur with hyperthyroidism.

Assess for orthostatic hypotension, which may occur in hypernatremia.

**EYES**

Ophthalmopathy is rarely found in elderly who are newly diagnosed with hyperthyroidism.

Visual problems may be a result of complications of diabetes.

**SKIN AND HAIR**

Assess for dry skin, poor skin turgor, and thin or fine hair. Some of these may occur with thyroid dysfunction. Persons with frequent yeast or fungal infections may have diabetes mellitus.

**MUSCULOSKELETAL**

Assess ability to perform ADL and other activities. Lack of energy, muscle weakness, and apathy occur with hypernatremia and thyroid and pancreatic dysfunction.

Arthralgias may occur with adrenal insufficiency. Fractures and loss of height may occur from osteoporosis secondary to decreased estrogen.

**GASTROINTESTINAL**

Assess for changes in bowel habits. Constipation may occur with hypothyroidism.

Diarrhea may occur with hyperthyroidism. Weight loss, nausea, and abdominal pain may occur with adrenal insufficiency. Anorexia and weight loss may occur with hypothyroidism and hyperthyroidism.

**PSYCHOSOCIAL**

Apathy, nervousness. Apathy is often the most apparent symptom of hyperthyroidism in an older adult. Depression and withdrawal are often found in persons with hypothyroidism.

The cause of psychological symptoms is unclear.

**COMMON RELATED DISORDERS IN ELDERS**

Hypothyroidism

Type 2 diabetes mellitus

## SUBJECTIVE DATA

A review of the normal functions of all hormones as described on the preceding pages reveals that they influence four broad domains: maintenance of a normal internal environment; energy production, storage, and utilization; growth and development; and reproductive and sexual function. Alterations in endocrine function lead to varied manifestations because of disruption in maintenance of a normal internal environment; inadequate energy production, stores, and utilization; abnormal growth and development; and abnormal reproductive and sexual function. Systemic assessment of multiple parameters is necessary to define the healthiness of a person's endocrine system or needs. The anatomical location of endocrine glands precludes their direct assessment. A thorough history from the patient or significant others is absolutely necessary. Special attention should be paid to the patient's history regarding fluid and nutritional intake, elimination pattern, energy level, perceptions of changes in body characteristics, reproductive and sexual function, and tolerance to stressors.

### FLUID/NUTRITIONAL INTAKE

Endocrine abnormalities can lead to alteration in fluid and food intake (increased or decreased) that may or may not be associated with weight loss or weight gain. Many endocrine problems are chronic and require long-term special diets and, at times, fluid restriction. Qualitative and quantitative assessment of food intake is necessary to determine the cause of weight loss or gain, adequacy of intake for normal metabolic needs, and adherence to any special diet. Having the patient list food and fluid taken on the previous day is an excellent way to assess fluid and nutritional intake. The history must include alcohol and snacks. The preferences of the patient with regard to types of food, as well as times of eating, are important in providing a diet that meets nutritional needs. Elements such as a pleasant environment, mouth care before meals, and small meals to decrease anorexia and nausea may be necessary. Assessment of how the patient is tolerating foods and fluids must be ongoing.

### ELIMINATION PATTERN

The endocrine system is involved in maintenance of water and electrolyte balance. The history should include information on the frequency, approximate amount, and color of urinary elimination. The presence of nocturia or dysuria is also noted. In endocrine disease, depending on the cause, there may be a history of increased output and increased thirst, or decreased output and increased weight. Some patients may be on diuretics, and their adherence to the therapy should be assessed. The frequency and color of bowel movements also are determined. Information concerning constipation or other changes in bowel habits that may be caused by changes in water balance, dietary intake, or sluggishness of the bowel may be elicited. Treatment of pathological conditions may include changes in diet and fluid intake that will influence elimination. The patient's previous pattern of elimination will help the nurse teach about needed changes such as decreasing fluid intake after dinner to decrease nocturia.

### ENERGY LEVEL

Because the endocrine system is directly involved in the metabolism (storage and utilization) of nutrients for energy, pathological conditions will usually decrease the person's energy level. Many patients will complain of "not being able to do their normal things." It is important to assess the person's energy level and to use this as a guide for helping plan activities of daily living. Some persons need help in adjusting their activities to allow for rest periods; they may need assistance in eliminating activities or in changing the ways they do activities to conserve energy.

Most endocrine problems can be well controlled so that permanent changes in lifestyle will not be necessary. Recovery may be slow, however, and the patient's physical status may be so impaired that, although the energy level may be normal, additional time will be required for complete recovery.

### PERCEPTIONS OF CHANGES IN BODY CHARACTERISTICS

Changes in hair distribution, body proportions, voice, skin pigmentation, and facial appearance may accompany problems of the endocrine system. A description of changes by patients or their significant others is important, because characteristics of persons vary so greatly and changes may not be so extensive or rapid that observation alone will pick them up.

The collection of information regarding changes in body characteristics is important not only in helping to define the physiological problem but also in identifying potential or present emotional or psychological problems. Some of the changes that occur with endocrine problems are irreversible even when problems are controlled. Body characteristics are part of the identity of the person, and the person may have problems dealing with the changes.

### REPRODUCTIVE AND SEXUAL FUNCTION

The endocrine system is extensively involved with reproductive functions. A thorough reproductive and sexual history must be obtained. Data regarding the menstrual cycle (onset, frequency of menses, duration, amount of flow), presence of problems with the cycle (e.g., menorrhagia), presence of erectile dysfunction, and any perceived problems with fertility should be obtained. The history should also include information about satisfaction with sexual relationships for two reasons. First, sometimes the first changes in reproductive functioning will manifest themselves as changes in sexual satisfaction. Second, reproductive changes may not be a problem for the patient if sexual satisfaction is maintained. For example, infertility may not be a concern if childbearing is not a desired outcome (see Chapter 46).

### TOLERANCE TO STRESSORS

The endocrine system helps the body respond to all types of physical and psychological stressors. The patient or significant others should be questioned in relation to the person's ability (or change in ability) to tolerate stressors. Such things as intolerance to heat and cold, increased frequency of infections, increased irritation, euphoria, depression, increased crying, or increased anger may be elicited. Depending on the person's ability to handle stressors, special environmental controls to decrease the chance of infection and to maintain a consistent physical and emotional environment may be necessary.

## OTHER SUBJECTIVE INFORMATION

Each endocrine problem has unique clinical manifestations, which are described in Chapters 34 and 35. As part of the history of a patient with a known diagnosis, the patient should be asked if continued signs and symptoms associated with the specific uncontrolled pathological condition are still present. In addition, information regarding whether the patient is experiencing any signs or symptoms of any uncontrolled endocrine pathological condition is elicited. The last area to be assessed concerns the patient's teaching-learning needs. The person's learning style, adherence to the prescribed therapeutic regimen, difficulty in carrying out the regimen, and other self-management skills are determined.

## OBJECTIVE DATA

The collection of objective data about the endocrine system may require a complete physical examination. The major areas in which abnormalities may be found are discussed next. Collection of these data requires a thorough inspection and use of the techniques of palpation and auscultation. (See Table 33-9 for a systematic approach for assessing endocrine dysfunction.)

Inspection should be used to assess the patient's growth and developmental status. Factors such as height, weight, body proportions, amount and distribution of muscle mass, fat distribution, skin pigmentation, and hair distribution should be assessed. A great variation in these parameters

**table 33-9** *Assessment Findings in Endocrine Disorders*

| System | Findings | Endocrine Dysfunction |
|---|---|---|
| Respiratory | Dyspnea | Hyperthyroidism, hypoparathyroidism |
| | Kussmaul's respirations<br>Acetone breath | Diabetes—ketoacidosis (DKA) |
| Neurological | Confusion | DKA, hyperparathyroidism, hypoglycemia, Cushing's syndrome |
| | Decreased mentation | Cushing's syndrome, hypothyroidism, hypoglycemia, DKA |
| | Decreased tone and reflexes | Hyperparathyroidism, hypothyroidism |
| | Spasms, positive Trousseau's and Chvostek's signs | Hypoparathyroidism |
| | Seizures | Hypoparathyroidism, adrenal insufficiency, hypoglycemia |
| | Hoarseness, speech changes | Acromegaly |
| | Blurred vision | Hypoglycemia, diabetes |
| | Exophthalmos, lid changes, increased temperature | Hyperthyroidism |
| | Decreased temperature | Hypothyroidism |
| Musculoskeletal | Weakness, fatigue | Acromegaly, hypoglycemia, hypothyroidism |
| | Muscle cramps | Hypoparathyroidism, adrenal insufficiency |
| | Muscle wasting | Cushing's syndrome |
| | Fractures, osteoporosis | Cushing's syndrome, hyperparathyroidism |
| Dermatological | Erythema, facial plethora, striae, thin skin, moon face, supraclavicular fat pads, thin hair | Cushing's syndrome |
| | Hyperpigmentation, vitiligo, poor skin turgor, dry mucous membranes | Adrenal insufficiency |
| | Pallor, coarse texture, decreased perspiration, cool and dry skin, puffy eyes, nonpitting edema, thin hair | Hypothyroidism |
| | Smooth texture, increased perspiration, flushing, warmth, goiter, onycholysis | Hyperthyroidism |
| Cardiovascular | Decreased temperature, cold intolerance, bradycardia | Hypothyroidism |
| | Increased temperature, heat intolerance, palpitations, diaphoresis, increased blood pressure, angina | Hyperthyroidism |
| Gastrointestinal/ Genitourinary | Constipation, decreased urine output, weight gain | Hypothyroidism |
| | Diarrhea, weight loss | Hyperthyroidism |
| | Polyuria, polydipsia, polyphagia | Diabetes |
| | Salt craving, diarrhea, decreased urine, weight loss | Adrenal insufficiency |
| Psychosocial | Depression | Adrenal insufficiency, Cushing's syndrome |

exists in the general population, and often the changes are not obvious. Inspection of family members for like characteristics provides information as to whether the characteristics seen in the patient are caused by heredity or pathophysiological alterations. The patient's alertness, responsiveness, and speech patterns can be assessed while the history is being collected.

The endocrine system plays a major role in growth and development, metabolism of food products, and regulation of sex hormones. All of these functions, if affected, cause changes in body characteristics. Some examples of specific changes are (1) dwarfism caused by thyroid and pituitary problems; (2) changes in fat distribution, producing buffalo hump and thickened girdle from adrenocortical excess; (3) presence of purplish striae instead of white striae because of adrenocortical excess; (4) muscle wasting with a wide variety of endocrine problems; and (5) change in sexual characteristics because of abnormalities of hormonal levels. All these changes can be identified during inspection.[9]

Inspection and palpation are used to check skin turgor, mucous membrane moisture, and jugular vein distension (JVD) and to check for the presence of edema. These data will give information about the fluid and electrolyte status of the person, which can be changed with almost any endocrine problem.

The following changes may be found:

1. In states of fluid depletion, as seen in uncontrolled diabetes mellitus, adrenocortical insufficiency, and possibly diabetes insipidus, the mucous membranes are sticky.
2. Edema, as might be seen in adrenocortical excess, can be graded from 1+ to 4+ (see Chapter 15).
3. Skin turgor can be checked on the forearm, on the forehead, or over the sternum. Note that decreased skin turgor is not a reliable indicator of fluid status in the elderly.
4. Abnormal JVD may be present with fluid overload.

Assessment of cardiovascular status is imperative. A minimal assessment includes orthostatic blood pressure and pulse. If fluid volume or electrolyte problems are present, a more extensive evaluation of factors such as rhythm and heart sounds will be necessary.

Of all the endocrine organs discussed, only the thyroid is routinely examined. In disease states, sometimes the pancreas and parathyroid gland can be palpated. The thyroid gland is usually examined along with examination of the head and neck. Palpation of the thyroid provides information about the size, shape, and symmetry of the gland and the presence of nodules or tenderness. Auscultation may be used to assess for bruits.

## DIAGNOSTIC TESTS

Endocrine dysfunction in most instances can be classified as resulting from hypersecretion or hyposecretion. The excess or deficient secretion can result from (1) primary dysfunction of any of the endocrine glands; (2) abnormal function of the pituitary gland, resulting in secondary thyroid, adrenal, or gonadal dysfunction; (3) abnormal endocrine gland functioning caused by a nonendocrine disease; (4) ectopic secretion of hormones by nonendocrine tissue; or (5) iatrogenic causes. Although most diseases can be classified into one of these categories, endocrine dysfunction also can result from abnormal receptor functioning or intracellular responses.

*guidelines for care*

**Preparing the Person for Diagnostic Tests**

- Physical preparation as ordered
- Explain purpose of test
- Explain what to expect before and during the test (include sensory information)
- Explain any special care after the test

Diagnostic tests are used to evaluate (1) the level of hormone in the blood (both basal and cyclic changes); (2) the adequacy of endocrine tissue in secreting hormone in response to exogenous stimulants; (3) the interrelationships among the hypothalamus, anterior pituitary gland, and other endocrine glands controlled by the anterior pituitary hormones; and (4) the various substrates controlled by the endocrine system.

Usually several tests are necessary in the evaluation of an endocrine gland and its functioning. Most of the tests of the endocrine system require taking samples of blood; some cause discomfort, and some require fasting. The nurse is responsible for preparing the patient appropriately. The routine physical preparation for any test will vary from institution to institution. Besides carrying out the physical preparation, the nurse teaches the patient as appropriate (see the Guidelines for Care Box).

Because the endocrine system affects fluid and electrolytes, patients with suspected pathological conditions or those being evaluated to establish total health status will have serum electrolytes evaluated. In this section specific diagnostic tests for evaluation of particular glands will be described. The diagnostic tests for each gland are discussed separately.

### PITUITARY FUNCTION TESTING

Pituitary gland malfunction can lead to a variety of symptoms, depending on which hormone is in excess or in deficit. The pituitary gland, as described previously, is interrelated with functions of the thyroid, the adrenal glands, and the gonads. The tests for the function of the pituitary with regard to TSH, ACTH, and gonadotropins are discussed when the diagnostic tests of these glands are outlined.

#### Radiological Tests

Pituitary malfunction may be associated with pituitary tumors, and skull x-ray films to assess the size of the pituitary gland are carried out. Computed tomography (CT) scanning or magnetic resonance imaging (MRI) may be used to demonstrate the presence of sella turcica masses.

#### Growth Hormone

The absence or deficit of growth hormone (GH) (somatotropin) leads to dramatic changes in appearance.

#### Laboratory tests

Assay of GH is possible. Growth hormone release follows a diurnal pattern; basal levels can best be determined in the morning, but they are usually less than μg/ml. Levels at other times are less than 10 ng/ml. Growth hormone secretion can be stimulated by L-dopa, bromocriptine, and hypoglycemia. The provocative tests are done as follows: (1) baseline levels of GH and glucose are determined; (2) glucose (100 mg orally); (3) GH and glucose serum levels are drawn at 0.5, 1, 2, and 3 hours. Growth hormone falls to very low levels between 0.5 and 2 hours after glucose administration. In adults with acromegaly, there is minimal or no suppression of GH.

#### Radiological tests

Diagnostic tests for abnormalities related to somatotropin include skeletal x-ray films to assess changes in bone structure.

### Prolactin

Prolactin excess is seen in the presence of some pituitary tumors, or it may be idiopathic. Prolactin deficiency may result in failure of postpartum lactation.

#### Laboratory tests

Levels of prolactin can be measured by radioassay; the normal level is generally 3 to 23 mg/ml depending on the laboratory. Provocative tests for prolactin with the use of chlorpromazine or TRH are available. The tests are done as follows: (1) basal levels of prolactin are measured; (2) TRH (500 μg IV) is given; and then (3) serum levels of prolactin are drawn at timed intervals.

### Antidiuretic Hormone

Absence of ADH leads to a disease called *diabetes insipidus.* The major symptom of this problem is an output of large quantities of dilute urine (greater than 7 to 11 L/day). Before diabetes insipidus can be conclusively diagnosed, the patient must be shown to have a deficiency in ADH, and the patient's kidneys must be able to respond to ADH. Exogenous sources of ADH have no effect if the patient's kidneys cannot respond. Exogenous ADH will increase the osmolality of the urine, whether the dilute urine is caused by excess intake of water or by diabetes insipidus. The differentiation is made between these two conditions by demonstrating response or lack of response to osmolality changes in the serum.

#### Laboratory tests

A water deprivation test is occasionally used if problems with ADH are suspected. Water is withheld for 4 to 18 hours, and the person's response to this deprivation is documented. A person without diabetes insipidus will respond with a rapid decrease in urine volume and an increase in urine osmolality. A patient with diabetes insipidus will have no decrease in volume and no increase in urine osmolality, but the serum osmolality will increase to more than 300 mOsm/kg. The person who cannot produce ADH is susceptible to vascular collapse, because the massive output of urine will continue unabated. Close monitoring for impending collapse during the test is required. Monitoring should include hourly vital signs, urine output, and specific gravity. If a weight loss greater than 3% of body weight occurs or if tachycardia or significant hypotension develops, the test should be terminated. The patient with psychogenic polydipsia may have extreme behavioral problems associated with the deprivation of water and will need emotional support during this period.

The water deprivation test may be followed by a vasopressin test to determine whether the kidney can respond to vasopressin (exogenous ADH). After 5 U of aqueous pitressin is given subcutaneously, urine osmolality should increase. Failure to show an increase in osmolality confirms the diagnosis of nephrogenic diabetes insipidus.[6]

## THYROID FUNCTION TESTING

Testing for thyroid function can be made at the hypothalamic, pituitary, thyroid, or serum levels. The major tests and their procedures, preparations, and interpretations are presented in Tables 33-10, 33-11, and 33-12.

### Laboratory Tests

The most commonly used tests are serum thyroxine ($T_4$), serum triiodothryronine resin uptake ($T_3$RU), serum thyroid-stimulating hormone (TSH), and free thyroxine index ($FT_4I$) (Table 33-10). Serum levels of $T_4$ and $T_3$ reflect total thyroid hormone concentration in the blood, both the metabolically active (free) portion and the inactive (bound) portion.

The largest part (99%) of $T_4$ and $T_3$ is bound to carrier proteins: thyroid-binding proteins (thyroid-binding globulin [TBG] and thyroid-binding albumin [TBA]). The carrier proteins have a greater affinity for $T_4$ than for $T_3$, allowing free $T_3$ to enter cells more rapidly.[11] The $T_3U$ ($T_3RU$, $RT_3U$) test indirectly measures whether unusual levels of thyroid-binding proteins are influencing the serum levels of $T_3$. The $FT_4I$ is calculated as the product of the result of the $T_3U$ and the $T_4$ level.[11] Usually, the order for an $FT_4I$ is written as an $F_7$ or $F_{12}$ test, which is really a $T_4$ test and $T_3U$ test with a calculated $FT_4I$. Because the $FT_4I$ is not affected by the TBG, it reflects hormonal status more accurately than does the total $T_4$.

Further laboratory studies may be done to determine functioning of the hypothalamic-pituitary-thyroid (HPT) axis and the level at which dysfunction exists. (See Table 33-11 for several provocative tests that may be used to stimulate or depress the HPT axis.)

### Radiological Tests

The most commonly used tests are thyroid ultrasound and thyroid scan (see Table 33-12 for details).

## PARATHYROID FUNCTION TESTING

The maintenance of normal calcium and phosphorus metabolism is under the control of other systems (musculoskeletal, GI, urinary) in addition to the parathyroid gland. When parathyroid function is assessed, the patient will also have diagnostic tests of these other systems. This is necessary to determine whether the problem with calcium and phosphorus metabolism is caused by

**table 33-10** *Tests of Thyroid Function*

| Function Test/Procedure and Preparation | Interpretation |
|---|---|
| **SERUM $T_4$ CONCENTRATION**<br>Radioassay of blood is done; no special preparation is needed. | Test measures circulating thyroxine that is bound to TBG and free $T_4$; normal values are 4.7-11 μg/dl. Hyperthyroidism and increased TBG such as occurs in pregnancy and estrogen therapy cause increased $T_4$ values. Hypothyroidism and decreased TBG, as seen with glucocorticoid therapy and hypoproteinemia, cause decreased $T_4$ values. |
| **FREE $T_4$ INDEX ($FT_4I$)**<br>Serum $T_4$ and $T_3U$ are measured. | $FT_4I$ is product of serum $T_4$ and $T_3U$; changes in TBG cause reciprocal alterations in serum $T_4$ and $T_3U$ so that $FT_4I$ stays normal. |
| **SERUM $T_3$ CONCENTRATIONS**<br>Radioassay of blood sample is done; no special preparation is needed. | Test measures circulating $T_3$ that is bound to TBG and free $T_3$; normal values are 110-230 ng/dl and are elevated in $T_3$ thyrotoxicosis; variations in TBG can influence test results as they do for serum $T_4$. |
| **SERUM TSH CONCENTRATION**<br>Radioassay of blood is done; no special preparation is needed. | Test measures circulating TSH; normal values are 5-10 ng/dl. Elevated levels reflect pituitary hypersecretion of TSH. |
| **TRIIODOTHYRONINE RESIN UPTAKE ($T_3U$)**<br>Blood sample is drawn; in laboratory, resin and radioactive $T_3$ are added to sample of blood. Radioactive $T_3$ will bind to unoccupied sites of TBG. Excessive radioactive $T_3$ will bind to resin. Radioactive counts are done on blood and resins to determine amount of $T_3$ (radioactive) bound to resin. | Normally 25% to 30% of radioactive $T_3$ will bind to resin; in hyperthyroidism, where there are increased amounts of endogenous thyroid hormone, value of amount binding to resin will be increased; in hypothyroidism, $T_3$ resin uptake will be low. This test is not a measure of the patient's endogenous $T_3$ level. Test is affected by total amount of TBG. In wasting diseases where amount of TBG may be decreased, reading may be falsely elevated. In conditions such as pregnancy and estrogen therapy, abnormal amounts of TBG may be available, and a false-low resin uptake may be obtained; phenytoin (Dilantin) and salicylates compete with thyroxine for TBG sites and may give false-negative $T_3$ resin uptake. |

**table 33-11** *Provocative Tests of Thyroid Function*

| Function Test/Procedure and Preparation | Interpretation |
|---|---|
| **TRH STIMULATION TEST**<br>TRH is given IV and then serum thyroid-stimulating hormone (TSH) levels are repeatedly measured. Patient may feel facial flushing, the urge to urinate, or nausea for 5 minutes after injection. These are self-limiting but not complications. | Normal serum TSH begins to rise at 10 minutes and peaks at 45 minutes; subnormal tests reflect diminished TSH reserve; supranormal response occurs in patients with hypothyroidism of thyroid origin; no response occurs in most patients with thyrotoxicosis except when it is caused by excess TSH. |
| **TSH STIMULATION TEST**<br>Baseline levels of radioactive iodine uptake (RAIU) and protein-bound iodine (PBI) are taken, TSH injection is given, and repeat RAIU and PBI levels are taken. | Test assists in differentiating between primary and secondary hypothyroidism; in primary hypothyroidism repeat level of RAIU and PBI stays the same; if they become normal, this indicates hypothyroidism caused by too little TSH (secondary). |
| **THYROID SUPPRESSION TEST**<br>RAIU test and serum $T_4$ levels are done. Patient is given thyroid hormone for 7-10 days, and RAIU and serum $T_4$ tests are repeated. | If euthyroid (normal), repeat RAIU and serum $T_4$ levels will be low; failure of hormone therapy to suppress RAIU and serum $T_4$ indicates hyperthyroidism. |

**table 33-12** *Radiographic Tests of Thyroid Gland*

| Function Test/Procedure and Preparation | Interpretation |
|---|---|
| **RADIOACTIVE IODINE UPTAKE (RAIU)** | |
| Tracer dose of radioactive iodine is given orally. At 2, 6, and 24 hours after administration, scintillation detector is placed over neck and amount of accumulated iodine is measured. Urine is collected for 24 hours; decreased amounts in urine indicate hyperthyroid state. No precautions necessary. | Normal thyroid will take up 5% to 35% of tracer dose. Increased uptake occurs in hyperthyroidism. Excess iodine in foods, cough medicine, x-ray media, other medications, and enriched iodine foods affect test by giving low readings. Diarrhea gives low readings from absorption of tracer dose. Decreased excretion with renal failure gives elevated readings. |
| **THYROID SCAN** | |
| Dose of radioactive iodine or labeled pertechnitate is given, and scintillation scan is done. Scanner is moved over thyroid, and a picture of distribution of radioactivity is recorded. No radiation precautions necessary. | Size, shape, and anatomic function of gland are assessed; areas of increased uptake are noted. |
| **THYROID ULTRASOUND** | |
| Thyroid is assessed by ultrasound. | Test is helpful in defining "cold" areas as cystic or solid. |

altered parathyroid metabolism or by other disease states. Calcium has a very important role in the maintenance of normal neuromuscular irritability. Because hypocalcemia can be lethal, the patient will be assessed and continually monitored for the presence of Trousseau's and Chvostek's signs when hypoparathyroidism is suspected. See Chapter 15. Increased neuromuscular irritability can result in carpopedal spasm, hypertonic flexion, or rigidity of the fingers or toes. This sign is seen in the fingers when a blood pressure cuff is inflated on the arm (Trousseau's sign). Tapping of the finger over the facial nerve can evoke a muscular tic on that side of the face (Chvostek's sign).

### Laboratory Tests

The specific tests of parathyroid function consist of serial laboratory determinations of serum calcium and phosphorus, urinary calcium, and serum alkaline phosphatase. Calcium and phosphorus are evenly proportional, so both must be measured. Normally, serum calcium levels are 8.0 to 10.5 mg/dl, serum phosphorus levels are 2.5 to 4.5 mg/dl, urinary calcium excretion in 24 hours is 1 to 300 mg (depending on diet and need), and serum alkaline phosphatase measures 30 to 85 IU/L.

## ADRENAL FUNCTION TESTING

The adrenal function tests can be divided into those designed to test cortical function and those designed to test medullary function.

### Adrenocortical Function Tests

Because the adrenal cortex affects so many physiological functions, tests that are diagnostic for many disorders may be ordered.

#### *Laboratory tests*

Analysis of blood to ascertain electrolyte balance, a glucose tolerance test to determine the ability of the patient to use carbohydrates, and a test of the ability of the renal tubules to concentrate and dilute urine will probably be done. In addition, x-ray films of the kidney area may be taken to ascertain the presence of adrenal tumors.

**table 33-13** *Diurnal Pattern of Serum Cortisol and Adrenocorticotropic Hormone (ACTH) Levels*

| Serum Values | 6 AM | 4 PM (or Later) |
|---|---|---|
| Cortisol | 6-28 ng/dl | 2-12 ng/dl |
| ACTH | 15-100 pg/ml | 50 pg/ml |

Diagnostic tests of adrenocortical function include tests of all three types of hormonal secretions. Plasma cortisol and ACTH follow a diurnal pattern. Each can be measured at 8 AM and 4 PM (or later) to ascertain whether the normal diurnal pattern is present. A high serum value of cortisol or ACTH and loss of the diurnal pattern are associated with hypercortisolism (Table 33-13). A below normal serum level of cortisol or a normal level of cortisol in a stressed patient indicates adrenal insufficiency. Adrenal insufficiency is confirmed by a blunted or absent response to ACTH. The rapid ACTH stimulation test is particularly useful in the critically ill patient. Plasma aldosterone, angiotensin II, and renin are measured to evaluate the renin-angiotensin-aldosterone system. Plasma levels of aldosterone are increased by dietary potassium loading, sodium restriction, and assumption of an upright position. Aldosterone levels may be measured before and after manipulating these factors. Plasma levels of androgens are also measured to evaluate the adrenal androgen system.

A 24-hour urine collection may also be analyzed for 17-ketosteroids (17-KS), 17-ketogenic steroids (17-KGS), and 17-hydroxycorticosteroids (17-OHCS). These compounds are metabolites of the hormones produced by the adrenal gland.

These 24-hour urine collections require special preservatives, and the nurse should know the institution's requirements and make sure the appropriate container is available.

In addition to these studies, other definitive tests are available to determine whether hypofunction or hyperfunction of the adrenal cortex is present and to establish whether the malfunction is caused by a primary adrenocortical problem or whether the malfunction is secondary to pituitary malfunction. These studies are described in Table 33-14.

## Adrenomedullary Function Tests

### Laboratory tests

The function of the adrenal medulla can be assessed by the assay of catecholamines in urine. Table 33-15 gives the normal values of 24-hour urine measurements. In pheochromocytoma, a catecholamine-secreting tumor, basal levels of plasma and urinary catecholamines are elevated; and, further, they are not suppressed by the oral administration of 300 mg of clonidine. Clonidine normally suppresses the secretion of catecholamines; hypotension, bradycardia, and somnolence may occur as side effects.

The *clonidine suppression* test is now more widely used than are pressor tests that manipulate the blood pressure.[6] This test yields fewer false-positive and false-negative results and is less risky. In the *histamine* test, 0.01 to 0.25 mg of histamine is administered intravenously; this can provoke a hypertensive crisis. In pheochromocytoma, a dramatic rise in blood pressure is seen. In the *Regitine* test, phentolamine (Regitine), 5 mg, is administered intravenously; this agent can provoke a hypotensive crisis. In pheochromocytoma the blood pressure drop is diagnostic when there is a decrease of 35 mm Hg systolic and 25 mm Hg diastolic. In either test, close monitoring is necessary and preparations should be made to treat a crisis if it develops.

### Radiographic tests

Because 10% of catecholamine-secreting tumors are extra-adrenal, radiographic tests are not limited to the adrenal gland and kidney. The $^{131}$I- or $^{123}$I-labeled metaiodobenzylguanidine (MIBG) scintigraphy may be the initial study done to locate a pheochromocytoma.[6] Other techniques to locate tumors and to plan surgical treatment may include CT, MRI, ultrasonography, arteriography, and retroperitoneal air sufflation.

**table 33-14** *Tests of Adrenocortical Function*

| Function Test/Procedure and Preparation | Interpretation |
|---|---|
| **SCREENING ACTH STIMULATION TEST; COSYNTROPIN TEST** | |
| Cosyntropin, 250 ng, is given IV and plasma cortisol level is measured before and 30-60 minutes after this dose. | Normally, plasma cortisol increases >18 μg/dl; this increase confirms a functional HPA axis and rules out adrenal insufficiency. |
| **SCREENING SUPPRESSION TEST; MINERALOCORTICOID SUPPRESSION TEST (VARIOUS TESTS ARE AVAILABLE)** | |
| Dexamethasone, 1 mg, is given orally at 12 PM. At 8 AM cortisol level is drawn. | Normally, cortisol should be less than 5 μg/dl. |
| Saline, 500 ml/hr for 4 hours, is infused IV. | Normally, saline infusion depresses plasma aldosterone to <8 μg/dl if patient has been on a sodium-restricted diet and to <5 μg/dl if patient has been on a normal-sodium diet. |
| An alternative is that patient is placed on normal-sodium diet (100 mEq) or high-sodium diet (200 mEq). After patient is in sodium balance, deoxycorticosterone acetate (DOCA) (10 mg q12h) is administered IM for 3-5 days. | Normal persons in sodium balance from diet will have a 70% decrease in aldosterone. |
| **ACTH STIMULATION TEST (VARIOUS TESTS AVAILABLE)** | |
| Synthetic adrenocorticotropic hormone (ACTH) is given in 500-1000 ml of normal saline at 2 U/24 hr; then 17-OHCS and plasma cortisol levels are measured; alternative is to infuse 25 units of ACTH over 8 hours on 2-3 days and measure 17-OHCS and plasma cortisol levels on these days. | Normally, 17-OHCS excretion increases to 25 mg/24 hr, and plasma cortisol increases to 40 μg/dl or greater; in patients with secondary adrenal insufficiency, the 17-OHCS rate is 3-20 mg/24 hr, and the cortisol level is 10-40 μg/dl. |
| **CORTISONE SUPPRESSION TEST** | |
| A 24-hour urine specimen for 17-OHCS is collected for baseline; dexamethasone, 0.5 mg, is given every 6 hours for 2 days; 24-hour urine is collected for these 2 days. | Dexamethasone suppresses pituitary secretion of ACTH and thus steroid levels; normally by second day of dexamethasone, 24-hour urinary level of OHCS should drop more than 50% below baseline. Patients with adrenocortical excess (primary) will not show decrease in 24-hour urine levels; patients with secondary adrenocortical excess will have drop, but less than 50%. |

NOTE: The ACTH stimulation test is not performed as often as it once was. The cosyntropin test is the most commonly performed test. The diagnostic value of the cortisone suppression test is currently being questioned.

## PANCREATIC ENDOCRINE FUNCTION TESTING

The major endocrine disorder of the pancreas is caused by disturbance in production, action, or metabolic rate of utilization of insulin. The relative lack of insulin leads to elevated blood glucose levels and the presence of glucose in the urine.

### Laboratory Tests

Tests to assess blood glucose levels are described in Table 33-16, and a more detailed explanation of them is given in Chapter 36. The glucose tolerance test (GTT) is no longer used to diagnose diabetes except in suspected gestational diabetes and acromegaly. The current diagnostic test for diabetes is the fasting serum glucose. According to Diabetes Complication and Control Trial (DCCT) and American Diabetes Association (ADA) guidelines, a level greater than 126 mg/dl on two separate occasions is diagnostic for diabetes.

The C-peptide test can be helpful in determining whether a patient is secreting insulin. This finding is particularly useful in a patient receiving exogenous insulin because exogenous insulin does not contain the C-peptide fragment.

Glycosylated proteins (proteins bonded with glucose) can be measured; the amount of glycosylation correlates with average blood glucose levels over the life span of the protein. For the glycosylated hemoglobin ($HbA_{1C}$) test, the life span is 9 to 12 weeks; the time is shorter for albumin and fructosamide. Glycosylated protein tests (usually $HbA_{1C}$) can be helpful in evaluating whether the current blood glucose level is a marked change from those in the past.

Laboratory tests of venous blood to measure fasting blood glucose, postprandial blood glucose, premeal blood glucose, and $HbA_{1C}$ are used periodically to evaluate the effectiveness of blood glucose control in treated persons with diabetes. Therapeutic goals are established for each patient individually; the goals may be set at normal blood glucose levels or higher. For example, goals might include a fasting blood sugar of 126 mg/dl or lower, blood glucose at other times of 180 mg/dl or lower, and $HbA_{1C}$ at every 3 months of 7 or less.[1]

In addition to laboratory tests of blood glucose, nurses use blood glucose monitors to measure capillary blood for frequent testing each day of patients in hospitals or nursing homes. Patients use capillary blood for self-blood glucose monitoring as an important part of daily self-management. The most common times for blood glucose monitoring are fasting, before meals (ac), and at bedtime (hs). (See Chapter 35 for information about teaching patients about the use of self-blood glucose monitoring.)

Testing of urine for glucose yields inaccurate findings, and urine tests have been supplanted by blood glucose monitoring in most instances. However, testing for glycosuria is part of a urinalysis. Several products for testing urine are still available. It is important to follow directions on the product label to ensure accuracy. The products vary in their sensitivity to glucose and ketones and in the ranges of glycosuria levels that they detect.

**table 33-15** *Urinary Tests of Adrenomedullary Secretions*

| Specific Tests | Normal Values |
|---|---|
| Epinephrine | 5-40 ng/24 hr |
| Norepinephrine | 10-80 ng/24 hr |
| Metanephrine | 24-96 ng/24 hr |
| Dopamine | 65-400 ng/24 hr |
| Vanillylmandelic acid (VMA) | 1-9 mg/24 hr |

## chapter SUMMARY

### ANATOMY AND PHYSIOLOGY

- Hormone levels are finely regulated by various types of feedback mechanisms.
- Many hormones display intrinsic rhythms that vary minute to minute, daily, or over longer periods.
- A hormone acts only on tissue that has an appropriate receptor for the hormone.
- Steroid hormones and thyroid hormones are lipid soluble and enter cells to combine with intracellular receptors.
- Other types of hormones (biogenic amines, small peptides, protein hormones, glycoproteins) are water soluble and combine with membrane receptors; the combination of hormone and membrane receptor stimulates a second messenger such as cAMP.
- The hypothalamus serves as a major link between the rest of the nervous system and the endocrine system by its control of the pituitary gland, as well as its communication with other parts of the brain and the autonomic nervous system.
- Posterior pituitary hormones, ADH, and oxytocin are synthesized in the hypothalamus and stored in the pituitary.
- Antidiuretic hormone controls serum osmolality, and oxytocin is involved in lactation and uterine contraction.
- The hypothalamus controls anterior pituitary gland function by synthesis of releasing or inhibiting hormones, including prolactin-inhibiting and prolactin-releasing hormones, growth hormone–releasing and growth hormone–inhibiting hormone, corticotropin-releasing hormone, gonadotropin-releasing hormone, and thyrotropin-releasing hormone.

**table 33-16** *Diagnostic Blood Tests for Pancreatic Endocrine Function*

| Function Test Procedure and Preparation | Interpretation |
|---|---|
| **FASTING BLOOD GLUCOSE (FBG)** | |
| NPO after midnight | Level >126 mg/dl on two separate occasions is diagnostic for diabetes mellitus. |
| **C-PEPTIDE TEST** | |
| Blood sample drawn (does not have to be fasting) | Normal values: 2-20 μg/ml. Levels of C-peptide fragment correlate with level of active insulin molecule endogenously secreted. |

- The anterior pituitary secretes six hormones: growth hormone, prolactin, follicle-stimulating hormone, luteinizing hormone, thyroid-stimulating hormone, and adrenocorticotropin. Hormone release is regulated by the hypothalamus and negative feedback.
- The thyroid gland consists of two cell types: follicle cells, which synthesize thyroid hormone; and C-cells, which synthesize calcitonin.
- Control of thyroid function is from the hypothalamus, the anterior pituitary gland, and external factors.
- Thyroid hormone alters protein, carbohydrate, and fat metabolism; calorigenesis; growth and development; cardiac, respiratory, musculoskeletal, neurological, and reproductive function; and function of the sympathetic nervous system.
- Calcitonin is involved in calcium homeostasis.
- The four small parathyroid glands lie on the posterior aspect of the thyroid; parathyroid hormone is responsible for maintaining serum calcium levels.
- The adrenal cortex gland secretes the adrenal androgens, aldosterone, and glucocorticoids. Androgens are involved in development of secondary sex characteristics. Aldosterone is a major controller of sodium balance and volume status. Glucocorticoids are involved in gluconeogenesis, protein catabolism, and lipolysis; are antiinflammatory; and suppress immune responsiveness, alter mood, and maintain emotional stability.
- Glucocorticoid production is controlled by the hypothalamus, the anterior pituitary gland, and external factors such as glucose level and physiological and psychological stressors. Aldosterone levels are controlled by the renin-angiotensin system.
- The adrenal medulla produces and secretes epinephrine and norepinephrine and works with the sympathetic nervous system in a coordinated response to stressors; all body systems are affected.
- The adrenomedullary sympathetic response is designed to stimulate organ systems that are necessary for life, such as the cardiovascular, respiratory, and neurological systems, and to inhibit systems such as the gastrointestinal, hepatic, and pancreatic systems.
- The endocrine functions of the pancreas are carried out by the islet cells.
- The β-cells secrete insulin, which works on muscle, hepatic, and fat cells to lower blood glucose, store carbohydrates and fat, and synthesize protein.
- The α-cells secrete glucagon, which elevates blood glucose and mobilizes fat. Glucagon works with cortisol, growth hormone, and epinephrine to counterbalance the effects of insulin.
- Aging alters endocrine functioning, specifically pituitary, adrenal, pancreatic, thyroid, and parathyroid functioning.
- Aging is associated with altered bone and calcium metabolism, hypothyroidism, and diabetes mellitus.
- Most disorders of the endocrine system result in hypersecretion or hyposecretion of hormones.

### SUBJECTIVE DATA

- Endocrine dysfunction affects fluid intake, nutritional intake, elimination, energy level, body characteristics, reproductive and sexual functioning, tolerance to stressors, and almost every physiological system.

### OBJECTIVE DATA

- An entire endocrine system history must be completed, along with a thorough head-to-toe physical examination.

### DIAGNOSTIC TESTS

- Diagnostic tests of the endocrine system focus on hormone levels; the interrelationships among the hypothalamus, the anterior pituitary gland, and other endocrine glands; or the substrates controlled by the hormone.

## References


1. American Diabetes Association: Standards of medical care for patients with diabetes mellitus (position statement), *Diabetes Care* 20(1):5-13, 1997.
2. Andreoli TE, Bennett JC, Carpenter CC, et al: *Cecil essentials of medicine,* ed 3, Philadelphia, 1993, WB Saunders.
3. Baxter JD: Introduction to endocrinology. In Greenspan FS, Strewler GJ, editors: *Basic and clinical endocrinology,* ed 5, Norwalk, Conn, 1997, Appleton & Lange.
4. Greenspan FS: The thyroid gland. In Greenspan FS, Strewler GJ, editors: *Basic and clinical endocrinology,* ed 5, Norwalk, Conn, 1997, Appleton & Lange.
5. Huether SE: Mechanisms of hormonal regulation. In McCance KL, Huether SE, editors: *Pathophysiology: the biologic basis for disease in adults and children,* ed 3, St Louis, 1998, Mosby.
6. Hintz RL: The pituitary gland and growth failure. In Lavin N, editor: *Manual of endocrinology and metabolism,* ed 2, Boston, 1994, Little, Brown.
7. Kaplan S: The newer uses of growth hormone in adults, *Adv Intern Med* 38:2287, 1993.
8. Locker FG: Hormonal regulation of calcium homeostasis, *Nurs Clin North Am* 31:797, 1996.
9. Loriaux TC: Endocrine assessment: red flags for those on the front lines, *Nurs Clin North Am* 31:695, 1996.
10. Porterfield SP: *Endocrine physiology,* St Louis, 1997, Mosby.
11. Rusterholtz A: Interpretation of diagnostic laboratory tests in selected endocrine disorders, *Nurs Clin North Am* 31:715, 1996.

chapter

# 34 MANAGEMENT OF PERSONS WITH Problems of the Pituitary, Thyroid, Parathyroid, and Adrenal Glands

JUNE HART ROMEO, KATHLEEN ZUPAN, and JANE F. MAREK

## objectives *After studying this chapter, the learner should be able to:*

1 Compare and contrast the pathophysiology of hypersecretion and hyposecretion of the anterior and posterior pituitary, thyroid, parathyroid, and adrenal glands.

2 Correlate the clinical manifestations, including history, physical examination, and diagnostic test findings, with hypersecretion and hyposecretion of the anterior and posterior pituitary, thyroid, parathyroid, and adrenal glands.

3 Synthesize a nursing plan of care, including identification of appropriate nursing diagnoses, patient outcomes, and interventions, for a patient with hypersecretion or hyposecretion of the anterior or posterior pituitary, thyroid, parathyroid, or adrenal gland.

4 Explain reasons for surgery of the pituitary, thyroid, parathyroid, or adrenal gland.

5 Formulate a nursing plan of care for an individual having surgery on the pituitary, thyroid, parathyroid, or adrenal gland.

6 Relate self-care skills needed by a patient receiving long-term hormonal replacement therapy for pituitary, thyroid, parathyroid, or adrenocortical insufficiency.

7 Develop a teaching plan for a patient receiving long-term hormonal replacement therapy for pituitary, thyroid, parathyroid, or adrenocortical insufficiency.

Alterations in function of the endocrine system result in a variety of physiological changes. Dysfunction of the endocrine system is serious and can be fatal because of the vital functions regulated by the hormones from the pituitary, thyroid, parathyroid, and adrenal glands. The result of most pathological processes affecting the endocrine glands is depression or elevation of blood levels of hormones.

Many types of pathological processes can result in destruction of endocrine tissue and decreased blood levels of hormones. Selected types of problems that result in decreased blood hormone levels include:

1. Destruction of glands by infiltrative processes, infarction, infection, autoimmune and immunological processes, and tumor
2. Abnormal embryonic development, resulting in structural problems or inadequate capacity for synthesis
3. Destruction of glands by surgical removal, radiation therapy, or trauma
4. Suppression of hormones by medications for specific medical conditions such as cardiac, psychiatric, or others

The target cells for the selected hormones can become nonresponsive to the hormones. Although in this type of problem the blood hormone levels may be normal or even high, the condition mimics those seen with depression of blood hormones.

Selected types of problems that result in increased blood levels of hormones include:

1. Hyperplasia or hypertrophy of endocrine glands
2. Benign or malignant tumor growth with capacity to secrete hormone
3. Stimulation of glands by trophic factors liberated from ectopic nonendocrine sites
4. Stimulation of hormonal production secondary to administration of certain medications for cardiovascular, psychiatric, neurological, and gastrointestinal diseases
5. Secretion of hormones by ectopic nonendocrine tissues
6. Exogenous administration of hormones
7. Decreased metabolism of hormones, resulting in their prolonged activity

For those endocrine glands controlled by the hypothalamus and pituitary gland, which include the thyroid and adrenocortical glands and the gonads, glandular disorders resulting in hypersecretion or hyposecretion can be classified as *primary, secondary,* or *tertiary*. Primary problems occur when the thyroid gland, adrenocortical gland, or gonads are diseased. Secondary dysfunction occurs when the problem results from anterior pituitary dysfunction, and tertiary problems arise from hypothalamic dysfunction.

Tumor growth can have an impact on the endocrine system as well. Although hormonal levels are often not immediately affected by the tumor growth, progressive growth can either destroy normal tissue, resulting in hyposecretion of hormones, or the tumor can be made up of secreting tissue, resulting in hypersecretion. Also, the treatment of the tumor by surgery, radiation, or drug therapy often results in iatrogenic depressed blood levels of hormones.

## PITUITARY GLAND

The hypothalamus and pituitary gland form a unit that controls the function of several endocrine glands—thyroid, adrenals, and gonads—as well as a wide range of physiological activities. This section describes the brain-endocrine interactions or *neuroendocrinology*. These actions and interactions constitute the regulatory mechanisms for virtually all physiological activities. These regulatory mechanisms are also important in pathology.

## HYPERFUNCTION OF THE PITUITARY GLAND

### Etiology

Hyperfunction of the anterior portion of the pituitary gland may involve one or more hormones. A cause from the pituitary gland itself is deemed *primary*. If the cause is from interference with the pituitary pathway (i.e., if the cause stems from the hypothalamus, for example), the problem is considered *secondary*. Tumors of the pituitary gland are common causes of hyperfunction. Pituitary hyperfunction also can result from pituitary hyperplasia. The cause of hyperplasia is not always known, but one hypothesis states that altered feedback signals cause the hypersecretion. Diminished feedback from target organ secretions can result in hyperplasia and hypersecretion.

### Epidemiology

The cause of pituitary tumors, or adenomas, is generally unknown. Pituitary adenomas are functioning or nonfunctioning, depending on whether or not they secrete a hormone. Most adenomas are benign, but some can become quite aggressive and grow to large sizes. Pituitary tumors are generally classified according to the hormone being secreted, for example, prolactinomas and growth hormone-secreting tumors. Pituitary adenomas are also classified according to tumor size (Box 34-1).

Recent advances in endocrinological and neuroradiological research allow earlier recognition and more successful treatment of pituitary adenomas. Prolactinomas are the most common type, accounting for approximately 60% of primary pituitary tumors.[11] Growth hormone (GH) hypersecretion will occur in about 20% of cases and adrenocorticotropin (ACTH) excess in 10%. Hypersecretion of thyroid-stimulating hormone (TSH), the gonadotropins, or alpha subunits is rare. Nonfunctional tumors represent only 10% of all pituitary adenomas, and some of these may in fact be gonadotropin-secreting or alpha subunit-secreting adenomas.[2]

Early clinical recognition of the endocrine effects of excessive pituitary secretion, particularly secondary hypogonadism caused by increased prolactin levels,[15,21] leads to earlier diagnosis of pituitary tumors. Late manifestations of pituitary hypersecretion include sellar enlargement, panhypopituitarism, and suprasellar extension with visual impairment.

**box 34-1** *Classification of Pituitary Adenomas*

| | |
|---|---|
| Enclosed | No invasion into the floor of the sella turcica |
| Invasive | Destruction of part or all of the sella turcica |
| Microadenoma | Enclosed tumors <10 mm in diameter |
| Macroadenoma | Enclosed tumors >10 mm in diameter; these tumors may show suprasellar extension |

### Pathophysiology

Pituitary adenomas may be defined as intrasellar adenomas less than 1 cm in diameter that present with manifestations of hormonal excess without sellar enlargement or extrasellar extension. *Panhypopituitarism* (insufficiency of pituitary hormones caused by damage or deficiency of the pituitary gland) does not occur, and these tumors are very successfully treated.

Pituitary macroadenomas are tumors larger than 1 cm in diameter and cause generalized sellar enlargement. Tumors 1 to 2 cm in diameter and confined to the sella turcica can usually be successfully treated; however, larger tumors and especially those with suprasellar, sphenoid sinus, or lateral extensions are much more difficult to manage and treat. Panhypopituitarism and visual loss increase in frequency with tumor size and suprasellar enlargement.

Alterations in physiological functioning that occur with pituitary tumors result from the presence of a space-occupying mass in the cranium and from the effects of the excessive secretion of hormones by functional neoplasms. In contrast, another alteration may result from the compression of glandular tissue by the tumor mass; this can cause a decrease in the secretion of one or more anterior pituitary hormones and is caused by a nonfunctional adenoma.

#### *Neurological alterations*

Neurological alterations occur because the growing tumor presses on the dura, diaphragm sellae, or adjacent structures. The optic chiasm lies anteriorly and superiorly, and tumors that extend upward may cause compression. In some patients, cranial nerves III, IV, and VI also may be involved with lateral extension of tumors. The most common signs of compression are visual field defects. *Bilateral hemianopsia* (blindness in half the visual field) is often identified during visual field testing in a routine eye examination. The tumor may involve the neighboring bony structures or the temporal or frontal lobe, and very large tumors may compress or infiltrate the hypothalamus.

Hemorrhage into the tumor or pituitary apoplexy (see p. 1063-1064) can cause a sudden increase in size, with rapid onset of various neurological signs and symptoms. Pituitary apoplexy may occur years after surgery and/or radiation therapy for the original tumor.

#### *Endocrine alterations*

Depending on which hormone the adenoma is secreting, a variety of effects may be seen (Box 34-2). This section focuses on hypersecretion of prolactin, GH, and gonadotropins (Table 34-1). The Nursing Management section that follows growth hormone hypersecretion is applicable to all patients with hyperpituitarism. The pathophysiological factors associated with increased secretion of ACTH or TSH are the same as those seen with adrenocortical hormone or thyroid hormone excess and are discussed in later sections.

### Collaborative Care Management

Pituitary adenomas are treated with surgery, radiation, or drugs to suppress hypersecretion by the adenoma. Goals of therapy are to correct hypersecretion of anterior pituitary hormones, to preserve normal secretion of other anterior pituitary hormones, and to remove or suppress the adenoma. These goals are usually achievable in patients with pituitary microadenomas. However, in patients who have macroadenomas, multiple therapies are often required and may be less successful.

Pituitary surgery is the initial therapy of choice by many surgeons, and the transsphenoidal microsurgical approach to the sella turcica is the procedure of choice.[20] Transfrontal craniotomy is required only in the occasional patient with massive

**table 34-1** *Gonadotropin Hypersecretion*

| | |
|---|---|
| INCIDENCE | Males more than females<br>Highest incidence in middle age |
| HORMONE SECRETED | Follicle-stimulating hormone (FSH) most common<br>Luteinizing hormone (LH) |
| CLINICAL MANIFESTATIONS | Usually none<br>Hypersecretion of only FSH can result in secondary hypogonadism<br>Patients will have history of normal pubertal development and fertility |

**box 34-2** *clinical manifestations*

***Pituitary Hormone–Secreting Tumors***

**NEUROLOGICAL**

1. Visual defects often first seen as losses in superior temporal quadrants with progression to hemianopia or scotomas and finally to total blindness
2. Headache
3. Somnolence
4. Rarely, signs of increased intracranial pressure (hydrocephalus, papilledema)
5. With very large tumors, disturbance in appetite, sleep, temperature regulation, and emotional balance because of hypothalamic involvement
6. Behavioral changes and seizures with expansion causing compression of the temporal or frontal lobe (very rare)

**ENDOCRINE**

**Prolactin Hypersecretion**

1. Females
   a. Menstrual disturbances, such as irregular menses, anovulatory periods, oligomenorrhea, or amenorrhea
   b. Infertility
   c. Galactorrhea
   d. Manifestations of ovarian steroid deficit, such as dyspareunia, vaginal mucosal atrophy, decreased vaginal lubrication, decreased libido
2. Males
   a. Decreased libido and possible erectile dysfunction
   b. Reduced sperm count and infertility
   c. Gynecomastia
   d. Galactorrhea
3. Both males and females: depressed levels of gonadal steroids

**Growth Hormone (GH) Hypersecretion (Acromegaly)**

1. Macroadenomas with resultant headache and visual changes
2. Changes in facial features (coarsening of features; increased size of nose, lips, and skin folds; prominence of supraorbital ridges; growth of mandible resulting in prognathism and widely spaced teeth; soft tissue growth resulting in facial puffiness)
3. Increased size of hands and feet (see Figure 34-1), weight gain
4. Deepening of voice from thickening of vocal cords
5. Increases in vertebral bodies resulting in thoracic kyphosis
6. Enlarged tongue, salivary glands, spleen, liver, heart, kidney, and other organs; cardiomegaly may result in increased blood pressure and signs and symptoms of congestive heart failure.
7. Elevated blood pressure even without cardiac failure
8. Snoring, sleep apnea, and respiratory failure
9. Dermatological changes: acne, increased sweating, oiliness, development of skin tags
10. Hypertrophy progressing to atrophy of skeletal muscles
11. Backache, arthralgia, or arthritis from joint damage and bony overgrowth
12. Peripheral nerve damage, such as carpal tunnel syndrome or neuropathies, from bony overgrowth and changes in nerve size
13. Impaired glucose tolerance progressing to diabetes mellitus
14. Changes in fat metabolism resulting in hyperlipidemia
15. General changes in mobility: presence of lethargy and fatigue
16. Osteoporosis
17. Radiographic findings indicative of bony proliferation in hands, feet, skull, ribs, and vertebrae
18. Electrolyte changes: increased urinary excretion of calcium; elevated blood phosphate level

suprasellar extension of the adenoma. In the transsphenoidal procedure, the surgeon approaches the pituitary from the nasal cavity through the sphenoid sinus, removes the anterior-inferior sellar floor, and incises the dura. The adenoma is removed. Normal pituitary tissue is identified and preserved when possible. Success rates approach 90% in patients with microadenomas. Complications, including postoperative hemorrhage, cerebrospinal fluid leak, meningitis, and visual impairment occur in less than 5% of patients and are most frequent in patients with large or massive tumors.[11] Transient diabetes insipidus lasting from several days to 2 weeks occurs in approximately 15% of patients. Permanent diabetes insipidus is rare. A transient form of the syndrome of inappropriate antidiuretic hormone (SIADH) with symptomatic hyponatremia occurs in 10% of patients.[14] Surgical hypopituitarism is rare in patients with microadenomas, but approaches 5% to 10% in patients with larger tumors. The perioperative management of such patients should include glucocorticoid administration in stress doses and postoperative assessment of daily weight, fluid balance, and electrolyte status.[14]

Pituitary radiation is usually reserved for patients with larger tumors who have had an incomplete resection of large pituitary adenomas. Conventional radiation using high-energy sources is most commonly used. The response to radiation therapy is slow, and 5 to 10 years may elapse before the full effect is realized. Treatment is ultimately successful in about 80% of people with acromegaly, but only about 55% to 60% of patients with Cushing's disease respond.[11] The response rate of patients with prolactinomas is not precisely known, but tumor progression is prevented in most patients. Morbidity with radiotherapy is minimal, although some patients experience adverse side effects including malaise and nausea. Hypopituitarism is common, and the incidence increases with time following radiotherapy; it develops in 50% to 60% of patients at 5 to 10 years.[2] Rare late complications include damage to the optic nerves and chiasm, seizures, and radionecrosis of brain tissue.

Heavy particle irradiation with alpha particles or protons is also used. An advantage of this technique is the ability to focus the radiation beam precisely, limiting the radiation exposure of surrounding structures. Disadvantages are the limited availability and the smaller radiation field, which precludes use of this technique in patients with tumors larger than 1.5 cm in diameter and in those with extrasellar extension. Responses to therapy are more rapid than with conventional radiation and occur within 2 years in most patients.[9] Successful responses are obtained in a majority of patients with acromegaly or Cushing's disease.[9] However, experience in patients with prolactinomas is limited.[9] Neurological damage and visual impairment are rare complications of heavy particle radiation, and hypopituitarism occurs in 20% to 50% of patients treated.[9]

Medical management of pituitary adenomas became feasible with the availability of bromocriptine, a dopamine agonist.[19] This drug is most successful in the treatment of hyperprolactinemia and is also useful in selected patients with acromegaly or Cushing's disease. Octreotide acetate, a somatostatin analog, is useful in the therapy of acromegaly and TSH-secreting adenomas.[6]

#### *Patient/family education*

The patient with a pituitary adenoma will need teaching and support to deal with a variety of issues including body image changes, anxiety, sexual functioning, activity intolerance, and home-going medications. The individual patient and type of tumor and treatment used will determine which issues are of priority. The family should be involved with teaching, so they will be better equipped to assist the patient at home.

If the patient has been treated surgically with transsphenoidal resection, activities causing increased intracranial pressure must be avoided. Bending over at the waist, blowing the nose forcefully, coughing, and straining with defecation can increase intracranial pressure. Teaching should include strategies to prevent constipation and avoidance of such activities.

Assistance may be needed with activities of daily living (ADL) because of generalized weakness or neurological deficits. The patient will generally need regular follow-up care to monitor progress and hormone levels.

No known primary prevention exists for pituitary tumors or pituitary hyperplasia. There is concern about nonmedical use and increased availability of GH, now produced by RNA recombinant gene technology. Research is exploring the effects of GH excess and long-term consequences of its use in healthy persons to increase height, to increase athletic ability, and to combat aging.

Erectile dysfunction in men younger than 65 years can be an early sign of pituitary hyperplasia. Prolactin and testosterone levels may be used for early screening. Screening examinations also can detect early visual field deficits from compression by tumors.

## PROLACTIN HYPERSECRETION

### Etiology/Epidemiology

Prolactin (PRL) hypersecretion is the most common endocrine abnormality caused by hypothalamic-pituitary disorders, and PRL is the hormone most commonly secreted in excess by pituitary adenomas. The understanding that PRL hypersecretion causes galactorrhea and gonadal dysfunction and the use of PRL measurements in screening such patients have permitted recognition of these PRL-secreting tumors before the development of sellar enlargement, hypopituitarism, or visual impairment.[11] Therefore, plasma PRL should be measured in patients with galactorrhea, suspected hypothalamic-pituitary axis dysfunction, or sellar enlargement and also in those with unexplained gonadal dysfunction including amenorrhea, infertility, decreased libido, or erectile dysfunction. The causes of prolactinemia are physiological, pathological, and pharmacological (Table 34-2).

### Pathophysiology

Normal serum prolactin levels are usually less than 20 ng/ml. Prolactin is a natural contraceptive (inhibits gonadotropin-releasing hormone) and is necessary for lactation.

**table 34-2** *Causes of Hyperprolactinemia*

| |
|---|
| **PHYSIOLOGICAL** |
| Sleep |
| Stress (physical and psychological) |
| Pregnancy, lactation |
| **PATHOLOGICAL** |
| Prolactinoma |
| Primary hypothyroidism |
| Chronic renal failure |
| Polycystic ovarian syndrome |
| Cushing's disease |
| Hypothyroidism |
| Acromegaly |
| Chest wall trauma |
| Spinal cord injury |
| Idiopathic |
| **PHARMACOLOGICAL** |
| Psychotropic agents |
| Neuroleptics: phenothiazine, chlorpromazine, haloperidol |
| Antidepressants |
| Tricyclics |
| Imipramine |
| Monoamine oxidase inhibitors |
| Anxiolytics |
| Benzodiazepines |
| Antiemetics |
| Metoclopramide |
| Sulpiride |
| Opiates |
| Methadone |
| Morphine |
| Gastrointestinal agents |
| Metoclopramide |
| Cisapride |
| Domperidone |
| $H_2$ blockers |
| Ranitidine |
| Cimetadine |
| Famotidine |
| Antihypertensive agents |
| Reserpine |
| Methyldopa |
| Calcium-channel blockers |
| Verapamil |
| Hormones |
| Estrogens |
| Thyrotropin-releasing hormone (TRH) |

The clinical manifestations of PRL excess are the same regardless of the cause. The classic features are galactorrhea and amenorrhea in women and galactorrhea and decreased libido or erectile dysfunction in men. Although the sex distribution of prolactinomas is essentially equal, microadenomas are much more common in women, presumably due to the earlier recognition of the endocrine consequences of PRL excess.

Pathophysiological mechanisms of prolactin hypersecretion include dopamine disorders, hypersecretion by pituitary tumors, hypothalamic thyrotropin-releasing hormone stimulation, neurogenic secretion triggered by chest irritation (rib fracture, thoracotomy, or herpes zoster) and decreased clearance of prolactin as seen in chronic renal failure. The secretion of prolactin by the pituitary is controlled chiefly by inhibitory factors of the hypothalamus, most importantly dopamine.

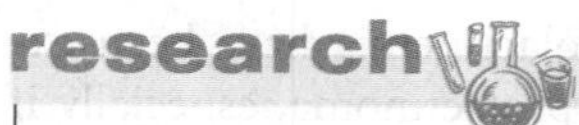

Reference: Romeo JH, Dombrowski RC, Aron DC, et al: Hyperprolactinemia and verapamil: prevalence, evidence for causality, and associated hypogonadism. *Clin Endocrinol* 45:571-575, 1996.

Increased prolactin levels have been associated with administration of the calcium channel blocker, verapamil, but the prevalence is not known. This cross-sectional study consisted of 463 male patients taking verapamil for control of hypertension. Exclusion criteria included persons taking medications known to elevate prolactin levels, persons with renal failure, and those with primary hypothyroidism. Control subjects were drawn from a random sample of eligible outpatients not taking verapamil. Serum prolactin was measured by Abbott Laboratories microparticle enzyme immunoassay, which reports for male patients a normal mean of 6.75 and a range of 1.58 to 23.12 ng/ml. The main outcome measures were (1) proportion of patients in each group with elevated serum prolactin levels and (2) mean serum prolactin level in each group. Prolactin levels were obtained for 463 subjects taking verapamil and 172 control subjects. The prevalence of hyperprolactinemia associated with verapamil use in this study was 8.6% compared with 2.9% in the control group. There was a significant association of hypogonadism in the patients with hyperprolactinemia. These clinical findings demonstrate the importance of a detailed drug history in the evaluation of hyperprolactinemia.

## Collaborative Care Management

The evaluation of patients with galactorrhea or unexplained gonadal dysfunction with normal or low plasma gonadotropin levels should include a history regarding menstrual status, pregnancy, fertility, sexual function, and symptoms of hypothyroidism or hypopituitarism. Current and previous use of medications, drugs, or estrogen therapy should be documented. Prolactin excess can result from pharmacological agents such as psychotropic agents, some antihypertensive drugs, estrogens, and opiates (Table 34-2 and Research Box).[2,15,16] Prolactin levels less than 150 ng/ml are more likely caused by medication than a tumor. With tumors, PRL levels may exceed 3000 ng/ml, although any level greater than 150 ng/ml is virtually diagnostic for adenoma. Basal PRL levels, gonadotropins, thyroid function tests, and TSH levels should be measured as well as serum testosterone level in men. Liver and kidney function should be assessed, and a pregnancy test should be performed in women with amenorrhea.

Patients with galactorrhea but normal menses may not have hyperprolactinemia and usually do not have prolactinomas. If the PRL level is normal, they may be reassured and followed with sequential PRL measurements.

When other causes of hyperprolactinemia have been excluded, the most likely cause is a prolactinoma, especially if there is associated hypogonadism. Since currently available suppression and stimulation tests do not distinguish PRL-secreting tumors from other causes of hyperprolactinemia, the diagnosis must be established by the assessment of both basal PRL levels and neuroradiological studies.[12] There is a general correlation between the PRL elevation and the size of the pituitary adenoma.

Satisfactory control of PRL hypersecretion, cessation of galactorrhea, and return to normal gonadal function can be achieved in most patients with PRL-secreting microadenomas.[12] The choice of surgical or medical therapy, however, remains controversial. All patients with PRL-secreting macroadenomas should be treated because of the risks of further tumor expansion, hypopituitarism, and visual impairment. Treatment of patients with microadenomas is also recommended to prevent early osteoporosis secondary to persisting hypogonadism and to restore fertility.[22]

Surgical treatment consists of resection of the adenoma with the transsphenoidal approach being the one of choice for microadenomas and some macroadenomas.[19,20] Transsphenoidal microsurgery is considerably less successful in restoring normal PRL secretion in patients with macroadenomas, and many clinicians would treat these patients with bromocriptine alone. The surgical outcome is directly related to tumor size and the basal PRL level. Surgery may be recommended, however, for decompression purposes if severe visual field defects are present. In patients with major suprasellar extension of the tumor, the transfrontal craniotomy may be the approach of choice. It must be followed by bromocriptine or radiation therapy, since residual tumor is virtually always present.

Medical treatment consists mainly of bromocriptine (2-bromo-$\alpha$-ergocryptine mesylate), a potent dopamine agonist that stimulates dopamine receptors and affects both the hypothalamic and pituitary levels. Bromocriptine is effective therapy for a PRL-secreting pituitary adenoma and directly inhibits PRL secretion by the tumor. The dosage is 2.5 to 10 mg/dl orally in divided doses. Side effects such as dizziness, postural hypotension, nausea, and occasional vomiting are common at the onset of therapy but usually resolve with continuation of the medication. Side effects can usually be avoided by starting with a low dose and gradually increasing the dose over days to weeks until the PRL level is suppressed to the normal range.[2,15]

Pergolide mesylate is a long-acting ergot derivative with dopaminergic properties that has been shown to reduce hypersecretion and shrink most PRL-secreting macroadenomas. More potent than bromocriptine, pergolide requires doses of 25 to 300 $\mu$g/dl to treat hyperprolactinemia. The side effects are similar to those of bromocriptine. Other dopamine agonists include quingolide and cabergoline, nonergot alkaloid-derived dopamine agonists, which are in clinical trials. These medications normalize PRL values in 70% to 80% of patients and may have fewer side effects than bromocriptine.

#### *Patient/family education*

The teaching needs of the patient with hyperprolactinemia are similar to those of persons with hyperfunction of the pituitary gland (see p. 1054).

## GROWTH HORMONE HYPERSECRETION

### Etiology

Excessive pituitary GH secretion can be secondary to abnormal hypothalamic function, but in most cases it is a primary pituitary disorder. Pituitary adenomas are present in virtually all patients with acromegaly and are usually greater than 1 cm in diameter. Hyperplasia alone is rare, and nonadenomatous anterior pituitary tissue does not exhibit somatotroph hyperplasia when examined histologically.

### Epidemiology

Acromegaly affects men and women equally, and the mean age at diagnosis is approximately 40 years. The duration of symptoms is usually 5 to 10 years before the diagnosis is established. Acromegaly is relatively uncommon; the incidence is approximately 4 cases per million persons.

Acromegaly is a chronic disabling and disfiguring disorder with increased late morbidity and morality if untreated. Causes of death include cardiomyopathy with congestive heart failure, hypertension, diabetes, and pulmonary infections. Acromegaly is also associated with an increased incidence of colon cancer caused by a GH-secreting pituitary adenoma in 98% of patients. Although spontaneous remissions have been described, the course is slowly progressive in the majority of cases.

### Pathophysiology

In acromegaly, chronic GH hypersecretion is usually related to a pituitary adenoma. The secretion remains episodic, although the number, amplitude, and duration of secretory episodes increase and occur randomly. The characteristic nocturnal surge is absent, and there are abnormal responses to suppression and stimulation. Therefore glucose suppressibility is lost, and GH stimulation by hypoglycemia is usually absent.

Thyrotropin-releasing hormone (TRH) and gonadotropin-releasing hormone (GnRH) may cause GH release, whereas these substances do not normally stimulate GH secretion. Dopamine and dopamine agonists such as bromocriptine, which normally stimulate GH secretion, paradoxically cause GH suppression in about 70% to 80% of patients with acromegaly.[2]

Most of the deleterious effects of chronic GH hypersecretion are caused by its stimulation of excessive amounts of insulin-like growth factor 1 (IGF-1; a protein secreted by the liver), and plasma levels of this are increased in acromegaly. The growth-promoting effects of IGF-1 lead to the characteristic proliferation of bone, cartilage, and soft tissues and increase in size of other organs to produce the classic clinical manifestations of acromegaly. The insulin resistance and carbohydrate intolerance seen in acromegaly appear to be direct effects of GH and not due to IGF-1 excess.

## Collaborative Care Management

Patients are generally referred to endocrinologists for diabetes or glucose intolerance, goiter, high blood pressure, and sexual disturbances or for the characteristic dysmorphic features of acromegaly, usually recognized by family doctors, rheumatologists, or dentists. Changes in physical appearance consist of coarsening of facial features with an enlarged nose, lips, and ears and prognathism, with abnormal spacing between the teeth leading to malocclusion. Progressive enlargement of the hands and feet, thickening of the skin, excessive sweating, cardiomegaly, hepatomegaly, hypertension, dysphasia from hypertrophy of the tongue, lowering of the voice pitch (caused by laryngeal hypertrophy), osteoarthritic pain, and carpal tunnel syndrome are other common symptoms of acromegaly (Figure 34-1).

When GH hypersecretion is present for many years, progressive cosmetic deformities and disabling degenerative arthritis occur, and the patient is seen with the typical acromegaly features. The majority of diagnoses are made via visual assessment of the patient.

### Diagnostic tests

Laboratory findings include postprandial plasma glucose elevations and elevated serum phosphorus (due to increased renal tubular resorption of phosphate) and hypercalciuria. These findings are directly due to effects of GH or IGF-1.

Plain films show sellar enlargement in 90% of patients. Thickening of the calvarium, enlargement of the frontal and maxillary sinuses, and enlargement of the jaw can also be seen. Radiographs of the hand show increased soft tissue bulk. Radiographs of the feet show similar changes, and there is increased thickness of the heel pad.

While diagnosis is usually clinically obvious and can be readily confirmed by assessment of GH secretion, other dynamic tests may also confirm the diagnosis. Suppression with oral glucose is the simplest and most specific dynamic test for acromegaly. IGF-1 measurement is also a confirmatory test. TRH stimulation tests can also contribute to the diagnosis.

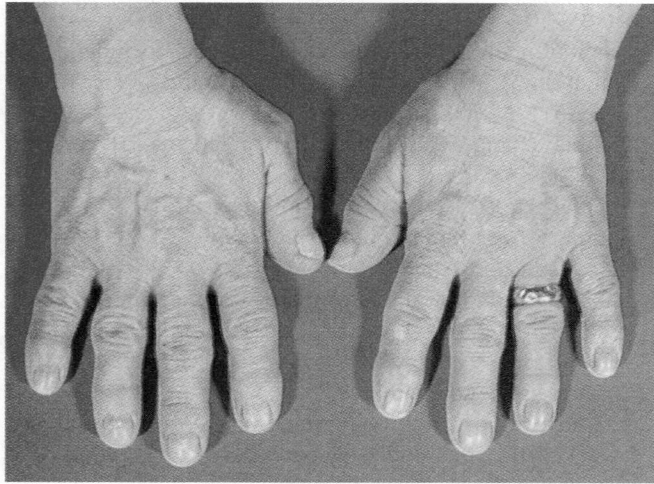

**fig. 34-1** The hands of the patient with acromegaly may appear broad and spade-like.

### Medications

Octreotide acetate, a long-acting somatostatin analog, is now available for the treatment of acromegaly and appears to be most useful in patients who have incomplete responses to surgery or irradiation.[6] Bromocriptine, a dopaminergic agonist, is also used for the treatment of acromegaly. Side effects, as previously mentioned include nausea, constipation, dizziness, and nasal congestion. Taking the medication with food improves tolerance. Pergolide has been used effectively but is not approved by the Food and Drug Administration (FDA) for use in acromegaly. Medications do not produce reduction in tumor size.

### Treatments

All patients with acromegaly should undergo therapy to halt progression of the disorder and to prevent late complications and excess mortality. The objectives of therapy are removal or destruction of the pituitary tumor, reversal of GH hypersecretion, and maintenance of normal anterior and posterior pituitary function. These are attainable in the majority of patients. The initial therapy of choice is transsphenoidal microsurgery because of its high success rate, rapid reduction of GH levels, low incidence of postoperative hypopituitarism, and low surgical morbidity. Conventional radiotherapy is also successful, although a much longer period is required to reduce GH levels to normal.

### Surgical management

As previously mentioned, transsphenoidal adenomectomy is the treatment of choice for GH-secreting adenomas. Surgical excision is curative in selected tumors in over 70% of patients. Some tumors require a frontal craniotomy (see Chapter 52). Complications of surgical intervention include transient diabetes insipidus, meningitis, infection, cerebrospinal fluid rhinorrhea, and hypopituitarism. Large and extensive tumors may not be resectable, and other therapy may be needed. Gamma knife surgery is used in some instances. Figure 34-2 illustrates the surgical incision made through the upper gingival mucosa, along one side of the nasal septum, and through the sphenoid sinus to the sella turcica.

### Diet

Dietary changes may be necessary for patients with acromegaly or Cushing's syndrome. Carbohydrate intolerance or frank diabetes mellitus may be associated with both these disorders. (See Chapter 35 for interventions related to dietary management of diabetes mellitus.) Congestive heart failure may occur in patients with acromegaly, and sodium and lipid restrictions may be necessary (see Chapter 26). The subsequent decrease in calcium levels may put the patient at higher risk for osteoporosis. Therefore, supplemental calcium may be required.

### Activity

No specific activity is prescribed for persons with pituitary tumors. Efforts should be made to maintain or improve the mobility of patients with acromegaly who have bone, muscle, or joint problems. Kyphosis and arthritis may impose problems with mobility and balance.

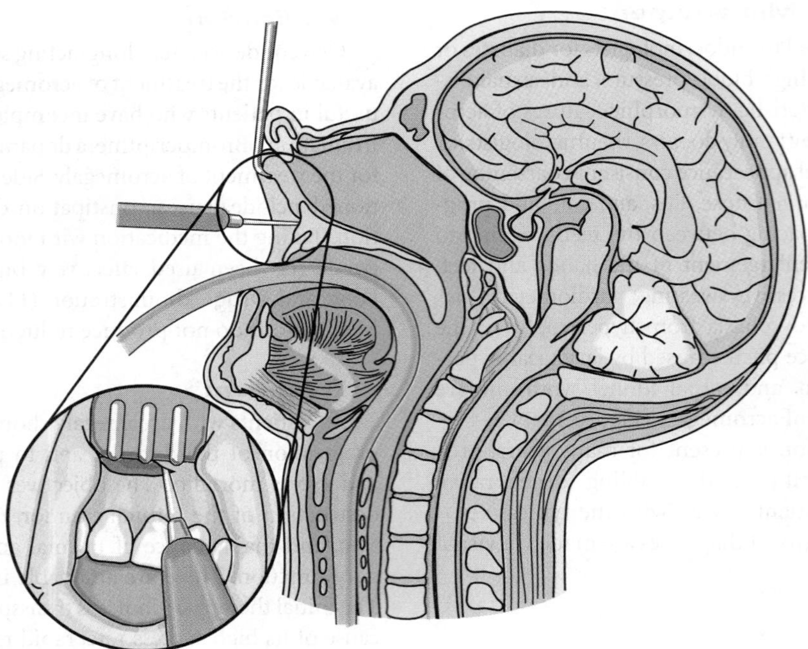

fig. 34-2 Diagram of transsphenoidal approach in anterior pituitary surgery with incision in the gingival mucosa.

### Referrals

The patient with acromegaly may benefit from physical or occupational therapy. The patient with visual loss may benefit from occupational therapy and visual rehabilitative services. Social work services can be helpful when an acute crisis or the burdens of chronic illness stress financial, personal, and family resources. A referral to a mental health professional is usually indicated to assist the patient in coping with the not insignificant physical changes in his or her appearance and people's reactions to those changes.

## NURSING MANAGEMENT

This Nursing Management section refers to the patient with acromegaly and all patients with hyperfunctioning of the pituitary gland.

## ■ ASSESSMENT

Assessment of the patient focuses on identification of manifestations and hormone hypersecretion and the effects on the patient's total health. Assessment should also include the psychological response of the patient to these major body changes.

### Subjective Data

Data to be collected to assess the patient with hypersecretion of the pituitary gland associated with pituitary tumor include:

- History of sensory alterations, particularly vision, as well as other peripheral sensory changes
- Discomforts: temporal or frontal headache of moderate intensity, arthralgia, backache
- History of changes in body appearance: coarsening of facial features; increases in ring, glove, or shoe size; increase in sweating or oiliness of skin
- History of change in energy level (lethargy or fatigue) or decrease in mobility
- Psychosocial concerns: behavioral changes such as anxiety, irritability, concerns about self-image
- History of menstrual changes in females, erectile dysfunction in males, changes in libido; infertility concerns
- Drug history: oral contraceptives, psychotropic drugs
- Knowledge level related to disorder, treatment, potential outcome of treatment

### Objective Data

Data about neurological and endocrine effects include:

- Functioning of cranial nerves II, III, IV, and VI (see Chapter 51)
- Retinal changes indicative of papilledema or elevated blood pressure
- Mental status: alertness and emotional status
- Peripheral nerve functioning (see Chapter 51)
- Body appearance and description
- Mobility and joint functioning (see Chapter 59)
- Vital signs: blood pressure, pulse, respirations, and temperature
- Body weight and height
- Presence of organomegaly, particularly cardiac and hepatic, and signs associated with these changes

## ■ NURSING DIAGNOSES

Nursing diagnoses are determined from analysis of patient data. Nursing diagnoses for the patient with hypersecretion of the anterior pituitary gland associated with pituitary tumor may include but are not limited to:

| Diagnostic Title | Possible Etiological Factors |
|---|---|
| **All Patients—Pretreatment** | |
| Anxiety | Uncertainty about cause of problem and outcomes of treatment; changes in physical appearance; sexual dysfunction; inability to conceive; changes in lifestyle |
| Knowledge deficit: disorder and treatment, expected outcomes, expected complications or side effects | New diagnoses and treatment |
| Pain | Headache from intracranial mass: from pressure on nerve roots and on nerves associated with changes in joints and vertebrae related to abnormal bone growth |
| Self-esteem disturbance | Changes in body characteristics and functions associated with hormonal excess, visual loss, sexual dysfunction, impaired mobility |
| Sensory/perceptual alterations: visual | Pressure on optic chiasma disrupting functioning of cranial nerve II or pressure on cranial nerves III, IV, and VI |
| **Patients with Prolactin-Secreting Tumors—Pretreatment** | |
| Knowledge deficit: disorder, treatment, relationship of disorder to sexual functioning | New diagnoses and treatment |
| Sexual dysfunction | Alteration in menstrual cycle, decreased libido, or impotence associated with increased secretion of prolactin |
| **Patients with GH-Secreting Tumors—Pretreatment** | |
| Knowledge deficit: disorder, treatment, effect of treatment on signs and symptoms | Newly diagnosed disorder and new treatment |
| Mobility, impaired physical | Pain from pressure on nerve roots |
| Pain | Pressure on nerves associated with changes in joints and vertebrae related to growth |
| **Patients with Any Type of Tumor Treated with Surgery** | |
| Fluid volume deficit, risk for | Disruption in normal antidiuretic hormone (ADH) secretion or adrenocortical functioning associated with surgical trauma |
| Gas exchange, impaired | Inadequate deep breathing; instructions not to cough and presence of nasal packing |
| Infection, risk for | Loss of barriers to organisms associated with disruption of external incision in mucous membrane from improper care; disruption of internal incision through dura associated with increased intracranial pressure (ICP) resulting in cerebrospinal fluid (CSF) leak |
| Knowledge deficit: expected outcomes, expected complications | New treatment, no previous exposure to information |
| **Patients with Any Type of Tumor Treated with Radiation** | |
| Injury, risk for | Inability to maintain homeostasis, cardiac output, respiratory functioning, and fluid and electrolyte balance associated with ACTH and/or TSH deficiency |
| Knowledge deficit: procedure, expected outcomes, potential complications | Newly prescribed treatment, no previous exposure to information |
| **Patients with Any Type of Tumor Treated with Drug Therapy** | |
| Knowledge deficit: drugs, self-administration techniques, expected results, potential side effects | Newly prescribed treatment so no previous exposure to information |

## ■ EXPECTED PATIENT OUTCOMES

Expected patient outcomes for the person with hypersecretion of the anterior pituitary gland associated with pituitary tumor may include but are not limited to the following.

### All Patients—Pretreatment

1. Describes anxiety level as tolerable and amount of sleep as adequate, and identifies one or more anxiety-reducing strategies.

2a. Explains nature of the disorder, how signs and symptoms relate to the disease, and how the disease will alter ADL.

b. Describes the purpose of each diagnostic test and special pretest and posttest requirements.

c. Explains (a) dietary regimen and plans to implement the regimen; (b) medications, including knowledge about the drug and administration, expected results, and potential side effects; (c) measures to relieve signs and symptoms, as appropriate; and (d) plans for follow-up care.

3. States headache is controlled by prescribed interventions and environmental modifications.
4. Talks positively about self when discussing body characteristics and functions that are reversible and those that will not change.
5. Is able to function independently in the hospital or at home.

### Patients with Prolactin-Secreting Tumors—Pretreatment

1. Has adequate knowledge, as evidenced by patient's and family's ability to describe disease process and goals of treatment.
2. Attains adequate knowledge, as evidenced by patient's and significant others' ability to describe how the sexual dysfunction relates to prolactin excess and what effects treatment has on sexual functioning.

### Patients with GH-Secreting Tumors—Pretreatment

1. Has adequate knowledge, as evidenced by patient's and significant others' ability to describe the effects of treatment on signs and symptoms.
2. Is independent in ADL and states ability to participate in all activities enjoyed.
3. States that interventions prescribed control back and joint discomfort and that discomfort does not limit activity.

### Patients with Any Type of Tumor Treated with Surgery

1. Exhibits physical signs of fluid balance:
   a. Returns to baseline weight.
   b. Has good skin turgor and moist mucous membranes.
   c. Has blood pressure and pulse within normal range.
   d. Has serum electrolytes and hematocrit within normal limits.
   e. Has urine specific gravity of 1.010 to 1.025.
   f. Has a fluid intake of 2500 to 3000 ml/day, orally or parenterally (unless restrictions are prescribed).
   g. Explains measures to prevent fluid deficit.
2. Has adequate gas exchange, as evidenced by:
   a. Normal ranges of arterial blood gas
   b. Results of pulse oximetry >95%
   c. Usual mental status and skin color
   d. Usual respiratory depth, rate, and effort
   e. Usual tolerance to activity
3. Remains free of infection, as evidenced by absence of persistent headache, of CSF leak, and of nuchal (nape of neck) rigidity.
4. Demonstrates knowledge of rationale for surgical intervention and expected outcomes of treatment.

### Patients with Any Type of Tumor Treated with Radiation

1. Is free of injuries because of patient's and significant others' ability to state signs and symptoms they should monitor for and report immediately.
2. Has adequate knowledge, as evidenced by patient's and significant other's ability to explain radiation procedure, expected outcomes, and potential complications.

### Patients with Any Type of Tumor Treated with Drug Therapy

1. Has adequate knowledge, as evidenced by patient's and significant others' ability to name drugs, state how to administer drugs, and describe the expected results and potential side effects.

## INTERVENTIONS

The patient with a hormonal excess caused by a secreting pituitary tumor will seek care for various reasons. These reasons include symptoms and signs such as frequent or persistent headache, visual changes, changes in body characteristics or function, or high anxiety.

### Reducing Anxiety

1. Assess anxiety level, particular stressors, and patient's use of stress-reducing strategies.
2. Provide clear instructions for and explanations of diagnostic tests and treatment measures.
3. Provide opportunity for the patient to express concerns and to use resources perceived as helpful.
4. Provide support as necessary to maintain optimal level of independence in ADL, decision making, and planning for discharge.

### Promoting Comfort

1. Monitor pain using pain scales and flow sheets (see Chapter 12) every 4 hours; assess for nonverbal signs of pain. Ask the patient to be specific about location and type of pain.
2. Assess for factors that increase or decrease pain.
3. Implement measures to reduce pain:
   a. Identify optimal pain schedule and administer prescribed analgesics; assess for response; anticipate and prevent common side effects.
   b. Assist with nonpharmacological measures for pain relief (e.g., music, massage, distraction, relaxation, imagery, heat or cold, and exercise).
4. Consult physician if pain-reducing measures fail to provide adequate pain relief.
5. Ensure adequate rest and sleep.

The patient may need immediate treatment for headache, such as mild nonnarcotic analgesics. Other helpful measures include sitting and lying with the head elevated. Relaxing in a dark room, listening to quiet music, meditation, and other types of relaxation may also help. The nurse needs to identify, in cooperation with the patient, measures that help relieve the headache. The patient with a GH-secreting tumor requires comfort measures to manage joint and back pain and impaired mobility. These measures may include nonnarcotic analgesics, warm baths, range-of-motion (ROM) exercises, and moist or dry heat.

### Minimizing Low Self-Esteem

1. Assess for factors posing a threat to self-esteem and for statements of negative self-appraisal.
2. Provide support for the patient in asking questions, in seeking information, in obtaining needed resources, and in making decisions about care.
3. Reassure patient about normalcy of individual responses to stressors.
4. Enable patient to maintain optimal level of independence in ADL and personal control.
5. Clarify patient knowledge about disease, its treatment, and anticipated effects on body appearance and functions.

The patient who has just learned of a tumor in the pituitary gland, enclosed within the skull, and who must make choices about type of treatment may be overwhelmed and feel helpless. Threats to self-esteem might be increased by visual disturbances, infertility, immobility, or changes in body appearance. Chronic or stable low self-esteem may be a usual attribute of the patient; however, stressors may induce low self-esteem in any person. Referral of the patient and his or her family to a Pituitary Support Group can provide an opportunity to learn how others have coped. The support group may be contacted at: The Pituitary Tumor Network Association, 16350 Ventura Boulevard, Suite 231, Encino, CA 91436; phone: (805) 499-9973. The Network will assist in contacting the local group.

### Preventing Fluid Volume Deficit

1. Assess risk factors for fluid deficit and correct when possible.
2. Measure weight daily before breakfast with the patient wearing the same clothing, with an empty bladder, and on same scale.
3. Monitor every 8 hours for signs of fluid deficit: decreased skin turgor, dryness of mucous membranes, postural hypotension, tachycardia, and extremes of specific gravity of urine. Monitor available laboratory reports: serum osmolality and sodium levels, and hematocrit.
4. Encourage fluid intake to 2500 to 3000 ml/day unless contraindicated; assess patient's preferences for types of fluids.
5. Maintain prescribed parenteral therapy.
6. Teach patient/family about diet and fluid needs and measures to prevent fluid deficit, as appropriate.

Fluid volume deficit is a potential problem in any patient during the postoperative period. However, the patient who has had a transsphenoidal adenectomy or hypophysectomy is at higher risk because inadequate release of ADH may cause diabetes insipidus. Diabetes insipidus usually develops within 24 hours and is usually temporary because ADH is produced in the hypothalamus, and adequate amounts can be released even if damage occurs to the posterior pituitary gland. Remissions may occur for up to 2 weeks, followed by a recurrence.[2]

Polyuria (urine output greater than 200 ml/hr) and continuously dilute urine (specific gravity of 1.000 to 1.005) are signs of diabetes insipidus. Intake and output measurements every 4 to 8 hours, specific gravity checks, daily weights, and assessment for complaints of thirst help identify the presence of diabetes insipidus. If a deficit in ADH does occur, treatment depends on the severity. Mild deficits may be treated by increasing intake of oral fluids sufficiently to satisfy thirst. In patients with severe ADH deficits or in those unable to tolerate oral fluids, vasopressin is administered. In the immediate postoperative period, aqueous vasopressin, given subcutaneously or intramuscularly, is the drug of choice if replacement therapy is necessary. Parenteral use of desmopressin is also reported as effective. Vasopressin is usually administered intranasally in the form of desmopressin acetate, a synthetic analog of the human hormone.

Although rare after adenectomy, ACTH deficiency resulting in glucocorticoid deficiency is a potential problem. ACTH deficiency can result in severe fluid volume deficit.

After a hypophysectomy, cortisol replacement is necessary to maintain life. Intravenous administration of a cortisol drug is started preoperatively. All patients should be monitored for potential glucocorticoid deficiency and early signs and symptoms of adrenal insufficiency. Monitoring should include assessment of the adequacy of ADH, as well as vital signs every 4 hours and observation of energy level, alertness, patient's stated feelings of well-being, and appetite. If abnormalities in these data are found, serum sodium, potassium, and glucose levels may be obtained. Increased urine output, hypotension while lying down, or orthostatic hypotension, persistent nausea, vomiting, fatigue and tiredness, hyponatremia, hyperkalemia, hypoglycemia, and acidosis indicate inadequate ACTH and glucocorticoid secretion. Hydrocortisone (Cortef) or other high-potency corticoids and fluid replacement are provided. If the deficit in ACTH is permanent, the patient will have to be treated as discussed later in this chapter for persons with chronic adrenal insufficiency.

### Promoting Gas Exchange

1. Monitor gas exchange status every 4 hours, including arterial blood gas (ABG) values (if needed), pulse oximetry, vital signs, mentation, and skin color. Signs of decreased gas exchange should be reported.
2. Place the patient in a semi-Fowler's position (or as ordered) to facilitate adequate ventilation. Turn patient every 2 hours.
3. Administer oxygen therapy as ordered.
4. Teach deep breathing, sighing, and mouth breathing and how to avoid coughing.
5. Initiate activities within limits of dyspnea and ABG values, increasing gradually as tolerated.

Because of the caution against coughing and the nasal packing necessitating mouth breathing, patients are at some risk for ineffective gas exchange. Patients should be instructed about mouth breathing and deep breathing exercises before surgery, have an opportunity for practice and a return demonstration, and then be monitored for compliance with deep breathing exercises at least every 2 hours for the first 1 to 3 postoperative days. Assessment of vital signs and breath sounds every 4 to 8 hours helps identify any impairment of air exchange. Maintenance of adequate fluid intake helps prevent drying of mucous secretions and the formation of mucous plugs.

### Preventing Infection

1. Use proper hand-washing technique before and after contact with the patient.
2. Assess for signs of infection every shift, including elevated temperature, rhinorrhea, nuchal rigidity, and persistent headache.
3. Assess for halo ring on each change of nasal sling dressing; send drainage to laboratory for glucose analysis if halo ring is present.
4. Provide frequent, gentle mouth rinsing with prescribed mouthwash or normal saline; use mouth care sponges for cleansing teeth. Avoid brushing teeth.
5. Teach patient the importance and methods of mouth care.

With transsphenoidal adenectomy, the sella turcica is entered from below through the sphenoid sinus, and the tumor is removed. An external incision is made between the upper gum and lip, and an internal incision is made through the sella turcica and dura. Preventing infection and maintaining the integrity of these incisions are nursing priorities. Oral incisional care consists of rinsing the mouth with saline or mouthwash and cleansing the teeth with a Toothette or cotton swab. Brushing the teeth and the use of dental floss is forbidden until the suture line heals.

Clear-liquids are given as soon as the patient is alert and no longer nauseated from the anesthetic. The diet is advanced as tolerated. Foods that could irritate the mucous membranes and disrupt the suture line must be avoided because of the mouth incision.

Increased ICP can disrupt the incision in the sella turcica and dura. After the tumor is resected, the sella turcica is packed with muscle or fat from the abdomen or thigh. (NOTE: It is important that the patient be prepared for this additional incision.) The floor of the sella turcica is reconstructed with bone or cartilage. This patching, although strong, can be disrupted by increased ICP, which causes pressure on the incisional site. Activities such as bending over, straining, coughing, sneezing, and blowing the nose are forbidden. The head of the patient's bed should be elevated at least 30° when the patient is reclining. In most cases, these interventions will prevent disruption of the patch and incision.

CSF leakage will occur if the patching and incision in the sella turcica are disrupted. The nurse monitors for signs and symptoms of such leakage. After surgery the patient's nose is packed for 24 to 48 hours, and a gauze sling is worn under the nose to absorb drainage. A CSF leak may be identified by:

1. Complaints of postnasal drip, even with the packing in place
2. Increased swallowing (observation or patient's report)
3. Appearance of a *halo ring* on the gauze sling (CSF is clear, and when mixed with serous fluid on gauze, will form a halo surrounding the serous drainage.)

Nasal drainage can be differentiated from CSF based on glucose content. Although the nurse can assess the glucose content of nasal drainage with Tes-Tape or a dipstick for glucose, fluid should be sent to a laboratory for confirmation. If a CSF leakage occurs or is suspected, bedrest with the patient's head elevated is reinstituted and maintained until the leakage is ruled out or stops. Occasionally, patients will have to return to surgery for repair of the leakage site in the sella turcica.

If a documented CSF leak occurs, the patient is at high risk for infection, including meningitis. Besides restricting the patient's activities to prevent or control a CSF leak, the nurse should monitor the patient for signs of an infection. Monitoring includes temperature checks at least every 4 hours and evaluation for presence of nuchal rigidity (see Chapter 52). Antibiotics should be administered as prescribed.

### Facilitating Learning (Perioperative Period)

The first objective of patient education is similar to that for any patient during the perioperative period (see Chapter 18). The second objective of perioperative education is to prepare the patient for discharge, to resume self-care, and to assume responsibility for follow-up care. The patient should know when to return to see the physician (usually within 1 to 2 weeks), again in 1 month, and then every 6 to 12 months. At the first follow-up visit the patient's hormonal status and general recovery from surgery are assessed. At the other visits, recurrence of the tumor and any newly developing hormonal deficits are assessed.

The third objective of patient education is to prepare the patient to manage any hormonal deficiencies that have occurred. If ADH or ACTH and glucocorticoid deficiency occurred postoperatively, diagnostic tests are done before the patient leaves the hospital to identify whether the deficiencies are permanent. If they are permanent, the patient needs the same education required by any patient with diabetes insipidus or adrenocortical insufficiency (see discussions later in this chapter).

If a deficiency of ACTH and glucocorticoid occurs, secretion of other hormones, such as TSH or gonadotropins, from the anterior pituitary gland may also be deficient. The adequacy of anterior pituitary secretion of these hormones is assessed before discharge and at the return visits. Diagnostic tests to evaluate hormonal status are performed 4 to 6 weeks postoperatively if no hormonal deficiencies develop.

The final objective of patient education is to reinforce care needs for irreversible changes in body appearance, joint and back pain, and visual problems. Information shared may include ways to minimize body changes with makeup and clothes, frequent showers to help control increased sweating and oily skin, pain management techniques (see Chapter 12), modification of activities to decrease stress and strain on the joints and back (see Chapter 61), and referral to the Society for the Visually Impaired.

### Promoting Comfort (Postoperative Period)

Incisional discomfort and headache may occur postoperatively and are treated with nonnarcotic analgesics or codeine. Persistent headaches may indicate meningitis and should be reported to the physician immediately. A firm mattress, ROM exercises, back massage, frequent ambulation, and heat may be used to help decrease back and joint discomfort in persons with GH-secreting tumors. Early ambulation helps to prevent deterioration in mobility and joint movement. Postoperatively the patient's vision should be monitored for changes. Rearranging the room so that necessary articles are placed in line with intact vision may be necessary (see Chapter 56). Although visual complications after transsphenoidal resection are rare, the visual pathway can be damaged during surgery or as a result of hemorrhage.

#### *Patient/family education*

Patients with pituitary hypersecretion may exhibit high anxiety levels in response to the body changes induced by neurological or endocrine alterations and uncertainty about diagnosis, treatment method, and effects of treatment. Particular stressors may include visual loss, infertility, sexual dysfunction, or immobility. Although some patients in whom neurological symptoms are diagnosed require immediate surgical treatment, most patients have a diagnostic workup in the outpatient setting and time to learn about their illness and its implications. The nurse can help the patient reduce stress by attending to the emotional impact of the illness. The major need of the patient at this stage of the illness is education. The patient and significant others need to know the following:

1. How the patient's symptoms relate to a pituitary tumor and hormone excess.
2. What is meant by the term *tumor;* some people automatically assume that tumor means cancer. These tumors are usually not malignant.
3. What diagnostic tests are planned, including blood tests; skull roentgenogram, computed tomography (CT) scan, or magnetic resonance imaging (MRI); and visual assessment.
4. What treatment is available for the tumor. Based on the signs and symptoms, the physician has a high index of suspicion for the type of tumor and potential treatment. This is the information that the physician shares at this time and the nurse reinforces.
5. Dietary instruction about prescribed changes as needed, and ways of meeting dietary requirements.
6. Medication therapy: hormonal agents used as *replacement therapy* (in diabetes insipidus, hypopituitarism, or insufficiency of cortisol, thyroxine [$T_4$], and/or sex hormones) and *hormonal suppressant drugs* (bromocriptine and octreotide).
7. How to perform subcutaneous injection if prescribed; the nurse should provide teaching and multiple opportunities for practice and return demonstration.
8. What outcomes are expected from the treatment, including reversibility or irreversibility of signs and symptoms.
9. Why follow-up care is important. The nurse should clarify the plans for follow-up care.

This knowledge assists the patient in dealing with physiological changes and should help relieve uncertainty and decrease anxiety. Usually teaching is done in an outpatient setting. The nurse can have a model of a brain available, which may help the patient better understand the pathology and treatment of his or her illness. Written material should be provided to reinforce the teaching. The nurse should also provide the name and telephone number of someone (nurse or physician) who can be contacted if the patient thinks of more questions.

## EVALUATION

To evaluate the effectiveness of nursing interventions, compare patient behaviors with those stated in the expected patient outcomes. Successful achievement of patient outcomes for the person with hypersecretion of the anterior pituitary gland associated with pituitary tumor is indicated by:

1. Reports that anxiety is at a tolerable level, uses anxiety-reducing strategies, and perceives ability to manage stressors.
2. Explains diagnostic and treatment effects and implications for self-management.
3. Reports that comfort is at an acceptable level.
4. Comments positively about self-attributes, abilities, and participation in activities to regain optimal functioning.

The patient and significant others need to know that changes in body characteristics and vision are not always reversible, but that progressive changes will be stopped. The nurse can assist the patient and family to cope with irreversible changes. Sexual dysfunction associated with prolactin excess is usually reversible. The patient must be assessed for the ability to maintain a safe environment if visual disturbances are present. Although severe visual disturbances rarely occur, interventions such as those discussed in Chapter 56 for the person with blindness may be necessary.

## SPECIAL ENVIRONMENTS FOR CARE

### Critical Care Management

The patient with a acromegaly or hypersecretory state of the pituitary gland would need critical care nursing only in the case of complications. If transsphenoidal resection of the tumor resulted in the development of meningitis or increased intracranial pressure, monitoring of the patient's intracranial pressure and overall status in an intensive care unit would be necessary. If the tumor required resection by craniotomy, the patient would be routinely admitted to an intensive care unit after surgery and then transferred to a regular nursing floor when the patient's condition stablilizes (see Chapter 52).

### Home Care Management

If significant neurological deficits develop as a result of tumor growth or surgical intervention, the patient may be transferred to a subacute unit for rehabilitation after discharge. Arthritic changes occur in the patient with long-standing acromegaly, and adaptations may need to be made to the home environment (see Chapter 61). A home health aid may be necessary for assistance with ADL. Assistance may be needed in administration of medications, particularly if the patient has any visual deficits. Ensuring safety is a priority, especially if the patient has limitations in musculoskeletal functioning or neurological deficits. The home environment should be assessed for potential safety hazards. In addition, the patient must have access to the physician or other health care provider for routing monitoring of hormonal levels.

## COMPLICATIONS

Common complications of pituitary tumors and their management have been discussed previously and are summarized in Box 34-3. In addition, *pituitary apoplexy* can occur. This syndrome is the result of a sudden enlargement of the tumor by hemorrhagic necrosis occurring from damage to the tumor's fragile vascular supply. Other causes of pituitary hemorrhage include head injury, pregnancy and delivery, long-term ventilatory support, meningoencephalitis, estrogen drug therapy, anticoagulation, and radiation therapy.

There is sudden onset of severe headache, vomiting, visual impairment, and altered mental and autonomic functioning

**box 34-3** *Complications of Pituitary Tumors*

**NEUROLOGICAL**

Compression of optic chiasm and/or other brain tissue; visual loss

After surgery: CSF leak, meningitis, increased ICP, neurological deficit, visual impairment

Pituitary apoplexy

Increased ICP

**ENDOCRINE**

Syndromes of excess hormone: acromegaly, Cushing's syndrome; suppression of gonadotropic hormones; infertility and/or sexual dysfunction

Iatrogenic syndromes of hormonal deficit: diabetes insipidus, adrenal insufficiency, hypopituitarism (deficit in one or more anterior pituitary hormones: ACTH, TSH, GH, or gonadotropin)

Recurrence of pituitary tumor

(hypotension or hyperthermia). Laboratory abnormalities include leukocytosis, xanthochromic or bloody CSF, and increased CSF pressure. Radiographic examination may show an enlarged sella turcica.

The treatment of these patients is still controversial. Most authorities agree that corticosteroids should be given to correct any adrenal insufficiency and decrease cerebral edema.[2,11,19] Most patients with visual or mental changes are treated with decompression surgery using a transsphenoidal approach. Many patients recover with normal endocrine function, but if deficiencies occur later, care is similar to that described for hypofunctioning states.

# ANTERIOR PITUITARY GLAND

## HYPOPITUITARISM

### Etiology

Several disorders can interfere with the function of the anterior pituitary gland and cause hyposecretion of one or more hormones or *hypopituitarism* (Box 34-4).

Hypopituitarism may be classified in a number of ways: isolated, partial, or panhypopituitary; transient or permanent; idiopathic or organic; and primary (pituitary) or secondary (affecting hypothalamic releasing factors).

Any combination of deficits of the six major hormones may occur. The aim of therapy is to restore normal function and may be accomplished in two ways: (1) administration of the target gland hormone, or (2) administration of the releasing factor of the absent or deficient pituitary hormone.

### Epidemiology

The incidence of hypopituitarism is unknown; more is known about the incidence of specific disease states, and these are discussed under the appropriate sections. Because prolactinomas are the most common pituitary tumors, one can assume that related gonadotropic insufficiency is the most common pituitary deficiency in adults.

**box 34-4** *Causes of Hypopituitarism*

Tumors: craniopharyngioma, primary central nervous system tumors, nonsecreting pituitary tumors

Ischemic changes: Sheehan's syndrome (ischemic changes following postpartum hemorrhage or infection resulting in shock)

Developmental abnormalities

Infections: viral encephalitis, bacteremia, tuberculosis

Autoimmune disorders

Radiation damage, particularly after treatment of secreting adenomas of pituitary gland

Trauma, including surgery

### Pathophysiology

In hypopituitarism the symptoms vary widely depending on the cause and the endocrine dysfunction present. If a tumor is the cause, the patient may have some of the symptoms previously described for secreting pituitary tumors. These include symptoms resulting from growth of a space-occupying lesion in the cranium, effects resulting from pressure on the optic chiasm, and potential disturbances of cranial nerves III, IV, and VI. If the tumor arises from regions surrounding the pituitary, such as Rathke's pouch (craniopharyngiomas), the hypothalamus, or the third ventricle, the neurological signs and symptoms will be more severe and include manifestations of increased ICP.

The endocrine dysfunction may be the result of hypothalamic damage or primary pituitary disease. The most frequent pathophysiological alteration results from lack of synthesis and secretion of gonadotropins. The symptoms associated with deficiency of individual anterior pituitary hormones are summarized in Figure 34-3. The patient with hypopituitarism exhibits all or only selected aspects of these deficiencies. Usually the pathological alteration progresses slowly.

The exact manifestations vary depending on the cause of the anterior pituitary problem and the type of hormonal deficiency. The major manifestations are listed in Box 34-5.

#### *Growth hormone (GH) deficiency*

While primarily a disease of children (covered in pediatric textbooks), a distinctive GH deficiency syndrome occurs in adults, characterized by abnormal body composition, impaired physical performance, and decreased quality of life. Early data indicate that treatment with relatively low doses of GH leads to increased lean body mass and decreased fat mass and an alteration in the circulating lipids. Edema has been shown to be a major side effect in the administration of GH to adults. Further studies are needed to better define this syndrome and to determine the optimal treatment for adults.

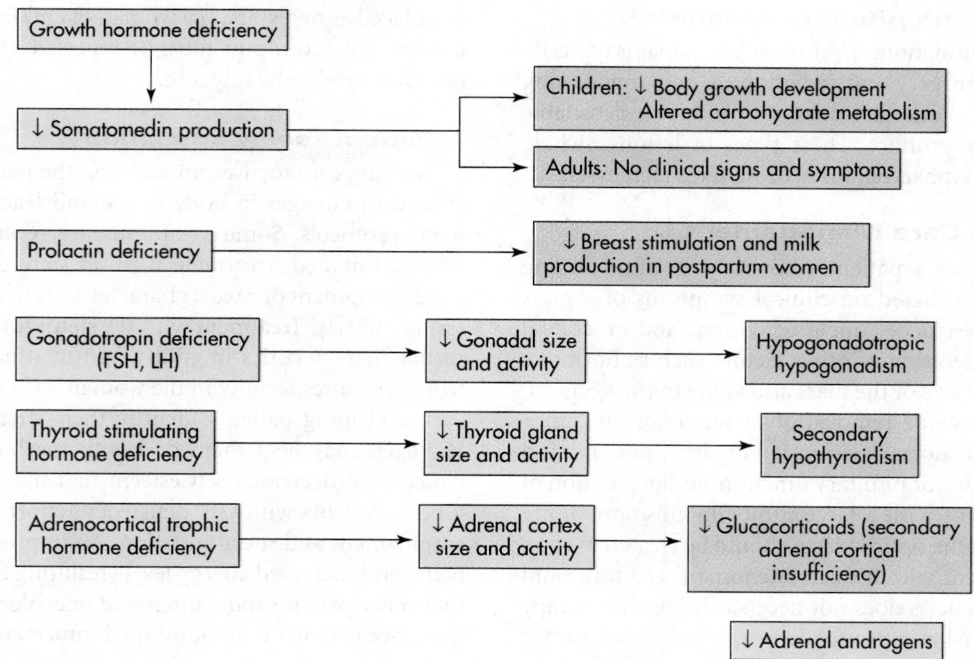


**fig. 34-3** Pathophysiological findings associated with individual anterior pituitary hormone deficiency.

### Thyroid-stimulating hormone deficiency

Thyroid stimulating hormone itself is not available for replacement therapy; therefore, a thyroid hormone preparation is used. L-Thyroxine is sufficient for replacement in most adults. Adults will generally require between 1.5 and 3.0 μg/kg/day. Monitoring of thyroxine levels, generally with the free $T_4$ blood test, is done on a regular basis as an evaluation of therapy. Because thyroxine is converted to triiodothyronine ($T_3$) in the periphery, circulating $T_3$ levels may also be monitored. It is important to evaluate the symptoms of hyperthyroidism, especially in elderly patients with cardiac disease. Side effects may include tachycardia, heat intolerance, weight loss, and a slow loss of calcium from bone that may cause significant and symptomatic osteoporosis in time. Because thyroid hormone replacement accelerates the metabolism of glucocorticoids, it is imperative that the status of the adrenal axis be determined before L-thyroxine therapy is begun. Replacement therapy may unmask an underlying cortisol deficiency and precipitate an adrenal crisis.

### Adrenocorticotropic hormone deficiency

Glucocorticoid deficiency is replaced with hydrocortisone or one of the more potent synthetic analogs. The replacement dosage of hydrocortisone averages 25 mg/day in divided doses, but varies considerably in individuals. Because the normal diurnal secretion of cortisol peaks in the early morning, two thirds of the dose is generally given in the morning and one third at night. Also, since cortisol is a primary stress hormone, it is imperative to augment these physiological doses when a patient is ill, injured, or undergoing anesthesia. For mild stress, such as a viral illness, the dose should be doubled or tripled. With more severe stress such as surgery, three- to fivefold increments should be administered. Patients with hypopituitarism should wear a Medic-Alert bracelet that states a need for hydrocortisone for emergency use (50 or 100 mg of hydrocortisone intramuscularly or intravenously). Intravenous hydrocortisone infusion should be continued at doses of 50 to 100 mg every 6 hours until resolution of the acute condition occurs. Cortisone, prednisone, and prednisolone are also used for replacement therapy. Side effects include those of mild Cushing's syndrome.

### Gonadotropin deficiency

The majority of patients with gonadotropin deficiency have a hypothalamic GnRH deficiency. For men, appropriate therapy is treatment with testosterone cypionate or testosterone enanthate (longer acting). Replacement therapy in adults should average 100 mg/week, generally given as 200 mg every 2 weeks or 300 mg every 3 weeks. Testosterone is given by deep intramuscular injection in the gluteus because of the viscosity of the solution. The deltoid is not an appropriate site for testosterone injection. The vastus lateralis may be used in persons with adequate musculature. An oral preparation of testosterone is available but is not in general use because of hepatotoxicity. Scrotal patches and body patches are also available. Testosterone deficiency in men can lead to osteoporosis and therefore should be considered in elderly men even if sexual function is not a priority with the patient.

### Prolactin deficiency

The only sign or symptom associated with prolactin deficiency is failure of postpartum lactation. Human prolactin is not available for therapeutic use, nor are there therapeutic indications for its replacement.

#### Nonfunctioning pituitary adenoma

Therapy for nonfunctioning pituitary adenomas is typically a combination of surgery and radiation. A non-functioning pituitary adenoma is one that does not produce a detectable level of a secretory product. These types of lesions include meningiomas, craniopharyngiomas, or Rathke's cleft cysts.

### Collaborative Care Management

The decision to treat a patient who has a nonfunctioning pituitary adenoma is based on clinical symptoms of a mass lesion including headache, impaired vision, and/or cranial nerve palsy. Consideration of other factors such as hormone deficiencies and the size of the mass also apply to the decision. Goals of therapy include removal of or reduction in tumor mass, restoration of normal vision if impaired, preservation of anterior and posterior pituitary function, and prevention of recurrence. A patient with a large tumor in close proximity to or impinging on the optic chiasm should be treated as soon as possible. A patient with a microadenoma (<10 mm) and no hormone deficiencies does not necessarily require therapy and may be followed as an outpatient to monitor the tumor for changes. Microadenomas are often discovered incidentally in patients undergoing a CT scan or MRI of the head for an unrelated reason. Options for treatment of symptomatic patients include surgical resection of the tumor (preferably via the transsphenoidal route) pituitary radiation, and in some circumstances, medical therapy with a dopamine agonist.

Medical management is focused on identifying patients with deficiency syndromes, treating the underlying problem, and supplying the appropriate hormonal replacement. The target gland hormone (thyroid, cortisol, or gonadal steroids) is replaced as necessary. If a woman of childbearing age desires fertility, gonadotropins must be replaced. However, prolactin does not need to be replaced.

#### Patient/family education

Nursing care focuses on assisting the patient to effectively cope with changes in body image and teaching about treatment protocols. Some symptoms are reversible once treatment is initiated. Treatment with sex steroids helps to initiate the development of sexual characteristics in the adolescent entering puberty. Treatment with sex steroids restores secondary sexual characteristics in adults, and treatment with gonadotropins restores fertility in the woman with normal menstrual cycles. Helping patients identify their strengths and coping strategies may help them deal with the body image disturbances and decreased self esteem that may result from their illness. Patients with GH deficiency report high rates of unemployment and social isolation. An improved sense of well-being and increased energy level (resulting from GH therapy) may make patients more interested in exploring coping strategies. (See Chapter 6 for additional information on coping.)

Patient education is another focus of care. The patient must be prepared for various diagnostic tests, including blood tests and roentgenograms, CT scans, or MRI of the head. If a tumor is the cause of the deficiency, the tumor is removed. Hormonal replacement and therapy with gonadal steroids and gonadotropins in adolescents and adults are individualized. The patient needs to be taught about prescribed medications. GHs are given subcutaneously. Gonadal steroids are given orally to restore sexual characteristics, and gonadotropin or clomiphene citrate is used in women to induce ovulation if

**box 34-5** *clinical manifestations*

#### Hypopituitarism

1. Manifestations based on cause, such as bacteremia, viral hepatitis, autoimmune disorders, and trauma
2. Manifestations such as vision changes, papilledema, or hydrocephalus if cause is tumor
3. Manifestations of gonadotropin deficiency
   a. Decreased serum levels of FSH, LH, and gonadal steroids
   b. Children—delayed puberty
   c. Adults
      (1) Women—oligomenorrhea or amenorrhea, uterine and vaginal atrophy, potential atrophy of breast tissue, loss of libido, decrease in body hair
      (2) Men—loss of libido, decreased sperm count, possible erectile dysfunction, decreased testicular size, decreased total body hair
4. Manifestations of GH deficiency
   a. Children
      (1) Stunted growth (below third percentile) with normal body proportions, excessive subcutaneous fat, poor muscle development
      (2) Immature facial features, immature voice
      (3) Slow growth of nails and thin hair
      (4) Delayed puberty but eventual normal sexual development
      (5) Decreased levels of GH
   b. Adults
      (1) Severe, short stature
      (2) Immature facies
      (3) Moderate obesity
      (4) Decreased muscle mass and weakness
      (5) Lassitude
      (6) Emotional lability
      (7) Decreased basal levels of GH or decreased response to provocative testing
      (8) Some persons may have normal GH levels with low level of somatomedins (IGF-I)
5. Manifestations of prolactin deficiency
   a. Failure to lactate in the postpartum woman
   b. Decreased serum levels of prolactin
6. Manifestations of TSH deficiency
   a. Signs and symptoms of secondary hypothyroidism
   b. Decreased serum level of TSH and thyroid hormone
7. Manifestations of ACTH deficiency
   a. Signs and symptoms of secondary ACTH insufficiency; *no hyperpigmentation*
   b. Decreased serum levels of ACTH, glucocorticoids, and adrenal androgens (aldosterone levels may be normal)

pregnancy is desired. Patients should be taught that steroids are effective in preventing premature bone demineralization. Patients who decline hormone therapy, particularly women, need to be monitored periodically for accelerated bone loss and must take adequate calcium.

If visual changes are present, care as described in Chapter 56 is necessary. In relation to sexual dysfunction, patient education about the cause of the problem and the replacement therapy described previously are the major interventions.

## POSTERIOR PITUITARY GLAND: HYPERFUNCTION

### SYNDROME OF INAPPROPRIATE ANTIDIURETIC HORMONE SECRETION

#### Etiology/Epidemiology

The syndrome of inappropriate antidiuretic hormone secretion (SIADH) occurs as a result of the excessive release of ADH (vasopressin), resulting in fluid and electrolyte imbalances. Many factors cause SIADH, which is also known as Schwartz-Bartter syndrome (Box 34-6). Approximately 80% of cases are associated with oat cell carcinoma of the lung.

#### Pathophysiology

In patients with SIADH, total body water increases because of water retention, and a hypoosmolar state results from hyponatremia. ADH release follows one of four patterns:

1. ADH release is erratic and unrelated to plasma osmolality.
2. ADH release varies with the plasma osmolality, but the osmostat has been reset, and ADH release occurs at a lower plasma osmolality.
3. ADH release is normal in response to a normal or elevated plasma osmolality, but ADH is not reduced as the plasma osmolality is lowered.
4. ADH release is normal, but the patient is more sensitive to the released ADH, or some "unmeasured factor" that increases water retention is released.

The abnormally released ADH or the increased sensitivity of cells to ADH increases the permeability of the distal renal tubules and collecting ducts to water, and water resorption by the kidney increases. Intravascular volume increases, but edema is not present, as would be seen in congestive heart failure (see Chapter 26) or cirrhosis (see Chapter 37). Edema does not occur because the volume expansion in SIADH results in *natriuresis* (urinary sodium excretion). Natriuresis is a result of enhanced glomerular filtration and decreased proximal tubular sodium reabsorption, even with hyponatremia.

It is important to note that a reduction in plasma sodium level from 139 to 119 mEq/L within 2 hours can result in death, compared with a gradual reduction to 99 mEq/L over 2 weeks, which results only in lethargy.

The following are guidelines to correlate a patient's symptoms with serum sodium levels:

1. Serum sodium levels less than 125 mEq/L can cause nausea and malaise.
2. Serum sodium levels between 115 and 120 mEq/L cause headache and lethargy, and obtundation may appear.
3. Seizures and coma are not usually seen until the plasma sodium concentration falls below 110 to 115 mEq/L.

The hyponatremia results in hypoosmolality and creates an osmolar gradient across the blood-brain barrier and other cellular membranes. This osmolar gradient results in water movement into the brain and other cells and cellular overhydration.

Box 34-7 summarizes clinical manifestations of SIADH.

#### Collaborative Care Management

Medical management of acute SIADH focuses on treating the etiological factor (e.g., carcinoma or infection) and

**box 34-6** *Etiological Factors Associated with SIADH*

Pulmonary disorders: malignant neoplasms (e.g., oat cell adenocarcinoma of lung), tuberculosis, ventilator patients receiving positive pressure, lung abscesses
Other malignancies: duodenum, pancreas, prostate lymphoma, sarcoma, leukemia, Hodgkin's lymphoma, non-Hodgkin's lymphoma
CNS disorders: tumors, infection, trauma, cerebrovascular accident, surgery
Endocrine disorders that result in hypovolemia and impaired free water excretion, particularly if associated with fluid replacement (adrenal insufficiency, anterior pituitary insufficiency)
Drugs such as clofibrate, chlorpropamide, thiazides, vincristine, cyclophosphamide, morphine, general anesthetic agents, opioids, tricyclic antidepressants, carbamazepine
Stressors: fear, acute infections, pain, anxiety, trauma, surgery

**box 34-7** ***clinical manifestations***

*SIADH*

**EARLY SYMPTOMS**

| | |
|---|---|
| Anorexia | Mild disorientation |
| Nausea | Malaise |
| Vomiting | Hostility |
| Weight gain | Anxiety |
| Muscle weakness | Uncooperativeness |
| Irritability | |

**LATE SYMPTOMS**

| | |
|---|---|
| Lethargy | Coma |
| Headache | Seizures |
| Decreased deep tendon reflexes | |

**FLUID AND ELECTROLYTE CHANGES**

Decreased plasma sodium and plasma osmolality
Increased urinary sodium and urinary osmolality
Decreased urinary volume
Absence of edema

correcting, or at least restoring toward normal, the plasma sodium level and plasma osmolality. Water restriction is the first priority of management. Water may be restricted to as little as 500 ml/day. Oral salt intake is increased if the patient is able to take oral nutrients.

Chronic SIADH and hyponatremia are first treated with water restriction. If water restriction alone cannot prevent hypoosmolality, pharmacological treatment is added. Demeclocycline, a tetracycline derivative, blocks the action of ADH on the renal tubule and collecting duct cells and decreases urine osmolality. Lithium carbonate and phenytoin have also been used to treat SIADH.

If the patient's plasma sodium level is less than 120 mEq/L and the patient is exhibiting central nervous system (CNS) manifestations such as nausea, vomiting, lethargy, and headaches, more rapid correction of the low plasma sodium level is necessary. This *severe hyponatremia* is treated with hypertonic saline (3% sodium chloride) and a loop diuretic such as furosemide (Lasix) or ethacrynic acid.[15,19] The goal of this therapy is not to return the plasma sodium level to normal but to increase it to 125 to 130 mEq/L or to administer enough sodium chloride to relieve symptoms or increase the plasma sodium by 25 mEq/L. This correction needs to be done cautiously because of potential complications from either too rapid or too slow correction.

Too rapid an increase in the plasma sodium level can produce a hypertonic plasma solution and a fluid shift from the intracellular to the extracellular compartment. A rapid fluid shift can result in central pontine myelinolysis, which is demyelination of the pons. This demyelination results in dysfunction of the nerve tracts that travel through or originate in the pons, causing bulbar palsies, quadriplegia, coma, and death. During treatment with hypertonic saline or loop diuretics, plasma osmolality and serum sodium are monitored every 2 to 4 hours. Note that 3% sodium chloride is used for sodium replacement, not for volume replacement.

Nursing care of the person with SIADH includes the following:

1. Perform assessment.
   a. Identify patients at high risk.
   b. For high-risk patients, monitor daily weights, daily intake and output, daily serum and urinary sodium levels and osmolality, vital signs, and neurological status every 4 hours. Report any decrease below normal in serum sodium (if the level is below 125 mEq/L, report laboratory results immediately), any signs of fluid retention (increased weight or decreased output), and any neurological changes (complaints of headaches or nausea or decreased responsiveness).
   c. For patients with diagnosed SIADH being treated aggressively with hypertonic sodium or loop diuretics, the frequency of monitoring is increased to every 1 to 2 hours. Any deterioration in neurological status is reported immediately.
   d. For patients with chronic SIADH, monitor weights daily to weekly and report any increases not attributed to dietary changes or any complaints of nausea, headache, or lethargy. Monitoring by the nurse in the outpatient department is the same as that described for high-risk patients.
2. Provide supportive care.
   a. Restrict fluids as prescribed.
   b. Control discomfort from thirst.
      (1) Space fluid intake throughout the 24-hour period.
      (2) Use ice chips, which allow more frequent relief of thirst with less fluid intake.
      (3) Provide frequent mouth care.
   c. Administer drugs or fluids as ordered.

#### Patient/family education

Patient and family teaching should include information about the following:

1. Review the purpose and management of fluid restriction.
2. Review self-monitoring required on a long-term basis (intake and output measurement, weight change).
3. Discuss drug therapy as appropriate.

Diuretics may be used long-term, and a high-sodium diet may be continued. In some patients, salt tablets are used with diuretics to replace urinary sodium losses and prevent volume depletion.

## DIABETES INSIPIDUS

### Etiology/Epidemiology

Pituitary diabetes insipidus (DI) results from lack of sufficient ADH either from inadequate levels of circulating ADH, insufficient pituitary release of ADH, or accelerated degradation of circulating ADH. The cause may be a central brain or pituitary tumor, head trauma, encephalitis, meningitis, hypophysectomy, or cranial surgery. The cause is often idiopathic. Nephrogenic DI is a second form of the disorder and results from failure of the renal tubules to respond to ADH. Chronic renal failure, sickle cell anemia, and Sjögren's syndrome are causes of nephrogenic DI. A rare hereditary form of nephrogenic DI can also occur. Diabetes insipidus may be transient or permanent. Postsurgical DI is discussed earlier in this chapter. Transient DI associated with pregnancy is caused by an excessive amount of placental secreted vasopressinase that neutralizes ADH activity.

### Pathophysiology

The lack of adequate ADH or an ineffective kidney response to ADH results in insufficient water reabsorption by the kidney. The loss of excessive water from the body (polyuria) stimulates the perception of thirst (polydipsia). If the problem is long-standing, diabetes insipidus can result in an increased bladder capacity and hydronephrosis. When inadequate water replacement occurs, CNS and vascular changes from hyperosmolality and volume depletion can occur. Box 34-8 lists clinical manifestations of DI.

### Collaborative Care Management

The person with pituitary DI is treated with vasopressin replacement; four preparations of ADH are available (Table 34-3). Vasopressin or its synthetic analogs bind with $V_2$ receptors in the renal tubule; vasopressin also binds with $V_1$ receptors found in smooth muscle of arterioles and other tissues. The action of ADH on $V_1$ receptors is responsible for pressor side effects of exogenous ADH (abdominal cramping, hypertension, and angina). These pressor effects occur because of vasoconstriction and are seen in all preparations except desmopressin (DDAVP), which acts only on $V_2$ receptors.[2] DDAVP is also much more potent in its antidiuretic effect and has a longer duration of action; thus, it is the drug of choice for chronic DI. For persons who have some residual pituitary function, chlorpropamide and clofibrate, which stimulate release of endogenous ADH, may be prescribed.

Temporary DI associated with head trauma or surgery is treated with aqueous vasopressin, 5 to 10 IU subcutaneously, until nasal administration of lysine or DDVP becomes appropriate. After transsphenoidal surgery, nasal packing and edematous nasal mucosa preclude using the nasal route for medications. In addition, the physician may choose the shorter-acting aqueous vasopressin until the hormonal status stabilizes. Administration of DDAVP by IM injection in the immediate postoperative period has been reported to be an alternative.[2]

The most common treatment for persons with nephrogenic DI is a low-sodium, low-protein diet and thiazide diuretics. The low-sodium diet and thiazide diuretics induce a mild volume depletion. This volume depletion enhances sodium chloride and water reabsorption in the proximal part of the kidney tubule, resulting in less water being delivered to the collecting tubules where ADH should be; therefore, less water is excreted. The diuretic also increases the osmolality of the medullary interstitial space and thus promotes more water resorption in collecting tubules that are less permeable because of inadequate ADH. The protein restriction helps control water loss by decreasing solute excretion. Nephrogenic DI can also be treated by administration of nonsteroidal antiinflammatory agents, which impair prostaglandin production in the kidney and increase urinary concentrating ability.

For patients with clinical evidence of hypernatremia, such as mental status changes and hyperthermia, replacement of water must be instituted. Fluid replacement is calculated by estimating the patient's water deficit and adding the insensible water loss and urinary loss. Fluid replacement must be done carefully over 48 hours to avoid cerebral edema, seizures, or even death. Too rapid correction of hypernatremia by fluid administration may result in the establishment of an osmotic gradient, with plasma osmolality being less than intracellular osmolality and the entry of water into the brain. The exact fluid administered will vary depending on the patient's needs. If pure water loss is present, free water is given orally or in the form of dextrose in water. If the patient is hypotensive as well as hypernatremic, isotonic saline is given until vascular volume is adequate, and then free water is given. If the patient has a slight sodium deficit together with a free water deficit, one-quarter strength sodium chloride is used. During fluid replacement, serial measurement of plasma sodium level and assessment of mental and circulatory status are required every 1 to 2 hours.

Nursing interventions for the person with DI focus on the following:

1. Maintain fluid and electrolyte balance.
   a. Monitor intake and output, daily weights, urine specific gravity, vital signs (orthostatic), skin turgor, and neurological status every 1 to 2 hours during the acute phase, then every 4 to 8 hours until discharge, and again on return to physician or outpatient clinic.
   b. Provide fluids; be sure patient can reach them.
2. Provide daily rest periods during the time when nocturia interferes with sleep.

**box 34-8** *clinical manifestations*

### *Diabetes Insipidus*

1. Polyuria: as much as 20 L of urine/day may be excreted; urine is dilute, with a specific gravity of 1.005 or less or an osmolality of 200 or less
2. Polydipsia secondary to increased thirst
3. Only slightly elevated serum osmolality because water intake is usually maintained
4. Abnormal results of tests for urine concentration
   a. Water deprivation test (see Chapter 33): no increase in urine concentration with either pituitary or nephrogenic DI
   b. ADH replacement: increase in urine osmolality with pituitary DI but no response with nephrogenic DI
5. Sleep disturbance from polyuria
6. Inadequate water replacement results in:
   a. Hyperosmolality: irritability, mental dullness, coma, hyperthermia
   b. Hypovolemia: hypotension, tachycardia, dry mucous membranes, poor skin turgor

**table 34-3** *Common Medications Used for Treatment of* ***Diabetes Insipidus***

| Drug | Action | Nursing Intervention |
|---|---|---|
| Arginine vasopressin* (vasopressins for injection), aqueous solution | 0.25-0.5 mg | SC, IM |
| Lysine vasopressin* (Lypressin, Diapid), aqueous solution | 3-8 doses/24 hr | Nasal spray |
| Pitressin tannate in oil* | 10-40 ng<br>1-3 doses/wk | IM |
| Desmopressin (DDAVP)†, parenteral solution | 5-10 ng dose; 1 or 2 doses/24 hr<br>1-2 ng dose; 1 or 2 doses/24 hr | Nasal instillation<br>IM |

*These preparations interact with $V_1$ and $V_2$ receptors; thus, pressor side effects can occur (abdominal cramping, hypertension, and angina).
†DDAVP interacts with $V_2$ receptors only; thus, pressor side effects do not occur.

***Patient/family education***

Patient and family teaching should include information about the following:

1. Diagnostic tests: purposes, procedures, and required monitoring (see Chapter 34)
2. Drug therapy
   a. Administration: dosage, route, and frequency
   b. Effectiveness: if nasal congestion occurs, drug effectiveness may decrease, and polyuria and thirst will occur
   c. Side effects: particularly signs of volume excess (weight gain, edema)

## THYROID GLAND

Disorders of the thyroid gland are relatively common endocrine problems second only to diabetes mellitus. Alterations in the thyroid gland may be associated with hypersecretion, hyposecretion, or normal secretion of thyroid hormone.

Hypertrophy of the thyroid gland *(goiter)* is associated with hyperthyroidism, hypothyroidism, or euthyroidism. A goiter causes a pronounced protuberance in the neck and occurs as a result of increased amounts of TSH or any substances that act as TSH (Figure 34-4).

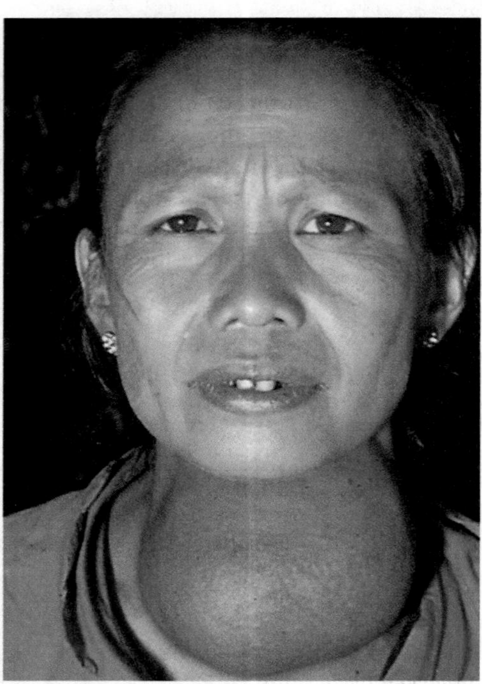

**fig. 34-4** Simple goiter.

## HYPERSECRETION OF THYROID HORMONE: HYPERTHYROIDISM

### Etiology

*Hyperthyroidism* is an increased production and secretion of thyroid hormone from the thyroid gland. *Thyrotoxicosis* is the clinical syndrome resulting from increased levels of thyroxine ($T_4$) or triiodothyronine ($T_3$). The numerous causes of hyperthyroidism are summarized in Table 34-4. Certain medications have been associated with hyperthyroidism (Research Box).

The most common cause of hyperthyroidism is Grave's disease, accounting for 60% to 90% of the incidence of hyperthyroidism.[17] *Graves' disease* is an autoimmune disorder characterized by one or more of the following: diffuse goiter, hyperthyroidism, infiltrative ophthalmopathy, and infiltrative dermopathy. Ophthalmopathy or dermopathy may occur without hyperthyroidism. There is a genetic component of Grave's disease, and it is associated with other autoimmune disorders including rheumatoid arthritis, pernicious anemia, and systemic lupus erythematosus.

Another common cause of hyperthyroidism is toxic multinodular goiter. *Toxic multinodular goiter* or Plummer's disease is a disorder characterized by the presence of many thyroid nodules and a milder form of hyperthyroidism than is seen with Graves' disease. Toxic multinodular goiter is more common in patients older than 50 years with long-standing multinodular disease. Unlike Graves' disease, it does not have an autoimmune basis.

### Epidemiology

Incidence rates of hyperthyroidism in adults have been estimated at 0.02% to 0.06%.[7] Community screening programs have shown prevalence rates of subclinical hyperthyroidism of about 1% but have not been successful in identifying a significant number of persons with unsuspected clinical hyperthyroidism. Because subclinical disease is usually not treated, screening in the wide community is not recommended.

**research**

Reference: Mechlis S et al: Amiodarone-induced thyroid gland dysfunction, *Am J Cardiol* 59:833-835, 1997.

The purpose of this study was to determine the effects of amiodarone on the thyroid gland. Of a population of 400 patients treated with amiodarone, 97 underwent thyroid function evaluation. Of these, 20 patients proved to be thyrotoxic and 16 hypothyroid. In thyrotoxic patients, symptoms developed 2 to 36 months after they started treatment with amiodarone, the most specific laboratory finding being a high total $T_3$ level. No antithyroid treatment proved useful. Thyroid function returned to normal 3 to 7 months after they stopped amiodarone therapy. In the hypothyroid group, a high TSH level was the most specific laboratory finding. These patients were treated with substitute therapy with or without withdrawal of amiodarone. The iodine content of the thyroid gland in part of the population taking amiodarone was measured by in vivo x-ray fluorescence. Patients in whom thyrotoxicosis developed showed especially high iodine content. During treatment with amiodarone, patients must be routinely monitored by thyroid function tests to detect hyper- and hypothyroidism. Nurses should be alert for the signs and symptoms of thyroid dysfunction in patients taking amiodarone.

Graves' disease is more common in women than in men, and although it may occur at any age, usually presents in the second or third decade.[17] Approximately 15% of persons in whom Graves' disease is diagnosed have a close relative with the disease. Additionally, about one half of the relatives of persons with Graves' disease have circulating thyroid autoantibodies.[7]

## Pathophysiology

### Hypermetabolism

In hyperthyroidism from any cause, the normal regulatory control of thyroid function is lost, resulting in an increased concentration of thyroid hormone and increased peripheral manifestations of thyroid hormone excess. Thyroid hormone increases metabolic rate and calorigenesis; alters protein, fat, and carbohydrate metabolism; directly stimulates some body systems, such as bone and bone marrow; and increases sympathetic (adrenergic) activity.

The pathophysiological factors just described are related to specific clinical manifestations, as noted in Table 34-5. The underlying pathophysiology of all manifestations of hyperthyroidism is not known. However, the effects of hyperthyroidism on body systems are well known and occur in large part because of the interaction of the hypermetabolic state, increased circulation, and adrenergic stimulation.

Tachycardia is present, and more severe illness can lead to atrial fibrillation, other dysrhythmias, angina, and congestive heart failure. In addition, thyroid storm can develop; this life-threatening crisis is discussed on p. 1079.

The typical patient with hyperthyroidism from any cause is nervous and has tremors, muscle weakness, fatigue, weight loss, and intolerance to heat. The patient usually demonstrates emotional lability and may give a history of insomnia, and in females, amenorrhea.

### Ophthalmopathy

In Graves' disease, ophthalmopathy may precede, coincide with, or follow hyperthyroidism. The changes may have an infiltrative or noninfiltrative cause. Both types of ophthalmopathy may be present. In infiltrative ophthalmopathy the retrobulbar connective tissue and extraocular muscle volume are expanded. This volume expansion occurs because of fluid retention resulting from the accumulation of glycosaminoglycans. The increase in tissue mass forces the eye forward (*proptosis*) up to the limits of the restraining action of the extraocular muscles (*exophthalmos*). The pressure in the retrobulbar space increases because of an increase in retrobulbar tissue and limited forward movement, causing periorbital and lid edema and pressure on the optic nerve. The stretched enlarged extraocular muscles do not function well.

Noninfiltrative changes occur due to the thyrotoxicosis and will usually resolve when the hyperthyroidism is treated. These changes, including lid retraction and lid lag, are due to sympathetic nervous system overstimulation resulting in contraction of the eyelid levator muscle.

Glycosaminoglycans and fluid accumulation also occurin the connective tissue in other parts of the body. This

**table 34-4** *Causes and Definitions of Types of Hyperthyroidism*

| Cause | Definition |
|---|---|
| Toxic diffuse goiter (Graves' disease) | See discussion in text. |
| Toxic multinodular goiter (Plummer's disease) | See discussion in text. |
| Toxic adenoma | Single or occasionally multiple adenomas of follicular cells that secrete and function independent of TSH. |
| Thyroiditis | Increased amount of $T_4$ and $T_3$ released during acute inflammatory process; transient hyperthyroid state followed by return to euthyroid state, and eventually to hypothyroid state as gland is destroyed by the recurring inflammatory exacerbations; hyperthyroid state usually requires no treatment. |
| $T_3$ thyrotoxicosis | $T_3$ level elevated but cause unknown; $T_4$ normal or low; should be suspected in patients who have normal $T_4$ but have signs and symptoms of thyrotoxicosis. |
| Hyperthyroidism caused by metastatic thyroid cancer | Rare because thyroid cancer cells do not usually concentrate iodine efficiently; may occur with large follicular carcinomas. |
| Pituitary hyperthyroidism | Rare; pituitary adenomas may secrete excess TSH; treatment involves removal of pituitary tumor. |
| Chorionic hyperthyroidism | Chorionic gonadotropin has weak thyrotropin activity; tumors such as choriocarcinoma, embryonal cell carcinoma, and hydatidiform mole have high concentrations of chorionic gonadotropins that can stimulate $T_4$ and $T_3$ secretion; hyperthyroidism disappears with treatment of tumor. |
| Struma ovarii | Ovarian dermoid tumor made up of thyroid tissue that secretes thyroid hormone. |
| Factitious hyperthyroidism | Results from ingestion of exogenous thyroid extracts. |
| Iodine-induced hyperthyroidism (Jod-Basedow) | Overproduction of thyroid hormone resulting from administration of supplemental iodine to a person with endemic goiter. |

**table 34-5** *Thyroid Gland: Normal Function, Pathological Alterations, and Clinical Manifestations*

| Normal Function | Hyperthyroidism | Clinical Manifestations |
|---|---|---|
| Regulates metabolic rate, calorigenesis, and oxygen consumption | Increased metabolic rate, heat production, and oxygen consumption: peripheral vasodilation, increased nutrient requirements | General: increased body temperature and intolerance to heat<br>Skin: warm, moist<br>Hair: fine, friable<br>Increased appetite |
| Regulates protein, fat, and carbohydrate (CHO) metabolism | Altered CHO, protein, and fat metabolism:<br>1. Increased protein synthesis, glycogenolysis, and lipolysis | Metabolic fatigue, increased appetite, weight loss, muscle weakness |
| | 2. Increased glucose absorption and degradation of insulin | Blood glucose levels may increase in patients with diabetes mellitus |
| | 3. Decreased lipid metabolism, especially lipid degradation | Decreased serum triglycerides and cholesterol |
| | 4. Hepatic dysfunction in severe cases | Signs of hepatic dysfunction |
| | 5. Increased intestinal motility | Increased frequency of stools |
| Sensitizes cells to catecholamines | Altered cardiovascular functioning<br>Hypermetabolic and adrenergic state: increased myocardial oxygen consumption, shortened systolic time intervals, increased cardiac output | Tachycardia, palpitations, increased blood pressure, dyspnea, angina, atrial fibrillation, congestive heart failure |
| Regulates rate of cellular functions; interacts with other hormones and systems | Increased and altered CNS function | Nervousness; restlessness; decreased attention span; insomnia; emotional lability; hyperkinesis; fine, rhythmic tremors of hands, tongue, and eyelids |
| Regulates bone resorption of calcium and phosphorylation of creatine | Increased excretion of calcium and phosphorus; sometimes associated with demineralization of bones | Hypercalcemia; mild osteoporosis; fractures; muscle weakness and wasting, most prominent in proximal muscles |
| Regulates reproductive system | Altered reproductive function, altered secretion and metabolism of gonadotropins and gonadal steroids | Prepubertal: delayed sexual development<br>Postpubertal: increased libido, altered menses, decreased fertility; failure to conceive |

**box 34-9** *Ophthalmopathy in Graves' Disease*

**SIGNS**

Bright-eyed stare: results from retraction of upper eyelid
Lid lag: on downward gaze, upper lid lags behind globe movement, and sclera seen between lid and limbus
Globe lag: globe lags behind lid with upward gaze
Lid movement: jerky and spasmodic
Eyes partly open when sleeping
Periorbital edema

**SYMPTOMS**

Sense of irritation and excessive tearing
Feeling of pressure behind eyes
Complaints of blurred or double vision, easy tiring of eyes

**COMPLICATIONS**

Corneal ulceration
Optic nerve involvement (optic neuropathy)
Myopathy of extraocular muscles

accumulation is particularly seen in the pretibial area. Box 34-9 lists other signs and symptoms of ophthalmopathy, and Figure 34-5 illustrates the eyes' appearance.

Research supports the contention that Graves' disease is caused by stimulation of the thyroid by IgG immunoglobulins. It is believed that the thyroid-related immunoglobulins are a heterogenous group of antibodies directed at varying sites within the thyroid cell membrane. These immunoglobulins are called *thyroid-stimulating immunoglobulins (TSIs)*. The cause of the abnormal development of immunoglobulins is unknown. Heredity, gender, and perhaps emotions have a role.[7]

### Goiter

A goiter results from increased stimulation of the thyroid gland by TSH or TSH-like substances. Goiters are seen in toxic diffuse goiter (Graves' disease), toxic multinodular goiter, pituitary hyperthyroidism (secondary hyperthyroidism), thyroiditis, $T_3$ thyrotoxicosis, iodine deficiency, excessive dietary goitrogens (some roots, seeds, and cabbage), medications with large amounts of iodine (amiodarone) (see the Research Box on p. 1070), and iodine-induced hyperthyroidism. Chorionic

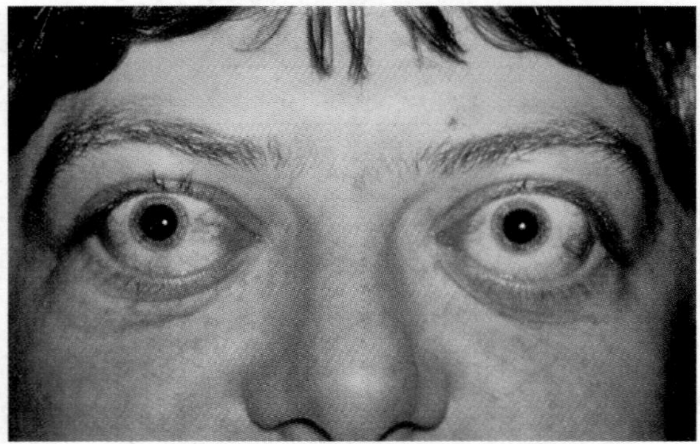

**fig. 34-5** Classic Graves' ophthalmopathy.

hyperthyroidism may or may not be associated with a goiter. In toxic adenomas, small well-defined nodules occur, whereas with cancer there are poorly defined nodules. Persons with hyperthyroidism resulting from struma ovarii and persons with factitious hyperthyroidism do not have goiters.

## Collaborative Care Management

The nurse works collaboratively with the physician to implement prescribed medical therapy. Because the nurse has a major role in discharge planning and patient teaching, these are discussed under nursing management. A sample Clinical Pathway for hyperthyroidism with atrial fibrillation is found on p. 1074-1075.

Medical therapy is designed to reduce the output of thyroid hormone and to antagonize the effects of thyroid hormone on peripheral tissue. Three treatment options are available although no therapy reverses the underlying autoimmune defect. Therapies include antithyroid drugs, radioactive iodine-131 (RAI), or surgery. Both surgery and RAI therapy have the potential side effect of hypothyroidism. Drug therapy is often used first to promote a euthyroid state before using ablation therapy in Graves' disease and multinodular goiter. However, RAI therapy is usually the first treatment in elderly persons with Graves' disease and is the most frequently used treatment in the United States. Surgery is reserved for large goiters and large, hot nodules and when RAI is contraindicated. RAI therapy is now generally considered safe in women of childbearing age, although many physicians prefer to try medications first.[7] Women of childbearing age might also prefer antithyroid medications (exception: iodides) or surgery instead of RAI therapy. The choice of therapeutic measures is individualized based on age, size of goiter, severity of hyperthyroidism, duration of illness, reproductive status, and cause of hyperthyroidism.

### *Diagnostic tests*

When hyperthyroidism is suspected, various diagnostic tests are necessary to confirm the diagnosis. (See Chapter 33 for a complete description of tests used.) The first tests done are measurement of serum $T_4$ and free $T_4$ or the free $T_4$ index. In most persons with hyperthyroidism, these levels are elevated. If these tests are not conclusive, measurements of serum $T_3$ level and free $T_3$ are done. In $T_3$ thyrotoxicosis, these levels are elevated with normal $T_4$ and free $T_4$ index.

TSH levels are measured and are low in most patients with hyperthyroidism if "sensitive" TSH assays of blood are used. (TSH levels would be high if there were a pituitary hypersecretory state.) The sensitive TSH assay differentiates low serum levels from normal levels of TSH (previous TSH assays were unable to do this). Radioactive iodine uptake (RAIU) is elevated in all types of hyperthyroidism except thyroiditis, factitious thyrotoxicosis, and struma ovarii. RAIU findings are inaccurate if the patient has received iodine in the past few weeks. Other tests, such as thyroid-binding globulin (TBG), may be used to calculate the $T_4$ index if the patient has recently received iodine. Further clarification of the hormonal status can be done with provocative testing; however, the sensitive TSH test has reduced the use of the TRH stimulation test or thyroid suppression tests. Patients with hyperthyroidism usually show a blunted TSH response to TRH and no suppression of RAIU with exogenous thyroid therapy. (See Chapter 33 for a description of radiographic tests that might be used in the diagnosis of hyperthyroidism.)

### *Medications*

Three classes of medications are used in the treatment of hyperthyroidism: the antithyroids, or *thioamides,* which inhibit the synthesis of thyroid hormones; the *iodides,* which primarily inhibit the release of thyroid hormones; and thyroid antagonists: *β-adrenergic blockers* (propranolol) and *calcium antagonists,* which antagonize the effects of thyroid hormone on body cells. The severity of the hyperthyroidism is a major factor in whether drugs from one, two, or three of these classes will be used in any given patient. Table 34-6 provides details for these drugs and alternate choices.

The thioamides propylthiouracil (PTU) and methimazole (Tapazole) are the most frequently used antithyroid drugs. Because the action of these drugs is slow, 2 to 4 weeks are required before improvement is noticeable. The onset of action is slow because these drugs block thyroid hormone synthesis and not the secretion of the hormone itself. The supply of hormone stored in the gland must be reduced before improvement is seen, and this takes from 2 to 4 weeks. The patient usually is given a relatively large dose of the antithyroid drug (PTU, 300 to 450 mg/day in three divided doses; methimazole, 30 to 45 mg/day in three divided doses). Then the dosage is gradually reduced to a level sufficient to maintain the euthyroid state (PTU, 100 to 150 mg/day, or methimazole, 10 to 15 mg/day, both given in divided doses). When antithyroid drugs are used as the primary therapy, they usually are continued for 6 to 18 months or longer. Approximately one half of those with Graves' disease will develop a spontaneous remission of their hyperthyroidism. Although it is impossible to predict which persons will go into remission, persons whose goiters decrease in size and who remain euthyroid as drug dosage is decreased are the most likely candidates. No guarantee exists that patients will remain in remission. The patient should see the physician regularly after drugs are discontinued so that early signs of recurrence can be detected.

## clinical pathway *Hyperthyroidism with Atrial Fibrillation*

DRG #: 300; EXPECTED LOS: 7

| | DAY OF ADMISSION<br>DAY 1 | DAY 2 | DAY 3 |
|---|---|---|---|
| DIAGNOSTIC TESTS | CBC; UA; SMA/18*; serum TSH and free $T_4$ index or free $T_4$ concentration; total $T_4$ or $T_3$ concentrations as necessary; ECG; C&S blood/UA/sputum if necessary; $O_2$ saturation on room air, ABGs if necessary | CBC; $O_2$ saturation on room air, ABGs if necessary | SMA/18,* ECG |
| MEDICATIONS | IV @ 30 ml/hr; propylthiouracil; antiatrial fibrillation medication (possibly including coumadin, propranolol, or calcium channel blockers); medication for CHF as necessary; eye drops OU q2hr prn for dryness; multivitamins; medication for rest/ sleep if necessary; stool softener | IV @ 30 ml/hr; propylthiouracil; antiatrial fibrillation medication; medication for CHF as necessary; eye drops OU q2hr prn for dryness; multivitamins; medication for rest/sleep if necessary; stool softener | IV @ 30 ml/hr; propylthiouracil; antiatrial fibrillation medication; medication for CHF as necessary; eye drops OU q2hr prn for dryness; multivitamins; medication for rest/sleep if necessary; stool softener |
| TREATMENTS | I&O q4hr; VS qhr 4 times then q2hr; $O_2$ prn; cardiac monitor; weight; record food intake; assess moisture to eyes q2hr; assess neuro-cardio-pul-circ systems q2hr 4 times then q4hr | I&O q8hr; VS q4hr; $O_2$ prn; cardiac monitor; weight; record food intake; assess moisture to eyes q2hr; assess neuro-cardio-pul-circ systems q4hr | I&O q8hr; VS q4hr; $O_2$ prn; cardiac monitor; weight; record food intake; assess moisture to eyes q2hr; assess neuro-cardio-pul-circ systems q4hr |
| DIET | Soft diet with high calories, protein, and CHO; serve 6 meals; NO STIMULANTS | Soft diet with high calories, protein, and CHO; serve 6 meals; NO STIMULANTS | Soft diet with high calories, protein, and CHO; serve 6 meals; NO STIMULANTS |
| ACTIVITY | Bedrest with BRP; minimize environmental stressors (keep room cool, calm, quiet; provide rest periods) | Bedrest with BRP; minimize environmental stressors | Up to chair qid; minimize environmental stressors |
| REFERRAL/ CONSULTATIONS | Social services | Dietary, home health if necessary | |

*Serum calcium, phosphorus, triglycerides, uric acid, creatinine, blood urea nitrogen (BUN), total bilirubin, alkaline phosphate, aspartate aminotransferase (AST) (formerly serum glutamic oxaloacetic transaminase [SGOT]), alanine aminotransferase (ALT) (formerly serum glutamic pyruvic transaminase [SGPT]), lactic dehydrogenase (LDH), total protein, albumin, sodium, potassium, chloride, total $CO_2$, glucose.

*CBC*, complete blood count; *UA*, urinalysis; *C&S*, culture and sensitivity; *ABGs*, arterial blood gases; *CHF*, congestive heart failure; *OU*, each eye; *CHO*, carbohydrates; *BRP*, bathroom privileges.

Patients who redevelop hyperthyroidism require drug therapy, RAI therapy, or surgery.

Patients are instructed to look for toxic signs of the drugs, such as fever, sore throat, and skin eruptions, or any signs of infection and to call their physician immediately if these signs appear. The signs of infection need to be reported immediately because they may indicate *agranulocytosis* (lack of production of granulocytes). If this occurs, the drugs are stopped immediately. Almost all patients recover from agranulocytosis; however, the patient must be treated with an alternative therapy.

The *β-adrenergic blockers*, such as propranolol (Inderal), are used to treat symptoms from increased sympathetic nervous system stimulation, such as tachycardia, dysrhythmias, and angina. These blockers reduce the signs and symptoms rapidly because they block β-receptors. Thus the cate-

| DAY 4 | DAY 5 | DAY 6 | DAY OF DISCHARGE DAY 7 |
|---|---|---|---|
| | CBC, SMA/18* | | |
| IV saline lock; adjust propylthiouracil, antiatrial fibrillation medication, and other medications for home use; eye drops OU q2hr prn for dryness; multivitamins; medication for rest/sleep prn; stool softener | IV saline lock; adjust propylthiouracil, antiatrial fibrillation medication, and other medications for home use; eye drops OU q4hr prn for dryness; multivitamins; medication for rest/sleep prn; stool softener | IV saline lock; adjust propylthiouracil, antiatrial fibrillation medication, and other medications for home use; eye drops OU q4hr prn for dryness; multivitamins; medication for rest/sleep prn; stool softener | Discontinue saline lock; continue propylthiouracil, antiatrial fibrillation medication, and other medications for home use; eye drops OU q4hr prn for dryness; multivitamins; medication for rest/sleep prn; stool softener; provide info for $^{131}$I radioactive isotope as outpatient in 6 wk |
| I&O q8hr; VS q6hr; discontinue $O_2$; cardiac monitor; weight; record food intake; assess moisture to eyes q4hr; assess neuro-cardio-pul-circ systems q6hr | Discontinue I&O; VS q8hr; weight; discontinue cardiac monitor; assess moisture to eyes q8hr; assess neuro-cardio-pul-circ systems q8hr | VS q8hr; weight; assess moisture to eyes q8hr; assess neuro-cardio-pul-circ systems q8hr | VS q8hr; weight; assess moisture to eyes q8hr; assess neuro-cardio-pul-circ systems q8hr |
| Regular diet with high calories, protein, and CHO; serve 6 meals; NO STIMULANTS | Regular diet with high calories, protein, and CHO; serve 6 meals; NO STIMULANTS | Regular diet with high calories, protein, and CHO; serve 6 meals; NO STIMULANTS | Regular diet with high calories, protein, and CHO; serve 6 meals; NO STIMULANTS |
| Up in room ad lib; minimize environmental stressors | Up in room ad lib | Up ad lib | Up ad lib |

cholamines, even if present, cannot stimulate the receptors. These agents block β-receptors on all organs in the body, producing widespread effects. The blocking of the actions of catecholamines helps to prevent critical complications of thyroid hormone excess.

β-Adrenergic blockers also improve tremors, restlessness, anxiety, and sometimes myopathy. Propranolol, 20 to 40 mg every 4 to 6 hours, may be given for symptom control except in persons with congestive heart failure or bronchial asthma. Worsening of these conditions can occur from the negative inotropic side effects of β-adrenergic blockers. Alternative drugs used to treat adrenergic symptoms include calcium antagonists or drugs that deplete catecholamines. These drugs have fewer negative inotropic side effects than do the β-blockers.[18]

### Treatments

**Radioactive iodine therapy.** RAI therapy with $^{131}$I is increasingly being used because it (1) can be given on an outpatient basis, (2) is safer for a wider range of patients, including elderly persons, who are poorer surgical risks, (3) can result in faster improvement in thyroid function than antithyroid drug therapy, and (4) although still controversial, can be used in women of childbearing age. RAI is given orally in

table 34-6 Common Medications Used in Treatment of **Hyperthyroidism**

| Class | Major Actions | Major Side Effects or Problems |
|---|---|---|
| **ANTITHYROIDS/THIOAMIDES** | | |
| Propylthiouracil (PTU)<br>Methimazole (Tapazole) | Inhibit biosynthesis of thyroid hormone<br>Stops production step of iodination<br>Inhibits conversion of $T_4$ to more active $T_3$ (PTU) | Agranulocytosis, hypersensitivity reactions |
| **THYROID BLOCKERS OR ANTAGONISTS** | | |
| Propranolol | $\beta$-Adrenergic blocking agent | Negative inotropic effects, hypotension, worsening of cardiac or airway disease<br>Hypotension |

one dose. The dosage is individualized, but on the average, it is 80 to 90 $\mu$Ci/g of thyroid tissue or equivalent to 6000 to 7000 rad. Although symptoms of hyperthyroidism will decrease in approximately 3 weeks, *a euthyroid state will not be achieved for 6 months.* The treatment must be repeated in about 20% of patients.

The RAI is eliminated after treatment (approximately 2 days). Because of this short excretion time, no tests are used to monitor RAI elimination from the body. RAI is excreted in urine, saliva, sweat, and feces. Standard Precautions should be maintained. Breastfeeding is not allowed for a few days.

Radiation precautions are dose dependent; instructions are individualized for each patient (see the Patient/Family Teaching Box). RAI is not used in pregnant women because of the potential teratogenic effects on the fetus; the placenta transports iodine easily. If RAI is used in women of childbearing years, pregnancy should be delayed for 6 months after therapy.

The major side effect of RAI therapy is hypothyroidism. Although different authorities[8,13] report different figures for the percentage of persons developing hypothyroidism each year after $^{131}$I therapy, eventually almost 100% of all persons become hypothyroid. Persons must be told about this complication before treatment; they are monitored for hypothyroidism, should know the signs and symptoms (see p. 1084), and must report their onset to the physician.

**patient/family teaching**

**The Person Receiving Radiation Therapy of the Thyroid Gland**

Flush the toilet two or three times after each use.
Increase intake of fluids to aid in RAI's excretion.
Use separate eating utensils and separate towels and washcloths; wash these and underclothes and bed linens separately.
Rinse bathroom sinks and tubs thoroughly after use, and wash hands carefully after using the bathroom.
Sleep alone for a few days, and avoid kissing and intercourse (although the amount of radiation in the patient's body is minimal).
Avoid prolonged physical contact with anyone.
Do not breastfeed.
Delay pregnancy for 6 months after therapy.

### Surgical management

Surgery is no longer the treatment of choice for patients with Graves' disease who have large goiters and whose thyroid glands have low RAIU. However, surgery is frequently still used as primary therapy for children. Surgery and/or treatment with antithyroid drugs is used in treating the pregnant woman with hyperthyroidism. RAI therapy is not used during pregnancy because iodine is a teratogenic agent,[7] and the placenta transports iodine easily. Surgery remains the treatment of choice for patients with thyroid cancers.

Surgical techniques include the removal of one lobe, 75% to 80% of the gland *(subtotal thyroidectomy)*, or removal of 100% of the gland *(total thyroidectomy)*. Subtotal thyroidectomy has an advantage over RAI therapy in that the incidence of hypothyroidism is much less. However, hyperthyroidism may occur from hypertrophy of the remaining tissue over time. The risks associated with thyroid surgery are minimal in patients treated by experienced surgeons. Nursing management of the patient undergoing thyroid surgery is discussed on p. 1092-1093.

### Diet

Increased food intake and weight loss are characteristic of untreated hyperthyroidism. Increased nutrient and calorie intake are necessary to meet the increased food requirements. Weight gain in the treated patient can signal the return of the euthyroid state in elderly patients.[7] While hyperthyroidism is present, caloric intake needs to be increased, with attention to appropriate distribution of calories from macronutrients. Supplemental vitamins and trace minerals may be prescribed.

### Activity

Activity may be self-limited because of the fatigue the patient experiences. Usually activity restrictions are not imposed unless the patient has symptoms of tachycardia, atrial fibrillation, or other cardiovascular problems. (See Chapter 25 for activity interventions for these problems.) Thyroid storm mandates complete bedrest and admission to an intensive care unit.

The patient is advised to rest. Symptoms of fatigue and insomnia may help patients accept and plan for rest periods during the day; however, hyperkinetic activity may make trying to rest at any one time very frustrating. Work requiring concentration for long periods may be difficult to perform. The patient may need assistance coping with activity restrictions that interfere with occupational and financial demands.

### Referrals

Concerns about personal, family, or financial resources may be identified. Decreased emotional stability and energy level may decrease ability to cope or solve problems. Barriers to compliance with treatment recommendations are explored carefully to maximize compliance and thereby prevent recurrence of symptoms or onset of thyroid storm. Appropriate patient-specific referrals are made.

# NURSING MANAGEMENT

## ASSESSMENT

As described, hyperthyroidism can affect almost every system of the body and cause major physiological and psychosocial problems.

### Subjective Data

Data to be collected to assess the patient with hyperthyroidism include:

- History of emotional and mental status changes
- Complaints of palpitations or chest pain
- Complaints of dyspnea, with or without exercise
- History of changes in hair, skin, nails, or amount of sweating
- Complaints of visual disturbances and irritations; reports of eyes tiring easily
- Appetite and history of nutritional intake and weight changes
- History of increased stool frequency and stool bulk
- History of intolerance to heat
- Complaints of weakness, fatigue, and decreased ability to complete ADL
- History of changes in menses or change in libido
- Knowledge: disease, treatment, care needs

### Objective Data

Data to be collected to assess the patient with hyperthyroidism include:

- Mental status changes: shortened attention span, emotional lability, hyperkinesia, tremor
- Cardiovascular status changes: increased systolic blood pressure, decreased diastolic pressure, tachycardia at rest, dysrhythmias, murmurs
- Skin and hair changes: warm, flushed, moist skin; dermopathy; fine, thinning hair
- Eye changes: lid lag, globe lag, diplopia, injection of conjunctiva, decreased acuity
- Nutritional/metabolic changes: decreased weight, increased appetite and intake, decreased serum triglycerides and cholesterol levels
- Musculoskeletal changes: muscle weakness, decreased muscle tone, difficulty rising from sitting position

Diagnostic test findings include:

1. Elevations of serum $T_3$, $T_4$, and $T_4$ index
2. Decreased serum levels of TSH measured by "sensitive" assay

Other tests may be used to interpret accurately the results of the above tests, as discussed in Chapter 33. One of the factors that can make $T_3$, $T_4$, and serum TSH levels poorly reflect true hormonal status is total binding proteins (TBG). Other factors are elevation of $T_3$ or $T_4$ and the suppression of TSH by acute or severe illness and the effects of drugs such as iodides.

## NURSING DIAGNOSES

Nursing diagnoses are determined from analysis of patient data. Nursing diagnoses for the person with hyperthyroidism may include but are not limited to:

| Diagnostic Title | Possible Etiological Factors |
|---|---|
| Activity intolerance, risk for | Muscle weakness and wasting associated with altered metabolism |
| Cardiac output, decreased | Dysrhythmias associated with increased sympathetic activity |
| Coping, ineffective (individual) | Altered processing of sensory input, decreased attention span, emotional lability |
| Home maintenance management, impaired | Delay between initiation of therapy and return of euthyroid state |
| Hyperthermia | Increased heat production greater than dissipation |
| Knowledge deficit: disease, treatment, outcomes, self-monitoring needs | Lack of familiarity with information |
| Nutrition, altered; less than body requirements | Increased metabolic needs |
| Sensory/perceptual alterations; visual | Disruption of function of optic nerves or extraocular muscles of eyes associated with infiltrative changes |
| Sleep pattern disturbance | Increased metabolic rate, restlessness |

## EXPECTED PATIENT OUTCOMES

Expected patient outcomes for the person with hyperthyroidism may include but are not limited to:

1. Demonstrates no further decrease in activity tolerance, and shows a gradual increase in activity over 2 to 3 months.
2. Shows evidence of adequate tissue perfusion and cardiac output: no change in mental status, breath sounds clear, no edema formation, heart rate within 20 beats of baseline, and gradual decrease in resting heart rate.

3. Shows effective coping:
   a. Rates self as less anxious or less stressed on a scale of 1 to 10, with 1 meaning no stress and 10 the worst stress.
   b. Lists three ways to cope with feelings.
4. Identifies home maintenance difficulties and methods to deal with difficulties until health stabilizes.
5. Has normal body temperature.
6. Describes how hyperthyroidism causes the signs and symptoms present, lists treatment options available, lists expected outcomes of treatment with realistic time frames, lists signs and symptoms requiring self-monitoring (signs/ symptoms of hypothyroidism, hyperthyroidism, agranulocytosis), and lists precautions to be observed if RAI therapy is used.
7. Does not lose more weight; weight will return to within 0.5 kg of preillness weight.
8. Does not complain of eye pain, diplopia, or decreased visual acuity.
9. Sleeps uninterrupted through the night, has rest periods during the day if needed.

## INTERVENTIONS

A Nursing Care Plan for a specific patient appears on p. 1080-1082 and highlights some of the care needs of persons with hyperthyroidism. Many patients with hyperthyroidism are managed outside the hospital setting.

### Providing Recuperative Care

As recovery ensues, the nurse must continue to provide interventions that address the outcomes related to hyperthyroidism. These include but are not limited to:

1. Promote adequate rest.
   a. Provide a quiet, comfortable environment.
   b. Provide back rubs.
   c. Use home remedies such as hot milk to assist in promoting sleep.
   d. Encourage quiet periods even if the patient does not sleep.
2. Maintain and increase activity tolerance.
   a. Encourage short walks if cardiac output is stable.
   b. Space activity between rest periods.
3. Maintain adequate nutrition intake.
   a. Monitor intake and output every 8 hours.
   b. Weigh daily.
   c. Monitor nutritional intake.
   d. Provide frequent high-protein, high-calorie meals.
4. Promote good eye care.
   a. Perform visual assessment every shift.
   b. Initiate appropriate measures such as using dark glasses, elevating the head of bed, using artificial tears, and taping the eyelids closed at various intervals.
   c. Report any new complaints immediately.
5. Facilitate improved coping; offer patients interventions to help them relax, such as music, back rubs, and distraction.
6. Enhance patient knowledge.

#### *Patient/family education*

The nurse can help the patient learn to incorporate the therapeutic regimen into ADL. In addition, the patient needs to plan how to achieve rest, adequate nutrition, and energy conservation at home and at work. The patient may explore with the physician the appropriate and recommended options of definitive treatment. The nurse can support information seeking about risks, benefits, consequences of the treatment, and the requirements for follow-up care. The patient's beliefs and desires need to be valued, and the patient should be supported in expressing any concerns to the physician. A common concern is the effect of environmental radiation if RAI therapy is an option.

The teaching plan should include information to allow the patient to:

1. Describe the disease and how it causes signs and symptoms.
2. Clarify treatment options.
3. List the expected outcomes, such as relief of symptoms in 4 weeks if the patient is receiving drug therapy, the need for drug therapy for extended periods, and the potential complications of therapy.
4. Explain each medication, purpose, dose and schedule, and side effects to report.
5. List precautions if the patient received RAI (see the Patient/Family Teaching Box, p. 1076).
6. List the signs and symptoms the patient must self-monitor.

Patients at risk should be taught preventive measures. Only two of the causes of hyperthyroidism are preventable: factitious (artificial) hyperthyroidism and iodine-induced hyperthyroidism. Primary prevention of factitious hyperthyroidism is possible through appropriate health teaching regarding safe measures for weight reduction and weight control. To prevent iodine-induced hyperthyroidism, persons with endemic goiter who are treated with supplemental iodine must be monitored very closely. Secondary prevention for persons with hyperthyroidism includes early detection of signs and symptoms and early prompt treatment to prevent disease progression. Screening is recommended in clinic patients with risk factors shown in the box below. The "sensitive" TSH assay of blood is used most often.[8] Prompt treatment and adequate follow-up can reduce the incidence and severity of complications of hyperthyroidism (tertiary prevention).

## EVALUATION

To evaluate the effectiveness of nursing interventions, compare patient behaviors with those stated in the expected patient outcomes. Successful achievement of patient outcomes for the person with hyperthyroidism is indicated by:

1. Reports increased energy level, activity endurance, and activity completion.
2. Has pulse rate less than 80 at rest.
3. Rates anxiety as reduced and tolerable.

**risk factors**

**Hyperthyroidism**

Family history of thyroid disease
Autoimmune disorders
Age older than 40 for women
Age older than 65

4. States plans for home maintenance that address rest and required resources.
5. Has temperature of 37.2 °C (99 °F) or below.
6. Describes dosage schedule, rationale, and importance of drug therapy.
7. Maintains weight or increases weekly by at least 0.5 kg.
8. Reports no visual problems or loss of visual acuity.
9. Reports adequate rest and sleep.

## GERONTOLOGICAL CONSIDERATIONS

1. Elderly patients have less clear-cut clinical findings of hyperthyroidism. There may be weight loss, fatigue, and irritability, but goiter, tachycardia, eye changes, or tremor may be absent. In fact, subclinical hyperthyroidism, or "apathetic" or "masked" hyperthyroidism, is typical in elderly persons.
2. Hyperthyroidism may be the cause of new onset atrial fibrillation.
3. Nonthyroid disease may or may not raise the serum $T_3$ and/or $T_4$ in elderly persons and may suppress serum TSH. Elderly persons typically have more than one chronic illness.
4. RAI therapy is the treatment of choice in elderly patients.
5. Common drug interactions with hyperthyroidism include increased metabolism of drugs typically taken by elderly persons: digoxin, theophylline, and warfarin.

## SPECIAL ENVIRONMENT OF CARE

### Critical Care Management

*Thyroid crisis* or *storm* is a medical emergency in which patients develop severe manifestations of the signs and symptoms of hyperthyroidism, including an elevated temperature, increased tachycardia or onset of dysrhythmias, worsening tremors and restlessness, worsening mental status including a delirious or psychotic state or coma, and sometimes reports of abdominal pain. Blood pressure and respiratory rate increase above baseline.

Thyroid storm is usually seen in persons with Graves' disease. Symptoms result from a severe increase in metabolism and are usually precipitated by a major stressor such as infection, trauma, or surgery. The use of medications to suppress thyroid activity before surgery decreases the risk of thyroid storm, since less hormone is released into the blood with manipulation of the gland. Thyroid crisis also may occur in a person who has been inadequately treated or who stops taking prescribed therapy.

Patients with thyroid storm must be hospitalized. The immediate focus of care is to lower the metabolic rate as fast as possible, remove the precipitating cause, and support physiological functioning. The typical therapeutic regimen is outlined in the Guidelines for Care Box. Note that the doses of medicines in the box are higher than those used in less critically ill patients. Doses of drugs are adjusted according to patient response. Patients may require continual monitoring during rapid treatment.

Priority interventions are focused on the management of the fever and the cardiovascular responses seen in thyroid storm. Atrial fibrillation is often the first cardiac alteration noted; other dysrhythmias are possible. Angina and congestive heart failure may occur in hyperthyroid patients in intensive care units; often these patients have underlying heart disease. Interventions include:

1. Maintain cardiac output.
   a. Monitor cardiovascular status every hour.
   b. Report any changes to the physician, such as increased tachycardia, dysrhythmias, or signs of congestive heart failure (see Chapter 26).
   c. Decrease cardiac workload by decreasing physical and emotional stressors.
2. Maintain normothermia.
   a. Monitor temperature every hour: report any elevations.
   b. Use external cooling devices as ordered.
   c. Maintain room temperature in cool range.

As the acute crisis subsides, continued attention should be paid to maintaining cardiac output and normal temperature.

### Home Care Management

The nurse focuses on assessment of the patient's and family's ability to manage the therapeutic regimen and to adapt resources to meet patient needs. The patient and family need to understand the therapy and expected results and to decide

**guidelines for care**

**The Person with Thyroid Crisis or Storm**

Monitor the patient's temperature, intake and output, neurological status, and cardiovascular status every hour.

Initiate an IV line for medications and fluids.

Administer increasing doses of oral propylthiouracil as ordered (200 to 300 mg every 6 hours may be given) after a loading dose of 800 to 1200 mg orally.

Administer iodide preparations as ordered. Sodium iodide given IV twice daily or an oral preparation may be ordered.

Administer dexamethasone, 2 mg IV every 6 hours. Glucocorticoids help to inhibit the release of thyroid hormone.

Administer propranolol, 20 to 80 mg PO or 2 to 10 mg IV, as ordered. Propranolol ($\beta$-adrenergic blocker) can worsen asthma or congestive heart failure because it constricts bronchial smooth muscles and causes a decrease in cardiac output.

Initiate measures to lower body temperature, including external cooling devices, cold baths, and acetaminophen. Salicylates are contraindicated because they inhibit thyroid hormone binding to protein carriers and thus increase free thyroid hormone levels.

Initiate other supportive therapy as ordered, including oxygen, cardiac glycosides, and treatment measures for the precipitating event.

Maintain a quiet, calm, cool, private environment until the crisis is over.

Maintain continuity of care.

Decrease stressors by use of patient education, comfort measures, or family support.

## nursing care plan *The Person with Hyperthyroidism*

**DATA** Mrs. T., a 28-year-old housewife, is admitted for diagnostic evaluation before a thyroidectomy, which is scheduled to be performed in 2 weeks. Graves' disease was diagnosed 2 days ago; hospitalization was delayed until child-care arrangements were made for her 6-year-old stepson. (She was married 3 months ago.) Initial therapy, started 2 days ago, is Tapazole and Lugol's solution. The ECG report is sinus tachycardia (rate 132).

The nursing history identified the following about the patient:

- She feels overwhelmed, cries frequently, and fears losing control of temper.
- She has lost 15 pounds in 2 months and is always hungry, although she is eating large amounts of food.
- She is bothered by heat, others' noisiness, and her own clumsiness.
- She expects medicine to make her feel better and dreads surgery.

The physical examination revealed the following:

- Blood pressure: 140/60; pulse: 132, respiration: 24
- Staring gaze of eyes with proptosis (equal bilaterally); lid lag and globe lag present; right eye slightly reddened
- Skin warm and perspiration present
- Increased muscle tone with weakness of lower extremities; quick muscle response to sudden noise; fine tremor of both hands
- Diffuse visible enlargement of thyroid
- Bruit present over thyroid

Collaborative nursing actions include those to prevent further environmental stressors that could make the patient more uncomfortable and increase her signs and symptoms.

Nursing actions include monitoring the following: temperature, pulse, respiration, blood pressure, weight, appetite, and tremulousness.

**NURSING DIAGNOSIS** *Decreased cardiac output related to increased sympathetic stimulation*

| expected patient outcomes | nursing interventions | rationale |
|---|---|---|
| Pulse rate is less than 20 above baseline during first 72 hours.<br>Pulse rate decreases gradually after 72 hours.<br>Cardiac dysrhythmias do not occur. | Assess vital signs, especially heart rate and rhythm, at least q4hr; if worsens, assess qhr.<br>Instruct patient to report palpitations, chest pain, and dizziness.<br>Assess daily weight, daily intake and output; assess for signs of edema, jugular vein distention, and pulmonary congestion q8hr.<br>Decrease known stressors; explain all interventions, and listen to patient.<br>Balance periods of activity with rest.<br>Administer prescribed drugs and monitor therapeutic response.<br>Report any changes to physician. | Early detection of atrial fibrillation or thyroid storm allows prompt treatment and prevents cardiovascular crisis. |

**NURSING DIAGNOSIS** *Ineffective individual coping related to personal vulnerability to environmental stimuli*

| expected patient outcomes | nursing interventions | rationale |
|---|---|---|
| Explains reason for change in behavior.<br>Decreases emotional lability.<br>Identifies at least one coping mechanism that will help during periods of nervousness. | Discuss reasons for emotional lability.<br>Maintain calm, relaxed environment.<br>Encourage visitors who are calm and will not upset Mrs. T.<br>Provide privacy (e.g., a single room).<br>Suggest that others avoid sharing distressing news with Mrs. T.<br>Explain all interventions.<br>Avoid stimulants such as coffee, caffeine, and alcohol.<br>Help Mrs. T. identify previous coping mechanisms or explore new ones.<br>Offer measures to help Mrs. T. relax.<br>Include family in discussions. | A supportive environment can reduce environmental stimuli and stressors and assist patient in coping. |

*Continued*

how to incorporate therapeutic requirements into daily life. The nurse can help the patient and family to:

1. Increase resources for home maintenance while fatigue is present.
2. Ensure adequate nutrition; monitor weight weekly.
3. Plan for increased rest periods during the day.
4. Plan strategies to manage insomnia, hyperkinesis, increased stool frequency, and heat intolerance.
5. Understand the importance of adherence to therapy and follow-up monitoring.

## The Person with Hyperthyroidism–cont'd

**NURSING DIAGNOSIS** *Altered nutrition: less than body requirements related to increased metabolic needs*

| expected patient outcomes | nursing interventions | rationale |
|---|---|---|
| Maintains normal weight.<br>Gains at least 0.5 kg/wk if weight below normal. | Monitor weight qod to weekly.<br>Monitor serum albumin, hemoglobin, and lymphocyte levels.<br>Help her plan for high-calorie, high-protein, high-carbohydrate diet with selection from all food groups.<br>Suggest six small meals per day or between-meal snacks. | Increased nutrient intake meets increased metabolic demand. |

**NURSING DIAGNOSIS** *Sensory/perceptual alterations (potential visual) related to infiltrative changes associated with Graves' disease*

| expected patient outcomes | nursing interventions | rationale |
|---|---|---|
| Vision does not worsen.<br>Explains measures to protect eyes. | Assess visual acuity, ability to close eyes, and photophobia.<br>Protect eyes from irritants:<br>**1.** Use patches or glasses when in high wind.<br>**2.** Use artificial tears, if prescribed.<br>**3.** Elevate head of bed at night.<br>Instruct patient not to lie prone.<br>If eyes do not close completely, check about using shields at night. | These measures can prevent corneal injury and minimize risk of loss of vision. |

**NURSING DIAGNOSIS** *Hyperthermia related to increased heat production greater than dissipation*

| expected patient outcomes | nursing interventions | rationale |
|---|---|---|
| States that she feels more comfortable.<br>Maintains normothermia. | Control environmental temperature for comfort (fans may be helpful).<br>Suggest that she take frequent showers.<br>Encourage adequate fluid intake and monitor fluid losses.<br>Monitor temperature q4hr. | These measures keep her comfortable by increasing heat loss. |

**NURSING DIAGNOSIS** *Activity intolerance related to generalized muscle weakness*

| expected patient outcomes | nursing interventions | rationale |
|---|---|---|
| States fatigue is decreased.<br>Maintains current activity level. | Assess activity schedule.<br>Suggest ways to modify activities that cause fatigue.<br>Identify activities that can be done by others until condition is controlled.<br>Schedule rest periods between activities.<br>Encourage activities that promote sleep at night.<br>At present, keep activities at current level. | Reduction of energy expenditure is necessary to reduce fatigue in persons with increased metabolism until treatment decreases metabolism. |

*Continued*

### COMPLICATIONS

Various ocular changes occur in Graves' disease. Patients usually have some degree of ophthalmopathy (see earlier discussion). In addition, more serious ocular conditions resulting from infiltrative changes may be present.

None of the therapy described previously directly attacks the basic pathophysiological process, that is, the infiltrative changes. The therapy does not inhibit the production of glycosaminoglycan in the retrobulbar tissue. Better understanding of this pathophysiological process will lead to

## The Person with Hyperthyroidism–cont'd

**NURSING DIAGNOSIS** *Impaired home maintenance management related to delay in initiation of therapy and stabilization of patient*

| expected patient outcome | nursing interventions | rationale |
|---|---|---|
| States plan for home maintenance management. | Assist her to identify home maintenance difficulties.<br>Assist her to identify persons who can provide temporary help.<br>Make referrals as needed, such as to social services.<br>Identify persons who can help monitor her compliance with medical regimen.<br>Help Mrs. T. plan own schedule to allow for rest.<br>Include husband and stepson in plan of care. | These measures increase resources available to Mrs. T. and reduce stress from inability to meet expectations of role. |

**NURSING DIAGNOSIS** *Knowledge deficit (disease, treatment, expected outcomes) related to new information and no previous exposure to information*

| expected patient outcomes | nursing interventions | rationale |
|---|---|---|
| Explains medical regimen and care needs. | Explain how and when to take prescribed medications.<br>Describe symptoms of infection to be reported to physician, such as sore throat or fever.<br>Describe ways to plan prescribed dietary intake.<br>Provide required teaching about care needs (comfort, sleep, and rest).<br>Explain the reason for the delay before surgery. | These measures increase likelihood of compliance with therapy used to achieve euthyroid state and optimal physical status before surgery. |

new treatment measures. (For a detailed discussion of the surgical eye procedures, the reader should refer to Chapter 56.)

## HYPOSECRETION OF THYROID HORMONE: HYPOTHYROIDISM

### Etiology

Hypothyroidism is a metabolic state resulting from a deficiency of thyroid hormone that may occur at any age. Congenital hypothyroidism results in a condition called *cretinism*. Hypothyroidism may result from the following:

1. Loss or atrophy of thyroid tissue: autoimmune thyroiditis, ablative therapy for hyperthyroidism, thyrotoxic drugs, congenital agenesis, maldevelopment, or radiation for head and neck malignancies
2. Loss of trophic stimulation: pituitary dysfunction (pituitary or secondary hypothyroidism) or hypothalamic dysfunction
3. Miscellaneous alterations: deficit in hormone biosynthesis, peripheral resistance to thyroid hormone, idiopathic factors, or environmental factors (iodine deficiency)

In the United States, the most frequent causes of hypothyroidism are autoimmune thyroiditis and ablative therapy, whereas in the world, iodine deficiency is the leading cause.

**box 34-10** *Goitrogenic Factors*

- Iodine deficiency
- Foods with goitrogenic factors: cabbage, turnips, soybeans
- Drugs: lithium, thiocarbamides, sulfonylureas
- Intrinsic abnormality in thyroid hormone synthesis

Goiter formation may occur as the pituitary gland secretes more TSH in response to lower levels of thyroid hormone in the blood. Over time the resultant enlargement of the gland (goiter) is unable to maintain sufficient hormonal output, and hypothyroidism develops.

#### Goiter

Any enlargement of the thyroid gland is called a *goiter*. If this enlargement is not associated with hyperthyroidism or hypohyroidism, cancer, or inflammation, it is referred to as a *simple goiter*. *Endemic goiters* refer to those that occur in a particular geographic region and from a common cause, such as iodine deficiency. *Sporadic goiter* describes those that occur sporadically in regions that are not the locus of endemic goi-

**table 34-7** *Thyroiditis: Types and Characteristics*

| TYPE | CHARACTERISTICS |
|---|---|
| **ACUTE THYROIDITIS** | |
| Acute pyogenic thyroiditis | Rare form of thyroiditis; results from infection of thyroid by pyogenic organism; symptoms include pain and tenderness in thyroid, dysphagia, fever, malaise; treated symptomatically. |
| **SUBACUTE NONSUPPURATIVE THYROIDITIS** | |
| De Quervain's thyroiditis<br>Granulomatous thyroiditis | Rare form of thyroiditis; results from viral infection of thyroid gland; may follow an upper respiratory infection; most often seen in 4th and 5th decades of life; symptoms include pain in thyroid, fever, hoarseness, dysphagia, palpitations, nervousness, lassitude, thyroid moderately enlarged; subsides in a few months; treatment usually symptomatic; aspirin for mild cases; glucocorticoids when disease unresponsive to other measures. |
| **SUBACUTE LYMPHOCYTIC THYROIDITIS** | |
| Painless thyroiditis<br>Lymphocytic thyroiditis | Form of thyroiditis increasing in frequency; etiological factor unknown but possible autoimmune factor; symptoms include self-limiting form of hyperthyroidism and nontender enlarged thyroid gland, which may be followed by hypothyroidism; treatment symptomatic during hyperthyroidism phase and may include $\beta$-adrenergic blockers but not propylthiouracil (not effective); monitor annually for hypothyroidism. |
| **CHRONIC THYROIDITIS** | |
| Hashimoto's thyroiditis | See text. |
| Riedel's thyroiditis | Rare form of thyroiditis; cause unknown; extensive fibrosis of gland occurs; symptoms include insidious onset; symptoms from compression of trachea, esophagus, and recurrent laryngeal nerve; gland enlarged, hard; hypothyroidism can occur; treatment is symptomatic with surgery for symptoms of compression; thyroid replacement for hypothyroidism. |

ters. (See Box 34-10 for goitrogenic factors.) In most cases of simple goiter in the United States, no extrinsic factors can be identified. Simple goiter is seen most frequently in females (3:1 ratio with males)[8] and occurs most often during pregnancy or adolescence. Goiter also occurs more frequently in particular families.[7]

#### Autoimmune disorders

Hashimoto's disease is the leading cause of hypothyroidism in the United States. Autoimmune changes in the thyroid gland occur often in persons older than age 60 and immunological changes lead to goiter, resulting in hypothyroidism. Early in the disease there may be hormonal imbalance or episodic hyperthyroidism because of inappropriate release of hormones from the thyroid gland. When atrophy occurs later, the condition is called *atrophic thyroiditis* and is more frequently found in elderly persons. Other forms of thyroiditis, acute and chronic, are described in Table 34-7.

#### Ablation therapy

Total thyroidectomy, hypophysectomy, and radiation therapy of the pituitary or thyroid gland cause *iatrogenic hypothyroidism.* Patients undergoing these treatments must take thyroid hormone replacement for life.

## Epidemiology

Hypothyroidism affects an estimated 1% of the population and is particularly underdiagnosed in elderly persons. Prevalence rates are greater in elderly women (10%) than in elderly men (2.3%). Hypothyroidism is detected in 1 of every 4000 to 5000 newborns.

## Pathophysiology

### Goiter

The patient with hypothyroidism may or may not have a goiter. An enlarged thyroid gland is seen when the disease results from thyroiditis, defective hormone biosynthesis, peripheral resistance to thyroid hormone, and environmental factors. All these conditions reduce thyroid hormone production, and as a result, TSH secretion is increased because of lack of negative feedback. Increased thyroid mass then results from the increased stimulation. In contrast, if hypothyroidism results from lack of TSH (secondary hypothyroidism), growth of the thyroid gland is not stimulated.

### Thyroiditis

The three types of thyroiditis (inflammation of the thyroid) are acute, subacute, and chronic. *Hashimoto's thyroiditis,* a form of chronic thyroiditis, is the most common form of thyroiditis and is described here. In Hashimoto's thyroiditis lymphocytes and antithyroid antibodies infiltrate the thyroid. The pathological changes support the belief that Hashimoto's thyroiditis is an autoimmune disease. It is generally believed that thyroiditis is one of the triad of autoimmune thyroid disorders that include Graves' disease and primary thyroid atrophy. The mechanisms for the autoimmunity are not understood, although significant association exists between Hashimoto's thyroiditis and specific haplotypes, as well as other autoimmune diseases.

The lymphocytic infiltration in Hashimoto's thyroiditis results in obliteration of thyroid follicles and fibrosis. The destruction of the gland decreases the serum levels of $T_4$ and $T_3$ and thus increases TSH. The increase in thyroid tissue is not usually associated with overproduction of thyroid hormone, although transient hyperthyroidism can occur early in the disease. The increase in thyroid tissue and hyperfunction help to maintain an euthyroid state for some time, but eventually hypothyroidism and atrophy will develop.

The major clinical finding in Hashimoto's thyroiditis is diffuse thyroid enlargement, found as a goiter on examination. The thyroid gland is firm and smooth, moves freely, and is usually painless. Both lobes are enlarged, but one lobe may be larger than the other. Some persons may experience dysphagia or choking.

### Hypometabolism

Regardless of the cause, a lack of thyroid hormone results in a general depression of basal metabolic rate and slows the development or functioning of almost every system of the body. Alterations in the integumentary, cardiovascular, nervous, musculoskeletal, alimentary, and reproductive systems are often seen. One major change is an accumulation of hyaluronic acids and alteration of ground substances producing mucinous edema *(myxedema)* and third-space fluid effusions. Figure 34-6 illustrates the puffiness characteristic of myxedema facies. In the periphery the edematous tissues feel thickened or "doughy." Table 34-8 lists the pathophysiological alterations seen in hypothyroidism and relates the clinical manifestations seen with each.

The manifestations of hypothyroidism in infants are not usually seen until several months after birth, when signs such as retardation of mental and physical development occur and are usually irreversible.

In adults, early signs and symptoms are vague and may go unrecognized. A typical clinical picture is as follows. Early complaints may consist of tiredness, lethargy, and weakness resulting in the inability to carry out a normal day's activities. Intolerance to cold and constipation develop. Menstrual cycle irregularity, menorrhagia, and inability to conceive may occur. Loss of libido may be noted by men or women. As the disease progresses, mental dysfunction occurs, appetite decreases, changes in physical characteristics are noted, muscle and joint discomforts are present, and chest pain occurs. If hypothyroidism is not treated, myxedema coma will develop.

### Myxedema coma

Myxedema coma represents the most severe form of hypothyroidism and ultimately can occur in any patient with untreated prolonged hypothyroidism. Precipitating factors include sedatives, narcotics, exposure to cold, surgery, infections, and trauma. The patient has all the classic symptoms of hypothyroidism and also is comatose and has severe hypothermia. (See Table 34-8 for further discussion.)

## Collaborative Care Management

### Diagnostic tests

Studies of thyroid function useful for diagnosing hypothyroidism include the serum free $T_4$ index and a "sensitive" serum TSH assay. As in hyperthyroidism, these tests may need to be repeated. Other tests may be needed to determine the true hormonal status (see Chapter 33).

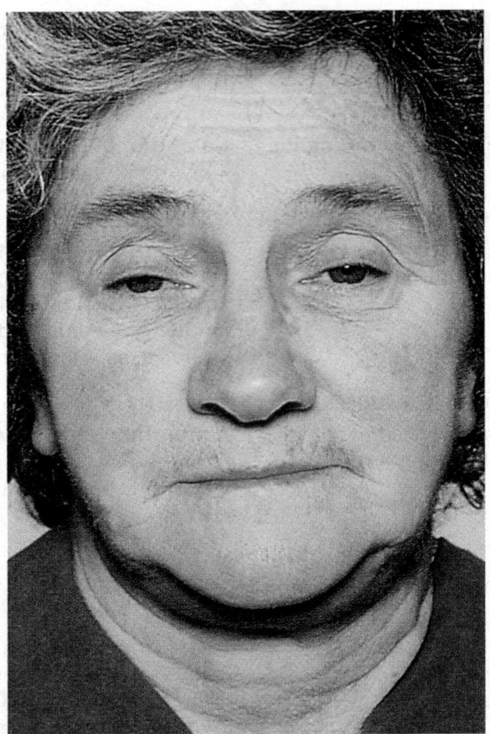

**fig. 34-6** Adult with hypothyroidism.

Decreased levels of $T_4$ and $T_3$ and an elevated TSH level can confirm the diagnosis of a patient who has primary thyroid hyposecretion and no other disease. Two factors may alter $T_3$, $T_4$, and TSH results: acuity of illness and presence of nonthyroid disease. In nonthyroid disease, there is a decreased conversion of $T_4$ to $T_3$. As a result, 70% of all patients in intensive care units have low serum levels of $T_3$ and normal TSH levels. As patients recover, levels of $T_3$ increase (low $T_3$ state). $T_4$ and TSH levels may also be affected by illness. When Hashimoto's disease is suspected, the physician will order thyroid antibody tests and perhaps a fine-needle biopsy to confirm the presence of chronic thyroiditis or to identify other pathological factors.

### Medications

**Goiter suppression.** Medical management of simple goiter is focused on removing the stimulus causing the increased thyroid mass. Suppression of the increase in TSH is necessary to correct the stimulus for growth of the thyroid gland. Correction also reduces the associated increase in turnover of iodine and the increased $T_4/T_3$ ratio in thyroid secretion.[18] With elevated TSH, the patient has remained euthyroid at the expense of the elevated TSH and an enlarged gland. If extrinsic factors such as goitrogenic drugs or foods are the cause, they are eliminated. Iodine deficiency, although very rare, is ruled out and replacement is instituted if appropriate.[18]

In most instances the cause of goiter is unknown, and therapy is directed at supplying exogenous hormone, which will inhibit TSH secretion. Similar therapy is used to suppress

**table 34-8** *Hypothyroidism: Normal Function, Pathological Alterations, and Clinical Manifestations*

| NORMAL FUNCTION | PATHOPHYSIOLOGICAL ALTERATIONS | CLINICAL MANIFESTATIONS |
|---|---|---|
| Regulates metabolic rate, calorigenesis, and oxygen consumption | Decreased metabolic rate, heat production, and oxygen consumption<br>May be vasoconstriction in periphery<br>Decreased nutrient requirements<br>Decreased sweat gland and sebaceous gland activity<br>Myxedema | General: decreased body temperature, intolerance to cold; hair: thin, dry; deepened voice; decreased appetite; dry, thickened, cool, pale, scaly skin<br>Myxedema facies: large tongue, peripheral edema, deepened voice |
| Regulates protein, fat, and carbohydrate metabolism | Altered carbohydrate, protein, and fat metabolism<br>Decreased protein synthesis, gluconeogenesis, and glycogen storage<br>Increased interstitial fluid with polysaccharide deposits and increased albumin content<br>Decreased glucose absorption and cellular uptake; decreased degradation of insulin<br>Decreased lipid metabolism, especially degradation of lipid<br>Decreased erythropoietin production<br>Hypercarotenemia | Metabolic: decreased appetite, weight gain (edema), slow wound healing<br>Myxedematous tissues: peripheral organs, tongue, vocal cords<br>Hypoalbuminemia<br>Decrease in blood glucose possible in patients with diabetes mellitus<br>Increased serum triglycerides and serum cholesterol<br>Anemia; yellow cast to skin and nails |
| Sensitizes cells to catecholamines | Altered cardiovascular functioning<br>Hypometabolic state, decreased inotropic and chronotropic effects on heart, polysaccharide infiltrate of myocardium<br>Decreased cardiac output, decreased contractility and rate<br>Increased interstitial fluid and third-space fluids | Cardiovascular: bradycardia, enlargement of heart, pericardial effusion, pleural effusion, decreased excretion of water load, hyponatremia, possible increased blood pressure |
| Regulates rate of cellular functions: multiple interactions of thyroid hormone with other hormones and systems | Altered CNS function<br>Altered reproductive function | CNS: apathy, slow slurred speech, lethargy, somnolence, coma, paresthesia, slow deep tendon reflexes<br>Reproductive: decreased libido, failure to conceive, changes in menses, anovulation in women, oligospermia and erectile dysfunction in men |

TSH secretion in goiter associated with Hashimoto's disease. Sodium L-thyroxine is usually necessary. The adequacy of the dosage in suppressing TSH secretion is verified by an RAIU test that should have a value of less than 5%. Surgery is sometimes necessary if suppression is not accomplished with other therapy. Surgery will result in hypothyroidism, requiring lifelong replacement of thyroid hormone.

**Replacement therapy.** Hypothyroidism is treated with replacement of thyroid hormone. Sodium levo-thyroxine (sodium L-thyroxine) is the standard treatment of choice. Other thyroid replacement therapies (triiodothyronine, desiccated thyroid hormone, and synthetic combinations of thyroid hormones) are no longer used. Drug therapy should be initiated slowly, particularly if the patient has heart dysfunction or is elderly. The initial daily dose usually should not exceed 12.5 to 25 $\mu$g of L-thyroxine. This dose is increased by increments of 25 to 50 $\mu$g every 2 to 4 weeks until a normal metabolic rate is attained.[7,8]

The optimal maintenance dose of replacement therapy varies and is determined by the patient's clinical state. The earliest clinical response is diuresis, resulting in weight loss and regression of puffiness. The pulse rate then increases, appetite improves, constipation is relieved, and mental and motor activity increase.

The major side effects of thyroid replacement therapy are (1) inadequate treatment, with the patient continuing to show signs and symptoms of hypothyroidism; (2) excessive treatment, resulting in signs and symptoms of hyperthyroidism; (3) increases in drug dose at too fast a rate, resulting in cardiac problems such as angina, palpitations, tachycardia, or cardiac failure; and (4) bone loss and decreased bone density. During the initiation of therapy, the physician sees the patient every 2 to 4 weeks. After the patient's condition stabilizes, thyroid hormone replacement should be monitored annually by tests such as serum free $T_4$ and TSH level.

### Treatments

Treatment of hypothyroidism consists of pharmacological therapy, as previously described. Surgery may be performed for large goiters (see discussion below).

### Surgical management

Thyroidectomy may be used to treat large goiters, particularly those compressing adjacent tissues. A very large goiter may displace or compress the esophagus or trachea and cause dysphagia, a choking sensation, or inspiratory stridor. Compression of the recurrent laryngeal nerve may lead to hoarseness, although this sign is more suggestive of cancer. Narrowing of the thoracic inlet decreases venous return from the head, neck, and upper limbs and results in venous engorgement. This obstruction is accentuated with elevation of the person's arms and results in dizziness and syncope (Pemberton's sign).

#### Diet

Adequate nutrition (well-balanced meals) is promoted for patients with hypothyroidism. Patients are advised to follow prescribed caloric intake to achieve goals of weight loss if indicated. If iodine deficiency or excessive intake of goitrogenic foods has been identified, instructions are given. In severe hypothyroidism, apathy, anorexia, and self-care deficit may combine to limit food intake, and attention must be given to achieve adequate intake. Fluid restriction and occasionally sodium modifications are necessary in severe hyponatremia.

#### Activity

Fatigue limits endurance in persons with hypothyroidism. Symptoms such as angina and dyspnea on exertion may occur with severe fatigue. Patients should be encouraged to increase activity gradually, building endurance and tolerance.

#### Referrals

Appropriate referrals might include home care nursing, physical therapy, and social services if family or personal resources are limited.

## NURSING MANAGEMENT

### ASSESSMENT

#### Subjective Data

Hypothyroidism affects every system of the body. Early manifestations will most likely be identified by a thorough history. The history should focus on assessing the following areas for changes:

- Changes in physical energy level and activity or mental/neurological status
- Changes in skin, hair (head or body), nails
- Presence of chest pain; occurrence of syncope
- Changes in appetite and weight with a typical nutrition intake
- Changes in bowel elimination
- Presence of discomfort: headache, muscle or joint pain, intolerance to cold
- Changes in sexual function:
  - (a) Women: changes in menses or libido, difficulty conceiving
  - (b) Men: changes in libido
- Knowledge level: dysfunction, diagnostic tests, treatment

#### Objective Data

Data are collected using a head-to-toe approach, with particular emphasis on the following systems. The nurse should assess the patient for signs of hypothyroidism:

- Mental status: intellectual functioning; memory; speech pattern; presence of somnolence, lethargy, or confusion
- Body weight and temperature
- Skin: pigmentation, temperature, presence of nonpitting edema
- Neck/hair: quality and quantity of head and body hair, thyroid examination
- Cardiovascular: pulse rate, blood pressure at rest and with exercise, heart size
- Respiratory: rate, breath sounds
- Abdomen: bowel sounds
- Motor: muscle strength, tone, and mass; ROM; deep tendon reflexes; joint movement

The first diagnostic studies ordered are $T_4$ level, free $T_4$ index, and TSH assay. In confirmed hypothyroidism, findings include:

1. Increased serum levels of TSH
2. Decreased $T_4$, $T_3$, free $T_4$, and free $T_4$ index

These tests may need to be repeated if findings are inconclusive, as discussed earlier.

To confirm Hashimoto's disease, test findings would include:

1. Presence of antithyroid antibodies
2. Chronic thyroiditis findings on pathology report of biopsy

### NURSING DIAGNOSES

Nursing diagnoses are determined from analysis of patient data. Nursing diagnoses for the person with hypothyroidism may include but are not limited to:

| Diagnostic Title | Possible Etiological Factors |
|---|---|
| Activity intolerance | Poor work capacity associated with poor cardiac function, decreased breathing capacity, and muscle stiffness |
| Body image disturbance | Change in appearance (weight gain, hair and skin changes), change in functioning (decreased mental and physical function) |
| Constipation | Decreased peristaltic action, decreased physical activity |
| Hypothermia | Decreased heat production associated with decreased metabolic rate |
| Knowledge deficit: disease, treatment, expected outcomes, self-monitoring, follow-up care | New interventions with no previous exposure to information |
| Nutrition, altered: more than body requirements | Decreased metabolic rate |
| Pain | Headache and joint pain associated with chronic thyroid problems |

| | |
|---|---|
| Self-care deficit, total (varies): bathing-hygiene, dressing-grooming, feeding, toileting | Inability to perform care associated with altered thought process and mental functioning |
| Sexual dysfunction | Alterations in menstrual cycle, ovulation, sperm production, and libido |
| Skin integrity, impaired | Mucinous deposits in skin, decreased circulation, immobility |
| Thought processes, impaired | Slowing of intellectual functions associated with chronic deficit of thyroid hormone |

## EXPECTED PATIENT OUTCOMES

Expected patient outcomes for the person with hypothyroidism may include but are not limited to:

1. Shows a gradual increase in activity tolerance over 2 to 3 months.
2. Relates body image changes to hypothyroidism and verbalizes that most changes are reversible.
3. Maintains a bowel pattern that was typical before onset of illness.
4. Maintains a body temperature of 36° to 37° C (96.8° to 98.6° F).
5. Patient and significant others are able to:
   a. Explain the disease in simple terms.
   b. Explain that treatment is lifelong drug therapy.
   c. Explain that treatment should reverse most signs and symptoms.
   d. Describe self-monitoring needs and planned follow-up.
6. Shows improvement in nutritional status, as evidenced by a gradual decrease in body weight.
7. States pain is controlled.
8. Meets self-care needs.
9. Understands that sexual function will increase as thyroid status returns to normal.
10. Has intact skin, as evidenced by no injuries and participation in decisions as much as possible.
11. Has no injuries and participates in decisions as much as possible, despite alteration in thought processes.

## INTERVENTIONS

The nursing interventions required by the patient with hypothyroidism vary greatly depending on the severity of disease.

### Providing Recuperative Care

Because the hypothyroid state is reversed slowly, the patient will not return to the premorbid health state for 2 to 3 months. Potential nursing interventions include:

1. Promote activity to the level of patient tolerance.
   a. At first the patient will have a very limited tolerance and may only be able to move around in the room. Activities should be increased gradually.
   b. Monitor the cardiovascular response to new activities. If the patient complains of chest pain or develops an unacceptable heart rate, stop the activity and then resume at a slower rate.
   c. Monitor blood pressure, pulse, and respirations before, during, and after each new activity.
2. Promote positive body image.
   a. Provide information that helps the patient and significant others understand the relationship of body changes to hypothyroidism.
   b. Educate about reversible body changes.
   c. Stress the positive changes that have occurred.
3. Promote normal bowel elimination.
   a. Monitor bowel elimination.
   b. Maintain adequate fluid intake.
   c. Increase bulk in the diet.
4. Treat hypothermia.
   a. Monitor temperature every 2 to 4 hours.
   b. Maintain an environmental temperature that is comfortable for the patient.
   c. Use blankets to increase body temperature if necessary.
5. Facilitate intake of a nutritional diet that is low in calories and includes food from all food groups.
6. Promote comfort.
   a. Use nonmedicinal comfort measures such as massage, cool or warm heat, and distraction to promote pain control.
   b. If medications are used, monitor the patient carefully. Patient will have a lower tolerance for sedative and depressant medications.
7. Provide for self-care needs. At first the patient may require complete care for hygiene, toileting, and dietary needs.
8. Facilitate patient's understanding of the relationship between the sexual problems and the hypothyroidism.
9. Maintain skin integrity.
   a. Monitor skin condition each shift.
   b. Institute preventive care measures such as sheepskin pads and soft sheets.
   c. If patient is unable to or does not turn by self, assist in turning every 2 hours.
10. Facilitate a safe environment and orientation to environment.
    a. Monitor neurological status every shift.
    b. Reorient the patient frequently, use resources such as current events, clocks, and newspapers.
    c. Maintain a safe environment: remove any clutter, keep bed low, and keep bed rails up.
    d. Check on patient frequently, especially at night, and use nightlights to prevent confusion.
    e. Inform significant others of relationship between mental status and hypothyroidism.
    f. Involve patient, as possible, in decisions about care.

### Patient/Family Education

The nurse helps the patient and family caregivers learn how to continue the plan of care after discharge. The importance of compliance with medications and follow-up care should be stressed. The teaching plan should include:

1. Nature of the disorder, diagnostic tests, and treatment; need for lifelong replacement therapy
2. Medications: dosage, method of administration, and side effects
3. Self-monitoring of vital signs, weight, skin integrity, and bowel function
4. Methods to prevent skin breakdown and constipation
5. Need for periods of rest alternating with activity
6. Need for continued follow-up care

The patient with a large goiter may need help with altered body image related to disfigurement. The goiter may be concealed by the use of scarves, high collars, and makeup. An open and trusting relationship is necessary so that the patient can share feelings and concerns.

### Health Promotion

Primary prevention of hypothyroidism is concerned with the prevention of iodine deficiency and its consequences. Iodine is necessary for proper growth and development of the brain of the fetus, infant, and child. Hypothyroidism from iodine deficiency is a global health problem and is recognized as the most important preventable cause of mental defects in the world. The World Health Organization estimates that more than 200 million people have goiter and 20 million have some degree of brain damage from the effects of iodine deficiency during pregnancy.[8]

People at risk for iodine deficiency live in geographic areas lacking iodine in soil and in the water supplies. In the United States the Great Lakes region is lacking in sufficient iodine. Foods grown in these areas also lack iodine. Public health measures can be used to increase iodine intake in diet through additives to salt, water, sauces, or oil. In the United States, iodized salt has been an effective means for reducing the incidence of goiter. Programs to educate the public about iodine intake and the use of iodized salt date from the 1920s.

Target populations for secondary prevention of hypothyroidism are newborn infants and persons older than age 60, especially women, and those persons with risk factors as listed in the box below. Screening of all newborns is done in the United States by the use of $T_4$ tests since symptoms of even severe hypothyroidism are seldom evident until the infant is several months old and irreversible damage has occurred. Prompt treatment of newborns with congenital deficiencies of thyroid hormone is necessary to prevent irreversible brain damage and dwarfism (cretinism).

**risk factors**

**Hypothyroidism**

History of thyroid disease
History of radiation to neck
Autoimmune disorders
Family history of thyroid disease
History of treatment with lithium, amiodarone, or iodine
Increased serum cholesterol

Screening of adults in clinics and hospitals can be done with either the serum assays of $T_4$ or TSH. The former test is less sensitive and less costly. Community-wide screening of older adults is rarely done because most hypothyroidism in older adults is subclinical, and there is no consensus about when to treat asymptomatic patients. Asymptomatic persons with elevated TSH and decreased $T_4$ serum levels should be followed and monitored at intervals.

Tertiary prevention includes iodide replacement in patients with iodine-deficient states and the administration of thyroid hormone to those with thyroid hormone deficiency. Efforts to increase compliance with thyroid hormone replacement drugs are important measures to prevent complications.

## EVALUATION

To evaluate the effectiveness of nursing interventions, compare patient behaviors with those stated in the expected patient outcomes. Successful achievement of patient outcomes for the person with hypothyroidism is indicated by:

1. Demonstrates increasing ability to ambulate and participate in ADL.
2. Attributes body changes to disease and its treatment.
3. Reports resumption of usual elimination patterns.
4. Maintains temperature between 36° and 37° C (96.8° to 98.6° F).
5. Patient and significant others accurately explain disease and need for lifelong intake of a thyroid drug even though symptoms will be alleviated.
6. Has weight decrease of no more than 2 kg/week (or by prescribed amount) after diuresis has occurred.
7. Reports absence of severe headache or joint pain.
8. Reports initiation and completion of increased number of self-care activities.
9. Explains how therapy should increase sexual function.
10. Has intact skin.
11. Experiences and reports no injuries.

## GERONTOLOGICAL CONSIDERATIONS

1. Assess for signs and symptoms of decreased alertness, decreased mobility, or increased susceptibility to cold, which may be signs and symptoms more typically noted with hypothyroidism in elderly persons.
2. Assess for signs of myxedema, as seen with untreated hypothyroidism.
3. Assess for signs of drug toxicity because of decreased metabolic activity from diminished endocrine function.
4. Assess for signs of infection because thymic activity is decreased.
5. Assist elderly patient to plan a way for remembering to take replacement therapy; without a plan, the apathetic patient may forget to take the thyroid hormone replacement.
6. Teach patient and significant others the following:
   a. Monitor for drug side effects.
   b. Report signs of angina or congestive heart failure, which may result from initial doses of thyroid hormone replacement.

c. Take precautions to avoid infections.
d. Take measures to prevent constipation, which often occurs with hypothyroidism, especially in elderly persons.

## SPECIAL ENVIRONMENTS FOR CARE

### Critical Care Management

Hypothyroid patients requiring intensive care are the rare patients with myxedema coma and those with respiratory failure and heart failure secondary to hypothyroidism. The most frequent cause of death in this population is respiratory failure. The mortality rate of patients with myxedema coma is very high because it occurs more often in older patients who have underlying vascular and pulmonary problems. Assessment and management priorities are focused on supporting respiratory and cardiac function.

Several factors seen in patients with severe hypothyroidism are significant in intensive care units:[18]

1. Respiratory function may be compromised by a large tongue and sleep apnea; respiratory effort may be decreased by hypoxic and hypercapneic ventilatory drives and respiratory muscle weakness.
2. Cardiac output is low as a result of bradycardia and a decrease in stroke volume; frank congestive heart failure usually occurs in patients who have an underlying cardiac disorder.
3. Metabolism of digoxin is slowed, so cardiac glycosides must be used cautiously.
4. Long-standing hypothyroidism can cause secondary adrenal insufficiency; stress doses of corticosteroids are recommended.
5. Early treatment of myxedema coma improves patient outcome. Myxedema coma is often a clinical diagnosis. Treatment often must start before laboratory test findings are conclusive.

Therapy for patients with myxedema coma includes supportive care (cardiovascular, respiratory, and fluid balance support), treatment of the underlying precipitating factor, and administration of thyroid hormone. Thyroid hormone is given intravenously. Usually, L-thyroxine, 2 μg/kg, is given as the initial dose, with an additional 100 μg every 24 hours. If adrenal insufficiency is known or suspected, plasma cortisol levels are measured. Treatment with hydrocortisone is started before the plasma cortisol levels are reported. Hydrocortisone (100 mg) is given intravenously and followed by doses of 50 mg every 6 hours. The dose is then tapered over 1 week. If the plasma cortisol levels are 20 μg/dl or greater, hydrocortisone is tapered sooner.[7] The patient is kept warm enough to avoid additional heat loss without overwarming to avoid vascular collapse. Tracheal intubation and mechanical ventilation may be necessary. Improvement is seen in 3 to 24 hours.

Nursing interventions include care of the comatose patient; surveillance of respiratory, cardiovascular, and fluid status; care of the patient with respiratory insufficiency; preventive care for problems of immobility; and assistance with the institution of the medical regimen.

### Home Care Management

Family involvement is usually necessary to ensure appropriate care and compliance with the therapeutic regimen in the elderly patient with myxedema. Fatigue may necessitate rearrangement of the home environment to avoid stair climbing until the patient regains endurance. A bedside commode can be obtained if the bathroom is a significant distance from the patient's room.

## COMPLICATIONS

Myxedema coma is a life-threatening complication of hypothyroidism (see p. 1084). Severe hypothyroidism is associated with respiratory failure, usually in the presence of myxedema coma. Chronic hypothyroidism may also result in cardiovascular disease. The patient should be monitored for any manifestations of heart disease and taught lifestyle changes (diet, exercise, smoking cessation, and maintenance of ideal weight) to decrease the risk of development of cardiovascular disease (see Chapter 25). Any symptoms of chest pain or difficulty breathing should be reported to the health care provider immediately.

Because the need for thyroid replacement is lifelong, the patient should be taught to recognize the signs and symptoms of hyperthyroidism, which may occur as a result of hormone replacement. The need for medical supervision and follow-up care is also lifelong.

## CANCER OF THE THYROID GLAND

### Etiology/Epidemiology

Cancer of the thyroid is less prevalent than other forms of cancer, and only a very small percentage of thyroid neoplasms are malignant (1% of invasive neoplasms).

Thyroid nodules occur in 4% of the population. One of 1000 nodules is malignant. The incidence of malignancy in nodules is much higher in children (50%) and the elderly. The female/male ratio of malignancy is 4:1. A history of radiation to the thyroid in amounts of 6.5 to 2000 rad is linked with a 7% incidence of thyroid cancer.[7,8] Papillary carcinoma accounts for 65% of thyroid malignancies[7,8] and is linked with radiation exposure. Thyroid lymphomas usually occur after 50 years and comprise 8% of thyroid cancers.

### Pathophysiology

Two general types of malignant neoplasms are found: those arising from follicular epithelium (papillary, follicular, medullary, and anaplastic) and those arising from parafollicular tissue. Non-Hodgkin's lymphomas can also develop in thyroid tissue. Table 34-9 presents characteristics for the five forms of primary malignant neoplasms of the thyroid.

### Collaborative Care Management

#### *Diagnostic tests*

Diagnosis of thyroid cancer has been simplified by the acceptance of fine-needle biopsy in obtaining tissue samples from solid tumors or fluid from cysts. Biopsy is most reliable for detecting papillary cancers and less reliable for detecting follicular cancers and other types; therefore

**table 34-9** *Characteristics of the Five Types of Thyroid Cancer*

| Characteristics | Cancers of Follicular Epithelium: Papillary | Follicular | Anaplastic | Thyroid Lymphoma | Cancer of Parafollicular Tissue: Medullary |
|---|---|---|---|---|---|
| Incidence of all thyroid cancers | 65% | 20% | 5% | 5% | 5% |
| Age | Young persons | After 40 | After 60 | After 40 | After 50 |
| Female/male ratio | 2-3:1 | 2-3:1 | F > M | F > M | F = M |
| Metastasis | By intraglandular lymphatics; slow-growing tumor | By blood vessels to distant sites (bone, lung, liver); occurs early | By direct invasion to adjacent structures; highly malignant | By lymphatic system; gland fixed to other structures | By intraglandular lymphatics and blood vessels |
| Prognosis | Good; rarely causes death in young persons if occult or intrathyroidal | Good if minimally invasive lesion | Prognosis varies with cell type; for giant cell, very poor (<6 months from diagnosis); for small cell, better (5-year survival rate of 20-50%) | Good | Moderate; 10-year survival is estimated as 2 of 3 persons |
| Symptoms | Asymptomatic | Goiter may have been present for years | Hoarseness, inspiratory stridor, pain, dysphagia (signs of invasion of adjacent areas) | May have long history of previous goiter; rapid enlargement of goiter, hoarseness, dysphagia, pressure sensation, dyspnea, some pain | Because tumor produces hormones, possible paraendocrine manifestations such as carcinoid syndrome, watery diarrhea, Cushing's syndrome |
| Tumor | Occult (<1.5 cm in diameter), intrathyroidal (>1.5 cm in diameter but does not extend through thyroid surface), and extrathyroidal (extends through thyroid surface); well differentiated; psammoma body found in 40% of tumors and virtually diagnostic of malignant nature; tumors appear as "cold" spots on thyroid scan | Well differentiated to poorly differentiated; cyst formation and calcification possible; tumors may appear as "hot" areas on thyroid scan | Two cell forms: giant cell and small cell | Usually of nodular histocytic form | Tumor of C cells of thyroid; not encapsulated; some appear as "cold" spots on thyroid scan; may produce ACTH, prostaglandin, or carcinoembryonic antigen |

*Continued*

follow-up open biopsy is done if pathological analysis is inconclusive. This procedure can be done in the office and allows earlier detection of malignancy. Many factors are now being studied to develop a consensus on the staging classification of thyroid malignancy. (See Chapter 11 for principles related to diagnosis, staging, and treatment of all malignancies.)

Three tests help differentiate benign and malignant nodules. Briefly, radionuclide imaging is based on the concept that cancer cells do not concentrate iodine and thus are labeled as "cold" on scans. Only 20% of "cold" nodules seen on thyroid scans are malignant. Ultrasound aids in differentiating cystic nodules (usually benign) from solid nodules. Thyroid suppression tests reveal whether the nodule decreases in size; if so,

**table 34-9** *Characteristics of the Five Types of Thyroid Cancer—cont'd*

| Characteristics | Cancers of Follicular Epithelium | | | Thyroid Lymphoma | Cancer of Parafollicular Tissue |
|---|---|---|---|---|---|
| | Papillary | Follicular | Anaplastic | | Medullary |
| Other | Growth partially dependent on TSH; thyroid hormone can cause regression of metastatic lesions; $^{131}$I may be used for nonresectable lesions; may have history of radiation therapy to head and neck | Suppressive thyroid therapy can cause regression of metastatic lesions; radiation therapy with $^{131}$I may be used when vascular invasion or metastasis present | — | Strong association with Hashimoto's thyroiditis; may have lymphoma at other sites | Occurs as a familial form as part of multiple endocrine neoplasia (MEN) type IIa or MEN IIb; in MEN IIa, there is medullary carcinoma, adrenomedullary hyperplasia, or bilateral pheochromocytomas and hyperparathyroidism; in MEN IIb, there is medullary carcinoma, bilateral pheochromocytomas, and an unusual phenotype with ganglioneuromas of eyelids, oral mucosa, tongue, and labia, marfanoid habitus; skeletal abnormalities; also occurs as a non-MEN familial form |

it is likely to be benign. Serum calcitonin and carcinoembryonic antigens may be measured and may be high in some patients with medullary carcinoma. Serum TSH levels are used as the first test to determine thyroid function. Most patients with thyroid cancer are euthyroid.

### Medications

Thyroid hormone is prescribed for replacement therapy and to suppress further cellular growth. Ablation therapy with radioactive iodine ($^{131}$I) is used primarily for epithelial tumors. The dosage depends upon the individual patient and tumor size. $^{131}$I therapy is frequently used after total thyroidectomy for follicular carcinoma. Chemotherapy, usually Adriamycin, is used to treat anaplastic thyroid cancer and for thyroid lymphomas.

### Treatments/surgical management

Medical management of persons with thyroid cancer includes use of all modalities of cancer treatment: surgery, radiation, hormonal suppression, and chemotherapy. For occult papillary cancer, treatment consists of lobectomy and isthmectomy followed by thyroid hormone suppression therapy (thyroid hormone preparation to suppress TSH). For extrathyroidal papillary carcinoma and invasive follicular carcinoma, total thyroidectomy followed by $^{131}$I therapy is frequently used. Removal of the entire thyroid gland in follicular carcinoma increases the effectiveness of treatment of distant metastasis with $^{131}$I. Follicular cancer does trap iodine but not nearly as well as normal thyroid tissue. A total thyroidectomy allows the metastatic tissue to trap the iodine without competition.

Treatment of intrathyroidal papillary carcinoma and noninvasive follicular carcinoma is more controversial. Some authorities recommend the conservative approach used for occult papillary carcinoma, and others recommend the approach used for extrathyroidal papillary and invasive follicular carcinoma.[7,8] For both papillary and follicular cancer, the involved lymph nodes are resected during surgery. Also, these patients may be seen every 2 to 3 months, and any recurrence is treated with $^{131}$I therapy. Suppressive thyroid hormone therapy and $^{131}$I therapy are frequently used.

Anaplastic thyroid cancer may be treated aggressively with surgery, radiation therapy, and chemotherapy. However, in many cases the cancer is too far advanced and only palliative surgery is done.[7,8]

Thyroid lymphoma usually is treated using radiation and chemotherapy; however, very small lymphomas may be treated surgically. Medullary carcinoma is treated with total thyroidectomy. These tumors do not respond to $^{131}$I therapy or thyroid hormone suppression. Recurrence and metastatic lesions have been treated with surgery and sometimes radiation therapy. Calcitonin levels can be used to monitor recurrence.

For some patients with certain tumors and lymph node involvement, a modified radical neck dissection is recommended. (See Chapter 31 for a discussion of neck dissection.)

## NURSING MANAGEMENT

Care of the patient with a thyroid nodule first focuses on helping the patient through the diagnostic process. Thyroid nodules occur frequently, and most are not cancerous. No one diagnostic test is completely reliable. Depending on patient characteristics and physician philosophy, various tests may be performed. The nurse prepares the patient for each test, focusing particularly on education.

### PREOPERATIVE CARE

The patient having thyroid surgery needs care focused on producing and maintaining a euthyroid state (see earlier sections on hyperthyroidism or hypothyroidism), if this is not already present. Patients with both hyperthyroidism and hypothyroidism have been treated medically for varying lengths of time to induce the euthyroid state, and this care must be continued. Because patients who have recently experienced alteration in thyroid hormone levels may have an altered nutritional status, extra attention should be paid to promoting and maintaining positive nitrogen balance.

The patient with previous abnormal thyroid hormone levels may still be having difficulty coping effectively. The patient with a diagnosis of cancer may be experiencing a major disruption in coping because of that diagnosis. Therefore the patient who is to have thyroid surgery requires a nonstressful environment (quiet room and calm, relaxed approach by staff). General measures to induce relaxation, such as back rubs, a consistent nurse, and a consistent schedule should be included in patient care.

Patient teaching regarding general preoperative and postoperative care (see Chapters 18 and 20) is given. The patient also needs to learn how to cough and to move the head and neck postoperatively without placing strain on the suture line. Thus the patient is taught preoperatively to support the neck by placing both hands behind the neck when moving the head or when coughing.

### POSTOPERATIVE CARE

Immediate interventions for postoperative care are listed in the Guidelines for Care Box. In addition to routine monitoring, the patient is checked for major complications that can occur after thyroid surgery: recurrent laryngeal nerve injury, hemorrhage, tetany, and respiratory obstruction. Signs of these complications are reported immediately to the surgeon. Although the signs of laryngeal nerve damage may be related to intubation during surgery, such hoarseness should clear

**guidelines for care**

**The Person After Thyroid Surgery**

1. Monitor for and report signs of complications.
   a. Laryngeal nerve damage; hoarseness, weak voice
   b. Hemorrhage or tissue swelling
      (1) Bleeding on dressing: check back of dressing by slipping hand gently under neck and shoulders
      (2) Choking sensation
      (3) Difficulty in coughing or swallowing
      (4) Sensation of dressing being too tight even after it is loosened
   c. Calcium deficiency (tetany)
      (1) Early signs: tingling around mouth or of toes and fingers, decreasing serum calcium levels
      (2) Later signs: positive Chvostek's and Trousseau's signs (see Chapter 15), grand mal seizures
   d. Respiratory distress associated with any of signs just listed
2. Provide emergency care.
   a. Keep emergency supplies readily available:
      (1) Tracheostomy set (for laryngeal nerve damage), oxygen and suction equipment, suture removal set (for respiratory obstruction from hemorrhage)
      (2) IV calcium gluconate or calcium chloride (for tetany)
   b. For acute respiratory distress:
      (1) Call for immediate medical help.
      (2) Raise head of bed.
      (3) Loosen dressing over incision.
      (4) Give calcium as ordered, if signs and symptoms of tetany are present.
      (5) If loosening the dressing does not relieve symptoms of respiratory distress and if medical help is not readily available, remove clips or sutures as instructed.
3. Provide comfort.
   a. Avoid tension on suture lines; encourage patient to support head when turning by placing both hands behind neck.
   b. Give prescribed analgesics as necessary.
4. Maintain nutritional status.
   a. Start soft foods as soon as tolerated (only fluids may be tolerated initially).
   b. Encourage a high-carbohydrate, high-protein diet.
5. Teach patient:
   a. ROM exercises to neck when suture line is healed to prevent permanent limitations
   b. Need for lifelong thyroid hormone replacement therapy after a total thyroidectomy
   c. Any special care measures related to the underlying disease
   d. Need for follow-up care

gradually. If hoarseness persists or worsens, it is reported immediately to the surgeon. Hoarseness may be a first sign of laryngeal nerve damage, which can result in vocal cord spasm and respiratory obstruction. An emergency tracheostomy may be necessary, and equipment for this should be available on the nursing unit.

The patient is monitored for hemorrhage for the first 12 to 24 hours postoperatively. Hemorrhage can result in incisional bleeding or in compression of the trachea or surrounding tissue. If hemorrhage causes compression, the patient will complain of signs of respiratory distress. If these signs should occur and if loosening of the dressing does not relieve respiratory distress, the physician or his or her designee may need to remove surgical clips or sutures. The patient may have to be taken back to surgery for ligation of the blood vessels and wound closure.

Although the occurrence of tetany is minimal, the parathyroid glands can be injured during surgery, or inflammation may block the normal release of parathyroid hormone. If the level of parathyroid hormone drops, symptoms of calcium deficiency can occur. If not treated promptly, calcium deficiency can result in contraction of the glottis, respiratory obstruction, and death. Tetany may appear from 1 to 7 days postoperatively. Treatment for calcium deficiency is calcium chloride or calcium gluconate given intravenously. Oral calcium is then necessary until normal parathyroid function returns.

The nurse must know that respiratory obstruction can occur from (1) recurrent laryngeal nerve damage causing vocal cord spasms that close off the larynx, (2) tracheal compression from hemorrhage, (3) tissue swelling, or (4) tetany. The nurse should be prepared to manage all these problems.

A patient who had surgery for hyperthyroidism, although treated to promote a euthyroid state before surgery, requires extra monitoring of cardiovascular and respiratory status after surgery to assist in early identification of any problems caused by the hyperthyroid state. During surgery with manipulation of the gland, extra hormone can be released, and this may precipitate a thyroid storm or crisis. If a total thyroidectomy was done, the patient needs to be monitored for signs of hypothyroidism (see p.1084), and replacement therapy should be started postoperatively.

## GERONTOLOGICAL CONSIDERATIONS

Thyroid nodules have been identified in 5% of persons older than age 60 years, and 90% of these nodules are found to be benign. The elderly person awaiting biopsy results will need emotional support during the time until diagnosis is final. The elderly person will need special consideration when undergoing surgical intervention (see Chapters 18 through 20).

## SPECIAL ENVIRONMENTS FOR CARE

### Critical Care Management

The person recovering from thyroidectomy or thyroid resection will only need intensive nursing care if complications such as hemorrhage or respiratory distress develop. The patient may require invasive monitoring to adequately assess fluid volume and cardiac status or may require ventilator support.

## COMPLICATIONS

As mentioned earlier, hemorrhage and respiratory distress are complications after thyroid surgery. Other complications associated with the procedure or anesthesia may occur (see Chapter 19). If hemorrhage occurs, the patient may have to be taken back to the operating room for ligation of bleeding vessels. In patients with severe respiratory distress, intubation for long-term ventilation or tracheostomy may be necessary (see Chapter 32).

# PARATHYROID GLAND

## HYPERSECRETION OF PARATHYROID HORMONE: PRIMARY HYPERPARATHYROIDISM

### Etiology

Primary hyperparathyroidism (PHPT) is being diagnosed with increased frequency because of the more frequent routine measurements of serum calcium levels.[13] An elevated serum calcium level is the key clinical feature of PHPT.

The most frequent cause of PHPT is benign adenomas (80% of persons), although hyperplasia and malignant tumors may also be causes. The cause of adenomas, hyperplasia, or malignant tumors is not known, but a history of earlier radiation of the neck has been reported in some patients.[1,13] There is no evidence that postmenopausal estrogen causes tumors of the parathyroid gland; however, it may unmask the effects of preexisting tumors.[1]

It is postulated that the "set point" at which ionized calcium inhibits parathyroid gland tissue may be increased so that the normal negative feedback control between calcium and parathyroid gland function is lost. A genetic component is present in some patients who have PHPT as part of the syndrome of multiple endocrine neoplasia, type I (MEN I) (PHPT is associated with islet cell tumors and pituitary adenoma) or part of MEN IIa (PHPT is associated with medullary thyroid carcinoma and pheochromocytoma).

### Epidemiology

PHPT is seen most frequently in women older than age 40 and is found in 2% of white women older than age 60. The incidence increases after age 50 in both men and women but is 2 to 4 times more common in women. Elderly women are at an increased risk. Routine testing of serum calcium levels has increased the identification of the disorder, particularly in asymptomatic persons. Most patients are asymptomatic or have mild symptoms of malaise, muscle weakness, and mental depression; they may have hypertension and mild osteoporosis. Before routine calcium screening, the typical picture was that of a patient with severe hypercalcemia, bone pain, and renal stones.

### Pathophysiology

The alteration in physiological functioning associated with PHPT is the result of one or two major problems:

1. The exaggeration of the normal effects of parathyroid hormone (PTH) on the skeletal, renal, and gastrointestinal (GI) systems
2. The associated hypercalcemia

The primary function of PTH is the maintenance of a normal serum level of calcium. Hypersecretion of PTH results in continual stimulation of target organs and elevates serum calcium. The normal negative feedback of serum calcium on PTH secretion is lost or ineffective. Increased PTH (1) increases bone resorption, (2) enhances the reabsorption of calcium from the glomerular filtrate, and (3) increases calcium absorption through the GI tract.

In the skeletal system, increased PTH increases bone resorption, resulting in osteopenia and, in very severe cases, cysts and fractures from osteitis fibrosa cystica. Joint changes also occur. In the renal system, increased PTH enhances the reabsorption of calcium from the glomerular filtrate, reabsorption of phosphate, and alteration in the excretion of bicarbonate. Production of activated vitamin D increases. Elevated PTH effects on the GI tract are indirect and occur through the action of vitamin D. The activated vitamin D results in increased calcium absorption through the GI tract.

The processes just described result in elevated serum calcium, which in itself leads to neurological, musculoskeletal, cardiac, GI, and renal alterations. The alterations in the various systems caused by hypercalcemia result in most of the clinical manifestations. The relationship between the pathophysiology of hyperparathyroidism and the clinical manifestations is presented in Table 34-10.

Because calcitonin from the C cells of the thyroid opposes the effect of PTH, it would be logical to assume that in response to the increased serum calcium, calcitonin secretion would increase. This is not seen in PHPT.

## Collaborative Care Management

### *Diagnostic tests*

An increased serum PTH level and persistent hypercalcemia are criteria for establishing the diagnosis of PHPT; other causes of hypercalcemia (Box 34-11) and increased

**table 34-10** *Hypersecretion of Parathyroid Hormone: Normal Function, Primary Pathophysiological Factors, and Clinical Manifestations*

| Normal Function | Pathophysiological Factors | Clinical Manifestations |
|---|---|---|
| Maintenance of normal serum calcium | Hypersecretion, continual stimulation of target organs | Increased serum calcium |
| Regulates bone resorption of calcium | Increased bone resorption resulting in osteopenia, cysts, and fractures (osteitis fibrosa cystica); bone formation increased but less than resorption | Bone pain, arthralgia, osteopenia |
| Regulates reabsorption of calcium from glomerular filtrate | Early in disease, hypocalciuria in response to increased blood calcium level; later, hypercalciuria as reabsorptive capacity is overwhelmed | Early, hypocalciuria; later, hypercalciuria and polyuria, polydipsia, urinary calculi, renal failure |
| Regulates phosphate and bicarbonate excretion in kidney tubule | Ineffective bicarbonate reabsorption and phosphate clearance | Hyperchloremic acidosis: anorexia, nausea, vomiting |
| Regulates calcium absorption in intestines; influenced by estrogen in women and activated vitamin D (1,25-dihydroxycholecalciferol, calcitriol) | Increased calcium absorption from intestines adds to hypercalcemia; increased gastrin secretion, increased calcitriol production | Hypercalcemia: possible peptic ulcer and pancreatitis |
| | | *Neuromuscular* |
| Calcium regulates pores of cell membranes, movement of sodium, and thus depolarization and resultant action potential in nerves and muscles | Hypercalcemia blocks cell membrane permeability and depresses nerve and muscle activity | Impaired mentation, apathy, lethargy, somnolence, coma, hypoactive reflexes, fasciculation of tongue, muscle weakness/aches (lower limbs more than upper) |
| | | *Cardiovascular* |
| | Depresses activity of cardiac muscle | Electrocardiographic changes: shortened QT intervals, dysrhythmias, hypertension |
| | | *Gastrointestinal* |
| | Slows intestinal motility | Anorexia, nausea and vomiting, constipation |

serum PTH must be ruled out. Another disorder (e.g., malignancy) may coexist with PHPT. Table 34-11 gives details of tests typically performed in parathyroid diseases. In addition to these tests, the physician studies x-rays of the renal and skeletal systems for evidence of PHPT complications, including urine stones, changes in bone density, and cysts or signs of demineralization in bone. If the patient is severely hypercalcemic, treatment is started before findings of most tests are received.

The control of elevated calcium levels is the first priority of treatment. Although the upper limits of blood calcium levels are 10.1 to 10.4 mg/dl (or those established by a laboratory), aggressive treatment may not be instituted until the patient becomes symptomatic or the calcium levels are 13 mg/dl or higher. The immediate treatment is normal saline infusion to ensure adequate hydration, lower serum calcium concentration, and to promote calcium clearance in the kidney tubule. In addition, the excretion of sodium enhances excretion of calcium. Patients often have a history of anorexia, nausea, and vomiting and thus are hypovolemic and require fluid replacement.

### Medications

Loop diuretics (furosemide or ethacrynic acid) are given intravenously or orally. Drugs that increase serum calcium (e.g., thiazides) are avoided. In a severe crisis, more potent anticalcemic drugs may be used. These increase urinary excretion of calcium, as do the loop diuretics, and they also inhibit bone resorption and/or intestinal absorption of calcium. Anticalcemic agents are toxic drugs, and their use is limited to one or two doses, if possible.

Plicamycin, a cytotoxic neoplastic agent, is also a very potent hypocalcemic agent. It acts as a vitamin D antagonist, inhibiting the action of parathyroid hormone on osteoclasts. Edetate disodium is a chelating agent, binding calcium in the blood so that the resultant complexes can be excreted in the urine. Nephrotoxicity has limited its use. Calcitonin (salmon) and dexamethasone are other choices of treatment, but their effectiveness is limited in PHPT. Dexamethasone is particularly effective in treating hypercalcemia related to bone malignancy.

**box 34-11** *Causes of Hypercalcemia (Other Than Hyperparathyroidism)*

- Malignancy
- Leukemia, lymphoma, multiple myeloma
- Vitamin D intoxication
- Hypervitaminosis A
- Granulomatous diseases
- Other endocrine disorders: thyrotoxicosis, adrenal insufficiency
- Milk-alkali syndrome
- Immobilization

**table 34-11** *Diagnostic Tests for Parathyroid Function*

| TEST | PROCEDURE | INTERPRETATION |
|---|---|---|
| **SERUM** | | |
| Total calcium 9.6-10.4 mg/dl | Blood sample | Measures both bound and ionized calcium; increased in PHPT; decreased in hypoparathyroidism or with low albumin |
| Phosphorus 2.8-4.5 mg/dl | Blood sample | Decreased with hypercalcemia and elevated in hypocalcemia and renal failure |
| Alkaline phosphatase 2-5 Bodansky units | Blood sample | Increased in bone demineralization and liver disease, and by certain drugs |
| PTH by radioimmunoassay | Blood sample | Elevated in hyperparathyroidism and decreased in hypoparathyroidism |
| **URINE** | | |
| Calcium | Collect single specimen | Decreased in hypoparathyroidism |
| Quantitative | 24-hour collection | Elevated in hyperparathyroidism |
| Phosphorus | 24-hour collection | Elevated in hypocalcemic states and PTH excess; decreased with PTH lack and renal failure |
| **FUNCTION TESTS** | | |
| Ellsworth-Howard excretion test (PTH infusion test) | Fasting required; 200 units of PTH extract administered IV; hourly urine collections | Normal response is 5-6 times increased urinary phosphate excretion; an increase of 10 times is found in hypoparathyroidism |
| Urinary cyclic adenosine monophosphate (cAMP) | Urine sample | High levels of AMP found in hyperparathyroidism |

In PHPT, serum phosphate levels are usually low. In this type of hypercalcemia, phosphates may be used as anticalcemic agents; however, caution is necessary. Phosphates lower serum calcium levels by inhibiting bone resorption, and if an acute elevation of serum phosphate occurs, calcium phosphate salts precipitate. Extensive precipitation of calcium phosphate salts can result in hypocalcemia, renal stones, and renal failure. Cautious use of phosphates includes oral rather than IV administration; careful monitoring of blood urea nitrogen (BUN), serum calcium, and phosphate levels; and monitoring for signs of hypocalcemia and renal stones. If medications are not effective or not appropriate for a particular patient, severe hypercalcemia can be treated by dialysis.

Once anticalcemic drug therapy is initiated, the high infusion rate of sodium chloride must be maintained. Electrolytes are replaced as necessary, and serum calcium, potassium, magnesium, and phosphate levels are monitored.

#### Treatments

Once the diagnosis has been made and hypercalcemia treated, options for treating PHPT are considered. Although surgical removal of the parathyroid glands is the therapy of choice, some controversy surrounds the selection of patients for surgery.[1,4] The issues involve whether to offer surgery to the asymptomatic patient or to the one who has mild symptoms and slight elevations of serum calcium.

Medical management, as an alternative to surgery, consists of continuing hydration, administration of the loop diuretics, replacement of electrolytes, and administration of sodium chloride, 300 to 400 mEq/24 hr. Patient follow-up is necessary to monitor serum calcium levels for worsening hypercalcemia and the onset of renal or bony lesions. Use of an anticalcemic agent sometimes is necessary. Medical management may be the only treatment used in patients who are not suitable candidates for surgery.

#### Surgical management

Before surgical intervention for hyperparathyroidism, abnormal parathyroid glands must be localized by one or more of the following tests: CT, ultrasound, radiothallium scanning, or MRI. The definitive treatment for primary hyperparathyroidism is surgery. The goal is to restore normal parathyroid function and avoid hypercalcemia or hypocalcemia. The amount of parathyroid tissue removed depends upon the appearance of each of the glands. If one or two enlarged glands are found, they are removed and the normal sized glands remain. If all four glands are enlarged, a subtotal parathyroidectomy (3½ glands) is performed.[4,13]

#### Diet

In the past, a calcium-restricted diet was ordered for patients with PHPT who were treated medically. At present, not all physicians prescribe low-calcium diets; some believe these diets reduce urinary excretion of calcium and should not be used.[10]

#### Activity

Activity is not restricted unless the patient has severe hypercalcemia and/or pathological bone conditions. In fact, maintaining activity is advised because stress on long bones helps reduce calcium resorption.

#### Referrals

Careful assessment should be made of the patient's and/or family caregiver's ability to manage the therapeutic regimen at home and to continue with required follow-up care. Appropriate referrals might include home nursing, physical therapy, and social services.

## NURSING MANAGEMENT

### ASSESSMENT

#### Subjective Data

Nursing assessment includes identifying the presence of signs and symptoms of hyperparathyroidism and the resultant hypercalcemia. Data to be collected to assess the patient with PHPT include:

- Mental status: history of change in mentation, personality, or alertness
- Skeletal system: presence of bone or joint pain
- Renal system
  - Changes in urine output, particularly polyuria or nocturia
  - Symptoms of renal colic or pyelonephritis
- GI system
  - Normal 24-hour intake
  - Symptoms of anorexia, nausea, vomiting
  - Changes in bowel elimination
- Neuromuscular system
  - Symptoms of fatigue or weakness
  - Changes in ability to carry out ADL
  - Presence of pruritus
  - Presence or absence of flank pain

#### Objective Data

Data to be collected to assess the patient with PHPT include:

- Mental status: short-term memory, affect, alertness, orientation
- Skeletal system: ROM, presence of excessive immobility
- Renal system: urine output, characteristics of urine
- GI system: fluid/food intake, bowel movements, bowel sounds, weight
- Neuromuscular system: muscle strength, peripheral sensory function, reflexes
- Cardiovascular system: blood pressure, pulse (rhythm, rate), electrocardiogram (ECG)

Results of tests indicative of PHPT include the following:

1. Laboratory tests
   a. Blood: elevated serum calcium, decreased serum phosphate, elevated PTH levels
   b. Urinary: elevated urinary cyclic adenosine monophosphate (cAMP)

2. Radiographic: abnormalities particularly noticeable in the phalanges, e.g., cysts or demineralization
3. Radiographic: renal abnormalities such as calculi

## ■ NURSING DIAGNOSES

Nursing diagnoses are determined from analysis of patient data. Nursing diagnoses for the person with PHPT may include but are not limited to:

| Diagnostic Title | Possible Etiological Factors |
|---|---|
| **For Patients Treated Medically on Long-Term Basis and Acutely Before Surgery** | |
| Injury (trauma), risk for | Muscular weakness, altered mental status, bone demineralization |
| Cardiac output, decreased | Dysrhythmias associated with altered electrical conduction |
| Pain | Bone changes, joint changes, potential renal colic and pruritus |
| Urinary elimination pattern, altered | Polyuria |
| Activity intolerance | Muscular weakness, decreased cardiac output associated with changes in electrical activity of heart |
| Nutrition, altered: less than body requirements | Anorexia, nausea, vomiting |
| Constipation | Decrease in GI motility |
| **For Patients After Surgery** | |
| Breathing pattern, ineffective | Tracheal obstruction associated with spasm of vocal cords or hemorrhage, laryngeal stridor associated with low serum calcium level, intraoperative laryngeal nerve damage, edema |
| Injury (trauma), risk for | Hemorrhage, increased neuromuscular excitability associated with low serum calcium level |
| Knowledge deficit: follow-up care after surgery | No previous exposure to information |

## ■ EXPECTED PATIENT OUTCOMES

Expected patient outcomes for the patient with PHPT include but are not limited to the following.

### For Patients Treated Medically on Long-Term Basis and Acutely Before Surgery

1. Reports no injuries; falls or dislodged arterial lines do not occur.
2. Maintains cardiac output, as evidenced by stable blood pressure; dysrhythmias or electrocardiogram (ECG) changes are detected.
3. States that pain reduction measures are effective; activities or self-care is not limited because of pain; signs of renal colic (bloody urine, pain, nausea) do not occur.
4. Output equals intake and is at least 2000 ml/day.
5. Activity level does not decrease; gradually increases activity, as evidenced by more ambulation.
6. Maintains normal nutritional status, as evidenced by maintenance of weight or, if necessary, a return to normal weight, with a gain of 1 to 2 lb/wk; the patient eats 75% to 100% of every meal.
7. Maintains normal patterns of bowel elimination (as established by assessment).

### For Patients After Surgery

1a. Maintains patent airway with clear breath sounds. No signs of respiratory distress, pulse oximetry and ABG values within normal limits.

b. Vital signs are within patient's normal range.

2. Is free from injury.
3. Verbalizes knowledge of treatment, expected outcomes, and plan for follow-up care.

## ■ INTERVENTIONS

Care of the patient depends on the treatment. This section describes the care during the acute preoperative period for patients treated medically. Nursing management of the postoperative patient is discussed at the end of this section.

### Promoting Safety

PHPT may increase the likelihood of the patient being injured in a fall because of weakness or because of changes in mental status. If altered mental functioning is present, patients are placed in an environment where they can be observed closely, measures to increase orientation are used, and side rails are kept up. Soft restraints may be necessary but should be the last alternative.

If weakness is a factor, the patient must be assisted when up, have nonskid slippers for ambulation, and be provided with a room that is free of unnecessary equipment. A gradual increase in activity or the incorporation of isometric exercise may increase endurance. A physical therapist may be helpful in planning an exercise strengthening program.

### Maintaining Cardiac Function

Hypercalcemia associated with PHPT presents a risk for decreased cardiac functioning. The patient is monitored frequently (every 2 to 4 hours) to detect early signs and is instructed to report any episodes of palpitations or vertigo. If dysfunction occurs, the patient may need to have continuous cardiac monitoring. The patient receiving digitalis therapy is monitored closely for digitalis toxicity because the myocardium is unusually sensitive to digitalis in the presence of hypercalcemia. The dose may be decreased.

### Promoting Comfort

The exact cause of patient discomfort must be identified. If bone or joint pain is present, proper positioning, support of joints and body parts, and gentleness in moving the patient are required. If renal colic is the cause of pain, the pain is severe and narcotics are necessary for relief; their effectiveness must be documented. Measures are taken to relieve pruritus as necessary (see Chapter 63); antihistamines or mild tranquilizers may be required.

### Promoting Urinary Elimination

The first intervention for alteration in urinary elimination is to increase the patient's fluid intake. Increased fluid intake decreases the urinary mineral concentration and thus decreases urinary stone formation. A fluid intake of at least 3 L/day should be the goal unless other physiological alterations such as cardiac or renal problems are present. Fluids are given throughout the 24 hours. The urine is strained through a gauze mesh to collect any small stones that pass, and the patient is monitored continually for recurrence of stone formation (see Chapter 44). Monitoring includes assessing intake and output and observing for the presence of flank pain from renal colic, hematuria, and nausea and vomiting.

### Promoting Activity

The patient with PHPT may have activity intolerance and needs to be involved in some weight-bearing activities that provide bone stress and help lower serum calcium levels. Thus a schedule of progressive activities is planned with the patient. Activities are spaced so fatigue is lessened. Goals should be established collaboratively with the patient to provide motivation and to increase activities gradually. The patient may need help bathing and with ADL.

### Promoting Nutrition

The patient is advised to avoid foods high in calcium (Box 34-12) to prevent hypercalcemia. The nurse should note that very few groups of food are high in calcium. Anorexia is often present, and measures such as environmental control of noxious stimuli, encouraging rest, and providing oral hygiene are taken to promote nutrition.

**box 34-12** *Foods High in Calcium*

| Food | Calcium |
|---|---|
| Almonds | 332 mg/1 cup |
| Blackstrap molasses | 137 mg/1 tbsp |
| Brazil nuts | 260 mg/1 cup |
| Broccoli spears | 132 mg/1 cup |
| Cabbage (cooked) | 220 mg/1 cup |
| Canned mackerel | 221 mg/3 oz |
| Cheese (blue cheese, cheddar, American) | About 100 to 150 mg/1 oz |
| Collard greens (cooked) | 289 mg/1 cup |
| Custard | 280 mg/1 cup |
| Dandelion greens (cooked) | 252 mg/1 cup |
| Egg | 27 mg/1 egg |
| Green beans | 80 mg/1 cup |
| Ice cream | 175 mg/1 cup |
| Ice milk | 292 mg/1 cup |
| Kale (cooked) | 147 mg/1 cup |
| Lima beans | 75 mg/1 cup |
| Macaroni (enriched) and cheese, baked | 398 mg/1 cup |
| Milk (whole, 2%, skim, buttermilk) | 290 mg/1 cup |
| Mustard greens (cooked) | 193 mg/1 cup |
| Oranges | 50 mg/1 orange |
| Oysters | 226 mg/1 cup |
| Peanut halves | 107 mg/1 cup |
| Pizza (cheese) | 107 mg/1 slice |
| Raisins | 124 mg/1 cup |
| Rhubarb (cooked) | 212 mg/1 cup |
| Salmon, pink, canned | 167 mg/3 oz |
| Sardines | 372 mg/3 oz |
| Spinach (drained solids) | 212 mg/1 cup |
| Turnip greens (cooked) | 250 mg/1 cup |
| White sauce, medium | 305 mg/1 cup |
| Yogurt | 295 mg/1 cup |

### Promoting Bowel Elimination

The patient's bowel movements are monitored because constipation is a major problem. Fluids, dietary fiber, and ambulation are increased for prevention of constipation. If preventive measures are ineffective, the physician may prescribe stool softeners or laxatives.

### Providing Postoperative Care

Most patients with PHPT are treated surgically. Postoperatively, the care requirements are very similar to those required after thyroidectomy. Potential physiological complications include hemorrhage, hypocalcemia, and airway obstruction. The patient's respiratory, cardiovascular, neurological, and fluid volume states are monitored routinely. A tracheostomy set should be immediately available for emergency use. The serum calcium level will decrease within 24 hours, and the patient is monitored for tetany. Parathyroid function usually returns to normal within 5 to 7 days after a partial parathyroidectomy because the remaining tissue resumes normal functioning.

If mild hypocalcemia occurs, oral calcium is given. Severe hypocalcemia can occur if there has been extensive bone demineralization. With the removal of the elevated PTH level, the calcium-deficient bones extract larger-than-normal quantities of calcium from the extracellular fluids. For patients with severe hypocalcemia, calcium chloride or calcium gluconate is given intravenously. These calcium preparations should be readily available for immediate administration if necessary. If permanent hypoparathyroidism results because the remaining tissue does not resume normal secretion or because a total parathyroidectomy is done, the patient will need continued treatment.

The Guidelines for Care Box outlines postoperative care after surgery of the parathyroid gland.

### Patient/Family Education

Patient and family teaching should include information about the following:

1. Assess knowledge of disease, diagnostic tests, therapeutic measures, barriers to learning, and information patient wants.
2. Provide dietary instruction about calcium, as needed, and help patient and family plan ways of meeting dietary requirements.
3. Teach patient about medication therapy (specify): name, purpose, dosage, side effects, signs and symptoms to report immediately, and special administration requirements. Provide written instructions.

**guidelines for care**

### The Person After Parathyroidectomy

**Assessment**

1. Monitor vital signs q2-4hr.
2. Monitor quality of voice and presence or absence of stridor, complaints of dyspnea, and choking sensation q1hr for 8 hours, then q2hr for 4 to 8 hours, and then q4hr.
3. Monitor serum calcium and the presence of signs of tetany and paresthesias.

**Nursing Diagnoses**

1. Breathing pattern, ineffective: tracheal obstruction associated with spasm of vocal cords or hemorrhage, laryngeal stridor associated with low serum calcium
2. Injury (trauma), risk for: hemorrhage, increased neuromuscular excitability associated with low serum calcium level
3. Knowledge deficit (follow-up care after surgery): no previous exposure to information

**Expected Patient Outcomes**

1. Maintains adequate air exchange, as evidenced by adequate breath sounds throughout lung field, pulse oximetry >95%, ABG values within normal range, and absence of signs of respiratory distress.
2. No injuries occur; shows no undetected changes in vital signs or neuromuscular excitability.
3. Patient and significant others can:
   a. Describe reason for frequent vital signs and neurological assessments.
   b. Describe symptoms they should report immediately.
   c. Describe plans for follow-up care.

**Interventions**

1. Have a tracheostomy set and IV calcium preparations readily available.
2. Report any sign of hemorrhage, hypocalcemia, or airway obstruction.
3. Assess mental status and motor strength.
4. Perform complete respiratory assessment. Keep head of bed elevated 30° to facilitate respiration. Encourage deep breathing, coughing, and turning q2-4hr.
5. Increase ambulation at patient's tolerance; take into account mental status and weakness.
6. Maintain fluid intake at prescribed level or enough to achieve 1000 ml or more if serum calcium levels are normal or 2000 ml or more if they are higher.
7. Teach patient and significant others about:
   a. Prescribed drugs
   b. Prescribed diet, if any
   c. Electrolyte replacement, if any
   d. Fluid intake requirements
   e. Wound care
   f. Symptoms to report: those indicating infection, hypocalcemia, or hypercalcemia
   g. Follow-up care requirements

4. Assess ability to perform skills of prescribed regimen (specify); provide teaching and multiple opportunities for practice and return demonstration.
5. Refer to community agencies (specify type) as needed, or provide patient and family with necessary information.
6. Clarify patient and family understanding about the need and plans for follow-up care.

Teaching can help the patient cope more effectively with changes. Frequent reexplanations may be required for the person with altered mental functioning. Anxiety may also interfere with the person's ability to learn and process information.

The family is included in the teaching. Because the patient's condition can be critical and may change rapidly, it may be helpful to plan with the family for daily formalized updates. Patients receiving medical therapy need instructions about comfort measures, safety, diet, activities, increased fluid intake, prevention of constipation, medications, and planned follow-up. Much of the care the patient required as an inpatient must be provided at home. Written and verbal instructions are helpful. Patients who have undergone surgery need the general teaching described in Chapter 18.

## ■ EVALUATION

To evaluate the effectiveness of nursing interventions, compare patient behaviors with those stated in the expected patient outcomes. Successful achievement of patient outcomes for the patient with PHTH is indicated by the following.

### For Patients Treated Medically on Long-Term Basis and Acutely Before Surgery

1. Reports no injuries.
2. Maintains stable blood pressure within acceptable parameters.
3. Reports no episodes of flank pain, bloody urine, or bone pain.
4. Output equals intake and is at least 2000 ml/24 hr.
5. Maintains activity level at baseline or increases.
6. Maintains weight at desired or prescribed level.
7. Reports bowel pattern restored to usual pattern and no rectal or abdominal discomfort.

### For Patients After Surgery

1a. Breath sounds are clear; if available, ABG values are within normal range; pulse oximetry is >95%.

b. Blood pressure, pulse, and respiratory rate remain within specific parameters that are normal for patient.

2. Reports no injury.
3. Patient verbalizes knowledge of symptoms, treatment rationales, and need for follow-up care.

## SPECIAL ENVIRONMENTS FOR CARE

### Critical Care Management

The indications for critical care nursing for the patient with hyperthyroidism are similar to those for the patient recovering from thyroid surgery. Intensive care monitoring and nursing are needed in the case of development of postoperative complications, including respiratory distress and hemorrhage.

## COMPLICATIONS

As mentioned earlier, complications after parathyroid resection include vocal cord spasm, hemorrhage, tracheal obstruction, laryngeal stridor, and laryngeal nerve damage. Hypocalcemia may also develop, and the nurse should be prepared to administer intravenous calcium if ordered. Surgical complications and sequelae are similar to those mentioned for thyroid resection.

Postoperatively, there is usually adequate parathyroid tissue to maintain calcium and phosphorus metabolism. If the remaining parathyroid gland is too small or nonfunctioning, some of the tissue removed can be implanted into the forearm. The excised gland must have been cryopreserved at the time of surgery to allow reimplantation.

## SECONDARY AND TERTIARY HYPERPARATHYROIDISM

### Etiology/Epidemiology

*Secondary hyperparathyroidism* is a disease characterized by excessive production of PTH resulting from chronic hypocalcemia. Malabsorption and chronic renal failure are two common causes of secondary hyperparathyroidism. Tertiary hyperparathyroidism is the result of long-standing secondary *hyperparathyroidism.* It is characterized by the development of autonomous parathyroid gland functioning that is not under normal homeostatic control mechanisms. When tertiary hyperparathyroidism occurs, the patient with chronic renal failure or malabsorption syndrome will develop hypercalcemia. In many instances, parathyroid hyperplasia will regress with removal of the chronic stimulus of hypocalcemia.

### Pathophysiology

In both secondary and tertiary hyperparathyroidism the calcium level is chronically low. In chronic renal failure the low calcium results from hyperphosphatemia, a decrease in production of activated vitamin D, and a decrease in calcium absorption. There also may be a decreased sensitivity of the bones to the action of PTH.[1,13] The low calcium level is a chronic stimulus to the parathyroid glands and results in their hyperplasia. The hyperplasia and excessive production of PTH are usually able to keep the calcium level close to normal, but at the expense of bone destruction. The bone lesions are characterized by osteomalacia, osteosclerosis, and osteitis fibrosa cystica.

### Collaborative Care Management

Treatment for secondary hyperparathyroidism is focused on decreasing the chronic stimulation of the parathyroid gland by improving the calcium level. In patients with malabsorption, calcium supplements and vitamin D are used. In patients with chronic renal failure, the treatment is first focused on (1) lowering the phosphorus level with a phosphorus-depleting agent such as aluminum hydroxide or calcium carbonate and (2) increasing the calcium level with calcium and vitamin D supplementation. There is concern about long-term use of aluminum hydroxide because of bone toxicity. If medical therapy does not lower the phosphorus level, thus elevating the calcium level and halting chronic stimulation of the parathyroid gland and bone destruction, a subtotal parathyroidectomy may be done.

If a single adenoma is the problem, it is removed. With hyperplasia, usually three complete glands and part of the fourth are removed. In hyperplasia a total parathyroidectomy sometimes is performed, with transplantation of some parathyroid tissue into the muscle of the forearm to avoid loss of function of the residual tissue in the neck resulting from vascular failure, which is a complication of surgery.

If no abnormal glands are found during the exploration of the neck, the search may be extended into the retroesophageal and retropharyngeal spaces to search for ectopic glandular tissue. Later surgical exploration may be necessary if no abnormal tissue is found during the initial surgery. This latter surgery is only carried out after localizing procedures are instituted. Subsequent surgery may require mediastinal exploration.

Serum calcium levels decline within 24 hours after successful surgery, and subnormal levels may be present for 4 to 5 days. Severe postoperative hypocalcemia may occur. The hypocalcemia may result from "hungry bone syndrome," which causes an increase in new bone formation. This syndrome is treated with calcium replacement. Most patients develop hypocalcemia because of temporary hypoparathyroidism. This is also treated with calcium replacement and usually resolves in 1 week. If permanent hypoparathyroidism occurs, the patient is treated as described below.

Treatment consists of hydration, diuretics, and restriction of calcium intake to prevent hypercalcemia until the gland returns to normal. In some patients the glandular hyperplasia does not regress, and a partial parathyroidectomy is necessary.

#### *Patient/family education*

The care for patients who undergo partial parathyroidectomies for secondary or tertiary hyperparathyroidism is the same as that for patients who have partial parathyroidectomies for primary hyperparathyroidism. Nurses have a major role in helping patients with malabsorption syndrome or chronic renal failure follow prescribed regimens so secondary or tertiary hyperparathyroidism is prevented.

## HYPOSECRETION OF PARATHYROID HORMONE: HYPOPARATHYROIDISM

### Etiology/Epidemiology

The causative factors of true hypoparathyroidism may be classified into three major categories: surgically induced, idiopathic, and functional.[4] Hypoparathyroidism occurs mainly from trauma of the anterior neck during surgery, particularly thyroid surgery, parathyroid surgery, or radical neck surgery. In rare instances, hypoparathyroidism may result from radioactive iodine therapy for hyperthyroidism of thyroid cancer. Idiopathic hypoparathyroidism is deficient hormone production from unknown causes. It may be seen at an early age and is probably the result of a genetic defect. There may be an autoimmune basis for early-age idiopathic hypoparathyroidism because many of these persons have abnormal antibodies directed against the parathyroid gland.[1,4] Late-onset idiopathic hypoparathyroidism has no known cause. Functional hypoparathyroidism is the result of chronic hypomagnesemia, which may be seen in malabsorption or alcoholism and appears to impair PTH release.

In *pseudohypoparathyroidism* the secretion and release of PTH are normal, but there is target tissue resistance to PTH. The cause of the resistance is unknown.

### Pathophysiology

A deficiency of or tissue resistance to PTH results in decreased bone resorption, decreased activation of vitamin D (and thus decreased intestinal absorption of calcium), increased renal excretion of calcium, and decreased renal excretion of phosphorus. The result is hypocalcemia and hyperphosphatemia. The major physiological alterations result from the effects of low calcium levels on neuromuscular irritability. Nerves show decreased thresholds of excitation, repeated responses to a single stimuli, and, in severe cases, continuous activity or muscular spasms *(tetany)*. Cardiac activity is altered. Calcification of basal ganglia and the lens of the eye may occur.

The severity of the hypocalcemia and the chronicity of the problem dictate the signs and symptoms seen with true hypoparathyroidism. In mild cases, which result in only slightly decreased serum calcium levels, the patient may be asymptomatic. In more severe cases, any or all of the clinical manifestations listed in Box 34-13 may be seen.

The patient with pseudohypoparathyroidism may have the same signs and symptoms as seen with true hypoparathyroidism. In addition, such patients may have skeletal and developmental abnormalities, including short stature, round face, short neck, stocky body, and discrete bone lesions. The most common bone lesion is unilateral or bilateral shortening of the fourth and fifth metacarpal and metatarsal bones. Mental retardation may also be present. The patient has low serum calcium and high serum phosphorus levels with normal to high PTH level on radioimmunoassay.

### Collaborative Care Management

The first priority of treatment is correcting calcium levels to prevent tetany. This is achieved by giving IV calcium gluconate or calcium chloride. Airway patency must be maintained. Maintenance of a calcium level of about 7 mg/dl usually prevents signs and symptoms such as laryngeal stridor and convulsions.

The cause of hypoparathyroidism is then identified, and long-term therapy is started as soon as possible. Normal serum calcium levels are maintained by supplemental dietary and elemental calcium, by dietary phosphate restriction and phosphate-binding agents such as aluminum hydroxide, and by vitamin D therapy to increase GI absorption of calcium. Vitamin D preparations include ergocalciferol (Drisdol, Geltabs), dihydrotachysterol (Hytakerol), or the cholecalciferol metabolites calcifediol (Calderol) or calcitriol (Rocaltrol).

It takes several weeks before the full effect of vitamin D therapy is seen. Major complications of therapy are vitamin D toxicity and renal calculi formation. Renal calculi can occur in the hypoparathyroid patient even in the presence of normal serum calcium because of excessive urinary calcium excretion in response to decreased levels of PTH. The patient is monitored at 6- to 12-month intervals to evaluate the effectiveness of treatment and to assess for side effects.

The patient may experience anxiety and ineffective breathing patterns as a result of the signs and symptoms of hypoparathyroidism. The nurse should be readily available to answer the patient's questions. The patient should be placed in a room so the nurses' station is visible. The patient's call light should be answered promptly. The nurse needs to follow up on any patient complaint. Hyperventilation, which can accompany anxiety, worsens the hypocalcemia because hyperventilation causes respiratory alkalosis, which in turn causes more of the ionized calcium to bind to serum protein. The decrease in ionized calcium exacerbates symptoms of hypocalcemia. Thus the patient should be supported to prevent hyperventilation. Keeping patients informed of their serum calcium levels will also help them feel in control and may lessen anxiety.

Patients are assessed for the following:

1. Chvostek's and Trousseau's signs (see Chapter 15)
2. Airway patency

**box 34-13** *True Hypoparathyroidism: Clinical Manifestations*

1. Neuromuscular manifestations: changes in nerve activity affect peripheral motor and sensory nerves
   a. Numbness and tingling (paresthesia) around mouth, tips of fingers, and sometimes in the feet
   b. Tetany with positive Chvostek's and Trousseau's signs (Chapter 15), spasms of wrists, fingers, and forearms or feet and toes
   c. Convulsions that may consist of tonic spasms of the total body or the more typical tonic-clonic activity
   d. Laryngeal stridor and dyspnea
   e. Other neurological signs: headache, papilledema, elevated CSF pressure, local signs that mimic a cerebral tumor; extrapyramidal neurological signs and symptoms, including gait changes, tremors, rigidity, and spasms; possible signs and symptoms of parkinsonism (see Chapter 53)
2. Emotional-mental manifestations: irritability, depression, anxiety, emotional lability, memory impairment, confusion, frank psychosis
3. Cardiovascular manifestations (effect of hypocalcemia)
   a. Prolonged QT and ST intervals and occasional dysrhythmias
   b. Resistance to effects of digitalis preparations
   c. Decreased cardiac output from congestive heart failure
4. Eye manifestations (calcification of lens)
   a. Cataract formation
   b. Eventual loss of all sight
5. Dental manifestations (depending on age of onset)
   a. Enamel defects seen on the tooth crown
   b. Delayed or absent tooth eruption
   c. Defective dental root formation
6. Integumentary manifestations: fragile nails, thin patchy hair, dry scaly skin, skin infections (usually candidiasis), vitiligo
7. GI manifestations: malabsorption, steatorrhea

3. Mental status: orientation
4. Emotional status: anxiety, irritability
5. Vital signs, particularly pulse rate and rhythm

Abnormal changes are reported immediately so that treatment can be instituted and convulsions prevented. The initiation of maintenance therapy does not immediately correct the physiology problem, and therapy is adjusted to maintain a normal serum calcium level without complications. Monitoring is continued during this period of adjustment and with any future changes.

A high priority for care is the maintenance of a safe environment. Seizure precautions such as padded bed rails, suctioning equipment, oxygen, a tracheostomy tray, and IV calcium must be readily available. The patient should be in a room that facilitates easy and frequent observation.

Protecting the patient from injury is an important nursing intervention. Safety precautions are particularly important if the patient has visual impairment. The environment is structured to allow the patient to function as independently as possible. If confusion or memory deficits are present, the patient is reoriented frequently. The room should be free of clutter. A chest restraint may be necessary.

#### *Patient/family education*

The potential for convulsions and spasms and the necessity for diagnostic tests and frequent monitoring need to be explained to the patient and significant others. The nurse must explain the relationships among the signs and symptoms, tests, monitoring, the disease, and each new intervention. Patient teaching includes the following:

1. Nature of the disease and need for long-term therapy
2. Medication administration
   a. Prescribed calcium, phosphate-binding agents, and vitamin D to be taken daily
   b. Monitor for signs of:
      (1) Ineffective treatment: recurrence of tetany
      (2) Signs of hypercalcemia: thirst, polyuria, lethargy, decreased muscle tone, constipation
      (3) Complications: renal stones (flank pain or pain radiating down into groin)
3. Need for continual follow-up care every 6 to 12 months
4. Dietary changes: increased calcium and decreased phosphorus

The nurse's role is to assist the patient and his or her family to understand and comply with the prescribed medical regimen. Dietary instruction should include a list of foods high in calcium but low in phosphorus. These include processed cheese, yogurt, and milk. The need for lifetime therapy for hypocalcemia should be emphasized. A medical alert-type bracelet might be encouraged in case of emergency. The patient and significant others should be taught to recognize the signs and symptoms of hypocalcemia, hypomagnesemia, and hypoparathyroidism. The nursing team also supports the patient and family during treatment and aids them in coping with anxiety and stress.

## ADRENAL GLAND

The adrenal gland is essential to life. Without the hormones cortisol and aldosterone produced in the adrenal cortex, the body's metabolic processes respond inadequately to even minimal physical and emotional stressors such as changes in temperature, exercise, or excitement. More severe stressors such as serious infections, surgery, or extreme anxiety would possibly result in shock and death.

The adrenal medulla secretes hormones that are also produced by the sympathetic nervous system although more slowly. Dysfunction of the adrenal gland can be manifested as increased or decreased function of the cortex or increased function of the medulla (Figure 34-7).

### HYPERFUNCTION OF THE ADRENAL CORTEX: CORTISOL EXCESS

#### Etiology

Excessive levels of glucocorticoids, whatever the cause, result in a constellation of symptoms known as *Cushing's syndrome* (Figure 34-8). The causes of Cushing's syndrome may be divided into three major groups.

1. Primary Cushing's syndrome: excessive cortisol production resulting from adrenal adenomas or carcinomas; also called *adrenal Cushing's syndrome*

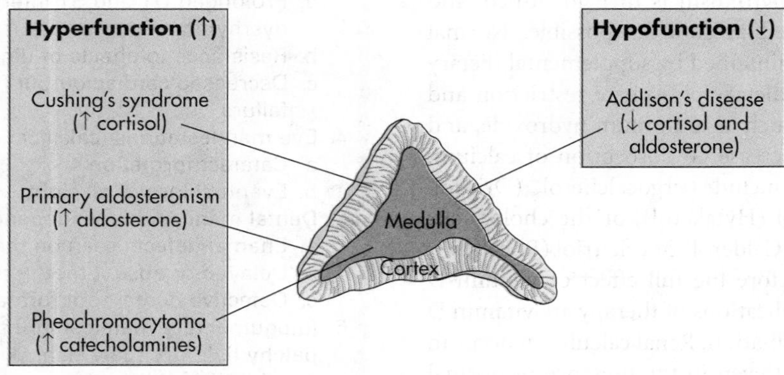


**fig. 34-7** Adrenal gland dysfunctions.

2. Secondary Cushing's syndrome: excessive cortisol production resulting from adrenal hyperplasia because of excessive ACTH production. The excessive ACTH production may result from either:
   a. Increased release of ACTH from the pituitary gland because of pituitary or hypothalamic problems; also called *Cushing's disease* or *pituitary Cushing's syndrome*
   b. Increased release of ACTH from ectopic nonpituitary sites such as bronchogenic carcinoma, pancreatic carcinoma, and bronchial adenoma; also called *ectopic Cushing's syndrome*
3. Iatrogenic Cushing's syndrome: excessive cortisol levels resulting from chronic glucocorticoid therapy

### Epidemiology

Ten million Americans receive glucocorticoid therapy each year. Although estimates of the incidence of iatrogenic Cushing's syndrome are imprecise, it is the most common cause of cortical excess. The second highest incidence of cortisol excess occurs with ectopic ACTH syndrome, estimated at 660 cases per 1 million persons per year, attributed to patients with small cell lung cancer. One percent of patients with lung cancer have ectopic ACTH syndrome.[3] In the past, ectopic ACTH syndrome was found more often in men than women; this pattern is changing as the number of women smokers increase. The incidence of Cushing's disease (ACTH-dependent cortisol excess) is estimated at 5 to 25 cases per 1 million persons per year. Women have a higher incidence than men of Cushing's disease, which occurs most frequently in women 25 to 45 years of age. The incidence of adrenal tumors is also higher in women than men (four to five times). There is no known explanation for the gender differences.

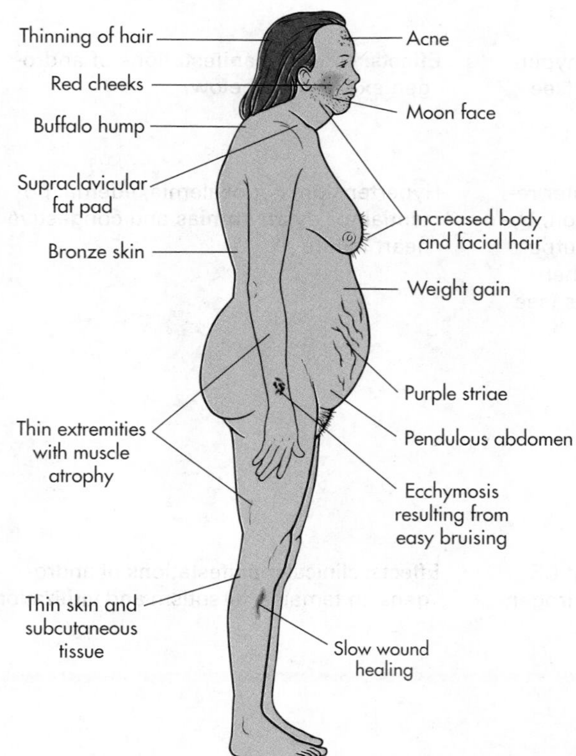


**fig. 34-8** Common characteristics of Cushing's syndrome.

### Pathophysiology

The major result of Cushing's syndrome is excessive production of cortisol. Early in the noniatrogenic disorders, the most prominent alteration is loss of the normal diurnal secretory pattern. With loss of the diurnal pattern, the morning level of cortisol production may not be abnormally elevated, but levels during the day do not show the normal decrease below the morning peak. At later stages, cortisol is elevated at all times.

The pathophysiological factors associated with cortisol excess primarily result from exaggeration of all the known actions of glucocorticoids and include alterations in the following:

1. Protein, fat, and carbohydrate metabolism
2. Inflammatory and immune response
3. Water and mineral metabolism
4. Emotional stability
5. Red blood cell (RBC) and platelet levels

Excessive cortisol may also disturb secretion of other anterior pituitary hormones (prolactin, thyrotropin, LH, and GH) and cause alterations in sleep patterns. Some of these alterations may contribute to the clinical picture.[2,3,5]

In many instances, cortisol excess is also associated with excessive production of androgen; this results in virilization in females. Adrenal tumors may secrete cortisol, androgens, and mineralocorticoids in various proportions. Depending on the hormone produced in excess, the patient will have (1) the clinical picture associated with Cushing's syndrome, (2) only the effects of androgen excess, (3) a clinical picture similar to that for hyperaldosteronism, or (4) any combination of these three.

Table 34-12 lists the normal function, pathophysiological alterations in function, and clinical manifestations of corticosteroid excess. Box 34-14 presents the pathophysiological alterations and clinical manifestations of corticosteroid excess.

### Collaborative Care Management

Medical management is focused on identifying the cause of the problem and removing the cause of cortisol excess, if possible. In iatrogenic Cushing's syndrome, care is focused on control of signs and symptoms if the chronic therapy cannot be terminated.

For patients with pituitary Cushing's syndrome resulting in adrenal hyperplasia, six therapeutic options are available (Table 34-13, p. 1106), although transsphenoidal removal of the pituitary tumor is the first line of therapy. When pituitary tumor removal is not possible or successful, other methods are used as adjunctive therapy.

For patients with the ectopic syndrome, the first line of therapy is to remove the source of the ectopic ACTH secretion. If this is not possible, drugs that inhibit cortisol production (Table 34-13) may be used. In some instances, when the

**table 34-12** *Hypersecretion of Glucocorticoids, Aldosterone, and Androgens (Cushing's Syndrome): Normal Function, Pathophysiological Alterations, and Clinical Manifestations*

| Normal Function | Pathophysiological Alterations | Clinical Manifestations |
|---|---|---|
| **GLUCOCORTICOIDS** | | |
| Organic metabolism<br>Protein catabolism<br>Gluconeogenesis<br>Changes in peripheral tissue sensitivity to insulin<br>Role in maintenance of blood glucose | Increased catabolism of protein (including bone matrix) and of fats: in particular, lipolysis and mobilization of fats<br>Increased blood glucose from glycogenolysis and gluconeogenesis | Hyperglycemia, onset of worsening of diabetes, osteoporosis, muscle wasting, purple striae, poor wound healing, easily bruised<br>Appearance: moon face, buffalo hump, central obesity, thin musculature |
| Negative feedback on secretion of ACTH | Variable effects on hypothalamic-pituitary-adrenal (HPA) axis: primary disease—suppression of ACTH; secondary (ACTH-dependent) and ectopic Cushing's syndrome (CS)—increased ACTH and melanocyte-stimulating hormone (MSH) | Hyperpigmentation seen in ACTH-dependent CS |
| Potentiate response to catecholamines | Increased catecholamine sensitivity; vasoconstriction increases peripheral resistance<br>In combination with alterations of aldosterone excess (see below), increases workload of heart | Hypertension and manifestations of altered aldosterone excess (see below) |
| Antiinflammation and immunosuppression | Increased susceptibility to infection, impaired localization (fibrin deposition) of infection | Increased incidence of infections, suppression of local signs of infection: redness, heat, edema, pain |
| Maintain emotional stability | Emotional instability | Mood swings, anxiety, depression, low tolerance for frustration; possible psychoses |
| Maintain fluid and electrolyte balance: effects similar to aldosterone (see below) | In ACTH-dependent CS, increased aldosterone secretion (see below); in primary CS, possibly minimal effects | Manifestations similar to those of aldosterone excess (see below) |
| Some androgenic effects | In ACTH-dependent CS with adrenal hyperplasia, excess of androgens present (see below) | Effects: clinical manifestations of androgen excess (see below) |
| **ALDOSTERONE** | | |
| Renin-angiotensin system is major controller of production.<br>Aldosterone acts at kidney tubules, particularly distal nephrons, to increase sodium reabsorption with consequent expansion of intravascular and extracellular fluid volume.<br>Potassium excretion is increased. | Abnormal increase in sodium and water retention; increased potassium excretion, hypervolemia, and increased cardiac output; cardiovascular effects heightened when combined with catecholamine effects (see above) | Hypertension, hypokalemia, edema; potential for dysrhythmias and congestive heart failure |
| **ANDROGENS** | | |
| Some role in establishment and maintenance of secondary sexual characteristics | Androgen excess; in ACTH-dependent CS with adrenal hyperplasia, excess androgen secretion present | Effects: clinical manifestations of androgens; in females, hirsutism and virilization |

**box 34-14** *Pathophysiological Alterations in Corticosteroid Excess*

**ALTERATION IN PROTEIN, FAT, AND CARBOHYDRATE METABOLISM**

**Altered Protein Metabolism**

Excessive catabolism of proteins results in loss of muscle mass, causing the following symptoms:

1. Muscle wasting, particularly of extremities, resulting in thin arms and legs, difficulty getting up from low chairs, difficulty climbing stairs, or generalized weakness and fatigue
2. Depletion of protein matrix of bone, resulting in osteoporosis, compression fractures of spine, backache, bone pain, and pathological fractures
3. Loss of collagen support of skin, resulting in thin, fragile skin that bruises easily, ecchymosis at trauma sites, and pink to purple cutaneous striae
4. Poor wound healing

**Altered Fat Metabolism**

Changes in fat metabolism cause obesity, with abnormal deposition of fat in face producing *moon face* (Figure 34-8), in intrascapular area producing the *buffalo hump,* and in mesenteric bed producing *truncal obesity.* Redistribution of fat with these characteristic features may be seen in patients without obesity. Body weight usually is increased.

**Altered Carbohydrate Metabolism**

Increased hepatic gluconeogenesis and impaired insulin use result in postprandial hyperglycemia and occasionally frank diabetes mellitus with all its signs and symptoms (see Chapter 35). Patients with concurrent diabetes mellitus may have worsening of signs and symptoms of their diabetes.

**ALTERATION IN INFLAMMATORY AND IMMUNE RESPONSE**

Cortisol excess results in decreased lymphocytes, particularly T lymphocytes; decreased cell-mediated immunity; increased neutrophils; and altered antibody activity. These changes make persons particularly vulnerable to viral and fungal infections. Depression in inflammatory and immune responsiveness results in opportunistic infections such as *Pneumocystis carinii* or other fungal infections. Early signs of infection, such as fever, may not be seen. Poor wound healing may also be related to infections.

**ALTERATIONS IN WATER AND MINERAL METABOLISM**

Cortisol itself possesses mineralocorticoid activity; therefore, cortisol excess results in characteristic signs and symptoms of increased mineralocorticoid activity even though level of aldosterone is normal. These include the following:

1. Sodium and water retention, which may accentuate body weight increase and may cause edema; serum sodium usually normal.
2. Hypertension, which is found in almost every patient with excessive cortisol and may be caused by increased volume or increased sensitivity of arterioles to circulating catecholamines.
3. Hypokalemia, hypochloremia, and metabolic alkalosis if cortisol excess is severe because of increased excretion of potassium and chloride (most often seen with ectopic Cushing's syndrome)
4. Increased calcium resorption from the bones and renal calculi from hypercalciuria (resulting in renal colic)

**ALTERATION IN EMOTIONAL STABILITY**

Various emotional changes may occur: from irritability and anxiety, to mild depression and poor concentration and memory, to severe depression and psychosis. Euphoria and sleep disorders are frequently noted.

**HEMATOLOGICAL ALTERATIONS**

Various changes in blood components, which occur as the result of excessive cortisol:

1. High to normal RBC count, hemoglobin, and hematocrit (may account in part for facial plethora [appearance of increased facial circulation])
2. Leukocytosis, lymphopenia, eosinopenia
3. Increases in various clotting factors and platelets, resulting in thromboembolic phenomena

**EXCESSIVE ANDROGEN ACTIVITY**

If excessive androgens are present, female patient exhibits virilization, which includes the following signs:

1. Hirsutism, manifested as fine, downy coat of hair on face and total body
2. Loss of scalp hair
3. Acne
4. Changes in menstrual cycle, varying from irregularities to oligomenorrhea to amenorrhea
5. Changes in libido

**OTHER FINDINGS**

Hyperpigmentation may be present and indicates elevation of ACTH, usually from ectopic site. ACTH has melanotrophic activity. Hyperpigmentation is seen on skin and mucous membranes.

site of ectopic ACTH cannot be found and the signs and symptoms cannot be controlled, bilateral adrenalectomy may be done.

For patients with adrenal tumors, the treatment of choice is tumor removal. See Box 34-15 for disorders that are treated with adrenalectomy. If the tumor is localized to one gland, a unilateral adrenalectomy is done. Excessive cortisol production by one gland causes negative feedback that results in a decrease in ACTH and subsequent atrophy of the unaffected gland. Thus the patient needs glucocorticoid replacement therapy for some time until normal function of the other adrenal gland returns. If the adrenocortical tumors are bilateral, bilateral adrenalectomy is done, and the patient will receive lifetime hormone replacement therapy. Immediately after bilateral adrenalectomy, the patient is depleted of both glucocorticoids and mineralocorticoids, and the patient

**table 34-13** *Medical Management of Patients with Pituitary Cushing's Syndrome*

| Treatment | Comments | Complications |
|---|---|---|
| Transsphenoidal adenectomy | First approach for pituitary tumors; preserves normal pituitary function; very successful for microadenomas; less successful for macroadenomas or invasive tumors | Complete recovery of gland requires a year or so; patients may require glucocorticoids for some time. |
| Transsphenoidal hypophysectomy | Gives 100% cure but removes total pituitary; may be used for invasive tumors or macroadenomas | Patient requires replacement therapy of glucocorticoids, thyroid hormone, gonadal steroids, and possibly ADH for life. |
| Radiation therapy by conventional methods, heavy particles of implants | Implants successful if no evidence of exact tumor found; conventional and heavy particle therapy used as adjunct to surgery | Complete remission not always possible; patient may develop hypopituitarism or damage to visual system. |
| Bilateral total adrenalectomy | Produces complete cure of signs and symptoms of cortisol excess; does not decrease ACTH | Replacement therapy of glucocorticoids and mineralocorticoids required for life; hyperpigmentation occurs because ACTH still elevated; visual problems result from a continually growing tumor (Nelson's syndrome). |
| Drug therapy (work at level of adrenal gland)<br>Aminoglutethimide (inhibits cholesterol synthesis)<br>Mitotane (inhibits cortisol production; can destroy gland)<br>Metyrapone (partially inhibits adrenal cortex steroid synthesis) | Used as adjunct to surgery of pituitary or radiation when complete remission not achieved; used for unresectable malignant tumors producing ACTH or unresectable adrenal carcinoma | All drugs have toxic effects; control symptoms but do not cure; can result in permanent adrenal insufficiency (mitotane); all patients require adrenal steroid replacement during therapy; patient can develop Nelson's syndrome because pituitary tumor remains. |
| Drug therapy (work at level of pituitary gland)<br>Cyproheptadine (serotonin antagonist that inhibits ACTH release) | Thus far used only in a few patients who have had recurrence after pituitary adenectomy | Effective only as long as drug is given; some patients show no response. |

**box 34-15** *Disorders That Respond to Adrenalectomy*

**UNILATERAL**
Single adrenocortical adenomas or carcinomas
Single adrenomedullary tumors

**BILATERAL**
Bilateral adrenal hyperplasia if other forms of therapy are ineffective
Bilateral adrenocortical adenomas or carcinomas
Bilateral adrenomedullary tumors
Removal of source of excessive cortisol secretion in response to ectopic ACTH secretions if ectopic site not controllable and Cushing's syndrome severe

who is not managed correctly will develop adrenal crisis (see p. 1118, 1121-1122).

### *Diagnostic tests*

Various diagnostic procedures are performed to confirm the diagnosis and differentiate among the various causes of cortisol excess. Positive test results, regardless of the cause, include the following (see Chapter 33 for a detailed discussion of these tests):

1. Elevated serum cortisol level or elevated excretion of urine free cortisol
2. Elevated urinary levels of 17-ketogenic steroids (17-KGS) and 17-hydroxycorticosteroids (17-OHCS)
3. Loss of diurnal rhythms of cortisol production
4. Loss of suppression of endogenous cortisol with the normal and screening cortisone suppression tests
5. Abnormalities in serum electrolyte concentrations, blood chemistry, and hematology, as described earlier

Secondary Cushing's syndrome from either pituitary disease or diseases that cause ectopic ACTH secretion results in elevated plasma ACTH, whereas persons with primary Cushing's syndrome have ACTH levels too low to measure. Pituitary and ectopic Cushing's syndromes are differentiated by response to the high-level dexamethasone suppression test (2 mg of dexamethasone given every 6 hours). Pituitary production of ACTH and thus of cortisol is suppressed with this high level of drug, whereas no suppression occurs in ectopic Cushing's syndrome. The presence of pituitary, ectopic, or adrenal tumors may be demonstrated by CT scans, ultra-

**box 34-16** *Factors Causing False-Positive Tests for Cortisol Excess*

**Persons with acute or chronic illnesses:** Acute stressors may result in high cortisol levels and abnormal dexamethasone tests; these tests must be repeated after patient's condition is stable.
**Obesity:** This results in high levels of urinary 17-OHCS and 17-KGS and abnormal screening suppression tests, but urine free cortisol, serum cortisol, and response to normal suppression test are normal.
**Pregnancy, estrogen therapy, and oral contraceptives:** Elevated estrogen associated with these states can increase serum cortisol and give abnormal results on a screening cortisol suppression test, but urine free cortisol and response to normal suppression test are normal.
**Alcoholism:** Alcoholics may have both clinical and diagnostic characteristics of Cushing's syndrome, but abstinence from alcohol reverses signs, symptoms, and abnormal test results.
**Depression:** Endogenous depression results in increased cortisol levels, loss of diurnal rhythm, increased urine free cortisol, increased urine 17-OHCS and 17-KGS, and abnormal suppression tests; however, patients with depression have increased cortisol in response to insulin-induced hypoglycemia, whereas patients with true Cushing's syndrome do not.

sound, and angiographic studies. To analyze the results of the diagnostic tests accurately, various factors that cause false-positive results must be eliminated (Box 34-16).

#### Medications

The previous discussion identified two classes of drugs used in treatment of cortisol excess: inhibitors of cortisol production and serotonin antagonists that may inhibit the release of ACTH (see Table 34-13). Pharmacological therapy may be combined with irradiation, especially if surgical intervention is contraindicated.

#### Treatments

Surgical intervention is a treatment option in some patients with cortisol excess. Surgical procedures include pituitary adenectomy or hypophysectomy, adrenal adenectomy, and unilateral or bilateral adrenalectomy. In addition, any of the various surgeries might be involved in removing an ectopic source of ACTH or cortisol. Ablative radiation therapy to the pituitary is an option if surgical intervention is unsuccessful or not desired. Irradiation is associated with many adverse effects, including radiation necrosis of the brain.

#### Diet

Diet modifications are prescribed according to individual patient needs. Calories, sodium, lipids, and cholesterol are commonly restricted. Depending on blood glucose patterns and the development of diabetes mellitus, dietary management of blood glucose levels may be appropriate.

#### Activity

The patient with untreated Cushing's syndrome has persistent fatigue and obesity and may have muscle weakness and/or pathological bone conditions. Maintenance of optimal activity is encouraged; activity restrictions are related to particular complications.

#### Referrals

Only through individual assessment of patient and family can the nurse learn their perceptions of issues related to the patient's health and the ease or difficulty they have in incorporating the medical regimen in daily living. Problems in home maintenance and role performance in the family and workplace may reveal a need to strengthen the resources available to the patient and/or family. Referral or consultation with social services, home nursing, or other services may be helpful.

## NURSING MANAGEMENT

## ■ ASSESSMENT

### Subjective Data

Data to be collected to assess the patient with cortisol excess include:

General data
Changes noted in body proportions, weight, hair distribution, pigmentation, bruising, delayed wound healing
History of discomfort, particularly back pain
History of frequent infections: skin, respiratory
Neurological data: changes noted in behavior, concentration, memory
Nutritional data
Usual 24-hour food/fluid intake
History of increase in thirst
Musculoskeletal data: complaints of weakness, fatigue, or difficulty doing normal activities
Elimination data: changes in urine output
Sexuality data
Females: changes in menstrual history, secondary sexual characteristics, libido, or feelings about self
Males: changes in libido, secondary sexual characteristics, or feelings about self
Knowledge level: condition, treatment, diagnostic tests

### Objective Data

Data to be collected to assess the patient with cortisol excess include:

General: body appearance (presence of moon facies, buffalo hump, truncal obesity, thin arms and legs, hyperpigmentation, striae, bruises, ecchymoses, fragile skin, facial plethora, unhealed wounds)
Neurological: affect and its appropriateness to situation, short-term memory, concentration
Cardiovascular: blood pressure, pulse, weight, presence of edema, jugular vein distention
Nutrition: intake of food and fluids

Musculoskeletal: muscle mass, strength, ability to stand up from a sitting position or do knee bends
Elimination: urine output, presence of glycosuria
Sexuality: female secondary sexual characteristics, body hair distribution, scalp hair changes, presence of acne

## NURSING DIAGNOSES

Nursing diagnoses are determined from analysis of patient data. Nursing diagnoses for the person with cortisol excess may include but are not limited to:

| Diagnostic Title | Possible Etiological Factors |
|---|---|
| **For Patients During Acute Period Before Definitive Treatment or if Definitive Treatment Not Possible** | |
| Activity intolerance | Muscle weakness, abnormal carbohydrate metabolism, abnormal electrolyte balance |
| Body image disturbance | Changes in body characteristics, change in functioning |
| Coping, ineffective (individual) | Inability to mount a normal physiological response to stressors, possible lack of learned coping strategies, emotional lability |
| Fluid volume excess | Abnormal retention of sodium and water |
| Infection, risk for | Inability to fight organisms because of depression of immune and inflammatory responsiveness |
| Injury (trauma), risk for | Falls associated with muscle weakness and bone changes |
| Nutrition, altered: more than body requirements | Increase in appetite with increased cortisol, alteration in metabolism |
| Pain | Demineralization of bone resulting in compression fractures |

## EXPECTED PATIENT OUTCOMES

Expected patient outcomes for the patient with cortisol excess may include but are not limited to the following.

### For Patients During Acute Period Before Definitive Treatment or If Definitive Treatment Is Not Possible

1. Improves activity tolerance as evidenced by maintenance of current activity level and a weekly increase in activity.
2. Has improved body image, as evidenced by speaking about self in positive terms.
3. Shows adequate coping, as evidenced by absence of signs of uncontrolled stress (restlessness, lack of attention, and increased heart rate or blood pressure).
4. Shows return of fluid volume to normal, as evidenced by elimination of signs of hemodilution or edema.
5. Detects early signs and symptoms of infections.
6. Does not fall or injure self.
7. Maintains adequate nutritional status, as evidenced by a gradual decrease in weight and a decrease in caloric intake.
8. States pain is controlled; activities are not limited because of pain.

## INTERVENTIONS

The patient with excessive cortisol secretion needs skilled nursing care. The patient can be critically ill. During the acute period, the primary focus of care is on the high-priority needs of supporting coping, restoring fluid balance, and preventing infections and injuries. In the more stable patient, these needs are still a focus of care, but the focus will expand to the other needs described by the additional nursing diagnoses listed earlier. (See the Guidelines for Care Box for pre- and postoperative nursing considerations.)

### Providing Physical Care

1. Decrease controllable stressors.
   a. Provide continuity of care.
   b. Explain all procedures slowly and carefully.
   c. Spend time with patient and listen carefully.
   d. Avoid sudden noises, temperature changes, drafts, and unnecessary invasion of privacy.
   e. Promote relaxation.
2. Monitor physiological coping ability.
   a. Ensure blood pressure and pulse remain stable.
   b. Take vital signs at least every 2 to 4 hours.
3. Control fluid volume excess.
   a. Restrict fluids as prescribed; distribute fluids throughout the 24 hours; use ice chips to prevent thirst.
   b. Provide a diet low in sodium as necessary.
   c. Provide potassium replacement as ordered, and increase intake of foods high in potassium.
   d. Monitor daily weight, intake and output every 4 to 8 hours, and laboratory values of sodium, potassium chloride, bicarbonate, and pH.
4. Prevent infection and falls.
   a. Monitor temperature every 4 hours.
   b. Assess mouth, lungs, and skin every shift for early signs of infection; report signs immediately.
   c. Limit staff and visitors with signs and symptoms of upper respiratory infections.
   d. Institute preventive care: sterile technique for invasive procedures; routine turning, coughing, and deep breathing every 2 hours; oral hygiene before breakfast, after meals, and at bedtime.

### Maintaining and Increasing Activity

As the patient begins to recover from the acute episode, the goal is to maintain the patient's current activity level. This requires assisting with some activities that require energy, such as bathing. In addition, the nurse should space the patient's activities and provide rest periods between them. When electrolyte and fluid balance and glucose metabolism have been stabilized, the patient's energy level will increase and more activities can be added gradually on a week-by-week basis.

### Promoting Nutritional Balance

Patients with cortisol excess are usually overweight. The nurse should provide a diet that restricts calories but is high in protein and that meets special needs based on glucose metabo-

**guidelines for care**

### The Person Undergoing Adrenal Surgery

**Preoperative**

1. Provide supportive care.
2. Assist patient with usual preoperative care.
3. Maintain nutritional status with a high-protein, prescribed-calorie diet with adequate minerals and vitamins.
4. Assist with correction of fluid and electrolyte imbalance.
5. Assist with hormonal therapy as prescribed.
6. Assist with measures used to prevent or treat crisis of adrenal hormonal excess or deficit.
7. Administer prescribed IV fluids and glucocorticoids before surgery.

**Postoperative**

1. Establish monitoring schedule to detect complications of surgery and:
   a. Adrenal crisis
   b. Blood pressure alterations
   c. Blood glucose alterations
   d. Fluid and electrolyte imbalances
2. Because the patient may have unusual activity intolerance, pace postoperative activities with alternate periods of rest and a gradual increase in self-care.
3. Provide measures to minimize effects of postural hypotension:
   a. Supply Ace bandages or elastic stockings.
   b. Assess effects of posture on blood pressure.
   c. Assist or accompany the patient during ambulation while blood pressure remains labile.
4. Provide measures to decrease risk of infection in the immunosuppressed patient (e.g., strict surgical asepsis, deep breathing, and avoiding contact with persons with infections).
5. Administer cortisol replacement as typically prescribed:
   a. IV route for the first 24 to 48 hours
   b. Oral route when patient is able to tolerate food by mouth
6. Administer mineralocorticosteroid (fludrocortisone) replacement, if prescribed; this is typically prescribed when cortisol replacement is less than 40 to 50 mg/24 hours in the patient with bilateral adrenalectomy.
7. Assist patient and family in learning about required hormonal replacement:
   a. Bilateral adrenalectomy—maintenance dose of cortisol and mineralocorticoids
   b. Unilateral adrenalectomy—doses of cortisol dependent on degree of suppression of HPA axis

lism. Because cortisol excess can increase appetite, patients need assistance in controlling calories; the approach to this is individualized. (See Chapter 3 for a discussion of techniques that can be used.) The patient's nutritional status should be monitored by checking weight, actual food intake, and blood glucose level. Blood glucose levels should be monitored every 4 to 8 hours until the patient's condition is stable.

### Promoting Comfort

Pain occurs because of demineralization of bones and compression fractures. Measures that can be used to promote comfort include (1) providing a mattress with good support, (2) giving back rubs to promote relaxation, and (3) using pain medications as appropriate. If these measures are unsuccessful, the nurse should consult the physician and physical therapist about other alternatives, including braces. Pain must be controlled so that ambulation and activity can be maintained.

### Promoting Positive Body Image

Another major focus of care is helping the patient deal with changes in body image, sexuality, and self-concept. Patients should know that some body changes are reversible with treatment. To help increase self-concept, patients are assisted in setting realistic goals. Clear explanations about changes in sexual characteristics and changes that will occur with treatment help patients to cope better.

#### *Patient/family education*

An assessment to determine what information the patient desires should be done initially. Education of patients and significant others is ongoing. The patient will need basic information regarding the care being given and restrictions such as diet and limitation of some visitors. Many diagnostic tests may be necessary, and careful explanations are given. Over time the patient needs information about the disease process and planned treatment, long-term care needs related to the disease process, and specific care for complications such as adrenal insufficiency, which can occur with some treatments.

#### *Health promotion*

Most causes of excessive cortisol production are not preventable except for the ectopic secretion of ACTH from bronchogenic carcinoma. Elimination of smoking would decrease the occurrence of bronchogenic carcinoma.

No screening tests are available for secondary prevention. Evaluation of adrenal function depends on the clinical suspicion of the primary health care provider.

Tertiary preventive activities should be a major focus of nursing care. Nurses should help patients deal with their chronic health problems, carry out self-monitoring practices to identify exacerbations early, and maintain their therapeutic regimens. These practices help prevent progression of problems. Patients receiving long-term glucocorticoid therapy are an important group for nurses to target for teaching. Through their patient educator roles, nurses can help patients carry out their therapy in the safest manner possible.

## ■ EVALUATION

To evaluate the effectiveness of nursing interventions, compare patient behaviors with those stated in the expected patient outcomes. Successful achievement of patient outcomes for the person with cortisol excess is indicated by:

1. Reports that activity level is increased from baseline.
2. Comments positively about self.
3. Shows no excessive restlessness.
4. Reports decreasing weight and a decrease in peripheral edema, if present.
5. Maintains body temperature within specified parameters.
6. Reports no injuries.
7. Discusses future plans, including ways to decrease food intake.
8. States pain is controlled and does not restrict activity.

## SPECIAL ENVIRONMENTS FOR CARE

### Critical Care Management

The person who has undergone adrenal surgery is usually managed in the intensive care unit postoperatively. The high risk for adrenal crisis and need for invasive monitoring to maintain fluid and electrolyte balance after adrenalectomy necessitates intensive care nursing.

Hemodynamic monitoring (central venous pressure, blood pressure, pulse, and at times pulmonary wedge pressure) is done continuously. In addition, daily serum electrolyte concentrations, blood glucose levels every 4 hours, daily weights, and hourly intake and output are monitored.

Intravenous cortisol replacement is continued for at least the first 24 hours postoperatively and usually for 48 hours. Fluids are given based on the clinical data and usually include saline/dextrose solutions. On the second day postoperatively, mineralocorticoids may be started. By the third day, the patient is usually able to tolerate oral glucocorticoids and a normal diet. If unusual weakness or anorexia, nausea, or vomiting occurs, glucocorticoids are increased. If unusual hypotension occurs, mineralocorticoids and fluids are adjusted appropriately.

A major complication of surgery is poor wound healing and infection caused by the effects of excess cortisol. Strict aseptic technique is used with wound care. Splinting the incision during coughing or turning prevents stress on the suture line and promotes comfort. Other postoperative needs are similar to those described for the patient with adrenal insufficiency (see the Nursing Care Plan). Replacement therapy is necessary throughout life.

For the patient who has had a unilateral adrenalectomy, monitoring, hormonal support, fluid therapy, and other care needs are the same during the immediate postoperative period as for the patient with a bilateral adrenalectomy. After the patient's condition has stabilized, and physiological and psychological crises have been successfully avoided, the glucocorticoid support is slowly withdrawn because eventually a single gland can maintain enough hormonal secretion for both daily living and additional stressors. When glucocorticoids are withdrawn, monitoring for signs and symptoms of adrenal insufficiency and crisis must be continued because the remaining gland may have atrophied and may not have fully recovered. If signs and symptoms occur, glucocorticoids are restarted and then again slowly withdrawn.

A patient who has chronic adrenal insufficiency and who needs surgery for an unrelated adrenal problem requires the preoperative and postoperative care just described. This information must be stressed to the patient.

## COMPLICATIONS

Persons with Cushing's syndrome caused by pituitary adenoma and treated by transsphenoidal resection may experience complications described for hyperpituitarism on p. 1063. Persons treated with adrenalectomy will require lifelong glucocorticoid and mineralocorticoid replacement therapy. Adrenal crisis is a potential complication (see p. 1118). Occasionally severe side effects are associated with treatment of ectopic ACTH-secreting tumors with radiation or chemotherapy (see Chapter 11). If pituitary irradiation is used, panhypopituitarism or pituitary dysfunction may result. The effects of excess cortisol on the musculoskeletal system may result in pathological fractures and avascular necrosis, necessitating total joint replacement in some patients.

## IATROGENIC CUSHING'S SYNDROME

### Etiology/Epidemiology

Iatrogenic Cushing's syndrome occurs when a patient takes large doses of exogenous glucocorticoids for their therapeutic antiinflammatory effects. As described in Chapter 33, the glucocorticoids have profound antiinflammatory and immunosuppressive effects. Because of these effects, glucocorticoids are frequently prescribed in therapeutic doses to suppress undesirable inflammatory reactions and immune responses. Box 34-17 presents examples of clinical situations in which glucocorticoids might be used for their antiinflammatory and immunosuppressive effects. See p. 1103 for epidemiological information about this most common cause of cortisol excess.

When glucocorticoids are given for any reason other than replacement therapy, the person receives dosages that will elevate the serum glucocorticoid level above normal. Adrenocorticosteroids used in this manner can cause problems when they are prescribed for long-term, continuous use and when they are withdrawn after long-term use. The total dosage and the duration of therapy determine the side effects. The larger the dose and the longer the time during which glucocorticoids are used, the greater the side effects.

### Pathophysiology

Long-term therapeutic doses of glucocorticoids can result in the full clinical picture of Cushing's syndrome. In other patients, the clinical presentation is atypical. Bone changes may be greater in iatrogenic Cushing's syndrome, and patients often develop vascular necrosis. Fluid and electrolyte disturbances may not be as severe because synthetic glucocorticoids possess less mineralocorticoid activity than natural glucocorticoids. Severe myopathy can occur. Peptic ulcers occur more often in patients who receive glucocorticoid therapy for more than 30 days.[3] Patients receiving glucocorticoid therapy are very susceptible to cataract formation, which is not seen in endogenous Cushing's syndrome. Patients

## nursing care plan The Person with Adrenal Insufficiency

**DATA** Mr. J. is admitted from the emergency room with complaints of feeling so tired that he is unable to get out of bed. He also complains of nausea, vomiting, and diarrhea and having no appetite. He gives a history of feeling poorly for the last 2 months with increasing fatigue. Mr. J. thought he just could not recover from the flu that had been prevalent in the winter. He is an accountant and had been working every day; he also believed that his work partly caused his fatigue.

Physical examination reveals the following:

- 52-year-old white man with "good tan" (NOTE: Mr. J. denies sun exposure)
- Looks ill
- Skin cool, sweaty
- Complains of lightheadedness when head of bed (HOB) elevated
- Lungs clear
- Heart rate—sinus tachycardia; jugular vein distention—flat when HOB elevated 15°
- Skin turgor poor; mucous membranes dry
- Blood pressure: lying, 90/60; sitting, 70/50
- Pulse, 110
- Respirations, 20
- Temperature, 36.5 °C
- Weight, 70 kg (lost 3 kg in last month)

Laboratory results were:

- White blood cells, 16,000
- Blood glucose, 60 mg/dl
- Sodium, 130 mEq/L
- Chloride, 86 mEq/L
- Hematocrit, 46%
- Hemoglobin, 15 g/dl
- BUN, 39 mg/dl
- Creatinine, 0.8 mg/dl
- Potassium, 5.4 mEq/L

**NURSING DIAGNOSIS** *Activity intolerance related to postural hypotension*

| expected patient outcome | nursing interventions | rationale |
|---|---|---|
| Increases activity level gradually. | Provide bedrest for first 24 hours.<br>Avoid any unnecessary activities, such as bathing, for first 12 hours.<br>Explain that when hormone level returns to normal, Mr. J. will feel stronger. | Activities should only be increased when serum glucocorticoid levels return to normal. |

**NURSING DIAGNOSIS** *Ineffective individual coping related to inability to mount normal response to stressors*

| expected patient outcome | nursing interventions | rationale |
|---|---|---|
| Stressors and signs of stress decrease. | Decrease stressors from noise, lights, and temperature changes.<br>Explain everything to Mr. J.<br>Maintain consistent persons caring for patient for first 24 hours.<br>Pad door to prevent slamming.<br>Set temperature to comfortable level.<br>Keep stressful news from reaching Mr. J.<br>If family members are comforting, have one stay with Mr. J.<br>Make sure family members are calm. | Because of lack of glucocorticoids, patient can not respond physiologically to any stressor; nurse should limit stressors. |

**NURSING DIAGNOSIS** *Fluid volume deficit related to inability to conserve fluid*

| expected patient outcomes | nursing interventions | rationale |
|---|---|---|
| Fluid intake is approximately 3000 ml/day.<br>Signs of fluid deficit decrease. | Monitor intake and output hourly.<br>Monitor blood pressure and pulse hourly until normal.<br>Weigh daily.<br>Monitor hematocrit, hemoglobin, and BUN daily.<br>Administer IV fluids (usually 5% dextrose in normal saline) as ordered.<br>Administer cortisol as ordered. | Surveillance will identify any problems with replacement therapy early so that solutions can be changed.<br>Fluid volume deficit results from excessive loss of sodium and water and lack of glucocorticoids. |

*Continued*

## The Person with Adrenal Insufficiency–cont'd

**NURSING DIAGNOSIS** *Risk for injury (trauma) related to weakness and hypoglycemia*

| expected patient outcome | nursing interventions | rationale |
|---|---|---|
| Experiences no injury. | Keep bed low.<br>Keep bed rails up.<br>Maintain quiet environment and consistent nurse for 24 hours.<br>Monitor blood glucose q4hr.<br>Instruct Mr. J. to stay in bed. | Hypoglycemia and weakness can lead to injury; nurse should provide safe environment. |

**NURSING DIAGNOSIS** *Knowledge deficit related to new problem with no previous exposure to information*

| expected patient outcome | nursing interventions | rationale |
|---|---|---|
| Mr. J. and significant others can explain what will happen over next 24 hours. | Explain all care to patient and family so that no unexpected event occurs.<br>Focus only on care to be given for next 24 hours.<br>Help Mr. J. and family know that his condition will be much more stable in 24 hours. | Mr. J. can only handle minimal knowledge, so limit to what must be provided in first 24 hours; knowledge helps to decrease stress. |

**box 34-17** *Therapeutic Use of Glucocorticoids: Clinical Situations*

1. Eye surgery or trauma: usually given as drops, ointment, or intraorbital; systemic effects minimal
2. Dermatological disorders: used as ointments; can have systemic effects if used over large part of body or used daily
3. Autoimmune diseases: rheumatoid arthritis, systemic lupus erythematosus, scleroderma
4. Hematological disorders: hemolytic anemia, thrombocytopenia, lymphomas, leukemias
5. Allergic reactions: anaphylaxis, contact dermatitis, transfusion reactions
6. GI disorders: ulcerative colitis, Crohn's disease, hepatitis
7. Nephrological disorders: nephrotic syndrome
8. Neurological disorders: head trauma and surgery, to prevent cerebral edema and increased intracranial pressure
9. Cardiopulmonary disorders: asthma, chronic obstructive pulmonary disease, myocarditis
10. Transplantations: renal, liver, heart, and $\beta$-cell transplantation
11. Other: part of many protocols for various malignancies

receiving long-term glucocorticoid therapy are very susceptible to all types of infection.

### Collaborative Care Management

A different type of problem, cortisol deficit, can occur when glucocorticoids are given for a prolonged period. They must be withdrawn slowly to prevent adrenal insufficiency. High blood levels of exogenous glucocorticoids cause negative feedback to the hypothalamus and anterior pituitary gland, and the production of corticotropin-releasing factor (CRF) and ACTH is suppressed, resulting in depression of the hypothalamic-pituitary-adrenal (HPA) axis and adrenal atrophy. Thus, if glucocorticoids are stopped suddenly, the patient develops signs and symptoms of adrenal insufficiency because of an inability to produce the glucocorticoids. It may take as long as 9 months for return of normal HPA function.[3]

To prevent depression of the HPA axis, some physicians prescribe every-other-day glucocorticoid therapy. In these instances, double the patient's daily dose is given at 8 AM every other day. The benefit of this schedule is that it allows the serum glucocorticoid level to drop low enough every other day to prevent the negative inhibition of the hypothalamus and the anterior pituitary gland. Thus, every other day the person has a normal secretion of endogenous CRF and ACTH and normal stimulation of the adrenal cortex, and atrophy of the adrenal cortex glands does not occur. Even though the glucocorticoid level drops low enough to prevent negative feedback, the antiinflammatory effect is not reduced. Even though every-other-day therapy should prevent HPA axis depression, the dose of glucocorticoids is still tapered when they are withdrawn. In some instances after withdrawal, the patient may be able to produce enough glucocorticoids to meet body needs in nonstressful times but may need additional glucocorticoids during increased stress.

Blood glucose levels may be monitored frequently, particularly if there is a family history of diabetes mellitus. If hyperglycemia develops, dietary control is necessary to control blood glucose levels. Some patients may develop type 1 diabetes (see Chapter 35).

Most persons experience an increase in appetite. If weight gain is a problem, a calorie-restricted diet may be necessary.

To prevent GI problems, steroids should be taken with food or antacids. Stools should be guaiac-tested regularly to monitor for early signs of GI irritations.

If fluid retention becomes a problem, a sodium-restricted diet is prescribed. The patient is weighed frequently, and the extremities are observed for signs of edema; changes are reported as soon as possible because diuretic therapy may be necessary. To prevent hypokalemia, the person should be consuming a diet high in potassium, and a potassium replacement may be prescribed unless some underlying condition results in potassium retention.

The effects of glucocorticoids on muscle wasting and bone demineralization can best be minimized by promoting a regular activity regimen incorporating weight bearing, adequate dietary protein, ambulation, and exercise. The patient should be taught to avoid potentially injurious activities.

The person receiving prolonged glucocorticoid therapy must avoid anyone with an infection. Because young children frequently have upper respiratory infections, close contact with them may have to be limited. Crowded, poorly ventilated environments should also be avoided. The patient is monitored constantly for signs of infection, and the primary caregiver should be notified immediately if any signs of infection occur.

Assessment of the patient's psychological and emotional status is important. Anxiety, depression, and mood swings are common problems.

To prevent adrenal insufficiency secondary to sudden withdrawal, patients taking glucocorticoids for a prolonged time must have the steroids withdrawn gradually to allow the HPA axis to recover. During the time the drug is being withdrawn, these patients should be monitored for signs and symptoms of adrenal insufficiency. If symptoms occur, withdrawal is slowed. To prevent sudden withdrawal in emergency situations, the patient should wear an identification bracelet or carry an identification card that states the name and dosage of the prescribed glucocorticoid. If the patient is ill or injured and requires emergency care, those treating the patient will be able to determine if more glucocorticoids are needed because of the increase in stressors; additional glucocorticoids can be given intravenously if they cannot be tolerated by mouth.

It may take some time for the adrenal cortex to recover sufficiently to respond to additional stressors after withdrawal of therapeutic doses of glucocorticoids. Therefore patients with a recent history of glucocorticoid therapy are monitored for manifestations of adrenal insufficiency, particularly at times of stress.

Although most of the emphasis in this section has been on care of patients receiving oral therapy, the information applies as well to those receiving prolonged steroid therapy intravenously or topically.

***Patient/family education***

Patients receiving prolonged therapeutic glucocorticoid therapy need considerable teaching to be able to manage therapy and to identify signs and symptoms of complications (see the Patient/Family Teaching Box). In addition, counseling is usually needed to help the patient cope with changes in appearance and behavior.

The disturbances associated with long-term therapeutic doses of glucocorticoids cannot be completely avoided, but they often can be minimized and complications avoided. The changes in body structure may not be avoidable. Patients should be aware of these side effects and be supported in dealing with these changes. Instructions on use of clothes and makeup may be incorporated into care.

The patient and significant others must be aware of potential changes in behavior that may occur. Usually, patients adjust to the therapy, but if behavior changes occur, the physician should be notified immediately. Written and verbal instructions should be given.

***patient/family teaching***

**The Person Receiving Long-Term Therapeutic Doses of Glucocorticoids**

1. Take drugs as prescribed.
   a. Do not miss a dose or stop medication suddenly.
   b. Drug must be withdrawn slowly under a physician's supervision.
   c. If nausea and vomiting occur and drug cannot be taken, notify physician immediately.
   d. Keep sufficient tablets on hand to avoid missing a dose.
   e. Take drug with food or antacids.
   f. With every-other-day therapy, take twice the normal dose every other day at 8 AM.
   g. If traveling, *carry* medications on person not in luggage (do not ship them).
2. Monitor self for and report side effects of weight gain, edema, behavior changes, GI bleeding, increased urination or thirst, or signs of infection.
3. Check blood glucose level if directed.
4. Prevent infections.
   a. Avoid persons, especially children, with infections.
   b. Avoid crowded, poorly ventilated places.
   c. Care for wounds carefully.
   d. Report signs of infection, which may include feelings of increased weakness, feeling poorly, and having less energy.
5. Maintain a nutritious diet, including foods from all food groups (see Chapter 3); follow directions for any prescribed diet (low calorie, high potassium, low sodium).
6. Carry out a regular exercise program; walking helps strengthen muscles and decrease bone problems.
7. Have yearly eye examinations.
8. Consult physicians regularly as instructed.

## HYPERFUNCTION OF ADRENAL CORTEX: ALDOSTERONE EXCESS

### Etiology/Epidemiology

Aldosterone excess, aldosteronism, can be either primary (Conn's syndrome) or secondary. *Primary aldosteronism* results from bilateral nodular hyperplasia or from a single aldosterone-producing adenoma. *Secondary aldosteronism* occurs frequently and results from the presence of exogenous conditions that stimulate the renin-angiotensin-aldosterone system (Box 34-18).

Primary aldosteronism is a rare disorder affecting approximately 2% of the hypertensive population. Twice as common in women as in men, it occurs most frequently in the third to fifth decades of life.

## Pathophysiology

In primary aldosteronism, excessive aldosterone is secreted and stimulates the reabsorption of sodium in the kidney in exchange for potassium and hydrogen. The increased sodium retention is accompanied by water retention and results in volume expansion and hypertension. The hypertension may result in ECG and radiological changes of left ventricular enlargement and in retinopathy. Although the extracellular volume is expanded, edema is not usually present. Headache is a typical clinical finding.

The loss of intracellular and extracellular potassium changes the excitability of muscle membrane, resulting in muscular weakness, intermittent paresthesia, and sometimes diminished deep tendon reflexes. Paralysis can also occur. A low potassium level can result in ECG changes, dysrhythmias, and hypersensitivity to digitalis preparations. Severely low levels of potassium result in loss of the concentrating ability by the kidney tubules, leading to increased water loss, polyuria, nocturia, and polydipsia. The increased loss of water by the kidney can result in hypernatremia. Excessive loss of hydrogen ions results in hypokalemic alkalosis, producing signs and symptoms of tetany.

Aldosterone secretion is high with low plasma renin activity. The aldosterone level does not decrease in response to sodium loading and does not increase in response to volume and sodium depletion or assuming the upright position.

Secondary aldosteronism results when increased renin secretion is stimulated by the various pathological factors. Usually the increased renin activity results from decreased perfusion pressure or decreased effective plasma volume to the kidney. The increased aldosteronism leads to hypokalemia and alkalosis. Hypertension may or may not be present, and some patients have edema. Sodium concentration is normal or low.

## Collaborative Care Management

### Diagnostic tests

Laboratory tests will reveal alterations in serum electrolytes. See Box 34-19 for common laboratory test results. Hypertension and hyperkalemia are key features.

### Medications

Electrolyte imbalance and volume excess are treated with potassium replacements and spironolactone or amiloride. Spironolactone is prescribed in doses as high as 200 to 400 mg/day and amiloride in doses of 20 to 40 mg/day. Spironolactone is a mineralocorticoid antagonist, which blocks the effect of aldosterone on the kidney tubule, and thus blocks the abnormal reabsorption of sodium and potassium excretion. Potassium is conserved with spironolactone. Amiloride also is a potassium-sparing diuretic.

### Treatments

If primary aldosteronism results from an aldosterone-secreting adenoma, the treatment of choice is surgical resection. Unilateral adrenalectomy is recommended.

For bilateral hyperplasia, medical treatment with sodium restriction, potassium replacement, and spironolactone is the treatment of choice. If the hypertension is not controlled by this treatment, traditional antihypertensive therapy is used. Some patients respond to suppression of aldosterone secretion by glucocorticoids.

In secondary aldosteronism, medical treatment for the abnormal sodium and water retention is sodium restriction, potassium replacement, and diuretics. In addition, treatment is focused on the underlying pathological factors.

### Diet

One of the dietary modifications used in the treatment of aldosteronism is sodium restriction. Potassium replacements are frequently ordered, so the patient should be instructed regarding potassium-rich foods. Salt substitutes frequently contain

**box 34-18** *Exogenous Causes of Secondary Aldosteronism*

- Cardiac failure
- Liver disease
- Nephrosis
- Renal artery stenosis
- Bartter's syndrome (hypertrophy and hyperplasia of the juxtaglomerular cells)
- Idiopathic cyclic edema
- Pregnancy
- Hypovolemic states
- Estrogen therapy

**box 34-19** *Laboratory Test Results with Primary Aldosteronism*

BLOOD TESTS

- Lower serum potassium level (hypokalemia)
- High serum sodium level (hypernatremia)
- Elevated serum bicarbonate level and pH (alkalosis)
- Low serum magnesium level (hypomagnesemia)
- Elevated plasma aldosterone with low plasma renin levels

URINE TESTS

- Low specific gravity (dilute urine)
- Increased urinary protein
- Increased urinary aldosterone

potassium and may be used in the diet. If surgical intervention is used in treatment, no dietary restrictions are necessary postoperatively, as aldosterone levels will return to normal.[19]

### Activity

The patient is encouraged to increase activity gradually; as potassium levels return to normal, weakness and fatigue should improve. The patient should be taught to avoid rapid changes in position to avoid postural hypotension. The patient should be monitored to prevent injury due to the paresthesias and visual disturbances that may occur.

### Referrals

The patient may benefit from a referral to a dietitian to reinforce dietary teaching. If the patient experiences adverse effects with spironolactone therapy, such as amenorrhea, hirsutism, or erectile dysfunction, counseling may be indicated. These side effects should be reported to the health care provider.

## NURSING MANAGEMENT

Nursing care is focused on assisting with implementation of medical therapy, monitoring for effectiveness of therapy, monitoring for side effects of therapy (e.g., fluid overload), and preventing or detecting complications that may result from the patient's changed mental status (particularly respiratory depression). Monitoring for fluid status may include vital signs taken as often as every 15 minutes, hourly intake and output, and daily weights. Temperature is monitored hourly because hyperpyrexia is often present.

## ■ ASSESSMENT

### Subjective Data

Data to be collected to assess the patient with aldosterone excess include:

History of weakness, paresthesias, palpitations
History of visual changes, headaches
History of polyuria, nocturia, polydipsia, kidney infections
Nutritional intake
History of edema, weight change
Knowledge of the disease, planned tests, therapy

### Objective Data

Data to be collected to assess the patient with aldosterone excess include:

Vital signs, especially blood pressure
Heart sounds, point of maximal impulse
Weight
24-hour fluid intake and output
Visual acuity
Muscle strength, deep tendon reflexes, sensory perception
Edema

## ■ NURSING DIAGNOSES

Nursing diagnoses are determined from analysis of patient data. Nursing diagnoses for the person with aldosterone excess (before surgery or while being treated medically only) may include but are not limited to:

| Diagnostic Title | Possible Etiological Factors |
|---|---|
| Activity intolerance | Muscle weakness and fatigue associated with electrolyte imbalance, especially hypokalemia |
| Fluid volume excess | Abnormal retention of sodium and water associated with increased aldosterone |
| Pain | Headache associated with hypertension |

## ■ EXPECTED PATIENT OUTCOMES

Expected patient outcomes for the person with aldosterone excess (before surgery or while being treated medically only) may include but are not limited to:

1. Shows improvement in activity tolerance as potassium level improves.
2. Maintains fluid balance, as evidenced by normal serum sodium levels.
3. Controls headaches.

## ■ INTERVENTIONS

Nursing interventions are focused on managing critical care, increasing activity tolerance, maintaining fluid balance, promoting comfort, and preparing for discharge.

### Increasing Activity Tolerance

Care is spaced to allow for rest periods. Activity is increased gradually, and as potassium is returned and maintained at a normal level, strength should increase. A high-potassium diet, potassium replacement, and spironolactone are given as prescribed.

### Maintaining Fluid Balance

The patient's fluid volume status is monitored by checking daily weights, intake and output, and serum electrolyte concentrations. A sodium-restricted diet may be necessary preoperatively, and a high-sodium diet may be necessary when surgery is performed. If the patient is treated medically, a long-term sodium-restricted diet is maintained.

### Promoting Comfort

Headache may be eased by the use of cold packs, relaxation therapy, and analgesics. Polydipsia may be controlled by making sure the patient has ready access to water and receives frequent oral hygiene.

### Patient/Family Education

Ongoing teaching is necessary and includes:

1. Preoperative
   a. Information about diagnostic tests and proposed surgery
   b. Need for long-term care
2. Postoperative
   a. Prescribed diet: may include a high-sodium diet to be followed for several weeks or longer

   b. Monitoring for unstable blood pressure and fluid volume deficit
3. Patient treated medically
   a. Medication (diuretics): dosage, frequency, and side effects
   b. Signs and symptoms of uncontrolled disease to be reported to physician

## ■ EVALUATION

To determine the effectiveness of nursing interventions, compare patient behaviors with those stated in the expected patient outcomes. Successful achievement of patient outcomes for the person with aldosterone excess is indicated by:

1. Reports increased initiation and completion of ADL.
2. Maintains serum sodium levels within normal limits, and has no edema.
3. Reports infrequent and mild headache.

## GERONTOLOGICAL CONSIDERATIONS

As mentioned earlier, primary aldosteronism is a relatively rare disorder, affecting approximately 2% of persons with hypertension. The elderly person should be monitored for secondary aldosteronism, which results from many conditions that stimulate increased renin secretion. An elderly patient who has cardiac or liver disease may be at increased risk for developing secondary aldosteronism.

## COMPLICATIONS

Potential complications include hypertension, hypokalemia, tetany, and alkalosis. Until the patient's condition stabilizes, vital signs are monitored at least every 4 hours. If hypertension is present, hourly monitoring of vital signs may be necessary. Increases in blood pressure are reported immediately and managed as directed. Cerebral dysfunction may indicate uncontrolled hypertension. Care is designed to prevent activities that increase blood pressure, such as the Valsalva maneuver, straining during defecation, or heavy exertion. If antihypertensive drugs are ordered, monitoring for side effects must be included.

Assessment of serum electrolyte concentrations (especially potassium) and the presence of weakness, cardiac dysrhythmias, and Chvostek's and Trousseau's signs should be ongoing (see Chapter 15). Hypertension remains a potential problem postoperatively for some time. It may take as long as 1 month for the patient to return to a normotensive state. In addition, hypoaldosteronism may occur postoperatively and result in sodium loss and potassium retention. A high sodium intake prevents sodium deficit in the postoperative period.

## HYPOFUNCTION OF THE ADRENAL CORTEX: CORTISOL INSUFFICIENCY

### Etiology/Epidemiology

Inadequate secretion of cortisol may occur as a result of (1) insufficient secretion of ACTH resulting from hypothalamic-pituitary disease (secondary adrenocortical insufficiency), (2) insufficient secretion of ACTH and adrenal atrophy resulting from suppression of hypothalamic-pituitary function by long-term exogenous glucocorticoids given in therapeutic doses (iatrogenic), or (3) destruction of the adrenal cortex itself (primary). Primary insufficiency, also called *Addison's disease,* can result from several causes (Box 34-20).

Iatrogenic adrenal insufficiency, resulting from glucocorticoid therapy, is the most frequent cause of adrenal insufficiency. In primary adrenocortical insufficiency, clinical signs of adrenocortical insufficiency develop when 90% of both glands is destroyed. Under stress, clinical signs may develop when a smaller amount of adrenal tissue is present. The most common causes of primary adrenocortical insufficiency are autoimmune destruction (70%) and tuberculosis (20%).

Autoimmune destruction is termed *idiopathic atrophy* of the adrenal gland; the disorder probably has a genetic component because it often occurs in families and is associated with specific haplotypes. It can be part of multiple endocrine defects caused by autoimmune processes, such as those associated with thyroid and parathyroid gland dysfunction.

### Pathophysiology

Adrenocortical insufficiency, whether primary or secondary, is a rare problem. However, adrenal insufficiency is life-threatening because the adrenocortical hormones are necessary for existence. The disorder can occur abruptly, as with hemorrhage and infarction, or slowly, as with idiopathic insufficiency. With slow progressive destruction, the adrenal cortex may initially be able to meet the hormonal needs of daily living, but when a stressor occurs, insufficiency becomes evident because the gland cannot meet the extra needs associated with the stress response.

Primary adrenocortical insufficiency deprives the body of both mineralocorticoids and glucocorticoids. These hormonal losses decrease the body's ability to retain sodium and secrete potassium. The loss of sodium decreases extracellular electrolytes and fluid volume. The decreased volume, along with decreased vascular tone, diminishes cardiac output and decreases renal perfusion. Excretion of waste products is inhibited.

The loss of glucocorticoids in primary adrenocortical insufficiency decreases hepatic gluconeogenesis and increases tissue glucose uptake. Muscle strength is lost. Various GI disor-

**box 34-20** *Causes of Addison's Disease*

- Idiopathic atrophy, probably caused by an autoimmune abnormality
- Infection of adrenal glands
- Infiltration of adrenal glands with cancer
- Impairment of blood flow from vasculitis or thrombosis
- Hemorrhage and infarction secondary to septicemia (Waterhouse-Friderichsen syndrome)
- Destruction of adrenal glands by chemicals such as mitotane
- Congenital hypoplasia
- Surgical removal of adrenal glands
- Metastases to adrenal glands

ders occur, and mental and emotional functioning and stability are impaired. The loss of negative feedback of glucocorticoids with pituitary secretion of ACTH results in uncontrolled ACTH release along with $\beta$-lipotropin. The $\beta$-lipotropin is hydrolyzed to $\beta$-melanocyte-stimulating hormone ($\beta$-MSH). Thus excessive amounts of ACTH and $\beta$-MSH are present in the serum. Various changes in sexual characteristics may result from a decrease in adrenal androgen or from the general debility associated with the insufficiency (Table 34-14).

Secondary adrenal insufficiency results in similar pathophysiological disturbances, except that the fluid and electrolyte imbalances are not usually as severe because the adrenal cortex can still produce mineralocorticoids (aldosterone) in response to the renin-angiotensin system. In addition, because ACTH secretion is diminished, no increase occurs in serum levels of $\beta$-MSH.

In chronic insufficiency the earliest symptoms are vague, and the clinical picture is not easy to recognize. Clinical

**table 34-14** *Hyposecretion of Glucocorticoids, Aldosterone, and Androgens (Addison's Disease): Normal Function, Primary Pathophysiological Alterations, and Clinical Manifestations*

| Normal Function | Pathophysiological Alterations | Clinical Manifestations |
|---|---|---|
| **GLUCOCORTICOIDS** | | |
| Organic metabolism<br>Protein catabolism<br>Fat metabolism<br>Gluconeogenesis<br>Changes peripheral tissue sensitivity to insulin<br>Role in maintenance of blood glucose | Inadequate metabolism of protein, carbohydrates, and fats; in particular, inadequate gluconeogenesis and glycogen stores<br>Increased insulin sensitivity in periphery | Potential low fasting blood glucose; inability to tolerate prolonged fasts; experiences hunger, weakness, lightheadedness; fatigue and weakness possibly extreme; nausea and vomiting leading to emaciation |
| Negative feedback on secretion of ACTH | Diminished negative feedback on secretion of ACTH; ACTH stimulates MSH | Hyperpigmentation particularly in areas exposed to light, pressure areas, hand creases, and buccal mucosa |
| Potentiate response to catecholamines | Diminished catecholamine activity; poor response to stressors | Hypovolemic shock, as seen by hypovolemia, hypotension, and tachycardia |
| Antiinflammation and immunosuppression | Poor response to any trauma, infection, or stress | May give history of many infections, frequent sick days, not ever really feeling well |
| Maintain emotional stability | Emotional lability | Mood changes: often depressed, lack of interest, sad, mild neuroses |
| Maintain fluid and electrolyte balance: effects similar to aldosterone (see below) | Effects similar to those seen with aldosterone deficiency, but if client produces aldosterone without glucocorticoids, pathophysiological effects not as severe (see below) | Effects similar but milder than those seen with aldosterone deficiency (see below) |
| Some androgenic effects | Androgen deficiency similar to that seen with decreased adrenal androgens (see below) | Clinical picture similar to that seen with decreased adrenal androgens (see below) |
| **ALDOSTERONE** | | |
| Renin-angiotensin system is major controller of production.<br>Aldosterone acts at kidney tubules, particularly distal nephrons, to increase sodium reabsorption with consequent expansion of intravascular and extracellular fluid volume.<br>Potassium excretion is increased. | Abnormal increase in water and sodium loss; abnormal potassium conservation; inadequate maintenance of blood volume, decreased cardiac output, and decreased blood pressure | Dehydration and hypovolemia (decreased weight, increased BUN, increased hematocrit, poor skin turgor); hyponatremia; hyperkalemia; decreased bicarbonate; acidosis; postural hypotension to shock; muscle weakness and fatigue |
| **ANDROGENS** | | |
| Some role in establishment and maintenance of secondary sexual characteristics | Androgen deficiency in females<br><br>Androgen deficiency in males | In females, loss of hair in axillae, pubis, and over lower extremity; may give history of menstrual irregularities<br>Loss of erectile function; loss of male escutcheon; decreased need to shave; decreased libido |

signs of acute and chronic insufficiency include those listed in Box 34-21.

*Adrenal crisis* (addisonian crisis) is a severe exacerbation of adrenal insufficiency, occurring in any person with chronic insufficiency regardless of the cause. Previously undiagnosed adrenal crisis is usually seen when a person undergoes a major stressor; it can also occur in a person who has abrupt withdrawal of therapeutic glucocorticoids. A person with poorly controlled adrenal insufficiency may develop addisonian crisis in response to a stressful situation. Adrenal hemorrhage may also precipitate a crisis in a previously well individual.

Severe hypovolemia (up to 20% of circulating volume can be lost) can lead quickly to hypovolemic shock, hypoperfusion, and lactic acidosis. Patients may experience mental status changes and coma, dysrhythmias, azotemia, and vascular collapse. Hyperkalemia and hyponatremia are present. Acute adrenal insufficiency is a life-threatening crisis and must be treated rapidly.

## Collaborative Care Management

### Diagnostic tests

Findings from diagnostic tests include:

1. Low serum sodium and glucose and high serum potassium levels
2. Increased serum BUN from hemoconcentration and decreased renal perfusion
3. Normal basal levels of cortisol may be noted; low to normal levels during acute illness indicate adrenocortical insufficiency.
4. Response to ACTH stimulation
   a. Low or no plasma cortisol with primary insufficiency
   b. Normal response to repeated stimulation with secondary insufficiency
5. Elevated ACTH serum levels with primary insufficiency
6. Abnormal ACTH response to metyrapone or hypoglycemia with secondary insufficiency

For patients having a known history of adrenal insufficiency or clinical symptoms of the disorder, treatment is begun with a minimum of testing. The short ACTH test is very helpful in confirming or ruling out adrenal insufficiency. Serum cortisol levels are measured at 0, 30, and 60 minutes after administration of ACTH (cosyntropin, 250 ng) intravenously. When a patient is severely stressed, baseline levels of serum cortisol less than 5 ng/dl are diagnostic, and levels less than 10 ng/dl suggest adrenal insufficiency. A blunted or absent elevation of serum cortisol at 30 and 60 minutes in response to the ACTH is diagnostic for adrenal insufficiency. (See Chapter 33 for details of this test and others used in evaluating ACTH and cortisol secretion.) The rapid or short ACTH test does not differentiate between primary and secondary adrenal insufficiency.

### Medications

Pharmacological treatment of adrenal crisis includes the following:

1. *Administration of glucocorticoids and mineralocorticoids.* Hydrocortisone, 100 to 200 mg, is given intravenously, first as a bolus and then as repeated doses every 8 hours in the pa-

**box 34-21** ***clinical manifestations***

***Adrenal Insufficiency***

1. Mental and emotional changes are some of earliest symptoms and may include lethargy, loss of vigor, depression, irritability, and loss of ability to concentrate. Patient can become increasingly apathetic and be unable to participate in any ADL.
2. Hypoglycemia occurs in about 50% of patients with adrenocortical insufficiency. Periods of fasting may exacerbate problem.
3. Weakness and fatigue are some of most common findings in adrenocortical insufficiency. At first, this may be episodic but can progress to general prostration. Muscle changes may be associated with muscle pain.
4. Anorexia, nausea, and vomiting are very common manifestations. Diarrhea or constipation may be present. Abdominal pain occurs frequently, and all patients experience weight loss.
5. Electrolyte changes include low serum sodium and high serum potassium levels. However, total body potassium is low because potassium moves out of cells in response to extracellular hypoosmolality. Some potassium is lost through the GI tract and kidney, and less potassium is taken in. Low serum sodium levels can result in dizziness, confusion, and neuromuscular irritability; some patients give history of salt craving. High serum potassium levels can result in ECG changes (peaked T wave and broadened QRS complex) (see Chapter 15) and, if very severe, cardiac standstill. Muscles become weaker, and flaccid paralysis can occur. Occasionally, high serum calcium levels may be present because of increased protein concentration associated with volume deficit.

   Along with the sodium deficit, a fluid volume deficit also occurs. Signs of dehydration, such as poor turgor, sunken eyeball, and dry mucous membranes, are present. Hypotension is seen initially with postural changes but eventually is always present. Complete vascular collapse (shock) may occur.
6. Hyperpigmentation is seen only in primary adrenocortical insufficiency when ACTH and possibly $\beta$-MSH are elevated. It appears as a bronzing seen with a normal suntan in light-skinned persons or generalized darkening in dark-skinned persons. The hyperpigmentation affects both exposed and unexposed skin areas, as well as mucous membranes, and is often exaggerated over pressure areas such as knuckles, knees, elbow, and ischial tuberosities. Palmar creases, thumbnails, and the dorsum of tongue may also show the unusual pigmentation.
7. Most females experience loss of body and axillary hair and menstrual changes. Menstrual changes may be related more to weight loss than to changes in adrenal androgens. Males experience erectile dysfunction, probably related to generalized debility associated with adrenocortical insufficiency.

tient with known adrenal insufficiency. In the patient with undiagnosed adrenal crisis, dexamethasone (Decadron), 4 to 10 mg, may be chosen instead of hydrocortisone because dexamethasone does not cross-react with cortisol, which can influence tests of cortisol function. Hydrocortisone has some mineralocorticoid activity, whereas dexamethasone does not; fludrocortisone (Florinef) is more likely needed when dexamethasone is prescribed.

2. *Initiation of volume replacement.* Volume replacement with IV normal saline is started immediately at a rapid rate (e.g., 500 to 1000 ml in the first hour and 2000 to 3000 ml in the next 2 to 3 hours). Typically, glucose is added to the first liter as 5% dextrose in normal saline.
3. *Administration of glucose.* The results of blood glucose testing can quickly determine whether additional IV glucose needs to be given. Patients are often nauseated and vomiting and may complain of abdominal pain, so food ingestion is not an appropriate source of glucose.
4. *Administration of vasopressors.* If glucocorticoid and fluid therapy do not improve vascular status, vasopressors may be started.

Chronic adrenal insufficiency is treated by hormone replacement. In primary insufficiency a glucocorticoid, usually cortisone, 37.5 mg daily (25 mg on awakening and 12.5 mg before 4 PM), or hydrocortisone (20 mg in the morning and 5 mg before 4 PM) and a mineralocorticoid, usually fludrocortisone (0.1 to 0.2 mg daily), are prescribed. Other forms of these drugs may be prescribed. If a different adrenocortical derivative with glucocorticoid properties (e.g., prednisone) is prescribed, the dosage is equivalent to the antiinflammatory potency of hydrocortisone. For example, the dosage of prednisone is approximately 10 mg/day. Table 34-15 presents a comparison of the antiinflammatory potency of the adrenocortical steroids relative to the glucocorticoid potency of hydrocortisone and the mineralocorticoid potency of desoxycorticosterone acetate. In secondary insufficiency, only glucocorticoid replacement is necessary.

The dose of glucocorticoids or mineralocorticoids is adjusted until the patient has no symptoms. The dosage of glucocorticoids is temporarily tripled or doubled in situations such as psychological stressors, vacations, infections, trauma, or dental work. When the stressors have dissipated, the dosage is returned to normal.

### Treatments

Identification of the precipitating factor and the initiation of treatment are carried out as rapidly as possible.

### Diet

Fluids are encouraged, and the patient's hydration status is continually monitored. Nursing interventions should include measures to decrease nausea, vomiting, and diarrhea in an effort to maintain fluid and nutritional balance. The patient should be weighed daily. A high-sodium and low-potassium diet is indicated.

### Activity

The patient will have muscular weakness until hormonal balance is restored. Adequate rest should be encouraged; increase activities gradually. Range of motion and isometric exercises should be encouraged until the patient is fully ambulatory. Assistance may be needed with ADL.

## NURSING MANAGEMENT

## ■ ASSESSMENT

Because the clinical manifestations in chronic adrenal insufficiency are subtle and affect a variety of systems, a thorough assessment is necessary.

See p. 1111-1112 for a Nursing Care Plan for the person with adrenal insufficiency.

### Subjective Data

Data to be collected to assess the patient with cortisol insufficiency include:

General: history of weakness, fatigue, muscle pain, dizziness, changes in behavior, lethargy, depression; attention or ability to do work and activities
Appearance: history of changes in pigmentation
Nutrition: history of anorexia, nausea, vomiting, salt craving, weight loss, and abdominal pain; usual 24-hour food/fluid intake
Elimination: history of changes in bowel habits; urine output
Sexual
Females: menstrual history, history of changes in body/axillary hair

**table 34-15** *Comparison of Antiinflammatory and Mineralocorticoid Potency of Derivatives of Adrenocorticosteroids*

| DRUG | ANTIINFLAMMATORY POTENCY* | MINERALOCORTICOID POTENCY† |
|---|---|---|
| Hydrocortisone (cortisol) | Potency = 1 | Potency 0.03 times that of DOca |
| Cortisone acetate | Potency 0.8 times that of hydrocortisone | Potency 0.03 times that of DOca |
| Prednisone | Potency 4 times that of hydrocortisone | Potency 0.04 times that of DOca |
| Methylprednisolone | Potency 6 times that of hydrocortisone | Potency 0.02 times that of DOca |
| Triamcinolone | Potency 5 times that of hydrocortisone | No mineralocorticoid activity |
| Dexamethasone | Potency 30 times that of hydrocortisone | Only mild natriuretic effect |
| Desoxycorticosterone | Zero antiinflammatory effect | Potency = 1 |
| Fludrocortisone | Potency 10 times that of hydrocortisone | Potency 4.2 times that of DOca |

*Potency relative to hydrocortisone, whose potency = 1.
†Potency relative to desoxycorticosterone acetate (DOca), whose potency = 1.

Males: history of erectile dysfunction
Knowledge: disease, treatment, expectations

### Objective Data

Data to be collected to assess the patient with cortisol insufficiency include:

Emotional-mental status: affect, attention, activity level
Integumentary status: hyperpigmentation, axillary/body hair distribution, skin turgor, eyeball softness
Cardiovascular status: blood pressure and pulse, especially with postural changes; heart rhythm
Gastrointestinal status: weight, 24-hour intake and output, abdominal tenderness
Musculoskeletal status: muscle strength; presence of wasting; ability to do ADL, rise up from sitting position, or walking

## NURSING DIAGNOSES

Nursing diagnoses are determined from analysis of patient data. Possible nursing diagnoses for the patient with cortisol insufficiency include but are not limited to:

| Diagnostic Title | Possible Etiological Factors |
|---|---|
| Activity intolerance | Muscle weakness, postural hypotension, electrolyte imbalance |
| Coping, ineffective (individual) | Inability to mount normal response to stressors, insufficient learned coping mechanisms |
| Fluid volume deficit | Sodium and water loss associated with deficiency of adrenal cortex hormones |
| Injury (trauma), risk for | Instability associated with weakness, electrolyte imbalance |
| Nutrition, altered: less than body requirements | Decreased intake associated with anorexia, nausea, vomiting |
| Pain | Abdominal discomfort |
| Self-esteem disturbance | Change in functional ability, change in body characteristics |

## EXPECTED PATIENT OUTCOMES

Expected patient outcomes for the person with cortisol insufficiency may include but are not limited to:

1. Improves activity tolerance, as evidenced by increased activity level.
2. Improves coping, as evidenced by no signs and symptoms of stress; avoids stressors when possible.
3. Maintains fluid intake of approximately 3000 ml/day, and signs of fluid deficit decrease.
4. Experiences no injuries.
5. Has improved nutritional status, as evidenced by increase in weight; eats and retains 100% of prescribed diet.
6. States pain is controlled.
7. Verbalizes increased perception of self-esteem, expresses positive self-appraisal, participates in decision making.

## INTERVENTIONS

Nursing care that relates to identified nursing diagnoses includes:

1. Promoting activity
   a. Limit activities until vascular volume is stable and blood pressure is normal.
   b. Gradually increase activity and monitor for fatigue and weakness.
   c. Schedule rest periods throughout the day.
2. Facilitating coping
   a. Provide a stressor-reduced environment: quiet, private room, controlled temperature; limit visitors but promote visits by persons who have a calming effect.
   b. Avoid surprises; explain everything carefully before proceeding with care.
   c. Use preventive measures for infection or trauma, such as sterile technique, coughing and deep breathing, and good skin care.
   d. Ensure continuity of care.
   e. Help patient identify daily stressors and ways to avoid and cope with them.
3. Promoting fluid balance
   a. Monitor for fluid deficit:
      (1) Weight every day
      (2) Intake and output every 1 to 8 hours
      (3) Laboratory values for signs of hemoconcentration every day
      (4) Skin turgor every 4 hours
      (5) Vital signs every 1 to 4 hours
   b. Report signs of increasing fluid deficit immediately.
   c. Maintain fluid intake at several liters a day.
   d. Provide diet with a "normal" sodium (approximately 4 g of sodium chloride) level.
4. Preventing injury
   a. Remove unnecessary equipment from room.
   b. Assist patient with ambulation.
   c. Use side rails as necessary and keep bed low to floor.
5. Promoting good nutrition
   a. After patient's condition is stable, provide a high-calorie diet incorporating foods from all food groups.
   b. Provide good oral hygiene before meals.
   c. Provide an environment conducive to eating.
6. Promoting comfort: back rubs and relaxation techniques; stress reduction
7. Improving self-esteem
   a. Help patient and significant others understand relationship between changes in self and the disease process; explain that physical changes are reversible.
   b. Help patient set short-term realistic goals.
   c. Compliment patient on accomplishments.
   d. Involve patient in decision making, even if patient is unable to perform physical activities.

#### *Patient/family education*

The initial teaching during the acute phase relates to proposed diagnostic tests and immediate interventions. After the patient's condition is stable, information is given about the disease and long-term needs. Instructions about replacement therapy are similar to those given to patients taking therapeutic doses of glucocorticoids, but some important differences exist (see the Patient/Family Teaching Box).

**patient/family teaching**

**The Person Taking Replacement Doses of Glucocorticoids and Mineralocorticoids**

1. Follow medication regimen.
   a. Take drugs with meals or snacks.
   b. Glucocorticoids: take ⅔ of dose at approximately 8 AM and ⅓ of dose at approximately 4 PM.
   c. Mineralocorticoids: take medication in the morning.
   d. Do not omit a drug dose.
   e. Keep sufficient medication on hand.
   f. If unable to retain oral form of drug, take parenteral form as instructed.
   g. Carry drugs on person or in carry-on luggage when traveling; do not ship drugs with luggage; make sure traveling companion knows how to give the injectable form of glucocorticoid.
   h. Carry extra doses in case of delays or illness.
2. Wear a Medic Alert bracelet or necklace that lists condition, drugs and dosage, and name and phone number of physician.
3. Monitor self for presence of increased stressors (fever, infections, dental work, accidents, or family or personal crises) and increase dose of glucocorticoids as instructed or consult physician (normal dose covers only daily needs; it does not provide for additional stressors).
4. Monitor self daily for signs and symptoms of insufficient drug therapy (anorexia, nausea, vomiting, weakness, depression, dizziness, polyuria, and weight loss) and report immediately (larger drug dose may be necessary).
5. Monitor self daily for signs and symptoms of excessive drug therapy (rapid weight gain, round face, edema, or hypertension) and report immediately (smaller drug dose may be necessary).
6. Eat a well-balanced diet, choosing foods from all food groups.
7. Maintain a regular schedule with adequate sleep, regular meals, and regular exercise (irregular health habits increase glucocorticoid needs).
8. Eliminate as many work and home confrontations as possible to decrease stress response that increases glucocorticoid needs.
9. See physician as instructed; consult as necessary if questions arise concerning therapy.

Surgery results in complete remission of symptoms in most patients; therefore discharge teaching for most patients is focused on helping the patient plan for resumption of normal activities, maintenance of an adequate diet, and follow-up care.

Additional teaching should include the effect of stressors on the disease and methods to reduce or eliminate stress. The patient and significant others should be able to describe:

1. Home medication program, the need for continued treatment if replacement is necessary, and situations that require an increase in medication dosage
2. Medical follow-up plan
3. Symptoms indicating adrenal crisis and the need for medical attention
4. Need for continual medical follow-up
5. Need to carry identification card with information concerning physician and current medication

Some physicians have the patient keep a parenteral form of cortisol at home and instruct significant others in its administration for emergency purposes. Patients may also carry a vial of hydrocortisone with a syringe for use when away from home.

## ■ EVALUATION

To determine the effectiveness of nursing interventions, compare patient behaviors with those stated in the expected patient outcomes. Successful achievement of patient outcomes for the person with cortisol insufficiency is indicated by:

1. Reports more activity tolerance.
2. Identifies at least three techniques that help in reducing stress responses.
3. Describes strategies to monitor fluid intake and to drink 3000 ml/24 hr.
4. Reports no injuries.
5. Eats 100% of planned caloric intake every 24 hours.
6. Reports no severe pain.
7. Verbalizes increased level of self-esteem, expresses positive self-appraisal, and participates in decision making.

## GERONTOLOGICAL CONSIDERATIONS

The feedback mechanisms involved in maintaining glucocorticoid levels are not affected by age. However, the decrease in the metabolic rate of the glucocorticoids is age-related. The amount of fibrous tissue in the gland increases, and the gland loses some weight after the age of 50. As liver and kidney function decline with age, the metabolic clearance of cortisol decreases.

Elderly persons may be at risk for iatrogenic adrenal insufficiency resulting from glucocorticoid therapy. Cancer may metastasize to the adrenal glands, resulting in insufficiency. In Japan, tuberculosis accounts for most cases of adrenal insufficiency.

## SPECIAL ENVIRONMENTS FOR CARE

### Critical Care Management

In critical care settings the most frequent acute adrenal insufficiency is caused by hemorrhage of the adrenal glands. Adrenal hemorrhage is associated with conditions of overwhelming sepsis, concurrent infections of human immunodeficiency virus (HIV), and other disorders.

Management priorities in adrenal crisis are restoration of fluid volume and electrolyte balance, administration of cortisol, administration of glucose, and support to patient and family. Frequent monitoring of the patient is necessary to detect changes, to evaluate effectiveness of therapy, to detect side effects of therapy (e.g., fluid overload), and to prevent or detect complications. Of particular concern are the changes in mental status and respiratory depression. Monitoring for fluid status may include vital signs taken as often as every 15 minutes, hourly intake and output, and daily weights. Temperature is monitored hourly because hyperpyrexia is often present. Hemodynamic monitoring may be used to help determine the exact amount of fluids needed. The fluid deficit is usually corrected in 4 to 6 hours.

Until the patient's condition is stabilized, serum values are monitored daily or more frequently as necessary. During the early phase of illness, a neurological assessment is made at least every 4 hours for signs of hyponatremia (dizziness, confusion, or neuromuscular irritability); this assessment can be done while the nurse is taking vital signs.

If serum potassium levels are elevated, the patient should be attached to a cardiac monitor to check for changes in T wave or QRS complexes or for changes in rhythm. The hyperkalemia usually disappears with cortisol and fluid therapy, and the patient may actually need potassium after the acute period. Until the serum potassium level returns to normal, the nurse should make sure the patient does not inadvertently receive potassium in IV fluids or medications. Measures to prevent infections and trauma, which can increase cell death and the liberation of potassium into the extracellular space, are incorporated into the nursing care.

Monitoring for signs and symptoms of hypoglycemia and monitoring of blood glucose levels are done on a routine basis, such as every 4 hours. Glucose is given in IV fluids as prescribed and, when food is allowed, snacks may be incorporated between meals to avoid long periods of fasting. If symptoms of hypoglycemia occur, the blood glucose is checked, if possible, and treatment is initiated for the hypoglycemia (see Chapter 35).

A focus of care is avoiding additional stressors. These patients should do absolutely nothing for themselves and should be protected from all stimuli and from exposure to infection. To decrease stressors, the same nurse should provide care for the first several hours, during which time the patient's condition stabilizes. One-to-one care may be necessary. To prevent aspiration, the patient is given nothing by mouth until nausea and vomiting subside and until mental status is normal. After several hours, oral liquids may be given, and oral glucocorticoids may be started within 48 hours. The patient may experience a severe headache that may be relieved by an ice bag.

After the patient's condition is stabilized, attention is focused on achieving an improved state of well-being and preparing for discharge; the plan of care is modified as the patient recovers from crisis to a state of chronic adrenal insufficiency. A sample Nursing Care Plan is presented on p. 1111-1112. Acute adrenal insufficiency or addisonian crisis is a potential complication for any patient with adrenal insufficiency.

#### Home Care Management

The patient will require lifelong therapy with both mineralocorticoids and glucocorticoids. In the event the medication cannot be taken orally, the patient must be taught to administer the medication intramuscularly. A family member or friend should also be taught the IM injection technique in case of emergency. A medical alert bracelet is also useful and can be purchased at most drugstores. In case of stress or minor illness, the patient will need to increase the dosage of hormones.

## COMPLICATIONS

The major complication of adrenal insufficiency, adrenal crisis, was discussed previously. Untreated minor illness and infections may result in adrenal crisis if additional cortisone is not administered. Adrenal crisis may result in cardiac arrest, renal failure, or death. Patients with unexplained weakness or confusion and a history of chronic disease that may be managed with corticosteroids should be assessed for the possibility of adrenal crisis. The patient may be unable to give an accurate medication history and a history of steroid use may be missed Hospitalization or surgical intervention may have depleted adrenocortical reserves.

## HYPERSECRETION OF THE ADRENAL MEDULLA: PHEOCHROMOCYTOMA

### Etiology/Epidemiology

Pheochromocytoma is a catecholamine-producing tumor of the sympatheticoadrenal medullary system that causes hypertension. An estimated 36,000 persons in the United States have pheochromocytoma. Although pheochromocytomas account for less than 1% of the cases of hypertension, they should be diagnosed because these persons can be cured. If a person with an undiagnosed pheochromocytoma has surgery or an accident, he or she may die from a hypertensive crisis.

A single benign adrenomedullary tumor is the most common pathological finding. Pheochromocytomas occur most frequently in the fourth and fifth decades of life and are slightly more common in women. Although pheochromocytomas may occur anywhere along the sympathetic nervous system trunk, 90% are found in the adrenal glands. The tendency to develop pheochromocytomas may be inherited and may be part of the MEN syndromes. Pheochromocytomas may be found in MEN IIa in association with hyperparathyroidism and medullary carcinoma or in MEN IIb in association with medullary thyroid carcinoma and multiple mucosal neuromas. Persons with MEN syndrome have a higher incidence of bilateral pheochromocytomas. Pheochromocytomas can also be malignant; the incidence may be as high as 25%.

#### Pathophysiology

Pheochromocytomas of the adrenal medulla release excessive amounts of catecholamines, both epinephrine and norepinephrine. A tumor of the sympathetic nervous system trunk releases excessive amounts of norepinephrine. The hormone release may be constant or episodic, producing constant or episodic clinical manifestations.

A paroxysm or crisis may be precipitated by any lifting, straining, bending, or exercise that increases intraabdominal pressure or moves abdominal contents. Palpation of the abdomen may also precipitate a paroxysm. Anxiety or stress does not usually precipitate an attack. In some patients, no precipitating factors can be identified. The frequency of paroxysms varies but usually increases as the disease progresses.

Release of norepinephrine causes an exaggeration of its effects on $\beta$-receptors, producing massive vasoconstriction. Release of epinephrine causes an exaggeration of its effects on $\beta$-receptors, producing cardiac-stimulating effects and alterations in metabolism. Release of dopamine alone may not produce any vascular symptoms.

Hypertension is the key feature of pheochromocytoma, occurring in 90% of patients. Two thirds of patients exhibit paroxysmal hypertension; the remaining one third of patients have sustained hypertension. The hypertension is resistant to treatment by traditional antihypertensive drugs. In addition, orthostatic hypotension is frequently present, resulting from a decrease in plasma volume and loss of tone of postural reflexes.

Other manifestations frequently present include:

1. Signs of cardiac stimulation: tachycardia, palpitation, chest pain, ECG changes, angina
2. Headaches that are throbbing, abrupt, and severe
3. Increased metabolic rate manifested by heat intolerance, sweating, fever, wasting of fat stores, and weight loss
4. Elevated blood glucose level
5. Nausea, vomiting, and epigastric pain
6. Tremors or weakness
7. Flushing
8. Pallor
9. Tachypnea
10. Nervousness or anxiety

Nephrosclerosis and retinopathy may result from uncontrolled sustained hypertension. Severe episodes of hypertension may cause cerebrovascular accident.

Most persons with malignant pheochromocytoma experience a progressively downhill course. Metastases to the lung, liver, brain, and bone are common. Most persons die from the tumors.

The diagnosis is confirmed by assays of catecholamines and their metabolites in urine (see Chapter 33). Pharmacological tests are used infrequently; these tests either demonstrate the dependence of the hypertension on catecholamines by evaluating response to an $\alpha$-receptor antagonist or provide a paroxysm. Both types of tests are very hazardous. Results of CT scans, arteriography, and venography are used to localize the tumor.

## Collaborative Care Management

Before surgery, treatment consists of controlling hypertension and symptoms of cardiac stimulation. An $\alpha$-adrenergic blocker such as phenoxybenzamine (usual dose, 10 to 20 mg every 6 to 8 hours) is given to help control blood pressure and paroxysms and to increase blood volume. This therapy is started 1 to 2 weeks before surgery. Phentolamine may also be given if hypertensive crisis occurs. A liberal salt diet is prescribed to restore blood volume. If necessary, saline and blood products are given 12 to 24 hours before surgery.

Tachycardia, dysrhythmias, sweating, and angina are controlled with a $\beta$-blocker such as propranolol. This is started only after $\alpha$-adrenergic blockade is established.

Surgical resection of the tumor is the treatment of choice. Postoperative management is focused on maintaining normal blood pressure. Immediately after surgery the patient may be hypertensive; this hypertension is first managed with diuretics and then with phentolamine if necessary. Later the patient may need fluid replacement for hypotension.

Some tumors are not resectable because of disseminated malignancy or other illnesses. Pheochromocytomas do not respond to radiotherapy or chemotherapy. However, bone metastases can be treated with radiation. The tumors are slow growing, and morbidity results from excessive catecholamine secretion. The disease is controlled with $\alpha$- and $\beta$-adrenergic blocking agents and $\alpha$-methyl-*p*-tyrosine, which reduces the production of catecholamines. Radioactive iobenguane sulfate and combined chemotherapy have been used successfully in selected patients.

Preoperatively, nursing care is focused on instituting measures to help stabilize the patient's hemodynamic status, monitor the clinical state, prepare the patient for tests and surgery, and prevent episodes of hypertension. Patients experiencing hypertensive crises should be in an intensive care unit because frequent cardiac, blood pressure, and neurological monitoring is required. If phentolamine infusion is necessary, the blood pressure is checked every 15 minutes, and the drug is given by controlled infusion at a rate to keep the blood pressure at a prescribed level. During this time the patient must be informed about planned diagnostic tests and planned treatment and is prepared for surgery. Activities that precipitate paroxysms, such as bending, Valsalva maneuver, palpating the abdomen, and lifting, should be limited.

The patient continues to need close monitoring of blood pressure, pulse, cardiac rhythm, neurological status, and the effectiveness of treatment postoperatively. After the hypertensive period, hypotension may occur; thus, nursing care is focused on continual monitoring and administration of fluids or plasma expanders as prescribed.

### *Patient/family education*

For patients treated medically or surgical patients without remission of symptoms, nursing care is focused on helping the patient attain the skills necessary for self-care. Patient teaching includes:

1. Knowledge about the disease and its relationship to the signs and symptoms
2. Medication regimen: purpose, dosage, expected effects, and side effects
3. Blood pressure self-measurement
4. Methods to prevent paroxysms: preventing constipation, avoiding Valsalva maneuver, and avoiding bending or flexion of the body
5. Importance of follow-up care
6. Wear medical alert bracelet or carry wallet card

Surgery results in complete remission of symptoms in most patients; therefore, discharge teaching for most patients is focused on helping the patient plan for resumption of normal activities, maintain an adequate diet, and follow-up with the physician.

## critical thinking QUESTIONS

**1** Miss G., 56 years old and previously in good health, is seen with complaints of fatigue, weight gain, lack of energy, and thinning hair. As you talk with her you sense she is mildly depressed. Analyze these data, draw conclusions about the patient's endocrine status, and form an opinion about a pathophysiological etiology for her health status. What diagnostic tests might you, as her nurse, be asked to facilitate? What are Miss G.'s educational needs at this time?

**2** Miss T., 38, has the diagnosis of adrenal dysfunction; rule out adrenal insufficiency. What questions or methods of inquiry would you use to facilitate differential diagnosis?

**3** Think about the implications of an endocrine disorder on body image and self-esteem. Plan strategies for improving a patient's adjustment/adaptation to a disorder such as Cushing's syndrome.

## chapter SUMMARY

- Various pathological processes, including tumor growth, hyperplasia, atrophy, autoimmune processes, infections, and ischemic changes, can affect the endocrine glands. The pathophysiological alteration that occurs in the endocrine glands can be classified as hypoactivity and hyposecretion or hyperactivity and hypersecretion.
- Endocrine dysfunction can also result from resistance to the action of a hormone at the level of the target cell; this type of problem mimics those seen with hyposecretion of hormone.
- Cancer of the endocrine glands can be made up of (1) secreting cells that result in hypersecretion or (2) nonsecreting cells that do not change hormone level or cause hyposecretion by depressing the function of normal tissue.

### ANTERIOR PITUITARY GLAND: HYPERPITUITARISM

- Hypersecretion of the anterior pituitary gland is usually of one hormone, prolactin, resulting in amenorrhea and galactorrhea and hypogonadism or GH, resulting in gigantism in children and acromegaly in adults.
- Hypersecretion of the anterior pituitary gland is usually caused by an adenoma; these adenomas can cause neurological problems, vision changes, or headache by compressing normal neural tissue.
- Prolactin-secreting tumors may be controlled by drug therapy or surgery, depending upon size and symptoms; GH-secreting tumors are resected, followed by radiation and/or drug therapy.
- Nursing care for the patient with a pituitary adenoma consists of (1) helping the patient deal with the irreversible changes (growth changes, bone changes in acromegaly, and possible visual changes); (2) helping the patient achieve a stable metabolic status before surgery; (3) preparing the patient for surgery; (4) caring for the patient after surgery, with a particular focus on monitoring fluid and electrolytes status, monitoring for signs of hormonal deficit (ADH or adrenocortical hormones), preventing increases in intracranial pressure and stress on the suture line, and preventing infection; and (5) preparing for home care.

### ANTERIOR PITUITARY GLAND: HYPOPITUITARISM

- Hyposecretion of the anterior pituitary gland can be of one hormone or all anterior pituitary hormones and ADH (panhypopituitarism).
- Hyposecretion of gonadotropins results in reproductive problems and hypogonadism; hyposecretion of prolactin results in problems in lactation in postpartum patients; hyposecretion of TSH results in hypothyroidism; and hyposecretion of ACTH results in adrenocortical insufficiency.

### POSTERIOR PITUITARY GLAND: HYPERFUNCTION

- SIADH results from hypersecretion of the posterior pituitary gland.
- SIADH causes abnormal water reabsorption, as well as hyponatremia and hypoosmolality, which cause fluid movement from the extracellular to the intracellular compartment and change electrical activity of nerves, potentially resulting in seizures.
- Nursing care for patients with SIADH is focused on increasing osmolality and sodium by water restriction, monitoring for and reporting critical changes (sodium <120 mEq/L, neurological changes), maintaining a safe environment, and patient education.
- Diabetes insipidus, a deficiency of ADH, results from posterior pituitary gland insufficiency.
- Although diabetes insipidus can cause volume deficit and hyponatremia, it usually does not because the thirst precipitated will cause increased fluid intake.
- Vasopressin in a nasal spray is used to treat permanent diabetes insipidus.

### HYPERSECRETION OF THYROID HORMONE: HYPERTHYROIDISM

- Hypersecretion of thyroid hormone most frequently results from Graves' disease, which is caused by an autoimmune process.
- Graves' disease can include hyperthyroidism, goiter, pretibial myxedema, and ophthalmopathy.
- Hyperthyroidism results in increased activity of the neurological system; increased GI motility; increased metabolism, heat production, and calorigenesis; increased cardiac activity; increased respiratory activity; and muscle wasting and weight loss. Many of these changes result from hyperactivity of the sympathetic nervous system.
- Thyroid crisis results from worsening hyperthyroidism when critical increases occur in metabolism, calorigenesis, and sympathetic stimulation.
- Hyperthyroidism is treated with antithyroid drugs or radiation therapy. Surgical resection is performed in rare cases. Use of radioactive iodine after stabilization of the patient's condition is the treatment of choice.
- The major nursing needs of the patient with hyperthyroidism include potential decrease in cardiac output, hyperthermia, activity intolerance, ineffective coping, home maintenance problems, nutritional problems, sleep pattern disturbances, visual deficits, nervousness, and anxiety.

- Treatment of hyperthyroidism does not generally result in immediate improvement; that is, the return to a euthyroid state may not be observed for 6 to 8 weeks.

## HYPOSECRETION OF THYROID GLAND: HYPOTHYROIDISM

- Hypothyroidism is seen most frequently in elderly women; has a slow, insidious onset; causes neurological, respiratory, cardiovascular, GI, and metabolic dysfunction; and requires lifelong hormonal replacement.
- Nursing interventions for patients with hypothyroidism focus on activity intolerance, body image disturbances, constipation, hypothermia, pain, self-care deficits, sexual dysfunction, impaired skin integrity, altered mental status, knowledge deficits, and depression.
- The problems of patients with hypothyroidism vary from minimal dysfunction to severe dysfunction, in which the patient requires complete care, is unresponsive, and may have respiratory failure and diminished cardiac reserve.
- Myxedema coma is critically depressed physiological function resulting from hypothyroidism.
- Hashimoto's thyroiditis is the most frequently occurring form of thyroiditis. It is an autoimmune disease and has exacerbations and remissions.
- With Hashimoto's thyroiditis the thyroid is enlarged, smooth, and painless. With disease progression, the thyroid is eventually destroyed and hypothyroidism occurs. During acute exacerbations, before the gland is destroyed, the patient can experience episodes of hyperthyroidism.
- A goiter is an enlargement of the thyroid gland. It can result from iodine deficiency, exposure to goitrogens, hypothyroidism, or hyperthyroidism.

## CANCER OF THE THYROID GLAND

- Cancer of the thyroid is more rare than other forms of cancer. It can be classified into one of five types: papillary, follicular, anaplastic, medullary, or thyroid lymphoma.
- The prognosis in thyroid cancer varies from very good for patients with papillary and follicular cancer to very poor (less than 6-month survival from diagnosis) for those with anaplastic tumors.
- Most cancers of the thyroid are treated with total thyroidectomy. Thus after surgery, the patient requires lifelong hormonal replacement therapy.
- Nursing interventions for patients with thyroid cancer focus on preparing them for diagnostic tests, preparing them for surgery, helping them to cope with the diagnosis, and caring for them postoperatively.
- The major nursing needs after thyroid surgery relate to monitoring for respiratory distress or any of its etiological factors: internal hemorrhage, which can cause compression on the trachea; laryngeal damage to the vocal cords and obstruction of the airway; or tetany, which can cause laryngeal spasms. Any signs of respiratory distress or its causes need to be reported immediately.
- The tetany results from damage to the parathyroid glands during thyroid surgery. The nurse should have an intravenous preparation of calcium available as well as a tracheostomy tray.

## HYPERSECRETION OF PARATHYROID HORMONE: HYPERPARATHYROIDISM

- Hyperparathyroidism can be primary, secondary, or tertiary: primary results from adenomas and hyperplasia; secondary from chronic hypocalcemia, which causes chronic stimulation of the parathyroid gland; and tertiary from the development of an autonomous parathyroid gland chronically stimulated by a hypocalcemic state.
- In primary hyperparathyroidism, continual bone resorption and changes in renal and GI processing of calcium occur. The results are hypercalcemia and changes in neurological, GI, and cardiac functioning. Renal stones can occur; bone density decreases.
- Secondary hyperparathyroidism is a compensatory process that maintains the plasma level of calcium at the expense of bones; chronic renal failure is a major cause.
- Hypercalcemia is treated before parathyroid surgery by hydration with normal saline, and diuretics such as furosemide or ethacrynic acid; thiazide diuretics are not used because they inhibit calcium excretion.
- Primary hyperparathyroidism is treated by surgery; three to three and one half glands are removed.
- The major complications after parathyroid surgery are hypocalcemia and laryngeal spasms from tetany and respiratory obstruction for compression of the trachea by hemorrhage or from laryngeal nerve damage.

## HYPOSECRETION OF PARATHYROID HORMONE: HYPOPARATHYROIDISM

- Hypoparathyroidism can result from trauma or surgery or be idiopathic.
- Hypoparathyroidism results in hypocalcemia, which leads to cardiac and neurological problems; the latter results from increased excitability of neurons.
- The treatment for hypoparathyroidism is vitamin D and calcium replacement.

## HYPERFUNCTION OF THE ADRENAL CORTEX: CORTISOL EXCESS

- Glucocorticoid excess (Cushing's syndrome) can result from excessive production of ACTH by the pituitary gland, excessive production of ACTH by ectopic tumors, excessive production of glucocorticoids by the adrenal glands, or intake of large doses of exogenous steroids.
- Glucocorticoid excess results in increased protein breakdown and muscle wasting, abnormal metabolism of fats with changes in fat stores and increased serum lipid levels, and increased glucose production. Abnormal retention of sodium and water with increased excretion of potassium and hydrogen ions also occurs. Bone demineralization results. Suppression of the immune system and the inflammatory response is a major result of glucocorticoid excess.
- Patients with glucocorticoid excess have fluid volume excess, hypernatremia, hypocalcemia, alkalosis, infections, muscle wasting, osteoporosis, hyperglycemia, peptic ulcers, mental changes, body changes (thin extremities, truncal obesity, moon face, and kyphosis), poor wound healing, and bruising.
- Nursing care for patients with Cushing's syndrome focuses on the nursing diagnoses of activity intolerance, disturbances in body image, ineffective coping, fluid volume excess, risk for infection and injury, nutrient excess, pain, and knowledge deficit.
- The most frequent cause of Cushing's syndrome is iatrogenic, and the treatment focuses on dealing with the signs and symptoms of glucocorticoid excess.
- When patients have been taking steroids long-term, drug therapy must be tapered as it is discontinued.

### HYPERFUNCTION OF THE ADRENAL CORTEX GLAND: ALDOSTERONE EXCESS

- Aldosterone excess results in sodium and water excess, volume expansion, hypokalemia, and hypertension.
- Treatment for aldosterone excess is designed to lower blood pressure using sodium restriction and spironolactone or amiloride diuretics or surgery.

### HYPOFUNCTION OF ADRENAL CORTEX

- Adrenocortical insufficiency is a medical emergency because the person is not able to mount a compensatory response to a major stressor. When glucocorticoids are deficient and a stressor is present, the person is unable to retain needed water and sodium, maintain blood pressure, and produce energy substrates (glucose, fatty acids).
- Patients deficient in glucocorticoids require lifetime replacement therapy. They must know what to monitor to identify signs of a deficit or an excess, must know when to take additional hormones, and must wear or carry appropriate identification.
- Hyperpigmentation occurs in patients with Cushing's syndrome resulting from increased ACTH and primary adrenocortical insufficiency, which is associated with increased ACTH.

### HYPERSECRETION OF ADRENAL MEDULLA

- Tumors of the adrenal medulla cause excessive production of catecholamines and are called pheochromocytomas.
- Hypertension, constant or paroxysmal, is the major sign of pheochromocytoma.
- Activities such as increased abdominal pressure, Valsalva maneuver, straining, and bending over can increase release of catecholamines and worsen hypertension in patients with pheochromocytoma.
- Surgery is the treatment of choice for patients with pheochromocytoma.

## References


1. Arnaud CD: The calciotropic hormones and metabolic bone disease. In Greenspan FS, Strewler GJ, editors: *Basic and clinical endocrinology,* ed 6, Norwalk, Conn, 1997, Appleton and Lange.
2. Aron DC, Findling MD, Tyrell JB: Hypothalamus and pituitary. In Greenspan FS, Strewler GJ, editors: *Basic and clinical endocrinology,* ed 6, Norwalk, Conn, 1997, Appleton and Lange.
3. Aron DC, Tyrell JB, editors: Cushing's syndrome, *Endocrinol Metab Clin North Am* 23:451, 1994.
4. Attie JN: Primary hyperparathyroidism. In Bardin CW, editor: *Current therapy in endocrinology and metabolism,* ed 5, St Louis, 1994, Mosby.
5. Danese RD, Aron DC: Cushing's syndrome and hypertension, *Endocrinol Metab Clin North Am* 23:299-324, 1992.
6. Ezzat S, et al: Octreotide treatment of acromegaly: a randomized, multicenter study, *Ann Intern Med* 117:7111, 1992.
7. Greenspan FS: The thyroid. In Greenspan FS, Strewler GJ, editors: *Basic and clinical endocrinology,* ed 6, Norwalk, Conn, 1997, Appleton and Lange.
8. Gregerman RI: Thyroid disorders. In Barker LD, Burton JR, Zieve PD, editors: *Principles of ambulatory medicine,* ed 4, Baltimore, 1995, Williams & Wilkins.
9. Hughes MN, Llamas KJ, Yelland ME, et al: Pituitary adenomas: long-term results for radiotherapy alone and post-operative radiotherapy, *Int J Radiat Oncol Biol Phys* 27:1035, 1993.
10. Locker FG: Hormone regulation of calcium homeostasis, *Nurs Clin North Am* 31:797-802, 1996.
11. Molitch ME: Neuroendocrinology. In Felig P, Baster JD, Frohman LA, editors: *Endocrinology and metabolism,* ed 3, New York, 1995, McGraw-Hill.
12. Molitch ME: Pathologic hyperprolactinemia, *Endocrinol Metab Clin North Am* 21:877, 1992.
13. Porterfield SP: *Endocrine physiology,* St Louis, 1997, Mosby.
14. Reeves WB, Andreoli TE: The posterior pituitary and water metabolism. In Wilson JD, Fowter DW, editors: *Williams' textbook of endocrinology,* ed 8, Philadelphia, 1992, WB Saunders.
15. Romeo JH: Hyperfunction and hypofunction in the anterior pituitary, *Nurs Clin North Am* 31(4):769-778, 1996.
16. Romeo JH, Dombrowski RC, Aron DC, et al: Hyperprolactinemia and verapamil: prevalence, evidence for causality, and associated hypogonadism, *Clin Endocrinol* 45:571-575, 1996.
17. Schilling JS: Hyperparathyroidism: diagnosis and management of Grave's disease, *Nurse Pract* 22(6):72-94, 1997.
18. Streff MM, Pachucki-Hyde LC: Management of the patient with thyroid disease, *Nurs Clin North Am* 31:779-795, 1996.
19. Styne DM: The therapy for hypothalamic-pituitary tumors, *Endocrinol Metab Clin North Am* 22:163, 1993.
20. Tindall GT, Oyesiku NM, Watts NB, et al: Transsphenoidal adenomectomy for growth hormone-secreting pituitary adenomas in acromegaly: outcome analysis and determinants of failure, *J Neurosurg* 78:203, 1993.
21. Whitcomb RW, Crowley WF Jr: Male hypogonadotropic hypogonadism, *Endocrinol Metab Clin North Am* 22:125, 1993.
22. Ybarra Y, Ade RA, Romeo JH: Osteoporosis in men: a review, *Nurs Clin North Am* 31(4):805-813, 1996.

chapter 35

# MANAGEMENT OF PERSONS WITH Diabetes Mellitus and Hypoglycemia

MARGARET M. ULCHAKER

## objectives

*After studying this chapter, the learner should be able to:*

1 Differentiate among type 1 diabetes mellitus (type 1 DM, previously called insulin-dependent diabetes mellitus), type 2 diabetes mellitus (type 2 DM, previously called non–insulin-dependent diabetes mellitus), and gestational diabetes mellitus (GDM).
2 Compare and contrast the epidemiological and etiological factors of type 1 DM and type 2 DM.
3 Differentiate the pathophysiological basis for type 1 DM from that for type 2 DM.
4 Describe the common manifestations of uncontrolled type 1 DM and type 2 DM.
5 Compare and contrast the comprehensive care of the individual with type 1 DM and type 2 DM.
6 Describe the pivotal role of dietary management and education in type 1 DM and type 2 DM.
7 Discuss the role of exercise in the treatment of type 1 DM and type 2 DM.
8 Describe physiological insulin regimens in type 1 DM.
9 Analyze the oral agents used in treatment of type 2 DM: mechanism of action, dosage ranges, metabolic effects, side effects, and contraindications.
10 Develop a nursing care plan, including nursing diagnoses, patient outcomes, and interventions, for an individual with stable diabetes mellitus.
11 Discuss sick-day management guidelines for the individual with diabetes mellitus.
12 Describe the surgical considerations for the individual with diabetes mellitus.
13 Discuss hypoglycemia as a consequence of diabetes management: causes, signs and symptoms, treatment, and prevention.
14 Differentiate the pathophysiology, clinical manifestations, and management of persons with diabetic ketoacidosis from persons with hyperglycemic hyperosmolar nonketotic coma.
15 Describe the chronic complications of diabetes mellitus, the relationship between metabolic control and the chronic complications, and the management of the complications.
16 Differentiate fasting and reactive hypoglycemia based on causes, clinical manifestations, and management.

## DIABETES MELLITUS

"Diabetes mellitus is a group of metabolic diseases characterized by hyperglycemia resulting from defects in insulin secretion, insulin action, or both."[6] The basis of the abnormalities in carbohydrate, protein, and fat metabolism in diabetes is the deficient action of insulin on the target tissues of skeletal muscle, adipose tissue, and the liver. Uncontrolled diabetes mellitus (DM) may result in long-term damage, dysfunction, and failure of various organs. Diabetes cannot be cured, but it *can* be controlled. Elliott Joslin, MD, who is considered to be the father of diabetes care, stated, "Diabetes is a serious disease and deserves the best effort of doctor and patient from beginning to end."[54]

By its very nature, DM can be significantly influenced by daily self-care. No other disease demands so much of the patient's own self-knowledge and skills. Thus the professional nurse has the challenge and responsibility to help patients gain the knowledge, skills, and attitudes necessary for self-care.

National (American Diabetes Association)[7] and international (World Health Organization/St. Vincent Declaration) Standards of Care for diabetes mellitus have been in existence for several years. These Standards of Care encompass diabetes evaluation, management, and education. Standards of care represent *minimum* levels of care to be provided and by no means represent excellence in care. Excellence has yet to be defined. Despite their publication and dissemination to both the health care community and patients alike, these protocols have yet to become standard practice. Fewer than 5% of patients with diabetes in the United States attend endocrinologists for diabetes care; primary care physicians provide the bulk of diabetes care, although the standards recommend care be delivered by an endocrinologist. Numerous studies demonstrate a large gap between current recommendations for diabetes care and actual practice patterns of primary care

**table 35-1** *Classification of Diabetes Mellitus and Other Disorders of Glucose Tolerance*

| Type | Defining Characteristics |
|---|---|
| Type 1 DM | |
| Immune mediated | Insulinopenic (insulin deficient) and dependent on exogenous insulin to sustain life<br>Onset generally before age 30, but may occur at any age, including the geriatric years<br>Generally lean, rarely obese<br>Variable rate of $\beta$-cell destruction<br>Clinical presentation usually rapid<br>In 85-90%, one or more of the following autoantibodies are present at the time when fasting hyperglycemia is initially detected:<br>Islet cell autoantibodies (ICA)<br>Insulin autoantibodies (IAA)<br>Glutamic acid decarboxylase autoantibodies (GAD)<br>Tyrosine phosphatase IA-2 or IA-2$\beta$ autoantibodies<br>Strong human leukocyte antigen (HLA) associations<br>Linkage to DQA and B genes<br>Influenced by DRB genes |
| Idiopathic diabetes | No immunological evidence for $\beta$-cell destruction<br>No HLA association<br>Strongly inherited<br>Most individuals affected are of African or Asian origin<br>Episodic ketoacidosis with varying degrees of insulin deficiency between episodes<br>The absolute requirement for exogenous insulin is episodic |
| Type 2 DM | No requirement for exogenous insulin to sustain life at least initially<br>Ranges from a picture of predominantly insulin resistance with mild relative insulin deficiency to a picture of more severe insulin secretory defects with insulin resistance<br>Usually obese; those who are not obese by traditional criteria usually have abdominal adiposity<br>Onset usually after age 40, but may occur at any age<br>No autoimmune or HLA association |
| Other | |
| Genetic defects of $\beta$-cell function | Previously termed *maturity onset diabetes of youth* (MODY)—impaired insulin secretion without defects in insulin action<br>Autosomal dominant inheritance<br>Abnormalities in three genetic loci have been determined to date |
| Genetic defects in insulin action | N/A |
| Diseases of the exocrine pancreas | Pancreatitis, trauma, infection, pancreatectomy, pancreatic carcinoma, cystic fibrosis, hemochromatosis |
| Endocrinopathies | Acromegaly, Cushing's syndrome, glucagonoma, pheochromocytoma |
| Drug-induced | Permanent destruction of $\beta$-cells (Vacor [rat poison], IV pentamidine)<br>Impairment of insulin action (nicotinic acid, glucocorticoids, thiazide diuretics)<br>Impairment of insulin secretion, thereby precipitating DM in an individual with insulin resistance (e.g., drug-induced hypokalemia) |
| Infections | Congenital rubella, cytomegalovirus |
| Uncommon forms: immune mediated | Stiff-man syndrome, anti-insulin receptor antibodies |
| Genetic syndromes associated with DM | Turner's syndrome, Down syndrome, Klinefelter's syndrome |
| Gestational DM | Pregnancy related |
| Impaired glucose tolerance (IGT) | Glucose levels are higher than normal but do not meet diagnostic criteria for DM<br>21 million individuals in United States<br>Generally obese<br>7% per year progression to overt type 2 DM<br>Insulin resistant and are at increased cardiovascular risk |
| Impaired fasting glucose | Fasting glucose levels higher than normal but lower than those in IGT or DM |

Adapted from American Diabetes Association, Expert Committee on the Diagnosis and Classification of Diabetes Mellitus: Report of the Expert Committee on the Diagnosis and Classification of Diabetes Mellitus, *Diabetes Care* 20(7):1183, 1997.

physicians.[48,50,65,66,81,124] Diabetes care by a dedicated specialty team, however, has been demonstrated to confer a survival advantage of up to 15 years.[64,122]

This chapter focuses on the two most common types of diabetes: type 1 DM and type 2 DM. However, much of the information applies to the other types.

## CLASSIFICATION

In July 1997 a new diagnostic and classification system for diabetes was published by the Expert Committee on the Diagnosis and Classification of Diabetes Mellitus of the American Diabetes Association (Table 35-1). This new system reflects the etiology and pathophysiology of diabetes, with the two major categories being type 1 diabetes mellitus (previously termed *insulin-dependent diabetes mellitus* or *juvenile-onset diabetes mellitus*) and type 2 diabetes mellitus (previously termed *non–insulin-dependent diabetes mellitus* or *maturity-onset diabetes mellitus*).[6] The previous system published by the National Diabetes Data Group of the National Institutes of Health in 1979 and accepted by the World Health Organization in 1980 was based to a large degree on the pharmacological therapy used (i.e., insulin-dependent DM or non–insulin-dependent DM).

Table 35-2 compares the characteristics of type 1 DM and type 2 DM. Both the classifications and their characteristics are important for the professional nurse in understanding this chapter.

## ETIOLOGY

The etiology of each type of diabetes mellitus is still unfolding. Table 35-3 identifies etiological factors of type 1 DM and type 2 DM. In relation to type 1 DM, genetics seem to have a permissive role that allows environmental factors, perhaps viruses, to trigger the onset of diabetes by stimulating an autoimmune response. (Individuals with a family history of diabetes are at high risk for type 2 DM.) A prior history of impaired glucose tolerance (IGT) or gestational diabetes mellitus (GDM), particularly in obese individuals, are risk factors for type 2 DM. Approximately 25% of individuals with IGT and up to 70% of individuals with GDM develop type 2 DM. Glucotoxicity, the toxic effects of hyperglycemia on the islets, may be another causal factor in precipitating type 2 DM. Insulin resistance has a role in the pathogenesis of type 2 DM. *Insulin resistance* is defined as the inability of the insulin-sensitive tissues (skeletal muscle, liver, and adipose tissue) to respond normally to insulin-stimulated glucose uptake.

## EPIDEMIOLOGY

In the United States, approximately 16 million individuals have diabetes, with half of them being undiagnosed. Diabetes mellitus is the sixth leading cause of death by disease in the United States. Diabetes cannot be cured. Diabetes, however, *can* be controlled. The prevalence of diagnosed individuals is slightly greater in women and also increases significantly with age (Box 35-1). Prevalence also varies with race and ethnicity (Table 35-4). Incidence indicates new cases of diabetes (see Box 35-1). Each year, approximately 625,000 new cases are diagnosed; approximately 595,000, or 95%, are type 2 DM. Each day, approximately 1700 individuals are diagnosed with diabetes.[76]

Figure 35-1 depicts the risks of major complications of diabetes when persons with diabetes are compared with nondiabetic persons. Additionally, as many as 50% of men with diabetes and 35% of women with diabetes have sexual problems from neuropathy.

**table 35-2** *Characteristics of Type 1 and Type 2 Diabetes Mellitus*

| Characteristics | Type 1 DM | Type 2 DM |
|---|---|---|
| Insulin status | Insulin secretion ↓ | Insulin secretion ↑, ↓, or normal |
| Age | Usually under 30 but may occur at any age | Usually over 40 but may occur at any age |
| Clinical presentation | Rapid | Slow |
| Body build | Lean or normal usually | 80-90% overweight |
| Family history | Weak | Strong |
| Islet cell antibodies | Present at onset in 85-90% | Absent |
| HLA association | Positive (DQA, B) | Negative |
| Incidence | 10% of total | 90% of total |
| Symptoms | Polyuria, polydipsia, polyphagia, weight loss | No symptoms or may have same symptoms as type 1<br>May have symptomatic complications when diagnosed |
| Ketones | Prone | Resistant except during infection or with stressors |
| Complications | Related to degree and duration of hyperglycemia<br>Not present at time of diagnosis | Related to degree and duration of hyperglycemia<br>May be present at diagnosis in 20% or more because of delay in diagnosis |
| Treatment | Insulin, diet, exercise | Diet, exercise, oral agents, insulin |
| Racial distribution | More common in whites | More common in African Americans and Hispanics<br>Highest in Native Americans |

**table 35-3** *Etiological Factors in Type 1 and Type 2 Diabetes Mellitus*

| Factors | Type 1 DM | Type 2 DM |
|---|---|---|
| Genetic | Associated with HLA antigens (particularly DQA and B genes) | Not associated with HLA antigens |
| Heredity | Unknown<br>Familial aggregates rare<br>Less than 50% concordance in monozygotic twins<br>Greater risk for child to develop type 1 if father has type 1 (6%) vs. mother having type 1 (3%) | Unknown except for class of genetic defects of $\beta$-cell destruction, which is inherited dominantly |
| Autoimmune basis | Strong autoimmune basis as seen by:<br>Insulitis (inflammation of the islets of Langerhans with lymphocytic infiltration)<br>Presence of autoantibodies to islet cells (ICA), insulin (IAA), glutamic acid decarboxylase (GAD), or tyrosine phosphatase | None |
| Environmental basis | Viral infections may be an environmental trigger; as counterregulatory hormones increase in response to stress of illness, the islets are unable to respond with the needed increased insulin secretion to maintain euglycemia | Modern lifestyle of poor eating and nutritional habits resulting in obesity and inactivity provides stimuli for those who are predisposed |

**box 35-1** *Definitions of Prevalence and Incidence*

- **Prevalence**—total number of people known to have the disease at a particular time
- **Incidence**—number of people diagnosed with a disease for the first time in the previous year (new cases)

**table 35-4** *Prevalence of Diabetes by Race/Ethnicity*

| Race/Ethnicity | Diagnosed and Undiagnosed (%) |
|---|---|
| White Americans | 6.2 |
| Cuban Americans | 9.1 |
| African Americans | 9.6 |
| Mexican Americans | 9.6 |
| Puerto Rican Americans | 10.9 |
| Native Americans | Ranges from 5 to 50 |
| Japanese Americans | Up to 20 |

Adapted from National Institute of Diabetes and Digestive and Kidney Diseases, National Diabetes Information Clearinghouse, National Institutes of Health: *Diabetes statistics,* NIH publication no 96-3926, 1995.

Diabetes is a disease that kills women more readily than men. A woman with diabetes has four times the risk of cardiovascular disease as compared with her nondiabetic counterpart. A man with diabetes has only twice the risk of cardiovascular disease as compared with his nondiabetic counterpart.

Diabetes is a costly disease in terms of not only morbidity and mortality, but dollars and cents. Total costs for diabetes in 1992 were $92 billion; $45 billion were direct costs and $47 billion were indirect costs.[76] The average annual cost per patient is 3.5 times higher for an individual with diabetes as compared with a nondiabetic individual.

## PATHOPHYSIOLOGY

The hallmark of diabetes is insulin deficiency, either absolute or relative. In absolute insulin deficiency, the pancreas produces either no insulin or very little insulin, as is seen in type 1 DM. In relative insulin deficiency, the pancreas produces either normal or excessive amounts of insulin, but the body is unable to use it effectively, such that glucose levels remain elevated. This latter defect is called *insulin resistance* and is seen in type 2 DM (Figure 35-2). Fundamentally, it is failure of the pancreas to produce enough insulin to overcome this insulin resistance that precipitates clinical type 2 DM in predisposed individuals.

This absolute or relative insulin deficiency results in significant abnormalities in the metabolism of the body fuels. The body needs fuel for all its functions, for building new tissue, and for repairing tissue. The fuel comes from the food that is ingested, which is composed of carbohydrates, proteins, and fats. It is important to understand and emphasize to patients that diabetes is not a disease of glucose alone, although the diagnostic criteria that have been devised use the serum glucose level as the marker for the diagnosis and control of the disease. Because the most common word used in the diabetes vocabulary is "sugar," it is understandable how patients with long-standing or new diabetes can believe that if sugar is eliminated from the diet, the battle is won. It is important that nurses help patients understand that diabetes is a disease that affects how the body utilizes all foods (carbohydrates, fats, and proteins).

## HORMONES

The hormones involved in glucose metabolism include those from the pancreas (insulin and glucagon) (Table 35-5), pituitary gland (growth hormone [GH] and adrenocorticotropic

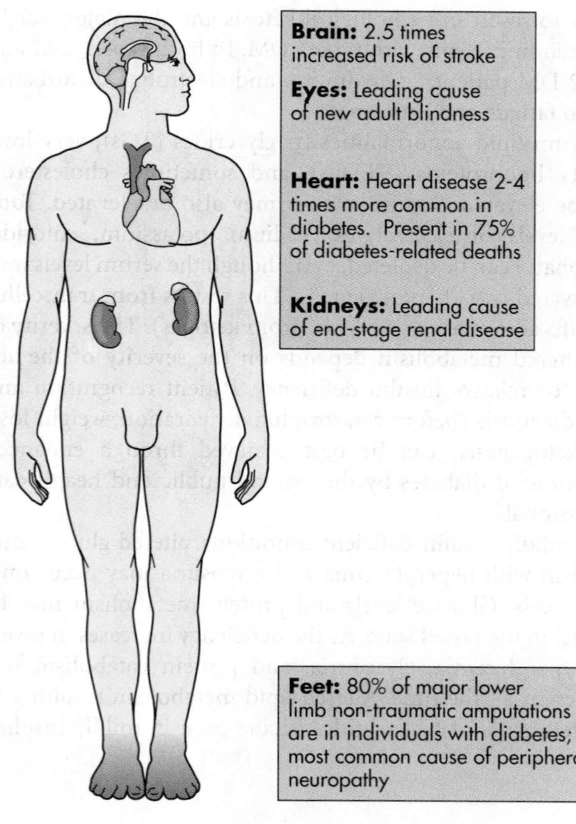
**Brain:** 2.5 times increased risk of stroke
**Eyes:** Leading cause of new adult blindness
**Heart:** Heart disease 2-4 times more common in diabetes. Present in 75% of diabetes-related deaths
**Kidneys:** Leading cause of end-stage renal disease
**Feet:** 80% of major lower limb non-traumatic amputations are in individuals with diabetes; most common cause of peripheral neuropathy

**fig. 35-1** Diabetes complications.

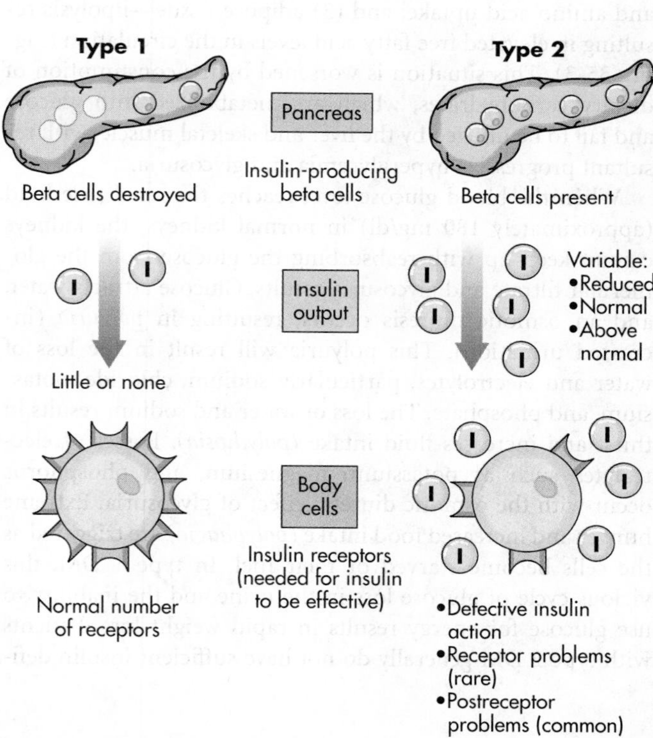
Type 1
Type 2
Pancreas
Insulin-producing beta cells
Beta cells destroyed
Beta cells present
Insulin output
Little or none
Variable:
•Reduced
•Normal
•Above normal
Body cells
Insulin receptors (needed for insulin to be effective)
Normal number of receptors
•Defective insulin action
•Receptor problems (rare)
•Postreceptor problems (common)

**fig. 35-2** Insulin defects in type 1 DM and type 2 DM.

**table 35-5** *Pancreatic Hormones*

| Insulin Promotes, Glucagon Inhibits | Insulin Inhibits, Glucagon Promotes |
|---|---|
| Glucose uptake into skeletal muscle and liver | Hyperglycemia |
| Glycogenesis (glycogen synthesis) | Gluconeogenesis (conversion of amino acids into glucose)<br>Glycogenolysis (glycogen breakdown) |
| Protein anabolism (protein synthesis) | Protein catabolism (protein breakdown) |
| Lipogenesis (fat synthesis and deposition) | Lipolysis (fat breakdown) |

NOTE: Insulin is the *only* hormone that lowers blood glucose levels.

**table 35-6** *Extrapancreatic Glucose-Elevating Hormones*

| Cortisol | Catecholamines | Growth Hormone |
|---|---|---|
| Gluconeogenesis | Glycogenolysis | Gluconeogenesis |
| Lipolysis | Lipolysis | Lipolysis |
| Secretion is controlled by pituitary ACTH; deficiency or excess affects glucose control | Inhibition of insulin release | Decreases glucose uptake into skeletal muscle |

hormone [ACTH]), adrenal cortex (cortisol), and autonomic nervous system (ANS) (norepinephrine) and adrenal medulla (epinephrine) (Table 35-6). Insulin is the only hormone that lowers blood glucose levels. The other hormones, called counterregulatory hormones, elevate blood glucose. Insulin is synthesized by the $\beta$-cells in the islets of Langerhans within the pancreas. Insulin ensures that the body is able to use glucose for energy. Insulin binds to insulin receptors on the surface of the insulin-sensitive tissues (skeletal muscle, liver, and adipose tissue). In response, a cascade of events occurs that allows glucose to move from the bloodstream into the cell. These events are called postreceptor events.

## CONSEQUENCES OF INSULIN DEFICIENCY: ABSOLUTE OR RELATIVE

The insulin-requiring organs are the liver, skeletal muscle, and adipose tissue. The consequences of either absolute or relative insulin deficiency at the level of these organs are as follows:

(1) liver—hyperglycemia, hypertriglyceridemia, and ketone production; (2) skeletal muscle—failure of glucose uptake and amino acid uptake; and (3) adipose tissue—lipolysis resulting in elevated free fatty acid levels in the circulation (Figure 35-3). This situation is worsened by the consumption of dietary carbohydrates, which are metabolized into glucose and fail to be utilized by the liver and skeletal muscle, with resultant progressive hyperglycemia and glycosuria.

When the blood glucose level reaches the renal threshold (approximately 180 mg/dl) in normal kidneys, the kidneys cannot keep up with reabsorbing the glucose from the glomerular filtrate and glycosuria results. Glucose attracts water, and an osmotic diuresis occurs, resulting in *polyuria* (increased urination). This polyuria will result in the loss of water and electrolytes, particularly sodium, chloride, potassium, and phosphate. The loss of water and sodium results in thirst and increases fluid intake *(polydipsia)*. Losses of electrolytes such as potassium, magnesium, and phosphorus occur with the osmotic diuretic effect of glycosuria. Extreme hunger and increased food intake *(polyphagia)* are triggered as the cells become starved of their fuel. In type 1 DM, this vicious cycle of glucose loss in the urine and the inability to use glucose for energy results in rapid weight loss. Patients with type 2 DM generally do not have sufficient insulin deficiency to result in pathological ketosis and the major weight loss seen in patients with type 1 DM. In both type 1 DM and type 2 DM patients, dehydration and electrolyte disturbance lead to fatigue and listlessness.

Serum lipid abnormalities (triglycerides [TGs], very-low-density lipoproteins [VLDLs], and sometimes cholesterol) may be elevated. Serum ketones may also be elevated. Total body levels of electrolytes (sodium, potassium, chloride, phosphate) can be depleted, even though the serum levels may be elevated (e.g., hyperkalemia). This results from transcellular shifts secondary to acidosis (from ketones). The severity of this altered metabolism depends on the severity of the absolute or relative insulin deficiency. Patient recognition and early diagnosis (before catastrophic dehydration, weight loss, and ketogenesis) can be best achieved through enhanced awareness of diabetes by the general public and health care professionals.

In mildly insulin-deficient conditions, altered glucose metabolism with hyperglycemia and glycosuria may occur only after meals. Glucose levels and protein metabolism may be normal in the fasted state. As the deficiency increases in severity, hyperglycemia, glycosuria, and protein catabolism will be present all the time. Altered lipid metabolism resulting in elevated levels of triglycerides occurs even in mildly insulin-

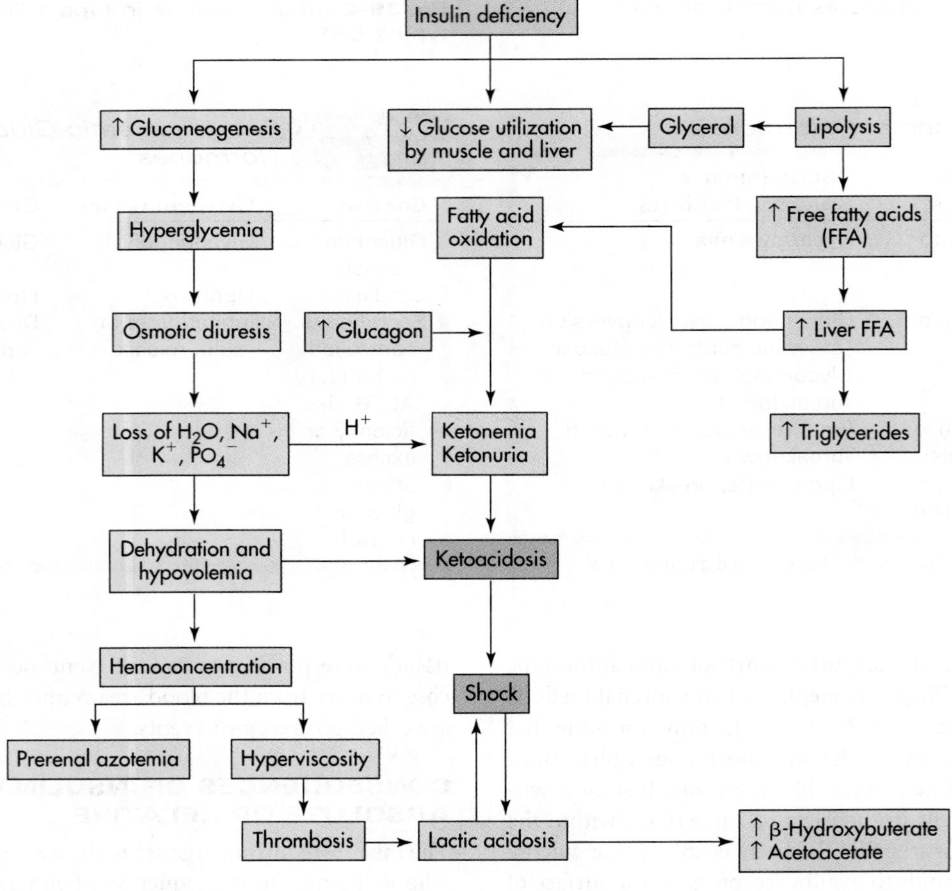


**fig. 35-3** Pathophysiology of insulin deficiency.

deficient states. Abnormally high production of ketones may be seen only in markedly insulin-deficient states and is usually present only in type 1 DM, but it can exist in type 2 DM in the settings of dehydration, electrolyte depletion, and significant hypertriglyceridemia.

If the alterations just described are not corrected or adequately controlled, acute and chronic complications can occur. Acutely, the patient can develop nausea and vomiting and other alterations, fluid and electrolyte problems worsen, and the patient's condition can advance to hyperglycemic coma or diabetic ketoacidosis (DKA). The mortality rate in DKA approaches 10%, and the mortality rate in hyperglycemic hyperosmolar nonketotic coma (HHNC) reaches 70%. Chronically, the patient can develop microvascular and macrovascular complications or neuropathy. These conditions are described later in this chapter.

The clinical manifestations of type 1 DM and type 2 DM appear in Box 35-2. The classic symptoms of diabetes, which are the "polys" *(polyuria, polydipsia, and polyphagia),* are nearly always present in type 1 DM and can be present in type 2 DM. However, many persons with type 2 DM have very subtle symptoms of acute metabolic changes or chronic complications.

When differentiating between type 1 DM and type 2 DM, most individuals are readily classified on the basis of age, body weight, and family history. Some elements of a patient's history may make diagnosis difficult (e.g., age 30 to 40 years, unavailable family history [adopted], and weight loss to less than 120% of ideal body weight). An understanding of the basic pathophysiology will readily clarify the situation. Pancreatic islet cell antibodies are positive in 85% to 90% of type 1 DM patients, and insulin levels will be low or subnormal. In a patient already being treated with insulin before a definitive diagnostic classification, a C-peptide level can provide clarification of endogenous insulin production. A molecule of C-peptide is generated when the insulin precursor molecule proinsulin, produced in the islet cells, is converted to insulin. Hence, for every molecule of insulin secreted by the pancreatic islets, a molecule of insulin is produced.

An important clue to correct classification of type 2 DM patients is the presence of other components of *syndrome X*—the syndrome originally described by Reaven in 1984, encompassing varying degrees of glucose intolerance, hypertension, hypertriglyceridemia, low high-density lipoprotein (HDL) cholesterol, abdominal obesity, hyperuricemia, and elevated levels of plasminogen activator inhibitor type 1. All are mediated and modulated by the control of insulin resistance.[89-91] Insulin resistance essentially blocks the normal uptake of glucose into these insulin-sensitive tissues. The earliest abnormality in glucose metabolism occurs in skeletal muscle, as insulin-mediated glucose uptake decreases. A compensatory hyperinsulinemia develops as the pancreatic islets try to increase production and secretion of insulin in an effort to maintain euglycemia. Eventually, pancreatic exhaustion occurs and the necessary insulin production falls off. Once the pancreas is no longer able to secrete enough insulin to overcome the insulin resistance, type 2 DM occurs.

**box 35-2** *clinical manifestations*

***Diabetes***

EARLY SYMPTOMS

Polyuria
Polydipsia
Polyphagia
Visual blurring
Fatigue
Weight loss

LATE SIGNS AND SYMPTOMS

Coma
Chronic complications

## COLLABORATIVE CARE MANAGEMENT

The expected length of hospitalization for patients with diabetes mellitus as determined by diagnosis-related groups (DRGs) is 5 to 6 days. In the past, patients with diabetes were often hospitalized to initiate management. This is done now only if the patient is experiencing acute metabolic decompensation. Patients need to establish goals with their health care team members for management of their diabetes. The foci of collaborative care are as follows:

1. Using diagnostic tests to determine the presence of diabetes mellitus or complications
2. Establishing goals related to level of daily control
3. Using medications, treatments, diet, and activities to manage diabetes on a day-to-day basis
4. Using medications, treatments, and diet to manage acute and chronic complications of diabetes
5. Working as a multidisciplinary team

The way to achieve the goal of metabolic control is through the use of medications, diet, activity, monitoring, and education. By its very nature, diabetes can be significantly influenced by each of these management components (Figure 35-4).

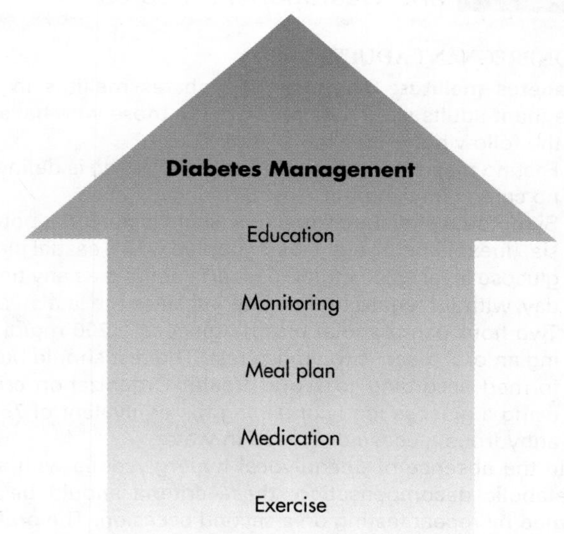


**fig. 35-4** Diabetes management.

## Diagnostic Tests

Diagnostic criteria for diabetes are found in Box 35-3. Frequent monitoring of diagnostic tests (blood glucose, lipids) is a method of assessing glycemic control.

The definition of control has changed dramatically over the years. Before the discovery of insulin in 1921, control was defined as the avoidance of early death or coma. The current definition of control is *normalcy*—normalization of not only glucose levels, but also of other metabolic parameters (Table 35-7).

The relationship of glycemic control to the development of microvascular (small blood vessel) complications of diabetes was debated for years, despite evidence gathered in a large retrospective study by Pirart[83] and smaller controlled studies, the KROC study[111] and Steno II,[57] which demonstrated a definite relationship. The control and complications issue, however, was put to rest and proved beyond doubt when results of the landmark Diabetes Control and Complications Trial (DCCT) were published in 1993.[110] The purpose of the DCCT was to examine the effect of two treatment regimens on the development and progression of complications. The DCCT was a 10-year, nationwide, multicenter randomized prospective clinical trial of over 1400 individuals with type 1 DM. Subjects were randomized to either conventional therapy or intensive therapy. Conventional therapy consisted of one or two insulin injections daily, random home blood glucose monitoring (HBGM), and clinic follow-up every 3 months. In contrast, intensive therapy consisted of three or more insulin injections daily or insulin pump therapy, HBGM before meals and at bedtime, and a more precise carbohydrate-consistent meal plan. Follow-up with the study diabetes team was every 1 to 2 months.

The DCCT was terminated 1 year early because the intensive therapy group had a statistically significant reduction in both (1) the development of and (2) the progression of microvascular complications (Table 35-8). The DCCT found that the lower the glycosylated hemoglobin (a marker of diabetes control), the lower the risk of complications. At no point did better blood glucose control not result in fewer complications. As a result of this landmark study, the American Diabetes Association (ADA) recommends intensive therapy for all individuals with type 1 DM, with few exceptions, such as advanced age and end-stage complications.[2,5]

Although the DCCT studied individuals with type 1 DM, the diabetes professional community believes there is no rea-

**table 35-7** *Goals for Control: Normalization of Metabolic Parameters*

| TARGET BLOOD GLUCOSE LEVELS IN THE NON-PREGNANT STATE: EUGLYCEMIA | |
|---|---|
| TIME | mg/dl |
| Fasting | 70-110 |
| 1 hour postprandially | <150 |
| 2 hours postprandially | <120 |
| 2 AM-4 AM | 70-110 |
| **TARGET LIPID LEVELS (ADULTS)*** | |
| PARAMETER | mg/dl |
| Total cholesterol | <200 |
| HDL cholesterol | >35 |
| LDL cholesterol | |
| Without vascular disease | <130 |
| With vascular disease | <100 |
| **TARGET BLOOD PRESSURE (ADULTS)†** | 130/85 mm Hg |

*NCEP Guidelines.[35,74]
†National High Blood Pressure Working Group.[75]

**box 35-3** *Diagnostic Criteria for Diabetes Mellitus, Impaired Glucose Tolerance, and Gestational Diabetes*

NONPREGNANT ADULTS

**Diabetes mellitus:** Diagnosis of diabetes mellitus in nonpregnant adults should be restricted to those who have one of the following:

1. Fasting plasma glucose ≥126 mg/dl. *Fasting* is defined as no caloric intake for at least 8 hours.
2. Symptoms of diabetes mellitus (such as polyuria, polydipsia, unexplained weight loss) coupled with a casual plasma glucose level ≥200 mg/dl. *Casual* is defined as any time of day, without regard to time interval since the last meal.
3. Two-hour postprandial plasma glucose ≥200 mg/dl during an oral glucose tolerance test. The test should be performed according to World Health Organization criteria using a glucose load containing the equivalent of 75 g of anhydrous glucose dissolved in water.

In the absence of unequivocal hyperglycemia with acute metabolic decompensation, these criteria should be confirmed by repeat testing on a second occasion. The oral glucose tolerance test is not recommended for routine clinical use. A normal glycosylated hemoglobin does not rule out the presence of diabetes, because the earliest defect is in postprandial control. Hence the glycosylated hemoglobin is not part of the diagnostic package.

**Impaired glucose tolerance:** Two-hour postprandial plasma glucose ≥140 mg/dl and less than or equal to 200 mg/dl during an oral glucose tolerance test. The test should be performed according to World Health Organization criteria using a glucose load containing the equivalent of 75 g of anhydrous glucose dissolved in water.

**Gestational diabetes:** After an oral glucose load of 100 g, gestational diabetes is diagnosed if two plasma glucose values equal or exceed the following:

- Fasting: 105 mg/dl
- 1 hour: 190 mg/dl
- 2 hour: 165 mg/dl
- 3 hour: 145 mg/dl

**Impaired fasting glucose:** Fasting plasma glucose level greater than 110 mg/dl and less than 126 mg/dl.

Adapted from Report of the Expert Committee on the Diagnosis and Classification of Diabetes Mellitus, *Diabetes Care* 20(7):1183, 1997.

son to presume that intensive therapy of type 2 DM would not yield similar results. Intensive therapy of type 2 DM, however, involves different regimens, aimed primarily at reducing insulin resistance. The Kumamoto Study of intensive insulin therapy in type 2 DM patients demonstrated a statistically significant relationship between control and complications comparable with the DCCT findings in type 1 DM patients.[78] The United Kingdom Prospective Diabetes Study (UKPDS), a multicenter trial of more than 5000 individuals with type 2 DM in the United Kingdom, is ongoing. Preliminary statistical analyses have also noted the relationship between improved glycemic control and a reduction in microvascular complications.[115]

### Blood parameters

**Short-term control.** Home blood glucose monitoring is a critical component of the treatment regimen for individuals with either type 1 DM or type 2 DM. Glucose levels are "vital signs" to individuals with diabetes. Home blood glucose monitoring is the only accurate measure of monitoring glucose control on a daily basis and allows the educated and motivated individual with diabetes to make any necessary changes in the diabetes regimen. Nonpregnant individuals with type 1 DM should ideally perform HBGM at least premeal and at bedtime. Frequency of HBGM in type 2 DM patients is determined by the treatment regimen and varies from once per week to several times per day. Results should be recorded in a logbook. A dilemma in HBGM in type 2 DM patients is that many third-party insurance carriers do not reimburse patients for home blood glucose monitoring equipment unless they are insulin treated—a very shortsighted approach.

Home blood glucose monitoring uses capillary whole blood obtained by a finger stick and correlates well with laboratory values when accurate techniques are used. Serum glucose values are approximately 10% lower than whole blood values (see the Guidelines for Care Box). The majority of available glucose meters use a "no blot" technique—the user does not blot or wipe the blood off the test strip. In HBGM with a meter, a drop of capillary blood is applied to a test strip containing either glucose oxidase or another chemical. A chemical reaction occurs, and the result is displayed on the meter. Test time varies between manufacturers, ranging from 20 seconds to 2 minutes. All marketed glucose meters must be approved by the U.S. Food and Drug Administration (USFDA) and yield accurate results when proper technique is used. Meters must be calibrated to each test strip lot according to manufacturers' specifications. The most common source of errors in HBGM results is user technique, followed by problems with the test strips. Because chemical is embedded in the test strip, any factor that can affect the chemical—light, heat, cold, humidity—will alter the result. Use of control solution is the only manner in which to test the accuracy of the strips. Control solution is glucose solution in a known concentration that yields a standard result. Each manufacturer produces its own solution. Unfortunately, control solution is often not readily available in pharmacies and is an additional cost to the individual, the insurance company, or both.

**Long-term control.** Long-term glycemic control is monitored by the glycosylated hemoglobin. The glycosylated hemoglobin reflects the average blood glucose level over a period of time. Glucose in the blood readily attaches to hemoglobin. Once attached, it remains so throughout the life span of the erythrocyte (90 to 120 days). The glycosylated hemoglobin provides an objective measure of control and is not influenced by age, sex, duration of diabetes, or very recent blood glucose levels. The total glycosylated hemoglobin reflects glycemic control over the past 3 months and is not affected by hemoglobin variants such as hemoglobin S found in sickle cell anemia. Fractions of the total, such as hemoglobin $A_1$ or hemoglobin $A_{1c}$, reflect glycemic control over similar time frames and are subject to influence by hemoglobin variants. A fructosamine level, reflecting control over the past 2 weeks, is

**table 35-8** *The DCCT: Reduction in Complication Risk with Intensive Therapy*

| Complication | % Risk Reduction |
|---|---|
| Clinically significant retinopathy | 76 |
| Severe retinopathy/laser surgery | 45 |
| Microalbuminuria | 35 |
| Albuminuria | 56 |
| Clinically significant neuropathy | 60 |

*Source:* The Diabetes Control and Complications Trial Research Group: The effect of intensive treatment of diabetes on the long-term complications in insulin-dependent diabetes mellitus, *N Engl J Med* 329:977, 1993.

**guidelines for care**

**Procedure for Capillary Blood Glucose Monitoring**

1. Verify meter calibration. If meter is not calibrated to current lot of strips, calibrate before using.
2. Use control solution when opening a new box or bottle of test strips or any time the glucose result does not make sense in the context of the clinical setting.
3. Cleanse finger with either soap and water or alcohol. If alcohol is used, wait for the finger to dry.
4. Place lancet in finger-stick device.
5. Prick finger.
6. Gently squeeze the finger to obtain an adequate sample of blood. NOTE: If alcohol was used to cleanse the finger, the first drop of blood must be discarded.
7. Follow the manufacturer's instructions to perform the test.
8. Discard in a hazardous waste receptacle the lancet, cap of the lancing device, and any other part of the equipment that may have been contaminated by blood.
9. Record the glucose result, noting the date, time, result, and action taken.

rarely used in the clinical setting. Glycosylated hemoglobin should be used in conjunction with HBGM results to assess glycemic control.

### Urine parameters

**Glucose monitoring.** Urine glucose monitoring is an antiquated method of assessing glycemic control. Glucose spills into the urine when serum glucose reaches the renal threshold (approximately 180 mg/dl). A urine glucose result always gives retrospective data, never current blood glucose levels. It only reflects, very indirectly, blood glucose levels hours before, when the renal threshold was exceeded. Urine glucose monitoring never tells a patient if he or she has a low blood glucose (≤660 mg/dl), a normal blood glucose (70 to 110 mg/dl), or even a moderately elevated blood glucose (>180 mg/dl). It only tells the patient if she or he had an excessively high blood glucose hours before. Urine glucose monitoring should no longer be used to assess glycemic control.

**Ketone monitoring.** Urine ketone monitoring should be performed by individuals with type 1 DM during illness and when HBGM results exceed 300 mg/dl. Test strips impregnated with acetoacetate are dipped into the urine. Test time varies depending on the manufacturer. Negative results are indicated by a beige color on the test strip. Urine ketones are positive at the trace level; as ketone levels rise, the color turns to deeper shades of purple. The presence of urine ketones is a dangerous sign in individuals with type 1 DM and requires prompt attention to insulin, diet, and fluid intake to avoid catastrophic DKA. Urine ketones should be monitored by individuals with type 2 DM during periods of illness. Ketones can be positive in a type 2 DM patient if there is significant hyperglycemia, hypertriglyceridemia, dehydration, and electrolyte depletion. As in a type 1 DM patient, positive urine ketones require prompt attention.

## MEDICATIONS AND TREATMENTS

Type 1 DM and type 2 DM are two separate and distinct pathophysiological entities. As a result, the pharmacological treatment regimen of type 1 DM differs significantly from that of type 2 DM.

### Type 1 DM: Insulin

Treatment of type 1 DM involves a triad: insulin, diet, and exercise. Because type 1 DM is characterized by insulinopenia, physiological insulin replacement is the first management component.

The discovery of insulin by Banting and Best in 1921 occupies a major place in medical history. Their "extract of pancreatic origin" became the *eau de vivre* of individuals with diabetes. Insulin products over the years have become increasingly pure and plentiful since January 11, 1921, when Leonard Thompson became the first individual treated with insulin.[16,101]

#### Properties of insulin

Three properties of insulin preparation may be identified in the prescription: source, strength, and type or kinetics.[41]

Animal-source insulins, extracts from pancreases of pigs or cows, have been discontinued from the U.S. market. Pork insulin most closely resembles human insulin, being only one amino acid different from human insulin; beef insulin has a three amino acid difference from human insulin. Human insulin is derived by recombinant DNA technology (Humulin from *Escherichia coli;* Novolin from *Saccharomyces cerevisiae* [bakers' yeast]) (Table 35-9). Because of its reduced antigenicity, human insulin is the insulin of choice (Figure 35-5). Individuals switching from animal-source to human-source insulin may require a dosage change and should consult their health care provider before making any changes. The strength of insulin in the United States is U-100: 100 units of insulin per milliliter of volume. A rare patient requiring very large doses of insulin may need U-500 insulin, which must be specially ordered. Insulins used to treat diabetes are detailed in Table 35-9.[82]

Insulins differ in speed of effect (onset), time of greatest action (peak), and how long they act (duration). Insulins are classified as quick, intermediate, and long acting. Dietary carbohydrate and activity must be coordinated with insulin action so that (1) insulin is available for optimal metabolism when the food that was eaten is absorbed, and (2) food is available while insulin is acting to prevent hypoglycemic reactions.

Two principles are useful in coordinating food and insulin:

1. Carbohydrate intake must be coordinated with insulin kinetics (action).
2. Regular or quick acting insulin requires that a supplemental snack of 15 g of carbohydrate be given to match the peak action of the insulin; for example, a 10 AM snack after a 7 AM injection of Regular insulin.

The nurse must clarify the insulin prescription in terms of the type, strength, and species. A change in any one of the properties may lead to differences in action. When the insulin

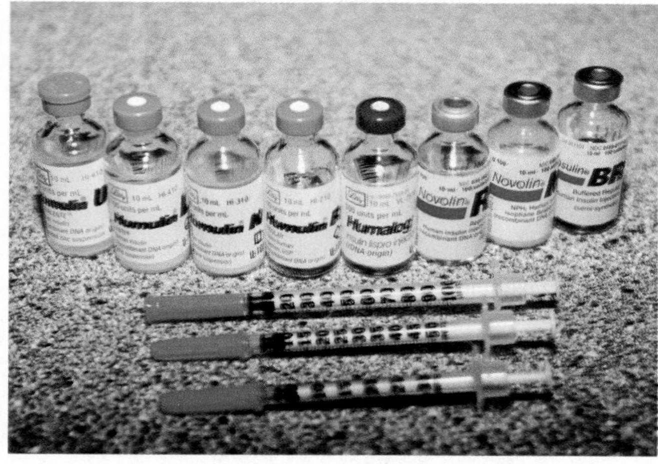

fig. 35-5 Human insulins.

**table 35-9** *Common Insulins for **Diabetes Mellitus***

| Type | Species | Onset (hr) | Peak (hr) | Duration (hr) | Retarding Agent | Appearance |
|---|---|---|---|---|---|---|
| **QUICK-ACTING INSULIN** | | | | | | |
| Lispro | Human | Immediate | 1 | 3-4 | None | Clear |
| Regular | Human | 0.5 | 2.5-5.0 | 6-8 | None | Clear |
| Regular (buffered) | Human | 0.5 | 1-3 | 6-8 | None | Clear |
| **INTERMEDIATE-ACTING INSULIN** | | | | | | |
| NPH | Human | 1.5 | 4-12 | 24 | Protamine sulfate<br>Zinc | Cloudy suspension |
| Lente | Human | 2.5 | 7-15 | 22 | Zinc | Turbid solution |
| **LONG-ACTING INSULIN** | | | | | | |
| Ultralente | Human | 4 | None | 28 | Zinc | Turbid solution |
| **COMBINATION INSULIN** | | | | | | |
| 70/30<br>70% NPH<br>30% Regular | Human | 0.5 | 2-12 | 24 | Protamine sulfate | Cloudy suspension |

NOTE: Beef and pork insulins have been discontinued from the U.S. market.

prescription is changed, careful patient monitoring is necessary to identify clinical effect.

### *Physiological replacement of insulin*

**Normal glucose metabolism.** In an individual without diabetes, insulin is secreted by the pancreas in two fashions: basal and prandial (Figure 35-6). Insulin is secreted in a basal fashion in the fasting state and between meals to control hepatic glucose output and disposal. In individuals without diabetes who live a "day life" (awake during the day and asleep at night), counterregulatory hormones are at their nadir between midnight and 2 AM; therefore blood glucose levels are at their lowest point. After 3 to 4 AM, the counterregulatory hormones rise, causing an increase in hepatic glucose output, which can continue until 10 or 11 AM. In a nondiabetic, in order to maintain euglycemia, the pancreas responds by increasing secretion of insulin by approximately 50% to maintain euglycemia. Prandial insulin is secreted by the nondiabetic pancreas in response to the ingestion of dietary carbohydrate. Native prandial insulin is secreted biphasically, with the first peak occurring in 1 minute and the second peak occurring in 6 minutes. The pancreas tailors the amount of insulin to the amount of carbohydrate ingested.

**Intensive insulin therapy regimens.** The challenge in the treatment of type 1 DM is physiological insulin replacement: one must "think like a pancreas." Joslin aptly described the challenge: "Insulin . . . is primarily a remedy for the wise and not the foolish, be they patients or doctors. Everyone knows it requires brains to live long with diabetes, but to use insulin successfully requires more brains."[54]

Intensive therapy employing multiple daily insulin injections has become the gold standard since the publication of

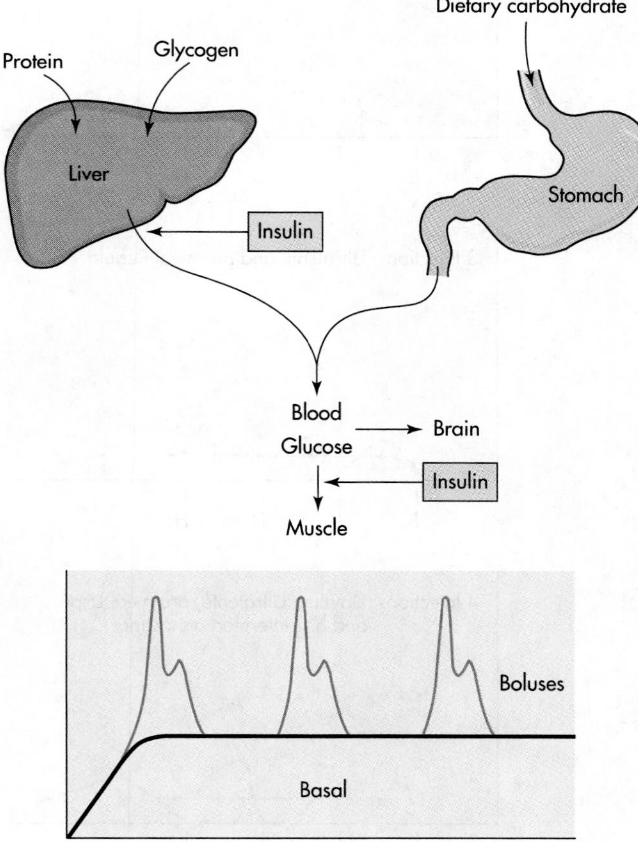


**fig. 35-6** Glucose metabolism.

the DCCT. Conventional therapies, which use once- and twice-daily insulin injection programs, are unphysiological, antiquated, and proven by the DCCT to be inferior care. The "split-mix" insulin regimen is one such regimen. If one strives for fasting blood glucoses consistently within the euglycemic range of 70 to 100 mg/dl with the "split-mix" program, an unacceptable incidence of nocturnal hypoglycemia occurs, because the predinner intermediate-acting insulin has its peak effect during the counterregulatory nadir (approximately 12 midnight to 2 AM) (Figure 35-7).

Premixed insulin (70/30) is a mixture of NPH and Regular insulins in a preset proportion—1 U of 70/30 insulin provides 0.7 U of NPH insulin and 0.3 U of Regular insulin. Premixed insulin does not permit fine-tuning of an insulin regimen and therefore has no role in the treatment of type 1 DM.

**Three injections per day: Regular or Lispro and intermediate-acting insulin (example follows with a daily insulin dose of 60 U).** Approximately two thirds of the total daily insulin dose (40 U) is given in the morning before breakfast, with one third of that dose (13 U) being given as

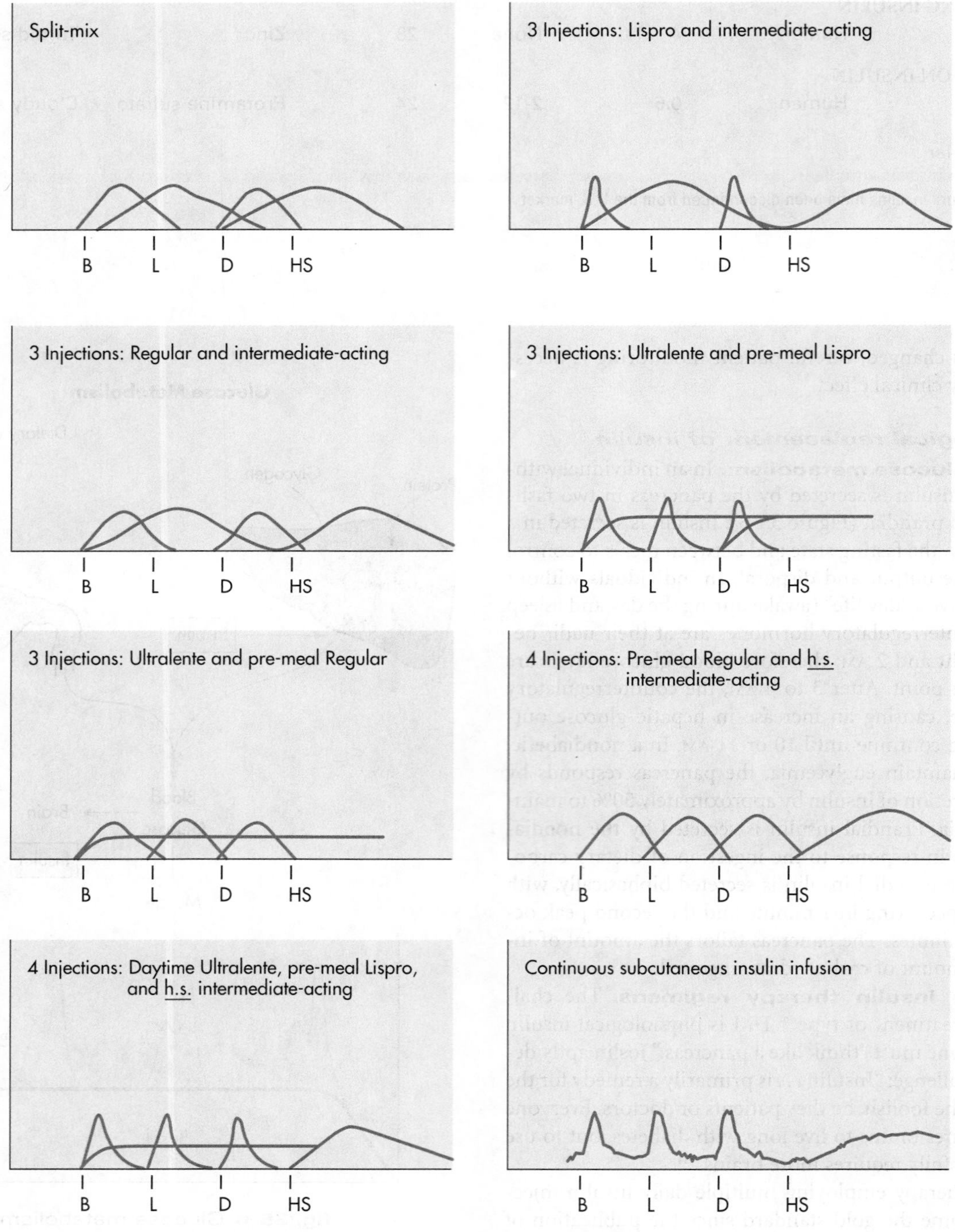


**fig. 35-7** Insulin delivery programs.

Regular or Lispro insulin; the remaining two thirds of that prebreakfast dose (27 U) is given as NPH or Lente. In the evening, the remaining one third of the total daily dose (20 U) is delivered: 50% (10 U) as Regular or Lispro insulin before dinner and 50% (10 U) as NPH or Lente at bedtime. This moving of the predinner NPH/Lente to bedtime (10 PM to 1 AM) moves the insulin peak to dawn and can reduce nocturnal hypoglycemia as much as fivefold. Therefore the dose is 13 U of Lispro and 27 U of NPH/Lente before breakfast, 10 U of Lispro before dinner, and 10 U of NPH/Lente at bedtime. The drawback of this insulin regimen is the lack of flexibility with regard to the timing of lunch caused by the emerging peak effect from the prebreakfast dose of NPH/Lente insulin (Figure 35-7).

**Three injections per day: Ultralente basal with premeal Regular or Lispro insulin.** In this program, approximately 50% of the total daily insulin dose is given as Ultralente, divided into two injections (before breakfast and before dinner). The Ultralente insulin acts as a basal insulin to control hepatic glucose output and disposal in the fasting state, and it is given regardless of whether or not dietary carbohydrate is consumed. Then, Regular or Lispro insulin is given before each meal, the dosage titrated to the amount of carbohydrate planned for the meal. This regimen provides a significant amount of flexibility in meal timing, and patients may compensate for addition or deletion of carbohydrate at each meal with the adjustment of the premeal insulin dose. Because of these advantages, this program is commonly termed *"the poor man's pump."* This regimen is not useful for treating the individual with a pronounced dawn hormonal surge (adolescents and pregnant women) and in individuals with long-standing diabetes in whom insulin kinetics may be erratic (see Figure 35-7).

**Four injections per day: premeal Regular and overnight NPH/Lente insulin.** Typically, approximately 20% of the total daily dose is given as NPH/Lente at bedtime (10 PM to 1 AM), with the remaining 80% of the total daily dose given as Regular insulin and distributed proportionately between the carbohydrate load at each of the three meals. This program is especially suited to patients with extremely labile diabetes when other programs fail. Patients with exuberant dawn phenomena are suitable candidates, as are patients who appear to have erratic or compromised absorption of longer-acting insulins. It must be remembered that the overnight NPH/Lente insulin dose does not cover the full 24-hour basal requirements. Therefore a portion of the premeal Regular insulin dose is covering the basal requirements. If individuals have longer than a 6-hour time span between injections of Regular insulin, they generally experience "insulin run-out hyperglycemia;" if the liver does not "see" insulin, it uncontrollably releases more glucose. The flexibility of this regimen in terms of fine-tuning of the dosage, as well as the ability to vary the interval between injection and meal to best control postprandial glucose, makes it an ideal program for the pregnant patient or for the patient with secondary diabetes caused by cystic fibrosis (see Figure 35-7).

**Four injections per day: prebreakfast Ultralente and Lispro, prelunch and predinner Lispro, overnight NPH/Lente insulin.** This program is ideal for individuals who use Lispro insulin, require flexibility, and have a significant dawn hormonal surge. The substitution of Lispro for Regular insulin in the previously described program would result in significant insulin run-out hyperglycemia because of the very short duration of action of Lispro. Insulin run-out hyperglycemia is eliminated with the addition of a small dose of Ultralente insulin before breakfast to control hepatic glucose output and disposal during the day, with the bedtime NPH/Lente insulin providing coverage of hepatic glucose output and disposal during the night (see Figure 35-7).

**Continuous subcutaneous insulin infusion (CSII)/insulin pump therapy.** Insulin pump therapy using a portable external insulin infusion pump offers the most physiological insulin delivery. The pump is preprogrammed to deliver varying basal rates hour by hour. For example, the pump can be programmed to deliver less insulin during the 12 midnight to 2 AM counterregulatory nadir and then to increase insulin delivery in the dawn hours, thus matching each individual's needs. The H-Tron Plus V100 by Disetronic has the capability of a different basal rate every hour. Before meals, the patient delivers a bolus of insulin matched to the carbohydrate content of the meal. In addition to being the most physiological insulin delivery system, an insulin pump is also the most flexible (see Figure 35-7).

Current insulin pumps are no larger than a pager (Figure 35-8). The ideal candidate for the pump is an individual who has failed to control diabetes on one of the aforementioned insulin programs, someone who is pregnant or contemplating pregnancy, or someone who desires increased daily flexibility. Disadvantages include the initial capital outlay ($4500) and maintenance supplies (although most insurance companies cover 70% to 100%), the continual presence of a needle or Teflon cannula placed subcutaneously in the abdomen, and the potential risk of sepsis. Attention to sterile technique and changing the infusion site every 48 hours minimize the risk of sepsis. The greatest risk is the potential for rapid-onset DKA if there is any interruption of insulin delivery via partial occlusion of the tubing, needle, or cannula or accidental removal of the

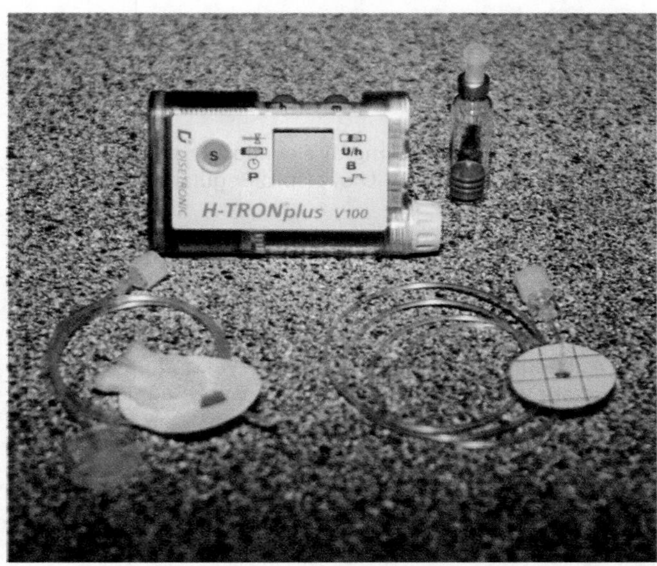


fig. 35-8 Insulin infusion pump and supplies.

needle or cannula. Because the pump uses only quick-acting insulin (Buffered Regular or Lispro), there is no intermediate- or long-acting insulin on board, thus rendering the patient at risk of rapid-onset DKA if insulin delivery is interrupted for any reason. A good safety net is to have patients with pumps change the infusion site if they have a finger-stick blood glucose greater than 300 mg/dl and they are unable to account for it by excess carbohydrate intake. Insulin pump therapy should be initiated only in an educated, motivated patient under the care of a diabetes team educated and skilled in pump therapy and offering 24-hour support of the patient.[2]

**Insulin algorithms as a component of intensive therapy.** An insulin algorithm is a plan for additional insulin to be administered for episodes of hyperglycemia; each patient should have an individualized plan. Via an algorithm, additional insulin is given over and above the baseline or usual insulin dose based on finger-stick blood glucose levels. For example, in a patient taking 0.5 to 0.8 U/kg of body weight, an additional unit of Lispro or Regular insulin would be expected to lower blood glucose by approximately 50 mg/dl (Box 35-4).[99]

Insulin algorithms must be differentiated from the obsolete "sliding scale," which unfortunately is still used. In a sliding scale, no baseline insulin is administered to control either hepatic glucose output and disposal or prandial needs; insulin is administered on a contingency basis every 4 to 6 hours based on the prevailing finger-stick blood glucose level (Box 35-5). In other words, with a sliding scale, quick-acting insulin is only given *after* hyperglycemia has already occurred. Not unexpectedly, sliding scale insulin results in hyperglycemia because of failure to control hepatic glucose output and disposal and prandial requirements. A health care team can readily precipitate nosocomial DKA by using sliding scale insulin.[86,98,116]

### Pharmacotherapy for Type 2 DM

Pharmacotherapy for type 2 DM can be directed at (1) decreasing insulin resistance and increasing insulin sensitization (metformin and troglitazone), (2) interfering with the digestion and absorption of dietary carbohydrate ($\alpha$-glucosidase inhibitors), and (3) augmenting insulin secretion and action (sulfonylureas) (Table 35-10). Insulin therapy is indicated in some instances for patients with type 2 DM.

#### Decreasing insulin resistance/increasing insulin sensitivity

Metformin (Glucophage) is a true insulin sensitizer, enhancing peripheral glucose utilization and decreasing hepatic glucose production. It is an antihyperglycemic agent; it has no effect on insulin secretion. Therefore, when used as monotherapy, it cannot induce hypoglycemia. Ideal candidates for treatment are overweight or obese type 2 DM patients. The potentially fatal side effect of lactic acidosis generally occurs only when metformin is used in contraindicated patients: those with renal insufficiency, liver disease, alcohol excess, or underlying hypoxic states (congestive heart failure, chronic obstructive pulmonary disease, significant asthma, or acute myocardial infarction).[17] Metformin should be discontinued 48 to 72 hours before (1) elective surgery that may require general anesthesia and (2) elective procedures using contrast materials (e.g., intravenous pyelogram, cardiac catheterization, barium enema), and it should not be restarted for 48 to 72 hours after the surgery or procedure. Adjustments in the individual's diabetes regimen will have to be made for this time period to maintain glycemic control.

Troglitazone (Rezulin), a thiazolidinedione, is a unique antihyperglycemic agent that binds to the peroxisome proliferator activated receptor-gamma (PPAR) nuclear receptor, amplifies the insulin signal, and reduces insulin requirements in insulin-treated type 2 DM patients. In addition to glucose-lowering properties, troglitazone has beneficial effects on the other components of Reaven's syndrome X and a side effect profile comparable with placebo. Uniquely, troglitazone can be safely used in patients with renal insufficiency without the need for dosage adjustment. Bioavailability is significantly enhanced by ingestion with food. The onset of glucose lowering is very gradual, such that individualized downward titration in insulin dosage in insulin-treated type 2 DM patients may not be needed for at least 2 weeks, and the maximum effect may not be seen for up to 8 weeks. Currently, troglitazone is approved only for use in insulin-treated type 2 DM patients. It is anticipated, however, that in the future it will be approved for a broad range of type 2 DM patients, either as monotherapy or in combination with metformin, acarbose, or sulfonylureas.[95]

**box 35-4** *Sample Algorithm for Hyperglycemia*

Premeal, for every 50 mg/dl elevation in blood glucose above 120 mg/dl, add 1 U of Lispro/Regular insulin to the baseline dose:

| BLOOD GLUCOSE | ADD LISPRO/REGULAR SC |
|---|---|
| ≥170 mg/dl | 1 U |
| ≥220 mg/dl | 2 U |
| ≥270 mg/dl | 3 U |

At bedtime, for every 50 mg/dl elevation in blood glucose above 150 mg/dl, add 1 U of Lispro/Regular insulin to the baseline dose:

| BLOOD GLUCOSE | ADD LISPRO/REGULAR SC |
|---|---|
| ≥200 mg/dl | 1 U |
| ≥250 mg/dl | 2 U |
| ≥300 mg/dl | 3 U |

**box 35-5** *Sample Sliding Scale*

Give *no* baseline insulin. Give Regular insulin every 4 hours based on finger-stick blood glucoses as follows:

| BLOOD GLUCOSE | GIVE REGULAR INSULIN SC |
|---|---|
| ≥200 mg/dl | 2 U |
| ≥250 mg/dl | 6 U |
| ≥300 mg/dl | 10 U |

### α-Glucosidase inhibition

α-Glucosidase inhibition by acarbose has a primary mode of action of decreasing postprandial blood glucoses via direct interference on the digestion and absorption of dietary carbohydrate. Acarbose is most commonly used as adjunctive therapy to metformin or sulfonylureas. Monotherapy with acarbose is an option in the newly diagnosed, mildly hyperglycemic type 2 DM patient. Increased intestinal gas formation is the most common side effect and improves with continued administration of acarbose. Acarbose needs to be

**table 35-10** *Common Oral Medications for Type 2 Diabetes Mellitus*

| PARAMETER | METFORMIN | TROGLITAZONE | SULFONYLUREAS | ACARBOSE |
|---|---|---|---|---|
| **Mode of action** | ↓ Hepatic glucose<br>↑ Skeletal muscle glucose utilization | ↓ Hepatic glucose<br>↑ Skeletal muscle glucose utilization | ↑ Insulin secretion<br>↓ Hepatic glucose production | α-glucosidase inhibition<br>↓ carbohydrate digestion and absorption from GI tract |
| **Glucose effects** | Fasting and postprandial | Fasting and postprandial | Fasting and postprandial | Postprandial |
| **Hypoglycemia as monotherapy** | No | No | Yes | No |
| **Weight gain** | No | Possible | Yes | No |
| **Insulin levels** | ↓ | ↓ | ↑ | ↓ |
| **Side effects** | GI (self-limiting symptoms of nausea, diarrhea, anorexia) | None; equal to placebo | Potential allergic reaction if sulfa allergy<br>Potential drug interactions (first-generation agents)<br>Syndrome of inappropriate antidiuretic hormone | GI (flatulence, abdominal distention, diarrhea) |
| **Lipid effects** | ↓ | ↓ | ↑ or ↓ | ↓ |
| **Starting dose for a 70 kg man** | 500 mg bid with meals | 200 mg qd with breakfast | Varies with each agent<br>Glyburide 2.5 mg qd<br>Glucotrol XL 5 mg qd<br>Glynase 3 mg qd<br>Amaryl 2 mg qd | 25 mg tid with first bite of each meal |
| **Maximum dose** | 850 mg tid with meals | 600 mg qd with breakfast | Varies with each agent<br>Glyburide 10 mg bid<br>Glucotrol XL 20 mg qd<br>Glynase 6 mg bid<br>Amaryl 8 mg qd | 100 mg tid with first bite of each meal |
| **Contraindications** | Type 1 diabetes<br>Renal dysfunction<br>Hepatic dysfunction<br>History of alcohol abuse<br>Chronic conditions associated with hypoxia (asthma, chronic obstructive pulmonary disease, congestive heart failure [CHF])<br>Acute conditions associated with potential for hypoxia (surgery, acute myocardial infarction, CHF)<br>Situations associated with potential renal dysfunction (e.g., IV contrast media) | Type 1 diabetes | Type 1 diabetes<br>Hepatic dysfunction | Type 1 diabetes<br>Inflammatory bowel disease<br>Bowel obstruction<br>Cirrhosis<br>Chronic conditions with maldigestion or malabsorption |

dosed with the first bite of the meal. Slow titration of acarbose to the maximum dosage of 100 mg three times daily minimizes the intestinal gas problem.

### Augmentation of insulin secretion

Sulfonylureas enhance insulin secretion and action. First-generation sulfonylureas (chlorpropamide, tolazamide, tolbutamide, acetohexamide), although efficacious, have a higher risk of side effects, such as sustained hypoglycemia, the cholpropamide flush (an Antabuse-like reaction), protein-binding interference with certain medications, and syndrome of inappropriate antidiuretic hormone (SIADH). The second- and third-generation sulfonylureas are preferred owing to their increased milligram potency, shorter duration of action, and better side effect profile. Prior concerns about possible cardiotoxicity of sulfonylureas related to the University Group Diabetes Program Study have generally disappeared, given the emergence of data to support the safety of these agents from the cardiovascular perspective.

### Insulin therapy

Insulin therapy in patients with type 2 DM remains controversial. Insulin therapy is indicated when patients are in a state of acute metabolic decompensation and are more insulin resistant because of the stress of illness. In these individuals, short-term insulin therapy can reestablish glycemic control and metabolic stability. Reevaluation of insulin secretory capacity via a C-peptide is important so that patients do not "inherit" insulin unnecessarily.[103-105]

In the individual with type 2 DM with a low-normal C-peptide or the lean individual with a normal C-peptide, insulin therapy will probably be needed, along with maintenance of diet, exercise, and oral agents. The use of bedtime insulin therapy with a single daily dosage of intermediate-acting insulin may be sufficient. The theory is that this bedtime dosage will maximally affect and control both the dawn hepatic glucose output and disposal and the peak insulin resistance. The bedtime insulin dose assists in achieving the best possible fasting blood glucose and minimizes glucotoxicity. Minimizing glucotoxicity maximizes the daytime pancreatic insulin secretory capability and minimizes the daytime insulin dose. Additionally, the appetite-stimulating effect of insulin is minimized, which assists weight control. Occasionally individuals may require multiple injections akin to a true type 1 DM patient. The exact needs of each patient may be determined based on the premeal and bedtime blood glucose levels.[103-105]

In contrast, insulin therapy in the C-peptide–positive overweight type 2 DM patient should be avoided if possible. Insulin is lipogenic, and the weight gain may further exacerbate the insulin-resistant state. Diet, exercise, and appropriate oral agents should be aggressively used before insulin therapy is contemplated. In such a patient requiring insulin, bedtime intermediate-acting insulin is the ideal starting point, along with the continuation of oral agent therapy. Combination therapy with oral agents usually helps maintain glycemic control with a lower insulin dosage.[103-105] Insulin therapy must not be viewed as a substitute for diet and exercise, but rather as an adjunct. Commonly, insulin therapy in the obese C-peptide–positive patient not only fails to improve glycemic control on a sustained basis, but also increases appetite, resulting in weight gain, increased hyperglycemia, and increased hyperinsulinemia, thus perpetuating the insulin-resistant state and the components of syndrome X.[89-91]

Insulin therapy will of course be necessary for the type 2 DM patient who becomes C-peptide negative ("burned out" type 2). Such individuals are usually lean, looking phenotypically more like an individual with type 1 DM. In these individuals, just as in type 1 DM patients, intensive insulin therapy with carbohydrate gram counting will be needed. It is also important to note that in the geriatric years, 10% of newly diagnosed individuals will have bona fide type 1 DM, again requiring intensive therapy and carbohydrate gram counting.[103-105]

Premixed insulin (70/30) has minimal value in the type 2 DM patient. The use of 70/30 insulin can result in an increase in appetite stimulation resulting from the Regular insulin component.

## Complications of Medication

### Insulin hypersensitivity

Hypersensitivity to insulin itself is uncommon. Rarely, an individual with a sulfa allergy will cross-react with NPH insulin, which contains protamine sulfate. A rare patient allergic to zinc may react to the Lente insulins. Patients may react to preservatives within insulin. A switch in insulin manufacturer may eliminate the latter problem. Insulin hypersensitivity reactions are generally local reactions, consisting of wheals at injection sites. However, systemic symptoms and anaphylaxis can occur. When systemic reactions occur, local reactions will also be present.

### Hypoglycemia

*Hypoglycemia,* defined as blood glucose less than 60 mg/dl, is a potential complication of therapy with insulin or oral hypoglycemic agents. Hypoglycemia is caused by a disturbance in the balance between insulin or sulfonylurea, carbohydrate, and activity (Box 35-6).

**Signs and symptoms.** The common signs and symptoms of hypoglycemia may be *adrenergic* (caused by activation

**box 35-6** *Causes of Hypoglycemia During Treatment with Exogenous Insulin or Oral Hypoglycemic Agents*

- Unphysiological insulin regimen
- Overdosage of insulin or sulfonylureas
- Inconsistent carbohydrate intake
- Omission of meal
- Omission of planned snack
- Uncompensated exercise
- End-stage renal disease
- End-stage liver disease
- Alcohol consumption

of the sympathetic nervous system) or *neuroglycopenic* (caused by depression of central nervous system activity as the brain perceives an insufficient supply of glucose) (Box 35-7). Adrenergic symptoms generally precede neuroglycopenic symptoms. The particular signs and symptoms in a given individual may vary with the absolute blood glucose level, the rapidity of the decrease in blood glucose level, and the duration of hypoglycemia. Additionally, signs and symptoms commonly vary throughout a given individual's life.

A rapid drop in plasma glucose results primarily in manifestations from increased sympathetic nervous system activity. In slow-developing hypoglycemia, as might be seen with long-acting insulin or with oral hypoglycemic agents, the central nervous system signs and symptoms predominate. If a rapid drop occurs and is allowed to persist, all signs and symptoms usually occur.

Hypoglycemia may occur during sleep. The only symptoms may be nightmares, sweating, restless sleep, headache on awakening, elevated fasting blood glucose, or feeling totally exhausted on awakening. Nighttime hypoglycemia may be part of the *Somogyi* effect (see p. 1161).

Individuals with long-standing diabetes may lose awareness of hypoglycemia and may have very low blood glucose levels before some, if any, symptoms occur. Research demonstrates that elimination of hypoglycemia can restore glucose transporter function and help restore hypoglycemia awareness.[27]

Patients with diabetes mellitus who are treated with $\beta$-adrenergic antagonists may be at special risk for hypoglycemia. The $\beta$-adrenergic agents block or inhibit the appearance of early signs and symptoms of hypoglycemia by blocking the sympathetic nervous system. In addition, these drugs prevent or block gluconeogenesis and glycogenolysis, thus inhibiting the normal endogenous response to hypoglycemia, making it more difficult to reverse the problem.

Signs and symptoms similar to those of hypoglycemia may occur when the blood glucose level is elevated and drops rapidly to a level that is still in an elevated range. The sudden rapid drop in blood sugar, regardless of the final level reached or the levels at which this occurred, is a stimulus for the physiological neuroendocrine response to stressors to come into play. Thus a patient whose glucose level drops rapidly from 500 mg/dl to 300 mg/dl may demonstrate the same signs and symptoms as a patient whose glucose drops to 30 mg/dl. Patients with uncontrolled diabetes may complain of feeling hypoglycemic, even though their plasma glucose levels are high.

This phenomenon should be discussed with patients with uncontrolled diabetes. They should be reassured that this "relative hypoglycemia" associated with improved glycemic control generally lasts only a few weeks.

**Severity.** Most hypoglycemia is mild and easily self-treated. The incidence of serious hypoglycemia (unconscious or near-unconscious) was shown to be increased with intensive therapy in the DCCT. In the vast majority of cases, however, the etiology of severe hypoglycemia results from patient error: inadequate carbohydrate intake at meals, missed snacks, and uncompensated activity.

**Diagnosis and treatment.** A finger-stick blood glucose should be obtained to verify hypoglycemia (blood glucose 60 mg/dl or lower). In a conscious patient, treatment consists of 15 g of quick-acting carbohydrate (e.g., three glucose tablets, 4 ounces of juice [no added sugar], three hard candies). Finger-stick blood glucose should be rechecked in 15 minutes. If blood glucose remains at 60 mg/dl or lower, the patient should self-treat again. If a glucose meter is not readily available, treatment should be taken regardless. In an unconscious patient, oral administration of glucose should never be attempted. In the hospital setting, one ampule of 50% dextrose should be given by intravenous push. Recovery is usually within 1 minute. In the outpatient setting, a significant other should inject 1 mg of glucagon subcutaneously; this causes the liver to release its glycogen store. The unconscious patient given subcutaneous glucagon generally regains consciousness in 10 to 20 minutes. After recovery, the patient should be given a snack of 45 g of carbohydrate to aid in replacing glycogen stores. Patients commonly are nauseated after receiving glucagon and may vomit. Seizures can occur when hypoglycemia is severe. If a seizure occurs, emergency personnel should be called to the scene immediately.

**Side effects of oral agents.** Oral agents may also cause hypoglycemia. Potential adverse effects of the oral agents are noted in Table 35-10.

## SURGICAL MANAGEMENT

Pancreas transplantation has been shown to be effective in improving the quality of life in persons with diabetes by eliminating the need for exogenous insulin, frequent blood glucose monitoring, and dietary restrictions.[3] However, there is no evidence that pancreas transplant prevents or slows progression

**box 35-7** *Signs and Symptoms of Hypoglycemia*

**ADRENERGIC SYMPTOMS**

Pallor
Diaphoresis
Tachycardia
Piloerection
Palpitations
Nervousness
Irritability
Sensation of coldness
Weakness
Trembling
Hunger

**NEUROGLYCOPENIC SYMPTOMS**

Headache
Mental confusion
Circumoral paresthesia
Fatigue
Incoherent speech
Coma
Diplopia
Emotional lability
Convulsions

of long-term complications of diabetes or that it prolongs life.[3] Pancreas transplant is indicated for persons with end-stage renal disease who are planning to or have had a kidney transplant. Pancreas transplant may be done at the time of kidney transplant or after kidney transplant. See Chapter 68 for further discussion of pancreas transplant.

## DIET

### Overview

Nutritional management is the cornerstone of therapy in all types of diabetes mellitus. Patients need to be referred early to a registered dietitian, preferably one who is also a certified diabetes educator (CDE), for nutritional education and the development of meal plans that are flexible and fit their lifestyles. Food issues are never simple to patients, and a good understanding from the beginning can often determine the success of their management. Patients are often fearful about what to put into their mouths. If this fear is not addressed through education, eating at first will be curtailed, but later all caution goes to the wind and it is difficult to make a new beginning. Here lies the rationale for an early referral to a dietitian. If no dietitian is available, the nurse should be able to give basic nutritional information to suffice until the patient can talk with a dietitian.

The current nutritional management for diabetes is to maintain reasonable weight and control blood glucose and lipid levels without compromising health. Current nutritional recommendations for people with diabetes are similar to those for healthy individuals without diabetes, as developed by the National Research Council, the American Heart Association, and the American Cancer Society (Box 35-8).[2,38,120]

Most persons need 25 kcal/kg of desired body weight (DBW) to maintain their weight and meet basic metabolic needs. With this as the basis, kilocalories are added or subtracted, based on activity level, age, and need to lose weight (Table 35-11).

Another dietary component that is manipulated is fiber. A high-fiber, high-carbohydrate diet has been shown to decrease insulin requirements and cholesterol, both fasting and postprandial glucose serum levels. Fiber can increase satiety, which might help with weight reduction. Fiber delays gastric emptying and decreases peak blood glucose, so when fiber is introduced into the diet, blood glucose should be monitored and insulin or any oral agents may need to be adjusted.

This dietary manipulation requires that 20 to 35 g of plant fiber be added to the diet each day.[2,10,11] Natural fiber is preferable to a commercial fiber supplement. A selection of high-fiber foods appears in Table 35-12. Research to define fully the benefits of a high-fiber diet and its side effects is ongoing. Adding fiber gradually helps minimize abdominal discomfort and flatulence. Increasing water intake also helps.

**box 35-8** *Target Nutritional Goals for Persons with Diabetes*

**CALORIES**

Sufficient to achieve and maintain as close to desirable body weight as possible

**CARBOHYDRATE**

Varies in relation to assessment and protein and fat intake; usually 45-60% calories

Liberalized individualized emphasis on total carbohydrate intake versus eliminating simple sugars only

Carbohydrate consistency at meals

Modest amounts of sucrose and other refined sugars may be acceptable contingent on metabolic control and body weight

**PROTEIN**

Usual dietary intake of protein is double the amount needed

Exact ideal percentage of total calories is unknown; however, usual intake is 12-20% of total calories

RDA is 0.8 g/kg body weight for adults; it is modified for children, pregnant and lactating women, elderly persons, and those with special medical conditions

Avoidance of excess dietary protein intake is important in renal disease

**FAT**

Usually ≤ 30% of total calories, but may be as high as 40%

Polyunsaturated fats, 6-8%

Saturated fats, 10%

Monounsaturated fats, remaining percentage

Cholesterol <300 mg/day

May need to be further modified, depending on lipid profile

**FIBER**

Up to 40 g/day

25 g/1000 kcal for low-calorie intakes

**ALTERNATIVE SWEETENERS**

Use of various nutritive and nonnutritive sweeteners is acceptable

**SODIUM**

≤3000 mg/day

Modified for special medical conditions (e.g., hypertension, edema)

**ALCOHOL**

≤2 equivalents per day

1 equivalent = 1.5 oz distilled liquor, 4 oz glass of wine, 12 oz glass of beer

**VITAMINS/MINERALS**

No evidence that diabetes mellitus influences need

### Principles of Dietary Management

If the person with diabetes mellitus has a nutritional history that incorporates the dietary recommendations described in the preceding section, few dietary changes will be needed. The diabetic diet is one that all persons should follow; however, given the dietary habits of most Americans, some dietary changes are usually necessary. Recommendations need to be made with the awareness that eating habits are difficult if not impossible to change overnight. Changes should be instituted gradually, and the nurse helps the patient adopt a diet that is as close to ideal as possible.

**table 35-11** *Guidelines for Estimating Calorie Requirements*

| LEVEL | ACTIVITIES | CALORIE REQUIREMENTS |
|---|---|---|
| Light, >55 years, obese, or inactive | Less than for "light" below | 10 calories/lb (22 kcal/kg) Desired body weight (DBW) |
| Light | Ambulating in hospital, washing clothes, walking 2.5 to 3 miles per hour, carpentry, electrical work, golfing, sailing | 10-12 calories/lb (22-26 kcal/kg) DBW |
| Moderate | Weeding and hoeing, bicycling, dancing, tennis, walking 3.5 to 4 miles per hour, scrubbing floors, work involving loading and stocking | 12-14 calories/lb (26-32 kcal/kg) DBW |
| Heavy | Climbing, walking uphill with a full load, basketball, football, swimming | 14-16 calories/lb (31-35 kcal/kg) DBW |
| Weight reduction | | Subtract 500 calories from total calories for the day for a 1 lb weight loss per week |

**table 35-12** *Fiber Content of Selected Foods*

| FOOD | SERVING SIZE | FIBER (g) |
|---|---|---|
| **BREADS/CEREALS** | | |
| 100% bran cereal | ½ cup | 10 |
| Kidney beans | ½ cup | 4.5 |
| Peas | ½ cup | 5.2 |
| Potatoes, white | 1 small | 3.8 |
| Rice, brown | ½ cup | 1.3 |
| Bread, whole-grain wheat | 1 slice | 2.7 |
| **FRUITS** | | |
| Apple, uncooked | 1 small | 3.9 |
| Orange | 1 small | 2.1 |
| Strawberries | ¾ cup | 2.4 |
| Peach | 1 medium | 1.0 |
| **COOKED VEGETABLES** | | |
| Beets | ½ cup | 1.7 |
| Broccoli | ½ cup | 2.6 |
| Carrots | ½ cup | 2.2 |
| Lettuce, uncooked | ½ cup | 0.5 |

To increase success, dietary planning should consider the following:

1. Religious, cultural, and personal preferences of the patient
2. Lifestyle components: family eating patterns, finances, and work schedule
3. Activity/rest patterns: amount, timing, and level of exercise, work, and sleep
4. Actions of prescribed hypoglycemic agents: onset, duration, and peak
5. Self-perception of desired body weight

Carbohydrates must be distributed on a consistent basis so that the blood level of nutrients matches the blood level of insulin or any oral hypoglycemic agent. Relative consistency in timing of meals is also important for the person who needs to lose weight. Distribution of carbohydrates helps prevent large increases in postprandial blood glucose and allows the blood glucose to return to the preprandial level before the next meal regardless of whether the patient is receiving a hypoglycemic agent.

## Systems for Learning and Maintaining Dietary Plans

Once the goals of nutritional therapy are established, patients are taught one of several methods for manipulating calories and food.

### Exchange system

The exchange system is the most widely used method. The American Dietetic Association and the American Diabetes Association have divided foods into six groups with exchange lists (or choices).[9] Each list is based on the amount of carbohydrate, protein, and fat contained in foods. There are six exchange lists: starch/bread, meat and meat substitutes, vegetables, fruit, milk, and fat. Each exchange list contains foods in specific serving sizes that contain approximately equal amounts of carbohydrates, proteins, fats, and calories. Because of this, these foods can be substituted, or exchanged, for one another. For example, in the fruit list, 1 apple = 12 cherries = ½ cup orange juice. What is important is using suggested serving size. Foods can be measured by tablespoons and measuring cups and meats by ounces. The exchange system offers a wide variety of foods and combinations of foods that can be eaten. Implementation of the system requires knowing the calorie, carbohydrate, protein, and fat content of different foods. Labels on food products, convenience foods, and special foods and recipe books list carbohydrate, protein, and fat content. The total number of exchanges for each day is determined from the total calorie, carbohydrate, fat, and protein prescription.

Once the dietary prescription has been made and the caloric amount decided, a meal plan such as the one shown in Figure 35-9 can be made. There are resources other than the one depicted in the figure. Some are simple and have pictures of foods and a place to write in the number of exchanges from each group to be used. Examples of other plans can be obtained from the American Diabetes Association.

It is important to maintain consistency with the distribution of exchanges and not to "borrow from lunch and add to dinner." The nutrition information in Box 35-9 is an example of what can be found on cereal boxes. In comparing the amounts of carbohydrate, protein, and fat to the exchange list, one serving, 1¼ cup of this cereal, would be equal to about 1⅓ bread exchanges.

**My Meal Plan**

Meal plan for: John Doe  Date: 8/16/98
Dietitian: Jane Smith  Phone: ______

| | Grams | Percent |
|---|---|---|
| Carbohydrate | 199 | 55 |
| Protein | 79 | 20 |
| Fat | 44 | 25 |
| Calories 1580 | | |

| Time | Meal plan | Menu ideas | Menu ideas |
|---|---|---|---|
| Breakfast | 2 Starch<br>Meat<br>Vegetable<br>1 Fruit<br>1 Milk<br>1 Fat | 1/2 Cup oatmeal, 1 slice whole grain toast<br><br><br>1/2 Banana<br>1 Cup skim milk<br>1 Tsp margarine | |
| | | | |
| Lunch | 2 Starch<br>2 Meat<br>1 Vegetable<br>1 Fruit<br>Milk<br>1 Fat | 2 Slices whole grain bread<br>2 Slices turkey breast (2oz)<br>1/2 Cup broccoli/cauliflower marinated in 1 tbsp low-calorie italian dressing (free food)<br>Apple<br><br>1 Tsp mayonnaise | Lettuce leaf, tomato slice (free) |
| Afternoon snack | 1 Starch<br>1 Meat | 3 Graham crackers<br>1 Tbsp peanut butter | |
| Dinner | 2 Starch<br>2 Meat<br>1 Vegetable<br>1 Fruit<br>Milk<br>1 Fat | 1 Large potato<br>Meatloaf (2oz)<br>1/2 Cup green beans<br>1 1/4 Cups fresh strawberries<br><br>1 Tsp margarine | Tossed salad with 1 tbsp low-calorie italian dressing (free food) |
| Bedtime snack | 1 Starch<br>1 Fat<br>1 Milk | 1/2 Bagel<br>1 Tbsp lite cream cheese<br>1 Cup skim milk | |

**fig. 35-9** Sample meal plan.

**box 35-9** *Nutrition Information per Serving*

Serving size. . . . . . . . . . . . . . . . . . . . . . 1 ounce (1¼ cup)
Serving per package . . . . . . . . . . . 20 (1-ounce servings)
Calories . . . . . . . . . . . . . . . . . . . . . . . . . . . . . . . . . . 110
Protein, grams . . . . . . . . . . . . . . . . . . . . . . . . . . . . . . . 4
Carbohydrate, grams . . . . . . . . . . . . . . . . . . . . . . . . . . 20
Sodium, milligrams . . . . . . . . . . . . . . . . . . . . . . . . . . 320
Percentage of vitamins and minerals listed next
Ingredients: Whole oat flour, wheat starch, salt, sugar, calcium carbonate, etc.

### *Food Guide Pyramid*

Another system that can be used to help patients with meal plans is the Food Guide Pyramid (Figure 35-10).[116] This guide recommends less meat and poultry than the exchange list does.

### *Points system*

Another system is point counting. With this system, foods are assigned points for number of calories and carbohydrate, protein, and fat content. The total daily food allowance is written as number of calorie and carbohydrate points, and the person is instructed to select foods according to a point distribution. This system is similar to the exchange list but is less well known.

### *Total gram counting of carbohydrate*

This system counts the amount of carbohydrate available in the total meal. Only carbohydrates are tracked. Some persons prefer this plan because they are directed to give insulin according to total carbohydrates. This system is becoming increasingly popular with intensive therapy programs.

Carbohydrate gram counting helps individuals understand the relationship between food ingested and blood glucose excursions.[45] One potential adverse effect of a total focus on carbohydrate gram counting is that patients may minimize carbohydrate intake and increase their intake of fat and protein, which is clearly undesirable.

Some individuals who have difficulty with the systems described are helped by being given a rigid menu plan that states the amount and type of food to eat or drink at each meal and snack. For example, the breakfast plan could be this: ½ grapefruit, 1 cup oatmeal, 1 slice toast with 1 teaspoon margarine, 1 cup 2% milk, and coffee. This system is used until the person is ready for more independence and advanced education.

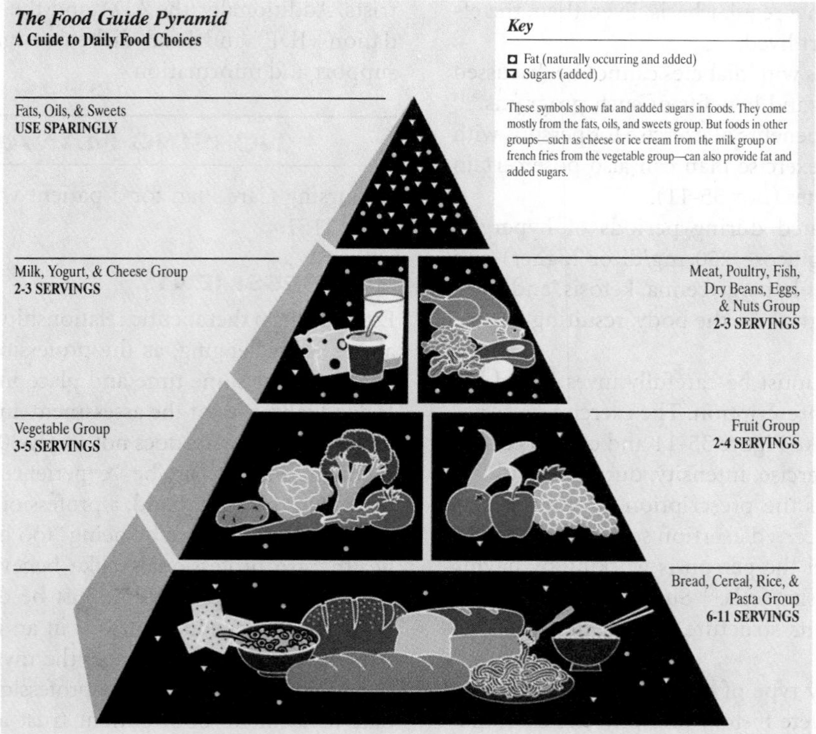

**fig. 35-10** Food Guide Pyramid.

## Dietetic Foods, Sweeteners, and Alcohol

The diabetic diet does not require the use of special or *dietetic* foods. Dietetic, diet, and dietary mean the same thing when used on labels. If used, these foods must be counted into the meal plan, because they are products that have had a substitution made and the substitution does not necessarily mean the product is low in calories or useful for people with diabetes.

Various sweeteners other than sugar are available in the United States, including saccharin, aspartame (Equal), acesulfame-K (Sunette), and sucralose (the first sugar substitute made from sugar). All these products are called low- or no-calorie sweeteners. Patients commonly ask how much of the sweeteners can be consumed safely. The accepted daily intake (ADI) is generous and is usually reported as an amount per kilogram of body weight (2.2 lb = 1 kg). For example, 50 mg/kg is the ADI for aspartame. For a 110-pound person this represents twelve 12-ounce cans of 100% aspartame-sweetened soda pop or 71 packets of Equal per day for a lifetime.

Other sweeteners that contain both carbohydrates and calories include fructose, sorbitol, and mannitol. Therefore all must be incorporated into the meal plan and are not "free foods." Sorbitol can lead to diarrhea from slow gastrointestinal absorption.

Alcohol does not furnish carbohydrate, protein, or fat, but it yields 7 kcal/g when metabolized and must be included in caloric calculations if weight loss is necessary. Some alcohol may be permitted, but the patient must be instructed about the caloric value of pure alcohol; the high carbohydrate content of beer, cordials, wine, and mixed drinks; the inhibiting effect of alcohol on gluconeogenesis with the possible precipitation of hypoglycemia; and the alcohol-induced increase in triglyceride levels.

The general rule is to allow a maximum of two drinks per day (1 drink equals 1½ oz of liquor, 5 oz of wine, or 12 oz of beer) and to consume alcohol with food. Lower carbohydrate alcohol (light beer, rum with diet cola) is preferable. Alcohol should never be consumed and calculated as part of the carbohydrate load of a meal. Hypoglycemia is especially common if alcohol is consumed without food, because the liver's priority is to metabolize alcohol and liver glucose output is then reduced.[14]

## ACTIVITY

In all persons with diabetes, activity is an important part of the medical management and deserves careful and thorough explanation before implementation. Physical activity has important physiological and psychological implications.

Exercise is a wonderful insulin sensitizer, enhancing glucose uptake into skeletal muscle. The exact mechanism is unknown, but it occurs in both type 1 DM and type 2 DM. An excellent example of insulin sensitization as a result of exercise is seen in children going away to summer camp. As a consequence of the insulin sensitization resulting from exercise, insulin doses can decrease 25%.[8]

Insulin resistance and excess weight are present in many persons with type 2 DM. Any type of therapy that decreases resistance and promotes weight loss has potential benefit. Exercise helps in both cases. Both clinical experience and various studies have shown exercise to be of value in both insulin resistance and weight loss. For maximal benefit, the exercise program should be done on a regular basis. Even then, the effect on glucose may be short lived.

Exercise plans for persons with diabetes cannot be discussed without exploring the risks and benefits of such programs.[8,13] Box 35-10 lists some of the benefits of exercise for persons with diabetes. Entering into an exercise plan can also pose certain risks for patients with diabetes (Box 35-11).

Exercise is contraindicated during periods of hyperglycemia (finger-stick blood glucose 250 mg/dl or higher) and ketosis. The combination of hyperglycemia, ketosis, and exercise exerts a physiological stress on the body, resulting in progressive hyperglycemia.

Both benefits and risks must be carefully investigated before launching an exercise prescription. The exercise prescription may look something like Figure 35-11 and consists of the following parts: type of exercise, intensity, duration, and frequency. The center part of the prescription is called a perceived exertion scale. A perceived exertion scale, developed by Borg, determines how hard the person is working by having a person rate how he or she feels.[83] Such a prescription is not always used; however, its structure gives better direction to patients.

Before entering into any type of exercise program, all patients should have a complete history and physical examination, with particular attention to the cardiovascular system and any existing long-term complications. An exercise stress electrocardiogram (ECG) is recommended for all patients over 35 years of age. By doing this test, silent ischemic heart disease and exaggerated hypertensive responses to exercise can be identified. Once the patient has been cleared for an exercise program, special precautions may be indicated. General guidelines for exercise are listed in the Guidelines for Care Box on p. 1150.

### REFERRALS

In some settings the nurse assumes responsibility for making referrals and consultations to other services. This depends on the area in which the nurse is working. In the hospital setting, frequent needs exist for referrals to ophthalmologists, diabetes nurse educators who are Certified Diabetes Educators (CDEs), registered dietitians who are CDEs, psychologists, and podiatrists. Additionally, the ADA and the Juvenile Diabetes Foundation (JDF) and local diabetes organizations may provide support and information.

## NURSING MANAGEMENT

A Nursing Care Plan for a patient with type 2 DM is found on p. 1151.

### ASSESSMENT

Establishing a therapeutic relationship with the patient with diabetes is challenging, as the professional nurse interacts with the patient at some time and place in the "diabetes life span." Individualization of the assessment and plan is critical. Having diabetes for 30 years does not imply 30 years of optimum management. People can be "experienced" at doing the wrong thing. On the other hand, a professional nurse must not insult a patient's intelligence by being "too basic." Many patients and health care professionals alike believe myths about diabetes (Box 35-12). These myths must be dispelled through education. The professional nurse is in an ideal position to educate patients and peers and dispel the myths of diabetes. The diabetes knowledge base of the professional nurse must be up to date to facilitate both patient trust and success (see the Research Box, p. 1150).

#### Subjective Data

Data to be collected to assess the patient with diabetes include:

- Psychosocial/emotional
- Perception of meaning of diagnosis and how it affects the person's life
- Future plans
- Day-to-day activities (work, social activities, family role, meals, etc.)
- Identification of life stressors
- Current coping strategies
- Support systems
- Level of education, literacy
- Knowledge level: concept of diabetes, effect of uncontrolled metabolic state, potential treatment

**box 35-10** *Benefits of Exercise for the Person with Diabetes*

- Improves insulin sensitivity
- Lowers blood glucose during and after exercise
- Improves lipid profile
- May improve some hypertension
- Increases energy expenditure
  - Assists with weight loss
  - Preserves lean body mass
- Promotes cardiovascular fitness
- Increases strength and flexibility
- Improves sense of well-being

From Horton ES: In Lebovitz HE, editor: *Therapy for diabetes mellitus and related disorders,* Alexandria, Va, 1991, American Diabetes Association.

**box 35-11** *Risks of Exercise for the Person with Diabetes*

- Precipitation or exacerbation of cardiovascular disease, angina, dysrhythmias, sudden death
- Hypoglycemia, if taking insulin or oral agents
  - Exercise-related hypoglycemia
  - Late-onset postexercise hypoglycemia
- Hyperglycemia after very strenuous exercise
- Worsening of long-term complications
  - Proliferative retinopathy
  - Peripheral neuropathy
  - Autonomic neuropathy

From Horton ES: In Lebovitz HE, editor: *Therapy for diabetes mellitus and related disorders,* Alexandria, Va, 1991, American Diabetes Association.

Family history: food buying, cooking, history of diabetes
Cardiovascular: drugs, history of blood pressure problems, chest pain or leg pain with exercise
Respiratory: smoking history, environmental hazards
Neuromuscular: history of changes in vision or speech, dizziness, confusion, headache, symptoms of neuropathy (tingling, numbness, pain at rest that disappears with activity)
Gastrointestinal: weight changes, history of gastrointestinal (GI) problems (indigestion, diarrhea, constipation)
Urinary: history of changes in urinary frequency or incontinence
Sexual function: women—menstrual history, history of changes noted with intercourse (if sexually active); men—problems with erectile dysfunction or amount of ejaculate (if sexually active)
Vision: history of blurring, decreased acuity, most recent eye examination
Financial security, insurance

## Objective Data

Data to be collected to assess the patient with diabetes include:
General: weight and height
Emotional/mental: emotional state, responsiveness, attention, alertness, comprehension, appropriateness of response
Neuromuscular: eyes—visual acuity (with and without glasses); motor—range of motion, muscle strength (both upper and lower extremities); sensory—touch, temperature, pain, vibratory sense (especially lower extremities), position sense, deep tendon reflexes
Cardiovascular: blood pressure (both lying and standing), peripheral pulses, ankle and brachial indices
Gastrointestinal: bowel sounds, masses
Urinary: output and fluid intake
Vagina: discharge, irritation
Skin: intactness, temperature, presence of lesions, moisture, hair distribution, texture (especially in lower extremities), turgor

Name: ______________________ Date: __________

Mode: (type of exercise)*

( ) Cycling ( ) Jumping rope
( ) Walking
( ) Swimming ( ) Other ______________
* Can change/rotate

Intensity: (how hard)

Perceived exertion scale

6
7 Very, very light
8
9 Very light
10
11 Fairly light
12
13 Somewhat hard
14
15 Hard
16
17 Very hard
18
19 Very, very hard
20

Duration: (how long)*

Slow (stretch-warm up) __________
Faster (training) __________
Slow (cooling down) __________
* Start slow and build up

Frequency: (how often)

| | Type of exercise | How often |
|---|---|---|
| Aerobic: | __________ | __________ |
| Other: | __________ | __________ |

Physician: ______________

**fig. 35-11** Sample exercise prescription.

**guidelines for care**

### Exercise Program for the Person with Diabetes

**EXERCISE TYPE**

Aerobic (low impact for type 2 DM)
Start with **light level.**

**EXERCISE SESSION**

Each session should eventually include:

1. 5-10 minutes of warm-up stretching and limbering exercises
2. 20-30 minutes of aerobic exercise and heart rate in target zone (as defined by physician) or perceived exertion rating
3. 15-20 minutes of light exercise and stretching to cool down

**EXERCISE FREQUENCY**

3 to 5 times per week

**SPECIAL PRECAUTIONS**

1. Consider the insulin/oral agent regimen (may need to ↓ insulin).
2. Consider the plan for food intake.
   Discuss with health care provider.
   May need to take extra carbohydrate before exercise.
3. Check blood glucose before, during and afterward (for baseline).
4. If glucose over 250 mg/dl, check urine ketones:
   If negative, okay to exercise.
   If positive, take insulin; do not exercise until ketones are negative.
5. Exercise should not cause shortness of breath and should be stopped with any onset of chest pain or dyspnea.
6. Carry diabetes ID card and bracelet.
7. Carry a source of easily absorbed carbohydrate (three glucose tablets or hard candies).
8. Do not exercise in extreme heat or cold.
9. Inspect feet daily and after exercise.

**PRECAUTIONS FOR SELECTED PERSONS**

1. Persons with insensitive feet should choose good shoes for walking and avoid running and jogging. Swimming and cycling may also be included.
2. Persons with proliferative retinopathy should avoid exercises associated with Valsalva maneuvers or that cause jarring and jolting of head or exercises with head in low position.
3. Persons with hypertension should avoid exercises associated with Valsalva maneuvers and exercises involving intense exercises of torso and arms. (Exercises involving the lower extremities are preferred.)

**box 35-12** *Myths of Diabetes*

1. Diabetes is just a touch of sugar.
2. My diabetes will always control me.
3. Symptom free means complication free.
4. Complications are inevitable.
5. If you have diabetes you are doomed to illness and early death.

**research**

Reference: Baxley SG, Brown ST, Pokorny ME, Swanson MS: Perceived competence and actual level of knowledge of diabetes mellitus among nurses, *J Nurs Staff Dev* 13(2):93, 1997.

Staff nurses in a rural 62-bed acute care hospital in the southeastern United States were surveyed on their perceived and actual level of knowledge of diabetes mellitus. Perception of diabetes knowledge was assessed by the Diabetes Self-Report Tool, a Likert-type scale; the mean knowledge score was 88%. The Diabetes Basic Knowledge Test measured actual knowledge; the mean score was 75%. Such a discrepancy between perceived and actual knowledge raises questions regarding competency validation in diabetes management.

### Diagnostic Test Findings

1. Blood/plasma glucose levels in the fasting state or postprandial state may be normal (euglycemia), high (hyperglycemia), or low (hypoglycemia).
2. Glycosylated hemoglobin may be normal or elevated.
3. Serum lipids may be normal or abnormal.
4. Urine ketones may be negative or positive.

## ■ NURSING DIAGNOSES

Nursing diagnoses are determined from analysis of patient data. Possible nursing diagnoses for the person with diabetes mellitus may include but are not limited to:

| Diagnostic Title | Possible Etiological Factors |
|---|---|
| Fluid volume deficit, risk for | Excess urination, limited access to fluids, inadequate knowledge |
| Fatigue | Inadequate nutrition (from glycemic state), muscle weakness |
| Infection, risk for | Elevated blood glucose |
| Nutrition, altered: less or more than body requirements | Alteration in metabolism, decreased nutrition, lack of knowledge |
| Fear | Long-term illness, taking insulin, lifestyle changes (loss of job) |
| Knowledge deficit: disease, drugs, self-care skills (insulin injection, HBGM), diet needs, activity needs | New information and skills; never exposed before |

## ■ EXPECTED PATIENT OUTCOMES

Expected patient outcomes for the patient with diabetes, based on the previous nursing diagnoses, may include but are not limited to:

1. Exhibits physical signs of fluid balance:
   a. Weight returns to patient's baseline weight.
   b. Skin turgor and mucous membranes are normal.

## nursing care plan Person with Diabetes Mellitus

**DATA** Mrs. F. is an obese, 72-year-old married woman with type 2 DM diagnosed 8 years ago. She was referred to a short-term ambulatory diabetes education program by her physician for instruction on insulin administration because blood glucose control had not been achieved with dietary measures alone or in conjunction with oral hypoglycemic agents.

The nursing history identified the following in Mrs. F.:

- She saw referral as necessary but perceived the need for insulin and her inability to control weight as personal failures.
- She maintained inconsistent sleep/activity schedule.
- She had accurate knowledge about dietary modifications and had participated successfully in several weight reduction programs with 20- to 40-pound weight loss each time.
- She did regular checks of feet and wore proper shoes.
- She did not exercise consistently.
- She has performed blood glucose monitoring on others and once or twice on herself.
- She stated that church activities were important to her; satisfactions were derived from church group socialization and it "keeps me busy."
- She feared that her husband would die suddenly at home. Two years ago, CPR had to be performed when he had a cardiac arrest at home.

Objective data included the following:

- Blood glucose (fasting), 220 mg/dl
- Weight, 200 pounds
- Height, 5′4″
- Blood pressure, 134/84
- Urine negative for microalbuminuria
- Peripheral pulses 1+
- Legs warm and dry, color even with rest of body
- Patellar and Achilles tendon reflexes 3+ (on 1 to 4 scale)
- Decreased perception to touch in lower extremities
- Decrease in vibration and pinprick sensation to great toe
- Vision 20/20 on Snellen chart eye examination.

Collaborative nursing actions included teaching Mrs. F. those measures that would help her achieve control of blood glucose (diet, insulin, exercise) and teaching her to detect, prevent, and treat hypoglycemic reactions.

**NURSING DIAGNOSIS** *Knowledge deficit: self-injections, care of equipment, and home monitoring of blood glucose related to lack of exposure to information*

| expected patient outcomes | nursing interventions | rationale |
|---|---|---|
| Independently administers injection to self. | Support patient as necessary to self-inject insulin. | Adults who perform this task have minimal discomfort and realize they are capable of giving own insulin. |
| Performs home blood glucose monitoring (HBGM) accurately. | Observe patient's skill in HBGM; correct as necessary. | Evaluation of patient technique is necessary to ensure accuracy. |
| Uses measurements obtained by HBGM to achieve fasting blood glucose below 100 mg/dl. | Review, with patient, effect of activity, dietary intake, and insulin on blood glucose. Instruct patient on frequency and timing of HBGM. | HBGM gives almost immediate feedback about previous behaviors and reinforces value of therapeutic measures. |
| Describes symptoms of hypoglycemia and knows how to treat. | Review, with patient, signs and symptoms and treatment measures for hypoglycemia. | This knowledge ensures that patient can safely give own insulin and decreases fear of reaction. |
| Describes how to care for insulin and supplies. | Review with patient information about care of insulin and supplies. | This knowledge ensures that insulin and equipment will be stable. |
| Describes how diet will be changed because of insulin. | Refer to dietitian for modification of diet necessary with insulin and verification of diet knowledge. | The dietitian is appropriate person to teach about diet. |

**NURSING DIAGNOSIS** *Altered health maintenance related to ineffective coping skills*

| expected patient outcome | nursing interventions | rationale |
|---|---|---|
| States at least one change that will improve blood glucose control. | Counsel patient about effects of stress, lack of exercise, and activity pattern on blood glucose. | Patient's understanding of how stress impairs health is necessary before change. |
| | Explore with Mrs. F. willingness and ability to change behaviors: sleep/activity, coping, and exercise. | Goals are more likely to be achieved if patient makes realistic choices after considering cost and benefits. |
| | Engage Mrs. F. in mutual problem solving; refrain from prescribing. | Increasing patients' sense of control can help with self-esteem and enhance attitudes toward change. |
| | Explore sources for long-term support in learning more effective coping skills. Suggest support groups:<br>1. For spouses of patients with myocardial infarctions (MI)<br>2. For weight loss and maintenance of weight loss<br>3. For exercise | Changing lifestyle, eating behaviors, and coping skills is very difficult; support over long periods is usually required. |

c. Blood pressure and pulse are within the patient's normal range.
d. Serum electrolytes and hematocrit are within normal limits.

The patient:

a. Has an oral fluid intake of 2500 to 3000 ml/day.
b. Explains how to prevent deficits.

2. Fatigue is improved:
   a. States fatigue level is decreased by a lower rating on a scale of 1 to 10 (1 = no fatigue, 10 = most fatigue).
   b. Verbalizes need to do regular home blood glucose monitoring in order to take action with high blood glucoses or low blood glucoses.
3. Risk for infection is decreased:
   a. Verbalizes need to do home blood glucose monitoring, the frequency of which is prescribed by the health care team.
   b. Identifies factors that increase blood glucose.
   c. Lists signs and symptoms of infection.
4. Exhibits signs of nutritional adequacy:
   a. Maintains weight, or loses or gains as appropriate.
   b. Blood glucose, glycosylated hemoglobin, and lipid measurements are moving toward normal.
   c. Food intake is distributed throughout the day.
5. Patient's fear is decreased:
   a. Expresses feelings about having diabetes.
   b. States coping strategies.
6. An adequate level of knowledge is attained:
   a. Verbalizes that diabetes is a disease in which the body is unable to use all foods properly because of lack of insulin or inability to use insulin.
   b. Demonstrates correctly how to give insulin.
   c. Demonstrates correctly how to monitor for blood glucose and urine ketones (knows when and whom to call for help).
   d. Verbalizes the definitions of hypoglycemia and hyperglycemia.
   e. Verbalizes symptoms and treatment of hypoglycemia.
   f. Verbalizes how to take oral agents and effects to report.
   g. Verbalizes dietary plan and ways to achieve dietary modifications.
   h. Verbalizes exercise plan, safety precautions, and what to report.

## INTERVENTIONS

### Improving Fluid Status

To improve fluid status, the patient's metabolic status needs to be improved, and the patient needs to ingest an adequate amount of fluids. Explore with the patient, using appropriate terminology, possible causes for loss of fluid (dehydration). Relate the fluid loss to the high blood glucose. Use terminology such as glucose attracts water, and when blood glucose is high, glucose goes out in the urine, pulling water with it, thus increasing urination. Relate increased thirst to nature's way of telling the person to drink more. If the person is not drinking, fluid losses will not be controlled. Relate symptoms of high blood glucose to the fluid loss. This illustration can help the patient visualize how to manage the diabetes using tools such as HBGM and testing for urine ketones. Teach the patient and family about diet, medications, and fluid needs. Teach HBGM and urine testing for ketones. Ensure that the patient has the telephone numbers of the physician and diabetes team for emergencies.

### Promoting Adequate Nutrition

The registered dietitian who is part of the health team is ideally responsible for the nutritional component of the educational program for the person with diabetes. The nurse, however, is also involved. A dietary history should be part of the nurse's initial assessment. Any pertinent data must be shared with other health team members, particularly the dietitian.

Because of the difficulty in changing food habits, the patient should be involved in setting goals for dietary changes. Compromises that may be necessary include the following:

1. Identifying an acceptable weight loss schedule for the obese person
2. Incorporating an alcoholic beverage into the daily plan, if desired
3. Distributing food in a different pattern (e.g., a large noon meal and a small evening meal)
4. Adding desserts to some meals

Information about cultural or social food habits that are identified in the dietary history need to be incorporated into the dietary plan. For example, it may be necessary to make accommodations for a vegetarian diet or for incorporation of fast foods in the diet.

The system for maintaining the dietary plan should be identified by the patient and the registered dietitian. The selected system is documented in the nursing care plan so that everyone involved uses the same terminology and food groupings. The mutually established goals, including compromises and sociocultural practices, are also documented so that the patient is not given conflicting information. Significant others should be included in the teaching.

After dietary goals are established, the nurse should help the patient apply dietary knowledge through the following:

1. Simulations in which the person chooses foods from the hospital menu, food models, or other learning tools
2. Patient participation in documenting food intake, blood and urine results, activity, and medications and in discussing how these interrelate

The patient's and significant other's satisfaction with the plan must be evaluated. Additional needs that are identified over time must be communicated to the dietitian so that they can be incorporated into the plan.

Skills that the patient should possess after the initial management period are (1) ability to manage the diet for stable condition over 1 week, (2) knowing who to contact if unusual events requiring adjustments occur, and (3) knowing how to handle sick days.

As individuals gain ability, they will be able to do the following:

1. Manage their diets on a daily basis, making adjustment for normal life changes
2. Select appropriate foods from restaurant menus or at social occasions
3. Manage dietary needs while traveling or for shift work

4. Manage dietary needs at unplanned social events (e.g., "happy hour" after work, unexpected business dinner, unexpected company)
5. Evaluate their success in dietary management through evaluating weight changes and glycosylated hemoglobin levels or through blood glucose self-monitoring
6. Make a conscious effort to include adequate vitamins and minerals, eliminate excess salt, decrease saturated fat intake, decrease caffeine intake
7. Keep up to date on new findings about dietary management and consult health team members about the new recommendations
8. Avoid "quack" recommendations
9. Manipulate diet, exercise, and medications together to cover a variety of daily situations
10. Work with others in the household to help them incorporate principles of healthy eating into the diet

### Decreasing Fatigue

Measures to improve metabolic control will improve fatigue. However, because the patient may have loss of muscle mass and be deconditioned, metabolic control will usually improve before the fatigue. Therefore the patient will need help in developing a schedule to promote graded increase in activity and adequate rest and sleep. The patient and the family need to understand the basis of the fatigue.

Teaching should include the following points:

1. Diabetes is a health condition in which the body is unable to use the body fuels of protein, fat, and carbohydrate properly because of insulin deficiency, improper insulin action, or both.
2. The metabolic abnormalities result in a loss of fluids and electrolytes.
3. Fatigue can result, which is reversible over time.

### Preventing Infection

Improvement in metabolic control is the primary way to prevent infections. The patient and significant others must understand the relationship of poor blood glucose control to infection. They must also understand that infection can worsen glycemic control. Awareness of the signs and symptoms of infections and management of sick days is critical (Box 35-13).

### Decreasing Fear

Before the patient is ready to accept self-care, the patient must learn to control his or her fears. The nurse should anticipate the presence of fears by asking straightforward questions about fear of impact of diagnosis on job, giving self-injections, or relationships with others. Possible conflicting factors such as lifestyle changes should be identified. The nurse needs to eliminate misconceptions that can increase fear. Patients must have permission to grieve for losses being experienced, must know that many individuals feel like they are "falling apart," and must know that with time they will get better and feel better. Referrals to clinical nurse specialists, psychologists, counselors, or clergy for emotional support will be necessary.

### Facilitating Learning

A major responsibility of the professional nurse is helping persons gain self-management skills for any chronic health

**box 35-13** *Sick Day Guidelines*

*When to call your physician/nurse about being sick or "out of sorts"* (just go through the checklist and check what you have):

____ If you are unable to keep down fluids/food
____ If you are unable to eat regular foods for more than 1 day
____ Signs of infection: redness, warmth, swelling, pus, tenderness any place
____ Symptoms of dehydration: dry mouth, fever, thirst, dry flushed skin, vomiting, abdominal pain, severe nausea, diarrhea, rapid breathing
____ Vomiting more than three times or diarrhea lasting longer than 6 hours
____ Increased urination and increased thirst
____ Have cough and bring up yellow or green material
____ Any symptoms getting worse
____ HBGM consistently elevated beyond specified levels
____ Fever present
____ Ketones present
____ Have any questions about how to take care of yourself and control your diabetes
____ Have questions about adjusting insulin/oral agents

*Information to have ready for physician/nurse when you call:*

____ Length of time you have been sick
____ Your temperature
____ What's bothering you (a list of symptoms)
____ Test results: urine ketones and blood glucose
____ Diabetes medication: type, time you take, and amount and what you have taken
____ Other medications you take; medication allergies; type, amount, time of medications recently taken
____ Pharmacy phone number

*Remember:*

1. Always take your insulin or oral agent.
2. Drink plenty of fluids, including broth.
3. Test urine ketones and blood glucose every 4 hours; record results.
4. Eat carbohydrates according to your meal plan; replace with liquids if necessary.
5. Know all your caregivers' phone numbers and names.

(When you get better, return to your normal eating plan and medication dosage. This information applies to *short-term* illness [1-2 days]. If you are unable to eat, or have vomiting or diarrhea, call immediately.)

problem through teaching and counseling. Self-management skills are probably the major determinant of how well the health problem is controlled and the quality of life maintained.[46] This is particularly true for persons with diabetes. Research supports the idea that patient education has a positive effect on patient outcomes.

The major problem confronting the nurse when dealing with the problem of knowledge deficit in the person with diabetes mellitus is, "What do I teach and how much do I teach?" The bottom line is that patients have to survive in the real world. This requires ability to perform day-to-day survival skills. *Always* validate that patients can perform survival/initial skills.

A "diabetes pretest" is an ideal format by which to assess a patient's fund of diabetes knowledge. The test should consist of questions that the patient, as well as the professional nurse, can correctly answer in order to deliver comprehensive care. Perhaps more important, a well-constructed test allows a patient to identify what he or she knows, or does not know, about diabetes. Remember, individuals can have "islands" of intelligence, and the diabetes island can be uninhabited.

The American Diabetes Association has suggested that diabetes education take place in three stages and is continuous:

1. Survival/initial stage
2. In-depth stage
3. Continuous stage

Stages 2 and 3 place emphasis on knowledge and skills needed to be completely self-sufficient in daily management and knowledge and skills needed to gain flexibility in management, insight, and self-determination. A tool such as the Professional Prompter Worksheet (Box 35-14) can help in facilitating learning. This tool provides the survival/initial knowledge that must be mastered by the person with type 1 DM or type 2 DM. The survival/initial information is identified on the tool. Other areas, such as dealing with complications and in-depth knowledge about hyperglycemia and ketoacidosis, are left for stages 2 and 3 teaching. The Professional Prompter Worksheet provides information on what to teach and on teaching strategies and available tools.

Many teaching tools are available from pharmaceutical companies. Nurses can access this information by contacting the professional or medical equipment representative for the institution or region in which they work. Teaching materials also are available from the American Diabetes Association. Almost every institution with a diabetes center will have materials similar to those listed on the Professional Prompter Worksheet that can be purchased or borrowed. The diabetes clinical nurse specialist is also a source of information and assistance.

## Managing Medications

### *Insulin knowledge*

Patients taking insulin should be able to name their prescribed type of insulin, their dose and the peak effects, and how the exercise regimen and diet are coordinated with the insulin. They should know insulin measurement (units) and the need for similarly calibrated syringes. In addition, they must know how to handle insulin needs on sick days.

### *Insulin self-administration*

For safe insulin administration, patients must know how to draw insulin into the syringe, mix two insulins (if pertinent), select and prepare the injection site, use consistent injection sites, rotate within those sites, and inject insulin. The essential teaching points are summarized on the Professional Prompter Worksheet (see Box 35-14). Most persons will have some fears related to self-injection. Repeated practice is necessary, so patients should be started on self-injections as soon as insulin treatment is deemed necessary.

**Preparing the insulin dose.** The patient is taught to rotate or roll the insulin vial of longer-acting insulin to return any precipitated particles to solution and to draw the required dose of insulin into the syringe using correct technique. Current insulin syringes have little or no dead space, thus eliminating a potential source of error. The procedure can be practiced using saline solution and a syringe.

Patient fear is greatly reduced if the nurse self-injects sterile saline, thus demonstrating no discomfort with injection. An ideal way for patients to learn is to have them self-administer either a saline or an insulin injection, rather than using the traditional sponge or orange; the physical resistance of a sponge or orange bears no resemblance to that of skin or subcutaneous tissue.

For the first injection, the nurse may elect to delay teaching about the preparation and focus first on self-injection. Adults may be better able to focus on preparing the syringe after experiencing self-injection.

**Mixing two insulins.** If the patient is using two insulins, they may be mixed in one syringe so that only one injection is necessary (see the Guidelines for Care Box). There are only a few instances in which insulins cannot be mixed. Crystalline zinc insulins (Lente and Ultralente) can be mixed together. The package insert of zinc insulins states that they cannot be mixed with other types of insulins. However, many practitioners permit patients to mix and inject immediately. The mix and inject immediately routine is the recommendation regardless of which insulins are being mixed together.

**guidelines for care**

**Mixing Two Insulins in One Syringe**

1. Gather equipment.
2. Wash hands.
3. Roll vial of longer acting insulin.
4. Cleanse tops of vials with alcohol.
5. Draw up air equivalent to dose of longer acting insulin, and inject the air into that vial. (Do not draw up this insulin.) Remove needle from vial.
6. Draw up air equivalent to dose of Lispro or Regular insulin, inject the air into the bottle, and withdraw the Lispro or Regular insulin to the correct dose. Remove all air, and readjust to correct dose. Remove needle.
7. Insert needle into vial of longer acting insulin, and draw up correct dose.
8. If an error is made, discard insulin in syringe and start over.

**box 35-14** *Professional Prompter Worksheet for Diabetes Education*

SI = Survival information/skills for type 1
SII = Survival information/skills for type 2

**SURVIVAL/INITIAL TEACHING**

| SURVIVAL/INITIAL SKILLS | TYPE 1 SURVIVAL/INITIAL SKILLS | TYPE 2 SURVIVAL/INITIAL SKILLS |
|---|---|---|
| 1. Concentrate on survival. These are the skills every patient must know before discharge. It is necessary, and patient cannot go further without this foundation.<br>2. Assess patient's knowledge via a pretest. | 1. Psychological and family.<br>2. Can patient give insulin correctly; i.e., see the increments, inject correctly, use proper sites, reuse syringe, know time action of insulin?<br>3. Monitor blood glucose and urine ketones.<br>4. Recognize and treat hypoglycemia. | 1. Psychological and family.<br>2. Explanation of what diabetes is—insulin resistance versus insulin deficiency.<br>3. Treatment with diet, oral agent, and insulin if necessary, or combination therapy.<br>4. Monitor blood glucose and urine ketones.<br>5. Recognize and treat hypoglycemia if on sulfonylureas or insulin. |

**TOOLS TO USE FOR SURVIVAL/INITIAL TEACHING**

- Barrier check
- Initial assessment
- Take-home Instruction Sheet
- American Diabetes Association (ADA) Curriculum Guidelines
- Refer to group class in local hospital
- Refer to specialty practice/center

**ASSESSMENT (SI & SII)**

Complete assessment, including diabetes knowledge

**BARRIERS (SI & SII)**

| DEFINE BARRIER | TEACHING TOOLS |
|---|---|
| 1. Fatigue/pain | 1. Give instructions another time. |
| 2. High anxiety | 2. Identify why and work on anxiety before proceeding. |
| 3. Blindness | 3. Audio material and devices. |
| | 4. Referral to specialty center. |

**OVERVIEW OF DIABETES (SII)**
**Patient Can Verbalize/Demonstrate**

1. Diabetes is a disease in which the body is unable to utilize carbohydrate foods properly due to lack of insulin or inability to use insulin.
2. Define high blood sugar in terms of blood glucose. Normal versus diabetes. List symptoms.
3. Define which type of diabetes the patient has.
4. Describe essential parts of diabetes management: Knowledge, self-care, meal planning, exercise, and medication. Know the effect each of these has on the blood glucose.
5. Know effect of activity on blood glucose.
6. Know effect of illness/stress on blood glucose.

**STRESS AND PSYCHOLOGICAL ADJUSTMENT (SI & SII)**
**Patient Can Verbalize/Demonstrate**

1. That patient has adapted to having diabetes.
2. That patient expresses feelings about having diabetes.
3. Acknowledges losses—grief process (fear, anxiety, denial, anger, bargaining, depression, acceptance). Discussion with nurse or social worker.

**FAMILY INVOLVEMENT AND SOCIAL SUPPORT (SI & SII)**
**Patient Can Verbalize/Demonstrate**

1. Family can identify one feeling a person with diabetes may experience.
2. Ways diabetes has affected the family.
3. A support person.

**NUTRITION (SI & SII)**
**Patient Can Verbalize/Demonstrate**

1. Individualized meal plan.
2. Reason for maintaining consistency (if appropriate) of: meal spacing, proper meal times, and snacks to avoid hypo/hyperglycemia.
3. Relationship of insulin or oral agent, activity, and calorie intake.
4. Diet changes for sick day management, exercise, use of alcohol, change in meal schedule, and restaurant dining.
5. The importance of attaining and maintaining ideal body weight.
6. Effects of dietary fiber.

Data from George Ann Eaks, RN, MN, CDE. From Cray Diabetes Center, University of Kansas Medical Center, Kansas City, KS.

*Continued*

**box 35-14** *Professional Prompter Worksheet for Diabetes Education—cont'd*

**EXERCISE AND ACTIVITY**
**Patient Can Verbalize/Demonstrate**

1. How exercise affects diabetes control.
2. Cautions and risks of exercise.
3. When one should not exercise.
4. Patient's personal exercise program.

**MEDICATIONS (SI & SII)**
**Patient Can Verbalize/Demonstrate**

*Insulin:*

1. What is function of insulin?
   - Quick, intermediate, or long acting.
2. Differentiation of insulin types.
3. Medication schedule—amounts and times taken.
4. Correct technique for insulin preparation:
   - Insulin to be injected is at room temperature.
   - Rotates bottle to mix (cloudy insulin).
   - Injects air.
   - Withdraws proper amount of insulin.
   - Rids syringe of air bubbles.
5. Correct technique for drawing up insulin, two types:
   - Rotates bottle to mix (cloudy) insulin.
   - Injects air into both bottles.
   - Withdraws clear (regular) insulin first.
   - Adds proper amount of second insulin.
6. Correct technique for insulin administration:
   - Cleans site with alcohol.
   - Gathers skin and inserts needle all the way.
   - Injects insulin, holding needle steady (needle should go in at 90° angle unless person is very thin).
   - Use of consistent sites, rotates within those sites (abdomen, arm, leg, buttocks).
7. Storage of insulin:
   - Best to store in refrigerator.
   - For travel okay at room temperature up to 1 month (57°-85° F).
8. Discard syringes in sealable can or special disposal unit.
9. Can cause hypoglycemia.

*Oral Agents:*

1. Action of oral agent.
2. Medication schedule—amount and *time* to be taken.
3. Need to eat 3 carbohydrate-consistent meals a day.
4. Can cause hypoglycemia.

**RELATIONSHIPS AMONG NUTRITION, EXERCISE, MEDICATION, AND BLOOD GLUCOSE LEVELS (SI & SII)**
**Patient Can Verbalize/Demonstrate**

1. Effect of food on blood glucose.
2. Effect of insulin oral agents on blood glucose.
3. Effect of oral agents on insulin resistance.
4. Effect of physical activity on blood glucose.
5. Effect of illness on blood sugar.

**MONITORING AND USE OF RESULTS (SI & SII)**
**Patient Can Verbalize/Demonstrate**

1. Explain need for monitoring glucose.
2. Normal range of blood glucose and acceptable targets.
3. Capillary blood glucose monitoring:
   - Loads and operates lancing device.
   - Holds arm down to the side to get better drop of blood.
   - Obtains large hanging drop of blood.
   - Places blood on strip properly.
   - Waits appropriate amount of time according to directions.
   - Reads visual and records results.
   - Uses meter (knows name of meter, strips to use, how to calibrate, use control solutions, how to clean, insert battery, and understand readout).
4. Checking urine ketones:
   - Knows how to do.
   - Knows when to do.
5. Knows when and whom to call for help.

**ACUTE COMPLICATIONS: HYPERGLYCEMIA**
**Patient Can Verbalize/Demonstrate**

1. Definition and cause of hyperglycemia.
2. Symptoms of hyperglycemia.
3. Illness and sick day rules:
   - What to do about insulin/oral agents when ill.
   - How often to check sugar and ketones.
   - When to call physician.
   - Sick day eating.

*Continued*

**box 35-14** *Professional Prompter Worksheet for Diabetes Education—cont'd*

**ACUTE COMPLICATIONS: HYPOGLYCEMIA (SI & SII)**
**Patient Can Verbalize/Demonstrate**

1. Definition and cause of hypoglycemia.
2. Symptoms of hypoglycemia.
3. Treatment of hypoglycemia (wears diabetes ID).
4. When to call physician, nurse practitioner.

**CHRONIC COMPLICATIONS**
**Patient Can Verbalize/Demonstrate**

1. Possible long-term complications.
2. Importance of prevention; primary role of glycemic control.
3. The organs/body systems at risk in diabetes:
   - Eyes
   - Blood vessels
   - Blood pressure
   - Feet
   - Kidneys
   - Neurological
   - Reproductive
4. Reasons for good foot care:
   - Daily cleansing and inspection/appropriate footwear
5. Reason for yearly dilated fundoscopic examination (and last date).
6. Need for blood pressure control.
   - Knows blood pressure goal.

**FOOT, SKIN, AND DENTAL CARE**
**Patient Can Verbalize/Demonstrate**

1. Importance of good health habits.
   - Dental
   - Skin
   - Feet
   - Signs of infection
   - Effect of smoking, alcohol, and drug abuse

**BEHAVIOR CHANGE STRATEGIES, GOAL SETTING, AND PROBLEM SOLVING**
**Patient Can Verbalize/Demonstrate**

1. The need for a planned system of medical care.
   - Follow-up and education
2. The benefits and responsibilities of goal setting for self-help care.
3. The importance of being well-informed, equal partners to make choices.

**USE OF HEALTH CARE SYSTEM AND COMMUNITY RESOURCES**
**Patient Can Verbalize/Demonstrate**

1. Resources that can help:
   - American Diabetes Association
   - Self-management classes
   - Services for the blind
   - Juvenile Diabetes Foundation
   - Local diabetes associations

**NECESSARY TAKE-HOME (SI & SII)**
**Patient Can Verbalize/Demonstrate**

1. Feel comfortable doing all skills under survival.
2. Know the skills and be able to simulate them in a normal day; i.e., take you through a day and list all diabetes-related activities as they would do them.
3. Know who to call, the telephone number, and when to call.
4. Have a return appointment card with health care provider name and phone number listed.
5. Have instructions written on:
   - *Take Home Instruction* form
   - *Choice to Better Daily Living* form
6. Have a schedule of the diabetes classes if patient chooses to attend them.
7. Have a meal plan—have patient seen by dietitian. If dietitian unavailable and you must instruct on meal plan, refer to section on nutrition.

Mixing two insulins in the same syringe is one of the more complex psychomotor skills the patient has to learn; therefore it needs to be started early. A major complication with mixing two insulins in one syringe is that each of the two vials of insulin can be contaminated with the insulin from the other vial. Cross-contamination can be avoided by always withdrawing from the Lispro or Regular insulin vial first, because injecting minute amounts of Lispro or Regular insulin into a vial of longer acting insulin is less problematic than the Lispro or Regular insulin contaminated with the longer acting insulin.

If the patient has difficulty mastering the skill of mixing two insulins, alternatives include the following:

1. Take two separate injections each time.
2. Have a family member, friend, or community health nurse prefill the syringes. A week's supply of a single type of insulin can be predrawn.

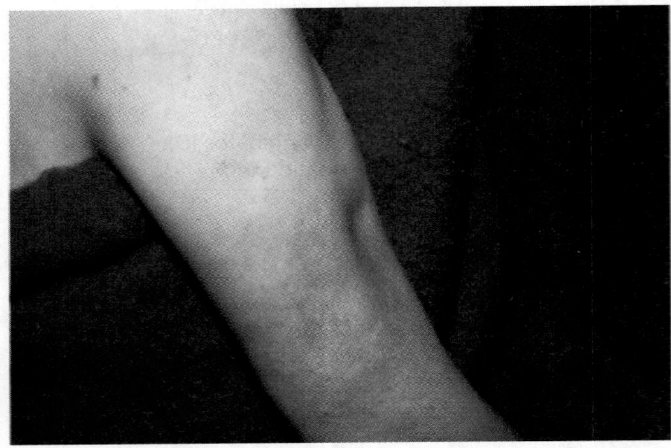

**fig. 35-12** Lipodystrophy of the arm.

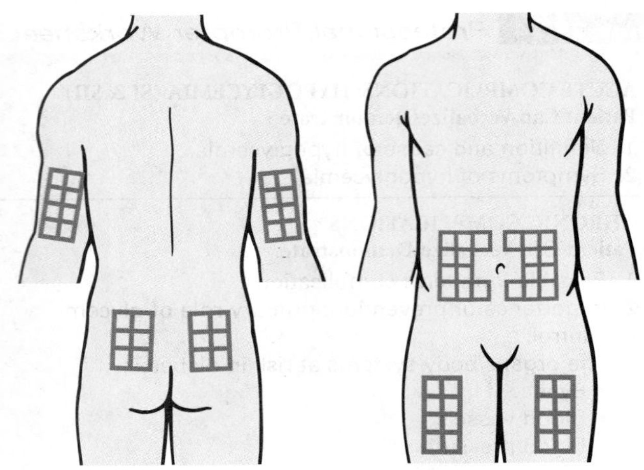

**fig. 35-13** Insulin injection sites.

**Injection sites.** Two principles govern injection sites: *consistency* and *rotation.* Consistent use of sites is critical because insulin absorption varies dramatically based on anatomical site. The upper abdomen provides the quickest absorption, followed by the arms, legs, and lower buttocks. Consistency with use of a specified injection site for a specified injection helps eliminate some variability in glucose levels. For example, use the abdomen for the prebreakfast injection, the arm for the predinner injection, and the buttocks for the bedtime injection. Then, rotation of injections among the designated anatomical sites helps prevent the development of lipodystrophy. Ideally, injections should be given 1 inch apart, while trying not to reuse an injection site within a 2- to 4-week period of time. The injection site should be cleansed with 70% isopropyl alcohol before use.

*Lipodystrophy* can occur with repeated injections, causing poor absorption of the medications. Two forms of lipodystrophy can occur: hypertrophy and atrophy. *Hypertrophy* is thickening of an injection site from development of fibrous scar tissue from repeated injections. A hypertrophic area is usually devoid of nerve endings, and the patient likes to reuse it because injections are painless, but absorption is erratic. *Atrophy* is loss of subcutaneous fat from unknown causes; however, an immunological process is implicated. Lipodystrophies may be partially caused by impurities in insulin; development of purified insulins has decreased this problem, but rotation of sites is still important (Figure 35-12).

**Selection and preparation of injection sites.** Any area of subcutaneous tissue can be used for injection. The recommended sites are illustrated in Figure 35-13.

The best site for the first injection is the abdomen. It is easy to work with and has the most rapid absorption, and absorption is not affected by physical activity.

**Injection of insulin.** Insulin should be administered subcutaneously. Historically, because of the longer needles used on glass syringes, the subcutaneous tissue was pinched up before injection. With the current insulin syringes, with needles from 0.25 to 0.5 inch long, there is no longer a need to pinch up the subcutaneous tissue, unless the patient is very thin or cachectic. Rather, the subcutaneous tissue should be gently gathered, or if the patient is obese, stretched tautly. With these shorter-needle syringes, the needle should be inserted at a 90° angle. There is no need for routine aspiration. Injections should produce little, if any, discomfort. Painful injections can be minimized by employing the techniques described in the Patient/Family Teaching Box.

All insulin syringe manufacturers recommend only a single use of each insulin syringe because sterility cannot be guaranteed otherwise. Syringes should never be shared between individuals. Many individuals with diabetes reuse their own insulin syringes until the needle dulls. Insulin has bacteriostatic additives that inhibit bacterial growth. With reuse of the syringe, however, the light coating of lubrication on the needle is lost, such that injections may be more uncomfortable. In patients who practice good hygiene and good injection technique, the reuse of syringes is safe and practical.[2]

Safe disposal of syringes and lancets used at home is critical. Procedures for at-home sharps disposal differ significantly from hospital techniques. Syringes should be made unable to be used by another individual and then disposed of safely. The needle, with cap on, of a standard insulin syringe can be easily broken off of the syringe. Then, both the needle and syringe should be placed in a hard-sided receptacle such as a coffee can or bleach bottle. Patients should call their local government office for information on disposal.

**Storage of insulin and other supplies and care of syringe.** Patients need to develop a home storage system for equipment and the currently used bottle of insulin and extra insulin. Insulin is stable for 30 days at room temperature; however, it is a good idea to have patients keep extra insulin in a refrigerator because room temperature differs from home to home. The current recommendation is to keep the currently used insulin bottle and the other supplies together at

**patient/family teaching**

**Steps to Eliminate Painful Insulin Injections**

1. Inject insulin that has been at room temperature for 15 minutes. Do not inject cold insulin.
2. Wait until the topical alcohol has dried before injecting insulin.
3. Keep muscles in the area of injection relaxed, not tensed.
4. Penetrate the skin quickly. Use the hinge-like action of the wrist to "dart" the needle in.
5. Do not change the direction of the needle on insertion or withdrawal.
6. Do not use dull needles.

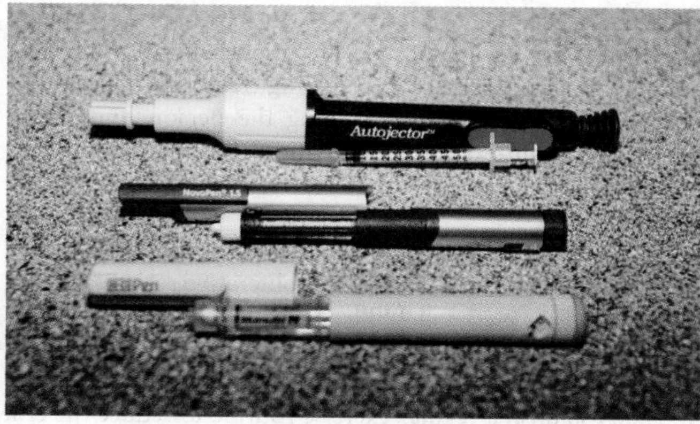


**fig. 35-14** Insulin injection aids.

room temperature and to store extra bottles of insulin in the refrigerator. Store prefilled syringes in the refrigerator with the needles facing upward. Equipment should be stored out of the reach of children.

Patients should always have an extra bottle of each type of insulin they use. Insulin has an expiration date, which should be checked at purchase; purchase only the amount that can be used before the expiration date. When traveling, insulin and supplies should be hand-carried to prevent loss. It is also recommended to bring twice as many supplies as one would anticipate using.

For persons unwilling or unable to use syringes, a variety of injection aids are available (Figure 35-14).[25] Pen devices for insulin delivery facilitate taking injections away from home. The Autojector by Ulster, an insulin injection aid, not only injects the needle, but also injects the insulin; it gives a virtually pain-free injection and retails for approximately $30. Jet spray injectors are also available but are expensive, retailing for approximately $300. Although these devices are designed to reduce discomfort and enhance insulin absorption, some patients actually find them more uncomfortable and report inconsistencies with insulin delivery caused by the variable pressure settings needed in different anatomical sites.

**Measures to assist the sensory-impaired person.** Adaptation of equipment may be necessary for the sensory-impaired person. A number of aids available for the visually handicapped are advertised in diabetes publications or are available from the American Federation of the Blind at 212-502-7600 or 212-947-1060 or from local sight agencies. Special syringes with plunger locks, attachable devices for locking the plunger, and attachable needle and insulin bottle guides to facilitate entry of the needle into the bottle can be purchased. Persons who have failing vision may also use a small magnifying adapter that can be clipped to a syringe.

Persons with poor vision may draw air instead of insulin into the syringe. They must be cautioned to invert the vial completely and insert the needle only a short distance. They are often advised to use only about two thirds of a vial of insulin. Some persons have a family member or a friend draw the last doses from a bottle of insulin. Another option is to know how long to use a vial before the level gets so low that the needle is not covered (e.g., 1000 U in vial—if the person is taking 40 U per day, he or she should stop using the vial on the twenty-second day unless assisted by a sighted person).

#### Oral agents

Patients taking oral agents must be equally prepared to handle their medication. Each patient must know the name of the medication, dose, peak effects, and how the diet and exercise regimens are coordinated with medication therapy. If taking sulfonylureas, patients must be educated about hypoglycemia symptoms and treatment. Patients must know how to handle illness. Oral agents should be kept out of the reach of children, at room temperature, and not exposed to direct sunlight. The medication should be hand-carried when traveling to decrease risk of loss.

### Managing Nutrition

Because diet is the cornerstone of treatment for the person with diabetes, it is important to be able to teach the patient information on the Professional Prompter Worksheet under nutrition (see Box 35-14). The registered dietitian should be the primary provider of meal planning and nutrition information. Nurses can help reinforce the individualized meal plan and must be aware of maintaining consistency of the carbohydrate content of meals. All diabetes teaching will interface with the relationship of insulin or oral agent, activity, and carbohydrate intake.

Weight is one of the major factors in monitoring diabetes control. Attaining and maintaining ideal body weight are major criteria in diabetes management, and these goals require the whole team's effort. Central to all nutrition management information that will help the patient is stressing the importance of following the meal plan. When patients are taking insulin, snacks may become a part of the treatment plan. See the section on dietary management earlier in this chapter.

## Providing Exercise Knowledge

Exercise is another major area of patient education for persons with diabetes mellitus. Nursing activities include obtaining an exercise history, helping the person understand and obtain a pre-exercise examination, and planning an enjoyable and safe exercise program. The nurse should do the following:

1. Help select an exercise that will not cause problems if conditions such as neuropathy or proliferative retinopathy are present.
2. Refer the patient to a podiatrist for correct footwear for the chosen exercise if applicable.
3. Help establish a regular exercise routine to reduce the risk of hypoglycemia.
4. Explain the components of a safe exercise program and the special needs of the person with diabetes.
5. Teach how to monitor cardiovascular tolerance (e.g., by pulse rate or level of exertion).
6. Identify the parameters to monitor before daily exercise (blood glucose level, ketone level, environmental temperature).
   a. Patient should not exercise if blood glucose is greater than 300 mg/dl or if there are ketones in the urine.
   b. If weather is hot, suggest exercising in an air-conditioned area, such as a shopping mall or gymnasium, or using an exercise bicycle to avoid dehydration.

See Boxes 35-10 and 35-11 on p. 1148 for the benefits and risks of exercise.

## Self-Monitoring of Metabolic Status

All individuals with diabetes should perform home blood glucose monitoring, if possible. Meters are affordable (less than $100), and most manufacturers provide discount coupons. These meters correlate well with venous samples when correct technique is used (see the Guidelines for Care Box, p. 1135). Meters are now small, with some the size of pens or credit cards. Visually read strips are not precise, and patients may "under-read" them because of the desire for a better blood glucose level. Urine glucose monitoring is imprecise and antiquated. Visually read strips and urine glucose monitoring are not a part of modern diabetes care. Urine ketone monitoring should be performed by individuals with diabetes when ill and when home blood glucose monitoring results exceed 300 mg/dl.

Although health professionals emphasize use of physiological parameters to monitor glucose status, patients continue to use symptoms as guides for self-regulation. In the presence of some chronic illnesses, even when patients are told the disease may be asymptomatic, they report that symptoms guide them. Health care providers must emphasize to patients the importance of performing a home blood glucose test to correlate a subjective symptom with an objective measure. Patients must be taught to act on objective data, not subjective data.

### *Patient teaching regarding self-monitoring*

Techniques for appropriate monitoring must be part of the teaching plan. Teaching should include knowledge about testing procedures, demonstrations, return demonstrations by patients, and information about what to do with the collected data. All patients should use a diary or log to record date, time, and monitoring results. Other diary notations may include medications, food intake, activity level, and illnesses so that the person can begin to see the relationship between blood glucose or urine ketone levels and the treatment regimen.

As patients gain flexibility and self-determination, they may manipulate insulin, diet, and exercise independently on the basis of monitoring results. Patients will progress toward more independence on the basis of ability, interest, and encouragement by caregivers.

## Managing Hypoglycemia

### *Overview*

Patients receiving insulin or sulfonylureas must be educated about hypoglycemia. Hypoglycemia is defined as a plasma blood glucose of 60 mg/dl or lower. Most hypoglycemia is mild and easily treated. Patients must know the following:

1. Causes of hypoglycemia (see Box 35-6)
2. Signs and symptoms of hypoglycemia (see Box 35-7)
3. Knowledge of appropriate treatment of hypoglycemia
4. How to obtain an identification card or Medic Alert bracelet or necklace and the importance of carrying or wearing it at all times
5. The importance of carrying a quickly absorbed glucose source
6. The importance of identifying why the hypoglycemic reaction occurred so that it can be avoided in the future

The signs and symptoms of hypoglycemia may be classified as adrenergic and neuroglycopenic (see Box 35-7). Treatment for conscious hypoglycemia is 15 g of fast-acting carbohydrate (Box 35-15).

Because hypoglycemia can occur suddenly, family members and friends should also learn the symptoms and how to handle a reaction. If a patient is awake but groggy, another person can be taught to assist with oral treatment—putting corn syrup, honey, or cake icing in the patient's mouth between the gum and cheek. This will be absorbed through the oral mucosa, and the patient will usually arouse sufficiently to take a glass of juice, milk, or sugar-sweetened coffee or tea.

Glucagon should be prescribed for all individuals with type 1 DM. Significant others should be educated in its proper

**box 35-15** *Carbohydrates (10 to 15 g) for Relief of Hypoglycemia*

½ cup pure fruit juice
6 oz. carbonated soda drink (Regular, not diet)
½ cup regular gelatin dessert, not diet
4 cubes or 2 packets of sugar
3 pieces of hard candy
3 glucose tablets

use. Prevention of hypoglycemia should be exercised by all patients. Information about hypoglycemia should be included as part of the survival skills during the initial management phase. A good time to teach about hypoglycemia is after teaching about insulin injection and self-monitoring has been completed. It is helpful to illustrate survival teaching using simulation and going through a typical day with patients, letting them guide you through all the diabetes-related activities in sequence. At this time, information about insulin reaction can be taught in relationship to time and action of insulin.

### Somogyi effect

The *Somogyi effect* is characterized by hyperglycemia after hypoglycemia. As is true with healthy persons without diabetes, the hypoglycemia in persons with diabetes stimulates the production of counterregulatory hormones (glucagon, glucocorticoids, growth hormone, epinephrine). These hormones promote glycogenolysis and gluconeogenesis. In individuals without diabetes the blood glucose level remains in the normal range because, as it minimally elevates within the normal range, insulin secretion is stimulated. In individuals with diabetes, the blood glucose rises to abnormally high levels because insulin secretion does not respond either at all or in the normal way. In some instances, the signs and symptoms of hypoglycemia are not obvious enough to be detected. In some instances, the hyperglycemia following the hypoglycemia is recognized in the early morning and may be mistaken for the *dawn phenomenon.* The assumption is made that the patient needs higher doses of insulin, but this treatment worsens the problem. Figure 35-15 illustrates this cycle.

The signs and symptoms of the Somogyi effect can be any of those normally associated with hypoglycemia, but commonly they consist only of nighttime sweats, nightmares, restless sleep, and a headache on arising (however, this can happen anytime). With both the Somogyi effect and the dawn phenomenon, there may be the presence of glycosuria, relatively normal blood glucose with positive ketones (remember that counterregulatory hormones stimulate lipolysis and $\beta$-oxidation of fats), and wide fluctuations in blood glucose unrelated to meals.

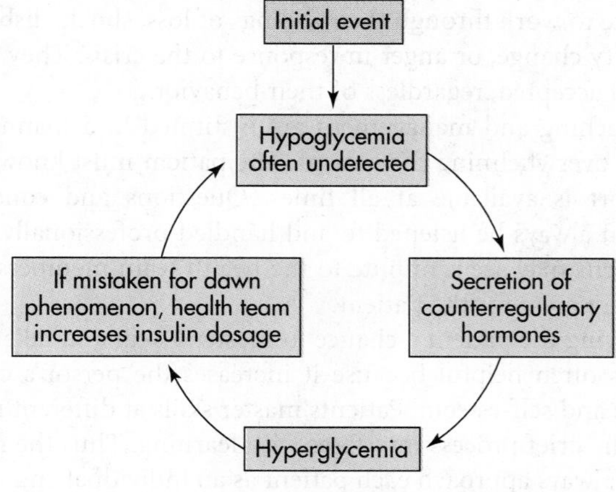


**fig. 35-15** Somogyi effect.

To differentiate the Somogyi effect from the dawn phenomenon, the patient should perform overnight home blood glucose monitoring at 2 AM and 4 AM. In the Somogyi effect, hypoglycemia will be identified and then followed by hyperglycemia. In the dawn phenomenon, there is no overnight hypoglycemia, but rather a consistent rise in blood glucose levels overnight. The Somogyi effect is treated by decreasing the dose of insulin precipitating the hypoglycemia. Treatment of the dawn phenomenon consists of increasing the dose of the insulin, which is affecting nocturnal glucose levels.

A primary nursing role is to document complaints of hypoglycemia, glucose intake, and laboratory results and to assess for complaints of night sweats, nightmares, and early-morning headaches. The nurse should also correlate these complaints and laboratory results with the meal times. Such data help identify the phenomenon.

## Providing Hygiene and Foot Care

### Hygiene

Persons with uncontrolled diabetes are at increased risk of infection. The effectiveness of the skin as a first line of defense can be diminished. Uncontrolled diabetes leads to loss of fat deposits under the skin, loss of glycogen, and catabolism of body proteins. Protein loss can hamper inflammatory response and wound healing and impair leukocyte function, migration of leukocytes to site of infection, phagocytosis, and bacterial killing, all of which are involved in combating infection. Circulatory impairments can also delay healing. The skin must be kept supple and as free of pathogenic organisms as possible. This is especially true in warm, moist areas that encourage growth of organisms (between the toes, under the breasts, and in the axillae and groin). It is extremely important that persons with diabetes carry out hygienic measures for prevention of infection daily, with special emphasis on foot care. They should seek medical attention immediately if an infection occurs.

### Foot care

Three major factors interact in foot problems in diabetes: neuropathy, ischemia, and sepsis. The need for foot care cannot be overemphasized. The patient's feet should be visually assessed at every follow-up visit (Box 35-16). Thorough assessment is required to identify patients at risk. Peripheral neuropathy must be assessed objectively by measuring sensation to pinprick, vibration, and temperature and by assessing deep tendon reflexes (see Box 35-16). Subjective sensations of paresthesias, pain, and numbness appear only after years of damage. The decreased ability to perceive a standard nylon filament pressure on the foot is a sign of advanced neuropathy with predisposition to foot ulceration.

Once protective sensory loss is determined, the risk of the patient's foot being injured can be categorized. A program

**box 35-16** *Assessment of Feet of the Person with Diabetes*

**Color:** Compare one foot with the other.
**Temperature:** Compare both feet with upper legs; assess for lines of demarcation.
**Sensory function:** Test for pinprick and vibratory sense.
**Reflexes:** Test Achilles and quadriceps tendon reflexes.
**Pulses:** Check dorsalis pedis and posterior tibial pulses (ankle-brachial indices should be performed by diabetes team).
**Lesions:** Examine for calluses, cuts, bruises, cracks, or infection.
**Self-care:** Discuss self-care regimen being used.

**table 35-13** *Risk Categories and Associated Footwear Guidelines*

| | Clinical Findings | Footwear Changes |
|---|---|---|
| Category 0 | Has protective sensation | Education on proper footwear |
| Category 1 | Has lost protective sensation | Add soft insole to shoe of proper contour and fit |
| Category 2 | Has lost protective sensation and has foot deformity | Depth footwear or custom shoe for severe deformity, molded insoles |
| Category 3 | Has lost protective sensation and has history of foot ulcer | Inspect type and condition of footwear and insoles at every visit |

From Coleman W: In Haire-Joshu D, editor: *Management of diabetes mellitus—perspectives of care across the life span,* St Louis, 1992, Mosby.

using the risk categories has been used for some years at the Hansen's Disease Center in Carville, Louisiana. The risk categories used by the team at Carville are listed in Table 35-13.

Ankle-brachial indices (ABIs) are part of clinical recommendations for assessment of vascular disease and risk.[79] A sphygmomanometer cuff of appropriate size is placed on the upper arm, above the antecubital, and using a handheld Doppler, the systolic pressure is auscultated at the radial artery. This procedure is repeated for the opposite arm. Then a cuff of appropriate size is placed on the lower leg proximal to the ankle. Using the Doppler, the systolic pressure is auscultated at both the dorsalis pedis (dorsum of foot) and the posterior tibial (medial and posterior to the malleolus). The procedure is repeated on the opposite leg. An index is calculated for each pedal site.

$$\frac{\text{Right dorsalis pedis pressure (mm Hg)}}{\text{Highest brachial pressure (mm Hg)}} = \frac{110}{180} = 0.61$$

An index greater than 1.2 is indicative of calcific disease. Calcification of blood vessels is common as a consequence of long-standing diabetes, which may be complicated by hypertension and dyslipidemia. An index below 0.9 signifies diminished blood flow and implies arterial disease. Abnormal results require a complete noninvasive lower extremity evaluation consisting of segmental pressures, pneumoplethysmography, and photoplethysmography for further assessment. The clinical importance of an ABI extends beyond the peripheral arterial tree. An isolated posterior tibial index carries a three-fold higher risk of all-cause mortality and a four-fold higher risk of coronary heart disease mortality.[28] The explanation is that when individuals with diabetes get vascular disease, it is generalized throughout the entire vascular tree. A reduced ABI is then a marker of systemic cardiovascular risk.

Each individual with diabetes is responsible for practicing preventive care on a daily basis through a thorough foot examination (see the Patient/Family Teaching Box). Podiatric consultation may be necessary for orthotics to relieve pressure areas and to treat calluses and corns. Extra-depth and custom-made shoes may be necessary and can be purchased in specialty stores. Medicare reimburses patients who meet certain foot problem criteria for a percentage of the cost of the shoes.

## Managing Concurrent Illnesses

All illnesses influence the status of diabetes control. In most instances, the person with diabetes needs increased insulin during a concurrent illness. A patient on oral agents may need an increased dosage or even temporary insulin therapy during a concurrent illness.

Unfortunately, many people mistakenly believe that if they cannot eat, they do not need to take the prescribed insulin or oral hypoglycemic agent. Patients with type 1 DM who fail to take insulin when they are sick commonly develop ketoacidosis. These persons must take carbohydrate in some form. Box 35-13 on p. 1153 presents data that patients must be taught related to managing concurrent illnesses.

## Assisting with Psychological Adjustment

Adjustment to a chronic illness such as diabetes is ongoing. The degree to which persons with diabetes mellitus adjust, as evidenced by taking control of the disease management, often depends on how well they adapt emotionally to their diagnosis.[61]

Helping the person begin to cope with chronic illness may be one of the first nursing care priorities. Patients must have a chance to work through their feelings of loss, shock, disbelief, identity change, or anger in response to the crisis. They need to feel accepted, regardless of their behavior.

Teaching and management are instituted in a manner to avoid overwhelming the patient. The patient must know that support is available at all times. Questions and concerns should always be listened to and handled professionally. The concerns may seem minute to the health team members, but they are great for the patient.

Giving the patient a chance to master a skill and take control is often helpful because it increases the person's confidence and self-esteem. Patients master skills at different rates, and the grief process interferes with learning. Thus the nurse must always approach each patient as an individual and move at the patient's pace. Because patients are not hospitalized as

**patient/family teaching**

### Foot Care for the Person with Diabetes

1. *Never* soak feet.
2. Wash feet daily and dry them well, paying attention to area between toes
3. Inspect feet daily. Look for the following:
   a. Color changes
   b. Swelling
   c. Cuts
   d. Cracks in the skin
   e. Redness
   f. Blisters
   g. Temperature changes
4. Never walk barefoot. Always wear shoes or slippers
5. Wear well-fitting shoes and clean socks.
6. After bathing, when toenails are soft, cut nails straight across. Do not cut into the corners. File edges smooth with an emery board. If you have visual problems, have someone else cut toenails for you.
7. If feet are dry, apply lotion or cream; do not put lotion between the toes.
8. Do not perform "bathroom surgery."
9. Do not self-treat corns, calluses, warts, or ingrown toenails. Consult a podiatrist.
10. Bath water should be no warmer than 90° F. Test water temperature on your inner forearm, just as you would a baby's bottle, before immersing hands or feet.
11. Do not use heating pads or hot water bottles.
12. Enhance your circulation by
    a. Not smoking
    b. Avoiding crossing legs when sitting
    c. Protecting your hands and feet when exposed to cold
    d. Avoiding tight elastic on socks
    e. Exercising
    f. Using sun screen
13. **Any foot problem is a medical emergency.** Consult your primary care provider, podiatrist, or diabetes team immediately if any foot problem arises. Delay in seeking care can cost you your feet.

long as they used to be, the community health nurse is often involved and must be informed before discharge regarding how well the patient is coping.

Family members and friends are included, as appropriate, to give them a better perspective of what the patient is dealing with. Local chapters of the American Diabetes Association and the Juvenile Diabetes Association sponsor support groups in some communities. Patients and families may find these groups helpful, both initially and over time.

As patients deal with chronic illness, they may deviate from parts of their regimens as a means of testing importance, either because of the effect on their lifestyle or because they do not know if the regimen is really necessary. If this behavior occurs, the nurse must show understanding and then help the patient get back on target with the therapeutic regimen. Health care team members should never be judgmental.

The behavior must be accepted without value judgment, and the cause of the deviation must be identified. The nurse must not assume that knowledge deficit is the cause of nonadherence; adherence to the diabetic regimen requires a large investment of the patient's energy and time, which may be difficult to do every day. The patient needs support to return to the regimen.

Depression commonly occurs with any chronic illness. Prevalence rates in individuals with diabetes may be as high as 32%.[43] The contributions of a behavioral psychologist or psychiatric clinical nurse specialist are important to assist in the many psychosocial aspects of diabetes mellitus.

Ultimately, patients are the final decision makers about self-care. The health team provides the teaching, the support, the guidance, and the counseling, but the patient makes the final decisions.

### Follow-up

Follow-up of patient teaching is usually accomplished in a clinic, physician's or nurse's office, or ambulatory education program and must be continuous, lifelong, and meet the identified patient needs. It is often incorporated into routine return visits for assessment of disease control and thus can be forgotten or missed when time is limited. The nurse responsible for this follow-up should identify the goals for each visit ahead of time so time is used effectively and the patient's teaching needs are met. Because of shortened hospital stays and because of the complexity of skills the patient with diabetes mellitus must master, outpatient follow-up is critical.

### Teaching Materials for Patient Education

The teaching needs described in the preceding sections are summarized in Box 35-14. In addition to planning and implementing an individualized teaching plan, the professional nurse is responsible for developing materials that can be used to complement or supplement any verbal exchanges. Written instructions should be provided for all parts of the diabetic education program so that the patient has a resource to consult at home. Culture-sensitive literature augments teaching.

The teaching materials available from the hospital's diabetes center, pharmaceutical companies, private clinics, various diabetes education programs, and local chapters of the American Diabetes Association are designed for the "typical" person; they must be evaluated for usefulness for a particular person. Streiff[106] found, from an evaluation of various printed materials for diabetic education, that a high school reading level was required; an evaluation of 106 adults revealed an average reading level of less than seventh grade (6.8). The patient's reading abilities must therefore be part of the initial assessment. Information about reading level and targeted population should be included when developing new materials.

### Economic Issues Related to Diabetes

Diabetes mellitus is an expensive disease for the patient and for society. Even the well-controlled person with stable diabetes and no complications will be affected by economics. The cost of the medications, syringes, and self-monitoring equipment alone may be prohibitive. Nurses need to be aware of this and economize wherever possible.

Another economic issue that nurses must be aware of is health insurance coverage. Many persons with diabetes do not have adequate coverage, because (1) the cost of private insurance may be prohibitive and (2) some companies will not insure people with diabetes. Also, many large companies are self-insured; they use their own funds to pay claims. Self-insurance is exempt from many of the laws regulating insurance companies, which could have a severe effect on the person with diabetes.[95] Prepaid capitation plans also have rules that may not adequately support the needs of persons with chronic illnesses. Therefore, even if a person is part of a group plan, the plan may be inadequate.

Nurses should either refer patients with diabetes to social workers or help them obtain information needed to evaluate insurance plans that may be available to them. Questions that patients need to ask include the following:

1. Is diabetes education covered?
2. Are routine visits to diabetes specialist, podiatrist, dietitian, and ophthalmologist covered?
3. Does the insurance cover glucose meters or external infusion pumps?
4. Will the cost of blood glucose test strips be covered?
5. Are syringes, alcohol pads, insulin, or oral hypoglycemic agents covered?
6. Is special footwear covered?
7. Are procedures and medications for complications covered?

Nurses will indirectly help patients with the economic issues related to insurance through patient education. However, nurses should also work on a societal level to promote adequate reimbursement (particularly for diabetes education) and to promote formation of "pooled-risk plans" as insurance alternatives.

The patient with diabetes also may have trouble obtaining other types of insurance, such as disability and life. Often the premiums can be prohibitive.

A third economic issue affected by diabetes is employment. Persons with diabetes may not qualify for some jobs because of poor vision or presence of peripheral vascular disease, which would interfere with walking, but they may also face discrimination. Problem areas include (1) the armed forces (diabetes makes the person ineligible; if onset occurs after acceptance, it may result in termination) and (2) law enforcement agencies, including the FBI. In regard to employment, both health care personnel and patients need to be familiar with the Americans with Disabilities Act.

Employment may also be limited because of inability to obtain necessary licenses. Individual drivers' licenses are not automatically withheld because of diabetes, but most states require a physician's statement to confirm the person's ability to drive safely, and the state can place restrictions on driving despite the physician's recommendation. The few studies that have been conducted do not support a major increase in motor vehicle accidents among people with diabetes.[96]

Persons who have type 1 DM or type 2 DM and are receiving insulin are prohibited from driving a commercial motor vehicle in interstate or foreign commerce.[96] Also, people who are being treated with medications for diabetes are, at present, prohibited from obtaining licenses to fly noncommercial airplanes. These restrictions may prevent persons from reporting their medications or cause them to avoid insulin, regardless of their clinical state. Saudek and Segal-Polin[96] reported no knowledge of restrictions on obtaining retail or professional licenses. The terms *prediabetes* and *chemical diabetes* should not be used; they are not diagnoses but can cause problems for patients.

### Patient Education

Joslin summarized the critical importance of patient education: "There is no disease in which an understanding by the patient of the methods of treatment avails as much."[54] Joslin told his patients, "therefore face the facts, accept the situation, study the disease, and become master of your fate"[54] (see the Research Box).

National and international Standards of Care for diabetes management and education have been published. Ideally, patient education is integrated with traditional medical care of patients with diabetes.[39] The American Diabetes Association and the American Association of Diabetes Educators (AADE) have worked closely over the past decade to improve the quality of diabetes education and management. The AADE and its certifying body, the National Certification Board for Diabetes Educators, are responsible for the certification of health care professionals as CDEs. These experts, primarily registered nurses and dietitians, practice in a variety of settings—private

**research**

Reference: Coonrod BA, Betschart J, Harris MI: Frequency and determinants of diabetes patient education among adults in the U.S. population, *Diabetes Care* 17(8):852, 1994.

The authors surveyed 2405 individuals at least 18 years of age with diabetes regarding attendance at a diabetes education class or program since diagnosis. Only 35.1% had ever attended such a class or program. Of individuals with insulin-dependent diabetes, 58.6% had done so; the percentages were 48.9% of insulin-treated individuals with non–insulin-dependent diabetes and 23.7% of non–insulin-treated individuals with non–insulin-dependent diabetes. Positive associations with diabetes education in individuals with non–insulin-dependent diabetes, regardless of insulin administration, were younger age, black race, residence in the midwestern United States, higher educational level, and presence of diabetes complications. Positive associations with diabetes education in non–insulin-treated individuals with non–insulin-dependent diabetes were increasing income, living alone, and not having a diabetes physician or not visiting one in the last year. Despite the fact that patient education has been recognized for its contribution to the reduction in morbidity and mortality of diabetes, many individuals, especially those with non–insulin-dependent diabetes, still do not receive such education.

practices, with physicians, and in hospitals—and are an excellent source for diabetes education. Local chapters of AADE are present in many major U.S. cities. To locate the nearest chapter call 1-800-TEAM-UP-4. The ADA has an accreditation process for diabetes education programs. Additionally, some states have similar accreditation programs.[2,4,108]

The use of CDEs and accredited programs is ideal, because they are formalized to address predefined areas of education (Box 35-17). However, nurses often find themselves in situations in which neither are present and in which they themselves are directly responsible for some or all of the diabetes education. Refer to Box 35-14 for details.

## Health Promotion/Prevention

Preventive health care for diabetes mellitus may be primary (prevention of the primary disease), secondary (early detection and control of the disease), or tertiary (control of complications).

*Healthy People 2000*[118] is a report of the U.S. Public Health Services that identifies goals for health care for the year 2000. These goals as related to diabetes are listed in the following preventive stages.

### Primary prevention

**Type 1 DM.** Primary prevention of type 1 DM is under active research in both basic science and clinical care. All type 1 DM prevention programs are experimental. Given that signs of autoimmunity can be detected for up to 10 years before the development of overt type 1 DM, studies look toward arresting the autoimmune process. Use of immunosuppressive agents such as cyclosporine, azathioprine, and niacinamide have been attempted with some encouraging results, but toxicity remains a concern. Research now focuses on the concept of islet cell rest using prophylactic insulin in individuals without overt type 1 DM, but who have positive islet cell antibodies. The underlying premise is that if an endocrine organ is "rested" by exogenous administration of the hormone, the autoimmune process can be halted. Pilot studies have been successful, and a nationwide clinical trial is now ongoing.

**Type 2 DM.** Primary prevention of type 2 DM takes on a very different focus. Obesity is a significant risk factor for type 2 DM. Abdominal or android obesity is characterized by the apple shape. Individuals with abdominal obesity have a high waist-hip ratio (>1.0). This ratio is calculated by measuring the circumference of the waist and dividing it by the measure of the circumference of the hips. In gynecoid or pear-shaped obesity, the weight distribution favors the hips, with a waist-hip ratio less than 1.0. Individuals with abdominal obesity are hyperinsulinemic and are at increased risk not only for type 2 DM, but for all components of syndrome X, as previously described.[89-91,121]

Primary prevention of type 2 DM involves identification and modification of risk factors (see the Risk Factors Box). Primary prevention should be directed toward lifestyle changes that include exercise, weight loss or weight control, and knowledge of risk factors. It is important that persons with diabetes be made aware of the familial tendencies and risks for siblings of the individual with either type of diabetes and that they be discussed (Table 35-14).[18,118,119] Current clinical trials are underway to look at halting the progression of IGT patients to overt DM with the oral agents troglitazone and metformin. The pilot studies have yielded promising results.

### Healthy People 2000

The surgeon general's report *Healthy People 2000*[119] established several goals that give the previously discussed primary prevention recommendations more momentum. One goal is to reduce overweight prevalence to not more than 20% among people aged 20 or older (baseline: 26% for people ages 20 through 74 in 1976-1980, 24% for men and 27% for women). For people aged 20 years and older, overweight is defined as body mass index (BMI) equal to or greater than 25. The BMI is calculated by dividing weight in kilograms by the square of height in meters. Another goal from *Healthy People 2000* that has relevance for prevention of type 2 DM pertains to exercise. The goal is to increase to at least 30% the proportion of people ages 6 years and older who engage regularly, preferably daily, in light to moderate physical activity for at least 30 minutes per day (baseline: 22% of people ages 18 and older were active for at least 30 minutes five or more times per week, and 12% were active seven or more times per week in 1985). Light to moderate physical activity requires sustained, rhythmic muscular movements; is at least equivalent to sustained walking; and is performed at less than 60% of maximal heart rate for age. Maximal heart rate equals about 220 beats per minute minus age. Examples of light to moderate physical activity include walking, swimming, cycling, dancing, gardening and yard work, various domestic and occupational activities, and games and other childhood pursuits.

The urgency of primary prevention is blatant when looking at the objective from *Healthy People 2000* to reduce diabetes-related deaths to no more than 34 per 100,000 people (age-adjusted baseline: 38 per 100,000 in 1986). Target populations for this goal are African Americans, Native Americans (including Alaskan Natives), Mexican Americans, and Puerto Ricans.[119] Cardiovascular disease is the leading cause of death among people with diabetes, accounting for more than half of all deaths. Health behaviors aimed at modifying the risk of cardiovascular disease by reducing cardiovascular

**risk factors**

**Type 2 Diabetes Mellitus**

Family history of diabetes
Obesity
Race (Native American, Hispanic, or African American)
Age
Previously identified IGT
Hypertension or hyperlipidemia
History of GDM or delivery of babies >9 pounds
Reactive hypoglycemia

**box 35-17** *Fifteen Content Areas of Diabetes Education*

1. *Overview of diabetes mellitus*
   - Definition of diabetes mellitus
   - Effects of alterations in metabolism of carbohydrates, proteins, and fats
   - Classification of diabetes (type 1, type 2, gestational, etc.)
2. *Stress and psychological adjustment*
   - Grieving and adaptation to living with a chronic disease
   - Expressing feelings openly
   - Unrealistic expectations
   - Effect of stress on metabolic control
   - Recognizing the need for professional help
   - Stress management
3. *Family involvement and social support*
   - Diabetes as a family challenge
   - Learning to recognize and work with adverse family dynamics
   - Need for support
4. *Nutrition*
   - Individualized meal plan to control weight, glucose, and lipids
   - Composition of the diet
   - Achieving and maintaining desired body weight and glucose control
   - Advice on alcohol use
   - Eating on special occasions
   - Reading and interpreting nutrition labels
5. *Exercise and activity*
   - Benefits/risks
   - Effects of exercise on therapeutic plan
   - Preparing for exercise (food and medication; companion)
   - Heart rate monitoring
   - Monitoring necessary before starting exercise
   - Monitoring necessary when establishing an exercise program
6. *Medications*
   - Goals of treatment
   - Oral agents
     - Action on blood glucose
     - Side effects
     - Drug interactions
   - Insulin
     - Action on blood glucose
     - Cautions (especially Somogyi effect)
     - Strengths/purities
     - Injection techniques
     - Complications of treatment: hypoglycemia, antibodies, lipodystrophy
   - Glucagon
     - How to buy, store, and use
7. *Monitoring and use of results*
   - Goals
   - Types of blood glucose monitoring available
   - Quality control of monitors
   - How to use blood glucose monitoring to achieve and maintain good glucose control: performing tests accurately, interpreting test results, frequency of testing, taking action appropriate to test results
   - Urine ketone testing
   - Glycosylated hemoglobin test: how to relate to average blood glucose level
8. *Relationships among nutrition, exercise, medication, and blood glucose levels*
   - Balancing nutrition, exercise, and medications
   - Adjusting each factor in relation to the others
   - Adjusting times of monitoring
   - Identify times for snacks
   - Effects of exercise on blood glucose
9. *Acute complications: hyperglycemia and hypoglycemia*
   - Definition of hyperglycemia and hypoglycemia
   - Prevention of each
   - Early recognition/treatment/record keeping
   - Hypoglycemia unawareness
   - Dawn phenomenon and Somogyi effect
   - What to do for diabetic ketoacidosis/hyperosmolar coma
   - Effects of illness on diabetes
   - Monitoring glucose/ketones
   - Sick day guidelines (including diet)
10. *Chronic complications: prevention, detection, and treatment*
    - Kinds of complications—microvascular and macrovascular, neuropathy
    - Examples of each kind of complication (especially those likely to occur in your population)
    - Possible causes of complication
    - Self-care for prevention or delay of complications
    - Coping strategies (support groups, counseling, stress management)
11. *Foot, skin, and dental care*
    - Daily self-care measures
    - Relationship of problems to diabetes care
    - The need for regular evaluation of feet and teeth
12. *Behavioral change strategies, goal setting, risk factor reduction, and problem solving*
    - Changing behaviors through goal setting
    - Rights of patient
    - Responsibility of patient
    - Patient-professional partnership in planning care
    - Taking care of self when sick
13. *Benefits, risks, and management options for improving glucose control*
    - DCCT results
    - Therapeutic care plans—maps to good health and quality of life
14. *Preconception care, pregnancy, and gestational diabetes*
15. *Use of health care systems and community resources*
    - Planned follow-up
    - Patient's responsibility
    - Names and telephone numbers of health care team members
    - Emergency care
    - Community resources
    - Planning for travel
    - Educational resources and need for continuing education
    - Insurance and employment regulations and reimbursement

With permission from American Diabetes Association: *Goals for diabetes education, clinical education program,* ed 2, Alexandria, Va; Task force to revise the national standards: National standards for diabetes self-management education programs, *Diabetes Care* 18(1):141, 1995.

**table 35-14** *Estimated Risk of Developing Diabetes Mellitus*

| Relationship to Person with Diabetes | Approximate Rate of Developing Diabetes |
|---|---|
| No diabetes in family | Type 1: 0.3% |
| Identical twin with type 1 | Type 1: 36% |
| One parent with type 1 | Type 1: 3% |
| Sibling with type 1 | Type 1: 3% |
| No diabetes in family | Type 2: 14% |
| Identical twin with type 2 | Type 2: almost 100% |
| One parent with type 2 | Type 2: 20-30% |
| Both parents with type 2 | Type 2: 35-55% |

Data from Bode BW et al: *DiabetesDek—how to control and manage diabetes mellitus,* Atlanta, 1992, Lifescan Infodek.

disease risk factors could have a major effect on morbidity and mortality from diabetes mellitus.

### *Secondary prevention*

**Type 1 DM.** Screening for type 1 DM is not recommended. From 85% to 90% of individuals with type 1 DM have autoantibodies at the time of initial fasting hyperglycemia. The presence of the autoantibodies before diagnosis identifies individuals at risk. First, the cutoff values for immune markers are not well established in the clinical setting outside of research trials. Second, there is no general consensus about the treatment if these antibodies are detected. Third, the incidence of type 1 DM is low, so routine testing of healthy children will identify only a small subset of "prediabetic" children. The cost-effectiveness, then, of screening for type 1 DM is low. The American Diabetes Association does not recommend screening for type 1 DM in either the general population or in higher-risk individuals (siblings of type 1 DM individuals) until clinical trials demonstrate the efficacy and safety of treatments to prevent or delay type 1 DM.[6]

**Type 2 DM.** On the other hand, the prevalence of undiagnosed type 2 DM is high, with as many as 8 million individuals in the United States undiagnosed. Individuals with components of syndrome X are in the high-risk group. Box 35-18 outlines The American Diabetes Association recommendations for screening for the presence of undiagnosed type 2 DM.[6]

### *Tertiary prevention*

Tertiary prevention is the major focus of diabetes management. Both chronic and acute complications occur often, and nurses who work with persons who have diabetes must be involved in tertiary prevention if complications are decreased. Another national goal for the year 2000 is to reduce the most severe complications of diabetes, as shown in Table 35-15. *Healthy People 2000* goals include reducing complications among people with diabetes as follows: end-stage renal disease, blindness, lower extremity amputation, perinatal mortality, and major congenital malformations.[119] Target populations are African Americans and Native Americans (including Alaskan Natives). The major emphasis of tertiary preventive education

**box 35-18** *Screening for Diabetes in Asymptomatic Individuals*

Screening for DM may be done via oral glucose tolerance test (OGTT) or with a fasting plasma glucose (FPG). In clinical settings, the FPG is preferred because of ease of testing, patient acceptance, convenience, and lower cost.

Screening for DM should be considered in any individual ≥45 years of age. If normal, screening should be repeated every 3 years.

Screening for DM should be considered at a younger age or be carried out more frequently in individuals who

- Have a first-degree relative with DM
- Are obese
  - Weight ≥120% of desirable body weight or
  - Body mass index (BMI) >25—Weight (kg) ÷ Height (meters squared)
- Belong to a high-risk DM ethnic population (Hispanic, Native American, African American)
- Are women with previously diagnosed GDM or those who have delivered a baby ≥9 lb
- Have hypertension
- Have a triglyceride level ≥200 mg/dl or an HDL cholesterol ≤35 mg/dl
- On previous testing have had impaired glucose tolerance (IGT) or impaired fasting glucose (IFG)

Adapted from American Diabetes Association, Expert Committee on the Diagnosis and Classification of Diabetes Mellitus: Report of the Expert Committee on the Diagnosis and Classification of Diabetes Mellitus, *Diabetes Care* 20(7):1183, 1997.

will be on the ability of nurses to counsel the patient about the early detection and interventions listed in Table 35-15.

The importance of patient education is clear, and the need for its availability was outlined in one of the goals of *Healthy People 2000.*[119] The goal is to increase to at least 40% the proportion of people with chronic and disabling conditions who receive formal patient education, including information about community and self-help resources, as an integral part of the management of their condition. (The specific target for the year 2000 for patient education of people with diabetes is 75%; the 1983-1984 baseline was 32% [classes] and 68% [counseling].) Target populations are African American and Hispanic persons with diabetes.[119]

## EVALUATION

To evaluate the effectiveness of nursing interventions, compare patient behaviors with those stated in the expected patient outcomes. Successful achievement of patient outcomes for the patient with diabetes is indicated by:

1. Fluid balance is improved:
   a. Weight has increased or decreased at about 2 pounds per week toward normal.
   b. Urination has returned to normal, and skin turgor shows no tenting.
   c. Blood pressure and pulse are normal and show no orthostatic changes.

**table 35-15** *Prevention of Long-Term Complications of Diabetes Mellitus*

| Complications | Early Detection | Early Intervention |
|---|---|---|
| Retinopathy | Dilated funduscopic examination | Care by an ophthalmologist or retinal specialist<br>Control of hyperglycemia<br>Control of hypertension |
| Nephropathy | Examination of urine for albumin or protein excretion<br>Measurement of serum creatinine and creatinine clearance | Control of hyperglycemia<br>Control of hypertension and other cardiovascular risk factors<br>Limiting protein intake<br>Avoiding nephrotoxic agents |
| Atherosclerosis | History of risk factors and symptoms<br>Examination: electrocardiogram and serum lipids measurements, peripheral pulses | Control of hyperglycemia<br>Control of hypertension<br>Weight control<br>Exercise<br>Control of lipids |
| Neuropathy | History of symptoms of pain, numbness, etc.<br>Examination: orthostatic blood pressures, muscle strength, reflexes, and sensory function | Control of hyperglycemia<br>Avoidance of neurotoxic agents<br>Education about the importance of routine evaluation, foot care, and specific treatment of neuropathy |
| Foot problems | History of symptoms of numbness, infection, and peripheral vascular insufficiency<br>Complete foot examination<br>Ankle-brachial indices | Control of hyperglycemia<br>Control of atherogenic risk<br>Education about the importance and methods of foot care<br>Referral to a podiatrist<br>Referral for orthotics/custom shoes |

Data from Herman W: *The prevention and treatment of complications of diabetes: a guide for primary care practitioners,* Atlanta, 1990, 6-1 to 6-4, US Department of Health and Human Services, Centers for Disease Control and Prevention.

   d. Sodium and chloride levels are normal, as well as hematocrit.

   The patient:

   a. Has an intake of fluid of about 2.5 liters.
   b. Describes correctly how to prevent dehydration.

2. Fatigue is improved:
   a. States that no fatigue is present.
   b. Demonstrates how to perform glucose monitoring correctly.
3. Risk for infection is decreased:
   a. States importance of checking glucose on regular basis.
   b. Correctly describes how infections affect blood glucose.
   c. Correctly lists signs and symptoms of infection.
4. Signs of nutritional adequacy are present:
   a. Maintains weight changes as listed previously.
   b. Has a glycosylated hemoglobin measurement that has decreased and serum lipid levels that have decreased.
   c. Appropriately describes food type, amount, and distribution.
5. Fear is decreased:
   a. States that fear is lessened.
   b. Explains way to obtain vocational rehabilitation.
6. An adequate level of knowledge is evidenced:
   a. Correctly describes the disease process of diabetes.
   b. Correctly demonstrates how to inject insulin and rotate sites.
   c. Correctly defines hypoglycemia.
   d. Correctly describes signs, symptoms, and treatment of hypoglycemia.
   e. Correctly describes dosage, time, and effects of oral hypoglycemic agents.
   f. Correctly describes exercise plan and safety precautions.

## NURSING MANAGEMENT OF THE PATIENT WITH DIABETES WHO IS UNDERGOING SURGERY

Most nurses working in acute care settings will provide care to the individual with diabetes who is undergoing surgery. Understanding patient concerns and the metabolic consequences of surgery will facilitate patient recovery.

In many instances, the greatest fear of the individual with diabetes who is admitted to the hospital is not the admitting medical problem, but the fear that his or her diabetes regimen and control will be tampered with and will deteriorate. This is a valid concern. Unfortunately, the diabetes team is not usually consulted for perioperative care. The admitting team or surgical team places the individual on sliding scale insulin on the grounds of uncertainty of oral intake. The truth, however, is that many of these health care providers are afraid of individuals with diabetes: afraid of euglycemia and the potential for hypoglycemia because of lack of knowledge. They would rather have the patient in the hyperglycemic range to decrease their personal anxiety. As previously discussed, placing any individual with diabetes on sliding scale insulin is the worst possible example for the patient, and as always, defies the pathophysiology of diabetes. Hyperglycemia will result; the patient will be labeled as "brittle." Nosocomial diabetic ketoacidosis (DKA) can be precipitated.[116] The consequences of hyperglycemia delay the recovery process and can, in fact, result in complications. Hyperglycemia is a poor metabolic state for recovery. Hyperglycemia, not the presence of diabetes, impairs leukocyte response to illness and thus impairs wound healing. Hyperglycemia is a hypercoagulable state and promotes thrombosis. As a member of the health care team, the professional nurse is in an ideal position to suggest consulting the patient's diabetes team to optimize the patient's recovery.

The perioperative management of the individual with diabetes may be complicated by antecedent suboptimal diabetes control and by the presence of preexisting complications such as hypertension, diabetic nephropathy, autonomic neuropathy, coronary artery disease, and systemic atherosclerosis.[125] Counterregulatory hormones increase during anesthesia, surgery, and recovery and result in hyperglycemia. Additionally, certain nonsurgical medical crises, such as congestive heart failure, result in an increase in counterregulatory hormones.

### Effects of Surgery on Metabolic Control of Diabetes

The person with diabetes mellitus faces the risk of developing hypoglycemia or hyperglycemia during the perioperative period. During the perioperative period, persons are not usually given anything by mouth and are given intravenous (IV) fluids. This decreases total carbohydrate intake and also decreases insulin needs; however, the effects of surgery on counterregulatory hormones usually increase the need for insulin. The stressors of surgery cause the release of glucocorticoids and catecholamines, which elevate blood glucose.

There are many ways to manage the person with diabetes during periods of fasting. To minimize the disruption in metabolic control, the person should be thoroughly regulated before surgery, and the surgery should be scheduled for early morning to minimize variations from normal control measures. Persons with diabetes are kept on their usual food, fluid, and medication routines until the night before surgery if possible.

### Management of Glucose Control During Surgery in Persons Treated with Insulin

Various protocols may be used to maintain glucose control in the person receiving insulin. Neither hyperglycemia nor hypoglycemia should be allowed to occur. One of the most commonly used perioperative protocols is starting an IV infusion of dextrose the morning of surgery and giving one half the usual insulin dose subcutaneously as intermediate-acting insulin. This insulin will cover hepatic glucose production during the intraoperative period and prevent hyperglycemia. If the surgery is long, blood glucose levels should be checked during surgery; insulin or extra glucose can be given as needed.

During the postoperative period, the person is maintained by IV glucose infusion until food can be taken. Insulin is given either by dividing the normal daily dose equally over a 24-hour period and giving it subcutaneously or by having a separate IV infusion of insulin fluids. If the person is receiving a standard dose of insulin, extra insulin may be administered via an algorithm based on finger-stick blood glucose checks every 4 to 6 hours. Inappropriately, some patients may receive no daily insulin dose and instead are given insulin based on the amount of blood glucose. This mode, a sliding scale, is unphysiological and antiquated, commonly results in hyperglycemia (even DKA), and should not be used.[116]

### Management of Glucose Control During Surgery in Persons Not Normally Receiving Insulin

Persons with diabetes who are not normally managed with insulin will receive an IV infusion of dextrose on the morning of surgery, after fasting during the night. Such patients may be able to meet their usual insulin needs with their endogenous insulin supply, but in times of stress they may require exogenous insulin. As mentioned earlier, patients with type 2 DM who are treated with metformin should have the drug discontinued 48 to 72 hours before elective surgery that may require general anesthesia. After surgery, blood glucose and urine ketone levels are checked every 4 to 6 hours; if hyperglycemia is present, exogenous insulin may need to be given.

### Management during Surgery of Persons Unable to Eat Prescribed Diet

All persons with diabetes, whether or not they are treated with insulin, should receive 125 to 250 g of carbohydrates per day until their normal diet is resumed. Fewer carbohydrates than this may result in starvation ketosis. The patient's normal diabetes regimen should be reinstituted as soon as possible. Blood glucose and urine ketone levels should be monitored frequently, even after the patient's usual diet and medication are resumed. The increase in catabolism because of the surgery will remain for some time, and additional insulin may still be needed. By the time patients are discharged, they should be back on their normal regimens. Other postoperative care measures are similar to those for all surgery patients. Initiation of these measures should prevent complications.

## GERONTOLOGICAL CONSIDERATIONS

The prevalence of diabetes mellitus increases with age because insulin resistance increases with advancing age. Diabetes mellitus prevalence estimates in individuals over 80 years of age are as high as 40%. An estimated 43% of all diabetic patients are in the geriatric age-group, rendering diabetes a major clinical problem. Accurate diagnosis of diabetes is a problem. Approximately 9.6% of the geriatric population has diagnosed DM, and an estimated near-equal percentage have undiagnosed DM. Furthermore, when one factors in the number of patients with IGT, the prevalence of abnormal glucose tolerance (IGT and DM) rises to 40% of the geriatric population. In elderly patients with hypertension and without diagnosed DM, 43.2% of patients had IGT and 11.6% had undiagnosed DM.[53] Even in this age-group, 10% of individuals with new-onset diabetes will have true type 1 DM requiring physiological insulin replacement. Even allowing for this latter fact, insulin resistance is very prevalent in the geriatric population, especially when one includes patients who have normal glucose tolerance because of compensatory hyperinsulinemia.

The etiology of geriatric insulin resistance is complex and may include genetic factors, obesity (increase in the ratio of fat body mass to lean body mass),[37,93] physical inactivity,[71] renal insufficiency, infections or illness, medications (corticosteroids, thiazide diuretics), and perhaps nutritional factors (increase in carbohydrate intake).[22] Insulin resistance at the cellular level may be due to decreased receptor number (accelerated degradation of receptors vs. recycling of receptors), molecular alterations affecting insulin binding to the receptor, and postreceptor defects.[37,93]

Worsening insulin resistance is not an inevitable consequence of aging and may be prevented by physical fitness,[113] control of obesity, good nutritional habits, and avoidance of medications that exacerbate insulin resistance (thiazide diuretics, beta blockers, corticosteroids). Clearly, lifestyle changes need to be made before the geriatric years as the primary preventive strategy. However, improvements are clearly attainable in later life, even in individuals who have developed overt diabetes.

Special considerations must be used when approaching the elderly patient (Box 35-19). Therapeutic principles need to be tailored to the elderly patient (Box 35-20).[109]

It is critical to note that diabetes may antedate a patient's advancement to the geriatric years or a patient may be diagnosed *de novo* in the geriatric years. Devastating diabetic complications plague these patients, such that early, accurate diagnosis and treatment are mandatory.[67] Unfortunately, because of the insidious onset of type 2 DM, the initial diabetes presentation in an elderly individual is often painful diabetic neuropathy or other diabetic complications without prior documentation of hyperglycemia.[15,44,73] The evidence to date supports glycemic control in the elderly to reduce the risk of chronic complications of DM.

## SPECIAL ENVIRONMENTS FOR CARE

### Critical Care Management

Patients experiencing hyperglycemic hyperosmolar nonketotic coma or severe diabetic ketoacidosis may need to be managed in a critical care environment. Both of these conditions are discussed in the following sections.

### Home Care Management

Given the current short hospital lengths of stay, short-term home care may be necessary for learning diabetes care survival skills, such as in the patient with severe visual impairment. Home care should not be used as a frank alternative to the professional nurse providing education within the hospital setting. The individual with diabetes should be immediately referred to the diabetes team for outpatient follow-up. Once diabetes survival skills have been mastered, the need for home care for diabetes is no longer present. Home care should not be used as an alternative to outpatient follow-up with the diabetes team. The individual with diabetes may require home care services for issues not pertaining to diabetes control, such as a nonhealing foot ulcer. The ultimate goal is to help the individual with diabetes maintain as much independence as possible while optimizing metabolic control and quality of life.

## COMPLICATIONS

The complications of DM are classified as acute and chronic. Acute complications include hypoglycemia, DKA, and hyperglycemic hyperosmolar nonketotic coma (HHNC). Information on hypoglycemia in individuals with DM was presented earlier in the chapter.

### Acute Complications

#### Diabetic ketoacidosis

*Diabetic ketoacidosis* is the extreme consequence of severe insulin deficiency at the insulin-sensitive tissues: adipose tissue, skeletal muscle, and liver (see Figure 36-3). Diabetic ketoacidosis can be precipitated by illness or omission of insulin. Insulin omission by the patient is a compliance issue; insulin omission by the health care team is inexcusable. Lack

**box 35-19** *Special Considerations for the Elderly Patient with Diabetes*

1. Accuracy of diagnosis
2. Accuracy of classification of diabetes; C-peptide level needed
3. Mental status; presence of depression or dementia
4. Visual acuity
5. Fine motor skills
6. Social support systems
7. Diabetes knowledge and education potential
8. Blood glucose monitoring: patient, family, friend
9. Diet and meal planning: may have poor or variable intake or compulsive overeating
10. Activity level: inactivity leads to weight gain and decreased insulin sensitivity
11. Increasing ratio of fat to lean body mass
12. Diabetic complications
13. Concurrent illnesses
14. Concurrent pharmacotherapy
15. Increased risk of adverse drug reaction

**box 35-20** *Therapeutic Principles in the Elderly Patient with Diabetes*

1. Set realistic goals for glycemic control in the context of age, general condition, and diabetic complications.
2. True type 1 DM patients should be treated with intensive therapy, i.e., multiple daily insulin injections and carbohydrate-consistent meal plan.
3. Avoid unnecessary insulin therapy.
4. Review potential for diet therapy with patient and family. A 5% to 10% weight reduction may be highly significant.
5. Increase physical activity safely whenever possible.
6. Use antihyperglycemic agents such as metformin, troglitazone, or acarbose if not contraindicated.
7. Use lower doses of sulfonylureas and monitor progress carefully. Glimeperide, with its reduced risk of hypoglycemia, may provide more safety.
8. Combination therapy with oral agents and insulin may be of value with selected patients.

of insulin at the adipocyte results in failure to suppress lipolysis, with resultant release of free fatty acids (FFAs) into the circulation and weight loss. The FFAs in turn serve as a substrate for the liver to synthesize triglyceride and ketone bodies. Lack of insulin at skeletal muscle results in (1) failure to take up glucose from the plasma and (2) protein catabolism with amino acid release into the circulation. These amino acids, in turn, may be used by the liver to make glucose (gluconeogenesis). Lack of insulin at the liver results in (1) glycogen breakdown to glucose (glycogenolysis) and (2) accelerated gluconeogenesis. This results in an outpouring of glucose into the circulation that cannot be used by the major consumer, skeletal muscle. Early in the course of insulin deficiency, this hyperglycemic state may be compounded by ingestion of dietary carbohydrate, which gets digested into glucose and is unable to be disposed.

Progressive hyperglycemia rapidly exceeds the renal threshold for glucose (approximately 180 mg/dl) and glycosuria results. Hyperglycemia may be as high as 1500 mg/dl. Glycosuria acts as an osmotic diuretic, resulting in dehydration, with water and electrolyte losses. An increase in thirst and oral fluid intake tends to minimize the severity of the dehydration early on; however, nausea and vomiting associated with progressive ketosis lead to rapidly worsening dehydration.

In the setting of insulin deficiency, high levels of FFAs, and high levels of counterregulatory hormones (especially glucagon), the liver will produce excessive amounts of ketone bodies. Ketone bodies are acidic and must be cleared from the circulation or buffered with alkali (bicarbonate) to prevent progressive lowering of the arterial pH and systemic acidosis. Early on, the ketones are cleared in the urine; however, with progressive dehydration and decreasing urine output, the production of ketone bodies rapidly exceeds renal clearance. Buffering with bicarbonate is another important mechanism to prevent systemic acidosis. However, this too has limited capacity, such that plasma bicarbonate levels fall, arterial pH falls, and acidosis worsens. Progressive ketosis is therefore associated with ketones in the urine, rising plasma ketones, lowering of plasma bicarbonate, and declining arterial pH. When plasma or urine ketones are measured, it is the later-appearing ketone acetoacetate that is measured, not the earlier-appearing ketone $\beta$-hydroxybutyrate. When DKA is resolving, it may falsely appear that DKA is actually worsening, as $\beta$-hydroxybutyrate is converted to acetoacetate.

Systemic acidosis is associated with transcellular shifts of ions, especially potassium, such that potassium comes out of the cells and the serum potassium value rises in the face of total body potassium depletion. Potassium depletion caused by renal losses may be compounded by gastrointestinal losses (vomiting and diarrhea).

Failure to recognize emerging and worsening DKA will result in progressive dehydration, ketosis, acidosis, circulatory collapse, tissue hypoxia, and shock. The advent of tissue hypoxia will result in lactate accumulation and superadded lactic acidosis, which dramatically decreases the rate of survival.

Treatment of DKA involves rehydration, insulin administration, and electrolyte repletion. Each medical institution will have its own protocol for DKA management. Basic principles are found in the following Guidelines for Care Box.

#### Hyperglycemic hyperosmolar nonketotic coma

Hyperglycemic hyperosmolar nonketotic coma is the acute complication of type 2 DM. The pathophysiology and clinical issues are similar to DKA, with the following exceptions. In HHNC:

1. Dehydration is profound, with fluid deficit as high as 8 to 9 L.
2. The degree of hyperglycemia is greater, with serum glucoses in the range of 600 to 2000 mg/dl.
3. The serum osmolarity is 350 mOsm/L or higher.
4. Ketosis is absent because affected individuals have adequate insulin secretion; remember, these individuals have type 2 DM.
5. An underlying central nervous system problem (e.g., underlying cerebrovascular disease) is usually present, which impairs the patient's thirst perception.
6. A concurrent illness is usually present.

Because of the aforementioned impairment in thirst perception, the patient does not have adequate oral fluid intake, resulting in the primary defect of profound dehydration. As a consequence of the profound dehydration, hemoconcentration and severe hyperglycemia occur. Polyuria disappears early because of the severe dehydration. Lethargy and somnolence may result.

Hyperglycemic hyperosmolar nonketotic coma is a medical emergency. The primary management of HHNC involves intravenous rehydration with hypotonic solutions (0.45 normal saline). Hypotonic solutions are indicated because the patient is hyperosmolar. As the patient is rehydrated, the hyperglycemia resolves. Intravenous insulin is generally not needed. Additionally, treatment of the precipitating illness is critical to patient survival, because the mortality rate approaches 70%.

### Chronic Complications

Chronic complications of diabetes are classified as microvascular (small blood vessel) and macrovascular (large blood vessel). They are a consequence of the duration and the degree of hyperglycemia. These changes result in diabetic retinopathy, diabetic nephropathy, peripheral and autonomic neuropathy, peripheral vascular disease, cerebrovascular disease, and coronary artery disease. Microvascular complications of diabetes rarely occur within the first 5 to 10 years after diagnosis of type 1 DM. They may, however, be present at the time of diagnosis with type 2 DM because of the slow, insidious onset of type 2 DM and resultant delay in diagnosis. Cigarette smoking increases the risk of the development and progression of every known complication of diabetes mellitus. Aggressive attempts at smoking cessation are critical.

#### Microvascular complications

**Diabetic retinopathy.** Diabetic retinopathy is the leading cause of new blindness among adults 20 to 74 years of age in the United States. Between 12,000 and 24,000 new cases

guidelines for care

**Diabetic Ketoacidosis: Management Principles and Priorities**

I. Monitoring
   A. Finger-stick blood glucoses q1h.
   B. Serum potassium initially and then q1h.
   C. Bicarbonate initially and q2h.
   D. Arterial blood gases initially and then q2-4h.
   E. ECG initially and prn.
   F. Additional monitoring may be needed pending patient status: continuous cardiac tracing, central venous pressure, Swan-Ganz catheter, nasogastric intubation, and indwelling urinary catheter.
   G. Intake and output.
II. IV rehydration
   A. The fluid deficit may be in excess of 6 L.
   B. Normal saline at 500 ml/hr for the first hour; then 250 ml/hr.
   C. Avoid hypotonic solutions (0.45% normal saline) because they may increase risk of cerebral edema.
III. IV insulin to control gluconeogenesis, lipolysis, and ketogenesis and to promote skeletal muscle glucose uptake
   A. Should be given as constant infusion. Start at rate of 0.1 U/kg of body weight. If no concern about IV volume (i.e., congestive heart failure) a more dilute solution is easier to titrate. Dilute as 50 ml Regular insulin in 500 ml normal saline; then 1 U = 10 ml. Titrate drip hourly by 0.1 U (1 ml) increments until glucose reaches goal of 70-150 mg/dl.
   B. IV bolus of Regular insulin has a half-life of 5 minutes and is of no value.
   C. When the patient begins to take oral fluids with carbohydrate, additional insulin must be given subcutaneously to match the carbohydrate load.
   D. When the patient is recovering and ready to eat, resume routine insulin program. Do not discontinue IV insulin infusion until 2 hours after subcutaneous insulin dosage to prevent loss of control of hepatic glucose output and disposal.
IV. Electrolyte repletion
   A. IV potassium once renal output is established:
      1. If serum $K^+$ is $\leq 3$ mEq/L, give 40-60 mEq/hr.
      2. If serum $K^+$ is 3-4 mEq/L, give 30 mEq/hr.
      3. If serum $K^+$ is 4-5 mEq/L, give 20 mEq/hr.
      4. If serum $K^+$ is $\geq 6$ mEq/L, withhold potassium replacement until serum $K^+$ is $\leq 6$ mEq/L.
   B. May give half as potassium chloride and half as potassium phosphate to also replace phosphate losses.
   C. May need magnesium replacement pending serum values.
   D. IV bicarbonate indicated only if arterial pH $\leq 7.0$ and patient has complicating medical problems such as hypotension, shock, or dysrhythmia. If given, should be by slow IV infusion. Goal is an arterial pH $\geq 7.0$. Concern with bicarbonate is association with the potentially fatal complication of cerebral edema.
V. White blood count with differential
   A. A leukocytosis may be present.
      1. Differentiate whether indicative of underlying sepsis vs. the leukocytosis with left shift commonly seen in DKA.
VI. Treat underlying cause (sepsis, myocardial infarction).
   A. In an individual with diabetes who acutely loses glycemic control, silent myocardial infarction must be ruled out.
VII. Patient education
   A. Educate the patient about prevention and early intervention.

of blindness from diabetic retinopathy occur each year.[76] A diagnosis of diabetic retinopathy results in an elevenfold increased risk of blindness as compared with the general population.[52] The DCCT demonstrated that intensive therapy resulted in a statistically significant decreased risk in the development and progression of retinopathy. Good visual acuity does not exclude significant retinopathy.

The earliest lesion is the microaneurysm in the retinal vessels. Having one dot-blot hemorrhage results in a twentyfold increased risk of blindness as compared with the general population.[52] Soft exudates, called "cotton wool spots," are areas of ischemia in the retina resulting from reduced retinal blood flow. Hard exudates are deposits of lipid on the retina, resulting from leaking retinal blood vessels. Early retinal changes, called *background retinopathy,* may progress to a more serious state, *proliferative retinopathy.*[55,114]

Proliferative retinopathy, or neovascular disease, results when the ischemic retina responds with the formation of new, fragile blood vessels on the retina. These fragile vessels bleed, causing vitreous hemorrhage (hemorrhage into the vitreous fluid of the eye) and sometimes result in retinal detachment. This hemorrhage can be repetitive and can lead to permanent visual loss. Early laser photocoagulation to seal off the leaking retinal vessels to preserve vision is now the standard based on the results of the Diabetic Retinopathy Study (DRS).[30] The DRS demonstrated a 60% statistically significant reduction in severe visual loss with the use of argon laser treatment. Laser photocoagulation does, however, destroy some normal retina in the process. Peripheral vision and night vision are most affected. However, without laser photocoagulation, progressive hemorrhage and subsequent blindness are inevitable. Laser photocoagulation is an outpatient surgical procedure performed in the ophthalmologist's office. In severe cases, the extent of vitreous hemorrhage necessitates a vitrectomy. In a vitrectomy, surgical instruments are placed into the eyeball and the hemorrhagic fluid is removed by suction and replaced with synthetic fluid. This inpatient surgical procedure is also vision preserving.[55,114]

Macular edema is a form of nonproliferative disease. Macular edema results from the leaking of fluid and lipid into the macula of the eye, resulting in edema. This is of concern because the macula is the part of the retina responsible for central vision. The Early Treatment Diabetic Retinopathy Study established the benefit of laser photocoagulation in macular edema with a 50% reduction in severe visual loss.[32]

An annual ophthalmological examination allows for early detection, diagnosis, and treatment of retinopathy.[2,7] An ophthalmologist is the specialist of choice and is preferred over an optometrist because of educational preparation and training.

The DCCT demonstrated that intensive therapy resulted in a significant decrease in the risk of development and progression of diabetic retinopathy. Additionally, blood pressure control is critical, because hypertension accelerates the development and progression of retinopathy.

**Diabetic nephropathy.** *Diabetic nephropathy* is the leading cause of end-stage renal disease in the United States, accounting for 36% of new cases. In 1992 alone, 19,790 new cases were diagnosed. In 1992, 56,059 individuals with diabetes were undergoing dialysis or transplantation treatment.[76]

The characteristic renal lesion is nodular glomerulosclerosis, called Kimmelstiel-Wilson syndrome. This involves nodular masses of laminated hyaline material that occur randomly throughout the kidney and is associated with proteinuria, edema, and hypertension. Kimmelstiel-Wilson lesions are seen only in diabetes mellitus and occur in 10% to 35% of individuals.

Laboratory abnormalities of renal disease generally do not occur until 10 years or more after onset of type 1 DM, but they may be present at diagnosis in type 2 DM. The natural history of diabetic nephropathy begins with early mesangial hypertrophy and hyperfiltration with an elevated glomerular filtration rate. Microscopic amounts of albumin in the urine, *microalbuminuria,* is the earliest laboratory abnormality and is asymptomatic. Microalbuminuria can be assessed via a radioimmunoassay on either a spot or timed urine collection. Microalbuminuria is present if the urinary albumin level is $\geq 30$ $\mu$g per milligram creatinine on a random urine specimen or if the excretion rate is $\geq 20$ $\mu$g/min ($\geq 30$ $\mu$g/24 hr) on a timed specimen.[1] Dipstick results are also available but are much less accurate. The development and progression of microalbuminuria can be reduced through meticulous glucose control, per the DCCT,[110] and blood pressure control, especially with angiotensin converting enzyme (ACE) inhibitors.

Microalbuminuria has additional significance. Individuals with microalbuminuria are at increased risk for retinopathy and autonomic neuropathy.[69] Microalbuminuria has poor prognostic implications in regard to both cardiovascular disease and mortality in both type 1 DM[80] and type 2 DM patients.[68]

Microalbuminuria may progress to albuminuria or clinical proteinuria ($\geq 300$ mg albumin/24 hr, which is equivalent to $\geq 500$ mg total protein/24 hr) and end-stage renal disease. Proteinuria also has poor prognostic implications in terms of cardiovascular disease and mortality rate in both type 1 DM[20,21] and type 2 DM patients.[63,77] Renal disease even at this point can remain asymptomatic, detectable only by objective measures.[88] Glycemic control still plays a role in reducing risks of progression.

A unifying hypothesis in microalbuminuria, albuminuria, proteinuria, and cardiovascular disease and mortality is the Steno hypothesis. The Steno hypothesis is based on the common cause, which appears to be endothelial dysfunction in a multitude of vascular beds in the body, with the resultant end-stage disease depending on the vascular bed involved.[29]

Hypertension is the factor that most often accelerates diabetic nephropathy. Aggressive blood pressure control decreases the rate of deterioration and improves survival.[23,40,97] Studies demonstrate that in an individual with diabetes, the lower the blood pressure within the normal range, the less albuminuria. Therefore a blood pressure of 132/74 results in less albuminuria than one of 140/80, and 122/66 results in less albuminuria than 132/74.

Angiotensin converting enzyme inhibitors have an important role in clinical proteinuria. The ACE inhibitor captopril is approved by the U.S. Food and Drug Administration (USFDA) for use in patients with clinical proteinuria to slow progression to end-stage renal disease, even in the absence of hypertension.[61] The use of ACE inhibitors in microalbuminuria is well studied with promising results and USFDA approval is pending.

Reduction in dietary protein intake may be of additional benefit, although clinical trials have not been conclusive. In patients with renal disease, a restriction to 0.8 mg of protein per kilogram of actual body weight is recommended.[70]

Clinical studies are ongoing in the use of an investigational drug (pimagedine) in diabetic nephropathy. Pimagedine, an inhibitor of glycosylation, has been shown in early trials to slow progression of diabetic nephropathy.

Unless aggressively treated, nephropathy rapidly progresses. End-stage renal disease may develop, requiring dialysis, transplantation, or both.

**Neuropathy.** *Diabetic neuropathy* affects 60% to 70% of individuals with diabetes.[76] The most common forms of neuropathy are peripheral and autonomic (Table 35-16).

***Symmetrical sensory peripheral polyneuropathy.*** In symmetrical sensory peripheral polyneuropathy, sensory changes and subsequent sensory loss occur symmetrically in a glove-and-stocking distribution. The lower extremities are generally affected first because they contain the longest nerves in the body; upper extremity involvement may follow. Comprehensive assessment of neuropathy is critical because even the patient with severe damage can remain asymptomatic. Abnormal sensations include paresthesias (pins and needles), numbness, and pain. Pain can range from minimal in the toes to sharp, stabbing, lancinating pain in a glove-and-stocking distribution. Abnormal sensations tend to worsen in the evening and may make it difficult for the patent to fall asleep. Even the light pressure of the bedsheet may be uncomfortable to the patient. Commonly, patients are unaware of sensory loss, so proper foot care is critical. In addition to sensory involvement, motor neurons may also be affected. The impairments occur slowly and are progressive.

**table 35-16** *Classification of Diabetic Neuropathy*

| Type | Signs and Symptoms |
|---|---|
| Peripheral sensory polyneuropathy | Classic symmetrical glove-and-stocking distribution |
| | Paresthesia |
| | Hyperesthesia |
| | Pain (characteristics vary; may be sharp, stabbing, lancinating, aching, etc.) |
| | Loss of sensation to pinprick, vibration, temperature |
| | Loss of deep tendon reflexes |
| | Muscle wasting and weakness |
| Autonomic | Orthostatic hypotension |
| | Cardiac denervation |
| | Anhidrosis |
| | Gustatory sweating |
| | Gastroparesis, with delayed gastric emptying, nausea, emesis |
| | Diarrhea |
| | Bladder atony |
| | Erectile dysfunction |
| Mononeuropathy | Cranial nerve palsy (III, IV, VI, and VII) |
| | Ulnar nerve palsy |
| | Carpal tunnel syndrome |
| Amyotrophy | Acute anterior thigh pain or numbness |
| | Weakness to hip flexion on examination |
| | Quadriceps wasting |
| Radiculopathy | Follows a dermatomal distribution on trunk |
| | Paresthesia |
| | Hyperesthesia |
| | Pain |
| | Numbness |

The DCCT demonstrated that intensive therapy resulted in a decreased risk of the development and progression of peripheral neuropathy.[110] Therefore glycemic control should be a priority in both prevention and treatment. Aldose reductase inhibitors have been studied in clinical trials but have not yet demonstrated improvement with a good safety profile, and none are approved by the USFDA. Further studies of aldose reductase inhibitors are ongoing. The efficacy of pimagedine is also being investigated in diabetic neuropathy.

***Painful peripheral neuropathy.*** Treatment of painful peripheral neuropathy revolves around the use of nonnarcotic agents. The neurotransmitter causing pain has been identified and is called substance P. The use of narcotics is frankly contraindicated in this chronic pain syndrome, because they fail to control pain and facilitate dependence. The last thing a patient with painful peripheral neuropathy needs is a narcotic addiction. Nonsteroidal antiinflammatory agents and acetaminophen are generally not efficacious in totally relieving neuropathy pain, but they may be helpful in some individuals. It is interesting to note that the majority of medications used to treat painful peripheral neuropathy do not have technical USFDA approval for that indication. Despite this, in the majority of patients with painful peripheral neuropathy, pain can be adequately controlled with one or more of the pharmacological agents detailed in Table 35-17.[123] New medications are under investigation for the treatment of painful peripheral neuropathy.

***Autonomic neuropathy.*** Damage to the autonomic nervous system may also occur, resulting in alterations in many body systems[3,123] (see Table 35-15). An easy and quick assessment of autonomic function is the R-R trend analysis. Using a special electrocardiograph machine, R-R trend analysis measures the variation in heart rate with deep breathing. In an individual with intact autonomic function, there is great variability in heart rate with deep breathing. Individuals with autonomic neuropathy lose that heart rate variability. A patient may experience none, some, or all of the dysfunctions. Commonly, the only symptom a patient may have is fatigue with exercise resulting from inability to increase heart rate to increase cardiac output. Another common symptom is dizziness on postural change. Autonomic neuropathy carries a poor prognosis, with up to a 50% 5-year mortality rate, generally because of silent ischemia resulting in silent myocardial infarctions or cardiac dysrhythmias.[34,87] Improvement in glycemic control can improve autonomic function.

***Mononeuropathy.*** Mononeuropathies have a vascular etiology, rather than a metabolic etiology. Vasculitis with subsequent ischemia or infarction of nerves is the cause. These neuropathies resolve spontaneously, usually within 6 to 8 weeks.[123]

Cranial nerve palsies occur more commonly in individuals with diabetes that in nondiabetic individuals. Onset is acute, and the course is self-limiting. A third cranial nerve palsy results in ptosis and restriction of ocular movement. Fourth and sixth cranial nerve palsies result in restriction of ocular movement. Seventh nerve palsies (Bell's palsy) result in a facial droop.[123]

An ulnar nerve palsy may be a result of a mononeuritis of acute onset or from nerve entrapment. Ulnar mononeuritis has an acute onset with pain and resolves spontaneously in 6 to 8 weeks, although the course is decreased with physical therapy. Nerve entrapment syndromes, in contrast, have a gradual onset and are associated with chronic pain. In the absence of interventions, they persist. Symptoms include numbness and pain to the affected hand and forearm. On examination, the patient may have weakness to abduction of the metacarpals and clawing of the fourth and fifth metacarpals from intrinsic muscle wasting as a result of denervation.[123] Once the etiology of the entrapment is determined (via electromyography [EMG], nerve conduction studies, ultrasound, magnetic resonance imaging, or vascular studies), intervention, commonly surgical, can then be undertaken.

Carpal tunnel syndrome is twice as common in individuals with diabetes as in nondiabetic individuals. Carpal tunnel syndrome is median nerve compression resulting from repeated trauma, metabolic changes, or edema within the carpal tunnel. Symptoms include paresthesias and numbness in the median nerve distribution. There may be weakness to the abductor pollicis brevis muscle, resulting in deceased thumb abduction. Significant muscle wasting can occur. Surgical intervention is indicated if symptoms persist or

**table 35-17** *Common Medications for **Painful Diabetic Neuropathy***

| Parameter | Propoxyphene with Darvon (Darvocet N-100) | Amitriptyline HCl (Elavil) | Carbamazepine (Tegretol) | Phenytoin (Dilantin) | Gabapentin (Neurontin) | Capsaicin (Zostrix) |
|---|---|---|---|---|---|---|
| Drug classification | Narcotic agonist analgesic | Tricyclic antidepressant | Anticonvulsant | Anticonvulsant | Anticonvulsant | Nonenamide<br>Topical analgesic |
| Benefit potential | High | High | Minimal to moderate | Questionable | High | Variable |
| Mode of action | Opiate agonist | Elevation in pain threshold | Unknown for analgesia | Unknown for analgesia | Unknown<br>? Inhibition of substance P | Extract of chili pepper<br>Inhibition of substance P |
| Starting dose | 1 tablet qid | Amitriptyline 10 mg 45 min before bedtime<br>Nortriptyline 25 mg 45 min before bedtime | 25 mg tid | 100 mg hs | 300 mg hs | Apply topically qid |
| Maximum dose | 2 tablets q4h | Amitriptyline 150 mg 45 min before bedtime<br>Nortriptyline 100 mg 45 min before bedtime | 100 mg tid | 100 mg qid | 600 mg qid | Apply topically 6 times daily |
| Precautions/Contraindications | Elevated hepatic transaminases<br>Known liver disease | Bradycardia<br>Clinically significant prostatic hypertrophy<br>Hypotension<br>Glaucoma<br>Hepatic or renal dysfunction | History of bone marrow suppression or disease<br>Monitor CBC/differential at baseline, 1 month, and every 3 months<br>Monitor blood levels | Impaired hepatic or renal function<br>Monitor blood levels | 300 mg is maximum dose to be used in setting of renal disease | Wash hands carefully after use<br>Avoid eyes and genitals |
| Side effects | Elevation in hepatic transaminases | Xerostomia<br>Bradycardia<br>Orthostatic hypotension<br>Urinary retention | Leukopenia<br>Thrombocytopenia<br>Pancytopenia<br>Aplastic anemia<br>Agranulocytosis | Gingival hyperplasia<br>Dizziness<br>Ataxia<br>Blood dyscrasias<br>Nephritis | Somnolence<br>Dizziness<br>Ataxia<br>Fatigue<br>Nystagmus<br>Leukopenia | Initial exacerbation of symptoms, release of substance P from neuronal endings |

clinical signs worsen, ideally before significant muscle atrophy. See Chapter 60 for further discussion of carpal tunnel syndrome.

***Amyotrophy.*** *Diabetic amyotrophy* is an acute event involving anterior thigh numbness or pain, which can be excruciating. Quadriceps muscle wasting and resultant weakness to hip flexion may occur within a few days. No specific diagnostic tests are indicated. Supportive therapy with nonnarcotic medication, as in painful peripheral neuropathy (see Table 35-17), and maintenance of walking are critical. Amyotrophy generally spontaneously resolves in 6 to 8 weeks, although severe cases may require 6 to 12 months.[3,123]

***Radiculopathy.*** Radiculopathy is sensory disturbance, loss of sensation or pain in a dermatomal distribution, which begins as an acute event; the discomfort can be excrutiating. As in amyotrophy, there are no specific diagnostic tests. On examination, there is loss of sensation to light touch, pinprick, and temperature along a dermatome of the trunk; the chest wall, the abdominal wall, or both may be affected. There may be a visible bulging to the chest or abdominal wall from acute denervation of the supporting musculature. Supportive therapy with nonnarcotic medication, as in painful peripheral neuropathy, is indicated (see Table 35-17). Radiculopathy generally spontaneously resolves after 6 to 8 weeks.[123]

### Macrovascular complications

Statistics of macrovascular disease comparing diabetic individuals with nondiabetic individuals are stunning. Cardiovascular disease is two to four times more prevalent in individuals with diabetes. Cardiovascular disease is present in 75% of diabetes-related deaths. Middle-aged individuals with diabetes have coronary disease death rates two to four times higher. The stroke risk in individuals with diabetes is 2 to 2.5 times higher.[76]

Individuals with diabetes develop the same macrovascular changes as nondiabetics. However, these changes occur at an earlier age, are more severe, and are more extensive in the vascular tree. Patients with type 2 DM have a higher rate than those with type 1 DM. Risk factors involved in the pathogenesis of macrovascular disease that must be aggressively addressed include dyslipidemia and hypertension.[72,126]

**Dyslipidemia.** Dyslipidemia affects an estimated 50% of individuals with diabetes. Elevated low-density lipoprotein (LDL) cholesterol, elevated triglycerides, and low high-density lipoprotein (HDL) cholesterol are risk factors for atherosclerosis. Because of insulin resistance, the lipid profile in the patient with type 2 DM is commonly characterized by hypertriglyceridemia and a low HDL cholesterol level with varying degrees of hypercholesterolemia. In type 1 DM, lipid disorders are generally seen only if there is a familial dyslipidemia or in the presence of renal disease. In diabetes, not only is the absolute LDL concentration important, but also qualitative abnormalities of the LDL particle, such as oxidation, glycation, and reduced LDL particle size (small, dense LDL), which make LDL more atherogenic.[42,107]

Data are available from clinical trials to support aggressive diagnosis and treatment in the individual with DM. The Scandinavian Simvastatin Survival Study (4S)[112] and the Cholesterol and Recurrent Events (CARE) trial,[94] two large randomized clinical trials of lowering LDL level as secondary prevention of coronary artery disease, have had a cohort of subjects with diabetes. The 4S demonstrated that diabetic subjects treated with simvastatin (20 mg or 40 mg) had a statistically significant lower risk of coronary heart disease death, nonfatal myocardial infarction, and any coronary heart disease event than their placebo-treated counterparts.[85] Impressively, this risk reduction was greater than that seen in the nondiabetic cohort. The CARE trial showed that diabetic subjects treated with pravastatin 40 mg had a statistically lower risk of coronary heart disease death, nonfatal myocardial infarction, coronary artery bypass graft, and angioplasty than their placebo-treated counterparts. Risk reduction in the diabetic subjects in the CARE trial was comparable with that in the nondiabetic cohort.[85] A randomized primary prevention trial, the West of Scotland Study,[102] demonstrated a reduction in events and mortality rates in the primary prevention of coronary artery disease. No subgroup analyses have yet been published on the subjects with diabetes. Aggressive screening, diagnosis, and treatment using the National Cholesterol Education Program Panel II (NCEP Panel II) guidelines[35,74] is critical to reduce morbidity and mortality.

**Hypertension.** Hypertension affects 60% to 65% of individuals with diabetes.[76] Hypertension in the patient with type 1 DM implies renal disease, microalbuminuria, or proteinuria, until proven otherwise. (In contrast, hypertension in the patient with type 2 DM can result from either coexistent renal disease or essential hypertension.) Regardless of the etiology, blood pressure must be aggressively monitored and hypertension diagnosed early because it exacerbates retinopathy, nephropathy, and macrovascular disease. The goal blood pressure in the individual with diabetes is 130/85 mm Hg.[75]

Lifestyle modification (weight loss, sodium restriction, exercise) should be the primary modality of treatment. When lifestyle modification fails, the pharmacological agent chosen should be metabolically neutral (i.e., not worsen insulin resistance or dyslipidemia or cause electrolyte disturbance). The ACE inhibitors are a good choice in a patient with microalbuminuria or proteinuria, calcium channel blockers are suitable for the patient with angina, and $\alpha$-blockers are a good choice in the male patient with concurrent benign prostatic hyperplasia. Because $\beta$-blockers and diuretics worsen insulin resistance, they should be avoided whenever possible. In the individual with diabetes, monotherapy is commonly unsuccessful, especially in the presence of nephropathy.[103-105]

## THE DIABETIC FOOT

Three major factors play a role in the diabetic foot: *neuropathy, ischemia,* and *sepsis.* Amputation commonly results.[58,59] Diabetes is responsible for almost 80% of major lower limb nontraumatic amputations in the United States.[56]

Sensory impairment leads to painless trauma and potential for ulceration. Motor impairment contributes to wasting of intrinsic muscles in the feet, resulting in foot deformity. Foot deformities alter the normal gait and pressure distribution. Friction and resultant callosities may develop and result in pressure necrosis and ulceration. Painless trauma can result in fractures in the ankle or forefoot and ultimately significant deformity, called a *Charcot* foot. Anhidrosis as a manifestation of autonomic neuropathy can result in excessive dryness and cracking of the skin, which also contributes to infection. Macrovascular and microvascular alterations produce tissue ischemia and may lead to sepsis. The triad of neuropathy, ischemia, and sepsis can result in gangrene and ultimately amputation. Gangrene may be classified as dry or wet. *Dry gangrene* occurs when tissue death is not associated with inflammatory changes. Aggressive glycemic control and hospitalization for IV antibiotics to limit spread of infection are necessary. Amputation of affected toes is often necessary. The area must be kept dry to prevent wet gangrene. *Wet gangrene* is gangrene coupled with inflammation; septicemia and shock may occur.

Podiatric care is critical to attain and maintain foot health. Proper toenail trimming and use of orthotic, extra-depth, extra-width, or custom-molded shoes can prevent ongoing trauma and ultimately the amputation associated with the diabetic foot.[58,59]

Prevention of microvascular disease, neuropathy, and macrovascular disease[33] should be a major focus of diabetes care. Thorough interim histories, interim physical examinations, and measurement of laboratory parameters will allow for early diagnosis, therefore allowing for early intervention and risk factor modification and prevention of end-stage disease.

## HYPOGLYCEMIA IN THE INDIVIDUAL WITHOUT DIABETES MELLITUS

Hypoglycemia in the nondiabetic person is characterized by subnormal plasma glucose, generally less than 50 mg/dl. It may be asymptomatic, may cause adrenergic symptoms (anxiety, irritability, palpitations, diaphoresis, pallor), or may cause neuroglycopenic symptoms with more severe hypoglycemia. Neuroglycopenic symptoms include mental confusion, seizures, and coma and may be associated with severe trauma (e.g., motor vehicle accidents). A firm diagnosis rests with the documentation of Whipple's triad: (1) appropriate signs and symptoms, (2) a documented subnormal blood glucose, and (3) response to normalization of blood glucose with carbohydrate ingestion.[36]

### CLASSIFICATION

Hypoglycemia may be broadly classified as either fasting or nonfasting (reactive) hypoglycemia. Fasting hypoglycemia generally results in neuroglycopenic symptoms, whereas reactive hypoglycemia is usually associated with more adrenergic symptoms. The etiology of each is generally entirely different.

#### Fasting Hypoglycemia

##### *Etiology*

The etiology of fasting hypoglycemia is presented in Box 35-21.

**box 35-21** *Etiology of Fasting Hypoglycemia*

**Insulin excess**
- Exogenous insulin surreptitously
- Sulfonylurea ingestion (accidental in individual without DM, surreptitious use, pharmacy dispensation error)
- Insulin-producing islet cell tumor (insulinoma) (benign or malignant)
- Islet hyperplasia
- Nesidioblastosis

**Decreased hepatic glucose production**
- Advanced renal disease
- Advanced liver disease
- Ethanol use, especially in the setting of poor nutrition
- Severe sepsis
- Severe malnutrition

**Counterregulatory hormone deficiencies**
- Hypopituitarism
- Adrenocorticotropic hormone (ACTH) deficiency
- Growth hormone deficiency
- Primary adrenal failure (Addison's disease)

**Hypothyroidism**—(rare)

**Non–islet cell tumors**—Mesenchymal tumors, generally clinically obvious, with limited life expectancy

**Autoimmune disease**—Antibodies that stimulate the insulin receptor (rare)

Adapted from Field JB: Hypoglycemia: definition, clinical presentations, classification, and laboratory tests, *Endocrinol Metab Clin North Am* 18(1):27, 1989.

##### *Collaborative care management*

Diagnosis of fasting hypoglycemia is performed in the hospital via a 72-hour fast to document a subnormal glucose with simultaneous increased insulin level and increased C-peptide level. Sulfonylurea levels are performed when indicated, especially when surreptitious use is suspected (Table 35-18). Surreptitious use of insulin or sulfonylureas is seen in psychiatric states as an attention-seeking ploy. Although uncommon, surreptitious use is certainly not rare, and it should be considered when the clinical scenario is not in keeping with an organic cause. Management of fasting hypoglycemia by surgical removal of the neoplasm, management of the underlying disease, or both.

##### *Patient/family education*

Patients using insulin or sulfonylureas surreptitiously should be educated regarding the deleterious effects and referred for counseling.

#### Reactive Hypoglycemia

##### *Etiology*

Reactive hypoglycemia generally occurs 3 to 5 hours after meals, related to either a primary delay in insulin secretion (idiopathic) or rapidly rising postprandial glucose related to rapid gastric emptying (postgastric surgery). Failure of the pancreas to keep pace with this rapidly rising postprandial glucose results in later insulin hypersecretion and hypoglycemia. Individuals with true idiopathic reactive hypoglycemia, reflecting an insulin secretory defect, are at increased risk of type 2 DM.

##### *Collaborative care management*

Reactive hypoglycemia is overdiagnosed as a result of Whipple's triad not being documented. Oral glucose tolerance testing is rarely indicated in the diagnosis of idiopathic reactive hypoglycemia. The diagnosis is best made by randomly documenting a blood glucose less than 50 mg/dl in association with signs and symptoms and prompt response to carbohydrate ingestion.[36,100] Indeed, oral glucose tolerance testing commonly results in post–glucose load blood glucoses of less than 50 mg/dl without signs and symptoms.[36]

**table 35-18** *Laboratory Parameters in Determining the Etiology of Fasting Hypoglycemia*

| Etiology | Laboratory Parameters |
|---|---|
| Insulinoma | ↑ Insulin<br>↑ C-peptide |
| Exogenous insulin | ↑ Insulin<br>↓ C-peptide |
| ? Sulfonylureas | ↑ Insulin<br>↑ C-peptide<br>No evidence of neoplasm or other cause |

Many individuals with underlying anxiety states are misdiagnosed with "hypoglycemia" with no documentation of a truly low blood glucose and are placed on unnecessarily ritualistic diets. These ritualistic diets are usually low in carbohydrate and high in protein and fat, with resultant weight gain and an adverse lipid profile. In the setting of true idiopathic hypoglycemia, this dietary approach is even more deleterious given these individuals' propensity to develop type 2 DM and syndrome X. (See Figure 35-16.)

### Patient/family education

Patient teaching needs focus on prevention of hypoglycemic episodes. The most logical management approach revolves around (1) delaying the postprandial glucose rise through increased dietary fiber and the use of complex carbohydrates and (2) enhancing insulin sensitivity through exercise and weight reduction toward desirable body weight.

## chapter SUMMARY

### CLASSIFICATION

- Diabetes mellitus is a complex metabolic disorder that may be clinically categorized in one of five different classifications. The two major classifications are type 1 diabetes mellitus and type 2 diabetes mellitus.

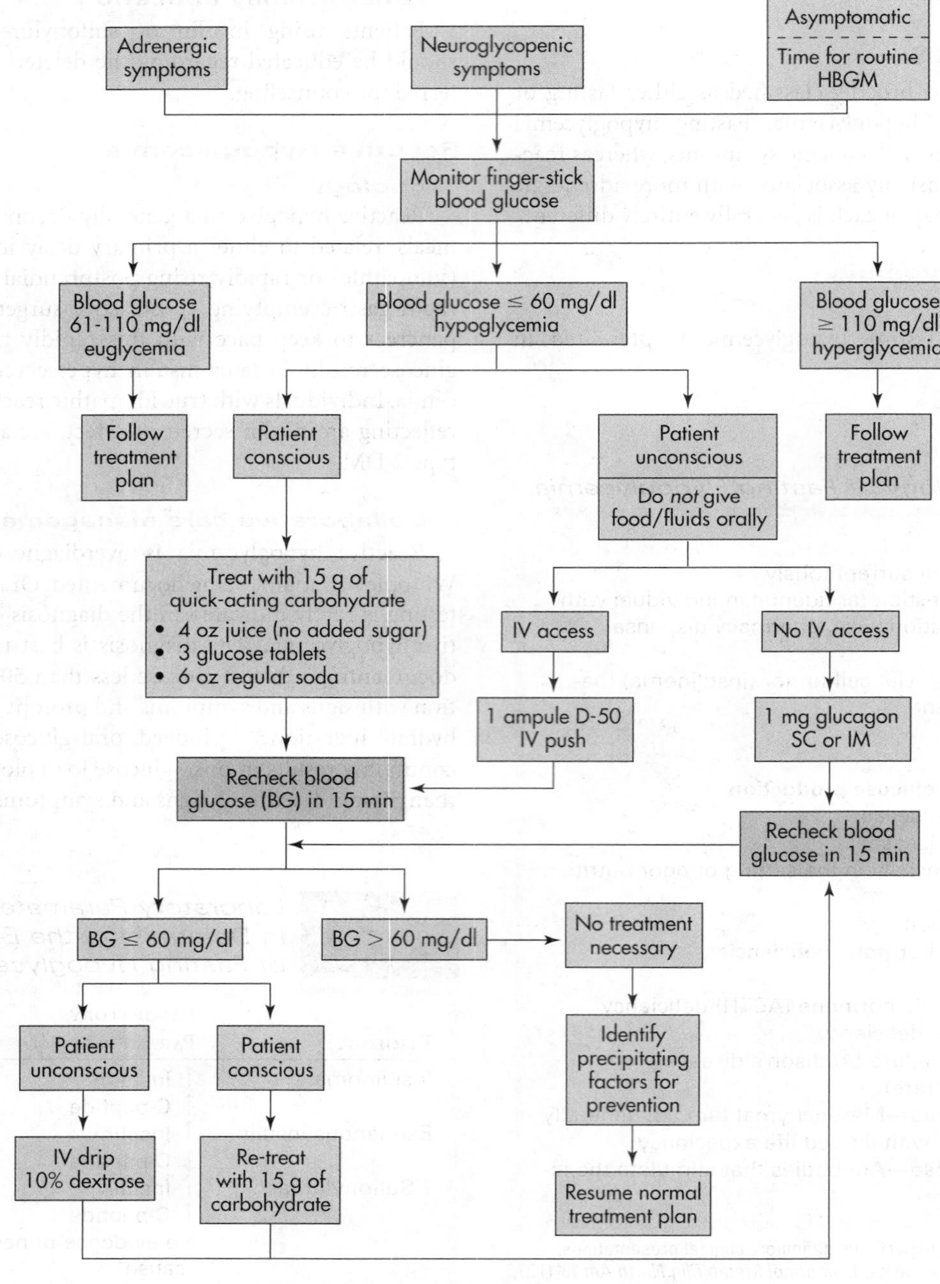


**fig. 35-16** Algorithm for treating hypoglycemia.

## ETIOLOGY

- Genetics, heredity, autoimmunity, and environmental factors have a role in the causes of type 1 DM.

## EPIDEMIOLOGY

- Type 2 DM occurs more often in Native Americans, Hispanics, African Americans, and elderly people.

## PATHOPHYSIOLOGY

- Insulin deficiency is a central feature of diabetes; insulin deficiency may be absolute, when $\beta$-cells do not secrete insulin, or relative, when $\beta$-cell defect and peripheral resistance to insulin are present.
- Insulin deficiency and hyperglycemia lead to many immediate alterations in metabolism, including hyperosmolarity and osmotic diuresis, glycosuria, cellular starvation, calorie loss, and increased fat metabolism and catabolism.
- The classic signs and symptoms of type 1 DM are polyuria, polydipsia, polyphagia, weight loss, weakness, and fatigue. Patients with type 1 DM may have these symptoms or signs and symptoms of diabetic ketoacidosis; patients with type 2 DM may have the same symptoms, except that they usually have weight gain instead of weight loss, or they may have signs and symptoms of hyperglycemic hyperosmolar nonketotic coma or vascular changes and neuropathy.

## PREVENTION

- Taking measures to prevent and treat obesity is the focus of primary prevention of type 2 DM; screening to detect undiagnosed cases (50%) is the focus of secondary prevention; detecting and preventing progression of complications is the focus of tertiary prevention.
- The five primary modalities of treatment for diabetes mellitus are diet, exercise, pharmacological agents, monitoring, and education.
- Dietary recommendations include calorie distribution of carbohydrate (40% to 60%); fat (usually ≤30% but may be as high as 40%), with restriction in saturated fat to 10%; protein (20%); and limitation of cholesterol and sodium.
- Exercise lowers blood glucose levels in most instances; it can worsen hyperglycemia if blood glucose levels are above 300 mg/dl or if exercise is intense. Exercise aids in cardiovascular fitness and weight reduction and maintenance, and it decreases peripheral resistance to insulin.

## COLLABORATIVE CARE MANAGEMENT

- Home blood glucose monitoring (HBGM) should be used by all individuals with DM. This technology has made it possible to achieve euglycemia in well-educated patients.
- Insulin is used in all individuals with type 1 DM and some with type 2 DM. Intensive therapy should be used in the majority of individuals with type 1 DM. Nurses and patients must be knowledgeable about the characteristics of the insulins.
- Oral agents are used in type 2 DM. They have multiple modes of action that may be complementary.
- Glycosylated hemoglobin is an indirect marker of glycemic control over the past 3 months. The lower the glycosylated hemoglobin, the greater the risk reduction for microvascular complications (DCCT).

## NURSING MANAGEMENT

- Assessment of the patient includes collecting objective data about metabolic status and assessing cardiovascular status, renal status, vision, and nerve function. The lower extremities should be examined carefully.
- Because patients must be responsible for diabetes management, nurses must assess the knowledge and coping skills of patients early after diagnosis so that appropriate education and counseling can proceed.
- A well-educated person will be assertive in describing special needs relating to patterns of food intake, exercise, monitoring, medication, and foot care.
- A well-constructed educational program for persons with diabetes mellitus has many components, including knowledge, skills, and attitudes for effective diabetes management.
- Diabetes education must be individualized and planned over time. Initial instruction should be restricted to survival/initial skills with plans for continued education.
- The impact of diagnosis of diabetes mellitus and living with this chronic illness may be expressed by patients emotionally, in concerns about the future, in family conflicts, and in noncompliance.
- The treatment of hypoglycemia must be prompt: in the conscious patient, 15 g of simple carbohydrate when blood glucose is ≤60 mg/dl confirmed or when symptoms are detected; in the unconscious patient, 1 ampule of 50% dextrose by IV push or 1 mg glucagon SC or IM. Generally, the first signs and symptoms are adrenergic symptoms; later neuroglycopenic symptoms appear. The signs and symptoms may be prolonged.
- Insulin or oral agents should not be omitted when short-term illness occurs. Carbohydrate in some form should continue to be consumed according to the meal plan. Increased frequency of HBGM with the addition of urine ketone monitoring is critical. Attention to the contraindications of metformin are especially important during intercurrent illness.
- Foot care includes daily inspection, measures to maintain integrity of skin, and prevention of injury. Referral to podiatric services is highly recommended. The patient should verbalize knowledge of feet at risk.
- Evaluation of nursing interventions includes assessment of whether the metabolic balance is improved, whether the patient has the requisite knowledge and coping skills for self-management, and whether appropriate referrals were made. The Professional Prompter Worksheet is a guide for nurses that outlines what to teach.
- Diabetes treatment is expensive but highly cost-effective in terms of reducing long-term complications and potentially reducing mortality rates. Persons with diabetes may have difficulty getting health insurance and certain jobs.

## NURSING MANAGEMENT OF THE PATIENT WITH DIABETES HAVING SURGERY

- Patients fasting or undergoing surgery require modifications of insulin and food intake and increased monitoring of metabolic status.

## COMPLICATIONS

- Diabetic ketoacidosis (DKA) and hyperglycemic hyperosmolar nonketotic coma (HHNC) are two life-threatening situations that occur in uncontrolled diabetes mellitus; they are usually precipitated by infection, stressors, or failure to follow regimen.
- Medical management of DKA and HHNC includes intensive fluid replacement, low-dose insulin infusion (IV insulin not necessary in all cases) and potassium replacement. The patient may also need phosphate and magnesium replacement.

- Hyperglycemia, from poorly controlled diabetes mellitus, is a major predictor of the development of microvascular lesions (nephropathy, retinopathy), macrovascular lesions (atherosclerotic disease), and neuropathy (autonomic and peripheral).
- Amputation of a limb may be necessary because of alterations in blood vessels and nerve trauma, tissue trauma, or infections occurring in persons with inadequate skin integrity and insensitivity to pain and pressure. Proper foot care, which helps prevent an infection, can reduce the chance of amputation.

### HYPOGLYCEMIC STATES

- Hypoglycemia can occur in individuals who do not have diabetes mellitus.
- Hypoglycemia can be classified as fasting (includes excessive insulin production from insulinomas) or reactive (hypoglycemia after a meal).
- The signs and symptoms of fasting or reactive hypoglycemia are caused by adrenergic activation and neuroglycopenia.
- As the year 2000 approaches, the prognosis for the individual with DM has never been better.
- We have a more in-depth understanding of the pathophysiology of DM, new medications, new technologies, and conclusive proof that glucose control prevents and delays the progression of microvascular complications.
- Health care teams should be teaming up for health and well-being.
- Diabetes can be controlled and complications prevented.

## References

1. Alzaid AA: Microalbuminuria in patients with NIDDM: an overview, *Diabetes Care* 19(1):79, 1996.
2. American Diabetes Association: Clinical practice recommendations 1997, *Diabetes Care* 20(suppl 1):S1-S70, 1997.
3. American Diabetes Association: Clinical practice recommendations 1995, *Diabetes Care* 18(suppl 1):1-96, 1995.
4. American Diabetes Association: *Diabetes—1991 vital statistics,* Alexandria, Va, 1991, American Diabetes Association.
5. American Diabetes Association: Implications of the Diabetes Control and Complications Trial, *Diabetes Care* 16(11):1517, 1993.
6. American Diabetes Association, Expert Committee on the Diagnosis and Classification of Diabetes Mellitus: Report of the Expert Committee On the Diagnosis and Classification of Diabetes Mellitus, *Diabetes Care* 20(7):1183, 1997.
7. American Diabetes Association: Standards of medical care for patients with diabetes mellitus, *Diabetes Care* 20(suppl 1):S5, 1996.
8. American Diabetes Association: *The health professional's guide to diabetes and exercise,* ed 1, Arlington, Va, 1995, American Diabetes Association.
9. American Diabetes Association and American Dietetic Association: *Exchange lists for meal planning,* Alexandria, Va, 1986, American Diabetes Association.
10. Anderson JW et al: Dietary fiber and diabetes, a comprehensive review and practical application, *J Am Diet Assoc* 87:1189, 1987.
11. Anderson J, Clark JT: The promise of fiber, *Diabetes Forecast* 40(12):47, 1987.
12. Baxley SG, Brown ST, Pokorny, ME, Swanson MS: Perceived competence and actual level of knowledge of diabetes mellitus among nurses, *J Nurs Staff Dev* 13(2):93, 1997.
13. Bell DS: Exercise for patients with diabetes. Benefits, risks, precautions, *Postgrad Med* 92(1):183, 1992.
14. Bell DS: Alcohol and the NIDDM patient, *Diabetes Care* 19(5):509, 1996.
15. Belmin J, Valensi P: Diabetic neuropathy in elderly patients. What can be done? *Drugs Aging* 8(6):416, 1996.
16. Bliss M: *The discovery of insulin,* Chicago, 1982, University of Chicago Press.
17. Blonde L, Guthrie RD, Sandberg MI: Metformin: an effective and safe agent for initial monotherapy in patients with non–insulin-dependent diabetes mellitus, *Endocrinologist* 6(6):431, 1996.
18. Bloomgarden ZT: Epidemiology, diagnosis, and treatment of type 2 diabetes—a meeting report, *Pract Diabetol* 12(2):4, 1993.
19. Bode BW et al: *DiabetesDek—how to control and manage diabetes mellitus,* Atlanta, Ga, 1992, Lifescan Infodek.
20. Borch-Johnsen K, Kragh AP, Deckert T: The effect of proteinuria on relative mortality in type 1 diabetes mellitus, *Diabetalogia* 28(8): 540, 1985.
21. Borch-Johnsen K, Kreiner S: Proteinuria: value as predictor of cardiovascular mortality in insulin-dependent diabetes mellitus, *BMJ* 294(6580):1651, 1987
22. Chen M, Bergman RN, Porte D Jr: Insulin resistance and beta cell dysfunction in aging: the importance of dietary carbohydrate, *J Clin Endocrinol Metab* 67(5):951, 1988.
23. Christensen CK, Mogensen CE: Effect of antihypertensive treatment of progression of incipient diabetic nephropathy, *Hypertension* 7(suppl 2):109, 1985.
24. Coleman W: Foot care and diabetes mellitus. In Haire-Joshu D, editor: *Management of diabetes mellitus—perspectives of care across the life span,* St Louis, 1992, Mosby.
25. Coonrod BA: Insulin syringes and pens: finding the best match for your patients' needs, *Clinical Diabetes* 15(3):114, 1997.
26. Coonrod BA, Betschart J, Harris MI: Frequency and determinants of diabetes patient education among adults in the U.S. population, *Diabetes Care* 17(8):852, 1994.
27. Cranston I, Lomas J, Maran A, et al: Restoration of hypoglycemia awareness in patients with long-duration insulin-dependent diabetes, *Lancet* 344(8918):283, 1974.
28. Criqui MH, Fronek A, Klauber MR, et al: The sensitivity, specificity, and predictive value of traditional clinical evaluation of peripheral arterial disease: results from noninvasive testing in a defined population, *Pathophysiology and Natural History—Peripheral Vascular Disease,* 71:516, 1985.
29. Deckert T, Feldt-Rasmussen B, Borch-Johnsen K, et al: Albuminuria reflects widespread vascular damage: the Steno hypothesis, *Diabetalogia* 32(4):219, 1989.
30. Diabetic Retinopathy Study Group: Photocoagulation treatment of proliferative diabetic retinopathy: clinical application of Diabetic Retinopathy Study (DRS) findings. DRS report no. 8, *Ophthalmology* 88:583, 1981.
31. Eaks GA: *Professional Prompter Worksheet,* Cray Diabetes Education Center, Kansas City, 1993, University of Kansas Medical Center.
32. Early Treatment Diabetic Retinopathy Study Research Group: Photocoagulation for diabetic macular edema, *Arch Ophthalmol* 103: 1796, 1985.
33. Eastman RC, Keen H: The impact of cardiovascular disease on people with diabetes: the potential for prevention, *Lancet* 350(suppl I): 29, 1997.
34. Ewing DJ, Campbell IW, Clarke BF: The natural history of diabetic autonomic neuropathy, *QJ Med* 49(193):95, 1980.
35. Expert Panel on Detection, Evaluation, and Treatment of High Blood Cholesterol in Adults: Summary of the second report of the National Cholesterol Education Program (NCEP) Expert Panel on Detection, Evaluation, and Treatment of High Blood Cholesterol in Adults (adult treatment panel II), *JAMA* 269:3015, 1993.
36. Field JB: Hypoglycemia: definition, clinical presentation, classification, and laboratory tests, *Endocrinol Metab Clin North Am* 18(1): 27, 1989.

37. Fink RI, Kolterman OG, Griffin J, Olefsky JM: Mechanisms of insulin resistance in aging, *J Clin Invest* 71(6):1523, 1983.
38. Franz MJ, Horton ES, Bantle JD, et al: Nutrition principles for the management of diabetes and related complications (technical review), *Diabetes Care* 17(5):490, 1994.
39. Funnell MM: Integrated approaches to the management of NIDDM patients, *Diabetes Spectrum* 9(1):55, 1996.
40. Gall MA, Borch-Johnsen K, Hougaard P, et al: Albuminuria and poor glycemic control predict mortality in NIDDM, *Diabetes* 44(11):1303, 1995.
41. Galloway JA, deShazo RD: Insulin chemistry and pharmacology: insulin allergy, resistance, and lipodystrophy. In Rifkin H, Porte D Jr, editors: *Ellenberg and Rifkin's diabetes mellitus, theory and practice,* ed 4, New York, 1990, Elsevier.
42. Garber AJ: Dyslipidemia as a risk factor for coronary artery disease in patients with diabetes, *Endocrine Practice* 3(4):244, 1997.
43. Gavard JA, Lustman PJ, Clouse RE: Prevalence of depression in adults with diabetes. An epidemiological evaluation, *Diabetes Care* 16(8):1167, 1993.
44. Greene DA: Acute and chronic complications of diabetes mellitus in older patients, *Am J Med* 80(5A):38, 1986.
45. Gregory RP, Davis DL: Use of carbohydrate counting for meal planning in type 1 diabetes, *Diabetes Educ* 20(5):406, 1994.
46. Guthrie DW, Guthrie RA: *Nursing management of diabetes mellitus,* ed 3, New York, 1991, Springer.
47. Hamera E et al: Self-regulation in individuals with type 2 diabetes, *Nurs Res* 37:363, 1988.
48. Hayes TM, Harries J: Randomised controlled trial of routine hospital care versus routine general practice care for type 2 diabetics, *BMJ* 289(6447):728, 1984.
49. Herman W: *The prevention and treatment of complications of diabetes mellitus—a guide for primary care practitioners,* Washington, DC, 1992, US Department of Health and Human Services, Public Health Service, Centers for Disease Control, National Center for Chronic Disease Prevention and Health Promotion, Division of Diabetes Translation, US Government Printing Office.
50. Ho M, Marger M, Beart J, et al: Is the quality of diabetes care better in a diabetes clinic or in a general medicine clinic? *Diabetes Care* 20(4):472, 1997.
51. Horton ES: Exercise. In Lebovitz HE, editor: *Therapy for diabetes mellitus and related disorders,* Alexandria, Va, 1991, American Diabetes Association.
52. Huang S: Diabetic retinopathy: prevention, diagnosis and vision preservation. Multidisciplinary management of diabetes mellitus in the post-DCCT era for primary care physicians and healthcare providers, Symposium sponsored by the Departments of Family Medicine and Medicine, Case Western Reserve University School of Medicine and University Hospitals of Cleveland, June 7, 1995, Cleveland, Ohio.
53. Johnson KC, Graney MJ, Applegate WB, et al: Prevalence of undiagnosed non–insulin-dependent diabetes mellitus and impaired glucose tolerance in a cohort of older persons with hypertension, *J Am Geriatr Soc* 45(6):695, 1997.
54. Joslin EP: *Diabetic manual,* ed 10, Philadelphia, 1959, Lea & Febiger.
55. Klein R, Klein BEK: Diabetic eye disease, *Lancet* 350(9072):197, 1997.
56. Kozak GP, Rowbotham JL: Diabetic foot disease: a major problem. In GP Kozak et al, editors *Management of diabetic foot problems,* Philadelphia, 1984, WB Saunders.
57. Lauritzen T et al: Continuous subcutaneous insulin (2-year Steno study data), *Lancet* 1:1445, 1983.
58. Lehto S, Ronnemaa T, Pyorala K, Laakso M: Risk factors predicting lower extremity amputation in patients with NIDDM, *Diabetes Care* 19(6):607, 1996.
59. Levin ME: Preventing amputation in the patient with diabetes, *Diabetes Care* 18(10):1383, 1995.
60. Levin ME, O'Neal LW, editors: *The diabetic foot,* St Louis, 1988, Mosby.
61. Lewis EJ, Hunsicker LG, Bain RP, Rohde RD for the Collaborative Study Group: The effect of angiotensin-converting-enzyme inhibition on diabetic nephropathy, *N Engl J Med* 329(20):1456, 1993.
62. Lloyd CE et al: Psychosocial factors and complications of IDDM, *Diabetes Care* 15(2):166, 1992.
63. MacLeod JM, Lutale J, Marshall SM: Albumin excretion and vascular deaths in NIDDM, *Diabetalogia* 38(5):610, 1995.
64. Mandrup-Poulson T: The Steno Diabetes Center, personal communication, 1992.
65. Marrero DG: Current effectiveness of diabetes health care in the U.S. How far from ideal? *Diabetes Reviews* 2:292, 1994.
66. Marrero DG: Evaluating the quality of care provided by primary care physicians to people with non–insulin-dependent diabetes mellitus, *Diabetes Spectrum* 9(1):30, 1996.
67. Meneilly GS, Tessier D: Diabetes in the elderly, *Diabet Med* 12(11): 949, 1995.
68. Mogensen CE: Microalbuminuria predicts clinical proteinuria and early mortality in maturity-onset diabetes, *N Engl J Med* 310(6): 356, 1984.
69. Molgard H, Christensen PD, Hermansen K, et al: Early recognition of autonomic dysfunction in microalbuminuria: significance for cardiovascular mortality in diabetes mellitus, *Diabetalogia* 37(8): 788, 1994.
70. Mudaliar SR, Henry RR: Role of glycemic control and protein restriction in clinical management of diabetic kidney disease, *Endocrine Practice* 2(3):220, 1996.
71. Myllynen P, Koivisto VA, Nikkila EA: Glucose intolerance and insulin resistance accompany immobilization, *Acta Med Scand* 222(1):75, 1987.
72. Nathan DM, Meigs J, Singer DE: The epidemiology of cardiovascular disease in type 2 diabetes mellitus: How sweet it is . . . or is it? *Lancet* 350(suppl I):4, 1997.
73. Nathan DM, Singer DE, Godine JE, Perlmuter LC: Non–insulin-dependent diabetes in older patients: complications and risk factors, *Am J Med* 81(5):837, 1986.
74. National Cholesterol Education Program: *Second report of the Expert Panel on Detection, Evaluation, and Treatment of High Blood Cholesterol Levels in Adults (adult treatment panel II),* NIH pub no 93-3095:0-5, Washington, DC, 1993, National Institutes of Health.
75. National High Blood Pressure Education Program Working Group: National High Blood Pressure Education Program Working Group report on hypertension in diabetes, *Hypertension* 23(2):145, discussions 159, 1994.
76. National Institute of Diabetes and Digestive and Kidney Diseases, National Diabetes Information Clearinghouse, National Institutes of Health: *Diabetes Statistics,* NIH pub no 96-3926, Washington, DC, 1995.
77. Niskanen LK, Penttila I, Paviainen M, Uusitupa MIJ: Evolution, risk factors, and prognostic implication of albuminuria in NIDDM, *Diabetes Care* 19(5):486, 1996.
78. Ohkubo Y, Kishikawa H, Araki E, et al: Intensive insulin therapy prevents the progression of diabetic microvascular complications in Japanese patients with non–insulin-dependent diabetes mellitus: a randomized prospective 6-year study, *Diabetes Res Clin Pract* 28: 103, 1995.
79. Orchard TJ, Strandness DE Jr: Assessment of peripheral vascular disease in diabetes. Report and recommendations of an international workshop sponsored by the American Heart Association and the American Diabetes Association, 18-20 September 1992 New Orleans, Louisiana, *Diabetes Care* 16(8):1199, 1995.
80. Parving HH, Hommel E, Mathiesen E, et al: Prevalence of microalbuminuria, arterial hypertension, retinopathy, and neuropathy

in patients with insulin-dependent diabetes, *BMJ* 296(6616):156, 1988.

81. Peters AL, Legorreta AD, Ossorio RC, Davidson MB: Quality of outpatient care provided to diabetic patients: a health maintenance organization experience, *Diabetes Care* 19(6):601, 1996.
82. *Physicians' Desk Reference,* ed 51, Montvale, NJ, 1997, Medical Economics.
83. Pirart J: Diabetes mellitus and its degenerative complications: a prospective study of 4400 patients observed between 1947 and 1973, *Diabetes Medicine* 3(2):97; 3(3):173; 3(4):245, 1977; *Diabetes Care* 1:168, 1978.
84. Pollock ML, Wilmore JH: *Exercise in health and disease—evaluation and prescription for prevention and rehabilitation,* ed 2, Philadelphia, 1990, WB Saunders.
85. Pyorala K, Pederson TR, Kjekshus J, et al, and the Scandinavian Simvastatin Survival Study (4S): Cholesterol lowering with simvastatin improves prognosis of diabetic patients with coronary heart disease: a subgroup analysis of the Scandinavian Simvastatin Survival Study (4S), *Diabetes Care* 20(4):614, 1997.
86. Queale WS, Seidler AJ, Brancati FL: Glycemic control and sliding scale insulin use in medical inpatients with diabetes mellitus, *Arch Intern Med* 157(5):545, 1997.
87. Rathmann W, Ziegler D, Jahnke M, et al: Mortality in diabetic patients with cardiovascular autonomic neuropathy, *Diabet Med* 10(9):820, 1993.
88. Reasner CA, DeFronzo RA: Diabetic nephropathy—can it be prevented? *Endocrine Practice* 2(3):220, 1996.
89. Reaven GM: Banting lecture 1988. Role of insulin resistance in human disease, *Diabetes* 37(12):1595, 1988.
90. Reaven GM: Role of insulin resistance in human disease (syndrome X): an expanded definition, *Annu Rev Med* 440:121, 1993.
91. Reaven GM: Syndrome X, *Clin Diabetes* 12:32, 1994.
92. Rifkin H, Porte D, editors: *Ellenberg and Rifkin's diabetes mellitus, theory and practice,* ed 4, New York, 1990, Elsevier.
93. Rowe JW, Minaker KL, Pallotta JA, Flier JS: Characterization of the insulin resistance of aging, *J Clin Invest* 71(6):1581, 1983.
94. Sacks FM, Pfeffer MA, Moye LA, et al, for the Cholesterol and Recurrent Events Trial Investigators: The effect of pravastatin on coronary events after myocardial infarction in patients with average cholesterol levels, *N Engl J Med* 335(14):1001, 1995.
95. Saltiel AR, Olefsky JM: Thiazolidinediones in the treatment of insulin resistance and type 2 diabetes, *Diabetes* 45(12):1661, 1996.
96. Saudek CD, Segai-Polin S: Economic aspects: insurance, employment, and licensing. In Rifkin H, Porte D, editors: *Ellenberg and Rifkin's diabetes mellitus, theory and practice,* ed 4, New York, 1990, Elsevier.
97. Sawicki PT, Muhlauser I, Didjurgeit U, et al: Intensified antihypertensive therapy is associated with improved survival in type 1 diabetic patients with nephropathy, *J Hypertension* 13(8):933, 1995.
98. Sawin CT: Action without benefit: the sliding scale of insulin use, *Arch Intern Med* 157(5):489, 1997.
99. Schade D, Santiago J, Skyler JS, Rizza R: Intensive insulin therapy, *Excerpta Medica,* 1983.
100. Service FJ: Hypoglycemia, including hypoglycemia in neonates and children. In DeGroot LJ, editor: *Endocrinology,* Philadelphia, 1995, WB Saunders.
101. Sheehan JP: The gift of insulin, *J Lab Clin Med* 115(2):267, 1990.
102. Shepherd J et al, for the West of Scotland Coronary Prevention Study Group: Prevention of coronary heart disease with pravastatin in men with hypercholesterolemia, *N Engl J Med* 333:1301, 1995.
103. Smith CK, Sheehan JP, Ulchaker MM: Diabetes mellitus. In Taylor RB, editor: *Fundamentals of family medicine,* New York, 1996, Springer.
104. Smith KC, Sheehan JP, Ulchaker MM: Diabetes mellitus. In Taylor RB, editor: *Family medicine: principles and practice,* ed 4, New York, 1993, Springer.
105. Smith KC, Sheehan JP, Ulchaker MM: Diabetes mellitus. In Taylor RB, editor: *Manual of family practice,* Boston, 1997, Little, Brown.
106. Streiff LD: Can clients understand our instructions? *Image J Nurs Sch* 18:48, 1986.
107. Syvanne M, Taskinen M: Lipids and lipoproteins as coronary risk factors in non–insulin-dependent diabetes mellitus, *Lancet* 350(suppl I):20, 1997.
108. Task Force to Revise the National Standards: National Standards for Diabetes Self-Management Education Programs, *Diabetes Care* 18(1):141, 1995.
109. Tattersall RB: Diabetes in the elderly—a neglected area, *Diabetologia* 27(2):167, 1984.
110. The Diabetes Control and Complications Trial Research Group: The effect of intensive treatment of diabetes on the long-term complications in insulin-dependent diabetes mellitus, *N Engl J Med* 329: 977, 1993.
111. The KROC collaborative study group: Blood glucose control and the evolution of diabetic retinopathy and albuminuria, *N Engl J Med* 311:364, 1984.
112. The Scandinavian Simvastatin Survival Study Group: Randomised trial of cholesterol lowering in 4444 patients with coronary heart disease: the Scandinavian Simvastatin Survival Study (4S), *Lancet* 344(8934):1383, 1994.
113. Tonino RP: Effect of physical training on the insulin resistance of aging, *Am J Physiol* 256(3 pt 1):E352, 1989.
114. Trobe JD: *The physician's guide to eye care,* San Francisco, 1993, American Academy of Ophthalmology.
115. UK Prospective Diabetes Study Group: UK prospective diabetes study XVI. Overview of 6 years' therapy of type 2 diabetes: a progressive disease, *Diabetes* 44(11):1249, 1995.
116. Ulchaker MM, Sheehan JP: Iatrogenic brittle diabetes: the hold-the-insulin decision, *Diabetes Educ* 17(2):111, 1991.
117. US Department of Agriculture/HNIS: *Food guide pyramid—a guide to daily food choices,* Washington, DC, 1992, USDA/HNIS.
118. US Department of Health and Human Services, US Public Health Service: *Diabetes in the United States: a strategy for prevention (map reference),* Washington, DC, 1992, National Center for Chronic Disease Control and Prevention, Division of Diabetes Translation, US Government Printing Office.
119. US Department of Health and Human Services, US Public Health Service: *Healthy people 2000: midcourse review and 1995 revisions,* Boston, 1995, Jones & Bartlett.
120. US Department of Agriculture, US Department of Health and Human Services: *Nutrition and your health: dietary guidelines for Americans,* ed 4, Hyattsville, Md, 1995, USDA Human Nutrition Information Service.
121. Vague J: The degree of masculine differentiation of obesities: a factor determining predisposition to diabetes, atherosclerosis, gout and uric calculour disease, *Am J Clin Nutr* 4:20, 1956.
122. Verlato G, Muggeo M, Bonora E, et al: Attending the diabetes center is associated with increased 5-year survival probability of diabetic patients: the Verona Diabetes Study, *Diabetes Care* 19(3):211, 1996.
123. Vinik AI, Milicevic Z: Recent advances in the diagnosis and treatment of diabetic neuropathy, *Endocrinologist* 6(6):443, 1996.
124. Weiner JP, Parente ST, Garnick DW, et al: Variation in office-based quality: a claims-based profile of care provided to Medicare patients with diabetes, *JAMA* 273(19):1503, 1995.
125. Wells S: Postoperative recovery: how diabetes complicates care, *J Cardiovasc Nurs* 7(4S):47, 1993.
126. Zimmet PZ, Alberti KGMM: The changing face of macrovascular disease in non–insulin-dependent diabetes mellitus: an epidemic in progress, *Lancet* 350(suppl I):1, 1997.

# chapter 36 ASSESSMENT OF THE Hepatic System

DEBERA JANE THOMAS

## objectives *After studying this chapter, the learner should be able to:*

1 Describe the normal anatomy and physiology of the liver.
2 Describe the role of the liver in metabolism and maintenance of energy balance.
3 Explain the basis for subjective and objective data that must be collected to identify problems of the hepatic system.
4 Relate the various laboratory and diagnostic tests used in identifying the pathophysiological states of the liver.
5 Synthesize a plan of care for patients undergoing the radiological and special tests used in diagnosing hepatic dysfunction.

The liver is the largest gland in the body and has 500 identified functions. Of primary importance is its role in metabolism and the maintenance of normal energy stores. Because the liver has so many functions, pathological conditions in the liver can cause a variety of problems that have an impact on the entire body.

## ANATOMY AND PHYSIOLOGY

### ANATOMY

The liver is one of the most complex organs in the body and weighs approximately 1.3 to 1.8 kg. The falciform ligament divides the liver into right and left lobes and provides attachment to the anterior abdominal wall (Figure 36-1).

The round ligament is a remnant of the umbilical vein and extends from the umbilicus to the inferior surface of the liver. Glisson capsule, a fibroelastic capsule containing blood vessels, lymphatics, and nerves, covers the liver.

Anatomically, the liver extends up under the ribs and is 4 to 8 cm in height at the midsternal line and 6 to 12 cm in height at the midclavicular line. The liver normally extends from the fifth intercostal space.

The liver is served by two separate blood supplies, and at any one time contains approximately 13% of the total blood supply of the body. The hepatic artery supplies oxygenated blood to the liver, and the portal vein carries nutrient-rich blood from the stomach and intestines. Approximately 75% of the blood flow is derived from the portal vein; thus the liver receives mostly unoxygenated blood (Figure 36-2). The remaining 25% is derived from the hepatic artery, which is highly oxygenated and supplies the hepatic cells.

The portal system is composed of veins, sinusoids, and hepatic veins, which drain the blood from the abdominal area of the digestive tract, spleen, pancreas, and gallbladder and carry it to the liver (Figure 36-3). Pressure in this system is normally 3 mm Hg.

The portal system empties into the inferior vena cava, which delivers blood to the right atrium. Portal hypertension is a rise in portal pressure to at least 10 mm Hg and can be caused by any disorder that obstructs or impedes blood flow through any portion of the portal system or vena cava. Elevated pressures in the portal system cause collateral vessels to open between the portal veins and the systemic veins, avoiding the obstructed portal vessels. These collateral vessels may develop in the esophagus, anterior abdominal wall, or rectum (Figure 36-3).

The liver is innervated by the sympathetic and parasympathetic nervous systems. Sympathetic fibers innervate the hepatic artery branches and the bile ducts. Parasympathetic innervation is supplied to the intrahepatic and extrahepatic biliary tract system. Stimulation of the sympathetic and parasympathetic nervous systems affects blood flow and the flow of bile within the biliary tract, but the function of the hepatic cells or parenchymal cells is not influenced.

The functional unit of the liver is the *liver lobule* (Figure 36-4). Each lobule is composed of multiple plates of hepatic cells. Between the individual cells of the cellular plate are biliary canaliculi, which empty into the bile ducts. The terminal bile ducts join to form the hepatic duct, which merges with the cystic duct of the gallbladder to form the common bile duct. Each side of the cellular plate contains a venous sinusoid, which receives blood from branches of the portal vein and hepatic artery. As blood flows through the sinusoids, substances can be exchanged between the hepatic cells and the blood.

The sinusoids are lined with phagocytic cells of the reticuloendothelial system (Kupffer cells). These cells remove bacteria and other foreign substances from the blood. Because the portal blood originates in the gastrointestinal (GI) tract, some bacteria or other foreign substances need to be removed.

The blood from the venous sinusoids empties into the central vein and then into the hepatic vein. The hepatic vein empties into the inferior vena cava.

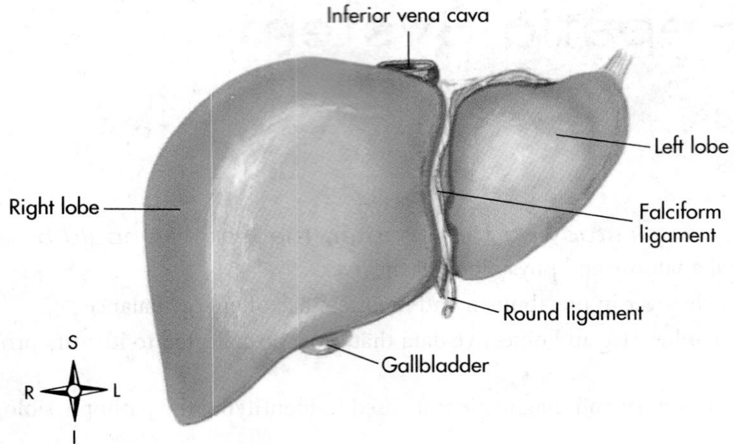


**fig. 36-1** Gross structure of the liver, anterior view.

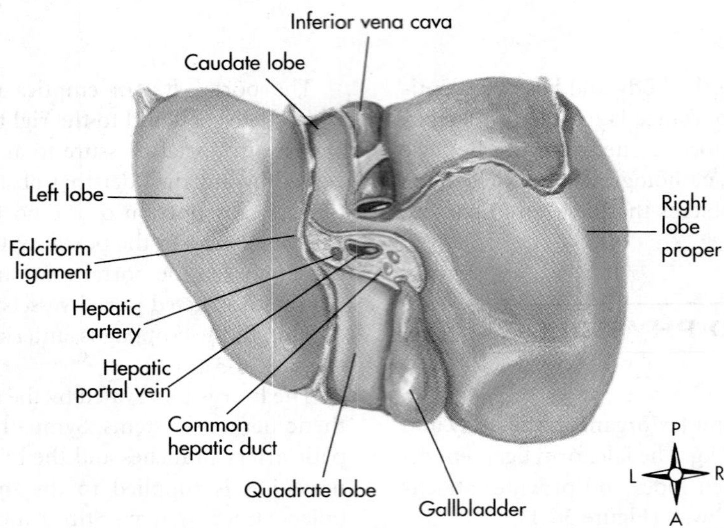


**fig. 36-2** Gross structure of the liver, inferior view.

## PHYSIOLOGY

The liver can be thought of as a metabolic factory and a waste disposal plant. As should be evident from the anatomical description of the blood and bile flow, the liver is ideally structured to carry out its multiple metabolic and waste disposal functions. The major functions of the liver are summarized in Box 36-1. Each of these functions is presented in more detail in the following sections.

### Carbohydrate, Protein, and Fat Metabolism

The liver has a significant role in the metabolism of each of the three major nutrients. The liver either oxidizes these components for energy, uses the nutrients to synthesize storage forms of substances for future use, or uses the nutrients to synthesize other essential compounds.

#### Carbohydrates

Immediately after meals, the liver extracts glucose, fructose, and galactose from the blood. These simple sugars are metabolized into glycogen *(glycogenesis)* to replenish liver stores. If the diet ingested is low in carbohydrates, the liver converts protein to glucose to replenish glycogen stores. If more carbohydrate is ingested than is needed to replenish glycogen stores or to supply energy, the excess carbohydrate is converted to fat *(lipogenesis)*. Between meals and during other fasting states, the liver assists in maintaining the blood glucose concentration. It does this by breaking down glycogen *(glycogenolysis)* or forming new glucose *(gluconeogenesis)*. The new glucose is made from amino acids, glycerol, and lactic acids. Through glycogenesis, lipogenesis, glycogenolysis, and gluconeogenesis processes, which are under hormonal control, the liver helps to maintain a normal blood glucose level, preventing high levels immediately after eating (postprandial) and hypoglycemia between meals or during other periods of fasting.

#### Proteins

The liver is vital to normal protein metabolism. It provides needed amino acids through transamination. *Transamination*

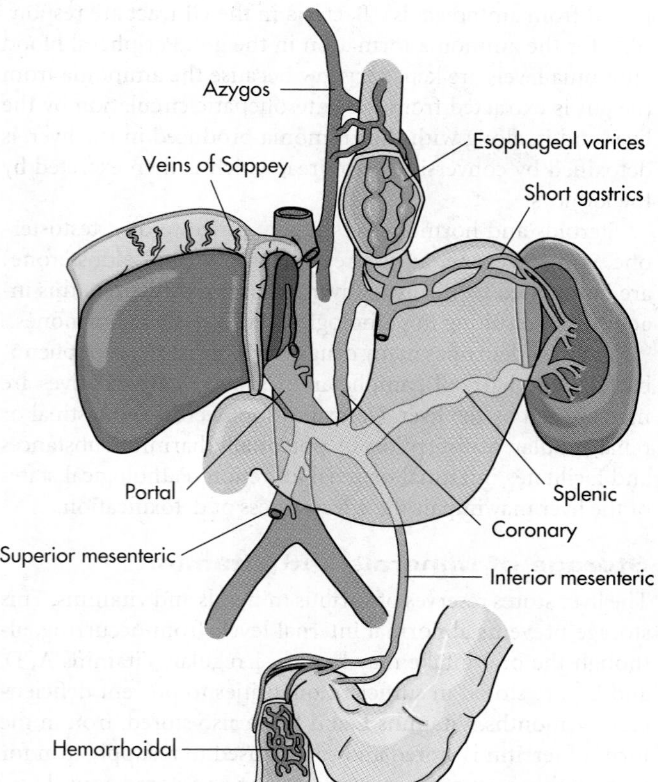


**fig. 36-3** Varices related to portal hypertension. Portal vein, its major tributaries, and the most important collateral veins between the portal and caval systems.

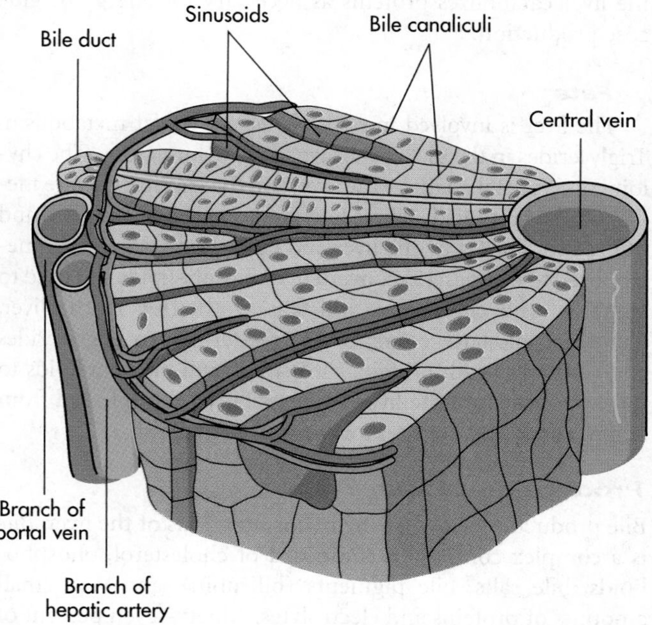


**fig. 36-4** Diagrammatical representation of a liver lobule. A central vein is located in the center of the lobule with plates of hepatic cells disposed radially. Branches of the portal vein and hepatic artery are located on the periphery of the lobule, and blood from both perfuses the sinusoids. Peripherally located bile ducts drain the bile canaliculi that run between the hepatocytes.

**box 36-1** *Summary of Liver Functions*

1. Carbohydrate, protein, and fat metabolism
   a. Carbohydrate metabolism
      (1) Glycogen formation and storage
      (2) Glucose formation from glycogen (glycogenolysis) and from amino acids, lactic acids, and glycerol (gluconeogenesis)
   b. Protein metabolism
      (1) Protein catabolism
      (2) Protein synthesis
         (a) Albumin
         (b) $\alpha$- and $\beta$-Globulins
         (c) Clotting factors
         (d) C-reactive protein
         (e) Transferrin
         (f) Enzymes
         (g) Ceruloplasmin
      (3) Formation of needed amino acids
   c. Fat metabolism
      (1) Oxidation of fatty acids for energy
      (2) Ketone formation
      (3) Synthesis of cholesterol and phospholipids
      (4) Formation of triglycerides from dietary lipids and excessive dietary carbohydrates and proteins
      (5) Formation of lipoproteins
2. Production of bile salts
3. Bilirubin metabolism
4. Detoxification of endogenous and exogenous substances
   a. Ammonia
   b. Steroids
   c. Drugs
5. Storage of minerals and vitamins
6. Blood reservoir

is the process of nitrogen metabolism in which the liver transfers an amino group ($NH_2$) to form nonessential amino acids. The liver also is the only source of some of the major plasma proteins. One of these major proteins is *albumin*, which is necessary for the maintenance of a normal internal environment and for fluid and electrolyte balance. Albumin, produced only in the liver, is responsible for maintaining colloid osmotic pressure and thus the proper distribution of fluids between the vascular and interstitial compartments.

The liver is the source of several clotting factors. It produces fibrinogen (factor I), prothrombin (factor II), factor V (proaccelerin), factor VII (serum prothrombin conversion accelerator), factor IX (Christmas factor), and factor X (Stuart or Stuart-Prower factor). The production of factors II, VII,

IX, and X requires vitamin K. Vitamin K is a fat-soluble vitamin and therefore requires adequate production and excretion of bile for its absorption. In addition to protein synthesis, the liver catabolizes proteins as necessary for energy or glucose production.

#### Fats

The liver is involved in multiple aspects of fat metabolism. Triglycerides in the diet are absorbed in chylomicrons. The chylomicrons are taken up by the liver, and the triglycerides are metabolized to fatty acids. These fatty acids may be (1) oxidized and utilized for energy by the liver and other body tissues; (2) metabolized to ketones; (3) converted to phospholipids; (4) used to combine with cholesterol, which is synthesized in the liver, to form cholesterol esters; or (5) reesterified to triglycerides and combined with protein, cholesterol, and phospholipids to form lipoproteins. The liver also uses fatty acids released from adipose tissue storage sites for these same processes.

### Production of Bile Salts

Bile production is one of the major functions of the liver. *Bile* is a complex compound composed of cholesterol, phospholipids, bile salts, bile pigments (bilirubin), and very small amounts of proteins and electrolytes. Ninety-seven percent of bile is water. Metabolites of drugs and other substances that need to be excreted may also be found in bile. Bile salts are necessary for the absorption of fats, cholesterol, and fat-soluble vitamins, particularly vitamin K. Bile is released from the liver and concentrated and stored in the gallbladder. The liver secretes approximately 700 ml of bile daily. The bile salts released during each meal are reabsorbed into the enterohepatic circulation and recycled two or three times during a meal. Bile is reabsorbed along the total intestinal tract, but the terminal ileum has a major role in its active reabsorption. If the terminal ileum is diseased or resected, reabsorption of bile does not occur and abnormal fat absorption results.

### Bilirubin Metabolism

Bilirubin is a byproduct of the heme portion of red blood cells and is released when these cells are destroyed. The released bilirubin is not water soluble (unconjugated). Unconjugated bilirubin is carried in the blood bound to albumin and other proteins. The liver extracts the unconjugated bilirubin from the blood and combines it with glucoronide into a water-soluble form (conjugated). The conjugated bilirubin is secreted into the bile and then enters the duodenum. In the GI tract, bilirubin is metabolized to urobilinogen. Urobilinogen is excreted in feces as stercobilin, giving feces its brown color, or it is reabsorbed. Most of the reabsorbed urobilinogen is extracted from the blood by the liver and recycled; some is excreted in the urine.

### Metabolic Detoxification

The liver has a prime role in metabolic detoxification or biotransformation of endogenous and exogenous substances. Ammonia ($NH_3$) is a major toxic product processed by the liver. Ammonia is produced in the gut and the liver from the deamination of amino acids (the removal of the amino group [$NH_2$] from amino acids). Bacteria in the GI tract are responsible for the ammonia formation in the gut. Peripheral blood ammonia levels are kept very low because the ammonia from the gut is extracted from the enterohepatic circulation by the liver and it, along with the ammonia produced in the liver, is detoxified by conversion into urea, which is then excreted by the kidneys.

Steroids and hormones (estrogen, progesterone, testosterone, corticosterone, antidiuretic hormone, and aldosterone) are inactivated by the liver. Liver diseases may depress this inactivation, resulting in pathological levels of these hormones.

The liver detoxifies many drugs; barbiturates (except phenobarbital and barbital), amphetamines, and many sedatives are metabolized by the liver. Detoxification decreases intestinal or renal tubular reabsorption of potentially harmful substances and facilitates intestinal or renal excretion. Pathological states of the liver may impair the effectiveness of detoxification.

### Storage of Minerals and Vitamins

The liver stores reserves of various minerals and vitamins. This storage prevents abnormal internal levels from occurring, although the oral intake may be very irregular. Vitamins A, D, and $B_{12}$ are stored in sufficient quantities to prevent deficiencies for months. Vitamins E and K are also stored. Iron in the form of ferritin is stored and can be used to resupply iron for hemoglobin formation as needed; copper is stored as well.

### Blood Reservoir

The liver, because of its tremendous vascular supply and sinusoidal system, can act as a reservoir for blood. When the venous vascular volume becomes greater than can be handled by the right side of the heart, the excess blood can be stored in the liver. In the event of hemorrhage, the liver can release blood to maintain systemic circulatory volume.

## PHYSIOLOGICAL CHANGES WITH AGING

As the body ages, the number and size of hepatic cells decrease, which results in an overall decrease in the size and weight of the liver. Conversely, the formation of fibrous tissue within the liver increases, resulting in decreased protein synthesis and possible changes in the production of enzymes that assist in the metabolism of drugs, particularly anticonvulsants, psychotropic drugs, and oral anticoagulants. The nurse should be alert to the signs and symptoms of drug toxicity even when the drugs are administered in normal doses because the decreased metabolism in the liver can cause an accumulation of the drug. (See the Gerontological Assessment Box). Although age-related changes in the hepatic system have not been fully studied, the common liver function tests usually show normal results in elderly persons unless a pathological condition exists.

## SUBJECTIVE DATA

A thorough history is necessary to assess adequately the health status of people with potential dysfunction of the hepatic system. These data assist in identifying immediate nursing needs and providing information necessary for helping patients to live with chronic problems of the hepatic system. Assessment focuses on comfort status; nutritional status; fluid and electrolyte status; elimination patterns; energy level; perception, motion, and cognition; and potential exposure to toxins, as well as general living conditions and lifestyle.

## COMFORT STATUS

Discomfort resulting from abdominal pain or *pruritus* (itching) may be one of the major problems of people with hepatic dysfunction. The person may complain of continuous upper abdominal discomfort or a dull ache in the upper right quadrant. The discomfort does not usually alter normal functioning, although it can cause ineffective breathing secondary to the abdominal pain. The discomfort is most significant in that it provides verification for the underlying pathological process. Comfort status may be altered because of the general body aching associated with acute viral infections of the hepatic system. Most distressing to the patient is the pruritus usually associated with jaundice, which may cause significant discomfort. The elevated serum bilirubin that occurs with jaundice causes capillary dilation in the skin, the source of the pruritus. In addition, bilirubin is an irritating substance to the chemosensitive area of the skin. The history should include an assessment of factors that worsen itching and of measures that help relieve it.

## NUTRITIONAL STATUS

People with hepatic dysfunction often experience alterations in nutritional status. Some hepatic problems result in anorexia, nausea, and vomiting. The patient should be questioned about the occurrence of such episodes. Assessment should include onset, precipitating factors, association with food or alcohol intake, and measures that provide relief.

Poor nutritional habits and malnutrition resulting from lifestyle patterns or food intolerances may be present. A useful method to assess the patient's nutritional status is to ask the patient what he or she has eaten in the past 24 hours and ascertain whether this is the typical eating pattern.

Alcohol use should also be assessed. Alcohol, which provides calories but has no nutrient value, may hide weight loss normally associated with malnutrition. In the case of chronic alcohol use, muscle mass may have decreased while the overall weight remained stable. In addition, weight loss may be masked by water retention.

People with chronic problems of the hepatic system often require treatment with special diets, such as low sodium, altered protein intake, and water restriction. The history should include information about food intolerances and food preferences.

## FLUID AND ELECTROLYTE STATUS

Hepatic dysfunction can be associated with volume deficit from nausea and vomiting or from acute bleeding with cirrhosis. Fluid volume excess typically occurs in people with hepatic dysfunction as a result of renal retention of sodium and water that is initiated by peripheral vasodilation. This expansion of the vascular space effectively decreases the circulating blood volume, which results in the release of renin, angiotensin, and aldosterone. These hormones increase sodium and water retention.

Another factor causing fluid volume excess is the hypoalbuminemia that is associated with liver disease. The hypoalbuminemia decreases the osmotic pressure in the vasculature, causing fluid to leave the vascular space and enter the interstitial space, resulting in edema. Levels of electrolytes, particularly sodium, potassium, hydrogen, and bicarbonate, can be elevated or decreased.

To establish the patient's needs, the history collected should include information about:

1. Normal fluid and food intake and output
2. Abnormal fluid and electrolyte losses, such as vomiting, diarrhea, or bleeding
3. Changes in weight, both losses and gains
4. Occurrence of signs and symptoms of fluid or electrolyte deficit, such as weakness, dizziness, syncope, and weight loss
5. Occurrence of signs and symptoms of fluid or electrolyte excess, such as edema in hands, feet, and legs; an increase in abdominal girth; and weight gain.

## ELIMINATION PATTERNS

Intestinal and urinary elimination may be altered in people with liver problems. If there is an obstruction of bile flow, the person may give a history of grayish-white or clay-colored stools and have dark amber, brown, or mahogany-colored urine. Blood in the urine or stools may be present. The nurse can test for occult blood in the urine by using a reagent strip and test the stool by performing a Hematest or guaiac test. A reported decrease in urine output or the occurrence of nocturia may result from sodium and water retention.

### gerontological assessment

**ASSESSMENT**

**Monitor Effects of Medications**

- Older patients seem to have more problems with both the therapeutic effects of medications and drug toxicity. This may be due in part to the decrease in hepatic circulation that accompanies aging as well as the decrease in the enzyme activity of the liver.
- Standard doses of medication published in a formulary may be too high for elderly patients. Most drug dosages are calculated for healthy white adult men.
- Polypharmacy occurs when the elderly patient receives multiple medications from multiple prescribers.

**Assess Nutritional Status**

- Because the liver has many functions that aim to maintain energy stores and metabolism, the elderly patient may show signs of fatigue if liver function has diminished enough to limit the available energy needed to support activities of daily living.

**COMMON DISORDERS IN ELDERS**

- Increased risk for drug toxicity
- Polypharmacy
- Malnutrition

### ENERGY LEVEL

Because of altered nutrient intake, abnormal fluid and electrolyte status, and increased metabolic needs, people with hepatic problems often report an activity intolerance to normal daily activities or simply fatigue. Weakness may be reported, and nursing care should be adjusted to provide for the patient's safety. As the underlying liver condition resolves, the fatigue and weakness may resolve. However, the patient and family must understand that the energy level may take a long time to return to normal.

### PERCEPTION, MOTION, AND COGNITION

Chronic health problems of the hepatic system can cause changes in neurological functioning, particularly in relation to the peripheral nervous system and higher cognitive functions. The patient should be asked about alterations in sensation in extremities, any noticeable changes in memory, episodes of forgetfulness or blackouts, and alterations in coordination or in the ability to do fine motor tasks. The onset of any alterations, pattern of changes (continuous or intermittent), and duration of any changes should be determined.

### EXPOSURE TO TOXINS

Hepatic dysfunction can be caused by various agents, such as alcohol, drugs, industrial chemicals, and viruses. A history of exposure to any toxins must be elicited. A drug and alcohol history is necessary to determine whether the patient has been exposed to these two hepatotoxins.

The drug history should focus on prescription, over-the-counter, and street drugs. For example, acetaminophen is a drug often used by adolescents to commit suicide and can cause severe liver damage in doses 10 times greater than the recommended dose. The liver damage is intensified by the combination of acetaminophen and alcohol. The alcohol history should focus on normal amount of intake and time since last intake. An occupational history helps to identify potential toxins in the work environment such as methylene chloride solvents. An environmental/social history might identify potential sources of viruses (see Box 36-2 for significant sources of contact with the hepatitis viruses). The environmental/social history also can help identify particular persons, factors, or places associated with substance abuse, if a problem exists. Data about persons, factors, or places associated with substance abuse are needed for long-term management of drug and alcohol abuse (see Chapter 14).

**box 36-2** *Health History Necessary to Identify Exposure to Hepatitis Viruses*

- Contact with persons with jaundice
- Travel or visits to environments with poor sanitation (e.g., camping trips, travel to developing countries)
- Ingestion of shellfish or raw fish
- History of recent ear or body piercing or tattooing
- History of recent blood transfusions
- Intravenous drug abuse (sharing of contaminated needles)
- Occupational exposure (e.g., health service personnel with frequent blood contact, personnel in daycare centers, personnel in centers of custodial care)
- History of hemodialysis
- History of multiple sex partners; male bisexual or male homosexual lifestyle

## OBJECTIVE DATA

To assess the functioning of the hepatic system completely, a thorough assessment of the total body is required. First, examination of the overall appearance of the patient is necessary. Does the patient appear chronically or acutely ill? Is the individual attentive, restless, or lethargic? Does the person appear nourished or malnourished? Is the skin jaundiced? Are the sclerae yellow? In a darker-skinned person, are the palms of the hands or soles of the feet jaundiced? Are the oral mucous membranes yellow? Are there any other signs of hepatic dysfunction, such as enlarged abdomen, palmar erythema, change in secondary sexual characteristics, bruises, muscle wasting, or edema? Petechiae and spider angiomas, usually on the nose, cheeks, or upper thorax, may be present.

After the general inspection, the assessment should focus on fluid status. Vital signs, including orthostatic changes, weight, temperature, skin turgor, mucous membrane moisture, presence of edema, and behavior changes should be assessed. To assess energy level and nutritional status, the patient's total muscle mass and muscle strength should be examined.

While performing the assessment note the patient's mental status, affect, and alertness. Note changes in facial expression, responsiveness, level of consciousness, and affect. Are there periods of confusion or disorientation? Is the affect appropriate for this situation? Because handwriting or the ability to draw a box, triangle, or square deteriorates with decreasing liver function, a sample of handwriting or a drawing of a geometric figure may be obtained from the patient.

After a general impression of the total patient is obtained, the assessment should focus on the abdomen. The abdomen is inspected for enlargement, presence of distended or dilated periumbilical veins (caput medusae), and ascites. *Ascites* is characterized by distention of the abdomen with tight, glistening skin, protruding umbilicus, and bulging flanks. Palpate or percuss the abdomen to ascertain the presence of a fluid wave and shifting dullness, which are indicative of ascites. Palpation and percussion are also used to assess for hepatic tenderness, size, and consistency and the presence of hepatic masses. The spleen often is enlarged in the patient with chronic hepatic dysfunction and should be percussed to determine the size and location; defer palpation because of the fragility of the enlarged spleen. Last, measure abdominal girth. Hemorrhoids caused by prolonged elevations in portal system pressure may be present.

## DIAGNOSTIC TESTS

Various tests help in assessing the status of the hepatic system. Many of the tests require taking samples of blood; other tests are more extensive and may cause discomfort; still others may require fasting. The nurse is responsible for preparing the patient for the tests. The physical preparation of the patient will vary from institution to institution, and the nurse must know the routine preparation. In addition to the physical preparation, the nurse carries out appropriate teaching and monitoring of the patient before, during, and after the diagnostic tests.

## LABORATORY TESTS

Multiple tests may be necessary to determine the extent and seriousness of hepatic disease. To be of benefit many tests require serial readings. The procedure, preparation, and interpretation of blood, stool, and urine studies used to evaluate liver function are summarized in Table 36-1.

## RADIOLOGICAL TESTS

Radiographic tests are used to assist in identifying the cause of hepatic dysfunction. Besides the examinations described in the following section, abdominal films, barium swallow, barium enema, and gastroscopy may be ordered (see Chapter 38). These tests help identify the presence of pathological GI conditions that may cause signs and symptoms similar to those found in hepatic dysfunction.

### Ultrasonography

Ultrasonography of the liver is done to assess jaundice of unknown etiology, hepatomegaly, or suspected tumors. Additional information obtained from ultrasound includes liver size, shape, and location; cysts; abscesses; and filling or dilation defects.

The preparation of the patient for ultrasonography is relatively simple. Usually the patient is not allowed to eat for 8 to 12 hours before the procedure, because bowel gas in the GI tract will interfere with the test. Any residual barium needs to be eliminated from the GI tract before the test. The patient must be well hydrated, because dehydration can decrease the ability of ultrasonography to distinguish between the liver and surrounding tissues.

### Computed Tomography Scan

Computed tomography (CT) scanning can also be used to assess patients with potential hepatic problems. It is helpful in identifying problems similar to those described for ultrasonography. Contrast medium can be used with the CT scan to intensify the appearance of vascular structures and hepatic parenchyma. The patient should eat nothing for 8 to 12 hours before the test; if contrast medium is to be used, the patient should be assessed for allergies to iodine or contrast media. Adequate hydration is necessary when a contrast medium is used. Barium studies should be done at least 4 days before the CT scan or after the scan because the barium can interfere with test results.

### Magnetic Resonance Imaging

Magnetic resonance imaging (MRI) is used to detect liver tumors. Because magnetic fields are used instead of radioactive isotopes to produce the image, no special preparation of the patient is necessary. It is important to inform the patient that this test is painless. The patient should be instructed to remove any jewelry, dentures and partial dentures if they contain metal, or any other item that contains metal, such as hairpins or limb prostheses. Patients should be assessed for claustrophobia before the procedure, because it may elicit this type of response. Contraindications to MRI include a pacemaker and titanium or stainless steel prosthetic implants or prosthetic heart valves.

### Radionuclide Imaging

The liver may be outlined by radionuclide imaging techniques. Selected radioisotopes are given intravenously. After the injection of the radioisotope, the patient is placed in the supine position, and a scintillation detector is passed over the abdomen in the area of the liver. The radiation coming from the isotopes immediately beneath the probe of the scanner is detected, amplified, and recorded. Scanning helps differentiate nonfunctioning areas from normal tissue and to identify hepatic tumors, cysts, and abscesses. Usually a nonfunctioning area will appear as an area of decreased activity. However, gallium-67 ($^{67}$Ga) is preferentially taken up by hepatocellular carcinomas and abscesses, and these areas will appear as areas of very heavy radioactivity. Adverse reactions to the radioisotopes used for radionuclide imaging are unusual, and the procedure is relatively safe. Discomfort is minimal. Only small amounts of radioactive material are given, and radiation precautions are *not* necessary. Only $^{67}$Ga scanning requires special preparation. $^{67}$Ga is excreted by the GI tract. To avoid absorption of the radioisotope by the GI contents, laxatives and enemas are prescribed. The toilet should be flushed twice for bowel movements after the $^{67}$Ga scanning to ensure the safety of the patient and others. Ultrasonography, CT scanning, and MRI have replaced radionuclide imaging in most instances of hepatic dysfunction.

### Angiography and Portal Pressure Measurements

Catheterization of the hepatic artery, portal venous system (by various routes), and hepatic vein allows the injection of a contrast medium and the visualization of the vascular supply of the hepatic system. Angiography determines the patency of the system and the presence of tumors, abscesses, collateral circulation, varices, and bleeding.

Portal and hepatic vein pressure (wedged hepatic vein pressure) can be measured. These readings may be done in conjunction with angiography or as a separate study. These measurements help in determining the degree of portal hypertension.

The presence of allergy to contrast media must be ascertained before angiography is done. After both angiography and pressure readings, the insertion site is observed for bleeding, and the patient's vital signs are checked every 15 minutes for 1 hour, every 30 minutes for 1 hour, every hour for 4 hours, and then if the patient is stable, every 4 hours. Bedrest is maintained for 24 to 48 hours after the test.

## SPECIAL TESTS

### Biopsy of the Liver

A liver biopsy may be used to aid in establishing the cause of liver disease. In this procedure a specially designed needle is inserted through the chest or abdominal wall into the liver,

**table 36-1** *Laboratory Tests of Liver Function*

| FUNCTION AND TEST | PROCEDURE AND PREPARATION | INTERPRETATION |
|---|---|---|
| **Fat metabolism** | | |
| Serum total cholesterol and cholesterol esters | Venipuncture; fasting may be required | Normal level is 140-220 mg/dl of blood; approximately 70% is cholesterol ester; in hepatocellular disease, amount of total serum cholesterol and cholesterol ester may be decreased; in obstructive biliary tract disease, total serum cholesterol is increased, but amount of esterified cholesterol is decreased; normal cholesterol levels rise with age. |
| Serum phospholipids | Venipuncture; no special preparation | Normal level is 150-250 mg/dl; serum phospholipids tend to be low in severe hepatocellular disease and high in obstructive biliary tract disease. |
| **Protein metabolism** | | |
| Total serum protein | Venipuncture; no special preparation | Normal level is 6-8 g/dl; measures all serum protein; may be normal in hepatocellular disease because increased serum globulin will replace decreased serum albumin; increased serum globulin is seen in chronic inflammatory disease, neoplastic diseases, and biliary obstruction. |
| Albumin | Venipuncture; no special preparation | Normal level is 3.4-5.0 g/dl; albumin made only in liver; in hepatocellular disease there may be a decrease in serum albumin level. |
| Protein electrophoresis | Venipuncture; no special preparation; protein fraction of blood will migrate in characteristic directions in electrical field; after separation of fractions, specimen stained, and densitometer used to measure amounts of various serum protein | Normal fractions in relation to total serum protein (100%) are albumin, 52-68%; $\alpha$-globulins, 12-17%; $\beta$-globulins, 7-15%; and immune serum globulins ($\gamma$-globulins), 9-19%; in severe hepatocellular damage, amount of albumin may be decreased; inflammatory processes of the liver may produce increased amounts of $\alpha_1$-globulins, neoplastic disease is associated with increased levels of $\alpha_2$-globulins, and some patients with obstructive biliary tract disease may have high levels of $\beta$-globulins. |
| Immunoglobulins | Venipuncture; no special preparation | Five classes of antibodies: IgA, IgG, IgM, IgF, and IgD; IgA and IgG are often increased in the presence of cirrhosis; IgG is elevated in the presence of chronic active hepatitis; biliary cirrhosis and hepatitis A cause an increase in the IgM component. |
| Blood urea nitrogen (BUN) | Venipuncture; no special preparation | Normal is 10-20 mg/dl; in severe hepatocellular disease if portal venous flow is obstructed, level may decrease; varies with dietary protein intake and fluid volume. |
| Serum prothrombin time (PT) | Venipuncture; no special preparation; reflects activity of extrinsic and common coagulation pathways, including prothrombin, fibrinogen, and factors V, VII, IX, and X | Normal PT is 12-15 sec; it is compared with a control level; the normal PT is calculated based on the institution's control and therefore may differ between institutions; may be expressed as International Normalized Ratio (INR); PT reflects activity of extrinsic and common coagulation pathways, including prothrombin, fibrinogen, and factors V, VII, IX, and X; PT may be increased in hepatocellular disease because of the inability of liver to produce clotting factors or in obstructive hepatic or biliary tract disease because of the malabsorption of vitamin K; persistence of abnormal PT after parenteral administration of vitamin K indicates hepatocellular damage. |
| Serum partial thromboplastin time (PTT) and activated partial thromboplastin time (APTT) | Venipuncture; no special preparation; reflects activity of intrinsic and common coagulation pathways | Normal PTT is 68-82 sec with standard technique, APTT is 32-46 sec; as with the PT, the normal value may differ between institutions depending on the control used; PTT reflects activity of intrinsic and common coagulation pathways; PTT and APTT will be increased in hepatocellular disease because of the inability of liver to produce clotting factors. |

*Continued*

**table 36-1** *Laboratory Tests of Liver Function—cont'd*

| FUNCTION AND TEST | PROCEDURE AND PREPARATION | INTERPRETATION |
|---|---|---|
| Blood ammonia levels | Venipuncture; may require fasting | Normal level is less than 75 μg/dl; may be elevated in severe hepatocellular disease because of obstruction of portal blood flow and rarely because of decreased urea synthesis. |
| Bilirubin metabolism | | |
| Total bilirubin<br>Conjugated (direct)<br>Unconjugated (indirect) | Venipuncture, no special preparation | Total serum bilirubin measures both conjugated and unconjugated bilirubin; normal total serum bilirubin values range from 0.1-1 mg/dl; conjugated bilirubin acts directly with diazo reagents; unconjugated bilirubin requires addition of methyl alcohol; thus the terms *direct* and *indirect;* conjugated bilirubin increases in the presence of hepatocellular or obstructive biliary tract disease; unconjugated bilirubin is elevated in the presence of increased hemolysis of red blood cells or hepatocellular disease. |
| Urine bilirubin | Spot urine specimen; no special preparation | Normally no bilirubin is excreted in urine; urine with abnormal bilirubin is mahogany colored and has a yellow foam when shaken *(foam test)*; unconjugated bilirubin even in excess is not excreted in urine because it is not water soluble; conjugated serum bilirubin levels greater than 0.4 mg/dl will lead to conjugated bilirubin being excreted in urine because it is water soluble and indicates hepatocellular or obstructive biliary tract disease; bilirubinuria may be present before jaundice. |
| Urine urobilinogen | 24-hr urine collection or 2-hr afternoon collection | Normally 0.2-1.2 units found in specimen; fresh urine urobilinogen is colorless; decreased amounts of urine urobilinogen found in obstructive biliary tract disease; increased amounts found in hepatocellular disease; alterations in intestinal flora by broad-spectrum antibiotics may change test. |
| Fecal urobilinogen | Stool specimen; no special preparation | Normally 90-280 mg/day; presence of fecal urobilinogen (stercobilin) gives stool brown color; absence of stercobilin causes stools to become clay (grayish white) to white colored; increased amounts of stercobilin found with increased hemolysis of red blood cells; absence of fecal stercobilin indicates obstructive biliary tract disease. |
| Serum enzymes | | |
| Asparate aminotransferase (AST), formerly called serum glutamic-oxaloacetic transaminase (SGOT)<br>Alanine aminotransferase (ALT), formerly called serum glutamic pyruvic transaminase (SGPT)<br>Lactic dehydrogenase (LDH)<br>γ-Glutamyl transpeptidase (GGT) (γ-glutamyltransferase) | Venipuncture; no special preparation | Normal values vary depending on measurement used; these enzymes are present in hepatic cells; with necrosis of hepatic cells, enzymes are released and elevated serum levels will be found; GGT is found in high levels in liver cells as well as kidneys; ALT is primarily present in liver cells; AST is also present in high levels in skeletal and heart muscle; LDH is also present in heart cells, kidney cells, skeletal muscle cells, and erythrocytes, but in each tissue the LDH enzyme has a characteristic composition: thus the tissue source of elevated serum LDH levels can be determined by isoenzyme tests; with the other three enzyme tests, necrosis of other organs must be ruled out; GGT is elevated early in liver disease, and elevation persists as long as cellular damage continues; GGT is routinely elevated in alcohol-induced liver disease, and increased levels are often seen before other abnormal test results occur. |

*Continued*

**table 36-1** *Laboratory Tests of Liver Function—cont'd*

| Function and Test | Procedure and Preparation | Interpretation |
|---|---|---|
| Alkaline phosphatase | Venipuncture; no special preparation | Normal values vary depending on measurement used; this enzyme originates in liver, bone, intestine, and placenta; alkaline phosphatase is slightly to moderately elevated in hepatocellular disease but extremely elevated in obstructive biliary tract and bone disease. |
| Antigens and antibodies of viral hepatitis | Venipuncture; no special preparation | Normally, no hepatitis antigens are found in the serum or other body fluids; *hepatitis A virus (HAV)* can be found in the stool during the last part of the incubation period and early prodromal phase; *IgM-class anti-HAV* appears in the acute and early convalescent period and is used to diagnose hepatitis A; *IgG-class anti-HAV* becomes detectable during the convalescent period and confers immunity; hepatitis B has many associated serum particles; complete *hepatitis B virus (HBV)* is also called Dane particle; a *core antigen ($HB_cAg$)* can be found in the liver, an *antibody (anti-$HB_c$)* can be found in the blood, and the presence of anti-$HB_c$ indicates past infection with HBV at some undefined time; a *surface antigen ($HB_sAg$)* and several subtypes and *antibody (anti-$HB_s$)* are also measurable; $HB_sAg$ is one of the antigens measured to diagnose hepatitis B, and its presence indicates infectivity; presence of anti-$HB_s$ indicates past infection and immunity to HBV, presence of passive antibodies from HBIG, or immune response from HBV vaccine; *hepatitis $B_e$ antigen ($HB_eAg$)* indicates high infectivity and its *antibody (anti-$HB_e$)* chronic infectivity; enzyme-linked immunosorbent assay (ELISA) has detected antibodies to hepatitis C (*anti-HCV*) in people who have been exposed to hepatitis C; however, the antibodies do not appear in most people until at least 5 months after exposure to the virus; an enterically transmitted virus that was previously related to hepatitis non-A non-B has been identified and labeled *hepatitis E (HEV); anti-HEV* has been detected using ELISA but is not available in the United States at this time.[1-3,5] |

and a small piece of tissue is removed for study. This procedure is contraindicated in a patient who has an infection of the right lower lobe of the lung, ascites, a blood dyscrasia, or a problem with blood clotting, as well as in any patient unable to cooperate by holding his or her breath. To avoid hemorrhage, vitamin K may be given parenterally for several days before and after the biopsy is performed. A biopsy usually is not done if the prothrombin time is below 40% of normal. The physician should explain the procedure to the patient, for example, the importance of being able to hold one's breath and remain absolutely still when the needle is introduced. Movement of the chest may cause the needle to slip and to tear the liver covering. Most hospitals require that the patient sign a written permission form for the procedure to be done. Food and fluids may be withheld for several hours preceding the test, and a sedative usually is given about 30 minutes before the biopsy.

A *liver biopsy* is performed as follows. The patient lies supine; the skin over the area selected (usually the eighth or ninth intercostal space) is cleansed and anesthetized with procaine hydrochloride. A nick is made in the skin with a sharp scalpel blade. Then the patient is instructed to take several deep breaths and then to hold his or her breath while the needle is introduced through the intercostal or subcostal tissues into the liver. The special needle assembly is rotated to separate a fragment of tissue and then is withdrawn. The specimen is placed into an appropriate container, which is labeled and sent to the pathology laboratory. A simple dressing is placed over the wound.

The dangers of liver biopsy are accidental penetration of blood vessels, causing hemorrhage, or accidental penetration of a biliary canniculi, causing a chemical peritonitis from leakage of bile into the abdominal cavity. After the procedure the nurse should assess the patient for signs of hypovolemia and shock. The patient's pulse and blood pressure should be monitored every 30 minutes for the first few hours after the procedure and then hourly for 24 hours. The patient's temperature should be taken at least every 4 hours to determine a baseline and detect peritonitis. The physician may order pressure applied to the biopsy site to help stop any bleeding. An effective way to apply pressure is to have the patient lie on the right side with a small pillow or folded bath blanket placed under the costal margin for several hours after the biopsy. Bedrest is maintained for 24 hours after the test.

### Paracentesis

A *paracentesis,* or peritoneal tap, can be done to remove peritoneal fluid (ascitic fluid) for cytological or other laboratory studies or to drain large volumes of ascitic fluid. When conditions such as respiratory distress, severe abdominal discomfort, or cardiac dysfunction are present because of the ascites, a paracentesis may be necessary. Repeated paracenteses are not the treatment of choice for controlling chronic, recurring ascites because of complications.

When paracentesis is performed, the skin is cleansed, and the abdominal wall is anesthetized. A long aspiration needle is inserted, and fluid is aspirated for diagnostic tests or drained as necessary. In preparation for the procedure, the patient is given a complete explanation and signs a consent form; the patient should void immediately before the procedure to diminish the risk of puncturing the bladder. Sterile technique must be maintained during the procedure.

The complications of paracentesis include peritonitis, if sterility is not maintained, and peritoneal bleeding resulting from trauma to blood vessels. The patient's vital signs, including temperature, urine output, and skin temperature and moisture, should be monitored for signs of peritonitis or bleeding. The patient's abdomen should be assessed for rigidity and his or her sensorium for confusion.

Removal of large amounts of fluid from the peritoneal space can result in hypovolemia and shock because additional fluid can shift from the intravascular compartment into the peritoneal cavity; this risk is minimal in the patient with cirrhosis and edema. Protein and potassium are commonly lost during paracentesis. The patient should be monitored for hypovolemia after the procedure. Data to be assessed include vital signs, mental status, urine output, skin temperature and moisture, and status of mucous membranes. Protein and potassium levels should also be monitored.

### Peritoneal Lavage

Peritoneal lavage may be used to assess damage to the liver from abdominal trauma in persons with altered states of consciousness who cannot give a satisfactory history. It may also be used in patients with abdominal trauma when unexplained hypotension is present, when unreliable physical examination results are present, or when the patient requires general anesthesia for other injuries.

Peritoneal lavage can be done by either the closed or open method. In the *closed method,* a peritoneal dialysis catheter is inserted, and the peritoneal space is aspirated for gross blood. If no gross blood is found, lavage is carried out with normal saline. In the *open method* the peritoneum is exposed completely and then opened enough to allow entry of a dialysis catheter. Again, gross blood is aspirated first, and if no blood is found, lavage is carried out.

Peritoneal lavage requires a complete explanation to the patient and significant others and informed consent. A nasogastric tube and Foley catheter are inserted before the procedure to prevent penetration of the intestines or bladder. In the closed method a local anesthetic is used, whereas in the open method general anesthesia is necessary. Postprocedural care involves monitoring for peritonitis and bleeding in patients who have closed peritoneal lavage. Patients who have open peritoneal lavage require general postanesthetic care (see Chapter 20).

## ENDOSCOPY

The hepatic system and gallbladder can be examined by several types of endoscopic procedures. The endoscope can be inserted directly through the peritoneum (peritoneoscopy), thus affording direct visualization of the abdominal organs and the taking of biopsy specimens. Esophagoscopy and gastroscopy can be used to diagnose esophageal varices or to perform injection sclerotherapy. An endoscopic retrograde cholangiopancreatography (ERCP) can be done to visualize and provide radiographic examination of the liver, gallbladder, and pancreas (see Chapter 38). All these procedures require that the patient be fasting at least 12 hours before the test. Before ERCP the patient should be asked about allergies or sensitivities to x-ray dye.

After the procedure, the nurse should assess the patient's ability to swallow. The patient's gag reflex may not return for 1 to 2 hours. After ERCP the patient should be monitored for signs of complications, which include perforation, sepsis, and pancreatitis. Vital signs are usually taken every 30 minutes and then hourly for 4 hours. IV sedation is frequently used during endoscopic procedures.

## chapter SUMMARY

### ANATOMY AND PHYSIOLOGY

- The liver is important for adequate energy production and waste disposal.

### SUBJECTIVE DATA

- Pathophysiological conditions of the liver result in discomfort, inadequate nutrition, fluid and electrolyte deficit or excess, bleeding, altered elimination, fatigue, and altered perception, cognitive, and motor functioning.

### OBJECTIVE DATA

- Pathophysiological conditions of the liver can result from exposure to various toxins, including drugs, alcohol, chemicals, and viruses.

## DIAGNOSTIC TESTS

- Liver dysfunction results in multiple abnormalities in blood studies that are used to help identify the pathophysiological state or other nursing needs.
- Radiologic, endoscopic, and other invasive tests are used to help in identifying the exact pathophysiological condition.

## References

1. American Medical Association: *Prevention, diagnosis, and management of viral hepatitis,* Chicago, 1996, AMA: Division of Health Science.
2. McMillan-Jackson M, Rymer TE: Viral hepatitis: anatomy of a diagnosis, *Am J Nurs* 94(1):43-48, 1994.
3. Moseley RH: Approach to the patient with abnormal liver chemistries. In Kelley WN, editor: *Textbook of internal medicine,* ed 3, Philadelphia, 1997, Lippincott–Raven.
4. Renkes J: GI endoscopy: managing the full scope of care, *Nursing 93* 23(6):50-55, 1993.
5. Siconolfi LA: Clarifying the complexity of liver function tests, *Nursing 95* 25(5):39-44, 1995.

chapter

# 37 MANAGEMENT OF PERSONS WITH Problems of the Hepatic System

DEBERA JANE THOMAS

## objectives *After studying this chapter, the learner should be able to:*

1 Anticipate the nursing care needs of patients with focal hepatocellular disorders.
2 Apply concepts of the pathophysiology of a variety of liver disorders to determine the signs and symptoms of each hepatic problem.
3 Contrast the differences between hepatitis A, B, C, D, and E.
4 Analyze the differences between toxic hepatitis and viral hepatitis.
5 Describe the pathophysiological basis for the clinical manifestations of cirrhosis and its complications.
6 Develop a plan of care for patients with diffuse hepatocellular disorders.

Because the liver is so complex and has so many functions, it is affected by many disorders that produce a variety of physiological and psychosocial problems for patients. The degree of illness in people with liver disease can range from critical, requiring intensive nursing care, to chronic, requiring home care. Some people with chronic liver disease require nursing interventions to assist them in making necessary changes in their lives that will help them control the problem and prevent disease progression. Some patients with chronic problems will have acute exacerbations when they will need intensive, total care. As the patient's condition is stabilized, the focus of nursing care is to promote self-management skills.

Severe liver problems can result from a variety of causes such as infective organisms, neoplastic growths, toxic agents, and trauma. The pathological states that result can be classified in several ways. In this chapter, disorders are classified as *focal hepatocellular disorders* (localized to one portion of the liver) and *diffuse hepatocellular disorders* (spread through a major portion of the liver) (Box 37-1).

## FOCAL HEPATOCELLULAR DISORDERS

Three of the more common focal hepatocellular disorders are discussed next.

### LIVER ABSCESS

#### Etiology

Liver abscesses may result from a variety of organisms, including *Escherichia coli, Staphylococcus, Streptococcus, Pseudomonas, Proteus,* and *Klebsiella.* In patients with depressed immune functioning, such as those with neutropenia or leukemia, systemic candidiases with multiple hepatic abscesses have been found. Many people with abscesses have multiple bacteria involved. *Entamoeba histolytica* is an important worldwide cause of amebic liver abscess and dysentery.

#### Epidemiology

Hepatic abscesses are uncommon in the United States but are associated with a high mortality. Amebic liver abscesses are common worldwide, particularly in countries with tropical and subtropical climates. In the United States, amebic liver abscesses occur occasionally in the temperate regions and in people who have traveled to topical climates.

#### Pathophysiology

Pyogenic abscesses can occur as either a singular large abscess or multiple small and/or microscopic abscesses. Amebic liver abscesses are typically large and singular.

Liver abscesses are usually a secondary site of infection. Pyogenic organisms originating in various areas of the body reach the liver through the biliary, vascular, or lymphatic systems. In addition, pyogenic organisms may be introduced by penetrating injuries to the liver or by direct continuous extension. In amebic abscesses, the vegetative form of the organism moves from the gut to the small portal vessels and into the hepatic tissue, where it becomes activated. The organisms cause necrosis of the liver tissue and abscess formation.

The abscess formation may disrupt hepatic function, but most of the altered physiological function is caused by the presence of an acute infective process. If liver abscesses are not identified, they continue to grow in size and can perforate into the pleural cavity, the peritoneal cavity, or the pericardial cavity. The major manifestations of liver abscess are caused by the infection rather than by changes in hepatic functioning. The person usually has history of not feeling well for several weeks. Common clinical manifestations are listed in Box 37-2.

**box 37-1** *Common Liver Disorders*

**FOCAL HEPATOCELLULAR DISORDERS**

Abscess
Trauma
Tumors

**DIFFUSE HEPATOCELLULAR DISORDERS**

Hepatitis
Cirrhosis
Sequelae of chronic diffuse hepatocellular disorders
- Portal hypertension
- Ascites
- Esophageal varices
- Portal-systemic encephalopathy
- Hepatorenal syndrome

**box 37-2** *clinical manifestations*

***Liver Abscess***

**SIGNS AND SYMPTOMS RESULTING FROM INFECTIOUS PROCESS**

Fever and chills (temperature between 102° F, [38.8° C] and 106° F [41.1° C])
Cough
Diaphoresis
Difficulty breathing
Abnormal breath sounds from pleural involvement
Right upper quadrant abdominal pain and tenderness
Anorexia
Nausea and vomiting
Clinical manifestations of peritonitis (see Box 37-3)

**SIGNS AND SYMPTOMS RESULTING FROM HEPATIC DYSFUNCTION**

Hepatomegaly
Jaundice and pruritus
Splenomegaly
Abdominal distention and ascites

The patient with *pyogenic abscesses,* particularly multiple small or microscopic abscesses, may have clinical manifestations of sepsis and septic shock. The patient with *amebic abscesses* may have signs and symptoms of intestinal amebiasis or give a history of previous intestinal signs and symptoms such as bloody, mucoid diarrhea; generalized abdominal pain; rectal tenesmus; dehydration; and hypotension. However, many patients with amebic abscess report no previous history of intestinal signs and symptoms.

## Collaborative Care Management

Diagnostic tests usually reveal leukocytosis and an elevated erythrocyte sedimentation rate caused by the infection and moderate elevation of serum alkaline phosphatase and minimal elevation of serum transaminases (aspartate aminotransferase [AST] and alanine aminotransferase [ALT]) from liver cell damage. Hyperbilirubinemia and hypoalbuminemia result from impaired liver function. In patients with amebic liver abscesses, serological laboratory tests such as immunoglobulins against antigens, indirect hemagglutination titers, complement fixation tests, and latex agglutination tests are highly diagnostic for amebic infection. Hepatic radioisotope scans, ultrasonic scanning, and computed tomography (CT) scans also are used in diagnosis and follow-up evaluation and reveal the presence of abscesses.

Metronidazole (Flagyl), chloroquine and dehydroemetine, or emetine are the drugs of choice for amebic abscesses. Empiric antimicrobial therapy is used initially for pyogenic abscesses with the specific type of antibiotic determined from the culture and sensitivity of the aspirate of the abscess. Acetaminophen is used to control fever, and fluid and electrolyte replacement is initiated as supportive therapy when needed.

For pyogenic abscesses, surgical drainage or needle aspiration may be necessary because the necrotic tissue walls off the abscess from the healthy liver tissue and makes it more difficult for antimicrobial therapy to reach the infection. Drainage of a pyogenic abscess is usually attempted only when there is a singular abscess. After an abscess has been located by ultrasound, arteriography, or CT scan, percutaneous aspiration can be attempted, usually under ultrasound guidance. After the application of a local anesthetic agent, the physician inserts a large-bore needle into the abscess, and the contents are aspirated. Complications for this procedure are similar to those of a liver biopsy, with hemorrhage being the most common. In the case of amebic abscesses, aspiration in not usually indicated because medications alone are very effective.

Patients with liver abscesses commonly complain of abdominal pain in the right upper quadrant. However, the pain can be described as shoulder pain. The patient may report nausea, vomiting, and anorexia.

There may be very few objective signs of liver abscess. Fever is common. A palpable mass in the right upper quadrant may be felt in some patients. Weight loss may result from the nausea, vomiting, and anorexia and the increased metabolic needs. Some patients may exhibit dyspnea and pleural pain if there is involvement of the diaphragm.

Nursing management focuses on (1) assisting with fluid and nutritional deficits, (2) controlling discomfort including dealing with pruritus if jaundice is present (see p. 1209, 1220), (3) assisting with the medical regimen (diagnostic tests and therapeutic measure), and (4) helping the patient attain appropriate knowledge for self-management. In the acute situation, nursing management may incorporate the care needs described for a patient with sepsis and septic shock (see Chapter 17) or severe intestinal colitis, appendicitis, and megacolon (see Chapter 41).

The first priority of care is to help with treatment of fluid volume deficit or shock, if present. The next priority is to provide comfort measures. The high temperature, episodes of chills and diaphoresis, pruritus, anorexia, and abdominal pain all cause discomfort. During periods of chills, adequate blankets to provide comfort without increasing temperature will be necessary. Cool sponge baths may help lower the temperature. The gown and bed linens should be changed if the patient is diaphoretic. Pruritus can be controlled with cool sponge baths, use of soft linens, prevention of dry skin, and cool environmental temperatures.

**box 37-3** clinical manifestations

**Peritonitis**

Abdominal tenderness
Rebound tenderness
Muscle rigidity or spasms
Decreased or absent bowel signs
Sometimes a fluid wave

Another aspect of care is to provide adequate fluids and nutrition. At first the patient may only tolerate IV fluids or at least need IV fluids to replace deficits. The effectiveness of these measures is evaluated by monitoring the patient's daily weight and skin turgor and assessing laboratory values for hemoconcentration or dilution. Food should be given in small amounts, and the patient's preferences should be incorporated to help overcome anorexia. Frequent oral hygiene (at least once every 2 hours) is necessary because fever and fluid loss cause drying of the mucous membranes and may worsen anorexia. The environment should be clean, free of odors, and relaxed.

In assisting with the medical regimen, the nurse is primarily involved with preparing patients physically for tests (instituting nothing by mouth status or other preparations as necessary, as described in Chapter 36 for the specific test). The patient and family also need appropriate education about the various tests (what will be done, the purpose of test, and special care necessary as described in Chapter 36). The nurse is involved in preparing those patients having surgical drainage of abscesses for surgery and providing appropriate postoperative care similar to that needed by any patient (see Chapter 20). The nurse also is involved in administering the prescribed antimicrobial and amebicidal agents. This involves not only appropriate administration but also monitoring for side effects.

### Patient/family education

Patient education for long-term care is also a major nursing responsibility. For some patients with liver abscesses, the medication may have to be taken for several weeks to several months. The patient must be instructed about the importance of continual adherence to the medication regimen. In addition, the patient should be instructed to report immediately any signs and symptoms of recurrence of infection (recurring chills, fever, or diaphoresis), of spread of infection (worsening abdominal pain or increased difficulty breathing), or of deteriorating liver function (e.g., jaundice or ascites), as well as any side effects of the medication. Instructions about the need for continual follow-up should be emphasized.

### Health promotion/prevention

For the person with amebic abscesses, prevention of recurrence is important. The nurse should help the patient identify potentially contaminated sources of food and water and help identify ways to decontaminate or avoid these sources, such as using iodine-releasing tablets in water and scalding of vegetables or eating only peeled fresh fruit.

**box 37-4** clinical manifestations

**Liver Trauma**

SIGNS OF SHOCK
Pale, cool, clammy skin
Diaphoresis
Hypotension
Tachycardia
Mental confusion

PENETRATING TRAUMA
Entry and sometimes exit wounds

BLUNT TRAUMA
Abdominal pain exaggerated by breathing
Shoulder pain indicating diaphragmatic irritation

# LIVER TRAUMA

## Etiology/Epidemiology

Because of its location and size, the liver is frequently subjected to trauma, which may be either penetrating (gunshot wounds or stab wounds) or blunt (collision with steering wheel during automobile accidents or falls). If the injury is severe, the liver may rupture, with severe internal hemorrhage.

## Pathophysiology

The pathophysiology varies with the type of liver injury. Injuries vary from a laceration and capsular tear with minimal parenchymal damage to liver rupture with extreme parenchymal damage and damage to the retrohepatic vasculature. Stab wounds often make a relatively superficial incision and may do no more damage than a needle biopsy of the liver. The liver receives 25% of the cardiac output and damage to the liver can result in hemorrhage and hypovolemic shock. Gunshot wounds and blunt trauma can result in severe hemorrhage leading to hypotension, shock, and peritonitis. Bile may also leak from the biliary canniculi and contaminate the peritoneal cavity causing *peritonitis* (Box 37-3). Less severe blunt trauma may result in subcapsular hematoma only.

The clinical manifestations of liver trauma vary with type of injury (Box 37-4). If peritoneal contamination from hemorrhage or bile has occurred, signs and symptoms of peritonitis may be present (see Box 37-3).

Late complications of liver trauma may include the following:

1. Severe hemorrhage resulting from disseminated intravascular coagulation that often accompanies shock during the total course of treatment
2. Degeneration and sloughing of segments of the liver that have had disrupted circulation with resultant hemorrhage
3. Intrahepatic abscess formation
4. Traumatic hepatic cyst formation
5. Infections of other areas of body after hepatic trauma
6. Subphrenic abscess formation
7. Biliary fistulas

The mortality for liver trauma has decreased over the years. The mortality depends on the type of injury (highest for blunt trauma because of the larger portion of liver damaged and because of other associated injuries), the severity of the injury (highest for those requiring resection of a large amount of liver), and the presence of associated injuries (increasing mortality with each additional injury to another organ).

### Collaborative Care Management

In some instances, the only sign of hepatic trauma is the presence of blood in peritoneal lavage (see Chapter 21 for a description of this test). Laboratory studies may reveal a decreasing hematocrit and hemoglobin from blood loss and leukocytosis from peritoneal infection and inflammation.

The immediate medical management for patients with suspected liver trauma is the same as that for any patient with intraabdominal trauma and includes the following:

1. Maintenance of airway
2. Hydration and intravenous fluids
3. Type and cross-match for blood replacement
4. Evaluation of laboratory assessments
5. Monitoring of intake and output
6. Mean arterial pressure monitoring
7. Treatment of shock with fluids, dextran, and blood components (see Chapter 17)
8. Immediate surgical exploration of the abdomen to detect the presence of abdominal hemorrhage, trauma to liver or other organs, presence of necrotic tissue, or presence of bile drainage
9. Treatment of peritonitis

The major focus of nursing care for the patient with suspected liver trauma is to establish and implement a systematic assessment of cardiovascular and fluid volume status, neurological status, and signs and symptoms of peritonitis (Guidelines for Care Box). This assessment is required from the moment the patient is first seen through the postoperative period.

**guidelines for care**

**Assessing the Person with Suspected Liver Trauma**

- Respiratory status (rate, breath sounds, pulse oximetry, and blood gases)
- Vital signs every 15 minutes (blood pressure, pulse)
- Mean arterial pressure every hour
- Other hemodynamic monitoring, such as intraarterial pressure monitoring and cardiac output measurements, as ordered
- Urine output and other fluid losses documented hourly
- Intake documented hourly
- Serum and urinary electrolytes and osmolality at least daily
- Hematocrit and hemoglobin daily
- Neurological checks for responsiveness and motion every hour
- Consciousness monitored every hour using Glasgow Coma Scale
- Skin temperature, color, and moisture every hour
- Bowel sounds, pain, and abdominal tenderness

The nurse also assists with the initiation of monitoring devices such as the Foley catheter and Dynamap (mean arterial pressure monitor), administration of fluids and blood, and collection of specimens for laboratory tests. The nurse should anticipate the possibility of surgery and prepare the patient and family for this procedure.

#### *Patient/family education*

The major nursing focus is to help the patient and family control their fear and anxiety by using simple explanations of all activities and maintaining a calm environment. Continuity of care is essential to minimizing fear and anxiety.

Providing information and support for the patient's family or significant others is another important aspect of care. A specific time should be set aside for the family and significant others to ask questions and verbalize their fears. Spiritual support is extremely important to many patients and their families and should be considered when planning care.

After the acute/critical period, which includes the postoperative period for some patients, continual monitoring as already described plus provision of emotional support for the patient and family are still needed. The patient will also need help with self-care, a gradual increase in activity, and comfort measures. The patient will need to be educated about the signs and symptoms of recurrent liver dysfunction. The importance of complying with follow-up care should be stressed.

## LIVER TUMORS

Liver neoplasms or tumors may be either benign or malignant. Benign lesions include hemangioma, cysts, and rarely, adenoma. Most benign tumors are asymptomatic, but occasionally they enlarge enough to become symptomatic. If they become symptomatic, surgical intervention may be required. The focus of this section is malignant neoplasms.

### Etiology

Malignant tumors are either primary or metastatic. The liver is highly vascular and is a common site for metastasis from the cancers of gastrointestinal (GI) tract, the lungs, the breasts, the kidneys, and malignant melanomas. Primary liver tumors arise in the liver cell (hepatocellular) or the bile duct cell (cholangiocellular), or they can be of mixed origin. The incidence of primary liver cancer is increased in people with chronic liver disease, particularly those with chronic hepatitis B. The risk of developing hepatocellular cancer is approximately 40 times greater in persons with alcohol-induced cirrhosis.

### Epidemiology

Hepatocellular tumors *(hepatomas)* are the most common type of primary liver cancer but account for only 1% to 2% of malignant tumors found at death in the United States. Primary liver cancer is one of the most common malignancies in other parts of the world, particularly in Africa. This geographical difference in incidence probably results from the prevalence of chronic liver disease from hepatitis B and nutritional deficiencies in other countries. Metastatic liver tumors occur 20 times more frequently than primary tumors and rank second only to cirrhosis as a cause of fatal liver disease in the United States. The prognosis for persons with liver cancer is poor; few persons are alive 5 years after diagnosis.

## Pathophysiology

Primary tumors arise from liver cells, bile ducts, or both. The lesions are multiple or singular, diffuse or nodular, and may involve a lobe or the entire liver. The cancerous cells compress the surrounding normal liver cells and invade the portal vein branches. Some cells infiltrate the gallbladder, mesentery, peritoneum, and diaphragm by direct extension. Primary cancers also tend to cause hemorrhage by extension into the vascular tissue of the liver and necrosis by depriving normal hepatic tissue of adequate circulation. The most common site for metastasis of the primary liver lesion is the lung, but metastasis can occur to the adrenal glands, spleen, vertebrae, kidney, ovary, or pancreas. Primary lesions grow rapidly, sometimes without signs or symptoms, and often the patient lives only a short time after the diagnosis.

Metastatic carcinoma of the liver varies from a few small nodules to large nodules. Adjacent nodules may eventually fuse and compress the surrounding liver tissue. Usually different parts of the liver are uniformly involved; thus liver biopsy may be a useful diagnostic aid.

The signs and symptoms of liver cancer depend on the size and extent of the tumor, the amount of hepatocellular damage, and the presence of liver failure. Box 37-5 lists clinical manifestations of liver cancer.

**box 37-5** *clinical manifestations*

### Liver Cancer

**EARLY SIGNS**

- Right upper quadrant mass
- Epigastric fullness
- Pain
- Fatigue
- Weight loss
- Changes in liver function tests

**LATER SIGNS**

- Fatigue
- Ascites
- Liver failure
- Fever
- Hepatic bruits
- Jaundice
- Variceal bleeding

**METASTATIC LIVER TUMORS**

- Fatigue
- Anorexia
- Weakness
- Weight loss followed by weight gain resulting from ascites
- Hepatomegaly
- Hepatic bruits
- Jaundice
- Portal-systemic encephalopathy

## Collaborative Care Management

### Diagnostic tests

Diagnostic tests include blood studies, radioisotope scans, magnetic resonance imaging, liver biopsy, ultrasonography, and CT scans. The blood studies may show an increased erythrocyte sedimentation rate associated with generalized inflammation of the liver; anemia resulting from increased metabolism and decreased food intake; hyperbilirubinemia; elevated alkaline phosphatase, AST, and ALT; decreased blood glucose; and hypoalbuminemia. The number of abnormalities depends on the severity of hepatocellular damage. A special test that is used to help diagnose primary liver carcinoma is serum concentrations of $\alpha$-fetoprotein (AFP). AFP in concentrations of 500 ng/ml to 5 mg/ml is found in up to 70% of patients with hepatocellular cancer and also in a small percentage of patients with metastatic carcinoma or viral hepatitis, but rarely at the same high levels. High levels that occur in any adult without obvious GI tract tumors strongly suggest primary liver cancer. Radioisotope and CT scans and ultrasonography may reveal lesions in the liver. A liver biopsy is necessary for definitive diagnosis of cancer.

### Medications

High-dose chemotherapy has been used to induce regression of primary and metastatic liver tumors. These chemotherapeutic agents, usually 5-fluorouracil and fluorodeoxyuridine, are given directly into the hepatic artery via a surgically implanted infusion pump. Arterial infusion allows more drug to be delivered directly to the tumor and decreases systemic effects.

### Treatments

Radiation therapy may be used to control pain, but it does not improve survival rates. Ligation of the hepatic artery decreases the oxygen delivered to the tumor and may help control the pain and diminish the mass of the tumor.

### Surgical management

For solitary primary tumors and some solitary metastatic tumors, surgery may be performed. The liver has remarkable regenerative capacity, which allows as much as 90% resection. Nursing management of the patient with a hepatic resection is discussed next. Orthotopic transplantation (removal of recipient's liver and replacement with a graft liver) has been performed for patients with primary liver tumors with varying success. Liver transplantation is discussed in Chapter 68.

### Diet

Special diet is necessary only if signs and symptoms of cirrhosis occur.

### Activity

Activity as tolerated is encouraged. The patient is encouraged to be as independent as possible.

### Referrals

Common referrals for patients with hepatic tumors include social services, cancer support groups, and cancer specialists.

### Assessment

#### Subjective data

Patients with liver tumors often experience epigastric fullness, fatigue, weight loss, and abdominal pain early in the course of their illness. Later, the fatigue becomes more pronounced, and patients may report weakness and anorexia.

#### Objective data

Objective signs of liver tumors are minimal until the disease is well advanced. As the disease progresses, the patient may become jaundiced, have ascites, and show signs of liver failure, including variceal bleeding and portal-systemic encephalopathy. Box 37-5 lists the clinical manifestations of liver cancer.

## NURSING MANAGEMENT OF THE PATIENT HAVING HEPATIC RESECTION

### ■ PREOPERATIVE CARE

For the patient having surgical resection of a hepatic tumor *(hepatic resection),* skilled perioperative care is necessary. Teaching about the preoperative preparation, the procedure itself, and postoperative care is needed (see Chapters 18-20). The patient may need vitamin K for defects in clotting factors, as well as other vitamins if deficits are present. Preparation of the bowel is the same as for intestinal surgery (see Chapter 41). If a blood volume deficit is present, blood will be given. The goal is to make the patient's physical condition as stable as possible before surgery.

### ■ POSTOPERATIVE CARE

Postoperatively the patient will require close monitoring. Sepsis is the most common complication. Hypovolemia from blood loss is also a complication. Vital signs should be monitored every 15 minutes until stable and then every hour. Dressings should be checked for oozing or bleeding. Intake and output, serum electrolytes, and hematocrit or hemoglobin levels are carefully monitored. Weights should be recorded daily. Assessment of the cardiorespiratory system (cardiac rhythm, breath sounds, and pulse oximetry) is also necessary. Temperature should also be monitored at least every 4 hours.

Assessment not only focuses on the potential for sepsis, hypovolemic shock, and cardiorespiratory complications, but should also include monitoring for decreased liver function (blood glucose, coagulation status, serum albumin levels, and neurological status). The nurse should anticipate the possibility of administering glucose, albumin, and blood. Restriction of protein is necessary if the patient is not able to adequately metabolize the ammonium released during the breakdown of proteins.

To promote turning and deep breathing, the nurse must ensure adequate pain control by giving the patient medications as ordered, splinting the incision, and positioning the patient properly (upright). Patient-controlled analgesia may be used to manage postoperative pain. Because most analgesics, narcotic and nonnarcotic, are metabolized in the liver, no "safe" analgesic exists for the patient with liver dysfunction, and the nurse should monitor closely for signs of toxicity.

The patient has nothing by mouth for several days and has a nasogastric tube attached to suction. Frequent mouth care every 2 hours and monitoring of the nasogastric suction are indicated. Oral intake is started on approximately the fifth postoperative day. Initially ice chips and clear liquids are given, and then the diet is advanced as tolerated based on appetite and bowel function. The patient needs adequate calories, protein, vitamins, and minerals. The nurse must monitor the patient for adequacy of intake by monitoring caloric intake. The patient's tolerance to protein nitrogenous waste products must be monitored. If the patient cannot metabolize protein adequately because of loss of liver tissue, a low-protein diet is necessary. If the patient can adequately detoxify ammonium, a high-protein diet is given.

After surgery, the patient initially dangles on the side of the bed and is out of bed by the first or second postoperative day. Close monitoring of vital signs, tolerance for activity, and respiratory status are required. The care of the patient undergoing hepatic resection is summarized in the Guidelines for Care Box.

**guidelines for care**

**The Person Undergoing Liver Resection**

**Preoperative Care**

Teaching
- Explain special postoperative procedures (nasogastric intubation and parenteral fluids for several days).
- Teach deep breathing exercises and leg exercises.
- Teach use of side rails to facilitate turning in bed without exerting pull on the abdominal muscles.

Preventing hemorrhage
- Give prescribed vitamin K.

Bowel preparation
- See Chapter 41.

**Postoperative Care**

Promoting oxygenation
- Encourage turning and deep breathing exercises.
- Encourage activity/ambulation as ordered.

Maintaining fluid and electrolyte balance
- Check dressings for oozing or bleeding.
- Maintain patency of GI tube.
- Maintain prescribed rate of parenteral fluids.
- Monitor for signs of fluid imbalance (daily weight changes, hematocrit, lung congestion, and dry skin and mucous membranes).

Promoting comfort
- Give analgesics on a regular basis during the first 48 hours to minimize severe pain.
- Give frequent oral hygiene until oral fluids are resumed.

Teaching
- Explain menu choices for a low-protein diet.
- Reinforce information about a low-sodium diet.

The patient should receive instructions concerning any dietary restrictions. The patient's liver function will be impaired for up to 6 months after surgery, and dietary protein and sodium are restricted. Corticosteroids are given to enhance regeneration and prevent fibrosis. If steroids are to be continued after discharge, the patient needs written and verbal instructions regarding dosage, purpose, administration, and side effects that need to be reported. The patient's activity tolerance will gradually increase. Activities such as heavy lifting should be avoided; generally, the patient should be instructed to lift no more than 5 to 10 pounds. Usually the patient uses his or her feeling of fatigue and tiredness as indicators of what can or cannot be done. The patient will not be able to assume all activities of daily living (ADL) immediately because of fatigue, and the nurse must assess whether self-care and home care needs can be met by the family or if outside help is necessary. Appropriate referrals should be made if necessary for home health care.

## GERONTOLOGICAL CONSIDERATIONS

Surgical resection of hepatic tumors is a commonly used treatment option. Surgical intervention poses a risk for all persons, but especially the elderly. (See Chapters 19 and 20 for perioperative needs of the elderly patient.) Changes in liver function associated with aging include decreased blood flow, decreased synthesis of cholesterol, and reduced bile storage. These normal changes may be more evident with destruction of liver tissue associated with tumors. There is evidence to suggest that aging affects the liver's ability to regenerate. This decrease in function is significant for persons undergoing hepatic resection. The elderly person is also susceptible to drug toxicity. Patients with impaired liver function should be monitored for toxic and adverse effects, which may indicate a need for a reduced dosage of certain drugs. This is especially true if chemotherapeutic agents are used as treatment. Fatigue and weakness, which are common symptoms associated with hepatic cancer, may be increased in the elderly patient, both as a result of aging or coexisting chronic disease.

## SPECIAL ENVIRONMENTS FOR CARE

### Home Care Management

#### *Care of the patient having chemotherapy*

Chemotherapy is increasingly being used to treat primary and metastatic tumors of the liver. Chemotherapy may be the treatment of choice if hepatic resection is not an option and may be given systemically or by infusion into the hepatic artery. Intraperitoneal chemotherapy has been used successfully in a limited number of patients. All chemotherapeutic agents have major side effects, and one of the major focuses of nursing is to help the patient and family deal with these side effects (see Chapter 11). Patients receiving hepatic chemotherapy will need to learn to care for an external infusion pump, as shown in Figure 37-1, or an internal pump, as shown in Figure 37-2.

**Hepatic arterial infusion.** Patients receiving chemotherapy through the hepatic artery have additional needs. Hepatic arterial infusion can be accomplished by one of two methods (see Chapter 11). In the first method, a percutaneous catheter is inserted into the hepatic artery using fluoroscopy. The catheter is attached to an external infusion pump that is filled with the appropriate chemotherapeutic agent and programmed to deliver the agent over a desired period. The catheter is removed after each drug treatment cycle. In the second method, a catheter is surgically inserted into the hepatic artery and connected to an implanted infusion pump (Figure 37-2).

The implanted pump can be filled with the correct amount of drug and programmed to deliver the chemotherapeutic agent over a desired time and at a desired dosage. Generally, pumps can deliver medication up to 14 days at a time. In chemotherapy-free intervals, the pump is filled with a heparin solution to maintain patency of the hepatic artery

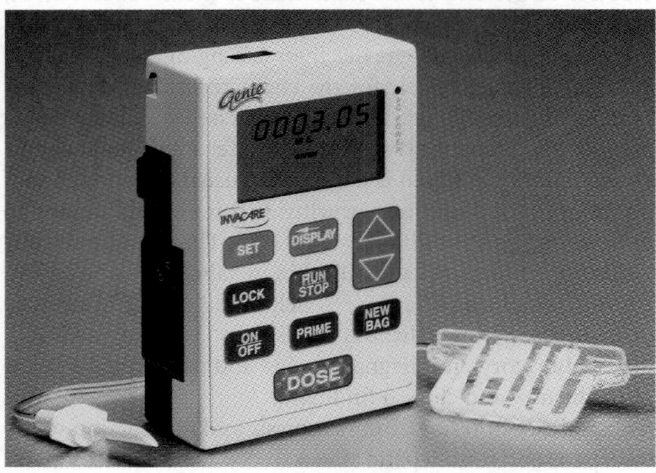


**fig. 37-1** External infusion pump. Lightweight battery-operated infusion pump for ambulatory patient. Flow rate is adjustable; power pack operates for 7 days before needing recharging.

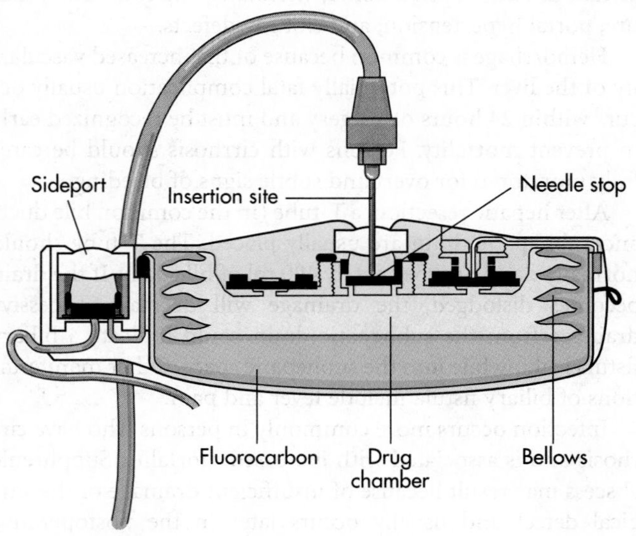


**fig. 37-2** Implantable infusion pump (Infusaid pump).

catheter. The chamber should be adequately filled to avoid complete emptying.

The implanted infusion pump allows the patient to be treated at home. The patient comes into an outpatient site at prescribed times for addition of drugs or heparin solution and a recheck of pump flow rate. The patient needs physical care before and after surgery similar to that for any patient having surgery (see Chapters 18 and 20) and instructions regarding self-care needs related to the chemotherapeutic agent being used (see Chapter 11 and a pharmacology text). The nurse also is involved in refilling the pump at the prescribed intervals.

## COMPLICATIONS

The poor prognosis associated with liver cancer is partially due to the late onset of definitive signs of disease. The cancer is usually far advanced at the time of diagnosis. If the cancer is untreated, death usually occurs within 6 to 8 weeks of diagnosis. As mentioned earlier, almost 50% of persons with hepatic cancer will have distant metastases to the lungs, bone, adrenal glands, and brain. Tumors spread rapidly within the liver and occlusion of the portal vein is common. Occlusion of the portal vein can lead to necrosis, rupture, and hemorrhage. As the cancer progresses, multiple body systems are affected, and complications arise. The cause of death in approximately 50% of patients with liver cancer is liver failure and hemorrhage. Other causes of death include pneumonia, malnutrition, and thromboemboli.

There are many complications associated with hepatic resection. Jaundice is common postoperatively, usually as a result of the inability of the remaining liver to utilize bile. Other causes of jaundice include multiple transfusions, vascular occlusion, and anoxia of hepatocytes during surgery. Jaundice usually resolves in approximately 10 days. If the jaundice persists, obstruction should be suspected. Major postoperative complications after hepatic resection include hemorrhage; biliary fistula; infection; subphrenic abscess; respiratory complications such as pneumonia, atelectasis, and respiratory failure; portal hypertension; and clotting defects.

Hemorrhage is common because of the increased vascularity of the liver. This potentially fatal complication usually occurs within 24 hours of surgery and must be recognized early to prevent mortality. Persons with cirrhosis should be carefully monitored for overt and subtle signs of bleeding.

After hepatic resection, a T-tube (in the common bile duct) and subhepatic drain are usually placed. The T-tube should normally drain approximately 400 ml of bile daily. If the drain becomes dislodged, the drainage will decrease. Excessive drainage from the subhepatic drain could indicate a biliary fistula leaking bile into the subhepatic space. Other manifestations of biliary fistula include fever and pain.

Infection occurs more commonly in persons who have cirrhosis and is associated with increased mortality. Subphrenic abscess may result because of insufficient drainage of the surgical defect and usually occurs later in the postoperative course. The proper placement and expected output of drainage tubes should be closely monitored in the postoperative period. An acute onset of sharp, piercing right upper quadrant pain and low-grade fever, and the presence of adventitious sounds in the lung bases suggest a subphrenic abscess.

Respiratory complications can arise because of the anatomical location of the surgical site. Persons are often reluctant to participate in pulmonary hygiene exercises due to incisional pain. Nursing care should be focused on preventing any respiratory complications (see Chapter 20).

Portal hypertension is another postoperative complication that results from the surgical alteration of venous blood flow in the remaining liver. This complication is usually transitory because the remaining liver has the potential to compensate and increase blood flow over time.

Coagulopathies usually develop during surgery, but may also occur postoperatively. The patient should be closely monitored for bleeding and nursing care should focus on preventing episodes of bleeding. Monitoring of central venous pressure is a good indicator of the fluid volume status. The prothrombin time is generally delayed in the first postoperative week, then gradually returns to normal.

Chemotherapy may be used in the person for whom surgery is not indicated. Refer to Chapter 11 for the complications associated with the use of chemotherapeutic agents.

Care for persons with advanced liver cancer is primarily supportive. Persons with advanced disease will often experience liver failure, ascites, infection, bleeding, pain, weight loss, anorexia, vomiting, weakness, and pneumonia. Both the patient and family should be informed about treatment plans and be assured that care will focus on promoting comfort.

# DIFFUSE HEPATOCELLULAR DISORDERS

*Jaundice* is a major problem in patients with diffuse hepatocellular disorders. It is caused by a disturbance in bilirubin metabolism. (See Chapter 36 for an explanation of bilirubin metabolism.) With jaundice, an excess of bilirubin in the blood is distributed to the skin, mucous membranes, sclerae, and other body fluids and tissues. This high total serum bilirubin level (usually greater than 2.5 mg/dl; normal: 0.5 to 1.0 mg/dl) is responsible for the characteristic yellow discoloration of these tissues. Bilirubin processed by the liver (extracted, conjugated, and secreted) is water soluble and can be excreted in urine, which is darker than usual. The presence of bilirubin in the skin causes pruritus (itching) in about 20% to 25% of the patients who have jaundice. The changes in concentration of bilirubin and bilirubin metabolites in the serum, urine, or stool (see Chapter 36) help in determining the type of jaundice. Serum bilirubin levels must be combined with other laboratory and diagnostic tests and interpreted in view of the history and clinical findings.

Jaundice can result from hemolysis and obstruction of extrahepatic and intrahepatic biliary ducts. Table 37-1 compares the different causes of jaundice. A common cause of *intrahepatic cholestasis* (stasis of bile within the small biliary canniculi of the liver) is drug reactions such as that from phenothiazines. Clay-colored (grayish-white) stools indicate that bile is

**table 37-1** *Types of Jaundice*

| CATEGORY | PATHOLOGY | POSSIBLE FINDINGS |
|---|---|---|
| **OBSTRUCTIVE** | | |
| Intrahepatic | Suppression of bile flow in canaliculi or small biliary ductiles (cholestasis) | Direct* bilirubin elevated; alkaline phosphatase elevated; no enlargement of bile ducts seen on scan or ultrasound |
| Extrahepatic (bile duct obstruction) | Obstruction of bile flow in large bile ducts, as in gallbladder disease | Direct* bilirubin elevated; alkaline phosphatase elevated; enlargement of bile ducts documented by scan, ultrasound; absence of urobilinogen in urine |
| **HEPATOCELLULAR** | Hepatocyte injury from toxins (toxic hepatitis), from viruses (viral hepatitis), or as part of syndrome of cirrhosis (all types) | Transaminases (ALT, AST) elevated 10- to 15-fold; both direct* and indirect† bilirubin may be elevated (direct more than indirect); prolonged prothrombin time |
| **HEMOLYTIC** | Excessive amounts of bilirubin are released from red blood cells (RBCs) as would be seen in sickle cell anemia or other hemolytic anemias; liver is unable to excrete bilirubin as rapidly as it forms | Usually mild elevation of total bilirubin (indirect more than direct) |

*"Direct" measures conjugated bilirubin.
†"Indirect" measures unconjugated bilirubin.

not reaching the intestine and suggest *extrahepatic obstruction* (obstruction of hepatic duct, gallbladder, or common bile duct). An absence of urobilinogen in the urine supports this inference because bile and bilirubin must reach the intestines for the normal formation of urobilinogen, some of which is usually excreted in the urine. Frequent causes of extrahepatic obstruction are gallstones lodged in the common bile duct, pancreatitis, and carcinoma of the head of the pancreas, all of which are discussed in Chapter 42.

In hepatocellular damage, there is interference with uptake, conjugation, and excretion of bilirubin into bile. Excretion is the most profoundly affected process, and a predominantly conjugated hyperbilirubinemia is seen. The level of jaundice does not correlate with the severity in hepatitis; but in persons with cirrhosis, jaundice suggests a poorer prognosis.

## HEPATITIS

Hepatitis is any acute inflammatory disease of the liver. Although the term *hepatitis* is most often used in conjunction with viral hepatitis, the disease can also be caused by bacteria or toxic injury to the liver.

Although some differences exist in the pathological and clinical phenomena of viral, bacterial, and toxic hepatitis, the clinical management of the person with any of these types of hepatitis is quite similar. The particular aspects of care for toxic and viral hepatitis are discussed next. It should be pointed out that almost any form of hepatitis can result in *postnecrotic cirrhosis,* unless the hepatitis responds to treatment.

### Toxic Hepatitis

#### Etiology

Because the liver has a primary role in the metabolism of foreign substances; many agents, including drugs, alcohol, industrial toxins, and plant poisons, can cause *toxic hepatitis* (Table 37-2). Many health care workers are concerned about hepatic injury caused by adverse drug reactions from the drugs they handle (especially those needing to be mixed from powder).

#### Epidemiology

Only a minor number of cases of acute hepatic disease in health care workers are the result of adverse drug reactions. However, up to 25% of *all* cases of fulminant hepatic failure are the result of adverse drug reactions.[14]

#### Classification of the hepatotoxins

The agents that produce hepatic injury are categorized into two major groups: *predictable (intrinsic)* hepatotoxins and *nonpredictable (idiosyncratic)* hepatotoxins. The predictable hepatotoxins are further divided into two subgroups: *direct* and *indirect* (Box 37-6). The selected agents listed in Table 37-2 have been classified according to type of hepatotoxin. As should be noted, most drugs are nonpredictable (idiosyncratic) hepatotoxins.

#### Pathophysiology

The morphological changes produced in the liver by the toxins vary, depending on the specific hepatotoxin. For example, carbon tetrachloride, tetracycline, and ethanol cause fatty infiltration and/or necrosis. Oral contraceptives, cholecystographic dyes, and chlorpromazine produce cholestasis and portal inflammation. Regardless of the morphological changes, some alteration in liver function occurs. The alteration may result in only minimal manifestations of altered liver function such as slightly elevated serum enzymes or major manifestations associated with terminal liver failure (see p. 1226-1233). Box 37-7 lists clinical manifestations of toxic hepatitis.

table 37-2 *Selected Hepatoxins and Class of Hepatotoxins*

| AGENTS | TYPE OF HEPATOTOXIN |
|---|---|
| **INDUSTRIAL TOXINS** | |
| Carbon tetrachloride and other chlorinated hydrocarbons | Predictable; direct |
| Yellow phosphorus | Predictable; direct |
| **PLANT POISONS** | |
| Mushroom poisoning (*Amanita phalloides* and related poisons) | Predictable; direct |
| **DRUGS** | |
| Ethanol | Predictable; indirect |
| Tetracycline | Predictable; indirect |
| Methotrexate | Predictable; indirect |
| L-Asparaginase | Predictable; indirect |
| Puromycin | Predictable; indirect |
| 6-Mercaptopurine | Predictable; indirect |
| Acetaminophen | Predictable; indirect |
| Mithramycin | Predictable; indirect |
| Urethane | Predictable; indirect |
| Halothane | Predictable; indirect |
| Cholecystographic dyes | Predictable; indirect |
| Rifamycin B | Predictable; indirect |
| Phenytoin | Nonpredictable |
| para-aminosalicylic acid (PAS) | Nonpredictable |
| Isoniazid (INH) | Nonpredictable |
| Chlorpromazine | Nonpredictable |
| Androgens and anabolic steroids | Nonpredictable |
| Chlorpropamide | Nonpredictable |
| Imipramine | Nonpredictable |
| Methyldopa | Nonpredictable |
| Monoamine oxidase inhibitors | Nonpredictable |
| Oral contraceptives | Nonpredictable |
| Sulfonamides | Nonpredictable |
| Allopurinol | Nonpredictable |
| Clindamycin | Nonpredictable |
| Erythromycin esters | Nonpredictable |
| Nitrofurantoin | Nonpredictable |
| Oxacillin | Nonpredictable |
| Estrogenic steroid | Nonpredictable |

#### Collaborative care management

Attention is focused on identifying the toxic agent and removing or eliminating it. Gastric lavage and cleansing of the bowel may be indicated to remove the hepatotoxin(s) from the intestinal tract. In some instances, there is a specific treatment for a particular hepatotoxin. For example, acetylcysteine, a mucolytic agent, can be given within 16 hours (immediately is preferred) of ingestion of an acetaminophen overdose. Acetylcysteine prevents hepatotoxicity by possibly maintaining or restoring glutathione levels or acting as an alternate substrate for the toxic metabolite of acetaminophen. The drug may be given orally or intravenously, although only the oral form has been approved for use in the United States. However, in most instances of toxic hepatitis, medical treatment is supportive and focused on particular manifestations, such as treatment of cirrhosis, portal-systemic encephalopathy, or accompanying renal failure. In patients with severe hepatotoxicity, liver transplantation may be necessary.

Nursing care for the person with toxic hepatitis is supportive. For the patient with acute toxic hepatitis, the nursing management in the acute care setting is focused on promoting comfort, maintaining normal fluid and electrolyte balance, promoting a well-balanced diet when food and fluid are allowed, and promoting rest as discussed in the section Viral Hepatitis. The nurse also assists with the implementation of any medical regimen. If cirrhosis develops or portal-systemic encephalopathy occurs, the patient may require all the interventions described for the patient with cirrhosis (see p. 1218-1225).

#### Patient/family education

The major focus for nursing management is in the community or other outpatient setting and is centered on the

box 37-6 *Classification of Hepatotoxins*

**PREDICTABLE HEPATOTOXINS**

Agents cause toxic hepatitis with predictable regularity and produce injury in a high percentage of persons exposed to them; occurrence of toxic hepatitis is dose dependent.

**NONPREDICTABLE HEPATOTOXINS**

Agents produce hepatic injury only in unusually susceptible persons and in only a small percentage of persons exposed to them; occurrence is not dose dependent.

**DIRECT PREDICTABLE HEPATOTOXINS**

Agents have direct effect on hepatic cells and organelles, producing structural changes that lead to metabolic defects.

**INDIRECT PREDICTABLE HEPATOTOXINS**

Agents first interfere with normal metabolic function, and this alteration in metabolic function produces structural changes.

box 37-7 *clinical manifestations*

***Toxic Hepatitis***

**EARLY MANIFESTATIONS**

- Anorexia
- Nausea and vomiting
- Lethargy
- Elevated ALT and AST levels

**LATER MANIFESTATIONS**

- Icterus
- Hepatomegaly
- Hepatic tenderness
- Dark urine
- Elevated serum bilirubin level
- Elevated urine bilirubin level

nursing diagnosis, potential for injury related to improper use of chemicals at home, exposure to chemicals in the work environment, or injudicious use of drugs or other materials.

**Primary prevention.** The nurse can assist in the prevention of toxic hepatitis by teaching the danger of injudicious use of materials that are known to be injurious to the liver. Emphasizing the need for a well-balanced diet with the recommended dietary requirements of nutrients and with minimal or no consumption of alcohol should be encouraged.

Because cleaning agents, solvents, and related substances sometimes contain products that are harmful to the liver, the public should read instructions on labels and should follow them explicitly. Dry cleaning fluids may contain carbon tetrachloride, which can cause liver injury if warnings to avoid inhalation of the fumes and to keep windows open are not heeded. If people must use these agents inside the home, a good practice is to open the windows wide; use the cleaning materials as quickly as possible; and then vacate the room, the apartment, or the house for several hours, leaving the windows open.

Many solvents used to remove paint and plastic material and to stain and finish woodwork contain injurious substances and should be used outdoors and not in the basement, since dangerous fumes may spread throughout the house. Cleaning agents and finishes for cars should be applied outdoors or in the garage with the door open. Nurses in industry have a responsibility to teach the importance of observing regulations to avoid industrial hazards. Nitrobenzene, tetrachloroethane, carbon disulfide, and dinitrotoluoyl are examples of injurious compounds used in industry.

**Secondary prevention.** Some drugs that are known to cause mild damage to the liver must be used therapeutically. However, the nurse should warn the public about the use of preparations available without prescription that can cause liver injury. Many drugs, prescription and nonprescription, reach the market before dangers resulting from their extensive use have been conclusively ruled out; for example, the prescription drug chlorpromazine, which was being widely used as a tranquilizer, has been found to cause stasis of bile in the canaliculi of the liver, which can lead to serious hepatic damage. A safe rule to follow is to avoid taking any medication except that specifically prescribed by a physician for a specific ailment.

## Viral Hepatitis

Viral hepatitis is by far the most important liver infection and is a major health problem in the United States and in many other countries. The term *viral hepatitis* is used to refer to several clinically similar but etiologically and epidemiologically distinct infections.

### Etiology

Five major categories of viruses have been identified as causing viral hepatitis: hepatitis A (HAV), hepatitis B (HBV), hepatitis C (HCV), hepatitis D (HDV or delta virus), and hepatitis E (HEV). Two other forms of hepatitis, hepatitis F and hepatitis G, have been identified but occur rarely.[7,12] Table 37-3 provides a summary of the modes of transmission for each viral type.

### Epidemiology

Viral hepatitis is a reportable disease in all states in the United States. Statistics from the Centers for Disease Control and Prevention (CDC) indicate that viral hepatitis is one of the most frequently reported infectious diseases in the United States. Native Americans and Native Alaskans have a high rate of endemic disease. The most common type of hepatitis worldwide is HAV, with 40% of the reported cases of hepatitis being caused by HAV.[11]

The incidence of HBV infection is reported to be about 5% of the world's population. Fifty-nine percent of the reported cases of HBV infection in the United States occur in heterosexuals with multiple sex partners, homosexual men, and IV drug users. The incidence of HBV infection in health care workers is about 3% of all reported cases.[3,6,16]

Twenty percent of all cases of viral hepatitis reported to the CDC are caused by HCV infection, and 50% to 80% of these persons will develop chronic hepatitis.[2] HDV is endemic among persons with HBV in areas around the Mediterranean and Middle East. HEV is extremely rare in the United States but occurs in epidemic proportions in areas of India. Cases of HEV have also been reported in Mexico, Asia, and Africa.[7,9,12]

Hepatitis in the vast majority of patients seen clinically is caused by HAV or HBV. Most cases of all types of hepatitis occur in young adults. Factors such as the viral agent, transmission, and high-risk groups vary for the five types of hepatitis. Table 37-3 summarizes the difference between the five types of hepatitis.

### Pathophysiology

Viral hepatitis causes diffuse inflammatory infiltration of hepatic tissue with mononuclear cells and local, spotty, or single cell necrosis. The liver cells may be very swollen. With typical viral hepatitis, there is no collapse of lobules, no loss of lobular architecture, and minimal or no fibrosis. Inflammation, degeneration, and regeneration occur simultaneously, distorting the normal lobular pattern and creating pressure within and around the portal vein areas and obstructing the bile channels. These changes are associated with elevated serum transaminase levels, prolonged prothrombin time, slightly elevated serum alkaline phosphatase level, and elevated bilirubin level.

The outcome of viral hepatitis is affected by such factors as the following:

1. Virulence of the virus
2. Amount of hepatic damage sustained
3. Natural individual barriers to damage and disease of the liver, such as immune status, nutritional status, and overall health of individual
4. Supportive individual care the patient receives

Most patients recover normal liver function, but the disease can progress to atypical life-threatening variants (Box 37-8). Chronic sequelae can occur with all types of hepatitis but are virtually absent with HAV and HEV. Because of the continual destruction of the liver in *chronic active hepatitis,* there are continual signs and symptoms of liver

**table 37-3** *Etiological/Epidemiological/Transmission Characteristics of Viral Hepatitis*

| Hepatitis A | Hepatitis B | Hepatitis C | Hepatitis D | Hepatitis E |
|---|---|---|---|---|
| **TRANSMISSION** | | | | |
| Fecal-oral | Parenteral/sexual/perinatal | Parenteral/sexual/perinatal | Superinfection or co-infection with chronic HBV | Fecal/oral |
| **INCUBATION PERIOD** | | | | |
| 2-6 wk | 4-24 wk | 2-20 wk | 4-24 wk | 2-8 wk |
| **VIRUS TYPE** | | | | |
| RNA picornavirus | DNA hepadenavirus | RNA flavirs | Defective RNA virus | Unclassified RNA virus |
| **DIAGNOSTIC SEROLOGICAL TESTS** | | | | |
| Acute phase: IgM anti-HAV<br>Lifetime: IgG anti-HAV | Acute phase: $HB_sAg$, anti-$HB_c$ IgM, $HB_eAg$<br>Lifetime: anti-$HB_s$; anti-$HB_c$ | Acute phase: anti-HCV<br>Life time: anti-HCV | Acute phase: anti-HDV | No tests available |
| **SECRETIONS THAT HAVE BEEN FOUND TO CONTAIN INFECTIVE AGENT** | | | | |
| Feces, blood | Blood/serous fluids, saliva, semen, urine, nasopharyngeal washings, feces, pleural fluid | Blood, semen | Blood | Feces |
| **INDICATION OF PROTECTIVE IMMUNITY** | | | | |
| IgG anti-HAV | anti-$HB_s$, total anti-$HB_c$ | None | None | None |
| **CHRONICITY** | | | | |
| None | 90% infants, 6-10% adults | 50-80% | 2-70% | None |
| **MORTALITY** | | | | |
| <1% | 1-2% | 1-2% | 2-20% | 1-2% |
| **HIGH-RISK GROUPS** | | | | |
| Travelers to developing countries; staff and clients in custodial care institutions (prison, daycare, nursing homes) | Household and sexual partners of HBV carriers; immigrants from HBV-endemic areas; IV drug users; clients and staff in custodial care institutions; sexually active gay men; patients on hemodialysis; health care workers with frequent contact with blood | Travelers to endemic areas; people receiving frequent blood transfusions; IV drug users; tattoos; organ transplant recipients; 40% report no risk factors | Same as for HBV | Immigrants and travelers to HEV-epidemic areas |
| **VACCINE AVAILABLE** | | | | |
| Yes | Yes | No | No | No |

impairment and histopathological changes on a liver biopsy. Chronic active hepatitis is usually indicative of a poor prognosis but can revert to an inactive form. *Chronic relapsing hepatitis* is characterized by the reappearance of symptoms and signs after recovery from an acute episode (usually within 6 months). *Chronic persistent hepatitis* refers to cases of hepatitis with a benign course in which all the signs and symptoms do not resolve in the usual time frame. The patient may be asymptomatic, except for minimal abnormalities in serum transaminase levels. There is no indication of progression to severe hepatic dysfunction, and eventually full recovery occurs.

The clinical manifestations of the various forms of hepatitis are generally not distinct from each other. An exception is

**box 37-8** *Atypical Life-Threatening Variants of Hepatitis*

| | |
|---|---|
| Fulminant viral hepatitis | Sudden, severe degeneration and atrophy of liver, resulting in hepatic failure |
| Subacute fatal viral hepatitis | Severe but slower degeneration of liver |
| Confluent hepatic necrosis—submassive or massive | Destruction of substantial groups of adjacent cells with necrosis of portions of a lobule (submassive) or entire lobule (massive); can result in chronic active disease or cirrhosis, but most patients will recover |

HAV, in which the manifestations may be more abrupt in onset. The signs and symptoms and abnormal diagnostic tests can be grouped into three phases: preicteric, icteric, and posticteric phases. Box 37-9 lists pathophysiology and related clinical manifestations.

### *Collaborative care management*

**Diagnostic tests.** Blood tests are done for viral antibodies and antigens and for actual viral particles (see Table 37-3). Elevations in the serum liver enzymes ALT and AST are present in hepatitis A and B. Liver function tests are monitored until normal.

**Medications.** Vitamin K is given if the prothrombin time is prolonged. Antihistamines are given for pruritus associated with jaundice, and antiemetics are given for nausea. Essentially, all analgesics are metabolized in the liver and therefore are given only sparingly in people with liver dysfunction. Fulminant viral hepatitis may be treated with corticosteroids, but this is controversial.

**Treatments.** Most persons infected with hepatitis are not hospitalized. Those requiring hospitalization include persons with serum bilirubin concentrations 10 mg/dl or greater than 10 times the normal. In persons with fulminating hepatitis, hospitalization and bedrest are indicated. Unnecessary medications, including all sedatives, are discontinued. Coagulation defects may be treated with the administration of fresh frozen plasma. The patient's intake and output are carefully monitored, and intravenous fluid containing electrolytes is administered. Vomiting and diarrhea may cause electrolyte imbalances, particularly hypokalemia.

**Diet.** If liver function is not impaired, a well-balanced diet is adequate. A low-fat, high-carbohydrate diet may be better tolerated. Protein (20 to 30 mg/day) and sodium are restricted if liver function is compromised. Abstinence from alcohol is essential.

**Activity.** Rest is the foundation of treatment for viral hepatitis. Activity can be increased as tolerated by the patient.

**Referrals.** Patients and their families may be referred to the local health department for information about viral hepatitis. Referral to a home health care agency may be indicated for persons not requiring hospitalization.

**box 37-9** *Pathophysiology and Clinical Manifestations of Viral Hepatitis*

| PATHOPHYSIOLOGY | CLINICAL MANIFESTATIONS |
|---|---|
| | **Preicteric and Icteric Phase** |
| Necrosis and inflammation of hepatic cells with decreased liver function | Elevated temperature, chills, nausea, vomiting, dyspepsia, anorexia; right upper quadrant tenderness and enlarged liver; fatigue, weakness, and malaise; enlarged lymph nodes; elevated serum transaminases (ALT and AST) and alkaline phosphatase |
| | **Preicteric Phase** |
| Circulating immune complexes and complement system activation | Arthralgia, headache, urticaria |
| | **Icteric Phase** |
| Impaired bilirubin metabolism and obstruction to bile flow | Jaundice with elevated total, conjugated, and unconjugated serum bilirubin; dark-amber urine with bilirubinuria and increased urobilinogen; light-brown to grayish-white stools (depending on the amount of bile obstruction); pruritus |
| | **Preicteric, Icteric, and Posticteric Phases** |
| Viral infection | Presence of viral antibodies, antigens, or virus particles |

## NURSING MANAGEMENT

### ■ ASSESSMENT

Nursing assessment focuses on identifying the changes related to viral hepatitis and sources of transmission that are controllable.

#### Subjective Data

Data to be included to assess the patient with viral hepatitis include:

- Presence of discomfort: headache, right upper abdominal quadrant tenderness, arthralgia, and pruritis
- Presence of GI alterations: history of anorexia, nausea, vomiting, or dyspepsia
- Changes in nutritional intake of food and fluids
- History of changes in weight
- History of episodes of fever, chills, or adenopathy
- Reports of weakness/malaise not relieved by rest
- History of potential exposure to hepatitis virus: work environment, child-care facilities, recent international travel, injections of illegal drugs, recent blood transfusions, contaminated food and water, recent sexual contact with infected person, homosexual or bisexual lifestyle
- Knowledge about the disease
- Length of time since onset of symptoms

### Objective Data

Data to be included to assess the patient with viral hepatitis include:

Skin/sclerae: adequacy of skin turgor, presence of jaundice or lesions from scratching; if jaundice is present, the nurse should assess the patient for the presence of petechiae or bruises
Lymph nodes: enlargement
Abdomen: liver enlargement or guarding in right upper quadrant
Documented nutritional and fluid intake and output
Temperature
Weight/height
Musculoskeletal: strength and ability to do activities

## NURSING DIAGNOSES

Nursing diagnoses are determined from analysis of patient data. Nursing diagnoses for the patient with viral hepatitis may include but are not limited to:

| Diagnostic Title | Possible Etiological Factors |
|---|---|
| Fatigue | Imbalance between energy level and demand, decreased rest, feeling of malaise |
| Activity intolerance | Fatigue, weakness |
| Fluid volume deficit, risk for | Vomiting, sweating, decreased intake, elevated temperature |
| Infection, risk for | Length of infectivity and transmission to others through blood and/or body fluids |
| Nutrition, altered: less than body requirements | Anorexia, inadequate intake, increased metabolic needs |
| Pain | Arthralgia, pruritis, headaches, abdominal tenderness |
| Health maintenance, altered | Lack of knowledge or indifference to "safe sex" practices, needle sharing |
| Skin integrity, risk for impaired | Jaundice, pruritis, scratching |
| Social isolation | Physical isolation, fear of others catching disease |
| Injury (trauma), risk for | Altered clotting or prothrombin time |

## EXPECTED PATIENT OUTCOMES

Expected patient outcomes for the person with viral hepatitis may include but are not limited to:

1. Is able to explain why fatigue occurs and indicates a decrease in fatigue, as evidenced by giving it a lower rating on a scale of 1 to 5, with 1 indicating no fatigue.
2. Slowly increases activity until former activity level is achieved.
3. Maintains good skin tone, stable weight, and adequate and balanced intake and output; demonstrates no significant orthostatic postural changes in blood pressure (decrease in systolic between lying and standing of $\leq$10 mm Hg) or pulse (increase in pulse between lying and standing of $\leq$10 beats/min).
4. Is able to demonstrate adequate isolation precautions while hospitalized and describes appropriate precautions for use at home.
5. Increases food intake until adequate in amount and content for body size.
6. Verbalizes that pain is controlled and/or rates pain on a scale from 1 (no pain) to 10 (severe pain).
7. Is able to explain safe sex practices and describe the risk of needle sharing (see Chapter 14).
8. Skin remains intact and free of lesions.
9. Expresses the feeling that isolation is not distressing and shares information that reveals he or she is being kept up to date about family affairs.
10. Does not experience undetected bleeding.

## INTERVENTIONS

The patient with hepatitis needs general supportive care that promotes rest, fluid balance, prevention of injury, prevention of spread of disease, adequate knowledge, adequate nutrition, comfort, prevention of impairment of skin integrity, and prevention of social isolation. If the patient with HBV or HDV infection has a history of multiple sex partners, counseling and patient education about safe sex practices, as described in Chapters 50 and 67, are necessary. If a history of illegal drug use is elicited, the patient needs the care described in Chapter 14. The spread of the human immunodeficiency virus (HIV) and the hepatitis virus can be stopped in users of IV drugs if the practice of sharing equipment ceases. Some persons have suggested that sterile needles/syringes should be distributed to persons who are addicted to IV drugs, and some communities are doing so.

### Monitoring Fatigue

The patient with hepatitis will need considerable rest during the acute phase of the illness. The level of physical activity allowed will be individually determined based on the amount of fatigue and severity of the disease. Rest periods should be interspersed throughout the day, and patient care should be scheduled to allow for uninterrupted periods for napping and relaxation.

### Increasing Activity Tolerance

The patient should be instructed to increase activity slowly as tolerated. An adequate diet will provide needed energy for increasing activity. If hepatic enzyme levels increase with resumption of near-normal activities, limitations on activity will be reimposed.

### Maintaining Fluid Intake and Nutritional Status

During the acute phase of the illness, the patient needs 3000 ml/day of fluids because of the increased fluid needs associated with febrile illness and vomiting. The fluid can usually be given orally if nausea and vomiting are not severe. When nausea and vomiting are severe, IV infusions are given. Intake, output, and weight should be monitored to assess the patient for adequacy of intake. Fluids such as fruit juices and carbonated beverages that provide both volume and nutrients are encouraged. Because patients with impaired liver function may not produce adequate levels of albumin and may not metabolize aldosterone, abnormal fluid retention can occur. Although abnormal retention of fluids is rare in acute viral hepatitis, the patient should be monitored for evidence of fluid overload.

No special dietary restrictions are required in most patients. The diet should be well balanced and provide adequate nutrients and calories based on the patient's size and age. The diet should be planned with the patient so that it is appealing. Frequent, small meals are usually better tolerated than larger meals. Fats may need to be restricted if poorly tolerated. Intolerance to fatty foods can occur if bile obstruction is severe. Frequent oral hygiene and the maintenance of a clean, pleasant environment may enhance appetite. Antiemetics may be used and should be given ½ hour before meals. Alcoholic beverages should be avoided, since they are metabolized in the liver.

### Preventing Spread of Infection

All patients with hepatitis require precautions to prevent spread of the virus. For patients with HAV, the following transmission-based or Standard Precautions are necessary:

1. Good hand washing by patient and staff
2. Wearing gloves when handling feces/urine
3. Wearing a gown when soiling of uniform is likely
4. Cleansing of toilet daily and use of private toilet
5. Having a private room (only if patient cannot take care of self regarding proper disposal of feces and urine)
6. Proper cleansing, bagging, and labeling of contaminated items such as bed linens and bedpans
7. Discarding contaminated items such as rectal thermometers

For the patient with HBV transmission-based or Standard Precautions are used and include the following:

1. Good hand washing by patient and staff
2. Wearing gloves when handling blood or body fluids
3. Wearing a gown, goggles, and/or mask when splattering of blood or body fluids is likely
4. Proper cleansing, bagging, and labeling of contaminated equipment and linens
5. Proper disposing of needles or any items exposed to the patient's blood or body fluids
6. Careful labeling of blood specimens to protect personnel working with them
7. Avoiding contamination of open cuts and mucous membranes with patient's blood or body fluid
8. Teaching patients to avoid sexual contact until results of liver function tests have returned to normal

At times the nurse in the hospital and particularly the nurse in the community are also involved in identifying patient contacts who will require prophylactic therapy.

Because HBV, HCV, HDV, and possibly HAV, as well as carrier states of some types of hepatitis, can be spread by contaminated needles and other equipment that comes in contact with infected blood and body fluids, disposable and nondisposable needles, syringes, and other equipment used in patient care must be handled with great care. Strict adherence to transmission-based and Standard Precautions is essential (see Chapter 10). Patients with viral hepatitis must be informed that they may never donate blood.

### Providing Comfort Measures and Promoting Skin Integrity

During the early phase of the illness, the patient may have headaches and arthralgia, resulting in discomfort. General comfort measures—relaxing baths, backrubs, fresh linen on the bed, and a quiet, dark environment—may ease the patient's discomfort. During the icteric phase of the illness, the presence of bile pigments in the skin may cause severe pruritus. The cause of pruritus is unknown, but it is aggravated by the presence of bile pigments in the skin and by tissue anoxia and dilation of capillaries. Pruritus can be exhausting and demoralizing to the patient.

Measures to control pruritus include the following:

1. Use of cool, light, nonrestrictive clothing and avoidance of clothes or blankets made of wool
2. Use of soft, dry, clean bedding; use of warm, not hot, tub baths
3. Application of emollient creams and lotions to skin; use of superfat soaps
4. Avoidance of activities that promote sweating and increase body temperature
5. Maintenance of a cool environment
6. Administration of antihistamines as ordered
7. Use of diversional activities such as reading, television, and radio to reduce the patient's perception of pruritus

The major aim of care is to prevent scratching with resultant injury to the skin. It is impossible for people with pruritus not to scratch. Sometimes the person may be given a soft cloth with which to rub the skin. The patient's fingernails should be kept short, and the patient's hands should be kept clean to decrease the likelihood of excoriation or infection, if scratching occurs.

### Supporting Health Maintenance

The nurse must provide an open and honest environment where frank discussions about dangerous sexual practices and drug use can be undertaken. The risk of contracting viral hepatitis through multiple sex partners should be addressed. Sharing of IV drug equipment should be discouraged, and alternatives, such as drug treatment, should be suggested.

### Promoting Social Interaction

The nurse must work with the patient and significant others so that they understand that the needed isolation does not prohibit social interaction and visiting. Fear of spread of the infection can lead others to avoid the patient. Proper teaching can ensure that both isolation and the patient's need for support from significant others are maintained.

### Preventing Injury

In a patient with a prolonged prothrombin time, bleeding may be a major problem. The patient should be assessed carefully for signs of bleeding. This includes monitoring the urine and stools for fresh or old blood, monitoring any incisions for recurrent bleeding, monitoring the skin for petechiae, monitoring vital signs, and monitoring prothrombin time, hematocrit, and hemoglobin. Minor procedures such as drawing of blood can result in hematoma formation, if precautions are not instituted. Care to prevent hematoma formation includes the following:

1. Planning so that all blood samples are collected at one time to avoid multiple punctures
2. Avoiding intramuscular and subcutaneous injections, if possible
3. Applying pressure to injection sites and venipuncture site for 5 minutes after the procedure

Other precautions to prevent bleeding include:

1. Using soft toothbrushes or swabs to avoid injury to gums and resultant bleeding, avoid the use of dental floss
2. Using electric razors instead of razor blades for shaving

Stool should be checked for occult blood.

If prothrombin time is prolonged, vitamin K may be administered.

### Patient/Family Education

A major focus of care is patient education. Most patients are treated at home for the duration of their illness. The nurse must prepare these persons for adequate home care by teaching them about the measures previously described for the provision of adequate rest, provision of adequate fluid and nutritional intake, relief of discomfort, identification of signs and symptoms of bleeding, and maintenance of adequate isolation. The patient must be able to detect changes indicating a worsening of his or her condition (e.g., increasing fatigue, uncontrolled nausea and vomiting, onset of bleeding, worsening of upper quadrant discomfort, and water retention) and be instructed to report these changes immediately.

All patients, whether treated in the hospital or at home, should understand that it may take several months or longer for complete recovery, and that they must be evaluated frequently for repeated assessment of blood studies to monitor their progress. Blood studies may be performed weekly for several weeks and then monthly until results return to normal. If blood studies do not show the expected improvement from the care being given, more invasive procedures, such as a liver biopsy, may be necessary. The patient will be followed for at least 1 year after liver function tests have returned to normal to ensure that relapse does not occur.

Patients and their families should be educated about appropriate preexposure and postexposure prophylaxis. Teaching should include methods to avoid transmission of infection.

#### Prevention

**Hepatitis A.** Postexposure prophylaxis is recommended for selected people who have had contact with a person known to be positive for HAV. Prophylaxis must be given *within* 2 weeks of exposure. Postexposure prophylaxis for the following people is recommended:

1. Close household and sexual contacts of people with HAV
2. Staff and attendees of daycare centers, if HAV is recognized among attendees or employees or two or more households of center attendees report cases; household members of families with children in diapers, if three or more families of attendees report cases
3. Residents and staff in institutions for custodial care who have close contact with people with HAV
4. Hospital staff who have close contacts with patients with HAV (only if outbreaks occur)
5. People exposed to a common source of infection (infected food or water), if identified within 2 weeks of exposure
6. Food handlers working with a handler in whom hepatitis A has been diagnosed; patrons of food establishments only treated in rare instances

**Hepatitis B.** Hepatitis B is a vaccine-preventable disease. As the cost of the vaccine decreases, worldwide use will become more realistic. The vaccine provides active immunity (HBV vaccine) and an immune globulin with high amounts of anti-$HB_s$ (HBIG). The HBV vaccine is used in both preexposure and postexposure prophylaxis.

HBV vaccine is given as a series of three intramuscular injections (deltoid in adults and children; anterolateral thigh muscles in infants and neonates), with the second and third doses given 1 and 6 months after the first dose. The vaccine has shown an efficacy of 85% to 95%.[10] The effect of the vaccine on the developing fetus is not known. Because HBV infection in pregnant women results in a severe infection in the mother and chronic infection in the infant and because the vaccine contains only noninfectious hepatitis B surface antigen ($HB_sAg$) particles, pregnancy should not be considered a contraindication for its use.

HBV vaccine causes *no adverse effects or benefits* in HBV carriers. Because HBV vaccine has no benefits for HBV carriers and because of the cost of the vaccination (approximately $110/person), prevaccination serological screening for anti-$HB_c$ and anti-$HB_s$ may be done to identify both carriers and previously infected noncarriers who have adequate immunity. The cost of screening is weighed against the cost of unnecessary but harmless vaccination to identify whether screening before vaccinating should be performed.

A strategy to interrupt the transmission of HBV was initiated in 1991. In an effort to prevent early childhood and eventually adolescent and adult infections, the routine vaccination of all infants born in the United States was recommended. In addition, vaccination of adolescents and adults at high risk was undertaken.[10] The cost effectiveness of this strategy has been studied (Research Box). Current CDC guidelines suggest vaccination of all infants and young children as part of the regular immunization schedule.

Preexposure vaccination against hepatitis B is recommended for everyone with highest priority for the following:

1. Health care workers at high risk for exposure (medical technologists or staff, phlebotomists, most nurses in acute and critical care settings, surgeons, pathologists, oncology and dialysis unit staff, dentists, oral surgeons, dental hygienists, laboratory and blood bank technicians, emergency medical technicians, and morticians)
2. Clients and staff of institutions for developmentally disabled

**research**

Reference: Margolis HS et al: Prevention of hepatitis B virus transmission by immunization: an economic analysis of current recommendations. *JAMA* 274:1201-1208, 1995.

The purpose of this study was to evaluate the effectiveness of prevention of hepatitis B virus transmission based on immunization strategies. Since 1991 strategies to interrupt the transmission of HBV virus in all age groups have been initiated. These included preventing perinatal infection, vaccinating all infants in successive birth cohorts, and vaccinating adolescents and adults who are at high risk and were not vaccinated as infants.

This study used a decision model to determine the effects of HBV immunization strategies. The main outcome measure evaluated was the lifetime of the cohort related to the number of infections, medical costs, and work loss costs of HBV-related liver disease for each strategy cohort compared with the outcome without immunization. Results indicated that prevention of perinatal infection and routine infant vaccination would lower the 4.8% lifetime risk of HBV infection by at least 68%, compared with a 45% risk reduction for adolescent vaccination. The strategies were not cost-saving in terms of direct medical costs, but were cost-saving from a societal perspective.

The authors concluded that continuing routine vaccination of infants would be cost-saving over a wide range of assumptions. Adolescent vaccination would be less cost-effective but would serve to protect those children who were not vaccinated as infants. The implications for nursing practice are in the area of community education programs that encourage the vaccination of infants and compliance with vaccination schedule recommendations.

3. Hemodialysis patients
4. Sexually active persons with multiple partners
5. IV drug users sharing needles
6. Frequent recipients of blood products, particularly patients with clotting disorders who receive frequent transfusions of clotting factors
7. Household and sexual contacts of HBV carriers
8. Some American populations, including infants, such as Alaskan Inuits, native Pacific islanders, and immigrants and refugees and their infants from areas where HBV is endemic, such as Eastern Asia; adoptees from countries with high HBV endemicity; and families of adoptees with positive $HB_sAg$ tests
9. Long-term correctional facility inmates
10. International travelers who plan to reside in areas with a high endemic incidence of HBV for 6 months or longer

Postexposure prophylaxis for HBV should be considered for the following:

1. Infants born to $HB_sAg$-positive mothers
2. Persons who have percutaneous or permucosal exposure to $HB_sAg$-positive blood
3. Persons who have sexual contact with $HB_sAg$-positive persons
4. Infants younger than 12 months old exposed to a primary caregiver who has acute HBV

Infants exposed perinatally are given HBIG at birth, and the HBV vaccination series is started at the same time, if possible. Persons who have percutaneous or permucosal exposure and are unvaccinated are also treated with HBIG, and the HBV vaccination series is started. If the exposed person has been vaccinated, he or she is checked for anti-$HB_s$ and given HBIG immediately plus a booster dose of HBV vaccination. The CDC also makes recommendations about prophylaxis after percutaneous or permucosal exposure from a source with unknown hepatitis B virus status.

**Hepatitis C and E.** Prophylaxis for HCV and HEV infections is not as effective as that for HBV. For travelers to countries where HEV occurs in endemic proportions, preventive health teaching is the best prophylactic measure. The value of immunoglobulin in this situation is unknown. For postexposure prophylaxis in persons exposed through breaks in the skin to blood from a patient with HCV, immunoglobulin may be given, but its value is questionable.[5]

**Hepatitis D.** HDV requires the presence of HBV; thus the preexposure and postexposure prophylaxes that are recommended for HBV should suffice to prevent delta hepatitis. Currently, no prophylaxis exists for preventing HDV infection in HBV carriers except health teaching.

The major activity that can assist in the general prevention of the spread of viral hepatitis is the use of Standard Precautions for all people. All feces, urine, blood, and other body fluids should be considered potentially infectious for a wide variety of organisms and disposed of properly. Nurses should educate others about the development of adequate sewage disposal systems to prevent contamination of food and water supplies that may result in endemic forms of HAV.

### *Health Promotion/Prevention*

***Healthy People 2000.*** *Healthy People 2000* goals regarding the reduction of the incidence of viral hepatitis were revised in 1995 (Box 37-10). Revisions also included reducing the number of cases of hepatitis A among international travelers to 1,119 from the 1987 baseline of 4,475.[18] Other high-risk groups are Native Americans and IV drug users. Currently, there are two HAV vaccines available, both containing inactivated virus.[4] However, use is limited due to cost and availability. HBV vaccine has the potential to dramatically decrease the incidence of HBV infection. *Healthy People 1995* revisions included increasing the use of hepatitis B vaccine among high-risk populations, including infants of hepatitis B surface antigen-positive mothers and occupationally exposed workers to at least 90%; and injecting drug users and men who have sex with men to at least 50%.[18] Health care workers have an increased risk of being infected with HBV. Reduction in the number of HBV cases will in part be accomplished by increasing to at least 90% the proportion of public health departments that provide adult HBV immunizations.[18]

**box 37-10** Healthy People 2000: *1995 Review and Revisions*

| **REDUCE VIRAL HEPATITIS AS FOLLOWS: (Per 100,000)** | **1987 Baseline** | **2000 Target** |
|---|---|---|
| Hepatitis B | 63.5 | 40.0 |
| Hepatitis A | 33.0 | 16.0 |
| Hepatitis C | 18.3 | 13.7 |
| **SPECIAL POPULATION TARGETS** | | |
| **Hepatitis B (Number of Cases)** | **1987 Baseline** | **2000 Target** |
| Injecting drug users | 44,348 | 7,932 |
| Heterosexually active people | 33,995 | 22,663 |
| Homosexual men | 13,598 | 4,568 |
| Children of Asians/Pacific Islanders | 10,817 | 1,500 |
| Occupationally exposed workers | 3,090 | 623 |
| Infants (chronic infections) | 6,012 | 1,111 |
| Alaska Natives (number of new carriers) | 15 | 1 |
| | **1992 Baseline** | **2000 Target** |
| African Americans (cases per 100,000) | 52.8 | 40 |
| **Hepatitis A (cases per 100,000)** | | |
| Hispanics | 53.8 | 27 |
| Native Americans/Alaska Natives | 256.0 | 128 |
| **Hepatitis C (cases per 100,000)** | | |
| Hispanics | 17.2 | 13 |

From US Department of Health and Human Services, Public Health Service: *Healthy People 2000: midcourse review and revisions.*

Since the identification of HCV, screening of blood products has reduced the incidence of post-transfusion hepatitis from hepatitis C to about 5% (Research Box).[16]

## ■ EVALUATION

To evaluate the effectiveness of nursing interventions, compare patient behaviors with those stated in the expected patient outcomes. Successful achievement of patient outcomes for the patient with viral hepatitis is indicated by:

1. States cause of fatigue, and that fatigue remains at a rating of 2 or less if rest periods are interspersed throughout the day.
2. Reports an increased activity level without an increase in fatigue.
3. Displays fluid volume balance by intake that equals output and is adequate for age and body size; has no orthostatic blood pressure changes; and weight is stable and within normal range.

4a. Describes isolation precautions for home, including using a separate bathroom from family if possible; flushing stool twice after using the toilet; handling own body secretions, not sharing razors, toothbrushes, and food or drinks; abstaining from sexual relationships until infection has subsided; and washing hands as appropriate.

b. Verbalizes understanding of blood tests; explains why isolation is necessary; identifies persons in household who may have been exposed to same source of infection from contaminated foods and fluids, hygiene practices, sharing of needles, or sexual relationships; explains need for high-

**research** 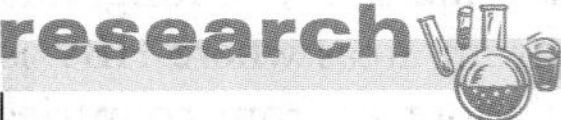

Reference: Cooksley WG, Butterworth LA: Hepatitis C virus infection in health care workers referred to a hepatitis clinic. *Med J Aust* 164:656-658, 1996.

The purpose of this research was to assess the method of acquisition of hepatitis C infection by health care workers. This study also examined the effect of HCV infection on the work practices of those health care workers who were infected.

The sample consisted of 33 health care workers who were referred to a hepatitis clinic for management of their HCV infection between 1990 and the end of 1994. The 12 men and 18 women ranged in age from 27 to 68 years. There were 6 physicians, 18 nurses, 2 scientists, and 7 others.

They were retrospectively assessed for the most likely method of infection. All underwent liver biopsy and measurement of HCV-RNA. After assessment it was found that only 30 had confirmed HCV infection. Only seven were thought to have occupationally acquired HCV infection. Liver biopsy indicated that only 1 had cirrhosis, and 12 had chronic hepatitis and fibrosis. Only 12 members of the sample continued to practice. The others had either retired, quit working, or modified their work practices.

The researchers concluded that very few health care workers acquire HCV infection from their employment situation. Recommendations included establishing guidelines in institutions to advise health care workers with HCV infection regarding methods to modify their work environment and practices to promote their health and the health of those they serve.

table 37-4 *Types of Cirrhosis*

| TYPE | ETIOLOGY | DESCRIPTION |
|---|---|---|
| Laënnec's cirrhosis (nutritional, portal, or alcoholic cirrhosis) | Alcoholism, malnutrition | Massive collagen formation occurs; liver in fatty and hepatitis stages is large and firm; in late state, it is small and nodular. |
| Postnecrotic cirrhosis | Massive necrosis from hepatotoxins, usually viral hepatitis | Liver is decreased in size with nodules and fibrous tissue. |
| Primary biliary cirrhosis | Inflammation of intrahepatic bile ductules resulting in biliary obstruction in liver and common bile duct; cholangitis (destruction of the intrahepatic bile ducts) of unknown etiology may occur; altered immune response suggested | Chronic impairment of bile drainage occurs; liver is first large, then becomes firm and nodular; jaundice is major symptom. Pruritus, hypercholesterolemia, cholestasis (blockage of bile flow), and malabsorption are common manifestations. |
| Cardiac cirrhosis | Right-sided congestive heart failure (CHF) | Liver is swollen, and changes are reversible if CHF is treated effectively; some fibrosis occurs with long-standing CHF. |
| Nonspecific, metabolic cirrhosis | Metabolic problems, infectious diseases, infiltrative diseases, GI diseases | Portal and liver fibrosis may develop; liver is enlarged and firm. |

protein, high-calorie, well-balanced diet, adequate rest, and avoidance of alcohol; explains hygiene practices, safe sex practices, and avoidance of sharing of needles to avoid future infections; and states plans for obtaining vaccinations for self and others as appropriate.

5. Verbalizes knowledge of nutritionally adequate diet, demonstrates adequate intake, and uses measures to enhance appetite.
6. States that itching and arthralgia are controlled and that no scratching, restlessness, or grimacing is present.
7. Correctly explains safe sex practices and dangers of sharing needles.
8. Displays intact skin.
9. Participates in social/family activities at level of ability.
10. Remains free from injury, hematocrit and hemoglobin levels remain within normal limits, prothrombin time is within normal limits, and no bleeding episodes occur.

## COMPLICATIONS

Potential complications of viral hepatitis include chronic active hepatitis with subsequent cirrhosis and liver failure. These complications are discussed in the following section.

## CIRRHOSIS OF THE LIVER

*Cirrhosis* of the liver is the term applied to chronic disease of the liver characterized by diffuse inflammation and fibrosis resulting in drastic structural changes and significant loss of liver function. The basic changes with cirrhosis are liver cell death and replacement of normal tissue by regeneration of cell mass and scar tissue that results in nodules of normal liver parenchyma surrounded by fibrous tissue and fat. These changes result in loss of function and distortion of the structure with a resultant obstruction of hepatic blood flow.

Cirrhosis of the liver can be classified in various ways. Table 37-4 lists the major types of cirrhosis based on a pathological classification.

### Etiology

As can be seen from Table 37-4, cirrhosis can result from liver disease secondary to intrahepatic and extrahepatic cholestasis, viral hepatitis, and other hepatotoxins (drugs and chemicals). Alcoholism and malnutrition are two major predisposing factors for development of Laënnec's cirrhosis. Less common causes of cirrhosis are right-sided congestive heart failure, hemochromatosis, Wilson's disease, glycogen storage disease, cystic fibrosis, and small bowel bypass. In some patients the cause is idiopathic.

### Epidemiology

*Postnecrotic* cirrhosis from hepatotoxins is the most common type of cirrhosis worldwide. *Laënnec's cirrhosis* is the most common type in North America and accounts for 75% of all cases of cirrhosis.

The role of alcohol in the development of cirrhosis is still under study. It is known, however, that approximately 15% of all alcoholics will develop cirrhosis and that the volume of alcohol rather than the type of alcohol is the important factor. Most persons with Laënnec's cirrhosis have a history of consumption of the equivalent of a pint of whiskey a day for 15 years.

Cirrhosis as a cause of death in the United States now ranks fourth in middle-aged men and women, accounting for 350,000 deaths each year. Cirrhosis can occur in any age group, but in the United States it is more common in 45- to 64-year-old white men and in nonwhites of both sexes.

### Pathophysiology

In Laënnec's cirrhosis caused by alcoholism and in other types of cirrhosis, fatty infiltration of the liver is the first alteration seen. This fatty infiltration is usually reversible if the causative factor (alcohol, malnutrition, or biliary obstruction) is halted or reversed. If the degenerative process continues, acute inflammation (alcoholic hepatitis) and cirrhosis result.

The result of any type of cirrhosis is loss of liver function and obstruction of hepatic portal blood flow. Alterations in physiology are usually seen late in the progression of the disease because of the large reserve capacity of the liver. As much as three fourths of the liver can be destroyed before physiological function is altered.

In the United States the pathophysiological changes seen most often are a result of both cirrhosis and long-term alcohol abuse. The relationships between normal functions of the liver and alterations seen in cirrhosis are presented in Table 37-5.

The fibrotic changes in the liver that result from continual destruction distort the hepatic structures and result in obstruction of splanchnic veins and portal blood flow. This obstruction can result in additional problems with fluid retention, including increasing edema, ascites, and hydrothorax. Increased portal pressure and splanchnic venous congestion result in splenomegaly and altered spleen function, which can cause leukopenia, thrombocytopenia, and anemia. Portal hypertension causes increased venous pressure, vascular hemostasis, varicose veins, hemorrhoids, and esophageal varices. (Figure 37-3, *A*, depicts the venous drainage of splanchnic organs, and Figure 37-3, *B*, depicts the massive ascites and dilated vasculature that can be seen in cirrhosis.)

A variety of signs and symptoms can be seen in persons with cirrhosis. The patient may exhibit any or all of the signs and symptoms. Most manifestations can be directly related to the pathophysiological changes (Table 37-5 and Figure 37-4). Box 37-11 lists clinical manifestations of cirrhosis.

## Collaborative Care Management

The goal for discharge of patients with cirrhosis as determined by diagnosis-related groups (DRGs) is 7 days. The nurse works collaboratively with the physician for implementation of prescribed medical therapy. Because the nurse has a major role in discharge planning and patient teaching, these are discussed under nursing management. A sample Clinical Pathway and Nursing Care Plan follows the Interventions section (p. 1219-1223).

### Diagnostic tests

The patient with cirrhosis will have various abnormalities in blood and urine laboratory data as depicted in Figure 37-4. Other studies, such as liver biopsy, CT scan, endoscopy, barium contrast, and angiography, may be done if the clinical manifestations are vague or inconsistent. The results of these later diagnostic tests depend on the complications the patient has developed.

### Medications

Drug therapy depends on the signs and symptoms the patient exhibits and includes the following medications: antihistamines for pruritus; potassium for hypokalemia; diuretics (particularly aldosterone antagonists for edema because the patient with cirrhosis does not catabolize aldosterone appropriately and has hyperaldosteronism); and folic acid, thiamine, and other vitamins and minerals for vitamin deficiency and anemia. Persons with alcoholism are particularly deficient in thiamine and folic acid because these water-soluble vitamins have been depleted and thus deficits occur rapidly with lack of intake of nutrients. Sodium and fluids are also usually restricted. Occasionally, albumin may be given for hypoalbuminemia; however, its effects last only a short time.

### Treatments

No specific medical management exists for the treatment of cirrhosis. Management is directed toward removal or treatment of causative factors such as alcoholism, biliary obstruction, infections, and cardiac problems and toward preventing additional liver damage. If ascites causes severe distress, para-

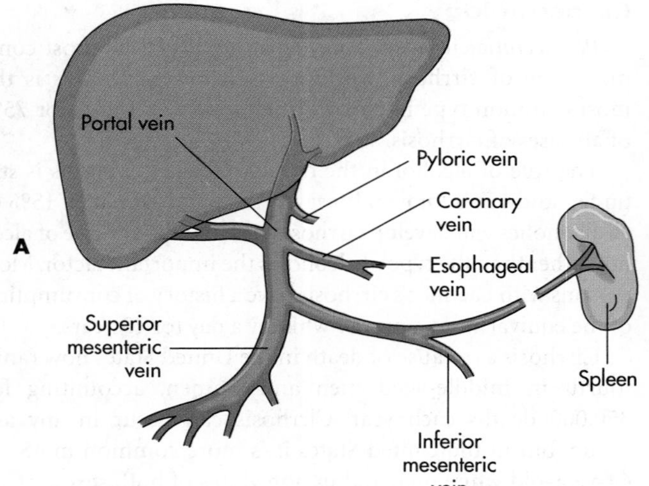


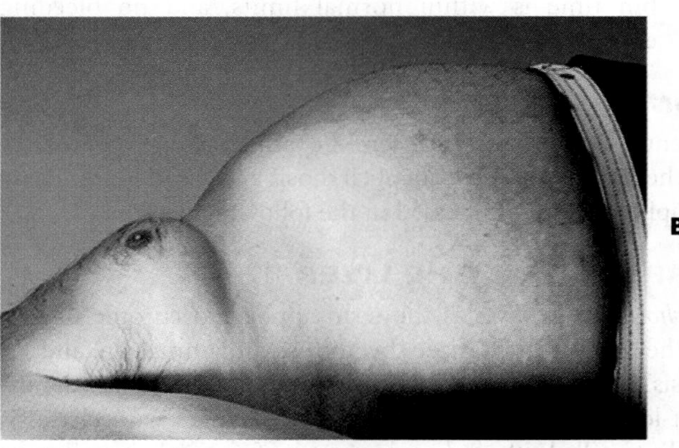


**fig. 37-3** **A,** Splanchnic veins. Venous drainage of splanchnic organs. When portal hypertension develops, other vessels can become engorged, leading to stasis and hypoxia of the respective organs. **B,** Ascites and gynecomastia associated with cirrhosis of the liver. Photograph taken after a paracentesis was performed.

**table 37-5** *Relationship Between Normal Liver Functions and Altered Functions Associated with Cirrhosis*

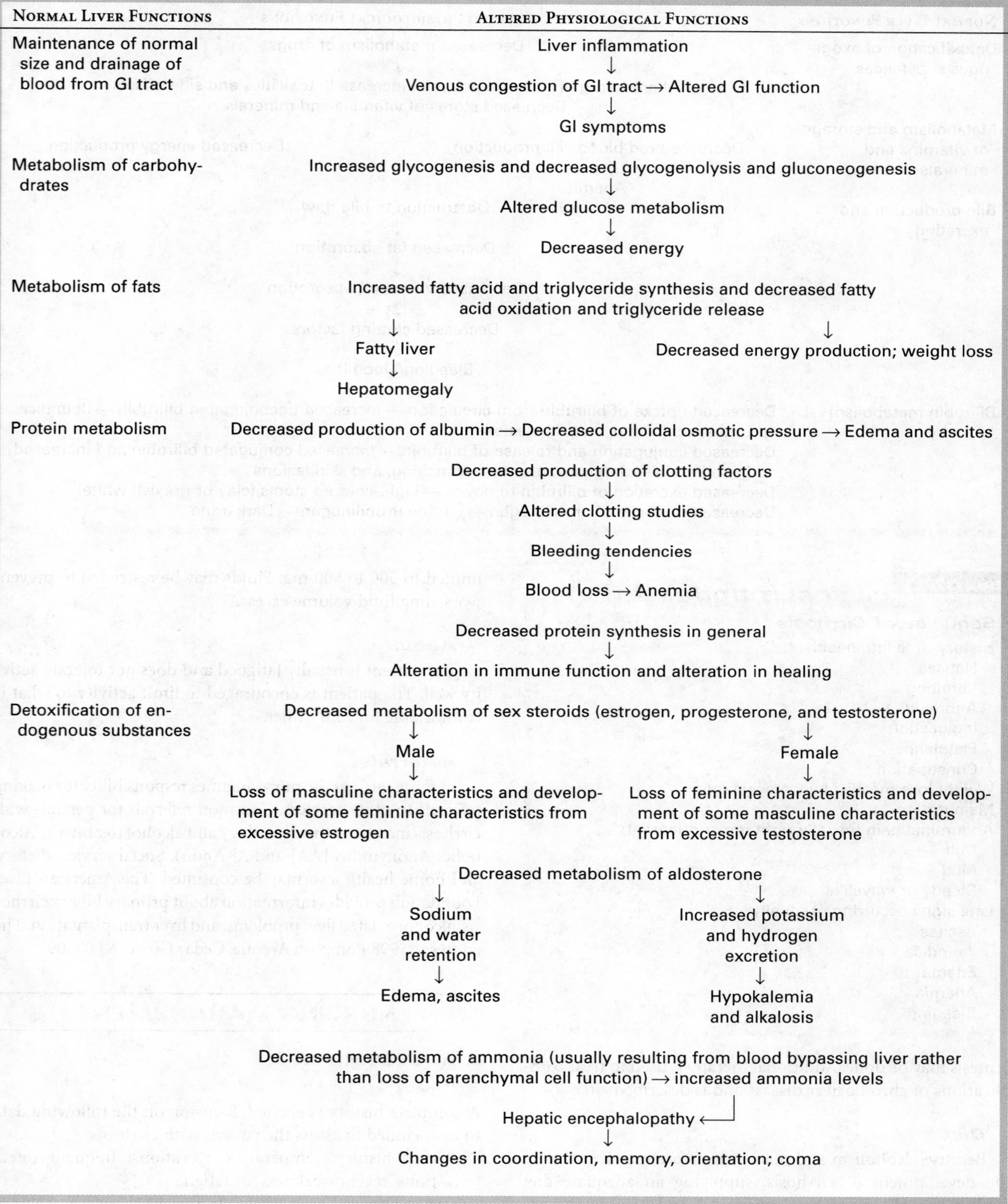

| NORMAL LIVER FUNCTIONS | ALTERED PHYSIOLOGICAL FUNCTIONS |
|---|---|
| Maintenance of normal size and drainage of blood from GI tract | Liver inflammation ↓ Venous congestion of GI tract → Altered GI function ↓ GI symptoms |
| Metabolism of carbohydrates | Increased glycogenesis and decreased glycogenolysis and gluconeogenesis ↓ Altered glucose metabolism ↓ Decreased energy |
| Metabolism of fats | Increased fatty acid and triglyceride synthesis and decreased fatty acid oxidation and triglyceride release ↓ Fatty liver ↓ Hepatomegaly; ↓ Decreased energy production; weight loss |
| Protein metabolism | Decreased production of albumin → Decreased colloidal osmotic pressure → Edema and ascites<br>Decreased production of clotting factors ↓ Altered clotting studies ↓ Bleeding tendencies ↓ Blood loss → Anemia<br>Decreased protein synthesis in general ↓ Alteration in immune function and alteration in healing |
| Detoxification of endogenous substances | Decreased metabolism of sex steroids (estrogen, progesterone, and testosterone)<br>↓ Male ↓ Loss of masculine characteristics and development of some feminine characteristics from excessive estrogen<br>↓ Female ↓ Loss of feminine characteristics and development of some masculine characteristics from excessive testosterone<br>Decreased metabolism of aldosterone<br>↓ Sodium and water retention ↓ Edema, ascites<br>↓ Increased potassium and hydrogen excretion ↓ Hypokalemia and alkalosis<br>Decreased metabolism of ammonia (usually resulting from blood bypassing liver rather than loss of parenchymal cell function) → increased ammonia levels ↓ Hepatic encephalopathy ↓ Changes in coordination, memory, orientation; coma |

*Continued*

**table 37-5** *Relationship Between Normal Liver Functions and Altered Functions Associated with Cirrhosis—cont'd*

| Normal Liver Functions | Altered Physiological Functions |
|---|---|
| Detoxification of exogenous substances | Decreased metabolism of drugs ↓ Altered drug effects and potential increase in toxicities and side effects |
| Metabolism and storage of vitamins and minerals | Decreased stores of vitamins and minerals ↙ Decreased red blood cell production ↓ Anemia; ↘ Decreased energy production |
| Bile production and excretion | Obstruction to bile flow ↓ Decreased fat absorption ↓ Decreased vitamin K absorption ↓ Decreased clotting factors ↓ Bleeding/blood loss |
| Bilirubin metabolism | Decreased uptake of bilirubin from circulation → Increased unconjugated bilirubin → Jaundice, pruritus, scratching, and skin lesions<br>Decreased conjugation and release of bilirubin → Increased conjugated bilirubin and increased urine bilirubin → Jaundice, pruritus, scratching, and skin lesions<br>Decreased excretion of bilirubin to bowel → Light-colored stools (clay or grayish white)<br>Decreased reuptake of urobilinogen → ↑ urine urobilinogen → Dark urine |

**box 37-11** *clinical manifestations*

***Sequelae of Cirrhosis***

- History of failing health
  - Nausea
  - Vomiting
  - Anorexia
  - Indigestion
  - Flatulence
  - Constipation
- Weight loss masked by water retention
- Malnutrition
- Abdominal pain (usually right upper quadrant)
  - Dull
  - Mild
  - Steady or wavelike
- Late signs occurring gradually
  - Ascites
  - Jaundice
  - Edema
  - Anemia
  - Bleeding

centesis may be done. Additional therapy is used to treat complications of chronic liver disease and is described later.

### *Diet*

Because alcoholism and malnutrition are major factors in the development of cirrhosis, supplying an adequate diet (well-balanced with normal nutrients) and helping the patient control alcohol intake are important. Vitamin supplements are usually prescribed. In the presence of ascites, a low-sodium diet is recommended. Daily intake of sodium is limited to 500 to 800 mg. Fluids may be restricted to prevent worsening fluid volume excess.

### *Activity*

The patient is usually fatigued and does not tolerate activity well. The patient is encouraged to limit activity to what is comfortable for him or her.

### *Referrals*

In some settings the nurse assumes responsibility for making referrals to other services. Common referrals for persons with cirrhosis include gastroenterology and alcohol treatment (Alcoholics Anonymous [AA] and Al-Anon). Social service, dietary, and home health also may be consulted. The American Liver Foundation provides information about primary biliary cirrhosis, alcohol-related liver problems, and liver transplantation. The address is: 998 Pompton Avenue, Cedar Grove, NJ 07009.

## NURSING MANAGEMENT

### ■ ASSESSMENT

#### Subjective Data

A complete history is elicited, focusing on the following data to be included to assess the patient with cirrhosis:

Recent history: temperature elevations; frequent infections, recent weakness, or fatigue

General body characteristics: history of changes in color of skin or sclera; history of skin marks such as bruising and hematomas; history of changes in secondary sex characteristics (external genitalia, body hair distribution, or

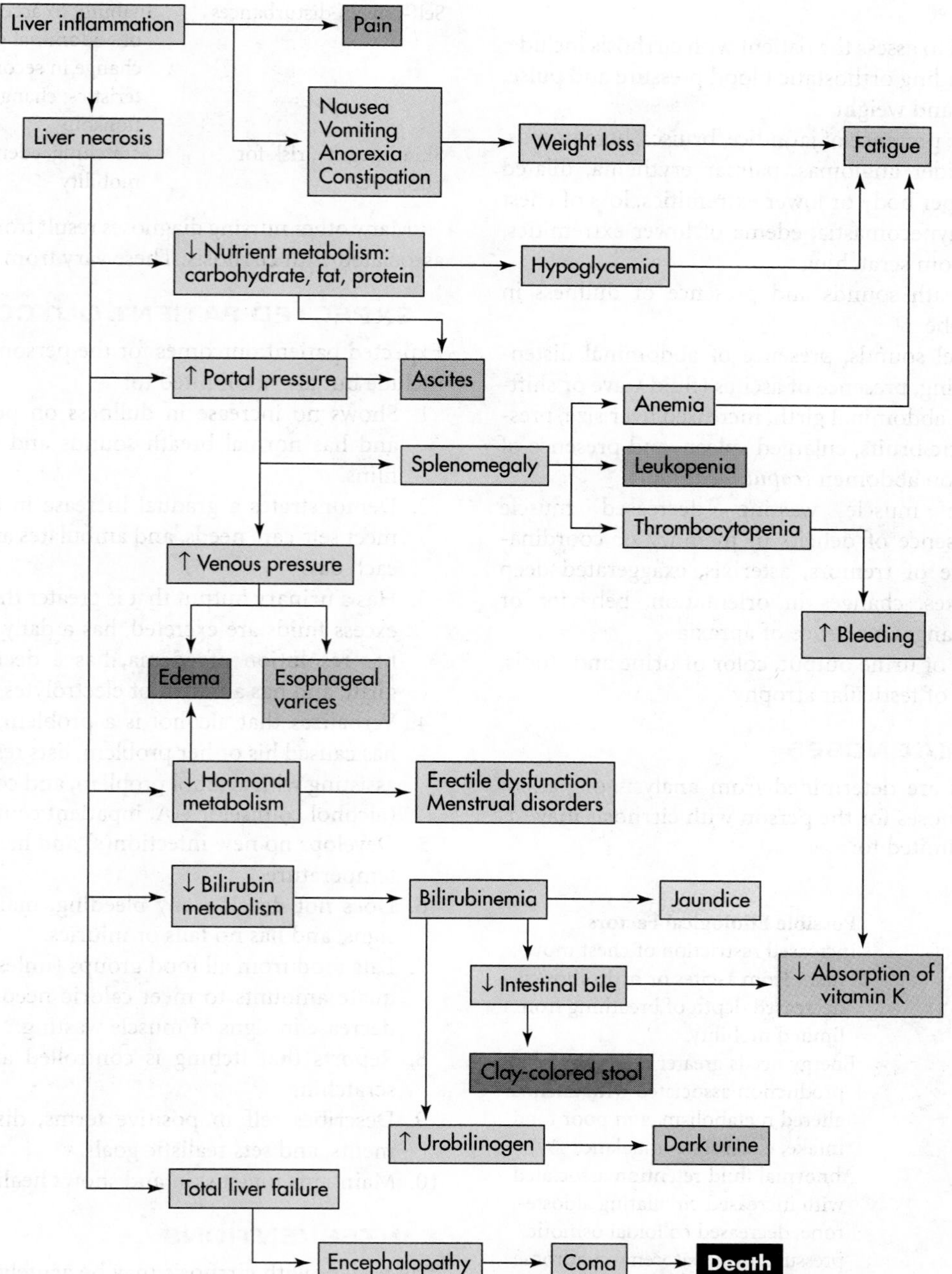


**fig. 37-4** Progression of liver cell failure. Pathophysiology of signs and symptoms that occur in cirrhosis. Note: process can be arrested if adequate liver regeneration occurs. Regeneration is rarely complete, and there is always some liver cell deficiency.

breast tissue); history of increase in abdominal girth (belt size); history of edema; any complaints of itching; muscle wasting

Social habits: drug and alcohol use, amount, factors that precipitate use, any attempts to quit, limitations on success, reasons for failure; last time patient had a drink; work environment

Nutritional history: daily 24-hour intake for past 1 to 3 days; history of recent change in appetite, anorexia, or weight loss

GI system: complaints of nausea, vomiting, anorexia, indigestion, flatulence, or abdominal tenderness

Elimination: history of any changes in amount or color of urine, changes in bowel movements, or changes in color of feces

Neuromuscular: any complaints of weakness or fatigue; history of decreased ability to do work; history of any changes in memory or coordination; any history of tremors

Sexuality: history of erectile dysfunction, decreased libido (men and women), or change in menstrual patterns

### Objective Data

Data to be included to assess the patient with cirrhosis include:

Vital signs, including orthostatic blood pressure and pulse, temperature, and weight

Skin and sclerae: presence of jaundice, bruises, hematomas, petechiae, spider angiomas, palmar erythema, dilated vessels on upper body or lower extremities, loss of chest hair (men), gynecomastia, edema of lower extremities, and lesions from scratching

Respiratory: breath sounds and presence of dullness in right lower lobe

Abdomen: bowel sounds, presence of abdominal distention or guarding, presence of ascites (fluid wave or shifting dullness), abdominal girth, increased liver size, presence of hepatic bruits, enlarged spleen, and presence of dilated veins on abdomen *(caput medusae)*

Neuromuscular: muscle wasting, decreased muscle strength, presence of deficits in memory or coordination, presence of tremors, asterixis, exaggerated deep tendon reflexes, changes in orientation, behavior or emotional changes, presence of apraxia

GI/GU: volume of urine output, color of urine and stools, and presence of testicular atrophy

## NURSING DIAGNOSES

Nursing diagnoses are determined from analysis of patient data. Nursing diagnoses for the person with cirrhosis may include but are not limited to:

| Diagnostic Title | Possible Etiological Factors |
|---|---|
| Breathing pattern, ineffective | Increased restriction of chest movement from ascites or hydrothorax; decreased depth of breathing from limited mobility |
| Fatigue | Energy needs greater than energy production associated with anemia, altered metabolism, and poor food intake; electrolyte imbalance |
| Fluid volume, excess | Abnormal fluid retention associated with increased circulating aldosterone, decreased colloidal osmotic pressure, or hepatorenal syndrome |
| Health maintenance, altered | Inability to make appropriate judgments because of alcoholism |
| Infection, risk for | Decreased immune competence associated with altered protein metabolism and alcoholism; loss of normal phagocytic function of liver or decreased leukocytes secondary to splenomegaly; alterations in external immune barriers (skin and GI mucosal integrity) |
| Injury (trauma), risk for | Alteration in clotting mechanism, enhancing bleeding; alteration in neurological function and strength that could lead to falls |
| Nutrition, altered: less than body requirements | Impaired metabolism, nausea, or decreased intake |
| Pain: itching | Enlarged liver and pruritus associated with jaundice |
| Self-esteem disturbances | Inability to accept physical changes of abdominal girth, jaundice, and change in secondary sexual characteristics; changes in roles and relationship |
| Skin integrity, risk for impaired | Scratching, edema, or impaired mobility |

Many other nursing diagnoses result from the complications associated with cirrhosis. These vary from patient to patient.

## EXPECTED PATIENT OUTCOMES

Expected patient outcomes for the person with cirrhosis may include but are not limited to:

1. Shows no increase in dullness on percussion of thorax and has normal breath sounds and normal chest x-ray films.
2. Demonstrates a gradual increase in activities, is able to meet self-care needs, and ambulates an increased amount each day.
3. Has a urinary output that is greater than fluid intake until excess fluids are excreted, has a daily decrease in weight, has resolution of edema, has a decrease of abdominal girth, and has a return of electrolytes to normal.
4. Verbalizes that alcohol is a problem, states that alcohol has caused his or her problem, lists resources available for assisting with alcohol problem, and contacts one resource (alcohol counselor, AA, inpatient center).
5. Develops no new infection(s) and has a return to normal temperature.
6. Does not develop any bleeding, maintains normal vital signs, and has no falls or injuries.
7. Eats food from all food groups (unless restricted) in adequate amounts to meet caloric needs and experiences a decrease in signs of muscle wasting.
8. Reports that itching is controlled and is not observed scratching.
9. Describes self in positive terms, discusses accomplishments, and sets realistic goals.
10. Maintains intact skin and shows healing of any lesions.

## INTERVENTIONS

The patient with cirrhosis may be acutely ill and may require critical nursing care or may be relatively free of acute problems and require teaching, counseling, and support. The nurse must set priorities for care on the basis of the patient's needs. Care for the various patient outcomes is described next and in the Nursing Care Plan on p. 1219-1221.

### Supporting Respiration

The patient with cirrhosis has decreased resistance to infection and may be particularly prone to respiratory infection because of the presence of a hydrothorax and/or shallow breathing. The patient may experience dyspnea because of pressure on the diaphragm from ascites.

A high Fowler's position may assist respiratory exchange. The patient for whom bedrest is prescribed should be encouraged to turn frequently and to take deep breaths to prevent stasis of secretions. Hydrothorax is sometimes treated

*Text continued on p. 1222*

# nursing care plan The Person with Cirrhosis

**DATA** Mr. S. is a 55-year-old salesman with portal hypertension who is admitted to the hospital with upper GI bleeding. Endoscopy revealed enlarged esophageal and upper gastric veins and a bleeding ulcer. One unit of packed red blood cells was given. Treatment orders included protein (20 g/day) and sodium (1000 mg/day) restrictions, fluid (1000 ml/day) restriction, neomycin (1 g every 4 hours), thiamine (1 ml intramuscularly), vitamin K subcutaneously once a day, and spironolactone (25 mg twice a day). A physical examination revealed slight jaundice of sclera and skin; ascites and peripheral edema; thin legs and arms and poor musculature; signs of increased estrogen; orientation to person, place, and time; blood pressure of 116/60 mm Hg; pulse of 90 beats/min; and respiration rate of 32.

The nursing history identified the following:

- Mr. S. has participated in AA for 1 year; he has not been drinking since then.
- Mr. S. has had influenza-like symptoms the past 2 weeks but continued with his busy schedule. He complains of fatigue, anorexia, and itching.

Collaborative nursing actions include interventions to prevent further impairment of physical status from hemorrhage and ammonia toxicity and to assist in treatment of the gastric ulcer and fluid excess. Nursing actions include monitoring for the following:

- Signs of hemorrhage: hematemesis, decreased blood pressure, tachycardia, restlessness, stools testing positive for guaiac, and cool, moist skin
- Signs of hepatic encephalopathy: change in mental status, asterixis, and change in handwriting, tremors

**NURSING DIAGNOSIS** *Fatigue related to muscle wasting, blood loss, and potential anemia*

| expected patient outcome | nursing interventions | rationale |
|---|---|---|
| Indicates on a weekly basis that he is less fatigued; shows improved rating of fatigue on a scale of 1 (no fatigue) to 10 (severe fatigue); shows a gradual increase in activities on a weekly basis. | Ensure or maintain bedrest as prescribed during the acute phase.<br>After acute phase, encourage increasing activity interspersed with rest periods as tolerated.<br>Intervene if patient shows fatigue after or during visits by family or friends.<br>Make sure diet is well balanced nutritionally and that patient takes calories, protein, and sodium within proper restrictions. | Graduated increase of activity is important to not overtax patient who has poor nutritional status and activity intolerance. |

**NURSING DIAGNOSIS** *Altered nutrition less than body requirements related to anorexia and flu-like symptoms*

| expected patient outcome | nursing interventions | rationale |
|---|---|---|
| Ingests required nutrients and adequate calories on a daily basis; signs of muscle wasting lessen. | Assess knowledge of nutrient needs.<br>On a daily basis, plan and implement well-balanced, high-carbohydrate, low-protein diet with adequate vitamins.<br>Decrease roughage in diet.<br>Encourage use of salt substitute or alternative seasonings (e.g., Mrs. Dash).<br>Give antiemetics as prescribed and mouth care if nausea is present.<br>Suggest six small, frequent meals daily.<br>Use measures that encourage eating, such as a clean environment and making sure patient is rested and comfortable.<br>Support continuation of AA activities while patient is hospitalized. | Food intake within prescribed limitation can influence liver regeneration; nursing measures can influence amount of intake in anorectic patient.<br>Low-roughage diet is necessary because of esophageal varices.<br>It is important that patient continue AA participation as he has for past year. AA representatives should be allowed to see patient as condition permits. |

**NURSING DIAGNOSIS** *Fluid volume excess related to impaired metabolism of aldosterone and hypoalbuminemia*

| expected patient outcomes | nursing interventions | rationale |
|---|---|---|
| Weight and abdominal girth decrease daily.<br>Edema resolves. | Monitor weight daily, blood pressure q4hr; assess edema every shift; and measure abdominal girth daily.<br>Monitor intake and output on every shift until excess fluid is excreted. | Diuresis in cirrhosis is undertaken slowly using very conservative measures because of the contracted intravascular fluid volume. Diuresis in excess can jeopardize renal perfusion |

Continued

## The Person with Cirrhosis—cont'd

**NURSING DIAGNOSIS** *Fluid volume excess related to impaired metabolism of aldosterone and hypoalbuminemia—cont'd*

| expected patient outcome | nursing interventions | rationale |
|---|---|---|
| Serum sodium and potassium levels remain within normal limits. | Teach patient rationale for sodium restriction when he or she shows interest.<br>Provide bedrest for ascites.<br>Give the patient prescribed diuretics.<br>Restrict fluids; provide those that are best tolerated, and space the fluids throughout 24 hours. | and precipitate portal-systemic encephalopathy, so careful monitoring is necessary. |

**NURSING DIAGNOSIS** *Ineffective breathing pattern related to ascites, immobility, and potential status of secretions*

| expected patient outcomes | nursing interventions | rationale |
|---|---|---|
| Dyspnea is decreased or does not worsen, as indicated on a scale of 1 (no dyspnea) to 5 (severe dyspnea).<br>Breath sounds are clear. | Monitor respirations and breath sounds q4hr.<br>Place in high Fowler's position.<br>Encourage patient resting in bed to turn frequently, q2hr.<br>Encourage deep breathing q2hr. | Nursing measures to encourage deep chest excursions are important when ascites and immobility are present. High Fowler's position can relieve pressure on diaphragm, which can decrease chance of stasis of secretions. |

**NURSING DIAGNOSIS** *Risk for impaired skin integrity related to immobility, poor nutrition, edema, and jaundice*

| expected patient outcome | nursing interventions | rationale |
|---|---|---|
| Skin remains intact. | Assess patient's skin daily for signs of possible breakdown.<br>Use measures such as flotation mattress and routine turning schedule to prevent skin breakdown.<br>Keep skin clean and moisturized. Clean and apply lotion every shift.<br>Keep nails short and clean.<br>Provide soft cloth to rub skin. | Patient has poor nutrition, edema, immobility; all these are risk factors for pressure ulcers requiring preventive care. Jaundice could lead to scratching and requires preventive care. |

**NURSING DIAGNOSIS** *Pain: itching related to jaundice and environmental stimuli*

| expected patient outcome | nursing interventions | rationale |
|---|---|---|
| States that he or she feels more comfortable and that itching is decreased. Patient not observed scratching. | Avoid heat and heavy clothing; provide a cool environment.<br>Apply antipruritic lotion as prescribed to skin as needed at least every shift.<br>Give patient prescribed antihistamines.<br>Use diversional activities such as music.<br>Keep patient's fingernails short and clean.<br>If patient must scratch, provide soft cloth to prevent excoriations.<br>Use tepid water for bathing. | Nursing measures relieve or lessen the effects of environmental stimuli, reduce itching, and promote comfort. |

**NURSING DIAGNOSIS** *Risk for infection related to immunosuppression*

| expected patient outcome | nursing interventions | rationale |
|---|---|---|
| Develops no infections; temperature remains normal. | Monitor patient for signs of infection every shift.<br>Use sterile technique for all invasive procedures. | Infections in patient with cirrhosis can be life-threatening because they can cause sepsis and precipitate liver failure, which may result in hepatic encephalopathy and septicemia. |

*Continued*

## The Person with Cirrhosis—cont'd

**NURSING DIAGNOSIS** *Risk for infection related to immunosuppression—cont'd*

| expected patient outcome | nursing interventions | rationale |
|---|---|---|
| | Encourage pulmonary hygiene, such as turning and deep breathing q1-2hr.<br>Restrict exposure to persons with infections. | Measures to prevent infection are essential in persons whose immune systems are suppressed.<br>Early detection is important for early treatment. |

**NURSING DIAGNOSIS** *Ineffective individual coping related to health crisis*

| expected patient outcome | nursing interventions | rationale |
|---|---|---|
| Describes at least one coping mechanism to deal with health crisis. | Assess patient's perception of health and present illness.<br>Identify and support patient's coping strategies, such as prayer, music, and conversation.<br>Listen actively if patient expresses feeling of powerlessness, fears, or spiritual distress. Plan time daily for listening.<br>Assess and facilitate family support. Meet with family or significant other on a scheduled basis. | Support of patient undergoing a health crisis can facilitate use of intrapersonal family resources. One can expect this patient to be discouraged and fearful. |

**NURSING DIAGNOSIS** *Risk for injury (bleeding, falls) related to decreased metabolic function of liver*

| expected patient outcomes | nursing interventions | rationale |
|---|---|---|
| No undetected bleeding occurs.<br><br>Vital signs return to normal.<br><br>No falls occur. | Monitor the following for bleeding: urine, stool, skin, and mucous membranes.<br>Check patient's vital signs q4hr and prothrombin and partial thromboplastin levels and thrombocytes daily.<br>Avoid injections if possible; apply pressure at all puncture sites for 5 minutes.<br>Give prescribed vitamin K.<br>Teach patient to use soft toothbrush, avoid use of dental floss, and to avoid straining or coughing.<br>Provide support when patient is ambulating to prevent falls.<br>Maintain safe environment. | Patient's esophageal varices and cirrhosis make him a candidate for bleeding and falls; surveillance is the major nursing focus, as well as decreasing precipitating factors. |

**NURSING DIAGNOSIS** *Self-esteem disturbance related to inability to accept physical changes of increased abdominal girth, jaundice, and change in secondary characteristics and potential changes in role*

| expected patient outcome | nursing interventions | rationale |
|---|---|---|
| Describes self in realistic terms, which include positive characteristics. | Encourage patient to participate in goal setting and decision making.<br>Help patient identify personal strengths and give positive feedback.<br>Assist family to understand patient's need for a positive self-concept and how they can help.<br>Assist patient to explore ways to diminish overt signs of jaundice and ascites and thus help body image. | Poor self-esteem can lead to poor coping, causing the patient to resume alcohol consumption. |

## clinical pathway Cirrhosis of Liver with Gastrointestinal Bleeding

DRG #: 202; expected LOS: 7

| | ADMIT TO ICU DAY OF ADMISSION DAY 1 | DAY 2 | DAY 3 |
|---|---|---|---|
| **Diagnostic Tests** | CBC, UA, SMA/18,* type and cross-match, PT/PTT, ABG | H&H, ABG, gastroscopy, hema-test stools | H&H, SMA/18,* hema-test stools |
| **Medications** | IVs, blood transfusions as indicated, IV cimetidine, antacids via NG tube after gavage | IVs, blood transfusions as indicated, IV cimetidine, acetaminophen PRN for fever and discomfort after sclerotherapy, antacids via NG tube | IVs, IV/PO cimetidine, Tylenol PRN for fever and discomfort, antacids, (?diuretics, $K^+$ replacement), multivitamins, folic acid, ferrous sulfate |
| **Treatments** | I&O q hr (including Foley and NG); VS q hr until stable, then q2hr; weight; measure abdominal girth; assess cardio-pul-neuro-circ systems q2hr; assess skin and mouth, give special care q2hr; NG gavage with NaCl for acute bleeding | I&O q hr (including Foley and NG); VS q2hr; weight; measure abdominal girth; assess cardio-pul-neuro-circ systems q2hr; assess skin and mouth, give special care q2hr; injection sclerotherapy as necessary | I&O q4hr (discontinue Foley and NG); VS q2hr; weight; measure abdominal girth; assess cardio-pul-neuro-circ systems q4hr; assess skin and mouth, give special care q2hr |
| **Diet** | NPO | NPO | Clear liquids and, as necessary, low sodium/protein and fluid restriction |
| **Activity** | Bedrest, T&DB q2hr | Bedrest, T&DB q2hr | Bedrest, up to bathroom with help, T&DB q2hr |
| **Referral/Consultation** | Gastroenterologist, other specialist as needed for other medical problems | | Social services, home health, dietary |

*ABG,* arterial blood gases; *CBC,* complete blood count; *CHO,* carbohydrate; *H&H,* hemoglobin and hematocrit; *I&O,* intake and output; *NG,* nasogastric; *PT,* prothrombin time; *PTT,* partial thromboplastin time; *T&DB,* turning and deep breathing; *UA,* urinalysis.
*Serum, calcium, phosphorus, triglycerides, uric acid, creatinine, blood urea nitrogen (BUN), total bilirubin, alkaline phosphate, aspartate aminotransferase (AST) (formerly serum glutamic oxaloacetic transaminase [SGOT]), alanine aminotransferase (ALT) (formerly serum glutamic oxaloacetic transaminase [SGPT]), lactic dehydrogenase (LDH), total protein, albumin, sodium, potassium, chloride, total $CO_2$, glucose.

with thoracentesis (see Chapter 32). The nurse should prepare the patient for this procedure, assist with the procedure, and monitor the patient's response during and after the procedure.

### Controlling Fatigue

Patients with cirrhosis have various levels of fatigue. The amount and type of activity encouraged depend on the individual's energy level, level of consciousness and coordination, and the presence of any complications of cirrhosis. If the patient has severe fluid excess and ascites or signs and symptoms of other complications, bedrest is usually required. When bedrest is required, special attention to skin care is necessary, particularly if the patient also has severe peripheral edema. Alternating pressure mattresses or flotation pads may be helpful. If bedrest is not required, the patient should be ambulated within the room or hall as tolerated. Level of tolerance is based on the patient's statement about the level of fatigue and/or pulse changes. (Pulse should not increase by more than 10 beats above baseline with activity.)

### Maintaining Fluid and Electrolyte Balance

Most patients with cirrhosis have sodium retention and hypokalemia. A great majority of patients have ascites, and some also have peripheral edema. The exact management of these depends on the patient's needs.

Potassium replacement will be given for hypokalemia. It is usually given orally, and the nurse should monitor the patient's serum $K^+$ values to verify that the patient is not developing hyperkalemia. Some patients with cirrhosis develop hepatorenal syndrome and have decreased renal function, which impairs the excretion of potassium, possibly resulting in hyperkalemia.

| TRANSFER OUT OF ICU DAY 4 | DAY 5 | DAY 6 | DAY OF DISCHARGE DAY 7 |
|---|---|---|---|
| Hema-test stools | H&H, hema-test stools | SMA/18* | CBC |
| IV to saline lock, PO cimetidine, Tylenol PRN for fever and discomfort, antacids, (?diuretics, $K^+$ replacement), multivitamins, folic acid, ferrous sulfate | IV saline lock, PO cimetidine, Tylenol PRN for fever and discomfort, antacids, (?diuretics, $K^+$ replacement), multivitamins, folic acid, ferrous sulfate | IV saline lock, PO cimetidine, discontinue acetaminophen, antacids, (?diuretics, $K^+$ replacement), multivitamins, folic acid, ferrous sulfate; adjust medications for home use. | Discontinue saline lock, continue cimetidine, antacids, vitamins, and other medications for home use |
| I&O q8hr; VS q6hr; weight; measure abdominal girth; assess cardio-pul-neuro-circ systems q8hr; assess skin and mouth, give special care q4hr. | I&O q8hr; VS q6hr; weight; measure abdominal girth; assess cardio-pul-neuro-circ systems q8hr; assess skin and mouth, give special care q4hr. | Discontinue I&O; VS q8hr; weight; measure abdominal girth; asses cardio-pul-neuro-circ systems q8hr; assess skin and mouth, give special care q6hr. | VS q8hr; weight; measure abdominal girth; assess cardio-pul-neuro-circ systems q8hr; assess skin and mouth, give special care q8hr. |
| Soft diet, high CHO and, as necessary, low sodium/protein and fluid restriction | Soft diet, high CHO and, as necessary, low sodium/protein and fluid restriction | Regular diet, high CHO and, as necessary, low sodium/protein and fluid restriction | Regular diet, high CHO and, as necessary, low sodium/protein and fluid restriction |
| Bedrest, up in chair twice with help | Up in chair 4 times with help, up walking in hall with help twice | Up ad lib, up walking in hallway with help 4 times | Up ad lib |
| | Chemical dependency counseling if appropriate | | |

Sodium imbalance and ascites are treated in several ways. Restriction of sodium aids greatly in limiting the formation of ascitic fluid. The basis for determining the amount of dietary restriction necessary to reduce sodium and water retention may initially be a collection of urine for 24 hours to determine sodium loss. Sodium is generally restricted to 1 g daily. The sodium restriction along with bedrest may relieve the ascites and edema.

If bedrest and sodium restriction do not improve ascites, diuretics may be used. Spironolactone A (Aldactone A), which inhibits the reabsorption of sodium in the distal tubules and promotes potassium retention by inhibiting the synthesis and renal effects of aldosterone, is frequently used. The therapy is adjusted on an individual basis. Sometimes furosemide (Lasix) or another diuretic is used with spironolactone. Because furosemide causes potassium excretion and can worsen hypokalemia, the patient's serum potassium level is monitored frequently, and the patient is observed for signs and symptoms of hypokalemia such as abdominal distention, nausea, vomiting, anorexia, decreased bowel sounds, weakness, or irregular pulse.

Removal of fluid through the kidneys has the advantage of not removing essential body protein, which can occur when fluid is removed from the abdominal cavity by paracentesis. However, diuretic therapy may cause serious side effects for the patient with cirrhosis. An extremely rapid diuresis can precipitate oliguria and uremia caused by the rapidly diminished blood volume. Ascites cannot be mobilized at rates greater than 500 ml/day or approximately 1 lb/day. Fluid losses in excess of 500 ml/day can result in the loss of nonascitic extracellular fluid. Infusions of albumin in 25-g units to promote retention of an adequate vascular volume may be given to prevent azotemia and encephalopathy by maintaining adequate perfusion to the kidneys and the brain and to promote diuresis. The administration of salt-poor albumin may expand the blood volume rapidly, and the patient should be monitored carefully for signs of congestive heart failure and pulmonary edema during and after administration.

Fluids are restricted if hyponatremia is caused by fluid retention. Fluid restriction is monitored closely because it may lead to decreased output and the hepatorenal syndrome (see p. 1233). When fluids are restricted, the nurse must work with the patient to provide fluids that are tolerated best and to spread the allotted fluids throughout the total 24 hours. Fluids will have to be distributed to provide some at each meal and some for required medicine. Some fluids should be given on all three shifts while the patient is hospitalized. At home the patient should distribute fluids over the waking hours.

To evaluate further the effectiveness of therapy, daily weighing is required. Measurements of abdominal girth assist in determining the gross amount of abdominal swelling. Patients need to be taught the importance of monitoring and reporting weight gain or a rapid increase in abdominal girth after discharge. When ascites is intractable to the therapies mentioned, other procedures such as a peritoneal venous shunt may be used. Peritoneal venous shunts are described in the section on Complications (see p. 1226).

### Helping the Patient Avoid Alcohol

A major nursing focus for many patients is helping them to deal with alcoholism. Helping patients cope with alcohol requires that they trust that the health team is interested in their well-being. The patient must admit that he or she has a drinking problem. Confrontation may sometimes be used to help the patient recognize the problem. (See Chapter 14 for a discussion of various techniques and support systems to assist persons with alcohol problems.)

### Preventing Infection

The loss of the normal phagocytic function of the liver and the leukopenia and malnutrition associated with cirrhosis require that precautions be taken to avoid infection. These precautions involve proper hand washing, observance of sterile technique with all invasive procedures, preventive respiratory care, and avoidance of contact with people with infections. The patient must be monitored carefully for the presence of infection, and any increase in temperature should be reported immediately so that appropriate measures can be taken.

### Preventing Bleeding and Falls

The patient with cirrhosis is at great risk for bleeding because of poor vitamin K absorption, impaired production of clotting factors, and thrombocytopenia. Esophageal varices and hemorrhoids can easily rupture, causing excessive bleeding. Nursing care should focus on monitoring for the presence of bleeding (Guidelines for Care Box) and instituting measures that decrease the risk of bleeding from trauma or injury to varices (Guidelines for Care Box). The information to be shared about diagnostic tests is described in Chapter 36. Treatment measures that will need to be explained include dietary restrictions (sodium and protein), fluid restrictions, diuretics, potassium supplements, and vitamin and mineral supplements. If bedrest is prescribed, the reason this is necessary must also be explained.

### Promoting Nutrition

Most patients with cirrhosis will require a well-balanced, high-protein, high-carbohydrate diet with adequate vitamins to provide nutrients for repair of the liver. When nausea is a problem, antiemetics should be given 30 minutes before meals to help increase food tolerance.

Sodium restriction is frequently necessary, and this restriction can make finding a palatable diet difficult. Salt substitutes and information on alternative seasonings may help.

The liver dysfunction and the presence of portal hypertension, which results in portal vessel blood being shunted around the liver, result in an impairment in the metabolism of ammonia. Ammonia, which originates from deamination of protein, is very toxic to the body. Protein restriction is necessary for the patient with cirrhosis who cannot metabolize ammonia, which would be evident by the onset of signs and symptoms of portal-systemic encephalopathy (see p. 1231).

Frequent oral hygiene and a pleasant environment should be provided to help increase food intake. The patient's food preferences should be incorporated into the diet. Food should be served in small, frequent amounts. Because persons with cirrhosis need increased calories but often have poor appetites, measures to increase calories without increasing the volume of food should be used. These measures include use of butter as a seasoning, adding dry milk to appropriate foods, and using gravies and sauces. The patient with cirrhosis has the same nutritional needs after discharge, and the person

**guidelines for care**

**Monitoring for Bleeding in the Person with Cirrhosis**

1. Monitor urine and stool for blood.
2. Check the patient's body daily for purpura, hematomas, and petechiae.
3. Check mouth, especially gums, carefully for signs of bleeding.
4. Check vital signs at least every 4 hours.
5. Monitor prothrombin time, partial thromboplastin time, and thrombocyte count frequently.

**guidelines for care**

**Decreasing the Risk of Bleeding**

1. Avoid all intramuscular and subcutaneous injections, if possible.
2. Use the smallest-gauge needle possible when giving an injection.
3. Apply pressure to injection sites and venous puncture sites for at least 5 minutes and to arterial puncture sites for at least 10 minutes.
4. Give vitamin K as ordered.
5. Use or instruct patient to use a soft-bristled toothbrush or cotton swabs for oral hygiene.
6. Instruct patient not to strain on defecation and to avoid vigorous blowing of nose or coughing.
7. Instruct patient to avoid foods (e.g., spicy, hot, or raw) that can traumatize esophageal varices.
8. Provide assistance to avoid falls.
9. Make sure that room is free of clutter, that floors are dry, and that shoes or slippers are worn to avoid injuries.

who shops and cooks for the patient must be included in the teaching. The patient's economic situation should be assessed to determine his or her ability to purchase the food required for the prescribed diet. A social service referral may be necessary to help the patient obtain financial assistance. For the person who eats out frequently, instruction about selecting appropriate meals from a restaurant menu is necessary. If the patient's meals are obtained through a service such as Meals on Wheels, arrangements can be made for some special dietary requirements.

### Controlling Pruritus

The management of pruritus is similar to that discussed earlier under care of patients with hepatitis (p. 1209, 1220).

### Promoting Positive Self-Esteem

The patient with cirrhosis may experience changes in body appearance and in roles and relationships. If the patient is not helped to establish or maintain positive self-esteem, this can add to the problem of alcoholism. The nurse is in a prime position to help promote positive self-esteem by giving the patient as much control as possible. Positive self-esteem can be facilitated by:

1. Involving the patient in goal setting
2. Allowing the patient to make as many decisions as possible
3. Giving positive feedback for accomplishments
4. Supporting the patient in times of failure, whatever the failure might be, including conflicts with family or friends or participation in drinking
5. Helping the patient recall past accomplishments
6. Helping significant others provide positive feedback
7. Helping the patient learn ways to disguise jaundice or ascites

### Providing Skin Care

Because of pruritus, malnutrition, and the edema often associated with cirrhosis, the patient is prone to skin lesions and pressure ulcer formation. Preventive nursing care to avoid skin breakdown, such as air mattresses, frequent turning, backrubs, and massage of bony prominences, should be instituted. Measures to prevent pruritus assist in preventing damage to the skin resulting from the patient's scratching.

### Patient/Family Teaching

All patients need to be prepared for diagnostic tests, to understand their treatment, and to learn to meet long-term care needs. Information should be given verbally and supplemented with written information, depending on the patient's physical status; the information may need to be repeated several times and given in small increments. Family members or significant others should be included so that they can help reinforce the information or participate in the patient's care. Long-term care usually requires major changes in lifestyle (diet, fluid intake, and alcohol cessation), and thus continual support is necessary. Specific information that the nurse may want to include in the teaching plan is highlighted in the Patient/Family Teaching Box.

### Health promotion/prevention

**Healthy People 2000.** The goal of *Healthy People 2000* is to reduce the number of deaths from cirrhosis to no more than 6 per 100,000 people, with African American men, Native Americans, and Alaskan Inuits being targeted populations.[17] Even though cirrhosis among African American and Native American men has decreased in the last decade, the death rate for nonwhite men is 70% higher than for white men.[17]

Progress towards *Healthy People 2000* goals has been made. Data gathered in 1993 show that deaths due to cirrhosis fell to 7.8 per 100,000 population.[15]

In the United States, programs aimed at the prevention of cirrhosis are designed primarily to control the ingestion of alcohol. The loss of time from work related to alcoholism is estimated to cost billions of dollars annually. Many large corporations have or are organizing programs to help employees control their alcohol intake (see Chapter 14).

### Secondary prevention

Early detection of cirrhosis is difficult because three fourths of the liver can be destroyed before signs of cirrhosis become evident. For this reason, cessation of alcohol intake is the focus of prevention.

## ■ EVALUATION

To evaluate the effectiveness of nursing interventions, compare patient behaviors with those stated in the expected patient outcomes. Successful achievement of patient outcomes for the patient with cirrhosis is indicated by:

1. Has clear breath sounds throughout lung fields and normal percussion results from thoracic cavity.

**patient/family teaching**

**The Person with Cirrhosis**

1. Avoidance of further hepatic damage: abstain from alcohol; abstain from any drugs not prescribed by physician, including over-the-counter drugs, such as analgesics or cold remedies; work environment hazards; home hazards
2. Dietary regimen (may include sodium and/or protein restrictions) should be well balanced and include sources high in protein such as milk, eggs, fish, and poultry
3. Fluid restriction if required; how to incorporate restrictions throughout the day
4. Signs and symptoms requiring immediate follow-up: weight gain; increased abdominal girth; recurrence of edema, fever, or bleeding (blood in urine, stool, or vomitus; epistaxis; cuts that continue to bleed); change in mental function or behavior
5. Measures that lessen chance of bleeding
6. Drug therapy (diuretics, potassium, and antihistamines)
7. Activity plan that promotes adequate rest
8. Care measures that help to control pruritus

2. Increases involvement in daily self-care activities and ambulation in hospital hallways.
3. Loses 1 to 2 lb/day until dry weight is reached; has decreasing edema, decreasing abdominal girth, and urine output of 500 to 1000 ml greater than intake until dry weight is reached.
4. States that alcohol is the cause of problem and is not controllable without some outside support, and attends one counseling session or one AA meeting.
5. Has normal body temperature and no indications of infections of any body organs or sites.
6. Shows normal prothrombin time and hematocrit, hemoglobin levels that are increasing, no orthostatic vital sign changes, and no falls, cuts, or other injuries.
7. Maintains adequate food intake to regain or keep weight as appropriate with incorporation of foods from all food groups and restriction of sodium and protein as necessary.
8. Shows no evidence of scratching, and states that itching is decreased and controlled.
9. Makes positive statements about self and realistic statements about future goals.
10. Maintains intact skin and appropriate healing of any lesions.

## GERONTOLOGICAL CONSIDERATIONS

The incidence of primary biliary cirrhosis (PBC) increases with age and peaks at age 50; the disease progresses until most patients are 60 to 70 years of age and thus is a serious problem in the elderly population. Liver transplantation is considered for persons with PBC when liver failure occurs. Advanced age is no longer an absolute contraindication for transplantation, but it is certainly controversial. Death usually results from complications of bleeding, ascites, or encephalopathy.

Cirrhosis develops in the last stage of the disease; the prognosis is poor then because of the complications associated with cirrhosis. Early symptoms are vague or absent. Late symptoms include jaundice, diarrhea, bone pain, bruising, night blindness, and gradual weight loss. Many symptoms are attributed to malabsorption of vitamins and nutrients. Skin manifestations, including thickening and darkening of the skin and pruritus, are common manifestations of PBC. Control of pruritus is especially important in the elderly patient because of skin changes associated with aging. The elderly person's skin is more fragile, and lesions may develop as a result from scratching. As the disease progresses, complications such as esophageal varices, ascites, and encephalopathy may develop. The elderly patient with anemia is at even greater risk from bleeding.

The blood flow to the liver decreases with aging. This physiological change may worsen the effects of hypotension on the liver. An episode of severe hypotension in the elderly patient may result in shock liver. Patients with preexisting right-sided heart failure may experience severe liver complications with a hypotensive episode. *Shock liver* results from ischemia of hepatic tissues and elevated liver enzymes, progressing to liver failure. Lactic acid levels increase and clotting factors decrease, with an increased risk of metabolic imbalance and hemorrhage. Patients should be monitored closely to avoid episodes of hypotension.

Encouraging a nutritionally adequate diet is an important intervention for the elderly patient. A low-fat diet and vitamin supplements are recommended.

Emotional support is necessary to assist the patient in living with a chronic disease. An assessment of the patient's support system and coping methods can assist the nurse in formulating a plan to reduce the patient's anxiety.

## SPECIAL ENVIRONMENTS FOR CARE

### Critical Care Management

Persons with cirrhosis will need critical care management usually if complications, such as hemorrhage, esophageal varices, and portal-systemic encephalopathy, develop (see section on Complications of Cirrhosis).

### Home Care Management

The home environment should be assessed for any alterations that may need to be made to accommodate the patient's long-term needs. The patient's bedroom and bathroom should ideally be on the same floor. If this is not possible, a portable commode, bedpan, or urinal may be substituted. Incontinence pads or adult-sized briefs may be needed in the case of incontinence. If the patient has ascites, raising the head of the bed to a high Fowler's position may be necessary to facilitate respirations. The head of the bed may be elevated with pillows, or the patient may be able to sleep in a reclining chair with a footrest. Alternatively, if resources permit, a hospital bed may be rented.

Environmental hazards should be eliminated, especially if the patient has any mental status changes. Because of clotting defects, the patient should be protected from injury. Maintenance of normal bowel function should be encouraged, particularly to avoid constipation, which could lead to rupture of hemorrhoids. The patient may also need assistance in the preparation of nutritionally adequate meals.

Before discharge, the patient and family should be taught to recognize the signs and symptoms of worsening liver function including increased abdominal girth, rapid weight gain, edema, signs of bleeding, and deteriorating mental status, which should be reported to the physician or home health nurse. Loss of libido, erectile dysfunction, sterility, and amenorrhea may occur, and the patient and his or her sexual partner should be counseled about these possibilities. The patient and family should be assessed for the capability to deal with a chronic illness. If the patient requires much assistance in ADL, the primary caregiver may need periodic relief from care responsibilities. Home health care assistance may be possible. All persons involved in the care of the patient are encouraged to share feelings and fears concerning the patient's illness.

## COMPLICATIONS

Persons with cirrhosis very frequently develop portal hypertension that can result in ascites, esophageal varices, and/or portal-systemic encephalopathy. Each of these major complications is discussed next.

## Portal Hypertension

As structural damage occurs, the portal vascular system may become obstructed. This obstruction to blood flow causes a rise in portal venous pressure and results in *portal hypertension.* The obstruction to portal blood flow can cause splenomegaly because of increased vascular pressure and venous congestion in the spleen, contribute to ascites by causing leakage of albumin and fluid from the vascular compartment of the liver into the peritoneal cavity, and cause the development of collateral channels of circulation that bypass the obstruction. Collateral channels are most likely to occur in the paraumbilical and the hemorrhoidal veins and at the cardia of the stomach extending into the esophagus.

### Collaborative care management

The nursing and medical management of portal hypertension is directed first to treatment of the consequences of portal hypertension: ascites and esophageal varices. The only way to achieve permanent lowering of portal pressure is surgical treatment to reduce blood flow through the obstructed portion of the portal system (see p. 1230). Because of the risks of the surgery and the frequent fatalities from hepatic failure after surgical treatment with a portacaval shunt, the shunt procedure is used only in persons who have esophageal varices (see p. 1228), have had bleeding from the varices, and do not respond to other therapy. Surgical care is discussed later in this chapter.

## Ascites

As mentioned earlier, *ascites* is one of the most frequent complications of cirrhosis of the liver and results in part from the portal hypertension. Other contributing factors are decreased hepatic synthesis of albumin, increased levels of aldosterone, and obstruction of hepatic lymph flow. Ascites may occur with or without peripheral edema. Because ascites is so frequently seen, the required therapy and nursing care were discussed earlier in the section related to general care needs of patients with cirrhosis. This section describes care related to use of a peritoneal venous shunt.

### Peritoneal venous shunt

In chronic and resistant ascites caused by cirrhosis, a LeVeen or Denver peritoneal venous shunt (PV shunt) may be used (Figure 37-5). The shunt allows for the continuous reinfusion of ascitic fluid into the venous system through a silicone catheter with a one-way pressure-sensitive valve. One end of the catheter is implanted in the peritoneal cavity, the tube is channeled through subcutaneous tissue to the superior vena cava, where the other end is implanted. The valve opens when there is a pressure differential greater than 3 mm of water between the peritoneal cavity and the vein in the thoracic cavity, allowing fluid to move from the peritoneal cavity into the superior vena cava.

People treated with a shunt may also receive furosemide therapy, and the two together have been successful in relieving ascites in some patients. Persons who have a shunt may still have severe problems, including disseminated intravascular coagulation, bleeding esophageal varices, and congestive heart failure.[8]

A modification of the original LeVeen peritoneal venous shunt, the Denver shunt, is sometimes used when severe ascites develops as a result of malignancy. Malignant ascites may contain particulate matter that can obstruct the flow of ascitic fluid through the tubing. The Denver shunt has a subcutaneous pump that can be compressed manually to irrigate the tubing. Increased comfort and improvement of renal and respiratory function have been reported with use of the Denver shunt.

After shunt implantation, dramatic changes, such as hemodilution of intravascular fluid, a decrease in abdominal girth, and an increase in renal output occur. As peritoneal fluid is removed, less of a pressure gradient exists between the peritoneal cavity and the superior vena cava; thus less fluid is removed. To force the valve open, deep breathing is encouraged at regular intervals (every 1 to 2 hours) with the patient supine.

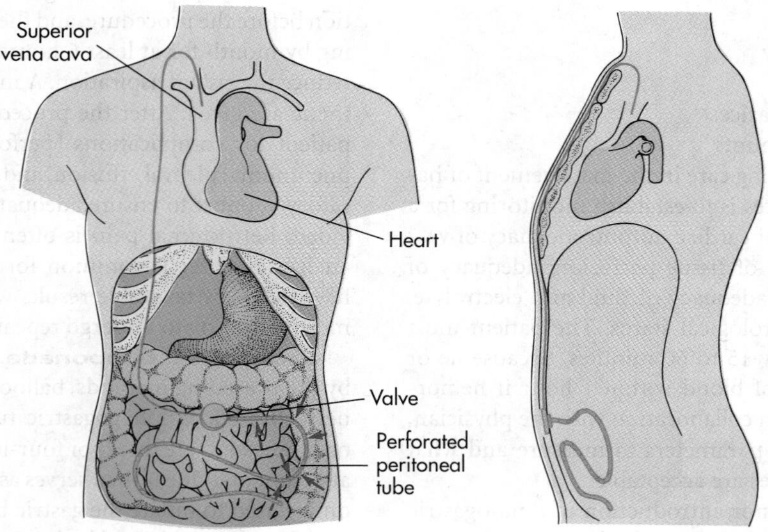


**fig. 37-5** LeVeen shunt, showing placement of catheter.

## Esophageal Varices

Bleeding esophageal varices are the most dangerous complication of portal hypertension. The mortality associated with variceal hemorrhage is 50%.[8] In portal hypertension, the azygos and vena cava veins become distended where they join the smaller vessels of the esophagus. Distention occurs because of the greater volume of blood flowing through these vessels as a result of higher pressure within the portal system. Normal portal pressure is about 9 mm Hg. The increased portal venous pressure causes the blood, which normally flows through the liver, to be forced into these other vessels (see Figure 37-3, *A*, for a diagram of the relationship between these various blood vessels). These small vessels cannot accommodate the increased blood volume and become tortuous and fragile. The changes in the structure of these vessels predispose them to injury by mechanical trauma from ingestion of coarse foods and acidic pepsin erosion, which may result in bleeding. Bleeding may also occur as a result of coughing, vomiting, sneezing, straining during defecation (Valsalva maneuver), or any physical exertion that increases abdominal venous pressure. The major clinical manifestation is upper GI bleeding. Bleeding is frequently abrupt and painless. If bleeding is slow, melena and decreasing hemoglobin and hematocrit levels may be the only signs. Severe hematemesis and resultant shock may follow, requiring emergency treatment. The patient exhibits signs and symptoms of hypovolemic shock (see Chapter 17) or may exhibit signs and symptoms of portal-systemic encephalopathy (see p. 1231).

### *Collaborative care management*

The first priority in medical management is to establish the source of GI bleeding. *Esophagoscopy* is the major diagnostic tool, and, if this is not possible, angiography is used. If severe hemorrhage is not present, barium studies or scans may be used. It must be remembered that in patients with cirrhosis, bleeding may be from other causes such as peptic ulcers and gastritis.

After diagnosis, the first line of therapy is to control bleeding and replace blood volume. Bleeding may be controlled with:

1. Gastric lavage
2. Pharmacological therapy
3. Injection sclerotherapy
4. Balloon tamponade of varices
5. Surgery—ligation and shunts

The first priority of nursing care in the management of patients with esophageal varices is to establish monitoring for a patent airway; parameters of cardiac output; adequacy of vascular volume; effectiveness of tissue perfusion; adequacy of hemostasis treatment; and adequacy of fluid and electrolyte, respiratory, renal, and neurological status. The patient must monitored frequently, every 15 to 60 minutes, because he or she can lose several units of blood within 1 hour if hemorrhage is severe. The nurse, in collaboration with the physician, decides what physiological parameters to measure and what minimal and maximal values are acceptable.

If the hemorrhage is minor, introduction of a nasogastric (NG) tube by the nurse or physician and administration of an antacid through the tube may be sufficient to control the hemorrhage. The NG tube removes gastric secretions, and the antacids neutralize gastric acids that may irritate esophageal varices. If hemorrhage is more severe, pharmacological therapy will be started. Pharmacological therapy includes administration of vasopressin, propranolol (Inderal), and octreotide (Sandostatin).

Vasopressin is given intravenously mixed in 120 to 200 ml of dextrose either intermittently or as a continuous infusion. It lowers portal pressure by causing splanchnic vasoconstriction and can thus stop or control esophageal bleeding. Side effects include abdominal cramping and pallor. Coronary artery vasoconstriction can occur, as well as mesenteric artery vasoconstriction; thus vasopressin must be used cautiously in persons with coronary artery disease and in elderly persons.[7,8]

Propranolol (Inderal), a $\beta$-adrenergic blocking agent, has been shown to reduce portal pressure and thus decrease esophageal bleeding in some people. These are conflicting data whether overall survival rates of patients treated with $\beta$-blockers is improved.[15]

Octreotide (Sandostatin) is frequently used to decrease total splanchnic flow and portal pressure.[15] Octreotide is a long-acting octapeptide that mimics the action of the hormone somatostatin. Octreotide is administered subcutaneously.

**Injection sclerotherapy.** For emergency treatment of acute bleeding esophageal varices or for long-term control and prevention of rebleeding, *injection sclerotherapy* or banding may be used. In this procedure the physician introduces a fiberoptic endoscope into the esophagus, identifies the bleeding site, and injects a sclerosing agent (sodium morrhuate, 5 ml) into the varices. This agent causes thromboses and sclerosis of the vessel and should result in hemostasis in 3 to 5 minutes. If hemostasis does not occur, a second injection may be given. The procedure may be repeated as necessary and can be performed while the varices are bleeding or as an elective procedure. Endoscopic therapy is ineffective in controlling bleeding from gastric varices. There are conflicting data regarding the effectiveness of chronic endoscopic therapy as a means of increasing survival rates of persons with bleeding esophageal varices.[15] The patient and significant others need an explanation before the procedure, and the patient should receive nothing by mouth for at least 6 hours before the the procedure to reduce the risk of aspiration. A mild sedative and a local anesthetic are given. After the procedure, the nurse monitors the patient for complications (perforated esophagus, aspiration pneumonia, pleural effusion, and worsening of ascites). Respiratory support to ensure adequate air exchange must be provided. Retrosternal pain is often present and is treated with analgesics; fever is common for several days. Some patients have had very favorable results with this procedure, but they must be willing to undergo repeated endoscopic sessions.

**Esophageal tamponade.** If bleeding is not controlled by the preceding methods, balloon tamponade of varices may be instituted. Esophagogastric tubes (Sengstaken-Blakemore or Minnesota) are three- or four-lumen tubes with two balloon attachments. One lumen serves as an NG suction tube, the second is used to inflate the gastric balloon, and the third is used to inflate the esophageal balloon (Figure 37-6). The Minnesota esophagogastric tamponade tube has a fourth lumen used for

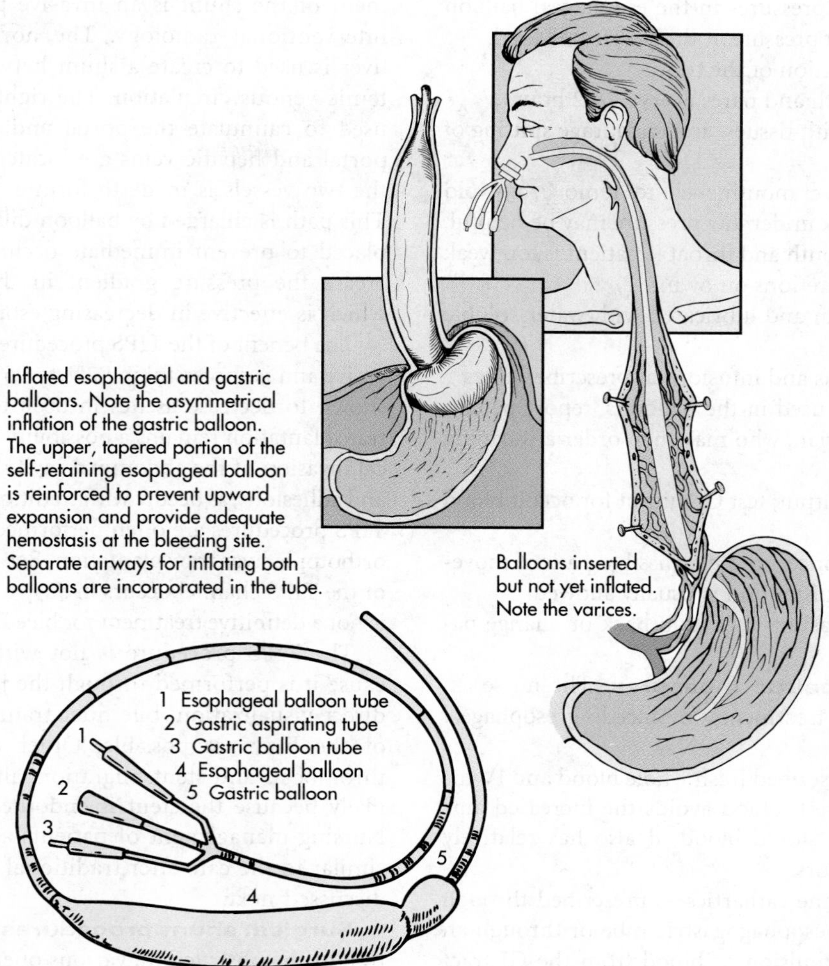
Inflated esophageal and gastric balloons. Note the asymmetrical inflation of the gastric balloon. The upper, tapered portion of the self-retaining esophageal balloon is reinforced to prevent upward expansion and provide adequate hemostasis at the bleeding site. Separate airways for inflating both balloons are incorporated in the tube.
Balloons inserted but not yet inflated. Note the varices.
1 Esophageal balloon tube
2 Gastric aspirating tube
3 Gastric balloon tube
4 Esophageal balloon
5 Gastric balloon
1
2
3
4
5

**fig. 37-6** Esophageal tamponade accomplished with a Sengstaken-Blakemore tube.

esophageal aspiration. The tube is passed by the physician through the nose into the stomach with the balloons deflated. When the tube is in the stomach, the gastric balloon is inflated and the lumen is clamped; the tube is then pulled out slowly so that the balloon is held tightly against the cardioesophageal junction. A football helmet-shaped device is used to provide traction on the tube, which keeps it in the proper position.

If bleeding continues after the gastric balloon is inflated, the esophageal balloon, which is connected by a Y tube to a manometer, is inflated to the amount of pressure designated by the physician and clamped. To stop the bleeding, the pressure must be greater than the patient's portal venous pressure. If bleeding is from esophageal varices rather than from the gastric mucosa, blood will no longer be aspirated from the stomach. If blood is still present, the stomach may be lavaged with a small amount of ice water, or a solution of iced alcohol and water may be circulated through the gastric balloon to provide vasoconstriction as well as pressure. The use of iced solutions to control bleeding is controversial, and some practitioners prefer the use of room-temperature fluids.

The NG lumen is usually connected to intermittent gastric suction, which permits easy appraisal of cessation of bleeding and also keeps the stomach empty. It is important to remove all blood from the stomach, because its presence may precipitate portal-systemic encephalopathy from ammonia produced from the digestion of protein in the blood.

The esophageal balloon can be left inflated for up to 48 hours without tissue damage. The fully inflated gastric balloon with traction compresses the stomach wall between the balloon and the diaphragm, causing ulceration of the gastric mucosa and severe discomfort. To offset the possibility of necrosis, the physician may release the traction on the gastric balloon and deflate the gastric balloon pressure periodically. If the gastric balloon ruptures (and the patient is not intubated), the entire tube may move and obstruct the airway; if the tube becomes dislodged, the esophageal balloon is immediately deflated, and the entire tube is removed. The major complication of the tube is ulceration.

Nursing care of the patient with esophageal tamponade includes the following:

1. Explain procedure and provide continued support to patient during the procedure.
2. Monitor vital signs every 15 minutes until blood pressure is stable, and then monitor hourly or every 2 hours.

3. Measure and record pressures in the esophageal balloon every hour; maintain pressure at the prescribed level.
4. Maintain proper position of the tube.
5. Provide care to mouth and nares every 1 to 2 hours
   a. Provide patient with tissues, and encourage spitting of saliva into tissues.
   b. Have patient rinse mouth well to remove any old blood; a Water Pik under low pressure may be helpful.
   c. *Gently* suction mouth and throat if patient is too weak to expectorate secretions on own.
   d. Keep nostrils clean and lubricated with water-soluble jelly.
6. Maintain transfusions and infusions at prescribed rates.
7. If iced solutions are used in the balloons, report patient chilling to the physician, who may then order a warming blanket.
8. Record intake and output; test GI output for occult blood (guaiac).
9. Consult physician concerning permissible patient movement; passive range of motion is usually allowed.
10. Provide comfort measures (e.g., rub back or change patient's position).

**Additional therapeutic measures.** The nurse assists with the following treatments for bleeding esophageal varices:

1. Administration of prescribed fresh whole blood and IV infusions. The use of fresh blood avoids the increased ammonia and citrate of stored blood; it also has relatively more coagulation factors.
2. Administration of saline cathartics as prescribed through the NG lumen of the esophagogastric tube or through an NG tube to hasten expulsion of blood from the GI tract and to prevent an increase in the production of ammonia. Enemas may also be ordered to decrease gut content and bacterial action on the blood.
3. Administration of lactulose or neomycin to prevent or decrease portal-systemic encephalopathy. Lactulose is a synthetic disaccharide degraded by bacteria in the lower intestines and is given either orally or by retention enema and promotes the excretion of ammonia in the stool by decreasing the pH of the bowel. Ammonia remains in its ionized state, which facilitates its movement from the blood to the stool. Bacterial growth is discouraged by the acidic environment.

   Neomycin is a broad-spectrum antibiotic that destroys the normal flora of the bowel. Bacteria in the bowel normally break down protein, including blood protein in the GI tract, producing ammonia. Therefore neomycin is given to decrease the protein breakdown by bacteria in the bowel.

**Shunt procedures.** A shunt procedure is one of the last measures used to treat bleeding esophageal varices. Portal decompression can be obtained by several shunt procedures, most of them requiring surgery. The mortality rate for shunt surgery is 5% to 15%, and if emergency shunt surgery is necessary, the mortality rate increases to 50%.

An alternative to the surgical shunt procedure is the *transjugular intrahepatic portosystemic shunt (TIPS)*. Placement of the shunt is an invasive procedure performed in interventional radiology. The normal vasculature of the liver is used to create a shunt between the portal and systemic venous circulation. The right internal jugular vein is used to cannulate the portal and hepatic veins. After the portal and hepatic veins are located, a connection between the two vessels is made to form a new path of blood flow. This path is enlarged by balloon dilation, and then a stent is placed to prevent immediate occlusion. The goal is to decrease the pressure gradient in the liver to 10 mm Hg, which is effective in decreasing esophageal bleeding.[1,8]

The benefit of the TIPS procedure is that it is minimally invasive and is successful in 92% to 96% of patients. It has been shown to decrease ascites in 80% to 90% of patients. Liver transplantation remains a possibility because there is no surgical invasion of the abdominal cavity with resultant scar tissue and adhesions, as occurs with traditional shunting procedures.[1] TIPS procedures are often performed while the patient awaits orthotopic liver transplantation. Because stenosis or occlusion of the TIPS channel occurs in 50% of patients within 1 year, it is not a definitive treatment for bleeding esophageal varices.[15]

The TIPS procedure is not without complications. Because it is performed through the jugular vein and without direct visualization, bile duct trauma and vascular trauma of the liver are possible. Other complications are stent thrombosis and stent migration, although migration is unlikely because the stent is endothelialized in 7 to 10 days. Nursing management of patients after a TIPS procedure is similar to the care after traditional shunt procedures and is discussed next.

**Surgical shunt procedures.** Depending on the location of the obstruction, various operative procedures may be used (Figure 37-7) to decrease the blood flow through the portal vascular system and thus decrease portal hypertension. Portal hypertension is lowered by shunting blood around the liver. The lowering of portal hypertension decreases the pressure in the esophageal vessels and the bleeding from the varices. Preoperatively, the patient's vascular volume is stabilized with fluids and blood as necessary. Vitamin K may be given to correct coagulation problems, antibiotics may be given prophylactically, and nutritional status is improved as much as possible.

General needs of postoperative patients are discussed in Chapter 20. In addition, the patient recovering from shunt placement needs the following nursing interventions:

1. Administering narcotics for pain (the amount given is usually decreased because most narcotics are metabolized in the liver); avoiding the use of sedatives because of their toxic effects on the diseased liver
2. Observing carefully for impending portal-systemic encephalopathy (beginning signs include mental confusion, slowness in response, and generally inappropriate behavior)
3. Monitoring for hemorrhage and signs of shock
4. Monitoring for signs of thrombosis at site of anastomosis (pain, distention, fever, and nausea)
5. Encouraging activity within the prescribed limits; starting leg and arm exercises on the first postoperative day

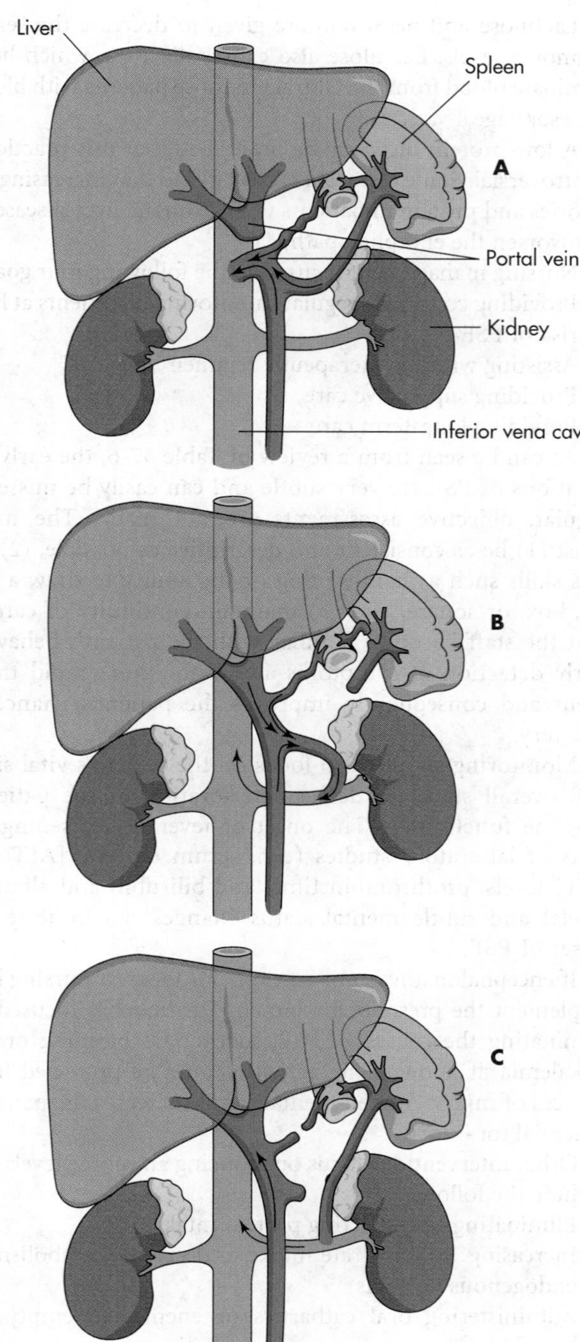


**fig. 37-7** Decompression procedures for portal hypertension: **A,** End-to-side portacaval shunt. **B,** Splenorenal shunt. **C,** Distal splenorenal shunt.

6. Monitoring the lower extremities for signs of edema; elevating the lower extremities if ordered to prevent edema formation (edema formation possible from the sudden increase of blood flow into the inferior vena cava)

All patients who have had a portal-systemic shunt are at risk for portal-systemic encephalopathy. The incidence of portal-systemic encephalopathy has been reported to be as high as 25% to 100% in patients undergoing portosystemic shunting.[15] Some patients will require lifelong restriction of protein because the shunted blood bypasses the liver and thus limits ammonia detoxification.

## Portal-Systemic Encephalopathy

*Portal-systemic encephalopathy (PSE),* also called hepatic encephalopathy or hepatic coma, is one of the major complications of cirrhosis. The onset of the condition may be acute or chronic.

PSE is a metabolic encephalopathy associated with liver failure that results from several metabolic derangements; a major cause is increased blood ammonia levels. Normally, ammonia, which is formed in the intestine from the breakdown of protein by intestinal bacteria, is carried directly to the liver and converted to urea through the Krebs-Henseleit cycle in the liver. In persons with liver failure, ammonia levels may be increased at the same time that the liver's detoxification ability is decreased or when blood is shunted past the liver. Many factors can increase ammonia levels.

A second hypothesis related to the onset of PSE has been called the "false-neurotransmitter hypothesis." Patients with PSE have increased levels of aromatic or short-chain amino acids (SCAAs) and a decrease in branched-chain amino acids (BCAAs). Normally, the liver clears SCAAs. With liver failure, they are not cleared, and the levels are increased. These SCAAs cross the blood-brain barrier. The SCAAs such as phenylalanine, trytophan, and tyrosine act as weak neurotransmitters and compete with regular neurotransmitters, resulting in an impairment of normal neurological function.

A third major cause in the onset of PSE is the presence of any of a number of metabolic derangements that may indirectly increase ammonia levels or depress liver function. *Hypokalemia* is a major metabolic factor precipitating PSE. As serum potassium decreases, it shifts from the cells in exchange for sodium and hydrogen. The shift of hydrogen ion into the intracellular compartment increases the acid level in the intracellular compartment and decreases the pH and increases the base in the extracellular compartment and the pH. The extracellular alkalosis increases liberation of $H^+$ from ammonium ($NH_4$) and the formation of ammonia ($NH_3$), which is gaseous and crosses readily into cells, where it accumulates and exerts toxic effects. Increased accumulation of base in the extracellular compartment from other causes can precipitate the same type of response.

Constipation may also increase formation and absorption of ammonia from the gut, or it may induce straining and thus precipitate bleeding from esophageal varices or hemorrhoids. Other metabolic factors such as exercise and infection may precipitate PSE by causing increased ammonia formation or decreased liver function.

A fourth major cause in the onset of PSE is increased central nervous system (CNS) sensitivity to depressants. Any hypoxic insult or sedative, which can increase the sensitivity of the CNS to any substance, can precipitate PSE. Common factors that can precipitate PSE are summarized in Box 37-12.

The manifestations of PSE vary and may occur quickly or gradually over the course of a few days. PSE results in alterations in the state of consciousness, intellectual function, behavior and personality, and neuromuscular function. These changes have been graded in four stages (Table 37-6).

### Collaborative care management

Medical management of PSE includes identifying the precipitating factors and treating them (hypokalemia, hemorrhage, and hypoxia), reducing serum ammonia levels, and providing supportive care.

Patients with PSE have abnormal liver function as described earlier for patients with cirrhosis. An elevated serum ammonia level provides the definitive diagnosis, but not all patients show an increase in ammonia. Therefore, treatment is determined by the signs and symptoms and not the serum ammonia level.

**box 37-12** *Common Factors Associated with Portal-Systemic Encephalopathy*

**FACTORS DEPRESSING CNS OR LIVER FUNCTION**

Hypoxia
- Secondary to hemorrhage and hypovolemic shock
- Secondary to morphine and other sedatives

Infections

Exercise
- In patients with chronic liver disease in whom coma is impending

Sedatives

Abdominal paracentesis
- Resulting in reduction of plasma volume

**FACTORS INCREASING LEVEL OF AMMONIA**

GI ammonia (old blood in bowel from GI hemorrhage)

High-protein intake

Transfusions, especially with stored blood because it contains more ammonia

Hypokalemia
- Secondary to thiazide diuretics
- Secondary to potassium loss from the bowel

Alkalosis secondary to hyperventilation or hypokalemia

Shunting of blood into systemic circulation without passing through hepatic sinusoids
- Natural collateral bypass of liver
- Surgical bypass of liver

Constipation

Lactulose and neomycin are given to decrease the serum ammonia levels. Lactulose also causes diarrhea, which helps eliminate blood from the GI tract in those patients with bleeding esophageal varices.

A low-protein diet may be prescribed, but this practice is controversial. Some researchers have found that increasing the calories and protein in patients with alcoholic liver disease do not worsen the encephalopathy.[8]

Nursing management focuses on the following four goals:

1. Providing continual, regular monitoring of patients at high risk of PSE
2. Assisting with the therapeutic regimen
3. Providing supportive care
4. Providing long-term care

As can be seen from a review of Table 37-6, the early indications of PSE are very subtle and can easily be missed if regular, objective assessments are not made. The nurse must (1) be as consistent and descriptive as possible, (2) assess skills such as handwriting or the ability to draw a circle, box, or square, and (3) maintain continuity of care so that the staff becomes familiar with the patient's behavior. Early detection of symptoms allows for more rapid treatment and consequently improves the patient's chance of recovery.

Monitoring should also focus on the patient's vital signs and overall status to detect deterioration of the patient's baseline functioning. The onset of fever or worsening results of laboratory studies (e.g., serum enzyme [ALT and AST] levels, prothrombin time, and bilirubin and albumin levels) and subtle mental status changes can indicate the onset of PSE.

If encephalopathy is present, a major focus of nursing is to implement the prescribed regimen. Treatment is focused on eliminating the causes of PSE, such as GI bleeding or hypokalemia, if known. The patient should be protected from sources of injury. Altered mental status increases the patient's potential for injury.

Other interventions focus on reducing ammonia levels and include the following:

1. Eliminating or restricting protein intake
2. Increasing carbohydrate intake to decrease metabolism of endogenous proteins
3. Administering oral cathartics or enemas to empty the bowel and decrease ammonia formation

**table 37-6** *Stages of Portal-Systemic Encephalopathy*

| Stage 1 (Prodromal) | Stage 2 (Impending) | Stage 3 (Stuporous) | Stage 4 (Coma) |
|---|---|---|---|
| Change in sleep pattern | Lethargy | Confused, somnolent | Unconscious |
| Slow response | Disorientation to time | Stupor, but arousable | No intellectual functioning |
| Shortened attention span | Impaired computation | Disorientation to place | Loss of deep tendon reflexes |
| Depressed or euphoric | Decreased inhibition | Anger, rage, paranoia | If responsive, only to deep pain |
| Irritable | Anxiety or apathy | Increased reflexes | Hyperventilation |
| Tremors | Inappropriate behavior | Clonus | Fetor hepaticus (musty, sweet breath odor) |
| Some incoordination | Speech slurred | Babinski reflex | Increased temperature and pulse rate |
| Writing impaired | Decreased reflexes | Asterixis | |
| | Ataxia | | |
| | Asterixis | | |

4. Administering intestinal antibiotics such as neomycin to kill bacteria in the GI tract
5. Administering lactulose

The patient with PSE is very ill and requires care for the prevention of respiratory problems (see Chapters 18 and 32). Ventilatory support may be required. Coughing is prohibited if the patient has esophageal varices. The patient also needs care to prevent skin breakdown that may be worsened by malnutrition, pruritus, ascites, and frequent stools or incontinence. Infection must be prevented. If PSE progresses to hepatic coma, nursing care is similar to that of any unconscious patient (see Chapter 22).

Many patients with PSE die of renal failure secondary to an inadequate circulating blood volume (hypovolemia). In some patients, renal function progressively deteriorates without any apparent cause. The treatment of PSE requires a careful balancing of fluid administration to maintain adequate perfusion of the kidney without creating an excessive load on the cardiovascular system. To monitor renal function adequately, an indwelling catheter is often inserted, especially if the patient is being maintained on intravenous fluids. Central venous pressure monitoring is also frequently used to determine fluid volume status.

Because most narcotics and sedatives must be detoxified by the liver, they are contraindicated in patients with impaired liver function. If a sedative must be used, drugs such as chlordiazepoxide (Librium), barbital, or phenobarbital, which are excreted by the kidney, are prescribed. If any sedatives, analgesics, or hypnotics are used, they should be given in less than normal doses, and the patient's response should be evaluated carefully.

Maintenance of adequate nutrition is a major nursing focus. A low-protein diet is often less palatable than a regular diet. Providing good oral hygiene, maintaining a pleasant clean environment, and serving small attractive meals may help increase appetite. A low-protein (20 to 40 g/day) diet may be prescribed indefinitely. Dietary or IV supplements that provide selected BCAAs and are lower in SCAAs may be used. Both oral and IV preparations are available commercially; these also contain carbohydrates. Vitamins and minerals are added as necessary.[8]

The patient and family will need instructions regarding dietary restrictions and how to take medications. They also must be taught to be alert for subtle changes in the patient's behavior that indicate worsening or onset of PSE and to seek medical attention immediately if the patient shows any of these behaviors.

## Hepatorenal Syndrome

Hepatorenal syndrome is a poorly understood complication of cirrhosis. It is characterized by sudden renal failure for no known cause in a patient with progressively worsening liver failure.

The pathogenesis of hepatorenal failure is uncertain but includes a marked decrease in renal cortex blood flow because of intrarenal vasoconstriction. The intrarenal vasoconstriction can possibly result from the following[8]:

1. An increase in renin
2. A decrease in prostaglandin production by the kidney
3. The release of endotoxin in the body because of liver failure
4. A change in sympathetic activity, causing vasoconstriction
5. The production of a vasoconstrictor by the diseased liver

The patient with hepatorenal failure has oliguria and azotemia. Blood pressure may be elevated or decreased. The patient complains of anorexia, fatigue, and weakness. Fluid retention leads to hyponatremia and a decrease in urine osmolality. The continual accumulation of waste products and alterations in fluid and electrolytes cause neurological changes that can resemble those of PSE. Blood pressure continues to drop. Hepatorenal failure has a very poor prognosis.

### *Collaborative care management*

The focus of management is to determine whether the oliguria is caused by decreased cardiac output, hepatorenal syndrome, or acute tubular necrosis. Any of these processes can occur in the person with cirrhosis. Once the diagnosis of hepatorenal syndrome is made, the management is designed to improve hepatic function and support renal function. Fluid and electrolytes are given to maintain hemodynamic status. Potentially nephrotoxic drugs such as neomycin are stopped. Some patients have shown improvement after a portacaval shunt has been implemented for other reasons, and others have shown improvement with a decrease in ascites. Liver transplantation is the major intervention for most patients. Liver transplantation and the related nursing care are discussed in Chapter 68. Hemodialysis has been successful in treating hyperkalemia. Continuous arteriovenous hemodialysis or ultrafiltration may be used to treat fluid overload and pulmonary edema. Note that these last treatments improve only symptoms and not the hepatorenal syndrome itself, because the basic problem is in the liver and not in the kidney.

## critical thinking QUESTIONS

1 Examine the scientific principles underlying the nursing management of individuals with cirrhosis of the liver, and determine those that could be applied or broadened to nursing care related to all types of liver disorders.

2 Differentiate the characteristics of hepatitis A from hepatitis B. Identify principles of preventing transmission that are universal to all types of hepatitis.

3 A patient with cirrhosis is admitted for bleeding esophageal varices and ascites. A TIPS procedure is planned. What information should be included in preparing the patient and family for this procedure?

## chapter SUMMARY

**FOCAL HEPATIC DISORDERS**

- Liver abscesses may be pyogenic and treated with broad-spectrum antibiotics and surgery, or they may be amebic and treated with amebicidal drugs.
- Metastatic tumors of the liver are 20 times more prevalent than primary tumors of the liver.
- Malignant lesions of the liver are treated with resection, palliative use of radiation, and chemotherapy by systemic routes or hepatic arterial infusion.

### DIFFUSE HEPATOCELLULAR DISORDERS

- The incidence of toxic hepatitis may be reduced by decreased use or proper use of toxins such as petroleum distillates.
- There are five types of viral hepatitis. Measures to control hepatitis A and E focus on hand washing, thus interrupting the fecal-oral route of transmission. The other three types are spread through blood and body fluid routes.
- Many tests use serological markers (antigens and antibodies) for differentiating the type of hepatitis; $HB_sAg$ is one test for HBV. HAV is detected by the presence of IgM class anti-HAV. HCV is detected by the presence of anti-HCV.
- The Centers for Disease Control and Prevention considers HBV to be the greatest occupational hazard for health care workers. Measures to decrease risk include HBV vaccination, hand washing, and Standard Precautions.
- Preexposure and postexposure prophylaxis for HAV and HBV infection include immune globulin (passive immunity for HAV) and HBIG (passive immunity for HBV) and HBV vaccine (active immunity for HBV) and a vaccine for HAV (active immunity for HAV.)
- Anorexia and influenza-like symptoms are often more acute in hepatitis B, but these symptoms occur in all types of hepatitis. They occur before icterus (jaundice) appears.
- Most persons with viral hepatitis recover within 6 months and have no residual liver damage. HBV and HCV infection may lead to a carrier state, atypical course of illness, chronic hepatitis, or cirrhosis.
- All types of jaundice involve increased serum levels of bilirubin. Hemolytic jaundice is a problem of excessive red blood cell breakdown; obstructive jaundice is associated with an elevation of conjugated bilirubin (direct) and an absence of urinary urobilinogen, and hepatocellular jaundice is often associated with elevated serum transaminase levels.
- In the United States, cirrhosis is most often a result of chronic alcoholism and is characterized by multiple abnormal hepatic function tests. Portal hypertension and bleeding esophageal varices are two life-threatening problems.
- The major focus of nursing care is on supporting the patient by dealing with problems related to altered liver function and helping patients deal with the alcoholism that is frequently the cause.
- The major complications of cirrhosis are portal hypertension, varices, ascites, portal-systemic encephalopathy, and hepatorenal syndrome.
- Varices are treated pharmacologically, with sclerotherapy, with balloon tamponade, and in some instances with shunting procedures.
- Ascitic fluid must be decreased slowly at a rate of no greater than 500 ml/day to prevent hypokalemia, elevated blood urea nitrogen, oliguria, and hepatic encephalopathy.
- Resistant ascites may be treated with transjugular intrahepatic portosystemic shunt.
- Hepatic encephalopathy causes subtle neurological changes that can be missed unless assessment focuses on collecting objective neurological data.
- Hepatic encephalopathy can be precipitated by increased ammonia from gastrointestinal bleeding or increased protein in the diet, by electrolyte imbalances such as hypokalemia and alkalosis, and by depressed central nervous system states such as hypoxia and sedation.
- Hepatic encephalopathy is treated with neomycin, lactulose, and a low-protein diet.
- Hepatorenal syndrome is renal failure from no known cause in persons with hepatic failure; it has a very poor prognosis.
- Liver transplantation is increasingly being performed for a variety of liver problems.
- Patient education is a major nursing intervention for most patients with diffuse liver disease because of the chronicity of the liver problems.

## References


1. Adams I, Soulen MC: TIPS: a new alternative for variceal bleeder, *Am J Crit Care* 2(3):196-201, 1993.
2. Caldwell SH, Dickson RC, Driscoll C, Sue M: Sexual, vertical and household transmission of hepatitis C, *Va Med Q* 122:270-274, 1995.
3. Conrad DA, Jensen HB: New and improved vaccines: promising weapons against varicella, hepatitis A and typhoid fever, *Postgrad Med* 100:113-125, 1996.
4. Cooksley WG, Butterworth LA: Hepatitis C virus infection in health care workers referred to a hepatitis clinic, *Med J Aust* 164:656-658, 1996.
5. Herreid JA: Hepatitis C: past, present, and future, *Medsurg Nurs* 4:179-187, 1995.
6. Hollinger FB: Comprehensive control (or elimination) of hepatitis B virus transmission in the United States, *Gut* 38(suppl 2):S24-S30, 1996.
7. Kowdley K: Update on therapy for hepatobiliary diseases, *Nurse Pract* 21:78-88, 1996.
8. Lucey MR: Approach to the patient with cirrhosis, portal hypertension, and end-stage liver disease. In Kelley W, editor: *Textbook of internal medicine,* ed 3, Philadelphia, 1997, Lippincott-Raven.
9. Margolis HS, et al: Prevention of hepatitis B virus transmission by immunization: an economic analysis of current recommendations, *JAMA* 274:1201-1208, 1995.
10. Mast EE, Krawczynski K: Hepatitis E: an overview, *Ann Rev Med* 47:257-266, 1996.
11. Moyer L, Warwick M, Mahoney FJ: Prevention of hepatitis A virus infection, *Am Fam Physician* 54:107-114, 1996.
12. Okoth FA: Viral hepatitis, *East Afr Med J* 73:308-312, 1996.
13. Pessoa MG, Wright TL: Hepatitis G: a virus in search of a disease, *Hepatology* 24:461-463, 1996.
14. Perrillo T, Regenstein F: Viral and immune hepatitis. In Kelley W, editor: *Textbook of internal medicine,* ed 3, Philadelphia, 1997, Lippincott-Raven.
15. Rakel, RE: *Conn's current therapy 1997,* Philadelphia, 1997, WB Saunders.
16. Ryan ME, Jones L, Miller D: Healthcare workers and bloodborne pathogens: knowledge, concerns, and practices, *Gastroenterol Nurs* 19:96-101, 1996.
17. US Department of Health and Human Services, Public Health Service: *Healthy people 2000: national health promotion and disease prevention objectives,* Washington, DC, 1990, US Government Printing Office.
18. US Department of Health and Human Services, Public Health Service: *Healthy people 2000: Midcourse review and 1995 revisions,* Sudbury, Mass, 1996, Jones and Bartlett.
19. US Preventive Services Task Force; Adult immunizations. In *Guide to clinical preventive services,* ed 2, Baltimore, 1996, Williams & Wilkins.

chapter

# 38 ASSESSMENT OF THE Gastrointestinal, Biliary, and Exocrine Pancreatic Systems

SHELLEY Y. HUFFSTUTLER and JUDITH K. SANDS

## objectives After studying this chapter, the learner should be able to:

1 Explain the functions of the mouth, esophagus, stomach, gallbladder, biliary ductal system, exocrine pancreas, and intestines.

2 Discuss the physiological changes that occur in the gastrointestinal system in response to aging.

3 Relate the subjective and objective data components of the nursing assessment of the gastrointestinal system.

4 Differentiate various data that may be obtained from the diagnostic tests used for problems of the gastrointestinal tract.

5 Explain the nursing responsibilities associated with common diagnostic tests used for problems of the gastrointestinal tract.

The gastrointestinal (GI) system, also termed the *digestive system* and *alimentary canal,* consists of the GI tract and its accessory organs. Its primary function is to convert ingested nutrients and fluids into a form that can be used by the cells of the body. This goal is accomplished through the processes of ingestion, digestion, and absorption. The second major function of the GI system is the storage and final excretion of the solid waste products of digestion. Proper functioning of the GI system is essential to the maintenance of proper nutrition and health.

## ANATOMY AND PHYSIOLOGY

The upper portion of the GI tract consists of those structures that aid in the ingestion and digestion of food. They include the mouth, esophagus, stomach, and duodenum, plus the related organs of the biliary system and exocrine pancreas. The lower GI tract consists of the small and large intestines, the rectum, and the anus. The structures of the GI system are illustrated in Figure 38-1. The GI system is primarily composed of a hollow, muscular tube approximately 9 m (30 feet) in length that stretches from the mouth to the anus.

Although the tube is located within the body, it is really an extension of the external environment. The walls of the GI tract successfully prevent most harmful agents from entering the body. The walls also prevent the escape of essential body fluids and materials. The composition of the walls is predominantly smooth muscle; however, the mouth and upper esophagus, along with a portion of the rectum and anus, consist of voluntary muscle.

### MOUTH

The mouth is made up of the lips, cheeks, tongue, hard and soft palates, teeth, and salivary glands (Figure 38-2). These structures begin the digestive process by mechanically breaking down and lubricating the food. Because digestive enzymes can function only on the exposed surfaces of food particles, the teeth begin the breakdown of food. No other portion of the GI system can perform the function of the teeth in their absence.

The lubrication of food is accomplished by the action of the watery and mucous secretions of the salivary, parotid, sublingual, and submandibular glands of the mouth. Saliva also contains ptyalin (amylase), which hydrolyzes starch to maltose. Small amounts of saliva, which contain IgA antibodies to many normal environmental microorganisms, are produced continually to keep the tissues of the mouth moist and clean. After chewing and moistening are completed, the muscular tongue pushes the food bolus back to the pharynx to initiate swallowing (deglutition).

### ESOPHAGUS

The esophagus begins at the lower end of the pharynx. It is a hollow, muscular tube 10 inches (25 cm) in length that lies behind the trachea, passes through the thorax, and connects the mouth and stomach. The upper third is composed of skeletal muscle, and the lower two thirds are smooth muscle. Both ends of the esophagus are protected by sphincters that help prevent the reflux of gastric contents. Both sphincters are normally closed, except during the act of swallowing.

The primary function of the esophagus is to move the food bolus by peristalsis from the pharynx to the stomach. No enzymes are secreted by the esophagus, and only mechanical digestion takes place. The secretion of mucus assists in the movement of the food bolus and protects the walls of the esophagus from abrasion by partially digested food.

Swallowing is a complex physiological mechanism that must be accomplished without compromising respiration. It consists of three phases: (1) the voluntary phase, in which the tongue forces the bolus of food into the pharynx; (2) the involuntary pharyngeal phase, in which the food moves into the upper esophagus; and (3) the esophageal phase, during which food moves from the pharynx down into the stomach. The esophageal muscles are activated by the glossopharyngeal and vagal nerves, which create rhythmic peristaltic waves that

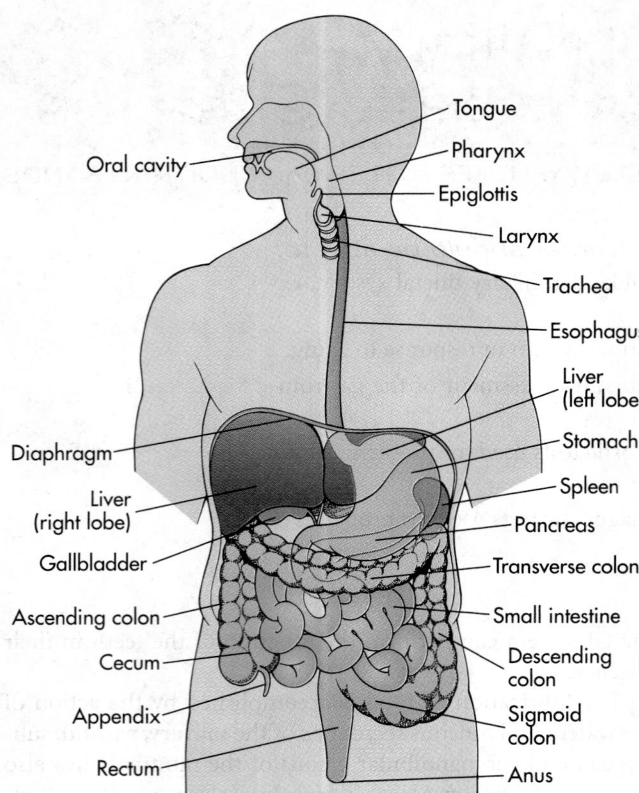


**fig. 38-1** The organs of the gastrointestinal system and related structures.

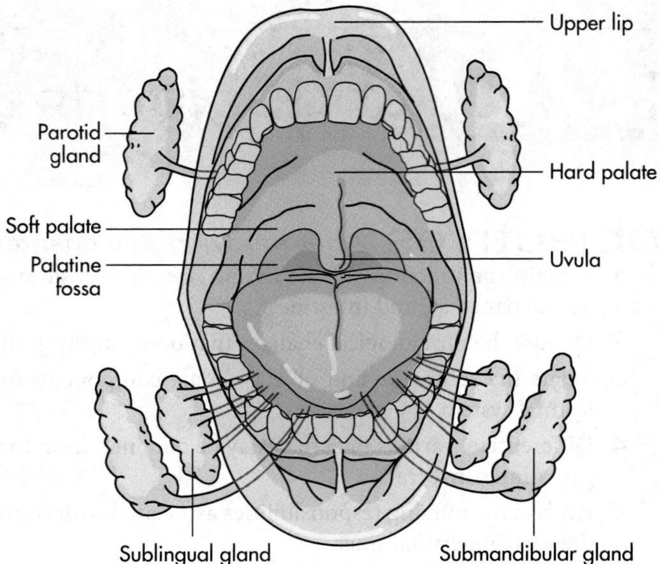


**fig. 38-2** The structures of the mouth.

propel the food toward the stomach. Food is prevented from passing into the trachea by the closing of the epiglottis and the opening of the esophagus.

## STOMACH

The stomach is roughly J shaped and lies in the upper abdomen to the left of midline. It is positioned to the left of the liver, to the right of the spleen, and posterior to both organs. It is a muscular pouch whose shape changes with its contents. Its three major regions are the fundus, body, and antrum. The cardiac sphincter protects the opening from the esophagus, and the pyloric sphincter protects the exit to the duodenum. The rugae, or longitudinal folds, of the stomach enable it to quadruple in size and increase from a resting volume of 50 ml to a capacity of approximately 1500 ml for food digestion without major changes in pressure. The stomach has an outer serous layer and three layers of smooth muscle. The outermost layer of smooth muscle is longitudinal, the middle layer is circular, and the inner layer is oblique (Figure 38-3). The rugae are found on the inner mucosal layer.

The stomach primarily serves as a reservoir but also has digestive and secretory functions. Food is stored in the stomach until partially digested. The fundus contains chief cells, which secrete digestive enzymes, and parietal cells, which secrete water, hydrochloric acid (HCl), and the intrinsic factor that is essential for the absorption of vitamin $B_{12}$. The HCl is responsible for the highly acidic medium of the stomach (pH of 0.9 to 1.5), which is needed to activate the enzymes that initiate protein digestion. This highly acidic pH also serves as a protective barrier, destroying most ingested microorgansims. Gastric acid secretion is under the control of parasympathetic stimulation via the vagus, as is the secretion of gastrin and histamine. Gastrin is a hormone secreted from endocrine cells in the gastric glands of the stomach in response to vagal stimulation and mechanical distention of the stomach. The secretion of histamine 2 ($H_2$) also increases gastric acid secretion. Approximately 2.0 to 2.5 L of gastric secretions are produced each day.

The gastric mucosa is covered by a thick mucous gel layer produced by the densely packed epithelial cells of the mucosa. The mucous layer is almost completely impermeable to hydrogen ions. The mucosal epithelial cells also secrete bicarbonate, which acts as a buffer and helps neutralize the acidic secretions. The combined actions of these two mechanisms are so effective that, although the gastric secretions have a pH of less than 2, the intraluminal pH of the mucosa is maintained at about 7.[19]

Gastric emptying is controlled by both hormonal and autonomic nervous system activity. Parasympathetic stimulation by the vagus nerve increases both peristalsis and secretion. Sympathetic stimulation inhibits them. The peristaltic contractions of the stomach propel the chyme toward the antrum and occur at a frequency of about three to five contractions per minute. The pylorus closes during antral contraction, and larger food particles are propelled back toward the body of the stomach for further mixing. Gastric contents are emptied into the duodenum *between* peristaltic contractions. Although the pylorus is not a true anatomical sphincter, it does help prevent the backflow of duodenal contents and bile salts into the stomach.[13]

## GALLBLADDER AND BILIARY DUCTAL SYSTEM

The gallbladder is a pear-shaped organ that lies on the inferior surface of the liver. It is composed of serous, muscular, and mucous coats and has a usual capacity of 50 ml, although it

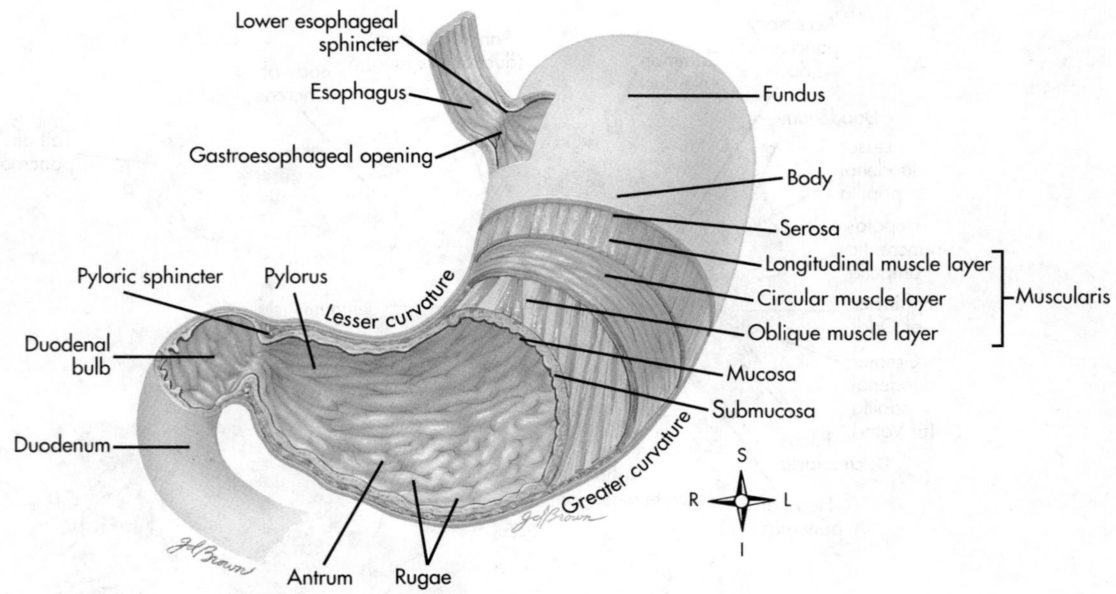


**fig. 38-3** The stomach.

can increase in size under normal conditions. Innervation of the gallbladder is from the parasympathetic and sympathetic nervous system. The cystic duct connects the gallbladder with the remaining structures of the ductal system—the hepatic ducts and common bile duct.

The major function of the gallbladder is to store and concentrate bile. Bile, which is formed in the liver, is excreted into the hepatic ducts, which unite to form the common bile duct. It passes behind the pancreas, is joined by the pancreatic duct, and empties into the duodenum. The sphincter of Oddi regulates the flow of bile into the duodenum. A second sphincter is located above the junction with the pancreatic duct and controls the flow of bile in the common bile duct. When this sphincter is closed, bile moves back into the gallbladder, where it is concentrated fivefold to tenfold. Because bile can be released directly into the duodenum from the liver, the gallbladder is not essential to life. Bile salts facilitate fat digestion by emulsifying fats for action by intestinal lipases and facilitate the absorption of fats, fat-soluble vitamins, and cholesterol.

The release of bile from the gallbladder or liver is controlled by cholecystokinin (CCK). Approximately 600 to 800 ml of bile is produced daily. The CCK is released from the walls of the duodenal intestinal mucosa when lipids, amino acids, and hydrogen ions enter the duodenum from the stomach. It travels by the blood to the gallbladder and causes contraction of the gallbladder's smooth musculature and relaxation of the sphincter at the end of the common bile duct (the sphincter of Oddi), so that bile can be emptied into the duodenum.

Most of the bile salts are reabsorbed from the intestine into the enterohepatic circulation and returned to the liver, where they can be recirculated. The system is so efficient that only 15% to 25% of the bile salt pool needs to be replaced by the liver each day.

## PANCREAS

The pancreas is an elongated, flattened organ located in the posterior abdomen, with its head lying within the curve of the duodenum and its tail resting against the spleen. The pancreas has both exocrine and endocrine functions. The exocrine functions are carried out by the acini cells and duct system, and the endocrine functions are carried out by islets of Langerhans cells (Figure 38-4). Exocrine functions will be discussed in this chapter. The endocrine functions have been previously discussed in Chapter 35.

The pancreas is divided into three parts, which are composed of lobules. The lobules are formed from groups of secretory cells termed *acini,* which drain into a ductal system that ultimately reaches the main pancreatic duct of Wirsung. This major duct extends the entire length of the gland. At the head of the pancreas the ductal secretions enter the duodenum through the ampulla of Vater. The sphincter of Oddi controls its opening.

Approximately 2 L of pancreatic secretions are produced daily. The ductal epithelium produces a balanced electrolyte secretion, and the acini secrete digestive enzymes in an inactive precursor state. The pancreatic secretions contain proteolytic enzymes, which break down protein; pancreatic amylase, which breaks down starch; and lipase, which hydrolyzes fat into glycerol and fatty acids. The pancreatic acini also produce an enzyme inhibitor that prevents the activation of the secretions until they reach the duodenum. The production of the pancreatic secretions is controlled by the action of the parasympathetic nervous system, gastrin, and hormones released from the duodenum during digestion.

## INTESTINES

The small intestine is about 2.5 cm (1 inch) wide and 6 m (20 feet) long and fills most of the abdomen. It consists of three parts—the duodenum, which connects to the stomach;

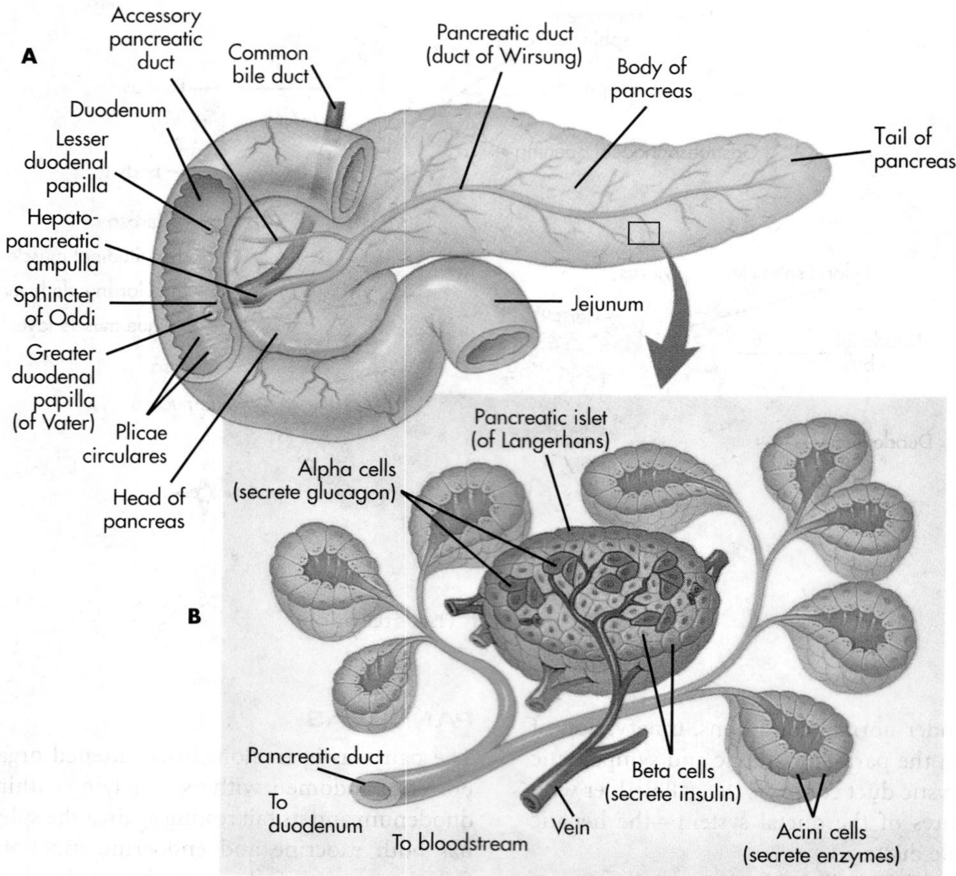


**fig. 38-4 A,** The pancreatic ductal system. **B,** Note both the endocrine and exocrine glandular cells of the pancreas.

the jejunum, or middle portion; and the ileum, which connects to the large intestine (see Figure 38-1).

The large intestine is about 6 cm (2.5 inches) wide and 1.5 m (5 feet) long. It also consists of three parts—the cecum, which connects to the small intestine; the colon; and the rectum. The ileocecal valve prevents backward flow of fecal contents from the large intestine to the small intestine. The vermiform appendix, which has no known function, is an appendage close to the ileocecal valve. The colon is subdivided into four sections—the ascending, transverse, descending, and sigmoid colons. The points at which the colon changes direction are named for adjacent organs—the liver (hepatic flexure) and the spleen (splenic flexure). The rectum is 17 to 20 cm (7 to 8 inches) long, ending in the 2 to 3 cm anal canal. The opening of the anus is controlled by a smooth muscle internal sphincter and a striated muscle external sphincter.

Table 38-1 summarizes the major digestive enzymes. The actions and stimuli for secretion of the major gastrointestinal hormones are presented in Table 38-2.

### Small Intestine

The primary functions of the small intestine are the digestion of food and the absorption of nutrients. This process occurs primarily in the jejunum and ileum. The duodenum contains the opening for the bile and pancreatic ducts, which allow bile and pancreatic secretions to enter the intestine. Mucus-producing glands are concentrated where gastric contents are emptied and digestive secretions enter the duodenum. The mucus helps protect the duodenum from the acids in the gastric chyme and the actions of the digestive enzymes.

Digestion begins in the mouth and stomach, but it takes place primarily in the small intestine. The intestinal mucosa is impermeable to most large molecules, so proteins, fats, and complex carbohydrates must be broken down into small particles before they can be absorbed. The intestinal mucosa also secretes surface enzymes that aid in digestion and about 2 L per day of serous fluid that acts as a diluting agent to facilitate absorption.

Carbohydrate digestion, which begins in the mouth, is completed in the small intestine as disaccharides are broken down into monosaccharides (glucose, fructose, and galactose) by the action of intestinal enzymes and pancreatic amylase. Protein digestion, which begins in the stomach, is completed as polypeptides are broken down into peptides and amino acids by the action of pancreatic trypsin. Fat digestion is accomplished by emulsification into small droplets by the action of bile and pancreatic lipase. The droplets are then further broken down into glycerol and fatty acids. The release of digestive secretions is stimulated by the hormones secretin and cholecystokinin (CCK) (also called pancreozymin), as well as by the action of the parasympathetic nervous system.

**table 38-1** *Digestive Enzymes*

| SOURCE | ACTION |
|---|---|
| **MOUTH** | |
| Pytalin (salivary amylase) | Breaks starch into maltose (polysaccharides to disaccharides) |
| **STOMACH** | |
| Gastric pepsin | Breaks protein into polypeptides |
| Gastric lipase | Digests butterfat |
| **PANCREAS** | |
| Pancreatic amylase | Breaks starch into maltose (polysaccharides to disaccharides) |
| Trypsin | Splits polypeptide chains |
| Pancreatic lipase | Splits emulsified fat into monoglycerides |
| **SMALL INTESTINE** | |
| Maltase | Breaks maltose into glucose |
| Dextrinase | Breaks alpha-limit dextrin to glucose |
| Lactase | Breaks lactose into galactose and glucose |
| Sucrase | Breaks sucrose into glucose and fructose |
| Enterokinase | Activates trypsin |
| Peptidases | Splits polypeptides into amino acids |
| Intestinal lipase | Splits neutral fats into glycerol and fatty acids |

**table 38-2** *Major Gastrointestinal Hormones*

| HORMONE | ACTION | STIMULUS FOR SECRETION |
|---|---|---|
| Gastrin | Stimulates secretion of gastric acid and pepsinogen; increases gastric blood flow; stimulates gastric smooth muscle contraction and motility | Secreted from antrum of stomach and duodenum in response to vagal stimulation, epinephrine, solutions of calcium salts, and alcohol; inhibited by an antral stomach pH of less than 2.5 |
| Secretin | Stimulates secretion of bicarbonate-containing solution by the pancreas and liver; inhibits gastric acid secretion and motility | Secreted by duodenum in response to low pH chyme (less than 3.0) entering the duodenum |
| Cholecystokinin | Stimulates the contraction of the gallbladder and the secretion of pancreatic enzymes; slows gastric emptying | Secreted in duodenum and jejunum in response to the presence of fatty and amino acids |
| Enterogastrone | Inhibits gastric secretion and motility; relaxes sphincter of Oddi | Secreted in duodenum in response to the presence of partially digested proteins and fats |

The inner mucosal surface of the small intestine is covered with millions of villi, which are the functional units for absorption. Each villus is equipped with a blind-end lymph vessel (lacteal) in its center, which is surrounded by capillaries, venules, and arterioles (Figure 38-5). These structures bring blood to the surface of the intestine and provide a network for absorption into the portal blood or lymphatic system.[13] Ninety percent of absorption occurs within the small intestine by either active transport or diffusion. Active transport requires a metabolic energy expenditure and is used to absorb amino acids, monosaccharides, sodium, and calcium. Fatty acids and water diffuse passively, primarily into the lymphatics.

The contents of the small intestine (chyme) are propelled toward the anus by regular peristaltic movements. Both segmental and propulsive movements occur. The segmental movements involve primarily the circular muscles of the intestine. Slow contractions move the chyme back and forth in small segments of the intestine (1 to 4 cm). This movement mixes the chyme and facilitates digestion and absorption. Segmental peristaltic movements increase after meals. The propulsive peristaltic movements involve intestinal segments of 10 to 20 cm in length.[19] Contraction occurs in the proximal segment, with relaxation in the distal segment. Chyme advances slowly and normally takes 3 to 10 hours to move from the stomach to the colon. Parasympathetic stimulation, primarily through branches of the vagus nerve, increases peristaltic activity. Sympathetic stimulation is primarily inhibitory.

## Large Intestine

Minimal chemical digestion takes place in the large intestine. It functions primarily to absorb water and electrolytes from the chyme and store the food waste (feces) until defecation.

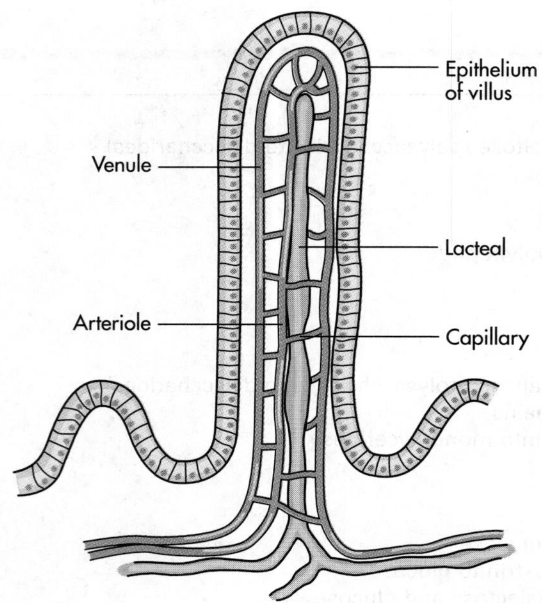


**fig. 38-5** The intestinal villus. Note the circulatory vessels surrounding the lacteal, which drains into the lymphatic system.

Reabsorption occurs predominantly in the right or ascending colon. The colon can absorb 6 to 8 times more fluid than is delivered to it daily, and only approximately 100 ml of fluid is left in the colon to be mixed with the fecal residue.

The large number of microorganisms found in the large intestine further break down the residual proteins that were not digested or absorbed in the small intestine. The breakdown of amino acids produces ammonia, which is converted to urea by the liver. These intestinal bacteria also play a vital role in the synthesis of vitamin K and some of the B vitamins. The only significant secretion of the colon is mucus, which protects the walls and helps the fecal matter adhere into a mass.

Approximately 450 ml of chyme reaches the cecum each day. The transit time in the large bowel is slow, taking about 12 hours to reach the rectum. The fecal contents in the colon are pushed forward by mass movements that occur only a few times each day. These mass movements are stimulated by gastrocolic reflexes initiated when food enters the duodenum from the stomach, especially after the first meal of the day.

The rectum is well innervated with sensory fibers. Parasympathetic fibers are responsible for the contraction of the rectum and relaxation of the internal sphincter of the anus. The defecation reflex occurs when feces enter the rectum. Afferent impulses are transmitted to the sacral segments of the spinal cord; subsequently, reflex impulses are transmitted back to the sigmoid and rectum, initiating relaxation of the internal anal sphincter.

## PHYSIOLOGICAL CHANGES WITH AGING

Gastrointestinal complaints are extremely common in elderly persons. Distinct changes occur in the GI system with aging, although these changes are incompletely understood. Although most of the aging-related changes do not interfere with normal functioning, it is important for nurses to be cognizant of the changes and incorporate appropriate modifications when planning care for the elderly population. Additionally, problems associated with other chronic illnesses such as diabetes require careful consideration because they are usually more important than the effects of aging itself.

In the mouth, teeth darken and may loosen or fracture, and the gums recede. Salivary gland output decreases, which causes mouth dryness and increased susceptibility to infection and tissue breakdown. Aging causes decreased motility and strength of peristalsis in the esophagus, but these changes appear to have minimal significance in healthy persons. Some deterioration in the lower esophageal sphincter may increase the frequency of esophageal reflux.[1]

Gastric motility and emptying diminish slightly but progressively with age, and gastric acid secretion also decreases steadily after age 50. Achlorhydria (absence of free HCl) is relatively common. These changes can produce minor problems in digestion but are usually asymptomatic. Chronic gastritis is common in elderly persons, but the condition is usually the result of bacterial colonization by *Helicobacter pylori* and not aging.[2]

No significant changes in biliary system morphology are associated with aging. However, the composition of the bile becomes increasingly lithogenic (likely to produce calculi), possibly related to an increase in biliary cholesterol; therefore the incidence of gallstones increases with each decade.[5]

The pancreas exhibits ductal hyperplasia and fibrosis with aging, but these changes are not necessarily associated with altered functioning. The output of pancreatic secretions steadily declines after age 40, but related problems with absorption have not been documented.

Aging-related changes in small intestinal function are important and can lead to poor nutrition even with adequate intake. Nutrient absorption is impaired, particularly the absorption of carbohydrates. Absorption of water-soluble vitamins remains intact, but the absorption of vitamin D is defective in many elderly persons, and the active transport of calcium is also impaired. Decreased production of secretory IgA can lead to an increase in the frequency and severity of infections.[4]

Chronic constipation is one of the most common complaints in elderly persons. Yet, the segmental mass movements and contractions of the large intestine have been found to be unchanged as long as the individual remains physically active. The incidence of both diverticula and polyps in the colon rises with age. There is a decrease in elasticity in the rectum and a steady decrease in the rectal volume, which can result in sphincter failure. However, the sensation of rectal fullness remains intact, and most problems with bowel incontinence in elderly persons are not attributable to the effects of aging.[3]

## SUBJECTIVE DATA

A thorough health history is necessary to adequately assess the health status of persons with potential dysfunction of the GI system.

### PATIENT/FAMILY HISTORY

The nurse asks the patient about previous GI problems, hospitalizations, and surgeries. This includes past and current med-

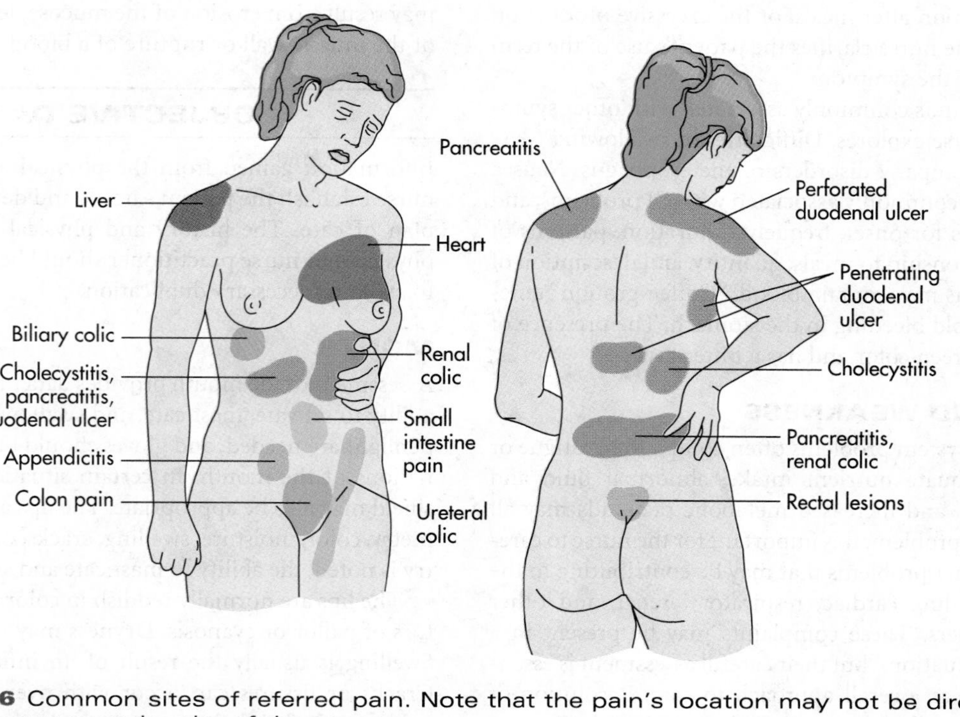

**fig. 38-6** Common sites of referred pain. Note that the pain's location may not be directly over or even near the site of the organ.

ication use, both over-the-counter and prescribed. The use of antacids and laxatives is particularly important. The nurse inquires about the presence of GI problems in the nuclear or extended family, including cancer and disorders such as inflammatory bowel disease, which have a documented hereditary link.

## DIET AND NUTRITION

The adequacy of the diet, in terms of both quality and quantity, can be quickly estimated through comparison of the diet with recommended food intake patterns. The nutritional assessment has particular significance in GI disorders, because it may reveal changes in eating patterns that are characteristic of specific illnesses or disorders. The nutritional assessment includes an exploration of usual eating patterns and any changes that may be the result of illness or specific symptoms. The assessment explores changes in appetite, food preferences and intolerances, food allergies, planned and unplanned changes in weight, adherence to special or therapeutic diets, and the use of dietary or vitamin supplements. A 24-hour dietary recall may be a useful tool to approximate caloric and specific nutrient intake and analyze the overall adequacy of the diet. Symptoms related to food intake should also be carefully assessed. Changes in appetite and the presence of such symptoms as dysphagia, nausea, and discomfort are carefully explored.

Lifestyle, economic, and cultural factors affecting nutrition are also assessed. Food has multiple social and emotional values for individuals that are distinct from its role in nutrition. Financial resources, access to food preparation and storage facilities, and religious or social beliefs may all influence both the quality and quantity of the diet. Lifestyle factors can have a direct or indirect effect on GI function. Gastrointestinal symptoms commonly develop in response to life stressors or worsen in response to those stressors. Open-ended questions are most effective for exploring beliefs and feelings about food.

Complete nutritional assessment includes an evaluation of the patient's use of sugar and salt substitutes, coffee, alcohol, and tobacco (both chewing and smoking). The presence of dentures is an essential consideration because dentures may significantly influence food selection and chewing.

## ABDOMINAL PAIN

Although pain is not an early or common manifestation of GI disease, it is frequently the reason individuals seek medical attention. The nurse assesses its onset, duration, character, location, and relationship to meals, stressful events, or activity. Pain may be experienced anywhere along the length of the GI tract in a specific localized pattern, a general nonspecific pattern, or referred to another somatic or skeletal region that shares the same nerve innervation[8] (Figure 38-6). Abdominal pain may be continuous, episodic, or associated with eating. The pain sensation is thought to arise from the distention or sudden contraction of a hollow viscus; therefore local stretching or traction on pain-sensitive structures will elicit the pain stimulus. The painful area may demonstrate local muscle guarding, which serves as a protective mechanism as the overlying muscles contract. The pain associated with pancreatic or biliary dysfunction is usually severe.

Abdominal pain or discomfort may be reported as heartburn, indigestion, or stomachache and requires further clarification. The pain may interfere with chewing or swallowing food. Specific foods, such as those that are spicy, very hot, or very cold; alcohol; or smoking may initiate or aggravate the pain. Abdominal pain may have been self-treated with a variety of over-the-counter preparations.

The term *indigestion* is commonly used by patients to describe heartburn (usually the result of reflux), uncomfortable fullness or distention after meals, or the excessive production of flatus (gas). The nurse clarifies the patient's use of the term and the nature of the symptom.

Abdominal pain is commonly associated with other symptoms that the nurse explores. Difficulties in swallowing (dysphagia) may accompany disorders of the esophagus. Nausea and vomiting are commonly associated with GI problems, and the nurse assesses for onset, frequency, duration, patterns of occurrence, relationship to meals, quantity, and description of the emesis. Emesis may contain blood. "Coffee-ground" emesis may indicate old bleeding in the stomach. The presence of bile produces a green color and has a bitter taste.

### FATIGUE AND WEAKNESS

Persons with GI system problems often complain of fatigue or weakness. Inadequate nutrient intake, abnormal fluid and electrolyte status, and increased metabolic demands may all contribute to the problem. It is important for the nurse to carefully consider other problems that may be contributing to the symptoms, including cardiac, respiratory, renal, and other metabolic disorders. These complaints may be present in a wide variety of situations, but their careful assessment is essential for planning an overall approach to care. Resolution of these problems usually takes time. Fatigue and weakness may also contribute to weight loss, particularly when associated with persistent anorexia, nausea, vomiting, or abdominal pain.

### ELIMINATION PATTERNS

Patterns of bowel elimination vary significantly among healthy individuals, and these patterns are commonly altered by GI system disorders. The nurse assesses the individual's usual elimination pattern and explores any changes that have occurred. The use of laxatives, suppositories, or other products to support bowel elimination is carefully assessed.

Changes in the normal pattern of bowel elimination may represent a physiological alteration, a pathological condition, or simply a change in normal diet and activity patterns. Constipation—defined as the presence of small, hard stools that are passed with difficulty at infrequent intervals—is a classic example. It may be a temporary response to inactivity and a diet change or a sign of bowel obstruction. Diarrhea and stools containing mucus, pus, and possibly undigested food may indicate enteritis or invasion by a parasite. Partial obstruction of the descending colon may produce small, ribbon-shaped stools, whereas no stool is passed if obstruction is complete. Constipation may also result from the administration of narcotics that slow peristalsis, and diarrhea can be the result of surgical interventions that remove significant bowel segments.

When fat absorption is abnormal, steatorrhea (bulky, foul-smelling, fatty stools) may occur. If biliary obstruction is present, the patient may give a history of clay-colored (grayish) stools. Bright red blood in the stool indicates lower GI bleeding. Blood from the upper GI tract is changed by digestive secretions, and the stool appears black and sticky (tarry). Sometimes the presence of blood in the GI tract acts as a powerful cathartic and may produce abrupt, severe diarrhea. Blood in the stool (melena) may be a recent or a chronic symptom and may result from erosion of the mucosa, leading to perforation of the muscle wall or rupture of a blood vessel.

## OBJECTIVE DATA

Information gained from the physical assessment helps the nurse establish the patient's needs and develop an appropriate plan of care. The history and physical examination by the physician or nurse practitioner should be used when available to avoid unnecessary duplication.

### MOUTH

Assessment of the mouth provides data indicating the patient's ability to salivate, masticate, and swallow. A tongue blade and penlight are needed, and gloves should be worn for all examinations of the mouth. In certain situations, a mask and eye shield may also be appropriate. The lips are observed for symmetry, color, moisture, swelling, cracks, or lesions. If asymmetry is noted, the ability to masticate and swallow is assessed.

The lips are normally reddish in color and are good indicators of pallor or cyanosis. Dryness may indicate dehydration. Swelling is usually the result of an inflammatory response. Cracks or fissures can occur with overdryness, exposure to cold, poorly fitting dentures, or a riboflavin deficiency. When cracks occur in the corners of the mouth they are referred to as angular stomatitis.

Lesions on the lips may be benign or malignant. A commonly encountered benign lesion is herpes simplex (cold sore, fever blister), which is caused by a virus and can create enough discomfort to limit mastication. The enamel surface of the teeth should be white but will darken with surface stains (tea, coffee, tobacco). Commonly found abnormalities of the teeth include caries, loose or broken teeth, and absence of some or all teeth. The gums—or gingivae—are normally pink, attach to the teeth, and fill the interdental surfaces. If the person is partially or completely edentulous (without teeth), the gingivae are examined for areas of redness caused by improperly fitting dentures, partial plates, or implants. The person is then asked to insert the dentures to assess correct fit and comfort for adequate mastication. Recession of the gum line is not uncommon in older individuals.

The buccal mucosa is light pink, although patchy pigmentation is seen in dark-skinned individuals. The mucosa is examined for moisture, white spots or patches, debris, areas of bleeding, or ulcers resulting from ill-fitting dentures or braces. Dryness and debris may indicate dehydration. White, curdy patches—which are removable with some effort—may be caused by candidiasis (thrush). White, nonremovable patches (leukoplakia); white plaques within red patches; or red, granular patches may be premalignant lesions and should be reported to the physician. A round or oval white ulcer surrounded by an area of redness is indicative of an aphthous ulcer (canker sore). (See Chapter 39.)

When the tongue is depressed with a tongue blade and the person says "Ah," the soft palate is observed for symmetry and the effective functioning of cranial nerve X (necessary for effective swallowing). The uvula, soft palate, tonsils, and posterior pharynx are observed for signs of inflammation. Tongue mobility and function are essential to mastication, taste, and swallowing. Normally, there is no limitation to movement in any direction, but the tongue will deviate to the paralyzed side with paralysis of the twelfth cranial nerve (hypoglossal). A thin, white coating and presence of large papillae on the dorsum of the tongue are normal findings. A thick coating indicates poor oral hygiene, and a smooth, red surface suggests a nutritional deficiency. The ventral surface is examined for leukoplakia, ulceration, or nodules, any of which may indicate malignancy.

Any distinctive odor of the breath is noted. A foul odor may occur after the ingestion of certain foods, with poor hygiene or oral infections, and with some metabolic dysfunctions such as diabetic ketoacidosis, liver disease, and bowel obstruction. Normally the mandible will slide forward and down without difficulty, and a "cracking" sound is audible when the mouth is opened widely. The interior of the mouth should also be carefully examined with a gloved finger to check for areas of tenderness, ulcers, and lumps.

## ABDOMEN

Examination of the abdomen determines the presence or absence of (1) tenderness, (2) organ enlargement, (3) masses, (4) spasm or rigidity of the abdominal muscles, and (5) fluid or air in the abdominal cavity. Physical examination of the abdomen is performed in the following order: inspection, auscultation, percussion, and palpation. Auscultation is performed before percussion and palpation, because the latter two may alter the frequency and intensity of bowel sounds.

The surface of the abdomen may be described anatomically in either four quadrants or nine regions (Figure 38-7). The patient should be in a supine position and as relaxed as possible. Bending the patient's knees slightly and placing a small pillow under the head can help the patient relax the abdominal muscles and make palpation easier. Good lighting should be available.

### Inspection

The skin of the abdomen is inspected for color, texture, scars, rashes, lesions, symmetry, contour, and visible peristalsis. The abdomen is normally flat but will be rounded in an obese person and may appear scaphoid in the thin or emaciated person. The integrity and turgor of the skin are reliable indicators of total body hydration.

Abdominal distention may be caused by air or fluid in the GI tract or fluid in the peritoneal space (ascites). Air may collect from swallowing or from gas produced by bacterial action in the bowel. Decreased peristalsis prevents the accumulated air from moving through the GI tract. Fluid may also accumulate from decreased peristalsis and be a symptom of partial or complete bowel obstruction. Ascites usually results from increased portal hypertension secondary to liver or heart disease.

Measurement of abdominal girth provides a baseline for the evaluation of any increase or decrease in size related to distention. A measuring tape is placed around the abdomen at the level of the umbilicus or 2.5 cm below, and the reading is taken. It is important to lightly mark the site for measurement on the patient's skin with a waterproof pen so that all subsequent measurements are taken at the same level for accurate evaluation.

Inspection will incorporate assessment for the presence of jaundice, which is a common symptom in biliary tract or liver disease. A slight aortic pulsation may be present in the epigastric area, but peristalsis is normally not visible. A summary of common findings from abdominal inspection is included in Table 38-3.

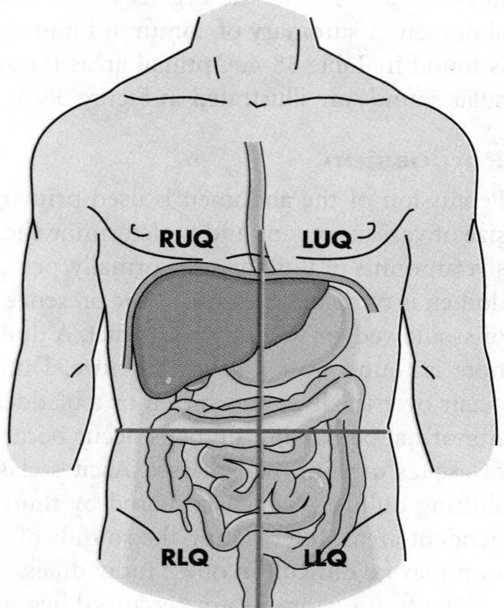


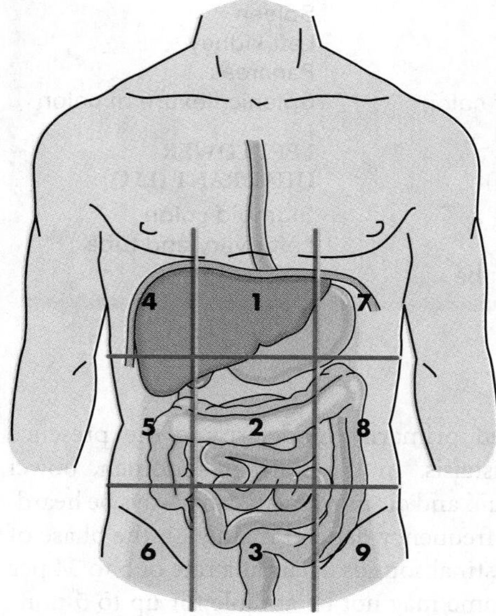


**fig. 38-7** Regions of the abdomen. *Left,* The abdomen divided into four quadrants. *Right,* The abdomen divided into nine topographical regions: *1,* Epigastrium; *2,* umbilical; *3,* suprapubic; *4,* right hypochondrium; *5,* right lumbar or flank; *6,* right inguinal or iliac; *7,* left hypochondrium; *8,* left lumbar or flank; *9,* left inguinal or iliac.

**table 38-3** *Common Findings from Abdominal Inspection*

| FINDING | INTERPRETATION |
|---|---|
| Scars or striae | May be result of pregnancy, obesity, ascites, tumors, edema, surgical procedures, or healed burned areas |
| Engorged veins | May be caused by obstruction of vena cava or portal vein and circulation from abdomen |
| Skin color | Observe for evidence of jaundice or inflammation (redness) |
| Visible peristalsis | May be caused by pyloric or intestinal obstruction; normally peristalsis not visible except for slow waves in thin persons |
| Visible pulsations | Normally slight pulsation of aorta, visible in epigastric region |
| Visible masses and altered contour | Observe for hernias, distention of ascites, and obesity; instructing patient to cough may bring out hernia "bulge" or elicit pain or discomfort in the abdomen; marked concavity may be caused by malnutrition |
| Spider angioma | Appear on upper portion of body and blanch with pressure; commonly result from liver disease |

**box 38-1** *Anatomical Location of Organs within Each Abdominal Quadrant*

| RIGHT UPPER QUADRANT (RUQ) | LEFT UPPER QUADRANT (LUQ) |
|---|---|
| Liver | Stomach |
| Gallbladder | Spleen |
| Duodenum | Left kidney |
| Right kidney | Pancreas |
| Hepatic flexure of colon | Splenic flexure of colon |
| **RIGHT LOWER QUADRANT (RLQ)** | **LEFT LOWER QUADRANT (LLQ)** |
| Cecum | Sigmoid colon |
| Appendix | Left ovary and tube |
| Right ovary and tube | |

## Auscultation

Auscultation is used primarily to determine the presence or absence of peristalsis. In the normal abdomen, bowel sounds caused by fluid and air movement can always be heard. Their intensity and frequency depend mainly on the phase of digestion. Most intestinal sounds occur at a rate of 5 to 34 per minute (although some may not be audible for up to 5 minutes) and are high pitched and gurgling in quality. A normal peristaltic wave produces audible sounds of air and fluid movement through the intestine. The sounds are the loudest to the right and below the umbilicus.[17]

**table 38-4** *Common Findings from Abdominal Auscultation*

| FINDING | INTERPRETATION |
|---|---|
| Absence of sounds in 5 minutes | Peritonitis, paralytic ileus, pneumonia, and hypokalemia |
| Repeated, high-pitched sounds occurring at frequent intervals | Increased peristalsis heard in gastroenteritis, early pyloric obstruction, early intestinal obstruction, and diarrhea |
| Bruit | Presence of abnormal sounds (turbulence of blood flow through partially occluded or diseased aorta or renal artery) |
| Hum and friction rub | Heard over liver and splenic areas, indicating an increased venous blood flow, possibly related to peritoneal inflammation |

Abnormalities may include either extreme. A virtual absence of normal sounds occurs when bowel motility is inhibited by inflammation or paralytic ileus. Exaggerated peristalsis produces waves of loud, gurgling sounds called borborygmi, which may result from infection or obstruction. Bowel sounds are auscultated by placing the diaphragm of the stethoscope lightly against the abdomen and listening to all quadrants systematically. It may take 5 full minutes to determine that bowel sounds are completely absent, but the absence of any bowel sounds in 2 minutes clearly indicates a problem.[10] Sounds that occur at a rate of about one per minute are hypoactive. The bell of the stethoscope may be used to auscultate for vascular sounds, such as bruits over the aorta and renal and iliac arteries.[11] These sounds are not normally present. Box 38-1 outlines the location of the organs within the quadrants of the abdomen. A summary of common findings from auscultation is found in Table 38-4. Optimal areas for auscultation of vascular sounds are illustrated in Figure 38-8.

## Percussion

Percussion of the abdomen is used primarily to confirm the size of various organs and to determine the presence of excessive amounts of fluid or air. Normally, percussion over the abdomen is tympanic because of the presence of a small amount of swallowed air within the GI tract. A dull or flat percussion note is found over a solid structure. Dull sounds normally occur over the liver and spleen or a bladder filled with urine. Abnormal percussion findings occur because of the presence of ascites or abnormal masses. Ascites classically produces a shifting dullness, which is caused by fluid movement to dependent areas. Interpreting the sounds of abdominal percussion may be difficult in obese individuals.

The four quadrants are percussed beginning with the thorax and moving downward systematically. The degree of tympany, from soft to pronounced, is recorded. Tympanic sounds should be heard beginning at the ninth interspace in the left upper quadrant of the abdomen.

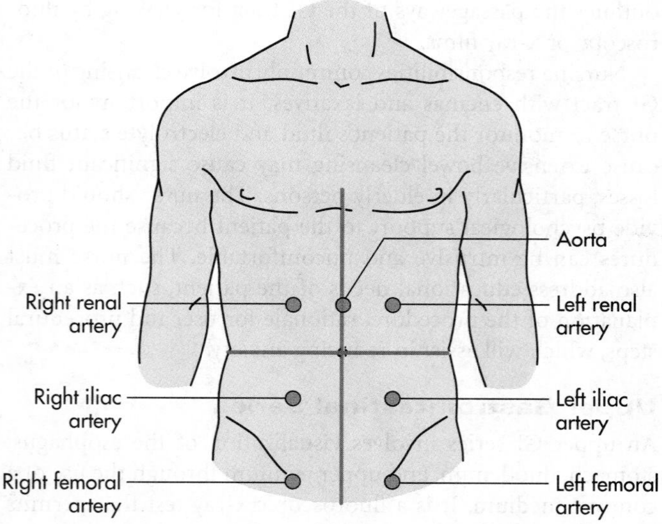

Aorta
Right renal artery
Left renal artery
Right iliac artery
Left iliac artery
Right femoral artery
Left femoral artery

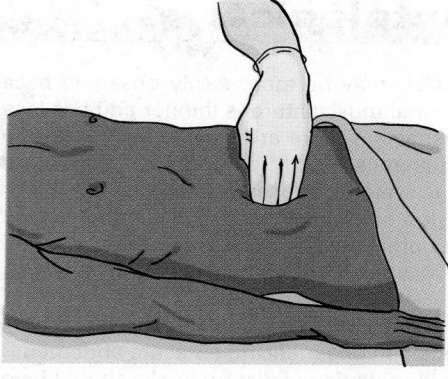

**fig. 38-8** Sites for auscultation of vascular sounds in the abdomen.

### Palpation

Palpation is of value in determining the outlines of the abdominal organs, determining the presence and characteristics of any abdominal masses, and identifying the presence of direct tenderness, guarding, rebound tenderness, and muscular rigidity. In the presence of gallbladder disease, normal palpation of the liver elicits sharp pain and a positive inspiratory arrest (Murphy's sign). The acute onset of pain causes the patient to stop inspiration abruptly, midway through the breath.[16]

Abnormal findings from palpation may include (1) direct tenderness over an organ capsule, (2) rebound tenderness (Blumberg's sign), (3) muscular rigidity, or (4) masses that may be felt if they are large enough or close enough to the surface. Distinction should be made between a distended abdomen that is firm to the touch and one that is soft to the touch.

Light palpation is used to elicit tenderness and cutaneous hypersensitivity. The nurse uses the pads of the fingertips, with the fingers together, and presses gently, depressing the abdominal wall about 1 cm. All quadrants are palpated using smooth movements.[6]

Deep palpation is used to delineate organs and masses and should be performed only by properly trained persons because improper technique can result in injury. The nurse again uses the palmar surface of the fingers but presses more deeply using a single- or two-handed technique. Rebound tenderness is tested by pressing slowly but firmly over the painful site. The fingers are then quickly withdrawn. Acute pain on withdrawal reflects peritoneal inflammation (positive Blumberg's sign).[9] This maneuver (illustrated in Figure 38-9) can be extremely painful and should never be performed unnecessarily.

## RECTUM

The normal perineal and perianal skin resembles the skin on the remainder of the body with no breaks in integrity. Abnormal findings may include pruritus ani, coccygeal or pilonidal sinus tract openings, fistulas, fissures, external hemorrhoids, or rectal prolapse. Internal hemorrhoids may appear when the patient bears down.

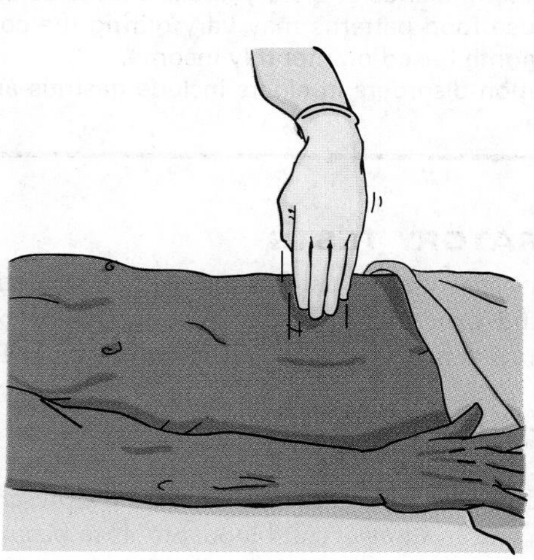

**fig. 38-9** Palpating for rebound tenderness.

Variations in assessment findings in elderly persons are summarized in the Gerontological Assessment Box. These are not abnormal findings and are common in this population.

## DIAGNOSTIC TESTS

Many of the examinations and tests performed for diagnosis of problems of the GI system are both time consuming and unpleasant. Several of the tests are intrusive procedures that are uncomfortable and embarrassing for the patient, which results in added stress for the patient. Representatives from the radiology department or laboratory may assume responsibility for instructing patients about diagnostic tests, because the tests will usually be performed on an outpatient basis. Most institutions also have prepared literature for the patient and family. It remains the nurse's responsibility to meet the educational and psychological needs of the patient by answering questions concerning the test procedure, rationale for its use, and specific test preparation in a caring manner. Diagnostic tests are sequenced to make the most effective use of time and equipment. The nurse ensures that the patient is prepared physically and mentally to avoid the preventable repetition of time-consuming and expensive tests.

## gerontological assessment

- Peristalsis may be more easily observed because the abdominal musculature is thinner and has less tone.
- On inspection there are usually increased deposits of subcutaneous fat on the abdomen because the ratio of fat to water increases with aging.
- Palpation of abdominal organs is often easier because the abdominal wall is softer and thinner. The liver and kidneys are most often palpable in the absence of obesity.
- Older adults often verbalize less pain than younger adults when experiencing an acute abdomen.
- Week-long diaries of dietary intake should be obtained because food patterns may vary during the course of the month based on monthly income.
- Common disorders in elders include gastritis and gallstones.

## LABORATORY TESTS

Numerous tests may be used as part of the evaluation of GI, biliary, and exocrine pancreas function. Major blood and urine tests that may be ordered are summarized in Table 38-5.

## STOOL EXAMINATION

Stool specimens are collected primarily for culture, determination of fat content, and examination for the presence of ova, parasites, and fresh or occult blood. Stools to be analyzed for the presence of bacteria (*Salmonella, Shigella,* and *Staphylococcus aureus*), ova, and parasites require that a fresh, warm specimen be received in the laboratory and may necessitate special collection procedures.

Fecal urobilinogen is responsible for the brown color of the stool. Biliary obstruction may cause decreased amounts to be present and turns the stool light or clay colored. These specimens should also be sent promptly to the laboratory because urobilinogen breaks down rapidly. Table 38-6 identifies other fecal color changes that may occur.

Detection of occult blood in the stool is useful in identifying bleeding in the GI tract. Occult blood may be identified by one of three tests—guaiac (Hemoccult), benzidine, or orthotoluidine (Occultest). The guaiac test is the least sensitive test and is often used to determine whether additional study is indicated. It does not require any special preparation. Meat, poultry, or fish can cause a false-positive test, and vitamin C in quantities of greater than 500 mg per day may cause a false-negative test; therefore these substances must be omitted from the diet for 3 days before testing with benzidine or orthotoluidine. Determination of fecal fat may be done as part of a workup for malabsorption. Elevations in fecal fat will be present with biliary or pancreatic obstructions and many intestinal malabsorption disorders.

## RADIOLOGICAL TESTS

Visualization of the GI tract may be performed by barium swallow, upper GI series, or barium enema. Barium is a radiopaque substance that, when ingested or given by enema, outlines the passageways of the GI tract for viewing by fluoroscopy or x-ray films.

Nursing responsibilities commonly involve cleansing of the GI tract with enemas and laxatives. It is important for the nurse to monitor the patient's fluid and electrolyte status because extensive bowel cleansing may cause significant fluid losses, particularly in elderly persons. The nurse should provide psychological support to the patient because the procedures can be intrusive and uncomfortable. The nurse must also address educational needs of the patient, such as an explanation of the procedure, rationale for use, and procedural steps, which will assist in reducing anxiety.

### Upper Gastrointestinal Series

An upper GI series involves visualization of the esophagus, stomach, duodenum, and upper jejunum through the use of a contrast medium. It is a fluoroscopic x-ray test that permits the examination of the structure, position, peristaltic activity, and motility of the organs. It can assist in the detection of tumors, ulceration, inflammation, abnormal anatomy, or malposition.

The procedure involves swallowing the contrast medium (usually barium), which is prepared in a milk shake form. Although it is flavored, the barium is unpleasant tasting and may cause vomiting. It is administered cold. The barium outlines the structures as it flows by gravity through the esophagus and stomach into the intestinal loops. Films are taken at intervals during the test, and the entire test takes about 45 minutes. The procedure may also be termed a *barium swallow* if only the function of the esophagus is to be evaluated. This shortened procedure takes about 15 minutes. If the small bowel is the primary focus of the test, it may be termed a *small bowel series.* The procedure is essentially the same, although it takes longer.

No special preparation is necessary before a GI series; however, the patient maintains nothing-by-mouth (NPO) status for at least 6 hours before the test. After an upper GI series, the patient is prescribed a laxative to hasten elimination of the barium; barium that remains in the colon may become hard and difficult to expel, leading to fecal impaction. The stool should return to the normal color (barium is white) after the barium is expelled.

### Barium Enema

A barium enema clearly outlines most of the large intestine through the use of a contrast medium. It is used to detect colon polyps, tumors, and chronic inflammatory bowel disease. If both an upper GI series and a barium enema are to be performed, the barium enema is done first, before barium from the upper GI series reaches the colon.

The procedure involves the instillation of barium through a rectal tube with an inflatable balloon to hold the barium in the colon. The patient is then placed in various positions while the radiologist observes on a monitor as the barium flows through the colon. The procedure takes about 30 minutes, and the instillation and retention of the barium cause the patient considerable embarrassment and discomfort.

**table 38-5** *Major GI, Biliary, and Exocrine Pancreas Blood and Urine Tests*

| Blood Test | Range of Normal Values | Description and Purpose |
|---|---|---|
| Stomach gastrin | <200 pg/ml (200 ng/L) | Gastrin is a gastric hormone that is a powerful stimulus for gastric acid secretion. Elevated levels are found in those with pernicious anemia and Zollinger-Ellison syndrome. |
| *Helicobacter pylori* | None | *Helicobacter pylori* detected in serum is a highly sensitive but less specific indicator of an active infection; *H. pylori* infection predisposes to peptic ulcer disease. |
| **BILIARY SYSTEM** | | |
| Total bilirubin | 0.1 to 1.0 mg/dl | Bilirubin is excreted in the bile. Obstruction in the biliary tract contributes primarily to a rise in conjugated (direct) values. |
| Conjugated (direct) | 0.1-0.3 mg/dl | |
| Unconjugated (indirect) | 0.1-0.8 mg/dl | |
| Alkaline phosphatase | 30-85 ImU/ml | Alkaline phosphatase is found in many tissues with high concentrations in bone, liver, and biliary tract epithelium. Obstructive biliary tract disease and carcinoma may cause significant elevations. |
| **PANCREAS** | | |
| Amylase | 80-150 Somogyi units | Amylase is secreted normally by the acinar cells of the pancreas. Damage to these cells or obstruction of the pancreatic duct causes the enzyme to be absorbed into the blood in significant quantities. It is a sensitive yet nonspecific test for pancreatic disease. |
| Lipase | 0-110 units/L | Lipase is a pancreatic enzyme normally secreted into the duodenum. It appears in the blood when damage occurs to the acinar cells. It is a specific test for pancreatic disease. |
| Calcium | 9.0-11.5 mg/dl | Calcium levels may be low in cases of severe pancreatitis or steatorrhea, because calcium soaps are formed from the sequestration of calcium by fat necrosis. |
| **INTESTINE** | | |
| Total protein (albumin/globulin) | Total protein: 6-8 g/dl<br>Albumin: 3.2-4.5 g/dl<br>Globulin: 2.3-3.4 g/dl | Although primarily a reflection of liver function, serum protein level is also a measure of nutrition. Malnourished patients have greatly decreased levels of blood protein. |
| D-xylose absorption test | Blood levels of 25-40 mg/dl 2 hr after ingestion | D-xylose is a monosaccharide that is easily absorbed by the normal intestine but not metabolized by the body. It does not require biliary or pancreatic function. D-xylose is administered orally and assists in the diagnosis of malabsorption. |
| Lactose tolerance test | Rise in blood glucose level of >20 mg/dl | An oral dose of lactose is administered. In the absence of intestinal lactase, the lactose is neither broken down nor absorbed and plasma glucose levels do not rise. The test assists in the diagnosis of lactose intolerance. |
| Carcinoembryonic antigen (CEA) | <5 ng/ml | CEA is a protein normally present in fetal gut tissue. It is typically elevated in persons with colorectal tumors. Although not useful as a screening tool, it is useful in determining prognosis and response to therapy. |
| **URINE** | | |
| 5-hydroxyindoleacetic acid (5-HIAA) | 2-9 mg/2 hr | Carcinoid tumors are serotonin secreting and are derived from neuroectoderm tissue—e.g., the appendix and intestine. These neurohormones are metabolized to 5-HIAA by the liver and excreted in the urine. |
| Urine bilirubin | None | Bilirubin is not normally excreted in the urine. Biliary stricture, inflammation, or stones may cause its presence. |
| Urobilinogen | 24-hr collection: 0.2-1.2 units<br>24-hr collection: 0.05-2.5 mg | A sensitive test for hepatic or biliary disease. Decreased levels are seen in those with biliary obstruction and pancreatic cancer. |
| Urine amylase | 10-80 amylase units/hr | A rise in level usually mimics the rise in serum amylase. The level remains elevated for 7-10 days, however, which allows for retrospective diagnosis. |

**table 38-6** *Interpretation of Feces Color*

| Color | Interpretation |
|---|---|
| White | Barium |
| Gray, tan (clay) | Lack of bile, biliary obstruction |
| Red | Lower gastrointestinal bleeding, food intake (e.g., beets) |
| Black | |
| Tarry | Upper GI bleeding |
| Dry | Rapid peristalsis with bile present |
| Green | Rapid peristalsis with bile present |

NOTE: Stool color may also vary in response to food intake and artificial colors in foods.

Preparation for a barium enema involves thorough cleansing of the bowel by laxatives, enemas, or both. Thorough preparation is essential because retained fecal material obscures the normal bowel anatomy. The patient may be asked to restrict dairy products and follow a liquid diet for 24 hours before the test. The patient typically maintains NPO status for at least 8 hours before the test. Laxatives are administered after the test with some barium preparations to facilitate the removal of the barium. The stools may be white tinged for several days. Inpatients are closely monitored for complications after the test, such as perforation of the bowel. Outpatients are instructed to report the development of abdominal pain and to monitor carefully for constipation.

### Ultrasonography

Ultrasonography involves the use of high-frequency sound waves that are transmitted into the abdomen and create echoes that vary with tissue density. The echoes bounce back to a transducer and are electronically converted into pictorial images of the organs. This reveals organ size, shape, and position and is extremely useful in diagnosing cysts, tumors, and stones. Ultrasonography has gradually become the procedure of choice for diagnosing gallbladder disease because it does not expose the patient to radiation. The procedure is both painless and safe.

Patient preparation is straightforward. The patient maintains NPO status for 8 to 12 hours before the test, because gas in the bowel may interfere with the results. If the gallbladder is the focus of the test, the patient is instructed to eat a low-fat meal the evening before the test so that bile will accumulate in the gallbladder, thereby enhancing visualization. The patient resumes a normal diet and activity after the test.

### Computed Tomography

Computed tomography (CT) can also be used to assess patients with gallbladder, biliary ductal system, or pancreatic problems. It is helpful in identifying problems similar to those described for ultrasonography. Multiple x-rays are passed through the abdomen. A computer reconstructs the data into two-dimensional images on a television screen. Still photographs can also be taken of the images. Contrast medium can be used with the CT scan to better visualize the biliary tract or to accentuate differences in tissue density of the pancreas. The test is comparable to ultrasonography in effectiveness. It is used less often because of its significantly higher cost and moderate radiation exposure for the patient. It is extremely useful with obese individuals, however, because increased tissue density limits the effectiveness of ultrasound transmission.[12]

The patient should maintain NPO status for 8 to 12 hours before the test. If contrast medium is to be used, the patient should be assessed for allergies to iodine, seafood, or contrast medium. Barium studies, if necessary, should be done at least 4 days before CT scan or after the scan, because the barium can interfere with test results. There are no special aftercare considerations. The patient may resume pretest diet and activity.

### Radionuclide Imaging

Gastrointestinal scintigraphy may be used to localize the site of GI bleeding. Endoscopy provides excellent visualization of gastric or esophageal bleeding, but other areas of the GI tract are much more difficult to visualize and pinpoint. An intravenous injection of $^{99m}$Tc sulfur colloid is administered. Pooling of the radionuclide will occur at the bleeding site.[7] No pretest preparation is required, and no discomfort is experienced. Patients in unstable condition may not be candidates for this test if they are unable to travel safely to the nuclear medicine department for the 30 minutes required for the test.

### Cholecystography

Oral cholecystography involves the radiographical examination of the gallbladder after the administration of a contrast medium. A normal liver will remove radiopaque drugs—such as iodoalphionic acid (Priodax), iopanoic acid (Telepaque), and iodipamide methylglucamine (Cholografin Meglumine)—from the bloodstream and store and concentrate them in the gallbladder. The dye-filled gallbladder shows on x-ray examination as a dense shadow. If no shadow is seen, this indicates a nonfunctioning gallbladder. Stones, which are not radiopaque, show as dark patches on the film. Visualization of the gallbladder depends on absorption of the dye through the intestinal tract, isolation of the medium by the liver, and a free passageway from the liver to the gallbladder.

Ultrasonography has gradually replaced this once commonly used test in the diagnosis of gallbladder disease. Cholecystography is primarily used today when the ultrasound picture is inconclusive.

Patient preparation involves instruction to eat a fat-free meal the evening before the test and to avoid all additional intake except water until the test is completed. The patient is carefully assessed for allergies to contrast dyes, seafood, or iodine. The radiopaque substance (usually iopanoic acid) is administered orally 2 to 3 hours after the evening meal. The dose is based on body weight, and the tablets are administered one at a time at 5- to 10-minute intervals with several swallows of water after each pill. Side effects of the iodine-based tablets may include abdominal cramping, vomiting, or diarrhea. The patient then maintains NPO status until the test. A high-fat food or drink may be administered during the procedure to stimulate emptying of the gallbladder. No specific care is indicated after the test.

### Cholangiography

Cholangiography involves the x-ray examination of bile ducts to demonstrate the presence of stones, strictures, or tumors. The radiopaque substance may be administered intravenously or injected directly into the common bile duct with a needle or catheter at the time of surgery. After surgery on the common bile duct, a radiopaque drug such as iodipamide methylglucamine instilled through a drainage tube such as the T tube to determine the patency of the duct before the tube is removed (T tube cholangiography). This dye also may be injected through the skin and abdominal wall directly into a bile duct within the main substance of the liver (percutaneous transhepatic cholangiography). The technique is useful in visualizing the location and extent of a pathological process, such as obstructive jaundice. It permits decompression of the liver for improved function. The procedure helps the surgeon identify the location of pathological processes before surgery, or it may indicate that surgery is not necessary. Complications from the test are rare, but include bile leakage leading to bile peritonitis or bleeding caused by accidental rupture of a blood vessel.

The patient maintains NPO status for about 8 hours before the test. The injection of the contrast medium may cause temporary pain or a feeling of pressure or epigastric fullness. The patient is carefully monitored for bleeding or adverse reactions to the dye. Vital signs are monitored, and the patient typically rests in bed for about 6 hours after the test, lying on the right side as much as possible. The needle insertion site is carefully monitored for signs of bleeding or infection.

## SPECIAL TESTS

### Esophageal Function Tests

Several diagnostic tests may be used to evaluate the functioning of the esophagus and aid in the diagnosis of esophageal reflux or motility problems. These tests can be performed by having the patient swallow two or three tiny tubes that are attached to an external transducer. Once the tubes are located in the stomach, they are slowly pulled back into the distal esophagus at varying levels. Lower esophageal sphincter pressure, swallowing activity, pH, and effectiveness of clearance can all be measured in about 30 to 45 minutes. However, 24-hour pH monitoring may be performed because it is considered the gold standard for the accurate diagnosis of esophageal reflux.

No special preparation is required for these tests. It is important to provide the following instructions to the patient: (1) remain NPO for 8 hours before the procedure(s); (2) avoid alcohol and smoking the day before; and (3) medications such as antacids, $H_2$-receptor antagonists, cholinergics, and anticholinergics should not be taken before the test(s). Sedation is not required but may be used if the patient experiences persistent choking or gagging during the procedure. After removal of the tubes, a mild sore throat is common.

#### Manometry

This test is used to measure the pressure in the lower esophageal sphincter and record the duration and sequence of peristaltic movements within the esophagus. Readings are taken at various levels in the esophagus with the patient at rest and during swallowing. Baseline sphincter pressure is normally about 20 mm Hg. The test is used primarily to diagnose esophageal reflux, but the graphic record of muscular activity during swallowing may also help document the presence of achalasia or esophageal spasm.[12]

#### pH monitoring

This test evaluates the competency of the lower esophageal sphincter (LES) by obtaining a single measurement of the esophageal pH. An electrode is placed above the LES and attached to a manometry catheter. Normally, the esophagus maintains a pH of more than 6. Serial measurements may be obtained by maintaining the electrode for a 24-hour period. The probe must be inserted transnasally and connected to a recording box similar to a Holter monitor that is worn about the waist. The patient can then be monitored at home while eating a normal diet. Twenty-four–hour pH monitoring is the most sensitive and specific diagnostic test for the presence of abnormal acid reflux.

#### Esophageal clearance test

In conjunction with the previous two tests, esophageal clearance tests evaluate the function of both the upper and lower esophageal sphincters along with the body of the esophagus in response to swallowing foods or fluids. Normally, esophageal function allows for the complete clearance of acid material from the esophagus in less than 10 swallows. Readings are recorded from the catheter tip to determine the rate and efficiency of acid clearance.

#### Acid perfusion test (Bernstein test)

Confusion surrounding the origin of heartburn symptoms is often resolved with the Bernstein test, which attempts to reproduce the pain. Small quantities of HCl are instilled into the distal esophagus by nasogastric tube. The test is positive if the acid produces pain. Saline is instilled to rinse out the acid, and an antacid may be administered to relieve the pain.

### Tests of Gastric Function

#### Gastric analysis (basal gastric secretion and gastric acid stimulation tests)

Examination of the fasting contents of the stomach may be used in establishing a diagnosis of gastric disease. The purpose is to quantify gastric acidity in the fasting and stimulated states. Abnormal secretion may be related to ulcers, malignancy, pernicious anemia, or Zollinger-Ellison syndrome. A nasogastric tube is inserted, and gastric contents are aspirated. Gastric contents may then be aspirated every 15 minutes for 90 minutes.

The patient is instructed to restrict food, fluid, and smoking for 8 to 12 hours before the test. The flow of gastric acid is then stimulated by betazole hydrochloride, histamine phosphate, or pentagastrin given subcutaneously. The person may experience side effects of the medication, including flushing, feeling of warmth, slight headache, or itching. Epinephrine is given to counteract the effects of histamine if sensitivity occurs.

#### *Tubeless gastric analysis (Diagnex blue test)*

Tubeless gastric analysis may be used for detection of gastric achlorhydria. The test will indicate the presence or absence of free hydrochloric acid but cannot be used to determine the *amount* of free hydrochloric acid, if any is present. For a tubeless gastric analysis, a gastric stimulant such as caffeine is given. One hour later, a cation exchange resin containing azure A is given orally with water on an empty stomach. If there is free hydrochloric acid in the stomach on the introduction of this resin, a substance will be released in the stomach that will be absorbed from the small intestine and excreted by the kidneys within 2 hours. Absence of detectable amounts of blue dye in the urine indicates that free hydrochloric acid probably was not secreted.

#### *Schilling test*

The Schilling test evaluates vitamin $B_{12}$ absorption. In the normal GI tract, vitamin $B_{12}$ combines with the intrinsic factor that is produced by the parietal cells in the gastric mucosa and is absorbed in the distal portion of the ileum. Pernicious anemia will develop if intrinsic factor is lacking or malabsorption exists. This is relevant in patients who have had the terminal ileum removed for diseases such as Crohn's disease. The test can identify problems of absorption.

The patient is administered an oral preparation of radioactive vitamin $B_{12}$, followed by an intramuscular injection of nonradioactive vitamin $B_{12}$ to saturate the tissue-binding sites. Urinary $B_{12}$ levels are measured after urine collection for 24 to 48 hours. With normal absorption of vitamin $B_{12}$, the ileum absorbs more vitamin $B_{12}$ than the body needs and excretes the excess into the urine. With impaired absorption of vitamin $B_{12}$, little or no vitamin $B_{12}$ is excreted into the urine. Intrinsic factor preparations may also be administered to differentiate intestinal problems from pernicious anemia.

The person is instructed to maintain NPO status for 8 to 12 hours before the test, except for water. Laxatives should not be used during the duration of the test, but no specific aftercare is indicated.

#### *Urea breath test*

Testing for *H. pylori* is technically difficult and expensive. The urea breath test (UBT) is based on the principle that the *H. pylori* organism is able to produce large amounts of urease, a surface enzyme that catalyzes the urea in gastric secretions into bicarbonate and ammonia. Patients are administered an oral solution of carbon isotope–labeled urea in water. If *H. pylori* is present in the stomach the urea is metabolized. The labeled bicarbonate is excreted in the form of labeled carbon dioxide, which can be collected and measured. The patient exhales into a balloon or other receptacle, and the carbon dioxide is measured with a scintillation counter. The sample can be collected 20 minutes after the solution is ingested. The test has minimal risks associated with radioactivity and is estimated to be 97% sensitive for *H. pylori* and 100% specific. Teaching is the essential component of patient preparation. No specific aftercare is needed.

### Biopsy

#### *Upper gastrointestinal biopsy*

A biopsy of the oral cavity or tongue may be done on any lesion or ulcerated area that requires a differential diagnosis. This procedure is usually performed with a local anesthetic. After the biopsy, the biopsy site is assessed for bleeding. Biopsy of the stomach is typically performed during fiberoptic endoscopy.

#### *Intestinal biopsy*

Biopsy of the small or large bowel may also be performed during the course of endoscopic examination to allow tissue analysis of lesions, polyps, or masses. A knife blade or snare is typically used to obtain the tissue sample. The procedure is not usually painful, although a feeling of pressure may be experienced. Bleeding from the site of the biopsy is uncommon. If bleeding does occur, the patient is instructed to report this to the physician and to curtail physical activity until examined by a physician.

### Endoscopy

Endoscopy allows for direct visualization of portions of the GI tract by means of a long, flexible, fiberoptic scope (Figure 38-10). Images are provided through an eyepiece or onto a video screen. The remote control tip moves in four directions. Endoscopy may be used for direct inspection, biopsy, and removal of polyps and stones.[14] Additionally, bleeding may be controlled through laser or photocoagulation or the injection of sclerosing agents. The upper GI tract may be visualized as far as the duodenum by insertion of a fiberscope through the mouth. A fiberscope inserted through the rectum

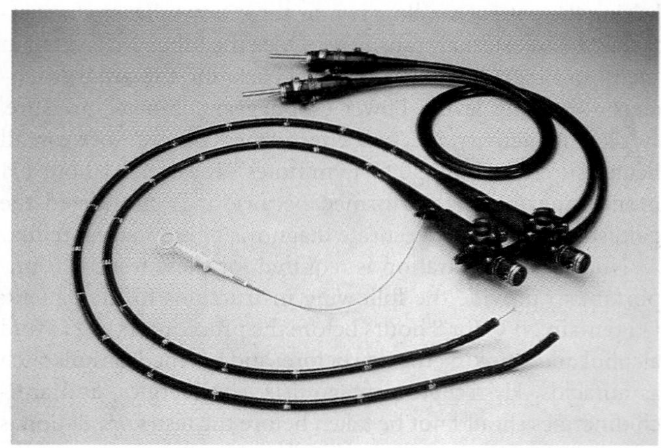

**fig. 38-10** Flexible colon fiberscopes.

is used for visualization of the rectum (proctoscopy), sigmoid colon (sigmoidoscopy), or the entire colon (colocoscopy).

Today, most endoscopic procedures are performed on an ambulatory basis, even with the elderly. Oral fiberscope insertion is uncomfortable and may precipitate gagging or choking despite the use of topical anesthetic sprays or gargles. Premedication with an IV sedative such as midazolam (Versed) or diazepam (Valium) or an analgesic such as meperidine (Demerol) is used. Thus the patient is conscious but sedated; amnesia is often experienced when high doses of these drugs are used.

### Esophagogastroduodenoscopy

Upper GI endoscopy may be limited to the esophagus (esophagoscopy), stomach (gastroscopy), or duodenum (duodenoscopy), or it may involve examination of the entire region (esophagogastroduodenoscopy [EGD]) (Figure 38-11). It is particularly useful for identifying the source of upper GI bleeding and for differentiating gastric malignancies from benign ulcers, and gastric ulcers from duodenal ulcers. Other uses include visualization of esophageal strictures, varices, tumors, achalasia, and hiatal hernias; and surgical removal of gastric polyps.

Preparation for an EGD involves instructing the patient to maintain NPO status for 8 hours before the test. Because air is typically introduced as the endoscope is advanced to improve visibility, the patient should be told that a feeling of pressure or fullness will likely be experienced. The entire test lasts about 15 to 30 minutes, unless additional treatments are planned.

After the procedure the patient is monitored carefully for signs of dyspnea, pain, bleeding, or acute dysphagia. Vital signs are taken every 30 minutes for 3 to 4 hours, and no oral food or fluids are administered until the nurse determines that the gag reflex is fully intact. Throat lozenges or saline gargles may be used to relieve sore throat after the test. Complications are rare but include aspiration, perforation, and bleeding.

### Endoscopic retrograde cholangiopancreatography

Endoscopic retrograde cholangiopancreatography (ERCP) also involves the oral insertion of an endoscope, but this device has a side-viewing tip and a cannula that can be maneuvered into the ampulla of Vater (Figure 38-12). Dye may be injected to outline the pancreatic and biliary ducts. The procedure may be combined with papillotomy to enlarge the sphincter and release gallstones.[18] Glucagon may be administered to minimize spasm in the duodenum and sphincter.

Care after the procedure is similar to that previously described following an EGD. The patient is monitored carefully for signs of abdominal pain, nausea, and vomiting, which might indicate the development of pancreatitis.

### Colonoscopy

Fiberoptic colonoscopy allows the examination of the entire colon in most patients. It may be used to evaluate benign and malignant growths, remove polyps, take biopsy specimens, and localize sites of bleeding. The colonoscope is 105 to 185 cm (42 to 72 inches) long.

Thorough bowel preparation is essential before the test, which is especially difficult for the elderly. The patient may

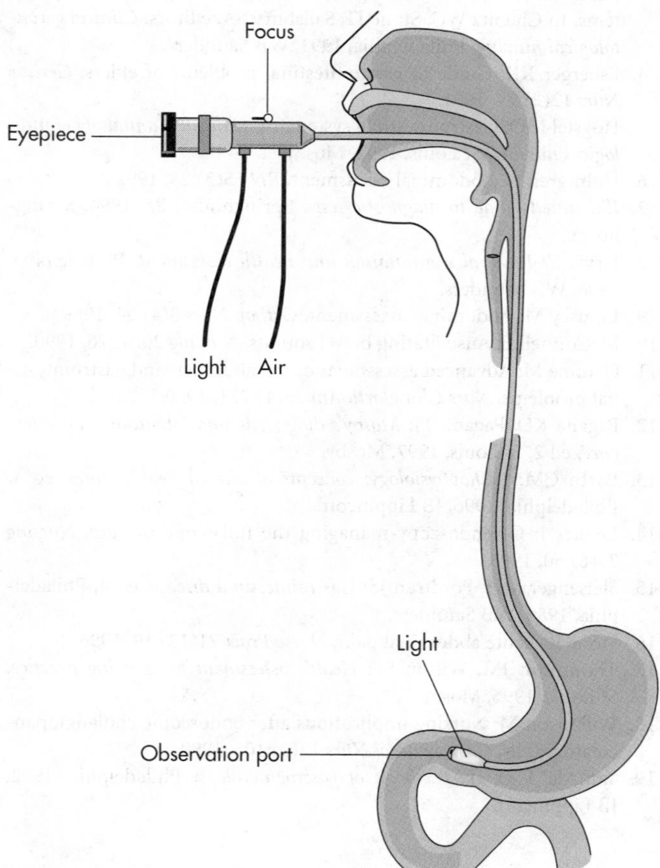


**fig. 38-11** Fiberoptic endoscopy of the stomach.

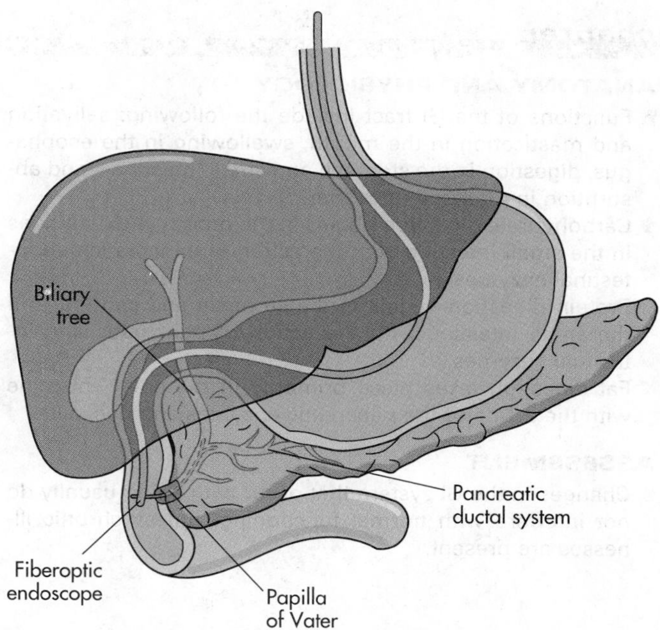


**fig. 38-12** Endoscopic retrograde cholangiopancreatography (ERCP).

receive a 2- to 3-day preparation involving a clear liquid diet, strong laxatives, and an enema the day of the test. A 1-day preparation with an oral osmotic solution has become standard because it reduces overall electrolyte loss. A gallon of polyethylene glycol (Colyte) solution is administered rapidly (8 ounces every 15 minutes) and induces a profuse watery diarrhea within 30 to 60 minutes, which lasts about 4 hours.[12] The patient is then NPO for about 8 hours before the test.

The procedure lasts for 20 to 60 minutes. Air is introduced as the colonoscope is inserted to increase visualization of the mucosa. The air commonly causes abdominal cramping.

Afterward, the nurse assumes responsibility for carefully monitoring the patient and ensuring full recovery from sedation. Any changes in vital signs or development of severe abdominal pain, rectal bleeding, or fever should be immediately reported to the physician. Additionally, arrangements for transportation home are important because the patient should not drive.

Sigmoidoscopy may be performed rather than colonoscopy. This procedure allows for visualization of the anus, rectum, and distal sigmoid colon. Approximately 75% of all polyps and tumors of the large intestine can be visualized with a flexible sigmoidoscope. Pretest preparation instructions vary widely. The patient may be instructed to prepare with a 2-day clear liquid diet and pretest fasting. Fleet enemas may be ordered, or a cleansing enema may be preferred. The knee-chest position and a strong urge to defecate that is produced by the larger-diameter sigmoidoscope make this both an uncomfortable and unpopular procedure for patients. Sedation is not usually employed.[7] Aftercare involves monitoring for distention, increased tenderness, and bleeding. The patient may initially pass large amounts of flatus from the instillation of air during the procedure. Slight rectal bleeding may occur if biopsies have been taken.

## chapter SUMMARY

### ANATOMY AND PHYSIOLOGY

- Functions of the GI tract include the following: salivation and mastication in the mouth, swallowing in the esophagus, digestion in the stomach and small intestines, and absorption in the large intestine.
- Carbohydrate digestion begins in the mouth and continues in the small intestine with the action of pancreatic and intestinal enzymes.
- Protein digestion begins in the stomach and continues in the small intestine with the action of pancreatic and intestinal enzymes.
- Fat digestion takes place primarily in the small intestine with the action of the pancreatic enzymes and bile salts.

### ASSESSMENT

- Changes in the GI system that occur with aging usually do not interfere with normal functioning, unless chronic illnesses are present.
- Subjective data for GI assessment include patient/family history; diet and nutrition; presence of abdominal pain, anorexia, or vomiting; fatigue and weakness; and elimination patterns.
- Objective data include assessment of the mouth, abdomen, and rectum.
- The abdomen is divided into either four quadrants or nine regions for assessment. Auscultation precedes percussion and palpation, because the assessment activities may alter the frequency and intensity of bowel sounds.

### DIAGNOSTIC TESTS

- Laboratory tests include analysis of stool and urine and a variety of blood tests.
- Major radiological tests include barium contrast studies of the entire GI tract, endoscopic examinations of the upper and lower GI tract, ultrasonography, and cholecystography.
- Endoscopy and ultrasonography are the mainstays of diagnosis in GI system disease.

## References


1. Altman DE: Changes in gastrointestinal, pancreatic, biliary and hepatic function with aging, *Gastroenterol Clin North Am* 19(2):227, 1990.
2. Barker LR, Burton JR, Zieve PD: *Principles of ambulatory medicine,* Baltimore, 1995, Williams & Wilkins.
3. Bell JE, Dixon L, Sehy YA: Physical assessment: the breast and the pulmonary, cardiovascular, gastrointestinal, and genitourinary systems. In Chenitz WC, Stone JT, Salisbury SA, editors: *Clinical gerontological nursing,* Philadelphia, 1991, WB Saunders.
4. Esberger KK: Guide to gastrointestinal problems of elders, *Geriatr Nurs* 12(2):74, 1991.
5. Hogstel MO: Gastrointestinal system. In *Clinical manual of gerontological nursing,* St Louis, 1992, Mosby.
6. Holmgren C: Abdominal assessment, *RN* 55(3):28, 1992.
7. *Illustrated guide to diagnostic tests,* Springhouse, Pa, 1994, Springhouse.
8. Jarvis C: *Physical examination and health assessment,* Philadelphia, 1996, WB Saunders.
9. Lindsey M: Abdominal assessment, *Orthop Nurs* 8(4):34, 1989.
10. McConnell E: Auscultating bowel sounds, *Nursing* 20(6):76, 1990.
11. O'Toole M: Advanced assessment of the abdomen and gastrointestinal problems, *Nurs Clin North Am* 25(4):771, 1990.
12. Pagana KD, Pagana TJ: *Mosby's diagnostic and laboratory test reference,* ed 2, St Louis, 1997, Mosby.
13. Porth CM: *Pathophysiology: concepts of altered health states,* ed 4, Philadelphia, 1996, JB Lippincott.
14. Renkes J: GI endoscopy-managing the full scope of care, *Nursing* 23(6):50, 1993.
15. Sleisenger MH, Fordtran JS: *Gastrointestinal disease,* ed 4, Philadelphia, 1989, WB Saunders.
16. Stone R: Acute abdominal pain, *Nurse Pract* 21(12):19, 1996.
17. Thompson JM, Wilson SF: *Health assessment for nursing practice,* St Louis, 1996, Mosby.
18. Wilkinson M: Nursing implications after endoscopic cholangiopancreatography, *Gastroenterol Nurs* 13(2):105, 1990.
19. Yamada T et al: *Textbook of gastroenterology,* Philadelphia, 1992, JB Lippincott.

# chapter 39 MANAGEMENT OF PERSONS WITH Problems of the Mouth and Esophagus

JUDITH K. SANDS

## objectives *After studying this chapter, the learner should be able to:*

1. Describe lifestyle modifications for the prevention of common oral and esophageal disorders.
2. Discuss the pathophysiology underlying common problems of the mouth and esophagus.
3. List the major clinical manifestations of common oral and esophageal disorders.
4. Discuss the collaborative care management of common problems of the mouth and esophagus.
5. Use the nursing process to describe nursing care of patients with major esophageal disorders.

Problems involving the mouth and esophagus include a number of common disorders that affect millions of individuals throughout the adult life span. The majority of the disorders are managed by the individual in the home and rarely involve admission to the acute care setting. The nurse's role includes patient and family education directed toward prevention and health promotion, as well as self-care management.

## PROBLEMS OF THE MOUTH

### TOOTH AND GUM DISEASE

Progressive tooth loss used to be considered a virtually inevitable consequence of aging. Advances in our understanding of dental health and new approaches to tooth maintenance have changed these perspectives substantially, and today major efforts are expended toward preserving natural teeth.

#### Etiology/Epidemiology

Tooth decay is by far the most common problem affecting the teeth. It is the result of a pathological process that causes the gradual destruction of the enamel and dentin of the teeth. Plaque formation is clearly the most important aspect of tooth decay, but familial tendency, poor oral hygiene, and poor health are also factors. A diet high in simple or refined sugars may also play a role.

The periodontium is the tissue that surrounds and supports the teeth. Disease affecting this structure is the most common cause of tooth loss in adults after age 50. At any time, an estimated 25% to 75% of the adult population with natural teeth has some evidence of the disease.[6] Bacterial plaque is again the most important contributor to the problem, but dental malocclusion, caries, dietary deficiencies, and systemic diseases such as diabetes may also play a role.

#### Pathophysiology

Plaque formation is the most important aspect of the decay process. Dental plaque is a soft mass composed of proliferating bacteria in a matrix of polysaccharides and salivary glycoproteins. It adheres to the teeth and is both transparent and colorless. Acids produced by the bacteria slowly decalcify the inorganic tooth enamel. Food, particularly carbohydrates, stimulates bacterial acid production. Simple sugars have the greatest effect. The plaque begins to collect on the teeth within 2 hours of eating, and the longer or more frequently carbohydrates are ingested, the longer it takes for the pH of the mouth to return to normal. Cavity formation is the visible clinical evidence of the progression of the decay process.

Gingivitis, the earliest form of periodontal disease, is characterized by color alterations in the gums, swelling, and easy bleeding. Inflammation causes the gingivae to separate from the tooth surface. Pockets form in the gingivae that can collect bacteria, food particles, and pus. As the process gradually worsens over time, the gums recede, the alveolar bone is resorbed, and the teeth loosen (Figure 39-1). Bleeding of the gums with normal toothbrushing is a common early sign. There is usually no pain.

#### Collaborative Care Management

Prevention is the most appropriate management strategy for both dental decay and periodontal disease. Most strategies should be instituted in childhood and continued throughout life. The *Healthy People 2000* goals related to oral health are summarized in Box 39-1.

Widespread fluoridation of water supplies has had significant positive effects in decreasing the incidence of tooth decay. Fluoride makes tooth enamel more resistant to acids and is commonly added to drinking water in many localities. It is widely available in toothpastes, dental rinses, and mouthwashes. Fluoride may also be applied in concentrated forms by a dentist. Sealants and bonding preparations may be applied in childhood to increase tooth resistance to decay.

Treatment of periodontal disease routinely includes the removal of decayed tooth structures and their replacement with restorative barriers. The presence of progressive gingivitis may require aggressive measures such as scaling or root planing to

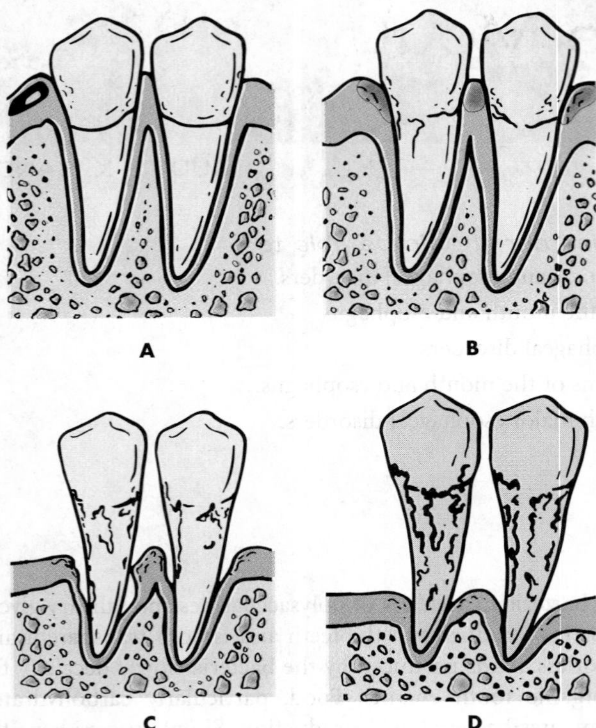


**fig. 39-1** The progression of periodontal disease. **A,** Calculus deposited on teeth at gum line. **B,** Gingivae become swollen and tender. **C,** Inflammation spreads, pockets develop between gums and gingivae, and gums recede. **D,** Alveolar bone is destroyed and teeth loosen.

control or correct the problem. If control is not possible the individual may face the need for tooth extraction and the fitting of dentures.

### *Patient/family education*

Good oral hygiene with frequent regular brushing and flossing is the mainstay of prevention for tooth and gum disease, and health care providers take every opportunity to reinforce this principle and instruct individuals in correct techniques. Regular checkups and professional cleaning aid in careful monitoring and early intervention. Restricting the amount of simple sugars in the diet is a standard recommendation, and adequate or supplemental vitamin C is believed to reduce plaque.

**box 39-1** Healthy People 2000 *Objectives Related to Oral Health*

1. Increase to at least 45% the proportion of people ages 35 through 44 who have never lost a permanent tooth because of dental caries or periodontal diseases.
2. Reduce to no more than 20% the proportion of people ages 65 and older who have lost all of their natural teeth.
3. Reduce the prevalence of gingivitis among people ages 35 through 44 to no more than 30%.
4. Reduce destructive periodontal diseases to a prevalence of no more than 15% among people ages 35 through 44.
5. Reduce deaths related to cancer of the oral cavity and pharynx to no more than 10.5 per 100,000 men ages 45 through 74 and 4.1 per 100,000 women ages 45 through 74.
6. Increase to at least 75% the proportion of people served by community water systems providing optimal levels of fluoride.
7. Increase use of professionally administered or self-administered topical or systemic (dietary) fluorides to at least 85% of people not receiving optimally fluoridated public water.
8. Extend to all long-term institutional facilities the requirement that oral examinations and services be provided no later than 90 days after entry into these facilities.
9. Increase to at least 70% the proportion of people ages 35 and older using the oral health care system during each year.
10. Extend requirement of the use of effective head, face, eye, and mouth protection to all organizations, agencies, and institutions sponsoring sporting and recreation events that pose risks of injury.
11. Reduce smokeless tobacco use by males aged 12-24 to a prevalence of no more than 4%.

From *Healthy People 2000: midcourse review and 1995 revisions,* US Department of Health and Human Services, Public Health Service, Washington, DC, 1996.

## MOUTH INFECTIONS

Any of the structures of the mouth may develop infections. The presence of infection can seriously affect the ability of the patient to adequately and comfortably ingest food and fluids by mouth.

### Etiology/Epidemiology

A wide variety of oral infections can develop, and minor oral ulcerations are a common problem. They may be primary disorders triggered by various bacteria and viruses, or they may occur secondary to vitamin deficiencies, other systemic diseases or treatments, or in response to local trauma or stress. Common examples include the following:

*Aphthous stomatitis (canker sore)* produces well-circumscribed ulcers on the soft tissues of the mouth, including the lips, tongue, insides of the cheeks, pharynx, and soft palate. The lesions are acutely painful but noncontagious and are of uncertain, although perhaps autoimmune, origin. Aphthous ulcers are a chronic problem in as much as 17% of the population and usually first appear in the teenage years.[9] Healing is usually achieved in 1 to 3 weeks.

*Herpes simplex* is an extremely common viral infection that produces characteristic blisters commonly called *cold sores* or *fever blisters.* The individual usually acquires the virus in early childhood. As many as 80% of the adult population may have been infected. The virus is harbored in a dormant state by cells in the sensory nerve ganglia. Reactivation of the virus can occur with emotional stress, fever, or exposure to cold or ultraviolet light. The lesions appear most commonly on the mucocu-

**table 39-1** *Mouth Infections*

| INFECTION | CLINICAL MANIFESTATIONS | COLLABORATIVE MANAGEMENT |
|---|---|---|
| Aphthous stomatitis (canker sore) | Painful, small ulceration on oral mucosa; heals in 1 to 3 weeks | Palliative: mouthwashes, hydrocortisone-antibiotic ointment; fluocinonide (Lidex) ointment in Orabase |
| Herpes simplex stomatitis (cold sore, fever blister) | Painful vesicles and ulcerations of mouth, lips, or edge of nose; may have prodromal itching or burning; fever, malaise, lymphadenopathy may occur | Palliative: mouthwashes, fluids, soft diet, topical or systemic acyclovir (Zovirax) in severe cases |
| Acute necrotizing ulcerative gingivitis (trench mouth) | Painful hemorrhagic gums with ulceration, foul mouth odor, fever, lymphadenopathy | Oral antibiotics, analgesics, topical hydrogen peroxide, good oral hygiene, referral to dentist for removal of plaque or tartar |
| Candidiasis (thrush) | Creamy white, curdlike patches closely adherent to mucosa; mucosa bleeds and ulcerates when patches scraped off; condition is painful | Oral nystatin, ketoconazole, clotrimazole; amphotericin B for the immunocompromised person |
| Parotitis | Fever, swelling, and pain in the glands with an abrupt onset | Local heat and cold, frequent oral hygiene, adequate hydration; broad-spectrum antibiotics occasionally needed<br>Salivary secretion is stimulated with lozenges, hard candies, and lemon slices |

taneous border junction of the lips in the formof small vesicles, which then erupt and form painful, shallow ulcers.

*Acute necrotizing ulcerative gingivitis (ANUG),* also called *trench mouth,* is an acute inflammatory gum disease caused by a tremendous proliferation of normal mouth flora, such as spirochetes and fusiform bacilli. It is commonly triggered by poor oral hygiene, nutritional deficiencies, alcoholism, infection, or immunocompromise. Individuals develop ulcerative lesions that are covered by a grayish pseudomembrane and surrounded by erythematous areas. It is not infectious.

*Candidiasis (thrush)* is caused by an increase in the level of *Candida albicans,* a yeastlike fungus normally found in the skin, gastrointestinal (GI) tract, vagina, and oral cavity. Overgrowth of the organism may result from antibiotic depletion of normal flora or immunosuppression from steroid therapy, chemotherapy, or human immunodeficiency virus (HIV) infection. The condition is painful and, if widespread, can interfere with oral nutrition.

*Parotitis* is an inflammation of the salivary or parotid glands. The viral inflammation known as mumps occurs primarily in the pediatric population, although it can occur in adults. Acute bacterial parotitis typically occurs in debilitated or elderly patients in whom dehydration, minimal oral intake, or medications have resulted in chronic dry mouth.

Poor oral hygiene may also play a role in parotitis. The acute form of the inflammation can also occur in postoperative patients as surgical mumps. As the natural secretions diminish, bacteria invade the gland. The causative organism is often *Staphylococcus,* and the infection may be serious. Sudden onset of pain and acute swelling typically occur, and the infection can become chronic and recurrent.

### Pathophysiology

The structure of the mouth causes many ulcerative diseases to have similar signs and symptoms. The mucosa throughout the mouth is thin, and evolving vesicles and bullae break open rapidly into ulcers. The ulcers are typically further traumatized by the teeth and can become readily infected by the abundant oral flora. Many of the causative organisms are the same as those that cause common skin infections. Clinical manifestations of common disorders are summarized in Table 39-1.

### Collaborative Care Management

Most oral infections are self-limiting and will heal spontaneously without the need for direct intervention. Supportive or palliative care with oral hygiene, mouthwashes, diet modification, and ointments is provided as outlined in Table 39-1. A variety of antibiotic and antiviral products may be used in selected situations. Oral hygiene is an essential part of the treatment of mouth infections and includes brushing and flossing, rinsing with mouthwashes, and modifying the diet to reduce irritation.

#### *Patient/family education*

Teaching is directed at self-care management because virtually all infections will be treated at home. The proper use of antibiotics, rinses, and ointments is discussed, as well as the importance of maintaining regular oral hygiene despite discomfort. Herpes virus lesions are contagious when present, and the importance of good hand washing is stressed. The patient is also provided with specific information about symptoms that would indicate complications requiring medical intervention.

## CANCER OF THE MOUTH

### Etiology

Cancer may develop on the lips, tongue, palate, floor of the mouth, or other portion of the oral cavity. The development of oral cancer is clearly linked to a history of smoking and alcohol consumption, and the risk increases strongly with heavy

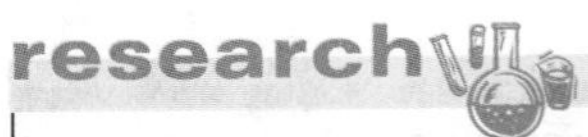

Reference: Vigneswaran N et al: Tobacco use and cancer: a reappraisal, *Oral Surg Oral Med Oral Pathol* 80(2):178, 1995.

This study reanalyzed the data concerning the use of smokeless tobacco and the risk of oral cancer. Smoking and alcohol use have been identified as the primary causes of oral cancer, and the risks have been assumed to transfer to the use of smokeless tobacco. This theory is supported by the frequent development of smoker's leukoplakia in smokeless tobacco users. These lesions have been assumed to be premalignant. Keratoses were found to be present in 60% of all smokeless tobacco users, but less than 3% of cases exhibited any degree of dysplasia versus more than 20% for comparable lesions in smokers. Malignancy occurred in approximately 1% of smokeless tobacco users in 5 years. The authors conclude that there may be other health issues of concern in the use of smokeless tobacco, but the risk of oral cancer is extremely low, particularly in comparison with the risk in smokers.

**box 39-2** *clinical manifestations*

***Oral Cancer***

Masses in the mouth or neck
Chronic ear pain
Enlarged lymph nodes (cervical nodes are commonly affected)
Discomfort or burning
Ulcer on lateral or ventral surface of the tongue or elsewhere
Dysphagia
Visible lesion on lips or elsewhere
Presence of erythroplakia (bright red velvety lesions)

NOTE: Many oral cancers are asymptomatic in the early stage.

use. Differentiating the unique effects of these two factors is difficult, but epidemiological studies seem to indicate that alcohol intake is the most significant factor.[8] The use of snuff or chewing tobacco rapidly produces characteristic lesions on the mucosa, which have been widely believed to be premalignant in nature. Research to date, however, has not been able to consistently demonstrate a causative link (see the Research Box). Additives and other compounds in the products may play a more significant role than the tobacco.

The combination of alcohol and smoking is theorized to cause a breakdown in the body's defense mechanisms, as evidenced by a decrease in the levels of immunoglobulin A (IgA). The role of viruses, particularly the herpes viruses, is also being thoroughly researched.

## Epidemiology

Oral cancers account for approximately 4% of cancers in men, 2% of cancers in women, and 3.5% of cancers overall. More than 90% of these cancers occur in persons over 45 years of age, and the incidence increases with age.

The incidence of oral cancer shows a significant variation worldwide with clear linkages to patterns of long-term alcohol and tobacco use. Disease development is most clearly linked to increasing age and the duration of exposure to significant risk factors.

## Pathophysiology

The vast majority of oral cancers arise from the squamous cells, which line the surface oral epithelium; epidermoid, basal cell, and other carcinomas also may arise. The majority of tumors arise on the lateral or ventral surfaces of the tongue, although rarely on the dorsal surface, and they commonly go unnoticed by the patient. A single ulcer is the typical pattern.

The tongue has an abundant vascular supply and lymphatic drainage channels, and spread of the cancer to adjacent structures may be rapid. Metastasis to the neck has already occurred in 60% of patients at the time the diagnosis is made. The mortality rate is high. The cure rate for cancer involving the lips, on the other hand, is high, because the lesion is so readily apparent. Early metastasis is rare, although rapid extension to the mandible or floor of the mouth is possible. Tumors that involve the parotid gland are usually benign, although those arising in the submaxillary glands have a high rate of malignancy and tend to grow rapidly.

Malignant lesions of the mouth may be asymptomatic and are usually difficult to detect in their early stages. Possible clinical manifestations are summarized in Box 39-2.

### Premalignant lesions

A large number of varied conditions and disorders can result in red and white mouth lesions. The vast majority are asymptomatic, and the primary issue is related to their degree of cancer-causing potential. Much research has been conducted, but only broad generalizations can be drawn at this time.

The term *leukoplakia* refers to white lesions that usually occur on the cheeks, lips, gingivae, and palate and cannot be characterized clinically or histologically as any other disease. They may take varied forms but are commonly associated with smoking and *Candida* infection. They are more common in males and individuals over 60 years of age. One classic variety, stomatitis nicotina (also called *smokers' patch*), is clearly linked to heavy smoking, with pipe smoking the most common form. These grayish-white lesions appear on the palate and are theorized to be related to the high heat exposure through the smoke. Although suggestive in appearance, the lesions disappear completely if the person stops smoking, and they are not generally related to an increased cancer risk unless found on the floor of the mouth. *Snuff dippers' lesion* is another classic form, and similar lesions commonly develop in response to friction trauma from ill-fitting dentures or from chronic cheek and lip biting. The lesions of erythroplakia are similar in many respects but are bright red and velvety in appearance. They need to be clearly differentiated from inflammatory lesions, are usually asymptomatic, and appear to be associated with a sig-

**guidelines for care**

**The Person with Radioactive Needle Implants in Oral Tissue**

**Implant Care**

1. Do not pull on the strings. Any movement could alter the placement or direction of the radiation or cause the needles to loosen.
2. Check needle patency several times each day.
3. Monitor linens, bed areas, and emesis basin for needles that may dislodge.
4. Ensure that a protective container is present in the room to contain any needles that might dislodge.

**Patient Care**

1. Assist with gentle oral hygiene q2h while awake.
2. Encourage the patient to avoid hot and cold foods and beverages, as well as smoking.
3. If the patient has dentures, encourage their removal at night for comfort. Assess gums for irritation and bleeding whenever dentures are removed.
4. Provide viscous lidocaine (Xylocaine) solutions or lozenges as needed when oral discomfort interferes with nutrition.
5. Provide the patient with an alternate means of communication; talking around implanted needles is usually difficult or impossible.
6. Assist the patient to implement the mouth care regimen prescribed by the physician.

nificantly higher risk of malignant transformation. The decision about which lesions to biopsy is a clinical judgment made on the basis of location, duration, risk factors, age of the patient, and presence of symptoms. Treatment decisions are generally made based on the biopsy results.

## Collaborative Care Management

### Diagnostic tests

Biopsy is the primary diagnostic test used in cases of suspected oral cancer. It may be used to evaluate lymph nodes, leukoplakia or erythroplakia lesions, ulcers, or neck masses that do not resolve spontaneously within 1 to 2 weeks. Ultrasonography is an excellent adjunct to evaluate masses that are close to the surface. Computed tomography (CT) scans may be used to evaluate deeper, less defined masses, and magnetic resonance imaging (MRI) is most useful in the effort to evaluate deep masses of inconclusive structure.

### Medications

Pharmacotherapy does not play a role in the treatment of oral cancer except to increase patient comfort and correct any concurrent or underlying infection.

### Treatments

Treatment of oral cancer depends on the location and staging of the tumor. Early-stage cancer is usually treated by either radiation or surgery, depending on the size and accessibility of the tumor. More invasive cancers may require both modalities, and advanced oral cancers are treated palliatively.

Early lesions are highly curable with radiation if they are confined to the mucosa, and the use of radiation prevents widespread tissue destruction. Radiation may be delivered by external beam or through the insertion of needles or seeds. If both radiation and surgery are planned, the radiation therapy is usually administered *after* the surgery, because irradiated tissue is more susceptible to infection and breakdown. The method and effects of the radiotherapy need to be fully explained to the patient before the start of treatment. Care of the patient with implanted radioactive needles in oral tissue is summarized in the Guidelines for Care Box. For a more complete discussion of radiotherapy and associated nursing care, see Chapter 11.

Secondary effects of radiation therapy to the mouth and neck include mucositis, xerostomia (dryness in mouth), and dental decay. The xerostomia begins 1 to 2 weeks after treatment is started and may persist throughout life. The dryness creates chronic discomfort and may cause a persistent unpleasant mouth odor. Alterations in taste and smell are also commonly reported.

Dental decay, especially at the gingival margins, results from decreased salivary secretion and altered pH of the saliva. Interventions to minimize tooth decay are initiated before the start of radiation therapy and include a conscientious tooth-care regimen using fluoride toothpaste, a soft toothbrush, and dental floss. Fluoride treatments may also be given.

### Surgical management

The treatment objective for oral cancer is cure, and adequate first-time treatment is the key. Several surgical options exist. Confined local excision is possible in some situations, but many of the procedures are radical in nature and involve extensive resection. Examples include partial mandibulectomy, partial (hemiglossectomy) or total (glossectomy) removal of the tongue, and resections of the floor of the mouth or buccal mucosa. Because oral cancers commonly metastasize early to the cervical lymph nodes, the surgical procedure usually also includes functional or radical neck dissection, with removal of the regional and deep cervical lymph nodes and their channels. In a functional dissection the lymph nodes and channels are removed but the other structures are preserved. In advanced cases the surgery may also include removal of the sternocleidomastoid muscle or other neck muscles, internal jugular vein, thyroid gland, submaxillary gland, and spinal accessory nerve (Figure 39-2).

The need to ensure sufficient excision can create significant aesthetic and functional problems for the patient, including speech, chewing and swallowing, and airway management. Reconstructive technology continues to improve, and the patient may be scheduled for reconstructive surgery at some future point.

### Diet

No specific diet modifications are associated with the treatment of oral cancer. The treatment approach selected, however, may necessitate modifications in food selection and feeding methods to maintain adequate nutrition. As previously

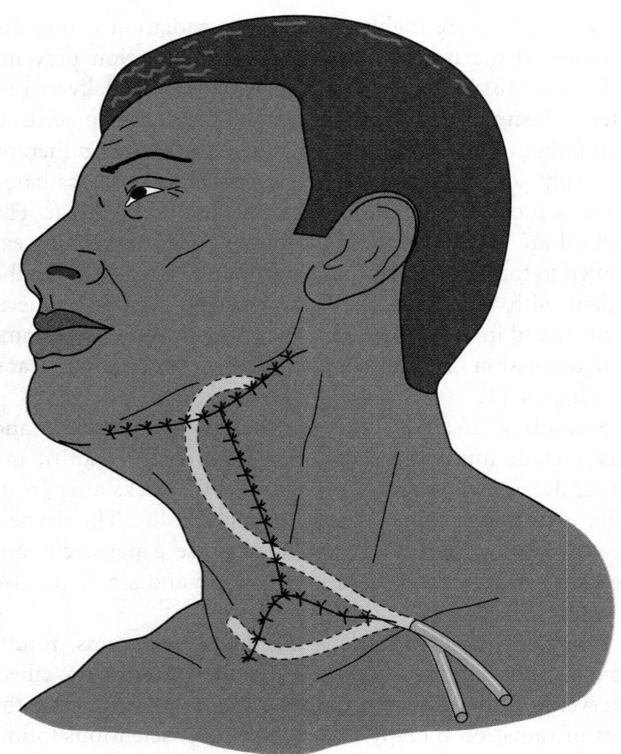

**fig. 39-2** Radical neck incision with drainage tubing in place.

discussed, high-dose radiation therapy commonly causes stomatitis or xerostomia, as well as changes in taste, which may be long term. Extensive oral surgery may radically alter the patient's ability to ingest, chew, or swallow food and fluid. Specific strategies are discussed under Promoting Nutrition on p. 1259.

#### *Activity*

Patients with oral cancer are encouraged to remain as active as possible. The only restrictions will be the fatigue associated with radiotherapy and surgery and the patient's willingness to resume daily activities.

#### *Referrals*

Common referrals for persons with oral cancer include speech and occupational therapy. Most forms of treatment at least temporarily interfere with the patient's oral communication. The dietitian and occupational therapist may also be involved in devising strategies to improve oral nutrition and assisting the patient to relearn chewing and swallowing after treatment.

## NURSING MANAGEMENT OF THE PATIENT UNDERGOING SURGERY FOR ORAL CANCER

### ■ PREOPERATIVE CARE

The mouth is thoroughly cleansed before surgery to reduce the number of bacteria present. Antibiotics may also be started at this time. Impressions of the palate and jaw will be made before radical surgery if prostheses are planned to replace resected tissue. The actual prosthesis is fitted when surgical healing is completed. The nurse provides the patient with careful explanations of all planned activities and treatments, with special attention to the feeding and communication adaptations that may be necessary in the immediate postoperative period. Emotional support in the preoperative period is an essential intervention; the changes the patient faces may be extensive. The remainder of the preparation is similar to that required before any major surgery (see Chapter 18).

### ■ POSTOPERATIVE CARE

Postoperative care of the patient focuses on promoting an adequate airway, mouth drainage, oral hygiene, comfort, nutrition, speech, and ongoing emotional support. Care of the patient after surgery for oral cancer is summarized in the Guidelines for Care Box on p. 1259.

#### Maintaining a Patent Airway

Removal of secretions is the primary concern immediately after surgery. Tissue and nerve trauma may impair the natural protective reflexes and leave the airway vulnerable. A side-lying position is used until the patient is fully alert, followed by a head-elevated Fowler's position. Oral suction is kept available at the bedside, and the nurse instructs the patient in its proper use. An emesis basin or gauze wicks may also be used to collect saliva. The nurse carefully monitors the airway, auscultates the lungs, and maintains the patency of any drainage tubes.

#### Facilitating Verbal Communication

The ability to speak is commonly lost for short or long periods after surgery, but if the vocal cords are intact, speech will eventually return. Phrasing questions initially in a yes-or-no format enables the patient to respond effectively with gestures, head nods, or simple sounds. The nurse validates all communication by repeating answers or questions before acting on perceived requests. Loud noises may be disturbing to the patient because the loss of oral tissue may create a channel that amplifies sound; the person should therefore be addressed in a soft, clear voice. As speech begins to return, the patient is encouraged to speak slowly and to use the throat rather than the lips to achieve clarity. Speech retraining may be necessary, and referrals for speech therapy are usually initiated. A tape recorder may be useful so that the person can hear his or her own voice and work on improvements.

#### Promoting Oral Hygiene

Good mouth care after surgery is essential for comfort, prevention of infection, and promotion of healing. Tooth brushing is usually contraindicated because of discomfort and potential trauma. Sterile equipment is used to prevent introduction of exogenous organisms. Patients are encouraged to assist in their oral hygiene as soon as possible.

Mouth irrigations are standard postoperative interventions and are performed every few hours and after feedings. Com-

**guidelines for care**

### The Person Undergoing Surgery for Oral Cancer

**Preoperative Care**

1. Clarify the patient's knowledge of changes expected after surgery
2. Explain expected postoperative measures (including suctioning, nasogastric tube)
3. Provide opportunities for the patient to begin to express feelings about changes in body image

**Postoperative Care**

1. Monitoring
   a. Assess facial movement for facial nerve damage (if parotid gland excised): ask the patient to raise the eyebrows, frown, smile, show the teeth, pucker the lips
   b. Assess the degree and character of drainage
      (1) Amount of drainage and presence of blood should be minimal
      (2) Hemorrhage may occur with wide resection of the tongue
2. Maintaining an adequate airway
   a. Place the patient in side-lying position initially
   b. Place the patient in Fowler's position when fully alert
   c. Suction the mouth (except for lip surgery)
   d. Gauze wick may be used to direct saliva into an emesis basin
   e. Maintain patency of drainage tubes, if used
3. Promoting oral hygiene and comfort
   a. Clean involved areas of the mouth with a cotton applicator moistened with hydrogen peroxide and saline
   b. Mouth irrigations
      (1) Use sterile equipment
      (2) Use a solution of sterile water, diluted hydrogen peroxide, normal saline, or sodium bicarbonate (avoid commercial mouthwashes)
      (3) Protect any dressings from getting wet
      (4) A catheter may be inserted along the side of the cheek and the solution injected with gentle pressure; a spray may also be used
      (5) Give analgesics as indicated (pain is *not* usually severe)
4. Promoting nutrition
   a. Tube feedings will be used initially with hemiglossectomy
   b. Oral fluids: place in back of throat with aseptic syringe or feeding cup with attached tubing
   c. Eating soft foods
      (1) Encourage the patient to feed self when possible
      (2) Teach the patient to drink clear water after all meals to cleanse the mouth
      (3) Avoid using a fork, which may traumatize new tissue
      (4) Avoid very hot or cold foods (hot foods irritate new tissue; cold foods may cause facial pain or paralyze oral functions)
5. Promoting speech
   a. Limit patient responses initially to *yes* or *no,* which can be answered by gestures
   b. When speech returns, encourage the patient to speak slowly
   c. Listen carefully and validate communication before acting on requests
   d. Speak in a soft, clear voice
   e. Refer the patient to a speech therapist if appropriate
6. Promoting a positive body image
   a. Prepare all visitors for visible outcomes of surgery
   b. Include the family in all teaching
   c. Encourage the patient to ventilate feelings about changes
   d. Encourage socialization with others

mercial mouthwashes are avoided in preference for sterile water, dilute peroxide and saline, or bicarbonate solutions. The solution is typically introduced into the mouth via a catheter, which is gently inserted along the cheek line, or with a spray. A cotton-tipped applicator moistened with peroxide and saline may be used to reach difficult or painful areas. The nurse encourages self-care and teaches the patient to use mirrors to increase visualization.

### Promoting Adequate Oral Nutrition

The problems that the patient faces related to oral nutrition after oral surgery depend entirely on the nature and extent of the surgical procedure. Chewing is difficult without an intact tongue, and the person often has a problem getting the food to the posterior pharynx. Sensation in the mouth is decreased, and the patient has difficulty locating the position of the food in the oral cavity. One method of eating is for the person to use the forefinger to push the food to the posterior pharynx.

A syringe or tube is commonly used to assist the patient to successfully direct fluids toward the back of the mouth. The tube may be placed and anchored by the surgeon at the time of surgery. Tube feeding is used while tissue healing takes place, and it may be a permanent approach to nutrition when extensive tissue removal is necessary.

Most patients can suction and feed themselves a few days after mouth surgery and are happier doing so. With practice, the patient develops confidence in self-care and is often more adept than the nurse in placing the catheter or tube in a position where fluids can be received into the mouth and swallowed without difficulty. A mirror often helps. Privacy is essential during the initial period. The patient should not be hurried and is observed very carefully to determine how much assistance is needed. Forks are *not* used, because they may traumatize healing tissues. Both very hot and very cold foods are avoided because they may irritate healing tissue or produce facial pain.

Patients are instructed to carefully rinse the mouth with clear water or with a prescribed solution after finishing each meal. Some patients experience persistent problems with choking or nasal regurgitation, which can significantly interfere with the social nature of meals.

### Facilitating Adaptation to Altered Body Image

Treatment for cancer of the mouth interferes with major oral functions such as eating and speaking and thus creates major changes in the person's life. Changes in the patient's ability to speak can occur, varying from minimal limitations to complete inability to speak, depending on the amount of tissue resected or destroyed. Eating patterns may be changed in terms of the consistency of foods, as well as methods of ingestion. Persistent drooling is a common problem. The person's facial appearance may also change, depending on the extent of tissue removed or destroyed, and even with reconstructive surgery, noticeable changes may be present.

Therefore one of the major problems that the person will have to cope with and adapt to is the change in body image. Patients need to know in advance the changes that will occur and the measures that will be taken to assist them during the adjustment period. The impact of the loss may be slightly minimized when the grieving process begins early. The full emotional impact of the loss, however, occurs after surgery.

Problems with speaking and eating can cause the patient to avoid interactions with family, friends, or strangers. Family members are included, if possible, in all teaching, and the nurse encourages them to include the patient in mealtimes and social occasions as soon as possible. Visiting is encouraged, but all visitors need to be prepared in advance concerning the visible changes and functional problems created by the surgery.

## GERONTOLOGICAL CONSIDERATIONS

Oral cancer develops primarily in response to the long-term use of alcohol and tobacco. Oral malignancies are most common in the elderly population. Therefore the importance of seeking prompt evaluation of any mouth lesion should be stressed with all elderly individuals.

Surgical intervention for oral cancer is typically radical, and it may be a significant stressor for an elderly person with less adaptive reserve. The need to learn new approaches to secretion removal, oral feeding, and communication may pose significant challenges to an older adult, particularly if psychomotor abilities are compromised by arthritis. Discharge planning needs to be carefully undertaken because social isolation may become a reality for elders who live alone. The nurse is an essential link in the process of identifying persons who will need home care assistance.

## SPECIAL ENVIRONMENTS FOR CARE

### Critical Care Management

The treatment of oral cancer will typically not necessitate critical care management. However, because the target population is older and may experience a wide variety of complicating chronic illnesses, temporary critical care support may be indicated in selected situations. Airway management and hemodynamic monitoring would be typical areas of concern.

### Home Care Management

Home care considerations are primarily related to the extent of the surgery and its impact on speech and oral nutrition. When wound healing is prolonged, the patient may need ongoing assistance or supervision in performing oral care or feedings. If nutritional needs are not being met, home administration of tube feedings or gastrostomy feedings may be initiated.

The nurse stresses the importance of maintaining scrupulous oral hygiene with ongoing care for the teeth and gums to prevent future complications. Regular dental screening will be important if radiation was used, particularly to ensure the proper fit of dentures. The cancer can recur, and the patient will be encouraged to use alcohol only in moderation and to quit smoking if at all possible. Ongoing work with a speech therapist is commonly necessary.

## COMPLICATIONS

Complications are primarily related to the progression of the original disease process or treatment-related problems. Tissue necrosis and severe pain can occur in advanced cancer of the mouth, either from failure of treatment or from death of tissue as a result of radiation. The patient usually experiences difficulty in swallowing, fear of choking, and the constant accumulation of foul-smelling secretions. The danger of severe and even fatal hemorrhage must always be considered. It is difficult to assist these patients to take sufficient nourishing fluids. A gastrostomy may be created to permit direct introduction of food into the stomach. Family members caring for the person at home may need considerable ongoing support to safely manage care.

# PROBLEMS OF THE ESOPHAGUS

## GASTROESOPHAGEAL REFLUX DISEASE

### Etiology

Gastroesophageal reflux disease (GERD) is a heterogeneous syndrome resulting from esophageal reflux. Most cases are attributed to the inappropriate relaxation of the lower esophageal sphincter (LES) in response to an unknown stimulus. Reflux allows gastric and duodenal contents to move back into the distal esophagus. The presence of a hiatal hernia, which displaces the LES into the thorax, was formerly commonly assumed to be the primary cause of GERD. However, hiatal hernia has subsequently been found to be a common condition in the adult population and, although most persons with hiatal hernias do experience reflux, the reverse has not been found to be true.[13] A number of environmental and physical factors have been identified that appear to influence the tone and contractility of the LES, and these may play an etiological role in some cases of GERD. The pressure of the LES is lowered by fatty foods, chocolate, cola, coffee, and tea; nicotine; drugs such as calcium channel blockers, theophylline, and possibly nonsteroidal antiinflammatory drugs (NSAIDs); elevated levels of estrogen and progesterone; and conditions that elevate intraabdominal pressure, such as obesity, pregnancy, or heavy lifting. Reflux is much more common in the postprandial state, and over 60% of reflux sufferers have delayed gastric emptying.[13]

## Epidemiology

Gastroesophageal reflux disease occurs in all age groups and is estimated to affect up to 45% of the population to some degree, which translates into greater than 60 million persons.[13,17] It produces daily symptoms in as much as 10% of the general population. It is theorized that the actual incidence of mild disease may be even higher, because many individuals simply accept reflux as an occasional mild problem that can be effectively self-treated. Fewer than 25% of all reflux sufferers ever consult a health care provider about it. There are no documented gender or cultural patterns associated with reflux, but elders experience decreased esophageal peristalsis and a higher incidence of hiatal hernia, which together increase the likelihood of reflux in this population.

## Pathophysiology

Two zones of high pressure, one at each end of the esophagus, normally prevent the reflux of gastric contents. The zones maintain a constant pressure and relax only during swallowing. Although they are termed the *upper esophageal sphincter* and *lower esophageal sphincter,* they are not really distinct anatomical structures. Esophageal reflux occurs when either gastric volume or intraabdominal pressure is elevated or when LES sphincter tone is decreased. Periodic reflux occurs normally in most persons and is usually asymptomatic.

The normal physiological response to occasional reflux is immediate swallowing. One or more rapid swallows induce peristatic contractions to clear the reflux and neutralize the acid with the bicarbonate-rich saliva. However, the esophagus has only a limited ability to withstand the damaging effects of acid reflux, and GERD will develop when frequent episodes of reflux break down the mucosal barrier and initiate an inflammatory response.

The degree of esophageal inflammation is related to the number, duration, and acidity or alkalinity of the reflux episodes. The effectiveness and efficiency of esophageal clearance also are important. Esophageal clearance is particularly important at night when the swallowing rate and salivation decrease by two thirds and a recumbent position interferes with clearance. An inflamed esophagus gradually loses its ability to clear refluxed material quickly and efficiently, and the duration of each episode gradually lengthens.

Hyperemia and erosion occur in the face of chronic inflammation. Minor capillary bleeding is common, although frank bleeding is rare. Repeated episodes of inflammation and healing can gradually produce a change in the epithelial tissue, which makes it more resistant to acid. However, the presence of this new tissue, termed *Barrett's epithelium,* is also associated with a higher risk of adenocarcinoma. Barrett's epithelium is estimated to be present in about 40% of symptomatic patients.[17] Over time, fibrotic tissue changes can also result in esophageal stricture, which can progressively impair normal swallowing.

The clinical manifestations of GERD are consistent in their nature, but they vary substantially in severity. The irritation of chronic reflux produces the primary symptom, which is heartburn (pyrosis). The pain is described as a substernal or retrosternal burning sensation that tends to radiate upward and may involve the neck, jaw, or back. The pain typically occurs 20 minutes to 2 hours after eating. An atypical pain pattern that closely mimics angina may also occur and needs to be carefully differentiated from true cardiac disease. The second major symptom of GERD is regurgitation, which is not associated with either belching or nausea. The individual experiences a feeling of warm fluid moving up the throat. If it reaches the pharynx, a sour or bitter taste is perceived. Water brash, a reflex salivary hypersecretion that does not have a bitter taste, occurs less commonly.

In severe cases GERD can produce dysphagia or odynophagia (painful swallowing). Belching and a feeling of flatulence are other common complaints. Nocturnal cough, wheezing, or hoarseness all may occur with reflux, and it is estimated that greater than 80% of adult asthmatics may have reflux. The frequency and severity of reflux episodes usually determine the severity of the symptoms. The clinical manifestations of GERD are summarized in Box 39-3.

## Collaborative Care Management

Patients with GERD are rarely admitted to the acute care setting unless they require surgery or experience serious complications. The problem is self-managed in the outpatient setting. The goal of treatment is to decrease the incidence of reflux and eliminate the symptoms.

### *Diagnostic tests*

Mild cases of GERD are diagnosed from the classic symptoms, and treatment is initiated based on the presumptive diagnosis. More involved cases may require other screening tools. The gold standard for diagnosis is 24-hour pH monitoring, which accurately records the number, duration, and severity of reflux episodes and is considered to be 85% sensitive. The esophageal motility and Bernstein tests can be performed in conjunction with pH monitoring to evaluate LES competence, quantify reflux episodes, and evaluate the response of the esophagus to acid infusion. These tests are described in more detail in Chapter 38. The barium swallow with fluoroscopy is widely used to document the presence of

**box 39-3** *clinical manifestations*

***Gastroesophageal Reflux Disease***

**Heartburn**—substernal or retrosternal burning sensation that may radiate to the back or jaw
NOTE: In some cases the pain may mimic angina
**Regurgitation** (not associated with nausea or belching)—a sour or bitter taste is perceived in the pharynx
**Water brash**—a reflex hypersecretion that does not have a bitter taste
**Frequent belching, flatulence**
**Dysphagia** or **odynophagia** (difficult or painful swallowing)—usually occurs only in severe cases
**Nocturnal cough, wheezing, hoarseness**

hiatal hernia, but it can demonstrate only gross disease. Endoscopy is rarely necessary to establish the diagnosis, but it is routinely performed to evaluate the presence and severity of esophagitis and to rule out malignancy.

### Medications

Drug therapy is an important aspect of GERD management, and it is usually initiated with the occasional use of antacids to control heartburn by the patient. Antacids are effective in dealing with occasional heartburn and usually produce prompt relief of symptoms. Either aluminum or magnesium products may be used, but combination mixtures such as Maalox and Mylanta are usually best tolerated because they minimize the incidence of common side effects such as diarrhea and constipation. Antacids were the mainstay of GERD treatment until the 1980s and are still effective for symptom management in mild disease. When they are incorporated into a formal treatment plan, antacids are given 1 and 3 hours after meals and at bedtime plus as needed for breakthrough heartburn discomfort. Alginates may be used as an alternative. Alginates (Gaviscon) combine alginic acid with an antacid, which forms a viscous foam that floats on top of the gastric contents. This theoretically creates a mechanical barrier to reflux and supposedly also limits acid contact with the mucosa when reflux occurs.

Frequent symptomatic reflux requires more aggressive management. A stepwise treatment plan usually begins with high doses of histamine ($H_2$) receptor antagonists such as cimetidine (Tagamet), ranitidine (Zantac), famotidine (Pepcid), or nizatidine (Axid). Although these drugs do not influence reflux directly, they reduce gastric acid secretion and provide symptomatic improvement. They also support tissue healing, although esophageal inflammation is much more difficult to heal than duodenal ulcers. The drugs are given at least twice daily because once-a-day dosing has been found to be ineffective. This reduces gastric acid secretion by 40% to 70%.[12] These drugs have demonstrated safety for long-term use.

Healing of severe GERD is difficult to achieve and sustain with $H_2$ receptor antagonists, and patients are increasingly being treated with a newer category of drugs, the proton pump inhibitors. Omeprazole (Prilosec) is the most widely used (see the Research Box). A single daily dose decreases acid secretion by 90% to 95% and supports prompt healing within 4 to 6 weeks.[13] Concern has existed about the long-term effects of prolonged acid suppression, and the use of these drugs remains restricted in the United States. No adverse effects have been reported in Europe, where proton pump inhibitors have been in use for years. Their use is being increasingly advocated for initial treatment, but concern exists that this represents overtreatment in many situations.[12]

Prokinetic drugs that increase the rate of gastric emptying have always been a logical part of GERD therapy, but both bethanechol (Urecholine) and metoclopramide (Reglan) are associated with multiple side effects that make them inappropriate for long-term use. Cisapride (Propulsid) has now been accepted for general use and appears to be an effective and well-tolerated drug. It can be used in addition to $H_2$ receptor antagonists or proton pump inhibitors. Drug therapy for GERD is summarized in Table 39-2.

**research**

Reference: Vigneri S et al: A comparison of five maintenance therapies for reflux esophagitis, *N Engl J Med* 333:1106, 1995.

Reflux esophagitis is a chronic disease with a high degree of relapse within 1 year of treatment. This study compared cisapride, ranitidine, and omeprazole in single-drug maintenance therapy and two combination drug maintenance therapies (ranitidine plus cisapride and omeprazole plus cisapride). The study involved 175 patients who had experienced relapse of reflux esophagitis indicated by endoscopy findings and return of symptoms. Follow-up visits were maintained at intervals of 8 weeks for 12 months.

Maintenance therapy with omeprazole alone or in combination with cisapride was found to be significantly more effective than the other approaches in preventing relapse. Omeprazole was concluded to be the drug of choice for initial and maintenance treatment of severe reflux esophagitis.

### Treatments

Gastroesophageal reflux disease is typically managed using a combination of drug therapy, lifestyle modification, and surgical intervention if necessary. There are no specific treatments included in the standard medical plan of care.

### Surgical management

Antireflux surgery is usually performed in patients with severe GERD who do not respond to aggressive medical management. However, as more is learned about the difficulties in healing esophagitis and the discouragingly high relapse rates, the use of surgery is again being explored as an earlier primary strategy in GERD. The question of long-term cost-effectiveness is also being raised because it appears that drug therapy must be maintained at high dosage levels almost indefinitely to prevent relapse. The application of laparoscopic techniques to fundoplication procedures is making surgical intervention for GERD a viable option in the hands of a skilled surgeon. The surgical procedures used are the same as those used to correct hiatal hernia and are discussed on p. 1266. They involve fundoplication, the wrapping and suturing of the gastric fundus around the esophagus, which reinforces the LES area and anchors it below the diaphragm.

### Diet

The modification of diet and eating patterns may significantly relieve symptoms in mild GERD. Certain foods have been demonstrated to affect LES pressure. Fatty foods, cola, coffee, tea, chocolate, onions, tomato-based products, and alcohol all decrease LES pressure and should be avoided. Adequate dietary protein stimulates the release of gastrin and cholecystokinin, which increase LES pressure. Spicy and acidic foods are usually restricted until healing occurs and then may be resumed

**table 39-2** *Common Medications for* ***Gastroesophageal Reflux Disease***

| DRUG | ACTION | NURSING INTERVENTION |
|---|---|---|
| **ANTIBIOTICS** | | |
| Antacids:<br>Aluminum or magnesium-based product | Neutralize gastric acids | Evaluate effectiveness<br>Monitor frequency of use<br>Monitor for constipation or diarrhea, and assist patient to adjust product use as needed |
| Antacid plus alginic acid:<br>Gaviscon | Neutralizes gastric acid; forms viscous foam that prevents reflux or buffers its effects | Same as for antacids |
| Histamine ($H_2$) receptor antagonists:<br>Cimetidine (Tagamet)<br>Ranitidine (Zantac)<br>Famotidine (Pepcid)<br>Nizatadine (Axid) | Reduce gastric acid secretion and support tissue healing | Instruct patient to take drugs with meals if ordered at intervals<br>Monitor for common side effects: fatigue, headache, diarrhea |
| Prokinetics:<br>Cisapride (Propulsid) | Increase LES pressure and enhance GI motility | Instruct patient to take drug no more than 15 minutes before eating<br>Monitor levels of drugs that require careful titration |
| Proton pump inhibitors:<br>Omeprazole (Prilosec)<br>Lansoprazole (Prevacid) | Inhibit enzyme system of gastric parietal cells and suppress gastric acid secretion by more than 90% | Instruct patient to take the drug before meals; monitor for side effects: abdominal cramping, headache, diarrhea |

if they do not produce pain. Weight loss and avoiding overeating may also reduce the frequency of reflux episodes.

### *Activity*

Activities that increase intraabdominal pressure and the likelihood of reflux are restricted. Lifting heavy objects, straining, constrictive clothing, and working in a stooped or bent-over position are all contraindicated.

### *Referrals*

Referrals are rarely necessary for persons with uncomplicated GERD, but the nurse may encourage the patient to seek assistance for weight loss or smoking cessation as indicated.

## NURSING MANAGEMENT

## ■ ASSESSMENT

### Subjective Data

Subjective data to be collected to assess the patient with gastroesophageal reflux disease include:

- Heartburn—severity and duration
- Regurgitation or water brash—presence and severity
- Diet and meal pattern
- Relationship of symptoms to food, meal pattern, and activity
- Dysphagia and odynophagia—presence and severity
- Belching or flatulence
- Nocturnal cough—presence and severity
- Use of over-the-counter medications, particularly antacids and $H_2$ receptor antagonists

### Objective Data

Objective data to be collected to assess the patient with gastroesophageal reflux disease include:

- Body weight
- Auscultation for signs of reflux aspiration
- Hoarseness or wheezing—day or night

## ■ NURSING DIAGNOSES

Nursing diagnoses are determined from analysis of patient data. Nursing diagnoses for the person with GERD may include but are not limited to:

| Diagnostic Title | Possible Etiological Factors |
|---|---|
| Pain | Acid reflux in the esophagus |
| Knowledge deficit | Diet and lifestyle modifications needed to control reflux |

## ■ EXPECTED PATIENT OUTCOMES

Expected patient outcomes for the patient with GERD may include but are not limited to:

1. Reports minimal or no episodes of heartburn
2. Can list diet and lifestyle changes that will control reflux and incorporates these changes into daily living

## ■ INTERVENTIONS

### Promoting Comfort

The nurse discusses the medication regimen with the patient and ensures that written information about the safe use and expected side effects of all medications is provided. The nurse encourages the patient to use antacids as ordered 1 hour before and 2 to 3 hours after meals and at bedtime during the healing phase of management. Either tablets or liquid preparations may be used. Most patients find tablets to be more portable and convenient. Antacids should not be restricted to an as-needed status for actual heartburn episodes. The nurse informs the patient about the common bowel problems that accompany extensive antacid therapy and suggests strategies such as alternating mixtures or using combination products to maintain a normal pattern of bowel elimination.

The nurse also explores the patient's use of other medications. Anticholinergics, calcium channel blockers, xanthine derivatives, and diazepam all appear to lower the LES pressure, and their use should be avoided.

### Patient/Family Education

#### *Promoting lifestyle changes*

Because reflux tends to be a chronic disease with a high tendency to relapse, lifestyle changes need to be permanent. With the ongoing development of newer and more potent pharmacological agents it is easy to overlook the value of traditional therapeutic measures, but they remain an integral part of effective GERD management. Treatment begins with lifestyle changes.

Teaching the patient to elevate the head of the bed 6 to 12 inches for sleep is the highest-priority lifestyle change. Nighttime reflux is the most difficult to manage. Wooden blocks have traditionally been recommended, but research indicates that the use of foam wedges can also achieve satisfactory results. The nurse must introduce this crucial intervention with tact and care, because a change affects both the patient and his or her sleeping partner.

The nurse will recommend other lifestyle changes, including avoiding increases in intraabdominal pressure caused by constrictive clothing, straining, lifting heavy weights, or working in a bent-over or stooped position. Smoking cessation is another critical and sensitive area. Smoking causes a rapid and significant drop in LES pressure and should be reduced or eliminated if at all possible. Evening smoking, particularly while resting in bed, is of particular concern. The combination of evening snacking and smoking receives the highest priority.

#### *Modifying the diet*

The patient is encouraged to eliminate or significantly reduce consumption of foods that have been shown to lower LES sphincter pressure. A low-fat diet with limited use of caffeine-containing beverages, such as tea, alcohol, and chocolate, is ideal. Adequate protein intake is encouraged for its LES sphincter–enhancing ability. The nurse explores barriers to adherence in the patient's usual diet pattern and involves the family if possible to support needed changes.

Patients are also encouraged to modify their basic meal pattern. Eating four to six small meals daily is recommended. Large meals increase gastric pressure and volume and delay gastric emptying. These factors increase the frequency and severity of reflux episodes. Avoiding evening snacking is particularly important. The individual should not eat for at least 3 hours before bedtime. Nighttime reflux, when both recumbency and inactivity dramatically decrease the effectiveness of esophageal clearance, is a serious problem in GERD that is significantly worsened by evening snacking.

Reducing body weight helps lower intraabdominal pressure and may be helpful for obese patients. Simple strategies such as eating slowly and chewing thoroughly facilitate digestion and reduce belching. The nurse works with the patient to carefully evaluate which strategies most effectively reduce the incidence and severity of symptoms.

Recommended diet and lifestyle changes for patients with GERD are summarized in the Guidelines for Care Box.

#### *Health Promotion/Prevention*

Primary prevention does not play a major role in GERD because the condition does not have readily identifiable preventable etiological factors. Standard preventive measures might include maintaining an optimal body weight and avoiding episodes of overeating, particularly at night. The most significant factor in secondary prevention is for health care professionals to directly inquire about a patient's experience with heartburn. Studies have shown that patients rarely report heartburn to their health care provider unless directly asked or until the symptoms have become severe.[12] If identified and recognized early, the disease may be more responsive to diet and lifestyle modification measures.

## ■ EVALUATION

To evaluate the effectiveness of nursing interventions, compare patient behaviors with those stated in the expected pa-

**guidelines for care**

**Diet and Lifestyle Modifications to Manage Gastroesophageal Reflux Disease**

**Diet**

Eat 4-6 small meals daily.
Follow a low-fat, adequate-protein diet.
Reduce intake of chocolate, tea, and all foods and beverages that contain caffeine.
Limit or eliminate alcohol intake.
Eat slowly, and chew food thoroughly.
Avoid evening snacking, and do not eat for 2-3 hr before bedtime.
Remain upright for 1-2 hr after meals when possible, and never eat in bed.
Avoid any food that directly produces heartburn.
Reduce overall body weight if indicated.

**Lifestyle**

Eliminate or drastically reduce smoking.
Avoid evening smoking, and never smoke in bed.
Avoid constrictive clothing over the abdomen.
Avoid activities that involve straining, heavy lifting, or working in a bent-over position.
Elevate the head of the bed at least 6-8 inches for sleep, using wooden blocks or a thick foam wedge.
Never sleep flat in bed.

tient outcomes. Successful achievement of patient outcomes for the patient with GERD is indicated by:

1. Experiences no heartburn episodes

2a. Knows dietary factors that increase reflux

b. Adopts specific lifestyle factors that reduce the incidence of reflux

## GERONTOLOGICAL CONSIDERATIONS

Esophageal function continues effectively into advanced age, but some decline in esophageal peristalsis is expected, and a decrease in saliva production impairs the efficiency of esophageal clearance. Even routine reflux becomes protracted and increases the risk of irritation. Elderly individuals need to be assessed for heartburn, because they are found to routinely underreport their symptoms. They also appear to be particularly vulnerable to alkaline reflux from the duodenum. Acid combined with bile and pancreatic juice is believed to be more damaging to the mucosa than acid alone. Alkaline reflux typically occurs at night and causes respiratory symptoms such as choking, paroxysmal coughing, and wheezing. Patients with frequent nighttime awakenings from coughing should be evaluated for GERD. The risk of aspiration is high. Treatment approaches are the same as those outlined for other forms of GERD.

## SPECIAL ENVIRONMENTS FOR CARE

### Critical Care Management

Gastroesophageal reflux disease is a common disorder that is self-managed almost exclusively in the home by the patient. Critical care management would be used only to treat severe complications such as aspiration pneumonia or hemorrhage.

### Home Care Management

The patient is in charge of the self-care regimen in the home. Written instructions are provided about all aspects of the plan to reinforce verbal teaching. The nurse involves the spouse or partner and family where possible, because changes in diet and meal patterns affect the entire family. Major lifestyle changes are not necessary, but even relatively minor regimen restrictions require planning and support if they are to be successful.

## COMPLICATIONS

If GERD is not successfully controlled, it can progress to serious and even life-threatening problems. Esophageal ulceration and hemorrhage may result from severe erosion, and chronic nighttime reflux is accompanied by a significant risk of aspiration. Adenocarcinoma can develop from the premalignant tissue termed Barrett's epithelium. Gradual or repeated scarring can permanently damage esophageal tissue and produce stricture.

# HIATAL HERNIA

## ETIOLOGY

The opening in the diaphragm that allows the esophagus to pass from the thorax to the abdomen is called the esophageal hiatus. Hiatal hernias (also called diaphragmatic hernias) develop when the distal esophagus, and possibly a portion of the stomach, move into the thorax through the hiatus. There are two major types. One type is the sliding hernia, which accounts for 90% of the total.[11] In these hernias the distal esophagus, gastric junction, and possibly a portion of the stomach are simply displaced upward into the thorax (Figure 39-3, *A*). The hernia is usually freely movable and slides back and forth in response to changes in position or abdominal pressure. Sliding hernias are believed to develop from muscle weakness in the esophageal hiatus, which undermines the supports. The defect is consistent with the aging process, although congenital weakness, trauma, surgery, or prolonged increases in intraabdominal pressure may also play a role.

The second and relatively unusual form of hiatal hernia is the paraesophageal, or rolling, hernia. The gastric junction remains anchored below the diaphragm, but the fundus of the stomach, and possibly portions or even all of the greater curvature, rolls into the thorax next to the esophagus (Figure 39-3, *B*). An anatomical defect may be the cause, but muscle weakening does not appear to play a major role.

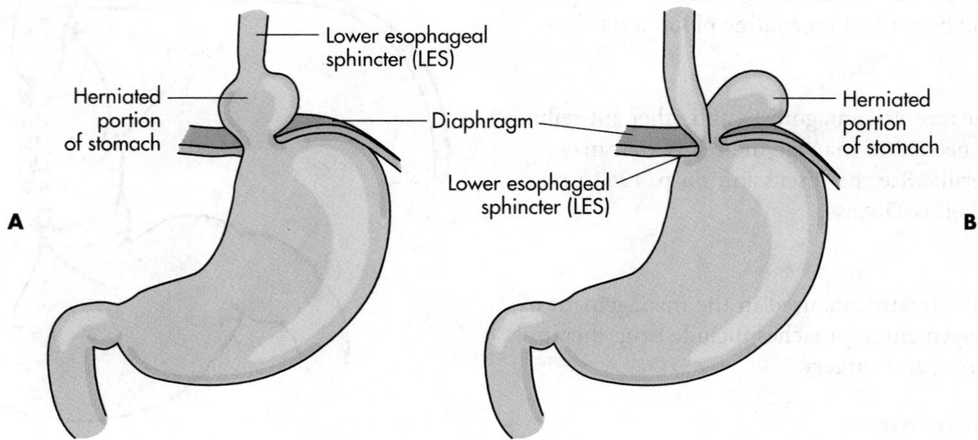


**fig. 39-3** Hiatal hernia. **A,** Sliding hernia. **B,** Paraesophageal hernia.

## EPIDEMIOLOGY

Hiatal hernias are common in the adult population. Their incidence is roughly estimated at 25% to 30% in the general population and as high as 60% in the over-60 age group.[11] Hiatal hernias affect women much more commonly than men, although their incidence increases in both sexes with aging.

## PATHOPHYSIOLOGY

Most individuals with hiatal hernias are completely asymptomatic. The development of symptoms is rare before middle age. Hiatal hernias are usually small, but their relative size is not necessarily related to the presence or severity of symptoms.

With sliding hernias the problems are rarely anatomical. The problems relate directly to the functional consequences of chronic reflux. Reflux occurs from the ongoing exposure of the LES to the low-pressure environment of the thorax where sphincter function is significantly impaired.

Reflux is rarely a concern with paraesophageal hernias, because the LES remains anchored below the diaphragm. However, the anatomical risks of volvulus, strangulation, and obstruction are high. In addition, venous obstruction in the herniated portion of the stomach causes the mucosa to become engorged and to ooze. Slow bleeding leads to the development of iron deficiency anemia, but significant bleeding or hemorrhage is rare.

Unless acute complications develop, most hiatal hernias are diagnosed as part of a workup for GERD. The clinical manifestations (see Box 39-3) and diagnostic tests are similar.

## COLLABORATIVE CARE MANAGEMENT

### Diagnostic Tests

The barium swallow with fluoroscopy is the most useful test for diagnosing hiatal hernia. Paraesophageal hernias are usually clearly visible, and sliding hernias can be easily demonstrated when the individual is moved into positions that increase intraabdominal pressure. Any or all of the tests used as part of a reflux workup may be used to evaluate the degree of esophageal damage (see Chapter 38). Additional findings in individuals with paraesophageal hernias may include low hemoglobin and hematocrit levels from chronic low-grade bleeding, which will be evident on routine blood tests.

### Medications

Antacids, histamine receptor antagonists, and other antireflux agents are used as needed to manage the reflux that may accompany hiatal hernia. See the discussion on p. 1262 under Gastroesophageal Reflux Disease.

### Treatments

There are no specific treatments used in the management of hiatal hernia. Management approaches include drug therapy, lifestyle modifications, and surgery.

### Surgical Management

Surgical correction of paraesophageal hernias is mandatory because the risk of serious complications is significant. The surgery consists of straightforward anatomical repair because there is no need to correct or modify LES function.

The repair of sliding hernias is more complex, because simple repair of the defect in the diaphragm rarely corrects the reflux problem. Restoring LES competence becomes a second major consideration. Several different surgical procedures exist, but each involves LES reinforcement through fundoplication, or wrapping of the stomach fundus around the LES zone.

The Nissen fundoplication (Figure 39-4) is the most commonly used procedure. The fundus of the stomach is wrapped a full 360 degrees around the lower esophagus to reinforce the LES. Both abdominal and thoracic approaches are used for the surgery with advantages and disadvantages to each. Laparoscopic fundoplication was first performed in 1991, and in skilled hands it has become a suitable alternative to an open procedure for selected patients.[19] Surgeons throughout the world are using and reporting on other procedures and techniques that utilize various degrees of fundoplication, posterior vs. anterior wrapping, and fixation to the diaphragm vs. the abdominal wall for stability. Fundoplication procedures are associated with a significant incidence of complications, and consensus does not yet exist about which procedures are most effective.

### Diet

The recommended diet modifications for hiatal hernia follow the general guidelines outlined in the section on antireflux therapy. The diet also focuses on reducing obesity if possible. Obesity can significantly increase intraabdominal pressure and worsen the severity of both the hernia and the symptoms of reflux.

### Activity

Activities that increase intraabdominal pressure and reflux are restricted as discussed under Gastroesophageal Reflux Disease (see p. 1263).

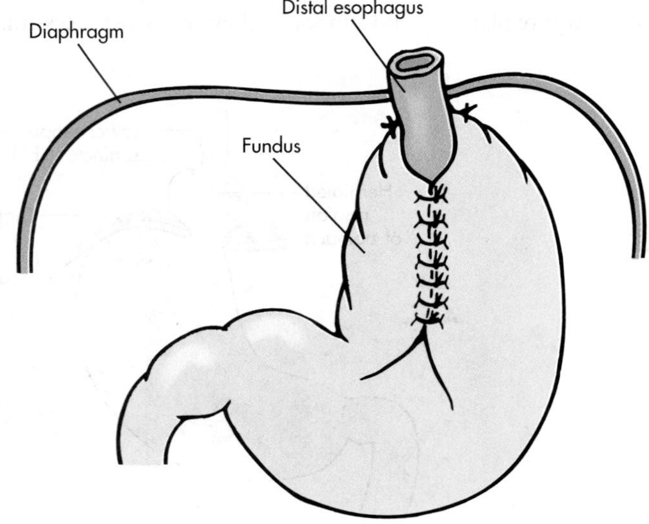


**fig. 39-4** Nissen fundoplication for repair of hiatal hernia.

### Referrals

Referrals are rarely necessary for the management of hiatal hernia, except possibly to assist the individual with weight loss and smoking cessation, which are critical components in managing reflux.

## NURSING MANAGEMENT OF THE PATIENT WITH HIATAL HERNIA SURGERY

### PREOPERATIVE CARE

Preoperative teaching focuses on instructing the patient in deep breathing, the correct use of an incentive spirometer, and splinting the incision effectively for coughing. The surgical approaches all involve the diaphragm, and pulmonary hygiene is essential in preventing respiratory complications. The high incision of open procedures makes pulmonary hygiene painful, and it is essential to discuss the plan and approach to pain management with the patient. If a thoracic approach is used, teaching will also include the management of chest tubes. Individuals who are overweight are encouraged to lose weight if possible before surgery, and smokers are encouraged to significantly reduce or eliminate their use of tobacco. The nurse also teaches the patient about the nasogastric (NG) tube that will be inserted during surgery with open procedures and the planned time frame for restarting oral feedings.

### POSTOPERATIVE CARE

#### Facilitating Airway Clearance

Prevention of respiratory complications is the primary postoperative consideration. The head of the bed is elevated 30 degrees to facilitate lung expansion. The nurse assists the patient out of bed as soon as possible and supports the incision for coughing. Regular lung auscultation, incentive spirometry, and chest physiotherapy are routinely employed. Adequate analgesia is essential to the success of the respiratory protocol. It should be provided via patient-controlled analgesia or through aggressive nursing management, particularly before ambulation or chest physiotherapy. Patients with a smoking or pulmonary disease history need to be managed even more aggressively.

Patients treated laparoscopically may remain in the hospital only overnight. Although their pain should be significantly less than that experienced by patients with major incisions, it is still essential that they be instructed in the importance of frequent deep breathing and effective coughing if needed.

#### Facilitating Swallowing

A large-diameter NG tube is usually inserted during surgery to prevent the fundoplication from being made too tight. The nurse monitors the tube postoperatively for secure anchoring and patency and regularly assesses the drainage, which should consist of normal yellowish-green gastric secretions within the first 8 hours after surgery. It should not contain fresh blood. It is essential that the stomach remain decompressed to prevent vomiting, which could disrupt the fundoplication sutures.

The NG tube is carefully placed by the surgeon and is usually neither moved nor repositioned. Orders concerning irrigation should be carefully followed. Sterile solutions are generally preferred in the early postoperative period. Frequent oral and nasal hygiene are important for comfort, because the large tube is irritating. An NG tube may not be used with the laparoscopic procedures.

The patient is offered oral fluids after peristalsis has been reestablished. Some surgeons prefer to use gastrostomy feedings to facilitate healing, but most patients progress to a near-normal diet within 6 weeks. Temporary dysphagia is almost universal because of the tight wrap around the LES. The food storage area of the stomach is also decreased. The nurse encourages the patient to eat multiple small meals throughout the day, gradually exploring tolerance to different foods and consistencies. Few foods need to be completely restricted. An upright position is also helpful. Support and encouragement during early feeding attempts are essential.

Many patients also experience temporary or persistent gas bloat from a decreased ability to belch as needed. The nurse teaches the patient to avoid carbonated beverages and gas-producing foods. Patients who swallow a lot of air need to eat and drink slowly and chew food thoroughly. Excess air in the stomach that cannot be relieved by belching produces significant abdominal discomfort. Frequent position changes and ambulation are often effective strategies for clearing air from the GI tract.

A Nursing Care Plan for patients undergoing hiatal hernia repair is found on p. 1268.

### GERONTOLOGICAL CONSIDERATIONS

The muscle weakness that develops in the esophageal hiatus is associated with aging. It is estimated that 60% of the over-60 age group is affected by hiatal hernia. The development of reflux symptoms in older individuals should be investigated and the possibility of hiatal hernia determined. The management, as outlined in the preceding discussion, is applicable to the elderly as well as the younger adult population. Primary considerations relate to the increased risk of surgical complications, particularly respiratory complications, and the need for vigilant postoperative nursing management.

### SPECIAL ENVIRONMENTS FOR CARE

#### Critical Care Management

Critical care management will rarely be needed for patients undergoing hiatal hernia repair. However, high-risk patients, particularly the elderly, can readily experience complications whenever major surgery is undertaken, particularly if a thoracic approach is used. In addition, although rare, esophageal hemorrhage accounts for up to 7% of all massive upper GI bleeds and can be life threatening.

#### Home Care Management

Minimal ongoing care is required after hiatal hernia surgery, but lifting and stair climbing will be restricted until healing is complete. Relatively few dietary restrictions are in place at discharge, but the patient should continue to incorporate measures

*Text continued on p. 1269*

## nursing care plan — Person Undergoing Hiatal Hernia Repair

**DATA** Mr. K. is a 56-year-old businessman with a 5-year history of progressively worsening heartburn. The pain is most severe at night. Recently he has noted the occurrence of regurgitation—sometimes of just "water" and other times of sour, acidic fluid. He has self-treated his problem with liquid antacid, but recently his wife has been urging him to seek medical help because he "always seems to be taking that stuff." He otherwise has an unremarkable medical history and considers himself to be in good health.

Mr. K.'s physician sent him for esophageal studies, which documented severe reflux. A barium swallow under fluoroscopy revealed a large sliding hiatal hernia, which shifted into the thorax with minimal position changes. An esophagoscopy revealed inflamed and minimally ulcerated tissue but no signs of cancer. The size of the hernia and rapid progression of his symptoms caused the physician to recommend surgical repair.

Mr. K. is admitted for hiatal hernia repair via Nissen fundoplication. In addition to the above data, the nursing history identified the following:

- Mr. K. has always been overweight and now carries about 40 extra pounds, concentrated in his abdomen.
- He has an almost 40-year history of cigarette smoking. He has made sincere efforts to cut down but still smokes about one-half pack per day.
- Mr. K. considers his job to be highly stressful. He gets frequent headaches for which he takes aspirin or ibuprofen, usually several days each week.
- He is a moderate social drinker, stating, "Food is my real vice. There is nothing I enjoy more than a big meal." He frequently snacks at night while reading or when relaxing in bed and watching TV.
- He is extremely anxious about the surgery because he has never been hospitalized before.

Collaborative nursing actions before surgery include preparing Mr. K. for his imminent surgery, including the following:

- Clarifying knowledge and expectations concerning surgery.
- Preparing Mr. K. for the expected postoperative care, particularly the importance of respiratory hygiene.
- Implementing preoperative orders and providing Mr. K. with support and reassurance.

Mr. K. is returned to the unit directly after surgery. The surgery was successful and uneventful. He has an NG tube connected to low suction and IVs with boluses of cimetidine and antibiotics. His incision is intact, with a Jackson Pratt drain. The planned abdominal approach was successful, and no chest tubes were used. He is groggy but alert when addressed by name and appears to be in significant pain.

**NURSING DIAGNOSIS** *Ineffective airway clearance related to incisional pain and limited mobility*

| expected patient outcome | nursing interventions | rationale |
|---|---|---|
| Maintains clear breath sounds and effectively coughs up secretions. | Maintain head of bed in a semi-Fowler's position (at least 30 degrees). | Drops diaphragm and lungs to facilitate ventilation. |
| | Perform pulmonary assessment q2-4h. | Assess for atelectasis and retained secretions. |
| | Monitor PCA pump or provide adequate narcotic analgesia. | Adequate pain control facilitates pulmonary hygiene and mobility. |
| | Supervise pulmonary hygiene q4h.<br>Incentive spirometry<br>Chest percussion and vibration<br>Deep breathing q1-2 h | Prevents atelectasis and facilitates expulsion of secretions. |
| | Assist with position changes and ambulation. | Movement and position changes facilitate expulsion of secretions and prevent atelectasis. |
| | Splint incisions for movement and position changes.<br>Medicate ½ hr before getting Mr. K. out of bed. | Pain control facilitates ability to deep breathe and cough. |

**NURSING DIAGNOSIS** *Impaired swallowing related to the functional changes of fundoplication surgery*

| expected patient outcome | nursing interventions | rationale |
|---|---|---|
| Successfully progresses from clear liquids to a normal diet without aspiration or discomfort. | Maintain initial NPO status and monitor patency of NG tube. | NG tube used is very large to support esophageal lumen. |
| | Do not irrigate or reposition the tube. | Stomach must remain decompressed to prevent vomiting. |
| | Report the incidence of any fresh blood in the drainage after 8 hr postop. | Tube movement or vomiting could disrupt the sutures. |
| | Offer frequent oral and nasal hygiene. | |
| | Initiate feedings with 30 ml of clear liquids once peristalsis is reestablished. | Fresh bleeding indicates incisional complications. |
| | Evaluate presence and severity of dysphagia. | The food storage area of the stomach is significantly reduced, and the fundoplication makes swallowing more difficult. |

*Continued*

## Person Undergoing Hiatal Hernia Repair–cont'd

**NURSING DIAGNOSIS** *Impaired swallowing related to the functional changes of fundoplication surgery—cont'd*

| expected patient outcome | nursing interventions | rationale |
|---|---|---|
| | Advance to multiple small feedings.<br>Progress from liquids to solids as patient tolerates.<br>Encourage thorough chewing of small food boluses. | Ability to swallow should improve slowly and steadily. |
| | Teach Mr. K. to avoid air swallowing and gas bloat. | The fundoplication usually makes belching difficult if not impossible. |
| | Avoid carbonated beverages, use of straws, and gas-producing foods.<br>Eat slowly and chew thoroughly.<br>Always eat sitting up.<br>Avoid excessive talking while eating.<br>Ambulate after meals. | Retained air and gas can produce significant abdominal discomfort. |

**NURSING DIAGNOSIS** *Altered health maintenance related to lack of knowledge concerning measures to prevent reflux*

| expected patient outcome | nursing interventions | rationale |
|---|---|---|
| Correctly identifies dietary and lifestyle changes to reduce the incidence of reflux. | Provide Mr. K. with instructions about diet modifications: | Fundoplication reduces the severity of reflux but does not eliminate it. |
| | Follow a low-fat diet and avoid excess tea, coffee, chocolate, and other caffeine-containing foods.<br>Strictly limit or eliminate alcohol intake. | Foods that lower the LES pressure should be avoided. |
| | Eat 4-6 small meals daily.<br>Eat slowly and chew food thoroughly.<br>Remain upright 1-2 hr after meals.<br>Never eat in bed. | Overloading the stomach increases the occurence of reflux. |
| | Avoid evening snacking.<br>Reduce overall body weight.<br>Avoid any food that induces heartburn. | Reflux is increased at night, so stomach needs to be empty at bedtime. |
| | Discuss lifestyle modifications that can reduce the incidence of reflux: | |
| | Enroll in a smoking cessation program. | Smoking decreases the LES pressure significantly and can induce reflux. |
| | Avoid activities such as straining, lifting, and stooping.<br>Avoid constrictive clothing. | Heavy lifting and straining increase abdominal pressure and can induce reflux. |
| | Never sleep flat in bed.<br>Elevate the head on a 6-inch foam wedge for sleep. | Reflux is more common and severe at night in the recumbent position. |
| | Use antacids for occasional heartburn. Report frequent or severe episodes. | Surgical repair rarely completely eliminates the incidence of reflux. |

designed to facilitate swallowing and prevent air accumulation. Even with successful surgery, reflux may continue to some degree, and antireflux diet and lifestyle modifications may need to continue indefinitely. This can be discouraging to the individual who anticipated a complete cure from the procedure.

### COMPLICATIONS

Routine complications of hiatal hernia surgery include persistent dysphagia and gas bloat. In some cases dilation may be necessary to support effective swallowing. The surgery is not always effective, and the individual may still face chronic and debilitating problems with gastroesophageal reflux.

## MOTILITY DISORDERS

Motility disorders of the esophagus are conditions in which the normal motor function of the esophagus is disturbed. The problem may be primary in the esophagus or secondary to another systemic disease. Selected regions or the entire length of the esophagus may be affected. The classic disorder is a failure

**box 39-4** *Motility Disorders Resulting in Dysphagia*

**PRIMARY ESOPHAGEAL DISORDERS**
Achalasia
Esophageal spasm
Effects of tumor or stricture

**NEUROMUSCULAR DISORDERS**
Cerebrovascular accident
Multiple sclerosis
Myasthenia gravis
Amyotrophic lateral sclerosis
Muscular dystrophy
Myopathies
Cranial nerve disease or trauma (V, IX, X)

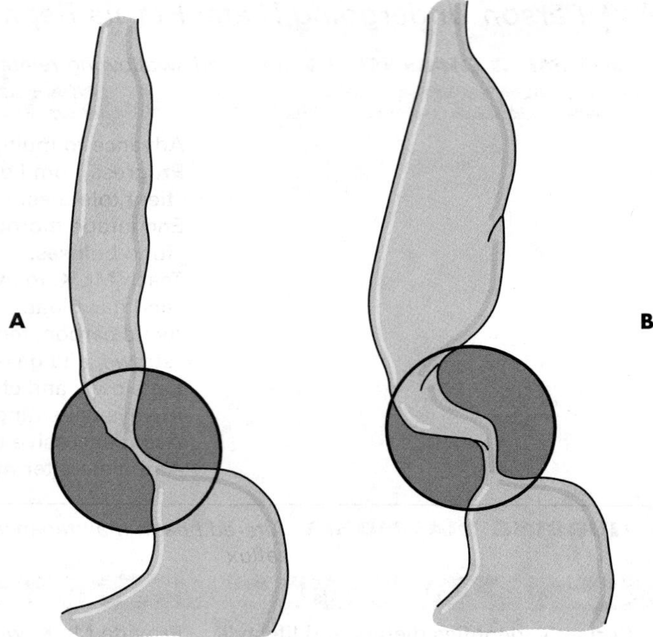

**fig. 39-5** Esophageal achalasia. **A,** Early stage showing narrowing of lower esophagus. **B,** Advanced stage showing dilated middle esophagus.

of the esophageal muscle to relax in synchrony, which can result in mechanical or functional obstruction to food passage. Failure to close adequately after swallowing can also occur, resulting in chronic reflux or regurgitation. Esophageal spasm is a common component of motility disorders, and the spasm is usually intense enough to mimic angina. Achalasia is the predominant primary disorder. Common neuromuscular disorders that can affect esophageal motility are summarized in Box 39-4.

## ACHALASIA

### Etiology/Epidemiology

Achalasia is a primary motility disorder of the esophagus in which the lower esophageal muscles and sphincter fail to relax appropriately in response to swallowing. The cause of the disorder is unknown, although a familial link is possible.[16] Achalasia usually develops in early or middle adulthood, although over one third of cases develop after age 60. Both sexes are affected about equally, and there appear to be no discernible cultural differences in incidence.

### Pathophysiology

Achalasia is theorized to result from a neuromuscular defect that is localized in the inner circular muscle layer of the esophagus. Degeneration of ganglion cells causes both a failure of peristalsis and severe muscle spasm. As the disease progresses, the portion of the esophagus around the constriction becomes dilated and the muscle walls hypertrophy (Figure 39-5). Although the severity of achalasia varies widely, the spasm may be so severe that little or no food can enter the stomach. In extreme cases the esophagus may hold a liter or more of food and fluid above the constricted area. Chronic and progressively worsening dysphagia is the classic symptom. Spasm may be provoked by cold or hot liquids or foods and worsened by stress or overeating. Ninety percent of patients experience some degree of dysphagia or spasm, and 70% experience slight to massive regurgitation of retained food.[16] A foul mouth odor from retention of food in the esophagus may be a chronic problem. The classic "bird's beak" narrowing plus dilation are readily observable with barium studies. Esophageal manometry reveals an elevated resting LES pressure, combined with diminished or absent peristaltic waves.

### Collaborative Care Management

Various categories of medications have been investigated in the attempt to lower esophageal pressure and relax the LES. Anticholinergics, nitrates, and calcium channel blockers have all been used, but none has proven to be of consistent value or effectiveness. Analgesics may be needed when pain is severe.

Esophageal dilation has been a mainstay of treatment for achalasia for centuries. Various techniques have been employed, but pneumatic balloon dilation is currently believed to be the most effective. The procedure involves passing polyurethane balloons on a catheter across the lower esophagus and then inflating the balloon to a predetermined volume. It is repeated as needed. Esophageal tearing is the primary concern, and the risk of perforation is small but serious. The success rate is 60% to 85%, and long-term relief is obtained for many patients.[16] Dilation is an outpatient procedure that can be repeated in 2 to 3 months if needed.

The surgical approach to achalasia involves esophagomyotomy, which uses longitudinal incisions to release the sphincter and facilitate passage of food. A success rate of 90% is reported with the surgery, which may use either a thoracic or an abdominal approach. Antireflux fundoplication may be included, based on surgeon preference. Surgery is usually recommended after two or three dilations have failed to provide lasting relief.

#### *Patient/family education*

Dysphagia is the primary challenge of motility disorders, and the nurse works with the patient and family to explore diet and lifestyle modifications that will best control it. Education begins with careful assessment of the scope and severity of the dysphagia, including the following:

- Swallowing ability with liquids vs. solids
- Response to foods of differing textures and temperatures
- Variability of the dysphagia (intermittent or constant)
- Response to stress, fatigue, and other activities
- Approaches used by the patient to manage the dysphagia and the degree of success

The nurse encourages the individual to experiment with various types and consistencies of foods and meal sizes to evaluate their influence on swallowing. Small, frequent, semisoft meals are usually best tolerated. Warm liquids are recommended, and extremes of temperature should be avoided because they usually worsen the spasm. The nurse also advises the patient to experiment with changing positions during eating. Some individuals can swallow more effectively if they arch their back. Use of the Valsalva's maneuver (bearing down with a closed glottis) while swallowing may help propel food beyond the LES. Nocturnal reflux of retained food and fluid presents a significant risk for aspiration. The nurse instructs the patient to sleep on a foam wedge or with the head of the bed elevated.

Patients who undergo dilation are carefully monitored for complications before discharge. The care after myotomy is similar to that provided after fundoplication (see p. 1267).

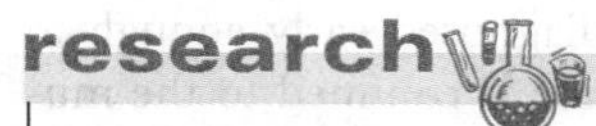

Reference: Chow WH et al: The relation of gastroesophageal reflux disease and its treatment to adenocarcinomas of the esophagus and gastric cardia, *JAMA* 242(6):474, 1995.

This study involved a medical records search of a sample of just under 200 patients newly diagnosed with adenocarcinoma of the esophagus and gastric cardia who were cared for in a large health care plan. Eighty-five percent of the patients were men, 82% were white, and the majority (62%) developed tumors in the gastric cardia versus 38% in the esophagus. The study controlled for smoking history, race, and body weight but still found a significant twofold or greater risk associated with a history of GERD, hiatal hernia, or esophageal ulcer. The risk was greater when the history of reflux was reported to be longer than 5 years.

The use of $H_2$ antagonists was not associated with a risk of cancer, but a large increase in risk was noted among persons taking four or more prescriptions. These findings appear to confirm the belief that long-standing GERD may predispose to adenocarcinoma, usually through the gradual process of dysplasia and cellular changes. The use of the standard medications does not appear to increase the risk of cancer, but cases that require polypharmacy, usually indicating refractory disease, have a sharply increased risk. The risk is believed to be primarily related to the presence of long-standing severe disease rather than the use of particular medications.

## ESOPHAGEAL CARCINOMA

### ETIOLOGY

Both benign and malignant tumors occur in the esophagus. Benign tumors, usually leiomyomas, are extremely rare and usually asymptomatic; they require no intervention unless symptoms necessitate local excision.

Malignant tumors of the esophagus are not common, but they assume increased importance because of their virulence. Esophageal cancer ranks twenty-fourth in the United States in incidence but thirteenth in mortality. Worldwide it has demonstrated variations in incidence within and between countries and regions, leading to the belief that environmental factors play a major role in its etiology.[10]

In the United States alcohol intake and tobacco use have been identified as the primary risk factors for esophageal cancer, and there is a clear dose-response and duration-of-use relationship.[18] Heavy alcohol use increases the risk threefold even without the synergistic effect of smoking, which can drive the incidence to six times that of the rest of the population.[10] The carcinogenic effects are clearly cumulative because the cancer typically appears in persons between 60 and 70 years of age. In certain areas of the world where esophageal cancer is common, the development of the tumor is linked to high levels of nitrosamines and other contaminants in the soil and foods. Diets that are chronically inadequate in fresh fruits, vegetables, vitamins, and certain proteins are also implicated.

The incidence of esophageal cancer is also high in selected regions of the world where the major risk factors do not apply, particularly in regions of Asia. The effects of opium smoking and the practice of consuming extremely hot beverages are also under investigation. The effects of chronic GERD and the development of Barrett's epithelium are also being studied (see the Research Box).

### EPIDEMIOLOGY

Despite statistically significant annual increases in the incidence of cancer of the esophagus over the past several decades, particularly among the African American population, the tumor still accounts for less than 2% of all newly diagnosed cancers and 7% of gastrointestinal tract cancers in the United States.[15]

However, low incidence statistics for esophageal cancer are unique to the United States and the Western world. Localized areas of China, the former Soviet Union, Iran, and southern Africa have such high incidence that 25% of all cancer deaths can be attributed to cancer of the esophagus in some regions.[10]

The disease typically affects men between the ages of 50 and 80 years. It occurs in men four times as often as in women and in African Americans four times as often as in whites.

The most disturbing epidemiological finding has been the steady rise in the incidence of adenocarcinoma, which has previously been rare. This cancer now accounts for between 20% and 40% of all cases and does not appear to be linked to the classic risk factors.[3,15] It is related instead to the presence of Barrett's epithelium, which forms in response to chronic reflux.

Cancer of the esophagus is almost always fatal, and this is particularly true in the African American population. The 5-year survival rate is less than 10%, and less than 5% of all cases are cured.[18] The median survival time after diagnosis is

10 months. The tumor is rarely diagnosed early enough to allow for effective treatment. Disease is confined to the mucosa or submucosa in less than 10% of cases.

## PATHOPHYSIOLOGY

Tumors may develop at any point along the length of the esophagus, but the majority occur in the middle and lower two thirds of the esophagus. Squamous cell tumors have typically predominated. They tend to develop in the middle third and are clearly related to the risk factors of smoking and alcohol use. Adenocarcinomas represent the remaining minority of tumors. These tend to develop in the lower third of the esophagus and may evolve from the Barrett's epithelium.

Barrett's epithelium is an acquired condition. The tissue changes occur in response to acid irritation over a period of months to 1 to 2 years. Barrett's epithelium is typically present for 20 to 30 years before malignant change occurs, but its presence increases the risk of cancer from 30 to 400 times.[1,3]

Esophageal tumors of all types appear to emerge as part of an initially slow process that begins with benign tissue changes. Local growth of the tumor is rapid, however, and early spread is common because of the rich lymphatic supply found in the esophagus. Tumors are characteristically intraluminal and ulcerating, with a tendency to encircle the esophageal wall, as well as extend up or down the length.

Spread of the carcinoma is by local invasion or through the bloodstream or lymphatics. Neoplasms of the upper and middle esophagus may extend into the pulmonary system and those of the lower esophagus into the diaphragm, vertebrae, or heart. Metastasis is present in about 80% of esophageal cancers at the time of diagnosis.

Ninety percent of the circumference of the esophagus is commonly involved before symptoms develop, and early diagnosis is rare. Tumors of less than 10 cm are considered to be small. Patients typically complain of symptoms related to reflux, dysphagia, or obstruction.

Pulmonary complications such as fistula formation or aspiration are common, and complete obstruction is inevitable without successful therapy. Box 39-5 summarizes the common clinical manifestations of esophageal cancer.

## COLLABORATIVE CARE MANAGEMENT

### Diagnostic Tests

The barium swallow with fluoroscopy is the primary diagnostic tool. Large masses will be clearly outlined. Endoscopy allows for direct visual inspection and biopsy for cytologic analysis. Computed tomography scans may be employed to evaluate the extent of the tumor.

### Medications

Primary treatment of esophageal cancer increasingly includes combinations of various antineoplastic agents. Chemotherapy is most effective when combined with radiation, surgery, or both and is commonly given before surgery to debulk a tumor. Chemotherapy plus radiation is a viable treatment alternative for palliation that preserves the integrity of the esophagus.

**box 39-5** *clinical manifestations*

***Esophageal Cancer***

- Early disease is largely asymptomatic
- Gradually progressive dysphagia
  - Usually not present until >60% of diameter is obstructed
  - Progresses typically from solids to liquids
  - Continuous, not intermittent
- Odynophagia—typically a steady, dull substernal pain
- Regurgitation—foul breath from retained food in esophagus
- Heartburn
- Anorexia
- Weight loss—up to 40 lb in 2-3 mo is common

### Treatments

Treatment decisions are based on the location and size of the tumor, degree of metastasis, and the individual's health status. Nonsurgical options are usually selected when the individual is unable or unwilling to undergo radical surgery. They focus on palliation of symptoms. Options include radiation therapy, dilation of strictures, and prosthesis insertion, as well as chemotherapy.

#### *Radiation therapy*

Radiation therapy is the treatment of choice for palliation. It reduces tumor size and gives consistent long-term symptom relief, but it may lead to debilitating stricture or stenosis, because esophageal tissue is extremely sensitive to radiation. The treatment is spread over 6 to 8 weeks to minimize the edema and epithelial desquamation, which often lead to acute esophagitis and odynophagia. Anorexia, nausea, and vomiting may also occur. Combining radiation and chemotherapy is thought to improve the results. Various protocols are being researched.

Palliative treatment of the tumor may also be accomplished by use of the neodymium:yttrium-aluminum-garnet (Nd:YAG) laser, which vaporizes a part of the tumor to open the esophageal lumen. The treatment is performed endoscopically and offers substantial relief of obstruction in over 90% of cases.[7]

#### *Dilation*

Esophageal dilation is performed as needed throughout therapy to relieve dysphagia resulting from either tumor obstruction or radiation stricture. The malignant esophageal tumor may be dilated safely by skilled physicians, and the treatment is employed as needed to preserve swallowing (see discussion under Achalasia, p. 1270).

#### *Prosthesis insertion*

A semirigid prosthesis may be inserted into the esophagus to bypass an obstruction or fistula. The procedure preserves swallowing and a patent esophagus, but it carries the significant risk of aspiration, dislodgement, or esophageal perforation, which occur in about 20% of those treated. The prosthesis disrupts the function of the LES and permits free reflux of gastric contents.

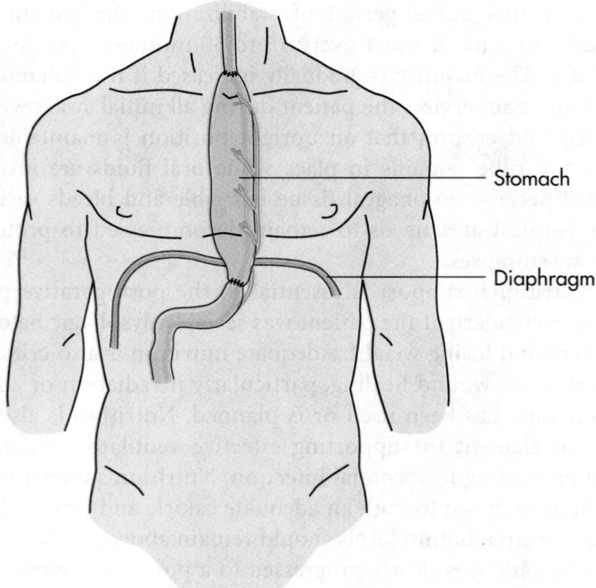


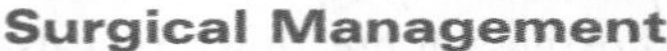

fig. 39-6 Esophagogastrostomy for esophageal cancer.

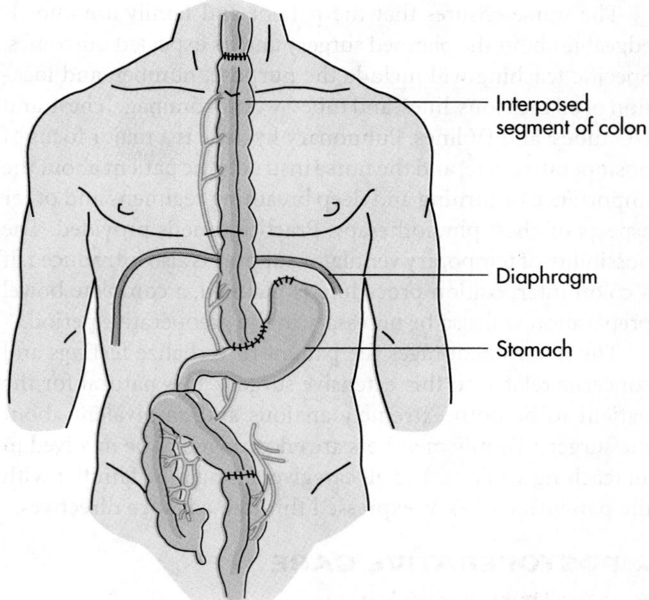


fig. 39-7 Esophagectomy with colon interposition.

### Surgical Management

Radical surgery is the only definitive treatment for esophageal cancer, and it is the treatment of choice for otherwise healthy individuals. The surgeries are extensive, with a high mortality rate, especially for patients with concurrent health problems. Disease survival rates are extremely low, even with radical procedures. Subtotal or total esophagectomy is usually required. Although several procedural options exist, the preferred surgery is the esophagogastrostomy, in which the diseased portion of the esophagus is removed, and the cervical stump is anastomosed to the stomach, which is drawn up into the thorax through the esophageal hiatus (Figure 39-6). This procedure is the simplest, but it still involves both laparotomy and thoracotomy incisions. If the tumor also involves the stomach, the surgeon may perform a colon interposition by substituting a portion of the right or left colon for the esophagus (Figure 39-7).

In addition to the usual complex surgical risks of shock, hemorrhage, and infection, these procedures also create a serious risk of leakage at the site of anastomosis, particularly with colon interposition. Anastomosis leakage occurs in up to 20% of cases.[18] Even when surgical healing is successful, the patient remains at serious risk for reflux and aspiration from the elimination of the sphincter protection of the LES.

### Diet

Maintaining adequate nutrition as the disease progresses is the primary consideration. The diet is modified as needed as dysphagia worsens. Tube or gastrostomy feedings and short-course hyperalimentation may all be needed at some point in the disease process.

### Activity

The individual is encouraged to remain as active as the condition and treatment allow. Positioning and activity restrictions are important for individuals experiencing frequent reflux or regurgitation. The nurse teaches the patient to remain upright for several hours after meals; to avoid all bending, stooping, or lifting; and to never lie down in a flat position. The head should always be elevated at least 30 to 45 degrees.

### Referrals

In some settings the nurse assumes responsibility for making referrals to other services. Nutritional support services are commonly needed to plan feeding approaches for the patient and to ensure adequate nutrients. Patients also commonly need significant assistance at home, particularly after radical surgery, and the nurse coordinates these referrals as part of the discharge planning.

## NURSING MANAGEMENT OF THE PATIENT WITH ESOPHAGOGASTROSTOMY SURGERY

### ■ PREOPERATIVE CARE

The duration of preoperative preparation is largely determined by the patient's nutritional status. Nutritional support is provided as needed via tube feedings or hyperalimentation. Most of this preparation will take place in the home setting. Intake and output, total daily calories, and body weight are all carefully monitored. The nurse encourages the patient to perform frequent mouth care to reduce the risk of postoperative infection, because the patient may be regurgitating retained food particles, blood, or pus from the tumor. Mouthwashes can help control foul mouth odors and make oral intake more palatable. Dental problems will also usually be corrected before surgery, particularly if radiation treatment is planned.

The nurse ensures that the patient and family are knowledgeable about the planned surgery and its expected outcomes. Specific teaching will include the purpose, number, and location of all incisions, lines, and tubes; wound drainage, chest, and NG tubes; and IV lines. Pulmonary hygiene is a major focus of postoperative care, and the nurse instructs the patient about the importance of turning and deep breathing regimens and other aspects of chest physiotherapy. Practice time is provided. The possibility of temporary ventilator support is also introduced. If a colon interposition procedure is planned, a complete bowel preparation will also be necessary in the preoperative period.

The nurse encourages the patient to verbalize feelings and concerns related to this extensive surgery. It is natural for the patient to be both extremely anxious and ambivalent about the surgery. Family members are encouraged to be involved in all teaching sessions, and all caregivers should be familiar with the patient's wishes as expressed through advance directives.

## ■ POSTOPERATIVE CARE

### Protecting the Airway

The patient receives routine but meticulous postoperative care, because the extensive nature of the surgery increases the risk of serious complications. Respiratory care is the highest priority. The patient typically remains intubated for the first 24 hours. Respiratory assessment is documented every 1 to 2 hours, and vigorous turning, deep breathing, coughing, and chest physiotherapy routines are used. Tracheal suctioning is avoided if possible. Adequate analgesia is essential to the achievement of respiratory goals. The nurse assists the patient to adequately splint major incisions for turning and coughing and ensures that appropriate narcotic analgesia is being provided, usually through patient-controlled analgesia (PCA) or epidural analgesia, which minimizes respiratory depression.

The patient is placed in a semi-Fowler's or high Fowler's position to support ventilation and prevent regurgitation and reflux. Supplemental oxygen is administered routinely, and blood gases or $O_2$ saturation is monitored. The nurse ensures the patency of the chest tubes and water seal drainage system.

The multiple incisions and drains significantly increase the potential for problems with wound healing. Anastomosis leakage is a serious complication that can compromise the airway and pulmonary gas exchange. The risk is highest 5 to 9 days after surgery. Prompt identification of leakage is essential. The nurse monitors for signs of inflammation, fever, or fluid accumulation. Pulmonary edema is a common problem, and the patient may be kept somewhat dry. Early symptoms of shock, such as tachycardia, tachypnea, or restlessness, may be the first warning signs.

### Promoting Adequate Nutrition

The patient is usually allowed nothing by mouth for 4 to 5 days until GI motility is fully reestablished. The NG tube is carefully secured and monitored frequently to prevent movement or dislodgement, which might disrupt the sutures at the anastomosis sites. The tube is *not* irrigated or repositioned. The initial NG drainage is bloody, but it should gradually resume a normal greenish-yellow color by the end of the first postoperative day. The continued presence of blood might indicate oozing at the suture line. Frequent oral hygiene is provided.

After this initial period of stabilization, the patient is given 3 to 5 ml of water every 15 to 30 minutes throughout the day. The quantity is gradually increased if it is tolerated. The nurse supervises the patient during all initial swallowing efforts and ensures that an upright position is maintained. The NG tube remains in place while oral fluids are introduced because esophageal tissue is friable and bleeds easily. The surgical area needs to remain decompressed to protect the anastomoses.

Nutritional support is essential in the postoperative period, particularly if the patient was severely dysphagic before surgery and losing weight. Adequate nutrition is also critical for effective wound healing, particularly if radiation or chemotherapy has been used or is planned. Nutrition is also a critical element in supporting effective ventilator weaning and preventing nosocomial infection. Nutrition support will include attention to both an adequate calorie and protein intake. Serum albumin levels should remain above 3.5.

The patient is slowly progressed to a pureed or semisolid diet if problems do not develop. The nurse assists the patient to carefully determine the amount and type of foods and fluids that can be safely and comfortably swallowed. Small meals are essential because the food storage area of the stomach is drastically decreased. Initially patients may experience a feeling of fullness in the chest or shortness of breath with meals. Adjusting meal size and progressing slowly usually alleviates these problems. The process of gradually resuming oral nutrition will continue into the postdischarge period and requires patience. Calorie counts and daily weights assist in the ongoing evaluation of the patient's nutritional status. The nurse will also stress the importance of eating only in an upright sitting position because the loss of the LES leaves the patient vulnerable to reflux aspiration.

### Promoting Coping

Despite the radical surgery, the patient with esophageal cancer still has a terminal illness and dramatically shortened life expectancy. Considerable psychological support is provided to the individual patient and family members in their efforts to cope with the diagnosis, prognosis, and physical limitations of the disease. Realistic planning is important, because the patient's condition will inevitably worsen. The nurse encourages the patient and family to talk about the situation together, make realistic plans, and seek out supports available in the community.

Guidelines for care of the patient undergoing esophagogastrostomy are summarized in the accompanying Guidelines for Care box on p. 1275.

## GERONTOLOGICAL CONSIDERATIONS

Cancer of the esophagus is usually identified in late middle age or in the elderly population. These patients have a high incidence of chronic health problems, which makes the risks of radical surgery more extensive. Postoperative complications are both more common and more severe. These patients are also less likely to have family and support networks to help them manage their care after discharge. The nurse must be vigilant in assessing the need for postdischarge assistance and initiating needed referrals.

guidelines for care

### The Person Undergoing Esophagogastrostomy

**Preoperative Care**

1. Encourage improved nutritional status
   a. High-protein, high-calorie diet if oral diet is possible.
   b. Total parenteral nutrition may be necessary for severe dysphagia or obstruction
2. Assist with frequent oral hygiene to minimize breath odor
3. Teach appropriate techniques for effective deep breathing and coughing and the importance of frequent pulmonary hygiene; have patient demonstrate respiratory exercises and how to splint the incision for coughing
4. Teach patient about all tubes and drains that will be used postop and how surgical pain will be managed

**Postoperative Care**

1. Promote good pulmonary ventilation
   a. Hourly deep breathing and coughing if needed
   b. Incentive spirometry and chest physical therapy as ordered
   c. Auscultate lung fields q2h (avoid tracheal suctioning if possible)
2. Maintain chest drainage system as prescribed
3. Provide for adequate analgesia by PCA or epidural catheter; monitor respiratory and neurological response
4. Maintain gastric drainage system
   a. Small amounts of blood may drain from nasogastric tube for 6 to 12 hr after surgery
   b. Do not disturb nasogastric tube (to prevent traction on suture line)
5. Maintain nutrition
   a. Start clear fluids at frequent intervals when oral intake is permitted
   b. Introduce soft foods gradually, and slowly progress to several small meals of bland foods
6. Prevent aspiration if LES is removed or disrupted
   a. Always raise the head of the bed for swallowing food or liquid
   b. Head of the bed must be elevated for sleeping
   c. Bending or stooping should be avoided
   d. Keep suction apparatus available at the bedside

## SPECIAL ENVIRONMENTS FOR CARE

### Critical Care Management

The radical surgery undertaken to treat cancer of the esophagus carries an extremely high risk of complication, particularly if the patient is frail and has chronic diseases affecting the cardiovascular or pulmonary systems. Critical care management may be necessary while the patient is intubated and ventilated or for close monitoring of hemodynamic stability. It may also be needed if the patient experiences severe anastomosis leakage in the postoperative period.

### Home Care Management

Most patients with cancer of the esophagus require a significant amount of assistance after discharge. Even without major postoperative complications, the patient will need to deal with ongoing respiratory care, wound healing concerns, and nutritional support. The care initiated in the hospital continues after discharge, and both the patient and family need to be well informed about its components. Essential concerns include pulmonary hygiene, which may include chest physiotherapy. Any surgery that removes or disrupts the LES necessitates constant care with positioning to protect the airway and prevent reflux or regurgitation. No anatomical protection remains, and the risk of aspiration is constant. Wound healing also remains a concern, and the incisions need to be inspected regularly for signs of infection. Nutritional recovery is ongoing. The patient and family will slowly explore the patient's range of food tolerance to meet nutrient needs. Home preparations of milk shakes or other supplements may be used to support nutrient intake. The family may also need to learn to manage tube feedings or hyperalimentation. The nurse encourages the family to seek out and use supports such as those available from the American Cancer Society and makes referral to community home care agencies as needed. Hospice referrals may be appropriate for patients with later-stage disease.

## COMPLICATIONS

Esophageal cancer is commonly a terminal illness, and complications are expected. Tumor regrowth may cause recurrent dysphagia and obstruction, and dilation may be needed for recurrent dysphagia. Weight loss may persist. The high risk of aspiration from regurgitation makes pulmonary complications common. Tumor regrowth, invasion, and metastasis can create problems with chronic pain, bleeding, and fistula development.

### critical thinking QUESTIONS

1. Mrs. Frost is a 79-year-old woman who has come to the medical clinic with a 6-month history of heartburn, which has been steadily increasing in both frequency and severity. She also reports frequent regurgitation of acidic fluid into the mouth. She has self-medicated with antacids, but they are no longer controlling the discomfort. She is 5 feet 4 inches tall and weighs 180 pounds. She is an avid gardener and spends long hours weeding and pruning. She laughs as you ask her to put on a gown for a physical examination, saying that it will take a few moments to get out of her corset.
   a. What specific factors in Mrs. Frost's presentation will you target to teach her how to better control esophageal reflux?
   b. What other data do you need to improve your understanding of her situation?
2. Ms. Perry is a 33-year-old mother of five who has come to the clinic for a prenatal examination for her sixth pregnancy. She is a single mother on Medicaid and does not have family in the area. As part of the oral examination you note that her teeth are in poor repair, her gums are reddened and receding, and there is a smoker's patch leukoplakia on her dorsal tongue surface, plus an ulcer on her inner cheek near a broken tooth.
   a. What specific assessment data do you need to complete your understanding of the situation?

b. Review the *Healthy People 2000* guidelines for oral health. What services are available in your community, and which services might be lacking to enable a client such as Ms. Perry to meet those goals?

3 Design a nursing research study to test the effectiveness of the lifestyle modifications recommended for patients with GERD.

## chapter SUMMARY

### DENTAL DISORDERS

- Oral health can be promoted by good nutrition, good oral hygiene, fluoridation of water supplies, regular dental examinations and care, and avoidance of alcohol and tobacco use.

### MOUTH INFECTIONS

- Common infections of the mouth include aphthous stomatitis (canker sore), herpes stomatitis (cold sore, fever blister), acute necrotizing ulcerative gingivitis, thrush, and parotitis.
- Oral hygiene is an essential part of the treatment of mouth infections and includes brushing and flossing, rinsing with mouthwashes, and modifying the diet to reduce irritation.

### CANCER OF THE MOUTH

- Contributing factors to cancer of the mouth include alcohol and heavy smoking.
- Carcinoma of the mouth can occur on the lips, the tongue and floor of the mouth, and in the salivary glands. Treatment is by surgery, radiation, or both.
- After surgery for oral cancer, the patient may have problems with verbal communication, eating, and mouth discomfort.

### PROBLEMS OF THE ESOPHAGUS

- Common esophageal disorders include gastroesophageal reflux, hiatal hernia, cancer, and motility disorders. Heartburn and dysphagia are common symptoms of esophageal disorders.
- Gastroesophageal reflux may result from an incompetent LES, obesity, or hiatal hernia. Heartburn is a major symptom. Management includes medications (antacids, histamine receptor antagonists, prokinetic agents, and proton pump inhibitors), lifestyle modifications (including sleeping with the head of the bed elevated and avoiding activities that increase intraabdominal pressure), diet changes (including avoiding fatty foods, caffeine, and chocolate), and hiatal hernia repair. Relapse is common.
- The two types of hiatal hernias are sliding and paraesophageal. They are usually asymptomatic but may cause problems with reflux.
- Hiatal hernias may be treated surgically if symptoms are severe. There are a variety of procedures, but all of them involve some form of fundoplication (wrapping the stomach fundus around the distal esophagus to reinforce the LES).
- Motility disorders create dysphagia and may cause spasm. Achalasia is a common primary motility disorder. Treatment includes dilation and myotomy.
- Risk factors for cancer of the esophagus include smoking and long-term, high-dose alcohol intake. Any person with dysphagia should consult a physician.
- Cancer of the esophagus has a poor prognosis, because metastasis is usually present when the diagnosis is made. Treatment is by surgery, radiation, and chemotherapy.
- Postoperative care for esophageal cancer includes promotion of pulmonary ventilation, maintenance of drainage systems, nutritional support, and monitoring wound healing.

## References

1. Bonelli L, GOSPE: Barrett's esophagus: results of a multicentric survey, *Endoscopy* 25(suppl):652, 1993.
2. Brightman VJ: Diseases of the tongue. In Lynch MA et al, editors: *Burket's oral medicine: diagnosis and treatment,* ed 9, Philadelphia, 1994, JB Lippincott.
3. Cameron AJ: Epidemiologic studies and the development of Barrett's esophagus, *Endoscopy* 25(suppl):635, 1993.
4. Campbell AD, Ferrara BE: Toupet partial fundoplication, *AORN J* 57(3):671, 1993.
5. Chow WH, et al: The relation of gastroesophageal reflux disease and its treatment to adenocarcinomas of the esophagus and gastric cardia, *JAMA* 274(6):474, 1995.
6. Coleman GC, Nelson JF: *Principles of oral diagnosis,* St Louis, 1993, Mosby.
7. Ellis P, Cunningham D: Management of carcinomas of the upper gastrointestinal tract, *BMJ* 308:834, 1994.
8. Epstein JB: Oral cancer. In Lynch MA et al, editors: *Burket's oral medicine: diagnosis and treatment,* ed 9, Philadelphia, 1994, JB Lippincott.
9. Greenberg MS: Salivary gland disease. In Lynch MA et al, editors: *Burket's oral medicine: diagnosis and treatment,* ed 9, Philadelphia, 1994, JB Lippincott.
10. Greenwald P, Kelloff G, Kalagher S, McDonald S: Research studies on chemoprevention of esophageal cancer at the United States National Cancer Institute, *Endoscopy* 25(suppl):617, 1993.
11. Haubrich WS: Diaphragmatic hernias. In Haubrich WS et al, editors: *Gastroenterology (Bockus),* vol 1, ed 5, Philadelphia, 1995, JB Lippincott.
12. Klinkenberg-Knol EC, Festen HPM, Meuwissen SGM: Pharmacological management of gastro-esophageal reflux disease, *Drugs* 49(5): 695, 1995.
13. Marshall JB: Severe gastroesophageal reflux disease, *Postgrad Med* 97(5):98, 1995.
14. Morton LS, Fromkes JJ: Gastroesophageal reflux disease: diagnosis and medical therapy, *Geriatrics* 48(3):60, 1993.
15. Munoz N: Epidemiologic aspects of esophageal cancer, *Endoscopy* 25(suppl):609, 1993.
16. Ouyang A, Cohen S: Motility disorders of the esophagus. In Haubrich WS et al, editors: *Gastroenterology (Bockus),* vol 1, ed 5, Philadelphia, 1995, JB Lippincott.
17. Robinson M: Gastroesophogeal reflux disease, *Postgrad Med* 95(2): 88, 1994.
18. Sideranko S: Esophagogastrectomy, *Crit Care Nurs Clin North Am* 5(1):177, 1993.
19. Stengel JM, Dirado R: Laparoscopic Nissen fundoplication to treat gastroesophageal reflux, *AORN J* 61(3):483, 1995.
20. Sterling TD, Rosenbaum WL, Weinkam JJ: Analysis of the relationship between smokeless tobacco and cancer based on data from the National Mortality Followback Survey, *J Clin Epidemiol* 45(3):223, 1992.
21. Department of Health and Human Services, Public Health Service: *Healthy people 2000: midcourse review and 1995 revisions,* Washington, DC, 1996, DHHS.
22. Vigneswaran N, Tilashalski K, Rodu B, Cole P: Tobacco use and cancer, *Oral Surg Oral Med Oral Pathol* 80(2):178, 1995.

chapter 40

# MANAGEMENT OF PERSONS WITH Problems of the Stomach and Duodenum

JUDITH K. SANDS

## objectives

*After studying this chapter, the learner should be able to:*

1. Discuss the etiology and epidemiology of common problems affecting the stomach and duodenum.
2. Describe the mechanisms of mucosal defense and breakdown and the roles of *Helicobacter pylori,* nonsteroidal antiinflammatory drug administration, and other risk factors in the development of peptic ulcer disease.
3. Compare the advantages and disadvantages of the medical and surgical management of peptic ulcer disease and its complications.
4. Describe appropriate nursing interventions for the management of peptic ulcer disease and its complications.
5. Explain the role of surgery in the management of morbid obesity.
6. Outline the medical and nursing management of gastric cancer.
7. Identify the essential nursing care associated with gastric surgery.

Problems related to the stomach are extremely common in American society. Many of these problems are episodic in nature and can easily be managed through temporary diet modification or self-medication in the home setting. Other stomach problems require aggressive medical or surgical intervention. Peptic ulcer disease and its complications are the primary foci of this chapter, but it also discusses the management of gastric cancer and the surgical management of severe obesity.

## GASTRITIS AND DYSPEPSIA

The terms *gastritis* and *dyspepsia* are used in a highly nonspecific manner by both laypersons and health care professionals. Gastritis refers to a diffuse or localized response of the gastric mucosa to injury or infection. It is a histological diagnosis.[33] The term *dyspepsia,* on the other hand, refers to a symptom complex of fullness, heartburn, bloating, and possibly nausea that is typically experienced after eating and may not be accompanied by any histological changes in the stomach or duodenum.[33] Dyspepsia affects millions of people on a regular or occasional basis. It can occur with specific clinical problems such as gastroesophageal reflux disease (GERD) (see Chapter 39), gastritis, peptic ulcer disease, or gastric cancer; but it can also be present when there is no demonstrable evidence of any underlying pathology. Dyspepsia syndrome is described in Box 40-1.

### ACUTE GASTRITIS

#### Etiology/Epidemiology

Acute gastritis is a short-term inflammatory process that can be initiated by numerous factors such as excess alcohol ingestion, drug effects, severe physical stress or trauma, ingestion of caustic or noxious substances, radiation exposure, and bacterial contamination of food or water with the toxins of organisms such as salmonella or staphylococci. Acute gastritis is predominantly an erosive process and is believed to be responsible for up to 10% to 30% of all episodes of gastrointestinal (GI) bleeding.

#### Pathophysiology

Acute gastritis develops when the protective mechanisms of the mucosa are overwhelmed by the presence of bacteria or irritating substances. Mucus is a poor protector against chemical injury. Regeneration of the gastric mucosa after injury is both prompt and efficient, however, and the disorder usually is self-limiting once the irritating agent is removed. Common symptoms include anorexia, nausea and vomiting, abdominal cramping or diarrhea, epigastric pain, and fever. Painless GI bleeding may occur and is more likely if the person uses aspirin or nonsteroidal antiinflammatory drugs (NSAIDs) regularly.

#### Collaborative Care Management

Most cases of acute gastritis are managed by removing the causative agent and supporting the patient while the mucosa heals itself. The person is usually put on nothing-by-mouth (NPO) status to support healing of the mucosa and then slowly advanced to liquids and a return to a normal diet. Antacids and histamine 2 ($H_2$) receptor antagonists may be administered to reduce acid secretion and increase comfort. Temporary intravenous fluid and electrolyte replacement may be indicated in severe cases, and the patient is monitored carefully for signs of bleeding.

##### *Patient/family education*

Bacterial food-borne illness has serious public health ramifications, and the nurse will provide preventive health teaching concerning safe food handling and preparation. The public

**box 40-1** *Dyspepsia Syndrome*

A syndrome of chronic dyspepsia is one of the most common GI complaints encountered in primary practice. The person experiences persistent or recurrent discomfort centered in the upper abdomen. There is no evidence of structural or biochemical abnormality, and the cause is unknown. Research findings to date indicate that individuals with dyspepsia syndrome have

- Normal rates of acid secretion
- Postprandial hypomotility and delayed gastric emptying in 25% to 50% of cases; cause unknown
- Increased sensitivity to gastric distention; cause unknown
- No identified link with life stress or personality profiles

SYMPTOMS

- Epigastric discomfort or pain
- Feeling of fullness or flatulence
- Early satiety
- Bloating or nausea

TREATMENT

There is no approved drug treatment.

- Histamine receptor antagonists may be used for ulcer-like pain.
- Antacids may be used for occasional heartburn or bloating symptoms.
- Prokinetic agents (cisapride [Propulsid]) are helpful in many cases.
- Diet and lifestyle changes are suggested:
  - Reducing dietary fat (fat prolongs digestion and may worsen bloating)
  - Eating smaller, more frequent meals
  - Avoiding foods that precipitate symptoms

health concerns related to food-borne illness are reflected in the *Healthy People 2000* goals related to food safety, which are summarized in Box 40-2. General measures to prevent food-related illness are presented in Box 40-3. The nurse will suggest that the patient resume a normal diet slowly, using only foods that minimize symptoms. A pattern of four to six small meals a day may initially be better tolerated. The nurse will also encourage the patient to avoid irritating foods, alcohol use, and smoking until recovery is complete. Follow-up with a health care provider is strongly recommended if the symptoms persist.

## CHRONIC GASTRITIS

### Etiology/Epidemiology

Chronic gastritis is a separate clinical entity that can be further subdivided into type A and type B. Its presence is usually a sign of some underlying disease process.

Type A is believed to be autoimmune in nature and involves all of the acid-secreting gastric tissue, particularly the tissue in the fundus. Circulating antibodies are produced that attack the gastric parietal cells and eventually may cause pernicious anemia from loss of the intrinsic factor.

The vast majority of cases are type B. Type B chronic gastritis is caused primarily by infection with *Helicobacter pylori* bacteria. The infection is usually acquired from contaminated food and water, and fecal-oral transmission is theorized. The prevalence of *H. pylori* infection increases with age. Less than 10% of persons in the United States are estimated to be infected with *H. pylori* at age 20, but at least 50% to 60% are infected by age 60.[35] The prevalence of *H. pylori* infection is inversely proportional to socioeconomic status, and the infection rate is nearly 100% by young adulthood in developing countries.[35] *Helicobacter pylori* plays a pivotal role in the development of peptic ulcer disease (discussed later in this chapter).

**box 40-2** Healthy People 2000 *Goals Related to Food Safety*

1. Reduce infections caused by key food-borne pathogens.
2. Reduce outbreaks of infections due to *Salmonella enteritidis* to fewer than 25 outbreaks yearly.
3. Increase to at least 75% the proportion of households in which principal food preparers routinely refrain from leaving perishable food out of the refrigerator for over 2 hours and wash cutting boards and utensils with soap after contact with raw meat and poultry.
4. Extend to at least 70% the proportion of states and territories that have implemented model food codes for institutional food operations and to at least 70% the proportion that have adopted the new uniform food protection code ("Unicode") that sets recommended standards for regulation of all food operations.

From US Department of Health and Human Services, Public Health Service: *Healthy People 2000: midcourse review and 1995 revisions,* Washington, DC, 1996, DHHS.

### Pathophysiology

Type A chronic gastritis results in a decrease in gastric secretions from an autoimmune attack on the parietal cells. The gastric glands gradually atrophy, and the mucosa thins and deteriorates. The disease is commonly nonerosive in nature and is differentiated by the histological appearance of the gastric mucosa. The progressive decline in parietal cell function leads steadily toward pernicious anemia. There are usually no symptoms until the destructive process is well advanced.

Type B chronic gastritis involves primarily the fundus and antrum of the stomach. There is less reduction in acid secretion, gastrin levels remain normal, and vitamin $B_{12}$ absorption is rarely impaired. As the condition progresses the mucosa increasingly atrophies, and acid secretion is reduced.

The diagnosis of type B chronic gastritis can be confirmed only by histological evaluation of a biopsy specimen. The diagnosis is challenging because the endoscopic appearance of the mucosa does not necessarily correlate with the histology. The diagnosis cannot be made on the basis of symptoms alone because most persons are asymptomatic after the initial acute infection, and those who experience symptoms report only the symptoms of general dyspepsia (see Box 40-1). There also does not appear to be any causal relationship between the presence of dyspepsia and the severity of the disease.[35]

**box 40-3** *Prevention of Food Poisoning*

1. Wash hands before handling food.
2. Do not thaw foods on the kitchen counter.
3. Keep meats, fish, poultry, mayonnaise, and cream-filled foods refrigerated.
4. Wash hands and utensils after contact with raw meat or poultry.
5. Never leave perishable foods unrefrigerated for more than 2 hours—less in hot weather.
6. Use a meat thermometer when cooking large pieces of meat, especially pork.
7. Stuff poultry immediately before roasting (warm stuffing is a good medium for bacterial growth).
8. Avoid slow cooling of meat and poultry.
9. Freeze or refrigerate leftovers promptly.
10. Can low-acid foods (foods other than tomatoes or fruits) under pressure to prevent botulism.
11. Discard any can that bulges.

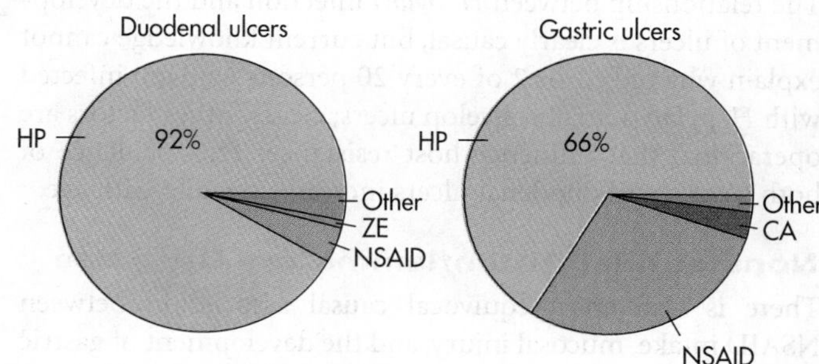


**fig. 40-1** The relationship of *Helicobacter pylori* infection to the development of peptic ulcer diease.

### Collaborative Care Management

Treatment of type A chronic gastritis focuses on management of the underlying systemic disease. Vitamin $B_{12}$ is administered if pernicious anemia occurs. The treatment of type B is less clear. Although caused almost exclusively by *H. pylori* infection, treatment of the infection is rarely recommended today unless the patient is extremely symptomatic or develops ulcers. Treatment of *H. pylori* infection is evolving rapidly. It currently involves the use of combinations of antibacterial agents to eradicate the organism. Symptomatic patients may also be treated with acid-reducing drugs, antacids, and sucralfate. Drug treatment of *H. pylori* is discussed under Peptic Ulcer Disease later in this chapter.

#### Patient/family education

The nurse instructs the patient in the safe use of any prescribed medications and how to manage expected side effects. The nurse stresses the importance of not using any over-the-counter medications, such as antacids and histamine receptor antagonists, in addition to, or instead of, those prescribed by the health care professional. If treatment is prescribed the nurse stresses the importance of completing the entire course of medications. Relapse is common with inadequate treatment, and drug-resistant strains of *H. pylori* are already being identified.

The nurse will also encourage the person to experiment with minor diet and lifestyle modifications that may reduce the incidence and severity of symptoms. These include reducing the intake of dietary fat to reduce postprandial bloating, eating smaller and more frequent meals, and avoiding known precipitators. Stress management techniques may be helpful to some individuals. The nurse will also emphasize the importance of seeking prompt evaluation if symptoms recur after treatment or if any symptoms of peptic ulcer disease develop.

## PEPTIC ULCER DISEASE

The last two decades have produced a revolution in our knowledge about peptic ulcer disease and its treatment. Traditional treatment approaches have been radically altered as we have increased our understanding of both mucosal aggressive forces and mucosal defensive forces and the factors that influence each. Although much progress has been made, peptic ulcer disease still absorbs up to $10 billion annually in direct care costs plus the additional toll in lost work and wages.[21] Medications alone consume more than $3 billion annually, and that figure is expected to escalate with the movement of traditional prescription ulcer drugs to the over-the-counter market.

### ETIOLOGY

Peptic ulcers were once believed to be the direct result of acid oversecretion in response to stressful life events. This assumption is reflected in the traditional treatment approaches, which emphasized acid neutralization and acid reduction. Although it is true that ulcers will not develop in the absence of acid, it is increasingly apparent that the primary etiological factors of ulcers relate to (1) infection by the organism *H. pylori,* which produces a chronic histological gastritis, and (2) the side effects of NSAID administration. These factors target the mucosal defenses of the stomach and duodenum and can eventually lead to ulceration in vulnerable people.

#### *Helicobacter pylori* Infection

The *H. pylori* bacteria is believed to be one of the most common pathogens in humankind. The stomach is its natural habitat. The organism causes most cases of chronic histological gastritis and is the primary etiological factor in the development of peptic ulcers not directly attributable to NSAID use.[13] Figure 40-1 shows the relationship between *H. pylori* infection and the incidence of peptic ulcers. The organism can be found in the gastric antrum of at least 90% of persons with duodenal ulcers and up to 70% of those with gastric ulcers.[12] The relationship between *H. pylori* infection and the development of ulcers is clearly causal, but current knowledge cannot explain why only 1 or 2 of every 20 persons who are infected with *H. pylori* actually develop ulcers; clearly other factors are operational that influence host resistance. The incidence of both gastric and duodenal ulcers increases steadily with age.

### Nonsteroidal Antiinflammatory Drug Use

There is also an unequivocal causal association between NSAID intake, mucosal injury, and the development of gastric ulcers (and, to a lesser degree, duodenal ulcers). The GI complications of NSAID use are increasingly being recognized as one of the most common and severe drug side effects in the United States.[17] The NSAIDs cause both local and systemic damage. Within 1 hour of taking a single dose of aspirin multiple subendothelial hemorrhages can be found in the stomach, and gastric erosion will develop within 24 hours if use is continued.[17] No relationship, however, has been established between the presence and severity of these superficial lesions and the development of ulcers. Although dramatic, these lesions appear to have little clinical significance in most patients. Most adverse effects of NSAIDs result from their inhibiting action on cyclooxygenase, an enzyme needed for the synthesis of endogenous prostaglandins. Prostaglandins are critical to the maintenance of the normal mucosal defenses.

The risk of ulcers associated with NSAID use is not predictable, and most NSAID users can derive benefit from their use without experiencing complications. The risk appears to be dose related, but problems can occur with even the smallest doses, especially with aspirin use. Ulcer risk is low in the under-50 age-group but rises rapidly over age 60. Approximately 2% to 4% of long-term NSAID users develop serious complications each year, and approximately 25% of NSAID users will develop ulcers. The NSAID-induced ulcers are believed to be directly responsible for 30% of upper GI bleeding episodes and approximately 30% of all ulcer-related deaths.[21] The concurrent presence of *H. pylori* infection in NSAID users does *not* appear to add to the risk of ulceration caused directly by the NSAIDs.

### Other Factors

Our knowledge of the etiology of ulcers is still evolving and various other factors appear to play a role, but their contribution to ulcer development is not clear. Twin studies point to a genetic role in ulcer development, but its specific nature is unknown. Ulcers also appear to demonstrate a familial clustering, but this effect may prove to be related to *H. pylori* exposure and infection. An observed link between duodenal ulcers and blood group O is currently believed to be associated with the improved ability of *H. pylori* to attach to the gastric epithelium when blood group antigens A and B are not present.

The role of both cigarette smoking and alcohol intake have been carefully explored. Although more study is needed, it would appear that a strong positive association exists between smoking and ulcer incidence, complications, recurrence, and mortality.[21] Current smokers are twice as likely as nonsmokers to develop ulcers, and the effects appear to be related to the amount smoked and duration. The pathology is not well identified, but smoking may increase the risk of infection with *H. pylori,* thereby acting as a cofactor. Smoking also plays a significant role in ulcer relapse. Although heavy smokers appear to have a higher incidence of peptic ulcer, quitting smoking has not been proven to affect the long-term course of the disease in a positive manner.

Alcohol is known to cause direct surface irritation of the gastric mucosa and can cause acute gastritis, but its role in ulcer development, if any, is unclear. Wine and beer are known to be potent secretagogues for acid secretion, but no etiological role in ulcers has been identified.

Diet has received a great deal of attention over the years and was once a focus of ulcer management, but no data currently support the theory that any diet causes ulcers, despite the frequent occurrence of dyspepsia symptoms in response to food. Tea, coffee, cola, and milk have all been identified as potent secretagogues, but no causal link to ulcers is apparent. The same appears to be true for spices. The role of dietary fiber in ulcer development is being explored in some regions of the world where the use of rice-based versus wheat-based diets appear to be associated with a lower incidence of peptic ulcers.

The role of stress in ulcer etiology, once believed to be pivotal, is also unknown. The relationship between intense physiological stress and acute hemorrhagic gastritis is well documented, but there is clearly no "ulcer personality" that plays an identifiable etiological role in ulcer development. However, ulcer incidence has been linked with the presence of several chronic diseases, most notably chronic obstructive pulmonary disease (COPD) and chronic renal failure. The exact etiological mechanisms remain undefined.

### Zollinger-Ellison Syndrome

Zollinger-Ellison syndrome is an ulceration syndrome of the duodenum or jejunum caused by a gastrinoma (gastrin-producing tumor). The tumor is commonly found in the non–insulin-producing islet cells of the pancreas. Most patients have a single tumor that eventually becomes malignant. This rare syndrome occurs more commonly in men, usually in early or middle adulthood.

The tumors produce an enormous quantity of gastrin, which massively overstimulates gastric acid secretion. The resulting ulcers usually do not respond to conventional therapy, and complications are common. Diarrhea is a common symptom. It is caused by a relative lack of the pancreatic lipase needed for fat digestion. The diagnosis of Zollinger-Ellison syndrome is differentiated from standard duodenal ulcers by radioimmunoassay measurements of high serum gastrin levels. A computed tomography (CT) scan may be used to localize the pancreatic tumor, and the tumor is removed if possible. The ulcers are treated as outlined for peptic ulcer disease.

## EPIDEMIOLOGY

The prevalence of peptic ulcer disease has changed dramatically over the last century. Duodenal ulcers were seldom encountered in the nineteenth century. Gastric ulcers were more common and occurred primarily in young women of low socioeconomic status.[25] They usually caused perforation. The incidence of peptic ulcer disease increased rapidly in the early 1900s and has become one of the most common human ailments. Four million Americans suffer from active disease in any given year, and over 500,000 new cases are diagnosed annually.[25] These figures actually represent a steady decline in duodenal ulcer incidence, which peaked in the 1950s, declined steadily until 1980, and now appears to have stabilized. The lifetime prevalence for men is about 10% to 14% and just slightly less for women.[25,32] This represents a 43% decrease in duodenal ulcer prevalence since the peak in the 1950s but a stable prevalence for gastric ulcers. The progressive aging of the population is in fact pushing the statistics for gastric ulcer steadily higher. Physician visits, hospitalizations, and the incidence of complications have all declined by greater than 50% in this period, and ulcer-related mortality has dropped over 30%.[21] No satisfactory explanation exists for these dramatic epidemiological swings in a relatively short period of time. It is theorized that some unidentified, possibly environmental factor was introduced in the early twentieth century that has now declined.

The changes in sex ratios have also been dramatic and baffling, and wide variation can still be found worldwide. The incidence of duodenal ulcers in men was about four times that of women during the peak period of the 1950s.[21] This incidence supported the theory that ulcer etiology was related to social and occupational stress. The current sex ratio is almost 1:1.[32] The ratio of duodenal to gastric ulcers has also steadily declined since the 1950s, from nearly 4:1 to almost 1:1. The prevalence for both types of ulcers increases steadily with age, peaking in the sixth decade. The overall mortality rate for ulcer is low, but it increases dramatically in persons over 75 years of age, particularly in elders who have gastric ulcers.[32]

Both regional and seasonal variations in ulcer incidence have been noted worldwide. No satisfactory explanation exists at present for any of these variations. Some researchers postulate that outbreaks of *H. pylori* may account for some of the variability, but this is purely speculative. As mentioned, an increased incidence is observed in persons with COPD, chronic renal failure, cirrhosis, and other chronic systemic diseases. Racial and cultural variations have also been noted, with gastric and duodenal ulcers occurring about equally in whites, but gastric ulcers being more common in African Americans and much more common in Hispanics.[32] See the Research Box for a summary of a recent national study on ulcer prevalence.

**research**

Reference: Sonnenberg A, Everhart JE: The prevalence of self reported peptic ulcer in the United States, *Am J Public Health* 86(2):200, 1996.

In 1989 a special questionnaire on digestive diseases was included in the annual National Health Interview Survey that reached 42,000 adults. The objective was to assess the pattern of peptic ulcer disease in the United States. The results showed some striking differences from past reported patterns. Lifetime prevalence for all ulcers was 10%. Occurrence of duodenal and peptic ulcers was equal. Prevalence rates were similar among men and women. An age-related rise in prevalence was noted, but it was less significant with gastric ulcers. Gastric and duodenal ulcers occurred about equally in whites, but gastric ulcers were more common in African Americans and strikingly more common in Hispanics. Inverse relationships were seen between education and income and the prevalence of gastric ulcers, and current smoking was strongly associated with each ulcer category. These findings indicate that the prevalence of peptic ulcer disease continues to show dramatic changes from patterns observed earlier in the century.

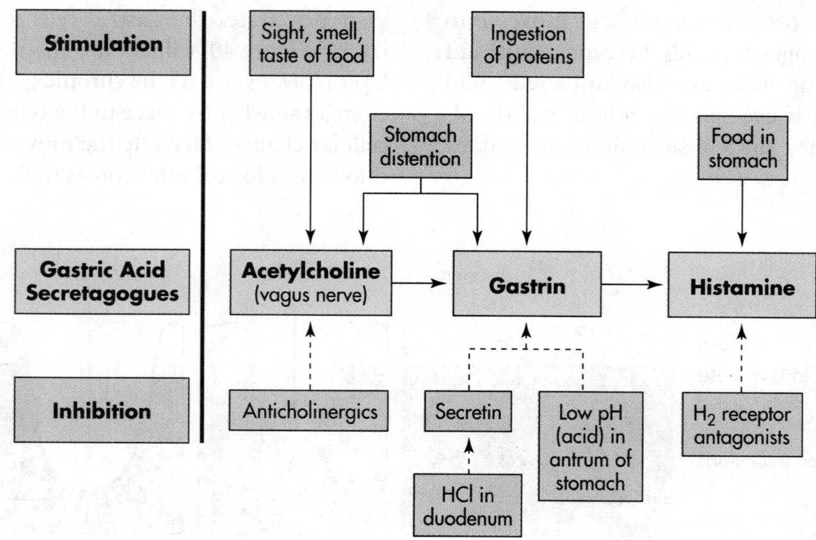


**fig. 40-2** Stimulation and inhibition of gastric acid.

## PATHOPHYSIOLOGY

The integrity of the gastric mucosa is maintained when a balance exists between the acid-secreting functions and mucosal protective functions of the stomach and duodenum. Peptic ulcers are present when a distinct crater is visible radiologically or endoscopically. The actual ulcer represents the endpoint of mucosal disruption.

### Acid Secretion

Acid secretion is controlled by endocrine, neural, and paracrine factors. Gastric acid is secreted by the parietal cells of the fundus of the stomach in response to gastrin (secreted by cells in the pyloric region), acetylcholine (cholinergic action of the vagus nerve), and histamine (found in cells throughout the gastric mucosa). There are two types of cellular receptors to histamine in the body. $H_1$ receptors are found in the cells of smooth muscle and capillaries, and they mediate smooth muscle contraction and capillary dilation. $H_2$ receptors are found in cells of the stomach and mediate secretion of hydrochloric acid (HCl). The process of stimulation and inhibition of gastric acid is illustrated in Figure 40-2.

Acid oversecretion had traditionally been assumed to be the major factor in ulcer development. This assumption is being challenged by the data indicating that the vast majority of duodenal ulcer patients have gastric acid secretory responses at rest and after meals that are identical to those in so-called normal individuals. Patients with gastric ulcers commonly have low levels of acid secretion, and the presence of *H. pylori* often decreases overall acid secretion.[21] The most common abnormality in acid secretion is a slight increase in the duration of acid secretion that is particularly apparent after meals, at rest, or at night.[36] The cause of these changes is basically unknown, although they can occasionally be attributed to an increase in parietal cell mass, which increases both gastric and peptic acid activity. Neither *H. pylori* nor NSAIDs increase the aggressive forces of acid secretion.

Some patients also exhibit an increased rate of gastric emptying. The ability of protein to buffer gastric acid is therefore impaired, and more unbuffered acid moves into the duodenum. These changes typically become significant only when the mucosal defenses are also impaired. Acid oversecretion alone rarely if ever plays a role in gastric ulcers. Figure 40-3 illustrates the classic lesions formed by peptic ulcer disease.

### Mucosal Defenses

The entire stomach and duodenum is covered by a 100 micrometers layer of mucus, which forms a gel that is 95% water and 5% glycoproteins. This layer is continuously both degraded and secreted. The gel protects the mucosa against shearing and mechanical injury, assists in the transport of food particles, retains water near the mucosa, and impedes the back diffusion of hydrogen ions. Few physical agents cause more than transient damage to the mucosa. The epithelial cells secrete bicarbonate into the mucous layer, which helps maintain a neutral pH immediately adjacent to the mucosa. The epithelial cells of the stomach are densely packed, which makes the stomach mucosa extremely resistant to injury, but the cells are less dense in the duodenum, which is therefore more susceptible. When minor injury occurs the surface epithelium is capable of quick repair by creating a "cap" of mucus and fibrin to increase the mucosal pH and repair the damage. An adequate mucosal blood flow at a normal pH is critical to the support of normal epithelial cell function. The combined effects of these defenses are so powerful that mucosal pH is maintained at a level greater than 6, even when the gastric luminal pH is as low as 1.5. Table 40-1 summarizes the major components of mucosal defense.

### Effects of *Helicobacter Pylori* Infection and Nonsteroidal Antiinflammatory Drugs

*Helicobacter pylori*-induced gastritis or peptic ulcer disease is associated with a decrease in duodenal bicarbonate secretion. The bacteria also contain proteases that can degrade mucus. Cytokines released by the organism cause inflammatory changes in the mucosa, and cytotoxins produced by *H. pylori* may cause epithelial cell injury and necrosis. It is theorized that different strains of *H. pylori* may differ in their ability to damage the cells, which would partially explain the erratic incidence and prevalence data for peptic ulcer disease.[2] *Helicobacter pylori* produces large amounts of urease, which allows the bacteria to split urea into ammonia. The organism then wraps itself in ammonia, protecting itself from stomach acid as it penetrates the gastric cells and weakens the mucous layer.[17] Figure 40-4 illustrates the penetration of the mucous layer by *H. pylori.* As the chronic gastritis persists, metaplastic changes slowly take place in the cells of the duodenum. These cellular changes facilitate the movement of *H. pylori* into the duodenum for colonization as well.

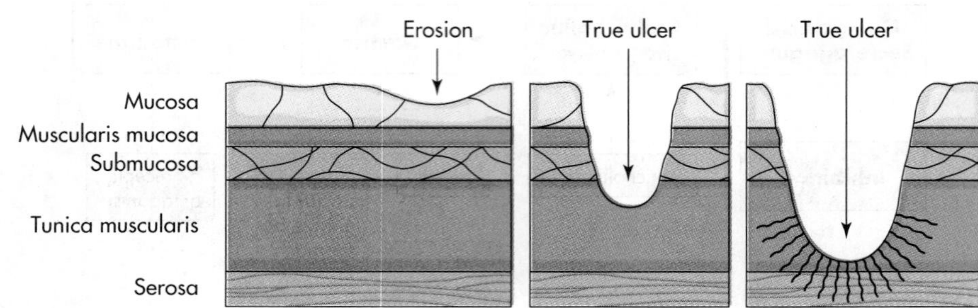


**fig. 40-3** Lesions caused by peptic ulcer disease.

Most NSAIDs are weak acids that can cause local mucosal irritation and inflammation, but their primary adverse effect on the stomach involves the inhibition of cyclooxygenase, an enzyme essential for the production of endogenous prostaglandins in the plasma and mucosa. Prostaglandins are critical in maintaining normal mucosal defenses. A deficit in prostaglandins results in decreased mucus and bicarbonate secretion, decreased mucosal blood flow, and a failure to inhibit gastric acid secretion. It also prevents the formation of the mucous "cap" that supports epithelial regeneration in the event of injury. Most gastric ulcers are localized in an area about 2 cm long on the antral side of the stomach along the lesser curvature where muscle fibers are prominent and blood supply is decreased. The major elements involved in the pathophysiology of peptic ulcers are presented in Figure 40-5.

Pain is the classic symptom associated with peptic ulcer disease, but its sensitivity and specificity as a marker is very low.[21] The pain traditionally has been attributed to the irritation of gastric acid over the eroded mucosa. During endoscopy, however, rubbing, cutting, and burning the mucosa produce little or no perceived pain in most individuals. Even

**table 40-1** *Mechanisms of Gastroduodenal Mucosal Defense*

| Level of Defense | Mechanism or Effect |
|---|---|
| Preepithelial | |
| Mucus/bicarbonate barrier | Provides a modest barrier to $H^+$ diffusion and other molecules |
| Mucoid cap | Develops in response to mucosal injury and provides a juxtamucosal alkaline or neutral microenvironment |
| Epithelial | |
| Restitution | Prompt reconstitution of surface epithelium by movement of existing cells over damaged area; impeded by ischemia, reduced $Ca^{2+}$, and acidosis |
| Acid-base transporters | Transport $HCO_3^-$ into the pH/mucous barrier and subepithelial tissues and extrude acid to prevent cellular acidification |
| Release of growth factors, prostaglandins, nitric oxide | Growth factors promote cell division; prostaglandins stimulate mucus and $HCO_3^-$ secretion and increase mucosal blood flow; nitric oxide increases mucosal blood flow |
| Subepithelial | |
| Mucosal blood flow | Delivers nutrients and buffers, especially $HCO_3^-$, to the surface epithelial cells |

Modified from McCance KL, Huether SE: *Pathophysiology: the biologic basis for disease in adults and children,* ed 3, St Louis, 1998, Mosby.

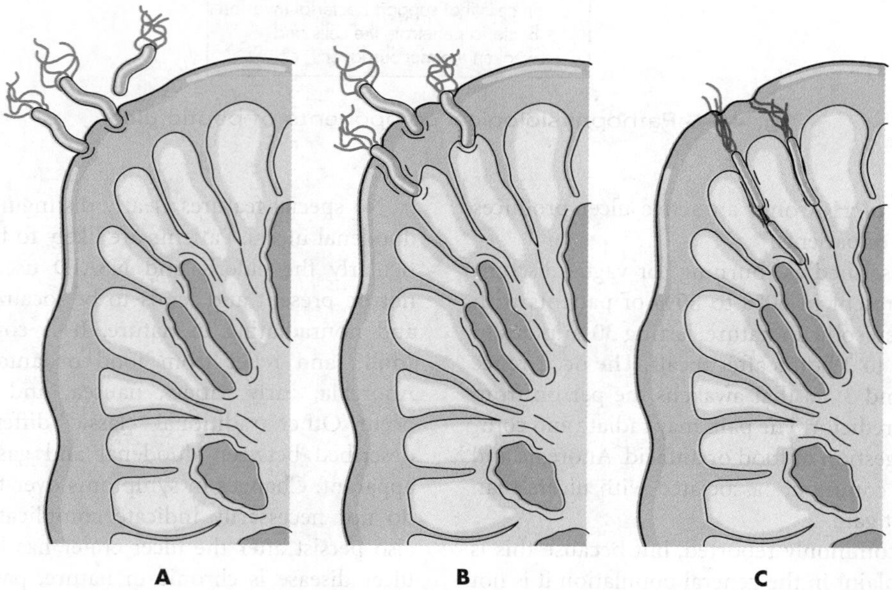


**fig. 40-4** Penetration of the mucosal layer by *H. pylori.* **A,** After penetration *H. pylori* forms clusters near membranes of surface epithelial cells. **B,** Some attach to the cell membrane. **C,** Others lodge between the epithelial cells.

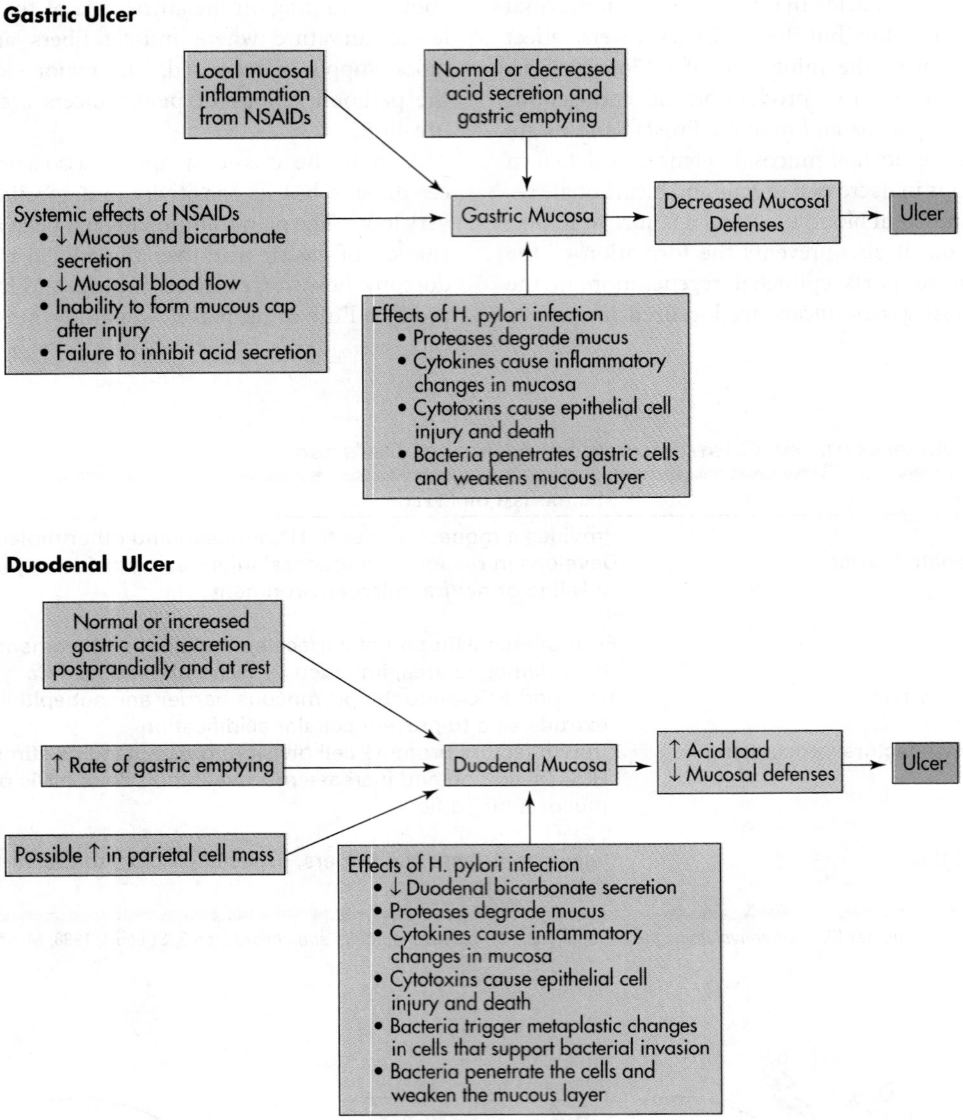

**Gastric Ulcer**

Local mucosal inflammation from NSAIDs

Normal or decreased acid secretion and gastric emptying

Systemic effects of NSAIDs
- ↓ Mucous and bicarbonate secretion
- ↓ Mucosal blood flow
- Inability to form mucous cap after injury
- Failure to inhibit acid secretion

Gastric Mucosa → Decreased Mucosal Defenses → Ulcer

Effects of H. pylori infection
- Proteases degrade mucus
- Cytokines cause inflammatory changes in mucosa
- Cytotoxins cause epithelial cell injury and death
- Bacteria penetrates gastric cells and weakens mucous layer

**Duodenal Ulcer**

Normal or increased gastric acid secretion postprandially and at rest

↑ Rate of gastric emptying

Possible ↑ in parietal cell mass

Duodenal Mucosa → ↑ Acid load ↓ Mucosal defenses → Ulcer

Effects of H. pylori infection
- ↓ Duodenal bicarbonate secretion
- Proteases degrade mucus
- Cytokines cause inflammatory changes in mucosa
- Cytotoxins cause epithelial cell injury and death
- Bacteria trigger metaplastic changes in cells that support bacterial invasion
- Bacteria penetrate the cells and weaken the mucous layer

**fig. 40-5** Pathophysiological components of peptic ulcer.

the direct instillation of HCl onto an active ulcer produces pain in less than 40% of patients.

Epigastric pain, described as "burning" or vague discomfort, is consistently present in 60% to 80% of patients with duodenal ulcers. It is episodic in nature, lasting 30 minutes to 2 hours, and occurs 1 to 3 hours after meals. The occurrence of pain between 12 and 3 AM that awakens the person from sleep is a fairly good predictor. The pain may radiate and commonly responds to ingestion of food or antacid. Anorexia and weight loss are more commonly associated with ulcers than are hunger and weight gain.

Dyspepsia is also commonly reported, but because this is such a common complaint in the general population it is not very helpful in distinguishing ulcers. Fewer than 30% of persons who experience chronic and severe dyspepsia are found to have ulcers on endoscopy, but many ulcer sufferers experience dyspepsia.

No special features clearly distinguish gastric ulcers from duodenal ulcers. Patients are likely to be asymptomatic, particularly the elderly and NSAID users. Pain may or may not be present and tends to be localized to the epigastrum and nonradiating in nature. It is commonly described as "dull," and relief from food or antacid is less common. Anorexia, early satiety, nausea, and weight loss may all occur. Other traditional "classic" differences that have been described between duodenal and gastric ulcers are rarely apparent. Changes in symptoms over time are common and do not necessarily indicate complications. Symptoms may also persist after the ulcer crater has healed. Because peptic ulcer disease is chronic in nature, patients may experience several episodes of symptoms that persist for 1 to 2 weeks at a time before a diagnosis is established. Clinical manifestations associated with peptic ulcer disease are summarized in Box 40-4.

**box 40-4** ***clinical manifestations***

***Duodenal and Gastric Ulcers***

Ulcers may be completely asymptomatic.

**DUODENAL ULCER**

**Pain**

- Episodic in nature lasting 30 min-2 hr
- Epigastric location near midline; may radiate around costal border to back
- Described as gnawing, burning, aching
- Occurs 1-3 hr after meals and at night (12-3 AM)
- Often relieved by food or antacid

**GASTRIC ULCER**

**Pain**

- Dull epigastric location near midline
- Early satiety
- Not usually relieved by food or antacid

**BOTH**

Dyspepsia syndrome: fullness, epigastric discomfort, vague nausea, distention, and bloating

Anorexia

Weight loss

## COLLABORATIVE CARE MANAGEMENT

### Diagnostic Tests

The diagnosis of peptic ulcer disease cannot be made from symptoms alone because they are nonspecific in many situations. Although an ulcer crater is readily identifiable with an upper GI series, a definitive diagnosis usually involves endoscopy with biopsy to rule out cancer, which typically causes an ulcer crater. Biopsy is required to accurately differentiate between benign and malignant ulcers. Gastric cancer is rare in young adults, but its incidence increases rapidly after the fifth decade.

*Helicobacter pylori* screening is increasingly being included in the diagnostic workup for ulcers. Several diagnostic options exist. Serological tests for specific IgG antibodies to the organism can reveal prior exposure to *H. pylori.* A rapid urase test establishes the presence of the organism but is prohibitively expensive for general use. The same applies to histological analysis of biopsy specimens. Urea breath tests are currently being tested for mass use. The patient ingests a capsule of carbon-labeled urea. In the presence of *H. pylori* the urea is hydrolyzed, releasing the labeled $CO_2$, which can be measured by spectrometry. See Chapter 38 for additional information about diagnostic testing.

### Medications

Advances in drug therapy have dramatically changed the management of peptic ulcer disease and significantly improved its effectiveness. A variety of choices exist, and the specific protocol for any particular patient is determined based on the preferences of the physician and the patient's unique profile. Drug therapy controls peptic ulcer symptoms effectively, often in a matter of days. It heals most ulcers completely within 8 weeks. However, ulcer relapse is a serious threat to long-term control. It is increasingly apparent that the presence of *H. pylori* is the major factor involved in ulcer recurrence, and any successful treatment must also consider the eradication of the infection.

Antacids, histamine 2 receptor antagonists, proton pump inhibitors, and cytoprotective agents are the primary choices for pharmacological management of ulcers. All are effective, but they vary substantially in cost, ease of administration, side effects, and patient acceptability.

#### *Antacids*

Antacids are weak bases that neutralize free hydrochloric acid to prevent irritation and permit mucosal healing. Antacids usually play a supporting role in ulcer therapy today and are used primarily for symptomatic relief. However, they can also heal ulcers, although at a slower rate than other products. The main disadvantage to antacid therapy is the frequency with which the antacids must be administered. Their effect is transitory, and they need to be administered 1 and 3 hours after meals and at bedtime. This is not a practical schedule for most patients, who are usually encouraged to use antacids during treatment on an as-needed basis.

Aluminum hydroxide antacid preparations are preferred; in addition to their acid-neutralizing effects, it is believed that they decrease pepsin activity and possibly stimulate prostaglandin synthesis. Administration in tablet rather than liquid form prolongs the buffering effect slightly and is recommended. Antacids should never be given concurrently with other ulcer drugs such as $H_2$ blockers because they will decrease drug absorption by 10% to 20%. Because aluminum hydroxide products used alone commonly cause constipation, they typically are combined with magnesium hydroxide for its laxative effect. Table 40-2 summarizes the commonly used antacids.

#### *Histamine receptor antagonists*

Histamine ($H_2$) receptor antagonists inhibit HCl secretion by binding to the $H_2$ receptors on stomach cells and blocking the release of histamine, which is a secretagogue for HCl. Gastric emptying is unaffected by their use.

Several different generations of $H_2$ receptor antagonists have been developed, but there is no clear evidence that one is bcst.[28] They vary in potency and cost but are equally effective in healing peptic ulcers after an average of 4 weeks of therapy.

Recommended dosage schedules have varied over the years. Most are now administered twice a day in divided doses or in one bedtime dose. Administering the drugs once a day at bedtime produces healing rates that are comparable to or better than those achieved with twice-a-day administration despite the short half-lives of the drugs. Suppression of nocturnal acid secretion appears to support rapid healing.[19]

There are few side effects, and these drugs have an excellent record of safety. Potential side effects may include diarrhea and abdominal cramps, as well as confusion, dizziness, and

**table 40-2** *Common Medications for* ***Ulcer Discomfort (Antacids)***

| Drug | Action | Nursing Intervention |
|---|---|---|
| **ALUMINUM PRODUCTS** | | |
| Amphojel<br>AlternaGEL<br>Alu-Cap<br>Basaljel | All antacids act by buffering excess acidity in the stomach to neutralize the pH. | All aluminum hydroxide antacids are constipating. Patients need to be taught to maintain regular bowel elimination.<br>Teach patient to use as needed for ulcer discomfort, but not at the same time as an $H_2$ receptor antagonist. |
| **COMBINATIONS OF ALUMINUM AND MAGNESIUM** | | |
| Maalox<br>Gaviscon<br>Riopan | | As above, but nonconstipating. |
| **CALCIUM PRODUCTS** | | |
| Alka-Mints<br>Tums<br>Rolaids | | As above, but only for short-term use.<br>Often severely constipating.<br>May cause acid rebound. |
| **ANTACIDS WITH SIMETHICONE** | | |
| Mylanta<br>Maalox Plus<br>Gelusil | | Simethicone is non–gas forming and can be recommended to patients with gas problems.<br>Nonconstipating. |

NOTE: Antacid tablets have a longer duration of effect than liquids and are recommended.

weakness, which are more common in elderly patients. The drugs in current use include the following:

- Cimetidine (Tagamet) is the oldest and least expensive drug. It also has the potential for multiple drug interactions and is not recommended in situations that necessitate multiple drug administration. Cimetidine has also been shown to have antiandrogenic effects that may cause gynecomastia, decreased libido, and impotence in some men. It is also known to cause confusion in the elderly.
- Ranitidine (Zantac) is more potent and usually has no side effects.
- Famotidine (Pepcid) is the drug of choice when the possibility of adverse reactions with other prescribed medications is a concern.
- Nizatidine (Axid) is the newest and most costly of $H_2$ receptor antagonists.

Cimetidine, ranitidine, and famotidine are all available in intravenous forms to address acute and emergency situations. Several of the histamine 2 receptor antagonists are also now available in nonprescription strength for over-the-counter purchase.

### *Proton pump inhibitors*

Omeprazole (Prilosec) is the most tested form of this newer category of drugs. It virtually eliminates acid secretion and is significantly more effective in healing duodenal ulcers than other medications. Its effectiveness in gastric ulcer management is less clear. The drug is not approved for long-term use at this time, which makes it inappropriate for maintenance administration. Clinically significant side effects are

**research**

Reference: Sung JJY et al: Antibacterial treatment of gastric ulcers associated with *Helicobacter pylori, N Engl J Med* 332(3):139, 1995.

This study sought to further delineate the role of *H. pylori* infection in the incidence of gastric ulcers by treating identified gastric ulcers with antibacterial therapy to the exclusion of acid reduction therapy. Patients with ulcers clearly attributed to the use of NSAIDs were excluded from the study.

One hundred qualified patients were randomly assigned to one of two treatment groups. Group one was treated with a week-long course of bismuth subcitrate, metronidazole, and tetracycline. Group two was treated for 4 weeks with omeprazole.

After 5 weeks *H. pylori* was successfully eradicated from 91% of patients in group one and 12% of patients in group two. After 9 weeks endoscopy showed a 95% rate of ulcer healing in group one and a 94% rate of healing in group two. However, 4 months after treatment was completed, recurrent ulceration was found in just one member of group one and in over 50% of group two. Two participants in group two also showed evidence of ulceration in the duodenum at that time. Both interventions were shown to be successful in ulcer healing, but *H. pylori* eradication was an essential component in preventing ulcer relapse.

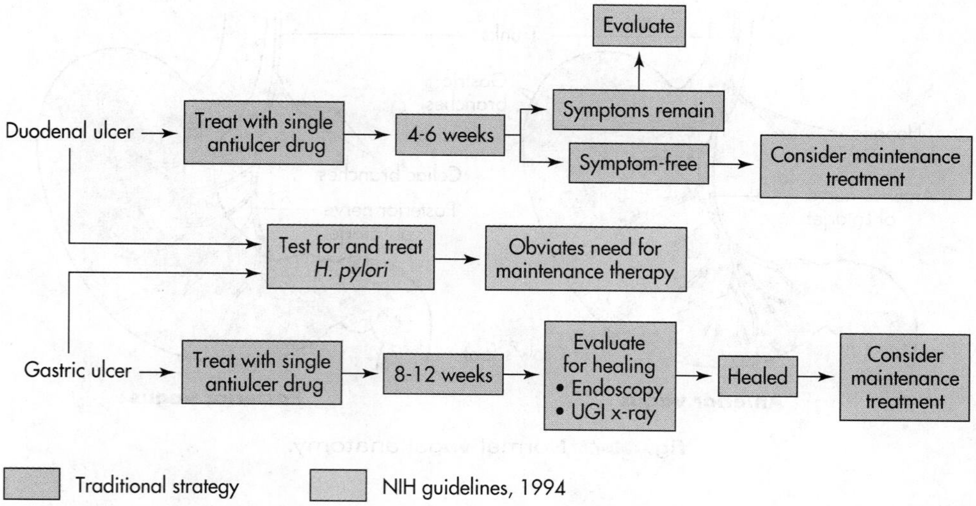

Duodenal ulcer → Treat with single antiulcer drug → 4-6 weeks → Symptoms remain → Evaluate
4-6 weeks → Symptom-free → Consider maintenance treatment
Duodenal ulcer → Test for and treat *H. pylori* → Obviates need for maintenance therapy
Gastric ulcer → Test for and treat *H. pylori*
Gastric ulcer → Treat with single antiulcer drug → 8-12 weeks → Evaluate for healing • Endoscopy • UGI x-ray → Healed → Consider maintenance treatment

Traditional strategy

NIH guidelines, 1994

**fig. 40-6** A comparison of traditional ulcer treatment with current National Institute of Health guidelines for managing *H. pylori* infection and ulceration.

rare. Omeprazole is also currently being used in the treatment of *H. pylori* infection. A second drug in this category, lansaprazole (Prevacid), has also been approved for use.

### Mucosal protective agents

Improved understanding of the etiology of peptic ulcers has shifted attention to the development and use of drugs designed to support the mucosal barrier. These include sucralfate (Carafate) and misoprostol (Cytotec).

**Sucralfate (Carafate).** Sucralfate originally was believed to coat an ulcer and provide a sealant protection against acid irritation. Additional research has indicated that it also acts as a cytoprotective agent and increases prostaglandin synthesis. It neither inhibits acid secretion nor neutralizes gastric acid, but it has an excellent record of ulcer healing. Its only common side effect is constipation.

The drug comes in a large tablet and must be taken orally, which limits its usefulness in certain situations. Combining sucralfate with an acid-suppressing agent does not significantly affect healing and is not recommended.

**Misoprostol (Cytotec).** Misoprostol and the newer drug enprostil are synthetic prostaglandin analogues that offer a new dimension to ulcer management. They enhance mucosal defenses by replacing gastric prostaglandins and also appear to have some antisecretory properties.[19]

In low doses they have a protective effect on the stomach but not the duodenum. These drugs are used at present primarily for the prevention of gastric ulcers in high-risk elderly patients who need to continue to take NSAIDs. The pain-relieving effectiveness of NSAIDs does not appear to be lessened by use of these drugs. Misoprostol commonly causes diarrhea and crampy abdominal pain, which are usually dose dependent. Administration after meals decreases side effects in many patients. The drug can induce abortion, and all sexually active women of childbearing age need to have a pregnancy test before beginning its use.

### Helicobacter pylori *drug treatment*

*Helicobacter pylori* infection is now recognized to be the main determinant of ulcer relapse (see the Research Box on p. 1286). Controversy continues, however, over exactly which patients need to be treated for the infection. Treatment advocates contend that immediate treatment of documented *H. pylori* infection in ulcer patients is cost-effective because the vast majority of ulcers will otherwise eventually relapse. Others recommend that *H. pylori* treatment be reserved for refractory lesions or patients who experience frequent relapses.

Drug protocols for the treatment of *H. pylori* infection continue to evolve with research and testing. The drug regimens in use have been complex and associated with multiple side effects that make patient adherence a serious concern. Treatment with any single agent has thus far proven to be ineffective, and the development of antibiotic-resistant strains of the organism are an increasing concern. A 1994 consensus conference sponsored by the National Institutes of Health (NIH) advocated a protocol that included 2 weeks of treatment with at least two antibiotics and bismuth compounds (Pepto-Bismol) plus 6 weeks of treatment with an $H_2$ receptor antagonist. Current recommendations include 2 weeks of treatment with a combination of omeprazole (Prilosec) and an antibiotic such as clarithromycin (Biaxin). Protocols will continue to change as research on effective treatment accumulates.

Successful treatment of the *H. pylori* infection reduces the incidence of ulcer relapse to well below 10%, and maintenance therapy with $H_2$ receptor antagonists or other drugs is usually unnecessary.[6] Figure 40-6 compares the traditional approach to ulcer treatment with the guidelines developed by NIH for treatment of *H. pylori* infection plus ulceration.

The release of the $H_2$ receptor antagonists for over-the-counter sale has added a new dimension to the diagnosis and pharmacological treatment of peptic ulcer disease. It is far too

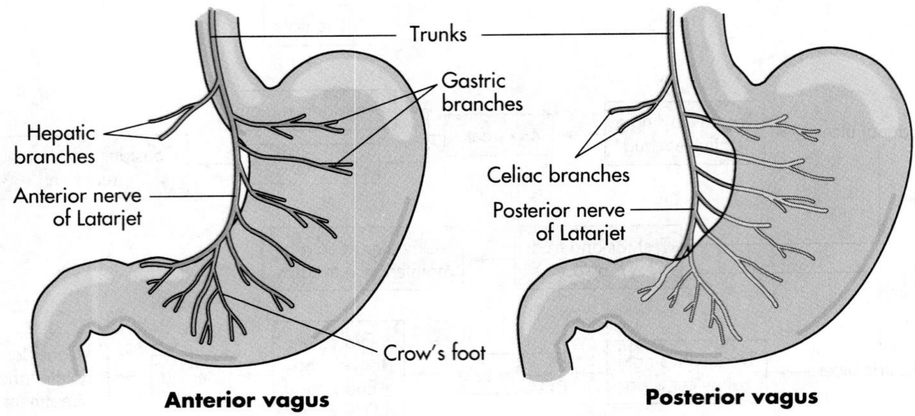


**fig. 40-7** Normal vagal anatomy.

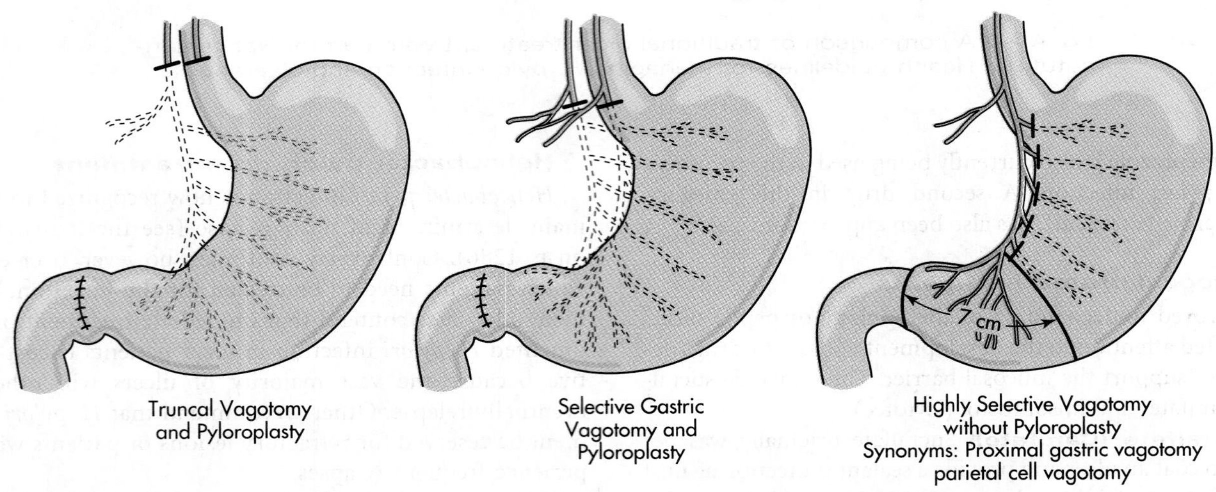


**fig. 40-8** Types of vagotomy with and without pyloroplasty.

early to measure the outcomes, but concern does exist that the as-needed and symptomatic use of over-the-counter drugs will delay the onset of effective treatment for many new-onset ulcer patients and increase the likelihood of relapses. Complete effective drug therapy is critical to the success of treatment, and this may be adversely affected by the use of over-the-counter agents.

### Treatments

Most peptic ulcers are responsive to the aggressive pharmacological approach already discussed. There are no routinely ordered treatments. If an ulcer should bleed, obstruct, or perforate, however, the management will shift dramatically. Treatments for these problems are discussed under Complications (see p. 1293).

### Surgical Management

The emergence of effective drug therapy for peptic ulcer disease has caused a massive change in the role of surgery in disease management. As effective treatment of *H. pylori* in patients with ulcer recurrence becomes more standard, it is anticipated that the need for elective surgery for ulcer management will be rare. Surgery is used primarily for the management of complications such as perforation and the treatment of the occasional intractable ulcer that is resistant to all standard therapy. Patients who require surgery to manage acute complications are usually older and frailer and commonly have significant comorbid conditions. The recommended procedures are highly technical, and the outcomes are strongly related to the skill of the surgeon performing the procedure. The rapid development of laparoscopic surgical techniques is also significantly altering the nature of ulcer surgery. Efforts are ongoing to refine and adapt vagotomy procedures for laparoscopic approaches. Such efforts add to the technical challenges of the surgery but significantly decrease patient recovery time.

Vagotomy, with or without drainage procedures, is the most commonly performed ulcer surgery today. Vagotomy procedures reduce acid production by decreasing cholinergic stimulation of the parietal cells and limiting the response to gastrin. The vagotomy procedure of choice is the highly selective vagotomy, which preserves the pylorus and almost abolishes the negative outcomes of dumping syndrome, diarrhea, and bilious vomiting. More aggressive procedures that include

**box 40-5** *Vagotomy Procedures for Management of Intractable Ulcers*

**TRUNCAL VAGOTOMY**

Severs the vagus nerve on the distal esophagus:

- Removes the cholinergic drive
- Reduces parietal cell sensitivity to gastrin
- Creates gastric stasis and poor gastric emptying and requires a drainage procedure (pyloroplasty)
- Affects motility of duodenum, biliary tract, and pancreas and is associated with multiple digestive complications

**SELECTIVE VAGOTOMY**

Divides and severs the vagal nerve branches to confine the effects to the stomach and preserve the function of the biliary tract, pancreas, and small intestine:

- Removes the cholinergic drive to the parietal cells
- Creates gastric stasis and poor gastric emptying and requires a drainage procedure (pyloroplasty)
- Technically difficult and outcomes are not significantly better than the truncal approach

**HIGHLY SELECTIVE VAGOTOMY**

Divides and severs the specific vagal nerve branches that supply the stomach while preserving those that supply the antrum and pylorus, biliary tract, pancreas, and intestine:

- Removes the cholinergic drive to the parietal cells
- Preserves innervation of the antrum and pylorus and does not require a drainage procedure
- Preserves extragastric function
- Minimizes digestive side effects
- Technically extremely difficult

various forms of partial gastrectomy are rarely recommended today. The various approaches to vagotomy are described in Box 40-5 and illustrated in Figures 40-7 and 40-8.

### Diet

The role of diet in peptic ulcer disease management has changed dramatically over the past 40 years. The Sippy and Hurst milk-based therapy was used for years in the belief that constantly diluting and neutralizing acid would facilitate ulcer healing. Although milk-based diets provide symptomatic relief, they do not influence healing. In fact, research has shown that the amino acids and calcium in milk actually act as secretagogues and increase acid secretion. Current management reflects the understanding that diet plays no defined role in ulcer etiology. Bland diets are not helpful in facilitating healing, and patients should simply be encouraged to eliminate or restrict specific foods that cause discomfort until healing occurs.

### Activity

Patients with ulcers do not need to restrict their activity in any particular way to support the healing of the ulcer. Most care is managed at home, and patients are able to continue with their usual activities while undergoing treatment. Adequate rest is encouraged because it appears to promote ulcer healing.

### Referrals

Consultation usually is not needed for management of uncomplicated ulcers. The nurse may encourage patients to seek community support for reducing alcohol intake and smoking. Surgical consultation may be indicated if ulcer complications develop.

## NURSING MANAGEMENT

### ASSESSMENT

#### Subjective Data

Subjective data to be collected to assess the patient with peptic ulcer disease include:

Pain: presence, location, severity, nature, and relationship to eating and sleeping
Medications being used
Ulcer agents (prescription or over-the-counter drugs)—frequency and pattern of use, effectiveness for symptom control
Aspirin, NSAIDs, or other ulcerogenic drugs
Dietary habits and meal patterns
Use of alcohol and smoking history
General lifestyle: work, leisure, exercise, stressors, usual coping measures
Knowledge of peptic ulcer disease: causes, treatment, complications

#### Objective Data

Objective data to be collected to assess the patient with peptic ulcer disease include:

Evidence of GI bleeding
Occult blood in stool
Decreased hemoglobin (Hgb), hematocrit (Hct), and red blood cell (RBC) counts
Weight loss or gain from baseline

### NURSING DIAGNOSES

Nursing diagnoses are determined from analysis of patient data. Nursing diagnoses for the person with peptic ulcer disease may include but are not limited to:

| Diagnostic Title | Possible Etiological Factors |
|---|---|
| Pain | Mucosal irritation and ulceration |
| Health maintenance, altered (risk for) | Lack of knowledge of disease process, treatment regimen, and signs and symptoms of complications |

### EXPECTED PATIENT OUTCOMES

Expected patient outcomes for the patient with peptic ulcer disease may include but are not limited to:

1. Describes pain as decreased, minimal, or absent
2. Describes components of disease management:
   a. Medication schedule and control of side effects
   b. Plans for follow-up care

c. Describes lifestyle factors that may facilitate ulcer healing and prevent recurrence
d. Eliminating or reducing smoking and alcohol intake
e. Balancing rest, exercise, and stress reduction
f. Modifying the diet to minimize known irritants
g. Accurately lists symptoms that indicate presence or development of complications

## INTERVENTIONS

### Relieving Pain

Taking prescribed medications as ordered is the major strategy for relieving ulcer pain. Drug therapy will control or eliminate the pain within a few days to a week, but peptic ulcer control is a long-term process. Successful self-care depends on a clear understanding of the purpose of each drug and the importance of adherence to the complete ulcer regimen, including follow-up. Most cases of ulcer relapse can be traced to nonadherence unless the initial treatment is inadequate or inappropriate (e.g., does not include *H. pylori* treatment).

#### *Patient/family education*

The nurse teaches the patient how to take prescribed medications in regard to meal times and discusses the management of common side effects that involve bowel function. Elderly patients and their families are encouraged to monitor for and report the incidence of any mental confusion or dizziness that may occur with cimetidine use. Patients are taught to never abruptly discontinue their use of antiulcer medications because of the danger of severe acid rebound. Antacids should never be taken with $H_2$ receptor antagonists because they significantly block absorption.

The patient is strongly cautioned to substitute the use of acetaminophen for other NSAIDs in routine pain and fever management. Over 70 million prescriptions for NSAIDs are written each day in addition to their routine over-the-counter use. Patients with chronic arthritis who need daily NSAID administration should be encouraged to explore the concurrent use of misoprostol (Cytotec) to minimize the risk of gastric ulceration. This is particularly important for older patients. When discontinuation of NSAIDs is not feasible, the nurse may also consult with the physician about the possible use of nonacetylated NSAIDs or one of the newer drugs that has less severe adverse effects on the stomach mucosa. Possible options include:

- Salsalate (Disalcid)
- Nabumetone (Relafen)
- Etodolac (Lodine)

The nurse will teach the patient and family that no special diet is needed to promote ulcer healing. The nurse encourages the patient to avoid any food that causes discomfort and to avoid overdistention of the stomach and binge eating. There is no research evidence that a pattern of small, frequent feedings is any more effective in ulcer management than a standard three-meal-a-day pattern, but overeating should be avoided. Eating slowly and chewing thoroughly prevent overdistention and reflux. Bedtime snacking may promote nighttime acid secretion and should be avoided.

The nurse may encourage the patient to limit the use of foods that have been shown to have a strong acid-stimulating effect, at least during the initial treatment period. These include coffee, tea, cola, and chocolate. Direct irritants such as spices and red and black pepper also should be limited.

The role of lifestyle or psychological stress in peptic ulcer disease is unclear, although mental and physical rest do appear to facilitate ulcer healing. The nurse encourages the patient to establish a pattern of regular exercise and to explore appropriate approaches to stress reduction at home and work. The accompanying Guidelines for Care Box summarizes the major points involved in teaching self-care management to the patient with peptic ulcer disease.

**guidelines for care**

**The Person with a Peptic Ulcer**

**Medications**

1. Know the dosage, administration, action, and side effects of all drugs in use.
2. Take all of prescribed drug, even when pain is relieved. It is essential to complete the full treatment.
3. Keep antacids available for use as needed, but do not take them at the same time as an $H_2$ receptor antagonist. Antacids should be taken 1 to 3 hours after meals, at bedtime, and as needed for pain.
4. Avoid the use of over-the-counter $H_2$ receptor antagonists.
5. Use acetaminophen for routine pain relief during treatment if needed. Avoid the use of all NSAIDs, including aspirin and ibuprofen.
6. If the treatment of arthritis or other chronic illness requires the ongoing use of NSAIDs, explore the use of misoprostol with health care provider.
7. Know the symptoms of ulcer recurrence and report them promptly to the health care provider.

**Diet**

1. Eat three balanced meals a day.
2. Eat between-meal snacks if this helps control pain. Avoid bedtime snacking because it increases nighttime acid secretion.
3. Eat slowly and chew foods thoroughly. Do not overeat.
4. Avoid any foods that increase discomfort.
5. Avoid the use of alcohol during treatment if possible. Never drink alcohol on an empty stomach.

**Smoking**

1. Stop smoking if possible.
2. Explore community support for smoking cessation or use of nicotine withdrawal patches.

**Stress Reduction**

1. Participate in recreation and hobbies that promote relaxation.
2. Participate in a moderate aerobic exercise program for promotion of well-being.
3. Provide for increased rest during healing.

### Health Promotion/Prevention

Ulcer relapse is a serious treatment problem. Although the initial peptic ulcer cannot usually be prevented, it is often possible to minimize the risk of relapse by effective *H. pylori* diagnosis and treatment. However, *H. pylori* drug treatment is often associated with multiple side effects. The nurse reinforces the patient's knowledge about the causal role of *H. pylori* in ulcer development and the importance of completing treatment to prevent relapse and the development of drug resistance. The importance of this treatment is reflected in a 1995 addition to the national *Healthy People 2000* goals to reduce the prevalence of peptic ulcer disease to no more than 18 per 1000 people aged 18 and older by preventing its recurrence.

The nurse cautions the patient about the use of over-the-counter $H_2$ receptor antagonists once therapy is completed. The return of pain may indicate that the ulcer treatment has been inadequate or that *H. pylori* treatment is indicated. Use of over-the-counter ulcer medications to manage symptoms could delay treatment or mask the development of complications.

The role of cigarette smoking in ulcer relapse is also clearly documented, and the nurse strongly encourages the patient to quit smoking. Referral to community smoking cessation programs should be made with consultation with the health care provider about the appropriateness of the various nicotine patch systems. The role of alcohol in ulcer relapse is less clear, but moderation is encouraged, and alcohol should never be ingested on an empty stomach because of its irritating effects on the mucosa. A Nursing Care Plan for a patient with a peptic ulcer is found on p. 1292.

## EVALUATION

To evaluate the effectiveness of nursing interventions, compare patient behaviors with those stated in the expected patient outcomes. Successful achievement of patient outcomes for the patient with peptic ulcer disease is indicated by:

1. States that ulcer pain is no longer present
2. Correctly describes medication schedule and management of side effects

## GERONTOLOGICAL CONSIDERATIONS

Although the incidence of peptic ulcer disease in the general population has been steadily declining, the incidence in elderly persons has shown a slight increase as the population ages. The elderly are also much more likely to be colonized by *H. pylori,* which contributes to an increased incidence of peptic ulcers in this population.

Hospitalization rates for elders with peptic ulcer disease also have risen steadily in the face of a continuing overall decline in hospitalization for the disease. Most of the complications and mortality associated with ulcers occur in elderly patients, with more than 80% of ulcer-related deaths in the over-65 age-group.

Peptic ulcer disease is clearly a more serious problem in elderly persons, and elderly persons are also more prone to complications. It is ironic that susceptibility to ulceration should increase at the exact time when normal basal acid secretion is in decline and moving toward achlorhydria.

The elderly experience frequent dyspepsia, which makes the diagnosis of ulcers more difficult. They are also less likely to seek medical attention for their symptoms. The frequent use of NSAIDs in this population for the management of chronic arthritis is another significant contributor to ulcer incidence. An estimated 1% of the total U.S. population uses NSAIDs daily, and the elderly are the most frequent users. From 2% to 4% of long-term NSAID users develop serious complications each year, and 30% of ulcer-related deaths can be attributed to NSAID use. If hemorrhage occurs, the seriousness is potentiated by the platelet inhibition associated with NSAID use.

Peptic ulcer disease often manifests in an atypical manner in elders. Symptoms tend to be more poorly defined and variable, and the standard pain characteristics commonly are not present. The discomfort, if present at all, often is poorly localized and vague, radiating in ways that cause confusion and overlap with angina, gallbladder disease, and dysphagia. Because early accurate diagnosis is rare, the ulcers tend to be larger at diagnosis, or patients are already exhibiting complications. The risk of serious complications is four times higher in the elderly, and most patients are completely asymptomatic until complications develop. Elderly women appear to be at particular risk.

The diagnosis and treatment of peptic ulcer disease in elders follow the same general guidelines outlined in the prior discussion. Elders are more likely to require aggressive *H. pylori* treatment to heal the ulcer and minimize relapse, and they are more likely to need maintenance therapy. Elders should be thoroughly assessed concerning their use of both prescription and over-the-counter NSAIDs and cautioned to eliminate use of these drugs if possible. Acetaminophen is considered to be a much safer alternative for occasional use than aspirin and most NSAIDs. Consideration should be given to the concurrent use of a synthetic prostaglandin such as misoprostol for this population.

## SPECIAL ENVIRONMENTS FOR CARE

### Critical Care Management

Critical care management is rarely indicated in peptic ulcer disease management. The vast majority of patients are successfully managed in a community or home setting. However, when complications occur, they tend to be emergent and potentially life threatening, and sophisticated critical care management may be essential. This is particularly true for the elderly. Common complications include upper GI bleeding or hemorrhage and perforation (discussed on p. 1293). These complications commonly require critical care management.

### Home Care Management

Standard management of peptic ulcer disease is achieved by the individual patient and family in a home-based self-care regimen. Adherence issues are important as they relate to

## nursing care plan *Person with Peptic Ulcer*

**DATA** Mr. J. is a single, 42-year-old computer operator with a history of duodenal ulcer 4 years ago. He has had periods of epigastric distress for the past month with partial relief from Maalox and over-the-counter cimetidine. He was admitted 2 days ago with hematemesis, tarry stools, faintness, and a blood pressure of 96/54 (usual 124/84). IV fluids were initiated, and an NG tube was inserted for lavage. When the bleeding persisted, an endoscopic examination was performed for local treatment of the recurrent duodenal ulcer. Antacids were administered hourly through the NG tube after the endoscopy. Cimetidine was administered by IV push.

Mr. J.'s blood pressure is now stable, and the NG tube was removed earlier today. He is taking oral fluids and has been started on a soft diet. The cimetidine has been changed to 30 mg with meals and at bedtime. Maalox 30 ml is ordered 1 hour and 3 hours after meals and as needed.

The nursing history also identified the following:

- Mr. J. is vague about the nature of peptic ulcer disease, its treatment, and potential complications.
- He takes aspirin fairly regularly for headaches caused by "computer eye strain."
- He smokes 1½ packs per day; he has tried several times unsuccessfully to quit.
- He spends two to three evenings a week at a local bar and "puts down quite a few beers."

Collaborative nursing actions include monitoring for the following:

- Signs of further hemorrhage: hematemesis; decreased blood pressure; restlessness; cool, moist skin; stools that show positive reaction to guaiac test.
- Signs of perforation: severe, sudden, sharp abdominal pain.

**NURSING DIAGNOSIS** *Epigastric pain related to mucosal irritation and ulceration*

| expected patient outcome | nursing interventions | rationale |
|---|---|---|
| States epigastric pain is decreased or absent. | Administer prescribed cimetidine with meals and at bedtime (8 AM, 12 noon, 5 PM, and 10 PM). | Cimetidine facilitates ulcer healing by decreasing gastric acid secretion; it is given with meals to inhibit food-stimulated HCl secretion. |
| | Give prescribed antacid 1 and 3 hr after meals (9 AM, 11 AM, 1 PM, 3 PM, 6 PM, and 8 PM) and as needed. | Antacids neutralize HCl and quickly reduce pain; they interfere with absorption of cimetidine if given concurrently. They must be given frequently because they are cleared rapidly from the stomach. |

**NURSING DIAGNOSIS** *Risk for altered health maintenance related to lack of knowledge of disease process, treatment regimen, and signs and symptoms of complications*

| expected patient outcome | nursing interventions | rationale |
|---|---|---|
| Accurately describes:<br>• Components of disease process<br>• Lifestyle modifications to facilitate ulcer healing<br>• Symptoms of complications<br>• Role of *H. pylori* in ulcer relapse | Encourage patient to avoid:<br>• Any food that causes pain.<br>• Foods that have a strong acid-stimulating effect, e.g., tea, coffee, chocolate, cola, and milk products. | Diet elements do not cause and cannot heal ulcers but can relieve discomfort. |
| | Teach patient the links between aspirin use and smoking on ulcer relapse.<br>• Encourage reduction of intake or use.<br>• Refer to community smoking cessation programs.<br>• Suggest substituting acetaminophen for aspirin or ibuprofen for occasional pain relief. | Aspirin and ibuprofen contribute to mucosal breakdown, and smoking appears to be related to an increased rate of ulcer relapse. |
| | • Avoid over-the-counter use of cimetidine. | Can mask ulcer relapse symptoms. |
| | Suggest eye examination or environmental modification to reduce eye strain. | Reduce stress level in daily lifestyle. |
| | Explore new patterns of recreation and stress-reduction techniques. | Ulcer recurrence is more common in patients with chronic anxiety and poor coping skills; stress reduction may aid in changing nonhealthful recreation patterns. |

*Continued*

## Person with Peptic Ulcer—cont'd

**NURSING DIAGNOSIS** *Risk for altered health maintenance related to lack of knowledge of disease process, treatment regimen, and signs and symptoms of complications*

| expected patient outcome | nursing interventions | rationale |
|---|---|---|
| | Explain side effects of prescribed medications and relationship to bowel elimination. | Antacids may have either a cathartic or constipating effect depending on their constituents; bowel elimination may need to be supported through diet changes. |
| | Reinforce importance of *H. pylori* treatment to relapse prevention. | *H. pylori* drug treatment creates multiple GI side effects that adversely affect treatment adherence.<br>Failure to adhere creates drug-resistant strains. |
| | Instruct Mr. J. to monitor for and report the following:<br>• Persistent epigastric pain<br>• Sudden severe abdominal pain<br>• Tarry stools<br>• Persistent vomiting<br>• Bloody or brown vomitus | These symptoms may indicate ulcer complications, e.g., GI bleeding, perforation, or obstruction. |

medication administration, the restriction of alcohol, and the cessation of smoking. The severity of symptoms provides an initial impetus for regimen compliance, but this effect is difficult to sustain once symptom control has been achieved. The nurse's teaching concerning the regimen and its rationale is essential to long-term success in management.

## COMPLICATIONS

The major complications of peptic ulcer disease are hemorrhage, perforation, and obstruction of the pyloric outlet.

### Hemorrhage

Acute upper GI bleeding results in over 300,000 hospital admissions each year, and peptic ulcer disease is responsible for about 50% of all cases.[31] The 10% associated mortality rate has generally remained stable throughout the years despite vast improvements in endoscopic diagnostic techniques for treatment. The mortality rate reflects the vulnerability of the elderly population, who commonly have comorbid conditions, and the fact that most upper GI bleeding–related deaths are actually caused by problems other than peptic ulcer disease. Although close to 80% of all bleeding episodes are self-limiting and will resolve spontaneously with only supportive care, bleeding is a serious complication that must be handled in an appropriate and timely manner. Massive bleeding should always be treated in an intensive care unit (ICU) setting if possible.[11]

The severity of ulcer bleeding ranges from slight oozing to frank profuse hemorrhage (Figure 40-9). The presence of occult blood in the stool, or tarry stools, indicates that enzymes in the GI tract have had time to oxidize the blood and to break down the blood proteins. Emesis that is dark or of coffee-ground appearance indicates that the blood has been in the stomach long enough for HCl to alter it. Bright-red bleeding indicates a very recent onset. Significant bleeding is almost always arterial in nature and originates from a single eroded vessel in the base of the ulcer. Small arteries typically are involved, but deep erosion (greater than 1 mm) may affect the larger arterial trunks. Clinical manifestations vary with the extent of the bleeding. The most common sign is hematemesis, although patients with duodenal ulcers may not exhibit any overt bleeding signs even with gastric aspiration if the pylorus successfully prevents duodenal reflux. They may experience melena.

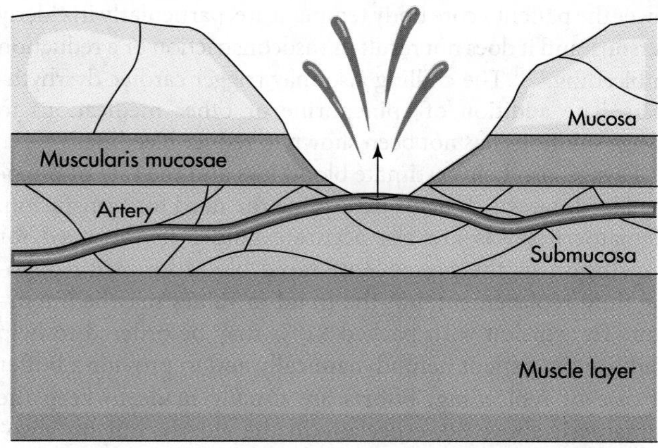


**fig. 40-9** Bleeding vessel at ulcer base occurs when ulcer erodes into artery.

Care begins with meticulous patient assessment to estimate the urgency of the situation. Careful vital sign assessment can yield early cues. Postural blood pressure changes of 10 mm Hg or a rise in pulse rate of more than 20 beats per minute indicates at least a 20% blood loss.[31] Anxiety and altered alertness may also be present. Shock will not occur until blood loss approximates 40% of the total volume. (See Chapter 17 for a more detailed discussion of shock assessment.) Initial care focuses on resuscitation efforts. A large-bore IV catheter is inserted, and normal saline is infused rapidly to sustain the systolic pressure above 100 mm Hg.

Hematemesis presents a serious risk for aspiration, particularly when large clots are present. Maintaining a patent airway is critical. The nurse turns the patient to the side and keeps the head of the bed elevated about 45 degrees unless the vital signs become unstable. Suction should be present at the bedside and used as needed to help clear the mouth. Mouth care after vomiting episodes is important for comfort.

Standard interventions for GI bleeding include the placement of a nasogastric (NG) tube to help determine the rate of ongoing blood loss and to facilitate gastric lavage. A large-bore NG tube allows the stomach to be cleared of excess blood and clots through lavage and prepares it for diagnostic endoscopy. Fluid is instilled in 500 to 1000 ml volumes and followed by gentle suction removal. This process is repeated until the returns are clear. Room temperature tap water is commonly used for lavage, although some centers still advocate the use of saline to minimize the risk of electrolyte washout.

Iced saline no longer is advised because it can significantly lower the patient's core body temperature, particularly in elderly persons, and it does not result in vasoconstriction or a reduction in bleeding.[23,31] The chilling also may trigger cardiac dysrhythmias. The addition of epinephrine or other medications to lavage solutions has not been shown to reduce bleeding.[31]

Lavage also helps estimate blood loss and the rate of ongoing bleeding, which helps determine the need for transfusion. Hematocrit levels are not accurate guides to the need for transfusion in the presence of rapid blood loss with ongoing fluid replacement, but the trend in values may be important. Transfusion with packed RBCs may be ordered to help stabilize the patient hemodynamically and to provide a buffer in case of rebleeding. Efforts are usually made to keep the hematocrit above 30, especially in the elderly, but no absolutes exist, and younger healthy people may tolerate much lower hematocrit values. Supplemental oxygen is also routinely administered.

Acute bleeding can be terrifying for the patient. The nurse maintains a calm and confident approach and remains at the bedside to provide reassurance to the patient. All interventions should be carefully explained. Ensuring warmth also is important. Gastric lavage, IV solutions, and chilled blood products can induce chilling and shivering. This will significantly increase the body's need for oxygen.

Drug therapy during an active bleeding episode usually involves the administration of an $H_2$ receptor antagonist IV. Omeprazole may be used as an alternative because it almost totally eliminates acid secretion. Although no studies have documented the effectiveness of these drugs in acute bleeding situations, it is assumed that reducing the acid load will promote rapid healing. Antacids and sucralfate are not used initially because they interfere with endoscopic evaluation.

Most bleeding episodes resolve spontaneously, and the situations that will require more definitive interventions cannot be predicted. Concern exists for both the control of the initial bleeding episode and the risk of rebleeding. Endoscopic evaluation is essential to isolate and evaluate the bleeding site. It is generally agreed that actively bleeding ulcers, either oozing or spurting, or the presence of visible vessels in the ulcer crater warrant further intervention.[23]

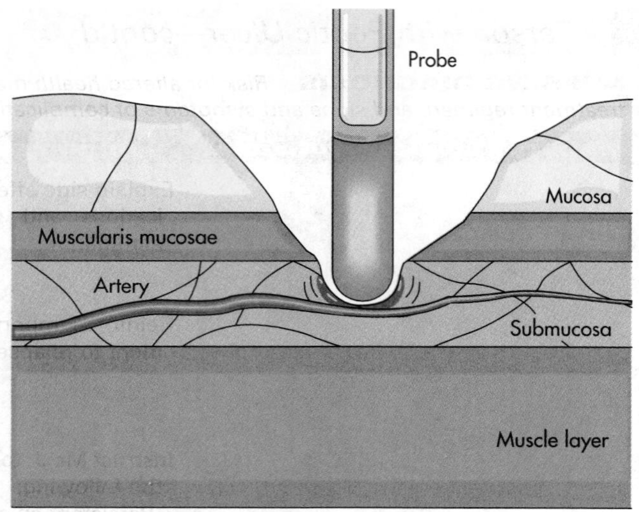


**fig. 40-10** Heater probe or bipolar electrode is used first for tamponade of bleeding vessel, then to bring about coagulation.

Therapeutic endoscopy may incorporate thermal coagulation of the bleeding vessel or injection therapy. Both approaches are consistently effective, and the choice is a clinical one. Thermal coagulation may be achieved through bipolar electrodes, heater probes, or laser therapy (Figure 40-10). Lasers produce excellent results, but they require extremely expensive equipment that can rarely be brought directly to the bedside, and they require a highly trained operator. The former methods are more efficient and cost-effective.

Injection therapy—with epinephrine, absolute alcohol, or other sclerosing agent—is an alternative primary or adjunct therapy. It is also the easiest and least expensive approach. Angiographic techniques that embolize the bleeding vessel with foreign materials can produce dramatic results, but they require extremely experienced and skilled angiographers.

Surgery is used only when all nonsurgical methods have been tried. Results are tied to the promptness of the decision to operate, and the outcomes deteriorate rapidly when surgery is delayed. Operative mortality ranges between 30% and 40%. Agreement does not exist concerning the procedure to use. Simple oversewing of the ulcer is quick and effective, but many surgeons advocate performing an acid reduction procedure (vagotomy) at the same time to reduce the risk of future bleeding.

guidelines for care

**The Person with Gastrointestinal Bleeding**

Establish at least one large-bore IV access:
- Instill normal saline or Ringer's lactate as ordered

Monitor vital signs frequently for signs of shock.
Start oxygen by nasal cannula as ordered:
- Extremely important in elderly persons

Draw blood for CBC, type, and crossmatch.
Insert NG tube and institute gastric lavage:
- Instill 250 ml room-temperature tap water
- Allow a 2 min dwell time
- Aspirate and evaluate the returns using a piston type of syringe
- Repeat as needed until returns are light colored and free of clots

Measure and record all output.
Raise head of bed 45 degrees if vital signs remain stable.
Turn vomiting patient on side to protect the airway.
Maintain the patient NPO.
Provide oral suction at bedside to help clear blood.
Provide mouth care after vomiting episodes.
Reassure patient and maintain a calm manner.
Administer IV $H_2$ receptor antagonist as ordered.
Administer blood products as ordered.
Prepare patient for therapeutic endoscopy.

The nursing role in the management of GI hemorrhage is largely collaborative and involves careful ongoing patient assessment, preventing complications, and support of the patient and family. The nurse establishes IV access and implements the fluid resuscitation and ongoing vital sign monitoring. The nurse is usually responsible for the gastric lavage. Management of the patient with GI bleeding is summarized in the accompanying Guidelines for Care Box, and a Clinical Pathway for the patient with a GI bleed is found on p. 1296.

### Perforation

Perforation involves the erosion of a peptic ulcer through the muscular wall of the stomach or duodenum, with spillage of gastric secretions into the abdominal cavity. It occurs six to eight times more commonly with duodenal ulcers than with gastric ulcers. A chemical peritonitis quickly develops from contact with the GI contents, and a bacterial peritonitis follows within 12 hours. The clinical presentation of perforation usually is dramatic in younger adults, but it may be subdued in elderly persons. This fact typically causes delays in seeking treatment and contributes to the high mortality rate associated with perforation in older patients, which runs as high as 35%. Perforations commonly seal spontaneously in younger adults but are less likely to do so in elderly persons.[29]

The classic clinical picture of ulcer perforation includes (1) severe, sharp abdominal pain; (2) an abdomen that becomes rigid, with rebound tenderness; (3) tachycardia, tachypnea, and diaphoresis; and (4) decreased bowel sounds. A perforation usually is diagnosed by the symptom pattern and supported by the finding of subdiaphragmatic free air on abdominal x-ray film.

Immediate care consists of establishing IV access to replace fluids and inserting an NG tube for drainage of the GI tract. High-dose antibiotics are usually administered in anticipation of sepsis. Effective management of pain is crucial.

The patient is kept in low Fowler's position in the attempt to contain the escaped secretions in a limited area of the abdomen. The nurse provides the patient with emotional support and reassurance, offers comfort measures, and attempts to prepare the patient for surgery.

Emergency surgery is the definitive treatment for perforation. Controversy exists over whether the surgery should simply repair the defect with oversewing and use of an omental patch or include definitive ulcer correction.[29] Truncal vagotomy and pyloroplasty may be performed in stable elderly patients in whom the risk of recurrence is believed to be high.

### Obstruction

Improved treatment of peptic ulcers has caused the incidence of gastric outlet obstruction to decline to the point of being rare. Obstruction can result from scar tissue formation but also from muscle obstruction and narrowing caused by spasm and inflammatory edema. It is usually associated with long-standing peptic ulcer disease.

The obstruction usually develops slowly, and the patient may initially experience dyspepsia symptoms, including anorexia and nausea, as the stomach fails to empty completely. Weight loss and malnutrition will develop if the diagnosis is delayed, and this is a common occurrence in elderly persons. Vomiting occurs when the chyme is completely unable to pass into the duodenum, which usually represents a narrowing of the normally 10 to 20 mm pyloric channel to less than 6 mm.[22]

The diagnosis of obstruction can be established by aspiration of stomach contents or abdominal x-ray films that show gastric distention and large fluid levels. Endoscopy is performed to rule out the presence of an obstructing tumor and may be used to treat uncomplicated obstructions.

The initial management of obstruction involves fluid and electrolyte replacement and gastric decompression with an NG tube. Aggressive therapy for the ulcer may be initiated first because obstruction is rarely an emergent condition. The obstruction may resolve sufficiently with ulcer healing to eliminate the need for surgical intervention. When surgery is needed a vagotomy-plus-drainage procedure is the procedure of choice to minimize postoperative digestive problems.[29] Even high-risk elders can generally tolerate this surgery if attention has been paid to careful preoperative stabilization.

## STRESS ULCERS

### ETIOLOGY/EPIDEMIOLOGY

The terms *stress-related mucosal damage* and *stress ulcer* refer to a syndrome characterized by the development of multiple diffuse gastric lesions and ulceration shortly after the

*Text continued on p. 1300*

## clinical pathway *Gastrointestinal Hemorrhage*

| | DAY 1 | DAY 2 | DAY 3 | DAY 4 | DAY 5 | DAY 6 |
|---|---|---|---|---|---|---|
| **Assessment** | | | | | | |
| ***Neurological/ psychological*** | Mental status • LOC • restlessness • subjective statement of fatigue & weakness • explore anxiety/coping skills • begin assessment of knowledge of health care problem & potential modifiable risk factors (smoking, diet, alcohol, stress, & exercise) • identify available & needed family/human/economic resources to resume independent self-care activities | Mental status • LOC • restlessness • subjective statement of fatigue & weakness • anxiety/coping skills • continue assessment of knowledge of health care problem & potential modifiable risk factors (alcohol, smoking, diet, stress, exercise) • collaborate w/social services re: available & needed family/human/economic resources to resume independent self-care activities | Mental status • restlessness • subjective statement of fatigue & weakness | Mental status • restlessness • subjective statement of fatigue & weakness | Mental status | Mental status |
| ***Pulmonary:*** | RR & pattern | RR & pattern | RR & pattern | RR & pattern | RR | RR |
| ***Cardiovascular:*** | HR & BP for hypovolemia & tachycardia • rhythm for dysrhythmias • narrow pulse pressure • pulses & capillary refill | HR & BP for hypovolemia & tachycardia • rhythm for dysrhythmias • narrow pulse pressure • pulses & capillary refill | HR & BP for hypovolemia & tachycardia • narrow pulse pressure • pulses & capillary refill | HR & BP for hypovolemia & tachycardia • BP for orthostatic changes • pulses & capillary refill | BP for orthostatic changes • pulses | BP for orthostatic changes • pulses |
| ***Gastrointestinal:*** | Mucous membranes for dryness • bowel sounds • abdominal pain (location, stage, level, & duration), cramps, distention • nausea • vomiting • stool for frequency, color, & form • daily wgt | Mucous membranes for dryness • bowel sounds • abdominal pain (location, stage, level, & duration), cramps, distention • nausea • vomiting • stool for frequency, color, & form • daily wgt | Mucous membranes for dryness • bowel sounds • abdominal pain (location, stage, level, & duration), cramps, distention • nausea • vomiting • stool for frequency, color, & form • daily wgt | Appetite & food tolerance • stool for frequency, color, & form • daily wgt | Appetite & food tolerance • stool for frequency, color, & form • daily wgt | Appetite and food tolerance • stool for frequency, color, & form • daily wgt |

| | DAY 1 | DAY 2 | DAY 3 | DAY 4 | DAY 5 | DAY 6 |
|---|---|---|---|---|---|---|
| *Genitourinary:* | I & O • UO > 30 ml/hr | I & O • UO > 30 ml/hr | I & O • UO > 30 ml/hr | I & O • UO > 30 ml/hr | UO qs | UO qs |
| *Integumentary:* | Skin turgor, temp, color, & integrity • presence of diaphoresis, petechiae, or spider angiomata | Skin turgor, temperature, color, & integrity • presence of diaphoresis, petechiae, or spider angiomata | Skin turgor, temp, color, & integrity • presence of diaphoresis, petechiae, or spider angiomata | Skin turgor, temp, color, & integrity • presence of diaphoresis, petechiae, or spider angiomata | Skin turgor & integrity | Skin turgor & integrity |
| **Focus** | Fluid resuscitation/ volume replacement • identify source of bleeding | Fluid resuscitation/ volume replacement • initiate PO fluid intake | Increase in PO fluid • progressive increase in activity • teaching | Teaching • increased independence in ADL • increased activity & diet tolerance | Discharge plan & teaching | Self-care & discharge |
| **Diagnostic Plan** | Chemistries • monitor Hct & hemoglobin q2-4h until stable • hemolytic profile w/platelets • coagulation studies • liver function tests • blood grouping & crossmatch • stool for occult blood • specific gravity qs *Consider:* urgent anoscopy, sigmoidoscopy, colonoscopy, or endoscopy (esophageal, stomach, duodenal) w/cautery/injection or biopsy • gastric secretion pH & occult blood q4h • $SaO_2$ pulse oximeter • cardiac monitor | CBC w/differential • continue monitoring Hct, hemoglobin, & electrolytes q6-8h until stable • repeat abnormal lab tests *Consider:* visceral (mesenteric) angiography • nuclear bleeding scan w/labeled red blood cells • gastric secretion analysis | Repeat any abnormal lab test(s) *Consider:* contrast x-ray to rule out underlying pathology • further coagulation studies | CBC w/differential • repeat abnormal lab tests | Repeat Hct & any lab study w/abnormal value | None |
| **Therapeutic Interventions** | Large-bore IV access • give 2 L IV NS/RL in 1-2 hr then 150-200 ml/hr (as tolerated) to keep UO > 30 ml/hr until stable • irrigate NGT q2h w/30 ml NS • NPO w/frequent oral care | Clamp NGT for 12 hrs • give sips of $H_2O$ PO • discontinue NGT if clamping tolerated • continue IV fluid hydration • start on clear fluids once | Discontinue NGT • decrease IV fluids as PO fluid intake increased to maintain UO > 30 ml/hr • progress diet from fluids to soft • change to PO meds | Discontinue IV • increased walking in hall • soft diet | Encourage activity & independence in ADL | Discharge • encourage lifestyle modifications |

From Birdsall C, Sperry SP: *Clinical paths in medical surgical practice,* St Louis, 1997, Mosby.
*LOC,* Level of consciousness; *NGT,* nasogastric tube; *ASA,* aspirin; *NS,* normal saline; *RL,* Ringer's lactate.

*Continued*

## *Gastrointestinal Hemorrhage—cont'd*

| | DAY 1 | DAY 2 | DAY 3 | DAY 4 | DAY 5 | DAY 6 |
|---|---|---|---|---|---|---|
| **Therapeutic Interventions—cont'd** | • bed rest • cardiac monitor • $O_2$ prn *Consider:* antacids • histamine $H_2$ receptor blocker • sucralfate • antibiotics (if ulcers suspected) • IV vasopressin • packed red blood cells (if Hct <25%) | NGT removed & no nausea • BRP w/assistance • assist w/hygiene | • get OOB to chair tid • walk in hall w/help bid • discontinue cardiac monitor & specific gravity *Consider:* oral iron, stool softener, & fiber supplement | | | |
| **Patient/Family Teaching/ Discharge Planning** | Explain initial treatment/ meds/fluids • instruct to call nurse for chest pain, SOB, dizziness, fast HR, diaphoresis, vomiting, diarrhea • explore potential precipitating factors (ASA, NSAID, smoking, alcohol, corticosteroids, family history, anticoagulants, prolonged retching) & document same • identify available & needed family/ human/economic resources to resume independent self-care activities • identify Pt/family coping mechanisms • initiate discharge plan • discuss plan for daily review of plan of care w/Pt/family | Explain need for adequate hydration • explain disease process • identify learning needs related to disease syndrome & document same • discuss potential lifestyle changes prn (alcohol, smoking cessation, diet, stress management, wgt reduction, exercise program) • reassure that responses (anxiety, subjective feelings of emotional lability or inability to concentrate, etc.) are a normal reaction • encourage verbalization of anxiety/fear • review, clarify, & confirm information given to date | Collaborate w/dietitian & initiate diet teaching • teach to get up slowly from lying position • teach signs of intestinal bleeding (hematemesis, melena, hematochezia) • review meds & food/drug interactions | Teach S & S of bleeding (thirst, frequent lip licking, lightheadedness, dizziness, weakness/ fatigue, impaired mental status, irritability, pallor, tremors, decrease in uo, dry skin & mucous membranes) • review meds, food/ drug interactions, appropriate health-seeking behaviors, & when to seek medical care | Review discharge plan, disease process, exercise plan, meds & drug/food interactions • value of relaxation techniques & health-seeking behaviors by modifying lifestyle prn (smoking, stress, alcohol, diet, aspirin, other meds, etc.) | Review appointment dates for physician visit & discharge plan |

| | DAY 1 | DAY 2 | DAY 3 | DAY 4 | DAY 5 | DAY 6 |
|---|---|---|---|---|---|---|
| **Expected Outcomes** | W/volume replacement, hemodynamic stability is restored • active bleeding stopped • UO > 30 ml/hr • verbalizes treatment plan | Tolerating PO fluids • plan for encouraging PO fluids documented • fluid & potassium in balance as evidenced by UO > 30 ml/hr, stable VS, & stable Hct & hemoglobin • decrease in anxiety | No parenteral therapy • increased tolerance of PO fluids & diet • nutritional assessment documented & calorie/protein needs identified • well hydrated • no bleeding • no abdominal distress • formed stools • independent ADL • verbalizes disease process & potential lifestyle changes | Ambulates without assistance & independent in ADL • verbalizes meds information • demonstrates improved appetite • states signs of intestinal bleeding (hematemesis, melena, hematochezia) & to report same (red or brown-tinged vomitus & maroon, red, bloody, or tarry stools) | Verbalizes diet restrictions (avoid foods that previously caused discomfort, high-acid foods, hot pepper, caffeine, highly spiced food, & alcohol) & need to prevent constipation while on oral iron • denies subjective feelings of anxiety • verbalizes appropriate concerns & fears • states S & S of bleeding (thirst, frequent lip licking, light-headedness, dizziness, weakness/fatigue, impaired mental status, irritability, pallor, tremors, decrease in urine output, dry skin & mucous membranes) & when to seek medical care | Verbalizes risk factors & health-seeking behaviors • states appointment date w/physican |
| **Trigger(s)** | S & S of new bleeding w/ hypotension, tachycardia, & UO <30 ml/hr | Persistent hypotension, tachycardia, or UO <30 ml/hr • nausea/vomiting/abdominal pain | Persistent hypotension, tachycardia, or UO <30 ml/hr • nausea/vomiting/abdominal pain | Pain, new bleeding, anorexia, decreased output • inability to maintain fluid & food intake needed for hydration & to meet caloric needs | Inadequate fluid or dietary intake | Inadequate fluid or dietary intake • unable to be independent in ADL |

onset of acute illness, trauma, or sepsis. The problem has been considered to be almost universal among patients in critical care settings. Research studies from the 1970s and 1980s showed the incidence of stress ulcers to be in excess of 80% of the critical care population and the incidence of bleeding to be nearly 20%.[14] Because GI hemorrhage in the critically ill is accompanied by a mortality rate of nearly 50%, these studies were used as the basis for the development of aggressive prevention protocols that have been implemented with virtually every critically ill patient. Outcome studies demonstrated the effectiveness of these aggressive interventions with antacids, $H_2$ receptor antagonists, and sucralfate in preventing most serious bleeding episodes.[4]

The assumptions underlying these stress ulcer protocols have been increasingly challenged in recent years because newer, rigorously designed research studies have failed to replicate the earlier findings.[9] It appears that the older studies failed to adequately differentiate between the presence of occult blood and the presence of clinically significant bleeding. Attention is now being directed toward the incidence of clinically significant bleeding, which appears to occur in about 6% of the critical care population.[9] This much lower incidence figure represents both more stringent criteria for "bleeding" but also improved overall care for critically ill patients. The mortality rate associated with significant bleeding remains high.

It is becoming accepted that not all ICU patients are at equal risk for stress ulcer bleeding. Efforts are ongoing to identify the factors that place patients at risk and conditions where the association with bleeding is high. Curling's duodenal ulcers have been recognized in conjunction with severe burns for many years, and Cushing's ulcer is clearly associated with central nervous system trauma. Other risks have been identified and are presented in the Risk Factors Box. The presence of multiple risk factors dramatically increases the odds of clinically significant bleeding.

## PATHOPHYSIOLOGY

The major factor that causes stress ulceration is a loss of the ability to maintain the integrity of the mucosa. The maintenance of mucosal homeostasis is a complex process involving mucus production, mucosal blood flow, prostaglandin secretion, bicarbonate production, and maintenance of the needed pH gradient. The stress state decreases gastric mucosal blood flow, and this event triggers a series of changes that ultimately result in mucosal breakdown. The epithelial cells of the mucosa are extremely sensitive to hypoxia, and the process of cellular necrosis can begin within minutes. Stress ulceration cannot occur without the presence of acid and pepsin, but overproduction of acid is rarely the cause of stress ulcers. In fact, acid secretion commonly is temporarily diminished in the acute stress state. Mucosal resistance therefore is believed to be the key.[14] The notable exceptions are Cushing's and Curling's ulcers, which are associated with massive increases in acid output, often exceeding 3 to 4 L per day.

Stress ulcer lesions tend to be more shallow than standard peptic ulcers, and there are usually multiple ulcerated areas rather than a single well-defined lesion. The proximal acid-secreting areas of the stomach are the prime targets. The classic presentation of stress ulcers is the development of painless bleeding within 3 to 7 days of admission.

***risk factors***

**Stress Ulcer Bleeding**

**Clinical Risk Factors**

Hypotension/shock
Respiratory failure/mechanical ventilation
Multiple trauma/major surgery
Severe burns over >30% of body surface area
Sepsis
Neurological injury/surgery
Hepatic/renal failure
Coagulopathy
NOTE: The presence of more than one risk factor dramatically increases the likelihood of significant bleeding.

## COLLABORATIVE CARE MANAGEMENT

The primary clinical dilemma in preventing and treating stress ulcers is determining which patients to treat prophylactically and in what way.[9] The traditional approach has been to treat all critical care patients preventively with antacids, histamine receptor antagonists, or sucralfate. Frequent monitoring of gastric pH is usually performed either by intermittent aspiration of gastric secretions or through the use of special NG tubes that have electrodes for continuous pH monitoring. The pH is usually kept above 3.5, although some advocate a higher level.

Increased individualization of care is now recommended by many researchers. Patients with multiple risk factors, and particularly patients who will need mechanical ventilation longer than 48 hours and those with demonstrable coagulopathies or neurological trauma, are recommended for preventive treatment.[9,11] Lower-risk patients may not need it. The unique patient situation also governs the choice of drugs. Sucralfate is emerging as the treatment option that appears to have the best outcomes with the least adverse characteristics.[9] The frequent and time-consuming administration needed for the use of antacids plus their major adverse effects on the GI tract make them a less desirable option in most situations. When the enteral route is impractical, continuous administration of IV ranitidine provides for the most constant pH control.

Concern has arisen that the prophylactic neutralization of gastric secretions may be leaving ICU patients vulnerable to nosocomial infection, particularly in the form of gram-negative pneumonias. These organisms can colonize the stomach within 2 to 5 days.[4] Design flaws in the available research have called some of the conclusions into question, and the use of mechanical ventilation is an independent risk factor for nosocomial infection, but sucralfate is increasingly being recommended as the primary agent for the prevention of stress ulcer, at least in part because it acts without altering the gastric pH. Much remains to be learned about the origins,

**research**

Reference: Hansson LE et al: The risk of stomach cancer in patients with gastric or duodenal ulcer disease, *N Engl J Med* 335:242, 1996.

This study explored the relationship between peptic ulcer, gastric ulcer, and gastric cancer. It followed the course of 29,000 patients with gastric ulcers, 24,500 patients with duodenal ulcers, and 4000 patients with both types discharged following hospital care in Sweden from 1965 to 1983. Patients were followed an average of 8.3 years. A risk of gastric cancer of twice the expected rate was found in patients with gastric ulcers; a risk at the expected rate for the general population was found for patients with prepyloric ulcers; and a decreased risk compared with the general population was found in patients with duodenal ulcers. No connection with the use of NSAIDs was found. Smoking increased the risk of cancer in all populations. The increased incidence of gastric cancer peaked in the first 3 years of follow-up and then leveled off.

prevention, and treatment of stress ulcers, but it is clear that meticulous bedside monitoring of patient status by skilled ICU nurses will continue to play an essential role in patient management.

### Patient/Family Education

Critically ill patients and families need to be kept informed about all aspects of the plan of care. This includes all measures aimed at the identification, prevention, or treatment of stress ulcers. The nurse is the primary liaison with the family and will need to keep them knowledgable about the rationale for all planned interventions.

Stress ulcer is not a problem that is familiar to most laypersons, and the nurse will need to lay the foundation for understanding all relevant care. The stresses of the situation may make it difficult for the patient and family to hear and process information, and time for reteaching should be planned as needed.

## CANCER OF THE STOMACH

### ETIOLOGY

The cause of cancer of the stomach remains unknown, yet its highly erratic worldwide incidence pattern suggests the involvement of multiple environmental, genetic, and possibly cultural factors.

Diet and living conditions appear to be the most significant aspects in etiology, and early life exposure is critical. High nitrate content in soil and water and diets high in smoked and preserved foods are believed to be causative. Nitrates and nitrites in foods are reduced to nitrosamines in the body, and a cascade of DNA changes can then occur that lead to cancer. Improved refrigeration and diets with fresh fruits and vegetables appear to decrease the risk, suggesting a possible protective role for vitamins A and C and carotene. The sharp decline in incidence rates in the United States since the 1950s is largely believed to be attributable to these factors.[11] No strong links have been found with alcohol or caffeine consumption, and although a smoking link is present, it is primarily with heavy smoking. Familial clustering of gastric cancer is occasionally observed, and an inverse relationship appears to exist between incidence and socioeconomic status.

**risk factors**

**Gastric Cancer**

Diets high in smoked and preserved foods, which contain nitrites and nitrates
Diets low in fresh fruits and vegetables
High nitrate content in the soil and water
History of heavy smoking
Presence of chronic gastritis and achlorhydria (10% of patients develop cancer within 15 years)
Age and sex (incidence increases steadily after age 40, male-to-female ratio is 2:1)

The development of gastric cancer is related to the presence of achlorhydria and pernicious anemia. It is estimated that 10% of patients with chronic gastritis will develop gastric cancer within 15 years, and thus the role of *H. pylori* is being carefully explored.[11] The pervasiveness of the infection worldwide makes it clear that *H. pylori* does not act alone in gastric cancer etiology. The presence of peptic ulcer disease is not considered to be a contributing factor (see the Research Box).

### EPIDEMIOLOGY

Cancer of the stomach was the most common malignant disease in the United States as recently as the 1940s. Since that time it has undergone a steady decline in incidence that is not readily explainable. It remains the second leading cause of cancer death worldwide behind lung cancer and exhibits tremendous variation from region to region. The mortality rate from gastric cancer in the United States has dropped from 22.5 to 6 per 100,000, as compared with Japan, where the rate is 70 per 100,000—the highest in the world.[18] The links to environmental factors appear clear because the risk to immigrants to the United States drops sharply by the second generation.[11]

Gastric cancer is rare before age 40, and the incidence increases sharply with age. The male-to-female ratio is about 2:1. Risk factors for gastric cancer are summarized in the Risk Factors Box. Most gastric cancers are found in the antral portion of the stomach, but the incidence of proximal tumors appears to be rising. Figure 40-11 illustrates typical sites of gastric cancer.

### PATHOPHYSIOLOGY

Gastric cancers are virtually all primary adenocarcinomas that are derived from the epithelium. They have been found traditionally in the pyloric and antral regions, particularly along the lesser curvature. There are numerous ways to

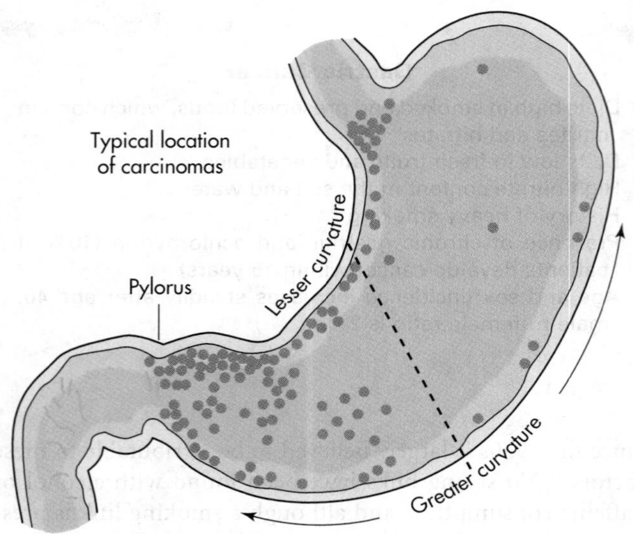


**fig. 40-11** Typical sites of gastric cancer.

classify gastric cancer, which manifests in a variety of forms. Histologically the cancer is classified as diffuse or intestinal. The intestinal form is associated with the presence of intestinal metaplasia in the stomach. This type of gastric cancer has been declining in incidence. The diffuse forms have shown little change in incidence. The disease is believed to begin locally in the mucosa and exhibits a long latency.

Gastric cancer may spread directly through the stomach wall into adjacent tissues; to the lymphatics; to the regional lymph nodes of the stomach; to the esophagus, spleen, pancreas, and liver; or through the bloodstream to the lungs or bones. Involvement of regional lymph nodes occurs early. Prognosis depends on the depth of invasion and extent of metastasis. Three fourths of patients with gastric carcinoma have metastases at the time of diagnosis.

Gastric cancer has an insidious onset. It is accompanied by vague nondescript dyspeptic symptoms that overlap with multiple benign disorders, including nonulcer dyspepsia and peptic ulcer disease.[18] Early diagnosis is therefore extremely rare. Pain does not usually develop until late in the disease. Marked cachexia and a palpable mass in the abdomen may be present at diagnosis. Possible clinical manifestation are presented in Box 40-6.

## COLLABORATIVE CARE MANAGEMENT

### Diagnostic Tests

Biopsy is considered to be the diagnostic procedure of choice when gastric cancer is suspected. Multiple specimens are obtained through endoscopy. Many gastric cancers can be located by barium contrast upper-GI x-ray films, but only biopsy can confirm the diagnosis. Computed tomography scanning and endoscopic ultrasonography also may be used to define the tumor and to search for distant metastasis.

**box 40-6** *clinical manifestations*

***Gastric Cancer***

Dyspepsia: early satiety, bloating, anorexia
Epigastric pain or burning (usually mild and relieved by antacids)
Mild nausea
Weight loss (may be rapid and severe)
Fatigue and weakness
Changes in bowel habits: constipation or diarrhea

NOTE: Gastric cancer typically is asymptomatic in early stages.

### Medications

Medications do not play a role in the management of gastric cancer except when chemotherapy is used. Adjuvant therapy guidelines for gastric cancer are not well developed, and the use of chemotherapy has not proved to be of clear benefit. Chemotherapy is, however, the mainstay of treatment for nonresectable tumors. Several new drug and combination chemotherapy-radiotherapy protocols are currently under investigation at major cancer research centers. Preoperative chemotherapy has shown some promise as an adjuvant to surgery.

Early diagnosis is crucial in gastric cancer, yet it is rarely achieved. Concern exists that the ready availability of $H_2$ receptor antagonists over the counter may further delay the diagnosis because early ulcerative lesions are commonly at least temporarily responsive to acid reduction.

### Treatments

Radiotherapy is being researched as a treatment option for gastric cancer. At present it shows little proved effectiveness. It usually is used in combination with chemotherapy for nonresectable or recurrent cancer cases, and its role in palliation of bone metastases is well recognized. Research studies are underway utilizing direct intraoperative radiotherapy and show promising results, but much additional research will be needed to test this approach.

### Surgical Management

The only potentially curative treatment for gastric cancer is surgical resection. The procedure of choice depends on the location and extent of the tumor. Most surgeons perform subtotal gastrectomies and attempt to remove all of the tumor (Figure 40-12). Total gastrectomy is not commonly used in the United States because of the serious digestive difficulties that may result. It also appears to have no positive effects on disease mortality. The extensive experience of Japanese surgeons with gastric cancer emphasizes the importance of performing more extensive lymph node dissections than have been standard in the United States. Physicians have been reluctant to adopt this aggressive approach and question its applicability for the U.S. population.

Tumors that are high in the cardia present more technical challenges to resection and anastomosis. Removal of other abdominal organs appears to have no positive impact at all on

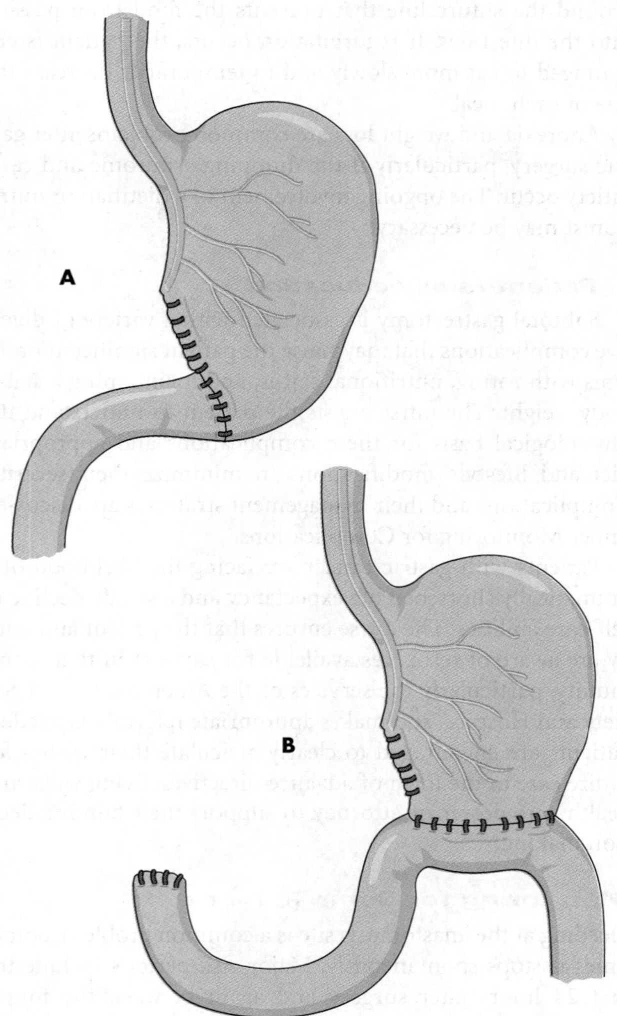


**fig. 40-12** Types of gastric resections with anastomoses. **A,** Billroth I anastomosis of gastric segment to duodenum. **B,** Billroth II, anastomosis of gastric segment to the proximal jejunum.

survival. Despite aggressive intervention, 5-year survival remains at 5% to 15%.

One specific form of gastric cancer termed *early gastric cancer* is limited to the mucosa and submucosa even when lymph node metastasis is present. These tumors are extremely responsive to surgical intervention and can have a 10-year survival rate as high as 80%. This form of gastric cancer is not commonly identified.

### Diet

There are no specific dietary considerations for the treatment of gastric cancer. Patients may experience severe weight loss and cachexia and eventually require nutritional support. If a patient experiences ulcer-related pain, the standard recommendations for avoiding spicy and irritating foods will be made. The patient is encouraged to work within the scope of individual preferences to maintain adequate nutrition. Patients who undergo gastric resection may develop significant problems with dumping syndrome and malabsorption. Management of these disorders is discussed on p. 1305.

### Activity

The patient with gastric cancer does not need to restrict activity in any way. Patients are encouraged to remain as active in their usual lifestyles as possible. Treatment for gastric cancer is rigorous and may take a significant toll on the patient's energy level and stamina. The nurse encourages patients to make any necessary modifications in their daily activities to accommodate the demands of the treatment protocol.

### Referrals

The treatment of resectable gastric cancer is primarily surgical. Referral to consultants usually is not necessary in the early period. The primary ongoing concerns are maintenance of desired weight and nutritional status. If digestion and absorption problems become severe, the patient may be referred to a nutritional support team for guidance and management.

## NURSING MANAGEMENT OF THE PATIENT WITH GASTRIC SURGERY

### ■ PREOPERATIVE CARE

Preoperative care focuses on ensuring that the patient is in the best nutritional state to support healing and on patient teaching. Correction of nutritional deficits may involve short-term parenteral nutrition if the patient is severely cachectic.

A high abdominal incision is standard with gastric surgery. This incision limits respiration and places the person at high risk for postoperative respiratory complications. The nurse focuses preoperative teaching on pulmonary hygiene and the importance of deep breathing, effective coughing, splinting the incision, frequent position changes, incentive spirometry, and chest physiotherapy if indicated. These teaching interventions are even more critical if the patient has a history of smoking. Planned methods for postoperative pain control will also be discussed.

Most patients undergoing gastric surgery have an NG tube in place for several days after surgery. The NG tube prevents trauma, reduces pressure on the suture lines, and minimizes gas and fluid accumulation from decreased postoperative peristalsis. The nurse teaches the patient about the NG tube and its purpose, the necessity for an initial NPO status, and the planned use of any other wound-drainage device.

Relieving anxiety is the final area addressed by the nurse in the preoperative period. Gastric cancer carries an extremely poor prognosis, and the threat of death will color the patient's ability to attend to teaching and participate in self-care. Accurate staging of the cancer is commonly not possible until surgical exploration is completed, and this adds an additional element of uncertainty to an already stressful situation. The nurse provides support and encourages the patient to verbalize any concerns.

## POSTOPERATIVE CARE

### Maintaining a Patent Airway and Ventilation

The patient who has had gastric surgery tends to lie still and breathe shallowly to limit incisional pain. Pain medications are provided frequently, or patient-controlled analgesia is used and monitored. Adequate pain management is essential to achieving respiratory goals. Turning, deep breathing, incentive spirometry, and ambulation are essential postoperative activities, and the nurse must ensure that the patient is comfortable enough to participate actively in self-care. A semi-Fowler's position assists with natural chest expansion. The nurse routinely auscultates the lungs to monitor pulmonary status and consistently encourages the patient in all pulmonary hygiene routines.

### Supporting Adequate Nutrition

The patient is given nothing by mouth until peristalsis resumes and initial surgical healing occurs. Drainage from the NG tube usually contains some blood for the first 6 to 12 hours, but the presence of bright-red blood, large amounts of blood, or excessive bloody drainage is reported to the surgeon at once. If the NG tube stops draining, the surgeon also is notified immediately because a buildup of gas or fluid can put pressure on the suture line, resulting in rupture or dislodgment of the sutures.

To protect the healing suture line, the nurse does not routinely irrigate or reposition the NG tube. Fluids are given parenterally until the tube is removed and the patient is able to drink sufficient fluids. The nurse offers or provides the patient with frequent mouth care. It is important for gastric drainage and urinary output to be accurately measured and recorded.

Fluids by mouth may be restricted for 12 to 24 hours after the NG tube is removed. Small amounts of fluid are then given frequently, and the patient is observed for signs of leakage, such as difficulty in breathing, pain, or rise in temperature. Foods are added as tolerated by the patient. The dietary regimen must be adapted to the individual, because some persons tolerate increasing amounts of food and fluids better than others.

When the cardia of the stomach has been removed, the patient may complain of nausea and vomiting. This problem is usually caused by irritation of the esophageal mucosa by the gastric juices that reflux into the esophagus when the patient lies down. The patient should never lie flat in bed and should avoid bending and stooping.

Early satiety is a common problem after gastric surgery. Regurgitation after meals also occurs and may be caused by eating too fast, eating too much, or postoperative edema around the suture line that prevents the food from passing into the intestines. If regurgitation occurs, the patient is encouraged to eat more slowly and to temporarily decrease the size of each meal.

Anorexia and weight loss are common problems after gastric surgery, particularly if the dumping syndrome and early satiety occur. The ongoing involvement of a dietitian or nutritionist may be necessary.

#### *Patient/family education*

Subtotal gastrectomy is associated with a variety of digestive complications that may cause the patient significant problems with eating, nutritional status, and maintaining a stable body weight. The nurse assists the patient to understand the physiological basis for these complications and appropriate diet and lifestyle modifications to minimize their severity. Complications and their management strategies are discussed under Monitoring for Complications.

Patients with gastric cancer are facing the likelihood of a dramatically shortened life expectancy and a steady decline in self-care abilities. The nurse ensures that the patient and family are aware of resources available for support in their community, particularly the services of the American Cancer Society and Hospice, and makes appropriate referrals as needed. Patients are encouraged to clearly articulate their wishes for future care in the form of advance directives, living wills, and health care power of attorney to support their family's decision making.

### Monitoring for Complications

Bleeding at the anastomosis site is a common problem. Sometimes it stops spontaneously. Major risk periods include the first 24 hours after surgery and again between the fourth and seventh days when nonhealing becomes apparent. The nurse carefully monitors the NG tube drainage for blood and avoids irrigating or repositioning the tube unless specifically ordered.

Any of the anastomosis sites are at risk for leakage in the early postoperative period. The blind-end duodenal stump that is created with a Billroth II (Figure 40-12) procedure appears to be particularly vulnerable. The nurse monitors for classic peritonitis symptoms such as severe abdominal pain, rigidity, and fever. Surgical drainage and closure are often necessary.

## GERONTOLOGICAL CONSIDERATIONS

Gastric cancer is rare before the age of 40 years and typically occurs in persons between 50 and 70 years of age. Therefore the entire discussion related to the collaborative management of gastric cancer is targeted primarily toward elderly persons who are most likely to be affected by this deadly disease process.

## SPECIAL ENVIRONMENTS FOR CARE

### Critical Care Management

Critical care management will rarely be needed in the management of gastric cancer. The disease prognosis is extremely poor, especially for advanced invasive disease, and only palliative treatment may be undertaken. Treatment is usually designed to relieve obstruction or pain. Anastomosis leakage is a serious complication of gastrectomy surgeries, and its occurrence might require critical care monitoring, particularly if patients have other chronic illnesses that increase their risks.

### Home Care Management

Home management will present a series of ongoing challenges for the patient and family. The dumping syndrome is the most common complication of the surgical treatment of gastric cancer, and the patient will need to make multiple dietary adjustments to control its symptoms. Nutritional support may become necessary in certain situations and will be essential if further active treatment is planned.

Pain control is a common home care issue for patients with advanced disease. The appropriate use of long-acting oral narcotics, transdermal patches, epidural catheters, and infusion pumps can make it possible for patients to remain comfortably in their home environments with home health or hospice support.

The greatest ongoing challenge is the knowledge of the terminal prognosis. The patient and family will need support and encouragement to deal effectively with a progressive and deteriorating situation. In many cases the disease is fatal within 1 year of diagnosis, and the patient's physical decline can be rapid and frightening.

## COMPLICATIONS

Gastrectomy is associated with several major digestive complications that will require ongoing management. These include dumping syndrome and malabsorption. Vitamin $B_{12}$ deficiency may also develop.

### Dumping Syndrome

*Dumping syndrome* is the term used for a group of unpleasant vasomotor and gastrointestinal symptoms that occur after gastric surgery in as many as 50% of patients. It is a complex process with several contributing causative factors. One major element is believed to be the rapid entry of hypertonic food directly into the upper small intestine without first undergoing the usual breakdown and dilution in the stomach. This causes distention, stimulates motility, and produces both an intense feeling of fullness and discomfort plus diarrhea. The undiluted chyme is highly hyperosmolar and causes an osmotic shift of fluid from the intravascular compartment into the intestine. This worsens the distention and triggers a systemic reaction of weakness, sweating, tachycardia, and possibly flushing. This reaction is called the early dumping syndrome and occurs within 1 hour of eating.

A second "late" dumping syndrome follows. Rapid absorption of glucose from the chyme results in hyperglycemia and provokes insulin secretion. The insulin secretion outlasts the hyperglycemia, which then swings to hypoglycemia and its associated anxiety, weakness, diaphoresis, palpitations, and faintness. These symptoms develop about 2 hours after eating.

Prevention is the most effective means of controlling dumping syndrome. The nurse instructs the patient to follow a moderate-fat, high-protein diet with limited carbohydrates. Simple sugars should be avoided completely. Fluids with meals are discouraged because they increase total volume. Lying down on the left side for 20 to 30 minutes after eating to delay gastric emptying is helpful for some patients. Anticholinergic or antispasmodic drugs may be effective in certain cases. Management of the dumping syndrome is summarized in the Guidelines for Care Box.

### Malabsorption

Malabsorption of fat may occur after gastric resection from decreased acid secretion, decreased availability of pancreatic enzymes, and increased upper gastrointestinal motility, which prevents adequate mixing of the chyme with biliary and pancreatic secretions. It is particularly troublesome after Billroth II procedures. The patient experiences steatorrhea, diarrhea, and weight loss. Deficiencies in fat-soluble vitamins may occur. Diet adjustments are made to test the patient's responsiveness to various amounts of dietary fat. Pancreatic enzymes or antispasmodic agents may be helpful.

The combined effects of dumping syndrome and steatorrhea can result in significant weight loss over a relatively short time. The patient is encouraged to monitor body weight at least weekly and to experiment with food supplements as tolerated to meet nutritional needs.

### Vitamin $B_{12}$ Deficiency

Gastrectomy procedures result in a partial or total loss of the intrinsic factor that is secreted by the parietal cells of

**guidelines for care**

**The Person with Dumping Syndrome**

**Clinical Manifestations**

Weakness
Dizziness
Diaphoresis
Tachycardia
Palpitations
Feeling of fullness or discomfort
Nausea
Diarrhea
Onset of symptoms occurs first within 1 hour of eating and may reoccur after 2 hours

**Management**

Prevention is the key:
- Small frequent meals
- Moderate-fat, high-protein diet
- Limited carbohydrates, no simple sugars
- Minimal liquids with meals
- Avoid very hot and very cold foods and beverages
- Rest on left side for 20-30 min after eating
- Anticholinergic or antispasmodic medications

the stomach. Intrinsic factor is essential to the absorption of vitamin $B_{12}$ in the intestine. Without its presence, the patient will gradually develop the symptoms of pernicious anemia, which can be fatal if not treated. The nurse teaches the patient about the vitamin deficiency and explains why oral vitamin replacement is not possible. A 100 to 200 $\mu g$ monthly injection of vitamin $B_{12}$ will prevent the deficiency. Replacement therapy will be lifelong. The digestive changes associated with gastrectomy also impair the absorption of both calcium and iron. Iron deficiency anemia commonly develops, and ferrous sulfate may be prescribed if tolerated. Over time the calcium deficiency could result in bone disease, especially in older postmenopausal women. Calcium supplementation has minimal effect. Box 40-7 summarizes the care provided to a patient undergoing gastric surgery.

**box 40-7** *Nursing Care of the Patient Undergoing Gastric Surgery*

**PREOPERATIVE CARE**

1. Teach deep breathing exercises.
2. Explain special postoperative measures: nasogastric tube and parenteral fluids until peristalsis returns.

**POSTOPERATIVE CARE**

1. Promote pulmonary ventilation.
   a. Position patient in mid or high Fowler's position.
   b. Encourage patient to turn and breathe deep at least q2h (or more frequently until ambulating well); splint or support incision with hands or folded towel during coughing if needed to clear secretions.
   c. Provide adequate analgesics during first few days; patient-controlled analgesia (PCA) is effective.
   d. Encourage ambulation.
   e. Provide good mouth care until oral fluids can be resumed.
2. Promote nutrition.
   a. Measure NG drainage accurately; monitor for blood in drainage. Do not irrigate or reposition tube unless ordered.
   b. Monitor for signs of leakage of anastomosis (dyspnea, pain, fever) when oral fluids are resumed.
   c. Add food in small amounts at frequent intervals until well tolerated.
   d. Monitor for early satiety and regurgitation.
   e. If regurgitation occurs, tell patient to eat less food at a slower pace.
   f. Report signs of dumping syndrome to physician (weakness, faintness, palpitations, diaphoresis, nausea, diarrhea).
   g. Monitor weight.
3. Provide patient/family education.
   a. Gradually increase amount of food each meal until able to eat 3 to 6 meals per day, if possible.
   b. If discomfort occurs after eating, decrease size of meals and amount of fluids with meals; eat more slowly.
   c. Avoid eating simple carbohydrates and concentrated sweets.
   d. Avoid stress during and immediately after meals; plan a rest period after eating. Lie on left side.
   e. Elevate head when lying down (if cardia of stomach removed).
   f. Monitor weight regularly.
   g. Report signs of complications: vomiting after meals, increasing feelings of abdominal fullness or weakness, hematemesis, tarry stools, persistent diarrhea.

## SURGICAL MANAGEMENT FOR SEVERE OBESITY

### ETIOLOGY/EPIDEMIOLOGY

Surgery for obesity is reserved for persons with severe obesity who have diligently tried other methods of weight control and failed. Opinions vary as to its appropriateness and effectiveness, but there is general consensus that it can be lifesaving if performed by a skillful surgeon under the right circumstances.

Obesity is a major general health problem in the industrialized world, and an estimated 25% of the adult population in the United States is overweight.[3] Surgical intervention is targeted at the approximately 3 million persons who can be considered to be severely obese, which is typically defined as at least 100 pounds over ideal weight.

### PATHOPHYSIOLOGY

Obesity has multiple effects on the body that often manifest as comorbid conditions. Obesity is listed as an independent risk factor for coronary artery disease and is also implicated in hypertension, reflux esophagitis, arthritis, stress incontinence, non–insulin-dependent diabetes mellitus, and sleep apnea. The psychosocial toll that is extracted from an obese individual by a society fixated on thinness and physical perfection is difficult to overestimate.

### COLLABORATIVE CARE MANAGEMENT

A variety of surgical procedures have been used in the treatment of clinically severe obesity, but most have been discontinued because they were ineffective or associated with an unacceptably high rate of complications. A 1991 NIH Consensus Conference on surgery for obesity endorsed two procedures: (1) vertical banded gastroplasty and (2) gastric bypass procedures (Roux-en Y bypass) of varying lengths. Both are effective, and the choice is largely based on physician preference and individual patient circumstances. Weight loss is typically greater with bypass, but so is the incidence of nutritional deficiencies.

Vertical banded gastroplasty involves the construction of a small pouch with a limited outlet along the lesser curvature of the stomach. This creates a gastric reservoir of about 15 ml that empties through the narrow channel into the residual stomach (see Figure 40-13). This procedure preserves the continuity of the GI tract and avoids nutritional deficiencies. Gastric bypass procedures involve the construction of a proximal stapled gastric pouch of approximately 15 ml whose outlet is

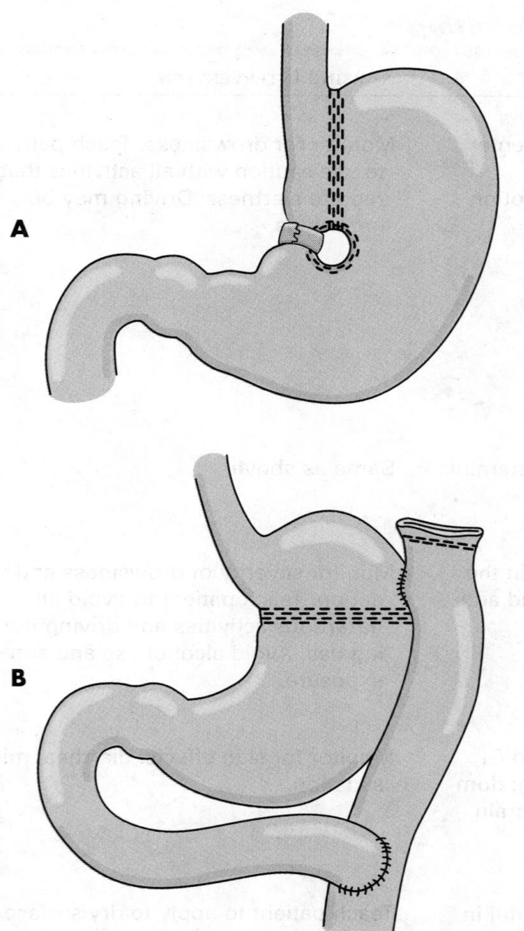


**fig. 40-13** Surgeries for clinically severe obesity. **A,** Vertical band gastroplasty with creation of a small gastric reservoir with limited outlet. **B,** Gastric bypass Roux-en Y with creation of a small proximal gastric reservoir with outlet connection to a Y-shaped limb of small bowel that bypasses the stomach.

connected by a 10 mm anastomosis to a 40 cm Y-shaped limb of small bowel that bypasses the stomach, duodenum, and proximal jejunum (see Figure 40-13). The small bowel limb may be of varying lengths. The development of sophisticated stapling techniques has significantly reduced the risks of anastomosis leakage and failure. Both procedures reduce food intake by prolonging satiety. The bypass procedure adds an element of malabsorption to the weight loss process.

Surgery for the severely obese is associated with an increased risk of general postoperative complications, but increasing technical surgical skill has reduced the mortality rate to about 1%.[3] Wound infections are the most common complication. Weight loss is greatest during the first 12 months and then tapers off and stabilizes, with weight typically about 30% to 40% above ideal body weight.[7] The care of these patients requires a multidisciplinary team approach, and patients usually undergo a careful selection process. Widely used criteria for these procedures include (1) age between 18 and 55 years, (2) at least 100 pounds over ideal body weight, (3) morbid obesity for at least 5 years, (4) evidence of serious dieting efforts, and (5) absence of major illnesses.

Postoperative care is similar to that provided to any patient after abdominal surgery, with particular attention to pulmonary hygiene and wound healing. The head of the bed is elevated 30 to 45 degrees to support respirations. Patient-controlled analgesia is useful because appropriate narcotic doses are more difficult to calculate in the obese person. The nurse carefully monitors wound healing and is alert to the increased risk of wound infection, dehiscence, or both.

### Patient/Family Education

An oral diet of clear liquids is resumed 2 to 3 days after surgery. The nurse teaches the patient about the dietary restrictions in food type and amount that need to be followed to prevent discomfort and the dumping syndrome. Small feedings are essential, and the patient is encouraged to avoid the consumption of soft, high-calorie foods that can be easily digested but that will block the planned weight loss of the surgery. Vitamin and iron supplements are prescribed because iron deficiency and other nutritional anemias are common.

The nurse encourages the patient to use peer support groups in the community to support continued weight loss. The surgical procedures are neither miracles nor panaceas. Patients often have unrealistic expectations about the effects of weight loss on their daily life success and happiness. Failure to achieve major changes can result in depression. To achieve maximum benefit from the surgery, the patient needs to explore and resolve food-related issues in daily life. As weight drops, aerobic exercise will become an essential component of continued weight loss and improved health and well-being.

## NAUSEA AND VOMITING

### ETIOLOGY/EPIDEMIOLOGY

Nausea and vomiting, which often occur together but may occur independently, are common and important GI symptoms. They are part of the body's protective mechanisms and are usually a response to chemical, bacterial, or viral insults to the body's integrity. They are present in a wide array of disorders and, if persistent, can lead to serious consequences. Chronic problems with nausea and vomiting may develop during pregnancy, in severe metabolic imbalances associated with uremia or alcoholism, and during cancer chemotherapy.

### PATHOPHYSIOLOGY

Nausea is a psychic experience that is difficult to define. It may be accompanied by weakness, hypersalivation, and diaphoresis. Gastric tone and peristalsis are typically slowed or absent. The neural pathways that control nausea are not

table 40-3 Common Medications for **Nausea and Vomiting**

| Drug | Action | Nursing Intervention |
|---|---|---|
| **ANTIHISTAMINES** | | |
| Buclizine hydrochloride (Bucladin-S)<br>Cyclizine hydrochloride (Marezine)<br>Meclizine (Antivert)<br>Diphenhydramine hydrochloride (Benadryl)<br>Dimenhydrinate (Dramamine, Dimetabs)<br>Hydroxyzine hydrochloride/hydroxyzine pamoate (Atarax, Vistaril) | Act on neurons in the vomiting center and the vestibular pathways<br>Used in morning sickness and motion sickness | Monitor for drowsiness. Teach patient to use caution with all activities that require alertness. Driving may be hazardous. |
| Promethazine (Phenergan) | Phenothiazine with strong antihistaminic activity | Same as above. |
| **ANTIDOPAMINERGICS** | | |
| Prochlorperazine (Compazine)<br>Thiethylperazine (Torecan)<br>Fluphenazine (Permitil)<br>Droperidol (Inapsine) | Antagonize dopamine receptors in the CTZ; also have antihistamine and anticholinergic effects | Monitor severity of drowsiness and sedation. Teach patient to avoid all hazardous activities and driving during use. Avoid alcohol use and sun exposure. |
| **BENZAMIDES** | | |
| Metoclopramide (Reglan)<br>Domperidone (Motilium)<br>Cisapride (Propulsid) | Complex actions in both CNS and GI tract; stimulate gastric emptying; domperidone does not cross blood-brain barrier | Monitor for side effects: diarrhea, mild sedation. |
| **ANTICHOLINERGICS** | | |
| Scopalamine (Transderm-Scōp) | Reduce neuron transmission; useful in motion sickness and postoperative nausea | Teach patient to apply to dry surface behind the ear. Use in advance of anticipated need. |
| **SEROTONIN ANTAGONISTS** | | |
| Ondansetron (Zofran)<br>Granisetron (Kytril) | Bind serotonin receptor sites along GI tract and afferent nerves | Monitor for side effects: diarrhea, headache. |
| **CANNABIS DERIVATIVES** | | |
| Dronabinol (Marinol) | Site of antiemetic action unknown | Teach patient to be alert to mood and behavior change. Drowsiness is common so driving should be avoided. Avoid concurrent alcohol use. |
| **MISCELLANEOUS** | | |
| Trimethobenzamide (Tigan) | Believed to act on CTZ; has weak antihistaminic action, similar to phenothiazines | Monitor for side effects: hypotension, diarrhea, irritation at injection site. Drowsiness is common. |
| Benzquinamide (Emete-Con) | Inhibits stimulation of the CTZ; similar activity to antihistamines and phenothiazines | Monitor for side effects: drowsiness, fluctuations in blood pressure. |

well identified but probably are the same general pathways that control vomiting.

Vomiting is a complex phenomenon that begins with rhythmic contractions of the respiratory and abdominal muscles and culminates in the forceful expulsion of gastric contents from the mouth. It may be accompanied by retching or dry heaves and should be distinguished from the classic regurgitation that may accompany gastroesophageal reflux.

The vomiting center is located in the medulla adjacent to the respiratory and salivary control centers and can be stimulated directly by the vagus nerve and sympathetic nervous system. Receptors can be found throughout the GI tract and internal organs that, when triggered by spasm or inflammation, can directly produce vomiting. Indirect stimulation can come from the chemoreceptor trigger zone (CTZ), which is located on the floor of the fourth ventricle and appears to act as an emetic chemoreceptor responding to chemical stimuli in the blood. A wide variety of medications and other substances can act on the CTZ in this manner. The CTZ may also mediate the response to nonchemical stimuli such as radiation and motion sickness.

There is strong evidence that dopamine receptors in the CTZ play a role in mediating vomiting.[26] The effects of other neurotransmitters are being studied. Activation of the CTZ causes a reflex loss in gastric tone and peristalsis resulting in delayed gastric emptying. The CTZ may also play a role in psychogenic vomiting, which occurs in response to specific sensations and situations.

Short-term episodic nausea and vomiting is distressing, but prolonged vomiting can have serious physiological effects. Prolonged and severe vomiting interferes with nutrition and causes fluid and electrolyte imbalance—specifically dehydration, metabolic alkalosis, and loss of potassium, chloride, and hydrogen ions. The act of vomiting strains the abdominal muscles and in postoperative patients may cause wound dehiscence. It can also result in Mallory-Weiss lacerations in the esophagus or stomach and trigger serious bleeding.

Vomiting is especially dangerous for anesthetized patients and persons in coma because they are likely to aspirate the vomitus into the lungs. Aspiration may cause atelectasis, pneumonitis, or asphyxia, especially in the elderly person whose protective reflexes work less efficiently.

## COLLABORATIVE CARE MANAGEMENT

The treatment of nausea and vomiting depends on the cause. Medications or other substances known to cause nausea and vomiting are discontinued if possible, and fluid and electrolyte imbalances are corrected. Fluids may be given intravenously if vomiting persists.

Antiemetic medications may be necessary. Drugs that are classified as antiemetics are theorized to function as a form of pharmacological blockade to stimuli that may trigger nausea and vomiting. Most of the drugs also are believed to have some direct sedative action on the CTZ. Antiemetics are prescribed orally if the patient is able to retain the tablets, but they often need to be given by rectal, IM, or IV routes. The choice of drug is governed by the specific clinical situation. Table 40-3 summarizes some of the commonly prescribed medications. Drug categories include the following:

*Antihistamines.* These drugs are believed to act on neurons in the vomiting center and in the vestibular pathways. They are effective in motion sickness and morning sickness management but have little known effect in gastrointestinal disorders. These drugs cause drowsiness and sedation.

*Antidopaminergics.* These drugs are believed to act by antagonizing dopamine receptors in the CTZ. They also have antihistamine and anticholinergic effects. They are effective in managing mild symptoms and are often first-line therapies. They have significant side effects, including drowsiness and sedation.

*Anticholinergics.* These drugs are useful in the management of motion sickness, but the common side effects of dry mouth, urinary retention, and drowsiness limit their use.

*Benzamides.* These dopaminergic antagonists are useful in preventing the vomiting associated with anesthetics and chemotherapeutic agents. They have complex effects in both the central nervous system and GI tract. Metoclopramide also stimulates gastric emptying. Domperidone does not cross the blood-brain barrier and causes fewer side effects. Cisapride increases gastric emptying but has no antidopaminergic effects.

*Serotonin antagonists.* This newer class of drugs avoids the central nervous system effects of many drugs and is extremely effective in controlling severe chemotherapy-induced and postoperative vomiting. The site of action is theorized to be receptor sites in the GI tract and along afferent nerves. A variety of drugs in this category are in active testing.

*Cannabis derivatives.* The antiemetic site of action is uncertain, but the active ingredient in marijuana is often useful in controlling chemotherapy-related nausea and vomiting. Side effects of drowsiness and dry mouth are common.

### Patient/Family Education

Nausea and vomiting can be extremely distressing and debilitating problems that severely interfere with quality of life. Effective management may involve drug therapy but also necessitates careful exploration of daily lifestyle strategies, including environmental modification and stress management. There are rarely quick answers or easy fixes. Acupuncture and acupressure techniques can produce dramatic results for some people. Control and prevention of dehydration are important because dehydration appears to worsen the cycle of nausea and vomiting. Liquids are usually better tolerated in the diet because they exit the stomach rapidly. Highly sweetened drinks should usually be avoided. Creamy and milk-based liquids are rarely well tolerated, and starches are generally better tolerated than fatty foods. Lean poultry is usually

## guidelines for care

### The Person with Nausea and Vomiting

**Safety and Comfort**

Keep head of bed elevated and emesis basin handy.
Protect airway with suction and positioning if patient is not alert.
Provide frequent mouth care.
Control sights and odors in room.
Reduce anxiety if possible.
Provide quiet or distraction on the basis of patient response.
Modify environmental stimuli (cool cloth, dim light), and evaluate response.
Provide ongoing patient support. Explore new strategies.

**Diet Modifications**

Maintain NPO if vomiting is severe.
Explore use of clear liquids:

- Serve liquids cool or room temperature.
- Try effervescent drinks and evaluate effect.
- Avoid fatty foods.
- Avoid highly sweetened foods and milk products.
- Encourage adequate fluids to prevent dehydration.
- Keep meals small, avoid overdistention.

**Drugs**

Administer medications before vomiting occurs, if possible.
Evaluate patient response to medications.
Maintain patient safety and assess for sedation or confusion.

the recommended source of protein. Guidelines for the management of nausea and vomiting are summarized in the accompanying Guidelines for Care Box.

## critical thinking QUESTIONS

**1** Your neighbor confides in you that he is afraid to go to the doctor because he fears he has stomach cancer. On further questioning you learn that he has had frequent episodes of indigestion and increased flatulence. He also comments that he has been under a lot of pressure at work, which has caused him to become nauseated on a few occasions. He does not have a family history of stomach cancer. What is the best approach to take in this situation?

**2** Ruth has had a gastroplasty for severe obesity and is going home in the morning. You are teaching her about home care. After your discussion Ruth comments, "I'm glad I'm going to lose weight without exercising. I really hate to exercise." Does Ruth require any further teaching, or is she ready for discharge?

**3** You are a nurse in a busy medical ICU where routine stress ulcer prophylaxis is the standard of care. Design a research project to test the effectiveness of routine prophylaxis. What patient criteria would you use for selection? How will you measure your outcomes?

## chapter SUMMARY

### GASTRITIS

- Gastritis may be acute or chronic. Acute gastritis results from severe irritation by chemicals, foods, drugs, or bacteria. Chronic gastritis is occasionally caused by an autoimmune process that results in atrophic problems but is usually related to chronic infection with *H. pylori* bacteria.

### PEPTIC ULCER DISEASE

- The overall incidence of peptic ulcer disease has declined. Duodenal ulcers still occur more commonly than gastric and are slightly more common in men.
- Peptic ulcer disease results from an imbalance in the aggressive acid-secreting forces and the mucosal protective forces. Most ulcers result from a breakdown of the gastric mucosa. Actual acid oversecretion is rare.
- *Helicobacter pylori* produces chronic gastritis and weakens the mucosa. It is considered to be the primary cause of duodenal ulcers and gastric ulcers not caused by NSAIDs. It is the most important cause of ulcer relapse.
- The use of NSAIDs plays a crucial role in the development of gastric ulcers because NSAIDs seriously impair the effectiveness of the mucosal defenses.
- Pain remains a classic symptom of ulcers and is located in the epigastrum. Duodenal ulcer pain commonly wakens the person at night and is relieved by food or antacid. Patients often report general dyspepsia symptoms that are not specific to ulcers. Many ulcers are asymptomatic.
- Drug therapy is the cornerstone of ulcer management. Histamine receptor antagonists, proton pump inhibitors, and sucralfate may all be used, supplemented by antacids for symptomatic relief.
- Misoprostol may be given to patients taking NSAIDs. It is a synthetic prostaglandin that supports the integrity of the gastric mucosal defenses.
- Controversy still exists about which patients should receive *H. pylori* treatment as part of their ulcer management. Treatment is becoming increasingly common.
- Nursing care of patients with peptic ulcers involves teaching about the medication regimen, fostering adherence, and exploring lifestyle changes to reduce recurrence risk (e.g., eliminating smoking).
- No special diet is required for ulcer healing. Patients are encouraged to avoid any foods that cause pain.
- The most common complication of peptic ulcer is hemorrhage; treatment consists of preventing or treating shock, gastric lavage, drugs for peptic ulcer therapy, and endoscopic treatment of the bleeding site. Surgery may be needed if bleeding persists.
- Perforation of an ulcer through the stomach wall is treated with parenteral fluids, nasogastric suction, antibiotic therapy, and surgery.

- Surgical treatment of peptic ulcers is rarely needed today except in the management of complications. Highly selective vagotomy and pyloroplasty are the most common procedures.

## STRESS ULCERS

- Stress ulcers can develop rapidly after major trauma, surgery, or other critical illness. Mucosal ischemia triggers the ulcerative cycle. Aggressive prevention with $H_2$ receptor antagonists or other drugs has been standard but is being increasingly questioned. It may be possible to improve risk assessment and avoid treating everyone. Sucralfate is emerging as the preferred drug for prevention.

## CANCER OF THE STOMACH

- The incidence of gastric cancer has declined significantly. Its cause is unknown but is related to the interplay of environmental factors such as smoking, diets high in nitrates and low in fresh fruits and vegetables, and genetic vulnerability.
- Most gastric tumors are incurable by the time symptoms appear. The mortality rate is extremely high. Surgical resection (partial gastrectomy) is the preferred treatment when curative resection is possible.
- Postoperative care after gastric surgery focuses on promoting ventilation, promoting nutrition, providing comfort, and teaching about self-care.
- Dumping syndrome is a postoperative complication that results from rapid entry of hyerosmolar chyme directly into the jejunum. There is also a sudden rise in blood glucose (from absorbed glucose) followed by hypoglycemia. Therapy consists of a low-carbohydrate, moderate-fat, and high-protein diet with fluids restricted between meals.

## SURGICAL TREATMENT FOR OBESITY

- Surgery for morbid obesity usually consists of gastroplasty or gastric bypass.

## NAUSEA AND VOMITING

- Nausea and vomiting is a complex problem that has physiological, cognitive, and emotional components. The vomiting center is located in the medulla and may be stimulated directly by the chemoreceptor trigger zone or indirectly by the cortex.
- Antiemetics are usually only partially effective in controlling nausea and vomiting. Nursing interventions focus on reducing anxiety, manipulating the environment, and experimenting with diet modifications.

## References


1. Achord JL: Nausea and vomiting. In Haubrich WS et al, editors: *Bockus gastroenterology,* ed 5, Philadelphia, 1995, WB Saunders.
2. Anderson ML: *Helicobacter pylori* infection, *Postgrad Med* 96(6):40, 1994.
3. Benotti PN, Forse A: The role of gastric surgery in the multidisciplinary management of severe obesity, *Am J Surg* 169:351, 1995.
4. Bezarro ER: Changing perspectives of the $H_2$ antagonists for stress ulcer prophylaxis, *Crit Care Nurs Clin North Am* 5(2):325, 1993.
5. Brozenec SA: Ulcer therapy update, *RN* 59(9):48, 1996.
6. Cerda JJ, Go MF, Loeb D, Westblom U: A revolution in peptic ulcer disease, *Patient Care* 28(9):19, 1994.
7. Consensus Development Conference Panel: Gastrointestinal surgery for severe obesity, *Ann Intern Med* 115(12):956, 1991.
8. Davis GR: Neoplasms of the stomach. In Sleisenger MH, Fordtran JS, editors: *Gastrointestinal disease,* ed 5, Philadelphia, 1993, WB Saunders.
9. DePriest JL: Stress ulcer prophylaxis, *Postgrad Med* 98(4):159, 1995.
10. Elder JB: Carcinoma of the stomach. In Haubrich WS et al, edi.tors: *Bockus gastroenterology,* ed 5, Philadelphia, 1995, WB Saunders.
11. Elta GH: Approach to the patient with gross gastrointestinal bleeding. In Yamada T, editor: *Textbook of gastroenterology,* ed 2, Philadelphia, 1995, JB Lippincott.
12. Fedotin MS: *Helicobacter pylori* and peptic ulcer disease, *Postgrad Med* 94(3):38, 1993.
13. Fennerty MB et al: Helicobacter pylori: *the new factor in management of ulcer disease,* Bethesda, Md, 1994, American Gastroenterological Association Foundation.
14. Fisher RL, Pipkin GA, Wood JR: Stress related mucosal disease, *Crit Care Clin* 11(2):323, 1995.
15. Hansson LE, Nyren O, Hsing AW, et al: The risk of stomach cancer in patients with gastric or duodenal ulcer disease, *N Engl J Med* 335:242, 1996.
16. Heatley RV, Wyatt JI: Gastritis and duodenitis. In Haubrich WS et al, editors: *Bockus gastroenterology,* ed 5, Philadelphia, 1995, WB Saunders.
17. Heigh RI: Use of NSAIDs, *Postgrad Med* 96(6):63, 1994.
18. Hendlisz A, Bleiberg H: Diagnosis and treatment of gastric cancer, *Drugs* 49(5):711, 1995.
19. Hixson LJ, Kelley CL, Jones WN, Tuohy CD: Current trends in the pharmacotherapy for peptic ulcer disease, *Arch Intern Med* 152:726, 1992.
20. Holt S: Over the counter histamine $H_2$ receptor antagonists, *Drugs* 47(1):1, 1994.
21. Isenberg JI, McQuaid KR, Laine L, Walsh JH: Acid peptic disorders. In Yamada T, editor: *Textbook of gastroenterology,* ed 2, Philadelphia, 1995, JB Lippincott.
22. Johnston D, Martin I: Surgical treatment of duodenal and gastric ulcer. In Haubrich WS et al, editors: *Bockus gastroenterology,* ed 5, Philadelphia, 1995, WB Saunders.
23. Kankaria AG, Fleischer DE: The critical care management of nonvariceal upper gastrointestinal bleeding, *Crit Care Clin* 11(2):347, 1995.
24. Koch KL: Approach to the patient with nausea and vomiting. In Yamada T, editor: *Textbook of gastroenterology,* ed 2, Philadelphia, 1995, JB Lippincott.
25. Lam SK, Hui WM, Ching CK: Peptic ulcer disease: epidemiology, pathogenesis, and etiology. In Haubrich WS et al, editors: *Bockus gastroenterology,* ed 5, Philadelphia, 1995, WB Saunders.
26. Lee M, Feldman M: Nausea and vomiting. In Sleisenger MH, Fordtran JS, editors: *Gastrointestinal disease,* ed 5, Philadelphia, 1993, WB Saunders.
27. Netchvolodoff CV: Refractory peptic lesions, *Postgrad Med* 93(4):143, 1993.
28. Parent K: Acid reduction in peptic ulcer disease, *Postgrad Med* 96(6):53, 1994.
29. Pounder RE, Fraser AG: Peptic ulcer disease: diagnosis, medical management and complications. In Haubrich WS et al, editors: *Bockus gastroenterology,* ed 5, Philadelphia, 1995, WB Saunders.
30. Prevost SS, Oberle A: Stress ulceration in the critically ill patient, *Crit Care Nurs Clin North Am* 75(4):853, 1993.

31. Qureshi WA, Netchvolodoff CV: Acute bleeding from peptic ulcers, *Postgrad Med* 93(4):167, 1993.
32. Sonnenberg A, Everhart JE: The prevalence of self reported peptic ulcer in the United States, *Am J Public Health* 86(2):200, 1996.
33. Talley NJ: Nonulcer dyspepsia. In Yamada T, editor: *Textbook of gastroenterology,* ed 2, Philadelphia, 1995, JB Lippincott.
34. Department of Health and Human Services, Public Health Service: *Healthy people 2000: midcourse review and 1995 revisions,* Washington, DC, 1996, DHHS.
35. Yardley JH, Hendrix TR: Gastritis, duodenitis and associated ulcerative lesions. In Yamada T, editor: *Textbook of gastroenterology,* ed 2, Philadelphia, 1995, JB Lippincott.
36. Ziller SA, Netchvolodoff CV: Uncomplicated peptic ulcer disease, *Postgrad Med* 93(4):126, 1993.

# chapter 41 MANAGEMENT OF PERSONS WITH Problems of the Intestines

JUDITH K. SANDS

## objectives

*After studying this chapter, the learner should be able to:*

1. Discuss lifestyle modifications for the management of constipation, diarrhea, and flatulence.
2. Compare the common forms of intestinal infections and their management.
3. Describe current pharmacological and nursing management of inflammatory bowel disease.
4. Discuss the use of enteral and parenteral feedings in the management of malabsorption and malnutrition.
5. Compare the pathophysiology of hernias, cancer, and volvulus as causes of bowel obstruction.
6. Discuss the nursing management of the patient with an ostomy.
7. Compare the various surgical approaches to the management of common anorectal disorders.
8. Discuss preoperative and postoperative care of the patient undergoing bowel surgery.

Disease and disorders that affect the intestines constitute major health problems in the United States. Digestion, absorption, and elimination may be affected. The scope of problems ranges from mild to life-threatening. The categories of intestinal disorders discussed in this chapter include problems of elimination, infectious and inflammatory bowel disease, malabsorption and malnutrition, bowel obstructions, and anorectal disorders.

## COMMON PROBLEMS OF ELIMINATION

### CONSTIPATION

#### Etiology/Epidemiology

The act of defecation is initiated when feces enter the rectum and is voluntarily controlled by contraction of the external anal sphincter. Most people have a regular pattern of defecation, but the pattern varies widely among persons, from three times a day to once every 2 or 3 days. The term *constipation* refers to an abnormal infrequency of defecation or the passage of abnormally hard stools or both. The term lacks precise definition because it has different meanings to different people. Almost everyone experiences occasional constipation, and it is a common complaint among elderly persons. Hundreds of millions of dollars are spent annually on over-the-counter products to support intestinal elimination. Many of these products are unnecessary; some are even harmful.

Constipation can be a functional consequence of endocrine and neurological diseases such as diabetes, hypothyroidism, multiple sclerosis, and Parkinson's disease. It is also an associated side effect of the use of narcotics, anticholinergic drugs, and a wide variety of specific drugs such as anticonvulsants and calcium channel blockers. In many adults, however, occasional constipation is the result of physical inactivity, stress, diet changes, lack of fluids, and failure to respond to the urge to defecate.[20]

Overuse of laxatives is a common problem in elders, who become laxative dependent and experience chronic constipation. If the urge to defecate is not heeded, it soon disappears, and the feces remain in the rectum. The urge to defecate occurs most frequently after meals, particularly breakfast, as a result of stimulation of the gastrocolic reflex from food entering the stomach. Common risk factors for constipation are summarized in the following Risk Factors Box.

#### Pathophysiology

Constipation may result from decreased motility of the colon or from retention of feces in the lower portion of the colon, or *rectum.* Dietary fiber increases the water content of the stool, and colonic motility is enhanced through the bacterial degradation of the fiber.

The longer the feces remain in the colon, the greater the amount of water reabsorbed and the drier the stool becomes. The stool is then more difficult to expel. Occasionally constipation is not detrimental to health, but habitual constipation leads to decreased intestinal muscle tone, increased use of Valsalva's maneuver as the person bears down in the attempt to pass the hardened stool, and an increased incidence of hemorrhoids.

Fecal impaction is a significant negative outcome in the institutionalized elderly in whom mental confusion and immobility may complicate the effective management of elimination. The development of megarectum can blunt rectal and anal sensation and lead to vicious cycles of impaction, spurious diarrhea, and fecal incontinence.

#### Collaborative Care Management

The treatment of constipation begins with a careful assessment of the nature, severity, and duration of the problem. Treatment is individualized to the unique needs of the patient

**risk factors**

**Constipation**

**Functional Disorders**

Diabetes mellitus
Hypothyroidism
Multiple sclerosis
Parkinson's disease
A wide variety of other neurogenic and collagen disorders

**Medications**

Aluminum-based and calcium-based antacids
Narcotics
Anticholinergics
Antidepressants/antipsychotics
Iron, calcium, and bismuth salts
Anticonvulsants
Calcium channel blockers

**Immobility**

Dehydration
Lack of dietary fiber
Confusion, disorientation
Interruption of normal bowel routines, stress

**research**

Reference: Hall GR et al: Managing constipation using a research based protocol, *Med Surg Nurs* 4(1):11-18, 1995.

This study involved the development and evaluation of a research-based protocol for managing bowel elimination in elderly patients on a vascular surgery unit at a large acute care hospital. Baseline data had indicated that 60% of patients experienced alterations in elimination requiring laxatives and/or enemas, and 34% developed impactions. Interventions for the study were developed in the areas of food intake, fluid intake, exercise, and hygiene (privacy and positioning for elimination). Interventions included adding a dietary fiber supplement, consuming 1500 to 2000 ml of fluid intake daily, ensuring privacy and an upright position if possible, and teaching abdominal exercises that could be practiced in bed. The fiber supplement was added to a special recipe of blueberry muffins and oatmeal raisin cookies developed for the study.

An assessment protocol for risk identification was implemented on admission. All high-risk patients were assigned to the protocol. They received dietitian visits, teaching about the use of fiber, encouragement to consume fluids with every nursing contact and exercise teaching. Staff were trained in the use of the protocol.

Unit continuous quality improvement was used to measure outcomes. Ninety percent of patients reported normal bowel function, and 95% required neither laxatives nor enemas. The incidence of constipation dropped from 60% to 9%, and the incidence of impaction was eliminated. All elements of the protocol were regularly used by staff except for the exercise component, which never was consistently reflected in practice.

and generally includes diet and fluid modifications, increased activity, establishment of regular toileting patterns, and use of emollients or fiber supplements as needed. The chronic use of stimulant laxatives is avoided if possible. Examples of drugs commonly used in the management of constipation are presented in Table 41-1.[26]

Hospitalization inevitably interferes with a person's normal patterns of exercise and eating. The nurse monitors all hospitalized patients for constipation and records all bowel elimination. For greatest success, bowel programs need to be initiated *before* problems with constipation arise. A plan to prevent problems with constipation should be initiated for any patient on bedrest or receiving frequent doses of opioids. (See the Research Box).

### *Patient/family education*

Teaching begins with ensuring patient understanding of the interplay between diet, fluids, activity, and stress and the occurrence of constipation. The nurse encourages patients to eat a high-fiber diet and to avoid highly refined foods. Bran may be used as a supplement in a limited way. Patients should attempt to drink at least 2500 to 3000 ml of fluid daily, unless their medical condition contraindicates a liberal fluid intake. Regular exercise and a planned daily time for defecation are important measures. The patient is instructed to manage occasional episodes of constipation with bulk laxatives or emollients if possible and to avoid the regular use of harsh laxatives or any type of enema.

## DIARRHEA

### Etiology/Epidemiology

Diarrhea is a major cause of morbidity in this country and remains a leading cause of death in developing nations, especially among infants and small children.[36] Diarrhea is also one of the classic symptoms of gastrointestinal disease and can be caused by a wide variety of agents and disorders. Diarrhea usually represents an increase in stool number and/or a change in consistency, but the diagnosis is based primarily on the consistency of the stool rather than the number of stools per day. There is a variety of ways to classify diarrhea that take into account the wide range of etiologies including infectious and inflammatory processes, malabsorption, and secretory diarrhea. Acute diarrhea, those cases continuing for less than 2 to 3 weeks, is usually self-limiting although supportive intervention may be necessary. Chronic diarrhea is usually related to changes in the gastrointestinal (GI) tract that alter the transport of fluids, electrolytes, and solids. See Box 41-1 for some of the common causes of diarrhea.

Acute diarrhea is by far the most common form and is usually caused by infectious agents. Improvements in sanitation, hygiene, and food handling practices have decreased the incidence of acute diarrhea in developed countries, but it is still a common occurrence. Oral fecal transmission from contaminated food and water or person-to-person contact is the most common cause. The contamination of food-preparation surfaces has been increasingly identified as a prime etiology.[19] Organisms can then proliferate rapidly when food is either in-

**table 41-1** *Common Medications for* ***Treatment of Constipation***

| Drug | Action | Intervention |
|---|---|---|
| **BULK FORMERS** | | |
| Psyllium (Metamucil)<br>Methylcellulose (Citrucil) | Polysaccharides and cellulose derivatives mix with intestinal fluids, swell, and stimulate peristalsis. | Ensure adequate fluid intake to prevent impaction or obstruction.<br>Take separately from prescribed drugs to avoid problems with absorption. |
| **STOOL SOFTENERS (EMOLLIENTS)** | | |
| Docusate sodium (Colace)<br>Docusate calcium (Surfak) | Docusate salts act as detergents in the intestine, reducing surface tension, which facilitates the incorporation of liquid and fat, softening the stool. | Preparations lose effectiveness with long-term use; patient should not rely on this measure alone. Discontinue if abdominal cramping occurs. |
| **LUBRICANTS** | | |
| Mineral oil | Soften fecal matter by lubricating the intestinal mucosa, facilitating easy stool passage.<br>Excessive use interferes with absorption of fat-soluble vitamins A, D, E, and K, leading to deficiency. | Do not take with meals or drugs because oil can impair absorption; swallow carefully to prevent lipid aspiration. |
| **HYPEROSMOLAR LAXATIVES** | | |
| Lactulose (Cephulac)<br>Polyethylene glycol (GoLYTELY)<br>Sorbitol | Nonabsorbable sugars are degraded by colonic bacteria and increase stool osmolarity. Fluid is drawn into the intestine, stimulating peristalsis. | Adjust dose and frequency of administration to control side effects and regulate defecation. Monitor for fluid and electrolyte imbalance if response is severe. |
| **SALINE LAXATIVES** | | |
| Magnesium citrate<br>Magnesium sulfate (epsom salts)<br>Magnesium hydroxide (milk of magnesia) | Cause osmotic retention of fluid which distends the colon and increases peristalsis. | Liquid preparations are more effective than tablets. Take with full glass of water. Monitor for fluid and electrolyte imbalance if response is severe. |
| **STIMULANT/IRRITANT LAXATIVES** | | |
| Cascara sagrada<br>Senna (Senokot)<br>Bisacodyl (Dulcolax)<br>Castor oil | Directly stimulate and irritate the intestine, promoting peristalsis. | Cramps and diarrhea can occur; monitor for fluid and electrolyte imbalance if reaction is severe. |
| **PROKINETIC AGENTS** | | |
| Cisapride (Propulsid) | Stimulates colonic motility in the proximal colon and improves rectal sensation. | Monitor for effectiveness. Drug has produced inconsistent results in chronic constipation. Monitor for side effects such as nausea and abdominal pain. Take at least 15 minutes before meals. |

adequately cooked or refrigerated. Risk factors for infectious diarrhea are identified in the box on p. 1316. Table 41-2 presents an overview of the major parasitic forms of acute diarrhea.

## Pathophysiology

Large-volume diarrhea is caused by a hypersecretion of water and electrolytes by the intestinal mucosa. This secretion occurs in response to the osmotic pressure exerted by nonabsorbed food particles in the chyme or from direct irritation of the mucosa. Peristalsis is increased, and the transit time through the intestine is significantly decreased. Increased peristalsis also may result from inflammation as mucosal cells hypersecrete water in the presence of infectious organisms. Diarrhea may be accompanied by severe abdominal cramping, tenesmus (persistent spasm) of the anal area, abdominal distention, and borborygmus (loud bowel sounds).

Fluid and electrolyte imbalances can quickly result from diarrhea, depending on its severity. Mild diarrhea in adults can lead to losses of sodium and potassium (causing metabolic alkalosis). Severe diarrhea causes dehydration, hyponatremia, hypokalemia, and metabolic acidosis (from the loss of large amounts of bicarbonate). Malnourished or elderly

**box 41-1** *Common Causes of Diarrhea*

**INFECTIONS**
Bacteria *(Escherichia coli, Salmonella, Shigella, Staphylococcus, Campylobacter jejuni)*
Viruses (rotavirus, human immunodeficiency virus [HIV])
Parasites (*Giardia, Cryptosporidium, Trichinella, Etamoeba histolytica,* hookworm)

**HYPERSENSITIVITY**
Food allergy

**AUTOIMMUNE DISEASE**
Ulcerative colitis, Crohn's disease
Graft vs. host disease

**EFFECTS OF CYTOTOXIC AGENTS**
Chemotherapy-induced mucositis
Radiation enteritis

**risk factors**

**Acute Diarrhea**

Recent travel to developing nations
Outdoor camping
Ingestion of raw meat, seafood, or shellfish
Eating at banquets, restaurants, picnics, or fast food establishments
Daycare placement or employment
Residence in institutions, nursing homes, prisons, or mental institutions
Homosexual lifestyle
Prostitution
IV drug abuse

persons tolerate severe diarrhea less well than do younger or well-nourished persons. Persistent diarrhea also readily leads to skin breakdown in the perianal region.

### Collaborative Care Management

The management of diarrhea involves the prevention of fluid and electrolyte imbalance, controlling the symptoms, and treating the underlying cause if possible. The risk of serious outcome or death is usually directly attributable to dehydration, and short-term hospitalization may be necessary to ensure adequate fluid replacement. Aggressive rehydration with oral replacement solutions is used if the person is alert and able to take oral fluids. Solutions such as the World Health Organization solution, Pedialyte, Resol, and Rehydralyte are preferred to fruit juices, soda, or even Gatorade because they have a balanced electrolyte composition plus glucose.[36]

Bowel rest is no longer routinely recommended as an approach to most cases of acute diarrhea as malnutrition can develop rapidly. Clear liquids are provided along with diets low in fiber but rich in sodium and glucose.[19] The use of antidiarrheal agents is variable. Motility-altering drugs are rarely given in infectious diarrhea because of the risk of worsening the colonization or invasion by the pathogen.[26] Bismuth subsalicylate is usually safe and can be helpful. Kaolin-pectin preparations are rarely helpful. Antibiotic therapy is also controversial and is reserved for patients with acute disease who do not promptly respond to conservative treatment.[26] The decision is based on the nature of the causative organism. Commonly used antidiarrheal medications are summarized in Table 41-3.

If patients are hospitalized with acute diarrhea, the nurse maintains an accurate record of diarrhea incidence and severity, estimates fluid losses, assesses for fluid and electrolyte disturbances, and promotes patient comfort. The prevention of perianal skin breakdown is an important nursing intervention. The nurse may need to assist a weakened patient in keeping the area clean and dry. Skin ointments and barriers (e.g., zinc oxide) are reapplied as needed after each episode of diarrhea. Sitz baths can be extremely comforting when perianal skin becomes irritated.

#### *Patient/family education*

Patient teaching primarily focuses on measures related to the preventable causes of acute diarrhea. Strict cleanliness in regard to all food preparation surfaces and utensils is critical. Care should be taken in defrosting and handling uncooked meat and ensuring prompt and adequate refrigeration of all foods. Avoiding raw meats and seafood and thoroughly cooking ground beef are essential. *Healthy People 2000* goals related to food safety and handling are presented in Chapter 40. Travelers are cautioned to exercise care in consuming local water, uncooked fruits, and raw vegetables. Thorough hand washing and personal hygiene practices are helpful preventative strategies for all forms of infectious diarrhea.

Two additional goals that relate directly to infectious diarrhea are:[47]

- Reduce outbreaks of infections due to *Salmonella enteritidis* to fewer than 25 outbreaks yearly.
- Reduce infections caused by key food-borne pathogens to incidences of no more than:

| Disease (per 100,000) | 1987 Baseline | 2000 Target |
|---|---|---|
| *Salmonella* species | 18.0 | 16.0 |
| *Campylobacter jejuni* | 50.0 | 25.0 |
| *Escherichia coli* O157 : H7 | 8.0 | 4.0 |
| *Listeria monocytogenes* | 0.7 | 0.5 |

## FECAL INCONTINENCE

### Etiology/Epidemiology

Fecal incontinence is a complex problem that has a variety of causes. The external anal sphincter may be relaxed, the voluntary control of defecation may be interrupted in the central nervous system, or messages may not be transmitted to the brain because of a lesion within or external pressure on the spinal cord. The disorders that cause breakdown of conscious control of defecation include cortical clouding or lesions, spinal cord lesions or trauma, and trauma to the anal sphincter (e.g., from fistula, abscess, or surgery).[31] Perineal relaxation and actual damage to the anal sphincter are often caused by injury from perineal surgery, childbirth, or anal intercourse.

**table 41-2** *Common Parasitic Infections That Cause Acute Diarrhea*

| Infection/Organism | Source | Pathophysiology | Clinical Manifestations | Treatment |
|---|---|---|---|---|
| Amebiasis/ *Entamoeba histolytica* | Direct person-to-person contact; contaminated water, milk, food; infection rates as high as 30% in tropical countries | Ingested cyst releases active trophozoite that invades and ulcerates intestinal mucosa. Can migrate to liver and cause abscesses. | Abdominal cramping; diarrhea (may be severe); flatulence; reappearance of symptoms at intervals of several months | Metronidazole (Flagyl) for 5-10 days often in combination with other amebicides |
| Giardiasis/ *Giardia lamblia* | Direct person-to-person contact; contaminated water; common cause of traveler's diarrhea | Ingested cyst releases active trophozoite that infects the small intestine. | Persistent watery diarrhea; abdominal cramping and bloating; malabsorption in severe cases | Usually self-limiting in 2-6 wk but may recur; quinacrine (Atabrine) or metronidazole (Flagyl) for at least 2 wk |
| Trichinosis/ *Trichinella spiralis* | Ingestion of undercooked pork and pork products | Larvae of roundworm infect the meat and mature in the intestine. Larvae are then released into blood and lymphatics and pass into striated muscle of the host where they encyst. | Early stage symptoms include nausea, anorexia, cramping, and diarrhea; muscle pain and fever develop in 2-8 weeks; can involve jaw, eyes, diaphragm, and heart | Symptomatic treatment with analgesics and anti-inflammatory drugs; use of mebendazole (Vermox) or thiabendazole (Mintezol) |
| Cryptosporidiosis/ *Cryptosporidum* | Parasite present in birds, fish, cattle, sheep, and spread by person-to-person contact and contaminated water | Organism is ingested and primarily affects the small intestine. It can affect the entire GI tract in immunocompromised persons. | Causes massive watery diarrhea, which may exceed 4 L/day; if persistent, malabsorption may develop; nausea and fatigue | No effective therapy; supportive treatment with fluid and electrolyte replacement used as infection is self-limiting in immunocompetent persons. |

**table 41-3** *Common Medications for* ***Treatment of Acute Diarrhea***

| Drug | Action | Intervention |
|---|---|---|
| **LOCAL ACTING** | | |
| Bismuth subsalicylate (Pepto-Bismol) | Mechanism not known<br>May bind bacterial toxins | Shake liquids well before using.<br>Bismuth products may turn the stool black. |
| Kaolin and pectin (Kaopectate) | Soothes the intestinal mucosa and increases absorption of water, nutrients, and electrolytes | Shake liquids well before using. No significant side effects exist. |
| **SYSTEMIC ACTING** | | |
| Loperamide (Imodium)<br>Tincture of opium (paregoric)<br>Diphenoxylate hydrochloride with atropine (Lomotil) | Acts systemically to reduce peristalsis and GI motility | Be aware that these drugs are part of the narcotic family; potential for addiction exists with paregoric.<br>Loperamide has few side effects and no associated physical dependence.<br>Lomotil has a low potential for dependency. Monitor patient response. Can enhance bacterial invasion and prolong excretion of the pathogen. Monitor for narcotic side effects: central nervous system depression, or respiratory depression. |

Relaxation of the sphincter usually increases with the general loss of muscle tone in aging. The normal changes that occur with aging are not of sufficient significance to cause incontinence, however, unless concurrent health problems predispose the patient to the disorder.[31]

### Pathophysiology

Normally the contents of the bowel are moved by mass movements toward the rectum. The rectum then stores the stool until defecation occurs. Distention of the rectum initiates nerve signals that are transmitted to the spinal cord and then back to the descending colon, initiating peristaltic waves that force more feces into the rectum. The internal anal sphincter relaxes, and if the external sphincter is also relaxed, defecation results. Defecation occurs as a reflex response to the distention of the rectal musculature, but this reflex can be voluntarily inhibited. Voluntary inhibition of defecation is learned in early childhood, and control typically lasts throughout life. Emptying of the rectum occurs when the external anal sphincter (under cortical control) relaxes, and the abdominal and pelvic muscles contract.

Reflex defecation continues to occur even in the presence of most upper or lower motor neuron lesions, because the musculature of the bowel contains its own nerve centers that respond to distention through peristalsis. Reflex defecation therefore often persists or can be stimulated even when motor paralysis is present. Defecation occurs primarily in response to mass peristaltic movements that follow meals or whenever the rectum becomes distended. Any physical, mental, or social problem that disrupts any aspect of this complex learned behavior can result in incontinence.[39]

### Collaborative Care Management

Biofeedback training is the cornerstone of therapy for patients who have motility disorders or sphincter damage that causes fecal incontinence.[39] The patient learns to tighten the external sphincter in response to manometric measurement of responses to rectal distention. This technique has demonstrated effectiveness with alert motivated patients.

Bowel training is the major approach used with patients who have cognitive and neurological problems resulting from stroke or other chronic diseases. If a person can sit on a toilet, it may be possible to achieve automatic defecation when a pattern of consistent timing, familiar surroundings, and controlled diet and fluid intake can be achieved. This approach allows many patients to defecate predictably and remain continent throughout the day. Surgical correction is possible for a small group of patients whose incontinence is related to structural problems of the rectum and anus.

#### *Patient/family education*

Bowel training requires significant amounts of time and effort on the part of the nursing staff, family, and patient. The nurse teaches the family about the training program and how they can assist and support the effort. Incontinence is a major issue in home care and frequently is cited as the most common cause for elderly persons to be admitted to nursing homes.

To plan the most effective approach the nurse gathers specific information concerning the person's general physical and cognitive condition, ability to contract the abdominal and perineal muscles on command, and awareness of the need or urge to defecate. Data are also collected about the nature and frequency of the incontinence problem, particularly its relationship to meals or other regular activities.

The nurse teaches the family about the importance of a high-fiber diet and ensuring that the patient consumes at least 2500 ml of fluid daily. The need for a regular stool softener or bulk former is evaluated. When an optimal time for defecation has been established, usually after breakfast, a glycerine suppository may be inserted to stimulate defecation.

Despite honest efforts by family members, staff, and patient, the fecal incontinence may remain uncontrolled. Efforts will then shift toward odor control, preventing skin breakdown, and supporting the patient's psychological integrity. Commercially available protective pants are expensive, but they can substantially reduce the burden of care for the family and provide the patient with a sense of security and dignity.

## ACUTE INFECTION/INFLAMMATION OF THE INTESTINES

### APPENDICITIS

#### Etiology/Epidemiology

The vermiform appendix is a small, fingerlike projection that is attached to the cecum usually just below the ileocecal valve (Figure 41-1). The appendix is approximately 10 cm (4 inches) long and has no clearly identified function. It is an integral part of the cecum and fills with chyme and empties by peristalsis along with the rest of the bowel.

Appendicitis is an acute inflammation of the appendix and is one of the most common surgical emergencies. The cause rarely is clear-cut, but the lumen of the appendix is quite small, making it vulnerable to incomplete emptying, distention by accumulated mucus secretion or obstruction, which can lead to infection. Obstruction by fecaliths (hardened feces) or foreign bodies and the presence of concurrent acute infectious diseases may also trigger the acute inflammatory response.

Appendicitis occurs most commonly in teenagers and young adults between the ages of 10 and 30 years. Only 10% of all cases occur after age 50. Appendicitis can occur at any age, however, and is an extremely serious condition in elders. Males are affected more commonly than females during the teenage and young adult years. Approximately 7% of the population is affected by the disorder at some point. Appendicitis increased steadily in incidence from the late nineteenth century to a peak in the 1950s. The incidence since 1950 has been steadily declining for poorly understood reasons. Appendicitis appears to occur more commonly in societies in which the diet is low in fiber and high in refined carbohydrates. The higher incidence of constipation associated with this diet pattern is theorized to increase the chance of developing obstructive fecaliths.

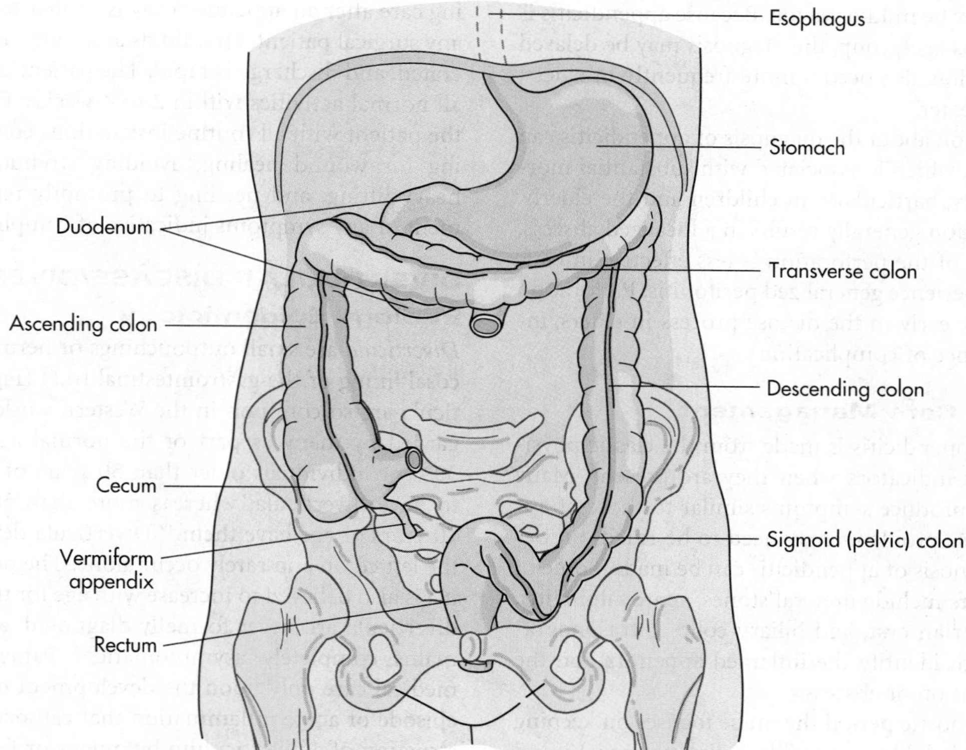


**fig. 41-1** The appendix at the beginning of the ascending colon.

## Pathophysiology

The inflammatory process of appendicitis can involve all or part of the appendix. Intraluminal pressure increases, leading to occlusion of the capillaries and venules and vascular engorgement. Bacterial invasion follows and microabscesses may develop in the appendiceal wall or surrounding tissue, which, unless treated, can progress to gangrene and perforation within 24 to 36 hours. If the inflammatory process develops fairly slowly, the infection may be successfully walled off in a local abscess. In more rapidly developing cases, the risk of rupture and acute peritonitis is quite high.

The classic clinical manifestation of appendicitis is abdominal pain that comes in waves. The pain starts in the epigastric or umbilical region but gradually becomes localized in the right lower quadrant of the abdomen. Localization at McBurney's point, halfway between the umbilicus and the anterior spine of the ileum (Figure 41-2) is considered classic. The pain is intermittent at first but becomes steady and severe over a short period. Pain frequently is accompanied by nausea, anorexia, and vomiting. Light palpation of the abdomen elicits pain in the right lower quadrant. Rebound tenderness is a common finding (see Chapter 38). The abdominal muscles overlying the area of inflammation in the right lower quadrant may feel tense as a result of voluntary rigidity. The person with appendicitis often lies on the side or back with knees flexed in an attempt to decrease muscle strain on the abdominal wall. Other symptoms may include temperature elevations in the range of 38° to 38.5° C (100.5° to 101.5° F) accompanied by an elevation

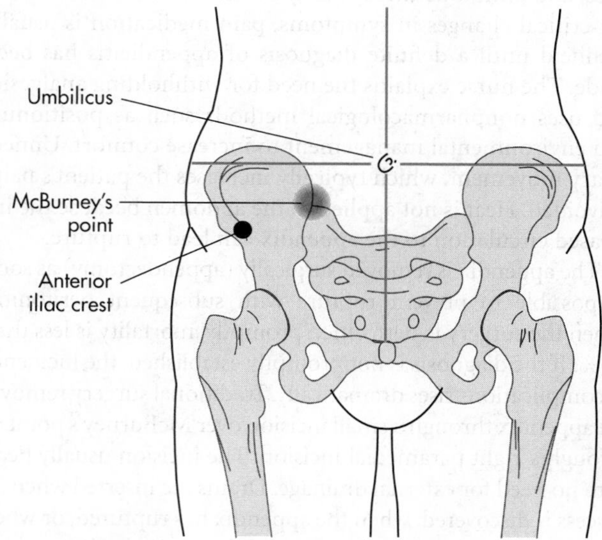


**fig. 41-2** McBurney's point, located halfway between the umbilicus and the anterior iliac crest in the right lower quadrant of the abdomen.

in white blood cell (WBC) count more than 10,000/mm³ and a neutrophil count more than 75%.

Patients with appendicitis may experience less well-defined local symptoms that can make prompt and accurate diagnosis a challenge. Elderly patients are less likely to experience classic acute symptoms. Their response to pain is decreased, and their symptoms may be mild or vague. Because appendicitis is relatively rare in this age-group, the diagnosis may be delayed or missed. Perforation also occurs more frequently in elders, and mortality is greater.

Delay or confusion about the diagnosis of appendicitis can lead to perforation, which is associated with substantial morbidity and mortality, particularly in children and the elderly. In adults a perforation generally results in a localized abscess. Local containment of the perforation is less effective in children who often experience generalized peritonitis. Perforation is believed to occur early in the disease process in elders, increasing the incidence of complications.

### Collaborative Care Management

The diagnosis of appendicitis is made from the classic physical and laboratory indicators when they are present. Many other diseases can produce symptoms similar to those of appendicitis, and these problems may need to be ruled out before a positive diagnosis of appendicitis can be made. Some of the related disorders include ureteral stones, acute salpingitis, regional ileitis, ovarian cyst, and biliary colic. Ultrasonography may be used to identify the inflamed appendix and the presence of perforation or abscess.

During the diagnostic period the nurse focuses on keeping the patient as comfortable as possible, relieving anxiety, and preparing the patient for surgery. The patient is placed on bedrest and given nothing by mouth. Administration of intravenous fluids is started to maintain fluid and electrolyte balance, and antibiotic therapy may be initiated. To avoid masking critical changes in symptoms, pain medication is usually withheld until a definite diagnosis of appendicitis has been made. The nurse explains the need for withholding analgesics and uses nonpharmacological methods such as positioning and environmental management to increase comfort. Unnecessary movement, which typically increases the patient's pain, is avoided. Heat is not applied to the abdomen because the increased circulation to the appendix can lead to rupture.

The appendix is removed surgically (appendectomy) as soon as possible to prevent rupture with subsequent peritonitis. When the surgery is performed promptly, mortality is less than 0.5%. If the diagnosis is not promptly established, the incidence of complications rises dramatically. Traditional surgery removes the appendix through a small incision over McBurney's point or through a right paramedial incision. The incision usually heals with no need for external drainage. Drains are inserted when an abscess is discovered, when the appendix has ruptured, or when the appendix is severely edematous and surrounded by a pocket of clear fluid. Bowel function usually returns to normal soon after surgery, and convalescence is short. Appendectomies can also be successfully performed laparoscopically, but the cost and length of stay parameters are not significantly altered although patients do report a decreased level of pain. Laparoscopic appendectomy does not appear to offer any significant improvement over traditional open surgery at this time.

#### *Patient/family education*

The nurse provides the patient with an overview of the planned surgery and postoperative care. Postoperative nursing care after an appendectomy is similar to that provided for any surgical patient. Oral fluids and foods are restarted as tolerated, and discharge is rapid. The patient usually can resume all normal activities within 2 to 4 weeks. The nurse provides the patient with all routine instructions concerning monitoring for wound healing, avoiding strenuous activities and heavy lifting, and needing to promptly report the development of any symptoms indicative of complications.

## DIVERTICULAR DISEASE/DIVERTICULITIS

### Etiology/Epidemiology

*Diverticula* are small outpouchings or herniations of the mucosal lining of the gastrointestinal tract (Figure 41-3). Diverticula are so common in the Western world that they are regarded by many as part of the normal aging process. Only 30% of individuals older than 50 years of age are estimated to have diverticula, whereas more than 50% of those over 70 years of age have them.[49] Diverticula develop primarily in the left colon and rarely occur alone. The number of diverticula is also believed to increase with age for the vast majority of diverticula are never formally diagnosed, and the person remains completely asymptomatic.[49] Patients typically seek medical care only upon the development of diverticulitis, an episode of acute inflammation that can occur from local obstruction of a diverticulum by mucus or fecal matter. Microperforation occurs from a process that is quite similar to appendicitis. In about 20% of persons with diverticula an episode of diverticulitis will develop at some point.

Diverticulosis has been described as a disease of Western civilization because of its high incidence in developed countries. The incidence of the disease shows wide geographic variations that are at least partly attributable to the quantity of nonabsorbable dietary fiber. The increased incidence of diverticular disease parallels the changes in Western diet that have occurred since the 1850s when the refinement of grains

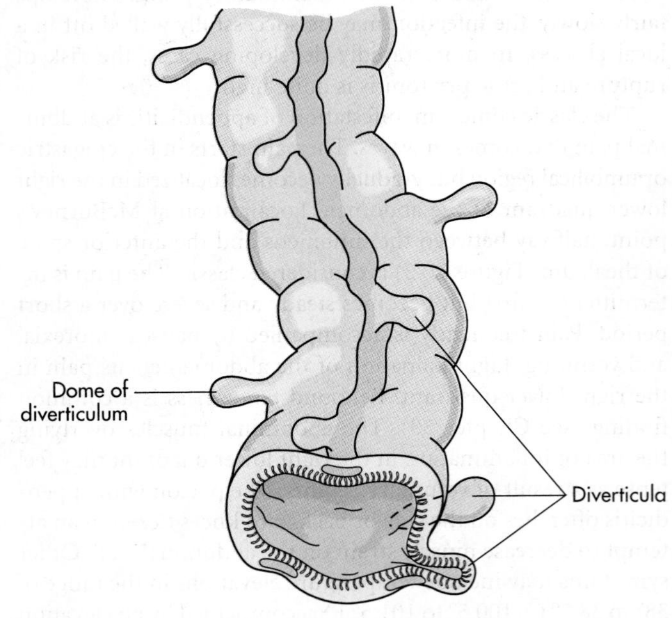


**fig. 41-3** Diverticuli in the colon.

became standard. The steady aging of the population is also reflected in these figures. Low-fiber diets have been shown to increase intraluminal pressure in the bowel, but aging also appears to change the composition of the bowel, which decreases its tensile strength.[49]

### Pathophysiology

The development of intestinal diverticula is theorized to be related to low fecal volume in the colon, increased intraluminal pressure, and decreased muscle strength in the colon wall. Diverticula tend to form at points in the colon wall where blood vessels penetrate the mucosal and muscular layers, creating points of relative weakness. It is theorized that increased muscular contractions in the sigmoid colon that are generated to push stool into the rectum increase both the thickness of the muscle and the intraluminal pressure. The weaker connective tissue then herniates between the circular muscle bands and forms the diverticula.

Diverticulitis frequently develops in a single diverticulum in response to irritation initiated by trapped fecal material. Blood supply to the area decreases, and bacteria proliferate in the obstructed diverticulum.[11] Perforation of the dome may occur which, if small, is usually quickly and effectively walled off. Larger perforations may progress to abscess formation or general peritonitis. Generalized inflammation can result in thickening and scarring of the bowel wall.

Diverticular disease is usually asymptomatic, but mild inflammation can trigger a nonspecific bowel dysfunction that resolves in a matter of hours or days. The clinical manifestations of diverticulitis reflect the inflammation of the diverticula or the development of complications. Crampy lower left quadrant abdominal pain accompanied by low-grade fever is a classic sign. The pain is triggered by muscle spasms of the sigmoid colon and is acute and persistent in nature. Nausea, vomiting, and a feeling of bloating are also common. The inflammatory process also frequently involves the bladder and causes urinary symptoms. The development of an abscess initiates the symptoms of localized peritonitis (see p. 1322). The traditional symptoms tend to be less pronounced or underreported by elders.

#### *Diverticular bleeding*

Diverticular disease is also one of the most common causes of lower GI bleeding.[8] The diverticula develop around a rich network of blood vessels, and as the vasa recta passes over the dome of the diverticulum it may be separated from the lumen of the colon only by the thin layer of mucosa. Episodes of acute bleeding occur in 20% of persons with diverticular disease.[11] The bleeding is abrupt and copious and not related to any identifiable precipitating event in most cases. The bleeding is self-limited and stops spontaneously in more than 80% of patients.[8]

#### *Meckel's diverticulum*

Meckel's diverticulum is a congenital abnormality in which a blind tube, similar in structure to the appendix, is present, which usually opens into the distal ileum near the ileocecal valve. The tube may be attached to the umbilicus by a fibrous band. It occurs in about 2% of the population and is more common in men. The anomaly usually remains asymptomatic but can become grossly inflamed later in life and require surgical excision.

### Collaborative Care Management

The preliminary diagnosis of diverticulitis may be made from the history and presenting symptoms. A computed tomographic scan or an abdominal ultrasound examination reveals the presence of an abscess. A barium enema will reveal the classic diverticular pouches and thickened muscle layers but is usually not performed until after the inflammation subsides.

An episode of diverticulitis is managed by resting the bowel. Hospitalization may be required in acute episodes. The patient is given nothing by mouth, and a regimen of intravenous fluids, antibiotics, analgesics, and anticholinergics (propantheline bromide [Pro-Banthine]) is started to reduce bowel spasm. Symptoms should subside within 48 to 72 hours. Mild cases can be effectively managed in the home environment.

Acute diverticulitis usually subsides with conservative medical management. In about 25% of patients, however, surgical intervention may be needed to deal with complications.[49] Surgical resection of the involved portion of the bowel may be necessary, particularly if abscesses need to be drained. An end-to-end anastomosis is performed if possible.

Nursing care during an acute episode is largely supportive and focused on patient comfort. The nurse teaches the patient the rationale for bedrest and bowel rest and the role these interventions play in bowel healing. The nurse monitors fluid and electrolyte balance and the status of the patient's pain. The patient is regularly assessed for signs of complications.

#### *Patient/family education*

Asymptomatic diverticulosis is managed by the prevention of constipation through the use of a high-fiber diet. Bulk-forming laxatives also may be used to increase the mass and water content of the stool. The nurse encourages the patient to maintain a liberal fluid intake of 2500 to 3000 ml/day and to ingest a diet that contains soft foods high in fiber, such as fruits, vegetables, and whole grains. The person is advised to avoid eating items such as nuts and seeds, which can become trapped in the diverticula and trigger inflammation. Small amounts of bran may be added to regular foods, or bulk-forming agents may be used daily to increase stool mass and softness, increase the diameter of the colon, and reduce intraluminal pressure associated with straining at hard stool. Diet suggestions for the patient with diverticular disease are summarized in the Patient/Family Teaching Box. High-fiber foods should not be consumed when symptoms of inflammation are present because they can be highly irritating to the mucosa. The patient also is encouraged to avoid activities that increase intraabdominal pressure. Weight loss may be recommended in the attempt to lower the baseline levels of intraabdominal pressure.

## PERITONITIS

### Etiology/Epidemiology

Peritonitis involves either a local or generalized inflammation of the peritoneum, the membranous lining of the abdomen that covers the viscera. Peritonitis may be primary or

**patient/family teaching**

**Diet Modifications for Diverticular Disease**

**Foods to Include**

Foods high in fiber with emphasis on cellulose and hemicellulose types:

| | |
|---|---|
| Wheat or oat bran | Lettuce |
| Whole grain breads and cereals | Peaches |
| | Prunes |
| Peas | Seedless grapes |
| Carrots | |

**Foods to Avoid**

Foods containing nuts and seeds or indigestible strings or threads:

| | |
|---|---|
| Cucumbers | Strawberries |
| Celery | Raspberries |
| Tomatoes | Figs |
| Corn/popcorn | Nuts and seeds (sesame, caraway) |

secondary, aseptic or septic, and acute or chronic. Primary peritonitis usually is caused by bacterial infection, whereas secondary peritonitis often results from trauma, surgical injury, or chemical irritation.

A ruptured appendix, perforated peptic ulcer, diverticulitis, pelvic inflammatory disease, urinary tract infection or trauma, bowel obstruction, and surgical complications are possible causes of primary peritonitis. Secondary bacterial invasion occurs within hours of the initiating event and is an important component of all forms of peritonitis. Common organisms for bacterial invasion include *E. coli,* streptococci, staphylococci, pneumococci, gonococci, *Klebsiella,* and *Pseudomonas.*

## Pathophysiology

The body uses natural barriers to attempt to control the inflammation associated with peritonitis. Adhesions form rapidly and may be successful in limiting involvement to only a portion of the abdominal cavity. The end result may be abscess development. Adhesions are more likely to develop in the lower portion of the abdomen. As healing progresses, the adhesions may shrink and virtually disappear, or they may persist as constrictions that bind the involved structures together, possibly creating intestinal obstruction.

The peritoneal lining serves as a semipermeable membrane lining that allows the flow of water and electrolytes between the bloodstream and peritoneal cavity. When peritonitis occurs, fluid can shift into the abdominal cavity at a rate of 300 to 500 ml/hr in response to the acute inflammation. The inflammatory process also shunts extra blood to the inflamed areas of the bowel to combat the secondary bacterial infection, and peristalsis typically ceases. The bowel increasingly becomes distended with gas and fluid. The circulatory, fluid, and electrolyte changes can rapidly become critical. Local reactions of the peritoneum include redness and inflammation and the production of large amounts of fluid that contains electrolytes and proteins. Hypovolemia, electrolyte imbalance, dehydration, and finally shock can develop. The loss of circulatory volume is proportional to the severity of peritoneal involvement. The fluid usually becomes purulent as the condition progresses and as the bacteria become more numerous. The bacteria also may enter the blood and cause septicemia.

The clinical manifestations of peritonitis are both local and systemic. They depend to some degree on the site and extent of the inflammation. Abdominal findings include local or diffuse pain and rebound tenderness. Guarding and rigidity are classic signs. Distention and paralytic ileus develop as the inflammation progresses. Systemic signs may include fever and elevated WBC count, nausea and vomiting, and symptoms of early shock such as tachycardia, tachypnea, oliguria, restlessness, weakness, pallor, and diaphoresis. The symptoms initially are much less severe in elderly persons, and the diagnosis may be overlooked until the condition is extremely serious. Patients receiving high doses of corticosteroids also may exhibit mild or ambiguous symptoms, making early diagnosis difficult.

## Collaborative Care Management

The diagnosis of peritonitis is made primarily on the basis of the symptom pattern, laboratory findings, and x-ray studies that may show abnormalities in gas and air patterns in the abdomen. Free air or fluid in the abdominal cavity is indicative of perforation. Specimens of blood and peritoneal fluid are obtained for culture before the initiation of antibiotic therapy. WBC counts frequently are elevated to 20,000/mm$^3$ or higher. Electrolyte values are carefully monitored.

The primary curative intervention for peritonitis is surgery to correct the underlying cause and remove infected material. Surgical healing is impaired if sepsis or ischemia occurs, and complications associated with wound healing are common. Peritoneal lavage with warm saline may be performed during surgery, followed by the insertion of drainage tubes to facilitate healing. Surgery may have to be delayed until the patient's condition can be medically stabilized.

The patient with peritonitis is critically ill and requires careful monitoring of all vital parameters. Placement in a critical care environment frequently is indicated. The nurse monitors vital signs and intake and output frequently and adjusts IV lines and medications as ordered. Fluid, electrolyte, and colloid replacement is the major focus of medical care. The fluid shifts that cause massive hypovolemia and shock need aggressive management. Broad-spectrum antibiotics against suspected organisms are administered and then adjusted as needed in response to culture and sensitivity reports.

A nasogastric tube is inserted to help relieve abdominal distention. Bedrest in a semi-Fowler's position is maintained to support ventilation and increase patient comfort. The nurse encourages the patient to deep breathe frequently because pain and distention can significantly impair ventilation. The nurse also provides comfort measures, including frequent mouth care, basic hygiene, and measures to reduce anxiety. Nutritional management with total parenteral nutrition (TPN) solutions may be necessary when sepsis is severe and recovery is expected to be prolonged. The overall mortality of patients with severe peritonitis is about 40%.

### Patient/family education

Peritonitis typically develops rapidly and creates a serious and frightening situation for the patient and family. The nurse reinforces teaching about the nature of the problem and its treatment and provides ongoing support and encouragement. The nurse teaches the patient the importance of routine respiratory care and encourages ambulation when tolerated. If the abdominal involvement is extensive, the patient may have multiple drains in place, and wound healing is complex. Careful teaching about wound management is important as recovery is frequently prolonged, and the patient is likely to be discharged with ongoing needs for wound care support from home health care services. Careful discharge preparation and referrals are critical.

## INFLAMMATORY BOWEL DISEASE

*Inflammatory bowel disease (IBD)* is an umbrella term used to describe conditions that are characterized by bowel inflammation. Crohn's disease and ulcerative colitis are the two major forms of IBD. They have distinctly different pathological characteristics but actually share many overlapping features. They are therefore presented together.

### Etiology

The etiology of IBD remains unknown despite extensive research. A clear familial link has been demonstrated, but no genetic markers have been isolated. First-degree relatives have a significantly increased risk of contracting IBD, and familial aggregations of cases are found.

Available data strongly support the theory that environmental factors play an important role in disease frequency and changes in incidence over time, but no clear answers have emerged from the research.[22] It seems probable that some factor that gains entry into the GI tract interacts with the bowel wall to produce the inflammatory changes of IBD, but no transmissible agent been found. Diet is an obvious explanation, but none of the extensive studies performed thus far supports diet as the etiology of IBD.[22] The erratic and constantly changing patterns of worldwide incidence remain tantalizing but unexplained. The influence of smoking provides a typical example. Smokers have a 2 to 4 times greater risk of contracting Crohn's disease than nonsmokers, and the risk does not appear to be dose dependent. Nonsmokers, however, appear to be at greater risk of contracting ulcerative colitis, and the apparent protective effect of cigarette smoking does appear to be dose dependent (Table 41-4).[43] Similar contradictory evidence confounds research into infectious etiologies of IBD as well. An apparent increased risk in women using oral contraceptives is seen in the statistics but remains an unproven link.

Stress and emotional factors once were believed to play an important etiological role in IBD, but research has shown no indication of a psychogenic cause.[15] IBD is clearly multifactorial in origin, and at this point it can simply be said that IBD occurs in susceptible people, probably based on genetic factors, with environmental agents acting as triggers to produce a disturbance in the function of the bowel wall.[44] Other environmental factors may influence the presentation and severity of the disease process as well as its tendency to relapse.

**table 41-4** Comparison of Ulcerative Colitis and Crohn's Disease

| Ulcerative Colitis | Crohn's Disease |
|---|---|
| **USUAL AREA AFFECTED** | |
| Left colon, rectum | Distal ileum, right colon<br>Can occur anywhere in GI tract |
| **EXTENT OF INVOLVEMENT** | |
| Diffuse areas, contiguous | Segmental areas, noncontiguous |
| **INFLAMMATION** | |
| Mostly mucosal | Transmural |
| **MUCOSAL APPEARANCE** | |
| Shallow mucosal ulcerations, edematous, superficial bleeding | Cobblestone effect, granulomas<br>Thickened walls, narrowed lumen |
| **COMPLICATIONS** | |
| Loss of absorption and elasticity<br>Replacement of mucosa by scar tissue<br>Development of pseudopolyps that may become malignant<br>Toxic megacolon<br>Hemorrhoids<br>Hemorrhage | Fistulas<br>Perianal disease<br>Strictures<br>Abscesses<br>Perforation<br>Anemia<br>Malabsorption of fat and fat-soluble vitamins |

### Epidemiology

Inflammatory bowel disease occurs worldwide with an annual incidence rate of approximately 3 to 20 new cases per 100,000 population.[7] The incidence is significantly higher in the United States, northern Europe, and the United Kingdom, and approximately 1 million Americans deal with the problem on a daily basis.[7]

IBD used to be extremely rare or nonexistent in many parts of the world, but its incidence has accelerated during the twentieth century. Ulcerative colitis used to occur much more commonly than Crohn's disease, but the incidence of Crohn's disease now equals and in some areas such as the United States and northern Europe even exceeds that of ulcerative colitis.[22] Incidence rates for both major forms of IBD are still increasing around the world but appear to have stabilized in the areas of highest risk.[7] It is difficult to know to what degree the steady increases in incidence can be attributed, at least in part, to improved disease recognition and diagnosis.

IBD is common among whites but less common in African Americans and Native Americans. One of the most unusual aspects of the incidence statistics is the higher incidence among American and European Jews. This higher incidence does not occur among native-born Israelis and appears to point to some as yet unidentified genetic and environmental interaction.[7]

No gender pattern is evident in racially mixed groups, but white women appear to be at particular risk. Although IBD can occur at any age, its peak period of onset is in young adulthood between the ages of 15 and 25 years. Another smaller peak occurs between 55 and 60 years in some countries. Risk factors for IBD are summarized in the box below.[7]

## Pathophysiology

Although inflammation is the hallmark of both Crohn's disease and ulcerative colitis, the two disorders have a markedly different effect on the intestinal tract. The diseases are distinguished largely by the nature of the inflammation, the location in the GI tract, the pattern of distribution, and the degree of mucosal penetration. See Table 41-4 for a comparison of the major pathophysiological features of each disease process.

**risk factors**

**Inflammatory Bowel Disease**

Age 15-25 years
White race
  Women at slightly higher risk
Jewish ancestry, but does not apply to native born Israelis
First-degree relative of person with IBD
Residence in the United States, Great Britain, northern Europe, and Scandinavia
Smoking history (Crohn's disease)
Nonsmoking status (ulcerative colitis)
Use of oral contraceptives (among white women)

Both forms of IBD are characterized by a pattern of exacerbation and remission. Although there is a great deal of overlap in the symptoms, ulcerative colitis and Crohn's disease have different characteristic features. Bowel problems and abdominal discomfort are also characteristic features of irritable bowel syndrome, which is summarized in Box 41-2.[42]

### Ulcerative colitis

Ulcerative colitis creates a diffuse continuous process of inflammation characterized by edema and shallow mucosal ulceration. It primarily affects the distal colorectal area, and about 30% of patients are seen with disease confined to this region.[21] More extensive disease is termed *left-sided* and affects about 40% of patients. It involves the colon up to the splenic flexure.[21] In severe disease the inflammatory process extends all the way to the hepatic flexure or ileocecal junction. The mucosa is very fragile and bleeds spontaneously or in response to minimal trauma. Over time it becomes increasingly thickened and edematous. The ulceration and healing process gradually result in scar tissue formation that may cause the colon to lose its normal elasticity and absorptive capability.[21] As normal mucosa is gradually replaced by scar tissue the colon becomes thickened, rigid, and pipelike. The mucosa also may undergo structural changes over time, forming pseudopolyps that can become malignant.

Rectal bleeding is usually the earliest symptom of mild ulcerative colitis. The classic diarrhea, which begins as disease involvement becomes more extensive, ranges in severity from 3 to 4 times daily to hourly and is small in volume, mushy in consistency, and liberally mixed with blood, mucus, and pus.[12] The inflammatory exudate and mucus secretion increase both

**box 41-2** *Irritable Bowel Syndrome*

Irritable bowel syndrome (spastic colon, mucous colitis) refers to a syndrome of abdominal pain and altered bowel habits—usually diarrhea—that occurs in the absence of any identifiable organic disease. The diagnosis is made only when other pathological conditions are ruled out.

ETIOLOGY/EPIDEMIOLOGY

- Unknown
- Much more common in women
- Related to stress and overindulgence in food
- Often linked to a history of physical or sexual abuse
- Onset typically during late adolescence to mid-thirties
- Most frequently encountered GI condition in medical practice

PATHOPHYSIOLOGY

- Major findings are rarely present
- Laboratory tests are typically normal, but colon spasticity can be visualized by x-ray and endoscopy
- Increased small bowel motility plus increased frequency and amplitude of large bowel contractions
- Symptom patterns include:
  (1) Spastic colon: colicky abdominal pain, periodic constipation, and diarrhea
  (2) Painless urgent diarrhea after meals

COLLABORATIVE CARE MANAGEMENT

Treatment involves lifestyle modifications and supportive care, e.g.,

- Diet modification
  - Avoid rich fatty foods
  - Avoid gas-producing foods
  - Avoid gastric stimulants such as alcohol and smoking
  - Test response of symptoms to the ingestion of a high-fiber diet
- Medications
  - Bulk-forming laxatives, e.g., psyllium
  - Antispasmodics, e.g., dicyclomine
  - Antidiarrheals, e.g., loperamide
  - Motility agents, e.g., cisapride
- Health promotion
  - Adequate rest, stress management
  - Regular aerobic exercise

the fecal solutes and water. The diarrhea is associated with significant urgency and left-sided abdominal pain that is colicky in nature and is relieved by emptying the bowel.[12]

As the scarring within the bowel progresses, the sensation of the urge to defecate is lost, leading to involuntary leakage of stool. With severe diarrhea there may be significant losses of fluids, sodium, potassium, bicarbonate, and calcium.

### Crohn's disease

Crohn's disease can occur anywhere in the GI tract, but is found most often in the proximal colon and ileocecal junction, making it a right-sided disease. Twenty five percent of patients experience disease confined to the colon.[22] The inflammation of Crohn's disease is transmural, affecting all layers of the intestinal wall. It follows a "skip" or "cobblestone" pattern in which affected areas are separated by normal tissue. Mucosal granulomas, luminal narrowing, thickening of the intestinal wall, mucosal nodularity, and ulceration are characteristic features.[44] The lesions may perforate and form fistulas that connect with the bladder, vagina, or other segments of the bowel or mesentery. Scar tissue may form as the lesions heal, preventing the normal absorption of nutrients, and strictures may form, causing intestinal obstruction. Mesenteric lymph nodes are enlarged and firm. Figure 41-4 illustrates several of the common complications of Crohn's disease.

Diarrhea also is a feature of Crohn's disease, but it reflects the location and severity of the inflammation. It is more likely to consist of three to five large semisolid stools daily that contain mucus and pus but no blood.[33] Steatorrhea may be present if the ulceration extends high in the small intestine. Fat-soluble vitamins—A, D, E, and K—may be poorly absorbed with marked steatorrhea.[33]

Severe abdominal pain that is colicky in nature and tenderness that is diffuse or localized in the right lower quadrant are characteristic of Crohn's disease.[33] A tender mass of thickened intestines may be palpable in the area. During an acute episode the symptoms may closely resemble those of appendicitis.

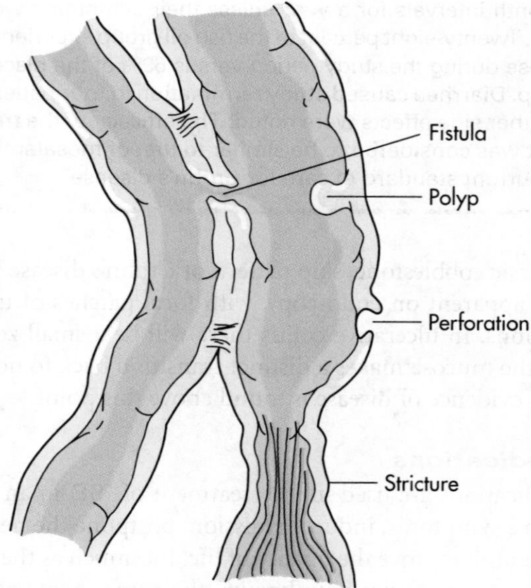


**fig. 41-4** Common complications of Crohn's disease.

### Extraintestinal and systemic symptoms of inflammatory bowel disease

Extraintestinal and systemic symptoms of IBD occur commonly and often complicate the patient's disease management. IBD can involve virtually every organ system. Although it is generally accepted that extraintestinal symptoms are systemic disorders, their etiology is not understood. They appear to reflect some type of generalized tissue vulnerability and usually are considered to be immunological phenomena.[22] They may precede or accompany the underlying bowel disorder. A patient with one extraintestinal manifestation has an increased risk of developing others.

Peripheral arthritis is the most common extraintestinal manifestation and occurs in 4% to 23% of patients with IBD.[12] It is migratory in nature, affects single joints in an asymmetric pattern, and primarily targets the hips, ankles, wrists, and elbows. A wide range of ocular problems may occur, for example, uveitis, corneal ulceration, and retinopathy. The incidence is about 4% to 10%.[33] Skin lesions are also common. A grouping of small bowel-related problems appears to be associated with Crohn's disease. Cholelithiasis, for example, has an incidence of 13% to 34% in patients with Crohn's disease versus 10% to 15% in the general population.[33]

In addition to the classic symptoms, IBD frequently causes anorexia, nausea, weakness, and malaise from the chronic inflammation. Weight loss is common and may result in nutritional deficiencies if the absorption capability of the bowel is significantly impaired. Intermittent fever and leukocytosis frequently accompany an exacerbation, and iron deficiency anemia may develop from both chronic mucosal bleeding and poor iron absorption. Patients are frequently pale and thin and look chronically ill. During disease exacerbations patients also have a significantly increased risk of developing kidney stones, primarily from the chronic fluid deficits. Classic clinical and extraintestinal manifestations of IBD are summarized in Box 41-3.

## Collaborative Care Management

### Diagnostic tests

The diagnosis of IBD begins with a careful history that includes the symptom pattern and its severity and duration. Many of the features of IBD overlap, and accurate diagnosis depends on establishing a constellation of contributory findings. A stool examination for leukocytes, parasites, blood, and culture are performed to rule out an infectious origin for the symptoms. Laboratory tests may include a complete blood count, erythrocyte sedimentation rate, and serum albumin measurement, although no laboratory study is diagnostic by itself.

A barium enema usually is ordered to evaluate the physical changes in the bowel; it provides accurate data about the structure of the colon, can be performed rapidly, and provides

**box 41-3** *clinical manifestations*

### *Inflammatory Bowel Disease*

**GENERAL**

Anorexia, nausea, and weight loss
Weakness and malaise
Fever and leukocytosis (a high fever and WBC >15,000/mm³ suggests an abscess)
Iron deficiency anemia

**SPECIFIC TO ULCERATIVE COLITIS**

Profuse diarrhea (15-20 stools per day)
Stools containing blood, mucus, and possibly pus
Abdominal cramping can be present before the bowel movement
Losses of fluid, sodium, potassium, bicarbonate, and calcium

**SPECIFIC TO CROHN'S DISEASE**

Three to five large, semisolid stools per day
Stools containing mucus and possibly pus but rarely blood
Steatorrhea if small bowel affected
Right lower quadrant cramping pain—may be severe and mimic appendicitis; diffuse rather than localized pain.

**EXTRAINTESTINAL MANIFESTATIONS**

**Arthritis (4%-23%)**
Involvement of large joints: hips, ankles, wrists, and elbows
Migratory and asymmetric incidence, nondeforming

**Ocular (4%-10%)**
Uveitis, episcleritis
Serous retinopathy

**Skin (3%-6%)**
Erythema nodosum: raised red tender nodules on anterior tibial surfaces
Pyoderma gangrenosum: painful necrotizing ulcerations most common on legs

**Hepatobiliary (4%-5%)**
Cholelithiasis
Fatty liver, cirrhosis
Cholangitis (70% of patients with cholangitis have ulcerative colitis)

**Renal (4%-23%)**
Kidney stones
Ureteral obstruction

a permanent record for future disease comparison. The classic "string lesions" of Crohn's disease are readily visible on barium enema.[44] These represent areas of extensive bowel narrowing and are often found in the terminal ileum.

An upper GI series also may be prescribed to evaluate small bowel involvement if Crohn's disease is suspected. Endoscopy procedures such as sigmoidoscopy or colonoscopy may be used to directly examine the nature and pattern of the inflammation. The presence of major perianal complications such as abscesses and fistulas are characteristic of Crohn's disease.[22]

**research**

Reference: Thomas GAO et al: Transdermal nicotine as maintenance therapy for ulcerative colitis, *N Engl J Med* 332(15):988-992, 1995.

This study was a controlled trial of the effect of transdermal nicotine on the maintenance of remission in patients with ulcerative colitis. The disease primarily affects nonsmokers, and patients who smoke often report improvement in their symptoms. The study involved 80 patients with ulcerative colitis who were in clinical remission. They were randomly assigned to groups and treated with either nicotine or placebo patches. Once patients achieved a maintenance level of 15 mg of nicotine their standard mesalamine treatment was gradually tapered. The pattern of relapse was then monitored over a period of 6 months.

Half of each group completed the full trial period. There was no significant difference in the number of relapses between the two groups. The time course for relapse was also almost identical. The study concluded that transdermal nicotine was ineffective in maintaining remission for the ulcerative colitis patients in this population.

**research**

Reference: Belluzzi A et al: Effect of an enteric coated fish oil preparation on relapses in Crohn's disease, *N Engl J Med* 334(24):1557-1560, 1996.

This study investigated the effects of a new enteric-coated fish oil preparation on the maintenance of remission in patients with Crohn's disease. A sample of 78 adult patients with Crohn's disease in clinical remission were randomly assigned to receive either three enteric-coated capsules of fish oil three times daily or a similar regimen with a placebo capsule. A special coating ensured that the capsules would dissolve in the small intestine. Patients were evaluated at 3-month intervals for a year unless their symptoms worsened. Twenty-eight percent of the fish oil group experienced relapse during the study period versus 69% of the placebo group. Diarrhea caused study termination in four patients. No other side effects were noted. The efficacy of the treatment was considered to be similar to that of mesalamine, the current standard of care for Crohn's disease.

The classic cobblestone, skip pattern of Crohn's disease is also readily apparent on endoscopy, with focal patches of ulcerative lesions. In ulcerative colitis there will be a small zone in which the mucosa makes a distinct transition back to normal, and no evidence of disease is found above this point.

#### *Medications*

Medications are used in the treatment of IBD in an effort to relieve symptoms, induce remission, postpone the need for surgery, and improve the quality of life. Inasmuch as the cause of IBD remains basically unknown, the components of drug therapy are empirically based on a combination of clinical trials and practical experience (see the Research Boxes).

Sulfasalazine (Azulfidine) was developed in the 1930s and first used for treating arthritis. Arthritis was believed to have an infectious origin, and sulfasalazine combined the proved effectiveness of aspirin with a sulfonamide antibiotic. Its use was quickly broadened to include IBD, and it has been a mainstay of treatment ever since. The exact mechanism of action of sulfasalazine is unknown, but its effectiveness is primarily attributed to the antiinflammatory effects of aspirin. It successfully induces and sustains remission in most patients with mild to moderate ulcerative colitis and mild Crohn's disease. Sulfasalazine is split by bacteria in the colon into its two components. 5-Acetylsalicylic acid (ASA) is poorly absorbed and thus maintains prolonged contact with the inflamed mucosa. Sulfapyridine, its second component, has no proved effectiveness against IBD and yet accounts for most of the troubling side effects.

Efforts have, therefore, focused on developing 5-ASA products that can be delivered intact to the colon without an additional carrier drug. Options include olsalazine (Dipentum), which is poorly absorbed in the small intestine and broken down in the colon by the action of the intestinal bacteria; and mesalamine (Pentasa, Asacol), which is coated with a pH-sensitive resin that only dissolves in a pH greater than 7 in the terminal ileum and proximal colon.[35] Sustained release granules of this product are also available.

These drugs are well tolerated if started in graduating doses and taken buffered with food. Toxicity appears to be minimal. The most common side effects include nausea, vomiting, and diarrhea. No particular agent has been shown to be superior. Sulfasalazine retains the advantage of being significantly less costly than the other preparations for patients who can tolerate the drug.

Sulfasalazine-derivative drugs also can be used topically for the 25% or more of patients with ulcerative colitis whose disease is confined to the rectal and sigmoid area. These drugs can be administered by enema, which provides for homogeneous delivery to the inflamed lower colon. Enemas provide high local concentrations of the drug, with minimal systemic absorption, and have been shown to be as effective as steroids in many situations. Suppository forms of the drugs also have been developed in the attempt to increase patient acceptability. Patients frequently find daily enemas to be unacceptable for long-term therapy. Medications commonly used to treat IBD are summarized in Table 41-5.

Corticosteroids also have played an important role in IBD management for many years. The potent antiinflammatory effects of steroids have proved effective in inducing remission in patients with moderate to severe Crohn's disease and severe ulcerative colitis. Although both local and systemic steroids are used, their widespread and severe side effects limit their long-term use. Steroids can be administered rectally, but most forms absorb readily from the rectal mucosa and produce systemic effects. A continuing research focus is on adapting the newer, less absorbable steroids such as budesonide and beclomethasone, which are currently used extensively in inhalers. Corticosteroids have a major role in the management of Crohn's disease, which is less responsive to sulfasalazine derivatives, but they have not been shown to maintain remission.

Potent immunosuppressive agents such as azathioprine (Imuran), mercaptopurine (Purinethol), and cyclosporine (Sandimmune) may be used in selected patients who cannot be successfully weaned from steroids. Long-term administration of corticosteroids is contraindicated because there does not appear to be a safe daily dose that does not eventually cause significant adverse side effects.[35] These potent immunosuppressive drugs have a slow onset of action and are not useful in acute situations, but they are effective in prolonging remission and are usually well tolerated.

Antibiotics have also been extensively explored. They do not appear to be effective in managing ulcerative colitis, but metronidazole (Flagyl) has been shown to be effective for mild Crohn's disease that is confined to the colon.[22,35] Antibiotics also are appropriate for severely ill patients at risk for infection and in situations in which bowel stricture causes stasis and bacterial overgrowth in the bowel.

Drug therapy for IBD also may include the use of antidiarrheal medications when a high degree of disease activity is present (Table 41-5). These drugs are administered for symptomatic relief, and an accurate record needs to be maintained of their administration and effectiveness in controlling symptoms. Vitamin supplements frequently are necessary, particularly when anorexia and nausea are present.

#### *Treatments*

No specific treatments are indicated for IBD management. Patients with primarily rectal involvement may follow a regimen of daily enema administration. Other prescribed treatments may be related to the management of skin breakdown or excoriation that may accompany severe diarrhea.

### *Surgical management*

**Crohn's disease.** Surgical intervention is avoided in Crohn's disease as much as possible because recurrence of the disease process in the same region is virtually inevitable.[40] Nevertheless more than 50% of patients will need surgery at least once during the course of their disease.[40] The major management challenge with Crohn's disease is the fact that it is stubbornly incurable even with aggressive medical or surgical intervention. Therefore surgical approaches to Crohn's disease focus on sparing and conserving as much of the bowel as possible, particularly when the small bowel is involved. The loss of more than 100 cm of bowel almost inevitably results in short bowel syndrome and persistent problems with malabsorption.[40] Segmental resection with reanastomosis has been the primary surgical approach. Surgeons typically resect the bowel 5 to 10 cm above and below the macroscopically visible disease. Recurrence symptoms appear at a rate of approximately 10% per year,[40] but they do not always necessitate repeat surgery. The primary indications for surgery include bowel obstruction, fistula, abscess, perforation, or hemorrhage.

Bowel strictures are a common complication of Crohn's disease that can cause acute bowel obstruction. The development

**table 41-5** *Common Medications for* ***Treatment of Inflammatory Bowel Disease***

| DRUG | ACTION | INTERVENTION |
|---|---|---|
| **AMINOSALICYLATES (ORAL)** | | |
| Sulfasalazine (Azulfidine) | Converted in colon to sulfapyridine and 5-aminosalicylic acid, which may exert an antiinflammatory effect, possibly through prostagladin inhibition | Assess for allergy to sulfonamides or aspirin.<br>Monitor for common side effects: anorexia, nausea, and vomiting, headache.<br>Teach patient to:<br>Take in divided doses.<br>Take with full glass of fluid or with food.<br>Maintain a liberal fluid intake (2500-3000 ml daily).<br>Report incidence of skin rash or other adverse effects. |
| Olsalazine (Dipentum) | As above without antibacterial action of sulfapyridine | Monitor for common side effects as above.<br>Also may cause mild to moderate diarrhea.<br>Teach patient to:<br>Take in divided doses.<br>Take with full glass of fluid or with food.<br>Maintain a liberal fluid intake (2500-3000 ml daily). |
| Mesalamine (Asacol, Pentasa) | Same as olsalazine | Teach patient to:<br>Take in divided doses.<br>Maintain a liberal fluid intake (2500-3000 ml daily).<br>Swallow tablets whole; do not chew or break outer coating. |
| **AMINOSALICYLATES (RECTAL)** | | |
| Mesalamine in suspension for retention enema<br>Mesalamine suppository | As above | Administer enema while patient positioned on left side and teach patient to retain as long as possible. |
| **CORTICOSTEROIDS (ORAL/IV)** | | |
| Prednisolone/ prednisone | Potent systemic antiinflammatory action | Teach patient to:<br>Take with food or fluid.<br>Monitor weight gain; assess for edema.<br>Have blood pressure checked regularly.<br>Be alert to signs of infection and report promptly.<br>Be aware that mood swings occur commonly.<br>Do not change dose or schedule or abruptly discontinue drug.<br>Maintain good personal hygiene; keep perianal area clean and dry. |
| **CORTICOSTEROIDS (RECTAL)** | | |
| Hydrocortisone<br>Intrarectal foam (Cortifoam)<br>Retention enema (Cortenema) | As above | As above |
| Budesonide enema | As above; rapid presystemic metabolism minimizes absorption | Administer enema while patient is positioned on left side and teach patient to retain as long as possible. Other interventions as above; side effects should be less. |

*Continued*

**table 41-5** *Common Medications for* ***Treatment of Inflammatory Bowel Disease***

| Drug | Action | Intervention |
|---|---|---|
| **IMMUNOSUPPRESSIVE AGENTS** | | |
| Mercaptopurine (Purinethol) | Potent systemic suppression of immune response; may take 4-6 mo for full effect | Teach patient to:<br>Report any signs of infection.<br>Be alert to easy bruising.<br>Return for laboratory work as scheduled.<br>Maintain liberal daily fluid intake (2500-3000 ml daily).<br>Take with food or after meals. |
| Azathioprine (Imuran) | As above | As above |
| Cyclosporine (Sandimmune) | As above; effects seen after several days | Oral solution may be mixed in glass and given with milk or orange juice at room temperature; avoid refrigeration.<br>Teach patient to:<br>Monitor blood pressure.<br>Report hematuria or any change in urinary function. |

of strictureplasty (Figure 41-5), which is analogous to pyloroplasty, enables surgeons to release the strictures without the need for major surgery.[13] The procedure can correct the obstruction without physical loss of the involved bowel segments. Strictured segments tend to be fibrous in nature rather than acutely inflamed and rarely obstruct again. It is theorized that the obstruction, rather than the stricture, triggers the acute inflammation, and that the bowel is able to resolve the inflammation once the obstruction is relieved. The nursing management of patients undergoing bowel resection is presented on p. 1354.

**Ulcerative colitis.** Surgical intervention may be selected for patients with ulcerative colitis whose disease cannot be satisfactorily controlled with standard medical management. The procedures are curative in nature and involve the removal of the entire colon. Surgery is also undertaken when acute complications such as hemorrhage or toxic megacolon develop or when the presence of cellular dysplasia indicates an unacceptably high risk of bowel cancer.[40] Most patients are able to achieve a high quality of health after surgery,[37] and the successful development of continent procedures has made the lifestyle challenges much less daunting (Research Box).

***Ileostomy.*** The Brook ileostomy procedure is the oldest colectomy procedure and remains the standard against which other procedures are measured.[34] The Brook procedure involves the removal of the colon, rectum, and anus, with permanent closure of the anus. The ileostomy is created when the end of the terminal ileum is brought out through the abdominal wall to form a stoma (Figure 41-6). Any colectomy procedure eliminates the ability of the colon to reabsorb fluid and electrolytes, and the ileostomy drainage is profuse and watery. The terminal ileum dilates over time and assumes some of the functions of the cecum. The volume of stool decreases, but a minimum of 300 to 800 ml of fluid is still lost in the stool each day along with substantial amounts of electrolytes, particularly sodium.[34] The person experiences chronic fluid deficit as the small intestine is unable to make adequate adjustments to fluid deficits, and any increase in fluid intake simply increases the volume of the ileostomy drainage.

The surgery cures the ulcerative colitis and eliminates the risk of colon cancer. However, the permanent ileostomy can create both physical and emotional complications for the patient. Malfunctioning of the ostomy is relatively common as poorly digested foods can easily cause obstruction. Fears of leakage, embarrassment from noise and odor, and negative effects on self-concept, body image, and sexuality are common problems.[14] Impotence can also occur after the surgery unless the surgeon is able to successfully dissect around the autonomic nerves in the pelvis.

***Continent ileostomy.*** In the late 1960s Dr. Nils Kock developed a surgical procedure to spare patients some of the challenges of traditional ileostomy. The procedure (the Kock pouch) involves the creation of an abdominal reservoir to store the feces by use of a piece of terminal ileum. A portion of the ileum is intussuscepted to form a nipple valve that lies flush with the abdomen (Figure 41-7). A catheter is used to empty the pouch, and a small dressing or adhesive bandage is worn over the stoma between emptyings. The pouch eventually can expand to hold about 500 ml.

Problems with the nipple valve are common and frequently require open laparotomy for repair. This plus the incidence of chronic inflammation in the pouch limits the usefulness of the procedure, and it is rarely recommended as a primary intervention.[34]

***Ileoanal anastomosis (ileorectostomy).*** The ileoanal anastomosis was the first colectomy procedure developed

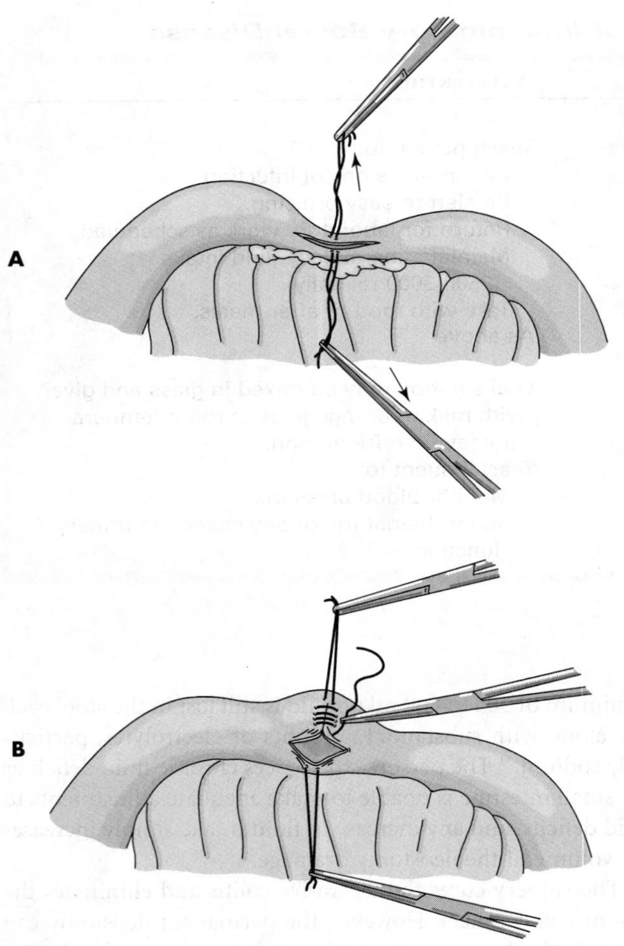


fig. 41-5 Strictureplasty. **A,** A linear incision is made at and beyond the stricture site. The site is spread open. **B,** The widened site is sutured closed.

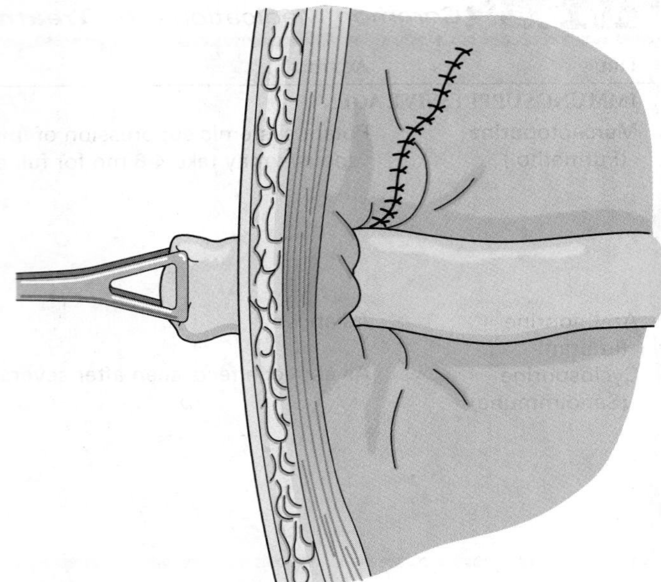

fig. 41-6 Construction of an ileostomy.

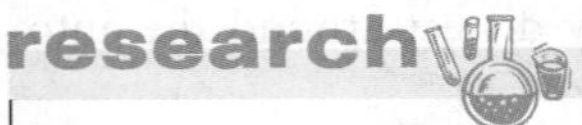

Reference: Provenzale D et al: Health related quality of life after ileoanal pull through, *Gastroenterology* 113(1):7-14, 1997.

The purpose of this study was to measure the "health-related quality of life" of patients after ileoanal pull through surgery. Health-related quality of life encompasses physical, psychosocial, and emotional functional status. The sample of 22 patients was drawn from all patients undergoing colectomy for IBD in 1 year at a major medical center. The sample was composed of 14 men and 8 women with a median age of 39 years.

A variety of measuring instruments was used. Overall health status and quality of life for the sample were reported as generally excellent and similar in most respects to the normal population. Sample patients exhibited a significantly better health status than a national sample of patients with IBD. They also exhibited significantly better psychosocial health. Quality of life was rated much higher than a comparison sample of patients with chronic gastroesophageal reflex disease, achalasia, or after esophagectomy.

that does not require any type of ileostomy. A 12- to 15-cm rectal stump is left after the colon is removed. The small intestine is inserted inside this rectal sleeve and anastomosed (Figure 41-8). The procedure is technically easier than the anal reservoir surgeries (see below), but it requires a large compliant rectum, which makes it inappropriate for some older adults. Complications related to the rectal stump are the primary drawbacks to the procedure.[13] The ulcerative colitis can recur in the rectal stump, which is also at significant risk for rectal cancer. Five to 50% of ulcerative colitis patients who undergo ileoanal anastomosis will need surgery at some point in the future to remove the rectal segment.[14] If the rectum remains disease free, however, its ability to reabsorb water and electrolytes results in a decreased volume of stool and an increased quality of life.[14] The procedure can also be used successfully for patients with Crohn's disease who have pancolitis.

***Ileoanal reservoir.*** The current procedure of choice for colectomy involves the creation of a pouch from the terminal ileum that is sutured directly to the anus.[14,34] The anal sphincter is left intact, which preserves continence, plus approximately 1 inch of rectum that is stripped of its mucosa to remove the last vestige of ulcerative colitis. A temporary loop colostomy is formed until healing of all anastomoses is complete, making this a two-stage procedure. The loop ileostomy usually can be closed within 3 to 4 months. Several different approaches to reservoir construction have been developed. A J-shaped anastomosis is shown in Figure 41-9. W- and S-shaped pouches are also used but the S-shaped pouch is large, and the distal limb may not empty effectively.[14]

Functional results continue to improve for up to 12 months after surgery, and most patients have three to eight bowel movements per day. Slight fecal incontinence is a problem—sometimes a persistent one and especially at night—but the

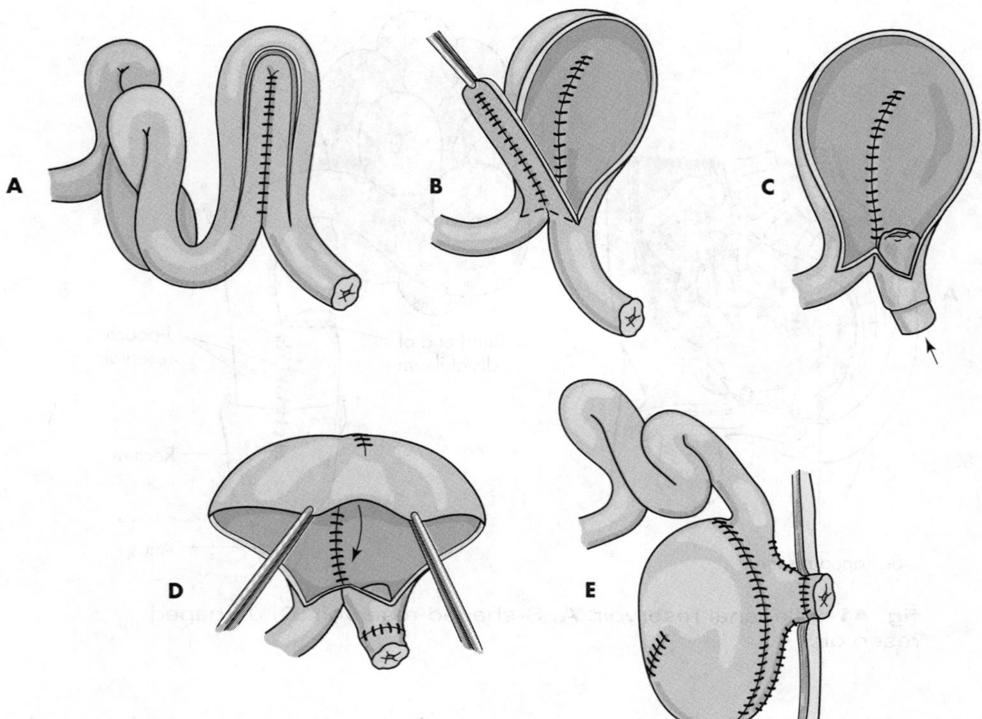


**fig. 41-7** Continent ileostomy (Kock pouch). **A,** Loop of bowel sewn together. **B,** Removal of anterior portion. **C,** Nipple valve made by pushing bowel back on itself. **D,** Pouch formation. **E,** End brought through stoma.

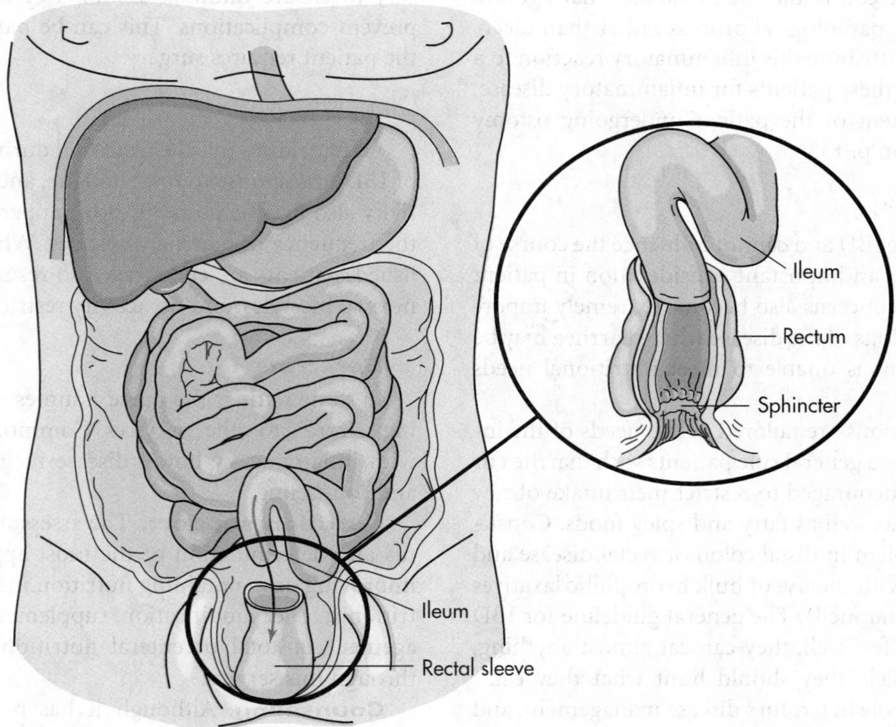


**fig. 41-8** Ileoanal anastomosis.

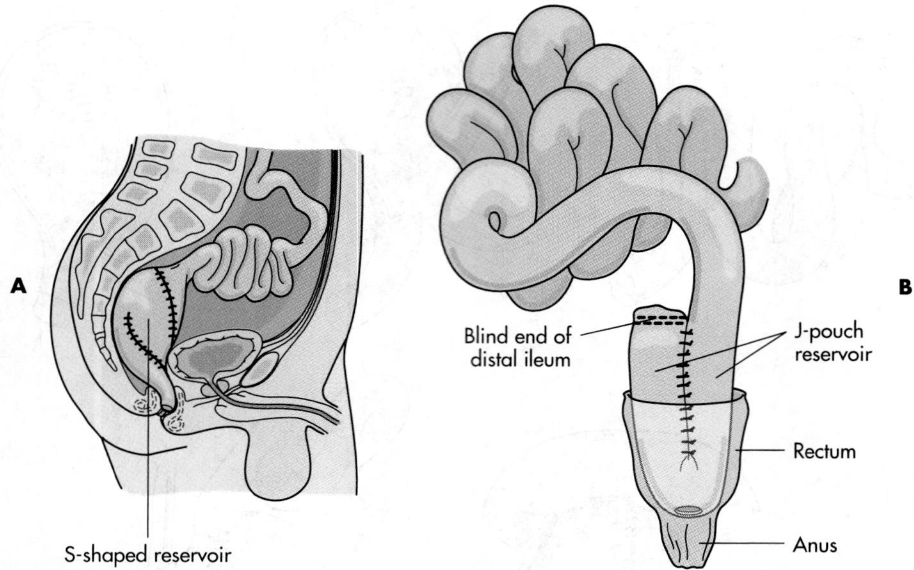


**fig. 41-9** Ileoanal reservoir. **A,** S-shaped reservoir. **B,** J-shaped reservoir.

normal manner of defecation makes this a popular procedure.[34] It usually is not used in persons older than 55 years who may experience anal sphincter deterioration related to aging.

The procedure is not without complications, and "pouchitis," acute inflammation within the reservoir, is a common chronic problem.[13] Pouchitis creates discomfort, bleeding, and increased output that is similar in many ways to the original disease process. This is attributed by some researchers to faulty diagnosis of the colitis and the possibility that Crohn's disease is the primary pathological process rather than ulcerative colitis.[14] Others attribute this inflammatory reaction to a general propensity of these patients for inflammatory disease.

Nursing management of the patient undergoing ostomy surgery is presented on p. 1336.

### Diet

Diet does not cause IBD and cannot influence the course of the disease, but diet is an important consideration in patient comfort. Nutritional concerns also become extremely important during exacerbations of the disease when diarrhea may be severe, and the patient is unable to meet nutritional needs through an oral diet.

Diet recommendations are tailored to the needs of the individual patient, but as a general rule patients with diarrhea or abdominal pain are encouraged to restrict their intake of raw fruits and vegetables as well as fatty and spicy foods. Constipation may be a problem in distal colon or rectal disease and usually is controlled with the use of bulk hydrophilic laxatives such as psyllium (Metamucil). The general guideline for IBD is that when patients feel well, they can eat almost anything, but when they feel sick, they should limit what they eat.[33] Bowel rest can play a role in Crohn's disease management, and elemental diets or supplements may be used. These preparations are completely digested and absorbed in the duodenum and ileum and place no demands on the large bowel. Recent attention has been focused on the possible suppressive effect of fish oil on the inflammatory process. Lactose intolerance is occasionally a problem in persons with IBD, and patients may be encouraged to evaluate the effect of restricting dairy products.

Acute exacerbations of IBD make it difficult to maintain adequate nutrition. Total parenteral nutrition may be necessary to ensure minimal amounts of essential nutrients and prevent complications. This can be particularly important if the patient requires surgery.

### Activity

Activity levels may be restricted during acute exacerbations of IBD in response to fever, fatigue, and malaise. Reduced activity also may be useful in slowing peristalsis and decreasing the frequency of diarrhea episodes. When remission is established, patients are encouraged to resume all aspects of their normal lifestyles, and no activity restrictions apply.

### Referrals

In some settings the nurse assumes responsibility for making referrals to other services. Common referrals for persons with inflammatory bowel disease include nutrition support and counseling.

**Nutrition support.** The assessment of nutritional status and determination of the most appropriate approach to improving or maintaining nutrition may involve a skilled nutritionist. Diet modification, supplement selection, and management of total parenteral nutrition may be coordinated through this service.

**Counseling.** Although it has been clearly established that neither stress nor personality is part of the etiology of inflammatory bowel disease, coping with the effects of IBD can put a tremendous strain on a person's adaptive abilities. Disease exacerbations may leave the patient particularly vulnerable to depression and even despair. Support services in this area can be extremely important. Patients and families should be routinely referred to the services of the National Foundation for Ileitis and Colitis.*

## NURSING MANAGEMENT

### ASSESSMENT

#### Subjective Data

Subjective data to be collected to assess the patient with IBD include:

- Patient's knowledge base and understanding of the disorder
- Pain: location, nature, severity, frequency; relationship to eating; measures used to self-treat
- Bowel elimination pattern: constipation or diarrhea, frequency of stools
- Nutritional status: usual meal pattern and intake; recent weight changes, food intolerances and allergies, appetite, fatigue or weakness, nausea
- Social relationships: support network; impact of illness on family, employment, lifestyle, and sexuality
- Perceived life stress and usual coping patterns
- Medications in current use: prescribed and over the counter; dosage and side effects; perceived effectiveness in managing disease and symptoms

#### Objective Data

Objective data to be collected to assess the patient with IBD include:

- Body weight
- Skin turgor and condition of mucous membranes
- Presence of fever
- Bowel sounds: presence and character
- Condition of perianal skin
- Composition of stools: presence of blood, fat, mucus and/or pus

### NURSING DIAGNOSES

Nursing diagnoses are determined from analysis of patient data. Nursing diagnoses for the patient with IBD may include but are not limited to:

| Diagnostic Title | Possible Etiological Factors |
|---|---|
| Pain, chronic | Inflammatory process in intestine |
| Diarrhea | Chronic inflammation in intestine |
| Nutrition, altered: less than body requirements | Anorexia and nausea, abdominal cramping with meals, malabsorption of food |
| Coping, ineffective (individual) | Persistent symptoms and lack of curative treatment |
| Health maintenance, altered | Lack of knowledge of condition, treatment, or recognition of complications |

*National Foundation for Ileitis and Colitis, 386 Park Ave South, New York, NY 10016-7374; (800) 932-2423.

### EXPECTED PATIENT OUTCOMES

Expected patient outcomes for the patient with IBD may include but are not limited to:

1a. Relates an improvement in frequency and severity of abdominal discomfort.
 b. Utilizes dietary and noninvasive pain-relief measures to manage pain.
2a. Has fewer episodes of diarrhea.
 b. Identifies dietary and activity factors that improve or worsen diarrhea.
 c. Lists the major signs and symptoms of dehydration and electrolyte imbalance.
3a. Follows a balanced, high-nutrient diet, avoiding foods that increase symptoms.
 b. Maintains desired weight or regains weight to desired goal at a rate of ½ to 1 pound per week.
 c. Achieves a positive nitrogen balance as evidenced by serum albumin level greater than 4 g/dl.
4a. Identifies factors that increase disease-related anxiety and stress.
 b. Verbalizes coping strategies and support mechanisms to handle problems.
5a. Describes nature of illness, prescribed therapy schedule, and side effects of all medications.
 b. Lists symptoms requiring medical attention.
 c. Identifies plans for ongoing medical follow-up.

### INTERVENTIONS

#### Promoting Comfort

The nurse encourages the patient to accurately document the character and severity of the pain and to determine its relationship to eating, drinking, and passing stool or flatus. Anticholinergic or antispasmodic medications such as propantheline bromide (Pro-Banthine) may be prescribed to reduce the cramping, but narcotics are not used because of their negative effect on peristalsis. A warm heating pad to the abdomen often is comforting but should not be used during acute exacerbations. The nurse assists the patient with position changes and encourages diversional activities and the practice of relaxation strategies. The nurse documents the patient's pain pattern and response to all interventions.

#### Controlling Diarrhea

Chronic diarrhea often becomes a focus of care during exacerbations of the disease process. Patients may feel trapped by the frequency and urgency of their need to defecate. The nurse encourages the person to keep accurate records of the frequency, severity, and character of each diarrhea episode, particularly if blood or pus is present.

The medication regimen is designed to control the inflammation and eventually the diarrhea, but this process may take days or weeks. Antidiarrheal agents such as loperamide may be used to slow peristalsis, and mucilloids such as Metamucil may add bulk to the stool and help reduce the frequency of defecation. The patient is encouraged to limit activity when diarrhea is severe and to lie down for 20 minutes after meals to limit peristalsis. Patients are encouraged to use the toilet or commode whenever possible, but a weak, acutely ill person may need to have a bedpan readily accessible. Room deodorizers may be necessary for odor control.

The anal region often becomes excoriated from the frequent stools. Painful anal fissures and fistulas may develop. The anal area needs to be kept clean and dry. Medicated wipes (such as Tucks) can provide greater comfort than toilet tissue. Sitz baths three times a day also promote comfort and cleanliness. Ointments such as Desitin or zinc oxide may be used to protect the perianal skin.

Profuse diarrhea can lead to severe losses of fluids and electrolytes. If the patient is consuming an oral diet, the nurse encourages a liberal fluid intake (at least 2500 to 3000 ml daily) and explores the patient's tolerance to solutions such as Gatorade, which can help replace lost electrolytes. It is important for the patient to understand that any increase in fluid intake will also increase output since the bowel is limited in its ability to reabsorb fluids. The nurse records accurate intake and output and monitors the patient's weight daily.

### Promoting Nutrition

During acute exacerbations of IBD, the patient usually is malnourished from anorexia, inflammation of the bowel, and malabsorption. The method of feeding depends on the type and extent of the disorder. With severe or extensive disease, especially when complications are present, the patient may be given nothing by mouth, and TPN may be instituted. Bowel rest can be very helpful in Crohn's disease but has no proved therapeutic benefit in ulcerative colitis.

Elemental feedings, similar to those given in tube feedings, are started as soon as possible; these feedings are absorbed rapidly in the upper GI tract, causing minimal demand on the colon. Palatability is a problem with the oral intake of elemental diets. Serving the fluids chilled and offering a variety of flavors increase patient acceptance. A low-residue, high-protein, high-calorie diet is then gradually introduced.

During periods of remission, patients are advised to continue to eat a well-balanced, high-caloric diet with a liberal fluid and salt intake to compensate for daily losses. Only those foods that are known to cause problems are restricted. The person with ulcerative colitis may need to avoid intestinal stimulants such as alcohol, caffeinated beverages, high-fat foods, and very high-fiber foods such as raw fruits and vegetables (cooked fruits and vegetables usually are better tolerated). Milk products may be poorly tolerated, and the nurse encourages the patient to evaluate the effect of milk product restriction on the severity of symptoms. Multivitamin and mineral supplements are used regularly.

### Promoting Effective Coping

Inflammatory bowel disease is characterized by periods of exacerbation and remission throughout the patient's adult life. It can significantly disrupt the patient's preferred lifestyle. Although emotions and stress do not play a role in disease etiology, they are believed to influence the severity and frequency of disease exacerbations. Frustration, depression, and a sense of powerlessness are common responses to the disease, and they may precipitate hostile or dependent behaviors. Patients frequently become preoccupied with their physical symptoms.

The nurse encourages the patient to become an active participant in all decisions related to disease management and to verbalize concerns and feelings related to the disease and treatment. The nurse provides the patient with information about local support groups and encourages involvement with the National Foundation for Ileitis and Colitis.

Fatigue is a common problem with IBD and can worsen the patient's psychological response to the disease. Fatigue is the result of increased energy demands from the inflammatory process and a decreased energy supply from inadequate nutrition and anemia. Planned rest periods should be included in daily activities. When the acute episode begins to subside, progressive activity is encouraged. During periods of remission the person is encouraged to participate in social activities but should not overexert to the point of fatigue. Sexual response also may be affected by IBD. Malnutrition and frequent diarrhea often lead to decreased libido, and the presence of an ileostomy may be associated with a sense of diminished sexual attractiveness. The nurse encourages the patient to express sex-related concerns and explore them openly with the spouse or partner. IBD support groups can be excellent resources for strategies to manage concerns over odor and leakage during sexual activity, particularly after colectomy surgery.

### Promoting Effective Self-Care

Accurate knowledge about the disease process and therapeutic modalities can be extremely influential in helping the patient achieve a sense of control. The nurse explores the patient's existing knowledge base about the cause, course, and prognosis of the disease, treatment options, and the identification and management of complications. Patient education materials are available from the National Foundation for Ileitis and Colitis. The nurse ensures that the patient understands the importance of careful adherence to the medication regimen and has a plan for scheduled medical follow-up. Guidelines for teaching the patient with IBD are summarized in the Patient/Family Teaching Box.

## EVALUATION

To evaluate the effectiveness of nursing interventions, compare patient behaviors with those stated in the expected patient outcomes. Successful achievement of patient outcomes for the patient with IBD is indicated by:

1a. States that abdominal pain is absent or less frequent and severe.
 b. Successfully uses noninvasive pain-relief strategies to manage abdominal pain.
2a. Reports fewer or no episodes of diarrhea.
 b. Successfully modifies diet to reduce diarrhea.
 c. Correctly identifies major warning signs of fluid and electrolyte imbalance (see Chapter 15).

### *patient/family teaching*

**The Person with Inflammatory Bowel Disease**

**Diet and Fluids**

Eat a high-calorie, well-balanced diet.
Avoid any foods that increase symptoms (e.g., fresh fruits and vegetables, fatty foods, spicy foods, and alcohol).
Assess the effect of dairy products on disease symptoms and limit use if appropriate.
Take a multivitamin/mineral supplement daily.
Ensure a liberal fluid intake—2500-3000 ml daily:
Drink Gatorade or other commercial products, if tolerated during flare-ups, to replace lost electrolytes.
Use salt liberally during disease flare-ups.

**Elimination**

Take medication as prescribed.
Keep rectal area clean and dry; use analgesic rectal ointment or sitz baths for rectal discomfort.
Consult with physician about the appropriateness of antidiarrheal agents or bulk laxatives when diarrhea is present.
Monitor weight daily during disease flare-ups.

**Rest and Coping**

Maintain a regular sleep schedule.
Schedule daily activities to avoid fatigue; take rest periods as necessary.
Use relaxation strategies when stress levels rise.
Discuss concerns with family or support person.
Attend local IBD support group if available.

**Health Maintenance**

Report signs requiring medical attention:
Change in pattern or severity of abdominal pain or diarrhea
Development of constipation
Change in stool character
Unusual discharge from rectum
Fever
Plan for regular follow-up care.

3a. Adheres to a high-calorie, well-balanced diet.
b. Maintains optimal body weight.
c. Achieves serum albumin levels within normal range.
4a. Identifies personal lifestyle factors that increase stress.
b. Uses community support mechanisms to enhance coping strategies.
5a. Accurately describes nature of illness and prescribed therapy, schedule, and side effects of medications.
b. Correctly lists symptoms needing medical attention.
c. Schedules appointments for follow-up care.

## GERONTOLOGICAL CONSIDERATIONS

Although both forms of inflammatory bowel disease typically begin in young adulthood, the onset can occur after age 60 years. The presentation, clinical course, and response to treatment generally are similar in both age-groups. The disease frequently takes the form of proctitis in elders, and local treatment usually is effective. Complications are more likely to be related to comorbidity problems than the primary IBD, but toxic megacolon occurs frequently. Once the disease is controlled, the person with ulcerative colitis is less likely to have a relapse, and the risk of disease-related cancer is minimal. Crohn's disease in elders tends to be localized in the distal colon and rectum, and generalized involvement is unusual. Because both forms of IBD tend to concentrate in the distal colon and rectum, the differential diagnosis may be unclear in elderly patients. This is particularly true if the disease does not have an acute onset.

Surgical intervention is avoided if possible because patients tend to experience an increased incidence of complications, although recurrence of Crohn's disease after surgery is not common in elders. Sphincter-sparing colectomy procedures are used less commonly in this population because it is more difficult to achieve adequate continence, particularly at night.

## SPECIAL ENVIRONMENTS FOR CARE

### Critical Care Management

Critical care management is not an expected part of the treatment of IBD. Most disease flare-ups can be successfully managed in the community setting. The development of complications may require hospitalization for replacement of fluids and electrolytes, provision of nutritional support through total parenteral nutrition, initiation of high-dose steroid or immunosuppressive therapy, and surgery. It is conceivable that critical care intervention would be needed in the management of such crises as perforation or toxic megacolon, especially in older patients, but these would not be a standard part of disease management.

### Home Care Management

The patient with inflammatory bowel disease has a chronic lifelong condition that will be primarily managed in the home with family support. Two particular situations may necessitate the involvement of home care supports. Patients may need short- or long-term home administration of TPN for nutrition support (see p. 1364). The monitoring of this therapy will involve home health nurses. In addition, patients who undergo ileostomy procedures will be referred to community enterostomal therapy services for ongoing teaching and follow-up. The patient will need to know where ostomy supplies can be purchased in the local community and is encouraged to contact a local ostomy support group for peer assistance.

## COMPLICATIONS

The primary complications of inflammatory bowel disease are hemorrhage, obstruction, perforation, toxic megacolon, and cellular dysplasia that can lead to cancer. The management of the first three is similar to that discussed elsewhere in this chapter. Toxic megacolon involves an extreme dilation of a segment of the diseased colon (frequently the transverse colon) that typically results in complete obstruction. The patient is at risk for toxic megacolon during acute exacerbations. The problem may develop after bowel preparation for a barium enema or other diagnostic test or from the negative effects of narcotics and anticholinergic drugs on peristalsis. Bacteria rapidly invade the inflamed tissue, creating the acute state. The condition may respond to conservative management or require surgical correction.

The development of cellular dysplasia and eventually carcinoma from the chronic irritation of ulcerative colitis has been a concern for many years. Patients who have had the disease for 7 to 10 or more years need routine surveillance inasmuch as dysplasia develops frequently. The risk of cancer increases exponentially after 10 years and is estimated to be 30 times that of the average 40- to 60-year-old person.[35] The risk of cancer is also greater with widespread than with localized disease. Colectomy eliminates the risk and may be recommended even when medical management is satisfactorily controlling the disease. Generally, patients who developed ulcerative colitis at a young age and who experience ongoing inflammation are at greatest risk. Dysplasia is estimated to be present in 50% to 80% of patients before the development of the cancer.[35] Sigmoidoscopy and colonoscopy are the primary tools for detecting dysplasia. Colonoscopy allows for improved visualization and greater accuracy of diagnosis. In general it is recommended that colectomy be performed if mass lesions or high-grade dysplasia is found; conservative management consists of repeat colonoscopy at 3-month intervals or less.

It was formerly believed that patients with Crohn's disease did not have an increased risk of cancer. This premise is no longer accepted, and research indicates a cancer incidence six times that of normal populations. The risk increases with the duration of the IBD disease process, and dysplasia usually appears at sites of severe disease involvement or at sites of stricture formation. Standards for the early detection of cancer in patients with Crohn's disease are still under study,[35] and recommendations for routine cancer surveillance do not currently exist.

## THE PATIENT UNDERGOING OSTOMY SURGERY

An ostomy may be created as a temporary or permanent approach to the management of a wide variety of bowel problems. Ostomies can be created from the ileum or at various sites within the large bowel (see Figures 41-6 and 41-10). Loop colostomies are generally temporary and allow for easy closure at a future point. Although each type of ostomy presents its own unique management problems, all ostomies challenge patients to maintain skin integrity and achieve effective self-care.

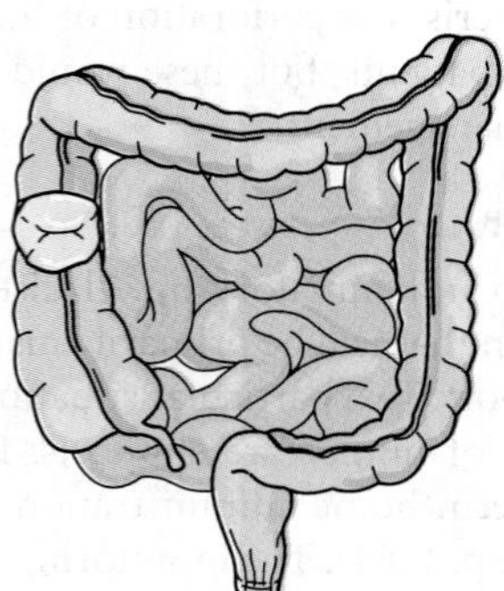

The **ascending colostomy** is done for right-sided tumors.

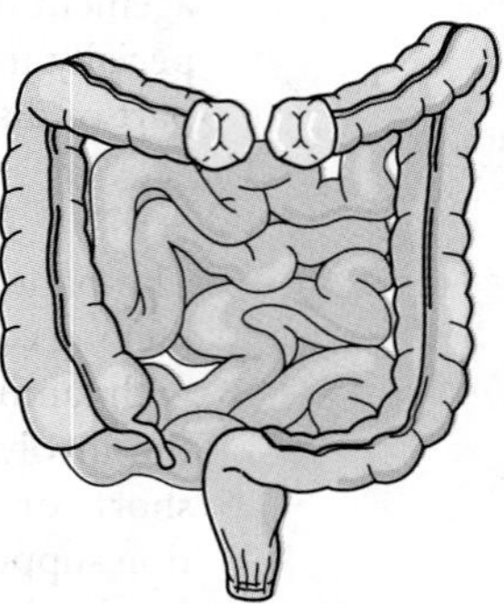

The **transverse (double-barreled) colostomy** is often used in such emergencies as intestinal obstruction or perforation because it can be created quickly. There are two stomas. The proximal one, closest to the small intestine, drains feces. The distal stoma drains mucus. Usually temporary.

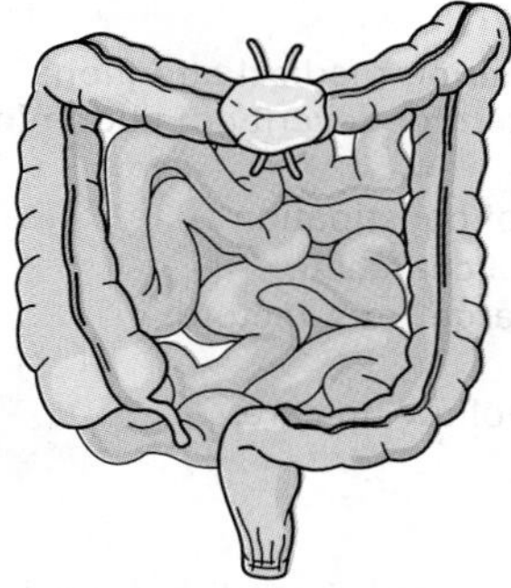

The **transverse loop colostomy** has two openings in the transverse colon, but one stoma. Usually temporary.

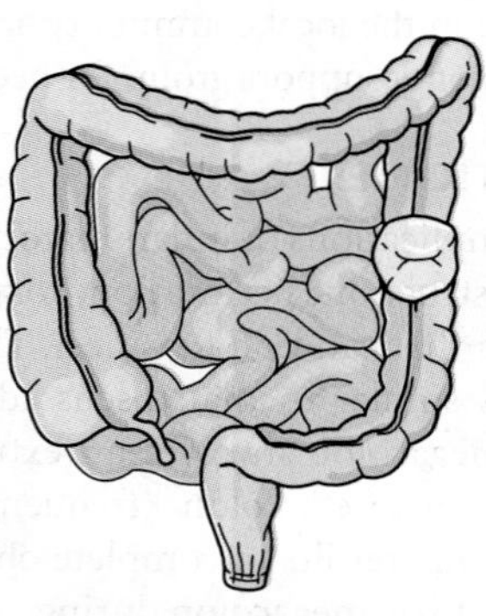

**Descending colostomy**

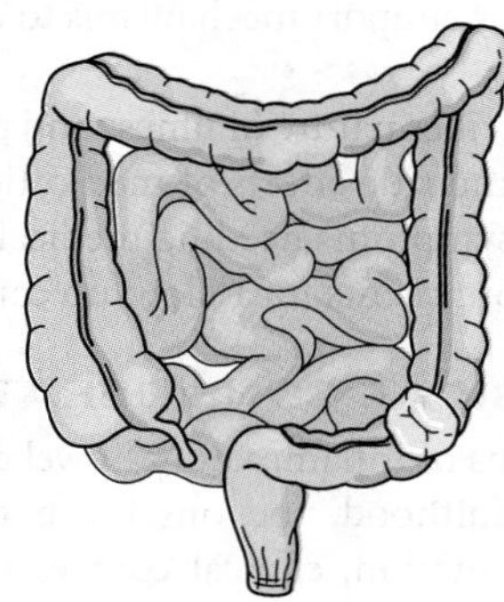

**Sigmoid colostomy**

**fig. 41-10** Types of colostomies.

## PREOPERATIVE CARE

Preoperative care focuses on patient teaching. The nurse assesses the patient's knowledge and understanding of the proposed surgery and its outcomes. This includes a brief overview of GI tract structure and function and the nature and functioning of the ostomy. Written materials are also provided that outline the components of the postoperative teaching plan. The enterostomal therapy nurse should be introduced at this time as it is essential for this advanced practice nurse to be involved in site selection and marking. Many common stoma complications can be avoided by appropriate site selection where the shape and contour of the skinfolds of the patient's abdomen in both a sitting and upright position are considered. The site should be visible to the patient when sitting or standing, lie within the rectus muscle, and be away from scars, bony prominences, and skinfolds. The patient's belt line also should be avoided. The stoma site frequently is the most significant factor influencing the patient's ability to maintain a good pouch seal and manage the ostomy independently after surgery.

Emotional preparation for ostomy surgery is extremely important. The nurse encourages the patient to verbalize feelings related to this radical change in body image and function. Validating the appropriateness of these concerns lays the foundation for an effective working relationship with the patient. The patient may need to progress through the grieving process, and if the person is in the shock state, specific factual teaching may be ineffective. The nurse offers acceptance of all feelings and reinforces the importance of open communication.

The preparation phase may include nutritional support and possibly TPN, if the patient's nutritional state is inadequate for surgery. The patient should know what to expect in the postoperative period. The nurse discusses the management of postoperative pain, the nature and appearance of all incisions and drains, and the purpose of the nasogastric (NG) tube and IV lines. Bowel cleansing also is performed and may include the use of enemas, laxatives, and antibiotics to reduce intestinal bacterial flora.

## POSTOPERATIVE CARE

The nurse provides general postoperative care. Nasogastric suction is usually maintained for 4 to 5 days after surgery, and the patient is given nothing by mouth to prevent distention or pressure on the suture lines.

### Maintaining Fluid and Electrolyte Balance

Attention to fluid and electrolyte balance is crucial for the person with an ileostomy. After surgery the fecal drainage from the ileostomy is liquid and may be constant. The patient will have fecal outputs ranging from 1000 to 1500 ml every 24 hours. This amount should begin to decrease slightly within 10 to 15 days as the terminal ileum begins to absorb more water, and the stool becomes thicker. The losses still are significant, however, and careful intake and output records are essential. The ileostomy patient becomes dehydrated easily. The stool may not thicken if the patient has had previous small bowel resections for Crohn's disease. The more intestine that has been resected, the greater the chance for a high-volume output of liquid stool. Some patients require medication to help decrease the output and control the loss of fluid.

The pouch may need to be emptied every 1 to 2 hours. Volumes in excess of 1500 ml per 24 hours are considered excessive. Fluid and electrolyte problems are usually not a major concern after colostomy surgery although it may take awhile to reestablish a normal pattern of elimination.

### Stoma Monitoring

The patient who has undergone ostomy surgery typically returns from surgery with an ostomy pouch system in place. The nurse observes the stoma regularly for redness and edema. Color reflects perfusion, and a dark, dusky, or brown-black stoma indicates ischemia and necrosis. Color changes should be reported immediately. Initial stoma edema is an expected response to surgical manipulation. The shape of the stoma will continue to change slightly throughout the day in response to peristalsis, and the pouch opening will need to be adjusted to accommodate the changing stoma size. Edema typically resolves in 5 to 7 days. A small amount of bleeding from the stoma is expected, but any significant bleeding should be reported to the surgeon immediately.

The abdominal incision and sutures anchoring the stoma are inspected for intactness. Some of the stoma mucosa may pull away from the abdominal skin before healing is complete. Superficial separations heal by granulation, but deeper separations may require packing or resuturing.

The stoma drainage consists initially of mucus and serosanguineous secretion. As peristalsis returns, flatus and fecal drainage begin, usually in 2 to 4 days. The pouch should be emptied when it is one-third to one-half full of stool or more frequently if excess gas is present.

A loop colostomy may be opened during surgery or in the patient's room 48 to 72 hours later. A cautery is used to open the bowel, which creates two openings, one proximal and one distal, in the one stoma (Figure 41-10). The nurse reassures the patient that the procedure causes no pain because the bowel has no sensory nerve endings for pain sensation. The procedure creates a distinct burning smell, however, and can be quite frightening. The nurse offers support and reassurance during the loop opening. The supporting rod for the loop is removed after 7 to 10 days when adhesions prevent the stoma from retracting into the incision.

### Managing the Perineal Wound

The abdominal perineal resection has been the gold standard for the treatment of rectal cancer for many years and is still the treatment of choice for managing highly invasive disease. Postoperative care is more complex because of the presence of a major perineal wound that may require up to 6 months to completely heal. The patient's convalescence is prolonged.

The perineal wound is created by the removal of the entire rectum and anus plus muscle and fatty tissue. The wound may be left open and loosely filled with packing. The large gap that is created gradually fills with granulation tissue. Wound irrigations and absorbent dressings are used until the wound closes. The perineal wound may instead be sutured closed with stab wounds formed for drainage and irrigation. The remaining pelvic organs shift slightly to fill the remaining space.

The perineal wound makes it difficult for the patient to sit or find a comfortable position. Foam pads or soft pillows may increase comfort while the patient is sitting. The nurse instructs the patient to avoid the use of air or rubber rings that separate the buttocks and stress the healing wound. The side-lying position usually is preferred. Phantom rectal sensations and itching may occur after healing. The origin of these sensations is unknown. Wound drainage initially is copious and serosanguineous and must be effectively removed to prevent infection and abscess formation. The drainage tubes may work passively by gravity or be attached to a suction apparatus. Wound irrigations, usually with normal saline, are initially performed by catheter, but the patient gradually may progress to a hand-held shower massage or Water Pik. The dressings are changed as needed. A T binder may be useful in holding the dressings in place in the perineum. Sitz baths may be substituted for irrigations once the patient is ambulatory, but a free flow of water on the perineal wound is preferred.

## Teaching for Self-Care

It is essential that the patient acquire basic ostomy self-care skills during the postoperative period. Successful self-care provides the foundation for both independence and a reintegration of body image that includes the ostomy. The nurse teaches the patient the principles of ostomy care, but also provides the patient with the opportunity to handle, assemble, and use all equipment. Time for practice is imperative. The process rarely can be completed during the hospitalization, particularly with elderly persons, and the nurse initiates referral to appropriate home health care and community ostomy services. Involvement of a family member or supportive friend can be helpful if acceptable to the patient.

### Stoma care

An ostomy pouch is placed over the new stoma at the conclusion of the surgery. Teaching begins with the first pouch change. The patient may or may not be ready to view the stoma, but the nurse gently encourages the patient to look at and touch it. The nurse briefly and factually explains each step of the procedure. The nurse reminds the patient that the stoma has no touch sensation, but the rest of the abdomen will still be tender and sore from the surgery. Surgical pain should be thoroughly controlled before any teaching session.

A systematic plan should be in place to guide teaching the colostomy regimen. Teaching sessions should be spaced throughout the hospitalization to allow for repetition and assimilation. Pouches are changed more frequently than needed

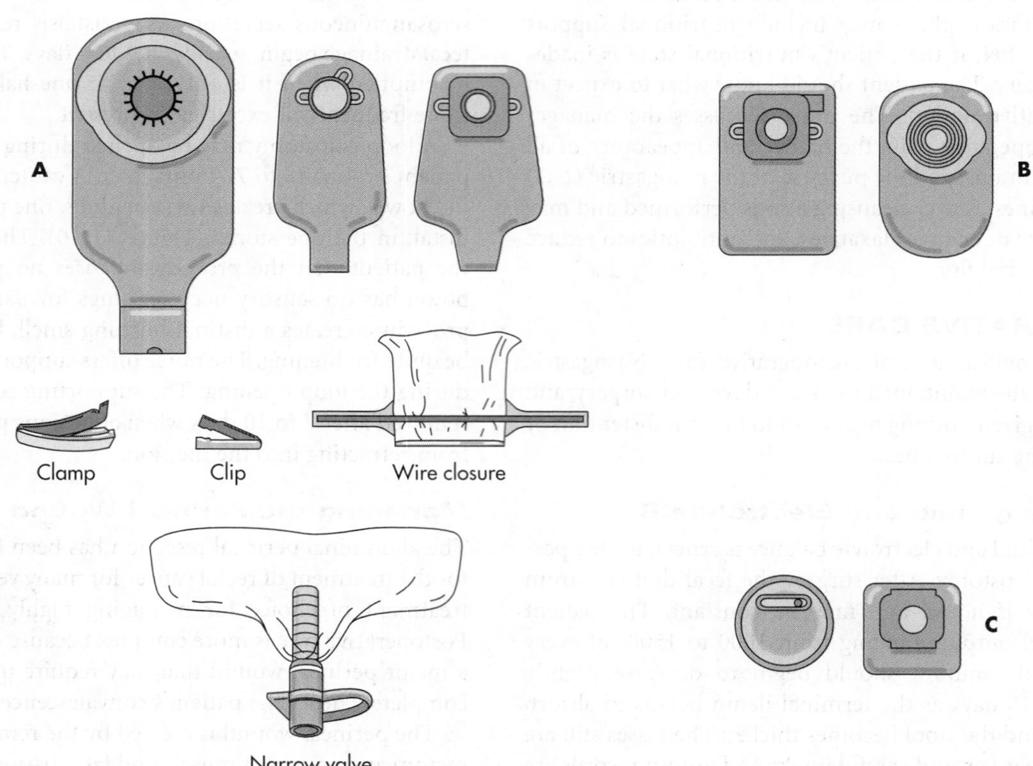


**fig. 41-11** Common ostomy pouch products, closures, and patches. **A,** Drainable pouches and pouch closures. **B,** Nondrainable pouches. **C,** Patches for regulated colostomies.

to allow for adequate practice time. Written instructions and resource materials are invaluable supplements to instruction by the nurse.

**Pouch selection.** An effective pouch system protects the skin, contains stool and odor, molds to the body's contours, allows for movement, and is inconspicuous under clothing. It is the most important aspect of ostomy management. Choices are based on ostomy type, size and contour of the abdomen, peristomal skin condition, financial considerations, and personal preferences.

Products for ostomy care are available in a variety of styles, shapes, and sizes. Disposable pouches are available in one- and two-piece systems, with skin barriers attached, and in a variety of materials (Figure 41-11). Reusable pouches are worn, cleaned, and worn again. Drainable pouches are easier to keep clean and are more economical than closed nondrainable pouches. They are available in one- and two-piece systems and in a variety of materials. Drainable colostomy pouches are changed every 3 to 7 days if there are no problems with leakage. The usual wearing time for an ileostomy pouch is 5 to 7 days with the pouch emptied every 4 to 6 hours.

A properly applied pouch system is odor-free except during changes. Persistent odor is usually the result of inadequate cleansing of the drainage spout or a poor pouch seal. Pin holes in a pouch destroy its odor-proof quality and should not be used to release gas. The drainage from an ileostomy is not strongly foul-smelling. A foul odor may indicate a problem such as infection or obstruction.

It is essential that the patient learn to properly measure the stoma to ensure a proper pouch fit. The pouch should closely surround the stoma but not press or rub against it. The stoma may shrink dramatically during the first week after surgery, and it will continue to change in size slightly throughout the first year. It is important for the patient to measure the stoma accurately during each pouch change in the first weeks after surgery. Cutouts of various diameters are included in the box of pouches. The skin barriers are cut approximately ⅛ inch larger than the stoma to accommodate stoma swelling. Later in the first year the stoma size is rechecked occasionally to ensure optimum fit. The pouch change procedure is outlined in more detail in the Guidelines for Care Box.

The nurse teaches the patient to change the pouch immediately if leakage occurs, and to establish a routine in which pouches are being changed before stool leakage occurs. The nurse instructs the patient to empty the pouch when it is one-third to one-half full. The pouch is changed during inactive times and before meals to minimize the chance of the intestine emptying during the change. The nurse instructs the patient to use each pouch change as an opportunity to carefully assess the stoma and peristomal skin.

The nurse ensures that the patient has adequate temporary supplies before discharge, a complete list of supplies that will be needed for home management, and information about where supplies can be obtained in the local community. A prescription may be needed for Medicare or insurance reimbursement.

**Skin care.** The drainage from an ileostomy is both continuous and erosive, and it is essential that the pouch be secure and properly fitted. Ileostomy drainage contains residual digestive enzymes that will quickly break down the peristomal skin if they are allowed to make contact with it. The use of a skin barrier with the pouch is an important means of protecting the peristomal skin (Figure 41-12).

Skin care is also important with colostomies. In addition to irritation from stool, the skin also can be damaged by an allergic reaction to the tape or skin barrier product, rough or frequent removal of pouch adhesives, or infection. The skin around the stoma should appear as healthy and normal as the remainder of the skin on the abdomen. Prevention of skin problems is always easier and less expensive than treatment. The most common peristomal skin infection is caused by *Candida albicans.* The skin becomes bright red with papular lesions. Dryness and scaling develop if the condition persists. The infection is treated with nystatin (Mycostatin) powder.

The use of a skin barrier is an important means of protecting the peristomal skin. Skin barriers come in several basic forms: powder, paste, washer, or wafer (Figure 41-12). Skin

**guidelines for care**

### Changing an Ostomy Pouch

**Stoma Measurement**

Use the measuring guide and sample diameters, and cut the ostomy appliance to fit—pattern should be ⅛ to ¼ inch larger than the stoma.

Use the same procedure to prepare the skin barrier. NOTE: The pouch opening is cut slightly larger than the skin barrier to prevent the paper from cutting the stoma.

**Removing Old Pouch**

Empty drainable pouch to prevent spills.

Disconnect pouch from skin wafer if two-piece system is used.

Gently peel the wafer away from the skin beginning at the top.

**Skin Care**

Cleanse the skin with warm water and dry thoroughly; use soap only if stool adheres to skin. Rinse thoroughly with water.

Assess peristomal skin and stoma carefully for signs of irritation or infection.

Pat peristomal skin dry thoroughly.

**Applying New Pouch**

Center the pouch opening over the stoma. Ask patient to tense abdominal muscles to make application easier.

Gently press into place and hold for at least 30 seconds to seal.

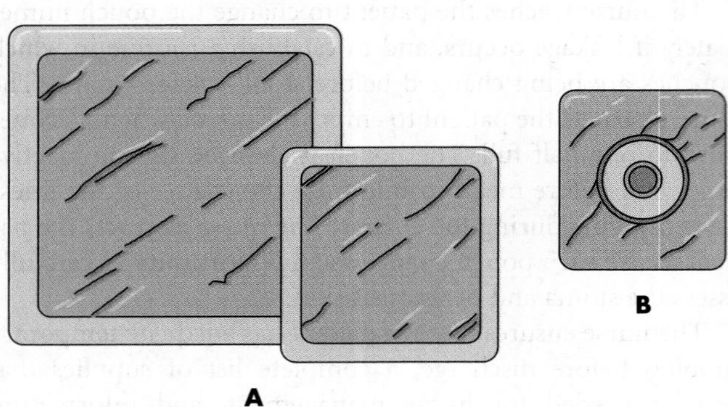


**fig. 41-12** Skin barrier products. **A,** Skin barriers. **B,** Wafer.

*guidelines for care*

**Ostomy Skin Care**

- When a pouch seal leaks, the pouch should be immediately changed, not taped. Stool held against the skin can quickly result in severe irritation.
- Pouches are removed gently, with one hand holding the skin in place to decrease pulling.
- The skin should be gently but thoroughly cleansed, rinsed, and patted dry.
- Peristomal hair should be trimmed but not shaved to prevent folliculitis.
- A skin barrier should be used to protect the peristomal skin from liquid stool.
- A skin sealant should be used under all tape.
- The patient should consult with an enterostomal therapist for specific care guidelines if skin problems occur.

barriers include products such as Karaya, Stomahesive (Convatec), Hollihesive (Hollister), ReliaSeal (Bard), Skin Barrier (Coloplast), and Mason Colly-Seal Disc. Skin barriers attached to the pouches are available as one- or two-piece systems, as well as single-use items that can be used with any pouch.

**Powder.** A pouch will not adhere to powder, cream, or ointment. If powder is applied to the skin, it must be sealed before applying the pouch. Karaya powder releases an acid that may sting irritated skin, but Stomadhesive powder works well.

**Paste.** Paste is available for use around the stoma, to fill in creases or folds, and to supplement skin barriers for a longer seal. The use of paste has made it easier to keep a pouch seal intact in poor locations.

**Skin barrier wafers.** These may be used with a variety of pouches and protect the skin from stool. The opening in the wafer is carefully measured so that it fits at the base of the stoma without rubbing into or onto the stoma.

**Skin sealants.** These come in sprays, liquids, gels, and wipes. These products seal in powders and coat the skin with a clear film; they are useful under pouch adhesives. When tape is removed from the skin the stratum corneum layer of the skin is also pulled off. If a skin sealant is used under the tape, the removal of the tape pulls off the skin sealant but leaves the skin intact.

Guidelines for skin care are summarized in the Guidelines for Care Box. If the peristomal skin becomes irritated, barrier powder may be applied to help dry moist irritation. The addition of barrier powder or a wafer to the usual pouching system allows for rapid healing. An enterostomal therapist should be consulted for the management of severe skin problems. The use of antacids or products that contain alcohol should be avoided inasmuch as they dry the skin and alter the pH, leaving it vulnerable to infection.

**Managing odor.** Ostomy pouches are made of odor-proof plastic, but a leaking seal or improperly cleaned pouch can emit an unpleasant ordor. The inside of the pouch should be rinsed with tepid water after emptying and the pouch outlet wiped with toilet paper. If the patient desires, deodorizing solutions and tablets may be placed in the pouch.

The nurse encourages the patient to eat a balanced diet and to chew foods slowly and thoroughly. No special diet is required; however, patients need to be informed about foods that increase gas and odor. Dairy products, highly seasoned foods, fish, and a variety of vegetables are known to increase the odor of the stool. Individual responses to gas-producing foods tend to be variable, with known exceptions such as beans, cabbage, and Brussels sprouts. The patient will need to experiment with diet modifications that reflect individual food tolerances. Closed pouches usually have a charcoal filter at the top that releases and deodorizes gas. Pouches should be opened to release accumulated gas but never pricked. A puncture in the pouch would create a constant odor problem.

### *Ostomy irrigation*

An ostomy irrigation is an enema given through the stoma to stimulate bowel emptying at a regular and convenient time. The procedure is no longer routinely recommended and is used only with sigmoid colostomies that expel formed stool. Irrigation is never a part of the routine management of an ileostomy because the drainage is continuous and semiliquid in nature. A patient who uses irrigations successfully may be able to dispense with a standard pouch and wear a stoma cap—a small adhesive pouch with an absorbent dressing. Because the ostomy continues to secrete mucus and release flatus, a gas filter is desirable.

If irrigations are planned, they are initiated about 5 to 7 days after surgery. The procedure is described in the following Guidelines for Care Box, and common equipment is illustrated in Figure 41-13. A variety of equipment is commercially available, and most sets include irrigating sleeves, a cone tip for insertion into the stoma, a bag to hold the solution, and clips to close the sleeve. The procedure is ideally taught in the bathroom. Cramping during an irrigation may be caused by instilling the water too rapidly or solutions that are too cold or too hot. The flow should be halted until cramping subsides.

### *Preventing ileostomy complications*

Excess loss of fluids can be a serious concern after ileostomy surgery, and the nurse instructs the patient that diarrhea accom-

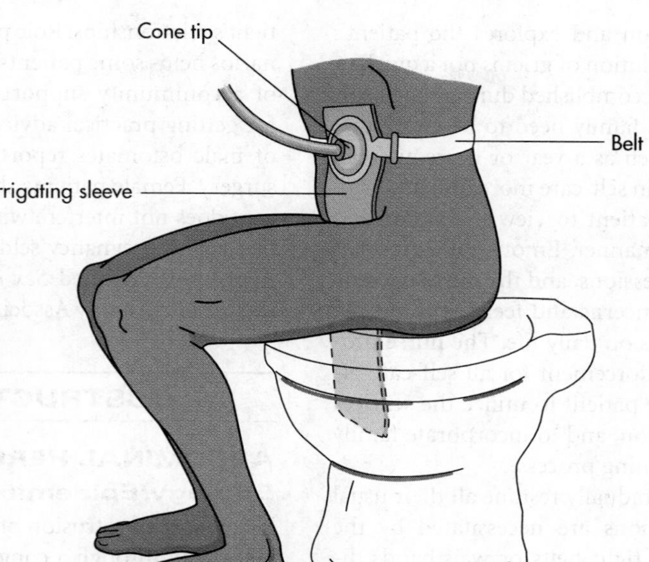


**fig. 41-13** Colostomy irrigation with person sitting on the toilet; irrigating sleeve drains into the toilet.

## guidelines for care

### Colostomy Irrigation

Assemble all equipment:
- Water container, irrigating sleeve, and belt
- Skin care items
- New pouch system, ready for use

Remove old pouch and dispose.
Clean the stoma and peristomal skin with water and assess.
Apply the irrigating sleeve and belt.
- Place open end of sleeve in toilet.

Fill irrigating container with 500 to 1000 ml of lukewarm tap water, and suspend container at shoulder height.
Run water through the tubing to remove air.
Gently insert the irrigating cone into stoma, and slowly start the flow of water. Catheters are inserted no more than 2 to 4 inches. Do not force. If cramping occurs, stop the irrigation and wait.
Allow approximately 15 to 20 minutes for stool to empty.
Rinse sleeve, dry the bottom, roll it up, and close off the end. Patient should go about regular activities for 30 to 45 minutes.
Remove sleeve, clean stoma, and apply new pouch.
Clean and store the irrigating equipment.

panied by nausea and vomiting can rapidly progress to dehydration. The nurse provides the patient with a list of signs of dehydration and electrolyte imbalance. Losses of sodium and potassium are of particular concern. The patient needs to know how to safely replace lost fluids and when to seek medical attention. Persons with ileostomies also may become dehydrated if they are given laxatives as preparations for diagnostic procedures.

Enteric-coated, time-released medications, or hard tablets may not be absorbed in a patient with an ileostomy and should not be used. Liquid or chewable forms of medications are preferred. Because the remaining ileum develops a bacterial flora, antibiotic therapy can cause diarrhea. Supplementation of vitamins A, D, E, and K is a standard measure inasmuch as colon absorption and synthesis are eliminated.

Ileostomy patients should be aware of the potential for obstruction. Obstruction usually is caused by a large mass of undigested food that becomes lodged at a narrow point in the bowel and blocks the intestinal lumen. After ileostomy surgery some persons discover that they can eat foods such as coconut, corn, or celery only in limited amounts.

If the ileostomy becomes obstructed, the person should get into a knee-chest position and gently massage the area below the stoma. Stomal edema will develop with a food blockage. The pouch should be changed and the opening enlarged to accommodate the swelling. Diarrhea usually follows the passage of the obstruction, and fluids must be replaced. Abdominal pain in the peristomal area generally is present for 3 to 5 days after the obstruction is relieved. If the obstruction is not relieved within a few hours, the physician should be notified. It may become necessary to gently irrigate the stoma with 30 to 50 ml of normal saline through a 14 or 16 F catheter with a bulb syringe. The procedure is repeated until the obstruction is relieved.

### Supporting a Positive Self-Concept

The formation of a stoma frequently is viewed as mutilating, and most patients need time and the support of others to work through their feelings. Removal of any part of the body involves a sense of loss and grief. The nurse encourages the patient to express these feelings of loss and makes no attempt to suppress them or minimize their validity. The nurse acknowledges the work involved in grief resolution and explores the patient's usual coping strategies. The resolution of grief is not a quick or easy process, and it will not be accomplished during the hospitalization. Both the patient and family need to be aware that grief resolution can take as much as a year or more and can make a return to independence in self-care more difficult.

The nurse encourages the patient to view the stoma and care for it in a matter-of-fact manner. Emotional support is incorporated into all self-care sessions, and the nurse encourages the patient to verbalize concerns and feelings about the stoma and its anticipated effects on daily life. The nurse provides positive support and reinforcement for all self-care efforts. The nurse encourages the patient to utilize the services of the United Ostomy Association, and to incorporate family members into the teaching-learning process.

Patients are encouraged to gradually resume all their usual activities. No clothing restrictions are necessitated by the stoma except the avoidance of tight belts or waistbands directly over it. Pouches hold well in baths and showers, and normal hygiene patterns may be resumed as soon as the incision is healed. There are no specific restrictions on exercise or recreational activities.

The nurse reminds the patient always to carry ostomy supplies when traveling and not to place them in checked luggage. The quality of water is of particular concern inasmuch as traveler's diarrhea could create serious problems.

### Preventing Sexual Dysfunction

Many patients will not directly verbalize their concerns about sexuality after ostomy surgery; thus it is usually necessary for the nurse to address the topic directly. The nurse provides the patient with specific suggestions for dealing with sexual concerns such as:

- Exploring positions for sexual activity that minimize stress and pressure on the pouch
- Emptying and cleaning the pouch before sexual activity
- Using a smaller-sized pouch or a pouch cover during sexual activity
- Use of a binder or special underwear to hold the pouch secure

The nurse encourages the patient to discuss sexual concerns with his or her partner. Silence and emotional distancing are common reactions, but they can be very destructive to the patient's relationships. Role playing or visualizing worst-case scenarios helps some patients to acknowledge their fears. The use of a community support group can be particularly helpful for getting practical advice about sexual matters. About 15% of male ostomates report a decrease in sexual activity after surgery. Female patients should be reassured that ostomy surgery does not interfere with contraception, pregnancy, or delivery; and pregnancy seldom produces stoma complications. A pamphlet entitled *Sex and the Ostomate* is available from the United Ostomy Association.*

## OBSTRUCTIVE DISORDERS

### ABDOMINAL HERNIAS

#### Etiology/Epidemiology

A *hernia* is a protrusion of an organ or structure from its normal cavity through a congenital or acquired defect, usually in the muscle of the abdominal wall. Depending on its location, the hernia may contain peritoneum, omentum, a loop of bowel, or a section of bladder. Inguinal and umbilical hernias usually result from congenital weakness of the muscle, whereas incisional hernias are usually a complication of surgery. Hernias can occur at any age and are more common in men and elders.

Hernias of the groin account for approximately 80% of all hernias and are the result of primary muscular defects. *Indirect hernias* represent more than 50% of all hernias and are much more common in men than in women. The higher incidence is probably explained by the need for the testes to pass through the inguinal ring during fetal development. Indirect inguinal hernias develop from weakness of the abdominal wall at the point where the spermatic cord emerges. A parallel weakness is found in the female from the emergence of the round ligament. Figure 41-14 illustrates the indirect inguinal hernia. The protruded bowel may rest in the inguinal canal or move down into the scrotum in men and, on rare occasions, into the labia in women.

*Direct inguinal hernias* pass through the posterior inguinal wall at a point of muscle weakness. They typically are caused by increased intraabdominal pressure. These hernias occur

*United Ostomy Association, 36 Executive Park Suite 120, Irvine, CA 92714; (800) 826-0826.

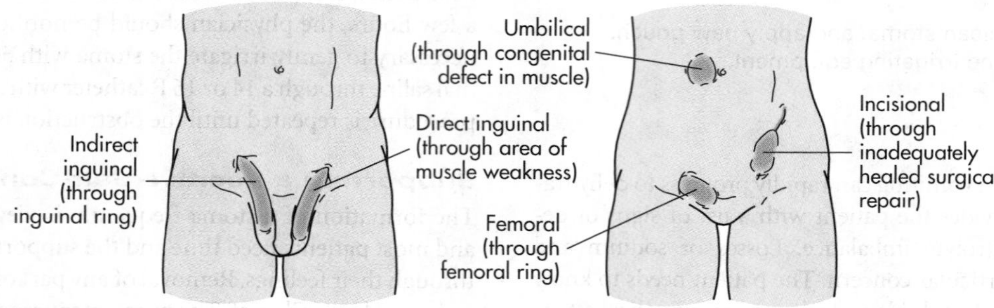


**fig. 41-14** Common sites of abdominal herniation.

most often in elderly men. They are the most technically difficult to repair and frequently recur after surgery.

*Femoral hernias* develop when a loop of intestine passes through the femoral ring and down the femoral canal. They appear as a round bulge below the inguinal ligament and are thought to be caused by changes related to pregnancy. Femoral hernias are rare in men.

Several other terms are used to describe abdominal hernias and reflect the severity of the problem. A *sliding hernia* moves freely in and out of the hernia sac. If the protruding structure requires manipulation to return it to its proper position, the hernia is termed *reducible.* If the protruding structure cannot be returned to its proper position, the hernia is called *irreducible.* The term *incarcerated* usually is reserved for an irreducible hernia in which bowel obstruction occurs. The size of the defect largely determines whether the hernia can be reduced. When the blood flow to the trapped segment is compromised by pressure from the surrounding muscle ring, the hernia is said to be *strangulated.* Intestinal obstruction occurs, and gangrene of the viscera can develop rapidly.

### Pathophysiology

The major pathological concern associated with hernias is the risk of strangulation and bowel obstruction. Once present, hernias tend to extend and the risk of major complications increases.

The person with a hernia typically has a lump in the groin, around the umbilicus, or protruding from an old surgical incision. The lump or swelling may always have been present, or it may have appeared suddenly after coughing, straining, lifting, or other vigorous exertion. Hernias frequently cause no other symptoms. The protrusion usually disappears when the person lies down, and reappears with standing, coughing, or lifting.

The person may perceive a vague discomfort as the hernia contents slide in and out of the abdominal defect, but little actual pain is experienced as long as the hernia is freely reducible. A "dragging" sensation or feeling of heaviness is common, especially with groin hernias. An irreducible hernia may become strangulated, causing severe pain and symptoms of intestinal obstruction such as nausea, vomiting, and distention. These complications require emergency surgery, and a portion of bowel may have to be resected.

### Collaborative Care Management

A diagnosis of hernia is readily established by reviewing the patient's history and results of the physical examination. Palpation of the herniated area reveals the contents of the sac as soft and nodular (omentum) or smooth and fluctuant (bowel). Fingertip palpation is used to feel the edges of the hernial ring and its contents by inserting the examining fingertip into the ring and feeling for the impulse as the person coughs.

Hernias should always be repaired by elective surgery if at all possible. Strangulation is an ever-present risk, and if it should occur, the surgical repair would need to be performed on an emergency basis. Attempts are generally not made to reduce strangulated hernias because of the high risk of rupture. The emergency surgery is accompanied by a high incidence of postoperative complications. The herniated tissues are returned to the abdominal cavity, and the defect in the fascia or muscle is closed with sutures *(herniorrhaphy).* To prevent recurrence of the hernia and to facilitate closure of the defect, a *hernioplasty* may be performed. This procedure uses fascia or a variety of synthetic materials to strengthen the muscle wall. Hernia surgery often is performed in ambulatory surgical centers with the patient under local or spinal anesthesia.

The patient is discharged directly home after the repair. Hernia repair may be performed by either open or laparoscopic methods. The results appear to be quite similar although laparoscopic surgery causes less pain and allows a more rapid return to normal activities. However, laparoscopic surgery is also significantly more expensive and necessitates the use of general anesthesia.[9] These factors have significantly limited the use of this technique for hernia repair.

Recovery from hernia repair usually is rapid and without incident. Standard postoperative interventions are used, but the nurse encourages the patient to deep breathe rather than cough. Fluid and food are resumed as tolerated. Ice bags are applied after inguinal hernia repair to minimize edema, particularly in the scrotum. A scrotal support or "jockey" style underwear may make initial ambulation easier and less painful. Fluids are encouraged, and IV infusions are continued until the patient is able to successfully empty the bladder.

#### *Patient/family education*

Discharge teaching includes the avoidance of any heavy lifting, pushing, or pulling for about 6 weeks. Driving and stair climbing initially are restricted. The nurse instructs the patient to monitor the incision for signs of infection. Postoperative ecchymosis should disappear in a few days. Stool softeners or bulk laxatives are prescribed to prevent straining at defecation. The nurse also reassures the patient that sexual functioning is not affected by the surgery and may be resumed once healing is complete.

## BOWEL OBSTRUCTION

### Etiology/Epidemiology

Normal functioning of the small and large intestines depends on an open lumen for the movement of intestinal contents as well as adequate circulation and nervous innervation to sustain rhythmic peristalsis. Any factor or condition that either narrows the intestinal passageway or interferes with peristalsis can result in bowel obstruction. Bowel obstruction occurs in both genders, all races, and at any point in the life span. It is the cause of about 20% of all cases of acute abdominal pain. Because bowel obstruction usually is a secondary effect of a primary problem, incidence statistics are unreliable. The close relationship of large bowel obstruction to cancer of the colon, and small bowel obstruction to abdominal surgery and adhesions creates a few clear patterns. Obstruction is more common in elderly persons, who are more vulnerable to colon cancer. The occurrence of volvulus obstruction also has been tied to chronic constipation in elders. Bowel obstructions commonly are classified as either mechanical (affecting the intestinal lumen) or nonmechanical (related to peristalsis) and can be either partial or complete.

### Causes of mechanical obstruction

**Adhesions.** Adhesions may form after abdominal surgery for unknown reasons, perhaps related to inflammatory responses in the healing bowel. Adhesions are the most common cause of small bowel obstruction, accounting for more than 70% of all cases.[25] In some persons the adhesions may become massive. The fibrous bands of scar tissue can loop over bowel segments, either causing the bowel to kink or compressing the loop (Figure 41-15).[25]

**Hernias.** A hernia can result in bowel obstruction if the abdominal wall defect through which the hernia protrudes becomes so tight that the bowel segment becomes strangulated. (See p. 1342 for a discussion of abdominal hernias.)

**Tumor.** A tumor mass will gradually restrict the internal lumen of the bowel as it enlarges. Eventually a fecal mass may be unable to pass through the constriction, leading to partial or complete obstruction. Bowel cancer accounts for approximately 60% of obstructions of the large intestine, with most occurring in the sigmoid colon.[25] (See p. 1347 for a discussion of bowel cancer.)

**Volvulus.** A twisting of the bowel upon itself, usually at least a full 180°, obstructing the intestinal lumen both proximally and distally, is called a *volvulus* (Figure 41-16). The acute obstruction can quickly result in bowel infarction and can be life-threatening as a result of necrosis, perforation, and peritonitis.

**Intussusception.** Intussusception involves a telescoping of the bowel on itself (Figure 41-16). The invagination occurs with peristalsis and in the adult often is triggered by the presence of a tumor mass. The bowel segment containing the mass is propelled by peristalsis into the adjacent bowel segment. Constriction is immediate, and strangulation of the trapped segment can develop.

Other possible causes of mechanical obstruction include fecal impaction, gallstones, and strictures resulting from diverticulitis and IBD.

### Causes of nonmechanical obstruction

**Paralytic ileus.** Adynamic or *paralytic ileus* results from a lack of peristaltic activity, usually as a result of neurogenic impairment. Ileus is a common temporary problem after abdominal surgery, particularly if the bowel has been extensively handled. If the absence of peristalsis persists for longer than 72 hours, the diagnosis of paralytic ileus is made.[25] In addition to direct irritation, paralytic ileus also can occur as a response to major trauma, sepsis, and electrolyte imbalances (particularly hypokalemia).

**Other.** A variety of other disorders can create a form of nonmechanical obstruction from failure to propel the intestinal contents. These are frequently chronic problems for the patient. Most cases result from a failure of nervous innervation such as multiple sclerosis, Parkinson's disease, or Hirschsprung's disease or from muscular problems that affect propulsion such as primary muscle or collagen diseases. Endocrine disorders such as diabetes mellitus are also associated with problems of GI motility. Although constipation is the more common manifestation of all of these disorders, chronic problems with bowel obstruction may also occur. Thrombosis

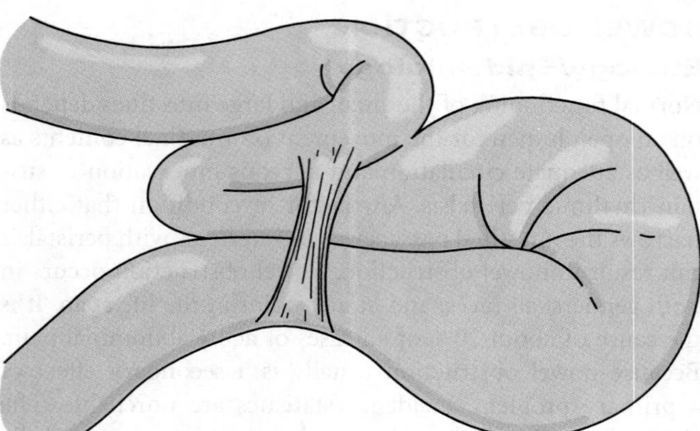

fig. 41-15 A band of adhesions causing intestinal obstruction in the small bowel.

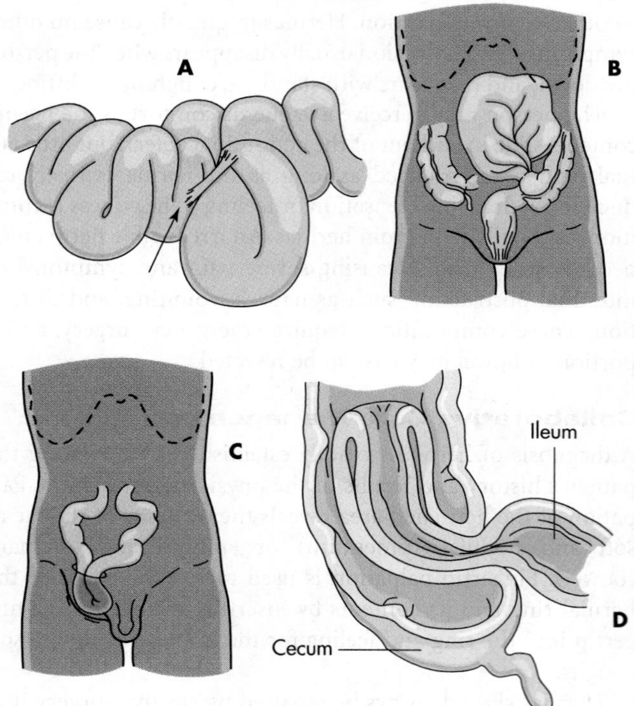


fig. 41-16 Common causes of intestinal obstruction. A, Constriction by adhesions. B, Volvulus of the sigmoid colon. C, Strangulated inguinal hernia. D, Ileocecal intussusception.

of the mesenteric arteries is a possible complication of heart disease in the elderly. It can create an abrupt ischemic episode that may necessitate surgical intervention to remove the affected bowel.

### Pathophysiology

Intestinal obstruction triggers a series of GI tract events whose clinical manifestations depend largely on the location of the obstruction and the degree of circulatory compromise. Approximately 7 to 10 L of electrolyte-rich fluid is secreted into the small intestine each day. In the normal bowel all but approximately 600 to 800 ml are reabsorbed before the chyme enters the cecum. About 200 ml is lost daily in the stool. Even when the forward movement of chyme is obstructed, GI secretion continues, at least initially.

A steadily worsening imbalance between secretion and absorption develops, and fluid and air accumulate proximal to the site of the obstruction. The mediators that trigger sustained secretion in the presence of obstruction have not been clearly identified. Progressive distention occurs with an increase in intraluminal pressure. The bowel wall becomes increasingly edematous, and venous drainage is impeded. Increased capillary permeability allows massive amounts of isotonic fluid to move from the plasma into the distended bowel, which begins to weep fluids from its surface into the peritoneum.[30]

Normal reabsorption processes in the bowel are blocked by the tissue edema and decreased mucosal blood flow. Gas accumulates in the bowel from both air swallowing and the action of intestinal bacteria on stagnant bowel contents. This worsens the abdominal distention.[30]

Vascular compromise is the most serious aspect of obstruction. Bowel ischemia breaks down the normal barrier to bacteria, and the stagnant and distended bowel becomes increasingly permeable to bacteria. Organisms can enter the peritoneal cavity and lead to peritonitis. Bacteria are normally sparse in the small bowel but accumulate rapidly during obstruction. *E. coli, Klebsiella,* and *Pseudomonas* are particularly prevalent, and the release of toxins can result in septic shock. The ischemic process can progress to gangrene and perforation. Submucosal hemorrhage and sloughing can also be a source of substantial blood loss.[30]

The loss of extracellular fluid can range from 2 to 6 L within 2 to 3 days of a mechanical bowel obstruction. The resulting hypovolemia may be mild or severe enough to compromise renal perfusion and induce dehydration, electrolyte imbalance, and shock. The concentration of the blood can result in vascular thrombosis. Mortality as a result of acute small bowel obstruction is 10% and rises to 30% for large bowel obstruction.[25] If the bowel is strangulated, these percentages increase to 20% in the small bowel and 60% in the large bowel.[25]

The clinical manifestations of bowel obstruction vary based on the exact site of the obstruction, but abdominal pain is a fairly universal symptom. Simple obstruction produces crampy and poorly localized pain. Its onset parallels the initial increase in peristalsis that raises intraluminal pressure in an attempt to clear the obstruction. Frequent, loud, high-pitched bowel sounds are often heard on auscultation. The pain typically lessens as the obstruction worsens. Smooth muscle atony decreases peristalsis and bowel sounds are diminished. The pain associated with bowel strangulation is constant and severe.

Nausea and vomiting are also common features, especially with obstructions that occur in the small intestine. Depending on the level of the obstruction, the vomiting can be profuse. Abdominal distention usually develops slowly although obstipation is common. Rising fever usually indicates the presence of dying bowel. Laboratory values typically reflect the progressive nature of the dehydration. The range of clinical manifestations that can occur with bowel obstruction is summarized in Box 41-4.

### Collaborative Care Management

Intestinal obstruction is diagnosed primarily from its clinical manifestations. In addition, abdominal radiographs generally show clear patterns of air and fluid entrapment in the obstructed area. Obstruction cannot be ruled out, however, by the presence of apparently normal x-ray findings.

There are no laboratory tests that can confirm or rule out a diagnosis of bowel obstruction. White blood cell (WBC) counts may be elevated in the presence of strangulation but

**box 41-4 clinical manifestations**

***Bowel Obstruction***

**PAIN**

Crampy in nature
Poorly localized
Severe, continuous pain with strangulation of the bowel

**NAUSEA AND VOMITING**

Presence and severity depends on the level of the obstruction
Can be profuse with proximal small bowel obstructions
May have fecal odor if the obstruction is in the distal small bowel
Occurs late if at all in most large bowel obstructions

**OBSTIPATION**

**ABDOMINAL DISTENTION**

Usually nontender
Slow to develop, especially with large bowel obstructions

**BOWEL SOUNDS**

Frequent and high-pitched early in the obstructive process
Decreased or absent late in the obstructive process

**FEVER**

Indicates the death of bowel tissue

**LABORATORY VALUES**

Reflective of dehydration and fluid shifts
- Decreased urine output
- Hemoconcentration
- Hypokalemia and hyponatremia

otherwise are normal. Once hypovolemia becomes severe, hemoconcentration elevates hemoglobin and hematocrit values and serum potassium levels typically fall.

The treatment of bowel obstruction is directed toward correcting the fluid and electrolyte imbalances, decompressing the GI tract, and preventing infection. A decision about the need for surgical correction is generally made within 48 hours depending on the patient's initial response to traditional interventions. Decompression is accomplished with nasogastric or intestinal intubation. This procedure usually is successful in removing gas and fluid. Decompression also typically relieves any associated vomiting and prevents aspiration. In patients with partial obstruction, decompression alone may relieve the problem.[2]

Analgesics are rarely used, even in the presence of moderate to severe abdominal pain. The negative effects of analgesics on peristalsis mitigate against their use, and the pattern and severity of the pain may be important in establishing a correct diagnosis. Antibiotics may be administered to counter the effects of the significant overgrowth of bacteria in the bowel.

NG tubes appear to accomplish the same outcomes as longer tubes, but some physicians still prefer to use intestinal tubes, particularly when the obstruction is in the small bowel. Intestinal tubes are longer (180 to 300 cm) and permit passage into the intestinal tract. They are constructed with a small balloon at the tip that, when filled with water or mercury, acts like a bolus of food and stimulates peristalsis. The tube advances in this way along the intestinal tract. Even in the absence of peristalsis, the weighted tip usually is able to pull the tube along. Intestinal tubes are avoided by some physicians because their insertion is more difficult and uncomfortable for the patient. Common examples of intestinal tubes (Figure 41-17) include the following:[2]

- *Cantor tube.* A single-lumen 300-cm tube with just one opening used for drainage; its balloon is injected with 4 to 5 ml of mercury before insertion of the tube.
- *Harris tube.* A single-lumen 180-cm tube with a metal tip; its single lumen is used for drainage or irrigation and is weighted with a prefilled mercury balloon.
- *Miller-Abbott tube.* A double-lumen 300-cm tube with markings to indicate how far it has passed. One lumen leads to the balloon, which is filled with mercury after it has been inserted; the second lumen has openings along its course to allow for drainage and irrigation.
- *Dennis tube.* A three-lumen 300-cm tube with one lumen for suction, one for irrigation or venting, and one for insertion of mercury into a distal balloon.

Guidelines for care of the person with an intestinal tube are presented in the box below.

**guidelines for care**

### The Person with an Intestinal Tube

#### Facilitating Movement of the Tube

Position patient:
- 2 hours on right side
- 2 hours on back with head elevated
- 2 hours on left side

Encourage ambulation once tube has passed the pylorus (assessed by radiograph).

Gently advance the tube 2-10 cm (1-4 inches) as ordered to provide slack for movement.

Do not tape tube until desired location has been reached; pin extra tubing to clothing.

#### Facilitating Drainage

Use intermittent low suction with single-lumen tubes to prevent mucosal injury.

Constant suction may be used with sump action tubes.

Use normal saline to irrigate tube if there is no drainage or patient becomes nauseated. (It is rarely possible to aspirate returns back through a long intestinal tube.)

#### Promoting Comfort

Tape tube securely to nostril once the desired location has been reached.

Pin tube to clothing to support its weight.

Apply water-soluble lubricant to nares for comfort and to prevent secretion crusting.

Provide frequent mouth care:
- Offer hard candy and occasional ice chips.
- Provide throat lozenges or saline rinses for sore throat.

Assess mucous membranes for signs of irritation or infection.

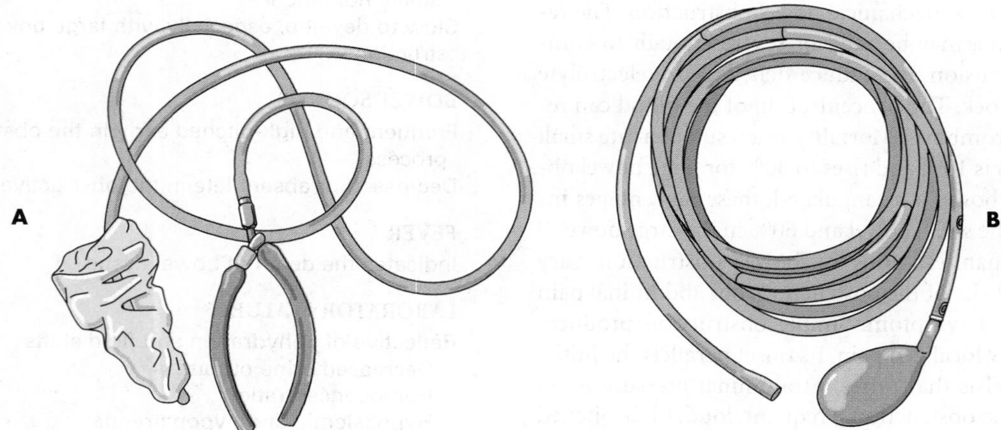


**fig. 41-17** Examples of intestinal tubes. **A,** Miller-Abbott tube. **B,** Cantor tube.

The treatment of nonmechanical obstruction and paralytic ileus is generally conservative and supportive. An NG tube may be inserted to decompress the stomach and relieve nausea and bloating, and careful attention is again paid to restoring and maintaining the balance of fluids and electrolytes. Careful monitoring for complications is ongoing. Promotility drugs are most likely to be useful in nonmechanical obstructive situations.

Nursing management focuses on careful monitoring of all physical parameters. The nurse monitors the patient's vital signs, urine output, and NG output frequently. Changes are compared with the symptoms of early shock (see Chapter 17). The nurse administers IV fluids as ordered and monitors for symptoms of electrolyte imbalance. Fluid replacement is provided for all patients with intestinal obstruction because fluid losses usually are significant. Supplemental potassium is added to IV lines as needed to compensate for losses through vomiting and fluid shifts.

Third spacing of fluids is typical with intestinal obstruction. The nurse assesses for edema and measures abdominal girth every 2 to 4 hours. Fluid losses trigger nagging thirst, and small amounts of ice chips may be comforting.

General comfort measures include positioning the patient with the head of the bed elevated to relieve abdominal pressure and providing frequent position changes. A side-lying position often is the most comfortable. Oral and nasal care are offered every 2 to 4 hours to counter the drying and irritating effects of the NG tube and nothing-by-mouth status.

The nurse regularly assesses the patient's pain. Analgesics rarely are given to patients with bowel obstruction until the diagnosis is established, and it is critical for the nurse to explore nonpharmacological measures to increase comfort. If the patient's pain increases significantly or shifts from a cramping to a constant character, it should be reported promptly. It may indicate strangulation or perforation of the bowel. A Nursing Care Plan for a patient with a bowel obstruction is found on p. 1348.

Surgical correction of mechanical bowel obstruction is often necessary after bowel decompression. Specific surgical procedures depend on the nature and location of the obstruction. Release of adhesions, bowel resection with reanastomosis or temporary colostomy, may all be used. The existence or development of bowel strangulation or vascular compromise necessitates that corrective surgery be performed on an emergency basis. Postoperative care is the same as that provided to any patient who undergoes major abdominal surgery. See the discussion on p. 1354-1355.

#### *Patient/family education*

The patient may be extremely anxious during the initial treatment period. It is important for the nurse to explain all tests, procedures, and planned care thoroughly. Support and reassurance are important, especially if corrective bowel surgery is planned.

The majority of large bowel obstructions affect older patients and are related to the presence of cancer. The nurse will need to assist the patient in dealing with the discomfort and anxiety of the obstruction as well as the diagnosis of cancer and the possible need for ostomy surgery. Both the patient and family are likely to feel overwhelmed and will need teaching and reteaching as they attempt to understand the diagnosis and treatment options.

Discharge planning is tailored to the unique needs of the patient. Recovery from intestinal obstruction may be prolonged or swift based on the location and severity of the obstruction and whether or not surgery was performed. Home care issues include wound healing, reestablishing a normal diet, and regular bowel habits. Teaching is provided concerning the prevention of constipation through a fiber-rich diet, adequate fluids, and exercise.

Patients who undergo colostomy surgery because of cancer or bowel complications need ongoing support and supervision as they adjust to new self-care patterns (see pages 1337-1342). Referral to a home health care agency is initiated.

## COLORECTAL CANCER

### Etiology

The available knowledge base about bowel cancer has expanded tremendously over the last decade, but the precise origins of bowel cancer remain elusive. Bowel cancer is currently categorized into three distinct forms, which reflect the evolving understanding of the interplay of environmental and genetic factors in the etiology of the disease. The incidence rates for bowel cancer vary substantially around the world, and these variations provided the early evidence of the importance of environmental factors in its etiology. The importance of genetic factors has been recognized more recently. The development and gradual carcinogenic transformation of bowel polyps and adenomas can now frequently be traced to specific gene mutations.

The role of genetics in bowel cancer was first recognized in a rare disorder, familial adenomatous polyposis. This autosomal dominant disorder causes the early development of multiple polyps in the colon and rectum. The incidence of bowel cancer in individuals with this disorder is nearly 100% by midlife.[46] Gardner's syndrome is one small subtype of this disorder that causes osseous as well as soft tissue tumors. A second disorder, familial nonpolyposis syndrome, is also an autosomal dominant disorder. It causes the development of only a small number of bowel polyps, but they demonstrate an extremely strong tendency to undergo malignant change in affected persons at a very young age. The malignant change is attributed to the presence of a mutant gene, which promotes mutations in other genes. The polyposis syndromes account for only 10% of all bowel cancers, but genetics is also believed to play an important role in the remaining 90% of so-called "sporadic" cases of colorectal cancer.[46]

Colorectal cancer usually develops as part of a slow and orderly change process in the bowel mucosa from polyp development to gradual malignant transformation in response to genetic signals. Most of the genetic changes involve the deletion of chromosome fragments, but the total number of mutations appears to be more significant than their specific placement or sequence.[45] A number of the mutations have

## nursing care plan *Person with a Bowel Obstruction*

**DATA** Mrs. R.L. is a 62-year-old woman who was admitted last night with a probable small bowel obstruction. She developed cramping upper abdominal pain at her office yesterday, which slowly but steadily worsened. She felt bloated and increasingly nauseated and thought that she was probably getting the flu. She went home and rested, but her condition did not improve, and during the evening she began vomiting. The vomiting temporarily relieved her pain, but the cycle would then repeat itself again at shorter and shorter intervals. Her family became frightened and insisted that she come to the emergency room.

Mrs. L. has been in good health. She has a stable, loving family and a job she enjoys. Her health history is unremarkable and includes only the removal of her appendix in her teens, the uncomplicated birth of three children, and an abdominal hysterectomy for dysfunctional uterine bleeding about 5 years ago.

On admission Mrs. L. had a temperature of 100° F (37.8° C), blood pressure of 110/60, and pulse of 88. She reported continued abdominal pain and a tight bloated feeling in her abdomen. Auscultation of the abdomen revealed diminished bowel sounds in the lower quadrants but high-pitched sounds in the upper quadrants. She was not passing gas per rectum and had not had a bowel movement for 2 days. She voided 90 ml of concentrated urine on admission. Abdominal x-rays revealed significant accumulation of gas and fluid in the intestine. Her blood work was normal except for a hematocrit of 40% and low normal values of sodium and potassium. The admission diagnosis was R/O small bowel obstruction, probably related to the development of adhesions.

An IV line was inserted for hydration, and Mrs. L. is to be given nothing by mouth except for small amounts of ice chips. She has bathroom privileges, but intake and output are to be strictly recorded. An NG tube was inserted to begin abdominal decompression, and a decision about the need for surgery will be made within 48 hours.

**NURSING DIAGNOSIS** *Pain related to distention of the bowel with fluid and gas*

| expected patient outcome | nursing interventions | rationale |
|---|---|---|
| States pain is steadily decreasing and remains within tolerable levels. | **1.** Assess the patient's pain level at least every 4 hours.<br>**a.** Assist patient to develop a pain-rating scale for evaluating changes.<br>**b.** Record patient's pain ratings on bedside flow sheet. | **1.** Pain presence and severity are important cues for identifying subtle changes in patient status. Worsening pain can indicate bowel ischemia or peritonitis.<br>**a.** Pain records demonstrate pattern changes over time. |
| | **2.** Administer prescribed analgesics and antiemetics as ordered. | **2.** Analagesics are frequently withheld until the diagnosis is established. Aggressive comfort measures are needed to help the patient gain control of the pain. Nausea and vomiting contribute significantly to general discomfort. |
| | **3.** Use nonpharmacologic comfort measures that are acceptable to the patient:<br>a. Hygiene and linen changes<br>b. Oral care<br>c. Back rubs and repositioning<br>d. Relaxation exercises or distraction | **3.** Analgesic administration is limited due to the adverse effect on peristalsis. Adjunct pain relief measures are therefore critical. |
| | **4.** Maintain patency and proper functioning of NG suction.<br>**a.** Attach to low intermittent suction as prescribed.<br>**b.** Irrigate or reposition tube as needed to maintain drainage. | **4.** Effectively decompressing the GI tract will decrease both fluid and gas distention. |
| | **5.** Position in a semi- to high Fowler's position.<br>**a.** Encourage frequent position changes.<br>**b.** Encourage patient to get out of bed once condition is stabilized. | **5.** An upright position relieves pressure in the abdomen and facilitates ventilation. Activity is important to help reestablish peristalsis. |
| | **6.** Provide frequent oral care.<br>**a.** Provide lubricant for lips. | **6.** NG intubation causes significant dryness and irritation of the oral mucous membranes. Oral care decreases thirst and helps relieve irritation and bad tastes. |

*Continued*

## Person with a Bowel Obstruction–cont'd

**NURSING DIAGNOSIS** *Risk for fluid volume deficit related to vomiting, NG suction, nothing-by-mouth status and fluid shifts in the GI tract*

| expected patient outcome | nursing interventions | rationale |
|---|---|---|
| Maintain fluid balance:<br>Stable body weight<br>Good skin turgor<br>Urine output >30 ml/hr<br>Stable vital signs | 1. Maintain accurate intake and output records.<br>a. Assess and record all NG aspirate. | 1. Intake and output provides initial data about the patient's fluid needs and degree of third spacing. |
| | 2. Maintain IV fluids at prescribed rate of flow. | 2. Obstruction causes significant fluid and electrolyte losses. Steady replacement helps prevent stressful fluid swings and decreases nausea. |
| | 3. Monitor weight daily. | 3. Body weight is the most accurate method of assessing fluid gains and losses. |
| | 4. Measure abdominal girth each shift until stabilized. | 4. Fluid and gas accumulation in GI tract can result in significant abdominal distention. |

**NURSING DIAGNOSIS** *Anxiety related to lack of knowledge concerning pathological cause of bowel obstruction and uncertainty over need for surgery*

| expected patient outcome | nursing interventions | rationale |
|---|---|---|
| Communicates concern about illness and treatment.<br>Verbalizes understanding of all planned interventions. | 1. Provide reassurance and comfort.<br>a. Spend time with patient and family.<br>b. Listen attentively. | 1. Interventions communicate a feeling of empathy and willingness to support patient through crisis. |
| | 2. Provide simple explanation of all tests and procedures. Correct misconceptions as needed. | 2. Accurate understandable information reduces unnecessary fears and restores a sense of control. |
| | 3. Encourage supportive involvement of the family.<br>a. Set aside time to address family concerns as well. | 3. When relationships are supportive, family involvement decreases fear and increases active coping. |

been identified, but none of them can currently be used for general screening. Although virtually all colon cancers appear to develop from polyps that gradually transform into adenomas, only about 5% of all colon adenomas ever become malignant.[45] It is clear that the process of genetic mutation is critical to the eventual development of cancer.

Environmental factors are believed to function as stimulants or enablers, which initiate the gene mutations that result in bowel cancer. Inherited factors probably increase the vulnerability of individuals to specific environmental factors. Diet is the environmental factor that has received the most attention in recent years. Because bowel cancer is significantly more common in industrialized societies, research has focused on the detrimental role of a diet that is low in fiber and high in fat, protein, and refined carbohydrates. It is theorized that harmless foodstuffs are transformed into metabolic and bacterial end products that act as carcinogens in the bowel. Low-fiber diets also increase colon transit time and increase the overall contact time of the bowel mucosa with these carcinogenic agents. Study results to date are inconsistent, inconclusive, and prone to bias; but the trends in diet research strongly suggest an important etiological role.[13]

Cigarette smoking is significantly associated with the formation of adenomas in the bowel. Both the amount and duration of the smoking history affect the incidence.[6] The regular use of aspirin appears to inhibit the formation of polyps, but research in this area is too new to support generalizations about aspirin's potential protective effects[18,46] (Research Box). The risk of colon cancer also is strongly associated with long-standing ulcerative colitis and granulomas. Risk factors for bowel cancer are summarized in the following box.

### Epidemiology

Cancer of the colon and rectum is the third most common type of cancer in men and second most common type in women, and it is the second most common cause of death from cancer in adults of both sexes. Approximately 150,000 new cases are diagnosed each year and 56,000 deaths are attributed to the disease annually.[46] In the United States this represents an annual incidence rate of 14 per 100,000 population. When bowel cancer is diagnosed in its early stage, 5-year survival rates of 90% or greater can be expected, but unfortunately many cases are diagnosed in advanced invasive stages for which 5-year survival rates hover around 40%.[46] Bowel cancer therefore is theoretically amenable to significant decreases in mortality through early diagnosis. This possibility is reflected in the *Healthy People 2000 goal* "to reduce the

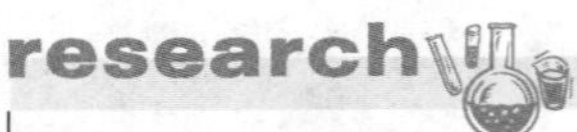

Reference: Giovannucci E et al: Aspirin and the risk of colorectal cancer in women, *N Engl J Med* 333(10):609-614, 1995.

This study attempted to determine the relationship between aspirin use and the risk of colon cancer. It used the large longitudinal study population that comprises the Nurses Health Study. Questionnaires were mailed at 2-year intervals from 1982 to 1992 after baseline health and medication use was established in 1980. Aspirin use was evaluated based on the average number of pills per week. Regular use was defined as 2 to 4 tablets per week. Users and nonusers in the sample were approximately equal in age, body mass, alcohol use, diet, and proportion of current and former smokers. Between 40% and 60% of the study population reported regular aspirin use with each follow-up.

During the period of the study a slight but not significantly lower risk of colon cancer was found among regular aspirin users. Women who reported being regular users of aspirin on three consecutive follow-ups, however, were found to have a 38% lower risk. A significant effect was seen at a use level of 4 to 6 aspirin tablets per week, but no further reduction in risk was seen with higher levels. Benefits of aspirin use did not become significant until after 10 years of regular use. The significance of risk reduction then continued to climb as use approached 20 years. The study appears to verify that a significantly decreased risk of colon cancer is associated with the use of 4 to 6 tablets of aspirin a week for 10 or more consecutive years.

## risk factors

### Colorectal Cancer

Age >50 years
Family history
- Colon cancer in two or more first-degree relatives
- Familial adenomatous polyposis syndrome

History of ulcerative colitis
- Risk appears 8-12 years after diagnosis

Colon polyps or adenomas
Cigarette smoking
- High pack-year history important

Diet low in fiber, high in fat
Obesity (nature of the risk is currently unknown)

incidence of colorectal cancer deaths from 14.4 per 100,000 to no more than 13.2 per 100,000 by the year 2000."[47]

The incidence of bowel cancer is clearly age related. Incidence rates rise slightly after age 40 and more sharply after age 50, and the mean age at onset is 63 to 67 years. All adults older than age 50 are considered to be at average risk for the disease.[29] Men are affected slightly more often than women, and whites are affected slightly more often than African Americans. Roughly 25% of persons report the incidence of bowel cancer in two or more first-degree relatives.[38]

The disease shows significant variations in incidence and mortality rates worldwide, but there have been only minor changes in these parameters in the United States in recent years. The incidence rates are significantly higher in the industrialized Western world than in Asia and Africa. The rates in immigrant families rapidly increase to match those of the larger society, however, again supporting a strong environmental link.

Figure 41-18 illustrates the pattern of incidence of colon cancer by site. The presence of adenomas is a significant risk factor, and adenomas appear to be distributed about equally above and below the splenic flexure. Adenomas with a malignant focus are more likely to be found in the distal colon; however the incidence of right colon cancer has been increasing slowly but steadily, particularly in women. The development of cancer in the small intestine is extremely rare and accounts for less than 1% of all GI tract malignant tumors.

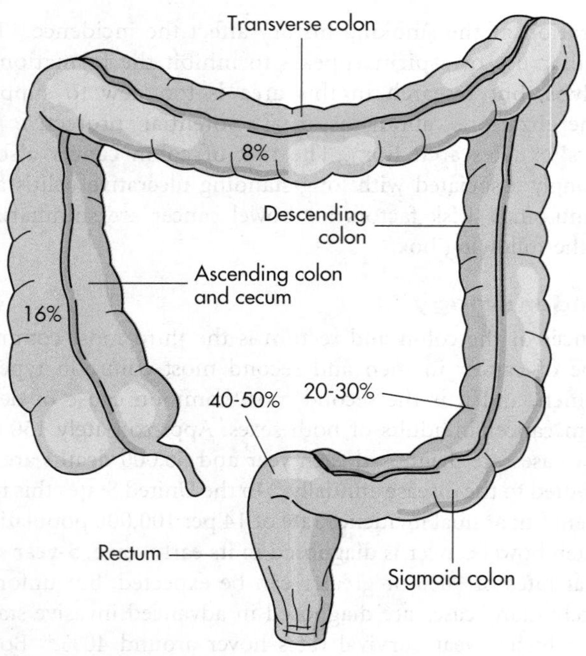


**fig. 41-18** Incidence of cancer in various segments of the colon and rectum.

### Pathophysiology

There is strong evidence that almost all bowel cancers arise from preexisting benign adenomatous colon polyps.[45] All adenomas are dysplastic by definition, and they are considered to be premalignant lesions even though only about 5% are believed to transform to malignancy.[45] At present there are few indicators to predict which small polyps are likely to mutate, but the severity of the dysplasia is clearly related to the size of the polyp. Malignancy is found in less than 1% of polyps which are less than 1 cm in diameter, but it is found in 10% of those greater than 2 cm in diameter.[45] The process of transformation is slow. It is theorized that it takes a 1-cm

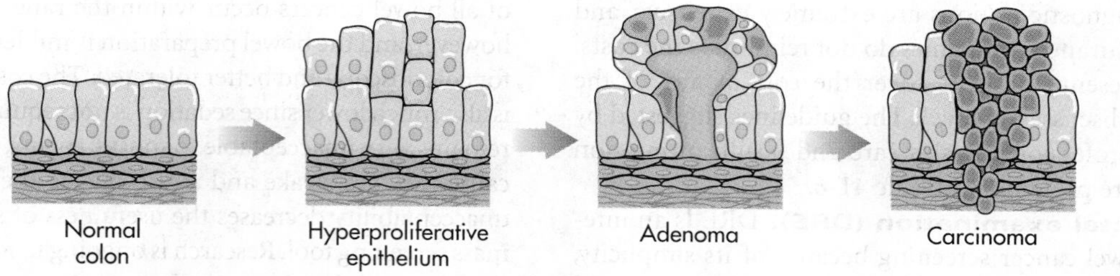

Normal colon
Hyperproliferative epithelium
Adenoma
Carcinoma

**fig. 41-19** The progression to malignancy in bowel cancer.

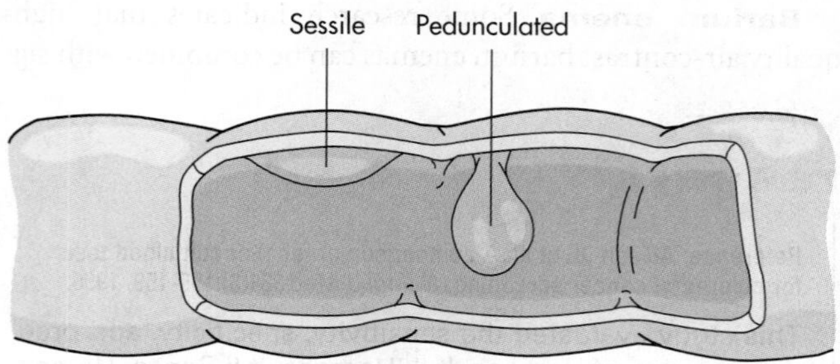


**fig. 41-20** Colon polyps.

polyp 7 years to progress to invasive adenocarcinoma (Figure 41-19).

Adenomas may present in various shapes and configurations. They are typically round and polypoid (sessile), but they also may be more elongated and have stalks (pedunculated) (Figure 41-20). Infrequently they appear as flat or even depressed. Over time the lesions penetrate the colon wall and extend into the surrounding tissue.

Cancer of the colon may spread by direct extension or through the lymphatic or circulatory systems. It may seed at distant points in the peritoneum or at distant points in the colon. The liver and lungs are the major organs of metastasis. Box 41-5 summarizes the Dukes' classification system used for colorectal cancer. Note that the stage of bowel cancer is determined by the degree of invasion of the tumor and not its size. Staging is used to establish the appropriate level of intervention and treatment. Persons with stage A disease have a 90% 5-year survival rate; those with stage D have less than a 5% 5-year survival rate.[46]

The clinical manifestations of colon cancer vary with the location of the tumor. There are usually no early symptoms and the disease is often diagnosed incidentally.[5] Cancer in the distal colon and rectum typically produces symptoms related to partial obstruction. The lesions are more likely to be annular, and they grow circumferentially, encircling the colon wall. The lumen becomes narrow and constricted. Obstruction occurs when formed stool is unable to pass through the narrowed lumen.

The patient may experience a change in bowel habits, a feeling of incomplete bowel emptying, or rectal bleeding. The bleeding may be overt or occult. Obstruction in the right colon is less common because of the semiliquid nature of the stool in this region. Abdominal pain usually accompanies larger lesions.

**box 41-5** *Dukes' Classification of Colorectal Cancer*

Stage A: confined to bowel mucosa
Stage B: invading muscle wall
Stage C: lymph node involvement
Stage D: metastases or locally unresectable tumor

**box 41-6** ***clinical manifestations***

***Bowel Cancer***

- Frequently asymptomatic and diagnosed incidentally
- Symptoms of partial bowel obstruction
  - Change in bowel habits, e.g., constipation or diarrhea
  - Pencil- or ribbon-shaped stool
  - Sensation of incomplete bowel emptying
- Gas or bloating
- Occult blood in the stool or rectal bleeding
- Weakness, fatigue, malaise, and anorexia
- Weight loss
- Abdominal pain

Weakness, malaise, anorexia, anemia, and weight loss are nonspecific symptoms that occur frequently in patients with colorectal cancer. The occurrence of weight loss often accompanies metastases. The tumor occasionally may perforate into the peritoneal cavity, and acute peritonitis occurs before the person notices any other signs of illness. The clinical manifestations of bowel cancer are summarized in Box 41-6.

## Collaborative Care Management

### *Diagnostic tests*

The diagnostic technology that is currently available has the theoretical capability to eliminate bowel cancer as a major cause of death. Early and accurate diagnosis for prompt treatment is the primary concern since most bowel cancers are slow growing and easily removed in their early stages. The challenge of early diagnosis is obviously enormous, however, since virtually all adults older than age 50 are considered to be at average risk and would need to be included in any mass screening program. Research is ongoing to attempt to determine the optimal tests and time intervals for bowel cancer screening.[10,38] The issue is of tremendous importance since some of the diagnostic options are extremely expensive, and most private insurance companies do not reimburse the costs. Medicare at present does not cover the cost of any of the screening tests discussed below.[10] The guidelines suggested by several major professional health care and health promotion organizations are presented in Table 41-6.

**Digital rectal examination (DRE).** DRE is an integral part of bowel cancer screening because of its simplicity, low cost, and general acceptability to patients. It is usually performed as part of a routine gynecological or prostate examination. Figure 41-18 illustrates the fact that up to 40% of all bowel cancers are found in the rectal region and may be within the reach of the examiner's finger.

**Fecal occult blood tests.** The use of fecal occult blood testing is based on the premise that evolving adenocarcinomas routinely bleed in amounts that are too small to be visible but can be readily detected in laboratory tests. The sensitivity of these tests is felt to be no more than 50% for cancerous lesions and less than 25% for adenomatous polyps. Both false-positive and false-negative results are frequently found.[1,46] Occult blood tests often yield false-negative results by missing cancers that were not bleeding at the time of testing and false-positive results for which no bleeding source is ever found. Diet and medication can both cause false-positive results. The false-positive rate averages 10% in most studies.[1] This is important from a cost perspective since patients whose test results are positive are virtually all referred for screening via colonoscopy. Fecal occult blood tests are included on most screening guidelines at least partly because of their relatively low cost and general acceptability to patients (Research Box). This trend is reflected in a recent amendment to the *Healthy People 2000* goals, which reads: "Increase to at least 50% the proportion of people aged 50 and older who have received fecal occult blood testing within the preceding 1 to 2 years, and to at least 40% those who have ever received proctosigmoidoscopy."[47]

**Sigmoidoscopy.** Flexible fiberoptic sigmoidoscopy allows for good endoscopic visualization of the rectum and descending colon, but cannot reach the proximal colon. Up to 70% of all bowel cancers occur within the range of sigmoidoscopy, however, and the bowel preparation is milder than that required for colonoscopy and better tolerated. The cost of sigmoidoscopy is also much lower since sedation is not required. Sigmoidoscopy remains very unacceptable to most patients, however, partly because they are awake and aware during the procedure, and its unacceptability decreases the usefulness of sigmoidoscopy as a mass screening tool. Research is ongoing to identify the maximal time interval for screening that can be recommended to low- and average-risk patients. Some studies indicate that 5- to 10-year intervals may be sufficient.

**Barium enema.** Some research indicates that high-quality air-contrast barium enemas can be combined with sig-

**research**

Reference: Allison JE et al: A comparison of fecal occult blood tests for colorectal cancer screening, *N Engl J Med* 334(3):155-159, 1996.

This study evaluated the sensitivity, specificity, and predictive value of Hemoccult II, Hemoccult II Sensa, HemeSelect, and the combination of Hemoccult II Sensa and HemeSelect in identifying the presence of colorectal cancer in a large population of adults older than age 50 considered to have an average risk for colon cancer. The population included 8000 adults who were balanced in sex, distributed evenly in age between 50 and over 70, and reflected the general population in race breakdown.

At least one fecal occult blood test was positive in 16% of the sample. Rates of positive response were 2.5% with Hemoccult II, 6% with HemeSelect, and 14% with Hemoccult II Sensa. Fifty-seven percent only exhibited a positive response with the Sensa test. Colonoscopy was used to determine specificity of the positive results, which were best correlated with results from the HemeSelect test. The study concluded that the Hemoccult II Sensa test had the highest sensitivity but lowest specificity. It was very likely to be influenced by diet and other factors. Therefore the best combination of sensitivity and specificity for colon cancer was achieved by the use of the combination of two products—Hemoccult II Sensa and HemeSelect.

**table 41-6** *Guidelines for Colorectal Cancer Screening*

| Organization(s) | Recommendations |
|---|---|
| American Cancer Society | Annual DRE beginning at age 40 |
| American Cancer Institute | Annual fecal occult blood test every 3-5 yr beginning at age 50 |
| American Gastroenterological Association | Flexible sigmoidoscopy every 3-5 yr beginning at age 50 |
| American College of Physicians | Flexible sigmoidoscopy, colonoscopy, or barium enema for patients 50-70 yr; repeat tests every 10 yr |
| American College of Obstetricians and Gynecologists | Annual fecal occult blood testing for all women older than age 40 |
| American Academy of Family Physicians | Flexible sigmoidoscopy and/or fecal occult blood testing beginning at age 50 |
| American College of Radiology | Barium enema every 3-5 yr |
| World Health Organization | Annual DRE and fecal occult blood testing beginning at age 50<br>Flexible sigmoidoscopy every 3-5 yr beginning at age 50<br>Colonoscopy after positive fecal blood tests |

moidoscopy and produce results that are comparable to those of colonoscopy for whole colon screening and yet still represent a cost savings.[10] Barium enemas are excellent for outlining large polyps but are relatively ineffective for polyps less than 1 cm in size. This combination of tests is generally highly unacceptable to patients.

**Colonoscopy.** Colonoscopy is considered to be the gold standard for bowel cancer diagnosis, but it is also extremely expensive, must be performed by highly trained professionals, requires patients to be sedated, and is associated with an extremely uncomfortable bowel preparation. A major advantage of colonoscopy is the fact that if small lesions are found, they can be immediately removed by a snare that is built directly into the endoscope (Figure 41-21). Treatment does not require a second step at some future point. At present, however, it would be virtually impossible to offer colonoscopy screening to the entire adult population older than 50 years of age. The optimal interval and frequency of screening by colonoscopy are not known. Some authorities believe that enormous gains could be achieved by screening the entire bowel once or perhaps twice in a lifetime.[45] Any of these tests would eventually have to be used with a huge population, which makes the potential cost staggering. It is clear that any recommendations concerning bowel cancer screening will incorporate social policy as well as medical research.

### Medications

Chemotherapy is not used as a primary treatment modality for bowel cancer, but it is used as part of adjuvant postoperative treatment for patients with advanced disease. Chemotherapy is primarily palliative in nature. 5-Fluorouracil (5-FU) is the drug with the most established record of effectiveness. Current research protocols combine the drugs

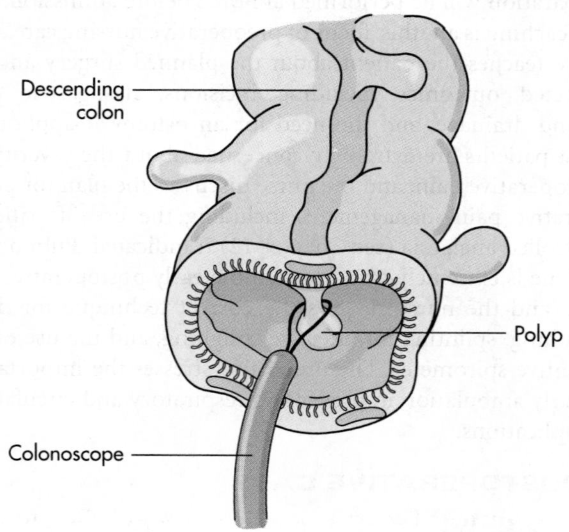


**fig. 41-21** Colonoscopy allows for both diagnosis and treatment during the same procedure. A built-in snare attachment can remove any polyps found during the examination.

levamisole or leukovorin with 5-FU to stimulate immune system function and minimize the damage to healthy cells. 5-FU is also used routinely as an adjunct to the newer sphincter-sparing surgeries, and the incidence of recurrences is significantly reduced. Chemotherapy may also be administered in combination with radiotherapy.

### Treatments

Radiation is rarely used in the treatment of colon cancer, but it plays an important role in the management of rectal cancer. Generally used postoperatively to reduce the chance of recurrence, radiation is also being used to shrink tumors preoperatively. External beam radiation or endocavitary irradiation, in which the radiation source is placed directly on the tumor, may be used. Radiation enteritis is a common complication during treatment, but the incidence of serious complications is only 5% to 6% at major centers.

### Surgical management

Surgery is the definitive treatment for colorectal cancer. It typically involves removal of the tumor, surrounding colon, and lymph nodes. When the tumor is located in the ascending, transverse, or descending colon, it usually is possible for the surgeon to perform a resection with end-to-end anastomosis that preserves the natural process of defecation. The specific type of surgery performed depends on the exact location and size of the tumor and the overall condition of the patient. The use of laparoscopic techniques for bowel resection is under careful study and has shown clear promise to reduce pain and recovery time in early stage cancers.[9]

There are no clear guidelines at this time concerning the use of local versus wide excision and whether or not extensive lymph node dissection should be performed. Local excision is used for Dukes' Stage A and some Stage B tumors. Wide excision plus adjuvant therapy is used for more aggressive disease.

Patients with tumors in the rectum were previously managed exclusively by removing the entire rectum and anus through a dual incision procedure called an *abdominoperineal resection.* The procedure necessitates permanent colostomy and leaves a significant perineal wound that heals slowly around active drains. The anus is sutured closed. Patients with early localized rectal cancers are now routinely offered the option of a sphincter-sparing procedure. Regional rectal resection is performed, and the rectum is reconstructed with the creation of a pouch as discussed on p. 1329 for ulcerative colitis.

The use of an anastomotic stapler has made these technically difficult procedures feasible. Low anterior resection through an abdominal incision has been used most extensively, but several other surgical approaches, for example, transanal approaches, are being used as well. The risk of rectal recurrence of the cancer is greater with this type of surgery. Therefore, adjuvant therapy with chemotherapy and external beam radiation is also provided.

The newer procedures have significantly reduced the need for permanent colostomies, but temporary colostomies are often created to allow for bowel rest and healing, particularly if bowel obstruction with inflammation occurred. Examples of various colostomy procedures are illustrated in Figure 41-10. General nursing care associated with ostomy management is discussed on p. 1337-1342.

### Diet

No special diet restrictions are ordered for patients with colorectal cancer. Anorexia and weight loss are common early symptoms, and concern may develop over the adequacy of the patient's nutritional status, especially with the elderly. The standard treatment approaches also may compromise the patient's nutritional status. Bowel surgery necessitates a period of nothing by mouth or limited oral intake. Aggressive chemotherapy may be accompanied by nausea and/or vomiting, and both external beam and endocavitary irradiation can trigger radiation enteritis.

Low levels of serum albumin are associated with a higher incidence of postoperative complications, especially in elders. It is essential to improve and sustain the patient's nutritional status during all planned treatments.

### Activity

The diagnosis of bowel cancer may affect the patient's activity level in several ways. Anemia and fatigue are common early signs of colon cancer. Severe anemia and fatigue frequently accompany aggressive chemotherapy and radiotherapy. Bowel surgery is initially very painful and significantly restricts the patient's activity. The patient is encouraged to modify and space activities throughout the day to remain involved in the usual activities of daily living. The patient is encouraged to remain as active as possible throughout all phases of treatment.

### Referrals

In some settings the nurse assumes responsibility for making referrals to other services. Common referrals for persons with bowel cancer include the following:

1. *Enterostomal therapy.* Some patients are still treated with surgical procedures that result in permanent ostomies, and it is essential that an enterostomal therapy specialist be involved in the patient's care from the point of admission.
2. *Nutrition support.* The involvement of a nutrition support team may be appropriate at any point in the treatment plan. The team may perform a detailed nutritional assessment and plan for the appropriate use of scheduled meals and supplements to meet the varying needs of the patient. Ensuring adequate protein and calories for healing is essential.

A sample Clinical Pathway for a patient undergoing colon resection is presented on p. 1356. It summarizes the general care discussed under collaborative and nursing management. Patients with uncomplicated cases are successfully restarted on oral feedings as soon as peristalsis is reestablished, and may be discharged as early as postoperative day 4. When a colostomy is necessary for any reason the patient's care will follow the principles discussed on p. was 1337-1342.

# NURSING MANAGEMENT OF THE PATIENT UNDERGOING BOWEL SURGERY FOR COLORECTAL CANCER

## ■ PREOPERATIVE CARE

Most preoperative care is completed in the community before the patient's admission. The diagnosis of cancer adds additional anxiety to the preoperative period and may make it difficult for the patient to understand and retain information about the planned surgery and the care that will be provided in the postoperative period. The nurse ensures that the patient has been adequately prepared for abdominal surgery and general anesthesia.

Bowel cleansing is required. This is accomplished by diet modification, mechanical cleansing, and pharmacological suppression of colon bacteria. The patient begins with a low-residue diet and moves toward clear liquids as surgery approaches. Boluses of vitamins K and C may be given to support clotting and wound healing in the postoperative period. The synthesis and absorption of these vitamins are impaired by the vigorous bowel preparation.

Preparation of the bowel for surgery may involve the use of either laxatives, enemas, or both. Bowel preparation is performed to cleanse the colon and suppress bacterial growth that might lead to infection in the postoperative period. A solution such as GoLYTELY (sodium sulfate and polyethylene glycol) provides for an osmotic cleansing of the entire bowel. Up to 4 L are administered orally in divided doses 10 to 15 minutes apart. The cleansing usually is complete in about 4 hours. Systemic or oral antibiotics also may be administered to reduce colonic bacteria. Oral neomycin is a standard preparation. If the patient is in good physical condition, bowel preparation will be performed at home before admission.

Teaching is another focus of preoperative nursing care. The nurse teaches the patient about the planned surgery and its expected outcomes including incisions, nasogastric and wound drainage, and the need for an ostomy if applicable. Most patients are extremely concerned about the severity of postoperative pain, and the nurse discusses the plan for postoperative pain management, including the use of patient-controlled analgesia (see Chapter 12) if indicated. Pulmonary hygiene is extremely important in the early postoperative period, and the nurse reviews the correct technique for deep breathing, splinting for effective coughing, and the use of an incentive spirometer. The nurse also stresses the importance of early ambulation in preventing respiratory and circulatory complications.

## ■ POSTOPERATIVE CARE

### Maintaining Fluid and Electrolyte Balance

The patient usually receives nothing by mouth for brief or extended periods after surgery and nasogastric suctioning may be in use. NG suctioning was formerly a standard intervention after any bowel surgery, but it is increasingly being either omitted entirely or terminated very quickly as studies have failed to demonstrate any difference in outcomes for patients who do not develop prolonged ileus.[13] If an NG tube is used, the output from the tube is carefully assessed and recorded, and the tube is irrigated as needed to maintain patency. The nurse evaluates intake and output balance, maintains IV fluids as ordered, records daily weight, and monitors for electrolyte imbalance. Monitoring continues as the patient is gradually advanced to a normal diet.

Early feeding has also become fairly standard, and patients may only be given nothing by mouth (NPO) for the first 24 hours.[50] The experience of early feeding after laparoscopic surgery has supported this approach. The importance of adequate nutrition for wound healing also supports this move away from a prolonged postoperative NPO period. The nurse carefully assesses the adequacy of the patient's oral intake as oral feeding is resumed.

### Promoting Ventilation

Incisional pain typically is severe with abdominal surgery, and pain can interfere with lung excursion. The nurse monitors the effectiveness of the patient-controlled analgesia system or ensures that adequate narcotic analgesia is provided to allow for early ambulation and regular deep breathing. The nurse auscultates regularly for signs of atelectasis and encourages the use of incentive spirometry to open the alveoli. Deep breathing must be performed hourly in the early postoperative days to prevent pulmonary complications.

### Supporting Peristalsis

Temporary paralytic ileus is an expected complication of bowel surgery in which manipulation of the intestines takes place. Prolonged ileus may indicate an abdominal abscess or obstruction. The passage of gas rectally indicates the beginning return of peristalsis. The nurse auscultates the patient's abdomen for bowel sounds every 4 hours and assesses for the movement of gas or presence of distention. Ambulation facilitates the return of peristalsis, and the nurse encourages the patient to be as active as possible. The diet and activity changes plus loss of bowel tissue that accompany resection may make it difficult for the patient to resume a normal elimination pattern. Diarrhea may occur initially, but it usually is temporary and self-limiting. The nurse teaches the patient to avoid constipation through regular exercise, adequate fluids, and adjusting the fiber content of the diet. Laxatives should be avoided if possible.

## GERONTOLOGICAL CONSIDERATIONS

The incidence of cancer of the bowel is strongly skewed toward the elderly population, and the entire discussion of the disease is really aimed at that population. The issues of comorbidity and general health, therefore, become extremely important. Healthy elders can withstand the rigors of treatment well, but the concurrent existence of other chronic health problems increases the risk for postoperative complications.

Early diagnosis frequently is difficult in the older population. Symptoms tend to be underreported and attributed to the effects of aging. This is particularly true concerning symptoms related to digestion and elimination. Chronic constipation is a frequent complaint in this population, and changes in bowel habits may not be reported until the disease is well established.

The challenges of learning an ostomy self-care regimen if needed also may be more significant for older persons who are acknowledged to have some difficulty in processing new information and learning new tasks. The presence of arthritis or failing vision may make it difficult for elders to acquire the psychomotor skills necessary for self-care. The teaching plan will need to be structured to address these concerns and probably will need to move at a slower pace.

## SPECIAL ENVIRONMENTS FOR CARE

### Critical Care Management

The standard diagnosis and treatment of bowel cancer will not necessitate the involvement of the critical care team unless serious complications develop. Advancing age has not been shown to be a factor in surgical management unless significant comorbid conditions complicate the patient's care. The rapid development of laparoscopic approaches to bowel surgery should lessen the associated pain and immobility and further decrease the incidence of complications. The use of sphincter-sparing surgeries has lessened the complexity of postoperative wound management and healing even though these surgeries are extremely difficult from a technical point of view.

### Home Care Management

As the acute care hospitalization phase of treatment continues to get shorter, home care considerations for patients with colorectal cancer become increasingly important. It is extremely unlikely that sufficient time will be available for the hospital-based nurse to ensure that the patient can be safely independent in self-care before discharge, especially if the patient is elderly and has a colostomy.

Discharge planning must begin at admission. The nurse assesses the patient's home environment and the supports that are available to meet physical and emotional needs. For elderly patients, particularly those who live alone, this assessment includes extended family and friendship networks. The involvement of a social worker may be helpful to determine insurance and financial qualifications for home care assistance (see the Research Box on p. 1358).

Referral for postdischarge assistance may be necessary. Plans for adjuvant treatment with radiation or chemotherapy will further deplete the patient's physical and emotional resources. The American Cancer Society can provide much-needed services and support, and direct referral should be made.

## COMPLICATIONS

Immediate complications related to bowel cancer are primarily surgical. The surgeries that have been described are extensive, and wound complications are a real risk, particularly for elderly patients and those with diabetes. Complications

## clinical pathway *Colectomy*

| HOSPITAL DAY | CONSULTS | TESTS | ACTIVITY/REST | MEDICAL INTERVENTIONS | MEDICATIONS | NUTRITION | NURSES' SIGNATURES |
|---|---|---|---|---|---|---|---|
| PTA or Day of Admittance<br>Date: ______ | Anesthesia | CBC<br>Urinalysis | Up ad lib | | Own, if any | NPO | ______ |
| Surgery<br>Date: ______ | | Lytes if NG<br>H&H or CBC | Up in PM to bathroom with help<br>If A-line: bedrest, turn, cough, deep breathe q2hr<br>Bedside commode with help | IV<br>JP tube(s)<br>NG suction<br>Foley<br>Possible A-line | Analgesics IM, IV, epidural<br>Antibiotics | NPO, I&O | ______<br>______<br>______ |
| Day 1<br>Date: ______ | | Lytes if NG<br>H&H or CBC | Walk in hall 4 times with assistance<br>If A-line: turn, cough, deep breathe q2hr when in bed<br>Up in chair | IV<br>JP tube(s)<br>NG to suction<br>Foley<br>A-line | Analgesics IM, IV, epidural<br>Antibiotics | NPO, I&O | ______<br>______<br>______ |
| Day 2<br>Date: ______ | If ordered, internist for resumption of usual meds | Lytes if NG<br>H&H or CBC | Walk in hall at least 4 times with help | JP tube(s)<br>NG to suction<br>Possible to go to clamping schedule, if ordered | Analgesics PO, IM, IV, epidural, antibiotics | NPO, I&O<br>Possible clear liquid (if ordered)<br>If total clamping scheduled (if ordered) | ______<br>______<br>______ |
| Day 3<br>Date: ______ | | | Walk in hall at least 4 times with help | Possible discontinue NG if ordered<br>Clamping schedule for NG if ordered<br>JP<br>IV | IV, PO, IM, epidural<br>Antibiotics | I&O<br>Clear liquid → full liquid late in day if tolerated clear liquids. | ______<br>______<br>______ |
| Day 4<br>Date: ______ | | | Walk in hall at least 4 times (self-ambulation) | Possible heparin well<br>JP tubes<br>Colostomy or ileostomy | Analgesics PO or IM<br>Antibiotics | Full liquid to diet as tolerated | ______<br>______<br>______ |
| Day 5<br>Date: ______ | | | Walk in hall at least 4 times (self-ambulation) | Possible heparin line<br>JP tube(s)<br>Colostomy or ileostomy | Analgesics PO<br>Antibiotics | Diet as tolerated | ______<br>______<br>______ |
| Day 6<br>Date: ______ | | | | Heparin line<br>Colostomy/ileostomy | | | ______ |

| HOSPITAL DAY | ASSESSMENT | DISCHARGE PLANNING | TEACHING | PSYCHOSOCIAL | SELF-CARE | NURSES' SIGNATURES |
|---|---|---|---|---|---|---|
| PTA or Day of Admittance<br>Date: ______ | Lung status<br>Location and nature of pain | | Reinforce preop teaching<br>Reassure and encourage patient that numerous people have ostomies and still enjoy active, happy and productive lives | Assess anxiety level | ADL | ______<br>______<br>______ |
| Surgery<br>Date: ______ | Lung status<br>Bowel sounds | | Reinforce postop teaching | Continue to assess anxiety level<br>Inform of colostomy/ileostomy immediately postop if one was constructed | Assisted ADL | ______<br>______<br>______ |
| Day 1<br>Date: ______ | Lung status<br>Bowel sounds | Assess at home needs | Continue to reinforce postop teaching | Continue to assess anxiety level<br>Patient to look at ostomy area during AM care and ostomy care; if no ostomy, look at incision area/dressing | Assisted ADL | ______<br>______<br>______ |
| Day 2<br>Date: ______ | Lung status<br>Bowel sounds | Assess at home needs<br>Ostomy to see patient if has ostomy. | Continue to reinforce postop teaching<br>Begin ostomy self-care teaching if has ostomy | Continue to assess anxiety level<br>Begin handling ostomy equipment, possibly refer patient to ostomy client if available to decrease sense of isolation | Assisted ADL | ______<br>______<br>______ |
| Day 3<br>Date: ______ | Lung status<br>Bowel sounds | Assess at home needs | Continue to reinforce postop and ostomy teaching<br>If path report indicates malignancy give 1-800-4-CANCER number to patient for access to more information | Continue to assess anxiety level<br>Patient may choose to look at incision when dressing is changed<br>Empty own ostomy pouch | Self ADL | ______<br>______<br>______ |
| Day 4<br>Date: ______ | Lung status<br>Bowel sounds | Assess at home needs | Continue to reinforce postop teaching<br>Continue ostomy teaching and assess patient response | Continue to assess anxiety level<br>Patient may choose to look at incision when dressing is changed<br>Empty own ostomy pouch | Self ADL | ______<br>______<br>______ |
| Day 5<br>Date: ______ | Lung status<br>Bowel sounds | Assess at home needs<br>Continue ostomy teaching, assess pt. response | Continue to reinforce postop teaching | Continue to assess anxiety level<br>Begin/continue self-care of stoma incl. changing bag, skin care per ostomy if appl. | Self ADL | ______<br>______<br>______ |
| Day 6<br>Date: ______ | Lung status<br>Bowel sounds | Assess at home needs<br>Continue ostomy teaching, assess pt. response | Ascertain that patient and family are competent to handle ostomy care (if applicable) | Continue to assess anxiety level<br>Continue assisted/self-care of stoma if appl. | Self ADL | ______<br>______<br>______ |

From: Cohen EL, Cesta TG: *Nursing case management,* ed 2, St Louis, 1997, Mosby.
*ADL,* Activities of daily living; *CBC,* complete blood count; *H&H,* hemoglobin and hematocrit; *I&O,* intake and output; *JP,* Jackson Pratt; *Lytes,* electrolytes; *NG,* nasogastric tube; *PTA,* prior to admission.

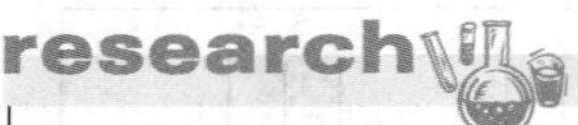

Reference: Galloway SC, Graydon JE: Uncertainty, symptom distress, and information needs after surgery for cancer of the colon, *Cancer Nurs* 19(2):112-117, 1996.

This study explored the concerns of 40 patients who underwent colon resection for cancer without ostomy formation. The purpose was to determine the relationships between uncertainty, symptom distress, and discharge information needs. The sample was evenly distributed between men and women, who ranged in age from 43 to 89 years. Patients were interviewed with a variety of questionnaires to measure symptom distress, learning needs, and uncertainty before discharge and again 7 to 9 weeks after discharge.

The study found that patients experienced a moderate amount of uncertainty related to their illness experience. Patients with more education exhibited significantly higher levels of uncertainty. Symptom distress was quite low with fatigue reported as the most troubling symptom. Before discharge patients exhibited a moderate number of information needs, primarily related to self-care. This need continued into the postdischarge assessment and manifested as informational concerns over home management. The highest needs were for information related to treatment and complications, activities of daily living, and enhancing quality of life. The higher the patient's uncertainty score, the greater was the need for information.

include infection, bleeding, anastomosis leakage, and fistula development. Close monitoring is required in the initial days and weeks.

Patients who undergo extensive lymph node dissection in the pelvic region frequently experience difficulties with urinary control and may develop sexual dysfunction from disruption of the nerve pathways. These problems may resolve with time or cause permanent disruption in the patient's lifestyle. The use of radiotherapy as an adjuvant therapy is frequently accompanied by mucosal inflammation that may result in severe and protracted diarrhea. When the patient has an ileoanal pouch, this inflammation can result in fecal incontinence. None of these problems can be readily resolved, and the patient and family will need ongoing support as they attempt to address these challenges in their daily lives.

Long-term concerns are primarily related to the risk of disease recurrence and metastasis. Ongoing disease surveillance is extremely important. Carcinoembryonic antigen is a tumor marker produced in the body in response to the presence of cancer and secreted into the circulation.[5] In some cases its levels can be used to monitor for recurrence, and it is an effective monitoring tool when the original cancer is more advanced at the time of diagnosis. Surveillance colonoscopy is typically performed at 3-year intervals unless the patient's clinical status warrants a shorter time interval. The prognosis is primarily related to the degree of invasiveness of the cancer at the time of diagnosis and initial treatment. Recurrent bowel cancer is often accompanied by chronic and severe pain, which makes patient comfort an ongoing and challenging goal.

**box 41-7** *Primary and Secondary Causes of Malabsorption*

**PRIMARY CAUSES**
Lactase deficiency
Celiac disease, tropical sprue

**SECONDARY CAUSES**
Subtotal gastrectomy
Ileal resection or bypass greater than 3 feet
Pancreatic disease: pancreatitis, cancer, cystic fibrosis
Liver or biliary disease or obstruction
Inflammatory bowel disease
Bacterial, viral, or parasitic infection of the bowel
Radiation enteritis
Allergy
Drug side effects: antibiotics, colchicine

## MALABSORPTION AND MALNUTRITION

### MALABSORPTION

#### Etiology/Epidemiology

The GI tract must be able to both break down ingested food and transport nutrients across the mucosa of the intestine to the bloodstream. Approximately 7 to 10 L of liquid chyme move through the GI tract daily, but reabsorption in the small intestine is so efficient that all but 600 to 800 ml of chyme are reabsorbed before reaching the ileocecal valve. The term *malabsorption* refers to a broad heterogeneous category of disorders that share the common feature of failure to assimilate one or more essential ingested nutrients.[23] It can result from the impaired function of any of the primary or accessory organs of digestion. The problem may be primarily structural in nature, involve a digestive alteration, or be related to impairment of nutrient transport across the mucosa, vasculature, or lymphatic system. The problem with absorption may relate to a primary disorder such as celiac disease or lactase deficiency; or it may develop secondary to surgery, inflammatory diseases, infections, or the administration of specific medications.[23] Examples of common causes of malabsorption are presented in Box 41-7.

#### Pathophysiology

Malabsorption syndrome is a group of signs and symptoms resulting from inadequate absorption of fat, protein, and/or carbohydrates in the small intestine. Fat malabsorption is the most common problem, but malabsorption can occur with any nutrient. The classic symptoms will vary somewhat based on the specific problem. Because fat-soluble vitamins (A, D, E, and K) require fat for absorption, decreased absorption of fat also typically results in a deficiency of these vitamins.

The characteristic sign of malabsorption syndrome is *steatorrhea,* excess loss of fat in the stool. The range of severity can be from minimal to overwhelming. The fat gives the stool a light, greasy, bulky, mushy appearance and a foul odor. The stools float because of their low specific gravity and high gas content. Stools may be limited to one bulky stool a day or may occur frequently. Steatorrhea causes flatulence with borborygmus (loud bowel sounds) and abdominal distention. The decreased fat absorption leads to weight loss, weakness, fatigue, and anorexia.

Signs and symptoms of concurrent vitamin deficiencies can include bleeding (ecchymosis and hematuria), bone pain, fractures, hypocalcemia, anemia, glossitis, cheilosis, muscle tenderness, peripheral neuritis, and dermatitis. Protein deficiency results in edema, hypoalbuminemia, and loss of muscle mass. The person with malabsorption syndrome usually appears pale and emaciated and has dry, scaly skin that may be hyperpigmented.

Major malabsorption disorders in adults include the following.

#### Gluten-sensitive enteropathy (celiac disease)

This familial disorder involves a permanent intolerance to fractions of gluten (wheat protein). It primarily affects whites and about 30% to 40% of those affected develop overt symptoms. Diarrhea is the primary symptom. Effective treatment involves the rigid and lifelong exclusion of gluten.

#### Tropical sprue

This syndrome primarily affects residents of and visitors to tropical areas. The cause is unknown although an infectious origin is theorized. Affected persons develop severe malnultrition and vitamin deficiencies from the protracted diarrhea. The disorder can be life threatening. Effective treatment involves both antibiotic therapy and folic acid replacement.

#### Short bowel syndrome

The small intestine has a tremendous functional reserve, but loss of more than 50% of its length can significantly reduce the amount of mucosal surface area available for absorbing nutrients. Symptom severity depends on the site and extent of small bowel loss. The loss of jejunum is best tolerated. Treatment is complex and may involve long-term parenteral nutrition, enteral feedings, and drugs to decrease peristalsis.

#### Disaccharide malabsorption

Congenital lactase deficiency is the most common form of genetic deficiency syndrome in humans. It affects more than 50% of the world's population and is particularly prevalent among non-Europeans. The milk intolerance may be mild or severe and is treated by diet restriction and/or enzyme supplement.

#### Protein-losing gastroenteropathy

This problem of excess loss of serum proteins is not a unique entity but is increasingly recognized as a part of a wide variety of disorders, e.g., IBD, pancreatic disease, and cystic fibrosis. Management is directed at effective control of the primary disorder.

### Collaborative Care Management

Medical treatment for malabsorption is based on the underlying cause. Nutrition is the major concern, and dietary intervention is the primary approach to management. Diet modifications are usually successful in compensating for the malabsorption on a daily basis, but more aggressive management with enteral or parenteral (TPN) feedings may be necessary during acute phases.

#### Patient/family education

The nurse assists the patient to incorporate needed dietary changes into the daily lifestyle and works with the family on strategies to promote adherence. The nurse ensures that the patient understands the rationale for all prescribed dietary and drug interventions. The severely malnourished person may require frequent gentle mouth care to increase comfort and prevent oral inflammations as well as skin care to prevent skin breakdown.

## PROTEIN-CALORIE MALNUTRITION

### Etiology/Epidemiology

Any condition that interferes with a person's ability to ingest, digest, or absorb nutrients can result in malnutrition. Acute and chronic illness, infection, and wound healing put enormous strain on the body's nutritional reserve. A poor nutritional state is a common problem in both acute and long-term care settings, and the problem of protein-calorie malnutrition has received increasing attention as the importance of nutrition to factors such as wound healing, immunocompetence, and ventilator weaning is acknowledged. The actual incidence of protein-calorie malnutrition is unknown, but some authors estimate that it may occur in up to 60% of hospitalized elders, 80% of elders in nursing homes, and 20% of outpatients. Box 41-8 identifies some of the typical causes of malnutrition in hospitalized patients.

### Pathophysiology

If a diet provides adequate carbohydrates and fats, the body uses these nutrients to meet its energy needs. When intake of these nutrients is inadequate, however, the body meets its energy needs by using body proteins. Most severely ill hospitalized adults experience a deficiency of all dietary elements. The process of protein synthesis in the body is constant. The body can synthesize certain amino acids from its stored pools, but it depends on ingested protein sources for others. Amino acids that are not used are excreted. Negative nitrogen balance occurs when more nitrogen (which is an end product of amino acid breakdown) is excreted than is ingested via dietary proteins.

Ongoing severe protein loss leads to decreases in both muscle and visceral mass. Cardiac output decreases, respiratory

**box 41-8** *Causes of Malnutrition in Hospitalized Patients*

**DECREASED INTAKE**

| | |
|---|---|
| Anorexia and nausea | Self-care deficits |
| NPO status | Dysphagia |
| Pain | Depression |
| Medication effects | |

**INCREASED LOSSES**

| | |
|---|---|
| Vomiting | Open wounds |
| Diarrhea | GI suctioning |

NOTE: Patients can lose 50 g of protein daily through an open weeping pressure ulcer

**INCREASED NEEDS**

| | |
|---|---|
| Fever | Trauma |
| Infection | Surgery |

muscles weaken, and malabsorption occurs in the GI tract. Immunocompetence is impaired, and the risk of infection increases. The greatest impairment is noted in cell-mediated immunity. The number of T cells declines. Weight loss, decreased muscle mass, and weakness are common, but the affected person may have few overt signs.

### Collaborative Care Management

The primary approach to malnutrition management is recognizing patients at risk, monitoring physical and laboratory parameters, and intervening with oral supplements, tube feedings, or TPN as indicated. Weight loss usually exceeds 15% of usual body weight. Serial measurements of serum albumin and transferrin levels are obtained. Albumin levels less than 3.5 g/dl indicate early malnutrition. Prealbumin levels are followed during treatment inasmuch as they provide an analysis of protein changes during the previous 48 hours. Total lymphocyte counts reflect a basic measure of immunity and should remain greater than $1800/mm^3$. A nutrition-support team, if available, will guide decision making concerning dietary supplements or replacements (see discussion of tube feedings and total parenteral nutrition below).

#### *Patient/family education*

The nurse teaches the patient and family about the disease and its planned management. Anemia-induced fatigue is common, and the nurse provides the patient with frequent rest periods and spaces needed treatments and activities throughout the day. A high-calorie, high-protein diet is encouraged if the patient can tolerate an oral diet. The nurse ensures that the environment is conducive to eating and arranges for small frequent feedings rather than large meals. It is essential that all nutritional planning incorporate the patient's food preferences and cultural habits as much as possible. The goal is to modify the diet just enough to keep the patient symptom free. The nurse keeps an accurate record of the patient's weight and records calorie counts if ordered. Care for the patient receiving tube feedings or total parenteral nutrition is discussed in the next section.

# ENTERAL AND PARENTERAL NUTRITION

## ENTERAL NUTRITION

Enteral nutrition involves the delivery of nutrients directly into the GI tract via tube feeding. It can be used to either supplement or replace oral nutrition in patients who cannot take in adequate amounts of nutrients by mouth. Enteral nutrition is used primarily for patients who have normal GI motility and absorption, although enteral feedings are increasingly being used successfully with critically ill patients who would not previously have been considered good candidates.[27] A safer alternative in many situations than TPN, enteral nutrition is also significantly less likely to cause sepsis and other complications. Other advantages of enteral feedings include the following:

- Preservation of normal sequence of intestinal and hepatic metabolism
- Maintenance of normal insulin : glucagon ratios
- Maintenance of lipoprotein synthesis by the intestinal mucosa and liver[27]

Tube feedings may be delivered to the stomach (nasogastric) or to the distal duodenum or proximal jejunum (nasointestinal). Nasointestinal feedings have become increasingly popular since it was established that the ileus resulting from acute illness or trauma only affects the stomach and colon.[27] The small intestine remains able to absorb nutrients. Long-term enteral nutrition is usually delivered with a permanent access, either into the stomach or jejunum.

### Enteral Feeding Tubes

A wide variety of containers, tubes, catheters, and delivery systems are available for use in enteral feedings. Enteral tubes are classified according to their composition, external diameter, length, and the presence or absence of a weighted tip. Most tubes are constructed of either polyurethane or silicone. The polyurethane tubes have a large internal diameter, which facilitates fluid flow.[28] Enteral feeding tubes range in diameter from 8 to 10 F (small bore), 12 to 14 F (medium bore), and 16 to 18 F (large bore).

Nasogastric feeding tubes can be used with patients who have intact gag and swallow reflexes and a competent lower esophageal sphincter to minimize reflux. Nasointestinal tubes are used for patients who are at risk for aspiration or who are experiencing acute stress-related gastric ileus.[28] They are typically small bore and have a weighted tip to help the tube move through the pylorus into the duodenum or jejunum. A monofilament or stainless steel stylet may be used with small bore tubes to guide insertion. A typical small bore feeding tube is shown in Figure 41-22.

#### *Gastrostomy*

Insertion of a gastrostomy tube is an alternative approach to enteral nutrition for patients who are unable to take oral nutrients for long periods. The gastrostomy tube is inserted surgically through an incision in the abdominal wall or endoscopically.

The percutaneous endoscopic gastrostomy (PEG) does not require incision into the abdominal cavity and is a safe and

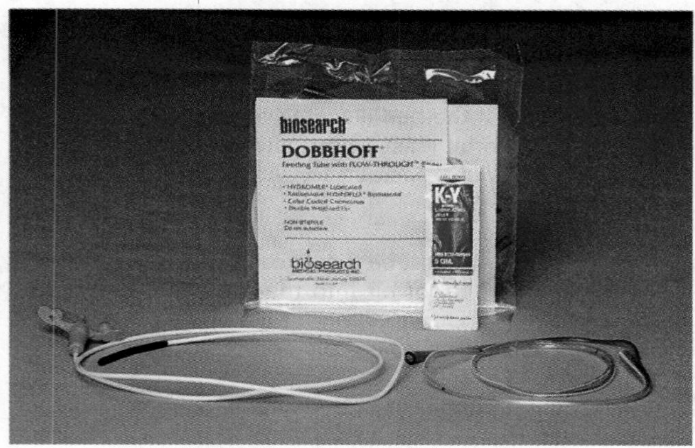


**fig. 41-22** Typical small-bore feeding tube.

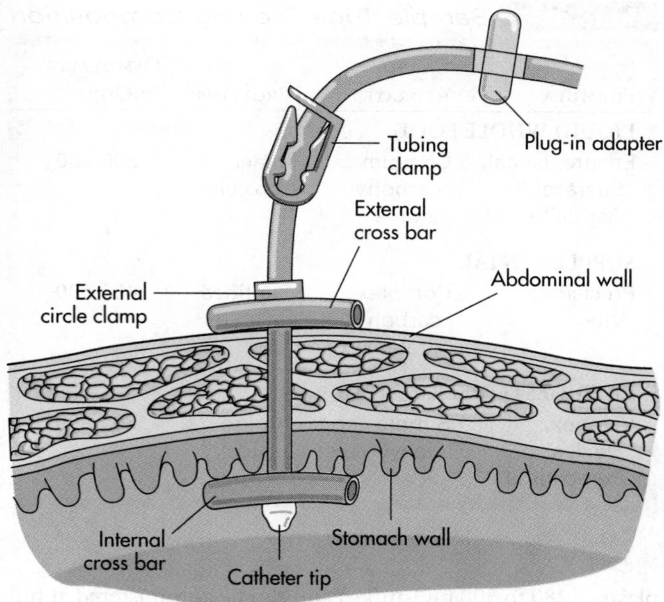


**fig. 41-23** A percutaneous endoscopic gastrostomy (PEG) tube in place in the stomach.

rapid method of creating a gastrostomy. It is performed via endoscopy and local anesthesia. A small incision is made on the skin of the abdomen, and a cannula is pushed through the abdominal and gastric walls into the stomach while the site is observed through a gastroscope. A long suture is threaded through the cannula, grasped, and pulled up through the endoscope, which is then removed. A specially prepared catheter is attached to the suture thread, and the catheter is then pulled back through the esophagus and stomach and out the abdominal wall. Internal and external dams hold the catheter in place. A jejunostomy tube may be inserted by a similar method (Figure 41-23).

The catheter used to create a gastrostomy usually is large in diameter (18 to 24 F). A Foley catheter can be used, which allows the balloon to serve as an anchor against the stomach wall. PEG tubes are smaller (12 to 16 F) and usually are anchored by a 1- to 2-inch cross-linked latex tube placed inside the stomach. A dressing is not generally used. Keeping the site open helps to prevent skin laceration, breakdown, and infection. The skin around the gastrostomy may be cleaned with hydrogen peroxide solution to remove crusts and rinsed with normal saline or water.

An alternate type of gastrostomy that does not require a tube and therefore lessens the chance of complications from tube irritation or obstruction may be used in certain situations. This "button" gastrostomy is constructed by making a small tube from the wall of the stomach and then pushing it in to form an intussusception valve. The "valve" is brought out flush with the skin surface to create a flat stoma. The valve prevents leakage of stomach contents; therefore no skin care or dressings are needed. A tube is inserted through the valve for feedings. The stoma can be closed at a later date.

### Enteral Feeding Solutions

Many types of feeding solutions are available to meet the multiple and diverse needs of patient populations. All formulas contain the essential nutrients, but they differ in the balance of nutrients as well as in the amount of digestion and absorption that is required to utilize them.

Protein usually is considered to be the most critical component of any formula. The solution may contain intact nutrients and resemble a purėed diet, but these products require normal levels of pancreatic enzymes to break down the protein for absorption. Formulas also may contain hydrolyzed proteins derived from meat, soy, and lactalbumin. These proteins have been predigested to dipeptides and free amino acids and do not require further digestion. GI absorption must be intact, however. Crystalline amino acid formulas are composed of amino acids that require no digestion and readily transport across the intestinal mucosa for easy absorption.

The major concerns in the carbohydrate content of feeding solutions relate to lactose content and total calorie needs. Increasing awareness of the pervasiveness of partial lactose intolerance has stimulated the development of formulas without a milk base. Carbohydrates in standard formulas are easily used as long as intestinal absorption remains intact. Components include starch and polysaccharides, disaccharides, and monosaccharides. Effective carbohydrate use also depends on the person having adequate amounts of insulin, glucagon, norepinephrine, and vitamins. Any imbalance or deficiency in these elements can impair absorption and produce watery diarrhea.

Fats in the formula provide a source for concentrated calories and essential fatty acids and serve as a carrier for fat-soluble vitamins. Fat digestion depends on pancreatic enzymes, bile salts, and normal intestinal flora. Short-, medium-, and long-chain fatty acids may be included in both saturated and polyunsaturated forms.

Caloric density (the number of calories per unit volume) is an extremely important consideration. High-density formulas tend to be more hypertonic and may contribute to diarrhea. Lower-density formulas require a larger volume of solution to provide needed nutrients, which may be an issue if fluids must be restricted.

Osmolality is another essential consideration for enteral solutions. Isotonic formulas approximate the osmolality of

**table 41-7** *Sample Tube Feeding Composition*

| Formula | Carbohydrate | Proteins | Osmolality (mOsm) |
|---|---|---|---|
| **LIQUID WHOLE FOOD** | | | |
| Ensure, Isocal, Sustacal, Osmolite | Complex carbohydrates | Intact proteins | 300-600 |
| **SUPPLEMENTAL** | | | |
| Precision, Vital | Complex carbohydrates | Peptides | 450-600 |
| **PREDIGESTED/ELEMENTAL** | | | |
| Vivonex, Flexical, Pregestimil | Simple carbohydrates | Amino acids | 500-800 |

plasma (280 to 300 mOsm/kg) and can be administered at full strength with the rate adjusted to patient tolerance. Adequate amounts of hypotonic fluids such as water are also essential to maintain the desired osmolality. The osmolality of enteral solutions is primarily a reflection of the concentration of proteins and carbohydrates. Hypertonic formulas typically have osmolalities ranging from 400 to 1100 mOsm/kg and need to be diluted initially or administered at an extremely slow rate until patient tolerance increases. Formulas with simple (predigested) proteins often have a higher osmolality, and patients receiving them need careful monitoring. Table 41-7 compares the various components of a few sample formulas. All formulas are supplemented with substantial quantities of essential vitamins and minerals.

### Enteral Feeding Techniques

Feeding schedules may be planned on a continuous, intermittent, or bolus basis. Continuous feedings are used for most short-term nutrition support situations because the volume of fluid delivered can be kept very low, which increases patient tolerance. This is ideal for nasointestinal delivery since the small intestine normally receives nutrients from the stomach in small volumes over several hours after a meal. Intermittent or bolus scheduling would significantly increase the risk of dumping syndrome and diarrhea. When long-term support is planned, an intermittent schedule with delivery of the feeding to the stomach best replicates a normal eating pattern. It also permits the patient to be free of the tube feeding for intervals throughout the day. Clinical decisions are based on the unique patient circumstances.

Residual volumes are checked before each intermittent feeding and at specified intervals, usually at least once a day, for patients receiving continuous feedings. Most institution protocols provide for holding an intermittent feeding if the residual is greater than 100 to 150 ml. Lower parameters are set for gastrostomies. With continuous feedings a residual of two times the amount of feeding delivered over the last hour would prompt a notification of the physician. Consensus does not exist over whether the aspirated fluid should be refed to the patient, although this is frequently recommended. The bag and tubing are thoroughly washed after each intermittent feeding and are discarded every 24 to 48 hours per institutional policy. Care of the patient receiving an enteral feeding is summarized in the Guidelines for Care Box.

**guidelines for care**

**The Person Receiving Enteral Tube Feedings**

Keep the head of the bed elevated at least 30° during all feedings and for at least 1 hour after discontinuation.
- Use high Fowler's position for intermittent feedings if permitted.

Verify tube placement.
- Check the length of tube that protrudes from the nose.
- Inject 10 to 30 ml of air into the tube and auscultate over the left upper quadrant of the abdomen.
- Aspirate secretions if possible and check the pH of the aspirate.
- Check the volume of the residual against ordered parameters.
- Refeed aspirated fluid per institution protocol.

Flush tube with 30 to 50 ml of water before initiating and at the end of the feeding or every 4 hours for continuous feedings.

Always flush the tube before and after medication administration.

Verify rate settings on the delivery pump.

Ensure that the tube is properly and securely taped and check for the presence of nasal irritation.

Record all administered volumes and residuals, including irrigation fluids, on intake and output records.

Cleanse delivery equipment after each use and discard per institution protocol (usually 24 to 48 hours).

**Intermittent (Bolus) Feedings**

Attach syringe to feeding tube.
- Elevate syringe 18 inches above the patient's head.
- Fill syringe with formula.
- Allow feeding to empty by gravity.
- Keep syringe filled to avoid infusion of air.

#### Managing complications

**Tube obstruction.** Feeding tube obstructions are relatively common problems. Pill fragments, formula residue adhering to the tube lumen, and formula/medication incompatibilities are common causes. The Guidelines for Care Box on the next page summarizes strategies to prevent tube clogging.

**Regurgitation/aspiration.** Pulmonary complications are the most dangerous problems associated with enteral feedings. A tube of any size may enter the tracheobronchial tree on insertion or migrate there with vigorous coughing or suctioning. Patients who are obtunded and have impaired cough or gag reflexes are at particular risk.

No method except chest x-ray is foolproof in verifying correct tube placement. Most institutions use several tests of tube placement. Proper taping of the tube to secure it in position and verifying the external length of the tube should be routinely performed. Instilling a small amount of air while si-

## guidelines for care

### Preventing Feeding Tube Obstruction

Use a polyurethane feeding tube if possible.

Flush the tube with at least 30 ml of water every 4 hours; do this before and after administering medications and before and after checking gastric residual volumes.

Use a controller pump to maintain a steady flow.

Administer all medications with care.

- Do not administer medications with the tube feeding running. Always flush first.
- Do not administer any enteric-coated, chewable, or sublingual drugs through the tube. Obtain liquid forms of medications if possible.
- Do not crush slow-release tablets. The beads from slow-release capsules may be flushed through the tube if size permits.
- Crush all tablets thoroughly into a fine powder. Do not open the package before crushing. Mix with 15 to 100 ml of water before administering.
- Time the administration of antacids around the other medications.
- Administer each drug separately; do not combine.
- Stop feedings for 15 to 30 minutes before administration if a drug needs to be given on an empty stomach.

Irrigate clogged tubes with water. If this is ineffective, Viokase or a declogging stylus may be used per institution policy. There is no evidence that cranberry juice is effective, and water is as effective as cola products.

multaneously auscultating the abdomen is a recommended test of tube placement even though sounds are readily transmitted throughout the abdomen, and this does not guarantee that the tube is located where the sounds are heard. Aspirating tube contents is more accurate, and pH testing of the aspirate can help to verify accurate placement (Research Box). However, small bore tubes often collapse easily, making aspiration difficult or impossible. The head of the bed is kept elevated 30 to 40° at all times if possible to decrease the risk of aspiration. The use of nasointestinal tubes with weighted tips for patients at risk for aspiration appears to decrease the incidence of reflux (Research Box).

**Diarrhea.** Diarrhea is the most commonly encountered complication of enteral feedings, and it may be caused by a variety of factors. Diarrhea may be directly related to the formula in use. Formulas with lactose, high-fat content, or low-fiber content have been implicated in the development of diarrhea. High osmolality also appears to be important, particularly with severely malnourished patients. Strategies may include the use of bulking agents, slow delivery rates, and formula dilution during the initial administration period.

It is essential that dehydration be prevented through adequate amounts of free water. The greater the formula's osmolality the more water is needed. Diarrhea may also be related to prescribed medications, such as antibiotics, H2-receptor antagonists, and elixirs containing sorbitol.

## research

Reference: Metheny N, Reed L, Berglund B, Wehrle MA: Visual characteristics of aspirates from feeding tubes as a method for predicting tube location, *Nurs Res* 43(5):282-287, 1994.

The purpose of this study was to describe the visual characteristics of aspirates from feeding tubes and determine the extent to which these characteristics can be used in determining feeding tube location. Fluid was aspirated from 880 feeding tubes, half from the stomach and half from the intestine. Eight samples were drawn from tubes that had inadvertently been placed in the respiratory tract. From this sample the researchers drew up a list of visual characteristics for each type of aspirate.

Professional color photographs were taken of 50 gastric and 50 intestinal aspirates and 6 respiratory aspirates. A convenience sample of 30 experienced critical care nurses was asked to predict tube location for each photograph based on the visual characteristics. They were then asked to go through the photographs again, classifying the samples with the aid of the list of visual characteristics prepared by the researchers. Correct classification was less than 70% on the uncued trial but rose to more than 90% with the aid of the list of aspirate characteristics. Aspirates from the respiratory tract could not be correctly classified with either method. The study concluded that visual characteristics can be useful in differentiating gastric from intestinal aspirates but should not be used as the main criteria for verifying tube placement. They are most useful when combined with pH measurements. Visual characteristics have little value in differentiating between GI and respiratory secretions.

## research

Reference: Mateo MA: Nursing management of enteral tube feedings, *Heart Lung* 25(4):318-323, 1996.

The purpose of this study was to describe the care provided to patients with enteral tube feedings. An investigator-developed questionnaire was distributed to a convenience sample of 235 acute and critical care nurses at a major medical center. The instrument contained questions about (1) checking the flow rate of feedings, (2) flushing the tube, (3) unclogging obstructed tubes, (4) checking residual volumes, and (5) administering medications.

The study found that there was a wide range in practice within this one institution. Frequency of rate checking ranged from 1 to 12 hours, and tubes were routinely flushed with sterile water, tap water, and saline. Flushing was used to attempt to unclog obstructed tubes and solutions in use included sterile water, carbonated beverages, and papain. Repositioning the tube and the use of air boluses were also reported. Residual volumes were checked fairly routinely every 4 hours, but half of the nurses reported discarding the residual and half readministered it. Tubes were consistently flushed after medication administration, but only half the nurses flushed tubes before administration and only 38% reported flushing between the administration of multiple medications.

Malnutrition, particularly hypoalbuminemia, is associated with a decrease in intestinal absorption and can contribute to diarrhea. This problem is corrected as the patient's nutritional status is improved, but it may require formula readjustment or direct replenishment of the serum albumin.

Bacterial contamination is a significant cause of diarrhea. Formula can become contaminated at any point in the preparation and delivery process. Formulas with higher osmolalities appear to be less likely to support bacterial growth. The length of time the formula hangs at room temperature also is a factor. Hospital-prepared formulas that contain milk are the most vulnerable. The Guidelines for Care Box summarizes measures to help reduce the risk of bacterial contamination of formula.

**Hyperglycemia.** Hyperglycemia may become a problem for patients who are receiving high-caloric density formulas and especially those taking corticosteroids. Elderly persons are at increased risk. Blood glucose monitoring may be used, and administration of sliding-scale insulin may be necessary.

## PARENTERAL NUTRITION

Parenteral nutrition (TPN) is a method of giving highly concentrated solutions intravenously to maintain a patient's nutritional balance when oral or enteral nutrition is not possible. TPN is indicated for patients when the GI tract is not functioning as a result of obstruction, acute inflammation, or malabsorption. It is also used for patients who are hypermetabolic from trauma or sepsis, who need to be given nothing by mouth for more than 5 to 7 days, who are unable to take adequate nutrients by mouth, and who experience severe side effects from radiation therapy or chemotherapy.[17] The increased recognition of the importance of adequate nutrition for healing has caused physicians to use parenteral nutrition as a therapeutic tool early in the management process.[17]

Parenteral nutrition is commonly administered through the central venous route, but it can be administered by peripheral vein as well. Peripheral solutions differ primarily in their glucose content, which generally does not exceed 10% because strongly hypertonic solutions can be extremely irritating to the peripheral veins. The peripheral solutions rely more on isotonic lipid emulsions as the main nonprotein calorie source. TPN usually is selected when a patient is expected to need extensive nutritional support over an extended period.

> **guidelines for care**
>
> **Preventing Bacterial Contamination of Tube Feeding Formulas**
>
> Use prefilled, ready-to-use sets if available.
> Follow strict aseptic technique in handling all components; good hand washing is essential.
> Use full-strength ready-to-use formula; dilution and reconstitution increase the chances of contamination.
> Rinse the delivery set with water before adding new formula.
> Hang commercially prepared formulas for no more than 8 to 12 hours (hospital-prepared formulas for no more than 6 hours).

### Central Venous Catheters

A variety of options exist for the delivery of TPN solutions. Central venous catheters allow for rapid mixing and dilution of strongly hypertonic solutions. Subclavian, tunneled, and implantable port catheters are available in single-lumen and multilumen forms. Central venous catheters and venous access devices are discussed and illustrated in Chapter 11. Infection is the primary concern related to the administration of TPN. It is believed that catheter contamination at the point of entry into the skin and migration of bacteria along the catheter are the major sources of TPN sepsis. Rigorous dressing care is essential, but there are wide variations in institutional protocols. Research is ongoing to determine the optimal interval for dressing changes and the effectiveness of the various dressing materials.

### Total Parenteral Nutrition

TPN solutions are complex formulas that provide all the known essential nutrients in quantities that will support wound healing, anabolism, weight gain or maintenance, and growth in children. All TPN solutions contain water, protein, carbohydrates, fat, vitamins, and trace elements. The various proportions of each element are individualized to the patient's unique clinical situation and needs.

Solutions used to deliver TPN usually consist of 25% to 35% dextrose, 3% to 5% amino acids, electrolytes, minerals, and vitamins. Intravenous fat emulsions in 10% to 20% concentrations also may be added. Dextrose and fat are given for their caloric value. The body uses them to meet its energy needs. This permits the administered amino acids to be utilized for anabolism. Fat provides twice the caloric value of dextrose, exerts minimal osmotic pressure, and prevents fatty acid deficiency. Regular insulin may be added to the solution or administered subcutaneously to support glucose utilization.

TPN solutions provide good culture media for bacteria. They are therefore prepared under strict aseptic conditions in the pharmacy under a laminar airflow hood. The solutions are kept refrigerated until ready for use and are left at room temperature for 30 minutes before administration. Prepared formulas ideally should be used within 24 hours to prevent contamination, but institutional protocols may vary slightly.

Solutions of TPN are initiated slowly and advanced as patient tolerance permits. Blood glucose levels are checked frequently at the beginning of treatment while endogenous insulin production adjusts to the increased glucose load. A steady infusion rate is ensured through the use of a pump controller. If TPN administration needs to be interrupted for any reason, infusions of 10% dextrose should be administered to prevent rebound hypoglycemia. TPN administration is gradually tapered before it is discontinued. Lipid emulsions may be mixed with the TPN solution, given through a separate peripheral IV line or through a Y connector in the main IV line.

The use of a 0.22-$\mu$m filter is recommended for administering all TPN solutions, but if lipids are also administered their large molecules require the use of a filter of at least 1.2 $\mu$m or larger. The effectiveness of filters in reducing the risk of bacterial contamination remains unproved, but they will trap crystals and air from the solution and tubing.[48]

#### Preventing complications

Complications of TPN include problems with the catheter, infection, and metabolic imbalances. Correct insertion and placement of the catheter are extremely important. Proper insertion prevents most problems related to pneumothorax or hemothorax, air embolism, brachial plexus injury, and thromboembolism.

Infection is a serious complication of TPN that cannot always be prevented. Strict aseptic technique during catheter insertion and subsequent care is essential. Vital signs are taken regularly, and the insertion site is monitored for tenderness, redness, and drainage. The onset of sepsis may be preceded by the development of unexplained hyperglycemia.

The major metabolic alteration associated with the use of TPN is glucose intolerance. Blood glucose levels must be carefully monitored through finger sticks. Insulin may be added to the TPN solution or administered on a sliding scale if needed. Severe osmotic diuresis can result from uncontrolled hyperglycemia and can lead rapidly to dehydration. Hypoglycemia is also a potential problem when the patient is being weaned from TPN or whenever the continuous infusion of solution is interrupted for any reason.

Other possible complications associated with TPN include fluid imbalances, electrolyte imbalances, and acid-base imbalances (primarily acidosis). Vitamin D deficiency and vitamin A excess also may occur. Serum electrolyte levels are monitored several times a week. Carbohydrate metabolism yields water and carbon dioxide. The increased production of carbon dioxide caused by concentrated glucose solutions can induce respiratory distress in patients with compromised pulmonary status. Abnormalities in liver function may also occur when patients receive high volumes of carbohydrate calories. The body converts the calories into intrahepatic fat, which results in liver dysfunction.

Directions for care of the patient receiving parenteral nutrition are summarized in the Guidelines for Care Box.

### Home IV Therapy

The administration of IV therapy in the home has expanded rapidly in the last decade as acute care facilities have worked aggressively to adapt high-techology interventions to the home setting. The cost savings can be dramatic. Antibiotics, hydration, and parenteral nutrition are the most common interventions. They may be a continuation of care initiated in a hospital or be initiated in the outpatient setting. To qualify for insurance or Medicare coverage these interventions must usually be long term rather than of short duration. See Box 41-9 for sample Medicare requirements.

Home administration of TPN has enabled thousands of patients to remain in their homes and out of the acute care

**guidelines for care**

### The Patient Receiving Parenteral Nutrition

If possible, do not use the TPN catheter for other purposes.

#### Preventing Infection

Maintain strict aseptic technique.

Keep solutions cold until ready for use, but allow solution to warm to room temperature before administration; use solutions within 24 to 36 hours.

—All additions to TPN solutions should be performed in laminar flow areas.

Change dressing according to institutional protocol.

—Follow strict aseptic technique in handling catheter, dressing, tubing, and solution.

Change administration sets every 24 hours or by institution protocol.

Monitor for signs of redness, swelling, or drainage at insertion site.

—Suspect sepsis if afebrile patient develops a fever.

#### Preventing Air Embolism

Tape all connections securely.

Clamp catheter before opening system.

Cover subclavian catheter insertion site with an air-occlusive dressing (covered with adhesive tape) or transparent polyurethane (Op-site) dressing.

Position patient as flat as possible for dressing and tubing changes.

Instruct patient to perform Valsalva's maneuver whenever catheter hub is open to the air.

#### Maintaining Fluid and Electrolyte Balance

Maintain a uniform infusion rate. Never abruptly discontinue solution administration.

- Use a pump for controlled delivery rates.
- Never exceed prescribed rate of administration; do not attempt to "catch up" if infusion falls behind schedule.
- Monitor for signs of *overhydration* (neck vein distention, cough, weight gain):
  - Weigh patient daily.
  - Record accurate intake and output.

#### Preventing Metabolic Imbalance

Monitor and report to physician signs of *hypoglycemia* (pallor, diaphoresis, tachycardia, hunger, trembling, behavioral changes):

- Administer 10% glucose solution if TPN must be interrupted for any reason

Monitor for signs of *hyperglycemia* (nausea, weakness, thirst, headache, rapid respirations):

- Check finger-stick blood glucose as ordered (every 6 hours initially and every day once stable).
- Administer sliding scale insulin as ordered.

#### Promoting Comfort

Provide for good oral hygiene.

Encourage ambulation and activities of daily living.

Monitor for "refeeding syndrome" when TPN is initiated (first 24 to 48 hours).

- Symptoms include respiratory depression, lethargy, confusion, and weakness.
- Syndrome results from the abrupt shift of electrolytes from the plasma to the intracellular compartment.

**box 41-9** *Sample Medicare Criteria for Home IV Therapy*

The patient must be homebound; i.e., unable to leave the home for work, shopping, or other self-care activities.
The planned TPN therapy must be at least 90 days in length.
TPN must be the patient's sole source of nutrition.
Documentation must exist that the patient is unable to absorb nutrition from the enteral route.

NOTE: Coverage is provided by Medicare Part B—Durable Medical Equipment Benefit.

setting. Advanced inflammatory bowel disease is the most common medical indication, but acquired immunodeficiency syndrome (AIDS) and cancer are other common diagnoses. Cost constraints put significant pressure on patients and families to learn to safely administer the TPN without the ongoing supervision of a home health nurse. In addition, with a well-structured teaching plan most families are able to successfully provide the needed care.

A nutrition-support team, if available, usually initiates the educational process before the patient's discharge. The nurse typically coordinates the home care team, which may include the physician, dietitian, social worker, pharmacist, and counselor or psychiatrist. Successful management demands a team approach. Patient teaching includes basic information about TPN; discussion about symptoms, problems, and complications; and practical planning concerning the acquisition of equipment, location and storage of supplies, and special telephone service to cover emergencies. A sample teaching plan for home TPN is outlined in the Patient/Family Teaching Box.

Recognizing and managing complications is another important aspect of the care plan. Common TPN complications and their management are outlined in Table 41-8. The nurse also needs to offer support and encouragement to the patient and family. Home TPN is a demanding therapy that requires a major time commitment. It is easy for caregivers to feel isolated and alone with the demands of the task.

Documentation is always a crucial issue in home care. Standard Medicare reimbursement is limited to 2 to 3 weeks of intermittent visits. Ongoing professional involvement by the home care nurse depends on clear documentation of exceptional circumstances that support the need for continued care.

## ANORECTAL DISORDERS

A variety of common disorders can affect the perianal area. Persons who experience anorectal disorders typically seek medical care for symptoms such as pain, tenderness, itching, or the development of rectal bleeding. Many of the disorders can be treated on an outpatient basis.

**patient/family teaching**

**Sample Teaching Plan for Home Total Parenteral Nutrition**

Review purpose and procedures for the home TPN regimen.
Validate presence of detailed written instructions for each procedure and piece of equipment.
Validate understanding of all home equipment:
- Provide additional instruction as needed inasmuch as equipment and supplies used in the hospital frequently differ from those available through home health care.

Validate aseptic technique and skills.
Evaluate adequacy of home refrigeration and supply storage.
Teach patient/family about ordering replacement supplies.
Establish record-keeping system for body weights, temperatures, finger sticks, and sliding-scale insulin if ordered.
Reinforce importance of aseptic technique and safe disposal of equipment.
Discuss troubleshooting of common equipment problems.
Review symptoms related to infection, air embolism, and other complications; provide written instructions of actions to be taken in the event of a complication.
Provide list of emergency telephone numbers.

## HEMORRHOIDS

### Etiology/Epidemiology

Hemorrhoids are masses of dilated blood vessels that lie beneath the lining of the skin in the anal canal. They are extremely common and estimated to be present in up to 50% of the population by age 50.[31] Hemorrhoids affect persons of all ages, but they typically cause more problems with increasing age. Pregnancy is a common condition for initiating or aggravating hemorrhoids. Other conditions associated with the development of hemorrhoids include obesity, congestive heart failure, and chronic liver disease, which results in portal hypertension. These conditions are all associated with persistent elevations in intraabdominal pressure. Sedentary occupations that involve long periods of sitting or standing also are implicated, although the exact mechanism is not known.

Hemorrhoids usually are classified into two types. Those that occur above the anal sphincter are termed *internal hemorrhoids* and those that occur below the anal sphincter are termed *external hemorrhoids* (Figure 41-24). Internal hemorrhoids are further classified by size, since size determines both the nature and severity of symptoms and the appropriate management.[31] A person can have both forms of hemorrhoids at the same time. Although hemorrhoids usually are a chronic health problem, they may cause acute episodes.

### Pathophysiology

Hemorrhoids traditionally have been viewed as varicose veins of the rectum. The superior hemorrhoidal veins contain no valves

**table 41-8** *Potential Problems of Home Total Parenteral Nutrition*

General Guidelines to Prevent Home TPN Problems:
- Wash hands thoroughly before any procedures.
- Wear gloves for all procedures, particularly if cuts, scrapes, or rashes are present on the hands.
- Keep all supplies dry and sterile during storage.
- Use aseptic technique for any procedures.

| Problem | Symptoms | Patient Instructions |
|---|---|---|
| Possible leak in internal catheter | Swelling of skin over catheter insertion site; sensations of pain, heat, burning near site | Call home health nurse or physician.<br>Do not use catheter to give fluids.<br>Tape the catheter securely to the skin so that it does not dangle.<br>Avoid rough contact or sports that could dislodge catheter. |
| Possible loose cap or leak in external catheter | Leak of blood from injection cap or catheter | Clamp catheter.<br>Change cap and heparin lock.<br>Call physician or go to emergency room for catheter repair. |
| Water intoxication | Puffy eyes, neck vein distention, increased urination, confusion | Contact physician and go to emergency room for laboratory tests. |
| Possible air embolism—air may be drawn into the vein if catheter is not clamped during cap change | Cough, shortness of breath, chest pain | If giving fluids, stop and place heparin lock on catheter.<br>Lie on left side.<br>Call physician or go to emergency room. |
| Skin infection or irritation | Redness, swelling, drainage, tenderness at exit site | Call home health nurse or physician.<br>Change bandage and clean daily. |
| Possible infection within the bloodstream | Chills, fever, fatigue, aches, weakness, hyperglycemia | Change the bandage and clean around the catheter if bandage gets wet or soiled.<br>Go to emergency room for tests. |

and are vulnerable to overdistention when the person is in an upright position. Additional studies have documented that hemorrhoids actually are composed of spongy vascular tissue or "cushions" with multiple direct arteriovenous connections.

External hemorrhoids are seen most often in young and middle-aged adults and can be detected by the affected person. The classic "skin tag" consists of small lumps of fibrous tissue and folds of anal skin that have been stretched by bulging of the hemorrhoids. They rarely bleed and only become truly symptomatic when they become thrombosed or rupture subcutaneously with hematoma formation. A thrombosed external hemorrhoid may occur suddenly after vigorous exercise or after a severe episode of diarrhea or constipation. The intense pain accompanying thrombosis is caused by the presence of multiple sensory nerve endings in the epithelial tissue that composes the hemorrhoid. Bluish skin-covered lumps are readily visible in the anal region.

Internal hemorrhoids are usually asymptomatic. Excessive engorgement and prolapse occur, but painless rectal bleeding is their most common feature. The person may notice spotting on the toilet tissue or occasional episodes of spurts of blood that accompany straining at stool. Although the blood loss typically is small, it can deplete iron reserves if it persists over a long period. Pain, which can be excruciating, occurs with prolapse and thrombosis.

Hemorrhoids of both types are basically asymptomatic unless complications occur. Routinely painful defecation accompanied by rectal bleeding is associated with anal fissure more

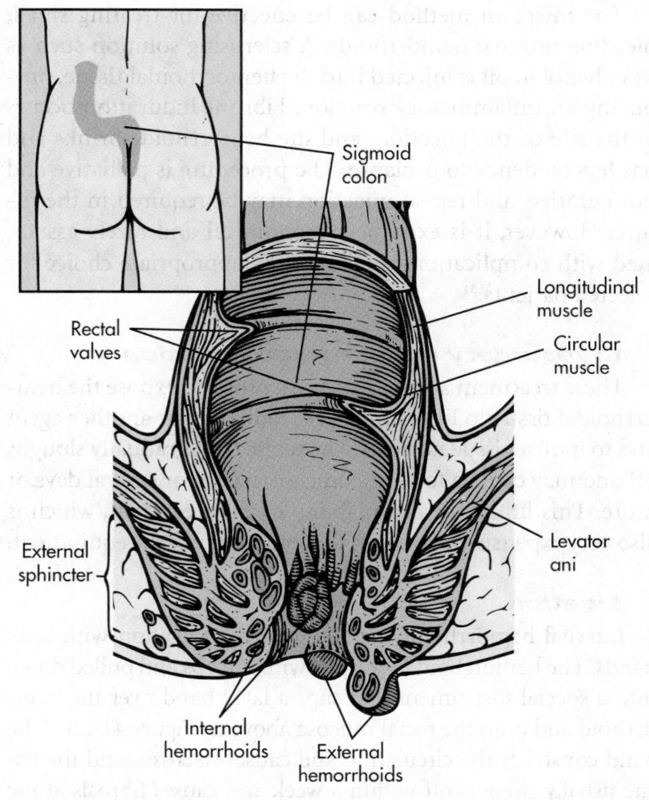


**fig. 41-24** Internal and external hemorrhoids.

often than with uncomplicated hemorrhoids. Perianal itching may occur with higher grade internal hemorrhoids, but other causes should also be explored. If a painful episode has occurred, the patient may develop problems with constipation in an effort to prevent pain or bleeding associated with defecation.

## Collaborative Care Management

The diagnosis of hemorrhoids is fairly straightforward. The person's presenting symptoms establish the initial diagnosis, which usually can be confirmed by inspection and digital palpation. Proctoscopy may be used to confirm the diagnosis, and middle-aged or older patients who are experiencing rectal bleeding may undergo colonoscopy to rule out cancer.

Both forms of hemorrhoids can be managed conservatively if the symptoms are not severe. Conservative management includes a high-fiber diet, bulk laxatives, warm sitz baths, and gentle cleansing. If severe pain, bleeding, or thrombosis are present, however, more definitive management may be indicated. A variety of options have been used over time including sclerotherapy, cryotherapy, bipolar diathermy, rubber band ligation, and surgical hemorrhoidectomy. Currently grades 2 and 3 internal hemorrhoids are treated by rubber band ligation and complicated grades 3 and 4 by surgery. Patients with prolapsed external hemorrhoids that are diagnosed promptly can be treated with scissors excision under local anesthesia. The wound is left open to heal by secondary intention. Complicated prolapses may require surgery.

### *Sclerotherapy*

The injection method can be effective for treating small, bleeding internal hemorrhoids. A sclerosing solution such as 5% phenol in oil is injected into the hemorrhoidal tissue, producing an inflammatory reaction. Fibrous induration occurs at the site of the injection, and the hemorrhoid shrinks and has less tendency to prolapse. The procedure is palliative and not curative, and repeat injection may be required in the future. However, it is extremely economical and rarely associated with complications, making it an appropriate choice for selected patients.[31]

### *Cryosurgery and photocoagulation*

These treatment approaches use a probe to expose the hemorrhoidal tissue to liquid nitrogen, radiation, or another agent and to induce tissue necrosis. The tissue then gradually sloughs off and may cause a foul-smelling discharge for several days or more. This limits the acceptability of the treatment, which is also very expensive because of the complexity of the equipment.

### *Ligation*

Internal hemorrhoids may be treated by ligation with latex bands. The hemorrhoid is grasped with forceps and pulled down into a special instrument that slips a latex band over the hemorrhoid and onto the rectal mucosa above it (Figure 41-25). The band constricts the circulation and causes necrosis, and the tissue usually sloughs off within a week and causes fibrosis at the site. An enema is given before the treatment to prevent a bowel movement for 24 hours and thus prevent straining that would cause the band to break or slip off. Local discomfort is usually minimal and can be successfully relieved by aspirin or acetaminophen and the use of sitz baths.

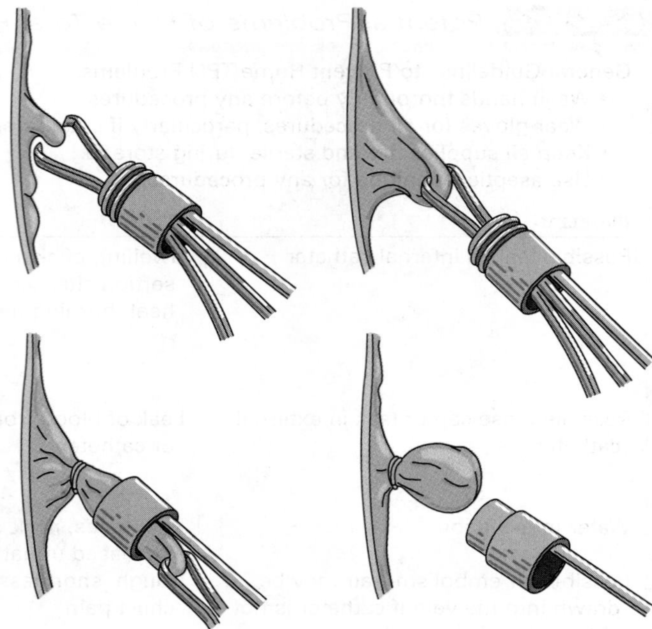

**fig. 41-25** Rubber band ligation of an internal hemorrhoid.

### *Hemorrhoidectomy*

Surgical excision (hemorrhoidectomy) is the treatment used for external or internal hemorrhoids that do not respond well to more conservative treatment or that must be treated on an emergency basis because of acute strangulation. The patient is often in extreme pain and may not be able to focus on the elements of preoperative teaching. Care of the patient after anorectal surgery is summarized in the Guidelines for Care Box.

### *Patient/family education*

Minor problems with hemorrhoids often can be successfully managed through a combination of strict personal hygiene and prevention of constipation and straining. The nurse encourages the patient to follow a high-residue diet rich in fruit and vegetable fiber. Bran may be added to ease stool passage. Liberal intake of fluids and regular exercise also are encouraged to promote normal bowel function. If necessary, a bulk-forming hydrophilic laxative may be added to the daily routine.

Local treatment promotes comfort during symptom flare-ups. The patient is instructed to apply ice, warm compresses, or analgesic ointments such as dibucaine (Nupercaine) to provide temporary relief from pain and reduce the edema around external or prolapsed internal hemorrhoids. Sitz baths also are extremely helpful in relieving pain. The nurse stresses the impor-

**guidelines for care**

### The Person Undergoing Anal/Rectal Surgery

**Preoperative Care**

Bowel preparation is standard, but an enema may not be prescribed if rectal pain is acute.

Stool softeners may be given to promote a soft stool before surgery.

**Postoperative Care**

***Promotion of comfort***

Administer analgesics as prescribed, especially before initial defecation (considerable rectal discomfort may be present).

Provide emotional support before and after first defecation.

Suggest side-lying position.

Provide sitz baths as ordered (monitor for hypotension secondary to dilation of pelvic blood vessels in early postoperative period).

***Promotion of elimination***

Administer prescribed stool softeners.

Encourage patient to defecate as soon as the inclination occurs (prevents strictures and preserves the normal anal lumen). Considerable anxiety is usually present.

Monitor for hypotension, dizziness, and faintness during first defecation.

If an enema must be given, use a small-bore rectal tube.

***Patient teaching***

Clean rectal area after each defecation until healing is complete (sitz bath is recommended).

Avoid constipation with a high-fiber diet, high-fluid intake, regular exercise, and regular time for defecation.

Use stool softeners until healing is complete.

Seek medical consultation for rectal bleeding, suppurative drainage, continued pain on defecation, or continued constipation despite preventive measures.

tance of good personal hygiene after defecation and thorough cleansing of the bath tubs or containers used for sitz baths.

## ANAL FISSURE, ABSCESS, AND FISTULA

### Etiology/Epidemiology

Anal fissures, fistulas, and abscesses are relatively common problems that develop from trauma or infection in the anorectal area. An anal fissure is an elongated laceration between the anal canal and the perianal skin. Fissures may be primary or secondary. Most primary fissures are idiopathic. Secondary fissures are associated with chronic constipation and the passage of hard stool, trauma, or the presence of chronic ulceration from inflammatory bowel disease. An anal abscess results most often from the obstruction of gland ducts in the anorectal region by feces, but they also may complicate the presence of a fissure. Stasis of duct contents results in acute infection that can spread to adjacent tissue. An anal fistula involves the development of an abnormal communication between the anal canal and skin outside the anus. The rupture and drainage from chronic infection of an abscess frequently causes an anal fistula.

**table 41-9** *Treatment Options for Anal Fissure, Abscess, and Fistula*

| Lesion | Clinical Manifestations | Medical Management |
|---|---|---|
| Fissure | | |
| Slitlike ulceration in epithelium of anal canal | Pain with defecation; bleeding; pruritus; constipation | Stool softeners; analgesic ointments; sitz bath; sphincterotomy or fissurectomy if medical therapy ineffective |
| Abscess | | |
| Abscess in tissue around anus | Persistent throbbing; anal pain with walking, sitting, defecation; systemic signs of infection | Incision and drainage of abscess |
| Fistula | | |
| Hollow track leading through anal tissue from anorectal canal through skin near anus | Purulent discharge near anus; pain; pruritus | Fistulotomy or fistulectomy |

### Pathophysiology

Most acute anal fissures are superficial and heal spontaneously or in response to conservative therapy. If healing does not occur, however, the fissure may cause significant bleeding or become infected. The infection of an abscess may be relatively minor and confined to a single rectal crypt or become widespread. Widespread infection or sepsis may develop in patients with immunodeficiencies. The development of a fistula may necessitate extensive surgical repair.

Pain is the primary problem associated with anal fissure and abscess. It can be severe and prolonged from pressure on the somatic nerves in the perianal area. Any position can be painful as the pain often is reflected. Constipation is inevitable because the patient attempts to avoid pain by preventing defecation. Local swelling, erythema, and acute tenderness accompany abscess development. Pruritus in the anal region frequently accompanies both fissure and fistula. When a fistula is present, the patient notices periodic purulent drainage, which stains undergarments.

### Collaborative Care Management

The degree of medical intervention necessary for anal fissures, abscesses, and fistulas depends on the exact nature and severity of the problem. Medical treatment options are outlined in Table 41-9. Initial nursing interventions for anal disorders focus on improving the patient's comfort level. This may include analgesics, sitz baths, and the local application of heat, cold, or astringent preparations such as witch hazel. These interventions also are important if the patient is undergoing surgical excision or repair. The repair of fistulas is technically more involved, and nursing interventions focus on restoring and maintaining skin integrity and ensuring adequate nutrition for healing.

#### *Patient/family education*

Patient education focuses on the prevention of recurrences. The nurse teaches the patient the importance of careful perianal hygiene and avoiding constipation. All standard measures are presented, including a diet rich in fiber, the selective addition of bran to the diet, adequate intake of fluids and exercise, and the use of stool softeners or bulk laxatives to prevent straining.

## *critical thinking* QUESTIONS

1 Ms. Butler has been in the hospital for more than 3 weeks. Her initial diagnosis was diverticulitis. However, she developed a perforation that led to peritonitis. While you were assisting her with a bath she asks why she became so sick and what will be done for her now. How could you best explain the complication of peritonitis and its treatment to her?

2 Jodi Washington is an 18-year-old first-year nursing student in whom ulcerative colitis has recently been diagnosed. She has lost 20 pounds in the last 8 weeks from persistent severe diarrhea, which occurs every 1 to 2 hours and causes occasional incontinence at night. She is fatigued and anorexic, but she desperately wants to continue with her education. What specific concerns would you anticipate that Jodi would have about her disease and treatment regimen? What modifications would you recommend that she make in her lifestyle to attempt to meet her goal? What resources would you refer her to?

3 You are Mr. Freeman's home health nurse and Mrs. Freeman calls you in a panic state. She tells you that Mr. Freeman's Groshong site is red and swollen. He has been running a fever of 101° F. What problem do you suspect, and what plan of action would you take to reduce their anxiety and address the problem?

## *chapter* SUMMARY

### COMMON BOWEL DYSFUNCTIONS

- Constipation refers to the passage of abnormally infrequent or hard stools. Although a wide variety of drug therapies exist, it is best managed by increasing dietary fibers, fluids, and exercise.
- Diarrhea refers to abnormally watery stools and may be caused by food allergies, GI infections, hypermetabolism, or malabsorption disorders. Medical treatment is aimed at correcting the underlying cause.

### ACUTE INFECTION/INFLAMMATION OF THE INTESTINES

- Appendicitis involves acute inflammation of the appendix. Its classic features include acute right lower quadrant abdominal pain and rebound tenderness at McBurney's point, anorexia, fever, and nausea.
- Peritonitis is an inflammation of the peritoneum. Loss of fluids into the peritoneal cavity leads to dehydration and shock; peristalsis may cease. Treatment consists of fluid replacement and antibiotic therapy; surgery may be necessary.
- Diverticular disease involves small outpouchings of the colon wall; diverticulitis is the associated inflammatory condition. It is related to chronic constipation and managed with a high-fiber diet and bulk laxatives. Surgical resection may be necessary.
- Parasitic infections of the intestine include amebiasis, giardiasis, and trichinosis. Treatment consists of appropriate antibiotics.

### INFLAMMATORY BOWEL DISEASE

- Ulcerative colitis primarily affects the rectum and left colon. Mucosal involvement is continuous and causes profuse diarrhea, which contains blood but rarely fat.
- Crohn's disease affects primarily the distal ileum but may occur anywhere in the GI tract. It involves all layers of the bowel and appears in scattered segmental sections. Fistulas and strictures are common. The frequent stools contain fat but rarely blood.
- Care of the patient with inflammatory bowel disease involves drug therapy with sulfasalazine and other antiinflammatory agents, comfort measures, and facilitation of coping.
- Total colectomy is curative for ulcerative colitis. Continent procedures that preserve the anal sphincter are used more commonly today than the traditional ileostomy.
- Surgery in Crohn's disease is used to treat strictures, fistulas, or perforation. The disease frequently recurs after surgery.

### INTESTINAL OBSTRUCTION

- Intestinal obstruction may result from inhibition of peristalsis (paralytic ileus) or from mechanical obstruction. Large amounts of fluid and electrolytes are lost from the circulation into the intestinal lumen, resulting in fluid and electrolyte imbalances and finally shock. Therapy consists of inserting an NG tube, restricting oral intake, and removing the source of obstruction, if possible. Surgery may be necessary.

### ABDOMINAL HERNIAS

- Hernias may occur in the inguinal, femoral, or umbilical areas. The treatment is surgical repair.

### COLORECTAL CANCER

- Risk factors for bowel cancer (the second most common form of cancer) are age 50 years or older; history of colon polyps or ulcerative colitis or a family history of colorectal cancer.
- Recommendations for early detection of colorectal cancer are not established. Options include digital rectal examination; occult blood stool test; sigmoidoscopy, and colonoscopy.
- Surgery for cancer of the colon and upper rectum usually consists of resection with anastomosis; cancer involving the lower rectum has traditionally involved abdominoperineal resection plus colostomy. Sphincter-sparing surgeries that avoid colostomy are being increasingly used for distal cancers.
- Care of the patient after bowel surgery includes breathing exercises to promote oxygenation, ensuring adequate fluid intake, monitoring for return of peristalsis, giving analgesics for pain, and teaching to avoid constipation.

- Types of ostomies include end stoma, loop stoma, and loop-end stoma.
- Care of a person with a colostomy or ileostomy includes preparing the person for the surgery, monitoring the stoma, promoting acceptance of body changes, teaching the person stoma care, and referring the person to community support services.
- A teaching plan for a person with an ostomy includes skin care, pouch care and changes, controlling odor, irrigation techniques, and supporting the patient's return to normal activities and sexuality.

## MALABSORPTION AND MALNUTRITION

- Malabsorption syndrome results from inadequate absorption of fat, protein, carbohydrates, and/or minerals in the small intestine. It can result from inflammatory diseases, allergic reactions, extensive GI surgery, pancreatic insufficiency, and failure of other GI organs. Diarrhea is the most common symptom.
- Tropical sprue is a malabsorption disorder that appears to have both nutritional and infectious origins; treatment consists of antibiotics and folic acid.
- Celiac disease results from an intolerance to gluten found in grains; treatment consists of a gluten-free diet.
- Adult lactase deficiency is the most common form of malabsorption in humans. Symptoms may be mild or severe.
- Protein-calorie malnutrition is an extremely common problem in acutely ill patients who cannot meet their daily nutrient needs.
- Persons with protein-calorie malnutrition may be fed orally, enterally, or parenterally.
- Tube feeding solutions differ in terms of carbohydrate or protein content, osmolality, consistency, palatability, and expense.
- TPN solutions are deposited into the superior vena cava. Less concentrated solutions can be given peripherally. Complications include infection, air embolism, electrolyte imbalances, overhydration, hyperglycemia, hypoglycemia, vitamin D deficiency, and vitamin A excess.
- Long-term TPN may be administered successfully in the home setting with careful teaching of the patient and caregiver.

## ANORECTAL DISORDERS

- Anorectal lesions include anal fissures, abscesses, fistulas, and hemorrhoids. Relief of discomfort may include measures to prevent constipation, analgesics, and sitz baths
- Care after anorectal surgery includes analgesics and sitz baths for comfort, stool softeners, and teaching to prevent constipation.

## References


1. Allison JE, Tekewa S, Ransom LJ, Adrain AL: A comparison of fecal occult blood tests for colorectal cancer screening, *N Engl J Med* 334(3):155-159, 1996.
2. Barnie DC, Currier J: What's that GI tube being used for? *RN* 58(8):45-48, 1995.
3. Belluzzi A, Brignola C, Campieri M, Pera A et al: Effect of an enteric coated fish oil preparation on relapses in Crohn's disease, *N Engl J Med* 334(24):1557-1560, 1996.
4. Bitton A, Peppercorn MA: Emergencies in inflammatory bowel disease, *Crit Care Clin* 11(2):513-527, 1995.
5. Bond JH, Volk EE, Wexner SD: Colorectal cancer: effective treatment, diligent follow-up, *Patient Care* 30(10):20-41, 1996.
6. Burris J, McGovern P: Mass colorectal cancer screening, *AAOHN J* 41(4):186-191, 1993.
7. Calkins BM, Mendelhoff AI: The epidemiology of idiopathic inflammatory bowel disease In Kirsner JB, Shorter RG, editors: *Inflammatory bowel disease,* Philadelphia, 1995, Lea & Febiger.
8. Catalano MF, Grace ND: Getting to the cause of rectal bleeding, *Patient Care* 30(19):32-59, 1996.
9. Deziel DJ, Swanstrom L, Turec K: Laparoscopy's changing state of the art, *Patient Care* 30(10):42-54, 1996.
10. Dominitz JA, McCormick LH, Rex DK: Colorectal cancer: latest approaches to prevention and screening, *Patient Care* 30(7):124-149, 1996.
11. Ellis DJ, Reinus JF: Lower intestinal hemorrhage, *Crit Care Clin* 11(2):369-387, 1995.
12. Farmer RG: Ulcerative colitis-clinical features, In Haubrich WS et al, editors: *Bockus gastroenterology,* ed 5, Philadelphia, 1995, WB Saunders.
13. Fazio VW: Surgery of the colon and rectum, *Am J Gastroenterol* 89(8):S106-S115, 1994.
14. Fazio VW: Ulcerative colitis—surgical management, In Haubrich WS et al, editors: *Bockus gastroenterology,* ed 5, Philadelphia, 1995, WB Saunders.
15. Fullwood A, Drossman DA: The relationship of psychiatric illness with gastrointestinal disease, *Annu Rev Med* 46:483-496, 1995.
16. Galloway SC, Graydon JE: Uncertainty, symptom distress and information needs after surgery for cancer of the colon, *Cancer Nurs* 19(2):112-117, 1996.
17. Gianino S, Seltzer R, Eisenberg P: The ABC's of TPN, *RN* 59(2):42-47, 1996.
18. Giovannucci E et al: Aspirin and the risk of colorectal cancer in women, *N Engl J Med* 333(10):609-614, 1995.
19. Gorbach SL: Infectious diarrhea and bacterial food poisoning, In Sleisenger MH, Fordtran JS, editors: *Gastrointestinal disease,* ed 5, Philadelphia, 1993, WB Saunders.
20. Hall GR et al: Managing constipation using a research based protocol, *Med Surg Nurs* 4(1):11-18, 1995.
21. Hamilton SR, Mocson BC: Ulcerative colitis—pathology. In Haubrich WS et al, editors: *Bockus gastroenterology,* ed 5, Philadelphia, 1995, WB Saunders.
22. Hanauer SB: Inflammatory bowel disease, *N Engl J Med* 334(13):841-846, 1996.
23. Kalser MH: Malabsorption syndromes—clinical features and evaluation. In Haubrich WS et al, editors: *Bockus gastroenterology,* ed 5, Philadelphia, 1995, WB Saunders.
24. Kinash RG, Fischer DG, Lukie BE, Carr TL: Coping patterns and related characteristics in patients with IBD, *Gastroenterol Nurs,* 15(8):9-16, 1993.
25. Livingstone AS, Sosa JL: Ileus and obstruction. In Haubrich WS et al, editors: *Bockus gastroenterology,* ed 5, Philadelphia, 1995, WB Saunders.
26. Mamel JJ: Clinical pharmacology of commonly used drugs in GI practice, part II, *Gastroenterol Nurs* 15(4):156-162, 1993.
27. Matarese LE: Rationale and efficacy of specialized enteral nutrition, *Nutr Clin Pract* 9(2):58-64, 1994.
28. Mateo MA: Nursing management of enteral tube feedings, *Heart Lung* 25(4):318-323, 1996.
29. Mayer RJ, Thomas P: Colon cancer: knowledge is power, *Harvard Health Lett* 20(12):4-6, 1995.
30. McConnell EA: Loosening the grip of intestinal obstruction, *Nursing* 24(3):34-41, 1994.
31. Metcalf A: Anorectal disorders, *Postgrad Med* 98(5):81, 1995.
32. Metheny N, Reed L, Berglund G, Wehrle MA: Visual characteristics of aspirates from feeding tubes as a method for predicting tube location, *Nurs Res* 43(5):282-287, 1994.

33. Meyers S: Crohn's disease—clinical features and diagnosis. In Haubrich WS et al, editors: *Bockus gastroenterology,* ed 5, Philadelphia, 1995, WB Saunders.
34. Pemberton JH, Phillips SF: Ileostomy and its alternatives. In Sleisenger MH, Fordtran JS, editors: *Gastrointestinal disease,* ed 5, Philadelphia, 1993, WB Saunders.
35. Penney C: Innovations in gastrointestinal diseases, *Practitioner* 238(10):694-699, 1994.
36. Powell DW. Approach to the patient with diarrhea. In Yamada T, editor: *Textbook of gastroenterology,* ed 2, Philadelphia, 1995, JB Lippincott.
37. Provenzale D et al: Health related quality of life after ileoanal pull through, *Gastroenterology* 113(1):7-14, 1997.
38. Ransohoff DF: The case for colorectal screening, *Hosp Pract* 29:25-32, 1994.
39. Rao SSC: Functional colonic and anorectal disorders, *Postgrad Med* 98(5):115-126, 1995.
40. Scott-Conner CEH: Current surgical management of inflammatory bowel disease, *South Med J* 87(12):1232-1241, 1994.
41. Shoji BT, Becker JM: Colorectal disease in the elderly patient, *Surg Clin North Am* 74(2):293-316, 1995.
42. Snape WJ: Irritable bowel syndrome. In Haubrich WS et al, editors: *Bockus gastroenterology,* ed 5, Philadelphia, 1995, WB Saunders.
43. Thomas GAO, Rhodes J, Mani V, Williams GT et al: Transdermal nicotine as maintenance therapy for ulcerative colitis, *N Engl J Med* 332(15):988-922, 1995.
44. Tooson JD, Varilek GW: Inflammatory diseases of the colon, *Postgrad Med* 98(5);46-74, 1995.
45. Toribara NW, Sleisenger MH: Screening for colorectal cancer, *N Engl J Med* 332(13):861-867, 1995.
46. Truszkowski JA, Summers RW: Colorectal neoplasms, *Postgrad Med* 98(5):97-112, 1995.
47. US Department of Health and Human Services: *Healthy People 2000: midcourse review and 1995 revisions,* Washington DC, 1996, US Government Printing Office.
48. Viall C: Taking the mystery out of TPN, *Nursing* 25(4):34-41, 1995.
49. Williams RA, Davis IP: Diverticular disease of the colon. In Haubrich WS et al, editors: *Bockus gastroenterology,* ed 5, Philadelphia, 1995, WB Saunders.
50. Witt ME: Current management of adults with colorectal cancer, *Med-Surg Nurs* 2(2):105-111, 1993.

http://www.mosby.com/MERLIN/medsurg_phipps

# chapter 42 MANAGEMENT OF PERSONS WITH Problems of the Gallbladder and Exocrine Pancreas

JUDITH K. SANDS

**objectives** *After studying this chapter, the learner should be able to:*

1. Describe the etiology, epidemiology, and pathophysiology of cholelithiasis, cholecystitis, and cancer of the biliary tract.
2. Compare treatment alternatives for biliary tract disease.
3. Describe the nursing care needs of patients with disorders of the biliary system.
4. List the causes of acute and chronic pancreatitis.
5. Explain the pathophysiological basis for signs and symptoms of acute and chronic pancreatitis and pancreatic tumors.
6. Discuss management approaches for acute and chronic pancreatitis.
7. Develop nursing diagnoses, patient outcomes, and plans of interventions for patients who have acute or chronic pancreatitis or cancer of the pancreas or who have had pancreatic surgery.

## PROBLEMS OF THE GALLBLADDER

The biliary system is affected by stones and obstruction, inflammation and infection, and cancer. Gallbladder disorders are extremely common and affect millions of adults every year.

### CHOLELITHIASIS/CHOLECYSTITIS/ CHOLEDOCHOLITHIASIS

#### Etiology

Gallstones can occur anywhere in the biliary tree. The term *cholelithiasis* refers to stone formation in the gallbladder and represents the most common biliary disorder. Either acute or chronic inflammation, termed *cholecystitis,* can result, usually precipitated by the presence of stones. When stones form in or migrate to the common bile duct the condition is termed *choledocholithiasis.* Figure 42-1 illustrates common sites for gallstones.

Eighty percent of gallstones are composed of cholesterol.[19] The remaining 20% are pigmented stones, which are further classified as black or brown.[19] Although the precise etiology of gallstones is unknown, the basic component of supersaturation of the bile with cholesterol is widely accepted. Because most healthy individuals experience supersaturation of the bile at various times without developing gallstones, it is clear that other factors are operational as well. Risk factors for gallstones have been well identified and include various clinical states associated with changes in cholesterol formation and excretion (Research Box). The risk factors for cholesterol gallstones are listed in the Risk Factors Box on the next page. The development of pigmented stones is linked to disease states such as cirrhosis, hemolytic disease, and chronic small bowel disease.[19]

#### Epidemiology

Cholelithiasis is a common health problem in the United States. Stones affect about 10% of men and 15% of women older than 55 years of age. An estimated 20 to 25 million adults have gallstones, and 1 million new cases are diagnosed annually.[19] Many, if not most, patients are asymptomatic, and it is theorized that a large number of cases remain undiagnosed. Ten percent of persons with gallstones develop symptoms within 5 years of diagnosis, and greater than 500,000 surgical procedures are performed each year at an annual treatment cost in excess of five billion dollars.[16] These figures make cholelithiasis and its associated disorders the most common and costly digestive disease. Cholelithiasis is two times more

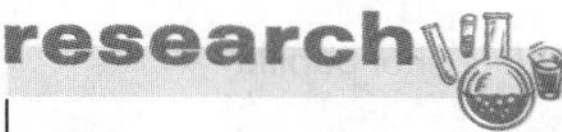


Reference: Everhart JE: Contributions of obesity and weight loss to gallstone disease, *Ann Intern Med* 119(10):1029-1035, 1993.

Obesity and the process of rapid weight loss are typically identified as significant risk factors for the development of gallstone disease. This study involved a data review of studies related to the prevalence of gallstone disease from 1966 to 1992. The data showed that obesity was a strong risk factor for gallstones in women, particularly during periods of rapid weight loss. Between 10% and 25% of obese persons will develop gallstones within a few months of beginning a very low-calorie diet, with perhaps one third of the total becoming symptomatic. The risk is less strong in men and most strong in persons with the highest body mass index and most rapid weight loss. Treatment with ursodeoxycholic acid (ursodiol) during weight loss effectively prevented the development of stones. The effect of various diets on the incidence of stone formation was not explored.

common in women, occurs most frequently in middle-aged and older persons, and affects American Indians, Mexican Americans, and whites more frequently than African Americans and Asians, although the incidence in Asians is increasing.

### Pathophysiology

Bile is primarily composed of water plus conjugated bilirubin, organic and inorganic ions, small amounts of proteins, and three lipids—bile salts, lecithin, and cholesterol. When the balance of these three lipids remains intact, cholesterol is held in solution. If the balance is upset, cholesterol can begin to precipitate. Cholesterol gallstone formation is enhanced by the production of a mucin glycoprotein, which traps cholesterol particles. Supersaturation of the bile with cholesterol also impairs gallbladder motility and contributes to stasis.

Cholesterol stones are hard, white or yellow-brown in color, radiolucent, and can be quite large (up to 4 cm). The stones most frequently occur in multiples but can be solitary. The process of stone formation is slow. Stones are theorized to grow steadily for 2 to 3 years and then stabilize in size.

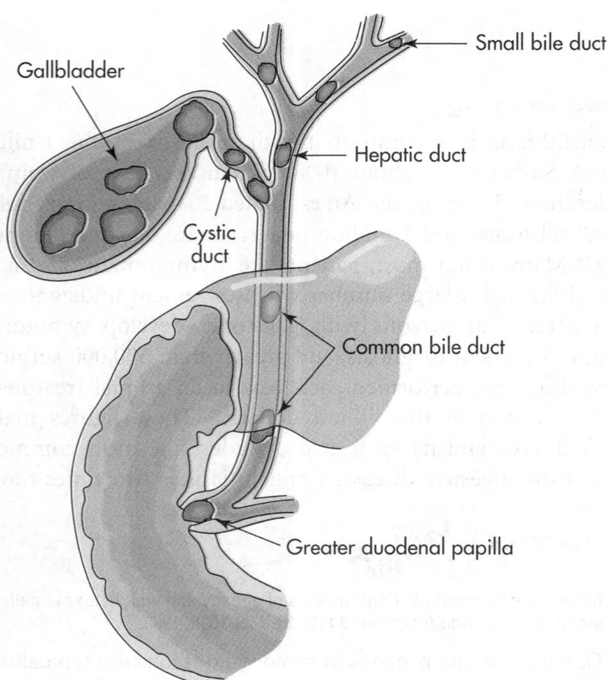


**fig. 42-1** Common sites of gallstones.

**risk factors**

**Cholesterol Gallstones**

- Obesity
- Middle age
- Pregnancy, multiparity, and the use of oral contraceptives
- Rapid weight loss (~5 pounds/wk)
- Hypercholesterolemia, use of anticholesterol medications
- Diseases of the ileum
- Gender (approximately twice as common in women)

Eighty-five percent of all stones are less than 2 cm in diameter. Most are found in the gallbladder, but it is estimated that 15% to 60% of persons older than age 60 who undergo surgery for gallstones also have stones in the common bile duct.[8]

Black pigmented stones form as the result of an increase in unconjugated bilirubin and calcium with a corresponding decrease in bile salts. Gallbladder motility may also be impaired. Brown stones develop in the intra- and extrahepatic ducts and are usually preceded by bacterial invasion.

Although most persons with gallstones are asymptomatic, cholecystitis can develop at any time, usually from a blockage of the cystic duct by the stone or from edema and spasm initiated by the presence or passage of the stone. In acute cholecystitis the gallbladder is enlarged and tense. A secondary bacterial infection can occur within several days and is the cause of most of the serious consequences of the disease.

Classic clinical manifestations of symptomatic gallstones include pain in the right upper quadrant (RUQ) of the abdomen, which is described as severe and steady. The pain frequently radiates to the right scapula or shoulder, has a sudden onset, and persists for about 1 to 3 hours.[8] It may awaken the patient at night or be associated with the consumption of a large or high-fat meal. Some patients experience nausea and vomiting and may be febrile. Chills and fever are more likely with acute cholecystitis. Patients are rarely jaundiced. Bowel sounds may be absent. Palpation of the RUQ causes a severe increase in pain and temporary inspiratory arrest *(Murphy's sign)*. The episode of cholecystitis usually subsides in 1 to 4 days. Clinical manifestations of cholecystitis are summarized in Box 42-1.

The diagnosis of gallstones is fairly straightforward when the classic symptoms are present. The diagnosis is more difficult when the symptoms are milder or reflect simply general dyspepsia. It is estimated that up to 25% of patients with irritable bowel syndrome or peptic ulcer disease also have gallstones, and the exact etiology of the patient's symptoms needs to be determined if possible.[8] Researchers theorize that many patients with "poor outcomes" after gallbladder surgery may actually reflect situations where the gallbladder was not really the source of the patient's dyspepsia.[8,19]

**box 42-1** *clinical manifestations*

***Cholecystitis***

- Sudden onset pain in the RUQ of the abdomen
  - Severe and steady in quality
  - Frequently radiates to the right scapula or shoulder
  - Persists for about 1 to 3 hours
  - May awaken the patient at night
  - May be associated with consumption of a large or fatty meal
- Anorexia, nausea, and possibly vomiting
- Mild to moderate fever
- Decreased or absent bowel sounds
- Acute abdominal tenderness and a positive Murphy's sign
- Elevated white blood cell count, slightly elevated serum bilirubin and alkaline phosphatase levels

Cholecystitis may become chronic after several acute attacks. Chronic cholecystitis, however, is usually the result of stone injuries to the gallbladder wall that cause scarring, thickening, and possibly ulceration. Bacterial infection may also be present. Patients with chronic disease often do not seek help until jaundice or other complications develop. Figure 42-2 shows the relationship between stone formation and associated outcomes in uncomplicated gallbladder disease.

## Collaborative Care Management

### Diagnostic tests

Ultrasonography is the primary diagnostic tool for identifying cholelithiasis. If the results of ultrasonography are inconclusive, oral cholecystography may be performed (Figure 42-3). Laboratory tests include white blood cell count, serum bilirubin, alkaline phosphatases, and liver function. Any additional diagnostic testing is performed to rule out other causes of gastrointestinal (GI) discomfort.

### Medications

Oral dissolution therapy with ursodeoxycholic acid (Actigall) may be prescribed for patients who are poor surgical risks or who refuse surgery. The drug gradually desaturates the bile, which allows space for the reuptake of the cholesterol in the stones. The treatment is only effective when stones are less than 1.5 to 2 cm in diameter. A full course of treatment takes from 1 to 3 years and is extremely expensive. Up to 50% of patients experience recurrences within 5 years.[19]

Direct dissolution therapy with methyl-*tert*-butyl ether is occasionally used in high-risk surgical patients. The drug is instilled through a percutaneous catheter, which is monitored fluoroscopically. Multiple drug instillations are required over 12 to 24 hours, which makes the treatment labor intensive for the physician and extremely expensive.

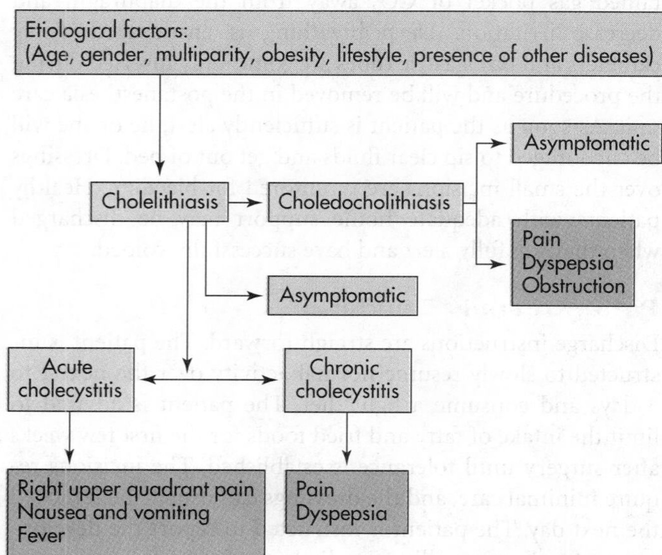


**fig. 42-2** The development of uncomplicated cholecystitis.

### Treatments

Extracorporeal shock wave lithotripsy was pioneered in Germany and adapted to the treatment of gallstones. Lithotripsy uses shock waves to disintegrate the stones. Extensive selection criteria limit the use of this treatment to a small number of patients with gallstones.[19] Patients must also undergo oral dissolution therapy after treatment to dissolve the stone fragments. Recurrence is a problem, and the treatment, including follow-up drug therapy, is five times more expensive than surgery. It is rarely a cost-effective option.[8]

Percutaneous drainage may be used as a primary treatment for patients with acute cholecystitis or to relieve inflammation and infection before surgery. The drainage tube is placed percutaneously using sonographic guidance. An operating scope may be introduced by dilating the tract to remove a stone. The procedure has good short-term results, but since the gallbladder remains intact, recurrence rates run as high as 50%.[19]

### Surgical management

Cholecystectomy was first performed in Berlin in 1882 and evolved into a procedure with excellent effectiveness and extremely low associated morbidity and mortality. It is the

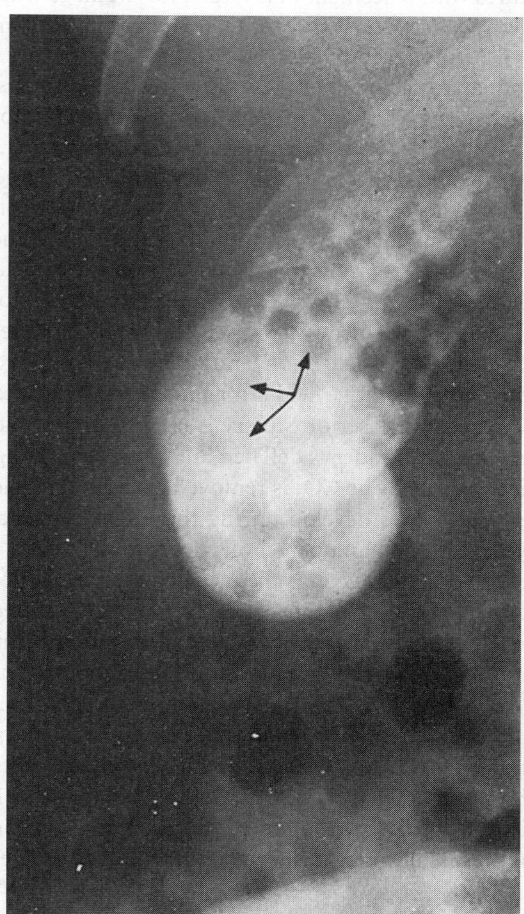

**fig. 42-3** Oral cholecystogram. Radiolucencies *(arrows)* are caused by gallstones.

second most common surgical procedure performed in the United States following cesarean section and serves as the standard against which other gallstone treatments are measured.[8] The main advantage of cholecystectomy is the fact that it stops the disease. The recurrence rate is zero. The main disadvantage has always been that it is major abdominal surgery with all of the associated pain and disability. Hospital stays averaged 3 to 7 days and recovery required 4 to 6 weeks.

Laparoscopic cholecystectomy was first performed in France in 1987 and in the United States in 1988, and by the early 1990s had revolutionized the care of patients with gallbladder disease.[16] Laparoscopic cholecystectomy offers several real advantages over traditional surgery. It is less invasive, which allows a shorter healing and recuperation time; there is less scarring; and, most importantly, the pain associated with the procedure is significantly reduced. The hospital stay is less than 24 hours, and patients can return to normal activities in 2 to 3 days. It is conservatively estimated that at least 80% of all cholecystectomies are being performed laparoscopically today, and the number continues to increase as surgical techniques improve. Acute infection is the only remaining contraindication. When the laparoscopic cholecystectomy was first introduced, the ability to explore the common bile duct was limited. This limitation necessitated the use of open cholecystectomy procedures with placement of a T-tube for drainage whenever stones were present or suspected to be present in the common bile duct. Surgical techniques have continued to improve, however, and laparoscopic approaches are now being successfully combined with endoscopic exploration and sphincterotomy to effectively treat patients with common bile duct stones.

Laparoscopic cholecystectomy is performed under general anesthesia. The procedure consists of the creation of four ½-inch incisions made at the umbilicus, midline in the epigastric region, in the right upper quadrant at the midclavicular line, and at the anterior axillary line. Three to 4 L of carbon dioxide gas are introduced to insufflate the abdomen and permit adequate visualization and the introduction of instruments. The operative field is magnified and projected on a videoscreen, and a laser or cautery is used to dissect the gallbladder. The gallbladder is deflated and removed through the umbilical incision. The $CO_2$ is removed at the end of the procedure. If problems develop during the procedure, it can be rapidly converted to an open cholecystectomy.

The skill of the surgeon is the primary determinant of outcomes. The slightly higher rate of bile duct injury associated with the procedure is usually attributable to inexperience with the technique. Laparoscopic cholecystectomy takes about 90 minutes and is more expensive than traditional open surgery. The short hospital stay and tremendous patient satisfaction with the procedure, however, clearly outweigh the higher surgical costs. The mild shoulder pain that patients may experience for up to 1 week is attributed to nerve irritation from distention and the $CO_2$ gas, but the discomfort is easily managed with mild analgesics.

#### Diet

No diet is known to prevent the formation of gallstones. Patients who are experiencing symptoms are encouraged to follow a low-fat diet and eat small meals until definitive therapy is completed. After treatment they can resume a normal diet.

#### Activity

There are no activity restrictions for persons with cholelithiasis, cholecystitis, or choledocholithiasis.

#### Referrals

Referrals would not generally be required for the management of uncomplicated gallstones unless a serious comorbid condition necessitated the involvement of additional professionals.

## NURSING MANAGEMENT OF THE PATIENT UNDERGOING LAPAROSCOPIC CHOLECYSTECTOMY

### PREOPERATIVE CARE

Patients will complete their preoperative preparation at home before their arrival on the day of surgery. The nurse will verify that the patient has had nothing by mouth (NPO) and completed any required bowel preparation. Preoperative teaching includes reviewing the scope and nature of the surgical procedure and the care that will be provided in the immediate postoperative period. The nurse also ensures that the patient understands that the expected pain is mild to moderate and can be successfully managed with standard analgesics.

### POSTOPERATIVE CARE

The patient will be closely monitored in the immediate postoperative period, and pain control will receive priority attention. A left side-lying Sims position can help to move the retained gas pocket of $CO_2$ away from the diaphragm and decrease irritation. Deep breathing is encouraged. Foley catheters and nasogastric tubes are commonly inserted during the procedure and will be removed in the postanesthesia care unit. As soon as the patient is sufficiently alert, he or she will be encouraged to sip clear fluids and get out of bed. Dressings over the small incisions are monitored for bleeding. Healthy patients with adequate home support may be discharged when they are fully alert and have successfully voided.

#### Patient/Family Education

Discharge instructions are straightforward. The patient is instructed to slowly resume normal activity over the next 2 to 3 days and consume a light diet. The patient is advised to limit the intake of fatty and fried foods for the first few weeks after surgery until tolerance is established. The incisions require minimal care, and the dressings can usually be removed the next day. The patient is instructed to report the development of redness, swelling, or discharge from any incision, as well as the onset of fever, pain, or tenderness in the abdomen. Heavy lifting should be avoided.

A Clinical Pathway for the patient undergoing laparoscopic cholecystectomy is shown below. The Guidelines for Care Box summarizes the care provided to a patient who undergoes traditional open cholecystectomy.

## GERONTOLOGICAL CONSIDERATIONS

Gallbladder disease is seen more frequently with advancing age but is treated in the same manner. Elderly persons may have more subtle symptoms and signs in the presence of cholecystitis. Thus they can develop bacteremia before they seek help. Because of the normal decrease in immune function with aging, they are at greater risk for septic shock. Elderly patients have more risks with surgery just because of their age.The laparoscopic cholecystectomy procedure is particularly effective in this age-group as it decreases the period of immobility and recovery substantially. Wound healing needs to be carefully monitored.

## clinical pathway *Laparoscopic Cholecystectomy Without Complications*

| | DAY OF SURGERY<br>DAY OF ADMISSION<br>DAY 1 | DAY OF DISCHARGE<br>DAY 2 |
|---|---|---|
| **Diagnostic Tests** | Preoperative: CBC, UA<br>Postoperative: Hgb and Hct | |
| **Medications** | PAR: IVs decreased to saline lock after nausea subsides; IV analgesic, then PO | Disc saline lock; PO analgesic |
| **Treatments** | PAR: I&O q shift; VS q4hr × 4, then q8hr; assess bowel sounds q4hr; check drainage on bandages q2hr | Disc I&O; VS q8hr; assess bowel sounds q8hr; remove bandages and reapply bandages after shower if necessary |
| **Diet** | NPO until nausea subsides, then clear liquids; advance to full liquids, low fat | Regular diet, low fat |
| **Activity** | Up in room with assistance about 6 to 10 hr after surgery; T & DB q2hr | Up ad lib, OK to shower |
| **Consultations** | | |

*DB,* Deep breathing; *Hct,* hematocrit; *Hgb,* hemoglobin; *PAR,* postanesthesia recovery; *UA,* urinalysis; *VS,* vital signs.

## guidelines for care

### The Person Undergoing Open Cholecystectomy

#### Preoperative

Teach patient the importance of frequent deep breathing and use of incentive spirometer because the high incision and RUQ pain predispose the patient to *atelectasis* and *right lower lobe pneumonia.*

Explain the types of biliary drainage tubes that are anticipated, if any.

Teach patient about the pain control plan to be used in the postoperative period.

#### Postoperative

Place patient in low Fowler's position; assist to change position frequently.

Urge patient to deep breathe at regular intervals (every 1 to 2 hours) and to cough if secretions are present until ambulating well. Assist patient to effectively splint the incision. Encourage use of incentive spirometer.

Give analgesics fairly liberally the first 2 to 3 days.

Use patient-controlled analgesia if possible. Meperidine (Demerol) has been the drug of choice because it is believed to minimize spasms in the bile ducts, but morphine is being used with increasing frequency.

Maintain a dry, intact dressing; usually a drain is inserted near the stump of the cystic duct; some serous fluid drainage is normal initially.

Encourage progressive ambulation when permitted.

Increase diet gradually to regular with fat content as tolerated (appetite and fat tolerance may be diminished if there is external biliary drainage).

#### Biliary Drainage

Connect any biliary drainage tubes to closed gravity drainage. See Figure 42-4 and the Guidelines for Care Box on p. 1378 for care of a T-tube.

Attach sufficient tubing so the patient can move without restriction.

Explain to patient the importance of avoiding kinks, clamping, or pulling of the tube.

Monitor the amount and color of drainage frequently; measure and record drainage at least every shift.

Report any signs of peritonitis (abdominal pain, rigidity, or fever) to the physician immediately.

Monitor color of urine and stools; stools will be grayish-white if bile is flowing out a drainage tube, but the normal color should gradually reappear as external drainage diminishes and disappears.

## SPECIAL ENVIRONMENTS FOR CARE

### Critical Care Management

Critical care management would not be anticipated for any phase of routine gallstone management. The surgical procedures have an excellent safety record and are associated with a less than 7% incidence of morbidity from any cause.

### Home Care Management

Cholecystectomy is the foundation of care for gallstones, and the procedure has become essentially same-day or overnight surgery. Self-care management at home is therefore expected. Most patients have no specific home care needs beyond routine monitoring of wound healing and the progressive return to usual activities.[17] For more complex procedures patients may be discharged from the hospital with a T-tube in place. Teaching concerning T-tube care is included in the Guidelines for Care Box. Elderly patients may need some additional assistance at home when they undergo same-day surgery. These needs are ideally identified and arranged before surgery.

**guidelines for care**

**Managing a T-Tube**

**Purpose**

A T-tube may be placed after surgical exploration of the common bile duct to preserve patency of the common duct and ensure drainage of bile until edema resolves and bile is effectively draining into the duodenum. The tube is usually connected to gravity drainage and can be converted to a leg bag to limit its restrictiveness and visibility. The patient may be discharged with the T-tube in place (see Figure 42-4).

**General Care**

- Attach the tube to gravity drainage. Ensure that sufficient tubing is in place to prevent pulling and restriction of movement.
  - Check drainage every 2 hours on the first day and at least once per shift on subsequent days.
  - Record output carefully. Initial drainage may be as much as 500 to 1000 ml per day, but this amount should steadily decrease as healing occurs.
- Follow physician's order for initiating clamping of the tube.
  - Monitor patient's response to clamping and record incidence of distress.
  - Unclamp the tube promptly if distress occurs.
- Monitor the color of the stool. Stool is initially clay-colored but regains pigmentation as bile again flows into the duodenum.
- Keep the skin clean and protected from bile drainage as bile is extremely irritating to the skin.
- Teach the patient to empty the bag and convert it to a leg bag if discharge with the T-tube is planned.
- Provide self-care teaching:
  - A daily shower is usually permitted.
  - A sterile dressing should be reapplied to the T-tube entry site each day.
  - Zinc oxide may be used to protect the skin from irritation.
  - Redness, swelling, or drainage from the site and the development of fever should be promptly reported to the physician.

## COMPLICATIONS

Transient mild diarrhea is the only adverse outcome that has been consistently linked to cholecystectomy. The most common complication of nonsurgical management of gallstone disease is recurrence, and it is clear that undiagnosed or inadequately treated gallbladder disease can result in serious and even life-threatening complications, including overwhelming sepsis and peritonitis. Chronic dyspepsia and subclinical malabsorption are often included as possible complications of cholecystectomy, but there is no concrete evidence that the reduction in the pool of bile salts and the loss of the reservoir function of the gallbladder increase the incidence of duodenal reflux or an alkaline shift in the gastric pH.[16] Some researchers suggest that these so-called "complications" may actually reflect situations in which the patient's original digestive symptoms were never related to the gallstones and therefore were not improved by their removal (Research Box).[5]

## PRIMARY SCLEROSING CHOLANGITIS

### Etiology/Epidemiology

Inflammation and scarring of the biliary tree occur most commonly as a result of gallstones and bile duct infection. Parasites are a common source of chronic duct infection in Asia and developing countries. When no cause for the bile duct injury can be found, the process is called *idiopathic* or *primary sclerosing cholangitis (PSC)*.

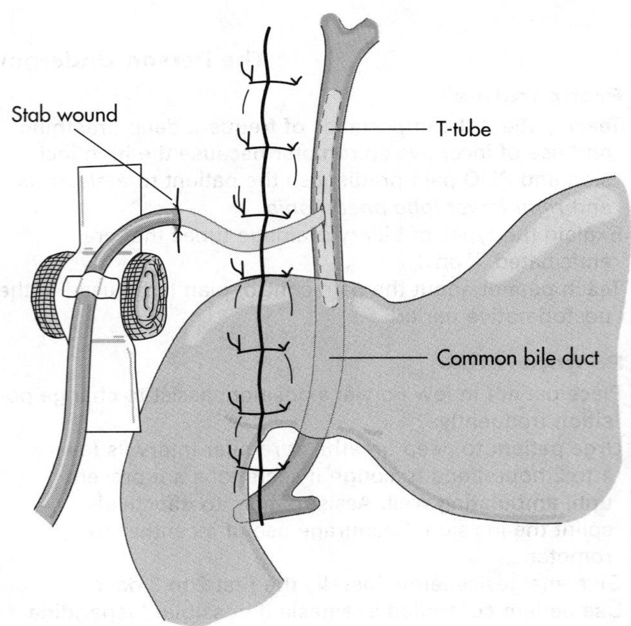


**fig. 42-4** Section of T-tube emerging from stab wound may be placed over roll of gauze anchored to skin with adhesive tape to prevent its lumen from being occluded by pressure.

The prevalence of PSC is unknown. Both genetic and immunological mechanisms are suspected in its development. The disease may occur alone but is generally associated with other disorders, most of which have a strong immunological component. The closest link is with inflammatory bowel disease (IBD), particularly ulcerative colitis. Of patients with PSC 70% have IBD, although PSC only occurs in 2% to 4% of all patients with IBD.[23] The PSC may precede the diagnosis of IBD or follow it from 1 to 20 years later. The patients are usually male, and PSC is diagnosed in early or middle adulthood, typically by the age of 45. PSC is the cause for about one third of all patients needing liver transplantation.

### Pathophysiology

Primary sclerosing cholangitis causes changes in and around the large bile ducts from inflammation, obstruction, and intra- and extrahepatic fibrosis. Strictures can usually be found in multiple locations. These strictures are short and diffusely distributed and alternate with normal or dilated segments of the ducts to create a beadlike appearance on x-ray. It is unusual for the gallbladder or cystic duct to be involved. Liver biopsy shows the combination of inflammation, fibrosis, proliferation, and ductal obliteration that confirms the presence of the disease. The disease proceeds in stages, and by stage 4, biliary cirrhosis is present (Chapter 37), making the diagnosis complex.

Many patients are asymptomatic in early stages. Others are seen with a combination of fatigue, fever, jaundice, abdominal pain, and weight loss. Persistent severe pruritis can be a particularly difficult aspect of the disease. Patients may experience recurrent attacks of cholangitis.

### Collaborative Care Management

The diagnosis of PSC is not easily established and is usually made as part of a workup for cholecystitis or general nonulcer dyspepsia. PSC causes elevated liver enzymes and serum bilirubin levels, but the elevations in alkaline phosphatase are considered to be a hallmark feature. Endoscopic retrograde cholangiopancreatography (ERCP) (Chapter 38) is used to visualize the biliary tree. Liver biopsy helps rule out other causes of the symptoms and assists in estimating the severity of the liver damage.

The prognosis of PSC largely depends on its clinical course, which can be highly unpredictable. The aggressiveness of the disease is influenced by the number and severity of infections and the development of complications related to cirrhosis. Death is usually the result of liver failure, bleeding, or sepsis, but timely intervention with a liver transplant can significantly alter the outcomes.[23] Survival is typically about 10 years.

Drug therapy is aimed at reducing biliary tree inflammation and preventing the scarring that leads to obstruction. Steroids and other immunosuppressive agents have not been effective, but the use of ursodeoxycholic acid has shown promise even though its mechanism of action in PSC remains unknown. Surgical procedures other than transplant have been effective for diffuse disease. Endoscopic treatment to remove stones, relieve obstruction, dilate ducts, and place stent tubes is ongoing but primarily in the form of clinical trials. Liver transplantation is the primary treatment option.

#### *Patient/family education*

The uncertain nature of PSC is one of its most difficult characteristics. Patients are instructed about the disease and its possible outcomes and are prepared for the possibility of the eventual need for liver transplant. Persistent jaundice may negatively affect body image, and chronic severe pruritis can be a daily nightmare. Some patients respond to cholestyramine resin, which theoretically binds the itch-triggering elements in the bile. The nurse also suggests that the patient experiment with common interventions that may lessen itching. Possible strategies are summarized in the Guidelines for Care Box. A low-fat diet is recommended to patients who develop problems with diarrhea or steatorrhea, and the fat

**research**

Reference: Fenster LF, Lonborg R, Thirlby RC, Traverso LW: What symptoms does cholecystectomy cure? *Am J Surg* 16(5):533-538, 1995.

This study attempted to evaluate the effectiveness of cholecystectomy in relieving presenting GI problems. Data were collected from 225 patients who underwent laparoscopic cholecystectomy. Eighty-two percent had documented gallstones before surgery, 91% experienced biliary-related pain, and 77% had both. Eighty-two percent also experienced related GI symptoms, e.g., bloating, gas, indigestion, and intolerance to fatty foods. The study results showed that documented gallstone-related pain was universally relieved by surgery, but pain was only relieved in 52% of those without documented gallstones (acalculous cholecystitis). And, although nonpain symptoms were extremely common in this population, surgery only relieved the related symptoms in approximately 44% of the patients.

**guidelines for care**

**Strategies to Control Pruritis**

- Avoid irritating clothing (wool or restrictive clothing).
- Use tepid water for bathing rather than hot.
  - Experiment with nonirritating soaps and detergents.
  - Pat skin dry after bathing or showering; do not rub.
- Apply emollient creams and lotions to dry skin regularly.
- Maintain a cool environment and ensure adequate amounts of humidity in the air.
- Avoid activities that increase body temperature or cause sweating.
- Experiment with treatments such as oatmeal baths.
- Keep the fingernails short and consider use of cotton gloves at night to minimize skin damage from scratching.
- Use antipruritic medications as ordered.

restriction usually promptly corrects the problem. Fat-soluble vitamin replacement is often needed.

## CARCINOMA OF THE BILIARY SYSTEM

### Etiology/Epidemiology

Primary tumors of the gallbladder are extremely rare in clinical practice, and their incidence may be declining because of prompt surgical intervention for gallbladder disease. The etiology is unknown. Gallbladder cancer occurs almost exclusively in persons older than 60 years of age and is twice as common in women.[23] High-risk groups for gallbladder disease in general have a slightly increased risk of gallbladder cancer.

Cancer can also develop in the bile ducts. This disease process also typically affects patients between 50 and 70 years of age. It demonstrates a striking link with the presence of inflammatory bowel disease.

### Pathophysiology

Carcinoma can occur anywhere in the biliary system. It has a very insidious onset and can metastasize by direct extension, through the lymphatics, and through the blood. Most patients have no symptoms that are referable to the gallbladder. Others have symptoms similar to those seen with cholelithiasis and cholecystitis because of obstruction and inflammation.

Intermittent pain in the upper abdomen is the most common symptom. Anorexia, nausea, vomiting, weight loss, and jaundice may also be present. The patient may have a palpable abdominal mass. Signs and symptoms indicative of metastasis to the liver or pancreas may also be present.[23] By the time gallbladder cancer produces symptoms it is usually incurable.

### Collaborative Care Management

Surgery is the primary treatment for cancer of the gallbladder. If the disease is diagnosed incidentally, it may be confined to the gallbladder and be curable with surgery. Cholecystectomy with wedge resection of 3 to 5 cm of normal liver plus lymph node dissection is usually performed. Survival for those with invasive disease is usually less than 2 years. Neither radiotherapy nor chemotherapy has thus far improved patient outcomes.

Treatment of bile duct cancer focuses on maintaining bile flow. Surgery may be used to divert bile flow to the jejunum, or stent tubes may be placed to attempt to maintain duct patency. When bile flow can be maintained, patients may live for several years after diagnosis.

#### *Patient/family education*

Nursing intervention is focused on assisting the patient to self-manage the symptoms and possibly care for bile drainage systems (see the Guidelines for Care Box on p. 1378). The remainder of care and teaching is generally supportive as the patient and family face an uncertain future and poor prognosis. General care of the cancer patient is discussed in Chapter 11.

# PROBLEMS OF THE PANCREAS

## ACUTE PANCREATITIS

### Etiology

Acute pancreatitis occurs when obstruction of the outflow of pancreatic secretions triggers acute inflammation in the gland. The obstruction can progress to necrosis of the pancreatic exocrine and endocrine cells and can involve either the large or small pancreatic ducts or both. The two major causes of acute pancreatitis in the United States are gallbladder disease and alcohol abuse.[11,23] Together they account for about 80% of all cases. Acute pancreatitis may be similar in presentation to chronic pancreatitis, but it represents a different pathological process.[11] Other rare causes of pancreatitis include abdominal or surgical trauma, obstruction of the gland by neoplastic growth, drug effects, a variety of infectious diseases, and other chronic diseases of the GI tract.

#### *Alcohol-related pancreatitis*

The role of alcohol in the development of acute pancreatitis is well recognized clinically but remains poorly explained. Alcohol is presumed to have a direct toxic effect on the pancreas in selected persons, probably through some genetic enzymatic abnormality. Extensive amounts of alcohol over a minimum period of several years are probably required to initiate the process. Alcohol also weakens cell membranes and makes the acinar cells more vulnerable to injury. It is also known to decrease the amount of trypsin inhibitor available, which again increases the susceptibility of the pancreas to injury. Alcohol is believed to initiate an asymptomatic pancreatitis in the organ before the first acute episode. Alcoholic patients also typically develop chronic disease once an acute episode has occurred, and the presence of chronic pancreatitis appears to make the pancreas even more vulnerable to the damaging effects of alcohol.[12,21,23] Recurrent episodes of acute pancreatitis are common.

#### *Biliary pancreatitis*

Transient obstruction of the ampulla of Vater by a gallstone is considered to be a major cause of biliary pancreatitis. Stones were found in the stool of more than 90% of patients with gallstone pancreatitis in some studies. The obstruction does not have to be prolonged to initiate acute inflammation. How the obstruction activates the pancreatic enzymes is not understood. The presence of tiny gallstones (microlithiasis or biliary sludge) too small to be identified by imaging studies, is believed to play a role. There is also considerable evidence that structural abnormalities that lead to narrowing at the sphincter of Oddi can be considered a cause of biliary pancreatitis. It is theorized that the various forms of obstruction can reverse the normal pancreatic pressure gradient. This would permit reflux of bile or duodenal contents into the pancreatic ducts and possibly even cause small duct rupture.[11]

Biliary pancreatitis begins acutely, but is likely to be mild in course and followed by rapid recovery. It can, however, in selected situations trigger massive pancreatic necrosis and lead to death. It rarely leads to chronic disease.

## Epidemiology

The incidence of acute pancreatitis has increased in recent years, but this increase may represent improved diagnostic capabilities rather than a true increase in cases. The current annual incidence is estimated to be 0.1 to 0.5 cases per 1000 population. Patients with biliary pancreatitis are likely to be 55 to 65 years of age and predominantly female, whereas patients with alcohol-related pancreatitis are usually slightly younger and predominantly male.

Acute pancreatitis may take a mild, severe, or fulminant course. Pancreatitis has a fulminant course in approximately 5% to 15% of all patients, and 20% to 60% of these patients will either die or face potentially lethal complications.[6] The overall mortality rate for pancreatitis remains at about 10% despite improved diagnosis and more aggressive treatment.

## Pathophysiology

The two major pathological varieties of acute pancreatitis are the (1) acute interstitial form and (2) acute hemorrhagic form. Although either form can be fatal, the interstitial form is often a milder disease.

The defining characteristic of acute interstitial pancreatitis is a diffusely swollen and inflamed pancreas, which retains its normal anatomic features. There are minimal or no areas of hemorrhage or necrosis in the gland. The interstitial spaces become grossly swollen by extracellular edema, and the ducts may contain purulent material. The acute hemorrhagic disease presents with a very different picture. The gland readily shows acute inflammation, hemorrhage, and marked tissue necrosis. Extensive fat necrosis is present in patients with fulminant disease, not just in the pancreas but throughout the abdominal and thoracic cavities and subcutaneous tissues.[23] Necrosis of vessels can cause significant loss of blood, and abscesses and infection form in areas of walled off necrotic tissue. Systemic complications such as fat emboli, hypotension, shock, and fluid overload are common.

Pancreatic juice normally contains only inactive forms of the proteolytic enzymes. The pancreas secretes a trypsin inhibitor specifically to prevent activation within the gland, because once trypsinogen is activated to trypsin it can then activate the other enzymes as well. Activation of the pancreatic enzymes before they reach the duodenum has long been recognized as a major component of the disease process. The mystery of acute pancreatitis is how that pathological sequence is initiated. The etiological roles of alcohol and biliary disease have been discussed, but they fail to fully explain the disease process.[22] Enzyme activation overwhelms all of the normal protective mechanisms of the pancreas and initiates a massive attack on the pancreatic tissues. Pancreatic autodigestion is initiated. Other systemic effects of the activated enzymes include:

- Activation of complement and kinin, producing increased vascular permeability and vasodilation
- Increased stickiness of the inflammatory leukocytes with the formation of emboli, which plug the microvasculature
- Initiation of consumptive coagulopathy, leading to disseminated intravascular coagulation
- Increased permeability causing massive movement of fluids, which leads to circulatory insufficiency
- Release of myocardial depressant factor, which further compromises cardiac function
- Activation of the renin-angiotension network, which impairs renal function in conjunction with circulatory insufficiency

Figure 42-5 outlines the major pathological events that can occur in acute pancreatitis.

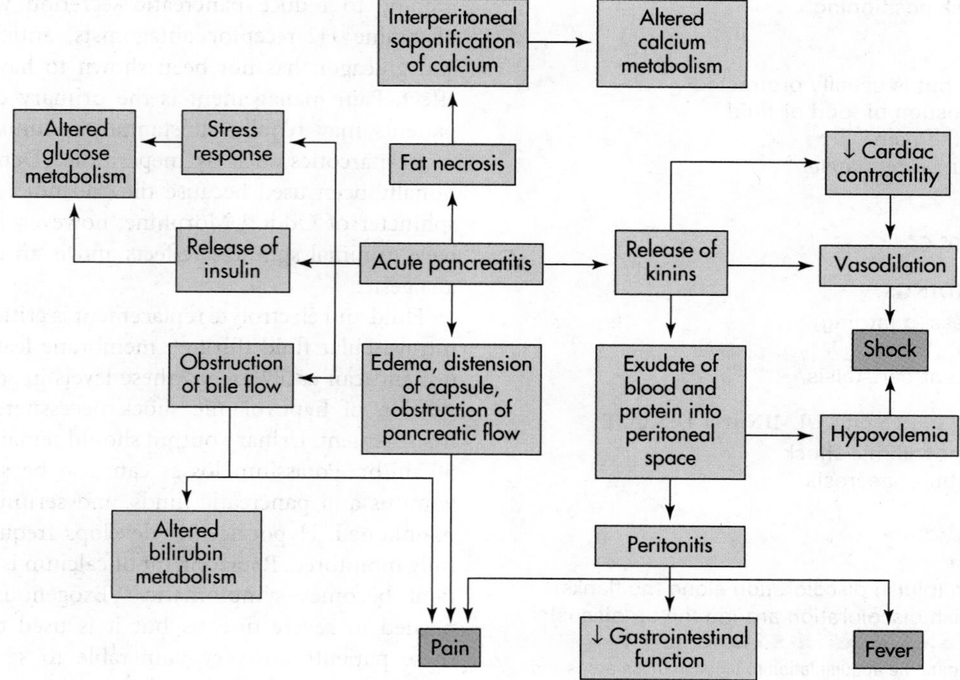


**fig. 42-5** Summary of major pathological events that occur in acute pancreatitis.

The clinical manifestations of acute pancreatitis vary somewhat according to the severity of the attack. Acute pain in the epigastric region is the hallmark feature of the disease. The pain is usually steady in nature and may radiate to the back. It is typically worsened by lying supine, and patients may curve their backs and draw their knees up toward the body in an attempt to diminish its intensity. The pain is variously attributed to stretching of the pancreatic capsule, obstruction of the biliary tree, and/or chemical burning of the peritoneum by activated enzymes. In more severe forms of the disease the pain may be agonizing.

Vomiting is a second common feature of acute pancreatitis. The severity of the vomiting varies and is typically worsened by the ingestion of food or fluid. Vomiting does not relieve the pain and may become protracted. Physical findings for patients with severe pancreatitis include abdominal tenderness and rigidity, progressive abdominal distention, and decreased bowel activity. Fever is common, but it rarely exceeds 39° C. Fulminant disease may progress to hypovolemic shock, ascites, acute tubular necrosis, and respiratory failure. The clinical manifestations of mild and severe pancreatitis are summarized in Box 42-2.

**box 42-2** *clinical manifestations*

### *Acute Pancreatitis*

PAIN
- Steady and severe in nature, excruciating in fulminant cases
- Located in the epigastric or umbilical region; may radiate to the back
- Worsened by lying supine; may be lessened by flexed knee, curved back positioning

VOMITING
- Varies in severity but is usually protracted
- Worsened by ingestion of food or fluid
- Does not relieve the pain
- Usually accompanied by nausea

FEVER
- Rarely exceeds 39° C.

ABDOMINAL FINDINGS
- Rigidity, tenderness, guarding
- Distention
- Decreased or absent peristalsis

ADDITIONAL FEATURES OF FULMINANT DISEASE
- Symptoms of hypovolemic shock
- Oliguria: acute tubular necrosis
- Ascites
- Jaundice
- Respiratory failure
- Grey Turner's sign (bluish discoloration along the flanks)*
- Cullen's sign (bluish discoloration around the umbilicus)*

*NOTE: These signs indicate the accumulation of blood in these areas and represent the presence of hemorrhagic pancreatitis.

## Collaborative Care Management

### *Diagnostic tests*

The diagnosis of acute pancreatitis is made initially from the measurement of the serum amylase level, which rises within a few hours of the onset of the disease. In mild disease it may only remain elevated for a few days. There is no apparent relationship between the severity of the disease and the height of the enzyme levels.[18] The levels of urinary amylase may also be measured if the patient sustains adequate kidney function. Serum lipase elevations are also diagnostic and persist for up to 5 to 7 days.[18] Neither amylase nor lipase elevations are exclusive to pancreatic disease, which complicates diagnosis in questionable cases.

Other laboratory findings commonly seen with acute pancreatitis include leukocytosis, hyperglycemia, which may reach levels as high as 500 to 900 mg/dl, and elevated liver function tests. Hypocalcemia may develop from the sequestering of calcium by fat necrosis in the abdomen, and this is usually a poor prognostic sign. It may occur in conjunction with low levels of both albumin and magnesium, especially in chronic alcoholics.

Computed tomographic (CT) scanning has become the gold standard for diagnosing acute pancreatitis, although it is actually not needed except for patients with severe disease and suspected complications. CT scans can estimate the size of the pancreas; identify cysts, abscesses, and masses; and with contrast medium can clearly diagnose hemorrhagic disease. Early in the diagnostic process abdominal x-rays may be taken to rule out ulcer perforation, and ultrasonography may be used to rule out the presence of gallstones.

### *Medications*

There is no drug treatment for acute pancreatitis. Drug therapy to reduce pancreatic secretion with somatostatin, histamine H2-receptor antagonists, anticholinergic agents, and glucagon has not been shown to have any therapeutic effect. Pain management is the primary consideration, and patients may require substantial amounts of opioids. Synthetic narcotics such as meperidine (Demerol) have traditionally been used because they do not cause spasm in the sphincter of Oddi.[11] Morphine, however, is now believed to have minimal sphincter effects and is an extremely effective analgesic.

Fluid and electrolyte replacement is critical since the loss of intravascular fluid through membrane leakage averages 4 to 6 L and can easily exceed these levels in severe cases.[3,23] Prevention of hypovolemic shock necessitates aggressive fluid management. Urinary output should remain at or above 30 to 50 ml/hr. Potassium losses can also be significant in both vomitus and pancreatic fluids, and serum levels need to be maintained. Hypocalcemia develops frequently and is carefully monitored. Replacement of calcium is initiated if the patient becomes symptomatic.[23] Exogenous insulin may be needed in severe disease, but it is used cautiously because these patients are very vulnerable to severe hypoglycemia from decreased glycogen and glucagon reserves.

### Treatments

There are no known treatments for pancreatitis. Medical therapy is directed at general supportive care for most patients with mild to moderate disease. The patient is generally given NPO. Nasogastric suctioning has frequently been used, but is probably not necessary unless the patient develops ileus or experiences persistent vomiting.

More aggressive and invasive interventions are available for patients who are at high risk for complications. The course of acute pancreatitis is not readily apparent, and several clinical prognostic rating scales have been developed to help clinicians identify patients at greatest risk. The older system uses the criteria of Ransom applied at admission and again within the first 48 hours. The modified Glasgow criteria are easier to apply clinically. These prognostic scoring systems are presented in Table 42-1.

Peritoneal lavage has been used in patients with severe pancreatitis in the attempt to remove toxic substances. Clinical trials have involved small numbers of patients, and results have been somewhat inconsistent, but a trend toward a decrease in deaths related to pancreatic infection has been observed. The removal of retained gallstones by ERCP reduces overall morbidity in the select group of patients in whom an obstructing stone can be identified.

### Surgical management

Surgery is not a routine part of the management of acute pancreatitis, but some procedures may be necessary to control related gallbladder problems, pseudocyst, or abscess. Necrotic tissue may also be resected. Patients requiring surgery typically have fulminant disease and are acutely ill. The discussion of surgical intervention is included under Complications on p. 1386.

### Diet

The patient is given nothing by mouth until the abdominal pain has subsided, and amylase levels return to normal. This practice, in theory, rests the pancreas and limits or stops the secretion of enzymes. Most patients do recover without complications or sequelae.[10] Oral fluids and feedings can usually be resumed within 3 to 7 days and gradually advanced to a normal diet once peristalsis is reestablished. There is no clinical proof of the need for a low-fat diet or any other dietary restrictions during recovery except for abstinence from alcohol.[6]

Total enteral or parenteral nutrition may be implemented for patients who are unable to eat for extended periods of time (Research Box). The early use of total parenteral nutrition (TPN) does not appear to affect outcomes of patients with mild pancreatitis, but its use significantly decreases morbidity and mortality in severe and fulminant disease.[11] Efforts are made to keep plasma albumin levels above 3.5 g/d and total protein values above 6.5g/d, thereby maintaining a positive nitrogen balance.[11]

### Activity

Bedrest is maintained during the acute phase of disease management to decrease the body's overall metabolic demands. Once the patient's condition has stabilized, activity can

**table 42-1** *Two Representative Prognostic Scoring Systems Used in Acute Pancreatitis*

| RANSOM | GLASGOW |
|---|---|
| **ADMISSION** | **WITHIN 48 HR OF ADMISSION** |
| Age >55 years | Age >55 years |
| WBC >20,000 cell/mm$^3$ | WBC >15,000 |
| LDH >350 IU/L | Glucose >180 mg/dl |
| AST >250 IU/L | BUN >45 mg/dl |
| Glucose >200 mg/dl | $Po_2$ <60 mm Hg |
| | Albumin <3.2 g/dl |
| **INITIAL 48 HR** | Calcium <8 mg/dl |
| Hematocrit decrease >10% | LDH >600 IU/L |
| BUN increase >5 mg/dl | |
| Calcium <8 mg/dl | |
| $Po_2$ <60 mm Hg | |
| Base deficit >4 | |
| Estimated fluid sequestration >6 L | |

Data from Ransom JAC et al: *Surg Gynecol Obstet* 143:209, 1976 and Neoptolemos VP et al: *Lancet* 2:979, 1988.
*WBC,* white blood cell count; *LDH,* lactic dehydrogenase; *AST,* aspartate aminotransferase; *BUN,* blood urea nitrogen.
NOTE: Presence of three or more factors indicates poor prognosis.

**research**

Reference: McClave SA et al: Comparison of the safety of early enteral vs. parenteral nutrition in mild acute pancreatitis, *J Parent Ent Nutr* 21(1):14-20, 1997.

This study was designed to compare the safety, cost, and effectiveness of two methods of nutrition support for patients with mild acute pancreatitis. The study involved 30 patients who were admitted with mild acute pancreatitis documented by the presence of pain and elevated serum amylase and lipase levels. Patients were randomly assigned on admission to receive either total enteral nutrition (TEN) via a nasointestinal tube or total parenteral nutrition (TPN) by central or peripheral catheter. Nutrition support was initiated within 48 hours of admission. No differences were noted between the groups on admission in mean age, Ransom criteria, APACHE score, or other prognostic screening tool.

No deaths occurred in either group. No differences were found in serial pain scores, the number of days before normalization of blood values occurred, serum albumin levels, or the incidence of nosocomial infection. The cost of TPN, however, was more than four times greater than the cost of TEN, and stress-induced glucose levels were significant in the TPN group. The study concluded that isocaloric/isonitrogenous TEN via nasointestinal tube appears to be a cost-effective alternative to intervention with TPN in this population.

be gradually increased based on the patient's tolerance. There are no long-term restrictions.

#### Referrals

Patients with acute pancreatitis are severely ill and may require the expertise of a variety of specialists during the treatment and recovery periods. Fulminant illness may necessitate critical care monitoring and consultation. This is particularly true for patients who develop respiratory complications such as adult respiratory distress syndrome (ARDS) or respiratory failure and require intubation and mechanical ventilation. The nutrition support team will be involved if TPN is initiated.

Any number of medical specialists may be consulted to manage emergency complications. The surgeon is often needed to drain abscesses, relieve obstruction, or debride necrotic tissue. An enterostomal therapist may be consulted if draining wounds are left open to heal by secondary intention.

In many patients alcohol abuse is the etiological stimulus of acute pancreatitis, and continuation of alcohol use will increase the risk of recurrent acute pancreatitis and chronic pancreatitis in the future. The nurse needs to be knowledgeable about resources available in the local community for supporting individuals who want to become and remain abstinent from alcohol. The severe nature of acute pancreatitis may serve as a stimulus for lifestyle change in some individuals. It is important to use this opportunity to refer the person for alcohol treatment if possible.

## NURSING MANAGEMENT

### ASSESSMENT

#### Subjective Data

Subjective data to be collected to assess the patient with acute pancreatitis include:

Pain: steady and severe in nature and quality; located in the epigastric or umbilical region, may radiate to back; worsens when patient is supine

Nausea and vomiting, usually severe and protracted; worsens by the ingestion of food or fluid; vomiting does not relieve pain

History of gallbladder disease; long-term high alcohol intake

#### Objective Data

Objective data to be collected to assess the patient with acute pancreatitis include:

General affect: patient looks distressed; sits with knees pulled toward abdomen

Fever, generally <39° C

Abdominal rigidity, distention, guarding, and tenderness

Diminished or absent bowel sounds

Signs of dehydration: falling urine output, decreased skin turgor, dry or sticky mucous membranes

Vital signs: evidence of hypovolemia; tachycardia, tachypnea, normal to low blood pressure, restlessness, and anxiety

Presence of Grey Turner's or Cullen's signs: bluish discoloration on flanks and/or around umbilicus

Jaundice

### NURSING DIAGNOSES

Nursing diagnoses are determined from analysis of patient data. Nursing diagnoses for the person with acute pancreatitis may include but are not limited to:

| Diagnostic Title | Possible Etiological Factors |
|---|---|
| Pain | Inflammation of pancreas or peritoneum |
| Fluid volume deficit | Vomiting, fluid shifts in abdomen |
| Nutrition, altered: less than body requirements | Nausea and vomiting; pain |
| Risk for impaired home maintenance management | Lack of knowledge about disease process and therapeutic regimen |
| Health maintenance, altered | Unhealthy lifestyle patterns, including alcoholism |

### EXPECTED PATIENT OUTCOMES

Expected patient outcomes for the person with acute pancreatitis may include but are not limited to:

1. States that pain is controlled and does not appear to be in pain (does not display distressed appearance, limited body movement, or limited activity).
2. Will have adequate fluid volume as demonstrated by normal blood pressure, absence of orthostatic changes, normal skin turgor, moist mucous membranes, and adequate urine output.
3. Will gradually resume a normal oral diet without discomfort and regains lost weight.
4. Patient and significant others will be able to:
   a. Describe the disease and the purpose of various interventions.
   b. Explain the relationship between the etiological factor (e.g., alcoholism or biliary disease) and pancreatitis.
   c. Explain plans for follow-up care.
5. Will assume safe and adequate health practices (e.g., controls alcoholism if present as an etiological condition of acute pancreatitis).

### INTERVENTIONS

#### Controlling Pain

Control of pain is a major priority, and either morphine or meperidine (Demerol) may be used. Critically ill patients may receive a continuous infusion of IV narcotics supplemented by boluses as needed for breakthrough pain. Patient-controlled analgesia should be used if feasible to allow for successful pain management.[14] The nurse will regularly and frequently assess the patient's level of pain and response to interventions. The physician will be consulted for needed changes in the regimen. An attitude occasionally encountered in caring for patients with alcohol-induced pancreatitis is that the patient is somehow "getting what he or she deserves," especially on repeat admission for recurrent disease. The nurse must serve as the patient's advocate in the system, documenting the severity of the pain and ensuring that an effective plan is in place to manage it.

Some patients find that the pain is decreased if they assume a sitting position with the trunk flexed, or a side-lying, knee-chest position with their knees drawn up to the abdomen. Epidural analgesia can be used if pain is persistent and not relieved by routine narcotic administration. Although the research is currently inconclusive most patients will be given nothing by mouth to "rest" the pancreas and decrease the autodigestive process. A nasogastric (NG) tube will be inserted to keep the stomach decompressed if vomiting is severe.

The nurse will also explore the use of a variety of nonpharmacological pain relief strategies with the patient, including distraction, imagery, massage, or back rub. The environment should also be kept quiet, comfortable, and conducive to rest. These measures are used in addition to, and not in place of, narcotic administration for pain control.

### Maintaining Fluid and Electrolyte Balance

As soon as the patient is admitted, the nurse should institute monitoring related to fluid and electrolyte status, cardiac output, and renal status. It is a critical need. Monitoring includes intake and output, vital signs, daily weights, abdominal girth, and all routine laboratory values with particular emphasis on potassium and calcium levels. Physical assessment will include assessing for signs of hypokalemia and hypocalcemia (see Chapter 15).

An indwelling Foley catheter may be necessary, since decreased renal function can occur in association with hypotension and shock. Monitoring parameters and frequency of monitoring will depend on the stability of the patient's condition. Fluids, electrolytes, colloids, or blood will be given as necessary.

Aggressive fluid replacement will necessitate establishing and maintaining large bore IV access. The nurse is responsible for administering the fluids and for monitoring the patient's response. The development of hypovolemic shock is of particular concern in the early days of the disease, and the nurse watches carefully for the early signs that could indicate the development of shock (see Chapter 17). The patient also is monitored for hyperglycemia, and checks of blood glucose should be performed four times a day. If severe hyperglycemia occurs, it may be treated with insulin.

### Promoting Adequate Nutrition

The patient will be given nothing by mouth and often has a nasogastric tube in place. Good oral hygiene will be necessary to decrease discomfort from NPO status and from the nasogastric tube. TPN may be used during the critical phase of the illness for patients with severe disease. When the acute symptoms decrease (3 to 5 days), oral fluids and food are restarted. The patient is given clear liquids and then slowly advanced toward a regular diet. Tolerance for oral feedings is carefully assessed as is the possibility of the return of pain. Frequent small meals are usually better tolerated in the early refeeding period. The only diet restriction that needs to be followed after discharge is the avoidance of alcohol.

### Patient/Family Education

Teaching the patient and significant others will be ongoing. At the beginning of hospitalization, the patient and significant others need basic information about the disease, the diagnostic tests, and the treatment. Because of the pain and the distress acute pancreatitis causes and because of the severity of the disease process, the patient and family may be experiencing tremendous anxiety. Therefore explanations and instructions should be brief and as simple as possible and may need to be repeated. Support and continuity of care also need to be provided to help decrease anxiety. Education will be directed toward preventing future attacks and maintaining a nutritious diet. The patient must know that any recurrence of signs and symptoms should be reported immediately. Follow-up care must be explained in detail.

### Health Promotion/Prevention

If unhealthy lifestyle patterns such as alcoholism are a cause of acute pancreatitis, the nurse must work with the patient on the problems. This care will not be instituted until the patient's condition is stabilized, but it must be introduced before the patient leaves the hospital. See Chapter 14 for further information on coping with alcoholism.

If the patient's pancreatitis is related to biliary disease, it will be important to stress the importance of treatment for gallstones. The episode of pancreatitis is frightening and could make the patient reluctant to undergo any further medical or surgical treatment. The nurse will reinforce the etiological role of biliary disease in the development of pancreatitis and encourage the patient to follow through on recommended treatment.

## ■ EVALUATION

To evaluate the effectiveness of nursing interventions, compare patient behaviors with those stated in the expected patient outcomes. Successful achievement of patient outcomes for the patient with acute pancreatitis is indicated by:

1a. States no pain.
 b. Does not splint, grimace, and breathe shallowly.
2. Has hemodynamic measures within normal limits and shows intake equal to output.
3a. Maintains NPO status as appropriate.
 b. Consumes a well-balanced diet without nausea, vomiting, or pain by discharge.
 c. Returns to normal weight.
4a. Appropriately describes the disease, tests, and planned interventions.
 b. Appropriately describes the relationship between etiological factors and the disease.
 c. Appropriately describes and selects well-balanced diet.
5a. Correctly identifies planned follow-up treatment for biliary disease.
 b. Makes commitment to treatment for alcoholism.

## GERONTOLOGICAL CONSIDERATIONS

Biliary disease becomes increasingly common as people age, and biliary disease-related pancreatitis is most likely to occur in the elderly patient. The severity of the disease is difficult to predict, but elderly patients with acute pancreatitis may become critically ill faster because of comorbid problems.

Elders are also more likely to develop complications related to their disease-enforced immobility as well as to the pancreatitis. Respiratory complications are of particular concern, and the elderly patient needs frequent respiratory assessment and aggressive pulmonary hygiene during the acute stage of the disease.

Infection is a common complication of pancreatitis (see discussion under Complications), and elderly patients are less able to withstand the stress imposed on the body by sepsis. The same is true for the development of hypovolemia and fluid shifts. These factors strain the cardiovascular system and may overwhelm the elderly patient's ability to adapt and respond.

## SPECIAL ENVIRONMENTS FOR CARE

### Critical Care Management

Although most patients with pancreatitis recover without any residual dysfunction, a minority experience life-threatening disease. These patients will be managed in a critical care unit. The nurse's major roles are collaborative with the physician and involve ongoing monitoring of all systems and the prevention or identification of complications.

Routine interventions will include hemodynamic monitoring and aggressive fluid support. Critically ill patients may also need cardiac support with drugs such as dopamine. A pulmonary artery catheter may be inserted to assess perfusion adequacy. Left ventricular dysfunction is a common problem.

The airway is compromised in several ways. Severe pain limits diaphragmatic excursion, and both shock and sepsis place extraordinary metabolic demands on the respiratory system that can progress into full-blown ARDS in some patients. Prompt intubation and mechanical ventilation will be crucial. Hypercoagulability increases the risk of pulmonary embolism. Management includes supplemental oxygen, suctioning as needed, and aggressive chest physiotherapy. Assessment is conducted hourly. Respiratory failure accounts for a disproportionate number of pancreatitis-related deaths.

In addition to the concerns addressed above, the critically ill patient with pancreatitis will receive TPN to support a positive nitrogen balance and may undergo peritoneal lavage through a peritoneal catheter. Other interventions will be directed at specific complications as they arise.

### Home Care Management

Most patients with acute pancreatitis recover spontaneously and can be discharged from the hospital within 1 to 2 weeks. Patient needs for home care will be minimal if complications did not develop. Normal activities are gradually resumed as strength and activity tolerance increase.

Patients with alcoholism present a unique challenge as even the pain and anxiety of acute pancreatitis may not be sufficient motivation for them to abstain from alcohol. The nurse will discuss the importance of abstinence with the patient and make referrals to community programs for alcohol treatment if the patient agrees. It is important to recognize, however, that the decision to continue drinking is a matter of personal choice. The nurse's role is to be certain that the patient has all of the information that he or she needs to make an informed decision about the future. A positive outcome cannot be guaranteed.

## COMPLICATIONS

About 25% of patients who have acute pancreatitis will develop complications, and most deaths associated with the disease occur in that group of patients. Complications may be local or systemic. The systemic complications tend to occur within the first week and have largely been discussed within the context of the fulminant disease process. These include complications such as hypovolemic shock, sepsis, renal failure, and ARDS. The major complications of acute pancreatitis are summarized in Box 42-3.

### Pseudocysts

Pancreatic fluid or exudate forms in up to 50% of patients with acute pancreatitis.[6] Pseudocysts are rounded collections of fluid enclosed in a fibrous capsule. This process occurs in only 5% to 10% of all patients.[6] Many pseudocysts resolve spontaneously over time, and intervention is not always warranted. However, pseudocysts can also become life threatening if they obstruct neighboring structures, rupture or hemor-

**box 42-3** *Major Complications of Acute Pancreatitis*

**CARDIOVASCULAR**
Hypotension/shock from hypovolemia or hypoalbuminemia

**HEMATOLOGICAL**
Leukocytosis from generalized inflammation or secondary infections, anemia from blood loss, disseminated intravascular coagulation (DIC) from unknown causes

**RESPIRATORY**
Atelectasis, pneumonia, pleural effusion, adult respiratory distress syndrome (ARDS)

**GASTROINTESTINAL**
GI bleeding

**PANCREATIC**
Pancreatic pseudocysts, pancreatic necrosis or phlegmon, pancreatic abscesses, pancreatic ascites

**RENAL**
Oliguria and acute tubular necrosis

**METABOLIC**
Hyperglycemia, hypocalcemia, hyperlipidemia

rhage, or become infected. A "wait and see" policy is generally followed, and the cysts are monitored regularly. Inflammatory exudate from the pancreas may form into an inflamed mass, which is called a *phlegmon*. Intervention is again not indicated unless bleeding or infection develops. As with pseudocysts the phlegmon may be drained, surgically debrided, or resected as needed.

### Pancreatic Infection

As treatment for systemic complications has improved, pancreatic infection has become the most frequent cause of serious morbidity and mortality associated with acute pancreatitis. Infection typically appears 8 to 20 days after the onset of pancreatitis and has a 100% mortality rate if untreated.[2] Infection usually develops in the areas of necrosis created by fulminant disease. The initial diagnosis of infection can be complicated by the fact that acute pancreatitis itself manifests with the common symptoms of inflammation and infection. Infection-related fever, however, typically exceeds 39° C, and the patient's clinical condition deteriorates.

CT scanning allows for the accurate identification of areas of necrosis, which can then be aspirated by CT-guided needle aspiration. Gram stain and culture can then identify the specific organisms responsible for the infection. Broad-spectrum antibiotics are initiated immediately, but definitive therapy requires percutaneous drainage or surgical debridement. Attempts to prevent the development of infection with the routine use of antibiotics have not proven to be effective, although imipenem (Primaxin) is able to effectively penetrate the capsule of the pancreas and shows promise.

Percutaneous drainage is used most effectively with infected pseudocysts because there is minimal particulate matter present that can clog the tubes. The traditional surgical approach had been to excise as much necrotic material as possible and then place multiple large-bore sump drains in the operative areas to remove infected material.[2] Continuous saline infusion and suction were needed to maintain tube patency. Many surgeons now recommend an open method in which the resected areas are packed, and the dressings are changed under anesthesia every 2 to 3 days until granulation is well underway. The abdomen is left open and eventually closes over an absorbable mesh barrier. A feeding tube is placed once granulation is underway. The development of fistulae can complicate the healing process.

### Chronic Pancreatitis

Patients with alcohol-induced acute pancreatitis are believed to already have asymptomatic chronic disease when they experience their first acute episode. If the patient continues to drink, the likelihood of recurrence is extremely high. Chronic pancreatitis is discussed below.

## CHRONIC PANCREATITIS

### Etiology/Epidemiology

Chronic pancreatitis is present when recurrent bouts of inflammation lead to progressive injury and scarring of pancreatic tissue with gradual fibrous replacement of the normal tissue.[21,23] The progressive degeneration of the gland makes chronic pancreatitis a separate disorder from recurrent acute pancreatitis in which pancreatic function essentially returns to normal when the inflammation subsides.[1,23] Chronic pancreatitis occurs almost exclusively in alcoholics and is more common in men. Other potential causes of chronic pancreatitis include neoplasms, structural problems, and, rarely, inflammatory problems such as inflammatory bowel disease and primary sclerosing cholangitis. Biliary tract disease remains the primary causative factor in acute recurrent pancreatitis.

### Pathophysiology

The basic pathological change of chronic pancreatitis is destruction of the exocrine parenchyma and replacement with fibrous tissue. This process is associated with varying degrees of duct dilatation. Scarring and fibrotic changes may occur throughout the pancreas or be limited to selected areas. Calcium salts may be deposited in both the ducts and the parenchyma, usually in areas of fat necrosis. Ductal obstruction occurs secondarily. The factors that influence the solubility of calcium in the calcium-rich pancreatic secretions are not well identified. As the process becomes increasingly severe the islets of Langerhans are also involved and destroyed.

The role of alcohol in both acute and chronic pancreatitis remains obscure. Alcohol appears to act as a direct toxin, but since only a minority of heavy drinkers develop problems, some genetic defect must also exist that allows alcohol to have such detrimental effects. The pathological nature of the alcohol-induced injury is believed to be similar to that occurring in acute pancreatitis. In addition there is evidence of small protein plugs in the acinar ductules. Secretions are more viscous and tend to form calcium-containing stones. Trypsinogen and other proteases are activated by poorly understood mechanisms.

The patient with chronic pancreatitis may initially have signs and symptoms identical to those described for the patient with acute pancreatitis, with *pain* being the major manifestation. The pain occurs in the right or left upper quadrant, in the back, or throughout the total abdomen. It is severe and constant and is not relieved by food ingestion or antacids. Nausea, vomiting, and abdominal distention may be present, but they are usually secondary to the pain.

In the alcoholic patient it is very difficult to decide where acute pancreatitis leaves off and chronic disease begins. Theoretically the dense fibrosis can entrap and alter the pancreatic nerves, affecting both sensory and motor functions.[1] It is possible that much of the pain is eventually related to this nerve entrapment, although the pain is not different in nature or severity from that which accompanies acute pancreatitis.[1] It is frequently worsened by eating and needs narcotic administration for control.

Pancreatic insufficiency begins once 80% of the pancreatic tissue is destroyed. Symptoms include diarrhea, which is often steatorrhea, and marked weight loss. Diabetes is common and may precede other clinical symptoms. Unique metabolic derangements in glucose metabolism create a strong vulnerability to hypoglycemia and a smaller need for insulin. Oral hypoglycemic agents are not effective. Malabsorption leads to clinical deficiency in vitamins E and $B_{12}$ and other fat-soluble vitamins, but patients rarely develop overt symptoms of deficiency.

A history of acute pancreatitis is the best diagnostic connection to chronic disease. Amylase and lipase levels will rise during recurrent attacks, and both fasting and postprandial hyperglycemia are usually present. Stool examination can quantify the severity of the steatorrhea and malabsorption. CT scanning is the basis of diagnosis and can demonstrate fibrosis, atrophy, duct dilatation, and calculi.

## Collaborative Care Management

Effective management of abdominal pain is the greatest challenge with chronic pancreatitis. Patients who continue to drink alcohol will continue to have pain, and even abstinence is eventually no guarantee of relief. Patients can usually adapt to the malabsorption and steatorrhea, but the persistent pain may lead to drug dependence and motivate the patient to undergo risky surgical procedures, which are frequently accompanied by poor outcomes and multiple complications.

Flare-ups of chronic pancreatitis are managed just like acute disease. Bowel rest is maintained, and attention is paid to managing the acute pain. Ongoing care involves the use of a low-fat diet and supplemental pancreatic enzymes. These extracts will increase the patient's body weight and improve absorption, increasing the patient's general sense of well-being. The recommended diet is high in protein and carbohydrates and may provide as much as 3000 to 6000 calories/day. The use of medium-chain triglycerides to improve the patient's nutritional state is being evaluated in several research trials. Fat-soluble vitamin replacement may also be indicated, and the management of diabetes often requires the use of insulin.

Chronic pancreatitis affects the small ducts of the pancreas and is not amenable to surgical correction. Surgical intervention is frequently used to attempt to relieve the chronic abdominal pain, but there are no proven surgical solutions. Extensive pancreatic resection or pancreatectomy may be performed in patients who are unable to refrain from drinking alcohol. Sympathectomy is occasionally performed to release the entrapped nerves.

The nurse serves as the patient's advocate in the search for comfort. Concerns about drug dependence must not be allowed to prevent the patient from receiving adequate and necessary analgesia. Health care providers can easily become exasperated with patients who are unable or unwilling to stop drinking and can begin to consider the pain of chronic pancreatitis as appropriate retribution for the patient's addiction. This attitude can seriously compromise the patient's care.

In some instances the patient has had negative experiences with pain management during previous hospitalizations for exacerbations and thus believes that analgesics are not being given because the health team does not care about him or her. The involvement of a pain management team is desirable if such services are available. See Chapter 12 for further discussion of pain management.

### *Patient/family education*

The role of alcohol in the etiology and progression of chronic pancreatitis is unequivocal, and yet many alcoholics find themselves unable or unwilling to abstain from alcohol use. The nurse consults with a substance abuse specialist to develop a consistent and appropriate approach for the patient's care and ensures that the patient has all the data necessary to make informed decisions about his or her present and future. Information concerning community resources for alcohol treatment should be current and accurate and offered to the patient. The involvement of the family is encouraged if the dynamics are supportive.

Family members and health care workers need to be helped to understand and accept that ultimately it is the patient's right to make fundamental decisions about his or her own care, even when these decisions do not appear to be in the patient's own best interests.

The patient also needs to learn how to modify the diet and use pancreatic enzyme replacement effectively to control diarrhea and maintain a stable weight. Timing of the medications is critical. The nurse teaches the patient to take the capsules 1 to 2 hours before, during, or after meals. Powders can be mixed directly with food. Patients are informed that these products frequently produce a bad taste and may alter the taste of foods. The patient is instructed to monitor the body's response to the supplements and consistently track weight changes. The anorexia and poor eating habits commonly associated with long-term alcohol use makes adherence to a high-protein, high-calorie diet difficult. The use of vitamin supplements is encouraged if recommended by the physician.

Patients who continue to drink alcohol will always be just one step away from their next flare-up or complication. The nurse provides the patient with written material that outlines the symptoms of complications and encourages the patient to adhere to the plan for continued follow up. A Nursing Care Plan for the patient with chronic pancreatitis is found on p. 1389.

# CANCER OF THE PANCREAS

## Etiology/Epidemiology

Cancer of the pancreas may arise from any of the elements of the pancreas, although most involve the ductal epithelium and are adenocarcinomas. Both benign and malignant tumors can also arise from the islet cells but these are rare.[15] Tumors of the islet cells usually retain some endocrine functions and tend to have a better prognosis than adenocarcinomas.

Pancreatic cancer usually occurs in persons older than 50 years of age, but it can develop at any point in the lifespan. It is much more common in men. The etiology is unknown, but an association has been noted with cigarette smoking and

## nursing care plan *Person with Chronic Pancreatitis*

**DATA** Mr. T. is a 52-year-old self-employed accountant with a 12-year history of acknowledged alcoholism. He experienced his first attack of acute pancreatitis 4 years ago and chronic pancreatitis has since been diagnosed. He is admitted now with another flare-up of the disease.

Mr. T. has made several efforts to stop drinking and has even undergone inpatient alcohol treatment. His longest period of sobriety has been about 6 months. Some life stressor has always precipitated his descent into alcohol dependency. His wife accompanies him to the hospital but is quick to say "I don't think that I can take much more of this. He's killing himself and nothing I say or do is changing that. I don't think I can stay around any longer watching him die. It hurts too much."

Mr. T.'s admission assessment shows a thin, poorly nourished man who appears older than his stated age. He reports the presence of:

- Acute abdominal pain that is generally localized in the mid-epigastric region and radiates to the back. He rates the pain as an 8 on a 10-point scale in severity.
- Steady and protracted vomiting that began late yesterday afternoon. He has had nothing to eat or drink for more than 12 hours.
- Large, soft, and foul-smelling stools that have been increasing in frequency and severity over the last few weeks. He has lost 12 pounds.
- A history of decreased alcohol use over the last 3 months. Mr. T says "I know no one will believe me but I've really been drinking much less. The pain starts so quickly when I drink that I have really been steadily decreasing my intake. I don't understand why this should happen now. What's the use? The doctor said the pain would stop if I stopped drinking so much and look at me now. Maybe I should just drink myself to death and get it over with."

Other data on admission include:

- Blood pressure is 94/60, pulse is 92, and respirations are 22 and shallow. Temperature is 99.8° F.
- Bloodwork shows the following abnormalities: hemoglobin of 10.2 g, red blood cell count of 2.9 million, $K^+$ of 3.0 mg/dl, serum calcium of 8.2 mg/dl, and glucose of 162 mg/dl.

Initial care orders include:

- IV of 1000 ml of 5% dextrose in $^1/_2$ N saline with 20 mEq of KCl at 125 ml/hr
- NPO
- Monitor intake and output, daily weight, and abdominal girth once daily
- Demerol 100 mg IM q 3 hr PRN for pain
- Insert NG tube and attach to low intermittent suction if vomiting persists past 4 PM
- Accucheck 4 times daily per protocol, call house officer if glucose >160
- Monitor closely for hypovolemic shock, electrolyte imbalance, delirium tremens (DTs)
- Call substance abuse resource counselor for DT protocol initiation if needed

**NURSING DIAGNOSIS** *Acute pain related to distention of pancreatic capsule and activation of pancreatic enzymes*

| expected patient outcome | nursing interventions | rationale |
|---|---|---|
| States pain is effectively controlled with pharmacological and nonpharmacological methods. | **1.** Assess pain levels frequently, especially before and after administration of analgesics. | **1.** Frequent assessment is essential to validate the nature and severity of the patient's pain experience. |
| | **a.** Document pain levels on flow sheet. | **a.** Recording on a flow sheet allows for a pattern of pain to be established and the effectiveness of pain control to be evaluated. |
| | **2.** Administer meperidine q3h as needed. | **2.** Synthetic narcotics are effective analgesics and do not cause spasm in the sphincter of Oddi. |
| | **a.** Encourage patient to use analgesics on a regular rather than PRN basis. | **a.** A regular time schedule of drug use allows for a steady blood level to be established. |
| | **b.** Validate your acceptance of the reality of the patient's pain and its severity. | **b.** Patients with chronic pancreatitis are frequently labeled "drug seekers" by staff. |
| | **c.** Evaluate effectiveness of the narcotic order. Collaborate with physician to make adjustments in dose or drug as needed. | **c.** Acute pain can be immobilizing. Morphine may be substituted for meperidine. |
| | **3.** Collaborate with Mr. T to determine the nonpharmacological methods that help to reduce his pain. | **3.** Nonpharmacological methods allow the patient a degree of control of the pain experience. |
| | **a.** Position him in a mid to high Fowler's position with his knees flexed. | **a.** This position is theorized to reduce tension on the abdomen. |
| | **b.** Explore his experience with strategies such as distraction, massage, relaxation, and guided imagery. | **b.** All of these can be effective methods of pain control, but the patient must have an open mind and be willing to experiment with new strategies. |

*Continued*

## Person with Chronic Pancreatitis–cont'd

**NURSING DIAGNOSIS** *Risk for fluid volume deficit related to vomiting, NPO status, hyperglycemia, and increased capillary permeability*

| expected patient outcome | nursing interventions | rationale |
|---|---|---|
| Maintains balance of fluids and electrolytes; intake and output are balanced; weight is stable. | 1. Assess fluid and electrolyte status each shift.<br>a. Maintain accurate intake and output.<br>b. Weigh daily.<br>c. Assess skin turgor and status of mucous membranes each shift.<br>d. Monitor cardiovascular response to fluid replacement.<br>e. Measure abdominal girth daily or as ordered. | 1. Patient is at risk for hypovolemic shock and dehydration. May lose 4 to 14 L of fluid into the abdomen. Fluid replacement is based on estimates of losses. A urine output of 30 to 50 ml/hr is essential to prevent the onset of acute tubular necrosis.<br>Fluid and gas accumulation in GI tract can result in significant abdominal distention. |
| | 2. Monitor blood glucose 4 times daily.<br>a. Administer sliding-scale insulin per protocol. | 2. Destruction of the beta cells and islets of Langerhans produces severe hyperglycemia. Because of the risk of labile hypoglycemia, insulin is not given unless glucose level continues to rise. |
| | 3. Monitor for hypokalemia and hypocalcemia:<br>• muscle weakness, cramping<br>• numbness and tingling in fingertips or around mouth; positive Chvostek's and Trousseau's sign | 3. Large amounts of potassium are lost through vomiting and in the pancreatic secretions; calcium is believed to bind with free fats and can drop to levels that increase neural excitability. |

**NURSING DIAGNOSIS** *Altered nutrition: less than body requirements related to vomiting, NPO status, and malabsorption caused by loss of function of pancreatic enzymes*

| expected patient outcome | nursing interventions | rationale |
|---|---|---|
| Receives sufficient nutrients by mouth or TPN to maintain stable body weight, keeps albumin levels above 3.8 g/dl, and produces normal stools. | 1. Maintain NPO status and bed rest until patient's condition stabilizes. | 1. NPO status is theorized to reduce the secretion of pancreatic enzymes. Bed rest decreases the body's metabolic rate. |
| | 2. Assess current nutritional and elimination status. | 2. Patients with chronic pancreatitis are often malnourished before the attack from alcoholism and malabsorption. |
| | 3. Monitor daily weight and serum protein and albumin levels. | 3. These parameters provide the best ongoing data about nutritional status. |
| | 4. Initiate TPN if NPO status needs to be protracted. | 4. If pain is not controlled promptly the rapid catabolism of the disease must be counteracted by TPN to prevent life-threatening complications. |
| | 5. Reinitiate oral feedings once abdominal pain is controlled and amylase/lipase levels stabilize. | 5. Once pain and enzyme levels are stable there is no contraindication to oral feeding, and the severity of malabsorption needs to be established. |
| | 6. Offer small, frequent feedings to the patient's tolerance; assess patient response.<br>a. Restrict fat in diet if steatorrhea persists. | 6. This feeding pattern minimizes distention and malabsorption symptoms.<br>a. Malabsorption primarily affects digestion of fats. |
| | 7. Evaluate composition and volume of stools. Adjust dose of pancreatic enzymes to achieve normal elimination. | 7. Malabsorption manifests itself as large-volume, greasy, foul-smelling stools. Adequate enzyme replacement will restore the stool to near normal. |

*Continued*

## Person with Chronic Pancreatitis–cont'd

**NURSING DIAGNOSIS** *Risk for ineffective management of therapeutic regimen related to inability to abstain from alcohol and inadequate knowledge of management of malabsorption and hyperglycemia*

| expected patient outcome | nursing interventions | rationale |
|---|---|---|
| Verbalizes understanding of disease process, role of alcohol, and pharmacological management of symptoms. Makes commitment to abstain from alcohol. | 1. Assess patient's current understanding of the disease process and the role of alcohol in its recurrence. | 1. This establishes a baseline for planning and intervention. |
| | 2. Assess patient's interest and commitment to abstain from alcohol.<br>a. Assess knowledge of community resources for treatment and support. Refer as appropriate. | 2. Patient has stated his attempts to decrease alcohol use. Wife has stated the end of her tolerance for his continued use of alcohol. |
| | 3. Assess for symptoms of DTs during first 48 to 72 hours. Consult with substance abuse specialist if needed. | 3. Patient may not be truthful about current level of use. Withdrawal carries a high mortality in acutely ill patients and necessitates specialty asisstance. |
| | 4. Teach patient correct use of pancreatic enzymes:<br>• Take with each meal and snack.<br>• Monitor weight and stool consistency to judge need for dosage adjustment. | 4. Malabsorption is permanent, and patient will develop serious nutrient deficiencies if enzymes are not adequately replaced. Dosage adjustments can be safely made by a well-informed patient. |
| | 5. Teach patient about the nature and planned management of diabetes.<br>a. Teach symptoms to report:<br>• Hyperglycemia: frequent urination, thirst, lethargy, abdominal cramping<br>• Hypoglycemia: anxiety, tachycardia, diaphoresis | 5. Insulin may be needed to control the diabetes of chronic pancreatitis, but hypoglycemia must be prevented. Patient will remain hyperglycemic but must know how to recognize ketoacidosis. |
| | 6. Encourage patient to make commitment to changing his lifestyle and gaining control of his disease and his life. | 6. Patients with chronic pancreatitis often have given up hope on themselves and their ability to influence the future. |

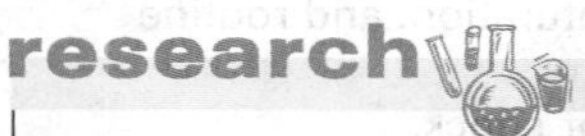

Reference: Price TF, Payne RL, Oberletiner MG: Familial pancreatic cancer in South Louisiana, *Cancer Nurs* 19(4):275-282, 1996.

This study explored a possible familial predisposition to pancreatic cancer among a Cajun heritage population in the Acadiana region of Louisiana. The study was descriptive in nature and used a questionnaire to explore cancer incidence and risk factors. Thirty-eight patients or family surrogates were enrolled from among the 140 possible cancer patients documented during the year of study. Sampling was difficult as patients rapidly became extremely ill or died. Of the sample sixty-five percent reported Cajun ancestry. They reported a total of 366 first-degree relatives of whom 44 had also developed pancreatic cancer. This represented an incidence rate far above national norms where pancreatic cancer accounts for only 2% of all new cancer diagnoses. The sample incidence rate was comparable to that of lung cancer. African Americans had the highest incidence (32 per 100,000 versus 17 per 100,000 nationwide). The incidence rate was also significantly increased for whites (18 per 100,000 versus 10 per 100,000 nationwide). Heavy prolonged cigarette smoking was shown to be a clear risk factor, which has been true in all samples. Although flawed by sampling difficulties, the study does appear to confirm the presence of a significant familial risk for pancreatic cancer in this unique population.

the presence of long-standing diabetes, especially in women. Incidences of familial clustering of cases point to a hereditary component (Research Box). A link with chronic pancreatitis has been suggested but remains unproven.

### Pathophysiology

Pancreatic cancers usually develop in the head of the gland and vary dramatically in size at the time of diagnosis. The tumor is usually deeply encased in normal tissue and is poorly demarcated. The common duct is often obstructed and distended by the presence of the tumor. Metastasis has almost always occurred before the tumor produces its first symptoms because there is no capsule surrounding the pancreas to prevent the growth and spread of the tumor. Direct extension of the lesion may cause its spread to the posterior wall of the stomach, the duodenal wall, the colon, and the common bile duct. Vital blood vessels in the area are also frequently involved.

Pain is the earliest and most common symptom of pancreatic cancer. The pain is usually described as epigastric in location and steady and severe in character. It occurs or is worsened by lying down and bears no relationship to meals. The pain is relentlessly progressive in nature. Weight loss frequently accompanies the pain and can be dramatic. Anorexia is also common. Jaundice and pruritis will typically develop when bile duct obstruction occurs. Diarrhea and/or steatorrhea develop fairly late in the disease. Diabetes may also develop.

## Collaborative Care Management

The diagnosis of pancreatic cancer is often first made based on the pattern of symptoms and then is confirmed through CT scanning. Guided needle biopsy may be performed at the same time. A histological diagnosis is important in planning care.[9]

Cancer of the pancreas is usually fatal within 6 months regardless of treatment. Less than 2% of patients survive 2 years. The treatment is generally surgical, although surgery has not been proven to improve survival. Obstruction is a common problem with large tumors involving the pancreatic head, and surgical bypass is frequently attempted. Procedures include gastrojejunostomy to bypass the duodenum and choledochojejunostomy to relieve biliary obstruction. Endoscopic placement of stent tubes to support biliary drainage is increasingly considered as an alternative to surgery. Stents may be placed internally or inserted for external drainage.

Surgeons who are attempting curative procedures may use the more aggressive Whipple procedure or total pancreatectomy (Figure 42-6). Neither radiotherapy nor chemotherapy alone has had any positive effects on the course of the disease, but combination protocols used in research trials appear to extend life expectancy to nearly 1 year.

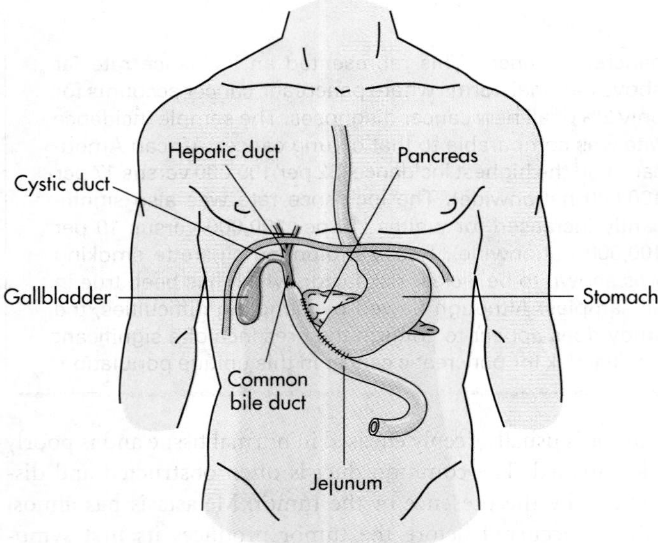


**fig. 42-6** Pancreatoduodenectomy (Whipple's procedure) with anastomosis.

### Patient/family education

Pain management is an ongoing challenge with pancreatic cancer and is often the primary determinant of quality of life. The nurse serves as the patient's advocate in the health care system to establish an effective pain management protocol and continuously adapt it to changes in the patient's condition. The nurse provides careful teaching about the use of narcotic analgesics and the inevitable development of tolerance and physical dependence (see Chapter 12). Instruction is also provided about expected side effects and their management. Other general measures are those provided to any patient with invasive cancer (see Chapter 11). Nursing care of the patient undergoing pancreatic surgery is summarized in the Guidelines for Care Box.

### guidelines for care

#### The Person Undergoing Pancreatic Surgery

**Preoperative Care**

Provide thorough teaching about planned surgical procedure and expected postoperative care.
Monitor prothrombin time and other clotting studies; vitamin K and other clotting factors may be administered.
Assess nutritional status. Administer TPN if ordered.

**Postoperative Care**

Monitor vital parameters every hour. Critical care placement is usually necessary.
- Check vital signs, intake and output, and hemodynamic parameters.
- Perform blood gas, oxygen saturation, and routine blood studies.
- Be alert to signs of bleeding or shock.
- Maintain urine output at 30 to 50 ml/hr.

Initiate pulmonary hygiene every hour with deep breathing, coughing as needed, and use of incentive spirometry.
Establish effective pain management regimen. Monitor every hour.
Monitor dressings and drainage tubes. Keep skin clear of drainage.
Maintain nutritional support with TPN.
- Initiate oral feedings with clear liquids. Advance as tolerated.
- Monitor blood glucose and administer insulin as ordered.
- Monitor patient's weight and the development of steatorrhea.
  - Administer pancreatic enzyme replacement as ordered.
  - Assess for signs of dumping syndrome (see Chapter 40).

Provide support for patient and family and initiate discharge planning.

## critical thinking QUESTIONS

1 Mrs. Blue has a T-tube present after an abdominal cholecystectomy. What may normally occur after the removal of her T-tube? What complication should the nurse be alert for? Why? How should he or she respond?

2 In what ways would your assessment findings for a person with chronic pancreatitis differ from those for a person with acute pancreatitis?

3 Mr. Ryan 77, is being treated for acute pancreatitis related to biliary obstruction. What aspect of this type of pancreatitis differs from acute alcohol-induced pancreatitis?

## chapter SUMMARY

### CHOLELITHIASIS/CHOLECYSTITIS/ CHOLEDOCHOLITHIASIS

- Cholelithiasis and cholecysitis are common health problems. Risk factors include obesity, female gender, multiparity, use of birth control pills, and middle age.
- Biliary tract surgery by laparoscopic cholecystectomy is the treatment of choice for gallbladder disease.
- If acute cholecystitis occurs, pain, nausea, and vomiting, and fluid and electrolyte problems may be of concern.
- Patient problems requiring nursing attention after open cholecystectomy include ineffective breathing pattern, pain, and management of the T-tube.

### PRIMARY SCLEROSING CHOLANGITIS

- Primary sclerosing cholangitis is usually idiopathic in etiology but frequently occurs in conjunction with IBD. There is no treatment, and most patients eventually require liver transplant.

### CARCINOMA OF THE BILIARY SYSTEM

- Carcinoma of the biliary system is insidious and can be asymptomatic until late in the disease.

### PANCREATIC DISORDERS

- Pancreatitis may be acute or chronic.
- Acute pancreatitis can result in critical fluid and electrolyte problems, metabolic disturbances, and pain.
- Most cases resolve spontaneously, but the mortality from hemorrhagic forms is high.
- Care in acute pancreatitis focuses on pain management, fluid resuscitation to prevent shock, resting the pancreas by NPO status, and collaborative monitoring for complications.
- Chronic pancreatitis is progressive and usually results from alcoholism. It is not reversible.
- Chronic pancreatitis results in pain, malabsorption and steatorrhea and possibly diabetes mellitus.
- Abstinence from alcohol use is the primary treatment objective in patients with chronic pancreatitis.
- Malabsorption is treated with the use of pancreatic enzyme supplements. Pain management is extremely difficult if the patient continues to drink alcohol.
- Cancer of the pancreas is insidious and has a very poor prognosis. In rare instances a pancreatoduodenectomy may be performed.

## References


1. Ambrose MS, Dreher HM: Pancreatitis—managing a flareup, *Nursing* 26(4):33-39, 1996.
2. Baker CC, Huynh T: Acute pancreatitis—surgical management, *Crit Care Clin* 11(2):311-322, 1995.
3. Domingues-Munoz JE, Malfertheiner P: Management of severe acute pancreatitis, *Gastroenterologist* 4:248-253, 1993.
4. Everhart JE: Contributions of obesity and weight loss to gallstone disease, *Ann Intern Med* 119(10): 1029-1035, 1993.
5. Fenster LF, Lonborg R, Thirlby RC, Traverso LW: What symptoms does cholecystectomy cure? *Am J Surg* 169(5): 533-538, 1995.
6. Forsmark CE, Toskes PP: Acute pancreatitis—medical management, *Crit Care Clin* 11(2):295-306, 1995.
7. Gauwitz DF: Endoscopic cholecystectomy: The patient friendly alternative, *Nursing* 20(12):58-59, 1992.
8. Ghiloni BW: Cholelithiasis: current treatment options, *Am Fam Physician* 48(5):762-768, 1993.
9. Greifzo S, Dest V: When the diagnosis is pancreatic cancer, *RN* 54(3):38-41, 1991.
10. Kohn CL, Brozenec S, Foster PF: Nutritional support for the patient with pancreatobiliary disease, *Crit Care Nurs Clin North Am* 5(1):37-45, 1993.
11. Krumberger JM: Acute pancreatitis, *Crit Care Nurs Clin North Am* 5(1):185-201, 1993.
12. Marshall JB: Acute pancreatitis: a review with an emphasis on new developments, *Arch Intern Med* 153(6):1185-1193, 1993.
13. McClave SA, Greene LM, Snider HL: Comparison of the safety of early enteral vs. parenteral nutrition in mild acute pancreatitis, *J Parenter Enteral Nutr* 21(1): 14-20, 1997.
14. McConnell E, Lewis LW: Managing the patient with pancreatitis, *Nursing 21*(11):98-102, 1991.
15. Murr MM et al: Pancreatic cancer, *CA: Cancer J Clin* 44(2):304-314, 1994.
16. National Institutes of Health: National Institutes of Health Consensus Development Conference Statement on Gallstones and Laparoscopic Cholecystectomy, *Am J Surg* 165(4): 390-398, 1993.
17. Ondrusek RS: Cholecystectomy: an update, *RN* 56(1):28-31, 1993.
18. Peterson KJ, Solie CJ: Interpreting lab values in pancreatitis, *Am J Nurs* 94(11):45A-B, 56F, 1994.
19. Price P, Hartranft TH: New trends in the treatment of calculus disease of the biliary tract, *J Am Board Fam Pract* 8(1):22-28, 1995.
20. Price TF, Payne RL, Oberleitner MG: Familial pancreatic cancer in South Louisiana, *Cancer Nurs* 19(4):272-282, 1996.
21. Sidhu SS, Tandon RK: The pathogenesis of chronic pancreatitis, *Postgrad Med* 71(2):67-70, 1995.
22. Smith A: When the pancreas fails, *Am J Nurs* 91(9):38-48, 1991.
23. Spiro HM: *Clinical Gastroenterology,* ed 4, New York, 1993, McGraw Hill.
24. Thompson C: Managing acute pancreatitis, *RN* 55(3):52-54, 1992.

chapter

# 43 ASSESSMENT OF THE Renal System

LYNN NOLAND

## objectives

*After studying this chapter, the learner should be able to:*

1. List the major functions of the kidney.
2. Describe the anatomy of the kidney.
3. Apply subjective and objective (including laboratory) data to assess renal function.
4. Relate significant urinary tract symptoms to their most likely etiology.
5. Identify potential etiologies for common abnormal urinalysis findings.
6. Describe guidelines for caring for patients after urological diagnostic procedures.

The kidneys are paired retroperitoneal organs that are integral to the maintenance of the body's homeostasis, or chemical and physical equilibrium. They produce and secrete hormones and enzymes that help regulate red blood cell production, blood pressure, and calcium and phosphate metabolism. By excreting metabolic end products and varying the excretion of water and solutes, the kidneys regulate body fluid volume, acidity, and electrolytes, thus maintaining normal body composition (Box 43-1).[3,9]

## ANATOMY AND PHYSIOLOGY

### ANATOMY

#### Upper Urinary Tract

The kidneys are two reddish-brown, lima bean-shaped organs that lie behind the parietal peritoneum against the posterior abdominal wall at the costovertebral angle. The kidneys lie on either side of the abdominal aorta, inferior vena cava (Figure 43-1), and lumbar spine between the twelfth thoracic and third lumbar vertebrae. The liver pushes the right kidney down to a level slightly lower than the left.

The kidneys are encased in a tough, white, fibrous coat known as the renal capsule. In addition, each kidney is surrounded by a mass of perinephric fat that provides protection against injury. An adrenal gland lies above each kidney within the perinephric fat. The renal fascia and surrounding organs help hold the kidneys in place. On the medial aspect of each kidney is a concave notch known as the hilum. The renal arteries and nerves enter, and the renal veins, lymphatics, and ureters exit the kidney at the hilum (Figure 43-2).

When the kidney is cut longitudinally and opened, three distinct areas can be seen: the cortex, medulla, and renal sinus (see Figure 43-2). The renal cortex is pale and has a granular appearance. Most parts of the nephron, the functional unit of the kidney, lie in this area.

The middle section, the renal medulla, contains 8 to 10 triangular wedges or pyramids. The bases of the pyramids face the cortex, and their apexes or renal papillae face the center of the kidney. The pyramids have a striated appearance because of the segment of the nephrons and collecting ducts located here.

The third section of the kidney is the renal sinus. It is a cavity almost completely filled with blood vessels and structures formed by the expanded upper end of the ureter. Before entering the kidney, the ureter dilates to form the renal pelvis. The renal pelvis branches into two or three calyces. Each major calyx branches into several minor calyces. The minor calyces collect the urine that drains from the collecting ducts.

The nephron is the functional unit of the kidney. Each kidney contains approximately 1 million nephrons. The two types of nephrons, cortical and juxtamedullary, are named according to the location of their glomeruli within the renal parenchyma. The cortical nephrons comprise 85% of the total nephrons and perform excretory and regulatory functions. The juxtamedullary nephrons make up the remaining 15% and play an important role in the concentration and dilution of urine by generating a steep interstitial fluid osmotic gradient between the cortex and deep medulla. The structures of the nephron involved in the process of urine formation include the renal corpuscle, the renal tubules, and the collecting duct (Figure 43-3). The renal corpuscle consists of the glomerulus and Bowman's capsule and is responsible for the formation of ultrafiltrate from the blood. The renal tubules consist of the proximal convoluted tubule, the

**box 43-1** *Functions of the Kidney*

- Regulation of body fluid volume and osmolality
- Regulation of electrolyte balance
- Regulation of acid-base balance
- Excretion of metabolic waste products, toxins, and foreign substances
- Production and secretion of hormones

NOTE: Additional related functions such as blood pressure regulation and red cell production occur as the result of the above.

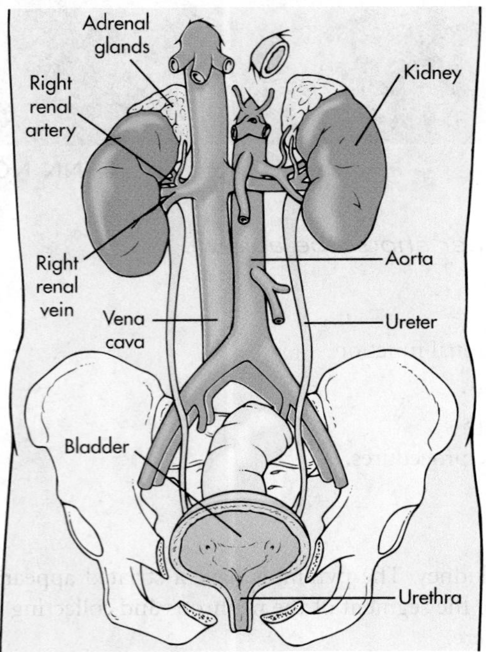

fig. 43-1 Organs and structures of the urinary system.

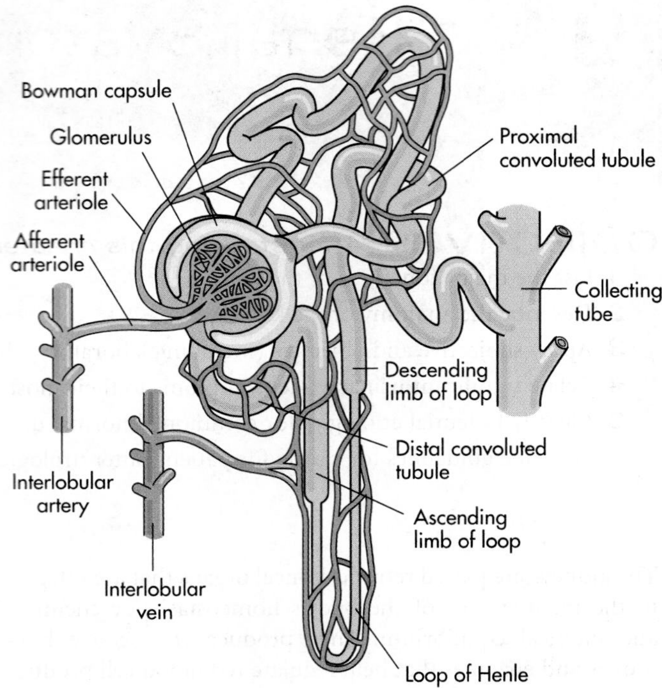

fig. 43-3 Nephron.

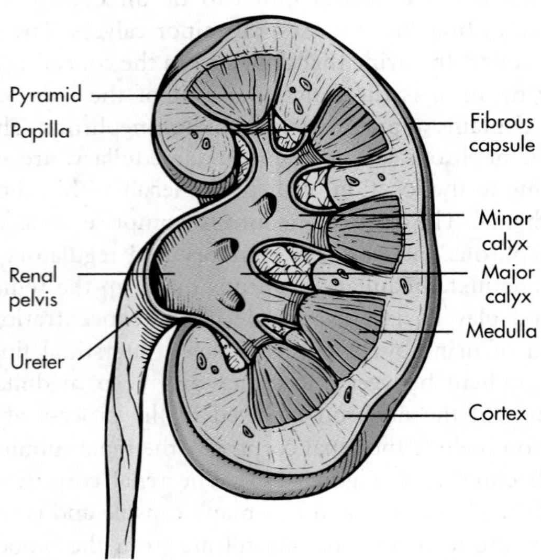

fig. 43-2 Frontal section of kidney.

loop of Henle, and the distal convoluted tubule and are responsible for the reabsorption and secretion that alter the volume and composition of the ultrafiltrate to form the final urine product. The collecting duct receives tubular fluid from many nephrons and transports the fluid from the cortex to the minor calyx.

The kidneys are highly vascular organs, receiving about 20% of the cardiac output in the resting state. Arterial blood is supplied by the renal arteries, which branch directly off the abdominal aorta (see Figure 43-1). Although 70% of human beings have one renal artery supplying each kidney, about 30% have one or more accessory renal arteries that also branch off the aorta and supply a portion of the kidney.

The renal artery branches into approximately five segmental arteries, dividing the kidney into vascular segments. The segmental arteries branch to form the lobar arteries that supply each pyramid. The lobar arteries then branch several more times so blood can move efficiently through each nephron. Each nephron actually has its own blood supply; blood enters the glomerulus through the afferent arteriole and exits through the efferent arteriole. Blood then flows through the peritubular capillaries that surround the nephron's tubules. Ultimately the peritubular capillaries empty into venules that return the filtered blood to the general circulation via the renal venous system.[2]

The ureters (see Figure 43-2) arise as extensions of the renal pelvis and empty into the bladder in an area known as the trigone (Figure 43-4). The trigone is a fold of mucous membrane that serves as a valve preventing the backflow or reflux of urine into the ureter when the bladder contracts. The ureters are composed of smooth muscle and are innervated by the sympathetic nervous system. The function of the ureters is to propel urine from the renal pelves to the bladder.

## Lower Urinary Tract

The bladder, located behind the symphysis pubis (see Figure 43-1), serves as a collecting bag for the urine. The mucous membrane lining of the bladder is arranged in folds called rugae. These rugae, together with the elasticity of the muscular walls, enable the bladder to distend to hold large amounts

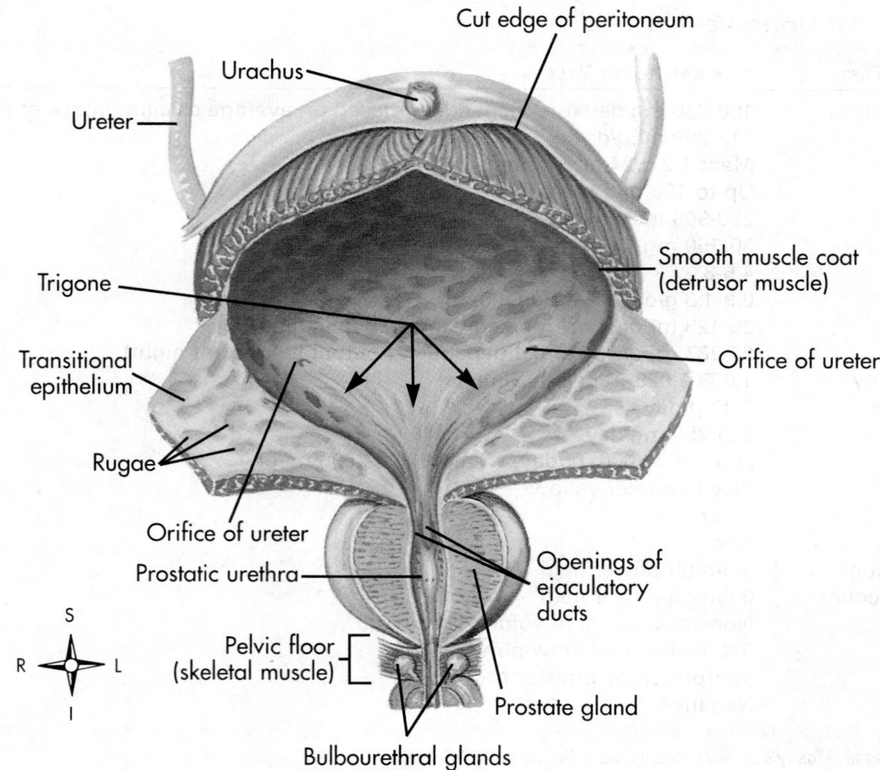


**fig. 43-4** Interior of urinary bladder and associated structures in the male.

of urine. A layer of skeletal muscle encircles the base of the bladder, forming the external urinary sphincter. Both the sympathetic and parasympathetic nervous systems innervate the bladder. The urethral sphincter, operating under voluntary control, allows the urine to pass into the urethra.

The urethra serves as the outlet for urine from the bladder. The male urethra is about 20 cm (8 in) in length, whereas the female urethra is about 4 cm (1.5 in) long. The urinary meatus is the opening through which urine exits the body.

The prostate gland is a roughly walnut size male reproductive gland that encircles the upper portion of the male urethra (Figure 43-4). The gland is doughnut-shaped with the urethra passing through the "hole." When the prostate is enlarged, the urethra is squeezed, obstructing the flow of urine. Numerous prostatic ducts empty into the urethra. Bacteria from urinary tract infections may travel up these ducts, causing inflammation and infection of the prostate.

## PHYSIOLOGY

A clear understanding of the physiology of the kidneys is essential to mastering the constellation of physiochemical changes that occur with renal failure. A short review of renal physiology follows.

### Ultrafiltration

Ultrafiltration is the renal process by which urine is formed. As blood passes through the capillary bed of the glomerulus, filtration of the plasma occurs. In this process of ultrafiltration, glomerular filtrate is formed. The volume of the glomerular filtrate approximates 180 L per day. Of this volume, 99% is reabsorbed by the kidneys. Because of this tremendous reabsorptive power of the kidneys, the average urinary output of an adult is only 1 to 2 L/day.

Ultrafiltration is measured as the glomerular filtration rate (GFR). Clinically GFR is defined as the amount of glomerular filtrate formed in 1 minute. The larger the body surface area is, the greater the GFR. The GFR in an average-sized adult is approximately 125 ml/min (7.5 L/hr). At this rate a volume of approximately 60 times the plasma volume is filtered each day. The average GFR of a woman is about 10% less than that of a man. Glomerular filtrate is formed by the same forces that affect fluid transport between vascular and interstitial spaces in other tissues of the body. These factors include hydrostatic pressure and oncotic pressure.

The kidneys receive approximately 20% of the cardiac output, resulting in renal blood flow rates of about 1200 ml/min. This rapid blood flow rate exceeds the metabolic and oxygen needs of the kidneys but facilitates efficient clearance of metabolic waste products. Therefore, severe or prolonged interruptions in cardiac output or renal perfusion profoundly affect the formation of urine, as well as the viability of the cells responsible for maintaining the consistency of the body's internal environment.

Urine formation actually begins when blood from the renal artery passes through a series of progressively smaller arteries and then enters the afferent arteriole of the nephron. It is in Bowman's capsule and the tubules that the ultrafiltrate begins

**table 43-1** *Normal Urine Values*

| Laboratory Test | Normal Adult Values |
|---|---|
| Calcium (24 hr) | 100-250 mg/day (diet dependent; based on average calcium intake of 600-800 mg/24 hr) |
| Chloride | 110-250 mEq/day |
| Creatinine | Men: 1-2 g/24 hr; women: 0.8-1.8 g/24 hr |
| Glucose | Up to 100 mg/24 hr |
| Osmolality | 250-900 mOsm/kg |
| Protein | 30-150 mg/24 hr (method dependent) |
| pH | 4.5-8 |
| Phosphorus | 0.9-1.3 g/day (diet dependent) |
| Potassium | 26-123 mEq/24 hr (markedly intake dependent) |
| Sodium | 27-287 mEq/24 hr (diet dependent; output is lower at night) |
| Specific gravity | 1.003-1.029 (range in SI units) |
| Urea nitrogen | 6-17 g/day |
| Uric acid | 250-750 mg/day |
| Volume | Men: 800-2000 ml/day; women: 800-1600 ml/day |
| Color | Pale to darker yellow |
| Clarity | Clear |
| Ketones | None |
| Red blood count | 0-5/high-power field |
| White blood count | 0-5/high-power field |
| Bacteria | None/occasional in voided specimen |
| Casts | 0-4 hyaline casts/low-power field |
| Crystals | Interpreted by physician |
| Culture | Negative |

Data from Thompson JM et al: *Mosby's clinical nursing,* ed 4, St Louis, 1997, Mosby.

**table 43-2** *Average Filtration and Reabsorption Values for Several Common Substances*

| Substance | Amount Filtered (per day) | Amount Excreted (per day) | Percent Reabsorbed |
|---|---|---|---|
| Water (L) | 180 | 1.8 | 99.0 |
| Sodium (g) | 630 | 3.2 | 99.5 |
| Glucose (g) | 180 | 0.0 | 100.0 |
| Urea (g) | 54 | 30.0 | 44.0 |
| Potassium (g) | 35 | 2.0 | 94.0 |
| Calcium (g) | 5 | 0.2 | 96.0 |
| Amino acids (g) | 10 | 0.3 | 97.0 |

to be transformed into urine.[3] Table 43-1 presents the normal composition of urine.

The ability of the kidney to conserve water and electrolytes is essential for survival. If conservation were not possible, a person would be volume and electrolyte depleted in 3 to 4 minutes. This miraculous ability for conservation occurs because of the kidney's tremendous reabsorptive capacity. Refer to Table 43-2 for a summary of the filtration and reabsorption values of common substances.

The proximal convoluted tubule reabsorbs 85% to 90% of the water in the ultrafiltrate; up to 80% of filtered sodium; and most of the filtered potassium, bicarbonate, chloride, phosphate, glucose, and amino acids. The distal convoluted tubule and collecting tubule produce the final urine.

Another mechanism that prevents water and electrolyte depletion is endocrine or hormonal response. See Table 43-3 for a description of hormones that affect sodium and water balance via their action on the kidney. Antidiuretic hormone (ADH) is a classic example of how hormonal influence regulates salt and water balance. ADH is a hormone produced by the hypothalamus and stored and released by the pituitary gland in response to changes in plasma osmolarity. Osmolarity refers to the concentration of ions in a solution, in this case in the blood. If water intake is low or if water loss is high, ADH is released, which causes the kidney to retain water. ADH acts on the distal portion of the nephron to enhance water permeability, thus allowing more water to be reclaimed from the ultrafiltrate in the tubules and returned to the blood. The result is reversal of the dehydrated state and maintenance of equilibrium.[1,9]

The kidneys maintain physiological equilibrium by controlling the fluid and solute composition of the blood. Three intricate processes are used: filtration, reabsorption, and secretion. Each part of the nephron is anatomically constructed to perform one or more of these processes. Filtration occurs in Bowman's capsule and reabsorption and secretion in the tubules and collecting duct. See Box 43-2 for a summary of the regions of the nephron and their primary functions. Briefly, equilibrium is maintained through effective ultrafiltration as summarized below.[1,2]

Blood enters the glomerular capillaries, and water and small molecules begin to be filtered out into Bowman's capsule through tiny pores in the capillary wall. The pore size restricts the size of molecule that can leave the blood. For example, blood cells are too large to filter, but urea is the correct

**table 43-3** *Hormones that Regulate NaCl and Water Reabsorption*

| Hormone | Major Stimulus | Nephron Site of Action | Effect on Transport |
|---|---|---|---|
| Angiotensin II | ↑ Renin | PT | ↑ NaCl and $H_2O$ reabsorption |
| Aldosterone | ↑ Angiotensin II, ↑ $[K^+]_p$ | TAL, DT/CD | ↑ NaCl and $H_2O$ reabsorption* |
| Atrial natriuretic peptide | ↑ BP, ↑ ECF | CD | ↓ $H_2O$ and NaCl reabsorption |
| Sympathetic nerves | ↓ ECF | PT, TAL, DT/CD | ↑ NaCl and $H_2O$ reabsorption* |
| Dopamine | ↑ ECF | PT | ↓ $H_2O$ and NaCl reabsorption |
| ADH | ↑ $P_{osm}$, ↓ ECF | TAL, DT/CD | ↓ NaCl and $H_2O$ reabsorption* |

From Berne RM, Levy MN: *Principles of physiology,* ed 2, St Louis, 1996, Mosby.
*PT,* proximal tubule; *TAL,* thick ascending limb; *DT/CD,* distal tubule and collecting duct; ↓ *ECF,* decrease in extracellular fluid volume; ↑ *ECF,* increase in extracellular fluid volume; ↑ *BP,* increase in blood pressure; ↑ $[K]_p$, increase in plasma $[K^+]$; ↑ $P_{osm}$, increase in plasma osmolality. All of the hormones listed act within minutes, except aldosterone, which exerts its action on NaCl reabsorption with a delay of 1 hour.
*Indicates that the effect on $H_2O$ reabsorption does not occur in TAL.

size to be filtered out of the blood. From Bowman's capsule the ultrafiltrate moves into the proximal tubule where most of the water, sodium, potassium, calcium, chloride, and bicarbonate filtered out in the capsule originally are reabsorbed and returned to the blood. Body waste products such as hydrogen ions, phosphate, and drugs and their metabolites are secreted from the blood in the proximal tubules.[1,2,8]

In both the descending and the ascending loops of Henle the ultrafiltrate is further refined as more sodium and water are reabsorbed, and magnesium is reclaimed from the tubules. Final adjustment in urine composition is made in the distal nephron, which includes the distal convoluted tubule and the collecting ducts. The primary solutes affected in this area are potassium, bicarbonate, hydrogen ions, and again, sodium and chloride. This final refinement of the urine is accomplished mostly by feedback mechanisms regulated by the hormones aldosterone and ADH. The filtrate or eventual urine becomes increasingly concentrated and acidic as it moves from the proximal to the distal tubules and finally into the collecting ducts. The final pH of the urine is usually between 5 and 6. The total amount of urine leaving the body is finally reduced to between 1 and 2 L. Considering the total blood volume filtered, an incredible amount of filtrate concentration occurs between the glomerulus and the ureter.[1,2] The nephron's intricate work successfully maintains the extracellular pH within a narrow range and finely tunes the fluid and electrolyte composition to sustain the complex delicate processes of the body. Figure 43-5 illustrates the mechanism of urine formation.

## Electrolyte Balance

There is a constant ebb and flow of electrolytes (electrically charged particles) along the anatomical path of the ultrafiltrate. Electrolytes are filtered out in the capsule only to be mostly reabsorbed in the proximal tubules. Ultimately their concentration is adjusted in the distal nephron under the influence of hormones (primarily aldosterone and ADH). The specific mechanisms for moving electrolytes across the tubular membranes are both passive and active. Passive movement of electrolytes occurs when there is a concentration difference of molecules across the semipermeable membrane; molecules move from an area of greater concentration to one of lesser concentration. Active movement of electrolytes or active transport requires the expenditure of energy and enables the movement of molecules regardless of concentration gradients. Active and passive movement allow the kidney to maintain optimal electrolyte balance, thereby ensuring proper cell function.

**box 43-2** *Regions of the Nephron and Their Primary Functions*

**Bowman's Capsule**
Filtration: Ultrafiltrate of plasma enters Bowman's capsule and flows into the proximal convoluted tubule

**Proximal Convoluted Tubule**
Obligatory reabsorption (approximately 66% of the glomerular filtrate): Sodium, potassium, chloride, bicarbonate, and other electrolytes; glucose; amino acids; water; and urea
Secretion: Hydrogen ions and some unwanted substances (drugs and toxins)

**Loop of Henle**
Reabsorption (approximately 25% of the glomerular filtrate): Chloride, sodium, and calcium ions; water; and urea

**Distal Convoluted Tubule**
Facilitatory reabsorption (approximately 9% of the glomerular filtrate): Sodium, chloride, bicarbonate, water, and urea
Secretion: Hydrogen, potassium, and ammonia

**Collecting Duct**
Facilitatory reabsorption: Water and urea
NOTE: Obligatory reabsorption depends on the maximum capacity of the tubular cells. It is not thought to be affected by hormonal mechanisms. Facilitatory reabsorption depends on hormones such as antidiuretic hormone, aldosterone, and atrial natriuretic peptide. Urea is absorbed passively wherever its concentration in the lumen increases as water leaves the tubule.

From Brundage D: *Renal disorders,* St Louis, 1992, Mosby.

## Maintenance of Acid Base Balance

For normal cell function, plasma pH must be maintained in a tight range, between 7.35 for venous blood and 7.45 for

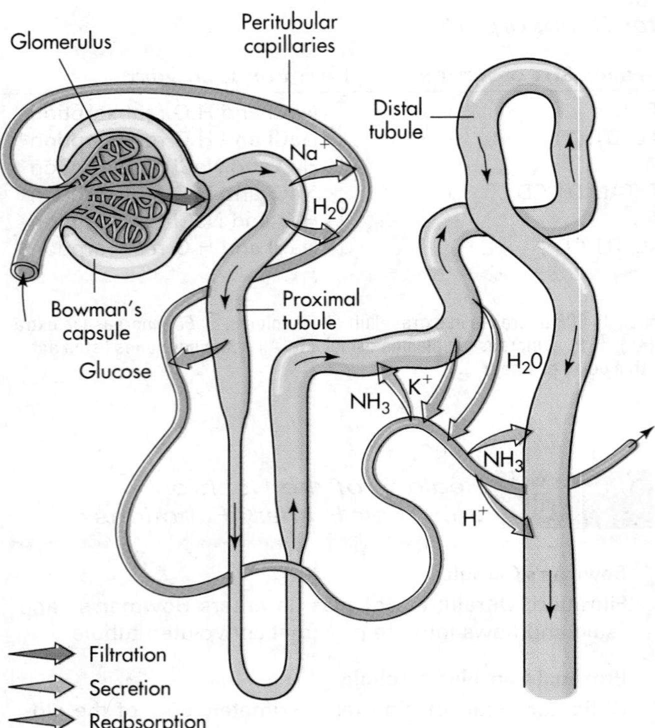


**fig. 43-5** Mechanism of urine formation. Diagram shows the mechanisms of urine formation and where they occur in the nephron: filtration, reabsorption, and secretion.

arterial blood. This balance is achieved by maintaining a blood bicarbonate to carbon dioxide ratio of 20:1. The respiratory system and the kidneys work together to maintain the ratio. The lungs contribute by varying the carbon dioxide content of the blood. The kidneys principally secrete or retain bicarbonate and hydrogen ions in response to the pH of the blood. These two substances must move in or out of the blood at precisely the right time for the pH to remain stable. The exchange is accomplished in both the proximal tubules and in the collecting ducts of the nephron. See Chapter 16 for further discussion of acid base balance.[1]

### Erythropoieisis

The kidneys play a crucial role in red blood cell production. They produce the enzyme, erythropoietin factor (EPF), that activates erythropoietin, a hormone manufactured by the liver. EPF is produced in response to the changes in renal blood flow that accompany many forms of serious renal disease. The role of erythropoietin is to stimulate the bone marrow to make more blood cells of all types, but especially red blood cells. Without this stimulus, patients with liver and kidney disease do not manufacture sufficient red blood cells and become anemic. A synthetic form of erythropoietin now allows patients to achieve near-normal production of erythrocytes and reverses chronic anemia. Constant blood transfusions can therefore be avoided.[1]

### Calcium and Phosphorus Regulation

Serum calcium and phosphorus regulation is one of the kidney's most important functions. Calcium is crucial for bone formation, cell division and growth, blood coagulation, hormone response, and cellular electrical activity. Phosphate is a component of all intermediates of glucose metabolism, a part of the structure of all high-energy transfer compounds such as adenosine triphosphate (ATP), and an integral part of the crystalline structure of bones. The kidneys are the major regulators of calcium/phosphorus balance. They accomplish this primarily by converting ingested or externally absorbed vitamin D to a more active form, 1,25-dihydroxyvitamin $D_3$. The kidney increases the conversion rate of this active molecule whenever serum calcium or phosphorus levels fall. The active vitamin D molecule in conjunction with parathyroid hormone causes increased absorption of calcium and phosphorus by the gut.[8]

### Blood Pressure Regulation

The kidneys play an active role in the regulation of blood pressure. They do so primarily by regulating plasma volume and vascular tone. Plasma volume is maintained by direct reabsorption of water and control of extracellular fluid composition.[1,9] For example, if a state of dehydration exists, aldosterone, an adrenal cortical hormone, is released. Aldosterone causes the kidney to conserve sodium, which in turn results in water reabsorption; thus the overall process aids in reversing dehydration.

Modification of vascular tone by the kidney also helps regulate blood pressure. This is accomplished primarily by the renin-angiotensin-aldosterone system. Renin is a hormone released by the juxtaglomerular apparatus of the nephron in response to sodium depletion, renal artery hypoperfusion, or stimulation of the renal nerves through the sympathetic pathway when blood pressure is low. Renin stimulates the conversion of angiotensinogen (a substance produced by the liver) to angiotensin I. Conversion of angiotensin I to angiotensin II by angiotensin-converting enzymes from the lung produces a powerful vasoconstriction and release of aldosterone. Both mechanisms elevate blood pressure.[1]

Prostaglandin and bradykinin, hormones produced by the kidney and other tissues, help elevate blood pressure as well. They are released in response to renal ischemia, the presence of ADH and angiotensin II, and sympathetic stimulation. Acting locally and rapidly inactivated, they provide an immediate mechanism for improving renal blood flow.[1,2]

### Excretion of Metabolic Wastes and Toxins

Metabolic wastes are excreted in the glomerular filtrate. Creatinine contained in the glomerular filtrate is excreted unchanged in the urine. Other wastes, such as urea, are excreted unchanged in the glomerular filtrate but undergo reabsorption during passage through the nephron. The amount of waste material excreted in urine is only a portion of that which was originally contained in the glomerular filtrate. As electrolytes are reabsorbed by the nephron, so are most waste materials. It is important to remember that most drugs are either excreted directly by the kidneys or first metabolized by the liver to inactive forms and then excreted by the kidneys. Because of the role of the kidneys in drug excretion, some drugs are contraindicated and the dose of others must be adjusted when renal function is impaired. Examples include many antibiotics, salicylates, and long-acting barbiturates.

### Micturition

Micturition (urination) is a complex sensory-motor process. Urine flows from the kidney pelvis and is propelled through the ureters by peristaltic action. About 200 to 300 ml of urine can collect in the bladder before the urge to void is felt. As the bladder wall is stretched, baroreceptors cause reflex stimulation of parasympathetic nerves to the bladder, resulting in bladder contractions. When the motor nerves to the external urinary sphincter are inhibited, the muscle relaxes, opening the sphincter and permitting urine to be expelled.

When the motor nerves to the external urinary sphincter are activated, the sphincter remains contracted. This allows for voluntary control of urination even if the bladder muscles are also contracting. In summary, micturition is the culmination of the kidney's responsibility for maintaining homeostasis. The end products of ultrafiltration are finally eliminated in this last step and equilibrium is maintained.

## PHYSIOLOGICAL CHANGES WITH AGING

A variety of changes occur in the kidney and urinary tract in response to aging. A direct relationship exists between blood supply to the kidneys and renal function. The rate of blood flow to the kidneys is about 5 to 10 times greater than that to the heart, liver, and brain. Glomerular capillary pressure, which is the force that promotes ultrafiltration, is controlled by blood flow to the kidneys. Therefore physiological alterations in the vascular bed can lead to changes in renal function.

Arteriosclerotic changes in renal arteries are the most common form of renovascular pathological conditions. Arteriosclerotic changes occur to some extent in the normal aging process. The degree of morphological change depends on the specific arteries affected and the extent of involvement within those arteries.

Aging also is known to cause predictable increases in both systolic and diastolic blood pressure. This slow increase in blood pressure begins early in life and continues through adulthood. This relationship between aging and increasing blood pressure is so well accepted that normal systolic blood pressure commonly is described as 100 mm Hg plus the person's age. Although not entirely accurate, this description does emphasize the effect of aging on blood pressure. Untreated hypertension further accelerates the development of atherosclerosis, which can lead to renal failure.

Prostatic hypertrophy is a common physiological change associated with aging discussed in detail in Chapter 49. Untreated prostatic hypertrophy results in urinary obstruction that can lead to renal failure. Aging women frequently develop problems with stress incontinence as muscle tone weakens and the pelvic organs put increasing pressure on the bladder and urethra.

**table 43-4** *Terms Used to Describe Common Urinary Tract Symptoms*

| Term | Description |
|---|---|
| Dysuria | Pain/burning with voiding |
| Frequency | Voids multiple times during the day either in large or small amounts |
| Nocturia | Awakens to void; abnormal when it occurs multiple times during the sleep cycle |
| Hematuria | Red blood cells in the urine; may be gross (visible to eye) or microscopic (detectable with urine screen and microscope) |
| Hesitancy | Difficulty initiating voiding |
| Polyuria | Urine output greater than 3000 ml/24 hr |
| Oliguria | Urine output less than 400 ml/24 hr |
| Anuria | Urine output less than 100 ml/24 hr |
| Urgency | The need to void immediately |
| Urine odor | Foul smell associated with urine |
| Frothing | Excessive foaming of urine |
| Myoglobinuria | Red-brown, at times black, pigment in the urine |

## SUBJECTIVE DATA

As in every aspect of clinical care, information obtained from the patient is the single most important element of assessment. Baseline subjective renal assessment begins with an assessment of the patient's overall state of health and perception of what constitutes good health, rather than a listing of documented health problems and comorbidities. The interview then explores any patient concerns or health problems, especially any urinary tract symptoms. See Table 43-4 for a list of terms used to describe common urological symptoms.

When a kidney problem is suspected, the nurse asks the patient directly about the symptoms listed in Table 43-4. See Table 43-5 for the clinical significance of symptoms. Special considerations in assessment of elderly patients are summarized in the Gerontological Assessment box.

### URINATION

Obtaining baseline data concerning the person's usual voiding patterns, such as the frequency and amount of urine with each void, is helpful when changes are anticipated. Persons who are admitted to a hospital or other nursing facility are questioned about their ability to carry out toileting independently. All persons should be questioned about any changes noted in voiding patterns. If changes have occurred, more detailed information must be obtained pertaining to onset, duration, and measures that the person has taken to deal with these problems.

When asking questions about urination, it is important to be aware that some persons may be somewhat reluctant to answer, either because of embarrassment or misunderstanding.

**table 43-5** *Clinical Significance of Urinary Tract Symptoms*

| Symptom | Clinical Significance |
|---|---|
| Dysuria | Urinary tract infection |
| Frequency | Urinary tract infection, retention, hyperglycemia with increased fluid intake, prostatic hypertrophy |
| Urgency | Urinary tract infection, bladder irritation, trauma, tumor |
| Nocturia | Diuretics, prostatic hypertrophy, renal failure/insufficiency, increased fluid intake, congestive heart failure |
| Hesitancy | Partial urethral obstruction, neurogenic bladder |
| Incontinence | Urinary tract infection, urethral obstruction, post-urinary catheter removal, central nervous system or spinal cord disease, postprostatectomy, laxity of perineal muscles in older women |
| Frothing | Presence of protein in the urine |
| Foul odor | Urinary tract infection |
| Polyuria | Diabetes mellitis, hormonal abnormality, diabetes insipidis, high output renal failure |
| Oliguria | Renal failure, urinary retention/obstruction |
| Anuria | Renal failure, total obstruction (trauma, mass) |
| Myoglobinuria | Muscle tissue breakdown following extreme physical exertion or massive trauma (myoglobin is muscle hemaglobin b); can result in renal failure |
| Hematuria | Renal calculi, urinary tract infection, inflammation of the kidney or bladder, trauma to the kidney or urinary tract, post-urinary catheter removal, menses |

A calm, matter-of-fact approach by the nurse helps put the person at ease. Many persons are not familiar with terms such as "voiding" or "urination," and more colloquial words may need to be used. The nurse should confirm that the person understands the questions, thus ensuring the validity of responses.

The nurse asks specific questions to elicit information regarding the presence of abnormal conditions. Patients are asked directly in nonmedical terms if they have any of the signs or symptoms outlined in Table 43-4. The more descriptive the question, the more likely the clinician is to obtain accurate usable information. For example, asking, "Do you have any problems with urination?" is less likely to elicit useful diagnostic information than asking questions such as: "Do you experience burning when you pass urine?" or "Do you have to get up at night to urinate; if so, how many times?" Questions such as "How many times do you pass your water in 24 hours?" "Do you pass less than 2 cups of urine a day?" "Does your urine look cloudy or bloody?" are also helpful. Essentially the nurse needs to develop questions that are designed to target all possible urinary tract symptoms as listed in Table 43-4. See Box 43-3 for a review of health history guidelines related to upper urinary tract disorders.

**gerontological assessment**

**ASSESSMENT**

Determine urinary habits, especially if patient has any difficulty with urinary control.

Assess for mobility problems, diuretic use, or mental changes that may contribute to functional (environmental) incontinence.

Assess for signs of urinary tract infections commonly experienced by elderly persons. Usual signs of fever and pain or burning with urination may be minimal or absent; confusion and anorexia may be the only symptoms.

Monitor kidney function when elders undergo extensive testing that may lead to dehydration, which can compromise marginal kidney function in some elderly persons.

**COMMON DISORDERS IN ELDERS**

Urinary incontinence
Urinary tract infections
Benign prostatic hyperplasia
Cancer of kidney, bladder, or prostate
Renal failure

## PAIN

Urinary tract pain deserves special emphasis, as the etiology can be medically serious and may require immediate attention to prevent complications. Pain associated with urinary tract disorders is referred to different anatomical locations depending upon the etiology and the innervation of the area affected. (See Chapter 44 for a discussion of specific disease processes that cause urinary tract pain.) For example, pain from inflammation or infection of the kidney is commonly referred to the costovertebral angle (CVA) of the back and is often referred to as "flank pain." Patients complaining of low back pain of renal etiology experience tenderness over the CVA area of the involved kidney when that area is tapped by the examiner's fist. The pain is often described as severe. If there is an infectious cause, these patients may also complain of lower urinary tract pain or dysuria.

Pain involving the ureter or upper urinary tract is also generally referred to the back and presents as vague chronic back pain. Bladder pain by contrast is often experienced as lower midabdominal pain. This type of pain might be described by someone who has a bladder infection. It would not be uncommon for it to be described as cramping or spasmodic in nature.[5]

It is important to remember that pain intensity will vary from person to person. For example, patients with peripheral neuropathy commonly seen in advanced diabetes or patients with paresthesias from spinal cord lesions may experience remote, decreased, or even no pain from renal or urinary tract disease. The nursing implication of this deviation is that pain cannot be relied upon as a warning sign of disease in this pop-

**box 43-3** *Health History Related to Upper Urinary Tract Disorders*

**Change in Usual Voiding Pattern**
Dysuria: Pain or burning on urination
Frequency of urination: Frequent voiding
Nocturia: Need to void at night
Polyuria: Excretion of unusually large amounts of urine
Oliguria: Decreased capacity to form and pass urine
Anuria: Inability to urinate, cessation of urine production
Questions: Onset and duration, pattern, severity, associated symptoms, efforts to treat and their outcome

**Pain**
Location: Kidney—flank, costovertebral angle
ureter—along course of ureter to groin
Questions: Character, intensity, onset and duration, precipitating factors, relieving factors, accompanying symptoms

**Change in Appearance of Urine**
Hematuria: Bright red bleeding, rusty brown, cola-colored, at beginning, end, or throughout voiding
Proteinuria: Deep yellow color, foamy
Color changes may be caused by food or drugs

**Passage of Stone**
May be a single stone or gravel-like material; may be associated with hematuria, fever, and pain

**Patient's Perception of Problem**
Determine the degree of concern about the symptom, and the patient's opinion as to its cause.

**Patient History Relating to Upper Urinary Tract Disorders**
Concurrent disorders
Medical history
- Infancy-childhood
- Previous disorders (urinary tract infection, kidney stones, other kidney disease)
- Serious injuries
- Hospitalizations, surgery
- Gynecological history
- Medication history: Current and recent prescription and nonprescription drugs taken
- Family history: Polycystic kidney disease, renal calculi, renal tubular acidosis, hypertension, diabetes mellitus, renal or bladder cancer
- Diet and nutritional state
- Sociocultural history
- Psychosocial history

From Brundage D: *Renal disorders,* St Louis, 1992, Mosby.

ulation. This means that the examiner should be fully aware of all comorbid conditions and their symptomatic presentation to successfully evaluate renal pain and function.

## OBJECTIVE DATA

Moderate or severe renal disease can cause significant observable pathological changes. For example, the quantity of urine excreted in 24 hours offers critical diagnostic data. Polyuria, oliguria, and anuria as described in Table 43-5 are all clinically significant and require further evaluation.

Obtaining an accurate assessment of urinary output is often difficult in a hospital setting. Urine may be inadvertently discarded, or the patient may void into the toilet. The nurse explains the importance of accurate urine collection. All staff members need to be aware of patients whose output is being measured. In some cases, such as patients in shock or acute renal failure, when it is essential to accurately assess urinary output, an indwelling urinary catheter may be inserted. The risks and benefits of inserting an indwelling urinary catheter always should be assessed before placement.

The actual appearance of the urine is clinically important as well. The urine is inspected for gross variations from normal. Normal urine varies in color from pale to deep yellow, depending on specific gravity. A very dark color suggests that urine may be concentrated (high specific gravity) or that there may be an increased excretion of bilirubin. Certain medications and foods also can change the color of urine.

Hematuria (blood in the urine) may be detected overtly or may be present microscopically. In gross hematuria the urine may be pink-tinged to cherry red. If blood is observed in the urine of a woman having her menstrual period, the vaginal orifice can be blocked with cotton balls and another specimen obtained to ascertain the source of the blood. Hematuria with pain may be the result of calculi, a clot from renal bleeding, or bladder infection.

Cloudy urine may result from precipitation of phosphate salts in an alkaline urine or from bacterial growth. A urinary or vaginal discharge also may give the urine a cloudy appearance.

The physical appearance of the patient with renal failure can change noticeably. For example, renal failure commonly causes edema of the eyelids, hands, feet, and ankles (or even the sacrum in chair- or bed-bound patients). The skin may be pale or even have a frosted appearance ("uremic frost") when the kidneys stop functioning completely. The breath may have an ammonia-like odor as waste products accumulate in the body. Renal failure is presented in detail in Chapter 45.

## DIAGNOSTIC TESTS

Special examinations of the urinary system are performed to identify the location and nature of existing disease. The accuracy of the test findings often depends on the cooperation of the patient in restricting or augmenting fluids and collecting specimens at designated times. The patient should be given clear, precise directions; written instructions are a valuable supplement to verbal directions.

Many of the diagnostic tests used to assess renal function can be performed on an ambulatory basis. Therefore it is important to make sure that the patient understand all instructions in preparation for the test. Some examinations must be performed with the patient under sedation; if so, the patient is instructed to make arrangements for someone to take him or her home after the procedure.

## LABORATORY TESTS

### Blood Tests

Several serum tests can be performed to evaluate kidney function. The two most common are tests for blood urea nitrogen (BUN) and creatinine levels. The kidney maintains serum levels of these two by-products of protein breakdown and muscle metabolism within a narrow range. Although they can fluctuate, the levels are still maintained within a predictable range as long as the kidneys function normally. Of the two, BUN varies the most because it can be influenced by a high-protein diet or events such as GI bleeding.

Creatinine remains relatively constant. With severe renal disease (acute or chronic renal failure or end-stage renal disease), the complete blood count (CBC), iron studies, and the complete blood chemistry analysis become altered as the kidney loses nephrons and the capacity to maintain homeostasis.

Blood tests used in the evaluation of renal function are summarized in Table 43-6.

**table 43-6** *Selected Renal Function Tests*

| Test | Normal Results | Purpose or Significance | Pretest Preparation/ Posttest Care |
|---|---|---|---|
| **Blood tests** | | | |
| Serum creatinine | Men: 0.85-1.5 mg/100 ml<br>Women: 0.7-1.25 mg/100 ml | Test indicates ability of kidneys to excrete creatinine.<br>Serum creatinine gives a rough estimate of GFR. | No specific preparation is needed for test.<br>Diet and metabolic rate have little effect on serum creatinine value. |
| BUN | 5-20 mg/100 ml | Test indicates ability of kidneys to excrete nitrogenous wastes. | BUN can be affected by high-protein diet, blood in GI tract, and catabolic state (injury, infection, fever, poor nutrition). |
| **Urine tests** | | | |
| Urine specific gravity | 1.010-1.026 | Test measures ability of kidneys to concentrate urine. | First morning void usually is in the high normal range in healthy person.<br>False high is caused by presence of radiographic dyes. |
| Urine osmolality | 500-800 mOsm/L | Test is excellent indication of renal function.<br>Osmolality is total concentration of particles in solution. | No special preparation needed. |
| Fishberg concentration test | Urine volume 300/ml/12 hr<br>Specific gravity of 1.024 or greater<br>Urine osmolality of 850 mOsm or greater | Test is used to determine ability of kidney to conserve fluid and to establish differential diagnosis for diabetes insipidus and psychogenic polydipsia. | No fluid can be taken during test period.<br>Test period is 8-12 hr, usually during night.<br>First morning void ensures maximal concentration.<br>Three hourly urine specimens are collected for volume, specific gravity, and osmolality after test period.<br>Patient should be observed for signs of vascular collapse. |
| Urine chemistry | Sodium: 100-260 mEq/24 hr<br>Potassium: 39-90 mg/24 hr<br>Calcium: 100-300 mg/24 hr | Urine electrolytes reflect ability of kidney to excrete and reabsorb electrolytes. | Abnormal results may be caused by disease processes other than renal disorders; for example, elevated urine calcium in hyperparathyroidism or prolonged immobilization. |
| Creatinine clearance | Men: 90-140 ml/min<br>Women: 85-125 ml/min | Results provide rate at which kidneys remove creatinine from the plasma.<br>Because diet and metabolic state have little influence on it, creatinine clearance provides a rough estimate of GFR. | See the Guidelines for Care Box on p. 1406 for collecting a timed urine specimen. |

## Urine Tests

### Urinalysis

A urinalysis is performed in two parts. The first part (the urine screen) consists of dipping a reagent strip into a clean-catch urine specimen and noting the color changes in each section of the strip. This may be followed by a microscopic examination, which is performed whenever the results from the urine screen are abnormal, or abnormalities are suspected. The examination focuses on analysis of urine sediment, the solid matter found in the urine after centrifuging. Normal urine contains almost no sediment. Interpretation of abnormal sediment is difficult, and the findings are carefully correlated with data from the patient history and physical. Table 43-7 summarizes normal and abnormal urinalysis findings.[7]

**Clean-catch urine specimens.** All urinalysis specimens should ideally be clean-catch specimens, but this is particularly important if a urinary tract infection is suspected. Guidelines for clean-catch urine collection are found in the Guidelines for Care Box. Specimens are ideally transported to the laboratory within 30 minutes or promptly refrigerated. Clean-catch specimens are also obtained for toxicological analysis (drugs or chemicals), cytology (abnormal cells), and pregnancy testing. A catheterized specimen may need to be obtained if midstream urine cannot be collected. However, catheterization should only be used if absolutely necessary. The risk of bacterial contamination is significant any time a catheter is placed in the bladder for any reason or any amount of time.

**Timed urine collection.** A timed urine collection involves pooling all the urine a patient excretes over a specific period of time. This test is often required for urological diagnosis. The duration of urine collections may vary from 2 to 24 hours, with 24-hour collections being the most common. The pooled urine specimen is examined for sugar, protein, sediment (blood cells and casts), 17-ketosteroids, electrolytes, catecholamines, and breakdown products of protein metabolism. These tests provide information on (1) the ability of the kidneys to excrete and conserve various solutes, (2) the production of various hormones that are excreted in the urine, (3) changes in the body's regulation of glucose metabolism, (4) identification of organisms difficult to recognize through routine urine cultures, and (5) the presence of abnormal cells and debris in the urine.

The accuracy of findings in a timed urine collection depends on proper collection of the specimen. Whether the specimen is to be obtained in the hospital or in the home, the person needs to be told exactly how to collect it. Instructions for collecting a timed urine specimen are found in the Guidelines for Care Box on the next page.

**guidelines for care**

**Collecting a Midstream Urine Specimen**

**Equipment Needed**

Sterile container for the urine
Three sponges (cotton or gauze) saturated with cleansing solution

**General Directions**

Touch only the outside of collecting container
Collect the urine in container well after urinary stream is started

**Special Directions**

***Female***

Keep labia separated throughout procedure
Cleanse the meatus with one front-to-back motion with each of the three cleansing sponges

***Male***

Retract the foreskin if man is uncircumcised
Cleanse the glans with each of the three cleansing sponges

**table 43-7** *Urinalysis Findings*

| TEST | NORMAL | ABNORMAL |
|---|---|---|
| Color | Amber-yellow | Red indicates hematuria (possibly urinary obstruction, renal calculi, tumor, renal failure, cystitis) |
| Clarity | Clear | Cloudy: debris, bacterial sediment (urinary infection) |
| pH | 4.6-8.0 (average 6.0) | Alkaline on standing or with urinary tract infection<br>Increased acidity with renal tubular acidosis |
| Specific gravity | 1.010-1.026 | Usually reflects fluid intake; the less the fluid intake, the higher the specific gravity<br>If specific gravity remains low (1.010-1.014), renal disease or pituitary disease (deficit of ADH) is suspected |
| Protein | 0-8 mg/dl | Proteinuria may occur with high-protein diet and exercise (particularly prolonged)<br>Seen in renal disease |
| Sugar | 0 | Glycosuria occurs after a high intake of sugar or with diabetes mellitus |
| Ketones | 0 | Ketonuria occurs with starvation and diabetic ketoacidosis |
| Red blood cells | 0-4 | Injury to kidney tissue (see Color, above) |
| White blood cells | 0-5 | Urinary tract infection (UTI) |
| Casts | 0 | UTI, renal disease |

### guidelines for care

#### Collecting a Timed Urine Specimen

1. Instruct the patient to empty the bladder and discard the urine at the appointed time to start the test.
2. Save the urine from all subsequent voidings.
3. Provide specific directions for storing the urine. Some specimens need to be kept cold during the collection period; some need preservatives, and some need no special care.
4. Instruct the patient to void into a separate receptacle before defecating to avoid contaminating the specimen.
5. Instruct the patient to empty the bladder and add the urine to the collection at the appointed time to end the test.
6. Send the designated amount (properly labeled) to the laboratory.
7. If an aliquot (5-10 ml sample of the total specimen) is the designated amount, (a) measure the total amount collected and record and (b) mix the specimen well before the aliquot is removed.

Timed urine tests also may involve collecting urine from more than one source. The person may pass urine from the urethra and also drain urine from a nephrostomy tube. In addition, urine may drain from ureteral catheters, with urine being collected separately from each kidney. Depending on the purpose of the test the urine collected from each source may be collected in separate containers or combined.

### Clearance Tests

When renal disease is suspected, the physician will want to determine the amount of damage, if any, that has already occurred. Clearance tests are the most practical and efficient way to identify losses in renal function. These tests measure the amount of blood that a person's kidneys can "clear" of a substance in a given amount of time. When the results are compared with normal values, changes in renal function become apparent. Clearance tests also are used to monitor the direction of change and the rate of change in renal function over time.

The creatinine clearance test is the most practical and widely used of all clearance tests. Creatinine is a substance that results from the breakdown of muscle tissue. Produced at a relatively fixed and uniform rate throughout the day, creatinine can be measured readily in the blood, and it is not influenced by dietary intake. Creatinine is excreted through the kidneys; it is filtered in the glomerulus and passes practically unchanged through the renal tubules. Creatinine is an ideal naturally occurring substance that, when blood and urine values are compared, allows an estimation of changes in glomerular filtration rates and overall kidney function. A person's creatinine clearance value is expressed in terms of milliliters per minute and is determined according to the following formula:

$$\text{Creatinine clearance (ml/min)} = \text{Urine volume (ml/min)} \times \frac{\text{Urine creatinine concentration (mg/ml)}}{\text{Plasma creatinine concentration (mg/ml)}}$$

The Coclcroft and Gault equation (CGE) may also be used to assess kidney function. No urine collection is necessary for the CGE. The equation is

$$\text{Creatinine clearance (ml/min)} = \frac{(140 - \text{age}) \times (\text{IBW}) \times 0.85 \text{ if female}}{72 \times \text{SCR}}$$

where IBW is ideal body weight (kg) (men = 50 kg + 2.3 kg/in. over 5 ft; women = 45.5 kg + 2.3 kg/in. over 5 ft) and SCR is serum creatinine

A morning-to-morning 24-hour urine collection is obtained. Immediately after the final urine specimen is collected, a blood specimen is drawn to determine the serum creatinine level. Both blood and urine specimens are sent together for analysis. Analysis of the total urine volume for the test period is essential to accurately determine renal function. If one void is accidentally discarded, the test must be repeated. The nurse must ensure accurate collection of all urine in the prescribed time. A shorter time period may be used in instances in which it is not possible to obtain an accurate 24-hour urine collection.

The sodium excretion test measures tubular function. Specifically, this test provides information about the kidney's ability to appropriately excrete or conserve sodium; in chronic renal failure either inappropriate retention or excretion of sodium can occur. Knowledge of urinary excretion of this electrolyte is helpful in calculating the patient's sodium intake requirements. Current and past sodium excretion studies are compared to determine changes in tubular function. The test is performed by analyzing the sodium content of a 24-hour urine collection.

## RADIOLOGICAL TESTS

A number of radiological examinations are used to visualize the urinary tract (Table 43-8). Because the kidneys lie retroperitoneally, any accumulation of flatus or feces in the intestine can obstruct the view on the x-ray film. To ensure adequate visualization, bowel cleansing is necessary before the x-ray films are taken.

X-ray films of the urinary tract may be ordered in conjunction with other abdominal studies. Visualizing the urinary system may be difficult if the patient has recently undergone barium studies. This problem can be prevented by performing urinary tract examinations before barium contrast studies of the GI tract.

## SPECIAL TESTS

### Evaluation of Bladder Function

#### *Measurement of residual urine*

Normally the bladder contains little or no urine after voiding; however, certain disease states prevent the bladder from emptying completely. Some common conditions associated with incomplete emptying of the bladder are benign prostatic hypertrophy, urethral strictures, and interruptions in bladder innervation (neurogenic bladder). Urine remaining in the bladder after voiding is called *residual urine.*

One way to determine the amount of residual urine is to catheterize the person immediately after voiding. This may be performed on a one-time basis or repeated with each void. The physician's order also needs to include a plan for establishing urinary drainage if the urine residual is large. If a large residual urine volume is suspected, a foley catheter may be used to determine the residual so it can be left in place in the bladder. Residual urine volumes of 50 ml or less indicate near-normal or returning bladder function.

**table 43-8** *Common Radiological and Special Tests of the Urinary Tract*

| Purpose | Procedure | Pretest Preparation/Posttest Care |
|---|---|---|
| **RETROGRADE PYELOGRAPHY** | | |
| Visualization of urinary tract | 1. Ureteral catheterization required<br>2. Radiopaque material (Hypaque, Renografin) gently injected<br>3. X-ray films taken of renal collecting structures | Patient may experience discomfort in region of kidneys as dye is injected.<br>Pain may be experienced if too large a volume of dye is injected and renal pelvis becomes distended. |
| **INTRAVENOUS PYELOGRAPHY (IVP)** | | |
| Determination of size and location of kidneys<br>Demonstration of presence of cysts or tumors<br>Outline of filling of renal pelvis<br>Outline of ureters and bladder | 1. X-ray film of abdomen (KUB) taken to identify size and position of kidneys<br>2. Radiopaque dye given intravenously<br>3. X-ray films of kidneys taken at 3-, 5-, 10-, and 20-min intervals | Bowel cleansing is required.<br>Inform patient that a feeling of warmth, flushing of the face, and a salty taste in the mouth may occur as the dye is injected.<br>Inform patient that numerous x-ray films are taken during the procedure; this does not indicate a problem.<br>Patient is assessed before the test for any history of allergy to iodine, shellfish, or dyes and is carefully monitored for signs and symptoms of a reaction to the dye, including respiratory distress, diaphoresis, urticaria, instability of vital signs, or unusual sensations. Emergency equipment should be available.<br>Fluids are forced after the test to help excrete the contrast material and prevent renal failure. |
| **KIDNEY, URETER, AND BLADDER (KUB) X-RAY FILMS** | | |
| Gross visualization of KUB<br>Location of calcifications and stones possible | X-ray plain film of abdominal region obtained | Bowel cleansing sometimes is ordered. |
| **CT SCAN** | | |
| Visualization of kidneys and renal circulation using an x-ray beam rotated around body | Whole body CT scanner segments kidneys<br>Can be performed with IV contrast dye | If dye is used, the same implications apply as listed for IVP. |
| **RENAL ANGIOGRAPHY** | | |
| Visualization of renal circulation<br>Particularly useful in evaluating renal artery stenosis | Similar to IVP; however, contrast dye often injected directly into femoral artery by passing a catheter through artery to level of renal arteries | Nursing implications are the same as for IVP.<br>Patient must be observed for dye-induced acute renal failure and bleeding at arterial puncture site, especially within first 4 hr. The pressure dressing should be checked for fresh bleeding. The puncture site should be checked for tenderness or swelling. Vital signs and distal pulses must be assessed frequently (q 15 min × 4 hr). Bedrest should be maintained for 8 hr after the procedure. |
| **ISOTOPE GFR** | | |
| Uses an isotope that is eliminated by the kidney to accurately measure GFR | Radioisotope injected and blood samples collected for 4-6 hr to track the clearance of the isotope | Reassure the patient that only trace doses of the isotope are used, and there is no risk related to radioactivity. |
| **ULTRASOUND** | | |
| Uses sound waves to determine the size and texture of the kidneys.<br>Can grossly differentiate cystic and solid masses | Sound waves reflect off the kidneys and computer interprets the different tissue densities | Procedure is painless and noninvasive.<br>A full bladder is required to delineate the abdominal structures. |

To avoid inserting a catheter an x-ray film examination of retained urine may be performed. A radiopaque substance is injected intravenously. As the dye is excreted in the urine, it passes into the bladder. A sufficient amount of urine containing the radiopaque material is allowed to accumulate in the bladder, and the person is then instructed to void. An x-ray film is taken. Any urine retained in the bladder will be visualized on the x-ray film. This means of determining residual urine is used in conjunction with other studies requiring visualization of the urinary tract.

#### *Cystometrography*

Cystometric examination is performed to evaluate bladder tone. The examination is indicated in the presence of incontinence or evidence of neurological dysfunction of the bladder. A Foley catheter is inserted before the examination. With the person in a supine position, a liter bag of normal saline or sterile distilled water and a cystometer are connected to the catheter. Fluid is instilled at a constant and specified rate; measurements of the pressure that the bladder musculature exerts on the fluid are recorded after the instillation of every 50 ml of fluid. The person is asked to report feelings of fullness, the need to void, and any urgency or discomfort. Fluid is instilled until urgency occurs or sensation is determined to be absent. During cystometric examination, bethanechol chloride (Urecholine), a cholinergic drug, may be administered to determine its effect on enhancing the tone of a flaccid bladder; or an anticholinergic medication may be given to assess relaxation in a hyperactive bladder. No specific care is required after cystometric examination.

Electromyography may also be used to evaluate sphincter tone and determine whether nerve pathways are intact.

### Renal Biopsy

Renal biopsy is potentially the most accurate diagnostic tool for determining the type and stage of a pathological condition involving the kidneys. This test aids in differentiating diagnoses, following the progression of disease processes, assisting in selection of therapy, and determining prognosis of the illness. The biopsy can be performed either through a skin puncture (percutaneous) or through an incision (open renal biopsy) over the kidney.

Because the kidney is such a vascular organ, hemorrhage after a biopsy is a potential threat. Throughout the procedure, care is taken to prevent and detect early blood loss. Before biopsy is performed, a thorough medical evaluation with particular attention to any abnormality in bleeding or coagulation time is completed. The patient's blood usually is typed and cross-matched for 2 units of blood; the blood is held for the patient until any threat of bleeding has passed. The risk of bleeding is greatest in the first 12 hours after biopsy.

Preparation before either type of biopsy includes discussing the procedure with the patient and answering any questions the patient may have. In most institutions the patient must sign a special permit before having the biopsy performed. The biopsy may be performed in the patient's room, the operating room, or in the radiology department.

The procedure for percutaneous (closed) renal biopsy is as follows. Before the biopsy, the patient is taken to the radiology department for localization of the kidney. This is accomplished with a plain film, a dye contrast film, or fluoroscopic location. The lower pole of the kidney is located and marked on the skin in ink. The lower pole is the site for obtaining the biopsy specimen because it contains the fewest number of blood vessels. The patient is then transported to the area where the biopsy will be performed. The biopsy may be performed blindly or with CT to guide the placement of the biopsy needle.

Sedation usually is not required except for patients who are restless and unable to relax sufficiently to follow instructions during the procedure. The patient is placed in a prone position over a sandbag or firm pillow. The physician identifies the location for biopsy, and a local anesthetic agent is injected. As the biopsy needle is inserted, the patient is instructed to take a breath and hold it because the kidneys move up and down with respiration. Pressure pain may be felt in the kidney region as the needle punctures the tough renal capsule. The needle is withdrawn immediately, and direct pressure is applied to the site for 20 minutes. A pressure dressing is then applied, and the patient is turned supine and kept flat for at least 4 hours. A small sandbag may be placed over the biopsy site to help prevent bleeding. The nursing care associated with renal biopsy is summarized in the Guidelines for Care Box.

An open biopsy carries less risk of hemorrhage and provides better visualization of the kidney. However, it is a more invasive procedure with associated risks of anesthesia, wound infection, and longer recovery time.

The procedure for an open biopsy is similar to that used in kidney surgery. The nursing care for this type of surgery is discussed in Chapter 44. Most biopsies are performed by the percutaneous method.

***guidelines for care***

**Care of the Person After Percutaneous Renal Biopsy**

1. Bedrest must be maintained with the patient flat, in a supine position, and motionless for 4 hours after the biopsy.
2. Coughing is avoided for first 4 hours after the biopsy.
3. Blood pressure and pulse should be taken on the following schedule:
   a. Every 15 minutes for 1 hour
   b. Every 30 minutes for 1 hour
   c. Every hour for additional 2 hours or until stable
   The responsible physician should be notified of increases in pulse of more than 10 to 20 beats/min above the baseline or decreases in blood pressure of more than 10 mm Hg, unless the physician instructs otherwise.
4. Bedrest should be maintained for 24 hours.
5. Urine is observed for hematuria for first 24 hours after the biopsy.
6. Patient should avoid heavy lifting for 10 days after the biopsy.

## ENDOSCOPY

Technological advances make it possible to visualize the urinary tract directly and indirectly. Endoscopies allow for assessment of both structure and function of the organs and tissues of the urinary tract. Visualization of the urinary tract is used not only for diagnosis but also for evaluation of the patient's response to therapy over time.

### Cystoscopy

Cystoscopy is the direct examination of the bladder with an instrument called a *cystoscope* (Figure 43-6). The cystoscope relies on a flexible optic fiber to provide illumination in the urinary tract. The instrument is attached to the illuminating source and then slowly passed through the urinary tract, enabling direct visualization of the urethra, ureteral orifices, and bladder. Informed consent is usually required before the procedure. The patient is asked to drink 2 to 3 L of fluid 2 hours before the procedure to ensure a continuous flow of urine in the event specimens need to be collected. If the patient is to receive general anesthesia, the fluids may be administered intravenously. If x-ray films are to be taken during the procedure, bowel preparation is ordered.

The cystoscopic examination may be performed with or without anesthesia. General anesthesia is rarely required for cystoscopy but may be used if the person is expected to be uncooperative, and the procedure is absolutely necessary. The need for painful manipulation during the procedure may also necessitate general anesthesia. In these instances, anesthesia reduces the possibility of urethral trauma or bladder perforation caused by the patient's sudden vigorous movement during the examination.

Much of the discomfort felt during this procedure is the result of contraction or spasm of the bladder sphincters; this can be decreased through deep-breathing exercises and general relaxation. A sedative such as diazepam (Valium) or midazolam (Versed) and a narcotic such as morphine or meperidine hydrochloride (Demerol) usually are given an hour before the examination. This type of analgesia is by far the most common option.

If the patient is relatively comfortable, the cystoscope should be passed with little pain, provided there is no obstruction in the urethra. A local anesthetic such as procaine (usually 4%) may be instilled into the urethra before insertion of the cystoscope.

When the patient is awake, passing the instrument is followed immediately by a strong desire to void. This occurs as a result of the pressure the instrument exerts against the internal sphincter. During the examination, the bladder is distended with normal saline for visualization. As the bladder becomes increasingly distended, the urge to void increases.

During cystoscopic examination a number of additional tests may be performed. *Cystography* involves the injection of a radiopaque dye such as methiodal (Skiodan) or air as a contrast medium to visualize the bladder and determine its size, shape, and irregularities. Bladder capacity can be measured through instillation of distilled water. A *voiding cystourethrogram* can reveal reflux of urine into the ureters on voiding, a bladder malfunction that can lead to pyelonephritis.

Ureteral catheterization (with a nylon, radiopaque, size 4F to 6F catheter) can be performed through the cystoscope. The catheter is inserted into the ureteral opening in the bladder, carefully advanced up the ureter, and into the renal pelvis (Figure 43-7). This procedure may involve one or both ureters. It is performed (1) when culture and analysis of urine from individual kidneys is required, (2) when tests of renal function are to be performed on the kidneys separately, and (3) when visualization of the urinary tract is desired, and intravenous pyelogram visualization has been inadequate,

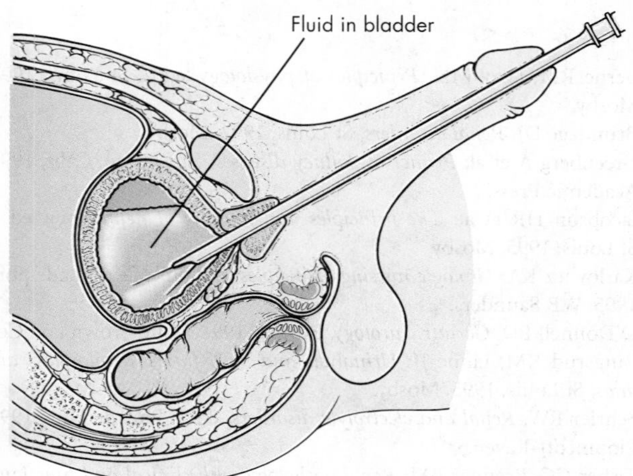


**fig. 43-6** Cystoscope inserted for examination of the bladder.

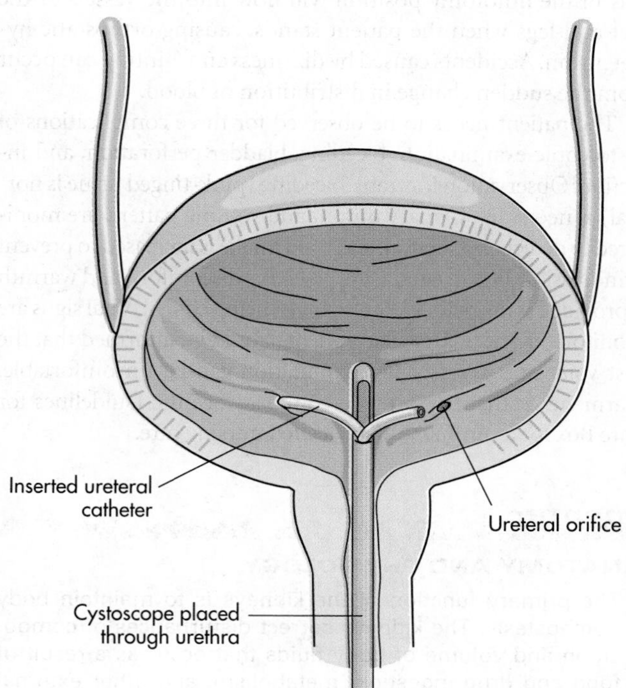


**fig. 43-7** Ureteral catheterization through cystoscope. Note ureteral catheter inserted into left orifice. Right ureteral catheter is ready to be inserted.

**guidelines for care**

### Care of the Person After Cystoscopy

1. If the procedure was done under general anesthesia or if a medication such as midazolam (Versed) has been used for relaxation and sedation, the first priority is to ensure that vital signs are stable and that the patient has a patent airway immediately postprocedure.
2. Ensure a comfortable transition to the recovery area. If patient does not have an indwelling catheter ask if he or she needs to void. If the patient does not void, check the bladder for distention and discomfort. If a catheter is in place and no urine is flowing, check the bladder for distention and the catheter and tubing for clots or kinking.
3. If the patient has a full bladder follow physician's order for catheterization. If the catheter is obstructed follow standard guidelines and orders for irrigation or catheter change.
4. Once urine is flowing check for signs of frank bleeding from the bladder. If the urine is grossly bloody, recheck pulse and blood pressure (and hematocrit if possible) and have the urologist evaluate whether this is expected bleeding or excessive bleeding. Note: Some bleeding is normal but excessive continuous bleeding indicates serious trauma to the bladder wall, perhaps even bladder perforation, and should be recognized and treated promptly. This complication is rare but possible.
5. Medicate for pain as ordered if vital signs permit. Pain should not be severe but might be mild to moderate once sedation wears off.
6. Explain to the patient and family that anytime an instrument is passed into the bladder it is possible that an infection might develop. Tell them to report any signs of infection or rebleeding. Describe these to the patient.
7. Monitor urine output and make sure that it is consistent with intake.
8. The patient is discharged when bleeding is minimal, and he or she is awake, voiding normally, and has stable vital signs. There may be mild pain with urination for a short time postprocedure.
9. Make sure that the patient has either a follow-up appointment or a number to call to reach the clinic or doctor.

obstruction is present, or sensitivity to intravenous radiopaque material is noted.

The nurse validates the person's understanding of the procedure as part of the pretest teaching. If local anesthesia is to be used, the nurse must be certain to describe what the patient can expect to feel during the procedure. The patient should not stand or walk alone immediately after cystoscopic examination because blood that has drained from the legs while the patient was in the lithotomy position will flow into the vessels of the feet and legs when the patient stands, causing orthostatic hypotension. Accidents caused by dizziness and fainting can occur from the sudden change in distribution of blood.

The patient needs to be observed for three complications of cystoscopic examination: bleeding, bladder perforation, and infection. Observation for frank bleeding (pink-tinged urine is normal) is necessary. Urinary output and voiding pattern are monitored to detect obstruction, and fluid intake is increased to prevent urine stasis. Mild analgesics are given for discomfort, and warmth is provided if the patient complains of being chilled. Vital signs are monitored as necessary. The patient should be informed that the first void after cystoscopic examination can be uncomfortable. Warm sitz baths may provide comfort. (See the Guidelines for Care Box for a summary of associated nursing care.)

## chapter SUMMARY

### ANATOMY AND PHYSIOLOGY

- The primary function of the kidneys is to maintain body homeostasis. The kidneys correct disturbances of composition and volume of body fluids that occur as a result of food and drug ingestion, metabolism, and other external factors.
- The kidneys regulate fluid, electrolyte, and acid-base balance; erythropoeisis; calcium and phosphorus balance; blood pressure; and excretion of metabolic wastes, toxins and drugs.

### SUBJECTIVE DATA

- In gathering data about urinary function, it is important to validate the person's understanding of all the questions asked, because many euphemisms exist about body elimination.

### DIAGNOSTIC TESTS

- The nurse must have a clear understanding of diagnostic tests to appropriately prepare and support the patient.
- The nurse must validate that the person understands all instructions related to diagnostic testing and provide written information whenever possible.

## References


1. Berne RM, Levy MN: *Principles of physiology,* ed 2, St Louis, 1996, Mosby.
2. Brundage DJ: *Renal disorders,* St Louis, 1992, Mosby.
3. Greenberg A et al: *Primer on kidney diseases,* San Diego, Calif, 1994, Academic Press.
4. Jacobson HR et al: *The principles and practice of nephrology,* ed 2, St Louis, 1995, Mosby.
5. Karlowicz KA: *Urologic nursing: principles and practice,* Philadelphia, 1995, WB Saunders.
6. O'Donnell PD: *Geriatric urology,* Boston, 1994, Little Brown and Co.
7. Ringsrud KM, Linné JJ: *Urinalysis and body fluids: a color text and atlas,* St Louis, 1995, Mosby.
8. Schrier RW: *Renal and electrolyte disorders,* ed 5, Philadelphia, 1997, Lippincott-Raven.
9. Tisher CC, Brenner BM: *Renal pathology with clinical and functional correlation,* ed 2, Philadelphia, 1994, Lippincott.

# chapter 44 MANAGEMENT OF PERSONS WITH Problems of the Kidney and Urinary Tract

DEBORAH K. MARANTIDES, JANE F. MAREK, and JACQUELINE MORGAN

## objectives

*After studying this chapter, the learner should be able to:*

1 Relate major health problems of the urinary system.
2 Discuss the pathophysiology and management of polycystic kidney disease.
3 Describe the etiology, pathophysiology, and management of lower urinary tract infections and pyelonephritis, including the importance of public awareness and patient teaching.
4 Compare glomerulonephritis and the nephrotic syndrome in relation to pathophysiology, clinical manifestations, and management.
5 Implement management strategies for persons requiring assisted drainage.
6 Correlate the pathophysiology of renal calculi with treatment strategies and nursing interventions for persons with renal calculi.
7 Compare different approaches to prostatectomy and the related nursing interventions.
8 Differentiate types of urinary incontinence and their management.
9 Develop a plan of care for patients undergoing urological surgery.
10 Compare and contrast the four types of urinary diversion procedures and management of urinary stomas.

A major cause of morbidity and a significant cause of mortality in the United States is disease of the urinary system. Mortality from disease of the urinary system is generally associated with damage to the interstitial kidney tissue. When a disease process involves the kidney, renal function is directly threatened. If disease is present in the urinary drainage system, it not only affects tissues at the site of the disease but it also can threaten renal function by two mechanisms: spread of the disease process or destruction of the kidney from obstruction of urine flow. The primary objective for treatment of disease in any part of the urinary tract should be early detection and adequate therapy focused on preserving or improving renal function; without renal function, life can be maintained for only a few days.

During the last two decades, some of the most striking developments in the treatment of urinary system diseases have evolved in both diagnosis and treatment. Advances in computed tomography (CT) and ultrasound have made major contributions to diagnosis. New technologies in membrane development have provided improved dialysis while surgical and immunological advances have greatly improved the success of transplantation.

Nurses can provide valuable assistance in significantly reducing morbidity related to the urinary system. This can be achieved by (1) increasing public awareness of preventive measures, (2) assisting in early detection of signs and symptoms of renal disease, (3) providing ongoing health teaching for persons with renal disease, and (4) providing long-term care to the growing population of chronically ill individuals with urinary tract disease. This chapter describes common disorders of the urinary system and their management.

## CONGENITAL DISORDERS

Structural malformation of the urinary collecting system occurs in about 10% to 15% of the population. These deviations range in severity from minor anomalies that do not require correction to those that are incompatible with life. Box 44-1 lists some of the congenital malformations that can potentially influence urinary function in adult life.

Details about the management of congenital disorders can be found in most pediatric nursing texts. However, renal cystic disorders contribute to significant adult morbidity and are discussed in this chapter.

### POLYCYSTIC KIDNEY DISEASE

#### Etiology

Renal cystic disorders encompass a relatively large group of diseases typified by the formation of one or more fluid-filled cavities within the kidneys. Cysts can arise in all parts of the kidney. Renal cysts may develop in utero, may be acquired after birth, and may be congenital or hereditary. Cysts may be slightly larger than a single nephron in their formative stage, or they may be so large as to compress the abdominal viscera. Renal cysts may be benign or may compromise function, causing renal failure. Cysts may be the primary renal disorder or may appear with nonrenal disorders.

#### Epidemiology

Polycystic kidney disease is the most common renal cystic disorder. The adult form of polycystic kidney disease (APKD) may be recognized in utero, shortly after birth, or after several decades of "normal" life. There is an autosomal dominant

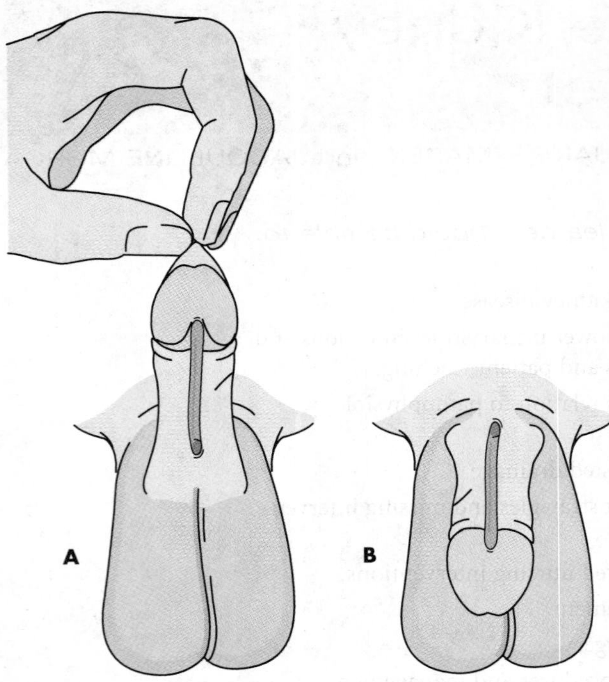


fig. 44-1 **A**, Hypospadias. **B**, Epispadias.

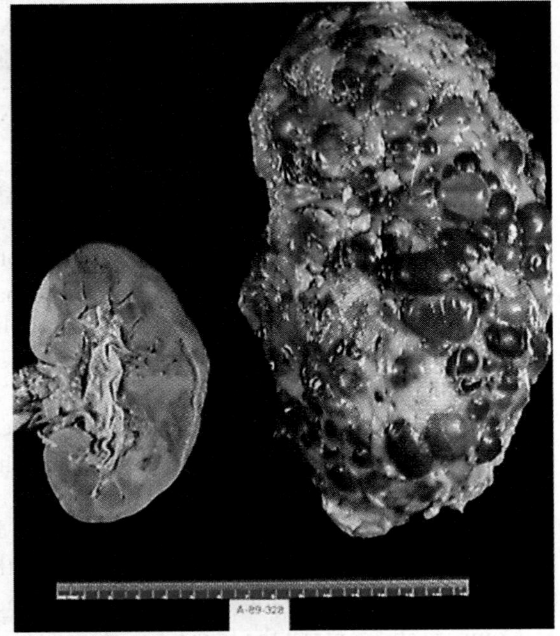


fig. 44-2 Polycystic kidneys.

**box 44-1** *Congenital Malformations of Urinary Tract*

| | |
|---|---|
| Duplication of ureters | Partial or complete |
| Hydroureters | Dilation of ureters |
| Exstrophy of urinary bladder | Eversion of bladder on outer abdominal wall |
| Hypospadias | Opening of urethra on underside of penis (Figure 44-1, *A*) |
| Epispadias | Opening of urethra on dorsum of penis (Figure 44-1, *B*) |

pattern of inheritance, although the gene for this disorder has a high degree of penetrance. In the United States, an estimated 1:500 to 1:1000 persons have APKD (200,000 to 400,000 people).[14]

### Pathophysiology

APKD is usually a bilateral disorder; that is, it affects both kidneys in 95% of patients.[21] Cysts are diffusely scattered through the renal parenchyma, with islands of normal tissue between the cysts (Figure 44-2). The cysts arise from all segments of the nephron and collecting system. The kidneys can be five times normal size and are studded with cysts of various sizes. As the cysts enlarge, they compress adjacent parenchyma, causing ischemia of surrounding tissue. Cystic enlargement also causes occlusion of the normal tubules. One of the most devastating features is that APKD undergoes relentless progression to end-stage renal failure in a high percentage of patients, usually in the fourth or fifth decade of life. Abnormalities may affect other organs: liver cysts occur in 20% to 40% of patients, 10% to 20% of patients have aneurysms of the cerebral artery or the abdominal aorta, and some patients develop pancreatic cysts. The cause of cyst formation is unknown, but researchers continue to explore the cytogenesis of the disease.[15]

Pain in one or both kidneys is the most common early sign in patients with APKD. The pain may be a dull aching, a vague sense of heaviness, or knife-like and stabbing. Medium-size blood vessels occasionally rupture and cause extravasation of blood either into cysts or into perinephric tissue. Hemorrhage may cause the cyst to rupture into the kidney pelvis and is associated with moderate to severe hematuria. Patients are prone to cyst infections and serious infections of the kidney parenchyma manifested by pain, fever, leukocytosis, pyuria, and positive blood and urine cultures. Hypertension develops in 60% to 70% of patients at some time in the course of the disease. Hypertension often antedates measurable functional renal impairment by several years. If hypertension is uncontrolled, renal destruction is accelerated. Serum and urine electrolyte levels, in addition to creatinine clearance tests, will provide data about renal function.

### Collaborative Care Management

The goals of management are to alleviate symptoms and slow the onset of renal dysfunction. Hypertension is closely monitored and controlled. Infections are treated vigorously because the scarring leads to further progression of the disease. Infection is difficult to eradicate and can lead to further destruction of kidney tissue. Antibiotic therapy is often instituted and should be given on time to ensure adequate blood levels. Urine output is closely monitored. Symptoms of uremia may be present when renal function has deteriorated to the point of end-stage renal disease.

Analgesic drugs may be necessary for control of flank pain associated with enlarged kidneys. Tepid baths will also provide comfort during infections. When urinary bleeding from ruptured cysts becomes severe, bedrest is often instituted.

Because polycystic disease is bilateral and leads to chronic renal failure, ongoing support and health teaching are essential nursing interventions. The patient is instructed to be alert to signs and symptoms of infection and bleeding. The emotional overtones of this illness can be severe for both the individual and the family. Challenges exist in helping the person deal with an illness on an individual basis when relatives have died of the same disease, and children have not yet developed symptoms. Counseling may be required about family health care and the individual's role in passing on a potentially fatal disease to children. Patients are instructed to monitor urine output and report changes to their physician.

Most patients require no modification in physical activity or lifestyle until they approach the end stage of their illness. Some patients are unusually susceptible to physical trauma to the abdomen. Cyst rupture has been caused by seat-belt constraints in automobiles and airplanes. This does not mean that patients are exempt from wearing seat belts, but they should be cautioned against strapping the lap belt too tightly across the abdomen. In male patients with massive kidneys, the use of suspenders for pants rather than constrictive belts is recommended. Patients with APKD should not participate in strenuous athletic events such as wrestling, boxing, football, and horseback riding. Although no evidence suggests that cyst rupture adversely affects renal function, the constant bouts of pain caused by cyst rupture can be avoided to some extent by tailoring the physical activity.

#### *Patient/family education*

Patients and their families should be instructed on the long-term complications and typical disease progression of APKD. It is important that the patient be able to identify early signs of infection so that treatment can begin as soon as possible.

Prevention is the key to decreasing the incidence of APKD. Prevention occurs only by prospectively identifying those with the disorder so that they may have the opportunity of determining whether to bear children. Because APKD is an autosomal disorder, patients with the gene may expect that each child will have a 50/50 chance of having the gene.

The family history is a crucial part of the counseling process; however, many family members are unwilling to reveal that they or other family members have had this disease. Guilt and denial are prominent coping patterns in these families. Often persons do not learn they have the APKD gene until beyond the childbearing period. Some believe it is advisable to evaluate all persons at risk for APKD. Recent studies using combined sonography and CT scanning indicate that the presence of the disease in young persons can probably be established with a 95% degree of certainty. For the individual found not to have renal disease, the future is clear: there is little chance the disease will be passed on. However, for the young person found to have early APKD, several socioeconomic problems have been identified. The most difficult problem is that nothing can be done to prevent the disease's progression. Second, the early discovery of a potentially disabling or life-threatening disease in a young person may affect future employability and insurability. These factors must be carefully discussed with the individual before screening for APKD.

## INFLAMMATORY DISORDERS

The kidneys are susceptible to inflammation caused by bacterial infection, altered immune response, drugs and other chemicals, toxins, and radiation. Inflammation may be acute or chronic. This section addresses the most common inflammatory disorders of the urinary system.

### LOWER URINARY TRACT INFECTIONS

Urinary tract infections (UTIs) are a significant source of morbidity in the United States and the most common bacterial infections in persons of all ages. These infections contribute to illness and also are significant in the development of chronic renal failure. Infection occurs in both acute and chronic stages in all portions of the urinary tract.

#### Etiology

Urinary tract infections result from pathogenic bacteria invading one or more urinary tract structure. See the risk factors listed in Table 44-1 for factors contributing to infection of the urinary tract. Although the great majority of uncomplicated UTIs are asymptomatic, a significant number warrant consideration as a health problem. UTIs account for more than 7 million office visits and more than 1 million hospital admissions in the United States annually.[16] Because untreated UTIs can lead to more serious problems, they must be taken seriously. Although routine screening for asymptomatic infection is needed, it is difficult to identify the specific groups at risk in whom detection and treatment yield significant improvement in health. As health care becomes more oriented toward prevention of health problems and specific target populations are better defined, the number of screening programs for asymptomatic UTIs should increase.

Structural and functional abnormalities of the urinary tract, obstruction to urine flow, and impaired bladder innervation promote UTI. Mechanisms that result in infection include urinary stasis that promotes a culture medium for bacterial growth, reflux of infected urine higher into the urinary tract, and increasing hydrostatic pressure.

Several chronic health problems (Table 44-1) predispose an individual to UTI by changing the metabolism of tissues, creating extrarenal obstruction, and altering the function and structure of kidney tissue.

Bladder catheterization is responsible for a large number of hospital-acquired UTIs. Approximately 50% of persons with indwelling catheters develop a UTI within 1 week of

**table 44-1** *Risk Factors Associated with Development of Urinary Tract Infections*

| Risk Factors | Common Examples |
|---|---|
| Female | Short urethra, close proximity to vagina and anus<br>Postmenopausal decrease in estrogen and loss of vaginal lactobacilli, which prevent infection<br>Pregnancy<br>Use of diaphragms |
| Structural abnormality | Strictures<br>Incompetent ureterovesical junction anomalies |
| Obstruction | Tumors<br>Prostatic hypertrophy<br>Calculi<br>Iatrogenic causes |
| Impaired bladder innervation | Congenital spinal cord malformation<br>Spinal cord injury<br>Multiple sclerosis<br>Urinary stasis |
| Chronic disease | Gout<br>Diabetes mellitus<br>Hypertension<br>Sickle cell disease<br>Polycystic kidney disease<br>Multiple myeloma<br>Glomerulonephritis<br>Immunosuppression |
| Instrumentation | Catheterization<br>Diagnostic procedures |
| Age | Incomplete bladder emptying<br>Decreased acidity of urine<br>Anemia<br>Malnutrition |

catheterization.[16] Catheterization, even when performed without a break in aseptic technique, results in a significant rate of bladder infection. *Escherichia coli* is responsible for 90% of uncomplicated UTIs.[16] Urinary tract infection makes up approximately 40% of all nosocomial infections. Drug-resistant strains of *Staphylococcus* and *Pseudomonas* along with various other organisms typically found in hospitals are also frequently those involved in nosocomial UTI. Prevention and control of all UTIs can be most significantly influenced through a lowering of the rate of nosocomial infection. Gram-negative aerobic organisms from the gastrointestinal tract are the most common cause of UTIs in immunocompromised persons.

Lower UTIs involve the urinary bladder *(cystitis)* and the urethra *(urethritis)*, and prostatitis. Upper UTIs may involve the kidney and renal pelvis *(pyelonephritis)*.

The mode of entry of bacteria into the genitourinary tract cannot always be traced with certainty. Four major pathways exist:

1. *Ascending infection* from the urethra is the most common cause of genitourinary tract infection in men and women. Because the female urethra is short and rectal bacteria tend to colonize the perineum and vaginal vestibule, females are especially susceptible to ascending UTI. Sexual intercourse has been shown to be a major precipitating factor of UTI in women. UTIs associated with sexual intercourse can develop as quickly as 12 hours after intercourse.[16]
2. *Hematogenous spread* occurs infrequently, with the exception of tuberculosis, renal abscesses, and perinephric abscesses. Bacteremia is more likely to complicate UTI when structural and functional abnormalities exist than when the urinary tract is normal.
3. *Lymphatogenous spread* is rare. Some researchers speculate that bacterial pathogens travel through the rectal and colonic lymphatics to the prostate and bladder and through the periuterine lymphatics to the female genitourinary tract.
4. *Direct extension* from another organ occurs with intraperitoneal abscesses, especially those associated with inflammatory bowel disease, fulminant pelvic inflammatory disease in women, paravesical abscesses, and genitourinary tract fistulas.

Pyelonephritis is discussed in greater detail on p. 1417-1418.

## Epidemiology

UTI occurs more frequently in females than males. Contributing factors include a shorter urethra with proximity to the vagina and rectum and the lack of prostatic fluid that provides protection from UTI for males. Infection rates for females are approximately 1% in school-aged girls. This rate increases to approximately 2.5% for women in the childbearing years and 20% in women aged 65 to 70. For persons older than 80 years, either living at home or in a chronic care facility, the incidence increases to 30%. Risk of infection also increases with increased sexual activity. Pregnancy is associated with an increased risk of UTI, and spontaneous resolving of infections is decreased during pregnancy. Infection of the lower urinary tract also increases the incidence of acute kidney infections as a result of ascending microorganisms.

## Pathophysiology

Most UTIs result from gram-negative organisms, such as *E. coli, Klebsiella, Proteus,* or *Pseudomonas,* that originate in the person's own intestinal tract and ascend through the urethra to the bladder. During micturition, urine may flow back up the ureters (vesicoureteral reflux) and carry bacteria from the bladder up through the ureters to the kidney pelvis (Table 44-2). Whenever urinary stasis occurs, such as with incomplete emptying of the bladder, renal calculi, or genitourinary obstructions, the bacteria have a greater opportunity to grow. Urinary stasis also promotes a more alkaline urine, which facilitates bacterial growth.

UTIs occur primarily when host resistance is impaired. The major factors preventing UTI are tissue integrity and blood supply. A break in the surface of the mucous membrane lining of the urinary tract permits the bacteria to invade tissue and cause infection. Breaks in tissue integrity result from erosions caused by tips from indwelling catheters, trauma, or rough-edged renal stones; from neoplasms; or from invasion of the tissue by parasites such as *Schistosoma.* In the bladder, blood supply to tissues can be compromised when the pressure

**table 44-2** *Normal Function, Pathophysiology, and Clinical Manifestations in Lower Urinary Tract Infection*

| Normal Function | Pathophysiology | Clinical Manifestations |
|---|---|---|
| Urine produced in kidneys flows unobstructed through urinary tract. Urine is sterile until it reaches urethra. | Urine stasis promotes bacterial growth. Bacteria may ascend urethra into bladder and ureters, leading to infection. Inflamed tissues may bleed. | Frequency, urgency, dysuria<br>Fever and chills<br>Hematuria<br>Bacteriuria |

within the bladder is greatly increased, as may occur with overdistention of the bladder, contracture of the bladder neck, or obstruction of the urethra by an enlarged prostate, metastatic growth, or urethral stricture.

Symptoms that bring the person with UTI to seek medical attention typically include frequency, urgency, dysuria (burning on urination), cloudy or foul-smelling urine, suprapubic discomfort, and hematuria. Upper UTIs and pyelonephritis are associated with fever, flank pain, costovertebral angle tenderness (CVA), nausea, and vomiting. Most persons, however, are asymptomatic or minimally symptomatic. In these persons the UTI is identified only on routine examination of the urine. Bacteriuria and positive urine cultures serve as the basis for diagnosing lower UTIs. Infection is indicated by growth of a single pathogen in excess of $1 \times 10^5$ organisms/ml of urine in a properly obtained and stored midstream specimen (Chapter 43).

## Collaborative Care Management

### Diagnostic tests

It is crucial that urine cultures be obtained before drug therapy is initiated to confirm the organism's sensitivity to antimicrobial medications and to decrease the development of resistant organisms. Twenty-four to 48 hours are required to obtain results of urine cultures. A broad-spectrum antibiotic may be prescribed until results are available. The urine should be recultured every few months during the following year to reconfirm urine sterility.

A more extensive urological workup, including an intravenous pyelogram (IVP) and a voiding cystogram, may be performed for men and young children after a repeated, or even first, UTI or when infection does not abate. This workup is performed on women when infection occurs repeatedly or cannot be resolved with treatment. The rationale for this extensive workup is that UTIs are not common in men and children. A significant portion of infection in these populations and in women with persistent infection involves a urinary tract abnormality.

### Medication

Medications typically used in the treatment of UTI (Table 44-3) include urinary tract antiseptics such as trimethoprim-sulfamethoxazole (TMP-SMX) or nitrofurantoin (Furadantin). Systemic antibiotics are also frequently prescribed. Sulfonamides are widely used and are usually effective against the organisms causing a large percentage of UTIs. Sulfonamides are relatively safe and are less likely than most systemic antibiotics to contribute to growth of resistant organisms.

For persons with chronic bacteriuria, urine-acidifying agents may be prescribed. The effect of these medications is to provide a less suitable environment for bacterial growth and to enhance the effectiveness of antibiotic and urinary antiseptics. When bacteriuria becomes constant, prophylaxis may be undertaken with antimicrobial drugs.

Patients with recurrent UTIs (two or more symptomatic UTIs within 6 months) may be treated with nitrofurantoin for 6 months to 2 years. Cephalexin has been used postcoitally to prevent infection. Some health care providers may prescribe intermittent self-treatment with a single or 3-day dose of TMP-SMX at the first symptoms of UTI.[16]

### Treatments

Additional treatment includes increasing fluid intake to 3 to 4 L/day unless contraindicated. Increased fluid intake helps to dilute the urine, lessen irritation and burning, and provide a continual flow of urine to minimize stasis and multiplication of bacteria in the urinary tract. Sitz baths may provide comfort for individuals with urethritis.

### Diet/activity

No special activity requirements are necessary. Regular intake of vitamin C in sufficient doses to be excreted in the urine can reduce bacterial growth. Vitamin C, when excreted in the urine, acidifies the urine; bacteria do not grow easily in acidic environments.[16] Cranberry juice is effective in preventing bacteria from adhering to the bladder wall. The patient should be advised to drink 2 to 3 glasses daily. Four to 8 weeks with a daily intake of 300 ml is required for effectiveness.

### Referrals

Referrals are not indicated in uncomplicated UTI. However, if UTIs are recurrent or complications develop, a urologist should be consulted for evaluation.

## NURSING MANAGEMENT

## ■ ASSESSMENT

### Subjective Data

The subjective data should include assessment of symptoms of frequency, urgency, and dysuria. Chills and fever may be present. Data should be collected on predisposing factors, such as the use of bubble baths or contraceptive jellies, and a history of previous infections.

**table 44-3** *Common Medications Used to Treat* ***Urinary Tract Infection***

| Drug | Action | Nursing Interventions |
|---|---|---|
| **ANTIINFECTIVES** | | |
| Trimethoprim-sulfamethoxazole (Bactrim, Septra) | Folate antagonist, enzymatic inhibition of bacterial synthesis | 1. Increase fluid intake to 1500 ml/day.<br>2. Monitor intake and output.<br>3. Observe for adverse reactions (rash, hives most common). |
| Nitrofurantoin (Macrodantin, Macrobid) | Interferes with bacterial enzyme systems | 1. Administer with food or milk.<br>2. Avoid exposure of the drug to light.<br>3. Space doses equally around the clock. |
| Ciprofloxacin (Cipro) | Inhibits DNA-gyrase, preventing bacterial DNA replication | 1. Instruct patient to avoid antacids.<br>2. Encourage intake of at least 1500 ml/day.<br>3. Monitor intake and output.<br>4. Assess for nausea, vomiting, and diarrhea. |
| Amoxicillin (Amoxil, Polymox, Trimox) | Inhibits mucoprotein synthesis in the cell wall of rapidly dividing bacteria | 1. Observe for urticaria or rash.<br>2. Assess renal, hepatic, and hematological function.<br>3. Administer around the clock without skipping doses. |
| **ANALGESICS** | | |
| Phenazopyridine (Pyridium, Urogesic, Pyridate) | Local anesthetic action on urinary mucosa | 1. Administer after meals.<br>2. Instruct patient that urine may turn orange and will stain fabrics.<br>3. Avoid prolonged use (>5 days). |
| **ANTICHOLINERGICS** | | |
| Propantheline bromide (Pro-Banthine) | Potent antimuscarinic activity, decreases bladder spasm | 1. Administer 1 hour before meals.<br>2. Do not crush medication.<br>3. Assess bowel sounds.<br>4. Assess for postural hypotension. |

### Objective Data

A urine culture is obtained because bacteriuria serves as the basis for diagnosis of lower UTI. The urine should also be tested for occult blood. Palpation of the abdomen and costovertebral angle for tenderness is also indicated. The patient should be assessed for the presence of fever.

## NURSING DIAGNOSES

Nursing diagnoses are determined from analysis of patient data. Nursing diagnoses for the person with UTI may include but are not limited to:

| Diagnostic Title | Possible Etiological Factors |
|---|---|
| Urinary elimination, altered | Urinary infection |
| Pain | Inflammation |
| Knowledge deficit | Lack of exposure/recall |

## EXPECTED PATIENT OUTCOMES

Expected patient outcomes for the person with UTI may include but are not limited to:

1a. Kidney function is stabilized or improved.
 b. Sterile urine or urine bacteria count is less than $1 \times 10^5$ organisms/ml of midstream urine.
2. States that symptoms of UTI are relieved.
3. Describes the following:
 a. Signs and symptoms of UTI.
 b. Rationale for and means of increasing fluid intake to 3 to 4 L/day.
 c. Risk factors for UTI.
 d. When and how to take prescribed medications.
 e. Plan for follow-up care, including urine cultures.

## INTERVENTIONS

### Facilitating Healing and Comfort

Antibiotic therapy must be given on time on a regular schedule to ensure adequate blood levels. If the patient is to undergo instrumentation, the nurse reinforces instructions about the specific procedure. Knowledge about potential sensations during instrumentation and deep breathing exercises during the procedure may assist in relaxing the patient.

Individuals with urethritis may experience perineal pain or itching in the perineum. Sitz baths may provide symptomatic relief.

### Patient/Family Education

Patient education concerning the specific problem and the requirements for drug therapy and follow-up care should increase compliance with drug regimens. Success depends directly on patient understanding and compliance and allows the patient to assist in overcoming this health problem. Female patients should be instructed about good perineal hygiene and to void after intercourse (Box 44-2).

### Health promotion/prevention

The most important defenses against UTI are large urine volume, free urine flow, and complete emptying of the bladder to prevent urinary stasis. Three considerations are important in preventing lower UTI: (1) preventing or minimizing morbidity that can accompany these infections, (2) preventing recurrence of the infection, and (3) preventing renal damage from untreated or inadequately treated ascending infections. Urinary catheterization should be performed only when absolutely necessary, and when inserted, the catheter should be removed as soon as possible. Persons with lower UTIs seek medical attention as a result of symptoms or are identified through routine urinalysis or screening. Education of the public (Box 44-2) and efforts of the health care community assist in decreasing the incidence of UTI and its complications.

## EVALUATION

To evaluate the effectiveness of nursing interventions, compare patient behaviors with those stated in the expected patient outcomes. Successful achievement of patient outcomes for the person with a UTI are indicated by:

1a. Kidney function does not deteriorate further, as demonstrated by follow-up tests.
b. Infection not present, as demonstrated by urine bacteria count less than $1 \times 10^5$ organisms/ml of midstream urine.
2. States that no pain, frequency, or urgency is present.
3. Correctly describes the following:
a. Signs and symptoms of UTI and need for prompt medical attention when they occur.
b. Rationale for increasing fluids to 3 to 4 L/day.
c. Risk factors for UTI.
d. Routine for taking prescribed medication with regard to dose, frequency, and length of therapy.
e. Follow-up care, including return visit to health care professional and repeat urine culture.

## GERONTOLOGICAL CONSIDERATIONS

An estimated 10% to 20% of persons 65 years and older have bacteriuria.[16] UTIs are the most common cause of bacterial sepsis in the older adult.[10] Structural changes of the urinary system associated with aging adds to susceptibility. Bladder muscles in the elderly woman may atrophy and weaken and men may have prostatic hypertrophy, both of which lead to incomplete bladder emptying and retention. The elderly patient who is incontinent and lacks the physical ability to adequately cleanse the perineum can also be at risk. Finally, older adults are more likely to have an indwelling catheter, which is a portal of entry for bacteria.

**box 44-2** *Information to Be Included in Public Education Programs About Urinary Tract Infection*

- Symptoms of UTI
- Need for prompt medical attention when symptoms of UTI occur
- Need to continue drug therapy even though symptoms abate
- Importance of follow-up care and repeat urine cultures
- Maintenance of fluid intake of 3 to 4 L/day if the person's health permits as increased fluid intake helps flush bacteria out of the urinary system
- Avoidance of bubble bath, powders, and harsh soaps in the perineal area
- Wearing of cotton underpants as nylon and synthetic fabrics do not allow ventilation and may facilitate bacterial growth
- Avoidance of tight-fitting pants that may irritate the urethra
- For women, importance of wiping the perineal area from front to back to prevent introducing bacteria into the urethra
- Need to shower instead of tub bath for persons with recurrent UTIs
- Need to increase fluid intake before and after sexual intercourse and empty the bladder immediately after intercourse
- Avoidance of urinary stasis by voiding approximately every 2 to 4 hours
- Need for regular intake of vitamin C or cranberry juice to help prevent UTIs

## SPECIAL ENVIRONMENTS FOR CARE

### Home Care Management

Many interventions for home care are aimed at preventing initial infections and/or recurrences. Patient education regarding risk factors is important. The client with a UTI needs the resources to fill prescriptions and return for follow-up visits. The patient may also require instructions to obtain a sterile urine specimen (see Chapter 43).

## COMPLICATIONS

The complications caused by untreated UTIs include sepsis and renal failure. Recurrent UTIs can cause scar tissue, leading to strictures and distention.

## PYELONEPHRITIS

### Etiology/Epidemiology

Pyelonephritis is an infectious inflammatory disease that involves both the parenchyma and the kidney pelvis. This infection usually begins in the lower urinary tract and ascends into the kidneys. Lower UTI may be asymptomatic, and kidney involvement may be the first indication of lower urinary tract disease. The diagnostic workup of a person with pyelonephritis often reveals previously unknown urinary tract obstruction or the presence of another chronic kidney disease. *E. coli* is the most common organism identified in pyelonephritis, and resistance to antibiotic therapy is rare. Other causes are gram-negative bacilli and enterococci. Pyelonephritis is most frequently associated with (1) cystitis, (2) pregnancy, or (3) obstruction, instrumentation, or trauma of the urinary tract. Pregnant women with bacteriuria are at significant risk for developing pyelonephritis. Other risk factors include septicemia and chronic health problems, including diabetes, analgesic abuse, polycystic kidney disease, and hypertensive kidney disease.

### Pathophysiology

Infection of the kidney occurs in both acute and chronic forms. Acute pyelonephritis may temporarily affect renal function, but rarely progresses to renal failure. Chronic pyelonephritis permanently destroys renal tissue through repeated inflammation and scarring (Table 44-4). The process of developing chronic renal failure from repeated kidney infections occurs over a number of years or after several extensive and fulminant infections. Pyelonephritis represents the original diagnosis in an estimated one-third of all persons with chronic renal failure.

Signs and symptoms of acute pyelonephritis may include those of lower UTI in addition to the following typical signs of inflammation: chills and fever, malaise, flank pain, CVA tenderness, and leukocytosis. Urinalysis demonstrates presence of white blood cells (WBCs), casts, and bacteria. In chronic pyelonephritis the only symptoms may be persistent bacteriuria until extensive scarring and atrophy result in renal insufficiency, as manifested by hypertension, increased blood urea nitrogen (BUN), and decreased creatinine clearance. The most significant efforts to prevent pyelonephritis are through early detection and adequate treatment of lower UTIs.

### Collaborative Care Management

Optimal treatment of pyelonephritis includes early detection of the bacterial infection through urine culture, antibacterial therapy based on identified sensitivities, and detection and treatment of any underlying systemic disease or urinary abnormality. The course of antibiotic therapy may extend over weeks. The urine is recultured 2 weeks after drug therapy has been discontinued and monthly for several months thereafter. If infection becomes chronic, maintenance drug therapy may continue indefinitely; the goal is to reduce and control the bacterial population of the urinary tract to prevent renal damage.

It is important to maintain sufficient urinary flow to remove byproducts of the inflammation and to prevent urinary stasis with further bacterial growth. Fluid intake of 3 L/day is encouraged in persons with normal excretory function.

During the acute phase the patient is encouraged to rest. Prescribed analgesics may be given for flank pain. Back massage often provides short-term relief of discomfort. Pain eases as the inflammation resolves.

#### *Patient/family education*

Persons with pyelonephritis may be treated at home; therefore patient teaching is important. Instruct the patient to:

1. Continue antibiotic therapy even after symptoms resolve.
2. Drink 3 L/day of fluids unless otherwise instructed.
3. Monitor urinary output; report to physician an output considerably less than fluid intake.
4. Weigh self daily; report a sudden weight gain to physician.
5. Take measures to prevent infection; report signs of urinary infection (increased flank pain, fever, chills, frequency, urgency) to physician.
6. Continue with medical follow-up and have follow-up urine cultures as instructed.

## TUBERCULOSIS OF THE KIDNEY

### Etiology/Epidemiology

*Mycobacterium tuberculosis* is the causative agent of renal tuberculosis. Renal tuberculosis is a secondary infection caused by pulmonary tuberculosis. Tuberculosis (TB), thought to be eradicated, is on the rise.[22] Risk factors for tuberculosis of the kidney are the same as for pulmonary tuberculosis (see Chapter 32). Tuberculosis of the kidney is acquired by hematogenous spread of the mycobacteria and is most common in men 20 to 40 years of age. An estimated 15% of persons with active pulmonary TB develop kidney involvement.[22]

### Pathophysiology

TB of the kidney occurs after the *M. tuberculosis* invades the kidney. Early in the disease the renal cortex or medulla is affected. Tissue damage is progressive and eventually the renal cortex can rupture into the renal pelvis and infection can spread via the mucosa to the remainder of the urinary tract.[22] If infection involves the ureters, strictures can develop, complicating the infection by causing an obstruction. In addition, blood supply will also be affected due to the destruction of kidney tissue by masses of the tubercles. Initially, collateral circulation may develop, but if the infection is left untreated, collateral circulation will become insufficient, and the kidney will become ischemic.

**table 44-4** *Normal Function, Pathophysiology, and Clinical Manifestations in Pyelonephritis*

| Normal Function | Pathophysiology | Clinical Manifestations |
|---|---|---|
| Fluid regulation<br>Electrolyte regulation<br>Blood pressure regulation<br>Excretion of metabolic wastes | Acute inflammation results in hyperemia and suppuration of tissues (inflammatory response).<br>Chronic inflammation results in scarring and atrophy, leading to chronic renal failure. | Acute: flank pain, fever, chills, malaise, leukocytosis, WBCs and bacteria in urine<br>Chronic: persistent bacteriuria; hypertension, ↑ BUN, ↓ creatinine clearance in late stages |

Signs and symptoms of renal tuberculosis are mild and usually include loss of appetite, unexplained weight loss, and intermittent fever. Hematuria may also be present. Diagnostic tests usually include screening for pulmonary tuberculosis. The patient will have a positive Mantoux skin test. Urine samples are also obtained and screened for the presence of *M. tuberculosis.*

### Collaborative Care Management

Treatment is usually involves antituberculosis medication (see Chapter 32). Medications typically used include isoniazid, rifampin, and ethambutol. Drug therapy is usually given for 9 to 24 months.

If the spread of infection has caused structural damage, a nephrectomy or urinary diversion may be necessary. These procedures are discussed in greater detail later in this chapter. Nursing care is focused on managing pain and discomfort and education regarding the medication regimen.

#### *Patient/family education*

Patients must be instructed to continue the entire course of medications even after symptoms subside. Educating the patient, family, and public regarding the risk factors and prevention of tuberculosis is essential. Prevention is primarily through the control of pulmonary tuberculosis by early detection and treatment (see Chapter 32).

## CHEMICAL-INDUCED NEPHRITIS

### Etiology/Epidemiology

Chemical-induced nephritis is an idiosyncratic reaction that results in damage to the kidney tubules and interstitium. This disease process was first noted in patients sensitive to the sulfonamides. Many other substances are now associated with chemical-induced nephritis, including those listed in Table 44-5.

### Pathophysiology

Chemical-induced nephritis usually begins within 15 days of exposure to the chemical. The inflammatory process disrupts the ability of the glomeruli to filter. Furthermore, the capillary membrane becomes permeable to plasma proteins and red blood cells (RBCs), which results in proteinuria and hematuria.

Signs and symptoms of nephritis include fever, eosinophilia, hematuria, mild proteinuria, and rash. Oliguria or urine output of 400 ml or less in a 24-hour period occurs in approximately 50% of all patients. Urinalysis is used to demonstrate protein or RBCs in the urine. Serum toxicology screening may identify the source of the nephritis.

**table 44-5** *Substances Associated with Chemical-Induced Nephritis*

| CATEGORY | SUBSTANCE |
|---|---|
| Solvents | Carbon tetrachloride<br>Methanol<br>Ethylene glycol |
| Heavy metals | Lead<br>Arsenic<br>Mercury |
| Antibiotics | Kanamycin<br>Gentamicin<br>Amphotericin B<br>Calistin<br>Neomycin<br>Phenazopyridine |
| Pesticides | |
| Poisonous mushrooms | |

### Collaborative Care Management

Medical management usually includes immediate withdrawal of the suspected chemical. Hemodialysis may be required to remove the nephrotoxins from the blood. Steroids are often administered because of their antiinflammatory effect. If renal function is severely compromised, dietary sodium and protein restrictions may be instituted.

The patient is assessed for fluid and electrolyte imbalance, including the presence of edema, blood pressure changes, and adventitious breath sounds. The person needs to know the rationale for maintenance of fluid balance and any sodium restrictions. Care is similar to that for the patient with acute renal failure (see Chapter 45).

#### *Patient/family education*

Education of the patient focuses on prevention. Patients should be instructed to keep solvents in well ventilated areas. All household chemicals should be clearly labeled.

Prevention of chemical-induced nephritis is best managed by identifying causative agents and removing them from the environment. Many people are exposed to these agents as a result of their medical regimen. The health care professional must be aware of these agents and the signs and symptoms associated with chemical-induced nephritis. With early detection and removal of the causative agent as soon as possible, the prognosis improves.

A major risk factor is industrial exposure to chemicals. Occupational health professionals should be aware of potential risks and should educate employees regarding appropriate preventive measures.

## ACUTE GLOMERULONEPHRITIS

### Etiology

Glomerulonephritis is a disease that affects the glomeruli of both kidneys. Etiological factors are many and varied; they include immunological reactions (systemic lupus erythematosus, streptococcal infection), vascular injury (hypertension), metabolic disease (diabetes mellitus), and disseminated intravascular coagulation. Glomerulonephritis exists in acute, latent, and chronic forms.

The most common form of acute glomerulonephritis occurs 2 to 3 weeks after a streptococcal infection. Common sites of the primary infection include the pharynx or tonsils and the skin (impetigo).

### Epidemiology

Preschool-aged and grade school-aged children are most likely to develop the illness. Of all individuals developing acute post-streptococcal glomerulonephritis, approximately 1% to 2% will develop end-stage renal failure requiring renal replacement therapy (dialysis or transplantation). Approximately 90% of children and 50% of adults with acute glomerulonephritis attain full recovery from illness, although recovery may require as long as 2 years.[1] The severity of the acute illness does not relate to the prognosis. Persons with mild illness may develop chronic disease, and those with severe illness may completely recover and have no recurrence of the illness.

### Pathophysiology

Acute post-streptococcal glomerulonephritis is a result of an antigen-antibody reaction with glomerular tissue that produces swelling and death of capillary cells. The antigen-antibody reaction activates the complement pathway (see Chapter 10), resulting in chemotaxis of polymorphonuclear leukocytes with release of lysosomal enzymes that attack the glomerular basement membrane. The response in the membrane is an increase in all three types of glomerular cells (endothelial, mesangial, and epithelial), causing an increase in membrane porosity with resultant proteinuria and hematuria. Renal function is depressed by scarring and obstruction of the circulation through the glomerulus.

Signs and symptoms reflect damage to the glomeruli, with leaking of protein and RBCs into the urine, and varying degrees of decreased glomerular filtration, with retention of metabolic waste products, sodium, and water (Box 44-3).

Typical patient complaints include shortness of breath, mild headache, weakness, anorexia, and flank pain. The usual signs associated with acute glomerulonephritis are proteinuria, hematuria, and azotemia.

### Collaborative Care Management

#### *Diagnostic tests*

Urinalysis provides important data, such as the presence of proteinuria, hematuria, and cell debris. Serum BUN and urine creatinine clearance tests indicate renal function status. Test to determine infection include erythrocyte sedimentation rate and antistreptolysin O titer. Urinary proteins are often analyzed to distinguish between nephrotic syndrome and glomerulonephritis.[1]

**box 44-3** *clinical manifestations*

***Acute Glomerulonephritis***

EARLY

Hematuria
Proteinuria
Azotemia
Increased urine specific gravity
Elevated erythrocyte sedimentation rate
Oliguria
Elevated antistreptolysin O titer

LATE

Circulatory congestion
Hypertension
Edema
End-stage renal failure

#### *Medications*

Persistent infection is treated promptly to help prevent an increase in antigen-antibody complex formation. Patients with post-streptococcal glomerulonephritis are given a course of prophylactic antibiotics; the drug of choice is penicillin. Prophylactic therapy may be continued for months after the acute phase of illness. Diuretic therapy is implemented when severe fluid overload develops. Elevated blood pressure is controlled by antihypertensive drugs only after fluid control has proved to be unsuccessful.

#### *Treatments*

No specific treatment exists for acute glomerulonephritis. General management is focused on prevention.

#### *Diet*

Fluid retention is often a problem and is managed by dietary sodium restrictions. Dietary protein is also restricted, usually to 1 to 1.2 g/kg/day when BUN and creatinine levels are elevated. It is important that the diet contain sufficient carbohydrates to prevent protein being used for energy, which will result in muscle wasting and nitrogen imbalance. Caloric requirements are 2500 to 3500 calories/ day. The patient should be monitored for weight loss, as loss of protein stores may occur. Potassium intake should be restricted if the glomerular filtration rate is less than 10 ml/min.

#### *Activity*

Bedrest is usually instituted until clinical signs of nephritis have resolved.

#### *Referrals*

Prolonged bedrest during acute glomerulonephritis may cause fatigue and impair performance of activities of daily living. Thus a referral for physical therapy for strengthening exercises may be beneficial after the acute phase of illness.

## NURSING MANAGEMENT

### ■ ASSESSMENT

#### Subjective Data

General questions to ask the patient include: Have you experienced shortness of breath, headaches, low back pain, weakness, nausea, vomiting, or anorexia? Have you noticed a change in your pattern of urination, either in frequency, color, or volume? Do you recall a recent infection or symptoms of a virus? Any recent weight gain or swelling?

#### Objective Data

Assessment data for the patient with acute glomerulonephritis include:

Vital signs: presence of fever, hypertension
Edema
Intake and output
Daily weights

## NURSING DIAGNOSES

Nursing diagnoses are determined from analysis of patient data. Nursing diagnoses for the person with acute glomerulonephritis may include but are not limited to:

| Diagnostic Title | Possible Etiological Factors |
|---|---|
| Fluid volume excess | Compromised regulatory mechanism, renal impairment |
| Infection, risk for | Decreased immune response |
| Coping, ineffective (individual) | Activity restrictions |
| Knowledge deficit | Lack of information |

## EXPECTED PATIENT OUTCOMES

Expected patient outcomes for the person with acute glomerulonephritis may include but are not limited to:

1. Achieves fluid balance; has fluid intake equal to output; shows decreased edema; maintains stable weight. Has renal function tests within normal limits.
2. Is free from infection.
3. Expresses concerns and feelings about restricted activity; does not express boredom with prolonged bedrest.
4. Describes the rationale for therapy, dietary restrictions, medication program, measures to prevent infection, and signs and symptoms requiring medical attention.

## INTERVENTIONS

### Maintaining Fluid Balance

Edema and fluid-overloading are anticipated and treated initially with dietary sodium and fluid restrictions. Sodium intake is usually restricted to 2 to 4 g/day, but the amount varies with the severity of fluid retention. Sodium restriction is maintained until dependent edema and circulatory overload are no longer present. Strict recording of fluid intake and output is necessary to determine the extent of fluid retention. The nurse should be constantly alert for signs and symptoms of fluid overload. Weigh the patient daily using correct procedure (see Chapter 15). Vital signs should be monitored every shift. The apical pulse should be assessed for dysrhythmias. The nurse should assess for jugular vein distention, indicating fluid overload and congestive heart failure. The lungs should be assessed for the presence of adventitious sounds. The nurse should assess for periorbital, pretibial, pedal, and sacral edema. Measure the circumference of edematous extremities to assess for changes in size. Antihypertensive and diuretic therapy is usually prescribed. Serum potassium levels should be monitored closely, especially for patients receiving diuretics that eliminate potassium. Hyperkalemia may occur with uremic symptoms.

### Preventing Infection

Mild infections may reactivate nephritis; therefore minimize the patient's exposure to infection, particularly persons with upper respiratory infections (URIs). If a URI is suspected, cultures are obtained, and when indicated, antibiotics are prescribed. When possible, avoid any procedures that may lead to nosocomial infection, such as catheterization.

### Facilitating Coping

Bedrest is prescribed during the acute phase of the illness. Ambulation is allowed when blood sedimentation rates and blood pressure are normal and edema abates. If ambulation causes an increase in proteinuria or hematuria, bedrest is reinstituted. Since the period of bedrest may be extensive, the nurse may need to continue to reinforce the importance of bedrest as the patient starts to feel better. The importance of diversional activities should not be ignored. When bedrest is reinstituted after a period of ambulation, the person may become depressed as a result of the perceived setback in recovery. Helping the patient express concerns can serve as the impetus for making realistic plans about the illness and its sequelae.

### Patient/Family Education

The recovery period for acute glomerulonephritis may be as long as 2 years; therefore patient teaching is important. Proteinuria, hematuria, and cellular debris may exist microscopically, even when other symptoms subside. Although fatigue may be present, these persons usually feel well; thus they often need to be convinced of the importance of follow-up care. Teaching includes:

1. Nature of the illness and effect of diet and fluids on fluid balance and sodium retention
2. Diet teaching regarding prescribed sodium and fluid restrictions (provide written information regarding sodium content of foods)
3. Medication regimen: dose, frequency, side effects, need to continue regimen as instructed by physician
4. Need to balance activities with rest if fatigue is present
5. Avoidance of infection, which may exacerbate the illness
6. Signs and symptoms indicating need for medical attention (hematuria, headache, edema, or hypertension)
7. Importance of follow-up care

#### *Health promotion/prevention*

Prevention of acute post-streptococcal glomerulonephritis involves prompt medical treatment of sore throats and upper respiratory infections. Cultures should be obtained, and antibiotics prescribed when indicated.

## EVALUATION

To evaluate the effectiveness of nursing interventions, compare patient behaviors with those stated in the expected patient outcomes. Successful achievement of patient outcomes for the patient with acute glomerulonephritis are indicated by:

1. Has decreased or absent edema or stable weight.
2. Has no infection.
3. Follows activity restrictions, participates in diversional activities, and does not express boredom.
4. Describes correctly the nature of the illness, dietary and fluid restrictions, the importance of preventing URIs, signs and symptoms to be reported to physician, and the importance of follow-up care.

## GERONTOLOGICAL CONSIDERATIONS

Because of pre-existing structural and age-related changes in the kidney, the elderly patient is at an increased risk for complications. Older adults are more likely to develop chronic glomerulonephritis. Treatment remains the same regardless of age.

### COMPLICATIONS

Besides the obvious complications such as sepsis from infection and renal failure due to extensive kidney damage, other complications may arise due to fluid overload. These fluid-related complications include congestive heart failure, pulmonary edema, and increased intracranial pressure. Each must be treated aggressively, and the patient may require critical care management. Cardiac glycosides may be prescribed to prevent congestive heart failure.

## CHRONIC GLOMERULONEPHRITIS

### Etiology/Epidemiology

Although chronic glomerulonephritis (CGN) may follow the acute disease, most persons have no history of the disease or source of predisposing infection. The course of CGN is extremely variable. Some persons with minimal impairment in renal function continue to feel well and show little progression of disease. The progression of renal deterioration may be insidious or rapid, resulting in end-stage renal disease.

### Pathophysiology

CGN is characterized by progressive destruction *(sclerosis)* of glomeruli and gradual loss of renal function. The glomeruli have varying degrees of hypercellularity and become sclerosed (hardened). The kidney decreases in size. Eventually there is tubular atrophy, chronic interstitial inflammation, and arteriosclerosis (Figure 44-3).

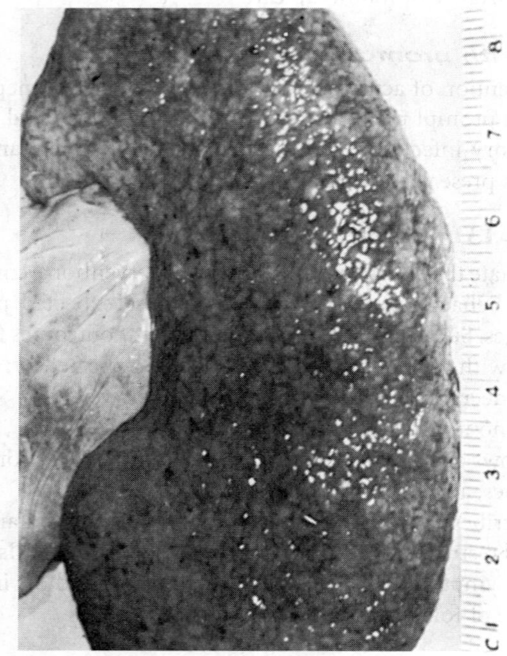

**fig. 44-3** End-stage chronic glomerulonephritis. Note pebbly surface corresponding to surviving hypertrophied nephrons and atrophy.

Various symptoms of renal dysfunction may lead the person to seek health care, including headache, especially in the morning; dyspnea on exertion; blurred vision; lassitude; and weakness or fatigue. Other signs of CGN include edema, nocturia, and weight loss.

Early in the disease process, urinalysis may reveal albumin, casts, and blood, despite normal renal function tests. The ability of the kidneys to regulate the internal environment will begin to decrease as more glomeruli become scarred, resulting in fewer functional nephrons. When few nephrons remain intact, hematuria and proteinuria decrease, the specific gravity of the urine becomes fixed at 1.010 (same as plasma), and the nonprotein nitrogen level in the blood increases.

### Collaborative Care Management

No specific therapy exists to arrest or reverse this disease process. Treatment of renal failure begins when the illness progresses to end stage renal disease (see Chapter 45).

With any exacerbation of hematuria, hypertension, and edema, the patient is returned to bedrest, and treatment similar to that for acute glomerulonephritis is instituted. Signs of pulmonary edema and congestive heart failure are closely monitored.

Women with CGN who become pregnant appear to be susceptible to toxemia and to spontaneous abortion. The woman who has had nephritis of any nature should be urged to see a physician if she plans to become pregnant. When pregnancy does occur, she should be followed closely by an obstetrician who specializes in high-risk pregnancies.

Care involves teaching the patient to live healthfully, to avoid infections, to eat a balanced diet within prescribed limits, to take prescribed medications appropriately, to maintain follow-up health care, and to report (to the physician) any exacerbation in signs or symptoms. If complications occur, specific treatment is symptomatic and supportive.

#### *Patient/family education*

Because predisposing factors have not been identified for CGN, no preventive measures can be instituted. Known infections should be treated promptly, as discussed under acute glomerulonephritis, to reduce the possibility of the acute disease progressing to CGN. Chronic diseases should be treated and controlled.

## NEPHROTIC SYNDROME

Nephrotic syndrome *(nephrosis)* is not a single disease entity but a constellation of symptoms including albuminuria, hypoalbuminemia, edema, hyperlipidemia, and lipuria. Nephrotic syndrome causes damage to the glomeruli with resultant proteinuria.

### Etiology

Nephrotic syndrome has been associated with allergic reactions (insect bites, pollen, acute glomerulonephritis), infections (herpes zoster), systemic disease (diabetes mellitus or sickle cell disease), circulatory problems (severe congestive heart failure or chronic constrictive pericarditis), cancers (Hodgkin's, lung, colon, and breast), renal transplantation, and pregnancy. Known glomerular disease is the most common precipitating event in adults. Fifty to 75% of adults with nephrosis develop renal failure within 5 years.[1] Many individuals will have periods of remission and exacerbation. Nephrosis may also exist be chronic. The etiology of nephrotic syndrome in children is usually idiopathic.

### Epidemiology

Nephrotic syndrome is seen most often in children with 70% to 80% of the cases diagnosed before the age of 16. The highest incidence of occurrence is between 6 and 8 years. Although nephrotic syndrome is not uncommon in adults, only 15% to 20% of cases are diagnosed after the age of 16.[6]

### Pathophysiology

The initial physiological change in nephrotic syndrome is a derangement of cells in the glomerular basement membrane, resulting in increased membrane porosity and significant proteinuria. As protein continues to be excreted, serum albumin is decreased (hypoalbuminemia), thus decreasing the serum osmotic pressure (Table 44-6). The capillary hydrostatic fluid pressure in all body tissues becomes greater than the capillary osmotic pressure, and generalized edema results (Figure 44-4). As fluid is lost into the tissues, the plasma volume decreases, stimulating secretion of aldosterone to retain more sodium and water, which decreases the glomerular filtration rate to retain water. This additional fluid also passes out of the capillaries into the tissue, leading to even greater edema.

Clinical manifestations of nephrotic syndrome include severe generalized edema *(anasarca)* pronounced proteinuria, hypoalbuminemia, and hyperlipidemia. Urine volumes and renal function may be either normal or greatly altered. Altered renal function and development of symptoms of renal failure occur as a result of progressing glomerulonephritis. Loss of appetite and fatigue are common. Women usually experience amenorrhea and other disturbances in the reproductive cycle.

### Collaborative Care Management

Treatment of nephrotic syndrome is focused on reducing albuminuria, controlling edema, and promoting general health.

#### Diagnostic tests

Laboratory tests include urinalysis for protein, casts, and erythrocytes and serum tests for protein and lipid analysis. Hyperlipidemia and elevated serum cholesterol, elevated triglyceride, and elevated low-density and very-low-density lipid levels are common findings. Periodic determinations of proteinuria and measures of renal function are performed to monitor response to treatment and level of kidney function. Renal biopsy is sometimes used to obtain a definitive diagnosis or the extent of kidney damage. Biopsy may reveal minimal to extensive changes including hypercellularity, changes in the epithelium, fatty deposits in the tubules, sclerosing of the glomeruli, and deposition of immunoglobins along the capillary walls. Persons with extensive damage generally do not respond to treatment and develop end-stage renal disease.

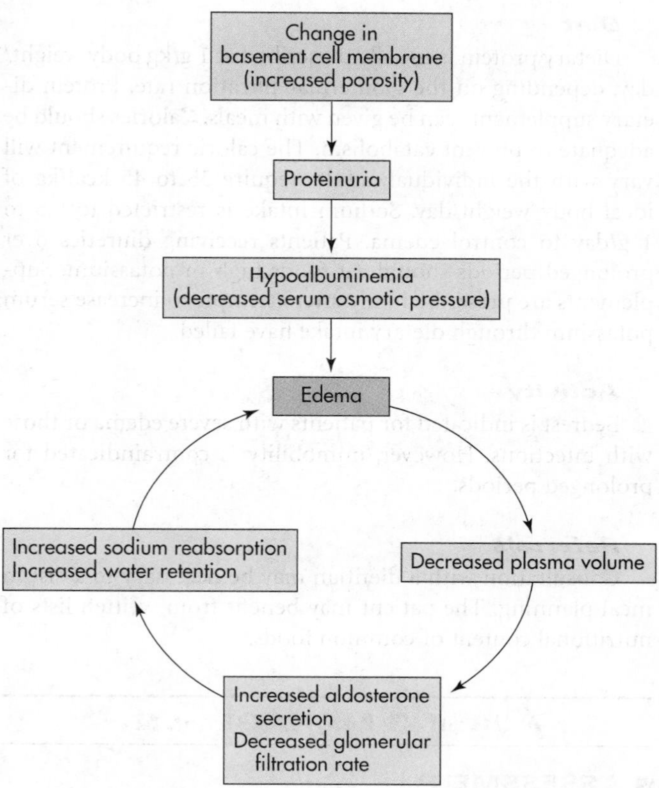


**fig. 44-4** Pathophysiological changes in nephrotic syndrome.

**table 44-6** *Normal Function, Pathophysiology, and Clinical Manifestations in Nephrotic Syndrome*

| Normal Function | Pathophysiology | Clinical Manifestations |
|---|---|---|
| Glomerular capillaries are impermeable to serum proteins. Plasma proteins create colloid osmotic pressure to retain intravascular fluid. | Glomerular capillaries become permeable to serum proteins, resulting in proteinuria and decreased serum osmotic pressure. Glomerular filtration rate decreases. | Severe generalized edema; pronounced proteinuria; hypoalbuminemia; hyperlipidemia |

### Medications

Corticosteroids may be useful in controlling the illness, but responses will vary. Approximately 50% to 60% of patients will have a relapse while tapering down steroid therapy. Prednisone is the drug of choice. Immunosuppressants are effective in stopping the proteinuria. Cyclophosphamide or azathioprine is used in patients unresponsive to steroids. Diuretics and infusions of salt-poor albumin are used cautiously to manage edema.[6]

### Treatments

No specific treatment exists for nephrotic syndrome. Prevention of infection is important because body defenses are impaired by protein losses and edematous tissues are susceptible to breakdown. Thoracentesis or paracentesis is indicated in patients with fluid accumulation in the pleural or abdominal cavities.

### Diet

Dietary protein is usually prescribed at 1 g/kg body weight/day, depending on the glomerular filtration rate. Protein dietary supplements can be given with meals. Calories should be adequate to prevent catabolism. The caloric requirement will vary with the individual; adults require 35 to 45 kcal/kg of ideal body weight/day. Sodium intake is restricted to 0.5 to 1 g/day to control edema. Patients receiving diuretics over prolonged periods should eat foods high in potassium. Supplements are prescribed only after attempts to increase serum potassium through dietary intake have failed.

### Activity

Bedrest is indicated for patients with severe edema or those with infections. However, immobility is contraindicated for prolonged periods.

### Referrals

Consultation with a dietitian may be necessary to assist in meal planning. The patient may benefit from written lists of nutritional content of common foods.

## NURSING MANAGEMENT

## ASSESSMENT

### Subjective Data

The subjective data are the same as those collected for glomerulonephritis (p. 1420).

### Objective Data

Specific assessment should include:

- Edema: amount, location, and degree of pitting
- Intake and output
- Daily weight
- Abdominal girth
- Condition of skin (severe edema may lead to skin breakdown)
- Respiratory status: signs of pulmonary edema
- Signs and symptoms of infection

## NURSING DIAGNOSES

Nursing diagnoses are determined from analysis of patient data. Nursing diagnoses for the person with nephrosis may include but are not limited to:

| Diagnostic Title | Possible Etiological Factors |
|---|---|
| Nutrition, altered: less than body requirements | Anorexia, edema |
| Infection, risk for | Decreased nutrition, immobility, edema |
| Knowledge deficit | Lack of exposure/recall |

## EXPECTED PATIENT OUTCOMES

1a. Eats a diet high in protein and calories and low in sodium.
 b. Maintains stable weight.
2a. Is free from infection.
 b. Maintains intact skin.
3. Describes dietary and drug therapy, measures to prevent infection, and symptoms requiring medical attention.

## INTERVENTIONS

### Promoting Nutrition

A sodium-restricted diet is usually prescribed. The protein prescription varies according to the amount of protein lost in the urine over 24 hours. Appetite is diminished as a result of fluid retention and decreased food palatability. Small, frequent feedings may be better tolerated. Vitamin supplements with iron may be prescribed. After the patient's food preferences are assessed, a diet plan should be developed with the dietitian. Whenever possible, the protein should be of high biological value (lean meat, fish, poultry, and dairy products).

Offer oral hygiene at regular intervals. Mouth care can help reduce the unpleasant metallic taste and breath odor that are partially responsible for the anorexia of renal failure.

Laboratory data, including serum protein, lipids, and calcium should be monitored to assess protein stores. The patient should be weighed daily.

### Preventing Infection

Persons with nephrosis need to focus on preventing infection because urinary protein losses impair body defenses. It is important to remember that corticosteroid use may mask the signs of infection. When infection is suspected, it is important to address the problem immediately. Specimens for culture and sensitivity should be obtained. Antibiotics should be administered at prescribed times to maintain therapeutic blood levels. Inform the patient of the importance of prescribed medications and the need to take all the antibiotic as directed. The patient should be protected against sources of infection. Invasive procedures should be avoided; when necessary, they should be performed under strict aseptic technique.

Edematous tissue is particularly susceptible to skin breakdown and infection. Careful positioning and frequent position changes may increase comfort while also protecting the skin. Air or water mattresses may increase comfort and relieve skin pressure. Males may develop scrotal edema; a scrotal support provides comfort and aids in reducing swelling.

### Patient/Family Education

Although nephrosis is often progressive, health teaching should focus on maintaining comfort. Teaching includes:

1. The effects of nephrotic syndrome on the kidneys and the possibility of the need for dialysis or renal transplant in the future.
2. Medication regimen: name, dose, actions, side effects, and the need to finish antibiotic prescription (as appropriate).
3. Nutrition: increased calories, adequate protein, and decreased sodium.
4. Self-assessment of fluid status, including signs and symptoms of hypovolemia and hypervolemia.
5. Signs and symptoms requiring medical attention: increased edema, dyspnea, fatigue, headache, and infection.
6. Promotion of good health habits to prevent infection, including nutritionally adequate diet, exercise, adequate rest and sleep, and avoidance of sources of infection.
7. Need for follow-up care to monitor renal function.

## ■ EVALUATION

To evaluate the effectiveness of nursing interventions, compare patient behaviors with those stated in the expected outcomes. Successful achievement of patient outcomes for the patient with nephrotic syndrome are indicated by:

1a. Eats meals high in calories and low in sodium and follows the protein prescription.
 b. Maintains stable weight.
2a. Shows no signs of infection.
 b. Maintains skin integrity.
3. Describes medication regimen, nutrition prescription, measures to assess fluid status, signs and symptoms requiring medical attention, the need for follow-up care, and complications of nephrotic syndrome.

## GERONTOLOGICAL CONSIDERATIONS

With age, interest in eating may decline because of changes in the sensory organs, which alter the taste of food. A major component of the treatment for nephrotic syndrome is maintaining a high-protein, low-sodium diet. Elderly persons may lack the resources to comply with the prescribed diet. In addition, older adults are more likely to have complications related to steroid therapy because of excess levels of circulating free glucocorticoids.

## COMPLICATIONS

Similar to glomerulonephritis, nephrotic syndrome can lead to renal failure and complications involving fluid overload in the periphery due to protein shifts. At the vascular level, the patient may become hypovolemic because of changes in osmotic pressure.

# VASCULAR DISORDERS

Vascular renal disease results from one of two processes: (1) disease of the main renal arteries or renal artery stenosis and (2) sclerosis of renal arterioles or nephrosclerosis.

## RENAL ARTERY STENOSIS

### Etiology/Epidemiology

Renal artery stenosis is the cause of approximately 5% of all cases of hypertension. Stenosis of the renal artery is usually classified as either arteriosclerosis or fibromuscular hyperplasia. In either case, the end result is a narrowing of the lumen of the arteries supplying the kidneys. Obstruction of the renal arteries can be caused by aneurysm, thrombosis, and emboli.

### Pathophysiology

Renal artery stenosis results in a major reduction in blood flow to the kidneys. This change in renal perfusion causes increased secretion of renin and activation of the renin-angiotensin-aldosterone system.[6] The end result is acceleration of hypertension, which, if untreated, leads to further pathological changes in the kidneys. Box 44-4 lists the signs of renal artery stenosis.

### Collaborative Care Management

Medical treatment includes vigorous antihypertensive therapy to control blood pressure. Beta blockers or angiotensin-converting enzyme inhibitors are used to manage hypertension. Analgesics are used to manage pain associated with vascular occlusion. Preventing pulmonary embolism is critical in persons with renal vein thromboses. Anticoagulants are indicated for patients with renal artery occlusion or renal vein thrombosis. When a well-defined lesion exists in the renal artery, angioplasty or surgical bypass of the stenotic area may be performed to improve circulation.[6] Persons with renal artery stenosis and hypertension that does not respond to medication may need a nephrectomy.

#### *Patient/family education*

Many patients have cardiac disease as well and should be educated on behaviors that lower cholesterol including maintaining a diet low in animal fat and increasing aerobic exercise. Patients should be instructed to monitor their blood pressure at home and to keep their health care provider apprised of

**box 44-4** *clinical manifestations*

***Renal Artery Stenosis***

- Abdominal bruits
- Hypertension
- Disparity in kidney size
- Delayed appearance of contrast medium in renal arteriogram
- Hyperconcentration of contrast media in kidney's calyceal system on intravenous pyelogram
- Lesion evidenced on renal arteriogram
- Increased serum creatinine level with captopril challenge
- Changes in blood flow on duplex Doppler ultrasonography
- Detection of change in blood flow within vessels on magnetic resonance imaging

their values. If anticoagulant therapy is prescribed, the patient and family should understand precautions to take to avoid injury and signs of excessive bleeding. Patients should be taught to recognize signs of decreasing renal function and to report these symptoms promptly to the health care provider.

## NEPHROSCLEROSIS

### Etiology/Epidemiology

Whereas renal artery stenosis results in hypertension, hypertension can cause nephrosclerosis or damage to the renal arteries, arterioles, and glomeruli. Hypertension is the second major cause of end-stage renal disease. An estimated 10% of individuals with essential hypertension will develop severe renal damage and approximately 1% will develop end-stage renal disease and die unless supportive care is provided.[6]

### Pathophysiology

The renal vasculature is affected in *benign* nephrosclerosis. The renal arterial vessels show thickening and narrowing of their lumina, and some glomerular capillaries are sclerosed and collapsed. Renal blood flow can be reduced as a result of these vascular changes. The renal tubules can also be affected, resulting in tubular atrophy. Signs and symptoms are usually mild and include mild proteinuria from glomerular damage. Nocturia may occur from moderate loss of tubular concentrating ability. Urinary casts may be present from tubular injury. Although the renal insufficiency is relatively mild, these patients are at risk for acute failure.

In *malignant* nephrosclerosis, the major changes are necrosis and thickening of the arterioles and glomerular capillaries and diffuse tubular loss and atrophy. Gross hematuria occurs with RBC casts, heavy proteinuria, and elevated plasma creatinine. Malignant nephrosclerosis is a medical emergency, and high blood pressure must be lowered to prevent permanent renal damage as well as damage to other vital organs.

Signs and symptoms of nephrosclerosis are the same as those for chronic renal failure (see Chapter 45). By the time the signs and symptoms develop, the disease has progressed to an extreme point. Deterioration in renal function progresses gradually. However, if an acute or malignant phase of hypertension occurs, the process may accelerate.

### Collaborative Care Management

Treatment of nephrosclerosis is focused on early detection and treatment of hypertension. Causative factors are sought, and treatment to lower blood pressure is initiated (see Chapter 25). When significant renal damage exists, stabilizing the person's current level of function or slowing deterioration of the kidney tissue is the goal. Control of hypertension is continued.

For hypertensive emergencies, potent vasodilators such as diazoxide and sodium nitroprusside are used. These IV medications usually act rapidly to lower blood pressure. Sodium nitroprusside is given as a continuous IV drip. Monitor the patient continuously for headache, hypotension, muscle twitching, tachycardia, restlessness, and retrosternal or abdominal pain.

Nursing management of patients with nephrosclerosis is the same as outlined for chronic renal failure (see Chapter 45). The goals for nursing care center around providing comfort and maintaining independence in daily living. During drug therapy, monitor the patient closely for tachycardia, hypotension, hyperglycemia, and marked sodium and water retention.

#### Patient/family education

Prevention is best accomplished by routine screening to detect hypertension and to provide adequate treatment and follow-up care. Identification of persons at risk for developing hypertension (age, race, obesity, diabetes mellitus, positive family history, smoking history, and lack of exercise) and implementation of teaching programs to institute lifestyle modifications are important preventive strategies.

Persons with nephrosclerosis need teaching regarding the treatment strategies (diet and medications) and the need for continuous follow-up care. Skills to monitor the effectiveness of treatment should be taught, including taking vital signs, measuring fluid intake and output, and recording weights. The patient and family should also understand the possibility of the need for dialysis or transplant in the future.

# OBSTRUCTIVE DISORDERS

Urinary tract obstruction can occur in any portion of the urinary tract from the urinary calyces to the meatus. Patients with obstructions have characteristic signs and symptoms, depending on the location and extent of the obstruction. Uncorrected urinary obstruction can lead to renal failure. This section describes the major concepts related to obstruction of the urinary system and the care of patients with obstructive disorders. Subsequent sections discuss specific obstructive disorders (renal calculi, urinary strictures, and tumors). Benign prostatic hypertrophy is discussed in Chapter 49.

## HYDRONEPHROSIS

### Etiology/Epidemiology

*Hydronephrosis* is the dilation of the renal pelvis and calyces with urine. Hydronephrosis may occur either unilaterally or bilaterally. Table 44-7 summarizes causes of obstruction of the urinary tract.

### Pathophysiology

Obstruction of any part of the urinary system from the kidney to the urethra will generate pressure that may cause functional and anatomic damage to the renal parenchyma. When any part of the urinary tract is obstructed, urine collects behind the obstruction, producing a dilation of the urinary collecting structures. Muscles of the affected area contract in an effort to push the urine around the obstruction. Partial obstruction may produce slow dilation of structures above the obstruction without functional impairment. As the obstruction increases, pressure builds up in the tubular system behind the obstruction, causing a backflow of urine and dilation of the ureter *(hydroureter)* (Figure 44-5). The urine

**table 44-7** *Causes of Urinary Tract Obstruction*

| LOCATION | MAJOR CAUSES |
|---|---|
| Lower urinary tract | Bladder neoplasms<br>Urethral strictures<br>Calculi<br>Tumors<br>Benign prostatic hypertrophy |
| Ureteral obstruction | Calculi<br>Trauma<br>Nephroptosis ("floating" or "dropped" kidney)<br>Enlarged lymph nodes<br>Lymphosarcoma<br>Reticulum cell sarcoma<br>Hodgkin's disease<br>Congenital anomaly |
| Kidney | Calculi<br>Ptosis<br>Polycystic kidney disease<br>Pregnancy (usually right-sided) |

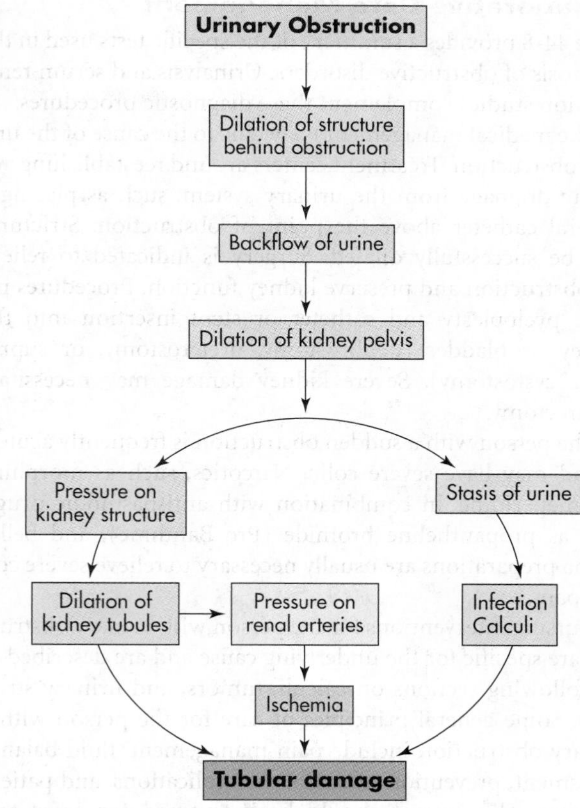


**fig. 44-5** Pathophysiology of uncorrected urinary obstruction.

backup eventually reaches the kidney, causing dilation of the kidney pelvis *(hydronephrosis)*. Pressure build-up in the renal pelvis leads to destruction of kidney tissue and eventually renal failure.

With obstruction, urine flow is decreased, even to the point of stagnation. This stagnant urine provides a culture medium for bacterial growth, and rarely is obstruction seen without some infection. The specific effects that occur with obstruction depend on the location, extent (partial or complete), and duration of the obstruction. Obstruction in the lower urinary tract causes bladder distention. If this is prolonged, muscle fibers become hypertrophied, and *diverticuli* (herniated sacs of bladder mucosa) develop between the hypertrophied muscle bands. Since the diverticulum holds stagnant urine, infection often occurs, and bladder stones may form.

Obstruction of the upper urinary tract can progress rapidly to hydronephrosis because of the small size of the ureters and kidney pelvis. Increased pressure causes partial ischemia between the renal cortex and medulla and the dilation of the renal tubules, leading to tubular damage. Urinary stasis in the dilated pelvis leads to infection and calculi, which add to the renal damage. Some urine can flow back up the renal tubules into the veins and lymphatics as a compensatory mechanism. The unaffected kidney then takes on increased elimination of waste products. With prolonged obstruction, the unaffected kidney hypertrophies and may function almost (80%) as effectively alone as both kidneys did before the obstruction. Obstruction of both kidneys leads to renal failure.

Hydronephrosis can occur without any symptoms as long as kidney function is adequate, and urine can drain. An acute upper urinary tract obstruction will cause pain, nausea, vomiting, local tenderness, spasm of the abdominal muscles, and a mass in the kidney region. The pain is caused by stretching of the tissues and by hyperperistalsis. Because the amount of pain is proportional to the rate of stretching, a slowly developing hydronephrosis may cause only a dull flank pain, whereas a sudden blockage of the ureter, e.g., from a stone, causes a severe stabbing *(colicky)* pain in the flank or abdomen. The pain may radiate to the genitalia and thigh and is caused by the increased peristaltic action of the smooth muscles of the ureter in an effort to dislodge the obstruction and force urine past it.

The nausea and vomiting frequently associated with acute obstruction are caused by a reflex reaction to the pain and will usually abate as soon as the pain is relieved. An extremely dilated kidney, however, may press on the stomach, causing continued gastrointestinal symptoms. If renal function has been seriously impaired, nausea and vomiting may indicate uremia. (See Chapter 45 for discussion of uremia and renal failure.)

When the bladder is distended from lower urinary tract obstruction, the person will experience lower abdominal discomfort and feel the need to void although voiding may not be possible. The bladder may be palpated above the symphysis pubis. With partial obstruction, as seen in benign prostatic hypertrophy, the patient first complains of increasing urinary frequency because the bladder fails to empty completely with each void and therefore refills more quickly to the amount that causes the urge to void (usually 250 to 500 ml). Nocturia, hematuria, and pyuria may also be present.

### Collaborative Care Management

Table 44-8 provides a summary of the specific tests used in the diagnosis of obstructive disorders. Urinalysis and serum renal function studies complement these diagnostic procedures.

The medical management is specific to the cause of the urinary obstruction. Treatment centers around reestablishing adequate drainage from the urinary system, such as placing a ureteral catheter above the point of obstruction. Strictures may be successfully dilated. Surgery is indicated to relieve the obstruction and preserve kidney function. Procedures include pyeloplasty and catheter or stent insertion into the kidney or bladder (nephrostomy, ureterostomy, or suprapubic cystostomy). Severe kidney damage may necessitate nephrectomy.

The person with a sudden obstruction is frequently acutely ill and may have severe colic. Narcotics, such as morphine and meperidine, in combination with antispasmodic drugs, such as propantheline bromide (Pro-Banthine), and belladonna preparations are usually necessary to relieve severe colicky pain.

Nursing interventions for the person with urinary obstruction are specific for the underlying cause and are described in the following sections on calculi, tumors, and urinary strictures. Some general principles of care for the person with a urinary obstruction include pain management, fluid balance assessment, prevention of urinary complications, and patient teaching. The patient should be monitored for signs and symptoms of infection.

#### *Patient/family education*

Patients and their families should be taught postoperative care of incisions and care and management of indwelling catheters if applicable. Information about the medication regimen, side effects of prescribed medications, diet and fluid restrictions, and signs and symptoms of infection and recurrent obstruction should be included in the teaching plan. Measures to prevent UTI should be stressed (see p. 1417).

## RENAL CALCULI

Urinary stones *(urolithiasis)* may develop at any level in the urinary system but are most frequently found within the kidney *(nephrolithiasis)*. Figure 44-6 illustrates the most common locations of calculi formation.

### Etiology

Renal calculi (stones) are crystallizations of minerals around an organic matrix such as pus, blood, or devitalized tissue. The mineral composition of renal calculi varies. Most stones consist of calcium salts (oxalates or phosphates) or

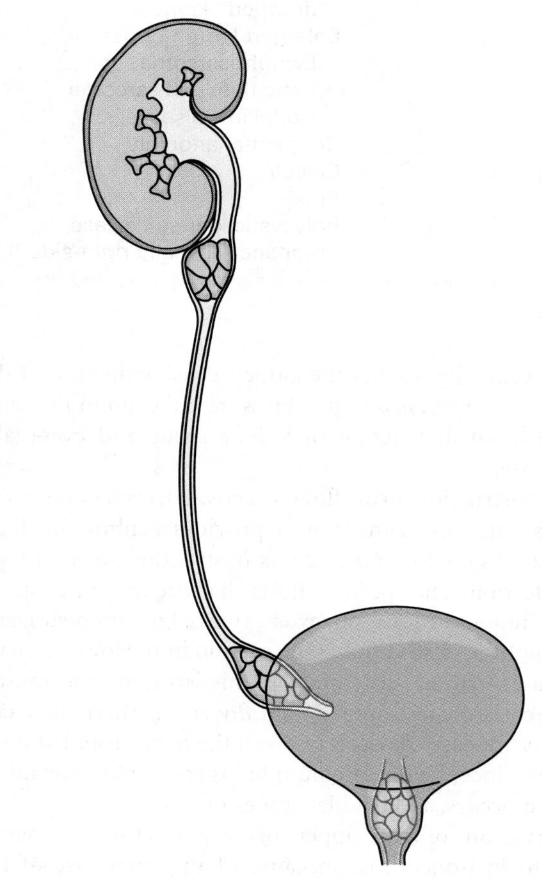

**fig. 44-6** Most common locations of renal calculi formation.

**table 44-8** *Summary of Tests Used for Diagnosis of Obstructive Disorders*

| | Renal Calculi | Renal Neoplasms | Prostatic Hypertrophy | Urethral Strictures |
|---|---|---|---|---|
| Cystoscopy | X | X | X | X* |
| Retrograde pyelography | X | X | | |
| Intravenous pyelography | X | X | X | X* |
| Kidney, ureters, and bladder (KUB) x-ray | X | X | | |
| Urethrography | | | X | X |
| Computed tomography | | X | | |
| Renal angiography | | X | | |
| Ultrasound | X | X | | |
| Renal biopsy | | X | | |

*Not always completed.

magnesium-ammonium phosphate; the remainder are cystine or uric acid stones.

No demonstrable cause can be found for more than half the renal stones that occur *(idiopathic)*. However, a major predisposing factor is the presence of UTI. Infection increases the presence of organic matter around which the minerals can precipitate and increases the alkalinity of the urine (by the production of ammonia). This results in precipitation of calcium phosphate and magnesium-ammonium phosphate. Stasis of urine also permits precipitation of organic matter and minerals. Other factors associated with the development of stones include long-term use of antacids, vitamin D, large doses of vitamin C, and calcium carbonate.

## Epidemiology

An estimated 1% of all people in the United States will develop urolithiasis. Most stones pass without medical intervention. About one third of the individuals who have recurrent upper urinary tract calculi will eventually have the affected kidney removed. An estimated 20% of persons with kidney stones seek medical attention.[20]

## Pathophysiology

Because most stones are calcium oxalates, anything that leads to hypercalciuria is a predisposing factor for renal stones (Table 44-9). In persons for whom no underlying pathological cause can be identified, hypercalciuria may result from increased calcium absorption from the intestine or from decreased reabsorption of calcium by the kidney tubules. These persons do not have hypercalcemia because the calcium is eliminated in the urine. See Table 44-9 for other contributing factors to renal stone formation.

Pain *(renal colic)* is the primary symptom in an acute episode of renal calculi. The location of the pain depends on the location of the renal stone. If the stone is in the kidney pelvis, the pain is caused by hydronephrosis and is more dull and constant in character, occurring primarily in the costovertebral angle. As the stone moves down the ureter, excruciating and intermittent pain is caused by spasm of the ureter and anoxia of the ureter wall from the pressure of the stone. The pain follows the anterior course of the ureter down to the suprapubic area and radiates to the external genitalia. Nausea and vomiting often accompany renal colic.

Patients frequently have two or three attacks of acute renal colic before the stone passes. This is probably because the stone becomes lodged at a narrow point in the ureter, causing temporary obstruction. The ureters are normally narrower at the ureteropelvic and ureterovesical junctions and at the point where they pass over the iliac crest into the pelvis. If the stone is to pass along the ureter by peristaltic action, the patient will have some pain.

Gross hematuria may occur if the stone has rough edges. Microhematuria is almost always present. Signs and symptoms of UTI (p. 1415) may also be present. Often a stone is "silent," causing no symptoms for years. This is especially true of very large stones that develop over a long period before resulting in symptoms. Extremely small smooth stones may be passed asymptomatically.

**table 44-9** *Renal Calculus Composition and Contributing Factors*

| Composition of Stone | Factors Contributing to Stone Formation |
|---|---|
| Calcium (oxalate and phosphate) | Hypercalcemia and/or hypercalciuria resulting from hyperparathyroidism, vitamin D intoxication, multiple myeloma, immobilization, severe bone disease, cancer, renal tubular acidosis, prolonged intake of steroids, and increased intake of calcium |
| Uric acid | High purine diet, gout, renal failure, blood dyscrasias, use of thiazide diuretics and alkylating agents |
| Cystine | Cystinuria resulting from genetic disorder of amino acid metabolism |
| Struvite (magnesium-ammonium phosphate) | Infection |

## Collaborative Care Management

### Diagnostic tests

Diagnostic studies performed to determine the presence of renal stones include kidney, ureters, and bladder (KUB) x-ray; IV or retrograde pyelography; ultrasound; CT; and cystoscopy. Additional studies include urinalysis and serum calcium and serum uric acid levels.

Because recurrence of renal calculi is common, additional studies are carried out after the acute episode has subsided. Successive determinations of serum calcium, phosphorus, protein, electrolytes, and uric acid levels are performed to identify the underlying disease that can influence stone formation. The urine pH is measured with a dipstick each time the patient voids to determine the urine acidity or alkalinity. A nitroprusside urine test may be performed to check for the presence of cystine. An accurate 24-hour urine specimen is collected to measure calcium, oxalate, phosphorus, and uric acid levels. The 24-hour urine specimen may be collected with the patient eating a normal diet or following a 3-day low-calcium, low-phosphorus diet.

### Medications

Sodium or potassium phosphate may be prescribed to decrease urinary calcium; these drugs are contraindicated if the kidney is infected. Thiazide diuretics, particularly hydrochlorothiazide, decrease the calcium content in the urine by increasing reabsorption of calcium in the renal tubules. Cellulose sodium phosphate (a cation exchange resin) can be administered with meals or can be used in conjunction with dietary restrictions to reduce formation of calcium oxalate and calcium phosphate nephrolithiasis.

Phosphate calculi develop in alkaline urine; therefore, their prevention depends on keeping the urine acidic and preventing UTIs. Cranberry juice can be taken (200 ml four times daily) to keep the urine acidic. Ascorbic acid may also be prescribed to acidify the urine.

Prophylaxis for uric acid stones consists of alkalinizing the urine by the administration of sodium bicarbonate or citrate solution. Allopurinol (Zyloprim) is usually prescribed to inhibit synthesis of uric acid. Cystine stones can be treated with penicillamine, which acts by combining with cystine to form a soluble compound.

### Treatments

About 90% of urinary calculi are passed spontaneously. If there is no infection or obstruction, the stone may be left in the ureter for several months. Fluids are prescribed at 2500 ml/day or more to promote passage of the stone and to prevent infection.

If the stone fails to pass, one or two ureteral catheters may be passed through a cystoscope up the ureter and left in place for 24 hours. The catheters dilate the ureter and when removed may allow the stone to pass into the bladder. If signs of infection are present, an attempt is made to pass a ureteral catheter past the stone into the renal pelvis. The catheter is left as a drain, to prevent the development of pyelonephritis. Patients with ureteral catheters are usually confined to bed to prevent catheter dislodgement.

Stones in the lower ureter may be removed by cystoscopic manipulation. General anesthesia may be required, and care is similar to that after cystoscopy (see Chapter 43).

**Percutaneous lithotripsy.** Percutaneous lithotripsy is a technique that requires a percutaneous nephrostomy tract created through an incision of ¼ to ½ inch over the kidney region. Anesthesia and x-ray are necessary for the procedure. A nephroscope is then passed through the tract, and a snare basket is used to retrieve the calculi. If the calculi cannot be removed, a lithotripter probe is used to break up the stone. Complications of the procedure are rare and include hemorrhage, urinoma, sepsis, and abscess. After the procedure the patient usually experiences pain similar to renal colic caused by manipulation of the kidney and ureters. Pain is controlled by administering narcotic analgesics. The patient may also have large amounts of drainage from the nephrostomy tract. Dressings should be changed frequently to prevent infection and skin breakdown. Urinary drainage from the incision may last for 3 to 4 days after the procedure. Patients usually receive a 2-week course of antibiotic therapy after lithotripsy.

**Extracorporeal shock wave lithotripsy.** With extracorporeal shock wave lithotripsy, the patient is submerged in a large tank of distilled water. Fluoroscopy or ultrasound is used for stone location. A shock wave electrode is placed at the bottom of the tank. The shock waves produced by the electrode fragment the renal stone. The shock waves are focused and directed at the stone by an alpha-dimensional radiographic scanning system and are keyed to follow the R wave of the patient's electrocardiogram.[20] The water bath allows passage of the shock waves into the body. Persons with pacemakers are not candidates for shock wave lithotripsy. Sedation and anesthesia may be necessary because of the pain from passage of each sound wave.

Modifications to lithotriptors have eliminated the need for a water bath and anesthesia. They use ultrasound to localize the stone and generate shock waves by a variety of mechanisms.

Immediately after the procedure, the patient may experience redness or bruising on the skin at the lithotripsy site. Pain may also be experienced in this region from the force of the ultrasonic shock waves. Pain is usually localized to the skin as a result of the shock waves entering the body. The patient can be discharged after the procedure if there are no complications. After lithotripsy, small particles are passed in the urine over the next several days. The patient is observed for signs of bleeding. Blood pressure is monitored frequently for the first several hours after the procedure. Urine output is also closely monitored for both quantity and quality. Initially blood may turn the urine cherry red to pink for the first several hours. The urine should then clear.

Pain resulting from passing fragments of the pulverized stone through the lower urinary tract occurs after lithotripsy. If large fragments of the stone are formed, a percutaneous nephrostomy may be performed to allow passage of the fragments. Narcotic analgesics are used to control pain. Pain may persist for up to 3 days after lithotripsy. The patient should be informed about the use of pain medications and signs requiring physician notification.

Occasionally, urinary obstruction may occur as a result of stone fragments blocking the flow of urine. The patient is instructed to observe the volume of urine output for several days after discharge. Daily weight should be obtained to detect urinary retention. Flank pain may also indicate urinary obstruction. When these symptoms are present, the patient should contact the physician immediately. Hematuria may occur due to local trauma.

**Candela laser therapy.** The Candela laser is a pulsed-dye laser system designed to break up calculi that have migrated to the lower ureters. The laser probe is inserted through a ureteroscope. A 2.4-mm flexible probe is used to decrease the minor ureteral injury often caused by a wider probe and ureteroscope. An advantage of the Candela laser system is that it spares the patient the discomfort and cost of lithotripsy or surgery.

### Surgical management

Surgical intervention is indicated when a large stone (greater than 1 cm) produces pain, obstruction, or infection. The procedure for removing a stone from the ureter is a *ureterolithotomy* (Figure 44-7, *C*). A radiograph is taken immediately preceding surgery so that the incision into the ureter is made directly over the stone. If the stone is in the lower third of the ureter, a rectus incision is made. If it is in the upper two thirds, a flank approach is used. If the patient has a ureteral stricture that causes stones to form, a plastic surgery procedure to relieve the stricture may be carried out as part of the procedure.

Removal of a stone through or from the renal pelvis is known as *pyelolithotomy* (Figure 44-7, *A*). Stones obstructing the ureteropelvic junction are removed, and the obstruction is relieved by pyeloplasty. Removal of a stone through the parenchyma is a *nephrolithotomy* (Figure 44-7, *B*). Occasion-

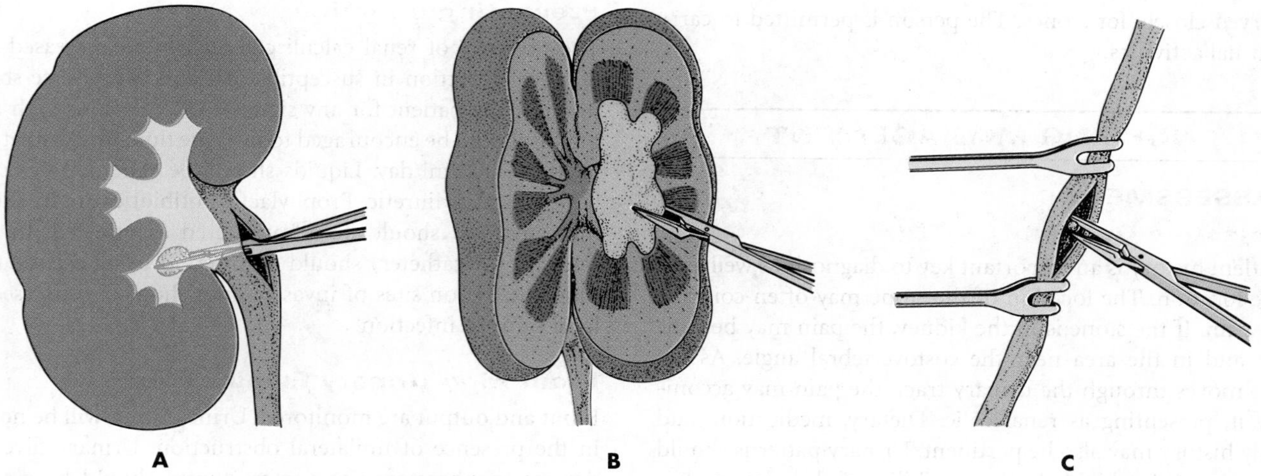


**fig. 44-7** Location and methods of removing renal calculi from upper urinary tract. **A,** Pyelolithotomy, removal of stone through renal pelvis. **B,** Nephrolithotomy, removal of staghorn calculus from renal parenchyma (kidney split). **C,** Ureterolithotomy, removal of stone from ureter.

ally, the kidney may have to be split from end to end (a kidney split) to remove the stone. Patients in whom such a split is performed are at risk for hemorrhage after surgery.

Bladder stones may be removed through a suprapubic incision, or they may be crushed with a lithotrite (stone crusher) that is passed transurethrally. This procedure is known as *litholapaxy.* After bladder stone removal, the bladder may be irrigated (intermittently or constantly) with an acid solution such as magnesium and sodium citrate (G solution) or hemiacidrin (Renacidin) to counteract the alkalinity caused by the infection and to help wash out the remaining particles of stone.

### Diet

Persons who have recurrent renal calculi benefit from ongoing prophylactic therapy determined by the type of stone being produced. For calcium stones, foods high in calcium are sometimes restricted.

Renal stone formation can often be controlled by regulating urinary pH. Table 44-10 provides a summary of diet principles applied to renal calculi. Persons at risk for developing calcium oxalate, calcium phosphate, or magnesium-ammonium phosphate stones may be placed on an acid-ash diet (Table 44-11) to promote excretion of an acid urine. Catheter irrigations using acetic acid solution or hemiacidrin help provide an acid environment and thus decrease precipitation of calcium and phosphate. Persons at risk for developing uric acid or cystine stones may be placed on an alkaline-ash diet because uric acid and cystine are soluble in an alkaline urine.

Fluid intake, preferably water, should be increased to 3500 to 4000 ml/24 hr. The patient should try to get up during the night at least once for a glass of water.

### Activity

A person who is up and moving is more likely to pass a stone than one who is in bed. The urine is strained and

**table 44-10** *Summary of Diet Principles in Renal Stone Disease*

| Stone Chemistry | Nutrition Modification | Diet Ash Urinary pH |
|---|---|---|
| Calcium | Low calcium (400 mg) | Acid ash |
| Phosphate | Low phosphorus (1-1.2 g) (milk, cheese, egg yolk, whole grains, legumes, nuts) | |
| Oxalate | Low oxalate <50 mg/day (tea, chocolate, nuts, spinach) | |
| Struvite ($MgNH_4PO_4$) | Low phosphorus (1-1.2 g) (associated with UTI) | Acid ash |
| Uric acid | Low purine (organ meats, shrimp, dried beans) | Alkaline ash |
| Cystine | Low methionine | Alkaline ash |

Data from Coe FL, Parks JH, Asplin JR: *N Engl J Med* 327(16):1141-1152, 1992.

**table 44-11** *Acid-Ash and Alkaline-Ash Food Groups Used to Control pH of Urine*

| Acid Ash | Alkaline Ash | Neutral |
|---|---|---|
| Meat | Milk | Sugars |
| Whole grains | Vegetables | Fats |
| Eggs | Fruit (except cranberries, blueberries, prunes, plums) | Beverages |
| Cheese | | Coffee |
| Cranberries, blueberries | | Tea |
| Prunes | | |
| Plums | | |

From Williams SR: *Nutrition and diet therapy,* ed 7, St Louis, 1993, Mosby.

observed closely for stones. The person is permitted to carry out usual activities.

## NURSING MANAGEMENT

### ASSESSMENT

#### Subjective Data

A patient history is an important key to diagnosis as well as to stone location. The location of the stone may often coincide with pain. If the stone is in the kidney, the pain may be constant and in the area near the costovertebral angle. As the stone moves through the urinary tract, the pain may accompany it, presenting as renal colic. Dietary, medication, and family history may also be pertinent. Urinary patterns should be investigated to highlight the possibility of obstruction: dysuria or voiding in small amounts followed by urgency. The patient may report episodes of nausea or vomiting.

#### Objective Data

Data to be collected to assess the person with renal calculi include:

Urine output
Presence of stones in urine
Vital signs, presence of fever
Flank tenderness
Costovertebral angle tenderness

### NURSING DIAGNOSES

Nursing diagnoses are determined from analysis of patient data. Nursing diagnoses for the patient with renal calculi include but are not limited to (see also the Nursing Care Plan):

| Diagnostic Title | Possible Etiological Factors |
|---|---|
| Pain | Presence and/or movement of stones |
| Infection, risk for | Urinary stasis, presence of stones |
| Altered urinary elimination | Obstruction from calculi |
| Anxiety | Home care and pain management |

### EXPECTED PATIENT OUTCOMES

Expected patient outcomes for the patient with renal calculi may include but are not limited to:

1. Reports pain controlled of 2 or less (scale of 1 to 10).
2. Is free of the signs and symptoms of infection.
3. Maintains urine output equal to intake.
4. Uses resources and support systems effectively.

### INTERVENTIONS

#### Pain

Renal colic is an excruciating type of pain. Morphine or other opiates are given in doses to control the pain. Antispasmodics, such as atropine or methantheline bromide (Banthine), may also be prescribed to relax the smooth muscles of the ureter and lessen pain from spasm. Relaxation techniques such as music therapy and guided imagery are also useful.

#### Preventing Infection

The presence of renal calculi can lead to an increased incidence of infection in susceptible patients. The nurse should monitor the patient for any signs of UTI. Persons with renal calculi should be encouraged to increase fluid intake to at least 3500 to 4000 ml/day. Liquids should be caffeine free as caffeine acts as a diuretic. Prophylactic antibiotics are frequently indicated and should be administered as directed. Invasive lines (IV or catheter) should be inserted using aseptic technique. Insertion sites of invasive lines should be assessed for local signs of infection.

#### Promoting Urinary Elimination

Input and output are monitored. Urine output will be normal in the presence of unilateral obstruction. Urinary diversion devices (nephrostomy or ureterostomy) should be assessed frequently for correct placement and patency. The tubing should be kept free of kinks to prevent reflux of urine. The patient should be assessed for an increase in occurrence and severity of pain. Additional radiographic studies may be needed to rule out obstruction.

The urine of all persons with relatively small stones should be strained. Urine can be strained easily by placing two opened 4 × 8-inch gauze sponges over a funnel. Stones vary in size and may be no larger than the head of a pin. The stones are saved for inspection by the physician and sent to the laboratory for analysis.

#### Decreasing Anxiety

Because of the abrupt nature and severity of pain due to renal calculi, fear and anxiety are commonplace. Careful assessment of the patient's anxiety level is necessary to guide future interventions and teaching. The patient should be encouraged to verbalize fears and concerns. The nurse should assist the patient in developing a support system and educate the patient on symptom management.

#### Patient/Family Education

The person who has had urinary calculi needs to know how to prevent development of further stones. Patient teaching includes:

1. Prevent UTIs.
   a. Drink at least 2500 ml of fluids/day.
   b. Avoid situations that lead to urinary stasis, if possible (e.g., long periods of inactivity).
2. Follow any dietary prescriptions.
3. Know name, dosage, and side effects of medications prescribed to acidify or alkalinize the urine.
4. Report to physician signs of recurrence of calculi (costovertebral pain or pain radiating to external genitalia).
5. Report to physician signs of UTI (burning on urination, frequency, urgency, or fever).

##### *Health promotion/prevention*

Measures can be taken to decrease the potential for renal stones in persons at high risk. Adequate hydration (intake of 2500 ml/day or more unless contraindicated) will help to prevent urinary stasis that can lead not only to stone formation

## nursing care plan: The Person with Renal Calculi Undergoing Placement of Nephrostomy Tube for Obstruction

**DATA** Mr. M. is a 57-year-old auto worker who complained of a sudden onset of severe right flank pain. His diagnosis is bilateral renal calculi with obstruction on the right side. A right nephrostomy tube has been placed to gravity drainage.

Mr. M. is married with two grown children living 10 miles away. His wife works full time as a legal secretary. Mr. M. is anxious about caring for his nephrostomy and voices concerns about pain management. His wife is concerned about the remaining stones blocking the other kidney.

The nursing assessment identified the following:

- Nephrostomy tube on right midback to gravity drain; urine in bag blood-tinged with some clots
- Small amount of crusted drainage on dressing; site without erythema
- Blood pressure 160/94; heart rate 100; temperature 98.2° F
- Patient guards right flank during examination
- Small pin-point granules seen in strained voided urine
- Wife at bedside states loudly, "He's not ready to go home; how will I manage?"

**NURSING DIAGNOSIS** *Pain related to renal calculi and placement of a nephrostomy tube*

| expected patient outcome | nursing interventions | rationale |
|---|---|---|
| Reports pain is controlled. | Assess location, severity, frequency, duration, and quality of pain. Use pain scale to rate patient's perception of pain. | Plan for appropriate interventions; collect baseline data to assess effectiveness of interventions. |
| | Apply warm compresses to flank area. | Decreases inflammation and promote relaxation. |
| | Administer analgesics as ordered. | Provide pain relief. |
| | Encourage use of relaxation techniques such as focused breathing, music, guided imagery. | Promote comfort and decreases narcotic use. |

**NURSING DIAGNOSIS** *Risk for infection related to urinary stasis and break in skin integrity, presence of nephrostomy tube*

| expected patient outcome | nursing interventions | rationale |
|---|---|---|
| Achieve wound healing, be free of purulent drainage, and no signs of urinary tract infection. | Assess temperature, nephrostomy site, frequency, urgency, and abdominal tenderness. | Changes in baseline examination will indicate signs of infection. |
| | Change nephrostomy dressing using aseptic technique as ordered and PRN. | Dressing change and keeping the site dry and covered decreases the potential for bacteria to contaminate the site and prevents skin breakdown. Wound assessment establishes baseline assessment and signs of local infection. |
| | Assess nephrostomy site for erythema, drainage, tenderness, induration, and swelling. | |
| | Note signs and symptoms of systemic infection: fever, chills, and diaphoresis. | Identify signs of systemic infection. |
| | Obtain tissue/fluid sample for culture and sensitivity. | Ensure effectiveness of antibiotic therapy. |
| | Maintain adequate hydration and voiding schedule. | Prevent bladder distention and urinary stasis. |
| | Administer prophylactic antibiotics as indicated. | Prevent susceptible infections. |

Continued

but also to UTI. Persons confined to bed should be encouraged to turn and move frequently, exercising arms and legs whenever possible. Urinary stasis can be prevented in immobile persons by frequent turning and position changes, including transferring the patient to a chair two to three times per day. Persons with indwelling catheters need scrupulous aseptic technique in catheter care to prevent infection and require adequate hydration and patent catheter drainage to flush away deposits at the catheter tip.

## ■ EVALUATION

To evaluate effectiveness of nursing interventions, compare patient behaviors with those stated in the expected patient outcomes. Successful achievement of patient outcomes for the patient with renal calculi is indicated by:

1. Reports pain is a <2 on a scale of 1 to 10.
2. Remains afebrile with no burning, urgency, or frequency of urination and temperature within normal limits. The invasive line site does not show signs of local infection.

## *The Person with Renal Calculi Undergoing Placement of Nephrostomy Tube for Obstruction—cont'd*

**NURSING DIAGNOSIS** *Altered urinary elimination related to the presence of renal calculi and the presence of a nephrostomy tube*

| expected patient outcome | nursing interventions | rationale |
|---|---|---|
| Maintain normal elimination pattern from the nephrostomy and voided urine output. | Assess input and output and presence of clots in nephrostomy collection bag. Strain all urine for calculi and send for analysis. | Deviations from normal indicate potential mechanical blockage. Determine treatment strategies. |
| | Encourage high fluid intake of 3500 to 4000 mL/24 hr. | Promote passage of stone, dilute urine. |
| | Assess and record any reports of dysuria, urgency, frequency, or incontinence. | Indications of infection or altered renal functioning are identified. |
| | Maintain patency and position of nephrostomy tube, avoid kinks in tubing, and keep bag in dependent position. | Prevent reflux of urine into kidney and dislodging of tube; allow for gravity drainage. |

**NURSING DIAGNOSIS** *Anxiety related to home management of the nephrostomy tube*

| expected patient outcome | nursing interventions | rationale |
|---|---|---|
| Use resources and support systems effectively. | Assess level of anxiety. | Provide a baseline for interventions. |
| Wife and Mr. M. report decreased level of anxiety and ability to independently care for nephrostomy tube. | Encourage patient/family to express fears and concerns. | Validate feelings and provides support. |
| | Assist patient to identify support system. | Decrease anxiety and identify previously effective coping skills. |
| | Instruct (demonstration and written instructions) patient and wife on care of nephrostomy tube. | Provide knowledge and decrease anxiety. |
| | Observe patient and wife performing care of nephrostomy tube. | Reinforcement builds confidence and decreases anxiety. |
| | Provide emergency numbers for home support. | Support mechanisms reduce anxiety. |

3. Has input equal to output; strained urine is free of stones.
4. Reports decrease in anxiety, has identified support systems, and is able to manage care independently.

### COMPLICATIONS

Complications occur as a result of untreated obstruction. If urine flow is not reestablished, severe pain and hydronephrosis with resultant renal failure may occur. Additionally, stasis of urine increases risk of infection.

## URETHRAL STRICTURES

### Etiology/Epidemiology

A *urethral stricture* is a narrowing or constriction of the lumen of the urethra. Urethral strictures can be congenital or acquired. Congenital urethral strictures can occur in isolation or in combination with other urinary tract anomalies. Acquired urethral stricture can result from trauma secondary to accident or instrumentation, infection (especially gonorrhea), muscle spasm, or pressure from the outside by adjacent structures or by growing tumors. Urethral strictures occur more often in men than women, primarily because of the length of the urethra.

### Pathophysiology

Narrowing of the urethra can result from chronic infection that leads to inflammation of the lining. The inflammation causes a hyperplasia of the lining, and the stricture develops. Trauma may completely sever the urethra. When the urethra is anastomosed, stricture frequently occurs at the surgical site. One of the leading causes of urethral stricture is a tumor that puts pressure against the exterior of the urethra, resulting in strictures of the lumen.

The first symptom of urethral stricture is usually a decrease in the urinary stream and difficulty initiating the stream. Other symptoms are those of UTI and urinary retention. Severe urethral strictures result in complete urinary obstruction, leading to the signs and symptoms of hydronephrosis (see p. 1426-1427).

### Collaborative Care Management

Urethral strictures are often repaired with urethroplasty. Strictures may also be corrected by dilation of the urethra. Dilation is accomplished by inserting splinting catheters into the urethra past the area of the stricture. The size of the splinting catheters can be increased to dilate the urethra.

#### Patient/family education

Education for the patient and family centers on recognition of early signs and symptoms of a decrease in urine stream and urine retention. Education should be focused on high-risk groups (persons with urinary tract cancers, frequent bladder infections, and a history of trauma to the structures of the urinary tract).

## TUMORS OF THE KIDNEY

### Etiology

Although the exact causes of renal cell carcinoma have not been identified, certain risk factors have been linked to the disease. The most common risk factor for all cancers of the urinary system is cigarette smoking. Occupational exposure to textile dyes, rubber, metallurgy, paint, and leather has been implicated in the development of renal cell carcinoma.[8]

### Epidemiology

Malignant renal tumors, primarily adenocarcinomas, account for 3% of all cancers. Small benign tumors (adenomas) may occur without causing significant damage or symptoms. Renal cell carcinomas rarely occur before the age of 30 years, are more often seen in the 40- to 70-year age range, and occur twice as often in men as in women.

### Pathophysiology

Renal carcinomas usually develop unilaterally but may occur bilaterally. In stage I the tumor margins are well defined (encapsulated) and compress the kidney parenchyma during growth rather than infiltrating the tissue. The upper pole of the kidney is usually involved, and the tumor is usually large at the time of diagnosis. In stage II the tumor invades the fat surrounding the kidney. Stage III consists of local metastasis either through direct extension or through the renal vein or lymphatics (lymph node involvement). Distant metastases during stage IV are primarily in the lungs or bone, but other areas, such as the liver, spleen, bone, opposite kidney, or brain, may also be involved.

Prognosis is based on the stage and advancement of the disease at diagnosis. Factors influencing the prognosis include the the overall health and nutritional status of the patient.

The kidney is more frequently affected by metastatic than primary cancers. Tumors usually originate in the lung and breast.

Painless hematuria is the most frequent sign of renal cell carcinoma. Unfortunately, the hematuria is often intermittent, lessening the person's concern and causing procrastination in seeking medical care. Any person with hematuria should have a should have a complete urological examination, since immediate investigation of the first signs of hematuria positively affect the prognosis. Other signs and symptoms include dull flank pain, flank mass, unexplained weight loss, fever, and polycythemia. Hypertension may also be present as a result of stimulation of the renin-angiotensin system.

An IVP may show a distortion of the renal outline, suggesting a kidney tumor. Small tumors in the parenchyma may not be apparent on a routine pyelogram but may be identified by renal ultrasound, CT scan (see Chapter 43) or magnetic resonance imaging (MRI). CT is also useful in differentiating between renal cell carcinoma and a renal cyst. Renal angiography may also be performed to differentiate a cyst from a tumor. Biopsy provides a definitive diagnosis.

### Collaborative Care Management

Unless the person is a poor surgical risk or has extensive metastases, the diseased kidney is removed *(nephrectomy)* through a transabdominal, flank, lumbar, or thoracoabdominal approach (Figure 44-8). The transabdominal and thoracoabdominal approaches are preferred to secure the renal artery and vein and to prevent any spread of malignant cells. *Radical nephrectomy,* includes the removal of the kidney, adrenal gland, proximal ureter, renal artery and vein, and surrounding fat and Gerota's fascia. Radical nephrectomy is performed to prevent metastases; radiation therapy may follow surgical intervention. In some instances, only a portion of a diseased kidney is removed *(partial nephrectomy).* If an entire kidney is removed, a drain may be placed to remove serous fluid from the space previously occupied by the kidney, but no urinary drainage occurs. Urinary drainage occurs with partial nephrectomy.

Radiation is used postoperatively for residual or recurrent tumors and is also beneficial for symptomatic bone metastases. The use of chemotherapeutic agents in combination with immunomodulating agents has shown some benefit. Interleukin 2 has shown some promise for the treatment of renal cell carcinoma, with partial to complete regression of tumor in clinical trials. The side effects of interleukin 2 can be severe and include severe hypotension, rigors, and anaphylaxis.[13] Hormonal therapy with progesterone, testosterone, and antiestrogens is useful in some patients. Five-year survival rates after treatment of stage I, II, and IIIA tumors are 70%.[4]

#### Patient/family education

If surgery is the treatment chosen, patient and family teaching will focus on perioperative instructions. Preoperative instructions may include a discussion of the type and length of surgery; type of anesthesia; and the need for an IV line, catheter, or other drains. Instructions in the use of an incentive spirometer are crucial because inadequate ventilation is a frequent problem postoperatively. The patient is informed of the pain medication routine: whether or not it will be offered or if it must be requested. A description of methods of decreasing pain, such as by splinting the incision, should be offered.

Management of the patient after nephrectomy is similar to that for persons undergoing major abdominal surgery and urinary diversion surgery (see Chapter 41 and p. 1446-1447).

Education for persons with nonsurgical treatment should focus on the disease process, treatment options, and expected outcomes. Many therapies for renal cell carcinoma are experimental. It is imperative that patients fully understand the risks and benefits of each option. The diagnosis of cancer is frightening for patients and their families. Information on support groups such as "I Can Cope" through the American Cancer Society will be helpful to persons facing cancer.

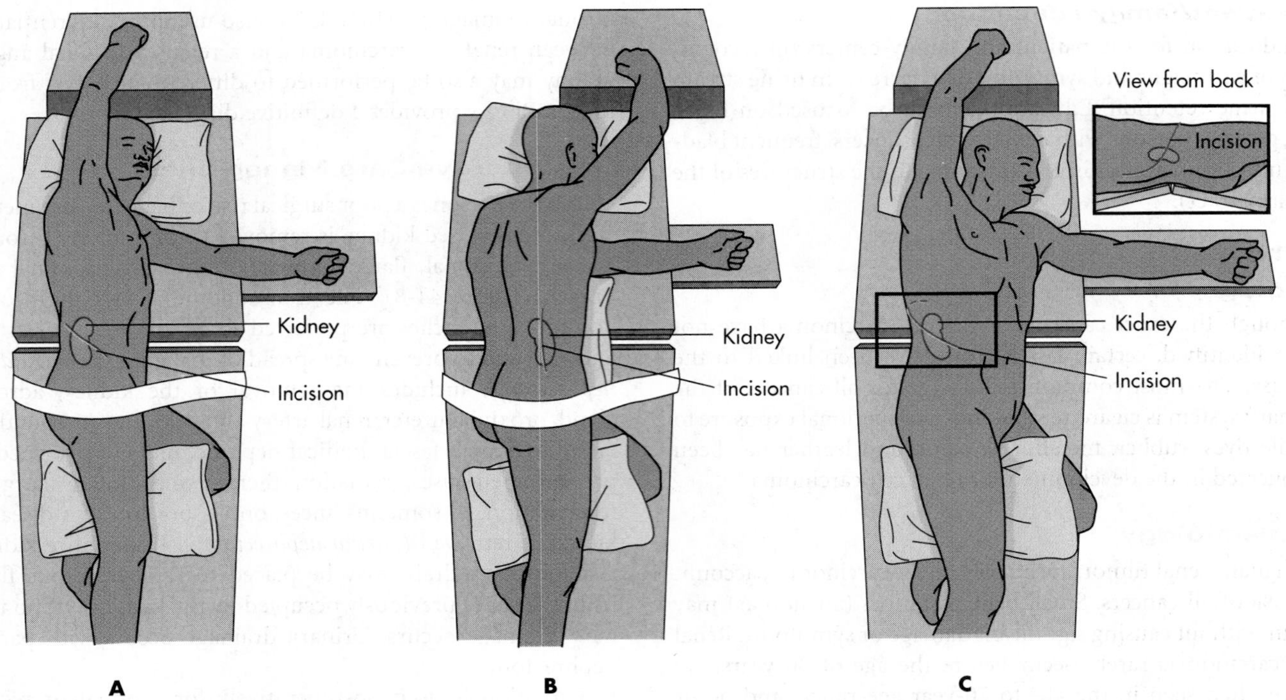


**fig. 44-8** Approaches to nephrectomy. **A,** Flank. **B,** Lumbar. **C,** Thoracoabdominal.

## TUMORS OF THE BLADDER

### Etiology/Epidemiology

The primary etiology of bladder cancer is exposure to aniline dyes used in the textile industry. Cigarette smoking is associated with an increase in bladder tumors. A 6- to 20-year latent period from exposure to tumor development is possible. Chronic bladder infections and renal calculi have also been identified as etiological agents of bladder tumors.[5]

The bladder is the most common site of cancer in the urinary tract. Cancer of the bladder occurs four times more often in males than in females, and multiple tumors are common. Most cases occur in men between 50 and 70 years of age. About 25% of patients have more than one lesion at the time of diagnosis. This figure increases to about 50% in persons with papilloma grade I carcinoma over a 5-year period. Approximately 40% of all tumors involve the trigone, and an additional 45% involve the posterior and lateral walls of the bladder. Ninety percent of bladder tumors are transitional cell carcinoma. The bladder is also the site of metastases from cervical and prostatic tumors.

### Pathophysiology

Tumors of the bladder range from small benign papillomas to large invasive carcinomas. Most neoplasms are of the transitional cell type because the urinary tract is covered with transitional epithelium. These neoplasms begin as papillomas; therefore, all papillomas of the bladder are considered premalignant and are removed when identified. Squamous cell carcinoma occurs less frequently (6% to 7%) and has a poorer prognosis. Other neoplasias include adenocarcinoma (which is often inoperable) and rhabdomyosarcoma (seen most frequently in infants).

Carcinomas of the bladder are graded and staged according to the definitions in Box 44-5. Grade I and II bladder tumors are usually superficial, whereas grade III and IV tumors are usually invasive in nature.

Painless hematuria is the first sign of a bladder tumor in most patients. It is usually intermit-tent, lessening the person's concern and delaying medical care. Hematuria may be accompanied by urgency and dysuria. Some patients are asymptomatic until obstruction occurs. Painless hematuria may also be seen in nonmalignant urinary tract disease and in cancer of the kidney; therefore, any hematuria should be investigated. Cystitis may be the first symptom of a bladder tumor, since the tumor acts as a foreign body in the bladder, causing inflammation. Symptoms of renal failure resulting from obstruction of the ureters is sometimes the reason for patients' seeking medical care. Vesicovaginal fistulas may occur before symptoms develop. The presence of renal failure or vesicovaginal fistula indicates a poor prognosis because they usually occur after the tumor has infiltrated widely.

### Collaborative Care Management

#### *Diagnostic tests*

Urinalysis that reveals blood in light of no other cause warrants further investigation via cystoscopy with cell analysis. Cytological analysis on a total voided urine sample should also be completed. IVP, CT scan, MRI, or ultrasound may also be done to evaluate surrounding tissue and organs. A chest

**box 44-5** *Grading and Staging of Advancement of Carcinomas of the Bladder*

| GRADES | DIFFERENTIATION |
|---|---|
| Grade I | Well differentiated |
| Grade II | Medially differentiated |
| Grade III | Poorly differentiated |
| Grade IV | Anaplastic |
| **STAGES** | **TISSUE INVOLVEMENT** |
| Stage O | Mucosa |
| Stage A | Submucosa |
| Stage B | Muscle |
| Stage C | Perivesical fat |
| Stage D | Lymph nodes |

x-ray and bone scan maybe ordered to rule out metastases. The serum carcinoembryonic antigen level is elevated.

Cytological examination of the urine may reveal malignant cells before the lesion can be visualized by cystoscopy. The diagnosis is established by cystoscopic visualization and biopsy of the bladder. Clinical determination of the invasiveness of the tumor is important in establishing a therapeutic regimen and in predicting the prognosis. Any person who has had a papilloma removed should have a cystoscopic examination every 3 months for 2 years and then less frequently if no new lesions are seen. Papillomas tend to recur without symptoms until they are far-advanced tumors. The necessity for frequent cystoscopies should be fully explained by the urologist and the explanation reinforced by the nurse.

### Medications

Chemotherapy is primarily palliative or used before radiation therapy. CMV (cisplatin, methotrexate, and vinblastine) with or without doxorubicin hydrochloride (Adriamycin) is the most frequently used therapy. Thiotepa may be instilled into the bladder as a topical treatment for noninvasive bladder cancer. Before instillation of thiotepa, the patient receives 8 to 12 hours of IV hydration. The dwell time for thiotepa is 12 hours, after which the drug is drained.

### Treatments

External cobalt radiation of large invasive tumors may be recommended before surgery to retard tumor growth. Supervoltage irradiation can be given when the patient physically cannot tolerate surgery. Radiation is not curative and has little value in patient management if the tumor is deemed inoperable. The goal of treatment is to preserve the bladder.[10] Internal radiation (radioisotopes or radon seeds) is rarely used because of the availability of external radiation. Radiation is also used for bony metastases.

### Surgical management

Small tumors with minimal tissue layer involvement may be adequately treated by endoscopic resection with *transurethral fulguration* or excision. A Foley catheter may be inserted after surgery. The urine may be pink-tinged, but not grossly bloody. Burning on urination may occur and is relieved by increasing fluid intake to dilute the urine. Heat applied over the bladder and sitz baths may provide relief. The patient is usually discharged within 1 to 2 days after surgery.

Partial removal of the bladder *(segmental resection)* is usually performed for tumors of the bladder dome. Bladder capacity will be small initially with a capacity of no more than 60 ml immediately after surgery. However, the elastic tissue of the bladder will regenerate, increasing bladder capacity to 200 to 400 ml within several months.

The decreased bladder size, is of major importance in the postoperative period. The patient will return from surgery with catheters draining the bladder both from a cystostomy and from the urethra to avoid obstruction of drainage. The bladder would become distended rapidly if obstruction occurred, resulting in disruption of the bladder suture line. Because bladder capacity is limited, the catheters usually cause severe bladder spasm. The urethral catheter is usually removed 3 weeks after surgery, but it may be left in place longer if the cystotomy wound is not healed.

As soon as the urethral catheter is removed, the patient becomes acutely aware of the small bladder capacity. Most patients will need to void at least every 20 minutes and be reassured that the bladder capacity will gradually increase. Total fluid intake should be 3000 ml throughout the day. Large quantities of fluid should not be ingested at one time, and fluids should be limited for several hours before going out.

Cystectomy is performed when the cancer appears curable. If the entire bladder is removed *(cystectomy)*, diversion of the urinary tract is necessary. Large amounts of surrounding tissue will also be removed if the tumor is malignant. A long, vertical abdominal incision is present, along with one or more pelvic drains. A nasogastric tube is inserted in the operating room, and the patient is given nothing by mouth until gastrointestinal function returns.

**Urinary diversion.** Urinary diversion procedures are required to treat malignancies of the urinary tract. Other indications for diversion procedures include birth defects, neurogenic bladder, chronic progressive pyelonephritis, and irreparable trauma to the urinary tract. A urinary diversion establishes an uninterrupted flow of urine, most often via a stoma. The flow of urine may be diverted at any level of the urinary system (see the Clinical Pathway). The most common urinary diversion procedure is the ileal or colon conduit. A surgical alternative that has an external stoma, the *continent urostomy,* has an internal reservoir made from intestine that holds urine. The stoma must be catheterized at regular intervals to drain the reservoir. The Kock continent ileal reservoir (Figure 44-9, p. 1444) is formed from loops of the small intestine. The ileocecal (or Indiana) pouch consists of portions of large intestine and ileum (Figure 44-10, p. 1444). Surgical techniques being studied consist of internal reservoirs anastomosed to the urethra.

Cutaneous ureterostomy is performed when the patient's physical condition prohibits more extensive surgical procedures. One or both ureters are excised from the bladder and

*Text continued on p. 1442*

## clinical pathway *Cystectomy**

**ATTENDING: POSTOP LOS 7 DAYS**
**MEDICAL DIAGNOSIS: ICD-9 CODE: 57.7x**
**Patient's/significant other's learning needs are identified and documented on PEP**

| | DATE:<br>CLINIC DAY | INT | DATE:<br>PREOP DAY | INT | DATE:<br>DOS | INT | DATE:<br>POD 1 & 2 | INT |
|---|---|---|---|---|---|---|---|---|
| INTERDISCIPLINARY COMMUNICATION (CONSULTS) | Schedule PFTs if COPD/para (10.0)<br>Schedule PAC if no preop day<br>Smoking cessation reference PRN (10.0) | | Anesthesia assmt<br>Stomal marking (ET) (5.0)<br>Home health (SW) (9.0)<br>OR/blood consent<br>Schedule OR<br>PFT if indicated (10.0)<br>Nutrition if hx pelvic radiation (7.0) | | Notify HO or arrival<br><br>Chaplain (8.0) | | ET (5.0)<br>SW discharge 9(.0)<br>RT if unable to wean $O_2$ (10.0)<br>PT PRN (6.0) | |
| ASSESSMENTS | High-risk screen (NSG)<br>ET—discharge plan | | Initiate database (RN)<br>Physical assmt (RN)<br>H&P (MD)<br>Discharge assmt (SW/RN)<br>Preprep weight (7.0) | | VS q1hr × 4, q2hr × 4, then q4hr<br>Urine output q4hr & notify HO if <30 ml/hr<br>Pain (1.0)<br>Epidural<br>Gastric pH q6hr<br>Protocols:<br>Preop 1.56<br>OR care 1.115<br>PACU care 1.164 | | VS q4 with $O_2$ sat (10.0)<br><br>Daily wt (7.0) | |
| DIAGNOSTICS (LABORATORY RADIOLOGY) | | | UA<br>Electrolytes<br>Type & screen<br>CBC & PLT<br>Chest x-ray<br>ECG per anesthesia protocol | | | | CBC & PLT<br><br>Chem 7 AM | |
| MEDICATIONS | Home meds<br>Multivitamin with iron 3 times/day | | GoLYTELY PO 1100 obtain wt previously<br>Erythromycin 1000 mg PO @ 1300, 1400, 2200<br>Neomycin 1000 mg PO @ 1300, 1400, 2200<br><br>$D_5$½NS IV @ 0000 150 ml/hr<br>Protocol 1.40<br><br>Neomycin 1% enema @ 2200<br><br>Benadryl 50 mg PO HS if needed<br>Home meds as ordered | | Cefoxitin 1 gm IVPB q8hr × 7 doses<br>Famotidine 20 mg IVPB q12hr<br>PCA: $MSO_4$ 1 mg q10min (max dose 6 mg) (1.2 acute pain) (1.79 IV opiates)<br>Ketorolac 15 mg IVP q6hr × 9 doses<br>Heparin flush 100 U IV q8hr PRN central line<br>Heparin 5000 U SQ q8hr (2.0)<br>Epidural–per APS 1.197<br>Epidural →<br>Phenergan 12.5 mg IV q30min × 3 PRN (then q6hr PRN)<br>Maalox 30 ml q4hr PRN for positive hem or pH <5<br>Benadryl 25 mg IVP QHS PRN<br>Tylenol suppository 650 mg PR for temperature >38.5° C<br>Cepstat Lozenges PRN | | →<br>→<br><br>→<br><br>→<br><br>→<br>2nd day change IV to $D_5$½NS with 20 KCl @ 100 ml/hr<br>→<br>→<br>→<br>→<br>→ | |

Courtesy University of Virginia Medical Center.
*Times are given by 24-hour clock.
*PEP,* Patient education plan; *PFTs,* pulmonary function tests; *HO,* house officer; *SW,* social worker; *COPD,* chronic obstructive pulmonary disease; *para,* paraplegic; *RT,* respiratory therapy; *PT,* physical therapy; *PAC,* preadmissions center; *IVPB,* intravenous piggyback; *OBR,* orthopedic bowel routine; *PCA,* patient-controlled analgesia; *D5½NS,* 5% dextrose in 0.5 N saline solution; *APS,* acute pain service; *SP,* Jackson-Pratt drain.

| DATE: POD 3 | INIT | DATE: POD 4 | INIT | DATE: POD 5 | INIT | DATE: POD 6 & 7 | INIT |
|---|---|---|---|---|---|---|---|
| | | HHR development (9.0) | | Solidify discharge plan: ET, SW & PT D/C needs identified (9.0)<br>HHR done (9.0) | | | |
| VS q8hr or as indicated<br>Continue to monitor sats q4hr × 2 after $O_2$ D/C (10.0)<br>→<br>Wound assmt | | →<br>→ | | →<br>Check BM (4.0)<br>→ | | | |
| | | CBC & PLT Chem 7 AM | | | | CBC Chem 7 AM | |
| → | | | | OBR if no BM (4.0) | | | |
| D/C Famotidine<br>Nizatidine 150 mg PO q12hr | | | | | | | |
| → | | D/C PCA Percocet #2 PO q4hr PRN (1.0) | | | | | |
| → | | → | | → | | → | |
| → | | | | | | | |
| | | D/C Epidural (1.0) | | | | | |
| D/C Maalox when NG out | | | | | | | |
| → | | → | | Benadryl 50 mg PO q HS PRN → | | → | |
| → | | → | | | | | |
| | | | | Tylenol 650 mg PO q4hr PRN → | | → | |
| → | | → | | | | | |

Continued

**clinical pathway** *Cystectomy—cont'd*

**ATTENDING: POSTOP LOS 7 DAYS**
**MEDICAL DIAGNOSIS: ICD-9 CODE: 57.7x**
**Patient's/significant other's learning needs are identified and documented on PEP**

| | DATE: CLINIC DAY | INIT | DATE: PREOP DAY | INIT | DATE: DOS | INIT | DATE: POD 1 & 2 | INIT |
|---|---|---|---|---|---|---|---|---|
| DRESSINGS, TUBES/DRAINS | | | Saline lock placed<br>Protocol 1.40<br>Start fluids by 2100<br>TEDS: Apply thigh high at hs preop (2.0) | | NG (1.43) to suction<br>Check dressing with VS. reinforce PRN<br>JP to bulb suction (1.41)<br>If continent voiding diversion<br>• stents to separate bag<br>• irrigate Foley with 30 ml NS q3hr—start in PACU<br>If catheterized continent diversion<br>• irrigate Malecot 30 ml NS q3hr—start in PACU<br>• stents to separate ostomy bags<br>If ileal conduit<br>• stents in ostomy bag | | →<br>Dressing off with wound assmt (3.0)<br>Ostomy supplies to room (5.0)<br>→ | |
| INTERVENTIONS/ TREATMENTS | | | Protocols:<br>1.5 Anxiety<br>Cystectomy POC 2.122 | | Hibiclens 4% bath 0500<br>Turn cough and deep breathe q2hr (10.0)<br>ICS while awake 10 × qhr (10.0)<br>$O_2$ per cannula to keep sats >90<br>Protocol 1.48 (10.0) | | →<br>Wean $O_2$ if sats >90 (10.0) | |
| ACTIVITY | | | As tolerated (6.0) | | Bedrest<br>Turn q2hr while in bed (6.0)<br>1.1 activity intolerance<br>1.103 ADL | | OOB to chair for 20 min × 2 (2.0) (6.0)<br>Walk into hallway POD 2 with assist (2.0) (6.0) | |
| NUTRITION | High-protein diet (7.0) until day of admission, then clear liquids | | Encourage fluids until NPO after midnight (7.0) | | NPO except hard candy (7.0) | | | |
| DISCHARGE PREPARATION | Discuss anticipated discharge plan with patient/family (include transportation | | Assess home situation (SW, RN) with patient/family | | Encourage open communication<br>1.5 Anxiety<br>1.210 Family coping | | Home health inpt visit as indicated (9.0) | |
| EDUCATIONAL ACTIVITIES | Educational material<br>Cystectomy information book given (8.0) | | Preop teaching 3.9<br>Pain management teaching booklet<br>Cystectomy educational plan | | Postop ICS reinforcement (10.0)<br>Review tubes with patient/family<br>Review pain meds (1.0)<br>PEPs 3.12 meds<br>3.21 anticoagulant therapy<br>Urinary diversion<br>Discuss operative outcome, preliminary plan with family (MD, RN)<br>Protocol 1.210 | | Give discharge sheets<br>Review teaching with patient/family | |

| DATE:<br>POD 3 | INIT | DATE:<br>POD 4 | INIT | DATE:<br>POD 5 | INIT | DATE:<br>POD 6 & 7 | INIT |
|---|---|---|---|---|---|---|---|
| D/C NG if + flatus (4.0)<br>→ | | One JP out if drainage <5 ml/8 hr<br>D/C central line as indicated<br>Convert IV to heparin lock<br>→ | | D/C heparin lock as indicated<br>→ | | Staples out<br>D/C JP day 6<br>Stents D/C day of discharge | |
| →<br>D/C $O_2$ (10.0) | | → | | → | | → | |
| Walk in hallway with assist × 2 (2.0) (6.0) | | Walk in hallway × 3 with assist (2.0) (6.0) | | Walk in hallway × 3 with or without assist (2.0) (6.0) | | Walk in hallway × 3 without assist (2.0) (6.0) | |
| IV fluids<br>NPO 8 hr after NG removed<br>Ice chip 30 ml max q1hr (7.0) | | Clear liquids (7.0) | | Reg diet (7.0) | | Reg diet (7.0) | |
| Ostomy supply resource identified (SW, RN) (5.0) | | HHR (NSG) (5.0) | | All discharge orders in MIS (MD)<br>Discharge plan complete, including patient transportation | | Discharge plans validated/ implemented (9.0) | |
| Begin ostomy teaching (ET) (5.0) | | Educational demonstration | | Ostomy care with staff assist<br>• Bag change<br>• Empty bag<br>• Night bag<br>• Patient irrigate with assistance (5.0) | | Patient/family member able to care for ostomy (5.0)<br>MIS med information sheets reviewed (pharmacy, RN)<br>Discharge teaching completed (RN)<br>Patient irrigate with RN observation | |

*Continued*

## clinical pathway *Cystectomy—cont'd*

**ATTENDING: POSTOP LOS 7 DAYS**
**MEDICAL DIAGNOSIS: ICD-9 CODE: 57.7x**
**Patient's/significant other's learning needs are identified and documented on PEP**

| | **Process and discharge outcomes** | |
|---|---|---|
| **Concern** | **Desired outcome** | **Data met/initials** |
| 1.0 Pain management | Verbalizes successful postop pain management | |
| | Ability to describe and manage pain needs | |
| | On discharge verbalizes ability to manage level of pain | |
| | Aware of implications of increased level of pain and who to notify after discharge | |
| 2.0 DVT | Free of all s/s of DVT | |
| | Aware of s/s of DVT and who to notify after discharge | |
| 3.0 Infection | Free of all s/s of infection | |
| | Aware of s/s of infection and who to notify after discharge | |
| 4.0 Bowel function | Bowel elimination maintained/restored to baseline | |
| 5.0 Ostomy care | Patient/family member able to demonstrate care of ostomy/tubes/drains and equipment | |
| | Home health referral completed | |
| 6.0 Mobility | Able to walk around unit 4 × with appropriate assistance on day 5 | |
| 7.0 Nutrition | Return to preop diet without GI distress | |
| | Able to describe high-protein foods | |
| | Able to describe maintaining intake of high-protein foods | |
| 8.0 Support group | Support group contact made available | |
| 9.0 Home health | Teaching communicated to home health agency in writing | |
| | Home health agency contacted | |
| 10.0 Respiratory function | Free of s/s of respiratory complication | |
| | Contact with smoking cessation program | |
| | | |

brought out through the skin, either on the flank or the anterior abdominal wall to create a small stoma. When both ureters are involved, each may be brought out to the skin surface separately, resulting in two stomas, or the ureters may be joined and brought out through the abdominal wall to form only one stoma. Initially after surgery, ureterostomy stomas are pink, but they will turn pale in several weeks. To avoid stenosis of the ureterostomy the ureters should be dilated during surgery. The complications associated with ureterostomy stoma stenosis are inadequate drainage of the kidney, resulting in hydronephrosis, infection, and progressive kidney damage. Urinary tract infection in persons with ureterostomy is common because of reflux of urine from the stoma to the kidney.

During the ileal conduit, ileal loop, or Bricker procedure, the ureters are excised from the bladder and transplanted into one end of a 15- to 20-cm (6- or 8-inch) segment of ileum that has been resected from the intestinal tract with its mesentery, which contains the blood supply. The remaining intestinal segments are anastomosed, and gastrointestinal function is expected to return to its normal preoperative state after healing. The end of the resected ileum into which the ureters

| ALTERED PATHWAY COURSE (note in progress notes) | |
|---|---|
| NOTE | DATE/SIGN |
| | |
| | |
| | |
| | |
| | |
| | |
| | |
| | |
| | |
| | |
| | |
| | |
| | |
| | |
| | |
| | |
| | |

| HOME EQUIPMENT/DISCHARGE | DATE/INITIAL |
|---|---|
| NEEDED: | PROVIDED: |
| Ostomy supplies | |
| If Malecot, irrigation setup | |
| Drain bag supplies | |
| If Foley, drain bag supplies | |
| Medication | |

are connected is sutured closed, and the other end is brought through the abdominal wall to the skin surface to create a stoma (Figure 44-11). The urinary bladder may be resected or left intact, depending on the reason for the diversion. The ileal segment functions as a passageway for urine rather than a reservoir.

The colon conduit (colonic loop) is performed similarly to an ileal conduit except that a segment of colon (ascending, descending, transverse, or sigmoid) instead of ileum acts as the conduit for the urine. The colon conduit has reduced the incidence of urinary reflux for some persons. Preoperative and postoperative nursing care and ongoing management are the same as those for ileal conduit surgery.

The continent urostomy (Kock or Indiana pouch, see Figures 44-9 and 44-10) consists of loops of intestine anastomosed together and then connected to the abdomen via the stomal segment. The anastomosed intestine is separated from the remaining intestine so gastrointestinal function occurs normally. For the Kock pouch, ureters from the kidney are connected to the pouch above a valve. This valve prevents urine from refluxing to the kidney. The urine stays in the reservoir because a second valve is placed in the intestinal

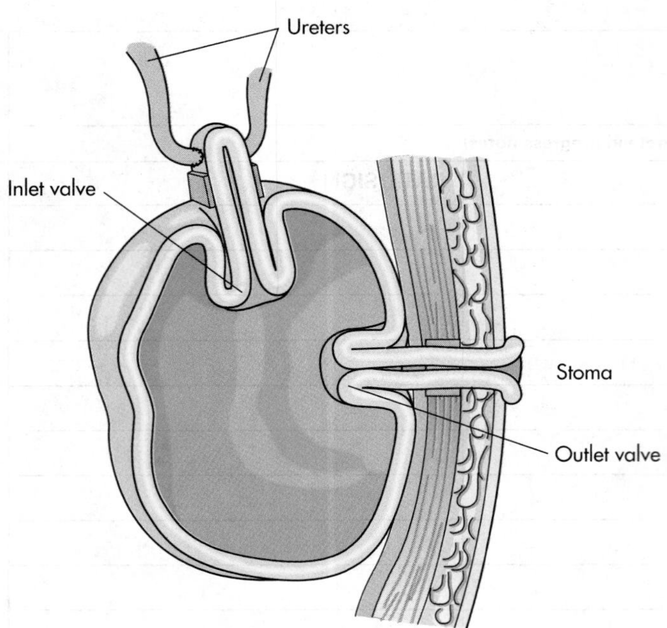


fig. 44-9 Kock continent ileal urinary reservoir.

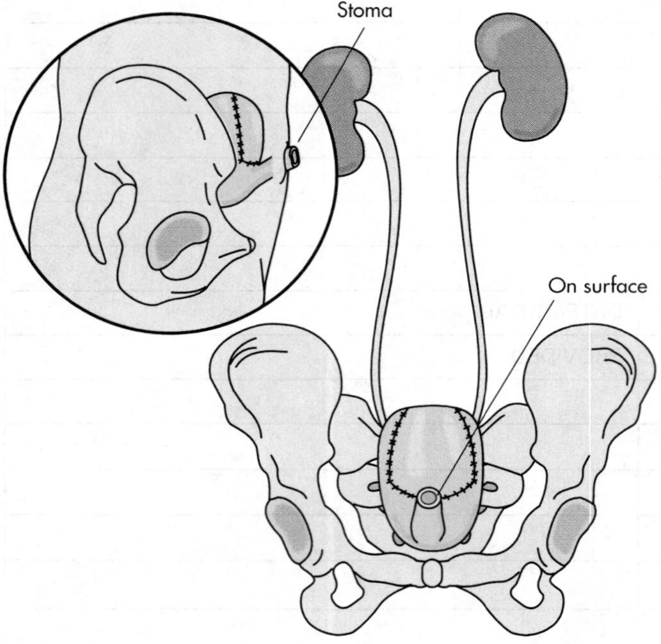


fig. 44-10 Ileocecal continent urinary reservoir (Indiana pouch).

segment leading to the stoma. This valve prevents the leakage of urine, thus maintaining continence.[9] For the ileocecal or Indiana pouch, the ureters are anastomosed to the colon portion of the reservoir in a manner to prevent reflux. The ileocecal valve is used to provide continence, and the section of ileum that extends from the intestinal reservoir to the skin is made narrower (plicated) to prevent urine leakage. The end of the intestinal segment is brought out onto the skin to form the stoma. The stoma for the continent urostomy is usually flush

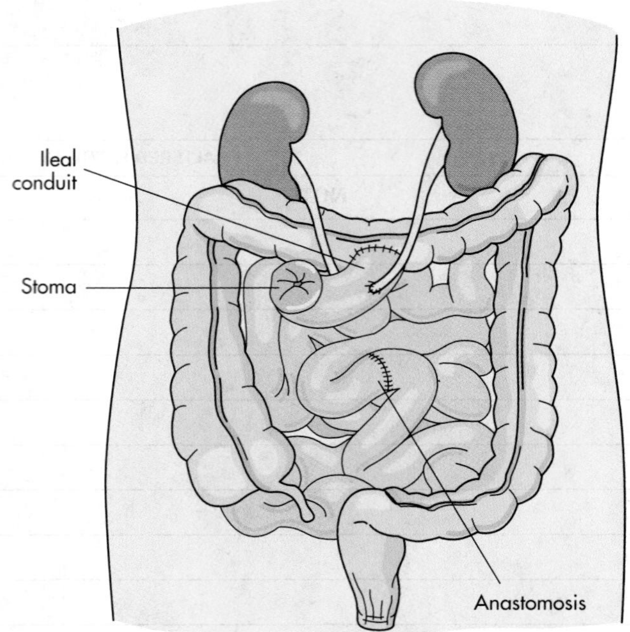


fig. 44-11 Ileal conduit or ileal loop.

to the skin and placed lower on the abdomen than the ileal conduit stoma.

The ileal conduit, colon conduit, and continent urostomy stomas should be a bright-red color. Early complications after surgery include breakdown of the anastomosis in the gastrointestinal tract, leakage from the ureteroileal or ureterosigmoid anastomosis, paralytic ileus, obstruction of the ureters, wound infection, mucocutaneous separation, and stomal necrosis. Complications that may occur after hospitalization include stomal problems (retraction, stenosis, or hernia) and urinary infections.

Any procedure for diversion of urine that results in an external stoma leads to a significant change in body image. Reactions may vary depending on the reason for the procedure, but virtually every person will require time and much nursing support while adapting to the altered means of urine elimination (Research Box).

### Diet

No specific dietary modifications are necessary for the patient with bladder cancer. Anorexia and nausea are problems that need to be addressed. High-caloric supplements are encouraged to prevent wasting. Fluid intake of at least 2 L/day is recommended to avoid dehydration. Substances that irritate the bladder should be avoided, including alcohol, tea, spices, and smoking.

### Activity

There are no specific activity restrictions related to treatment. Activity should be encouraged to promote the patient's well-being and return to activities of daily living.

### Referrals

The care of the patient after radical cystectomy should be approached in a multidisciplinary manner. An enterostomal

**research**

Reference: Raleigh E, Berry M, Monte J: A comparison of adjustments to urinary diversions: a pilot study, *J Wound, Ostomy Incontinence Nurs* 22(1):58-63, 1995.

The purpose of this pilot study was to evaluate patients' adjustment to different types of urinary diversions. A comparison between the traditional ileal conduit and a continent conduit was done. The researchers also evaluated illness-related dysfunction related to the urinary diversion. The patient population consisted of male patients who had undergone urinary diversion 10 to 30 months before the study. An equal number of patients were in each group. One group had the traditional ileal conduit; the other group had the continent conduit. Data were collected by mailing a questionnaire, which included the Sickness Impact Profile (SIP). Both groups reported the degree of illness-related dysfunction, which included incontinence and erectile dysfunction. There were no significant differences in results of the SIP from both groups. Both groups reported erectile dysfunction, but few had sought treatment. The group with the ileal conduit reported a larger dissatisfaction with social interaction. The implications for nursing include the need for support for patients undergoing any urinary diversion procedure and the need for education on the possible long-term complications and alterations on lifestyle that these procedures can generate. The impact on sexual functioning and social interaction needs to be addressed preoperatively. Further research including studies with a larger sample are needed.

therapist should be consulted to provide teaching on pouch and ostomy care. Home care will be involved to provide supplies for pouch care.[7] The American Cancer Society is a resource for all cancer patients and may provide supplies free of charge to patients. Another resource for patients is the United Ostomy Association, which has branches in most major cities. Sexual counseling and information on sperm banking may be indicated for some patients.

## NURSING MANAGEMENT OF THE PATIENT WITH URINARY DIVERSION SURGERY

### PREOPERATIVE CARE

Subjective data should include the patient's thoughts and feelings regarding the urinary diversion. Information on the patient's lifestyle, occupation, and family roles will help the nurse plan appropriate interventions. The patient is prepared preoperatively as for any other surgical procedure (see Chapter 18).

#### Counseling and Teaching

When the physician tells the person of the probable need for a urinary diversion, the first reaction is likely to be disbelief and disappointment. The reason for the surgery may influence the reaction. Time to grieve is essential, and the nurse can be a source of support during this time. Persons who have been well informed about the surgical procedure as well as the postoperative period and long-term management goals are generally better able to adjust to the entire experience than those who do not receive such preparation. When a urinary diversion is contemplated, the patient will have many questions. Accurate honest answers must be given at this time.

A person with a urinary diversion will need time to adjust to the change in body appearance, to the loss of the usual pattern of elimination, to the presence of an external pouch or an internal reservoir, and to the presence of a stoma. An opportunity should be provided for the patient to explore feelings and to begin to cope with all the changes. Postoperative instruction in the care of the stoma is started early; mastering stomal care enhances the person's self-confidence and acceptance of the stoma.

The enterostomal therapy nurse specializes in the care of and instruction to persons who have or will have an ostomy. If possible, a preoperative meeting with the patient and enterostomal therapy nurse should be arranged. In addition to providing information, the enterostomal therapy nurse can select and mark the site for the placement of the stoma. If time permits, a meeting with the patient and a representative from the United Ostomy Association can be arranged. The United Ostomy Association has trained volunteers who have coped well with an ostomy and are willing to visit patients and provide support, reassurance, and personal experiences. A postoperative or home visit can be arranged.

The nurse's goals for preoperative teaching must reflect the patient's needs. However, certain basic information must be included. The patient should understand the surgical procedure and should know whether a pouch will have to be worn postoperatively.

Preoperative instruction also involves preparing the person for the appearance of the stoma. The patient should be told that the stoma will be red, that the tissue is similar to the mucosal lining of the mouth, and that it will not be painful. A simple drawing supplements and clarifies explanations of the surgical procedure. The patient should be given the definition of terms such as *stoma, urostomy,* and *pouch.*

Booklets designed for the person having a urinary diversion may be given to the patient preoperatively. Some persons need this additional information to assist them in accepting the surgery. Others may be unable to review written materials until after surgery.

Finally, a brief description of the management of the urostomy is given. The patient with a ileal or colon conduit is informed of the need to wear the pouch, the frequency of changing and emptying the pouch, and the function of the urinary stoma. Patients undergoing continent urostomy procedures are informed of the need to catheterize the stoma at regular intervals and to irrigate the internal reservoir to remove mucus. Assurance is given that the nurse will provide stoma care immediately after surgery and that the patient will be assisted to master self-care before discharge.

Before an ileal or colon conduit diversion or a continent urostomy diversion, a complete cleansing of the bowel is required. Bowel preparation reduces the possibility of fecal contamination when the bowel is resected and used to form the conduit or internal reservoir. The cleansing routine consists of a low-residue diet for 2 days preoperatively followed by a clear liquid diet for 24 hours before surgery and nothing by mouth after midnight the night before surgery. Large-volume oral bowel cleansing solutions (GoLYTELY or Colyte) or a special laxative and fluid program may be prescribed the day before surgery. Cleansing enemas may be ordered to supplement the clean-out procedure. Intestinal antibiotics such as erythromycin or neomycin may also be administered orally.

Determination of the exact placement for the stoma should be made by the surgeon and/or the enterostomal therapy nurse. The stoma for the ileal conduit is usually constructed on the right side of the abdomen, below the waist, and within the rectus muscle. The continent urostomy stoma is placed lower on the right or left side of the abdomen because a flat surface for a pouch is not needed. Selection of the site is ideally made before surgery and should include evaluation of the proposed site when the patient is lying, sitting, and standing. Since smooth, even skin surrounding the stoma is important for optimal adherence of the pouch, it is important that the site selected is free of scars, skin folds, and bony prominences.

## POSTOPERATIVE CARE

The basic needs of the patient requiring urological surgery are the same as those of any other surgical patient (see Chapter 20). Special emphasis must be placed on promotion of ventilation and adequate urine output, prevention of distention and hemorrhage, and attention to drainage tubes and dressings (Guidelines for Care Box).

After an ileal or colon conduit procedure, stents are usually in place in the stoma for 1 week to 10 days to promote urinary drainage. The person with a continent urostomy will usually have a catheter and/or stents in the stoma sutured in place to allow drainage from the reservoir. A drain tube is placed into the pelvic area for drainage of blood and surgical fluids. The newly created internal reservoir must be protected from overdistention to prevent leakage at the anastomoses.

A nasogastric tube with suction will be used until effective intestinal peristalsis has returned. The nasogastric tube is maintained to prevent pressure on the intestinal anastomosis. The patient may have nothing by mouth until peristalsis returns. IV fluids are given until adequate intake of oral liquids is tolerated. Once peristalsis resumes, clear liquids are started and the diet is advanced gradually.

### Maintaining Skin Integrity

With any type of urinary diversion, care must be taken to prevent urine leakage onto the surrounding skin and abdominal incision. For the ileal or colon conduit, a transparent pouch is placed around the stoma in the operating room. This allows visualization of the stoma, catheter or stents, and stoma sutures. The stoma should be bright pink or red. Any evidence of gray or black discoloration is reported to the surgeon, since this may indicate decreased circulation, which leads to necrosis of the stoma. Careful assessment of the stoma that is in contact with a catheter is imperative because improper positioning of a catheter may exert pressure on the stoma mucosa, leading to necrosis. The pouch is changed within 24 to 48 hours after surgery to allow for better visualization and assessment of the stoma and the peristomal skin.

In the early postoperative period, the pouch is positioned so that it drains to the side of the bed, facilitating drainage and emptying of the pouch. The urostomy pouch has a valve at the bottom that permits emptying. Drain tubing and a collection bag can be attached to the valve of the pouch to allow continuous drainage in the postoperative period (Figure 44-12). The

**guidelines for care**

**The Person After Urological Surgery**

1. Promote ventilation.
   a. Encourage breathing exercises.
   b. Encourage self-turning in bed frequently.
   c. Encourage ambulation.
2. Monitor patency and output of urinary catheters.
3. Prevent complications.
   a. Change wet dressings to protect skin.
   b. Restrict food and oral fluids if bowel sounds are absent.
   c. Encourage fluids to 3000 ml/day when permitted.
   d. Monitor for bright-red blood on dressings or in urine.
4. Administer analgesics to control pain.

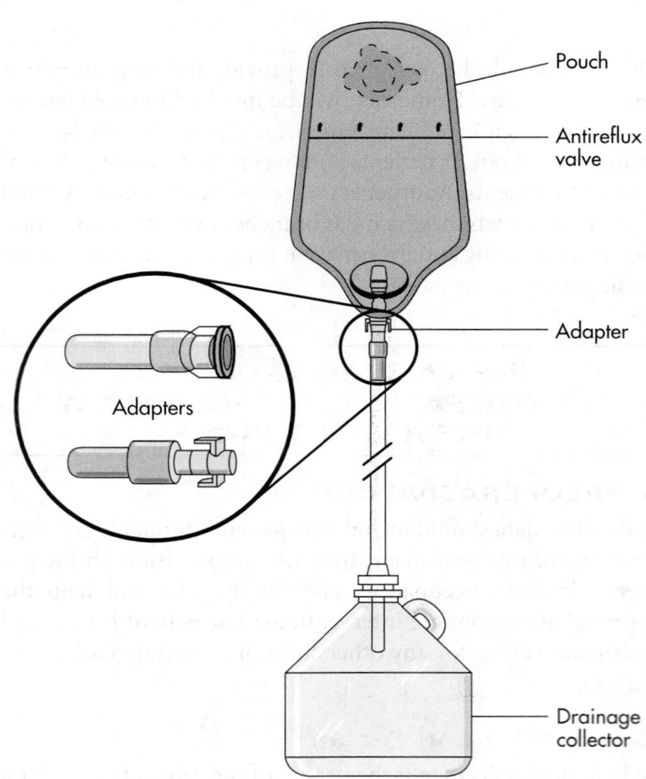


fig. 44-12 Urostomy pouch connected to continuous drainage.

procedure for changing the pouch is outlined in the Guidelines for Care Box.

### Monitoring Urine Output

After any type of urinary diversion, urine output must be carefully monitored. Edema of the stoma or of the ureteral anastomosis site may prevent urine drainage, leading to hydronephrosis or a break in the anastomosis. Other complications that may first be detected by decreased urine output include dehydration, obstruction of the ureters, or compromised renal function.

Decreased urine output is associated with symptoms of peritonitis (fever, abdominal distention, and pain). These symptoms should alert the nurse to the possibility of intraperitoneal leakage caused by a leak at either the intestinal or the ureterointestinal anastomosis. If this occurs, emergency surgery is required to repair the leak.

The color and nature of the urine are also noted. Blood in the urine is expected in the immediate postoperative period with gradual clearing. Mucus, a normal discharge from the intestinal segment, is usually secreted from an ileal or colon conduit or continent urostomy. The abdominal incision is observed *at least daily* for healing of the suture line.

**guidelines for care**

**Changing a Urinary Pouch**

1. Explain procedure to patient, being sure to include sensory information.
2. Assemble all supplies.
3. Empty the pouch and gently remove the pouch from the skin.
4. Cleanse the peristomal skin with mild soap and water. Rinse and pat dry. Wash mucous secretions off the stoma gently.
5. Place a rolled piece of gauze or cotton balls over the stomal opening to absorb draining urine while caring for the skin.
6. Measure the diameter of the stoma, and cut a corresponding opening in the skin barrier and the pouch or select the corresponding size of precut pouch.
7. Apply skin sealant around the stoma if desired. Allow the area to dry completely.
8. Attach the pouch to the skin barrier. The pouch and skin barrier may be applied to the skin separately or together. In the early postoperative period, it is easier to attach the pouch to the skin barrier and then apply the system in one piece to the skin.
9. Apply the pouch and skin barrier around the stoma, keeping the adhesive area free of wrinkles or creases. Press gently but firmly into place. The valve at the bottom of the pouch must be closed or attached to drain tubing and a collection bag.

### Patient/Family Education

Postoperative instruction is started as soon as the patient feels able to participate in urostomy care. During the active phases of teaching, the pouch is removed more often than is recommended after discharge. The patient (or caregiver) should learn how to manage the assembly and apply and empty the selected pouch.

Postoperatively, the edema of the stoma begins to subside within 7 days, but the stoma continues to decrease gradually in size for the next 6 to 8 weeks. Therefore, before discharge, the patient is taught how to measure the stoma and how to adjust the pouch size to accommodate the smaller stoma. Too large an opening can lead to skin problems for persons with an ileal or colon conduit. Too small an opening may restrict circulation or cause trauma to the stoma. The opening should be no more than 2 to 3 mm larger than the stoma.

Several types of pouches are available (Figures 44-13 and 44-14). All have two things in common: a pouch to collect the urine and an outlet or valve at the bottom for easy emptying every 3 to 4 hours. The basic types of pouches are (1) semidisposable pouches that fit onto a permanent disk or faceplate and (2) one-piece or two-piece disposable pouches that are discarded after use. The pouches adhere to the body with a skin barrier to form a watertight seal. The type of pouch selected depends on the patient's preference, body build, and special needs, such as physical or visual impairment. The enterostomal therapy nurse can assist the patient in the assessment and selection of the appropriate pouch.

#### *Health promotion/prevention*

Known factors predisposing to bladder cancer are exposure to the chemicals $\beta$-naphthylamine and xenylamine, infestation with *Schistosoma haematobium,* and cigarette

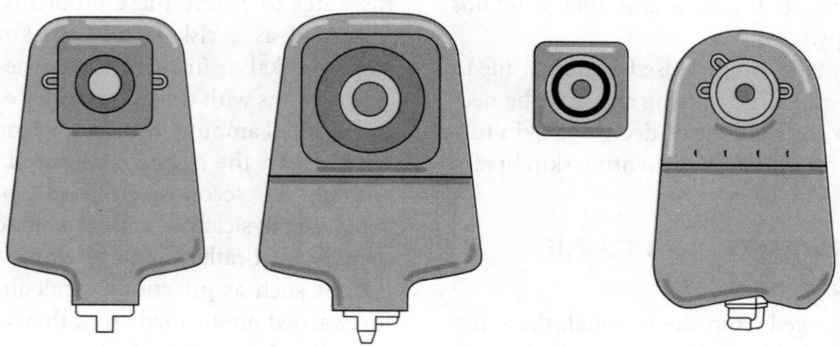

**fig. 44-13** Disposable one- and two-piece pouches.

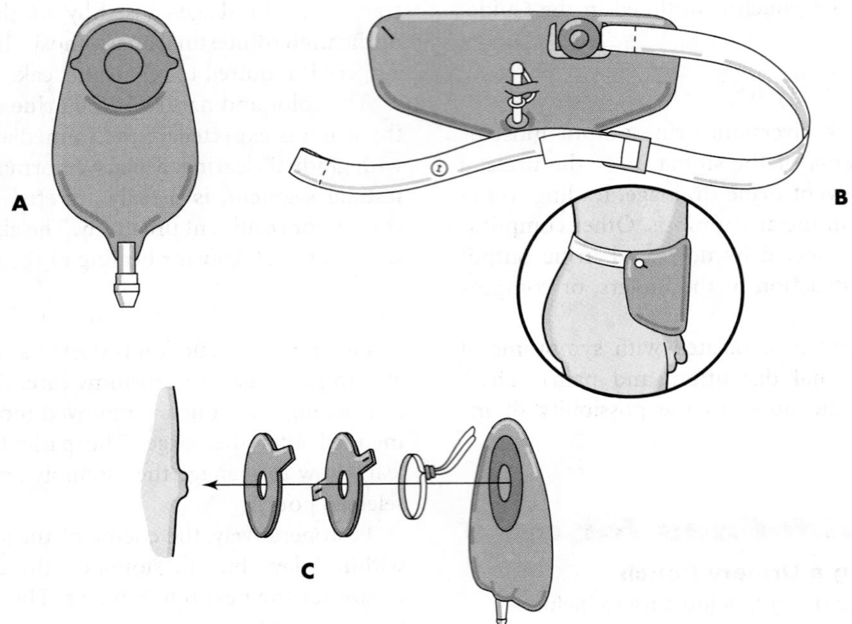


fig. 44-14 Reusable pouches: A, One-piece pouch. B, One-piece nonadhesive pouch. C, Two-piece reusable faceplate and reusable or disposable pouch.

smoking. Therefore, exposure to these substances should be avoided. Smoking is also a risk factor for developing bladder cancer. Smoking cessation programs should be encouraged for all tobacco users.

Most persons can wear a pouch for 3 to 5 days between changes. An interval longer than 7 days should be discouraged because of the risk of infection. An appropriate schedule that eliminates leakage and provides the best skin protection needs to be determined. For example, if the pouch tends to show signs of impending leakage or skin redness on the fifth day, it should be changed every 3 to 4 days—before leakage and skin problems occur. This individualized schedule provides security and prevents skin problems.

## GERONTOLOGICAL CONSIDERATIONS

The older adult is at greater risk for developing cancer of the bladder. The disease is most common in the 50- to 70-year-old age group.[5] Radiation and chemotherapy are not well tolerated by the geriatric patient because of decreases in skin turgor and the inability to tolerate the large amounts of liquids necessary for chemotherapy.

Allowances need to be made for decreased dexterity due to arthritis in the older patient. Home nursing care may be necessary to manage ostomy care. Because of decreased skin turgor, pouches may be difficult to fit and preventing skin breakdown may be a challenge.

## SPECIAL ENVIRONMENTS FOR CARE

### Home Health Management

Before the patient is discharged from the hospital, the nurse must be certain that the individual can manage the urinary drainage and can detect any deviations from normal. A return visit or an opportunity for telephone consultation with the primary nurse involved in the teaching or the enterostomal therapy nurse is extremely helpful. The majority of patients with bladder cancer undergoing urinary diversion will require home nursing care for stoma and pouch maintenance.

## COMPLICATIONS

The person with a urinary diversion is at greater risk for UTI because of the shorter distance from the urinary diversion to the kidneys. The patient must be taught the signs and symptoms of UTI (cloudy urine, blood in urine, strong odor to urine, flank pain, fever, and malaise). Urine cultures are correctly obtained by catheter from the ileal or colon conduit stoma. A specimen taken from the pouch is likely to be contaminated. A pouch with an antireflux valve is recommended to reduce infection from bacteria found in the pouch.

Problems with the peristomal skin include erythema and irritation from contact with urine, candidal infections, allergic dermatitis, and pseudoverrucous lesions. Table 44-12 lists measures to relieve these problems. Urine pH has also been identified as a risk factor for skin breakdown around the stoma.[5] Alkaline urine increases the risk of hyperkeratosis.[11]

Problems with the stoma include bleeding, stenosis, or hernia. A small amount of bleeding from the stomal mucosa may occur when the stoma is cleansed. Bleeding generally stops within a few seconds. If bleeding persists or is unusually severe, the physician is notified. Blood that originates from the urinary tract rather than the stoma may be related to complications such as infection or calculi. Patients also need to be forewarned about medicines that will discolor the urine; for example, doxorubicin (Adriamycin) will produce red urine. Peristomal hernia is treated by surgery; however, some pa-

**table 44-12** *Peristomal Skin Problems*

| PROBLEM | DESCRIPTION | THERAPY |
|---|---|---|
| Erythema | Redness from contact with urine | Correct pouch opening for better fit around stoma. Change pouch system if leakage occurs. |
| Candidal infection | Red rash surrounding stoma | Administer antifungal powder. |
| Allergic skin reaction | Redness, weeping | Change pouch system. Eliminate offending products. If severe, refer patient to dermatologist. |
| Pseudoverrucous lesions | Raised, painful, wartlike areas next to stoma | Cover exposed skin by recalibrating stomal opening. Protect affected skin area. |

Modified from Hampton BG, Bryant RA: *Ostomies and continent diversions,* St Louis, 1992, Mosby.

tients may elect not to have the hernia repaired. The pouch opening may need to be adjusted or enlarged to accommodate the stoma.

Electrolyte imbalance may develop if the urine is retained in the conduit because of stomal or loop stenosis. The conduit mucosa reabsorbs chloride from the urine, and the patient may develop a metabolic hyperchloremic acidosis. A person with optimal renal function has no difficulty excreting the reabsorbed chloride. When renal function is compromised, the patient is more likely to develop electrolyte problems. This reabsorption can also occur in those with internal reservoirs because the urine is retained within the internal pouch until the stoma is catheterized and the urine drained.[11] Follow-up urological care visits and electrolyte studies are imperative.

## TRAUMA TO THE URINARY TRACT

Assessing the integrity of the urinary tract must be part of the evaluation of any person with traumatic injury to the lower trunk. Injuries particularly related to the urinary tract damage include fractures of the pelvis, penetrating blows to the body, and blunt trauma.

### ETIOLOGY/EPIDEMIOLOGY

Pelvic fractures may result in bladder perforation and urethral tearing. A sharp blow to the body, particularly to the lower back, may result in contusion, tearing, or rupture of a kidney (Figure 44-15).

### PATHOPHYSIOLOGY

Urine output may be scant or absent after trauma to the urinary tract. Urine, if present, may be bloody, and symptoms of peritonitis may appear. The first symptoms of trauma to the kidney usually are hematuria and pain or tenderness of the upper abdominal quadrant and flank on the involved side. Signs of shock may be present if hemorrhage is extensive.

Diagnostic tests used to facilitate diagnosis of trauma to the urinary tract include KUB, cystogram, IVP, renal angiography, and CT scan. Laboratory tests include serial urinalysis and hemoglobin, BUN, and creatinine levels.

### COLLABORATIVE CARE MANAGEMENT

Treatment of injuries is focused on stabilizing the patient and surgically repairing any perforations or lacerations of the urinary tract. Initial treatment includes controlling bleeding, preventing shock, and promoting urinary drainage. A cystotomy may be performed to provide urinary drainage when injuries involve the bladder or urethra. Vital signs, fluid balance records, and hematocrit levels are monitored to assess bleeding. Complaints of pain may indicate ureteral colic, signifying obstruction of the ureter by a clot. Surgery is required to control severe hemorrhage; otherwise the kidney is allowed to heal spontaneously. Bedrest is maintained until gross hematuria resolves; thereafter, activity progresses according to tolerance and absence of hematuria.

When urethral injuries are suspected, great care must be taken when inserting urinary catheters to prevent further urethral injury. A urologist may need to insert the catheter during a retrograde urethrogram or cystogram (see Chapter 43).

A kidney may become loosened and "float" or become displaced *(nephroptosis).* If symptoms of obstruction occur, the kidney may be sutured to its anatomical site *(nephropexy).* Postoperatively the patient's hips are elevated to prevent tension on the suture line.

Nephrectomy may be indicated depending on the severity of the trauma. Adequate waste removal can be maintained by the remaining kidney or by less than half of one functioning kidney.

#### *Patient/family education*

Education for the patient with renal trauma focuses on treatment and surgical management. Much of the patient's concern depends on the type of surgery and cause of the trauma. Because the surgery will temporarily or permanently alter urinary elimination, the person will be concerned about the degree of change that will occur. Care of the person following nephrectomy is similar to that for persons with abdominal or urinary diversion procedures (see Chapter 41 and p. 1446-1448).

Trauma to the kidney is often associated with blunt trauma suffered as a result of motor vehicle accidents, contact sports, and falls. Teaching should include preventive strategies such as wearing a seat belt when in an automobile, following safety rules when riding a bicycle or walking, and wearing protective equipment when participating in contact sports. Persons with one kidney should be cautioned regarding participation in contact sports.

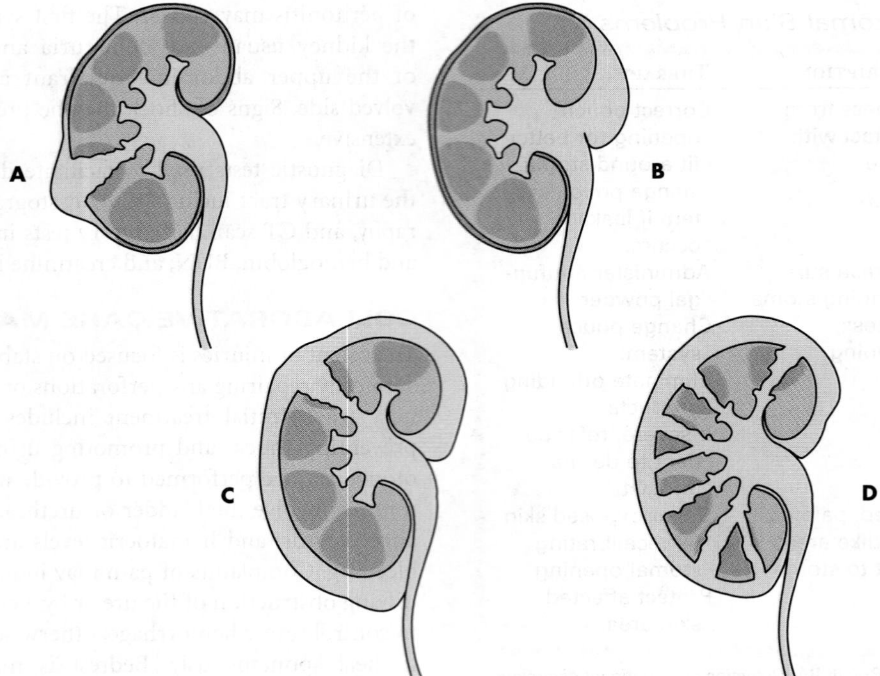


**fig. 44-15** Four degrees of renal trauma. **A,** Urine is extravasating from split in renal parenchyma but confined under renal capsule. **B,** Urine is extravasating through tear in renal pelvis. **C,** Urine is extravasating through rent in kidney and capsule and surrounds kidney and renal pelvis. **D,** Kidney is shattered, and urine is extravasating in all areas.

## URINARY RETENTION

Urinary retention is the inability to empty the bladder. The kidneys are producing sufficient urine, but the person is unable to expel the urine from the bladder.

### ETIOLOGY

Causes of urinary retention are either mechanical or functional. Mechanical causes may be congenital or acquired and include anatomic blockage of urine flow in the lower urinary tract. Functional causes include impairment of urine flow in the absence of mechanical obstruction. Box 44-6 summarizes causes of urinary retention.

### EPIDEMIOLOGY

The incidence of urinary retention is unknown. Because of the multifactorial etiology of urinary retention, it is difficult to predict the frequency of occurrence.

### PATHOPHYSIOLOGY

An inability to void results from blockage of the urethra. The end result and primary feature of urinary retention is inability to void. The bladder becomes distended with urine and is sometimes displaced to either side of the midline. Percussion over a full bladder produces a "kettle drum" sound. Discomfort occurs from pressure of the bladder on other organs, and the person has an urge to urinate. Restlessness and diaphoresis also may occur with a full bladder.

Voiding 25 to 50 ml of urine at frequent intervals often indicates retention with overflow. The intravesicular pressure increases as the bladder continues to fill with urine. As the bladder overfills, the restraining capability of the sphincter is taxed. A small amount of urine flows out of the bladder to reduce the intravesicular pressure to the level where the sphincter can control the flow of urine once again. The patient may state that the bladder continues to feel full. As the bladder fills again, the cycle is repeated. The urine specific gravity is nor-

**box 44-6** *Causes of Urinary Retention*

**MECHANICAL CAUSES**

**Congenital**
- Urethral stricture
- Urinary tract malformation
- Spinal cord malformation

**Acquired**
- Calculus
- Inflammation
- Trauma
- Tumor
- Hyperplasia
- Pregnancy

**FUNCTIONAL CAUSES**
- Neurogenic bladder dysfunction
- Ureterovesical reflux
- Decreased peristaltic activity of the ureter
- Detrusor muscle atrophy
- Anxiety, i.e., fear of pain after surgery
- Medications, i.e., anesthetics, narcotics, sedatives, and antihistamines

mal or high in the presence of retention with overflow because the kidney's ability to produce urine is not impaired.

## COLLABORATIVE CARE MANAGEMENT

Urinary retention is a urological emergency and, if untreated, can lead to kidney damage. Interventions for urinary retention are aimed at reestablishing urine flow.

### Diagnostic Tests

The diagnosis of urinary retention is based on determining the amount of residual urine after voiding attempts. Urine yield of 250 to 300 ml after catheterization is indicative of retention. Post-void residual should be less than 25% the person's total bladder capacity. To avoid the risk of urinary tract infection with catheterization, bladder scans are being used at the bedside. Bladder scans are similar to ultrasound technology. With this device, the amount of urine remaining in the bladder after voiding can be determined by noninvasive measures.[17] Cystoscopy is performed if obstruction is suspected.

### Medications

Medication use in urinary retention is determined by the etiology. Retention due to sensory/neurological problems may be treated with cholinergic medications. This group of medications stimulate bladder contraction and should not be used if obstruction is suspected. Bethanecol chloride (Urecholine) may be prescribed to initiate voiding by stimulating the detrusor muscle of the bladder. Retention from prostate enlargement is discussed in Chapter 49.

### Treatments

#### *Direct bladder drainage: cystostomy tube*

When obstruction occurs below the bladder, continuous drainage must be provided to prevent damage to the kidney. One means of providing drainage is by the use of a *cystostomy* tube (usually a Foley, Malecot, or Pezzar catheter), which is placed directly into the bladder through a suprapubic incision. This method is usually used when the urethra is completely obstructed or when the prolonged use of a urethral catheter is contraindicated. During surgery, a cystostomy tube and a small urethral catheter will be inserted to drain the bladder. Both catheters must be monitored for patency. Once patency is assured, it is not necessary to record the output from each catheter separately, since both tubes drain the bladder. The catheters will not necessarily drain equal amounts of urine. Securely anchoring these catheters is necessary to prevent them from slipping out of position.

### Surgical Management

#### *Drainage of kidney, pelvis, and ureters*

If a ureter becomes obstructed, a catheter must be placed directly into the renal pelvis. This prevents kidney damage that otherwise would occur as pressure increases because of continued urine formation. When a ureter is completely obstructed, a *nephrostomy* or *pyelostomy* tube may be inserted (surgically or under guidance of a radiologist) into the renal pelvis (Figure 44-16). The surgical incision is located laterally and posteriorly in the kidney region. Catheters used as nephrostomy or pyelostomy tubes are usually of the Pezzar (mushroom) or Malecot (batwing) types. An alternate form of drainage for a ureteral obstruction is the surgical placement of a ureterostomy tube (a whistle-tip or multi-eyed Robinson catheter, size 6F or 8F) passed through an incision in the upper outer quadrant of the abdomen into the ureter above the obstruction. The catheter is then passed through the ureter to the renal pelvis.

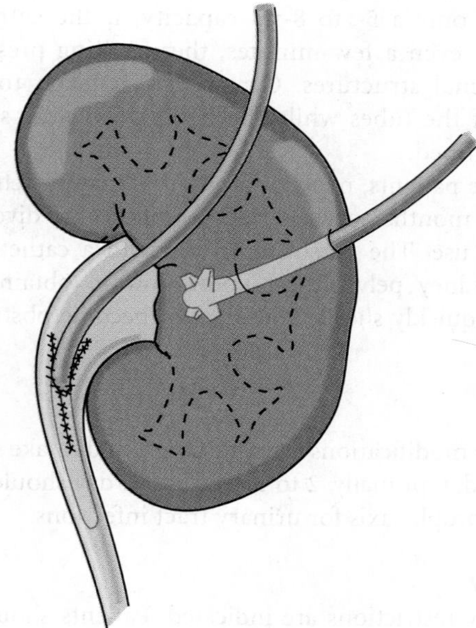

**fig. 44-16** Placement of stent after repair of ureteropelvic stricture. Note use of nephrostomy tube for urinary drainage during healing of anastomosis.

If the ureter is unobstructed or partially obstructed, the renal pelvis may be drained by a ureteral catheter, which is passed up the ureter to the renal pelvis through a cystoscope. Ureteral catheterization is performed before gynecological and lower abdominal surgery when there is danger of not recognizing and accidentally injuring the ureter during the operation. Ureteral catheterization is also used after surgery involving the ureters to prevent stricture as the ureter heals. When used for this purpose, the catheter is referred to as a *stent* (Figure 44-16). Whether it is expected to drain urine will depend on its relation to other catheters used.

The nephrostomy and ureteral catheters must be firmly anchored to prevent accidental dislodging and trauma to the tissues. The openings made for these tubes are essentially fistulas that rapidly decrease in size on removal of the catheter. Even 30 minutes after removal of this type of catheter, it is often impossible to reinsert a similar-sized tube. When a catheter is inserted during surgery, it is usually sutured in place and affixed to the skin. When not sutured in place, the tube should be anchored to the skin at two points using adhesive, with some slack in the tubing between the anchor points.

Unobstructed drainage of catheters leading to the renal pelvis is of the utmost importance. The normal renal pelvis has only a 5- to 8-ml capacity; if the catheter obstructs for even a few minutes, the resulting pressure can damage renal structures. Care must be taken to prevent kinking of the tubes while the patient is in the side-lying position in bed.

In some patients, nephrostomy tubes may be left in place for several months, serving as a form of urinary diversion for long-term use. The person at home with a catheter draining the kidney pelvis must know how to obtain medical assistance quickly should the catheter become obstructed or dislodged.

### Diet

No dietary modifications are necessary. Fluid intake should be encouraged. Optimally, 2 to 3 L of liquid/day should be consumed as prophylaxis for urinary tract infections.

### Activity

No activity restrictions are indicated. Patients should be instructed not to obstruct the tubing if a nephrostomy is in place. Patients should also keep drainage bags empty during activity to avoid strain on the drainage tubes.

### Referrals

Home health care support may be necessary for intermittent catheterization. Additionally, an enterostomal therapist may be needed to manage nephrostomy sites and prevent skin breakdown. Community resources include the United Ostomy Association and the American Urological Association.

# NURSING MANAGEMENT

## ASSESSMENT

Persons experiencing urinary retention may be unable to void any urine (retention) or may void small amounts of overflow urine but be unable to empty the bladder completely (retention with overflow). Urine remaining in the bladder is a good medium for bacterial growth, leading to UTI.

### Subjective Data

Data to be collected to assess the person with urinary retention include:

- Voiding pattern
- Pain or burning on urination (probable UTI)
- Sense of need to void or bladder fullness immediately after voiding (retention with overflow)

### Objective Data

Data to be collected to assess the person with urinary retention include:

- Frequency of voiding and volume of each void
- Characteristics of urine (color, clarity, and odor)
- Palpation of bladder above symphysis pubis after voiding
- Comparison of fluid intake versus output

## NURSING DIAGNOSES

Nursing diagnoses are determined from analysis of patient data. Nursing diagnoses for the person with urinary retention may include but are not limited to:

| Diagnostic Title | Possible Etiological Factors |
|---|---|
| Urinary retention | Obstruction, position for voiding, immobility, inability to initiate stream |
| Infection, risk for | Indwelling catheter |
| Knowledge deficit | Lack of exposure/recall |

## EXPECTED PATIENT OUTCOMES

Expected patient outcomes for the person with urinary retention may include but are not limited to:

1a. Voids several times a day in adequate amounts.
 b. States that bladder feels empty.
 c. Does nor have a palpable bladder after voiding.
2a. No signs of UTI are present.
 b. Catheter drains freely, if in place.
3a. Describes signs of retention or UTI (for indwelling catheter).
 b. Describes need to maintain fluid intake.

## INTERVENTIONS

### Promoting Micturition

Before catheterization, noninvasive measures are attempted to stimulate voiding of urine. These measures may include assuming a position that facilitates voiding (positional stimuli: male standing upright; female sitting upright), running water (auditory stimuli), or pouring water over the perineum or placing the patient's hands in water (tactile stimuli). Sitting in lukewarm water may help relax the urinary sphincters. Providing privacy and encouraging use of the bathroom whenever possible also help to promote voiding. The patient can be taught to "double void" to promote complete bladder emptying. After voiding, the patient attempts a second void 5 minutes later to completely empty the bladder.

### Facilitating Assisted Urinary Drainage/Preventing Infection

Urinary catheterization is used in a variety of clinical situations in both acute and chronic care. Major reasons for catheter drainage are to:

1. Relieve temporary anatomic or physiological obstruction.
2. Permit healing of the urinary system postoperatively.
3. Permit accurate measurement of urine output in severely ill patients.
4. Relieve inability to void.
5. Achieve continence.
6. Prevent retention of urine in persons with neurogenic bladder.
7. Permit irrigation to prevent obstruction or urine flow.

Reestablishing urine flow is an immediate treatment goal for obstruction. The type of catheter used to provide drainage in the presence of obstruction will depend on the location of the blockage. Table 44-13 summarizes the use of specific types of catheters.

### Urethral Drainage

Urethral catheterization is the most common means of draining the bladder. The Foley catheter is most frequently used for this purpose. *Catheterization is the major cause of UTIs,* and strict asepsis must be practiced during insertion and in assembling the drainage equipment. The need for urethral catheterization must be carefully evaluated and should never be undertaken for nursing convenience.

If the nurse finds it difficult to insert the catheter, the procedure is discontinued and the physician is notified. Traumatic catheterization predisposes the patient to UTIs, formation of urethral strictures, and bleeding. In patients who have urethral disorders, resistance may be encountered with a standard catheter; special equipment, such as catheter directors or filiform catheters, may be needed. Catheterization after urological surgery and the use of specialized catheter equipment are not nursing procedures.

The urethral catheter is changed when it is in danger of becoming obstructed by sediment within its lumen. Before discharge, the person going home with an indwelling urethral catheter needs to learn to change the catheter or have a family member demonstrate the ability to insert a catheter.

### Intermittent Catheter Drainage

Intermittent catheterization of the urinary bladder is used in the treatment of neurogenic bladder dysfunction secondary to spinal cord trauma, birth defects, urinary retention, and some chronic diseases.

Periodic complete emptying of the bladder eliminates residual urine (an excellent culture medium for bacteria) and maintains a good blood supply to the bladder wall by avoiding high intrabladder pressures.

Individuals are evaluated for the appropriateness of this form of management by the urologist. The potential for success should be evaluated, using input from the nurse, psychologist, social worker, and other involved health care professionals. Teaching, however, is generally a nursing responsibility. An individual catheterization regimen is planned using either clean or sterile technique as appropriate. The goals of intermittent catheterization are generally to prevent urinary retention and its sequelae (UTI and kidney damage) and to achieve continence. The patient needs to know the expectations of the treatment plan to promote cooperation.

Even though the clean technique is suitable for home use, sterile technique is necessary during hospitalization to decrease the possibility of hospital-acquired infection. When hospitalized, the patient who customarily performs self-catheterization may continue to use clean technique, but preferably a sterile catheter will be used each time. Specimens for culture must be obtained by the usual sterile catheterization technique to avoid contamination of the specimen. The patient is informed why sterile precautions are necessary in the hospital setting.

A size 14F catheter is generally used for an adult. A special silicone catheter without a balloon is used for intermittent catheterization. The volume of urine obtained with each catheterization is recorded so the catheterization schedule can be adjusted as needed. The adult bladder should not be permitted to hold more than 300 ml to 500 ml at any time, since greater amounts lead to overdistention of the bladder and increased susceptibility to infection. The frequency of catheterization is determined by the amount of residual urine.

After voiding, the patient performs self-catheterization to determine the amount of residual urine. A large amount of residual urine (>100 ml) indicates the need for more frequent catheterization. Self-catheterization is usually done every 4 to 6 hours, depending on the patient's schedule and fluid intake. Catheterization is rarely required during the night with the exception being the patient receiving IV fluids.

#### Patient/family education

The person needs to understand the rationale for intermittent catheter drainage and for regularity of bladder emptying (Patient/Family Teaching Box). Basic anatomy of the genitalia and urinary tract should be illustrated for the patient to alleviate fears of causing damage by misplacement of the catheter.

Most persons require much support during the actual teaching but usually become comfortable with the procedure. Initially, a mirror is used to teach women where to place the catheter. The woman should learn to catheterize while sitting on the commode, using palpation to locate the urethral meatus. Men may sit or stand for self-catheterization. It is important that men use generous amounts of lubricant to avoid urethral irritation; women generally do not require lubrication. Family members may be taught catheterization if the patient is unable to perform self-catheterization. Clean technique has been shown to be effective in home use (see the Research Box).

**table 44-13** *Types of Catheters*

| Type of Catheter | Description | Use |
|---|---|---|
| Whistle-tip | Open slant end | Hematuria or blood clots in urine |
| Robinson | Closed end, multiple lumen | Intermittent catheterization |
| Foley | Balloon (5 or 30 ml) to secure catheter in bladder | Constant drainage |
| Coudé | Tapered curved end | Suspected prostatic hypertrophy |
| Ureteral | 4F to 6F size (urethral catheters are usually 14F to 16F) | Drain ureters |
| Malecot | Batwing-shaped tip | Drain renal pelvis, nephrostomy drainage |
| Pezzar | Mushroom-shaped tip | Drain renal pelvis, nephrostomy drainage |

## patient/family teaching

### The Person with Intermittent Catheterization

The patient or family can:

1. Explain the need for adequate fluid intake, approximately 30 ml/kg of body weight.
2. Explain the reason for the intermittent catheter drainage.
3. State the need for regular, periodic, complete emptying of the bladder.
4. Demonstrate self-catheterization using clean technique unless sterile technique is prescribed.
5. Describe how to adapt the catheterization routine to the individual lifestyle.
6. State how to obtain needed supplies.
7. Describe symptoms of UTI requiring medical care.
8. State plans for ongoing urological care.

## research

Reference: Duffy L et al: Clean intermittent catheterization: safe, cost-effective bladder management for male residents of VA nursing homes, *J Am Geriatr Soc* 43(8):865-878, 1995.

The purpose of this study was to determine the incidence of urinary tract infection in male patients undergoing intermittent urinary catheterization. The sample consisted of 80 male residents of three VA long-term care facilities. The sample was randomly divided into two groups. One group was taught self-catheterization using clean technique. The second group was catheterized by the nursing staff using sterile technique. Blood and urine samples were analyzed at predetermined points. All incidences of urinary tract infections were also documented. No significant differences were found between the two groups in the number of infections, the amount of time elapsing before the first infection, or the types of organisms cultured. There was a significant difference in cost in terms of supplies and nursing time in the sterile catheterization group. The implication for nursing is that teaching self-catheterization to hospitalized patients is a cost-effective and safe bladder management technique for some patients. Clean technique is a reasonable, cost-effective alternative to traditional sterile intermittent catheterization procedures.

For the patient with an indwelling catheter, instruction on catheter maintenance should be reviewed. For home care, the person or care provider must be helped to understand the importance of cleanliness of the catheter and genitalia. Instructions should include the following:

- Good hand washing before and after working with the catheter
- Twice-daily cleansing of the meatal-catheter junction with soap and water
- Minimizing disconnection of the catheter and drainage tubing

The tubing is disconnected at night to change from a leg bag to the overnight drainage bag and again in the morning to resume leg-bag drainage. The drainage bag should hold at least 2000 ml for overnight collection. To lessen contamination, the caregiver is taught to wash the hands and then wipe the catheter and tubing with 70% alcohol before disconnection and reconnection. The disconnected ends of the drainage bags are protected with sterile gauze secured in place with a rubber band or protected with a connector cap. The drainage system should be kept as clean as possible by daily washing with soap and water. Teaching also includes the need to keep the drainage collection bag at a level lower than the cavity being drained to prevent urine reflux.

Persons requiring catheter drainage at home on a temporary or permanent basis must be able to safely maintain the urinary drainage system. A family member is instructed in all necessary care in case the patient is unable to perform care. Written instructions are provided. Teaching includes care of the catheter and drainage system as previously described. A written list of needed specific supplies and where they can be obtained is helpful to avoid confusion.

The person needs to be well informed about adaptations that can be made with the urinary drainage system to allow a return to an optimal level of activity. A shower or tub bath with a catheter in place is generally permitted unless there is an unhealed surgical incision. The adhesive tape holding the catheter in place needs to be replaced after bathing. Leg bags are available in a variety of sizes and are concealed by clothing. Men or women do not need to remove an indwelling catheter before intercourse. This information should be included in all teaching because patients may hesitate to ask. The man can fold the indwelling catheter over the penis to facilitate insertion during intercourse.

The person with a urinary catheter of any type needs follow-up medical care. Instructions include the need to contact the physician if back pain, fever, or other urinary tract symptoms are present. Educating the patient about signs and symptoms of urinary retention, changes in the color and clarity of the urine, and incontinence and dysuria is undertaken when bladder drainage is discontinued. Often the first indicators of dysfunction are subjective comments from the patient. This information enhances detection of early recurrence of urinary drainage problems.

## EVALUATION

To evaluate the effectiveness of nursing interventions, compare patient behaviors with those stated in the expected patient outcomes. Successful achievement of patient outcomes for the patient with urinary retention is indicated by:

1a. Voids several times a day in amounts of 150 to 400 ml/void.
 b. Bladder is not palpable after voiding.
2. Has no signs of UTI (fever, back pain, or increased serum WBC count). If catheter is in place, it drains freely.
3a. Describes signs of urinary retention or UTI (for indwelling catheter) to be reported to physician.
 b. Describes need to maintain fluid intake of 2000 to 2500 ml/day.

## GERONTOLOGICAL CONSIDERATIONS

Older patients are more at risk for urinary retention because of decreased bladder tone and increased incidence of chronic disease. Structural changes in bladder muscle tone and prostatic enlargement in men play a key role. Although treatment options remain the same, the geriatric patient must be fully evaluated regarding the ability to take part in treatment plans. Because of decreases in dexterity and sensory function, such as eyesight, catheterization and catheter care may be difficult.

## SPECIAL ENVIRONMENTS FOR CARE

### Home Care Management

Clean (not sterile) catheterization technique usually is prescribed for home use. Hand washing is required before each catheterization, and the meatal area is cleansed with soap and water. After the catheter is inserted and the bladder is drained, the catheter is removed, washed with soap and water, and dried on a clean surface. Once dry, the catheter is stored in a closed container for the next use. The catheter is reused until it becomes either too soft or too hard to be directed properly.

If sterile catheterization technique is needed for home use, careful explanation of sterile technique and sterilization of equipment must be given. More time is needed for the person to learn sterile technique.

If the hospital or outpatient teaching time is short, follow-up may be required by a home health care nurse to help the person adapt the catheterization routine to life routines and to assist with any difficulties the patient may be having. Ongoing urological care is essential, with periodic urine cultures.

## COMPLICATIONS

Complications from treatment of urinary retention are related to catheterization. It is normal to note some dribbling of urine for a few hours after a urethral catheter has been removed because of dilation of the sphincter muscles by the catheter. Dribbling of urine that persists longer than a few hours should be reported to the physician; this symptom may indicate damage to the sphincters. In determining the type of intervention necessary to reestablish bladder control, information about the nature of the incontinence is gathered. Incontinence is described as complete (constant dribbling) or occurring only on urgency or stress. Assessment should include whether incontinence is present in all positions (lying, sitting, and standing). If muscular weakness of the sphincters is the major problem, incontinence is least likely to occur when the person is in a prone position and most likely to be a problem when the person is standing or walking. Perineal exercises (p. 1462) may help to regain control of voiding.

Another problem that may arise after removal of a catheter is inability to void. The patient is encouraged to drink fluids and then attempt to void. The nurse carefully assesses the patient's bladder for distention. Efforts are made to provide comfortable positioning and privacy to facilitate voiding. A patient with adequate fluid intake should void within 8 hours. Patients with edema of the bladder neck may require temporary catheter reinsertion to facilitate urinary drainage.

*Cystitis* (inflammation of the bladder) may develop after catheter removal because of incomplete emptying of the bladder as muscle tone is being reestablished. Any abnormalities in color, odor, or sediment in the urine are reported.

# URINARY INCONTINENCE

## ETIOLOGY

Urinary incontinence is the involuntary unpredictable expulsion of urine from the bladder and is encountered in several temporary and permanent conditions (Table 44-14). *Functional incontinence* results from a variety of factors including urinary tract dysfunction, environmental causes (no toilet facilities), and locomotor and cognitive factors. Causes include pathological, anatomical, or physiological factors affecting the urinary tract, as well as external factors. Many of these factors are reversible, such as infection, atrophic vaginitis, acute confusional states, restrictions in mobility, fecal impaction, medical conditions that cause polyuria or nocturia, and drug side effects. Inability to control urination is a problem that frequently leads to emotional distress and can seriously impair a person's social activities. Incontinence must be managed in a way that makes the person feel both physically and emotionally comfortable and socially acceptable.[9]

Three distinct types of urinary incontinence are described in the literature. The exact pattern of incontinence may vary among patients; however, incontinence can be categorized into one of these three types: stress, urge, or overflow.

*Stress incontinence* occurs as a result of incompetence of the bladder outlet or urethral closure. The patient experiences a loss of 50 ml or less of urine as a result of increased abdominal pressure. Because of this incompetence, any activity leading to an increase in intraabdominal pressure on the bladder can result in urinary incontinence. Activities leading to stress incontinence include lifting, exercising, coughing, sneezing, or laughing.

*Urge incontinence* is the involuntary loss of urine associated with an abrupt and strong desire to void (urgency). *Motor urge incontinence* is caused by detrusor muscle instability; *sensory urge incontinence* is caused by hypersensitivity of the bladder. The incontinence occurs as a result of uninhibited detrusor contractions. When active detrusor contractions overcome urethral resistance, urine leakage occurs. This type of incontinence is seen in patients with multiple sclerosis or after a cerebrovascular accident (stroke).

Involuntary loss of urine associated with overdistention of the bladder is called *overflow incontinence.* It may have a variety of presentations, including frequent or constant dribbling or have urge or stress incontinence symptoms. Overflow incontinence can result from spinal cord injury, stroke, or diabetic neuropathy or after radical pelvic surgery.

## EPIDEMIOLOGY

More than 10 million Americans have urinary incontinence. It is estimated that more than $10 billion a year are spent in managing patients with incontinence. As the U.S. population continues to age, the incidence of incontinence will increase. For noninstitutionalized persons older than 60 years, the incidence ranges from 15% to 30%, with women having twice the

**table 44-14** *Major Causes of Urinary Incontinence*

| Cause of Urinary Incontinence | Factors Involved | | | | |
|---|---|---|---|---|---|
| | Awareness of Need to Void | Cortical Ability to Inhibit Voiding | Reflex Arc | Bladder Response to Filling | Result |
| Cerebral clouding | Impaired | Impaired | Intact | Normal | Uncontrolled voiding because of reflex response |
| Infection | Intact | Intact, but overcome by strong reflex response | Abnormally stimulated | Heightened | Voiding because of strong reflex response (urgency) |
| Disturbance of central nervous system pathways (cortical lesions) | Diminished | Impaired | Intact | Heightened | Voiding because of reflex response |
| Disturbance of urethrobladder reflex | | | | | |
| Upper motor neuron lesion | Destroyed | Destroyed | Intact but deranged | Heightened | Voiding because of reflex response |
| Lower motor neuron lesion | Destroyed | Destroyed | Destroyed or impaired | Diminished to absent | Distention or incomplete emptying |
| Tissue damage | Intact | Intact, but not functional because of poor muscle response | Intact | Normal | Loss of control of voiding because of muscular impairment |

incidence of men. Among the more than 1.5 million nursing facility residents, the incidence is greater than 50%. Because of underdiagnosis and underreporting, the problem of urinary incontinence may be even more widespread. See Table 44-15 for risk factors related to urinary incontinence.

## PATHOPHYSIOLOGY

### Physiology of Urinary Continence

Bladder sphincter control is necessary for urinary continence. Such control requires normal voluntary and involuntary muscle action coordinated by a normal urethrobladder reflex. As the bladder fills, the pressure within the bladder gradually increases. The detrusor muscle within the bladder wall responds by relaxing to accommodate the greater volume. When the bladder has filled to capacity, usually between 400 and 500 ml of urine, the parasympathetic stretch receptors located within the bladder wall are stimulated. The stimuli are transmitted through afferent fibers of the reflex arc for micturition. Impulses are then carried through the efferent fibers of the reflex arc to the bladder, causing contraction of the detrusor muscle. The internal sphincter, which is normally closed, reciprocally opens, and urine enters the posterior urethra. Relaxation of the external sphincter and perineal muscles follows, and urine is released. Completion of this reflex arc can be interrupted and voiding postponed through release of inhibitory impulses from the cortical center, which results in voluntary contrac-

**table 44-15** *Risk Factors for Urinary Incontinence*

| Type | Example |
|---|---|
| Stress | Loss of urethrovesicular junction in women |
| | Urethral irritation from infection or radiation after prostatectomy |
| | Obesity |
| | Sphincter incompetence |
| | Pelvic relaxation |
| Urge | Alzheimer's disease |
| | Parkinson's disease |
| | Multiple sclerosis |
| | UTIs |
| | Arthritis |
| | Stroke |
| | Medications: hypnotics, tranquilizers, sedatives, diuretics |
| Overflow | Retention with bladder distention |
| | Fecal impaction |
| | Benign prostatic hyperplasia |
| Reflex | Spinal cord injury |
| Psychological | Altered mental status |
| Environmental | Physical disabilities |
| | Physical barriers |

tion of the external sphincter. If any part of this complex control system is interrupted, urinary incontinence will result.

### Disturbances of Cerebral Control

Cerebral clouding is most common in elderly persons. In many instances the person is incontinent because of a lack of awareness of a full bladder. This type of incontinence is often not associated with any definite pathological problem at the cerebral level. Cerebral clouding also occurs in acutely ill persons—as a result of dulled cerebration as a function of the illness. These patients may not have the energy to exercise voluntary control of bladder function. Likewise, a comatose patient is incontinent because of loss of ability to control voluntary use of the external sphincter. As soon as urine is released into the posterior urethra on bladder filling, the bladder contracts and empties. This is why voiding sometimes occurs when a patient is under anesthesia.

Disturbance of the central nervous system pathways may occur in diseases such as cerebral embolus, cerebral hemorrhage, brain tumor, meningitis, or traumatic injury of the brain. Adequate voluntary (cortical or cerebral) control of bladder function is prevented in these situations. Urgency incontinence may be present as a result of the inability to inhibit completion of the urethrobladder reflex by the higher centers.

### Disturbances of Urethrobladder Reflex

Disturbance of the urethrobladder reflex may result from lesions of the spinal cord or damage to peripheral nerves of the bladder. Urethrobladder reflex may be seen in persons with spinal cord malformations, injuries, or tumors and in those with compression of the spinal cord caused by fractures of the vertebrae, herniated disk, metastatic tumor, or postoperative edema of the spinal cord. This type of difficulty can result in two types of responses known as *neurogenic bladder*: *automatic* and *flaccid.* The person with a neurogenic bladder has no control over bladder function.

Lesions above the S2 level of the spinal cord or impairment of the cerebrocortical centers do not destroy the reflex arc for voiding, although they may affect control. Such lesions destroy the potential for cortical control to inhibit the reflex. The result is an "upper motor neuron" or "automatic" bladder. The bladder is hypertonic and has a small capacity of usually less than 150 ml. The increased detrusor tone and increased sensitivity to small amounts of urine present in the bladder result in precipitous voiding and the potential for vesicoureteral reflex.

Damage to nerves in the cauda equina or sacral segments of the spinal cord may cause destruction of the reflex arc by interruption of the afferent, efferent, or central components. The result is a "lower motor neuron" or "flaccid" bladder. The bladder is hypotonic with large capacities, sometimes of 750 ml or more. Overflow incontinence, retention of residual urine, and the potential for vesicoureteral reflux are problems imposed by a hypotonic bladder.

### Bladder Disturbances

Overflow incontinence is caused by overdistention of the bladder. This type of incontinence may result from an underactive or a contractile detrusor muscle or from bladder outlet or urethral obstruction, leading to overdistention and overflow.

Infection anywhere in the urinary tract may lead to incontinence, since bacteria in the urine irritate the bladder mucosa. The resulting inflammation stimulates the urethrobladder reflex abnormally.

Tissue damage to the sphincters of the bladder from instrumentation, surgery, trauma, scarring from urethral infection, lesions involving the sphincter, or relaxation of the perineal structures may cause urinary incontinence. The latter cause of incontinence is seen occasionally after childbirth. The problem is local in nature and does not involve the nervous system.

### Relaxed Musculature

Stress incontinence is seen primarily in women who have relaxed pelvic musculature, but may also occur in men after prostatectomy. When bladder pressure is suddenly increased, urine enters the proximal third of the urethra, then returns to the bladder when pressure is decreased after exertion. Some of the urine escapes through the urethra.

### Psychogenic Disturbances

Some individuals derive secondary gains by feigning incontinence. This is typically seen in children and young adults. Even if psychogenic causes are suspected, a complete diagnostic workup must be done to rule out organic causes.[3]

## Collaborative Care Management

#### Diagnostic tests

Urinary incontinence can be diagnosed by a variety of urodynamic examinations. A cystometrogram and electromyogram are done to evaluate the detrusor muscle of the bladder as well as sphincter and perineal activity. An ultrasound of the bladder, cystoscopy, and IVP are also done to assess the structures and functioning of the urinary tract.

#### Medications

Medication management for the treatment of incontinence is based on the identified etiology of the incontinence. Table 44-16 lists some of the more common medications. These medications need to be used cautiously in older adults. Bladder outlet obstruction should be ruled out before use of medications.

#### Treatments

Treatment protocols and algorithms have been established by the U.S. Department of Health and Human Services for the management of the incontinent adult. Treatments can be categorized as behavioral, pharmacological, and surgical. A combination of therapies is often used. Behavioral techniques include bladder training, timed voiding, prompted voiding, and pelvic muscle exercises.

Biofeedback, vaginal cone retention, and electrical stimulation can be used in conjunction with behavioral techniques. Vaginal cones are used in addition to pelvic muscle exercises. A weighted cone is inserted vaginally, and the woman

table 44-16 Common Medications for *Urinary Incontinence*

| Drug | Action | Nursing Interventions |
|---|---|---|
| **ESTROGENS (Premarin, Estratab, Estrace)** | | |
| Quinestradiol<br>Piperazine estrone<br>Estriol | Binds to proteins responsible for estrogen effects; relieves atrophic vaginitis and restores urethral suppleness. | Explain risk of blood clots.<br>Review signs of thrombophlebitis.<br>Encourage smoking cessation programs. |
| **ANTICHOLINERGIC AGENTS** | | |
| Propantheline (Pro-Bantine)<br>Oxybutynin (Ditropan)<br>Dicyclomine (Bentyl) | Decreases the spasticity of the bladder; direct smooth muscle relaxation of bladder. | Avoid use in patients with glaucoma.<br>May cause postural hypotension. Instruct patient to change positions slowly.<br>Assess bowel sounds. |
| **CHOLINERGIC AGENTS** | | |
| Bethanecol (Urecholine)<br>Neostigmine (Prostigmine) | Treats flaccid bladder by simulating contractions of the bladder. | Administer medication on an empty stomach.<br>Monitor vital signs and intake and output.<br>Instruct patient to ambulate with caution. |
| **ALPHA-ADRENERGIC BLOCKERS** | | |
| Prazosin (Minipress)<br>Phenoxybenzamine (Dibenzyline)<br>Phenylpropanolamine | Reduces spasticity of the bladder neck. | Monitor orthostatic vital signs.<br>Monitor I/O and daily weights.<br>Instruct patient to avoid OTC medications unless instructed by physician. |
| **SYMPATHOMIMETICS** | | |
| Ephedrine<br>Phenylephrine (Neo-Synephrine) | Increases bladder neck and urethral tone. | Monitor for dysrhythmias, assess vital signs.<br>Instruct patient on potential side effects of dizziness, headache, or dyspnea. |
| **ALPHA-ADRENERGIC AGONISTS** | | |
| Phenylpropanolamine<br>Imipramine (Tofranil) | Increases urethral resistance. | Administer several hours before bedtime.<br>Instruct patients to avoid caffeine-containing beverages. |
| **CALCIUM CHANNEL BLOCKERS** | Reduces detrusor contractions. | Monitor blood pressure and heart rate.<br>Assess for orthostatic hypotension.<br>Monitor intake and output. |

is instructed to contract the pelvic muscles and retain the cone for up to 15 minutes twice daily. Electrical stimulation of the pelvic viscera, pelvic muscles, or nerves has been effective in management of bladder and urethral dysfunction in persons with or without neurological dysfunction.

#### *Urgency*

Incontinence caused by UTI is generally temporary, responding to treatment of the UTI by systemic antibiotics. Specific causes of infection such as obstruction must be identified and corrected when possible. Provisions must be made for adequate fluid intake of 3000 ml or more per day unless contraindicated by the person's medical condition.

The person who has a brain tumor, meningitis, or traumatic injury to the brain that prevents adequate voluntary control of bladder function may benefit from a bladder retraining program. If the person's condition or response prohibits such a program, an internal or external drainage device should be used.

#### *Neurogenic bladder dysfunction*

Persons with spinal cord injuries experience a transitory period of "spinal shock" in which urinary retention occurs (see Chapter 54). An indwelling catheter is placed to facilitate urinary drainage and prevent overdistention of the bladder. After the acute stage, management depends on the exact nature of any residual neurogenic bladder dysfunction. Persons with a lesion above the sacral segments and with an intact urethrobladder reflex may initiate voiding by pinching or stroking trigger areas of the thighs or suprapubic area. In persons with a lower motor neuron lesion, the use of the Credé method, which consists of exerting manual pressure over the bladder, may provide more complete bladder emptying. The appropriateness of this technique must be determined by the physician, based on the person's complete urological status. An increasing number of persons with neurogenic bladder dysfunction are being taught intermittent self-catheterization using clean technique to prevent infection and manage incontinence. Maintenance of a regular schedule for catheterization is stressed, and the frequency is determined on an individual basis.

For patients with spinal cord injuries at T6 or above, urinary retention or a blocked urinary catheter can lead to *autonomic dysreflexia.* This potentially fatal complication presents with hypertension; a pounding headache; flushing, goose-flesh (cutis anserina); and diaphoresis above the level of injury[12] (see Chapter 54).

## Surgical Management

### Sphincter dysfunction

For men, periurethral bulking injections (the injection of collagen) can increase urethral compression, especially in persons who have had pelvic radiation therapy. This procedure has been effective in treating male incontinence due to sphincter insufficiency. Repair of a sphincter that has been cut is almost impossible. When the external sphincter has been damaged, the person will be incontinent on urgency. A voiding schedule can be planned so that voiding occurs before the bladder is full enough to exert sufficient pressure to open the internal sphincter involuntarily. When the internal sphincter is damaged, the person may have no acute feeling of the need to void. Here the problem is not one of incontinence but of retention. To ensure routine emptying of the bladder, a regular voiding schedule is necessary. If both sphincters are damaged, total incontinence will occur.

### Stress incontinence

Surgery may be indicated for severe stress incontinence. A *vesicourethropexy* (Marshall-Marchetti procedure) consists of fixation of the urethra to the fascia of the rectus muscle of the abdomen with support given to the neck of the bladder. A suprapubic incision is usually made, but a transvaginal approach may be used if scar tissue is around the urethra from vaginal surgery. A urethral catheter is inserted postoperatively and maintained for 5 to 6 days. The urine may be pink, but the urethral catheter is not usually irrigated. The person may have difficulty voiding immediately after the indwelling catheter is removed. The woman is observed for signs of vaginal bleeding. Straining and the Valsalva maneuver should be avoided until healing has occurred, and mild laxatives may be given to prevent straining from constipation. Surgeons differ in the amount of activity permitted in the early postoperative period.

Less invasive is the *Stamey* (or needle suspension) procedure, a suspension of the bladder neck by sutures passed adjacent to the ureterovesical junction. A small incision is made above and lateral to the symphysis pubis. The needles are introduced suprapubically by endoscopy, and the positions are checked by cystoscopy before suturing. The procedure is then repeated on the opposite side. A percutaneous suprapubic catheter is inserted after the suturing; the catheter is removed when spontaneous voiding occurs, which may take several days. Postoperative discomfort is minimal. Antibiotics are given for 2 weeks postoperatively. The patient should refrain from sexual intercourse for about 1 to 2 months.

### Artificial sphincter

An artificial urinary sphincter may be used to achieve continence when other methods have failed. A hydraulically activated sphincter mechanism is placed around the urethra or bladder neck. The sphincter is made to open and close at will by squeezing one of two bulbs implanted under the skin of the labia or scrotum (Figure 44-17). Postoperative nursing care of the person with such an implant includes observation for and reporting of fever or pain on inflation of the device, swelling of the genitalia, and recurrence of incontinence. Complications of the procedure include erosion of the urethra, abscess, cellulitis, and mechanical malfunctions in the system. Men have had more success with the artificial sphincter than women.

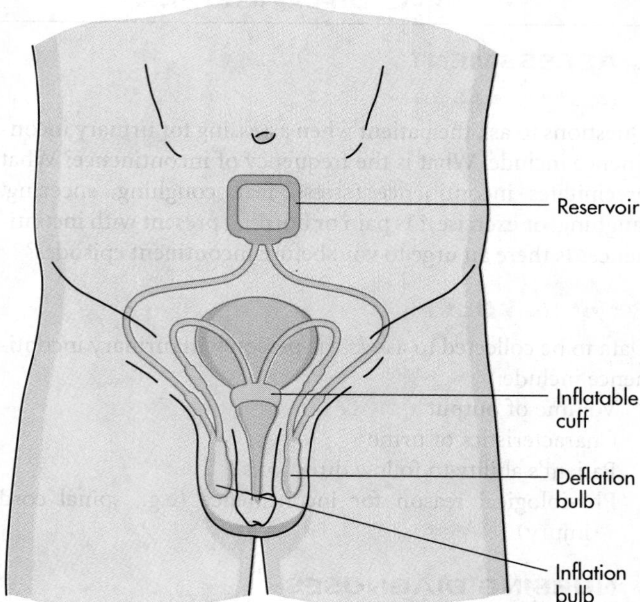


**fig. 44-17** Artificial bladder sphincter. Compression and release of inflation pump bulb inflates cuff surrounding urethra, stopping urine flow. Compression and release of deflation pump bulb deflates inflatable cuff, returning fluid to storage reservoir. This releases urethral constriction, permitting urine to flow.

## Diet

Nutritional alterations for the patient with urinary incontinence involve the scheduling of fluid intake as well as avoidance of bladder stimulants such as alcohol, chocolate, and coffee. Fluid intake after dinner should be reduced or avoided.

## Referrals

Patients with urinary incontinence should be referred to a urologist for management. Rehabilitation programs for bladder training are also useful for the patient with urinary incontinence. Community support programs are available in many areas. These programs are often sponsored by companies marketing products used for incontinence management. Local hospital newsletters are a good source for programs related to incontinence management.

The U.S. Department of Health and Human Resources published Clinical Practice Guidelines for adults with incontinence. Publications are available for health care professionals and lay persons.

## NURSING MANAGEMENT

### ASSESSMENT

#### Subjective Data

Questions to ask the patient when assessing for urinary incontinence include: What is the frequency of incontinence? What precipitates incontinence (stress, fear, coughing, sneezing, laughing, or exercise)? Is pain or burning present with incontinence? Is there an urge to void before incontinent episodes?

#### Objective Data

Data to be collected to assess the person with urinary incontinence include:

Volume of output
Characteristics of urine
Patient's ability to follow directions
Physiological reason for incontinence (e.g., spinal cord injury)

### NURSING DIAGNOSES

Nursing diagnoses are determined from analysis of patient data. Several nursing diagnoses could be made for the incontinent patient for which the interventions are not specific for urinary incontinence and thus are not discussed in this section. These nursing diagnoses include skin integrity, impaired; body image disturbance; social isolation; self-bathing hygiene deficit; mobility, impaired physical; and coping, ineffective individual. Nursing diagnoses specific for the incontinent patient may include but are not limited to:

| Diagnostic Title | Possible Etiological Factors |
|---|---|
| Incontinence | Relaxed pelvic muscles, altered environment, sensory deficit, neurological impairment, overdistention, decreased bladder capacity |
| Self-esteem, situational low | Loss of urinary control |
| Knowledge deficit | Lack of exposure/recall |

### EXPECTED PATIENT OUTCOMES

Expected patient outcomes for the person with urinary incontinence may include but are not limited to:

1. Achieves optimal urinary control.
2a. Verbalizes feelings and concerns without self-deprecating statements.
 b. Socializes with others.
3a. Demonstrates perineal exercises (if appropriate).
 b. Describes actions to control voiding (as appropriate), measures to maintain skin integrity, and plans for follow-up care.

### INTERVENTIONS

#### Assisting with Urinary Control

##### *Bladder retraining*

When incontinence is caused by dulled cerebration, confusion, or acute illness, control can usually be established if a persistent bladder retraining schedule is carried out. A voiding schedule is developed and strictly adhered to until the person gradually relearns to recognize and react appropriately to the urge to void. A successful program (Box 44-7), leading to complete rehabilitation or continence, requires mental competence of the individual. Otherwise, someone else must always remind the person to follow the schedule.

People ordinarily void on awakening, before retiring, and before or after meals. Consuming caffeinated beverages such as coffee creates a diuretic effect and the urge to void occurs in about 30 minutes. Using this knowledge, the nurse can begin to set up a schedule for placing the person on a bedpan or taking the person to the toilet. Then if a record is kept for a few days of the times the person voids involuntarily, it is usually possible to determine the normal voiding pattern. If the schedule based on the pattern of incontinence is not successful, toileting every 1 to 2 hours should be carried out on a 24-hour basis.

During the retraining program, mobilization of the individual, attention to the position assumed for voiding, and adequate fluid intake contribute to reduction of the possibility of infection. Complete emptying of the bladder eliminates the possibility of residual urine acting as a medium for bacterial growth, and a high fluid intake provides for internal bladder irrigation.

When possible, toileting should be carried out in surroundings that will remind the person of the voiding function; that is, the person should be taken to the bathroom to use the toilet. If this is not possible, a bedside commode can be an adequate substitute. Many men can void into a urinal more easily if allowed to stand at the bedside. The use of a bedpan is unfamiliar and distasteful to most persons, but in instances where women must remain in bed, voiding into a bedpan can be facilitated if the head of the bed is rolled up as high as allowed. This position is more consistent with the position normally assumed for voiding and facilitates complete emptying of the bladder. Few persons can void adequately in the supine position.

Providing adequate amounts of fluids, a minimum of 3000 ml/day, is necessary to ensure that adequate amounts of urine are produced and present in the bladder to stimulate the voiding reflex at the proper times. Fluids may be given at scheduled times, the largest portion being given during the day before 4 PM to decrease the frequency of voiding through the night. Persons with restricted fluid intake because of medical problems should receive the prescribed amount of fluid.[2]

**box 44-7** *Bladder Retraining*

- Establish patient's usual voiding patterns.
- Plan toileting based on the patient's usual pattern; assist patient as necessary.
- Plan toileting for every 1 to 2 hours (if no voiding pattern can be determined).
- Encourage patient to use normal toilet position.
- Encourage patient to empty bladder completely.
- Provide for a fluid intake of 3000 ml/day for adequate urine volume.
- Schedule majority of fluid intake before 4 PM.

### Catheterization

Occasionally, the use of an indwelling catheter for the incontinent patient is justified. Reasons include the need to protect a surgical incision or to permit healing of a pressure ulcer in the area. Indwelling catheterization, however, presents many potential dangers, such as UTI, urethritis, epididymitis, and urethral fistulas. All other means to manage the incontinence should be tried before resorting to catheterization.

### External urinary drainage

For a man, external drainage can be accomplished with a condom catheter. Several commercial products are available. The following is an alternative method to purchasing external drainage devices. Select a condom of the correct size. Puncture a hole in the closed end of the condom with an applicator stick. Attach the punctured end of the condom to a firm rubber or plastic drainage tube with either a 3-mm (⅛-inch) piece of rubber tubing or a strip of adhesive tape (Figure 44-18). Before applying the condom, clean and dry the penis thoroughly and check for edema, skin breaks, or discoloration. Invert the condom and roll it onto the penis. There should be no roll at the top that could cause constriction. At least 2.5 cm (1 inch) of the condom should remain between the meatus and drainage tube to allow for penile erection. There should not be so much slack as to cause twisting and subsequent interference with drainage. Elastoplast is then applied over the condom and around the penis (never touching the skin). *Under no circumstances should adhesive tape be used.* The Elastoplast must not be constricting.

The external catheter should be removed daily and the skin washed and inspected. Frequent assessment is necessary to determine whether edema or irritation is present and to ensure proper drainage. This is especially important in men with loss of sensation. The external device is attached to straight drainage or to a leg bag.

For persons who need external catheter drainage indefinitely, a rubber urinary appliance (sometimes called an *incontinence urinal*) may be used (Figure 44-19). Several models are available, and the one best suited to the person's needs is selected. Two appliances are recommended to allow for cleaning and drying of one device while using the other. They should be washed in mild soap, turned inside out, and thoroughly dried before application.

Most persons prefer to manage their own incontinence if they are at all able to do so. The nurse supports and encourages this, offering assistance as necessary and instruction in basic principles of skin care, equipment selection, and maintenance. The choice of management method should take into account the person's ability to manage as independently as possible.[4]

## Maintaining Skin Integrity

If none of the previous measures is appropriate or successful, nursing goals of assisting the person to remain clean, free of odor, and free of pressure sores may require external urinary protection. Incontinence leading to skin breakdown may result in sepsis, increased length of hospitalization, and increased costs.[4] The type varies with the person's gender, functional status, and physical status.

Those who are unconscious or incapacitated by critical illness depend on the nursing staff to manage their incontinence by protective pants or external catheter drainage. Others

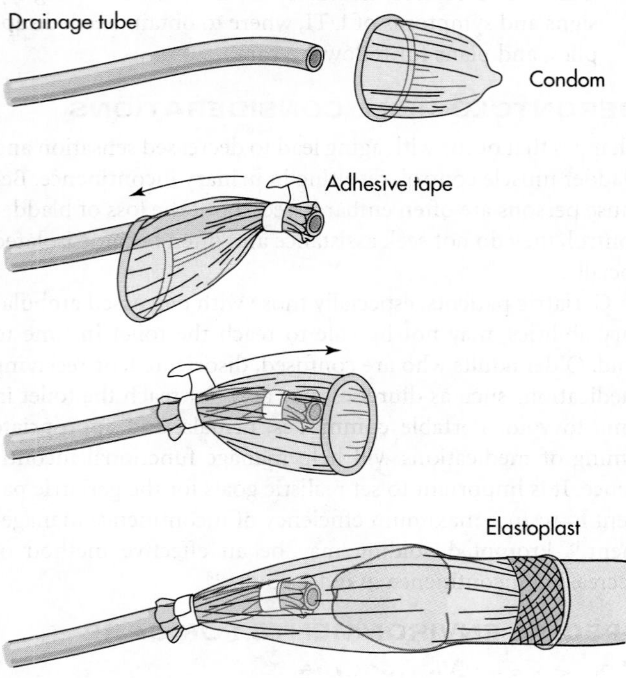


**fig. 44-18** One method of making an external drainage apparatus.

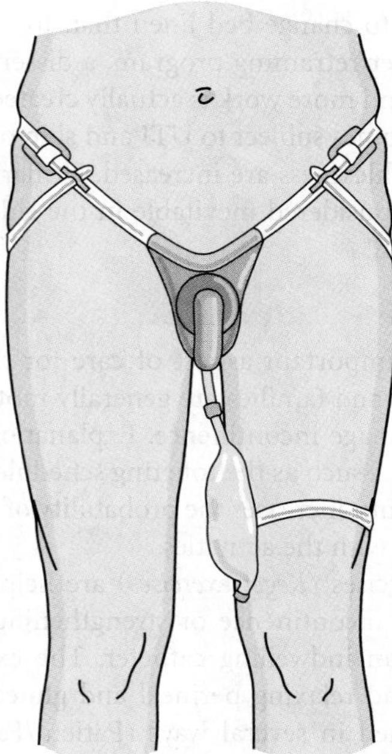

**fig. 44-19** Rubber urinary appliance. Bag is emptied by drain valve at bottom of bag.

may be capable of some or all of their own management. Men and women may wear protective waterproof pants lined by disposable or washable absorbent pads. Adult briefs are available commercially, but they are quite bulky under clothing. Skin breakdown is a problem due to decreased air circulation. A resourceful person may be able to improvise equipment that is as comfortable and is less costly than commercially available pants. Zippers, Velcro, elastic, and a variety of waterproof materials may be used. Bedding and furniture can be protected with waterproof materials such as commercially available squares of absorbent cellucotton backed with light plastic.

Whatever the type of padding, liners, or pants used, frequent changing is required for skin protection and comfort. The perineal and genital areas are thoroughly washed with soap and water and dried well at each changing. If possible, the person bathes in a tub of warm water at least once a day. Periodic exposure of the perineal area to air is beneficial. A moisture barrier product (e.g., A&D ointment) helps protect the skin. Zinc oxide powder can be applied to lessen irritation. Excess amounts of powder are avoided, since this will cake on the skin and cause irritation. Deodorant sprays for use on dressings and liners are valuable, but they may cause skin irritation in persons who develop a hypersensitivity to them. Deodorant room fresheners may be helpful if the odor is strong.

If the person can be up, a favorite chair can be equipped with a commode seat. Special commode wheelchairs are also available, making it possible for the person to be more comfortable and to socially interact with others.

### Promoting Self-Esteem

Persons who are incontinent may feel isolated from their families and familiar surroundings. They may also have decreased self-esteem. These patients frequently respond well to mobilization in bladder retraining programs. When nurses believe that it is easier to change bed linen than to establish an appropriate bladder retraining program, a disservice is done to the individual and more work is actually created for the nurse. The person becomes subject to UTI and skin breakdown, and feelings of worthlessness are increased. Urinary incontinence should not be considered inevitable in the elderly or institutionalized person!

### Patient/Family Education

Teaching is an important aspect of care for the incontinent person. Patients and families are generally motivated to learn measures to manage incontinence. Explanation of the rationale for activities, such as the toileting schedule, mobility, and fluid requirements, increases the probability of the person following through with the activities.

Perineal exercises *(Kegel exercises)* are helpful in controlling mild stress incontinence or strengthening muscles after withdrawal of an indwelling catheter. The exercises consist of tightening and relaxing perineal and gluteal muscles and can be performed in several ways (Patient/Family Teaching Box). Stress incontinence in women can be prevented if perineal exercises are taught before and after childbirth. These exercises also may be included as part of the health teaching of any woman.

**patient/family teaching**

**Perineal Exercises**

1. Tighten the perineal muscles as if to prevent voiding; hold for 3 seconds, then relax.
2. Inhale through pursed lips while tightening perineal muscles.
3. Bear down as if to have a bowel movement. Relax then tighten perineal muscles.
4. Hold a pencil in the fold between the buttock and thigh.
5. Sit on the toilet with knees held wide apart. Start and stop the urinary stream.

Additional teaching includes care of any drainage system, measures to maintain skin integrity, signs and symptoms of UTI (frequency or dysuria) that should be reported to the physician, and how to obtain and maintain any needed supplies and equipment (commode, protective padding, and drainage systems). The family or significant other should be included in the teaching.

## ■ EVALUATION

To evaluate the effectiveness of nursing interventions, compare patient behaviors with those stated in the expected outcomes. Successful achievement of patient outcomes for the patient with urinary incontinence is indicated by the following:

1. Achieves urinary continence through bladder retraining (if appropriate) or uses a drainage system or padding.

2a. Describes self in positive terms.
b. Socializes with others.

3a. Correctly demonstrates perineal exercises (if appropriate).
b. Correctly describes measures to maintain skin integrity, signs and symptoms of UTI, where to obtain needed supplies, and plans for follow-up care.

## GERONTOLOGICAL CONSIDERATIONS

Changes that occur with aging lead to decreased sensation and bladder muscle control, resulting in urinary incontinence. Because persons are often embarrassed about the loss of bladder control, they do not seek assistance and often become isolated socially.

Geriatric patients, especially those with decreased ambulatory abilities, may not be able to reach the toilet in time to void. Older adults who are confused, disoriented, or receiving medications such as diuretics may also not reach the toilet in time to void. Portable commodes, urinals, and appropriate timing of medications will help manage functional incontinence. It is important to set realistic goals for the geriatric patient to restore maximum efficiency of incontinence management.[19] Prompted voiding may be an effective method of decreasing incontinence in older adults.[18]

## SPECIAL ENVIRONMENTS FOR CARE

### Home Care Management

The incontinent patient may require supplies and equipment for home use. The home care nurse can evaluate the patient's home environment for ease of access to bathrooms, potential impediments to ambulation, and the need for supplemental equipment. The home nurse can also provide support for the family and reinforce patient teaching regarding incontinence.

## COMPLICATIONS

The incontinent patient is at a high risk for developing skin breakdown. Any break in the integrity of the skin can greatly increase the risk of serious infection. Another complication of incontinence is depression related to the social isolation.

## critical thinking QUESTIONS

**1** A 55-year-old man is seen by his health care provider with a history of voiding cherry-colored urine. He also reports fatigue and anorexia. His history is also significant for smoking 3 packs of cigarettes a day since age 18. What do these assessment findings suggest? Which diagnostic test should be ordered for this patient? What nursing measures are needed to prepare the patient for these tests?

**2** An unconscious man is admitted after a severe auto accident. He has blood around his meatus and his prostate is palpable and floating. What additional assessment data should you obtain? What is the expected diagnosis? What additional diagnostic test would you anticipate to confirm this diagnosis? What are some medical and nursing treatment options?

**3** M.J.'s older sister recently developed chronic renal failure as a result of polycystic kidney disease. M.J. is very concerned because she has three teenaged children and fears they will develop renal failure. Are M.J.'s concerns warranted, since neither she nor her children have any symptoms of kidney disease? What interventions are appropriate on M.J.'s behalf?

**4** After outpatient surgery; Mr. C. reports that he needs to urinate. The nurse provides privacy and gives him a urinal. He voids about 50 ml of urine. About an hour later, he again reports of needing to urinate and voids only 30 ml of urine. What is your assessment of this situation and what should the nurse do? Why is urinary retention considered a urological emergency?

**5** A patient has had recurring bouts of renal calculi. The stone composition is oxalate and calcium. He is a slightly overweight accountant who spends at least 11 hours at the office seated at the computer. He admits to eating fast food on the run and frequently does not take breaks throughout the day due to his rigorous meeting schedule. What modifications in his lifestyle should be suggested? What complications could develop? Develop a teaching plan for this patient.

## chapter SUMMARY

- The major health problems of the urinary system include congenital, inflammatory, vascular, and obstructive disorders; urinary incontinence; and trauma to the urinary tract.

### CONGENITAL DISORDERS

- Polycystic kidney disease is an inherited disease in which cysts form in the kidneys and enlarge and rupture, causing scarring with loss of kidney function. Treatment is symptomatic with control of infection.

### INFLAMMATORY DISORDERS

- Chronic health problems predisposing to urinary tract infections (UTIs) include diabetes mellitus, gout, hypertension, polycystic kidney disease, multiple myeloma, and glomerulonephritis.
- UTIs may occur in the lower urinary tract (most common) or ascend into the kidney (pyelonephritis).
- The most important defenses against UTI are large urine volume, unobstructed flow, and complete emptying of the bladder to prevent urinary stasis.
- It is essential to teach the patient receiving antibiotic therapy for UTI to continue antibiotics for the entire prescribed course even if symptoms resolve.
- Acute glomerulonephritis usually follows a streptococcal infection and is a result of an antigen-antibody reaction; the significant effect is loss of glomerular basement membrane porosity. Proteinuria, hematuria, and fluid retention result. Management consists of bedrest, maintenance of fluid balance, and prevention of infection.
- Chronic glomerulonephritis may follow the acute disease or may develop from unknown causes; it is characterized by slow, progressive glomerular destruction terminating in renal failure. No specific therapy exists; patients are taught to live with their disease and report signs of exacerbation.
- Nephrotic syndrome is a constellation of symptoms (severe generalized edema, pronounced proteinuria, hypoalbuminemia, and hyperlipidemia) resulting from kidney damage; it often progresses to kidney failure. Management consists of administering steroids and diuretics, promoting comfort (because of fatigue and massive edema), encouraging a restricted protein and sodium diet, and teaching the patient self-care.

### VASCULAR DISORDERS

- Vascular disorders include renal artery stenosis characterized by hypertension and nephrosclerosis caused by hypertension; treatment consists of control of hypertension and correction of the stenosis.

### OBSTRUCTIVE DISORDERS

- Disorders that may obstruct the urinary tract include urinary calculi, tumors of the kidney or bladder, prostatic hypertrophy, or urethral strictures. Backup of urine causes hydronephrosis, leading to kidney damage. General interventions include monitoring for signs of additional obstruction, promoting fluid balance and comfort, preventing urinary complications, and patient teaching.
- Urinary retention is the inability to empty the bladder; small amounts of urine voided frequently may result from retention with overflow; causes may be mechanical or functional. Methods of urinary drainage include urethral catheter drainage, direct bladder drainage with a cystostomy tube, and catheter drainage of kidney pelvis and ureters. Intermittent catheter drainage can be taught to the patient for home care of urinary retention.
- The most common urinary stones are calcium oxalate; the stones cause renal colic from urine backup or from irritation or stretching of the ureters. If the stone does not pass spontaneously and is causing symptoms or damage, it must be removed surgically or broken up by lithotripsy or laser treatment.
- Recurrence of some renal stones can be controlled by an alkaline-ash or acid-ash diet (depending on the type of stone).

- Bladder cancer is more common than malignant renal tumors; both are removed surgically. If the entire bladder is removed, permanent urinary diversion is necessary.

## UROLOGICAL SURGERY

- Postoperative care for patients having urological surgery includes promoting ventilation, monitoring urine output, observing for signs of distention and hemorrhage, protecting the skin from urinary drainage through the incision, and patient teaching.
- Two types of urinary diversion procedures include ileal or colon conduit and continent urostomy.
- Postoperative care after a urinary diversion procedure includes maintaining skin integrity, monitoring urine output, promoting body image, and facilitating learning the use and care of pouches.

## URINARY INCONTINENCE

- Urinary incontinence is not a normal part of aging; whenever urinary incontinence is present, the cause should be thoroughly investigated.
- Major types of urinary incontinence include stress, urge, and overflow incontinence; two other forms are reflex and total incontinence. Control largely depends on cause. Stress incontinence may be controlled surgically. Nursing interventions include teaching perineal exercises and bladder retraining. Keeping the person dry is of utmost importance; waterproof pants or external urinary drainage may be used when control is inadequate.

## References


1. Adhikar M: Comparison of noninvasive methods for distinguishing steroid-sensitive nephrotic syndrome from focal glomerulonephritis, *J Lab Clin Med* 129(1):47-52, 1997.
2. Cliner J: A nursing management protocol for incontinence, *Rehabil Nurs,* St Louis, 1994, Mosby.
3. Coe FL: Alterations in urinary function. In Isselbacher et al, editors: *Harrison's principles of internal medicine,* ed 13, New York, 1994, McGraw-Hill.
4. Connor P, Kooker B: Nurse's knowledge, attitudes and practices in managing urinary incontinence in the acute care setting, *Med/Surg Nurs* 5(2):87-92, 1996.
5. Frank IN, Graham SD, Nabors WL: Urologic and male genital cancers. In Murphy G et al, editors: *Textbook of clinical oncology,* ed 2, Atlanta, 1995, American Cancer Society.
6. Glasscock RJ, Brenner BM: The major glomerulopathies. In Isselbacher et al, editors: *Harrison's principles of internal medicine,* ed 13, New York, 1994, McGraw-Hill.
7. Golden T, Ratliff C: Development and implementation of a clinical pathway for radical cystectomy and urinary system reconstruction, *J Wound Ostomy Continence Nurs* 24(2):72-78, 1997.
8. Hald D, Aehring T, Razor B: the pathogenesis and management of urethral malignancies. *J Wound Ostomy Continence Nurs* 23(3):144-149, 1996.
9. Hamptom BG, Bryant RA: *Ostomies and continent diversions,* St Louis, 1992, Mosby.
10. Holmes H: *Mastering geriatric care,* Philadelphia, 1997, Springhouse.
11. Klein E: Options in the surgical treatment of bladder cancer, *J Enterostomal Ther Nurs* 19(4):122-125, 1992.
12. Latham L: When spinal cord injury complicates medical/surgical nursing care, *RN* August, pp 26-30, 1994.
13. Letzig M, Conway A: Interleukin 2 therapy for renal cell carcinoma: indication, effects, and nursing implications, *Crit Care Nurs* 16(5): 22-26, 1996.
14. McAninch JW: Disorders of the kidneys. In Tanagho EA, McAninch JW, editors: *Smiths's general urology,* East Norwalk, Conn, 1995, Appleton & Lange.
15. McCarthy S, McCullen M: Autosomal dominant polycystic kidney disease: pathophysiology and treatment, *ANNA J* 24(1):45-63, 1997.
16. Marchiondo, K: A new look at urinary tract infection, *Am J Nurs* 98(3):34-39, 1998.
17. Moore D, Edwards K: Using portable bladder scans to reduce the incidence of nosocomial UTI, *Med/Surg Nurs* 16(1):39-43, 1997.
18. Ouslander J et al: Predictors of successful prompted voiding among incontinent nursing home residents, *JAMA* 73(17):1366-1370, 1995.
19. Resnick B et al: Geriatric rehabilitation: nursing interventions and outcomes focusing on urinary function and knowledge of medications, *Rehabil Nurs* 21(3):142-147, 1996.
20. Shellenbarger T, Krouse A: Treating and preventing kidney stones, *Med/Surg Nurs* 3(5):389-394, 1994.
21. Spirnak JP, Resnick MI: Urinary stones. In Tanagho EA, McAninch JW, editors: *Smith's general urology,* East Norwalk, Conn, 1995, Appleton & Lange.
22. Vincenti FG, Amend WJC: Diagnosis of medical renal diseases. In Tanagho EA, McAninch JW, editors: *Smith's general urology,* East Norwalk, Conn, 1995, Appleton & Lange.
23. Wiseman K: TB: an old disease with a new face, *ANNA J* 22(6):541-546, 1995.

chapter 45

# MANAGEMENT OF PERSONS WITH Renal Failure

DEBORAH K. MARANTIDES, JANE F. MAREK, JACQUELINE MORGAN, and MARILYN ROSSMAN BARTUCCI

## objectives *After studying this chapter, the learner should be able to:*

1. Analyze the pathophysiological changes and clinical manifestations of acute and chronic renal failure.
2. Compare and contrast the medical and nursing management of patients during the oliguric and diuretic phases of acute renal failure.
3. Explain the benefits of continuous renal replacement therapy for patients with renal failure.
4. Relate treatment goals for patients with chronic renal failure.
5. Describe the physiological principles of dialysis.
6. Compare and contrast nursing assessment and management of patients undergoing hemodialysis, peritoneal dialysis, and kidney transplantation.

## INTRODUCTION

Renal failure is one of the most significant causes of death and disability throughout the world. More than 15 million persons in the United States alone are estimated to have renal disease.[8] The kidneys perform a large number of life-sustaining functions including filtration of waste from the blood, maintenance of acid-base balance, and regulation of blood pressure. Due to the complexity of kidney function, renal failure affects all body systems.

The kidneys have a tremendous ability to adapt to a decreasing number of functioning nephrons. With less than 25% of the original nephrons functioning, the kidneys are able to excrete waste products and maintain fluid and electrolyte balance.[17] As renal failure develops, laboratory tests reflect the changes in homeostasis, and the person appears clinically ill. The person in renal failure cannot independently sustain life.

Renal failure may be *acute* in onset (developing in hours to days) or *chronic* (developing slowly and progressively over a course of several years). When renal failure occurs suddenly, as within a few days, biochemical changes are often dramatic, and the person has little time to adjust to these changes. The person becomes very ill and is frequently treated in a critical care area.

In chronic renal failure, the kidney is progressively destroyed over the course of several months or years. The control of symptoms and preservation of function can be achievable goals. Kidney function may be preserved by dietary adjustment, medication, and health promotion. As renal function continues to deteriorate, dialysis or transplantation becomes necessary to maintain life.

*Renal insufficiency* exists when a significant loss of renal function occurs but enough functioning remains to maintain an internal environment consistent with life. Renal insufficiency generally refers to a decline in renal function to approximately 25% of normal function or a glomerular filtration rate (GFR) of 25 to 30 ml/min. When renal insufficiency exists, any additional physiological stressor, such as illness, dietary indiscretion, or nephrotoxic drugs, can lead to renal failure. The individual experiencing renal insufficiency may appear and feel well, even though laboratory data reflect deterioration in renal function. Renal insufficiency occurs as a phase in gradually but chronically progressive renal disease.

*Uremia* is a syndrome of renal failure characterized by elevated blood urea nitrogen (BUN) and creatinine levels. This syndrome (also referred to as *uremic syndrome*) is characterized by fatigue, anorexia, nausea, vomiting, pruritus, and neurological manifestations.

*Azotemia* is defined as an increase in serum urea and creatinine levels. The person with azotemia does not manifest symptoms of renal failure. Azotemia and uremia are sometimes inappropriately used synonymously. Both terms refer to the build up of nitrogenous waste products in the blood, which may contribute to the confusion regarding these two terms.

## ACUTE RENAL FAILURE

### ETIOLOGY

Renal failure refers to a significant loss of renal function; when only 10% of renal function remains, the person is considered to have *end-stage renal disease (ESRD)*.

*Acute renal failure (ARF)* is an abrupt decline in kidney function as defined by increases in BUN and plasma creatinine levels. Urine output is generally less than 40 ml/hr (oliguria) but may be normal or even increased. ARF can be further divided into prerenal, intrarenal or intrinsic, and postrenal etiologies.

Prerenal causes of ARF accounts for 55% to 70% of cases and is caused by intravascular volume depletion, decreased cardiac output, or vascular failure secondary to vasodilation or obstruction. Intrarenal causes account for 25% to 40% of cases of ARF. Intrarenal failure is caused by damage to the kidney tissues and structures and includes tubular necrosis, nephrotoxicity, and alterations in renal blood flow. Postrenal failure (approximately 5% of cases) is generally caused by obstruction of urine flow between the kidney and the urethral meatus. Box 45-1 outlines the causes for the development of acute renal failure.

## EPIDEMIOLOGY

Acute renal failure is a common problem, occurring in approximately 5% of hospitalized patients and up to 30% of patients admitted to intensive care areas. ARF is one of the leading causes of inpatient mortality. Oliguria accounts for 50% of cases of ARF and has a mortality of up to 80%.[2] Recovery from an episode of ARF depends on the underlying illness, the patient's condition, and management during the period of renal shut-down. Mortality associated with ARF approaches 50%. Acute tubular necrosis (ATN) is the cause of approximately 90% of all cases of intrinsic ARF. Although recovery statistics indicate that the kidney may regenerate more completely after toxic injury than after ischemic injury, follow-up studies of persons several years after episodes of ATN show normal or near-normal renal function.

For those in whom ARF has been caused by glomerular disease or severe infection of the kidneys, the prognosis may not be as favorable. Return of renal function is determined by the extent of scarring and obliteration of functional nephrons that occurred during the acute episode of kidney failure.

**box 45-1** *Causes of Acute Renal Failure*

**PRERENAL**
**Hypovolemia**
Hemorrhage
Dehydration
Vomiting
Gastric suction
Diabetes insipidus
Diabetes mellitus
Wound drainage
Cirrhosis
Diarrhea
Inappropriate use of diuretics
Diaphoresis
Burns
Peritonitis

**Decreased Cardiac Output**
Congestive heart failure
Myocardial infarction
Tamponade
Dysrhythmias

**Systemic Vasodilation**
Sepsis
Acidosis
Anaphylaxis

**Hypotension/Hypoperfusion**
Cardiac failure
Shock

**INTRARENAL (INTRINSIC)**
**Tubule/Nephron Damage**
Acute tubular necrosis (most common cause)
Glomerulonephritis
Rhabdomyolosis

**Vascular Changes**
Coagulopathies
Malignant hypertension
Sclerosis
Stenosis

**Nephrotoxins**
Antibiotics (gentamicin, tobramycin, amphotericin B, polymyxin B, neomycin, kanamycin, vancomycin
Chemicals (carbon tetrachloride, lead)
Heavy metals (arsenic, mercury)
Iodinated radiographic contrast media (IVP dye)
Drug-induced interstitial nephritis (nonsteroidal antiinflammatory agents, tetracyclines, furosemide, thiazides, phenytoin, penicillins, sulfonamides, cephalosporins)

**POSTRENAL**
**Ureteral and Bladder Neck Obstruction**
Calculi
Neoplasms
Prostatic hyperplasia

## PATHOPHYSIOLOGY

The kidneys receive approximately one fourth of the cardiac output; therefore they are very sensitive to alterations in perfusion. Most cases of ARF are caused by an ischemic episode. Ischemia causes nephron damage, although maintenance of fluid and electrolyte balance is possible with only 25% of nephrons functioning. A urinary output of at least 400 ml/day is necessary for adequate excretion of wastes. The decreased GFR that occurs in ARF is responsible for the increased BUN and serum creatinine levels.

The kidneys' response to hypoperfusion is the release of renin and an adaptive response to maintain perfusion to the glomerular bed. ARF develops when these adaptive responses are ineffective in maintaining normal kidney function.

The pathophysiology of ARF is not completely understood. Nephrotoxic factors and ischemia may produce acute renal failure.

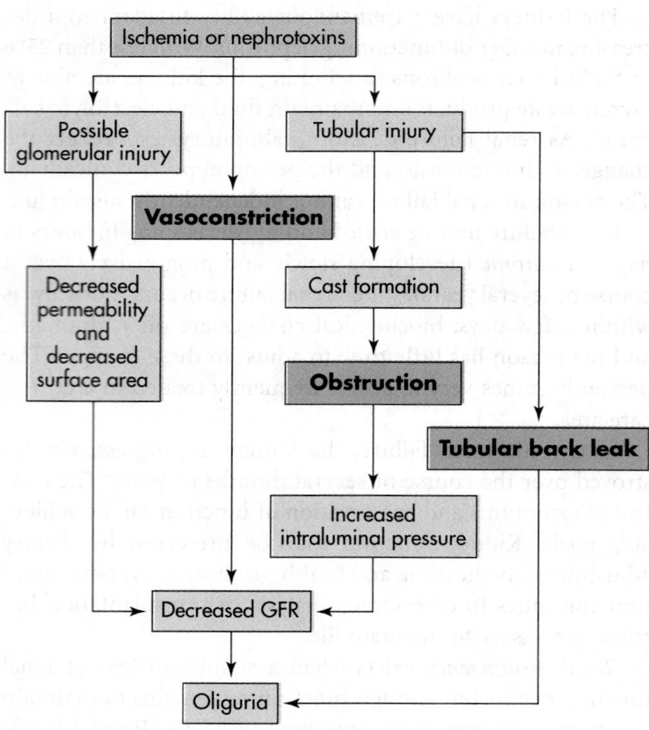


**fig. 45-1** Pathogenesis of acute renal failure.

Although a variety of conditions contribute to the development of ARF, ATN is the most common. ATN is classified as postischemic or nephrotoxic.

Ischemic events causing ATN occur most commonly after surgery (Box 45-1). Ischemia results in inflammation and causes cell swelling, injury, and necrosis along any part of the nephron. Necrosis associated with nephrotoxicity is generally limited to the proximal tubules.

There are three theories explaining the oliguria associated with ATN (Figure 45-1 and Table 45-1). Oliguria probably occurs as a result of a combination of all three mechanisms.

## Phases

Acute renal failure can be divided into four phases: onset, oliguric, diuretic, and recovery. The *onset* is the initial phase of injury to the kidney. Reversal or prevention of kidney dysfunction is possible at this stage by early intervention. The *oliguric* phase follows within 1 day of the onset. Major problems during the oliguric phase include inability to excrete fluid loads, regulate electrolytes, and excrete metabolic waste products. During the *diuretic* phase, large amounts of fluid (4 to 5 L/day) and electrolytes are lost. The *recovery* phase may last up to 12 months. Most patients are left with some residual renal dysfunction (Table 45-2).

Because of decreased kidney function, fluids are retained in the body, resulting in fluid overload and edema (see Chapter 15). When fluid overload is excessive, congestive heart failure and pulmonary edema may occur. Hypertension accompanies ARF when the person is hypervolemic.

Inability to excrete fluid loads leads to decreased urine output. Either oliguria or anuria (urine output less than 100 ml/day) may be present, although oliguria is more common. Classically, the patient in ARF shows a decrease in urine output to between 50 and 400 ml/day within 1 to 2 days. The urine specific gravity is low (1.010), and the osmolality of the urine approaches that of the person's serum (280 to 320 mOsm). Specific gravity and urine osmolality remain within this fixed range because the tubules have lost the ability to excrete sodium and water.[8]

**table 45-1** *Pathophysiological Theories of Oliguria of ATN*

| THEORY | PATHOPHYSIOLOGY |
|---|---|
| Tubular obstruction | Tubular necrosis causes cell sloughing or ischemic edema, which results in tubular obstruction. The GFR is decreased as a result of the obstruction. |
| Back leak | The GFR remains normal while tubular reabsorption of filtrate is increased. Ischemia is the underlying cause. |
| Alterations in renal blood flow | Exact mechanism is unknown. Ischemia may be responsible for changes in glomerular permeability and a fall in the GFR. Arteriolar constriction may be associated with the release of angiotensin II. |

The three major electrolyte problems are hyperkalemia, hyponatremia, and metabolic acidosis.

### Potassium imbalance

In the normal individual, the potassium ion is exchanged in the distal convoluted tubule of the nephron for either sodium or hydrogen ions; healthy persons cannot conserve the potassium ion. However, in the individual with ARF in whom many tubular cells are no longer functioning, no mechanism exists to remove potassium from the body. *Hyperkalemia* (the most sudden hazard in oliguric ARF) is said to exist when the serum concentration of this ion reaches a level of 5.5 mEq/L or higher. Serum concentrations of 7 to 10 mEq/L can be quickly reached in ARF and are incompatible with normal cardiac function and life.

The most reliable indicators of potassium toxicity are electrocardiography and laboratory determinations of serum potassium. Occasionally, neuromuscular symptoms such as paresthesias and paralysis (distal to proximal) are seen.[21] Changes in the patient's pulse are not reliable indicators of the amount of potassium excess.

### Sodium imbalance

Hyponatremia in ARF most often develops with overhydration. The oliguric patient cannot excrete large volumes of urine; as the administration of sodium-free or low-sodium intravenous or oral fluids continues, the serum is diluted, and the serum concentration of sodium falls.

Hyponatremia is accompanied or caused by hypervolemia. In the acutely ill patient, the situation typically occurs when the person receives numerous drugs and fluids in an attempt to treat coexisting life-threatening problems. When the volume of drugs and fluids cannot be reduced to a safe level, dialysis is required to remove the excess fluid and restore sodium balance.

Signs and symptoms of hyponatremia include warm, moist, flushed skin; muscle weakness; muscle twitching; and mental status changes such as confusion, delirium, coma, and convulsions. Serum sodium concentrations are less than 130 mEq/L. The hematocrit and hemoglobin values fall suddenly in the absence of bleeding because of hemodilution.

Increases in the total body content of sodium also occur in ARF when the patient is receiving medications high in sodium content and excess sodium in the diet. Edema and increasing blood pressure indicate retention of sodium and water, even though the serum sodium concentration is normal or below normal.

### Metabolic acidosis

Acidosis develops when hydrogen ion secretion and bicarbonate ion production diminish in the tubules. The pH of the blood decreases, the carbon dioxide content decreases, and central nervous system symptoms of drowsiness progressing to stupor and coma may appear (see Chapter 16). Although

**table 45-2** *Phases of Acute Renal Failure*

| Phase | Physiological Effect | Symptoms | Duration |
|---|---|---|---|
| **ONSET** | Initial phase of injury; hypotension, ischemia, hypovolemia | Subtle | Hours to days |
| **OLIGURIC** (Urine output <400 ml/24 hr or Urine output <30 ml/24 hr) | Inability to excrete metabolic wastes: increased serum urea nitrogen and creatinine; BUN may increase 20 mg/dl/day | Nausea, vomiting; drowsiness, confusion; coma; gastrointestinal bleeding; asterixis; pericarditis | 1-3 weeks, may extend to several weeks in older patients |
| | Inability to regulate electrolytes: hyperkalemia, hyponatremia, acidosis, hypocalcemia, hyperphosphatemia<br>Inability to excrete fluid loads: fluid overload, hypervolemia<br>Hematological dysfunction: anemia, platelet dysfunction, leukopenia<br>May still require dialysis | Nausea, vomiting; cardiac dysrhythmias, electrocardiogram changes; Kussmaul's breathing; drowsiness, confusion; coma; edema; congestive heart failure; pulmonary edema; neck vein distention; hypertension; fatigue; bleeding; infection | Duration also dependent upon type of toxic injury and duration of ischemia |
| **DIURETIC** (Urine output >1000 ml/24 hr) | Increased production of urine (deficit in concentrating ability of tubules and osmotic diuretic effect of high BUN); slowly increasing excretion of metabolic wastes; hypovolemia; loss of sodium; loss of potassium; high BUN initially; BUN gradually returns to baseline | Urine output of up to 4-5 L/day; postural hypotension; tachycardia; improving mental alertness and activity; weight loss; thirst; dry mucous membranes; decreased skin turgor | 2-6 weeks after onset of oliguria; duration varies |
| **RECOVERY** | Kidneys returning to normal functioning, some residual renal insufficiency; 30% of patients do not attain full recovery of GFR | Decreased energy levels | 3-12 months |

the lungs cannot totally compensate for the increasing acid load, they help determine the rate at which acidosis develops and the frequency or need for dialysis. In compensating for increased metabolic acid loads, the lungs attempt to excrete more carbon dioxide. Kussmaul's breathing is noted.

### Inability to Excrete Metabolic Wastes

Decreased kidney function alters the body's ability to eliminate metabolic waste products, producing the typical signs and symptoms of uremia. BUN and serum creatinine values rise sharply. In the person who has already sustained illness and trauma, BUN values may increase at a rate of 30 mg/dl/day. Signs and symptoms include neurological manifestations such as confusion, convulsions, coma, and asterixis. Gastrointestinal bleeding may result from uremic gastritis or colitis. Decreased cellular immunity causes an increased risk of infections. Bruising and bleeding result from changes in blood coagulation factors. Pericarditis is thought to develop as a result of pericardial irritation from accumulated metabolic wastes. A pericardial friction rub may be present on auscultation.

The increased output associated with the diuretic phase indicates that the damaged nephrons are healing and are able to begin excreting urine. Daily urine volume increases slowly, although within 1 to 2 days, diuresis up to or exceeding 4 to 5 L/day may occur. Although fluid can be excreted, the kidneys are not yet healed. Often the person is unable to excrete proportional amounts of waste products, and BUN and creatinine may rise or remain elevated as urine volume increases. At times, excessive excretion of sodium and potassium occurs during diuresis. Complete recovery of renal function is slow and requires weeks to months. Renal function is normal or near normal when the kidney can both concentrate and dilute urine, control serum electrolytes, and excrete nitrogenous wastes.

## COLLABORATIVE CARE MANAGEMENT

### Diagnostic Tests

When alterations in kidney function are suspected, an evaluation of BUN, creatinine, and electrolytes is indicated. Also, an urinalysis is beneficial to determine specific gravity, osmolality, and urine sodium content. Additional studies such as creatinine clearance, blood chemistry, complete blood count (CBC), arterial blood gases, and urine protein are indicated. See Table 45-3 for laboratory values in acute renal failure.

**table 45-3** *Laboratory Values in Acute Renal Failure*

| Finding | Prerenal | Intrarenal | Postrenal |
|---|---|---|---|
| **BLOOD VALUE** | | | |
| BUN | Increases | Increases | Increases |
| Creatinine | Normal | Increases | Increases |
| BUN/Creatinine ratio | 20:1 or greater (increased) | 10:1 or less (not increased because both values elevated) | Normal to slightly increased |
| **URINE VALUE** | | | |
| Urea | Decreases | Decreases | Decreases |
| Creatinine | ≈ normal | Decreases | Decreases |
| Specific gravity | 1.020 or more (increased) | Fixed and may be high | Variable |
| Volume | Oliguria | Nonoliguria or oliguria | Oliguria/polyuria |
| Osmolality | 400 mOsm or more (increases) | 250-350 mOsm (low and fixed, similar to plasma osmolality) | Anuria<br>Variable: increases or similar to plasma osmolality |

From Beare PG, Myers JL: *Adult health nursing,* ed 3, St Louis, 1998, Mosby.

Radiographic examinations of the kidney and surrounding structures are also useful in determining possible causes of ARF, particularly in postrenal failure. Ultrasonography, computed tomography (CT), intravenous pyelography (IVP), and magnetic resonance imaging can be done to rule out obstructive causes of renal failure. These procedures also determine the size and thickness of the kidneys. Enlarged kidneys may represent hydronephrosis. To visualize stones, a plain film of the abdomen may be helpful. Cystoscopy can be performed to visualize obstructions. If the etiology of ARF is unknown, a renal biopsy can help determine the cause.

### Medications

The use of medications in the treatment of ARF is determined by the underlying cause and the presenting symptoms. Hypovolemia is treated with hypotonic solutions such as 0.45% saline. If hypovolemia is due to blood or plasma loss, packed red blood cells and isotonic saline are administered. Volume replacement rates must match volume losses on a 1:1 basis. Loop diuretics are used to manage potassium levels. Doses of up to 320 mg/day of furosemide may be required to produce adequate diuresis.

Renal failure from nephrotoxins or ischemia is treated with agents that increase renal blood flow. These include renal-dose dopamine, mannitol, and loop diuretics. Inflammatory states as in acute glomerulonephritis are treated with glucocorticosteroids.

Patients with impaired renal function may have altered responses to therapeutic doses of many medications. Uremia alters the protein-binding sites, absorption, distribution, and metabolism of many drugs. Nonsteroidal antiinflammatory drugs and angiotensin-converting enzyme (ACE) inhibitors are contraindicated in patients with ARF.

### Treatments

When conservative management is not effective, dialysis is required. *Dialysis,* the process by which waste products in the blood are filtered through a semipermeable membrane, is indicated when the patient with ARF is fluid overloaded and/or has rapidly progressive azotemia, hyperkalemia, and metabolic acidosis. Three methods of dialysis are used: hemodialysis (see p. 1482), peritoneal dialysis (see p. 1482), and continuous renal replacement therapy.

#### Continuous renal replacement therapy

Continuous renal replacement therapy (CRRT) provides continuous (8 to 24 hours or more) ultrafiltration of extracellular fluid and clearance of uremic toxins. It must be administered in a critical care setting. This therapy does not require the use of a hemodialysis machine; instead it relies on the patient's own blood pressure to power the system. The ultrafiltration system is composed of arterial and venous tubing, the hemofilter, and an ultrafiltration collection receptacle. The success of CRRT depends on the maintenance of blood flow through the hemofilter. Both arterial and venous vascular access are required. Blood flows up to 200 ml/min can be obtained using an external arteriovenous shunt or percutaneous femoral catheter. In most patients, a mean arterial blood pressure of 60 mm Hg is required to maintain adequate blood flow (Figure 45-2).[21]

During CRRT, water, electrolytes, and other solutes are removed as the patient's blood passes over the semipermeable membrane in the hemofilter. The resulting ultrafiltrate is a protein-free fluid with solute and electrolyte concentrations similar to plasma. The plasma proteins and cellular components of the blood remain in the hemofilter circuit and return to the venous circulation. The mass transfer of water and solutes across a semipermeable membrane is a result of convection and diffusion. The convection forces applied across the hemofilter depend primarily on the patient's arterial blood pressure. The higher the blood pressure, the greater is the hydrostatic pressure within the hemofilter. Diffusion is the process by which solutes are passively transported across a semipermeable membrane and depends on the presence of a concentration gradient across the membrane. In CRRT, a

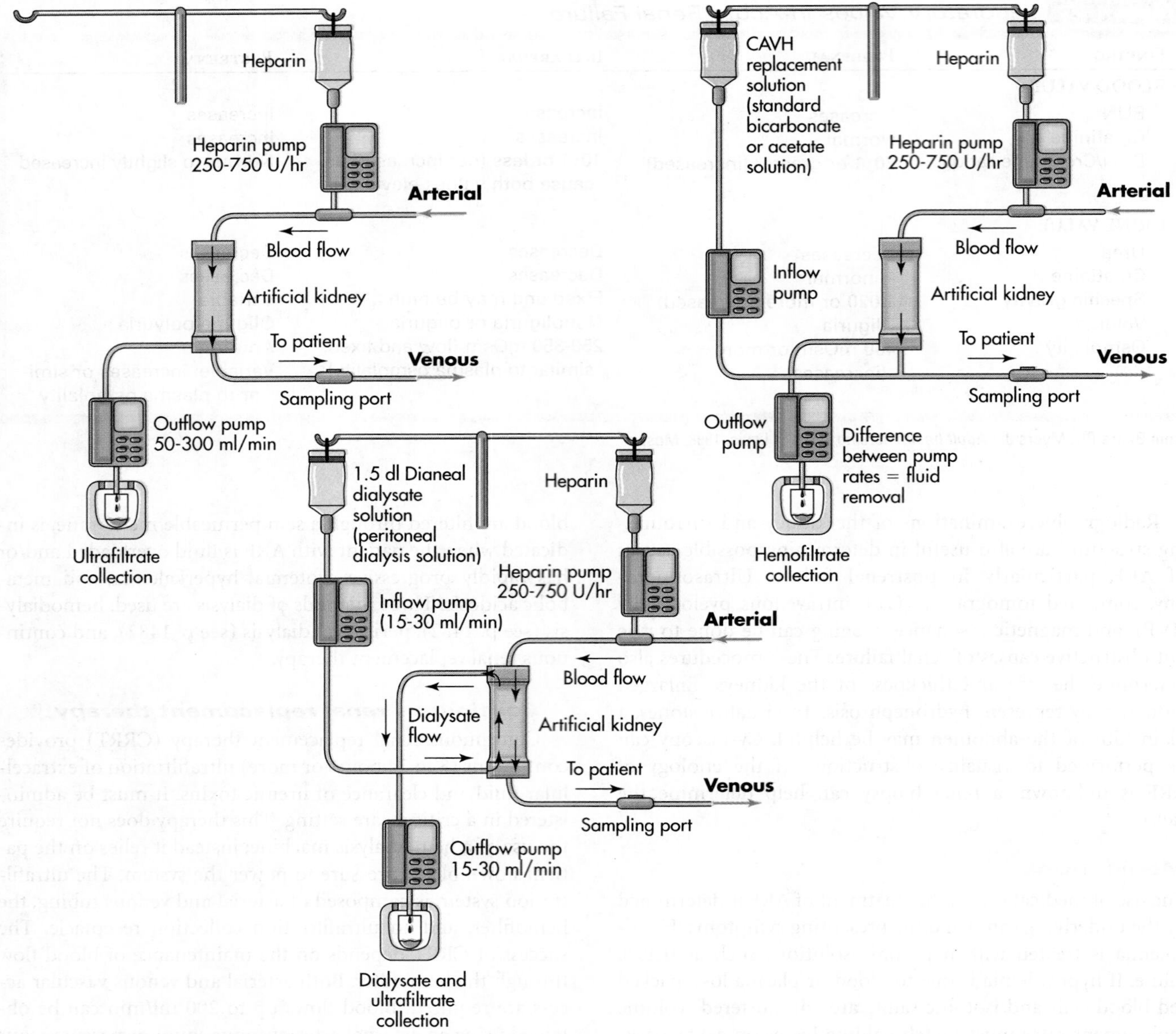


**fig. 45-2** Continuous renal replacement therapy. **A**, SCUF system setup. **B**, CAVH system setup. **C**, CAVHD system setup.

concentration gradient is established by infusing dialysate into the non–blood side of the hemofilter.

Removal of plasma water and electrolytes by CRRT is a gradual process that closely resembles the kidney's normal function. Because the process is gradual, rapid fluctuations in fluid and electrolyte status do not occur. Therefore CRRT is recommended for patients with ARF who are too hemodynamically unstable to tolerate hemodialysis or peritoneal dialysis. Patients who may benefit from CRRT are those with advanced cardiac disease, metabolic acidosis, abdominal wounds, cerebral edema, or sepsis.

Five variations of CRRT are in use: slow continuous ultrafiltration, continuous arteriovenous hemofiltration, continuous venovenous hemofiltration, continuous arteriovenous hemodialysis, and continuous venovenous hemodialysis. Each of these is designed to meet the renal replacement needs of a specific group of patients.

*Slow continuous ultrafiltration (SCUF)* slowly removes small amounts of plasma water and solutes at a rate of 150 to 300 ml/hr and is used to control fluid balance. SCUF is highly effective in patients with severe congestive heart failure who do not respond to diuretic therapy. Fluid removal by ultrafiltration can achieve significant preload reduction in these patients. This method is unsuitable for patients with ARF who are azotemic or have significant electrolyte abnormalities, because only small amounts of solutes are removed.

*Continuous arteriovenous hemofiltration (CAVH)* removes large amounts of plasma water and solutes at rates of 400 to

800 ml/hr. Control of fluid volume and electrolyte balance is achieved through large-volume fluid exchanges. Hourly ultrafiltrate loss is replaced by prescribed amounts of a sterile intravenous electrolyte solution. CAVH provides a mechanism of diluting the patient's plasma by selective replacement of solutes. It can be used as the primary dialysis therapy. Patients with ARF and mild to moderate azotemia and electrolyte disturbances can have CAVH as the primary method of dialysis.

*Continuous venovenous hemofiltration* is based on the principles of both SCUF and CAVH. Venous access is obtained with a double-lumen catheter, and the blood is pumped through a hemofilter.

*Continuous arteriovenous hemodialysis (CAVHD)* combines the convective transport of CAVH with diffusion dialysis. Sterile dialysate fluid is infused into the ultrafiltration compartment of the hemofilter. The dialysate flows countercurrent to the blood flow, which increases diffusion of solutes from the blood to the ultrafiltration compartment. Solute removal is much greater than in CAVH. CAVHD can be used as primary dialysis therapy in a wide variety of critically ill patients, including patients with ARF who have severe azotemia, electrolyte imbalances, and acid-base disturbances.

*Continuous venovenous hemodialysis (CVVH)* is the most recently developed mode of CRRT. The benefit of this mode is it does not require arterial access. Similar to CAVHD, it uses a pump to move dialysate opposite the blood flow to remove solute and fluid continuously. CVVH also minimizes effects on hemodynamic status.

The goals of nursing management for patients undergoing CRRT are optimization of the patient's fluid volume and hemodynamic status, maintenance of ultrafiltration system patency, prevention of blood loss from line disconnection, and prevention of infection. Emotional support is important for the patient and family while in a critical care setting.

During the diuretic phase, medical management centers around maintaining adequate fluid balance and regulating electrolytes. Even though the patient may be excreting large volumes of urine, dialysis may still be necessary to control electrolyte balance adequately. Protein restrictions are continued until BUN and serum creatinine levels decline.

### Diet

Dietary management is important for patients with all types of renal failure. Close collaboration between nurses, dietitians, and physicians is necessary to institute a diet that provides enough calories to avoid catabolism while preventing a surplus of nitrogen. Catabolism will lead to an increased BUN level because of the breakdown of muscle for protein. Generally, protein is restricted to 0.5 g/kg of body weight per day. Carbohydrate intake should be maintained at around 100 g/day. Sodium and potassium are restricted, as is free water in patients for whom hyponatremia is an issue. Dietary supplements are usually prescribed. Patients who are unable to take in sufficient nutrients may be candidates for total parenteral nutrition and administration of fat emulsions, which provide a nonprotein source of calories (see Chapter 40).

### Activity

The patient with ARF will experience fatigue and activity intolerance. Anemia may contribute to the fatigue. The acutely ill patient may need bedrest to decrease metabolic needs. A gradual resumption of activities will occur as kidney function improves. Frequent rest periods should be encouraged. As the patient's energy level increases, walking should be encouraged as an aerobic exercise.

### Referrals

A nutrition consultation is beneficial to establish the patient's caloric needs. Several agencies offer educational materials and resources for patients with kidney dysfunction. Examples include the National Kidney Foundation, 2 Park Ave., New York, NY 10006 and the American Kidney Fund, 7315 Wisconsin Ave., 203E, Bethesda, MD 20014.

## NURSING MANAGEMENT

## ■ ASSESSMENT

### Subjective Data

Data to be collected from the person with ARF or his or her significant other include:

- Voiding patterns, including any recent changes
- Weight gain (fluid retention)
- Nausea and vomiting
- Patient and family history of renal disease or trauma
- Medication use (prescription and over the counter)
- Recent surgery, anesthesia, or trauma
- Muscle weakness
- Mental status changes
- History of hypertension
- Exposure to nephrotoxins
- Medical history
- History of fatigue or lethargy
- Changes in bowel habits
- History of nausea or vomiting
- Presence of flank pain

### Objective Data

Objective data include:

- Amount of urine excreted in 24 hours
- Blood pressure, particularly postural changes
- Fluid status: presence of peripheral, periorbital, or sacral edema; lung sounds; skin turgor; daily weight
- Halitosis as a result of acidosis and/or ammonia secretion
- Mental status changes
- Pulse rate and rhythm
- Weight (compare to ideal body weight)
- Ecchymosis
- Pallor
- Muscle weakness
- Tachycardia

## NURSING DIAGNOSES

Nursing diagnoses are determined from analysis of patient data. Nursing diagnoses for the person with ARF may include but are not limited to:

| Diagnostic Title | Possible Etiological Factors |
|---|---|
| Fluid volume deficit/excess | Abnormal fluid loss, compromised regulatory mechanism |
| Nutrition, altered: less than body requirements | Anorexia, nausea, restricted diet |
| Activity intolerance | Biochemical alterations |
| Injury, risk for | Sensorimotor deficits, mental confusion |
| Infection, risk for | Decreased nutrition, decreased immune response |
| Coping, ineffective (individual) | Changes in health status |
| Knowledge deficit | Lack of exposure/recall |

## EXPECTED PATIENT OUTCOMES

Expected patient outcomes for the person with ARF during the oliguric phase may include but are not limited to:

1. Maintains fluid volume, electrolytes, and waste products at a functional level as evidenced by:
   a. Shows no pulmonary edema; has no or controls peripheral edema.
   b. Controls blood pressure (range between 140/90 and 100/60 mm Hg).
   c. Controls electrolyte balance: sodium 125 to 145 mEq/L, potassium 3.0 to 6.0 mEq/L, and bicarbonate greater than 14 mEq/L.
   d. Controls protein catabolism: BUN less than 100 mg/dl, creatinine less than 12 mg/dl, and absence of skin breakdown.
2. Verbalizes knowledge of a diet high in calories and fat and restricted in protein and potassium.
3. Reports increase in activity tolerance and decrease in fatigue.
4. Is free from injury.
5. Is free from infection.
6. Describes alternative ways of coping.
7. Verbalizes knowledge of nature of illness, diet therapy, signs and symptoms to be reported to physician, and plans for follow-up care.

## INTERVENTIONS

Nursing care focuses on three broad objectives: (1) monitoring for signs of fluid overload, (2) maintaining the patient's energy expenditure at a level compatible with the individual's state of health, and (3) controlling or helping to control fluid intake (Guidelines for Care Box).

### Maintaining Fluid and Electrolyte Balance

Control of fluids is essential during the oliguric phase of ARF because of the deceased ability of the kidneys to excrete urine. All observations about the patient's state of hydration need to be recorded so that hour-to-hour and day-to-day comparisons can

**guidelines for care**

**The Person with Acute Renal Failure**

1. Maintaining fluid and electrolyte balance
   a. Maintain fluid restrictions.
   b. Monitor intravenous fluids carefully.
   c. Keep accurate records of intake and output.
   d. Weigh patient daily.
   e. Monitor vital signs frequently, including postural signs.
   f. Assess fluid status of patient frequently.
   g. Administer phosphate-binding medications as prescribed.
   h. Monitor serum electrolytes.
   i. During diuretic phase:
      (1) Assess for changes in mental status indicative of low serum levels.
      (2) Assess for presence of irregular apical pulse indicative of hypokalemia.
2. Maintaining nutrition
   a. Provide fluid in small amounts during oliguric phase; ginger ale and other effervescent soft drinks may be tolerated better than other fluids.
   b. Provide a diet:
      (1) Restricted in protein, as prescribed.
      (2) High in carbohydrates and fat during protein restriction.
      (3) Low in potassium during hyperkalemia and high in potassium during hypokalemia.
   c. Take measures to relieve nausea (antiemetics and comfort measures).
3. Maintaining rest/activity balance
   a. Maintain bedrest in the acute phase.
   b. Assist patient with activities of daily living to conserve energy.
   c. Promote early ambulation when renal status permits.
   d. Provide for planned rest periods.
4. Preventing injury
   a. Assess orientation; reorient confused patient.
   b. During bedrest, keep side rails raised and use padded rails as necessary.
   c. When patient is ambulatory, assess motor skills and monitor ambulation; assist patient as necessary.
   d. Assess patient for signs of bleeding.
   e. Protect patient from bleeding: instruct patient to use soft toothbrush; perform guaiac tests on stool, emesis, and nasogastric returns.
5. Preventing infection
   a. Avoid sources of infection; limit visitors to well adults.
   b. Assess for signs and symptoms of infection.
   c. Maintain asepsis for indwelling lines or catheters.
   d. Perform pulmonary hygiene.
   e. Turn weak or immobile patients every 2 hours and as needed.
   f. Provide meticulous skin care.
   g. Bathe patient with superfat soap.
   h. Administer prescribed antipruritic agents.
6. Facilitating coping
   a. Encourage development of nurse-patient relationship to assist patient to express feelings as desired.
   b. Promote patient independence.
   c. Assist patient to explore alternative ways of coping.

be made. Any finding indicating fluid retention is reported to the health care provider. Edema can first be noted in dependent areas such as the feet and legs, in the presacral area, and around the eyes (periorbital). It is important to remember, however, that edema may not be detected until the person has gained 5 to 10 pounds (2 to 5 kg) in fluid. The person is observed carefully for signs of pulmonary edema and congestive heart failure (see Chapter 26).

Central venous lines or arterial monitoring lines will help provide data for short-term comparisons in managing the fluid balance of the critically ill person. Positioning and activity are determined daily based on assessment of the person's energy level and ability to breath adequately.

All fluid (parenteral and oral) input must total only slightly more than daily output if severe overhydration is to be avoided. Devices that allow precise control of intravenous fluids help avoid fluid overload when giving parenteral fluids to anuric or oliguric patients. Accuracy in fluid balance records is essential.

### Promoting Nutrition

Most patients with ARF are too ill to tolerate oral feedings. Oral intake can exacerbate nausea as a result of the altered biochemical environment and accompanying gastrointestinal tract irritation. If the patient is able tolerate oral feedings, dietary protein and potassium are restricted to modest amounts, thus increasing protein available for tissue building and increasing the palatability of the diet without leading to metabolic waste buildup or hyperkalemia.

A high-carbohydrate, high-fat diet is encouraged. Calories in the form of carbohydrates and fats provide energy and spare body protein stores, thus decreasing nonprotein nitrogen production. The body recycles urea to synthesize amino acids for protein building so that some regeneration of tissues can occur even though protein intake is curtailed.

### Promoting Rest/Activity Balance

The patient will need strict bedrest in the acute phase to decrease metabolic activity. Assistance will be needed with activities of daily living (ADL). Rest periods are encouraged to conserve patient energy. As renal function improves, progressive ambulation is indicated.

### Preventing Injury

The patient with ARF is weak, may be confused, and may have visual changes, thus increasing risk of falls. The amount of supervision required during daily care must be assessed continually and appropriate actions taken to prevent injury. The confused, agitated, or restless patient must be protected from injury; keep side rails elevated and pad them if necessary. To allay patient/family anxiety, explain the rationale for the mental status changes (electrolyte imbalance and uremia) (see Chapter 9). Meticulous skin care should be provided to prevent skin breakdown from edema.

Bleeding may occur from changes in blood coagulation factors. Nursing interventions should include measures to prevent and detect bleeding. (Further information on protection from bleeding can be found in Chapter 29.)

### Preventing Infection

Infection leads to tissue breakdown with production of metabolic wastes, which are difficult to eliminate for the patient with ARF. Aseptic technique must be maintained during all treatments, especially with invasive lines and catheters. Sources of infection should be avoided. Pruritus frequently occurs and may lead to skin lesions from scratching. Measures to relieve pruritus include bathing the patient with a superfat soap and administering prescribed antipruritics as necessary.

In compensating for increased metabolic acid loads, the lungs attempt to excrete more carbon dioxide. Pulmonary hygiene measures should be carried out to maximize this pathway for acid excretion, to maintain maximal lung expansion, and to prevent atelectasis.

### Promoting Coping

During the oliguric phase of illness, the biochemical alterations may affect not only the level of awareness but also the patient's personality. Family members and occasionally the patient will be aware of these changes, such as faltering memory or an inability to think clearly. Reassure the patient and family that mental capacities will return with recovery of kidney function. Structuring the environment and activities may help with coping in the initial phase. The nurse can assist the patient to explore feelings concerning the nature of the illness and find effective ways of coping.

### Patient/Family Education

Most of the patient teaching takes place after the acute phase of the illness is over; the patient is usually more receptive to teaching at this time. Items to include in the teaching plan are listed in the Patient/Family Teaching Box.

**patient/family teaching**

**The Person with Acute Renal Failure**

1. Cause of renal failure and problems with recurrent failures
2. Identification of preventable environmental or health factors contributing to the illness, such as hypertension and nephrotoxic drugs
3. Prescribed medication regimen, including name of medication, dosage, reason for taking, desired and adverse effects
4. Prescribed dietary regimen
5. Explanation of risk of hypokalemia and reportable symptoms (muscle weakness, anorexia, nausea and vomiting, lethargy)
6. Signs and symptoms of returning renal failure (decreased urine output without decreased fluid intake, signs of fluid retention, and increased weight)
7. Signs and symptoms of infection; methods to avoid infection
8. Need for ongoing follow-up care
9. Options for future; explanation of transplantation and dialysis if these are a possibility

### *Health promotion/prevention*

**Primary prevention.** The incidence of ARF can be reduced by the identification and control of environmental risk factors. A significant factor in preventive care is the control of nephrotoxic drugs. Attempts to control the distribution and identification of nephrotoxic drugs and chemicals are primarily accomplished through the Food and Drug Administration (FDA). Identification of nephrotoxic drugs and chemicals, enforced labeling of these substances, and drug dispensing only by prescription are examples of the FDA's attempts to promote public health. Proper labeling and storage of potentially toxic drugs and chemicals in the home can further reduce the number of accidental ingestions of nephrotoxic substances. Cleaners and solvents should be used in well-ventilated areas.

**Secondary prevention.** Prevention of ARF includes increased medical supervision of persons with sore throats and upper respiratory infections and detection and treatment of individuals with bacteriuria and obstructive disease of the urinary system. The greatest incidence of ARF occurs in persons with major trauma, extensive burns, surgery of the heart or large blood vessels, massive blood loss, and severe myocardial infarction. Frequent monitoring of urine output and detection of excessive losses of body fluid of these patients can help to identify instances of inadequate renal perfusion before renal failure develops.

## ■ EVALUATION

To evaluate the effectiveness of nursing interventions, compare patient behaviors with those stated in the expected patient outcomes. Successful achievement of patient outcomes for the patient with ARF is indicated by:

1. Fluid balance normal, electrolytes and waste products are at functional level.
   a. No signs of respiratory distress, pulmonary or peripheral edema.
   b. Blood pressures range between 140/90 and 100/60.
   c. Serum electrolytes are controlled: sodium 125 to 145 mEq/L, potassium 3.0 to 6.0 mEq/L, and bicarbonate greater than 14 mEq/L.
   d. Protein catabolism is controlled: BUN less than 100 mg/dl, creatinine less than 12 mg/dl, and absence of skin breakdown.
2. Eats diet high in calories and fat and restricted in protein and potassium.
3. Reports increased energy and rest.
4. No falls or bleeding occurs; is free from injury.
5. Is free from infection.
6. Uses effective methods of coping; manages ADL to full extent of ability.
7. Verbalizes knowledge of ARF, diet therapy, signs and symptoms to be reported to physician, and plans for follow-up care.

## GERONTOLOGICAL CONSIDERATIONS

Mortality in acute renal failure is greatest in the elderly population partially because of the prevalence of heart disease, hypertension, and diabetes in this population. Chronic illness and polypharmacy in the aging population can tax the kidneys. Early signs of ARF are vague and may be attributed to other causes. In the older person, signs of acute infection may be absent or diminished. Changes in mental status related to electrolyte imbalances may be attributed to early signs of dementia. In elderly men, decreased urine output, a sign of renal failure, may be mistakenly attributed to benign prostatic hypertrophy.

Although the treatment for acute renal failure remains the same regardless of the patient's age, treatment strategies are not tolerated easily in the older adult. Intravascular volume overload is particularly difficult to treat because of the increased risk of congestive heart failure. Older patients are much more likely to succumb to the severity of ARF because of an increased risk of complications such as pneumonia and sepsis.

## SPECIAL ENVIRONMENTS FOR CARE

### Critical Care Management

Most patients in the acute stages of ARF will be cared for in the intensive care unit because of the need for constant monitoring of blood pressure, electrocardiogram, pulmonary status, and mental status. Many patients will require mechanical ventilation and hemodynamic monitoring via a Swan-Ganz catheter to monitor intravascular fluid volume.

Patients who cannot tolerate hemodialysis because of hemodynamic instability may be treated with CRRT (see p. 1469). These patients require one-to-one nursing care to continuously monitor blood pressure, administer and titrate medications, and maintain the patency of the system. The type of CRRT chosen is patient specific and is selected after careful assessment of hemodynamic status, fluid and electrolyte balance, and laboratory and clinical manifestations.

### Home Care Management

The home needs of the patient recovering from acute renal failure vary depending on the success of therapy. If progressing well through the recovery phase, the patient may be discharged from the hospital with instructions to follow-up with his or her health care provider. Patients must be alert to early signs and symptoms of renal failure. It may be necessary for a visiting nurse to monitor hemodynamic status. Mental status should also be assessed to alert the nurse of early changes in electrolyte balance. Patients may also be discharged with a venous/arterial access device and will need assistance with dressing changes, care of the device, and monitoring for signs of infection.

## COMPLICATIONS

The leading complication of ARF is the development of chronic renal failure. Approximately 50% of patients will have some impairment of glomerular filtration. About 5% will never regain kidney function and will require long-term hemodialysis or renal transplantation. An additional 5% will slowly develop chronic renal failure after initial recovery.[3]

# CHRONIC RENAL FAILURE

## ETIOLOGY

Chronic renal failure (CRF) exists when the kidneys are no longer capable of maintaining an internal environment that is consistent with life and damage to the kidneys is irreversible. For most individuals, the transition from health to a state of chronic or permanent illness is a slow process that may occur over a number of years. Recurrent infections and exacerbations of nephritis, obstruction of the urinary tract, systemic disease, and destruction of blood vessels from diabetes and longstanding hypertension can lead to scarring in the kidney and progressive loss of renal function (Box 45-2). Some individuals, however, develop total irreversible loss of renal function acutely. Such loss of renal function usually develops in a few hours or days and follows direct traumatic kidney insult. The leading causes of ESRD in order of occurrence are (1) diabetes mellitus 32%, (2) hypertension 28%, and (3) glomerulonephritis 15%.

## EPIDEMIOLOGY

Chronic renal failure remains a significant health problem in the United States. More than 200,000 people have ESRD, and the number increases annually by 7%. The disease can affect persons of all ages, but the peak incidence is between 20 and 64 years of age.

Until the 1970s, treatment for end-stage renal disease was cost-prohibitive to many patients. At the present time, private insurance as well as government programs subsidize most treatments for CRF.[1] Medicare benefits were extended to persons with ESRD by legislation passed in 1973.

## PATHOPHYSIOLOGY

Chronic renal failure differs from acute renal failure in that the damage to the kidneys is progressive and irreversible. Progression of CRF is through four stages: decreased renal reserve, renal insufficiency, renal failure, and ESRD (Box 45-3). However, in practice, these stages are not sharply differentiated. Severe symptoms occur at the renal failure stage. As many as 50% of nephrons are destroyed before renal deficits are apparent.

The specific pathophysiological mechanisms depend on the underlying disease causing the destruction of the kidney. The following general pathophysiological mechanism summarizes these changes. During chronic renal failure, some of the nephrons (including the glomeruli and tubules) are thought to remain intact while others are destroyed *(intact nephron hypothesis)*. The intact nephrons hypertrophy and produce an increased volume of filtrate with increased tubular reabsorption despite a decreased GFR. This adaptive method permits the kidney to function until about three fourths of the nephrons are destroyed. The solute load then becomes greater than can be reabsorbed, producing an osmotic diuresis with polyuria and thirst. Eventually, as more nephrons are damaged, oliguria occurs, resulting in retention of waste products.

Although the clinical course of chronic renal failure varies, some common features exist. Signs and symptoms result from disordered fluid and electrolyte balance, alterations in regulatory functions of the body, and retention of solutes. Anemia results from impaired red blood cell (RBC) production because of decreased secretion of erythropoietin by the kidney. Patients may report lethargy, dizziness, and fatigue. In

**box 45-2** *Causes of Chronic Renal Failure*

**GLOMERULAR DYSFUNCTION**
Glomerulonephritis
Diabetic nephropathy
Hypertensive nephrosclerosis

**SYSTEMIC DISEASE**
Sickle cell anemia
Scleroderma
Polyarteritis nodosa
Systemic lupus erythematosus
Human immunodeficiency virus-associated nephropathy
Vasculitis

**URINARY TRACT OBSTRUCTION**
Prostatic and bladder tumors
Lymphadenopathy
Ureteral obstruction
Calculi

**OTHER**
Chronic pyelonephritis
Nephrotic syndrome
Polycystic kidney disease
Renal infarction
Cyclosporin nephrotoxicity
Multiple myeloma

**box 45-3** *Stages of Chronic Renal Failure*

**DECREASED RENAL RESERVE (RENAL IMPAIRMENT)**
40-75% loss of nephron function
GFR 40%-50% of normal
BUN and serum creatinine levels normal
Patient asymptomatic

**RENAL INSUFFICIENCY**
75-80% loss of nephron function
GFR 20%-40% of normal
BUN and serum creatinine levels begin to rise
Mild anemia; mild azotemia, which worsens with physiological stress
Nocturia, polyuria

**RENAL FAILURE**
GFR 10%-20% of normal
BUN and serum creatinine levels increase
Anemia, azotemia, metabolic acidosis
Urine specific gravity low
Polyuria, nocturia
Symptoms of renal failure

**END-STAGE RENAL DISEASE (ESRD)**
>85% loss of nephron function
GFR <10% of normal
BUN and serum creatinine at high levels
Anemia, azotemia, metabolic acidosis
Urine specific gravity fixed at 1.010
Oliguria
Symptoms of renal failure

addition, the life span of RBCs is shortened as a result of uremia and superimposed nutritional anemia resulting from dietary restrictions. Azotemia and acidosis are present, and potassium and hydrogen ion excretion is impaired. Fluid and sodium balance is abnormal and may involve either abnormal retention or secretion of sodium and water; therefore urine volume can be increased, normal, or decreased.[23]

Hyperuricemia is a common finding in ESRD although the varied serum levels of uric acid do not seem to have a definite relationship with the level of kidney function. Increased levels of serum phosphate are characteristic, and calcium levels may be low or normal. These findings result from decreased renal excretion of phosphate and a simultaneous reduction in ionized serum calcium. Through increased production of parathormone, the body may reestablish a normal serum calcium level, at the expense of the bone matrix.

Hypertension may or may not be present. As ESRD develops, blood pressure is elevated because of increased total body water, a renally released vasopressor, and inadequately secreted vasodepressors. Glucose intolerance may be seen, although usually not of sufficient severity to warrant treatment. The rising blood glucose level appears to be the result of an altered biochemical environment produced by the failing kidneys and does not signify the development of diabetes mellitus. As renal failure progresses, the patient develops increased pigmentation of the skin; the skin becomes sallow or brownish in color. *Uremic frost* is a pale deposit of crystals on the skin caused by kidney failure and uremia. Metabolic waste products, unable to be excreted by the kidney, are instead excreted through the small capillaries of the skin. With more advanced and insufficiently treated renal failure, the patient may develop muscular twitching, numbness in the feet and legs, pericarditis, and pleuritis. These signs usually resolve when the patient is treated by dietary modifications, medication, and/or dialysis.

The symptoms of uremia usually develop so slowly that the patient and family often cannot identify the time of onset. Symptoms of azotemia develop, which include lethargy, headaches, physical and mental fatigue, weight loss, irritability, and depression. Anorexia, persistent nausea and vomiting, shortness of breath, and pitting edema are symptomatic of severe loss of renal function. Pruritus may be present. All body systems are affected by CRF (Table 45-4).

**table 45-4** *Body System Manifestations in Chronic Renal Failure*

| CAUSES | SIGNS/SYMPTOMS | ASSESSMENT PARAMETERS |
|---|---|---|
| **HEMATOPOIETIC SYSTEM** | | |
| Decreased erythropoietin by the kidney | Anemia | Hematocrit |
| Decreased survival time of RBCs | Fatigue | Hemoglobin |
| Bleeding | Defects in platelet function | Platelet count |
| Blood loss during dialysis | Thrombocytopenia | Observe for bruising, hematemesis, or melena |
| Mild thrombocytopenia | Ecchymosis | |
| Decreased activity of platelets | Bleeding | |
| **CARDIOVASCULAR SYSTEM** | | |
| Fluid overload | Hypervolemia | Vital signs |
| Renin-angiotensin mechanism | Hypertension | Body weight |
| Fluid overload, anemia | Tachycardia | Electrocardiogram |
| Chronic hypertension | Dysrhythmias | Heart sounds |
| Calcification of soft tissues | Congestive heart failure | Monitor electrolytes |
| Uremic toxins in pericardial fluid | Pericarditis | Assess for pain |
| Fibrin formation on epicardium | | |
| **RESPIRATORY SYSTEM** | | |
| Compensatory mechanisms for metabolic acidosis | Tachypnea | Respiratory assessment |
| | Kussmaul's respirations | Arterial blood gas results |
| Uremic toxins | Uremic fetor (or uremic halitosis) | Inspection of oral mucosa |
| Uremic lung | Tenacious sputum | Vital signs |
| Fluid overload | Pain with coughing | Pulse oximetry |
| | Elevated temperature | |
| | Hilar pneumonitis | |
| | Pleural friction rub | |
| | Pulmonary edema | |
| **GASTROINTESTINAL SYSTEM** | | |
| Change in platelet activity | Anorexia | Monitor intake and output |
| Serum uremic toxins | Nausea and vomiting | Hematocrit |
| Electrolyte imbalances | Gastrointestinal bleeding | Hemoglobin |
| Urea converted to ammonia by saliva | Abdominal distention | Guaiac test for all stools |
| | Diarrhea | Assess quality of stools |
| | Constipation | Assess for abdominal pain |

*Continued*

As ESRD develops, most women note changes in their menstrual cycle. Bleeding may occur at more widely spaced intervals, may be heavier or lighter in flow than normal, or may cease altogether. This obvious change in reproductive cycle is usually accompanied by changes in fertility. Ovulation may occur normally or may occur only a few times a year. Pregnancy in uremic women is of much lower incidence than in the normal population. ESRD cannot be used as an effective method of birth control. In men, erectile dysfunction may occur as chronic renal failure progresses toward ESRD. Dialysis or more vigorous treatment of uremia is indicated to return or maximize reproductive function. It should be stressed that sexual activity of some persons with chronic renal failure may remain quite normal even though changes occur in reproductive ability.

The point at which the patient becomes obviously symptomatic and displays signs typical of renal failure occurs when approximately 80% to 90% of renal function has been lost (Figure 45-3). At this level of renal function, creatinine clearance values will fall to 10 ml/min or less.

Hypertriglyceridemia occurs in approximately 30% to 70% of persons with CRF. Atherosclerosis may develop as a result of an elevated ratio of high-density lipoproteins (HDL) to low-density lipoproteins (LDL). The production of HDL decreases because of decreased lipolytic activity caused by uremia.

Catabolism and proteinuria contribute to the negative nitrogen balance common in CRF. Muscle mass diminishes. Proteinuria adds to kidney damage by increasing inflammation.

## COLLABORATIVE CARE MANAGEMENT

### Diagnostic Tests

Because of the multisystemic effects of CRF, many serious abnormalities in laboratory values are characteristic of persons with CRF. Serum creatinine levels are essential in the evaluation of renal function. Increased levels of creatinine are seen only when a significant number of nephrons are destroyed, resulting in impaired creatinine excretion. A 12- or 24-hour urinary creatinine clearance test evaluates renal function and

**table 45-4** *Body System Manifestations in Chronic Renal Failure—cont'd*

| Causes | Signs/Symptoms | Assessment Parameters |
|---|---|---|
| **NEUROLOGICAL SYSTEM** | | |
| Uremic toxins | Lethargy, confusion | Level of orientation |
| Electrolyte imbalances | Convulsions | Level of consciousness |
| Cerebral swelling resulting from fluid shifting | Stupor, coma | Reflexes |
| | Sleep disturbances | Electroencephalogram |
| | Unusual behavior | Electrolyte levels |
| | Asterixis | |
| | Muscle irritability | |
| **SKELETAL SYSTEM** | | |
| Decreased calcium absorption | Renal osteodystrophy | Serum phosphorus |
| Decreased phosphate excretion | Renal rickets | Serum calcium |
| | Joint pain | Assess for joint pain |
| | Retarded growth | |
| **SKIN** | | |
| Anemia | Pallor | Observe for bruising |
| Pigment retained | Pigmentation | Assess color of skin |
| Decreased size of sweat glands | Pruritus | Assess integrity of skin |
| Decreased activity of oil glands | Ecchymosis | Observe for scratching |
| Dry skin; phosphate deposits | Excoriation | |
| Excretion of metabolic waste products through the skin | Uremic frost | |
| **GENITOURINARY SYSTEM** | | |
| Damaged nephrons | Decreased urine output | Monitor intake and output |
| | Decreased urine specific gravity | Serum creatinine |
| | Proteinuria | BUN |
| | Casts and cells in urine | Serum electrolytes |
| | Decreased urine sodium | Urine specific gravity |
| | | Urine electrolytes |
| **REPRODUCTIVE SYSTEM** | | |
| Hormonal abnormalities | Infertility | Monitor intake and output |
| Anemia | Decreased libido | Monitor vital signs |
| Hypertension | Erectile dysfunction | Hematocrit |
| Malnutrition | Amenorrhea | Hemoglobin |
| Medications | Delayed puberty | |

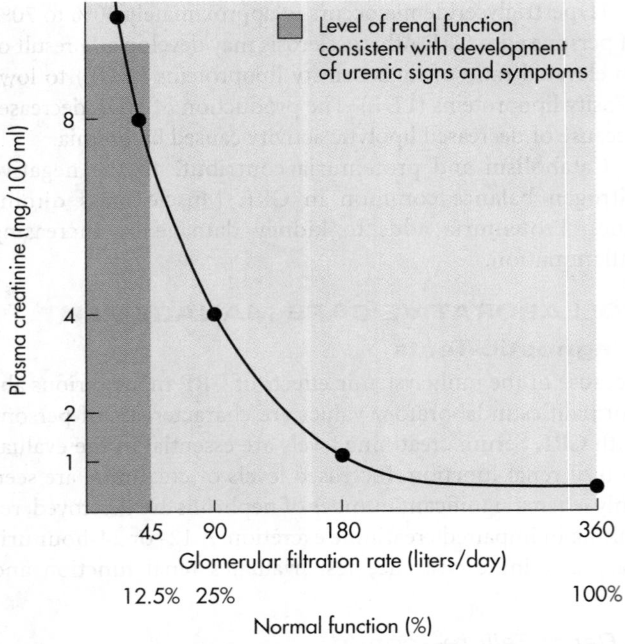


**fig. 45-3** Glomerular filtration and plasma creatinine levels.

determines the degree of dysfunction. This test is the most specific indicator of renal function. The creatinine clearance rate is equal to the GFR. Measurements of serum and urinary creatinine levels and urine volume are necessary to complete the test. A creatinine clearance less than 10 ml/min is indicative of severe renal impairment. Renal creatinine clearance is calculated based on 24-hour urine results (including serum and urinary levels) and data on body weight and height.

The BUN to creatinine ratio is also useful in evaluating renal function. The creatinine level will change only in response to renal dysfunction, while the BUN level will change in response to dehydration or protein breakdown.

Blood chemistry analysis, CBC, and urinalysis are performed to evaluate the degree of impairment in patients with CRF (Table 45-5). Urinary output declines with the progression of renal failure; hence urinalysis may not provide as much information as other laboratory tests.

Radiographic examinations are of little use in the evaluation of the patient with ESRD. A kidney, ureters, and bladder (KUB) film can evaluate kidney size, shape, and position. The patient with ESRD will often have atrophic kidneys. Ultrasound or CT may be ordered to evaluate possible obstruction. CT is preferably performed without contrast because of the nephrotoxicity potential of the contrast agent.

### Medications

Initial management of patients with CRF is focused on controlling symptoms, preventing complications, and delaying the progression of renal failure (see Box 45-4 for treatment goals). Medications are used to control blood pressure, regulate electrolytes, and control intravascular fluid volume.

Hypertension is controlled by the use of ACE inhibitors. Calcium channel blockers and β-blockers are also used if blood pressure cannot be controlled with a single agent. Immunosuppressive therapy is instituted in patients with glomerulonephritis.[3] Intravascular fluid volume is regulated by the use of diuretics.[18]

Electrolyte imbalances are corrected by the use of sodium bicarbonate for metabolic acidosis. Hyperkalemia is treated with a combination of insulin and dextrose or sodium poly-

**table 45-5** *Laboratory Findings in Chronic Renal Failure*

| Test | Normal Values | Findings in CRF |
|---|---|---|
| **SERUM CREATININE** | | |
| Male | 0.6-1.5 mg/dl | Elevated |
| Female | 0.5-1.1 mg/dl | >4 mg/dl indicates significant renal impairment |
| Elderly | Decreased (due to decreased muscle mass) | May rise to 30 mg/dl before symptoms appear |
| **BUN** | 7-20 mg/dl | |
| Elderly | 8-21 mg/dl | Values >100 mg/dl indicate severe renal impairment* |
| **BLOOD CHEMISTRY** | | |
| Sodium | 135-145 mEq/L | Decreased |
| Potassium | 3.5-5 mEq/L | Increased |
| Calcium | | |
| Total | 8.5-10.5 mg/dl | Decreased |
| Ionized | 4.5-5.6 mg/dl | |
| Phosphorus | 2.7-4.5 mg/dl | Increased |
| Magnesium | 1.2-1.9 mEq/L | Increased |
| Serum pH | 7.35-7.45 | Decreased (metabolic acidosis) or normal |
| Serum bicarbonate | 22-26 mEq/L | Decreased |
| **COMPLETE BLOOD COUNT** | | |
| Hemoglobin | | |
| Male | 10-17 g/dl | Decreased |
| Female | 11.5-15.5 g/dl | |
| Elderly | Decreased | |
| Hematocrit | | |
| Male | 39-49% | Decreased (may rise to near normal with epoetin therapy) |
| Female | 33-43% | |
| Elderly | Decreased | |
| **CREATININE CLEARANCE** | | |
| Male | 70-150 ml/min | Decreased |
| Female | 85-130 ml/min | Findings <10 ml/min indicative of renal impairment |
| Elderly | Decreased up to 30% in absence of renal disease | Decrease reflects decreases in GFR |
| **URIC ACID (SERUM)** | | |
| Male | 2.1-8.5 mg/dl | Increased |
| Female | 2.0-6.8 mg/dl | Findings >12 mg/dl indicate serious renal impairment |
| Elderly | 3.5-8.5 mg/dl | |

*Increased levels dependent on protein intake, liver disease, and hydration status.

**box 45-4** *Treatment Goals for the Person with Chronic Renal Failure*

1. Stabilization of the internal environment as demonstrated by:
   a. Mental alertness, attention span, and appropriate interactions
   b. Absence or control of peripheral and pulmonary edema
   c. Control of electrolyte balance within the following limits:

| | |
|---|---|
| Sodium | 125 to 145 mEq/L |
| Potassium | 3-6 mEq/L |
| Bicarbonate | >15 mEq/L |
| Calcium | 9-11 mg/dl |
| Phosphate | 3-5 mg/dl |

   d. Serum albumin >2 g/dl
   e. Control of protein catabolism and protein metabolic wastes as indicated by the following parameters:

| | |
|---|---|
| Urea nitrogen | <100 mg/dl |
| Creatinine | <10 mg/dl |
| Uric acid | <12 mg/dl |

   f. Absence of joint inflammation and pain
   g. Control of anemia

| | |
|---|---|
| Hematocrit | ≥33% |
| Ferritin | >50-100 ng/ml |
| Iron saturation | >20% |

2. Absence of infection
3. Absence of bleeding
4. Blood pressure controlled at <140/90 mm Hg sitting, <10 mm Hg postural change on standing
5. Control of coexisting disease including:
   a. Heart failure
   b. Anemia
   c. Dehydration
6. Absence of toxicity from inadequately excreted medications
7. Nutrient intake sufficient to maintain positive nitrogen balance
8. Anorexia and nausea controlled
9. Pruritus controlled

styrene sulfonate (Kayexalate). Calcium and phosphorus levels are maintained by the use of phosphate-binding agents, calcium supplements, and vitamin D.

## Treatments

### Fluid control

Changes in the ability to regulate sodium and water excretion are often the first clinical signs of renal failure. The ability to excrete sodium and water can vary considerably from one patient with chronic renal failure to the next. Although volume problems for most patients involve hypervolemia resulting from a marked inability to excrete sodium and water, some patients are unable to conserve these substances and hypovolemia results. With marked inability either to excrete or conserve body fluid, the patient can develop severe fluid imbalances in a relatively short time. Fluid imbalances are identified, and an intake of sodium and water equivalent to the amount of these substances excreted in a 24-hour period is prescribed. The desired effect is to maintain the person in a normotensive, normovolemic state.

### Electrolyte control

**Hyperkalemia.** Hyperkalemia is defined as a plasma potassium ($K^+$) level greater than 5.5 mEq/L, although the level at which hyperkalemic complications occur may vary depending on the steady-state value for a given patient. Potassium retention occurs in chronic renal failure because of a direct reduction in nephron excretory ability. Hyperkalemia can be controlled by decreasing dietary intake of foods high in potassium, such as citrus fruits, green leafy vegetables, and salt substitutes. Hemodialysis with a zero $K^+$ dialysate bath rapidly removes $K^+$ from the body and may be used in severe situations. Exchange resins, such as sodium polystyrene sulfonate, are also effective in removing $K^+$ from the body. The resin exchanges sodium ions for $K^+$ and calcium in the gastrointestinal tract. It can be given either as an oral preparation or by retention enema. It is usually given with sorbitol to enhance $K^+$ loss via the bowel. A 25-g dose removes approximately 12.5 to 25 mEq of $K^+$. The use of a retention enema is slower and requires 1 to 2 hours before onset of action.[10]

**Metabolic acidosis.** Metabolic acidosis occurs because the damaged kidneys are unable to excrete the normal load of acids generated by metabolism. When the GFR drops 30% to 40%, metabolic acidosis begins to develop primarily because of a reduced capacity of the distal tubules to produce ammonia and impaired reabsorption of bicarbonate. Although there is continued hydrogen ion retention and bicarbonate loss, the plasma pH is maintained at a level compatible with life by other buffering mechanisms, particularly the bone salts.

**Hypocalcemia/hyperphosphatemia.** When the kidneys fail, the ability to excrete phosphorus decreases. This cycle of hypocalcemia/hyperphosphatemia results in significant bone demineralization. Several factors are responsible for these imbalances. In a state of acidosis, there is dissolution of the alkaline salts of bone to serve as buffers because the kidney is no longer able to maintain acid-base balance. As a result, calcium and phosphorus are released into the bloodstream. Reduced glomerular filtration and excretion of inorganic phosphate lead to an elevation of plasma phosphate with a concomitant decrease in serum calcium. Decreased serum calcium concentrations stimulate the secretion of parathyroid hormone (PTH), which results in resorption of calcium from the bones. Under normal circumstances, PTH inhibits tubular reabsorption of phosphates. The kidneys are also unable to complete the synthesis of vitamin D to its active form, 1,25-dihydroxycholecalciferol, which is necessary for absorption of calcium from the gastrointestinal tract and deposition of calcium in the bones. This acquired resistance to vitamin D decreases calcium absorption, permits retention of phosphorus, and contributes to secondary hyperparathyroidism. The result of these complex disturbances is growth arrest or retardation in children and bone pain and deformities known as *renal osteodystrophy* in adults.[14] The aim of treatment is to decrease the serum phosphorus levels. This can be accomplished by restricting dietary phosphorus intake (eliminating dairy products and restricting protein) and using phosphate binders. The reduction of serum phosphorus toward normal is often associated with a small increase in serum calcium, a fall in serum PTH, and a reduced incidence of overt secondary hyperparathyroidism.

The goal of therapy with phosphate-binding agents is to reduce serum phosphorus to normal or near-normal levels. In dialysis patients, predialysis serum phosphorus levels are ideally maintained between 4.5 and 6 mg/dl, and phosphate binders should be taken with each meal. The available agents for intestinal phosphate binding include the aluminum-containing gels (AlternaGEL, Alu-Cap, Amphojel, and Basaljel), calcium carbonate, and calcium acetate. The aluminum-containing gels have been most widely used. Because aluminum absorbed from these compounds can accumulate in renal failure patients, they should be used as a last resort. Calcium carbonate in doses of 4 to 12 g daily with meals is an available alternative. The risks and side effects include hypercalcemia and diarrhea. If the calcium carbonate is given with meals, less calcium is absorbed and the risk of hypercalcemia is reduced.[6] It is critical that nurses adjust the medication times to coincide with meal delivery to enhance phosphate binding and minimize calcium absorption.

Some patients may benefit from the administration of the active form of vitamin D (calcitriol, 0.25 $\mu$g daily). Indications for use include adequate control of serum phosphorus, hypocalcemia, bone pain or myopathy, and rising serum alkaline phosphatase concentration.[9]

### Treatment of concurrent disorders

**Anemia.** Anemia universally accompanies chronic renal disease. Hematocrit values of 16% to 22% were not uncommon in the days before epoetin alfa (EPO). The introduction and subsequent clinical success of EPO, the recombinant form of human erythropoietin, have confirmed this hormone's primary role in regulating the erythropoietic cascade. Patients treated with this agent have an increase in hematocrit, a decrease in the need for blood transfusions, and improved energy levels. This increase in hematocrit enables the patient with CRF to carry out normal daily activities.

EPO is administered subcutaneously, three times a week, in a calculated dose of 50 U/kg of body weight. It is usually administered during a scheduled dialysis treatment. Patients who are in a predialysis state, receiving peritoneal dialysis, or receiving other home dialysis regimens learn to self-administer the drug at home. The medication is irritating to the subcutaneous tissue and causes a transient burning discomfort on administration.

Iron is a necessary component of erythropoiesis, and therapy with EPO will be hindered if patients do not have adequate iron stores. Iron stores should be evaluated before and during therapy. Iron deficiency may occur with EPO as a result of an internal shift of iron from stores to RBCs during the acute correction of anemia. The external loss of RBC iron during both the acute and maintenance phases of therapy contributes to iron deficiency. Because iron is necessary for continued RBC production, virtually all patients receiving EPO eventually require supplemental iron. Patients should be instructed that iron's adverse effects on the gastrointestinal tract, nausea and constipation, can be avoided or minimized by taking iron on a full stomach and by adding a stool softener or laxative to the medication regimen. Furthermore, simultaneous ingestion of iron and phosphate binders should be avoided because phosphate binders impede the absorption of oral iron.

Folate and vitamin $B_{12}$ are important cofactors in the production of RBCs and play a role in the formation and development of deoxyribonucleic acid (DNA). Shortages of these vitamins will hinder the formation of DNA and thus RBCs. Folate can be taken orally at a dose of 1 mg/day, and vitamin $B_{12}$ can be replaced with a monthly intramuscular injection of 100 to 1000 $\mu$g based on the vitamin $B_{12}$ blood level.

Blood pressure may rise during EPO therapy, especially during the early stage of treatment when the hematocrit is rising. About 25% of patients require initiation of, or an increase in antihypertensive therapy. Regulating a dialysis patient's blood pressure involves reevaluating dietary sodium intake, the dialysis prescription, and antihypertensive medications.

Therapy with EPO resulting in an increase in hematocrit and a decrease in plasma volume can affect dialysis efficiency. In such cases the patient may require increases in blood flow rates and treatment time or changes in membrane type and size. Patients may also require increases in anticoagulation during dialysis.

Stimulation of renal and extrarenal EPO production can be achieved by the administration of androgens. Before EPO, androgens were the mainstay in the treatment of the anemia of ESRD. Parenteral preparations, such as nandrolone decanoate (Deca-Durabolin) or testosterone propionate, are very effective. They are given in doses of 1 to 4 mg/kg of body weight once a week and then titrated down by increasing the dose interval. The use of androgens is associated with side effects, including hirsutism, acne, and cholestasis.

**Gastrointestinal disturbances.** In patients with uremia, disturbances in fluid, electrolyte, and waste composition of body fluids produce changes in osmotic gradients in all cells. When these changes occur in the cells of the gastrointestinal (GI) tract, anorexia, nausea, and vomiting result. Persons with uremia are subject to bleeding of the GI tract. Urea is broken down to ammonia by the action of intestinal bacteria. Because ammonia is a mucosal irritant, ulceration and bleeding can occur. Persons with chronic renal disease also have decreased salivary flow. The smell and taste of ammonia due to urea breakdown increases anorexia. Treatment includes vinegar mouthwashes to neutralize ammonia and antacids every 2 to 4 hours to decrease GI irritation. Dietary control of uremia helps to control disturbances in fluid, electrolyte, and water composition of body fluids and thus helps to control nausea and vomiting.

### Dialysis

Chronic intermittent hemodialysis was first used for the treatment of CRF in 1960. Before the early 1960s, hemodialysis was reserved for the treatment of ARF. Once renal failure was determined to be irreversible, hemodialysis was withdrawn. Many industrialized countries throughout the world continue to withdraw dialysis after irreversible renal failure is confirmed.

In 1972, the US Congress enacted legislation that provides some payment of health care costs for all US citizens with ESRD. Under this legislation, any person with CRF is provided benefits under Medicare. As a result of this legislation, many persons are able to live longer by undergoing chronic hemodialysis.

Many technological advances have been made in the treatment of persons with ESRD. Drastic changes in artificial kidneys allow for more efficient and comfortable hemodialysis treatments. Advances in the development of dialysis machines allow individuals the convenience of treatment in their own homes. Other developments in peritoneal dialysis permit patients to treat themselves with continuous peritoneal and intermittent peritoneal dialysis. Home dialysis provides persons with the opportunity to have more control over meeting their own health care needs.

Dialysis involves the movement of fluid and particles across a semipermeable membrane. It is a treatment that can help restore fluid and electrolyte balance, control acid-base balance, and remove waste and toxic material from the body. This treatment can sustain life successfully in both acute and chronic situations where substitution for or augmentation of normal renal function is needed. Specifically, dialysis is used to remove excessive amounts of drugs and toxins in poisonings, to correct serious electrolyte and acid-base imbalances, to maintain kidney function when renal shutdown occurs as a result of transfusion reactions, to replace renal function temporarily in persons with acute renal failure, and to permanently substitute for the loss of renal function in persons with ESR.

**Physiological principles of dialysis.** Dialysis is based on three principles: diffusion, osmosis, and ultrafiltration (Figure 45-4). *Diffusion* involves the movement of particles from an area of greater to an area of lesser concentration. In the body, this usually occurs across a semipermeable membrane. Diffusion is involved in the clearance of solute from the patient's body in both hemodialysis and peritoneal dialysis. Diffusion results in the movement of urea, creatinine, and uric acid from the patient's blood into the dialysate. This solution contains fewer particles to be removed from the bloodstream and high concentrations of particles to be added to the blood (Figure 45-5). Because the dialysate contains no protein waste products, the concentration of these substances in the blood

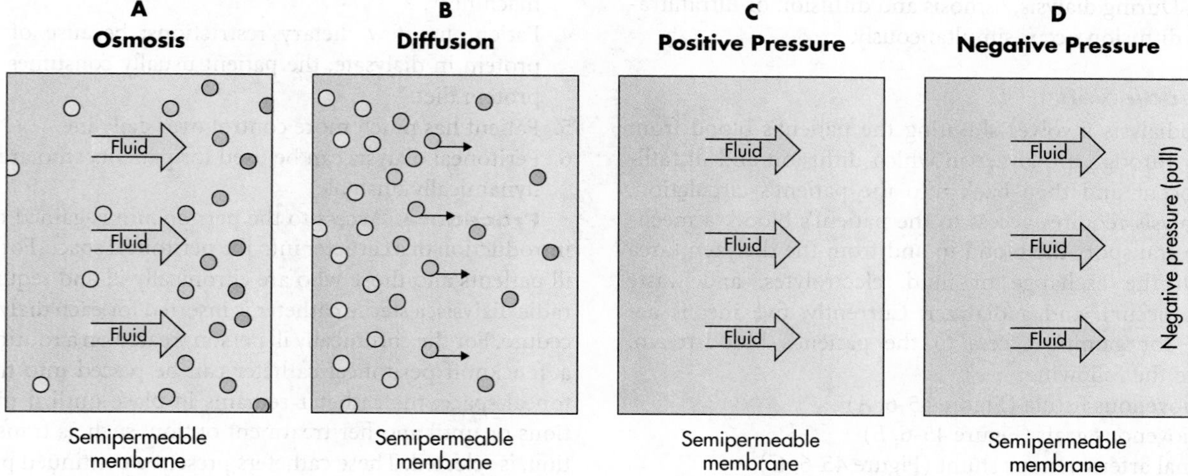


**fig. 45-4** Dialysis is based on principles of osmosis **(A)**, diffusion **(B)**, and ultrafiltration. Ultrafiltration occurs when either positive pressure **(C)** or negative pressure **(D)** is placed on the system. Ultrafiltration can be maximized by simultaneously exerting both positive and negative pressure on the system.

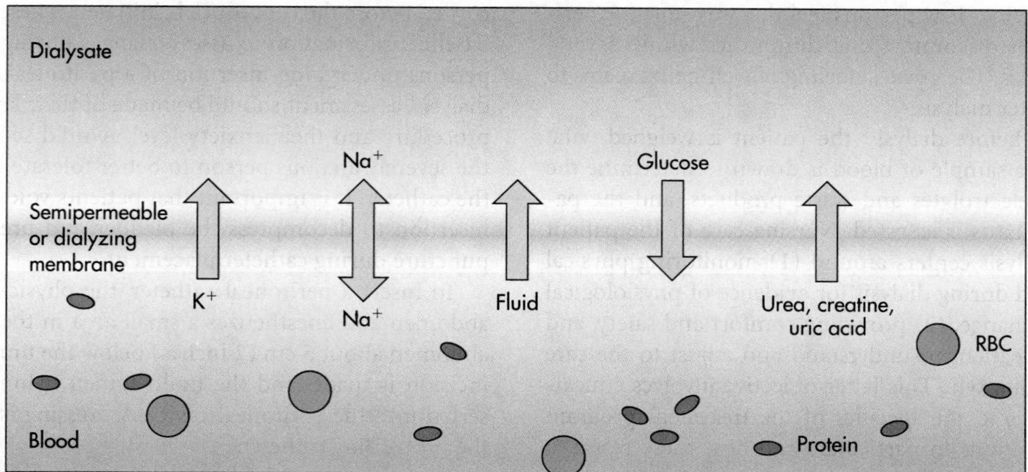


**fig. 45-5** Osmosis and diffusion in dialysis. Net movement of major particles and fluid is illustrated.

will decrease because of random movement of the particles across the semipermeable membrane into the dialysate. The same principle applies to the movement of potassium ions. Although the concentration of RBCs and protein is high in blood, these molecules are quite large and do not diffuse through the membrane pores; thus they are not lost from the blood.

*Osmosis* involves the movement of water across a semipermeable membrane from an area of lesser to an area of greater concentration (osmolality) of particles. Osmosis is responsible for movement of extra fluid from the patient, particularly in peritoneal dialysis. Figure 45-5 shows that glucose has been added to the dialysate to make its particle concentration greater than that of the patient's blood. Fluid will then move through the pores of the membrane from the patient's blood to the dialysate.

*Ultrafiltration* involves the movement of fluid across a semipermeable membrane as a result of an artificially created pressure gradient. Ultrafiltration is more efficient than osmosis for removal of fluid and is used in hemodialysis for this purpose. During dialysis, osmosis and diffusion or ultrafiltration and diffusion occur simultaneously.

### Hemodialysis

Hemodialysis involves shunting the patient's blood from the body through a dialyzer in which diffusion and ultrafiltration occur and then back into the patient's circulation. Hemodialysis requires access to the patient's blood, a mechanism to transport the blood to and from the dialyzen (area in which the exchange of fluid, electrolytes, and waste products occur), and a dialyzer. Currently, five means are available for gaining access to the patient's bloodstream. These are the following:

1. Arteriovenous fistula (Figure 45-6, *A*)
2. Arteriovenous graft (Figure 45-6, *B*)
3. External arteriovenous shunt (Figure 45-6, *C*)
4. Femoral vein catheterization (Figure 45-6, *D*)
5. Subclavian vein catheterization (Figure 45-6, *E*)

The indications and nursing implications for each type of access are summarized in Table 45-6.

Many patients expect to leave the dialysis treatment with a feeling of well-being. Few persons feel this way; most experience some minor discomfort that diminishes within several hours after dialysis. The greatest feeling of well-being seems to occur the day after dialysis.

Immediately before dialysis, the patient is weighed, vital signs are taken, a sample of blood is drawn to determine the level of serum electrolytes and waste products, and the patient's physical status is assessed. Nursing care of the patient during hemodialysis centers around (1) monitoring physical status before and during dialysis for evidence of physiological imbalance and change, (2) providing comfort and safety, and (3) helping the patient to understand and adjust to the care and changes in lifestyle. This latter objective involves educating the person as to the specifics of the treatment program (diet and medications in particular) and how these relate to altered kidney function. The person is encouraged to express concerns and feelings, and attempts must be made to help the individual work through these feelings. If dialysis is performed at home, the patient and dialysis partner must be able to institute all the care described. See the Nursing Care Plan on p. 1485-1486.

### Peritoneal dialysis

In peritoneal dialysis the dialyzing fluid is instilled into the peritoneal cavity, and the peritoneum becomes the dialyzing membrane (see Figure 45-7). Compared with hemodialysis treatments, which last 2 to 4 hours, peritoneal dialysis can be continuous for up to 36 hours or done intermittently in the hospital setting. The procedure, once instituted, becomes largely a nursing responsibility. Peritoneal dialysis is used to treat acute and chronic renal failure. It can be performed in the hospital or at home.

The major advantages of peritoneal dialysis include the following:

1. It provides a steady state of blood chemistry values.
2. Patient can readily be taught the process.
3. Patient can dialyze alone in any location without need for machinery.
4. Patient has few dietary restrictions; because of loss of protein in dialysate, the patient usually consumes a high-protein diet.
5. Patient has much more control over daily life.
6. Peritoneal dialysis can be used for patients who are hemodynamically unstable.

**Procedure.** Access to the peritoneum is gained through introduction of a catheter into the peritoneal space. For acutely ill patients and those who are chronically ill and require sporadic dialysis, a sterile catheter is inserted for each dialysis procedure. For the chronically ill person treated on a routine basis, a Tenckhoff peritoneal catheter can be placed into the peritoneal space; the catheter remains in place until it malfunctions or until another treatment option, such as transplantation, is selected. These catheters present a continued potential entrance for organisms into the peritoneum. Each patient must be thoroughly instructed in the care of the catheter and the signs and symptoms indicative of local or peritoneal infection. These must be reported to the physician.

For all patients, weight, blood pressure, and pulse are recorded before the procedure is initiated. These values serve as baseline information to assess changes during treatment. For persons undergoing insertion of a peritoneal catheter before dialysis, assessment should be made of their knowledge of the procedure and their anxiety level. A mild sedative may help the severely anxious person to better tolerate the insertion of the catheter. It is important that patients void before catheter insertion to decompress the bladder and prevent accidental puncture during catheter placement.

To insert a peritoneal catheter, the physician cleanses the abdomen and anesthetizes a small area in the midline of the abdomen about 5 cm (2 inches) below the umbilicus. A small incision is made, and the multi-lumen nylon catheter is inserted into the peritoneal cavity. A dressing is placed around the protruding catheter.

Approximately 2 L of sterile dialysate, which is warmed to body temperature, is attached by tubing to the catheter and allowed to run into the peritoneal cavity as rapidly as possi-

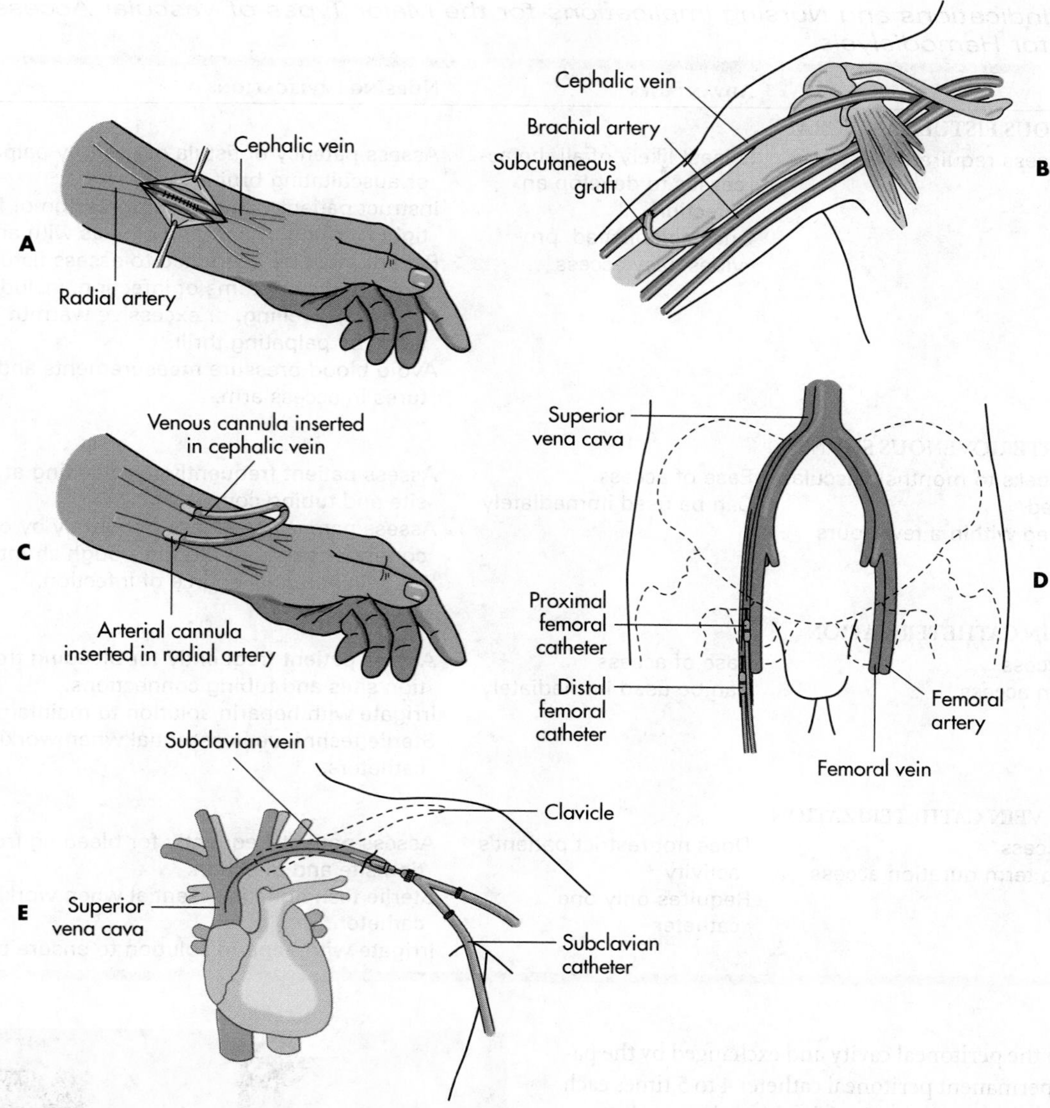


**fig. 45-6** Frequently used means for gaining vascular access for hemodialysis include **A,** arteriovenous fistula; **B,** arteriovenous graft; **C,** external arteriovenous shunt; **D,** femoral vein catheterization; and **E,** subclavian vein catheterization.

ble. This usually takes about 10 minutes. The tubing is then clamped. The maximal osmosis of fluid and diffusion of particles into the dialysate occurs in 20 to 30 minutes. At the end of the dwell time (amount of time the dialysate is left in the peritoneal cavity), the tubing is unclamped, and the fluid is allowed to flow by gravity from the abdomen. Fluid should drain in a steady stream. Drainage time should average about 10 to 15 minutes. The first drainage may be pink tinged as a result of the trauma of catheter insertion; however, drainage should clear with the second or third cycle. At no time should fluid draining from the abdomen be grossly bloody. After fluid has drained from the abdomen, another cycle is started immediately. Dialysis is initiated for the person with a permanent catheter by carefully cleansing the catheter and surrounding skin with a bactericidal agent before the catheter is connected to the dialysate line. After the infusion of dialysate has been completed, the permanent catheter is again cleansed and a sterile cap is applied to the tip.[4]

If the procedure is temporary, the catheter is removed, and the incision is covered with a dry, sterile dressing. The small abdominal wound from the catheter should heal completely in 1 to 2 days (Guidelines for Care Box on p. 1487).

**Other approaches to peritoneal dialysis.** Several advances in the management of patients with chronic ESRD have led to two variations of peritoneal dialysis. The emphasis of continuous ambulatory peritoneal dialysis and continuous cyclic peritoneal dialysis is for home and self-dialysis.

*Continuous ambulatory peritoneal dialysis (CAPD)* is one method of self-dialysis that is practical, is relatively inexpensive when compared with hemodialysis, and promotes independence. Basically, CAPD involves continuous contact of dialysate with the peritoneal membrane. Approximately 2 L of dialysate

**table 45-6** *Indications and Nursing Implications for the Major Types of Vascular Access for Hemodialysis*

| Indications | Advantages | Nursing Implications |
|---|---|---|
| **ARTERIOVENOUS FISTULA AND GRAFT** | | |
| Permanent access required | Is least likely of all the accesses to develop an infection<br>Once established, provides easy access | Assess patency of fistula or graft by palpating thrill or auscultating bruit.<br>Instruct patient to avoid compression of fistula by tight clothing or carrying objects with arm bent.<br>Patient must be instructed to assess fistula for signs and symptoms of infection, including pain, redness, swelling, or excessive warmth and patency by palpating thrill.<br>Avoid blood pressure measurements and venipunctures in access arm. |
| **EXTERNAL ARTERIOVENOUS SHUNT** | | |
| Long term (weeks to months) vascular access needed<br>Access required within a few hours | Ease of access<br>Can be used immediately | Assess patient frequently for bleeding at insertion site and tubing connections.<br>Assess patency of access frequently by observing continuous flow of blood through shunt.<br>Shunt is potential source of infection. |
| **FEMORAL VEIN CATHETERIZATION** | | |
| Immediate access<br>Short duration access | Ease of access<br>Can be used immediately | Assess patient frequently for bleeding from insertion sites and tubing connections.<br>Irrigate with heparin solution to maintain patency.<br>Sterile technique is essential when working with catheters. |
| **SUBCLAVIAN VEIN CATHETERIZATION** | | |
| Immediate access<br>Short- or long term duration access | Does not restrict patient's activity<br>Requires only one catheter | Assess patient frequently for bleeding from insertion site and infection.<br>Sterile technique is essential when working with catheter.<br>Irrigate with heparin solution to ensure patency. |

is maintained in the peritoneal cavity and exchanged by the patient through a permanent peritoneal catheter 4 to 5 times each day. No special equipment is required for the exchanges, but patient education is imperative (see p. 1494). This allows the patient to lead a fairly normal life. Exchanges can take place at home or at work by connecting an empty bag to the catheter and opening a clamp to allow drainage. A full dialysate bag is then instilled, and the patient has completed an exchange.

The second method is *continuous cyclic peritoneal dialysis (CCPD)*. CCPD differs from CAPD in that a machine known as a cycler is used to instill and drain dialysate from the patient (Figure 45-7). The machine has a series of clamps that are timer-controlled. The timers open and close the clamps in sequence to allow for instillation and drainage of dialysate from the patient. The cycle times for patients with chronic renal failure generally allow for the patient to be dialyzed in 6 to 8 hours. A patient, therefore, can connect to the cycler at bedtime, set the machine, and undergo dialysis while sleeping. Several alarms are built into the cycler to protect the patient from malfunctions such as dialysate that is too hot or cold, long or short dwell times, improper return of fluid, and changes in catheter pressures. The greatest advantage of CAPD and CCPD over other forms of dialysis is the unprecedented freedom the patient has in managing his or her own care.

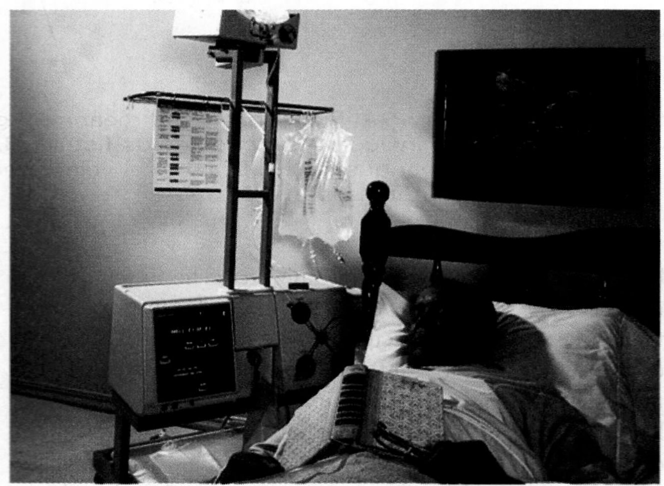

**fig. 45-7** Automated peritoneal dialysis cycler, which is used while the patient is sleeping at night.

### *Evaluating dialysis effectiveness*

*Kinetic modeling,* or prescription dialysis, is a tool developed by dialysis practitioners in the last decade to compute how much hemodialysis an individual needs. Kinetic modeling monitors the effectiveness of the delivered prescription.

## nursing care plan — The Person with Chronic Glomerulonephritis and Renal Failure Undergoing Dialysis

**DATA** Mr. D. is a 52-year-old high-school teacher with a 10-year history of chronic glomerulonephritis. He worked full time until 3 months ago, when his renal disease progressed to end-stage disease requiring hemodialysis. He has been depressed and confided in the nurse that he seems to be losing control over his life.

Mr. D. is married with three active adolescent children, who were accustomed to him attending their sports activities. Mr. D. can no longer attend these activities because of fatigue and limited mobility.

Because of financial hardship, his wife started working full time as a salesclerk. She no longer finds time to play bridge with friends.

The nursing assessment identified the following:

- His dialysis schedule is three times weekly with 4-hour treatments each time.
- He has an arteriovenous fistula in his left arm.
- His blood pressures ranged from 190/110 to 180/100 before dialysis and 120/70 to 100/64 after the second hour of treatment.
- He often develops a headache and becomes agitated during dialysis.

**NURSING DIAGNOSIS** *Fluid volume excess related to fluid accumulation since last dyalysis*

| expected patient outcome | nursing interventions | rationale |
|---|---|---|
| Maintains fluid volume status within established parameters. | Assess weight, lungs, and extremities for presence of edema. | Determine fluid volume status as a guideline for determining treatment parameters. |
| | Monitor intake and output and vital signs. | |
| | Monitor laboratory values: BUN; serum creatinine, sodium, potassium, calcium, magnesium, and phosphorous levels; hemoglobin and hematocrit. | Nitrogenous wastes and electrolytes accumulate between treatments; anemia is a continuing problem with chronic renal failure and blood losses associated with dialysis. |

**NURSING DIAGNOSIS** *Fluid volume deficit related to rapid fluid removal during dialysis and potential blood loss*

| expected patient outcome | nursing interventions | rationale |
|---|---|---|
| Does not exhibit signs of hypovolemia. | Monitor intake and output and vital signs during dialysis. | Recognize shifts in fluid balance. |
| | Monitor effects of anticoagulant therapy every hour during dialysis. | Anticoagulant therapy is necessary to prevent clotting in the dialysis tubing. |
| | Monitor blood clotting time hourly during dialysis. | The hourly checking of clotting time helps to prevent excessive bleeding in patient. |
| | Minimize blood loss by: | |
| | Careful drawing of blood samples for clotting times. | |
| | Returning all blood from hemodialysis machine to patient at end of treatment. | Careful returning of all blood to patient helps prevent worsening of anemia, which is a part of chronic renal failure. |
| | Applying pressure to fistula puncture point sites at end of dialysis. | |
| | Monitor weight during dialysis to prevent weight loss greater than 3-4 kg during treatment. | Prevent hypovolemia. |

**NURSING DIAGNOSIS** *Risk for infection related to invasive procedure and possible blood transfusion requirements.*

| expected patient outcome | nursing interventions | rationale |
|---|---|---|
| Does not develop an infection. | Identify Mr. D.'s hepatitis B and C virus and HIV status; follow Standard Precautions for exposure to blood and body fluids. | Protect patient and nurse. |
| | Use sterile technique to start and stop procedure for shunt or fistula care. | Protect patient from potential sources of infection during procedure. |
| | Assess sites for signs of infection. | |
| | Monitor temperature and WBC. | Detect infection; small elevations in temperature may reflect significant infection. |
| | Follow routine testing policies for hepatitis B and C and HIV antibodies for patients and staff. | Identify change in status; patients are monitored monthly and staff yearly. |

Continued

## The Person with Chronic Glomerulonephritis and Renal Failure Undergoing Dialysis—cont'd

**NURSING DIAGNOSIS** *Body image disturbance related to chronic renal failure requiring machine dependency*

| expected patient outcome | nursing interventions | rationale |
|---|---|---|
| Mr. D. and family accept the changes in body image that are part of chronic renal failure requiring dialysis. | Observe Mr. D.'s response to chronic illness, altered renal function, and other body alterations. | People vary greatly in their response to such life changes. |
| | Recognize response to dependence on a machine. | Patient may feel helpless and hopeless, deny reality, and personalize the machine or accept it as a necessity. |
| | Support strengths, self-confidence, determination, and motivation to live. | Dialysis patients are not disabled in all aspects of life. |
| | Be aware of changes in social involvement; help him develop or continue interests beyond dialysis and return to as normal a life as possible. | Patient may participate in fewer social-recreational activities, experience lifestyle changes, and withdraw because of being different. |
| | Be alert to excessive concerns with losses, depression, self-neglect, noncompliance with medical regimen, possibility of suicide; try to keep communication open; encourage questions. | Suicide is possible, and Mr. D. has access to several methods that could be used to commit suicide. |
| | Be aware of effect that loss of libido, erectile dysfunction, decreased orgasm has on patient's marital and sexual life. | |
| | Refer for psychological counseling as appropriate. | |
| | Try to help him develop realistic expectations of dialysis. | Hemodialysis does not reverse all signs and symptoms of chronic renal disease, and this may be difficult for Mr. D. to accept. |

**NURSING DIAGNOSIS** *Impaired thought processes related to dialysis disequilibrium syndrome or dialysis dementia*

| expected patient outcome | nursing interventions | rationale |
|---|---|---|
| Has no alteration in thought processes. | Monitor during and toward end of dialysis for headaches, nausea, vomiting, and agitation. | These signs indicate uneven or too rapid removal of fluid, electrolytes, and nitrogenous wastes that most often occurs toward the end of treatment. |
| | Monitor speech during dialysis; observe for myoclonus and change in behavior. | These signs may appear first during hemodialysis. |

**NURSING DIAGNOSIS** *Altered family processes related to need for hemodialysis*

| expected patient outcome | nursing interventions | rationale |
|---|---|---|
| Mr. D. and family have adjusted to his lifetime need to receive hemodialysis and are prepared for his dialysis treatments to be given in the community dialysis center. | Recognize the impact that chronic renal failure and hemodialysis has on the family. | Disruption, expense, and considerable alterations in time commitments may occur. |
| | Explore with patient and family the demands that his illness has made on family. | Patient outcomes affect the family's ability to cope and vice versa. |
| | Support coping skills of patient and family, and assist them in exploring alternatives. | |
| | Explore with patient his feelings about no longer being the family "bread-winner." | |
| | Prepare patient and family for community dialysis center by reviewing location of center and introducing them to a representative from the center who will review policies and procedures with them. | Mr. D. may have separation anxiety about moving to a new environment. Preparing patient and family in advance will give them time to work through feelings about the change. |
| | Support patient and family to express fears that they may have about leaving a familiar environment and staff for a new and unknown setting. | Meeting someone from the dialysis center can help allay fears about the unknown. |

## guidelines for care

### Peritoneal Dialysis

A. Regulating fluid volume and drainage
   1. Assess vital signs.
   2. Monitor mental status.
   3. Record fluid balance after each cycle.
   4. Turn patient side to side to facilitate drainage.
   5. Elevate head of bed.
   6. Apply firm pressure with both hands on top of abdomen if flow of dialysate stops.

B. Promoting comfort
   1. Administer analgesics as ordered.
   2. Provide diversional activities.
   3. Encourage side to side movement.
   4. Assist with oral care and feeding.

C. Preventing complications
   1. Assess respiratory effort.
   2. Encourage frequent small meals.
   3. Use aseptic technique.
   4. Culture dialysate as directed.
   5. Monitor temperature.
   6. Observe for nausea, vomiting, abdominal tenderness, and cloudy outflow.

Hemodialysis is usually prescribed by nephrologists based on the mathematical formula *Kt/V.* This formulation includes individual patient parameters of dialyzer clearance *(K),* time of dialysis *(t),* and volume of urea distribution *(V),* In addition, the normalized protein catabolic rate of the individual patient must be determined and periodically reassessed. Using serum urea levels as the kinetic factor, practitioners are able to determine an expected outcome of treatment. A *Kt/V* equal to 1.0 represents adequate dialysis. *Kt/V* less than 1.0 indicates the need for more dialysis time or a change in dialyzer. A peritoneal dialysis patient may need to increase the number of dialysis exchanges.

## Surgical Management

### *Kidney transplantation*

The advantage of kidney transplantation is the reversal of many of the pathophysiological changes associated with renal failure. It also eliminates the dependence on dialysis and the need for dietary restrictions, provides the opportunity to return to normal life activities, and is more cost-effective than dialysis after the first year.

Although transplant procedures are expensive, the current success rates have made transplantation a cost-effective treatment option compared with traditional medical management. A patient undergoing chronic hemodialysis costs the federal government, through Medicare, about $40,000/yr. The cost of a kidney transplant is approximately $40,000 for the first year and $5,000/yr for follow-up care. If the transplanted kidney functions for 5 years (the actual rate approaches 75%), the cost is $60,000 as opposed to $200,000 for 5-year chronic hemodialysis. Other financial factors that increase the cost-effectiveness of transplantation are the potential earning power of the transplant recipient and the discontinuation of disability benefits previously required. In short, transplantation is a therapy that can restore dignity and quality to the lives of patients and families dealing with ESRD and provides the potential for patients to become productive members of society again. (For a discussion of the methods of kidney transplantation and required care requirements, see Chapter 68.)

## Diet

The goals of diet therapy are to (1) reduce the quantity of metabolic waste that requires excretion by the kidney, (2) provide sufficient calories and protein for growth and repair while limiting excretory demands on the kidney, (3) minimize metabolic bone disease, and (4) minimize fluid and electrolyte disturbances. The dietary protein restriction is calculated at 1 to 1.5 g/kg of ideal body weight. Adequate protein intake is reflected by a BUN/creatinine ratio of 10 : 1. Excessive intake of protein results in nausea and vomiting, apathy, weakness, and neurological symptoms. Insufficient protein intake results in lowered serum albumin level, muscle wasting, edema, and weight loss. Two thirds of the total protein consumed should be protein of high biological value, that is, containing the essential amino acids.

Ample calories are obtained from carbohydrates and fats because they do not require renal excretion of their metabolic by-products. This spares protein for growth and repair. Catabolism of existing protein stores liberates nitrogenous wastes. For this reason, sources of potential infection, such as indwelling catheters, are avoided. When infection is noted, it is immediately treated.

## Activity

A patient undergoing hemodialysis must remain in a chair or in bed during dialysis because of the attachment to the machine. A patient with CAPD has more freedom during dialysis because the dialysate is in the abdominal cavity. However, the patient must cycle therapy over the 24-hour time frame; thus he or she must schedule their day around treatments.

Otherwise there are no activity restrictions or recommendations for the patient with ESRD, and patients should be encouraged to continue with their normal activities. Only 25% of Americans with ESRD are employed. These numbers are in part due to the fact many persons with ESRD are older than 65 years of age. Thus the Life Options Rehabilitation Advisory Council has suggested the five E's— encouragement, evaluation, employment, exercise, and education—for persons with ESRD.[7]

## Referrals

A patient with ESRD should be referred to a dietitian for education about meeting nutritional requirements and diet planning. ESRD patients may also need referrals to home health care to supervise treatments, provide dialysis supplies, and perform venipunctures. Social service referrals may be required to assist patients with financial concerns. Occupational and physical therapy is indicated to maximize independent functioning of the patient with ESRD.

## NURSING MANAGEMENT

### ASSESSMENT

The nursing assessment of the patient with chronic renal failure is extremely complex. The assessment must include physical, psychological, and social parameters. The basis of this assessment is the same as that described in Chapter 43 for the patient with suspected renal problems. The initial nursing history and physical assessment must elicit adequate information to generate the appropriate nursing diagnoses. An example of a comprehensive nursing history is found in Figure 45-8 and an example of a physical assessment in Figure 45-9.

The extent and nature of subsequent assessments are determined by the medical regimen, nursing diagnoses, and patient condition. The frequency of assessment is a function of the medical regimen and stability of the patient. For example, the patient being managed conservatively may be able to go several months without follow-up assessments. On the other hand, the hemodialysis patient will require a thorough assessment with each treatment.

#### Subjective Data

The initial nursing history and physical assessment must elicit adequate information to generate the appropriate nursing diagnoses. The history must be comprehensive and include not

**Hemodialysis Nursing Notes**
Admission History
(Inpatient)/Patient Notes (Outpatient)

| Date | Hour | | | | | |
|---|---|---|---|---|---|---|
| | | **I.** | **Perception of Illness** | | | |
| | | | Why, initially, did you come to the hospital? | | | |
| | | | What does the doctor plan for you while you are here? | | | |
| | | | What do you expect to happen to you when you start dialysis? | | | |
| | | **II.** | **History of Past Illness (Include dates and hospitalizations)** | | | |
| | | Medications | Dose | Frequency | Last Dose Taken | Reason for Taking |
| | | | | | | |
| | | | Do you receive any special treatments or exercises? | | | |
| | | **III.** | **Activity** | | | |
| | | | Do you have difficulty walking or getting in and out of a chair? | | | |
| | | | Can you climb stairs? | | | |
| | | | Are you employed? | | | |
| | | | What are your usual daytime activities? | | | |
| | | | What are your recreational interests? | | | |
| | | **IV.** | **Nutrition** | | | |
| | | | Are you on a special diet? | | | |
| | | | Do you have difficulty following a diet? | | | |
| | | | How many meals do you eat a day? | | | |
| | | **V.** | **Sleep Habits** | | | |
| | | | Do you sleep through the night at home? | | | |
| | | | What helps in getting to sleep at night? | | | |
| | | | What are your usual sleeping habits? | | | |

Continued

**fig. 45-8** Hemodialysis nursing notes: admission history.

only information on physical symptoms, but also on patient lifestyle. Health maintenance behaviors as well as the home environment should be explored to determine the consequences of various treatment options. The patient should report feelings of fatigue, nausea, pruritus, and lethargy.

### Objective Data

Objective data to be collected include vital signs, input and output, heart and lung sounds, mental status, and signs of pain. The skin should be assessed for increased pigmentation and signs of peripheral edema. Daily weight should also be part of the objective assessment.

## NURSING DIAGNOSES

Nursing diagnoses are determined from analysis of patient data. Nursing diagnoses for the person with chronic renal failure may include but are not limited to:

| Diagnostic Title | Possible Etiological Factors |
|---|---|
| Fluid volume excess | Compromised regulatory mechanism |
| Nutrition, altered: less than body requirements | Anorexia, nausea, decreased salivary flow, bad taste, pain |
| Infection, risk for | Compromised immune response |
| Injury, risk for | Sensorimotor deficits, lack of awareness of environmental hazards, decreased level of consciousness |
| Fatigue | Uremia, anemia, insomnia |
| Pain: muscle cramping, pruritus, ocular irritation | Sodium depletion, uremia |
| Coping, ineffective (individual) | Situational crisis |
| Self-esteem, situational low | Changes in body appearance, change in social involvement |
| Knowledge deficit | Lack of exposure/recall |

| Date | Hour | | |
|---|---|---|---|
| | | **VI. Elimination** | |
| | | How often do you urinate? | |
| | | Do you have any difficulty with urination? | |
| | | Frequency | Pain on urination |
| | | Urgency | Other |
| | | Have you ever had urinary tract infections? | |
| | | 24-hour urine output | cc/24 hr |
| | | Color of urine? | |
| | | What are your usual bowel habits? | |
| | | Do you have difficulty with diarrhea or constipation? | |
| | | How often do you use enemas or laxatives? | |
| | | **VII. Reproductive System** | |
| | | When was your most recent menses? | |
| | | Have you recently had a change in menses? | |
| | | Have you had any changes in sexual function recently? | |
| | | Do you have any concerns about reproductive or sexual functions? | |
| | | **VIII. Social** | |
| | | Do you live with anyone? | |
| | | Upon whom do you rely when you need help? | |
| | | In what type of dwelling do you live? | |
| | | Do you have to climb stairs? | |
| | | Financial resources/insurance | |

Admitting Nurse ______________________

**fig. 45-8, cont'd** Hemodialysis nursing notes: admission history.

(Inpatient)/Patient Notes (Outpatient)

| Date | Hour | | | | |
|---|---|---|---|---|---|
| | | A) | **Vital Signs** | | |
| | | | Temperature | | |
| | | | Pulses | Apical | |
| | | | | Radial | |
| | | | | Rhythm | |
| | | | Weight | | |
| | | | Height | | |
| | | B) | **Cardiopulmonary** | | |
| | | | Vascular access | | |
| | | | Peripheral pulses: | Right | Left |
| | | | Radial | | |
| | | | Femoral | | |
| | | | Popliteal | | |
| | | | Pedal | | |
| | | | Peripheral edema? | | |
| | | | Periorbital edema? | | |
| | | | Friction rub? | | |
| | | | Neck vein distention? | | |
| | | | Cough? | Sputum? | Smoking habits? |
| | | | Adventitious breath sounds? | | |
| | | | Shortness of breath? | | |
| | | | Orthopnea | | |
| | | C) | **Neuromuscular** | | |
| | | | Orientation | | |
| | | | Level of alertness and responsiveness? | | |
| | | | Muscle tone and strength, symmetry? | | |
| | | | Weakness or loss of function of extremities? | | |
| | | | Balance | | |
| | | | Numbness, tingling, or tremors? | | |
| | | | Patient experiencing difficulties with: | | |
| | | | Sight | | |
| | | | Speech | | |
| | | | Touch | | |
| | | | Taste/Smell | | |

*Continued*

**fig. 45-9** Hemodialysis nursing notes: admission assessment.

| Date | Hour | |
|---|---|---|
| | | **D) Skin** |
| | | Color |
| | | Turgor |
| | | Temperature |
| | | Lesions |
| | | Condition of nails |
| | | **E) General** |
| | | Presence of: |
| | | Nausea |
| | | Vomiting |
| | | Headache |
| | | Blurring of vision |
| | | Ability to perform ADL |

Admitting Nurse ______________

**fig. 45-9, cont'd** Hemodialysis nursing notes: admission history.

## EXPECTED PATIENT OUTCOMES

Expected patient outcomes for the person with chronic renal failure vary depending on the course of the disorder and the identified nursing diagnoses. Expected patient outcomes may include but are not limited to:

1. Exhibits no signs of respiratory distress, peripheral edema, hypertension, or other signs and symptoms indicating fluid and electrolyte imbalance.
2. Explains dietary plan, including fluid, protein, potassium, and sodium restrictions.
3. Shows no signs of infection; skin remains intact.
4. Is free from injury.
5. Reports feeling more rested and less fatigued.
6. Has no muscle cramping, itching, or ocular irritation.
7. Describes methods of effective coping; exhibits ability to perform ADL and desired activities independently.
8. States satisfaction with life and self.
9. Verbalizes knowledge of nature of illness, treatment regimen, and plans for follow-up care.

## INTERVENTIONS

Because the condition of the person with chronic renal failure can vary, nursing care focuses on the specific identified nursing diagnoses. Most persons, however, require some help or teaching to maintain fluid and electrolyte balance; prevent infection or injury; promote comfort, rest, and sleep; and cope with the effects of renal failure (see the Guidelines for Care Box).

### Maintaining Fluid and Electrolyte Balance

The person with chronic renal failure must learn how to identify signs of imbalances, take fluids in the prescribed amounts, and eat within the prescribed limits. This requires careful monitoring of intake and output.

Controlling sodium intake can be an extremely challenging problem for both the nurse and the patient. Any sudden increase in weight indicates accumulating fluid, and the source of this fluid must be discussed with the patient. When the patient is not acutely ill and is responsible for diet restrictions, the problem can be often traced to excess sodium ingestion, which produces thirst. In helping to avoid this cycle of sodium-driven thirst leading to increased fluid ingestion and overhydration, the patient is taught about the amount of sodium and fluid allowed in the diet and restrictions to observe when purchasing prepared foods. The words "sodium" and "salt" should be checked on all food labels. Salt substitutes should be avoided by all patients with chronic renal failure because these substitutes contain large amounts of potassium.

Sometimes the patient is unable to explain his or her increasing thirst and sodium ingestion. At this point the question of home self-medication is raised. The person may be taking over-the-counter antacids that are high in sodium. If the cause of the hypervolemia cannot be identified, the patient is asked to list all foods and fluids ingested over the previous 3 days. This list can be used to uncover dietary indiscretions as well as serve as a teaching tool to reinforce the prescribed diet.

**guidelines for care**

**The Person with Chronic Renal Failure**

1. Maintain fluid and electrolyte balance.
   a. Monitor for fluid and electrolyte excess.
      (1) Assess intake and output every 8 hours.
      (2) Weigh patient every day.
      (3) Assess presence and extent of edema.
      (4) Auscultate breath sounds.
      (5) Monitor cardiac rhythm and blood pressure every 8 hours.
      (6) Assess level of consciousness every 8 hours.
   b. Encourage patient to remain within prescribed fluid restrictions.
   c. Provide small quantities of fluid spaced over the day to stay within fluid restrictions.
   d. Encourage a diet high in carbohydrates and within the prescribed sodium, potassium, phosphorus, and protein limits.
   e. Administer phosphate-binding agents with meals as prescribed.
2. Prevent infection and injury.
   a. Promote meticulous skin care.
   b. Encourage activity within prescribed limits but avoid fatigue.
   c. Protect confused person from injury.
   d. Protect person from exposure to infectious agents.
   e. Maintain good medical/surgical asepsis during treatments and procedures.
   f. Avoid aspirin products.
   g. Encourage use of soft toothbrush.
3. Promote comfort.
   a. Medicate patient as needed for pain.
   b. Medicate with prescribed antipruritics, use emollient baths, keep skin moist, and control environmental temperature to modify pruritus.
   c. Encourage use of damp cloth to keep lips moist; give good oral hygiene.
   d. Encourage rest for fatigue; however, encourage self-care as tolerated.
   e. Provide calm, supportive atmosphere.
4. Assist with coping in lifestyle and self-concept.
   a. Promote hope.
   b. Provide opportunity for patient to express feelings about self.
   c. Identify available community resources.

### Facilitating Nutrition

Persons usually need help planning diets within the prescribed sodium, potassium, phosphorus, and protein limits. Modifying the diet to the individual's preferences can help to maintain intake of food. Dietary teaching and meal planning can be approached using an exchange system similar to that used for persons with diabetes.

Complying with a modified diet can be promoted through attempts to decrease emotional tension at the dinner table. Food that is attractively arranged and well-flavored is also likely to promote the appetite. Herbs and other flavorings can add variety to foods that are prepared without sodium. When the GI tract is ulcerated, bland foods may be tried in an attempt to increase ingestion of food.

### Preventing Infection and Injury

Tissue breakdown leads to infection. Extensive tissue damage can cause an elevation in serum potassium and must be avoided. Potassium is largely an intracellular cation, and extensive tissue damage can liberate a lethal amount of this ion into the system of the person with chronic renal failure. Edematous skin poses a high risk for skin breakdown; therefore, meticulous skin care is important. Patients with chronic renal failure should avoid others with infections; avoid fatigue, which lowers body resistance; and seek medical attention when symptoms of infections, GI bleeding, or other problems first appear.

The risk of constipation is also high in persons with chronic renal failure because of the fluid restrictions. Stool softeners or laxatives may be needed.

Other important nursing activities include helping the patient to control blood loss. A soft toothbrush is recommended for oral care. The patient is instructed to observe for melena and to report this without delay to the physician. Aspirin should be avoided because it is normally excreted by the kidneys and may rapidly build to toxic levels and prolong bleeding time. NSAIDs should also be avoided.

The buildup of osmotically active particles and fluid in the body that occurs with azotemia produces changes in the cells of the brain that may lead to confusion and impairment in decision-making ability. Fluid accumulation and hypertension can produce visual changes. The person's environment is assessed for potential for injury. At times the person may need help in limiting activities to a level commensurate with mental processes and level of awareness. For example, blurred vision and delayed reaction time contraindicate driving a motor vehicle.

### Promoting Comfort, Rest, and Sleep

The patient with chronic renal failure rarely has acute, sharp pain; however, these persons are subject to a wide variety of chronic discomforts, including pruritus, muscle cramping, headaches, ocular irritation, insomnia, and bone pain.

Most patients with ESRD develop pruritus and describe a sensation of deep itching. Itching is largely symptomatic, and measures that are effective in controlling it vary from person to person. Reducing levels of serum phosphorus with phosphate-binding preparations decreases itching for most patients. Medications such as trimeprazine tartrate (Temaril) may be effective for some patients. Keeping the skin moist and supple through use of lotions and bath oils, controlling the room temperature during sleep to prevent excessive warmth, and bathing with emollients or a vinegar solution are measures alone or in combination that may provide some relief from itching. Since emotional stress seems to increase the itching, helping the patient verbalize feelings may provide resolution of conflict and help decrease itching. The urge to scratch the skin is acute in some patients. Because scratching is often vigorous, injury to the skin with subsequent infection can result. Fingernails are trimmed closely. Instead of fingernails, a soft cloth should be used to scratch the skin.

Muscle cramping in the lower extremities and hands is common in renal failure. Often, cramping can be correlated with sodium depletion. Primary treatment for muscle cramping involves controlling the state of uremia and fluid and electrolyte balance. Temporary measures of heat and massage are effective for some persons. Quinine sulfate, 325 mg at bedtime, often prevents cramping.

Ocular irritation in chronic renal failure is caused by calcium deposits in the conjunctiva that cause burning and watering of the eyes. Treatment involves controlling the plasma phosphate level through administration of oral phosphate-binding preparations. "Artificial tears" (methylcellulose) placed in the conjunctival sac every few hours also help to reduce irritation.

Insomnia and chronic daytime fatigue are common complaints of persons with chronic renal failure. This alteration of normal sleep patterns has been attributed to a variety of causes. These include (1) recurring preoccupation with thoughts concerning the disease state and resultant changes in lifestyle, (2) pruritus, and (3) the state of uremia itself. Reduction of high serum levels of urea nitrogen and creatinine through decreasing dietary intake of protein or dialysis may bring sleep patterns back to normal. When control of uremia fails to cure insomnia, mild central nervous system depressants may be prescribed.

The severely anemic person will experience extreme fatigue and shortness of breath. The lack of RBCs creates an inability to transport sufficient oxygen to cells for energy production. The anemic person may be unable to work or play without extended rest periods. Rest periods should be taken early enough in the day to prevent sleeplessness at night.

General comfort at bedtime is needed to induce sleep and is especially important when sleeping problems arise. Comfort measures include tepid baths, pursuing quiet activities an hour or two before bedtime, controlling itching, or relaxation techniques.

### Facilitating Coping with Changes in Lifestyle and Feelings Regarding Self

The goals of therapy for patients with ESRD include not only the preservation of the patient's life in the presence of ESRD, but also restoration of optimal quality of life. There is broad agreement that patients' quality of life is related to their function in the physical/medical, ADL, psychological, and social/occupational dimensions.[22]

Optimal psychosocial care of patients with chronic renal failure requires careful and sophisticated psychosocial patient assessment. This assessment is accomplished as a collaborative effort of the physician, nurse, and social worker. Common psychological problems include dysphoric moods (anxiety, depression, frustration, and anger), impaired body image (with a perceived loss of physical attractiveness), impaired self-esteem, and suicidal crises.

Noncompliance with the treatment regimen is a common behavioral problem; this may include treatment participation, diet and fluid restriction, and medication noncompliance as well as noncompliance with other medical diagnostic and therapeutic procedures. Several factors contribute to noncompliance: the intrusive and demanding aspects of chronic dialysis regimen, strong feelings of frustration and depression, a strong desire to maintain control over one's life and deny the unpleasant personal reality of chronic illness, a need to indirectly express anger toward staff members, and attempts to balance health concerns with a short-term need for pleasure. Interventions that may effectively reverse significant patient noncompliance include (1) providing further information about the rationale for treatment procedures or restrictions, (2) helping the patient regain as much constructive control as possible over life's activities, (3) communicating with staff members to gather information and to design and implement a program to reward increased patient compliance, and (4) working with family members to educate them and enlist their support.

Social problems in ESRD patients include strains in intimate relationships, loss of vocational function, and restriction of social and leisure activities (see the Research Box). The introduction of a serious life-threatening illness such as ESRD is an added stress dimension to the already enormous demands placed on the contemporary family system. Role changes are common in families; spouses often take on the role responsibilities of the sick partner while maintaining their own role. This leads to reduced rest and leisure for the spouse and lowers physical reserve. Major adjustments in thinking and living must be made, and at the same time, relationships must be maintained and nurtured. Nursing staff must be aware that additional social support for patients may need to be provided by professional caregivers, especially when family members take little responsibility for either physical and/or emotional support. Caregiving staff may be viewed as important "significant others" for the ESRD patient.

Vocational dysfunction is a result of decreased physical capacities, the time-intensive requirements of dialysis, depression and cognitive impairment, governmental policies about reimbursement for dialysis medical care, and the reluctance of employers to hire individuals with kidney disease. The problems of vocational function are quite complex, particularly for patients with limited skills and whose work previously involved manual labor. Implications for nursing and social work consist of identifying patients beginning dialysis and providing vocational counseling.

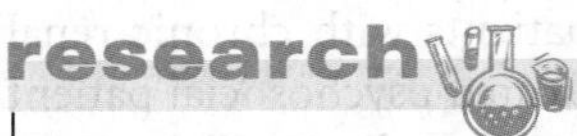

Reference: Rowe MA: The impact of internal and external resources on functional outcomes in chronic illness, *Res Nurs Health,* 19:485-497, 1996.

The purpose of this study was to determine if the use of internal and/or external resources could prevent or lessen negative consequences of physiological stress in chronic illness. Resource theory was used to determine if internal (psychological) and external (social support) resources could alter the relationship between physiological stress and decreased functional outcomes (distress). Several hypotheses were generated:

- Resources improve functional outcomes.
- In the presence of resources, stress will have a diminished effect on functional outcomes.
- High stress and low resources will result in poorer functional outcomes.
- Stressful situations negatively affect levels of resources.
- During stress, lack of resources will have a negative impact on functional outcomes.

The sample consisted of 112 adult end-stage renal patients receiving dialysis or renal transplant. Data were collected by questionnaire at 3 points during the study. The results did not support the hypothesis that functional outcomes are influenced by internal and external factors. This study did support the influence of physiological factors on functional outcomes. These findings may help nurses choose appropriate interventions based on desired functional outcomes.

## patient/family teaching

### The Person with Chronic Renal Failure

1. Relationships between symptoms and their causes
2. Relationships among diet, fluid restriction, medication, and blood chemistry values
3. Preventive health care measures: oral hygiene, prevention of infection, avoidance of bleeding
4. Dietary regimen, including fluid restrictions
   a. Prescribed sodium, potassium, phosphorus, and protein restrictions
   b. Label reading and identifying nutritional content of foods
   c. Use of small, frequent feedings to maintain nutrient intake when anorexic or nauseated
   d. Fluid prescription and sources of fluid in diet
   e. Avoidance of salt substitutes containing potassium
5. Monitoring for fluid excess
   a. Accurate measurement and recording of intake and output
   b. Monitoring for weight gain and edema
6. Medications
   a. Actions, doses, purpose, and side effects of prescribed medications
   b. Avoidance of over-the-counter drugs, especially aspirin, cold medications, and nonsteroidal antiinflammatory drugs
7. Planning for gradual increase in physical activity, including rest periods to conserve energy
8. Measures to control pruritus
9. Planning for follow-up health care
   a. Symptoms requiring immediate medical attention: changes in urine output, edema, weight gain, dyspnea, infection, increased symptoms of uremia
   b. Need for continual medical follow-up

### Patient/Family Education

The person with ESRD presents a unique opportunity for the nurse to promote optimal health through teaching and counseling. Important points to be included in patient teaching are listed in the Patient/Family Teaching Box.

The teaching plan for persons undergoing hemodialysis should include:

1. The process of hemodialysis and relationship to body needs
2. Information necessary to care for vascular access devices including infection and clotting
3. Appropriate care of arteriovenous access
4. Common side effects of treatment, means of controlling mild symptoms, and means of obtaining medical attention for severe or persistent complications
5. Changes in medication schedule required before and after dialysis
6. A work and activity schedule as physical capabilities permit

An example of a teaching care plan for the person receiving hemodialysis is illustrated in Box 45-5.

The teaching requirements for the patient undergoing peritoneal dialysis is consistent with the teaching plan for hemodialysis. However, the patient will need to be instructed in the specific details of the process of peritoneal dialysis. If the patient will undergo continuous ambulatory dialysis, training should be accomplished in a home-training center that is equipped to assist the patient in dealing with home care.

The teaching plan should include the following:

1. The process of dialysis and how the dialysis relates to the patient's body needs
2. Signs and symptoms of infection of the peritoneal cavity or catheter site and where to obtain care if these occur
3. Appropriate care of the permanent peritoneal catheter
4. Common side effects of treatment, means of controlling mild symptoms, and means of obtaining medical attention for severe or persistent complications
5. Changes in medication schedule required before and after dialysis
6. A work and activity schedule as physical capabilities permit

**box 45-5** *Example of a Teaching Plan for the Person Undergoing Hemodialysis*

| Date | Hour | Teaching/learning | RN signature |
|---|---|---|---|
| | | Chronic renal failure being treated by hemodialysis | |
| | | | |
| Start | Stop | Plan | |
| | | 1. Introduce patient to hemodialysis unit using available printed material and a visit to unit when appropriate. | |
| | | 2. Explain normal kidney function. | |
| | | 3. Explain kidney failure specific to patient's pathophysiology: | |
| | | a. Types | |
| | | b. Causes | |
| | | 4. Explain and reinforce medication regimen: | |
| | | a. Purpose of each prescribed medication | |
| | | b. Common side effects | |
| | | c. Dose and times of each medication | |
| | | d. Prescription filling procedure | |
| | | 5. Reinforce dietary instruction: | |
| | | a. Protein | |
| | | b. Potassium | |
| | | c. Sodium | |
| | | d. Fluids | |
| | | e. Calories | |
| | | 6. Instruct patient about need for and care of vascular access: | |
| | | a. Procedure for assessing presence of thrill and bruit; who to notify if thrill or bruit is absent | |
| | | b. Guarding against constriction of fistula; that is, sleeping on arm or wearing tight clothing | |
| | | c. Hygiene and removing dressing after dialysis | |
| | | d. Signs and symptoms of infection; that is, redness, swelling, or tenderness | |
| | | e. Measures to control hemorrhage should it develop while away from dialysis unit | |
| | | 7. Instruct patient about process of hemodialysis: | |
| | | a. Explain principles of dialysis in sufficient detail for learning level of patient. | |
| | | b. Describe hemodialysis in full detail to patient. | |
| | | c. Explain common sights and sounds of dialysis unit to patient. | |
| | | d. Describe common complications of hemodialysis to patient as well as usual treatments: | |
| | | (1) Hypotension | |
| | | (2) Nausea | |
| | | (3) Vomiting | |
| | | (4) Cramping | |
| | | 8. Instruct patient in interpretation of laboratory data and effects of hemodialysis, diet, and medications on these values. | |
| | | 9. Introduce patient to alternative modes of treatment of end-stage renal disease: | |
| | | a. Free-standing hemodialysis centers | |
| | | b. Self-dialysis (home) | |
| | | c. Peritoneal dialysis | |
| | | d. Transplantation | |

*Continued*

**box 45-5** *Example of a Teaching Plan for the Person Undergoing Hemodialysis—cont'd*

| Date | Status of problems at discharge | |
|---|---|---|
| | | |
| | | |
| Date | Patient knowledge | |
| | | |
| | | |
| | | |
| Date | Follow-up plan | |
| | | |
| | | |
| | | |
| | | |
| | | |
| | | |
| | RN signature ____________ | |

### *Health promotion/prevention*

**Primary prevention.** Obstruction and infection of the urinary tract and hypertensive disease are common and often asymptomatic causes of kidney damage and renal failure. A significant reduction in the incidence of chronic renal failure can be effected through increasing attention to general health promotion. Yearly physical examinations in which blood pressure is measured, urinalysis is performed, and the person is questioned about dysuria or urinary tract pain assist in early detection of diseases that may lead to chronic renal failure. Meticulous blood glucose control in diabetic persons is critical to reducing renal failure.

**Secondary prevention.** General health maintenance can reduce the number of individuals who progress from renal insufficiency to frank renal failure. The aim of care is to adequately treat medical problems and closely supervise the person's health status in times of stress (for example, infection or pregnancy).

***Healthy People 2000.*** A risk-reduction objective listed in *Healthy People 2000* of the US Public Health Service and Department of Health and Human Services that relates to ESRD is as follows: Reduce the incidence of end-stage renal disease as a complication of diabetes to 1.4 per 1000 from a 1988 baseline of 1.5 per 1000.[20] The 1995 review of objectives also identified special target populations for reduction of the incidence of ESRD. These populations included African Americans, Native Americans, and Native Alaskans.

The year 2000 goals are as follows: Reduce the incidence of ESRD due to diabetes in African Americans to 2.0 per 1000 and in Native Americans/Alaska Natives to 1.9 per 1000. (Baseline is 2.2 per 1000 and 2.1 per 1000 in 1983 to 1986.)[20]

## ■ EVALUATION

To evaluate the effectiveness of nursing interventions, compare patient behaviors with those stated in the expected patient outcomes. Successful achievement of patient outcomes for the patient with chronic renal failure is indicated by:

1. Lacks respiratory distress, peripheral edema, hypertension, or other signs of fluid and electrolyte imbalance.
2. Correctly explains dietary plan, including fluid, protein, potassium, and sodium restrictions.
3. Shows no signs of infection; skin remains intact.
4. Is free from injury.
5. States feeling more rested and less fatigued.
6. States that no muscle cramping, itching, or ocular irritation is present.
7. Demonstrates effective coping and ability to perform ADL and desired activities independently.
8. States satisfaction with life and self.
9. Correctly describes nature of illness, treatment regimen, and plans for follow-up care.

## GERONTOLOGICAL CONSIDERATIONS

The elderly patient with ESRD is more likely to develop complications due to age-related stressors placed on the kidneys. The GFR decreases 10% every 10 years after the age of 50 years. The geriatric patient is more likely to experience renal insufficiency, predominantly related to atherosclerosis.[13]

Older adults often have multiple risk factors such as diabetes and hypertension, which increase the risk of renal failure. Once faced with ESRD, all persons, particularly the elderly, need to consider their overall health when choosing a treatment option.

The patient's home environment and resources must be evaluated to determine the best treatment options. Obstacles for the elderly may be lack of transportation to a dialysis center. Lack of motor skills or a chronic illness such as osteoarthritis may prohibit elderly patients from performing home dialysis.

Options for the elderly patient include home health care or extended-care facilities. Agencies such as Help on Wheels offer transportation for patients free of charge to and from dialysis treatments. The federal government has recognized the difficulties the elderly patient with ESRD may face and has mandated a home visit for Medicare patients be made if patients are sent home while still receiving dialysis.[15] Complications are also more common among the elderly population.

## COMPLICATIONS

Many of the complications of ESRD and its treatments have been discussed. Fluid and electrolyte imbalances, shock, sepsis, and bleeding have been described previously. Other complications of CRF include anemia, hypertension, hyperkalemia, congestive heart failure, pulmonary edema, pericarditis, atherosclerosis, peptic ulcer disease, osteodystrophy, peripheral neuropathy, and metabolic encephalopathy.

Treatment options for CRF place the patient at risk for developing other complications. Those treated with hemodialysis often require multiple hospital admissions for problems with vascular access devices.[19] Infection, clotting, and displacement lead to a need for additional surgical intervention, making proper care of these devices crucial.

The patient treated with CAPD is at risk for infection from improper technique, manipulation of the catheter, and from exit-site care of the dialysis catheter. Many patients have expressed concern over the need for education on proper site care.[5] Research does not support the effectiveness of a particular protocol over others.[5] Peritonitis is an ever-present threat during peritoneal dialysis. Aseptic technique must be strictly maintained during insertion of the catheter and throughout the procedure. Care should be taken to avoid contaminating the solution or the tubing when dialysate solution is hung. Cultures of the dialysate fluid are performed routinely to rule out infection. The patient should be assessed for signs of peritonitis and be taught to recognize the symptoms at home. Signs of peritonitis include an elevated temperature, chills, tenderness, or abdominal pain, nausea and vomiting, and cloudy outflow of solution. If these signs develop, the patient should contact the health care provider immediately.

## SPECIAL ENVIRONMENTS FOR CARE

### Critical Care Management

The patient with ESRD will require critical care management if severe complications develop from the disease or therapy for renal failure. The treatment will depend upon the clinical manifestations, and the patient may require ventilatory and circulatory support.

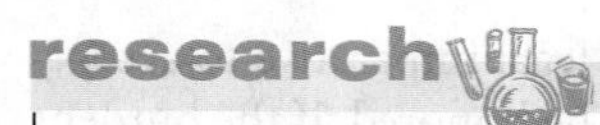

Reference: Friesen D: A descriptive study of home dialysis spouses, *Dialysis Transplant* 26(5):310-345, 1997.

The purpose of this study was to gather and evaluate data regarding the experiences and perceptions of spouses of home dialysis patients. The sample consisted of eight spouses ranging in age from 33 to 66. Data were collected by taped interviews. Questions covered the areas of level of involvement and level of resentment. Four categories were developed: The doer, the minimal assistant, the joint partner, and the nonparticipant. No spouses fell into the nonparticipant category. The doer spouses were older (40 to 50), female, no children at home, and married an average of 27 years. These spouses reported feelings of resentment tempered by a strong marital commitment. The minimal assistant group were in their thirties, married an average of 13 years, and had children living at home. These spouses had a high degree of resentment, social isolation, and overall dissatisfaction with the marriage. The joint partners were between 36 and 66 years of age and married between 13 and 36 years. These couples shared the duties of home dialysis equally and were more successful incorporating home dialysis into their lives. These couples stated that their marriage was strengthened by this commitment to do dialysis at home. The indications for nursing include the importance of assessing family support, communication patterns, and willingness to help as part of the screening process for complicated home therapies such as dialysis. Nurses need to communicate the importance of marital support groups for families dealing with chronic illness.

### Home Care Management

The home environment is a key issue when evaluating the feasibility of home care for the person with renal failure. Home peritoneal dialysis requires space and can turn a home into a hospital clinic.

Safety and cleanliness must be of top priority. Patients receiving CAPD will need to have dialysis equipment readily available. The cycler is currently being used in home CAPD.[12] The cycler requires little hands-on manipulation and allows for dialysis to take place continuously during the night, which permits freedom from dialysis during the day. Because of the increased amount of equipment, the patient requires additional teaching about the use of the cycler, including troubleshooting guidelines. Home management of dialysis can be a strain on families and requires a high degree of commitment (Research Box).

### Hospice Care

Approximately 15% to 20% of dialysis patients voluntarily choose to discontinue dialysis. Because patient autonomy in the United States is the overriding legal imperative to accepting treatment, patient wishes must be honored. If the burdens of a life with impaired quality are so great that continuation of therapy offers no benefit but only prolongs a miserable existence, then discontinuing dialysis is reasonable. This is not considered suicide by the major religious groups (Protestant, Catholic, Jewish, Muslim, and Buddhist). Patients are very apprehensive about the process of dying; they fear pain and discomfort. Nurses can assure patients and families that death from uremia is generally quiet, peaceful, and without pain or discomfort. Hospice care is very helpful for patients who wish to remain at home.[7]

As the patient dies, it is unreasonable to continue fluid and dietary restrictions. Many patients wish to enjoy favorite foods previously denied them; this wish should be honored. As the uremia progresses, patients will restrict their own intake. The goals of nursing care are maintaining comfort and safety and providing the opportunity for patient and family to express their feelings and arrive at some degree of emotional comfort.

In providing physical comfort, frequent turning and repositioning are necessary to prevent skin excoriation and breakdown. Oral care is extremely important, because mouth sores, once developed, will not heal. Mineral oil is an acceptable protective lubricant for the alert patient; a water-soluble lubricant with a vegetable base (such as K-Y jelly) is preferable for the unresponsive patient. Hydrogen peroxide is helpful in removing blood from the mouth and nose. A vinegar mouthwash neutralizes the ammonia.

As death approaches and the patient's level of awareness and ability to control the environment decreases, it becomes the responsibility of the nursing staff to provide safety. (Chapter 52 describes the specific care required for the unconscious patient.)

Providing an opportunity for the patient and family to talk about their feelings is one of the more important aspects of nursing care. Thoughts concerning death and concern about treatments can produce considerable anxiety. The wishes of the patient and family regarding spiritual counseling should be determined. Through demonstrating interest in individual needs and providing comfort measures, the nurse can do much to help the patient and family through the process of dying. (For further information on loss, grief, and dying, see Chapter 8.)

## critical thinking QUESTIONS

1. A 65-year-old man is seen at your clinic with complaints of voiding in small amounts and constant feelings of urgency despite having voided. He also complains of bouts of incontinence. His post-void residual volume is 300 ml. Both BUN and creatinine levels are elevated. What are some risk factors that may contribute to this patient's problem? What diagnostic examinations might be ordered? He is admitted for renal failure to a general medical unit. His blood pressure is stable. What nursing interventions are appropriate? What are treatment options?
2. A 31-year-old woman with streptococcal pneumonia is admitted. She was treated for strep throat last month with penicillin but did not take the entire course of antibiotics. She is now in the intensive care unit and showing signs of ARF. Her BUN and creatinine levels are elevated, and she has 5 to 10 ml of urine output per shift despite treatment with fluids and dopamine. What may have contributed to the cause of the ARF? What treatment options should be considered? Describe the appropriate nursing interventions.
3. A 50-year-old female patient receiving CAPD enters the emergency room with complaints of severe abdominal pain and cramping. She is nauseated and febrile. Her CAPD catheter site is red and swollen. Her white blood cell count is elevated. What do you suspect her diagnosis to be? Will she receive her dialysis while she has these symptoms? If so, how will dialysis be accomplished?
4. Mr. R., 39, is an exterminator. He is admitted to the hospital for persistent flank pain and denies urinary frequency, urgency, or pain. He has had no recent illnesses or injuries except for a sore throat 3 weeks ago that subsided without treatment. His family history is positive for hypertension and diabetes. He is currently taking no medication. What risk factors does Mr. R. have for the development of renal disease?
5. Mrs. G., 57, has a 10-year history of systemic lupus erythematosus. She has been treated intermittently with prednisone to control symptoms. Her disease has been slowly progressive but has not interfered with her ability to work. Mrs. G is married with two adult daughters. She is 5 feet 4 inches tall and normally weighs 132 pounds. Does Mrs. G. have any significant risk factors for renal failure? If so, what? Explain how lupus can affect her renal status.

## chapter SUMMARY

- Renal failure is a state of total or nearly total loss of the kidney's ability to excrete waste products and to maintain fluid and electrolyte balance.

### ACUTE RENAL FAILURE

- Signs and symptoms indicating the onset of ARF appear rapidly and are a direct result of retention of fluids, metabolic wastes, and inability to regulate electrolytes.
- The oliguric phase of ARF is characterized by inability to excrete fluid loads (oliguria), hyperkalemia, hyponatremia, metabolic acidosis, and uremia. The diuretic phase is characterized by excessive diuresis with loss of sodium and potassium; BUN remains elevated, then decreases slowly.
- Nursing care during the oliguric phase of ARF includes monitoring and controlling fluid intake, controlling protein and potassium intake, encouraging a high-carbohydrate, high-fat diet, promoting rest/activity balance, and prevent-

ing injury and infection. During the diuretic phase, monitoring of fluid and electrolyte balance continues, activity is encouraged, and learning is facilitated.

**CHRONIC RENAL FAILURE**

- Chronic renal failure represents progressive and irreversible kidney damage. It is characterized by altered fluid and electrolyte balance and regulatory body functions and by retention of nitrogenous wastes (uremia).
- Chronic renal failure can be treated by conservative medical management, CRRT, hemodialysis, peritoneal dialysis or its variations (CAPD and CCPD), or kidney transplantation.
- Nursing interventions for chronic renal failure include maintaining fluid and electrolyte balance, preventing infection and injury, promoting comfort, facilitating coping with lifestyle changes and feelings regarding self, and facilitating teaching.

**DIALYSIS**

- Dialysis involves movement of fluid and particles across a semipermeable membrane by diffusion, osmosis, and ultrafiltration. Hemodialysis involves shunting the patient's blood through a dialyzer to exchange fluids, electrolytes, and waste materials. With peritoneal dialysis, the peritoneum becomes the dialyzing membrane.
- Nursing care for hemodialysis includes preventing hypovolemia, shock, disequilibrium phenomenon, and blood loss; promoting comfort; maintaining activity and nutrition; and facilitating learning.
- Nursing care for peritoneal dialysis includes regulating fluid volume and drainage, promoting comfort, preventing complications, and facilitating learning.

**KIDNEY TRANSPLANTATION**

- Kidney transplantation restores normal kidney function, eliminates dependence on dialysis, and is less expensive than dialysis after the first year.

## References


1. Blanford N: Renal transplantation: a case study of the ideal, *Crit Care Nurse* 13(1):45-55, 1993.
2. Brady HR, Brenner BM: Acute renal failure. In Isselbacher KJ et al, editors: *Harrison's principles of internal medicine,* ed 13, New York, 1994, McGraw-Hill.
3. Brenner BM, Lazarus JM: Chronic renal failure. In Isselbacher KJ et al, editors: *Harrison's principles of internal medicine,* ed 13, New York, 1994, McGraw-Hill.
4. Catts L: Renal disorders and their management. In Urden, Lough, Stacy, editors: *Priorities in critical care,* St Louis, 1996, Mosby.
5. Chaing H, Liu H: An exploration of the factors influencing the needs for CAPD patients, an abstract, *Nursing Res* 3(2):106-116, 1996.
6. Emmett M, Hootkins R: Phosphorus binders. In Nissenson AR, Fine RN, editors: *Dialysis therapy,* St Louis, 1993, Mosby.
7. Foulks C: Ethical dilemmas in dialysis: to initiate or withdraw therapy. In Nissenson AR, Fine RN, editors: *Dialysis therapy,* St Louis, 1993, Mosby.
8. Guyton AC, Hall JE: *Textbook of medical physiology,* Philadelphia, 1996, WB Saunders.
9. Hodsman AB: Use of vitamin D sterols in the management of renal osteodystrophy. In Nissenson AR, Fine RN, editors: *Dialysis therapy,* St Louis, 1993, Mosby.
10. Keen M: Patients with fluid and electrolyte disturbances. In Clochesy J et al, editors: *Critical care nursing,* Philadelphia, 1996, WB Saunders.
11. King B: Preserving renal function, *RN* 60(8):34-39, 1997.
12. Llach F: Differential diagnosis of renal osteodystrophy. In Nissenson AR, Fine RN, editors: *Dialysis therapy,* St Louis, 1993, Mosby.
13. Newman L, Hanslik T, Tessman M: Cost effective automated peritoneal dialysis for the patient with average to low transport: an 8-10 L mixed APD/CAPD regimen, *ANNA J* 21(5):271-273, 1994.
14. Olivera J: Post surgical acute renal failure: which patients are at risk, *J Crit Care Illness* 9(7):673-685, 1994.
15. Peschman P: Renal physiology. In Clochesy J et al, editors: *Critical care nursing,* Philadelphia, 1996, WB Saunders.
16. Pescola G, Akhavan I, Carion G: Urinary creatinine excretion in the ICU; low excretion does not mean inadequate collection, *Am J Crit Care* 2(6):462-466, 1993.
17. Ponferrada L et al: Home visit effectiveness for peritoneal dialysis patients, *ANNA J* 20(3):333-336, 1993.
18. Price C: Issues related to care of the critically ill patient with end stage renal disease, *Crit Care Nurse* 3(3):585-595, 1992.
19. Stark J: Dialysis choices: turning the tide in acute renal failure, *Nursing 97* 27(2):41-46, 1997.
20. US Department of Health and Human Services, Public Health Service: *Healthy People 2000: midcourse review and 1995 revisions,* Washington, DC, 1990 US Government Printing Office.
21. Whittaker A: Patients with acute renal failure. In Clochesy J et al, editors: *Critical care nursing,* Philadelphia, 1993, WB Saunders.
22. Wolcott DL: Psychosocial rehabilitation of adult dialysis patients. In Nissenson AR, Fine RN, editors: *Dialysis therapy,* St Louis, 1993, Mosby.
23. Yarian S: Patients with end-stage renal disease. In Clochesy J et al, editors: *Critical care nursing,* Philadelphia, 1996, WB Saunders.

# chapter 46 ASSESSMENT OF THE Reproductive System and Sexuality

JOAN SHETTIG

## objectives

*After studying this chapter, the learner should be able to:*

1 Describe the structures and functions of the male and female reproductive systems.
2 Explain the functions of the major hormones that control the reproductive systems.
3 Describe age-related changes in the reproductive systems.
4 Identify data related to the reproductive system and sexual function that should be obtained from a patient history.
5 Discuss diagnostic and laboratory tests used in identifying reproductive tract problems and related nursing interventions.

Conditions affecting healthful functioning of the reproductive systems of men and women take a high toll in loss of life and acute and chronic physical and emotional stress. The nurse has a responsibility to assist in general health education, to refer patients for appropriate health care, and to understand the treatment available and the nursing care needed when disease develops. A sound knowledge of the structure and function of the reproductive system is essential to the assessment process.

## ANATOMY AND PHYSIOLOGY

### PELVIS

The bones of the pelvis are shown in Figure 46-1. The pelvis is the weight-bearing structure of the upper body and trunk. The pelvic bones consist of the innominate bones, the sacrum, and the coccyx. The two innominate bones are made up of the pubic bone, ilium, and ischium. Anteriorly, the pubic bones join at the symphysis pubis. The inferior borders of the pubic bones and symphysis form an inverted V, called the pubic arch. The sacrum and coccyx come together at the sacrococcygeal joint, which is movable.

The pelvis is divided into two parts (the true and the false pelvis) by a bony ridge called the pelvic brim (Figure 46-2). The false pelvis is the broad, expanded portion above the pelvic brim. The narrow part below the pelvic brim is the true pelvis. The true pelvis is further described as having an inlet and an outlet. The inlet is located at the pelvic brim, and the outlet is at the base of the pelvis. The iliac spines mark the midpoint between the inlet and the outlet. The distances between the bones of the true pelvis have special significance during childbirth, since it is through this bony canal that the baby must pass to be born.

There are four basic pelvic types: gynecoid, anthropoid, android, and platypelloid. The gynecoid, or typical female pelvis, occurs in the majority of women and is wider and more shallow and therefore especially suited for childbirth. The android, or typical male pelvis, is heart shaped and is characterized by a narrow subpubic angle and straight sacrum. Pelvic types vary by age, race, and gender. True pelvic types are rare; most pelves are a combination of two types, e.g., gynecoid and android. The major differences between the pelves of men and women are in the contour of the pelvis and thickness of the bones.

### FEMALE GENITAL SYSTEM

#### External Structures

Figure 46-3 shows the external female genitalia. The external genitalia, known collectively as the vulva or pudendum, consist of the mons pubis (mons veneris), labia majora, labia minora, clitoris, prepuce, frenulum, vestibule, urethral meatus, Skene's (paraurethral) glands, vaginal orifice, hymen, fossa navicularis, Bartholin's (vulvovaginal) glands, fourchet, perineum, and escutcheon. The *escutcheon* is the triangular pubic hair pattern from the upper portion of the pubic bone to the lateral areas of the labia majora. The *mons pubis* is the rounded area in front of the symphysis pubis. It consists of a collection of fatty tissue beneath the skin and is covered with hair after puberty.

The *labia majora* are two prominent, longitudinal folds of tissue extending back from the mons pubis. The labia are thicker in front, gradually become thinner as they extend back, and appear to flatten out as they merge with the adjacent tissues in the area of the perineum. The labia majora have two surfaces. The outer surface is covered by a thin layer of skin containing hair follicles and sebaceous and sweat glands. The inner surfaces are smooth, lack hair, and are supplied with many sebaceous follicles. The labia are homologous to the male scrotum.

The *labia minora* are two smaller folds of tissue parallel to the labia majora and sometimes concealed between the folds of the labia majora. In sexually active women and in women who have borne children, the labia minora may project beyond the labia majora. The labia minora join near the prepuce, which covers the clitoris, extend backward to enclose the urethral and vaginal openings, and merge with the labia

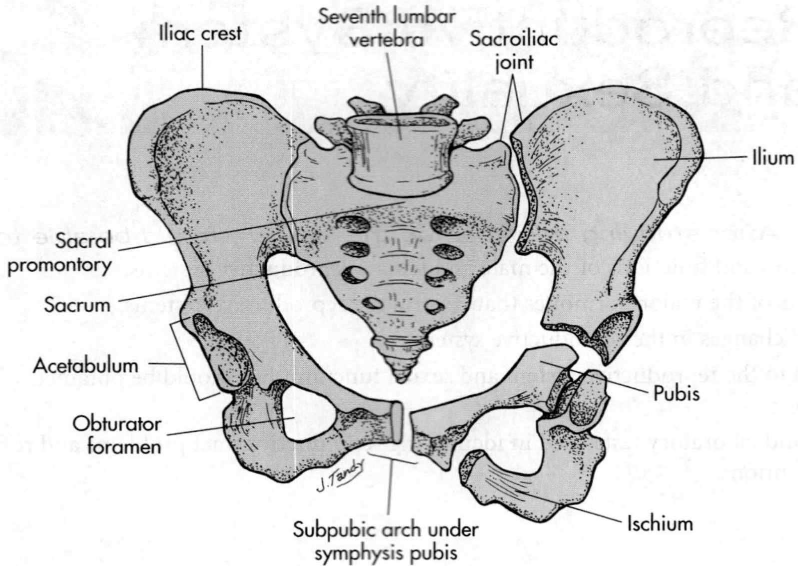


**fig. 46-1** Adult female pelvis.

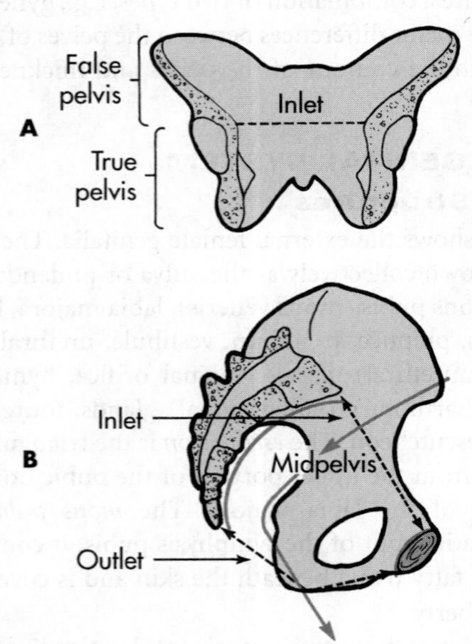


**fig. 46-2** Female pelvis. **A,** Cavity of the false pelvis is a shallow basin above the inlet; the true pelvis is a deeper cavity below the inlet. **B,** Cavity of the true pelvis is an irregularly curved canal *(arrows)*.

majora in the perineum. The labia minora are made up of connective and elastic tissue and contain little fatty tissue. Sweat glands and hair follicles are absent from the labia minora, but sebaceous glands are present.

The *clitoris* is situated near the anterior folds of the labia minora. The glans of the clitoris is a small, rounded area consisting of erectile tissue enclosed in a layer of fibrous membrane. Although it is often said to be homologous to the penis in males because it consists of the glans, corpus, and crura, the clitoris is unique in that its sole physiological functions are initiation and elevation of sexual tension levels. The clitoris both receives and transforms sexual stimuli. Sexual stimulation initiates a process whereby the clitoris becomes enlarged, erect, and very sensitive to sexual stimuli. Female orgasm can occur from stimulation of the clitoris but also results from stimulation of other sites.

The *vestibule* is a boat-shaped fossa formed between the labia minora, clitoris, and fourchet. The *fossa navicularis* is a small depression between the fourchet and hymen. On opening the labia minora, the vaginal and urethral orifices can be seen.

The *hymen* is a thin membrane that partially covers the vaginal orifice or introitus. It can be broken or avulsed by coitus, digital examination, tampon use, vigorous exercise, or surgery. Remnants of the hymen remain after avulsion and form an irregular border around the vagina.

The paraurethral or *Skene's glands* are located on either side of the urethral meatus and drain the multiple urethral glands. The *Bartholin's glands* secrete a lubricating mucus needed for intercourse and are located near the vaginal opening on either side of the labia. The Skene's and Bartholin's glands are usually not visible or palpable unless infected. If infected, the glands are enlarged, erythematous, and painful.

The *perineum* is the area between the vagina and anus. It is composed of muscles and subdermal and dermal tissue.

Appearance of the external genitalia varies with age. Before puberty, there is no pubic hair, and the labia minora is larger than the labia majora. Sexual maturation in girls usually begins between 8½ and 13 years. With the onset of menopause and gradual withdrawal of hormones, the external genitalia again become less prominent, and the pubic hair begins to thin. In elderly women, the mons pubis is thinner secondary to the loss of the fat pad, and the clitoris and labia become smaller. See p. 1513 for reproductive physical changes related to aging.

### Internal Organs

The female internal reproductive organs are shown in Figures 46-4 and 46-5. The internal reproductive organs are lo-

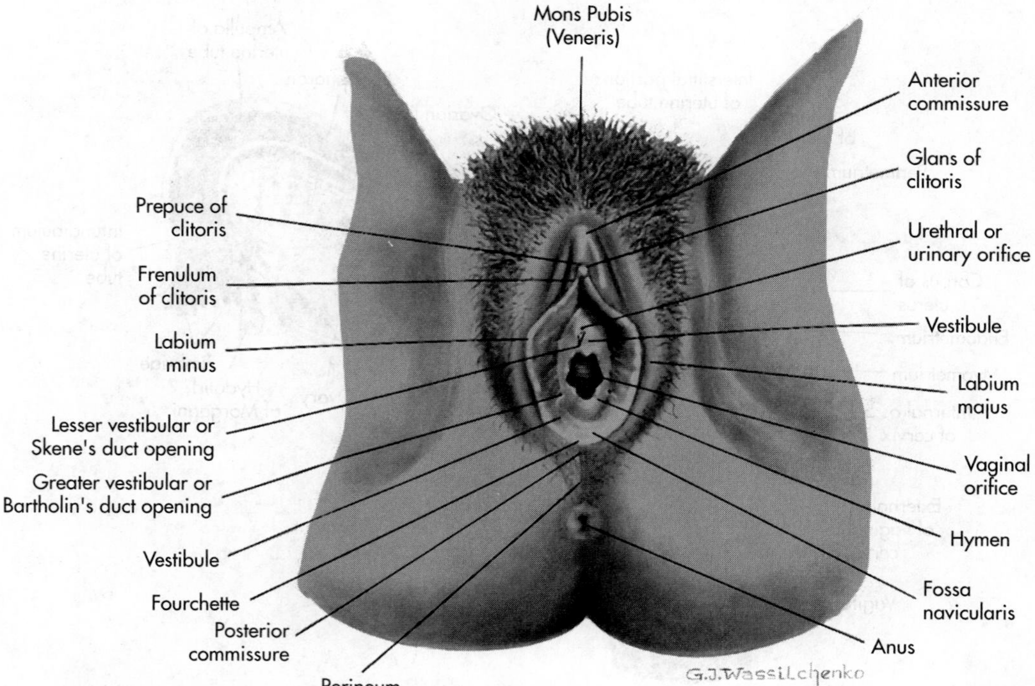


**fig. 46-3** External female genitals.

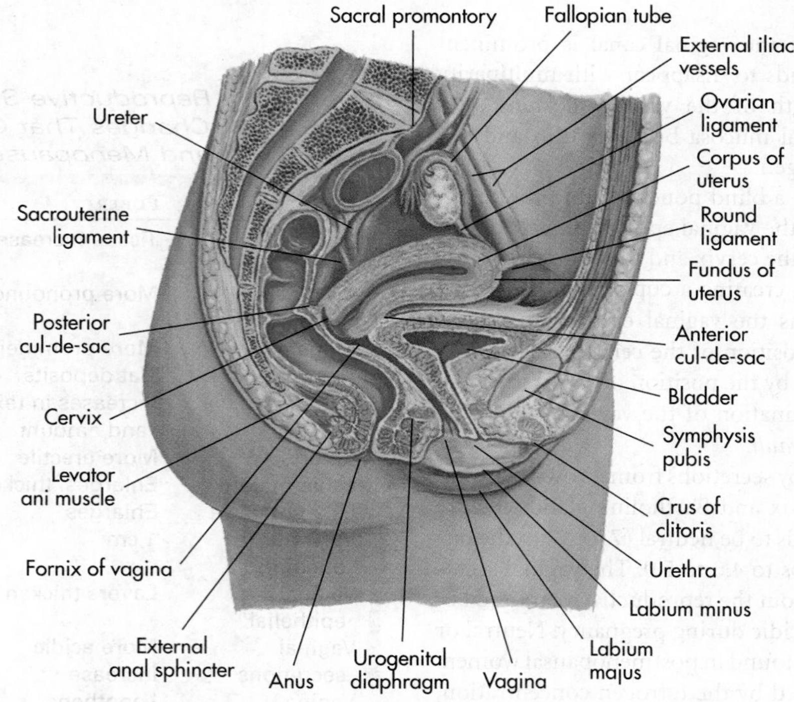


**fig. 46-4** Midsagittal view of the female pelvic organs.

cated in the true pelvis and remain there unless a disease process or pregnancy increase their size.

### *Vagina*

The *vagina* is a soft, tubular structure that extends upward and back from the vaginal opening connecting the vulva with the cervix and uterus. Located between the rectum and urethra, the vagina receives the penis during intercourse, allows for childbirth, and permits discharge of the menstrual flow. The length of the vaginal canal varies, and the posterior wall is longer (8 to 9 cm) than the anterior wall (6 to 8 cm).

The vagina is lined with pink mucous membrane arranged in transverse folds called *rugae*. The rugae make it possible for the vagina to distend and stretch during coitus and childbirth.

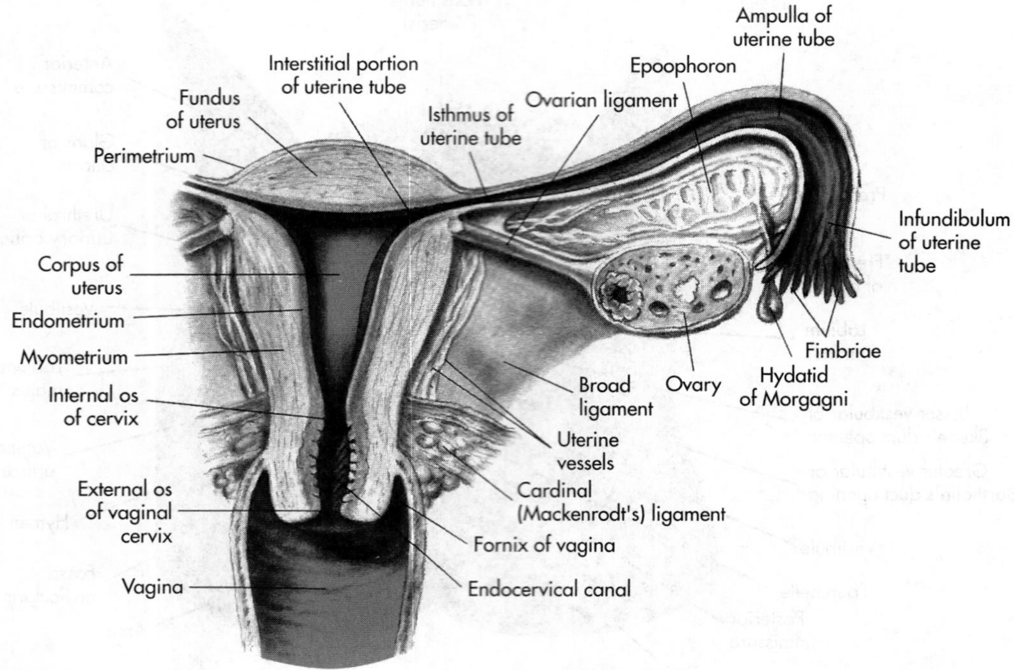


**fig. 46-5** Cross section of uterus, adnexa, and upper vagina.

The rugated appearance of the vaginal canal is prominent during adolescence and tends to disappear with multiparity and menopause. The length of the vagina shortens after menopause, and the vaginal mucosa becomes thin and dry due to the decrease in estrogen.

The vaginal walls end in a blind pouch around the cervix called the *fornix.* Note that the vaginal epithelium is continuous with the epithelium of the cervix and that the cervix projects into the upper vagina, creating a cup shape. The cervix has the same pink color as the vaginal epithelium, but is smoother in texture. The position of the cervix varies somewhat and can be influenced by the position of the uterus. The groove formed by the termination of the vagina around the cervix is called the *vaginal vault.*

The vagina is lubricated by secretions from its own cells and by secretions from the cervix and Bartholin's glands. Before puberty, the vaginal pH tends to be neutral (7.0). With the onset of puberty, the pH drops to 4.0 to 5.0. The vaginal secretions remain acidic throughout the reproductive years and become even more strongly acidic during pregnancy. Neutral or alkaline values are normally found in postmenopausal women. Acidity is strongly influenced by the estrogen concentration, which controls the glycogen levels of the cells. The normal vaginal flora, Döderlein's bacilli, interact with the secreted glycogen to produce lactic acid and maintain an acid pH.

The vaginal pH can be influenced by personal hygiene measures such as douches, deodorant tampons, and bubble baths or by pathogenic bacteria. Any change in vaginal pH decreases the natural vaginal defenses and increases the risk of infection. See Table 46-1 for additional physical changes that occur at puberty and at menopause.

**table 46-1** *Reproductive System Physical Changes That Occur at Puberty and Menopause*

| | Puberty | Menopause* |
|---|---|---|
| Breasts | Tissue increases | Smaller, less elastic |
| Nipple and areola | More pronounced | Smaller, flatter |
| Mons pubis | More prominent, fat deposits | Thinner, loss of fat pad |
| Pubic hair | Increases in texture and amount | Sparse, gray |
| Clitoris | More erectile | Smaller |
| Labia majora | Enlarges, thickens | Smaller |
| Labia manora | Enlarges | Thinner |
| Vaginal opening | 1 cm | Smaller |
| Vaginal epithelial | Layers thicken | Thin, pale, more fragile |
| Vaginal secretions | More acidic<br>Increase | Less acidic<br>Decrease |
| Vagina | Lengthens | Shortens, narrows |
| Uterus | Increases in size | Decreases in size |
| Endometrial lining | Thickens | Thins |
| Ovaries | Increase in size | Shrink to 1-2 cm, no longer palpable |

*Changes may be influenced by hormone replacement therapy.

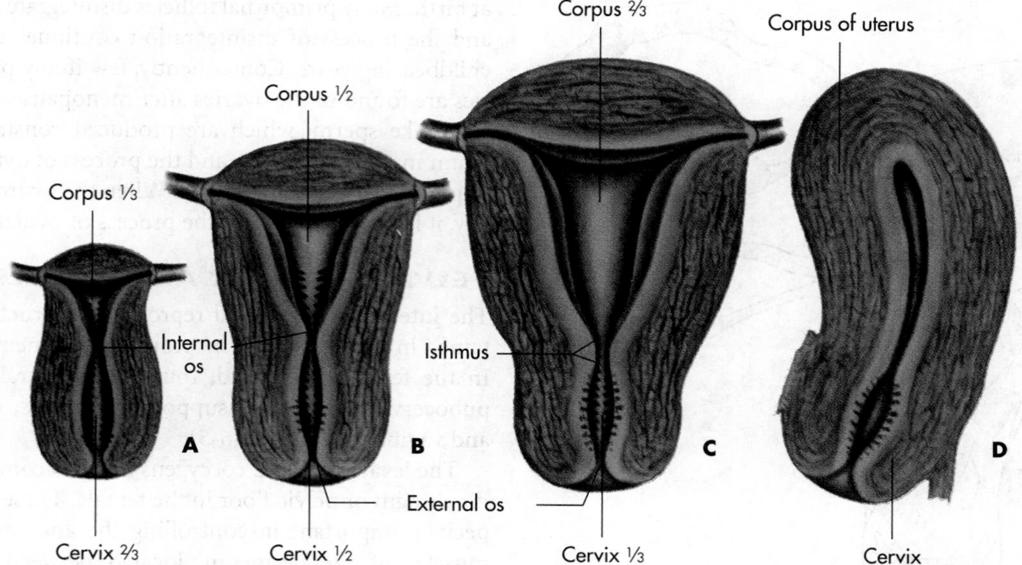


**fig. 46-6** Comparative sizes of uteri at various stages of development. **A,** Prepubertal; **B,** adult nulliparous; **C,** adult multiparous; **D,** lateral view, adult multiparous. The fractions give the relative proportion of the size of the corpus and the cervix.

### Uterus

The uterus is a hollow, muscular organ located between the urinary bladder and rectum. Its three portions are the *fundus, corpus* (body), and the *cervix.* The fundus is the thick muscular region above the insertion of the fallopian tubes. The corpus is the main portion of the uterus and is joined to the cervix by an isthmus of constricted tissue. The cervix is the narrow lower segment that terminates in the vagina and is the "neck of the uterus." The size of the uterus decreases from the fundus to the cervix, creating a triangular, pear-shaped appearance. The size of the uterus varies among women, ranging from 5.5 to 9 cm long, 3.5 to 6 cm wide, and 2 to 4 cm thick in nonparous women. All dimensions may be 2 to 3 cm larger in multiparous women (Figure 46-6).

The position of the uterus is subject to considerable variation. The uterus is usually anteverted and slightly anteflexed, although it may be retroverted, retroflexed, or in midposition. The body of the uterus is normally bent forward over the bladder so that the fundus is behind the symphysis pubis. The uterus is in direct contact with the bladder and may also touch the rectum, sigmoid colon, and small intestines. The cervix curves forward. During pregnancy, the uterus changes remarkably in size, shape, structure, and position and returns to its prepregnancy state within 6 to 8 weeks after delivery.

The outer surfaces of the uterus are covered by peritoneum, which is reflected from the abdominal wall. The anterior and posterior reflections of the peritoneum join at the sides to enclose the fallopian tubes and ovaries. Reflection of the peritoneum over the top of the pelvic organs creates spaces between the uterus and bladder anteriorly and the uterus and rectum posteriorly. The posterior space is known as the *cul-de-sac of Douglas* and is a common entry site for culdoscopy, culpotomy, and surgical drainage of the peritoneal cavity.

The uterus has three functional layers: the parametrium, which is the peritoneal and fascial outer layer; the myometrium, which is the middle muscular layer; and the endometrium, which is the uterine lining. The cavity of the uterus is continuous with the cervical canal and has an average capacity of 3 to 8 ml. Near the fundus, the uterus opens into the lumen of the fallopian tubes. Thus a direct route exists from the vagina through the cervix, uterus, and fallopian tubes to the peritoneum.

The cervix is firm, smooth, and round. It is primarily made up of elastic and fibrous connective tissue and smooth muscle. The *external os* is located in the center of the vaginal portion of the cervix. Extending upward from the external os is the cervical canal, which averages 2 to 3 cm in length. The cervical canal terminates as it joins the corpus, and the junction of the cervical canal and the corpus is termed the *internal cervical os.* The cervix secretes mucus to facilitate transport of sperm, dilates during labor, and provides a channel for discharge of the menstrual flow. Figure 46-7 illustrates the changes that occur in the uterus after menopause.

### Fallopian tubes

The fallopian tubes are two narrow, muscular canals ranging from 8 to 14 cm in length. They extend outward from the corpus near the fundus and are enclosed in the folds of the broad ligaments. The tubes are divided into three portions: the *isthmus* is the proximal portion of the tube; the *ampulla* is the longer, middle portion where fertilization usually occurs; and the distal portion of the tube is the *infundibulum,* which terminates in fimbria (see Figure 46-5).

The fallopian tubes serve as a site for union of the ovum and sperm, and transport the ovum to the uterus. The walls of the fallopian tubes contain smooth muscles that possess peristaltic properties. The fallopian tubes are lined with a mucous

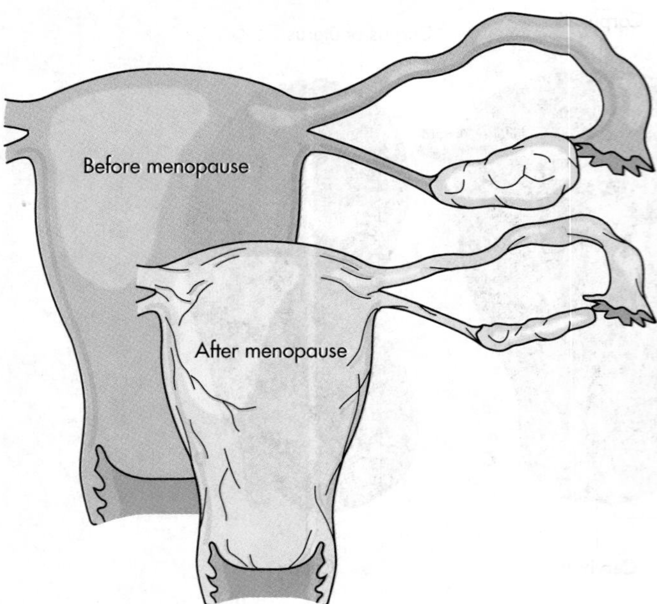


**fig. 46-7** Uterus and ovary before and after menopause.

membrane that contains cilia. At the time of ovulation, both the peristaltic and ciliary action increase and provide the mechanism for ovum transport.

### Ovaries

The ovaries are endocrine glands as well as reproductive organs. The two almond-shaped ovaries, ranging from 3 to 4 cm long, 2 cm wide, and 1 to 2 cm thick, lie near the fimbriae of the fallopian tubes. The ovaries are partly enclosed by the broad ligaments. Each ovary contains an outer portion (cortex) and an inner portion (medulla). The term *adnexa* refers to the ovaries, fallopian tubes, and supporting tissues. The ovaries store primordial follicles, produce mature ova, and produce and secrete estrogen, progesterone, and androgens.

The ovaries undergo physical changes in position, size, and shape during the life span. At birth, the ovaries are very small and are located in the false pelvis. Between infancy and puberty, the ovaries increase in size and descend into the true pelvis. During the childbearing years, the ovaries appear long and flat and have a nodular surface caused by the presence of follicles. During pregnancy, the ovaries are lifted out of the pelvis by the enlarging uterus, but they descend back into the pelvis after childbirth. After menopause, the ovaries undergo rapid regressive changes, decrease in size, and become wrinkled. In most postmenopausal women, the ovaries are so small that they cannot be palpated during vaginal examination.

After puberty, the surfaces of the ovaries are covered by connective tissue fibers that form a layer called the *tunica albuginea*. Immediately below the connective tissue is the ovarian cortex containing many minute vesicles, the primordial follicles. Each follicle contains an undeveloped ovum having the capacity to respond to stimulation by pituitary hormones. Each ovary contains an estimated 500,000 primordial follicles at birth. Many primordial follicles disintegrate before puberty, and the process of disintegration continues throughout the childbearing years. Consequently, few if any primordial follicles are found in the ovaries after menopause.

Unlike sperm, which are produced constantly, only one ovum matures at a time, and the process of ovum maturation requires an average of 28 days. When the ovum reaches maturity, it leaves the ovary by the process of ovulation.

## PELVIC LIGAMENT AND MUSCLES

The internal and external reproductive structures are maintained in their positions by groups of ligaments and muscles. In the female, the broad, round, uterosacral, cardinal, and pubocervical ligaments support the uterus, ovaries, cervix, and vagina (see Figure 46-5).

The levator ani and coccygeus muscles comprise the pelvic diaphragm or pelvic floor in the female. These muscles are especially important in controlling the anus and vagina. The muscles of the perineum, located between the anus and vagina, commonly called the perineal body or perineal center, reinforce the support provided by the levator ani and coccygeus muscles. The perineal body and pelvic diaphragm support the pelvic organs and external genitalia from below. Figure 46-8 illustrates the perineal muscles of the male and female.

## BLOOD, LYMPH, AND NERVE SUPPLY

In males and females, the organs of reproduction are supplied with blood from the aorta as it branches and divides into the internal iliac (hypogastric) artery. The ovarian and uterine arteries anastomose to furnish the ovaries with blood. The arteries are paired and bilateral and have multiple collaterals. The arteries thread their way through an interwoven mesh of large veins to reach the pelvic reproductive organs, giving off numerous branches and providing a rich blood supply. The venous drainage empties into the vena cava.

In both males and females, lymphatic drainage of the external and internal organs of reproduction is extensive. Nerve supply is derived from both sympathetic and parasympathetic fibers of the autonomic nervous system. In the female, the pudendal nerve and its branches supply the majority of the motor and sensory fibers of the muscles and skin of the vulvar region. The pudendal nerve arises from the second, third, and fourth sacral roots. In the male, the motor segment of the pudendal nerve innervates the urinary sphincter, and the sensory portion supplies the glans penis and urethra.

## BREASTS

The female breasts are accessory structures of the reproductive system meant to nourish the infant after birth (Figure 46-9). They are paired mammary glands located between the second and sixth ribs, the edge of the sternum, and the midaxillary line. They develop in response to hormonal stimulation from the hypothalamus, pituitary gland, and ovaries.

The tissue of the breast has three primary components: an interconnected network of glandular and ductal tissue, fibrous tissue, and fat. The proportion of each tissue is a reflec-

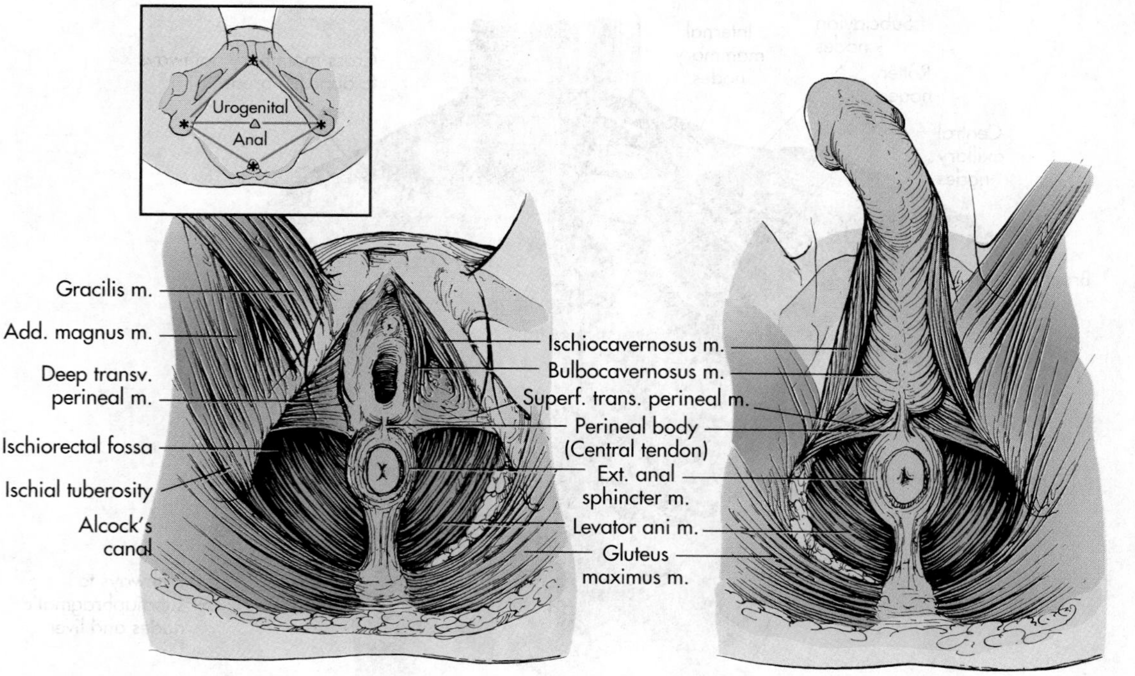

**fig. 46-8** The superficial muscles of the male and female perineum.

tion of the individual woman's genetic make-up, age, obstetric history, and weight. The breast is supported by Cooper's suspensory ligaments, which attach to the underlying muscles.

The nipple is the primary external structure of the breast and arises from the center of the pigmented areola. The elevations on the areola are small, round sebaceous glands termed *Montgomery's glands*. They are believed to secrete a fatty substance that offers some protection to the nipple during breastfeeding.

Internally, each mature breast is composed of 15 to 25 lobes arranged radially around the breast and separated from each other by fatty tissue. Each lobe is composed of several lobules, which in turn are composed of numerous alveoli. Each alveolus is connected by a duct to a larger lactiferous duct from the lobule, which join to form one duct from each lobe and then converge at the nipple. Just before the nipple, the ducts expand into sinuses, which serve as reservoirs. The epithelial linings of the alveoli synthesize and secrete the components of breast milk in response to stimulation by prolactin from the pituitary.

The breasts receive an abundant blood supply from the internal mammary and lateral thoracic arteries. Their venous drainage connects to the superior vena cava. They contain an extensive lymph drainage network originating within the breast and draining radially into the axillary and subclavian nodal system. Drainage from the axillary region empties into the jugular and subclavian veins. This short and direct route assumes significance in the metastasis of breast cancer (Figure 46-10).

Many women experience noticeable changes in their breasts in response to the menstrual cycle. The breasts may enlarge and become tender or nodular in the premenstrual period in response to the increasing levels of estrogen and progesterone. The cellular growth regresses after menstruation, and water retention is relieved.

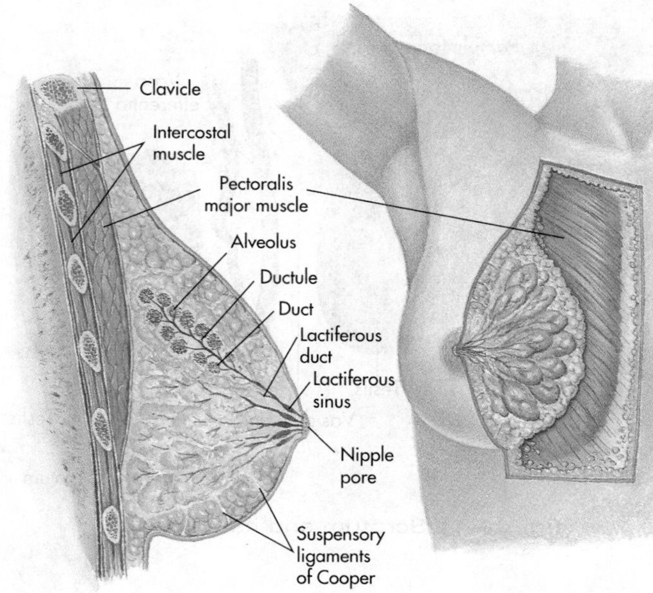


**fig. 46-9** Anatomy of the breast, showing position and major structures.

## MALE GENITAL SYSTEM

The male reproductive organs and associated structures are shown in Figure 46-11. The male reproductive organs produce

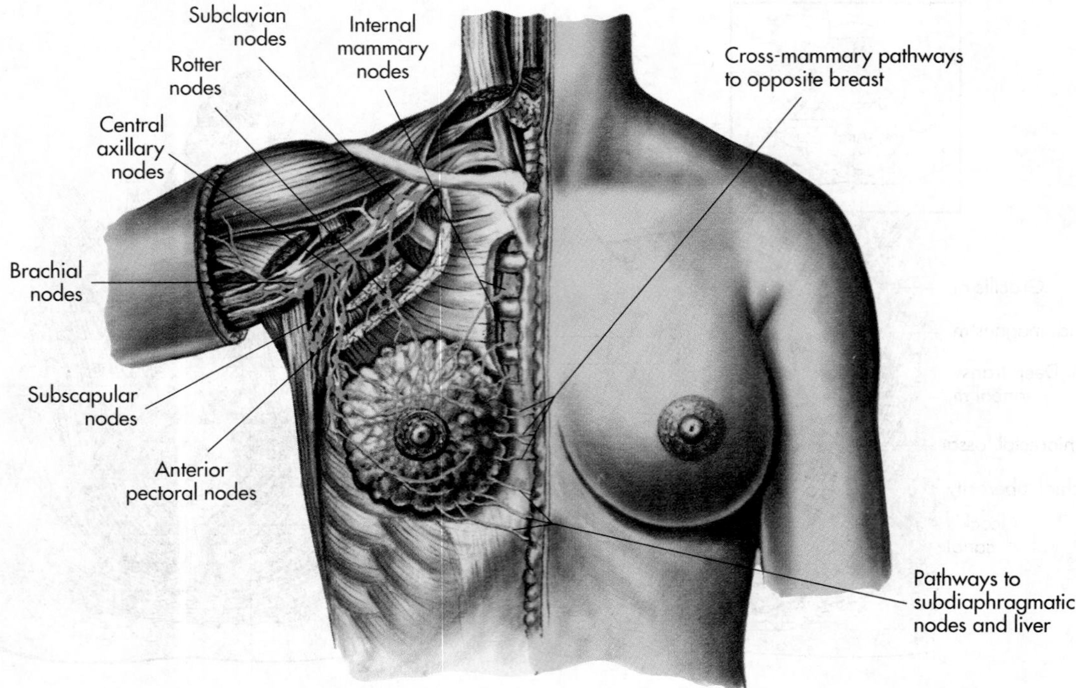


**fig. 46-10** Lymphatic drainage of breast.

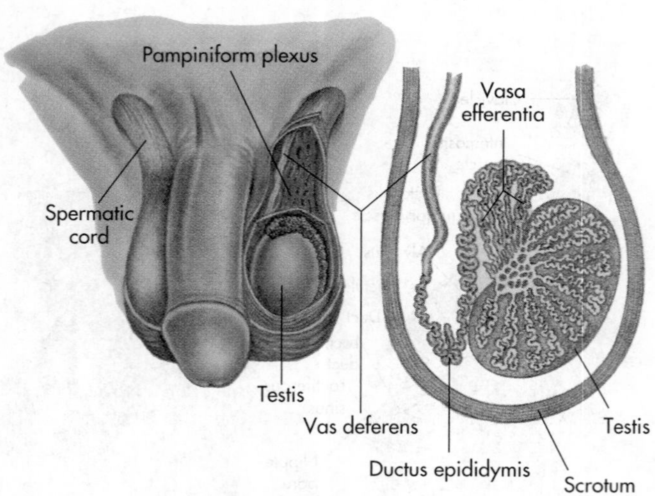


**fig. 46-11** Scrotum and its contents.

sperm, suspend the sperm in a liquid, and deliver the sperm into the vagina to fertilize an ovum. They also secrete male hormones, the androgens. The male genitalia include the penis, scrotum, and testes.

## External Structures

### *Penis*

The penis is a conduit for elimination of ejaculate and urine through the urethral opening. It can be divided into two parts; the pendulous portion or *corpus*, and the perineal portion or *radix* (root). The penis consists of three erectile columns of cavernous tissue. The two corpora cavernosa form the dorsum and sides of the penis. The corpus spongiosum forms the ventral side. In the root of the penis, the spongiosum is bulbous and is called the bulb of the penis. The corpus spongiosum continues distally and expands at the end of the penis to the glands or balanus. The urethra is encircled by the corpus spongiosum, and at the distal end there is a slitlike opening or *meatus*.

The glans covers the distal third of the corpus of the penis. The dorsum and lateral sides of the glans are called the *corona*. The dorsal surface of the glans meets the corpus in the neck of the penis or (retroglandular) *sulcus*.

The corpus of the penis is covered with a thin skin that contains no fat, is darker than body skin, and has redundant tissue, which allows for erection. In an uncircumcised male, the skin at the glans is folded over on itself to form the *prepuce* or foreskin.

Under the skin of the penis, the body of the penis is covered with the dartos layer, which is continuous with the fascia of the anterior abdominal wall, the scrotum, and the perineum. Contained within this layer are the superficial dorsal veins. The deep fascia of the penis, or Buck's fascia, contain the neurovascular bundle.

The root of the penis is attached to the abdominal wall through a thickening and extension of the dartos and Buck's fascia. In addition, the root is covered by the bulbocavernous muscle. This muscle also contains the perineal artery, vein, and nerve, and the pudendal artery, vein, and nerve.

The venous and arterial blood supply to the penis is complex. Several pairs of arteries supply blood (Figure 46-12), but the main arterial source is the internal pudendal artery, which

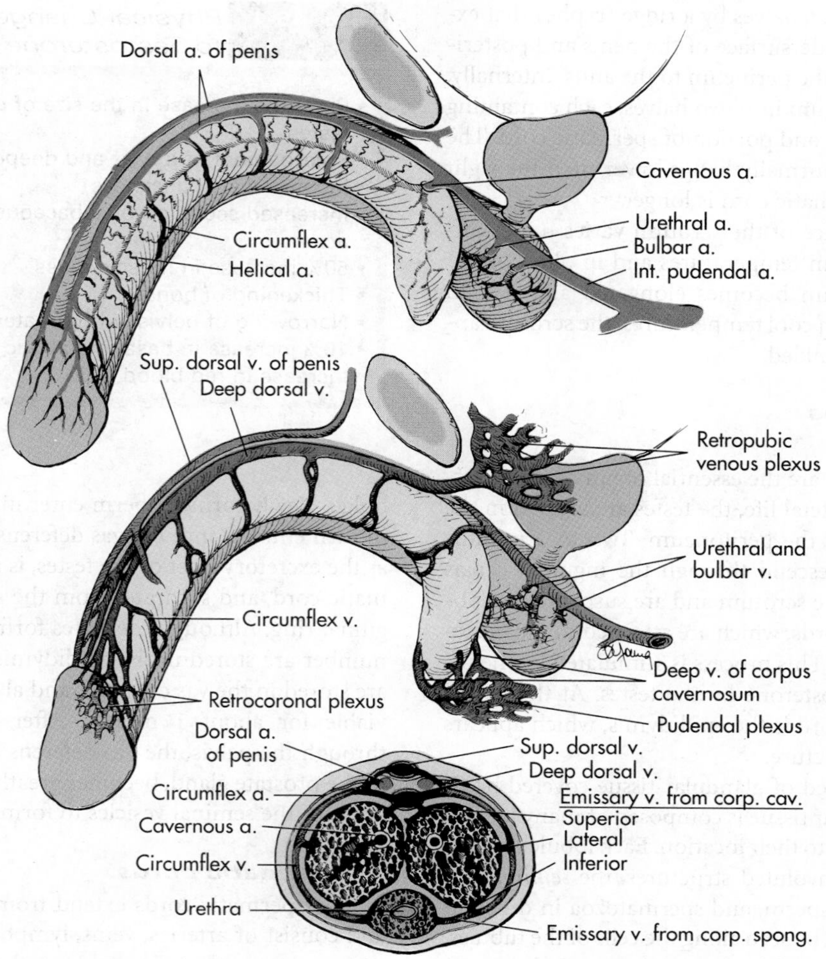


**fig. 46-12** Illustration of vasculature of penis.

branches to form the cavernous, bulbar, urethral, and dorsal arteries. These arteries continue to branch to form the vascular complex of the corpora cavernosa.

The venous drainage includes the superficial dorsal veins in the dartos tunic, the deep dorsal vein under Buck's fascia, and the deep or cavernous veins of the corpus cavernosum. The deep dorsal vein branches to form multiple circumflex veins. The corpus spongiosum is drained via the emissary veins through the urethral and bulbar veins, and the corpora cavernosa drain through the deep dorsal vein or cavernous veins.

In order for the penis to deposit sperm into the vagina an erection must occur. The two types of erections are reflexogenic and psychogenic. Reflexogenic erections follow local stimulation, while psychogenic erections follow stimulation of erotic centers in the brain. Erection and ejaculation are mediated by the sympathetic nervous system, but the exact mechanism is unknown. During erection, the corpora cavernosa and the corpus spongiosum vascular spaces fill with blood, which transforms the penis into a firm organ.

Ejaculation is a two-part process—emission and ejaculation. In the first phase, secretions from the periurethral glands, seminal vesicle, and prostate move into the posterior urethra. Through peristalsis, sperm from the vas deferens is also moved into the posterior urethra.

During ejaculation, the internal sphincter of the bladder closes, the external urethral sphincter relaxes, and ejaculate is expelled by contraction of the perineal and bulbourethral muscles. The typical emission is 3 to 4 ml and contains fluid from the prostate and seminal vesicles and 200 to 400 million spermatoza. After ejaculation, the penis returns to a flaccid state in 1 to 2 minutes.

### Scrotum

The scrotum is a cutaneous pouch that covers and protects the testes and spermatic cords. Because the testes are surrounded by serous membrane and are suspended in the cavity of the scrotum, the testes are capable of being moved about readily. The ease of movement within the scrotum protects the testes against injury.

The skin of the scrotum is thin, brownish, and very elastic because it contains rugae. Because of the rugae, the scrotum distends readily and may become greatly enlarged when edema is present. The scrotal skin is covered by thinly scattered hair and contains sebaceous follicles. The surface of the scrotum is divided into two halves by a ridge (raphe) that extends anteriorly to the undersurface of the penis and posteriorly along the midline of the perineum to the anus. Internally, a septum divides the scrotum into two halves, each containing a testis and its epididymis and portion of spermatic cord. The left side of the scrotum normally hangs lower than the right side because the left spermatic cord is longer.

The external appearance of the scrotum varies under different conditions. In warm temperatures and in older or debilitated men, the scrotum becomes elongated and flat. In young, healthy men and in cool temperatures, the scrotum appears short and more wrinkled.

## Internal Structures

### Testes

The oval-shaped testes are the essential organ of reproduction in the male. During fetal life, the testes are located in the abdominal cavity behind the peritoneum. Two to 3 months before birth the testes descend through the inguinal canals and inguinal rings into the scrotum and are suspended in position by the spermatic cords, which are attached to the posterior borders of the testes. This process is stimulated by the increased secretion of testosterone by the testes. At the lateral edge of each spermatic cord is the epididymis, which appears as a narrow flattened structure.

The testes are composed of glandular tissue covered by fibrous tissue. The glandular tissue is composed of many lobules differing in size according to their location. Each lobule consists of 600 to 1200 small, convoluted structures, the *seminiferous tubules* that produce the sperm, and spermatozoa in different stages of development can be seen along the cells of the tubules.

After puberty, the lining of the seminiferous tubules forms sperm continually. In a young man sperm is produced at a rate of 120 million/day. Each mature sperm has a whiplike tail that makes free movement possible, but the sperm are passive within the testes. The fluids produced within the seminal vesicles and prostate gland suspend the sperm and cause them to become active and motile.

In addition to producing sperm, the testes function as an endocrine gland. The male androgen hormones are stimulated by gonadotropin-releasing hormone (GnRH) from the hypothalamus. GnRH stimulates the anterior pituitary gland to secrete luteinizing hormone (LH) and follicle-stimulating hormone (FSH). LH stimulates testosterone production in the testes and FSH stimulates sperm development. The testes produce testosterone, dihydrotestosterone, and androstenedione. Testosterone is produced in much greater amounts than the other hormones and is therefore considered the most important testicular hormone.

Testosterone production increases greatly at puberty. This increase causes several changes in the male body, including an increase in the size of the penis and scrotum, hair growth on the pubis and face, and voice changes. See Box 46-1 for physical changes in males related to testosterone.

**box 46-1** *Physical Changes Related to Testosterone*

- Eightfold increase in the size of penis, scrotum, and testes
- Enlargement of larynx and deepening of voice
- Increased skin thickness
- Increased secretion of sebaceous glands, may cause acne
- 50% increase in muscle mass
- Thickening of bones
- Narrowing of pelvis, with greater strength
- 10% increase in basal metabolic rate
- Increase in red blood cells

### Epididymis/vas deferens

The comma-shaped epididymis is located at the lateral edge of the posterior segment of the testes where it creates a bulge. Newly formed sperm enter into the epididymis, which in turn empties into the vas deferens. The vas deferens serves as the excretory duct of the testes, is a constituent of the spermatic cord, and separates from the spermatic cord at the inguinal ring. Although the testes form the sperm, only a small number are stored in the epididymis. The majority of sperm are stored in the vas deferens, and although inactive, they stay viable for about 1 month. After taking a complex path through the pelvis, the vas deferens descends, enters the base of the prostate gland, becomes greatly narrowed, and joins the ducts of the seminal vesicles to form the ejaculatory duct.

### Spermatic cords

The spermatic cords extend from the deep inguinal rings and consist of arteries, veins, lymphatics, nerves, and the excretory duct of the testes held together by the spermatic fascia. At the deep inguinal rings the structures of the spermatic cords converge with the structures of the testes, pass through the inguinal canals, emerge through the superficial inguinal rings, and pass downward into the scrotum.

### Seminal vesicles

The seminal vesicles are two lobulated, membranous pouches, 5 to 10 cm long, located between the bladder and the rectum. They secrete fluid that is added to the secretions of the testes. This fluid contains fructose, citric acid, prostaglandins, and fibrinogen, which add to the bulk of the ejaculate. The fructose provides nutrients to the ejaculated sperm; the prostaglandins react with cervical mucous to make it more receptive and probably help to propel the sperm to the fallopian tubes.

The lower end of each seminal vesicle becomes constricted into a straight duct and joins the vas deferens to form the ejaculatory duct. The ejaculatory duct begins at the base of the prostate gland, runs posteriorly and downward, and enters the prostate gland in the midline. In the prostate gland, the ejaculatory duct opens into the prostatic portion of the urethra.

### Prostate gland

The prostate gland is located below the internal urethral orifice, behind the symphysis pubis, and close to the rectal wall, extending around the beginning of the urethra. Enveloped in a firm adherent capsule, the prostate gland grows to the size and shape of a walnut during puberty and weighs about 20 g. Internally, the prostate gland is partly muscular and partly glandular. The glandular substance consists of numerous follicular pouches that open into long canals and join to form 12 to 20 small excretory ducts. Prostatic ducts open into the prostatic portion of the urethra, thus adding the prostatic secretion to the seminal fluid. The prostatic secretion is a thin, white fluid that helps lower the pH of the fluid from the vas deferens and enhance motility and fertility of the sperm.

#### Cowper's glands

Cowper's (bulbourethral) glands are two small, round bodies located at the sides and to the back of the membranous portion of the urethra. Each gland has an excretory duct that opens into the urethra. The main excretory duct of a Cowper's gland represents the joining of many ducts from its internal glandular tissue. Cowper's glands secrete an alkaline substance into the semen to counteract vaginal and urethral acidity.

## ENDOCRINE FUNCTIONS

### Female Hormones

The major hormones produced by the ovaries are estrogen and progesterone. *Estrogen* is responsible for the development of secondary sex characteristics at puberty. After puberty, estrogen primarily causes development of the endometrium in preparation for implantation of a fertilized ovum. *Progesterone* enhances the action of estrogen on the endometrium. The ovaries depend on stimulation from pituitary hormones to fulfill their functions.

### Male Hormones

In males, secretion of the androgenic hormones increases at puberty, resulting in the appearance of secondary sex characteristics and production of mature sperm. *Testosterone* is the androgen most closely related to reproduction, since it specifically stimulates maturation of sperm and is responsible for maintaining the reproductive organs in a functional state. Testosterone secretion is closely related to pituitary gland function. The rate of secretion of testosterone is determined by levels of luteinizing hormone in the blood.

### Menstruation

*Menarche* is the term used to designate the onset of *menstruation*, and it reflects the time when reproduction is first possible. The onset of menarche reflects a girl's age, heredity, general health, weight, and nutritional status and cannot be accurately predicted. The average age at menarche has decreased significantly over the past 100 years and is now 12.5 to 12.8 years, with a normal range from 9.1 to 17.7 years. It is believed that a critical body weight (47.8 kg, or 105 pounds) and shift in body composition to a greater percentage of fat (from 16.0% to 23.5%) must be attained for the average girl to reach menarche.

#### Menstrual cycle

The menstrual cycle includes a complex series of uterine and ovarian changes that result in menstruation. The uterine cycle includes the menstrual, proliferative, and secretory phases that correspond to specific phases of the ovarian cycle as illustrated in Figure 46-13. Both cycles require an average of 28 days. The first day of menstrual flow is considered to be the first day of the menstrual cycle. Normal variation exists in the intervals between menstrual periods, but most cycles occur within a range of 26 to 36 days and last for 3 to 7 days. The greatest variance typically occurs during the perimenarchal and perimenopausal years. The smooth functioning of the menstrual cycle depends on complex relationships among the central nervous system, anterior pituitary, ovaries, and uterus.

**Menstrual phase.** During the menstrual phase of the cycle, the endometrium breaks down and is shed. The production of estrogen and progesterone stops before the onset of menstrual flow, which results in rupture of uterine capillaries and necrosis of endometrial tissue. The menstrual phase of the cycle lasts an average of 4 days. Menstrual fluid does not clot unless it is retained in the uterus or vagina for a prolonged time. It is believed that the endometrium produces an anticoagulant that prevents the clotting of blood in the uterus.

**Proliferative phase.** When menstruation ceases, the proliferative phase begins, extends over the next 14 days, and ends with ovulation. During the proliferative (ovarian follicular) phase, the pituitary gland secretes increasing amounts of FSH, which stimulates a primordial follicle to develop into a mature graafian follicle containing a mature ovum. Because the graafian follicle produces estrogen, FSH is essential for estrogen production. While increasing in size, the graafian follicle moves toward the surface of the ovary, where it appears as a blisterlike structure. Finally, the graafian follicle ruptures (ovulation), allowing the ovum to enter the fallopian tube and be carried in the direction of the uterus.

As the graafian follicle matures, it secretes increasing amounts of estrogen. Estrogen causes the endometrium to become thicker and softer as it prepares for implantation of a fertilized ovum. Estrogen also causes the cervical mucus to increase in quantity and attain a clear, elastic state that permits sperm to enter the cervix more readily. The high level of estrogen also suppresses pituitary release of FSH and triggers release of LH. A sharp rise in LH levels occurs 12 to 24 hours before ovulation, followed by a peak level about 8 hours after ovulation.

On the day of ovulation, about 25% of women experience pain in the lower abdomen on the side of ovulation. This pain is referred to as *mittelschmerz* and is probably a result of peritoneal irritation from follicular fluid or blood released from the ovary with the ovum.

**Secretory phase.** The proliferative phase ends with ovulation and the secretory phase begins, lasting for approximately 10 to 14 days. The secretory (ovarian luteal) phase is the least variable part of the menstrual cycle. Irregular menstrual cycles are usually related to variations in the menstrual or proliferative phases.

Under the influence of LH, the corpus luteum forms in the ovary at the site of the ruptured graafian follicle and produces progesterone. Progesterone further alters the endometrium by stimulating growth of cells and circulation of blood to the

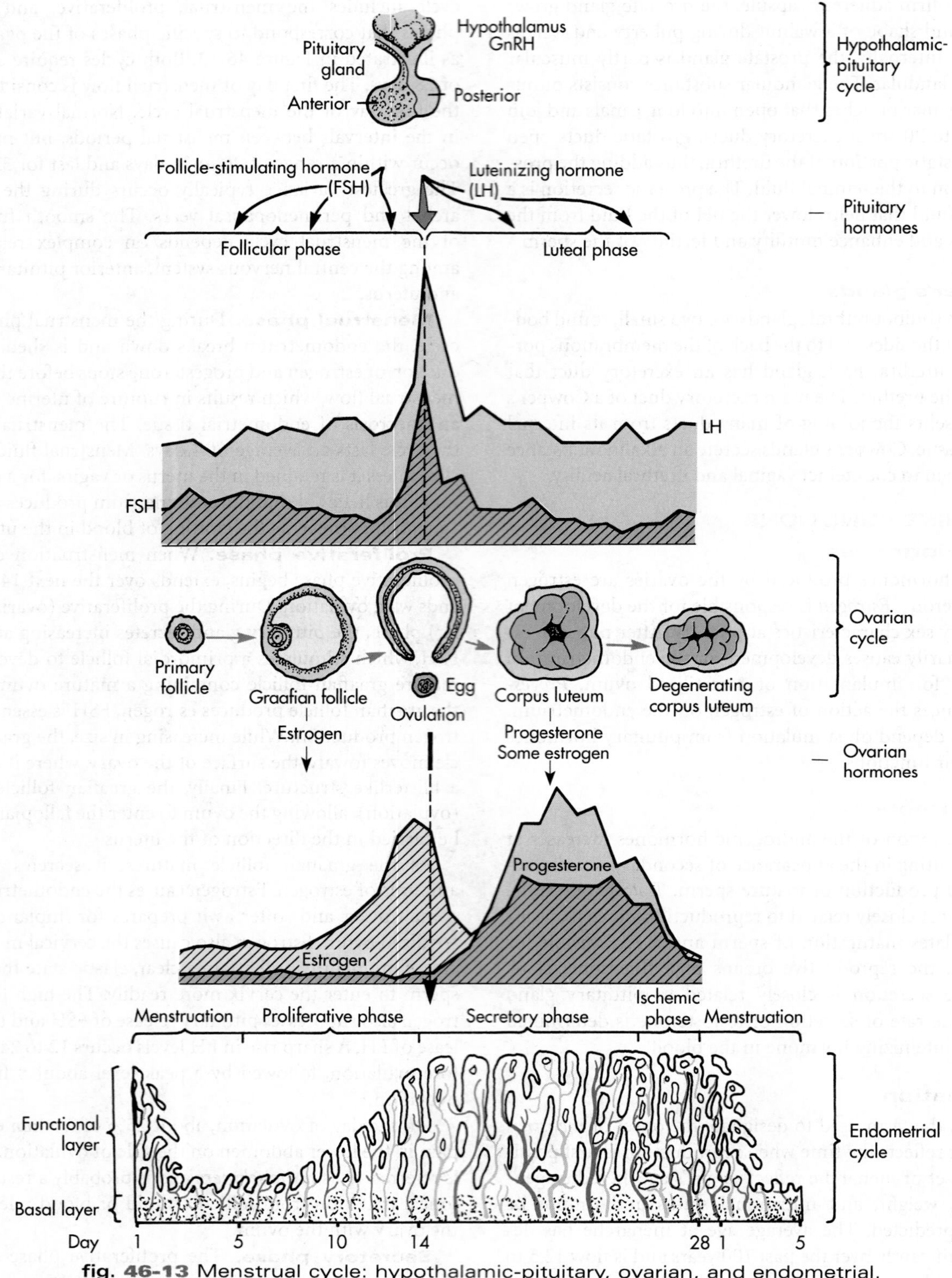


**fig. 46-13** Menstrual cycle: hypothalamic-pituitary, ovarian, and endometrial.

uterus. With these additional endometrial changes, the uterine environment is prepared for implantation of a fertilized ovum.

If pregnancy occurs, the corpus luteum remains secretory by the action of human chorionic gonadotropin (HCG), which the placenta produces within 1 week of conception. By 6 to 8 weeks after conception, the placenta is developed and assumes the function of secreting progesterone to maintain the endometrium. If pregnancy does not occur, the corpus luteum degenerates in about 10 days, progesterone secretion drops significantly, and the endometrium degenerates; menstruation results, and the cycle begins again.

### Menopause

The medical term *menopause* refers to a single, specific physical event in a woman's life—the occurrence of the last menstrual period. As such, it is an event that can be diagnosed only retrospectively, usually after 1 year has passed without spontaneous bleeding. In reality, the term is used much more broadly to refer to the 12- to 18-month *climacteric* or *transitional phase* between the end of reproductive ability and the beginning of the nonreproductive phase. Increasingly, menopause research has expanded to include the entire perimenopausal period, which may extend from age 35 to as old as 60 years of age. This is the period in which physical changes can be clearly linked to altered levels of hormones.

Natural menopause may occur in women between the ages of 35 and 60 years of age. The average age is 49 to 51 years in Western societies. This average has remained quite stable over time, despite fairly significant changes in the average age of onset for menstruation. Twenty five percent of all women experience menopause before age 45, 50% between 45 and 50 years of age, and 25% after age 50. Menopause may be artificially induced by surgical removal or irradiation of the ovaries, severe infections, and the effects of certain chemotherapeutic agents. The removal of the uterus, hysterectomy, results in a cessation of menses but does not itself result in menopause, as long as the ovaries are left intact.

The changes of menopause are primarily related to a gradual decline in ovarian production of estrogen. Although menopause is defined by a cessation of menses, the process is rarely abrupt. Over a period of years, the menses become more scanty and may become irregular or spaced further apart until they eventually stop. The ovaries produce three different forms of estrogen. Estriol is produced during pregnancy. Estradiol is produced in the ovulatory follicle and is the primary estrogen of premenopausal women. The third form, estrone, is a by-product of the metabolism of estradiol and is also produced and held in adipose tissue. It is the primary postmenopausal estrogen and has a potency of only one tenth that of estradiol. Cellular estrogen receptors are found in organs throughout the body, so a decline in estrogen triggers a wide variety of potential symptoms. The severity of symptoms is thought to be related to the rapidity of changes in estrogen level and may be mediated somewhat by the fat content of the body. Women with higher fat stores in their bodies will retain a storage pool of estrogen to buffer them through the early transition period. Commonly reported symptoms of menopause are summarized in Box 46-2.

**box 46-2 Common Menopausal Symptoms**

**VASOMOTOR**
Hot flashes
Hot flushes
Perspiration
Palpitations

**VAGINAL**
Dryness
Vulvar itching or burning
Dyspareunia

**URINARY**
Frequency or urgency
Stress incontinence

**PSYCHOLOGICAL**
Sleep disorders/insomnia
Irritability
Mood swings
Depression

## PHYSIOLOGICAL CHANGES WITH AGING

The major physiological changes that occur in the female reproductive tract with aging are related to the process of menopause, which is discussed above. When ovulation ceases the production of progesterone is halted, and estrogen levels decrease. These two primary hormone changes are responsible for most aging-related changes in the uterus, ovaries, and vagina. The ovaries atrophy and become nonpalpable within 3 to 5 years of menopause. The uterus also decreases in size. The vagina decreases in width and length, and the entrance narrows. The mucosal lining becomes thinner, and vaginal secretions are diminished. Externally the mons pubis decreases in fullness and the labia majora and minora decrease in size. Pubic hair becomes thinner and turns gray or white. Muscle weakness in the pelvis can lead to cystocele, rectocele, or uterine prolapse and may cause problems related to stress incontinence. The woman's capacity for sexual response, however, remains intact.

The primary changes in the male reproductive tract are also related to hormone changes. With increasing age testosterone secretion declines and appears to level off around age 60. This causes a decrease in the size and firmness of the penis and testes. The scrotum is more pendulous in appearance and has fewer rugae. Although some spermatogenesis continues throughout life, the seminal fluid decreases in amount and force of ejaculation decreases. The prostate gland typically hypertrophies and an increase in bladder neck tone creates problems with urinary retention. The pelvic muscles decrease in strength and the pubic hair thins and turns gray or white. The capacity for sexual response remains intact in healthy men and fertility, although diminished, does remain intact.

Aging-related changes occur at different rates and to varying degrees, and in general the changes are gradual. The Gerontological Assessment Box on the next page outlines variations in the process of assessment appropriate for use with elders and identifies common health problems that develop in the aging population.

# SUBJECTIVE DATA

## HISTORY

A reproductive history may be gathered as part of a complete health history or during an episodic examination. As with any nursing history, questions should be asked in a nonjudgmental manner, using open-ended questions.

### Chief Complaint

Subjective data may be organized through a review of systems or by a history of the chief complaint with a system review. For example, a sexually transmitted disease (STD) can mimic a urinary tract infection; therefore information about both the urinary and reproductive systems is important. The chief complaint is further broken down by the critical characteristics of the symptoms including location, character/qual-

## gerontological assessment

**ASSESSMENT**

Determine meaning of sexuality to patient; age does not imply loss of sexuality.

Assess for problems engaging in sexual intercourse because of disability or disease.

Determine frequency of regular gynecological examination in elderly women; some women are not aware that these examinations should be continued after menopause.

Assess for signs of vaginitis (vaginal pruritus and discharge).

Assess for signs of cystocele or rectocele (urinary incontinence and low back pain).

Assist older woman to position of comfort for pelvic examination if lithotomy position is not possible.

Encourage woman to change positions slowly after pelvic examination as orthostatic hypotension may occur.

Inquire directly about dysuria problems or difficulty urinating in elderly men. Assess knowledge and understanding of common prostate problems.

**COMMON DISORDERS IN ELDERS**

Vaginitis
Hernias
Uterine prolapse
Cystocele, rectocele
Cancer of cervix, uterus, breast, prostate

ity, quantity/severity, timing, setting, aggravating or relieving factors, associated factors, and the client's perception of the problem.

### Sexual Activity

Questions about sexual activity need to be routinely asked to screen for sexual problems, sexual assault, and risk for unplanned pregnancy or STDs. Screening for sexual abuse or sexual assault needs to be a routine part of the health history. Sexual preference can be determined by asking forthrightly, "Do you have sex with a man, a woman, or both?" Many experts also recommend recording the number of current and past sexual partners to determine risk status for STDs. Although the risk of exposure to STDs certainly increases with the number of partners, sexual activity with one partner in a nonmonogamous relationship also carries risk. Therefore determining if a client is sexually active, practices safer sex behaviors, or recently changed sexual partners is probably more significant than the number of partners.

### Female Genitourinary Assessment

Genitourinary health histories for women generally include data about the urinary system, menstruation, sexual activity, contraceptive use, pregnancies, and history of gynecological problems or surgeries. Although not part of the reproductive system, breast health is usually assessed during a routine gynecological visit. As previously noted, it is important to screen for physical abuse and sexual abuse and sexual assault. In-

**Abuse Assessment Screen**

1. Have you ever been emotionally or physically abused by your partner or someone important to you?

Yes ☐
No ☐

2. Within the last year, have you been hit, slapped, kicked, or otherwise physically hurt by someone?

Yes ☐
No ☐

If **Yes**, by whom ______________

Number of times ______________

Mark the area of injury on body map.

3. Within the last year, has anyone forced you to have sexual activities?

If **Yes**, who ______________

Number of times ______________

4. Are you afraid of your partner or anyone you listed above?

Yes ☐
No ☐

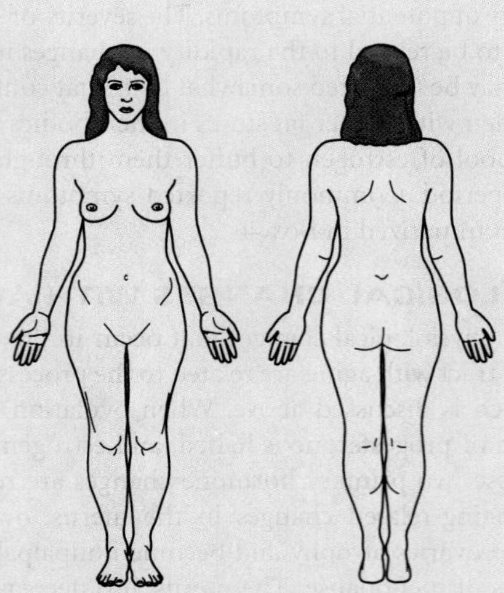

**fig. 46-14** Sample screening tool for abuse.

cluding questions that address these issues in assessment tools ensures that these issues are not excluded or missed. See Figure 46-14 for abuse assessment sample questions.

The assessment interview can be tailored to the age of the client. For example, a middle-aged woman can be questioned about perimenopausal symptoms, whereas older women should be screened for postmenopausal bleeding.

The method of contraception used and the client's satisfaction with the method need to be assessed. Screening for proper use of contraceptives can easily be accomplished during the assessment. Screening for common complications or serious side effects is also possible. The following outline summarizes the interview items, symptoms, and health promotion activities to be included in the assessment.

### *Female breast and genitourinary history*

1. Current breast health
2. Problems with breasts
   - Pain/tenderness
   - Lumps
   - Skin dimpling
   - Lesions or changes in the skin
   - Discharge from the nipples
3. Current genitourinary health
4. Urinary symptoms including infections and voiding dysfunction
   - Dysuria
   - Frequency
   - Urgency
   - Hematuria
   - Nocturia
   - True incontinence (loss of urine without warning)
   - Stress incontinence (loss of urine with cough or sneeze)
5. Menstrual history
   - Age at menarche (first menses)
   - Last menstrual period
   - Interval or frequency; regular or irregular
   - Duration
   - Menstrual flow: light, medium, or heavy (number of pads or tampons used in a specified time period)
   - Menorrhagia (increased amount or duration of flow)
   - Dysmenorrhea (pain with menstruation): frequency and severity
   - Bleeding between periods
   - Postcoital bleeding (bleeding after intercourse)
   - Postmenopausal bleeding: essential to assess for any bleeding since menopause to screen for endometrial cancer
   - Premenstrual syndrome symptoms: irritability, depression, weight gain, headaches, breast tenderness, and breast swelling
6. Obstetrical history
   - Number of pregnancies (gravida)
   - Pregnancy outcomes
     Term: number of births between 37 and 42 weeks of pregnancy
     Premature: number of births before 37 weeks of pregnancy
     Living: number of living children
     Abortions: spontaneous or elective
   - Types of deliveries: vaginal, forceps, or cesarean
7. Perimenopausal symptoms
   - Hot flashes/flushes
   - Headaches
   - Night sweats
   - Vaginal dryness
   - Mood swings
   - Numbness and tingling
8. Vulvovaginal problems
   - Discharge: color, amount, and odor
   - Vaginal itching
   - Lesions or lumps
   - Dyspareunia (pain with intercourse)
   - Vaginismus (spasms of muscles around vagina)
   - History of STDs
9. Sexual health
   - Sexually active: monogamous versus multiple partners; male/female/both
   - Satisfaction or problems related to sexual activity
   - Changes in ability to engage in sex: vaginal dryness, female sexual arousal disorder, inhibited orgasm, or pain with intercourse
10. Health promotion practices
    - Contraceptive choice, proper use of method, satisfaction, and side effects
    - Pelvic examinations: last Pap smear and results
    - Condom use
    - Breast self-examination
    - Vulva self-examination
    - Mammogram
    - Personal hygiene: douche, bubble baths, use of tampons, and feminine sprays
11. Family history
    - Breast cancer
    - Cervical, ovarian, or endometrial cancer
    - Diethylstilbestrol (DES) use; NOTE: Use of DES was decreased in the late 1960s and banned in 1971.

## Male Genitourinary Assessment

A male genitourinary history includes current health status as well as past medical history. Depending on the age of the patient, the interview can be tailored to screen for specific age-related problems. For example, prostate enlargement occurs in older men, and therefore it is necessary to screen for factors such as urinary retention, straining, and hesitancy. Data can be collected about the bladder, kidney function, the penis and testes, possible hernias, sexual health, and health promotion activities. The following outline summarizes symptoms and health promotion behaviors to be included in the assessment.

### *Male genitourinary history*

1. Current genitourinary health status
2. Screen for urinary symptoms including infections, voiding dysfunction, or prostate problems
   - Dysuria (pain with urination)
   - Frequency

- Urgency
- Hematuria
- Nocturia
- Urinary retention
- Straining
- Hesitancy
- Change in force/caliber of stream
- Dribbling
- History of prostate problems
- History of urinary tract infections

3. Screen for incontinence
   - True (loss of urine without warning)
   - Stress (loss of urine with cough/sneeze)
4. Screen for problems with penis such as skin lesions, cancer, or STDs
   - Pain
   - Lesions or sores
   - Discharge
   - History of STDs
5. Screen for problems with testes such as torsion, cancer, or infection and problems with the scrotum such as hydrocele, hernia, or varicocele
   - Lump or swelling in testes
   - Bulge or swelling in scrotum
   - Change in size of scrotum
   - History of hernia
6. Assess sexual health
   - Sexually active: monogamous versus multiple partners, male/female/both
   - Satisfactions with or problems related to sexual activity

## OBJECTIVE DATA

Physical examination of the breasts or genitourinary system may cause embarrassment for the patient. If this is the first breast, pelvic, or testicular examination, ignorance about the process may also cause fear. Before the examination it is important for the nurse to inquire if the patient has previously had an examination of this nature. If it is the first examination, take the time to explain the process, review normal anatomy, and teach self-examination of the breasts or testes. Pictures, three-dimensional anatomical models, and examples of equipment such as a speculum aid in the educational process.

### BREAST EXAMINATION

#### Female Breast

In a menstruating female, the ideal time to examine the breasts is several days after menstruation when they are less tender and nodular. In nonmenstruating females the timing of the examination is less important. Examination of the breasts begins with inspection of the skin and areola. The examination should be performed in both the sitting and supine position. See Figure 46-15 for a sample examination.

With the woman's hands at her sides, inspect the breasts for symmetry and the skin for dimpling, puckering, scaling, scars, or discharge from the nipples. A dimple, pucker, or retraction in breast tissue may indicate an underlying chest wall lesion. Scaly skin or nipple tissue can be seen in eczema of the breast or Paget's disease. While the woman slowly raises her hands over her head, observe for signs of retractions. Ask the woman to put her hands on her waist and flex her shoulders and elbows. Observe for puckering or retractions and for symmetrical movement. Women with large breasts should lean forward. The breast should move smoothly without signs of adhesions to the chest wall.

The breasts and axilla can be palpated in both sitting and supine positions. Bimanual palpation of large breasts is easily accomplished while the client is sitting. It should be repeated in a supine position. Before the the client lies down, palpate the supraclavicular and axillary lymph nodes for size, shape, mobility, or tenderness. The majority of the breast lymphatics drain toward the axilla.

When the client is supine, place a small pillow or towel under the shoulder of the breast to be examined. Ask the woman to raise her arm over her head as this helps flatten the breast tissue. The breast can be palpated in a circular, pie-shaped, or vertical pattern. The breast tissue is systematically palpated using the pads of three fingers. It is important to palpate the entire breast, including the tail of Spence in the upper outer quadrant near the axilla. The consistency of the breast tissue and the presence of any tenderness, lumps, or nodules are noted. If a nodule is identified, its location, size in centimeters, shape, and consistency are noted.

The nipple is palpated for underlying masses or tumors, and the nipple is gently squeezed to check for masses or discharge. A milky discharge may be related to pregnancy, lactation, hormones, or drugs. A nonmilky discharge may indicate a pathological condition. The process is then repeated on the opposite breast.

#### Male Breast

The male breast can be easily and quickly examined during a routine physical examination. Although rare, breast cancer does occur in males, most frequently in the areolar area. The examination is initiated with inspection of the skin and areolae. The presence of any swelling, retractions, or lesions is noted. The breast, areola, and axilla are then palpated for masses.

### ABDOMINAL EXAMINATION

Physical assessment of the reproductive organs includes a standard assessment of the lower abdomen (see Chapter 38). Any localized areas of prominence are noted since these may indicate enlargement of the reproductive organs or adjacent structures. The skin of the abdomen and pubic area is inspected for amount, distribution, and character of hair; abnormal pigmentation; and lesions. Abdominal muscle tone is assessed by having the patient cough or raise the head. See p. 1520 for a further description of hernia assessment.

Auscultation of the abdomen for bowel sounds and bruits should precede palpation. After auscultation, percussion of the abdomen is completed to identify any enlarged organ, tumor, or masses. A tumor, such as an ovarian cyst or uterine myoma, produces a dull, flat, tone. Because the reproductive organs in the female are normally situated in the pelvic cavity,

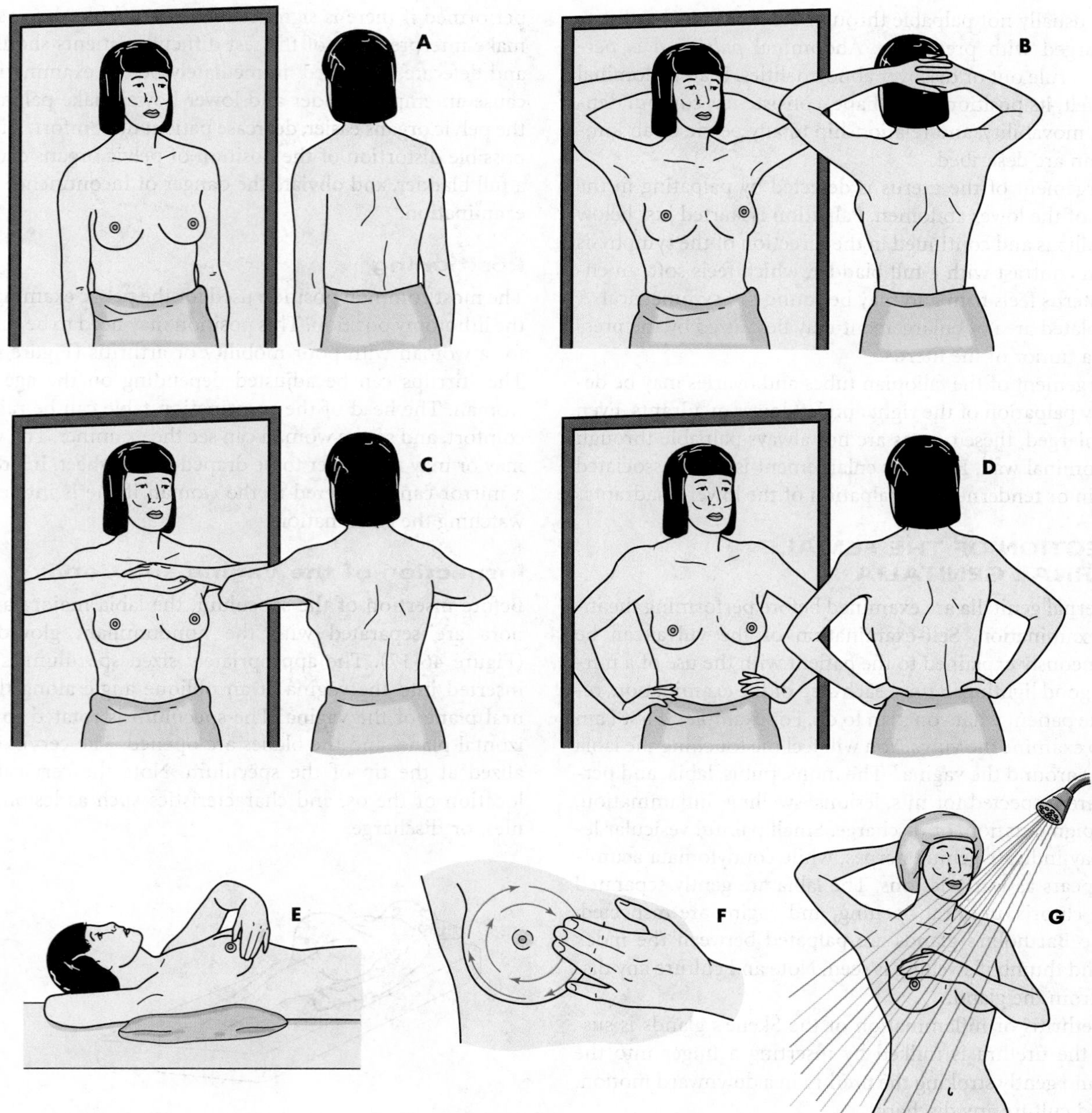


**fig. 46-15** Breast self-examination (BSE). **A,** Stand in front of a mirror where you can see yourself from head to waist in good light. Observe your breasts from the front, then from the right and left sides, in each position described as follows. With arms at your side notice the normal size, shape, color, contour, veins, nipple, and other characteristics of each breast. **B,** Raise your arms above your head; both breasts should rise when the arms are lifted. **C,** With your hands in front of you at shoulder height, press your palms firmly against each other to contract the chest wall muscles. Notice the manner in which your breasts move during position changes. **D,** Put your hands on your hips, squeeze your shoulders inward, and lean slightly forward and down. Look to see that the breasts appear normal for you. **E,** Lie down with one hand under your head and a pillow or folded towel under the scapula of the side you will be examining. **F,** Bring your three middle fingers of the other hand together, and using the flat part of the fingers, move in small concentric circles. It usually takes three circles to cover all breast tissue. Include the tail of the breast and axilla. Palpate areola; inspect and gently squeeze nipples to check for discharge. Move the nipples from side to side for mobility. Repeat for other breast. **G,** Repeat this technique during bath and shower, when soap and water allow fingers to glide easily over skin.

they are usually not palpable through the abdominal wall unless enlarged with pregnancy. Abdominal *palpation* is performed to rule out or discover abnormalities. If an abdominal mass is felt, its position, size, shape, consistency, contour, tenderness, movability, and relationship to any pelvic or abdominal organ are described.

Enlargement of the uterus is detected by palpating in the midline of the lower abdomen. Palpation is started just below the umbilicus and continued in the direction of the symphysis pubis. In contrast with a full bladder, which feels soft, an enlarged uterus feels firm and may be round or asymmetrical. A firm, isolated area of enlargement may be caused by the presence of a tumor of the uterus.

Enlargement of the fallopian tubes and ovaries may be detected by palpation of the right and left lower quadrants. Even when enlarged, these organs are not always palpable through the abdominal wall. However enlargement is often associated with pain or tenderness on palpation of the lower quadrants.

## INSPECTION OF THE FEMALE EXTERNAL GENITALIA

The external genitalia are examined before performing the internal examination. Self-examination of the vulva can be simultaneously explained to the patient with the use of a mirror and good lighting. Before each step of the examination, remind the patient what you plan to do. For example, "First I am going to examine the vulva. You will feel me touching the labia (or skin) around the vagina." The mons, pubis, labia, and perineum are inspected for nits, lesions, swelling, inflammation, altered pigmentation, or discharge. Small painful vesicular lesions may indicate genital herpes, while condylomata acuminata appears as warty lesions. The labia are gently separated and the clitoris, urethral opening, and vagina are inspected. Next the Bartholin's glands are palpated between the index finger and thumb if swelling is seen. Note and culture any discharge from the gland.

If urethritis or inflammation of the Skene's glands is suspected, the urethra is milked by inserting a finger into the vagina and gently stroking the urethra in a downward motion. Note and culture any discharge.

## PELVIC EXAMINATION

The pelvic examination is frequently a stressful event for the patient. The nurse can help the woman overcome pain, embarrassment, and anxiety by establishing a relaxed, positive atmosphere and addressing the woman's questions and concerns. Visual aids are useful when a pelvic examination is to be performed for the first time. Models of the pelvic organs and pamphlets assist with the presentation of information about the purpose of the examination, what is done, and what to expect. The nurse or examiner explains the procedure and answers questions before the patient is undressed and on the examination table.

Women who are scheduled for pelvic examination should be advised to avoid douching, sexual intercourse, and applying any vaginal preparations (medicinal or deodorant) for at least 24 hours before examination. A Pap smear should not be performed if there is significant menstrual bleeding as it will make interpretation of the test difficult. Patients should void and defecate, if needed, immediately before examination because an empty bladder and lower bowel make palpation of the pelvic organs easier, decrease patient discomfort, eliminate possible distortion of the position of pelvic organs caused by a full bladder, and obviate the danger of incontinence during examination.

### Positioning

The most common position used for the pelvic examination is the lithotomy position. This position may need to be modified for a woman with poor mobility or arthritis (Figure 46-16). The stirrups can be adjusted depending on the age of the woman. The head of the examination table can be raised for comfort, and so the woman can see the examiner. The woman may or may not prefer to be draped with a sheet. In addition, a mirror can be offered to the woman if she is interested in watching the examination.

### Inspection of the Vagina and Cervix

Before insertion of the speculum, the labia majora and minora are separated with the nondominant gloved hand (Figure 46-17). The appropriately sized speculum is gently inserted into the vagina at an oblique angle along the natural plane of the vagina. The speculum is rotated to a horizontal plane, and the blades are opened. The cervix is visualized at the tip of the speculum. Note the cervical color, location of the os, and characteristics such as lesions, nodules, or discharge.

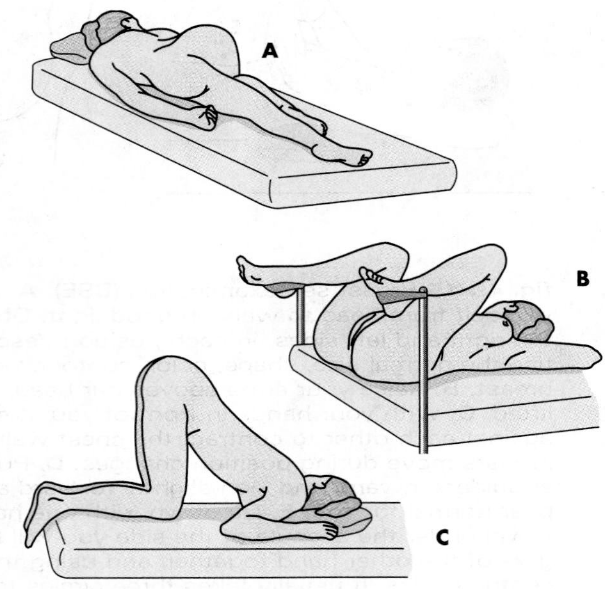


**fig. 46-16** Various positions that can be assumed for examination of rectum and vagina. **A,** Sims' (lateral) position. Note position of left arm and right leg. **B,** Lithotomy position. Note position of buttocks on edge of examining table and support of feet. **C,** Knee-chest (genupectoral) position. Note placement of shoulders and head.

The Pap smear, culture specimen for *Chlamydia* and gonorrhea, and wet mount specimens can be obtained at this time. Some authorities recommend performing the Pap smear before collecting specimens for culture. The presence of endocervical cells on the Pap smear is considered the gold standard for an adequate Pap test, as the majority of cervical cancers develop at the junction of the squamous epithelium and the columnar epithelium of the endocervix. The best specimen can be obtained by using an endocervical brush and an Aer's type spatula. However, some facilities use a cotton-tipped swab for the endocervical sample. In addition, the quality of the Pap smear specimen may be improved if the spatula is used to collect the smear, followed by the cytobrush.

With the long end of the spatula in the os, the spatula is rotated circumferentially around the os. The specimen is transferred immediately to a slide. The cytobrush is inserted into the endocervical os and rotated 360°. The specimen is then "unrolled" onto a glass slide. The specimens are fixed immediately with a spray or alcohol solution. *Chlamydia* and gonorrhea cultures can now be collected with the appropriate swabs.

On bimanual examination, the ovaries are normally slightly tender to palpation and are not always palpable, especially in obese women. When palpable, healthy ovaries feel smooth and oval in shape. Any irregular, firm palpable mass in the area of the fallopian tubes and ovaries indicates a possible deviation from normal. Because the ovaries atrophy during menopause, any mass felt in the areas of the ovaries in postmenopausal women is usually a sign of a problem.

The rectovaginal examination is performed to confirm uterine position, reassess the adnexal areas, follow-up on complaints of pain or bleeding, and determine rectal sphincter tone. The woman is told that it may be uncomfortable, and she may feel as though she has to have a bowel movement. Hemorrhoids, fistulas, and fissures can be observed.

After the pelvic examination, a woman may need assistance removing lubricating jelly or discharge from her genitalia, removing her legs from the stirrups, and getting down from the

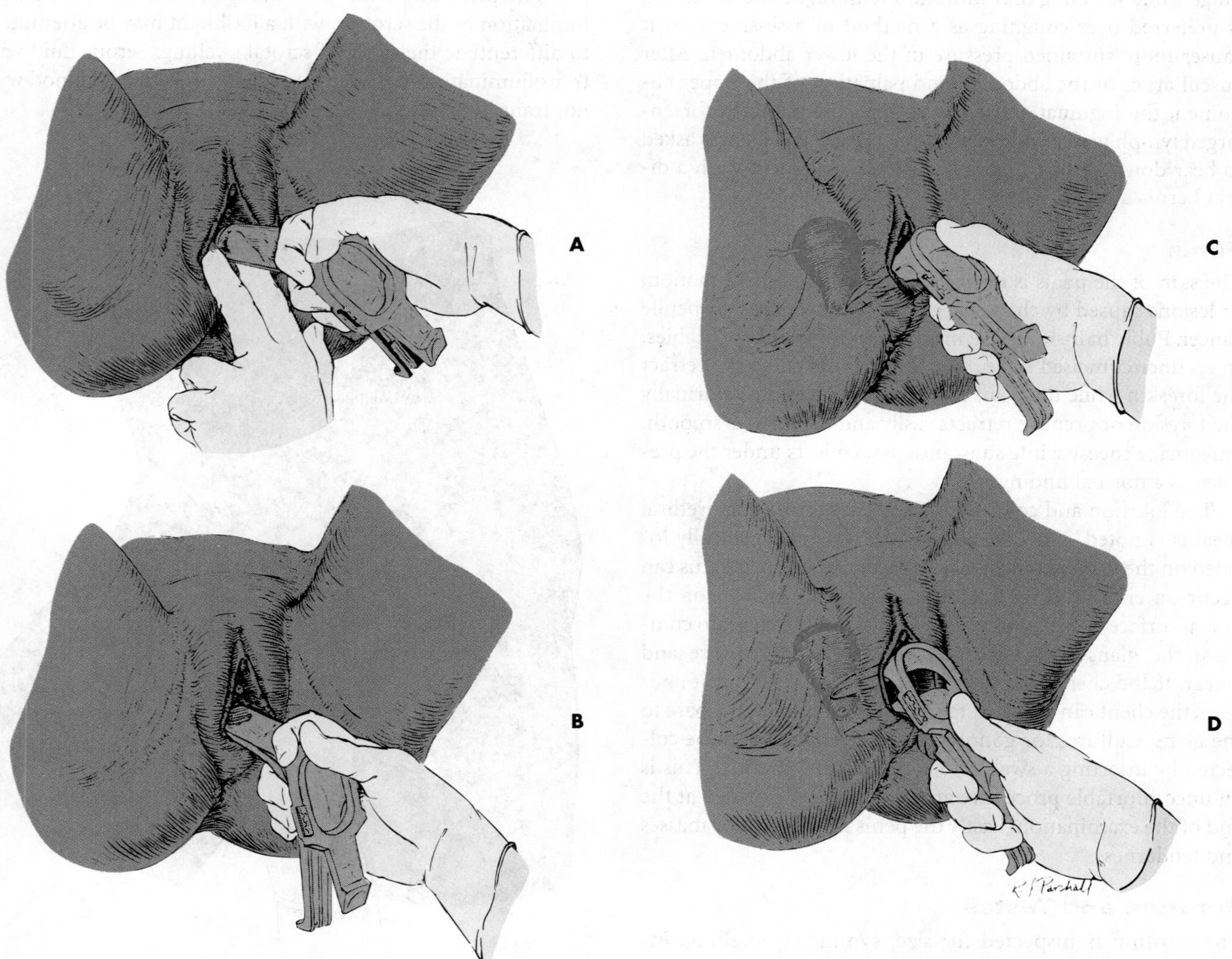


**fig. 46-17** Procedure for speculum examination. **A,** Opening of introitus. **B,** Oblique insertion of speculum. **C,** Final placement of speculum. **D,** Opening of speculum blades.

table. If a bloody discharge is present, a sanitary pad is provided. Elderly women merit careful assistance after pelvic examination because positions such as the knee-chest and lithotomy positions may alter the normal circulation of blood sufficiently to cause blood pressure changes or faintness.

## PHYSICAL EXAMINATION OF THE MALE GENITALIA

Physical examination of the male genitalia includes inspection, auscultation, and palpation of the lower abdomen; inspection and palpation of the external genitalia; and palpation of the prostate gland by rectal examination.

### Positioning

Depending on the patient's age, the external genitalia can be examined after the abdominal examination with the client in the supine or standing position. However, the patient should be in a standing position to evaluate hernias. The inguinal and femoral areas are inspected for any bulges or masses, and the patient is asked to bear down as the area is reinspected. A bulge while straining may indicate a femoral hernia. Straining is preferred over coughing as a method of assessment, as it causes more sustained pressure in the lower abdomen. After auscultation of the abdomen and palpation of the upper abdomen, the inguinal and femoral areas are palpated for enlarged lymph nodes and hernias. Once again the client is asked to bear down and the inguinal region is palpated. With a direct hernia a bulge will be felt.

### Penis

The skin of the penis is inspected for swelling, inflammation, or lesions caused by chancres, genital warts, herpes, or penile cancer. Pubic hair should be inspected for nits, lice, or scabies. In an uncircumcised male, the patient is instructed to retract the foreskin while the glans is inspected for lesions. Normally the foreskin or prepuce retracts easily and the glans is smooth. Smegma, a cheesy white substance that collects under the prepuce, is a normal finding.

The location and color of any discharge from the urethral meatus is noted. The urethral meatus is usually centrally located on the glans. Congenital displacement of the meatus can occur on either the ventral surface (hypospadius) or on the dorsal surface (epispadius) of the penis. Ask the client to compress the glans and collect any discharge for culture and smear. If the client has complained of discharge but none is seen, the client can be asked to milk the penis from the base to the glans. Cultures for gonorrhea and *Chlamydia* can be collected by inserting a swab 2 to 4 cm into the urethra. This is an uncomfortable procedure and should be performed at the end of the examination. Lastly the penis is palpated for masses and tenderness.

### Scrotum and Testes

The scrotum is inspected for size, symmetry, swelling, inflammation, and/or lesions. The left testis is lower than the right, which causes the scrotum to appear asymmetrical under normal conditions. Scrotal size is also determined by room temperature and age. In warm temperatures the dartos muscles relax, and the testes are more pendulous. Likewise, with age the dartos muscles atrophy, which also causes a pendulous appearance. Marked asymmetry can be caused by an undescended testicle, indirect hernia, hydrocele, tumor, or edema.

Palpation of the scrotum is necessary to distinguish between enlargement caused by a mass and swelling caused by the collection of fluid. The size, shape, and consistency of the testes are noted by palpating the testes between the thumb and first two fingers. The testes feel smooth and firm, are oval, and move freely. Any painless hard nodule should be further investigated as it may indicate testicular cancer. The epididymis and spermatic cord are palpated from the testes to the inguinal ring. At this time, the examination for hernia is repeated by invaginating the scrotal skin with the index finger to the external inguinal ring (Figure 46-18). The patient is asked to strain; the presence of a hernia will produce a bulge or tap. A load test can be done at this time if the hernia is not palpated despite complaints of hernia symptoms. Finally, transillumination of the scrotum with a flashlight may be attempted to differentiate the cause of scrotal swelling. Serous fluid will transilluminate and produce a red glow. Tissue and blood will not transilluminate.

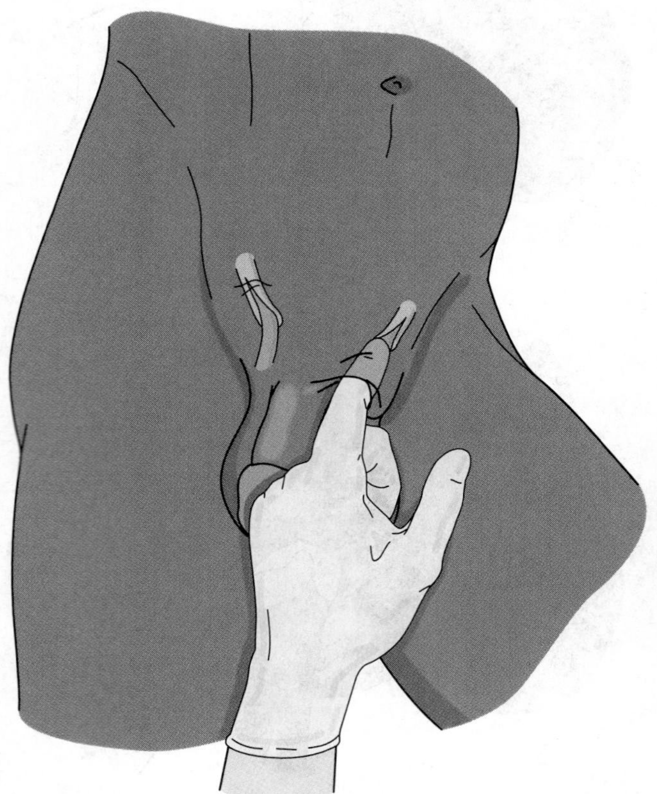

**fig. 46-18** Palpation of inguinal area for hernias.

## Prostate

The prostate gland is palpated by means of a rectal examination with the patient standing with hips flexed over an examination table or in a side-lying position (Figure 46-19). Before the examination advise the man that he may feel as though he needs to have a bowel movement. The patient is asked to bear down while a lubricated index finger is gently inserted into the anal canal and then the rectum. The prostate and seminal vesicles are palpated. The size, shape, and consistency of the lobes and median sulcus of the prostate are noted. The normal prostate is 2.5 by 4 cm, smooth, heart shaped, rubbery, and nontender.

Rectal examination is the most important step in the diagnosis of prostatic disease, especially carcinoma. Cancer of the prostate gland may start as a localized, hard nodule, which is palpable by rectal examination, before proceeding to an

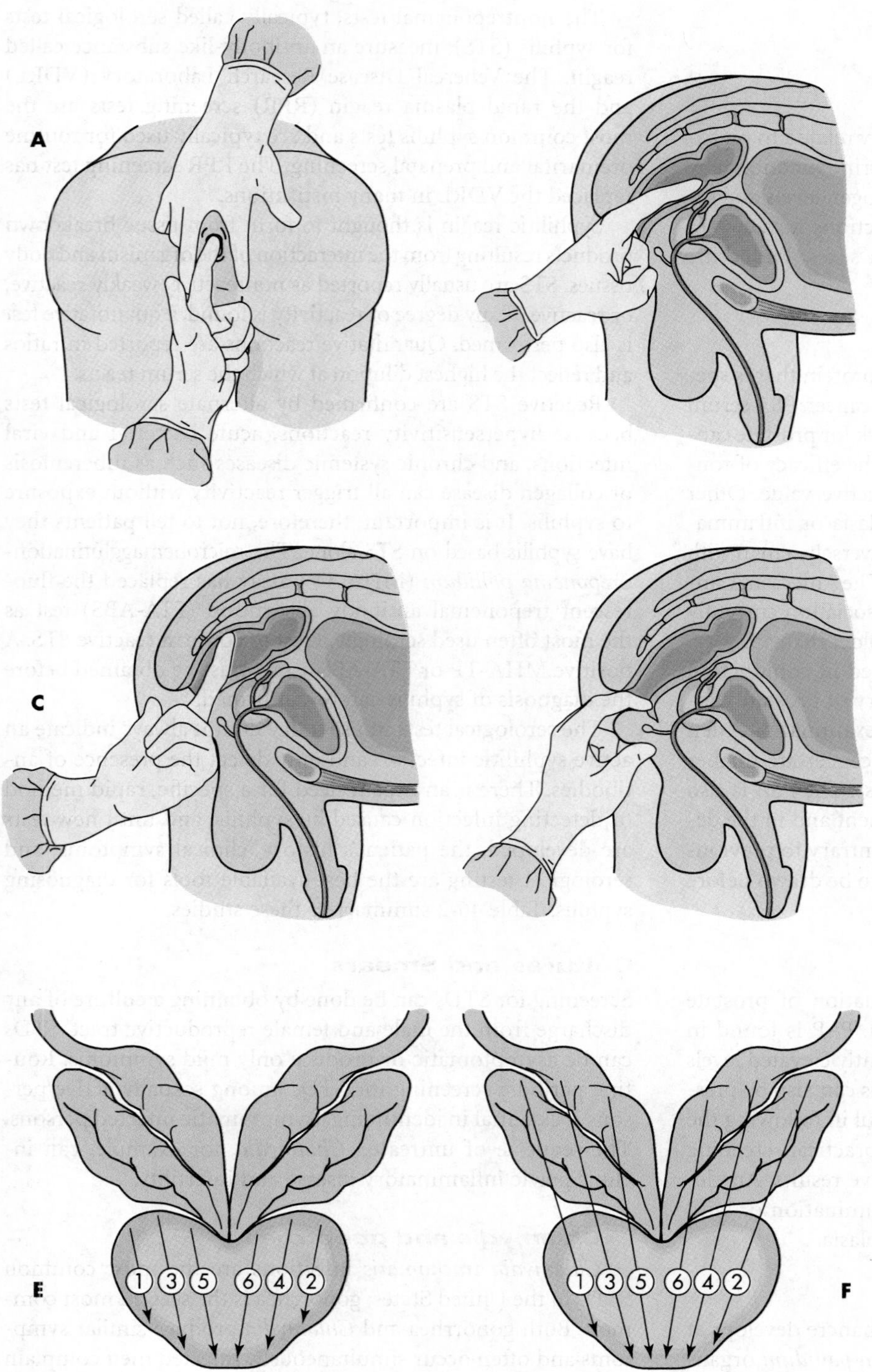


**fig. 46-19** Rectal examination. **A,** Introduction of protected, well-lubricated finger. **B,** Palpation of prostate gland and seminal vesicles, lateral view. **C,** Palpation of anterior surface of sacrum and coccyx. **D,** Palpation of Cowper's glands. **E,** Massage of prostate gland for specimen collection or treatment; order of strokes is indicated by gradually working toward center (verumontanum). **F,** Massage of seminal vesicles and prostate gland.

advanced stage. For this reason, it is recommended that all men, especially those older than age 50 years, have a rectal examination at least once a year.

## DIAGNOSTIC TESTS

Many diagnostic tests are useful in providing data about the reproductive system. They include blood and urine tests, cytological tests, radiological tests, biopsies, and endoscopic procedures.

### LABORATORY TESTS

#### Blood and Urine Tests

##### Endocrine testing

Because the endocrine system is so closely related to reproductive function, almost any study of endocrine function may be ordered, including determination of estrogen levels and secretion in women and 24-hour urine collections for ketosteroids and pituitary gonadotropins in both sexes. Endocrine system tests are presented in Chapter 33.

##### Prostate-specific antigen

Prostate-specific antigen (PSA) is a glycoprotein that is specific to the prostate gland but not to prostate cancer. PSA serum levels are currently used to identify men at risk for prostate cancer, although much controversy exists over the efficacy of routine PSA screening because of its low predictive value. Other conditions such as benign prostatic hyperplasia or inflammation can also cause an elevated PSA level. Conversely, a man with prostate cancer can have a normal PSA level. The American Cancer Society and the American Urological Association currently recommend annual PSA testing for all men older than 50.

The PSA is most valuable when evaluated in conjunction with the patient's symptoms, a family history of prostate cancer, and the findings of the digital rectal examination. Men who are believed to be at risk for prostate cancer are further evaluated by transrectal ultrasound or biopsy. The PSA is also valuable in evaluating the efficacy of treatment and in the detection of recurrence of prostate cancer. Contrary to previous belief blood for the PSA test does not have to be drawn before the rectal examination.

##### Prostatic acid phosphatase

Another glycoprotein used in the evaluation of prostate cancer is prostatic acid phosphatase (PAP). PAP is found in the epithelium of the prostate, and persistently elevated levels may indicate metastasis, although metastasis can also be present with a normal PAP level. Although useful in following the course of prostate cancer, the test is not a practical screening test because of the high rate of false-positive results. An elevated PAP level can occur after a rectal examination or with either prostatitis or benign prostatic hyperplasia.

##### Syphilis studies

During the primary stage of syphilis a chancre develops at the site of initial exposure to the *Treponema pallidum* organism, usually on the genitals, mouth, or lips within 1 to 3 weeks of exposure. Dark field examination of the chancre scrapings may reveal the *T. palladum* spirochete. A negative scraping does not necessarily rule out syphilis, however, as the specimen may have been inadequate.

Serological testing can also be used to detect syphilis because two identifiable antibodies appear in the blood 1 to 4 months after syphilis is contracted. Two types of tests, treponemal and nontreponemal, are presently available. The tests differ in the type of antibody measured and in the antigen used to detect antibodies.

The nontreponemal tests, typically called serological tests for syphilis (STS), measure an antibody-like substance called reagin. The Venereal Disease Research Laboratory (VDRL) and the rapid plasma reagin (RPR) screening tests are the most common syphilis tests and are typically used for routine premarital and prenatal screening. The RPR screening test has replaced the VDRL in many institutions.

Syphilitic reagin is thought to form from tissue breakdown products resulting from the interaction of the organism and body tissues. STS are usually reported as nonreactive, weakly reactive, or reactive. If any degree of reactivity is found, a quantitative test is also performed. Quantitative reactions are reported in ratios and reflect the highest dilution at which the serum reacts.

Reactive STS are confirmed by alternate serological tests because hypersensitivity reactions, acute bacterial and viral infections, and chronic systemic diseases such as tuberculosis or collagen disease can all trigger reactivity without exposure to syphilis. It is important, therefore, not to tell patients they have syphilis based on STS alone. The microhemagglutination-*Treponema pallidum* (MHA-TP) assay has replaced the fluorescent treponemal antibody absorption (FTA-ABS) test as the most often used serological test to confirm reactive STS. A positive MHA-TP or FTA-ABS assay must be obtained before the diagnosis of syphilis can be confirmed.

The serological tests in use today do not always indicate an active syphilitic infection and only detect the presence of antibodies. There is an urgent need for a specific, rapid method of detecting infection caused by syphilis, and until new tests are developed, the patient's history, clinical symptoms, and serological testing are the best available tools for diagnosing syphilis. Table 46-2 summarizes these studies.

#### Cultures and Smears

Screening for STDs can be done by obtaining a culture of any discharge from the male and female reproductive tract. STDs can be asymptomatic or produce only mild symptoms. Routine periodic screening for STDs among sexually active persons is essential in identifying asymptomatic infected persons. The sequelae of untreated *Chlamydia*, for example, can include pelvic inflammatory disease and infertility.

##### Chlamydia and gonorrhea

*Chlamydia trachomatis* infections are the most common STDs in the United States; gonorrhea is the second most common. Both gonorrhea and *Chlamydia* produce similar symptoms and often occur simultaneously. Infected men complain of urethral discharge and dysuria. Women may note postcoital

**table 46-2** *Diagnostic Studies for Syphilis* (Treponema pallidum)

| Diagnostic Test | Description | Pretest/Posttest Care |
|---|---|---|
| Dark field examination | Superficial scrapings of chancre to diagnose syphilis in primary stage as serology tests are not always positive for 14-21 days after contact. | Scrape base of chancre, transport to laboratory on glass slide with cover slip. Avoid contact with specimen. |
| **NONTREPONEMAL SEROLOGICAL TESTS** | | |
| VDRL (Venereal Disease Research Laboratory) | Serum test used as screening test. Confirm positive results with FTA-ABS or MHA-TP; results are positive 1-3 weeks after chancre; in primary syphilis titer is ≥1:32. Titers ↓ after treatment. | Some laboratories require patient to be NPO. No alcohol consumed 24 hr before test. |
| RPR (rapid plasma reagin) screening test | Serum test used as screening test. Confirm positive results as above. | None |
| **TREPONEMAL SEROLOGICAL TESTS** | | |
| MHA-TP (microhemagglutination-*Treponema pallidum*) | Serum test used to confirm positive RPR or VDRL. Remains positive for life. False-positives can occur. | None |
| FTA-ABS (fluorescent treponemal antibody absorption) | Serum test used to confirm positive RPR or VDRL. False-positives can occur. | None |

bleeding or an increase in vaginal discharge or have mucopurulent cervicitis.

Testing for *C. trachomatis* has evolved in recent years to include culture, direct antigen detection, and nucleic acid amplification techniques using either polymerase or ligase chain reactions. Culture is considered the gold standard in *Chlamydia* testing as it has 100% specificity. However, it is expensive and technically difficult and requires several days to complete. *Chlamydia* culture is usually reserved for children or victims of sexual abuse.[9,18]

Nonculture testing for *Chlamydia* is not as specific as the culture method, but it is cheaper and easier to complete. Direct antigen fluorescent antibody detection uses visualization of *Chlamydia* elementary bodies whereas enzyme immunoassay uses spectrophotometry to identify color changes in the elementary bodies. These tests have a sensitivity of about 70% and a specificity of about 96% to 99%.[9,18]

Nucleic acid amplification tests include polymerase chain reaction (PCR), ligase chain reaction (LCR), and direct probe. The direct DNA probe test screens for both *C. trachomatis* and *Neisseria gonorrhoeae* with one culture. In women, a swab is inserted 1 to 1.5 cm into the endocervical canal for 30 seconds and rotated several times before removal. A smaller urethral swab is used to obtain a culture in men. The male patient is advised not to urinate for at least 2 hours before the culture. The swab is inserted 2 to 4 cm into the urethra and rotated gently for 2 to 3 seconds.

One advantage of the PCR and LCR methods is the ability to screen urine for the presence of *C. trachomatis*. Multiple studies have demonstrated that first-voided urine (FVU) samples from both men and women are reliable tests for *Chlamydia*.[3,4,16,17] FVU samples are easier to collect than cervical and urethral swabs and can be easily used for screening.[16] However, these tests require complex equipment and may only be available at large hospitals.

### Herpes simplex virus

Genital herpes is a sexually transmitted disease most frequently caused by herpes simplex virus type 2 (HSV-2), although it can also be caused by herpes simplex virus type 1 (HSV-1), previously thought to only cause cold sores. Primary genital HSV is characterized by multiple, painful genital blisters and flulike symptoms. Diagnosis can be confirmed by physical examination, culture for herpes, Pap smear, and serology testing for HSV antibodies. A culture is obtained by rubbing a suspicious lesion with a cotton- or Dacron-tipped swab and then inserting it into a transport medium. A final culture report may take 7 days.

### Wet mounts

Vaginal discharge can be easily examined microscopically for the presence of *Gardnerella vaginalis, Trichomonas,* and *Candida*. During a pelvic examination vaginal discharge is collected with a cotton swab and mixed with saline on a clear slide. The specimen is covered with a cover slip and examined under a microscope for bacteria, white blood cells, "clue" cells (stippled epithelial cells), and trichomonads. Several drops of 10% potassium hydroxide are then added to the slide, and it is reexamined for a positive whiff test and *Candida*. Potassium hydroxide causes the epithelial cells to lyse and in cases of yeast infections release hyphae. In bacterial vaginitis, vaginal discharge that is mixed with potassium hydroxide produces a fishy smell or positive whiff test. See Table 46-3 for interpretation of wet mounts.

### Prostatic smear

For a prostatic smear the prostate is first massaged during a digital rectal examination and any discharge, is collected. If no discharge is expressed, the first urine sample after the examination is collected. Although some cases of tuberculosis and cancer can be detected by this method the use of the

**table 46-3** *Wet Mount Interpretations*

| | NORMAL | BACTERIAL VAGINOSIS | *CANDIDA* | *TRICHOMONAS* | ATROPHIC |
|---|---|---|---|---|---|
| Symptoms | None | Thin, gray, discharge; malodorous, pruritis can be present | Thick, white, curd-like discharge; pruritis | Increased, thin, frothy, yellow discharge; pruritis | Vulvar and vaginal dryness |
| pH | 3.5-4.1 | 5-6 | 3.5-4.5 | 6-7 | 7.0 |
| Microscopic findings | Lactobacilli | Clue cells, bacteria | Budding yeast | Increased WBCs, trichomonads | Increased WBCs, parabasal and intermediate cells |
| KOH | No findings | Positive whiff test, fishy odor | Budding yeast, pseudohyphae | No findings | No findings |

WBCs, white blood cells.

prostatic smear has declined in recent years. Findings from the digital rectal examination, PSA levels, and biopsy are used to diagnose prostate cancer.

## Cytology

### Pap smear

The Pap smear is a screening test for abnormal cervical cells including cancer. It is designed to determine who needs further evaluation and the type of evaluation needed. Pap smears can also identify vaginal infections such as *Trichomonas* and human papillomavirus, as well as evaluate hormone status.

The accuracy of the Pap test depends on the quality of the sample and the reliability of the laboratory interpreting the test. Results of 10% to 40% of tests are estimated to be reported as false negative due in part to inadequate specimens or misdiagnosis on the part of the cytologist.

Several new systems have been developed to improve the reliability of Pap smear samples and therefore reduce the incidence of false-negative results. The speculoscopy has been shown to improve the identification of abnormal cervical lesions during a pelvic examination. In speculoscopy, a chemiluminescent light is attached to the blade of a speculum. Once the Pap smear is obtained, the cervix and vagina are washed with 5% acetic acid. Using 400× magnification, the cervix is examined for areas of distinct acetowhite areas, which indicate cervical pathological changes.[20] The use of speculoscopy, combined with Pap smears, identifies more cervical lesions than Pap smears alone.[20]

The preparation of the Pap smear slide or specimen can also lead to false-negative results. Traditionally, Pap smear samples are rolled or scraped across a slide and sprayed with a fixative. The thin-layer preparation (ThinPrep, Cytic Corp) is a new slide preparation method developed to reduce the effects of air-drying distortion, excessive blood or mucus, or a thick layer of cells.[15] After the Pap smear sample is obtained, the collection device is rinsed in a bottle of preservative solution. A slide is prepared from the suspended cells and screened by a cytologist in a conventional manner. The ThinPrep slides produce an evenly distributed sample without obscuring artifacts, which is easier to interpret. The ThinPrep method is associated with an increase in the number of cervical lesions identified as well as better Pap samples.[15]

A new system has also been developed to rescreen Pap smears initially reported as negative or normal. The AutoPap 300 QC computer is a high-speed image processing computer with the ability to analyze the specimen for size, shape, density, and color of cells. Any Pap smear with abnormalities is reexamined by a cytologist. The misinterpretation of Pap smears should decline with this process.

The American Cancer Society recommends that all women who are or have been sexually active or who are at least 18 years of age have an annual Pap smear for 3 consecutive years and then every 3 years until middle age. A woman should not douche, take a tub bath, use vaginal medications or deodorants, or have sexual intercourse for at least 24 hours before the test. Some physicians request a 48-hour delay before the test. Pap smears are preferably obtained 5 to 6 days after menstruation, since menses makes interpretation difficult and may camouflage atypical cells. Infections can also interfere with hormonal cytology. Pap smears should be delayed for at least 1 month after use of topical antibiotics, which produce rapid, heavy shedding of cells. Many women experience slight vaginal bleeding after a Pap smear has been taken. They should be advised that this is expected, but that any bleeding in excess of spotting should be reported to the health care provider.

The results of Pap smears have been reclassified in recent years. Several classification systems were used in the past including the Numerical System, the Dysplasia Cytologic Classification, and the Cervical Intraepithelial Neoplasia System. See Table 46-4 for a comparison of Pap smear classifications and treatment recommendations. The Bethesda System is preferred because it provides better communication between the cytologist and the clinician. The Bethesda System evaluates the adequacy of the sample, e.g., satisfactory or not satisfactory for interpretation, and provides a general classification of normal or abnormal and a descriptive diagnosis of the Pap smear. While the classification system may vary, all clinicians agree it is important to monitor Pap smears and ensure

**table 46-4** *Pap Smear Classifications and Action*

| Numerical System | Dysplasia Cytological Classification | Cervical Intraepithelial Neoplasia (CIN) | Bethesda System | Action |
|---|---|---|---|---|
| Class I | Negative squamous metaplasia | No designation | Negative | Repeat annually |
| Class II | Atypical squamous cells | No designation | Atypical squamous cells | Treat infection, repeat Pap |
| Class III | Mild dysplasia<br>Moderate dysplasia | CIN I<br>CIN II | Low-grade squamous lesion | Treat infection, repeat Pap in 8-12 weeks; colposcopy |
| Class IV | Severe dysplasia<br>Carcinoma in situ | CIN III | High-grade squamous lesion | Colposcopy, biopsy, treatment |
| Class V | Invasive cancer | Invasive cancer | Invasive cancer | Colposcopy, biopsy, treat with conization, hysterectomy |

Adapted from Younkin EQ, Davis MS: *Women's health, a primary care clinical guide.* Norwalk, 1994, Appleton & Lange; Worthington S, Rubin M: Nurse-midwifery evaluation and management of cervical pathology and the colposcopic examination, *J Nurse Midwifery* 38(2, suppl):36S-41S, 1993.

proper follow-up including treatment of vaginal infections and colposcopy if necessary.

## RADIOLOGICAL TESTS

Diagnostic radiographic studies including computed tomography (CT), magnetic resonance imaging (MRI), mammography, and ultrasonography of the male and female reproductive system are used to identify soft tissue and bony abnormalities, to diagnose tumors and masses, and to diagnose infertility problems. Patient preparation and aftercare associated with the use of CT and MRI tests are similar to those described for other body systems and are not repeated here.

### Ultrasonography

Ultrasonography (ultrasound) has become a useful diagnostic tool for persons with reproductive system problems. It can be used to locate pelvic masses, intrauterine devices, ectopic pregnancies, and prostatic neoplasms. Transvaginal ultrasonography provides improved picture clarity compared with transabdominal sonography. Transvaginal sonography is currently being used to inspect and assess the uterus, ovaries, fallopian tubes, and extragenital structures (Box 46-3). A transducer is inserted a few centimeters into the vagina while the patient is in a lithotomy position. Vaginal probes are inserted into a sterile sheath before patient use. The transvaginal probe is also used to guide procedures involving needle puncture, such as ova retrieval for in vitro fertilization.

**box 46-3** *Uses of Transvaginal Sonography*

**UTERUS**
- Size, position
- Inspection of myometrium and endometrial lining
- Detection of malformations
- Identification of small fibroids
- Early pregnancy determination
- Early fetal heartbeats

**OVARIES**
- Size, texture, location
- Monitoring follicular growth
- Evaluation of ovulation
- Identification of corpus luteum
- Identification of tumors and structural deformities
- Follicular aspiration

**FALLOPIAN TUBES**
- Diagnosis of tubal pathological changes
- Detection of tuboovarian abscess
- Early recognition of tubal pregnancy

**EXTRAGENITAL STRUCTURES**
- Evaluation of free pelvic fluid
- Detection of pelvic blood clots

#### *Transrectal ultrasonography*

Transrectal ultrasonography (TRUS) may be used as part of a workup for benign prostatic enlargement or prostate cancer. The procedure is preceded by a rectal examination and possibly an enema. A transrectal probe is inserted 8 to 9 cm into the rectum. TRUS is valuable in evaluating the size of the prostate, determining the response of a prostate tumor to treatment, and guiding placement of needles for biopsy. However, TRUS is not sensitive enough to be used alone for the diagnosis of cancer because the numbers of false-negative and false-positive results are too high.

### Hysterosalpingography

Hysterosalpingography involves radiographic visualization of the uterine cavity and fallopian tubes after the injection of contrast material through the cervix. The test is useful in the evaluation of uterine tumors, tubal obstructions, and abnormalities. The procedure is usually performed in the radiology department, and the patient is placed in a lithotomy position on a fluoroscopy table. A plastic speculum is inserted into the vagina rather than a metal one, to allow for better visualization. A cannula is filled with a water-soluble contrast material, which is injected slowly under direct fluoroscopy. The hysterosalpingogram has largely replaced the older Rubin test, which was associated with numerous false-negative and false-positive results. The patient is assessed for allergy to iodine dye or shellfish although allergic reactions are rare, since the contrast material is not injected intravenously. The bowel may be cleansed with laxatives, suppositories, or enemas before the the test, but no food or fluid restrictions are needed. The patient may be given a sedative or antispasmodic agent before the test. The patient is advised that she may feel menstrual-type cramping and that she may experience shoulder pain caused by subphrenic irritation from the dye as it leaks into the peritoneal cavity.

After the procedure, the nurse assesses the patient for nausea, faintness, and discomfort. Analgesics may be prescribed. The patient is instructed to apply a perineal pad, since vaginal drainage may be present for 1 to 2 days after the test, and the radiopaque dye may stain clothing. The patient should report any signs of infection such as fever, increased pulse rate, or pain to the health care provider.

### Mammography/Xeromammography

Mammography is a radiological study of the breast used to evaluate differences in the density of tissue, particularly small or poorly defined masses or nodules. It is capable of detecting many breast cancers that are too small to be palpated on physical examination. Mammograms are most effective in older women who have a higher percentage of fatty tissue in their breasts, which creates a greater contrast density on x-ray film. The density of benign cysts and malignant tumors may be similar, but their appearance is usually quite different. Suspicious lesions may be referred for needle aspiration or biopsy.

Recommendations for mammography screening are under constant evaluation and revision. Currently it is recommended that a woman have a single baseline mammogram taken between ages 35 and 40. Routine screening is then undertaken at the advice of the physician, considering all known and suspected risk factors for breast cancer (see Chapter 48). Recommendations from various groups are contradictory and reflect political and economic pressures as well as research outcomes. Some sources believe that low-risk women can delay further screening until age 50. Others recommend mammography every 1 to 2 years for women in their forties. General consensus does exist concerning the appropriateness of annual screening after age 50.

No special preparation is required before a mammogram, but the woman should be instructed to avoid using deodorant, cream, or powder, which can mimic calcium clusters on x-ray film. Pretest teaching about the test is critical, since most women are highly anxious about the examination and the possibility of breast cancer. The woman is positioned standing next to the x-ray machine, and one breast at a time is placed between the platform and film plate. Most women experience some degree of discomfort from the breast compression. At least two views of each breast are taken.

Aftercare involves providing clear information concerning how and when the results of the test will be communicated to the patient. Most centers use this opportunity to reinforce skill and understanding of the purpose, technique, and timing of breast self-examination as well.

The xeromammogram provides an x-ray image with a much lower dose of radiation than that required for a traditional mammogram. The images are recorded on paper rather than film. The technique has become increasingly popular because the high contrast result is easier to read and may be more accurate.

## SPECIAL TESTS

### Pregnancy Tests

Laboratory tests for pregnancy first became available in the 1920s. They involved the injection of a urine specimen into a laboratory animal. Because of their relative lack of sensitivity and procedural difficulty, this type of test is no longer used. Most of the frequently used pregnancy tests are based on the fact that human chorionic gonadotropin (hCG) is present in the blood and urine of pregnant women.

Since the 1960s several commercial immunological tests for pregnancy have become available (Ortho, Hylan, Abbott, and Roche are manufacturers). Depending on the specific test blood or urine specimens are used. Results are obtained within 2 minutes to 2 hours. The newer tests can detect as little as 25 mIU/ml of hCG as early as 3 to 4 days after implantation. First morning urine specimens provide the best sample. Do-it-yourself pregnancy tests are available to women over the counter. These tests are sensitive and easy to perform.

The radioreceptor assay test for pregnancy is rapid and reliable. It is extremely accurate, and serial blood samples may be used to determine the viability of the pregnancy or identify molar or ectopic pregnancies. Serum hCG levels double approximately every 2 days until the 10th week of pregnancy. In men and nonpregnant women the normal hCG level is less than 5 mIU/ml. At 2 weeks gestation the value is 50 to 500 mIU/ml. In ectopic pregnancies the level increases at a slower rate.

### Schiller's Test

Schiller's test is a simple test that reveals the presence of atypical cervical cells. A solution of 3.5% iodine or Lugol's solution is applied to the cervix. Atypical cells, both malignant and benign, do not contain glycogen and will fail to stain. Early cancerous lesions and benign lesions, such as cervicitis, may appear as glistening areas of a lighter color than surrounding tissue. Biopsies can then obtained from these targeted areas. The test is used infrequently because colposcopy is a more accurate method of obtaining the same information.

### Biopsies

#### *Cervical biopsy*

A cervical biopsy is performed to obtain a tissue specimen for pathological examination. It is almost always performed with culposcopic direction. Although bleeding is minimal, the biopsy is ideally performed shortly after the menses when the cervix is less vascular. A punch biopsy can be safely performed as an office procedure without the use of anesthesia because the cervix has few pain receptors. The woman is instructed to leave the packing or tampon in place for 8 to 24 hours and report the incidence of excessive bleeding.

### Conization of cervix

Conization of the cervix may be performed as a diagnostic or therapeutic measure. It is typically performed in an outpatient setting with the woman under local anesthesia. A cone-shaped portion of the cervix containing the suspected malignant or infected tissue is removed. Bleeding from the site of conization is greater than that occurring from punch biopsy. If the bleeding is excessive or if hemorrhage seems likely, the cervix is sutured to control blood loss. Oozing is controlled by packing, which is kept in place for 24 to 48 hours. The patient is instructed to rest and avoid heavy lifting for at least 3 days. She should be informed that her next two or three menstrual periods may be heavy and prolonged.

### Endometrial biopsy

Although an ideal method for screening for endometrial cancer has not been developed, a variety of methods are now in use. Less than one half of women with uterine cancer have an abnormal Pap test at diagnosis. Cells rarely exfoliate from the endometrium in the early stages of the cancer, making this an unsatisfactory method of screening and diagnosis. The best results are obtained when cervical aspiration is performed as part of the Pap test.

Endometrial cells obtained by aspiration smear show malignant changes 75% to 90% of the time when uterine cancer exists. A small cannula is inserted through the cervix into the uterine cavity, and suction is applied by means of a syringe attached to the cannula. The specimen obtained is prepared as for a Pap smear.

Endometrial biopsy can be used to diagnose cancer; evaluate bleeding, polyps, or inflammatory conditions; and determine whether ovulation has occurred by assessing the effects of estrogen or progesterone on the endometrium. It is performed by introducing a small curette into the uterus and obtaining several strips of endometrial tissue. The specimens are taken from several sites in the uterine cavity to increase the chances of obtaining malignant cells. The biopsy method is considered to be about 90% accurate in diagnosing endometrial cancer.

Complications include perforation of the uterus, uterine bleeding, interference with early pregnancy, and infection. Any temperature elevation after the biopsy should be reported to the physician because this procedure may activate pelvic inflammatory disease. The patient is advised to wear a pad after the procedure because some vaginal bleeding is expected. If excessive bleeding occurs, the physician should be notified. The patient is advised that douching and intercourse should be avoided for 72 hours after the biopsy. The patient is encouraged to rest during the next 24 hours and avoid heavy lifting to prevent uterine hemorrhage.

### Breast biopsy

It is widely accepted that most breast masses need to be evaluated for cancer. Biopsy can differentiate fibrocystic lesions, fibroadenomas, and intraductal papillomas. Three major approaches are in use. An excisional biopsy removes the mass for pathological evaluation. An incisional biopsy samples some of the tissue from the mass, and an aspiration biopsy involves the removal of fluid or tissue from the mass through a large-bore needle. The aspiration method is in widespread use. Bloody fluid aspirated from the mass indicates the possibility of cancer. If nothing can be aspirated, the mass is considered to be solid and needs to be evaluated via the incisional route. Breast biopsies are usually performed in ambulatory settings with the patient under local anesthesia. It is crucial that the woman clearly understand what procedure is planned, the anesthesia to be used, and the sensations she may experience during the procedure. Aftercare is straightforward. The incision site is assessed for bleeding, edema, or infection. Mild analgesics are provided for discomfort. Numbness at the biopsy site may persist for months.

### Needle biopsy of prostate

A needle aspiration biopsy of the prostate is performed to retrieve cells for histological study. The procedure is usually performed at the same time as cystoscopy but can also be done as an office procedure with the patient under local anesthesia. Either a transrectal or a transperineal approach is used.

A transrectal approach uses guided ultrasound to identify biopsy sites (Figure 46-20). Before the procedure a digital rectal examination is performed to locate the suspicious lesions. A condom-covered ultrasound transducer is inserted into the rectum, and tissue samples are collected from suspicious lesions and other areas of the prostate.

Aspiration may be repeated several times in different locations to sample the tissue adequately. This method is thought

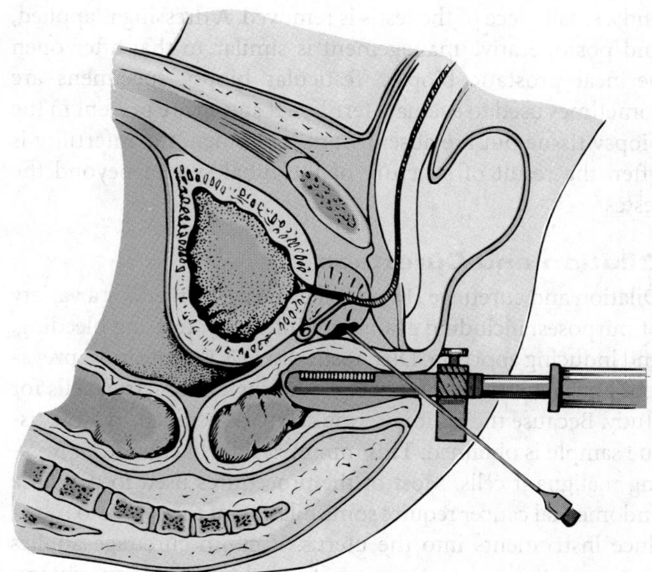

**fig. 46-20** Diagram demonstrating transrectal biopsy with transrectal ultrasound.

to be slightly more accurate than the transperineal approach, which involves insertion of the needle through the perineum into the prostate using the examiner's finger, which is placed in the rectum, as a guide.

Patient preparation for prostatic biopsy may include bowel cleansing if a rectal approach is used. Sepsis is a rare but potentially life-threatening complication. Prophylactic antibiotics are usually prescribed before and after the procedure. The patient may also experience transient hematuria and rectal bleeding. The patient should be advised to promptly report a temperature of greater than 100° F, chills, or difficulty voiding.

#### *Open perineal biopsy*

To obtain a specimen of tissue by open perineal biopsy, a small incision is made in the perineum between the anus and the scrotum. This technique gives the greatest accuracy because the suspect lesion can be clearly identified, and multiple specimens can be taken from the prostate gland. The procedure requires regional or general anesthesia.

A dressing is applied to the biopsy site and can be held in place for about 24 hours with a two-tailed binder. The patient is instructed to wipe from front to back after defecation so as not to contaminate the incision. Perineal irrigation is sometimes advised for both cleanliness and comfort. Unless the physician prescribes a solution, warm water poured from front to back over the incision can be used. After the sutures are removed, sitz baths may be used and add much to the patient's general comfort. The man is instructed to promptly report any signs of infection to the physician.

#### *Testicular biopsy*

Smears or biopsy specimens from the testes can be obtained by the needle method or by an incision made through the scrotum. Most often an incision is used. After a local anesthetic has been administered, a small incision about 2.5 cm long is made, and a small piece of the testis is removed. A dressing is applied, and postoperative management is similar to that after open perineal prostatic biopsy. Testicular biopsy specimens are sometimes used to evaluate fertility. If sperm are present in the biopsy tissue but are absent from the semen, the infertility is often the result of stricture of the tubal system beyond the testes.

### Dilation and Curettage

Dilation and curettage (D & C) may be performed for a variety of purposes, including evaluating infertility, treating bleeding, and inducing abortion. Diagnostically, D & C is the most prevalent and preferred method for obtaining endometrial cells for study. Because the entire uterine cavity is "scraped," a large tissue sample is obtained. This minimizes the likelihood of missing malignant cells. Most of the procedures used to diagnose endometrial cancer require some dilation of the cervix to introduce instruments into the uterus. Vacuum curettage applies suction to the entire uterine cavity to obtain tissue specimens. Vacuum curettage is considered to be at least as good as conventional biopsy for diagnosing endometrial cancer.

**guidelines for care**

**After Dilation and Curettage**

1. Apply a perineal pad to absorb the expected drainage.
2. Take vital signs every 15 minutes until stable.
3. Monitor bleeding every 15 minutes for 2 hours; if active bleeding continues, monitor every hour for about 8 hours.
4. Record each pad change and amount of blood loss in estimated milliliters (60 ml saturates a perineal pad).
5. Monitor urine output.
6. Give mild analgesics as prescribed; report immediately any abdominal pain that is continuous, sharp, and not relieved by analgesics (may indicate perforation of uterus).
7. Encourage ambulation when patient is awake and vital signs are stable.

**box 46-4** *Endoscopic Procedures for Visualization of Pelvic Organs*

COLPOSCOPY
Visualization of vagina and cervix under low-power magnification

CULDOSCOPY
Insertion of culdoscope through posterior vaginal vault into cul-de-sac of Douglas for visualization of fallopian tubes and ovaries (Figure 46-21)

FALLOPOSCOPY
Transcervical endoscopic examination of fallopian tubes

HYSTEROSCOPY
Insertion of hysteroscope through cervix for visualization of inside of uterus

LAPAROSCOPY
Insertion of laparoscope (patient under local or general anesthesia) through small incision in abdominal wall (inferior margin of umbilicus), which is insufflated with carbon dioxide; permits visualization of all pelvic organs (Figure 46-22)

For a D & C, metal dilators of graduated sizes are inserted into the cervical canal. Once the cervix is dilated, sharp curettes are used to remove endometrial tissue. The major complications of a D & C are hemorrhage and perforation of the uterus. Postoperative care is summarized in the Guidelines for Care Box. Most women are discharged on the day of the procedure. Normal daily activities can be resumed, but vigorous exercise is discouraged. Sexual intercourse may be resumed when the woman feels comfortable. The menstrual cycle usually is not disturbed by a D & C, and all vaginal bleeding should disap-

**table 46-5** *Examinations for Infertility*

| Gender | Tests | Data Obtained |
|---|---|---|
| Male | Multiple semen examination | Determine presence, number, and motility of sperm |
| | Testicular biopsy if sperm count low or absent | Presence of sperm indicates obstruction of vas deferens |
| Female | Basal body temperature chart | Determine that ovulation is occurring |
| | Postcoital test of cervical secretions | Measure ability of sperm to penetrate cervical mucus and remain active, and measure quality of the mucus |
| | Endometrial biopsy, serum progesterone and estradiol levels, laparoscopic inspection of ovaries | Determine whether ovulation is occurring (if in question) |
| | Laparoscopy | Determine patency of fallopian tubes |
| | Hysterosalpingography (x-ray film after insertion of contrast media) | Determine patency of uterus and fallopian tubes |
| Male/female | Hormonal tests | Determine whether the problem is hormonal |

**table 46-6** *Diagnostic Studies of Male and Female Reproductive Systems—Fertility Studies*

| Test | Description | Pretest and Posttest Care |
|---|---|---|
| Semen analysis | Semen is assessed for volume (2-5 ml), viscosity, sperm count (>20 million/ml), sperm motility (60% motile), and percentage of abnormal sperm (60% with normal structure). | Instruct patient to bring in fresh specimen within 2 hr after ejaculation. Protect specimen from cold. Instruct patient that specimen is to be collected after abstaining from intercourse for 2-5 days. |
| Basal body temperature assessment | This measurement indicates indirectly whether ovulation has occurred. (Temperature rises at ovulation and remains elevated during secretory phase of normal menstrual cycle.) | Instruct patient to take her temperature using special basal temperature thermometer (calibrated in tenths of degrees) every morning before getting out of bed. Tell her to record temperature on graph. |
| Sim-Huhner test (postcoital cervical mucus test or cervical mucus sperm penetration test) | Mucus sample from cervix is examined within 2-8 hr after intercourse. Total number of sperm is assessed in relation to number of live sperm. This test is performed to determine whether cervical mucus is "hostile" to passage of sperm from vagina into uterus. | Instruct couple to have intercourse at estimated time of ovulation and be present for test within 2-3 hr after intercourse. Instruct woman not to use vaginal lubrication, douche, or bathe until after examination. Instruct woman to remain in bed for 15 min after coitus. Study should be performed after 3 days of sexual abstinence. |

Modified from Lewis SM et al: *Medical-surgical nursing: assessment and management of clinical problems,* ed 4, St Louis, 1996, Mosby.

pear in a week to 10 days. Women are advised to report the recurrence of bright-red blood or the development of a vaginal discharge with an unpleasant odor.

### Infertility Tests

The purposes of an infertility evaluation are to establish the cause of infertility, give a prognosis for future fertility, provide a basis for medical or surgical treatment, and assist the couple to accept their diagnosis, treatment, and future options. The assessment and intervention can be physically painful as well as emotionally and economically stressful.

A full description of an infertility workup is beyond the scope of this discussion. Examinations and diagnostic studies used in infertility evaluation are listed in Table 46-5 and are summarized in Table 46-6.

### Endoscopy

The pelvic organs and surrounding tissues can be visualized directly by endoscopy. The procedures by which this can be accomplished are colposcopy, culdoscopy, laparoscopy (peritoneoscopy), hysteroscopy, and falloposcopy (Box 46-4). Most of the procedures can be performed on an outpatient basis even if general anesthesia is used. Culposcopy is used to augment a detailed examination of the vagina and cervix or to guide cervical biopsy. The associated care is the same as that for other types of cervical biopsy. The use of culdoscopy (Figure 46-21) is declining because laparoscopy has become a standard diagnostic and treatment intervention. Hysteroscopy is frequently performed as part of a D & C to allow the physician to inspect the inside of the uterus before scraping or treatment. In the male, cystoscopic examination allows the physician to inspect the condition of the urethra and bladder

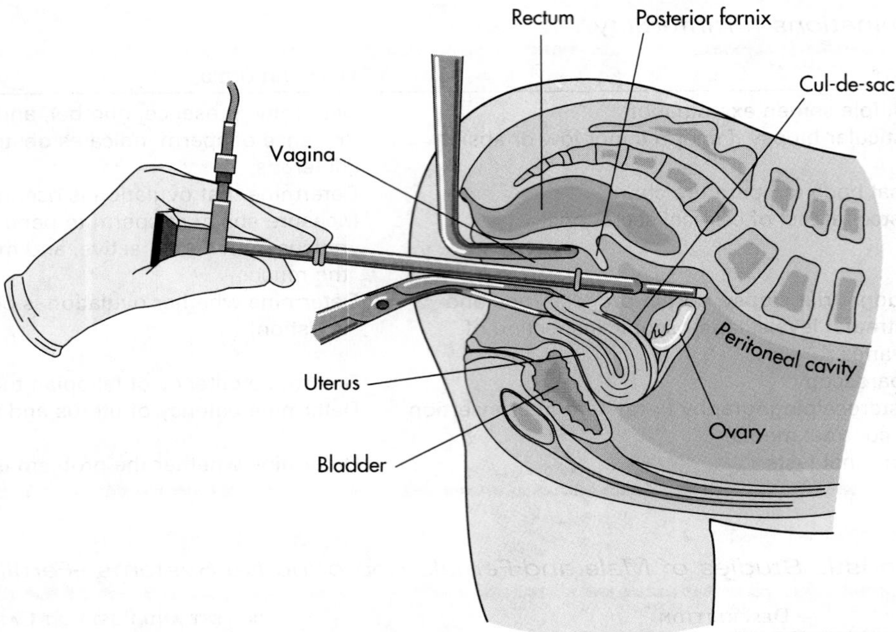


**fig. 46-21** With patient in knee-chest position, culdoscope is inserted through posterior fornix of vagina into cul-de-sac of Douglas. Note that ovaries can be seen.

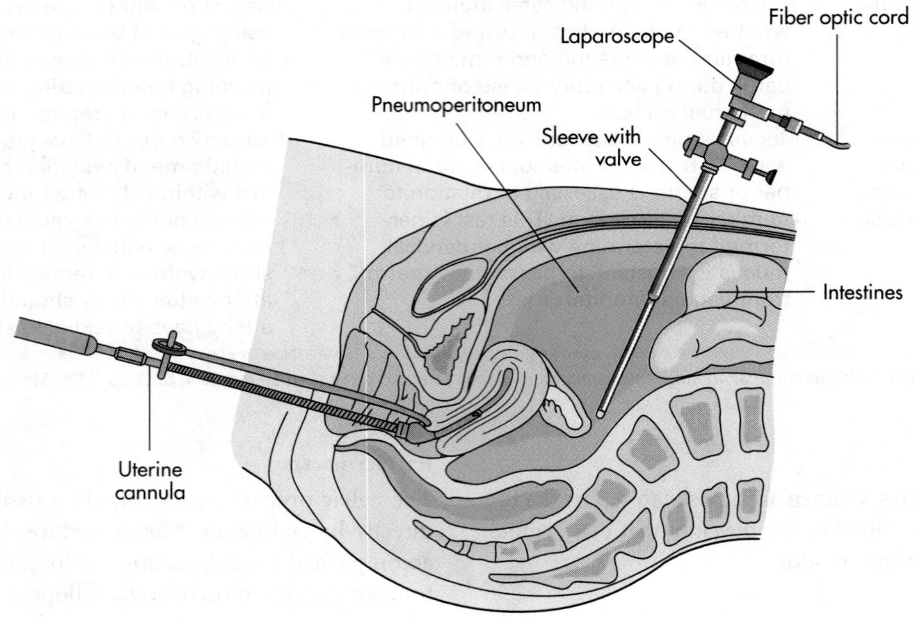


**fig. 46-22** Schema of gynecological laparoscopy.

mucosa and to detect prostatic encroachment on the urethra (see Chapter 49).

Laparoscopy (pelvic endoscopy or peritoneoscopy) may be used to inspect the outer surface of the uterus, fallopian tubes, and ovaries (Figure 46-22). A laparoscope is inserted through the abdominal wall through a small incision in the subumbilical area. The peritoneal cavity is filled with 3 to 4 L of carbon dioxide to separate the abdominal wall from the viscera and increase visualization. The laparoscope is then inserted to conduct the planned procedure. Laparoscopy may also be used for tubal sterilization, for lysis of adhesions, for biopsy, and in various infertility procedures. General anesthesia is typically used. At the end of the procedure, the carbon dioxide is removed, but referred pain to the shoulder from gaseous irritation of the diaphragm and phrenic nerve often occurs. The Patient/Family Teaching Box summarizes nursing care.

**patient/family teaching**

**Discharge Instructions After Routine Laparoscopy**

1. Rest for the next 24 hours before resuming normal activities.
2. Avoid sexual intercourse until after postoperative visit with physician.
3. Discomfort may be experienced in shoulder and upper abdominal area. Take oral pain medications as prescribed.
4. Call the physician if abdominal pain increases, if temperature elevates, if abnormal vaginal bleeding occurs, or if there is increased redness, swelling, soreness, or foul drainage at wound sites before first postoperative visit.
5. Wound dressings may be removed in 24 hours, and showering is permitted.
6. Resume regular diet and drink plenty of fluids.

Air may enter the abdominal cavity during the procedure and cause discomfort; a prone position with a pillow under the abdomen may increase the woman's comfort. The woman is instructed to avoid douching and intercourse for about 1 week after a culdoscopy. Complications such as hemorrhage and infection are rare, but women are cautioned to report fever or pain in the lower abdomen.

## chapter SUMMARY

### ANATOMY AND PHYSIOLOGY

- Major external structures of the female genital system include the mons pubis, labia majora, labia minora, clitoris, prepuce, frenulum, vestibule, urethral meatus, Skene's glands, vaginal orifice, hymen, fossa navicularis, Bartholin's glands, fourchet, perineum, and escutcheon.
- Major female internal reproductive organs are the vagina, uterus, fallopian tubes, and ovaries.
- The male genital system includes the testes, spermatic cords, vas deferens, seminal vesicles, ejaculatory ducts, penis, scrotum, prostate glands, and bulbourethral glands.
- The menstrual cycle is divided into phases according to uterine or ovarian changes. The ovarian cycle consists of the follicular and luteal phase, whereas the uterine cycle consists of the menstrual, proliferative, and secretory phases.
- Menstrual cycle function depends on the interrelationship of the central nervous system, anterior pituitary, ovaries, and uterus.

### SUBJECTIVE DATA

- An extensive history including the patient's complaint in detail, medications and allergies, reproductive health history, and family, personal and sexual history is collected.

### OBJECTIVE DATA

- The physical examination of female and male reproductive systems requires use of special positioning and extensive palpation, both requiring clear explanations.
- Preparation of the woman for a pelvic examination includes use of models, films, and visual aids, explanation of the procedure and answering questions, sharing information about sensations she will feel, draping or nondraping per the patient's request, and explanation of what is being done and findings during the examination.

### DIAGNOSTIC TESTS

- Laboratory tests used to assess reproductive health include tests for syphilis and *Chlamydia*, Pap smear, endocrine studies, and smears and cultures from various sites.
- Radiological tests used to assess reproductive health include ultrasonography, CT scan, and MRI.
- Screening tests for endometrial cancer include aspiration smear, endometrial biopsy, vacuum curettage, and D & C.
- Endoscopic procedures to assess reproductive health include colposcopy, culdoscopy, laparoscopy, hysteroscopy, and falloposcopy.
- Special tests for assessing reproductive health in men include prostatic smear, needle biopsies, open perineal biopsy, testicular smears and biopsy specimens, enzyme tests, and endoscopy.

## References


1. Berek JS, Adashi EY, Hillard PA: *Novak's gynecology,* ed 12, Baltimore, 1996, William & Wilkins.
2. Campbell J, Humphreys J: *Nursing care of survivors of family violence,* St Louis, 1993, Mosby.
3. Chernesky M et al: Ability of commercial ligase chain reaction and PCR assays to diagnose *Chlamydia trachomatis* infections in men by testing first-void urine, *J Clin Microbiol* 35(4):982-986, 1997.
4. Chernesky M et al: Diagnosis of *Chlamydia trachomatis* urethral infection in symptomatic and asymptomatic men by testing first-void urine in a ligase chain reaction assay, *J Infect Dis* 170(6):1308-1311, 1994.
5. *Clinician's handbook of preventive services: putting prevention into practice,* Washington, DC, 1994, US Department of Health and Human Services, Public Health Service.
6. Eisenberger D, Herenandes E, Tener T, Atkinson BF: Order of endocervical and ectocervical cytologic sampling and the quality of the Papanicolaou smear, *Obstet Gynecol* 90(5):755-758, 1997.
7. Emster V: Mammography screening for woman aged 40-49—a guidelines saga and a clarion call for informed decision making, *Am J Public Health* 87(7):1103-1106, 1997.
8. Evers JLH, Heineman MJ: *Gynecology, a clinical atlas,* St Louis, 1990, Mosby.
9. Ferreira N: Sexually transmitted *Chlamydia trachomatis, Nurse Pract Forum* 8(2):70-76, 1997.
10. Gillenwater JY, Grayhack JT, Howards SS, Duckett JW: *Adult and pediatric urology,* ed 3, St Louis, 1996, Mosby.
11. Guyton AC: *Textbook of medical physiology,* ed 8, Philadelphia, 1991, WB Saunders.
12. Henry JB: *Clinical diagnosis and management by laboratory methods,* ed 19, Philadelphia, 1996, WB Saunders.
13. Isacson C, Kurman RJ: The Bethesda system: a new classification for managing pap smears, *Contemp OB/GYN* 6(1):67-74, 1995.
14. Jarvis C: *Physical examination and health assessment,* ed 2, Philadelphia, 1995, WB Saunders.
15. Lee KR et al: Comparison of conventional Papanicolaou smears and a fluid-based, thin-layer system for cervical cancer screening, *Obstet Gynecol* 90(2):278-284, 1997.
16. Mouton J, et al: Detection of *Chlamydia trachomatis* in male and female urine specimens by using the amplified *Chlamydia trachomatis* test, *J Clin Microbiol* 35(6):1369-1372, 1997.

17. Paukku M, Puolakkainen M, Apter D, Hirvonen S, Paavonen J: First void urine testing for *Chlamydia trachomatis* by polymerase chain reaction in asymptomatic women, *Sexually Transmitted Dis* 24(6):343-346, 1997.
18. Peterson E: Laboratory detection of *Chlamydia trachomatis, West J Med* 167(1):36, 1997.
19. Tietz NW, editor: *Clinical guide to laboratory tests*, ed 3, Philadelphia, 1995, WB Saunders.
20. Wertlake PT, Francus K, Newkirk GR, Groesbeck PP: Effectiveness of the Papanicolaou smear and speculoscopy as compared with the Pap smear alone: a community based clinical trial, *Obstet Gynecol* 90(3):421-427, 1997.
21. Worthington S, Rubin M: Nurse-midwifery evaluation and management of cervical pathology and the colposcopic examination, *J Nurse Midwifery* 38(2, suppl):36S-41S, 1993.
22. Younkin EQ, Davis MS: *Women's health, a primary care clinical guide*, Norwalk, Conn, 1994, Appleton & Lange.

chapter 47

# MANAGEMENT OF WOMEN WITH Reproductive Problems

SALLY REEL and JO ANN LIERMAN

## objectives

*After studying this chapter, the learner should be able to:*

1. Discuss the collaborative management of common infectious diseases of the female reproductive tract.
2. Discuss the etiologies of various disorders of menstruation.
3. Compare the preoperative and postoperative care provided to women undergoing structural repair of a cystocele or rectocele versus the care provided for hysterectomy.
4. Outline the patient teaching provided to women undergoing intracavitary radiotherapy to the female reproductive tract.
5. Discuss the nursing responsibilities associated with caring for women undergoing sterilization or experiencing problems with fertility.

Diseases and disorders of the female reproductive system threaten the physical and emotional health of millions of women each year. Infectious processes and disorders of menstruation are common and pervasive problems. Malignant neoplasms destroy childbearing potential and end numerous lives each year. Some of the problems presented in this chapter can be prevented, many of the disorders are treatable, and some can be cured. Disorders affecting the female reproductive system are important national health concerns and are reflected in the *Healthy People 2000* goals as summarized in Box 47-1.

## INFECTIOUS PROCESSES

### VAGINITIS

#### Etiology/Epidemiology

Although the vulva and vagina are relatively resistant to infection, vaginitis is one of the most common problems for which women seek medical care. Although the symptoms of vaginal discharge, vulvar pruritis, tissue irritation and inflammation, and burning are associated with several vaginal infections, most cases result from an infection involving one of three organisms: *Candida albicans, Trichomonas vaginalis,* and *Gardnerella vaginalis. Candida* and *Trichomonas* each account for about 25% of all cases, and *Gardnerella* accounts for the rest.[4,21] Other bacteria (including those causing sexually transmitted diseases, such as *Chlamydia* and *Neisseria gonorrhoeae*), fungi, viruses, parasites, allergens, and foreign bodies are all potential causes.[4]

Bacterial vaginosis is the most common cause of vaginal discharge. Bacterial vaginosis is not a typical infectious process, but occurs from an overgrowth of bacteria that are considered to be normal flora in the vagina. *Gardnerella vaginalis* is the most common cause.[4] *Gardnerella* vaginosis occurs primarily in sexually active women and is rare in women who are not sexually active.[4,34]

#### Pathophysiology

The vagina is normally protected from infection by its acid pH and the presence of normal flora such as Döderlein's bacillus. Any factor that alters the normal vaginal physiology may predispose to infection. If the pH or vaginal mucosa is altered or the woman's resistance is decreased by aging-related changes, stress, or disease, her risk of infection increases. The use of antibiotics, which destroy the normal protective flora of the vagina, also increases the risk of infection.

Diseases causing immunocompromise, such as human immunodeficiency virus (HIV), or alteration in carbohydrate metabolism, such as diabetes mellitus, can also alter the vaginal ecosystem, leading to infection.[4] The use of steroids, which suppress the immune response, also increases the risk.

**box 47-1** Healthy People 2000 *Goals Related to Female Reproductive Problems*

1. Reduce the prevalence of *Chlamydia trachomatis* infections among young women (under the age of 25 years) to no more than 5%.
2. Reduce the incidence of pelvic inflammatory disease, as measured by a reduction in hospitalizations for pelvic inflammatory disease, to no more than 100 per 100,000 women of age 15 to 44 years and a reduction in the number of initial visits to physicians for pelvic inflammatory disease to no more than 290,000.
3. Increase to at least 95% the proportion of women age 18 years and older who have ever received a Pap test and to at least 85% those who received a Pap test within the preceding 1 to 3 years.
4. Ensure that Pap tests meet quality standards by monitoring and certifying all cytology laboratories.
5. Reduce deaths from cancer of the uterine cervix to no more than 1.3 per 100,000 women.

From US Department of Health and Human Services, Public Health Service: *Healthy People 2000: National health promotion and disease prevention objectives,* Washington DC, 1990, US Government Printing Office.

Many organisms proliferate in a more alkaline environment, which becomes important for postmenopausal women, who experience a decrease in normal vaginal secretions and a rise in vaginal pH caused by a decline in estrogen levels. Vaginitis can also be caused by tissue injury from foreign objects such as tampons or by chemical irritation from douches, which make tissues more susceptible to invasion by organisms. Different organisms are associated with specific types of discharge and symptom patterns, but pruritus is an extremely common symptom regardless of the cause and commonly is severe. Table 47-1 presents a comparison of different forms of vaginitis. Risk factors for infection are listed in the Risk Factors Box.

### Collaborative Care Management

The diagnosis of vaginitis is made by microscopic analysis of the vaginal secretions (e.g., KOH analysis, wet smear, or Gram's stain) and culture of the discharge. Serological testing and urine culture may also be used. The management of vaginitis is primarily pharmacological, and drug treatment is outlined in Table 47-1.

Many of these drugs are available as over-the-counter preparations, but women are advised to seek diagnosis from their primary health care provider for an initial episode of vaginitis if symptoms do not subside after one course of over-the-counter treatment.

The drugs may be administered orally or by ointment, cream, or suppository. Women are informed that the use of metronidazole (Flagyl) causes urine to turn a dark reddish brown. It also causes numerous gastrointestinal (GI) side effects that may be reduced by taking the drug with meals. The

**risk factors**

**Infections of the Vulva and Vagina**

- Pregnancy
- Age—premenarche and postmenopause
- Low estrogen levels
- Dermatological allergies
- Diabetes mellitus
- Oral contraceptive use
- Inadequate hygiene
- Douching
- Treatment with broad-spectrum antibiotics
- Use of vaginal contraceptives—foams, inserts
- Intercourse with infected partner
- Frequent intercourse with multiple partners
- Tight, nonabsorbent, and heat-retaining clothing

**table 47-1** *Common Causes, Clinical Manifestations, and Treatment of Vaginitis*

| Cause | Clinical Manifestations | Treatment |
|---|---|---|
| Infections | | |
| *Candida albicans* (20-30% of all vaginal infections) | White, curdlike, cheesy discharge; characteristic patches on vaginal walls and cervix; itching; inflamed vagina and cervix | Clotrimazole (Mycelex, Lotrimin) I applicator intravaginally qHS for 7 days<br>Miconazole (Monistat) cream intravaginally qHS for 7 days<br>Tioconazole 6.5% (Vagistat 1) intravaginally qHS for 1 dose<br>Fluconazole (Diflucan) one tablet orally stat<br>Nystatin (Mycostatin) suppositories daily or bid for 14 days |
| *Trichomonas vaginalis* (20-30% of all vaginitis) | Yellowish to greenish, frothy, copious discharge: "strawberry spots" on cervix, foul odor, severe burning, itching, and dyspareunia | Metronidazole (Flagyl) orally for 7 days or 2 g stat for both partners<br>Symptomatic therapy |
| *Gardnerella*-associated bacterial vaginosis | Grayish white, homogeneous discharge; scant amount; fishy or foul odor | Oral antibiotics: ampicillin for 5 days, metronidazole (Flagyl) for 7 days<br>Metronidazole (Flagyl) 2 g stat; clindamycin (Cleocin) for 7 days; intravaginal treatment with metronidazole (MetroGel) 1 applicator bid for 5 days; clindamycin phosphate 2% vaginal cream (Cleocin) 1 applicator qHS for 7 days |
| Foreign body | Blood-tinged serosanguineous or purulent discharge; usually foul odor, discharge may be thick or thin | Removal of object; antibiotics specific to secondary infection |
| Allergens or irritants | Increase in usual type and amount secretions; itching, burning, rash | Removal of possible allergen or irritant; topical steroid ointment as needed |

Modified from Bychkov V, Isaacs J: *Pathology in the practice of gynecology,* St Louis, 1995, Mosby; Hawkins J, Roberto-Nichols D, Stanley-Haney J: *Protocols for nurse practitioners in gynecologic settings,* New York, 1995, Tiresias Press.

use of alcohol can trigger an Antabuse-like reaction of severe nausea, vomiting, and abdominal distress and should be avoided during treatment and for 48 hours after completing the medication.

#### *Patient/family education*

Women have self-managed vaginitis for generations, and a number of alternative treatments are in common use. The nurse explores the woman's use of alternative therapies, ensures that the treatment is not contraindicated for the specific causative organism, and provides the woman with specific instructions about the safe and appropriate use of soaks, irrigations, and douches in vaginitis treatment.

Nursing management focuses primarily on the appropriate use of prescribed therapy and measures to prevent reinfection. The nurse instructs the woman to cleanse the genital area thoroughly with soap and water and dry well before applying any medication. The hands should be washed carefully before and after treatment.

The nurse advises the woman to remain recumbent for 30 minutes after insertion of a suppository or cream to facilitate absorption and prevent loss from the vagina. Tampons should be avoided during treatment. If vaginal drainage is present, the woman is encouraged to wear a minipad. Sitz baths can be comforting. The woman is instructed to refrain from intercourse while the infection is being treated, and the male partner should use a condom until all symptoms of inflammation have resolved.

Prevention of reinfection is an important consideration, because vaginitis can easily become a recurrent problem. The nurse discusses the various lifestyle modifications that can be made to reduce the incidence of vaginal infection. The accompanying Guidelines for Care Box summarizes these measures.

**guidelines for care**

**Preventing Vaginal Infection**

1. Cleanse the genital area thoroughly with mild soap and water daily.
   a. Wipe genital area from front to back after bowel movements.
   b. Avoid use of vaginal irritants (e.g., harsh deodorant and perfumed soap, deodorant sprays, douches).
   c. Avoid routine douching, which can alter the vaginal pH.
2. Use underwear with cotton crotch and change panties daily; avoid use of any clothing that is tight in the crotch or thighs. Avoid wearing underpants while sleeping.
3. Assess sexual partners for any sign of infection (e.g., discharge, lesions, reddened areas on genitals).
   a. Use a barrier method of contraception.
   b. Avoid any sexual practice that is painful or abrasive.
   c. Avoid anal genital intercourse.
   d. Cleanse genital area of self and partner and void before and after intercourse.
4. Change tampons or napkins frequently during menstruation.
5. Treat athlete's foot and "jock itch" with over-the-counter antifungals.
6. Consider using vitamin C 500 mg PO bid to increase the acidity of vaginal secretions.
7. Recognize the signs of infection and respond promptly.

## CERVICITIS

### Etiology/Epidemiology

The term *cervicitis* includes a number of conditions characterized by inflammation and infection of the cervix. In the past, a distinction was made between acute and chronic cervicitis. Clinically, it is difficult to distinguish these differences without microcellular evaluation.[35] Cervicitis has been linked with cervical cancer.

### Pathophysiology

Gonococci, streptococci, staphylococci, herpesvirus, and chlamydiae all can cause cervicitis. *Chlamydia* is the most common cause of infection.[35] Leukorrhea may be the only sign, and the amount may not be significant. On examination, the cervix is grossly erythematous and edematous, and there is usually a mucoid purulent discharge, but the amount may be so small that the patient does not notice it. The woman commonly has no subjective signs but may report pruritus, burning, lower abdominal pain, or dyspareunia. Symptoms of a urinary tract infection may also be present. Cervical stenosis, salpingitis, and infertility are possible sequelae of chronic disease.[35]

### Collaborative Care Management

Vaginitis, if present, is treated first. The cervix is cultured, and appropriate pharmacological therapy is initiated.

Gonococcal cervicitis is treated with one dose of ceftriaxone IM, plus oral doxycycline for 7 days, and one dose of oral azithromycin to treat concurrent chlamydial infection.[34] See Chapter 50 for a more thorough discussion of the treatment of sexually transmitted diseases (STDs). Other organisms may be treated as outlined in the section on vaginitis. If the woman's cervicitis does not respond to antibiotics, cryosurgery or laser therapy may be necessary.[35]

#### *Patient/family education*

Cryosurgery is a safe outpatient procedure. Women are told that a watery discharge is common after treatment but it resolves in several weeks. Healing is usually complete within 6 weeks.[35] Women are also told that they may experience mild to moderate cramping during the procedure.[7] The prevention of cervicitis includes those measures outlined in the above Guidelines for Care Box, because many cases of cervicitis develop from vaginal infection.

## BARTHOLINITIS (BARTHOLIN'S CYSTS)

### Etiology/Epidemiology

Bartholin's cysts are one of the most common disorders of the vulva. They result from obstruction of a duct, which may become infected. Thickened mucus, stenosis, or mechanical trauma may initiate the process.

### Pathophysiology

The infection usually is unilateral but can be bilateral. *Neisseria gonorrhoeae* is the most common infecting organism.[8] The secretory function of the gland continues, and the duct fills up with fluid, producing severe inflammation, enlargement of the gland, and tissue edema. The area becomes tender, and even walking may be difficult. The pain is constant, and dyspareunia can be severe. The abscess may rupture, resulting in temporary symptom relief, but it usually re-forms. Occasionally, the acute inflammation resolves, leaving scar tissue that can form a cyst. The cyst usually is nontender but may interfere with ambulation or intercourse.

### Collaborative Care Management

Cultures are taken, and the woman is treated for any underlying infectious process. If the cysts are symptomatic, incision and drainage may be performed. The cysts tend to recur, and a permanent opening for drainage of the gland may need to be constructed by placing a tiny WORD catheter through a stab wound into the cyst cavity. The catheter remains in the cyst for 3 to 4 weeks until healing has occurred and a new duct has formed. This procedure is also useful when infection is present. Laser therapy can also be used to remove the cyst.[27] Total gland excision may be performed in older women who have suffered repeated abscesses or when cancer is suspected.

#### *Patient/family education*

Nursing interventions focus on comfort. Mild analgesics and sitz baths help relieve pain. Because most procedures are performed on an outpatient basis, the nurse instructs the woman on the safe use of these interventions at home and reinforces the need to report any signs of infection.

## PELVIC INFLAMMATORY DISEASE

### Etiology/Epidemiology

*Pelvic inflammatory disease (PID)* is a general term that refers to acute, subacute, recurrent, or chronic infection of the reproductive organs, pelvic peritoneum, veins, or connective tissue. The infection may be confined to just one structure or be widespread.

More than 1 million cases of PID are diagnosed annually in women of reproductive age in the United States, and nearly 150,000 women become infertile annually as a complication of PID.[17,38,40] An estimated 4.2 billion dollars is spent annually to treat pelvic infections.[30] Sexually active adolescents have a greatly increased risk of contracting the disease.

Pelvic inflammatory disease is rare during pregnancy and in premenarchal, postmenopausal, and celibate women.[40] It occurs in women using intrauterine devices (IUDs) more often than in women using other forms of contraception.

The risk factors for PID are the same as those for STDs (see Chapter 50). Known risk factors include low socioeconomic status, early onset of sexual activity, multiple sex partners, frequent douching (three or more times per month), cigarette smoking, and a prior history of sexually transmitted disease.[33,40] Surgery on the reproductive organs, childbearing, and abortion all lower the woman's resistance to infection and provide portals of entry for pathogens.

### Pathophysiology

The routes of pelvic infection are illustrated in Figure 47-1. Pathogenic organisms usually are introduced from outside the body and pass up the cervical canal into the uterus. Common causative organisms include gonococci, *Chlamydia, Haemophilus,* and streptococci. There is growing evidence that the presence of bacterial vaginosis also increases the risk of acquiring a pelvic infection.[37] The causative organisms invade the pelvis by way of the fallopian tubes or through the uterine veins or lymphatics. Many of the pathogens lodge in the fallopian tubes and create an acute or chronic inflammatory reaction. Purulent material collects in the tubes, adhesions and strictures form, and steril-

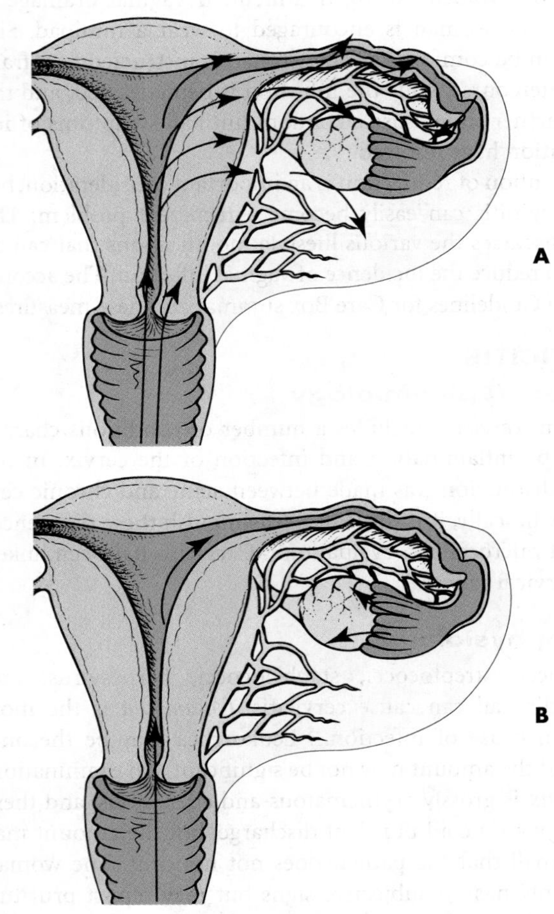


**fig. 47-1** Common routes of the spread of pelvic inflammatory disease. **A,** Direct spread of bacterial infection other than *Neisseria gonorrhoeae*. **B,** Direct spread of *Neisseria gonorrhoeae*.

ity, which is one of the most serious consequences of PID, may occur. Partial obstruction of the tubes may predispose a woman to ectopic pregnancy because the fertilized ovum cannot reach the uterus. Inflammatory adhesions become so severe that surgical removal of the uterus, tubes, and ovaries may be necessary. The infection usually remains localized in the lower abdomen and pelvis, although abscesses may form.

Clinical manifestations of acute PID include severe abdominal pain, lower abdominal cramping, intermenstrual bleeding, dyspareunia, fever and chills, malaise, nausea, and vomiting. A sensation of pelvic pressure and back pain may also be present, as well as a foul-smelling, purulent vaginal discharge. Symptoms often appear after the onset or cessation of menses.[30] Abdominal palpation reveals pain and tenderness in the lower quadrants of the abdomen, which is confirmed on pelvic examination. Masses may be felt, indicating enlargement of the fallopian tubes or ovaries or the presence of an abscess.

### Collaborative Care Management

Diagnostic studies include white cell counts and culture of any purulent secretions. A laparoscopy may be ordered to visualize pelvic structures and accomplish drainage of abscesses and lysis of obstructing adhesions. Ultrasonography may be used to evaluate masses.

Treatment is aimed at eradicating the infection and preventing complications. Hospitalization may be necessary if the woman is acutely ill. Broad-spectrum antibiotics are used until drug sensitivities are determined. Salpingectomy may be necessary if an abscess is found, and more radical surgery is performed if all the reproductive organs have been compromised by the infection.[9,17,40] If the woman has an IUD, it is removed.

Nursing interventions are largely supportive. Bedrest in a semi-Fowler's position is recommended to assist with pelvic drainage. Heat applied to the abdomen may be comforting, but tub or sitz baths should be avoided during the period of active infection. The vaginal discharge is copious and commonly purulent and may cause pruritus and excoriation. Other nursing measures include managing fever, monitoring vital signs, monitoring intake and output, and providing emotional support.

#### *Patient/family education*

The nurse instructs the woman to cleanse the perineal region every 3 to 4 hours and maintain scrupulous hygiene after urination and defecation. Tampons should not be used, and drainage pads should be changed frequently. A minimum of 3000 ml of fluids daily is recommended. Women treated as outpatients are reminded of the importance of seeking appropriate follow-up because PID can have serious lifelong consequences for fertility. The woman's sexual partner may be treated with antibiotics at the same time. The importance of using condoms to prevent reinfection or future infections is stressed.

## TOXIC SHOCK SYNDROME

### Etiology/Epidemiology

Toxic shock syndrome (TSS) is a severe disease caused by strains of staphylococci that produce a unique epidermal toxin. It can occur in any situation in which staphylococcal organisms can be harbored, but it is most clearly associated with women during menstruation, particularly women who use tampons. Toxic shock syndrome has occurred in infants, children, and men and has been associated with a variety of surgical procedures, including gynecological, urological, and orthopedic procedures. Women at increased risk include those who use superabsorbent tampons, insert tampons with their fingers, or have chronic vaginal infections or herpes genitalis. The overall incidence is currently about 6.2 per 100,000, which is a dramatic decrease since the link with tampon use was made in the early 1980s.[30]

### Pathophysiology

The exact mechanism by which staphylococcal toxins gain access to the circulatory system is unknown. The role of tampons also remains unclear. They may cause mucosal damage, but it is theorized that superabsorbent tampons obstruct the vagina and cause retrograde menstruation with peritoneal absorption of bacteria or toxins. The use of a diaphragm during menstruation creates a similar risk. Tampons may also cause an increase in aerobic bacteria from oxygen trapped in the interfibrous spaces. The longer a tampon is left in place, the greater the risk for TSS. The mortality rate is 3% to 6%.[30]

The onset of symptoms is usually abrupt, with fever, vomiting, watery diarrhea, headache, and myalgia. The patient will appear acutely ill with a fever near 39° C or higher, and the syndrome can progress to hypotensive shock within hours. An erythematous, sunburnlike rash develops over the face, proximal extremities, and trunk, and both the conjunctiva and the pharynx become erythematous. Muscle and abdominal tenderness commonly are present, but if neck rigidity, headache, or disorientation occurs, a lumbar puncture usually is performed to rule out meningitis.[30] Prompt diagnosis is critical, and these symptoms occurring in a menstruating woman using tampons are thoroughly explored.

### Collaborative Care Management

Diagnostic tests for TSS include a complete blood screen and cultures of the blood, throat, urine, vaginal secretions, and possibly cerebrospinal fluid. Vaginal cultures usually show penicillinase-producing *Staphylococcus aureus.* The cornerstone of medical care is beta-lactamase-resistant antibiotics such as nafcillin, cefoxitin, cefazolin, and cephalothin.[30] Penicillinase-resistant agents, antistaphylococcal agents, and corticosteroids may all be used. Aggressive fluid and electrolyte management is indicated if the patient shows signs of shock. Mechanical ventilation may be necessary if adult respiratory distress syndrome develops. The management of shock is discussed in detail in Chapter 17. Nursing care revolves around careful monitoring and supportive care similar to that offered any critically ill patient (see Chapter 22).

#### *Patient/family education*

If the woman is wearing a tampon, it should be removed immediately. Approximately 30% of women who develop TSS experience recurrences. The greatest risk for recurrence is during the first three menstrual periods after treatment. Recurrent episodes are usually less severe than the initial one. Women can almost entirely eliminate the risk of TSS by avoiding tampon use. In addition, the nurse instructs women about the importance of careful perineal hygiene, avoiding douching, and limiting the use of a contraceptive diaphragm to no more than 24 hours at one time.

## DISORDERS OF MENSTRUATION

Almost all women experience a problem with their menstrual cycle at some point in their reproductive years. Problems produce a variety of symptoms that may be directly or indirectly related to the pelvic organs. Most problems are self-managed and are rarely brought to a physician's attention unless they become severe or persistent.

### DYSMENORRHEA

#### Etiology/Epidemiology

Dysmenorrhea involves uterine pain with menstruation and is commonly called menstrual cramps. Primary dysmenorrhea is not associated with pelvic pathology and occurs in the absence of any organic disease. Its severity usually declines after pregnancy or by age 30. Secondary dysmenorrhea occurs in response to organic disease such as PID, endometriosis, leiomyomas (uterine fibroids), and IUD use.

Primary dysmenorrhea affects about 50% to 75% of menstruating women. About 10% have severe dysmenorrhea causing incapacitation. It is most severe in women in their late teens and early twenties and usually decreases with age.[11,24] Studies in industry and schools have shown dysmenorrhea to be the greatest single cause of absenteeism among women, and it is one of the most common health problems for which women seek treatment. Possible linkages between dysmenorrhea and factors such as fatigue, lack of exercise, anemia, and anxiety have been studied without clear conclusions.

#### Pathophysiology

Several factors contribute to the pain of primary dysmenorrhea, including high levels of uterine prostaglandins, abnormal uterine activity, uterine exposure to estrogen during the second phase of the menstrual cycle, and psychological and emotional factors.[11,24] The exact mechanism by which prostaglandins cause dysmenorrhea is not understood. What causes some women to have excess prostaglandins or increased sensitivity to them also remains in question, but women with dysmenorrhea have been found to have concentrations up to four times higher than those in women without pain.

The pain of primary dysmenorrhea typically occurs on the first or second day of the menses. It is usually described as colicky, cramping pain in the lower abdomen that may be perceived as minor, controllable with mild analgesics, or incapacitating. Backache and other systemic symptoms, particularly involving the GI tract, may also occur. The related symptoms are also thought to result from systemic prostaglandin absorption.[11]

#### Collaborative Care Management

Primary dysmenorrhea is treated with prostaglandin inhibitors, which block prostaglandin synthesis and metabolism. Nonsteroidal antiinflammatory drugs (NSAIDs) are effective for many women because these drugs inhibit prostaglandin synthesis.[24] Table 47-2 summarizes some treatment options. Oral contraceptives suppress ovulation and reduce menstrual fluid prostaglandin levels and are helpful in some cases.[11]

Treatment of secondary dysmenorrhea is aimed at correcting the underlying organic cause. Options include both pharmacological and surgical interventions.

#### *Patient/family education*

Women rarely seek professional help for mild primary dysmenorrhea. However, women who are consistently unable to engage in normal activities because of menstrual pain should be encouraged to seek medical care. The nurse instructs the patient that NSAIDs are most effective when taken at the

**table 47-2** *Common Medications for* ***Primary Dysmenorrhea***

| Drug | Action | Nursing Intervention |
|---|---|---|
| Ibuprofen (Motrin, Rufen, Advil, Nuprin, Pamprin-IB) | NSAIDs block prostaglandin synthesis, and have significant antiinflammatory, antipyretic, and analgesic effects | Teach patient to: • Take drug on an empty stomach unless GI irritation develops • Report the occurrence of any unexplained bleeding (e.g., menorrhagia, epistaxis) • Avoid concurrent use of aspirin or acetaminophen |
| Mefenamic acid (Ponstel) | Same as ibuprofen | Same as for ibuprofen, but the drug can be taken with meals or antacids to decrease gastric irritation; do not take for more than 7 days |
| Naproxen (Naprosyn/Anaprox) | Same as ibuprofen | Same as for ibuprofen |
| Ketoprofen (Actron, Orudis) | Same as ibuprofen | Same as for ibuprofen |

onset of the menses before pain becomes severe, and can be buffered with food or antacid if GI irritation occurs.

The nurse also encourages the woman to ensure adequate rest, nutrition, and exercise. Constipation should be avoided. If pain occurs, the nurse can suggest that the woman (1) use local heat, which helps dilate the blood vessels and relieve ischemia, and (2) use progressive relaxation strategies.

## AMENORRHEA

### Etiology/Epidemiology

Amenorrhea refers to the absence of menstruation. Primary amenorrhea exists if the first menses has not occurred by age 16. It usually results from a genetic, endocrine, or congenital developmental defect and is often associated with disorders of pubertal development.[2]

Secondary amenorrhea exists when a previously menstruating woman ceases to menstruate for more than 3 to 6 months (3 months in a woman with a history of regular menstrual cycles). Skipping an occasional single period is normal. Pregnancy is the most common cause of secondary amenorrhea.

Secondary amenorrhea is usually a response to environmental variables, such as excessive exercise or severe stress, or to an acquired pathology, such as altered function of the hypothalamus, pituitary gland, ovaries, thyroid, or adrenal gland.[10] Secondary amenorrhea can also be a side effect of some medications, and women who take oral contraceptives may experience amenorrhea for up to 6 months after discontinuing the pill.

### Pathophysiology

Prolonged secondary amenorrhea is common among certain groups of conditioned athletes, such as gymnasts and long-distance runners, because normal menarche is believed to require approximately 17% body fat.[2] A weight loss of 10% to 15% of total body weight can also result in amenorrhea.

The consequences of prolonged amenorrhea are not fully known, but strong evidence indicates that it is detrimental to bone density and can hasten the development of osteoporosis. A woman who does not ovulate may also develop endometrial cancer, breast disease, or dysfunctional uterine bleeding and will be infertile.

### Collaborative Care Management

The diagnostic workup for amenorrhea includes a detailed history and careful examination of the reproductive system. Pregnancy should be ruled out as a possible cause. The treatment depends on the cause. An organic problem is corrected if possible. Hormone therapy may be required.

#### *Patient/family education*

The nurse teaches the woman about the problem, its causes, and the diagnostic studies planned. Teaching may include information about weight gain, stress reduction, and reducing the energy drain of strenuous exercise. Women may need counseling and support to deal with feelings of threat to their self-concept and concerns over fertility that may be caused by the amenorrhea.

## PREMENSTRUAL SYNDROME

### Etiology/Epidemiology

*Premenstrual syndrome (PMS)* is defined as a cluster of distressing physical and behavioral symptoms that occur in the second half of the menstrual cycle and are followed by a symptom-free period. Anecdotal and research data report the prevalence of PMS to be anywhere from 10% to 30%[23] of menstruating women. About 5% experience severe symptoms. The peak prevalence for PMS occurs in the thirties, with a slight decline noted in the forties.

The etiology of PMS is unknown. Researchers theorize that it is the result of a wide variety of hormonal, psychological, and nutritional factors.[23] Research is ongoing.

### Pathophysiology

Symptoms of PMS are many and varied and may range in severity from mild to severe. The symptoms are not well defined and involve multiple body systems. The lack of a proven etiology makes it difficult to track a cause-and-effect relationship for physiological changes and observed or reported symptoms. The symptoms appear only in the luteal phase of the menstrual cycle and disappear completely with menopause. Table 47-3 presents common symptoms, possible etiologies, and associated treatment.

### Collaborative Care Management

No objective means of diagnosing PMS exists, and the diagnosis is primarily established by exclusion. A woman is considered to have PMS if her symptoms interfere with activities of daily

**research**

Reference: Taylor DL: Evaluating therapeutic change in symptom severity at the level of the individual woman experiencing severe PMS, *Image* 26(1):25, 1994.

Premenstrual syndrome is estimated to affect approximately 30% to 40% of reproductive-age women to a moderate or severe degree. The purpose of this study was to determine the effectiveness of a multimodal intervention program in relieving the symptom severity and distress of women experiencing severe PMS.

Five women with severe PMS were recruited from a specialty clinic treating PMS. They were followed over a period of about 7 months. The women were asked to complete a health diary menstrual symptom severity list daily for three complete cycles to establish the pattern and severity of their symptoms. This was followed by a 7-week intervention program including information presentation, diet change, exercise, and stress reduction strategies presented in a supportive group environment. The women then completed the assessment tool over three additional complete menstrual cycles.

A menstrual pattern of symptoms was clearly seen for four women but not the fifth. The intervention program was successful in reducing symptom severity in three of the five women and symptom distress in the others. The researcher emphasizes the importance of long-term research with this population and the uniqueness of both symptom patterns and individual responses.

**table 47-3** *Premenstrual Syndrome—Symptoms, Possible Etiology, and Treatment*

| Symptoms | Possible Etiology | Traditional Therapy | Nontraditional Therapy for PMS |
|---|---|---|---|
| Anxiety:<br>Nervous tension<br>Mood swings<br>Irritability | High serum estrogen<br>Low serum progesterone<br>Elevated adrenal androgens<br>Possible disturbance of thyroid axis | Progesterone; vitamin $B_6$; limit dairy products intake; increase outdoor exercise; lorazepam | Validation<br>Education<br>Exercise<br>Family therapy<br>Peer support groups<br>Stress management<br>Assertiveness training<br>Sex and marital therapy |
| Water-related symptoms:<br>Weight gain<br>Swelling of extremities<br>Breast tenderness<br>Abdominal bloating | High serum aldosterone<br>Retention of sodium and water<br>Decreased colloid osmotic pressure in abdomen | Restrict intake of salt, coffee, tea, cola, chocolate; $B_6$; primrose oil; spironolactone; antiprostaglandins; oral contraceptives | |
| Cravings:<br>Craving for sweets<br>Increased appetite | Increased carbohydrate tolerance<br>Low red cell magnesium levels | Restrict free sugar, sodium, animal fat intake; substitute complex carbohydrate for simple sugars | |
| Headache<br>Heart pounding<br>Fatigue<br>Dizziness or faintness | | | |
| Depression:<br>Forgetfulness<br>Crying<br>Confusion<br>Insomnia | High serum estrogen<br>Low serum progesterone<br>Elevated adrenal androgens<br>Possible disturbance of thyroid axis | Increase intake of foods high in B vitamins and magnesium (green leafy vegetables, legumes, whole-grain cereals) | |

Modified from DeCherney A, Pernoll ML: *Current obstetric and gynecologic diagnosis and treatment,* ed 8, East Norwalk, Conn, 1994, Appleton & Lange; Nikolai TF et al: *J Clin Endocrinol Metab* 70:1108, 1990; and Ryan KJ, Berkowitz R, Barbieri RL: *Kistner's gynecology: principles and practices,* ed 6, Chicago, 1995, Year Book.

living. Symptoms that occur in three consecutive menstrual cycles confirm the diagnosis. A careful clinical history is critical, and the woman is asked to keep accurate records of dates for (1) her menstrual period and (2) occurrence of symptoms and their exact nature and severity (see the Research Box on the previous page).

Table 47-3 outlines suggested therapies for typically occurring groups of symptoms. Numerous treatments have been suggested, including both pharmacological and nonpharmacological strategies, but no treatment has proven to be effective in all cases. The use of oral contraceptives produces symptoms similar to PMS in some women but also relieves symptoms in some women diagnosed with the disorder. Treatments attempt to reduce the number and severity of symptoms and restore the woman's psychological health.

### Patient/family education

The nurse helps the woman and her family understand the possible causes of the syndrome and the rationale for any planned treatments. Simple lifestyle modifications can reduce symptoms and improve the woman's overall well-being. Regular aerobic exercise is strongly recommended, because exercise results in a release of endorphins, which can elevate the mood. The nurse encourages the woman to avoid fatigue, because it exaggerates the symptoms of PMS. This is particularly important in the premenstrual period. Stress management techniques are also strongly recommended. The Patient/Family Teaching Box summarizes patient teaching related to PMS. The nurse can refer interested patients and families to the National Center for PMS and Menstrual Disorders, 15 Smith Road, Bedford, NH 03102; or the National PMS Society, P.O. Box 11467, Durham, NC 27703.

**patient/family teaching**

**The Woman with Premenstrual Syndrome**

1. Teach possible causes of condition and treatments.
2. Teach relaxation techniques.
3. Teach patient to do the following:
   - Avoid stressful activities during the premenstrual period.
   - Ensure adequate rest, especially during premenstrual period. Fatigue exaggerates symptoms.
   - Take medications as prescribed and explain rationale.
   - Reduce or eliminate smoking and alcohol consumption.
   - Reduce or eliminate consumption of caffeine.
   - Follow a regular exercise program.
   - Eat a well-balanced diet with adequate protein and a reduced intake of salt and refined sugars.
   - Incorporate stress-reducing strategies into daily lifestyle.

## DYSFUNCTIONAL UTERINE BLEEDING

### Etiology/Epidemiology

*Dysfunctional uterine bleeding (DUB)* is defined as excessive or irregular uterine bleeding with no demonstrable cause. It can

**table 47-4** *Causes of Dysfunctional Uterine Bleeding During Childbearing and Postmenopausal Years*

| TYPE | CAUSES |
|---|---|
| **Menorrhagia**—Prolonged profuse menstrual flow during the regular period | Submucous myomas, pregnancy complications, adenomyosis, endometrial hyperplasias, malignant tumors, hypothyroidism |
| **Metrorrhagia**—Bleeding between periods | Endometrial polyps, endometrial and cervical cancer, exogenous estrogen administration |
| **Polymenorrhea**—Increased frequency of menstruation | Anovulation; shortened luteal phase |
| **Cryptomenorrhea**—Unusually light menstrual flow | Hymenal or cervical stenosis, Asherman's syndrome (uterine synechiae), oral contraceptives |
| **Menometrorrhagia**—Bleeding at irregular intervals | Any condition causing intermenstrual bleeding; sudden onset is indication of malignant tumors or complications of pregnancy |
| **Oligomenorrhea**—Menstrual periods more than 35 days apart | Anovulation from endocrine causes (pregnancy, menopause) or systemic (excessive weight loss); estrogen-secreting tumors |
| **Dysfunctional uterine bleeding**—Abnormal bleeding without known organic cause | Unknown |

take many forms, including excessive flow, prolonged duration of menses, and intermenstrual bleeding.

Dysfunctional bleeding may be caused by a variety of factors. Table 47-4 lists and defines various types of DUB with associated etiologies. Endocrine abnormalities are the most common, although the likely causes differ in women of childbearing age and postmenopausal women.[14] Some systemic diseases can cause DUB. Liver disease may interfere with estrogen metabolism, and blood dyscrasias can produce spontaneous bleeding. DUB related to the menstrual cycle is usually anovulatory and painless and generally occurs at the extremes of menstrual life, when disturbances of ovarian function are common. In perimenopausal and postmenopausal women, DUB is commonly associated with uterine cancer.

### Pathophysiology

Dysfunctional uterine bleeding may occur between or during the menstrual periods. When menorrhagia is present, the woman may soak a tampon or pad every 1 to 2 hours for a week or more. The exact cause of the anovulatory episode is not understood, but it may represent a dysfunction of the hypothalamic-pituitary-ovarian axis that results in continuing estrogen stimulation of the endometrium. The endometrium outgrows its blood supply, partially breaks down, and is sloughed in an irregular manner. Anovulation may also result from thyroid or adrenal abnormalities.[14]

### Collaborative Care Management

The diagnostic workup for DUB begins with a thorough history of the frequency, amount, and duration of bleeding. Laboratory tests may include blood counts to estimate blood loss, pregnancy tests, thyroid studies, ovulation tests, and coagulation studies. Papanicolaou (Pap) smears, pelvic examinations, ultrasonography, endometrial biopsy, and sonohysterography may be employed to assess for structural problems and cancer (see Chapter 46).

The cause of the bleeding guides medical care. In the absence of an organic cause, the preferred treatment is usually conservative. Pharmacological options to stop heavy bleeding or reduce future blood loss in subsequent menstrual cycles include the use of estrogens, progestins, NSAIDs, antifibrinolytic agents, and gonadotropin-releasing hormone agonists such as danazol. Hysterectomy may be necessary for those women whose bleeding cannot be controlled with hormones, who are symptomatically anemic, and whose lifestyle is compromised by persistent bleeding.[14]

#### *Patient/family education*

Because most care for DUB is provided in the outpatient setting, the nursing role is largely educational. The impact of chronic excessive bleeding on a woman's lifestyle can be profound. The nurse teaches the woman to accurately assess the amount of bleeding in terms of number of pads or tampons, type of pad or tampon, and degree of saturation. The nurse helps the woman set up and maintain an accurate record of the bleeding in the form of a diary. The nurse also encourages the woman to express her concerns and fears. Anxiety related to infertility or fear of cancer can be intense but remain unexpressed.

## ENDOMETRIOSIS

### Etiology/Epidemiology

Endometriosis is a condition in which endometrial cells that normally line the uterus are seeded throughout the pelvis. Endometriosis typically affects women during their childbearing years. Although the age-specific prevalence is unknown, it is estimated that the incidence is 7% in the general female population.[24] The incidence in infertile women is 30% to 50%.[24]

The etiology of endometriosis remains unknown, but there are multiple theories and lines of research. The condition may be hereditary, because it occurs more often in women whose mothers had the disorder. Theories include the congenital presence of endometrial cells out of their normal location, the transfer of endometrial cells by means of the blood or lymph system, and reflux of menstrual fluid containing endometrial cells up the fallopian tubes and into the pelvic cavity. A more recent theory suggests a possible immune mechanism in the etiology of endometriosis.[20]

### Pathophysiology

With each menstrual period, the seeded endometrial cells are stimulated by ovarian hormones and bleed into the surrounding tissues, causing an inflammatory response. Encased blood may lead to palpable masses known as chocolate cysts. Occasionally the cysts rupture and spread endometrial cells deeper into the pelvis. Repeated inflammation and healing may create adhesions severe enough to fuse pelvic organs or cause bowel or bladder strictures.

The ovaries are the most common site of involvement, and the process is usually bilateral (Figure 47-2). The pelvic peritoneum; the anterior and posterior cul-de-sac; and the uterosacral, round, and broad ligaments are other common sites.

Endometriosis progresses gradually and usually does not produce symptoms until the woman is 30 to 40 years of age. The classic feature is menstrual pain and discomfort that becomes progressively worse. Other possible symptoms include abdominal pain, dyspareunia, irregular menses, bowel problems, and urinary dysfunction. Pelvic examination often reveals a fixed, retroverted uterus that is enlarged, tender, and nodular. Occasionally, the disease is far advanced but causes no symptoms, and it may first be diagnosed as part of a workup for infertility.

### Collaborative Care Management

Laparoscopy is the only definitive method of diagnosing endometriosis. The endoscopy is used to carefully map and describe the extent of disease involvement, and biopsies of suspicious tissue can be obtained during the procedure. Ultrasound may be helpful in differentiating solid from cystic lesions, but is of little value otherwise. Magnetic resonance imaging (MRI) is also of little value in either detecting or staging the disease. A newer approach involves the use of cancer antigen 125 (CA-125) as a chemical marker, because the levels of this antigen are elevated in most patients with endometriosis and continue to rise as the disease progresses.[20] The marker is not specific to endometriosis, however, and can be used only to follow the course of the disease.

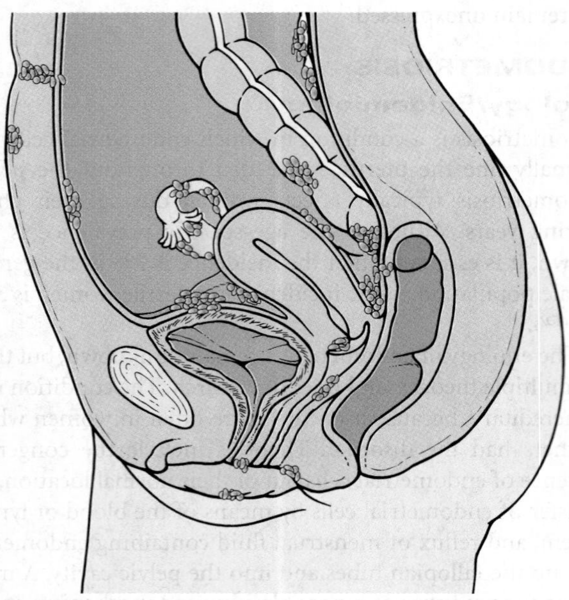

fig. 47-2 Common sites of endometriosis.

Because the cause of endometriosis is not understood, treatment is highly individualized. In rare cases, endometriosis disappears spontaneously. Pregnancy appears to slow the progression of the condition because menstruation is halted during pregnancy and lactation. Some women remain asymptomatic after pregnancy. A couple may be encouraged to attempt pregnancy if children are desired, because the fertility rate is low and continues to deteriorate with time. Mild cases may be managed with mild analgesics and regular monitoring.

Oral contraceptives with minimal estrogen and high levels of progestins may be used to produce endometrial atropy. Disadvantages to this approach include irregular bleeding and symptoms such as nausea, fatigue, and depression. Drugs with antigonadotropic action such as danazol may be used to suppress ovarian activity. Danazol stops endometrial proliferation, prevents ovulation, and produces atrophy of the ectopic endometrial tissue.

The major drawbacks to the treatment are its high cost and the occurrence of common side effects such as hot flashes, depression, and weight gain. Gonadotropin-releasing hormone (GnRH) analogs (leuprolide [Lupron Depot]) are an even more expensive approach to treatment. These drugs induce a hypoestrogenic state and result in amenorrhea. Side effects mimic the symptoms of menopause. A steady osteoporotic loss in bone density limits the duration of possible treatment.

Surgical intervention may be necessary if the disorder does not respond to drug therapy. Conservative approaches that attempt to preserve the woman's fertility include lysis of adhesions and destruction of pockets of implanted endometrial tissues by means of laparoscopic laser surgery. More radical surgery involves the removal of the uterus, tubes, and possibly the ovaries. Ovarian function is preserved if at all possible. The onset of menopause halts the disorder.

#### *Patient/family education*

Because most care for women with endometriosis is delivered in the community, the nurse's role is largely educational and supportive. The nurse reassures the woman that endometriosis can be treated. The nurse teaches about the prescribed drugs and the management of side effects. Strategies to manage chronic pain are particularly important. The importance of ongoing care and follow-up is reinforced. Referral to support groups may be beneficial. This is particularly important if infertility related to the endometriosis is diagnosed. Two excellent organizations are The Endometriosis Association, 8585 North 76th Place, Milwaukee, WI 53223; and Resolve Incorporated, 5 Water St., Arlington, MA 02174.

# STRUCTURAL PROBLEMS

## UTERINE DISPLACEMENT/PROLAPSE

### Etiology/Epidemiology

The uterus may undergo minor displacement in ways that are considered to be normal variations with little or no clinical effects (Figure 47-3). Retroversion is the most common variation and occurs in about 20% of women. Uterine prolapse represents a severe uterine problem in which the uterus protrudes through the pelvic floor aperture or genital hiatus. It is usually associated with a cystocele or rectocele. Uterine prolapse occurs most often in multiparous Caucasian women as a response to injuries to the muscles and fascia of the pelvis incurred during childbirth. Systemic conditions such as obesity and chronic pulmonary disease, and local conditions, such as ascites and uterine or ovarian tumors, are other potential causes. Chronic coughing, constipation, genetic predisposition, and estrogen deprivation after menopause can also contribute to prolapse.[39] Prolapse usually develops gradually, suggesting that the effects of aging play a major role. As the uterus begins to drop, the vaginal walls become relaxed and the bladder may herniate into the vagina (cystocele), or the rectal wall may herniate into the vagina (rectocele). These structural problems are illustrated in Figure 47-3. Both conditions may occur simultaneously. Cystoceles are common, and the woman may remain completely asymptomatic until after menopause. Estrogen helps maintain adequate blood flow and tone of the paravaginal tissues, and its loss results in atrophic changes that render the tissues more subject to prolapse.

### Pathophysiology

Variations in the normal position of the uterus or prolapse can result from congenital or acquired abnormalities of the pelvic support structures. Acquired weaknesses occur after childbirth, surgery, and closely spaced pregnancies and in response to obesity and the loss of tissue elasticity with aging. The severity of the prolapse is designated by degree. In a first-degree prolapse, the cervix is still within the vagina. In a second-degree prolapse, the cervix protrudes from the vaginal orifice. In a third-degree prolapse, the entire uterus, suspended by its stretched ligaments, hangs below the vaginal orifice. Before menopause the uterus hypertrophies and is engorged and flabby. The vaginal mucosa thickens, and stasis ulcers may develop. Anterior and posterior vaginal wall relaxation often accompany prolapse, allowing for the development of cystocele or rectocele. Older women may have these conditions for years before seeking medical attention.

Patients with first-degree prolapse experience few symptoms but may report sensations of heaviness or fullness and a feeling that something is falling out of the vagina. In more severe prolapse, when the cervix protrudes at the introitus, the patient may complain of feeling like she is sitting on a ball. With severe prolapse, the woman is clearly aware of the mass. Vaginal bleeding, discharge, and infection may be present.[12] Leukorrhea or menometrorrhagia may develop in premenopausal women with prolapse as a result of uterine engorgement. After menopause, discharge and bleeding with prolapse usually result from infection and ulceration.

The woman with a cystocele may complain of urinary incontinence accompanying any activity that increases intraabdominal pressure, such as coughing, laughing, or lifting. The patient with a rectocele may complain of chronic constipation and develop hemorrhoids.

### Collaborative Care Management

Uterine prolapse can be readily identified on pelvic examination. If a cystocele is present, the vaginal outlet is relaxed with a thin-walled, smooth, bulging mass present in the anterior vaginal wall below the cervix. The mass descends when the patient is asked to bear down. If a rectocele is present, palpation of the vaginal area reveals a thin-walled rectovaginal septum projecting into the vagina. Many women are found to have both a cystocele and a rectocele.

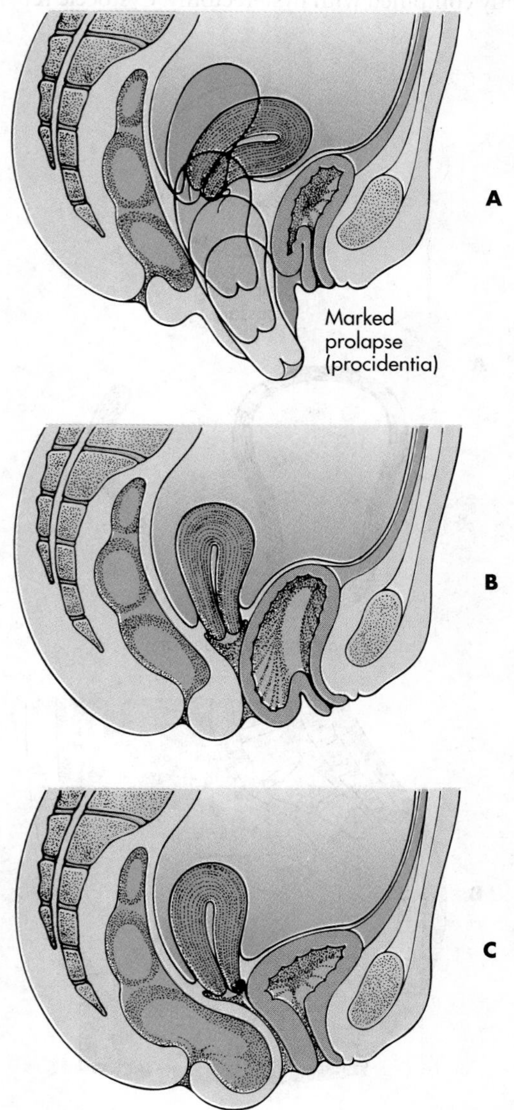


fig. 47-3 A, Uterine prolapse. B, Cystocele, C, Rectocele.

Postmenopausal women with first-degree prolapses are treated with estrogen therapy to maintain the tone and integrity of the pelvic floor muscles. Exercise therapy is suggested for all women. (Exercises for the pelvic floor are discussed under patient/family education. If pain or bleeding occurs, the uterus may be manually repositioned and supported by the insertion of a vaginal pessary (Figure 47-4). Pessaries are devices made of hard rubber or plastic that maintain the uterus in a forward position by exerting pressure on the ligaments attached to the posterior wall of the cervix.

Conservative treatment with estrogen, exercise, and a pessary may also be employed for a cystocele or rectocele if the woman experiences only mild symptoms. Surgery to repair cystoceles, rectoceles, and more advanced prolapses is undertaken when symptoms significantly interfere with the patient's lifestyle. The procedures designed to tighten the vaginal wall are termed *anterior* and *posterior colporrhaphy.* They are frequently combined with hysterectomy. Cystocele repair may be done abdominally and combined with a urethrovesical suspension procedure called a Marshall-Marchetti-Krantz procedure to correct stress incontinence.

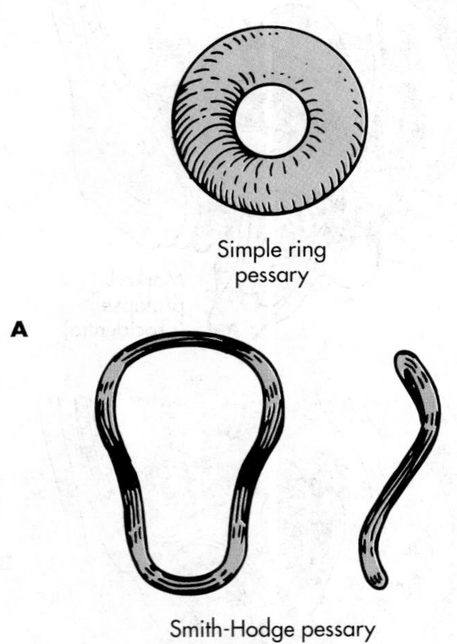


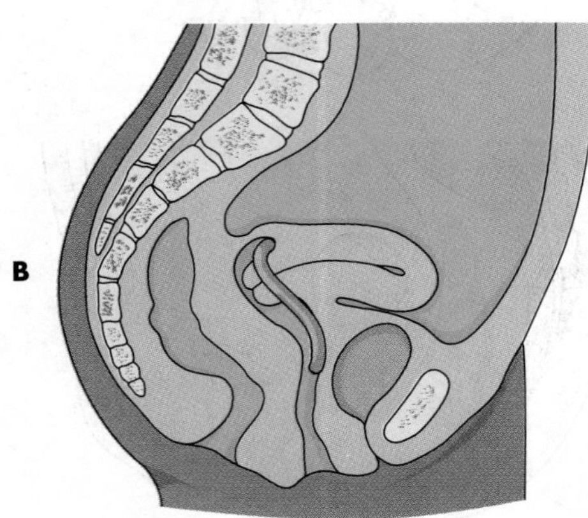


**fig. 47-4 A,** Examples of pessaries (simple ring, Smith-Hodge). **B,** Pessary in place to hold posterior vaginal fornix and, with it, attached cervix wall backward and upward in pelvis.

### *Patient/family education*

Exercise teaching is an important nursing intervention for any patient with a uterine displacement or prolapse. Kegel perineal exercises are the mainstay. The woman is instructed to tighten the muscles of the perineum as if to stop the flow of urine, maintain the tension for 5 seconds at a time, and repeat the exercise in sets of 10. The exercise is repeated 10 to 12 times daily. Knee-chest exercises are used less often but may be ordered to stretch or strengthen the pelvic ligaments. Corrective exercises for poor posture may also be prescribed.

The nurse encourages obese patients to lose weight to reduce intraabdominal pressure. Chronic cough and chronic

## guidelines for care

### The Woman Undergoing Vaginal Surgery

1. Provide perineal care after each voiding or defecation:
   a. Pour sterile normal saline over vulva and perineum.
   b. Cleanse perineum as needed with sterile cotton balls; cleanse away from vagina toward rectum.
   c. Dry perineum as needed with sterile cotton balls.
2. Encourage sitz baths after sutures are removed.
3. If douches are ordered during immediate postoperative period:
   a. Use sterile equipment and sterile solution.
   b. Insert douche nozzle very gently and rotate carefully.
4. Avoid pressure on suture line:
   a. Prevent a full bladder; keep urinary catheter patent.
   b. Use measures to prevent constipation.
   c. Teach patient to avoid the Valsalva's maneuver.
   d. Keep patient flat or in low Fowler's position in bed.
5. Provide an ice pack for perineal discomfort (covered, sealed plastic bags or gloves make an acceptable pack).
6. Encourage leg exercises.
7. Encourage deep breathing.
8. Monitor intake and output.
9. Note characteristics of urine and stool.

## patient/family teaching

### Discharge Preparation After Vaginal Surgery

1. Perform daily douches and tub baths as prescribed.
2. Avoid straining at stool.
3. Use stool softeners and laxatives as prescribed.
4. Avoid lifting for 6 weeks.
5. Avoid sexual intercourse until physician gives permission (usually about 6 weeks).
6. Avoid jarring activities.
7. Avoid prolonged standing, walking, or sitting. Continue leg exercises for 6 weeks.
8. Vaginal sensation may be lost for several months postoperatively, but sensation will return.
9. Eat a high-fiber diet and drink 3000 ml of fluids daily.

constipation are also corrected, because these conditions contribute to weakness of the muscular wall.

Women fitted with a pessary need to be taught how to insert it and withdraw it if the device becomes displaced or uncomfortable. Pessaries are removed and cleaned once every few weeks or months as recommended by the physician. If the pessary is neglected, it can cause infection or fistula. Women who undergo anterior colporrhaphy are instructed to refrain from heavy lifting, straining, and strenuous exercise for 3 months. Sexual intercourse may be resumed after about 3 weeks. Guidelines for care following vaginal surgery and patient/family teaching in preparation for discharge are presented in the boxes on p. 1544.

## FISTULAS

### Etiology/Epidemiology

A fistula is an abnormal tunnel-like opening between hollow internal organs or between an organ and the exterior of the body. Fistulas can develop from a variety of causes but are usually the result of surgery, childbirth, trauma, or radiation therapy.

The name of the fistula indicates the connecting structures. Fistulas can develop between the vagina and the rectum (rectovaginal), bladder (vesicovaginal), or urethra (urethrovaginal). They are illustrated in Figure 47-5. Vesicovaginal fistulas are the most common, followed by rectovaginal.

### Pathophysiology

Conditions that cause fistulas to form typically compromise the blood supply and cause tissue damage. Tissue sloughs, and a channel gradually develops between the affected tissue and the vagina.[18] The result is a constant leak of urine or escape of flatus and fecal material through the vagina. This is highly distressing to the patient and creates an offensive odor. The drainage excoriates and irritates the vaginal and vulvar tissue.

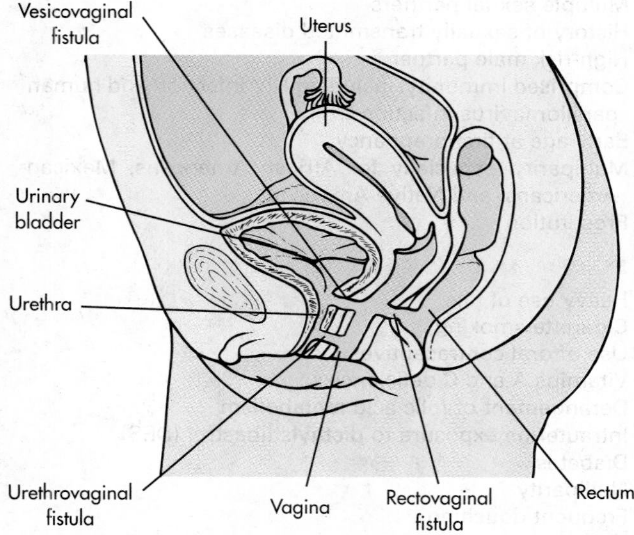


**fig. 47-5** Common fistulas involving the vagina.

### Collaborative Care Management

Fistulas are diagnosed primarily through pelvic examination. A fistulogram, which involves the injection of dye into the vagina, may be used to assess the exact location and severity of the fistula. Small fistulas may heal spontaneously if the tissue is allowed to rest. Surgery is otherwise necessary to close the fistula tract. Tissue inflammation and edema must be treated first, and this can take months. Either anterior or posterior colporrhaphy may be used. It may be necessary to temporarily divert the urinary or fecal stream in complex situations. A Foley, ureteral, or nephrostomy catheter is used to keep the area well drained and is left in place for weeks in some patients. With urinary diversion, many urinary fistulas are able to heal spontaneously.[22] Bowel rest contributes to healing of rectovaginal fistulas, and the patient may be placed on total parenteral nutrition (TPN).[22] A diverting colostomy may also be performed if surgical intervention is necessary.

Postoperative care focuses on tissue healing. A small amount of serosanguineous drainage is expected, but the patient is carefully monitored for evidence of continued fecal or urinary drainage. Douches may be ordered, and the nurse administers them gently and at low pressure to protect healing tissue. Bedrest is often enforced for several days.

#### *Patient/family education*

If the fistula is being conservatively managed, nursing intervention focuses on comfort and the prevention of infection. The nurse teaches the woman that a chlorine solution makes an effective deodorizing douche, and this solution is also excellent for perineal irrigation. A solution of 5 ml of household bleach to 1 L of water is appropriate. Douching should be performed at low pressure to prevent forcing the solution through the fistula tract. Sitz baths and careful cleansing with mild soap and water are also helpful. Although protective pads may be worn, the nurse stresses that cleansing must be repeated at regular intervals to prevent skin breakdown and odor.

Surgical repair is not always successful, and repeat procedures may be needed. The risk of infection is constantly present, and the nurse anticipates that the patient may become anxious and depressed about her situation. The nurse encourages the patient to verbalize her concerns and seek support from family and friends.

# BENIGN AND MALIGNANT NEOPLASMS OF THE FEMALE REPRODUCTIVE TRACT

## NEOPLASMS OF THE CERVIX

### Cervical Polyps

#### *Etiology/epidemiology*

Cervical polyps are relatively common and account for about 4% of gynecological conditions. The two main types are (1) endocervical from the canal in the opening of the cervix and (2) ectocervical from the lower portion that protrudes into the vagina. Endocervical polyps tend to occur in middle-aged multiparous women. Ectocervical polyps are found most often in postmenopausal women.

Although most cervical polyps are benign, some cervical cancers manifest as a polypoid mass. Fewer than 1% will become malignant.[19] Polyps are thought to arise from hyperplasia, possibly in response to chronic inflammation, abnormal responses to hormonal stimulation, or localized vascular congestion. Hyperestrinism is thought to play a major role.

#### Pathophysiology

Most polyps are asymptomatic and discovered on routine pelvic examination. Endocervical polyps are usually reddish purple to cherry red, smooth, soft growths that may vary in size from a few millimeters to 2 or 3 cm in diameter and length. They are usually attached to the mucosa by a narrow pedicle and may be single or multiple in number. Ectocervical polyps are pale or flesh colored, round or elongated, and often attach with a broad pedicle. Most polypoid structures are vascular, and both types of polyps may become infected and necrotic at the tip.[19] Their classic symptom is intermenstrual bleeding, particularly after intercourse or douching. Leukorrhea may be present. The chronic irritation and bleeding can lead to cervicitis, endometritis, or even salpingitis.

#### Collaborative care management

Cervical polyps are usually diagnosed by direct inspection and can be removed safely in a physician's office. The procedure causes minimal bleeding, but if bleeding should occur, it can be controlled by electrical or chemical cautery. All the excised tissue is sent for pathological examination. Antibiotics may be given prophylactically, particularly if there is any evidence of tissue necrosis or cervicitis. Simple removal of polyps is usually curative.[19]

**Patient/family education.** The nurse encourages the woman to rest and avoid strenuous activity after polyp removal. A perineal pad can be provided to absorb drainage. The nurse instructs the woman to report any significant bleeding or signs of infection. The nurse instructs her to avoid tampon use, douches, and sexual intercourse for about a week while healing takes place.

### Cancer of the Cervix

#### Etiology

Although the cause of carcinoma of the cervix remains unknown, a close association exists between early and frequent sexual contact with multiple partners and cervical viral infection, particularly the human papillomavirus (HPV). The HPV has been isolated in the vast majority of precancerous and cancerous changes of the cervix. It is spread predominantly through sexual contact.[6,35]

Studies have found a high incidence of cancer of the cervix in prostitutes. There is also an increased incidence in multiparous women, particularly African Americans, Mexican Americans, and Native Americans. Socioeconomic factors include poverty, early marriage, and early childbearing. Smoking, particularly long-term, high-intensity use, is now also considered a potential risk factor. Although high levels of tobacco mutagens are found in the cervical mucus of women who smoke, these mutagens have not been proven to cause cancer. It appears that the more a woman smokes, the greater is her risk of acquiring an HPV infection, which may explain the smoking risk factor. The two variables may also work as cofactors in the development of the disease.[35]

Immunosuppression also increases the risk of cervical cancer, and studies indicate that women positive for HIV are at high risk for cervical cancer and have a poorer disease prognosis. Sexually transmitted diseases are also linked with atypical cell transformation. Dietary factors include deficiencies of vitamins A and C and derangement in folic acid metabolism. The Risk Factors Box lists known and potential risk factors associated with the development of cervical cancer.

#### Epidemiology

Cervical cancer is the seventh most common type of cancer in women following breast, colorectal, lung, endometrial, and ovarian cancers and lymphoma. Pap smear screening has significantly reduced the mortality rate associated with cervical cancer in the United States, but 4600 women still die annually of cervical cancer in the United States and another 15,000 women are diagnosed with invasive forms of the disease each year. Cancer of the cervix is the leading cause of cancer deaths among women in underdeveloped countries with inadequate cervical cancer screening programs.

There has been a general decline in the incidence of cervical cancer in the United States, although the overall incidence of Pap smear abnormalities has risen rapidly over the past 2 decades. Cervical carcinoma in situ, a precancerous noninvasive stage, is now the most common form diagnosed and peaks in incidence between the ages of 25 and 35. Preinvasive

**risk factors**

**Cervical Cancer**

RISK FACTORS

Low socioeconomic status
Early age at first coitus
Multiple sexual partners
History of sexually transmitted diseases
High-risk male partner
Comprised immunity, including HIV infection and human papillomavirus infection
Early age at first pregnancy
Multiparity, especially for African Americans, Mexican Americans, and Native Americans
Prostitution

POTENTIAL RISK FACTORS

Heavy use of talc
Cigarette smoking
Use of oral contraceptives
Vitamins A and C deficiencies
Derangement of folic acid metabolism
Intrauterine exposure to diethylstilbestrol (DES)
Diabetes
Nulliparity
Frequent douching

lesions seem to occur in some populations at a very early age, perhaps related to the sexual practices of teenagers. The incidence of invasive cervical cancer increases with age. Cost-effective mass screening is of critical importance because over 95% of cervical cancers are curable in their early stages.[15,25] In a typical Pap screening program up to 5% of all smears exhibit some degree of abnormality.[15,35] The Patient/Family Teaching Box summarizes recommendations for preventing cervical cancer.

### Pathophysiology

Ninety-five percent of all cervical cancers are squamous cell, arising from the epidermal layer of the cervix. Cell dysplasia indicates the presence of a precursor lesion, typically called *cervical intraepithelial neoplasia (CIN)*, which has been divided into the following three stages:

CIN I: mild to moderate dysplasia
CIN II: moderate to severe dysplasia
CIN III: severe dysplasia to carcinoma in situ

Women diagnosed with dysplasia may experience disease regression, persistence, or a progression to carcinoma. There are usually no signs or symptoms of dysplasia, and the diagnosis is based on cytologic findings. Early detection is important to ensure positive outcomes. Routine Pap screening begins once a woman engages in regular intercourse or turns 18 years old. The frequency of Pap smear screening is still being debated. The American College of Obstetrics and Gynecology in conjunction with the American Cancer Society recommend that every woman be screened annually until three consecutive negative smears are obtained.[35] The screening interval can then be lengthened at the provider's discretion. All abnormal smears should be followed up with colposcopy and biopsy to further investigate cellular change.[15]

Cervical cancer spreads through the blood, by direct extension, and lymph invasion. As the lymph nodes grow larger, venous flow is obstructed, and leg edema, ureteral obstruction, or hydronephrosis may occur. Hematogenous spread can occur to the lungs, mediastinum, liver, and bone.[15] Prognosis is based on the stage of the disease, depth of invasion, and vascular involvement of the tumor.

Cervical cancer is asymptomatic in the early stages. As the disease progresses, the woman may experience a slight watery vaginal discharge and occasional bloody spotting, especially after intercourse. With advanced disease, a foul-smelling discharge may develop from sloughing of the epithelial tissue. Pain is usually a late sign and can involve the pelvis, flank, lower back, and abdomen. The growing tumor may place pressure on the rectum and bladder, causing irritation and discharge. Hemorrhage is possible with advanced infiltrative tumors, which may also erode the walls of adjacent organs and create fistulas. Box 47-2 presents the clinical manifestations of cervical cancer.

### Collaborative care management

**Diagnostic tests.** The diagnosis of cervical cancer can be confirmed only by biopsy. The Pap smear is a screening test but not a diagnostic tool. The two most common methods for obtaining a cervical biopsy are by conization or punch biopsy. Punch biopsies can easily be performed in the physician's office. Conization is performed diagnostically whenever a question exists about the presence of invasive disease.[35] Colposcopy allows for microscopic examination of the cervix and improves the accuracy of the biopsy process.[3] The widespread use of colposcopy has reduced the need for cone biopsies in the United States. Cervical conization, however, can also be used therapeutically to remove the entire lesion and remains a valuable tool for preserving a woman's fertility. Cone biopsy is illustrated in Figure 47-6.

Computed tomography (CT) scans, intravenous pyelography (IVP), cystoscopy, proctosigmoidoscopy, and barium studies of the lower GI tract are all possible diagnostic adjuncts. During the staging workup, the nurse ensures that the woman has all the information necessary to understand the tests and their rationale. Anxiety is typically high until the extent and invasiveness of the cancer can be determined.

**Medications.** Chemotherapy has not played a significant role in the management of cervical cancer. Squamous cell

#### patient/family teaching

**Prevention of Cervical Cancer**

Reinforce the importance of condom use during sex to limit transmission of STDs and genital viruses
Encourage adolescent girls to delay the onset of sexual activity and limit the number of their sex partners
Teach the importance of prompt and effective treatment of vaginal or cervical infections
Stress the importance of following American Cancer Society Guidelines for Pap screening:
- Annually for sexually active women 18 and older
- At intervals recommended by health care provider once a pattern of three annual negative tests is established
- Annually throughout life for women who are considered to be at high risk

#### box 47-2 clinical manifestations

***Cervical Cancer***

**EARLY SYMPTOMS**

Thin, watery vaginal discharge
Bloody spotting after coitus or douching
Metrorrhagia
Postmenopausal bleeding
Polymenorrhea

**LATE SYMPTOMS**

Dark, foul-smelling vaginal discharge
Pelvic, abdominal, or back pain
Flank pain
Weight loss
Anorexia
Anemia
Leg edema
Dysuria
Rectal bleeding

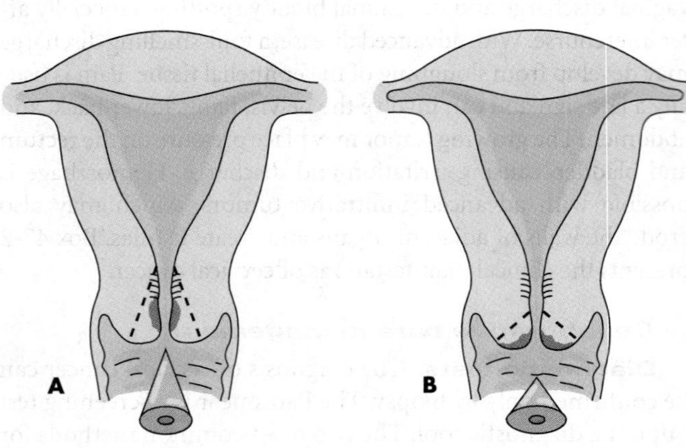


**fig. 47-6 A,** Cone biopsy for endocervical disease. Limits of lesion were not seen colposcopically. **B,** Cone biopsy for cervical intraepithethial neoplasia (CIN) of exocervix. Limits of lesion were identified colposcopically.

**table 47-6** *Summary of Treatment Options for Cervical Cancer*

| Clinical Stage | Treatment Options | 5-Year Survival (%) |
|---|---|---|
| Stage 0 (CIN) | Cryosurgery, conization, laser surgery, hysterectomy | 95-100 |
| Stage Ia | Simple hysterectomy or radiation (cesium implant) | 95-100 |
| Stage Ib | Radical hysterectomy with nodes or radiotherapy (external and implant) | 75-85 |
| Stage IIa | Radical hysterectomy with nodes or radiotherapy | 65-80 |
| Stage IIb | Radiation | 50-65 |
| Stage III | Radiation | 30-40 |
| Stage IV | Radiation, exenteration, chemotherapy | 5-15 |

**table 47-5** *Clinical Stages in Carcinoma of the Cervix Uteri (FIGO System)*

| Stage | Involvement |
|---|---|
| Stage 0 | Carcinoma in situ (CIN), intraepithelial carcinoma. |
| Stage I | Carcinoma is strictly confined to the cervix (extension to the corpus should be disregarded). |
| Stage Ia | Preclinical carcinomas of the cervix; that is, those diagnosed only by microscopy. |
| Stage Ia1 | Minimal microscopically evident stromal invasion. |
| Stage Ia2 | Lesions detected microscopically that can be measured. The upper limit of the measurement should not show a depth of invasion of more than 5 mm taken from the base of the epithelium, either surface or glandular, from which it originates, and a second dimension, the horizontal spread, must not exceed 7 mm. Larger lesions should be staged as Ib. |
| Stage Ib | Lesions of greater dimensions than stage Ia2, whether seen clinically or not. Preformed space involvement should not alter the staging but should be specifically recorded so as to determine whether it should affect treatment decisions in the future. |
| Stage II | Involvement of the vagina but not the lower third, or infiltration of the parametria but not out to the sidewall |
| Stage IIa | Involvement of the vagina but no evidence of parametrial involvement. |
| Stage IIb | Infiltration of the parametria but not out to the sidewall. |
| Stage III | Involvement of the lower third of the vagina or extension to the pelvic sidewall. All cases with a hydronephrosis or nonfunctioning kidney should be included, unless they are known to be attributable to other cause. |
| Stage IIIa | Involvement of the lower third of the vagina but not out to the pelvic sidewall if the parametria are involved. |
| Stage IIIb | Extension onto the pelvic sidewall or hydronephrosis or nonfunctional kidney. |
| Stage IV | Extension outside the reproductive tract. |
| Stage IVa | Involvement of the mucosa of the bladder or rectum. |
| Stage IVb | Distant metastasis or disease outside the true pelvis. |

From DiSaia PJ, Creasman WT: *Clinical gynecologic oncology,* ed 4, St Louis, 1993, Mosby.

cancers tend to be relatively unresponsive to drug treatment. Recurrent cancers tend to reappear in areas previously irradiated where the tissue is fibrotic and relatively avascular, making it difficult to obtain high tissue concentrations of the drugs. However, research protocols have been developed that administer chemotherapy *before* other treatments when advanced disease is present.[35] Chemotherapy treatment appears to drastically reduce the size of the tumor. Chemotherapeutic agents are usually administered in combinations. (Nursing care related to chemotherapy is discussed in Chapter 11.)

**Treatments.** Cervical cancer is treated according to the stage of the disease (Table 47-5). Figure 47-7 illustrates the extent of anatomical involvement represented by each stage. Carcinoma in situ may be treated by excisional conization, cryosurgery or laser surgery, particularly if the woman wants to have more children. Hysterectomy may be chosen if fertility is not an issue. More invasive cancer is treated with increasingly extensive surgical procedures or radiotherapy. Table 47-6 summarizes the major treatment options for various stages of cervical cancer and their associated long-term survival projections.

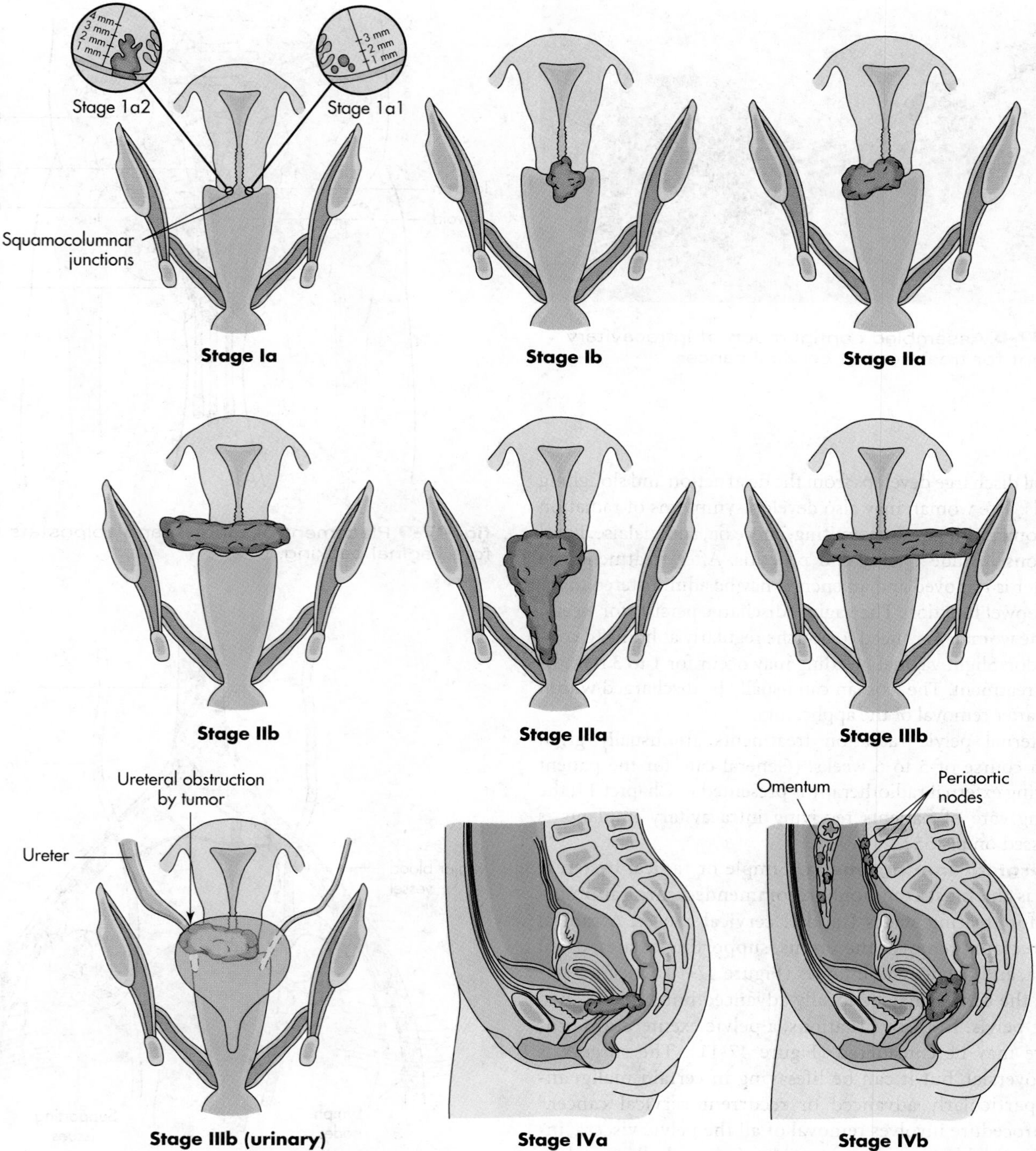


**fig. 47-7** FIGO staging and classification of cancer of cervix.

***Radiotherapy.*** When radiotherapy is used in the treatment of cervical cancer, it may consist of external pelvic irradiation or intracavitary implants (Figures 47-8 and 47-9). Intracavitary implants are usually left in place for 24 to 72 hours. (The use of radiotherapy as a cancer treatment is discussed in detail in Chapter 11.)

During treatment with an intracavitary implant, it is important that all untreated tissues remain in their normal positions and not come in close contact with the radioactive substance. The bowel is cleansed before therapy, and the woman is maintained on a low-residue diet during treatment to prevent bowel distention with defecation. A Foley catheter is typically inserted to keep the bladder small and decompressed. Gauze packing may be used in the vagina to support the rectum and bladder away from the treatment field. The woman is kept flat in bed during treatment to prevent dislodgement of the radioactive substance. The exact position of the implants can be verified by x-ray film.

The presence of the implant in the cervix may stimulate uterine contractions that may become severe. A foul-smelling

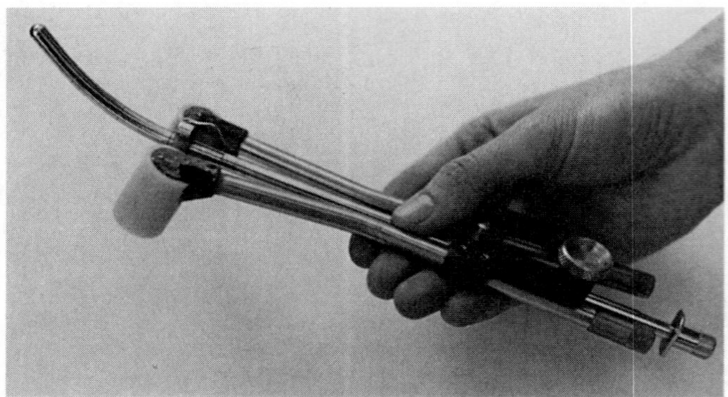

fig. 47-8 Assembled configuration of intracavitary implant for treatment of cervical cancer.

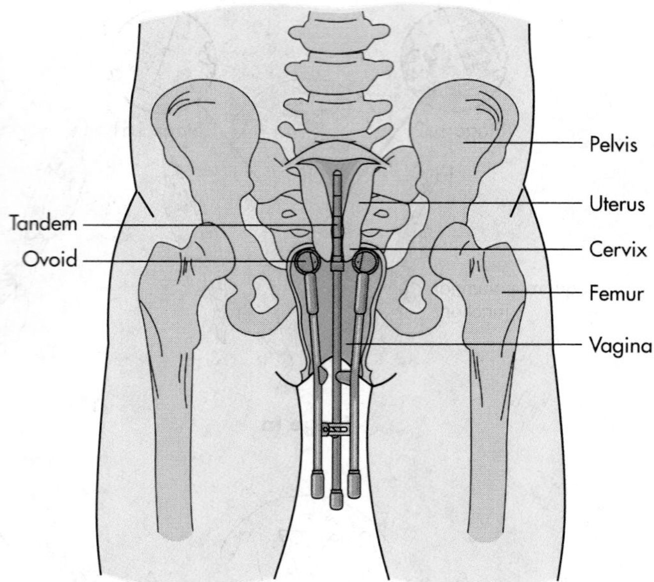


fig. 47-9 Placement of tandem and colpostats before vaginal packing.

vaginal discharge develops from the destruction and sloughing of cells. The woman may also develop symptoms of radiation syndrome, with nausea, vomiting, anorexia, and malaise. Local reactions include cystitis and proctitis. After treatment, the catheter is removed and an enema may be administered to restore bowel function. The vaginal discharge persists for weeks, and the woman may need to douche regularly at home to control odor. Slight vaginal bleeding may occur for 1 to 3 months after treatment. The woman can usually be discharged within 1 day after removal of the applicators.

External pelvic radiation treatments are usually given over a course of 5 to 6 weeks. (General care for the patient receiving external radiotherapy is presented in Chapter 11; the nursing care of patients receiving intracavitary implants is discussed on p. 1552.)

**Surgical management.** Simple or radical hysterectomy is the most commonly recommended surgical procedure for treating stages I and II cervical cancer. A radical hysterectomy removes the uterus, supporting tissues, distal vagina, and pelvic lymph nodes (Figure 47-10). In some patients the cancer may be locally advanced but still confined to the pelvis. In these situations, a pelvic exenteration procedure may be considered (Figure 47-11). The surgery is controversial, but it can be lifesaving in certain malignancies, particularly advanced or recurrent cervical cancer.[3] The procedure involves removal of all the pelvic viscera, including the bladder, rectosigmoid colon, and all reproductive organs. Five-year survival rates after this radical surgery range from 20% to 62%. The procedure is contraindicated if the disease has spread beyond the pelvis. Improved operative techniques support the possibility of reconstructive surgery to create a neovagina. This can be done at the time of surgery or as a second surgery later. Figure 47-12 illustrates an approach to vaginal reconstruction.

Nursing care of the patient undergoing hysterectomy is presented on p. 1557. Women undergoing exenteration receive this standard care but also receive care for an abdominal-perineal resection of the bowel and an ileoconduit or a continent urinary diversion. The extensive nature of the surgery usually necessitates at least a short stay in a critical care unit. Clear and honest teaching is a prerequisite for this surgery. Women need to be fully aware of the nature and consequences of the procedures in terms of both body appearance and function. Complications are numerous, occurring in 25% to 50% of all patients, and usually involve the urinary and GI systems. Fistula formation is a common problem.

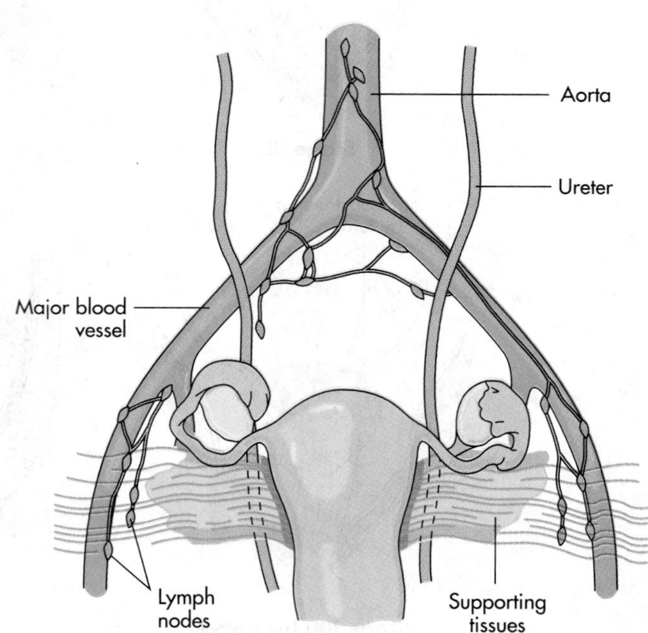


fig. 47-10 Radical hysterectomy includes removal of uterus, nearby supporting tissues, uppermost part of vagina, and pelvic lymph nodes.

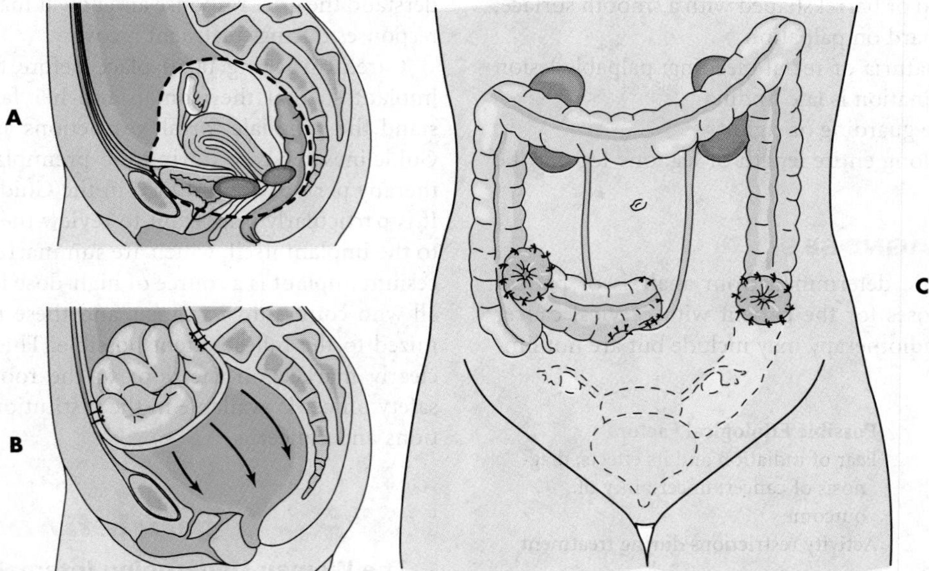


fig. 47-11 **A,** Lateral view of recurrent cancer involving cervix and upper vagina with extension into bladder and rectum. Stippled area is tissue to be removed by exenteration. **B,** Lateral view after pelvic viscera have been removed. Omental "carpet" is used to keep intestines out of pelvis during immediate postoperative period. With time, omental "carpet" will descend into pelvis, and "carpet" will adhere to pelvic floor. **C,** Urinary conduit and colostomy diversion after exenteration. Dotted areas of sigmoid colon, bladder, and internal genitalia have been removed.

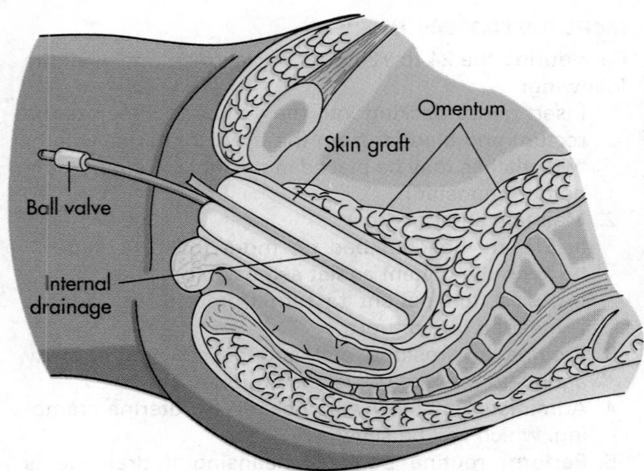


fig. 47-12 Vaginal reconstruction with skin graft. Omentum is placed in pelvis and sutured to rectum posteriorly and sigmoid colon laterally to create a "pocket" for neovagina. Two split-thickness skin grafts are harvested, sutured together over a Heyer-Schulte stent, and inserted into newly created pelvic space.

**Diet.** No special diet is required for a patient who has cancer of the cervix. Any change in diet is usually made in response to the side effects of radiation, chemotherapy, or surgical interventions.

**Activity.** No activity restrictions are required by the diagnosis. Sexual activity may be restricted temporarily after biopsy, radiation treatment, or surgery. General activity restrictions are made in response to the short-term requirements of specific treatments.

**Referrals.** In some settings the nurse assumes responsibility for making referrals to other services. The nurse may need to initiate a referral to an enterostomal therapist for stomal care if the patient undergoes pelvic exenteration. Sexual dysfunction as a result of disease or treatment may necessitate a psychiatric or sexual counseling referral.

## NURSING MANAGEMENT

### ■ ASSESSMENT

#### Subjective Data

Subjective data to be collected to assess the patient with cervical cancer include:

Vaginal discharge: thin and watery advancing to dark and foul smelling; spotting or intermittent metrorrhagia; increased amount or duration of menstrual flow

Pain: generalized abdominal discomfort; pelvic, back, flank, or leg pain; pain with intercourse

Elimination: dysuria or constipation

General complaints: anorexia, weight loss, fatigue

#### Objective Data

Objective data to be collected to assess the patient with cervical cancer include:

Cervix: colposcopic examination showing erosion of epithelium, obvious lesion; foul-smelling discharge; cervix may be enlarged or barrel shaped with a smooth surface; consistency is hard on palpation

Elimination: hematuria or rectal bleeding; palpable lesion on rectal examination is late finding

Abdomen: muscle guarding or rigidity

Edema: present along entire length of leg; one leg may be larger

## NURSING DIAGNOSES

Nursing diagnoses are determined from analysis of patient data. Nursing diagnoses for the patient with cervical cancer being treated with radiotherapy may include but are not limited to:

| Diagnostic Title | Possible Etiological Factors |
|---|---|
| Anxiety | Fear of radiation and its effects; diagnosis of cancer; uncertainty of outcome |
| Self-care: bathing-toileting deficit | Activity restrictions during treatment |
| Social isolation | Isolation and safety precautions necessitated by implant |
| Health maintenance, altered (risk for) | Insufficient knowledge about home care requirements |

## EXPECTED PATIENT OUTCOMES

Expected patient outcomes for the patient with cervical cancer being treated with radiotherapy may include but are not limited to:

1a. Verbalizes rationale for precautions followed by both staff and visitors
 b. Communicates feelings about diagnosis and treatment
 c. Expresses less anxiety about treatment and future outcomes
2. Adapts self-care tasks to activity restrictions and accepts assistance as needed
3a. Interacts with staff and visitors within the established safety guidelines
 b. Uses appropriate diversional activities
4a. Accurately describes components of home care and need for follow-up monitoring
 b. Demonstrates competency in care skills such as vaginal dilation and perineal cleansing
 c. Correctly identifies signs and symptoms of complications

## INTERVENTIONS

### Reducing Anxiety

A cancer diagnosis can produce a barrage of negative feelings in the patient that commonly escalate during the overwhelming diagnosis and staging period. The nurse encourages the woman to talk about her feelings and concerns and supports the need to ventilate emotions through anger or crying. As anxiety is controlled, effective teaching can begin concerning the condition, treatment options, and expected side effects. The nurse should assess the meaning of the diagnosis to the patient and her significant others, clarify misconceptions, and provide reliable information to enhance their understanding. Both the patient and spouse or significant other need to understand the grief response and how it may affect the woman's responses during treatment recovery.

Careful teaching takes place before the insertion of the implant so that the woman and her family clearly understand the rationale for all restrictions and safety measures. Guidelines for care during the preimplantation and radiotherapy periods are outlined in the Guidelines for Care Box. It is particularly important to review the precautions related to the implant itself, which are summarized in Box 47-3. The cesium implant is a source of high-dose ionizing radiation to all who come into its range, and these risks must be minimized to the fullest extent possible. The radiation hazard is clearly marked on the door to the room, and a radiation safety officer is available in the institution to deal with questions and concerns.

**guidelines for care**

### The Woman Undergoing Internal Radiotherapy

#### PREIMPLANTATION

Care before the insertion of the radioactive implant usually includes the following:

1. Provide cleansing enema to empty the bowel.
2. Insert Foley catheter to keep the bladder empty and small during treatment.
3. Provide Betadine douche, and shave pubic area if ordered.

#### IMPLANTATION PERIOD

Care during the 24 to 72 hours of treatment includes the following:

1. Insert gauze packing into the vagina to separate the rectum and bladder from the irradiated area. One or two stitches may be placed in the labia to support the holder in position.
2. Maintain strict bedrest.
   a. Elevate head of bed no more than 20 degrees. Keep the patient as flat as possible.
   b. Assist the patient to turn from side to side as needed for comfort.
3. Provide low-residue diet and possibly antimotility agents to prevent bowel distention.
4. Administer analgesics as needed for uterine cramping, which can be severe.
5. Perform routine perineal cleansing if drainage is present; provide room deodorizer if discharge is foul smelling.
6. Ensure a minimum fluid intake of 2500 ml daily.
7. Visit patient frequently from room doorway for emotional support.
8. Provide diversional activities appropriate to activity restrictions.
9. Monitor implant for proper placement; keep long-handled forceps and a lead-lined container in the room in case of dislodgement.
10. Monitor for complications:
    a. Infection: increased vaginal redness or swelling; increasingly dark, foul-smelling drainage; cloudy urine; fever
    b. Thrombophlebitis: painful leg swelling; positive Homans' sign

### Promoting Self-Care

The activity restrictions outlined in the Guidelines for Care Box for women undergoing internal radiotherapy must be followed carefully during the treatment period to prevent accidental dislodgement of the device or movement of the implant that endangers normal tissue. It is critical that the woman understand the rationale for all restrictions to promote adherence with the treatment plan. The nurse supports self-care and ensures that all needed articles are kept within easy reach, but assistance may be necessary because the woman must remain on flat bed rest. Hourly turning is encouraged, and back rubs may help relieve some of the discomforts of bedrest. The foul-smelling vaginal discharge may be both physically irritating and embarrassing. The nurse assists with frequent perineal hygiene and provides a room deodorizer.

Comfort is another concern during treatment. The uterine cramping can become severe, and comfort is ensured by the administration of NSAIDs or narcotic analgesics as needed. Regularly scheduled doses can help keep the discomfort under control. Patients may develop symptoms of radiation syndrome that make nutrition difficult. The nurse encourages the patient to maintain a fluid intake of 2500 to 3000 ml daily, even in the face of anorexia and nausea, and administers antiemetics as needed.

An adequate fluid intake is essential to prevent irritation of the bladder that can become severe. Phlebothrombosis is another concern during bedrest, and the nurse teaches the woman range-of-motion and isometric exercises that support venous return and encourages her to perform them 10 times each hour.

### Preventing Social Isolation

The woman receiving intracavitary radiation often feels alienated and depressed. The nurse spends time talking with the patient but must remain at a safe distance and observe the time restrictions for safety. Family members are also encouraged to visit, following the same guidelines. Children or pregnant women should not visit during treatment.

Strict bedrest rapidly creates a boring and uncomfortable situation for the patient. The nurse attempts to create a pleasant, odor-free environment. Self-care items are kept within easy reach, and diversional activities are provided for the patient, such as reading materials, music, telephone, and television. The nursing staff maintain frequent contact with the patient, checking on her at least hourly, and ensure that her call bell is within easy reach.

### Patient/Family Education

#### *Teaching home care skills*

The hospitalization period for intracavitary radiotherapy is short, and the patient is discharged soon after the removal of the implant. The woman must learn several self-care skills for home management and be aware of the signs and symptoms of potential complications. Radiotherapy causes fatigue, vaginal stenosis, loss of vaginal lubrication, and induced menopause.

The vaginal discharge often continues for weeks, and the woman may need to douche at least twice daily as long as discharge and odor persist. The nurse cannot assume that the woman has experience with douching and reviews the technique and precautions in detail. Some vaginal bleeding may also persist for a few months after treatment, and the woman should receive information from her physician about acceptable amounts of bleeding. Local application of estrogen cream may prevent bleeding.

The cesium implant causes vaginal narrowing and fibrosis. Regular vaginal dilation is essential to minimize these effects. If the woman has a spouse or sexual partner, regular sexual intercourse, usually at least three times per week, is one method of minimizing stenosis. The woman may prefer to use a manual obturator to dilate the vagina. The importance of this intervention is explained to women who are not sexually active as well. Even routine pelvic examination can become difficult or almost impossible if the vagina becomes severely stenosed. Dilation should be performed at least three times a week for 1 year after treatment. The obturator is lubricated before use and washed carefully with soap and water after each use. A vinegar and water douche may be ordered after treatment. The nurse informs the woman that slight bleeding may occur after dilation for up to a year.

Sexual intercourse may be resumed about 3 weeks after discharge, but the woman is instructed to use a water-soluble lubricant for comfort because vaginal secretions will be decreased or absent. The woman's partner is included in all discussions about sexual activity if the woman is comfortable with her partner's presence.

Other self-care teaching includes gradually increasing activity, maintaining a liberal fluid intake to prevent urological problems, and adjusting the diet to prevent bowel problems. Either constipation or diarrhea may occur in response to the radiation, and these problems may persist for months after treatment. The nurse also teaches the woman about

**box 47-3** *Radiation Precautions for Internal Radiotherapy*

1. Time at the bedside is limited—each contact should last no more than 30 minutes.
2. Children and pregnant women/staff should not visit during treatment.
3. Staff members should wear a dosimeter during every patient contact to monitor radiation exposure.
4. Lead shield may be installed at the side and foot of the bed.
5. Staff should use the principles of distance, time, and shielding in all contacts with the patient.
6. Implant is always handled by means of long-handled forceps, never with the hands. A lead-lined container should be present in the room for use if the implant dislodges.
7. A sign that clearly identifies the radiation hazard is posted on the room door.
8. A contact number for the radiation safety officer of the institution should be posted on the warning sign.

symptoms that indicate complications. The woman should promptly report unusually heavy discharge, foul-smelling urine, low-grade fever, persistent bowel problems, or pain. Radiotherapy can cause fistulas in the pelvis, both in the early posttreatment period and in the future. Written materials can be helpful resources for the woman at home. The importance of follow-up care and monitoring is emphasized.

## EVALUATION

To evaluate the effectiveness of nursing interventions, compare patient behaviors with those stated in the expected patient outcomes. Successful achievement of patient outcomes for the patient with cervical cancer receiving radiotherapy is indicated by:

1. a. Correctly explains the rationale for all radiation and activity restrictions
   b. Communicates feelings to partner, family, or staff
   c. States that anxiety is minimal or absent
2. Performs self-care activities independently or with the use of appropriate assistance
3. a. Regularly interacts with family, friends, and staff
   b. Uses books, hobbies, music, and television to break up the day
4. a. Correctly describes home care regimen and planned pattern for follow-up care
   b. Correctly demonstrates perineal care and use of an obturator for dilation
   c. Correctly describes signs of complications that need to be reported

## GERONTOLOGICAL CONSIDERATIONS

Cancer of the cervix occurs in women of all ages. Early diagnosis is critical and is an ongoing challenge in older women. After the childbearing years, many women stop having routine gynecological examinations. Pap smear screening for elderly women remains controversial, and current screening guidelines reflect no upper age limit. Symptoms are often discounted or attributed to the multiple effects of aging on the reproductive tract. Therefore it is less likely that cervical cancer will be detected in the early and curable stages. Elderly women are less able to withstand the rigors of radical surgery, are more prone to complications of treatment, and often experience exaggerated tissue responses to radiotherapy. It is critical that teaching and outreach be provided to this population about the ongoing importance of Pap smear screening for cancer because the incidence and mortality rates for cervical cancer in the United States are highest among elderly women.

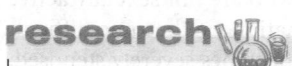

Reference: Corney R et al: The care of patients undergoing surgery for gynaecological cancer: the need for information, emotional support and counseling, *J Adv Nurs* 17(6):667, 1992.

In this study, 105 patients who had undergone major gynecological surgery for carcinoma of the cervix or vulva in the past 5 years were interviewed. A high proportion of the women were still found to be depressed and anxious when interviewed, and most reported chronic sexual problems. The women were asked if they had received enough information regarding their illness and its treatment; a high proportion would have liked to have had more information on the aftereffects of the surgery, including physical, sexual, and emotional aspects. Many of the younger women would have wanted their partner to have been included in the discussions, and 25% of the 40 partners who responded to a questionnaire stated they would have liked more information on the illness and its treatment. The women also indicated their needs for emotional support, discussion, and counseling.

## SPECIAL ENVIRONMENTS FOR CARE

### Critical Care Management

Women undergoing treatment for cancer of the cervix do not usually need critical care support except for women undergoing radical surgery. Total pelvic exenteration procedures are a complex assault on the body and involve extensive urinary and bowel diversion procedures. Short-term postoperative critical care monitoring is usually indicated, particularly for older patients and women who have concurrent major organ system diseases.

### Home Care Management

Much of the diagnostic and conservative treatment for cervical cancer takes place in an outpatient environment. Even hospitalization for radiotherapy extends only for the duration of the implant placement. It is therefore critical that the woman be an informed partner in her own care. Extensive teaching needs to be provided, with full understanding that the anxiety associated with the diagnosis of cancer and its treatment will make it difficult for the woman to hear and process much of the information (see the Research Box). Repeat sessions and written reference materials are critical. Formal home care services are rarely used or needed, so the goal of knowledgeable self-care becomes even more critical. The woman's partner is included in teaching sessions if possible, because the disease and treatment have significant potential impact on the couple's sexual activities, at least in the short term. The nurse ensures that the woman has the name and phone number of all appropriate support groups and services available in her home community.

## COMPLICATIONS

The primary complications of cervical cancer and its treatment have been outlined in the discussion. Recurrence and metastasis of the cancer are the primary concerns. The diagnosis can compromise the woman's body image, sexuality, and fertility. Implant therapy results in radiation-induced menopause, which adds to the challenge of keeping the vagina dilated, supple, and lubricated for intercourse. The presence of prolonged vaginal discharge does not promote the resumption of sexual activity, and the couple's relationship can deteriorate from communication problems and mixed messages between the partners. The woman must also cope with odor and drainage that can compromise her image of herself as a desirable sexual being. Physical complications such as fistula formation, tissue fibrosis, and inflammatory bowel problems are addressed in the discharge teaching, but the woman typically finds herself alone at home dealing with the reality of all of the changes. The nurse again stresses the importance of peer support.

## NEOPLASMS OF THE UTERUS

### Uterine Leiomyomas (Fibroids)

#### Etiology

Leiomyomas (myomas) are benign tumors of muscle cell origin that contain varying amounts of fibrous tissue. The etiology of leiomyomas is not completely understood. The stimulus for growth is unclear but is thought to be related to estrogen, because leiomyomas are rare before menarche and often decrease in size after menopause. The tumors often enlarge during pregnancy and with the use of oral contraceptives. Women who smoke tend to be relatively estrogen deficient and have been found to have a lower incidence of leiomyomas. The tumors can reach enormous proportions, weighing as much as 50 pounds. Malignant transformation is rare, occurring in less than 0.5% of myomas.[26,41]

#### Epidemiology

Leiomyomas are the most common type of pelvic tumor, developing in 20% to 25% of women during their reproductive years.[26] Leiomyomas occur more frequently in African-American women, and by the fifth decade of life, as many as 50% of African-American women will have leiomyomata.[26] They occasionally are found in the fallopian tubes or round ligament, and approximately 5% originate from the cervix.

#### Pathophysiology

Leiomyomas originate in the myometrium and are classified by their anatomical location (Figure 47-13). Submucous myomas lie just beneath the endometrium and compress it as they grow. They can develop a pedicle and protrude into the uterine cavity or even through the cervical canal. Intramural myomas lie within the uterine muscle, and subserous tumors lie at the serosal surface of the uterus or may bulge outward from the myometrium. These external tumors also tend to become pedunculated.

Most leiomyomas are asymptomatic and may go undetected even when large in size, particularly if the woman is obese.[41] The development of symptoms depends on the location, size, and condition of the tumor. Menorrhagia is the most common symptom. Bleeding can result from distortion and congestion of surrounding vessels or ulceration of the overlying endometrium. Bleeding usually takes the form of premenstrual spotting or prolonged light bleeding after the menses. Metrorrhagia is associated with venous thrombosis or necrosis on the surface of the tumor, particularly if it extrudes through the cervix. The blood loss may be significant enough to create an iron deficiency anemia that does not respond to iron therapy.[41]

Pain is not a characteristic symptom, although it can result from tumor degeneration or with myometrial contractions that attempt to expel the myoma from the uterus. If the pedicle stalk becomes twisted, it can cause sudden, severe pain. Women often report a sensation of heaviness in the pelvis or a "bearing down" feeling, especially with large tumors. The tumor may cause pelvic circulatory congestion and create backache, constipation, or dysmenorrhea. The woman even may notice an increase in abdominal girth.

Leiomyomas interfere with fertility by blocking the opening of the fallopian tubes, inducing spontaneous abortion, or obstructing the cervical canal, making delivery hazardous. Sudden growth of a myoma after menopause is considered to be a classic sign of leiomyosarcoma, which necessitates hysterectomy.

Anemia is associated with chronic blood loss, but women may also exhibit erythrocytosis. Although the etiology is unclear, it is speculated that compression of the ureters may increase ureteral back pressure and stimulate the production of erythropoietin by the kidneys.[41] Clinical manifestations of leiomyomas are summarized in Box 47-4.

**box 47-4 clinical manifestations**

***Leiomyomas***

NOTE: Most leiomyomas are asymptomatic.

- Premenstrual spotting
- Prolonged postmenstrual light bleeding
- Sensation of heaviness in the pelvis; can cause backache or constipation
- Iron deficiency anemia
- Metrorrhagia (sudden-onset pain indicates a complication)

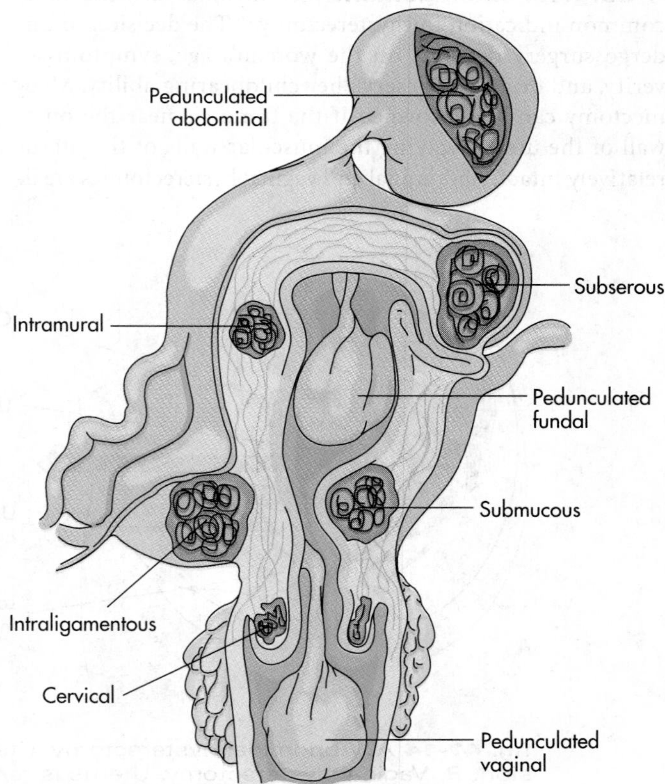


**fig. 47-13** Myomas of the uterus.

### Collaborative care management

**Diagnostic tests.** Myomas often can be detected by routine pelvic examination when the uterus is displaced and irregular nodules are felt on the uterine surface. Diagnosis is confirmed through the use of MRI, CT scan, pelvic sonography, and hysterography or hysteroscopy. These tests are used to determine the size and placement of the tumor(s) and evaluate the degree of urological compression.

**Medications.** Drug therapy does not play a major role in the management of leiomyomas. However, GnRH agonists may be used to reduce the level of circulating estrogens and shrink the tumor. The GnRH agonists are able to reduce tumor size by as much as 90%, but their effect is temporary. These drugs may be used in perimenopausal women to avoid the need for surgery because the tumors are known to regress after menopause. The GnRH agonists are also prescribed preoperatively to reduce the incidence and severity of postoperative bleeding. Reducing the tumor size also may permit the use of a vaginal approach for the hysterectomy rather than an abdominal and decrease recovery time.

**Treatments.** Small, asymptomatic myomas are simply monitored. The myomas tend to shrink as estrogen levels begin to decline. If a patient is experiencing bleeding an endometrial biopsy may be performed to verify the diagnosis and rule out cancer. Submucous myomas may be resected via the cervical canal using the hysteroscope and laser therapy as an outpatient procedure.

**Surgical management.** Leiomyomas are the most common indication for hysterectomy.[26] The decision to undergo surgery depends on the woman's age, symptom severity, and desire to preserve her childbearing ability. Myomectomy can be performed if the tumor is near the outer wall of the uterus, leaving the muscular walls of the uterus relatively intact. Abdominal and vaginal hysterectomies are illustrated in Figure 47-14. Various gynecological surgical procedures are defined in Box 47-5.

**Diet.** Diet therapy does not play a role in the management of leiomyomas.

**Activity.** A woman's usual pattern of activity does not need to be altered by the presence of leiomyoma.

The development of anemia often causes fatigue and activity intolerance. Women who experience pelvic heaviness or backache may also curtail their activities in response to their symptoms.

**box 47-5** *Surgeries of the Female Reproductive System*

**Oophorectomy**—Removal of an ovary
**Salpingectomy**—Removal of a fallopian tube
**Bilateral salpingo-oophorectomy (BSO or Bil S&O)**—Removal of both ovaries and fallopian tubes
**Total hysterectomy**—Removal of the entire uterus, including the cervix; may be referred to as a TAH (total abdominal hysterectomy). Procedure can be done vaginally or abdominally
**Subtotal hysterectomy**—Removal of the uterus except for the cervix; rarely done today
**Hystero-oophorectomy**—Removal of the uterus and an ovary
**Hysterosalpingectomy**—Removal of the uterus and a fallopian tube
**Total abdominal hysterectomy and bilateral salpingo-oophorectomy**—Removal of the entire uterus and both fallopian tubes and ovaries (also called TAH-BSO). The term *panhysterectomy* has been used previously to refer to this type of surgery
**Radical hysterectomy (Wertheim procedure)**—TAH-BSO, partial vaginectomy, and dissection of the lymph nodes in the pelvis

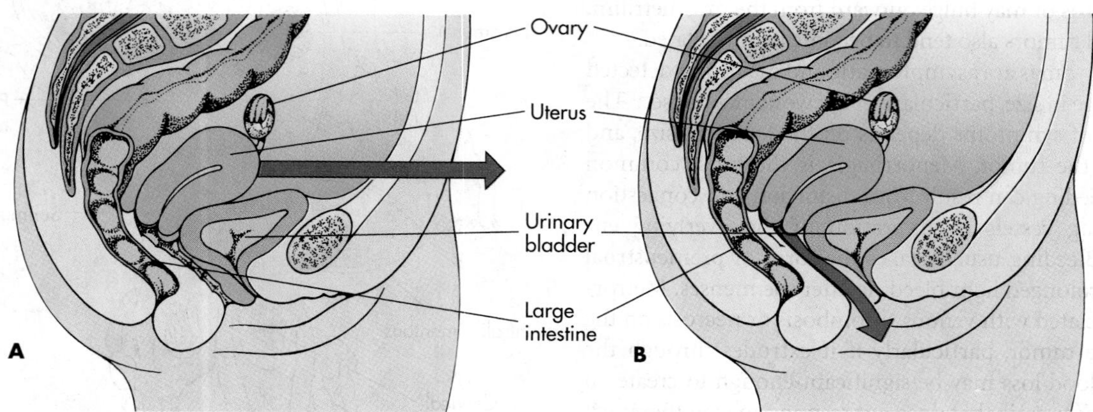


**fig. 47-14 A,** Abdominal hysterectomy. Uterus is removed through an abdominal incision. **B,** Vaginal hysterectomy. Uterus is removed through vagina and there is no abdominal incision.

**Referrals.** Unless the situation becomes complex, a patient with leiomyoma generally does not need multidisciplinary referral.

## NURSING MANAGEMENT OF THE PATIENT UNDERGOING HYSTERECTOMY FOR LEIOMYOMA

### ■ PREOPERATIVE CARE

Hysterectomy is used as a treatment for a variety of reproductive tract problems in addition to leiomyoma, including cancer of the cervix, uterus, and ovaries; and structural problems such as severe prolapse. Both vaginal and abdominal approaches are used (see the Research Box).

Most women are familiar with the term *fibroids* but have little real understanding of their development, treatment, or relationship with estrogen levels. Preoperative teaching is essential and usually is initiated in the physician's office or by the preadmissions team. The nurse verifies that teaching has been provided and that the woman can accurately describe the planned surgery and associated care. The nurse then clarifies and reinforces that teaching as needed, thoroughly discussing the plans for pain management and the importance of early and frequent ambulation.

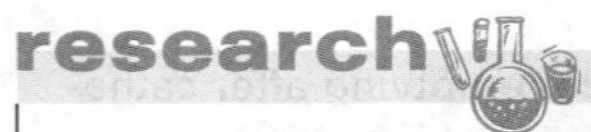

Reference: Dorsey JH et al: Costs and charges associated with three alternative techniques of hysterectomy, *N Engl J Med* 335(7):476, 1996.

Laparoscopic assisted vaginal hysterectomy has achieved increasing popularity in recent years. This study compared the costs, hospital charges, and use of resources associated with the three major surgical approaches to hysterectomy: (1) total vaginal hysterectomy, (2) total abdominal hysterectomy, and (3) laparoscopic assisted vaginal hysterectomy. The study included approximately 1000 patients who underwent hysterectomy during a 1-year period at a major metropolitan medical center. Patients being concurrently treated for major secondary disorders or undergoing radical hysterectomy were excluded from the study. Ninety-six surgeons performed the surgeries.

The study used a retrospective chart to audit process and assigned costs to each of the elements of the procedure and hospital care. Fifty-four percent of the women had abdominal procedures, 20% vaginal, and 26% laparoscopic assisted procedures. Results of the study showed that patients undergoing laparoscopic assisted vaginal hysterectomy had significantly shorter hospital stays (averaging 2.6 days). However, the mean total charges associated with the procedure were estimated to be $1032 higher than for abdominal procedures and $1895 higher than for vaginal procedures, despite the shorter stay. All associated costs were higher, primarily related to longer operating room times and the use of two setups to support both the vaginal and laparoscopic work.

Physical preparation for surgery typically includes bowel preparation with an enema or laxative the day before the procedure to empty and cleanse the bowel. A Betadine douche may also be prescribed, or the physician may order the woman to insert a Betadine-soaked tampon 12 hours before the surgery. Ferrous sulfate therapy may be prescribed several weeks before surgery if the woman is anemic from chronic blood loss.

### ■ POSTOPERATIVE CARE

Much of the postoperative care provided after hysterectomy is similar to that provided after any major surgery (see Chapter 20). Unique aspects of care are addressed here.

#### Promoting Activity

Ambulation begins on the day of surgery or the first postoperative day, and the nurse encourages regular brief periods of ambulation throughout the day. Ambulation supports oxygenation through natural deep breathing, assists in the prompt elimination of residual anesthetic, stimulates the return of peristalsis, and supports venous return. Venous pooling and pelvic congestion are common complications after hysterectomy because of the inflammatory response to the trauma of surgery. This is particularly true if the lithotomy position was used during surgery. The risk of thromboembolism is significant, and the physician may order subcutaneous heparin injections. Routine interventions include applying compression stockings, encouraging leg and foot flexion and extension exercises every 2 hours, and avoiding positioning the patient with the knees bent. Elevating the legs at intervals throughout the day may be helpful also. Routine monitoring for pain or swelling in the calf is included in the ongoing assessment.

#### Supporting Urinary Elimination

Urinary problems are common after hysterectomy. The woman who undergoes vaginal hysterectomy may have a catheter left in place for 24 hours to allow for resolution of edema around the urethra. The catheter is typically removed on the first postoperative day, but many women experience some difficulty in voiding spontaneously or emptying the bladder completely. Bladder problems are particularly troublesome in elderly women who have weakened muscles and decreased sensitivity to the neurological stimuli for voiding.[3] Suppressed immune functioning also makes them more vulnerable to infection.

#### Supporting Return of Peristalsis

Peristalsis is typically suppressed after hysterectomy, particularly if an abdominal approach with extensive handling of the GI organs was used. Gaseous distention is one of the most common and troublesome postoperative complaints. The woman typically receives nothing by mouth until bowel sounds return, and intravenous fluids are continued until she is taking oral fluids well. If problems do not occur, the patient moves quickly from a liquid to a regular diet. When paralytic ileus is severe, a nasogastric tube may be placed to relieve gaseous pressure. Frequent ambulation is encouraged as the most reliable means of stimulating peristaltic activity. The woman's potassium level is monitored to ensure that hypokalemia does not contribute to the ileus.

### Providing Emotional Support

Hysterectomy may be accompanied by emotional upset and ambivalence concerning the loss of reproductive ability, but this is not always the case. Many women are equally concerned about the effects of the surgery on femininity and sexuality. Postoperatively, almost all women experience some degree of depression for several days and may be inexplicably tearful. Grieving for losses is both appropriate and important, and the nurse encourages the woman to deal honestly with her emotions. Family members need to be informed about these expected responses, and partners may need to be encouraged to offer the patient specific reassurance and understanding during this time. Women are instructed to avoid intercourse until the vaginal vault is satisfactorily healed. This usually takes about 6 weeks. Satisfactory sexual relations can then be reestablished, but many women need to adjust to changes in the nature of pelvic sensations and stimuli during sex.

The accompanying Guidelines for Care Box summarizes the nursing care for the hysterectomy patient. A sample Nursing Care Plan for a woman undergoing hysterectomy for cervical cancer begins on p. 1559. A Clinical Pathway for a patient undergoing total abdominal hysterectomy begins on p. 1564.

## GERONTOLOGICAL CONSIDERATIONS

Leiomyomas typically develop in middle-aged women and are rarely a significant problem in postmenopausal women. However, estrogen replacement therapy will continue to stimulate the growth of a myoma. There are no major differences in treatment approaches for older women, and most older women tolerate hysterectomy extremely well. Older patients need to be carefully monitored because complications are more common in this age group, especially after abdominal surgery.

## SPECIAL ENVIRONMENTS FOR CARE

### Critical Care Management

Critical care management would rarely be indicated in the standard treatment of leiomyomas unless a woman developed severe and unexpected complications or had severe concurrent health problems in other major organ systems.

### Home Care Management

Patients are rapidly discharged to their home environments, especially following vaginal hysterectomy. They rarely need home health support unless complications develop. The nurse provides thorough teaching about care of the incision and the signs of wound infection. Ileus can be an ongoing problem, and patients are instructed to contact their physician if abdominal distention, nausea, or vomiting develops. Stool softeners, liberal fluids, and diet modifications are used until a normal bowel pattern is reestablished.

## COMPLICATIONS

The complications of hysterectomy are typically those associated with any major surgery and the use of general anesthesia. They have been discussed under the nursing interventions. Wound healing, ileus, constipation, and urinary dysfunction are the primary concerns.

**guidelines for care**

**The Woman Undergoing Hysterectomy**

**PREOPERATIVE CARE**

Verify patient understanding of the procedure and anticipated care.
Administer prescribed enemas, laxatives, and douches.
Verify completion of prescribed skin preparation.
Promote circulation and oxygenation.
- Apply antiembolic hose.
- Teach deep breathing, effective coughing, use of incentive spirometer, how to splint abdomen, and how to change positions.
- Teach leg and feet exercises.
- Teach how to use PCA for pain control.
- Encourage expression of feelings and concerns.

**POSTOPERATIVE CARE**

Promote comfort.
- Administer analgesics and encourage PCA use.
- Administer antiemetics as needed.

Promote circulation and oxygenation.
- Encourage turning, deep breathing, coughing, and use of incentive spirometer.
- Encourage leg and feet exercises every hour while in bed.
- Maintain use of antiembolic hose as ordered.
- Encourage frequent ambulation.
- Assess for signs of thromboembolism.

Maintain fluid and electrolyte balance.
- Accurately record all output and drainage.

Promote elimination.
- Monitor effectiveness of bladder emptying after catheter removal. Catheterize for residual if ordered.
- Monitor for signs of returning peristalsis.
- Encourage frequent ambulation and a liberal fluid intake.
- Teach diet modifications to prevent constipation.

Provide discharge teaching.
- Teach signs of urinary tract infection.
- Provide teaching regarding incision care.
- Instruct patient to avoid heavy lifting, prolonged sitting, and long car rides.
- Tell patient to refrain from coitus for about 6 weeks and not to douche unless prescribed by her physician. Vaginal bleeding or discharge may persist for up to 6 weeks.
- Help patient anticipate the occurrence of mood swings and emotional lability during healing.

### Cancer of the Endometrium

#### Etiology/epidemiology

Cancer of the endometrium (uterine corpus) is the most common form of gynecological cancer, and it primarily affects women over 50 years of age. It rarely occurs before age 40, and the average woman is 61 years old at the time of diagnosis.[26] Endometrial cancer is twice as common as ovarian cancer and

## nursing care plan — Woman After Hysterectomy for Cervical Cancer

**DATA** Mrs. Conn, age 42, saw her gynecologist 2 weeks ago because of bleeding between periods and occasional postcoital bleeding. The result of her Pap smear 5 years previously had been negative. The Pap smear this time was positive, and a cervical biopsy confirmed cancer of the cervix, stage I. She was admitted yesterday for a total hysterectomy.

Admission notes indicate that Mrs. Conn is married and has two teenagers, a boy and a girl. Her husband accompanied her to the hospital and appears to be supportive. Mrs. Conn is a bank teller and likes to read, knit, and watch TV. She has varicose veins but states these do not bother her. Her preoperative concerns centered mainly on the cancer: "I hope they get it all." She also stated, "Well, at least I hadn't planned any more children. My boy joked and said, 'You're going to be neutered like our cat was!' I wonder how it feels to be so-called neutered. I hope it won't affect my sex life." The nurse explored Mrs. Conn's knowledge of the surgery and explained that the surgery would not physically affect sexual relationships.

Mrs. Conn returned from the recovery room alert with an IV infusing and stable vital signs. The dressing was dry. She is receiving morphine sulfate (MS) per a patient-controlled analgesia (PCA) pump at 1 mg/hr with a bolus of 1 mg available every 8 minutes.

Nursing assessment includes monitoring the following parameters:

- Vital signs
- Breath sounds
- Urine output
- Fluid intake
- Patency of dressing
- Respiratory rate
- Pain status

**NURSING DIAGNOSIS** *Pain related to abdominal incision*

| expected patient outcome | nursing interventions | rationale |
|---|---|---|
| States she is feeling more comfortable within 1-2 hours after comfort measures are initiated. | Maintain analgesic infusion so analgesics given on a regular basis for first 24 hours. | Giving the analgesic regularly will prevent severe pain and thus be more effective. |
| | Encourage frequent changes of position in bed and early ambulation. | Activity decreases pain by increasing circulation and reducing muscle tension; ambulation will also encourage peristalsis, decreasing intensity of gas pains. |
| | Assess adequacy of pain relief q 2-4 hrs. | |
| | Encourage use of PCA bolus to maintain comfort. | |

**NURSING DIAGNOSIS** *Risk for self-esteem disturbance related to loss of uterus and concern about sexuality*

| expected patient outcomes | nursing interventions | rationale |
|---|---|---|
| Verbalizes concerns about loss of uterus. | Provide patient opportunities to express feelings and concerns about loss of uterus. Assess significant others' concerns and perceptions of body changes. | Patient may feel freer to talk about her feelings if opportunities are provided. Validates perceptions. Helps patient and significant other to ventilate doubts and resolve concerns. |
| | Provide factual information regarding anticipated bodily changes; include significant other if possible. | Provides accurate information and corrects misconceptions. |
| | Be empathetic about patient's feelings, which may include grief, guilt, shame, or remorse. | Feelings associated with grief may also be expressed when grieving over loss of a body part. |
| | Encourage her to continue activities associated with femininity, such as fixing hair, makeup, wearing own apparel. | Feelings of femininity will emphasize "feminine" rather than "neuter," and that she herself has not changed. |
| Makes plans for resuming her role. | Help her make plans for resumption of former activities. | If life pattern is not changed, her thoughts about her body changes may diminish. |

**NURSING DIAGNOSIS** *Risk for constipation related to surgical manipulation of bowel, pain medication, and immobility*

| expected patient outcome | nursing interventions | rationale |
|---|---|---|
| Stool is soft and formed. | Monitor stool characteristics and frequency. | Helps form basis of an effective treatment plan. |
| | Encourage ambulation q4h. | Ambulation promotes peristalsis. |
| | Assess abdomen for presence and quality of bowel sounds. | Peristalsis may be decreased from handling of pelvic viscera; helps determine flatus buildup. |

Continued

## Woman After Hysterectomy for Cervical Cancer–cont'd

**NURSING DIAGNOSIS** *Risk for constipation related to surgical manipulation of bowel, pain medication, and immobility—cont'd*

| expected patient outcome | nursing interventions | rationale |
|---|---|---|
| | Encourage oral fluids when permitted. | Hydration will promote a soft stool. |
| | Teach patient to avoid straining at stool. | Increases abdominal pain and can increase bleeding. |

**NURSING DIAGNOSIS** *Altered patterns of urinary elimination related to loss of bladder tone, pain with muscle contraction, and discomfort from urinating position*

| expected patient outcome | nursing interventions | rationale |
|---|---|---|
| Voids spontaneously and empties bladder completely. | Monitor urine output until she reestablishes a normal voiding pattern. | Handling of bladder during pelvic surgery may decrease bladder muscle tone, leading to urinary retention. Accurate I&O records detect inadequate emptying of bladder. |
| | Encourage patient to void q2h. | Promotes optimal bladder tone and prevents distention. |
| | Monitor for distention above symphysis pubis and for lower abdominal discomfort other than incisional pain, q4h. | Detects bladder distention and degree of fullness. |
| | Provide privacy during attempts to urinate. | Promotes elimination. |
| | Catheterize for residual urine as ordered. | Residual urine in bladder provides good medium for bacterial growth. |
| | Teach perineal care. | Helps prevent urinary tract infections. |

**NURSING DIAGNOSIS** *Risk for altered peripheral tissue perfusion related to pelvic venous stasis from surgery*

| expected patient outcome | nursing interventions | rationale |
|---|---|---|
| Normal circulation is present without development of thrombus, emboli, or leg or thigh pain. | Monitor for discomfort in legs/thighs or sudden dyspnea; assess for Homans' sign; check warmth, color, blanching of lower extremities q8h. | Early detection will ensure early treatment of phlebothrombosis. |
| | Encourage patient to lie completely flat in bed for short periods q4h for 24 hours, then q4h until ambulating well. | Lying flat for periods of time will help blood return from the pelvic veins. |
| | Encourage leg exercises and frequent turning in bed until ambulating well. | Exercises promote venous return (muscle pumps). |
| | Avoid elevating knees or placing pillows under knees; encourage patient to keep knees flat when in bed; minimize use of high Fowler's position. | Pressure on popliteal veins or sharp knee flexion may increase venous stasis. |
| | Provide antiembolic stockings or apply intermittent pneumatic compression stockings. | Antiembolic stockings help prevent venous stasis. Mrs. Conn is at higher risk for phlebothrombosis because of varicose veins (sluggish circulation) and sedentary life pattern. |
| | Encourage ambulation. | Ambulation promotes venous return by contracting muscles to compress veins. |

*Continued*

## Woman After Hysterectomy for Cervical Cancer–cont'd

**NURSING DIAGNOSIS** *Risk for impaired health maintenance related to lack of knowledge concerning self-care after discharge.*

| expected patient outcome | nursing interventions | rationale |
|---|---|---|
| Describes self-care accurately. | Teach patient: | |
| | 1. When activities can be resumed (see text). | Activities are resumed gradually to permit healing; heavy activities are avoided for 6-8 weeks. |
| | 2. Signs of phlebothrombosis to be monitored and reported. | Phlebothrombosis may occur 7-10 days postoperatively, after patient goes home. |
| | 3. Signs of vaginal bleeding to be reported (excessive or persistent); possibility of slight vaginal discharge for 1-2 weeks. | Bleeding could indicate impaired healing. |
| | 4. Bathing and light activity permitted after hospital discharge. | |
| | 5. Avoid driving car for 2-4 weeks, especially with standard shift. | |
| | 6. Avoid heavy activity and active sports for 4-6 weeks. | |
| | 7. Need for medical follow-up. | |
| | Include significant other if possible. | Promotes compliance with discharge teaching. |
| | Reinforce the preoperative explanations of the surgery and effect on sexual relationships; include significant other if possible. | Preoperative anxiety may have decreased her awareness; hysterectomy does not interfere with satisfactory sexual relationships. |
| | Find out what she has told her daughter about regular Pap smears. | Regular Pap smears enhance early detection of cervical cancer. |
| | Suggest she use support hose in her job as a bank teller. | Preventive measure for phlebothrombosis because of her varicose veins. |

three times more common than cervical cancer. The estimated annual incidence of endometrial cancer is 33,000 cases with an associated mortality of 4000 cases.[26]

Multiple risk factors have been identified in addition to age. These include obesity, diabetes, nulliparity, late menopause (after age 52), use of estrogen replacement therapy (ERT), and the use of tamoxifen for breast cancer. The risk of endometrial cancer among women taking ERT appears to be limited to unopposed estrogen products.[26] Adding progesterone to the therapy appears to eliminate the risk, and women receiving combined estrogen-progesterone products actually have a lower total risk of endometrial cancer than do women who are not receiving ERT.

### Pathophysiology

Uterine hyperplasia is somewhat analogous to dysplasia of the cervix. Some lesions revert to normal, some persist as hyperplasia, and a few progress to endometrial adenocarcinoma. Unfortunately, unlike cervical dysplasia, no reliable, widely available screening method for endometrial hyperplasia exists. Most women with this condition are diagnosed when they seek medical care for abnormal uterine bleeding. The diagnosis of endometrial hyperplasia can be made only by pathological examination of uterine tissue.

Endometrial cancer is an excellent example of an estrogen-dependent lesion. The underlying pathological process involves overgrowth of the uterine endometrium in response to an estrogen-dominant hormonal environment. The estrogen may come from the ovaries or from another source (e.g., hormone replacement therapy after menopause).[3]

Abnormal vaginal bleeding is the most common symptom, occurring in 90% of cases.[29] Occasionally women have a purulent, blood-tinged discharge. Pain is a late symptom and usually occurs with metastatic disease.[3]

### Collaborative care management

Cancer of the endometrium is a slow-growing form of cancer and is very responsive to treatment if detected early. High-risk women may have endometrial tissue samples taken periodically. Tissue samples may be acquired in a variety of ways, as outlined in Table 47-7.

**table 47-7** *Methods for Detection of Endometrial Cancer*

| Method | Effectiveness (%) |
|---|---|
| Endometrial aspirations | 70-80 |
| Endometrial washings | 80-90 |
| Dilation and curettage (fractional) | 85-90 |
| Pap smear | 45-50 |
| Combination of above | 90 |

**table 47-8** *Stages of Cancer of the Endometrium*

| Stage | Involvement |
|---|---|
| I | Confined to corpus |
| II | Involves corpus and cervix |
| III | Extends outside corpus but not outside pelvis (vaginal wall but not bladder or rectum) |
| IV | Involves bladder, rectum, or outside pelvis |

Endometrial cancer is treated according to its stage. Table 47-8 outlines the staging criteria. The most common treatment is total abdominal hysterectomy with bilateral salpingo-oophorectomy (TAH-BSO). Radiation and surgery often are combined to treat early-stage disease. In high-risk stage I disease, patients often receive postoperative radiation, whereas in more advanced stages the radiation may be given preoperatively to shrink the tumor and reduce the risk of local infection.[3] Radiotherapy is used as a primary modality if the woman is a poor risk for surgery or refuses surgery.

Hormonal therapy and chemotherapy often are added for stage III or IV disease. Progestins have been successfully used for years. They may be administered in a daily oral dose or by weekly intramuscular injection. Chemotherapy with doxorubicin, cyclophosphamide, and cisplatin, individually or in combination, has had mixed results.

**Patient/family education.** The nursing care associated with hysterectomy and radiotherapy has been discussed previously. Nurses play a major role in health teaching about the importance of careful evaluation of all dysfunctional uterine bleeding in the postmenopausal population. This single factor is the most important strategy for identifying endometrial cancer in a treatable stage.

## Gestational Trophoblastic Neoplasia

### *Etiology/epidemiology*

*Gestational trophoblastic neoplasia (GTN)* is the term used to describe choriocarcinoma and related diseases such as hydatidiform mole and invasive mole. The etiology of GTN is not thoroughly understood. The hydatidiform mole often precedes malignant diseases.

The risk of hydatidiform mole varies significantly in different regions of the world, being 10 times more prevalent in the Far East than the United States. Both nutrition and socioeconomic factors have been correlated. Risk factors for molar pregnancy include age (under 20 and over 40) and geographical residence in Mexico or Southeast Asia. Choriocarcinoma risk factors are similar.[28]

### *Pathophysiology*

Gestational trophoblastic neoplasia is an abnormal pregnancy characterized by a degeneration, or abnormal growth, of the trophoblastic tissue of the placenta, usually in the absence of an intact fetus. It produces a serum marker, human chorionic gonadotropin (HCG), whose levels are directly related to the number of tumor cells.

Early stages of GTN may be similar to normal pregnancy. As the disease progresses, most women experience uterine bleeding. Rapid uterine growth occurs, often accompanied by nausea and vomiting.

### *Collaborative care management*

The diagnosis of GTN usually is accomplished by ultrasonography, amniography, and analysis of HCG levels. Other diagnostic tests may be employed to rule out the presence of metastasis.

Suction curettage is the most common method used for evacuation of a molar pregnancy, although hysterectomy may be selected if the woman does not desire future pregnancies. Intravenous oxytocin may be used to assist in expulsion of tissue, which is then sent for extensive pathological analysis. Human chorionic gonadotropin titers are monitored after treatment to assess for recurrence. The woman is advised to postpone pregnancy for at least a year, because pregnancy will cause a rise in HCG levels.[3] Chemotherapy is used in the treatment of recurrent or persistent disease; GTN is extremely sensitive to chemotherapy and is considered to be one of the most curable gynecological malignancies. A 100% cure rate can be expected with low-risk nonmetastatic disease, and even patients with high-risk GTN are successfully treated in more than 70% of cases.[5]

**Patient/family education.** Nursing care of the woman undergoing hysterectomy has been discussed previously. It is essential to address the social and emotional impact of the disease process in the overall plan of care. Patient and family teaching includes an overview of this rather strange disease process, implications for future pregnancies, the effect of chemotherapy on future children, and the need for effective contraception during the first year after diagnosis.

# NEOPLASMS OF THE OVARIES

## Ovarian Cysts

### *Etiology/epidemiology*

Many types of benign tumors affect the ovaries; 80% are classified in the epithelial group, which includes serous, mucinous, endometrial, and mesonephroid lesions. Epithelial tumors are composed of supporting connective tissue and ovarian stroma but also have the capacity to alter the woman's hormonal status. Other types of ovarian neoplasms include simple cysts and nonneoplastic cysts originating in the graafian follicle. Nearly 80% of ovarian tumors are discovered during routine pelvic examination and are asymptomatic.

**box 47-6** *Characteristics of Various Types of Benign Ovarian Cysts and Tumors*

**CYSTS**

**Follicular Cysts**

Most common form of cysts
Frequently multiple; range in size from a few millimeters to as large as 15 cm in diameter
Depend on gonadotropin for growth
Occur during menstrual years and usually resolve spontaneously
May cause menstrual irregularities if blood estrogen elevated

**Corpus Luteum Cysts**

Less common variety
Associated with normal ovarian function or elevated progesterone
Average diameter 4 cm
May appear purplish red from bleeding within corpus luteum
May cause delayed menstrual bleeding from progesterone secretion; menorrhagia common

**Theca Lutein Cysts**

Least common variety
Usually bilateral and produce significant ovarian enlargement, up to 30 cm in diameter
Develop from prolonged or excessive stimulation by gonadotropins
Associated with hydatidiform mole 50% of the time and choriocarcinomas 10% of the time

**EPITHELIAL TUMORS**

**Serous Tumors**

Found in all age groups
Can be extremely large, filling pelvis or abdomen

**Mucinous Tumors**

Occur in second to third decade of life
May be bilateral
Can reach spectacular size; largest form

**Endometroid Tumors**

Small lesions, purplish blue in color
Large tumors called "chocolate cysts" because they contain brownish fluid
Very low malignancy potential

**Mesonephroid Tumors**

Usually multifocal
Involve peritoneal surfaces and may cause intestinal or urinary tract complications
Characterized by papillary proliferations without mitotic activity

Women between ages 45 and 60 are at greatest risk. Each of the various tumor types tends to affect a different age group and behave in a different way.

### Pathophysiology

Benign cysts and tumors develop from a variety of physiological imbalances. Elevated levels of luteinizing hormone may cause hyperstimulation of the ovaries. Follicular cysts depend on gonadotropins for growth and generally occur during the menstrual years and resolve spontaneously. Simple cysts occur commonly during menopause. Box 47-6 summarizes the characteristics of various common types of ovarian cysts and tumors.

Most ovarian tumors are asymptomatic for long periods or produce only nonspecific symptoms. Menstrual irregularities may be present when hormonal imbalance exists. Dull, unilateral, lower quadrant pain may occur, especially as the cyst grows in size, but overt pain is an unusual symptom. Fatigue or a sense of heaviness in the pelvis also may occur. Ascites and increasing abdominal girth have been reported in slender women. Large tumors may cause symptoms of pelvic pressure, such as urinary frequency and constipation.

### Collaborative care management

Palpation of the reproductive organs during pelvic examination commonly reveals the presence of any mass or enlargement of the ovary (Figure 47-15, p. 1566). Any mass palpated in a postmenopausal woman requires further investigation, because the ovaries normally atrophy after menopause. Ultrasonography may be employed to distinguish functional from neoplastic cysts. A CT scan is capable of distinguishing solid tumors, cysts, and ascites, but laparoscopy may be performed to confirm the diagnosis.

Many ovarian cysts resolve spontaneously. If the cyst does not decrease in size, oral contraceptives may be prescribed to shrink it. Surgery is usually recommended only when the cyst is larger than 8 cm or occurs after menopause or before puberty. A cystectomy rather than oophorectomy will be performed if possible.

**Patient/family education.** The woman is reminded of the importance of follow-up care to continue to monitor the tumor's size. Most women are extremely anxious concerning the effects of the tumor on fertility and should be reassured that even oophorectomy does not reduce childbearing potential as long as the second ovary is healthy. If both ovaries are removed, the woman undergoes surgical menopause and needs to receive information concerning estrogen replacement therapy.

## Cancer of the Ovary

### Etiology/epidemiology

Malignant neoplasms of the ovaries occur at all ages, including infancy and childhood. Cancer of the ovary is the fifth most common cancer in women in the United States and has

## clinical pathway *Total Abdominal Hysterectomy*

| | DAY 1 (OR) | DAY 2 | DAY 3 | DAY 4 |
|---|---|---|---|---|
| **ASSESSMENT** *Neurological/ Psychological:* | Mental status • pain via pain scale (severity, quality, location, duration, radiation) • standard for recovery from anesthesia • explore anxiety/coping skills • begin assessment of health care problem • identify available & needed family/human/economic resources to resume independent self-care activities. | Mental status • pain via pain scale (severity, quality, location, duration, radiation) • continue to explore anxiety/coping skills • continue to assess knowledge of health care problem • collaborate w/ social services to identify available & needed family/human/economic resources to resume independent self-care activities. | Mental status • pain via pain scale • continue to explore anxiety/coping skills. | Mental status • pain via pain scale • continue to explore anxiety/coping skills. |
| *Pulmonary:* | Breath sounds. | Breath sounds. | Breath sounds. | Breath sounds. |
| *Cardiovascular:* | VS per postop standard • capillary refill • pulses • Homans' sign. | HR • BP • pulses • Homans' sign. | HR • BP • pulses • Homans' sign. | HR • BP • Homans' sign. |
| *Gastrointestinal:* | Mucous membranes • nausea, vomiting • bowel sounds. | Mucous membranes • nausea, vomiting • bowel sounds • BM. | Nausea, vomiting • BM. | BM. |
| *Genitourinary:* | I & Q • UO > 30 ml/hr • presence of vaginal bleeding/discharge (amt/color/odor). | I & O • UO > 30 ml/hr • presence of vaginal bleeding/discharge (amt/color/odor). | UO qs • bladder distention • presence of vaginal bleeding/discharge (amt/color/odor). | UO qs • presence of vaginal bleeding/discharge (amt/color/odor). |
| *Integumentary:* | Skin turgor, temp, color, & integrity. | Skin turgor, temp, color, & integrity. | Skin turgor & integrity. | Skin integrity. |
| *Surgical Wound:* | Dsg/incision line • amt & type of drainage • S & S of bleeding/hematoma/edema/redness/heat. | Dsg/incision line • amt & type of drainage • S & S of bleeding/hematoma/edema/redness/heat. | Dsg/incision line • amt & type of drainage • S & S of bleeding/hematoma/edema/redness/heat. | Dsg/incision line • amt & type of drainage • S & S of bleeding/hematoma/edema/redness/heat. |
| **FOCUS** | Hemodynamic stability • pain control. | Hemodynamic stability • pain control. | Self-care • discharge plan. | Discharge. |
| **DIAGNOSTIC PLAN** | Postop Hct @ 6 PM | Postop Hct @ 6 PM | Repeat abnormal lab tests. | None. |
| **THERAPEUTIC INTERVENTIONS** | IV fluids to maintain UO >30 ml/hr • antibiotic • analgesic (IV/IM) • antiemetic • NPO, then progress to ice chips (8 hr postop), then clear liquids (16 hr postop) • perineal care & fresh pad q4hr | Continue IV therapy to maintain UO > 30 ml/hr until 6 PM, then discontinue IV line • remove Foley catheter • assist w/ voiding q3hr until voiding independently & in qs • full regular diet | Independent in ADL. | Independent ADL • discharge. |

| | DAY 1 (OR) | DAY 2 | DAY 3 | DAY 4 |
|---|---|---|---|---|
| | • support stockings • cough, deep breathe, & incentive spirometer q2-4h while awake • encourage ankle dorsiflexion exercises q1-2h while awake • OOB to chair this evening & ambulate w/assistance around room • assist w/hygiene. | • encourage PO fluids & document plan for same • OOB & ambulating in hall independently • reapply support stockings bid. *Consider:* iron • Milk of Magnesia/stool softener. | | |
| **PATIENT/FAMILY TEACHING/ DISCHARGE PLANNING** | Teach use of pain scale & review meds available for pain & anxiety • reassure that responses (anxiety, etc.) are a normal reaction • begin to explore threats to femininity/sexuality if Pt appears ready to discuss same • teach to splint incision w/hands, to cough & deep breathe & use incentive spirometer & to do ankle dorsiflexion & extension exercises • review treatment plan • initiate discharge plan • discuss plan for daily review of plan of care w/Pt/family. | Teach wound care (cleanse per standard & apply DSD) • teach to apply support stockings • review discharge plan & home care needs • review, clarify, & confirm information given to date. | Teach self-care strategies (no douche, no Tampax, no sex, no heavy lifting, no vigorous exercise, no prolonged sitting, & no driving for 6 wk or as surgeon indicates) • to expect a small amt of old brown-colored vaginal drainage • to notify surgeon of fever, sudden bright red blood, change in amt/color/odor of drainage, or leg pain/redness/swelling • review wound care, discharge plan, & home care needs • clarify & confirm information given to date • allow time for verbalization of feelings. | Review discharge plan, self-care strategies, S & S to report to physician. |
| **EXPECTED OUTCOMES** | Hemodynamically stable w/no signs of hematoma formation • verbalizes relief of pain w/ analgesia • acknowledges availability of analgesic/anxiolytic, plan of care, & need to communicate w/nurse if S & S of anxiety & fear become overwhelming (subjective feelings, emotional lability, or inability to concentrate) • demonstrates use of incentive spirometer. | Uses fewer doses of prn meds as evidenced by pain scale $< 3$ (0-10) • demonstrates how to splint incision w/hands & cough, deep breathe, & use incentive spirometer • demonstrates ankle dorsiflexion & extension exercises • ambulates freely • verbalizes appropriate anxiety & fears related to surgery. | Urine clear amber & qs • normal BM • verbalizes meds & food/drug interactions • demonstrates wound care & how to apply support stockings • states will notify surgeon for S & S of infection/phlebitis. | Demonstrates wound care • verbalizes self-care strategies, vaginal drainage expectations, S & S to report to physician • states appointment date w/physician • pain well controlled as evidenced by pain scale $< 3$ (0-10). |
| **TRIGGER(S)** | Hemodynamic instability • nausea & vomiting. | Persistent nausea & vomiting • UO $< 30$ ml/hr. | Persistent nausea & vomiting. | Unable to provide self-care. |

From Birdsall C, Sperry S: *Clinical paths in medical surgical nursing,* St Louis, 1997, Mosby.

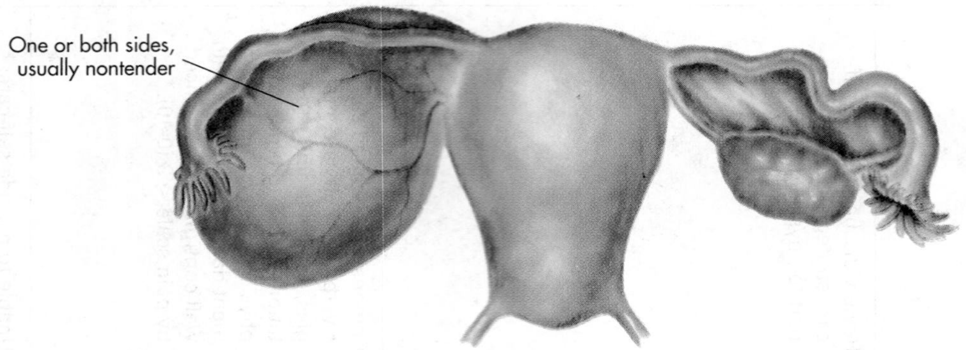


fig. 47-15 Ovarian cyst.

the highest mortality rate of the gynecological cancers. Overall, about 22,000 new cases are diagnosed each year, and about 60% of these patients die within 5 years of diagnosis because the disease is usually widespread before it is diagnosed.[3]

The etiology of ovarian cancer is not understood, but several factors appear to be associated with its incidence. Age is an important factor, and the disease occurs most commonly in the fifth and sixth decades of life. Hereditary, endocrine, environmental, dietary factors, and viral agents have all been implicated in the etiology of cancer of the ovary. Those at highest risk appear to be middle-class and upper-class women, nulliparous women, and women who have not used oral contraceptives.[3] Early age at first pregnancy, early menopause, and the use of oral contraceptives appear to have a protective effect. If a woman has had breast cancer, her chances of developing ovarian cancer double. Incidence rates are high in industrialized areas, which points to environmental influences. Exposure to talc and asbestos, diets high in meat and animal fat, and high milk consumption all appear to be linked to a higher incidence. The fat content of the milk appears to be the important variable. A slight familial link has been found, and unusual clusters of breast and ovarian cancers in family groups have been identified.[32]

The survival rate is 87% when the disease is diagnosed and treated early, but only about 23% of cases are detected in localized stages. Survival rates for women with regional and distant metastases are 39% and 19%, respectively.[2]

### Pathophysiology

*Ovarian cancer* is a broad term that can be divided into many categories depending on the cell type of origin. The major histological types occur in distinctive age ranges. The four main types are described in Table 47-9. Malignant germ cell tumors are most common in women under age 20, whereas epithelial cancers are primarily seen in women over age 50 and account for approximately 90% of all ovarian malignancies.[3]

The clinical manifestations of advancing disease include pelvic discomfort, low back pain, weight change, abdominal pain, nausea and vomiting, constipation, and urinary frequency. Any ovarian enlargement should be evaluated for malignancy. Palpable ovaries in premenarchal or postmenopausal women are abnormal physical findings.

**table 47-9** *Classification of Ovarian Neoplasms*

| Source of Neoplasm | Examples |
|---|---|
| Epithelium | Serous, mucinous, endometroid |
| Germ cell | Teratoma (mature and immature), dysgerminoma |
| Gonadal stroma | Granulosa (theca, Sertoli's, Leydig's cells) |
| Mesenchyme | Fibroma, lymphoma, sarcoma |

### Collaborative care management

The early diagnosis of an ovarian neoplasm usually occurs by chance rather than successful screening. No useful screening test exists at present for widespread use. Even ultrasonography, CT scanning, and MRI are not sufficiently specific to distinguish between benign and malignant tumors.

Although the use of transvaginal ultrasonography improves the recognition of early malignancies, both abdominal and transvaginal ultrasound are usually inadequate to confirm the diagnosis. CA-125, a tumor marker produced by tissues derived from the coelomic epithelium, is produced by about 80% of epithelial tumors,[32] but because other tumors also produce the marker and false-negative results are common, the test is not specific enough to be diagnostic. A variety of other tests may be employed in the search for metastasis.

Laparotomy is the primary tool for both diagnosis and staging. Ovarian cancer is surgically staged rather than clinically staged; Table 47-10 presents the staging system. Surgery is the primary therapeutic approach and usually involves total abdominal hysterectomy with bilateral salpingectomyoophorectomy. Ascitic fluid or washings are submitted for cytology. All the tissue of the pelvis is carefully assessed, and biopsies of any suspicious tissue are sent for analysis.

**table 47-10** *Stages of Cancer of the Ovary*

| STAGE | INVOLVEMENT |
|---|---|
| I | Limited to ovaries |
| II | Involving one or both ovaries with pelvic extension |
| III | Involving one or both ovaries with intraperitoneal metastasis outside pelvis or positive lymph nodes |
| IV | Involving one or both ovaries with distant metastasis (e.g., liver, lungs) |

Adjuvant therapy is often employed based on the stage of the disease. Chemotherapy is typically used for stage I disease, and various combinations of agents are under investigation. Patients with stage II disease may be treated with instillation of radioactive phosphorus ($^{32}P$) into the peritoneum, external irradiation, or combined chemotherapy. Patients with stages III and IV disease undergo surgical attempts to remove as much tumor as possible. This intervention appears to be directly related to survival. Surgery is followed by aggressive combination chemotherapy.

**Patient/family education.** The patient receives the standard postoperative teaching appropriate for any major abdominal surgery. Patient teaching concerning the diagnosis, surgery, and adjuvant therapy for ovarian cancer is an integral aspect of nursing care. Support and education are offered to the patient and family throughout each aspect of diagnosis and treatment. Cancer of the ovary carries a poor prognosis, and the woman and her family will need ongoing support.

## NEOPLASMS OF THE VULVA

### Cancer of the Vulva

#### *Etiology/epidemiology*

Vulvar cancer is rare, and invasive disease accounts for just 5% of malignancies of the female genital tract. It is a disease that primarily affects older women with a mean age at onset of 61 years.[36] Preinvasive disease (vulvar carcinoma in situ) is occurring more commonly in younger women, possibly because of factors such as exposure to human papillomavirus and HIV. Three times as many whites are affected as blacks. Parity does not seem to play a role in the incidence.

The exact etiology of cancer of the vulva is still unknown. Etiological factors are believed to include STDs involving the vulva and the use of tight-fitting apparel or nylon undergarments, perineal deodorants, and trauma. Herpes, syphilis, and other lesions have all been associated with the development of carcinoma. Immunosuppression, diabetes, smoking, and hypertension also have been linked, but a cause-and-effect relationship has not been established.

#### *Pathophysiology*

Most cancers of the vulva are squamous in origin (90%). The initial lesion often arises from an area of intraepithelial neoplasia, which can eventually form a firm nodule and ulcerate. The diagnosis of vulvar cancer can be made only by biopsy and histological tissue examination.

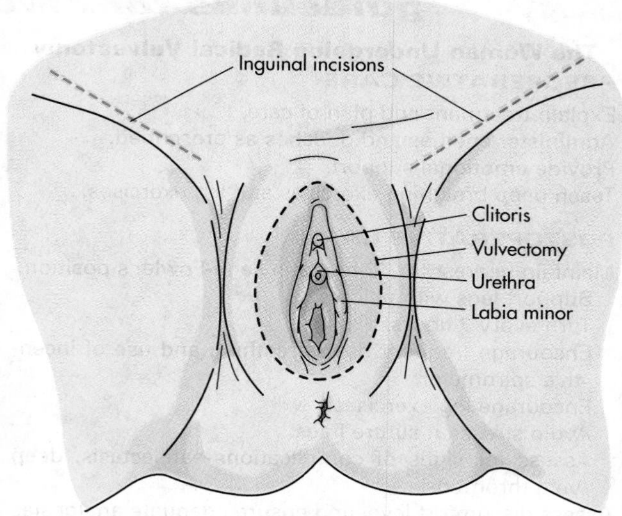


**fig. 47-16** Vulvectomy with operative incision lines shown. Note groin incisions.

The lesion can develop anywhere on the vulva, but 70% of lesions arise on the labia. The lesion is usually localized and well demarcated. Common clinical manifestations include vulvar itching and burning.

#### *Collaborative care management*

Treatment of carcinoma of the vulva varies significantly based on the location and extent of the disease. Preinvasive disease is usually treated surgically, although colposcopy-guided laser therapy has become more common.[36] Carcinoma in situ may also be treated nonsurgically with topical 5-fluorouracil (1% Efudex) applied daily, but long-term results are unknown. The standard treatment for invasive carcinoma has been radical vulvectomy, although the procedure has been modified for women with certain types of lesions to make it less mutilating. Radical vulvectomy involves excision of the mons pubis, terminal portion of the urethra, and vagina; excision of portions of the round ligaments and saphenous veins; and selected lymph node dissection (Figure 47-16). Radical surgery achieves a 70% to 80% 5-year survival rate.[3] Radiation treatment for advanced disease is being researched.[26] Chemotherapy has not proved useful.[36]

Complications related to radical vulvectomy include wound infection and disruption because the wounds are typically left open to heal by secondary intention. Delayed complications include stenosis of the vagina from scar tissue formation, pelvic muscle relaxation leading to stress incontinence, and swelling of the legs from obstructive lymphangitis.

Postoperative care focuses initially on comfort. Because of the widespread tissue destruction, the inguinal suture line is very tight and extremely uncomfortable. The woman needs frequent assistance to achieve a comfortable position. Wound breakdown is often a problem. The vulvar wound is usually left open, and sitz baths, whirlpool therapy, and topical agents may be used to support healing.

**guidelines for care**

**The Woman Undergoing Radical Vulvectomy**

**PREOPERATIVE CARE**

Explain treatment and plan of care.
Administer enemas and douches as prescribed.
Provide emotional support.
Teach deep breathing exercises and leg exercises.

**POSTOPERATIVE CARE**

Maintain bedrest for 72 hours in semi-Fowler's position.
- Support legs with pillows.
- Turn every 2 hours.
- Encourage frequent deep breathing and use of incentive spirometer.
- Encourage leg exercises.
- Avoid stress on suture lines.
- Assess for signs of complications—atelectasis, deep vein thrombosis.

Assess discomfort level and ensure adequate analgesia.
- Use a PCA pump if possible to allow patient to control dosage.

Monitor wound healing.
- Provide perineal hygiene and give sitz baths when ordered; keep perineum dry.
- Cleanse wound bid and after defecation.
- Maintain patency of Foley catheter.

Provide low-residue diet.
Provide diversional activities.
Encourage expression of feelings.

**DISCHARGE TEACHING**

Use support hose for 6 months; elevate legs frequently.
Can resume sexual activity in 4 to 6 weeks.
Discuss possible need for lubrication and position changes with coitus; genital numbness may be present.
Avoid straining with defecation.
Discuss signs and symptoms of complications to report to physician.
Note the possible altered directional flow of urine.

**Patient/family education.** The nurse teaches the patient that despite meticulous care the wounds heal very slowly and complications may occur. The nurse encourages the woman to express her feelings concerning this difficult and disfiguring surgery. The woman is reassured that sexual intercourse usually can be resumed after complete wound healing has occurred—usually at least 6 weeks. Lymphedema in the legs is treated with compression stockings for at least 6 months after surgery. The warning signs of other complications are discussed with the woman before discharge. The Guidelines for Care Box summarizes nursing care for patients experiencing radical vulvectomy.

## STERILIZATION

### ETIOLOGY/EPIDEMIOLOGY

Voluntary sterilization is the most commonly used method of fertility control for married couples over 30 years of age and is the most widely used contraceptive method worldwide. In the United States about 1 million sterilization procedures are performed annually; approximately one third of these are performed on men.[3] The primary reasons given are the desire to limit family size and the desire to be free of the risk of pregnancy with advancing age.

About 1% of sterilized women subsequently request reversal. The rate of successful reversal is approximately 75% after laparoscopic band procedures. Microsurgical techniques are used, and the surgery typically involves an end-to-end anastomosis of the ligated tubes. Success depends partly on the nature of the original surgery, and successful reversal occurs in only 40% to 60% of all cases (Table 47-11).[3]

### PATHOPHYSIOLOGY

Tubal sterilization terminates a woman's ability to bear children but does not alter ovarian hormone secretion or menstrual functioning. Artificial menopause is not induced, and the ability to enjoy intercourse should not be impaired. Women appear to have little regret after the surgery if they understand what to expect during and after the procedure and are able to express their feelings and have their questions answered before surgery. Occasionally, however, women who are ambivalent about the choice or have preexisting self-esteem issues develop psychological problems after sterilization.

### COLLABORATIVE CARE MANAGEMENT

Tubal sterilization was first performed in 1823, and since that time more than 200 different techniques for the procedure have been developed. Most methods involve the mechanical removal of a part of the female reproductive system so that the sperm and ovum cannot unite. Table 47-11 summarizes available methods of sterilization. Minilaparotomy and laparoscopy are by far the most common.

In the minilaparotomy, a small (2 to 3 cm) transverse abdominal incision is made about 3 cm above the pubis and the peritoneal cavity is entered. The fallopian tubes are located, and a portion of each tube is elevated and ligated at the base. The free ends may be tied off or cauterized. Minilaparotomy is an ambulatory procedure performed under local anesthesia.

Laparoscopic tubal sterilization is more common and requires only a small subumbilical incision for insertion of the laparoscope. A segment of each tube is coagulated by application of an electric current. Clips or rings may also be applied to the tube. The procedure is brief and safe and is performed under local anesthesia.

The laws governing sterilization vary from state to state and have undergone many changes over the years. In general, the surgery may be performed if written, informed consent is given by a woman capable of giving permission. Patients using federal funds for payment must be at least 21 years of age, and there may be a prescribed waiting period for patients using Medicaid funds.

#### Patient/Family Education

Patient teaching is the foundation of nursing care. The discussion of sterilization methods should be based on

**table 47-11** *Methods of Tubal Sterilization for Women*

| Description | Comments |
|---|---|
| **ABDOMINAL** | |
| **Minilaparotomy** | |
| Ligation or cutting of fallopian tubes under direct vision through small abdominal incision | Local or general anesthesia<br>Complications: wound infection, hematoma, bladder injury<br>Advantages: good chance for sterility reversal |
| **Laparoscopy** | |
| Electrocoagulation of segment of fallopian tubes by laparoscopy through small abdominal incision | Local or general anesthesia<br>Advantages: minimal discomfort, short procedure |
| **VAGINAL** | |
| **Culpotomy** | |
| Ligation or cutting of fallopian tube through small incision in cul-de-sac of Douglas | Local, spinal, or general anesthesia<br>Higher complication rate than laparoscopy (infection, hemorrhage) |
| **Culdoscopy** | |
| Electrocoagulation of segment of fallopian tubes by culdoscope through small incision in cul-de-sac of Douglas | Local anesthesia<br>Higher complication rate than laparoscopy |

the federal government's informed consent guidelines (Box 47-7). The nurse confirms that the woman understands the nature and consequences of the surgical procedure. The facts concerning reversibility, including current success rates, are discussed. Many people equate sterilization with a loss of femininity, and even women who know the difference may appreciate reassurance.

Postoperatively, the woman is instructed to rest for 24 to 48 hours after the procedure and avoid all heavy lifting and strenuous exercise for 1 week. The nurse instructs the woman to abstain from sexual intercourse until the wound is completely healed and to report any signs of fever, incisional bleeding, or persistent abdominal pain to the physician. (Care of the woman after a laparoscopic procedure is discussed in Chapter 46.)

## INFERTILITY

The term *infertility* refers to the inability to achieve a pregnancy within a stipulated period of time, usually 1 year. The problem may be considered primary if the couple has never conceived or secondary if conception was successfully achieved in the past.

**box 47-7** *Informed Consent Guidelines (Federal) Relating to Sterilization*

1. Choice is made by patient. No pressures are placed on choice (e.g., loss of welfare benefits, wrath of health care provider).
2. Benefits and risks of sterilization are described:
   a. Benefits: permanent, no further costs or decision making
   b. Risks: usual surgical risks, possibility of future pregnancy (i.e., not 100% effective)
3. Alternative contraceptive methods are described.
4. Patient is encouraged to ask questions.
5. Patient may withdraw from using the method without penalty.
6. Explanations are given about the entire sterilization procedure, costs, and possible side effects (effects of hormones, weight changes, menstrual changes, sexual response).
7. Written instructions and risk factors are given to patient.
8. A written consent to the procedure is signed by patient and witnessed.

### ETIOLOGY/EPIDEMIOLOGY

An estimated 10% to 15% of all couples in the United States are infertile. This number reflects both delayed childbearing and an increase in the number of women between the ages of 25 and 44 years.[31] Infertility is most often attributed to women, but about 40% of cases result from male infertility and 20% from both partners.[31] More couples today are seeking infertility treatment, despite its high costs. Approximately 50% of the couples who undergo assessment and treatment for infertility successfully conceive.[3]

From 80% to 90% of all women become pregnant within 1 year when they practice unprotected intercourse. Fertility in women is low during the early teenage years, peaks in the midtwenties, and declines after age 30. Approximately 33% of women who delay pregnancy until after age 35 experience problems with infertility. This rate increases to 60% after age 40. Fertility in men also reaches its peak in the midtwenties and subsequently declines, but the decrease is much less significant than in women. The frequency of coitus is another recognized variable in fertility because increased frequency appears to enhance sperm motility.

### PATHOPHYSIOLOGY

Three basic categories of infertility account for 95% of reproductive dysfunction: anovulation,[3] anatomical defects of the female genital tract, and abnormal sperm production. See Box 47-8 for common causes of infertility in men and women. No cause can be found in 10% to 20% of cases.

Ovulatory dysfunction is a leading cause of infertility. It can result from a malfunction at any point in the hormonal feedback system. Fallopian tube obstruction is a common structural defect. Acute salpingitis from gonorrhea or chlamydial infection is the most common cause of this obstruction. Pelvic infections, use of IUDs, and endometriosis can also cause fallopian tube obstruction.

Infection may destroy the glands that secrete the thin, watery mucus essential for sperm survival and migration. Estrogen deficiency may decrease the volume and quality of the cervical mucus. Anomalies of the uterus, including the presence of leiomyomas, may interfere with successful implantation.

Problems of sperm production account for about 40% of infertility cases.[3] Various causes of male infertility are outlined in Box 47-8.

A number of studies suggest that tobacco may be a causal factor in infertility. Nicotine appears to adversely affect tubal transport and implantation. Mycoplasma, which causes cervicitis, may contribute to infertility, and the role of other viruses is under investigation. Dietary deficiencies are known to adversely affect secretion of pituitary gonadotropins, and strenuous exercise such as running more than 10 miles per week has been implicated in infertility, either through its caloric demands or the effects of endorphins on the pituitary.

Infertility can produce profound psychological effects. When couples find themselves unable to have children, the trauma can affect every aspect of their lives and marriage. The experience of diagnosis and treatment can be an emotional roller coaster of raised expectations and dashed hopes.

## COLLABORATIVE CARE MANAGEMENT

The purposes of an infertility evaluation are to establish the cause of infertility and provide a basis for determining medical or surgical treatment options. The process can be physically painful, as well as emotionally and economically stressful. The various diagnostic tests used in the diagnosis of infertility are discussed in Chapter 46 and summarized in Table 47-12.

Artificial insemination is a simple, safe, inexpensive, and highly successful infertility treatment when male infertility is the cause. Semen may be deposited by a cervical-vaginal route, intracervically, or intrauterine. A few drops of semen are injected as close to the time of ovulation as possible. Treatment may use the partner's semen (homologous) or donor semen (heterologous). The fertility of donors is carefully de-

**box 47-8** *Causes of Infertility*

**FEMALE**

1. Developmental: uterine abnormalities
2. Endocrine: pituitary, thyroid, and adrenal dysfunctions, ovarian dysfunctions (inhibit maturation and release of ova)
3. Diseases: PID (especially from gonococcus), fallopian tube obstructions, diseases of cervix and uterus that inhibit passage of active sperm
4. Other: malnutrition, severe anemia, anxiety

**MALE**

1. Developmental: undescended testes, other congenital anomalies (inhibit development of sperm)
2. Endocrine: hormonal deficiencies (pituitary, thyroid, adrenal) (inhibit development of sperm)
3. Diseases: testicular destruction from disease, orchitis from mumps, prostatitis
4. Other: excessive smoking, fatigue, alcohol, excessive heat (hot baths), marijuana use

**BOTH FEMALE AND MALE**

1. Diseases: STDs, cancer-causing obstructions (inhibit transport of ovum or sperm)
2. Other: immunological incompatibility (inhibit sperm penetration of ovum), marital problems
3. Diethylstilbestrol exposure in utero (suggested but not proved as a cause of male infertility)

**table 47-12** *Diagnostic Testing for Infertility*

| Gender | Tests | Data Obtained |
|---|---|---|
| Male | Semen analysis | Determine presence, number, and motility of sperm |
| | Testicular biopsy if sperm count low or absent | Presence of sperm indicates obstruction of vas deferens |
| Female | Basal body temperature chart | Determine that ovulation is occurring |
| | Postcoital test of cervical secretions | Measure ability of sperm to penetrate cervical mucus and remain active; determine quality of mucus |
| | Endometrial biopsy | Determine whether ovulation is occurring (if in question) |
| | Laparoscopy | Examine the pelvis and determine patency of fallopian tubes |
| | Hysterosalpingography (x-ray film after insertion of contrast media) | Determine patency of uterus and fallopian tubes |
| Male/female | Hormonal tests | Determine whether problem is hormonal |

termined, and the sperm are screened for HIV. This can be an emotional topic for some couples and may induce strong reactions.

In the last decade a virtual explosion of reproductive technology has occurred. These procedures, known as assisted reproductive technologies (ARTs), are expensive and rarely covered by insurance plans in the United States.[3,13] Box 47-9 summarizes other, less commonly employed approaches to infertility.

The correction of structural problems is undertaken first if feasible. Transcervical balloon tuboplasty (TBT) may be performed to correct blocked or scarred fallopian tubes. A modified cardiovascular balloon is passed into the fallopian tube and inflated to clear the occlusion.

A variety of drugs can be used to induce or support ovulation. Clomiphene citrate (Clomid, Serophene) is used for women with intact pituitary function. Pergonal and Metrodin are used when patients have pituitary dysfunction, HCG may be used to trigger the release of mature follicles, and progesterone preparations may be used for luteal phase support. The drugs may also be combined.

Multiple births can occur with ovulatory induction therapy. The onset of low abdominal pain can indicate the development of an ovarian cyst or cyst rupture. The woman is informed of the multiple-drug side effects, which include hot flashes, emotional lability and depression, fatigue, nausea, and bloating.

Problems of sperm production are addressed by first eliminating alterations of thermoregulation. Optimal sperm production occurs at temperatures approximately 1° to 3° F below body temperature. The man is instructed to avoid sitting for long periods of time in hot tubs, wearing tight clothes that pull the testicles against the body, and sitting for long periods of time with poor heat dispersion. Clomid can also be used to stimulate sperm production, but it is successful only about 20% of the time.[3]

Traditional drug therapy may be combined with intrauterine insemination (IUI). This approach has achieved a success rate comparable with that of in vitro fertilization, approximately 20%.

**box 47-9** *Alternative Approaches to Infertility Management*

**IN VITRO FERTILIZATION AND EMBRYO TRANSFER**

One or more ova are recovered from the ovarian follicles and fertilized with the partner's sperm in a Petri dish. Oocyte retrieval is performed by means of ultrasound-guided needle aspiration. The cleaved ova are placed in the patient's uterus through a small catheter about 48 hours after retrieval. Pregnancy rates are related to the number of embryos placed and vary from 18% to 30%.

**GAMETE INTRAFALLOPIAN TRANSFER (GIFT)**

Oocytes aspirated from follicles are mixed with washed sperm and placed in the uterine tube via laparoscopy. This approach appears to achieve a higher pregnancy rate than in vitro fertilization. The preembryo travels toward the uterus, following the natural timetable for implantation in 4 days.

**ZYGOTE INTRAFALLOPIAN TRANSFER (ZIFT) AND TUBAL EMBRYO TRANSFER (TET)**

These procedures are similar to GIFT except transfer to the fallopian tubes occurs at the zygote stage, about 16 to 18 hours after oocyte insemination. TET involves transfer of embryos into the fallopian tube around 40 to 48 hours after oocyte insemination.

**SURROGATE MOTHERS**

Surrogate mothers are women who contract to conceive by artificial insemination and give the baby to the semen donor after delivery. Many social and legal implications with the process have received recent attention through some extremely public lawsuits over custody of the child.

**OVUM TRANSFER**

A donor provides the ovum, which is fertilized with the partner's sperm. The embryo is transferred to the infertile woman's uterus after about 5 days via a small catheter. Pregnancy rates have been as high as 25% to 50%.

### Patient/Family Education

Infertility can produce profound psychological effects. The nurse is challenged to assist couples to be active participants in the entire infertility workup and treatment plan, carefully exploring their own feelings about the limits they wish to set on the attempt to become pregnant. Sexual dysfunction often occurs, because this formerly pleasurable and spontaneous private activity becomes a public process to be dissected and often used as a measure of their success or failure concerning pregnancy. The nurse encourages the honest expression of feelings and provides time for dealing with the couple's intense feelings during treatment.

Nurses also play an important role in promoting fertility. Patient teaching aimed at preventing infection of the pelvic organs, particularly with gonorrhea and chlamydia, is critical. Salpingitis is often the first overt sign of gonorrhea infection and can result in obstruction of the fallopian tubes. Early diagnosis and effective treatment of all vaginal and cervical infections is critical. The nurse encourages the use of barrier contraceptives, which help reduce the risk of infection, and encourages the woman to limit the number of her sexual partners. Women with ovarian and hormonal problems commonly experience symptoms such as menstrual irregularities. Many of these problems can be successfully managed with hormone therapy if identified early before problems with infertility develop.

**critical thinking QUESTIONS**

1 You have been asked to speak to a group of high school students about women's health issues. How would you address the issues of personal

responsibility related to the development of PID, cervical cancer, and infertility?

**2** Megan Jeffries is completing intracavitary radiation treatment for early cervical cancer. You are beginning her discharge teaching related to vaginal fibrosis when she breaks into tears. She says, "How will we ever resume sexual intercourse? I stink, this drainage is disgusting, and my husband will never find me attractive again." How will you respond?

**3** Of the following individuals, who is at *highest* risk for developing a vaginal infection? (1) A 22-year-old nulliparous woman taking oral contraceptives; (2) a 35-year-old pregnant woman who has diabetes and is receiving ampicillin for a leg ulcer; or (3) a 49-year-old premenopausal woman using vaginal creams and suppositories for birth control. Why?

**4** A 38-year-old woman is admitted to the emergency department with a fever of 102° F and a sunburn-type skin reaction of the face. What should be the nurse's *first* assessment priority?

## chapter SUMMARY

### INFECTIOUS PROCESSES

- Many organisms play a role in the development of infections of the vulva and vagina. Women may be predisposed to infection as a result of malnutrition, aging, and decreased resistance.
- The clinical manifestations of vaginal infections include tissue inflammation; discharge from the vagina, urethra, or Bartholin's glands; and pruritus. Each organism also produces signs and symptoms specific to that organism.
- Associated risk factors for vaginal infections include pregnancy, premenarchal age, menopausal and postmenopausal status, allergies, diabetes, oral contraceptives, inadequate hygiene, excessive douching or use of vaginal inserts, treatment with broad-spectrum antibiotics, and intercourse with an infected partner.
- *Candida albicans* causes most cases of fungal vaginitis. Approximately 25% of women are colonized with the organism, but it becomes an opportunistic pathogen only when the normal ecosystem of the vagina is disturbed.
- Treatment of vaginal infections involves oral or intravaginal antibiotic therapy. Many drugs are now available as over-the-counter agents.
- Pelvic inflammatory disease is an infectious process involving the fallopian tubes, ovaries, pelvic peritoneum, pelvic veins, or pelvic connective tissue.
- Women need to be informed about methods to prevent infection, how to recognize infection in their sexual partners, and what to do when they suspect infection has occurred. Prompt treatment is essential.
- Signs and symptoms of acute PID include severe abdominal pain, lower abdominal cramps, intermenstrual spotting, dyspareunia, fever and chills, malaise, nausea and vomiting, and a foul-smelling purulent vaginal discharge.
- Women with TSS are treated with beta-lactamase–resistant antistaphylococcal antibiotics for 10 to 14 days.

### DISORDERS OF MENSTRUATION

- The menstrual cycle is usually 26 to 36 days but may be altered by changes in climate, changes in working hours, emotional trauma, fatigue, exercise, illness, and surgery.
- Premenstrual syndrome occurs in about 40% of all menstruating women; symptoms include behavioral changes, fatigue, signs of water and sodium retention, palpitations, headache, increased appetite, joint pain, and backache.
- Primary dysmenorrhea is caused by high levels of prostaglandin and can be treated with antiprostaglandins, many of which are now available without a prescription.
- Amenorrhea is classified as primary or secondary and results from a variety of causes.

### STRUCTURAL PROBLEMS

- Nonsurgical care for a patient with a cystocele or rectocele includes teaching Kegel exercises, diet management to decrease weight, prevention of constipation, psychological support, and possible instruction about use and care of a pessary.
- Postoperative nursing care after vaginal or perineal surgery includes perineal care after elimination, use of sitz baths, prevention of constipation, maintaining patency of Foley catheter, ice packs for perineal discomfort, and avoidance of Valsalva's maneuver.

### BENIGN AND MALIGNANT NEOPLASMS OF THE FEMALE REPRODUCTIVE TRACT

- Factors placing the woman at risk for developing cancer of the cervix include first coitus at an early age, multiple sexual partners, low socioeconomic group, and exposure to herpesvirus type 2.
- The incidence of and death rate associated with invasive cervical cancer can continue to be reduced through adequate screening using the Pap smear.
- Treatment for invasive cancer of the cervix depends on the stage of the disease. Surgery and radiation therapy are the most commonly used methods.
- Factors placing the woman at risk for developing cancer of the endometrium include obesity, nulliparity, late menopause, diabetes mellitus, hypertension, and the use of exogenous estrogens.
- Any postmenopausal woman with vaginal bleeding should be encouraged to seek medical advice.
- Treatment for endometrial cancer usually involves abdominal hysterectomy.
- No known risk factors are associated with ovarian cancer; nonspecific risk factors include family history and environmental factors.
- Treatment for ovarian cancer usually includes extensive debulking surgery followed by chemotherapy.
- The usual treatment for invasive cancer of the vulva is a radical vulvectomy.

### STERILIZATION

- Sterilization is the most widely used contraceptive method worldwide. Methods of female sterilization include abdominal tubal sterilization by minilaparotomy and laparoscopy and vaginal tubal sterilization (rarely performed) by culpotomy and culdoscopy.

## INFERTILITY

- Infertility affects 10% to 15% of all couples in the United States. Tests for men include multiple semen examination, hormonal tests, and testicular biopsy. Tests for women include the basal body temperature chart, postcoital test, endometrial biopsy, laparoscopy, hysterosalpingography, and hormonal tests.
- The incidence of infertility gradually increases in women after age 30.
- In the United States, approximately 10% to 15% of cases of infertility are caused by anovulation, 30% to 40% by an abnormality of semen production, 30% to 40% by pelvic disease, 10% to 15% by abnormalities of sperm transport through the cervical canal, and about 5% by uncommon causes.
- The technique of in vitro fertilization with embryo transfer is now being widely used to treat infertile couples.

## References


1. Baker V, Andreyko J: Amenorrhea. In Brown J, Crombleholme W, editors: *Handbook of gynecology and obstetrics,* Norwalk, Conn, 1993, Appleton & Lange.
2. Barbieri R, Ryan K: The menstrual cycle. In Ryan J, Berkowitz R, Barbieri R, editors: *Kistner's gynecology,* ed 6, St Louis, 1995, Mosby.
3. Beckman C et al: *Obstetrics and gynecology,* Baltimore, 1995, Williams & Wilkins.
4. Bengtson J: The vagina. In Ryan K, Berkowitz R, Barbieri R, editors: *Kistner's gynecology,* ed 6, St Louis, 1995, Mosby.
5. Berkowitz R, Goldstein D: Gestational trophoblastic diseases. In Ryan K, Berkowitz R, Barbieri R, editors: *Kistner's gynecology,* ed 6, St Louis, 1995, Mosby.
6. Bollen L et al: Human papilloma-virus DNA after treatment of cervical dysplasia: low prevalence in normal cytologic smears, *Cancer* 77(12):2538, 1996.
7. Brown J, Crombleholme W: *Handbook of gynecology and obstetrics,* Norwalk, Conn, 1993, Appleton & Lange.
8. Bychkov V, Isaacs J: *Pathology in the practice of gynecology,* St Louis, 1995, Mosby.
9. Centers for Disease Control and Prevention: 1998 Guidelines for treatment of sexually transmitted diseases, *MMWR* 47:RR-1, 1998.
10. Clark-Coller T: Dysfunctional uterine bleeding and amenorrhea: differential diagnosis and management, *J Nurse Midwife* 36(1):49, 1991.
11. Darwood M: Pelvic pain and dysmenorrhea. In Jacobs A, Gast M, editors: *Practical gynecology,* Norwalk, Conn, 1994, Appleton & Lange.
12. Dorr C: Relaxation of pelvic support. In DeCherney A, Pernoll M, editors: *Current obstetric and gynecologic diagnosis and treatment,* ed 8, Norwalk, Conn, 1994, Appleton & Lange.
13. Gast M: Evaluation of the infertile couple. In Jacobs A, Gast M, editors: *Practical gynecology,* Norwalk, Conn, 1994, Appleton & Lange.
14. Gerbic M: Complications of menstruation: abnormal uterine bleeding. In DeCherney A, Pernoll M, editors: *Current obstetric and gynecologic diagnosis and treatment,* ed 8, Norwalk, Conn, 1994, Appleton & Lange.
15. Goodman A, Hill E: Premalignant and malignant disorders of the uterine cervix. In DeCherney A, Pernoll M, editors: *Current obstetric and gynecologic diagnosis and treatment,* ed 8, Norwalk, Conn, 1994, Appleton & Lange.
16. Hawkins J, Roberto-Nichols D, Stanley-Haney J: *Protocols for nurse practitioners in gynecologic settings,* New York, 1995, Tiresias Press.
17. Hemsell D: Pelvic infections. In Jacobs A, Gast M, editors: *Practical gynecology,* Norwalk, Conn, 1994, Appleton & Lange.
18. Herzog T, Match D: Complications of gynecologic surgery. In Jacobs A, Gast M, editors: *Practical gynecology,* Norwalk, Conn, 1994, Appleton & Lange.
19. Hill E, Pernoll M: Benign disorders of the uterine cervix. In DeCherney A, Pernoll M, editors: *Current obstetric and gynecologic diagnosis and treatment,* ed 8, Norwalk, Conn, 1994, Appleton & Lange.
20. Hornstein M, Barbieri R: Endometriosis. In Ryan J, Berkowitz R, Barbieri R, editors: *Kistner's gynecology,* ed 6, St Louis, 1995, Mosby.
21. Kaufman R: Diseases of the vulva and vagina. In Lemcke D et al, editors: *Primary care of women,* Norwalk, Conn, 1995, Appleton & Lange.
22. Khan Z, Nagler H, Johnson M: Urogynecology. In Jacobs A, Gast M, editors: *Practical gynecology,* Norwalk, Conn, 1994, Appleton & Lange.
23. Klock S: Psychosomatic issues in obstetrics and gynecology. In Ryan J, Berkowitz R, Barbieri R, editors: *Kistner's gynecology,* ed 6, St Louis, 1995, Mosby.
24. Klotz M: Dysmenorrhea, endometriosis and pelvic pain. In Lemcke D et al, editors: *Primary care of women,* Norwalk, Conn, 1995, Appleton & Lange.
25. Muntz H: Cervical cancer screening and management of the abnormal Papanicolaou smear. In Lemcke D et al, editors: *Primary care of women,* Norwalk, Conn, 1995, Appleton & Lange.
26. Muto M, Friedman A: The uterine corpus. In Ryan K, Berkowitz R, Barbieri R, editors: *Kistner's gynecology,* ed 6, St Louis, 1995, Mosby.
27. Nichols D, Randall C: *Vaginal surgery,* Baltimore, 1996, Williams & Wilkins.
28. O'Quinn A, Barnard D: Gestational trophoblastic disease. In DeCherney A, Pernoll M, editors: *Current obstetric and gynecologic diagnosis and treatment,* ed 8, Norwalk, Conn, 1994, Appleton & Lange.
29. Pearl M: Endometrial cancer. In Brown J, Crombleholme W, editors: *Handbook of gynecology and obstetrics,* Norwalk, Conn, 1993, Appleton & Lange.
30. Ramin S, Wendel G, Hemsell D: Sexually transmitted diseases and pelvic infections. In DeCherney A, Pernoll M, editors: *Current obstetric and gynecologic diagnosis and treatment,* ed 8, Norwalk, Conn, 1994, Appleton & Lange.
31. Rein M, Schiff I: Evaluation of the infertile couple. In Ryan K, Berkowitz R, Barbieri R, editors: *Kistner's gynecology,* ed 6, St Louis, 1995, Mosby.
32. Rice L, Barbieri R: The ovary. In Ryan K, Berkowitz R, Barbieri R, editors: *Kistner's gynecology,* ed 6, St Louis, 1995, Mosby.
33. Scholes D, Dailing J, Stergachis A: Current cigarette smoking and risk of acute pelvic inflammatory disease, *Am J Public Health* 82:1352, 1992.
34. Schwartz B: Benign vaginal and cervical disorders. In Jacobs A, Gast M, editors: *Practical gynecology,* Norwalk, Conn, 1994, Appleton & Lange.
35. Sheets E, Goodman H: The cervix. In Ryan K, Berkowitz R, Barbieri R, editors: *Kistner's gynecology,* ed 6, St Louis, 1995, Mosby.
36. Sillman F, Muta M: The vulva. In Ryan K, Berkowitz R, Barbieri R, editors: *Kistner's gynecology,* ed 6, St Louis, 1995, Mosby.
37. Sweet R: Acute salpingitis and treatment. In Mead P, Hager W, editors: *Infection protocols for obstetrics and gynecology,* Montvale, NJ, 1992, Medical Economics.

38. Sweet R: Role of bacterial vaginosis in pelvic inflammatory disease, *Clin Infect Dis* 20(suppl 2):271, 1995.
39. Tishman V: Disorders of pelvic support. In Brown J, Crombleholme W, editors: *Handbook of gynecology and obstetrics,* Norwalk, Conn, 1993, Appleton & Lange.
40. Tuomala R: Gynecologic infections. In Ryan K, Berkowitz R, Barbieri R, editors: *Kistner's gynecology,* St Louis, 1995, Mosby.
41. Wexler A, Pernoll M: Benign disorders of the uterine corpus. In DeCherney A, Pernoll M, editors: *Current obstetric and gynecologic diagnosis and treatment,* ed 8, Norwalk, Conn, 1994, Appleton & Lange.
42. Williams D, Drews M: Assisted reproductive technologies. In Jacobs A, Gast M, editors: *Practical gynecology,* Norwalk, Conn, 1994, Appleton & Lange.

chapter 48

# MANAGEMENT OF PERSONS WITH Problems of the Breast

GLADYS E. DETERS

## objectives After studying this chapter, the learner should be able to:

1. Recognize the differences between benign breast conditions and breast cancer.
2. Analyze the patient's risk factor profile for developing breast cancer.
3. Describe early detection methods and diagnostic tests for breast evaluation.
4. Describe the technique of breast self-examination.
5. Discuss the advantages and disadvantages of surgery, chemotherapy, radiotherapy, and hormonal therapy in the treatment of breast cancer.
6. Describe the types of breast preservation and reconstruction procedures available.
7. Demonstrate how to correctly perform postmastectomy exercises.
8. Discuss the role of Reach to Recovery volunteers in the patient's adjustment to mastectomy surgery.
9. Compare the treatments for common benign breast conditions.

This chapter discusses the collaborative management of both breast cancer and other cystic and inflammatory breast conditions. Breast cancer is by far the most important of these disorders, and it is presented first. The nonmalignant conditions are discussed later in the chapter, followed by problems that affect the male breast.

## MALIGNANT CONDITIONS OF THE BREAST

### ETIOLOGY

For more than 30 years breast cancer has been the most prevalent and feared cancer in women and has caused the most cancer-related deaths each year. The incidence of breast cancer continues to rise, partly as a result of the steady aging of the population, and partly because of improved diagnostic technology. The mortality rates associated with breast cancer have changed little since 1930 despite advances in treatment modalities, but the alarming increase in lung cancer deaths now makes lung cancer the leading cause of cancer death in women.

The underlying cause of breast cancer is still unknown but a number of risk factors have been identified. These risk factors are discussed below. Hopefully, ongoing research efforts will reveal additional risk factors that have a role in breast cancer development.

#### Age and Gender

Women today have a 1 in 8 chance of developing breast cancer in their lifetime. As is the case with most malignant conditions, the incidence of breast cancer increases with age.[2] The disease is diagnosed most frequently in women older than 50 years. The reason for this age-related increase is thought to be the increased probability of mutagenic changes occurring over a longer life span rather than any instability inherent in aging cells.[29] Another reason that elderly women are at greater risk is related to present population figures. Elderly women outnumber younger women, and the gap is expected to widen. Breast cancer is almost exclusively a disease affecting women. Only 1,400 of the 180,200 new cases of breast cancer anticipated in 1997 are predicted to involve men.[2]

Breast cancer occurring within family members has been recognized for centuries, but the first documented cases were recorded in 1866. Inherited breast cancer accounts for about 5% to 10% of all breast cancer cases. The presence of inherited breast cancer is demonstrated by the incidence in first-degree relatives: mother, daughter, or sister. The risk increases if the first-degree relative had a history of premenopausal breast cancer or bilateral disease. When both conditions occur (premenopausal and bilateral disease), the risk to a first-degree relative increases 1.5- to 2-fold, including the risk of also developing bilateral disease.[23] Inherited breast cancer develops at an earlier age than the noninherited type.

In 1990 the first susceptibility gene for inherited breast cancer was located on chromosome 17q. The gene, referred to as *BRCA I,* is transmitted through the autosomal dominant pattern of inheritance, meaning that 50% of children of carriers will inherit the mutation. Isolation of *BRCA I* was accomplished through research on families with documented histories of inherited breast and/or ovarian cancer, especially in younger women.[32] For women who inherit *BRCA I* the risk of developing breast cancer is approximately 50% before age 50 and 80% by age 65. Their risk of developing ovarian cancer is estimated to be approximately 10% by age 60.[32] Ongoing genetic research on *BRCA I* and the recently discovered *BRCA II* will provide more definitive data on inherited breast cancer and how to treat and counsel families about this most sensitive and serious health problem. The characteristics of inherited breast cancer are listed in Box 48-1.

The development of noninherited breast cancer is considered to be a two-step process. The first step involves a change in cell structure or function, followed by a second event that promotes another change in the cell and causes it to become malignant. In hereditary breast cancer the inherited cell may already be in an altered state (first step) and require only one event to change it to a cancer cell.[48]

### Menstrual and Reproductive History

The risk of breast cancer is increased when menstruation begins at an early age (11 to 12 years) and extends to a late menopause (about age 55) age. The probability of mutagenic changes taking place from an intermediate phase to a malignant phase is more likely when the menstrual cycle spans more than 30 years.

Women who have never been pregnant (nulliparity) or who had their first child after the age of 30 years are at an increased risk of breast cancer. Women aged 30 to 35 years in their first full-term pregnancy are at greater risk for breast cancer than women who deliver for the first time at 18 years of age or younger. The implication is that a full-term pregnancy at an early age promotes changes in breast development that protect the breast from cancer. Breast development begins at menarche; however, full differentiation of mammary gland epithelium is not complete until a full-term pregnancy completes the developmental process. In addition, the longer the menstrual history the longer the dividing ductal cells are exposed to hormonal stimulation.[32] Pregnancy itself is not considered a risk factor for breast cancer development. However breast cancer is the most common malignancy found in pregnancy and accounts for about 2.5% of cases diagnosed.[38]

### Hormones and Oral Contraception

Hormonal replacement therapy at menopause has created a great deal of concern and controversy because of the increased incidence of breast cancer associated with it. Some reports indicate a 40% increased risk, especially in older women who have been receiving a medication regimen such as Premarin for many years. Combining estrogen with progesterone to alleviate the risk of endometrial cancer has not diminished the breast cancer risk and may, in fact, have increased it.[11,23,43]

An association between the use of oral contraceptives (OCs) and the risk of breast cancer is not clear at this time. The report from a nationwide, case-controlled study by the Cancer and Steroid Hormone Study (1983) concluded that women 20 to 54 years of age who had used OCs had the same breast cancer risk as women who had never used OCs. Other more recent findings also indicate no increased risk of breast cancer associated with ever having used OCs. However findings indicate a small increased risk of breast cancer if OCs are begun at an early age (within 5 years of menarche) and are taken continually for 10 or more years.[54] More research is needed to settle this issue.

**box 48-1 Characteristics of Inherited Breast Cancer**

- Occurs at an early age (premenopausal)
- Incidence of bilateral disease increased
- First-degree relative (mother, daughter, sister) with the disease
- Personal history of breast cancer in one breast, which increases the risk of developing it in the second breast

Modified from Smith P: *Semin Oncol Nurs* 8(4):258-264, 1992.

### Diet and Body Weight

The consumption of a diet high in animal fat has long been considered a breast cancer risk. This claim is largely unproved. Some large cohort studies indicate that there is no relationship between the total amount of fat intake and breast cancer in premenopausal and postmenopausal women.[55] Although a diet high in fat is not thought to be a causative factor in breast cancer development, some animal studies suggest that fat may be a promoter of cells being transformed from a normal to a malignant state.[10]

Obesity also has been considered a factor in breast cancer development. Although no positive correlation has as yet been established, obesity can have a stimulating effect on breast cancer growth. Estrogen is stored in body adipose tissue. Some breast cancers are estrogen receptor positive (ER+), meaning that estrogen will stimulate breast cancer cell growth. Therefore the more body adipose tissue present, the more estrogen will be available to attach to ER+ cancer cells. In the postmenopausal woman, androgens in adipose tissue can be converted to estrogen and become a source for stimulating cancer growth and spread. Recent studies have shown that the pattern of body-fat distribution (high waist-to-hip ratio) in postmenopausal women can influence their risk for breast cancer. In fact, there is a high correlation of breast cancer associated with obesity that has a high waist-to-hip ratio, low parity, and greater age at first pregnancy in postmenopausal women with a family history of breast cancer. Until there is more concrete evidence of a correlation between fat intake, obesity, and breast cancer, women should be advised to limit dietary fat intake and maintain optimum body weight.

### Benign Breast Disease

Fibrocystic disease, a benign condition, is considered to be a risk for breast cancer but usually only when it is related to hyperplasia (increased cellular proliferation). When hyperplasia is not present, the risk is linked to detection of lesions. Unless a woman performs monthly breast self-examination and knows the normal feel of her own breast, new lesions or hyperplastic changes may go undetected. Cystic breast disease is discussed in more depth later in this chapter.[10]

### Radiation Hazard

The survivors of the bombing at Nagasaski and Hiroshima have provided data on the effects of radiation exposure and breast cancer development. Young women who were exposed to the radiation show an increased incidence of breast cancer compared with older women (older than 39 years of age) exposed to the same degree of radiation.[29] Women who have had repeated fluoroscopic examinations of the chest or radiation as a treatment for mastitis also have demonstrated an increased incidence of breast cancer later in life. The box below reviews the risk factors associated with breast cancer development.

## EPIDEMIOLOGY

A comparison of the estimated cancer incidence and death rate figures reveal that breast cancer accounts for about one third (31%) of all cancers detected in women and 17% of all cancer-related deaths.[7] Despite advances in detection and treatment the annual death rates as a result of breast cancer have changed little since 1930, as seen in Figure 48-1.

Breast cancer recognizes neither national boundaries nor racial/ethnic groups. It is a worldwide problem, especially in the United States and Western Europe, where breast cancer

**risk factors**

**Breast Cancer**

| Factor | Risk | Comment |
|---|---|---|
| Female gender | Increased | 99% of all breast cancers occur in women and 1% in men. |
| History of a previous breast cancer | Increased | The risk of developing a cancer in the opposite breast is five times greater than for the average population at risk. |
| Age >40 | Increased | Incidence increases with age and peaks in the fifth decade. |
| Menstrual history | | |
| Early menarche or late menopause or both | Increased | The risk of breast cancer rises as the interval between menarche and menopause increases; shortening the interval by castration reduces the risk, especially if performed in women younger than 35 years of age. |
| Reproductive history | | |
| Nulliparity<br>First child born after 30 years of age | Increased | Childless women have an increased risk as do women who bear their first child near or after the age of 30 years. |
| Family history: | | |
| Mother or sister or both | Increased | Risk increases two to three times if a mother or sister has had breast cancer and is further increased if the relative was diagnosed during the premenopausal state and if the cancer was bilateral. |
| Diet | Controversial | Animal data and description epidemiology of breast cancer incidence strongly suggest an association of dietary factors, specifically a high-fat diet, with an increased risk of breast cancer. The National Academy of Sciences recommends decreasing total fat intake to 30% of available calories. |
| Alcohol | Unknown | A suggested small increase in risk with moderate alcohol consumption has been reported, although limitations in methodology have been cited, and results require confirmation. |
| Obesity | Controversial | Weight, height, obesity, and increased body mass have been reported to be associated with an increased risk of breast cancer. |
| Ionizing radiation | Increased | Three groups of women who received low-level radiation exposure demonstrated an increased breast cancer risk, which was particularly notable if the exposure occurred in the early years (<30 years). |
| Benign breast disease | None | Fibrocystic breast disease is not associated with breast cancer. However, biopsy-proven atypical hyperplasia is associated with an increased risk. |
| Oral contraceptives | None | There is no evidence yet to suggest a causal relationship between oral contraceptives and incidence of and survival from breast cancer. |
| Exogenous hormones | Controversial | Several studies report no link with replacement hormones and breast cancer, and those that do appear to identify only subsets of patients at risk: those who have taken replacement estrogens for very long periods of time and those who have taken large cumulative doses. |

Modified from Baird SB et al: *Cancer nursing: a comprehensive textbook,* Philadelphia, 1991, WB Saunders.

incidence and mortality rates are the highest. The reason for this occurrence has been debated without any consensus. One theory is that these countries are highly industrialized and therefore more economically and socially advantaged than some of the developing countries. As a consequence of this affluence, the dietary pattern of ingesting more expensive animal food (red meat high in fat) may be implicated as a causative factor (see preceding discussion of diet and obesity).

As industrialization proceeds in these developing countries the risk of exposure to environmental wastes and pollutants also increases. Although this theory is merely speculative, it is known that when women emigrate from third-world countries and the Far East to the United States and other Western countries, their rate of breast cancer incidence rises, possibly because of changes in eating patterns.

Although breast cancer is predominantly a disease of white women, the incidence and mortality among African-American women have been increasing. In the most recent 5-year data collection period (1989 to 1993), the age-adjusted breast cancer mortality rates fell about 6% in white women but rose 1% in African-American women (Figure 48-2). The underlying reason for the rise is not genetic but related to the fact that more black women live at or near the poverty level, have less basic education and educational opportunities, and have limited access to health care programs such as early screening and detection programs.[8] In black women breast cancer is more frequently diagnosed at a later stage of disease because they neither participate in nor are encouraged to participate in early detection and treatment programs.[53] Black women also have poorer survival rates than do white women, even when stage of disease is adjusted for.

In 1992 the federal government proposed health care-related objectives for the nation in *Healthy People 2000*.[51] Included in the objectives are those specifically related to breast cancer, which are found in Box 48-2. Because the mortality rate from breast cancer has declined little during the past 60 years even with improved detection and treatment methods, these objectives are well worth achieving.

## Prognostic Factors

Several factors are used to determine the overall prognosis at the time of diagnosis of breast cancer. These include the num-

**box 48-2** Healthy People 2000 *Objectives to Reduce Breast Cancer Mortality*

1. Reduce breast cancer deaths to no more than 20.6 per 100,000 women by the year 2000.
2. Increase, to at least 80%, the proportion of women 40 years of age and older who have had a clinical breast examination and mammogram and to at least 60% those aged 50 and older who have received them within the preceding 1 to 2 years.

From US Department of Health and Human Services, Public Health Service: *Healthy People 2000: summary report*, 1992.

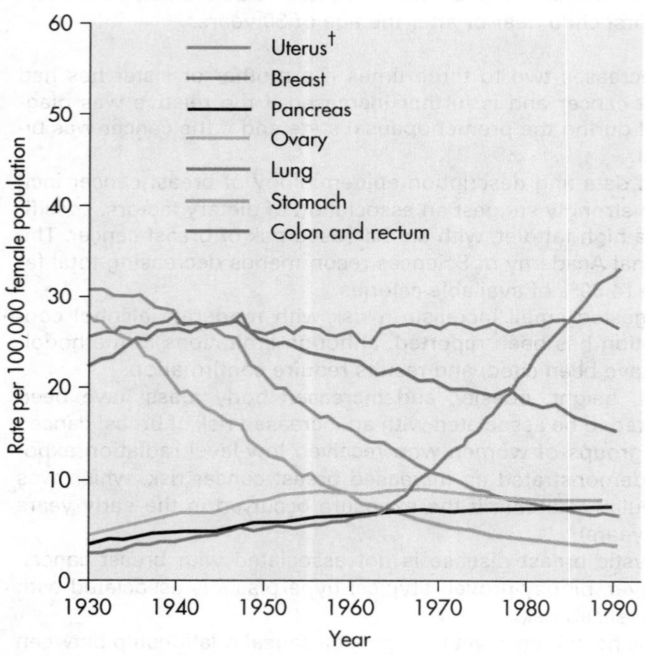


**fig. 48-1** Age-adjusted cancer death rates: females by site, United States, 1930-1992.

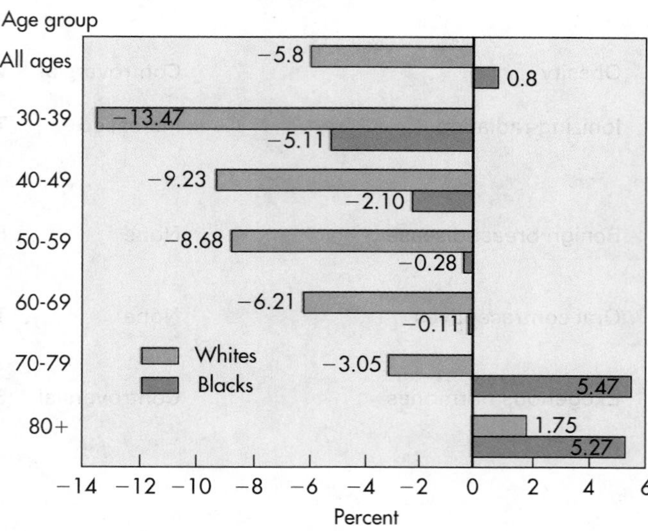


**fig. 48-2** Breast cancer mortality trends by age and race.

ber of axillary nodes involved, tumor size, and hormone receptor status.

### Axillary node involvement

Because metastasis to the lymph nodes is common, the number of axillary nodes involved has long been used as a predictor of breast cancer outcome. As the number of nodes involved increases, the chance of distant metastasis increases and prognosis worsens. If four or more nodes are involved, each additional node adds to the risk of recurrence after initial treatment.[36]

### Tumor size

Smaller tumor size at diagnosis is associated with fewer positive nodes involved and less metastasis. Women with tumors 2 cm or less in size and without node involvement have the best prognostic outcome.

### Cell activity and hormone receptor status

The fraction of tumor cells in the synthesis (S) phase of cell division is now widely used as a predictor of recurrence and long-term survival. A high S-phase is associated with a fast-growing tumor and a short disease-free survival time. (See Chapter 11 for a more detailed discussion on cell kinetics.)

Estrogen receptors (ER) and progesterone receptors (PR) are well-recognized predictors of long-term survival in women with breast cancer. The presence of 10 or more receptors on a cell indicates a positive (+) status. An ER+ or PR+ tumor is associated with a more favorable prognosis and a longer disease-free survival time.[34]

A major advantage of an ER+ or PR+ tumor lies in the ability to use hormonal manipulation to treat the tumor if and when the breast cancer advances to stage III or metastasis occurs. Approximately 78% of ER+ or PR+ tumors respond positively to hormonal therapy.[31]

## Staging of Breast Cancer

Staging of breast cancer incorporates the primary tumor, regional nodes, and metastasis (TNM) classification as shown in Box 48-3. Treatment decisions are based on the stage of the breast cancer, as well as those factors already discussed.

## PATHOPHYSIOLOGY

Tumors of the breast arise in the epithelial cells of either ductal or lobular tissue and are referred to as *carcinomas.* A number of histological subtypes also have been identified but are not as commonly seen, nor are they as invasive as ductal and lobular carcinomas. When the tumor is confined within a duct or a lobule and has not invaded surrounding tissue, it is considered *localized* or in situ carcinoma of the breast. *Infiltrative* ductal or lobular carcinomas are tumors that have spread directly into surrounding tissue and may have distant metastases if they have penetrated the axillary or internal mammary nodes or the systemic circulation.

The breast is served by an extensive lymphatic drainage system: central axillary, pectoral (anterior), subscapular (posterior), and lateral nodes. The ipsilateral axillary nodes drain up to 75% of lymph from the breast. Additional drainage flows upward to the infraclavicular and supraclavicular lymph nodes.[28] The normal lymphatic system and directional flow are shown in Figure 48-3.

**box 48-3** *Staging of Breast Cancer*

**T—PRIMARY TUMOR SIZE**

| | |
|---|---|
| TX | Primary tumor cannot be assessed |
| T0 | No evidence of primary tumor |
| Tis | Carcinoma in situ: intraductal carcinoma, lobular carcinoma in situ, or Paget's disease of the nipple with node |
| T1 | Tumor 2 cm or less in greatest dimension |
| T2 | Tumor more than 2 cm but not more than 5 cm in greatest dimension |
| T3 | Tumor more than 5 cm in greatest dimension |
| T4 | Tumor of any size with direct extension to chest wall or skin |

NOTE: Paget's disease associated with a tumor is classified according to the size of the tumor

**N—REGIONAL LYMPH NODES**

| | |
|---|---|
| NX | Regional lymph nodes cannot be assessed (e.g., previously removed) |
| N0 | No regional lymph node metastasis |
| N1 | Metastasis to movable ipsilateral axillary lymph node(s) |
| N2 | Metastasis to ipsilateral axillary lymph node(s) fixed to one another or to other structures |
| N3 | Metastasis to ipsilateral internal mammary lymph node(s) |

**M—DISTANT METASTASIS**

| | |
|---|---|
| MX | Presence of distant metastasis cannot be assessed |
| M0 | No distant metastasis |
| M1 | Distant metastasis (includes metastasis to ipsilateral, supraclavicular lymph node[s]) |

**STAGE GROUPING**

| | | | |
|---|---|---|---|
| Stage 0 | Tis | N0 | M0 |
| Stage I | T1 | N0 | M0 |
| Stage IIa | T0 | N0 | M0 |
| | T1 | N1 | M0 |
| | T2 | N0 | M0 |
| Stage IIB | T2 | N1 | M0 |
| | T3 | N0 | M0 |
| Stage IIIA | T0 | N2 | M0 |
| | T1 | N2 | M0 |
| | T2 | N2 | M0 |
| | T3 | N1 | M0 |
| | T3 | N2 | M0 |
| Stage IIIB | T4 | Any N | M0 |
| | Any T | N3 | M0 |
| Stage IV | Any T | Any N | M1 |

From Beahrs OH, Hutter RV, Kennedy BJ, editors: *AJCC Cancer staging data forms,* ed 4, Philadelphia, 1992, JB Lippincott.

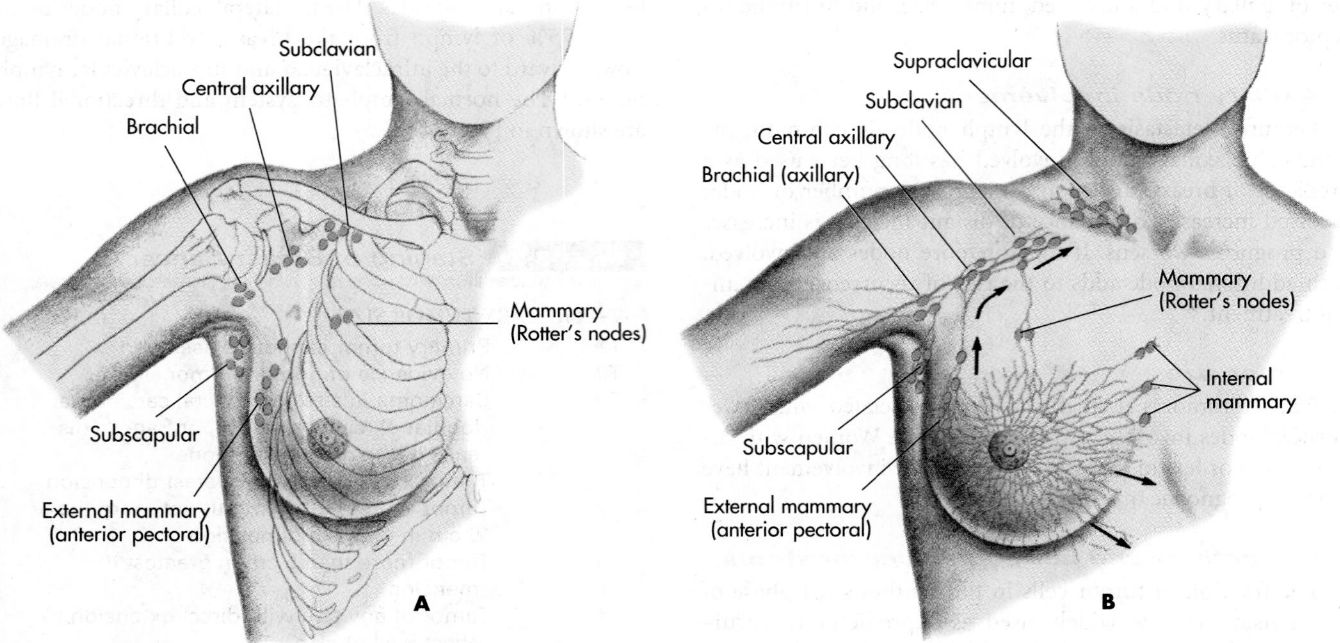


**fig. 48-3** **A**, Lymph nodes of the axilla. **B**, Lymphatic drainage of the breast.

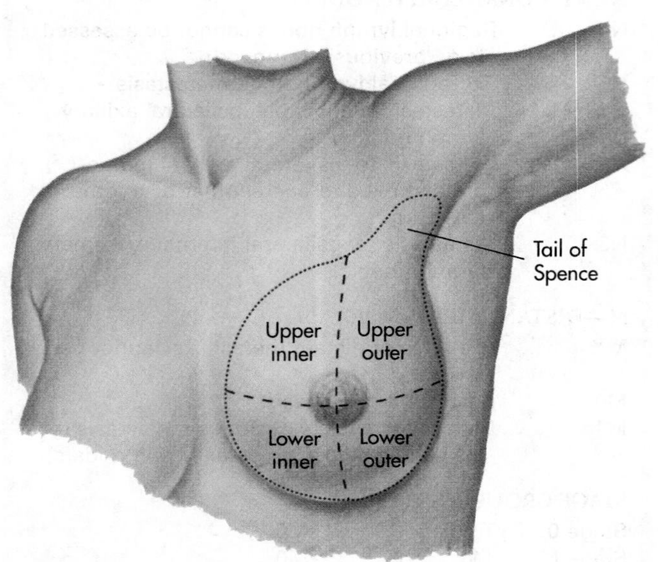


**fig. 48-4** Quadrants of left breast and axillary tail of Spence. Most tumors develop in the upper outer quadrant.

The breast is divided into four quadrants, as shown in Figure 48-4. Most breast tumors are located in the upper outer quadrant, but they can occur in any area of the breast. Of the invasive breast tumors, infiltrative ductal carcinoma is the most prevalent histological cell type, followed by infiltrating lobular carcinomas. Subtypes of each of these histological cell types comprise the remainder of breast tumors. Table 48-1 reviews selected histological types of breast cancer.

Paget's disease, an eczema-like inflammatory process affecting the nipple and aerola, may progress from an epidermal condition to an intraductal carcinoma of the breast. It can be accompanied by a palpable lump. Paget's disease of the breast accounts for less than 5% of breast cancers.[5]

### Clinical Manifestations

Early-stage cancer of the breast (symptomless) can be detected only on physical examination of the breast or by mammogram and is difficult to differentiate from benign tumors. With more advanced tumors a variety of signs and symptoms are helpful in differentiating a benign tumor from a malignant tumor. Benign tumors generally have well-defined edges, are encapsulated, and are freely movable. The shape of a malignant tumor is more difficult to define and is less mobile on palpation, usually the result of the tumor becoming "fixed" and adhering to the chest wall. As the tumor infiltrates into surrounding tissue, it can cause retraction of the overlying skin and create what is referred to as dimpling. The nipple also may be retracted or deviated at an odd angle from the same growth pattern. A peau d'orange breast sign indicates lymphatic obstruction from tumor growth with resulting edema. The breast resembles an orange peel with large prominent pores. These signs are more ominous, and usually reflect advanced disease. The clinical manifestations of breast cancer are found in Box 48-4.

## COLLABORATIVE CARE MANAGEMENT

The management of breast cancer is both complex and controversial. Treatment options are ever changing and influenced by new and better surgical techniques, new cytotoxic drug combinations, and more accurate knowledge of breast cancer growth and dissemination.

**table 48-1** *Selected Histological Types of Breast Cancer*

| Type | Incidence (%) | Characteristics | Prognosis |
|---|---|---|---|
| Infiltrating ductal carcinoma | 70 | Stony hard mass; gritty texture; may appear bilaterally | Poor; common involvement of axillary nodes |
| Medullary carcinoma | 5-7 | Soft mass; often reaches large size; may be circumscribed | Favorable |
| Mucinous, or colloid, carcinoma | 3 | Slow growing; can reach large size; may occur with other tumor type | Good if tumor is predominately mucinous |
| Invasive lobular carcinoma | 5 | Multicentricity common; may involve both breasts | Similar to ductal types |
| Paget's disease | 3 | Scaly, eczematoid nipple with burning, itching, discharge; two thirds have palpable, underlying mass | Related to histological type of underlying tumor |
| Inflammatory breast cancer | <1 | Skin red, warm, indurated, with obstructive lymphangitis (peau d'orange appearance) | Poor; often presents with palpable nodes and evidence of metastasis |
| Lobular carcinoma in situ | 2.5 | Usually found as incidental finding in benign breast specimens (high risk for development of invasive cancer in future) | Good |

From Entreken N: Breast cancer. In Clark JC, McGee RF: *Oncology Nursing Society core curriculum for oncology nursing,* ed 2, Philadelphia, 1992, WB Saunders.

**box 48-4** *clinical manifestations*

***Breast Cancer***

Lump that is
- Irregular, star-shaped
- Firm to hard in consistency
- Fixed, not mobile
- Poorly defined or demarcated
- Usually not tender, but can occasionally cause discomfort
- Single

Presence of skin or nipple retraction
Nipple discharge
Peau d'orange appearance (dimpling) of the skin

NOTE: Most breast tumors identified by mammography are completely without discernible symptoms.

## Diagnostic Tests

When a breast lump has been found, the exact nature of the lesion must be determined. The presence of a benign lesion, such as a fibroadenoma, cyst, or fibrocystic breast disease, must be ruled out. Characteristic features of benign lesions are presented later in the chapter. Most breast lesions are benign; however, only histological examination of tissue from the lesion will determine the true nature of the disease process.

### Noninvasive diagnostic tests

Monthly breast self-examination (BSE) is recommended by the American Cancer Society as an early detection method. However, its true value in detecting breast cancer at an early stage and decreasing breast cancer mortality has not been fully determined. Although 90% of all breast lesions are first detected by the woman herself, the practice of BSE has not resulted in more women performing the examination on a regular schedule. Some studies reveal that even though women recognize the importance of BSE and can perform it accurately, only about 25% of women practice it monthly.[15] Barriers that deter women from regular practice of BSE include forgetfulness, fear of finding a lump each time the examination is performed, being unaware of their personal breast cancer risk, and fear of mutilating surgery. Educating women about the importance of regular monthly self-examination and teaching the proper technique are essential to early detection and intervention (see Chapter 46).

At the present time *mammography* is the best diagnostic tool available to detect breast tumors. A mammogram can detect breast lesions before they become palpable on physical examination (1 cm) or before they can be seen on conventional roentgenogram (see the Research Box on p. 1582).

The recent increase in breast cancer incidence has been at least partially attributed to the increased use of mammography and its detection of cancer in an earlier, localized stage. Many women, however, are still reluctant to undergo mammographic examination. The most frequent barriers cited for not complying with health care provider recommended examinations or for nonparticipation in screening programs are cost of the examination (no insurance coverage or only partial coverage), fear of radiation exposure, pain during the procedure, no regular family health care provider who recommends the examination, and no family history of breast cancer (therefore seeing no need for a mammogram).

The accuracy of a mammogram depends on obtaining two views using sufficient compression of the breast. Compression is required to decrease breast thickness, thus allowing a reduced radiation dose. In addition, compression keeps the breast from moving and results in a more accurate image with less radiation

**research**

Reference: Benedict S, Williams RD, Hoomani J: Method of discovery of breast cancer, *Cancer Practi* 4(3):147-155, 1996.

One in eight American women will develop breast cancer in her lifetime. The three recommended means of discovering breast cancer are by BSE, professional clinical examination, and mammography. The purpose of this retrospective, descriptive study was to determine which methods of detection were most frequently used by a sample of 51 women in whom breast cancer was diagnosed. The mean age of participants was 53.7 years. Ten participants knew of a positive family history for breast cancer.

A recall questionnaire was administered, asking the participants about their use of BSE, mammography, and clinical examination. In the year before the diagnosis of breast cancer, clinical breast examination ($n = 37$) was the detection method most used, followed by monthly BSE ($n = 27$), and lastly, mammography ($n = 20$). Only 10 of the women 40 years of age and older followed all American Cancer Society (ACS) guidelines for breast cancer detection.

The actual discovery of the breast tumor occurred most often via mammogram ($n = 20$), followed by BSE ($n = 18$). Only three cancers were detected by clinical breast examination, and seven women found the breast mass during incidental palpation. Three lesions were found by the husband/lover by palpation.

Few women in this study used all three of the ACS recommended methods of breast cancer detection despite repeated exposure to information about their importance in breast cancer detection.

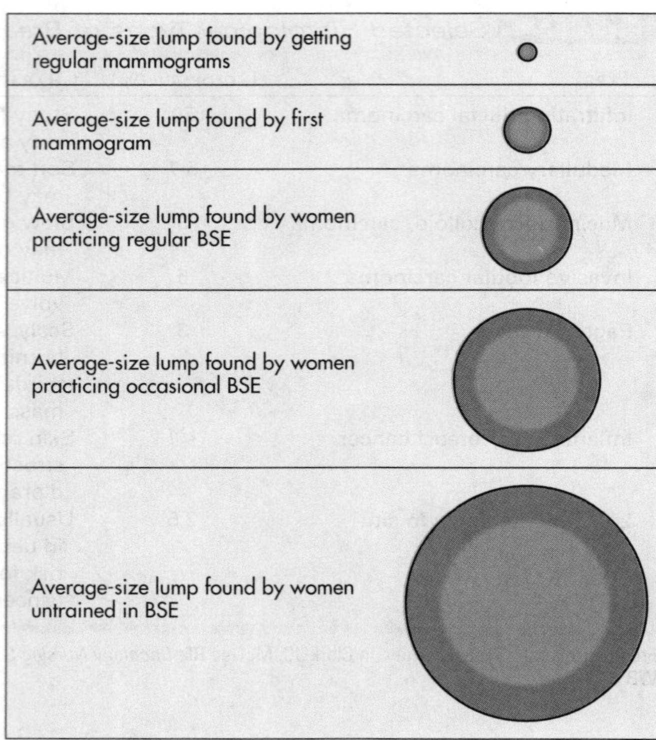


**fig. 48-5** Relative sizes of tumors detected by various detection methods, as reported by the Breast Health Program of New York.

scatter.[14] When accurately performed and read by an experienced radiologist, a mammogram can detect the presence of a lesion 2 to 4 years before it is large enough to be detected by conventional x-ray film or palpated on physical examination.[3] The major limitation of mammography is its inability to differentiate between malignant and benign lesions. It is estimated that of the lesions identified by mammogram and suspicious enough to biopsy, only 25% to 35% are malignant.[14] Figure 48-5 compares the average size of a lesion discovered by a woman on BSE and one capable of being detected on mammogram. See Chapter 46 for a detailed discussion of mammography.

Digital mammography is now being developed. It is expected to produce a better image and to more accurately distinguish between malignant and benign tumors. Figure 48-6 shows a mammogram with a malignant lesion.

*Ultrasound* also can be used as a noninvasive test to determine the size of a lesion and differentiate a fluid-filled cyst from a solid lesion. An ultrasound examination, which does not require the use of radiation, is a safer diagnostic tool than mammography for the initial evaluation of a breast lesion in a young, pregnant, or lactating woman.[14]

### Invasive diagnostic tests

Most breast tumors are not malignant; however, an accurate diagnosis cannot be made until tissue from the tumor is examined for histological cell type. Therefore when a tumor mass is discovered, whether on physical examination or mammogram, an invasive procedure, such as needle biopsy or excisional or incisional biopsy, is required.

*Fine-needle aspiration* can differentiate cysts versus other solid tumor masses. The contents of a cyst range from clear aspirate to bloody or even black fluid. The fluid generally is sent for cytological examination and may be helpful in the identification of histological cell type. A cytological examination is never used alone as a diagnostic tool for cancer because of the chance of both false-positive and false-negative reports.

*Tru-cut needle biopsy* is a useful diagnostic test. When performed correctly, it can provide a central core of tissue from a tumor that can be examined by a pathologist. This type of biopsy is helpful in differentiating the presence of fatty necrosis or localized infection from tumor.[5]

*Excisional* or *incisional biopsies* can be performed with the patient under local anesthesia in an outpatient department or a physician's office. Biopsies of deep lesions in a large breast are better performed in an operating suite. Tissue specimens are examined for cell type. If the lesion is malignant, the estrogen and progesterone receptor status should be determined at the same time. This information is important because the ER and PR status helps determine treatment choices.

### Other diagnostic tests

Breast cancer has a predilection to metastasize to bones; therefore, a bone scan and bone marrow biopsy may be or-

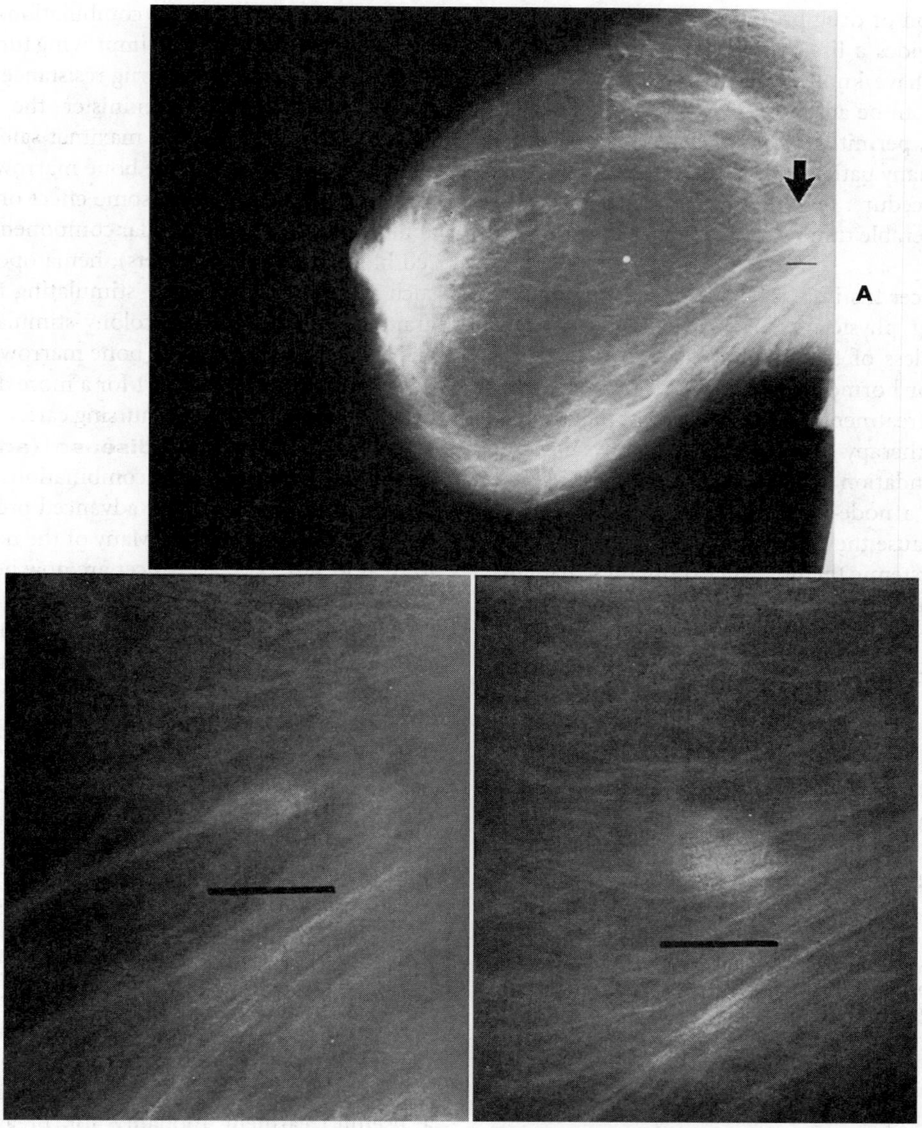

**fig. 48-6** Mammogram of patient with area of density indicating carcinoma. A small nodule *(arrow)* in a large fatty breast **(A)** was oval in shape with ill-defined margins **(B)**. The nodule increased in size over a 12-month interval. Black line represents 10-mm measure.

dered. Positive findings on these tests indicate the presence of widespread disease and a poorer prognosis. A liver scan may be indicated when results of liver function tests are abnormal. A chest x-ray film reveals lung status before any surgical intervention and also shows the presence of metastasis.

## Medications

The role of systemic drug therapy in the treatment of breast cancer (chemotherapy and endocrine therapy) is to either eradicate or impede the growth of micrometastatic disease.

### Chemotherapy

**Stages I and II disease (localized).** As a result of improved diagnostic tests, breast cancer is being discovered earlier and in a more localized stage, frequently without nodal involvement. It is estimated that more than 90% of women with tumors 1 cm or less and without nodal involvement can be expected to achieve long-term disease-free survival.[41] However, because the tumor cells of breast cancer are heterogeneous in nature—meaning there is no uniformity of cells and the cells are subject to changes with each cell generation—even localized, node-negative tumors can and frequently do recur. The presence of micrometastasis may be undetected at the time of initial treatment. When micrometastasis is present, changes (mutations) can occur in the tumor cells, making them resistant to the effects of chemotherapeutic agents even though tumor sensitivity to drug therapy is greatest when the tumor burden is small. Thus it is not always possible to predict with confidence that all tumors 1 cm or less without node involvement are "cured" with initial local/regional treatment.

The early introduction of drug protocols is now being advocated. Box 48-5 provides a list of chemotherapy agents and drug protocols that have known cytotoxic effects on breast cancer. These drugs can be administered at the time of diagnosis, before surgery, permitting surgical lumpectomy as the initial treatment in many patients rather than the more extensive mastectomy procedure. Preoperative chemotherapy also can make larger inoperable tumors more amenable to surgical removal.

The National Cancer Institute (NCI) issued a drug update in 1989 encouraging physicians to treat *all node-negative* breast cancer, regardless of the woman's age with combination chemotherapy or hormonal therapy with tamoxifen for 2 years after initial treatment with mastectomy or lumpectomy and radiation therapy. The reluctance of physicians to follow this recommendation is based on data suggesting that not all women with a node-negative status need additional systemic therapy because they are already "cured." It is feared that the additional systemic therapy will expose these patients to unnecessary side effects and to long-term sequelae of the therapy such as permanent amenorrhea. Clinical trials are therefore being conducted to determine specific subsets of node-negative breast cancers that will benefit most from this additional treatment modality.

At present there are few new chemotherapeutic agents useful in the treatment of breast cancer. Therefore treatment approaches that use established agents in new ways are being investigated. Alternating drug combinations may be more effective in treating breast cancer than using a single drug protocol. The use of various combinations of drugs (Box 48-5) also may prove beneficial in improving tumor cell sensitivity to drug therapy by reducing drug resistance. Another new treatment approach is to administer the prescribed chemotherapeutic agents at their maximal safe dosage levels while providing a "rescue" for the bone marrow. Because most chemotherapeutic drugs have some effect on the bone marrow's ability to produce vital cellular components (white blood cells, red blood cells, and platelets), hematopoietic growth factors such as granulocyte colony-stimulating factors (G-CSF) and granulocyte-macrophage colony-stimulating factors (GM-CSF) are given to stimulate bone marrow recovery after high-dose therapy. See Chapter 11 for a more detailed discussion of chemotherapy and related nursing care.

**Stages III and IV disease (advanced).** Chemotherapy with multiple drug combinations has been used in the treatment of recurrent and advanced breast cancer for many years with positive results. Many of the newer modalities used to treat localized breast cancer are now being used to treat recurrent and advanced disease as well.

Paclitaxel (Taxol) and docetaxel (Taxotere, a semisynthetic toxoid) are now considered first-line therapy for patients with locally advanced or metastatic breast cancer in whom anthracycline-based therapy (doxorubicin) has failed or who have a recurrence during anthracycline-based therapy.[18] Both paclitaxel and docetaxel have the ability to prevent cellular mitosis by disrupting microtubules, cellular structure, and intracellular activity.[40] These new cytotoxic agents give patients with metastatic breast cancer other treatment options.

The use of chemotherapy continues to generate many unanswered questions, such as optimal drug combinations, optimal dosage, and length of treatment. These are just a few of the concerns currently being addressed in clinical trials.

**box 48-5** *Chemotherapy Agents and Protocols Effective for Treating Breast Cancer*

**SINGLE AGENTS**

Cyclophosphamide
Melphalan
Thiotepa
Doxorubicin*
Epirubicin*

**PROTOCOLS USING VARIOUS AGENTS**

| | |
|---|---|
| CMF† | Cyclophosphamide, methotrexate, 5-fluorouracil |
| CPF | Cyclophosphamide, prednisone, 5-fluorouracil |
| CMF/VA | Cyclophosphamide, methotrexate, 5-fluorouracil, vincristine, doxorubicin |
| CMF/VP | Cyclophosphamide, methotrexate, 5-fluorouracil, vincristine, prednisone |
| AC | Doxorubicin, cyclophosphamide |
| FAC | 5-Fluorouracil, doxorubicin, cyclophosphamide |
| FEC | 5-Fluorouracil, epirubicin, cyclophosphamide |
| LMF | Melphalan, methotrexate, 5-fluorouracil |

*Anthracyclines. Doxorubicin is the most effective agent in the treatment of advanced breast cancer.
†This protocol has had the most use and is considered a standard regimen.

### Hormonal therapy

**Stages I and II disease.** Hormonal therapy has been a useful treatment modality for breast cancer for many decades. Whereas chemotherapy acts on rapidly dividing cells to achieve its effects, hormonal therapy targets cells that are dependent on estrogen for growth. The underlying reason for the success of hormonal therapy was not known until the development of bioassay methods that revealed the presence of estrogen receptors on the tumor cell surface. Before this discovery it was known only that surgical removal of the ovaries interfered in some way with breast cancer growth. One in three premenopausal women with advanced breast cancer who had their ovaries removed showed a delay in cancer growth or a disease-free interval.[30] Research revealed that tumors that are ER rich (>10) grow in response to stimulation by estrogen and are classified as ER+. It was theorized that if the level of circulating estrogen was removed or decreased, the growth of ER+ tumors could be impeded and disease-free interval and survival time increased. However estrogen ablation through oophorectomy also induced menopause, as the primary source of estrogen is the ovaries. Hot flashes, vaginal dryness, a rise in plasma lipids, atherosclerosis, and osteoporosis resulted. To counteract these menopausal effects, antiestrogen drug research led to the development of the antiestrogen drug tamoxifen. Tamoxifen is a nonsteroidal drug that competes for the estradiol-binding site on the ER+ cell, thus removing the stimulus (estrogen) for tumor growth. Although tamoxifen is most effective on ER+ breast cancer, it also affects (but to a lesser degree) ER− tumors as well. Tamoxifen is now considered the hormonal therapy of choice for both premenopausal and postmenopausal women.[30]

Tamoxifen is now being used in early-stage breast cancers in women with both node-negative and node-positive tumors. Data indicate that both groups have a decreased recurrence rate and better long-term survival of 25% and 16%, respectively.[24] The greatest benefits are in women 50 years of age and older.

**Stages III and IV disease.** Hormonal therapy is a mainstay of treatment for advanced breast cancer, especially for women with ER+ tumors and lymph node involvement. The higher the estrogen level, the better the response to the drug. Tamoxifen has been used either alone or in combination with chemotherapeutic agents. When used alone, it has fewer of the side effects such as hair loss and nausea that accompany chemotherapy drugs.

The length of treatment with tamoxifen is still a debatable question. Although 2 years of tamoxifen therapy is considered to be safe after surgical intervention, longer therapeutic value is questionable.[24] Analysis of data from the National Surgical Adjuvant Breast and Bowel Project found that tamoxifen increased the risk of development of endometrial cancer 2- to 3-fold in women receiving it compared with women with breast cancer not treated with tamoxifen.[21] Other side effects of therapy include symptoms similar to those of menopause (hot flashes, irregular menstrual periods, nausea, fluid retention, and vaginal discharge). The usefulness of tamoxifen as a breast cancer prevention agent in high-risk women needs further research.

Until more data become available and standard treatment protocols can be agreed on for both chemotherapy and hormonal manipulation, the patient and her physician will need to discuss each modality for its known advantages and disadvantages and select the one that meets each woman's individual needs and concerns.

## Treatments

### Radiation therapy

**Stages I and II disease.** Radiation to the breast after preservation surgery (lumpectomy) is now considered to be standard therapy in the United States.[36] Radiation to the breast eradicates tumor cells left behind after manipulation and handling of the tumor during surgery. The total recommended radiation dose is 4500 to 5000 cGy over 6 to 7 weeks. A booster dose of up to 1000 cGy may be prescribed with the use of either implants or external beam irradiation (Figure 48-7). The risk of local recurrence is minimal after this protocol. Tumors of less than 1 cm generally are not treated with radiation after breast preservation surgery because the risk of metastasis is minimal, and prognosis is considered excellent (see discussion under Medications on early-stage breast cancer). Although radiation after conservative surgery is widely used, some large breast tumors may be irradiated before surgery to facilitate easier surgical removal. Close medical follow-up is important after conservative surgery and radiation. Recommended guidelines include a breast physical examination every 3 to 4 months for 2 years, twice a year for 5 years, and then yearly. A mammogram is recommended 4 to 5 months after radiation and then annually.[1]

When the breast is irradiated, the side effects include skin reactions (redness, dryness, and itching), edema, mild tenderness, and fatigue. Fatigue is the result of bone marrow suppression from radiation to the thorax. The adult sternum, ribs, and thoracic vertebrae contain more than one third of the total body bone marrow (sternum 3%, ribs 16%, and thoracic vertebrae 16%). When these areas are within the treatment port, even when shielding devices are in place, some bone marrow function will be destroyed, and full recovery takes up to 6 months or more.[45] Patient instruction for dealing with the side effects of anemia and increased vulnerability to infection is vital to achieve patient compliance in completing treatment with the total prescribed radiation dose.

**Local recurrence.** Local recurrence of breast cancer usually occurs within 2 to 8 years after the initial diagnosis and treatment. Approximately 80% occur within 3 years. Generally the earlier the recurrence, the graver the prognosis. When recurrence follows conservative surgery and radiation therapy, mastectomy alone or with adjunct systemic therapy is recommended.

Tissue subjected to radiation therapy given at a dose intended for a "cure" does not respond well to repeated radiation exposure. This is because of the changes that occur in the vascular bed after initial radiation treatment, which results in a reduced blood and oxygen supply to the irradiated tissue. Radiation therapy works best on tissue with a good blood supply and a high oxygen saturation content. Complications of repeated radiation therapy include fibrotic changes to the lung, tissue necrosis, and rib fractures.

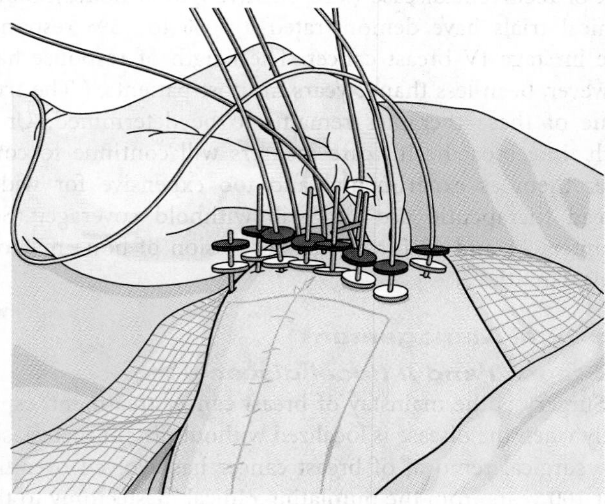

**fig. 48-7** Interstitial "booster" radiation therapy for breast cancer using iridium needles.

**Stages III and IV disease.** The role of radiation therapy in advanced breast cancer usually is palliative. Breast cancer has the propensity to metastasize to bone, which is a major source of pain. Bone involvement can result in pathological fractures of the spinal vertebrae, causing compression on nerve roots and the spinal cord. Radiation therapy can help to alleviate the discomfort from these complications. Metastasis from breast cancer often causes lymphatic obstruction and may result in pleural effusion. In addition, metastasis frequently involves other vital organ systems such as the lung and liver. Radiation therapy frequently is used to treat these metastatic lesions. When radiation is prescribed, the patient requires information and instruction on the rationale for the therapy and any specific care measures that will be necessary during treatment. It is important that the patient be aware that the radiation treatments will not cure the disease but can provide pain relief and improve quality of life. (See Chapter 11 for a more thorough discussion of radiation therapy in the treatment of cancer.)

#### Bone marrow transplantation

The use of bone marrow transplantation (BMT), a therapy developed for treatment of hematological cancers, is now showing promise as a treatment for solid tumors such as breast cancer. Two sources of marrow cells are being investigated: the patient's own marrow (autologous BMT) and the patient's circulating blood stem cells (peripheral blood stem cell transplantation [PBSCT]). BMT and PBSCT are able to "rescue" the breast cancer patient's bone marrow after ablation by high-dose chemotherapy or radiation therapy.[12] High-dose chemotherapy is administered to kill all tumor cells, and then the destroyed bone marrow is rescued with the patient's own healthy marrow or peripheral stem cells. Once the stem cells from either source are reintroduced into the patient's circulation, they migrate to the bone marrow and begin new marrow engraftment.

These procedures have demonstrated efficacy in women with metastatic breast cancer or in those who are at high risk of recurrent disease (>10 positive lymph nodes). Some clinical trials have demonstrated a 50% to 75% response rate in stage IV breast cancer. The length of response has, however, been less than 2 years in most patients.[37] The true value of these therapies remains to be determined. Until such time most health care insurers will continue to consider them as experimental and too expensive for widespread therapeutic use and will withhold coverage. (See Chapters 11 and 68 for further discussion of bone marrow transplantation.)

### Surgical Management

#### Stages I and II (local disease)

Surgery is the mainstay of breast cancer treatment, especially when the disease is localized without distant metastasis. The surgical removal of breast cancer has evolved over the past 100 years from the mutilating radical mastectomy to the more conservative surgical approaches in use today. Halsted introduced the radical procedure (removal of the entire breast, skin, chest wall muscles, and axillary lymph nodes) in the mistaken belief that as a breast tumor grows, it will spread in an orderly manner from the tumor core outward to all adjacent tissue and lymph nodes in its path. Unfortunately, this surgical procedure became the standard form of treatment for breast cancer for more than 70 years. Today, after years of clinical trials, surgery using less extensive tissue removal is now the rule.

When primary, localized breast cancer (less than 2 to 4 cm and no metastasis) is diagnosed, two surgical options may be offered: modified radical mastectomy, with or without breast reconstruction, or breast sparing (lumpectomy) procedures. The goal of both modified radical mastectomy and lumpectomy is to control local/regional disease, to accurately stage the disease so that patients at high risk for recurrence are identified, and to provide the best chance for long-term survival, in addition to achieving the best cosmetic result. The overall long-term survival rates for the two surgical methods are approximately the same.[57]

Modified radical mastectomy is now considered the standard form of mastectomy surgery. This procedure involves the removal of the whole breast, some fatty tissue, and dissection of the axillary lymph nodes. The pectoral muscles and surrounding nerves are left intact. The cosmetic result avoids the devastating chest wall defects, shoulder and arm limitations, and skin graft requirements that accompanied the more radical procedure. The modified surgery, however, is significantly more extensive than the breast-sparing procedures.

Breast-sparing procedures, known as partial mastectomy, wedge resection, or lumpectomy, involve the least removal of breast tissue and, therefore, have the best cosmesis. The tumor is removed, including a margin of normal tissue. The pathologist usually examines the specimen immediately to be sure that the margins around the tumor are cancer free. If not, a wider excision is required. A separate incision is used to determine axillary node involvement. Breast-sparing treatment for local disease is followed in 2 to 4 weeks by radiation therapy when wound healing is complete. The decision to include irradiation after breast-sparing procedures is a result of studies that showed that in up to 50% of patients some residual tumor cells were still present after tumor removal.[1] Breast-sparing surgery is not advised for all stage I and II disease. Contraindications are listed in Box 48-6.

Both modified radical mastectomy and lumpectomy include axillary lymph-node dissection because metastatic dissemination takes place primarily through these nodes. The number of diseased nodes (three to four) directly correlates with the risk of recurrent disease after initial treatment and with overall prognosis.[22] The level of lymph node dissection (sampling versus levels I, II, and III dissection) has been debated for many years. Low axillary dissection (level I) is the removal of an entire bloc of nodes in the area from the latissimus dorsi muscle laterally to the medial pectoralis muscle. Levels II and III dissection remove en bloc nodes from the middle to the entire axillary node chain, respectively (Figure 48-8). Approximately 80% of axillary nodes are found within a level I to II dissection, with the remainder in level III.

**box 48-6** *Contraindications for Use of Breast-Sparing Procedures*[1,34,52,56]

Pregnancy: first and second trimesters preclude the use of radiation therapy
Locally advanced or inflammatory breast cancer
Multiple lesions located in separate quadrants of the breast or diffuse malignant or indeterminate-appearing microcalcifications
Prior irradiation of the breast
History of collagen-vascular disease, which is recognized as having poor tolerance to the effects of radiation therapy
Tumor size: large tumor in a small breast, which will not allow adequate resection of tumor
Breast size: large pendulous breasts, which are difficult to irradiate; small breasts, which may result in an unacceptable cosmetic outcome
Location of tumor: tumors that are located beneath the nipple necessitate removal of the nipple-areola complex, which has questionable value compared with mastectomy

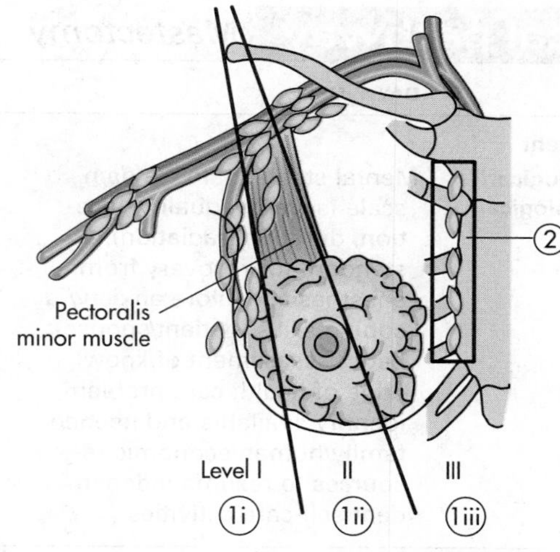


**fig. 48-8** Regional axillary lymph nodes demonstrating levels I, II, and III node dissection.

There is now general agreement that when axillary nodes are negative for cancer, a level I to II dissection, is adequate. If nodes are positive for disease,[6] a complete level III dissection is advised. *Sampling* involves the removal of one to several nodes from the lower axilla without any defined boundary and is not recommended even though "skipped" metastasis (i.e., negative nodes in a level I dissection while level III nodes are positive for tumor) is considered a rare occurrence.

### Stages III and IV disease

Surgery for advanced breast cancer includes mastectomy in combination with systemic chemotherapy or hormonal therapy. A Clinical Pathway for a patient undergoing mastectomy for breast cancer is found on p. 1588.

### Breast reconstruction

Two types of procedures are available for breast reconstruction: implants and autogenous tissue flaps. Implants, in their simplest form, are soft sacs filled with silicone gel that are placed in a pocket beneath the pectoralis major muscle and held in place by the pectoralis major, anterior serratus, and upper rectus abdominis muscles. The size and shape of the implant are matched to the size of the remaining breast. A second type of implant is called a tissue expander prosthesis. The expandable implant is placed in the manner just described by means of a single empty sac or a double-lumen sac.[9] The expander sac is filled with 100 to 200 ml of sterile saline at the time of surgery and then with 30 to 100 ml weekly until the desired size of breast is reached. The sterile saline is added to the expander sac through a needle inserted into a subcutaneous access port. The gradual expansion of the implant stretches the size of the pocket, thus giving size and shape to the new breast. Maximal expansion takes several months to achieve, at which time the prosthesis is removed and replaced by a silicone-filled implant. Newer expander sacs are available that do not need to be replaced unless a complication such as infection requires their removal. No activity restrictions are necessary during the expansion period, and pain and discomfort are usually easily controlled.

The use of silicone implants is not without complications or controversy. Complications include fibrous capsular contractions around the implant causing pain, tenderness, and fixation of the implant to the chest wall. Infection is a rare cause for implant removal. Debate about the effects of silicone on a woman's health resulted in the Food and Drug Administration's (FDA) restricting its use to those women undergoing breast reconstruction for cancer in 1992. Although silicone is not believed to be a health risk, this restriction is in place until more definitive data are available on its safety. An FDA review of saline-filled implants is scheduled in 1998 following several years of prospective studies.[9]

Nipple reconstruction, using tissue obtained from the opposite nipple-areola complex or skin from the upper portion of the inner thigh, requires a second surgical procedure after breast reconstruction. The use of a dermal tattoo that can match normal breast pigment is an alternative method of nipple formation.

The use of autogenous tissue flaps is a second means of breast reconstruction that can be performed at the time of mastectomy or at a later date. Tissue flaps eliminate the need for an implant unless insufficient tissue is available to form a breast of dimensions equal to the remaining normal breast. Performing immediate breast reconstruction avoids the cost of a second hospitalization and surgery and loss of time from normal activities. Flaps used include latissimus dorsi musculocutaneous tissue from the upper portion of the back to create a breast or transverse rectus abdominis myocutaneous (TRAM) tissue from the lower portion of the abdomen. A major disadvantage of the latissimus dorsi flap is the visible scar left on the back. A

## clinical pathway *Mastectomy*

| | DAY 1 (OR) | DAY 2 | DAY 3 |
|---|---|---|---|
| **Assessment** | | | |
| **Neurological/ Psychological** | Mental status; pain via pain scale (severity, quality, location, duration, radiation); standard for recovery from anesthesia; explore anxiety/coping skills (patient/spouse); begin assessment of knowledge of health care problem; identify available and needed family/human/economic resources to resume independent self-care activities | Mental status; pain via pain scale (severity, quality, location, duration, radiation); continue to explore anxiety/coping skills (patient/spouse); continue assessment of knowledge of health care problem; collaborate with social services to identify available and needed family/human/economic resources to resume independent self-care activities | Mental status; pain via pain scale; continue to explore anxiety/coping skills (patient/spouse) |
| **Pulmonary** | Breath sounds | Breath sounds | Breath sounds |
| **Cardiovascular** | VS per postop standard; capillary refill; pulses; Homans' sign. | HR; BP; pulses; Homans' sign | HR; BP; pulses; Homans' sign |
| **Gastrointestinal** | Mucous membranes; nausea; vomiting; bowel sounds | Mucous membranes; stool | Mucous membranes; stool |
| **Genitourinary** | I&O; UO qs | UO qs | UO qs |
| **Integumentary** | Skin turgor, temperature, color, integrity | Skin turgor and integrity | Skin turgor and integrity |
| **Surgical Wound** | Surgical drain (Jackson-Pratt/Hemovac) to self-suction; dsg/incision line; amount and type of drainage; S&S of bleeding/hematoma/edema/redness/heat | Surgical drain (Jackson-Pratt/Hemovac) to self-suction; dsg/incision line; amount and type of drainage; dsg; S&S of bleeding/hematoma/edema/redness/heat | Surgical drain (Jackson-Pratt/Hemovac) to self-suction; dsg/incision line; amount and type of drainage; dsg; S&S of bleeding/hematoma/edema/redness/heat |
| **Musculoskeletal** | Measure circumference of affected arm above elbow and compare with preop baseline | Measure circumference of affected arm above elbow and compare with preop baseline | Measure circumference of affected arm above elbow and compare with preop baseline |
| **Focus** | Hemodynamic stability; pain control | Self-care; pain control | Discharge |
| **Diagnostic Plan** | Postop Hct @ 6 PM | Repeat Hct | None |
| **Therapeutic Interventions** | Full fluid diet as tolerated this evening, then progress diet to regular; force fluids to 1500 ml by 10 PM; keep affected arm and hand elevated on pillow with elbow higher than shoulder; notify surgeon if arm circumference increases or S&S of lymphedema appear; cough, deep breathe, and use incentive spirometer q2-4h while awake; elastic support stockings; assist with getting up the first time; OOB to chair this evening and ambulate with assistance around room; assist with hygiene; *Consider:* arm sling. | After surgical dsg debulked, cleanse and cover wound with DSD daily; initiate hand and elbow exercises; full regular diet; OOB and ambulate in hall; reapply support stockings bid; social services to coordinate Reach to Recovery volunteer visit | Independent ADL; discharge |

From Birdsall C, Sperry SP: *Clinical paths in medical surgical practice,* St Louis, 1997, Mosby.

*Continued*

## Mastectomy—cont'd

| | DAY 1 (OR) | DAY 2 | DAY 3 |
|---|---|---|---|
| **Patient/Family Teaching/ Discharge Planning** | Teach use of pain scale and review meds available for pain and anxiety; reassure that responses (anxiety/fear, etc.) are a normal reaction; begin to explore threats to femininity/ self-esteem if patient appears ready to discuss same; teach to use incentive spirometer, to limit movement of affected arm and shoulder for 24 hr, to keep arm and shoulder elevated on pillows to facilitate drainage, to empty and measure surgical drain reservoir; review treatment plan; initiate discharge plan; discuss plan for daily review of plan of care with patient/family | Remove surgical dsg and encourage patient to look at wound (allow time in an attempt to have patient share concerns of self-image/ femininity before discharge); review how to empty and measure surgical drain reservoir and teach wound care (cleanse per standard and apply DSD); teach to apply support stockings and to do hand and elbow exercises (squeeze ball, open and close fist, flex and extend wrist and elbow) 10 × q2h while awake; introduce Reach to Recovery program, verify that volunteer will arrange a visit and leave patient pamphlet about exercise at bedside; review discharge plan and home care needs; review, clarify, and confirm information given to date | Review discharge plan; teach wound self-care (empty and record drain volume, cleanse and apply DSD, keep incision and drain dry until drain removed (7-10 days postop); teach that nerve-related numbness/tingling of arm and breast will gradually disappear; teach strategies to protect arm (no BP, injections, or blood tests; no constricting clothes, jewelry, wristwatch; no stretching, straining, or lifting packages/ pocketbook; do not allow arm to be dependent); to prevent a frozen shoulder, explain that a long-term, vigorous outpatient exercise program will be initiated; tell to notify physician if drainage changes (increase in volume/odor) and S&S of bleeding/hematoma/lymphedema/ redness/heat appear |
| **Expected Outcomes** | Hemodynamic stability with no signs of hematoma formation; verbalizes relief of pain with analgesia; acknowledges availability of analgesic/anxiolytic, plan of care, and need to communicate with nurse if S&S of anxiety and fear become overwhelming (subjective feelings, emotional lability, or inability to concentrate); demonstrates use of incentive spirometer; participates in self-care. | Voids qs; normal stool; uses fewer doses of prn meds as evidenced by pain scale <3 (0-10); demonstrates correct arm position to facilitate drainage; ambulates freely; verbalizes discharge plan, meds, and drug/food interactions; verbalizes appropriate anxiety and fears related to surgery; demonstrates how to empty and measure surgical drain reservoir | Demonstrates self-care of wound and drain; verbalizes planned exercises per teaching plan; states appointment date with physician; pain well controlled as evidenced by pain scale <3 (0-10); verbalizes health-seeking behaviors (nutrition, fluids, daily exercise, monthly breast self-exam, and annual mammogram); verbalizes community resources and support groups available |
| **Trigger(s)** | Hemodynamic instability from bleeding; hematoma formation | Reluctance to participate in self-care activities, especially wound care | Unable to be independent in ADL |

Consults for Consideration: (Date and initial when completed) Social Services ________ Dietary Dept. ________ Oncology CNS ________ Reach to Recovery ________ Home Care ________

TRAM flap has the advantage of using tissue that is similar in elasticity to normal breast tissue and is available in sufficient quantity to construct a new breast of equal size and shape of the uninvolved breast. An additional advantage is that the abdominal scar can be easily hidden.[33] Nipple reconstruction is performed in the same manner as already described. Figure 48-9 shows the three types of breast-reconstruction methods.

When mastectomy without breast reconstruction is chosen as the option, a breast prosthesis is necessary. For some women this may not be viewed as a problem. Others find the need for prostheses an uncomfortable nuisance and a constant reminder of their breast cancer experience. Some women describe feeling "out of balance" when wearing the prosthesis compared with the weight of the opposite normal breast. They also may feel confined in their choice of clothing or participation in physical activities. These kinds of concerns may prompt women to undergo breast reconstruction many months or years after selecting mastectomy alone. Some surgeons believe that a wait of 3 to 6 months is beneficial before reconstruction surgery. This delay permits recovery from the initial surgery and potential postoperative complications such as infection, hematoma formation, and lymphedema.

## Diet

Maintenance of good nutrition is essential for all patients with cancer. Dietary requirements include an increase in calories, carbohydrate (CHO), and protein. Body energy demands are known to increase with cancer, and more energy is necessary to withstand the potentially debilitating side effects of treatment. A diet high in calories and CHO spares body protein, necessary for tissue and wound repair, from being broken down for energy needs.

Good dietary management and patient education are especially important for the person with breast cancer. This diagnosis can evoke great emotional stress, and its treatment can affect appetite and nutrition in many ways.

All of the prescribed treatment options—surgery, radiation therapy, chemotherapy, and hormonal therapy, as well as adjunct medication and activity restrictions—affect body nutritional needs and maintenance to some degree. Table 48-2 provides an overview of nutritional problems generated by various cancer treatment options and the interventions commonly used to treat them.

## Activity

The activity level of the patient with breast cancer depends on several factors: extent of the disease process, type of treatment used, phase within the treatment modality, and state of physical and emotional adjustment. The patient is encouraged to engage in any activity for which she feels able and finds enjoyable. At least 8 hours of sleep each night and incorporation of rest periods throughout the day are advisable, especially in the immediate postoperative period and during chemotherapy or radiation therapy. Sexual activity is not contraindicated and can be resumed as desired.

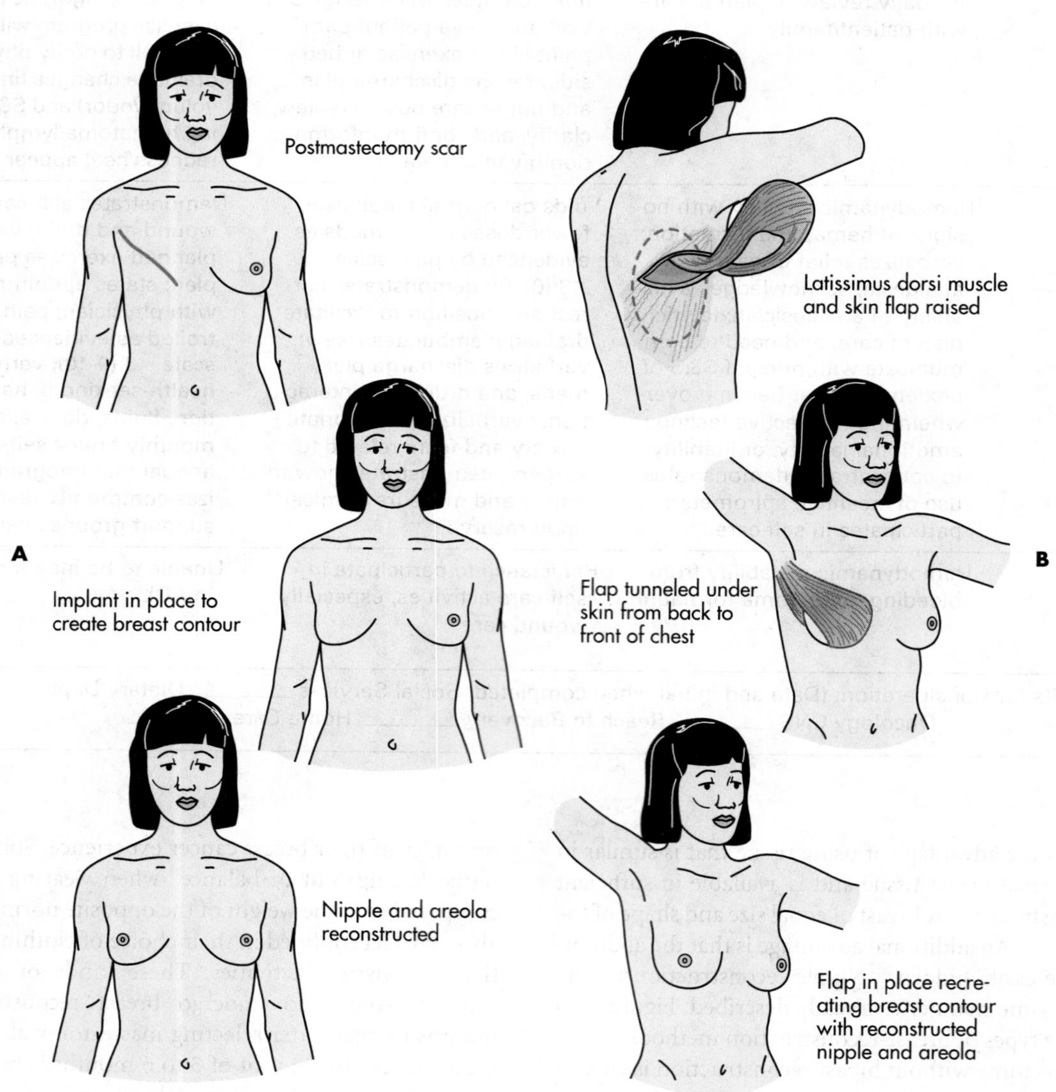


**fig. 48-9** Three types of breast reconstruction procedures. **A,** "Simple" implant placement. **B,** "Latissimus dorsi" reconstruction.

*Continued*

### Referrals

During the period of diagnosis and treatment, the patient may be referred by her primary physician to breast cancer specialists: surgeons and medical or radiation oncologists. The rationale for the referrals should be thoroughly discussed with the woman and her family. If breast reconstruction is to be performed at the time of mastectomy, a plastic surgeon will evaluate the patient's situation in regard to which procedure can be most easily performed and will best meet her needs. When radiation therapy or chemotherapy is to be part of the treatment plan, a referral to an expert in these areas is common practice. Often it is the woman herself who initiates a referral or consultation in the effort to obtain a "second opinion" regarding her breast cancer diagnosis and treatment. Second opinions should be encouraged and names of appropriate medical experts provided. This ensures the patient "peace of mind" and confidence that the diagnosis and prescribed treatment are in fact appropriate.

# NURSING MANAGEMENT OF THE PATIENT UNDERGOING MASTECTOMY

## PREOPERATIVE CARE

### Assisting with Treatment Decisions

The discovery of a breast "lump" elicits one of the most powerful and distressing emotional reactions that a woman of any age can experience. Anxiety and stress levels are high. Nurses caring for patients during this critical time (discovering the tumor, undergoing diagnostic tests, making treatment decisions) need to be cognizant of the impact

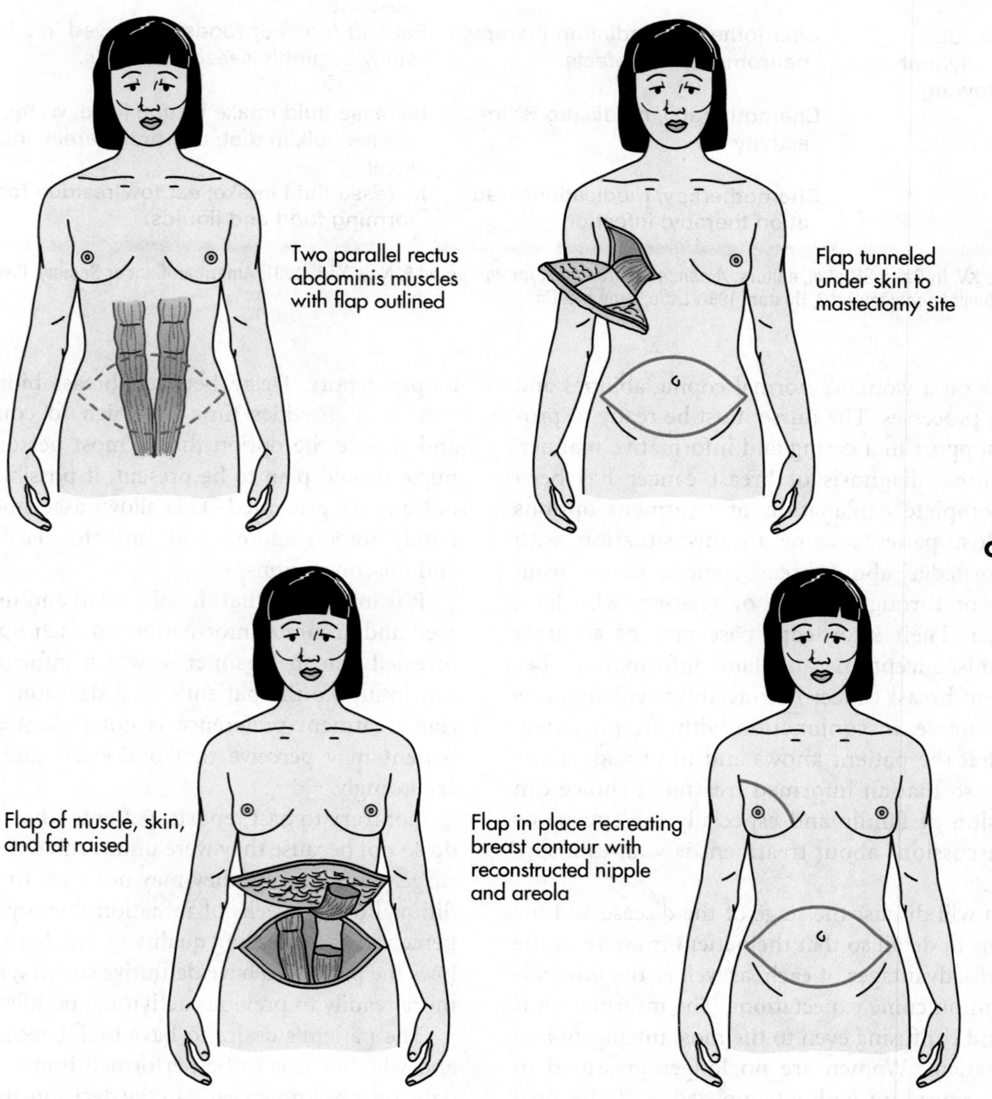


**fig. 48-9 cont'd** C, "Rectus abdominis" reconstruction.

**table 48-2** *Plan of Care for Treatment-Induced Nutritional Problems*

| Nutritional Problem Generated | Treatment Options Involved and Stress-Related Factors | Interventions |
|---|---|---|
| Oral | | |
| Stomatitis (mouth sores) | Chemotherapy, radiation therapy | Eliminate acidic, salty, and spicy foods; abstain from alcohol and tobacco; use good oral hygiene. |
| Anorexia | Chemotherapy, radiation therapy, emotional distress | Provide small, frequent high-caloric meals; make meal time an enjoyable occasion; avoid noxious odors. |
| Xerostomia (dry mouth) | Chemotherapy, radiation therapy, medications; mouth breathing | Ensure adequate fluid intake; suck on hard candies; use artificial saliva; moisten mouth with water, using a dropper or syringe if necessary. |
| Abnormal taste | Chemotherapy, radiation therapy, medications | Avoid offensive foods (red meat); mask bad taste by adding wine/beer to soups and sauces; marinate meats; use more and stronger seasonings; serve cold or room-temperature food; drink more liquids; add tartness with lemon juice or vinegar; remedy dental problems. |
| Nausea and vomiting | Chemotherapy, surgery, radiation therapy, narcotics; behavioral factors (anticipatory vomiting) | Use antiemetics as needed; withhold food before chemotherapy or radiation treatment: eliminate offensive foods; avoid noxious odors; avoid food preparation if possible. |
| Dysphagia (difficult swallowing), odynophagia (painful swallowing) | Chemotherapy, radiation therapy; neuromuscular defects | Eat soft foods or foods processed in a blender; avoid spicy or highly seasoned foods. |
| Constipation | Chemotherapy, medications; inactivity | Increase fluid intake (prune juice, water, coffee); increase bulk in diet; use bran cereal, increase activity level. |
| Diarrhea | Chemotherapy, medications, radiation therapy; infection | Increase fluid intake; eat low-residue foods; avoid gas-forming food and liquids. |

Modified from Baraie KV: In Baird SB et al, editors: *A cancer source book for nurses,* ed 6, New York, 1991, American Cancer Society; Casciato DA, Lowitz BB, editors: *Manual of clinical oncology,* ed 2, Boston, 1992, Little, Brown & Co.

these events have on a woman's normal coping abilities and decision-making processes. The nurse must be ready to provide emotional support in a caring and informative manner.

Once a definitive diagnosis of breast cancer has been established, a complete explanation of treatment options must follow. Most patients come to this situation with some prior knowledge about breast cancer, either from media exposure or through friends or relatives who have had breast cancer. Their knowledge base may be accurate or laden with misconceptions and false information. Because treatment of breast cancer is constantly evolving, it is essential for the nurse, in conjunction with the physician, to determine what the patient knows and to provide accurate information so that an informed treatment choice can be made. Inclusion of family and especially the spouse or partner in all discussions about treatment is vital to a successful outcome.

The physician will discuss the stage of the disease and the treatment options in detail so that the patient is aware of the advantages and disadvantages of each, as well as the immediate and long-term outcome expectations. The information is often complex and confusing even to the most intelligent and well-informed patient. Women are no longer pressured to select a surgical procedure without knowledge of the final biopsy report. Delay between breast biopsy and definitive treatment provides time in which to consider the options and choose the option that is most personally suitable. The nurse should plan to be present, if possible, when treatment options are presented. This allows assessment of patient and family understanding and time to clarify misinformation and misconceptions.

It is important that the physician and nurse provide unbiased and accurate information on each option. Studies have revealed that the manner in which information is presented can influence the patient's final decision. Even when physician treatment preference is not indicated or solicited, the patient may perceive that one exists and make her choice accordingly.[7,25,26]

Contrary to past reports, patients who choose mastectomy do so not because they were uninformed about breast-sparing surgery but because they may not wish to go through an additional 6 to 7 weeks of radiation therapy. Radiation may be perceived as decreasing quality of life. Mastectomy surgery allows the patient to have definitive surgery, recover, and return more readily to previous activities and lifestyle.

The patient's desire to have breast reconstruction surgery and whether it is to be performed immediately or at a later date must be known early in the decision-making process. Immediate reconstruction allows for shorter incisions and less skin removal by preserving breast landmarks and results in more balance and symmetry between the reconstructed breast and the remaining breast. Immediate reconstruction also has the advantage of requiring only one hospital stay, one anesthesia, and one rehabilitation.[9] Delayed reconstruction, while giving the woman more time to decide on all options, lacks all of the advantages mentioned above.

Financial concerns also can influence treatment decisions. The most recent information on the cost of a modified radical mastectomy in the United States, including hospital costs and physician fees, is about $6000.[4] If the patient has health insurance, generally she can be assured that costs for both mastectomy and breast reconstruction surgery are covered.

### Assisting with the Grieving Process

The diagnosis of breast cancer is extremely traumatic, but contrary to common belief, most women cope well with surgery and the loss of a breast. Most women state that they are not concerned about body image or sexuality when the decision on surgical procedure (lumpectomy versus mastectomy) is being made. Their most immediate concern is to have the cancer eradicated from the body. It may not be until after the mastectomy surgery that issues related to body image and sexuality arise. Therefore during the presurgical phase of treatment, it is essential for the nurse and physician to determine what impact breast cancer and total or partial loss of a breast will have on the patient's self-esteem and perceived sexuality. The loss of a breast can engender feelings similar to those caused by limb amputation. Reactions include anger, depression, denial, and withdrawal. Grieving for the lost body part is normal, and the patient should be permitted time to work through her grief. The nurse should offer reassurance that the expression of grief is "OK" behavior and is accepted and understood by staff members. It is important that family members be made aware of the grieving process and encouraged to provide emotional support to the woman for as long as it is needed. Patients with problems regarding intimate relationships and sexuality should be referred for counseling. Characteristics of women at higher risk for self-esteem problems and poor sexual adjustment after mastectomy are listed in Box 48-7. Women without partners may benefit from referral to a support group of women similar to themselves. Advancing age does not exempt a woman from concerns over self-esteem and sexuality, and elders should be included in all interventions and referrals for assistance. The spouse or partner should be present, if at all possible, during all discussion about sexual concerns so that his anxieties can be addressed as well.

Referral to the ACS's Reach to Recovery program provides another means of assisting the patient to work through her grief and anxieties after breast cancer surgery. A Reach to Recovery volunteer is a woman who has had breast cancer and has undergone successful surgery and rehabilitation. These volunteers have personal knowledge of the problems and fears faced by the patient. If possible, the volunteer is matched to the patient by age and type of surgery undergone. The volunteer is able to answer questions about rehabilitation, as well as types of prostheses and brassieres and where these items can be purchased. If the patient has not yet undergone breast-reconstructive surgery, the volunteer will provide the patient with a temporary breast prosthesis and will demonstrate its use. In addition, the volunteer will provide pamphlets that illustrate the prescribed rehabilitative exercises, as well as a rope and ball used for some of these activities. If breast reconstruction has been performed at the time of mastectomy, the volunteer will be able to address the expected cosmetic outcome and any rehabilitation concerns expressed by the patient. Figure 48-10 shows some common types of breast prostheses available.

**box 48-7** *Women at Risk for Sexual and Self-Esteem Problems After Loss of Breast*

1. Reported lack of support from a loving spouse or partner
2. Existence of an unhappy, unstable, intimate relationship
3. Desire to conceive more children if still in the childbearing years
4. Past sexual problems
5. History of sexual abuse such as rape or incest

From Schover LR: *CA Cancer J Clin* 41(2):112-120, 1991.

### Promoting Patient Participation in the Treatment Plan

The focus of nursing during the preoperative period is to provide teaching in regard to what the patient can expect after surgery. Instruction for the patient undergoing mastectomy and lymph node dissection includes a review of the expected incision line and the type of dressing, drains, and drainage collection device anticipated. If breast reconstruction is to be performed immediately, the location of the donor tissue is indicated (upper back area or lower abdomen). The use of pictures or diagrams similar to those shown on p. 1590-1591 will facilitate patient understanding. If an implant is to be inserted, the nurse clarifies position and placement guidelines. The patient is informed that movement of the arm and shoulder on the affected side will be limited for the first 24 hours and that the arm and hand will be elevated on a pillow to facilitate lymphatic and venous drainage. A return demonstration of breathing exercises and turning techniques prepares the patient to actively participate in postoperative recovery. (For a more extensive discussion of preoperative patient preparation see Chapter 18.)

## POSTOPERATIVE CARE

The focus of postoperative care after breast surgery is to provide physical comfort, maintain nutritional support, prevent

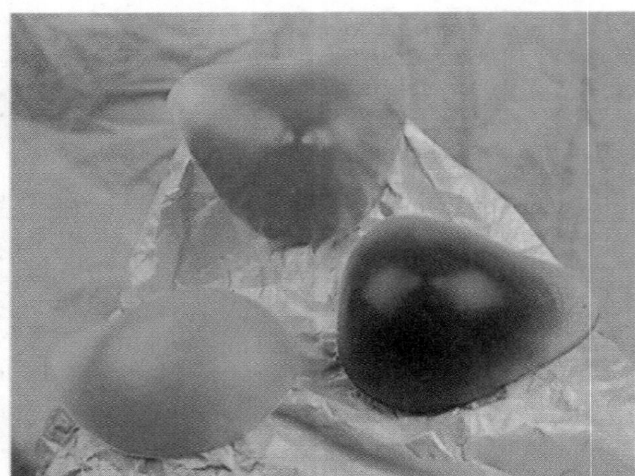

fig. 48-10 Examples of common silicone breast prostheses.

complications, and prepare the patient for discharge and successful home management. Adequate information must be provided so that the patient has full understanding of each intervention and the degree of participation required of her to make a successful transition from hospital to home management.

### Managing Pain

Surgical pain following mastectomy results from the transverse incision that usually extends from the sternum to the axilla. In addition, discomfort may result from either trauma or transection of thoracic and intercostal nerves and from fluid collection in the chest wall or at the site of the lymph node dissection. If the patient has had immediate breast reconstruction using the TRAM flap procedure, abdominal pain will be an added factor to consider in pain management.

Pain relief is managed after mastectomy surgery by the administration of prescribed analgesics and comfort measures. The amount of discomfort experienced varies with the individual patient and her degree of pain tolerance. Most patients are relatively pain free by the time of discharge, requiring only a mild analgesic. Thorough assessment of the patient's pain level and prompt administration of analgesic ensure both pain relief and adequate sleep and rest. Patient-controlled analgesia can be an effective intervention. Maintaining physical comfort also helps diminish the high stress level seen in the immediate postoperative period. Medicating the patient before activities such as turning or getting out of bed for the first time is advisable.

Instructing the patient to get out of bed from the unaffected side lessens pain and tension on the operative site. Providing support to the affected side for the first few days after surgery is necessary because movement of the affected arm and shoulder is restricted for at least 24 hours. The patient is informed that she may feel "out of balance" initially because of the weight of the dressing and the presence of the drainage collection apparatus. Temporary use of a sling on the affected arm during ambulation, if approved by the physician, provides comfort and support by lessening strain on the shoulder and prevents the accumulation of dependent lymphatic and venous stasis.

Abdominal pain after a TRAM flap procedure is best controlled with epidural or intravenous morphine. Morphine is less likely to cause nausea and vomiting than other narcotics.[27] This is an important consideration since nausea and vomiting can put a strain on the abdominal sutures and cause wound separation, dehiscence, and infection. Maintaining a semi-Fowler's position with the knees flexed and elevated also reduces pressure on the abdomen. An abdominal binder may be ordered to provide added support during ambulation.[27] Abdominal drainage devices are checked at least every 1 to 2 hours for proper function and for the amount and type of drainage. Excessive bright red drainage may indicate hemorrhage, while little to no return may indicate obstruction of the drain or drainage apparatus. The occurrence of either is promptly reported to the physician.

When nerves are cut or traumatized within the operative field, the patient may experience sensory changes such as numbness, tingling, changes in skin sensitivity of the chest wall, and even phantom breast sensations. The patient is informed that these changes are common and expected outcomes after surgery. The nurse can assure the patient that nerve-related discomforts gradually decrease and usually cease within a few months.

### Preventing Infection

Fluid collection in the chest wall or at the axillary node dissection site can be a source of infection. The build-up of lymphedema can be a secondary source. Lymphedema usually is a transitory event until collateral lymph channels are formed. When measures are not implemented to increase lymphatic flow, fibrosis can occur within the system, and lymphedema becomes an irreversible condition. The chronic collection of fluid and any subsequent injury to the involved extremity can result in infection.[35]

After the initial dressing change by the physician, the nurse performs wound care and dressing changes as needed, noting the condition of the wound and observing for signs of infection (redness, swelling, drainage, odor, increased discomfort, and fever). Proper placement of drains and drainage collection devices can prevent fluid collection and stasis. The nurse assesses the devices (Hemovac, Jackson-Pratt) for placement and for the amount and type of drainage. When the drain and drainage-collection device are functioning properly, the amount of fluid around the incision is minimal. The patient is instructed to avoid touching the dressing and drainage device, unless she is changing the dressing or measuring output.

When immediate breast reconstruction is performed, the hospital stay will be between 2 and 7 days depending on the extent of reconstruction (simple implant, tissue expander, or autologous tissue reconstruction).[1] If reconstruction involves the use of a tissue flap, such as a TRAM flap, it is important to observe for tissue perfusion, flap color, temperature, and capillary refill the first 2 days after surgery.[19]

When breast reconstruction is performed by the placement of a tissue expander, the patient will probably experience pulling and stretching sensations of the overlying muscles. This discomfort is caused when the expander pouch is filled with 100 to 300 ml of saline solution during surgery. Discomfort will gradually subside as the muscles adjust to their new length.

## Promoting Mobility of the Arm and Shoulder

One of the priority nursing interventions after mastectomy surgery is to maintain elevation of the affected arm and hand on pillows so that they are higher than the elbow and the elbow is higher than the shoulder. This strategy must be performed while the patient is in bed or sitting in a chair so that venous and lymphatic pooling are prevented.[20] The nurse monitors for lymphatic and venous stasis by measuring the circumference of the affected arm 6 inches above and below the elbow and comparing results with a preoperative baseline measurement and with the unaffected arm. The affected arm is kept relatively immobile for 24 hours to decrease any strain on the incision line. Hand exercises may be started, consisting of squeezing a ball, opening and closing the fist, and flexing and extending the wrist and elbow several times each hour. These exercises help facilitate lymphatic flow. More rigorous range-of-motion exercises for the arm and shoulder are initiated at the discretion of the physician. Some exercises are delayed 7 to 10 days until the sutures and drains have been removed. Figure 48-11 presents an overview of exercises prescribed after mastectomy surgery (see also Box 48-8, p. 1598).

## Patient/Family Education

Before discharge, the patient is instructed about wound care management, exercise guidelines and sensory change precautions, assessment and management of lymphedema, and prevention of trauma and infection. The Patient/Family Teaching Box on p. 1599 provides an overview of some general discharge instructions.

### Teaching wound care management

Having the patient perform wound care before discharge is a major nursing goal. Instruction includes aseptic technique, care of drains, the signs and symptoms of infection, and frequency of dressing change. Because hospital stay is limited and is generally a time of high stress and anxiety, all verbal teaching should be accompanied by simple, clearly written instructions. At least one return demonstration of the care ensures that the patient understands the procedure and performs it correctly. Dressing change is necessary at least once a day to examine the incision site for signs of infection and to ensure that the drainage device is working satisfactorily. The wound should be kept dry inasmuch as infection is more likely to develop in a warm, moist environment. The patient is instructed that once the sutures and drains are removed, usually in 7 to 10 days, the physician will indicate whether the incision requires any further dressing or can be left open.

### Instruction for arm/shoulder exercises

At the time of discharge the patient will still have restrictions on the type and amount of exercise permitted for the affected arm and shoulder. Squeezing a ball and bending and flexing the wrist and elbow of the affected arm are continued at home. The more rigorous exercises meant to restore full range of motion to the shoulder are delayed until the drain and sutures are removed. The physician will then prescribe a gradual increase in the amount and type of exercises to be performed (such as wall climbing or combing hair). Some of these exercises are described in Box 48-8. Performance of these exercises several times daily helps to restore full range of motion to the arm and shoulder, thus preventing a "frozen shoulder" from lack of normal movement. The exercises will, in addition, facilitate the development of collateral lymphatic channels and prevent lymphedema.

If the patient has had reconstructive surgery, she is cautioned to avoid heavy lifting (more than 10 lb) for 6 weeks. This time frame ensures that complete healing will have occurred and strain on the incision line will be minimal. A well-fitted brassiere will provide support and normal alignment of the newly formed breast. When the patient has sensory changes because of transection or trauma to nerves at the time of surgery, some side effects may persist well after discharge. Although most sensory problems resolve within 1 year, some may persist and can cause atrophy of muscles that move the shoulder on the affected side. The patient should be alert to any signs and symptoms of impaired shoulder mobility and report them immediately.

### Assessment and management of lymphedema

Instructions on how to assess for the presence of lymphedema and how to avoid its occurrence are very important. The nurse stresses the importance of the prescribed rehabilitative exercises and teaches the patient to avoid placing the affected extremity in a dependent position for extended periods. Compliance with these instructions helps to prevent the chronic form of lymphedema, which can occur soon after discharge or many months afterward. Some edema may be present at discharge, especially if lymph node dissection was performed. The greater the number of nodes removed, the greater the chance of edema. As the wound heals and the prescribed exercises are performed, the edema usually subsides.

Demonstration of the proper technique to measure arm circumference and a method to record arm measurements enables the patient to quickly recognize the presence of a problem and report it immediately. When edema is present, the patient is instructed to keep the affected extremity elevated as much as possible. If edema persists or increases, the physician should be notified. Treatment may include the application of an elastic bandage to the entire extremity, as well as continued elevation and range of motion exercises.

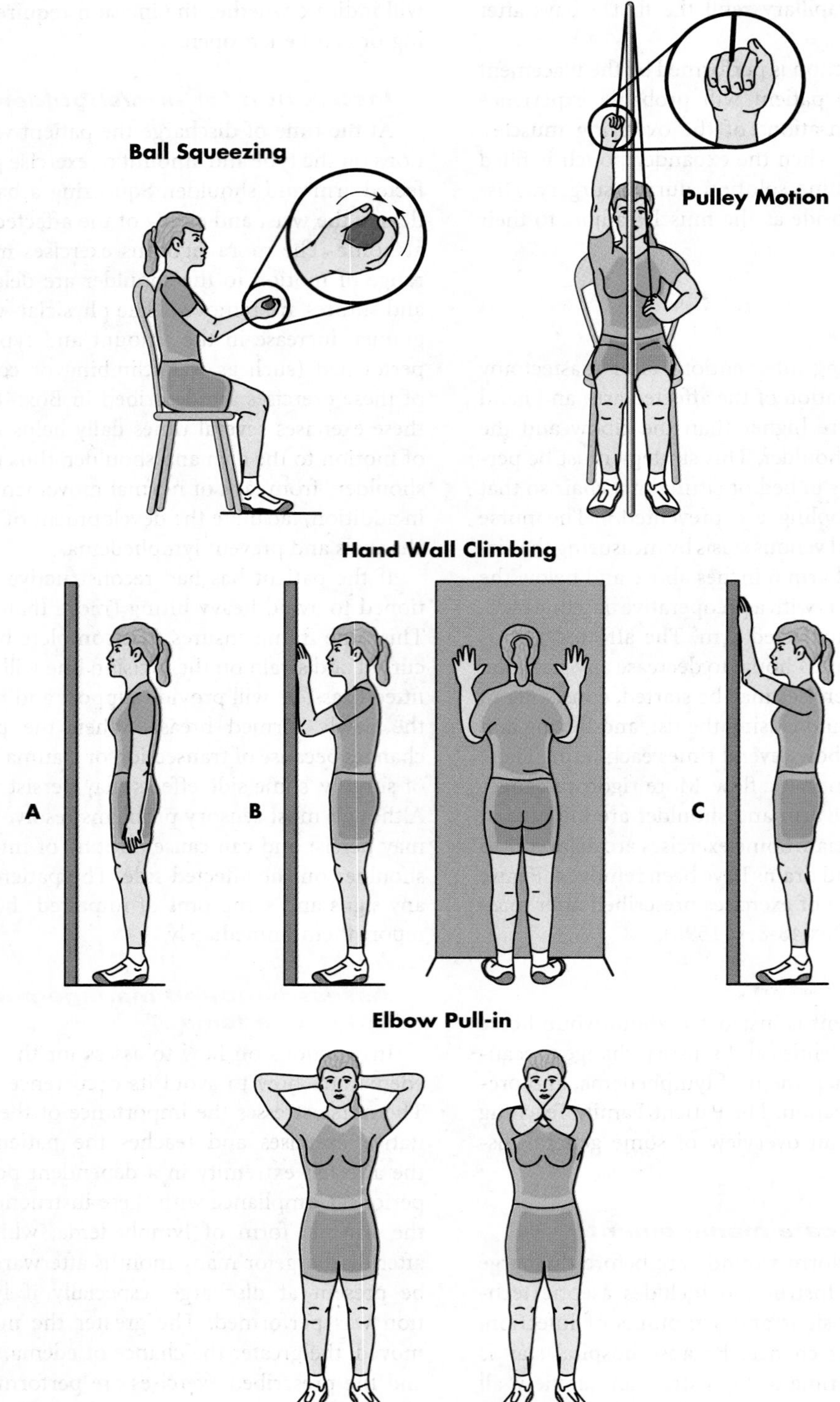


fig. 48-11 Arm and shoulder exercises commonly prescribed for patients after mastectomy surgery.

***Strategies to prevent trauma and infection***

The patient who has had breast surgery involving a level II or III lymph node dissection must be vigilant in avoiding trauma and infection to the affected arm. Protecting the arm and hand is essential because lymphatic circulation has been compromised by the removal of axillary lymph nodes. Radiation therapy is also known to interfere with the ability of the lymph nodes to remove foreign substances and destroy bacteria. Thus node dissection and radiation therapy can both lead to lymphatic dysfunction. Infectious agents can easily enter the lymphatic system from cuts, scratches, or burns. Special instructions to avoid these complications are listed in the Guidelines for Care Box, p. 1599. The patient must understand that these precautions need to be followed for the rest of her life.

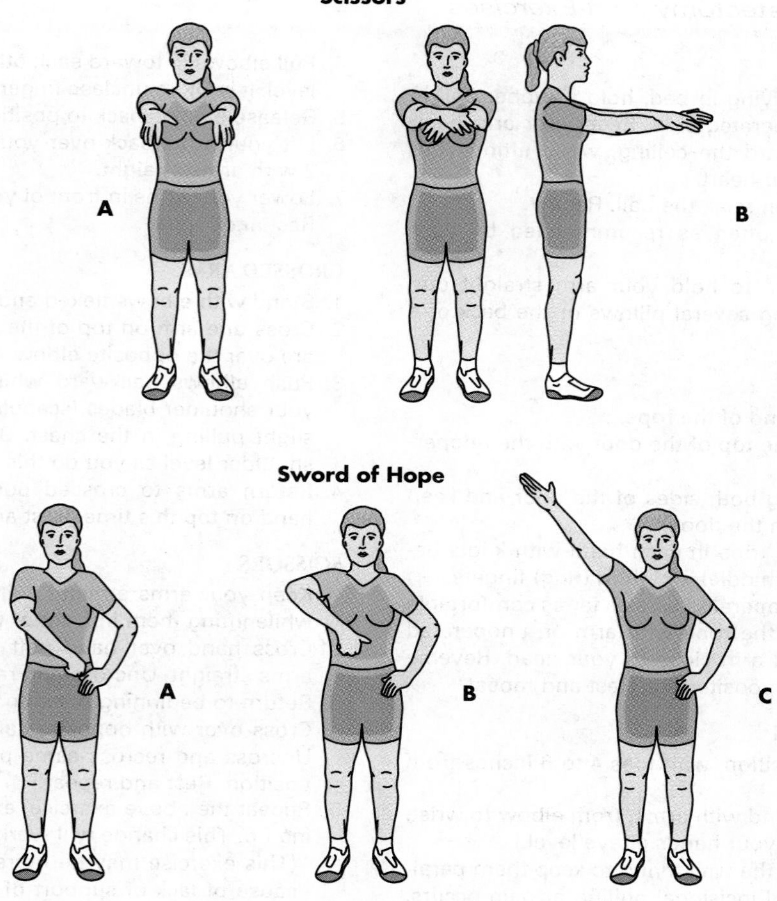


fig. 48-11 cont'd.

## Health Promotion/Prevention

The ultimate goal of primary prevention is to prevent a disease from occurring. Although many risk factors for breast cancer have been identified (see the Risk Factors Box, p. 1577) the specific cause is unknown. Women, even with knowledge of their own personal risk factors, cannot control risks such as age, gender, family, and menstrual or reproductive history. The risk of breast cancer may be reduced, however, through diet control, weight reduction, and avoidance of prolonged use of oral contraceptives and/or exogenous hormones.

Secondary prevention is used to detect a disease process in its early stage so it can be successfully treated or cured. Important measures to detect breast cancer in an early localized stage include monthly BSE, and mammographic examination as directed by a physician or as part of a mammography screening program. The ACS has designated physical examination of the breast and use of mammography as the approved basic detection methods for breast cancer. The criteria are listed in the Guidelines for Care Box on p. 1599.

A more recent secondary prevention method involves the establishment of breast cancer centers across the United States. The focus of these centers is to provide care for women with breast problems, whether benign or malignant. A major emphasis is education on risk-factor reduction, performance of breast examinations, teaching BSE techniques, and initiating referrals for screening, diagnosis, and treatment.[13] Ultimately these centers hope to detect more breast cancer in the early localized stage. Another positive outgrowth of the centers is the empowerment and education of a woman to take a more active role in promoting her own personal breast health care.

A Nursing Care Plan for a patient with breast cancer undergoing mastectomy and immediate breast reconstruction with a TRAM flap can be found on p. 1600-1602.

## GERONTOLOGICAL CONSIDERATIONS

Nearly one half of all breast cancers occur in women older than 65 years of age. Advanced-stage breast cancer is more often detected in elderly women than in their younger counterparts. One reason for this unfortunate occurrence may be that elderly women tend to receive less instruction on BSE technique and less encouragement to perform it on a regular schedule. Many older women are reluctant to touch and examine their breasts even with appropriate teaching. In addition, elderly women may not be aware of their increased vulnerability to cancer, especially breast cancer, nor know the suspicious signs and symptoms that they should report to the physician.

Changes occurring in the breast as a result of aging—such as fibrosis, calcification, shrinkage, and loss of subcutaneous

**box 48-8** *Postmastectomy Arm Exercises*

**BALL SQUEEZING**

1. Standing, sitting, or lying in bed, hold a rubber ball in your hand on the operated side. Keep your arm bent, with your palm toward the ceiling, while lifting your hand higher than your heart.
2. First squeeze and then relax the ball. Repeat.
3. Do this exercise as often as recommended by your doctor.
4. If it is uncomfortable to hold your arm straight out, support the arm using several pillows or the back of a chair.

**PULLEY MOTION**

1. Place knots at each end of the rope.
2. Toss the rope over the top of the door with the unoperated arm.
3. Sit with legs hugging both sides of the door and keep feet firmly planted on the floor.
4. Hold the ends of the rope in each hand with knots between your second (middle) and third (ring) fingers.
5. Slowly raise arm on operated side as far as comfortable by pulling down on the rope with arm on unoperated side; keep the raised arm close to your head. Reverse the motion to raise opposite arm. Rest and repeat.

**HAND WALL CLIMBING**

1. Start in standard position, with toes 4 to 6 inches from and facing the wall.
2. Bend elbows and stand with arms, from elbow to wrist, against the wall and your hands at eye level.
3. Work both hands up the wall trying to keep them parallel to each other until incisional pulling or pain occurs. Mark the spot you reach so progress can be checked.
4. Work hands down to shoulder level. Move feet and body closer to wall as comfort allows and reach requires.
5. Return to standard position. Rest and repeat. (It will relax you a bit if you rest your head against the wall.)
6. Once you reach your goal, push your fingers against the wall.

**ELBOW PULL-IN**

1. While sitting or standing, clasp fingers in front of you with elbows straight.
2. Raise your arms slowly over your head, keeping your arms straight. At first you may not be able to raise your arms over your head, but keep trying.
3. Bend elbows and bring hands behind your neck, keeping your fingers clasped together. Try to push your elbows backward so they are in a horizontal line with your shoulders.
4. Pull elbows in toward each other until they touch at chin level. It is OK to unclasp fingers to let your elbows touch.
5. Release elbows back to position in step 3.
6. Lift your arms back over your head to position in step 2 with arms straight.
7. Lower your arms in front of you to the starting position. Rest and repeat.

**CROSSED ARM**

1. Stand with elbows flexed and raised to shoulder level.
2. Cross one arm on top of the other arm so your fingers are over the opposite elbow.
3. Push elbows backward while attempting to squeeze your shoulder blades (scapula) together. You will feel a slight pulling in the chest. Be sure to keep elbows at shoulder level as you do this exercise.
4. Return arms to crossed position but place opposite hand on top this time. Rest and repeat.

**SCISSORS**

1. Keep your arms straight, with palms toward the floor, while lifting them in front of you to shoulder height.
2. Cross hand over hand (left over right) while keeping arms straight. Uncross and recross same position.
3. Return to beginning position.
4. Cross over with opposite hand on top—right over left. Uncross and recross same position. Return to starting position. Rest and repeat.
5. Repeat the above exercise, except start with palms facing up. This change will work different muscles.
   (This exercise may be more difficult to do at first because of lack of support of the extended arm. It may be better to do the CROSSED ARM exercise in the beginning.)

**SWORD OF HOPE**

1. Place the hand of your unoperated side on your hip. Make a fist with your hand on the operated side. Place your fist on the opposite hip with the thumb touching the hip. Raise your elbow slightly.
2. Lift your hand in a diagonal line from your hip to the breast area on the opposite side while keeping your elbow flexed.
3. Open your hand, palm up, as you straighten your arm over your head continuing the diagonal line.
4. Reverse the movements from position in step 3, step 2, step 1. Rest and repeat.
   (It may be recommended to do this exercise with the arm of the unoperated side for the first week before starting with the arm of the operated side.)

From *Reach to Recovery, exercises after breast surgery,* no 4668-PS, Atlanta, 1996. Reprinted by the permission of the American Cancer Society, Inc.

fat—may cause confusion regarding changes that are normal for aging and those that may indicate a possible malignant condition. Women with arthritis may have difficulty performing BSE and may discontinue the practice altogether.

Other factors that affect early diagnosis of cancer and successful treatment may be related to the socioeconomic status of elders. Retirement with reduced financial resources and the lack of health insurance beyond Medicare/Medicaid may deter elderly women from seeking medical care for a breast lump. Financial concerns about ability to pay for long-term chemotherapy or radiation therapy may cause elders to terminate treatment. Becoming a burden, both physically and financially, on their families is frequently a concern of the elderly patient with cancer.

Elderly women may also be offered fewer breast cancer treatment options. Mastectomy, rather than the conserva-

*Text continued on p. 1602*

**patient/family teaching**

### Discharge Instructions After Breast Cancer Surgery

**DRESSINGS**

**Incision**

There will be a dry gauze dressing over the incision when you leave the hospital. It is not necessary to change this dressing until you return to see the doctor.

**Drain Site**

A small dry dressing will be around the site where the drain is placed. Often there is some leakage of fluid around the drain. Check the gauze dressing for drainage and change if soiled. Some leakage is normal, but if the dressing becomes soaked more than once a day, call your doctor.

**Drains**

Your nurse has shown you how to empty the reservoir from your drain and how to measure the volume of drainage. You should empty the drain twice a day and record the measurements.

Drains are generally removed when drainage is about 30 ml in 24 hours.

Drains are often removed at the same time as the stitches, generally 7 to 10 days after surgery.

**BATHING**

Sponge baths or tub baths, making certain that the area of the drain and incision stay dry, are permitted. You may shower after the stitches and drains are removed.

**HAND AND ARM CARE**

You can begin using your arm for normal activities such as eating or combing your hair. Exercises involving the wrist, hand, and elbow such as flexing your fingers, circular wrist motions, and touching hand to shoulder are very good. More strenuous exercises can usually be resumed after the drains have been removed.

**COMFORT**

Some discomfort or mild pain is expected after surgery. Within 4 to 5 days most women have no need for medication or require something only at bedtime.

Numbness in the area of the surgery and along the inner side of the arm from the armpit to the elbow occurs in virtually all patients. It is a result of injury to the nerves that provide sensation to the skin in those areas. Women have described sensations such as heaviness, pain, tingling, burning, and "pins and needles." These sensations change over the months and usually resolve by 1 year.

**SUPPORT AND INFORMATION**

Pamphlets on exercises, hand and arm care, and general facts about breast cancer are available from your nurse or volunteer visitor. The American Cancer Society has volunteers who have had surgery similar to yours and are available to visit you.

From Knobf MT: In Baird SB: *Cancer nursing: a comprehensive textbook*, Philadelphia, 1991, WB Saunders.

**guidelines for care**

### Precautions After Mastectomy

Ensure that the affected arm is never used for blood pressure, injections, or venipunctures.

Wear no constricting clothing or jewelry, including wrist watch, on affected arm.

Do not carry heavy objects (pocketbook, packages) in affected arm.

Wear rubber gloves when washing dishes.

Use unaffected arm when removing items from hot oven, or protect by wearing a padded glove pot holder.

Use a thimble when sewing; wash needle pricks and cover as necessary.

Take care when trimming finger nails and cuticles; avoid using scissors for this task.

Use softening lotions or creams to keep skin in soft; supple condition.

Outdoor activities:

- Wear gloves when gardening.
- Avoid sunburn—wear protective clothing or use sunscreen liberally.
- Use insect repellent when in an area where biting or stinging insects may be located.
- Tend to cuts and scratches immediately by washing and applying protective covering.

**guidelines for care**

### American Cancer Society Guidelines for Breast Cancer Screening in Asymptomatic Clients

| Test or Examination | Age | Recommendation |
|---|---|---|
| Breast self-examination | Older than 20 | Monthly |
| Breast physical examination | 20-40 | Every 3 years |
| Mammogram | Older than 40 | Yearly |

American Cancer Society Revised Guidelines, June 12, 1997.

## nursing care plan *Person with Breast Cancer Undergoing Mastectomy and Immediate Breast Reconstruction with a TRAM Flap*

**DATA** Mrs. J. is a widowed 53-year-old white female supervisor at the phone company who has been admitted to the surgical unit with a diagnosis of cancer of the left breast. Mrs. J. had her annual mammogram 1 week before admission, at which time a 2-cm lesion was revealed. Her local medical doctor referred her to a surgeon who performed a tru-cut needle biopsy. The tissue report indicated that the lesion was an infiltrative ductal carcinoma. Treatment options were discussed with Mrs. J. in the presence of her children, daughters aged 20 and 17, respectively. Since the lesion was small and in a localized stage (stage I-II), Mrs. J. was offered the choice of either breast-sparing surgery (lumpectomy) followed by radiation therapy or a modified radical mastectomy and breast reconstruction, immediate or delayed. Mrs. J., after discussion with her daughters and older sister, indicated she did not want a silicone implant due to the possible physical problems she had heard about. She opted to have a mastectomy and immediate reconstruction using the TRAM flap procedure. Mrs. J. was referred to a plastic surgeon who would perform the TRAM flap portion of the surgery in conjunction with the general surgeon. Construction of a new areola and nipple is planned to take place after surgical healing has been achieved. Surgery is scheduled for the following morning. Routine preoperative orders include complete blood count (CBC), urinalysis, electrocardiogram (ECG), and chest x-ray; bowel preparation, and nothing by mouth (NPO) after midnight. Nursing orders include assessing Mrs. J.'s understanding of the impending surgical procedure, any concerns or fears not previously discussed, preoperative teaching regarding turning and breathing techniques, need for a nasogastric tube (optional), Foley catheter, incentive spirometer, and antiembolism hose; the method of pain control (patient-controlled analgesia [PCA] pump); nutrition plan (NPO to clear liquids to regular food as tolerated); positioning and mobility postoperatively; and Mrs. J.'s expected involvement in her postoperative recovery. The nurse will initiate a referral to Reach to Recovery for a visit by a volunteer who has had TRAM flap reconstruction.

The nursing history revealed the following:

- Mrs. J. performs monthly BSE and has a yearly mammogram.
- She has no known family history of breast cancer in first-degree relatives (mother or sisters).
- She has excellent family support available, and company health insurance provides complete coverage for surgical reconstruction.
- Although Mrs. J. is in good general health, does not smoke, and only drinks alcohol socially, she is about 25 pounds overweight and is involved in no regular exercise activity.
- Mrs. J. has 2 pints of her own blood reserved to be administered as needed during the surgical procedure.

Collaborative nursing actions include monitoring for the following:

- Signs of infection: redness, swelling, purulent drainage, pain at site, and elevated temperature
- Signs of neurovascular changes in the TRAM flap: decreased capillary refill, warmth, increased swelling, and loss of sensation

**NURSING DIAGNOSIS** *Knowledge deficit related to expected physical and cosmetic changes after mastectomy and TRAM flap breast reconstruction*

| expected patient outcome | nursing interventions | rationale |
|---|---|---|
| Patient will be able to discuss: | | |
| Location of donor site and after effects | Clarify location of TRAM flap from site in lower abdomen and fact that removal of muscle flap will result in some abdominal weakness and an abdominal scar. | This information provides a knowledge base to enable full understanding of the procedure and compliance in the treatment. |
| Lengthy course of recovery and rehabilitation | Reinforce that surgery will take about 7 hours to complete; hospitalization will be 6 to 7 days; employment can be resumed in about 6 weeks. A second operation will be needed to construct new areola/nipple. | Prepare patient for the need to continue therapy as an outpatient. |
| Expected appearance of new breast mound | Show pictures of breast mound. Indicate mound will have feelings of sensation and pressure. Breast size will be similar if adequate abdominal tissue is available. | Provide realistic expectation of new breast. |
| Activity/mobility limitations | Physician will permit very gradual increase in exercise/activities over a 3-month period. | Long-term compliance will be needed to attain presurgery strength and activity tolerance. |
| Benefits of visit from a Reach to Recovery Volunteer | Initiate referral to ACS Reach to Recovery Program for visit from a volunteer who has had a mastectomy with TRAM flap reconstruction. | Provide support from a woman with the same diagnosis and surgical reconstruction. |

*Continued*

## Person with Breast Cancer Undergoing Mastectomy and Immediate Breast Reconstruction with a TRAM Flap–cont'd

**NURSING DIAGNOSIS** *Altered tissue perfusion to affected arm and TRAM flap secondary to compromised circulation or lymphatic drainage*

| expected patient outcome | nursing interventions | rationale |
|---|---|---|
| Patient does not experience circulatory dysfunction at flap or lymphatic stasis | Assess flap q1hr × 24 hours then q2-4hr for capillary refill, color, warmth, edema, and decreased sensation. Use Doppler if necessary. | Ensure viability of flap blood supply. |
| | Perform neurovascular checks to affected arm q1h × 24 hours then q2-4hr. Teach patient how to perform when able to participate. | Lymphedema may be present with axillary node dissection. Lymphedema causes pressure on peripheral nerves, leading to cool, pale extremity, diminished pulse, and poor movement. |
| | Check drainage devices at TRAM flap and axillary area for patency, amount, color, and consistency each shift. Document changes and report to physician. | Increased drainage may indicate that drain is improperly placed or obstructed, leading to lymphedema or impaired circulation at flap. |

**NURSING DIAGNOSIS** *Pain from surgical procedure*

| expected patient outcome | nursing interventions | rationale |
|---|---|---|
| Patient will be pain free | Assess comfort level and document | Freedom from pain promotes patient cooperation and compliance with plan of care. |
| | Administer prescribed analgesic to provide maximum level of comfort. If using PCA pump, assess ability to use correctly. | Provide patient with some control in pain management. |
| | Elevate affected arm on pillow as directed. | Promote lymphatic and venous return and help prevent lymphedema. |
| | Position in semi-Fowler's position with knees flexed and elevated on a pillow when in bed. Use abdominal binder if ordered. Assist with turning and ambulation. | Reduce strain on abdominal incision; promote healing and competency of abdominal muscles necessary in the performance of daily activities. |
| | Restrict upper extremity exercise/activity until permitted by physician (about 10 days postoperatively). Secure drainage devices properly (2 at breast and 2 in abdominal wound). Check function q2hr. Drainage becomes clear as healing progresses. | Avoid hematoma or seroma formation and pressure on incision line and reduce potential for infection. |

**NURSING DIAGNOSIS** *Risk for infection related to mastectomy, axillary node dissection, abdominal wound, and invasive equipment (IV lines, catheter, drains)*

| expected patient outcomes | nursing interventions | rationale |
|---|---|---|
| Patient will be free of infection<br>Can discuss signs and symptoms of infection to report | Assist with performing deep breathing, turning q2hr, incentive spirometer. Splint abdomen for coughing. Encourage early ambulation as permitted. | Prevent inadequate respiratory efforts and pooling of secretions that cause respiratory infection. |
| | Assess for signs and symptoms of infection (elevation of temperature, redness, swelling, pain, and purulent drainage). | Provide for early recognition and treatment. |
| | Perform drain care using sterile technique. Teach patient how to perform before discharge and need for good hand washing. Monitor invasive equipment as a cause of infection. Document and report findings to physician | Promote patient involvement and self-care ability before discharge. |

Continued

## Person with Breast Cancer Undergoing Mastectomy and Immediate Breast Reconstruction with a TRAM Flap–cont'd

**NURSING DIAGNOSIS** *Risk for infection related to mastectomy, axillary node dissection, abdominal wound, and invasive equipment (IV lines, catheter, drains)—cont'd*

| expected patient outcomes | nursing interventions | rationale |
|---|---|---|
| | Post sign in room alerting staff *not* to use affected arm for blood pressure, injections, venipuncture, and IV lines. Inform patient of guidelines to follow to protect self from infection after mastectomy and lymph node dissection (see p. 1599). | Lymph node dissection disrupts lymphatic function. An inflated blood pressure cuff can obstruct lymph flow through channels and increase damage. Injections and venipunctures cause breaks in skin and provide a source for infection. |

**NURSING DIAGNOSIS** *Altered home maintenance related to lack of knowledge for long-term recovery and health maintenance*

| expected patient outcome | nursing interventions | rationale |
|---|---|---|
| Patient will discuss specific instructions related to exercise, wound care, activity limits to ensure recovery and total rehabilitation | Teach wound care and care of drainage devices after discharge. | Demonstration/return demonstration and written instructions give the patient/family confidence in their ability to perform self-care at home. |
| | Instruct on limitations for resuming full activities until permitted by physician. No lifting of any item more than 10 lb, no full range of motion exercises to affected arm and shoulder until complete wound healing (4-6 weeks). Sexual activity may be resumed; however, participation should be more passive in nature. New breast should be protected from pressure until healed. | Information will prevent complications from occurring and ensure good recovery/rehabilitation. |
| | Reinforce technique of breast self-examination and encourage monthly adherence. Discuss value of periodic mammograms to new and remaining breast. Involve patient's daughters in teaching of BSE and the need for mammograms as directed by their primary care physician. | Provides a means of prevention and of detecting recurrence of breast cancer. Family history is now a risk factor for daughters in family. |

tive surgical lumpectomy procedure, is frequently the only surgical treatment advised for elderly women, even those with early, localized disease and negative nodes.

The nurse must encourage the elderly woman to participate in cancer screening and detection programs, have a yearly mammogram, and perform monthly BSE. The nurse should also act as a patient advocate when treatment options are being presented and advised.

## SPECIAL ENVIRONMENTS FOR CARE

### Critical Care Management

The critical care setting is seldom used for the care of early-stage breast cancer patients. An exception may be a patient with a comorbid condition, such as diabetes or emphysema, that could complicate normal recovery and require more intensive nursing care. The elderly patient is a more likely candidate to have a chronic or acute comorbid condition that would benefit from close nursing and medical management.

### Home Care Management

For most women the home has become the setting in which recovery and rehabilitation after breast cancer treatment take place. Women who will receive additional treatment with radiation or chemotherapy should be provided with information about when and where treatment will begin and why it is necessary to keep all follow-up appointments. If a tissue expander was used for breast reconstruction, the nurse provides the patient with information about the timing of subsequent injections of saline solution into the implant. The nurse advises the woman that the procedure is uncomfortable because the muscle overlying the expander is stretched immediately after each injection. Once the muscle has been stretched to the desired size, the expander may be removed or left in place over the implant. If an autogenous tissue flap was created, nipple reconstruction may be planned after the operative site has healed.

Unfortunately, breast cancer can recur or develop in the remaining breast. Therefore, the nurse determines the patient's knowledge and skill in the performance of BSE. If necessary the proper procedure should be demonstrated and a pamphlet on BSE provided. Because breast cancer has a tendency to recur at the incision line, the nurse teaches the patient how to assess this area. Follow-up mammograms are an integral part of long-term care. The necessity for these examinations cannot be overstressed.

The ACS is an important resource for all cancer patients. Reach to Recovery volunteers are always available to meet with patients after discharge to answer questions and address concerns. Some will make home visits, accompany the patient in purchasing a permanent prosthesis and brassiere, and talk about breast-reconstruction issues. Other ACS volunteer groups, such as I Can Cope, are helpful for persons who have gone through a cancer experience and are successfully coping with life after cancer. Family members frequently find needed support from this group as well.

### COMPLICATIONS

The woman who has undergone treatment for breast cancer will always live with the fear of recurrent disease even when the cancer was found and treated in an early, localized stage (Research Box). Recurrent disease can develop within months of initial treatment or many years later. It is important that all women, regardless of age or stage of disease, be reminded to report the presence of symptoms such as bone pain or changes at the incision site, which could indicate disease recurrence or the presence of distant metastasis.

A chronic form of lymphedema may occur at any time after breast surgery, especially when large numbers of lymph nodes were removed. These women must always be on guard for signs of increasing edema. When the affected arm circumference exceeds that of the unaffected arm by 10% or more, the beginning of the irreversible and chronic form of the condition may have occurred. This is a serious problem that may require hospitalization and the use of a compression sleeve with intermittent pressure to force the edema fluid from the affected arm. These sleeves permit a uniform movement of the fluid that cannot be achieved with an elastic wrap. Antibiotics, salt and fluid restrictions, and in some cases, diuretic therapy have been used to treat chronic lymphedema.

The threat of trauma and infection after mastectomy and node dissection is ever present and requires that the woman comply with the aforementioned precautions. If signs and symptoms of trauma or infection occur, the woman is advised to inform her physician immediately so that appropriate measures can be instituted.

## NONMALIGNANT CONDITIONS OF THE BREAST

Benign breast disease is common and accounts for about 90% of all breast problems. Because there is no universally accepted classification system for benign disorders, the term *fibrocystic disease* has been used as an umbrella category into which most benign disorders are placed. This has resulted in confusion in diagnosing and treating patients with benign conditions.

**research**

Reference: Northouse LL, Laten, D, Reddy P: Adjustment of women and their husbands to recurrent breast cancer, *Res Nurs Health* 18:515-524, 1995.

The recurrence of breast cancer is an extremely stressful event, and both patients and families report shock, worry, and increased feelings of uncertainty. The purpose of this study was to determine if differences exist between a woman and her spouse in the areas of adjustment, amount of support perceived, symptom distress, feelings of hopelessness, and uncertainty after recurrence of breast cancer. Eighty-one women and 74 husbands participated in the study. Most women had undergone a modified radical mastectomy and approximately 3 years had elapsed since the initial diagnosis.

Results of the study indicate that there were both similarities and differences in patient and spouse responses. Women were very surprised when breast cancer recurred and reported the recurrence as more stressful than the initial cancer diagnosis. On the other hand, husbands were somewhat surprised at the recurrence, but were less stressed than at the initial diagnosis. Responses related to feelings of hopelessness and assessment of symptom distress were similar. Differences did exist in the perceived degree of support received. Women reported higher levels of social support, especially from family and friends that their husbands. Husbands reported more uncertainty at the time of recurrence than was felt by their wives.

Implications from the study include the need for health professionals to perform psychosocial assessments on both women and their spouses at the time of cancer recurrence to better understand each person's response to this stressful event. Interventions are needed that consider each partner's concerns, as well as those shared by both.

### CYSTIC BREAST DISEASE

#### Etiology/Epidemiology

The underlying cause of cystic breast disease is not fully known. Changes in the breast are cyclic and thought to be caused by hormonal imbalance or the exaggerated response of breast tissue to ovarian hormones. Breast tenderness is more pronounced during or before menstruation. Cystic breast disease is most common in nulliparous women between the ages of 40 and 50 years but can occur at any age. Occurrence is least frequent after menopause.

#### Pathophysiology

A number of commonalities are seen in cystic disease regardless of the diagnostic name used. Changes once thought to be abnormal such as microcysts, apocrine change, adenosis, fibrosis, and varying degrees of hyperplasia are now recognized as part of the involutional process of the breast. These changes include the presence of lumps of varying size, nipple discharge, and breast pain (mastodynia). Cystic lesions are soft, well demarcated, and freely movable. The process is almost always bilateral, with most lesions located in the left breast. The cysts may contain clear, milky, straw-colored, or yellow to dark brown fluid. Occasionally the contents may be blood-tinged. The common clinical manifestations of fibroadenomas and fibrocystic disease of the breast are compared in Table 48-3.

### Collaborative Care Management

The woman who discovers a mass or masses in her breast should seek the advice of a health care provider who will decide whether aspiration or biopsy should be performed. A needle aspiration generally confirms the presence of a cyst. Because the presence of nodular tissue in the breast makes the early detection of malignant lesions more difficult, some physicians suggest periodic mammograms to detect any changes. There is no evidence to suggest that cystic disease predisposes the woman to the development of a malignant lesion; but these women are at more risk than those without cystic disease.

The limitation or exclusion of methylxanthines (a class of chemicals found in coffee, tea, cola, and chocolate) is frequently recommended as a means of controlling cystic disease, but there is no research evidence that methylxanthines cause either benign or malignant breast disease.

Vitamin therapy, especially vitamin E, may have some anticancer properties, but again, no conclusive evidence exists that vitamin E therapy reduces the risk of cancer or relieves the distress of cystic breast disease. Danazol, an attenuated androgen, has some demonstrated therapeutic properties that decrease breast pain, feelings of heaviness, and tenderness in patients with cystic disease.[56] Studies of tamoxifen are ongoing. Some women with cystic disease have reported results that range from some regression of lesions to the complete disappearance of breast pain with tamoxifen use, but its appropriateness for cystic breast disease has not been established.

#### *Patient/family education*

The role of the nurse in the care of patients with benign breast disorders is primarily that of educator and facilitator. The nurse should be knowledgeable about benign conditions, understand their medical management, be able to provide and clarify information, and support the patient, emotionally and physically, through diagnosis and treatment.

Hospitalization is seldom required for the treatment of cystic breast disease. The nurse teaches BSE to those women who are not familiar with it and stresses its use every month. Women should be taught to recognize through touch their normal breast tissue and the location and size of any lesions present. They should report significant changes that differ from the normal cyclic fluctuations or that appear at a different time in the menstrual cycle. The use of a mild analgesic and wearing a firm supportive brassiere may provide comfort and reduce pain on movement. The use of warm, moist heat also may be beneficial to relieve aching pain. Eliminating caffeine consumption and decreasing salt content before menstruation to relieve bloating and weight gain can be recommended. The woman is advised to consult her health care provider before using vitamin E as a therapeutic intervention, so its beneficial effects, if any, can be professionally monitored. Side effects of vitamin E use are few.

## FIBROADENOMA

### Etiology/Epidemiology

*Fibroadenomas,* or adenofibromas, are the most common benign breast neoplasms. The tumors occur most often in women younger than 25 years of age; some lesions become evident by age 15. Fibroadenomas usually are firm, rubbery, round, freely movable, nontender, and encapsulated; they may be multiple and bilateral. Tumor size ranges from 1 to 3 cm. A "giant" fibroma is the most common lesion seen in the adolescent breast.

### Pathophysiology

Fibroadenomas are tumors of fibroblastic and epithelial origin thought to be caused by hyperestrinism. They are estrogen-dependent and associated with menstrual irregularities.[50] Tumors are slow growing and often are stimulated by pregnancy and lactation. Regression may occur after delivery. Fibroadenomas tend to regress at menopause and become hyalinized. "Giant" fibroadenomas grow very rapidly to 10 to 12 cm in diameter but are not more prone to malignant change than smaller lesions. Dimpling or nipple retraction is not associated with fibroadenomas.[50]

### Collaborative Care Management

Surgical removal is the standard treatment for fibroadenomas. Many can be removed under local anesthesia in an outpatient setting. Although the tumor is examined for definitive patho-

**table 48-3** *Clinical Manifestations of Fibroadenomas and Fibrocystic Disease of the Breast*

| | Fibroadenoma | Fibrocystic Disease |
|---|---|---|
| Likely age | 15-20, can occur up to 55 | 30-55, decreases after menopause |
| Shape | Round, lobular | Round, lobular |
| Consistency | Usually firm, can be soft | Firm to soft, rubbery |
| Demarcation | Well demarcated, clear margins | Well demarcated |
| Number | Usually single | Multiple usually, may be single |
| Mobility | Very mobile, slippery | Mobile |
| Tenderness | Usually none | Tender, increases before menses |
| Skin retraction | None | None |
| Pattern of growth | Grows quickly and constantly | Size may increase or decrease rapidly |
| Risk to health | None: benign; must diagnose by biopsy | Benign, though general lumpiness may mask other cancerous lumps |

From Jarvis C: *Physical examination and health assessment,* Philadelphia, 1992, WB Saunders.

logical characteristics, the association between fibroadenomas and cancer is very weak.

#### Patient/family education

When the woman discovers a breast mass, her primary concern is always a diagnosis of cancer. Reassurance that most breast lesions are not malignant should be avoided. Only the final pathology report will provide this reassurance. Before the surgical removal of the fibroadenoma, the nurse prepares the woman for the type of surgery to be performed, what to expect during the procedure, and how to care for the incision afterward. Practice of BSE should be encouraged, as well as the reporting of any unusual changes found during the examination.

## INFLAMMATORY LESIONS

### Mammary Duct Ectasia

#### Etiology/epidemiology

Mammary duct ectasia, also referred to as plasma cell mastitis, is a benign condition of unknown etiology. Some investigators believe an anaerobic bacteria may be implicated. Another causative factor may be bacterial infection that results from stasis of fluid in the large ducts of the breast. Age is the primary risk factor for duct ectasia, with a mean age ranging from 45 to 55 years. Breast pain and a palpable mass are typical symptoms in premenopausal women, nipple discharge predominates in perimenopausal women, and nipple retractions secondary to periductal fibrosis are more often noted in postmenopausal women.

#### Pathophysiology

Mammary duct ectasia involves inflammation of the ducts behind the nipple, duct enlargement, and a collection of cellular debris and fluid in the involved ducts. As the inflammatory response resolves, the ducts become fibrotic and dilated. Nipple discharge usually is bilateral and ranges from serous to thick, sticky, or pastelike. Drainage may be green, greenish brown, or blood-stained. Nipple itching, suggestive of Paget's disease, may accompany transient pain in the subareolar and inner quadrants of the breast. On palpation, the areolar area may feel wormlike; the nipple may be red and swollen or flat and retracted. The condition is not associated with breastfeeding.

#### Collaborative care management

Treatment varies depending on the severity of the problem. Because of the chronic nature of this problem, most women are monitored with routine physical examination of the breast. The symptoms of mammary duct ectasia may engender the fear of malignant disease in the patient. Once the benign nature of this chronic condition is affirmed, fears generally are dispelled, and most women are able to deal with their symptoms. Although there is no cure for mammary duct ectasia, antibiotics are prescribed for acute inflammatory episodes, such as the development of an abscess. If the chronic discharge can no longer be tolerated, surgical excision of the retroareolar ducts is performed.

**Patient/family education.** The nurse must be cognizant of the chronic yet benign nature of this condition and offer support and understanding care. The woman is taught how to cleanse the breast to minimize the risk of infection. Good hand washing and personal hygiene measures are stressed. Wearing a supportive yet nonconfining brassiere padded with sterile gauze and changing the bra daily or as necessary helps prevent abscess formation. The nurse teaches the woman the signs and symptoms indicative of abscess that should be reported immediately.

### Acute Mastitis and Abscess

#### Etiology/epidemiology

There are two forms of mastitis: acute and chronic. The acute form is a rare condition almost always found in breastfeeding mothers during the first 4 months of lactation.[28] It occurs most frequently from *Staphylococcus aureus* or *Staphylococcus epidermidis* infection that spreads from a break in the skin surface of the nipple to underlying breast tissue. It may be confined to only one quadrant of the breast. Symptoms include a fissured nipple, fever, chill, localized tenderness, and erythema. Purulent discharge from the nipple is usually not observed.

The chronic form of mastitis can follow acute mastitis or have a slow and insidious onset. Both acute and chronic mastitis are caused by the same bacterial agents. The chronic form occurs more often in older women, and the symptoms can mimic inflammatory breast cancer. The infection usually arises in the sweat or sebaceous glands and spreads to the breast. Symptoms of chronic mastitis include a painful breast mass that involves the nipple and areola and a low-grade fever.

#### Pathophysiology

In both acute and chronic mastitis there is edema and congestion of the periductal and interlobular stromata. The ducts are distended from the accumulation of neutrophils and retained secretions. If an abscess forms, its central core may be necrotic and contain creamy, yellow exudate. Fibrosis of the involved tissue can develop after treatment. Both the acute and chronic forms of mastitis can mimic inflammatory breast carcinoma, but recent lactation usually excludes the acute form from the need for further evaluation.

#### Collaborative care management

Acute mastitis is easy to diagnose in a nursing mother. Treatment with antibiotics resolves the infectious process. In older women, because the condition has similarities to inflammatory breast carcinoma, incision and drainage of the inflammatory exudate are performed to determine the cause. Antibiotics can then be prescribed.

**Patient/family education.** When acute mastitis is the result of an infection during lactation, most women immediately stop breastfeeding. Women should be informed that discontinuing breastfeeding is not always necessary or advisable. The infant is not affected by sucking on the involved breasts, and antibiotic therapy is not required.[49] Continued breastfeeding is believed reduce the pain and lessen the volume of milk that can be a source for bacterial growth. If breastfeeding is discontinued, the woman is instructed to keep her breasts as empty as possible by pumping. If the breast is not emptied, it will become engorged, and pain will increase.

The woman is instructed to complete the entire course of antibiotics and not discontinue them when symptoms are relieved. Because the infection generally does not originate in the breast, teaching about personal hygiene measures is important. The older woman with mastitis may be anxious about a diagnosis of cancer. Emotional support and frank discussion of her concerns are provided until the aspiration biopsy results are known.

Both acute and chronic mastitis resolve with antibiotic therapy, rest, and the application of local heat. Discomfort generally is relieved by analgesics.

## MALE BREAST PROBLEMS

### GYNECOMASTIA

#### Etiology/Epidemiology

Gynecomastia is a common disorder of the male breast. This condition is estimated to occur in up to 70% of pubertal boys during the time of rapid testicular growth between the ages of 12 and 15 years. Symptoms include a firm, circular, disklike, circumscribed, tender mass beneath the areola, usually bilateral at onset. In adolescent boys the condition is transient and lasts for approximately 12 to 24 months. Gynecomastia is seen again in men aged 45 years and older, with 40% of elderly men having some degree of the condition.[44] Gynecomastia is seen in obese men because obesity increases the rate of conversion of androgens to estrogen in patients with cirrhosis of the liver, because of the incomplete hepatic clearance of estrogen. Gynecomastia may develop in men who are receiving drugs such as estrogen, cimetidine, certain antibiotics (isoniazid), antihypertensive agents (reserpine and methyldopa), calcium channel blockers, and digoxin.[17]

#### Pathophysiology

Gynecomastia is caused by hormonal imbalance. As a result of the large estrogen secretion, hyperplasia (overdevelopment) of the stromata and ducts in the mammary glands occurs. The primary cause of gynecomastia in the older man is the aging process. As men age, the plasma testosterone concentration declines at the same time that the plasma testosterone-estrogen level increases. Thus less free testosterone is available.

#### Collaborative Care Management

When gynecomastia occurs and the condition cannot be attributed to rapid testicular growth (teenaged boys), to treatment with estrogen therapy (middle-aged men), or to hepatic dysfunction, a human chorionic gonadotropin-beta subunit (hCG-$\beta$) level should be obtained. This finding assists in ruling out a malignant testicular germ cell condition, which can manifest with gynecomastia and an elevated hCG-$\beta$ level. Chest and mediastinal roentgenograms and a careful testes examination are also included in the evaluation. In older men the physician may suggest obtaining a breast biopsy specimen because this age group is more prone to male breast cancer. Surgery is used for cosmesis only when the gynecomastia persists over a long period of time and is not associated with an underlying disease process.

##### *Patient/family education*

The nurse who cares for men with gynecomastia must offer sympathetic understanding. Most men are intensely embarrassed about the condition because enlarged breasts constitute a serious assault on the male self-image. The condition is visible whenever the man removes his shirt for work or recreation and frequently results in taunts and jokes. Similar problems exist for the man who undergoes mastectomy for breast cancer and is visibly asymmetrical. The problems and needs of these patients have not been fully recognized.

Patients who are treated with hormonal therapy for prostate cancer should be warned that gynecomastia is one of the side effects of treatment. Treatment of cancer takes priority over breast enlargement, but it may still constitute a psychological stress for the man. Elderly men should be informed that with normal aging, breast enlargement may occur. If the man is obese and elderly, the enlargement may be more pronounced. The nurse should be aware of the variety of drugs, other than hormones, that can increase male breast size. Men should be forewarned of this side effect.

### MALE BREAST CANCER

#### Etiology/Epidemiology

Breast cancer in men is relatively uncommon, accounting for approximately 1% (1,400) of the 181,600 new cases of breast cancer that were predicted for 1997.[42] The presentation, diagnosis, and treatments are similar to those for women with the disease.

The epidemiological characteristics of male breast cancer reveal an incidence rate that increases with age, usually occurring 5 to 10 years later than breast cancer in women. The average age at the time of diagnosis is 63.[1] A family history places men at increased risk for breast cancer.

#### Pathophysiology

Approximately 80% of breast cancers in men are ER+, with ductal infiltrating carcinoma being the predominant histological cell type.[1] Bioassay for the presence of estrogen and progesterone receptors is performed at the time of biopsy. Tumor staging is based on the TNM system.

Physical examination, mammography, fine-needle aspiration, and incisional or excisional biopsy are standard diagnostic procedures. The presence of advanced disease at the time of initial diagnosis is common, largely due to delays in seeking medical evaluation that average 10 to 18 months.[16] Gynecomastia caused by drug, alcohol, or hormone ingestion can be differentiated from a malignant lesion by both physical examination and mammogram. Fine-needle aspiration of the lesion may also be used to different gynecomastia from a malignancy. Gynecomastia generally is bilateral, whereas a malignant lesion generally occurs in a single breast.

The symptoms commonly seen at the time of diagnosis include a firm mass directly beneath the nipple in the subareolar area, most frequently in the left breast. A lesion in the upper outer quadrant is the next most frequent location for tumor growth. Bloody nipple discharge with nipple inversion is common. Evidence of Paget's disease of the nipple (eczema), itching, ulceration, and local tenderness also may be present. Metastasis may occur to bone, the lungs, and the liver.

### Collaborative Care Management

Treatment for a primary localized tumor is modified radical mastectomy with node dissection. Breast-sparing procedures are not often used because of the belief that men do not have the psychological need for this body image-sparing procedure. In addition, the typical location of the lesion in the subareolar area requires that the nipple be removed along with a tumor-free margin of tissue. Thus breast-preservation procedures cannot be safely used. Radiation therapy may be prescribed before or after surgery for control of micrometastasis or to prevent local recurrence, but radiation has no value in increasing long-term disease-free survival time.[16] When axillary nodes are involved in the disease process, systemic adjuvant therapy (chemotherapy or hormonal) is advised.

Recurrent or advanced disease is highly amenable to palliative therapy with hormonal manipulation inasmuch as most tumors are ER+. In the past orchiectomy or adrenalectomy followed by hypophysectomy was used to eliminate the source of estrogen in the body. Today the antiestrogen drug tamoxifen is the treatment of choice because it eliminates the need for surgical intervention. Chemotherapy protocols such as cyclophosphamide, methotrexate, and 5-fluorouracil (CMF), and 5-fluorouracil, Adriamycin (doxorubicin), and cyclophosphamide (FAC) may be prescribed. Antiandrogenic drugs such as flutamide and cyproterone acetate are under investigation for their usefulness in treating male breast cancer.[16]

#### *Patient/family education*

The nursing management of the man with breast cancer reflects the basic principles outlined earlier in the chapter. However, a man in whom breast cancer is diagnosed faces unique psychosocial stressors that the nurse needs to address on an individual basis. The long delays in diagnosis may reflect in part a basic disbelief that this "female problem" can be occurring. A subtheme of embarrassment needs to be identified, if present, and acknowledged. The threats of cancer remain present, however, and the treatment is aggressive. The use of tamoxifen has reduced the need for palliative surgeries such as orchiectomy, with their accompanying assault on male self-concept and body image. The male patient treated for breast cancer is an uncommon occurrence; however, the nurse will need to be sensitive to his unique needs and tailor the standard surgical care routines to the individual situation.

## critical thinking QUESTIONS

**1** Mrs. Allen, 50, is recovering from a modified radical mastectomy for stage II ductal carcinoma. All lymph nodes were negative. The physician is recommending a combination of chemotherapy and tamoxifen therapy. Discuss the ethical implications of adjuvant therapy for node-negative patients.

**2** Mrs. Lopez underwent a modified radical mastectomy and has been receiving weekly chemotherapy treatments, which have left her fatigued and weak. She tells you that she has decided to quit chemotherapy because, "I have four children to look after, my husband already works two jobs, and he can't be expected to manage the house also. I can't be much of a wife to him since this surgery anyway—the least I can do is meet my responsibilities as a mother." You know that 6 more months of chemotherapy have been planned. What major concerns do you have for Mrs. Lopez, and what interventions would you plan to help her?

**3** Use the research information presented in the chapter to support the importance of BSE as a diagnostic tool for breast cancer in light of the increasing sophistication of mammography screening.

## chapter SUMMARY

### MALIGNANT CONDITIONS OF THE BREAST

- Factors placing a woman at high risk for breast cancer include age, personal or family history of breast cancer, parity, and environmental agents.
- Breast cancers can be detected early with regular breast self-examination (BSE), physical examination, and mammograms.
- It appears that BSE skills are regularly practiced by women who are taught to look and feel for what is normal for them. This approach lessens their anxiety about finding "cancer" (pathological changes) each month, which discourages many from doing BSE regularly.
- Therapy for breast cancer depends on various factors, including histopathology, hormonal status, location and size of tumor, local or regional metastasis, and the woman's lifestyle.
- In the rehabilitation phase after breast cancer, women are working through the loss of a breast and its significance, learning to do wound care, initiating postmastectomy/lumpectomy exercises, mobilizing support systems, and pursuing prosthesis and clothing styles and possibly reconstruction options, if appropriate.
- Radiation therapy for women with breast cancer can last up to 6 weeks. Teaching includes mechanisms of radiation therapy's effect on cells, common side effects, and management of side effects and symptoms. Interstitial therapy requires additional support and teaching on the isolating aspects imposed by radiation policies.
- Teaching the woman with breast cancer about chemotherapy includes information on medications and mechanisms for managing and monitoring side effects and symptoms.

### NONMALIGNANT CONDITIONS OF THE BREAST

- Common benign conditions of the breast include cystic breast disease, fibroadenoma, inflammatory breast conditions, and male gynecomastia.

## References

1. Abeloff MD, Lichter AS, Niederhuber JE, Pierce LJ, Aziz DC: Breast. In Abeloff MD et al, editors: *Clinical oncology,* New York, 1995, Churchill Livingstone, Inc.
2. American Cancer Society: *1997 cancer facts and figures,* New York, 1997, The Society.
3. Andolina VF, Lille SL, Willison KM: *Mammographic imaging: a practical guide,* Philadelphia, 1992, JB Lippincott.

4. Anonymous: Average charges for modified radical mastectomies, *Oncology* 5(3):51-58, 1991.
5. Baker RR, Niederhuber J: Clinical management of a palpable breast mass. In Baker RR, Niederhuber J, editors: *The operative management of breast disease,* Philadelphia, 1992, WB Saunders.
6. Bargen PI, Heerdt AS, Moore MP, Petrek JA: Breast conservation therapy for invasive carcinoma of the breast, *Curr Probl Surg* 32(3):1991-2048, 1995.
7. Bilodeau BA, Degner LF: Information needs, sources of information, and decisional roles in women with breast cancer, *Oncol Nurs Forum* 23(4):691-700, 1996.
8. Boring CC, Squires TS, Heath CW: Cancer statistics for African Americans, *CA Cancer J Clin* 43(1):7-26, 1992.
9. Bostwick J: Breast reconstruction following mastectomy, *CA Cancer J Clin* 45(5):289-304, 1995.
10. Boyd NF: Nutrition and breast cancer, *J Natl Cancer Inst* 85(1):6-7, 1993.
11. Brinton LA, Schairer C: Estrogen replacement therapy and breast cancer risk, *Epidemiol Rev* 15(1):66-79, 1993.
12. Buchsel PC, Engelking C: Breast cancer treatment: the role of autologous stem cell support, *Innovations Oncol Nurs* 9(4):2-6, 1993.
13. Coleman C: Breast cancer team: roles, conflicts, interfaces, *Innovations Oncol Nurs* 8(3):2-6, 1992.
14. Conant EF, Maidment DA: Breast cancer imaging, *Sci Am* Jan/Feb:22-31, 1996.
15. Cope DG: Self-esteem and the practice of breast self examination, *West J Nurs Res* 14(5):618-631, 1992.
16. Dodd DG: American Cancer Society Guidelines on screening for breast cancer: an overview, *CA Cancer J Clin* 42(3):177-180, 1992.
17. Eberlein TJ: Gynecomastia. In Harris JR et al, editors: *Breast diseases,* ed 2, Philadelphia, 1991, JB Lippincott.
18. Eisenhauer EA: Docetaxel: current status and future prospects, *J Clin Oncol* 13(12):2865-2868, 1995.
19. Ellis C: Nursing care for the mastectomy patient who has immediate TRAM flap breast reconstruction, *Nurs Interventions Oncol* 5(1):10-13, 1993.
20. Entreken N: Breast cancer. In Clark JC, McGee RF: *Oncology Nursing Society core curriculum for oncology nursing,* ed 2, Philadelphia, 1992, WB Saunders.
21. Fisher B, Constantino J, Redmond C et al: Endometrial cancer in tamoxifen treated breast cancer patients: findings from the National Surgical Adjuvant Breast and Bowel Project (NSABP) B-14, *J Natl Cancer Inst* 86(7):527-537, 1994.
22. Freireich EJ: Toll of malignancies, past and present, *Hosp Pract* 28(3): 109-126, 1993.
23. Harris JR, Lippman ME, Veronesi U, Willett W: Breast cancer, *N Engl J Med* 327(5):319-328, 1992.
24. Hortobagyi GN, Buzdar AU: Current status of adjuvant systemic therapy for primary breast cancer: progress and controversy, *CA Cancer J Clin* 45(4):199-226, 1995.
25. Hughes KK: Decision making by patients with breast cancer: the role of information in treatment selection, *Oncol Nurs Forum* 20(4):623-628, 1993.
26. Hughes KK: Psychosocial and functional status of breast cancer patients, *Cancer Nurs* 16(3):222-229, 1993.
27. Ivey CL, Gordon SI: Breast reconstruction: new image, new hope, *RN* 57(7):48-53, 1994.
28. Jarvis C: Breast and regional lymphatics. In Jarvis C, editor: *Physical examination and health assessment,* Philadelphia, 1992, WB Saunders.
29. Johnson S: The causes of breast cancer. In Fentiman IS, editor: *Detection and treatment of early breast cancer,* ed 2, Philadelphia, 1990, JB Lippincott.
30. Jordan VC: Targeted hormone therapy for breast cancer, *Hosp Pract* 28(3):55-62, 1993.
31. Kardinal CG: Chemotherapy of breast cancer. In Perry MC, editor: *The chemotherapy source book,* Baltimore, 1992, Williams & Wilkins.
32. King MC, Rowell S, Love SM: Inherited breast and ovarian cancer: what are the risks? what are the choices? *JAMA* 269(15):1975-1980, 1993.
33. Kroll SS: Mastectomy with immediate autogenous tissue reconstruction, *MD Anderson Case Rep Rev* 5:8-10, 1993.
34. Mansour EG, Ravion PM, Dressler L: Prognostic factors in early breast cancer, *Cancer* 74(1 suppl):381-400, 1994.
35. McGrath EB: Lymphedema. In Dow KH, Hilderly LJ: *Nursing care in radiation oncology,* Philadelphia, 1992, WB Saunders.
36. Moore MP, Kinne DW: The surgical management of primary invasive breast cancer, *CA Cancer J Clin* 45(5):279-288, 1995.
37. Myers SE, Williams SF: Role of high-dose chemotherapy and autologous stem cell support in treatment of breast cancer, *Hematol Oncol Clin North Am* 7(3):631-644, 1993.
38. Nettleton J, Long J, Juban D, Wu R, Shaeffer J, El-Mahdi A: Breast cancer during pregnancy: quantifying the risk of treatment delay, *Obstet Gynecol* 87(3):414-418, 1996.
39. NIH Consensus Conference: Treatment of early-stage breast cancer, *JAMA* 265(3):391-395, 1991.
40. Noone MH, Fioravanti SG: Taxol: past, present, and future, *Oncol Nurs* 1(4):1-12, 1994.
41. Overmayer BA: Chemotherapy in the management of breast cancer, *Cleve Clin J Med* 62(1):36-52, 1995.
42. Parker SL, Tong T, Balden S, Wingo PA: Cancer statistics 1996, *CA Cancer J Clin* 46(1):5-28, 1996.
43. Peterson HB, Wingo PA: Breast cancer and the pill, *Patient Care* 11(2):67-82, 1992.
44. Powell DE, Stellilag CB, editors: *The diagnosis and detection of breast disease,* St Louis, 1994, Mosby.
45. Recht A, Hayes DF, Harris JR: The use of adjuvant therapy in patients treated with conservative surgery and radiotherapy. In Henderson IC, editor: *Adjuvant therapy of breast cancer,* Boston, 1992, Kluwer Academic Publishers.
46. Schover LR: The impact of breast cancer on sexuality, body image, and intimate relationships, *CA Cancer J Clin* 41(2):112-120, 1991.
47. Sellers TA et al: Effect of family history, body fat distribution, and reproductive factors on the risk of postmenopausal breast cancer, *N Engl J Med* 326 (20):1323-1329, 1992.
48. Silliman RA et al: Review breast cancer care in old age: what we know, don't know, and do, *J Natl Cancer Inst* 85(3):190-196, 1993.
49. Smith BL: Duct ectasia, periductal mastitis, and breast infections. In Harris JR et al, editors: *Breast diseases,* ed 2, Philadelphia, 1991, JB Lippincott.
50. Smith BL: Fibroadenomas. In Harris JR et al, editors: *Breast diseases,* ed 2, Philadelphia, 1991, JB Lippincott.
51. US Department of Health and Human Services, Public Health Service: *Healthy People 2000: summary report,* Boston, 1992, Jones & Bartlett.
52. Varricchio C, editor: *A cancer source book for nurses,* ed 7, Atlanta, 1997, The American Cancer Society, Inc.
53. Wells BL, Horn JW: Stage at diagnosis in breast cancer: race and socioeconomic factors, *Am J Public Health* 82(10):1383-1385, 1992.
54. White E, Malone KE, Weiss N, Daling JR: Breast cancer among young U.S. women in relation to oral contraceptive use, *J Natl Cancer Inst* 88(7):505-514, 1996.
55. Willett WC et al: Dietary fat and fiber in relation to risk of breast cancer: an 8 year follow-up, *JAMA* 268(15):2037-2044, 1992.
56. Wilson BA, Shanson MT, Stang CL: *Nurses' drug guide,* Norwalk, 1996, Appleton & Lange.
57. Winchester DP, Cox JD: Standards for breast conservation treatment, *CA Cancer J Clin* 42(3):134-162, 1992.

chapter 49

# MANAGEMENT OF MEN WITH Reproductive Problems

CAROLYN W. EDDINS

**objectives** *After studying this chapter, the learner should be able to:*

1. Describe the process of infectious diseases specific to men's reproductive health.
2. Compare the nursing care associated with benign and malignant neoplasms that are specific to men's reproductive health.
3. Describe expected patient outcomes for each condition discussed.
4. Identify teaching needs of the patient with impotence.
5. Compare the common causes of impotence, both physical and psychological.
6. Discuss nursing interventions related to the structural and infectious problems presented.

Men's reproductive health care is one dimension of an emerging specialty area of nursing practice, men's health. Traditionally, problems of the male reproductive system have been viewed only as problems of urination or fertility. As with women, men have unique biological and social health care needs. Often the complexity of the male reproductive system and the multiple psychosocial needs of the patient have been minimized in today's health care system. Consequently, myths and knowledge deficits related to the specifics of sexual function are common in the male population. It is important to provide health care that is sensitive to the unique problems of the male. This chapter focuses on those unique care needs.

The information in this chapter is divided into sections according to specific organ structures and functions of the male reproductive system. The focus is on the most common health problems of the male reproductive system. Particular emphasis is placed on common infections, problems of the prostate gland, and impotence. Table 49-1 summarizes the problems affecting men's reproductive health discussed in this chapter. Sexually transmitted diseases are presented in Chapter 50. Figure 49-1 illustrates the male reproductive organs and associated structures.

## PROBLEMS OF THE TESTES AND RELATED STRUCTURES

The scrotal sac contains the testes, epididymis, and part of the spermatic cord; other associated structures include nerve, lymphatic, and vascular networks (Figure 49-2). These structures are responsible for the production and storage of sperm and provide the pathway for ejaculation. The testes are also involved in hormonal production, primarily of testosterone. Consequently, any disorders related to these structures have the potential to affect male fertility adversely, as well as interfere with testosterone production.

Pathologies of these structures include problems with swelling, twisting of cords, trauma, and carcinomas. The testes are particularly sensitive to changes in scrotal environment, such as fluctuations in temperature and blood flow. Infection is also a common problem. Accurately differentiating between pathologies related to infection versus structural problems or neoplasms can facilitate timely therapy and positively affect the patient's prognosis.

### EPIDIDYMITIS

#### Etiology/Epidemiology

The epididymis is a convoluted tubular structure within the scrotal sac that acts as a reservoir for sperm. While in this structure, sperm mature and become fertile and mobile. Epididymitis is an acute inflammatory process within the epididymis and is the most common intrascrotal inflammation in adult males. In the United States, epididymitis accounts for more than 600,000 visits per year to health care providers. Epididymitis is responsible for 20% of all urological admissions in the military population. It is also the cause of more lost work days than any other disease in the military.[18] This inflammation is rarely seen in children and occurs infrequently in the elderly adult male.

Inflammation of the epididymis most often is caused by an ascending infection via the ejaculatory duct through the vas deferens into the epididymis. There are three means of introduction of the infection into the duct system. First, infection may be introduced when surgical or diagnostic procedures are performed. This occurs more frequently among males less than 15 years old and in those over 45 years old. The most common organism for contamination in these age groups is *Escherichia coli.* Second, structural malformations or developmental structural insufficiencies in the child may contribute to problems of urinary reflux. Reflux of sterile or infected urine causes a chemical irritation in the epididymis and is another common cause of inflammation.

Finally, in the adult male between the ages of 19 and 35, sexual transmission is the most common means of infection. The pathogens most likely to cause epididymitis in heterosexual males are *Chlamydia trichomatis* and *Neisseria gonorrhoeae.* In homosexual males, the most common

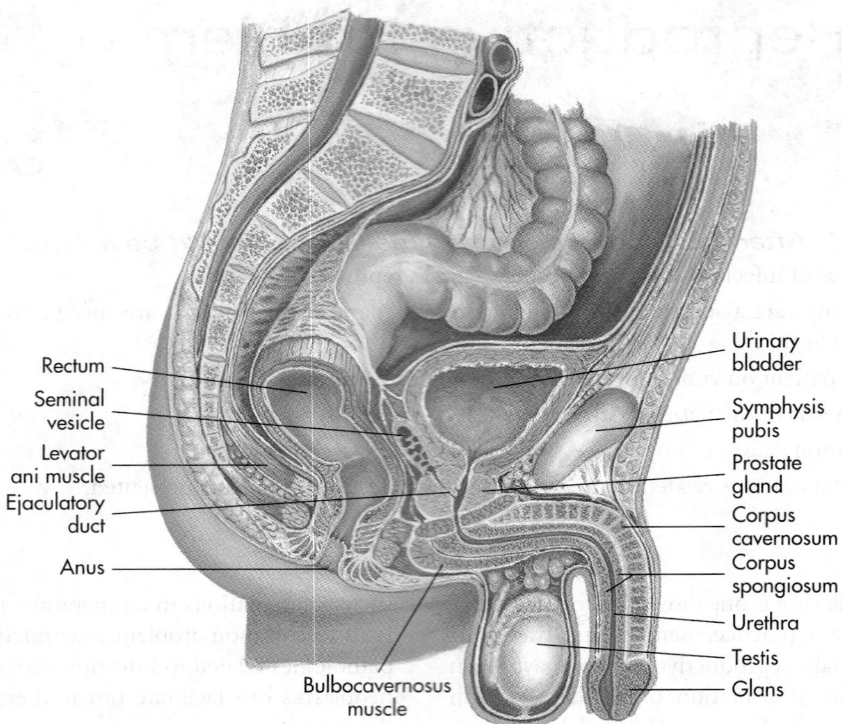


**fig. 49-1** Male reproductive organs and associated structures.

**table 49-1** *Major Problems Affecting the Male Reproductive System*

| PROBLEMS | SCROTUM | TESTES | PROSTATE | PENIS |
|---|---|---|---|---|
| Structural/mechanical | Hydrocele<br>Varicocele<br>Spermatocele | Torsion | Benign prostatic hypertrophy | Epispadias<br>Hyperspadias<br>Priapism |
| Infection | Epididymitis | Orchitis | Prostatitis | Staphylococcus aureus and others beneath foreskin |
| Cancer | | Seminomatous<br>Nonseminomatous | Prostatic | Penile |
| Impotence | | Infertility<br>Decline in spermatogenesis | Decline in prostatic fluid or fluid loss | Loss of erectile function |

pathogens are the ones that would be found in the anal canal, *E. coli* and *Haemophilus influenzae.*[14] (For more information on sexually transmitted diseases and the associated pathogens, see Chapter 50.)

## Pathophysiology

Epididymitis results from inflammation of the epididymis and scrotal sac. Fluid accumulates in the scrotal sac as an inflammatory response to the infectious process. Excess fluid loss into the interstitial space of the scrotal sac can lead to diminished blood flow, nerve damage, and resultant pain and swelling. Inflammatory fluids also can form pockets of pus called abscesses. Heat generated from the inflammatory process can negatively affect the testicular function of spermatogenesis. Consequently, complications of epididymitis include testicular infarction, chronic pain from nerve damage, abscess formation, and infertility.

The most common clinical manifestations are severe tenderness, pain in the scrotal area, and noticeable swelling of one or both sides of the scrotum. The onset of the pain may be insidious, gradually increasing over hours or days. The scrotal swelling can cause pain on ambulation and discomfort that is exacerbated by wearing restrictive clothing. Men with epididymitis often walk with a type of "waddle" to help spare the scrotum from rubbing up against the thighs or clothing. Elevation of the scrotum will

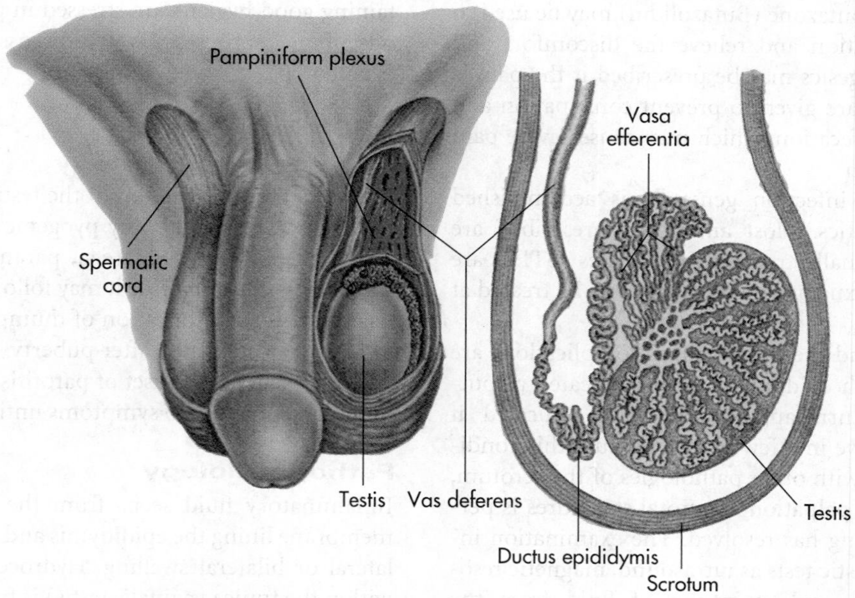


**fig. 49-2** The scrotum and its contents.

reduce the pain (Prehn's sign). Other symptoms include an increase in temperature of the scrotum and sometimes a systemic rise in temperature. A urethral discharge may also be present, with the color and consistency varying according to the type of causative organism. Urethritis is often associated with epididymitis, and the associated symptoms include burning on urination, frequency, urgency, and general malaise.

## Collaborative Care Management

Assessment of the patient with symptoms of epididymitis should include a sexual history. For young children, it should include questions to determine possible sexual abuse and any history of recent urinary examinations or instrumentation. In the elderly male, questions focus on history or symptoms of urinary obstruction or recent urinary examinations.

Prompt diagnosis is essential to decrease the risk of complications. Urinalysis is used to differentiate epididymitis from emergency conditions such as testicular torsion (see later discussion). If epididymitis is present, the urinalysis usually shows an increased white blood cell (WBC) count and the presence of bacteria. Urine and urethral cultures are needed to determine the specific causative organism and its sensitivity to various antibiotics, as well as to provide information for needed drug therapies.

Other diagnostic tests to detect epididymitis focus on changes in blood flow to the inflamed scrotum. An initial increase in blood flow to the area would indicate inflammation and/or infection, whereas other conditions resulting in swelling might impede blood flow. Scrotal ultrasound is a noninvasive diagnostic measure used when urinalysis and cultures are not conclusive. Ultrasound for this condition is usually done serially over minutes to hours. Any indication of reduced blood flow to the affected side usually indicates a more serious condition or a complication of epididymitis. Radionuclide scanning can also be performed when the diagnosis is questionable. These scans are more sensitive than ultrasound and generally show increased blood perfusion to the affected side of the scrotum if epididymitis is present.

The nature of the patient's pain is assessed; whether the pain is bilateral or unilateral, and if the pain is of sudden onset or has developed over hours or days. The nurse also notes if the pain is relieved by elevating the scrotum. Any symptoms of dysuria are documented, such as burning, frequency, urgency, fever, and general malaise. A recent history of urethral discharge or change in the discharge is important to help determine the possible type of causative organism. The color, consistency, and amount of any discharge are documented.

The patient is also observed for the classic "waddle," or a somewhat rolling gait, indicating that the patient is attempting to protect his scrotum. Swelling of the scrotum is documented, as well as whether it is on one or both sides. Palpation of the scrotum at this time is generally deferred to avoid causing severe pain.

For patients with chronic recurrent epididymitis, aspiration of fluid from the epididymis can be performed. It is a more direct method of determining the causative agent than routine cultures. This diagnostic method is rarely used, however, unless a chronic condition has been verified.

Treatment of epididymitis usually consists of pain management, medications to treat the infection, and supportive care. Nonsteroidal antiinflammatory drugs (NSAIDs), such as ibuprofen, or oxyphenbutazone (Butazolidin) may be used to decrease the inflammation and relieve the discomfort and swelling. Narcotic analgesics may be prescribed if the pain is severe. Stool softeners are given to prevent constipation and reduce straining on defecation, which may cause severe pain in the inflamed scrotum.

Eradication of the infection generally is accomplished by giving oral antibiotics. Most antibiotics prescribed are broad spectrum. If sexually transmitted diseases (STDs) are present, the patient's sexual partners also should be treated at the same time.

Unless high fever and the potential for complications are present, most men with epididymitis can be treated as outpatients. Frequent return appointments are indicated if swelling does not resolve in a few weeks. Because this condition can be associated with other pathologies of the scrotum, a more comprehensive palpation of scrotal structures is performed after the swelling has resolved. The examination incorporates such diagnostic tests as ultrasound, magnetic resonance imaging (MRI), and aspiration of fluid from the scrotum.

#### *Patient/family education*

Patient education initially focuses on comfort measures that will reduce the swelling of the scrotum. Bedrest with the scrotum elevated on a towel, application of ice packs, and the use of scrotal supports when the swelling is less severe decrease the discomfort caused by the heavy sensation resulting from the enlarged scrotum (Figure 49-3). Bedrest is maintained until the patient is pain free, then a scrotal support is worn for approximately 6 weeks. The patient is instructed to avoid work that would strain the lower abdomen and scrotal area.

Because STDs are the most common causes of epididymitis, it is important for the patient to be educated about prevention. The importance of using condoms and of maintaining good hygiene are stressed in patient teaching. (Methods of preventing STDs are discussed more completely in Chapter 50).

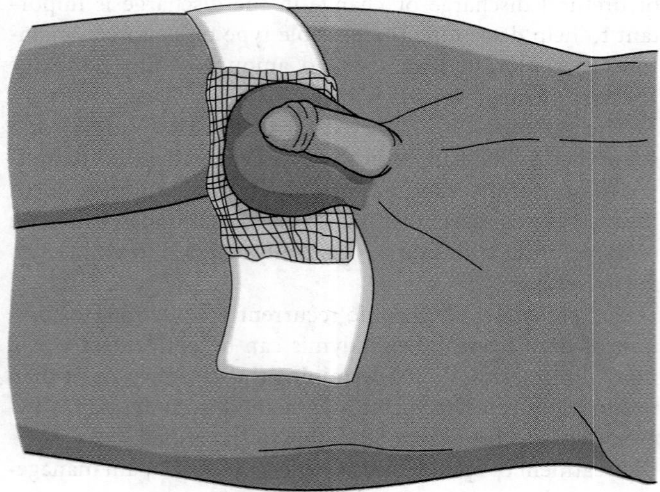

**fig. 49-3** A simple scrotal support.

## ORCHITIS

### Etiology/Epidemiology

Inflammation or infection of the testicle is known as orchitis. Orchitis may be caused by pyogenic bacteria, gonococci, tubercle bacilli, or viruses (e.g., paramyxovirus, the agent responsible for mumps), or it may follow any septicemia. Orchitis occurs as a complication of mumps in approximately 20% of all cases contracted after puberty. Symptoms may develop 4 to 6 days after the onset of parotitis. If the case of mumps is mild, there may be no symptoms until the onset of orchitis.[25]

### Pathophysiology

Inflammatory fluid seeps from the testicle into the serous membrane lining the epididymis and the testicle to create unilateral or bilateral swelling. Hydrocele (a collection of fluid within the tunica vaginalis testis) is frequently associated with orchitis. The signs and symptoms of orchitis are the same as those of epididymitis. However, because orchitis is caused by a systemic infectious process rather than a localized infection, more systemic symptoms are present. Consequently, the patient may also have clinical manifestations of nausea, vomiting, and pain radiating to the inguinal canal.

As a result of inflammation and fibrosis, some degree of testicular atrophy occurs in 50% of patients. The atrophy of the testes may lead to sterility. Unless both testes are severely involved, however, infertility is rare.

### Collaborative Care Management

Any postpubertal boy or man who is exposed to mumps usually is given gamma globulin immediately unless he has already had mumps or been vaccinated for the disease. If there is any doubt, gamma globulin usually is given. Gammaglobulin may not prevent mumps, but the disease is usually less severe and less likely to cause complications. Broad-spectrum antibiotics are given for common bacterial causes.

If hydrocele is present, the fluid may be aspirated to reduce pressure on the testes. If the hydrocele is surgically tapped within the first 2 days, the potential for testicular atrophy is decreased; however, a tap should only be done when edema is persistent because a chance exists that surgical decompression may exacerbate the inflammation.

#### *Patient/family education*

Patient education focuses on measures to reduce discomfort from gonadal swelling and alleviate systemic symptoms. During the acute phase of gonadal swelling, the scrotum may be supported with the same methods used for the patient with epididymitis. Warm or cold compresses may be applied to help reduce swelling and increase comfort. Antibiotics are administered for bacterial causes. Rest and an increased fluid intake are encouraged for all patients. Anti-inflammatory medication is given to help reduce pain and swelling.

## TESTICULAR TORSION

### Etiology/Epidemiology

Testicular torsion is a condition in which testicular circulation is acutely impaired by the twisting of the spermatic cord. Torsion may follow activities that put a sudden pull on the cremasteric muscle, such as jumping into cold water, blunt trauma, or bicycle riding. It may also occur at night when there is less gravitational pull from the testes on the cord, allowing more movement and consequent twisting.

Approximately 1 in 4000 males under age 25 years experiences torsion. Testicular torsion is most common between ages 12 and 18 years but can occur at any age. Forty percent of the cases reported occur spontaneously, awakening the male at night.[25,26]

### Pathophysiology

Torsion interrupts the blood supply to the testes, leading to ischemia and severe unrelieved pain that may be aggravated by manual elevation of the affected side. The scrotum is swollen, tender, and red. The affected side is usually elevated because the twisting and shortening of the cord pull up the testicle. The cremasteric reflex, elicited by stroking the inner aspect of the thigh to cause reflex refraction of the testicle, is usually absent on the side of the suspected torsion. Although the scrotum appears infected because of the swelling and redness, both urinalysis and blood tests are typically normal. Fever is rarely present. Absence of pain after a time may indicate infarction and necrosis. Gangrene may be a serious sequela.

Testicular viability after torsion is directly related to the duration of the torsion episode. If torsion has occurred for less than 4 hours, there is an 80% salvage rate for the testicle. If more than 12 hours have elapsed, the salvage rate is 20%. Early recognition and treatment are imperative if the testicle is to be preserved.[26] Table 49-2 lists assessment criteria to help differentiate torsion from epididymitis.

### Collaborative Care Management

Diagnostic studies for testicular torsion may include an orchiogram, or testicular scan, which is performed in the nuclear medicine department. This scan qualitatively measures the blood flow to the testis. Diminished or obstructed blood flow distinguishes torsion from an inflammatory process such as epididymitis. Doppler studies can also help to identify reduced blood flow and diagnose torsion.

Detorsion (a process of untwisting the spermatic cord) can be attempted manually. If detorsion is unsuccessful, surgical intervention is imperative within 6 to 12 hours to maintain viability of the testis. Even so, the testis may atrophy. Unless gangrenous, the testis is not excised, since it may still produce hormones, even if spermatogenesis is destroyed. The testis is fixed surgically to the scrotal wall (orchiopexy) to prevent recurrence. The contralateral testis is usually fixed prophylactically at the same time.

If the testicle is gangrenous or found to be nonviable after surgical detorsion, an orchiectomy (removal of the testicle) is carried out. If orchiectomy is performed, a testicular prosthesis is usually inserted.

Nursing care after orchiopexy and orchiectomy is similar. Ice bags and scrotal elevation may be ordered to reduce swelling. The nurse continues to monitor the patient for signs of testicular necrosis and fever in the case of orchiopexy. A small Penrose drain may be placed in the scrotum, which will necessitate dressing changes.

#### *Patient/family education*

After scrotal surgery, the patient should be instructed to limit stair climbing to two flights and not to lift or carry heavy objects for 4 weeks. He is instructed to refrain from sexual

**table 49-2** *A Comparison of Testicular Torsion and Epididymitis*

| TORSION | EPIDIDYMITIS |
|---|---|
| **AGE** | |
| First year through adolescence; most common age, 12-18 years | Adolescence and later |
| **ONSET** | |
| Acute | May be gradual |
| **SIGNS AND SYMPTOMS** | |
| **Pain** | |
| Localized to testis and radiates to groin and lower abdomen; severe in nature; similar episodes of self-limiting pains not unusual | Usually localized to epididymis and testis, sometimes to groin; increasing severity of pain; similar episodes of self-limiting pains rare |
| **Fever** | |
| Rare | Common |
| **Vomiting** | |
| Common | Rare |
| **Dysuria** | |
| Rare | Common |
| **PHYSICAL EXAMINATION** | |
| Testis may be in elevated position with abnormal lie; testis will be swollen and tender; epididymis also may be tender | Epididymis will be firm, tender, and swollen; testis may be normal or tender |
| **Cremasteric Reflex** | |
| Usually negative | Usually positive |
| **Prehn's Sign** | |
| Pain constant | Pain decreased |
| **Urethral Discharge** | |
| Not found | Common with sexually acquired infections |
| **URINALYSIS** | |
| Usually normal | Pyuria common |

activity for 6 weeks. The use of a scrotal support for at least 3 weeks is recommended to control edema. Sitz baths may help relieve any discomfort.

Body image disturbances may include fears of castration (orchiectomy), loss of masculinity, sterility, and impotence. The nurse provides specific information about the physiological changes resulting from testicular atrophy or surgical removal of the testicle. The patient is still able to have an erection after trauma or surgery to the testicles. Fertility may or may not be affected if there is still a remaining healthy testicle. Counseling on alternative means of conception may be suggested. The patient is reminded that the appearance of the scrotum will not be altered if a testicular prosthesis is inserted after orchiectomy.

## TESTICULAR CANCER

### Etiology/Epidemiology

The causes of testicular cancer are still unknown. A wide range of genetic and environmental causes are being explored. Chemical carcinogens, trauma, and orchitis all are theorized to initiate malignant changes. Since there is a greater incidence of testicular cancer in men who live in rural areas, environmental triggers are also suspected. Possible congenital etiologies include familial predisposition, gonadal dysgenesis (developmental abnormality), and cryptorchidism (failure of the testis to descend at birth). There is a 40% greater risk of testicular cancer in men who have a history of cryptorchidism.

Cancer of the testis is the leading cause of death from cancer in the 15- to 35-year-old age group. Two to three men per 100,000 have testicular cancer, but the number is increasing. The age groups that are most prone to testicular cancer are infants, men between 20 and 40 years, and men over age 60. Testicular cancer is more common in white than in African-American males. If it is detected and treated early, there is a 90% to 100% chance of cure. Unfortunately, approximately half the cases are found in advanced stages.[17] If testicular cancer remains untreated, death often occurs within 2 to 3 years.

### Pathophysiology

Testicular neoplasms are divided into two classifications: germinal and nongerminal. Germinal cancers make up 90% to 95% of all testicular neoplasms and are further divided into two groups: seminomatous (40%) and nonseminomatous (60%) tumors. In addition, tumors with mixed cell types can occur.

The determination of cell type is crucial for treatment. The diagnostic workup includes chest x-ray, computed tomograms (CT scans), intravenous pyelogram, skeletal surveys if the patient's alkaline phosphatase is elevated, and lymphangiography. Biopsy of the testis is contraindicated because of the highly metastatic character of testicular carcinoma. Manipulation and invasion of the cancer could cause it to seed to other areas. Laboratory tests include evaluation of alpha fetoprotein (AFP) and the beta subunit of human chorionic gonadotropin (beta-HCG). AFP and HCG are considered markers that indicate the presence of nonseminomatous disease, although a small number of men (less than 10%) with diagnosed seminoma will also have elevations in some of these marker hormones.[17] No one combination of elevated and normal markers specifically indicates testicular neoplasm. However, changes that occur in the laboratory values of these markers help to monitor the effectiveness of therapeutic interventions. The markers are monitored throughout the course of therapy.

Clinical manifestations of testicular cancer are often subtle and go unnoticed by the male until he notices a feeling of heaviness or dragging in the lower abdomen and groin area. A lump or swelling may be present, which is usually nontender and painless. Other symptoms are nonspecific, such as back pain, weight loss, and fatigue. Testicular tumors are often rapidly growing. Some complex tumors have been reported to double in size in a few days.[13]

### Collaborative Care Management

In any suspected case of testicular cancer, the testis is usually removed immediately. Men who are at higher risk for testicular cancer due to cryptorchidism may be encouraged to undergo orchiectomy as a prophylactic measure. Orchiectomy consists of en bloc excision of the spermatic cord, the contents of the inguinal canal, and the testis with the tunicae attached. The adjacent area is explored for metastases. The specimens are then examined to determine the cancer cell type. Staging of the disease (Box 49-1), as well as pathological findings, determines the course of treatment.

The two major cancer cell types in testicular cancer are seminomatous and nonseminomatous. Seminoma is highly responsive to radiation therapy. For stage I seminoma, irradiation is administered to the retroperitoneal nodes. In stage II, irradiation of the mediastinal and supraclavicular nodes is added. Chemotherapy is added for stage III. If tumor markers are present or elevated after irradiation, nonseminomatous involvement must be suspected. Seminoma can metastasize into a different type of cancer. A second primary lesion can develop in the remaining testis. The prognosis in that case is the same as if it were the first lesion.

Nonseminomatous neoplasms are radioresistant. Therefore retroperitoneal lymphadenectomy or radical node dissection is performed immediately. If the nodes are free of metastases, careful follow-up every 2 months is mandatory. Chemotherapy is given for clinical, radiological, or tumor marker evidence of metastasis. If the lymph node dissection is positive, the patient has stage II disease. Cyclic combination chemotherapy is administered over 2 years. In stage III, intensive cyclic combination chemotherapy is instituted for 10 to 12 months, followed by surgical excision of all metastatic sites. Drugs used in combination therapy include cisplatin, vinblastine, and bleomycin.

**box 49-1** *Staging of Testicular Neoplasia*

| | |
|---|---|
| Stage I | No metastasis; confined to testis |
| Stage II | Metastasis to retroperitoneal lymph nodes or other subdiaphragmatic areas |
| Stage III | Metastasis to mediastinal and supraclavicular nodes or other areas above diaphragm |

Nongerminal testicular tumors are rare. Treatment consists of various combinations of the four modes of treatment (orchiectomy, radiation, lymphadenectomy, chemotherapy) used in germinal neoplasms. Table 49-3 lists treatments for testicular cancer based on tumor type.

Seminoma has the best prognosis of any of the germinal neoplasms. Five-year survival rates are 95% to 100% for stage I, 70% to 90% for stage II, and 50% to 70% for stage III. Relapses are more common in patients with advanced stage cancer and thus chemotherapy with radiation are used to achieve a higher rate of sustained remission. For nonseminomatous neoplasms, 5-year survival rates are 90% for stage I, 60% to 85% for stage II, and 30% to 40% for stage III.[13]

### Patient/family education

Patient teaching focuses on the planned treatment and its expected side effects. Radiotherapy and chemotherapy are discussed in Chapter 11. Although the normal testis is shielded during external radiation, it is exposed to radiation scattered from the abdomen and thighs. The nurse explains to the patient that a period of 70 days is required to determine if spermatogenesis has been affected. Spermatogenesis may be decreased for 7 months to 5 years or more. The patient is encouraged to seek genetic counseling related to questions about the effects of radiation on sperm and consequently the possibility of genetic defects. Sperm banking before treatment is often recommended.

The nurse explains the effects of orchiectomy on fertility. Orchiectomy alone does not result in infertility if the contralateral testis is normal. The remaining testis undergoes hyperplasia, producing sufficient testosterone to maintain sexual function, drive, and sexual characteristics.

After a radical node dissection, there is danger of hemorrhage. Vigorous movement may be contraindicated, since nodes may have been resected from around many large abdominal vessels, but routine turning and leg and arm movement are essential to prevent postoperative pneumonia and thrombosis.

Pain and swelling of the scrotum are treated with pain medications, elevation of the scrotum when the patient is supine, and scrotal support when the patient is ambulating. Application of a warm or cool compress may also provide comfort, and decrease swelling.

Even though prosthetic testes are used to lessen the change in the physical appearance of the scrotum, the patient is usually very aware of the loss of a sexual organ. The nurse needs to explore the emotional affect that this loss has on the patient, and provide support and possible referral for counseling.

After a retroperitoneal lymphadenectomy, 90% of patients experience a decreased ejaculatory ability. Decreased ejaculation results from a disruption of the sympathetic nervous system pathways. The nurse informs the patient that ejaculation is independent of other sexual functions and that orgasm is still possible. The sexual partner should also be invited to learn about these changes in function.

Follow-up visits are often scheduled monthly for the first year after surgery to have serum tumor markers drawn, chest x-ray films, and possibly a CT scan. The interval between visits increases to 2 months for 2 more years to continue monitoring for signs of cancer recurrence.

The nurse also teaches the patient how to perform monthly testicular self-examination. Testicular self-examination should be performed by all males starting at puberty. Because men are at greatest risk for testicular cancer between the ages of 18 and 38 years, teaching needs to be targeted to this age group. Males should be taught to examine each testicle and spermata cord monthly. Any changes in morphology should be reported to a physician. Figure 49-4 illustrates the testicular self-examination.

**table 49-3** Treatment of Testicular Cancer Based on Tumor Type

| Stage | Tumor Type | Treatment |
|---|---|---|
| 0 | Benign | Surveillance |
| I | Seminomatous | Orchiectomy<br>Radiation therapy |
| | Nonseminomatous | Orchiectomy<br>Modified retroperitoneal lymph node dissection<br>Radiation therapy |
| II | Seminomatous | Orchiectomy<br>Radiation |
| | Nonseminomatous | Orchiectomy<br>Radiation therapy/ modified or full retroperitoneal lymph node dissection |
| III | Seminomatous | Combination chemotherapy/full retroperitoneal lymph node dissection |
| | Nonseminomatous | Combination chemotherapy/full retroperitoneal lymph node dissection |

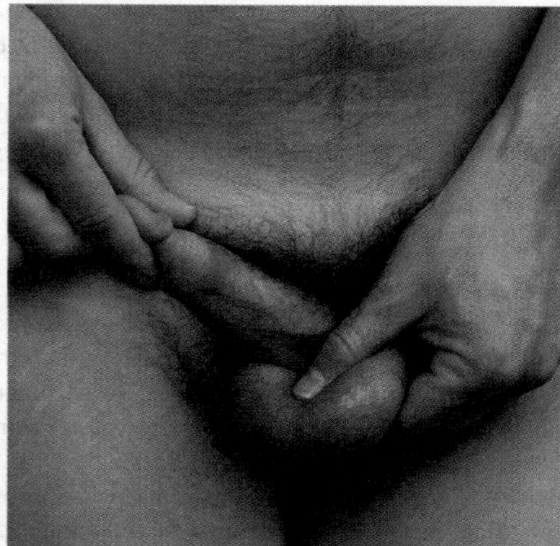

**fig. 49-4** Testicular self-examination. Examination is performed after a shower when the testicles are relaxed, descended, and easier to palpate. The man thoroughly palpates each testicle. Lumps are usually painless and circumscribed.

## PROBLEMS OF THE PROSTATE

Infection of the prostate occurs infrequently, but it can result in chronic problems that are difficult to eradicate. Prostatitis can cause long term discomfort and problems with fertility. Besides infections, benign prostatic hypertrophy and prostate cancer are the most common pathologies that affect the male reproductive system.

### PROSTATITIS

#### Etiology/Epidemiology

Prostatitis is one of the more common inflammations of the male reproductive system. It is most often seen in young and middle-aged men. The two common types of prostatitis are bacterial and nonbacterial. Nonbacterial prostatitis is the most common type. The organism of infection often cannot be identified. *Chlamydia trachomatis* has been suspected as the cause in many cases of nonbacterial prostatitis. Some nonbacterial inflammations may be attributed to allergic or antibody-antigen reactions.

Bacterial prostatitis can be acute or chronic. It is often caused by the same bacteria that cause urinary tract infections (UTIs), such as *E. coli* and *Pseudomonas.* Ascending UTIs or reflux of infected urine may be the route of bacterial contamination. Urethral instrumentation has also been cited as a source of bacterial infection.

#### Pathophysiology

The prostate gland becomes swollen, inflamed, and painful because of either a bacterial infection or other inflammatory process. The prostate surrounds the urethra and, when it becomes swollen, can compress the urethra and cause urinary obstruction. Men with prostatitis typically complain of changes in voiding patterns, such as difficulty starting the stream or the need to strain on urination. Low back pain, pelvic pain, and perineal pain are other common symptoms. Pain during or after ejaculation may also be experienced. In addition, the patient with bacterial prostatitis frequently complains of symptoms of UTIs that can include urgency, frequency, painful urination, and hematuria. Bacterial infection of the prostate typically causes fever, chills, and general fatigue.

#### Collaborative Care Management

Urine cultures are usually obtained to determine the organisms causing bacterial prostatitis. Cultures of prostatic secretions can verify a diagnosis of bacterial infection. Patients with nonbacterial prostatitis usually have negative urine cultures, but prostatic secretions can show an increased number of leukocytes and fat-containing macrophages.[7]

Treatment is conservative and consists of antibiotics for 30 days to prevent chronic infection, forced fluids, physical rest, stool softeners to decrease irritation of the prostate from hard feces, and local application of heat by sitz baths. Prompt treatment of prostatitis may prevent edema and resultant urinary obstruction. Urethral straight or indwelling catheterization is avoided if possible because of the risk of epididymitis. Suprapubic drainage will be established if necessary. Prostatic massage may be used to eliminate residual pus pockets, but it is contraindicated during the acute phase because of the risk of bacteremia.

Recurrent episodes of acute prostatitis may cause fibrotic tissue to form. The fibrosis causes a hardening of the prostate, which may initially be confused with carcinoma. In the granulomatous form of prostatitis, the enlargement may take 3 to 6 months to resolve.

Inadequate treatment of acute infection can result in chronic prostatitis. A subacute infection may also develop into a chronic prostatitis that remains asymptomatic. Therefore, prostatic secretions should be examined routinely to detect infection and to prevent complications such as acute or chronic cystitis, pyelonephritis, or epididymitis. It is believed that inflammation permits entry of antibiotics that normally do not diffuse into the prostatic fluid. They can be used during an acute infection but are ineffective in a chronic condition. Antibiotics that may diffuse into the prostatic fluid and be helpful include trimethoprim/sulfamethoxazole, carbenicillin, and ciprofloxacin.[13] Occasionally prostatic abscesses complicate the clinical course and may have to be drained surgically. If prostate calculi are present, they also may be infected. Antibiotics are ineffective against calculi, and surgical excision is required. Prostatectomy may be necessary to eradicate the infection.

##### *Patient/family education*

Patient teaching focuses on how to reduce the effects of swelling of the prostate. The patient is taught how to take warm sitz baths, use antiinflammatory medications, and avoid allergy-producing foods that may be exacerbating the inflammation.

The patient should refrain from sexual activity until the antibiotic has started to work, approximately 2 weeks into therapy. After 2 weeks regular ejaculation is encouraged to promote "flushing" of the prostate gland. The antibiotic must be taken for the entire prescribed time, even if the symptoms have been relieved sooner. Avoiding the use of alcohol and over-the-counter drugs (e.g., decongestants) can help prevent exacerbation of the symptoms of urinary obstruction. The continued use of stool softeners can decrease irritation to the inflamed prostate during defecation.

### BENIGN PROSTATIC HYPERTROPHY (HYPERPLASIA)

#### Etiology

The prostate gland, located below the bladder, surrounds the urethra and is responsible for contributing to ejaculatory fluid. During puberty, the prostate grows rapidly. After puberty, growth tapers off by age 30 years. Changes in the size of the gland next occur after age 50 when the gland begins to atrophy and become nodular. Benign prostatic hypertrophy (hyperplasia, BPH) is an enlargement of portions of this gland that eventually causes problems with urination. Parts of the gland may atrophy, whereas other parts become large and nodular. BPH is a common problem in men over age 50.

The changes in the size and shape of the prostate are associated with increased androgen levels. There is a greater concentration of dihydrotestosterone in males with BPH. Studies have shown that BPH does not occur in males castrated before puberty and that BPH does not progress after castration. Males without the enzyme 5-alpha-reductase cannot convert testosterone to dihydrotestosterone and also do not develop BPH.[2,19]

## Epidemiology

BPH is the most common problem of the male reproductive system. It occurs in at least 50% of all men over 50 years of age and 75% of men over 70 years. Symptomatic disease typically occurs in men in their mid 60s, although not all men with enlarged prostates develop symptoms, and symptomatic disease can occur as early as age 30. Symptoms appear slightly earlier in African American men.[4] An estimated 30% of men with symptomatic disease will eventually need surgery. The presence of benign prostatic hypertrophy does not appear to predispose a man to the development of cancer in the gland. BPH most often develops in the inner portions of the gland while cancer typically arises in the outer portions.

## Pathophysiology

The changes that occur in the prostate gland of older men can create a number of problems with the associated urinary system. When the enlarged nodular tissue of the prostate impinges on the urethra, the urethra elongates and compresses, causing obstruction of urinary flow. This can result in a compensatory hypertrophy of the bands of bladder muscles. This in turn increases the trabeculation (contouring) of the bladder wall, providing pockets for urinary retention. These trabeculated areas show up on ultrasound. Because of the muscular thickening, the bladder has less capacity. Muscle tone can diminish over time. Consequently, the bladder cannot empty completely at each voiding (residual urine); the urine becomes alkaline from stasis and is a fertile medium for bacterial growth.

These urethral and bladder changes can result in symptoms of urinary obstruction and irritation. Often the symptoms of obstruction are gradual and not noticed by the male until acute urinary retention occurs. Symptoms of gradual obstruction include a decrease in the urinary stream with less force on urination and often dribbling at the end of voiding. Other related symptoms include hesitancy, a difficulty in starting the stream, intermittency, and inability to maintain a constant stream. The patient may also complain of a sense of incomplete emptying of the bladder. Straining and urinary retention are the symptoms that often convince the patient to seek medical attention.

Symptoms of irritation often accompany the obstructive problems. Nocturia from incomplete emptying is common. Dysuria, urgency, and urge incontinence are symptoms associated with loss of muscle tone in the bladder and changes in the angle of the bladder neck. The patient also may have symptoms of UTI because of incomplete emptying and the increased risk of infection. As the prostate enlarges, so does the vasculature, and when straining takes place, these vessels may break and cause hematuria. Urinalysis and culture and sensitivity tests are routinely done to screen for blood and possible UTIs. Box 49-2 summarizes the typical clinical manifestations of BPH.

Other problems that can arise from BPH are kidney disorders caused by backflow of urine. Hydronephrosis and pyelonephritis are possible sequelae to urinary obstruction. Anemia may also occur if blood loss is severe or as a result of secondary renal insufficiency.

## Collaborative Care Management

### Diagnostic tests

Diagnostic tests for BPH include tests of renal function. These include monitoring changes in blood urea nitrogen (BUN), creatinine, proteinuria, specific gravity, hematuria, and increases in WBC. Other diseases that result in outflow obstruction need to be ruled out. Prostate cancer, bladder neck contracture, urethral stricture, bladder calculi, bladder cancer, inflammatory prostatitis, and neurogenic bladder are all problems that have similar symptoms. Prostate specific antigen (PSA), a blood test, is often performed on men 50 years and older (see Chapter 46 and the discussion under prostate cancer on p. 1624). It provides a rough estimate of the volume of the prostate.

Besides the urinary and blood tests already mentioned, endoscopic procedures may be performed. Cystourethroscopy is used to assess for outflow obstruction, measure the length of the urethra, and visualize the extent of bladder involvement. Uroflowmetry is a noninvasive procedure that can evaluate bladder emptying. An intravenous pyelogram (IVP) can be performed to outline the urinary tract. Sequential x-ray films are taken to assess the anatomy of the upper urinary tract, check for calculi (stones), and evaluate the degree of bladder emptying. IVPs are not routinely ordered for evaluation of BPH unless hematuria is present. Measuring postvoid residual urine is an easy but invasive technique that can also assess bladder emptying.

### Medications

Medications used to treat BPH are aimed at either reducing the size of the prostate gland or relaxing the tissue to decrease pressure on the urethra. Finasteride (Proscar) inhibits the

**box 49-2 clinical manifestations**

**Benign Prostatic Hypertrophy**

- Prostate gland enlarges, becomes more nodular
- Straining on urination
- Hesitancy in starting urine flow
- Decreased urine stream
- Postvoid dribbling
- Nocturia
- Dysuria
- Blood in urine
- Urgency

activity of 5-alpha-reductase so that it cannot turn testosterone into dihydrotestosterone, and consequently Proscar can reduce the prostate size.[20] Often the therapeutic effects of finasteride are not noticed for several months because of the time required to demonstrate an appreciable difference in the size of the prostate. Even though this drug actually changes the size of the prostate, it may not always help the symptoms of urinary retention. The urethra may remain compressed because the nodular growth in that immediate area may not shrink sufficiently to affect the flow of urine positively. It seems to be most effective in the treatment of large prostates. Adverse drug effects include decreased libido, impotence, and ejaculation disorders.

Other drugs are used to relax muscles and reduce straining on urination. These drugs tend to be effective in treating prostate glands of any size. Drugs include selective or nonselective alpha blockers. Selective blockers are prazosin (Minipress), doxazosin, and terazosin (Hytrin). Nonselective alpha blockers such as phenoxybenzamine (Dibenzyline) tend to have more severe side effects. The main side effects of all these drugs are orthostatic hypotension and fatigue. They are usually taken in the evening to reduce nocturnal symptoms of BPH. Alternative medicine approaches are also being used to both prevent and treat BPH. Dietary supplements and the use of botanicals such as saw palmetto are reported to reduce the symptoms of BPH. Research is ongoing.

Certain medications can exacerbate the symptoms of urinary retention because of their effects on the muscles of the bladder and urethral sphincter and should be avoided. Drugs that affect muscle function include anticholinergics and antidepressants. Tranquilizers and decongestants also can have side effects of urinary retention.

### Treatments

No specific treatment exists for mild BPH besides medication and some dietary restrictions. Patients are routinely monitored for signs of subtle changes in kidney function, which may initially be diagnosed by the use of blood tests. The phrase "watchful waiting" often is used to describe the monitoring of the condition with regular checkups.

### Surgical management

For patients with recurrent and obstructive problems caused by BPH, surgery is often the treatment of choice. The decision for surgery is based on the severity of urinary symptoms, presence of UTI, and the degree of physiological changes. Surgery removes the nodular gland tissue but leaves the capsule of the prostate gland intact. Males who undergo this treatment are typically symptom free for at least 8 years, after which there is a 5% to 15% retreatment rate.

**Transurethral prostatectomy.** Transurethral prostatic resection (TURP) is performed when the major glandular enlargement exists in the medial lobe that directly surrounds the urethra. There must be a relatively small amount of tissue requiring resection so that excess bleeding will not occur and the time required to complete the surgery will not be prolonged. A TURP may be performed with the patient under general or spinal anesthesia.

Two different surgical approaches can be used to remove a portion of the prostate gland through the urethra. The first uses a resectoscope and the second uses a Vaportrode®. A resectoscope (an instrument similar to a cystoscope but equipped with a cutting and cauterization loop attached to an electric current) is passed through the urethra. The bladder and urethra are continuously irrigated during the procedure. Tiny pieces of tissue are cut away, and the bleeding points are sealed by cauterization (Figure 49-5).

Another technique used for TURP is a microwave technique that burns the area. The tissue sloughs, creating a larger lumen in the urethra. This "microwave" procedure, done with a Vaportrode®, results in less postprocedural bleeding and usually takes less time. Postoperative care for both procedures is similar except the Vaportrode® rarely requires bladder irrigation.

After a resectoscope TURP, a large three-way Foley catheter may be inserted into the bladder. (The decision to insert a Foley catheter depends on the amount of bleeding expected after the procedure.) A large-size catheter is used to facilitate removal of clots from the bladder. After the retention balloon of the catheter is inflated, the catheter is pulled down so that the balloon rests in the prostatic fossa and supports hemostasis. Traction may be applied to the Foley catheter to increase pressure on the operative area to control bleeding (hemorrhage is a potential complication). Because the catheter balloon exerts pressure on the internal sphincter of the bladder, the patient may continually feel the urge to void. If the catheter is draining properly, the strongest of these sensations usually passes momentarily. Attempting to void around the catheter causes the bladder muscles to contract and results in a painful "bladder spasm." As the nerve endings become

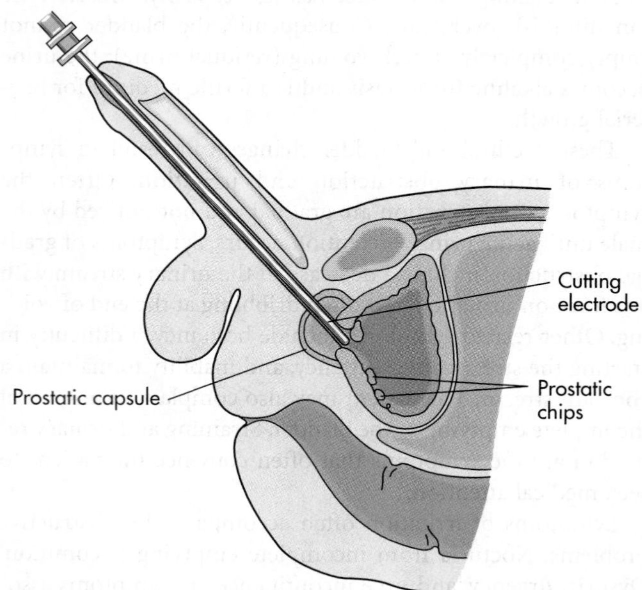


**fig. 49-5** Transurethral resection of prostate gland by means of resectoscope. Note enlarged prostate gland surrounding urethra and tiny pieces of prostatic tissue that have been cut away.

fatigued, the frequency and severity of spasms decrease. This usually occurs within 24 to 48 hours.

A constant bladder irrigation may be used to prevent excessive clotting or clot retention. This irrigation is usually performed via a three way Foley and IV drip apparatus and uses a GU irrigating solution. The use of the Vaportrode® technique decreases the incidence of bleeding and clot formation after surgery and limits the need for postoperative bladder irrigation. Typically patients treated by this method are in the hospital for 24 to 48 hours, with only a Foley catheter and IV infusion used postoperatively. Constant bladder irrigation following resectoscope TURP usually is discontinued within 24 to 48 hours if no clots are draining from the bladder.

Patients can develop water intoxication, formerly known as transurethral resection (TUR) syndrome, as a result of excessive irrigating solution being absorbed during surgery. Cerebral edema may result, which creates a medical emergency. Confusion and agitation may be the first signs of this condition. The patient may not be able to void after removal of the catheter because of urethral edema. When this occurs, the catheter may need to be reinserted. Continence is carefully assessed because the internal and external sphincters lie above and below the prostate, close to the operative area, and may have been damaged during surgery.

About 2 weeks after TURP, when desiccated tissue is sloughed out, a secondary hemorrhage can occur. The patient, who is home at this time, must contact the physician immediately if bleeding occurs.

Persistent bladder discomfort, bladder spasms, or failure of a catheter to drain properly usually signifies one of the following serious complications, which requires immediate medical attention: (1) hemorrhage and clot retention, (2) displacement of the catheter, or (3) unsuspected perforation of the bladder during surgery.

Long-term complications of TURP occur in approximately 18% of patients. These complications include problems with potency and a "change" in orgasms. Fertility can be affected because of retrograde ejaculation, which affects sperm viability and turns the urine cloudy. Other problems include chronic incontinence, which occurs in about 3% of all patients, and urethral strictures, which are rare.[12]

#### Diet

Alcohol can exacerbate incontinence and should be avoided. Dietary supplements of zinc and essential fatty acids are sometimes recommended, if the patient has deficiencies. These nutritional supplements are thought to help reduce nocturnal urinary symptoms.

Saw palmetto, a palm extract that inhibits the effect of dihydrotestosterone on the prostate gland, is being researched as an herbal approach to reducing the size of the prostate. It is given in a pill form and at present is considered an over-the-counter dietary supplement.

#### Activity

The man with BPH does not need to restrict his normal activity in any way. Frequent emptying of the bladder and avoiding bladder distention are important to prevent hypertrophy of the bladder. Avoiding straining and lifting heavy weights will help prevent hemorrhage resulting from strain on the increased vasculature in the prostate.

#### Referrals

In some settings the nurse assumes responsibility for making referrals to other services. Referrals for persons with BPH are rarely needed because of the temporary nature of any complications associated with the therapies.

## NURSING MANAGEMENT OF THE PATIENT UNDERGOING TURP

### ■ PREOPERATIVE CARE

A thorough preoperative assessment of the patient undergoing TURP enables the nurse to anticipate problems that put the patient at risk for complications. A baseline description of the patient's presurgical symptoms is documented. This information is used to compare the symptoms pre- and post-surgical intervention, as well as to follow long-term improvement of the patient. See Table 49-4 for a standardized format for collecting important assessment information.

Medication information is of particular importance for the patient undergoing surgery to this very vascular organ. Bleeding can be a common postoperative problem and the nurse carefully assesses the patient for a history of problems that can affect clotting times such as anemias. Information on the patient's use of over-the-counter medications that impair clotting, such as ASA and NSAIDs, is documented. The use of prescription NSAIDs and anticoagulants, such as Coumadin, is also crucial information.

Bowel elimination also is assessed before surgery. Constipation and hard stool can significantly increase the patient's discomfort in the postoperative period, and straining during defecation can cause pressure and pain to the prostate gland and also exacerbate bleeding. If the patient is laxative dependent before surgery, he will need some form of stool softener or laxative to prevent constipation after surgery.

The nurse assesses the patient's knowledge of the purpose for the surgery and the effects of the TURP on urinary elimination, sexual functioning, and fertility. Teaching about the effects of local or general anesthesia is provided preoperatively (see Chapter 18). In addition the nurse informs the patient about the three-way Foley catheter and bladder irrigation system that may be used postoperatively. The patient is informed that his urine may appear a red or pink color for several days after the procedure, and that this is a normal result of the manipulation of the prostate. Pain management is always a concern with surgical patients, and the nurse instructs the patient about the discomfort associated with bladder spasms and the presence of a large catheter and how this discomfort will be managed. Without an external incision of any kind, the TURP procedure is not associated with any significant incisional discomfort.

**table 49-4** *American Urological Association (AUA) Symptom Index*

| | AUA Symptom Score (Circle One Number on Each Line) | | | | | |
|---|---|---|---|---|---|---|
| Questions to Be Answered | Not at All | Less Than One Time in Five | Less Than Half the Time | About Half the Time | More Than Half the Time | Almost Always |
| Over the past month, how often have you had a sensation of not emptying your bladder completely after you finished urinating? | 0 | 1 | 2 | 3 | 4 | 5 |
| Over the past month, how often have you had to urinate again less than 2 hours after you finished urinating? | 0 | 1 | 2 | 3 | 4 | 5 |
| Over the past month, how often have you found you stopped and started again several times when you urinated? | 0 | 1 | 2 | 3 | 4 | 5 |
| Over the past month, how often have you found it difficult to postpone urination? | 0 | 1 | 2 | 3 | 4 | 5 |
| Over the past month, how often have you had a weak urinary stream? | 0 | 1 | 2 | 3 | 4 | 5 |
| Over the past month, how often have you had to push or strain to begin urination? | 0 | 1 | 2 | 3 | 4 | 5 |
| Over the past month, how many times did you most typically get up to urinate from the time you went to bed at night until the time you got up in the morning? | 0 | 1 | 2 | 3 | 4 | 5 |
| Sum of seven circled numbers (AUA Symptom Score): ______ | | | | | | |

Adapted from Benign prostatic hyperplasia: diagnosis and treatment, Rockville, Md, 1994, Department of Health and Human Services, AHCPR Pub No 94-0582. Mild = 0 to 7; moderate = 8 to 19; severe = 20 to 35.

## POSTOPERATIVE CARE

Nursing management of the patient following traditional resectoscope surgery is discussed below and summarized in the Guidelines for Care Box, p. 1621. A Nursing Care Plan can be found on p. 1622.

### Promoting Adequate Urine Elimination

The first 24 to 48 hours after prostatectomy surgery are critical in maintaining patency of the catheter or restoring spontaneous voiding. The chance of blood clots forming and interfering with the flow of urine is greatest at this time. If a bladder irrigation is being used, the flow rate of the irrigation must be set so that the urine remains free from clots and remains a light red to pink color. If a dark-red color is noted, the flow of the fluid needs to be increased. The nurse is responsible for regulating the flow of the irrigation in response to the color and consistency of the urine output. If bleeding persists despite the increased rate of irrigation the physician is notified promptly.

The intake and output record documents the urine output compared with the flow of the irrigation solution. The output should be at least 50 ml per hour greater than the hourly flow of the irrigation. Less urine output indicates a possible obstruction. All tubing is first checked for patency, and if no equipment problem can be determined manual irrigations using a 50 ml syringe may be ordered to help clear the catheter of clots.

Because irrigation solutions may be used in large quantities, there is a potential risk for water intoxication. The patient may absorb excess amounts of the irrigation fluid, and problems of hyponatremia, and other electrolyte imbalances may occur. The nurse assesses the patient for symptoms of elevated blood pressure, decreased pulse rate, confusion, and nausea. The nurse treats the hyponatremia as ordered by the physician. This often includes infusions of hypertonic saline and the use of diuretics such as furosemide (Lasix).

### Controlling Discomfort from Bladder Spasms and Straining

Narcotics may be given to lessen the pain sensation of bladder spasms but they are frequently unnecessary. Belladonna and opium (B & O) suppositories are most often prescribed to reduce bladder spasm. These soft suppositories do not cause pain or damage to the fragile tissue around the rectum, which may have been involved in the surgical procedure. Encouraging fluids, at least 8 to 10 full glasses of fluid per day, helps to flush the system and reduce irritation that causes spasms. Frequent voiding after the catheter has been removed also decreases irritation that causes spasms.

To prevent straining during defecation, which can put pressure on the recently traumatized tissues of the perineum, the patient is encouraged to use stool softeners or take mild laxatives and maintain a well-hydrated state to promote painless defecation.

### Preventing Infection

Intravenous antibiotics or oral antibiotics often are administered in the first few days after surgery. The patient is again en-

**guidelines for care**

**Postoperative Care for the Person Undergoing Prostatic Surgery**

1. Maintain patency of catheter system.
2. Monitor appearance of urine: red to light pink (24 hours) to amber (3 days).
3. Monitor patient for signs of water intoxication after TURP (confusion, agitation, warm moist skin, anorexia, nausea, vomiting).
4. Instruct patient not to try to void around catheter; explain feeling of needing to void from pressure of catheter.
5. Avoid use of enemas and rectal thermometers.
6. Give prescribed medications (analgesics, antispasmodics) as needed; tell patient spasms will decrease in intensity and severity within 24 to 48 hours.
7. After catheter removal:
   a. Monitor for signs of urinary retention.
   b. Monitor for continence; teach perineal exercises if dribbling occurs.
   c. Encourage increased fluids and frequent voiding.
8. Change dressings frequently around suprapubic wounds after suprapubic prostatectomy to prevent skin maceration.
9. Give patient opportunities to discuss feelings about sexuality and possible incontinence.
10. Teach patient to:
    a. Avoid vigorous exercise, heavy lifting (over 20 pounds), and sexual intercourse for at least 3 weeks.
    b. Avoid driving for 2 weeks.
    c. Avoid straining with defecation; use stool softeners or mild laxatives if needed.
    d. Drink at least 2500 ml of fluids per day to prevent urinary stasis and infection and to keep stools soft.
    e. Notify physician if urinary stream diminishes or if bleeding occurs.

couraged to increase his fluid intake to promote flushing of the system and help prevent urinary stasis and decrease the chances of infection. The nurse reviews the symptoms of UTI, which the man should report to his physician.

### Relieving Anxiety

The patient is told that most men have some temporary difficulty with continence after any type of prostatectomy. The man should understand that this is normal but will improve. Teaching perineal exercises such as Kegel exercises (see Chapter 44) can be helpful in controlling voiding. Frequent voiding can help reduce problems of dribbling. The nurse provides specific suggestions about absorptive devices and specialty underwear products that can be used for the temporary control of incontinence as needed.

The surgeries used to treat BPH do not usually affect the man's ability to have an erection. The patient needs to be reassured that there is a difference between infertility and impotence. Depending on the amount of prostate removed, fertility can be minimally or greatly reduced. Also, if the patient has continued retrograde emission of prostatic fluid even after several months, fertility will remain diminished.

The nurse must not assume that because males with BPH routinely are older, fertility is not an issue. Even if the man is not planning on having children, fertility is often closely associated with sexuality. The nurse may need to provide opportunities for the patient to express these concerns. Reminding the patient that the ability to have an erection is unchanged is often helpful. The ability to experience orgasm is also intact. The patient is cautioned that he may still be fertile, and use of birth control may still be necessary to prevent unwanted pregnancies.

## GERONTOLOGICAL CONSIDERATIONS

Benign prostatic hypertrophy rarely affects men before late middle age. Therefore, all of the preceding discussion clearly relates to an older population. Elderly patients withstand surgical intervention very well and do not have a significantly increased rate of problems postoperatively if they are in good general health. The new developments in treatment, which have decreased the invasiveness and length of the procedures, have also clearly benefited older patients.

## SPECIAL ENVIRONMENTS FOR CARE

### Critical Care Management

TURP surgery is on the verge of becoming a one-day outpatient procedure. Critical care management is therefore clearly not an expected part of the management plan for any patient. It would be used only if the patient experienced a catastrophic response to the surgical experience, perhaps an acute hemorrhage.

### Home Care Management

After any prostatectomy surgery, the patient is instructed to avoid heavy lifting and climbing more than two flights of stairs. The patient should avoid sexual activity for at least 3 weeks, and should not drive for 2 weeks.

The patient is instructed to watch for and report any sign of infection. The patient should also watch for blood or clots in the urine and any change in the urine stream. The patient rarely leaves the hospital with a Foley catheter but if the catheter must remain in place after discharge, the nurse provides instructions for Foley care. (See the discussion under prostate cancer on p. 1629). Mild analgesics, antibiotics, and stool softeners are often prescribed, and information on their use and side effects is provided.

The nurse teaches the patient to avoid the use of alcohol and over-the-counter medications such as antihistamines that increase the risk of urinary retention. The man is reminded to void at regular intervals and avoid straining and physical activities that create excessive abdominal or perineal pressure.

## COMPLICATIONS

The major complications of TURP surgery already have been presented in the overview of surgical management. They can include problems with bleeding, sexuality, fertility, and incontinence. Most patients, however, tolerate the surgery

## nursing care plan | *Person with TURP for Benign Prostatic Hypertrophy*

**DATA** Mr. J. is a 67-year-old retired married automobile mechanic. His physician has diagnosed benign prostatic hypertrophy. Mr. J. has undergone medical examinations on an outpatient basis and has never been admitted to the hospital. He is slightly obese. On admission his blood pressure is 140/90. He denies any history of hypertension. He takes only over-the-counter Tylenol for infrequent headaches. He had a TURP performed today.

**NURSING DIAGNOSIS** *Altered urinary elimination related to surgery*

| expected patient outcome | nursing interventions | rationale |
|---|---|---|
| Urine output is greater than 50 ml/hr | 1. Monitor urine output and characteristics.<br>2. Maintain constant bladder irrigation (CBI) as prescribed during first 24 hours.<br>3. Maintain patency of indwelling urinary catheter:<br>a. Irrigate manually as prescribed to keep catheter free of clots.<br>b. Maintain straight-line closed drainage system.<br>4. Encourage high fluid intake (2500 to 3000 ml/day) to promote increased urine flow.<br>5. After catheter is removed, monitor for signs of retention. | Ensure adequate bladder emptying. There is a potential for reabsorption of water from the bladder, so output must be carefully monitored. Clots may obstruct drainage catheter and must be detected early. |

**NURSING DIAGNOSIS** *Pain related to bladder spasm*

| expected patient outcome | nursing interventions | rationale |
|---|---|---|
| States feeling more comfortable. | 1. Check the catheter to ensure patency.<br>2. Teach patient not to try to void around catheter.<br>3. Monitor patient at regular intervals for 48 hours to identify early signs of bladder spasms.<br>4. Give prescribed medications (analgesics, antispasmodics).<br>5. Tell patient spasms will decrease in intensity and frequency within 24 to 48 hours. | Bladder spasm frequently follows urological procedures. Forcing voiding will encourage spasms. Antispasmodics may offer best relief by elimination or reduction of spasm. |

**NURSING DIAGNOSIS** *Risk for fluid volume excess related to absorption of irrigating fluid*

| expected patient outcome | nursing interventions | rationale |
|---|---|---|
| Does not exhibit signs of water intoxication. | 1. Monitor patient for signs of water intoxication during first 24 hours: confusion, agitation, warm moist skin, anorexia, nausea, vomiting, and low serum $Na^+$ level.<br>2. Monitor fluid intake (oral, IV, CBI) and output. | Irrigation fluid may be reabsorbed through bladder wall, resulting in water intoxication. |

**NURSING DIAGNOSIS** *Risk for infection/injury (hemorrhage) related to surgery*

| expected patient outcome | nursing interventions | rationale |
|---|---|---|
| Does not exhibit signs of infection or hemorrhage. | 1. Monitor vital signs; report signs of shock or fever.<br>2. Monitor appearance of urine for persistent bright-red color rather than expected light red/pink color beyond first few hours postoperatively.<br>3. Teach patient to avoid Valsalva maneuver, which may initiate prostatic bleeding. | Change in vital signs may alert nurse to infection. Bleeding is common after TURP and must be monitored closely. |

*Continued*

## Person with TURP for Benign Prostatic Hypertrophy—cont'd

**NURSING DIAGNOSIS** *Risk for infection/injury (hemorrhage) related to surgery—cont'd*

| expected patient outcome | nursing interventions | rationale |
|---|---|---|
| | 4. Avoid use of rectal thermometers, rectal examinations, or enemas for at least 1 week.<br>5. Maintain strict asepsis of urinary drainage system; irrigate only when necessary.<br>6. Encourage high fluid intake. | |

**NURSING DIAGNOSIS** *Risk for stress or urge incontinence related to catheter use*

| expected patient outcome | nursing interventions | rationale |
|---|---|---|
| Achieves urinary continence. | 1. Assess patient for dribbling after catheter is removed.<br>2. If dribbling occurs:<br>a. Tell patient this is a common occurrence but that continence will return.<br>b. Teach patient perineal exercises (Kegel).<br>3. Explain use of devices and pads for temporary incontinence. | Dribbling may occur after TURP but should resolve. Perineal exercises strengthen sphincter tone. |

**NURSING DIAGNOSIS** *Risk for sexual dysfunction related to surgery*

| expected patient outcome | nursing interventions | rationale |
|---|---|---|
| Describes possible effects of TURP on sexual functioning. | 1. Give patient opportunities to discuss feelings about the effects of prostatectomy on sexual intercourse.<br>2. Provide information as necessary:<br>a. Probable return of previous level of functioning.<br>b. Occurrence of retrograde ejaculation (first urine after intercourse may have a milky appearance).<br>c. Avoid sexual intercourse for 3 to 4 weeks after surgery. | Sexual functioning usually returns to presurgical level. Patients often need to be encouraged to discuss their concerns about the effects of surgery on sexual intercourse. |

**NURSING DIAGNOSIS** *Knowledge deficit (activity restriction, prevention of complications) related to lack of information*

| expected patient outcome | nursing interventions | rationale |
|---|---|---|
| Describes activity restrictions and medical follow-up. | 1. Teach patient:<br>a. Avoidance of heavy activities for 3 to 4 weeks.<br>b. Avoidance of straining during defecation for 4 to 6 weeks; use stool softeners or laxatives as necessary. | By adequately educating patient about postsurgical routine and restrictions, the nurse can help ensure compliance with the medical regimen. |
| | c. Drink 10 or more 8 oz glasses of fluid every day. | Help flush out system to prevent stasis. |
| | d. Do not drive for 2 weeks.<br>e. Be alert to the possibility of bleeding (the highest incidence is about 2 weeks after surgery when tissue sloughing occurs). Patient should contact his physician immediately if bleeding or urinary obstruction occurs. | Avoid straining perineal muscles to decrease pain and risk of bleeding. |

extremely well and are able to resume their normal lifestyle without ongoing difficulties.

## CANCER OF THE PROSTATE

### Etiology

Cancer of the prostate is the most common cancer in adult American men, but its etiology remains basically unknown. The tumors typically arise in areas of the gland that are atrophic rather than hyperplastic, but the process is not fully understood.

Factors that may affect the development of prostate cancer include hormonal changes and viral infections. Hormonal influences have been proved clinically to be a cancer risk factor, since men castrated before puberty do not develop prostate cancer. Hormonal changes during aging are the reason that prostate cancer is seen almost exclusively in men over age 40. A direct viral etiology has not been proved, but a strain of cytomegalovirus isolated from the prostate gland can produce malignant transformation in prostate tissue in the laboratory setting.[11] In addition, positive antibody titers to herpes simplex and cytomegalovirus have been found in men with prostate cancer.

Environmental influences may increase the risk for prostate cancer. Immigrants from countries with a low incidence of prostate cancer have demonstrated an increased incidence after living in a country with a high incidence of prostate cancer.[24] Other risk factors include a history of multiple sexual partners, episodes of STDs, the presence of cervical cancer in sexual partners, and industrial exposure to cadmium.

### Epidemiology

Prostate cancer has the highest incidence rate and second highest mortality rate of all cancers affecting men in the United States.[4] Prostate cancer rarely occurs before age 40, the incidence increases sharply with age, and there is a clear familial risk. African Americans have the highest incidence of prostate cancer in the world. Although white men in the United States have a lower incidence than African-American men; white American males have a rate higher than men in other parts of the world.[9]

### Pathophysiology

Cancer of the prostate often starts as a discrete, localized hard nodule in an area of senile atrophy. It is most often caused by an adenosarcoma that arises in the peripheral regions of the gland. Seventy-five percent of prostate cancers arise in the peripheral zone (outer area of gland, contiguous with the capsule), 20% in the transitional zone (midportion of gland), and 10% in the central zone surrounding the urethra. Because the growth is generally on the outer portion of the gland, compression of the urethra and subsequent voiding symptoms are not common until late in the disease. Nonurinary symptoms, if present, are often so ambiguous that the disease often is not diagnosed until it is well advanced.[23]

The cancer readily can spread outside of the capsule boundaries and be disseminated through the lymphatic and vascular systems. The most common sites of metastasis are the bones of the pelvis; lumbar and thoracic spine; femur; and ribs. Organ involvement (lung, liver, kidneys) usually is not seen until the late stages of the disease.

Because the posterior of the prostate gland is adjacent to the rectal wall, the tumor may be detected by rectal examination before symptoms appear. On physical examination, prostate cancer may present as a discrete or diffuse area of increased firmness. Unfortunately, up to 40% of cancers arise anterior to the midline of the prostate gland and consequently cannot be felt on rectal examination.[23]

Blood screening for prostate specific antigen (PSA) measures the elevation of a glycoprotein secreted by the prostate, and is used to help identify possible cancers. (See the Research Boxes below and on p. 1625.) Factors that can influence PSA levels are identified in Box 49-3. Epithelial cells in the ductal system of the prostate gland also secrete acid phosphatase. If acid phosphatase is found in serum blood tests, it usually indicates that prostatic tissue has spread beyond the capsule of the gland.

**research**

Reference: Cantor SB et al: Prostate cancer screening: a decision analysis, J Fam Pract 41(1):33-41, 1995.

Screening for prostate cancer remains controversial because it has not been demonstrated that early diagnosis increases either survival or quality of life. This study used a decision analysis to evaluate the effectiveness of annual screening of men 50 years of age and older. A model was created using probability and outcome data from the medical literature and tested with a pilot sample of 10 disease-free middle-aged men from a family practice. Probability variables included elements such as disease prevalence, disease stage, survival rates, and the specificity of tests such as PSA, digital rectal examination, transrectal ultrasound, and biopsy. The acceptability and impact of treatment-related effects such as impotence and incontinence were explored with the sample participants.

The decision analysis concluded that based on the variables identified prostate cancer screening for asymptomatic men is not recommended. When life expectancy is the only consideration, screening may extend a patient's life expectancy slightly, but when quality of life factors were included screening was not indicated. It is important to recognize that only patient-related variables and not the cost of mass screening were considered as variables in this decision model.

**box 49-3** *Factors That Affect PSA Levels*

**Race:** African Americans have higher PSA levels.
**Age:** Older adults have increased PSA levels.
**BPH:** Prostatic hypertrophy increases the gland volume and the PSA level.
**Manipulation of the prostate,** e.g., instrumentation, elevates PSA level.
**Sexual orgasm** within 24 hours elevates PSA level.

Prostate cancer can spread slowly or aggressively. The biological aggressiveness of malignant tumors depends at least in part on the degree of differentiation of the cells (see Chapter 11). Most prostatic malignancies are defined as adenocarcinomas or sarcomas. It is frequently difficult to determine the severity or extent of the tumor because multiple tumor sites may be present with varying degrees of cell differentiation.

Clinical manifestations of prostate cancer may include complaints of stiffness, back pain, and occasionally pathological fractures. The symptoms may also mimic those of BPH, with urinary outflow obstruction or severe bladder irritation with no signs of infection. Often there are no symptoms in the initial stages of prostate cancer (Box 49-4).

## Collaborative Care Management

### *Diagnostic tests*

Because symptoms are often ambiguous, regular screening for prostate cancer is very important. A combination of diagnostic tests is now used to improve the accuracy of prostate cancer detection. Blood screens, rectal examination, and ultrasound techniques all help in early detection. High-risk patients, with histories of multiple sexual partners, STDs, and certain viral infections, should be given special attention in screening routines.[11] See the Research Box on p. 1626.

It is recommended that all men over the age of 40 have an annual rectal examination. Hard nodular areas felt on the prostate at the time of the digital rectal examination (DRE) are often indicative of cancer.

Even before disease is noted on the rectal examination, the blood screening test for PSA may show that there is a possible prostatic cancer. Blood screening is often done serially because a rise in PSA or a consistently high PSA is more reliable than a single assay. Because PSA levels can rise with inflammation, benign hypertrophy, or irritation as well as in response to cancer, PSA screening is performed in conjunction with other diagnostic procedures. Knowledge of prostate size, along with PSA levels, provides a more definitive diagnosis than PSA alone. PSA is now routinely drawn starting at age 50 as part of physical examinations, and before and after biopsies or surgery on the prostate gland. Serial levels can be followed after the test or treatment to detect recurrence of the cancer. The laboratory parameters for significant PSA values are still being studied. Table 49-5 compares the efficacy of various diagnostic tests.

Transrectal ultrasound (TRUS) aids in the screening of nonpalpable tumors. It may also be used to help direct the physician in biopsy of palpable tumors so that these tumors can be graded and staged. TRUS allows greater accuracy in tumor localization and needle placement than using digital rectal examinations to help guide the biopsy. Biopsy of any firm or nodular area is necessary to confirm the diagnosis of prostate cancer. The biopsy procedure may be done in a office setting or minor surgery operating rooms. The biopsy can be done with the patient under local anesthesia or light general

**research**

Reference: Schwartz KL et al: Prostate specific antigen in a community screening program, J Fam Pract 41(2):163-168, 1995.

Prostate-specific antigen has proven utility in monitoring the progress of prostate cancer and the patient's response to therapy, but its value as a screening tool for prostate cancer remains unproven. This study used data from a major community-based health screening program to determine the predictors of participation in PSA screening and the predictors of PSA level in men who had a PSA screening test. The study explored whether age, race/ethnicity, and subsequent diagnosis with prostate cancer influenced the likelihood of screening. The study included 14,000 men, of whom 6,000 had PSA screening as part of the screening initiative.

Men who underwent PSA screening had a higher median income and were predominantly white. They also were clustered in the age range of 50 to 69 years. A statistically significant association was found between age and PSA levels, and age accounted for most of the variation in levels. No relationship was found between PSA values and race. The results indicate that a single elevated PSA level could easily lead to unnecessary testing. The sensitivity of PSA screening is not yet at a point where it can serve as the primary method of mass screening. Too many other variables are still operational in each individual patient, but refining PSA reference values by age appears to be an important strategy for increasing the sensitivity of the test.

**box 49-4** ***clinical manifestations***

***Prostate Cancer***

- Often no symptoms if cancer is confined to the gland
- Symptoms of urinary obstruction
- Symptoms of urinary tract infection
- Low back pain, malaise, aching in legs, and hip pain if cancer has metastasized

**table 49-5** *Diagnostic Tests for Prostate Cancer*

| Procedure | Screening Value | Staging Value |
|---|---|---|
| Digital rectal examination (DRE) | +++ | + |
| Prostate-specific antigen (PSA) | ++++ | +++ |
| Transrectal ultrasound (TRUS) | ++ | ++ |
| Prostatic acid phosphatase (PAP) | | |
| Automated radioimmunoassay | – | – |
| Enzymatic method | – | +++ |
| Radionuclide bone scan | – | +++ |
| Pelvic computed tomography (CT) | – | ++ |
| Endorectal magnetic resonance imaging (MRI) | – | +++ |
| Lymphadenectomy | – | +++++ |

Data courtesy of Gerald L. Andriole, Jr., MD.

**research**

Reference: Millon-Underwood S: Factors influencing early detection of prostate cancer, Appl Nurs Res 5(1):30-31, 1992.

This study was undertaken to determine why many men never have rectal examinations or other forms of screening done for prostate cancer. Millon-Underwood hypothesizes that interest in prostate screening was influenced by the man's belief that he was susceptible to prostate cancer and/or to his belief that screening was beneficial. A questionnaire that measured the beliefs and attitudes about screening and susceptibility was administered to a sample of 90 men, ranging in age from 39 to 78 years.

Of the 90 subjects, 88% believed that screening would help prevent advanced prostate cancers, and 61% thought that rectal examinations for screening were important but too embarrassing. Less than half the subjects had a rectal examination for prostate cancer. Thirty-six percent of the subjects believed that the screening could cause needless worry.

The study also found that men who believed that health screening was important were more likely to have prostate screening done. The men who thought that their health was too good to worry about screening were less likely to have screening done.

Because there was a significant correlation between the men's beliefs of susceptibility to prostate cancer and their willingness to be screened, the study concluded that attitudes and beliefs need to be addressed by nurses to help the patient take advantage of health screening.

anesthesia. If combined with ultrasound, a probe is placed in the rectum; otherwise, the surgeon uses a digital technique to guide the procedure. The needle biopsy can be performed by either a transperineal or transrectal route, depending on the physician's choice.

**Staging.** A system of staging prostate cancer has been developed to classify the location, size, and spread of the tumor and guide treatment decisions. For example, a tumor that is confined to the capsuled gland and is not clinically discernible is termed a stage A. If the tumor is confined to the gland but is a larger size, it may be staged as an A1 (Box 49-5). Staging helps determine prognosis and provides the basis for treatment recommendations. Stage A and B lesions are confined to the prostatic capsule and have a good prognosis. Higher numeric values and/or letter values of C or D have a poorer prognosis.

Treatment decisions are based on both the results of the staging and the Gleason rating scale. The Gleason grading scale is used to rank the correlation between the extent of tissue differentiation and the patient's prognosis. The Gleason system of grading has total scores ranging from 2 to 10. Two biopsy sites are used in testing, and the scores of each (which range from 1 to 5) are added together to obtain the total score of 2 to 10. The lower the score, the less aggressive is the cancer and the better the prognosis.

Patient preparation for prostate biopsy focuses on providing an optimal environment for visualization, preventing complications, and baseline data gathering for follow-up. Rectal cleansing by enema or oral laxative is often done before the procedure as a means of preventing potential infection. Preprocedural antibiotics are used and may be continued for several days after the procedure. The patient may be NPO or permitted to eat a light breakfast before the biopsy. The extreme vascularity of the prostate gland increases the risk of bleeding, and coagulation profiles usually are drawn before the procedure. Patients are taken off any anticoagulants and drugs such as aspirin at least 48 hours before the test.

**box 49-5** *Duke's System of Staging of Prostatic Neoplasia*

| | |
|---|---|
| Stage A | Microscopic lesions found in prostate gland removed because of benign hypertrophy |
| Stage B | Nodules confined to prostate gland: no capsular adherence or urethral involvement; normal serum acid phosphatase level |
| Stage C | Carcinoma involving prostatic capsule, seminal vesicles, urethra, bladder, and pelvic lymph nodes, or a malignant tumor of a lesser extent with elevated serum acid phosphatase level |
| Stage D | Findings as in stage III plus evidence of extrapelvic lesions or osseous involvement |

### *Medications*

**Hormone therapy.** When cancer of the prostate is inoperable, or when signs of metastasis occur after surgery, pharmacological treatment is given. Many patients experience dramatic improvement with hormonal therapy that may last for 10 years or more. Usually, the response is quite good for about 1 year, and then the patient's condition begins to deteriorate.[6] Because a large portion of the growth in prostate cancer is testosterone dependent, medication is used to block the production or action of this hormone. The testicles produce testosterone when stimulated by the release of hormones from the pituitary gland. Therefore, drugs that inhibit the release of these pituitary hormones are often first choice therapies. Hormone analogs such as leupolide (Lupron) and goserelin (Zoladex) are given monthly by IM injection.

In conjunction with drugs that inhibit the production of testosterone, antiandrogenic drugs are given to inhibit the action of testosterone produced by the adrenal glands. Examples of antiandrogen drugs include flutamide (Eulexin) and megestrol acetate (Megace). Side effects of both of these classes of drugs can include impotence, hot flashes, nausea and vomiting, chemical hepatitis, and diarrhea.

### *Treatments*

**Radiation therapy.** Radiation is used to treat localized tumors confined to the inside of the prostate capsule, or if a patient cannot tolerate or chooses not to undergo surgery. Radiation may be delivered by external beam or by implant. The testes are shielded during external radiation. Iodine retropubic prostatic implantation may be used initially or after failure of external radiation therapy. Complications of $^{125}I$ implantation include blood loss from multiple needle punctures during implantation, deep vein thrombosis, pulmonary emboli, hematomas, and abscesses.[9] Impotence from radiation develops over time as a result of scar tissue formation. There is a greater risk of complications if radioactive implants are used after external beam radiation. Irritability of the bladder caused by radioactive implants can produce urinary symptoms.

**Cryosurgical ablation of the prostate.** Cryosurgical ablation of the prostate is used to treat localized tumors or as an alternative to radiation therapy. This surgery uses a cryoprobe to freeze and destroy the cancerous prostate tissue (see Figure 49-6). A suprapubic catheter and urethral catheter are inserted as a method of directing warming fluid to areas that need to be protected from the freezing procedure. However, the freezing process still irritates surrounding tissue, with resultant urethral and scrotal edema. The scrotum becomes bruised and can swell to the size of a grapefruit. Impotence is a complication in approximately 70% of these patients.[3,15]

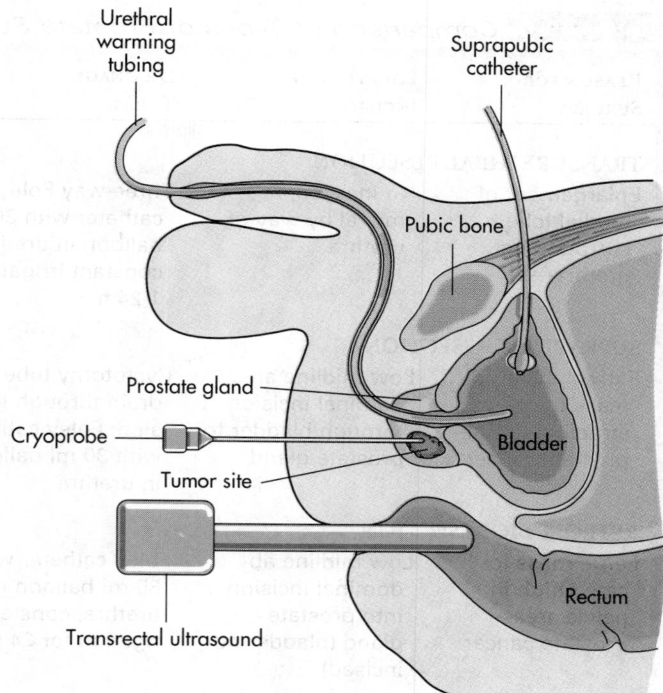


**fig. 49-6** Sketch showing the male genitourinary system and the relationship of the cryoprobe to the transrectal ultrasound transducer.

### Surgical management

A radical resection of the prostate gland usually is curative for patients with stage A or B prostate cancer. The entire prostate gland, including the capsule and the adjacent tissue, is removed. The remaining urethra then is anastomosed to the bladder neck. The surgery is accomplished by using a suprapubic, retropubic, or perineal approach. The suprapubic and retropubic approaches use a low midline incision, and the perineal approach uses a perineal incision. The patient has a Foley catheter in place for a period of days to several weeks, depending on the approach used by the physician, and if the patient is at risk for delayed healing because of previous radiation therapy. Table 49-6 compares the different surgical methods, and Figure 49-7 on p. 1629 illustrates the placement of drains and incisions.

**Suprapubic prostatectomy.** In the suprapubic resection, the prostate gland is removed from the urethra by way of the bladder; this type of resection is performed when a large mass of tissue must be resected. Some type of hemostatic agent is placed in the prostatic fossa, and urine is drained by Foley catheter, cystotomy tube, or both.

Hemorrhage is a possible complication, and the precautions are the same as those taken after TURP. Since some oozing of blood from the prostatic fossa occurs, continuous bladder irrigations may be ordered for the first 24 hours.

Cystotomy tubes are usually removed 3 to 4 days postoperatively; urethral catheters generally remain until the suprapubic wound is well healed. After the urethral catheter has been removed, the nursing care of the patient is similar to that for the patient undergoing TURP. If the suprapubic wound should reopen and drain, a urethral catheter is usually reinserted.

**Retropubic prostatectomy.** In a retropubic prostatectomy, a low abdominal incision similar to that used for suprapubic prostatectomy is made, but the bladder is not opened. The bladder is retracted, and the prostatic tissue removed through an incision in the anterior prostatic capsule. A large-diameter Foley catheter is inserted. Hemorrhage and infection are potential complications, but the sphincter muscles are not damaged, and the patient rarely has difficulty voiding. Nerve-sparing surgeries are the treatment of choice if the patient has less invasive cancer.[11]

**Perineal prostatectomy.** The perineal approach results in a draining incision in the perineal area. Often a penrose drain is placed to help direct the serous drainage from the wound site. The bladder remains intact during this surgery. Nerves that control urinary continence and penile erection may be damaged with this surgical approach. Also muscles and nerves around the rectal sheath can be traumatized. Consequently these patients may have difficulty with bladder and bowel continence as well as impotence. Nerve-sparing approaches are being successfully used with perineal approaches as well, but the surgery is technically difficult.

**Orchiectomy.** When symptoms of obstruction begin, a bilateral orchiectomy (castration) may be performed. This procedure is technically minor and is often performed using local anesthesia, but it may cause the patient considerable emotional distress. The man's permission for sterilization must be obtained. If he is married, he is usually urged to discuss the procedure with his wife. This surgery eliminates the testicular source of male hormones and seems to cause regression of the cancer or at least slow its growth. Very seldom, a hypophysectomy may be performed to further reduce hormonal stimulation.

### Diet

No therapeutic diet exists for patients with prostate cancer. A high-fiber, low-fat diet is recommended because men from

**table 49-6** *Comparison of Types of Prostate Surgery*

| Reason for Surgery | Location of Incision | Drainage Tubes | Bladder Spasms | Dressing | Complications |
|---|---|---|---|---|---|
| **TRANSURETHRAL RESECTION** | | | | | |
| Enlargement of medial lobe surrounding urethra—BPH | No incision; removal by way of urethra | Three-way Foley catheter with 30 ml balloon in urethra; constant irrigation 1-24 hr | Yes | None | Hemorrhage; water intoxication; incontinence; obstruction |
| **SUPRAPUBIC RESECTION** | | | | | |
| Extremely large mass of obstructing tissue—prostate cancer | Low midline abdominal incision through bladder to prostate gland | Cystotomy tube or drain through incision; Foley catheter with 30 ml balloon in urethra | Yes | Abdominal dressing easily soaked with urinary drainage | Hemorrhage; obstruction; wound infection; impotence; sterility |
| **RETROPUBIC RESECTION** | | | | | |
| Large mass located high in pelvic area—prostate cancer | Low midline abdominal incision into prostate gland (bladder not incised) | Foley catheter with 30 ml balloon in urethra, constant irrigation for 24 hr | Few | Abdominal dressing; no urinary drainage | Hemorrhage; obstruction; wound infection; impotence; sterility |
| **PERINEAL RESECTION** | | | | | |
| Large mass located low in pelvic area—prostate cancer | Incision between scrotum and rectum | Foley catheter with 30 ml balloon in urethra; perineal drain | Few | Perineal dressing; no urinary drainage | Hemorrhage; obstruction; wound infection; impotence; sterility; incontinence |
| **RADICAL PERINEAL RESECTION** | | | | | |
| Mass extends beyond the capsule; includes lymph node dissection—prostate cancer | Large perineal incision between scrotum and rectum | Foley catheter with 30 ml balloon in urethra; drain in incision | Few | Perineal dressing; no urinary drainage | Urinary incontinence; wound infection; impotence; sterility |

countries that routinely eat this type of diet have a lower incidence of prostate cancer. There is now clinical evidence that diet can play a role in preventing or slowing the growth of prostate cancer. A diet high in lycopene (a substance found in tomatoes) can reduce the risk of prostate cancer.[1] Diets are routinely modified if the patient is to have surgery. Increasing fluid intake after prostate surgery helps to prevent problems with constipation.

### *Activity*

If the patient has undergone radiation therapy or prostatic surgery, he should limit heavy lifting or straining. The patient should not drive a vehicle for 2 weeks after surgery. If the Foley catheter has been left in place at the time of discharge, the patient is cautioned not to engage in any activity that could pull or put strain on the catheter.

### *Referrals*

Because many of the therapeutic interventions affect the patient's fertility and ability to have an erection, a specialist in sexual therapy or counseling may be helpful to the patient. Sometimes patients are also interested in family-planning counseling for alternative means of conceiving children. If persistent urinary incontinence is a problem, nurses specializing in the care of incontinent patients (enterostomal therapy nurses) may be consulted. The American Cancer Society can help the patient deal with the emotional issues related to the diagnosis of cancer, as well as provide information on a variety of helpful resources.

## NURSING MANAGEMENT OF THE PATIENT WITH PROSTATE CANCER UNDERGOING PERINEAL PROSTATECTOMY

### ■ PREOPERATIVE CARE

If the patient is to have a perineal approach in surgery, he is given a bowel preparation, which may include enemas, cathartics, and sulfasalazine (Azulfidine) or neomycin preopera-

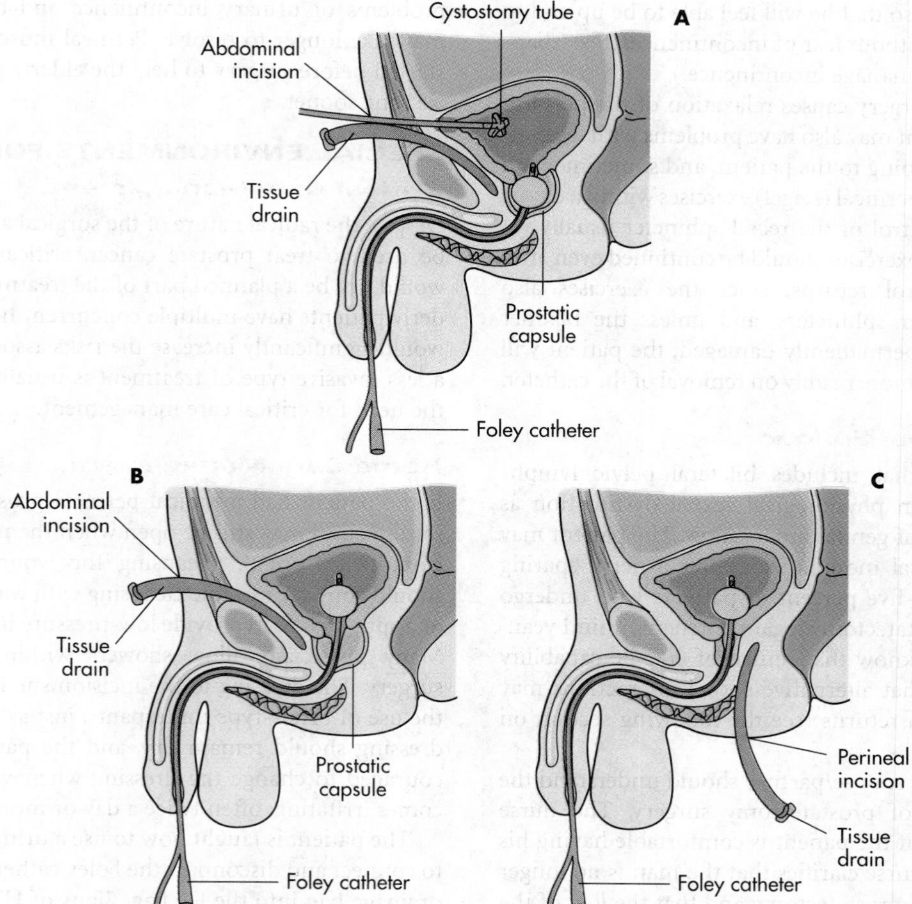


**fig. 49-7** Three types of prostatectomies. **A,** Suprapubic: note placement of inflated Foley catheter in prostatic fossa. **B,** Retropubic. **C,** Radical perineal: note tissue drain placed in incision between scrotum and rectum.

tively and only clear fluids the day before surgery to prevent fecal contamination of the operative site. The remainder of the preoperative care is similar to that described under benign prostatic hyperplasia.

## POSTOPERATIVE CARE

### Caring for the Perineal Wound

The care of the perineal wound consists of monitoring for possible urine leaks, hemorrhage, and signs of infection. Drains may be placed in the incision, and the wound may be left partially open to heal by secondary intention. Often the patient wears a Fuller shield or briefs-type underwear to support the dressing on the perineal incision. Open wounds may drain copious amounts and frequent dressing changes are usually necessary. The use of a "donut" or "Life Saver" cushion may be used to relieve pressure on the incision site while sitting. The use of rectal thermometers, rectal tubes, and suppositories is avoided to prevent injury to the fragile perineal area.

When solid food is permitted, a low-residue diet may be given until wound healing is well advanced. Camphorated tincture of opium may be prescribed to inhibit bowel action in the first postoperative week to prevent contamination of the incision.

### Restoring Urinary and Bowel Continence

A large amount of urinary drainage on the perineal dressing for a number of hours is not unusual. This can be managed by the use of an ostomy bag around the dressing. The urinary drainage should decrease rapidly. The amount of bleeding in the urine should not be the same as after suprapubic prostatic surgery. Since the catheter is not being used for hemostasis, the patient usually experiences less bladder spasm. The catheter is used both for urinary drainage and as a splint for the urethral anastomosis; therefore, care should be taken that it does not become dislodged or blocked. Clinically, the risk of blockage from clots is greatest during the first hour. The catheter may be irrigated intermittently or continuously as ordered by the physician. The catheter is usually left in the bladder for at least 2 to 3 weeks.

Temporary urinary incontinence is often a problem with patients who have had any type of radical prostatectomy. The patient needs to be encouraged, and provisions should be made to keep him dry so that he will feel able to be up and to socialize with others without fear of incontinence. (See Chapter 44 for strategies to manage incontinence.)

Because perineal surgery causes relaxation of the perineal musculature, the patient may also have problems with fecal incontinence. It is disturbing to the patient, and sometimes can be avoided by starting perineal (Kegel) exercises within a day or two after surgery. Control of the rectal sphincter usually returns readily. Perineal exercises should be continued even after rectal sphincter control returns, since the exercises also strengthen the bladder sphincters, and unless the bladder sphincters have been permanently damaged, the patient will regain urinary control more readily on removal of the catheter.

### Promoting Sexual Function

Total prostatectomy that includes bilateral pelvic lymphadectomy can result in physiological sexual dysfunction as a result of disruption of genital innervation. The patient may be impotent for several months even after a nerve-sparing prostatectomy. Ninety-five percent of patients who undergo the nerve-sparing prostatectomy regain potency within 1 year.[6] The patient needs to know that return of erectile capability may be delayed and that alternative sexual interactions may be used until function returns (see the following section on impotence).

The patient and his spouse/partner should understand the sexual consequences of prostatectomy surgery. The nurse teaches both partners if the patient is comfortable having his partner present. The nurse clarifies that the man is no longer fertile after any radical prostatectomy and that the loss of the prostate gland interrupts the flow of semen and he will not ejaculate. However, the ability to have an erection will gradually return, and he can still experience orgasm.

### Dealing with Grief

Patients who have stage A or B prostate cancer have an excellent survival rate. It is important to remind patients that prostate cancer is very different from many other forms of cancer, since even men with stage C prostate cancer often have a long survival rate. Prostate cancer is usually slow growing, and many elderly men do not die of their prostate cancer but from other causes. The fear of cancer must be acknowledged, however, and the patient needs time and encouragement to express these fears. If surgery has resulted in impotence the patient will need to be supported through his grief over the loss of sexuality. For more information on the grieving process related to cancer, see Chapter 11.

## GERONTOLOGICAL CONSIDERATIONS

Because prostatic cancer is often slow growing, treatment options for elderly patients may be more palliative in nature. Radical prostatectomies do not necessarily prolong life for elderly patients. Consequently, radiation or measures to decrease the size of the prostate (e.g., TUR) to relieve symptoms of urinary obstruction may be the treatment of choice rather than the radical prostatectomy.

If surgery is performed, healing times may be prolonged. The perineal muscles of the elderly patient are weaker, and problems of urinary incontinence and bowel incontinence may take longer to resolve. Perineal muscle exercises may be started before surgery to help the elderly patient regain muscle tone sooner.

## SPECIAL ENVIRONMENTS FOR CARE

### Critical Care Management

Despite the radical nature of the surgical approaches that may be used to treat prostate cancer, critical care management would not be a planned part of the treatment approach. If elderly patients have multiple concurrent health problems that would significantly increase the risks associated with surgery, a less invasive type of treatment is usually selected, negating the need for critical care management.

### Home Care Management

If the patient had a radical perineal prostatectomy, the perineal wound may still be open when the patient is discharged from the hospital. Cleansing the wound after defecation should consist of simple cleansing with water and possible use of a spray bottle to provide low-pressure irrigation to the area. Many physicians allow showers within the first week of surgery. The dressing to the incision site is held in place with the use of briefs-type underpants, just as in the hospital. The dressing should remain dry, and the patient should be encouraged to change the dressing whenever the drainage becomes irritating, often twice a day or more.

The patient is taught how to use a urinary leg bag and how to connect and disconnect the Foley catheter from the bedside drainage bag into the leg bag. Signs of UTI are taught to the patient, and he is told to notify his physician if any signs of infection occur. The catheter insertion site at the penis should be washed once a day with water and/or a mild soap if desired. The catheter needs to remain securely anchored to the thigh or abdomen to avoid pulling. Perineal exercises to promote the return of urinary continence when the catheter is removed should be practiced on a regular basis at home.

Reminding the patient that bowel incontinence may still be a problem for a few days when he returns home is important. The patient should have easy access to a bathroom. Instructing the patient to use the commode a few hours after meals may help to promote bowel continence.

## COMPLICATIONS

Complications of radical prostatectomy for prostate cancer include, but are not limited to, hemorrhage, urinary and bowel incontinence, infertility, impotence, and leakage at the anastomotic site of the urethra and bladder. Prostate cancer may metastasize to local organs such as the lymph nodes, bowel, and bladder. Sites of distant metastasis include the liver, spine, and lungs.

# PROBLEMS OF THE PENIS

Structural problems of the penis are typically related to the head of the penis and the foreskin. The head of the penis is susceptible to diseases caused by irritation, cancer, and trauma. The foreskin can also be a source of structural difficulties that can affect urination, cause pain, and interfere with blood flow to the penis. Functional problems of the penis primarily involve disorders of erection. Impotence is discussed later in the chapter. The anatomy of the penis is illustrated in Figure 49-8.

## PHIMOSIS AND PARAPHIMOSIS

### Etiology/Epidemiology

Phimosis is a condition in which the opening of the prepuce or foreskin is unable to be retracted behind the glans. The condition may be congenital or acquired as a result of inflammation or infection.

Paraphimosis, conversely, is a condition in which the prepuce is retracted over the glans and forms a constriction at the base of the glans (Figure 49-9). This is usually a result of manipulation of the foreskin over the glans and failure to return it to cover the glans. This condition is most often seen in children or in men with changes in mental status that predispose them to memory loss or with decreased sensation in the penis.

### Pathophysiology

The inability to retract the foreskin may interfere with adequate hygiene. Consequently, urine and smegma may be trapped in the preputial sac, resulting in irritation and predisposing the glans to infection. Chronic irritation may be a cause of penile carcinoma. Healing of the irritation or infection causes scar tissue formation, which can worsen the acquired phimosis. If the constriction of the foreskin at the head of the penis is severe enough, it causes urinary obstruction and painful urination.

Constriction is also a major problem with paraphimosis. The constriction at the base of the glans usually results in swelling of the glans. If the swelling is not reduced, blood vessels to the glans are compressed, reducing flow. Inadequate blood flow can result in necrosis of the glans.

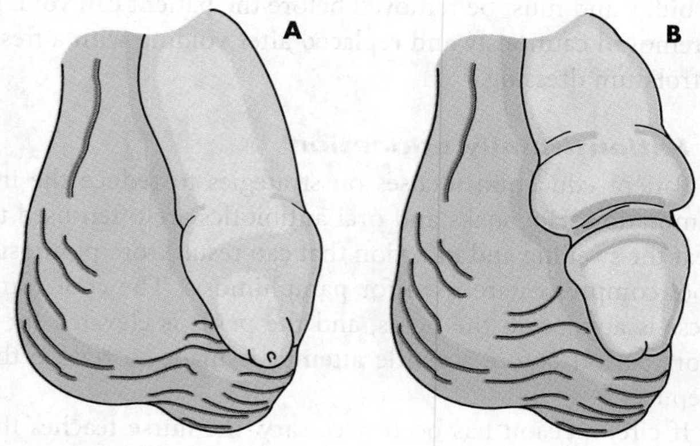


**fig. 49-9 A,** Phimosis; note pinpoint opening of foreskin. **B,** Paraphimosis; note foreskin is retracted but has become constricting band around penis.

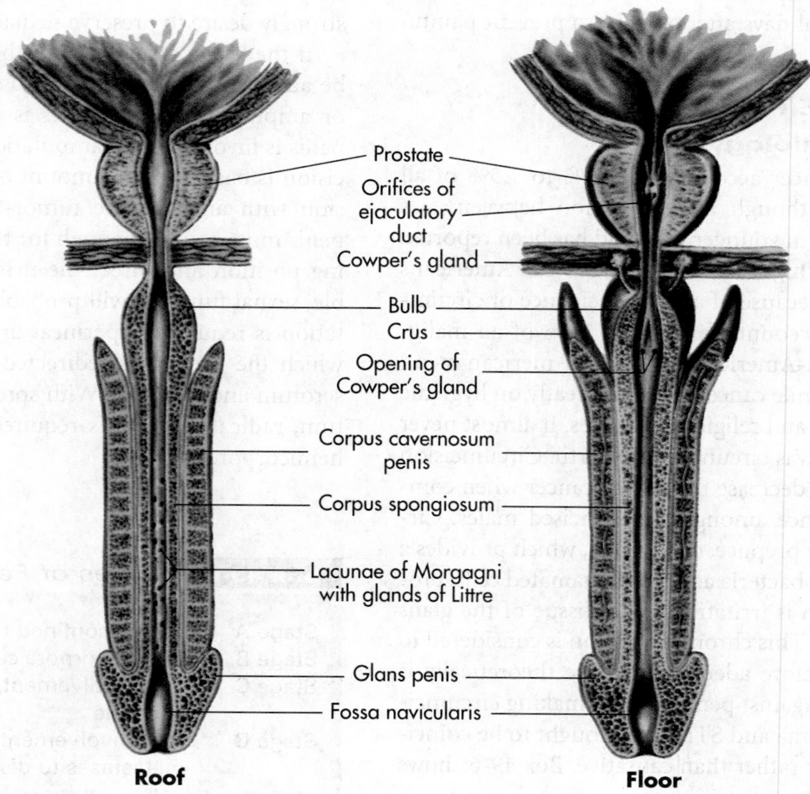


**fig. 49-8** Anatomy of the penis.

### Collaborative Care Management

Treatment for severe cases of phimosis may consist of incisions in the foreskin to reduce the contracture and widen the opening. Congenital phimosis may be successfully treated by gentle repeated stretching of the foreskin over the glans. Circumcision may be performed if the prepuce cannot be satisfactorily retracted.

Circumcision is done to prevent recurrence of paraphimosis. When the penis is circumcised, the wound is covered with gauze generously impregnated with petrolatum. Bleeding usually is controlled by applying a pressure dressing that may be bulky and must be removed before the patient can void. It is removed cautiously and replaced after voiding with a fresh petrolatum dressing.

#### *Patient/family education*

Patient education focuses on strategies to reduce the inflammation. Hot soaks and oral antibiotics are often used to treat the swelling and infection that can result from phimosis. Cool compresses are used for paraphimosis. The cool compress is applied to the penis, and the penis is elevated for a short period before a gentle attempt is made to reduce the prepuce.

If circumcision has been necessary, the nurse teaches the patient how to change the petrolatum dressing and observe for signs of infection. The nurse also instructs the patient to be alert for signs of bleeding. If severe bleeding occurs, a firm dressing should be applied to the penis, and the patient should be taken to the physician's office or the emergency room. If bleeding persists it may be necessary to resuture the wound. An estrogen preparation may be prescribed for the adult patient for several days after surgery to prevent painful erections.

## CANCER OF THE PENIS

### Etiology/Epidemiology

In America, penile cancer accounts for 0.5% to 1.5% of all male malignancies. Although most common between ages 50 and 70, it can occur in younger men and has been reported in children.[8] There is a higher incidence in African Americans than whites, possibly because of a lower incidence of circumcision. Penile cancer accounts for 10% to 20% of all malignancies among African-American and Asian-American men.[8]

The incidence of penile cancer depends greatly on hygienic standards and cultural and religious practices. It almost never occurs in a male who was circumcised at birth. Circumcision after puberty does not decrease the risk of cancer when compared with the incidence among uncircumcised males. Circumcision removes the prepuce, or foreskin, which provides a haven for bacteria. The bacteria act on desquamated cells, producing smegma, which is irritating to the tissue of the glans penis and the prepuce. This chronic irritation is considered to be carcinogenic. Therefore adequate hygiene theoretically is sufficient prophylaxis against penile cancer, making circumcision unnecessary. Trauma and STDs are thought to be coincidental to penile cancer rather than causative. Box 49-6 shows the stages of penile cancer.

### Pathophysiology

Penile cancer starts as a small lesion usually on or under the prepuce and extends until the entire glans and shaft are involved. The initial lesion may assume a variety of forms. It may appear as a small bump, resemble a pimple or wart, or occur as a nonhealing ulcer with the edges rolled inward. The latter is associated with earlier metastases and a poorer 5-year survival.

The most common (95%) type of malignancy is squamous cell carcinoma. Phimosis, which is present in 25% to 75% of patients with penile cancer, may obscure the lesion. The lesion may then cause erosion through the prepuce, resulting in a foul odor and discharge. Bleeding may or may not be present. Urethral and bladder involvement are rare. Eventually the disease can become autoamputative. If left untreated, death occurs in 2 to 3 years.

Clinical manifestations of penile cancer include weakness, fatigue, malaise, and weight loss. Men may complain of itching and burning under the prepuce and an occasional foul discharge. A 1-year delay before seeking treatment occurs in 15% to 50% of cases. Biopsy is performed to establish the diagnosis; however, benign penile lesions occur infrequently.

Metastasis usually occurs at the regional femoral and iliac nodes and is associated with a significantly worse prognosis. Five-year survival with inguinal node involvement is 20% to 25%.

### Collaborative Care Management

Treatment is usually surgical. Radiation therapy is indicated only in patients who have small superficial lesions and strongly desire to preserve sexual function.

If the lesion is confined to the prepuce, circumcision may be adequate. If the lesion is on the glans, partial penectomy or amputation of the penis is required. If the shaft of the penis is involved, total amputation may be necessary. The decision is based on the amount of penis remaining after excision with an adequate tumor-free margin. The remaining penis must be long enough for the patient to void in a standing position and direct the urinary stream. If this is possible, sexual function will probably be retained. If total amputation is required, a perineal urethrostomy is performed, in which the urethra is redirected to an opening between the scrotum and the anus. With spread of the cancer to the scrotum, radical removal is required, either hemipelvectomy or hemicorporectomy.

**box 49-6** *Stages of Penile Cancer*

|  |  |
|---|---|
| Stage A | Lesions confined to glans or foreskin |
| Stage B | Shaft or corpora cavernosa invaded by tumor |
| Stage C | Shaft involvement; lymph nodes involved but operable |
| Stage D | Shaft involvement; lymph nodes inoperable; metastases to distant sites |

Approximately one third of men with penile cancer have metastatic nodal disease at the time of initial diagnosis. Radiation therapy is used as adjuvant therapy at all stages. Lymphadenectomy is indicated for lymph node involvement. Accurate detection of metastases is difficult, since enlarged lymph nodes may be free of cancerous tissue, whereas normal-sized lymph nodes may contain metastatic lesions.

Chemotherapeutic agents have been used with some success, particularly in patients with stages A and B disease. Agents include high-dose methotrexate, bleomycin, and cisplatin. Because of the rarity of the disease, large-scale clinical studies to evaluate chemotherapeutic agents are lacking. Methotrexate has been somewhat successful. If the disease is confined to the penis, 5-year survival is 80% to 85% with amputation. With metastasis to the lymph nodes, it is only 20%.

#### Patient/family education

The nurse teaches the patient about the potential side effects of radiation in the perineal area. Radiation in this location can cause the skin to become dry, itchy, and sensitive. Special gels that are safe to use during radiation may be applied to the affected area.

Urethral strictures can develop several months to years after radiation therapy. The nurse informs the patient of symptoms of urethral stricture, which include difficulty starting or stopping the urine flow, frequent UTIs, and nocturia. Bowel patterns may change during radiation therapy and for up to several weeks. Effects of chemotherapy and nursing interventions are discussed in Chapter 11.

The emotional devastation of a diagnosis of penile cancer is difficult to overestimate. The proposed surgery may be unthinkable to the patient, who is frequently in a state of shock. The scope of support and sexual counseling needed by this patient is beyond the expertise of most nurses. The patient is referred for sexual counseling with experts who can clearly explain his options. Some patients with a urethrostomy have experienced orgasm and ejaculation after stimulation of the perineal, scrotal, and testicular regions.

## IMPOTENCE/ERECTILE DYSFUNCTION

### Etiology

Impotence is the inability of a man to have an erection firm enough or sustain an erection long enough for satisfactory intercourse. The term *satisfactory* is defined by the couple involved and may vary from couple to couple. The ability to have an erection depends not only on a healthy psychological state, but also on adequately functioning neurological, vascular, and hormonal systems. The brain is the controlling organ for sexual arousal. The brain perceives sexual stimuli and controls the physiological changes that occur during arousal. The two fundamental causes of impotence are physical and psychological.

Physical causes include changes in blood flow to the penis and neurogenic dysfunctions. Diseases such as diabetes, lupus, and rheumatoid arthritis can damage blood vessels and cause obstruction of blood flow in the penis. Anemia and dehydration can cause insufficient blood volumes to maintain an erection. Cardiac diseases and antihypertensive drugs can interfere with the capillary blood pressure.[22]

A wide variety of disorders that affect neurological functioning (e.g., spinal cord injury, diabetes, renal failure, MS, and Parkinson's disease) can interfere with erectile function. Changes in testosterone levels can affect the male sex drive. Aging affects the level of testosterone, and sexual function usually declines somewhat with advancing age.

Other causes of impotence include surgical procedures that interfere with both blood engorgement and neurogenic innervation of the penis, and prescription drugs that produce the side effect of impotence.

Psychological impotence can be attributed to many factors, such as long-term stressors, fears, anxiety, anger, and frustrations. "Performance anxiety," a fear of not performing well during sexual intercourse, is common. Fatigue also influences the ability to have an erection (see the Risk Factors Box).

### Epidemiology

Most men occasionally experience impotence. Short-term impotence can be caused by fatigue, stress, anxiety, or the use of alcohol or other drugs. Until recently, psychological problems were considered to be the cause of 90% of impotence cases. Now, physical causes have been found in 85% of cases. One in every 10 males in the United States has continuing or chronic impotence.[16] The tremendous anxiety produced by occasional or chronic impotence worsens the problem, even when the underlying disorder is physical in nature.

### Pathophysiology

Inability of the brain to respond to sexual stimuli can interrupt the signals to the parasympathetic nervous system that release a transmitter substance causing the small arteries in the penis to dilate. The result is insufficient blood flow to fill the network of sinusoids inside the corpora cavernosa (erectile chambers) that cause the penis to enlarge and become firm. When the blood volume in the erectile chambers is inadequate, they

**risk factors**

**Impotence**

- Stress
- Fatigue
- Drug effects, e.g., antihypertensive agents, beta blockers, or alcohol
- Diabetes mellitus
- Vascular disease, e.g., hypertension or peripheral vascular disease
- Neurological disorders, e.g., multiple sclerosis or spinal cord injury
- Effects of colorectal, cystectomy, or selected prostatectomy procedures
- Trauma to the perineal area
- Psychological factors

cannot create enough pressure to block blood return. Blood drains from the penis, and an erection cannot be maintained.

The sympathetic nervous system controls both orgasm and ejaculation. These two functions therefore can occur without an erection. After ejaculation, or when sexual stimulation diminishes, the arteries in the penis constrict, reducing blood flow, and the veins expand to allow disengorgement. Box 49-7 summarizes the clinical manifestations of impotence.

## Collaborative Care Management

### Diagnostic tests

Diagnostic tests for impotence include complete blood count, urinalysis, BUN, creatinine, and fasting blood sugars. These tests help rule out entities such as anemia, renal disease, and diabetes as possible causative factors. Other blood tests include cholesterol levels and hormonal studies.

Nocturnal monitoring of penile tumescence is also performed. This test involves the man wearing a device around the penis at night that can gauge normal nocturnal engorgement of the penis. Results indicate the ability of the penis to enlarge and become firm.

Invasive studies are ordered only when other testing measures are inconclusive. Arteriograms (dye injections to study blood flow) and cavernosometry, which measures pressures and blood vessel responses in the erectile chambers, are sometimes performed.

Psychological testing is also performed, which ideally also includes the man's partner.

### Medications

Several new medications for impotence are under development. Sildenafil (Viagra) has been released for use and attracted national attention. A phosphodiesterase inhibitor, Viagra promotes local vasodilation and has demonstrated 50% to 70% effectiveness during clinical trials. All oral agents still require sexual stimulation for the patient to achieve an erection. Viagra can lower the blood pressure significantly and has resulted in cardiac arrest in a few cases when taken in combination with nitrates. Other side effects include headache and gastrointestinal disturbances.

Topical agents are occasionally used to enhance venous congestion of the penis. These drugs can support an erection over a period of hours. Nitroglycerin ointment is an example of a topical vasodilator. Topical and oral agents are often combined with other therapies to treat impotence.

Hormonal therapy is prescribed for the 2% of the impotent population who have a low serum testosterone or an elevated serum prolactin level. Testosterone is given either intramuscularly or transdermally to avoid the hepatotoxicity of the oral preparations. Testosterone can stimulate growth of normal prostatic tissue, promote metastasis of prostatic cancer, stop sperm production, and cause fluid retention and therefore must be used cautiously.

Vasodilators can induce penile erections by means of increased arterial blood flow, sinusoidal relaxation, and increased venous resistance. The drugs generally used are a papaverine and phentolamine combination injected by the patient into the corpus cavernosum of the penis, or inserted into the tip of the penis via suppository. Drug combinations may include prostaglandin E (PGE). Once the drug is injected or inserted, the penis becomes turgid within 5 to 10 minutes, and the erection may last up to 2 hours. Response rate is about 100% for those with neurogenic impotence and 60% to 70% for those with vascular problems.[21] Test doses are given initially to determine the appropriate drug dosage for each patient. Dosages range from .05 to 1.5 ml of the combination drug. Side effects include dizziness, facial flushing, hypotension, and priapism (an erection that lasts longer than 4 to 6 hours; see Box 49-8).

Many medications have side effects that inhibit erectile function. Modifying the dosage, changing the brand, or trying an alternative medication can be helpful for many patients.

### Treatments

External vacuum devices are sometimes used to achieve an erection for a short time. These devices are cylinders that fit over the penis and use a suction pump to pull blood into the penis. A band is applied to the proximal aspect of the penis when an erection is achieved to impede the venous return. The erection may be maintained for approximately 30 minutes. The devices can be used daily and have minimal side effects if used properly. These devices are contraindicated for patients with bleeding disorders, sickle cell anemia, and severe circulatory compromise.

Counseling and sexual therapy classes may be suggested for patients who have identified psychological impotence. They may also be suggested for men dealing with the problem of impotence and the need to find alternative measures for sexual fulfillment.

**box 49-7** *clinical manifestations*

***Impotence***

- Inability to have an erection
- Inability to sustain an erection
- Inability to have an erection firm enough for penetration (incomplete erection)

**box 49-8** *Priapism*

Priapism is a painful condition, characterized by prolonged erection (>4 to 6 hours). Penile ischemia can result, causing permanent impotence or necrosis of the penis.

Etiology

- Caused by either prolonged venous occlusion or arterial blood engorgement
- Possible side effect of some impotence therapies

Treatment

- Treatment is directed at the specific cause.
- Options include administration of alpha agonists directly into the corpora cavernosa, and IV therapy to reestablish acid-base balance.
- Pain management is a high priority.

### Surgical management

Vascular reconstructive surgery may be helpful for the approximately 5% of impotent men who have problems with venous leakage. Venous leakage is defined as the inability to maintain an erection for more than about 2 minutes. The surgery may include the microscopic reconstruction of arterial vessels or removal of some veins to slow the draining of blood from the penis. These surgeries have a limited success rate of only 30% to 50%.[22] There is also a high rate of relapse because of arteriosclerosis and the continued development of incompetent veins. Complications of vascular surgery include numbness of the penile skin, shortened length, curvature, and hematoma formation.

A penile prosthesis may be implanted to treat organic erectile dysfunction. There are two types of penile prostheses. One type consists of two sponge-filled silicone rods, which are implanted in the corpora cavernosa. They support the penis in a constant semierect position. Another method, which more closely simulates an actual erection, is the inflatable penile prosthesis (Figure 49-10). This consists of two inflatable rods inserted into either side of the penis. The rods are connected to a reservoir that allows fluid to flow in or out of them when the man presses on a pump device inserted in the thigh or scrotum.

Both types of prostheses are implanted surgically and do not interfere with normal urinary elimination. The silicone implants are inserted through perineal or penile incisions and the inflatable prostheses through perineal and abdominal incisions. Penile edema is minimal, but scrotal edema may occur with the inflatable type. Pain may be severe during the first week, and mild pain may continue for several weeks after surgery. As with any prosthetic device, the man needs to integrate the device successfully into his body image and sexual relationship.[5] Table 49-7 compares treatment options for erectile dysfunction.

### Diet

A well-balanced diet is recommended for men with impotence. No studies have proved that any vitamin or mineral supplements specifically enhance the male's ability to have an erection. However, some foods are considered to be aphrodisiacs in various cultures, including oysters, avocados, and bull testicles. Obesity can interfere with erectile functioning. Low-fat reducing diets are recommended for patients who are overweight.

### Activity

Men who are in better physical condition often have more endurance and may fatigue less quickly when engaging in sexual activity. However, no specific exercise plan is known to have any positive effect on erectile function.

### Referrals

In some settings the nurse assumes responsibility for making referrals to other services. Common referrals for a man with impotence include certified sex therapists, social workers, and family counselors.

## NURSING MANAGEMENT

## ■ ASSESSMENT

### Subjective Data

Data to be collected to assess the patient with impotence include:

- History of sexual dysfunction
- Partner's view of sexual history
- Ability to have an erection: type, length of time penis remains engorged
- Length of time sexual functioning has been a concern
- Presence of psychosocial stressors
- History of physical diseases; especially vascular and neurogenic
- History of surgeries; especially TURP, prostatectomy, cystectomy
- Treatment approaches tried to alleviate the problem

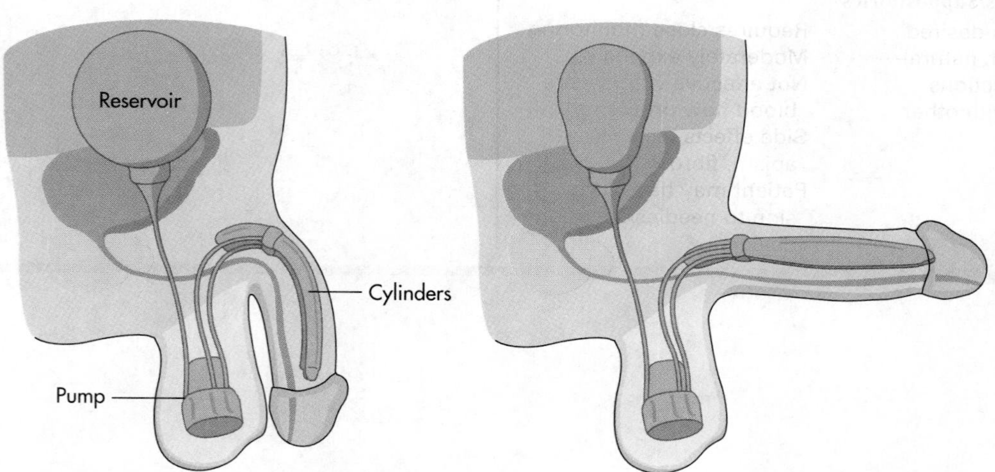


**fig. 49-10** The Scott Inflatable Prosthesis has both erect and flaccid positions designed to mimic normal erectile function.

**table 49-7** *Treatment Options for Male Sexual Dysfunction*

| Advantages | Disadvantages |
|---|---|
| **NONSURGICAL** | |
| **Oral Medications (sildenafil [Viagra], alprostadil)** | |
| Increases libido<br>Inexpensive<br>Minimal side effects<br>Can be used with other options | Newly released and still in trials, 50-70% effective<br>Side effects include headache, diarrhea<br>Contraindicated for concurrent use with nitrates |
| **Hormonal Therapy (Testosterone)** | |
| Increases libido<br>Inexpensive<br>Does not interfere with other treatment options<br>Widely available | Limited effectiveness (10% to 15%)<br>Contraindicated with prostate cancer<br>Must be taken on long-term basis<br>Side effects include fluid retention, liver damage |
| **External Vacuum Devices** | |
| Easy to understand<br>Inexpensive<br>Safe, reversible<br>Can be used with other treatment options | Requires preparation<br>Long-term effects not known<br>Side effects include bruising, pain<br>Requires manual dexterity |
| **Sexual Devices** | |
| Inexpensive<br>Easy to understand<br>May enhance foreplay/orgasm | Does not produce satisfactory erection<br>May not fit into value system<br>Inaccessibility |
| **Counseling** | |
| Involves partner<br>Can be used with other treatment options<br>May improve other psychosocial issues | Limited effectiveness<br>Long-standing problems may be difficult to treat |
| **Penile Injections/Suppositories** | |
| Use only when desired<br>Produces rapid, natural-appearing erections<br>Can be used with other treatments<br>Minimal pain | Requires close monitoring<br>Moderately expensive<br>Not effective with severe blood flow problems<br>Side effects include priapism, fibrosis<br>Patient may have aversion to needles/insertion device |
| **SURGICAL** | |
| **Vascular Reconstructive Surgery** | |
| Possibility of restoration to normal function<br>Natural appearance | Expensive<br>Technically difficult surgery<br>Low long-term success rate (30-50%)<br>High relapse rate |
| **Inflatable Prosthesis** | |
| Natural-looking erection<br>No preparation time<br>Use as desired<br>Increases girth of penis<br>No concealment problem | Device failure<br>Requires manual dexterity<br>May require removal/reimplant<br>Expensive<br>Risk of infection, erosion |
| **Self-contained Inflatable Prosthesis** | |
| Natural-looking erection<br>No preparation time<br>Use as desired<br>No concealment problem<br>Simpler surgery than that for full inflatable prosthesis | Device failure<br>Requires manual dexterity<br>May require removal/reimplant<br>Expensive<br>Risk of infection, erosion<br>Does not increase girth |
| **Semirigid/Malleable Prosthesis** | |
| Simple surgery<br>No moving parts<br>Least expensive implant<br>Use as desired | May be difficult to conceal<br>Does not increase girth of penis<br>Expensive<br>Risk of infection/erosion<br>May require removal/reimplant |

### Objective Data

Data to be collected to assess the patient with impotence include:

Sensory deficits: manual dexterity and visual acuity needed for many treatment options

General assessment of sexual organs to note any obvious deformity, or structural defects.

## ■ NURSING DIAGNOSES

Nursing diagnoses are determined from analysis of patient data. Nursing diagnoses for the patient with impotence may include but are not limited to:

| Diagnostic Title | Possible Etiological Factors |
|---|---|
| Sexual dysfunction (impotence) | Difficulty in attaining or maintaining an erection |
| Anxiety | Sexual performance |

## ■ EXPECTED PATIENT OUTCOMES

Expected patient outcomes for the patient with impotence may include but are not limited to:

1a. Identifies alternative methods of sexual intimacy that will provide a positive sexual interaction.

b. Demonstrates the effective use of devices to obtain an erection.

2. Demonstrates a relaxed positive attitude about sexual performance.

## ■ INTERVENTIONS

### Identifying Alternatives

Helping the patient choose sexual therapy options by providing accurate and up-to-date information is an important part of nursing care for the patient with impotence. Myths and erroneous information are common obstacles in sexual rehabilitation. The patient is informed of the physiological and psychological aspects of erectile function. The use of external devices and medications is reviewed, including their modes of action, side effects, and contraindications. Early referral to advanced practice nurses and other specialists is usually appropriate.

#### *Penile injections*

The nurse may be responsible for teaching the patient to administer penile injections. These patients need to be followed in an office or clinic on a regular basis. Systemic complications of the injections include orthostatic hypotension and dizziness. Local complications include pain, hematoma, edema, decreased glandular sensation, fibrosis, and priapism. Priapism may be reversed by application of ice, manual masturbation, injection of epinephrine, or the use of antihistamines. If priapism persists longer than 4 to 6 hours, the patient should notify his physician.

Injection sites are to the lateral sides of the penis and should be rotated, and injection into the urethra should be avoided. Applying pressure to the injection site can help decrease the possibility of fibrosis. The patient is instructed not to use injections more than twice a week. Liver enzyme levels should be monitored about every 3 months. If liver function studies are elevated or fibrosis is noted on the penis, it usually is recommended that the injections be discontinued. The drug should be kept in the refrigerator to avoid degeneration of the solution. Dosages can be altered if initial results are not satisfactory.

#### *External vacuum devices*

Vacuum devices come in one size with ring seals at the end that are different diameters to accommodate individual erection size. The patient is taught to use the device and make sure that the seals are the appropriate size to ensure sufficient vacuum to the penis. The vascular ring is applied once the penis is engorged and should only be left on for approximately 30 minutes to prevent possible vascular damage. The nurse involves both partners in the teaching session if possible. Couples need to discuss in advance how sexual activity may be modified comfortably with the use of the device.

The vacuum device may be used every day if desired. Complications include pulling of scrotal tissue, hematoma, inability to achieve or maintain the erection, and discomfort with the vascular ring. These complications can usually be managed by adjusting the procedure or switching to a different product. Blocked or retrograde ejaculation may also occur. Orgasm should not be affected. The patient is encouraged to schedule ongoing medical support to help him cope with this altered sexual pattern.

#### *Penile implants*

Infection rates are generally low with penile implant surgery. Antibiotics may be administered a few days before surgery and for a week after surgery to prevent infection. The patient also may be told to perform a Hibiciens prewash before surgery, to decrease the chance of infection. The nurse instructs the patient to take all antibiotics and report any symptoms of infection, such as unusual swelling, redness, excessive pain, or drainage around the incision sites.

To prevent the device from eroding through the penile skin, the patient is instructed to avoid sexual intercourse for at least 6 to 8 weeks after surgery. When sexual activity resumes, the patient is instructed to use a water-soluble lubricant. The patient needs to avoid wearing tight-fitting clothing and sitting with the legs crossed or in other positions that put pressure or cause friction to the penis.

The nurse teaches the patient that his erections will not necessarily be any larger than before surgery. The nurse includes the partner in teaching sessions if possible. The implant does not affect a man's sex drive or interfere with penile sensation. The patient should be able to have an orgasm and ejaculate with the implant in place. Patients with inflatable implants need to be instructed on how to inflate and deflate the prosthesis.

### Reducing Performance-Related Anxiety

Sexual counseling usually is offered in conjunction with other forms of treatment for the impotent patient. The nurse is often the person to encourage patients to avail themselves of counseling opportunities. The nurse helps the patient understand his needs and explains the general nature of sexual counseling, as patients often have misconceptions concerning the treatment. The nurse provides some specific examples of exercises used during sexual counseling and explains how partner communication can be enhanced.

## ■ EVALUATION

To evaluate the effectiveness of nursing interventions, compare patient behaviors with those stated in the expected patient outcomes. Successful achievement of patient outcomes for the patient with impotence is indicated by:

1a. Capable of engaging in sexual intimacy with a significant other that is a positive experience for both partners; statements by both partners indicate personal growth and closeness.

b. Is able to use devices to obtain an erection correctly and safely.

2. States he feels more relaxed and more positive about sexual performance.

## GERONTOLOGICAL CONSIDERATIONS

The nurse should not assume that elders do not have sexual needs. Impotence in the elderly patient is often caused by narrowing of the blood vessels and consequently decreased blood flow to the penis. Most healthy males can obtain an erection even at an advanced age. Often the elderly male needs more and prolonged stimulation than his younger counterpart to have an erection. The nurse can inform patients and their partners of the need for longer "foreplay" with the older male.

## SPECIAL ENVIRONMENTS FOR CARE

### Critical Care Management

Critical care does not play a role in the management of impotence. The treatment is largely based in the outpatient setting and surgery would not be recommended for any man who was not in good general health.

### Home Care Management

If the patient had surgical treatment for impotence, any signs of infection or erosion of the penile implant should be immediately reported to the physician. Often, when the patient uses the penile erectile devices for the first few times at home, questions arise. Patients need to be discharged with explicit instructions about whom to contact with concerns and phone numbers for resource persons.

## COMPLICATIONS

Complications of penile implant surgery include malfunction of the device, infection, and erosion of the prosthesis through the penis. Complications of injections and mechanical erectile devices include possible priapism and circulatory occlusions to the penis, causing tissue necrosis.

# VASECTOMY: MALE STERILIZATION

## ETIOLOGY/EPIDEMIOLOGY

Voluntary sterilization has become increasingly acceptable to both men and women as a method of preventing pregnancy. It is the most frequently used method of fertility control for married couples over 30 years of age and is the most widely used contraceptive method worldwide, protecting approximately 100 million couples. It has been estimated that more than 13.7 million adults have been sterilized in the United States and 100 million worldwide. Each year, 500,000 to 1 million American men have vasectomies.[10]

The primary reason given by both men and women for wishing sterilization is a desire to limit family size. More frequently than women, men give as an important reason for sterilization their wish for an effective contraceptive that does not interfere with sexual pleasure. Also, men express concern over the health of their sex partners. Some men believe that the "pill" is actually or potentially harmful to the woman.

The laws governing sterilization vary from state to state and have undergone many changes. In general, if the surgery does not violate specific state provisions and if written informed consent is given by a man or woman legally capable of giving permission, the surgery can be performed. Because sterilization is a permanent method of contraception, informed consent is absolutely necessary before the procedure.

## PATHOPHYSIOLOGY

Bilateral vasectomy is the surgical procedure used for male sterilization. Vasectomy interrupts the continuity of the vas deferens, and sperm are prevented from being ejaculated with other components of the semen. However, sperm still are produced, and the ejaculate is not noticeably diminished in amount. Residual fertility may be present for a variable period because of existing sperm in the semen beyond the point of occlusion of the vas deferens. Sperm gradually disappear from the ejaculate; thus conception is possible in the immediate postoperative period.

After vasectomy, antibodies to sperm develop in about 50% to 66% of men. No relationship has been found in humans between the presence of sperm antibodies and any systemic pathological condition. It is hypothesized that antisperm antibodies may result in circulating immune complexes that exacerbate atherosclerosis, but this has not been proven in human studies.

## COLLABORATIVE CARE MANAGEMENT

At least 11 different techniques for vasectomy exist. Bilateral partial vasectomy is the surgical method used most often. Because of its safety and simplicity, the procedure can be performed on an outpatient basis using a local anesthetic. A small incision is made in the scrotum to expose the sheath of the vas deferens. The sheath is opened, and a 0.63 to 1.27 cm segment of the vas deferens is removed. The severed ends of the vas deferens are then ligated or coagulated to ensure sterility. The incision is then sutured closed.

Complications after vasectomy are rare and usually minor. Bruising, mild edema, and mild discomfort are common and usually subside without treatment. Infection of the wound occurs in about 3% of patients. Hematoma, epididymitis, and granuloma formation can occur. The incidence of failure as a result of recanalization (reanastamosis) is reported to be 0% to 6%. The cause of spontaneous recanalization is unknown, but duplication of the vas deferens has occasionally occurred. A preoperative specimen of semen is examined to serve as a baseline for monitoring sperm disappearance after surgery.

Research is ongoing concerning techniques to reverse vasectomy and restore fertility. A vasovasostomy attempts to rejoin the severed ends of the vas deferens. Success is measured by the presence of sperm in semen specimens after reconstruction. Reports of success in restoring fertility range from 29% to 85%.

### Patient/Family Education

Patient education focuses on ensuring that the patient has made a careful and informed decision concerning sterilization. Teaching is based on the federal government's informed consent guidelines (see Chapter 47). The nature and consequences of the surgery are explained to the patient. It is important to emphasize that the sterilization procedure does nothing to increase or decrease sexual performance or enjoyment, but simply removes the risk of pregnancy. Visual aids and models can be of great value in explaining the surgery to patients.

Every effort is made to ensure that the decision for sterilization is not based on a lack of knowledge concerning other options for contraception. Most patients are satisfied with the results of vasectomy, but emotional difficulties can be experienced, as sterilization affects both partners.

The facts concerning reversibility, including current success rates, are discussed. In the case of vasectomy, the chance of recanalization and return of fertility should be pointed out. The man or couple must also be informed that sterility occurs progressively rather than immediately after vasectomy, and alternate methods of contraception need to be utilized until sterility is achieved. Men are taught to expect slight swelling of the scrotum, minor pain, and a small amount of bleeding after surgery. Ice to the scrotal area, sitz baths, and rest will ameliorate these discomforts. Any signs of infection should be reported promptly to the physician for evaluation and treatment.

It is important for the man to schedule follow-up semen analysis. A sperm count usually is taken 4 weeks after vasectomy. Two consecutive sperm-free specimens are necessary before the man can be considered sterile. Reanastomosis of the vas deferens is suspected if sperm fail to disappear from the ejaculate, if there is an increase in sperm in the semen after two successive sperm counts, or if motile sperm are found in the semen 3 months after vasectomy.

## critical thinking QUESTIONS

1 Mr. W. is a 40-year-old patient who is post-orchiectomy and radical node dissection for a nonseminomatous neoplasm. The nurse identifies hemorrhage, atelectasis, thrombosis, and paralytic ileus as potential complications of the surgery. Discuss preventive nursing measures for these potential complications specifically with regard to activity.

2 As a community health nurse in an industrial company. Ms. L. is designing a program to teach men in the company about reproductive health. Develop an outline depicting the priority diseases and preventative measures she might teach.

3 Mr. A., 59, is admitted to the hospital complaining of difficulty urinating. The ER physician orders routine urinalysis, CBC, and chemistry profile. Outline questions designed to help differentiate the cause of these symptoms.

## chapter SUMMARY

### PROBLEMS OF THE TESTES AND RELATED STRUCTURES

- Epididymitis is the most common intrascrotal inflammation. It affects men between ages 19 and 35 and is typically caused by an ascending infection acquired sexually.
- Epididymitis causes acute scrotal pain and swelling. Treatment involves antibiotics, antiinflammatories, and supportive care.
- Orchitis involves infection of a testicle by a bacteria or virus or as a complication of mumps.
- Testicular torsion occurs when testicular circulation is acutely impaired by a sudden twisting of the spermatic cord. Prompt treatment is essential to preserve the testicle.
- Testicular cancer is the leading cause of cancer death in men ages 15 to 35. It is 90% to 100% curable if diagnosed early.
- Testicular cancer is treated with surgical orchiectomy. Regular testicular self-examination should be taught to all young adult men.

### PROBLEMS OF THE PROSTATE

- Prostatitis is a common inflammation in young and middle-aged adults. It is treated with antibiotics and supportive care.
- Benign prostatic hyperplasia develops in mid-life, probably in response to increased androgen levels. Symptoms include urinary hesitancy, urgency, decreased stream, straining, and dysuria.
- Treatment of benign prostatic hypertrophy (BPH) involves transurethral prostatic resection (TURP). Early BPH may be treated by medication that either reduces the gland size or eases the obstructive process.
- Postdischarge care after TURP involves encouraging a liberal fluid intake, preventing straining at stool, restricting activity, and reassuring the patient that potency is rarely affected by the surgery, although sterility is common.
- Prostate cancer is the most common cancer site in men and the second leading cause of cancer death in men.
- Prostate cancer is associated with aging and frequently starts as a discrete hard nodule that may be asymptomatic.

- Prostate cancer tends to grow slowly in elderly men. Curative treatment options include radical prostatectomy or radiation therapy by implant or external beam. Both approaches can result in sterility and impotence, and surgery causes temporary problems with incontinence.

## PROBLEMS OF THE PENIS

- Phimosis and paraphimosis involve the inability to move the foreskin freely across the glans penis. Treatment involves relieving constriction and may involve circumcision.
- Penile cancer is rare but typically develops in the late middle-age years, possibly from chronic bacterial irritation. The treatment is surgical.
- Impotence may have psychologic, neural, vascular, and drug-related causes. Treatment involves vasodilator injections, medication adjustments, external vacuum devices, and penile prostheses.

## VASECTOMY: MALE STERILIZATION

- Sterilization is the most common method of contraception for married couples over age 30. The procedure is simple, carries few risks, and is performed on an outpatient basis.

## References


1. American Cancer Society: Guidelines on diet, nutrition, and cancer prevention. CA: *A Cancer Journal for Clinicians* 46(6):325-341, 1996.
2. Agency for Health Care Policy and Research, Public Health Service: Benign prostatic hyperplasia: diagnosis and treatment, Clinical Practice Guidelines, No 8, US Department of Health and Human Services, 1994.
3. Brenner AR, Krenzer ME: Update on cryosurgical ablation for prostate cancer, *Am J Nurs* 95(4):44-49, 1995.
4. Bruskewitz R, Cassel C: Benign prostatic hyperplasia: intervene or wait? *Hosp Pract* 27(8);99-115, 1992.
5. Bryant R, Boarini J: Treatment options for men with sexual dysfunction, *JET* 19(4):131-142, 1992.
6. D'Elia FL, Yomella LG: Prostate cancer update, *Compr Therapy* 21(1):35-40, 1995.
7. Donovan DA, Nicholas PK: Prostatitis: diagnosis and treatment in primary care, *Nurse Pract* 22(4):144-156, 1997.
8. Gordon SI, Brenden MA, Wyble JS, Ivey CL: When the Dx is penile cancer, *RN* 60(3), 41-44, 1997.
9. Greifzu S, Tiedemann D: Prostate cancer: the pros and cons of treatment, *RN* 58(6):22-26, 1995.
10. Hans JM, Butta PG, Giruin S: A comprehensive and efficient process for counseling patients desiring sterilization, *Nurse Pract* 22(6):52-66, 1997.
11. Held JL, Osborne, DM, Volpe H, and Waldman A: Cancer of the prostate: treatment and nursing implications, *Oncol Nurs Forum* 21(9):1517-1529, 1994.
12. Hicks RJ, Cook JB: Managing patients with benign prostatic hyperplasia, *Am Fam Physician* 52(1):135-142, 1995.
13. Higgs D: The patient with testicular cancer: nursing management of chemotherapy, *Oncol Nurs Forum* 17(2):243-249, 1990.
14. Kaler S: Epididymitis in the young adult male, *Nurse Pract* 15(5):10-16, 1990.
15. Keetch DW, Moore S, Shea L: Crysosurgical ablation of the prostate, *AORN* 61(5):807-820, 1995.
16. Kuritzky L: Solutions for patients with erectile dysfunction, *Hospital Practice* 30(12):24G-24K, 1995.
17. Lasater S: Testicular cancer, a perioperative challenge, *AORN* 51(2): 513-526, 1990.
18. Lewis AG et al: Evaluation of acute scrotum in the emergency department, *J Pediatric Surgery* 30(2):277-281, 1995.
19. McConnell JD: Benign prostatic hyperplasia: hormonal treatment, *Urologic Clinics of North America* 22(2):387-399, 1995.
20. Miller CA: New medication for the treatment of benign prostatic hyperplasia, *Geriatric Nursing* 14(2):111-112, 1993.
21. Moore S et al: Nerve sparing prostatectomy, *Am Nurs* 92(4):59-64, 1992.
22. Montorsi F et al: Pharmacological management of erectile dysfunction, *Drugs* 50(3):465-479, 1995.
23. O'Keefe M, Hunt DK: Assessment and treatment of impotence, *Med Clin North America* 79(2):415-433, 1995.
24. Pobursky J: Prostate cancer: detection and treatment options, *Today's OR Nurse* 17(3):5-9, 1995.
25. Roehrborn CG: The Agency for Health Care Policy and Research: Clinical Guidelines for the diagnosis and treatment of benign prostatic hyperplasia, *Urologic Clinics of North America* 22(2):445-453, 1995.
26. Samm BJ, Dmochowski RR: Urologic emergencies. Trauma injuries and conditions affecting the penis, scrotum and testicles, *Post Graduate Medicine* 100(4):187, 1996.
27. Tonetti J, Tonetti J: Testicular torsion or acute epididymitis? Diagnosis and treatment, *J Emergency Nursing* 16(2):96-98, 1990.

chapter

# 50 MANAGEMENT OF PERSONS WITH Sexually Transmitted Diseases

WILMA J. PHIPPS and KIMBERLY ADAMS-DAVIS

## objectives *After studying this chapter, the learner should be able to:*

1. Define sexually transmitted diseases (STDs).
2. Describe the transmission, prevention, and control of STDs.
3. List the causative agent, incubation period, signs and symptoms, medical therapy, and long-term effects of gonorrhea, syphilis, herpes genitalis, and chlamydia infection.
4. Describe the subjective and objective data to be collected from a person suspected of having any STDs.
5. Write a teaching plan for a unit on the prevention of STDs for a sex education course for adolescents.

## ETIOLOGY

Sexually transmitted diseases (STDs) are diseases that usually are or can be transmitted from one person to another with heterosexual or homosexual intercourse or intimate contact with the genitalia, mouth, or rectum. Because the causative organisms survive only briefly outside a warm, moist environment, there is almost no way to contract STDs from toilet seats, towels, or bed linens. Although STDs are not usually transmitted in public restrooms, conditions caused by fungi, bacteria, and lice can be transmitted from water in unclean toilet bowls. Women using a conventional toilet expose the vaginal and anal area to pathogens that can be introduced by the backsplash of contaminated toilet water.

There are some notable exceptions to sexual transmission. During pregnancy the fetus may become infected in utero by placental transmission, and the neonate may acquire congenital syphilis or be stillborn. Infants of mothers with gonorrhea may contract an infection of the eyes (ophthalmia neonatorum) during birth, and unless treated, it can lead to permanent blindness.

Until the 1980s only five venereal diseases (syphilis, gonorrhea, chancroid, lymphogranuloma venereum, and granuloma inguinale) were regularly monitored. In the 1980s several diseases were added to the list of STDs. These include *Chlamydia trachomatis*, genital herpes, human papillomavirus, genital mycoplasmas, cytomegalovirus, hepatitis B, vaginitis, enteric infections, and ectoparasitic disease.[27]

Early in the 1980s the human immunodeficiency virus (HIV) was identified, and acquired immunodeficiency syndrome (AIDS) emerged as a major STD. Because of the profound effect of AIDS on the immune system, Chapter 67 is devoted to its discussion.

The diseases classified as STDs and their causative organisms are listed in Table 50-1. Because of improved laboratory and epidemiological methods, the prevalence, modes of transmission, and clinical consequences of these newer STDs are better understood than in earlier decades. In addition, many of the newly recognized STDs have become epidemic or hyperendemic as a consequence of changing sexual behavioral patterns. Not only has the incidence of many STDs increased, but also, for agents with multiple modes of transmission (e.g., hepatitis B virus, enteric pathogens), the proportion of infections that are transmitted sexually has increased. In addition to the immediate consequences of STDs there are the recognized effects on maternal and infant morbidity, as well as on human reproduction and fertility.

All states require that each case of syphilis, gonorrhea, hepatitis A, hepatitis B, and AIDS be reported to the state or local health officer. Most states also require the reporting of chancroid, granuloma inguinale, and lymphogranuloma venereum. Herpes genitalis, trichomoniasis, and candidiasis do not need to be reported in any state. The true incidence of STDs is not known because of variable reporting requirements and also because many cases are not reported by the clinicians who treat them.

## EPIDEMIOLOGY

In the United States almost 12 million cases of STDs occur yearly, 86% of them in persons ages 15 to 29 years of age. By 21 years of age, approximately one out of every five young persons has undergone treatment for an STD. Because only some teenagers are sexually active, this amounts to an effective rate of at least 25% among those who are sexually active.[27]

Most STDs exhibit "biological sexism": in addition to the immediate consequences of STDs, there are serious complications, most of which have the greatest impact on women and children. The most serious complications are pelvic inflammatory disease (PID), sterility, ectopic pregnancy, blindness, cancer associated with the human papillomavirus, fetal and infant deaths, birth defects, and mental retardation. The populations most affected are medically underserved persons, poor persons, and racial and ethnic minorities.[27] The total societal costs of STDs exceed $315 billion annually, with the cost of PID and PID-associated ectopic pregnancy and infertility alone exceeding $2.6 billion.[27]

In explaining the trends of reported cases of STDs in the United States, three changes occurring since the 1960s are often referred to in the literature. The first of these concerns the use of antibiotics and changes in the antibiotic susceptibility of pathogenic organisms. The widespread, perhaps indiscriminate, use of penicillin and other antibiotics in the late 1940s and early 1950s parallels the decline in both syphilis and gonorrhea. It is said that the organisms developed a greater resistance to antibiotics over time and that antibiotics have therefore become less effective than previously. No firm evidence indicates a decrease in effectiveness of penicillin against syphilis. However, the gonococcus tends to develop resistance to antibiotics, and this has been increasing.

A second explanation for the rise in incidence of STDs is that they are more likely to occur if a social system is permissive. During times of war and other catastrophes, it is easier for agencies to control interpersonal behavior, whereas in times of peace and absence of national crisis, civil liberties tend to flourish. The incidence curve of syphilis and gonorrhea after the years of World War II seems to support this thesis.

The third explanation centers around sexual behavior patterns and includes permissiveness. Concern has been expressed particularly about the prevalence of gonorrhea among adolescents and young adults who are considered to be promiscuous. In fact, rates for gonorrhea show young adults of 20 to 24 years of age accounted for 40% of reported cases of gonorrhea, whereas persons 15 to 19 years of age accounted for 25% of cases. The highest morbidity rate for males was in the 20- to 24-year age group; for females it was in the 15- to 19-year age group.

The preceding discussion makes an assumption of sexual promiscuity and, in doing so, requires acknowledgment of advances in contraceptive technology, especially "the pill." These social changes are often referred to as the three *P*'s (permissiveness, promiscuity, and the pill). The underlying idea is that, with the advent of antibiotics and the pill, people began to lose fear of untreated venereal disease and pregnancy and that sexual promiscuity increased significantly, leading to increased exposure to infection. According to Hatcher et al.[10] the type of contraception chosen has a direct impact on STD risk.

If the definition of promiscuity is that sexual relations are not restricted to one partner, studies show that patients diagnosed in clinics as having STDs are not promiscuous. In one study 66.4% of patients having an STD named only one sexual contact.[6] It must be realized, however, that persons may hesitate to admit to having more than one sex partner for any number of reasons. Most unmarried persons admit to practicing "serial monogamy," which is a mutually faithful sexual relationship with one person for short periods of time. The practice of serial monogamy increases the number of lifetime sexual partners, thereby increasing the risk for contracting STDs.[10]

In the past, prostitution was considered a major force in the transmission of STDs. Before World War II it was estimated that approximately 75% of all STDs in the United States could be traced to prostitutes and that at least 10% of all prostitutes had contracted an STD at least once. Today fewer than 5% of patients with syphilis can be classed as prostitutes. Also, most persons with gonorrhea are single and under 25 years of age, and most clients of prostitutes are usually older, married men. *Chlamydia trachomatis* and herpes are two STDs that are common in middle-class America.

Before 1960 homosexuals were rarely mentioned in the literature as carriers of STDs. Since the early 1970s much more attention has been given to the risk of STDs among homosexual and bisexual men. Homosexual men carry pathogens in the rectum and colon, including gonococcus, *Giardia,* ameba, *Shigella,* and *Campylobacter.* Although lesbians are at low risk for contracting STDs and gay males are at higher risk, it is important to note that sexual orientation does not determine individual forms of sexual behavior.

The condom was the main method of contraception used before the advent of antibiotics and oral contraceptives. Use of the condom is believed to have prevented the spread of STDs by providing a mechanical barrier to the organisms. The pill revolutionized contraceptive practices, and it is known that estrogen alters the vaginal and cervical ecology, predisposing it to infection.

Two events during the 1980s and 1990s bear mentioning:

1. The designation of AIDS as an STD put other STDs in competition with it for attention and resources.[23]
2. Studies of the sociodemographic and geographic distribution of gonorrhea clearly indicate that the transmission of gonorrhea is predicated on the existence of small groups of persons who share common sociodemographic, behavioral, and geographic characteristics of a so-called core group. This concept was verified empirically in such diverse locations as New York State; Colorado Springs, Colorado; Dade County, Florida; and Liverpool, England. With the understanding of a core group pattern comes the opportunity to design intervention programs tailored to the group at risk.[23]

## PATHOPHYSIOLOGY

Although many persons with STDs may be asymptomatic, others commonly have genital lesions, genital itching or burning, changes in vaginal discharge, lower abdominal pain, penile discharge, or pain with intercourse.

**table 50-1** *Sexually Transmitted Diseases*

| Type of Organism | Disease |
|---|---|
| Bacteria | Gonorrhea, chancroid, granuloma inguinale, bacterial vaginosis |
| Spirochete | Syphilis |
| *Chlamydia* | Nongonococcal urethritis, epididymitis, cervicitis, pelvic inflammatory disease (PID), lymphogranuloma venereum |
| Virus | Herpes genitalis, hepatitis B, cytomegalovirus, AIDS, condylomata acuminata, molluscum contagiosum |
| Protozoa | Trichomoniasis |
| Fungi | Candidiasis |
| Parasites | Pediculosis pubis, scabies |

## COLLABORATIVE CARE MANAGEMENT

### Diagnostic Tests

Specific diagnostic tests are used to establish the diagnosis of each of these diseases. Diagnostic tests will be discussed under the specific disease later in this chapter.

### Medications

Treatment depends on the causative organisms identified through the history, physical examination, and diagnostic tests and is discussed in detail in the following pages. It is not unusual for an individual to harbor two or more organisms simultaneously. See Table 50-2 for standard treatment modalities for gonorrhea, syphilis, chlamydia, condylomata acuminata, and genital herpes.

## NURSING MANAGEMENT

## ■ ASSESSMENT

### Subjective Data

Data to be collected to assess the patient suspected of having any STD include:

Exposure to STD contact, including HIV
Prior STD history, treatment

**table 50-2** *Selected Sexually Transmitted Diseases*

| Incubation Period | Signs and Symptoms | Medical Therapy |
|---|---|---|
| **GONORRHEA** | | |
| Men: 3-30 days<br>Women: 3 days to an indefinite period | Men: purulent urethral discharge, dysuria, epididymitis, prostatitis<br>Women: asymptomatic in early stages: cervicitis with purulent discharge, bartholinitis, salpingitis | Ceftriaxone, 125 mg IM in a single dose, plus doxycycline, 100 mg PO bid for 7 days, or cefixime, 400 mg PO, plus doxycycline, 100 mg PO bid for 7 days, or ciprofloxacin, 500 mg PO in single dose, plus doxycycline, 10 mg PO bid for 7 days, or ofloxacin, 400 mg PO, plus doxycycline, 10 mg PO bid for 7 days (individuals with gonorrhea are concurrently treated for chlamydia). |
| **SYPHILIS** | | |
| 3 wk (9 days to 3 mo) | Positive serological tests, chancre in stage I | Benzathine penicillin G, 2.4 million units IM. |
| **HERPES GENITALIS** | | |
| 3-14 days | Vesicles that rupture and form ulcerations, pain, inguinal lymph node enlargement, dysuria, flulike symptoms | Herpes primary occurrence: acyclovir 200 mg PO 5 × 3 × 7-10 days; recurrence: acyclovir 200 mg PO 5 × days; suppression: acyclovir 200 mg PO bid for 1 year<br>Diet: Usually no dietary modications or restrictions during the treatment of STDs<br>Activity: No standard activity limitations<br>Referrals: Pregnant women with STDs may be referred to obstetricians for treatment. Persons with resistant strains of STDs may be referred to public health officials or infectious disease specialists. |
| **CHLAMYDIA** | | |
| 5-10 days or longer | Women: painful or difficult urination, abnormal vaginal discharge or bleeding, pain or bleeding with coitus, irregular menses; one third are asymptomatic<br>Men: testicular pain, nonspecific urethritis or epididymitis | Doxycycline, 100 mg PO bid for 7 days, or azithromycin, 1 g PO in a single dose. |
| **CONDYLOMATA ACUMINATA (GENITAL WARTS)** | | |
| 1-6 mo | Horny papules on vulva, vagina, cervix, perineum, anal canal, urethra, glans penis | Pharmocological therapies: Podofilox 0.5% solution and 80-90% trichloroacetic/bichloroacetic acid; intralesional interferon; surgical treatment: laser, cryotherapy, electrocautery, or loop electrosurgical excision procedure. |

Sexual orientation: "Have you been having sex with men, women, or both?"
Relationship of onset of symptoms to last sexual intercourse
Number of sexual partners in the past 2 months

Women are questioned about last menstrual period (LMP), vaginal discharge, vulvar itching, dysuria, urinary urgency, lower abdominal pain, rectal symptoms, sore throat, genital lesions, skin rashes or itching, and menstrual periods.

Heterosexual, gay, and bisexual men are questioned about urethral discharge, dysuria, genital lesions, skin rashes, itching, testicular pain, and sore throat. Gay and bisexual men are also asked about rectal symptoms such as pain, bleeding, discharge, and diarrhea.

If hepatitis is also suspected, the person is questioned about dark-colored urine, clay-colored stools, fatigue, and jaundice.

### Objective Data

Data to be collected to assess the patient suspected of having any STD include:

- Inspection and palpation of the integumentary system, reproductive system, and anorectal area
- Examination for women includes the following:
  - Inspection of skin of lower abdomen, inguinal area, hands, palms, and forearms
  - Inspection of pubic hair for lice and mites
  - Inspection and palpation of external genitalia, including perineum and anus
  - Speculum examination of vagina and cervix
  - Bimanual examination of the uterus and adnexa
  - Palpation for inguinal and femoral lymphadenopathy
  - Inspection of mouth and throat, including tonsils
  - Pregnancy test for all women of childbearing age
- Examination of heterosexual men includes the following:
  - Inspection of the skin and pubic hair
  - Inspection of the penis, including the meatus, with retraction of the foreskin and "milking" of the urethra
  - Palpation of the scrotum
- Examination of homosexual or bisexual men is the same as for heterosexual men plus the following:
  - Inspection of the mouth, throat including the tonsils, and anorectal area
  - Anoscopic examination if there are rectal symptoms

## NURSING DIAGNOSES

Nursing diagnoses are determined from analysis of patient data. Nursing diagnoses for the person with any STD may include but are not limited to:

| Diagnostic Title | Possible Etiological Factors |
|---|---|
| Knowledge deficit | Lack of exposure/recall, information misinterpretation, lack of familiarity with information sources about STDs |
| Health maintenance, altered | Lack of knowledge, cultural practices, lack of material resources |

## EXPECTED PATIENT OUTCOMES

Expected patient outcomes for the person with any STD may include but are not limited to:

1a. Person and partner can explain the etiology and factors contributing to the STD.
b. Person and partner can state the name, dosage, and schedule of administration of drug therapy, as well as its possible side effects.
c. Person and partner can explain the need for adherence to the entire treatment regimen.
d. Person and partner can state the reasons for abstaining from sexual activity during the infectious stages of the STD.
e. Person and partner can state effects of the STD on the reproductive system of oneself and one's partner.
f. Person and partner can state indications for seeking immediate health care if signs and symptoms reappear.
g. Person and partner can explain necessity for treatment of sexual partner or partners.
h. Person and partner can accept the occurrence of the STD.
i. Person and partner can explain how to prevent the transmission of STDs by using safer sex practices, including the type of condom to use, when and how to apply it, and how to remove it.[10] Recommendations on the proper use of condoms to prevent transmission of STDs can be found in Box 50-1.

2a. Person and partner describe resources necessary to achieve health.
b. Person and partner recognize personal strengths and weaknesses.
c. Person and partner participate actively in health maintenance activities.

## INTERVENTIONS

The following interventions apply to the person with any STD.

### Patient/Family Education

The nurse's first responsibility in STD control is to educate persons who have a sexually transmitted infection or may develop one. Nurses must be knowledgeable about the most prevalent diseases, the signs and symptoms, methods used in diagnosis, treatments used, and where individuals can obtain help and information. They also can influence the knowledge and attitudes of their colleagues and peers toward STD and its control. Nurses can exert influence in the community by taking an active role in education programs. Perhaps the best way to reduce the risk of STD is for persons who are sexually active to limit their number of sexual partners. Sexual activity with different partners increases the risk of infection.

Preventive measures such as washing or showering with soap and water, urinating after sexual intercourse, and using a condom are recommended but are no guarantee against STD. Good laundry and personal hygiene practices also may help reduce risk.

Before nurses can be effective in working with persons who have STDs, they must confront their own feelings and attitudes about STDs. The person is often young, fearful of pain, and unaccustomed to surroundings in a clinic or physician's office. Young people especially fear that their families and friends may learn they have an STD.

**box 50-1** *Recommendations from the CDC for the Use of Condoms*

The following recommendations for proper use of condoms to reduce the transmission of STDs are based on current information:

1. Latex condoms should be used, because they offer greater protection against viral STDs than natural membrane condoms.
2. Condoms should be stored in a cool, dry place out of direct sunlight.
3. Condoms in damaged packages or those that show obvious signs of age (e.g., those that are brittle, sticky, or discolored) should not be used. They cannot be relied on to prevent infection.
4. Condoms should be handled with care to prevent puncture.
5. The condom should be put on the erect penis (either partner can do this) before the penis comes into contact with the woman's genitals to prevent exposure to fluids that may contain infectious agents. Hold the tip of the condom and unroll it onto the erect penis, leaving ½ inch of space at the tip to collect semen, yet ensuring that no air is trapped in the tip of the condom.
6. Adequate lubrication should be used. If exogenous lubrication is needed, only water-based lubricants should be used. Petroleum- or oil-based lubricants (e.g., petroleum jelly, cooking oils, shortening, and lotions) should not be used, because they weaken the latex of the condom.
7. Use of condoms containing spermicides may provide some additional protection against STDs. However, vaginal use of spermicides along with condoms is likely to provide greater protection.
8. If a condom breaks, it should be replaced immediately. If ejaculation occurs after condom breaks, the immediate use of a vaginal spermicide has been suggested. However, the protective value of post-ejaculation application of spermicide in reducing the risk of STD transmission is unknown.
9. After ejaculation, care should be taken so that the condom does not slip off the penis before withdrawal; the base of the condom should be held while withdrawing. The penis should be withdrawn while still erect.
10. Condoms should never be reused.

Modified from Hatcher PA et al: *Contraceptive technology,* ed 16, New York, 1994, Irvington.

Once the diagnosis, tentative or conclusive, is made, focus should first be placed on obtaining a cure and preventing complications and reinfection. Many people know that the treatment for syphilis and gonorrhea is penicillin, but they may not be fully informed about this and other aspects of treatment. Because some of the diseases respond to penicillin or other antibiotics, many people believe that all genital infections can be cured easily, and this is not so. Some people believe that antibiotics not only cure an infection but also produce immunity against reinfection. Persons receiving an antibiotic or other medications for STDs must be informed of the action of the drug, its duration of effectiveness, side effects, chances of cure, and the need for follow-up. They need to be advised that treatment failures do occur and that reinfection rates are high. Return visits for tests of cure should be encouraged whenever possible, because adequacy of treatment of all of the STDs is evaluated best by laboratory analysis for the specific organism.

Many persons focus on how the diseases are spread rather than on the consequences of having an infection. For single persons, contracting an STD and securing help mean they must admit to sexual activity, and some of them may feel guilty. Their self-esteem may be threatened by what has happened to them. Persons with an STD have not only a physical but also a social, an emotional, and perhaps an economic problem. They need constructive and comprehensive help. The nurse who is successful in working with persons who have an STD is one who can create an atmosphere of trust in which the person feels free to discuss all aspects of the problem.

Persons who seek help recognize that they have a problem; they want to get better and stay well. Because of this they are highly motivated to do what is necessary, receptive to information and advice, and attentive when advice is given. Nurses can take advantage of the patient's readiness to learn and motivation to improve and maintain health.

Persons treated for sexually transmitted diseases need information about self-care. To understand their therapy and to responsibly engage in self-care, they must be informed about the sexual nature of the infection, how it is transmitted, and the possibility of reinfection and infection of their sexual partner or partners. The person needs to know that it is important for sexual partners to be checked for signs of infection, to be advised of what the signs are, and to have a culture for asymptomatic infection. The person should be advised to abstain from intercourse until cured. It also should be stressed that condoms should be used to prevent infection or reinfection if persons persist in engaging in intercourse even when advised not to.

Teaching about hygiene and personal health practices is beneficial in reducing the chances of secondary infection, recurrence, and infections of various types in the future. Frequent bathing and hand washing are indicated. It is known that many of the organisms causing STDs are destroyed by soap and water. For women, douching is contraindicated unless it is prescribed for the purpose of applying heat or applying medication. All women should be informed that, for personal cleanliness, frequent douching at any time is not advisable, because this may disturb the vaginal and cervical environments and predispose the woman to infection. If douching is prescribed by the physician, the woman should be instructed in the procedure.

If the lesions are present on body surfaces, the person should be instructed in their care. Unless contraindicated, a hot bath is taken two or three times per day, and lesions are kept as dry as possible between baths. Both men and women should be advised to wear cotton underwear, and women should be advised to avoid wearing pantyhose, because they tend to trap moisture and prevent circulation of air to the genitalia. Unless lotions, creams, or ointments are specifically prescribed as local medications, the patient should not apply them to any of the lesions associated with an STD.

Genital self-examination (GSE) is important for sexually active persons. Inspecting skin, mouth, genitalia, and perianal areas for lesions and discharges is recommended. Self-inspection helps the person become educated about the signs and symptoms of STDs and how to look for them. In addition, people can learn to casually inspect their partners during the initial period of lovemaking to identify any signs of STDs. Urinating after sexual activity can be helpful in cleansing the urethra of organisms.

Opportunities for promoting healthy attitudes about sexual activity and STDs frequently arise. These topics are approached tactfully and with consideration of the person's feelings. Adolescents especially require an approach that indicates understanding balanced with the ability to help them set limits. They need to understand that they are responsible for their own bodies and they do not have to give in to sexual pressures. It is well documented, however, that the strongest influence on teenagers comes from their peer group. For this reason, discussion with groups of teenagers about their sexual responsibilities may be helpful. In the climate of the 1990s there should be no doubt that abstinence is the only absolute way to prevent STD. If a teen elects to be sexually active he or she needs to understand that the consequences of unprotected sex may include unwanted pregnancy and/or STD. Monogamous relationships and the proper use of condoms should be stressed for those who are sexually active.

As mentioned earlier, a problem among sexually active teenagers and young adults is serial monogamy. When questioned about their sexual activities, most of them consider themselves to be monogamous, but the monogamy lasts for only a few weeks or months. Thus they are not having sex with more than one person in a time span, but are going from one short-term relationship to another without concern about their partners' sexual histories.

### Health Promotion/Prevention

Prevention and control measures for STDs include three levels of prevention. *Primary prevention* is directed at preventing the disease. This includes educating uninfected persons so that they can take responsibility for their own health and not expose themselves to an infected person; identification and treatment of exposed persons who are asymptomatic; interviewing persons with infection for identification of contacts, examination, and preventive treatment of contacts; educational programs for the public; and active involvement of professionals in programs of control. The goal of these efforts includes eradication of the reservoir of disease in the population. *Secondary prevention* is directed toward screening, early diagnosis, and treatment. *Tertiary prevention* focuses on the following: (1) prevention of complications, (2) supporting and counseling infected persons to receive treatment, and (3) asking infected persons to notify their sexual partners so that they can be examined and treated if infected.

In the prevention and control of STDs, especially gonorrhea, emphasis was once placed on interviewing for information regarding sexual contacts. The named contacts were sought out for examination and treatment. People knowledgeable about the required reporting to the local health department of some of the diseases were hesitant to name their sexual contacts. Young people often feared that their parents and the parents of the sexual partner(s) would find out about their infection. Minors need to know that they can probably obtain treatment without parental consent. Presently most states permit health care providers to treat minors for STDs without obtaining parental consent, and several states are proposing changes in existing legislation that restricts treatment of minors. People also may perceive reporting of STDs as a threat from an official agency and may hesitate to name their contacts out of a sense of protection if they do not know that no punishment is involved.

Interviewing the patient about his or her contacts is done at the time of the initial visit in the event that the patient does not return for follow-up. It is probably best that this interview take place after the patient is examined, the type of infection is determined, and the treatment is prescribed. If assessment is accompanied by information giving, the person should be better informed about STDs and how they are treated and be more willing and able to give information about sexual contacts.

Interviewing for contacts involves two aspects. The patient is first asked to name sexual contacts. Second, the patient is interviewed for cluster suspects, who are friends or acquaintances who may have been exposed to the same contacts or who have symptoms of an STD.

Because one focus of STD control is increasing self-referrals, the patient is asked to inform her or his sexual partner(s) (partner notification) to come in for examination and treatment. Confidentiality is stressed. There is reason to believe that individuals do not name all their contacts at the time of the first interview and that a reinterview will usually result in additional names of contacts. Because of the understandable reluctance of many people to name their sexual partner(s), the patient may be given the responsibility of informing the contacts and advising them of their need for treatment. (The contacts are not named, but instead cards that permit both examination and treatment without identification are given to the contacts by the patient.) Local health departments cooperate in locating, examining, and treating these contacts as necessary.

Whenever possible, the sexual partners of the infected person are located and advised to have an examination and tests as soon as possible. If the sexual partner or partners do not have symptoms of infection at the time of the first examination, treatment is instituted to abort infection. Giving preventive treatment to named contacts who have no clinical evidence of infection has gained acceptance in the United States, and there are indications that this same approach is being used more often in management of patients with "minor" STDs.

### *Healthy People 2000*

*Healthy People 2000* established several goals related to the reduction of STDs to be achieved by the year 2000. The progress in meeting these goals was reviewed in 1994 and 1995 and new goals established where indicated. Table 50-3 summarizes the findings related to gonorrhea, chlamydia, syphilis, genital herpes, and genital warts.[27,28]

Risk reduction objectives to help achieve the year 2000 goals include:

1. A reduction of the number of adolescents who have engaged in sexual intercourse by age 15 from a baseline of 27% to 33% to no more than 15%
2. A reduction of the number of adolescents who have engaged in sexual intercourse by age 17 from a baseline of 50% to 66% to no more than 40%
3. Increasing the number of unmarried sexually active persons who report using a condom at last sexual intercourse to 50% from a baseline of 19%

The special population targets for objective 3 appear in Table 50-4.

To achieve these important goals, changes need to occur in agencies that deliver primary health care, such as family planning clinics, maternal and child health clinics, drug treatment centers, and primary care clinics that screen, diagnose, treat, counsel, and provide (or refer for) partner notification services for HIV infection and bacterial STDs (gonorrhea, syphilis, and chlamydia). The Centers for Disease Control and Prevention (CDC) wants the goals to occur in at least 50% of the health care agencies as compared with 40% of family planning clinics for 1989.

Another need to achieve the objectives relates to education of the young. The CDC recommends that instruction in STD prevention be included in the curricula of all middle and secondary schools, preferably as part of quality school health education.

In addition, the CDC wants to increase to at least 90% the proportion of primary health care providers treating patients with STDs who correctly manage cases, as measured by their use of appropriate types and amounts of therapy. The baseline was 70% in 1988. The success of this objective will be monitored by the number of women treated for gonorrhea and PID. For example, one study found that only 10% of primary care providers assessed the sexual behavior of their patients. Also, a large proportion of providers did not prescribe combination antibiotics to treat polymicrobial PID.

It is essential to identify persons who may be infected and to get them under treatment so that they can be adequately treated and the transmission of the STD is stopped within the community. Proper treatment also helps prevent complications among those already infected.[27]

Even though the provider may be involved in the notification process, it is crucial that infected persons be supported and coached so that they can do partner notification themselves. This is especially so because provider referral is labor intensive, and current resources (budget constraints) may not allow health departments to notify all persons named by infected persons. Partner notification should help the infected person internalize the need to assume more responsibility for his or her health and for the well-being of sexual partners.[27]

After a review in 1995 of the progress made in achieving the goals set for the year 2000, two additional goals were added:

1. Increase to at least 40% the proportion of sexually active adolescents age 17 years and younger who have not had sexual intercourse for the previous 3 months
2. Increase to at least 90% the percentage of students who receive HIV and other STD information, education, or counseling on their college or university campus

**table 50-3** *Progress Made in Attaining Goals Set for Reduction of STDs by Healthy People 2000*

| Disease | Year 2000 Goal | 1995 Progress in Meeting Goal | Revised Year 2000 Goal |
|---|---|---|---|
| Gonorrhea | No more than 225 cases per 100,000 people | 149.5 cases per 100,000, 24 states below year 2000 goal | 100 cases per 100,000 persons |
| *Chlamydia trachomatis* | No more than 100,000 persons measured by decrease in nongonococcal urethritis | 290.29 cases per 100,000 persons, increased from 215 cases per 100,000 persons in 1988 | None |
| Syphilis (primary and secondary) | No more than 10 cases per 100,000 persons | 6.3 cases per 100,000 persons, 33 states below year 2000 goal | 4 cases per 100,000 persons |
| Genital herpes | No more than 138,000 cases per 100,000 persons | Number of cases increased 40% | 138,500 cases per 100,000 persons |
| Condylomata acuminata | No more than 246,500 cases per 100,000 persons | Number of cases decreased 283% | None |

**table 50-4** *Special Population Targets for Condom Use*

| Use of Condoms | 1988 Baseline | 2000 Target | 1995 Progress |
|---|---|---|---|
| Sexually active young women aged 15-19 yr (by their partners) | 25% | 60% | 48.6% |
| Sexually active young men aged 15-19 yr | 57% | 75% | 60.5% |
| Intravenous drug abusers | — | 75% | Not available |

## EVALUATION

Evaluation is based on the expected patient outcomes. Questions to be asked include the person's and partner's ability to:

1a. State the factors that contributed to the present infection with STD (multiple sexual partners, not using a condom)
b. State the drug therapy to be followed, including name of drug, dosage, schedule of administration, and side effects
c. Explain why the therapy must be taken without interruption (to prevent resistant strains of organisms from developing)
d. State why he or she should not engage in sexual activity while the STD is infectious
e. State effects of STDs that may develop in the reproductive system of either partner
f. State signs and symptoms (fever, pain, discharge) that indicate the need for immediate health care
g. Verbalize understanding of the necessity of treatment for his or her sexual partner or partners
h. Verbalize that she or he has an STD, and identify ways to prevent further STD infections
i. Explain what is meant by practicing "safer sex," including what type of condom to use, when and how to apply it, and how to remove it
j. Describe resources necessary to achieve health
k. Recognize personal strengths and weaknesses

2. Participate actively in health maintenance activities

## GONORRHEA

### Etiology/Epidemiology

Gonorrhea, often referred to as GC or the clap by lay people, is caused by *Neisseria gonorrhoeae.* Gonorrhea is of great concern, because persons with it often have another STD such as chlamydia or HIV. They also have a high reinfection rate and serious residual effects. The incubation period is 3 to 30 days in men and 3 days to an indefinite period in women.

The incidence of gonorrhea in the United States has declined rapidly since the 1980s (Figures 50-1 through 50-3). In men, the rate decreased from 179.8 per 100,000 in 1994 to 158.6 per 100,000 in 1995. In women the rate dropped from 150.7 per 100,000 in 1994 to 140.3 per 100,000 in 1995. In 1995 gonorrhea rates declined slightly among almost all racial and ethnic groups. The only exception was among Hispanics.[4]

This decline is believed to be due to fear of AIDS and concerted health education efforts.[12] The incidence of gonorrhea declined more than 95% among homosexual men and 50% among heterosexual men and women.[12] However, the rates are still high in urban inner cities where sex is exchanged for drugs and in other areas of the world. The World Health Organization has estimated that 35 million cases of gonorrhea occurred in 1990, second only to *C. trachomatis.*[12] The incidence of gonorrhea is believed to be much higher than shown, because it is known that the cases of many patients treated by private physicians are never reported to public health authorities and therefore are not reflected in the statistics. It is gen-

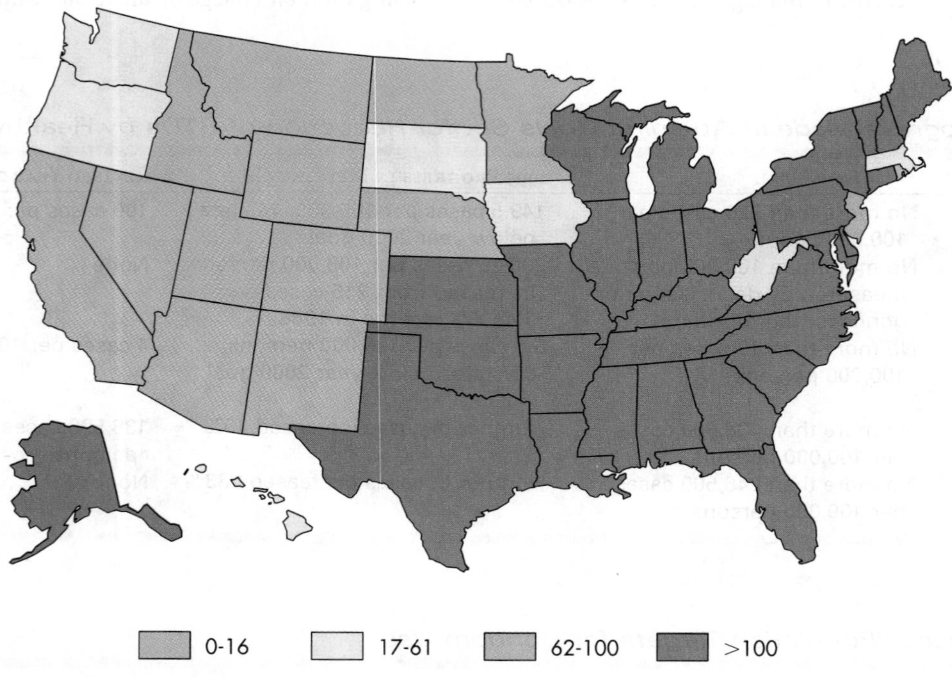

Gonorrhea—Reported cases
0-16
17-61
62-100
>100
NOTE: The Year 2000 Objective is ≤100 per 100,000 population.
The overall U.S. gonorrhea rate in 1995 was 149.5 per 100,000 population; 24 states reported gonorrhea rates that were below the revised *Healthy People 2000* national objective.

**fig. 50-1** Reported cases of gonorrhea per 100,000 population, United States, 1995.

erally accepted that only 25% to 50% of cases treated by private physicians are reported. In addition, women have few if any signs or symptoms of gonorrhea and thus are often not diagnosed. For this reason it is commonly believed that the actual number of cases per year in the United States is probably more than 2 million.

Asymptomatic persons or those with few symptoms are an important reservoir for infection, because they usually remain untreated. As many as 10% to 40% of gonorrheal infections in men are asymptomatic, and in women as many as 80% of infections are asymptomatic. Homosexual men can harbor reservoirs of anorectal and pharyngeal infections.

Young adults 20 to 24 years of age are at highest risk of acquiring gonorrhea, with the next highest rates found among teenagers 15 to 19 years of age. In fact, 1 of every 30 teenagers in this age-group will acquire gonorrhea each year.

It is estimated that the total cost of gonorrhea in the United States is several billion dollars yearly. Women and their offspring suffer the major physical, emotional, and economic burden. Pelvic inflammatory disease occurs in 10% to 20% of

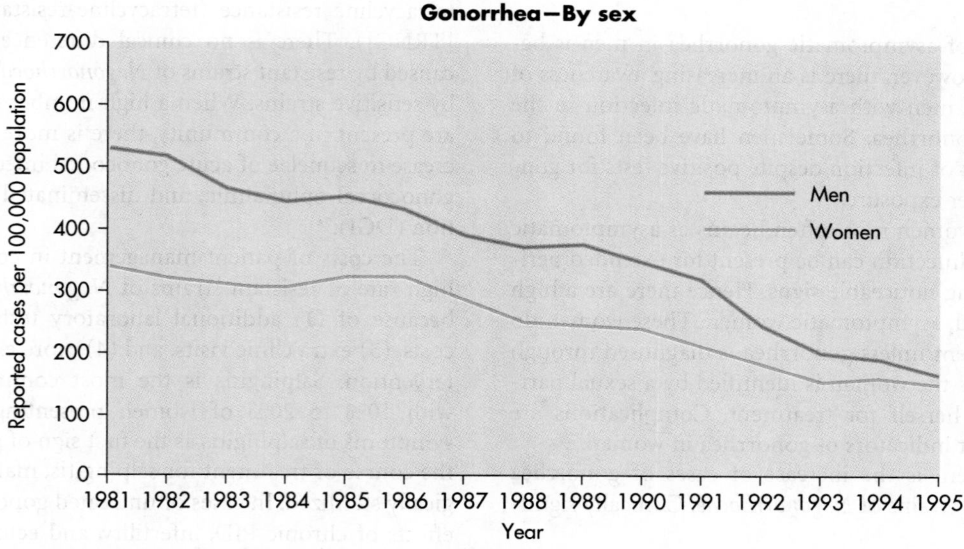


In 1995, the reported rate of gonorrhea in the United States continued to decline. In men, the rate decreased from 179.8 per 100,000 cases in 1994 to 158.6 in 1995; in women, it dropped from 150.7 per 100,000 cases in 1994 to 140.3 in 1995.

**fig. 50-2** Reported cases of gonorrhea per 100,000 population by sex, United States, 1981-1995.

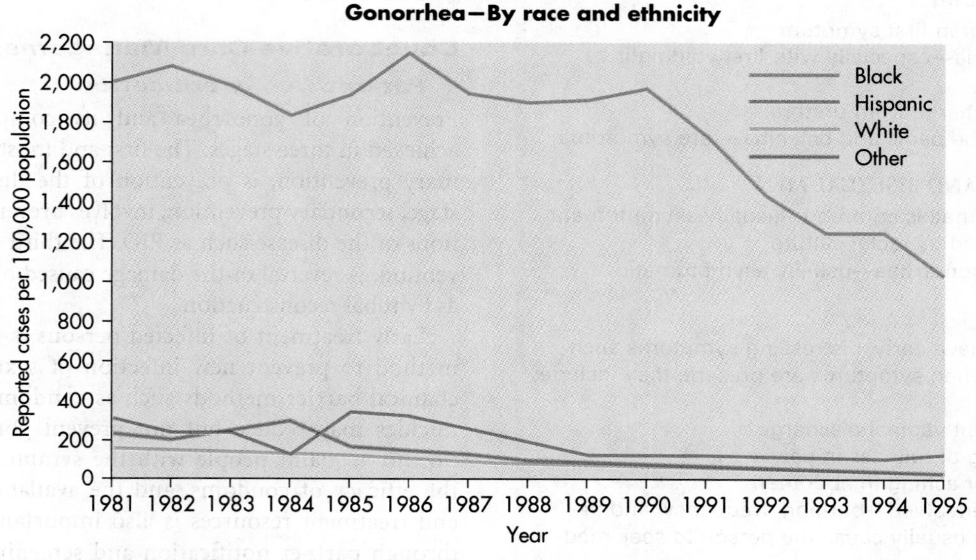


In 1995, gonorrhea rates decreased slightly among all racial and ethnic groups. The only exception occurred among Hispanics.

**fig. 50-3** Reported cases of gonorrhea per 100,000 population by race and ethnicity, United States, 1981-1995.

women with gonorrhea. Even when treated, these women are likely to suffer from recurrent salpingitis, ectopic pregnancy, infertility, and menstrual abnormalities and may face surgical removal of the pelvic organs, as well as fetal loss.

## Pathophysiology

The most common signs and symptoms are listed in Box 50-2. In men the gonococcus is introduced into the anterior urethra during sexual activity. Because most men are diagnosed and treated early, complications and residual effects of gonorrhea are uncommon among men. Sterility from orchitis or epididymitis can occur as a residual effect, but this is rare.

The incidence of asymptomatic gonorrhea in men is believed to be low; however, there is an increasing awareness of the importance of men with asymptomatic infection in the transmission of gonorrhea. Some men have been found to have no symptoms of infection despite positive tests for gonorrhea 2 weeks after exposure.

Gonorrhea in women most often begins as asymptomatic cervicitis, and the infection can be present for extended periods without causing noticeable signs. Hence there are a high number of infected, asymptomatic women. These women do not receive treatment unless gonorrhea is diagnosed through screening or unless the woman is identified by a sexual partner and presents herself for treatment. Complications are commonly the first indicators of gonorrhea in women.

A major problem is the increase of cases of gonorrhea caused by resistant strains of *N. gonorrhoeae.* Clinically significant resistance to the three widely used classes of drugs—the penicillins, the tetracyclines, and the aminoglycosides—has been reported. Plasma-mediated resistance to penicillin (penicillinase-producing *N. gonorrhoeae*) first emerged in 1976.

Resistant strains of the gonococcus can be plasma mediated, chromosomally mediated, or both, and many varieties have been identified. The three most important in terms of public health are (1) plasma-mediated resistance to penicillin (plasma-resistant *N. gonorrhoeae* [PRNG]); (2) chromosomally mediated resistance to penicillin, tetracycline, spectinamycin, or others (chromosomally mediated resistant *N. gonorrhoeae* [CMRNG]); and (3) plasma-mediated, high-level tetracycline resistance (tetracycline-resistant *N. gonorrhoeae* [TRNG]). There is no clinical difference in the infections caused by resistant strains of *N. gonorrhoeae* and those caused by sensitive strains. When a high number of resistant strains are present in a community, there is more likely to be an increase in sequelae of acute gonococcal infections such as PID, gonococcal ophthalmia, and disseminated gonococcal infection (DGI).[5a]

The costs of patient management in communities with a high rate of resistant strains of *N. gonorrhoeae* are increased because of (1) additional laboratory tests, (2) added drug costs, (3) extra clinic visits, and (4) more extensive disease intervention. Salpingitis is the most common complication, with 10% to 20% of women presenting themselves with symptoms of salpingitis as the first sign of gonorrhea. During the course of treatment for salpingitis, many women are surgically sterilized. In cases of untreated gonorrhea, the residual effects of chronic PID, infertility, and ectopic pregnancy are well known.

Other complications of untreated gonorrhea in both men and women include dermatitis, carditis, meningitis, and arthritis. The incidence of these complications is higher among women because of the prolonged period of infection without symptoms.

### box 50-2 Signs and Symptoms of Gonorrhea

**HETEROSEXUAL MEN**

1. Urethritis—often first symptom
2. Severe dysuria—especially with first voiding in morning
3. Purulent discharge from urethra
4. Swelling of the penis and balanitis—rare symptoms

**HOMOSEXUAL AND BISEXUAL MEN**

1. Rectal gonorrhea is common—usually asymptomatic and discovered by rectal culture
2. Pharyngeal gonorrhea—usually asymptomatic

**WOMEN**

Women rarely have early, distressing symptoms such as men have. When symptoms are present, they include the following:

1. Slight purulent vaginal discharge
2. Vague feeling of fullness in pelvis
3. Discomfort or aching in abdomen
4. If bladder is involved—burning, frequency, and urgency, which usually cause the person to seek medical attention

The first three symptoms are so slight that they may be ignored by the person.

## Collaborative Care Management

### Patient/family education

Prevention of gonorrhea and its complications can be achieved in three stages. The first and most crucial stage, primary prevention, is prevention of the disease. The second stage, secondary prevention, involves prevention of complications of the disease such as PID. The third stage, tertiary prevention, is reversal of the damage caused by the disease, such as by tubal reconstruction.

Early treatment of infected persons is the most effective method to prevent new infection of sexual partners. Mechanical barrier methods such as condoms used with spermicides may reduce but not prevent gonorrhea.[12] Education to acquaint people with the symptoms of gonorrhea, the efficacy of condoms, and the availability of diagnostic and treatment resources is also important. Early detection through partner notification and screening can reduce the serious complications of gonorrhea. There is no effective vaccine for gonorrhea, although clinical trials have been attempted.[12]

Some physicians believe that all persons with gonorrhea should be treated for chlamydia even though there are no signs or symptoms of it. No therapy for both diseases is effective when given in a single dose. It is generally accepted that all patients with gonorrhea should be offered testing and counseling for HIV.

## SYPHILIS

### Etiology/Epidemiology

Syphilis is caused by a spirochete, *Treponema pallidum,* that gains entry into the body through either the mucous membrane or skin during intercourse. The organism is readily destroyed by physical and chemical agents, including heat, drying, and mild disinfectants such as soap and water.

The incubation period for syphilis is usually 3 weeks. However, symptoms can appear as early as 9 days or as long as 3 months after exposure, which is the case for rectal infections in homosexual men.

The incidence rate for syphilis reached an all-time high during World War II, with 575,593 cases being reported in 1943. Incidence rates dropped sharply in the 1950s and began to rise again in the 1960s. This rise continued to increase annually, peaking in 1977, then leveling off in 1986, and dramatically increasing in the late 1980s.

In 1990 there was a dramatic increase in the number of cases of infectious syphilis (primary and secondary), with 50,233 cases being reported.[11] This was the single largest yearly total since 1948 (Figures 50-4 and 50-5). Since 1990 the number of cases has declined yearly. In men, the rate decreased from 8.4 per 100,000 in 1994 to 6.8 per 100,000 in 1995. In women, the rate decreased from 7.5 per 100,000 in 1994 to 5.8 per 100,000 in 1995. However, the rate for African Americans (46.2 cases per 100,000 population) was 58 times greater than for non-Hispanic whites.[4]

The trends for early congenital syphilis have paralelled the trends for primary and secondary syphilis among women. Factors thought to contribute to the level of early congenital syphilis are (1) an increase in the incidence of early infectious syphilis among pregnant women, (2) lack of available prenatal care, and (3) failure of the prenatal system to provide timely serological testing and prompt follow-up.

In addition, it is believed that the greatest percentage of cases of syphilis go unreported, and thus the incidence is much greater than the figures indicate.

### Pathophysiology

The signs and symptoms of the four stages of syphilis are listed in Table 50-5. If syphilis is adequately diagnosed and

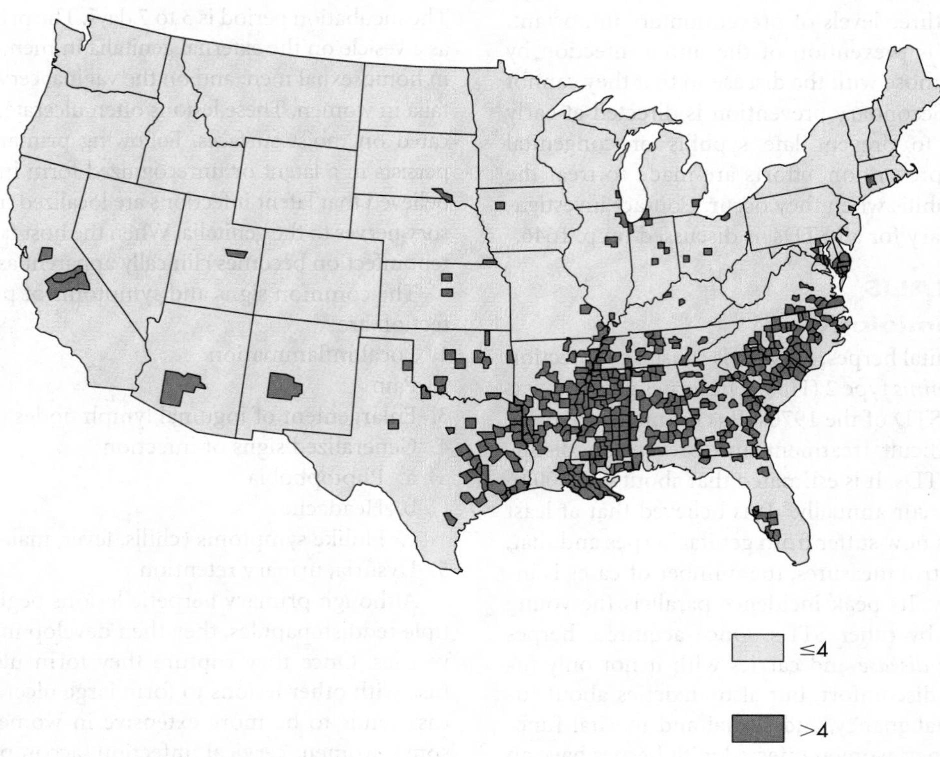


**fig. 50-4** Counties with primary and secondary syphilis rates above or at the national health objective for 2000 of four cases per 100,000 population, United States, 1997.

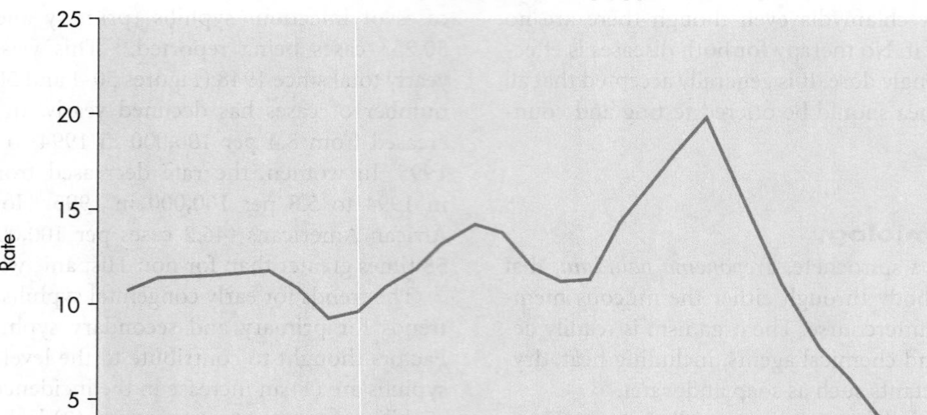


**fig. 50-5** Primary and secondary syphilis rates per 100,000 population by year, United States, 1970-1997.

treated during the primary stage, the other stages can be prevented.

### Collaborative Care Management

#### *Patient/family education*

As with gonorrhea, three levels of prevention are important. Primary prevention is prevention of the initial infection by finding and treating those with the disease so that they cannot spread it to others. Secondary prevention is directed at early treatment of cases to prevent late syphilis or congenital syphilis. In tertiary prevention, efforts are made to treat the complications of syphilis when they occur. Contact investigation, which is necessary for all STDs, is discussed on p. 1646.

## HERPES GENITALIS

### Etiology/Epidemiology

Herpes genitalis (genital herpes, HSV-2) is caused by infection with *Herpesvirus hominis* type 2 (HSV-2). Herpes genitalis was the most important STD of the 1970s. Its chronicity, frequent recurrences, and difficult treatment and prevention distinguish it from other STDs. It is estimated that about 400,000 to 600,000 new cases occur annually.[5] It is believed that at least one in six Americans now suffer from genital herpes and that, because of poor control measures, the number of cases is increasing dramatically. Its peak incidence parallels the young age-groups affected by other STDs. Once acquired, herpes genitalis is a *lifelong disease* and carries with it not only intense and recurrent discomfort, but also anxieties about future childbearing, malignancy, and sexual and marital function. In early pregnancy, women infected with herpes have an increased chance of miscarriage. Because genital herpetic lesions endanger the fetus during delivery, cesarean delivery is often necessary. Genital herpes has also been associated with cervical cancer. It is now generally accepted that HSV-2 is spread by sexual contact.

### Pathophysiology

The incubation period is 3 to 7 days. The primary lesion appears as a vesicle on the external genitalia in men; often in the rectum in homosexual men; and on the vagina, cervix, or external genitalia in women. These lesions often ulcerate, especially when located on moist surfaces. Following primary herpes, the virus persists in a latent or unrecognized form in most patients. It is believed that latent infections are localized in the ganglia of sensory nerves to the genitalia. When the host factors favor it, the latent infection becomes clinically apparent as recurrent herpes.

The common signs and symptoms of primary herpetic infection are

1. Local inflammation
2. Pain
3. Enlargement of inguinal lymph nodes
4. Generalized signs of infection
    a. Photophobia
    b. Headache
    c. Flulike symptoms (chills, fever, malaise)
5. Dysuria, urinary retention

Although primary herpetic lesions begin as single or multiple reddish papules, they then develop into clear, fluid-filled vesicles. Once they rupture they form ulcerations that may fuse with other lesions to form large ulcerated areas. The disease tends to be more extensive in women than in men. In some women cervical infection accompanies the external lesions, and in certain cases it may be the only infected site. Cervical involvement may be mild or severe with extensive

**table 50-5** *Stages of Syphilis*

| Primary | Secondary | Latent | Late |
|---|---|---|---|
| **DURATION** | | | |
| 2-8 wk | Appears 2-4 wk after chancre appears; extends over 2-4 yr | 5-20 yr | Terminal if not treated |
| **SIGNS AND SYMPTOMS** | | | |
| Hard sore or pimple on vulva or penis that breaks and forms painless, draining *chancre;* may be a single chancre or groups of more than one; may be present also on lips, tongue, hands, rectum, or nipples; chancre heals, leaving almost invisible scar | Depends on site; low-grade fever, headache, anorexia, weight loss, anemia, sore throat, hoarseness, reddened and sore eyes, jaundice with or without hepatitis, aching of joints, muscles, long bones; sores on body or generalized fine rash; condylomata acuminata (venereal warts) on rectum or genitalia | No clinical signs | Tumorlike mass *(gumma)* on any area of body; damage to heart valves and blood vessels; meningitis; paralysis; lack of coordination; paresis; insomnia; confusion; delusions; impaired judgment; slurred speech |
| **COMMUNICABILITY** | | | |
| Exudates from lesions and chancre are highly contagious | Exudates from lesions highly contagious; blood contains organisms | Contagious for about 2 yr; not contagious to others after that; blood contains organisms; may be transmitted placentally to fetus | Noncontagious; spinal fluid may contain organisms |

ulceration and pus. Genital lesions often worsen during the first 10 to 15 days but usually heal within 3 to 4 weeks. These symptoms usually lead the individual to seek medical attention.

Vaginal discharge is common among women, and discharge from the urethra is usual in men who have primary infections. Urinary tract involvement may occur and is reflected in symptoms of dysuria or urinary retention. The lesions can cause severe pain, requiring hospitalization for parenteral analgesia. Subclinical infections in which patients are unaware of any problem occur in only about 10% of the cases of genital herpes.

Unfortunately, about 75% of all patients have at least one recurrence. Fortunately, recurrent infections are usually milder and of shorter duration than primary infections and usually produce local rather than systemic reaction. The patient experiencing a recurrent infection often has prodromal signs of paresthesia and burning at the site where the lesion will erupt. Factors known to predispose to recurrent infection include fever, emotional upsets, premenstrual states, and overexposure to heat and sunshine. Although the mode of recurrent infection is not clear, it has been theorized that during primary infection the virus ascends sensory nerve sheaths, localizing in corresponding nerve ganglia, and that when the environment becomes favorable, the virus is reactivated. Recurrent herpes usually begins with an abnormal sensation or itching of a localized genital area. Lesions of recurrent infections usually occur at the site of the primary infection. Herpes encephalitis may also occur.

### Collaborative Care Management

#### *Patient/family education*

Persons with herpes should abstain from sexual contact while the lesions are present and for 10 days after the lesions heal. Risk of transmission during asymptomatic periods is unknown. Some experts advise using condoms to prevent transmission of the disease.

Because herpes genitalis is a recurrent disease with no cure, persons infected with the virus require considerable support. Some infected persons withdraw from an active social life rather than face the possibility of making a commitment that will require them to share knowledge of their disease with another person. For this reason, in some communities support groups have been formed for persons who have herpes genitalis.

## CHLAMYDIAL INFECTION

### Etiology/Epidemiology

*Chlamydia trachomatis* is caused by the gram-negative obligate *C. trachomatis.* Chlamydial infection is recognized as the most prevalent of the STDs in the United States (Figure 50-6). Because it is not a reportable disease, the actual number of cases is unknown. It is estimated, however, that each year more than 4 million Americans experience epidemic chlamydial infections. Age, number of sex partners, socioeconomic status, and sexual orientation are predictors of infection with *C. trachomatis.*[6]

1. *Age.* Infection rates are two to three times higher in sexually active women under age 20 years than in those over age

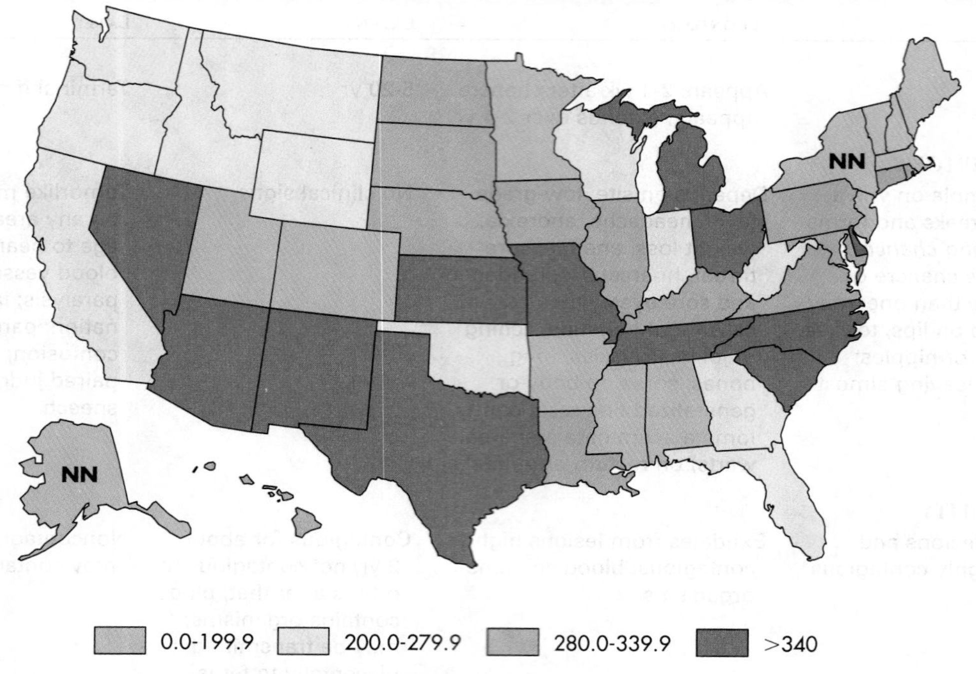
Chlamydia—Reported cases among women
NN
NN
0.0-199.9
200.0-279.9
280.0-339.9
>340
In 1995, the chlamydia rate among women was 290.29 cases per 100,000 population. The rates for men are not presented, as reporting for men is much more limited than it is for women.

**fig. 50-6** Reported cases of chlamydia among women per 100,000 population, United States, 1995.

20 years. The rates for women between 20 and 29 years of age are considerably higher than for women over age 30 years. The rates of urethral infection are higher for teenage males than for adult men.

2. *Number of sex partners.* Persons with several sex partners are at higher risk of infection.
3. *Socioeconomic status.* Some studies have shown that persons of lower socioeconomic status are at increased risk for infection with *C. trachomatis.*
4. *Sexual preference.* The prevalence of urethral chlamydial infection among homosexual men is one third that among heterosexual men. However, 4% to 8% of homosexual men seen in STD clinics have rectal chlamydia infection.

Chlamydial infections are responsible for about 20% to 30% of diagnosed pelvic inflammatory disease (PID) cases, and it is estimated that about 11,000 women each year become involuntarily sterilized and 36,000 suffer ectopic pregnancies as a result of this organism.[26] Chlamydial infections can be transmitted to infants during delivery, causing conjunctivitis and pneumonia in many.

*Chlamydia trachomatis* is the leading cause of pneumonia in infants less than 6 months of age. The rate of infection with pneumonia is 3 to 10 per 1000 live births and may go as high as 50 to 60 per 1000 in areas where *C. trachomatis* is epidemic. The organism has superseded *N. gonorrhoeae* as a cause of neonatal conjunctivitis.[10]

The incidence of chlamydia is highest in young, promiscuous, indigent, unmarried women who live in the inner city and in those who have had a prior history of STD.

### Pathophysiology

*Chlamydia trachomatis* is an intracellular parasite that has specific requirements for adenosine triphosphate (ATP) and amino acids. There are two stages in the life cycle of the organism. In stage 1, the infective stage, the elementary body attaches to the host cell and is ingested by phagocytosis. In stage 2, the elementary body undergoes metamorphosis to become a reticulate or initial body. This is the metabolic phase of the life cycle. The initial body duplicates by binary fission and changes into the elementary body. The host cell, which contains the elementary bodies, undergoes lysis, liberating infectious organisms that are capable of reinfecting new cells.[26]

Serotypes L1, L2, and L3 are responsible for lymphogranuloma venereum, which is common in South America and the Far East.

Serotypes D through K cause chlamydial infections. It is estimated that between 20% and 40% of sexually active women have been exposed to the bacterium and have antibody titers to *C. trachomatis.*[26] Table 50-6 shows how the infection can be transmitted between male and female sexual partners and from women to infants. It also lists the various ways the disease is manifested in men, women, and infants.

**table 50-6** Chlamydia Trachomatis *Infections*

| MALES | FEMALES | INFANTS |
|---|---|---|
| **TRANSMISSION** | | |
| Males ⟷ | Females ⟶ | Infants |
| **INFECTIONS** | | |
| Urethritis | Cervicitis | Conjunctivitis |
| Postgonococcal urethritis | Urethritis | Pneumonia |
| Proctitis | Proctitis | Asymptomatic pharyngeal carriage |
| Conjunctivitis | Conjunctivitis | Asymptomatic gastrointestinal carriage |
| Pharyngitis | Pharyngitis | |
| Subclinical lymphogranuloma venereum | Subclinical lymphogranuloma venereum | |
| **COMPLICATIONS** | | |
| Epididymitis | Salpingitis | |
| Prostatitis | Endometritis | |
| Reiter's syndrome | Perihepatitis | |
| Sterility | Ectopic pregnancy | |
| Rectal strictures* | Infertility | |
| | Vulvar/rectal carcinoma* | |
| | Rectal strictures* | |

From Centers for Disease Control and Prevention: *Chlamydia trachomatis* infections, policy guidelines for prevention and control, *MMWR* 35(suppl):54, 1985.
*Associated with lymphogranuloma venereum.

## Collaborative Care Management

### *Patient/family education*

It is important that the patient encourage sexual partner(s) to seek care as soon as possible to avoid reinfection of the patient and complications in the partner. Patients who are sexually active should be advised to wear condoms or use spermicides to reduce reinfection. Social and emotional support of these patients is as important as it is with any person with an STD (see p. 1645).

# LYMPHOGRANULOMA VENEREUM

## Etiology/Epidemiology

Lymphogranuloma venereum is a systemic STD caused by serotypes L1, L2, and L3 of *C. trachomatis*. Other species of *Chlamydia* are the causative organisms of trachoma and psittacosis. The disease is contracted by vaginal, anal, or oral intercourse; primary inoculation with the organism may occur at any site involved in close contact. The incubation period is 3 to 30 days. Lymphadenitis of regional lymph nodes draining the site of primary infection occurs, and the disease spreads by way of the lymphatic system.

Lymphogranuloma venereum is most prevalent in the tropics. It is endemic in parts of Africa, Southeast Asia, India, the Caribbean, and South America.[19] In the United States it is found most often in the southern states, but epidemiological studies are necessary to determine its true incidence. Recent reports indicate that there are about 500 to 1000 cases annually in the United States. The symptoms of lymphogranuloma venereum resemble those of other STDs, and its reported incidence may not be accurate for this reason.

## Pathophysiology

The three clinical phases of infection in lymphogranuloma venereum are (1) inoculation and appearance of the primary lesions, (2) lymphatic spread and generalized symptoms, and (3) late complications. In individual cases any one of the phases may be absent or go unnoticed.

The *primary lesion*, which is *transient, appears as a papule, small erosion, or vesicle*. The most common sites of the primary lesion are the prepuce and glans in men and the vagina and cervix in women. Because it is painless, the primary lesion may go unnoticed, especially in women. Localized edema may be present. If the rectum is infected, a bloody discharge is followed by a mucopurulent discharge, diarrhea, and cramping.

Involvement of the lymphatics occurs 1 to 4 weeks after the appearance of the primary lesion. If the primary lesion is on the penis, anal margin, clitoris, or upper vulva, the superficial inguinal lymph nodes are involved. Infection of the vagina or cervix as the primary site produces involvement of the deep iliac and anorectal lymph nodes. The large lymph nodes or *buboes* that appear are firm and lobular. The skin over the superficial nodes is bluish red and adheres to the nodes.

The first indication of infection in most patients is a feeling of stiffness and aching in the groin followed by swelling in the inguinal area. Symptoms of nongonococcal urethritis may be present. Constitutional symptoms of infection may or may not appear at this time. The involved lymph nodes may suppurate, causing extensive scarring. Obstruction of the lymphatics may result, leading to chronic edema and ulceration. Lymphatic spread of the infection is accompanied by generalized symptoms. Mild to severe fever, malaise, nausea, and vomiting may occur. Abdominal pain, symptoms of cystitis, and urinary retention are common when pelvic lymph nodes are involved. Acute proctocolitis is common in homosexual men.

Among the most severe complications of lymphogranuloma venereum are development of perianal abscesses, rectovaginal or rectovesical fistulas, and rectal strictures. In the last clinical phase, generalized infection is indicated by blood values showing anemia, leukocytosis, and an elevated sedimentation rate.

## Collaborative Care Management

### *Patient/family education*

These patients may require much counseling and teaching as they deal with their disease. Because the fluctuant lymph nodes may be disturbing to the patient's self-image, social and emotional support is extremely important. See p. 1645 for more discussion of these topics.

## CHANCROID

### Etiology/Epidemiology

Chancroid is an STD caused by a gram-negative bacillus, *Haemophilus ducreyi.* Before 1980 fewer than 1000 cases were reported yearly in the United States. Since then the number of reported cases has increased to 4000 to 5000 cases yearly.[25] Since the early 1980s epidemics associated with prostitutes have occurred in Boston, New York City, Dallas, Florida, and Orange County, California.

Although it is found worldwide, chancroid is most prevalent in tropical and semitropical areas in the Orient, the West Indies, and North Africa. In areas where it is endemic, chancroid is transmitted primarily by prostitutes who infect a large group of men. Many of these women have minimal symptoms and do not seek treatment. Men, however, usually develop severe symptoms and seek treatment because of pain and the appearance of an ulcer that causes them to cease sexual activity.[25]

The disease occurs more often in men and more often among nonwhites. It is possible that returning military personnel may have introduced the disease into areas where it did not previously exist. The incubation period varies from 1 to 14 days and averages 4 to 5 days.

Chancroid has been established as a cofactor for HIV transmission, and a high rate of HIV infection among patients with chancroid has been reported in the United States and other countries. As many as 10% of patients with chancroid may be coinfected with *T. pallidum* or HSV.[7]

### Pathophysiology

The initial lesions are acutely tender genital ulcers, lymphadenopathy, and tender buboes. The buboes, which are fluctuant inguinal node masses, may suppurate and lead to abscesses. Exudate from the ulcers or aspirate from the buboes is stained, and a "school-of-fish" pattern may be noted on microscopic examination by someone experienced in interpretation.[25]

In women the lesions of chancroid are most often found on the labia, anus, clitoris, vagina, and cervix. A few women do not have any lesions but may have signs of mild vaginitis. In men the lesions appear on the prepuce, glans, or shaft of the penis.

The ulcers found in chancroid are typically ragged and irregular. They are highly infectious, and autoimmunity may occur, resulting in multiple lesions. The ulcers appear excavated; have a granulating, purulent surface; and are painful. Often, edema of the surrounding tissues is present. Involvement of the inguinal lymph nodes occurs in about 50% of all cases of chancroid within 2 weeks after appearance of the primary lesion. The buboes are most often unilateral, painful, and spheric in shape. The skin over the buboes is inflamed. The buboes tend to become softer as abscesses form. These abscesses in turn may suppurate and rupture, further spreading the infection. Generalized symptoms of infection usually appear when inguinal abscesses form.

### Collaborative Care Management

#### Patient/family education

Follow-up is essential, because treatment failure can occur. The individual is taught to report any signs or symptoms that persist or worsen during treatment and to abstain from sexual activity until all lesions are healed. Proper use of a condom should also be stressed (see Box 50-1).

## GRANULOMA INGUINALE (DONOVANOSIS)

### Etiology/Epidemiology

Granuloma inguinale, or granuloma venereum, is believed to be most often transmitted by sexual contact, although nonsexual transmission has been reported. The infection is caused by a gram-negative bacillus, *Calymmatobacterium (Donovania) granulomatis,* widely referred to as *Donovan bacillus.* The organism is related to *Klebsiella.*

Donovanosis is common in tropical and subtropical areas and rarely occurs in the United States. It is most common in South Africa, Southeast India, New Guinea, and the Caribbean. The disease is mildly contagious and probably requires repeated exposures for spread of infection. Predisposing factors are poorly understood. The disease is more common in men than women and is especially common among homosexual men. The incubation period varies from several days to several months.[18]

### Pathophysiology

Lesions appear on the genitalia and in the perianal area. The most common sites of lesions are the prepuce and glans in men and the vagina and labia in women. The infection first appears with development of subcutaneous nodules. These elevated areas eventually ulcerate, producing sharply defined, painless lesions. The ulcers enlarge slowly and bleed on contact. With ulceration the infection tends to spread along the pubic region. Involvement of the lymph nodes is uncommon but can occur and produce occlusion of the lymphatics, resulting in elephantiasis.

### Collaborative Care Management

#### Patient/family education

Clinician follow-up of anyone diagnosed with granuloma inguinale is extremely important, due to the possibility of treatment failure. All persons should be advised to abstain from sexual activity until all sexual partners complete a course of treatment.

## CONDYLOMATA ACUMINATA (GENITAL WARTS)

### Etiology/Epidemiology

Genital warts caused by the human papillomavirus (HPV) are important because of their possible role in the development of cervical cancer.[8a,22,29] They are sexually transmitted and are the most commonly recognized clinical signs of genital HPV infections. Genital warts caused by HPV are the most commonly diagnosed viral disease in both the United States and the United Kingdom.

Epidemiological and molecular biological evidence support the assumption that genital infections by HPV are closely linked to invasive cervical cancer and cervical cellular changes (dysplasia).[21]

Between 500,000 and 1 million cases of genital warts occur per year in the United States. They are the leading cause of office visits.

### Pathophysiology

Genital warts occur in or around the vulva, vagina, cervix, perineum, anal canal, urethra, and glans penis. They enlarge during pregnancy and may cause hemorrhage or obstruction during delivery. The disease is most common in adolescent girls and young women. The HPV can remain dormant for decades before recurrences appear.

### Collaborative Care Management

#### Patient/family education

Because a diagnosis of HPV has been linked to an increased risk for cervical cancer, the patient is advised to have an annual Pap smear. More frequent Pap smears are sometimes recommended. Malignant changes may not be evident for 5 to 40 years.[22]

Prevention of HPV should be stressed. It includes (1) avoiding sexual relationships with persons in known high-risk groups, (2) using latex condoms if having sexual intercourse, and (3) avoiding anal intercourse.

The CDC does not recommend a cesarean birth to prevent transmission of HPV to newborns. Cesarean delivery may be indicated for warts obstructing the pelvic outlet or if a vaginal birth would cause excessive bleeding of the warts.

## TRICHOMONIASIS

### Etiology/Epidemiology

A protozoan, *Trichomonas vaginalis,* is the causative organism of trichomoniasis. Evidence suggests that the incubation period ranges between 4 and 28 days.[13] There are an estimated 3 million cases of trichomoniasis annually in the United States, and *T. vaginalis* organisms are found in 3% to 15% of women under the care of private physicians, 13% to 23% of women attending gynecological clinics, and 50% of women who have gonorrhea. It is most often sexually transmitted but can be transmitted by fomites such as towels, toilet seats, and so on. The parasite commonly exists in vaginal and cervical secretions and in seminal fluid. It is estimated that one of five females will have a trichomonal infection during her lifetime.

### Pathophysiology

Trichomoniasis is commonly viewed as an innocuous infection, yet there are serious implications for health. During the postpartum period in women who have trichomoniasis, the rate of persistent fever, prolonged vaginal discharge, and endometritis is twice as high as in women who do not harbor the organism. About 90% of patients with trichomoniasis have cervical erosions and leukorrhea, and it has been suggested that chronic irritation may predispose to cervical cancer. Interpretation of cervical cytology, as in the Pap test, is unreliable in the presence of trichomoniasis, because the infection causes inflammation of cervical cells. Unless the Pap test is repeated after the infection has cleared, cancer of the cervix may be missed. Trichomoniasis results in urethritis and causes prostatitis in men 40% of the time. Reversible sterility can occur as a result of inhibition of sperm motility by toxins produced by the organism.

### Collaborative Care Management

#### Patient/family education

The CDC recommends that both partners be treated simultaneously with metronidazole to prevent reinfection by the untreated partner at a later date. Vaginal inserts of metronidazole in the woman alone are less effective. The drug is known to cross the placental barrier. For this reason it is not given to pregnant women until after the first trimester.

## BACTERIAL VAGINOSIS

### Etiology/Epidemiology

Bacterial vaginosis is the most common vaginal infection among women of childbearing age.[2] Recent studies have linked it with preterm labor, infections of amniotic fluid, postpartum uterine infections, and PID. It is characterized by an overgrowth of normal flora resulting from the introduction of other flora and altered vaginal pH related to sexual activity or poor hygienic practices.

### Pathophysiology

Bacterial vaginosis infection is characterized by a small amount of homogeneous gray or grayish white discharge. The discharge usually has a disagreeable odor, and because it is less irritating than discharges caused by other organisms, pruritus is mild or absent. On inspection the vaginal walls are slightly reddened, and the discharge appears to adhere to the mucosal lining.

### Collaborative Care Management

#### Patient/family education

Self-care measures should be emphasized. These include use of condoms for 4 to 6 weeks after diagnosis, limiting hygienic douching to vinegar and water, and wiping from front to back after voiding.

## HEPATITIS B VIRUS

### Etiology/Epidemiology

Hepatitis B virus (HBV) is a DNA virus that causes acute and chronic hepatitis, cirrhosis, and hepatocellular carcinoma. There are more than 300 million persons infected worldwide. The risk of developing HBV infection is greatest in infants at birth and declines with age.[13] The chronic carrier rate in the United States is 0.1% to 0.5% of the population. The rate is considerably higher in other parts of the world. For example, the carrier rate in Asia may exceed 10%, and in isolated communities, such as Australian aborigine communities, the rate may be as high as 85%.[13]

Transmission of HBV is primarily through blood or intimate contact (usually sexual). Transmission from mother to neonates occurs in 70% to 90% of mothers positive for hepatitis B e antigen (HBeAg). HBeAg-negative mothers have a 10% to 40% risk of infecting their neonates. Hepatitis B virus is transmitted sexually, and risk factors include multiple sexual partners, a history of STD, and homosexuality, especially with receptive anal intercourse. It is also transmitted parenterally by drug abusers who share needles and by needle sticks by health care workers. It is not transmitted by blood transfusion because for more than 20 years all donors have been screened for hepatitis B surface antigen (HBsAg). Other risk factors include patients on hemodialysis and those who are institutionalized.[13] Between 30% and 40% of patients with HBV infection in the United States deny any of the risk factors, and the source of their infection may never be known.

### Pathophysiology

The hepatitis caused by HBV results in the same symptoms seen in other types of hepatitis. The liver is inflamed, and the patient may have jaundice, anorexia, slight fever, and gastrointestinal upset. For more information see Chapter 37.

### Collaborative Care Management

#### *Patient/family education*

The CDC recommends vaccination for persons identified as being at high risk, including residents of correctional or long-term care facilities, persons seeking treatment for an STD, prostitutes, homosexuals, and promiscuous heterosexuals. The CDC also recommends that all children regardless of their exposure risk be vaccinated against HBV. The vaccine is given at birth, 1 month, and 6 months. If serum HBsAg is not detected after 5 to 7 years, a booster dose of the vaccine should be considered. Vaccination is also recommended for all health care workers because of the possibility of needle sticks.

The CDC also recommends that postexposure prophylactic treatment with hepatitis B immune globulin (HBIG) should be considered in the following situations: sexual contact with a person who has active hepatitis B or who contracts hepatitis B and sexual contact with a hepatitis B carrier (blood test positive for HBsAg). The prophylactic treatment should be given within 14 days of sexual contact.

Because pregnant women can transmit HBV to their infants at delivery, HBIG and hepatitis B vaccine are given to the infant after birth. All pregnant women should be screened during their first obstetric visit for the presence of HBsAg. If they are HBsAg positive, their newborns should be given HBIG as soon as possible after birth and subsequently immunized with hepatitis B vaccine. The HBIG is also given to health care workers who suffer a needle stick. For more information about hepatitis see Chapter 37.

## OTHER SEXUALLY TRANSMITTED DISEASES

In addition to those diseases already discussed, pediculosis pubis, molluscum contagiosum, and scabies are considered to be STDs.

Pediculosis pubis, also known as "crabs," is caused by pubic lice. Although lice can be transmitted by bedding or clothing, they are often transmitted during sexual contact. They produce erythematous, itchy papules. The lice adhere to hair around the pubic area, anus, abdomen, and thighs. Diagnosis is made by observation of lice or microscopic observation of nits at the base of pubic hairs. Recommended treatment is 1% Kwell lotion or shampoo. One treatment per episode is necessary, but itching may persist.

Molluscum contagiosum is a viral infection, manifested by papular lesions on the abdomen, thighs, and genitals. Although molluscum contagiosum may be transmitted via fomites, its transmission is primarily sexual in adults. Diagnosis is often made on sight of the characteristic lesion. A punch biopsy may be used for diagnostic evaluation if visual diagnosis is uncertain. There is no effective medical treatment. If only a few lesions are present the core of the lesions may by surgically excised. Multiple lesions may be treated with cryotherapy. Most often patients are advised to allow the lesions to resolve spontaneously.[2]

Scabies, caused by mites known as *Sarcoptes scabiei*, is transmitted by close body contact, bedding, and clothing. Diagnosis is made from linear burrows, often characterized by a reddened papule containing the mite. Common sites are finger webs, wrists, elbows, ankles, and the penis. Nocturnal itching is common. A one-time use of 1% Kwell shampoo is recommended. Family, household, and sexual contacts should also be treated.

## *critical thinking* QUESTIONS

1. You have been requested to give a presentation on STDs to several health education classes at a local high school. What information should you be prepared to discuss? If you are limited to 45 minutes, what information do you think is most important to cover and why?
2. Explain why the incidence of STDs is growing among American teens. How might the care of a teenager who has an STD differ from that of an adult with the same disease?
3. Discuss the social and economic factors that affect the spread of STDs.
4. What social interventions may be needed to facilitate a decrease in the incidence and prevalence of STDs?

## *chapter* SUMMARY

### ETIOLOGY/EPIDEMIOLOGY

- The term *sexually transmitted diseases* refers to diseases that are usually transmitted by heterosexual or homosexual contact.
- The five classic STDs are gonorrhea, syphilis, chancroid, lymphogranuloma venereum, and granuloma inguinale.
- In the 1980s *C. trachomatis,* genital herpes, human papillomavirus, genital mycoplasmas, cytomegalovirus, hepatitis B virus, enteric infections, and ectoparasitic disease were added to the list of STDs.

- Three changes have affected the incidence of STDs in the United States since World War II: (1) antibiotics and antibiotic resistance, (2) social permissiveness, and (3) sexual behavior patterns.
- The highest incidence of STDs is in young adults and adolescents. This is believed to be because of permissiveness, promiscuity, and the pill.

### SEXUAL TRANSMISSION

- Partner notification (formerly called contact investigation) is important in identifying persons who may have been exposed to an STD and in trying to identify the source of the infection.
- Latex condoms are recommended to prevent the transmission of STDs. They are recommended because they provide greater protection against viral STDs than natural membrane condoms.

### GONORRHEA

- A major concern in the treatment of gonorrhea is the increased resistance of the organism to penicillin and other antibiotics.
- Gonorrhea in women is often asymptomatic and is diagnosed only when complications such as salpingitis occur.

### SYPHILIS

- In 1990 the reported cases of primary and secondary syphilis were the highest they had been since 1948. The number of cases has declined yearly since 1990. The rates are highest for African Americans.
- The drug of choice in the treatment of syphilis is penicillin G benzathine (2.4 million units IM).

### HERPES GENITALIS

- Herpes genitalis is a lifelong disease with no cure. It can be transmitted to the fetus during delivery and thus cesarean delivery is often recommended.
- Treatment for herpes genitalis is symptomatic, and acyclovir is prescribed, 20 mg orally 5 times per day for 5 days. It does not prevent recurrences.

### CHLAMYDIAL INFECTION

- *Chlamydia trachomatis* infections are recognized as the most prevalent STD in the United States.
- *Chlamydia trachomatis* can be spread between sexual partners during intercourse and from mothers to infants.
- Chlamydial infections are most common in women under the age of 20 years. They are also more common in persons who have several sexual partners.
- The treatment of choice for chlamydial infections is doxycycline, 500 mg twice daily for 7 days, or azithromycin, 1 g orally in a single dose.

### HUMAN PAPILLOMAVIRUS

- Condylomata acuminata (genital warts) is caused by HPV; it is most common in adolescent girls and young women.
- Genital warts are of particular concern, because they can undergo malignant changes after a latent period of 5 to 40 years.

### HEPATITIS B VIRUS

- In the United States HBV is most often transmitted by sexual contact.
- The CDC recommends that all persons at high risk for HBV be vaccinated. This includes health care workers because of the possibility of needle sticks.

## References


1. American Social Health Association: *STD counseling and treatment guide,* Research Triangle Park, NC, 1995, ASHA.
2. Bennett EC: Vaginitis and sexually transmitted diseases. In Youngkin EQ, Davis MS, editors: *Women's health: a primary care guide,* Norwalk, Conn, 1994, Appleton & Lange.
3. Bolon G et al: Syphilis: are you missing it? *Patient Care* p 126, Oct., 1993.
4. Centers for Disease Control and Prevention (CDC): Summary of notifiable diseases, United States, 1995, *MMWR* 44(53):1, 1996.
5. Centers for Disease Control and Prevention (CDC): Guidelines for treatment of sexually transmitted diseases, *MMWR* (RR-1), 1998.

5a. Centers for Disease Control and Prevention (CDC): Floroquinolone-resistant *Neisseria* gonorrhorae *MMWR* 47(20):405, 1998.

6. Centers for Disease Control and Prevention (CDC): Recommendations for prevention and management of *Chlamydia trachomatis* infections, *MMWR* 41:1, 1993.
7. Centers for Disease Control and Prevention (CDC): Special focus: surveillance for sexually transmitted diseases, *MMWR* 42:1, 1993.
8. Cox JT: Epidemiology of cervical intraepithelial neoplasia: the role of human papillomavirus, *Baillieres Clin Obstet Gynaecol* 9(1):1, 1995.

8a. Frisch M et al: Sexually transmitted infection as a cause of anal cancer, *N Engl J Med* 337(19):1350, 1997.

9. Guttmacher Institute: *Facts in brief: STDs in the United States,* New York, Guttmacher Institute, 1994.
10. Hatcher RA, Trusel J, Stewart F et al: *Contraceptive technology,* ed 16, New York, 1994, Irvington.
11. Hicks CS: Syphilis. In Rakel RE, editor: *Conn's current therapy 1996,* Philadelphia, 1996, WB Saunders.
12. Judson NJ: Gonorrhea. In Rakel RE, editor: *Conn's current therapy 1996,* Philadelphia, 1996, WB Saunders.
13. Lembo T: Acute and chronic viral hepatitis. In Rakel RE, editor: *Conn's current therapy 1996,* Philadelphia, 1996, WB Saunders.
14. Munoz A et al: The causal link between human papillomavirus and invasive cervical cancer: a population case-control study in Colombia and Spain, *Int J Cancer* 52:743, 1992.
15. Quinn TC et al: Epidemiologic and microbiologic correlates of *Chlamydia trachomatis* infection in sexual partnerships, *JAMA* 276(21):1737, 1996.
16. Reed BD: Vulvovaginitis. In Rakel RE, editor: *Conn's current therapy 1996,* Philadelphia, 1996, WB Saunders.
17. Rockley PF, Giannelli VF: Viral diseases of the skin. In Rakel RE, editor: *Conn's current therapy 1996,* Philadelphia, 1996, WB Saunders.
18. Rosen T: Granuloma inguinale. In Rakel RE, editor: *Conn's current therapy 1996,* Philadelphia, 1996, WB Saunders.
19. Rosen T: Lymphogranuloma venereum. In Rackel RE, editor: *Conn's current therapy 1996,* Philadelphia, 1996, WB Saunders.
20. Sacks SI et al: Patient-initiated, twice daily oral famciclovir for early recurrent genital herpes, *JAMA* 276:44, 1996.
21. Schiffman MH et al: Epidemiological evidence showing that human papillomavirus causes most cervical intraepithelial neoplasia, *J Natl Cancer Inst* 85(12):958, 1993.
22. Schiffman MH, Vittorio C: Epidemiology of human papillomaviruses, *Dermatol Clin* 13:561, 1995.

22a. Sun XW: Human papillomavirus infection in women infected with human immunodeficiency virus, *N Engl J Med* 337(19):1343, 1997.

23. Those other STDs, *Am J Public Health* 81(10):1250, 1991 (editorial).

24. Trofotter KF: Condylomata acuminata (genital warts). In Rakel RE, editor: *Conn's current therapy 1996,* Philadelphia, 1996, WB Saunders.
25. Tyndal M: Chancroid. In Rakel RE, editor: *Conn's current therapy 1996,* Philadelphia, 1996, WB Saunders.
26. Workowski KA: *Chlamydia trachomatis* infection. In Rakel RE, editor: *Conn's current therapy 1996,* Philadelphia, 1996, WB Saunders.
27. US Department of Health and Human Services, Public Health Service: *Healthy people 2000: national health promotion and disease prevention objectives,* Washington, DC, 1990, US Government Printing Office.
28. US Department of Health and Human Services, Public Health Service: *Healthy people 2000: midcourse review and 1995 revisions,* Washington, DC, 1990, US Government Printing Office.

# chapter 51 ASSESSMENT OF THE Nervous System

SHELLEY YERGER HUFFSTUTLER

## objectives *After studying this chapter, the learner should be able to:*

**1** State the four general kinds of functions of the nervous system.
**2** Describe the three parts of a neuron.
**3** Define the following terms: differential permeability, excitability, polarization, depolarization, action potential, and synapse.
**4** Differentiate between the two major divisions of the nervous system.
**5** Discuss the three main areas of the brain and at least two functions of each part.
**6** Explain the parts and functions of the four parts of the cerebral cortex.
**7** Explain possible symptoms a patient may manifest with pathology in the frontal lobe.
**8** Discuss the meningeal layers of the brain.
**9** Describe the circulation provided to the brain.
**10** Analyze physiological changes that occur in the nervous system with aging.
**11** Describe the parts of the neurological assessment that are assessed through the history.
**12** Differentiate between aphasia and dysarthria.
**13** Discuss the importance of each of the 12 cranial nerves.
**14** Describe diagnostic procedures used to evaluate neurological disease.

The ability to conduct an accurate neurological assessment depends on the nurse's knowledge of neuroanatomy and neurophysiology and skill in recognizing and interpreting subtle deviations from normal. This chapter contains an overview of neurological structure and function, tools for neurological assessment, and common neurological diagnostic tests. The complexity of the nervous system limits the depth of information that can be presented here, and the reader is referred to standard texts in anatomy and physiology for greater detail.

## ANATOMY AND PHYSIOLOGY

The nervous system, like an electrical conduction system, coordinates and controls all activities of the body. Broadly, the nervous system carries out four general functions:

1. Receives stimuli or information from the internal and external environments over varied afferent, or sensory, pathways
2. Communicates information between distant parts of the body (periphery) to the central nervous system
3. Computes or processes the information received at various reflex (spinal cord) and conscious (higher brain) levels to determine responses appropriate to existing situations
4. Transmits information rapidly over varied efferent or motor pathways to effector organs for body action, control or modification

Macroscopically, the nervous system is divided into two major divisions, the central nervous system and the peripheral nervous system.

### NEURON

The single neuron is the basic structural and functional unit of the nervous system. It shares all of the basic biological and biochemical properties of other body cells and is highly specialized and differentiated. The single neuron acts as a miniature nervous system and has properties specialized for its electrical function.

Neuroglial cells serve as adjuncts to the neurons providing nourishment, support, and protection. They make up almost half of the microscopic structures of the brain and spinal cord. Four different types of neuroglial cells have been identified, each with different functions (Table 51-1). Neuroglial cells divide and multiply by mitosis and can serve as a source for tumors of the nervous system.

Microscopically, the neuron consists of a cell body, or soma, with two extensions that project from it, a dendritic tree and an elongated cylindrical axon. A cell membrane encloses the outer boundary of the soma, dendrites, and axon, thus separating the inside from the outside of the cell. The presence of a large surface area of cell membrane makes it suitable to receive a large number of synaptic contacts at one time (Figure 51-1). The axon is specialized for the transmission of information along its extension away from the cell body to adjacent neurons; the dendrite or dendrites are specialized for receiving information from axon terminals at special sites called synapses. (It should be noted that the word axon is used in various ways. It may be used to describe the extension of one cell or the extension of several cells making up a nerve.) See Figure 51-2 for types of neurons.

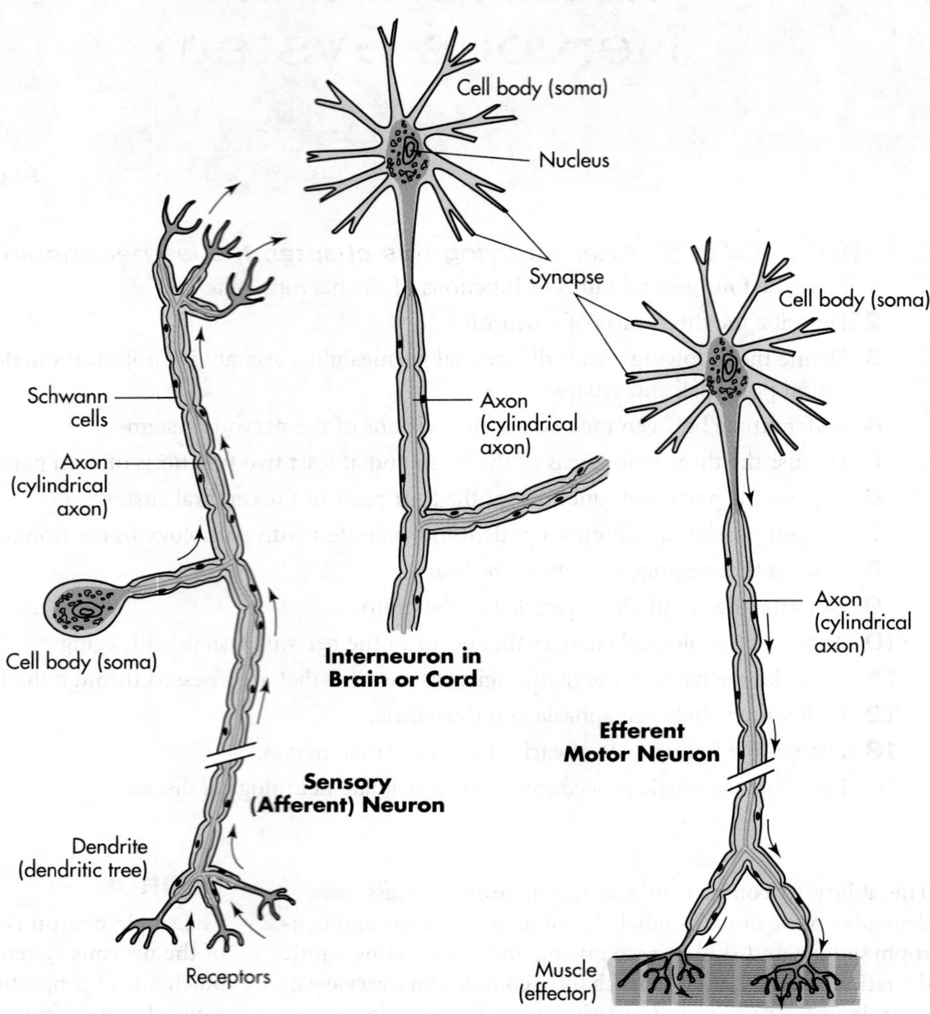


**fig. 51-1** Diagram of neurons showing the cell body (soma), dendrites, and axon. Direction of impulse conduction indicated by arrows.

**table 51-1** *Neuroglial Cells*

| Type of Cell | Function |
|---|---|
| Astrocyte | Maintain chemical environment for conduction and transmission of impulses |
| Ependyma | Produce cerebrospinal fluid |
| Microglia | Part of process of phagocytosis |
| Oligodendroglia | Produce lipid-protein complex that forms myelin |

## Cell Membrane

Many of the most important functional properties of the neuron lie within the cell membrane itself. Structurally, the membrane is made up of lipids and proteins and has the property of translocating materials across itself. The membrane exhibits differential permeability. For example, the membrane is permeable to oxygen, carbon dioxide, and certain inorganic ions, but impermeable to organic compounds (proteins) and other inorganic ions. This differential permeability results in a characteristic ionic distribution. The inside of the neuron contains a high concentration of proteins and potassium ($K^+$), whereas the outside of the cell is high in sodium ($Na^+$). This unequal distribution, or gradient, of $K^+$ and $Na^+$ across the membrane is supported by the presence of an active sodium-potassium pump within the membrane. The pump requires metabolic energy for rapid movement of sodium and potassium across the membrane, and this produces an electrical potential difference, or charge, between the inside and the outside of the cell. The magnitude of the potential difference is a function of the ratio of charged particles on opposite sides of the membrane and is called the resting membrane potential (resting potential). Thus, in the resting state, all neurons possess a potential for action and are said to be polarized. This resting potential is small, −60 mV, with the inside of the cell being electrically negative compared with the outside of the cell.

## Excitability

The neuron also exhibits the property of "excitability," which means that the resting potential is unstable under certain conditions. For example, a neuronal membrane becomes unstable when subjected to stimulation, application of chemicals, or

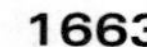

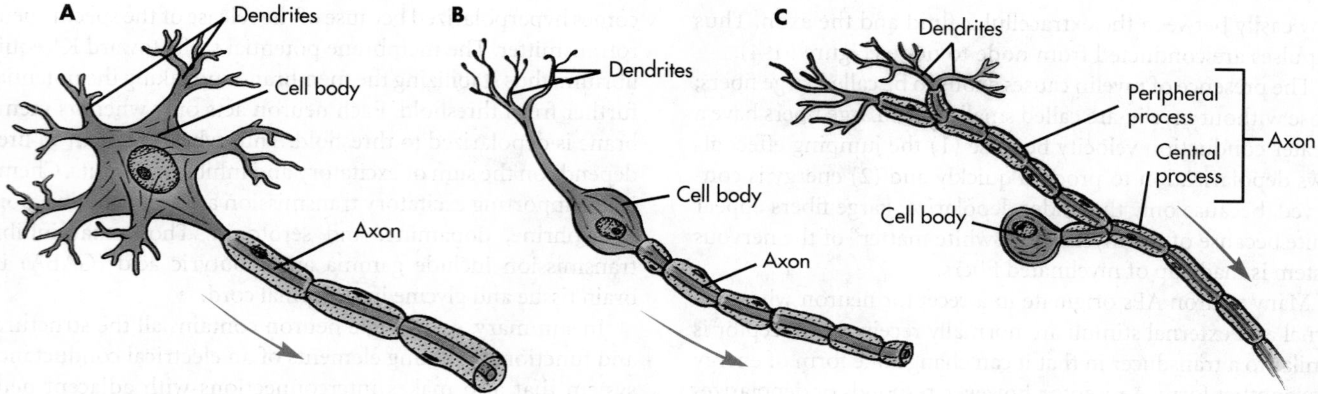


**fig. 51-2** Structural classification of neurons. **A,** Multipolar neuron: neuron with multiple extensions from the cell body. **B,** Bipolar neuron: neuron with exactly two extensions from the cell body. **C,** Unipolar neuron: neuron with only one extension from the cell body. The central process is an axon; the peripheral process is a modified axon with branched dendrites at its extremity. (The arrows show the direction of impulse travel.)

mechanical damage. This instability gives rise to the generation of action potentials (APs), which is a capacity unique to excitable cells. Action potentials transmit information within the nervous system and are therefore the basic phenomenon underlying all nervous system functions.

An AP occurs when a neuron is stimulated, which results in a significant increase in membrane permeability to $Na^+$. $Na^+$ quickly moves to the inside of the membrane through membrane pores or channels. These ions carry a sufficiently large positive charge to overwhelm the normal resting potential. A positive state develops within the cell and depolarization occurs (Figure 51-3).

Almost instantaneously the membrane pores return to being virtually impermeable to $Na^+$ while $K^+$ moves to the outside of the cell. Active transport then restores $Na^+$ and $K^+$ back to the original state. These mechanisms result in the disappearance of the internal positive state and a return to the normal resting potential, a phase called repolarization. These two phases together form the AP. An entire AP occurs within 1 to 2 ms.

When an action potential is generated it proceeds automatically to completion, independent of the property of the stimulus that initiated the depolarization. In other words, a strong stimulus does not give rise to a larger AP; the AP proceeds to completion in an "all-or-none" fashion. The AP is also spread, or propagated, over the entire membrane without a decrease in its velocity. The propagation velocity is related to the size of the axon (the larger the diameter, the higher the velocity) and to the presence or absence of myelin.

## Myelin

Myelin is an excellent insulator of axons. The myelin sheath is deposited around the axons by Schwann cells, and this sheath may be as thick as the axon itself. Myelin prevents almost all ion flow across the axon and its membrane. However, at distances approximately 1 mm apart the sheath is interrupted by nodes of Ranvier. At these small, uninsulated areas, ions can

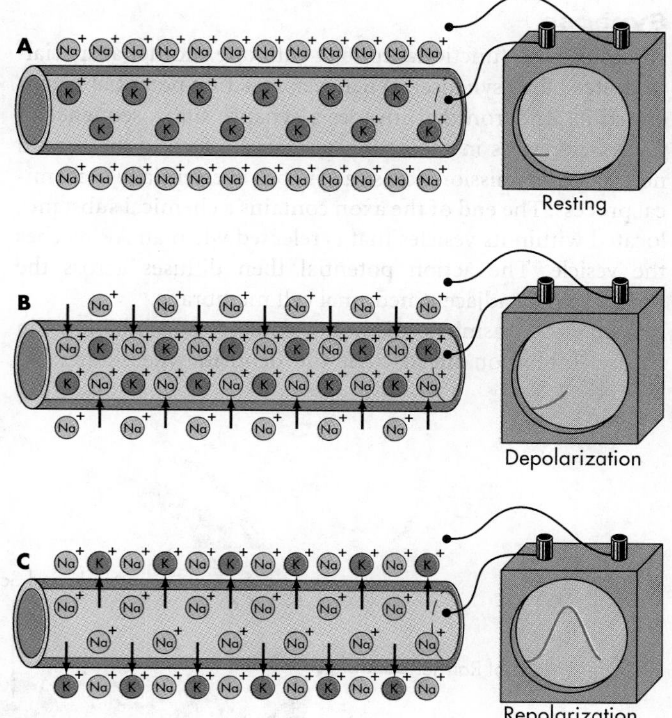


**fig. 51-3** Depolarization and repolarization. **A,** Resting membrane potential (RMP) results from an excess of positive ions on the outer surface of the plasma membrane. More $Na^+$ ions are on the outside of the membrane than $K^+$ ions are on the inside of the membrane. **B,** Depolarization of a membrane occurs when $Na^+$ channels open, allowing $Na^+$ to move to an area of lower concentration (and more negative charge) *inside* the cell—reversing the polarity to an inside-positive state. **C,** Repolarization of a membrane occurs when $K^+$ channels then open, allowing $K^+$ to move to an area of lower concentration (and more negative charge) *outside* the cell—reversing the polarity back to an inside-negative state. Each voltmeter records the changing membrane potential as a red line.

flow easily between the extracellular fluid and the axon. Thus impulses are conducted from node to node (Figure 51-4).

The presence of myelin causes axons to be called large fibers; those without myelin are called small fibers. Large fibers have a greater conduction velocity because (1) the jumping effect allows depolarization to proceed quickly and (2) energy is conserved, because only the nodes depolarize. Large fibers appear white because of the myelin; the "white matter" of the nervous system is made up of myelinated fibers.

Many neuron APs originate in a receptor neuron where internal and external stimuli are normally received. A receptor is similar to a transducer in that it can change one form of energy into another form. A receptor, however, responds or depolarizes to only one type of stimulus. For example, the retina of the eye responds only to the stimulus of light. Therefore the receptor neuron may initiate depolarization but only in response to a specific stimulus. The receptor neuron obeys the all-or-none theory, and a strong stimulus makes the receptor neuron fire more action potentials per unit of time than does a weak stimulus.

### Synapse

Neurons make functional contact with one another at specialized sites called synapses. Whenever an action potential is generated in a neuron that invades a synapse site, a sequence of processes results in the action potential affecting the second neuron. Transmission across a synapse is essentially a chemical process. The end of the axon contains a chemical substance located within its vesicles that is released when an AP reaches the vesicle. The action potential then diffuses across the synapse to the adjacent neuronal cell membrane.

Synaptic transmission is both excitatory and inhibitory in nature. Inhibition means that the dendritic membrane becomes hyperpolarized because of the release of the specific neurotransmitter. The membrane potential shifts toward $K^+$ equilibrium, thus stabilizing the membrane and taking the potential further from threshold. Each neuron acts only when its membrane is depolarized to threshold. Thus whether a neuron fires depends on the sum of excitatory and inhibitory inputs. Chemicals supporting excitatory transmission are acetylcholine, norepinephrine, dopamine, and serotonin. Those that inhibit transmission include gamma aminobutyric acid (GABA) in brain tissue and glycine in the spinal cord.

In summary, each single neuron contains all the structural and functional building elements of an electrical conductance system that also makes interconnections with adjacent neurons at synapses. Collectively, the neurons are organized into larger and larger units that serve to coordinate all the activities of the body.

## DIVISIONS OF THE NERVOUS SYSTEM

### Central Nervous System

The central nervous system (CNS) is made up of collections of neurons and their connections organized within the brain and spinal cord. Areas of the brain and spinal cord are distinguished where cell bodies are concentrated into nuclei, and groups of axons run in tracts that interconnect the parts. The connections determine the capability of each collection of neurons and are organized into circuits. Some circuits are simple and composed of relatively few neurons; others are highly complex. A single neuron may be a component of a number of different neuronal circuits and thus play a role in different functions.

Structurally, the brain and spinal cord are continuous and are protectively housed within the skull and vertebral column. When injured, centrally located neuron cell bodies are unable

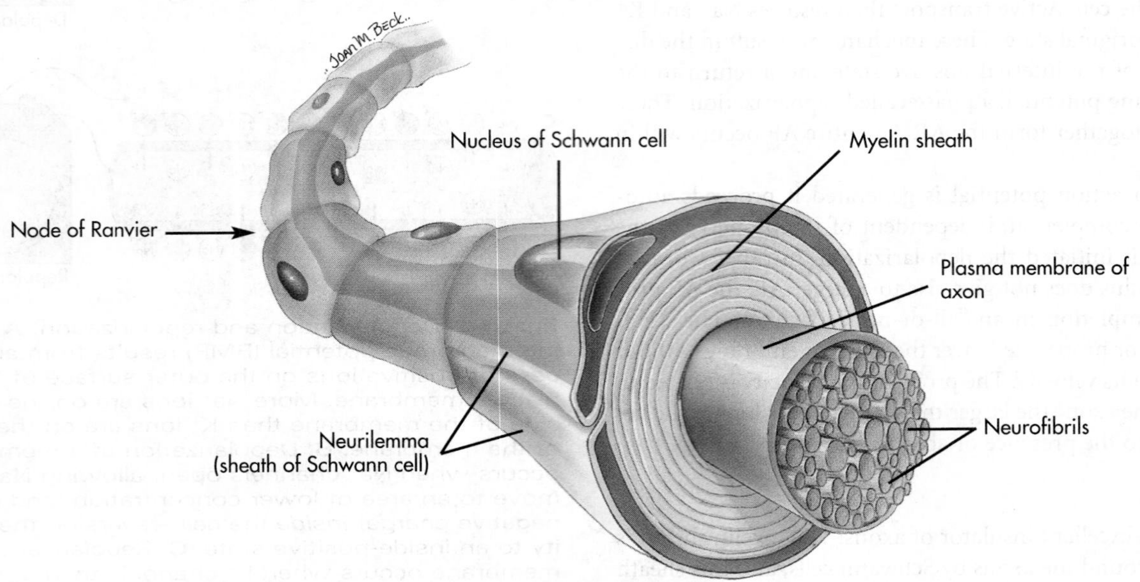


**fig. 51-4** Diagram of a nerve fiber and its coverings. This myelinated axon is located outside the central nervous system. Myelin is produced in concentric layers by the Schwann cell. The neurilemma is the outer sheath of the Schwann cell and is indented by successive nodes of Ranvier.

to reproduce themselves. However, nerve endings can regenerate because of the presence of neurilemma that covers all peripheral nerves and is believed to contain openings through which axonal regrowth occurs.

A blood-brain barrier exists in the nervous system that limits the free movement of substances from the blood to the brain tissue. The neurological sheath, as well as capillaries that have thickened basement membranes, slows the process of diffusion between the blood and the brain. The barrier is selective, allowing entry of fluid, gases, and small molecular substances, while preventing the entry of toxic substances, plasma protein, and large molecules.

### Meninges

The meninges are the coverings of the nervous tissue in the brain and spinal cord. The three fibrous coverings (dura mater, arachnoid, and pia mater) help support, protect, and nourish the brain and spinal cord (Figure 51-5). The outermost layer is the dura mater, a tough membrane consisting of two layers. This meningeal layer sends four processes deep into the cranium that form fibrous compartments for portions of the brain. These are the falx cerebri, the tentorium cerebelli, the falx cerebelli, and the diaphragma sellae.

The arachnoid, the delicate membrane lying beneath the dura, covers the brain more loosely. Projections called the arachnoid villi extend into the overlying dura. The pia mater, innermost of the meninges, is a vascular membrane having many small plexuses of blood vessels. The pia mater follows the course of the penetrating blood vessels as they dip into the substance of the brain.

These three coverings are also found in the spinal cord. The spinal cord arachnoid expands to surround the cauda equina; thus the subarachnoid space ends at S2 in the adult and is widest caudally. The spinal cord pia mater is thicker and less vascular than that of the cranium. The three meningeal layers give rise to three potential spaces. The spaces are epidural (external to the dura); subdural (between dura and arachnoid); and subarachnoid (between arachnoid and pia mater).

### Brain

The brain (encephalon) is grossly divided rostrally to caudally into four main areas: the cerebrum, diencephalon (thalamus, hypothalamus), brainstem (midbrain, pons, and medulla), and cerebellum (Figure 51-6). Each area carries out unique functions.

**Cerebrum.** The cerebrum, or cerebral cortex, is composed of two frontal lobes, two parietal lobes, two temporal lobes, and two occipital lobes. Each cerebral lobe is named from its overlying cranial bones (Figure 51-7) and carries out one or more functions as listed in Table 51-2. The cerebral cortex is separated into two hemispheres (left and right) by the falx cerebri.

Each of the hemispheres is further divided into the respective lobes by folds in the cerebral cortex called fissures or sulci. The frontal lobe is separated from the parietal lobe by the fissure of Rolando (also called the central sulcus) and from the temporal lobe by the sylvian fissure. It is separated from the occipital lobe by the parieto-occipital fissure. The temporal lobe lies below the sylvian fissure.

The cortex of the cerebrum is approximately 0.25 inch thick. It controls over 14 billion neurons, receives and analyzes all impulses, controls voluntary movement, and stores knowledge of all impulses received.

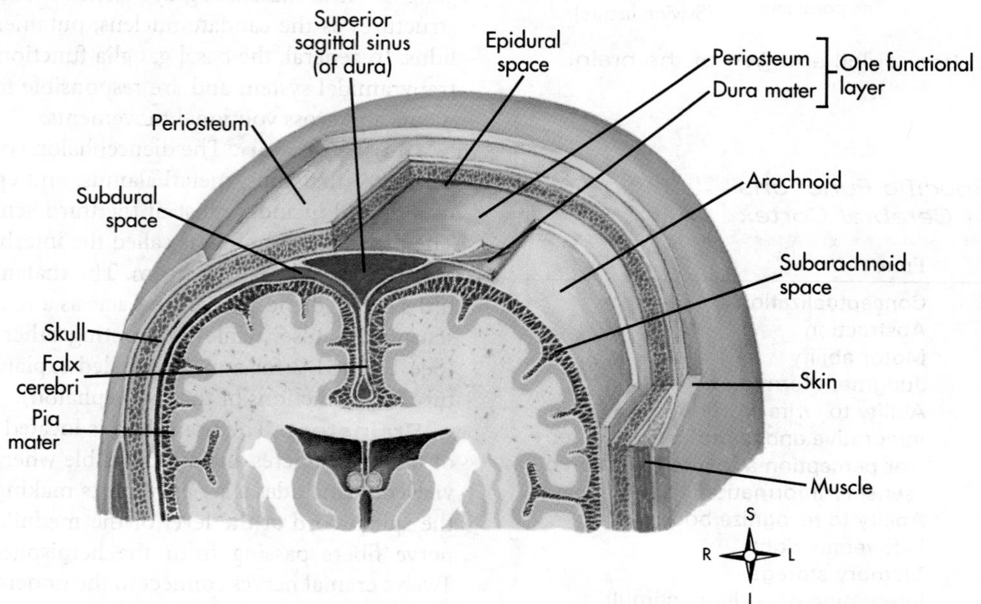


**fig. 51-5** Meningeal layers of the brain.

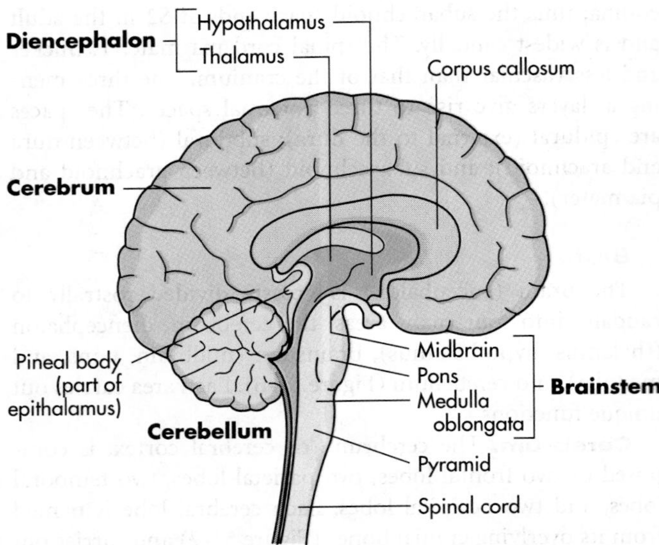


**fig. 51-6** Major structures of the brain.

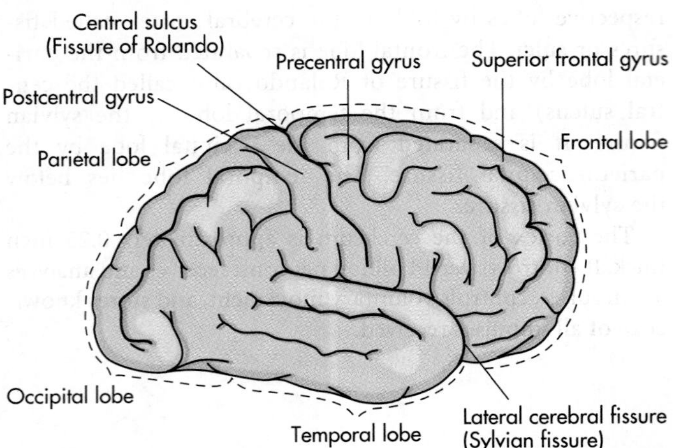


**fig. 51-7** Lobes, sulci, and gyri of the brain.

| table 51-2 Specific Functions of Cerebral Cortex | |
|---|---|
| LOBE | FUNCTION |
| Frontal | Conceptualization<br>Abstraction<br>Motor ability<br>Judgment formation<br>Ability to write words |
| Parietal | Integrative and coordinating center for perception and interpretation of sensory information<br>Ability to recognize body parts<br>Left versus right |
| Temporal | Memory storage<br>Integration of auditory stimuli |
| Occipital | Visual center<br>Understanding of written material |

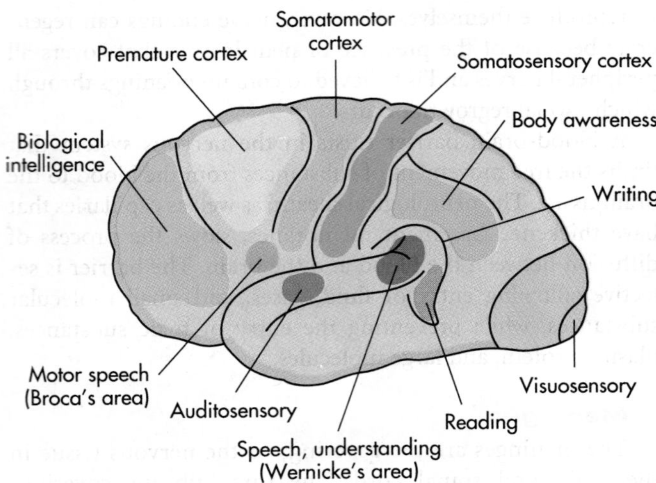


**fig. 51-8** Lateral view of cerebral cortex with identification of major cortical areas.

Speech is a function of the dominant hemisphere, which for all right-handed people and most left-handed people is the left side. The two identified speech centers are Broca's area and Wernicke's area (Figure 51-8). Broca's area is located in the lateral, inferior portion of the frontal lobe adjacent to the motor cortex and its projections. This area appears to control verbal, expressive speech. Wernicke's area is located in the posterior part of the superior temporal convolution and may extend to adjacent portions of the parietal lobe. This area is responsible for the reception and understanding of language. Other areas of the brain that are involved in speech include an area in the frontal lobe, which governs the ability to write words, and an area in the occipital lobe, which governs the ability to understand written material (see Figure 51-8 for important cortical areas).[10]

Deep within the cerebrum are structures called the basal ganglia. These masses of gray matter (cell bodies) include such structures as the caudate nucleus, putamen, and globus pallidus. In general, the basal ganglia function as part of the extrapyramidal system and are responsible for postural adjustments and gross volitional movements.

**Diencephalon.** The diencephalon consists of the hypothalamus, thalamus, metathalamus, and epithalamus. It surrounds and includes most of the third ventricle of the brain. The diencephalon often is called the interbrain because it lies directly beneath the cerebrum. The thalamus composes four fifths of the diencephalon and acts as a relay station for some sensory impulses while interpreting other sensory impulses. (See Table 51-3 for a more detailed explanation of the structures and functions of the diencephalon).

**Brainstem.** The brainstem is located deep in the center of the hemispheres and is not visible when the intact brain is viewed. It includes a series of parts making connections with the spinal cord at the level of the medulla, and it carries all nerve fibers passing from the hemispheres and the cord. Twelve cranial nerves connect to the undersurface of the brain (Figure 51-9), mostly on the brainstem.

The brainstem is made up of several structures, including the midbrain, pons, and medulla oblongata, (See Table 51-3

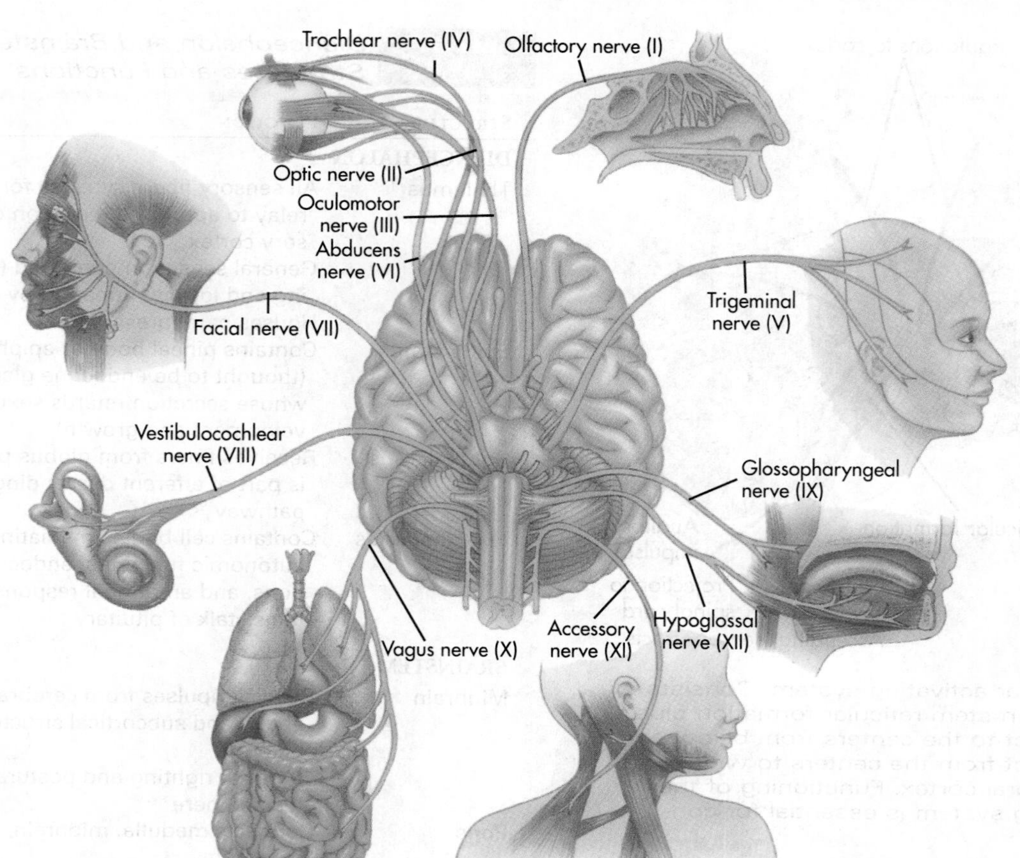


**fig. 51-9** Cranial nerves. Ventral surface of the brain showing attachment of the cranial nerves.

for a more detailed explanation of the structures and functions of the brainstem.)

Of special importance is the core of tissue extending throughout the entire brainstem. This is called the reticular activating system (Figure 51-10). This interconnected network of cells has important integrating centers for respiration, cardiovascular function, afferent and motor systems, and state of consciousness. Increased stimulation leads to wakefulness, and decreased stimulation results in sleepiness.

**Cerebellum.** The cerebellum is located in the posterior cranial fossa, just below the posterior cerebrum, and contains short and long tracts. The short tracts act as connections of nuclei within the cerebellum; the long tracts enter and exit through three peduncles, the inferior, middle, and superior. The inferior peduncle connects the cerebellum with the medulla, the middle peduncle connects the cerebellum with the pons, and the superior peduncle connects the cerebellum with the midbrain (Figure 51-11, p. 1669).

The cerebellum has three main functions related to monitoring and making corrective adjustments of body movements:

1. Keep persons oriented in space and maintain truncal equilibrium
2. Control antigravity muscles
3. Check or halt volitional movements

### *Circulation of the brain and spinal cord*

The blood supply for the brain derives from the aortic arch via the right innominate, left common carotid, and left subclavian arteries (Figure 51-12) and includes both conducting and penetrating vessels. The conducting arteries are (1) the internal carotids, which supply most of the cerebral hemispheres, basal ganglia, and the upper two thirds of the diencephalon; and (2) the vertebral arteries, which supply the brainstem, the lower one third of the diencephalon, the cerebellum, and the occipital lobes. These two systems anastomose at the circle of Willis, which is formed by the interconnection of the internal carotid, anterior cerebral, anterior communicating, and posterior communicating arteries as shown in Figure 51-13 on p. 1670. The circle of Willis provides equal circulation to both sides of the brain and helps compensate for alterations in blood flow and blood pressure. If one side of the circle of Willis is unable to supply adequate blood, the other side supports blood flow to the area normally supplied by the damaged side (Figure 51-13). The parts of the brain supplied by each of these vessels are listed in Table 51-4.

The penetrating vessels enter the brain at right angles after branching off from the conducting vessels. These vessels supply nutrients to the neurons and brain tissue. The venous system of the brain is unique in that the cerebral veins have no

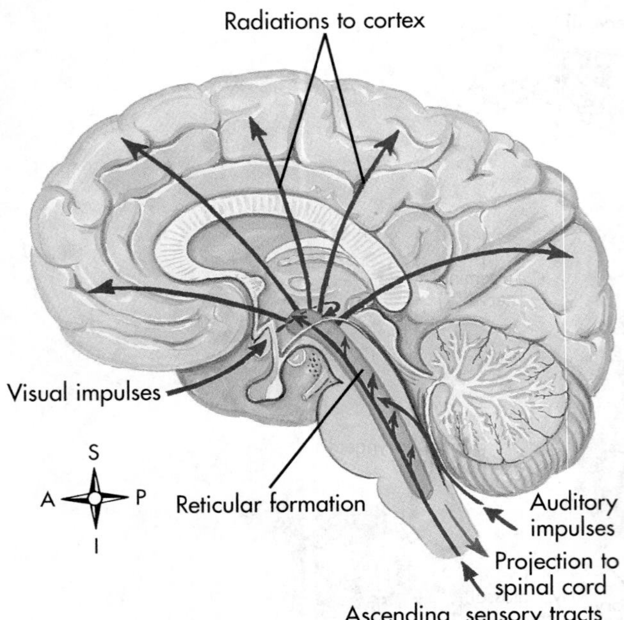


fig. 51-10 Reticular activating system. Consists of centers in the brain stem reticular formation plus fibers that conduct to the centers from below and fibers that conduct from the centers to widespread areas of the cerebral cortex. Functioning of the reticular activating system is essential for consciousness.

valves. All veins of the brain terminate in dural sinuses or reservoirs, which eventually empty into the superior vena cava by means of the jugular veins.

Circulation in the brain possesses special characteristics. The systemic circulation favors the central nervous system over all other body parts. This helps provide a constant supply of nutrients (glucose and oxygen) to nervous tissue. The brain's vessels also possess the ability to maintain a constant blood flow through autoregulation. In the presence of increased blood pressure, cerebral vessels constrict, decreasing blood flow and preventing possible tissue damage. Conversely, in the presence of decreased blood pressure, cerebral vessels dilate to increase flow. Cerebral vessels also react to biochemical changes. Elevated carbon dioxide content causes notable vasodilation of cerebral vessels; hypoxia and elevated hydrogen ion concentration also cause vasodilation. These autoregulatory mechanisms become less responsive with increasing age and in the presence of arteriosclerosis.

The blood supply to the spinal cord comes from the spinal artery and two radicular arteries. The spinal artery arises from the vertebral arteries, whereas the radicular arteries arise from the aorta.

### *Cerebrospinal fluid*

Cerebrospinal fluid (CSF) is found in the ventricles of the brain, in the central canal of the spinal cord, and in the

**table 51-3** *Diencephalon and Brainstem Structures and Functions*

| Structure | Function |
|---|---|
| **DIENCEPHALON** | |
| Thalamus | All sensory fibers synapse for final relay to appropriate portion of sensory cortex<br>General sensation perceived (meaning and locality imparted by cortex)<br>Houses pain threshold |
| Epithalamus | Contains pineal body or epiphysis (thought to be endocrine gland whose secretion retards sexual development and growth) |
| Subthalamus | Receives fibers from globus pallidus, is part of efferent descending pathway |
| Hypothalamus | Contains cell bodies mediating most autonomic functions, endocrine functions, and emotional responses; contains stalk of pituitary |
| **BRAINSTEM** | |
| Midbrain | Relays impulses from cerebral cortex above and subcortical structures below<br>Origin of righting and postural reflex located here |
| Pons | Connects medulla, midbrain, and cerebrum<br>Contains pneumotaxic center—controls rhythmic quality of respirations |
| Medulla | Connects with central canal or spinal cord<br>Vital centers of cardiac, respiration, vasomotor control, as well as swallowing and hiccoughing; gag and cough reflexes |

**table 51-4** *Circulation of the Brain*

| Vessel | Part of Brain Supplied |
|---|---|
| **INTERNAL CAROTID ARTERIES** | |
| Anterior cerebral | Medial surface of the frontal and parietal lobes<br>Basal ganglia<br>Parts of the internal capsule and corpus callosum |
| Middle cerebral | Lateral surface of parietal, frontal and temporal lobes<br>Precentral (motor) gyri<br>Postcentral (sensory) gyri |
| **VERTEBRAL ARTERIES** | |
| Basilar | Brainstem<br>Cerebellum |
| Posterior cerebral | Parts of temporal and occipital lobe<br>Vestibular organs<br>Cochlear apparatus |

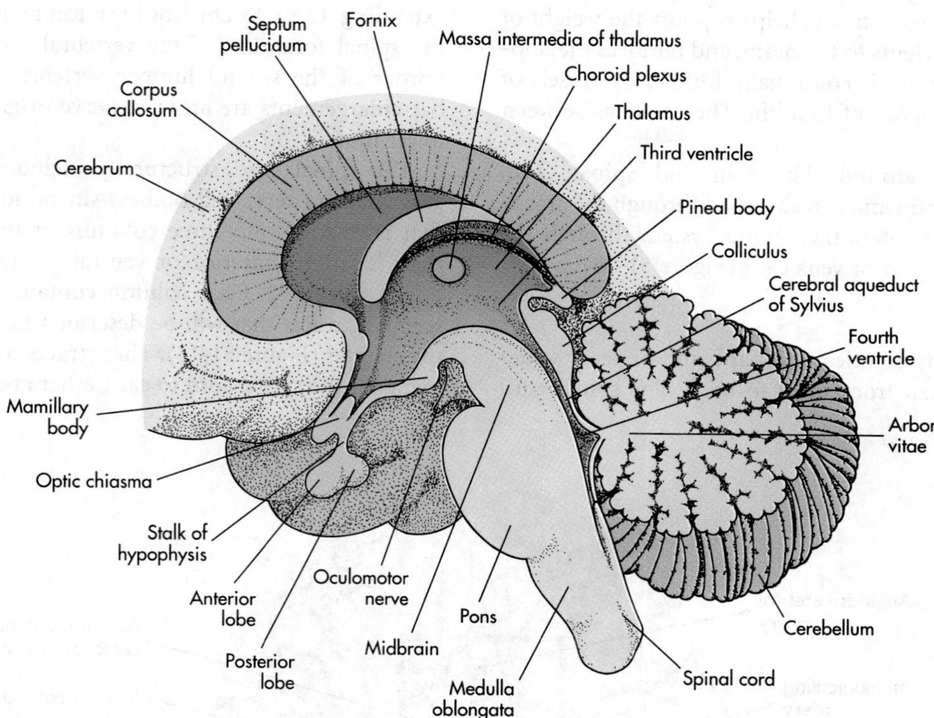


**fig. 51-11** Sagittal section through midline of brain showing continuity of brain and spinal cord.

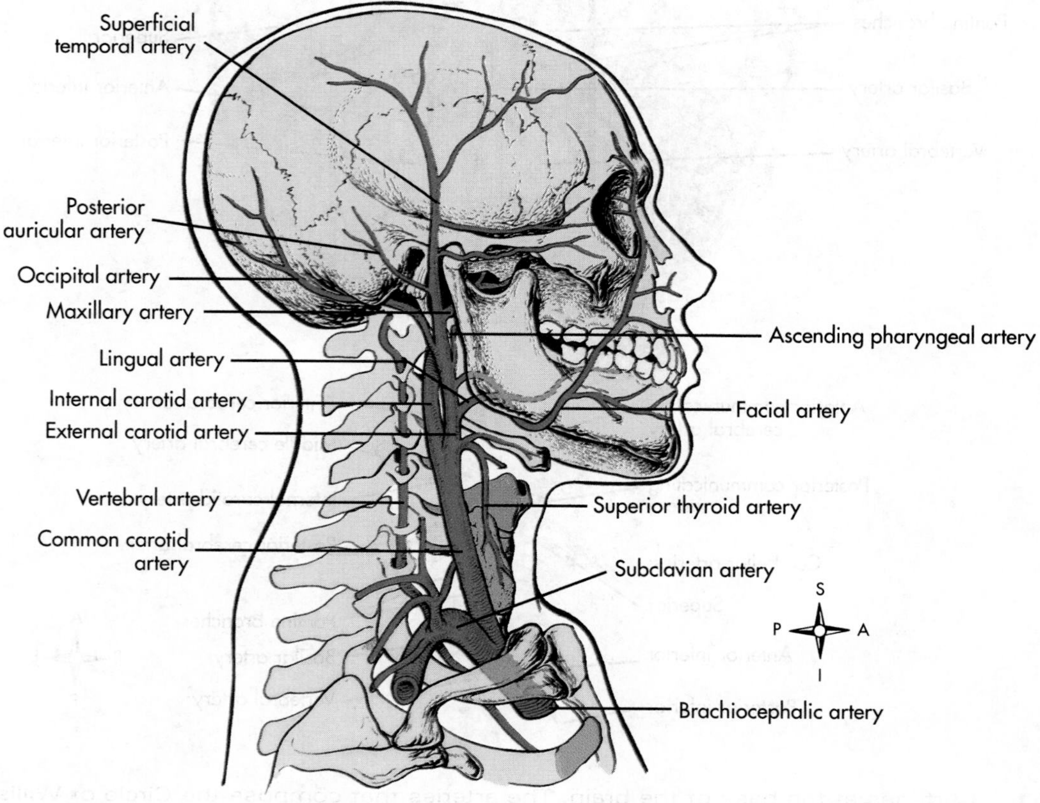


**fig. 51-12** Major arteries of the head and neck.

subarachnoid space. The CSF serves four purposes: it acts as a fluid cushion for nervous tissue, helps support the weight of the brain, carries nutrients to the brain, and removes metabolites. Cerebrospinal fluid is continually formed by vessels of the choroid plexus at a rate of 18 ml/hr. The adult has between 90 and 150 ml of CSF.

After circulating around the brain and spinal cord, CSF returns to the brain and is reabsorbed through the arachnoid villi. Then CSF enters the venous system through the jugular veins to the superior vena cava (Figure 51-14).

### Spinal cord

The spinal cord is elliptical in shape and appears wider from side to side than from front to back. The spinal cord forms a continuous structure with the medulla oblongata extending 42 to 45 cm from the foramen magnum through the spinal foramina of the vertebral column to the upper border of the second lumbar vertebra. Cervical and lumbar enlargements are areas of nerve origin to the upper and lower limbs.

The spinal cord structurally includes H-shaped central gray matter (nerve cell bodies) surrounded by white matter that is divided into three columns or funiculi according to their location (anterior or ventral, lateral, and posterior or dorsal columns). Each column contains ascending and descending tracts that will be described in more detail later in the chapter (Figure 51-15). These tracts connect different segments of the spinal cord to each other and connect the spinal

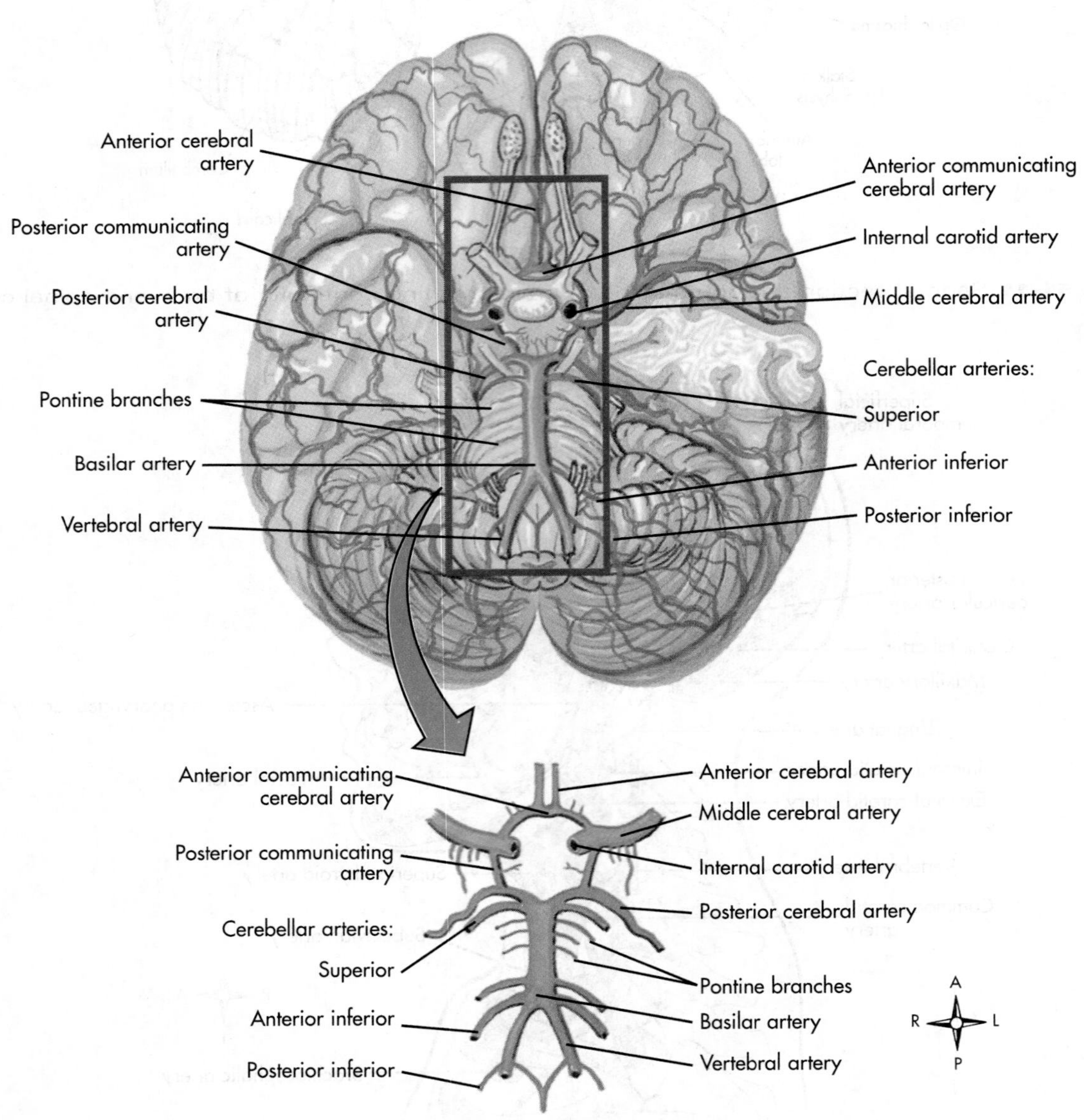


**fig. 51-13** Arteries at the base of the brain. The arteries that compose the Circle of Willis are the two anterior cerebral arteries joined to each other by the anterior communicating cerebral artery and to the posterior cerebral arteries by the posterior communicating arteries.

cord with the brain. The names of the tracts usually indicate the point of origin by the first part of the name and the endpoint by the last part of the name (Table 51-5).

The spinal cord is also the site of reflex pathways. Reflexes are an example of the simplest neuronal circuit and do not require relay to the brain for action. A reflex consists of a specific stereotyped motor response to an adequate sensory stimulus. The response may involve skeletal muscle movement or glandular secretion. A reflex may involve only two neurons as in a simple monosynaptic reflex arch that occurs with the knee-jerk reflex. A brisk tap over a partially stretched knee tendon stimulates sensory nerve endings within the tendons; subsequently, the stimulus travels over a sensory nerve fiber within a peripheral nerve toward the spinal cord where it synapses with a central motor neuron (anterior horn cell). The impulse is transmitted down the motor nerve (over the anterior nerve root of the spinal nerve or peripheral nerve) and across the neuromuscular junction to stimulate

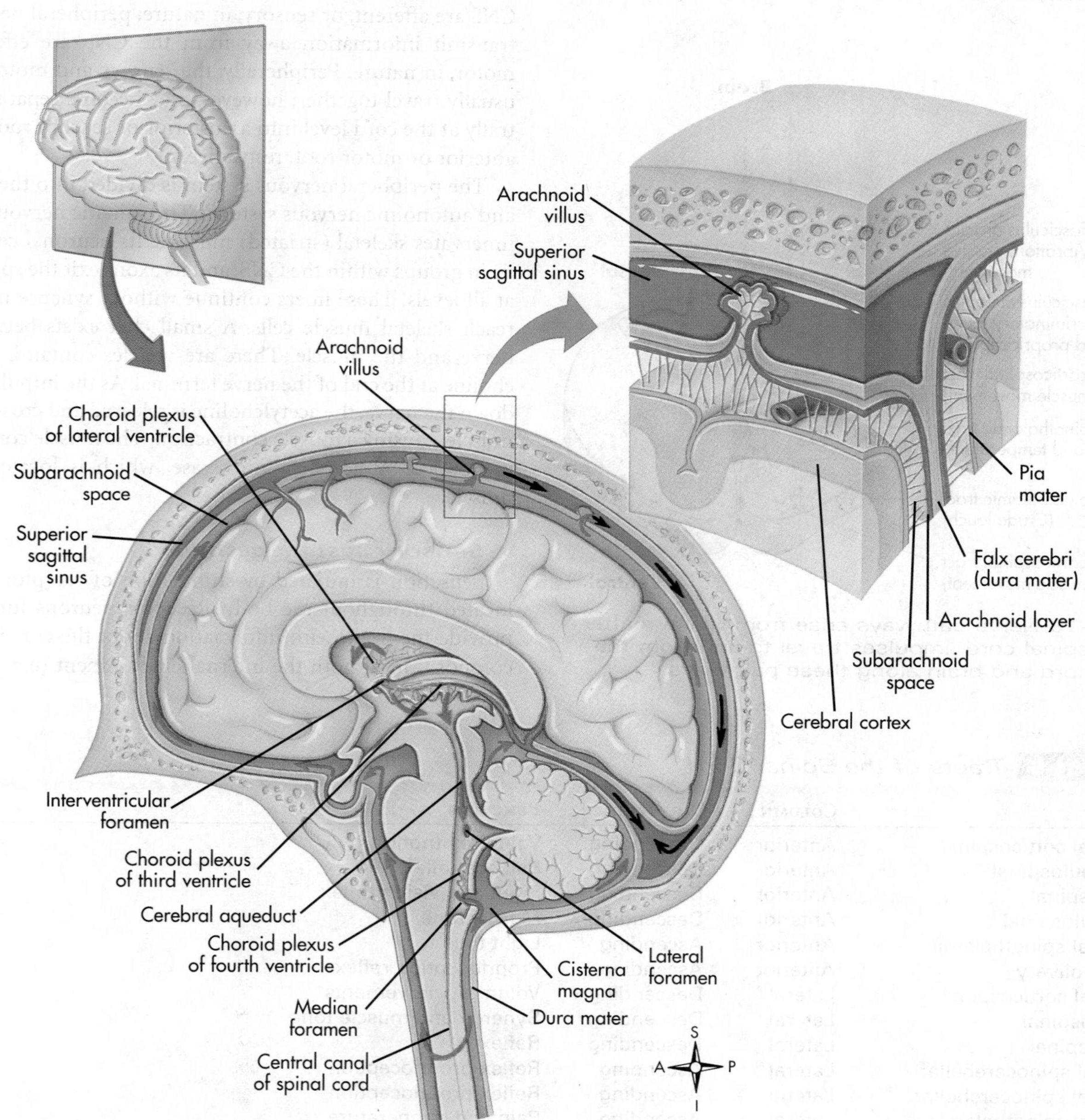


**fig. 51-14** Flow of cerebrospinal fluid. The fluid produced by filtration of blood by the choroid plexus of each ventricle flows inferiorly through the lateral ventricles, interventricular foramen, third ventricle, cerebral aqueduct, fourth ventricle, and subarachnoid space and to the blood.

the muscle to contract. Figure 51-16 shows the reflex arc. A reflex may involve only one spinal cord level, as in the knee-jerk reflex; one or a few spinal cord levels (segmental reflexes); or structures in the brain that influence the spinal cord (supraspinal reflexes).

### Peripheral Nervous System

The peripheral nervous system (PNS) is basically a set of communication channels located outside the central nervous system. Peripheral nerves are bundles of individual nerves that are either sensory, motor, or mixed (having both sensory and motor fibers). Structurally, the PNS consists of 12 pairs of cranial nerves and 31 pairs of spinal nerves. The cranial nerves carry impulses to and from the brain. They originate mainly in the brainstem, except for the first nerve (olfactory), which arises in the olfactory bulb. (See Table 51-9 on p. 1679 for an explanation of the functions of each cranial nerve.)

Spinal nerves are composed of a dorsal and ventral root. They correspond to the spinal cord segment from which they arise—8 cervical, 12 thoracic, 5 lumbar, 5 sacral, and 1 coccygeal (the first pair of cervical spinal nerves come off the cord above C1). From L3 to S5, the spinal nerves branch out to form the cauda equina (Figure 51-17).

Peripheral nerves that transmit information toward the CNS are afferent, or sensory, in nature; peripheral nerves that transmit information away from the CNS are efferent, or motor, in nature. Peripherally, the sensory and motor nerves usually travel together; however, they become separated centrally at the cord level into a posterior or sensory root and an anterior or motor root, respectively.

The peripheral nervous system is divided into the somatic and autonomic nervous systems. The somatic nervous system innervates skeletal (striated) muscles. Its neuronal cell bodies lie in groups within the CNS, and its axons exit the spinal cord at all levels. These fibers continue without synapse until they reach skeletal muscle cells. A small cleft exists between the nerve and the muscle. There are vesicles containing acetylcholine at the end of the nerve terminal. As the impulse moves down the nerve, the acetylcholine is released and crosses to the muscle, causing a muscle contraction. The muscle contraction is stopped by acetylcholinesterase, which is located in the muscle.

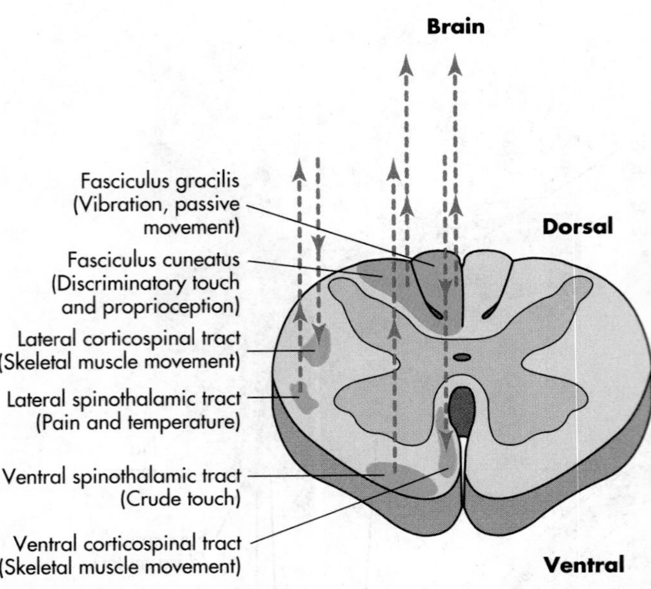


**fig. 51-15** Nerve pathways arise from white matter of the spinal cord. Impulses travel to and from the spinal cord and brain along these pathways.

#### *Sensory system pathways*

Sensation is initiated by stimulation of receptor neurons located throughout the body. Receptor neurons function to provide the brain with information about the condition and composition of both the internal environment (e.g., position

**table 51-5** *Tracts of the Spinal Cord*

| Tract | Column | Direction | Function |
|---|---|---|---|
| Ventral corticospinal | Anterior | Descending | Voluntary motion |
| Vestibulospinal | Anterior | Descending | Balance reflex |
| Tectospinal | Anterior | Descending | Sight and vision reflex |
| Reticulospinal | Anterior | Descending | Muscle tone |
| Ventral spinothalamic | Anterior | Ascending | Light touch |
| Spinoolivary | Anterior | Ascending | Proprioception reflex |
| Lateral corticospinal | Lateral | Descending | Voluntary movements |
| Rubrospinal | Lateral | Descending | Synergy and muscle tone |
| Olivospinal | Lateral | Descending | Reflex |
| Dorsal spinocerebellar | Lateral | Ascending | Reflex proprioception |
| Ventral spinocerebellar | Lateral | Ascending | Reflex proprioception |
| Lateral spinothalamic | Lateral | Ascending | Pain and temperature |
| Spinotectal | Lateral | Ascending | Reflex |
| Fasciculus interfascicularis | Posterior | Descending | Integration and association |
| Septomarginal fascicularis | Posterior | Descending | Integration and association |
| Fasiculus gracilis | Posterior | Ascending | Vibration, passive movement, joint, and two-point movement |
| Fasiculus cuneatus | Posterior | Ascending | Vibration, passive movement, joint, and two-point movement |

[proprioception] and action [enteroception] of body parts) and the external environment (exteroception). The latter is achieved through the eyes, ears, nose, skin, and tongue. The general sensory system by which this information is conveyed includes (1) receptor neurons responsive to special stimuli from both the internal and external environments, (2) posterior roots of the peripheral or afferent sensory nerves carrying nerve impulses toward the central nervous system, (3) ascending or sensory tracts within the spinal cord and upper brain centers, and (4) sensory areas of the cerebral cortex where stimuli are perceived and localized.

From the receptor neuron, the sensory impulse travels to the spinal cord along the afferent fibers, enters the spinal cord through the posterior root, and proceeds along either the spinothalamic tracts or the posterior columns. The pathway followed is specific to the sensation. For example, nerve fibers conducting the sensations of pain and temperature pass into the posterior horn of the spinal cord, synapse with a secondary sensory neuron, cross immediately to the contralateral side of the cord, and continue upward as the lateral spinothalamic tract. These fibers arrive at the thalamus, synapse with a third sensory neuron, and terminate in the appropriate area of the sensory cortex.

Sensations for crude touch follow a similar pathway to that for pain and temperature but ascend the spinal cord as the ventral spinothalamic tract. Impulses travel to the thalamus where they synapse with a third sensory neuron and terminate in the appropriate area of the sensory cortex. Sensations of fine touch, deep touch and pressure, vibration, and proprioception arrive at the spinal cord and are conducted by the posterior columns (fasciculus gracilis or fasciculus cuneatus) to the level of the medulla before synapsing with a second neuron, crossing over to the contralateral side, and continuing to the thalamus. At this location, they synapse with a third sensory neuron that terminates at the appropriate area of the sensory cortex (Figure 51-18).

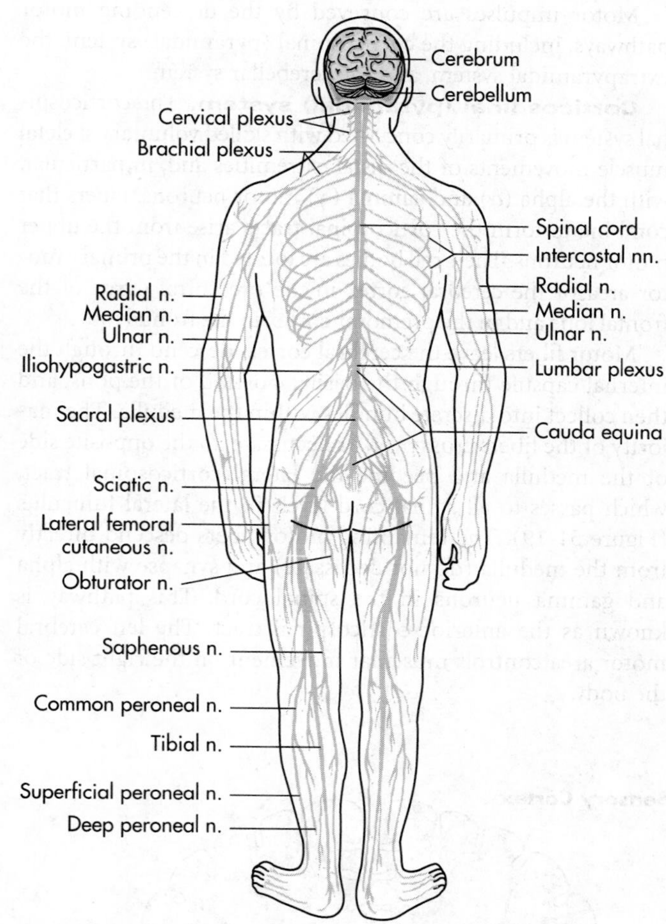


**fig. 51-17** The central and peripheral divisions of the nervous system. The central nervous system (CNS) consists of the brain and spinal cord. The peripheral nervous system is composed of the cranial and spinal nerves.

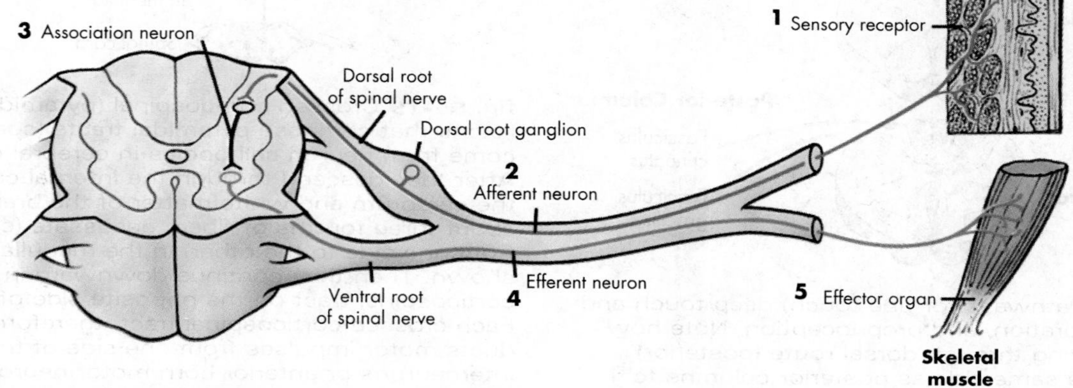


**fig. 51-16** Basic diagram of a reflex arc, including the (1) sensory receptor, (2) afferent neuron, (3) association neuron, (4) efferent neuron, and (5) effector organ.

### Motor system pathways

Motor impulses are conveyed by the descending motor pathways, including the corticospinal (pyramidal) system, the extrapyramidal system, and the cerebellar system.

**Corticospinal (pyramidal) system.** The corticospinal system is primarily concerned with skilled voluntary skeletal muscle movements of the distal extremities and, in particular, with the alpha ($\alpha$) and gamma ($\gamma$) motor neurons. Fibers that combine to form the corticospinal tracts arise from the upper motor neurons. Their cell bodies are located in the primary motor area of the cerebral cortex in the precentral gyrus of the frontal lobe and in the premotor cortex in the frontal lobe.

Motor fibers leave the cerebral cortex, descend through the internal capsule through the basilar portion of the pons, and then collect into discrete bundles within the medulla. The majority of the fibers cross over, or decussate, to the opposite side of the medulla and become the lateral corticospinal tract, which passes to all spinal cord levels in the lateral funiculus (Figure 51-19). The remaining motor fibers descend directly from the medulla (do not decussate) and synapse with alpha and gamma neurons in the spinal cord. This pathway is known as the anterior corticospinal tract. The left cerebral motor area controls muscular movement on the right side of the body.

Motor fibers synapse with large anterior horn cells in the spinal cord. These cells are the lower motor neurons and are responsible for providing the final direct link or final common pathway with muscles. Thus skeletal muscle activity is the result of the net influence of upper motor neurons on the alpha and gamma motor neurons through the anterior horn cells (lower motor neurons) in the spinal cord.

**Extrapyramidal system.** The extrapyramidal tracts are complex and provide separate pathways between the cortex, basal ganglia, brainstem, and spinal cord. Extrapyramidal tracts include all descending motor pathways other than the corticospinal tract (indicating that they do not pass through the medulla). These tracts are named from point of origin to termination. The extrapyramidal tracts collectively assist in maintaining muscle tone and the control of gross automatic skeletal muscle movements. Some tracts facilitate extensor activity and inhibit flexor activity (lateral vestibulospinal tract

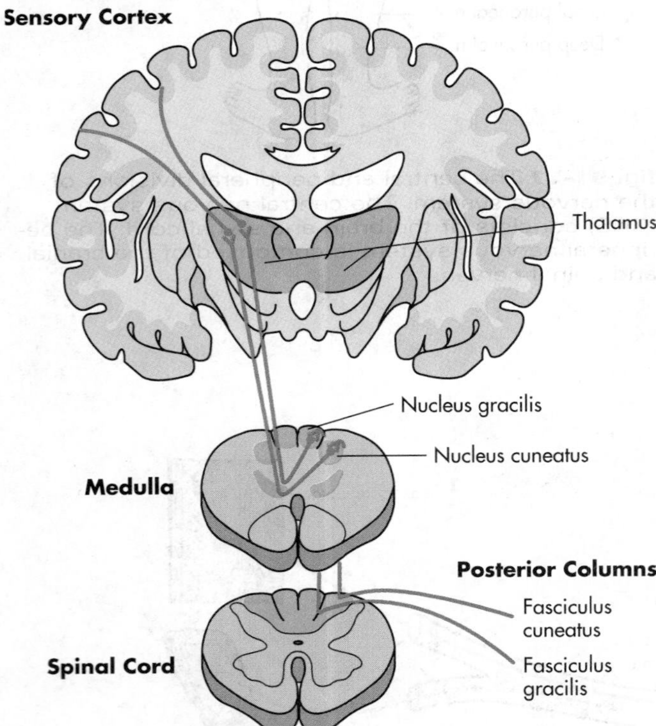


**fig. 51-18** Pathways for fine touch, deep touch and pressure, vibration, and proprioception. Note how stimuli entering through dorsal route (posterior) travel on the same side as posterior columns to medulla where they cross to the opposite side, ascend to the thalamus, and end in somasthetic area where perception occurs.

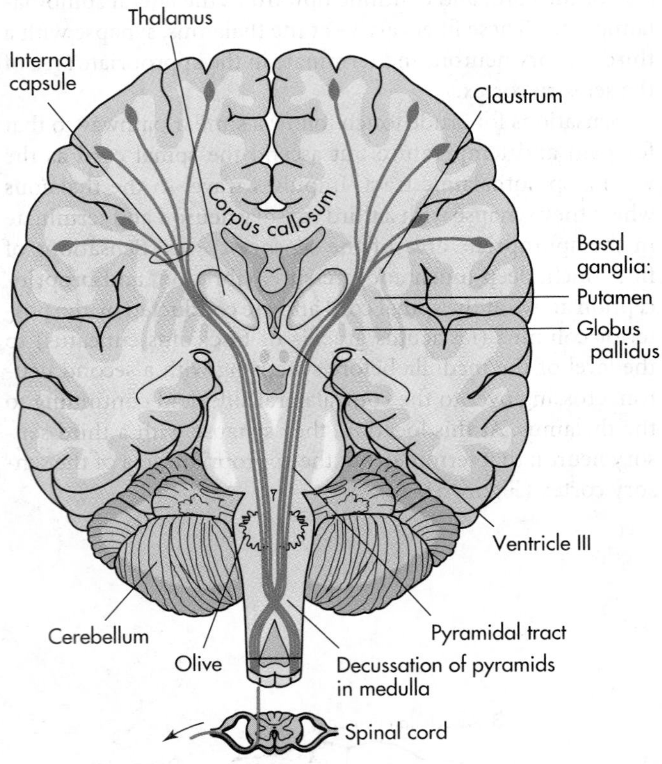


**fig. 51-19** Crossed corticospinal (pyramidal) tracts. Axons that compose pyramidal tracts (corticospinal) come from neuron cell bodies in cerebral cortex. After they descend through the internal capsule of the cerebrum and white matter of the brainstem, about three fourths of fibers decussate (cross over from one side to the other) in the medulla, as shown. Then they continue downward in the lateral corticospinal tract on the opposite side of cord. Each crossed corticospinal tract, therefore, conducts motor impulses from one side of the brain to interneurons or anterior horn motor neurons on the opposite side of the cord. Therefore, impulses from one side of cerebrum cause movements of opposite side of the body.

and pontine reticulospinal tract); others facilitate flexor activity and inhibit extensor activity (lateral corticospinal tract and rubrospinal tract).

**Cerebellar system.** The cerebellum coordinates the action of muscle groups and controls their contractions so that movements are performed smoothly and accurately. Voluntary movements can proceed without the cerebellum, but movements would be clumsy and uncoordinated (asynergia and cerebellar ataxia). The cerebellum receives tactile, auditory, and visual sensory stimuli and contains feedback circuits to all descending motor pathways. The functioning of the cerebellum allows nerve impulses to be returned to the same region from which they originated. The cerebellar cortex can detect any errors in muscle synergy and return the proper messages to adjust muscular control within the body.

Visceral efferent motor pathways mediate the action of involuntary, or smooth, muscles located within walls of tubes, hollow organs, the heart, and the glands. Most viscera are supplied by both excitatory and inhibitory fibers.

**Effectors.** Effectors may be considered as the cells of the body that "do something" by interacting with the internal and external environments and following the commands of the nervous system. The two classes of effectors are muscles and glands; both are transducers and capable of converting one form of energy into another. Effectors, like nerve tissue, are excitable tissues and are able to generate action potentials. The nervous system controls muscles and glands by directly turning them on or by altering their level of spontaneous activity through a neuron-to-effector chemical communication system.

### Autonomic Nervous System

The autonomic nervous system regulates automatic body functions, usually in an effort to preserve homeostasis. Fibers of the autonomic nervous system synapse once after leaving the CNS and before arriving at the neuroeffector junction. The site of this synapse is called a ganglion, and its neurotransmitter is acetylcholine. The autonomic nervous system is further divided into the sympathetic nervous system (adrenergic), which functions to maintain homeostasis and to provide defense against stressors, and the parasympathetic nervous system (cholinergic), which is responsible for conserving and restoring vegetative functions (Table 51-6).

Fibers leaving the ganglia finally synapse at the effector organ. The neurotransmitter for the postganglionic synapse of the parasympathetic nervous system is acetylcholine; the neurotransmitter for the postganglionic synapse of the sympathetic nervous system is norepinephrine.

### Physiological Changes with Aging

Changes in the nervous system occur with normal aging. However, it must be stressed that normal aging is not equated with senility or Alzheimer's disease. The healthy older person continues to function mentally at a high level into advanced age.

The changes in the nervous system associated with aging include the loss of brain cells with actual loss of brain weight. The nerve cell loss usually is diffuse and gradual. The gyri of the brain surface also atrophy, causing widening and deepening of the spaces between the gyri. Other changes include a decrease in blood flow to the brain. The ability of the brain to autoregulate its blood supply decreases with increased age.

The control of the autonomic nervous system over various functions of the body is unpredictable and labile in the elderly, but some changes do occur. In addition, velocity of nerve impulses decreases, which slows sensory and motor conduction, with sensory conduction decreasing faster than motor. This occurs especially in peripheral nerves. See the Gerontological Assessment Box for assessment of changes commonly found in elderly patients.

## SUBJECTIVE DATA

Although neurological assessment usually is completed in phases and depends on the condition of the person and the urgency of the situation, several aspects of the neurological examination contain largely subjective data.[2,6,9] Assessment of mental status, level of consciousness, language

**table 51-6** *Parasympathetic and Sympathetic Nervous System Influence*

| Organ System | Parasympathetic Influence | Sympathetic Influence |
|---|---|---|
| Heart | Decreases rate | Increases rate |
| Blood vessels | Dilates visceral and brain vessels | Constricts |
| Lungs | Constricts bronchi | Dilates bronchi |
| Gastrointestinal | Increases peristalsis | Decreases peristalsis |
| Gastric and salivary secretions | Increases | Decreases |
| Anal sphincter | Opens | Closes |
| Liver | Not applicable | Stimulates glycogen |
| Adrenal medulla | Not applicable | Stimulates production of epinephrine |
| Bladder | Contracts bladder | Relaxes bladder |
| | Opens sphincter | Closes sphincter |
| Eyes | Constricts pupil | Dilates pupil |
| | Accommodates for near vision | Accommodates for far vision |
| Skin | Not applicable | "Goose flesh" |

## gerontological assessment

Deep tendon reflexes are less brisk. Ankle jerks are commonly lost; those in the upper extremities are usually present. Aging people often find it difficult to relax their limbs; always support the limb when eliciting reflexes.

Loss of the sensation of vibration at the ankle malleolus is common after age 65. Position sense in the big toe may be absent, but this is less common.

Gait may be slower and more deliberate; also, the gait may deviate slightly from a midline path because of decreased coordination.

A decrease in muscle bulk often occurs and is most apparent in the hands. The hand muscles appear wasted; however, grip strength remains relatively good.

Cranial nerves mediating taste and smell may show some decline in function.

Senile tremors occasionally occur and are considered benign.

Some aging adults show a slower response to requests, especially to those calling for coordination of movements.

**COMMON DISORDERS IN ELDERS**

Stroke
Falls
Vision and hearing changes
Memory loss
Burns

and speech, perceptual status, and sensory status are discussed in this chapter. Levels of consciousness are discussed in Chapter 52.

## HISTORY

As in other specialties, a careful history precedes physical examination. The person is asked to give a time account of the illness including the onset and progression, as well as the nature of symptoms. It is particularly important to note the speed of onset, frequency of remissions (if any), and any diurnal patterns or intensity changes in symptoms. Symptoms that require further assessment are complaints of pain, headache, seizures, vertigo, numbness, visual changes, and weakness. Identification of specific patterns of symptoms may provide pertinent diagnostic information about the pathological process.

Information is collected about family members and their relationships and interactions, ethnic background, housing, recreational interests, occupation, education, coping mechanisms, dependence-independence characteristics, and how the person manages usual activities of daily living. Particular attention should be paid to reports of any recent changes in the person's usual behaviors, such as increased irritability or memory loss. A family health history and developmental history also are included.

During the course of the neurological examination, some of the observations made during the history may be confirmed. A skillfully taken history often holds the key to diagnosis.[3]

## MENTAL STATUS

Specific abnormalities of higher cerebral function are particularly significant in determining the presence of organic brain disease; therefore clinical observation of mental function is important.

Changes in the level of consciousness (LOC) can be the most sensitive indicator of a person's level of neurological function. The functional components of consciousness are arousal (alertness) and awareness (content) of self and environment. Arousal is mainly controlled by brainstem activity, including the reticular activating system (RAS). Awareness requires an intact cerebral cortex and association fibers. Thus the state of consciousness depends on the interactions between the brainstem and cerebral hemispheres.

Arousal is assessed by eye opening. A spontaneous opening of the eyes should occur when a person is spoken to by the examiner. A painful stimulus can be applied to determine whether the arousal mechanism is intact if eye opening does not occur with verbal and auditory stimuli. Awareness is assessed by determining the patient's orientation to self and environment. Assessment of person, place, and time (day, month, year) is the most effective method to evaluate awareness.[5,14]

The assessment of mood and behavior also is included in a mental examination, because a particular mood may be associated with a specific disease. For example, emotional lability often is seen in bilateral (diffuse) brain disease, where the mood shifts easily and quickly from one extreme to the other. Euphoria is a superficial elevation of mood accompanied by unconcern even in the presence of threatening events. It needs to be determined whether the person's mood is appropriate to the topic of conversation. Personality changes with the appearance of violent temper and aggressive behavior may occur with destructive lesions of the inferior frontal parts of the limbic system. Such behaviors can be validated by family and friends.

The individual's knowledge and vocabulary are tested in reference to common knowledge of current events. The ability to think abstractly may be tested by asking the person to explain the meaning of a proverb. Calculation is tested by examining the ability to serially subtract 7 from 100. Dyscalculia is the inability to solve simple problems. Recent memory loss is more common in brain disease than is remote memory loss. The findings of these gross tests may indicate the need for more definitive tests of mental function.

## LANGUAGE AND SPEECH

Language ability is concentrated in a cortical field that includes parts of the temporal lobe, the temporoparietal-occipital junction, the frontal lobe of the dominant (usually the left) hemisphere, and the occipital lobes. Lesions in any of these areas will produce some impairment of language ability.

To assess language and speech, it is important to distinguish between aphasia and dysarthria. *Aphasia* is the general term for impairment of language function; it represents a disorder of symbolic language. *Dysarthria,* on the other hand, is

**table 51-7** *Types of Aphasia*

| Type | Definition | Site of Lesion |
|---|---|---|
| **MOTOR (EXPRESSIVE)** | Impairment of ability to speak and write. Patient can understand written and spoken words. | Insula and surrounding region including Broca's motor area. |
| Anomic | Inability to name objects, qualities, and conditions although speech is fluent | Area of angular gyrus |
| Fluent | Speech is well articulated and grammatically correct but is lacking in content and meaning | |
| Nonfluent | Problems in selecting, organizing, and initiating speech patterns<br>May also affect writing | Motor cortex at Broca's area |
| **SENSORY (RECEPTIVE)** | Impairment of ability to understand written or spoken language | Disease of auditory and visual word centers |
| Wernicke's | As above | Wernicke's area of left hemisphere |
| **MIXED APHASIA** | Combined expressive and receptive aphasia deficits | Damage to various speech and language areas |
| **GLOBAL APHASIA** | Total aphasia involving all functions that make up speech and communication<br>Few if any intact language skills | Severe damage to speech areas |

an indistinctness in word articulation or enunciation resulting from interference with the peripheral speech mechanisms (e.g., the muscles of the tongue, palate, pharynx, or lips).[13] Gross assessment of speech and language is made while the history is being taken.

### Aphasia

Several different types of aphasia have been identified: (1) fluent, (2) nonfluent, and (3) global. Although one type often predominates, one or more of the other types is commonly detected to some degree. (See Table 51-7 for further information on the aphasias.) Aphasic problems can be detected by assessing spontaneous speech and by asking the examinee to follow simple commands, written and oral; to read and interpret newspaper stories; or to write down thoughts.

### Dysarthria

The ability to produce speech is tested through the detection of weakness or incoordination of muscles used in articulating speech. Limitations are observed during cranial nerve testing, particularly in cranial nerves V, VII, IX, X, and XII. Involvement of the motor component of these nerves may produce alterations in phonation, resonance, and articulation. The examiner asks the individual to produce different speech sounds to localize the problem.

Dysarthrias are usually noticed during ordinary conversation or by having the person repeat a difficult phrase such as "Methodist Episcopal" or "third riding artillery brigade." Dysarthrias may be manifested by a single alteration or a variety of alterations, and there are characteristic changes in particular diseases. For example, in cerebellar disease, speech is often thick with a prolongation of speech sounds occurring at intervals (scanning). In parkinsonism, speech is characterized by a decrease in loudness and a change in vocal emphasis patterns that makes sounds seem monotonous.

## PERCEPTION

Sensation is integrated and interpreted in the sensory cortex, especially in the parietal lobe. It is important for the nurse to recognize perceptual problems, because they can be more difficult to deal with than changes in the patient's ability to move or sense. Disorders of perception commonly involve spatial-temporal relationships or the perception of self.[1,11]

The ability to recognize objects through any of the special senses is known as gnosia. Lesions involving a specific association area of the cortex produce a specific type of agnosia (absence of this ability). One type of ability often tested is stereognosis, the ability to perceive an object's nature and form by touch. This is assessed by asking the person to identify familiar objects placed in the hand one at a time while keeping the eyes closed.

Apraxia is another perceptual problem often seen. This is the inability to perform skilled, purposeful movements in the absence of motor, sensory, or coordination losses. (See Table 51-8 for different types of apraxia.)

### Sensory Status

Accurate assessment of sensory function depends on the person's cooperation, alertness, and responsiveness. The person should be relaxed and have the eyes closed during all portions of the sensory examination to avoid receiving visual clues. Also, sensation should be tested side to side and distally to proximally.

Both superficial and deep sensation are tested on the trunk and extremities. Areas of sensory loss or abnormality are mapped out on a body diagram according to the distribution

**table 51-8** *Apraxia*

| Type | Impairment Produced | Lesion Site |
|---|---|---|
| Constructional | Impairment in producing designs in two or three dimensions<br>Involves copying, drawing, or constructing | Occipitoparietal lobe of either hemisphere |
| Dressing | Inability to dress oneself accurately<br>Makes mistakes, as putting clothes on backwards, upside-down, inside-out, or putting both legs in the same pant leg | Occipital or parietal lobe usually in nondominant hemisphere |
| Motor | Loss of kinesthetic memory patterns, which results in patient's inability to perform a purposeful motor task although it is understood | Frontal lobe of either hemisphere, precentral gyrus |
| Idiomotor | Inability to imitate gestures or perform a purposeful motor task on command<br>May be able to do task spontaneously | Parietal lobe of dominant hemisphere, supramarginal gyrus |
| Ideational | Inability to carry out activities automatically or on command because of inability to understand the concept of the act | Parietal lobe of dominant hemisphere or diffuse brain damage as in arteriosclerosis |

of the spinal dermatomes and peripheral nerves (see Figure 51-17). A dermatome, or skin segment, may be thought of as the area of skin supplied by one dorsal root of a cutaneous nerve. An area in which sensation is absent (anesthesia) is differentiated from areas in which sensation is intensified (hyperesthesia) or lessened (hypesthesia or hypoesthesia). Paresthesia is an abnormal sensation that is perceived as burning, prickly, or itching.

### *Pain, temperature, and touch*

Superficial pain perception is assessed by stimulating an area by pinprick and asking the person to report discomfort. Sharp and dull objects can be alternated for increased discrimination. Deep pain can be assessed by multiple means, some of which have the potential of causing tissue injury. It is necessary to assess deep pain only when the person has a decreased level of consciousness. Deep pain can be assessed by applying pressure over the nailbeds or supraorbitally. Pressure may also be applied over bony areas, such as the sternum. Nailbed pressure is applied by placing a pen or similar object on the nailbed and squeezing it between the examiner's thumb and forefinger (Figure 51-20). Deep pain may also be elicited by squeezing the trapezius muscle. Pinching and pricking may damage tissues and are avoided whenever possible.[7]

Crude touch may be assessed by touching an area with cotton and requesting that the person indicate when the touch is felt. Temperature is tested by touching particular areas with warm to hot and cool to cold objects and asking the person to state the sensations felt. Because pain and temperature have the same nerve pathway (lateral spinothalamic), testing for temperature can be eliminated in the routine examination if the tests for pain perception are normal.

### *Motion and position*

Proprioceptive fibers (fasciculus gracilis and fasciculus cuneatus) transmit sensory impulses from muscles, tendons, ligaments, and joints. This results in an awareness of the position of one's limbs in space (kinesthetic sense). Proprioception is tested by the examiner's grasping the sides of the person's distal phalanx and moving it up and down. If proprioception is intact, the person reports correctly the direction in which the joint is being moved. Proprioceptive abilities can also be assessed by the Romberg test, in which the person is asked to stand erect with the feet together and the eyes closed. A positive test occurs when the person loses balance, which indicates a pathological condition.

Vibration is tested by placing a low-frequency tuning fork on a bony prominence of each extremity and assessing the person's ability to feel it.

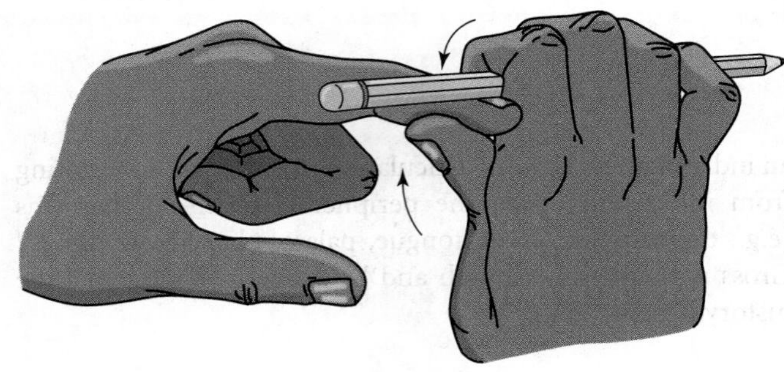

**fig. 51-20** Nailbed pressure stimulation using pencil.

## OBJECTIVE DATA

The sequence of the neurological examination varies with the examiner, but it should be one that ensures completeness without exhausting the person being examined. The examination depends largely on inspection and palpation and only occasionally on percussion. Auscultation may be used to detect related vascular abnormalities. Initially, functions may be tested grossly, followed by definitive testing

**table 51-9** *The Cranial Nerves and Their Functions*

| Cranial Nerves | Function |
|---|---|
| Olfactory (I) | Sensory: smell reception and interpretation |
| Optic (II) | Sensory: visual acuity and visual fields |
| Oculomotor (III) | Motor: raise eyelids, most extraocular movements |
| | Parasympathetic: pupillary constriction, change lens shape |
| Trochlear (IV) | Motor: downward, inward eye movement |
| Trigeminal (V) | Motor: jaw opening and clenching, chewing and mastication |
| | Sensory: sensation to cornea, iris, lacrimal glands, conjunctiva eyelids, forehead, nose, nasal and mouth mucosa, teeth, tongue, ear, facial skin |
| Abducens (VI) | Motor: lateral eye movement |
| Facial (VII) | Motor: movement of facial expression muscles except jaw, close eyes, labial speech sounds (b, m, w, and rounded vowels) |
| | Sensory: taste—anterior two thirds of tongue, sensation to pharynx |
| Acoustic (VIII) | Parasympathetic: secretion of saliva and tears |
| Glossopharyngeal (IX) | Sensory: hearing and equilibrium |
| | Motor: voluntary muscles for swallowing and phonation |
| | Sensory: sensation of nasopharynx, gag reflex, taste—posterior one third of tongue |
| | Parasympathetic: secretion of salivary glands, carotid reflex |
| Vagus (X) | Motor: voluntary muscles of phonation (guttural speech sounds) and swallowing |
| | Sensory: sensation behind ear and part of external ear canal |
| | Parasympathetic: secretion of digestive enzymes; peristalsis; carotid reflex; involuntary action of heart, lungs, and digestive tract |
| Spinal accessory (XI) | Motor: turn head, shrug shoulders, some actions for phonation |
| Hypoglossal (XII) | Motor: tongue movement for speech sound articulation (l, t, n) and swallowing |

From Seidel HM et al: *Mosby's guide to physical examination,* ed 3, St Louis, 1995, Mosby.

should an abnormality be identified. Equipment commonly used in a neurological examination is listed in Box 51-1.

**box 51-1** *Equipment Needed to Perform a Neurological Examination*

1. Compass
2. Cotton applicators
3. Diagram of dermatomes
4. Dynamometer
5. Flashlight
6. Miscellaneous items of varied shapes and sizes (coin, key, marble)
7. Ophthalmoscope
8. Otoscope
9. Colored pencil
10. Pins with sharp and blunt ends
11. Printed page
12. Reflex hammer
13. Tape measure
14. Tongue depressors
15. Tuning fork
16. Snellen chart
17. Stoppered vials containing:
    a. Peppermint, oil of cloves, coffee, soap (smell)
    b. Sugar, salt, vinegar, quinine (taste)
    c. Cold and hot water (temperature)
18. Watch with second hand

## CRANIAL NERVES

The 12 cranial nerves may be tested in numbered sequence (Table 51-9). Some nurses prefer to test at the same time those cranial nerves with similar function, such as voluntary motor function, visceral motor function, and special sensory or general sensory functions. It should be recalled, however, that some cranial nerves have both motor and sensory functions.[7]

### Cranial Nerve I (Olfactory)

The function of cranial nerve I is purely sensory, namely, smell. Special receptors located within the superior or uppermost part of each nasal chamber transmit neural impulses over the olfactory bulbs to the olfactory nerves in the area of the central cortex concerned with olfaction. When testing this cranial nerve the nurse asks if the patient smells an odor. If yes the patient is asked to name the odor. Awareness of an odor must be differentiated from the ability to name a specific substance. Anosmia (absence of smell) or hyposmia (decreased sensitivity of the sense of smell) is often associated with complaints of lack of taste, even though tests may demonstrate that sense to be intact. Anosmia is caused by varied lesions involving any part of the olfactory pathways.

### Cranial Nerve II (Optic)

The function of cranial nerve II is purely sensory, namely, sight or vision. When the retina is stimulated, nerve impulses are transmitted over the optic nerves (extending from the optic disc to the chiasm), and the optic tracts with the radiations terminating in the visual cortex of the occipital lobes. As shown in Figure 51-21, the medial (nasal) fibers of each optic nerve cross at the chiasm to the opposite side of the brain, whereas the lateral (temporal) fibers remain uncrossed. Thus fibers of the left optic tract contain fibers from only the left half of each retina and carry impulses to the left occipital lobe; fibers of the right optic tract contain fibers from only the right half of each retina and carry impulses to the right occipital lobe. Optic nerve function is assessed in relation to visual acuity, visual fields, and the appearance of the fundus. Each eye is tested separately.

### Visual acuity

Visual acuity is mediated by the cones of the retina. Central vision is grossly tested by reading newspaper print. Distance visual acuity is assessed through the use of the Snellen chart (see Chapter 55). Individuals with vision impairment are tested to determine light perception (LP), hand movement (HM), and finger count (FC).

### Visual fields

Field of vision is defined as the range in which objects are visible when vision is fixed in one direction. The field of vision thus relates to peripheral vision, or indirect vision. As in visual acuity, normality depends on the intactness of all parts of the visual pathway of the eye. The visual fields are tested grossly by confrontation techniques. A confrontation technique involves moving an object into the periphery of each of the quadrants of the eye. The person is instructed to cover one eye and fix the other eye on a point straight ahead. The patient reports when the moving object is first detected at the edge of each visual field. The examiner's finger may be used as the moving object. Visual fields may be altered in a variety of central nervous system diseases, such as neoplasia and vascular disease. Ocular disease such as glaucoma is a major cause. Damage to one optic nerve anterior to the chiasm affects only the field of the involved eye. Lesions at the chiasm or posterior to it produce a variety of bilateral visual field defects as shown in Figure 51-21. For example, compression of the optic chiasm damages the crossing fibers from the nasal retina and causes bitemporal hemianopsia, or the loss of vision in the temporal halves of each eye. Loss of vision in the corresponding halves of both visual fields produces homonymous hemianopsia, which can be further designated as right or left.

### Ocular fundus

The ocular fundus is defined as that portion of the interior of the eyeball that lies posterior to the lens. It includes the optic disc, blood vessels, retina, and macula. Examination, although painless in the normal eye, does require cooperation from the person being examined and is performed with an ophthalmoscope.

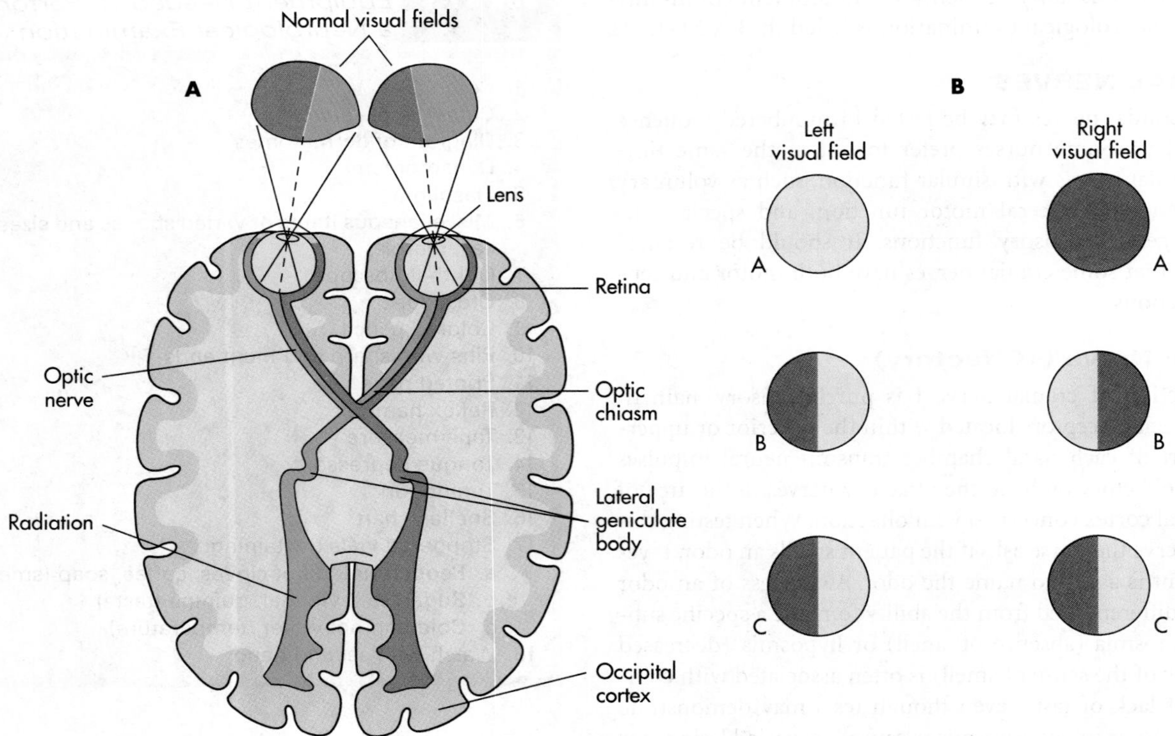


**fig. 51-21 A,** Visual pathways showing partial decussation of optic chiasm. Normal visual fields show reversal of light rays from the temporal and nasal sides to receptors in the retina. **B,** Abnormal visual fields. *A,* Normal left field of vision with loss of vision in right field as a result of complete lesion of right optic nerve. *B,* Loss of vision in temporal half of both fields as a result of lesion of optic chiasm (bitemporal hemianopia). *C,* Loss of vision in nasal field of right eye and temporal field of left eye caused by lesion of right optic tract (homonymous hemianopia).

### Examination and interpretation of ophthalmoscopic findings

The optic disc (papilla) is normally the most prominent structure visible; it is the center of observation from which the funduscopic examination proceeds. The optic disc is the area where the blood vessels and nerve fibers enter and exit from the eyeball (Figure 51-22). The normal characteristics of the optic disc are presented in Table 51-10.

The disc is examined in detail to assess size, shape, margins, and color. There can be excessive pallor or redness. Swelling of the optic disc, or papilledema, may be caused by active inflammation or passive congestion. Papilledema that results from passive congestion or increased intracranial pressure is also called a choked disc. Optic atrophy indicates partial or complete destruction of the optic nerve. It is associated with decreased visual acuity and with a change in the color of the disc to a lighter pink or gray. The largest blood vessels visible in the fundus, the central retinal artery and central retinal vein, branch throughout the retina. The retina is the only site in the human body where the microcirculation can be viewed directly.

## Cranial Nerve III (Oculomotor), Cranial Nerve IV (Trochlear), and Cranial Nerve VI (Abducens)

Cranial nerves III, IV, and VI are motor nerves that arise from the brainstem and innervate the six extraocular muscles attached to the eyeball. These muscles function as a group in the coordinated movement of each eyeball in the six cardinal fields of gaze, giving the eye both straight and rotary movement. The four straight, or rectus, muscles are the superior, inferior, lateral, and medial rectus muscles. The two slanting, or oblique, muscles are the superior and inferior (Figure 51-23).

Each muscle is coordinated with one in the other eye. This ensures that when the two eyes move their axes always remain parallel (conjugate movement). Parallel axes are important to present the brain with only one visual image with a binocular system. A single image is possible because the eyes move as a pair.

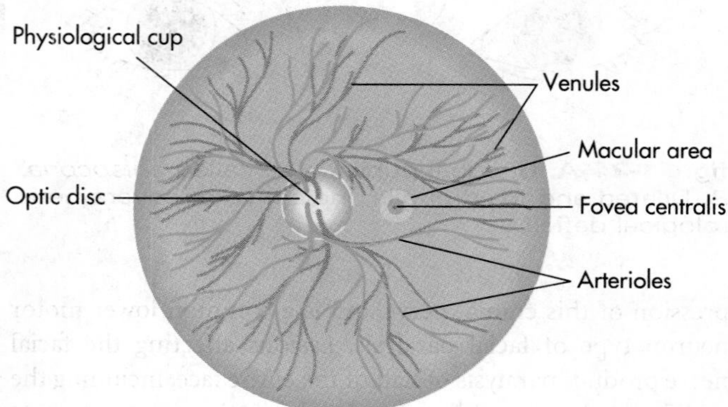


**fig. 51-22** Structures of the left eye as visualized through the ophthalmoscope.

### Extraocular movements

Eye movements are tested by covering one eye and following the examiner's finger in all fields of gaze with the uncovered eye while keeping the head stationary. Limitation of movement in any direction is noted, as well as actual paralysis (ophthalmoplegia). If one of the extraocular muscles is paralyzed, the eye is unable to deviate fully into the corresponding field of gaze.

Conjugate movements of the eyes also are tested by asking the person to look as far as possible to either side, then up and down, and then obliquely, as shown in Figure 51-23. The examiner observes for parallel movements of the eyes in each direction or any deviation from normal.

Double vision (diplopia), squint (strabismus), and involuntary rhythmic movements of the eyeballs (nystagmus) may indicate weakness of some of the extraocular muscles because of deficits of the motor nerves. Ptosis, or drooping of the upper eyelid over the globe, may be caused by damage to the oculomotor nerve. Normally, the upper lid minimally overlaps the iris as the person moves the eyes downward. The person with ptosis is unable to raise the lid voluntarily.

**Pupils.** Each pupil should be inspected first as to size and then as to shape and equality. Argyll Robertson pupils, for example, are constricted and do not react to light, although they react to accommodation for near objects. Pupil inequality, or anisocoria, may assist in diagnosis of some neurological diseases (Figure 51-24, *A*). The pupil is normally round, centrally placed, regular in outline, and equal in size to the other pupil. However, unequal pupils are found in approximately 25% of the normal population. Thus the briskness of the pupillary response is the more important part of the assessment.

**Direct light reflex.** The examiner darkens the room and focuses a small beam of light directly into each pupil. Normally, the pupil constricts quickly when a light is focused on the retina. Constriction is reported to be especially brisk in young people and those with blue eyes. After a head injury a dilated, fixed pupil may be observed on the side of the cranial injury (Figure 51-24, B). A slow or sluggish pupil occurs as the pupil contracts slowly or imperfectly and relaxes immediately.[8]

**Consensual light reflex.** Observations include inspection for constriction of the pupil opposite the one directly stimulated. As a result of the decussation (crossing) of nerve fibers both in the optic chiasm and in the pretectal area,

**table 51-10** *Normal Characteristics of the Optic Disc*

| | |
|---|---|
| Size | 1.5 mm |
| Shape | Flat round or vertically oval |
| Margins | Sharply defined |
| Color | Creamy red with a small whitish depression in the center (physiological cup) |

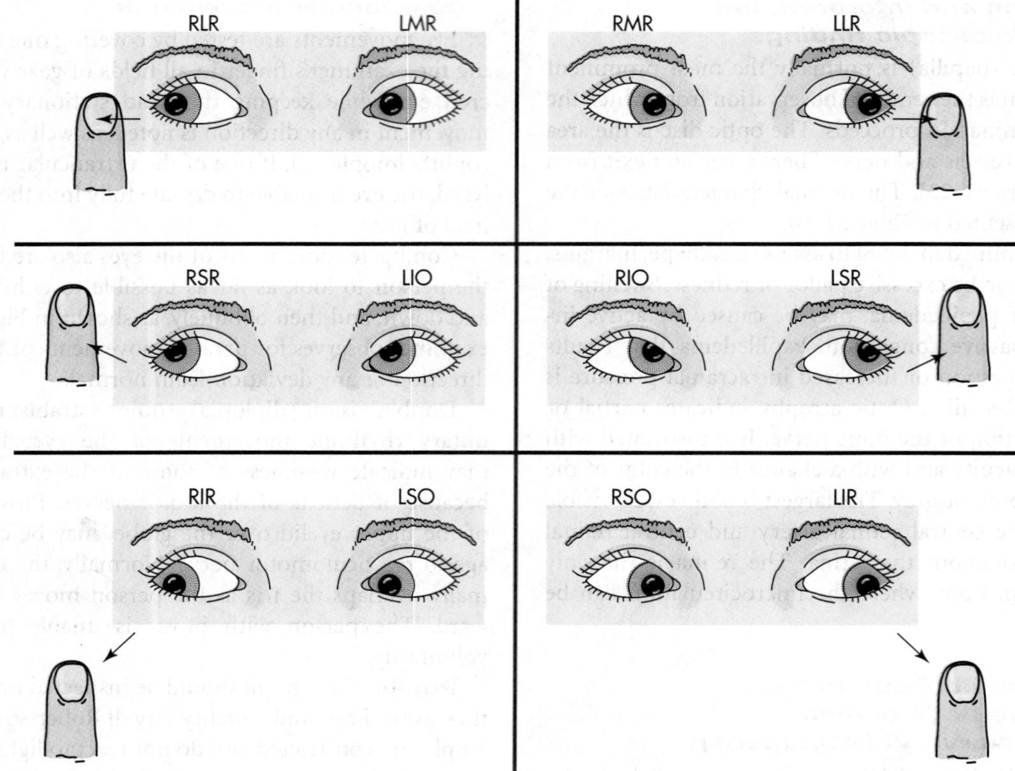


**fig. 51-23** Examination of extraocular muscles. Note that two muscles are involved in each cardinal direction. *R,* right; *L,* left; *LR,* lateral rectus; *MR,* medial rectus; *SR,* superior rectus; *IO,* inferior oblique; *IR,* inferior rectus; *SO,* superior oblique.

both the homolateral and contralateral pupil normally react to light.

### Cranial Nerve V (Trigeminal)

Cranial nerve V is a mixed nerve with motor and sensory components. It is the largest cranial nerve. The motor part innervates the temporal and masseter muscles; the sensory part supplies the cornea, face, head, and mucous membranes of the nose and mouth.

If muscle weakness is present the opened jaw tends to deviate to the side opposite the weakened muscles. The sensory components supplying the face are tested for touch, pain, and temperature. Bilateral corneal reflexes may also be assessed. Normally, the person blinks laterally. This is an especially important reflex to assess in persons with decreased levels of consciousness because the absence of the blink reflex can result in corneal damage.

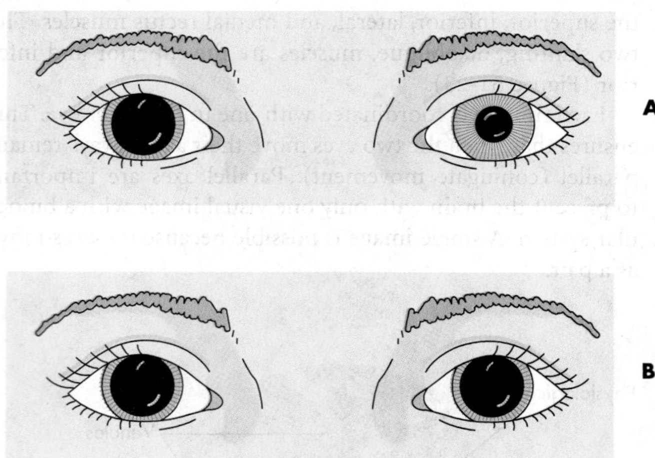


**fig. 51-24 A,** Unequal pupils, also called *anisocoria.* **B,** Dilated and fixed pupils, indicative of severe neurological deficit.

### Cranial Nerve VII (Facial)

Cranial nerve VII is a mixed nerve that is concerned with facial movement and the sensation of taste. The inability to smile, close both eyes tightly, look upward, wrinkle the forehead, show the teeth, purse the lips, and blow out the cheeks constitutes weakness or paralysis of facial muscles innervated by this nerve. Special attention is given to asymmetry. Distinction must be made between central and peripheral neurological involvement. Peripheral involvement is caused by compression of this cranial nerve and is a common lower motor neuron type of facial paralysis. Lesions affecting the facial nerve produce paralysis of half of the entire face, including the eyelids, forehead, and lips. Forehead function remains intact in central or upper motor neuron lesions and suggests that the lesion lies somewhere on the path from the cerebral cortex to the nucleus of the facial nerve.

The sensation of taste is tested by placing salty, sweet, bitter, and sour substances, in turn, on the side of the protruded tongue for identification. A loss of taste over the anterior two thirds of the tongue is present when this nerve is diseased, as occurs in mastoid canal lesions.

### Cranial Nerve VIII (Acoustic)

Cranial nerve VIII is composed of a cochlear division related to hearing and a vestibular division related to equilibrium. The cochlear portion is tested grossly by having the person listen and identify whispered words. A more complete examination, including bone and air conduction of sound, involves assessment with a tuning fork and audiometric testing (Chapter 57).

Disease of the cochlea is characterized by nerve deafness (perception deafness), which is usually the result of disease of the peripheral nerve. The ability to hear is lost or impaired. It also may occur from central lesions involving the acoustic nerve and nerve pathways in the brainstem and temporal lobe.

The vestibular portion of the acoustic nerve may be tested in a variety of ways. In the past-pointing test, the person is asked to raise the arms and bring the index finger down on the examiner's finger with the arm outstretched, first with the eyes open and then with the eyes closed. Normally, the person's finger touches the examiner's without difficulty. In vestibular disease, the finger points to one side or the other consistently. The person is also assessed for the presence of nystagmus "to-and-fro" movements of the eyeballs on horizontal and vertical planes, as they look to the side and upward. True nystagmus is characterized by sustained movement of the eyeball including a fast jerk to the side of the deviation and a slow jerk back to the midline. The vestibular portion of the acoustic nerve commonly is affected in diseases of the central nervous system, and the most important symptom is vertigo.

### Cranial Nerve IX (Glossopharyngeal) and Cranial Nerve X (Vagus)

Cranial nerves IX and X are tested together. The chief function of cranial nerve IX is sensory to the pharynx and taste to the posterior third of the tongue. Both nerves supply the posterior pharyngeal wall, and normally when the wall is touched there is prompt contraction of these muscles on both sides, with or without gagging. This test is thus unreliable for either nerve alone. Because cranial nerve X is the chief motor nerve to the soft palatal, pharyngeal, and laryngeal muscles, assessment includes testing voice and cough sounds. In unilateral involvement of the motor portion of the vagus nerve the voice is harsh and nasal. When the person says "ah," the soft palate does not stay in the midline but deviates to the intact side. Bilateral involvement produces more severe speech problems; swallowing is difficult (dysphagia), and fluids regurgitate through the nose because of palatal and pharyngeal involvement. Sensory function of the vagus usually is not tested.

### Cranial Nerve XI (Spinal Accessory)

Cranial nerve XI is a motor nerve that supplies the sternocleidomastoid muscle and the upper part of the trapezius muscles. The muscles are assessed for weakness and paralysis.

### Cranial Nerve XII (Hypoglossal)

Cranial nerve XII is a purely motor nerve. The person's tongue is first inspected at rest. Any asymmetry, unilaterality, decreased bulk, deviations, or fasciculations (fine twitching) are noted. When this nerve is involved, the tongue deviates toward the side of the lesion. In an upper motor neuron lesion the tongue is affected on the side opposite the lesion (contralateral). Atrophy of the tongue is shown through wrinkling and loss of substance on the affected side.

## MOTOR STATUS

Function of the motor system is assessed through gait and stance, muscle strength, muscle tonus, coordination, involuntary movements, and muscle stretch reflexes.

### Gait and Stance

Gait and stance are complex activities that require muscle strength, coordination, balance, proprioception, and vision. Gait, or walking, and associated movements give considerable information about motor status. Changes in gait may be characteristic of a specific neurological disease. Ataxia is a general term meaning lack of coordination in performing a planned, purposeful motion such as walking. Ataxia can be caused by disturbance of position sense or by cerebellar or other diseases. To evaluate gait the person is asked to walk freely and naturally and then walk heel to toe in a straight-line, tandem walk, because this exaggerates any abnormalities. To evaluate stance, the person is asked to perform the Romberg test standing with the feet close together, first with eyes open and then with eyes closed. Patients with problems of proprioception have difficulty maintaining balance with their eyes closed; patients with cerebellar disease have difficulty even with their eyes open.

A variety of distinctive gaits characterize specific neurological disorders. The hemiparetic gait seen in upper motor neuron disease is characterized by circumduction of the affected leg and inversion of the foot. Persons with Parkinson's disease walk with a slow, shuffling gait, and as they start walking, an increase in rapidity occurs until they are almost running (propulsive). They also have difficulty stopping, and deviation in the center of gravity causes retropulsion or lateropulsion. In addition, loss of associated movements of the arms in walking is noticeable. Persons with cerebellar disease, on the other hand, walk with a wide-based, staggering gait.

Muscle strength, or power, is assessed systematically, including trunk and extremity muscles. One common assessment of muscle strength is asking the patient to grasp both hands of the nurse and squeeze them simultaneously. The nurse compares the squeezing ability of one hand with the other. Assessment of muscular strength of the feet can be performed by plantar flexion and dorsiflexion. During manual testing of these and other muscle groups, the person attempts to resist the force applied by the nurse in moving the muscles. Impairment of any specific muscle is identified by the nurse as to distribution and degree of muscle weakness.

The person may also be tested for drift by asking the person to hold the arms straight out for 20 to 30 seconds with palms up and eyes closed. Hemiparesis is suggested when there is pronation of one forearm or a downward drift of the arm.

Motor evaluation may include all major muscles. Hemiplegia is complete paralysis of one half of the body (linear), whereas hemiparesis is weakness or incomplete paralysis. Paraplegia is paralysis of the lower extremities, and quadriplegia is paralysis of the four extremities.

### Muscle Tonus

Resting skeletal muscles have a certain number of fibers that are always partially contracted because of continual stimulation to receptors of certain reflex arcs, especially the stretch reflex. The minimal degree of contraction exhibited by a muscle at rest is called muscle tone. When some of the lower motor neurons or afferent fibers innervating neuromuscular spindles are injured, there is a reduction in the stimulation of a muscle and a concomitant loss of tone referred to as hypotonia. In contrast, a muscle with increased tone is hypertonic.

To test muscle tonus the nurse passively moves the person's limbs through a full range of motion. A skilled examiner can differentiate hypertonic from hypotonic muscles. Hypertonic extremities tend to stay in fixed positions and feel firm; hypotonic extremities assume a position governed by gravity. Overextension and overflexion are found in hypertonia; resistance to passive movement increases rapidly and then suddenly gives way to pyramidal spasticity, or clasp-knife rigidity. A steady, passive resistance throughout the full range of motion is characteristic of parkinsonian rigidity; the combination of passive resistance and parkinsonian tremor with small regular jerks is called cogwheel rigidity. In decorticate rigidity the upper limbs are flexed and pronated and the lower limbs are extended. In decerebrate rigidity, however, the upper limbs are extended.

### Coordination

Coordination of muscle movements, or the ability to perform skilled motor acts, may be impaired at any level of the motor system. However, the cerebellum is primarily responsible for control, so that movements take place in a smooth and precise manner. Disturbance in cerebellar function may result in ataxia, difficulty in controlling the range of muscular movement (dysmetria), and an inability to alternate rapid opposite and successive movements (adiadochokinesia). Simple motor activities are evaluated by asking the person to perform rapid rhythmic movements, such as the nose-finger-nose test, which requires the individual to alternately touch the nose and the tip of the nurse's finger, or the knee pat (pronation-supination).

### Involuntary Movements

Involuntary movements are also assessed and described during neurological examination. It is important to observe the location of muscles involved, amplitude of movement, speed of onset, duration of contraction and relaxation, and rhythm. The effects of posture, rest, sleep, distraction, voluntary movements, and emotional stress on involuntary movement are determined. Emotional stress usually increases involuntary movements, and they may subside during sleep. Abnormal movements may be the result of organic disease or may be psychosomatic in origin.

Tremor consists of rhythmic to-and-fro movements, usually of small amplitude. They are the result of alternate contractions of opposing groups of muscles, are continuous while the patient is awake, and may or may not be present during sleep. Chorea consists of short, sharp, rapid movements, usually of small excursion and irregular; movements occur in different parts of the body and persist during sleep. Hemiballismus is a variation of chorea in which movement is confined to one side of the body and affects the limbs to a great extent. Athetosis consists of slow, sinuous, and more sustained movements that may be of considerable amplitude; movements occur in the neck and trunk, as well as the extremities. Myoclonus consists of irregular, abrupt, and arrhythmic contractions of a muscle or a group of muscles in the extremities, trunk, or face.

### Reflexes

A reflex is a predictable response that results from a nerve input over a reflex arc. The term reflex is typically used to describe involuntary responses. Although all muscles can be made to undergo reflex contraction, many are not tested clinically.[15]

The stretch (myotatic) reflex is a two-neuron (monosynaptic) reflex arc. A well-known example is the knee-jerk reflex, or patellar reflex, which is produced by tapping the patellar tendon of the relaxed quadriceps femoris muscle (Figure 51-25). Such a reflex is described as ipsilateral because the response occurs on the same side of the body and spinal cord where the stimulus is received. Tapping on the patellar tendon elicits a stretching of the quadriceps tendon and its muscles along with some neuromuscular spindles within the muscle and generates nerve impulses. Afferent fibers convey these nerve impulses to the L2-L3 vertebral level of the spinal cord. The afferent neurons synapse with the lower motor neurons, which are large spinal neurons. Axons carry the impulse rapidly to the motor end plates of the quadriceps muscle, which stimulates contraction and extension of the lower leg.

Any abnormal reflex response may indicate a disorder of the nervous system. Hyporeflexia occurs when a reflex is less responsive than normal resulting from a lesion of the lower motor neurons; hyperreflexia, a reflex more responsive than normal, occurs from lesions in upper motor pathways. Some of the more common diagnostic reflexes tested are listed in Table 51-11.

Assessment of reflexes requires an experienced examiner, a reflex hammer, and a relaxed patient. The reflex is elicited by striking the hammer onto the muscle's insertion tendon. Comparison of right and left sides should reveal equal responses. The reflex response is graded on a subjective, four-point scale that requires clinical practice to use accurately (Table 51-12). If the reflex response fails to appear on the first attempt, the nurse encourages the person to relax by varying position or increases the strength of the hammer blow.

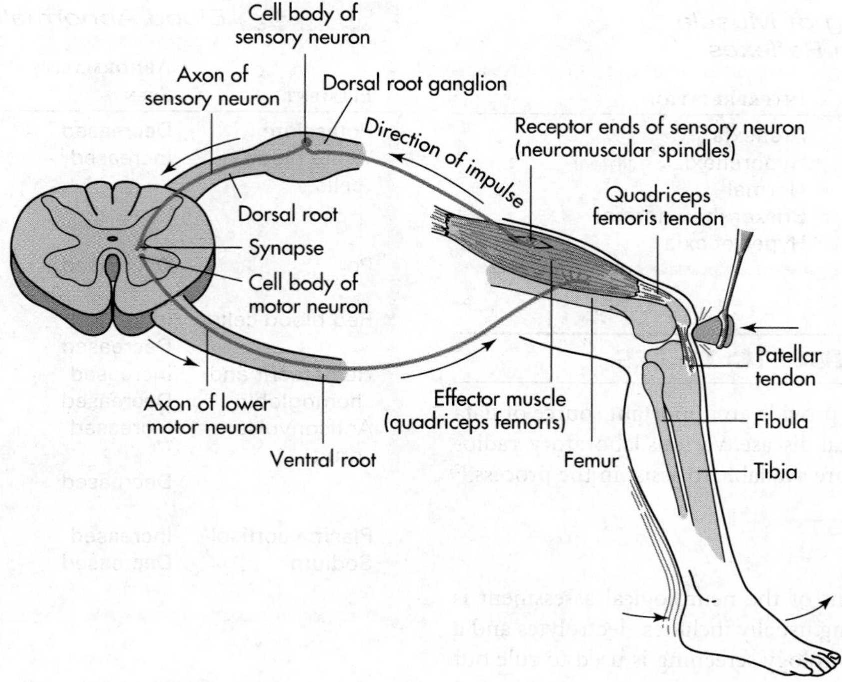


**fig. 51-25** The two-neuron patellar reflex, or "knee jerk."

**table 51-11** *Some Diagnostic Reflexes of the Central Nervous System*

| Reflex | Description | Indication |
|---|---|---|
| Abdominal reflex | Anterior stroking of the sides of lower torso causes contraction of abdominal muscles. | Absence of reflex indicates lesions of peripheral nerves or in reflex centers in lower thoracic segments of spinal cord; may also indicate multiple sclerosis. |
| Archilles reflex (ankle jerk) | Tapping of calcaneal (Achilles) tendon of soleus and gastrocnemius muscles causes both muscles to contract, producing plantar flexion of foot. | Absence of reflex may indicate damage to nerves innervating posterior leg muscles or to lumbosacral neurons; may also indicate chronic diabetes, alcoholism, syphilis, subarachnoid hemorrhage. |
| Biceps reflex | Tapping of biceps tendon in elbow produces contraction of brachialis and biceps muscles, producing flexion at elbow. | Absence of reflex may indicate damage at the C5 or C6 vertebral level. |
| Brudzinski's reflex | Forceful flexion of neck produces flexion of legs, thighs. | Reflex indicates irritation of meninges. |
| Kernig's reflex | Flexion of hip, with knee straight and patient lying on back, produces flexion of knee. | Reflex indicates irritation of meninges or herniated intervertebral disk. |
| Patellar reflex (knee jerk) | Tapping of patellar tendon causes contraction of quadriceps femoris muscle, producing upward jerk of leg. | Absence of reflex may indicate damage at the L2, L3, or L4 vertebral level; may also indicate chronic diabetes, syphilis. |
| Plantar reflex | Stroking of the lateral part of sole causes toes to curl down. If corticospinal damage, great toe flexes upward and other toes fan out (Babinski's sign). | Reflex indicates damage to upper motor neurons. Normal in children less than 1 year old. |
| Triceps reflex | Tapping of triceps tendon at elbow causes contraction of triceps muscle, producing extension at elbow. | Absence of reflex may indicate damage at C6, C7, or C8 vertebral level. |

**table 51-12** *Grading of Muscle Stretch Reflexes*

| Scale | Interpretation |
|---|---|
| 0 | Areflexia |
| 1+ | Hyporeflexia |
| 2+ | Normal |
| 3+ | Brisker than normal |
| 4+ | Hyperreflexia |

**table 51-13** *Blood Abnormalities*

| Element | Abnormality Seen | Possible Reason |
|---|---|---|
| Potassium | Decreased | Poor dietary intake |
| White blood cells | Increased | Infection such as meningitis |
| | | Common steroid effect |
| $Po_2$ | Decreased | Increased intracranial pressure |
| Red blood cells | Increased | Dehydration |
| | Decreased | Anemia |
| Hematocrit and hemoglobin | Increased | Dehydration |
| | Decreased | Anemia |
| Anticonvulsant drug | Increased | Toxicity or patient overdose |
| | Decreased | Patient not taking drug |
| Plasma cortisol | Increased | Acute head injury |
| Sodium | Decreased | Inappropriate antidiuretic hormone |

## DIAGNOSTIC TESTS

Relevant diagnostic tests provide an important source of data in diagnosing neurological disease. Various laboratory, radiological, and special tests are available to assist in the process.[12]

### LABORATORY TESTS

#### Blood

An important component of the neurological assessment is blood screening. Screening usually includes electrolytes and a complete blood count. Serology screening is used to rule out syphilis, which in its tertiary form may cause neurological symptoms. Arterial blood gases offer valuable information regarding oxygen and carbon dioxide levels. Additionally, drug levels may be drawn, which can give the practitioner a sense of the way a person metabolizes the drug and the person's compliance with the medication regimen. Abnormalities in any of the blood studies may be indicative of neurological disease. (See Table 51-13 for some specific abnormalities.)

#### Urine

Urine output and electrolyte excretion are easily influenced by cranial surgery and trauma. This is especially true if the pituitary gland is involved. (See Table 51-14 for possible alterations in urinary results.)

#### Cerebrospinal Fluid

Cerebrospinal fluid (CSF) is a clear fluid that is formed in the third, fourth, and lateral ventricles of the brain. Samples are obtained through either a lumbar or cisternal puncture and examined for any increase or decrease in its normal constituents and for foreign substances such as pathogenic organisms and blood.

Spinal fluid normally is under slight positive pressure; 75 to 180 mm $H_2O$ is considered normal. The pressure is measured on a manometer when a lumbar puncture is performed.

Normally each milliliter of spinal fluid contains up to eight lymphocytes. An increase in the number of cells may indicate infection. Tuberculosis and viral infections may cause an increase in lymphocytes; an increase in polymorphonuclear leukocytes from pyogenic infections may cause the CSF to become cloudy. Likewise, an alteration in CSF components may occur from bacterial infections, such as tuberculosis meningitis, which lower CSF glucose and chloride levels. Degenerative diseases and tumors usually cause an increased protein level in the CSF. (See Table 51-15 for normal values of CSF.)

Another test of CSF useful in diagnosing neurosyphilis or multiple sclerosis is the colloidal gold test. Cerebrospinal fluid is abnormal in about 90% of patients with multiple sclerosis, including CSF pleocytosis and abnormal gamma globulins as demonstrated by electrophoresis. Additionally, a culture of CSF may be obtained to assist in organism detection in an ill patient. Cerebrospinal fluid testing for syphilis is important because blood tests are often negative whereas CSF tests are positive.

Blood in the spinal fluid indicates hemorrhage into the ventricular system. It may be caused by a fracture at the base of the skull that has torn blood vessels or by the rupture of a blood vessel (e.g., with a congenital aneurysm). Occasionally, the first specimen of CSF contains blood from the trauma of the lumbar puncture. Therefore the specimens of CSF are numbered and the first vial is not used to determine the cell count.

### RADIOLOGICAL TESTS

Multiple radiological procedures of the brain and spinal cord may be performed, including plain radiographs, special contrast studies of the ventricular system and the cerebral vessels, and computed tomography.

#### Routine or Plain Radiographs

Plain radiographs of the brain and spinal cord are commonly used as diagnostic tests because they are safe and easily available. They can detect any developmental, traumatic, or degenerative bone abnormalities.

#### Computed Tomography

Computed tomography (CT) scans can provide 100% more information than conventional radiographs, and they provide enhanced image detail. A series of images are x-rayed, and each of the images is derived from a specific layer of brain tis-

**table 51-14** *Urine Abnormalities*

| Element | Abnormality Seen | Possible Reason |
|---|---|---|
| Urinary output | Decreased amount | Metabolic problem<br>Kidney failure |
| | Increased amount | Diabetes insipidus |
| Specific gravity | Decreased | Diabetes insipidus |
| | Increased | Dehydration |
| Glucose and acetone | Present | Steroid effect—possible chemical diabetes |
| Sodium | Increased amount | Inappropriate antidiuretic hormone<br>Diabetes insipidus |

**table 51-15** *Normal Values of Cerebrospinal Fluid*

| | |
|---|---|
| Pressure | 75 to 180 mm $H_2O$ |
| Glucose | 50 to 80 mg/dl |
| Chloride | 118 to 132 mEq/L |
| Protein | 20 to 50 mg/dl |
| Gamma globulin | 3% to 9% |
| Lymphocytes | 0 to 5/ml |

sue. The brain is thus scanned in successive layers by a narrow beam of x-rays.

Data are collected in x-ray and printout form, and information is also stored for future use. By comparing tissue densities found on the CT scan with norms, abnormalities can be detected. Tumor masses, infarctions, and displacement of bone and ventricles can be accurately detected. The CT scan is particularly efficient in detecting brain neoplasia and cerebrovascular lesions.

No special physical preparation is required. The patient should be informed that the CT scan is painless with the exception of insertion of an intravenous access before the procedure for installation of contrast medium. Patients should be assessed for allergies. The length of the procedure will extend from 30 to 60 minutes depending on the use of contrast medium. The patient must be supine with the head positioned in a rubber head holder.

After the completion of the CT scan, the nurse monitors the patient for any signs of increased intracranial pressure (if dye was used). If the patient becomes disoriented as a result of the test, reassurance should be given and the patient protected from injury.

### Brain Scan

The brain scan is a relatively safe and painless procedure that is useful in detecting cerebral pathology using radioactive isotopes and a scanner. The patient is given an intravenous injection of a radionucleotide, and the radioactivity is traced with a gamma scintillation camera or scanner, which converts the rays into images displayed on an oscilloscope screen. The underlying principle of the brain scan is that radionucleotide can penetrate the brain only through a disruption in the blood-brain barrier and subsequently collects in abnormal brain tissue.

Nursing care is primarily focused on the educational needs of the patient. The patient is informed that the injection of radioactive material causes burning at the insertion site, but no dangers are associated with its administration. The patient is told that the scanner oscillates back and forth around the patient's head during the scan and creates some loud noises. All jewelry and metal objects need to be removed before the procedure, which typically takes 45 minutes.

### Myelography

Myelography is performed by introduction of either a gas or a radiopaque liquid into the spinal subarachnoid space following a lumbar or cisternal puncture. Radiographs are taken to assist in the identification of lesions in the intradural or extradural compartments of the spinal canal. Fluoroscopically, the flow of the dye is monitored through the subarachnoid space.

The patient assumes a side-lying position with flexion of the head and knees or sits upright with the head flexed onto the chest. Following a lumbar puncture, dye or air is injected into the spinal canal. Oil-based dyes are aspirated at the completion of the test while the patient is positioned upright to prevent the flow of dye above the level of the spine, which would cause meningeal irritation. Water-based dyes such as Amipaque are absorbed into the bloodstream and require no special considerations.

Food and fluids are restricted for approximately 4 to 8 hours before the procedure. The nurse assesses for any history of allergies to iodine or dyes; the patient is asked to sign a consent form and remove all jewelry and metal objects. Medications such as phenothiazines and tricyclic antidepressants are restricted for 48 hours before the procedure if a water-soluble dye is used. A sedative may be given to relax the patient immediately before the procedure.

After the procedure, the patient must lie supine for several hours if an oil-based dye was used. In contrast, the patient assumes a semirecumbent position with the head elevated 30 to 60 degrees for 24 hours if a water-based dye was injected. These interventions attempt to decrease the incidence of headaches, nausea and vomiting, and seizures in the post-test period. Complaints of neck stiffness or pain with neck flexion are immediately reported to the physician because these symptoms may indicate meningeal irritation. Other nursing interventions include monitoring vital signs and encouraging a liberal fluid intake. The patient is usually able to resume usual diet and activities the following day.

### Cerebral Angiography (Angiogram)

Cerebral angiography involves the injection of a contrast medium into the cerebral arterial circulation, which assists in determining the etiology of strokes, seizures, headaches, and motor weakness. A catheter is inserted into the femoral artery (the most common entry site) and advanced to the carotid and cerebral vessels. Serial films are taken as the dye circulates throughout the cerebral circulation.

The nurse informs the patient that the procedure takes 1 to 2 hours and that a feeling of warmth often occurs after dye injection. The nurse carefully assesses for any allergies to iodine, seafood, or contrast medium. The patient is kept on nothing-by-mouth (NPO) status for 6 to 10 hours before the procedure. Informed consent is required, and jewelry, dentures, and hearing aids are removed before the angiogram. A sedative may be ordered before the test.

The patient remains on bed rest for 12 to 24 hours; however, the duration of bed rest varies among institutions. Vital signs, distal pulses, intake and output, and hemostasis at the insertion site are monitored.

### Digital Subtraction Angiography

Digital subtraction angiography (DSA) is a method of radiographically studying blood vessels and is particularly useful when the area of study is blocked by bone. Intravenous DSA is often preferred over cerebral angiography because less radiation is used, the procedure is cheaper, and there is a lower incidence of serious complications. Images of target areas are taken before and after injection of the dye. Pictures are digitized, stored, and compared in a computer that subtracts anything common between the before (mask) and after (contrast) images.

Patient education needs are addressed by the nurse before the procedure. The patient needs to lie completely still and is assessed carefully for potential allergy related to the contrast medium. After the procedure the insertion site is monitored for bleeding, and neurovascular checks are performed based on institution protocols.

## SPECIAL TESTS

Other tests can be important in determining the nature of neurological symptoms. These include the lumbar puncture, electroencephalogram, and electromyogram.

### Lumbar Puncture

The lumbar puncture is performed to measure pressure and obtain CSF for examination. However, it is not typically performed in the presence of increased intracranial pressure or a suspected brain tumor because of the risk of brainstem herniation into the foramen magnum.

Needle insertion is below the level of the spinal cord at the L4-L5 or L5-S1 interspaces (Figure 51-26). After removal of the inner needle, CSF is collected and measurement of pressure is performed. Queckenstedt's test is routinely performed to assess for subarachnoid blockage by compressing each jugular vein one at a time for approximately 10 seconds while monitoring for changes in spinal fluid pressures.

No dietary or fluid restrictions are required before the test. A consent form must be signed, and a sedative may be ordered. The patient is encouraged to empty the bowel and bladder and is assisted either to a fetal position near the edge of the bed or to sit upright on the side of the bed with the chest and head extended toward the knees. Sensations of pressure or brief pain may be experienced as the spinal needle is inserted.

The patient is instructed to lie in a prone position with a pillow under the abdomen after the procedure to increase intraabdominal pressure. The patient is encouraged to rest in bed, but no specific duration of bed rest is ordered. Nursing interventions include monitoring the insertion site for swelling, redness, and drainage. Signs of complications such as neck stiffness, irritability, and changes in level of consciousness or vital signs are reported immediately to the physician. A postlumbar puncture headache can occur from several hours to days after the procedure. The headache is treated with analgesics and bed rest in a quiet, darkened room.[12]

### Electroencephalography

The electroencephalogram (EEG) amplifies and records the electrical activity of the brain (brain waves) by the attachment of electrodes to the scalp. Any spikes, slowed activity, or asymmetrical rhythms on the EEG are abnormal. Electroencephalography is typically indicated in all patients who experience unexplained confusion, loss of consciousness, or seizure activity. The EEG is also used to establish brain death.

The nurse informs the patient that the test is painless and offers reassurance that the EEG is not a form of shock therapy.

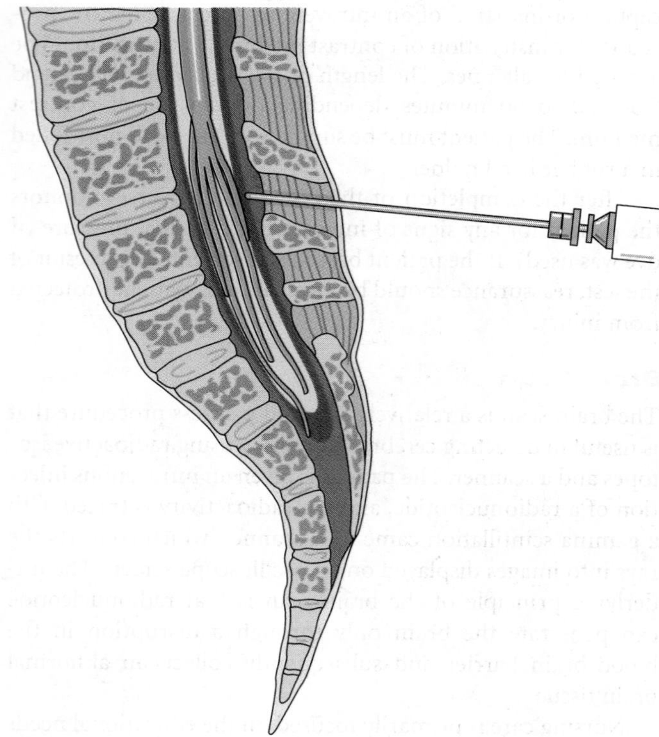

fig. 51-26 Position and angle of the needle when lumbar puncture is performed. Note that the needle is in the fourth lumbar interspace below the level of the spinal cord.

Colas, teas, and coffees are avoided the morning of the EEG because consumption of these beverages produces a stimulating effect. The patient's hair should be clean and free of hair sprays, gels, and lotions. The patient is instructed to be quiet and move minimally during the test; EEG recordings can be altered even with opening of the eyes. Medications are usually not withheld before the test, but protocols vary.

### Electromyography

The electromyogram (EMG) measures the electrical activity of muscles and records the variations of electrical potential (voltage) detected by a needle electrode inserted into skeletal muscles. The electrical activity can be heard over a loudspeaker and viewed on an oscilloscope and a graph simultaneously. No electrical activity can be detected in muscles at rest, but action potentials can be detected during movement. However, in motor disease abnormal electrical activity of various types appears in resting muscles. An EMG provides direct evidence of motor dysfunction and can be used to detect a dysfunction in the motor neuron, the neuromuscular junction, or muscle fibers. This is particularly helpful in the detection of lower motor neuron disease, primary muscle disease, and defects in the transmission of electrical impulses at the neuromuscular junction.

The patient is assured that there is no risk of electrocution from the needle. The sensation of needle insertion is similar to an intramuscular injection. Informed consent is required. After the procedure the patient may be encouraged to rest, and the nurse observes for any bleeding at the insertion sites.

### Magnetic Resonance Imaging

Magnetic resonance imaging (MRI) uses an electromagnet to detect radio frequency pulses from the alignment of hydrogen protons in the magnetic field. Computers convert the electromagnetic echo into images. Because contrast media are not employed, yet excellent visualization of tissue is provided, MRIs have become exceedingly popular. There is an increased sensitivity to tissue variations with MRI. Lesions such as brainstem tumors and brain abscesses that are not identified by CT scans can often be detected by MRI.[4,10]

The patient is informed that the MRI is painless and requires no special preparation. A supine position is assumed, and the patient is asked to lie still. The machine produces a "beating" noise, and earplugs are offered if the noise becomes bothersome. Jewelry is removed before the test; it is important to note whether the patient has surgical or orthopedic clips and heart valves because the MRI can cause displacement.

## chapter SUMMARY

### ANATOMY AND PHYSIOLOGY

- Neurological assessment depends on the examiner's knowledge of neuroanatomy and physiology and ability to recognize and interpret subtle deviations from normal.
- The nervous system coordinates and controls all activities of the body.
- The four general functions of the nervous system include receiving stimuli or information, communicating information, computing or processing the information, and transmitting information.
- The basic structural and functional unit of the nervous system is the neuron, which is composed of a cell body (soma), a dendritic tree, a cylindrical axon, and the cell membrane.
- The axon transmits information away from the cell body to adjacent neurons, whereas the dendrites communicate information to the cell body.
- The nervous system is divided into two major divisions: the central nervous system (CNS) and the peripheral nervous system (PNS).
- The CNS is made up of collections of neurons and their connections organized within the brain and spinal cord.
- The parts of the brain are the cerebrum, brainstem (midbrain, pons, and medulla), diencephalon (thalamus and hypothalamus), and cerebellum, each of which carries out specific functions.
- The blood-brain barrier is a phenomenon that limits the free movement of substances from the blood to the brain tissue.
- Cerebrospinal fluid cushions nervous tissue, helps support the weight of the brain, carries nutrients to the brain, and removes metabolites.
- The meninges are the coverings of the nervous tissue in the brain and spinal cord that help support, protect, and nourish the brain and spinal cord.
- Three potential spaces are associated with the meninges: epidural, subdural, and subarachnoid.
- The PNS is a set of communication channels located outside the CNS.
- The autonomic nervous system regulates autonomic body functions, usually in an effort to preserve homeostasis.

### ASSESSMENT

- Subjective data collected during the neurological examination include mental status, level of consciousness, language and speech, perceptual status, and sensory status.
- Objective data collection focuses on assessment of the 12 cranial nerves and function of the motor system (gait and stance, muscle strength and tonus, coordination, involuntary movements, and deep tendon reflexes).

### DIAGNOSTIC TESTS

- Diagnostic testing provides valuable data about neurological status. Laboratory tests, along with a variety of radiological and nonradiological tests, contribute significantly to the assessment process.

## References


1. Baggerly J: Sensory perceptual problems following stroke: the invisible deficits, Nurs Clin North Am 26(4):997, 1991.
2. Barker E, Moore E: Neurological assessment, RN 55(4):28, 1992.
3. Barker L, Burton J, Zieve P: Principles of ambulatory medicine, ed 4, Baltimore, 1995, Williams & Wilkins.
4. Beare P, Myers J: Adult health nursing, ed 3, St Louis, 1998, Mosby.
5. Cummings JL: The mental status examination, Hosp Pract 28(3):56, 1993.
6. Dykes P: Minding the five P's of neurovascular assessment, Am J Nurs 93(6):38, 1993.

7. Jarvis C: Physical examination and health assessment, ed 2, Philadelphia, 1996, WB Saunders.
8. Long B et al: Medical-surgical nursing: a nursing process approach, ed 3, St Louis, 1993, Mosby.
9. Lower J: Rapid neuro assessment, Am J Nurs 92(6):38, 1992.
10. O'Hanlon-Nichols T: Intracranial tumors, Am J Nurs 96(4):38, 1996.
11. Olson E: Perceptual deficits affecting the stroke patient, Rebabil Nurs 16(4):212, 1991.
12. Pagana KD, Pagana TJ: Mosby's diagnostic and laboratory test reference, ed 3, St Louis, 1997, Mosby.
13. Phipps MA: Assessment of neurological deficits in stroke: acute-care and rehabilitation implications, Nurs Clin North Am 26(4):957, 1991.
14. Specht DM: Cerebral edema: bringing the brain back down to size, Nursing 25(1):34, 1995.
15. Thibodeau GA, Patton KT: Anatomy and physiology, ed 3, St Louis, 1996, Mosby.

chapter 52

# MANAGEMENT OF PERSONS WITH Traumatic, Neoplastic, and Related Problems of the Brain

MARY VORDER BRUEGGE and LISA W. FORSYTH

## objectives *After studying this chapter, the learner should be able to:*

1 Identify at least four causes of altered level of consciousness.
2 Describe three assessment parameters for the person with altered level of consciousness.
3 Outline four nursing strategies to prevent increases in intracranial pressure.
4 Explain the significance of cerebral perfusion pressure in the patient with increased intracranial pressure.
5 Describe nursing assessment of the patient with a head injury.
6 Develop a plan of care for the patient with a severe head injury.
7 List at least three different types of primary brain tumors.
8 Outline preoperative and postoperative nursing care for the patient undergoing craniotomy for a brain tumor.
9 Describe the actions of medications used to prevent and treat migraine.
10 Differentiate among migraine, cluster, and tension headache.
11 Teach a patient how to keep a headache diary.
12 Differentiate between partial and generalized seizures.
13 List at least three anticonvulsants.
14 Describe the emergent management of status epilepticus.
15 List three infectious agents that cause meningitis.
16 Design a plan of care for a patient with meningitis.

This chapter discusses the care of persons with traumatic, neoplastic, and related problems of the central nervous system. The discussions of altered level of consciousness and increased intracranial pressure apply to the understanding and management of multiple neurological conditions. The remaining sections present specific disease processes such as headache, epilepsy, intracranial tumors, craniocerebral trauma, and infections and inflammations of the nervous system.

## ALTERED LEVEL OF CONSCIOUSNESS

### ETIOLOGY

Consciousness and coma exist at opposite ends of a spectrum. Full consciousness is a state of awareness and ability to respond optimally to one's environment. Coma is the opposite, a state of total absence of awareness and ability to respond even when stimulated. A wide range of awareness and responsiveness exists between these two extremes (Figure 52-1). The labels used to identify the various points along the continuum are arbitrary and do not reflect any universal agreement as to the nature of consciousness. Terms such as *lethargy* or *stupor* may be interpreted differently by different health care professionals.[3] Box 52-1 provides definitions for terms used to describe level of consciousness (LOC).

Consciousness has two primary components: arousal and content. Arousal is a function of the brainstem pathways that govern wakefulness, particularly the reticular activating system (RAS). Content is the sum of multiple interconnected cerebral hemisphere functions, including thought, behavior, language, and expression.[32] Disruptions in arousal, content, or both can alter the individual's LOC.

The two general causes for altered LOC are structural and metabolic. Structural causes include physical lesions interrupting neuronal pathways in the cortex or brainstem. Metabolic causes, such as hypoglycemia or hypoxia, involve alterations in the cellular environment affecting the function of neurons. Box 52-2 lists examples of both structural and metabolic causes of altered LOC.

The patient's LOC may fluctuate, and it is essential that there be clear communication and documentation of each assessment so practitioners can recognize changes and trends in the patient's condition. Thorough documentation of a patient's LOC includes both the patient's response and the stimulation needed to obtain the response. This objective information about the patient's response to a specific stimuli allows other practitioners to reproduce the same results. For example, "Patient opens eyes and answers questions when his name is called" provides clearer and more useful information than simply documenting "Patient is lethargic."

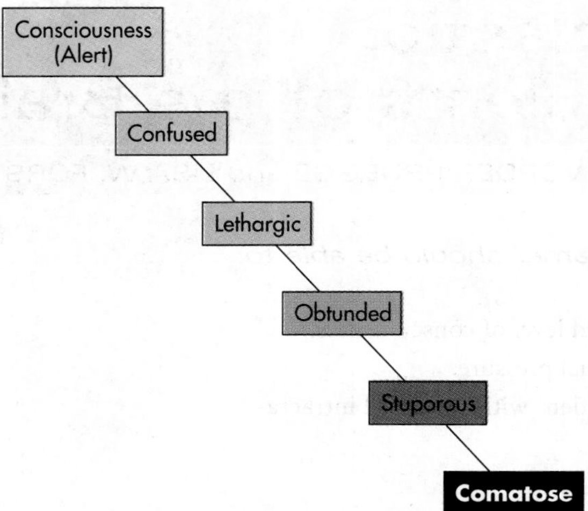


fig. 52-1 Continuum of consciousness.

**box 52-1 Altered Level of Consciousness Terminology**

*Alert:* attends to environment, responds appropriately to commands and questions with minimal stimulation
*Confused:* disoriented to surroundings, may have impaired judgment, may need cues to respond to commands
*Lethargic:* drowsy, needs gentle verbal or touch stimulation to initiate response
*Obtunded:* responds slowly to external stimulation, needs repeated stimulation to maintain attention and response to the environment
*Stuporous:* responds only minimally with vigorous stimulation, may only mutter or moan as a verbal response
*Comatose:* no observable response to any external stimuli

**box 52-2 Possible Causes of Decreased Level of Consciousness**

1. Structural causes
   a. Trauma (concussion, contusion, traumatic intracerebral hemorrhage, subdural hematoma, epidural hematoma, cerebral edema)
   b. Vascular disease (infarction, intracerebral hemorrhage, subarachnoid hemorrhage)
   c. Infections (meningitis, encephalitis, abscess)
   d. Neoplasms (primary brain tumors, metastatic tumors)
2. Metabolic causes
   a. Systemic metabolic derangements (hypoglycemia, diabetic ketoacidosis, hyperglycemic nonketotic hyperosmolar states, uremia, hepatic encephalopathy, hyponatremia, myxedema)
   b. Hypoxic encephalopathies (severe congestive heart failure, chronic obstructive pulmonary disease with exacerbation, severe anemia, prolonged hypertension)
   c. Toxicity (heavy metals, carbon monoxide, and drugs—especially opiates, barbiturates, and alcohol)
   d. Extremes of body temperature (heatstroke, hypothermia)
   e. Deficiency states (Wernicke's encephalopathy)
   f. Seizures

Three unique conditions of altered LOC demonstrate the complexity of the physiology of consciousness. A *persistent vegetative state* is a condition that can develop after a severe brain injury. Patients in this state experience eye opening and sleep-wake cycles that indicate arousal but demonstrate no cognitive function. In other words, these patients possess intact "vegetative" functions of the brainstem, such as respiratory drive, brainstem reflexes, and some functions of the RAS, but have no cognitive functions to enable them to interact voluntarily with their environment.

*Locked-in syndrome* is a condition in which the motor pathways in the brainstem are destroyed, but the RAS and higher cognitive functions remain intact. In this state, patients are unable to move or speak as a result of destruction of the motor pathways that control those functions, but they are capable of interacting with their environment. The motor functions of blinking and extraocular movements are usually spared because those pathways lie above the level of the pons. Locked-in patients therefore can communicate with eye movements and are capable of full arousal and receptive content.

*Brain death* is the third unique alteration in LOC with specific physiological features. Severely brain-injured patients are considered to be brain dead if they meet strict criteria set forth by state law. The laws governing brain death may vary by state, but most include criteria such as known cause of coma so that reversible causes, such as drug overdose or hypothermia, can be ruled out; unresponsive to external stimuli; absent brainstem reflexes; and absent respiratory effort in the presence of hypercapnea. These criteria are crucial because they do not include the classic layperson's criterion for death—an absent heartbeat. The definition of brain death becomes particularly important in situations involving tissue and organ donation (see Chapter 68).

## EPIDEMIOLOGY

The number of people experiencing altered LOC is not known, but its multiple etiologies clearly indicate that it is a common problem in clinical practice. Patients of all ages may experience altered levels of consciousness, and it may be present for brief periods of time or long term.

## PATHOPHYSIOLOGY

Full consciousness is a product of many delicate interactions within the nervous system. Arousal is a function of the RAS.[1,32] Fibers from the upper brainstem, thalamus, and hypothalamus receive input from sensory pathways in the brain and peripheral nervous system. The RAS fibers supply stimulation to the cerebral hemispheres to initiate and maintain arousal. When a person is aroused, or awake, he or she is ready to respond to the environment. The cerebral cortex also provides feedback to the RAS to modulate and regulate the information sent to the cortex. See Chapter 51 for a further description of the function of the RAS.

**box 52-3** *Sensory-Perceptual Alterations Associated with Changes in Level of Consciousness*

*Hallucinations:* subjective sensory perceptions that occur in the absence of relevant external stimuli; may be auditory, visual, tactile, or somatic
*Delusions:* false, fixed, personal beliefs that are not shared by others
*Illusions:* misinterpretations of real external stimuli

**box 52-4** *clinical manifestations*

**Altered Level of Consciousness**

Decreased wakefulness
Decreased attention to surrounding environment
Confusion
Hallucinations
Illusions
Disorientation
Agitation
Poor memory
Decreased ability to carry out activities of daily living
Decreased mobility
Incontinence

The ability to consciously respond to the environment is a function of the cerebral hemispheres. The cerebral cortex, diencephalon, and upper brainstem act together to control voluntary motor function, language, memory, and emotion. These higher-level cognitive functions represent the content portion of consciousness. A person needs both arousal, or wakefulness, and content to be considered fully conscious.

Disruptions to the nervous system controlling consciousness can be structural or metabolic. See Box 52-2 for examples. Structural lesions, such as a tumor or stroke, disrupt pathways of nerve transmission and produce specific, localized neurological deficits that reflect the location of the lesion. Metabolic causes, such as hypoglycemia or drug overdose, affect the biochemical environment of the brain and alter cellular function. Altered LOC resulting from metabolic changes usually produces global, nonlocalized neurological deficits.

Patients with selected sensory-perceptual alterations also may experience altered LOC. Patients experiencing hallucinations, agitation, and delirium are often found to have underlying problems such as hypoxia or medication interactions that disturb the metabolic environment of the brain. See Box 52-3 for a listing of sensory-perceptual alterations associated with altered LOC and Box 52-4 for clinical manifestations associated with altered LOC. Chapter 9 discusses the management of changes in LOC related to sensory-perceptual alterations.

## COLLABORATIVE CARE MANAGEMENT

### Diagnostic Tests

Diagnostic evaluation of altered LOC includes searching for the structural or metabolic etiology of the changes. The workup includes a detailed history, extensive neurological examination, radiological examination, and laboratory testing.

In the emergency setting, a rapid evaluation of life-threatening causes of reduced consciousness is carried out. Blood is drawn to assess electrolyte balance, glucose levels, and blood oxygen concentration. Blood levels of narcotics, sedatives, and other drugs cannot be immediately obtained, so naloxone may be administered as an antidote if narcotic overdose is suspected. A head computed tomography (CT) scan may be obtained to rule out the presence of space-occupying lesions with possible increased intracranial pressure (ICP). Interventions to protect the airway and support breathing and circulation are initiated while further diagnostic testing is done.

In the emergent setting diagnostic tests can be subdivided into those tests that evaluate possible structural lesions and those that evaluate possible metabolic causes of altered LOC. Box 52-5 summarizes the range of diagnostic testing for alterations in LOC.

While diagnostic test results are pending or tests are being scheduled, a detailed history is obtained and a physical examination is performed. The history is obtained from the patient when possible, and also from family, significant others, prehospital care providers, and home care providers, as appropriate.

A detailed neurological examination will also be performed and will follow the standard neurological assessment format of mental status, motor and sensory examination, and cranial nerve examination. The data from the neurological examination is perhaps the most important part of diagnostic testing for alterations in LOC. See Chapter 51 for details of a complete neurological examination. The items discussed next are specific to the evaluation of altered states of consciousness. The examination may be initially performed by a physician and then repeated on an ongoing basis by the nurse.

**box 52-5** *Diagnostic Testing for Altered Level of Consciousness*

**STRUCTURAL TESTS**
Skull x-rays
Electroencephalography
Computerized tomography of the head
Cerebral angiogram
Magnetic resonance imaging
Evoked potentials

**METABOLIC TESTS**
Complete blood count
Urinalysis
Electrolytes (includes glucose, blood urea nitrogen, creatinine)
Calcium
Liver function studies
Cardiac enzymes
Serum osmolarity
Lumbar puncture
Arterial blood gases
Toxicology screens for drugs of abuse (opiates, alcohol, barbiturates, antidepressants)

A mental status examination includes an overall assessment of consciousness and the patient's ability to remain awake and attentive and participate in the examination. Orientation, cognitive functions, and language are included in the mental status examination. Often subtle changes in orientation are the first indications of altered LOC. Patients with altered LOC may be disoriented to varying degrees. Orientation to date is usually lost first as patients experience disruption of their usual routines and may not have access to newspapers, calendars, television, and radio. The examiner asks the patient about the day, month, and year. If a patient cannot name a specific date, the examiner asks about the season or recent holidays for a more general response. Orientation to place may be lost, especially if the patient is in unfamiliar surroundings or has been transferred from one facility to another. If a patient cannot name the exact, current location, the examiner asks the patient what kind of place he or she is in (for instance, a hospital, hotel, grocery store). If the patient can look around at medical equipment, staff uniforms, and hospital logos and still not be able to correctly answer a question about place, the patient is considered to be disoriented with an impaired ability to reason and use information. This may affect patient teaching and the patient's ability to participate in self-care. Only with significant cognitive or language impairment are patients unable to state or respond to their names. It is important to clarify what name the patient is used to hearing and to use this name during interactions with the patient. Some patients may not respond to their given name but will respond to a familiar nickname. It is important to remember that orientation is only a small part of the overall mental status examination. Patients may be able to correctly guess or to memorize the correct answers to basic orientation questions. Interactions with the patient during the rest of the neurological examination provide important information about the patient's ability to think clearly, reason, and have insight into his or her illness.

Assessment of altered LOC includes attention, a component of mental status not often covered in the usual neurological examination. The examiner assesses the patient's ability to focus, or concentrate, on the examination and his or her distractibility. Irritability, restlessness, and boredom are also assessed. These may all be signs of cerebral dysfunction.

The time span associated with the altered LOC can be important in differentiating between delirium and dementia. Delirium develops over a short period, and its duration is usually brief. Because delirium is usually caused by an underlying organic disease process, the altered LOC may resolve when the underlying disease is treated. Dementia is not associated with reduced arousal or wakefulness, but it impairs intellectual functioning, memory, orientation, and the ability to care for self. Dementia develops slowly, is usually progressive, and is a chronic, irreversible state.

Motor examination is the next section of the neurological examination. The assessment of strength and coordination is described in Chapter 51. The patient with reduced LOC is examined for reflexive or pathological responses of the motor system. When patients have marked reductions in LOC, the examiner may need to use some degree of noxious stimuli to obtain a response. The examiner begins with verbal stimuli such as calling the patient's name or asking the patient to follow some simple command. A slightly stronger stimulus would be touching the patient's shoulder and gently tapping or shaking the patient while calling his or her name.

Some patients require a painful stimulus. Pressing on the sternum, pinching the trapezius muscle at the junction of the shoulder and neck, applying supraorbital ridge pressure, or applying pressure to the fingernail beds serve as common painful stimuli. The examiner documents both the stimulus used and the patient's response so that the next examiner can duplicate the examination to accurately assess for changes in the patient's status.

The patient who reacts to the painful stimulus and attempts to push the examiner away is said to "localize to pain." If the patient grimaces or demonstrates nonpurposeful movement, he or she is said to "withdraw to pain."

Lesions in the cerebral hemispheres below the primary motor cortex may result in pathological motor responses and cause abnormal flexor or extensor posturing. Abnormal flexion of the arms at the elbow, wrist, and hand with concurrent extension of the legs is called decorticate posturing. Lesions in the motor pathways of the midbrain or upper pons may cause abnormal extension of the arms with hyperpronation of the forearm, which is called decerebrate posturing. Abnormal motor postures are shown in Figure 52-2.

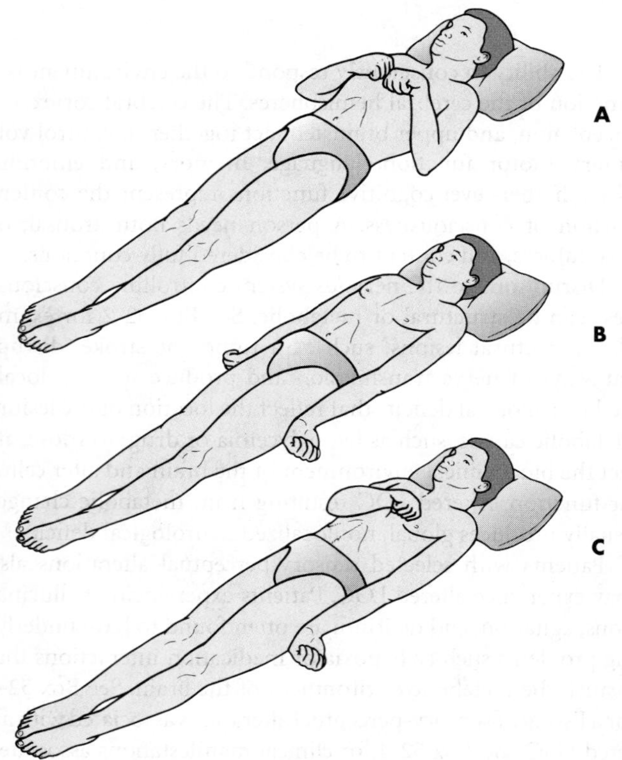


**fig. 52-2** Decorticate and decerebrate posturing. **A,** Decorticate response. Flexion of arms, wrists, and fingers with adduction in upper extremities. Extension, internal rotation, and plantar flexion in lower extremities. **B,** Decerebrate response. All four extremities in rigid extension, with hyperpronation of forearms and plantar extension of feet. **C,** Decorticate response on right side of body and decerebrate response on left side of body.

The sensory part of the neurological examination may reveal deficits that affect a cognitively impaired patient's ability to function. Patients with the sensory-perceptual deficit of hemiparesis after a stroke may neglect, or not attend to, the affected side.

The last portion of the neurological examination is the cranial nerve examination. Several specific cranial nerve reflexes are particularly important in assessing altered LOC. Protective reflexes, including gag, corneal, and cough, are checked to assess the patient's ability to protect herself or himself from injury and aspiration (see Chapter 51).

The oculocephalic and oculovestibular reflexes are not part of a normal neurological examination but are performed to assess the extent of brainstem pathology. The oculocephalic reflex (doll's eyes) is tested by holding the person's eyelids open and rotating the head quickly to one side and then to the opposite side. With an intact brainstem, the eyes move in the opposite direction to the head turning. This is considered to be a positive or normal response (Figure 52-3). If a person has a brainstem lesion the eyes passively follow the head movement.[32] This is one of the tests used to determine brain death.

The oculovestibular reflex (calorics) is tested by stimulating the semicircular canals of the ear with ice water. The patient is positioned supine with the head of the bed elevated 30 degrees. The eyelids of the unresponsive patient are then held open while the ear canals are irrigated with 50 ml of ice water. A normal response indicating intact function of cranial nerves III, VI, and VIII is conjugate eye movements toward the side being irrigated followed by rapid nystagmus to the opposite side (Figure 52-4). Absent or dysconjugate eye movement

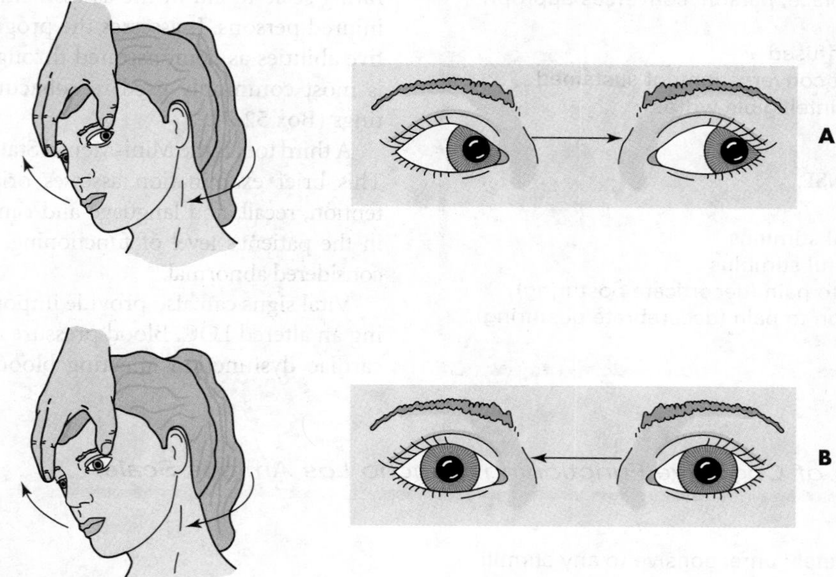


**fig. 52-3** Oculocephalic reflex testing. **A,** The normal response. Eyes move to the left as the head is briskly rotated to the right. **B,** Abnormal response. The eyes do not move as the head is turned, passively following the head.

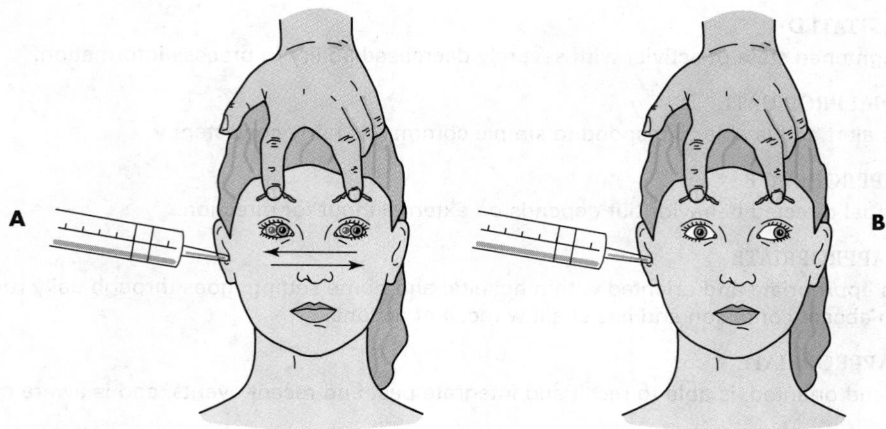


**fig. 52-4** Test for oculovestibular reflex response (caloric ice water test). **A,** In the normal response, the individual's eyes slowly move toward the side being irrigated, followed by rapid conjugate eye movements to the opposite side as shown. **B,** Dysconjugate or asymmetrical eye movements would be abnormal.

indicates brainstem damage. This test is also used for brain death determination.

The detailed neurological examination provides the foundation for assessment of the patient with altered LOC, but health care providers use a variety of scales to standardize the ongoing evaluation of a patient's functioning. Examples include the Glasgow Coma Scale (GCS), the Ranchos Los Amigos Levels of Cognitive Functioning, and the Mini-Mental State Examination. The GCS was developed to evaluate headinjured patients but can be used with a wide variety of neurological patients (Box 52-6).[42] The patient's total score is a sum of scores from three scales: eye opening, verbal response, and motor response. Numbers are given to the patient's best response in each area, and notations are made if a scale is not able to be evaluated, such as "eyes swollen shut" or "intubated, unable to test verbal score." The GCS does not take the place of a comprehensive neurological examination, but the results can be graphed and used to identify trends in the patient's overall function and predict outcomes.

Another widely used scale is the Ranchos Los Amigos Levels of Cognitive Functioning. It was developed as a behavioral rating scale to aid in the assessment and treatment of brain-injured persons. It assesses the progressive recovery of cognitive abilities as demonstrated through behavioral change and is most commonly used in subacute and rehabilitation settings (Box 52-7).

A third tool is the Mini-Mental State Examination (Box 52-8). This brief examination assesses orientation, registration, attention, recall, and language and can be used to follow trends in the patient's level of functioning. A total score below 24 is considered abnormal.[15]

Vital signs can also provide important information regarding an altered LOC. Blood pressure and heart rate may reflect cardiac dysfunction affecting blood flow to the brain. The

**box 52-6** *Glasgow Coma Scale*

**EYE OPENING**

4 Spontaneously open
3 Open to verbal request
2 Open with painful stimuli
1 No opening

**BEST VERBAL RESPONSE**

5 Oriented to time, place, person; converses appropriately
4 Converses, but confused
3 Words spoken, but conversation not sustained
2 Sounds made, no intelligible words
1 No response

**BEST MOTOR RESPONSE**

6 Obeys commands
5 Localizes to painful stimulus
4 Withdraws to painful stimulus
3 Abnormal flexion to pain (decorticate posturing)
2 Abnormal extension to pain (decerebrate posturing)
1 No response

**box 52-7** *Levels of Cognitive Functioning (Rancho Los Amigos Scale)*

**I. NO RESPONSE**
Patient is completely unresponsive to any stimuli.

**II. GENERALIZED RESPONSE**
Patient reacts inconsistently and nonpurposefully to stimuli in nonspecific manner.

**III. LOCALIZED RESPONSE**
Patient reacts specifically but inconsistently to stimuli.

**IV. CONFUSED—AGITATED**
Patient is in heightened state of activity with severely decreased ability to process information.

**V. CONFUSED—INAPPROPRIATE**
Patient appears alert and is able to respond to simple commands fairly consistently.

**VI. CONFUSED—APPROPRIATE**
Patient shows goal-directed behavior but depends on external input for direction.

**VII. AUTOMATIC—APPROPRIATE**
Patient appears appropriate and oriented within hospital and home setting, goes through daily routine automatically, with minimal to absent confusion and has shallow recall of actions.

**VIII. PURPOSEFUL-APPROPRIATE**
Patient is alert and oriented, is able to recall and integrate past and recent events, and is aware of and responsive to culture.

From Malkmus D et al: *Rehabilitation of the head-injured adult—comprehensive cognitive management,* Downey, Calif, 1980, Professional Staff Association of Rancho Los Amigos Medical Center, Adult Brain Inquiry Service.

patient's respiratory rate and pattern are helpful in localizing lesions in the central nervous system. Table 52-1 and Figure 52-5 give examples of abnormal respiratory patterns that result from neurological problems.

### Medications

Medications used in the treatment of altered LOC are prescribed for the underlying disease process or to control specific symptoms. Naloxone may be given to reverse the effects of narcotic overdose. Flumazenil is a benzodiazepine antagonist, used to reverse the effects of overdoses of drugs such as diazepam or lorazepam. If seizures are the cause of decreased LOC, anticonvulsants are administered to treat actual seizures and prevent future ones. A variety of medications may be administered to treat increased intracranial pressure, a common cause of altered LOC. These drugs are discussed on p. 1706.

### Treatments

Treatments for patients with altered LOC usually fall under the umbrella of nursing management. They are discussed in the section on nursing interventions.

### Surgical Management

If the cause of the patient's altered LOC is a space-occupying lesion, surgical removal of the mass may improve the patient's LOC. If the lesion has been present long enough to damage surrounding tissue, some residual deficit may remain. An example would be a patient with a subdural hematoma who becomes more alert and able to follow commands after the hematoma is evacuated. See the sections on craniocerebral trauma and brain tumors for a further discussion of surgical management.

### Diet

A patient's swallowing ability is carefully assessed before any decision is made about diet. Patients with decreased gag and cough reflexes, oral motor weaknesses, and decreased LOC may be candidates for placement of an enteral feeding tube to deliver nutrients and medications.

### Activity

Activity restrictions are rare for the patient with altered LOC unless precautions are in place to reduce ICP. Safety is the highest priority. Patients with altered LOC may easily become disoriented in unfamiliar surroundings and are at risk for both falls and wandering off. Patients with decreased mobility require assistance with range of motion, turning and bed mobility, and positioning.

### Referrals

Nurses often coordinate referrals to other disciplines for patients with complex care needs. Specific patient needs

**box 52-8** *Mini-Mental State Examination*

| Possible score | Actual score | |
|---|---|---|
| | | **Orientation** |
| 5 | ______ | What is the year? Season? Month? Day? Date? |
| 5 | ______ | Where are we (state, county, city, hospital, floor)? |
| | | **Registration** |
| 3 | ______ | Name three objects: 1 second to say each. Ask the patient all three after you have said them. (Give one point for each correct answer.) Repeat the objects until the patient has learned all three objects. Count trials and record. |
| | | **Attention and Calculation** |
| 5 | ______ | Serial 7's. Give one point for each correct answer. Ask the patient to count backward from 100 by 7's. Stop after 5 answers. Alternative is to spell "world" backward. |
| | | **Recall** |
| 3 | ______ | Ask for the three objects repeated above. (Give one point for each correct answer.) |
| | | **Language** |
| 9 | ______ | Display a pencil and a watch. Ask patient to identify them. (2 points) |
| | ______ | Repeat "No ifs, ands, or buts." (1 point) |
| | ______ | Follow a three-stage command. "Take a paper in your right hand, fold it in half, and put it on the floor." (3 points) |
| | ______ | Read and obey. "Close your eyes." (1 point) |
| | ______ | Write a sentence. (1 point) |
| | ______ | Copy design as shown. (1 point) |
| 30 total | ______ | **Total score** |

**CLOSE YOUR EYES**

Adapted from Folstein MF, Folstein SE, McHugh PR: Mini-Mental State: a practical method for grading the cognitive state of patients for the clinician, *J Psych Res* 12(3):189, 1975.

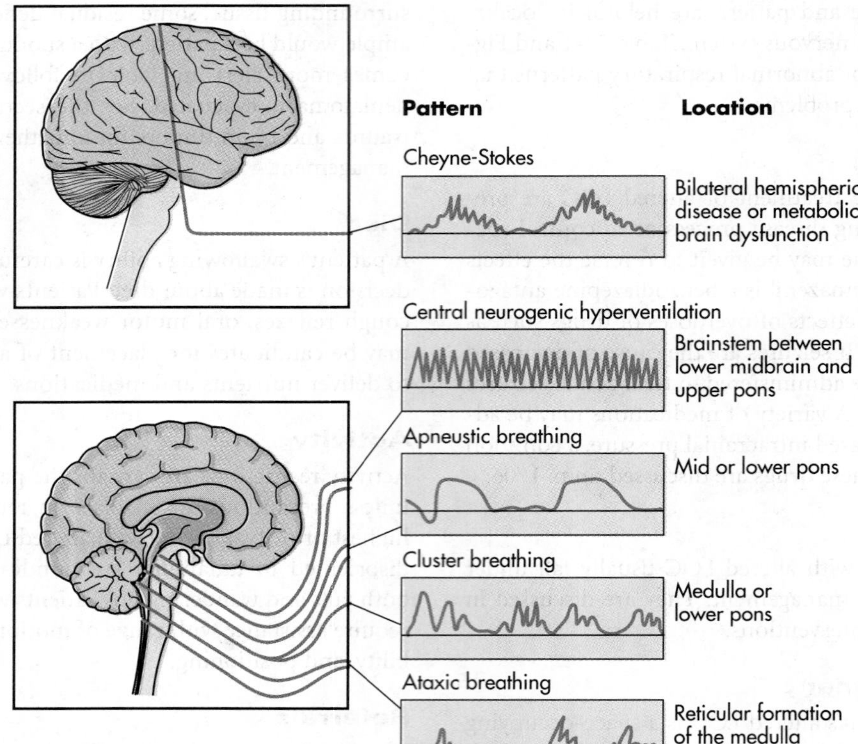


**fig. 52-5** Abnormal respiratory patterns with corresponding level of central nervous system activity.

**table 52-1** *Respiratory Patterns*

| RESPIRATORY PATTERN | DESCRIPTION OF PATTERN | SIGNIFICANCE |
|---|---|---|
| Cheyne-Stokes | Rhythmic crescendo and decrescendo of rate and depth of respiration, includes brief periods of apnea | Usually seen with bilateral deep cerebral lesions or some cerebellar lesions |
| Central neurogenic hyperventilation | Very deep, very rapid respirations with no apneic periods | Usually seen with lesions of the midbrain and pons |
| Apneustic | Prolonged inspiratory or expiratory pause of 2-3 seconds | Usually seen in lesions of the mid to lower pons |
| Cluster breathing | Clusters of irregular, gasping respirations separated by long periods of apnea | Usually seen in lesions of the lower pons or upper medulla |
| Ataxic respirations | Irregular, random pattern of deep and shallow respirations with irregular apneic periods | Usually seen in lesions of the medulla |

From Thelan LA et al: *Critical care nursing,* ed 2, St Louis, 1994, Mosby.

determine the nature and extent of referrals. Discharge planning and counseling are performed by social workers in many inpatient settings. Physical and occupational therapists offer services to patients with motor, sensory, or self-care deficits. Speech therapists can assist the patient and family with communication and swallowing difficulties. Respiratory therapists collaborate with nursing and other disciplines to help protect the patient's airway and improve gas exchange. Nurses in outpatient or community settings will use community resources to assist patients and families with home care needs.

## NURSING MANAGEMENT

### ASSESSMENT

#### Subjective Data

Nursing management begins with a detailed history as outlined previously. Specific factors to assess in a patient experiencing an altered level of consciousness include:

When the change in LOC was first noticed
Onset—sudden or slowly progressive
Patient and family awareness and understanding of the symptoms

- Ability to think, think abstractly, calculate, and make everyday decisions
- Recent history of falls, infection, or other trauma
- Medications in use—prescription and over-the-counter drugs; alcohol use
- Visual changes
- Other symptoms (pain, fever, nausea, headache)

### Objective Data

The most important objective data are reflected in the results of the complete neurological examination, which is a collaborative responsibility of both medicine and nursing:

- Motor status, presence of posturing
- Sensory status
- Cranial nerve assessment, protective reflexes
- Breathing pattern
- Oxygenation status
- Laboratory results (electrolytes, hemoglobin [Hgb], hematocrit [Hct], glucose, blood urea nitrogen [BUN], creatinine)
- Drug levels

## NURSING DIAGNOSES

Nursing diagnoses are determined from analysis of patient data. Nursing diagnoses for the patient with altered LOC may include but are not limited to:

| Diagnostic Title | Possible Etiological Factors |
|---|---|
| Ineffective breathing pattern | Neuromuscular impairment, cognitive impairment |
| Altered tissue perfusion, cerebral | Decreased or altered blood flow |
| Altered thought processes | Structural or metabolic imbalance |
| Ineffective thermoregulation | Impaired regulatory mechanisms |
| Risk for injury | Sensory/motor deficits, loss of integrative functions |
| Impaired physical mobility | Neuromuscular impairment |
| Altered nutrition, less than body requirements | Decreased alertness, chewing/swallowing difficulties |
| Bowel incontinence | Perceptual or cognitive impairment |
| Altered urinary elimination | Neuromuscular impairment |
| Impaired health maintenance | Perceptual or cognitive impairment, loss of motor skills |
| Risk for impaired skin integrity | Impaired mobility, nutrition, pressure or shearing forces |
| Ineffective family coping | Temporary family disorganization, crisis, role changes |
| Knowledge deficit: disorder, plan for treatment or rehabilitation | Lack of exposure, resources |

## EXPECTED PATIENT OUTCOMES

Expected patient outcomes for the patient with altered level of consciousness may include but are not limited to:

1. Maintains effective breathing pattern
2. Maintains adequate systemic blood pressure to perfuse the brain
3. Maintains coherent thought processes, is not confused
4. Maintains body temperature within normal limits
5. Safety precautions in place, does not experience injury
6. Maintains highest possible mobility with use of assistive devices and assistance of others
7. Consumes adequate balanced nutrients to maintain a stable body weight
8. Maintains a regular pattern of bowel elimination without constipation, diarrhea, or incontinence
9. Maintains urinary continence with or without external continence device
10. Participates in self-care to the maximum degree possible
11. Skin integrity maintained, no evidence of redness or breakdown
12. Family actively participates in all decision making and planning for patient's care, uses coping strategies to adapt to family role changes
13. Patient and family indicate understanding of diagnosis and treatment plan

## INTERVENTIONS

### Supporting Effective Ventilation and Perfusion

It is important for the nurse to closely monitor the breathing patterns of the patient with an altered LOC. The patient may require assistance in keeping the airway clear, including the use of suctioning when warranted. The nurse positions the patient on either side and keeps the head of the bed elevated to at least 30 degrees to facilitate an open airway. Patients with swallowing difficulties may require additional precautions to prevent aspiration. The patient may simply need reminders to take small bites and swallow carefully or need to have a feeding tube inserted until swallowing ability improves. Changes in breathing pattern can also provide insight into the nature and extent of the patient's neurological problems (see Table 52-1).

Patients with decreased LOC may not be able to turn themselves to mobilize pulmonary secretions or prevent atelectasis. The nurse assists patients to turn, encourages hourly deep breathing, and encourages the use of incentive spirometers. Patients with significant LOC reductions may hypoventilate and require supplemental oxygen or mechanical ventilation to maintain adequate oxygenation and prevent hypercapnea. The effectiveness of the patient's gas exchange can be evaluated with pulse oximetry and arterial blood gases. Pulse oximetry monitors oxygen saturation but cannot provide information about carbon dioxide exchange or blood pH, which require arterial blood gas sampling. The nurse checks breath sounds to evaluate the effectiveness of the patient's respiratory effort and pattern. The presence of decreased breath sounds indicates the potential for atelectasis and hypoventilation. Hypoxia or hypercapnea may result in increased intracranial pressure and further impair the patient's LOC.

### Supporting Tissue Perfusion

Some patients with altered LOC have impaired cerebral tissue perfusion. Decreased perfusion may be a result of increased intracranial pressure (discussed later in this chapter) or decreased cardiac output and reduced systemic blood pressure.

The nurse ensures that the patient receives adequate hydration to maintain blood volume and support blood pressure. The nurse works collaboratively with the physician to develop a medication plan that supports cardiac function and sustains the blood pressure at levels that ensure optimal peripheral and cerebral circulation.

Assisting patients to change position at least every 2 hours enhances circulation and venous return. The nurse also ensures that clothing, bedclothes, and body position do not constrict circulation. Immobile patients have impaired circulation at dependent sites. Passive or active range of motion is implemented to support blood flow and restore circulation to pressure-occluded or dependent sites. Elastic stockings or intermittent compression sleeves may be applied to prevent venous pooling and thrombus formation in the legs.

### Supporting Orientation

Patients with neurological impairments may have a variety of sensory-perceptual problems that need to be taken into account when planning care. Patients with visual field deficits need to have objects placed within their functioning field of vision and learn to compensate for visual field losses by turning their head to maximize their functional range of vision. Alternating eye patches may be helpful for patients experiencing diplopia. Eye patches restore vision to a single image and allow the patient to read, reach for objects, and ambulate more safely.

Patients with hearing loss need adaptive devices or additional visual sources of information to participate in self-care. The nurse ensures that hearing aids work and are fitted properly. Notations are made on the chart to indicate that a patient is hard of hearing so that a lack of response to questions or instructions is not interpreted as disorientation or cognitive impairment. The nurse can also ensure that the environment does not contain unnecessary background noise that can interfere with the patient's attempts to hear and communicate.

Patients with peripheral sensory losses such as hemiparesis may not attend to the affected body parts, a condition termed *neglect.* The nurse helps the patient use the affected extremity during routine care and assists with positioning it to prevent contractures, skin breakdown, or injury. Sensory loss on the face can affect the patient's ability to chew and swallow. Food or medications can unknowingly become pocketed in the cheek and later cause choking or aspiration. The nurse carefully checks the patient's mouth after meals and medication administration and removes any pocketed food.

Patients with sensory-perceptual alterations can easily misinterpret environmental stimuli, leading to confusion. The nurse gives special consideration to arranging the patient's environment to minimize confusion or altered thought processes. Large-print calendars and clocks within view can help maintain time orientation. Familiar pictures or objects from home provide a link to family and friends. Adequate lighting helps visually impaired patients see who is entering the room and may prevent the misinterpretation of shadows or unfamiliar objects. Lights should be kept to a minimum at night to promote sleep. The use of night-lights ensures sufficient light for the patient to find the call bell or get to the bathroom without falling while still promoting restful sleep. A quiet, restful environment requires the nurse to carefully eliminate unnecessary noise. Some patients want background music on to "drown out" other noise around them. The nurse carefully explains unfamiliar elements in the environment that can be confusing to the patient, such as infusion pumps or beeps from monitoring equipment. (See Chapter 9 for a further discussion of the assessment and management of confusion.)

Communicating with the confused patient requires patience and consistency. The nurse speaks quietly and slowly, using simple sentences or phrases to explain all care. It is important to speak to patients before touching them and to request only one action at a time. If the patient can read, a schedule of activities can remind the patient of events that will occur during the day. Consistent caregivers help the patient recognize familiar faces.

A patient's altered LOC can be frightening to family members, who need to understand why the patient is behaving in a confused manner. The nurse encourages the family to participate in planning and delivering the patient's care. Family members are often helpful in explaining how the patient reacts to unfamiliar settings and in identifying strategies that are likely to be successful in reorienting the patient. Guidelines for care of the confused person are summarized in the accompanying box.

### Maintaining Normal Body Temperature

Patients with severely reduced LOC are unable to communicate that they are too cold or too warm, and the nurse must ensure that the patient maintains a stable body temperature. If the patient becomes febrile, the nurse initiates an assessment for potential sources of infection. Fever can also be caused by damage to the hypothalamus. Treatment for any fever includes treatment of infection, antipyretic medication, tepid baths, and lowering the room temperature. Patients with neurological impairment can also become hypothermic. The nurse carefully uses heat lamps, warmed blankets, and an in-

**guidelines for care**

**The Person with Confusion or Disorientation**

1. Promote communication
   a. Touch may be useful to establish communication
   b. Use calm, quiet, and unhurried voice to talk to patient
   c. Talk slowly and distinctly and use short sentences
   d. Face patient when talking and stay within conversational range
2. Promote orientation
   a. Explain procedures in advance
   b. Environment should be well lighted
   c. Keep large calendar and clock in view
   d. Introduce self when caring for patient
   e. Keep sensory stimulation to a minimum
   f. Provide consistency in staff caring for patient
   g. Keep decision making to a minimum
3. Support family

crease in the room temperature to help restore the patient's temperature to the normal range.

### Preventing Injury

Numerous nursing activities are geared toward providing a safe environment for the patient experiencing an altered level of consciousness. The nurse inspects the patient's environment for equipment that may present a hazard. Call bells should be left within reach and the patient instructed how to use the device. Adaptive call bells are available for patients with limited motor abilities. When patients are unable to care for themselves, the nursing staff provides hygiene, eye care, and skin care to protect sensitive tissue. Seizure precautions may be implemented for patients with a demonstrated history or suspected risk of seizures.

Patients with limited mobility also present safety risks. Some patients may need a "seat belt" or slide cushion to prevent them from slipping or falling out of chairs. Confused patients may attempt to climb out of bed or wander off, but physical restraints should be used only as a last resort. Restraints have been shown to increase patient agitation and actually increase the risk of injury. See Chapter 9 for a discussion of "restraint-free" care.

The bed is kept in the low position. The nurse changes the patient's position frequently and provides frequent opportunities to meet elimination needs. Assisting the patient to be out of bed as much as desired may prevent the patient from trying to get up on his or her own. This behavior cannot always be prevented but is sometimes a response to muscle aches, thirst, the need to urinate, or simple loneliness. Frequent visits and monitoring are essential. Electronic monitoring systems can be useful for patients who wander. These systems alert the staff when a patient moves outside the monitored area.

### Promoting Mobility

The nurse positions patients and performs range-of-motion exercise to prevent contractures and other musculoskeletal complications in patients who are unable to move themselves. Changes of position also help patients mobilize pulmonary secretions. Getting patients out of bed and assisting them with ambulation supports weight bearing on the long bones and slows the demineralization associated with bed rest. An upright posture also improves the patient's ability to interact with the environment. The physical therapist may recommend specific activities to promote mobility and supply adaptive equipment, such as walkers, canes, or wheelchairs.

### Supporting Nutrition

A decreased LOC makes it difficult for patients to meet their ongoing nutritional needs, particularly if they also have swallowing difficulties. Adequate nutrition is essential to prevent infection and protect tissue integrity. The nurse keeps records of the patient's food and fluid intake so that accurate assessments can be made. The nurse works with the dietitian to determine the best diet to meet patient needs. If the patient is unable to maintain an adequate oral intake, enteral feedings may be started. Nasogastric tubes can be used for short-term feeding. If the need is believed to be long term, a gastrostomy, PEG, or jejunostomy tube is placed (see Chapter 41). Daily or weekly weights are obtained to monitor the patient's status.

### Promoting Bowel Elimination

Patients with altered LOC need to be started on a bowel program, especially if they are on bed rest with the tendency to become constipated or impacted. The nurse uses preventive measures such as stool softeners, fiber added to tube feedings or diet, and additional hydration to prevent constipation. The patient is offered the bedpan or placed on a commode at times close to the patient's usual time for elimination, such as in the morning after breakfast. If constipation is suspected, the nurse checks the patient for impaction and gently removes the stool if needed. Mild laxatives or suppositories can also be used to treat constipation, but enemas are used only as a last resort because of their tendency to completely disrupt the normal elimination pattern.

The need for communication among the nursing staff about the patient's bowel function is especially important. Bowel movements must be carefully recorded as to time, amount, and consistency for the nurse to make appropriate judgments about the need for laxatives and enemas.

### Supporting Urinary Elimination

Indwelling catheters may be used in the acute care setting if frequent monitoring of urine output is required. They should not be used for long-term management if possible because of the high risk of chronic infection. A condom catheter can be used for incontinent male patients. Female patients may require the ongoing use of an indwelling catheter. Patients with some neurological conditions experience urinary retention and require either an indwelling catheter or intermittent catheterization. When patients are able to communicate their needs, the nurse attempts to establish a regular schedule for bladder emptying that eliminates the need for catheters or diapers.

### Maintaining Skin Integrity

Patients with altered LOC are prone to skin breakdown. Agitated patients may accidentally abrade their skin or bruise themselves if not protected. Immobilized patients need frequent position changes and skin that is kept clean and free of excess moisture, but well lubricated to prevent dryness. Patients on prolonged bed rest or with actual skin breakdown require special pressure-relief mattresses. Providing adequate nutrition and hydration contributes greatly to the maintenance of skin integrity. The nurse carefully assesses the patient's skin during hygiene and position changes and protects the patient's skin from friction and shearing forces during position changes or when assisting the patient out of bed.

### Facilitating Self-Care

Patients with altered LOC may be unable to meet their own hygiene needs. Some patients may simply require assistance with activities of daily living such as supervision or verbal cueing during bathing or dressing. Others require the complete support of the nursing staff to complete hygiene activities. Performing self-care is an important part of rehabilitation. This may include bathing, hair shampoo, mouth care, eye care, and nail care. The nurse gives special attention to the skin in the axilla and perineal area and any skin folds that might retain moisture, such as the skin under the breast. These areas are particularly vulnerable to breakdown and infection with yeast and other organisms.

### Supporting the Family

Patients with altered LOC may be unaware of the severity of their situation, but the family is acutely aware. This awareness creates great anxiety and stress related to the crisis of a sudden illness or injury. The family may also need to make decisions about the patient's care for which they may feel unprepared. The nurse listens carefully to family members' concerns and assesses their ability to cope. The nurse clarifies which family member usually helps the patient make health care decisions. The nurse then explores what information that person needs to make current decisions and asks if the patient has a living will or advanced directive that can be used to guide decision making.

It is also important to find out what resources the family uses for support. Extended family, neighbors, and church friends are possible sources of support. The nurse ensures that the family is aware of other resources that are available, such as chaplains, social workers, and community groups appropriate to the patient's illness.

The nurse explains the hospital routines and surroundings to the patient and family to make the environment seem less foreign and unfamiliar. The family is directed to a quiet place where they can sit, make phone calls, and wait while the patient is being cared for. When family members are in the patient's room, the nurse provides them with chairs and encourages them to touch and talk to the patient. Some institutions allow families to participate in care delivery. When the family leaves the hospital, they should be given a phone number that they can use to check on the patient's progress and talk to the nurse or the patient, if he or she is able.

### Patient/Family Education

Altered LOC may leave patients with deficits that will profoundly affect many aspects of their lives and independence. Patients may not be independent because they have motor, sensory, or cognitive deficits that create safety concerns and interfere with their ability to be independent.

The patient's educational background and current cognitive abilities will affect her or his ability to be involved in the education process. The patient and family will need education about the diagnostic process and results, the treatment options, and how the treatment plan will be carried out. As care is delivered, the nurse provides the patient and family with feedback about the progress of the treatments, as well as any changes that are made in the plan of care. Discharge planning involves the identification of community resources and making appropriate referrals to ensure continuity of care. The nurse prepares a teaching plan to prepare the family for any care that the family will need to provide to the patient at home after discharge.

#### *Health promotion/prevention*

Specific disease processes that cause altered levels of consciousness cannot always be prevented. Altered LOC resulting from medication side effects and other situational factors may be prevented by altering or eliminating the causative factor. See Chapter 9 for further discussion of strategies to prevent changes in level of consciousness.

## ■ EVALUATION

Evaluation of care is an ongoing process. The current assessment is compared with the expected patient outcomes. Successful achievement of outcomes for the patient with an altered LOC is indicated by:

1. No evidence of aspiration, strong cough, clear breath sounds, respiratory rate of 12 to 20 per minute, and pulse oximetry above 90%
2. Systemic blood pressure and cerebral perfusion pressure within normal ranges
3. Alert and oriented to the surroundings, no evidence of confusion
4. Body temperature within normal limits
5. No sign of physical injury, environment is uncluttered
6. Uses assistive devices as needed to move about in the environment
7. Takes a balanced oral diet, maintains stable body weight
8. Uses diet, fluids, and stool softeners to maintain regular bowel elimination
9. Follows bladder training program to maintain continence
10. Uses adaptive aids and assistive equipment to maintain self-care in activities of daily living (ADL)
11. Skin intact without evidence of redness or breakdown
12. Family uses coping strategies to plan effectively for patient's care
13. Patient and family participate in planning for care after discharge

## GERONTOLOGICAL CONSIDERATIONS

The healthy gerontological patient should not experience memory loss, dementia, depression, or a decrease in LOC. Any of these changes is considered to be unexpected and should be investigated and treated. Older adults do experience a reduction in the speed of their reflexes, and they are prone to decreases in vision and hearing that may affect their ability to interact with those around them. These sensory losses are usually treatable and need to be addressed so that the patient can participate fully in education and self-care activities.

The older adult is more likely to experience multiple medical problems and therefore is more likely to be taking multiple medications. Medication interactions or sensitivity to side effects may account for some alterations in cognition and awareness in elders.

## SPECIAL ENVIRONMENTS FOR CARE

### Critical Care Management

The critical care environment can have serious effects on the patient with altered level of consciousness. An emergent admission to a critical care unit can be frightening and confusing if the high-tech environment is not carefully explained to the patient and family. Sedation and pain medication may be given to help patients tolerate the discomfort of invasive lines, endotracheal tubes, and mechanical ventilation. Careful assessment must be ongoing to ensure that the patient receives sufficient medication to be comfortable but is not oversedated, masking changes in LOC. Other measures to increase comfort may be implemented such as frequent repositioning, back rubs, or allowing the patient to choose soothing music or favorite TV shows.

For long-term patients in the intensive care unit (ICU), the noise and constant stimulation can lead to an altered LOC termed *ICU psychosis*. The patient becomes confused and agitated without discernible physiological cause. Altering the patient's plan of care to include adequate periods of uninterrupted sleep at night and decreasing meaningless stimulation such as monitor alarms or intercom use may help alleviate this problem. Having the patient decide how and when some of his or her care is done and grouping care activities so that the patient may rest in between allows the patient some control over care. Adequate pain control is also important.

### Home Care Management

Providing care to homebound patients has become increasingly common and high tech. Supplemental oxygen and respiratory therapy treatments can now be arranged for short- or long-term care at home. Intravenous fluids and medication can be administered in the home setting. Enteral or parenteral nutrition is also provided for long-term patients at home. When a patient with altered level of consciousness needs ongoing nursing care at home, the nursing staff of the inpatient setting carefully assesses the patient's needs and the available resources in the community for care, family support, and respite care. If home care needs to be provided by the family, the nursing staff is also responsible for ensuring their knowledge and skill before discharge.

## COMPLICATIONS

Complications of altered levels of consciousness are discussed under the specific disease process causing the condition. Many complications are related to immobility or the failure to meet basic care needs. The student is referred to a basic nursing text for a thorough discussion of the patient care that is provided to those unable to care for themselves. General guidelines for care of a patient with decreased LOC are summarized in the Guidelines for Care Box on p. 1704.

# INCREASED INTRACRANIAL PRESSURE

## ETIOLOGY/EPIDEMIOLOGY

Increased intracranial pressure (ICP) is a pathological process common to many neurological conditions. The intracranial volume is composed of brain tissue (85%), intracranial blood volume (5%), and cerebrospinal fluid (CSF) (10%). Any increase in the volume of any of these contents, singly or in combination, results in an increase in ICP because the cranial vault is rigid and nonexpandable. Any lesion that increases one or more of the intracranial contents is called a space-occupying lesion.[21] Common examples are listed in Box 52-9. Increased ICP is a common concern with a number of neurological conditions, but no data are available concerning the incidence or distribution of this condition.

## PATHOPHYSIOLOGY

The cranial vault is a rigid, closed compartment. The intracranial contents of brain, blood, and CSF occupy the skull fully and exist in a dynamic equilibrium under normal conditions. The Monro-Kellie hypothesis states that conditions that increase one or more of the intracranial contents must cause a reciprocal change in the remaining contents or an increase in ICP will occur.[21] As the intracranial volume increases, compensatory mechanisms take place. Cerebrospinal fluid–filled spaces can be compressed and CSF redistributed to the lumbar cistern to reduce intracranial CSF volumes. Intracranial blood vessels, especially the veins, can be compressed by surrounding brain tissue and displace intracranial blood volume. These compensatory mechanisms initially are able to accommodate a growing intracranial volume without significant increases in ICP, but these mechanisms are quickly exhausted if the intracranial volume continues to increase.

When the volume within the skull overwhelms the compensatory mechanisms, intracranial pressure begins to rise. See Figure 52-6 for the pressure-volume curve. Small increases in pressure occur in response to initial increases in volume. As

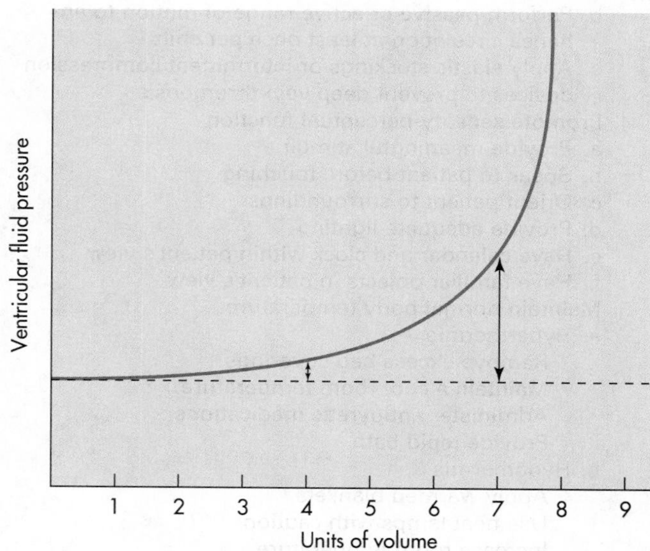


**fig. 52-6** Intracranial volume-pressure curve. Note that for the addition of any given unit of volume (abscissa) a markedly different rise in pressure occurs, depending on location (flat or steep portion) on the curve. Thus adding one unit of volume at the second arrow results in nearly four times the increase in pressure from the same volume at the first arrow.

compensatory mechanisms fail, additional increases in volume cause dramatic increases in ICP. Normal ICP is between 0 and 15 mm Hg. Pressures over 20 mm Hg are considered to be increased ICP.

As pressure within the skull increases, the cerebral blood vessels may be compressed, causing a reduction in cerebral blood flow. Inadequate perfusion initiates a vicious cycle, causing the partial carbon dioxide pressure ($P_{CO_2}$) to increase and the partial oxygen pressure ($P_{O_2}$) and pH to decrease. Cerebral arterioles have the ability to autoregulate, which allows them to dilate or constrict to maintain a constant blood supply to the brain. Changes such as an increasing $P_{CO_2}$ or decreasing pH cause vasodilation of the cerebral blood vessels and an increase in intracranial blood volume, which contributes to further increases in ICP. Autoregulation works when the mean arterial pressure (MAP) is between 50 mm Hg and 150 mm Hg and when the metabolic environment of the brain is normal. Severe anoxia and hypotensive states cause autoregulation to fail, subjecting the brain's blood supply to the wide variations of systemic blood pressure.

Cerebral perfusion pressure (CPP) is a parameter used to monitor the adequacy of blood flow to the brain in the face of increased ICP. As ICP increases, blood vessels may be com-

**box 52-9** *Space-Occupying Lesions*

| | |
|---|---|
| Edema caused by contusions or infarctions | Intracerebral hematoma |
| Subdural hematoma | Tumors |
| Epidural hematoma | Abcesses |
| | Hydrocephalus |

**guidelines for care**

### The Person with Decreased Level of Consciousness or Coma

1. Protect the airway and promote gas exchange
   a. Turn side-to-side q2h.
   b. Encourage coughing and deep breathing every hour while awake
   c. Suction oral and pharyngeal airway prn
   d. Monitor oxygen saturation and blood gases
2. Promote cerebral tissue perfusion
   a. Maintain hydration, prevent hypovolemia
   b. Monitor effects of antihypertensive, antiarrhythmic medications and promote adequate cardiac output and systemic blood pressure.
3. Promote tissue perfusion
   a. Turn q2h
   b. Perform passive or active range of motion to enhance circulation at least once per shift
   c. Apply elastic stockings or intermittent compression devices to prevent deep vein thrombosis
4. Promote sensory-perceptual function
   a. Provide meaningful stimuli
   b. Speak to patient before touching
   c. Orient patient to surroundings
   d. Provide adequate lighting
   e. Have calendar and clock within patient's view
   f. Have familiar objects in patient's view
5. Maintain normal body temperature
   a. Hyperthermia
      Remove excess bed coverings
      Maintain a cool room temperature
      Administer antipyretic medications
      Provide tepid bath
   b. Hypothermia
      Apply warmed blankets
      Use heat lamps with caution
      Increase room temperature
6. Prevent injury
   a. Keep a call bell within reach
   b. Implement seizure precautions as needed
   c. Provide eye care to prevent corneal damage at least once per shift
   d. Apply restraints only as last resort, with physician's order
7. Promote mobility
   a. Perform active or passive range of motion every shift
   b. Assist patient with ambulation or position changes
8. Maintain nutrition
   a. Record Intake to assess quantity and quality
   b. Assist patient with feeding and swallowing safely, with instructions to take small bites and chew carefully
   c. Administer enteral feedings at recommended rate for needs
   d. Weigh patient daily or weekly to assess gain or loss
9. Maintain regular bowel function
   a. Provide adequate hydration
   b. Ensure adequate fiber in diet or tube feedings
   c. Administer stool softeners as needed
10. Maintain bladder continence
   a. Remove indwelling catheters as soon as possible
   b. Provide regular toileting to prevent incontinence
11. Maintain hygiene
   a. Assist patient with ADL as needed
   b. If patient is unable to care for self, provide bath, mouth, eye, and skin care regularly
   c. Shampoo patient's hair as needed
12. Maintain skin integrity
   a. Reposition patient at least every 2 hours
   b. Use lotion or other skin moisturizers to prevent dry skin
   c. Keep sheets dry, free of wrinkles
   d. If skin breakdown is present or if patient is at high risk, use pressure-relief device
   e. Avoid shearing and friction when moving patient
13. Supporting family coping
   a. Assess family for usual coping skills and resources used
   b. Introduce family to new resources available for support
   c. Listen and address family concerns and provide needed information
   d. Teach patient care skills needed for home care to family

pressed, reducing blood flow to the brain. Systemic blood pressure needs to be high enough to overcome the ICP and deliver sufficient oxygen and glucose to brain tissues. The CPP is measured by subtracting ICP from MAP. The formula is CPP = MAP − ICP.

The actual brain structures can also be affected by increased ICP. The brain is surrounded and divided into compartments within the skull by the dura mater. The presence of edema or space-occupying lesions may cause brain tissue to shift or herniate. Subfalcial, or cingulate, herniation occurs when the brain is forced under the falx cerebri that separates the cerebral hemispheres. Uncal herniation occurs when the uncal portions of the temporal lobes shift over the edge of the tentorium cerebelli. Transforamenal herniation occurs when the brainstem is forced downward through the foramen magnum.

Increased ICP produces multiple signs and symptoms. Decreased level of consciousness is the earliest and most sensitive sign of increasing ICP. Altered blood flow and therefore an altered cerebral metabolic environment reduce the brain's ability to respond to stimuli. (See the section on altered level of consciousness.)

Pupillary responses are controlled by the oculomotor nerve (cranial nerve III), which carries motor fibers for pupil constriction and eyelid opening. The oculomotor nerve is compressed by the herniating uncal portion of the temporal lobe. Dilation of the ipsilateral pupil occurs when the herniation is limited to one hemisphere. If ICP continues to rise and herniation increases, bilateral pupil dilation and fixation occur. If the nerve has only been stretched, pupil dilation with slowed constriction may be seen. A pupil that is fixed and dilated sometimes is referred to as a blown pupil.

The effect of ICP on blood pressure and pulse is variable. Hypoxia or decreased pH may cause the arterioles to autoregulate and dilate the cerebral blood vessels to improve blood flow, further increasing ICP. Autoregulation fails at high ICP ranges because the vessels cannot dilate against the pressure of the surrounding brain tissue. Ischemia in the vasomotor center excites vasoconstrictor fibers throughout the body, causing an increase in systolic blood pressure. The vasomotor center also sends parasympathetic impulses via the vagus nerve to slow the heart rate. A rising systolic blood pressure, widened pulse pressure, and slow heart rate are referred to as Cushing's response and are classic indicators of increased ICP. When the pressure on the brainstem is increased and the vasomotor center is no longer able to function, a drop in blood pressure and an increase in heart rate are seen as the patient's condition deteriorates.[21]

Herniation also produces respiratory dysrhythmias that correspond to the level of brainstem compression. An irregular respiratory pattern or periods of apnea are significant. Cushing's triad is made up of slowed respirations, a slow pulse, and a rising systolic blood pressure. Patients with decreasing LOC may have difficulty keeping the airway clear and may have shallow or slowed respirations that contribute to hypoxia or hypercarbia, which, in turn, increase vasodilation and contribute to increased ICP.

Failure of the thermoregulatory center because of compression is a late sign of increased ICP. The most common manifestation of this failure is a fever without a clear source of infection. Hyperthermia, in turn, increases the metabolic needs of the already compromised brain tissues and further increases ICP.

Compression of motor and sensory tracts between the primary motor and sensory areas in the frontal and parietal lobes and the peripheral nervous system leads to contralateral loss of motor and sensory function. When disruptions to motor pathways become severe the patient may exhibit posturing, described earlier in the section on altered levels of consciousness. Motor inhibitory fibers from the frontal lobes are blocked, resulting in hyperactive deep tendon reflexes. Damage to the corticospinal tracts will also cause positive Babinski's reflexes.

The optic nerve attaches to the eye at the optic disc. The meninges surround the optic nerve and its attachment to the eye. As ICP increases, the resulting pressure is transmitted to the eyes through the CSF in the subarachnoid space and to the optic disc, causing papilledema (choked disc). This may be a late sign of increased ICP. Other visual acuity changes are related to pressure on or shifting of optic pathways within the brain.

Headache is often an early nonspecific symptom of increased ICP. It is thought to result from tension on intracranial blood vessels. Vomiting may occur, but it is more common in children with increased ICP. See Box 52-10 for common clinical manifestations of increased ICP.

**box 52-10** *clinical manifestations*

***Increased Intracranial Pressure***

**EARLY SIGNS**

- Decreasing level of consciousness
  - Earliest and most sensitive sign
- Headache that increases in intensity with coughing, straining
- Pupillary changes
  - Dilation with slowed constriction
  - Visual disturbances such as diplopia
  - Ptosis
- Contralateral motor or sensory losses

**LATE SIGNS**

- Further decreases in level of consciousness
- Changes in vital signs
  - Rise in systolic blood pressure
  - Decrease in diastolic blood pressure
  - Widened pulse pressure
  - Slow pulse
- Respiratory dysrhythmias
  - Shallow, slowed respirations
  - Irregular patterns or periods of apnea
  - Hiccups
- Fever without a clear source of infection
- Vomiting (more common in children)
- Decerebrate or decorticate posturing

## COLLABORATIVE CARE MANAGEMENT

Patient outcomes for increased ICP are related to the underlying disease process. The collaborative care of the patient is aimed at controlling and reducing the increased ICP and preventing neurological damage from herniation. The diagnosis of increased ICP is most accurately made when the pressure is measured by one of several available devices. However, monitoring devices may not be immediately available, and the diagnosis can be made with careful neurological examination and ongoing assessment.

A head CT can show structural changes associated with increased ICP. Space-occupying lesions and sites of edema can be located. A reduction in the size of the CSF-filled spaces called cisterns at the base of the skull indicates shunting of CSF out of the skull as a compensatory mechanism. Any shifting of brain tissue at herniation sites can be identified.[29]

Baseline and subsequent neurological checks are an integral part of the ongoing assessment of the patient's condition. Patients with identified neurological deficits warrant frequent assessment. Refer to the section on altered LOC and Chapter 51 for further assessment parameters.

Several methods have been developed to directly measure ICP. An intraventricular catheter, also called a ventriculostomy, is inserted through a small hole in the skull and through the brain directly into one of the lateral ventricles. The catheter is connected to a sterile drainage system with a three-way stopcock that allows simultaneous monitoring of pressures via a transducer connected to a bedside monitor and drainage of CSF. Another method employs a fiberoptic monitor. The fiberoptic device measures changes in the amount of light reflected from a pressure-sensitive diaphragm in the catheter tip. This device can be placed directly into the brain parenchyma, subarachnoid space, epidural space or into a ventricle. The fiberoptic cable is connected to a precalibrated monitor that displays the numerical value of ICP. These special monitors can also be connected to the bedside monitor for waveform display. A third form of ICP monitor is the subarachnoid bolt. The hollow, threaded bolt is inserted through a burr hole in the skull into a small opening in the dura and into the subarachnoid space. The bolt is connected via a fluid-filled tubing to a transducer leveled at the approximate location of the lateral ventricles. A fourth device uses strain gauge technology to detect pressure changes. Thin, pressure-sensitive cables are placed into the epidural or parenchymal spaces. See Figures 52-7 and 52-8 for illustrations of various ICP monitors.

Medications used to treat increased ICP are selected to treat the underlying pathological process. Osmotic diuretics such as intravenous mannitol or urea promote fluid removal from edematous brain tissue. Corticosteroids such as dexamethasone may be used to reduce the edema associated with

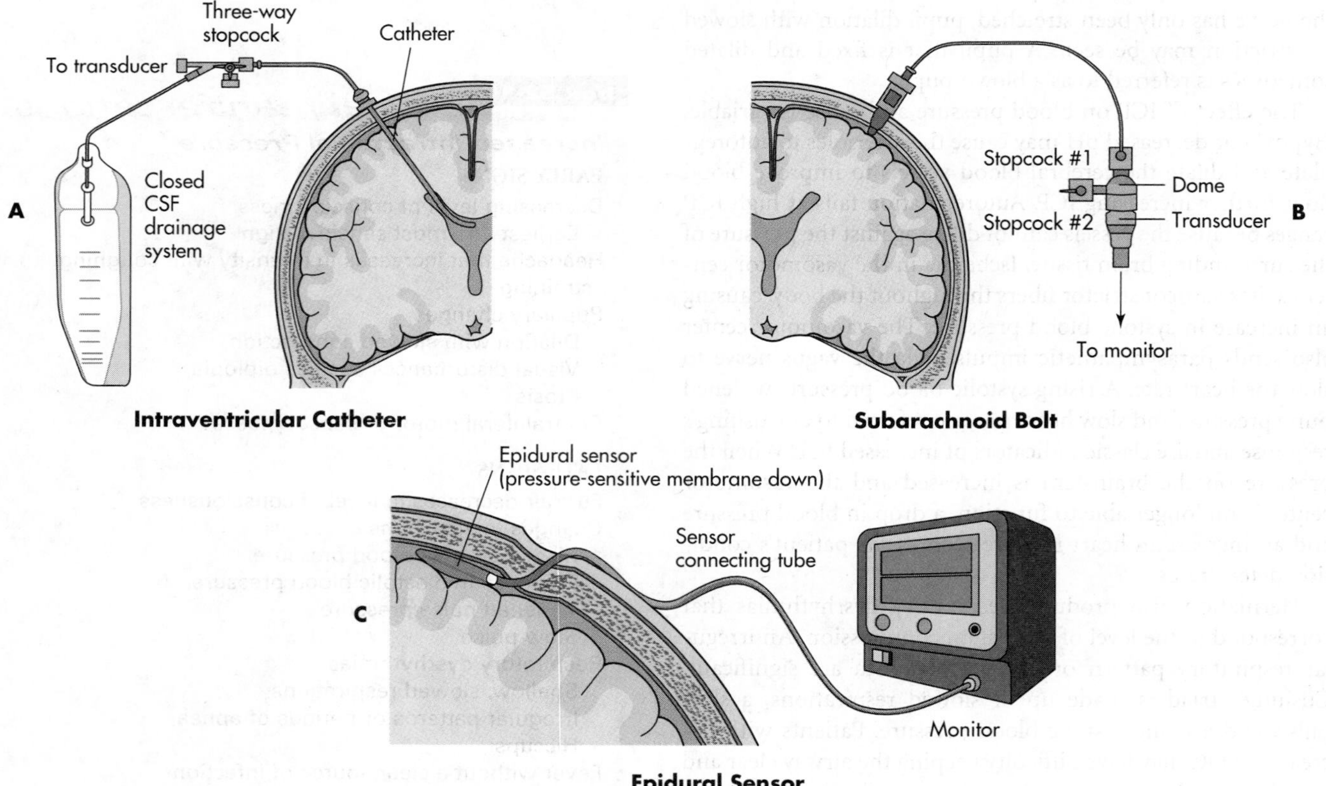


**fig. 52-7 A,** Intraventricular catheter monitoring system with a closed CSF drainage system. **B,** Subarachnoid bolt monitoring system. **C,** Epidural monitoring system.

tumors or abscesses. Narcotics and sedative medications are used cautiously because of their respiratory depressant effects. Narcotics and sedatives may also alter the patient's ability to cooperate with an accurate neurological examination. Anticonvulsant medication may also be prescribed to prevent seizures. Antibiotics are prescribed if the patient has an ICP monitoring device in place.[46,51]

Barbiturate coma is occasionally used for patients who are refractory to conventional management of elevated ICP. Large doses of barbiturates, usually pentobarbital, are given to reduce ICP and slow the cerebral metabolic rate in order to minimize the damage caused by ICP-induced ischemia. The use of barbiturate coma is associated with numerous side effects such as hypotension that require vasoactive drug treatment (e.g., dopamine infusion).[26] The high doses of barbiturate obscure the accuracy of any neurological assessment for the duration of the coma. Some sources recommend decreasing the dose of the barbiturate intermittently to allow for patient assessment.[26]

Surgical interventions are also aimed at correcting the underlying cause of the increase in ICP. Mass lesions such as tumors, abscesses, or hematomas are surgically removed. Excess CSF can be removed with a surgically placed ventriculostomy. If hydrocephalus becomes a chronic problem, a shunt from the lateral ventricle to the peritoneum can be placed for long-term removal of CSF. On rare occasions, a decompressive craniectomy may be performed to remove part of the skull, allowing the edematous brain to expand. The bone can be replaced at a later date after the edema has resolved.[21]

Hyperventilation of the intubated patient causes a decrease in $Pa_{CO_2}$, which causes vasoconstriction of cerebral blood vessels. This intervention is used commonly to temporarily help control ICP. However, if severe reductions in $Pa_{CO_2}$ continue, vasoconstriction can lead to ischemia. A balance is sought that keeps the $Pa_{CO_2}$ in the low-normal range of 30 to 35 mm Hg to prevent hypercapnea and subsequent vasodilation but does not reduce $Pa_{CO_2}$ to a level that causes vasoconstriction-induced brain ischemia.[9,17]

Control of activity plays an important role in the treatment of increased ICP. The pressure inside the skull is dynamic and changes in response to shifts in blood flow, CSF movement, and brain tissue edema. When compensatory mechanisms are intact, transient increases in ICP are brief and promptly return to baseline normal values at the end of the activity or treatment. When compensatory mechanisms have been exhausted, however, the rise in ICP may be more dramatic and take longer to return to normal. The patient's ICP response to any and all activities and treatments is therefore monitored, and activities are restricted as needed.

The patient's neck is kept in alignment to promote venous drainage through the jugular veins (see the Research Box).[50] In some cases, a cervical collar may be used to maintain this alignment. The head of the bed may also be elevated to promote

**research**

Reference: Williams A, Coyne SM: Effects of neck position on intracranial pressure, *Am J Crit Care* 2(1):68, 1993.

The investigators studied the effects of head rotation and neck flexion on ICP. Patients with ICP monitors in place but no previously elevated ICPs were manually positioned with their necks in flexion or in right or left rotation. Both rotating the head (to either side) and flexion resulted in significantly higher ICP readings than maintaining the head in neutral position. These data support previous research that patients at risk for increased ICP should be positioned with the neck in neutral alignment.

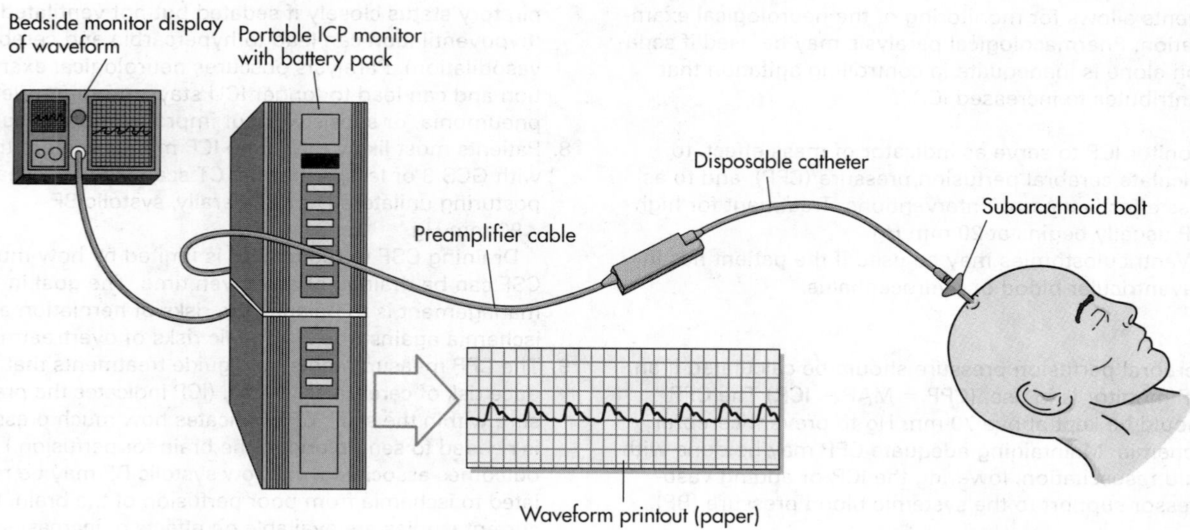


**fig. 52-8** Fiberoptic monitoring system using the subarachnoid bolt *(patient),* disposable catheter connected to preamplifier cable with continuous visual ICP waveform display on the bedside monitor *(upper left),* and a continuous digital readout of ICP *(lower monitor)* with ICP waveform printout.

venous drainage from the skull.[51] Activity that increases intrathoracic or intraabdominal pressure such as coughing, straining to have a bowel movement, or moving in bed may also increase ICP by interfering with venous drainage from the brain.[33,51] Some spontaneous patient activities such as shivering, vomiting, agitation, or abnormal posturing also contribute to increased ICP. If increases in ICP become severe during these activities and do not promptly return to baseline after the activity, the patient may be sedated to decrease activity.

Nurses need to carefully time and coordinate the patient's care to prevent prolonged increases in ICP. Activities such as bathing and position changes may need to be alternated with rest periods to allow time for the patient's ICP to return to baseline after activity.[45] Endotracheal suctioning contributes to increases in ICP because of increases in intrathoracic pressure and changes in oxygen and carbon dioxide levels. Preoxygenation and hyperventilation before suctioning the ventilated patient with increased ICP will minimize this problem. See the accompanying Guidelines for Care Box.

### Patient/Family Education

Neurological problems and their complications, such as increased ICP, are often confusing and frightening for patients and their families. Patients are more likely to cooperate with

**guidelines for care**

**The Patient with Increased Intracranial Pressure**

| INTERVENTION | RATIONALE |
|---|---|
| 1. Avoid hypotension (systolic blood pressure <90 mm Hg) and hypoxia ($Pa_{O_2}$ <60). | 1. Studies have shown that hypotension and hypoxia are two of the five most powerful predictors of poor outcome. |
| 2. Elevate head of bed (check to see if spine films have been done and cleared for raising head of bed). | 2. Promotes cerebral venous outflow. (Cerebral veins have no valves to promote forward flow.) |
| 3. Avoid jugular venous outflow obstruction. (Keep neck midline, cervical collar or endotracheal tube tape not too tight, check with increasing edema.) | 3. Promotes cerebral venous outflow. |
| 4. Prevent or avoid coughing, Valsalva's maneuver, hip flexion, high levels of positive end-expiratory pressure. | 4. Intrathoracic and intraabdominal pressure increases are transmitted to cerebral circulation by venous system when venous outflow is impeded. |
| 5. Maintain normothermia. Work up and treat fever promptly. | 5. Fever does not directly increase ICP but increases cerebral metabolic needs in injured brain. Hypothermia may lower ICP but does not positively affect outcome and presents some risk to patient. (Hypothermia is a second-tier treatment.) |
| 6. Prevent seizures. Phenytoin is used to prevent early posttraumatic seizures. Fosphenytoin is a new prodrug of phenytoin that causes fewer side effects when given IV and may be given in some circumstances. | 6. Seizures do not directly increase ICP but may precipitate adverse conditions in injured brain such as changes in oxygen delivery and cerebral metabolic needs. |
| 7. Prevent or treat agitation. Search for causes of agitation such as hypoxia or pain. Sedation with short-acting agents allows for monitoring of the neurological examination. Pharmacological paralysis may be used if sedation alone is inadequate in controlling agitation that contributes to increased ICP. | 7. Agitation or posturing may increase intrathoracic or intraabdominal pressure and increase ICP. Monitor respiratory status closely if sedated but not ventilated (hypoventilation can lead to hypercarbia and cerebrovasodilation). Paralysis obscures neurological examination and can lead to longer ICU stays, more frequent pneumonia, or sepsis without improved outcomes. |
| 8. Monitor ICP to serve as indicator of mass effect, to calculate cerebral perfusion pressure (CPP), and to assess effectiveness of interventions. Treatment for high ICP usually begins at 20 mm Hg.<br>Ventriculostomies may be used if the patient has intraventricular blood or hydrocephalus. | 8. Patients most likely to require ICP monitoring are those with GCS 8 or less, abnormal CT scan, age >40 years, posturing unilaterally or bilaterally, systolic BP <90 mm Hg.<br>Draining CSF to reduce ICP is limited by how much CSF can be drained at any given time. The goal in ICP management is to balance the risks of herniation and ischemia against the iatrogenic risks of overtreatment. |
| 9. Cerebral perfusion pressure should be calculated if an ICP monitor is in use. (CPP = MAP − ICP.) The CPP should be kept above 70 mm Hg to prevent cerebral ischemia. Maintaining adequate CPP may be done with fluid resuscitation, lowering the ICP, or adding vasopressor support to the systemic blood pressure (BP). | 9. The CPP measurements help guide treatments that reduce risk of cerebral ischemia. (ICP indicates the pressure within the skull; CPP indicates how much pressure is needed to send blood to the brain for perfusion.) Poor outcomes associated with low systolic BP may be related to ischemia from poor perfusion of the brain. No current studies are available on effects of increasing BP with vasopressors on the neurological outcome (second-tier treatment). |

Adapted from Bullock MR, Povlishock JT: Guidelines for the management of severe head injury, *J Neurotrauma* 13(11):639, 1996.

Continued

frequent neurological checks if the reason for them is explained. Patient and family education should include information about the underlying disease process and its relationship to increased ICP. As treatments and medications are introduced, the nurse explains their purpose to the patient and family. When patients are unable to care for themselves, the nurse can include the family in providing care as long the patient does not experience increases in ICP.

## HEADACHE

### ETIOLOGY/EPIDEMIOLOGY

Headache is a common symptom of many neurological conditions and is also a separate disease process. Headaches are classified by the International Headache Society as primary or secondary.[41] Primary headaches are not associated with any other known pathological cause. Examples of primary headaches are migraine, tension, and cluster headaches. Secondary headaches are caused by a known pathology such as meningitis, tumors, or subarachnoid hemorrhage. This section focuses on the care of the patient with a primary headache.[19]

Migraines occur more often in women than men and most commonly begin between adolescence and age 40. They demonstrate a strong hereditary pattern, but no specific genetic link has been identified.[5] Tension headaches can occur at any age and are associated with stress. No epidemiological pattern has been identified for cluster headaches.

### PATHOPHYSIOLOGY

The pathophysiology of headache is not fully understood. Some structures of the head are incapable of sensing pain. The structures that are capable of feeling pain are skin, muscles, periosteum of the skull, eyes, ears, nasal cavities and sinuses, meninges, cerebral blood vessels, and cranial nerves with sensory function. Pain is caused by traction, stretching, or movement of structures or by vasodilation of blood vessels. Serotonin is the primary neurotransmitter found in the pathways involved in headache, but its role is not fully understood.

Migraines are believed to be caused when cerebral blood vessels narrow and blood flow is reduced to some areas of the brain. The initial vasoconstriction is followed by significant vasodilation and inflammation of the blood vessels, which triggers a release of serotonin and causes the headache.[28] Migraines vary in duration, frequency, and intensity from patient to patient and from episode to episode in the same patient.

Cluster headaches are thought to be similar to migraines but the episodes are brief, usually lasting 45 minutes or less. They occur in "cluster" periods of weeks or months. Tension headaches are the result of stress induced muscle tension over the neck, scalp, and face of the patient. These headaches are

**guidelines for care**

**The Patient with Increased Intracranial Pressure—cont'd**

| INTERVENTION | RATIONALE |
|---|---|
| 10. Mannitol: osmotic diuretic used to treat cerebral edema. Usually given in bolus doses of 0.25 to 1.0 g/kg. Need to monitor for serum osmolarity of greater than 310 to 320 mOsm/L and effect of fluid and electrolyte shifts. Can contribute to dehydration, decrease in BP and CPP. | 10. Injured brain may lack intact blood-brain barrier in some areas, making mannitol less effective. Mannitol also has rheologic effects of increasing RBC deformability, decreasing blood viscosity, and improving blood flow (which improves flow to ischemic brain). |
| 11. Surgical Intervention: surgical evacuation of hematomas or skull fracture repair. On some rare occasions a piece of skull may be removed and left off to allow the brain more room to swell (craniectomy). | 11. Evacuation of hematomas (subdural or epidural) lessens mass effect but does not remove the cerebral edema. Intracerebral hemorrhages are not usually evacuated. Craniectomies present risk and are used as last resort treatment (second-tier). |
| 12. Hyperventilation. May be used initially in resuscitation when information about ICP is not readily available. May be used acutely for herniation. In general, ventilated patients will have their setting adjusted to keep $PCO_2$ between 30 and 35 mm Hg. Hyperventilating (and hyperoxygenating) patients before, during, and after endotracheal suctioning is still recommended to reduce the adverse effects of sudden rises in ICP with coughing and suctioning. | 12. Hyperventilation works by causing cerebrovasoconstriction, reducing cerebral blood volume. But this also reduces cerebral blood flow to the brain, risking ischemia. Limiting the use of hyperventilation may improve neurological recovery or at least reduce ischemic damage. Studies are still needed to determine if patients who hyperventilate themselves should be paralyzed or sedated to prevent this. |
| 13. Barbiturates may be used but have significant complications. Work by reducing cerebral metabolic needs and cerebral blood flow. Monitoring of EEG burst suppression is suggested. | 13. Used for refractory ICP treatment. Suppression of nervous system leads to hypotension, peripheral vasodilation, loss of neurological examination, loss of protective reflexes. Patient will require central venous and perhaps pulmonary artery (PA) monitoring and vasopressor support. Patients on barbiturate therapy have increased risk of infection. Pentobarbital, phenobarbital, or thiopental may be used. |

associated with the stresses of daily life. Table 52-2 compares the three major types of primary headaches.

Some headaches are preceded by prodromal signs and symptoms called aurae. The aura occurs before the acute attack and may include visual field defects such as "flashing lights," photophobia, confusion, or paresthesias. Aurae typically last an hour or more. These symptoms are associated with the reduction in cerebral blood flow that precedes the vasodilation of the migraine.[18]

## COLLABORATIVE CARE MANAGEMENT

The diagnosis of headache is made from the patient's history. Careful questioning can help rule out headaches caused by other illnesses. Headache caused by subarachnoid hemorrhage is sudden, severe, and generalized. Meningitis headaches are also generalized and severe and may radiate down the neck. Brain tumors can also cause headaches that may be related to increased ICP. These headaches may occur more often with straining, coughing, exertion, or sudden movement. A careful history is obtained and a physical examination is performed to rule out other disease processes that include headache as a symptom. Imaging studies such as CT and magnetic resonance imaging (MRI) are not usually done unless symptoms suggestive of other neurological processes are present.

Assessment parameters for headache are outlined in Box 52-11. The International Headache Society has developed specific criteria for the diagnosis of primary headache.[41] The criteria include presence or absence of aura, presence or absence of nausea or vomiting, frequency, duration, location, aggravating factors such as exercise, severity of pain, and presence of photophobia. Characteristic migraine symptoms include headaches that are preceded by aura, are slow in onset, and build in intensity. Migraines are also accompanied by other symptoms such as nausea and vomiting or photophobia.

The patient may be asked to keep a headache diary in which the patient records events surrounding the occurrence of headache such as food intake, sleep pattern, stressful events, stage of the menstrual cycle, and medication use. By providing clues to headache triggers, the diary aids in the design of an individual plan of care to prevent future attacks.

Medications for the treatment of headache fall into two broad categories: symptom relief and prevention. Symptomatic relief for mild, infrequent headache pain can usually be found with ibuprofen, propoxyphene, or codeine. Sumatriptan, a serotonin receptor agonist that causes vasoconstriction, is the first-line drug for treating a migraine headache. It can be given by mouth or subcutaneously and is administered at the first sign or symptom of the attack. Ergot alkaloids, such as dihydroergotamine mesylate and ergotamine, are other drugs used to cause cerebral vasoconstriction and abort the attack. Narcotics are rarely used for headache pain because of concerns over drug dependency. Antiemetics such as prometha-

**table 52-2** *Comparison of Migraine, Cluster, and Tension Headaches*

| Onset | Frequency/Duration | Pattern | Prodromal Associated Symptoms | Treatment |
|---|---|---|---|---|
| **MIGRAINE HEADACHES** | | | | |
| Occur at any age<br>Strongly hereditary<br>More common in women than men | Episodic; tend to occur with stress or life crisis<br>Last hours to days | Occur slowly; pain becomes severe, with one side of head affected more than other | Prodromal: vision field defects, confusion, paresthesias<br>Associated: nausea, vomiting, chills, fatigue, irritability, sweating, edema | Ergotamine tartrate<br>Propranolol<br>Nonnarcotic analgesics<br>Relaxation techniques |
| **CLUSTER HEADACHES** | | | | |
| Early adulthood; precipitated by alcohol or nitrate use<br>More common in older men | Episodes clustered together in quick succession for few days or weeks with remissions that last for months<br>Last minutes to a few hours | Intense, throbbing, deep, often unilateral pain; begins in infraorbital region and spread to head and neck | Prodromal: usually none<br>Associated: flushing, tearing of eyes, nasal stuffiness, sweating, swelling of temporal vessels | Narcotic analgesics during acute phase, often given intramuscularly |
| **TENSION HEADACHES** | | | | |
| Often in adolescence; related to tension or anxiety<br>No family history | Episodic; vary with stress<br>Duration is variable, can be constant | Dull, constant, aggravating pain; vary in intensity; usually bilateral and involve neck and shoulders; pain may be poorly defined | Prodromal: usually none<br>Associated: sustained contraction of head and neck muscles<br>Not aggravated by activity | Nonnarcotic analgesics<br>Relaxation techniques<br>Amitriptyline (Elavil) |

zine or metoclopramide may be given to relieve associated symptoms of nausea and vomiting.

Other drugs are used to prevent migraines. Propranolol is a beta blocker that inhibits vasodilation of cerebral blood vessels and inhibits the uptake of serotonin. Amitriptyline is a tricyclic antidepressant used to block the uptake of catecholamines and serotonin. Hydrochlorothiazide or other diuretics may be given in low doses to prevent fluid retention that can lead to migraines. Table 52-3 presents an overview of drugs commonly used to treat headache.

Other treatments for headache also attempt to prevent the attack or provide symptomatic relief. About one third of patients with migraine can be helped with biofeedback or relaxation techniques.[5] For patients who already have a headache,

**box 52-11** *Headache Assessment*

**Headache characteristics:** Time of onset, location, frequency, severity, duration, quality (deep, superficial, steady, throbbing, stabbing, burning), situations or activities that make the headache better or worse

**Presence of an aura:** Duration, relation to onset of pain

**Associated symptoms occurring before, during, or after a headache:** Nausea, vomiting, photophobia, visual disturbances, dizziness, incoordination, redness of the eye, facial symptoms (sweating, paleness, flushing), fatigue or sleepiness, mood swings, weakness, paresthesia

**Potential precipitating factors:** Change in eating pattern, dietary substances (e.g., tyramine, nitrates), relationship to menstrual cycle, sexual intercourse, pregnancy, menopause, psychosocial stressors, change in sleep pattern, weather changes, hot or cold wind, altitude, lights, smog

**Activities of daily living patterns:** Eating, sleeping, exercise, relaxation

**Drug history:** Over-the-counter and prescribed headache medications, other medications (nitroglycerine, reserpine, birth control pills, vitamin A, indomethacin, hormone replacement), alcohol and drug use, smoking history

**Medical history:** Asthma; peptic ulcer; motion sickness; head injury; seizure disorder; sleepwalking; Raynaud's disease; irritable bowel syndrome; infertility; skin problems; pain in neck, head, or throat; abdominal distress; anxiety; depression; insomnia

**Family history:** History of headache and other medical problems

NOTE: A headache daily diary must include complete description of each headache, precipitating events, associated symptoms, and, in women, the relationship to the menstrual cycle.

Adapted from Barker E: *Neuroscience nursing*, St Louis, 1994, Mosby.

**table 52-3** *Common Medications for* ***Headache***

| Drug | Action | Nursing Interventions |
|---|---|---|
| **SYMPTOMATIC TREATMENT** | | |
| Ergot alkaloids<br>Ergotamine tartrate (Cafergot)<br>Dihydroergotamine (D.H.E. 45) | Causes cerebral vasoconstriction<br>Decreases pulsation of cranial arteries | Take as soon as migraine symptoms begin.<br>Nausea is a common side effect; patients may need to also use antiemetics<br>Ergots have a cumulative effect: use sparingly and monitor for signs of ergotism—numbness and tingling, weakness, muscle pain |
| Metoclopramide (Reglan) | Increases gastrointestinal motility to decrease the incidence of nausea and vomiting | Patient should avoid driving or other hazardous activity after taking drug |
| Sumatriptan (Imitrex) | Serotonin receptor agonist, causes vasoconstriction | Contraindicated in pregnancy, coronary artery disease. Teach patient to take drug at first sign of a headache |
| **PROPHYLAXIS** | | |
| Beta blockers<br>Propranolol (Inderal)<br>Nadolol (Corgard)<br>Atenolol (Tenormin)<br>Timolol (Betimol)<br>Metoprolol (Lopressor) | Inhibit vasodilation and serotonin uptake; propranolol is the first drug of choice for prophylaxis of migraines | May cause cardiac dysfunction; monitor for bradycardia, orthostatic hypotension, lethargy, depression |
| Tricyclic antidepressants<br>Amitriptyline (Elavil) | Block uptake of serotonin and catecholamines<br>Most effective for migraine-associated tension headaches | May cause dry mouth, drowsiness, and urinary retention |
| Methysergide (Sansert) | Alternative if beta blockers are not tolerated | Used for migraine prophylaxis |

lying quietly in a darkened room and additional sleep offer some relief from pain.

Once the patient has kept a headache diary, it may be possible to identify certain foods or activities that trigger headache. Headache triggers can be confirmed by excluding them from the diet altogether and monitoring the patient for the recurrence of symptoms. Foods that have been shown to cause cerebrovasodilation in migraine patients are nitrites, nitrates, tyramines, alcohol, monosodium glutamate, and caffeine. Nicotine has also been associated with an increased incidence of headache, and it is advisable for the patient to quit smoking and avoid the use of nicotine gum or patches.[5] A high salt intake may lead to fluid retention and is a known problem for some women who experience migraines around the time of their menstrual cycle. Oral contraceptives should not be used by migraine sufferers. There is a recognized correlation between oral contraceptive use and an increase in migraine incidence.[19]

Fasting increases serotonin turnover in the brain, which can lead to vasodilation and trigger a headache. The nurse can assist the patient to identify foods that should be eliminated or reduced in the diet, refer the patient to a smoking cessation program, and encourage the patient to eat small, frequent meals to avoid fluctuations in glucose and serotonin levels.

Vigorous activity has been associated with triggering migraine headaches.[19] However, moderate exercise should not act as a trigger. Exercise is clearly associated with lowering stress and contributing to an overall sense of well-being. During the actual headache, patients benefit from rest until medication and other treatments take effect.

### Patient/Family Education

The nurse may refer the patient to a dietitian if the patient needs guidance regarding dietary changes to prevent headache. Referrals may be made for biofeedback or relaxation training to prevent stress-induced head pain. In addition, there may be local support groups for sufferers of headache. The National Headache Foundation provides consumer health information for persons with headache.

Patients with headache commonly worry that their headache is a symptom of some other serious disease. The nurse encourages the patient to accurately report all signs and symptoms and provides education that assists the patient and family to satisfactorily prevent and treat headaches. Identification of triggers is just a first step. The patient must then make lifestyle changes to avoid these triggers. The nurse teaches the patient how to appropriately use all medications. Drugs prescribed to prevent migraine need to be taken on a regular schedule, without missing doses. Drugs prescribed to treat headache symptoms need to be available and taken as soon as the patient becomes aware of symptoms or the presence of an aura.

# EPILEPSY

## ETIOLOGY/EPIDEMIOLOGY

Epilepsy is a chronic disorder surrounded by many myths and misconceptions. Recent advances in the understanding and treatment of epilepsy have improved societal attitudes toward this condition, but the diagnosis still represents a social stigma for many patients. A seizure is an abnormal, paroxysmal electrical discharge from the cerebral cortex. Seizures are clinically seen as alterations in sensation, behavior, movement, perception, or consciousness. Symptoms are related to the area of the cortex involved. Epilepsy is defined as recurrent, stereotypical seizures.[30]

An estimated 2 million people in the United States have epilepsy, and approximately 125,000 new cases are diagnosed each year. Thirty percent of newly diagnosed patients are less than 18 years old. The prevalence of epilepsy in persons over 65 years old is 1%. When no identifiable cause for epilepsy can be found the seizures are termed *idiopathic,* and idiopathic epilepsy accounts for 70% of all cases. The remaining 30% of cases are related to a known cause, such as central nervous system structural lesions. Risk factors for developing epilepsy in adulthood include lesions within the central nervous system (e.g., traumatic brain injury), meningitis or encephalitis, cerebral tumors, and stroke.[30] Initial seizures in children are commonly fever related.

Any condition that causes cerebral irritation or alters the biochemical environment of the brain can result in seizures. The risk of having an isolated seizure during one's lifetime is thought to be about 10%.[30] Seizures can occur as a result of a wide range of metabolic derangements that affect the central nervous system, and if the underlying condition is corrected the seizures do not recur. These seizures are not epilepsy. Genetics clearly plays a role in some forms of epilepsy. Common risk factors for epilepsy are listed in the accompanying box.

## PATHOPHYSIOLOGY

A seizure can be caused by any process that disrupts the cell membrane stability of a neuron. The point at which the cell membrane becomes destabilized and an uncontrolled electrical discharge begins is known as the seizure threshold. Some people have lower seizure thresholds than others and are therefore more prone to seizures.

**risk factors**

**Epilepsy**

- Anoxia
- Cerebral palsy
- Perinatal problems (toxemia, difficult delivery, low birth weight, hypoxia)
- Congenital central nervous system defects
- Mental retardation
- Febrile conditions
- Family history of epilepsy
- Head trauma
- Central nervous system infections
- Central nervous system tumors
- Cerebrovascular disease
- Alcohol or drug abuse
- Metabolic disturbances
- Exposure to toxins
- Degenerative diseases (Alzheimer's disease)

In 1981 the International League Against Epilepsy proposed a revised classification for epileptic seizures (Table 52-4). The major categories are partial (also called focal), generalized, and unclassified. Further subdivisions within the categories are based on the person's clinical behaviors during the ictal and interictal times. Ictal refers to the time during the seizure. Interictal refers to the time between seizure activity. Postictal refers to the time immediately after a seizure as the patient recovers.

Partial seizures do not always affect consciousness. Simple partial seizures have less motor, sensory, and consciousness involvement because they are limited to a smaller area of the brain. The wider the area of cerebral cortex affected, the more clinical symptoms are seen. With simple partial seizures a patient may have uncontrolled movement of an extremity or a portion of the face. He or she will be able to interact with others during the seizure and will remember the event afterwards. Complex partial seizures affect consciousness. The patient may recall the presence of an aura, which is a warning sensation that occurs before the seizure. Patients having complex partial seizures often exhibit automatisms (automatic behaviors) such as lip smacking, chewing, rubbing, or picking at clothes. These behaviors are not voluntary, because consciousness is impaired. Some complex partial seizures spread to larger areas of the cortex and become generalized tonic-clonic seizures. These are different than tonic-clonic seizures in which the initial seizure behavior is generalized.

Generalized seizures impair consciousness from the start. Absence seizures do not include motor signs and may last less than 1 minute, making them difficult to detect. These seizures are often seen in children and may be initially thought of as "daydreaming." There is no postictal state, and absence seizures can occur many times a day.

Tonic-clonic seizures have a tonic phase, during which the muscles become rigid, and then a clonic phase, which involves rhythmic muscle jerking. As the muscles of the trunk and diaphragm become rigid, the air moving past the vocal cords creates a "cry." Once the diaphragm is contracted, the patient is unable to breathe. If the seizure lasts long enough, the patient may become cyanotic. Bladder and bowel muscles are also affected, and the patient may experience incontinence.

Other generalized seizures include myoclonic and atonic types. Myoclonic seizures cause one or several muscles to jerk, often causing the patient to fall. Atonic seizures cause a brief loss of tone in one or more muscles, causing the patient to drop things or fall. They cause only a brief loss of consciousness and no postictal state. The patient is able get up right away unless he or she is injured from the fall.

Postictal states represent periods of recovery from the seizure. The brain must recover from the intense burst of electrical activity. The length of the postictal period varies from patient to patient. Patients may have some degree of confusion, lethargy, or an inability to follow commands or speak clearly during this period. In some rare cases, the patient may experience a prolonged period of weakness involving one or

**table 52-4** *Classification of Epileptic Seizures*

| Type of Seizure | Effect on Consciousness | Signs and Symptoms | Postictal State |
|---|---|---|---|
| **PARTIAL SEIZURES** | | | |
| Simple partial (focal) | Not impaired | Focal twitching of extremity<br>Speech arrest<br>Special visual sensations (e.g., seeing lights), feeling of fear or doom | No |
| Complex partial (formerly psychomotor or temporal lobe seizures) | Impaired | May begin as simple partial and progress to complex<br>Automatic behavior (e.g. lip smacking, chewing, or picking at clothes) | Yes |
| Complex partial generalizing to generalized tonic-clonic seizures | Impaired | Begins as complex partial as above, then progresses to tonic-clonic as described below | Yes |
| **GENERALIZED SEIZURES** | | | |
| Absence (formerly petit mal) | Impaired | Brief loss of consciousness, staring, unresponsive | No |
| Tonic-clonic (formerly grand mal) | Impaired | Tonic phase involves rigidity of all muscles, followed by clonic phase, which involves rhythmic jerking of muscles, possibly tongue biting and urinary and fecal incontinence<br>May be any combination of tonic and clonic movements | Yes |
| Atonic | Impaired for only a few seconds | Brief loss of muscle tone, which may cause patient to fall or drop something; referred to as drop attacks | No |
| Myoclonic | Impaired for only a few seconds or not at all | Brief jerking of a muscle group, which may cause the patient to fall | No |

more extremities called Todd's paralysis. Although not permanent, the "paralysis" may persist beyond the postictal period of confusion or fatigue.

Status epilepticus is an episode of seizure activity lasting at least 30 minutes, or repeated seizures without full recovery between seizures. Seizures cause a marked increase in cerebral metabolic activity and demands. These demands may outpace the delivery of oxygen and nutrients from the cerebral blood flow. Prolonged seizures can lead to cellular exhaustion and destruction and lead to death if not effectively treated.[11]

## COLLABORATIVE CARE MANAGEMENT

The diagnosis of epilepsy is made from a careful history and physical examination supplemented by selected diagnostic tests. The history should include the following:

- Family history of seizures
- Perinatal history (for childhood-onset seizures)
- Childhood illnesses, including febrile seizures
- Age at seizure onset
- History of head trauma
- Central nervous system infections
- Central nervous system tumors
- Stroke
- Degenerative nervous system diseases (multiple sclerosis, Alzheimer's disease)

A thorough description of the seizure itself is also obtained, including the following:

- Description of the aura, if any (preseizure sensation or feeling)
- Precipitating factors such as lack of sleep, alcohol intake, emotional stress, excess caffeine, time of day, menses
- Description of patient's behavior from beginning of the seizure to the end, especially if the motor signs started in one part of the body and spread to another part (jacksonian march)
- Length of the seizure
- Length of the postictal recovery period and behavior during this phase
- Incidence of incontinence
- Frequency of the seizures (if more than one) and interval between them

A physical examination is performed to evaluate the patient for possible neurological disease that could cause seizures. A CT scan or MRI may be ordered to check for structural lesions. Laboratory tests, including electrolytes, creatinine, BUN, arterial blood gases, and toxicology screens, are done to rule out metabolic causes for seizures.

An electroencephalogram (EEG) is performed after the history and physical. The EEG may be recorded during a brief outpatient test, overnight, or after 12 to 24 hours of sleep deprivation. The EEG can help identify the location, or foci, of the seizures and their pattern of spread, if any, over the cortex. However, an EEG can identify a seizure only if one occurs during the test. A normal EEG does not rule out the possibility of a past or future seizure. In some cases, patients may be monitored for several days as an inpatient.

Antiepileptic drugs (AEDs) are used to control seizures. These drugs are also called anticonvulsants. See Table 52-5 for the most commonly used AEDs. Once the patient is established on the medication, drug levels are tested to ensure that the patient has achieved a therapeutic level. While specific values have been established for therapeutic levels, the appropriate dose for any patient is one that prevents seizures but does not cause toxicity, even if the blood level is higher than the established norm. In the past, patients continued on anticonvulsant therapy for life. Today, the physician may attempt to wean the patient from the medication if the patient has remained seizure free for 1 to 2 years. A common side effect of most AEDs is drowsiness or other mental status changes. These side effects may interfere with the patient's social life or work. Multiple changes in drug or dose may be needed to achieve the best seizure control with the fewest side effects.

Because of the emergent nature of status epilepticus, slightly different medications are used. Benzodiazepines are used to rapidly terminate the seizure activity while a loading dose of anticonvulsants is administered. Anticonvulsants take longer to achieve a therapeutic blood level. See the Guidelines for Care Box below and the Nursing Care Plan on p. 1716.

The nurse institutes seizure precautions to protect the patient from injury if the patient's seizures are not well controlled or if the patient has a new illness or injury that predisposes her or him to a lower seizure threshold. In most hospitals,

***guidelines for care***

### The Patient in Status Epilepticus

1. Protect airway and provide oxygen. Position the patient on side to prevent aspiration. Place an oral airway if the teeth are not clenched. Administer oxygen by mask. If respiratory depression occurs from seizures or medication used to control seizures, intubation may be necessary.
2. Establish IV access for medication delivery and fluids.
3. Draw blood for electrolytes, arterial blood gases, and toxicology to rule out metabolic causes for seizures.
4. Administer benzodiazepines, usually lorazepam (Ativan) 4 to 8 mg over 2 to 4 minutes or diazepam (Valium) 5 to 20 mg over 5 to 10 minutes to stop seizures. These drugs are fast acting and will control seizures until anticonvulsant drugs reach therapeutic levels.
5. Administer anticonvulsants, usually phenytoin (Dilantin) 15 to 20 mg/kg in normal saline at 50 mg/min maximum rate at the same time as the benzodiazepines to begin establishing therapeutic levels. Dilantin can cause significant hypotension and cardiac dysrhythmias. Place the patient on a monitor during loading doses.
6. Continue the search for an underlying cause of seizures.

seizure precautions include keeping side rails up and padded if the patient has tonic-clonic seizures, assembling suction at the bedside, disabling locks on bathroom and room doors, and avoiding taking oral temperatures with glass thermometers.

Nurses need to be able to act quickly when a patient has a seizure. The nurse makes careful observations in order to document the seizure accurately. The patient is reassured that help is near if it is needed. If the seizure generalizes or begins as a generalized seizure, the nurse acts to protect the patient from injury. No attempt is made to restrain the patient, because this could cause injury. The nurse protects the patient from hitting his or her extremities or head on furniture or bed rails by moving them or padding obstructions. Nothing is forced into the patient's mouth. Patients having a tonic-clonic seizure will not have effective air exchange during the seizure, but a patient cannot "swallow" his or her own tongue. Patients may, however, occlude their airway by flexing their neck or clenching their jaw. After the seizure, the nurse gently clears oral secretions, positions the patient to open the airway, and administers oxygen if needed. After securing the airway, the nurse assesses the patient for injuries such as abrasions, bruises, or evidence of tongue biting that might have occurred during the seizure. The duration of the postictal phase is assessed and documented, including how much time elapses between the end of the seizure and when the patient can follow commands and answer questions. Someone should remain with the patient until he or she becomes fully responsive to the surroundings.[10]

There are no specific dietary restrictions for the patient with epilepsy. If the patient can identify certain foods that trigger seizures, these may be eliminated from the diet. These foods may include caffeine, chocolate, and alcohol. The intake of

**table 52-5** *Common Medications for **Epilepsy***

| Drug | Action | Nursing Interventions |
|---|---|---|
| **HYDANTOINS** | | |
| Phenytoin (Dilantin) | Blocks synaptic potentiation and propagation of electrical discharge in the motor cortex.<br>Blocks sodium transport and stabilizes membrane sensitivity.<br>Used alone or in combination to manage tonic-clonic, simple partial, and complex partial seizures.<br>Therapeutic range is 10-20 mg/L. Takes at least 7-14 days to establish. | Monitor for common side effects including nystagmus, ataxia, fatigue, drowsiness, and cognitive impairment.<br>Gastrointestinal symptoms (e.g., nausea, anorexia, vomiting) are common. Drug may be given with meals.<br>Gingival hyperplasia is a common side effect. Patients are taught the importance of scrupulous oral hygiene.<br>Regular follow-up for monitoring is encouraged. |
| **BARBITURATES** | | |
| Phenobarbital (Luminal) | Depresses postsynaptic excitatory discharge.<br>Used to manage tonic-clonic, simple partial, and complex partial seizures and status epilepticus. | Monitor for side effects, which include sedation, drowsiness, and depression. |
| **SUCCINIMIDES** | | |
| Ethosuximide (Zarontin) | Depresses motor cortex and raises threshold to stimuli.<br>Used to manage absence seizures. | Monitor for side effects (e.g., anorexia, nausea, vomiting, and drowsiness).<br>Caution patient to never abruptly discontinue the drug. Can precipitate status epilepticus. |
| **OTHER** | | |
| Carbamazepine (Tegretol) | Believed to reduce polysynaptic responses and block synaptic potentiation.<br>Used to manage tonic-clonic, simple partial, and complex partial seizures. | Monitor for side effects (e.g., drowsiness, dizziness, headache, anorexia, nausea, and vomiting). Side effects tend to decrease in severity over time.<br>Regular follow-up is encouraged because drug can cause rare but severe bone marrow toxicities. |
| Valproic acid (Depakene) | Increases levels of gamma-aminobutyric acid for membrane stabilization.<br>Used to manage absence seizures or in combination with other drugs for tonic-clonic and complex partial seizures. | Monitor for side effects (e.g., anorexia, nausea, and vomiting).<br>Teach patient to take drug with meals.<br>Central nervous system side effects such as drowsiness, tremor, and ataxia.<br>Regular follow-up is encouraged because drug may cause liver dysfunction and blood dyscrasias. |

## nursing care plan *Person with Status Epilepticus*

**DATA** Mr. F. is a 29-year-old man with a history of seizures. He experiences complex partial seizures that occasionally generalize to tonic-clonic seizures. He takes phenytoin (Dilantin) 300 mg qhs and carbamazepine (Tegretol) 200 mg tid to control his seizures. Despite good compliance with medications, he has about four or five seizures a year.

Today, after mowing the lawn, he was putting the lawn mower away and his wife heard him fall in the garage. She found him having a tonic-clonic seizure. The first seizure lasted 2 minutes, and she turned him on his side and moved tools in the garage away from him to protect him. He began to seize again and after 5 more minutes of generalized seizure activity his wife called the rescue squad. By the time he got to the emergency department he had been seizing for 25 minutes without any recovery between the first and second seizure.

Oxygen by mask was started. An IV was established, and 0.9% saline was started. Blood was drawn for electrolytes, toxicology, and anticonvulsant levels. Lorazepam 2 mg IV was given every 4 minutes for four doses for a total of 8 mg. Phenytoin (Dilantin) 1000 mg was hung in saline to infuse over 1 hour.

After the fourth dose of lorazepam was given, the seizure stopped, but his respiratory rate was 6/min and his oxygen saturation was 85%. His blood pressure (BP) was 85/50 mm Hg. He was electively intubated and ventilated and admitted to the intensive care unit (ICU).

One hour after admission to the ICU he was localizing to pain stimuli but not following commands. His Dilantin bolus infused, and his BP rose to 110/70, respiratory rate 8, no breaths above the ventilator. Breath sounds were clear bilaterally and oxygen saturation was 99% on 40% $FIO_2$.

**NURSING DIAGNOSIS** *Risk for injury related to seizure activity*

| expected patient outcome | nursing interventions | rationale |
|---|---|---|
| Patient will not experience injury during seizure or postictal period. | **1.** Implement seizure precautions.<br>**a.** Pad side rails.<br>**b.** Keep side rails up and bed in low position.<br>**c.** Monitor frequently.<br>**d.** Ensure rapid access to oxygen, suction, and other emergency equipment. | **1.** All seizure precautions are designed to minimize environmental risks to the patient in the event of a seizure and to ensure prompt access to emergency care as needed. |
| | **2.** Administer antiepileptic drugs (AEDs) as ordered.<br>**a.** Monitor patient response.<br>**b.** Insert nasogastric tube to administer Tegretol if needed. | **2.** Aggressive drug therapy is the key to halting the seizures. Tegretol cannot be administered IV. |

**NURSING DIAGNOSIS** *Fluid volume deficit related to altered mental status and sudden losses*

| expected patient outcome | nursing interventions | rationale |
|---|---|---|
| Patient will maintain a balanced intake and output and a blood pressure within normal limits. | **1.** Maintain NPO status until fully awake. | **1.** Aspiration is a risk until patient is fully alert with protective reflexes intact. |
| | **2.** Administer IV fluids as indicated. | **2.** Blood pressure must be supported during crisis period. |
| | **3.** Monitor vital signs frequently. | **3.** Phenytoin increases the risk of hypotension. |
| | **4.** Monitor intake and output levels. | **4.** Outdoor work before admission may have precipitated a fluid deficit. |

alcohol is recommended only in moderation because alcohol intake is associated with a lower seizure threshold.

Most patients with epilepsy can achieve satisfactory control of their disease through the use of pharmacological agents. For intractable epilepsy, however, additional testing to locate specific epileptogenic foci may be done so that the dysfunctional tissue can be surgically removed. Patients selected for this procedure are those whose seizures have not been controlled despite the use of multiple medications.

### Patient/Family Education

Patients and their families must learn to cope with a chronic illness that greatly affects their everyday life and independence. The Epilepsy Foundation of America is a patient-focused organization providing education and support for patients and their families. Local chapters can provide information about services available in the community, and the nurse encourages the patient to use this important resource.

Epilepsy was once believed to be of supernatural origin, and perhaps for this reason it has been thought of as evil or "wrong" in the public mind. No disease has been more carefully concealed within families than epilepsy. Attitudes toward persons with epilepsy have been gradually changing, but old prejudices continue to exist.

Education regarding the causes of epilepsy will greatly dispel the myth that persons with epilepsy are "possessed" or evil.

**research**

Reference: Dilorio C, Henry M: Self management in persons with epilepsy, *J Neurosci Nurs* 27(6):338, 1995.

Persons with epilepsy were surveyed to determine the extent to which they use recommended self-management strategies to control their epilepsy. Most respondents reported compliance with medications but less adherence with other safety practices such as not climbing ladders, getting enough rest, or eating properly. These findings suggest topics for nursing practice as additional topics for patient education plans.

With adequate medication control, the patient with epilepsy can lead a normal life. The nurse helps the patient understand the importance of adhering to the medication regimen and avoiding precipitating factors for their seizures. Self-care is an ongoing challenge (see the Research Box). Medications are prescribed and adjusted to achieve the best control of seizures without evidence of drug toxicity. The timing of doses can be altered to fit the patient's lifestyle and prevent missed doses.

The nurse stresses the importance of carrying some form of identification with information about the seizure disorder and all prescribed medications in case strangers must provide first aid in the event of a seizure or accident. If the patient feels comfortable sharing the information, a colleague at work or school can be informed about the disease and instructed about what to do in the event of a seizure.

Safety is a primary consideration for the patient with epilepsy. Activity is not generally restricted unless it puts the patient at risk of injury should a seizure occur. But a history of epilepsy does limit the patient's options in terms of employment, because employers must carefully consider their own liability in case of seizure activity on the job. Each state also has laws defining driver's licensing for persons with a seizure history. Driving may be permitted once a patient has been seizure free on medication for a period of time, often as much as 1 to 2 years.

# INTRACRANIAL TUMORS

## ETIOLOGY

Primary intracranial tumors arise from the support cells of brain tissues rather than from the neurons. These tumors invade or displace brain tissue as they grow and lead to neurological symptoms. They are therefore referred to as brain tumors. Brain tumors are generally believed to be the result of a change in the genetic control of cellular growth, leading to abnormal cell mutations and a loss of organized cell growth.[21] Both benign and malignant tumors occur, but this differentiation has less meaning for intracranial tumors than for other types of tissue. A histologically "benign" tumor can be surgically inaccessible, continue to grow, and cause increasing dysfunction ranging from increasing ICP to death.

Some intracranial tumors are graded I to IV reflecting the nature of the cellular changes. The more abnormal and anaplastic the tumor cells are, the higher the grade.[29] Highly malignant grades III and IV astrocytomas are the most common type of brain tumors, but a wide variety of tumors exist (Table 52-6).

## EPIDEMIOLOGY

The annual incidence of primary brain tumors is about 17,500 cases. An approximately equal number of secondary or metastatic tumors also occur each year. Brain tumors affect people of all ages with two peak periods of incidence—early childhood and the fifth to seventh decades of life.

Children are primarily affected by infratentorial tumors of the posterior fossa, such as medulloblastomas. Adults are most commonly affected by the various forms of gliomas. Gliomas and neuromas are more common in males, while meningiomas and pituitary adenomas are more common in females.

## PATHOPHYSIOLOGY

### Types of Tumors

Brain tumors are named for the tissues from which they arise. The more common ones are gliomas, meningiomas, pituitary adenomas, and acoustic neuromas (see Table 52-6). Gliomas account for about 45% of all brain tumors and arise from the connective tissue, the glia cells, of the brain. In adults gliomas primarily infiltrate the tissues of the cerebral hemisphere and are not encapsulated, making it difficult to excise them. They grow rapidly, and most persons do not survive longer than a few years after diagnosis. The less malignant gliomas are low-grade astrocytomas and oligodendrogliomas. Ependymomas arise from cells lining the ventricular system. The most malignant and rapidly growing forms of gliomas are the glioblastoma mulitiforme and medulloblastoma. Gliomas may start as one grade and rapidly become more malignant, especially if left untreated.[25]

The meningiomas, which account for 15% of all primary brain tumors, arise from the meningeal coverings of the brain. They occur most commonly in the meninges over the cerebral hemispheres in the parasagittal region along the ridge of the sphenoid bone and in the anterior fossa near the olfactory groove or sella turcica. When located in the posterior fossa, they arise from the cerebellopontine angle, from the tentorium, or rarely from the region of the foramen magnum. Meningiomas are usually benign, but they may undergo malignant changes or be found in a location that makes surgery impossible without causing significant neurological damage.

Acoustic neuromas constitute about 7% of all primary brain tumors. These tumors grow from the sheath covering the eighth cranial nerve, and the patient exhibits symptoms such as hearing loss or balance disturbance if the vestibular portion of the nerve is compressed. If the tumor becomes large, surrounding structures such as the trigeminal and facial nerves may also be involved causing additional neurological symptoms.

Pituitary adenomas make up about 7% of brain tumors. These tumors are considered benign but may be difficult to completely remove because of their location in the sella turcica and close proximity to the pituitary gland. Symptoms include hormonal changes, such as acromegaly from increased growth hormone production. Visual symptoms may develop

**table 52-6** *Types of Brain Tumors Occurring in Adults*

| TYPE AND INCIDENCE | PATHOLOGY |
|---|---|
| **GLIOMAS: NONENCAPSULATED, TEND TO INFILTRATE BRAIN TISSUE** | |
| Astrocytomas (grades I and II)—10%<br>Glioblastoma multiforme (also called astrocytoma grades III and IV)—20%<br>Oligodendroglioma (grades I to IV)—5%<br>Ependymoma (grades I to IV)—6%<br>Medulloblastoma—4% | Arise in any part of brain connective tissue; infiltrate primarily cerebral hemisphere tissue; not so well outlined as to be incised completely; grow rapidly—most persons live months to years; tumors assigned grade from 1 to 4, with 4 the most malignant |
| **TUMORS FROM SUPPORT STRUCTURES** | |
| Meningiomas—15% | Arise from meningeal coverings of brain; usually benign but may undergo malignant changes; usually encapsulated, and surgical cure possible; recurrence possible |
| Neuromas (acoustic neuroma, schwannoma)—7% | Arise from Schwann cells inside auditory meatus on vestibular portion of third cranial nerve; usually benign but may undergo cellular change and become malignant; will regrow if not completely excised; surgical resection often difficult because of location |
| Pituitary adenoma—7% | Arise from various tissues; surgical approach usually successful; recurrence possible |
| **DEVELOPMENTAL (CONGENITAL TUMORS)** | |
| Dermoid, epidermoid, craniopharyngioma—4% | Arise from embryonic tissue in various sites in the brain; success of surgical resection dependent on location and invasiveness |
| Angiomas—4% | Arise from vascular structures; usually difficult to resect |
| **METASTATIC TUMORS—18%** | Cancer cells spread to brain via circulatory system; surgical resection very difficult; even with treatment, prognosis is very poor; survival beyond 1 or 2 years is uncommon |

if the tumor expands beyond the sella turcica and compresses the optic chiasm, which crosses above the pituitary.

Metastatic tumors that have primary sites in the lung, kidney, breast, colon, and other organs account for about 18% of all intracranial tumors. Primary brain tumors, conversely, rarely metastasize to other organs. See Table 52-6 for a review of types of brain tumors.

### Clinical Manifestations

Brain tumors produce a wide range of neurological symptoms based on their size, location, and invasive qualities. Locally, the tumor invades, displaces, and destroys brain tissue, producing symptoms related to the functions of that particular site (Boxes 52-12 and 52-13). They also exert direct pressure on nerve structures, causing degeneration and interference with local circulation. Local edema develops, which interferes with nerve transmission and exerts a mass effect.

An intracranial tumor of any type can cause an increase in ICP. The increased ICP is transmitted throughout the brain and ventricular system and can produce additional symptoms such as headache, confusion, and papilledema. (See the section on increased ICP earlier in this chapter.)

Some tumors expand and displace the structures of the ventricular system, leading to partial obstruction of the flow of cerebrospinal fluid and eventually hydrocephalus. Cerebrospinal fluid is produced in the two lateral ventricles, flows through the third ventricle, through the aqueduct of Sylvius into the fourth ventricle, and then through the foramen of Luschka and foramen of Magendie out into the central canal of the spinal cord. It is distributed over the surface of the brain in the subarachnoid space until it is reabsorbed in the arachnoid granulations of the sagittal sinus. If the flow is disrupted at any point in the system, CSF builds up and causes the ventricles to dilate. Dilated ventricles exert outward pressure on the brain, increasing the ICP. One specific type of tumor, the ependymomas, originates in the ependymal cells that line the ventricular system.

Tumors occurring above the tentorium may disrupt brain function and lead to seizures. If the tumor is small and has not caused other symptoms, a seizure may be the first symptom that brings the person to medical attention.

## COLLABORATIVE CARE MANAGEMENT

The nurse works collaboratively with other members of the health care team to implement the prescribed medical therapy. Because the nurse has a major role in discharge planning and patient teaching, these are discussed in the section on nursing management.

### Diagnostic Tests

The CT scan is the most commonly used test to diagnose and evaluate brain tumors and their effect on surrounding brain

**box 52-12** clinical manifestations

***Intracranial Tumors***

Symptoms can be generalized, as well as specific to the tumor location and the structures of the brain that are compressed.

- "Pressure" headaches (generalized or periorbital)
- Nausea and vomiting unrelated to food intake
- Symptoms of increased intracranial pressure
- Visual changes:
  - Blurred vision
  - Diplopia (with third, fourth, and sixth nerve compression)
  - Visual field alterations (with tumor compression of the optic chiasm or optic pathways)
  - Enlarged blind spot related to papilledema
- Seizures
- Weakness or hemiparesis (when the tumor affects the motor cortex)
- Speech difficulty (when the tumor affects the language area in the dominant hemisphere)
- Alterations in level of consciousness (with a midbrain tumor)
- Personality changes (with frontal tumors)

**box 52-13** *Symptoms of Tumors Found in Specific Brain Lobes*

**FRONTAL LOBE**
Personality disturbances (range from subtle personality changes to obvious psychotic behavior)
Inappropriate affect
Motor dysfunction
Aphasia (expressive, motor)
Seizures

**OCCIPITAL LOBE**
Visual disturbances
Headache, seizures

**TEMPORAL LOBE**
Olfactory, visual, or gustatory hallucinations
Complex partial seizures with automatic behavior
Aphasia (receptive, sensory)

**PARIETAL LOBE**
Inability to replicate pictures
Loss of right-left discrimination
Seizures
Paresthesias
Sensory-perceptual deficits

tissue. A cerebral angiogram may be performed if the tumor is situated near major blood vessels, and information is needed regarding feeding vessels to plan the optimal surgical route. Magnetic resonance imaging is also used, particularly for tumors of the posterior fossa, where MRI can provide more detail than CT.

### Medications

Drug therapy is used in the management of brain tumors, both to treat the tumor with chemotherapy and to manage symptoms. A wide variety of chemotherapeutic agents are used, usually in combination protocols. Chemotherapy may be delivered by the standard intravenous route, but the tight junctions of the blood-brain barrier make it difficult to achieve therapeutic levels of the drugs in the brain tumor. Intrathecal administration delivers the drug directly into the central nervous system, but the distribution of the drug to the tumor is still uneven. The use of an Ommaya reservoir allows for the delivery of drugs into the lateral ventricle (Figure 52-9). Newer, controlled-release polymer "wafers" allow for the delivery of chemotherapy by diffusion directly into the tumor cavity. These wafers are implanted in the cavity at the time of tumor resection and are left in place to gradually degrade after the drug has been delivered.[39]

Drug therapy also plays a significant role in symptom management. Most patients receive a corticosteroid such as dexamethasone to help control cerebral edema around the tumor site. The effects are temporary, and steroids are usually tapered after a month or less. A histamine receptor antagonist such as ranitidine or famotidine may be administered along with the steroid to decrease the risk of peptic ulcer formation.

Anticonvulsant medication will also be initiated to prevent the development of seizures. Phenytoin (Dilantin) is the drug of choice, because carbamazepine (Tegretol) is known to cause bone marrow suppression. See Table 52-7 for a review of medications used to manage symptoms in patients with intracranial tumors.

### Treatments

Radiation therapy is another nonsurgical treatment used in the management of brain tumors. Radiation is usually administered after surgical resection of the tumor; however, it may be used as the primary therapy if the tumor is considered inaccessible.[38] Metastatic lesions and medulloblastomas are the most responsive to radiation. Radiation is used postoperatively in the treatment of most gliomas because the infiltrative nature of these tumors makes them extremely difficult to completely remove surgically.

Most patients respond well to radiotherapy, but some patients experience severe radiation-induced cerebral edema that is not controllable with steroids. These patients may develop symptoms of compromised brain function. Most brain tumors are invasive, and the radiation is administered to a large area of the brain, increasing the risk of cell damage and necrosis in the surrounding normal brain tissue.

Stereotaxic radiation, or "gamma knife" therapy, is an alternative form of radiotherapy available at selected centers. It is used to noninvasively treat deep-seated tumors that are inaccessible to conventional surgery. Using a stereotaxic frame fixed to the patient's head, beams of radiation can be concentrated and directed at small areas of brain tissue known to be malignant. This minimizes the radiation

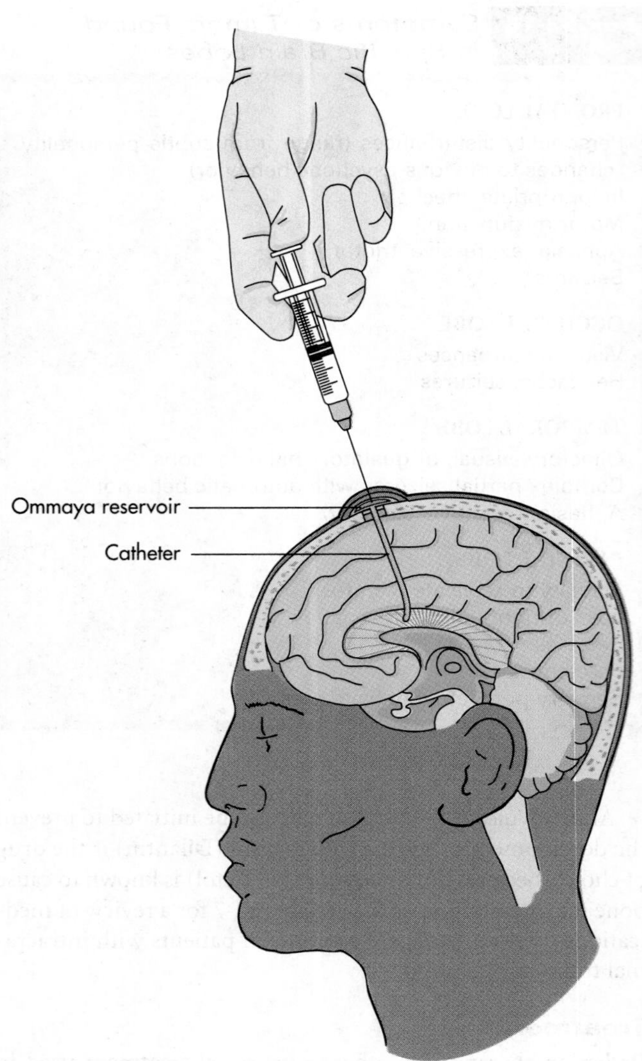


**fig. 52-9** The Ommaya reservoir. The reservoir is a mushroom-shaped device with an attached catheter that is implanted into the lateral ventricle through a burr hole. A silicone injection dome rests over the burr hole under the scalp. Drugs can be injected directly into the reservoir with a syringe.

damage to surrounding normal brain tissue. The final effects of treatment are not known for several weeks because the irradiated area responds slowly to the treatment.[38]

Other techniques that have been developed to treat brain tumors include the use of both hypothermia and hyperthermia. Hypothermia and controlled hypotensive states are used during surgery to make access to tumors less harmful to normal brain tissue. Hyperthermia is used to destroy tumor cells.[39]

Another treatment for brain tumors that is performed as an adjunct to surgery is the neuroradiological procedure called embolization. A cerebral angiogram identifies feeding blood vessels to a tumor, usually a meningioma. These vessels are then embolized by introducing a material that blocks blood flow through the vessel. Reduced blood flow to the meningioma enables the surgeon to resect the tumor with less blood loss.[37] Similar treatments are being used in preparation for surgery to remove or repair aneurysms and arteriovenous malformations.

### Surgical Management

Surgery is the treatment of choice for most intracranial tumors. Surgery is used to establish the histological tissue diagnosis and to either debulk or completely resect the tumor if possible. If the tumor is slow growing, the surgical procedure may keep the patient symptom free for years, even when the resection is not complete. Surgery may also be used more emergently to deal with obstructions to the flow of cerebrospinal fluid, which can cause increased ICP and hydrocephalus.

### Diet

No special diet is prescribed for the patient with a brain tumor. Rather, the patient's diet is modified as needed to reflect the patient's LOC and ability to swallow and protect the airway and prevent aspiration. A speech pathologist may be consulted if the patient is experiencing swallowing difficulties.

### Activity

The patient is encouraged to remain as active as possible. The only contraindication to normal activity is the presence of increased ICP, which necessitates keeping the patient as quiet as possible. Physical and occupational therapists may be involved in planning and implementing an activity program for the patient.

**table 52-7** *Common Medications for **Management of Brain Tumor Symptoms***

| Drug | Action | Nursing Intervention |
|---|---|---|
| Phenytoin (Dilantin) | Prevents seizures | Assess for gingival hyperplasia<br>Administer drug on schedule<br>Assess for signs of toxicity and rash |
| Dexamethasone (Decadron Phosphate) | Reduces cerebral edema | Monitor for increased blood glucose<br>Taper dosage after long-term therapy |
| Laxatives/stool softeners | Prevents constipation | Monitor for fecal impaction<br>Instruct patient not to strain |
| Famotidine (Pepcid)<br>Ranitidine (Zantac) | Decreases gastric acid secretion | Usually safe and without significant side effects |

### Referrals

Nursing assessment determines the patient's and family's need for specific referrals. Patients who undergo surgery or other treatments for brain tumors may require the services of physical, occupational, and speech therapists as they recover and attempt to compensate for residual deficits. Referrals for home care and community support help the patient return home and continue therapy started in the hospital setting. The prognosis for patients with malignant brain tumors is guarded, and both patient and family will need ongoing support to deal with both the psychological and physical complications of the illness and its treatment. Referral to the services of the American Cancer Society is always an appropriate first step.

## INTRACRANIAL SURGERY

A surgical opening through the skull is known as a craniotomy. This procedure is used to treat any pathology requiring surgical intervention within the cranial cavity. Persons with tumors, strokes, subarachnoid hemorrhage, and trauma requiring surgical repair may all undergo craniotomies. The basic preparation of the patient before surgery and care in the immediate postoperative period are virtually the same, regardless of the underlying condition. Unique aspects of care are discussed with the specific pathology. This section discusses the management of patients undergoing craniotomy for resection of a brain tumor.

The surgical site depends on the anatomical location of the lesion. The incision is usually made behind the hairline so that the scar will be hidden once the patient's hair grows back. A portion of the skull bone is removed, placed aside during the surgery, and replaced at the end of the procedure. On rare occasions the bone is not replaced, such as with depressed skull fractures or if the brain is severely swollen after trauma. When the bone is left off, the surgery is called a craniectomy. If possible, the bone is saved, stored in a bone bank, and replaced at a later date. Cranioplasty surgery, repair of a cranial defect, may be done with saved bone or with substitute acrylic bonelike materials.

Once the bone is off, the dura mater is opened, allowing access to the brain. At the end of the case, the dura will be carefully closed with sutures to prevent CSF from leaking while the dura heals.

Tumors involving the pituitary gland that do not extend outside the sella turcica may be removed by means of a transphenoidal approach. An incision is made beneath the nose under the upper lip, and access to the sella turcica is gained through an opening at the rear of the sphenoid sinus. After the surgery, packing is placed in the nose and a fat graft from the abdomen is used to close the defect in the dura.[25] With this type of surgery, recovery is rapid, tissue damage in the brain is minimized, and the patient has no loss of hair or external cranial incision.

The possibility of neurological deficits after surgery must be considered, and the surgeon discusses this possibility with the patient and family. The location of the lesion and the overall health of the patient are important considerations in evaluating the patient's risks. A clear discussion of risks, presented in lay terms, is a necessary component of the process of informed consent.

## NURSING MANAGEMENT OF THE PERSON UNDERGOING INTRACRANIAL SURGERY

### PREOPERATIVE CARE

A baseline neurological assessment is performed and documented by the nurse before surgery. A written surgical consent is obtained from the patient if he or she is able to understand and give consent. If the patient is unable to give consent, the next of kin is consulted. Even if the patient is able to give consent, the nurse will involve both the patient and family in all preoperative teaching. Both patient and family have concerns and fears related to the surgery and postoperative care. Specific fears may include a permanent change in appearance or behavior, dependency, or death. Psychological support of the patient and family is a priority nursing intervention. The nursing staff must provide sufficient time for the family to ask questions that will allay their fears. The patient or family may wish to see a spiritual counselor before surgery.

All treatments and procedures are carefully explained to the patient even if the person does not seem to fully understand. Shaving of the operative site is usually performed in the operating room. The hair is saved in case the patient wishes to have a wig made. Some surgeons prefer to shave only the area directly around the surgical site; other surgeons shave the entire head. Preoperative sedatives and narcotics are rarely administered to avoid depressing the patient's LOC.

Family members need to know where they may wait during surgery, approximately how long the surgery will take, and where the patient will go after surgery. If the patient is going to be in an intensive care unit after surgery, the patient or family may want a brief tour of the unit before surgery to become familiar with the environment.[40] Guidelines for preoperative care of the person undergoing intracranial surgery are summarized in the accompanying box.

**guidelines for care**

**Preoperative Care of the Person Having Intracranial Surgery**

1. Baseline data of neurological and physiological status are recorded.
2. Patient and family are encouraged to verbalize fears.
3. Treatments and procedures are explained fully, even if unsure whether patient understands.
4. If head is shaved, it usually is done in the operating room.
5. An antiseptic shampoo may be ordered the night before surgery and repeated in morning.
6. If hair is shaved, it is saved and given to patient or family.
7. Family is prepared for appearance of patient after surgery:
   - Head dressing
   - Edema and ecchymosis of face common
   - Possible decrease in mental status

## POSTOPERATIVE CARE

### Monitoring Vital Functions

In the immediate postoperative period, frequent monitoring is performed to assess for subtle changes in the patient's neurological status that might indicate complications that can be treated promptly. The patient is assessed regularly for signs of increased ICP. The frequency of assessments depends on the patient's condition.

Any changes in the patient's vital signs, LOC, cranial nerve examination, or motor examination are reported at once to the physician. Subtle changes in behavior such as restlessness can indicate increased ICP or bleeding into the surgical site that might require further investigation or immediate corrective surgery.

An ICP monitor may be placed at the time of surgery. The monitor allows for direct monitoring of ICP and CPP (see p. 1706). Because the manipulation of brain tissue at the time of surgery can cause cerebral edema postoperatively, precautions are taken to prevent activity-related changes in the patient's ICP. Coughing and vomiting are prevented if possible because they increase ICP. Suctioning, if permitted, is performed in short, limited passes of the suction catheter to limit coughing and associated hypoxia. Deep breathing exercises and incentive spirometry are encouraged but are not followed by forceful coughing.

### Preventing Injury

Most patients are started on anticonvulsant therapy preoperatively to prevent postoperative seizures. Seizure precautions are maintained during the immediate postoperative period, and blood levels of the anticonvulsant are checked frequently. Care must be taken to protect confused or agitated patients from injuring themselves by pulling at catheters, ICP monitors, or head dressings. Ventricular catheters can be taped securely and wrapped in bulky dressings, and a stockinette can be loosely tied under the patient's chin to keep a head dressing in place. As a last resort, and with a physician's order, restraints can be applied. The nurse attempts to use the least restrictive device possible because struggling against restraints increases the patient's ICP. Commercially available hand "mittens" prevent patients from using their fingers to pick at dressings or tubes but still allow arm movement and enable the nurse to assess the patient's skin and circulation in the affected hand.

### Caring for the Incision

Usually the craniotomy incision is covered with gauze dressings, wrapped securely around the head. The head dressing is inspected regularly for amount and type of drainage. Serosanguineous drainage on the dressing is measured and marked so it can be accurately evaluated over time. Yellowish drainage is reported immediately to the physician because it might indicate a CSF leak. Individual surgeons usually have preferences about changing head dressings. It is not uncommon for the head dressing to be removed after 3 days and the incision left open to the air. Sutures or staples are removed after approximately 7 days. When the dressings are removed, the scalp can be gently cleansed with half-strength hydrogen peroxide and saline to remove any residual dried blood. A loose head covering, similar to the caps worn by operating room (OR) staff, may be used to protect the incision, to help remind the patient not to scratch the incision, and to improve the patient's appearance until his or her hair grows back. Head scarves or wigs are preferred by some patients and are available for both men and women. The patient who has had a piece of bone removed will have a depression in the scalp and should be warned of the danger of bumping the head in this area. These patients are usually provided with a helmet to lessen the danger of brain injury.

### Promoting Nutrition

Fluid intake and output are accurately recorded. Fluids can be resumed as soon as the patient has bowel sounds, is alert, and has intact protective gag, swallow, and cough reflexes to drink safely. Intravenous fluids are used to supplement oral intake until the patient can take in 2000 to 2500 ml per day.

### Promoting Elimination

Urine output is usually monitored with an indwelling catheter for the first day or two postoperatively. The specific gravity of the urine is checked at least twice a day or more often if the patient is suspected of having diabetes insipidus (DI). Although DI occurs most commonly after pituitary surgery, it can also occur after head trauma or intracranial surgery (see the discussion of DI on p. 1724).

Stool softeners are given to prevent constipation and straining during defecation. Laxatives or suppositories may be used as needed to treat constipation.

### Promoting Comfort

Patients may complain of headache after intracranial surgery because of manipulation of the coverings of the brain. Medication given to treat headache is usually short acting to reduce the effects of central nervous system depression that might obscure the patient's neurological examination. Other measures to promote comfort include treating nausea, keeping bright lights and loud noises to a minimum, and assisting the patient with hygiene, turning, and repositioning.

### Promoting Mobility

The postcraniotomy patient may be allowed out of bed on the first postoperative day. If the patient has been on bed rest for more than a few days, deconditioning may have occurred. The patient is helped to sit on the edge of the bed and dangle his or her legs over the side. The nurse monitors the patient for postural hypotension or difficulty maintaining balance in the sitting position. Patients with motor or sensory deficits require additional support getting up to a chair or ambulating for the first few times. Early mobility prevents the complications associated with bed rest and helps the patient return to normal activity before discharge. Guidelines for care of the person after intracranial surgery are summarized in the box on p. 1723.

**guidelines for care**

**Postoperative Care of the Person After Intracranial Surgery**

1. Perform monitoring:
   a. Assess neurological status, including ability to move, level of orientation and alertness, and pupil checks.
   b. Assess degree and character of drainage.
      (1) Amount of drainage and bleeding should be minimal.
      (2) Initial head dressing can be reinforced as necessary.
      (3) Often incision is left open to air after first several days.
2. Promote mobility:
   a. Turning to either side is permitted.
   b. If supratentorial surgery was performed, the head of the bed is kept elevated at least 30 degrees.
   c. Early ambulation is encouraged to prevent complications of bed rest. Observe carefully for signs of postural hypotension; raise head of bed gradually; patient should always sit on edge of bed before standing.
3. Promote decreased intracranial pressure:
   a. Space nursing activities to allow patient to rest between them.
   b. Coughing and vomiting should be avoided.
   c. Suctioning should be performed only as necessary, and then gently and cautiously.
4. Protect safety of patient:
   a. Use soft hand restraints if restraints are necessary.
   b. Use mittens as alternative to restraints. Change mitt q4h—provide range of motion to hand at this time.
   c. Keep side rails up at all times.
5. Promote electrolyte balance:
   a. Perform accurate intake and output with measurement of specific gravity. Do frequent testing for blood glucose.
   b. Have patient resume oral diet as soon as possible; assess for difficulty in swallowing or absence of gag reflex.
   c. Monitor electrolytes for evidence of abnormalities.
6. Promote comfort:
   a. Medicate for comfort with codeine sulfate or nonnarcotic analgesic.
   b. Ice cap for headache may be helpful.

## GERONTOLOGICAL CONSIDERATIONS

The older adult having intracranial surgery has a few special needs, both preoperatively and postoperatively. It is important to differentiate between deficits related to the brain tumor and those related to other disease processes. For example, the patient may have underlying weakness from a prior stroke or unrelated orthopedic problem. The older patient may have underlying cardiac or pulmonary dysfunction that requires special preparation before surgery such as adjustment in blood pressure medications and review of pulmonary function. The patient with a significant medical history may spend the first postoperative night in the ICU for close monitoring.

Older patients may be slower to recover postoperatively. Patients with significant cerebrovascular disease are at greater risk for hemorrhage or ischemic stroke as a result of intracranial vessel manipulation. Cerebrovascular disease can also compromise collateral circulation and cause ischemic damage during or after intracranial surgery.

## SPECIAL ENVIRONMENTS FOR CARE

### Critical Care Management

Patients having a craniotomy for tumor resection may spend a brief time in the ICU after surgery. The critical care environment provides close monitoring of hemodynamic changes that may result from extensive neurosurgery. Once the patient recovers from anesthesia and is breathing effectively without assistance, he or she will be extubated. When stable, usually within 24 hours, the patient is transferred to a regular patient unit.

### Home Care Management

In preparing the patient for discharge, the nurse will assess the patient's continued needs for care at home. In cooperation with the patient and family, the nurse will help arrange any nursing or rehabilitation therapy needed after discharge. Short hospital stays ensure that patients are likely to have continuing care needs after discharge. Rehabilitation after surgery often takes months, and it is important for the nurse to ensure that services have been arranged for the patient before discharge.

## COMPLICATIONS

### Hydrocephalus

If the normal flow of cerebrospinal fluid becomes obstructed, the result is hydrocephalus. When the obstruction occurs between the ventricles, the CSF cannot flow out of the ventricular system and around the surface of the brain. This is called noncommunicating hydrocephalus. When CSF cannot be reabsorbed via the arachnoid granulations in the sagittal sinus because of obstruction, the resulting condition is called communicating hydrocephalus. The arachnoid granulations can become obstructed by blood or proteins produced by infection in the CSF.

Acute hydrocephalus may require a ventriculostomy. A small catheter is placed into the lateral ventricle via a frontal opening in the skull known as a burr hole. The catheter is connected to an external drainage system that monitors ICP and allows for drainage of CSF. The tubing and drainage system must be kept closed and sterile. If drainage appears to stop, the neurosurgeon is notified immediately. Ventriculostomies are left in place for only a few days to minimize the chance of infection. If the patient requires continued drainage of CSF, a shunt will be placed to replace the external drain (Figure 52-10). The different types of shunts are named for their point of origin and termination and include the following:

1. Ventricular-peritoneal
2. Lumbar-peritoneal
3. Ventricular-jugular
4. Cyst-peritoneal

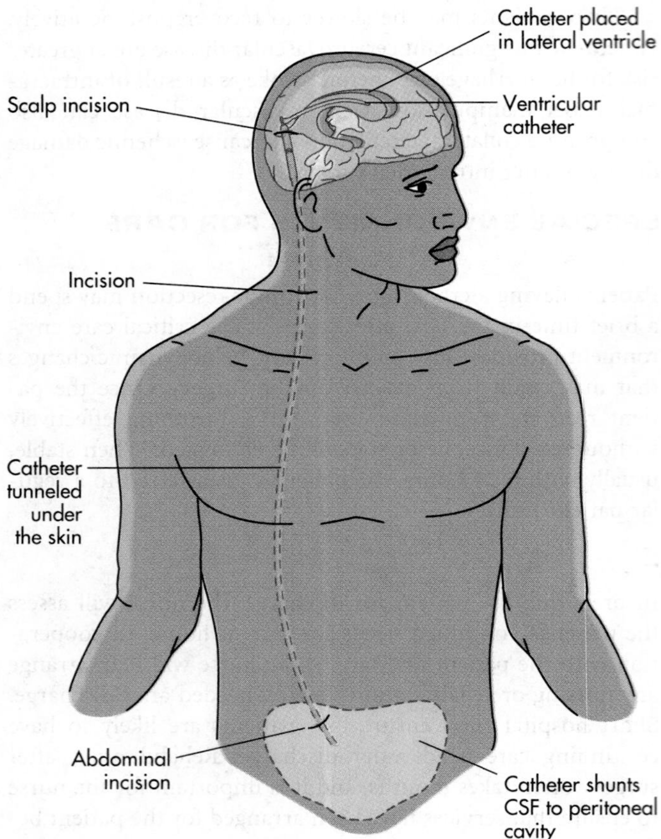


**fig. 52-10** Patient with ventriculoperitoneal (VP) shunt.

When a shunt is placed, excessive CSF is shunted away from the central nervous system and into either the peritoneal cavity or, occasionally, into the venous system, where it is reabsorbed. Shunts may include special valves or access reservoirs at the point where the catheter leaves the skull. These valves or reservoirs help control the volume and pressure of CSF leaving the ventricular system. Guidelines for care of the patient undergoing shunt placement are summarized in the accompanying box.

### Respiratory Failure

Respiratory arrest may occur after posterior fossa surgery as a result of edema in the brainstem and the inability to protect the airway with the cough or gag reflexes. Any irregularity of respiration, reduction in pulse oximetry, or onset of dyspnea is reported at once. Equipment is kept ready to support ventilation, including intubation if necessary.

### Cerebrospinal Fluid Leak

Any opening of the dura, whether from trauma or surgery, predisposes the patient to a CSF leak. The nurse monitors the patient for clear fluid oozing from the suture line or clear drainage on the head dressing. If the patient had surgery via a transphenoidal approach, the nurse also checks for clear fluid draining from the nose. A dural leak allows CSF to escape and provides a pathway for bacteria to enter the brain, causing meningitis (see p. 1733).

**guidelines for care**

**The Person Undergoing Shunt Placement**

1. Perform monitoring:
   a. Assess neurological status frequently for any decrease in mental status.
   b. Observe for symptoms of subdural hematoma, one of the possible side effects of the surgery.
   c. Monitor for symptoms of overdrainage, as evidenced by headache, especially when patient is sitting upright or standing.
   d. Assess degree and character of drainage:
      (1) Amount of drainage and bleeding should be minimal.
      (2) Reinforce dressing as needed.
      (3) Often incisional areas are left open to air after several days.
2. Maintain gastrointestinal status:
   a. Check frequently for signs of paralytic ileus; manipulation of the bowel that occurs with the placement of the shunt's peritoneal segment can predispose the patient to ileus.
   b. Patient usually is given nothing by mouth for first day, and then clear liquids are started.
   c. Regular diet is resumed as soon as good bowel sounds are present and patient tolerates liquids.
3. Maintain comfort:
   a. Patient may need frequent pain medication because of involvement of abdominal area.
   b. Keep pressure off incisional sites.
4. Promote mobility:
   a. Turning to either side is permitted.
   b. Raise head of bed gradually when mobilizing patient.
   c. Patient is encouraged to ambulate as much as possible to encourage adaptation to decreased intracranial pressure.

Cerebrospinal fluid leaks usually heal spontaneously and do not require surgical intervention to close the leak. The head of the bed is kept elevated to reduce CSF pressure at the site of the leak. Occasionally a lumbar drain is placed to remove small amounts of CSF and further reduce CSF pressure at the leak site. The patient is told not to blow his or her nose and to restrict activities that would increase ICP and force CSF out of the leak. Antibiotics are administered until the leak is resolved.

### Diabetes Insipidus and Syndrome of Inappropriate Antidiuretic Hormone

Patients undergoing surgery to the pituitary region are at risk for DI. Antidiuretic hormone (ADH) is made and stored in this area. Surgery, trauma, or cerebral edema from almost any neurological condition can disrupt the delicate balance of this fluid regulatory mechanism.

Diabetes insipidus occurs when there is insufficient ADH to cause the renal tubules to reabsorb water. Large quantities of very dilute urine are excreted, and the patient is at risk for severe dehydration. Serum sodium levels and osmolarity rise from the loss of fluid (Box 52-14). Treatment involves fluid replacement and administration of synthetic ADH in the form

**box 52-14** *Laboratory Parameters and Treatment of Diabetes Insipidus and Syndrome of Inappropriate Antidiuretic Hormone*

| PARAMETERS | DIABETES INSIPIDUS | SYNDROME OF INAPPROPRIATE ANTIDIURETIC HORMONE |
|---|---|---|
| Urine specific gravity | 1.001 to 1.005 | 1.030 or more |
| Serum osmolarity | High | Low |
| Serum Na | High | Low |
| Urine output | Very high | Low |
| Treatment | Fluid replacement<br>DDAVP 0.1 to 0.4 ml intranasally q12-24h<br>Aqueous vasopressin 5 to 10 U SQ q3-6h | Fluid restriction<br>Lasix for diuresis<br>Demeclocyline 300 mg qid |

of desmopressin acetate, DDAVP, or aqueous vasopressin. The condition is usually self-limiting.

The syndrome of inappropriate ADH (SIADH) can also occur as a complication of intracranial surgery and is in direct contrast to DI. Patients with damage to the hypothalamus, almost any central nervous system disorder, bronchogenic carcinoma, or pulmonary disease all may develop SIADH. In this syndrome, too much ADH is secreted, causing the renal tubules to reabsorb excess amounts of water. The patient's urine output is low, there is generalized weight gain, and the patient's serum sodium and osmolarity are low due to the dilutional effects of water retention (see Box 52-14). The treatment for SIADH is fluid restriction, often to 1500 ml of fluid per day or less. If the patient is receiving IV fluids, normal saline is given to provide additional sodium. On rare occasions, hypertonic saline of 3% may be administered under close monitoring. The problem is usually self-limiting. In severe cases the drug demeclocycline may be given to suppress the effects of ADH on the renal tubule.

### Corneal Abrasions

Positioning of the patient during intracranial surgery may expose the patient to the risk of corneal abrasion. Trauma, dysfunction, or surgery in the area of the seventh cranial nerve, which controls the ability to close the eye, also predisposes the patient to this complication. The nurse inspects the patient's eyes for redness and ability to blink and keeps the eyes moist. If the corneal reflex is absent, lubricating eyedrops or eye ointment are used to keep the eyes moist (see the Research Box). Patients may need teaching to continue this precaution after discharge. This intervention is extremely important with patients experiencing severe impairments of LOC. Abrasion is a serious complication that can rapidly progress to severe eye infection.

### Gastric Ulceration

Neurosurgical procedures predispose the patient to gastric ulceration, commonly called Cushing's ulcers. The underlying pathology is not well understood but is thought to be a massive stress response. In addition to the stress response, most neurosurgical patients are placed on steroids, which increase gastric secretions and can contribute to gastric irritation and ulceration. Patients are usually placed on a histamine $H_2$ blocker such as ranitidine or famotidine as a preventive measure. If a nasogastric tube is in place, the pH of the gastric secretions can be monitored and antacids or sucralfate can be administered to protect the gastric mucosa.

**research** 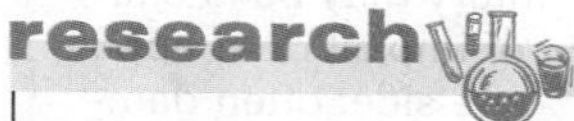

Reference: Cortese D, Capp L, McKinley S: Moisture chamber versus lubrication for the prevention of corneal epithelial breakdown, *Am J Crit Care* 4(6):425, 1995.

The authors compared the effectiveness of two eye care treatments on the prevention of corneal breakdown. One patient group received lubricating drops and another group had their eyes covered from brow to cheek with a clear polyethylene film taped in place. Eight of 30 patients with lubricating drops had corneal abrasions compared with one in the group with the moisture chamber.

## CRANIOCEREBRAL TRAUMA

### ETIOLOGY

Craniocerebral trauma may result from injury to the scalp, skull, and brain tissues, either singly or collectively. Variables that influence the extent of the injury to the head include the following:

- Status of the head at impact—moving or still
- Location and direction of the impact
- Rate of energy transfer
- Surface area involved in the energy transfer

Injuries vary from minor scalp wounds to concussions and open skull fractures with severe brain injury. The amount of obvious external damage does not necessarily reflect the seriousness of the injury. Serious craniocerebral damage can occur in the absence of obvious external injury.

Contusions, abrasions, and lacerations of the scalp may occur (Table 52-8). Lacerations of the scalp bleed profusely because of the scalp's rich blood supply and the poor vasoconstrictive abilities of these vessels. Hematomas that form under the surface of the scalp may obscure underlying skull fractures. The initial injury from head trauma is called the primary trauma. Secondary trauma occurs from the body's

**table 52-8** *Damage of Brain Tissue Caused by Trauma*

| Characteristics | Structural Alteration | Effects |
|---|---|---|
| **CONCUSSION** | | |
| Characterized by immediate and transitory impairment of neurological function caused by mechanical force | No | May be loss of consciousness that is instant or delayed; usually reversible |
| **CONTUSION** | | |
| Likened to bruising with extravasation of blood cells | Yes | Injury may be at site of impact or at opposite side; often damage is to cortex |
| **LACERATION** | | |
| Tearing of tissues caused by sharp fragment or shearing force | Yes | Hemorrhage is serious complication |

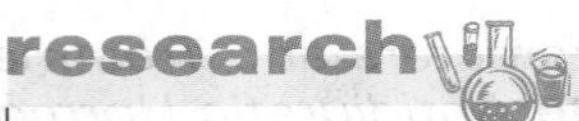

Reference: Kuthy S et al: After the party's over: evaluation of a drinking and driving prevention program, *J Neurosci Nurs* 27(5):274, 1995.

The authors studied the effectiveness of an educational program, designed for high school students, about the consequences of drinking and driving. A 20-minute slide presentation discussed actual patients who had suffered severe head injury or spinal cord injury as a result of motor vehicle accidents. A questionnaire was given to students immediately after the program and again 1 month later to determine student behaviors related to drinking and driving. A significant change in driving behaviors was reported. The study demonstrates the effectiveness of nursing-sponsored community outreach to educate others about ways to prevent head and spinal cord injuries.

response to the initial injury. Examples of secondary injuries are edema, hematoma formation, hydrocephalus, and infection.

## EPIDEMIOLOGY

Craniocerebral trauma, or traumatic brain injury (TBI), causes death and serious disability in persons of all ages. In the United States, TBI results in 500,000 hospitalizations per year. About 120,000 of those are classified as severe brain injuries. Approximately 75,000 to 90,000 persons die annually from such trauma.[31] Motor vehicle accidents are the cause of about 50% of TBIs, falls cause 21%, assaults and violence cause 12%, sports-related injuries make up 10%, and alcohol is implicated in a significant percentage of all injuries (see the Research Box).[44] Both morbidity and mortality rates are higher in males. Head injury is the second most common cause of major neurological deficits and the major cause of death in persons between ages 1 and 35 years. In some states the repeal of laws requiring motorcyclists to wear helmets has resulted in an increase in death and injury from TBI sustained in motorcycle accidents. Motorcycle accidents pose added risk for injury because of the body's exposure to direct force and fewer protective devices.

## PATHOPHYSIOLOGY

### Mechanisms of Injury

Mechanisms of trauma to the head are of three general types: deformation, acceleration-deceleration, and rotation (Figure 52-11). Deformation results from the transmission of energy to the skull. If the energy is sufficient, the skull is deformed or fractured. Acceleration-deceleration injuries typically occur when the accelerating skull, moving in a motor vehicle, suddenly decelerates when it hits an immobile object such as the steering wheel or windshield. The brain injury that results is often termed *coup–contra coup* because the brain first strikes the skull in the direction of movement, and then rebounds and strikes the inner surface of the skull in the opposite direction. The damage from such injuries is highly variable, depending on the speed of acceleration and deceleration. Rotational forces also distort the brain and can cause tension, stretching, and diffuse shearing of brain tissues. Often the forces of acceleration-deceleration and rotation occur together, affecting both the brain and spinal cord.

### Skull Fractures

Skull fractures are a common form of primary craniocerebral trauma. Fractures of the skull may be linear, comminuted, depressed, or basilar. Linear skull fractures appear as a fine line on skull x-ray. If the fracture crosses the path of the meningeal artery, arterial bleeding above the dura can occur, resulting in an epidural hematoma. Comminuted or depressed skull fractures involve bone displacement, sometimes down into the brain tissue itself. If the dura is torn, a CSF leak may occur.

Basilar skull fractures are particularly serious because the vital centers, cranial nerves, and nerve pathways may be permanently damaged. If the injury creates a direct communication between the cranial cavity and the middle ear or the sinuses, meningitis or a brain abscess may develop. Bleeding from the nose and the ears suggests a basilar fracture. Serosanguineous drainage from the ears or nose may also contain CSF. Drainage is tested for the presence of glucose and positive results are reported immediately. Other signs suggestive of basilar skull fracture include hemotympanum; bruising over the mastoid process, which is called Battle's sign; and periorbital ecchymosis, which is called raccoon eyes (Figure 52-12). The latter two signs may not be evident for 24 hours after injury.

### Concussion and Contusion

Another primary brain injury is a concussion, which is characterized by an immediate and transitory impairment

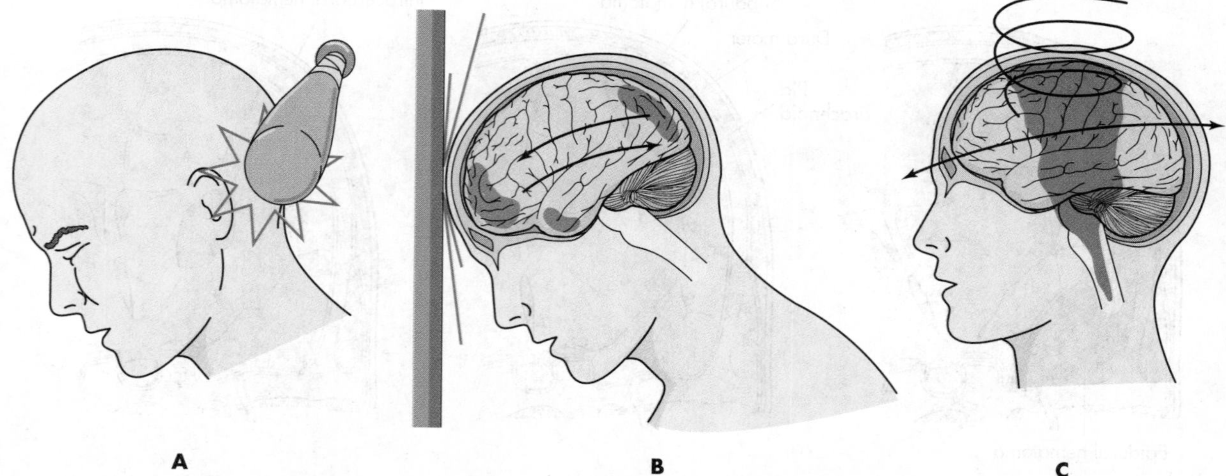


fig. 52-11 Mechanisms of injury. A, Deformation. B, Acceleration-deceleration. C, Rotation.

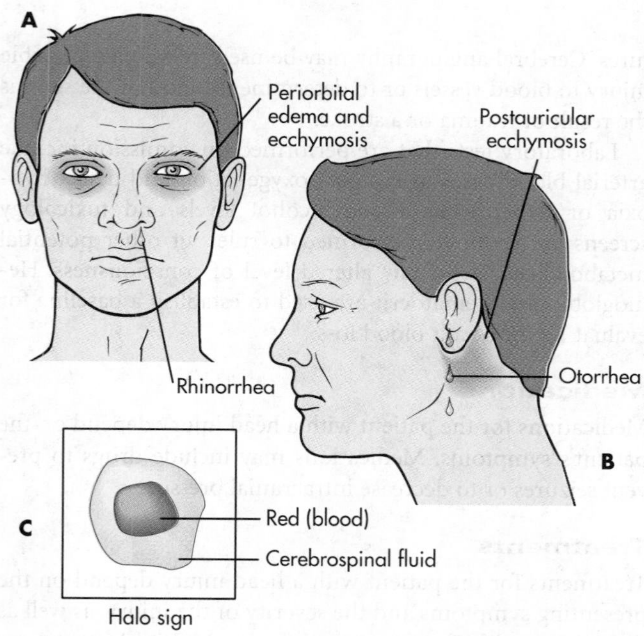


fig. 52-12 A, Racoon eyes and rhinorrhea. B, Battle's sign (postauricular ecchymosis) with otorrhea. C, Halo or ring sign. Drainage containing CSF forms a ring or halo as it dries on a gauze pad.

of neurological function caused by mechanical force. Although no structural neurological changes are evident, current research indicates that there may be a correlation between the concussion of minor head injury and subsequent cognitive impairments.[47] A loss of consciousness may occur that is instant or delayed, and the person usually recovers rapidly. Any person who exhibits an alteration in consciousness after a blow to the head should be closely observed after the injury, because the extent of the damage is not always immediately apparent. Postconcussion symptoms may develop and include headache, dizziness, fatigue, memory impairment, and impaired concentration. Diffuse axonal injury (DAI) is caused by rapid movement of the brain during which delicate axons are stretched and damaged. This damage interferes with nervous transmission and can cause extensive diffuse deficits.[48]

A contusion is a structural alteration characterized by the extravasation of blood into the brain. It can be likened to bruising without tearing of tissues. The contusion may be at the site of impact or on the opposite side, a coup–contra coup injury. Contusions often damage the cerebral cortex. Laceration of the brain and its blood vessels can occur with severe contusions and may be caused by a sharp fragment or object or a shearing force. On CT scan, small, petechial-like areas of bleeding can be seen.

## Secondary Injury

Secondary injury occurs as a result of the body's response to the initial trauma. Examples include cerebral edema, increased ICP, and hematoma formation. In response to local injury, bleeding, and systemic disturbances in circulation that result in hypoxia, the brain becomes edematous. Cell damage and systemic hypoxia cause cell membranes to fail, leading to cytotoxic edema. Cells lining the blood vessels are damaged and the capillaries become more permeable, allowing fluid to leak out into the interstitial space. This is called vasogenic edema and contributes to increased ICP, as discussed earlier in this chapter. Most deaths from head injury occur as a result of increased ICP rather than from the initial injury itself.

Hematoma formation is another type of secondary injury (Figure 52-13). An epidural hematoma forms as blood collects between the dura and the skull. Because bleeding in this area is usually caused by laceration of the middle meningeal artery, it is capable of producing rapid clot formation. Bleeding needs to be controlled promptly and the blood evacuated or

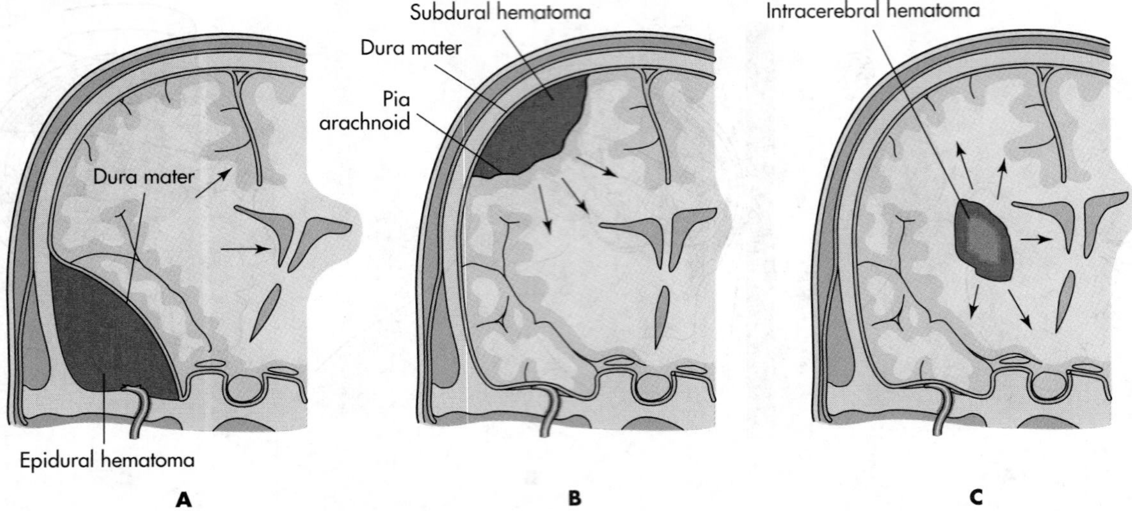


**fig. 52-13** Cerebral hematomas. **A,** Epidural hematoma. **B,** Subdural hematoma. **C,** Intracerebral hematoma. *Arrows* indicate direction of pressure generated by hematoma.

life-threatening neurological deterioration occurs. Common sites for epidural hematoma formation include basilar and temporal skull fractures. The nurse should be alert for signs of epidural hematoma when injuries occur in these sites.

A subdural hematoma forms as venous blood collects below the dural surface but above the brain. Because the bleeding is under venous pressure, the hematoma forms relatively slowly. However, the clot causes pressure on the brain surface and eventually displaces brain tissue if it becomes large enough. Subdural hematomas are divided into acute, subacute, and chronic varieties. Acute subdural hematomas develop within 48 hours of injury and have an organized clot. Subacute subdural hematomas develop within 3 days to 2 weeks after injury. The clot may have begun to lyse and become more fluid as the body attempts to break the clot down and remove it. The chronic subdural hematoma causes symptoms about 3 weeks to months after the injury. The damaged area is filled with fluid instead of an organized clot. Acute and subacute hematomas present a greater threat to neurological function because of the rapidity of symptom development. Chronic subdural hematomas may have evolved over a longer period of time, and the symptoms manifest as less acute neurological deficits.

A third type of hematoma is the intracerebral hematoma, which is common after a hemorrhagic stroke. The blood collects within the brain parenchyma itself. Symptoms are related to the area of the brain where the clot forms.

## COLLABORATIVE CARE MANAGEMENT

### Diagnostic Tests

Diagnostic procedures are performed as necessary and often include CT scans, skull x-rays, and possibly cerebral angiography. The CT scan evaluates for hematomas, edema, or damage from skull fractures. Skull x-rays assess for skull or facial fractures. Cerebral angiography may be used to evaluate possible injury to blood vessels or to determine if blood in the skull is the result of trauma or a stroke.

Laboratory tests that are performed on admission include arterial blood gases to evaluate oxygenation and detect hypoxia or hypercarbia. Blood alcohol levels and toxicology screens are routinely performed to rule out other potential metabolic causes for any altered level of consciousness. Hemoglobin and hematocrit are used to establish a baseline for evaluating for occult blood loss.

### Medications

Medications for the patient with a head injury depend on the patient's symptoms. Medications may include drugs to prevent seizures or to decrease intracranial pressure.

### Treatments

Treatments for the patient with a head injury depend on the presenting symptoms and the severity of the injury, as well as the presence of other systemic injuries. Multiple trauma are commonly present. The patient may be intubated to protect the airway and to provide hyperventilation as a treatment for increasing intracranial pressure.

### Surgical Management

If the head injury causes hematoma formation, surgical intervention may be necessary. Craniotomies are performed to remove both epidural and subdural hematomas and repair the source of bleeding. If edema is present, the dura is closed surgically, but the bone may be left out temporarily to allow room for anticipated brain expansion. The bone will be replaced when the edema subsides. Patients with craniectomies (bone removal) will need to wear a helmet for protection when they are out of bed.

### Diet

No special diet is prescribed for the patient with a head injury. The diet is determined largely by the patient's condition. If, after several days, the patient is unable to take in sufficient nutrients by mouth, enteral or parenteral nutrition will be initiated.

### Activity

The patient's activity level is determined by her or his neurological status. Safety is the primary concern. The patient with motor, sensory, or cognitive deficits may need supervision and assistance to prevent injury.

### Referrals

In some settings the nurse assumes responsibility for making referrals to other services. For the patient with a head injury this may include a dietitian, social worker, and physical and occupational therapists. The family is often aided by a referral to the local chapter of the Head Injury Foundation or another support group.

# NURSING MANAGEMENT

## ■ ASSESSMENT

### Subjective Data

Subjective data to be collected to assess the head-injured patient who is conscious include:

- Patient's understanding of injury and resulting pathological consequences
- Patient's ability to understand
- Information about nature of injury—how it happened
- Presence of headache, nausea, or vomiting
- Presence of diplopia or other visual problems
- Unusual sensations (paresthesias, ringing in ears)
- History of bleeding from ears, nose, eyes, or mouth
- History of loss of consciousness, duration

### Objective Data

Objective data to be collected to assess the patient with head injury include:

- Respiratory status (patency of the airway, ability to cough, need for intubation and mechanical ventilation)
- Arterial blood gases
- Level of consciousness, alertness, orientation
- Pupils—size, equality, reactivity
- Motor status
- Vital signs
- Presence of bleeding
- Presence of vomiting
- Presence of discharge from ears or nose
- Speech pattern abnormalities
- Battle's sign (ecchymosis behind the ears; indicates a basilar skull fracture)
- Raccoon eyes (ecchymosis and swelling around the eyes; indicates possible orbital fracture)

## ■ NURSING DIAGNOSES

Nursing diagnoses are determined from analysis of patient data. Nursing diagnoses for the patient with a head injury may include but are not limited to:

| Diagnostic Title | Possible Etiological Factors |
|---|---|
| Ineffective breathing pattern | Central nervous system disturbance, trauma |
| Tissue perfusion, altered (cerebral) | Decreased blood flow (arterial), increased ICP |
| Thermoregulation, ineffective | Trauma to vital control centers |
| Fluid volume excess or deficit | Dysfunction of pituitary secretion of ADH |
| Infection, risk for | Loss of cerebral protection, immobility |
| Activity intolerance | Sensory, motor deficits |
| Coping, ineffective family: compromised | Crisis of injury, uncertain outcomes |
| Knowledge deficit (knowledge of head injury) | Lack of exposure/recall to pathology, treatment plan |

## ■ EXPECTED PATIENT OUTCOMES

Expected patient outcomes for the patient with a head injury may include but are not limited to:

1. Maintains ventilation as indicated by pulse oximetry readings above 90%
2. Maintains cerebral perfusion as indicated by the absence of signs or symptoms of increased ICP
3. Maintains temperature within the range of 97.5° to 99.5° F
4. Does not develop edema or dehydration
5. Remains free of infection
6. Returns to preinjury activity level
7. Family member or significant other verbalizes adequate coping
8. Patient and family members able to verbalize knowledge of head injury, treatment, and rehabilitation

## ■ INTERVENTIONS

### Promoting Adequate Ventilation

One of the most common complications of severe head injury is respiratory failure. Cerebral anoxia, which is a sequela of respiratory failure, is a leading cause of death in head-injured patients. The patient with respiratory failure may have hypoxia, hypercapnia, hypotension, and dyspnea. Intubation and mechanical ventilation are commonly necessary.

Arterial blood gas levels and pH are checked frequently to determine the adequacy of respiratory exchange. Pulse oximetry may be used as a less invasive means of monitoring the patient's oxygenation status. Alert patients are reminded to deep breathe frequently, but coughing is not encouraged because of the risk of increasing intracranial pressure. Suctioning is used only if absolutely necessary to ensure a patent airway, and the nurse carefully hyperventilates and hyperoxygenates the patient before suctioning to minimize the adverse effects on intracranial pressure.

### Controlling Intracranial Pressure

Increased intracranial pressure is a major concern in patients with head injury, and the nurse is responsible for ongoing patient monitoring. Interventions to control increasing ICP are discussed on p. 1706.

### Maintaining Vital Signs and Temperature Control

Vital signs are taken frequently until the patient's condition stabilizes. Patients with head injury may have experienced trauma to other body systems and are at risk for shock. See sections on altered LOC and ICP for changes in vital signs related to severe head trauma. Patients with fever are worked up to identify possible sources of infection. Once cultures are sent the patient may be treated with appropriate antibiotics and antipyretics to increase comfort. Tepid sponge baths or other more aggressive measures of reducing body temperature such as cooling blankets are used as a last resort to control acute hyperthermia when the brain's thermoregulation completely fails.

### Monitoring Fluid and Electrolyte Balance

Intake and output are carefully measured and recorded. The specific gravity of the urine is also measured and recorded if diabetes insipidus is suspected. These measurements may be performed hourly when the patient's condition is unstable.

Fluid intake will be prescribed according to the patient's need for blood pressure support, replacement of gastrointestinal losses from suctioning, or to balance urine output. Fluids may be given parenterally, by feeding tube, or by mouth depending on the patient's condition. The nurse uses caution in administering fluids orally because the patient may have difficulty with vomiting and aspiration. The patient's urine output is also carefully monitored to assess the response to osmotic diuretics such as mannitol.

An indwelling catheter is essential when giving mannitol because of the large amounts of urine produced and the need to measure output accurately. The presence of an indwelling catheter increases the risk of urinary tract infection, and the catheter should be removed as soon as possible.

Careful monitoring of electrolytes is also necessary. Several types of sodium imbalances are known to occur after head injury. Natriuresis, or increased urinary excretion of sodium, is common. This is attributed to the SIADH with an increased plasma level of ADH, serum hyponatremia, and hypoosmolarity, which aggravates cerebral edema. Hypernatremia, or cerebral sodium retention, also may occur. No specific variations in potassium or chloride levels have been noted. Plasma cortisol levels also are elevated in acute head injury. Serum levels of BUN, pH, electrolytes, and urinary electrolyte levels are checked frequently.

### Preventing Infection

The patient's ears and nose are observed carefully for signs of blood or serous drainage, which may indicate that the meninges have been torn (common in basal skull fractures) and that spinal fluid is escaping. Drainage from the nose can be tested for glucose to help differentiate CSF from mucus. Drainage can also be blotted on a gauze pad. CSF forms a halo on the gauze as it dries. No attempt should be made to clean these orifices. Usually the flow of cerebrospinal fluid subsides spontaneously. Meningitis is a possible complication whenever a tear in the dura allows communication between the nose and ears and the brain. Antibiotics are started immediately if a patient is suspected to be at risk.

If a leak is suspected, the patient is instructed not to cough, sneeze, or blow the nose. These activities may, in addition to contributing to the development of meningitis, enable air to enter the cranial cavity, where it may increase symptoms of intracranial pressure.

Nasal suctioning is not used to remove secretions, and neither nasogastric nor nasotracheal tubes are used with any patient suspected of having a leak because of the risk of causing further damage or introducing infection.

### Resuming Activities

The duration of convalescence depends entirely on how much damage has been done and how rapid recovery has been. Patients are usually encouraged to resume normal activities as soon as possible. Headache and occasional dizziness may be present for several months after a head injury, but gradually resolve. Loss of memory and initiative may also persist for a time. Neuropsychological testing can be used to identify subtle cognitive deficits to help guide rehabilitation.

Some persons require intensive rehabilitation, and others fail to make a satisfactory recovery and are left with serious functional deficits. Complete recovery from head injury is most likely in persons younger than 20 years of age. Persons between the ages of 20 and 50 years who remain in a coma longer than 2 weeks rarely recover.

### Providing Emotional Support

The patient with a head injury may lose cognitive functions and memory and develop behavioral problems associated with lack of judgment and restlessness. Emotional support is important for both the patient and family caregivers, because both are likely to experience significant frustration in the situation. These patients need firm but gentle care, with specific guidelines for appropriate behavior.

The nurse encourages the patient and family to focus on short-term gains rather than long-term goals to avoid becoming discouraged with the slow pace of progress. Head injury support groups can be extremely helpful to the family as they learn to cope with the patient's behavior and deficits. The nurse also reinforces the importance of regular respite care for the family caregivers.

### Patient/Family Education

A patient with a head injury may be evaluated in the emergency department but not admitted to the hospital. The families of these patients need teaching about monitoring for complications. A sample set of instructions is presented in the Patient/Family Teaching Box.

Teaching for the head-injured patient who is left with deficits is targeted to the patient's and family's unique strengths and deficits. The rehabilitation principles used will be similar to those discussed in Chapters 53 and 54 for patients with stroke, spinal cord injury, or degenerative neurological diseases.

**patient/family teaching**

**Monitoring the Person with a Minor Head Injury**

Patient should be awakened periodically through the first 24 hours to be sure he or she can wake up easily. Also, for the first 24 to 48 hours, the family should watch carefully for the following warning signs:

1. Vomiting, often with force behind it
2. Unusual sleepiness, dizziness and loss of balance, or falling
3. Complaint of seeing two of everything or blurry objects; jerking movements of the eyes
4. Bleeding or discharge from nose or ears
5. A slight headache may be expected; however, if it worsens and the patient complains of feeling even worse when moving about, it should be reported
6. Seizures—any twitching or movements of arms or legs that the patient is not able to control
7. Any behavior or symptom that is not normal for the individual
8. Change in speech or ability to converse

*Call a physician at once* if any of these signs are observed. Call either your personal physician or emergency services.

Few illnesses tax the entire physical and emotional resources of the patient's family as do neurological problems. It is imperative that the family participate in all long-term planning for the patient. Family members may have severe emotional reactions to the patient's injury and difficulties in adjustment that may require the assistance of a specially trained person such as a psychiatrist. Both patients and families need time to work through their feelings. Sometimes, neither the patient nor family can grasp the enormity of the diagnosis and may need weeks or months to cope with the reality of the patient's losses.

Even the person who has suffered a mild head injury may experience long-term effects. These most often include cognitive problems such as difficulty with concentration and loss of memory. Recovery of intellectual functioning often is delayed and may be manifested in the inability to keep a job or manage the challenges of daily living.

If the patient with neurological disease has severe personality changes, aphasia, or convulsions, the family may even be afraid of the patient, and they may make tactless remarks in front of the patient. The nurse carefully assesses the family's understanding of the situation. This assessment provides an opportunity for the nurse to interpret the patient's actions and responses so that the family may better understand and support the patient. Chapter 7 provides a more comprehensive overview of the nature and scope of the rehabilitation process. The Guidelines for Care Box summarizes the major elements involved in the care of a person who has experienced a head injury.

**guidelines for care**

**The Person with a Closed Head Injury**

1. Promote rest:
   a. Provide quiet environment.
   b. Observe frequently.
   c. Administer anticonvulsants as ordered.
   d. Medicate for pain as necessary.
2. Maintain temperature:
   a. Give tepid sponge baths if hyperthermic.
   b. Administer antipyretics as ordered.
   c. Use hypothermia blanket if ordered.
   d. Reduce or increase temperature in patient's room as needed.
3. Promote adequate respiration:
   a. Suction only as necessary to provide adequate airway.
   b. Elevate head of bed to 30 degrees.
   c. Administer supplemental oxygen if ordered.
   d. Place patient in side-lying position.
4. Observe for drainage from ears or nose:
   a. Make no attempt to clean out orifice.
   b. Do not suction nose if drainage is present.
   c. Have patient avoid coughing, sneezing, or blowing nose.
   d. Test drainage for presence of CSF and report immediately if present.
5. Control cerebral edema:
   a. Administer diuretics as ordered.
   b. Elevate head of bed to 30 degrees.
   c. Perform neurological checks as ordered.
6. Maintain electrolyte balance:
   a. Observe for inappropriate ADH or DI.
   b. Monitor electrolytes.
7. Maintain elimination:
   a. Keep accurate intake and output record.
   b. Restrict fluid if ordered.
   c. Monitor output.
   d. Remove catheter as soon as possible.
8. Provide emotional support:
   a. Give specific guidelines for appropriate behaviors.
   b. Give positive feedback.
   c. Allow patient adequate time to complete tasks.

### Health promotion/prevention

Traumatic head injuries can often be prevented. Primary prevention focuses on reducing the incidence of head injury through improved environmental safety and is a major focus of *Healthy People 2000* (Box 52-15). Secondary prevention is aimed at prompt and accurate diagnosis and treatment of injuries to minimize the damage and limit the incidence of complications. Public information campaigns focus on reducing risk and the importance of thorough evaluation of all head injuries.

Much can be done in terms of primary prevention of head injuries. Factors that can influence the incidence of head injury include the following:

1. Use of seat belts, passive restraints, and air bags in automobiles
2. Use of helmets when riding motorcycles, snowmobiles, or bicycles
3. Practice of firearm safety and gun control
4. Minimal use of alcohol and drugs

**box 52-15** Healthy People 2000 *Goals Related to Head Injury*

- Reduce deaths caused by motor vehicle crashes to no more than 1.9 per 100 million vehicle miles traveled and 16.8 per 100,000 persons.
- Reduce deaths from falls and fall-related injuries to no more than 2.3 per 100,000 persons.
- Reduce nonfatal head injuries so that hospitalizations for this condition are no more than 106 per 100,000 persons.

From US Department of Health and Human Services, Public Health Service: *Healthy People 2000: National health promotion and disease prevention objectives,* Washington DC, 1990, US Government Printing Office.

5. Not driving after taking drugs or drinking alcohol
6. Improving home environmental safety features (e.g., securing throw rugs, removing clutter on stairs, installing grab bars in bathrooms, and increasing lighting)

## EVALUATION

To evaluate the effectiveness of nursing interventions, compare patient behaviors with those stated in the expected patient outcomes. Successful achievement of patient outcomes for the patient with a head injury is indicated by:

1. Pulse oximetry readings above 90%, with regular and unlabored respirations
2. Absence of signs and symptoms of increased ICP
3. Body temperature between 97.5° and 99.5° F
4. Fluid intake of at least 1500 ml/day
   a. Balanced urine output
   b. Normal electrolyte and BUN values
   c. Stable weight, neither loss nor gain
5. Free of infection
6. Can ambulate, transfer, or move freely in a wheelchair
7. Family member or significant other states ability to cope with injury of loved one: absence of excessive crying, inability to sleep, appetite disturbances, and other signs of increased stress
8. Family or significant other correctly explains pathology of head injury and associated care

## GERONTOLOGICAL CONSIDERATIONS

The older patient may have preexisting conditions that contribute to injury. Altered gait, balance, and reflexes make the older patient more prone to falls. Osteoporosis can increase the risk, frequency, and severity of fractures of the skull and face. Syncope, hypotension, and cardiac dysrythmias can also lead to falls. Patients receiving anticoagulation therapy are more likely to develop hematomas after falls.

Elderly persons with significant medical histories who experience a moderate to severe head injury have less physiological reserve to survive the acute period of resuscitation.[22] The assessment of patients with a known degenerative disorder is complicated by the need to differentiate between pretrauma abnormalities and those of the trauma itself. Patients with sensory losses resulting from aging, such as vision or hearing losses, may have a more difficult time participating in therapy. An elderly patient who was barely independent before a nervous system trauma may not be able to regain independence even when the residual deficits are minor.

Nurses can educate patients and families in ways to keep the older population safe from injuries that rob them of their independence and health. Environmental modifications to remove hazards, mobility aids, sensory enhancement aids, and therapy can help the older patient retain strength and mobility.

## SPECIAL ENVIRONMENTS FOR CARE

### Critical Care Management

The patient with a mild or moderate head injury will probably not require critical care. Patients with multisystem trauma and those needing intubation and ventilation are admitted to a critical care setting. Initial management of the patient focuses on resuscitation and stabilization. The full trauma evaluation is then completed to identify occult injuries. Effective ventilation is established, and circulatory support is initiated to ensure perfusion to the injured brain.

During the acute phase of recovery the patient's intracranial pressure is monitored and treated as necessary. Ventilatory support is maintained and then gradually withdrawn as the patient recovers from his or her injuries. As the patient becomes more stable, less invasive monitoring is required and the patient is encouraged to participate in more of the activities of daily living. In rare instances, the patient may need prolonged ventilatory support but is otherwise stable. In this case, rehabilitation begins in the critical care setting.

The patient and family require a great deal of support during the critical care period. Trauma is unexpected, and families need to cope with sudden changes in their lives, as well as the threat of losing a loved one. Helping a family cope during the crisis phase is a major nursing responsibility in the ICU and is continued throughout the patient's recovery. Research has identified that the families of the critically ill list information about the patient's condition and access to the patient as their most important needs during this stressful time.[15]

### Home Care Management

Patients with moderate head injuries may be sent home to continue their rehabilitation on an outpatient basis. Hospital-based nurses assist families to identify resources in the patient's community. Resource selection is based on the patient's ability to perform self-care and the family's resources and supports to provide the needed care and support.

Patients with more severe head injuries may need long-term care at home. These services provide supportive rather than restorative care. The care needs of head-injured patients are enormous because they include physical, psychological, and cognitive challenges. Families need enormous support when providing this care long term.

## COMPLICATIONS

There are a wide range of potential complications from head injury. Complications related to immobility include atelectasis, risk of pneumonia, cardiovascular deconditioning, skin breakdown, muscle atrophy, and constipation. Patients are

**table 52-9** *Organisms That Cause Central Nervous System Infections*

| Disease | Organism | Comments |
|---|---|---|
| Pneumococcal meningitis | *Streptococcus pneumoniae* | Gram-positive diplococci; most common type in adults, especially if history of pneumonia, sinus infection, trauma |
| *Haemophilus influenzae* meningitis | *Haemophilus influenzae* | Gram-negative cocci; most common in children, especially if history of upper respiratory infection or ear infection |
| Meningococcal meningitis | *Neisseria meningitidis* | Gram-negative diplococci; highest incidence in children or young adults; may have petechial rash; about 10% develop overwhelming septicemia |
| California encephalitis | Arbovirus of California, mosquito borne | Aseptic meningitis or encephalitis |
| St. Louis encephalitis | St. Louis encephalitis virus, mosquito borne | Encephalitis or aseptic meningitis |

also at risk for infection from breaks in the body's natural defenses. Invasive monitoring devices and IV lines, urinary catheters, and endotracheal tubes all breach the body's natural defenses and increase the risk of infection. If the patient has a skull fracture with a dural tear, meningitis is also a risk.

Head-injured patients are also at risk for complications related to the neurological injury. Some patients become prone to seizures and need lifelong anticonvulsant therapy. Other patients develop obstructions to CSF flow and need to be treated for hydrocephalus. Autonomic responses to the injury may increase stomach acid production and place the patient at risk for ulcer formation. The nurse works collaboratively to identify possible complications and develop plans for prevention and treatment.

## INFECTIONS AND INFLAMMATION

The nervous system may be attacked by a variety of bacteria and viruses. The infection may wall off and create an abscess, or the meninges and sometimes the brain itself may become involved. Organisms reach the nervous system by various routes. Chronic otitis media, sinusitis and mastoiditis, and fracture of any bone adjacent to the meninges can be the source of infection. Some organisms, such as the tubercle bacillus, reach the nervous system by means of the blood or the lymph system. Infection also can occur as a complication of invasive procedures such as lumbar puncture. The exact route by which some infectious agents reach the central nervous system is not known. Two of the more common central nervous system infections, meningitis and encephalitis, are discussed next.

### MENINGITIS

#### Etiology/Epidemiology

Bacterial meningitis affects the leptomeninges, the pia and arachnoid layers, and the CSF. The most common pathogens causing meningitis are *Haemophilus influenzae, Neisseria meningitidis,* and *Streptococcus pneumoniae.* The causative organisms vary significantly at different ages. *Haemophilus* is common in young children and often follows an upper respiratory infection or ear infection. *Neisseria* has its highest incidence in children and young adults and can cause an overwhelming septicemia. *Streptococcus pneumoniae* causes the pneumococcal form of meningitis, which is common in adults.

The incidence of meningitis is fairly constant throughout the year but typically declines during the summer months. The infection has associated risks of serious adverse complications. It is therefore specifically targeted in the *Healthy People 2000* goals to *reduce bacterial meningitis to no more than 4.7 cases per 100,000 people.*

Viral meningitis, also called aseptic meningitis, is an inflammation of the meninges. Caused by viral or nonviral sources, the disease is usually self-limiting and does not require extensive treatment. Enteroviruses and mumps are the most common causative agents.

#### Pathophysiology

Organisms and viruses reach the nervous system by many routes. The most common route is the bloodstream, and bacteria in the nasopharynx may enter the bloodstream during an upper respiratory infection. Once organisms reach the brain, the CSF in the subarachnoid spaces and the pia-arachnoid membrane become infected. The infection then spreads rapidly throughout the meninges and eventually invades the ventricles. Pathological alterations include hyperemia of the meningeal vessels, edema of brain tissue, increased intracranial pressure, and a generalized inflammatory reaction with exudation of white blood cells into the subarachnoid spaces. Hydrocephalus may be caused by exudate blocking the small passages between the ventricles. Table 52-9 presents some of the common organisms that cause central nervous system infections.

#### Collaborative Care Management

The diagnosis of meningitis involves culturing the CSF, which is obtained by lumbar puncture or from a ventriculostomy. A CT scan may also be performed to rule out other pathology.

Meningitis can cause a medical emergency. The onset is usually sudden and characterized by severe headache, stiffness of the neck, irritability, malaise, and restlessness. Nausea, vomiting, delirium, and complete disorientation may develop quickly. Kernig's sign (the inability of the patient to extend the legs when the knee is flexed at the hip) usually is present, and Brudzinski's sign (the hip and knee flex when the patient's neck is flexed) may also be present (Figure 52-14). Fever and tachycardia are also present. The causative organism can usually be isolated from the spinal fluid, which is cloudy if a pyogenic organism is present. The CSF pressure is also usually elevated along with the protein level in the CSF. The glucose content is usually decreased.

Treatment for bacterial infections consists of antibiotic therapy for the causative organism as determined by culture of the CSF. Parenteral antibiotics are administered for at least 10 days. The antibiotic may be given directly into the spinal canal (intrathecally). The use of hyperosmolar agents or steroids may be necessary to decrease cerebral edema. Anticonvulsants may be administered to prevent or control seizures.

Respiratory isolation is required for meningococcal infections only until the pathogen can no longer be cultured from the nasopharynx, usually after 24 hours of antibiotic therapy. If the patient develops hydrocephalus as a result of the meningitis, a shunt may need to be inserted to facilitate the flow of CSF.

General treatment measures include supportive care to control and reduce fever, balance fluids and electrolytes, and promote comfort. The headache can be severe, and the patient's fever may remain high throughout the illness. Acetaminophen (Tylenol) is typically given to reduce the fever and relieve the headache. Ice packs may increase the patient's comfort. Patients who are experiencing photophobia will be more comfortable in a darkened room. The nurse monitors the patient frequently, avoiding unnecessary stimulation and touching. Lights and noise are minimized as much as possible. Seizure precautions are instituted, and tepid baths may be necessary to control the patient's fever.

### *Patient/family education*

The patient and family often have questions regarding how the disease started and the plan for treatment. The extent of symptoms varies greatly from patient to patient. Some patients are mildly affected and need primarily supportive care. Others are more severely affected and may need critical care support. The nurse helps prepare the family for the possibility that the disease could prove fatal or leave the patient with residual deficits.

## ENCEPHALITIS

### Etiology/Epidemiology

Encephalitis is an acute infection of the brain parenchyma and meninges caused by bacteria, viruses, or fungi. Viral infection is the most common, typically caused by the arboviruses or herpes simplex. A wide variety of viruses, indigenous to various geographical areas, are capable of causing the disease if they gain access to the brain. Eastern equine encephalitis is the most serious, although least common, form. The most significant outbreak of encephalitis in the United States followed the influenza epidemic of 1918 and involved von Economo's

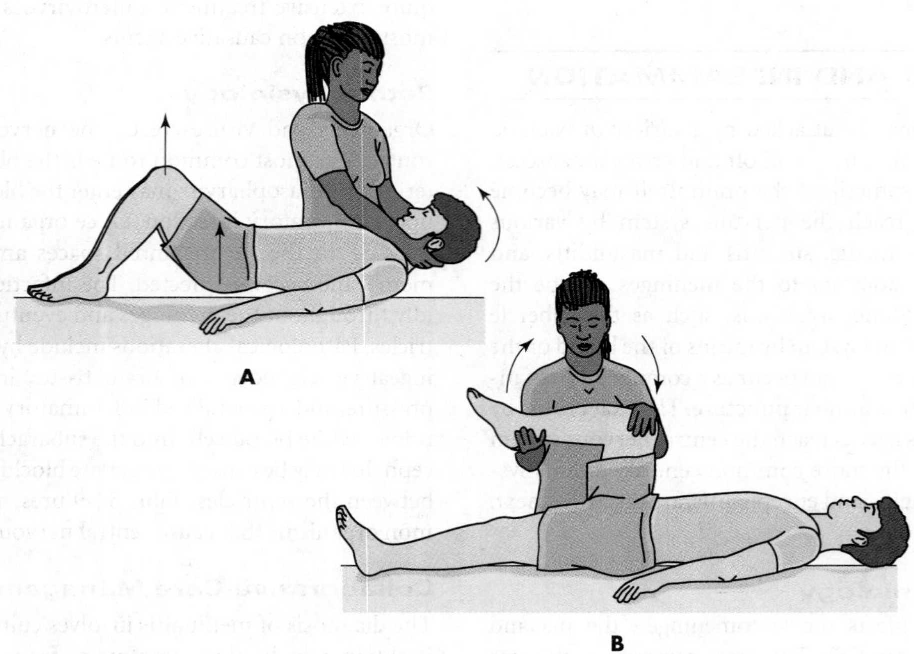


**fig. 52-14 A,** Brudzinsi's sign is elicited as the examiner passively flexes the patient's head and neck. A positive sign is indicated by the involuntary flexion of the hips and legs. **B,** Kernig's sign is the inability to extend the leg when the thigh is flexed onto the abdomen and is elicited by flexing the patient's upper leg at the hip to a 90° angle and then attempting to extend the leg at the knee. The sign is present if the patient cannot extend the leg or complains of hamstring pain.

disease. This particular form of encephalitis has not reappeared since 1926.

### Pathophysiology

Encephalitis causes degenerative changes in the nerve cells of the brain and produces scattered areas of inflammation and necrosis. Some inflammation of the meninges is also typically present. The symptoms vary significantly from virus to virus but often include fever, headache, seizures, stiff neck, and a declining level of consciousness that can progress from lethargy and restlessness to coma. A wide variety of local neurological signs can also be present. The mortality rate for encephalitis also varies substantially, but most patients experience some degree of residual deficit. Deficits include decreased cognitive functioning, personality changes, paralysis, and dementia. Patients can also be left deaf and blind.

### Collaborative Care Management

Encephalitis is diagnosed primarily from the clinical picture, serology assays, and analysis of the CSF. Antiviral medications such as acyclovir are effective for some forms of the disease, but treatment is otherwise largely supportive and symptomatic. Prompt initiation of acyclovir therapy has reduced the mortality rate for herpesvirus infections from up to 80% to less than 28%.

Analgesics may be prescribed for the headache and neck pain that accompany the disease. Steroids are administered to suppress inflammation, and anticonvulsants are used to control seizures. In severe cases of encephalitis, dramatic increases in pressure can result from brain herniation or cause widespread areas of cell necrosis.

#### *Patient/family education*

The needs of the patient and family for education and support are similar to those outlined for patients with meningitis, particularly when the patient is seriously ill. The fear associated with the disease and the uncertainty of the outcome necessitate frequent interventions and ongoing support from the nurse. It is essential that the nurse include the family in all decisions about the patient's care.

## critical thinking QUESTIONS

**1** Patricia is a 34-year-old woman admitted after having a tonic-clonic seizure. What would you assess during her postictal phase? What safety precautions would you take?

**2** Bruce is a 40-year-old patient with meningitis, admitted to your unit and started on antibiotics. He complains of photophobia. Is there cause for concern? What would you do to resolve this problem?

**3** Your assessment of a patient with a recent head injury reveals unequal pupils and less motor movement on the right side. An emergent CT scan shows a subdural hematoma on the left. How would you prepare this patient for the OR? What would you explain to the family?

**4** A patient with a left side acoustic neuroma is admitted to your unit postoperatively. The eighth cranial nerve was damaged during the surgery. Why is that expected? How will you communicate with this patient?

## chapter SUMMARY

### ALTERED LEVEL OF CONSCIOUSNESS

- Consciousness is the state of awareness and ability to respond to one's environment.
- Altered level of consciousness can be caused by structural or metabolic problems.
- Safety is a primary consideration when caring for a patient with altered LOC.

### INCREASED INTRACRANIAL PRESSURE

- An increase in the volume of any of the three cranial contents, singly or in combination, results in increased ICP when compensatory mechanisms are exhausted.
- Cerebral perfusion pressure is the pressure required to supply adequate blood flow to the brain in the presence of increased ICP.
- The most sensitive indicator of increasing ICP is a change in LOC.

### HEADACHE

- Migraine headaches are vascular in origin.
- Drugs that interfere with the vasoconstriction and vasodilation of cerebral blood vessels are effective in aborting migraine headaches.
- Headache diaries are an important strategy in helping patients design individualized treatment plans.

### EPILEPSY

- A seizure is an abnormal, paroxysmal electrical discharge from the cerebral cortex.
- Seizures can be partial or generalized.
- The primary goals of the care of the patient with epilepsy are patient teaching for medication compliance and safety practices.

### INTRACRANIAL TUMORS

- Brain tumors generally arise from the tissues surrounding or supporting the brain, such as the meninges or the glial cells.
- Brain tumors are difficult to treat because they often invade brain tissue or their position makes surgical excision difficult.
- The surgical opening of the skull for removal of any mass, such as tumor, hematoma, or abscess, is called a craniotomy.

### CRANIOCEREBRAL TRAUMA

- Trauma can involve the scalp, skull, and brain in any combination.
- Damage is classified as primary, occurring at the time of impact, or secondary, occurring later as the body responds to the initial injury.
- Subdural hematomas are usually venous in origin and lie between the dura and the brain.
- Epidural hematomas are usually arterial in origin and lie between the skull and the dura.

**INFECTIONS**

- Infections that can affect the brain include meningitis and encephalitis.
- The brain may be affected by infections that are caused by a variety of organisms and viruses and also may be affected by toxic reactions to bacterial and viral disease.

## References


1. Alguire PC: Rapid evaluation of comatose patients, *Postgrad Med* 87(6):223, 1990.
2. American Brain Tumor Association: *A primer of brain tumors,* Des Plaines, Ill, 1996.
3. American Congress of Rehabilitation Medicine: Recommendations for use of uniform nomenclature pertinent to patients with severe alterations in consciousness, *Arch Phys Med Rehabil* 76(2):205, 1995.
4. Barker FG II, Israel MA: The molecular biology of brain tumors, *Neurol Clin* 13(4):701, 1995.
5. Bernat JL, Ferrante JA: Helping your patient cope with migraine, *Patient Care* 26(7):44, 1992.
6. Boring CC et al: Cancer statistics, *CA Cancer J Clin* 43(1):7, 1993.
7. Broderson JM: Surgical options for brain tumor treatment, *Crit Care Nurs Clin North Am* 7(1):91, 1995.
8. Bronstein KS: Epidemiology and classification of brain tumors, *Crit Care Nurs Clin North Am* 7(1):79, 1995.
9. Bullock MR, Povlishock JT: Guidelines for the management of severe head injury, *J Neurotrauma* 13(11):639, 1996.
10. Callanan M: Seizures and epilepsy. In Barker E, editor: *Neuroscience nursing,* St Louis, 1994, Mosby.
11. Chang CWJ, Bleck TP: Status epilepticus, *Neurol Clin* 13(3):529, 1995.
12. Crosby LJ, Parsons LC: Cerebrovascular response of closed head-injury patients to a standardized endotracheal tube suctioning and manual hyperventilation procedure, *J Neurosci Nurs* 24(1):40, 1992.
13. Devinsky O, Yerby MS: Women with epilepsy: reproduction and effects of pregnancy on epilepsy, *Neurol Clin* 12(3):479, 1994.
14. Dodson WE et al: Status epilepticus, *Patient Care* 26(11):100, 1992.
15. Folstein MF, Folstein SE, McHugh PR: Mini-Mental State: a practical method for grading the cognitive state of patients for the clinician, *J Psychiatr Res* 12(3):189, 1975.
16. Fountaine DK: Effect of sensory alterations. In Clochesy JM et al, editors: *Critical care nursing,* Philadelphia, 1993, WB Saunders.
17. Geraci E, Geraci T: A look at recent hyperventilation studies: outcomes and recommendations for early use in the head-injured patient, *J Neurosci Nurs* 28(4):222, 1996.
18. Goadsby PJ: Current concepts of the pathophysiology of migraine, *Neurol Clin* 15(1):27, 1997.
19. Grossman RI et al: Severe headache: initial measures, *Patient Care* 27(9):124, 1993.
20. Hilton G: Seizure disorders in adults: evaluation and management of new onset seizures, *Nurse Pract* 22(9):42, 1997.
21. Hickey JV: *The clinical practice of neurological and neurosurgical nursing,* ed 4, Philadelphia, 1997, JB Lippincott.
22. Hickey M: Psychosocial needs of families. In Clochesy JM et al, editors: *Critical care nursing,* Philadelphia, 1993, WB Saunders.
23. Jastremski CA: Traumatic brain injury, assessment and treatment, *Crit Care Nurs Clin North Am* 6(3):473, 1994.
24. Kraay CR: Intracranial pressure monitoring. In Clochesy JM et al, editors: *Critical care nursing,* Philadelphia, 1993, WB Saunders.
25. Laws E, Thapar K: Brain tumors, *CA Cancer J Clin* 43(5):263, 1993.
26. Lee MW et al: The efficacy of barbiturate coma in the management of uncontrolled intracranial hypertension following neurosurgical trauma, *J Neurotrauma* 11(3):325, 1994.
27. McNew CD, Hunt S, Warner LS: How to help your patient with epilepsy, *Nursing* 27(9):57, 1997.
28. Mathews NT: Serotonin 1D (5-HT) agonists and other agents in acute migraine, *Neurol Clin* 15(1):61, 1997.
29. Murphy G: Cancer statistics, 1995, *CA Cancer J Clin* 45(1):12, 1995.
30. National Institutes of Health Consensus Development Conference Statement: Surgery for epilepsy, *Epilepsia* 31(6):806, 1990.
31. Pieper DR, Valadka AB, Marsh C: Surgical management of patients with severe head injuries, *AORN J* 63(5):854, 1996.
32. Plum F, Posner JB: *The diagnosis of stupor and coma,* ed 3, Philadelphia, 1982, FA Davis.
33. Prociuk JL: Management of cerebral oxygen supply-demand balance in blunt head injury, *Crit Care Nurse* 15(4):38, 1995.
34. Commission on Classification and Terminology of International League Against Epilepsy: Proposal for classification of epilepsies and epileptic syndromes, *Epilepsia* 22(4):489, 1981.
35. Ricci M, Barker E: Pain and headache. In Barker E, editor: *Neuroscience nursing,* St Louis, 1994, Mosby.
36. Richmond TS: Intracranial pressure monitoring, *AACN Clin Issues Crit Care Nurs* 4(1):148, 1993.
37. Schwartz RB: Neuroradiology of brain tumors, *Neurol Clin* 13(4):723, 1995.
38. Shrieve DC, Loeffler JS: Advances in radiation therapy for brain tumors, *Neurol Clin* 13(4):773, 1995.
39. Sipos EP, Brem H: New delivery systems for brain tumor therapy, *Neurol Clin* 13(4):813, 1995.
40. Stewart-Amidei C et al: Quality of life in the neuro-oncology patient: a symposium, *J Neurosci Nurs* 27(4):219, 1995.
41. Solomon S: Diagnosis of primary headache disorders, validity of the IHS criteria in clinical practice, *Neurol Clin* 15(1):15, 1997.
42. Teasdale G, Jennett B: Assessment of coma and impaired consciousness, a practical scale, *Lancet* 2(7872):81, 1974.
43. Tfelt-Hansen P: Prophylactic pharmacotherapy of migraine: some practical guidelines, *Neurol Clin* 15(1):153, 1997.
44. US Department of Health and Human Services, Public Health Service: *Healthy people 2000: national health promotion and disease prevention objectives,* DHHS pub no (PHS) 91-50212, Washington, DC, 1990, US Government Printing Office.
45. Vos H: Making headway with intracranial hypertension, *Am J Nurs* 93(2):28, 1993.
46. Walleck CA: Preventing secondary brain injury, *AACN Clin Issues Crit Care Nurs* 3(1):19, 1992.
47. Walleck C: Patients with head injury and brain dysfunction. In Clochesy JM et al, editors: *Critical care nursing,* Philadelphia, 1993, WB Saunders.
48. Walleck C, Mooney K: Neurotrauma: head injury. In Barker E, editor: *Neuroscience nursing,* St Louis, 1994, Mosby.
49. Wijdicks EF: Determining brain death in adults, *Neurology* 45(5):1003, 1995.
50. Williams A, Coyne SM: Effects of neck position on intracranial pressure, *Am J Crit Care* 2:68, 1993.
51. Winkelman C: Advances in managing increased intracranial pressure: a decade of selected research, *AACN Clin Issues Crit Care Nurs* 5(1):9, 1994.

chapter 53

# MANAGEMENT OF PERSONS WITH Vascular, Degenerative, and Autoimmune Problems of the Brain

JUDITH K. SANDS and CAROL LYNN MAXWELL-THOMPSON

## objectives *After studying this chapter, the learner should be able to:*

1 Identify the major risk factors for ischemic and hemorrhagic stroke.
2 Correlate stroke pathology with its major clinical manifestations.
3 Compare transient ischemic attacks and reversible ischemic neurological deficits, and right versus left hemisphere strokes.
4 Develop specific assessment strategies for identifying the primary communication and sensory perceptual deficits of stroke.
5 Discuss the rationale for antiplatelet therapy, reperfusion therapy, and carotid endarterectomy in the management of cerebrovascular disease and stroke.
6 Develop nursing interventions to assist patients to regain self-care independence after stroke.
7 Describe nursing interventions to prevent the musculoskeletal and nutritional complications of stroke.
8 Develop a family teaching plan to manage the communication, cognitive, behavioral, and emotional outcomes of stroke.
9 Compare the treatment options for aneurysms and arteriovenous malformations.
10 Compare the major degenerative and autoimmune neurological disorders in terms of incidence, populations affected, and primary pathology.
11 Describe the pharmacological management of myasthenia gravis and Parkinson's disease.
12 Compare the major nursing interventions used to manage mobility, self-care, nutrition, bowel and bladder, and risk of injury concerns for each of the major degenerative and autoimmune neurological disorders.

This chapter presents the management of vascular, degenerative, and autoimmune disorders affecting the brain. Cerebrovascular accident is by far the most important of these disorders because of its incidence statistics and extensive residual deficits, which challenge patients, families, and health care providers. Numerous autoimmune and degenerative disorders could be included in the chapter discussion, but only the most common of these disorders are presented. All of them have complex associated care needs, but they all share the common goal of maximizing the patient's independence in self-care for as long as possible and supporting overall coping. These disorders are managed by a multidisciplinary team, but the nurse is commonly called on to serve as the case manager, coordinating needed services.

## CEREBROVASCULAR DISEASE

Cerebrovascular disease refers to any pathological process involving the blood vessels of the brain. It is the most common neurological disorder in adults and is the third-leading cause of death in the United States, behind heart disease and cancer. The heterogeneous category of cerebrovascular disease encompasses two major types of disorders, ischemic and hemorrhagic, each of which can produce either temporary or permanent deficits in neurological functioning. Major problems in either category create a syndrome of neurological deficits that reflect impairment of oxygenation to a specific area of the brain. This syndrome is usually referred to as a cerebrovascular accident or stroke. Although strokes can have either an ischemic or a hemorrhagic origin, the following discussion is primarily directed toward the management of ischemic strokes, which are by far the most common form. Hemorrhagic strokes are discussed later in the chapter under the heading of aneurysms and other structural vascular problems.

## CEREBROVASCULAR ACCIDENT/STROKE

### Etiology

A cerebrovascular accident (CVA) can be defined as a neurological deficit that has a sudden onset and lasts over 24 hours. Ischemic strokes account for an estimated 85% of the total, and this percentage can be further broken down into strokes resulting from atherosclerotic disease (20%), cardiogenic or embolic sources (20%), idiopathic (30%), and other causes (15%).[2] These categories are described in Box 53-1. Hemorrhagic strokes are typically classified by the location of the bleeding. Subarachnoid strokes occur from bleeding into the subarachnoid space, and intracerebral strokes occur from bleeding into the brain tissue itself. Subarachnoid bleeding is

**box 53-1** *Etiologies of Ischemic Strokes*

ATHEROSCLEROTIC
Atherosclerosis affects both the large extracranial and intracranial arteries. The lumen of the vessel narrows and can be a target site for thrombus formation. Transient ischemic attacks occur in about half of patients before the stroke.

SMALL PENETRATING ARTERY THROMBOSIS/LACUNAR
Thrombosis of a small penetrating brain artery causes a small damaged area of tissue in the deep white matter structures of the brain, called a lacuna. Lacunae typically occur in the basal ganglia, internal capsule, pons, or thalamus.

CARDIOGENIC/EMBOLIC
Most of these strokes are the result of emboli, usually of cardiac origin, that break off and travel in the arterial circulation until they reach a vessel that is too narrow to allow further passage. Atrial fibrillation is the most common cause of the emboli.

OTHER
Ischemic strokes can also result from vasospasm, inflammation, coagulation disorders, and the effects of drug abuse, particularly cocaine.

IDIOPATHIC
No identifiable cause is established in up to 30% of all ischemic strokes.

**risk factors**

**Stroke**

**Age**
From 60% to 75% of all strokes occur in persons over 65 years of age.

**Sex**
Men have a slightly increased incidence of stroke, possibly because of poorer control of hypertension and heart disease.

**Race**
African Americans are twice as likely to develop thrombotic strokes and three times more likely to develop hemorrhagic strokes. Whether this is truly a race-related risk is unknown.

**Hypertension**
Hypertension is a major risk factor for stroke, particularly in combination with atherosclerosis. The improved diagnosis and treatment of hypertension have decreased the incidence and mortality of stroke over the last two decades.

**Heart Disease**
Heart disease is a major contributor to stroke both from atherosclerosis and as a common source of emboli.

**Diabetes**
Diabetes is associated with an accelerated rate of microvascular and macrovascular changes that contribute to atherosclerosis.

**Other**
Cigarette smoking
Oral contraceptive use (especially if also a smoker)
Alcohol intake
Family history of transient ischemic attack or cerebrovascular accident
*Obesity
*Sedentary lifestyle
*Elevated serum cholesterol and triglycerides

*These factors are less well studied but are believed to contribute to stroke.

usually the result of the rupture of a cerebral aneurysm or arteriovenous malformation, whereas intracerebral bleeds result from the rupture of a small artery, often a deep penetrating vessel, and are often related to poorly controlled hypertension.

### Risk factors

Both modifiable and nonmodifiable risk factors are associated with stroke. The nonmodifiable risks of age, gender, sex, and race are discussed under Epidemiology and summarized in the Risk Factors Box. In addition, hypertension, cardiac disease, diabetes mellitus, and blood lipid abnormalities can all increase the risk of stroke, particularly when they are present in combination. Improvements in community outreach efforts for the diagnosis and treatment of hypertension have had a significant positive effect on reducing stroke incidence and mortality over the last several decades.[9] The presence of atherosclerosis elsewhere in the body is presumed to also influence the cerebral vessels. Patients who have preexisting heart disease have a clearly increased risk, as do patients with diabetes mellitus, which accelerates the processes of atherosclerosis and arteriosclerosis in the blood vessels. Most of the other lifestyle factors associated with an increased risk of heart disease, however, have not been clearly demonstrated to influence the etiology of stroke.[16]

## Epidemiology

Although a significant decrease in stroke incidence and mortality has occurred over the last two decades, stroke remains the third-leading cause of death in the United States. An estimated 500,000 first-time strokes occur each year, with a 25% to 33% associated fatality rate.[2] The mortality rate has declined about 33% since 1980, but stroke leaves about 25% of its victims with mental or physical disabilities that require ongoing assistance with activities of daily living (ADL).[16] This creates a pool of more than 2 million people who are currently partially or totally disabled from stroke, and this number is expected to rise as the population continues to age. The importance of stroke as a national health concern is reflected in its addition to the *Healthy People 2000* goals as part of the 1995 evaluation and midcourse corrections project. The health status objective is "to reduce stroke deaths to no more than 20 per 100,000 people."

Stroke has profound social and economic consequences for the person, family, and community. Direct and indirect care

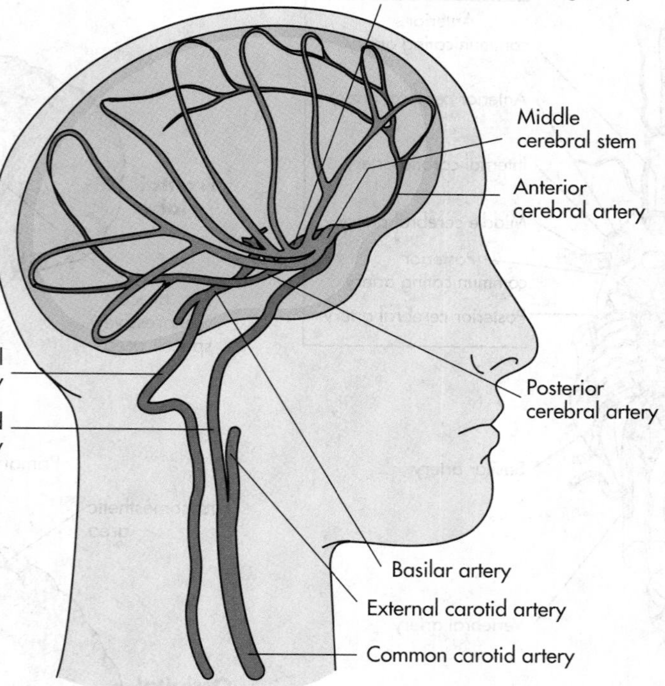

Posterior communicating artery
Middle cerebral stem
Anterior cerebral artery
Vertebral artery
Internal carotid artery
Posterior cerebral artery
Basilar artery
External carotid artery
Common carotid artery

**fig. 53-1** The major arteries that supply the brain. The internal carotids branch to supply the anterior portions of the brain. The vertebral arteries supply the posterior portions.

costs for stroke management and ongoing care are estimated at 25 to 30 billion dollars.[2] The obvious economic impact of stroke is reflected in the rapid proliferation of clinical pathways for case management of stroke patients. These pathways attempt to clearly delineate the specifics of care to be provided at each stage of rehabilitation. The social and emotional tolls are more difficult to quantify but are readily apparent to anyone whose family has been touched by stroke.

From 60% to 75% of all strokes occur in persons over 65 years of age.[2] The remaining 25% to 40% affect younger persons. Strokes are slightly more common in men than in women. African Americans are twice as likely to experience ischemic strokes and three times more likely to experience hemorrhagic strokes than whites. It is unclear whether this increased incidence is directly related to racial factors or reflects generally poorer diagnosis and treatment of hypertension, heart disease, and diabetes in this population, particularly male African Americans. Some incidence and mortality variations have also been noted worldwide, particularly in Japan. The meaning of these differences is not clear.

## Pathophysiology

The brain must receive a steady supply of nutrients from the blood because it has no capacity to store either oxygen or glucose. It is supplied with blood from two major pairs of vessels, the internal carotids and the vertebrals. The carotids supply the anterior portions of the brain, including most of the hemispheres except for the occipital lobes (Figure 53-1). The vertebrals join together to become the basilar artery and supply the posterior portions of the brain, including the cerebellum, brainstem, and occipital lobes. The Circle of Willis is the region of the brain in which the branches of the basilar and internal carotid artieries join, creating a circular network, which in theory allows blood to circulate from one hemisphere to the other and from the anterior to the posterior portions of the brain (Figure 53-2). Functionally, however, the circulations of the two hemispheres usually remain separate. The circle is composed of the middle cerebral arteries; the anterior cerebral arteries; the anterior communicating artery, which connects the anterior cerebrals; the posterior cerebral arteries; and the posterior communicating arteries, which connect the middle cerebrals with the posterior cerebrals, thus uniting the two systems. Figure 53-3 illustrates the major areas of the brain supplied by these cerebral vessels.

The complex processes of cerebral autoregulation maintain blood flow to the brain at a fairly constant rate of 750 ml per minute. The cerebral vessels dilate and constrict in response to changes in blood pressure and carbon dioxide tension. Ischemia can cause primary death of cerebral cells or cerebral infarction, which creates a core of necrotic tissue. The ischemia, in a process similar to that seen after myocardial infarction, also causes a second area of tissue damage in which cells are temporarily unable to function but may remain viable. A complex cascade of biochemical changes occurs in response to the ischemia, and this process is the target of intense current research.[13] When the components of the ischemic response can be accurately mapped it may be possible to prevent or

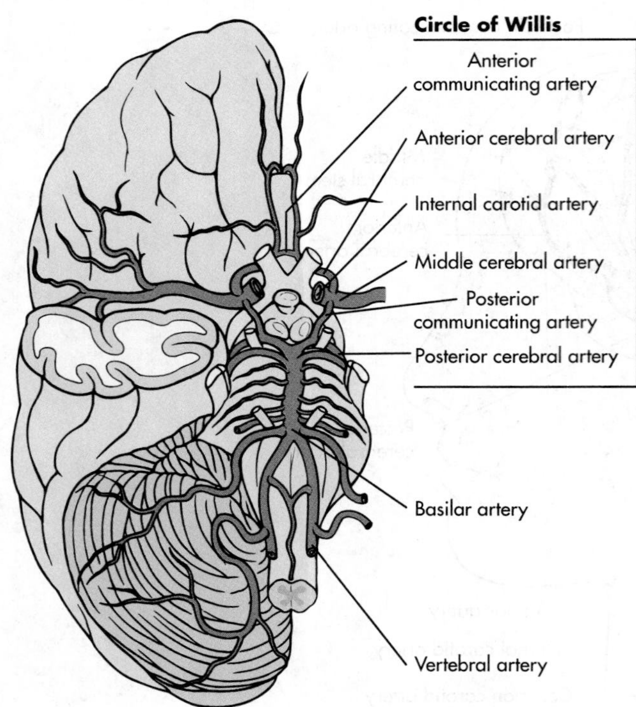


fig. 53-2 The Circle of Willis as seen from below the brain.

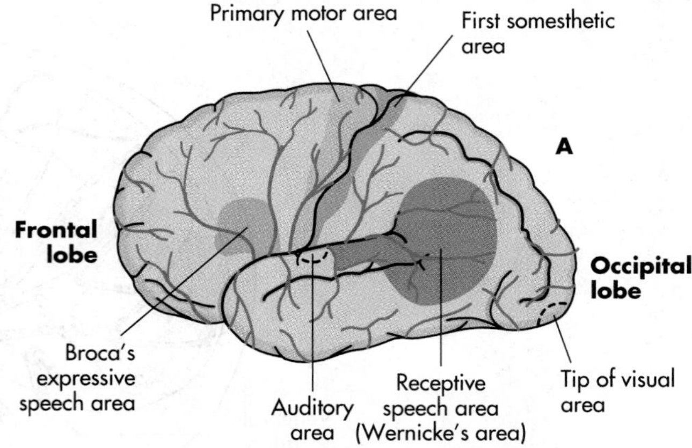


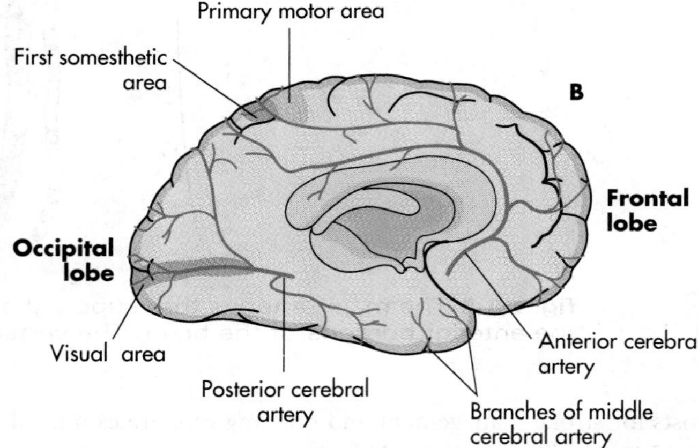


fig. 53-3 A, Distribution of the middle cerebral artery on the lateral surface of the brain. B, Distribution of the anterior and posterior cerebral arteries on the medial surface of the brain.

reverse its effects. Ischemia is known to cause the following disparate responses:[13]

- Impaired movement of calcium and potassium. High levels of calcium are believed to trigger the activation of enzymes that attack neuron cell membranes.
- The accumulation of oxygen free radicals, which further disrupt calcium metabolism.
- The presence of glucose in low-perfusion areas enhances lactate production, which worsens cellular damage and acidosis.
- An influx of fluid-activated white cells and coagulation factors further clog the microcirculation.

The pathophysiology associated with hemorrhagic strokes is primarily related to an abrupt rise in intracranial pressure and ischemia followed by cerebral edema. With intracerebral bleeding blood is forced into the adjacent brain tissue where a hematoma forms. The compression of tissue then extends the ischemic damage and can even result in brain tissue displacement or herniation. The pathophysiological process of elevated intracranial pressure is described in Chapter 52.

### Clinical manifestations

The specific neurological deficits that are produced by stroke reflect the location and severity of the ischemia and the adequacy of the collateral circulation in the region. Many of the features overlap with other forms of brain injury. A number of specific syndromes have been identified that reflect the involvement of specific vessels and the areas of the brain that they serve, but in clinical practice it is unusual to see these syndromes in their pure forms. Box 53-2 outlines a few of the major syndromes and their associated neurological deficits. The two vessels affected most commonly are the middle cerebral artery and the internal carotid artery.

The term *stroke* commonly evokes a classic mental picture of specific disabilities, but a wide variety of presentations can occur. Commonly encountered symptoms are summarized in Box 53-3. Each of the major types of stroke is associated with a fairly typical onset and course of symptoms. A stroke caused by a thrombus occurs during sleep or rest more than 60% of the time. This may be related to the decline in baseline blood pressure that occurs at rest or to increases in blood viscosity that develop during sleep periods. Symptoms may develop abruptly or progress over a period of hours depending on how much blood is able to move through the obstructed vessel lumen. The symptoms usually peak within 72 hours and then demonstrate some improvement as the cerebral edema resolves. Embolic and hemorrhagic strokes are more likely to develop suddenly and progress rapidly over minutes or hours. There is rarely any prior warning. Patients with embolic strokes usually remain conscious during the event, but a decreased level of alertness is expected during the first few days following any type of stroke.

The term *stroke in evolution* may be used to describe an ischemic stroke whose symptoms develop progressively over a

**box 53-2** *Characteristics of Major Stroke Syndromes*

**MIDDLE CEREBRAL ARTERY (MCA) SYNDROME (MOST COMMON OCCLUSION)**

If blockage of the main stem of the MCA occurs, the infarction can affect most of the hemisphere, because the MCA accounts for about 80% of the blood supply to the cerebral hemispheres.

- Contralateral hemiparesis or hemiplegia—arm affected more severely than the leg
- Contralateral sensory impairment over same area affected by hemiplegia (proprioception, touch)
- Unilateral neglect or inattention (if nondominant hemisphere)
- Aphasia (if dominant hemisphere)
- Homonymous hemianopia

**INTERNAL CAROTID ARTERY (ICA) SYNDROME**

- Contralateral hemiparesis or hemiplegia
- Contralateral sensory losses
- Aphasia (if dominant hemisphere)

The symptoms of MCA and ICA strokes are almost identical, but if blockage of the main stem of the MCA occurs (see above), the deficits can be profound, because cerebral edema is usually extensive.

**VERTEBROBASILAR ARTERY SYNDROMES**

Occlusion of the vessels in this system creates unique symptoms that reflect the perfusion of the cerebellum and brain stem:

- Ataxia, clumsiness
- Dysphagia and dysarthria
- Dizziness and nystagmus
- Bilateral motor and sensory deficits
- Facial weakness and numbness

period of hours or days. This pattern is most characteristic of a gradually enlarging thrombus. *Completed stroke* is a term used to describe a situation in which no further deterioration in function has occurred over a 2- to 3-day period. Active rehabilitation usually begins as soon as an ischemic stroke is considered to be complete.

**Transient ischemic attack.** A transient ischemic attack (TIA) is a brief episode of neurological deficit that resolves without any residual effect. The episode may last for seconds, minutes, or hours, but the average duration is 10 minutes and the vast majority resolve within an hour. By definition, the symptoms must resolve within 24 hours. The term *reversible ischemic neurological deficit (RIND)* may be used if the deficit persists beyond 24 hours but then resolves over a period of days with no permanent deficits.[17] Some authorities believe that a RIND event may actually be a completed stroke that is mild enough to leave no residual deficits.

Transient ischemic attacks are generally considered to be warning signs of an impending ischemic problem and usually reflect advanced atherosclerotic disease. It is theorized that TIAs may be caused by microemboli that break off from atherosclerotic plaque lesions. However, TIAs can also be triggered by events that temporarily decrease blood flow to the affected area of the brain, such as vasospasm.

**box 53-3** ***clinical manifestations***

***Stroke***

**NOTE: Specific symptoms will reflect the site and severity of ischemic damage. The following is a general listing of common deficits. See also Box 53-2 for specific deficits associated with ischemia in individual cerebral vessels.**

**MOTOR**

Hemiparesis or hemiplegia of the side of the body opposite the site of ischemia
- Initially flaccid, progressing to spastic

Dysphagia
- Swallowing reflex may also be impaired

Dysarthria

**BOWEL AND BLADDER**

Frequency, urgency, and urinary incontinence
- Potential for bladder retraining is good if cognitively intact

Constipation
- Related more to immobility than to the physical effects of stroke

**LANGUAGE**

Nonfluent aphasia (also known as motor/expressive aphasia)—difficulty or inability to express self verbally
Fluent aphasia (also known as sensory/receptive aphasia)—difficulty or inability to comprehend speech
Alexia—inability to understand the written word
Agraphia—inability to express self in writing

**SENSORY-PERCEPTUAL**

Diminished response to superficial sensation
- Touch, pain, pressure, heat, and cold

Diminished proprioception
- Knowledge of position of body parts in the environment

Visual deficits
- Decreased acuity
- Diplopia
- Homonymous hemianopia (see Figure 53-4, p. 1743)

Perceptual (see Box 53-5, p. 1743)
- Unilateral neglect syndrome
- Distorted body image
- Apraxia—inability to carry out learned voluntary acts
- Agnosia—inability to recognize familiar objects through sight, sound, or touch
- Anosognosia—inability to recognize or denial of a physical deficit
- Possible deficits in
  - Telling time
  - Judging distance
  - Right-left discrimination
  - Memory of locations, objects

**COGNITIVE-EMOTIONAL**

Emotional lability and unpredictability
- Behavior may be socially inappropriate (e.g., crying jags, swearing)

Depression
Memory loss
Short attention span, easy distractability
Loss of reasoning, judgment, and abstract thinking ability

An estimated one third of persons who experience a TIA will have future episodes, one third will have no future episodes, and about one third will have a stroke within 2 years. TIAs may also recur repetitively over days, weeks, and even years without progressing to stroke.[17] The unique symptoms produced by the TIA are specific to the vessel involved and can usually be traced to involvement of the carotid supply or that of the vertebral arteries. There is tremendous variety in the range of possible symptoms. Common symptoms of TIAs are summarized in Box 53-4.

**Motor deficits.** Motor symptoms are the most widely recognized clinical manifestations of stroke. Compromise of the motor pathways can affect the initiation of movement, strength of movement, integration of movement, muscle tone, and reflex activity. The classic symptoms are hemiparesis or hemiplegia on the side of the body oppo-site the site of cerebral ischemia. Most patients are initially hyporeflexic and then progress to hyperreflexia and spasticity as recovery progresses. The upper and lower extremities may be affected to different degrees. Motor deficits also commonly impair swallowing and produce weakness in the muscles of speech.

**Bowel and bladder deficits.** Frequency, urgency, and incontinence are common problems in the initial days after stroke, but the reflex arc remains intact, as does at least a partial sensation of bladder filling. The stroke lesion usually affects only half of the motor and sensory control of the bladder, which makes effective continence rehabilitation a reasonable goal. The extent of motor deficit and the presence of cognitive deficits influence the degree of success. If extended indwelling catheterization can be avoided there is a good chance of successful bladder retraining. The problems that develop with bowel elimination are more related to cognitive losses and immobility than the physical effects of the stroke. Constipation is the most common problem.

**Communication deficits.** The ability to communicate is a complex process that involves receiving and effectively processing the written or spoken word and being able to communicate appropriately both verbally and in writing. The left hemisphere is dominant for language in all right-handed and many left-handed individuals. Broca's area, which is located at the inferior gyrus of the frontal lobe, is critical for the motor control of speech. Wernicke's area, which is located in the temporal lobe on the superior temporal gyrus, is responsible for auditory association (Figure 53-3). When the dominant hemisphere is affected stroke can create a language disorder termed *aphasia,* which can be subdivided and classified in several ways. Nonfluent aphasia is an expressive, primarily motor disorder involving Broca's area. Patients will have difficulty expressing thoughts because Broca's area contains the memory for motor patterns of speech. The deficits may range from difficulty finding the desired word to oral communication that is restricted to single-word responses. The ability to understand language usually remains intact, although many patients with aphasia have mixed patterns of abilities and disabilities. Agraphia, the inability to express ideas in writing, may or may not be present.

A fluent aphasia is a receptive, primarily sensory disorder involving Wernicke's area. The patient may speak fluently but be unable to comprehend speech. The patient's use of language is often full of errors, although automatic social responses such as yes, no, and fine are used appropriately. Either agraphia or alexia, the inability to understand the written word, may also be present. Global aphasia reflects damage to both regions of the brain and may result in the inability to either understand or use language. The presence of dysarthria can complicate the picture of aphasia.

**Sensory-perceptual deficits.** Perception is a complex process of recognizing and interpreting environmental stimuli. The right side of the brain, and the parietal lobe in particular, plays a significant role in perception. Sensory-perceptual deficits are common following stroke and can take a variety of forms. Straightforward sensory losses manifest as a diminished response to superficial sensations such as touch, temperature, heat, and cold. These create a substantial risk for injury.

Visual deficits may complicate environmental management and commonly occur because the visual pathways pass through most of the cerebral hemispheres. These may manifest as decreased visual acuity or diplopia, but more commonly manifest as some degree of homonymous hemianopsia—loss of vision in a portion of the visual field of each eye. (See Figure 53-4 for a comparison of the visual deficits created by ischemic damage at different portions of the visual pathway.)

The more subtle perceptual problems that occur with stroke may initially be overlooked but can be profoundly disturbing to the family because of their more bizarre manifestations. Proprioceptive knowledge of the position of body parts in the environment may be affected, which contributes to perceived clumsiness and the potential for injury.[29] Distortions of

**box 53-4** ***clinical manifestations***

***Transient Ischemic Attacks***

**SYMPTOMS RELATED TO CAROTID INVOLVEMENT**

- Visual disturbances
  - Temporary blindness in one eye
  - Blurred vision
- Motor disturbances
  - Hemiparesis
  - Localized motor deficits in face or extremities
- Sensory disturbances
  - Hemianesthesia
  - Sensory deficits in face or extremities

**SYMPTOMS RELATED TO VERTEBRAL INVOLVEMENT**

- Motor disturbances
  - Ataxia
  - Dysarthria
  - Dysphagia
  - Unilateral or bilateral weakness
- Visual disturbances
  - Diplopia
  - Bilateral blindness
- Other
  - Brief lapses in level of consciousness
  - Sensory disturbance
  - Dizziness, vertigo
  - Tinnitus

body image, lack of ability to accurately judge spatial relationships, apparent denial of the physical effects of the stroke, and the loss of ability to identify or use familiar objects correctly, particularly to complete learned tasks essential for self-care, can all be present to some degree. These deficits are outlined in Box 53-5.

**Cognitive-emotional deficits.** Patients commonly demonstrate a loss of control over their emotions following a stroke. Their emotional responses can be exaggerated, flattened, or inappropriate and are usually unpredictable. Depression occurs in most patients and is compounded by frustration over the losses in functional abilities and

**box 53-5** *Perceptual Deficits Caused by Stroke*

**UNILATERAL NEGLECT SYNDROME**
A distortion in body image in which the patient ignores the affected side of the body

**ANOSOGNOSIA**
Apparent unawareness or denial of any loss or deficit in physical functioning

**LOSS OF PROPRIOCEPTIVE SKILLS**
Lack of awareness of where various body parts are in relationship to each other and the environment

**AGNOSIA**
Inability to recognize a familiar object by use of the senses
- Visual agnosia
- Auditory agnosia
- Tactile agnosia

**APRAXIA**
Loss of ability to carry out a learned sequence of movements or use objects correctly when paralysis is not present
Constructional: may not be able to sequence a planned act necessary for activities of daily living (e.g., dressing, brushing teeth, combing hair)

**SPATIAL RELATIONSHIPS**
Loss of ability to judge distance or size or localize objects in space
Impaired right-left discrimination

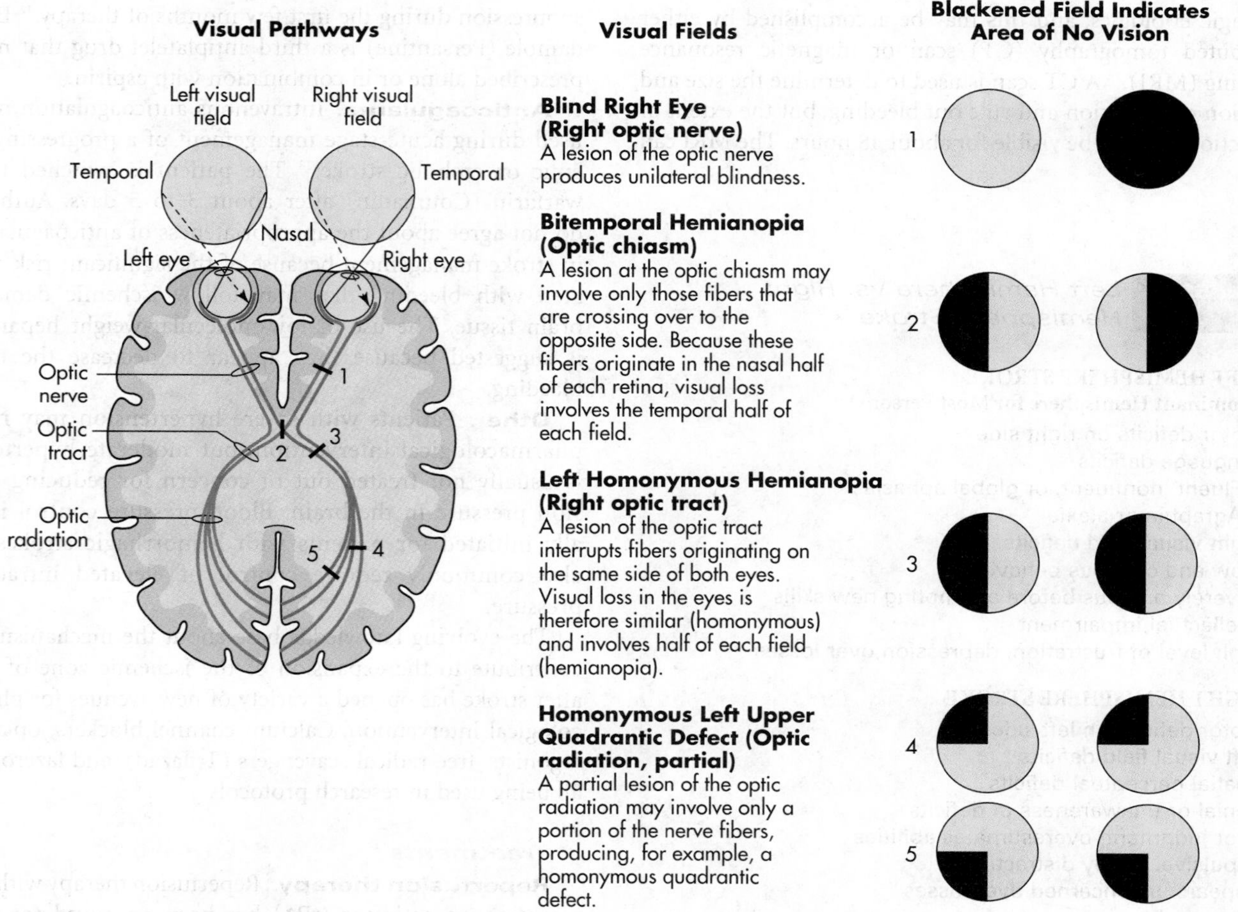

Visual Pathways
Left visual field
Right visual field
Temporal
Temporal
Nasal
Left eye
Right eye
Optic nerve
Optic tract
Optic radiation
1
2
3
4
5
Visual Fields
Blackened Field Indicates Area of No Vision
Blind Right Eye (Right optic nerve)
A lesion of the optic nerve produces unilateral blindness.
Bitemporal Hemianopia (Optic chiasm)
A lesion at the optic chiasm may involve only those fibers that are crossing over to the opposite side. Because these fibers originate in the nasal half of each retina, visual loss involves the temporal half of each field.
Left Homonymous Hemianopia (Right optic tract)
A lesion of the optic tract interrupts fibers originating on the same side of both eyes. Visual loss in the eyes is therefore similar (homonymous) and involves half of each field (hemianopia).
Homonymous Left Upper Quadrantic Defect (Optic radiation, partial)
A partial lesion of the optic radiation may involve only a portion of the nerve fibers, producing, for example, a homonymous quadrantic defect.


**fig. 53-4** Visual field defects produced by selected lesions in the visual pathways.

communication. It is often difficult to distinguish between normal emotional responses and those related to emotional lability. Uncontrolled anger or tears can be frightening symptoms for families. Stress and fatigue may increase the unpredictability and severity of the patient's emotional responses.

Memory and judgment are also commonly compromised by stroke, although these losses may not be readily apparent in the early days of recovery. A short attention span with easy distractibility may be present, which interferes with self-care learning. The ability to reason and think abstractly may be significantly altered, which can deepen the depressive response to stroke as patients must come to terms with the extent of their losses.

**Effects of laterality.** As our understanding of the functions of each side of the brain continues to increase, some predictions about the effects of stroke injury to each hemisphere are possible. The effects of left hemisphere versus right hemisphere stroke for individuals who are left hemisphere dominant (all right-handed individuals and many left-handed persons) are summarized in Box 53-6.

**box 53-6** *Left Hemisphere vs. Right Hemisphere Stroke*

**LEFT HEMISPHERE STROKE**
**(Dominant Hemisphere for Most Persons)**
- Motor deficits on right side
- Language deficits
  - Fluent, nonfluent, or global aphasia
  - Agraphia or alexia
- Right visual field deficits
- Slow and cautious behavior
- Severely anxious before attempting new skills
- Intellectual impairment
- High level of frustration, depression over losses

**RIGHT HEMISPHERE STROKE**
- Motor deficits on left side
- Left visual field deficits
- Spatial perceptual deficits
- Denial or unawareness of deficits
- Poor judgment, overestimates abilities
- Impulsive, highly distractible
- Appears unconcerned over losses

## Collaborative Care Management

### Diagnostic tests

A stroke is initially diagnosed by means of a careful history and physical examination. Aggressive early intervention to attempt reperfusion of the ischemic portions of the brain necessitates a rapid differentiation between ischemic and hemorrhagic etiologies, and this may be accomplished by either computed tomography (CT) scan or magnetic resonance imaging (MRI).[28] A CT scan is used to determine the size and location of the lesion and rule out bleeding, but the extent of infarction will not be visible for about 48 hours. The MRI can demonstrate the ischemic zone within the first few hours following stroke, but its high cost and limited accessibility usually make MRI the second diagnostic option.

A variety of other tests may also be used to identify other problems that may have contributed to the stroke. These might include a cardiac workup to rule out the possibility of cardiogenic emboli. Carotid Doppler or ultrasonography may be performed to rule out or evaluate the degree of carotid stenosis. Angiography may be used to localize and evaluate a bleeding site if a hemorrhagic stroke has occurred. No laboratory tests confirm the presence of stroke, but routine blood work will be performed to assess the patient's baseline status and provide a framework for anticoagulation if needed.

### Medications

Platelet aggregation inhibitor drugs are the mainstay of drug therapy for stroke. Aspirin is the most extensively used drug. It can be used in the management of TIAs or following ischemic strokes. Aspirin has been shown to reduce platelet adhesiveness and prevent the progression of a stroke in evolution, as well as recurrence after an initial stroke. Even in low doses, however, some patients are unable to tolerate the long-term use of aspirin, and its use increases the risk of peptic ulcer disease. Ticlopidine (Ticlid) has been shown in some studies to be a more effective agent for secondary stroke prevention, but patients need to be monitored for bone marrow suppression during the first few months of therapy.[32] Dipyridamole (Persantine) is a third antiplatelet drug that may be prescribed alone or in combination with aspirin.

**Anticoagulants.** Intravenous anticoagulation may be used during acute-stage management of a progressing ischemic or embolic stroke.[28] The patient is switched to oral warfarin (Coumadin) after about 3 to 5 days. Authorities do not agree about the appropriateness of anticoagulant use in stroke management because of the significant risk associated with bleeding that may follow ischemic damage to brain tissue. The use of low-molecular-weight heparinoids is suggested because they appear to decrease the risk of bleeding.

**Other.** Patients with severe hypertension may require pharmacological intervention, but moderate hypertension is usually not treated out of concern for reducing perfusion pressure in the brain. Blood pressure control is usually initiated for patients with hemorrhagic strokes, who also commonly require control of elevated intracranial pressure.

The evolving knowledge base about the mechanisms that contribute to the expansion of the ischemic zone of injury after stroke has opened a variety of new avenues for pharmacological intervention. Calcium channel blockers, opiate antagonists, free radical scavengers (Trilazad), and lazeroids are all being used in research protocols.

### Treatments

**Reperfusion therapy.** Reperfusion therapy with tissue plasminogen activator (tPA) has been approved for use in selected stroke patients and represents one of the first major efforts to intervene and minimize the effects of ischemic damage. The same principles that guide the use of tPA following acute myocardial infarction also apply to its use in stroke.[27] The risk of major bleeding is a serious concern, and only thrombotic and embolic strokes can be approached this way. The risk of bleeding appears to be minimized if the tPA is administered within the first 3 hours following the onset of symptoms. If tPA is administered to necrotic tissue the damage to the brain can worsen, so the window of opportunity is extremely narrow.[11] Patients are carefully screened for risk factors because the risk of generalized bleeding from fibrinolysis is significant. Successful treatment with tPA has been shown to dramatically decrease the severity of the residual deficits of stroke.

**Hypervolemic-hyperdilution therapy.** Maintaining adequate and stable cerebral perfusion is an essential goal of early stroke management. As discussed previously, no effort is made to reduce moderate hypertension, and blood pressure stability is supported. Hypervolemia and hyperdilution can be achieved by the administration of saline and perhaps albumin.[28] This treatment supports a sustained blood pressure, promotes vasodilation of the cerebral vessels, and thereby maximizes perfusion to the brain.

### Surgical management

Carotid endarterectomy is the primary surgical intervention used in stroke management. It is targeted at stroke prevention primarily for patients with symptomatic carotid stenosis. Endarterectomy carefully removes the plaque after the artery has been clamped both above and below the obstruction (Figure 53-5). Circulation to the brain on the affected side is maintained through the vertebrobasilar arterial system with supplemental flow through a temporary bypass shunt. Despite these precautions the greatest risks associated with the procedure relate to compromised cerebral blood flow, especially if carotid stenosis is present on both sides. Embolization of plaque and microthrombi resulting from the surgical manipulation increase the risk of additional strokes and are the primary postoperative concerns. Intervention is usually reserved for patients with greater than a 70% carotid blockage.[13]

Care in the postoperative period relates to blood pressure instability, which usually persists for about 12 to 24 hours and causes concern for the development of both hypertension and hypotension. The sudden restoration of blood flow through a significantly obstructed carotid can in itself result in hemorrhage, and the increased perfusion may initially overwhelm the brain's ability to effectively autoregulate. In appropriate surgical candidates carotid endarterectomy significantly reduces the risk of stroke. See the Guidelines for Care Box for a listing of the major nursing care considerations. A Clinical Pathway for a patient undergoing carotid endarterectomy is found on p. 1746.

Bypass surgeries are also attempted in selected situations. They are primarily performed to support perfusion to regions served by the middle cerebral artery, but outcome studies have shown equivocal results at this time.

### Diet

The patient is usually placed on nothing-by-mouth (NPO) status on admission and is maintained NPO until stabilization has occurred and a thorough evaluation of swallowing can be performed. Protecting the airway from the risk of aspiration of food, fluid, and secretions is the primary concern.[3] Intact gag and swallow reflexes are essential prerequisites for oral feedings, and their presence

*Text continued on p. 1749*

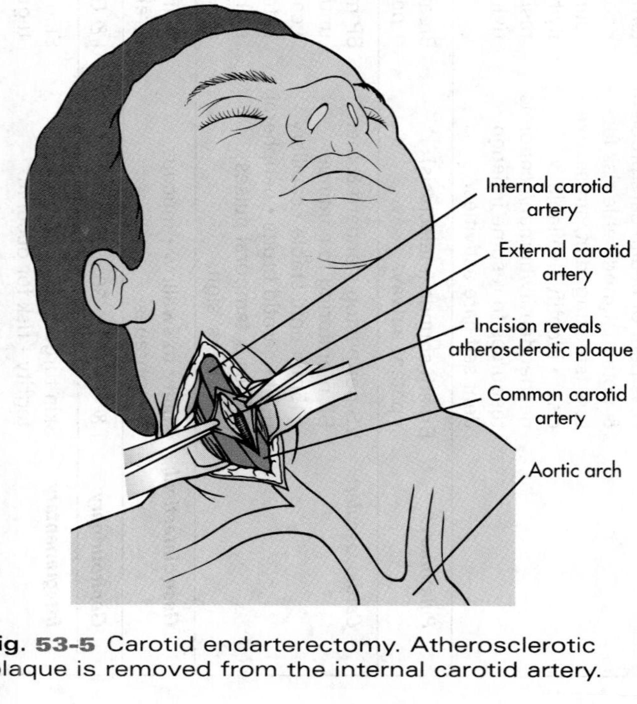

Internal carotid artery
External carotid artery
Incision reveals atherosclerotic plaque
Common carotid artery
Aortic arch

**fig. 53-5** Carotid endarterectomy. Atherosclerotic plaque is removed from the internal carotid artery.

## guidelines for care

### The Person Undergoing Carotid Endarterectomy

Postoperative nursing care focuses on monitoring and the early identification of potential complications. Primary areas include the following:

**Vital Signs**

Monitor vital signs q1-2h
- Blood pressure instability is anticipated in the first 12-24 hours
- Report incidence of blood pressure fluctuations above or below established parameters immediately

**Monitoring for Complications**

Monitor neurological status through frequent neurological checks
- Evaluate cranial nerves, particularly facial and vagus

Monitor for dysrhythmias and assess for incidence of chest pain

Monitor for signs of reperfusion injury
- Worsening or recurring stroke symptoms
- Signs of increasing intracranial pressure

Monitor incision site for patency, drainage

**clinical pathway** *Carotid Artery Endarterectomy*

| | DAY 1 (OR) | DAY 2 | DAY 3 | DAY 4 |
|---|---|---|---|---|
| **Assessment** | | | | |
| ***Neurological/ Psychological:*** | Mental status • LOC/confusion • headache • vision • pupils (size, shape, reaction) • facial symmetry (smile/facial/eye ptosis) • ability to follow directions, speak (quality & tone of voice/hoarseness), & swallow • tongue movement • sensory loss • motor weakness (tingling, paralysis) • pain via pain scale (severity, quality, location, duration, radiation) • standard for recovery from anesthesia (local or general) • raise arms to horizontal position • risk for falls • explore anxiety/coping skills • begin assessment of health care problem & potential modifiable risk factors (smoking, diet, stress, exercise) • identify available & needed family/human/economic resources to resume independent self-care activities. | Mental status • LOC/confusion • headache • vision • pupils (size, shape, reaction) • facial symmetry (smile/facial/eye ptosis) • ability to follow directions, speak (quality & tone of voice/hoarseness), & swallow • tongue movement • sensory loss • motor weakness (tingling, paralysis) • pain via pain scale (severity, quality, location, duration, radiation) • raise arms to horizontal position • risk for falls • continue to explore anxiety/coping skills • continue assessment of health care problem & potential modifiable risk factors (smoking, diet, stress, exercise) • collaborate w/social services to identify available & needed family/human/economic resources to resume independent self-care activities. | Mental status • vision • pupils (size, shape, reaction) • facial symmetry (smile/facial/eye ptosis) • ability to follow directions, speak (quality & tone of voice/hoarseness), & swallow • tongue movement • raise arms to horizontal position • continue to explore anxiety/coping skills | Mental status • ability to follow directions |
| ***Pulmonary:*** | Breath sounds (atelectasis) • patent airway. | Breath sounds (atelectasis) • patent airway. | Breath sounds | Breath sounds |
| ***Cardiovascular:*** | VS per postop standard & then BP monitoring to continue q15min until stable • capillary refill • carotid bruits • peripheral pulses & temporal pulses • Homans' sign. | BP monitoring to continue q15min until stable • capillary refill • carotid bruits • peripheral pulses & temporal pulses • Homans' sign. | HR & BP • peripheral & temporal pulses • Homans' sign. | HR & BP • peripheral & temporal pulses • Homans' sign. |
| ***Gastrointestinal:*** | Ability to swallow • mucous membranes. | Ability to swallow • mucous membranes. | Tolerance of diet. | Tolerance of diet. |
| ***Genitourinary:*** | I & O • UO > 30 ml/h. | I & O • UO > 30 ml/h. | UO qs. | UO qs. |
| ***Integumentary:*** | Skin turgor, temp, color, & integrity • risk for decubiti. | Skin turgor, temp, color, & integrity • risk for decubiti. | Skin turgor & integrity. | Skin turgor & integrity. |

| | DAY 1 (OR) | DAY 2 | DAY 3 | DAY 4 |
|---|---|---|---|---|
| ***Surgery Wound:*** | Dsg/incision line • amt & type of drainage • S & S of bleeding/ hematoma/edema/redness/heat • assess area under neck & shoulders for blood • neck swelling. | Dsg/incision line • amt & type of drainage • S & S of bleeding/ hematoma/edema/redness/heat • assess area under neck & shoulders for blood • neck swelling. | Dsg/incision line • amt & type of drainage • S & S of bleeding/ hematoma/edema/redness/ heat. | Dsg/incision line • amt & type of drainage • S & S of bleeding/hematoma/edema/redness/heat. |
| **Focus** | Hemodynamic stability • maintain airway • pain control. | Hemodynamic stability • pain control. | Improved PO fluid & food intake • teaching • initiate definitive treatment plan for therapeutic regimen for self-care. | Discharge • teaching • self-care. |
| **Diagnostic Plan** | Postop electrolytes & HCT @ 6 PM. | Repeat abnormal lab tests. *Consider:* repeat HCT. | Repeat abnormal lab test(s). | None. |
| **Therapeutic Interventions** | IV fluids to maintain BP systolic range of 100-160 mm/Hg & UO >30 ml/h • call physician if BP <100 mm/Hg systolic for 5 min & institute vasopressor-medicated infusion per standard • call physician if BP >160 mm Hg for 5 min & institute NTG or sodium nitroprusside-medicated infusion per standard • antibiotic • analgesic • use Doppler prn for temporal pulse assessment • NPO then progress to clear liquids (8 h postop) if swallowing intact • cough, deep breathe, & incentive spirometer q2-4h while awake • bedrest • assist w/turning q2h to maintain skin integrity unless BP labile • lotion to both heels & reapply heel protectors tid while in bed • encourage ankle dorsiflexion exercises q1-2h while awake • assist w/hygiene • elastic support stockings. | Continue IV therapy to maintain systolic BP within 100-160 range • continue w/ meds & treatments • progress diet to regular • encourage PO fluids & document plan for same • stool softener • OOB to chair tid unless BP labile. | Discontinue IV fluids • heplock line • independent w/ hygiene • progressive activity as tolerated • encourage participation in hygiene & wound care • OOB ad lib • walk in hall × 4. | Independent ADL • discharge. |

From Birdsall C, Sperry S: *Clinical paths in medical-surgical practice,* St Louis, 1997, Mosby.

Continued

## Carotid Artery Endarterectomy—cont'd

| | DAY 1 (OR) | DAY 2 | DAY 3 | DAY 4 |
|---|---|---|---|---|
| **Patient/Family Teaching/ Discharge Planning—cont'd** | Teach use of pain scale & review meds available for pain & anxiety • reassure that responses (anxiety, etc.) are a normal reaction • initiate discharge plan • teach to cough, deep breathe, & use incentive spirometer & ankle dorsiflexion & extension exercises • discuss plan for daily review of plan of care w/patient/ family. | Teach adequate hydration to ensure UO >50 ml/h & to apply support stockings • identify learning needs & discuss potential lifestyle changes prn (smoking, diet, stress, weight, exercise) & document same • teach nutritional needs, carotid disease, & treatment plan. | Teach self-care strategies (no heavy lifting, no vigorous exercise, no prolonged sitting, no driving for 2 wk or as surgeon indicates) • teach S & S to report to physician (fever, drainage, redness, swelling, tenderness of back or calves) • review discharge plan & home care needs • clarify & confirm information given to date • allow time for verbalization of feelings • review meds & med/food interactions • review knowledge of health care problem & potential modifiable risk factors (smoking, diet, stress, exercise). | Review discharge plan, self-care strategies, S & S to report to physician, & to see physician in 3 wk • review appropriate health-seeking behaviors & need to modify lifestyle prn. |
| **Expected Outcomes** | Hemodynamically stable & UO >30 ml/h • assists w/ turning • verbalizes relief of pain w/ analgesia • acknowledges availability of analgesic/anxiolytic, plan of care, & need to communicate w/ nurse if S & S of anxiety & fear become overwhelming (subjective feelings, emotional lability, or inability to concentrate) • demonstrates coughing, deep breathing, & use of incentive spirometer. | Demonstrates how to cough, deep breathe, & use incentive spirometer effectively • demonstrates ankle dorsiflexion & extension exercises • BP stable within range w/ fluid support • verbalizes relief of pain w/ PO analgesia as evidenced by pain scale <3 (0-10) • acknowledges availability of analgesics/anxiolytics prn but denies anxiety • verbalizes appropriate anxiety & fears related to surgery • home care referral complete. | Voids independently & in qs • verbalizes meds & food/drug interactions • states will notify surgeon for S & S of infection/phlebitis • normal BM • uses fewer doses of prn meds as evidenced by pain scale <2 (0-10) • parenteral therapy discontinued • independent in ADL • acknowledges potential lifestyle changes & appropriate concerns & fears • social services screening documented • demonstrates applying support stockings. | Verbalizes self-care strategies & S & S to report to physician • states appointment date w/ physician • pain well controlled as evidenced by pain scale <2 (0-10) • social services referral to home care or outpatient follow-up documented • ambulates without assistance & independent in ADL • normal BM • verbalizes risk factors & health-seeking behaviors. |
| **Trigger(s)** | Hemodynamic instability • respiratory distress • neuro deficit (new). | Hemodynamic instability • neuro deficit • unable to get OOB. | Unable to tolerate fluids/food/ activity. | Unable to be independent in self-care. |

and strength will be closely monitored. The process of swallowing is complex and requires the coordination of several structures and muscle groups. If the patient is unable to ingest an oral diet, tube feedings may be initiated to prevent excessive catabolism and resultant malnutrition. A nasogastric route is initially used, and either continuous or intermittent feedings may be used. The standard concerns related to formula hyperosmolality and problems with dehydration and diarrhea will exist (see Chapter 41). A percutaneous gastrostomy may be needed for long-term management. Nutritional concerns are discussed further in the nursing management section.

#### Activity

Patients who have experienced an intracerebral hemorrhage require bedrest until the risk of rebleeding is minimized and intracranial pressure stabilizes. Patients who have experienced an ischemic stroke are mobilized into active rehabilitation as soon as the stroke has stabilized, usually within 48 hours.[24] A multidisciplinary team of physical and occupational therapy specialists and nurses will then collaboratively plan the patient's self-care rehabilitation. Preventing immobility-associated problems is a major focus of intervention.

#### Referrals

Stroke rehabilitation is truly a multidisciplinary collaborative effort. A nursing case management approach can be extremely effective in ensuring that discharge planning is initiated in a timely fashion and that appropriate arrangements are made for assistance through home health care, short-term residential rehabilitation, or long-term care through a nursing facility. This process will involve the direction of the physician, the coordination of the nurse case manager, and the active involvement of professionals from physical, occupational, and speech therapy and social and dietary services.

## NURSING MANAGEMENT

### ASSESSMENT

#### Subjective Data

Subjective data to be collected include:

- Health history, including hypertension and its management, history of coronary artery disease (CAD), diabetes, and history of TIA (symptoms, frequency, workup, and treatment, if any)
- Medications in use, both prescription and over-the-counter drugs
- Smoking history
- Circumstances surrounding the stroke
- Onset, nature, and severity of symptoms
- Presence of headache—nature and location
- Visual ability—acuity, diplopia, blurred vision
- Ability to concentrate and follow commands, memory
- Emotional/affective response
- Level of consciousness, response to tactile stimuli
- Family and social support network, financial and insurance status

#### Objective Data

Objective data to be collected include:

- Motor strength—presence and severity of paresis or paralysis
- Coordination—gait, balance
- Ability to communicate (speak and understand speech)
- Cranial nerve assessment, including gag and swallow reflex, facial movement, tongue movement, and eye blink
- Bowel and bladder control or incontinence

### NURSING DIAGNOSES

Nursing diagnoses are determined from analysis of patient data. Nursing diagnoses for the patient with a stroke may include but are not limited to:

| Diagnostic Title | Possible Etiological Factors |
|---|---|
| Altered cerebral tissue perfusion | Interruption of arterial blood flow |
| Risk for disuse syndrome | Hemiparesis or hemiplegia |
| Self-care deficit: feeding, bathing hygiene, toileting | Neuromuscular and sensory-perceptual impairments |
| Impaired swallowing | Oral and neck muscle weakness |
| Impaired verbal communication | Residual aphasia |
| Sensory-perceptual alterations (visual, tactile) | Altered sensory reception, transmission, and integration |
| Urinary incontinence | Altered neurological stimulation |
| Impaired adjustment | Residual disability necessitating changes in lifestyle and independence |

### EXPECTED PATIENT OUTCOMES

Expected patient outcomes for the patient with a stroke may include but are not limited to:

1. Maintains cerebral perfusion as indicated by the absence of signs of increased intracranial pressure and stable vital signs
2a. Transfers independently from bed to chair/wheelchair
b. Remains free of the complications of disuse as evidenced by full range of motion and intact skin
3. Uses adapted equipment and strategies to regain independence in ADL
4a. Is able to tolerate food and fluid without choking or aspiration
b. Ingests sufficient nutrients to maintain a stable weight and meet the body's baseline nutritional needs
5. Uses alternative methods of communication effectively to communicate needs
6. Compensates for visual and spatial perception impairments and remains free of injury
7. Regains urinary continence
8. Participates in appropriate socialization and in making plans for future care

## INTERVENTIONS

### Monitoring Cerebral Perfusion

Immediately after the patient's admission the focus of nursing care is on monitoring the patient's neurological status and preventing complications while simultaneously assessing the severity of the stroke. Maintaining a patent airway is essential to support oxygenation and cerebral perfusion. The patient is placed on bedrest with the head of the bed elevated about 30 degrees and positioned to prevent the tongue from falling back and partially obstructing the airway. Supplemental oxygen may be administered. Vital signs and neurological checks are performed regularly to rule out the presence of increasing intracranial pressure. The environment is kept as quiet and restful as possible, and all activities that are known to increase intracranial pressure, such as coughing, straining, lying prone, isometric muscle contraction, emotional upset, and abrupt head or neck flexion, are avoided or minimized. See Chapter 52 for a more thorough discussion of the management of changes in intracranial pressure and Chapter 51 for a thorough review of neurological assessment.

### Preventing the Complications of Immobility and Disuse

#### Positioning

The mobility impairments associated with stroke place patients, especially elderly patients, at high risk for a variety of complications related to disuse. The rehabilitation plan incorporates active physical therapy, but the nurse needs to incorporate a variety of interventions into the patient's daily care routines. Appropriate positioning is a key concern. Positioning is fundamental to preventing complications such as contractures and skin breakdown. The challenge of positioning is increased by the presence of sensory impairments, flaccidity or spasticity of muscle groups, and the need to minimize the time the patient spends lying on the paralyzed side. The patient is assisted to change positions every 2 hours and encouraged to move independently in bed as soon as possible. The affected arm is positioned with the hand elevated above the wrist and the wrist above the elbow to support venous return and minimize edema.[22]

Special care must be taken to avoid excess pressure or pull on the shoulder joint, which is extremely vulnerable to joint subluxation and adduction contractures. The shoulder is positioned in a neutral position with support as needed from positioning devices. Pillows, rolled towels, and sandbags are used as needed to support normal body alignment with particular attention to preventing external rotation of the hip. The heels should be elevated off the mattress to avoid pressure injury, and foot positioning aids such as boots and high-top sneakers may be used to decrease the incidence of footdrop. The use of a footboard to support positioning is no longer recommended because it is believed to stimulate plantar flexion. The same principle applies to the affected hand. Resting splints are often necessary to prevent contractures in the hand when spasticity is present, but rolled washcloths are avoided because they stimulate the grasp reflex. Firm hand splints are preferred. The supine position is also avoided for any patient who has a diminished or absent gag reflex to minimize the risk of aspiration. A side-lying position with the head of the bed elevated 10 to 20 degrees is preferred. Accomplishing these basic care goals is both labor intensive and time consuming for the nursing staff, and they must be recognized as high-priority interventions.

Skin care is another essential aspect of positioning. Pressure devices such as 4-inch foam mattresses and elbow and heel protectors are standard, and the nurse assesses the patient for signs of pressure, shearing, or friction damage during each repositioning. Once the patient is out of bed attention shifts to pressure reduction in chairs and preventing injury related to dragging and pulling on the affected extremities. Arm and shoulder supports when the patient is out of bed are important.

#### Exercise

The return of motor impulses is significant for the future use of the affected part, but it also presents new challenges. Most stroke patients are initially flaccid on the affected side (stage 1) but within a few days begin to exhibit signs of muscle spasticity (stage 2). If flaccidity persists the chances of return of functioning decrease substantially.[10] Muscles that draw the limbs toward the midline become very active because the adductor and flexor muscles are stronger than opposing muscles. The arm may be held tightly adducted against the body and the affected lower limb may be held inward and adducted to, or even beyond, the midline. Without regular preventive exercise the heel cord shortens, the heel may be lifted off the ground, and the knee becomes bent.[12] In the upper extremity the elbow flexes into a bent position, the wrist is flexed, and the fingers curl into palmar flexion. Contractures will develop rapidly if preventive measures are not instituted promptly and consistently. The use of resting splints may become necessary (Figure 53-6).

The third stage of recovery is termed *synergy* and develops after several weeks. In synergy the flexion of a single muscle group results in simultaneous flexion of a broader group of muscles such as the elbow, wrist, hand, and fingers. Over time synergy can resolve into a nearly normal pattern of movement, although residual muscle weakness is almost always present. The patterns of recovery are unpredictable, however, and not uniform. The arm and hand recover sooner than the leg but rarely to the same extent. Recovery may also stop at any stage and progress no further.

Physical therapy is usually consulted to develop the overall exercise plan.[36] Range-of-motion exercise for all joints is the foundation of the plan. The exercise is initially passive but will progress as soon as possible to active exercise of the unaffected side and assisted exercise of the affected side. Balance training is another important step. Patients may expe-

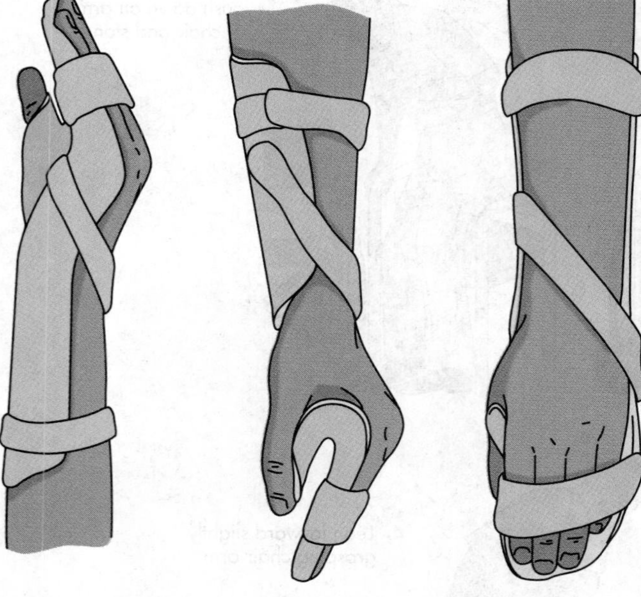

**fig. 53-6** Volar resting splint provides support to wrist, thumb, and fingers of patient following CVA, maintaining them in position of extension.

rience problems with proprioception, dizziness, and sensory-perceptual deficits that will make it difficult to control movement even when they have adequate muscle strength and coordination. Voluntary muscles lose tone rapidly with bedrest, which makes fatigue an additional challenge during early rehabilitation. Patients need frequent reminders and assistance to sit straight and focus on maintaining a balanced posture.

Learning to make safe transfers to a chair or wheelchair is the next step. The chair is placed next to the patient's unaffected side. The patient stands and faces the chair and then turns and sits down after the unaffected arm has been placed on the distant chair arm. The nurse is positioned on the patient's affected side during transfers and can use a safety or transfer belt around the patient's waist to provide needed support and stability without ever needing to grasp or pull on the affected arm. If the patient's knees should buckle, the nurse can quickly move in front of the patient and block the unaffected knee so that it locks in position. The chair should provide firm support and have a high back and arms. A lapboard, pillow, or other device can provide additional support to the affected arm and shoulder. As strength and balance improve the hemiplegic patient can be taught to transfer independently (Figure 53-7).

The same basic principles guide the gradual move to ambulation. Early ambulation promotes vasomotor tone and has strong positive psychological effects on both the patient and the family. Correct walking patterns must be established early because incorrect patterns are difficult and sometimes impossible to change. A sideward shuffle should be prevented. A walker, crutch, or four-point cane may be helpful, and the affected arm can be placed in a sling for support during ambulation. Ambulation retraining begins between the parallel bars in physical therapy, but on-unit practice time will provide essential reinforcement. The use of a safety belt can enable the nurse or therapist to provide additional support and stability.

**box 53-7** *Application of Bobath Rehabilitation Principles*

1. The use of both sides of the body is emphasized during activities of daily living and other activities.
2. Weight bearing on the affected side is encouraged during sitting and standing.
3. Movement toward the affected side is encouraged.
4. Positioning is accomplished in opposition to the patterns of spasticity.
5. The patient is consistently encouraged to straighten the trunk and neck to normalize body tone and posture.

In some rehabilitation settings the Bobath neurodevelopmental technique has been found to be useful in stroke rehabilitation. This approach seeks to normalize muscle tone, posture, and movement and promote bilateral functioning.[22] Therapy seeks to redirect short-term memory toward an appreciation of normal movement of the paralyzed side. When a Bobath approach is used transfers are made to the affected *and* unaffected sides to promote bilateral functioning. Other principles of Bobath rehabilitation are presented in Box 53-7.

### Promoting Independence in Self-Care

Efforts to regain independence in self-care activities require the collaboration of the physical and occupational therapist, nurse, patient, and family (see the Research Box, p. 1753). A plan is designed for the patient by the physical and occupational therapists and then is implemented by the nursing staff and family. The plan is developed after thorough assessment of the patient's motor skills and deficits, as well as the cognitive and sensory-perceptual problems that will support or complicate rehabilitation. Rehabilitation seeks to help patients relearn lost skills and compensate for temporary or permanent losses.

Each new skill is demonstrated, and then the patient practices with ongoing support and encouragement from the nursing staff and family. Families need to be incorporated into all teaching so they understand how to support independence rather than dependence. Providing extra time for activities is essential. Most motivated patients with moderate impairments can relearn the skills needed to complete basic ADL.

Assistive devices play a major role in regaining self-care independence because accomplishing basic tasks with only one hand is both challenging and frustrating. A wide variety of

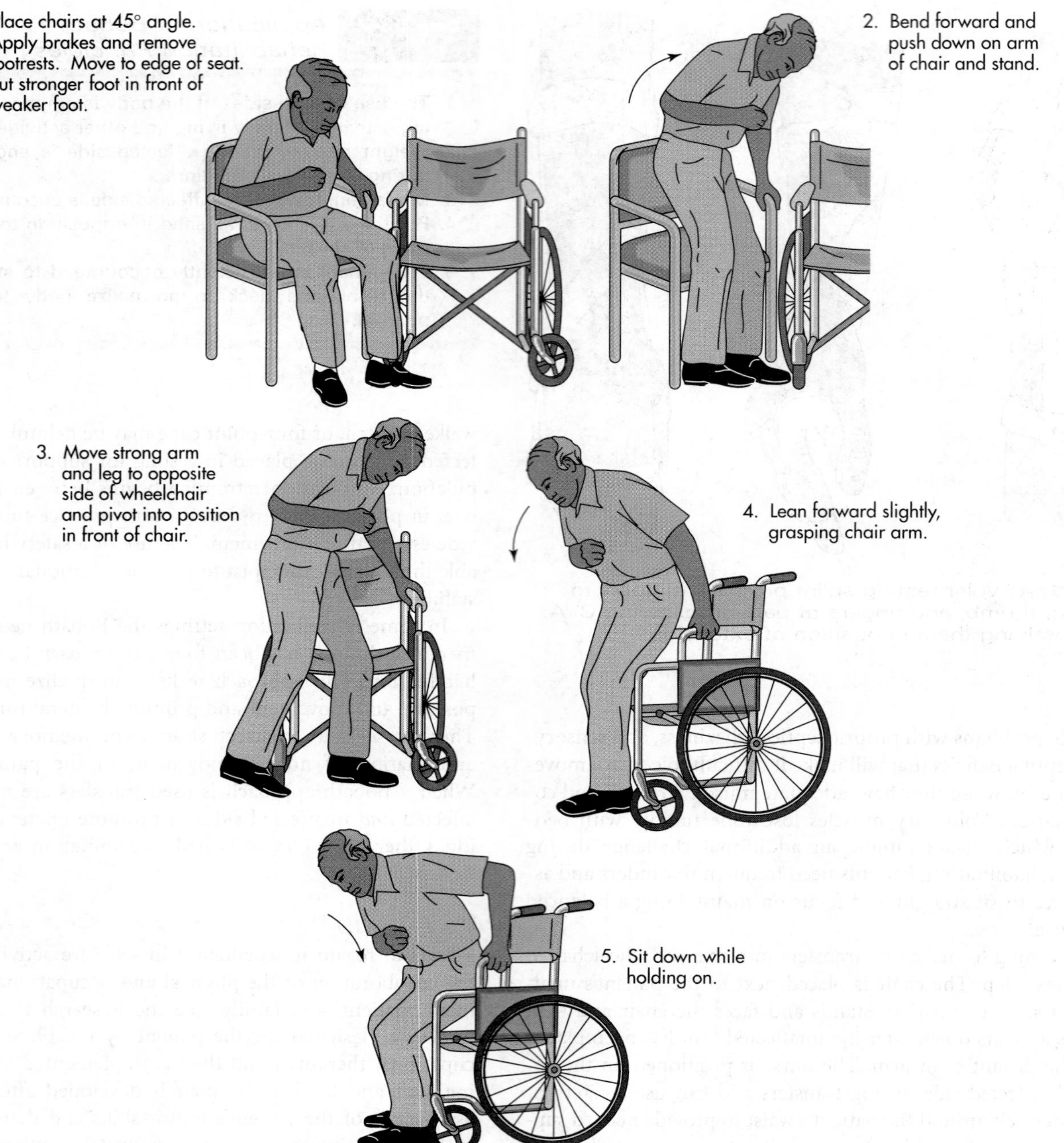

1. Place chairs at 45° angle. Apply brakes and remove footrests. Move to edge of seat. Put stronger foot in front of weaker foot.
2. Bend forward and push down on arm of chair and stand.
3. Move strong arm and leg to opposite side of wheelchair and pivot into position in front of chair.
4. Lean forward slightly, grasping chair arm.
5. Sit down while holding on.


**fig. 53-7** Doing a standing transfer from a chair to a wheelchair.

devices exist to assist patients with eating and dressing, and the nurse can help the patient and family think of simple modifications that can promote independence, such as slip-on shoes, Velcro closures, loose pullover shirts, and elastic-waisted pants (Figure 53-8).[36] Patients are encouraged to dress in simple workout-type clothes rather than pajamas and gowns as soon as active rehabilitation is started (Figure 53-9).

## Promoting Safe Swallowing and Adequate Nutrition

The protective swallowing and gag reflexes usually return within a few days after the stroke, but the patient may have ongoing problems managing the complex act of swallowing. A number of cranial nerves are involved in this process. The presence of facial drooping or asymmetry, drooling, and a weak voice are strong indicators of swallowing difficulties. The gag and swallow reflexes are carefully assessed, and an occupational or speech therapist may be consulted to establish a management plan.[18] The act of swallowing can be grossly assessed by placing the thumb and index finger on either side of the patient's Adam's apple and feeling for a symmetrical elevation of the larynx when the patient attempts to swallow. Even if swallowing is intact, the patient may still be at risk for aspiration because of easy distractability. A quiet environment for eating where the patient can concentrate on effective swallowing is preferred. Oral reminders to "think swal-

## research

Reference: Hinkle JL, Forbes E: Pilot project on functional outcome in stroke, *J Neurosci Nurs* 28(1):13, 1996.

This pilot study compared the outcomes of stroke patients who were cared for on an acute stroke unit with the outcomes of patients who received care on a routine medical surgical unit. Eighty-eight patients were included, with 68 on the acute unit and 20 on the general unit. Functional outcomes included such variables as walking, personal hygiene, and dressing. Patient abilities were rated with a variety of activities of daily living scales developed for the rehabilitation field.

The study found that the patients who were admitted to the general care units were younger and less functionally impaired at admission than patients on the stroke unit, yet they made less progress during their hospitalization in terms of functional gains. The study was small in size and the patients were not randomly assigned to the study groups, but the results were interpreted to indicate that functional gains for patients cared for in specialty acute care stroke units were greater than those achieved by patients in general care environments.

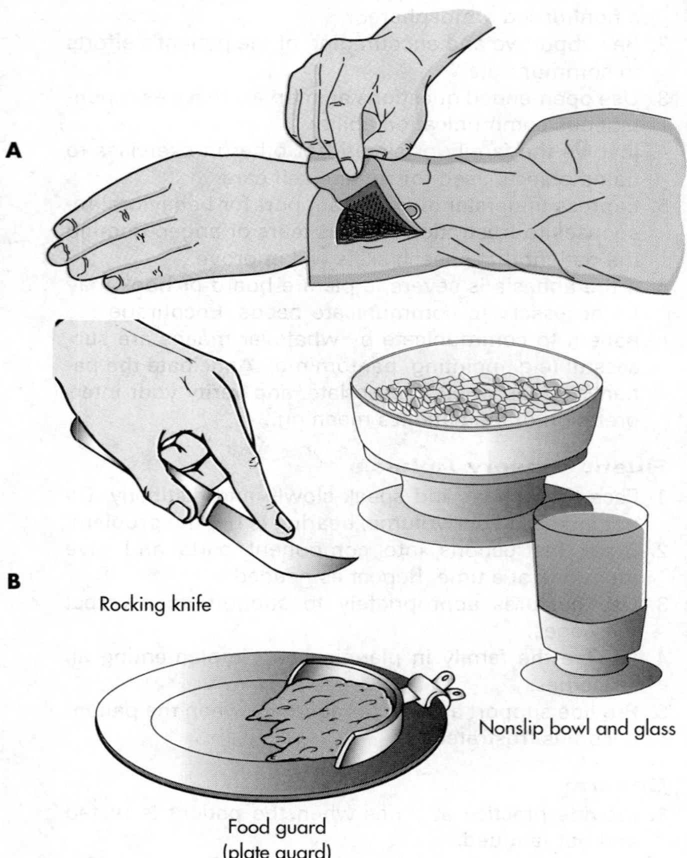


**fig. 53-8** Assistive devices for self-care. **A,** Velcro closure on shirtsleeve. **B,** Assistive devices for eating.

## guidelines for care

### The Patient with Impaired Swallowing

1. Place the patient upright in bed or preferably sitting in a chair for meals.
2. Offer mouth care before meals to stimulate saliva flow. Strong-tasting or salty liquids also stimulate saliva flow.
3. Position the patient's head and neck slightly forward with the chin tucked in to prevent premature movement of food to the back of the mouth before it is adequately chewed.
4. Experiment with food texture. Most patients tolerate a mechanically soft diet better than liquids. Avoid thin liquids. Consider adding a thickener to liquids if they are poorly tolerated.
5. Encourage the patient to take small bites and chew food thoroughly.
6. If hemiplegia is present, food should be placed in the unaffected side of the mouth. If "pocketing" of food occurs on the affected side, instruct the patient to sweep the affected side with a finger after each bite. Teach the patient to clean the affected side of the mouth with gauze wipes and perform mouth care after meals. Retained food causes mouth odors, infection, and tooth or gum disease.
7. Position foods within the patient's visual field if hemianopia is present (see Figure 53-10, p. 1756).
8. Keep an accurate intake and output record until the patient is drinking sufficient liquids daily. IV supplementation may initially be needed.
9. Monitor the patient's weight weekly. Add supplements to diet or liquids to increase calorie and nutrient intake.

low" and encouragement are also helpful.[18] The nurse should never give anything by mouth to a patient whose swallowing has not been thoroughly evaluated because the patient can aspirate without the usual accompanying coughing or choking if protective reflexes are not intact.[3] Specific strategies for approaching the problems of swallowing and nutrition in patients following stroke are presented in the Guidelines for Care Box above.

### Supporting Communication

Communication problems following stroke may include both aphasia and dysarthria. Each person reacts to language problems differently, but anger and frustration are common. Some patients become easily discouraged when they encounter problems and may quickly refuse to speak. This can progress to complete withdrawal from social interactions, even with family and close friends. Family members may be at a loss as to how to respond to the patient's problems and may even encourage the patient to avoid frustration by not trying to communicate. Embarrassment at the person's attempts at speech is common.

A speech therapist is an integral part of the patient's rehabilitation plan, but the nurse can do much to reinforce that learning and help the family be an active part of the rehabilitation team. The patient needs frequent and meaningful

**Putting on a Pullover Garment**

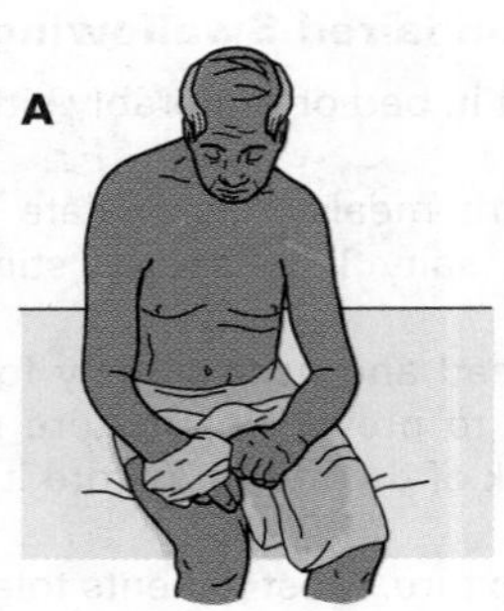
A

Put strong hand through outside of armhole for weak hand and gather up garment with strong hand. Then pull weak hand and arm through the inside of garment and out the armhole.

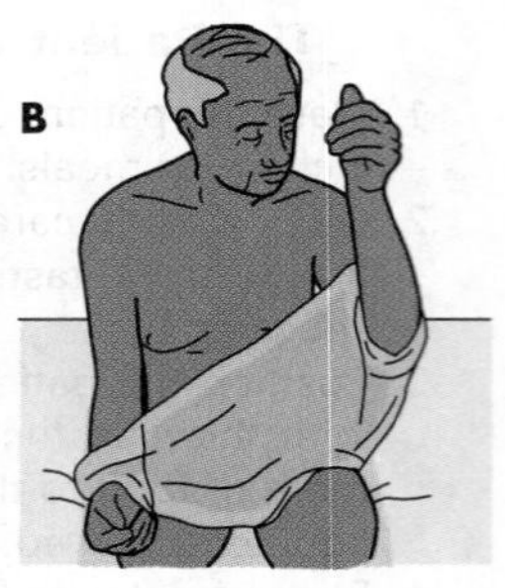
B

Put strong arm through the other armhole.

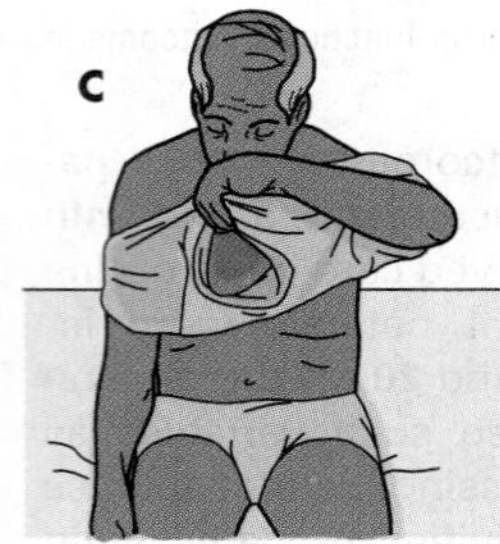
C

Put the neck of the garment over your head.

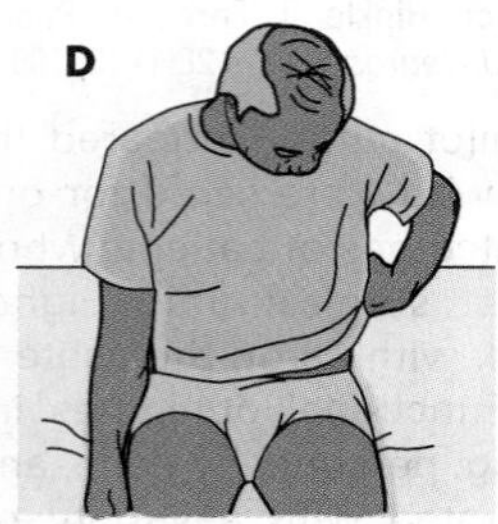
D

Pull down and adjust.

**fig. 53-9** Putting on a pullover garment.

communication and ample time to practice in a nonstressful environment. Sitting down and spending time with the patient conveys interest and willingness to make communication a priority. Practice sessions should focus on concrete topics related to self-care needs, and the family can be consulted about specific areas of interest to the patient.[21] Patients with fluent forms of aphasia may have baffling abilities to sing, recite poetry or bible verses, or swear creatively. These actions can be extremely troubling to family members, who need to understand the organic basis of the behavior. Specific strategies for assisting patients with aphasia are summarized in the Guidelines for Care Box at right.

## Compensating for Sensory-Perceptual Deficits

A wide variety of sensory-perceptual deficits may be present following stroke, particularly strokes involving the right hemisphere. These deficits make it more difficult for patients to react appropriately to their environment. Deficits that involve proprioception, depth, and distance perception can present serious risks of injury as the patient becomes more active. These deficits are of particular concern when a patient also experiences denial of the stroke limitations and approaches activities with impulsive self-confidence. Until the exact nature and severity of the deficits are determined the nursing staff provides increased supervision during all activities to ensure patient safety. The room should be kept as free of clutter as possible, but familiar personal objects from home can often help the patient stay oriented to the environment. Frequent verbal cueing can also help patients stay focused on the task at hand.[29] Providing consistent caretakers improves ongoing assessment and evaluation and supports implementation of a consistent plan of care to address the patient's unique deficits. Accurate documentation can be extremely valuable in evaluating outcomes and planning for future services. Specific interventions designed to address the major sensory-perceptual deficits are presented in the Guidelines for Care Box on p. 1755.

## guidelines for care

### The Patient with Aphasia

**Nonfluent Expressive Aphasia**

1. Allow the patient adequate time to respond. Establish a nonhurried atmosphere.
2. Be supportive and encouraging of the patient's efforts to communicate.
3. Use open-ended questions at intervals to assess spontaneous communication ability.
4. Involve the family or significant other in exercises to name objects used for routine self-care.
5. Express understanding and support for behavioral responses to frustration such as tears or anger. Remind the patient that speech skills will improve.
6. If the aphasia is severe, a picture board or book may be necessary to communicate needs. Encourage the patient to communicate by whatever means are successful (e.g., pointing, pantomime). Anticipate the patient's needs when appropriate, and verify your interpretation of the patient's meaning.

**Fluent Sensory Aphasia**

1. Face the patient and speak slowly and distinctly. Do not increase your volume; hearing is not the problem.
2. Break instructions into component parts and give them one at a time. Repeat as needed.
3. Use gestures appropriately to support your verbal messages.
4. Involve the family in planning and implementing all strategies.
5. Provide support and encouragement when the patient becomes frustrated.

**General**

1. Provide practice at times when the patient is rested and not fatigued.
2. Offer liberal praise and reinforcement for efforts. Remind patient and family that small gains can still be made months into the rehabilitation process.

## guidelines for care

### The Patient with Sensory-Perceptual Deficits

#### Hemianopia (Loss of Vision in a Portion of the Visual Field)

1. Approach the patient from the side of intact vision.
2. Position the patient in the room so that her or his intact visual field faces the door if possible.
3. Teach the patient to move the head from side to side (scan) to compensate for diminished visual fields. Scanning is also important with meals (see Figure 53-10).
4. Place objects needed for self-care within the patient's intact visual fields.

#### Denial/Neglect and Body Image Distortions

1. Encourage the patient to look at and touch the affected side. Verbally remind the patient to check the position and safety of the affected side during activity.
2. Lightly touch and stimulate the affected side during care.
3. Provide gentle but consistent reminders to include the affected side in care (e.g., bathing, dressing).
4. Monitor the affected side for injuries when the patient is out of bed. A sling may be used to protect the affected side during ambulation.
5. Use a full-length mirror to assist the patient to reintegrate an intact body image and to assist with posture and balance.
6. Assist the family to understand the nature of the patient's behavior.

#### Agnosia/Apraxia

1. Encourage the patient to use all senses to compensate for problems in object recognition.
2. Practice the recognition and naming of commonly used objects, and encourage the family to participate in the relearning process.
3. Encourage the patient to participate in self-care.
4. Correct the misuse of any object or task, guiding the patient's hand if necessary.
5. Continue to verbally cue the patient about the correct use of any objects or self-care tasks.
6. Be aware that memory deficits may make frequent reteaching necessary.
7. Explain the nature of all deficits to the family.

### Restoring Continence

Problems with urinary continence are common after stroke, but the chances for restoring continence are good because half of the innervation and control pathways to the bladder remain intact. The primary problem is poor bladder control. Efforts should be made to support normal bladder elimination and minimize the use of a Foley catheter if possible, even though this usually increases the amount of nursing care the patient requires.[6] Long-term catheterization commonly results in urinary tract infection and makes regaining voluntary control more difficult. An adequate daily fluid intake is essential, although it may be necessary to restrict evening fluids to avoid nighttime incontinence. The patient is assisted to a commode every 2 hours and encouraged to empty the bladder. Efforts are made to keep the patient as dry as possible, and the skin is monitored frequently for signs of redness or irritation. The patient is verbally encouraged to maintain continence, and the family is enlisted in the total effort. Every effort is made to communicate to the patient the expectation that continence can and will be regained. The importance of continence cannot be overestimated because achieving continence is often the single most important variable in a family's decision about whether or not an elderly stroke patient can be successfully cared for at home.

Constipation is the most common bowel problem after stroke. Regaining bowel continence is a reasonable expectation for most patients if a pattern of constipation, impaction, and diarrhea is not permitted to develop. The nurse needs to carefully monitor the patient's bowel elimination pattern and ensure that the patient receives adequate daily fluid. A bowel program of stool softeners, fiber laxatives, and suppositories should be implemented at admission and modified as needed to support bowel regularity.[6] Following the patient's normal daily pattern for elimination can also be helpful.

### Promoting Effective Coping

The effects of stroke are usually life altering and can be devastating to the patient and family. Depression and despair are normal responses to stroke. In addition the patient may experience significant difficulty in responding appropriately to any situation. The patient may be extremely emotional and cry easily. Behavior may be significantly different from the patient's prestroke baseline, and the patient may exhibit significant emotional lability. The patient's tolerance to stress is usually diminished.

These emotional changes are distressing and commonly embarrassing to the spouse and family. Families need to be helped to understand that these behaviors are outcomes of the stroke and are not volitional acts by the patient. Distraction and shifting the patient's attention can be successful strategies for assisting the patient to regain control. The nurse teaches the family not to become sidetracked attempting to explain or interpret the behavior and to avoid feeling responsible for causing it. Emotional responses typically become more stable with time.

### Patient/Family Education

The greatest challenges for the patient and family occur after the patient has survived the initial acute stroke period. Married couples often express the view that the stroke has happened to both of them because the threat to their established way of life is so profound. The patient and family need to be included in all explanations of interventions and procedures as well as provided with realistic appraisals of the patient's future status and deficits. Most people have a basic understanding of stroke and its classic manifestations, but this knowledge is rarely sufficient to understand the unique situation at hand. The nurse uses every opportunity for teaching and encourages the family to be involved in the patient's actual care within the scope of their comfort level.

The acute care phase of stroke management is brief, and the family will need assistance to make decisions about the

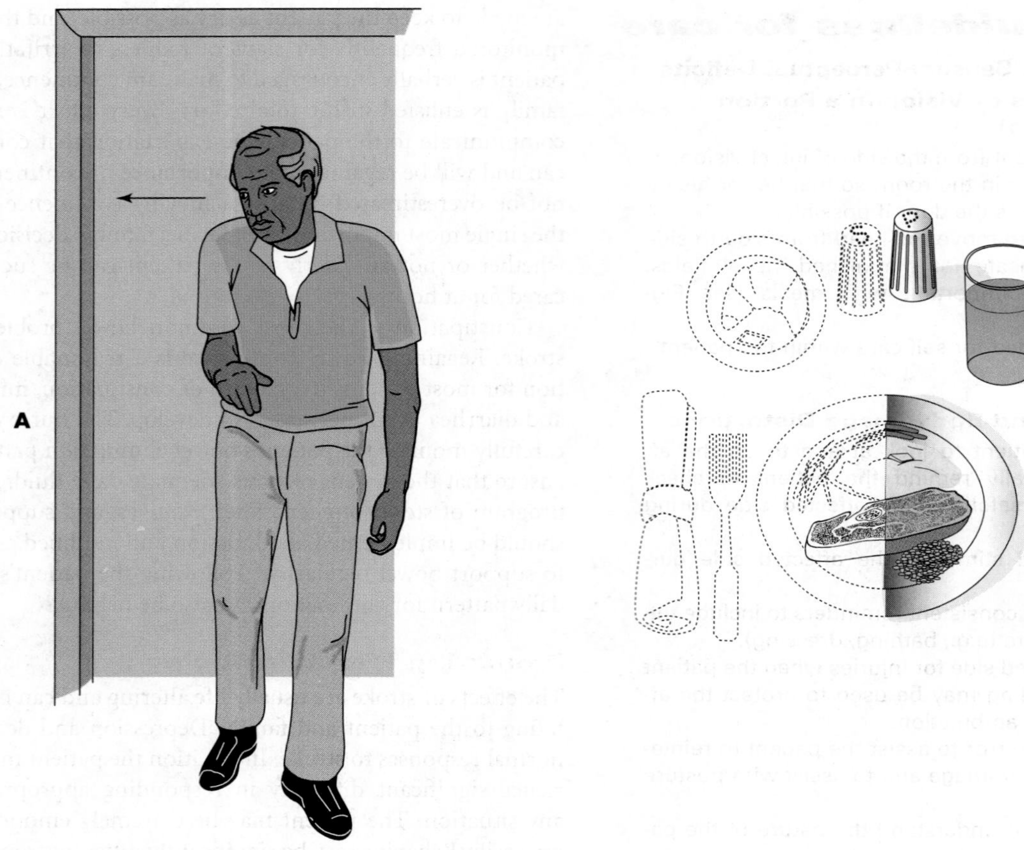


**fig. 53-10** Spatial and perceptual deficits in stroke. **A,** Patient is instructed to look toward the affected side when walking to avoid bumping into things. **B,** With homonymous hemianopsia, the patient is unable to see the left side of the tray and may ignore the items on that side.

next phases of care for the patient. A social service referral is usually helpful.[36] A lifetime of family dynamics and history complicate the efforts to make reasonable and rational decisions about bringing a patient home or seeking long-term nursing home placement. The financial consequences of either decision can be devastating. Ongoing and sometimes severe deficits are common after stroke, and most patients require some degree of supervision and assistance. This support may be needed on a temporary or permanent basis. Stroke support groups and resources such as the American Heart Association and National Stroke Association can be useful sources of information and referral services.

Recent years have seen an increased emphasis on aggressive stroke rehabilitation, but this also can increase the pressure on the family to attempt to manage the patient's care at home. Decision making about care is difficult, and the nurse attempts to support all parties, facilitate communication, and ensure that the family has all of the information they need. Involvement in the patient's daily care may assist the family to have a more realistic picture of the patient's needs for assistance and their ability to provide such support at home. Chapter 7 provides additional information about the challenges of rehabilitation. The nurse may need to remind the family that regular respite for caregivers is an essential component of the overall plan.

### Health promotion/prevention

Increased attention to high blood pressure diagnosis and control has been successful in reducing the mortality and morbidity of stroke. These outreach efforts need to continue to expand, especially for the African American population. Reducing cardiac risk factors, normalizing body weight, smoking cessation, and diabetes management can all positively affect stroke statistics. High-risk patients will usually be placed on antiplatelet agents, as will most patients who experience TIA. Compliance with these medication regimens can reduce stroke incidence. All patients who experience TIA are encouraged to undergo a workup to establish whether their symptoms are attributable to carotid stenosis that could possibly be surgically reversed. Finally, the population is being encouraged to consider stroke as a form of "brain attack," viewed as a corollary of heart attack, in which early intervention can be critical in limiting the extent of ischemic damage. This may not prevent the stroke itself, but it can limit the scope of its devastation.

## EVALUATION

To evaluate the effectiveness of nursing interventions, compare patient behaviors with those stated in the expected patient outcomes. Successful achievement of patient outcomes for the patient with a stroke is indicated by:

1. Maintains stable vital signs and has no signs of increased intracranial pressure
2. Is able to move and transfer using adaptive equipment as needed; maintains an intact skin; no evidence of joint contracture
3. Performs ADL independently with the use of adaptive equipment
4. Consumes a balanced oral diet without choking or aspiration and maintains a stable body weight
5. Communicates needs effectively
6. Uses techniques to compensate for perceptual deficits and remains free of injury
7. Maintains bladder and bowel continence
8. Participates with family in social interaction and planning for future care needs

## GERONTOLOGICAL CONSIDERATIONS

The majority of all strokes affect the older population, and it is anticipated that the ongoing aging of the population will cause the incidence statistics to continue to increase. It is difficult to overestimate the impact of even a mild stroke on an elder's ability to maintain an independent lifestyle. The burdens for the spouse and family can be sudden and completely overwhelming. Even a mild stroke may require the complete restructuring of daily living patterns. In more severe strokes long-term institutionalization is commonly necessary. Even when the physical consequences are limited, the cognitive, emotional, and behavioral effects of stroke may still change the patient in small but significant ways.

The nature and scope of stroke rehabilitation are usually prescribed within the managed care framework. The nurse will play a crucial role in assisting patients to gain access to needed services and move appropriately through the established care pathway. Stroke care for elders necessitates multidisciplinary collaborative management and will continue to challenge the health care team to develop strategies to address the multiple areas of concern.

## SPECIAL ENVIRONMENTS FOR CARE

### Critical Care Management

Ischemic stroke management rarely necessitates admission to a critical care unit, although some institutions have specialized stroke units to increase the quality and accuracy of patient monitoring. Hemorrhagic strokes, however, commonly create life-threatening situations that require management in critical care environments. This is particularly true for patients whose cerebral bleeding is the result of aneurysm rupture. These patients require aggressive management of increasing intracranial pressure to minimize extension of the damage. Older patients who have experienced nonaneurysmal intracerebral bleeding will usually be transferred to general care as soon as CT scans confirm that the bleeding has stopped.

### Home Care Management

The challenges of reintegrating the stroke patient back into community and home care are substantial and have been previously discussed under each nursing diagnosis. The financial costs and resource challenges for the patient and family, community services, and insurers can be enormous. Few diagnoses are as initially overwhelming as stroke or create as many challenges for ongoing care and support. The nurse will usually serve as the patient's care coordinator, initiating discharge planning, assisting the family to plan and implement necessary structural modifications in the home, and making referrals for the delivery of needed care in the home.

## COMPLICATIONS

The list of possible complications of stroke is almost endless. The stroke may result in death or profound neurological injury. With less severe strokes, the initial acute period may be complicated by respiratory problems related to aspiration and atelectasis. Other disuse-related complications include skin breakdown, deep vein thrombosis, muscle atrophy, and joint contracture. Urinary tract infection may result from the use of Foley catheters, and both constipation and impaction may result from immobility. Patients are at high risk for environmental injury from a variety of physical and cognitive impairments, and the consequences of communication impairments can isolate the patient from full and active participation in the world. Furthermore, for each complication the patient experiences, there is the very real possibility that additional problems will develop for the family and support network. Prevention of these multiple complications is addressed in the collaborative care and nursing management sections.

## CEREBRAL ANEURYSM AND ARTERIOVENOUS MALFORMATION

### Etiology/Epidemiology

A cerebral aneurysm is a thin-walled outpouching or dilation of an artery of the brain. These aneurysms typically develop at points of bifurcation of the blood vessels, and the vessels of the circle of Willis are affected most often. If the aneurysm ruptures, bleeding into the subarachnoid space usually ensues. This is termed a *subarachnoid hemorrhage (SAH).* Aneurysms can be classified by their shape as follows (Figure 53-11):

- Berry aneurysm: berry shaped with a neck or stem
- Saccular aneurysm: any aneurysm that has a saccular outpouching
- Fusiform aneurysm: an outpouching of a vessel wall without a stem
- Dissecting aneurysm: the intimal layer pulls away from the medial layer of the artery and blood is forced between the two layers

Aneurysms are also classified by size:

- Small: up to 15 mm

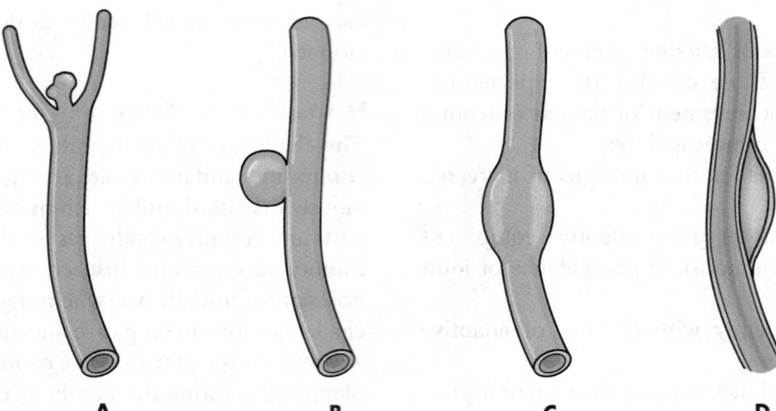


**fig. 53-11** Types of aneurysms. **A,** Berry aneurysm. **B,** Saccular aneurysm. **C,** Fusiform aneurysm. **D,** Dissecting aneurysm.

- Large: from 15 to 25 mm
- Giant: from 25 to 50 mm
- Super giant: greater than 50 mm

An estimated 10 to 15 million people in the United States have cerebral aneurysms, but most of these aneurysms are extremely small and remain asymptomatic throughout the person's life. Approximately 30,000 persons experience subarachnoid hemorrhage each year related to aneurysmal bleeding, and the outcome for these individuals remains poor.[13] From 20% to 40% die at the time of rupture. Subarachnoid hemorrhage primarily affects the 35- to 60-year-old age-group and is more common in women than men by a ratio of 3 : 2.

A congenital developmental weakness in the artery has long been believed to play a major role in the etiology of aneurysms. Research suggests that aneurysms develop as a result of degenerative vascular disease of the intima. Hypertension may predispose to aneurysm development, and head trauma, bacterial and fungal infections, and atherosclerosis are all clearly implicated. Because multiple aneurysms are occasionally found in family groups, a genetic factor is being explored.

Arteriovenous malformations (AVMs) are also commonly diagnosed for the first time when the patient has signs of acute cerebral bleeding, but the nature of the problem is different. Arteriovenous malformations are among the more common developmental cerebrovascular malformations and are composed of a tangled mass of arteries and veins that lack a capillary network. Blood is directly shunted from the arteries to the veins. Arteriovenous malformations may form anywhere but are commonly found in the distribution of the middle cerebral artery. Most patients develop symptoms for the first time between the ages of 20 and 40 years. The annual incidence of AVMs is about 3 per 100,000, which represents 9% of all intracerebral hemorrhages and 1% of all strokes.

### Pathophysiology

When a cerebral aneurysm ruptures, blood at high pressure is forced out into the tissue, usually into the subarachnoid space. In some situations, however, blood is forced into the brain substance itself, resulting in an intracerebral hemorrhage. The amount of blood lost is usually small because acute vasoconstriction occurs in adjacent vessels, and rising tissue pressure helps seal the bleeding site while fibrin and platelets initiate clot formation.

The pathology of AVM develops over time. The lack of a capillary network between the arteries and veins results in lower resistance in the arteries and the need for the veins to continually expand to handle the additional blood flow. Brain tissue within the AVM suffers degenerative changes. The patient may become steadily more symptomatic over time or have an active intracerebral hemorrhage.

Many patients are completely asymptomatic before the hemorrhage of either an aneurysm or AVM. The classic symptom is a sudden-onset violent headache, usually described as the "worst headache of my life." Immediate loss of consciousness may occur from the abrupt rise in intracranial pressure. Focal or widespread symptoms of an acute stroke will develop. In addition, the blood itself is a noxious agent and irritates the blood vessels, meninges, and brain as it hemolyzes. Arterial spasms are triggered by the blood and the release of vasoactive substances, which can further decrease cerebral perfusion. Arteriovenous malformations also commonly manifest first as an acute hemorrhage, but some patients experience warning signs such as persistent unilateral headache or the onset of seizures.

### Collaborative Care Management

The diagnosis of cerebral aneurysms and AVMs is usually made from the symptom pattern and the findings of CT scanning, which demonstrate the bleeding. Once the diagnosis is made, cerebral angiography is used to visualize the major cerebral vessels, identify the specific characteristics of the aneurysm or AVM, and determine the presence and severity of vasospasm.

Surgical repair is the treatment of choice if anatomically and technically feasible. The surgery will be performed as soon as possible after an initial period of stabilization and workup. Surgery was previously delayed for about 2 weeks after SAH, but studies have demonstrated improved outcomes with earlier intervention. Patients whose aneurysms are graded as I to III by an aneurysm classification system are the best candidates for early surgical intervention (Box 53-8).

The surgical approach depends on the location and size of the aneurysm. A berry aneurysm is usually clipped or ligated around the stem, whereas other types of aneurysms may be wrapped to support the weakened vessel and induce scarring around the wrapping (Figure 53-12). Balloon therapy involves the insertion and inflation of a small silicone catheter with a balloon to occlude either the aneurysm or parent vessel. These latter procedures are still considered to be experimental.

Surgery for AVMs is extremely difficult from a technical perspective and may involve ligation or occlusion of feeder vessels. Surgery may be preceded by attempts to embolize feeder vessels with liquid polymerizing agents, gelfoam particles, and microcoils. These experimental approaches progressively reduce the blood flow to the AVM. Gamma knife surgery may be used for certain inaccessible lesions (see Chapter 52).

The rehabilitative aspects of the care provided to patients with aneurysms and AVMs is similar to that previously discussed for stroke. However, initial management focuses on efforts to stabilize the patient and prevent the risk of rebleeding. The focus of medical management is on maintaining a stable cerebral perfusion pressure by sustaining systolic blood pressure in the 150 mm Hg range and intervening to prevent rebleeding and manage vasospasm. Despite years of clinical use, antifibrinolytics such as aminocaproic acid (Amicar) remain controversial because of the serious risk of thrombus formation. These agents delay the lysis of the clot that forms at the bleeding site and reduce the risk of rebleeding.

Vasospasm complicates the course of significant numbers of persons who survive initial aneurysm hemorrhage. Vasospasm occurs in about 30% of patients and peaks in incidence at 7 to 10 days postbleed.[19] Treatment is directed at increasing cerebral perfusion by administering crystalloid and colloid solutions to expand the intravascular volume and keep the vessels dilated. A calcium channel blocker is also routinely given to enhance collateral blood flow. Steroid use is widespread but remains controversial.

The focus of nursing care is careful patient monitoring and implementation of aneurysm bleeding precautions. The purpose of these precautions is to maintain a stable perfusion pressure. The rigor of aneurysm precautions has been decreased in recent years because concern has arisen over the development of sensory deprivation and related behavioral and cognitive impairments. Basic principles of care are outlined in the following Guidelines for Care Box and are similar to those used for the management of increased intracranial pressure. Care after neurosurgery is described in Chapter 52.

### *Patient/family education*

Aneurysm or AVM bleeding creates a sudden and potentially life-threatening crisis for the patient and family. The nurse plays an essential role in explaining all needed care routines, especially when a patient is in a critical care environment. The fear and anxiety can easily overwhelm the family's ability to learn and retain information. Participating in informed consent concerning high-risk surgical interventions can be particularly overwhelming. The nurse attempts to bridge the gap between the neurosurgical team and the patient and family, providing concrete explanations and support as needed. The rationale for all treatments and

**box 53-8** *A Grading System for Symptoms and Neurological Deficit after Subarachnoid Hemorrhage*

| | |
|---|---|
| Grade I—minimal bleed | Asymptomatic or minimal headache, slight nuchal rigidity |
| Grade II—mild bleed | Moderate to severe headache, nuchal rigidity, minimal neurological deficits |
| Grade III—moderate bleed | Drowsiness, confusion, mild focal neurological deficits |
| Grade IV—moderate to severe bleed | Stupor, moderate to severe hemiparesis, early decerebrate posturing |
| Grade V—severe bleed | Deep coma, decerebrate rigidity, disruption of vegetative functions |

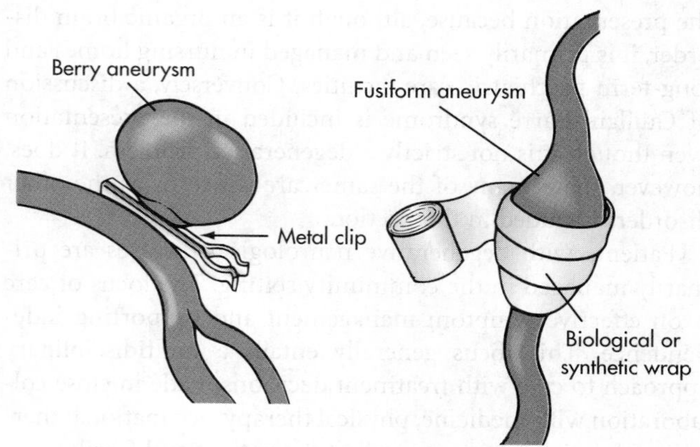


**fig. 53-12** Clipping and wrapping of aneurysms.

**guidelines for care**

**The Patient on Aneurysm Precautions**

1. Place the patient in a quiet private room without a telephone.
2. Maintain bed rest with the head of the bead elevated about 30 degrees. Some surgeons now permit bathroom privileges for selected patients. If the patient is allowed out of bed, stress the importance of not bending over (e.g., to pick up slippers or dropped objects).
3. Restrict visitors to close family or significant others and keep visits short. Prevent contact with visitors who upset or excite the patient.
4. Encourage quiet, restful activities such as reading or listening to quiet music. Television may be permitted if it does not excite the patient.
5. Keep the room slightly darkened and avoid bright artificial light.
6. Use stool softeners to prevent straining at stool.
7. Discourage isometric contraction and use of Valsalva's maneuver (e.g., coughing, dragging self up in bed by the elbows, holding the breath during painful interventions such as venipuncture). Avoid the use of restraints.
8. Provide gentle assistance with all needed care.
9. Administer analgesics as needed for headache.
10. Monitor patient carefully for any changes in alertness or mental status.

restrictions is carefully explained, and the family is incorporated into the patient's care whenever it is safe and feasible to do so. Referral for social service and spiritual support may also be appropriate.

## DEGENERATIVE DISEASES

Degenerative neurological disease includes a variety of neurological disorders in which breakdown or progressive dysfunction of nerve cells exists. Only the most common of these disorders is discussed here. Alzheimer's disease is not included in the presentation because, although it is an organic brain disorder, it is primarily seen and managed in nursing homes and long-term psychiatric care facilities. Conversely, a discussion of Guillain-Barré syndrome is included in the presentation even though it is not strictly a degenerative problem. It does, however, share many of the same care concerns as the other disorders included in this section.

Patients with degenerative neurological diseases are primarily managed in the community setting. The focus of care is on effective symptom management and supporting independence. This focus generally entails a multidisciplinary approach to care with treatment decisions made in close collaboration with medicine, physical therapy, occupational therapy, and social services, as well as the patient and family.

Degenerative diseases typically cause a slowly progressive loss of independence. The patient must be assisted to maintain a balance between the goal of independent self-care and acceptance of appropriate self-help aids and devices, or the need for direct assistance. Patients and families are forced to constantly adjust to changes in the patient's health status and cope with a future reality of declining abilities. The patient's and family's psychosocial responses to these losses are often as important as the physical challenges of the disease process. The nurse's role is usually focused on both ongoing patient education and support. Being knowledgeable about the disease process and treatment options allows the patient to effectively manage the environment and plan appropriately for the future. A major role for nurses is supporting the patient's and family's coping resources and remaining alert and open to quality-of-life issues as they arise. Community support groups can be extremely helpful to patients and their families in dealing with both today's challenges and future crises.

### MULTIPLE SCLEROSIS

#### Etiology/Epidemiology

Multiple sclerosis (MS) is a chronic degenerative neuromuscular disease that is characterized by inflammation of the white matter of the central nervous system. The etiology of MS is unknown, although an underlying viral infection has been suggested as a cause. A slow viral infection is theorized to either directly cause the inflammation of the white matter or to trigger an autoimmune response that produces antibodies that result in the destruction of the myelin. Immunological abnormalities are clearly part of the disease profile. Other autoimmune theories include the possibility that autosensitization occurs in response to an antigen on the myelin membrane, or that a cell-mediated immune reaction triggers the demyelination process.

An estimated 250,000 to 500,000 persons in the United States have MS. The highest incidence is in young adults between the ages of 20 and 40 years, and women are affected slightly more often than men.[20] Genetic makeup is implicated because the disease occurs 15 times more often in first-degree relatives of persons with MS than in the general population. Epidemiological studies consistently demonstrate a higher incidence in colder northern latitudes.

Multiple sclerosis is typically discussed as a single disease process, but it actually manifests in a variety of patterns, and in a significant minority of patients the disease causes little or no disability. Sclerotic lesions are even discovered on autopsy or by incidental scanning in individuals who are or were completely asymptomatic. Patients with more aggressive forms of the disease are obviously more likely to be hospitalized and have come to symbolize the disease for many health care professionals. Multiple sclerosis is classified into four distinct disease courses:[20]

- *Relapsing/remitting disease (65% of all cases).* Disease exacerbations occur over 1 to 2 weeks and then gradually resolve over 4 to 8 weeks, usually returning the patient to baseline or near-baseline functioning.
- *Relapsing/progressive disease (15% of all cases).* Disease exacerbations occur, but the patient does not return to baseline and is left with increasing amounts of residual disability.

- *Chronic progressive disease (20% of all cases).* Disease is characterized primarily by spinal cord and cerebellar symptoms, which are progressive and rarely remit.
- *Stable MS.* This term is used to describe patients who have not experienced a disease relapse or functional deterioration in the past year.

## Pathophysiology

Multiple sclerosis causes scattered demyelination of the white matter of the central nervous system. Research evidence suggests that viral infection initiates the autoimmune response that results in demyelination. The acute inflammation reduces the thickness of the myelin sheath that surrounds the axons and nerve fibers, and impulse conduction is slowed or blocked (Figure 53-13). Astrocytes or scavenger cells then remove the damaged myelin and scar tissue forms over the damaged areas. Natural healing may restore some of the function of the myelin, or the lesions may continue to interfere with nerve conduction. This partial healing accounts for the transitory nature of early disease symptoms. Eventually the nerve fibers may degenerate so that permanent damage occurs and overt disabilities increase. The blood-brain barrier usually protects the brain from immune cell activity. In MS, however, this barrier is breached, and activated T cells, antibodies, and macrophages attack the fatty myelin sheath and the oligodendrocytes that produce it. The central nervous system damage is thought to be caused by a delayed type of hypersensitivity response, a cell-mediated immune response.

The course of MS is highly variable and unpredictable. Sites of inflammatory demyelination can occur virtually anywhere in the brain and spinal cord, and MS produces a greater range of signs and symptoms than any other neurological disease.[35] Events that can precipitate a relapse of the disease include emotional stress, fever, hot and humid weather, infection, and fatigue. Viral infections are again implicated in disease exacerbations. Early relapses may last just a day or two but typically become more prolonged as the disease progresses. The list of possible symptoms associated with MS is summarized in Box 53-9. Classic symptom categories include sensory, motor, cerebellar, and neurobehavioral. Visual problems and fatigue are common early symptoms. Clinically silent relapses can also occur and are evident on MRI scans in patients with relapsing remitting and relapsing progressive disease even in the absence of overt clinical symptoms.

## Collaborative Care Management

The wide variety of initial symptoms and their transitory nature make the diagnosis of MS a challenge. There is no single reliable diagnostic test for the disease, and diagnosis often requires more than one episode of symptoms. Magnetic resonance imaging is extremely sensitive to white matter lesions and is useful in locating specific sites of demyelination. When gadolinium is administered during the MRI, it is even possible to distinguish between old and new lesions. Nevertheless the diagnosis of MS remains a clinical one established by ruling out other neurological causes of the symptoms.

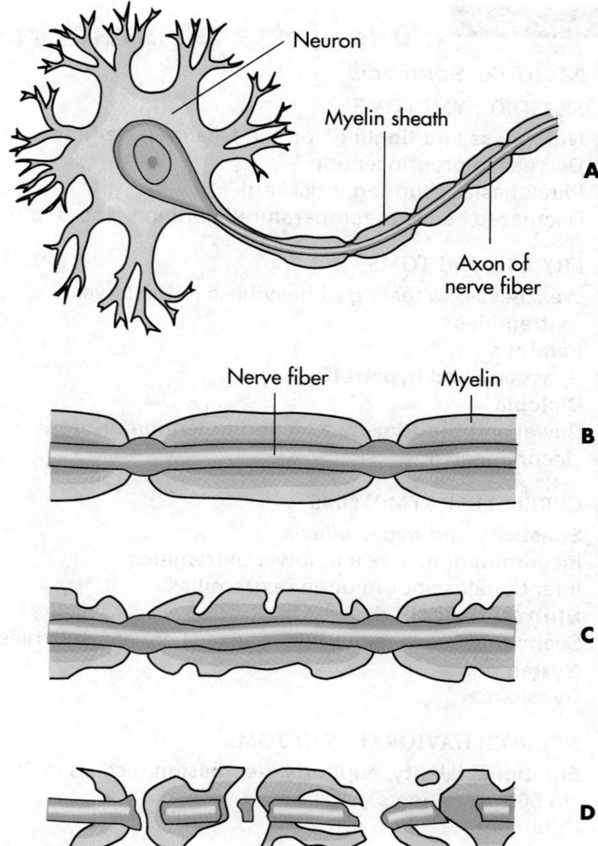


**fig. 53-13** The process of demyelination. **A** and **B** depict a normal nerve cell and axon with myelin. **C** and **D** show the slow disintegration of myelin, resulting in a disruption in axon function.

Laboratory testing will show an increase in activated T4 lymphocytes and immune globulin G (IgG) content. Oligoclonal bands of IgG are commonly isolated from the cerebrospinal fluid (CSF). Myelin basic protein, which is found in the myelin sheath, is liberated during an acute attack and can be measured by radioimmunoassay. Finally, visual, auditory, and somatosensory evoked potentials will be performed to assess nerve conduction.

Drug therapy is used in the management of MS to treat an acute attack, decrease the number and frequency of relapses, and support symptom management. The basic premise of all drug therapy approaches is to decrease the inflammation and destruction of the myelin sheaths.[35] Some patients fail to respond to or respond poorly to drug therapy, and most approaches remain part of ongoing disease research studies. Drug therapy that is aimed at influencing the frequency and severity of relapses is summarized in Box 53-10. The development of recombinant forms of interferon-beta has offered patients with relapsing remitting forms of MS a new drug therapy. Interferons have the ability to "interfere" with viral infections, but their mode of action in MS is not clear. Studies suggest that interferon-beta inhibits the number of lymphocytes

box 53-9 *clinical manifestations*

***Multiple Sclerosis***

SENSORY SYMPTOMS

**Numbness and tingling*** on the face or extremities
Decreased proprioception
Paresthesias (burning, prickling)
Decreased sense of temperature, vibration, and depth

MOTOR SYMPTOMS

Weakness or a feeling of heaviness in the lower extremities
Paralysis
**Spasticity and hyperreflexia**
**Diplopia**
Bowel and **bladder** dysfunction (retention or urge incontinence)

CEREBELLAR SYMPTOMS

**Spasticity and hyperreflexia**
**Incoordination,** ataxia in lower extremities
Intentional tremor in upper extremities
**Slurred speech,** dysarthria
Scanning speech (slow, with pauses between syllables)
Nystagmus
Dysphagia

NEUROBEHAVIORAL SYMPTOMS

**Emotional lability,** euphoria, **depression** (occurs in 30% to 50% of patients)
Irritability
Apathy
Poor judgment, inability to problem solve effectively
Loss of short-term memory

OTHER

**Optic neuritis** (visual clouding, visual field deficits)
Impotence, sexual dysfunction
**Fatigue** (extremely common, ranges from mild to disabling)

*Commonly occurring symptoms are highlighted in **boldface.**

box 53-10 *Drug Therapy for Multiple Sclerosis*

**Reducing the Frequency or Severity of Relapses**

ACUTE EXACERBATIONS

Short course of high-dose corticosteroids:
- Methylprednisolone (Medrol) IV daily for 3 to 7 days with or without a follow-up taper of oral prednisone
- Oral prednisone tapered over 2 to 4 weeks
- Corticotropin (ACTH) by IV infusion or IM injection gradually tapered over 2 to 4 weeks

DECREASING RELAPSES

- Interferon beta-1b (Betaseron) by SQ injection
- Interferon beta-1a (Avonex) by SQ injection
- Copolymer 1, an injectable polymer that appears to have some effectiveness if started early in the disease; effectiveness has not been proven
- Azathioprine (Imuran), an antiinflammatory and immunosuppressive agent; effectiveness is unproven

NOTE: Most drugs are effective for just one or two forms of MS.

HALTING DISEASE PROGRESSION

Administration of selected immunosuppressive agents has shown some positive benefit in progressive disease. Drugs in use include the following:
- Cyclophosphamide (Cytoxan)
- Cyclosporine (Sandimmune)
- Cladribine (Leustatin)
- Total lymphoid radiation
- Oral myelin (currently in clinical trials)

migrating to the central nervous system and suppresses production of macrophages. These are the first agents developed that can decrease the frequency and severity of MS exacerbations.

A wide variety of additional drugs may be used for symptom management. These include drugs to reduce tremor, spasticity, bladder dysfunction, and depression. Commonly used drugs are summarized in Box 53-11. Plasmapheresis has been used experimentally during exacerbations.[31] The treatment removes antibodies from the plasma in the hope of decreasing the severity of the inflammation. Results are unpredictable.

The goal of all collaborative interventions for MS is to keep the patient as independent as possible for as long as possible. Care is managed in the home setting except for short-term hospitalizations to treat disease exacerbations. A multidisciplinary team approach to care is essential, and the nurse commonly acts as the case manager. Physical therapy plays a crucial role. Range-of-motion and muscle strengthening exercises are important to maintain intact function of uninvolved nerves. Gait retraining is essential when spasticity or ataxia is present, and the patient may need to be fitted with assistive or supportive devices for safety. Stretching exercises are useful in balancing mild spasticity. Range-of-motion exercise assumes greater importance as the need to prevent contracture develops.

#### *Patient/family education*

Multiple sclerosis challenges patients and their families with its unpredictability and uncertainty. The threat of relapse and potential for loss of function are virtually always present. These threats assume even greater magnitude for patients who may be in their young or middle adult years and at their height of productivity. Enormous pressure is placed on the patient's ability to maintain normal daily activities, pursue a career, establish relationships, marry, and make responsible reproductive decisions.[26] The uncertainty can be paralyzing to some patients and overwhelming to partners and families. Patient and family education plays a critical

**box 53-11 Drug Therapy for Multiple Sclerosis**

**Managing Symptoms**

**SPASTICITY**
Baclofen (Lioresal)
Dantrolene (Dantrium)
Diazepam (Valium)

**TREMORS**
Hydroxyzine (Vistaril)
Isoniazid (INH)
Trihexyphenidyl (Artane)
Primidone (Mysoline)

**SPASTIC BLADDER AND URGE INCONTINENCE**
Oxybutynin (Ditropan)
Imipramine (Tofranil)
Propantheline (Pro-Banthine)

**URINARY RETENTION**
Bethanechol chloride (Urecholine)

**ANTIDEPRESSANTS**
Amitriptyline (Elavil)
Imipramine (Tofranil)
Trazodone (Desyrel)
Fluoxetine (Prozac)
Paroxetine (Paxil)
Sertraline (Zoloft)

**FATIGUE**
Amantadine hydrochloride (Symmetrel)
Pemoline (Cylert)

**OTHER**
Stool softeners
Laxatives

role in assisting them to understand the disease process and how to prevent or minimize relapses if possible (see the Research Box).

Multiple sclerosis is a crippling rather than a fatal disease process, and patients and families need to adapt and cope with the disease over many years. The nurse assumes major responsibility for coordinating patient education. The goal is to help the patient effectively manage self-care to minimize the need for hospitalization and recurrences. The nurse encourages MS patients to maintain a general health-promoting lifestyle.[26] This includes remaining active in normal daily activities to the limits of their energy tolerance and balancing activity with adequate rest to effectively manage fatigue. The nurse stresses the use of energy conservation techniques, and an occupational therapist may be consulted about the use of appropriate self-help devices and aids. Chronic fatigue can be one of the disease's most debilitating features, and patients must become skilled at interpreting their body's responses and avoiding overexertion.

**research**

Reference: Good DM, Bower, DA, Einsporn RL: Social support: gender differences in multiple sclerosis spousal caregivers, *J Neurosci Nurs* 27(5):305, 1995.

Social support has long been recognized as a key factor in family adaptation to long-term caregiving roles. This study attempted to determine if there were gender differences in the social support of spousal caregivers for patients with multiple sclerosis. The convenience sample consisted of 65 caregivers who were about evenly split between males and females. Data were collected about caregiver social support, the level of disability of the spouse with MS, and demographic data about age, length and quality of the marriage, and so on using a variety of scales.

Both social networks and social support were evaluated. Social networks refer to the number and type of relationships a person has; social support evaluates the nature and value of social interactions. Caregivers were primarily over 50 years of age, and their marriages were of greater than 25 years' duration. Female caregivers were found to have significantly more social resources than male caregivers. When problems occurred, the female caregivers used friends and self-help groups as primary resources. Male caregivers turned to children, other relatives, and their spouse more frequently. Female caregivers also reported a significantly greater level of perceived social support than did male caregivers. In both groups the presence of additional family members and demands in the family unit significantly decreased the caregivers' social life and participation in activities beyond the home.

The nurse instructs the patient on the importance of maintaining optimal nutrition. Patients with MS should eat a well-balanced diet that includes all five food groups. Natural fiber is encouraged to promote bowel regularity. Vitamin C is administered to acidify the urine and help prevent urinary tract infection. Low-fat diets that limit the amount of animal fat are recommended by some researchers because some polyunsaturated vegetable fatty acids are used by the body to produce myelin.

Patients with sensory losses need instruction about environmental safety.[35] They need to use their eyes if possible to protect their extremities from trauma related to heat, cold, and pressure. Patients with diplopia often find that an eye patch is helpful. The nurse teaches the patient about the effect of heat, especially moist heat, on symptoms. When body temperature rises the nerves may decrease or cease transmission, and symptoms can escalate dramatically. Hot baths, showers, hot tubs, steam baths, and saunas should all be avoided. Fever, stress, and infection can cause the same effect. Chilling can also exacerbate symptoms. Female patients should be informed that pregnancy often exacerbates the disease, and they should be supported in their decision making about childbearing.

Bladder problems are extremely common in progressive disease. Drug therapy can be helpful in controlling symptoms, and the nurse instructs the patient about the effective use of prescribed medications. Urinary tract infection is a common cause of morbidity in MS and cannot always be prevented. A high daily fluid intake is important, and the nurse instructs the patient about the symptoms of infection that need to be reported to the health care provider. An intermittent catheterization program can be helpful for some patients with severe bladder problems. Bowel problems are best managed by the intake of adequate fluids and a high-fiber diet to establish a regular pattern of elimination.

If the patient progresses to permanent disabilities a variety of additional interventions may be necessary. Referral to support groups such as the Multiple Sclerosis Association of America and the National Multiple Sclerosis Society can be helpful to both patients and families. Coping resources will need to expand to adapt to the challenges posed by the steady loss of self-care abilities. Multiple changes may be required in family, occupational, and social roles. Changes in sexual patterns and abilities for couples should not be ignored. Families will also need ongoing support to deal with the cognitive and behavioral changes that may accompany MS. They need to understand that these symptoms, although often extremely troubling and frightening, are organic and disease related.

## PARKINSON'S DISEASE

### Etiology/Epidemiology

Parkinson's disease is a chronic degenerative disorder that primarily affects the neurons of the basal ganglia. First described in 1817 by James Parkinson, Parkinson's disease is currently one of the more common diseases of the nervous system. An estimated 100 to 150 persons per 100,000 population, or about 50,000 new cases, are diagnosed annually.[13] About 1.5 million persons are currently living with the disease.

Parkinson's disease affects men and women about equally and usually occurs after the age of 50 with a median age of onset of about 55 years. A number of theories of causation for Parkinson's disease are being tested, but the actual etiology remains unknown. A genetic component has recently been proposed. The disease usually begins insidiously and then progresses. Primary Parkinson's disease is idiopathic, but a variety of other categories exist. Symptoms of Parkinson's disease may develop in response to the use of antipsychotic or neuroleptic agents; following an encephalitis infection; in response to brain trauma, tumors, hydrocephalus, or ischemia; in association with rare metabolic disorders; and in response to arteriosclerosis. Neurotoxins such as cyanide, manganese, and carbon monoxide have also been proposed as possible causes of the disease. Most cases are the primary idiopathic variety.

### Pathophysiology

The primary pathology of Parkinson's disease involves degenerative changes in the substantia nigra, which is an area within the basal ganglia. Destruction of the dopaminergic neurons in the substantia nigra significantly reduces the amount of available striatal dopamine.[13] Dopamine and acetylcholine are primary neurotransmitters that are responsible for controlling and refining motor movements and have opposing effects. Dopamine has inhibitory effects and acetylcholine has excitatory effects. When the excitatory activity of acetylcholine is inadequately balanced by dopamine, an individual has difficulty controlling or initiating voluntary movements. Cellular degeneration in Parkinson's disease also leads to impairment of the extrapyramidal tracts that control semiautomatic and coordinated movements.

Clinical manifestations of Parkinson's disease do not usually occur until about 70% of the affected neurons are destroyed. The disease begins insidiously and usually progresses so slowly that the person is seldom able to recall its onset. A faint tremor is a common early symptom that may be attributed to the aging process. (See Figure 53-14). The mnemonic TRAP, an acronym often used to label the classic four major disease manifestations, stands for tremor, rigidity, akinesia/bradykinesia, and postural instability.[10] The disease is often categorized based on the nature and severity of the patient's symptoms. The major disease manifestations are described in more detail in Box 53-12 and illustrated in Figure 53-15.

There are also numerous secondary disease manifestations. Patients usually experience generalized weakness and fatigue, difficulty with fine motor movements, loss of facial expression, difficulty chewing and swallowing, and voice changes. Many patients, particularly older adults, also experience cognitive losses involving memory, problem solving, and visual-spatial deficits.[10] There is no explanation for these cognitive losses at present, and many persons with Parkinson's disease remain cognitively intact despite major clinical manifestations of the disease. A decline in cognitive functioning is *not* universal.

Depression is seen in over 50% of patients and is often present before the development of the classic disease symptoms.[13] Many other signs and symptoms, primarily related to

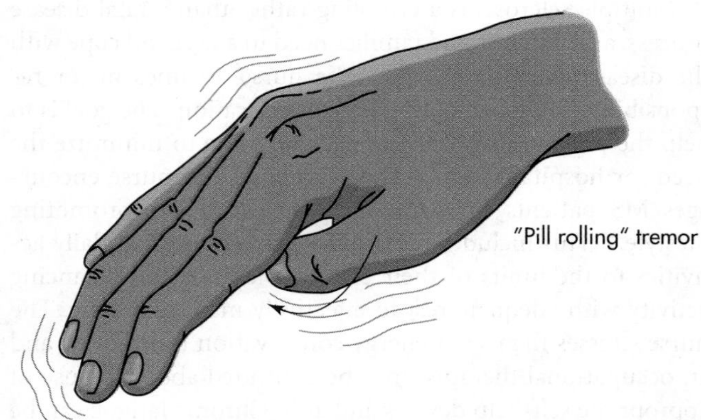


**fig. 53-14** The classic tremor of Parkinson's disease. The movement of the thumb across the palm gives it a "pill rolling" appearance. The tremor is present at rest and may be relieved by movement.

**box 53-12** *"Classic" Clinical Manifestations of Parkinson's Disease*

**TREMOR** (see Figure 53-14)
- Most recognized and least disabling symptom
- Present in 75% of patients
- Nonintentional, present at rest but usually not during sleep
- Characterized by rhythmic movements of 4 or 5 cycles per second
  - Movement of the thumb across the palm gives a "pill-rolling" character
  - Tremor also seen in limbs, jaw, lips, lower facial muscles, and head

**RIGIDITY**
- Muscles feel stiff and require increased effort to move
- Discomfort or pain may be perceived in muscle when rigidity is severe
- "Cogwheel" rigidity refers to ratchetlike rhythmic contractions of the muscle that occur when the limbs are passively stretched

**BRADYKINESIA/AKINESIA**
- Slowness of active movement
- Difficulty initiating movement
- Often the most disabling symptom; interferes with ADL and predisposes patient to complications related to constipation, circulatory stasis, skin breakdown, and other related complications of immobility

**POSTURAL INSTABILITY**
- Changes in gait
  - Tendency to walk forward on the toes with small shuffling steps
  - Once initiated, movement may accelerate almost to a trot
  - Festination may occur, which propels the patient either forward or backward propulsively until falling is almost inevitable
- Changes in balance
  - Stooped-over posture when erect (see Figure 53-15)
  - Arms are semiflexed and do not swing with walking
  - Difficulty maintaining balance and sitting erect
  - Cannot "right" or brace self to prevent falling when balance is lost

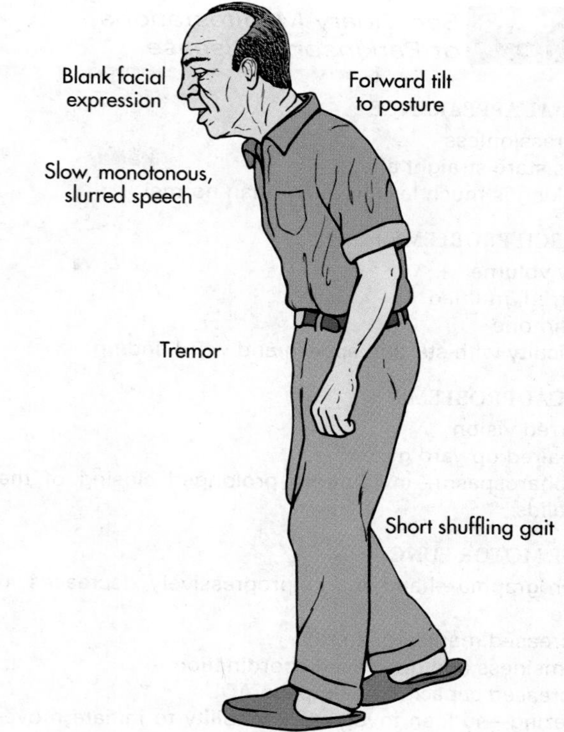


**fig. 53-15** Characteristic appearance of a patient with Parkinson's disease.

autonomic nervous system dysfunction, may also be present. The major examples of secondary symptoms of Parkinson's disease are presented in Box 53-13. All symptoms typically worsen with stress and fatigue.

## Collaborative Care Management

The diagnosis of Parkinson's disease is made clinically from the patient's history and symptoms. No definitive diagnostic test exists, and the diagnosis may be confirmed primarily from the patient's response to medication.

Parkinson's disease can neither be stopped nor cured, but developments in drug therapy over the last 30 years have resulted in enormous progress in the area of symptom control. In addition, general supportive care and education are provided to assist the patient to effectively manage disease manifestations in the home setting. Supportive care is primarily directed at supporting independence in self-care, developing coping resources, and ensuring safety. Multidisciplinary involvement of specialists such as physical, occupational, and speech therapists can help create a daily regimen that is effective in slowing the rate of disability.

Drug therapy for Parkinson's disease involves the potential use of five different classes of drugs. Each drug program is individually designed and reflects the patient's age, symptom severity, and lifestyle. All treatment decisions are made collaboratively with the patient and family, who need to be carefully instructed about the advantages, disadvantages, and predicted side effects of each option. Drug categories include the following:

*Anticholinergics.* These drugs are typically used in conjunction with levodopa or for patients who cannot tolerate levodopa. They have been used in the treatment of Parkinson's disease for almost a century. They antagonize the excitatory effects of the cholinergic neurons and have some effect in relieving muscle rigidity. Although somewhat selective in action they still produce general anticholinergic side effects in the patient and may not be well tolerated. Trihexyphenidyl (Artane) and benztropine mesylate (Cogentin) are two traditional drugs in this category.

**box 53-13** *Secondary Manifestations of Parkinson's Disease*

**FACIAL APPEARANCE**
Expressionless
Eyes stare straight ahead
Blinking is much less frequent than normal

**SPEECH PROBLEMS**
Low volume
Slurred, muffled
Monotone
Difficulty with starting speech and word finding

**VISUAL PROBLEMS**
Blurred vision
Impaired upward gaze
Blepharospasm—involuntary prolonged closing of the eyelids

**FINE MOTOR FUNCTION**
Micrographia—handwriting progressively decreases in size
Decreased manual dexterity
Clumsiness and decreased coordination
Decreased capacity to complete ADL
Freezing—sudden involuntary inability to initiate movement. Can occur during movement or inactivity

**AUTONOMIC DISTURBANCE**
Constipation (hypomotility and prolonged gastric emptying)
Urinary frequency or hesitancy
Orthostatic hypotension (dizziness, fainting, syncope)
Dysphagia (neuromuscular incoordination)
Drooling (results from decreased swallowing)
Oily skin
Excessive perspiration

**COGNITIVE/BEHAVIORAL**
Depression occurs in more than 50% of patients
Slowed responsiveness
Memory deficits
Visual-spatial deficits
Dementia

*Levodopa.* Levodopa is a precursor of dopamine that is able to cross the blood-brain barrier. Once present in the brain it is converted to dopamine by the action of the enzyme dopa decarboxylase. This enzyme is also found outside of the central nervous system and acts on the levodopa wherever it is encountered. Most patients are therefore given Sinemet, which is a combination of levodopa and carbidopa. Carbidopa blocks the conversion of levodopa in the peripheral tissues. This ensures that more of the drug reaches the brain and increases its effectiveness. Combining the two drugs usually permits a reduction in the dose of levodopa, which helps control the multiple drug side effects.

The effectiveness of levodopa gradually decreases over time, which may necessitate gradual increases in the dose to sustain its beneficial effects. Sensitivity to drug side effects also increases, however, which limits the ability to continue to increase the dose.[4] Some patients experience unpredictable responses to levodopa, including an "on-off" phenomenon. Motor function can fluctuate in a matter of minutes from active and ambulatory to severe motor freeze-ups. "Drug holidays" are recommended by some authorities for patients on prolonged levodopa therapy. Patients are admitted to the hospital and completely withdrawn from their medication. Although symptoms will exacerbate dramatically, it is usually possible to restart the levodopa after about a week at a much lower dosage.

The use of levodopa is associated with a wide variety of side effects and potential toxicities. Major drug effects are listed in Table 53-1. Points to be included in patient education are summarized in the Patient/Family Teaching Box.

*Antiviral agents.* Amantadine hydrochloride (Symmetrel) is an antiviral agent with known antiparkinsonian action. It blocks the reuptake of catecholamines, which allows dopamine to accumulate at synaptic sites. The drug's effectiveness is usually limited to about 3 months, and drug holidays do not prolong sensitivity to the drug's effects.

*Dopamine agonists.* Dopamine agonists stimulate dopamine receptors in the brain. They help prevent or minimize the fluctuations in motor response that occur in Parkinson's disease. Bromocriptine (Parlodel) and pergolide (Permax) are two forms in use.

*Monoamine oxidase B inhibitors.* Selegiline (Eldepryl) may be used in the early stages of Parkinson's disease. It blocks the metabolism of dopamine and often delays the need for levodopa therapy. This drug directly targets the disease process and not just its symptoms.

A variety of experimental approaches have been or are being tried in the management of Parkinson's disease. Stereotactic surgery was used in the 1960s before the synthesis of levodopa. It is again being studied in the management of severe tremor and rigidity in young patients.[10] Selected portions of the basal ganglia or thalamus are destroyed to relieve intractable tremors. Case histories demonstrate positive outcomes in severe cases. Experimental approaches have also included autotransplantation of tissue from the adrenal medulla, where dopamine is produced peripherally. This therapy is based on the hope that the transplanted tissue will be able to produce dopamine in the brain. Embryonic tissue transfer has also been performed.

### Patient/family education

Parkinson's disease is primarily managed in the home setting, and the nurse's primary role is to educate the patient and family effectively for the challenges of self-care. Patients and families need a thorough understanding of the disease process, appropriate self-care strategies, and signs that indicate medication failure or toxicity.[8] The purpose of all interventions is to keep the patient as independent as possible in the face of a progressive decline in function. Teaching, support, and encouragement will be needed throughout the course of the disease (see the Research Boxes on p. 1768). A Nursing Care Plan for a patient with Parkinson's disease is found on p. 1770.

**table 53-1 Common Medications for Parkinson's Disease**

| Drugs | Action | Nursing Interventions |
|---|---|---|
| Anticholinergics—trihexyphenidyl (Artane), benztropine (Cogentin), biperiden (Akineton) | Antagonize the transmission of acetylcholine in the central nervous system; most effective in decreasing rigidity; selective action but still have systemic anticholinergic effects | Monitor the incidence and severity of side effects: dry mouth, constipation, urinary retention, dysarthria, blurred vision, changes in memory, confusion. |
| Antivirals—amantadine (Symmetrel) | Block the reuptake and storage of catecholamines, allowing for the accumulation of dopamine | Positive effects may not last beyond 3 months. Monitor for effectiveness and severity of side effects (e.g., mental confusion, visual disturbances). |
| Levodopa—carbidopa-levodopa (Sinemet) | Restores deficient dopamine to the brain; carbidopa blocks peripheral conversion of levodopa | Monitor for side effects (e.g., nausea and vomiting, orthostatic hypotension, dry mouth, constipation, sleep disturbances, confusion, hallucinations). See teaching guidelines in the Patient/Family Teaching Box. |
| Dopamine agonists—bromocriptine (Parlodel), pergolide (Permax) | Directly stimulate dopamine receptors and increase the effect of levodopa; minimize fluctuations in drug response | Monitor for side effects, which are similar to levodopa. Mental dysfunction is common. |
| Monoamine oxidase B inhibitor—selegiline (Eldepryl) | Blocks the metabolism of dopamine; may slow the underlying disease process | Monitor for incidence of orthostatic hypotension. Do not exceed prescribed dose. May be given in combination with levodopa as the disease progresses. |

**patient/family teaching**

### Guidelines for the Safe Use of Levodopa

1. Levodopa is best absorbed on an empty stomach. If nausea occurs it can be taken with food.
2. Dry mouth is a common side effect. Chewing gum and hard candy can counter this effect.
3. Depression and mood swings may occur. Report the incidence of these or other cognitive-behavioral changes such as insomnia, agitation, or confusion to the health care provider.
4. Avoid the use of alcohol or minimize alcohol intake. It is believed to antagonize the effects of levodopa.
5. Avoid protein ingestion near the times for medication administration. Some protein amino acids are believed to inhibit the absorption of levodopa. A pattern of a low-protein breakfast and lunch with a high-protein dinner has improved symptoms in selected patients.
6. Be alert to the possibility of orthostatic hypotension. Change positions slowly. Avoid steam baths, saunas, and hot tubs. Experiment with the use of support stockings to support venous return.
7. Avoid vitamin supplementation with products that contain vitamin $B_6$ (pyridoxine). Pyridoxine increases the conversion of levodopa in the liver, which decreases the amount available for conversion to dopamine in the brain.
8. Consult with primary care provider and pharmacist about the use of all other drugs. Levodopa has multiple adverse drug interactions.

The nurse teaches the patient and family about the management of rigidity. Activity and exercise promote independence and reduce the risks of injury and complications. A physical therapist should be consulted to establish an initial activity plan and teach the patient and family range-of-motion exercises. These exercises are performed several times each day to relieve stiffness and prevent joint contracture.

Massage and muscle stretching are also effective strategies for reducing rigidity. Strategies for managing gait problems and preventing injury during ambulation can also be taught. A wide-based stance helps maintain balance for ambulation. Holding the hands clasped behind the back when walking may help the patient keep the spine erect and counter the problems created by the arms hanging stiffly at the sides.

The nurse emphasizes the importance of correct posture. Lying on a firm bed without a pillow during rest periods may help prevent the spine from bending forward, and lying in the prone position at intervals is also helpful. The use of assistive devices to prevent injury and support mobility is also explored. Patients with severe resting tremor may find that holding an object or placing the hands firmly along the arms of a chair when sitting may reduce its severity.

Environmental safety is another ongoing concern. The nurse can assist the patient and family to evaluate their home environment for risks posed by scatter rugs, clutter, or poor lighting. Simple home adaptations such as raised toilet seats and grab bars in the bathroom can significantly improve patient safety. Episodes of akinesia (freeze-ups) are more difficult to manage. The nurse reminds the patient to change positions frequently and avoid sitting in one position for extended periods. The use of firm supportive chairs with arms and practicing rocking movements to initiate large movements such as rising from a chair can be helpful for some patients.

Patients with Parkinson's disease face a wide variety of other daily disease-related challenges depending on the unique presentation and severity of their disease process. General teaching guidelines for patients with Parkinson's disease are summarized in the following Patient/Family Teaching Box. Patients and families will need ongoing support and encouragement because the

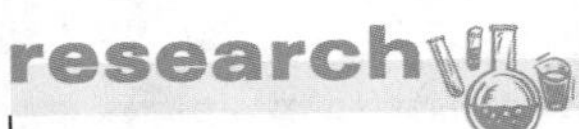

Reference: Vernon GM, Jenkins M: Health maintenance behaviors in advanced Parkinson's disease, *J Neurosci Nurs* 27(4):229, 1995.

This pilot study attempted to describe the health maintenance behaviors engaged in by a sample of patients with advanced Parkinson's disease. A convenience sample was used that consisted of 30 patients who responded to questions concerning their health maintenance and disease prevention activities.

Study findings demonstrated that the patients in this sample behaved in ways that were similar to the national patterns identified by the U.S. Preventive Task Force. In fact, in 11 of the 12 categories these patients exhibited increased frequency of participation, perhaps reflecting their frequent contact with health care providers. Study behaviors included such elements as seat belt use, Pap smears, mammograms, immunizations, and health promotion activities such as exercise and adherence to a low-fat diet. Interestingly, behaviors that have the lowest rate of goal attainment among the general population also were found to be low in the study population, even when they represented an important target area for disease management, such as exercise.

research

Reference: Dowling GA: Sleep in older women with Parkinson's disease, *J Neurosci Nurs* 27(6):355, 1995.

This study sought to compare the sleep patterns of female patients with Parkinson's disease with other women of the same age. A convenience sample of 45 women volunteers was recruited. The group was about equally split between women with Parkinson's disease and healthy subjects. Several sleep questionnaires were administered to gather data for the study.

Study results indicated that overall the women with Parkinson's disease tended to sleep more during the day and less at night than their counterparts. Both exhibited similar 12- and 24-hour sleep periodicities and sleep characteristics, but women with Parkinson's disease expressed less satisfaction with their sleep. The women with Parkinson's disease also exhibited significantly more mood disturbance, which was consistent with the presence of borderline clinical depression, and were significantly more impaired in their abilities to carry out the activities of daily living.

burden of caregiving is heavy and will become steadily more severe as the patient's condition worsens. They may profit from referral to the National Parkinson Foundation or American Parkinson Disease Association. All persons involved with caring for an individual with Parkinson's disease should be aware of the possibility of cognitive changes and deterioration, as well as the frequency with which patients develop severe depression. Pharmacological intervention may be necessary, and information about this disease complication should be provided to the family.

**patient/family teaching**

### The Person with Parkinson's Disease

#### Activity and Exercise

Perform range-of-motion exercise to all joints three times daily.

Massage and stretch muscles to reduce stiffness.

Use a broad base of support when ambulating. Consciously lift and place the feet when ambulating.

Pay attention to posture. Try walking with the hands clasped behind the back.

Explore the use of assistive devices.

Avoid staying in one position for prolonged periods. Alter position regularly.

#### Safety

Examine the home environment for risks of injury.

Modify the environment to improve lighting and remove hazards.

Consider installing devices such as raised toilet seats and grab bars.

Change positions slowly if orthostatic hypotension develops.

Be alert to the effects of heat, stress, and excitement on symptom severity.

#### Nutrition

Monitor weight once a week.

Evaluate dysphagia and modify diet to increase ease of chewing and swallowing if appropriate.

Practice swallowing and take small bites.

Provide an unhurried atmosphere and allow additional time for meals.

Follow a plan of small, frequent meals if fatigue is a problem during meals.

Avoid eating high-protein meals at times of medication administration.

Do not use vitamin supplements containing pyridoxine (vitamin $B_6$).

Ensure adequate fiber and fluid intake to prevent constipation.

Manage drooling problems with soft cloths.

#### Elimination

Monitor bowel elimination pattern.

Use diet, exercise, and fluids to ensure regularity if possible.

Use stool softeners if needed.

Keep a urinal or commode at the bedside.

Respond promptly to the urge to urinate, and be sure to empty the bladder at least every 2 to 4 hours. Bradykinesia can result in episodes of incontinence.

#### Cognitive/Behavioral

Monitor for depression. Report its presence to health care provider.

Monitor for changes in sleep pattern, disordered thoughts, and the development of agitation, confusion, or hallucinations. Report these symptoms promptly.

#### Communication

Exercise the voice regularly by singing or reading aloud.

Attempt to project the voice and alter volume and pitch.

Consult a speech therapist if vocal problems are severe.

# MYASTHENIA GRAVIS

## Etiology/Epidemiology

Myasthenia gravis (MG) is a rare chronic disease that affects the myoneural junction. Although its exact etiology is unknown, MG is widely believed to result from an autoimmune response that destroys a variable number of acetylcholine receptors (AChR) at the myoneural junction. This results in the classic disease features of weakness and fatigue of selected voluntary muscles. Estimates of the incidence of MG vary from 1:10,000 to 1:40,000, or approximately 25,000 to 100,000 individuals in the United States. Myasthenia gravis is bimodal in incidence.[15] It affects primarily young women who are 20 to 40 years of age and primarily men who are 60 to 80 years of age. Infants of affected mothers may exhibit symptoms at birth, but the symptoms generally disappear within a few weeks. The thymus gland has long been believed to play a role in the autoimmune process of MG because thymic hyperplasia is seen in as many as 80% of MG patients and 15% have thymic tumors.[15] However, the exact role of the thymus gland in the disease is not understood.

## Pathophysiology

Effective muscle contraction is contingent on adequate amounts of acetylcholine (ACh), a neuromuscular transmitter, being available at the postsynaptic membrane to generate an action potential that can spread along the length of the muscle and culminate in muscle contraction. Mitochondria in the motor nerve axons synthesize ACh, which is released when the nerve is stimulated. The ACh crosses the myoneural junction and binds with an acetylcholine receptor on the postsynaptic membrane to initiate the action potential (Figure 53-16). Acetylcholinesterase (AChE) is also released into the synaptic cleft. The AChE breaks down the ACh, which limits the duration of the muscle contraction. The number of AChR sites is significantly reduced in persons with MG as a result of the destructive effects of an antibody-mediated autoimmune attack that specifically targets the AChR sites. As a result, the stimuli may lack sufficient amplitude to trigger an effective action potential in some muscle fibers. The strength of muscle response is weakened, and with repeated stimuli the amount of ACh steadily decreases, resulting in muscle fatigue.

The severity of MG is directly related to the number of AChR sites involved.[15] Muscle biopsy can demonstrate the normal number of sites being reduced by as much as two thirds. The disease can be classified based either on the severity of the clinical symptoms or the course of the disease (Box 53-14). The onset of MG is usually gradual, and the disease may elude diagnosis for a prolonged period if it is not considered as a possible cause of the patient's symptoms. The course of the disease is also highly variable, as is commonly true with autoimmune disorders.

The classic symptoms of MG are muscle weakness and generalized fatigue, which occur in more than 80% of patients. Ptosis and diplopia are common early findings, and the disease is occasionally limited to the eye muscles.[15] Muscles innervated by the cranial nerves are often affected, and it may be impossible for the patient to keep the mouth closed or to chew

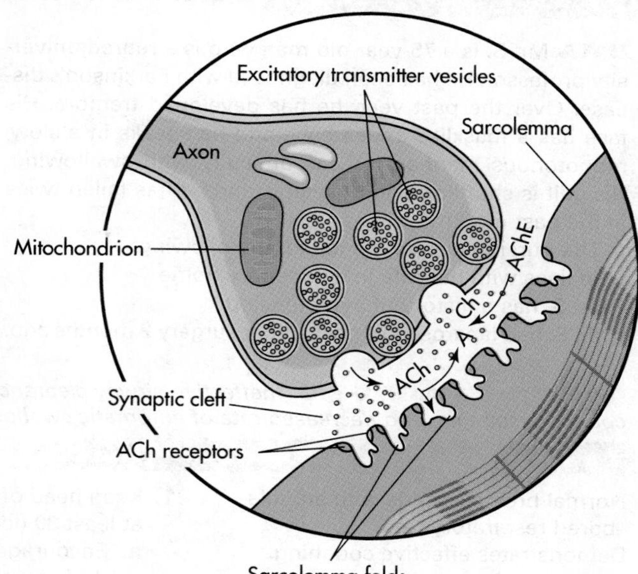


**fig. 53-16** Normal myoneural junction. ACh released from the nerve initiates the muscle contraction. Acetylcholinesterase (AChE) breaks down ACh, limiting the duration of contraction.

**box 53-14** *A Classification System for Myasthenia Gravis*

Type 1—Ocular myasthenia
Type 2A—Mild
Type 2B—Severe
Type 3—Fulminating/acute
Type 4—Chronic, late severe

and swallow for extended periods. The mobility of the facial muscles is also affected, and the face may take on an expressionless appearance (Figure 53-17, p. 1774). Attempts to smile may result in the classic myasthenic "snarl." The patient's voice is often weak, and as fatigue sets in it may become difficult for the patient even to swallow saliva effectively. Weakness of the neck tends to cause the head to fall forward.

Weakness of the arm and hand muscles may first become apparent during self-care activities such as shaving or combing the hair. Symptoms develop rapidly, but early in the course of the disease they also are relieved easily with rest. As the disease progresses fatigue becomes evident with less and less exertion. The muscles of the trunk and lower limbs may also become involved, creating difficulties with walking and even sitting.[15] The distal muscles are rarely affected as severely as the proximal muscles. During a disease exacerbation muscle weakness of the intercostals and diaphragm may become so severe that intubation and mechanical ventilation are necessary. Exacerbations of the disease can be triggered by upper respiratory infection, emotional stress, secondary illness,

*Text continued on p. 1773*

## nursing care plan *Person with Parkinson's Disease*

**DATA** Mr. S. is a 75-year-old man who is a retired university professor. He has been diagnosed with Parkinson's disease. Over the past year, he has developed tremors. His face has a masklike appearance and he speaks in a slow, monotonous manner. He has difficulty with swallowing. His gait is shuffling and unsteady, and he has fallen twice in the past month.

The nursing history identified the following:

- He lives with his wife in a two-story home.
- Mr. S. has a history of hypertension.
- Mr. S. had laparoscopic gallbladder surgery 2 months ago.

Nursing actions should include monitoring for the following:

- Aspiration precautions: monitoring patient closely at mealtime
- Safety precautions to prevent falling
- Assessing for adverse reactions to medications

The following care plan is adapted from Delgado JM, Billo JM: Care of the patient with Parkinson's disease: surgical and nursing interventions, *J Neurosci Nurs* 20(3):142, 1988.

**NURSING DIAGNOSIS** *Ineffective airway clearance related to rigidity of truncal muscles resulting in an impaired cough, dysphagia, and decreased rate of automatic swallowing*

| expected patient outcome | nursing interventions | rationale |
|---|---|---|
| Normal breath sounds with an unlabored respiratory rate.<br>Demonstrates effective coughing. | **1.** Keep head of bed (HOB) elevated at least 30 degrees.<br>**a.** Encourage to be out of bed during waking hours.<br>**b.** Clear excess saliva: encourage swallowing of secretions if gag reflex intact; remove excess secretions with tissue or suction machine. | **1.** With increased salivation and decreased cough and gag reflexes, the chance of aspiration and respiratory complications is increased. |
| | **2.** Encourage deep coughing q1h when sedentary.<br>**a.** Remind of or assist with proper body alignment.<br>**b.** Monitor ventilatory status and respiratory rate and effort; auscultate breath sounds, assess for alterations in level of consciousness. | **2.** Early interventions can prevent complications.<br>**a.** Assessment of respiratory status is necessary to assess the flow of air and to detect any adventitious sounds. |
| | **3.** Assess ability to cough, gag, and swallow.<br>**a.** If cough and gag reflexes are intact, avoid thin, warm liquids such as coffee and soup—use thickeners as needed.<br>**b.** Take precautions during feedings: check gag reflex before feeding; position upright in chair, or in bed with HOB elevated 90 degrees; have suction equipment available at bedside. | **3.** Dysphagia precautions are essential to prevent aspiration. |

**NURSING DIAGNOSIS** *Risk for injury related to decreased postural reflexes; frequent falls; orthostatic hypotension; akinesia; rigidity, propulsive, and retropulsive gaits*

| expected patient outcome | nursing interventions | rationale |
|---|---|---|
| Patient and family express understanding of injury potential.<br>Does not experience falls.<br>Uses assistive devices to avoid injury. | **1.** Assess orthostatic blood pressure, pulse, and presence of dizziness immediately after changing to upright position.<br>**a.** Change positions slowly. | **1.** Assess response of cardiovascular system to position changes.<br>**a.** Reduces orthostatic BP changes. |
| | **2.** Use side bars in bathrooms, hand rails in hallways, chairs with backs and arm rests.<br>**a.** Use gait belt for assisted transfers. | **2.** Safety devices decrease the risk of falls. |

Continued

## Person with Parkinson's Disease—cont'd

**NURSING DIAGNOSIS** *Risk for injury related to decreased postural reflexes; frequent falls; orthostatic hypotension, akinesia; rigidity, propulsive, and retropulsive gaits—cont'd*

| expected patient outcome | nursing interventions | rationale |
|---|---|---|
| | **3.** Choose a clear path for walking; avoid crowds, narrow doorways, fast turns, uneven surfaces, and scatter rugs. | **3.** Environment is modified to reduce the hazards that can contribute to falls. |
| | **4.** When turning, walk in a wide arc instead of pivoting.<br>**a.** If balance unsteady when walking, nurse should grasp patient's hands (nurse's and patient's arms extended) and walk backward.<br>**b.** Use closed-heeled, supportive shoes or slippers.<br>**c.** Repeatedly remind patient to maintain upright position when ambulating (tendency to flex excessively at knee and hop).<br>**d.** Stop occasionally to slow down walking speed (festinating gait).<br>**e.** Repeatedly remind patient to maintain wide-based gait (12 to 15 inches).<br>**f.** Chest restraint or loose bedsheet around midriff while up in chair.<br>**g.** Place call button, telephone, etc. within reach.<br>**h.** Both side rails up while in bed. | **4.** Rigidity makes sudden turns difficult. Balance can easily be lost. Patient must actively compensate for loss of previously automatic movements. Exercise increases muscle strength and independence. |

**NURSING DIAGNOSIS** *Alteration in communication, oral and written, related to micrographia, decreased volume, monotone speech*

| expected patient outcome | nursing interventions | rationale |
|---|---|---|
| Demonstrates effective communication.<br>Uses alternative methods of communication. | **1.** Assess ability to speak, read, and write (micrographia, decreased speech tone and volume occur due to tremors and rigidity). | **1.** Patients with Parkinson's disease have limited movement of facial muscles, causing difficulty speaking clearly. |
| | **2.** Reduce environmental noise.<br>**a.** Encourage patient to speak slowly and pause to breathe between words.<br>**b.** Ask patient to repeat unclear words.<br>**c.** Watch patient's lips for clues.<br>**d.** Teach patient to express ideas in short phrases or sentences.<br>**e.** Teach patient to organize thoughts and plan what he or she will say.<br>**f.** Teach patient to exaggerate pronunciation of words.<br>**g.** Do not interrupt patient (spontaneous speech may take time).<br>**h.** Encourage patient to use facial expressions while speaking.<br>**i.** Encourage patient to talk for 10 to 15 minutes each day with staff or family. Singing can also be helpful. | **2.** Teaching the patient these exercises and interventions will enhance articulation and communication, reduce environmental distraction, and increase attentiveness of caregivers. |

*Continued*

## Person with Parkinson's Disease—cont'd

**NURSING DIAGNOSIS** *Alteration in communication, oral and written, related to micrographia, decreased volume, monotone speech—cont'd*

| expected patient outcome | nursing interventions | rationale |
| --- | --- | --- |
| | **j.** Encourage writing when antiparkinsonian medications are at peak effectiveness.<br>**k.** If speech is unintelligible, teach patient and family to use alternative means of communication such as pointing to objects and using a communication board. | |

**NURSING DIAGNOSIS** *Constipation related to decreased fluid intake, decreased peristalsis, and side effects of medications*

| expected patient outcome | nursing interventions | rationale |
| --- | --- | --- |
| Maintains a daily bowel elimination pattern of soft, formed stool. | **1.** Assess patient's bowel regularity (bowel movement every 3 to 5 days may be normal for this patient population). | **1.** Monitoring the bowel elimination pattern is essential to identify patterns and evaluate the effectiveness of interventions. |
| | **2.** If medically stable, increase fluid intake to 2 to 3 L per day.<br>**a.** Encourage consumption of high-fiber foods.<br>**b.** Encourage regular schedule (gastrocolic reflex may be helpful after meals).<br>**c.** Provide ample time to defecate.<br>**d.** Use bathroom or bedside commode instead of bedpan.<br>**e.** Increase physical mobility.<br>**f.** When regularity cannot be established through diet and exercise, training program with suppositories may be established.<br>**g.** To promote adequate bowel tone, laxatives and enemas should not be used unless absolutely necessary. | **2.** A well-balanced diet that is high in fiber content with adequate fluid intake stimulates peristalsis and elimination. Using a bathroom or bedside commode for proper positioning allows gravity and the abdominal muscles to promote elimination. |

**NURSING DIAGNOSIS** *Altered nutrition: less than body requirements related to decreased gag, decreased cough, dysphagia, difficulty chewing*

| expected patient outcome | nursing interventions | rationale |
| --- | --- | --- |
| Maintains adequate balanced nutrient intake and a stable weight. | **1.** Provide small, frequent, high-calorie meals.<br>**a.** Allow adequate time to eat.<br>**b.** Minimize distractions.<br>**c.** Provide thick, cold foods to promote easy swallowing (ice cream, shakes, frozen liquid supplements).<br>**d.** Consult dietitian.<br>**e.** Give oral care before and after meals. | **1.** Parkinson's disease is associated with eating difficulties related to difficulty in swallowing and in hand-to-mouth coordination. |
| | **2.** Assess daily caloric intake.<br>**a.** Record weight every third day.<br>**b.** Schedule medications so that peak time coincides with meals.<br>**c.** Encourage family to bring patient's favorite meals from home. | **2.** Monitor nutrient intake and body weight over time. |

Continued

### *Person with Parkinson's Disease—cont'd*

**NURSING DIAGNOSIS** *Self-care deficit (feeding, dressing, bathing, grooming) related to akinesia, decreased postural reflexes, tremor*

| expected patient outcome | nursing interventions | rationale |
|---|---|---|
| Remains independent in the activities of daily living with the use of appropriate self-help aids. | **1.** Occupational and physical therapy consultation for adaptive equipment: feeding (padded utensils and plate guards); bathing (sponge mitts); dressing (Velcro straps).<br>**a.** Encourage use of chairs and commodes with elevated seats. | **1.** Multidisciplinary planning facilitates access to all needed services. |
| | **2.** Provide unhurried atmosphere and allow time for completion of tasks.<br>**a.** Foster independence as much and as long as possible.<br>**b.** Provide encouragement if problems arise and provide support for achievements. | **2.** It is crucial that the Parkinson's disease patient be supported to maintain independence in self-care as long as possible. Deterioration is progressive. |
| | **3.** Perform active or passive range of motion to all extremities.<br>**a.** If joints are rigidly flexed or extended, apply slight pressure at joint with palm of your hand, while attempting to exercise joint by slowly moving extremity distal to joint with other hand. | **3.** Muscle rigidity can quickly progress to joint contracture. |
| | **4.** Encourage patient to actively swing arms to improve balance and decrease tremor.<br>**a.** If patient becomes "stuck" while ambulating, face patient; either hold patient's hands or have patient hold your shoulders or waist with both hands; "rock" patient slightly from side to side. | **4.** Bradykinesia is a classic sign of Parkinson's disease. Episodes of akinesia or freeze-up can occur in which patient is unable to initiate movement. |

trauma, surgery, pregnancy, and even menstruation. There is no accompanying sensory loss in the affected areas.

A rare condition exists called Eaton-Lambert syndrome that can mimic the symptoms of classic MG. It is found almost exclusively in individuals with oat cell carcinoma of the lung. It is therefore important that this rare possibility be excluded in the diagnostic process for MG.

## Collaborative Care Management

The diagnosis of MG is first established presumptively from the patient's history and symptoms and then is confirmed through laboratory testing. A positive Tensilon test is usually considered to be diagnostic. In this test edrophonium (Tensilon), a short-acting anticholinesterase, is administered IV. A patient with MG experiences a brief but significant increase in muscle strength in previously weakened muscles in response to the drug, and this response is considered to be a positive test.[15] The AChR antibody titers are elevated in the vast majority of patients with MG, and electromyogram (EMG) results are considered to be 99% sensitive in diagnosing MG. The EMG can detect transmission delay or failure in muscle fibers that are repetitively stimulated. An MRI may be performed to evaluate thymus gland involvement.

There is no known cure for MG, but drug therapy is effective in managing symptoms in most patients. Individual responses vary tremendously, however, and an individualized treatment plan needs to be collaboratively developed for each patient. The management of MG primarily takes place in the community, and it is essential for patients to be well informed about self-care management of their disease. Patients may require hospitalization in rare circumstances to manage disease crises, but the bulk of care and treatment takes place in the home.

Drug therapy with acetylcholinesterase inhibitor agents is the cornerstone of MG treatment, but these drugs do not in any way reverse the actual disease process. By blocking the action of AChE in the myoneural junction more ACh is made available for receptor site binding.[7] Pyridostigmine (Mestinon) is the most commonly used drug. Its use is associated with multiple side effects (Box 53-15), and an individualized dosage schedule needs to be established that allows the patient to receive maximum benefit

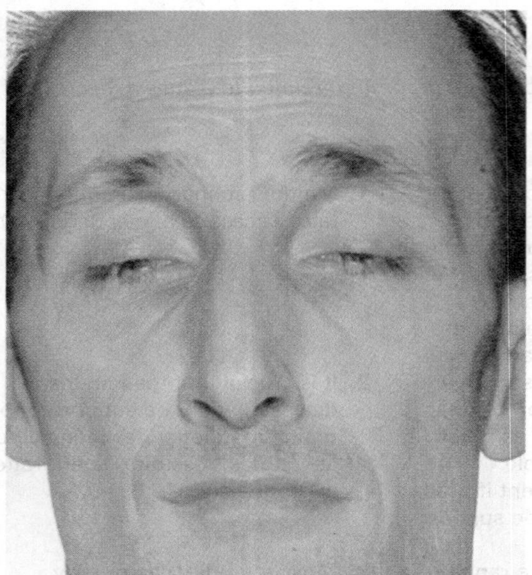

fig. 53-17 Facial appearance in myasthenia gravis. Note ptosis, lack of expression, and wrinkled brow.

**box 53-15** *Side Effects of Mestinon Therapy*

**MUSCARINIC EFFECTS (Effects on Smooth Muscle and Glands)**
Gastrointestinal distress, heartburn
Nausea and vomiting
Increased peristalsis, abdominal cramping, diarrhea
Bradycardia
Increased bronchial secretions, bronchoconstriction/bronchospasm
Excess salivation
Sweating
Pupil miosis
Weakness

**NICOTINIC EFFECTS (Effects on Skeletal Muscle)**
Muscle twitching (fasciculations) and spasms
Profound muscle weakness

from the drug while keeping the side effects within tolerable limits. The drug peaks in about 2 hours and its duration of effect is 3 to 6 hours, so its administration must be carefully timed to support specific muscle group activities such as chewing and swallowing at mealtimes. Atropine is the antidote for Mestinon and should be available to treat adverse side effects. The patient may be permitted to slightly adjust the dosage and time of administration within stated parameters to meet the fluctuating needs and demands of daily living.

Other treatment approaches for MG target the disease process itself. Long-term immunosuppression with corticosteroids, azathioprine, or cyclosporine may be prescribed for patients who do not respond well to cholinesterase inhibitors or develop disabling ocular or generalized MG. The potential benefits of this treatment must be carefully weighed against the risks of long-term immunosuppression. Prednisone is the drug of choice and produces improvement in 70% to 80% of patients, but it is often difficult to sustain the improvements when the drug is tapered. Azathioprine (Imuran) has been shown to reduce the number of circulating AChR antibodies, but improvement may not be noticed for months. Cyclosporine acts by decreasing T cell function and also decreases circulating AChR antibodies. These drugs may also be used in conjunction with plasmapheresis to treat a serious disease exacerbation.

Plasmapheresis or intravenous immunoglobulin (IVIG) administration provide for short-term immunomodulation. During plasmapheresis the patient's plasma is removed and replaced with albumin or fresh frozen plasma. The AChR antibodies are removed in the process.[13] Improvements can be dramatic but are often temporary. Intravenous immunoglobulin is also used to treat disease exacerbations, and although its action is not understood, it has produced dramatic improvement in some MG patients. It is theorized that human immunoglobulins may react with antigens in the plasma and decrease the formation of the targeted antibodies.

The role of the thymus gland in MG has intrigued researchers for years. A thymectomy results in symptom remission in about 40% of patients. It appears to be most effective when performed in patients under 40 years of age who have had symptomatic MG for less than 5 years.

### *Myasthenic and cholinergic crises*

Patients with MG are vulnerable to two crisis situations that may result in dramatic symptom exacerbation and the need for acute ventilatory support. A myasthenic crisis represents an acute exacerbation of the disease process and may occur in response to stress, trauma, or infection. Problems with breathing and swallowing can rapidly progress to life-threatening levels, and intubation is usually performed when the patient's vital capacity drops below 1 L.[3] Mechanical ventilation is continued until the patient shows some signs of return of muscle strength. Cholinesterase inhibitor drugs are gradually restarted in an effort to once again find an effective balance.

A cholinergic crisis represents a toxic response to medication. The muscarinic side effects develop slowly, but as toxic levels are reached, severe nicotinic effects can rapidly appear. The patient experiences profound weakness, copious respiratory secretions, and respiratory failure, which again may require intubation and mechanical ventilation. In this crisis the cholinesterase drug is temporarily stopped and then gradually restarted and retitrated. A Tensilon test can be used to differentiate between the two forms of crisis. If no improvement is seen with the administration of Tensilon or if symptoms worsen, a cholinergic crisis can be assumed.

Acute care nurses are most likely to encounter patients with MG during an episode of disease exacerbation or crisis. Nursing care involves meticulous monitoring and implementing respiratory support. The nurse regularly monitors the severity of the patient's ptosis, the degree of swallowing impairment, hand strength, and voice quality. Respiratory rate and quality, the patient's ability to cough to clear the airway, and the use of accessory muscles are standard assessments. The patient's subjective assessment of breathlessness is also crucial, but decisions about intubation are generally made based on vital capacity measurements. Patients who are weak enough to require intubation require total care and interventions to prevent the complications of immobility.[7] Temporary placement in intensive care may be necessary. The experience of crisis is extremely frightening for the patient, who will need ongoing support and reassurance during the acute period. Patients and families dealing with any stage of the disease may profit from referral to the Myasthenia Gravis Foundation.

#### Patient/family education

Self-care is the foundation of care for MG, and education of the patient and family is its most critical component. Respiratory complications are the most serious disease threat, and knowledgeable self-care can positively affect their frequency and severity.[13] The medication regimen is also commonly adjusted by the patient within preset parameters, and the patient needs to be extremely knowledgeable about safe drug administration and the management of side effects.[7] Box 53-15 outlines the major side effects associated with the use of Mestinon, and principles of patient teaching for MG are summarized in the Patient/Family Teaching Box.

**patient/family teaching**

**The Patient with Myasthenia Gravis**

1. Use Mestinon safely and appropriately:
   a. Take the drug with food or fluid.
   b. Take the drug before meals to permit maximum effect for chewing and swallowing.
   c. Adjust drug dosage and time of administration within set parameters in response to individual pattern of weakness.
   d. Do not take any other medication, including over-the-counter products, without prior approval of health care provider or pharmacist. Many drugs can compromise neuromuscular transmission and will worsen MG symptoms (e.g., local anesthetics, aminoglycosides, beta blockers, and calcium channel blockers).
2. Modify diet as needed in response to swallowing problems.
   a. A soft diet is usually well tolerated.
   b. Eat slowly and take small bites.
3. Balance rest and activity throughout the day in response to weakness.
   a. Plan for additional rest periods.
   b. Seek out energy conservation strategies for routine activities.
4. Keep Medic Alert identification with you at all times.
5. Know the symptoms of cholinergic and myasthenic crisis and contact physician promptly.
6. Be alert to disease response to periods of stress, infection, temperature extremes, and hormonal swings (e.g., menstruation or pregnancy).

## AMYOTROPHIC LATERAL SCLEROSIS

### Etiology/Epidemiology

Amyotrophic lateral sclerosis (ALS), or motor neuron disease (MND), is a chronic and rapidly progressive motor neuron disease that eventually weakens and paralyzes the respiratory muscles, resulting in death. It is also referred to as Lou Gehrig's disease after the New York Yankee baseball player who died from the disease.

Amyotrophic lateral sclerosis is a rare disease that occurs in 2 or 3 persons per 100,000 annually. Men have a higher incidence of ALS than women. The average age at onset is from 40 to 70 years. The cause is unknown, but theories of causation include exposure to heavy metals, viral infection, lymphoma, gammopathy, and hexosaminidase A deficiency. Amyotrophic lateral sclerosis has also occurred in association with infection by the HIV virus.[13] Approximately 10% of ALS patients inherit an autosomal dominant gene that can result in the disease. Other theories of etiology include autoimmune destruction and neurotransmitter depletion.[13]

### Pathophysiology

The term *amyotrophic* refers to the weakness and atrophy that occur from the degeneration of the alpha or lower motor neurons. Alpha motor neurons originate in the anterior horn of the spinal cord, and their axons connect the central nervous system with the voluntary muscles. They are essential for motor function and innervate the voluntary skeletal muscles. Lateral sclerosis refers to the hardness of the spinal cord that is typically found in patients with the disorder. Amyotrophic lateral sclerosis involves degeneration of both cortical and alpha motor neurons of the final pathway. Cortical or upper motor neurons originate in the upper regions of the brain. The neurons of the brainstem are primarily affected by ALS. The axons of the upper motor neurons synapse in the descending corticospinal or pyramidal tract to the alpha or lower motor neurons.

Amyotrophic lateral sclerosis causes progressive degeneration of both the upper and lower motor neurons from demyelination and scar tissue formation. The disease gradually destroys motor pathways but leaves sensation and mental status intact. Lower motor neurons are usually affected first, resulting in muscle weakness and atrophy. The muscles of the upper body are affected much earlier than the legs. Patients may notice that they drop items or have a decreased ability to perform tasks that require fine motor skills. Other early symptoms include muscle atrophy, fasciculations and fibrillations of the muscles, and decreased tendon reflexes. Muscle cramping and generalized fatigue are also common. The disease is relentlessly progressive and eventually involves the upper motor neurons, which causes increased weakness and spasticity in affected muscles. Hyperactive reflexes, jaw clonus, tongue fasciculations, and a positive Babinski's reflex may be present. As the muscles of the neck, pharynx, and larynx become increasingly involved, slurring of the voice occurs, which gradually worsens to dysarthria and dysphagia. Paralysis is inevitable, and death usually results from pneumonia and respiratory failure within 5 years of diagnosis.

### Collaborative Care Management

Amyotrophic lateral sclerosis is diagnosed by a process of elimination because no definitive diagnostic test exists. Muscle biopsies may be performed to determine the source of muscle weakness, and an EMG will show muscle denervation, fibrillation, and fasciculation, which are closely associated with ALS. Blood studies typically show elevations in the levels of creatine phosphokinase.

There is no cure for ALS, and treatment is primarily directed toward symptom relief. Riluzole (Rilutek) has recently been approved for use in ALS treatment. Its action is unknown, but it is believed to have a neuroprotective effect and to extend the lives of ALS patients by a few months. Specific interventions are directed at managing complications as they arise. The focus of nursing care is on supporting the self-care abilities of the patient and the coping resources of the entire family. General interventions are targeted at maintaining good general health, supporting nutrition, promoting adequate sleep, appropriately balancing activity and rest, and introducing the use of self-help devices as they become appropriate. Physical therapy targets both the muscle weakness and spasticity, and occupational therapy assesses the need for adapted equipment and assistive devices.

As ALS progresses, it is increasingly important to maintain a patent airway. Aspiration is a common concern and makes it increasingly difficult to meet the patient's nutritional needs with oral feedings. A gastrostomy may be needed to support nutrition.

#### *Patient/family education*

Both the patient and family need specific teaching concerning airway protection. The patient is taught to use a tucked-chin position while eating or drinking to encourage more effective swallowing and to always be in an upright position for meals. If the patient's cough is weak, it may be necessary to keep suction equipment at the bedside during meals to assist in clearing the mouth if needed. The patient is taught how to manage oral suctioning independently if possible.

Disease education is an important ongoing nursing responsibility. The reality of progressive physical deterioration can easily become overwhelming for both the patient and the family. Health care providers assist patients and families to make decisions about the types of interventions that will be used as the disease progresses. One of the most difficult decisions involves the use of a ventilator as respiratory muscles weaken. Death commonly results from aspiration, infection, or respiratory failure, and decision making in this area is essential. The issues need to be addressed before a respiratory crisis occurs, and the participants need to receive nonjudgemental support for whatever decision they make. Patients also need to be clearly aware that they can change their minds as the reality of their situation becomes apparent. The need for long-term ventilatory support may be accepted and incorporated into daily care or completely rejected. The inevitability of complete dependency is made clear. Referral to local or regional support groups for ALS patients and families may be helpful. The patient remains alert throughout the course of the disease, and most patients experience significant fear and anxiety over both the reality of today and the uncertainty of the future. Respite care for families who are caring for ALS patients at home needs to be addressed and legitimized, because the burden of caregiving can be overwhelming. Involvement with hospice services can be of tremendous aid to both patients and families. The nurse plays an important role in assisting patients and families to deal with loss and grief (see Chapter 8).

## GUILLAIN-BARRÉ SYNDROME

### Etiology/Epidemiology

Guillain-Barré syndrome (GBS) is an acute inflammatory polyneuropathy characterized by varying degrees of motor weakness or paralysis. It primarily affects the motor component of the cranial and spinal nerves and is known by a variety of other names, including postinfectious polyneuritis, acute inflammatory polyradiculopathy, and idiopathic polyneuritis. It is a rare disorder with an incidence of 1.5 to 1.9 per 100,000 population.[13] The etiology of the disorder is unknown, but it is believed in most cases to be an autoimmune response to a viral infection. The onset of GBS usually occurs 1 to 3 weeks after an illness, infection, or immunization and commonly follows an upper respiratory infection.

The syndrome is seen worldwide and affects all ages and races, but it appears to be most frequent in whites over 45 years of age.[13] It received a great deal of attention when numerous cases were identified as a sequela of immunization for swine flu during the 1970s. The syndrome is usually rapidly progressive and can advance to full paralysis. Improved respiratory management has significantly decreased the mortality rate associated with the disease, and most patients recover. The mortality rate for GBS remains higher in the elderly.

### Pathophysiology

In GBS an immune-mediated response triggers destruction of the myelin sheath surrounding the peripheral nerves, nerve roots, root ganglia, and spinal cord. Collections of lymphocytes and macrophages are believed to be responsible for the myelin stripping. Demyelination occurs between the nodes of Ranvier, which impairs or blocks the transmission of impulses from node to node. The nerve axons are generally spared and recovery takes place, although the process of remyelination occurs slowly.[23] In severe forms of the disease wallerian degeneration occurs that involves the axons, making recovery slower and more difficult. In a small percentage of patients the disease does not resolve and becomes chronic or recurrent.

There are four major forms of GBS. Each reflects a different degree of peripheral nerve involvement.

- Ascending GBS is the most common form. Weakness and numbness begin in the legs and progress upward. Fifty percent of the patients experience respiratory insufficiency. Sensory involvement is also usually present.
- Pure motor GBS is similar to the ascending form, but no sensory involvement is present. It is usually a milder form of the disease.
- Descending GBS begins with weakness in the muscles controlled by the cranial nerves and then progresses downward. The respiratory system is quickly impaired. Sensory involvement is present.
- Miller Fisher syndrome, a variant of GBS, is rare and primarily involves the eyes, loss of reflexes, and severe ataxia.

The patient with GBS has symmetrical muscle weakness and flaccid motor paralysis. The paralysis usually starts in the lower extremities and ascends upward to include the thorax, upper extremities, and face. Cranial nerves may also be affected, and the facial nerve is the most commonly involved. When the seventh, ninth, and tenth cranial nerves are involved, the patient may have difficulty swallowing, speaking, and breathing.[23] The vital centers in the medulla oblongata may also be affected, and involvement of the vagus nerve may explain the autonomic dysfunction that is commonly seen with the syndrome.

Pain and paresthesias are present when sensory nerves are involved. Tingling or a pins and needles sensation is common. Either a heightened sensitivity to touch or numbness may occur, and about 25% of patients experience pain.[25] The pain is usually experienced as a cramping in the extremities but can become severe enough to require analgesics.

Autonomic dysfunction is now recognized as a common problem with GBS and may include dysrhythmias, blood pressure instability, tachycardia or bradycardia, flushing, sweating, urinary retention, and paralytic ileus. Guillain-Barré syndrome does not affect the patient's level of consciousness, alertness, or cognitive functioning.[23] The patient is alert and aware throughout the course of the disease and is acutely vulnerable to sensory deprivation problems from the decrease in environmental stimuli.

Guillain-Barré syndrome generally progresses through three stages. The initial period lasts from 1 to 3 weeks and ends when no further physical deterioration occurs. A plateau period follows, which lasts from a few day to a few weeks. The recovery period can last from 6 months to well over 1 year. The remyelination of damaged nerves occurs during the recovery phase. Permanent deficits may remain.

## Collaborative Care Management

The diagnosis of GBS is made from the clinical presentation supported by a history of recent viral infection, elevations in the levels of protein in the CSF, and the results of EMG studies. The management of GBS is largely supportive and aimed at preventing complications until the recovery process can begin.[23] Respiratory support is always the priority intervention. Corticosteroid therapy is often used to attempt to reduce the autoimmune inflammation, but steroids have not been conclusively proven to be of benefit in GBS. Positive outcomes have been achieved with the use of plasmapheresis during the first 1 to 2 weeks after disease onset. With plasmapheresis, blood is removed and filtered of antibodies, immunoglobulins, fibrinogens, and other proteins. The filtered blood is then mixed with an isotonic solution or fresh frozen plasma and returned to the patient.

Respiratory failure from neuromuscular weakness is common in GBS. Continuous monitoring of vital capacity, tidal volume, or minute volume is performed, and intubation with mechanical ventilation is generally initiated when the patient's vital capacity falls below a preset optimal level, usually about 1.0 to 1.5 L for an average-size adult.[3] The need for long-term ventilatory support necessitates a tracheostomy. Atelectasis and pneumonia are common complications. Intensive care placement may be necessary for weeks, and meticulous supportive care is needed. Rigorous assessment of motor, sensory, and cranial nerve status is ongoing.

Patients can lose weight rapidly with GBS, and nutritional support is a priority concern. Complete immobility can cause a rapid loss of muscle mass.[13] Nutritional support is crucial for patients who need to be weaned from mechanical ventilation. Tube feedings may be used, but if the patient also experiences autonomic dysfunction and paralytic ileus, total parenteral nutrition (TPN) may need to be implemented.

Supportive care also addresses the range of concerns related to partial or total immobility and loss of self-care abilities. Interventions include standard measures for preventing skin breakdown and maintaining range of motion in all joints. The risk of deep vein thrombosis (DVT) and pulmonary embolus is high, and low-dose anticoagulant therapy may be initiated.[25] A regular bowel program is established, and either indwelling or intermittent catheterization is implemented. A thorough rehabilitation plan will be established as soon as the patient begins to recover. Physical therapy is initiated with safeguards to prevent excessive fatigue, which can prolong the patient's recovery.[25]

It is critical to remember that the patient remains alert, aware, and cognitively intact throughout the course of GBS. Sleep disturbances are extremely common and can contribute to sensory deprivation or overload symptoms in patients who are maintained in intensive care unit settings for protracted periods of time. The patient needs meaningful stimulation and communication and should be included in care decisions as much as possible even if eyebrow raising or eye blinks are the full extent of the patient's ability to communicate. Family members are also encouraged to participate in care activities to their level of tolerance.

### Patient/family education

Guillain-Barré syndrome is a terrifying and mysterious disease process for the patient and family. It is often difficult to convince the patient and family that recovery from GBS is not just possible but expected. Teaching about the disease and its management is an important nursing responsibility. Reteaching of basic principles is commonly necessary. The nursing staff also need to encourage the patient and family to remain optimistic about the future. Each stage of GBS increases the anxiety level of an alert patient, particularly the need for intubation. It is difficult for patients to communicate their needs for position changes, pain relief, and restful sleep. The slow pace of recovery may cause the patient and family to become discouraged about the future. Once patients are moved from the intensive care unit setting they lose the constant support and care of the critical care nurses and may become extremely fearful about the ability of nurses on less acute units to adequately meet their needs. The patient's care manager needs to carefully coordinate care services to ensure that all transitions are as smooth and anxiety free as possible. Referral for community-based care and rehabilitation may also be needed.

## critical thinking QUESTIONS

1 You are caring for Mr. Martin, who was admitted 2 days ago with a left hemisphere ischemic stroke. You were told during report that he has "some aphasia." What kinds of assessment activities would you plan to thoroughly evaluate the nature and extent of his communication problems?

2 Mrs. Gomez has experienced a right hemisphere stroke, and you suspect that she may be vulnerable to sensory-perceptual deficits.
   a. How would you assess the presence and severity of problems such as hemianopia, unilateral neglect, or agnosia?
   b. What effects might her right-sided stroke have on your plan for compensating for these deficits?

3 The nursing diagnosis of risk for altered nutrition: less than daily requirements might apply to patients with Parkinson's disease and myasthenia gravis.
   a. How would your nursing interventions related to nutrition be the same for these two disorders?
   b. How would your interventions differ?

4 Jane Schwartz is admitted for an acute exacerbation of her myasthenia gravis. You gave her a dose of Mestinon at 11:30 AM before lunch. It is now 1:00 PM and she is reporting dramatically increased weakness, cramping, gastrointestinal upset, and difficulty swallowing her saliva.
   a. Is this likely to be a myasthenic or a cholinergic crisis? Support your choice.
   b. How could the two forms of crisis be differentiated?

## chapter SUMMARY

### CEREBROVASCULAR DISEASE

- Stroke is the most common disease of the nervous system and the third-leading cause of death in the United States.
- Strokes have ischemic and hemorrhagic etiologies. Thrombi and emboli are the most common forms of ischemic strokes. Hemorrhagic strokes can be caused by vessel rupture, aneurysms, and AVMs.
- Over 75% of strokes affect elders, and the middle cerebral artery is the blood vessel affected most commonly.
- Risk factors for stroke include advancing age, hypertension, heart disease, and diabetes mellitus. Men are affected slightly more often, and African Americans have a significantly increased risk of stroke.
- A TIA is a brief episode of cerebral ischemia that warns the patient of an underlying pathological condition. It may include virtually any focal neurological symptom and persists for less than 24 hours, usually less than 1 hour.
- A stroke causes a core of necrotic tissue surrounded by a much wider zone of ischemia where the tissue is potentially viable.
- Clinical manifestations of stroke vary based on the location of the ischemia but typically include hemiparesis or hemiplegia, sensory deficits, cognitive-perceptual problems, communication deficits, and problems with bowel and bladder control.
- Aphasia is a disorder of language (speech, reading, writing, understanding) caused by damage to the speech-controlling areas of the brain. Nonfluent aphasia is expressive and affects speech and writing. Fluent aphasia is sensory in nature and affects understanding and reading.
- Strokes are diagnosed by the presence of classic symptoms and CT scan, which can determine whether the damage is ischemic or hemorrhagic.
- Antiplatelet therapy with aspirin or ticlopidine (Ticlid) is used to prevent TIAs from progressing to stroke or to prevent stroke recurrence. Reperfusion therapy is attempted for some ischemic strokes.
- Carotid endarterectomy may be performed if the source of ischemia is stenosis in the internal carotids.
- Initial care of the stroke patient focuses on stabilization and prevention of complications.
- Active rehabilitation begins within a few days for ischemic strokes. It teaches the patient to compensate for motor losses and adapt self-care activities to residual functions.
- A major focus of nursing intervention is prevention of the complications of immobility.

- Safe swallowing is the foundation of adequate nutrition. Patients are taught to sweep pocketed food from the affected side of the mouth after they eat.
- Patients with aphasia need extra time for responding and should be encouraged to practice speaking. Families need to be incorporated into the rehabilitation plan.
- Sensory-perceptual deficits create significant risks for environmental safety. Modifications of the environment are essential.
- Patients are often emotionally labile after stroke. This is challenging and upsetting for families.
- Cerebral aneurysms and arteriovenous malformations are common causes of intracerebral hemorrhage. The preferred treatment is surgical.
- Outcomes of intracerebral hemorrhage are often poor. Care is similar to that required following ischemic stroke.

## DEGENERATIVE DISEASES

- Multiple sclerosis is a chronic autoimmune disorder involving patchy demyelination of the white matter of the central nervous system.
- Multiple sclerosis follows a variety of courses. Many patients experience minimal disability after many years. Others progress quickly to disability. There is no known cure.
- Parkinson's disease involves a deficiency of dopamine in the basal ganglia and produces multiple movement problems. Classic symptoms include rigidity, tremor, and bradykinesia.
- Symptoms of Parkinson's disease are managed by the administration of a levodopa product. Treatment is symptomatic.
- Myasthenia gravis is a neurological disease in which nerve impulses fail to cross the myoneural junction.
- Myasthenia gravis is managed by the administration of Mestinon, which supports muscle function.
- Both cholinergic and myasthenic crises may occur. Respiratory failure is the primary challenge.
- Amyotrophic lateral sclerosis is a degenerative, fatal disorder of the voluntary muscles. Death occurs from failure of the respiratory system.
- Guillain-Barré syndrome is an acute demyelinating disorder that may follow an upper respiratory illness. It is characterized by ascending weakness or paralysis that may cause total paralysis and respiratory failure. The deficits are reversible.

## References


1. Ackerman L: Interventions related to neurologic care, *Nurs Clin North Am* 27(2):325, 1992.
2. American Heart Association: *1993 heart and stroke facts,* Dallas, 1994, American Heart Association.
3. Calliano C: Guarding against aspiration complications, *Nursing* 25(6):52, 1995.
4. Cerrato PL: Nutrition support. Diet therapy helps this drug work better, *RN* 54(2):71, 1991.
5. Cochran I, Flynn CA, Goetz G et al: Stroke care—piecing together the long term picture, *Nursing* 24(6):34, 1994.
6. Cochran JW, Kessler ES, Wittenborn R: Neurologic disease: five scenarios to manage, *Patient Care* 28(10):32, 1994.
7. Donohoe KM: Nursing care of the patient with myasthenia gravis, *Neurol Clin* 12(2):369, 1994.
8. Dowling GA: Sleep in older women with Parkinson's disease, *J Neurosci Nurs* 27(6):355, 1995.
9. Easton JD: Preventing stroke: an overview of medical and surgical options. In *Healthcare information projects; reducing the odds of stroke,* New York, 1995, McGraw-Hill.
10. Fitzsimmons B, Bunting LK: Parkinson's disease, *Nurs Clin North Am* 28(4):807, 1993.
11. Gwynn M: TPA in acute stroke—risk or reprieve? *J Neurosci Nurs* 25(3):180, 1993.
12. Hayn MA, Fisher TR: Stroke rehab, *Nursing* 27(3):40, 1997.
13. Hickey J: *The clinical practice of neurological and neurosurgical nursing,* ed 4, Philadelphia, 1997, Lippincott-Raven.
14. Hickey J: Myasthenic crisis—your assessment counts, *RN* 54(5):54, 1991.
15. Hopkins LC: Clinical features of myasthenia gravis, *Neurol Clin* 12(2):243, 1994.
16. Jacob D et al: The US decline in stroke mortality: what does ecological analysis tell us? *Am J Public Health* 82(12):1596, 1992.
17. Kane-Carlsen PA: Managing patients with TIAs, *Nursing* 22(1):34, 1992.
18. Lugger KE: Dysphagia in the elderly stroke patient, *J Neurosci Nurs* 26(2):78, 1994.
19. Mayberg MR, Batjer HH, Dacey R, Diringer M: Guidelines for the management of aneurysmal subarachnoid hemorrhage, *Stroke* 25(11):2315, 1994.
20. Mitchell G: Update on multiple sclerosis therapy, *Med Clin North Am* 77(1):231, 1993.
21. Moore K: Stroke, the long road back, *RN* 57(3):50, 1994.
22. Moore K, Trifiletti E: Stroke—the first critical days, *RN* 57(2):22, 1994.
23. Morgan SP: A passage through paralysis, *Am J Nurs* 91(10):70, 1991.
24. Mower DM: Brain attack—treating acute ischemic CVA, *Nursing* 27(3):35, 1997.
25. Murray DP: Impaired mobility: Guillain-Barré syndrome, *J Neurosci Nurs* 25(2):100, 1993.
26. Murray TJ: The psychosocial aspects of multiple sclerosis, *Neurol Clin* 13(1):197, 1995.
27. National Institute of Neurological Disorders and Stroke tPA Stroke Study Group: Tissue plasminogin activator for acute ischemic stroke, *N Engl J Med* 333(24):1581, 1995.
28. National Stroke Association: Stroke—the first six hours, *Stroke Clinical Updates* (spec ed) 4(1):3, 1993.
29. Olson E: Perceptual deficits affecting the stroke patient, *Rehabil Nurs* 16(4):212, 1991.
30. Rankin J: The nursing diagnosis: swallowing, impaired and bedside assessment of swallowing in neurologically involved cases, *J Neurosci Nurs* 24(2):117, 1992.
31. Ross AP: Nursing interventions for persons receiving immunosuppressive therapies for demyelinating pathology, *Nurs Clin North Am* 28(4):829, 1993.
32. Ruoff GE: Initial antiplatelet therapy for stroke prevention. In *Healthcare information projects: Reducing the odds of stroke,* New York, 1995, McGraw-Hill.
33. Tidwell J: Pulmonary management of the ALS patient, *J Neurosci Nurs* 25(6):337, 1993.
34. Vernon GM, Jenkins M: Health maintenance behaviors in advanced Parkinson's disease, *J Neurosci Nurs* 27(4):229, 1995.
35. Weiner HL, Hohol MJ, Khoury SJ et al: Therapy for multiple sclerosis, *Neurol Clin* 13(1):173, 1995.
36. Wojner AW: Optimizing ischemic stroke outcome: an interdisciplinary approach to post stroke rehabilitation in acute care, *Crit Care Nurs Q* 19(2):47, 1996.

# chapter 54 MANAGEMENT OF PERSONS WITH Problems of the Spinal Cord and Peripheral Nerves

JUDITH K. SANDS

## objectives

*After studying this chapter, the learner should be able to:*

1 Discuss the demographics of spinal cord injury and the major targets for risk factor reduction.

2 Describe how the pathophysiology of secondary injury extends the damage that results from spinal cord injury.

3 Link the clinical manifestations of both spinal shock and autonomic dysreflexia with the specific physiological consequences of spinal cord injury.

4 Differentiate between the effects of UMN and LMN injury on muscle function, bowel and bladder function, and sexuality after spinal cord injury (SCI).

5 Discuss the options available for medical and surgical management of the common problems of SCI including compression, malalignment, and instability of the spine.

6 Describe the nursing management of the patient with SCI with a focus on skin care, bowel and bladder care, and patient and family teaching and support.

7 Outline a standard protocol for preventing and/or treating autonomic dysreflexia.

8 Contrast the care provided to patients with SCI with that required by patients with spinal tumors.

9 Compare the clinical manifestations and nursing interventions for the patient with trigeminal neuralgia versus Bell's palsy.

This chapter presents an overview of the collaborative management of problems involving the spinal cord and peripheral nerves. The multidisciplinary challenges of spinal cord injury are the major focus of the discussion. Spinal cord injury is not a common problem, but its complexity and impact on the patient's life make it an enormous management concern in all phases of care from emergency to long-term rehabilitation. The remaining problems included in the chapter are relatively rare and often lack definitive therapy. Guillain-Barré syndrome, which affects the peripheral nervous system is included in the presentation of chronic neurological problems in Chapter 53. The pathophysiology of spinal cord and peripheral nerve injuries is complex, and the reader is also referred to Chapter 51 for a review of the associated anatomy and physiology.

## SPINAL CORD INJURY

### Etiology

The spinal column is a circular bony ring that provides excellent protection for the spinal cord from most low-intensity injury. The vertebrae are dense bony structures with multiple articulations that provide for a wide range of head and neck movement, but these articulations also create points of weakness that are vulnerable to a variety of types of injury. The close anatomical proximity of the spinal cord to the vertebrae, muscles, and ligaments increases the chance that injury to any of the supporting structures will also result in injury to the cord itself. Spinal injuries occur most commonly when excessive force is exerted on the spinal column, resulting in excessive flexion, hyperextension, compression, or rotation. Events that cause abrupt forceful acceleration and deceleration are common initiating factors.

Injuries to the spinal cord can be classified in a variety of ways that take into account damage to both the vertebrae and the underlying spinal cord. Most injuries are the result of sudden and often violent external trauma, but persons who have chronic conditions affecting the vertebrae such as stenosis, arthritis, or osteoporosis are also at a high risk for injury.

#### *Mechanisms of injury*

Hyperflexion injuries (Figure 54-1) are frequently the result of sudden deceleration as might be experienced in a head-on collision or from a severe blow to the back of the head. The head and neck are forcibly hyperflexed and then may be snapped backward into forced hyperextension. These injuries are typically seen in the C5-6 area of the cervical spine. They may result in fracture of the vertebra, dislocation, and or tearing of the posterior ligaments.

Hyperextension injuries (Figure 54-2) are frequently acceleration injuries as are seen in rear-end collisions or as the result of falls in which the chin is forcibly struck. These injuries tend to cause significant damage because the downward and backward arc of the head's movement is so great. C4-5 is the area of the spine most commonly affected.

Compression injuries cause the vertebra to squash or burst (Figure 54-3). They usually involve high velocity and affect both the cervical and thoracolumbar regions of the spine.

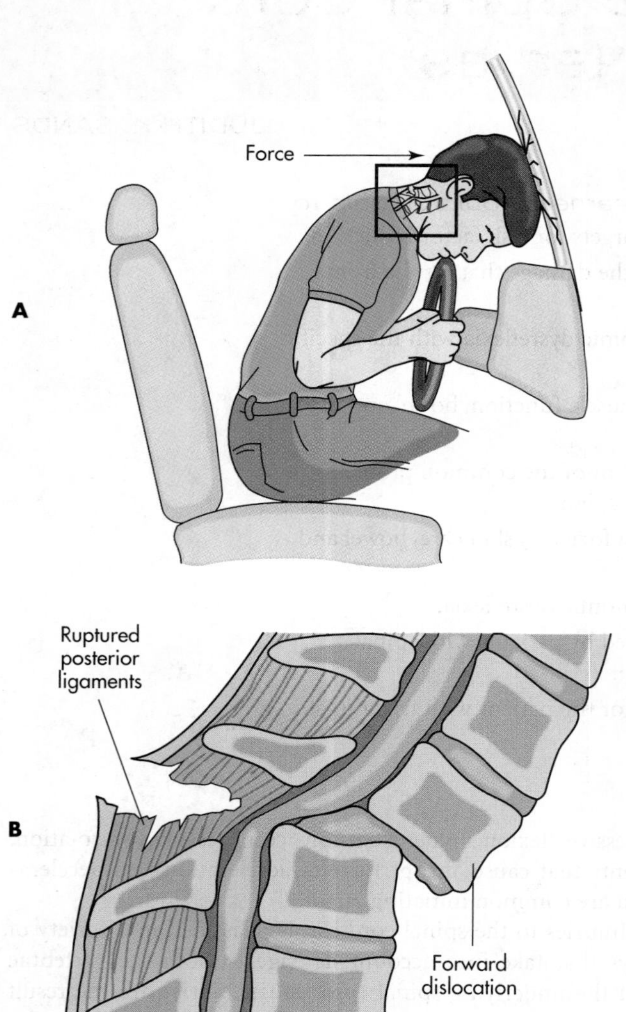


**fig. 54-1** Hyperflexion injury. If hyperflexion occurs in the cervical spine **(A)**, it can result in tearing or rupture of the posterior ligaments **(B)**, with resulting fracture or dislocation in the anterior spine.

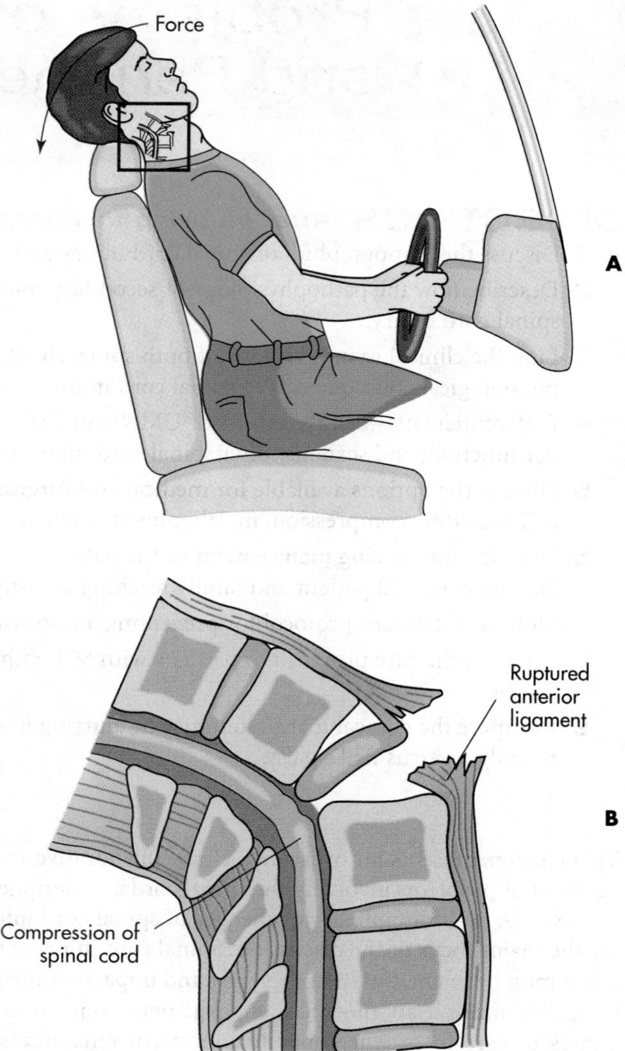


**fig. 54-2** Hyperextension injury. If hyperextension occurs in the cervical spine **(A)**, it can result in rupture or tearing of the anterior ligaments **(B)**, with dislocation or compression in the posterior spine.

Blows to the top of the head and forceful landing on the feet or buttocks can result in compression injury.

Rotational injuries are caused by extreme lateral flexion or twisting of the head and neck (Figure 54-4). The tearing of ligaments can easily result in dislocation as well as fracture, and soft tissue damage frequently complicates the primary injury. The result can be a highly unstable spinal injury. Many spinal cord injuries involve more than one type of directional force.

The injuries that can affect the spinal cord itself are described in Box 54-1. The problems of concussion, contusion, and laceration follow similar patterns to those described for head injury in Chapter 52. Penetrating injuries occur when knives, bullets, or other objects penetrate the spinal column. The object may fracture the vertebra creating bone fragments and splinters or may directly enter the spinal cord. These injuries are most common in the thoracic and lumbar spine. Complete transection, severing of the spinal cord, is a relatively rare initial outcome of spinal trauma as the protective layers of the cord are quite strong. However, many patients are seen with a clinical picture of complete transection as the result of secondary injury. A spinal cord injury is termed *complete* when there is a total loss of motor and sensory function below the level of the injury. Complete injuries are more common in the thoracic spine because the spinal canal is quite narrow in that region. An *incomplete* lesion is one in which there is some preservation of motor and or sensory function below the level of the injury.

### *Spinal cord syndromes*

Several unique and specific syndromes can occur after spinal cord injury. They represent specific types of localized

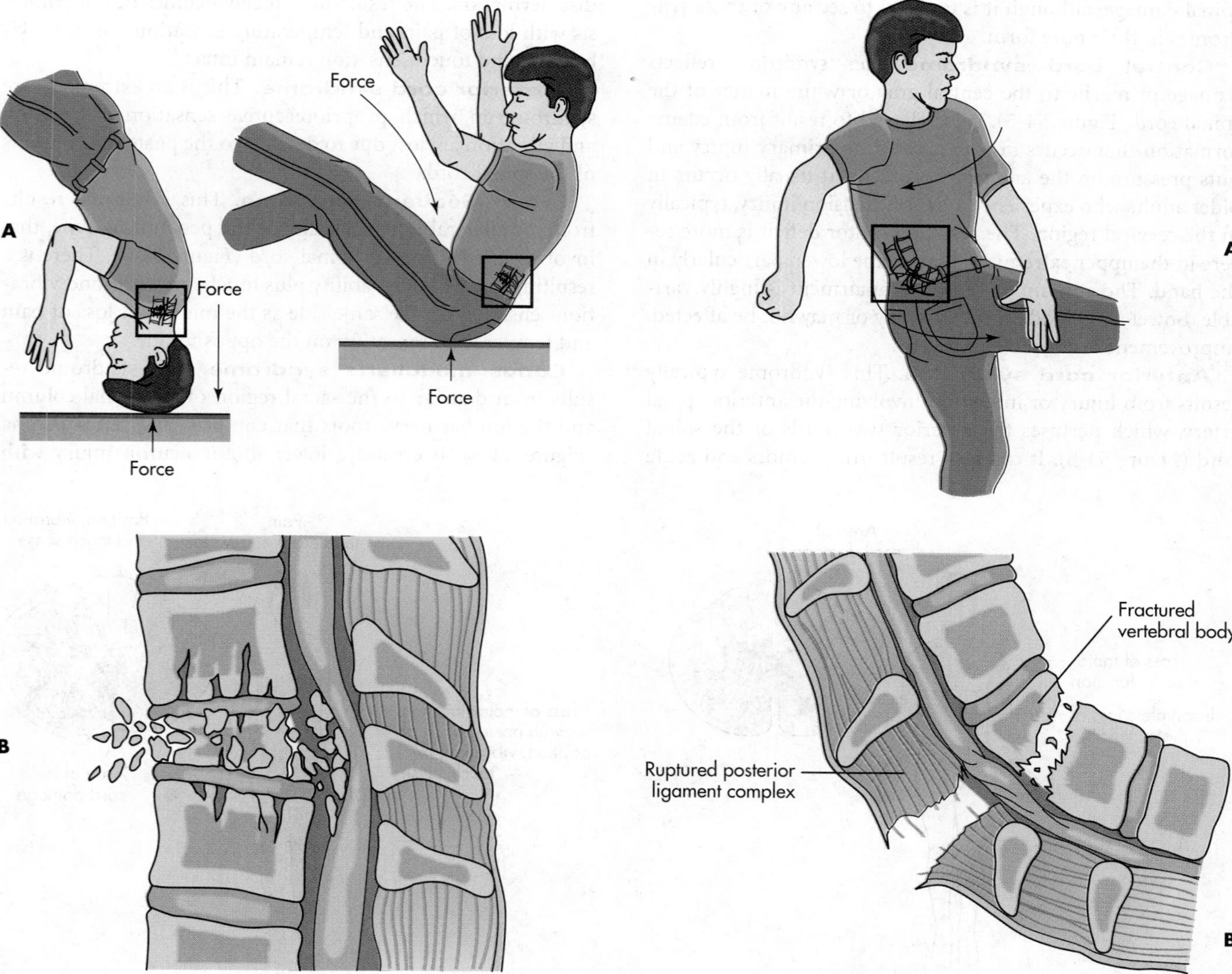


**fig. 54-3** Compression injury. Excessive direct force to either the cervical or lumbar spine **(A)** can result in shattering of the vertebra **(B)**.

**fig. 54-4** Rotational injury. When rotational force occurs **(A)**, it is frequently accompanied by tearing and/or fracture of the ligaments **(B)**.

**box 54-1** *Types of Spinal Cord Damage*

**CORD CONCUSSION**

The cord is severely jarred or squeezed as is frequently seen with sports-related injuries, e.g., football. No identifiable pathological changes are detectable in the cord but a temporary loss of motor or sensory function, or both, can occur. The dysfunction usually resolves spontaneously within 24-48 hours.

**CORD CONTUSION**

This injury is frequently caused by compression. Bleeding into the cord results in bruising and edema. The extent of damage reflects the adequacy of the overall perfusion to the cord and the severity of the inflammatory response.

**CORD LACERATION**

An actual tear occurs in the cord which results in permanent injury since the neurons of the central nervous system do not regenerate. Contusion, edema and compression will all usually be present and complicate the damage.

**CORD TRANSECTION**

A complete or incomplete severing of the spinal cord with loss of neurological function below the level of the injury. The cord segment identified reflects the lowest cord segment in which neurological function is preserved.

spinal damage, although it is unusual to see any of these syndromes in their pure form.

**Central cord syndrome.** This syndrome reflects damage primarily to the central gray or white matter of the spinal cord (Figure 54-5). It is believed to result from edema formation that occurs in response to the primary injury and puts pressure on the anterior horn cells. It usually occurs in older adults who experience a hyperextension injury, typically in the cervical region. The resulting motor deficit is more severe in the upper extremities than in the lower, particularly in the hand. The amount of sensory impairment is highly variable. Bowel and bladder function may or may not be affected. Improvement over time is expected.

**Anterior cord syndrome.** This syndrome typically results from injury or infarction involving the anterior spinal artery, which perfuses the anterior two thirds of the spinal cord (Figure 54-6). It can also result from tumors and acute disc herniation. The resultant damage includes motor paralysis with loss of pain and temperature sensation. Position, vibration, and touch sensation remain intact.

**Posterior cord syndrome.** This is an extremely rare syndrome in which proprioreceptive sensation of position and vibration are lost due to damage to the posterior columns of the spinal cord.

**Brown-Séquard syndrome.** This syndrome results from a unilateral injury, usually of the penetrating type, that involves just half of the spinal cord (Figure 54-7). There is a resulting loss of motor ability plus touch, pressure, and vibration sensation on the same side as the injury but loss of pain and temperature sensation on the opposite side.

**Conus medullaris syndrome.** This syndrome results from damage to the sacral region of the spinal column and the lumbar nerve roots that comprise the cauda equina (Figure 54-8). It creates a lower motor neuron injury with

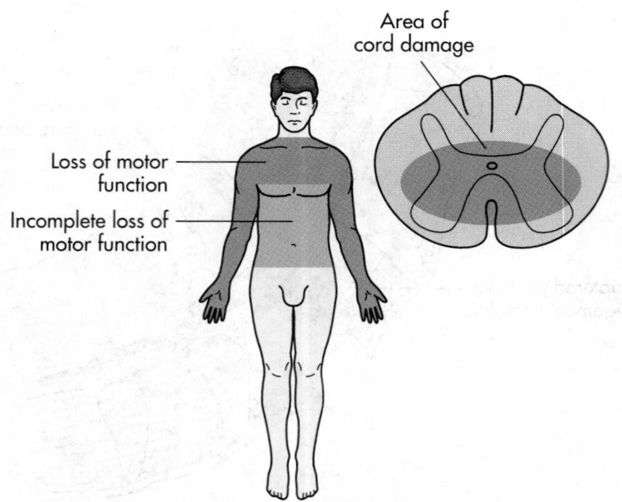


**fig. 54-5** Central cord syndrome.

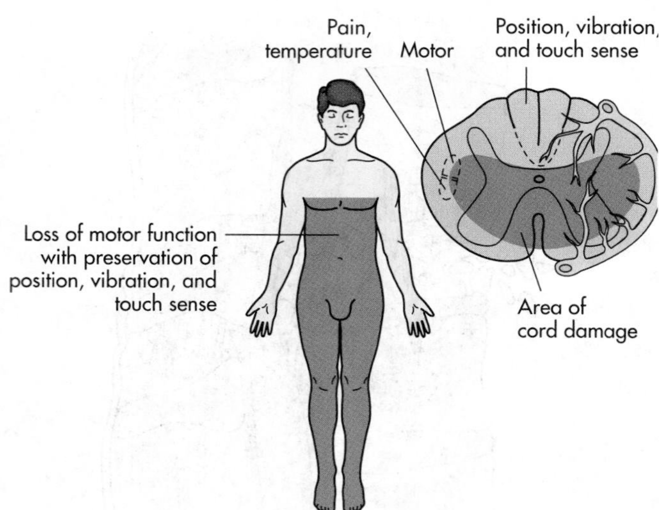


**fig. 54-6** Anterior cord syndrome.

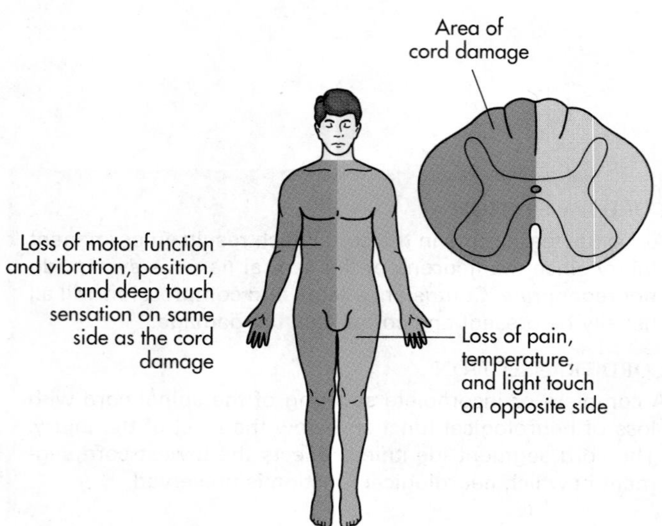


**fig. 54-7** Brown-Séquard syndrome.

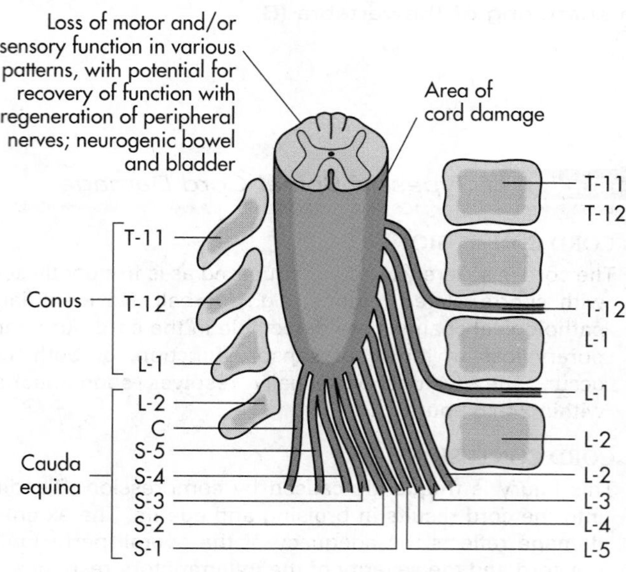


**fig. 54-8** Conus medullaris and cauda equina syndrome.

flaccid paralysis of the bowel and bladder and loss of sexual function. Motor function in the legs and feet may be affected to various degrees, but sensory involvement is rarely present.

## Epidemiology

Spinal cord injuries (SCIs) are catastrophic crises whose incidence has remained fairly stable in recent years. The 10,000 new injuries occurring each year have produced an estimated 200,000 to 500,000 individuals living with the consequences of SCI in the United States.[22] Age and sex are the primary risk factors. Greater than 80% of all persons affected are male, and greater than 60% of SCIs occur in persons between 15 and 25 years of age. Nineteen is the most prevalent age for injury. Of all SCIs, 48% result from motor vehicle accidents. Falls cause 20%, sports injuries (primarily diving accidents) 14%, and trauma 15% (gunshots, stabbings, etc.).[22] Alcohol and/or drug use is present in the majority of the "accidental" injuries. Falls are the most common cause of SCI in the elderly. Risk factors for SCI are summarized in the box. Accidents are such a significant cause of devastating spinal injuries that their incidence is targeted in the *Healthy People 2000* goals (Box 54-2).

Slightly more than 50% of all new SCIs involve injury to the cervical spine although the incidence of tetraplegia as an outcome has dropped slightly, possibly as a result of improved on-site emergency care and the increasing use of air bags in cars. Thoracic injuries account for an additional one third of all injuries.

The treatment and rehabilitation of patients with spinal cord injuries is a relatively recent phenomena. SCI was long considered to be an untreatable injury, and the associated mortality ran as high as 85% up to the 1940s. World War II stimulated a tremendous upsurge of research into approaches for managing spinal cord injuries, and the mortality rate today has dropped to about 3% to 4%. However, SCI remains a multidisciplinary challenge of huge dimensions, which consumes many billions of dollars annually to treat and support those affected by it. And, since life expectancy for persons with SCI is close to the norm for other adults, the demands for supportive care are truly lifelong.

**risk factors**

**Spinal Cord Injury**

**Age**

More than 60% of SCIs occur in persons 15-25 years of age

Elderly persons experience the most fall-related injuries

**Sex**

Males are affected four times as often as females

**Alcohol/Drug Use**

Substance use is present in the majority of motor vehicle accidents that result in SCI, as well as in many other accidents, diving incidents, and episodes of violent trauma

## Pathophysiology

Trauma to the spinal cord produces both primary and secondary injury processes. The primary damage results from the initial mechanical insult and is usually irreversible. Bruising and compression are the most common types of injury. The cord is rarely transected at the time of primary injury, but the initial insult initiates a self-destructive process that frequently results in a worsening of the injury. This is primarily the result of a progressive slowing of blood flow to the cord.

The primary compression, stretching, jarring, or tearing of the spinal cord causes small hemorrhages in the gray matter of the cord. Edema causes the blood flow to the cord to slow in a matter of minutes. Hypoxia develops rapidly, which often leads to tissue necrosis.

Secondary cord injury results from the body's natural responses to injury and inflammation, which can have dramatic negative consequences for the spinal cord. Capillary permeability increases in response to trauma, which allows fluid to move into the interstitial spaces. Edema impairs the microcirculation and worsens the ischemia. The developing hypoxia stimulates the release of vasoactive substances such as catecholamines, histamines, and endorphins from the injured tissue, which further decrease blood flow in the microcirculation and may induce vasospasm.[3] Proteolytic and lipolytic enzymes are also released from the injured cells, which can clog the microcirculation and worsen the edema, ischemia, and necrosis. The enzymes actively work to clear cellular debris, which can include removal of neural tissue that is then incapable of regeneration. This secondary injury process can destroy the full thickness of the spinal cord at the level of injury and further extend its effects several cord segments above and below the original level of injury. The process of secondary injury is initiated immediately after the original insult and progresses rapidly. Blood flow to the injured spinal cord is further compromised by the onset of spinal shock.

### *Spinal shock*

Spinal shock represents a temporary but profound disruption of spinal cord function, which occurs immediately

**box 54-2 Healthy People 2000 *Goals Related to Spinal Cord Injury***

Reduce nonfatal spinal cord injuries and resultant hospitalizations to no more than 5/100,000 people.

Increase use of occupant protection systems, such as safety belts, inflatable safety restraints, and child safety seats to at least 85% of motor vehicle occupants.

Increase use of helmets to at least 80% of motorcyclists and at least 50% of bicyclists.

Extend to the 50 states laws requiring safety belt and motorcycle helmet use for all ages.

Enact in the 50 state laws requiring that new handguns be designed to minimize the likelihood of discharge by children.

From US Department of Health and Human Services: *Healthy People 2000—1995, midcourse review and revision,* Washington, DC, 1996, US Government Printing Office.

after injury, typically within 30 to 60 minutes. It is a state of areflexia characterized by the loss of all neurological function below the level of the injury. Spinal shock causes a complete loss of motor, sensory, reflex, and autonomic functioning. The severity of spinal shock varies depending on the extent and level of the primary injury, but injuries at T6 or above usually result in more severe forms.

Spinal shock is the direct result of the neuronal injury and is not preventable. The normal functioning of the spinal cord is dependent on a constant low-level axonal stimulation from the higher centers in the brain, which keeps the cord neurons in a state of excitability or readiness. Without this stimulation the resting excitability of the cord is dramatically reduced. Over time the spinal neurons gradually regain their excitability, which ends the period of spinal shock. The duration of spinal shock varies greatly with an average of 1 to 6 weeks. The gradual reappearance of reflex activity signals the resolution of the spinal shock period. The clinical manifestations of spinal shock are summarized in Box 54-3.

Injury above the thoracic outflow of the sympathetic nervous system (T6-7) disconnects the sympathetic nervous system from control by higher centers in the brainstem. Therefore, the vasoconstrictive message from the medulla cannot be transmitted, and sympathetic tone is lost. Widespread venous pooling occurs in the lower extremities and splanchnic circulation, which results in hypotension, and can be severe. The unopposed parasympathetic stimulation of the vagus in the absence of the cardiac accelerator impulses causes an extreme bradycardia. This helps to distinguish spinal neurogenic shock from hypovolemic shock, which is also commonly associated with trauma. The vasodilation causes the skin to feel warm and dry but also permits significant heat loss to occur. The body is unable to use either sweating or shivering as a means to control body temperature. These hemodynamic characteristics of neurogenic shock peak in the first 3 to 4 days and then gradually taper off and stabilize over 10 days to 2 weeks. Orthostatic hypotension, however, may persist for months. The clinical manifestations of spinal shock, summarized in Box 54-3, are also the initial symptoms of spinal cord injury in general.

**box 54-3** *clinical manifestations*

***Spinal Shock***

- Flaccid paralysis
  - Affects all skeletal muscles below the level of injury
- Loss of spinal reflex activity
  - Paralytic ileus
  - Loss of bowel and bladder tone
- Sensory loss below the level of injury
  - Pain, temperature, touch, pressure, and proprioreceptive senses
  - Somatic and visceral sensation
- Bradycardia (results from unopposed parasympathetic vagal slowing of the heart)
- Hypotension (results from venous pooling in lower extremities and splanchnic circulation, related to loss of vasomotor tone)
- Loss of temperature control
  - Warm, dry skin
  - Inability to shiver or perspire
  - Poikilothermia: the body assumes the temperature of the external environment

### Clinical manifestations

The clinical manifestations of spinal cord injury are dependent on the level of the injury and whether the injury is complete or incomplete. The terms *paraplegia* and *tetraplegia* are used to describe the functional consequences of SCI. Tetraplegia is recommended in place of the former "quadraplegia."[1] The American Spinal Injury Association defines *tetraplegia* as "the impairment or loss of motor and/or sensory function in cervical segments of the cord due to damage of neural elements within the spinal canal. The arms, trunk, legs and pelvic organs are affected."[1] *Paraplegia* refers to a similar impairment affecting thoracic, lumbar, or sacral segments of the cord.

The functional losses and residual functions that characterize injuries at specific spinal segments are summarized in Table 54-1. The sensory dermatomes are illustrated in Figure 54-9. The sparing of even one spinal segment can have significant impact on the patient's future self-care potential, particularly in the cervical spine.

**Respiratory system effects.** The effects of spinal cord injury on respiratory function are of critical importance, particularly with cervical injuries. All ventilatory muscles receive their innervation from the spinal cord. Disturbance of respiratory function in injuries below T6 is minimal, but respiratory compromise becomes significant above this level. The loss of the intercostal muscles (T1 through T7) prevents adequate expansion of the rib cage and decreases alveolar ventilation by as much as 60%.[10] Both the intercostal and abdominal muscles (T6 through T12) are essential for adequate and effective coughing.

The most immediate threat of a cervical injury is hypoventilation. The action of the diaphragm is controlled by the phrenic nerve and accounts for 50% to 60% of an individual's vital capacity. Phrenic nerve innervation occurs at C3 through C5 with the C4 root being most critical.[16] Therefore, injury above C4 necessitates intubation and mechanical ventilation. The accessory muscles are innervated from C2 through C8, and injuries in this area reduce their ability to assist in the effort of breathing.

**Effects of upper motor neuron or lower motor neuron injury.** The effects of SCI are primarily determined by the level of injury, but injury to upper versus lower motor neurons is also an important consideration in outcome, particularly when the effects of injury on bowel, bladder, and sexual function are considered. Lower motor neurons (LMNs) (Figure 54-10, p. 1789) consist of the large anterior horn cells located in the anterior gray matter of the spinal cord or the motor cranial nuclei of the brainstem. Each anterior horn cell has a long axon that exits the cord via the anterior spinal root and extends out to a peripheral nerve (Chapter 51). When a lesion involves some part of the LMN, it characteristically

**table 54-1** *Physical Effects and Functional Outcomes of SCI*

| Level of Injury | Motor/Sensory Effects | Functional Potential |
|---|---|---|
| C1 through C3 | No voluntary movement or sensation below the level of the injury<br>Remaining function in the trapezius, sternomastoid, and platysma muscles allowing head and neck movement with varying degree of control<br>Diaphragm and intercostal muscles paralyzed<br>Sensory losses include occipital region of head, ears, and some areas of face (Figure 54-9) | Ventilator-dependent<br>Completely dependent for care<br>Limited mobility potential with voice-, chin-, or breath-controlled wheelchair |
| C4 | As above but neck accessory muscle function intact plus potential for partial function of diaphragm<br>Some shoulder movement | May be able to breathe without ventilator for intervals<br>May have limited self-feeding ability with adaptive sling |
| C5 | Deltoid and biceps function present, which adds shoulder strength, elbow flexion, and good control of head and neck<br>Unopposed trapezius and levator scapulae action may cause shoulders to elevate<br>Full sensation to head, neck, upper back, and chest and lateral parts of upper arms<br>Phrenic nerve intact to diaphragm | Independent breathing, but poor lung capacity<br>Tidal volume 300 ml<br>Improved hand-to-mouth coordination permitting self-feeding, oral care, dressing of upper body, all with assistive aids<br>Dependent in other areas of care<br>Needs assistance to transfer<br>Electric wheelchair for mobility |
| C6 | Action of brachioradialis added, permitting wrist dorsiflexion and some grasp; some wrist extension<br>Unopposed action of biceps and deltoids pulls the arms into abducted forearm flexed position<br>Sensation present over lateral aspects of entire arm, thumb, and index finger | Independence in feeding and grooming, with adaptive equipment<br>Can assist with dressing, transfers, and elimination<br>Independence with manual wheelchair<br>Can drive a car with hand controls |
| C7 | Diaphragm and accessories can compensate for losses of intercostal and abdominal muscles and support normal breathing<br>Elbow flexion and extension present; wrist flexion and some finger control<br>Sensation to middle finger and part of ring finger | Potential for independent living<br>Can achieve independence in feeding, bathing, dressing, transfer, wheelchair mobility, and elimination care |
| C8 | Addition of adductor and internal rotator muscles balance muscle function and eliminate abnormal arm and shoulder positions<br>Full sensation to hand; finger flexion | Moderate to full control of shoulders, arm, wrist, and fingers<br>Should be able to live independently |
| T1 through T5 | No voluntary movement or sensation below the level of the injury<br>Full control of upper extremities<br>Some intercostal and thoracic muscle function<br>Sensation intact to arms and midchest/midback | Pulmonary function within acceptable norms; tidal volume 500-700 ml<br>Independent in self-care; manual wheelchair<br>Potential for full-time employment |
| T6 through T10 | Increasing control over abdominal and trunk muscles<br>Sensation steadily increasing to level of umbilicus and midback | Balance improves with each segment of abdominal muscles<br>No interference with respiratory function<br>Full independence in care; manual wheelchair<br>Employment reasonable expectation, can participate in sports activities |
| T11 through L5 | Progressively adds function of hip flexors, knee extension, knee flexion, and ankle dorsiflexion<br>Slight foot movement added at L4<br>Sensation intact to lower abdomen, hips, anterior surface of legs, selected sections on posterior of legs (Figure 54-9)<br>No sensation present in groin, genitals, anus, or portions of buttocks | Independent in self-care<br>Ambulation with long leg braces possible, but tires easily |
| S1 through S5 | Progressive return of full control to legs, ankles, and feet<br>Progressive control of bowel, bladder, and sexual function. Sensory function to groin, anus, and posterior aspects of legs and feet | Independent in self-care<br>Independent ambulation; short braces may be used for support |

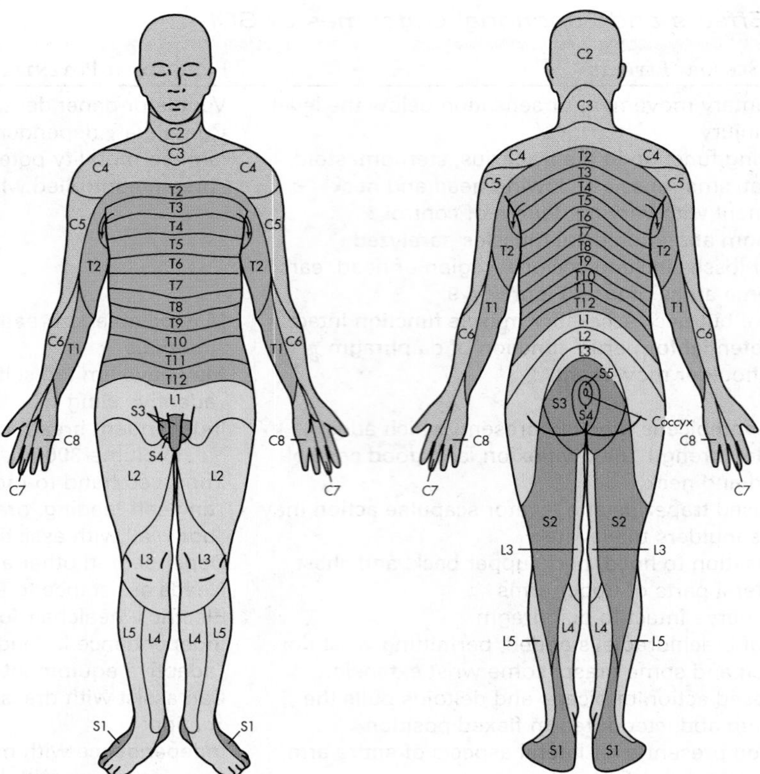


fig. 54-9 Sensory dermatomes.

results in flaccid muscle weakness or paralysis, loss of reflex activity, and atrophy of the involved muscles.

Upper motor neurons (UMNs) (Figure 54-10) originate in the motor strip of the cerebral cortex and in multiple brainstem nuclei, and they eventually synapse with LMNs in the spinal cord. Any lesion that destroys UMNs or interferes with their influence over LMNs is called an *upper motor neuron injury.* Initially, the muscles affected by a UMN injury are flaccid (hypotonic) and hyporeflexic. This period of hypotonicity persists for a variable period of time, but gradually the reflex arcs become increasingly reactive in the absence of UMN modulation. Voluntary muscle function is lost, but hyperreflexia of all cord segments occurs with increased muscle tone and spasticity in response to muscle stretch or autonomic or noxious stimuli.

The principles of upper and lower motor neuron injury apply to skeletal muscles below the level of spinal cord injury, but they are also important determinants of residual bowel, bladder, and sexual functioning. The micturition reflex center is located in the conus medullaris at S2 through S4 and is linked to the detrusor muscle of the bladder by sensory and motor fibers in the pelvic nerves.[6] Injury above this level affects the UMN control of micturition. The micturition center remains functional, as does the internal sphincter, but they are no longer under voluntary control. The reflex arc is intact but the voluntary coordinated control of urination is lost. After the period of spinal shock, as spinal reflex activity resumes, a spastic automatic bladder develops. The person is unable to sense bladder fullness or an urge to void, and the bladder fills and empties spontaneously. An LMN injury below T12 directly affects the micturition center and results in an autonomous flaccid bladder. The reflex arc is no longer intact. The person is unaware of bladder distention, and the reflex center and both urinary sphincters are nonfunctional. The bladder can easily overdistend, and urinary retention, infection, and overflow incontinence are common.

The spinal defecation reflex center is also located at S2 through S4, and similar types of outcomes accompany injury to this area of the spinal cord. Injuries affecting the UMNs cause a loss of voluntary control over the external anal sphincter. The ascending impulses are blocked, and the person cannot feel rectal fullness nor the urge to defecate. The reflex center is intact, however, and continues to exert tone. This results in spastic bowel dysfunction, but the intact reflexes are capable of triggering regular evacuation of the bowel. Injuries below T12 affect the LMN and create flaccid bowel dysfunction. No tone exists, and incontinence can occur at any time.

Similar principles govern the outcomes of spinal cord injury on sexual functioning. SCI at any level abolishes the communication between the genitals and higher brain centers, but the sexual reflex center, which controls erection in males and spontaneous lubrication in females, is affected differently by upper versus lower motor neuron injuries.[14] The reflex center is located between S2 and S4. Psychogenic sexual responses are

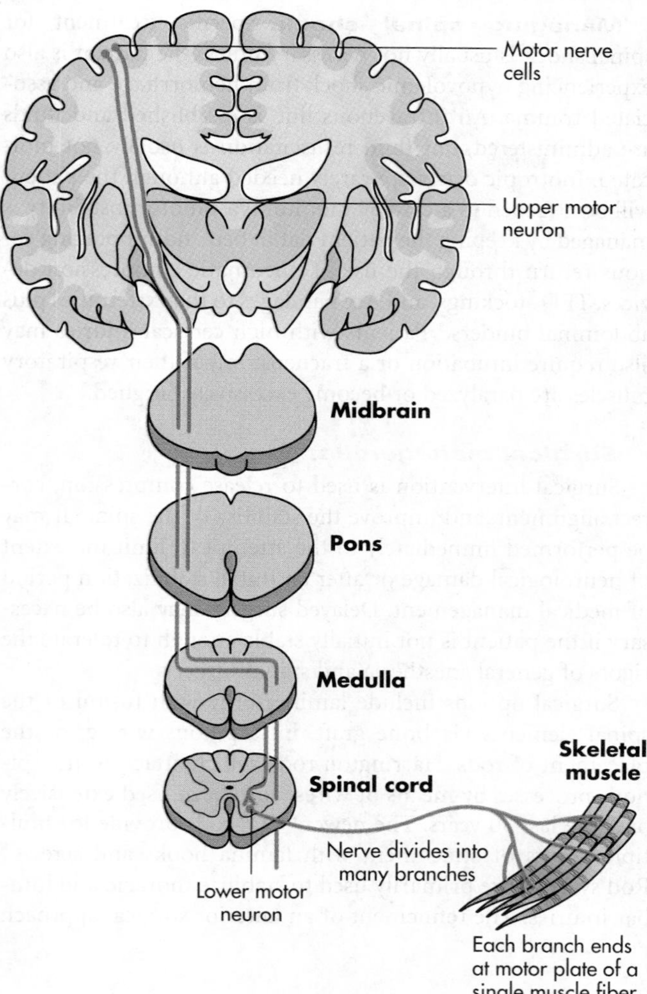


**fig. 54-10** Upper and lower motor neurons.

not possible with injuries above T12, but reflex erections are usually possible although the usefulness of these erections for sexual activity is usually governed by their duration. The higher the level of injury the more likely a man is to be able to perform sexually. The reflex center is blocked when injuries occur below T12 and no physical sexual response occurs.[14] Sex drive remains intact, but ejaculation is rare after any SCI. The experience of orgasm is possible, but patients usually report it as being different from before the injury. Women with SCI can continue to perform sexually although again the experience of orgasm is altered. Fertility is decreased in males but remains intact in females once the menstrual cycle is reestablished.

## Collaborative Care Management

### Diagnostic tests

Spinal cord injury is initially diagnosed on the basis of the presenting clinical symptoms. Emergency services policies mandate that all trauma patients be treated as potentially having a spinal cord injury until this risk can be ruled out. Approximately 5% of major trauma patients have unstable cervical spines, and as many as two thirds of these patients have no initial neurological deficits.[3] Standard x-rays can reveal the presence of fracture and/or dislocation of the vertebral bodies or spinal processes in the cervical region quite clearly, but they are less effective in identifying injuries to the thoracic spine.

The initial assessment roughly establishes the extent of injury and provides a baseline for evaluating symptoms related to secondary injury. A systematic assessment of the movement and strength of all major muscle groups is performed and documented. Baseline vital capacity is a critical value. A digital rectal examination is performed to determine whether or not the injury appears to be "complete." Any voluntary contraction of the perianal muscles, or perception of the examiner's finger indicates the presence of an incomplete injury and carries a much more favorable prognosis. A complete sensory evaluation of proprioception, pinprick, and response to light touch is also performed and recorded for each dermatome.

Both computed tomography (CT) and magnetic resonance imaging (MRI) scanning may be used to accurately evaluate the extent of injury. CT scans can reveal the exact anatomy of any bony injury and are useful in the patient who has neurological symptoms but negative x-rays. MRI shows bone poorly but provides excellent visualization of spinal cord damage related to hemorrhage, contusion, or compression. The patient's clinical status and restricted movement may make MRI scanning impractical in the acute period after injury.

### Medications

As research steadily reveals the complex mechanisms involved in the process of secondary injury after SCI, multiple research protocols have been developed to attempt to minimize or reverse the consequences of secondary injury. Only one approach has received widespread endorsement. The administration of high-dose IV bolus methylprednisolone within the first 8 hours of injury followed by a continuous infusion for the first 24 hours has resulted in significant long-term improvements in sensory and motor function. Numerous other drugs have been used, but none has demonstrated effectiveness.[11,19] Research protocols include the use of:

- Reserpine—depletes catecholamines
- Levodopa—competes for norepinephrine
- Naloxone—counters the release of catecholamines
- Mannitol—creates an osmotic diuresis
- Droperidol—blocks catecholamines

Each of these drug protocols specifically targets one of the primary mechanisms of secondary injury.

### Treatments

Immediate medical care after SCI begins in the field at the site of injury and is focused on stabilizing the spinal column. The need for decompression and realignment can then be determined by diagnostic testing. The greatest concerns for instability exist with injuries to the cervical spine, which is capable of extensive movement. The spine from T1 through T10 has little intrinsic movement and is inherently quite stable. Instability becomes a concern again with injuries from

T11 through L2 that may affect one or more of the nerve fibers of the cauda equina.[9,20]

Decompression and stabilization procedures may need to take place on an emergency basis if the patient's neurological status continues to deteriorate. Both surgical and nonsurgical approaches to stabilization are available. Surgical options are discussed below. Hard cervical collars (Figure 54-11) and backboards are used in the field to stabilize the spine during rescue efforts and transport.[3] The incidence of complete injuries has decreased from 50% to 39% over the last decade due at least in part to improved field care, which limits secondary compression injury to the nerve roots.

Most patients who do not require surgery are managed with skeletal traction and/or immobilization. Immobilization with a halo device is the most common approach. Traditional cervical traction is used much less frequently than in the past because early surgical intervention is used so successfully. Cervical traction devices such as Crutchfield or Vinke tongs (Figure 54-12) are rarely used and when necessary are used on an extremely short-term basis. The halo device may be used to apply traction weight or with an attached vest to stabilize the spine for healing (Figure 54-13).

The halo device is applied under local anesthesia and consists of a metal ring that is attached to the skull by means of two anterior and two posterior pins. External vertical rods attach the halo to the body vest. The device provides for complete external immobilization of the head and neck without flexion, extension, or rotation movements.[14] Patients with halos can be managed in standard hospital beds and be mobilized into active rehabilitation as soon as they are hemodynamically stable. The length of stay in the acute care setting after SCI has therefore been dramatically decreased. Guidelines for Care of the patient in a halo device are summarized in the box on the next page. Bedrest alone may be sufficient to provide immobilization for lower thoracic and lumbar injuries. If additional stabilization is needed, braces, corsets or a fiberglass shell may be used.

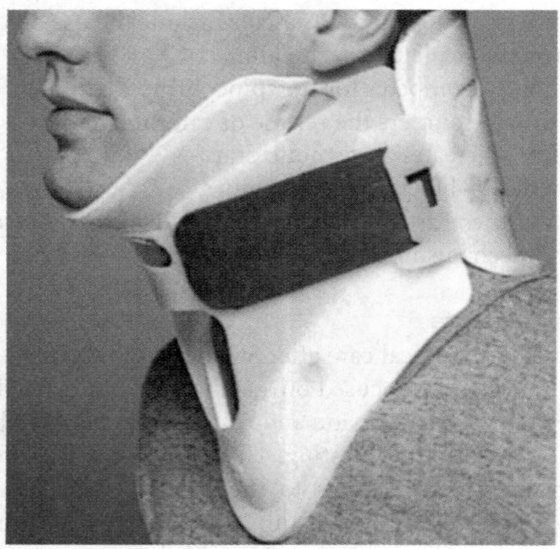

**fig. 54-11** Rigid cervical collar.

**Managing spinal shock.** Specific treatment for spinal shock is usually not necessary unless the patient is also experiencing hypovolemic shock from hemorrhage and associated trauma. An intravenous line is established and fluids are administered, but fluid resuscitation is usually not indicated. Inotropic drugs are rarely needed although the patient will be attached to a cardiac monitor. Vasomotor instability is managed by keeping the patient flat in bed and supporting venous return through the use of pneumatic compression devices, TED stockings, and Ace bandages to the extremities plus abdominal binders.[3] Patients with high cervical injuries may also require intubation or a tracheostomy if their respiratory muscles are paralyzed or become excessively fatigued.

### *Surgical management*

Surgical intervention is used to release compression, correct alignment, and improve the stability of the spine. It may be performed immediately in the attempt to limit the extent of neurological damage or after an initial stabilization period of medical management. Delayed surgery may also be necessary if the patient is not initially stable enough to tolerate the rigors of general anesthesia and spinal surgery.

Surgical options include laminectomy with fusion of the spinal elements via bone graft, intraspinous wiring, or the placement of rods. Harrington rods, which attach to the spinous processes by means of wires, have been used extensively over the last 30 years. The newer "CD" rods provide for multiple points of attachment with lamina hooks and screws.[8] Rod systems are primarily used to stabilize thoracic and lumbar injuries. The refinement of an anterior surgical approach

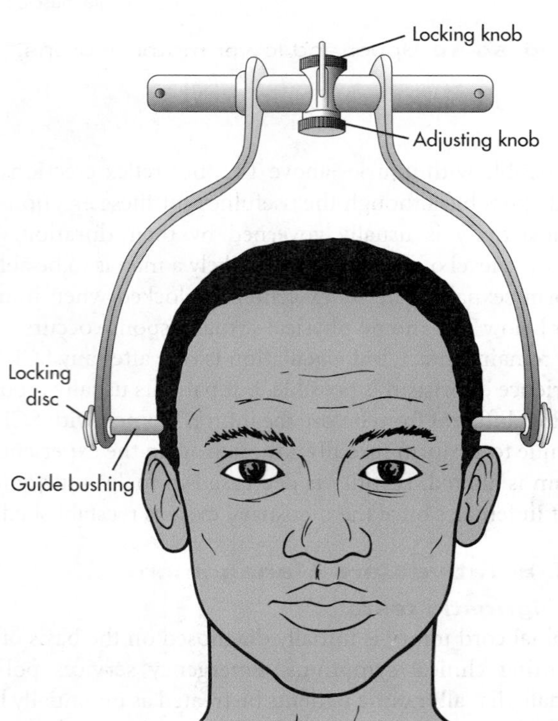


**fig. 54-12** Vinke cervical tongs.

for surgery involving the cervical spine has made cervical surgery much safer. It can now be performed much earlier in the acute management period. An anterior approach is particularly effective for removing disc material or bone fragments from the injured area. Cervical surgery can also be performed with the stabilizing halo device in place.

### Diet

Ileus develops after SCI as part of the process of spinal shock and persists for a variable length of time. The patient is given nothing by mouth and a nasogastric (NG) tube is usually inserted to reduce abdominal distention and prevent aspiration. The SCI triggers a profound metabolic stress response, which is often significantly greater than seems warranted by the severity of tissue damage. Energy needs are increased by as much as 50% after SCI. Glycogen stores are tapped to meet the body's immediate needs, but these reserves are typically exhausted within 24 hours. The body turns next to fats and proteins, which then are unavailable for tissue building and repair. A state of protein calorie malnutrition can develop within 3 to 5 days after SCI that may require intervention with total parenteral nutrition. A minimum of 2000 calories is needed daily, and patients lose weight easily. Once the rehabilitation period is underway daily caloric intake is adjusted to maintain a stable body weight.

The development of stress ulcers is also a significant concern in the early days after SCI. The risk of overt hemorrhage is about 6% and is highest in patients with cervical injuries.[22] Histamine receptor blockers are routinely administered, and the pH of all gastric secretions is carefully monitored. Antacids may be administered through the NG tube.

### Activity

Most of the progress in the management of SCI over the last 40 years has come from the development of treatment approaches that foster an early return to activity, e.g., halo devices. Bedrest with the patient lying flat is maintained in the initial spinal shock period, but patients are gotten out of bed and into aggressive multidisciplinary rehabilitation as soon as spinal stability and alignment are assured, and vasomotor status is stabilized. Mobility interventions both help to prevent the complications of immobility and disuse and establish appropriate and attainable self-care goals.

### Referrals

The management of patients with spinal cord injuries is truly a multidisciplinary effort. The nurse may serve as the case manager and coordinate the implementation of a critical pathway for care. At a minimum the patient's care will necessitate the involvement of physical therapy, occupational therapy, and social work resources. Depending on the level and severity of the injury the patient's care may also involve respiratory therapy, nutrition support, and spiritual counseling resources. Nurse specialists coordinate

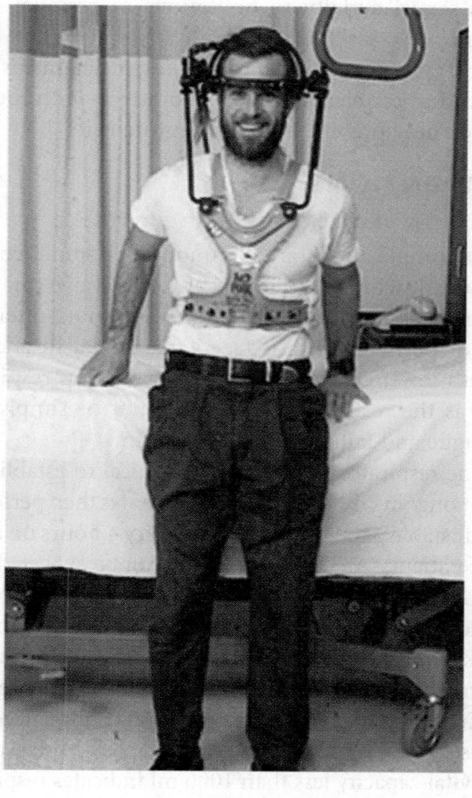

**fig. 54-13** Halo fixation device with vest jacket.

**guidelines for care**

#### The Patient in a Halo with Vest

**Managing the Halo**

- Inspect the pins and pin sites each shift.
  - Be sure that all pins are tight.
  - Provide pin care if ordered.
  - Inspect the margins of the vest for signs of skin irritation.
  - Provide skin care to all areas affected by the halo and vest.
  - Replace or add to vest padding as needed to prevent skin irritation.
- Support the vest when the patient is in bed.

**Ensuring Patient Comfort**

- Keep rubber caps on the tips of the halo ring to minimize excessive sound magnification.
- Provide mild analgesics for headache or discomfort at the pin insertion sites.
- Turn and reposition the patient every 2 hours.

**General Care Considerations**

- Adjust the patient's diet to compensate for swallowing difficulties and discomfort.
- Implement standard measures to minimize the complications of immobility:
  - Bowel and bladder care
  - Deep breathing and coughing
  - Skin care
  - Prevention of DVT

the family education efforts, but families are also referred to resources in their home communities for care, education, and support.

## NURSING MANAGEMENT

### ASSESSMENT

#### Subjective Data

Data to be collected to assess the patient with a spinal cord injury include:

- Information about the nature of the injury and how it happened
- History of loss of consciousness
- Level of consciousness
- Patient's understanding of injury and the resulting deficits
- Presence and severity of dyspnea
- Baseline sensory evaluation
- Level of sensory loss/intactness: pain, touch, pressure, proprioception, and temperature
- Presence of paresthesias or other abnormal sensations
- Presence, quality, location, and severity of pain
- Time of last urination and defecation

#### Objective Data

Data to be collected to assess the patient with a spinal cord injury include:

- Baseline respiratory status
  - Rate and pattern
  - Tidal volume/vital capacity
  - Abdominal breathing
  - Use of accessory muscles
- Baseline vital signs
  - Apical pulse and blood pressure
  - Body temperature
- Baseline motor evaluation
  - Level of injury, motor strength, and movement
  - Presence/absence of spinal reflexes
- Baseline skin assessment
  - Signs of redness, pressure, or breakdown
- Positioning and alignment of spinal column
- Presence and severity of bladder distention

### NURSING DIAGNOSES

Nursing diagnoses are determined from analysis of patient data. Nursing diagnoses for the patient with a spinal cord injury may include but are not limited to:

| Diagnostic Title | Possible Etiological Factors |
|---|---|
| Breathing pattern, ineffective | Neuromuscular weakness/paralysis of intercostal muscles |
| Airway clearance, ineffective | Paralysis of intercostal/abdominal muscles |
| Cardiac output, decreased | Decreased venous return with pooling of blood in the peripheral circulation |
| Thermoregulation, ineffective | Autonomic dysfunction and loss of ability to shiver or perspire |
| Disuse syndrome | Paralysis and required treatment immobilization |
| Impaired skin integrity, risk for | Sensory losses and physical immobilization |
| Urinary retention | Atonic flaccid bladder |
| Constipation | Atonic bowel and immobility |
| Sexuality patterns, altered | Physical effects of injury on sexual response |
| Family processes, altered | Crisis of injury and loss of self-care capacity |

### EXPECTED PATIENT OUTCOMES

Expected patient outcomes for the patient with a spinal cord injury may include but are not limited to:

1. Maintains a tidal volume >7 to 10 ml/kg, respiratory rate <25/min, and vital capacity >15 to 20 ml/kg. Verbalizes an absence of dyspnea.
2. Coughs effectively and lungs are clear to auscultation.
3. Is hemodynamically stable with a heart rate >60/min, and no occurrence of orthostatic hypotension.
4. Maintains a stable body temperature of ~98° F (36.6° C).
5. Maintains full range of motion in all joints. No objective sign of deep vein thrombosis (DVT) or pulmonary embolus.
6. Maintains intact skin.
7. Establishes an intermittent catheterization program that ensures urine volumes of <400 ml/catheterization. Maintains a balanced intake and output.
8. Establishes a regular pattern of bowel evacuation without incidence of impaction or incontinence.
9. Adapts sexual activity to limitations of residual sexual function.
10. Demonstrates the ability to use coping mechanisms effectively and to problem solve collaboratively with the family concerning present status and future care.

### INTERVENTIONS

#### Maintaining Adequate Ventilation

Respiratory complications are common after spinal cord injury. Any patient with a cord injury at C4 or above can be expected to need assistance to maintain respiration, often on a long-term or permanent basis (see Table 54-1). In addition, patients with lower cervical injuries may develop respiratory difficulties as the result of secondary injury or simply from gradual fatigue and failure of the diaphragm.

A baseline respiratory assessment is critical to establish parameters for ongoing monitoring. Assessment is then performed hourly on unstable patients and at least every 4 hours on apparently stable patients. At a minimum, SCI can be expected to result in hypoventilation. Paradoxical respirations may also occur when the action of the intercostal muscles is lost. The thoracic cage collapses on inspiration as the diaphragm descends and expands when the diaphragm ascends. This reversed breathing pattern is tiring and inefficient in meeting the body's needs.

The nurse closely monitors either vital capacity, tidal volume, or both. A vital capacity less than 1000 ml indicates respiratory insufficiency and a higher risk of complications. A vital capacity less than 500 ml usually indicates a need to intubate,[1] particularly if the patient's respiratory rate is greater than 30/min, or if paradoxical breathing patterns are present.[12] The physician may decide to intervene earlier if the baseline assessment reveals a history of smoking or pulmonary allergy, or a history of chronic pulmonary disease that could further compromise the patient's respiratory reserve.

Supplemental oxygen is routinely administered, and the nurse monitors pulse oximetry values and the results of serial blood gas assessments. A $Po_2$ less than 80 mm Hg or a $Pco_2$ greater than 45 mm Hg is a clear indicator of the need for intubation and supportive ventilation. A tracheostomy is performed to make patient management easier if the need for extended ventilator support is anticipated. The use of fenestrated or "talking" tracheostomy tubes enables the patient to communicate. Deep breathing remains a critical intervention for patients who do not require intubation, and the nurse helps the patient use an incentive spirometer every 1 to 2 hours while awake to expand the alveoli and support adequate gas exchange.

### Promoting Secretion Removal

Pneumonia is a leading cause of death in the acute stage following SCI. Therefore, effective secretion management is a nursing care priority. Effective coughing requires the intercostal and abdominal muscles to build up sufficient pressure in the thorax so that air can be vigorously expelled. These muscles are typically affected by high thoracic and cervical injuries, and the patient loses the ability to cough and clear the airway. Adequate humidity and hydration are assured to keep secretions thin, and chest physiotherapy is generally used to help the patient move the secretions. Frequent position changes are also important, but the positioning limitations of SCI make this extremely difficult in the early management period. To compensate for the inability to change positions, many centers use special beds such as the kinetic treatment table (Rotorest Bed), which continually turn the patient through a maximal arc of about 120° (Figure 54-14). The constant movement benefits both circulation and ventilation.

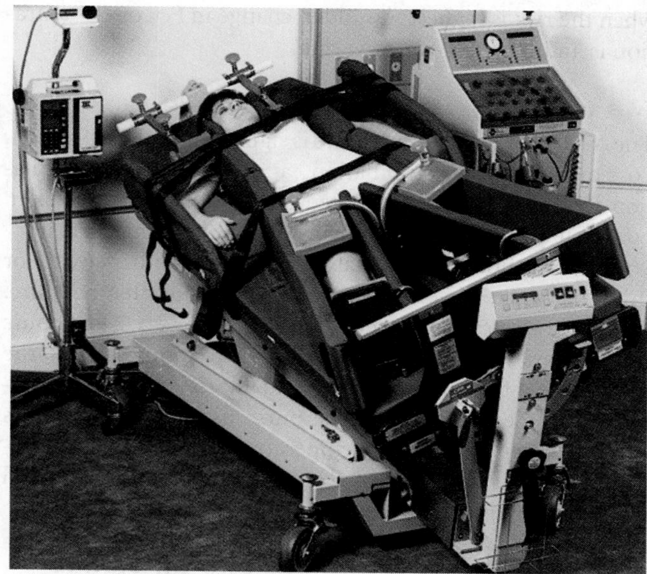

**fig. 54-14** The Rotorest Kinetic treatment table. This oscillating bed keeps the patient's spine in proper alignment yet slowly turns the patient through an arc of about 120° every 1 to 2 hours.

The nurse performs endotracheal suctioning as needed, especially if the cough reflex is weak. A moist-sounding but unproductive cough clearly indicates the need to assist in airway clearance. Suctioning can trigger a vasovagal response in patients with spinal cord injuries, which can result in profound bradycardia. This can be life threatening, especially during the unstable period of spinal shock. The patient is attached to a cardiac monitor, and the nurse carefully hyperoxygenates the patient before suctioning. All patients with weakened coughing ability are assisted to cough through the technique of "quad coughing," which is essentially an adaptation of the Heimlich maneuver. The nurse's hand is placed between the patient's umbilicus and xyphoid. The nurse pushes vigorously inward and upward as the patient exhales to support coughing and secretion removal.

### Supporting Cardiac Output

The patient is often hemodynamically unstable during the period of spinal shock. The bradycardia of spinal shock does not usually require intervention unless heart rate drops precipitously during movement or suctioning. Atropine may be given to block the vagal suppression of heart rate in this situation. Orthostatic hypotension can, however, be severe. Patients are usually stable as long as they lie in a flat supine position, but they frequently develop severe blood pressure instability with position changes. The move from a supine to a vertical position causes an immediate redistribution of about 500 ml of blood.[8] The patient with a spinal cord injury lacks the ability to vasconstrict the peripheral vessels to compensate for the fluid shifts and is likely to faint if moved precipitously.

The patient is initially managed in a flat supine position. Some combination of Ace wraps, TED stockings, pneumatic compression devices, and abdominal binders are used to support venous return.[5] The use of a Rotorest type bed also supports movement and circulation in the extremities. As spinal shock resolves, the patient is very gradually moved toward an upright position.[20] This is accomplished slowly and in tiny increments, increasing the angle of the head of the bed a few degrees at a time. The nurse carefully monitors the patient's response to each position change.

Deep vein thrombosis is another common adverse outcome of the prolonged venous pooling associated with spinal cord injury. An estimated 14% to 100% of patients with SCI develop DVT. The risk is high, but diagnosis is difficult because the patient is unaware of pain or tenderness, and the clinical evaluation is unreliable as much as 50% of the time. The nurse monitors calf and thigh circumference at least daily and assesses the skin for discoloration or warmth each time the TED stockings or other support devices are removed for skin care.[3] Doppler ultrasound can be a useful bedside diagnostic aid. The nurse also performs range-of-motion exercise each shift and avoids putting the patient in any position that results in pressure behind the knee. Pulmonary emboli occur in about 5% of patients with SCI, and subcutaneous heparin may be administered during the first 2 to 3 weeks postinjury when the risk is highest. A sudden change in $Po_2$ or $O_2$ saturation is an important warning sign.

### Maintaining a Stable Body Temperature

The control of body temperature is significantly altered by SCI. Loss of sympathetic stimulation causes widespread vasodilation with an ongoing associated heat loss through the skin. Loss of upper motor neuron control by the thermoregulatory center of the brain means that the body can neither sweat nor shiver below the level of the injury to adjust body temperature. The nurse assesses the patient's temperature every 2 to 4 hours and ensures that minimal temperature variations occur in the environment because the body gradually assumes the temperature of the environment.[8] The nurse uses extra blankets as needed to keep the patient's temperature around 98° F. The patient and family are instructed about the risks of chilling and especially the risks of overheating in hot weather.

### Preventing the Complications of Disuse

Current approaches to the management of SCI are based on early mobility and minimizing the multiple problems related to disuse. Early mobilization is important regardless of the level of injury. Mobilization initially includes active and passive range-of-motion exercise and position changes to prevent contractures and pressure damage to the skin. Mat exercises and resistive exercises are initiated to increase strength and endurance in the muscles that remain under voluntary control. Rehabilitation increasingly involves wheelchair activities although orthostatic hypotension may limit the ability of the patient to tolerate an upright position. A tilt table is used in therapy, and a reclining wheelchair may be used until the patient is able to tolerate a sitting position.

Weight-bearing activities become extremely important in minimizing the osteoporosis associated with long-term immobility. As calcium slowly leaves the bone matrix, it becomes more porous increasing the risk of pathological fracture. Hypercalcemia is a potential problem that primarily affects adolescents with SCI. The bone remodeling process becomes so unbalanced that clinical hypercalcemia may occur along with the attendant risk of kidney stones. Fifteen to 20% of patients experience excess bone deposits around the joints, which can severely limit range of motion.[20] The cause of these bone deposits is unknown.

Disuse complications are a significant priority for nursing care while the patient is hospitalized. The nurse assesses joint range of motion every day and performs range of motion exercise at least twice daily. Range of motion becomes increasingly important because muscle spasticity develops over time, and the frequency of exercise may need to be increased. Most joint deformities in a paralyzed person are preventable. The nurse carefully positions the limbs in normal anatomical positions. Knee flexion contractures and footdrop are severe complications following SCI that must be prevented. A flexion contracture in the knee joint interferes significantly with the patient's potential to bear weight in an upright position and accomplish transfers successfully. Patients with sufficient residual function will learn to accomplish transfers from bed to wheelchair and how to propel a wheelchair independently (Figures 54-15 and 54-16). Specific instruction is initiated by the physical medicine team and then practiced in the unit under nursing supervision. Prolonged sitting can also result in contractures and hip deformities. Positioning the patient in a prone position at intervals, if possible, can help to counteract this type of problem.

The entire multidisciplinary team works collaboratively to assist the patient to compensate for the losses resulting from the SCI and restore a maximal level of self-care ability. Patients with high cervical cord injuries need daily care for the rest of their lives, but patients with injuries as high as C7-8 have the potential for some degree of independent living.[22] The rehabilitation process is hard physical work as the patient attempts to build strength in the remaining muscle groups. Occupational therapists typically coordinate the efforts to obtain appropriate assistive devices and to teach the patient to successfully use them to support independence.

### Protecting the Skin

As the largest organ of the body the skin is also the most vulnerable to damage related to spinal cord injury. The loss of sensory input and restricted mobility combine to create a lifelong threat of injury to the skin. Pressure-related skin injury is the primary concern, but shearing forces are also important as patients struggle to regain self-care abilities. Skin protection is an ongoing management problem.

Care for the skin begins immediately after injury. Microscopic tissue changes related to local ischemia can occur in less than 30 minutes.[15] The skin is further compromised by the hemodynamic instability of the spinal shock period with significant venous pooling and inadequate tissue perfusion. Pressure injury to the skin is frequently initiated during the time when the patient is strapped to a rigid backboard. The nurse pads bony prominences if patient transport or diagnostic scanning prolong the backboard phase of initial care.

The use of special beds such as the Rotorest decrease pressure-related concerns significantly during the acute phase. As the patient's condition stabilizes the regular hospital bed may be used, but a minimum of a 4-inch foam antipressure mattress should be used.

Inspection and pressure reduction are the two mainstays of preventive skin care. These strategies are initially implemented by the nurse, but the responsibility for skin protection is transferred to the patient as soon as possible to the patient. Frequent changes of position are essential throughout the day. They are especially important once the patient is out of bed in a sitting position. Pressure-relieving pads should always be used in wheelchairs. The nurse teaches the patient to perform weight shifts at frequent intervals. Depending on the patient's mobility limitations weight shifts may include wheelchair pushups to relieve pressure on the buttocks, leaning alternately over the sides of the wheelchair to shift weight, or brief rest periods with the wheelchair in a full reclining position.[27] The importance of these routines cannot be overemphasized, as the development of open pressure ulcers creates serious management challenges. Pressure ulcers are extremely difficult to heal in patients with SCI and adversely affect the quality of the person's life.

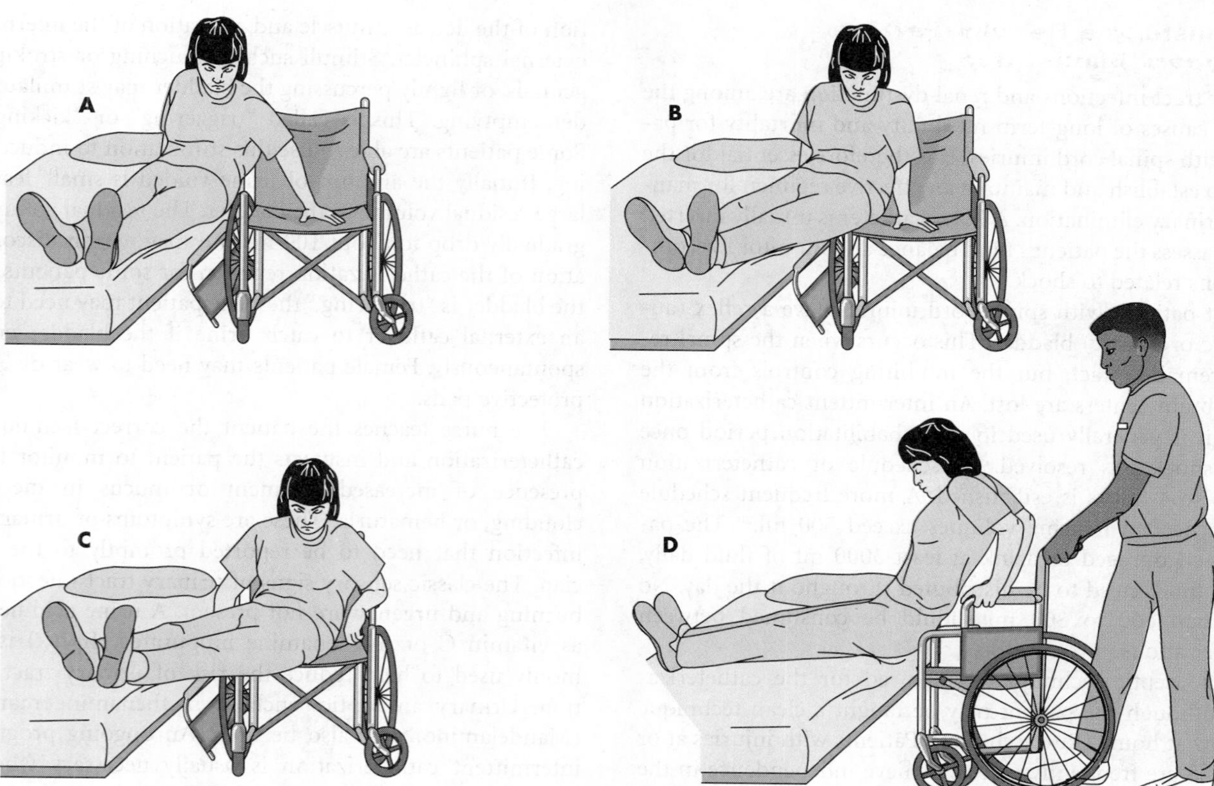


fig. 54-15 Two methods for patient with paraplegia and strong upper extremities to transfer from bed to chair. With one method: A, patient moves sideways (note wheelchair, with right armrest removed, placed next to bed); B, then patient uses her arms to lift trunk into chair seat; and C, patient settles her hips comfortably into chair; she will then swing footrests into place and lift her legs from bed. D, Second method involves patient pushing backward off bed into chair.

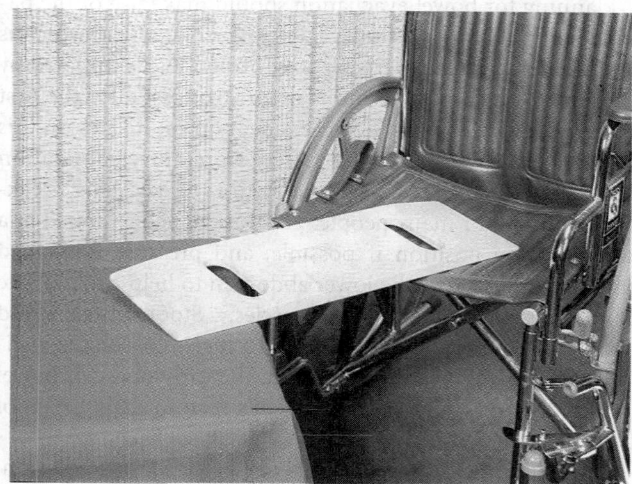

fig. 54-16 Patient with paraplegia whose upper extremity strength is not yet developed can use a sliding board to transfer from bed to chair. Board provides a firm surface on which to move, and trunk is supported by board through the move.

Inspection is the second essential intervention. Pressure causes a period of sustained ischemia for the skin. Reddened areas that do not blanch within 20 to 30 minutes are serious warning signs of pressure damage. The nurse initiates routine skin inspection with each change of position and then teaches the patient to accomplish this task if possible with the use of mirrors or other devices.

The nurse avoids the use of items such as incontinence pads that hold moisture close to the skin. The patient's skin is kept clean, but overdrying through frequent washing or the use of harsh soaps is avoided. The temperature of bath water is carefully monitored, and heating pads and hot water bottles are not used during care. If the patient's care regimen includes the use of braces or splints, a layer of thin cloth should always be worn between the brace and the skin. The nurse ensures that the patient and family receive specific instructions about the proper use and care of each piece of assistive equipment so that secondary injury does not occur. Subcutaneous and intramuscular injections into affected tissue are also avoided if at all possible.

## Establishing a Regular Pattern of Urinary Elimination

Urinary tract infections and renal dysfunction are among the leading causes of long-term morbidity and mortality for patients with spinal cord injuries. It is therefore essential for the nurse to establish and maintain an effective regimen for managing urinary elimination. A Foley catheter is initially inserted to help assess the patient's fluid balance and monitor for complications related to shock.

Most patients with spinal cord injuries have a reflex (autonomic or spastic) bladder. This occurs when the spinal reflexes remain intact, but the inhibiting controls from the higher brain centers are lost. An intermittent catheterization program is generally used in the rehabilitation period once spinal shock has resolved.[6] A schedule of catheterization every 3 to 4 hours is established. A more frequent schedule may be needed if urine volumes exceed 500 ml.[20] The patient is encouraged to drink at least 3000 ml of fluid daily, but the fluids need to be distributed throughout the day. No more than 600 to 800 ml should be consumed between catheterizations.

Strict aseptic technique is followed for the catheterizations, although the patient may be taught a clean technique to follow at home (Research Box). Patients with injuries at or below C8 are frequently able to achieve independence in the management of their urinary elimination. With a spastic bladder stimulation of the bladder wall can lead to contraction of the detrusor muscle and relaxation of the internal and external sphincter. Stimuli such as touching or stroking the genitals, or lightly percussing the bladder may stimulate bladder emptying. This is called "triggering" or "kicking off." Some patients are able to use this stimulation to induce voiding. Initially the amount of urine voided is small, leaving a large residual volume in the bladder. The residual volume can gradually drop to about 100 ml and may permit discontinuation of the catheterization regimen for some patients. Once the bladder is "triggering," the male patient may need to wear an external catheter to catch urine if the bladder empties spontaneously. Female patients may need to wear disposable protective pads.

The nurse teaches the patient the correct technique for catheterization and instructs the patient to monitor for the presence of increased sediment or mucus in the urine, clouding, or hematuria. These are symptoms of urinary tract infection that need to be reported promptly to the physician. The classic sensory signs of urinary tract infection, i.e., burning and urgency are not present. A urine acidifier such as vitamin C or methenamine hippurate (Hiprex) is commonly used to help reduce the risk of urinary tract infection. Urinary antiseptics such as methenamine mandelate (Mandelamine) may also be used. An ongoing program of intermittent catheterization is usually necessary when patients have atonic bladders resulting from lower motor neuron damage.

### research

Reference: Prieto-Fingerhut T, Banovac K, Lynne CM: A study comparing sterile and nonsterile urethral catheterization in patients with spinal cord injury, *Rehabil Nurs* 22(6):299-301, 1997.

This study compared the outcomes of sterile and clean intermittent catheterization programs for a group of 29 SCI patients. The entire sample of patients had neurogenic bladders and were studied during admission to a rehabilitation center. They were randomly assigned to one of the two groups. The sterile catheterization group used a closed sterile system, and the clean technique group used a red rubber catheter that was cleaned after each use and changed once a week.

Urine samples were obtained on a weekly basis. The rate of urinary tract infection was 28% for the patients using sterile catheters and 42% for the group using clean catheters. In both cases the most common pathogen was *Escherichia coli.* The cost of antibiotic management for the sterile catheter group was only 43% of the cost for the clean catheter group; however, the sterile kits cost 371% more than the costs for the rubber catheters. The sterile program had a net cost 277% more than the nonsterile program. The data did not achieve statistical significance because of the small sample size.

The researchers conclude that differences do exist in outcomes for patients using sterile versus nonsterile catheter programs. However, these outcomes need to be carefully weighed within the total context of morbidity and cost of care for long-term management.

## Promoting Regular Bowel Elimination

The nurse is also responsible for developing an effective bowel elimination program. Most patients with spinal cord injuries are able to regain and maintain continence with an effective bowel program. With most spinal cord injuries the neural innervation that is located in the bowel wall remains intact although injuries above T6 eliminate the patient's ability to bear down using the abdominal muscles.

Planning for bowel evacuation should make use of the patient's normal body rhythms. The gastrocolic reflex, which is responsible for strong peristaltic contractions, is initiated by a meal and warm liquids and is often strongest after the first meal of the day. Planned bowel evacuation capitalizes on this factor. The nurse assesses the patient's preinjury elimination pattern and establishes an acceptable time of day. After breakfast is optimal for many people. The patient is positioned in a natural sitting position if possible, and pressure is applied with the hands across the lower abdomen to help compensate for the loss of the abdominal muscles.[22] Stool softeners and suppositories are generally used, and a high-fiber diet is instituted if the patient can tolerate it. In the early phase of bowel training the nurse checks the patient's rectum daily for stool to prevent impaction.

Digital stimulation is generally used to initiate defecation. The nurse gently inserts a lubricated gloved index finger into the rectum to dilate the anal sphincter. Anesthetic ointments are used to minimize the spastic reflex responses that digital stimulation can initiate in the rectum. Suppositories and small volume enemas may be used during the training period to stimulate defecation if digital stimulation alone is ineffective.[8] Stool frequency and consistency are monitored and used to evaluate the effectiveness of the bowel program. Once a regular pattern has been established digital stimulation alone plus the ongoing management of diet and fluids may be sufficient to maintain regular bowel elimination. The bowel program should be acceptable and manageable for the patient to use at home after discharge. Many patients can achieve independence in bowel management, but if assistance is required it is important for the nurse to be aware that the patient's spouse may not be the appropriate person to assume this responsibility. Bowel management can significantly impede the ability of the spouse to view the patient again as a sexual partner.

### Supporting Sexual Function

Spinal cord injury has profound effects on a person's ability to function sexually, and concerns about sexuality are a critical area for nursing intervention. The nurse provides the patient with accurate and specific information about the effects of the injury on sexual response and performance.[27] This information needs to be provided to every SCI patient along with written reference materials to supplement the teaching. Generally, the higher the injury the more normal sexual functioning can be. Sacral injuries are the only SCIs that eliminate a man's ability to achieve any type of erection.

Effective nursing intervention in the area of sexuality requires far more than simple factual information. The nurse must explore each individual's sexual beliefs and practices and establish the parameters for acceptable sexual activity. Although it is true that most patients with an SCI are able to engage in satisfying sexual activity with a cooperative partner, clearly not all sexual alternatives are acceptable to every patient and partner. The nurse also emphasizes to patients that sexuality encompasses far more than just intercourse.

Most men with spinal cord injuries are not able to experience psychogenic erections (those that occur in response to sexual thoughts), but they are usually capable of reflexogenic erections. Reflex erections occur from direct stimulation of the genitalia, but may also result from stroking the inner thigh, rectal stimulation, or manipulation of a urinary catheter. The ability to ejaculate is usually not present or may occur in a retrograde fashion; but orgasm, with a perceived release of tension, is possible. Patients often report that although extensive sensory loss is present, there is heightened sensitivity in the remaining intact tissue. The woman with a spinal cord injury is able to participate fully in sexual activity, but may not experience orgasm. Women also frequently require the application of a water-soluble lubricant to replace natural lubricating fluids.

The nurse stresses that spontaneous sexual activity is rarely possible or successful after SCI and that open communication between the partners is essential. Men with indwelling catheters can either remove the catheter just before sexual activity or fold it back on the penis where the catheter can provide extra support for the erection. Women who have a Foley catheter can also leave it in place if desired. The bowel should be empty before intercourse to prevent the possibility of reflex emptying.

A variety of sexual resources exist for men whose reflex erections do not last long enough to engage in sexual activity. These include implants, injections, and vacuum pumps as discussed under impotence in Chapter 49. Nurses who are uncomfortable discussing sexual matters with patients should ensure that referrals are made to advanced practice nurses or other appropriate resources.

Most men with SCI experience infertility or low sperm counts, but this needs to be verified by laboratory analysis before sterility can be assumed. Women with spinal cord injuries, however, typically retain their ability to conceive. The menstrual cycle is initially interrupted by the injury, but then resumes after about 4 to 6 months, reestablishing fertility. Birth control counseling is therefore essential. Pregnancy can proceed safely, and infants can be successfully delivered vaginally although there is an increased incidence of urinary tract problems and autonomic dysreflexia during both pregnancy and labor (see p. 1799).

### Supporting Family Coping Resources

Spinal cord injury has devastating effects on the patient and the entire family unit. A wide range of emotional responses are experienced by each person. Roles and relationships are abruptly and often permanently altered by the injury, and the family's sense of the future is shattered. The rapid pace and intensity of the initial rehabilitation period propel the patient and family at breakneck speed toward an unclear and often frightening future. The nurse needs to be aware of the range of possible responses to crisis and be skillful in assisting patients and families to progress toward effective coping.

Grieving is an essential task for both patient and family. The patient grieves the loss of functional abilities, and family members grieve the loss of the family unit as it was before the injury.[1] Each person will move through the stages of grief at a different pace. Family members are often so focused on being positive and supportive of the patient that they fail to acknowledge their own needs. The nurse plays a pivotal role in helping each person deal openly and honestly with these complex feelings.

In addition to the obvious psychological challenges of SCI, the patient is also dealing with massive changes in the level of sensory input received from the body, and the limited world that results from immobility. The patient is confronted with the helplessness and lack of control exemplified by being unable to perform self-care or possibly even change positions. The reality of total dependency can be overwhelming. The range of emotional responses is virtually unlimited but frequently includes intense anger, fear, and depression. Acting-out behaviors are expected at some point in the rehabilitation experience. The physical, emotional, and financial impact of the patient's injury also becomes increasingly clear to the family, who may need to face an indefinite future of extensive caregiving responsibility. This can be particularly difficult when the injury affects a teenager or young adult and when alcohol or drug use contributed to the injury.

The nurse uses the principles of crisis theory to attempt to assist patients and families in coping. Shock and disbelief dominate the first stage of care when the focus is on survival. As the physical crisis stabilizes, denial typically appears. The denial may be focused on the permanence of the situation or on some specific part of the injury such as the inability to walk.[8] The nurse does not attempt to break the denial but attempts to focus the patient and family on the here and now and on actions and interventions that are necessary to meet the challenges of the present. As the reaction stage is entered the full range of emotional responses may be encountered, but severe depression alternating with anger is an extremely common pattern.[22] Encouraging verbalization and providing consistent support are important nursing interventions. Consistent caregivers are highly desirable, and the nurse must accept the patient's behavior without being judgmental. Multidisciplinary resources are used to ensure that the patient and family receive the support they need.

Reaching the resolution stage of grief over the injury and its outcomes may take years and is frequently not accomplished. However, the patient will usually gradually become an active participant in both care and rehabilitation outcomes. The patient is then supported in making decisions and assuming some control in structuring care. Early mobilization is a key strategy for effectively moving the patient past denial and reaction. The nurse reminds the patient and family that aggressive rehabilitation accomplishes good functional outcomes after even severe SCI, and almost 90% of SCI patients do return to their home settings.

## EVALUATION

To evaluate the effectiveness of nursing interventions, compare patient behaviors with those stated in the expected patient outcomes. Successful achievement of patient outcomes for the patient with a spinal cord injury is indicated by:

1. Maintains spontaneous and adequate ventilation and experiences neither dyspnea nor hypoxia.
2. Utilizes quad assisted coughing to adequately clear the airway.
3. Maintains stable vital signs without incidence of orthostatic hypotension.
4. Adjusts clothing and environmental conditions to maintain a body temperature ~98° F (36.8° C).
5. Easily moves joints through their full range of motion; uses wheelchair and other assistive devices to support mobility.
6. Uses pressure-relieving devices and frequent weight shifts to maintain an intact skin.
7. Implements a spontaneous voiding or intermittent catheterization program to effectively empty the bladder and minimize episodes of incontinence.
8. Uses a bowel program to evacuate soft formed stool daily or every other day without episodes of incontinence.
9. Speaks openly with partner about sexual effects of the SCI and refers to self as a sexual being.
10. Actively engages in the rehabilitation process and plans collaboratively with the family for the future.

## GERONTOLOGICAL CONSIDERATIONS

Spinal cord injury is a devastating and life-altering process at any point in a person's life. While most SCIs occur in young adults, about 20% occur in persons older than 65 years of age. These are usually the result of falls and often reflect the weakening of vertebra related to osteoporosis. The challenges of SCI that have been outlined in the prior discussion can be even more overwhelming for the older person. Elders experience a higher mortality related to respiratory failure, aspiration, and pneumonia and have more difficulty compensating for the other consequences of spinal shock. The incidence of deep vein thrombosis and related pulmonary emboli is higher, and they are also frequently more severe than in younger individuals

The functional losses of SCI are also often more severe for elders. Concurrent health problems make complications more common and reduce self-care potential. Elders with spinal cord injuries are less likely to achieve rehabilitation goals and are more likely to be placed in long-term custodial care.

## SPECIAL ENVIRONMENTS FOR CARE

### Critical Care Management

Critical care plays a significant role in the initial management of patients with spinal cord injuries, particularly injuries involving the cervical region of the cord. Motor vehicle accidents are the most common cause of SCIs, and these accidents frequently involve multiple trauma and not SCI alone. Patients may be managed in surgical intensive care units or in specialized neurological care areas.

Critical care monitoring and management are particularly important with unstable spinal injuries, especially if cervical traction is used to stabilize the spine. The use of special beds such as the kinetic treatment table also requires constant nursing assessment and monitoring. Critical care assessment is also needed to monitor the patient's ongoing respiratory effort and appropriately time the need for intubation and mechanical ventilation.

Critical care monitoring is essential to manage the complex hemodynamic instability that results when both hypovolemic and spinal shock occur together. Hemodynamic monitoring is frequently required to adequately assess fluid balance and cardiac output (see Chapters 17 and 22). The presence of head trauma adds the additional challenge of intracranial pressure management to this already complex situation.

### Home Care Management

The aim of the aggressive multidisciplinary rehabilitation approach provided to patients with SCI is to restore the maximum possible self-care potential and to return the patient to his home environment. In the current world of managed care the patient's acute care hospital stay is likely to be quite brief (Research Box). The patient is transferred to an acute rehabilitation setting as soon as he or she is hemodynamically stable, and problems of malalignment and spinal instability have been resolved. The patient is likely to be transferred at least one or two more times to facilities that focus on long-term rehabilitation.

**research**

Reference: Hart KA, Rintala DH, Fuhrer MJ: Educational interests of individuals with spinal cord injury living in the community: medical, sexuality, and wellness topics, *Rehabil Nurs* 21(2):82-90, 1996.

This study attempted to identify the educational topics of interest to persons with SCI living in the community. Short hospital stays mean that most patients are discharged before receiving education about all topics of concern for future management of the SCI. Shifting educational efforts to the community is an important need. The study was conducted under the auspices of a large Baylor College of Medicine study of the life status of persons with SCI and included 590 persons recruited from the metropolitan areas around Houston and Galveston, Texas. Contacts were made by telephone interview.

Topics related to medical issues, sexuality, and wellness were included in the study. Greater than 40% of the sample expressed significant interest in education related to bladder and kidney problems, testing of nerve and muscle function, pain, spasticity, sexuality issues, exercise programs, and stress reduction. Contractures, dysreflexia, family planning, alcohol and drug use, and smoking cessation were not topics of interest to the sample. Participants had a mean age of 38 years and had lived with their SCI for almost 10 years. The researchers concluded that this technique is a reasonable one for identifying topics of interest for education and that these topics are appropriate to address in community-based education programs.

**research**

Reference: Richmond TS, Metcalf J, Daly M: Requirement for nursing care services and associated costs in acute spinal cord injury, *J Neurosci Nurs* 27(1):47-51, 1995.

This descriptive study analyzed the requirement for professional nursing care and nursing care costs of patients with acute SCI. A convenience sample of 50 patients was obtained from admissions to a major medical center. The sample consisted of 26 quadraplegic, 5 ventilator-dependent quadraplegic, and 19 paraplegic patients. The researchers interviewed the patients and nurse caregivers daily and reviewed the patients' charts to obtain a clear picture of care needs and care provided.

A few patients in the sample had prolonged hospitalizations, which skewed the sample data, and the research was reported as "median" figures. There was no significant difference in length of stay between the three groups of patients. The overall length of stay was 16 days with 4 days spent in the intensive care unit and 11 days in a intermediate care unit. Care needs and associated costs of nursing care varied significantly between the groups, however, with the ventilator-dependent patients receiving the most professional care. The median number of care hours was 143.

The researchers conclude that length of stay is an inadequate measure to reflect the intensity and cost of nursing care required by patients with acute spinal cord injury and encourage "unbundling" the professional care costs from the flat hospital charges to more accurately reflect the level and intensity of care provided.

Case management is essential after SCI, and the nurse is the ideal professional to serve as case manager for patients with spinal cord injuries. Social services and community resources need to be involved from the time of the patient's admission to allow for thoughtful planning about placements and to acquire the equipment and skills needed to provide care for the patient at home. Social services are also essential to assist the family in dealing with the maze of financial costs and insurance coverage. Discharge planning must truly begin at admission even though the patient and family's shock and disbelief will make it difficult for them to play an active role in the early planning (Research Box).

Most patients require long-term rehabilitation. However, it is important to remember that 90% of patients with SCI *do* return to the home setting, but the path to this destination is neither straight nor easily traveled. The problems of SCI are lifelong and do not resolve. Effective management is focused on long-term physical and psychosocial support to minimize the incidence and severity of complications.

## COMPLICATIONS

The patient with a spinal cord injury is vulnerable to a wide range of complications, primarily related to immobility. Fecal impaction, pulmonary infections, contractures, skin breakdown, and urinary tract infection are all common complications. Much of the patient's daily routine is aimed at preventing their occurrence. Although these complications are usually not fatal, they can necessitate frequent readmission to the acute care setting, dramatically increase the cost of care, and significantly impair the patient's ability to function independently.

### Autonomic Dysreflexia

Autonomic dysreflexia is a unique complication of SCI that occurs in patients with cord injuries at T6 or above. The problem is most common with cervical injuries. Autonomic dysreflexia is an exaggerated sympathetic response, which results in uncontrolled paroxysmal hypertension.[9] The spinal nerves that innervate the preganglionic neurons of the sympathetic nervous system emerge from the thoracic and lumbar regions of the spine. The thoracic chain has primary control over vascular resistance. When injuries affect the upper cord, the sympathetic nervous system is shut off from the control of higher centers in the brain. During the period of spinal shock the sympathetic nervous system simply does not function below the level of the injury. As the hemodynamic instability gradually resolves, the sympathetic nervous system regains function but in an uncontrolled manner. If autonomic dysreflexia is triggered, a group of stimuli produce a massive sympathetic reflex discharge that causes reflex vasoconstriction. The rise in blood pressure distends the baroreceptors in the carotid sinus and aortic arch, which remain intact. These baroreceptors cause vasodilation in the vessels above the cord injury and stimulate the vagus to slow the heart in an attempt to reduce the blood pressure. The intense sympathetic response continues below the level of the injury, however, because the inhibitive impulses from the higher centers are blocked. The blood vessels remain constricted, and extreme hypertension persists (Figure 54-17).

The clinical manifestations of autonomic dysreflexia are summarized in Box 54-4. Paroxysmal hypertension is the classic defining feature, and the blood pressure can rapidly reach life-threatening levels.[20] The hypertension is accompanied by a pounding headache, nausea, and blurred vision. Vasodilation above the injury level results in skin flushing and profuse perspiration in those areas. The continuing vasoconstriction in areas below the level of the injury results in pallor and coolness of the skin along with piloerection (goosebumps). Vagal stimulation causes severe bradycardia. Patients experience variations in the symptom pattern but are usually able to promptly recognize their own unique pattern of symptoms.

The abnormal stimuli that trigger autonomic dysreflexia arise from localized areas below the level of injury. Although a variety of stimuli can trigger the response (Box 54-5), the most common cause is some form of visceral stimulation—a distended bladder or stool in the rectum. A full bladder triggers 80% of all cases.

Autonomic dysreflexia is a medical emergency that can result in stroke, blindness, or death. The major goal is to prevent episodes from occurring, primarily by maintaining an effective regimen for bladder and bowel evacuation to prevent overdistention. If the syndrome occurs, however, prompt treatment is essential. The patient is immediately placed in an upright position, which causes orthostatic changes that lower the blood pressure. Vital signs are monitored as frequently as every 5 minutes. TED stockings, Ace wraps, abdominal binders, and pneumatic compression stockings are all removed to promote venous pooling and reduce blood return to the heart.[8] If the patient has a urinary catheter, its patency is immediately checked. If the patient is using an intermittent catheterization routine, the bladder is immediately catheterized. If the dysreflexia does not respond immediately, the nurse next checks the patient's rectum for the presence of stool. If it is necessary to remove stool from the rectum, dibucaine (Nupercaine) ointment or another anesthetic ointment

**box 54-4** *clinical manifestations*

**Autonomic Dysreflexia**

- Extreme hypertension
- Pounding headache
- Blurred vision, nausea
- Bradycardia
- Profuse sweating above the level of the injury
- Flushed skin on the face and neck
- Nasal congestion
- Piloerection below the level of the injury
- Cool mottled skin below the level of the injury

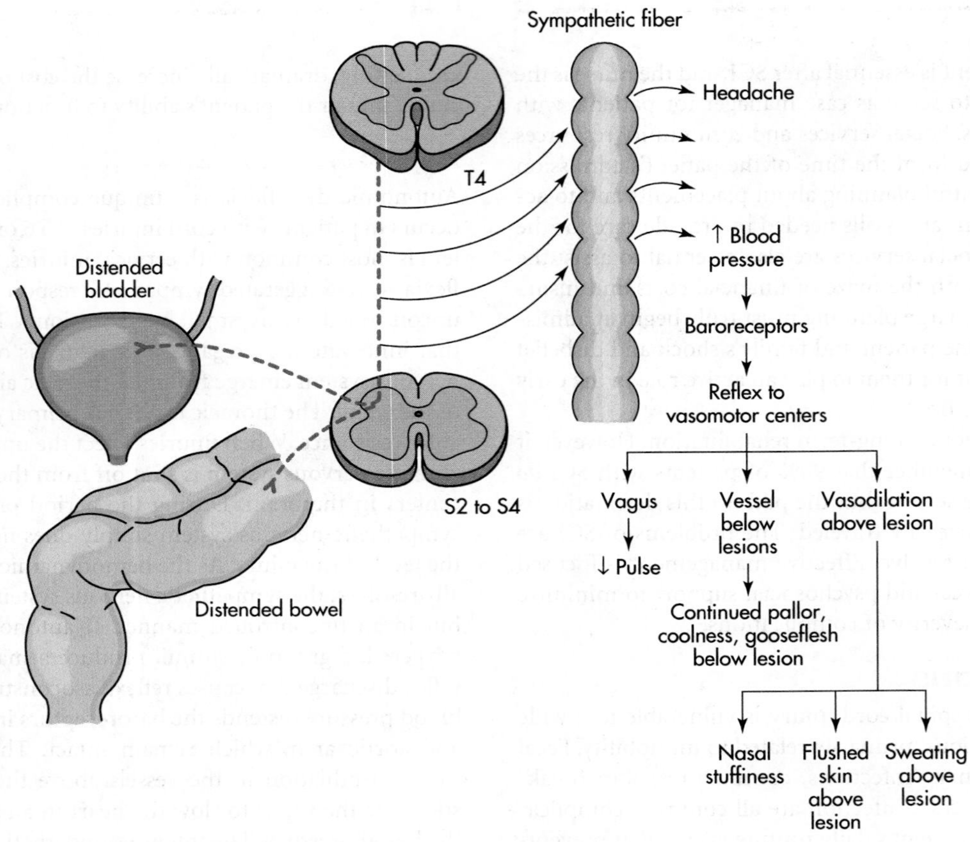


**fig. 54-17** Pictorial diagram of cause of autonomic dysreflexia and results.

should be applied before inserting the finger. This prevents triggering of another visceral stimulus and worsening the dysreflexia. If the triggering stimulus cannot be promptly identified and removed by these measures, most SCI unit protocols call for the prompt administration of emergency medications to lower the blood pressure, e.g., reserpine, hydralazine, guanethidine, nitroprusside, or diazoxide. Guidelines for the care of the patient experiencing autonomic dysreflexia are summarized in the accompanying box.

It is important to recognize that patients only become vulnerable to autonomic dysreflexia once the period of spinal shock has been completely resolved. The two problems do not occur together. Once spinal reflexes begin to return, the risk of dysreflexia grows. Up to 80% of patients at risk will develop dysreflexia within the first year after injury, although it has been known to occur for the first time up to several years after the initial injury. The incidence and severity of dysreflexia typically decrease over time.

### Spasticity

Muscle spasticity can become a serious concern for patients whose spinal cord injuries affect the upper portions of the spinal cord. Spinal reflex activity begins to reappear with the resolution of spinal shock. This reflex activity is not under the voluntary control of higher brain centers, but it is frequently interpreted by both patients and families as a sign of returning function, especially if the patient is experiencing extreme denial of the consequences of the SCI. The heightened muscle responsiveness adds resting tone to the flaccid muscles and often makes it easier to move the patient and prevent muscle wasting, but spasticity also creates safety concerns and heightens the risk for contractures.[27] Flexor spasticity develops first so the initial risk is for flexion contractures. If flexion contractures are not successfully prevented, they significantly limit the patient's rehabilitation and self-care potential. Extensor spasticity develops at a later point. Both sustained (tonic) and intermittent (clonic) spasticity can occur. Most patients experience a peak of spasticity within the first year after injury, which then stabilizes within about 2 years.

Positioning and exercise are the two primary interventions for managing spasticity. The frequency of passive range-of-motion exercise is increased to at least four times daily as general muscle stiffness tends to worsen the spasticity. The nurse limits the amount of incidental tactile stimulation while providing care and handles the patient's limbs in a gentle yet firm manner. The patient's position needs to be changed at least every 2 hours, and the joints are carefully positioned to prevent contracture development. Splints may be needed to support optimal positioning in vulnerable limbs. The involvement of physical and occupational therapists to establish an exercise plan and design effective splinting devices is essential. Noxious stimuli are avoided where possible as spasticity is triggered by many of the same factors that cause autonomic dysreflexia (see Box 54-5). Spasticity that does not respond to these general measures may require the use of muscle relaxant medications such as baclofen (Lioresal), dantrolene (Dantrium), or diazepam (Valium).[24,25] In severe cases surgical intervention with rhizotomy or a similar procedure may be necessary.

### Pain

Pain is a multifactorial sensory experience that is difficult to understand and manage. It is particularly challenging in the patient with a spinal cord injury who has experienced profound sensory losses from the injury. Pain in the early postinjury period is usually related to the fracture and soft tissue damage of the initial trauma. This pain usually responds well

**box 54-5 Common Precipitating Factors for Autonomic Dysreflexia**

- Bladder distention (80% of all cases)
- Distended bowel
- Local pressure or irritation (especially to the penis, groin, or sacrum); pressure ulcers
- Constrictive clothing
- Catheterization of bladder; digital stimulation of rectum/anus
- Exposure to hot or cold stimuli or drafts
- Abdominal or pelvic distention or infection
  - Menstruation
  - Urinary tract infection
  - Urinary calculi
  - Sexual activity, ejaculation
  - Gastritis, peptic ulcers, or gallstones
  - Labor contractions
- Muscle spasticity or pain

**guidelines for care**

**The Patient with Autonomic Dysreflexia**

1. Elevate the head of the bed to a sitting position if possible.
2. Monitor the blood pressure and apical pulse q2-5 min until the episode resolves.
3. Check the patency of the retention catheter if present.
   Ensure that it is not kinked or plugged. Insert new catheter as needed.
   Catheterize immediately if a retention catheter is not in place.
4. If dysreflexia persists, check for bowel impaction.
   If stool is present, apply an anesthetic agent to the rectum and anal area and monitor response.
   Stool can be gently removed once the blood pressure is lowered.
5. Initiate drug therapy as outlined in care protocols if blood pressure does not respond and notify the physician promptly.
6. If no cause can be identified:
   Change the patient's position.
   Send a urine specimen for culture and sensitivity.
   Assess the skin carefully for signs of irritation or breakdown.
7. Remain with the patient to provide support, reassurance, and needed explanations.

to traditional measures and decreases dramatically once the spine is decompressed, realigned, and stabilized.

Chronic pain syndromes can develop after SCI and become extremely difficult management issues. These syndromes are more common with injuries that affect the lower portions of the spine, particularly those involving the cauda equina, and occur most frequently when the injury is incomplete. Most develop within the first 6 months after the injury. Three typical chronic pain syndromes occur, and each is managed differently.

*Radicular* pain is caused by specific spinal nerve roots and produces an aching or shooting pain along the path of the nerve. Mild cases are managed fairly successfully with anticonvulsant drugs such as carbamazepine (Tegretol).[24] *Visceral* pain is poorly localized and creates a burning or aching pain that diffuses throughout the abdomen or pelvis. *Central* pain is also diffuse in nature and creates a general burning sensation that is aggravated by movement or touch. Both of the latter forms of chronic pain are theorized to occur from the abnormal firing of pain neurons, possibly because of the absence of normal input that helps the nerves to maintain a steady state. These forms of pain are more responsive to management strategies such as transcutaneous electrical nerve stimulation (TENS) units or the use of tricyclic antidepressant medications such as imipramine (Tofranil). See Chapter 12 for an in-depth discussion of various forms of pain and their management. These are complex problems, and patients benefit from the involvement of a pain management team. It is also crucial for the patient to be reassured that the nurse accepts the reality of the pain experience as reported and that the nurse will collaborate with the patient and multidisciplinary care team to find acceptable management strategies.

## TUMORS OF THE SPINAL CORD

### Etiology/Epidemiology

Both primary and secondary tumors affect the spinal cord. Primary tumors arise from the substance of the cord and meninges or from the surrounding bone or blood vessels. The etiology of these tumors is unknown. About 90% of primary spinal tumors are extramedullary, outside the spinal cord, while less than 10% are intramedullary, arising within the substance of the spinal cord (Figure 54-18). Fifty-five percent of the extramedullary tumors are neurofibromas and meningiomas. Vascular tumors, sarcomas, and chordomas each represent a small percentage of the remainder. Fifty percent of spinal tumors occur in the thoracic region, 30% in the cervical region, and 20% in the lumbar area.[8,30] Primary spinal tumors are relatively rare, accounting for only 0.5% of all newly diagnosed tumors and 10% to 15% of central nervous system tumors. Risk factors are unknown although spinal tumors occur primarily in adults in the 20- to 50-year-old age group and affect both sexes about equally.

Secondary spinal cord tumors are metastatic in nature and can be attributed to primary tumors in other organs of the body. Secondary tumors occur fairly commonly from primary sites in the lungs, breast, prostate, colon, and uterus. Most secondary tumors are located in the epidural space in the lower thoracic spine and rarely infiltrate the spinal cord itself. The damage results mainly from spinal cord compression.

### Pathophysiology

The pathological consequences of spinal cord tumors are primarily related to the effects of compression. Infiltration and invasion are much less common. Pressure can cause irritation of the spinal nerve roots, displacement of the cord, interruption of perfusion, and obstruction of the flow of cerebrospinal fluid. Compression also interferes with the normal physiology of the spinal cord and causes tissue edema. The specific signs and symptoms relate to the specific level affected by the tumor.[7] The patient may experience sensory or motor problems or both. The rate of tumor growth is also important. Slow-growing tumors allow time for the spinal cord to adapt and may produce no symptoms until quite advanced. A rapidly growing tumor, particularly one composed of dense tissue, allows minimal time for compensation and triggers significant amounts of responsive edema.

The general symptoms of spinal cord tumors include pain, motor and sensory deficits, and bowel and bladder dysfunction. Pain, with or without accompanying neurological deficits, is the first symptom in the vast majority of patients with metastatic tumors. The pain may be localized, which is common when the tumor affects the vertebra, or radiate along the path of the involved spinal nerve root. The pain varies in intensity from mild to severe. Sensory losses reflect the exact anatomic location of the compression within the cord and may be accompanied by weakness or paralysis in the same nerve distribution. Tumors are a common cause of anterior cord syndrome as discussed on p. 1784.

### Collaborative Care Management

The diagnosis of a spinal cord tumor begins with a detailed history and neurological examination. The diagnostic test of choice is the enhanced MRI scan, although CT scanning and myelography may also be used. MRI is able to clearly visualize tumors in the vertebral bodies as well as those within the cord itself. Treatment usually includes a combination of approaches and is aimed at preserving neurological function.

Surgical intervention is the treatment of choice for most types of spinal cord tumor, and primary extramedullary tumors are often treated with surgery alone.[13] Intramedullary and metastatic tumors usually require a multiple modality approach. Surgery for metastatic lesions is typically focused on decompression of the spinal cord and debulking of the tumor to improve the patient's quality of life.

Radiation therapy is the primary approach for the management of intramedullary tumors whose invasive growth patterns make complete surgical excision impossible. Radiation is also used as a palliative strategy to relieve pain and compression in patients with advanced disease. Patients who survive for 12 to 18 months after high-dose radiation therapy are at extremely high risk for developing a radiation myelopathy that involves chronic and progressive sensory impairments progressing to motor involvement and eventually spastic paraplegia.[7] New approaches to the delivery of radiation

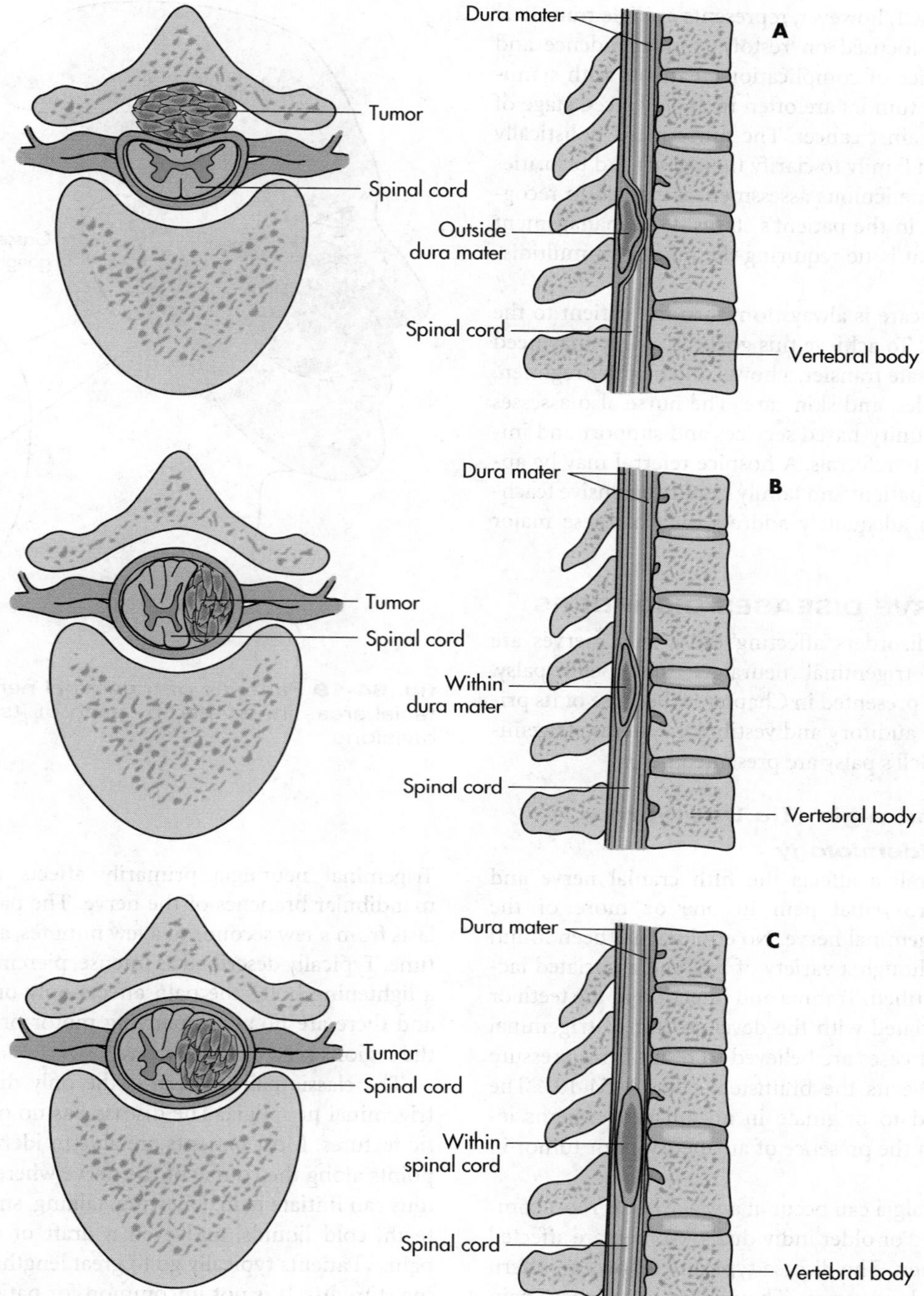


**fig. 54-18** Spinal tumors. **A,** Extradural tumors—outside the dura mater. **B,** Subdural tumors—within the dura mater. **C,** Intramedullary tumors—within the spinal cord.

are being researched. Chemotherapy has little documented effectiveness in the management of spinal tumors although adjunctive hormonal treatment may be useful when the primary cancer site is the breast or prostate gland.

Edema is present with most tumors involving the spinal cord, and minimizing edema is one standard treatment goal. Corticosteroids, usually dexamethasone (Decadron), are administered. Immobilization is a priority if the spine is unstable. Immobilization may involve simple bedrest with the patient in correct alignment or the use of cervical collars and trunk braces. Surgical stabilization may become necessary.

### *Patient/family education*

Some of the nursing care priorities for patients with spinal tumors overlap with those discussed under spinal cord injury. This is particularly true for the management of bowel and bladder problems. SCI, however, represents a single traumatic injury, and care is focused on restoring independence and limiting the incidence of complications. Patients with symptomatic spinal cord tumors are often in an advanced stage of a complex battle against cancer. The nurse plans holistically with the patient and family to clarify their goals and priorities for care. Ongoing meticulous assessment is critical to recognize subtle changes in the patient's status. Pain management may be an important issue requiring the input of a multidisciplinary pain team.

A major goal of care is always to return the patient to the home environment. To achieve this goal the family may need to learn to manage safe transfer, a bowel and bladder regimen, positioning principles, and skin care. The nurse also assesses the need for community-based services and support and initiates the appropriate referrals. A hospice referral may be appropriate. Both the patient and family require extensive teaching and support to adequately address each of these major areas of concern.

## CRANIAL NERVE DISEASES/DISORDERS

The three classic disorders affecting the cranial nerves are Ménière's disease, trigeminal neuralgia, and Bell's palsy. Ménière's disease is presented in Chapter 58 because of its primary effects on the auditory and vestibular systems. Trigeminal neuralgia and Bell's palsy are presented here.

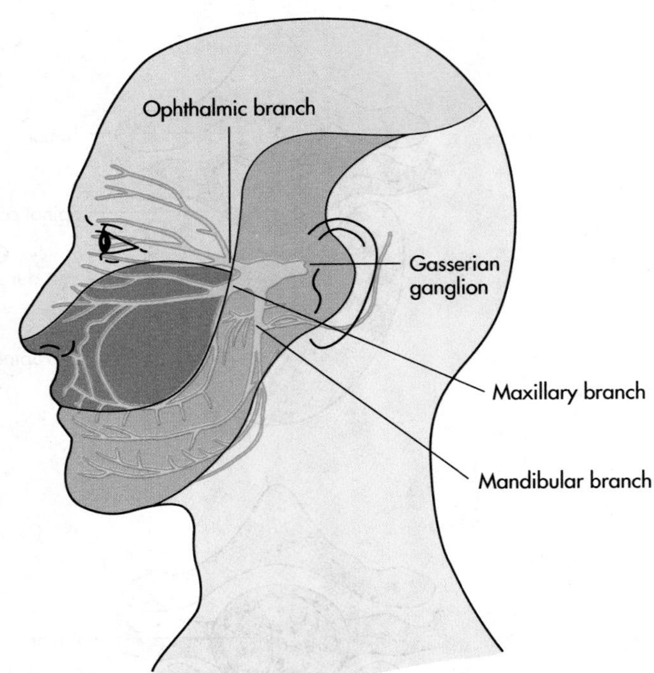


**fig. 54-19** Pathway of trigeminal nerve and the facial areas innervated by each of its three main divisions.

### Trigeminal Neuralgia (Tic Douloureux)

#### *Etiology/epidemiology*

Trigeminal neuralgia affects the fifth cranial nerve and causes intense paroxysmal pain in one or more of the branches of the trigeminal nerve. No etiology has been found for the disorder although a variety of risk and associated factors have been identified. Trauma and infection in the teeth or jaw are often associated with the development of trigeminal neuralgia, but most cases are believed to result from pressure on the nerve as it exits the brainstem (Figure 54-19). The pressure is believed to originate in an adjacent atherosclerotic artery or from the presence of an aneurysm or tumor in the area.

Trigeminal neuralgia can occur at any age but is most common in middle-aged or older individuals. Women are affected more often than men. The disease typically follows a pattern of exacerbation and remission. The patient experiences pain episodes over a period of weeks or months, and then the disease undergoes a spontaneous remission of variable length.[8] The remissions tend to become shorter in duration as the patient ages. The incidence and severity of the pain can have a significant negative impact on the patient's quality of life and even on the ability to maintain self-care and adequate nutrition.

#### *Pathophysiology*

The trigeminal nerve exits the pons and merges into the gasserian ganglion before it separates into its three major branches (Figure 54-19). The trigeminal nerve is the largest of the cranial nerves and has both motor and sensory fibers. Trigeminal neuralgia primarily affects the maxillary and mandibular branches of the nerve. The pain occurs abruptly, lasts from a few seconds to a few minutes, and can recur at any time. Typically described as intense, piercing, burning, or "like a lightening bolt," the pain affects only one side of the face, and there are no accompanying motor or sensory deficits in the regions served by the nerve.

The classic pain pattern is the only diagnostic feature of trigeminal neuralgia. The disease has no other clear diagnostic features. Most patients are able to identify specific trigger points along the course of the nerve where the slightest stimulus can initiate pain. Chewing, talking, smiling, brushing the teeth, cold liquids, and even a draft of air can trigger the pain.[17] Patients typically go to great lengths to avoid a triggering stimulus. It is not uncommon for patients to socially isolate themselves or neglect routine personal hygiene such as washing the face, brushing the teeth, or shaving in the effort to avoid pain. Significant weight loss can occur if chewing is a triggering stimulus.

#### *Collaborative care management*

There is no definitive treatment for trigeminal neuralgia. Treatment attempts to prevent or block the pain episodes in the most minimally invasive way. Drug therapy is tried first and may include anticonvulsants, analgesics, and tranquilizers. Carbamazepine (Tegretol) is the drug of choice. It is usually successful in lessening the frequency and duration of the pain episodes, but it may not be able to eliminate them.

Phenytoin (Dilantin), clonazepam (Klonopin), or baclofen (Lioresal) may all be tried if carbamazepine is ineffective.

In patients with refractory disease alcohol or phenol may be injected into one or more branches of the nerve. This treatment successfully blocks pain episodes for up to 18 months, but also results in complete anesthesia to the areas supplied by the nerve, which makes it unacceptable to many patients.[8] Patients with uncontrolled pain often require surgery, and a variety of procedures have been used. The most common involves percutaneous electrocoagulation of the nerve roots, which provides lasting pain relief with minimal destruction of the other sensory functions of the nerve. The procedure is performed under conscious sedation. Increasingly surgeons are using a posterior fossa craniotomy to visualize the trigeminal nerve and relieve any pressure that may be exerted by adjacent blood vessels.

**Patient/family education.** The presence of trigeminal neuralgia can have devastating outcomes for the patient's daily lifestyle. The nurse assesses the patient's response to the disease process and ensures that both the patient and family have accurate information about the disease and the various treatment options. Medication teaching is particularly important, as anticonvulsants and muscle relaxants may affect the patient's alertness and safety during routine daily activities.[18] Carbamazapine can cause myelosuppression and follow-up blood analysis is important. The nurse assists the patient to explore ways to minimize triggering episodes and to modify the diet as needed to maintain a stable body weight. Alternatives for oral hygiene may also need to be explored.

Neurological assessments help determine the presence and severity of any motor or sensory compromise in the postoperative period. If pain sensation is lost or diminished, the patient is instructed to avoid rubbing the eye on the affected side and to inspect it regularly for signs of irritation or infection. Regular dental follow-up is also necessary if the protective pain warning sign is absent. The patient also needs to adjust the diet in response to any residual deficits in sensation or chewing. A Nursing Care Plan for a patient with trigeminal neuralgia is found on p. 1806.

## Bell's Palsy

### Etiology/epidemiology

Bell's palsy involves an acute paralysis of cranial nerve VII, the facial nerve. The etiology of the disease is unknown, but it is generally believed to be a type of localized inflammatory reaction. The disease usually affects adults between 20 and 60 years of age, and the incidence in men and women is about equal. More than 80% of patients recover completely over a period of a few weeks or months and experience no residual effects although recovery depends on nerve regeneration.

### Pathophysiology

The facial nerve is primarily composed of motor nerves that innervate the muscles of expression on the face. Sensory branches supply the anterior two thirds of the tongue. Bell's palsy is characterized by a rapid weakening or paralysis of the facial muscles on one side of the face, which creates a masklike appearance. The eye on the affected side tears constantly, and the person has difficulty swallowing secretions (Figure 54-20). The paralysis may develop over a period of 24 to 36 hours or be fully present when a patient wakens from sleep. The diagnosis is established from the history and classic presenting symptoms.

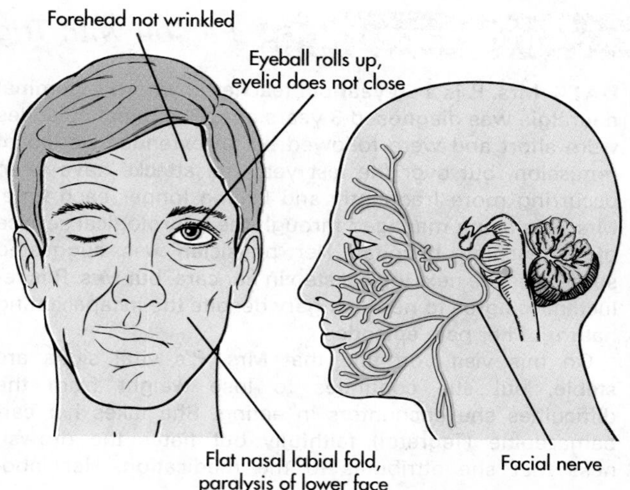


**fig. 54-20** Bell's palsy.

### Collaborative care management

There is no definitive treatment for Bell's palsy, but prednisone is usually given in the first week of treatment to suppress inflammation. Analgesics may be administered for pain management. Other supportive interventions include heat, massage, and electrical nerve stimulation.

**Patient/family education.** Because most patients with Bell's palsy can be adequately managed in the community setting, the nurse focuses on offering support and educating the patient and family about the disease process. The nurse provides instruction concerning the safe use of steroid medication and significant side effects to report. The nurse also teaches the patient to safely use heat, massage, and TENS therapy in the home. The patient is taught the importance of protecting the eyes from injury and infection related to excessive dryness. Artificial tears are recommended, and the eye should be patched or taped to protect it from abrasion and light damage.[29] As nerve function begins to return, the patient is instructed in facial exercises to help regain facial muscle tone.

## PERIPHERAL NERVE TRAUMA

### Etiology/Epidemiology

The peripheral nerves are vulnerable to injury from all the causes that damage other body tissues including athletic injuries, vehicular accidents, mechanical and equipment injury, and acts of violence. The mechanisms of injury are similar to those discussed under spinal cord injury and include partial and complete transection, contusion, compression, ischemia,

## nursing care plan | *Person with Trigeminal Neuralgia*

**DATA** Mrs. P. is a 56-year-old teacher in whom trigeminal neuralgia was diagnosed 3 years ago. The initial episodes were short and were followed by an extended period of remission, but over the last year the attacks have been occurring more frequently and lasting longer each time. Mrs. P. is being managed through the neurological service of a teaching hospital. Her physician has suggested surgery as the next logical step in her care, but Mrs. P. is reluctant to agree to neurosurgery despite the incapacitating nature of her pain episodes.

On this visit you find that Mrs. P.'s vital signs are stable, but she continues to lose weight from the difficulties she encounters in eating. She takes her carbamazepine (Tegretol) faithfully but hates the drowsiness that she attributes to the medication. Her laboratory values show no changes. Other pertinent data include:

- She had to take disability retirement this year due to the pain episodes.
- Her voice is low and hard to understand and she barely opens her mouth to speak.
- Her facial expression and affect are blank. Mrs. P. shows no emotion and does not smile. Her body language is tense and anxious.
- A foul breath odor is noticeable during conversation. Her general appearance is more unkempt than on prior visits.
- She states that she rarely leaves the house anymore except for doctor's appointments and generally keeps her phone unplugged.

**NURSING DIAGNOSIS** *Pain related to activation of trigger zones along the nerve pathway*

| expected patient outcome | nursing interventions | rationale |
|---|---|---|
| Pain episodes are less severe and less frequent. | Assess current pain management strategies and their effectiveness:<br>Pharmacological<br>Nonpharmacological | Establish baseline for measuring effectiveness of new strategies. |
| | Assess patient's knowledge of specific trigger activities for pain, e.g., chewing, talking, smiling/laughing, heat and cold, drafts, pressure, grooming activities, and mouth care. | Identify factors that can be manipulated in pain control interventions. |
| | Explore acceptability of cognitive and behavioral strategies to use in pain management, e.g., relaxation, imagery, and distraction. | Patient must believe that nonpharmacological strategies can be effective adjuncts to pain management. |
| | Consult with physician and pain management service concerning options for drug therapy. | Chronic pain necessitates a multidisciplinary approach to management. |
| | Encourage patient to take medication at regular intervals and to use analgesics at first hint of pain. | Steady blood levels increase drug effectiveness, and analgesics work more effectively if administered before pain reaches severe levels. |

**NURSING DIAGNOSIS** *Altered nutrition, less than body requirements related to fear of triggering pain with chewing.*

| expected patient outcome | nursing interventions | rationale |
|---|---|---|
| Adjusts diet effectively to maintain stable body weight. | Complete 24-hour recall assessment of dietary intake. | Provides objective data to assess balance and adequacy of diet. |
| | Explore modifications in diet to increase nutrient intake, e.g., consistency, texture, liquid supplements, adding skim milk powders to foods:<br>Avoid empty calories.<br>Add a liquid multivitamin supplement.<br>Ensure adequate fluids. | An inadequate diet can be supplemented with powders and formulas to increase nutrient base without increasing volume substantially. |
| | Assist patient to explore ways to avoid pain while eating:<br>Use soft foods and liquids as needed.<br>Avoid hot and cold foods/liquids.<br>Place food on the unaffected side of the mouth. | Success in avoiding pain will allow patient to consume more nutrients. |

*Continued*

## Person with Trigeminal Neuralgia—cont'd

**NURSING DIAGNOSIS** *Altered nutrition, less than body requirements related to fear of triggering pain with chewing—cont'd*

| expected patient outcome | nursing interventions | rationale |
|---|---|---|
| | Involve dietitian in planning. | Dietitian has expert knowledge base about community access to appropriate supplements. |
| | Instruct patient to weigh self weekly and maintain weight record. | Helps track progress in meeting nutritional goals. |

**NURSING DIAGNOSIS** *Altered mucous membranes related to inadequate oral hygiene secondary to fear of triggering pain*

| expected patient outcome | nursing interventions | rationale |
|---|---|---|
| Adapts oral care routines to maintain health of teeth and tissues yet avoid pain. | Inspect oral tissue on each visit. | Provides baseline for evaluation of progress or problems. |
| | Assess patient's current practice for oral care and evaluate effectiveness. | Provides baseline for planning interventions. |
| | Explore alternatives for oral care with patient, e.g., swabs, Water Pik, and mouthwashes. | Provides patient with alternatives to meet self-care goals. |
| | Encourage patient to carefully rinse mouth after eating. | Helps reduce mouth odor from retained food particles. |
| | Encourage patient to perform oral hygiene between pain episodes. | Uses pain-free intervals. |
| | Refer patient to dentist for regular assessment and care. | Infection in teeth or mouth is a common trigger for increased pain episodes. |

and stretch trauma. Peripheral nerves however, possess the potential to regenerate after injury if the conditions are favorable. Specific epidemiological data are not available concerning peripheral nerve injuries; but the median, ulnar, and radial nerves of the arm and the femoral, peroneal, and sciatic nerves of the legs are affected most commonly.

### Pathophysiology

When a peripheral nerve is completely transected, several degenerative processes occur. Swelling of the axon fibers initiates a degenerative process that progresses proximally back toward the nerve cell body. The distal nerve also degenerates and retracts (Wallerian degeneration). The axon and myelin sheath fragment and a phagocytic process is triggered to remove the breakdown products. A corresponding loss of motor and sensory function occurs distal to the injury. When repair and recovery are possible, the Schwann cells of the neurolemma proliferate from both sides of the injury to form neurolemma cords, which act as guide wires for the regenerating axon. The axon cylinder generates multiple tiny buds or sprouts in a random pattern. If some of the sprouts are successful in using the neurolemma cords to cross the transected gap, they achieve union with the distal stump.[8] The rate of growth for a regenerating sprout is 1 to 4 mm/day. Successfully realigned nerves then remyelinate and regrow to nearly their former size. The conduction velocity of regenerated nerves is typically about 80% of normal, and the chances for functional return are good. With transection injuries microsurgical realignment is usually necessary to support the regenerative process (Figure 54-21).

The clinical signs and symptoms resulting from peripheral nerve damage depend on the exact location of the injury and the specific function of the involved nerve or nerves. Because peripheral nerves contain both sensory and motor components, deficits may exist in both areas distal to the site. Motor alterations include lower motor neuron signs such as flaccid paralysis and muscle wasting in the muscles innervated by the affected nerves. Autonomic and trophic changes are also present after injury. Damage to sympathetic fibers creates an initial warm phase in which the affected area is dry and warm to the touch and flushed in appearance. A cold phase may follow in several weeks in which the extremity becomes cold and cyanotic.

### Collaborative Care Management

Peripheral nerve injuries are diagnosed primarily from the injury history and presenting symptoms. Electromyography may be used to determine the degree of connection between the nerve and muscle. Treatment options are individualized to the specific situation. Immobilization is frequently used to support healing. Surgical intervention is used to reapproximate transected nerve fibers, but little agreement exists about

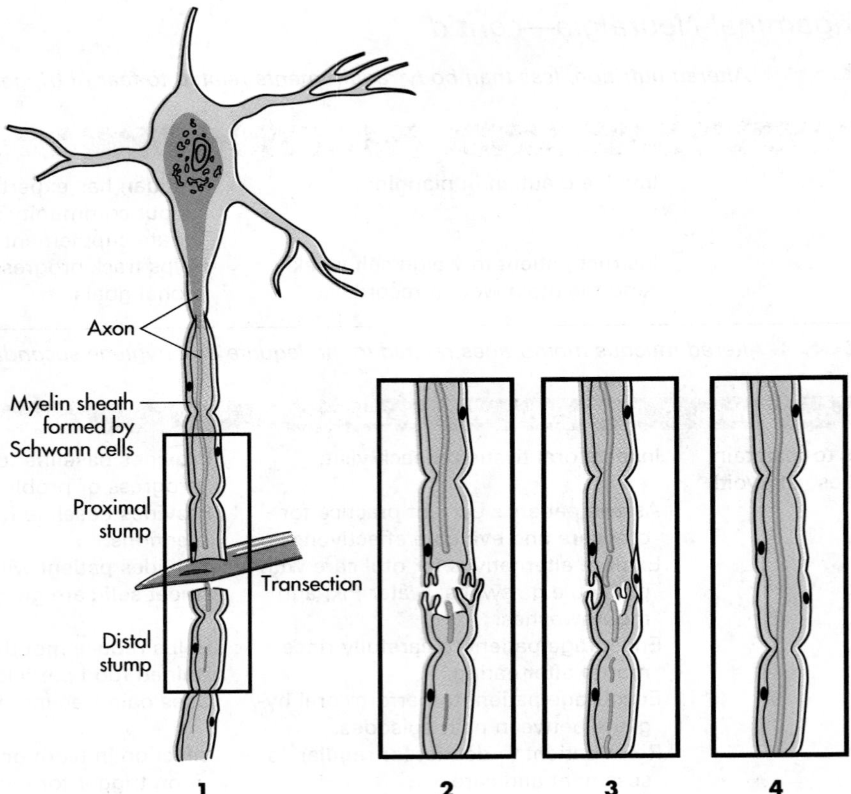


**1** After nerve transection, degeneration and retraction of the distal stump occur within 24 hours.

**2** Healing begins as Schwann cells of the neurolemma proliferate from both proximal and distal stumps, forming neurolemmal cords that will guide the regenerating axon.

**3** Some unmyelinated axon sprouts that are generated from the proximal stump find their way to the distal stump, guided by the neurolemmal cords.

**4** The axon regrows and remyelinates.

**fig. 54-21** The process of repair and regeneration of a peripheral nerve.

the optimal timing for surgical repair, which may take place at any time from several weeks to 2 months after the original injury. Microsurgical techniques now allow for earlier intervention, but the timing of surgery remains a clinical judgment. One of the many surgical challenges is the fact that the severed portions of the nerve retract and form scar tissue at their tips, which must be removed before reanastomosis. The remaining nerve is often shorter than desired and may require that the patient's limb be immobilized in a flexed position with a splint or cast during the healing process. Nerve grafts are increasingly being used when the nerve segments are short.

A physical therapy program is initiated as soon as possible after the injury since the loss of nervous innervation causes the muscles to begin to atrophy virtually immediately. Physical therapy is critical and includes range of motion, resistive exercise, splints and braces to support positioning, and electrical nerve stimulation to the muscles to minimize atrophic changes. The hypotonic muscles are unable to successfully balance their opposing muscles, i.e., flexors versus extensors, and the risk of contracture is high. Positioning in neutral or counter positions is essential to help prevent joint deformities. If the associated tendons are allowed to shorten, the contracture will be permanent.

### *Patient/family education*

The rehabilitation process after peripheral nerve injury is prolonged and carries no guarantees. The nurse reinforces the rationale for all components of the treatment plan and the importance of adherence to the regimen. Ongoing support and encouragement are essential as the patient and family may become discouraged at the pace of progress and the cost of treatment. The nurse instructs the patient about safety measures to compensate for any sensory losses. Thorough visual assessment of all affected areas is essential. The nurse teaches the patient to carefully protect the affected areas from damage related to temperature extremes.

The nurse also emphasizes the importance of skin care to the affected areas. In the cold phase after injury the skin is fragile and vulnerable to injury. Daily inspection and gentle cleansing are critical. Lanolin creams or cocoa butter may be used to counteract dryness and scaling. Pain management is also critical because unmanaged pain can seriously limit the rehabilitation effort. Multiple adaptations in self-care skills may be necessary during the treatment and rehabilitation periods, and the nurse assists the patient to acquire and effectively use needed assistive devices.

## critical thinking QUESTIONS

**1** Kevin Mitchell is a 19-year-old adolescent with a C8 spinal cord injury. He was injured 3 months ago and is in active rehabilitation. He has recently developed muscle spasticity, which is becoming increasingly severe. What *nursing* interventions can you implement to attempt to reduce the spasticity?

**2** You are working in an acute spinal cord injury rehabilitation unit. Two of your patients are 23-year-old William Nabor who suffered a T8 injury and 32-year-old Julie Bateman, who suffered a C6 injury. In planning your day how will your priorities for these two patient be the same? How will they be different? Why?

**3** Chantel Lincoln suffered an L2 spinal cord injury. She has been complaining of increasing levels of intense burning pain shooting through her legs and lower back. A fellow nursing student asks you if you think that Chantel really has pain, or if she is just trying to get pain medication as a way of coping with her disability. "After all, spinal cord injury results in a loss of sensation below the level of the injury, doesn't it?" How would you respond to your friend? Support your answer.

## chapter SUMMARY

### SPINAL CORD INJURY

- Spinal cord injury can result whenever excessive force is applied to the cord or supporting structures. Excessive flexion, extension, compression or rotation of the spinal column may result in concussion, contusion, laceration, or transection of the spinal cord.
- SCI primarily results from motor vehicle accidents, falls, sports injuries, and violence. About 10,000 new injuries occur each year. Sixty percent of these affect persons between 15 to 25 years of age, and 80% of them involve males.
- The physiological effects of SCI are the result of the initial injury plus secondary damage caused by edema, vasoconstriction, and hypoxia, which worsen the effects of the initial injury.
- Spinal shock occurs immediately after SCI. All neurological function below the level of the injury is lost. Flaccid paralysis, areflexia, flaccid dysfunction of the bowel and bladder, and loss of sympathetic tone of the blood vessels are its major characteristics.
- The clinical manifestations of SCI reflect the level of the injury. Respiratory impairment is a significant concern with cervical injuries.
- The effects of SCI also reflect damage to UMNs versus LMNs. This is particularly important with bowel, bladder, and sexual functioning.
- Lower motor neurons consist of large anterior horn cells located in the anterior gray matter of the spinal cord. Upper motor neurons originate in the motor strip of the cerebral cortex and in multiple brainstem nuclei.
- Initial medical care for SCI focuses on stabilizing the spine, relieving compression, and restoring alignment. These goals may be accomplished by the use of traction, halo devices, or surgical intervention with laminectomy, fusion, or the placement of rods.
- Supporting ventilation is a primary concern of early care. Injuries at C4 or above usually require intubation and mechanical ventilation. Quad assistive coughing is often necessary to clear secretions in the absence of the abdominal muscles.
- Hemodynamic instability is a major concern during the period of spinal shock. The patient is kept flat in bed and Ace wraps, TEDs, abdominal binders, and pneumatic compression devices may all be used to support venous return.
- The major principles for care after SCI are early mobilization, prevention of complications, and maximization of self-care potential. This effort is multidisciplinary in nature.
- Physical and occupational therapy focus on muscle strengthening and self-care adaptations to promote independence.
- Maintaining an intact skin is a major nursing priority. Interventions include meticulous frequent inspection, weight shifts, and the use of appropriate pressure-relieving devices.
- Urinary elimination is managed by intermittent catheterization unless adequate bladder emptying can be achieved by automatic voiding. Preventing infection is an ongoing concern.
- Bowel continence is achieved by a regimen of stool softeners, suppositories, digital stimulation, and conditioning. Continence is achievable.
- Sexual functioning is compromised after SCI. Men with UMN lesions can achieve reflex erections, which may be sufficient to support intercourse, but ejaculation usually does not occur. Male fertility is diminished, but women can conceive and safely carry an infant to full term.
- SCI represents a major crisis for both patients and families. They all need to move through the stages of grieving. Ninety percent of patients with SCI return to their home setting.
- Autonomic dysreflexia is a serious complication of SCI above T6. It is an exaggerated sympathetic response, which usually occurs from visceral stimuli such as a full bladder or bowel. It creates severe paroxysmal hypertension and bradycardia, which can be life threatening.
- Patient teaching about autonomic dysreflexia focuses on prevention. If an episode occurs, standard protocols call for immediately placing the patient in an upright position and attempting to relieve the stimulus through catheterization or removing stool from the rectum. If these measures are unsuccessful, emergency medications are given to lower the blood pressure.

- Spasticity develops with UMN lesions once the spinal shock period has resolved. Spasticity adds useful tone to muscles but is often severe enough to require drug therapy.

## SPINAL TUMORS

- Tumors affecting the spinal cord may arise from the cord and adjacent structures or represent metastasis from a primary source elsewhere in the body. Most spinal tumors are metastatic.
- Damage from tumors is related to spinal cord compression and reflects both the tissue density of the tumor and its growth rate. Many tumors create anterior or central cord syndromes.
- Treatment options for spinal tumors include surgery and radiation therapy. The main goal is to remove the tumor or relieve the compression on the cord without affecting overall cord function.

## CRANIAL NERVE DISORDERS

- Trigeminal neuralgia is a disease of unknown etiology that affects the fifth cranial nerve. It creates spasms of severe pain along the nerve pathway and can become disabling.
- Treatment of trigeminal neuralgia includes the use of anticonvulsants, muscle relaxants, injection of phenol or alcohol into the nerve, or surgery to interrupt nerve pathways or relieve pressure.
- Bell's palsy affects cranial nerve VII and results in temporary acute paralysis of the facial nerve muscles on one side of the face. Bell's palsy is of unknown etiology and has no known treatment. The damage is usually reversible over a period of weeks, and care is generally supportive.

## PERIPHERAL NERVE TRAUMA

- Trauma to the peripheral nerves follows many of the principles of primary and secondary injury that apply to SCI. Nerve regeneration is possible, however, under optimal conditions.
- Treatment may involve immobilization or immobilization plus surgery to support nerve regeneration.

## References


1. American Association of Spinal Cord Injury Nurses: Standards of spinal cord injury nursing practice, *SCI Nurs* 11(1):33-37, 1994.
2. Campbell SK, Almeida GL, Penn RD, Corcos DM: The effects of intrathecally administered baclofen on function in patients with spasticity, *Phys Ther* 75(5):352-362, 1995.
3. Chiles BW, Cooper PR: Acute spinal injury, *N Engl J Med* 334(8):514-520, 1996.
4. Dyck PJ, Haase G, May M: When you suspect Bell's palsy, *Patient Care* 26(1):151-168, 1992.
5. Gilbert M, Counsell CM: Coordinated care for the SCI patient, *SCI Nurs* 13(3):87-89, 1995.
6. Halm MA: Elimination concerns with acute spinal cord trauma, *Crit Care Nurs Clin North Am* 2(3):385-398, 1990.
7. Held JL: Identifying spinal cord compression, *Nursing* 24(5):28-29, 1994.
8. Hickey JV: *Clinical practice of neurological and neurosurgical nursing,* ed 4, Philadelphia, 1997, JB Lippincott.
9. Huston CJ, Boelman R: Autonomic dysreflexia, *Am J Nurs* 95(6):55, 1995.
10. Jackson AB, Groomes TE: Incidence of respiratory complications following spinal cord injury, *Arch Phys Med Rehabil* 75(3):270-275, 1994.
11. Kidd PS: Emergency management of spinal cord injuries, *Crit Care Nurs Clin North Am* 2(3):349-356, 1990.
12. Kocan MJ: Pulmonary considerations in the critical care phase, *Crit Care Nurs Clin North Am* 2(3):369-374, 1990.
13. Kuric J: Spinal cord tumors, *Crit Care Nurs Clin North Am* 7(1):151-157, 1995.
14. Laskowski-Jones L: Acute SCI: how to minimize the damage, *Am J Nurs* 93(12):22-31, 1993.
15. Lehman CA: Risk factors for pressure ulcers in the spinal cord injured in the community, *SCI Nurs* 12(4):110-114, 1995.
16. Lemons VR, Wagner FC Jr: Respiratory complications after cervical spinal cord injury, *Spine* 19(20):2315-2320, 1994.
17. Levins TT: Bell's palsy versus trigeminal neuralgia questioned, *J Emerg Nurs* 20(2):86-87, 1994.
18. McConaghy DJ: Trigeminal neuralgia: a personal review and nursing implications, *J Neurosci Nurs* 26(2):85-90, 1994.
19. Maybuch D, Lee A, Butler D: High dose methylprednisolone after spinal cord injury, *Crit Care Nurs* 14(4):69-72, 77-78, 1994.
20. Nolan S: Current trends in the management of acute spinal cord injury, *Crit Care Nurs Q* 17(1):64-78, 1994.
21. Polos J: The power of nursing, *Rehabil Injury* 19(1):42-43, 1994.
22. Richmond TS: Spinal cord injury, *Nurs Clin North Am* 25(1):57-69, 1990.
23. Segatore M, Miller M: Understanding chronic pain after spinal cord injury, *J Neurosci Nurs* 26(4):230-236, 1994.
24. Segatore M, Miller M: The pharmacotherapy of spinal spasticity, a decade of progress. I. Theoretical aspects, *SCI Nurs* 11(3):66-69, 1995.
25. Segatore M, Miller M: The pharmacotherapy of spinal spasticity, a decade of progress II. Therapeutics, *SCI Nurs* 12(1):2-7, 1995.
26. Spoltore TA, O'Brien AM: Rehabilitation of the spinal cord injured patient, *Orthop Nurs* 14(3):7-16, 1995.
27. Thomason SS: Preventing and detecting unique complications in the spinal cord injured, *Home Healthcare Nurse* 8(5):16-21, 1990.
28. Weir AM et al: Bell's palsy: the effect on self-image, mood state and social activity, *Clin Rehabil* 9(2):121-125, 1995.
29. Wollenberg SP: Primary care diagnosis and management of Bell's palsy, *Nurse Pract* 18(12):15-19, 1994.

chapter 55

# ASSESSMENT OF THE Visual System

BARBARA ASTLE and MARION ALLEN

**objectives** *After studying this chapter, the learner should be able to:*

1. Describe the structure and function of the eye.
2. Identify the normal physiological and anatomic ocular changes that occur with aging.
3. Identify the subjective and objective data that should be obtained when assessing the eye.
4. Discuss the nursing interventions and patient teaching associated with common ocular diagnostic tests.

Orientation to our world is primarily visual. We learn much about our environment and ourselves through our eyes. Practically every behavior is affected by the visual sense. One hears a noise and looks in the direction from which it came. Something touches our body, and we look to see what it was. Vision contributes meaning and pleasure to the human experience.

Assessment of the visual system is an integral part of the nurse's role. Visual screening is conducted with persons of all ages and in all settings, and most eye disorders are identified by nurses and physicians in schools, industry, outpatient clinics, or ophthalmologists' offices. Admission to the hospital is usually limited to medical or surgical treatment that cannot routinely be accomplished on an outpatient basis.

Because persons with eye problems usually are managed on an outpatient basis, visual impairment is usually not the major diagnosis of persons for whom the nurse is providing care. However, visual impairment is frequently present and may be undiagnosed. Therefore nurses should routinely assess visual ability, especially in persons who have systemic diseases that affect vision or who are taking medications with known visual side effects.

## ANATOMY AND PHYSIOLOGY OF THE EYE

### LAYERS OF THE EYE

The eyeball has three main coats or layers (Figure 55-1). The tough outer layer consists of the *opaque sclera* (white) and the *transparent cornea.* These structures are joined at the *corneoscleral sulcus* or *limbus.* The middle vascular layer or *uvea* is composed of three parts: the *choroid,* the *ciliary body,* and the *iris,* which contains an opening in its center called the *pupil.*

The *retina,* the third and innermost layer of the eye, is composed of two parts: a sensory portion and a layer of pigmented epithelium. The sensory portion contains the photoreceptors (rods and cones). These photoreceptors synapse in the retina with bipolar neurons and then with ganglion neurons, and these become the fibers of the optic nerve that pass visual information to the brain.

The *cones,* which are less numerous than the rods, are mainly concentrated near the center of the retina in an area termed the *macula* (Figure 55-2). They are considered to be the receptors for bright daylight and color vision and allow us to see sharp images. The *rods,* which are found mostly in the periphery of the retina, are receptors for dim or night vision. Rods contain rhodopsin, a photosensitive protein that rapidly becomes depleted in bright light. The slow regeneration of rhodopsin, which depends on the presence of vitamin A, explains the time needed to adjust from a bright to a dim light.

### CHAMBERS OF THE EYE

The interior of the *eyeball* is divided into two compartments (anterior and posterior). The anterior compartment includes the space from the back of the cornea to the lens, and the posterior compartment is the space from the posterior surface of the lens to the retina.

The anterior compartment is further subdivided into an anterior chamber (between the cornea and the iris) and a posterior chamber (between the iris and the lens). This compartment is filled with a clear liquid called *aqueous humor,* whose purpose is to nourish and bathe the lens and cornea. Produced by the ciliary body in the posterior chamber, aqueous humor flows through the pupil into the anterior chamber and leaves the eye through the filtration structures at the junction of the iris and cornea (anterior chamber angle). The filtration structures consist of the trabecular meshwork and an encircling tubular channel into which the aqueous humor drains (Schlemm's canal).

Schlemm's canal has several exit channels that empty into the scleral and episcleral veins. Aqueous humor passes through these exit channels and eventually is absorbed into general circulation (Figure 55-3).

The posterior compartment is the larger of the two and is filled with a clear gel-like substance called the *vitreous humor.* The structure of the vitreous humor can be pictured as fine collagen fibers crossing one another to form a scaffolding that helps to maintain the shape of the eyeball. This fibrous network

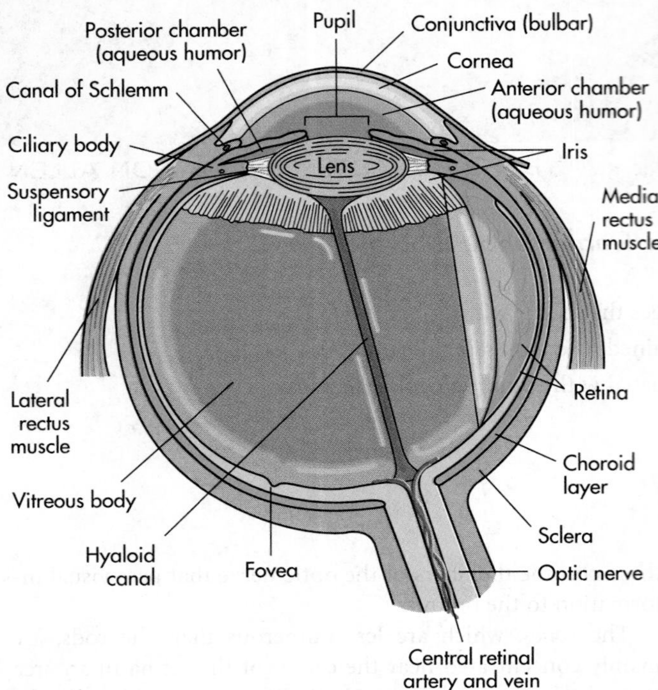


fig. 55-1 Horizontal section through the left eye.

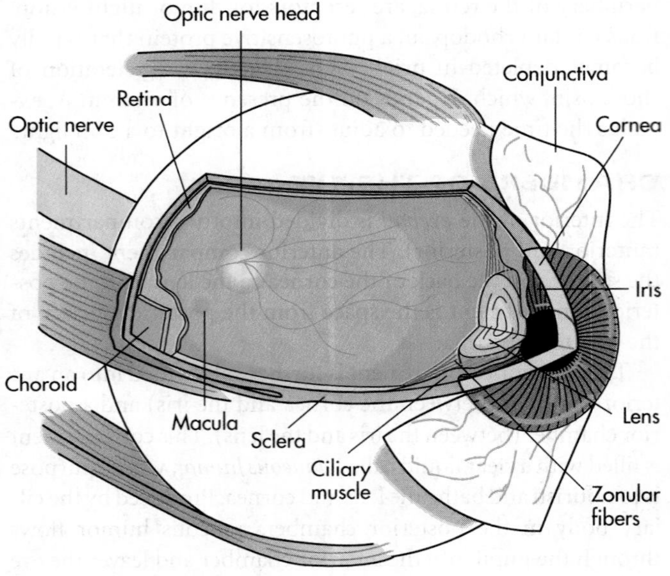


fig. 55-2 Cutaway section of the eye.

becomes more dense toward the outermost portion of the vitreous humor, particularly in the areas of strong attachment between the vitreous humor and retina. These attachments occur at the anterior edge of the retina, the optic disc, the equator of the eye, and the macula. The vitreous humor is clear, thus allowing transmission of light posteriorly to the retina.

## LENS

The lens is a transparent biconvex structure located directly behind the iris and pupil. It is attached to the ciliary body by multiple suspensory ligaments called *zonules.* The lens, which

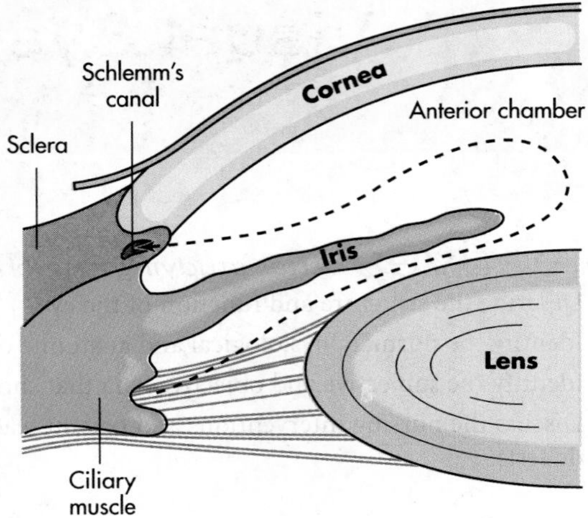


fig. 55-3 Flow of aqueous humor. Aqueous humor is largely produced by the ciliary processes in the posterior chamber; it flows into the anterior chamber and leaves the eye through Schlemm's canal.

is the fine-focusing mechanism for the eye, allows a clear image to be focused on the retina.

## EYE MUSCLES

There are two types of eye muscles: extrinsic and intrinsic. The six extraocular muscles are extrinsic voluntary muscles that control the extraocular movements of each eye (Table 55-1 and Figure 55-4). The lateral and medial rectus muscles control outturning (abduction) and inturning (adduction), respectively, with the remaining four. The rectus muscles move the eye up and down and toward the nose while the oblique muscles also control up and down movement plus movement toward the ear. The simultaneous actions of the muscles of each eye are integrated by the brain.

The intrinsic involuntary muscles within the eye are the ciliary muscles (in the ciliary body), which control the shape of the lens, and the sphincter and dilator pupillae muscles in the iris, which control pupil size and consequently the amount of light that enters the eye.

## EYELIDS AND CONJUNCTIVA

The *eyelids* (palpebrae) are made up of thin layers of skin, muscle, fibrous tissue, and mucous membrane. The main purposes of the eyelids are to protect the eye from external irritation, spread tears over the front of the eye, and interrupt and restrict the amount of light entering the eye. The *conjunctiva,* the mucous membrane lining of the eyelid (palpebral conjunctiva) that extends over the anterior sclera (bulbar conjunctiva), is of particular significance. This membrane and its blood vessels provide nutrients, antibodies, and leukocytes to the avascular cornea. The conjunctiva and glands within the eyelid secrete mucus and oil, which help keep the cornea moist and clear and decrease friction when the lids close.

## LACRIMAL SYSTEM

The lacrimal system consists of the *lacrimal gland* and a *tear drainage system* (Figure 55-5). The lacrimal gland produces

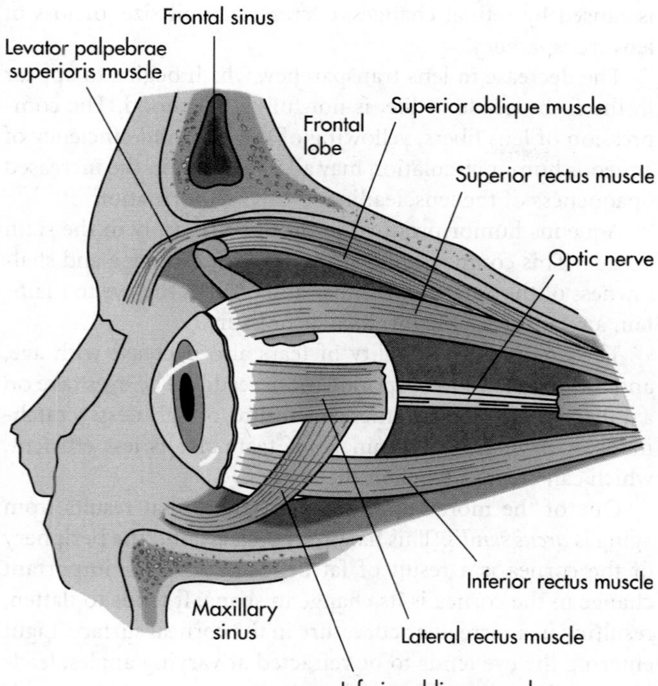


**fig. 55-4** Extrinsic muscles of the eye. Both oblique muscles insert behind the equator of the globe. The inferior oblique muscle passes inferiorly to the body of the inferior rectus muscle but beneath the lateral rectus muscle.

the tears that flow across the eye and enter the drainage system nasally. Each time the eyelids blink, the tears are pumped by the blinking action and flow across the surface of the eyes. The tears flow through small holes in the eyelids (puncti) and ducts (canaliculi) to the lacrimal sac. They then drain into the nasolacrimal duct through the opening of the inferior meatus of the nasal cavity. Tears keep the surface of the eye and conjunctiva moistened and lubricated. Tears also contain an enzyme that functions as an antibacterial agent.

## ORBIT

The eye rests within the confines of the bony orbit. This orbit is a cone-shaped cavity formed by the union of cranial and facial bones. The eyeball itself occupies only about one fifth of the space of the orbit. The remainder is filled with the lacrimal gland, muscles, blood vessels, nerves, and fatty tissue. This fatty tissue serves as a protective cushion for the eye. The optic nerve exits the orbit posteriorly, transmitting visual information from the eye to the brain.

## PHYSIOLOGY OF VISION

Light rays entering the eye are bent *(refracted)* as they pass over the curved surfaces of the cornea and through the various (more posterior) structures of the eye (aqueous humor, lens, and vitreous humor) to focus on the retina. The cornea provides the major refractive change for light entering the eye, with the lens providing the fine focus for light transmitted posteriorly to the retina.

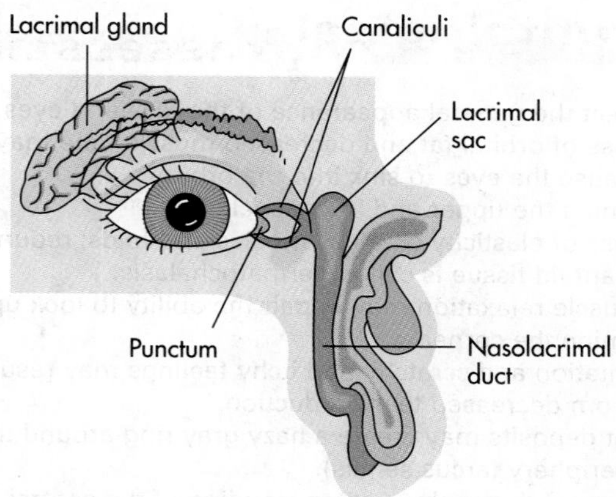


**fig. 55-5** Lacrimal system.

**table 55-1** *Extrinsic Muscles*

| Name | Function |
|---|---|
| Superior rectus | Rotates eye upward and toward the nose |
| Inferior rectus | Rotates eye downward and toward the nose |
| Lateral rectus | Moves eye toward the temporal side |
| Medial rectus | Moves eye toward the nose |
| Inferior oblique | Rotates eye upward and toward the temporal side |
| Superior oblique | Rotates eye downward and toward the temporal side |

The eye can adjust *(accommodation)* to seeing objects at various distances by the flattening or thickening of the lens. Near vision requires contraction of the ciliary muscles in the ciliary body. This contraction allows the ciliary muscle to move forward and relaxes the zonules attached to the lens. The lens then bulges to bend the light rays more acutely so the rays focus on the retina. Accommodation also is facilitated by changing the size of the pupil. With near vision, the iris constricts the pupil to force light rays to pass through the shortened but thicker lens. The pupils also constrict with bright lights to protect the retina from intense stimulation.

Light rays are absorbed by photoreceptors on the retina, changed to electrical activity, and transmitted via the optic nerve to the visual cortex areas of the brain for processing. The fibers of the optic nerve (cranial nerve II; see Chapter 51) divide at the optic chiasm; the medial portion of each nerve crosses to the opposite side, and the impulses are then transmitted to the visual cortex. In this way, visual information received by each eye is transmitted simultaneously to both sides of the brain. Bilateral vision provides depth perception.

## PHYSIOLOGICAL CHANGES WITH AGING

Aging affects many aspects of visual function, both physiological and anatomic.[9] Decreased flexibility and elasticity of the lens lead to one of the first noted signs of aging—the

### gerontological assessment

Inspect the general appearance of the face and eyes.
- Loss of orbital fat and decreased muscle tone may cause the eyes to sink into the orbit.

Examine the upper and lower eyelids.
- Loss of elasticity creates wrinkles and folds; redundant lid tissue is called dermatochalasis.
- Muscle relaxation may impair the ability to look up.

Examine the cornea.
- Irritation and scratchy and itchy feelings may result from decreased tear production.
- Fat deposits may create a hazy gray ring around the periphery (arcus senilis).
- Corneal dystrophy creates clouding of the central cornea.

Examine the size of the pupil.
- Pupillary size typically decreases with age.

Examine the lens.
- Yellow discoloration may be present, which can progress to cataract formation.

Examine the retina with an ophthalmoscope.
- The effects of diabetes, hypertension, and macular degeneration are often evident in hemorrhages, exudates, and abnormal areas of pigmentation.

Perform vision screening.
- Normal aging is associated with refractory changes, senile miosis, and decreased visual acuity.

Explore the impact of any change in vision or color perception on the patient's ability to perform activities of daily living and engage in desired pursuits.

**COMMON DISORDERS IN ELDERS**

Corneal dystrophy
Glaucoma
Cataract
Diabetic retinopathy
Macular degeneration/macular hole

decreased ability of the eye to focus (accommodate) for near and detailed work *(presbyopia)*.

With the aging process an older person's color vision declines and contributes to impaired depth perception.[6] This causes greater difficulty in distinguishing among colors at the blue end of the spectrum; however warm colors are easier to differentiate. A smaller pupil *(senile miosis)* adds to this distortion of color. It also affects the amount of light that reaches the peripheral retina and the ability of the person to adapt to dim light and darkness. As a result, the older person has impaired night vision. Persons older than 60 years of age need about twice as much light to see as they did when they were 20.

This increase in the amount of light needed for close work can also create problems with glare. Glare, a veil-like luminance superimposed on the retinal image, masks and reduces the brightness of objects in the visual field.[9] Glare is related to increased light scatter in the eye caused by corneal, scleral, lens, and vitreal changes.

The field of vision also begins to decrease with age, affecting the breadth of vision. It is uncertain whether this decrease is caused by retinal changes, decreased pupil size, or loss of lens transparency.

The decrease in lens transparency, which begins to appear in the fifth decade of life, is not fully understood. The compression of lens fibers, yellowing of the lens, and efficiency of aqueous humor circulation may all play a part in the increased opaqueness of the lens, leading to cataract formation.

Aqueous humor production drops off sharply in the sixth decade. This compensates for the reduced drainage and shallowness of the anterior chamber and enables the eye to maintain a relatively stable intraocular pressure.[8]

The quantity and quality of tears also decrease with age, and the tears tend to evaporate more readily. The eyes take on a duller appearance, and there is a feeling of tightness, scratchiness, or dryness. The drainage of tears also is less efficient, which can create a block in the system.

One of the more common eye changes that results from aging is *arcus senilis.* This hazy gray ring around the periphery of the cornea is a result of fat deposits. Another important change in the cornea is its change in shape. It tends to flatten, resulting in an irregular curvature in the corneal surface. Light entering the eye tends to be refracted at varying angles, leading to a distorted and blurred image (astigmatism). Appropriate changes in eye assessment for elderly persons is summarized in the Gerontological Assessment Box.

## ASSESSMENT

### SUBJECTIVE DATA

A complete visual assessment consists of a careful patient interview combined with a physical assessment of the eye structures. General areas explored during the interview include the patient's assessment of his or her vision and any recent changes in visual acuity, whether glasses or contacts are used, and the date of the last professional eye examination. The presence and severity of common eye symptoms such as blurred vision, "floaters," dry scratchy eyes, burning, or chronic headache are explored. The interview allows the nurse to also explore the person's health promotion practices in regard to use of protective eyewear, particularly for occupational exposure. Any history of head trauma, loss of consciousness, or direct eye trauma or infection is important to explore.

Because many eye disorders are inherited, a family history is essential. Questions are directed specifically to a family history of cataracts, glaucoma, diabetes, hypertension, poor vision that could not be corrected with glasses, or blindness. A personal medical history is also obtained, with particular attention to all medications in current use.

### OBJECTIVE DATA

The tissues of the eye are for the most part transparent, making abnormalities easily detectable. Ocular manifestations of systemic disease also can be identified. In addition, the vascular system (retinal vascular system) and cranial nerve (optic nerve) of the eye can be visualized on examination. Assessment includes inspection of the external structures and gross measures of visual acuity. More complete eye examinations, such as electrophysiological studies of the retina and other fundus examinations, are performed by physicians in conjunction with specially trained nurses or technicians. A basic assessment of the eye and vision is summarized in Table 55-2.

## Inspection of External Structures

The nurse first inspects the general appearance of the face and eyes of the patient. The presence of an abnormal protrusion or bulging of an eye is called *exophthalmia* or *exophthalmos*. In elderly persons the eyes tend to sink into the orbit *(enopthalmos)*, caused primarily by the loss of orbital fat.

The eyelids are assessed for color, texture, mobility, and position. The lids should be able to close completely to prevent drying of the conjunctiva and cornea. Any swelling, redness, or discharge is noted. If one upper lid seems to be lower than the other, or "droops," *ptosis* of the eyelid may be present. If ptosis is present in both eyes, the upper lid is noted to be in an abnormally low position, covering the upper portion or more of the iris. Ptosis may be the result of extreme debility or neuromuscular disease. Extreme ptosis can interfere with vision by covering the pupil.

As the person ages, the eyelids become thinner and less elastic and positional defects may occur. In addition to ptosis, ectropion, entropion, and dermatochalasis may be present. *Ectropion* is eversion of the lower lid. It is usually bilateral, and symptoms include tearing and irritation. *Entropion* is the turning in of the eyelids. The person experiences a foreign body sensation caused by the eyelashes rubbing against the cornea. *Dermatochalasis* is a redundancy of upper or lower lid tissues. This usually occurs from loss of elasticity and results in wrinkles and drooping folds.

The conjunctiva of the lower lid is examined by pulling downward on the lid as the person looks upward (Figure 55-6). To examine the conjunctiva of the upper lid, the lid must be everted (Figure 55-7).

The lacrimal gland normally is not observable. Enlargement of the gland may occur in certain disorders that cause inflammation of the eye. This may be most evident when the upper lid is everted.

Small blood vessels normally are visible in the conjunctiva. The sclera shows through the conjunctiva and has a shiny porcelain-like appearance. Dilation of blood vessels of the conjunctiva may indicate disease of the cornea or disease within the eye. Spontaneous small hemorrhages may occur beneath the conjunctiva in the normal eye. A yellow discoloration of the sclera indicates jaundice.

The cornea, which is normally visible except for surface reflections, must be smooth and transparent for good vision. It should look shiny and bright when examined with a penlight. Moving the light and directing it from the side, the examiner looks for abrasions and opacities. If the cornea is clear, the iris and pupils should be clearly visible.

Defects in the epithelium of the cornea may be demonstrated with the use of topical dyes. Contact lenses should be removed before dye instillation because the dye tends to stain soft lenses. The dye is put in the conjunctiva by drops or by touching the conjunctiva with a moistened strip of filter paper that has been impregnated with the dye. Injured tissue absorbs the dye allowing visualization of foreign bodies, abrasions, and inflammation of the cornea. After the test, the nurse cleans the dye from the patient's face with a moist tissue.

**table 55-2** *Basic Assessment of the Eye and Vision*

| | |
|---|---|
| Facial and ocular expression | Prominence of eyes; alert or dull expression |
| Eyelids and conjunctiva | Symmetry, presence of edema, ptosis, itching, redness, discharges, blinking, equality, growths |
| Lacrimal system | Tears, swelling, growths |
| Sclera | Color |
| Cornea | Clarity |
| Anterior chamber | Depth, presence of blood/pus |
| Iris and pupils | Irregularities in color, shape, size |
| Pupillary reflex | |
| Light | Constriction of pupil in response to light in that eye (direct light reaction); equal amount of constriction in the other eye (consensual light reaction) |
| Accommodation | Convergence of eyes and constriction of pupil as gaze shifts from far to near object |
| Lens | Transparent or opaque |
| Peripheral vision | Ability to see movements and objects well on both sides of field of vision |
| Acuity with and without glasses | Ability to read newsprint, clocks on wall, and name tags and to recognize faces at bedside and at door |
| Supportive aids | Glasses, contact lenses, prosthesis |

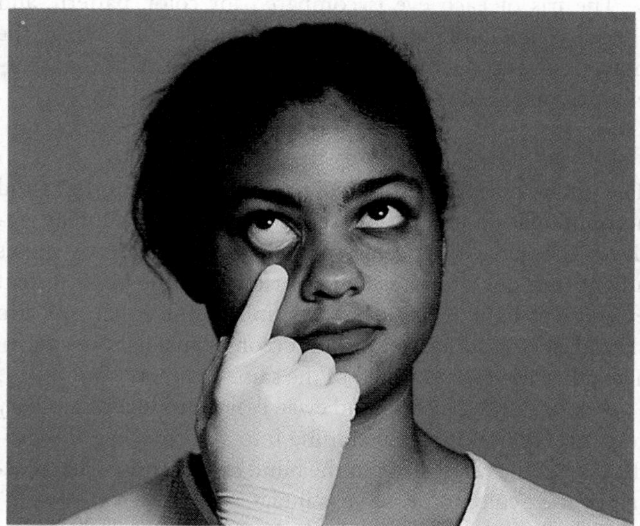

**fig. 55-6** Eversion of lower eyelid by drawing margin downward as subject looks upward.

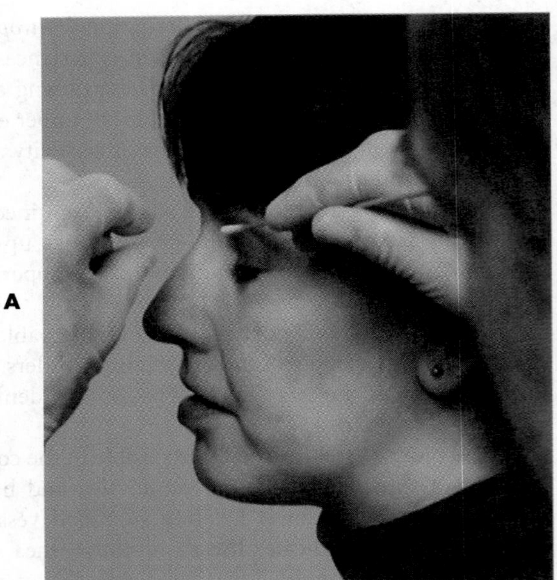


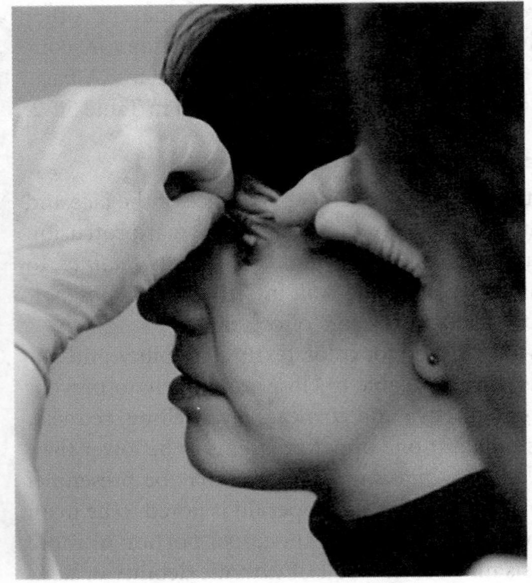


**fig. 55-7** Eversion of upper eyelid. Patient is instructed to look downward, and lashes of upper eyelid are grasped between thumb and index finger. **A,** Cotton-tipped applicator is placed at level of tarsal fold. **B,** Eyelid is folded back on applicator while patient continues to look downward.

Occasionally, a physician may have the nurse perform a *tear test* (Schirmer test). This test is performed to verify abnormal tear production (dry eyes). The nurse explains the procedure to patients and informs them that the test may be uncomfortable but is not painful. The quantity of tears is measured with a strip of filter paper, folded and hooked over the lower lid and left in place for approximately 5 minutes. The extent to which the filter paper is soaked with tears is then measured.

The anterior chamber is examined. The anterior chamber is bathed in aqueous humor and has a normal depth of 3 to 3.5 mm. Blood and purulent matter in the anterior chamber may interfere with vision. When blood is observed in the anterior chamber, the condition is called a *hyphema; hypopyon* is when purulent matter accumulates in the anterior chamber.

The iris of each eye is compared for color, pattern, and shape. When looking through the pupillary opening, the nurse is also inspecting the lens, which is normally transparent. An opaque lens is termed a *cataract.*

## Pupillary Reflexes

The pupils normally are equal, round, and react to light and accommodation (PERRLA). When assessing the pupillary reflexes, the nurse approaches from the side and quickly shines a light into one eye, causing constriction of the pupil in that eye (direct light reaction). The pupil of the other eye also should constrict the same amount (consensual light reaction). The other eye is then tested in the same manner.

A light shining into a blind eye will not produce a pupillary response; however, a light shining into a normal eye will produce a pupillary response in the blind eye by consensual reaction if the oculomotor nerve is intact.[2]

The pupillary reflex can also be tested by having the person focus on an object that is moved directly toward the nose. When the person focuses on the near object, the pupils of both eyes should constrict (near reaction, reaction in accommodation). The examiner looks for the presence of a response and whether the response is equal in both eyes. Loss of pupillary reflexes when sight is present is caused by neurological disease.

## Assessment of Vision

Visual acuity means acuteness or sharpness of vision and includes measurement of distance and near vision. Visual acuity can vary with attention, intelligence, and physical conditions such as lighting.[11]

### Distance vision

Distance vision usually is determined by the use of a Snellen chart (Figure 55-8, *A*), with the person standing 20 feet (6 m) from the chart. The chart consists of rows of letters, numbers, or other characters arranged with the larger ones at the top and the smaller ones at the bottom. The uppermost letter on the chart is scaled so that it can be read by the normal eye at 200 feet, and the successive rows are scaled so that they can be read at 100, 70, 50, 40, 30, 20, 15, and 10 feet, respectively. Visual acuity is expressed as a fraction, and a reading of 20/20 is considered normal. The upper figure refers to the distance of the person from the chart, and the lower figure indicates the distance at which a normal eye can read the line. Each eye is tested separately, using a piece of stiff paper or a plastic occluder to cover the eye not being tested. The person is tested with and without distance lenses, and the results are recorded.

For preschool children, illiterate adults, and others unable to read the English alphabet, a modified Snellen chart may be used (Figure 55-8, *B*). A block E is shown in varying positions, and the person is asked to indicate in which direction the "legs" or "fingers" of the E point. A variety of other visual acuity testing charts are available for measuring visual acuity in

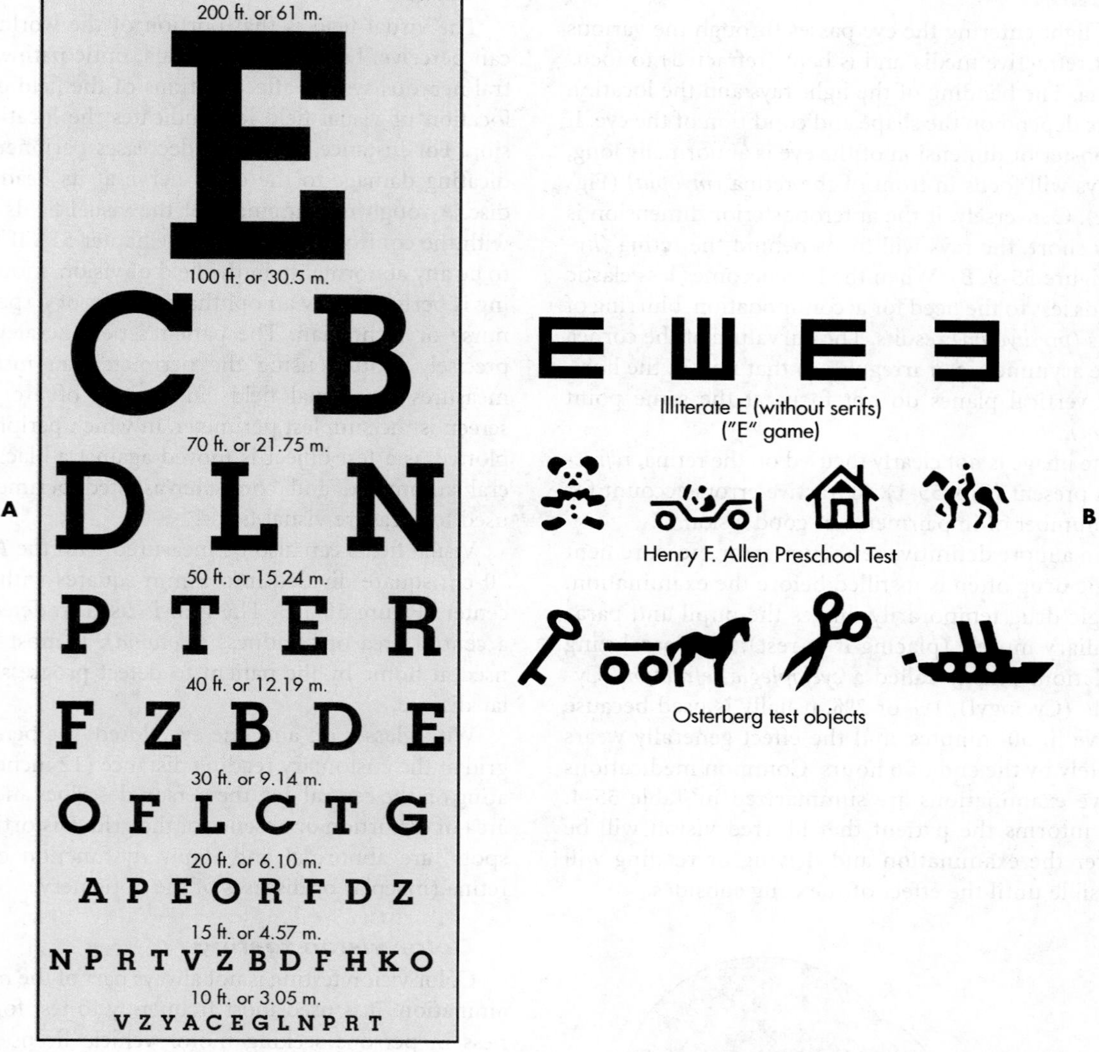


**fig. 55-8** **A,** Snellen chart used in vision screening. **B,** Symbols used in testing distance vision in children and illiterate adults.

preschool children (Figure 55-8, *B*), including the Allen charts with various silhouetted pictures, such as a telephone, that the child is asked to identify.

### Near vision

Near vision can be tested with the use of a Jaeger chart or newsprint. The Jaeger chart is a card containing varying sizes of print that is held 14 inches (35 cm) from the eye. The score obtained can be expressed in Snellen, metric, and percentage figures.

For persons unable to read letters visual acuity can be assessed by asking them to count the number of the nurse's fingers that they can see held in front of their eyes. Some persons may not be able to count fingers but can see hand movement. Still others may be able to tell only the direction from which light is coming (light projection) or just respond to light flashed in their eyes (light perception). Table 55-3 outlines some examples of visual acuity measurements.

**table 55-3** *Examples of Visual Acuity Measurement*

| Measurement | Meaning |
|---|---|
| 20/20 | Normal |
| 20/40-2 | Missed two letters of the 20/40 line |
| 10/400 | At 10 ft, reads line that normal eye sees at 400 ft |
| CF/2 ft | Counts fingers at 2 ft |
| HM/3 ft | Sees hand movement at 3 ft |
| LP/Proj. | Light perception with projection |
| NLP | No light perception |

Any person with vision less than 20/30 OD (right eye) or OS (left eye) or with a two-line difference between eyes should be referred to an ophthalmologist for further testing and treatment as the Snellen, block E, and Jaegar chart examinations provide only basic screening test data.

### Refraction

A ray of light entering the eye passes through the various transparent refractive media and is bent (refracted) to focus on the retina. The bending of the light rays and the location of the image depend on the shape and condition of the eye. If the anteroposterior dimension of the eye is abnormally long, the light rays will focus in front of the retina *(myopia)* (Figure 55-9, *A*). Conversely, if the anteroposterior dimension is abnormally short, the rays will focus behind the retina *(hyperopia)* (Figure 55-9, *B*). When the lens becomes less elastic and responds less to the need for accommodation, blurring of near objects *(presbyopia)* results. The curvature of the cornea also may be asymmetric or irregular so that rays in the horizontal and vertical planes do not focus at the same point *(astigmatism)*.

When the image is not clearly focused on the retina, *refractive error* is present (Box 55-1). Refractive errors account for the largest number of impairments of good vision.

To obtain a more definitive refractive error measurement a cycloplegic drug often is instilled before the examination. A cycloplegic drug temporarily dilates the pupil and paralyzes the ciliary muscle (placing it at rest), thus paralyzing accommodation. This is called a *cycloplegic refraction.* Cyclopentolate (Cyclogyl), 1% or 2%, usually is used because it is effective in 30 minutes, and the effect generally wears off completely by the end of 6 hours. Common medications used for eye examinations are summarized in Table 55-4. The nurse informs the patient that blurred vision will be present after the examination and driving or reading will not be possible until the effect of the drug subsides.

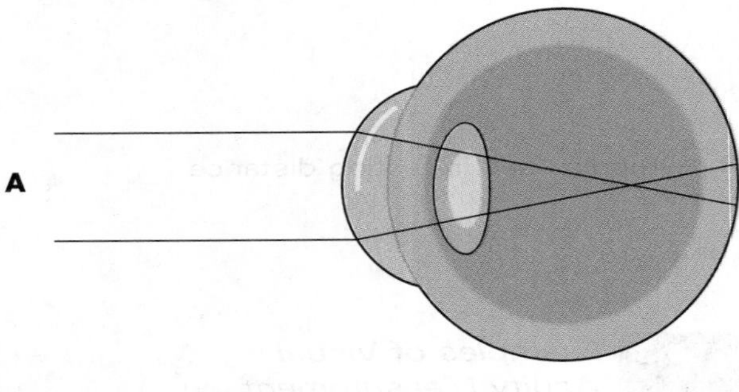


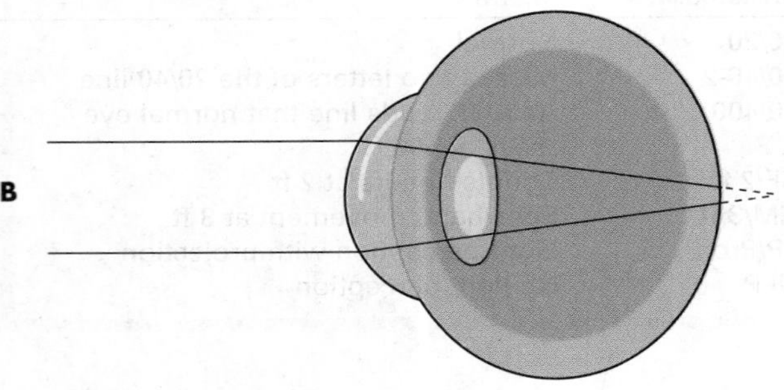


**fig. 55-9** Two major types of refractive errors. **A,** Myopia. Parallel light rays come to a focus in front of the retina. **B,** Hyperopia. Parallel light rays come to a focus behind the retina.

### Visual fields

The visual field is that portion of the world that the eye can perceive. Lesions of the retina, optic pathways, and central nervous system affect sections of the field of vision. The location of visual field loss indicates the location of the lesion. For instance, glaucoma decreases peripheral vision, indicating damage to the optic nerve at its head or the optic disc. A rough measurement of the visual fields can be made with the confrontation test (see Chapter 51). If there appears to be any abnormality in the field of vision, more precise testing is performed by an ophthalmologist or a specially trained nurse or technician. The patient's peripheral vision can be precisely plotted using the perimeter, an instrument that measures the visual fields in degrees of arc. The tangent screen is the simplest perimeter, in which peripheral vision is plotted as a test object is moved against a black screen. Several automated and computer-assisted perimeters are also used to measure visual fields.

Visual fields can also be measured with the Amsler grid, a 20-cm square divided into 5-mm squares with a dot in the center (Figure 55-10). The grid is used to detect and follow a central area of blindness *(scotoma)*. It most commonly is used at home by the patient to detect progression of macular disease.

With glasses on and one eye closed, the person holds the grid at the customary reading distance (12 inches). While fixating on the central dot, the person describes and outlines any area of distortion or absence of the grid. Distortions or "blind spots" are abnormal and imply dysfunction of the central retina (macula) or diseases of the optic nerve.

### Color vision testing

Color vision testing is not always part of the normal eye examination. It is used most frequently to test for color blindness in persons seeking motor vehicle licenses or jobs for which color discrimination is important. Color vision deficiencies occur as a hereditary defect in both men (7%) and women (0.5%). Nutritional deficiencies, drug toxicities,

**box 55-1** Terms Describing Refraction

| Term | Description |
|---|---|
| Accommodation | Ability to adjust between far and near objects |
| Emmetropia | Normal eye; light rays focus on retina |
| Ametropia | Refractive error; light rays do not focus on retina |
| Myopia | Nearsightedness; light rays focus in front of retina |
| Hyperopia | Farsightedness; light rays focus behind retina |
| Presbyopia | Hyperopia from loss of lens elasticity because of aging |
| Astigmatism | Irregular curvature of cornea; light rays do not focus at same point |

and various disorders of the optic nerve and fovea centralis also can alter color perception.

There are both gross and sensitive measures of color vision. A common test consists of color plates on which numbers are outlined in primary colors and surrounded by confusion colors. The person with a color vision problem is unable to recognize the figure. The more sensitive tests involve hue discrimination. One such test consists of 84 chips of color that are matched in terms of increasing hue.

### Assessment of Ocular Movements

Ocular movements are evaluated to determine whether the eyes are moving in a synchronous manner. Muscle imbalances and cranial nerve damage also can be detected.

To test ocular muscles the nurse and patient sit facing each other. The patient looks straight ahead, and a penlight is shined on the cornea. The corneal light reflex should be in exactly the same position on each pupil. The nurse then covers one of the person's eyes while the person looks at the light. When the cover is quickly removed, the nurse notes whether that eye moves to regain fixation on the light. Movement may indicate a drift of the eye behind the cover, which can indicate muscle imbalances.

To evaluate possible weaknesses of individual extraocular muscles, muscle testing can be performed in six cardinal fields of gaze, as well as straight ahead. The reader is referred to Chapter 51 for more detailed information about assessment of ocular movements.

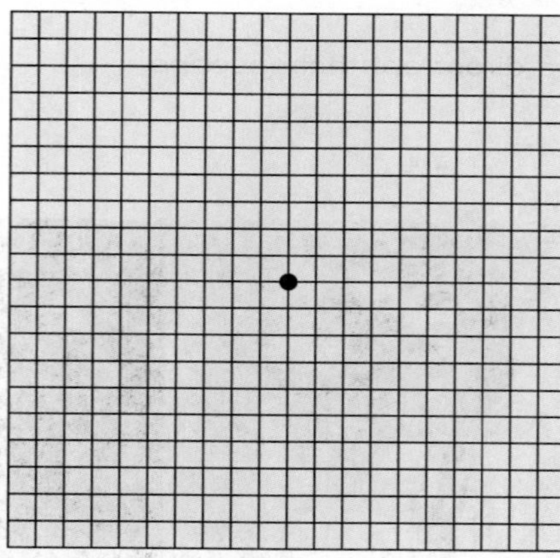

**fig. 55-10** The Amsler grid.

### Inspection of Internal Structures

#### *Ophthalmoscopy*

The fundus of the eye is examined with a hand-held instrument called an *ophthalmoscope,* which magnifies the view of the back of the eye so that the optic nerve, retina, blood vessels, and macula can be seen through the pupil (Figure 55-11). The examiner may use either the direct (Figure 55-12) or the indirect (Figure 55-13) method of ophthalmoscopic examination. The indirect ophthalmoscope allows the examiner to view the retina stereoscopically, thus allowing a wide-angle, three-dimensional view. This method provides visualization of the ocular fundus as far as the ora serrata (anterior margin of the retina). The indirect method, which requires a great degree of skill, normally is performed by an ophthalmologist. Nurses trained to perform an ophthalmoscopic examination use the direct method, the more commonly used approach. Because the entire retina cannot be visualized at one time, the examiner moves the ophthalmoscope until the entire fundus is visualized.

Difficulty in perceiving the fundus may be caused by interference with the light penetrating the eye as a result of intraocular inflammation, corneal scarring, or cataract. Data obtained from visualization of the fundus may indicate eye disease (cupping of the disc in glaucoma) or systemic disease

**table 55-4** *Eye Medications Commonly Used for Diagnostic Purposes*

| Drug | Action | Intervention |
|---|---|---|
| Mydriatics (eyedrops): phenylephrine hydrochloride (Neo-Synephrine, Mydrin) | Pupil dilation by blocking the responses to the sphincter muscle of the iris from cholinergic stimulation | Evaluate the effectiveness (dark-eyed individuals usually require more drops to achieve the dilation required).<br>Use is contraindicated in patients with a history of narrow or closed anterior chamber angles as may precipitate an increase intraocular pressure or angle closure attack.<br>Monitor for temporary blurred vision—caution patients about driving or operating machinery until vision improves.<br>Monitor for photophobia, and instruct patient to wear dark glasses in the sunlight or brightly lit rooms as needed. |
| Cycloplegics (eyedrops): atropine sulfate, cyclopentolate hydrochloride, homatropine hydrobromide, topicamide | Pupil dilation, but also blocks accommodation by paralyzing the ciliary muscles | Same as for mydriatics. |

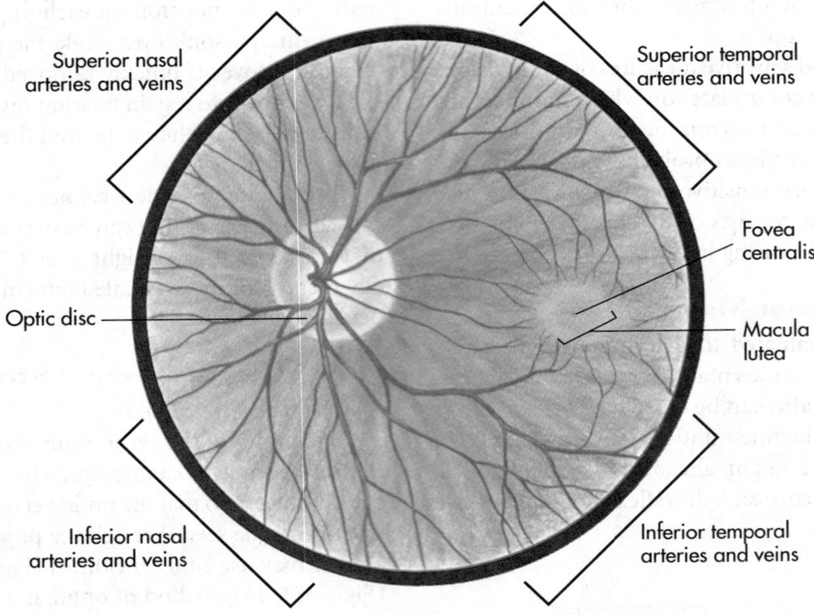


**fig. 55-11** A normal right fundus as seen through a direct ophthalmoscope.

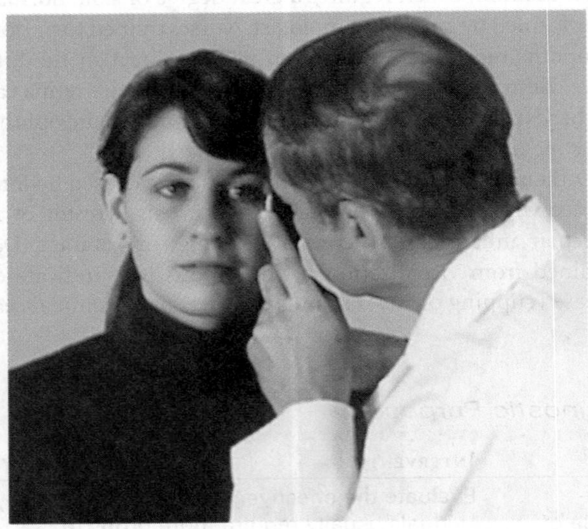

**fig. 55-12** Direct method of ophthalmoscopic examination.

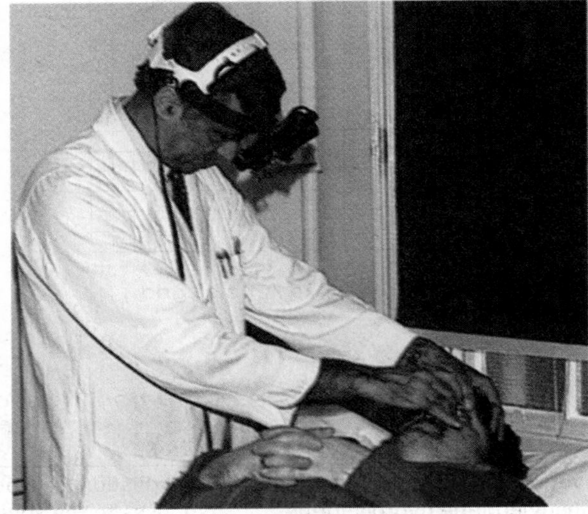

**fig. 55-13** Indirect method of ophthalmoscopic examination.

(arteriosclerosis or hypertension). Hemorrhages in deep retinal layers occur in advanced hypertension, severe renal disease, certain collagen diseases, advanced diabetes, and blood dyscrasias.

#### *Slit-lamp examination of the fundus*

The anterior segment of the eye can be examined with a slit-lamp, an instrument that combines a microscope and a light source. By adjusting the lens, the examiner can test for such problems as corneal ulcerations, lens changes, foreign bodies in the vitreous, or retinal changes.

### Estimation of Intraocular Pressure

An instrument known as a *tonometer* is used to measure ocular tension and is helpful in detecting early glaucoma. The most common tonometer in general use is that of Schiøtz. The procedure is performed with the patient lying down or in the chair with the head back and looking upward at some fixed point. The eye may be anesthetized, after which the tonometer is placed on the cornea (Figure 55-14). While the weight of the tonometer is supported by the cornea, the amount of indentation that the instrument makes in the cornea is measured on the attached scale. This reading is used to

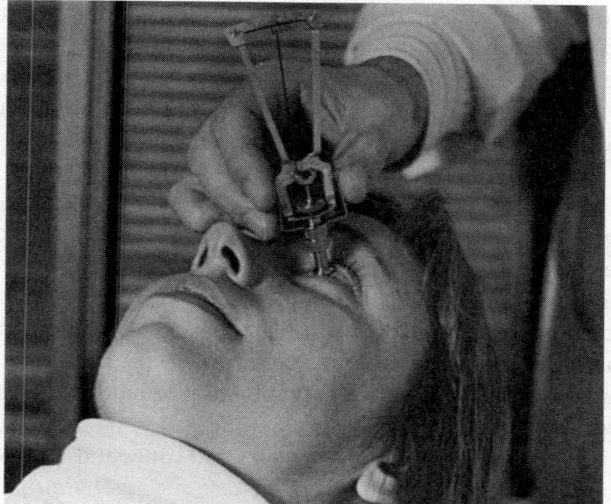

fig. 55-14 Measurement of intraocular pressure with Schiøtz tonometer.

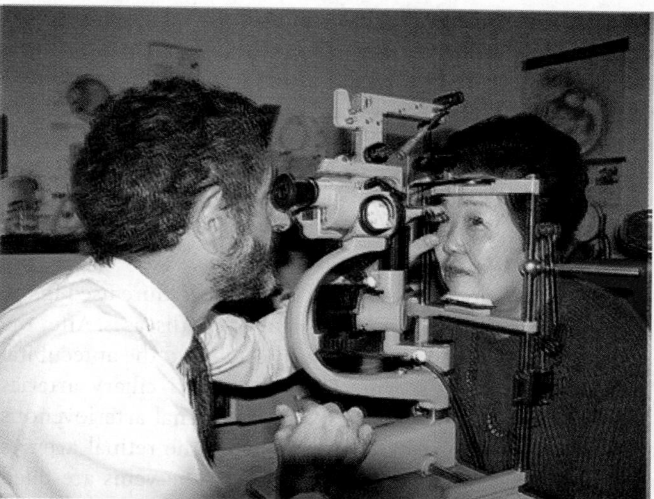

fig. 55-15 Measurement of intraocular pressure with applanation tonometer.

determine the pressure within the eye. Readings over 24 torr (Schiøtz) suggest glaucoma, but tests usually are repeated because temporary increases sometimes are caused by occurrences such as emotional stress. The *applanation tonometer* (Goldmann) is more accurate in estimating intraocular pressure and is frequently attached to the slit-lamp (Figure 55-15). Instead of indenting the eye, a small area of the cornea is flattened to counterbalance a spring-loaded measuring device, and the pressure is measured directly.

Noncontact tonometers are also available for measuring intraocular pressure. They use a puff of air to flatten a circular area of the cornea, thus bypassing the necessity for physical contact between the tonometer and the eye. For this test the eye does not need to be anesthetized.

## DIAGNOSTIC TESTS

### LABORATORY TESTS

Neither blood nor urine tests play a significant role in the evaluation of problems related to the eye, although they are used extensively to evaluate other systemic disorders such as diabetes that may be causing visual symptoms.

### RADIOLOGICAL TESTS

Several radiological procedures are used to aid in the diagnosis of eye conditions. These include plain x-ray films, computed tomography (CT) scans, and magnetic resonance imaging (MRI).

#### Plain X-Ray Films

Plain x-ray films of the orbit are used to assist in the diagnosis of orbital fractures and tumors. Right and left oblique views and a lateral view of the affected side usually provide the needed information.

#### Computed Tomography Scan

The CT scan is a rapid, safe, and noninvasive technique for the investigation of serial sections of the orbit and eye. The globe, lens, vitreous humor, optic nerve, extraocular muscles, visual pathway, and brain can all be evaluated. The CT scan is valuable in the diagnosis of orbital disease, retrobulbar tumors, intraocular eye masses, and intracranial disease and can be augmented by the injection of contrast material that increases the density of inflammatory or vascular lesions.[11] The nurse's primary responsibilities relate to careful pretest patient teaching.

#### Magnetic Resonance Imaging

MRI is a noninvasive technique that uses a high magnetic field to evaluate the brain, orbit, and eye. MRI provides better definition of tissues and fluids in the brain and eye than can be achieved with a CT scan. It is particularly helpful in identifying edema.[12] The nurse explains the procedure and carefully prepares the patient for the noises and sensations experienced during the test.

### SPECIAL TESTS

#### Ultrasonography

Ultrasonography is a noninvasive test that uses high-frequency sound waves to outline and detect intraocular and orbital structures and measure the distance between them. Various abnormalities, such as retinal masses and detachments, intraocular foreign bodies, and changes in the orbit, can be easily delineated by this test. Two types of ultrasonography, A-scan and B-scan, are used in ophthalmology. The A-scan is useful in differentiating between benign and malignant tumors and measuring the axial length of the eyeball, a value that is needed to calculate the power of an intraocular lens for implantation after a cataract extraction. The B-scan provides a two-dimensional image that helps visualize tumors, retinal detachments, swollen muscles, or inflamed tissue. The nurse gives the patient information about the procedure itself and any sensory effects. In both scans, a probe is placed on the front of the eye (or on the closed eyelid), sound waves are delivered, and measurements are recorded on the screen of the oscilloscope. The test is not uncomfortable although anesthetic drops may be instilled if the probe is applied directly to the eye.

## Fluorescein Angiography

Fluorescein angiography is a specialized procedure used in the diagnosis, monitoring, and treatment of eye diseases. After the pupil is dilated, fluorescein dye is injected into the antecubital fossa of the patient's arm. The retinal and ciliary arteries transmit the dye into the eyes, and the retinal arteriovenous circulation is visualized. The dye reaches the retinal arteries 10 to 16 seconds after the injection, and the veins are filled within 25 seconds. To provide a permanent record of this circulation, photographs are taken with a specially designed camera called a *fundus camera.* The camera is equipped with an optical system for viewing the retina and a light flash system for illumination and is mounted on a stand similar to that for a slit-lamp. The patient sits in a chair with the chin placed in the chin rest and the forehead against a bar while a rapid series of photographs are taken to capture the movement of the dye through the retinal arteriovenous circulation. This test may take as long as 1 hour to complete. When the photographs are assessed, they provide definitive information about any avascular obstruction, the growth of new vessels (neovascularization), microaneurysms, abnormal capillary permeability, and defects in the pigmented layer of the retina.

Fluorescein angiography is a relatively safe procedure with few untoward effects. The patient is assessed for any allergies or previous reaction to dye. Those with a history of hay fever or asthma may be given a small test dose before the entire dose is injected.[1] Although rare, a severe allergic reaction can occur.

The nurse explains the procedure, obtains an informed consent, and explains the need to keep the head still during the test. The nurse warns the patient that a dazzle effect may occur from the frequent camera flashes. Mydriatic eye drops are instilled to dilate the pupils, facilitating visualization of the fundus. Some patients experience transient nausea or vomiting as the dye is injected.

Patients are informed that it may require several minutes for the dazzle effect to resolve after the test. The nurse also informs the patient that yellowing of the skin, especially in persons with fair complexions, and a fluorescent orange or green discoloration of the urine usually is present for 24 hours. Patients are encouraged to drink increased amounts of fluids to promote excretion of the dye. The pupils remain dilated for a few hours, and the patient should avoid bright light and wear sunglasses when outdoors until the pupils return to normal.

## Electrophysiology Examinations

There are four electrophysiology examinations performed in ophthalmology: electroretinogram (ERG), electrooculogram (EOG), dark adaptometry, and visual evoked potential. The main purpose of these examinations is to assess the function of the visual pathway from the photoreceptors of the retina to the visual cortex of the brain. Electrophysiological testing is useful in diagnosing retinal vascular occlusions, toxic drug exposure, inherited retinal diseases, and intraocular foreign bodies.[4]

### Electroretinogram

ERG is a process of graphing the electrical response from the retina that occurs as a consequence of light stimulation. In this test the pupil is dilated, a topical anesthetic is applied, and a corneal electrode is placed on the cornea using a contact lens. A grounding electrode is placed on the ear. Lights at various intensities and intervals are then flashed and the nervous response graphed.

ERG tests the function of the rods and cones and is helpful in evaluating widespread retinal disease such as *retinitis pigmentosa.* The visual potential of an eye that has a dense cataract or other opacification also can be assessed with ERG. However, normal results do not rule out the presence of macular or optic nerve disease. The patient is told the nature of the test and the steps of the procedure. A demonstration of the flashing lights often is helpful. The test does not require any special follow-up care.

### Electrooculogram

EOG measures the difference in the electrical potential between the front and back of the eye (retina) in response to periods of dark and light. The preparation of the patient requires that skin electrodes be placed on the lateral and medial canthi of both eyes. Corneal contact lenses are not required.

### Dark adaptometry

Dark adaptometry measures the universal phenomenon of dark adaptation. Normally, when a person is placed in a room and the lights are suddenly turned out, the eyes gradually become more sensitive and vision in the darkness improves over time. For this test, the patient is placed in a totally darkened room with a dark adaptometer machine. The patient is then exposed to a standardized level of light for a specified period of time. The light is gradually dimmed until total darkness is restored. Patients respond to the various intensities of light to which they are exposed by pushing a button on the machine.

### Visual evoked potential

Visual evoked potential is a measurement of visual function monitored at the level of the occipital cortex with scalp electrodes that evaluate the integrity of the visual pathways from the optic nerve to the occipital cortex. Stimulation of the retina with light changes the electrical activity of the cortex. Through various computer processes, the electrical activity associated with this stimulation of the retina is summed and shown as a measurable electrical wave. Optic neuritis, demyelinating disease, and optic atrophy can alter this wave. For these electrophysiological tests, the nurse explains the procedures, indicating that they are pain free and require no special follow-up.

## *chapter* SUMMARY

### ANATOMY AND PHYSIOLOGY OF THE EYE

- The eye has three main layers: the outer layer, made up of the sclera and cornea; the uvea, consisting of the choroid, ciliary body, and iris; and the innermost layer, or the retina.
- Visual changes that occur with aging include presbyopia, decreased ability to tolerate glare, decreased peripheral fields, decreased ability to adapt to dim light and darkness, and a decrease in the quantity and quality of tears.

### ASSESSMENT

- A complete history—including a family history of eye problems and the presence of any systemic diseases—is necessary in assessing a person's eyes and vision.
- Objective data required when doing an ocular nursing assessment include assessment of visual acuity, visual fields, pupillary reflexes, and ocular movement, as well as inspection of internal structures and an estimation of intraocular pressure.

### DIAGNOSTIC TESTS

- Radiological tests used to aid diagnosis of eye problems include x-ray films, CT scans, and MRIs.
- Electrodiagnostic examinations are used mainly to evaluate retinal and optic nerve diseases.
- The main nursing responsibility is to explain diagnostic tests, including any discomfort or alteration in vision that may be experienced.

## References

1. Anand R: Fluorescein angiography. I. Technique and normal study, *J Ophthal Nurs Technol* 8:48-52, 1989.
2. Bates B, Heokelman RD, Thompson JB: *A guide to physical examination and history taking,* ed 6, Philadelphia, 1995, JB Lippincott.
3. Ebersole P, Hess P: Toward healthy aging: human needs and nursing response, ed 4, St Louis, 1994 Mosby.
4. Follmer BA, Smith SC: Electrophysiology testing and the ophthalmic registered nurse, *INSIGHT* 19(4):12-18, 1994.
5. Hunt L: Ophthalmic nursing assessment, *INSIGHT* 17(3):9-11, 1992.
6. Hunt L: Aging and the visual system, *INSIGHT* 18(3):6-7, 18, 1993.
7. Jakobiec FA, Azar D, editors: *International ophthalmology clinics: pediatric ophthalmology,* Boston, 1992, Little, Brown & Co.
8. Kapperud MJ: *The aging eye: a guide for nurses,* St Paul, Minn, 1983, The Minnesota Society for the Prevention of Blindness and Preservation of Hearing.
9. Kelly JS: Visual impairment among older people, *Br J Nurs* 2(2):110-116, 1993.
10. Mrochuk J: Introduction to diagnostic ophthalmic ultrasound for nurses in ophthalmology, *J Ophthal Nurs Technol* 9:234-239, 1990.
11. Newell F: *Ophthalmology: principles and concepts,* ed 8, St Louis, 1996, Mosby.
12. Wirtschafter JD, Berman EL, McDonald CS: *Magnetic resonance imaging and computed tomography: clinical neuro-orbital anatomy,* San Francisco, 1992, American Academy of Ophthalmology.

# chapter 56 MANAGEMENT OF PERSONS WITH Problems of the Eye

BARBARA ASTLE and MARION ALLEN

## objectives *After studying this chapter, the learner should be able to:*

1 Discuss the etiologies of the common forms of visual impairment.
2 Compare the pathophysiology of common eye inflammations and infections.
3 Describe the emergency treatment of eye injury.
4 Discuss the collaborative management of glaucoma.
5 Compare the preoperative and postoperative care of patients undergoing surgery for cataracts and retinal detachment.
6 Outline the effects of diabetes, hypertension, and human immunodeficiency virus on the eye.

Eye disease and blindness affect millions of people throughout the world. In the United States nearly 11.5 million persons have some degree of visual impairment, and approximately 1.5 million persons do not have useful vision in one or both eyes. This chapter discusses the major causes of visual impairment, common eye infections and injuries, and the management of major eye disorders such as glaucoma and cataracts. The nurse plays a significant role in the collaborative care of patients experiencing eye disorders and also has an important role in educating the general public about primary and secondary prevention strategies to maintain eye health.

## VISUAL IMPAIRMENT

### ETIOLOGY/EPIDEMIOLOGY

Visual impairment ranges in severity from diminished visual acuity to total blindness. Legal blindness is defined in the United States as: (1) a visual acuity, with maximal correction, of 20/200 or less and/or (2) a visual field reduction to a range of 20° (compared with a normal range of about 180°). This is an arbitrary definition that was established early in the century to identify individuals who would need public assistance to function in society. The definition is not accepted or used worldwide.

An estimated 1 million persons in the United States are legally blind, and most of these persons are older than 65 years of age. Almost 80 million Americans have a disorder of one or both eyes, and this figure does not include the additional millions of persons with straightforward refractive errors who require the use of corrective lenses to participate fully in daily activities. These figures make visual impairment one of the most common disorders affecting adults in this country. Uncorrected vision problems have a negative impact on school and work performance and contribute to injury. Loss of vision limits the individual's interaction with the environment and reduces the range and variety of experiences available. Personal care, home maintenance, social interaction, and interpersonal communication are all affected.

Visual impairment has numerous causes, and preventable blindness is a major worldwide health problem. Refractive errors are by far the most common problem, but numerous other nutritional, infectious, metabolic, and systemic disorders adversely affect the function of the eye. Nutritional deficiencies are a major global health concern. A lack of adequate vitamin A and B complex can cause changes within the retina, cornea, and conjunctiva. Night blindness is a classic outcome of vitamin A deficiency, and optic neuritis can result from deficits of vitamin B, especially in alcoholics. Infection, e.g., trachoma, is another common cause of visual impairment and causes blindness in millions of persons in developing countries. Macular degeneration, a disease of the aging retina, is the leading cause of blindness in the elderly. Twenty to 30% of persons between 75 and 85 years of age are affected. The leading causes of visual impairment/blindness in the United States include glaucoma, cataract, and macular degeneration.

The eye can also be adversely affected by a variety of systemic diseases (Table 56-1). The exophthalmos associated with Graves' disease is one of the most visible examples; and visual field problems are common outcomes of cerebrovascular accidents. The demyelination associated with multiple sclerosis also frequently affects the eye. Retinopathy is a complication of vascular disease, particularly uncontrolled hypertension, and is frequently both progressive and irreversible (see Chapter 27). Cytomegalovirus (CMV) retinopathy has become a serious complication associated with the severe immunocompromise of acquired immunodeficiency syndrome (AIDS). Diabetic retinopathy is perhaps the most important example. Laser treatment has proven effective in treating these

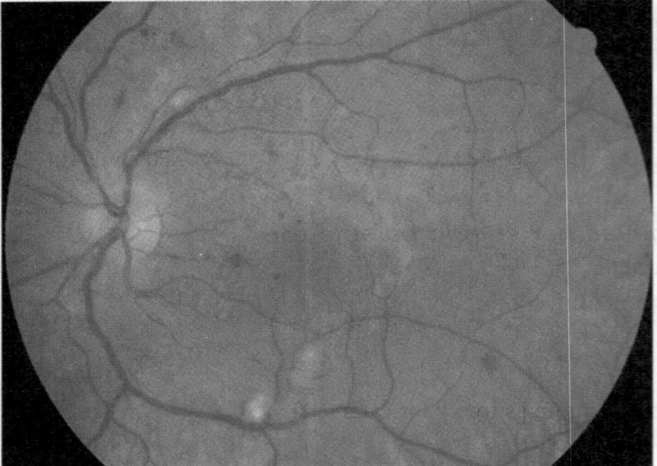

**fig. 56-1** Diabetic retinopathy with cotton wool spots (exudates) below the macula.

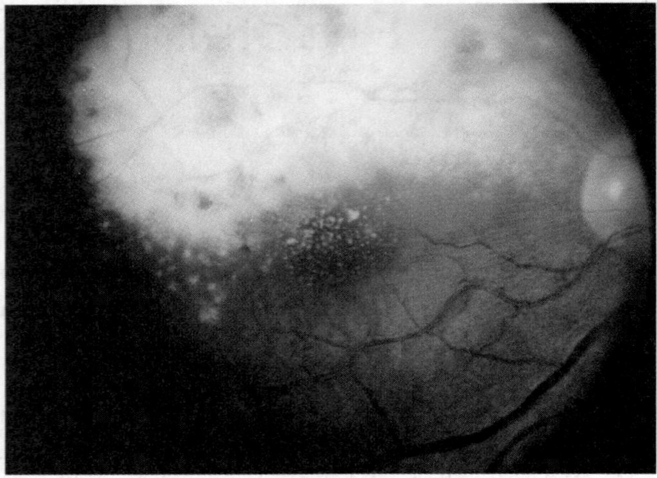

**fig. 56-2** CMV retinitis infiltrating the superior retina.

**table 56-1** *Eye Manifestations of Systemic Diseases*

| Disorder | Effect on the Eyes |
|---|---|
| **VASCULAR DISORDERS** | |
| Hypertension | Persistent uncontrolled hypertension can cause hemorrhage, edema, and exudates in the retina. Retinal arteries narrow, causing degenerative changes. |
| Cerebrovascular accident | Depending on the location of the stroke, the patient may experience hemianopsia or blindness. |
| Sickle cell disease | This can cause neovascularization, arterial occlusions, or retinal hemorrhage. |
| **NEUROLOGICAL DISORDERS** | |
| Multiple sclerosis | Demyelination can result in optic neuritis, diplopia, and nystagmus. |
| **ENDOCRINE DISORDERS** | |
| Graves' disease | Accumulation of fat and fluid in the retro-ocular tissue can produce exophthalmos (protrusion of the eye) and lid retraction. |
| Diabetic retinopathy | Retinal capillary walls thicken and develop microaneurysms. Retinal veins widen and become tortuous (Figure 56-1). Small hemorrhages occur, which leave scars that decrease vision.<br>As the disease worsens, neovascularization occurs, and the new vessels grow into the vitreous humor. These vessels are vulnerable to both obstruction and rupture. Vision decreases and "floaters" are perceived in the eye. |
| **CONNECTIVE TISSUE DISORDERS** | |
| Rheumatoid arthritis, systemic lupus erythematosus | Neovascularization, inflammation of the cornea, sclera, or uveal tract occur. |
| **AIDS-RELATED DISORDERS** | |
| Herpes zoster ophthalmicus | Herpes can invade the cornea and create ulceration that is potentially blinding. |
| CMV | CMV affects an estimated 20% of AIDS patients. It spreads rapidly through the cells of the retina and the blood vessels and can totally destroy the retina (Figure 56-2). |
| Kaposi's sarcoma | The lesions of Kaposi's sarcoma can affect the skin of the eyelids and conjunctiva or the orbit itself. |

retinal changes in early stages, but steady progression toward blindness is still common in diabetic patients, particularly those with uncontrolled or brittle disease (see Chapter 35). Treatment options for diabetic retinopathy are summarized in Box 56-1.

## PATHOPHYSIOLOGY

### Refractive Disorders

Refractive disorders include irregularities of the corneal curvature, length, and shape of the eye as well as the focusing ability of the lens. There are three main types of refractive dis-

**box 56-1** *Treatment Options for Diabetic Retinopathy*

**PHOTOCOAGULATION**

A laser is used to direct energy onto selected spots on the retina. Irritation and scarring of the peripheral retina appear to decrease the ischemia that triggers the pathological neovascularization process. The risk of blindness is reduced by 60% with this treatment. Retinopathy becomes inactive, and new vessels stop appearing.

**VITRECTOMY**

A technically difficult procedure in which bloody vitreous humor is removed from the posterior chamber along with scar tissue, which frequently causes the retina to detach. The vitreous is replaced with a saline solution, silicone oil, perflurocarbon liquid, or an air-gas mixture. The oils can be left in place after surgery.

NOTE: Tight glucose control is considered to be the most effective strategy for preventing or limiting the incidence of all diabetic complications, including retinopathy.

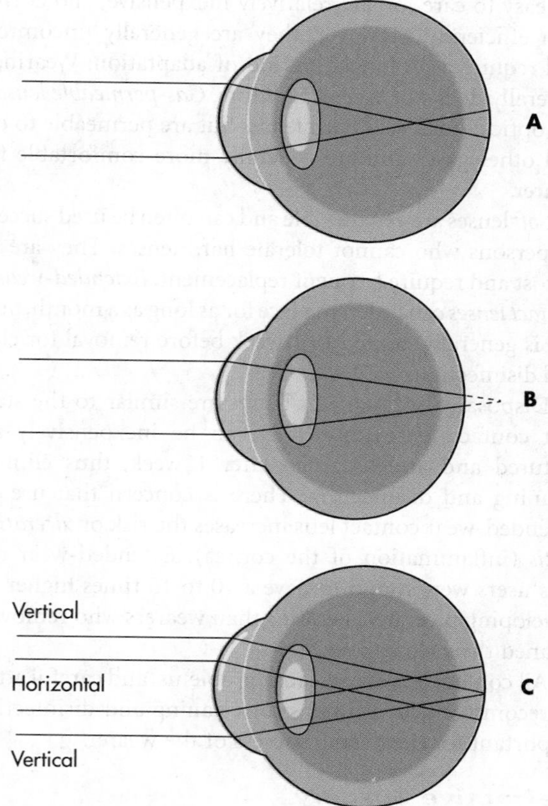


**fig. 56-3** Three types of refractive errors. **A,** Myopic eye. Parallel rays of light are brought to a focus in front of the retina. **B,** Hyperopic eye. Parallel rays of light come to a focus behind the retina in the unaccommodative eye. **C,** Simple myopic astigmatism. The vertical bundle of rays is focused on the retina; the horizontal rays are focused in front of the retina.

orders (Figure 56-3). The major symptoms of all three disorders include blurred vision and headache.

*Myopia* or nearsightedness occurs when parallel rays of light focus in front of the retina as the person looks at a distant object. *Hyperopia* or farsightedness occurs when light rays focus in back of the retina as the individual looks at a near object. A shortened eyeball may contribute to the problem. An *astigmatism* is caused by an unequal curvature of the cornea. Light rays are bent unevenly and do not focus on a single spot on the retina. *Presbyopia* is a common problem associated with aging. The lens loses elasticity making it more difficult to focus on near objects.

## Macular Degeneration

Degenerative changes occur in the thin layer of blood vessels that arise in the retina and extend into the choroid and their membrane cover. Both neovascular (exudative or wet) and non-neovascular (nonexudative or dry) forms occur. In neovascular degeneration there is a sudden proliferation of new fragile blood vessels in the macular area that tend to leak and damage the macula. Scarring occurs and functional losses progress rapidly. The neovascular form of macular degeneration occurs in only 5% to 10% of all patients, but it is responsible for about 80% of the severe vision loss attributed to the disease. The non-neovascular form of macular degeneration is more common. Degeneration occurs from the deposit of waste products and slow atrophy of the choroid, retina, and pigment epithelium.

Macular degeneration causes a variety of symptoms including visual blurring and distortion and usually causes some degree of central vision loss and a decreased ability to distinguish colors. Early signs and progression of the disease can be readily detected with the use of the Amsler grid (see Chapter 55). The individual perceives dark spots, missing areas, and distorted wavy lines. Intravenous fluorescein angiography may be used to visualize or confirm the extent of neovascularization if vessel leakage is suspected.

# COLLABORATIVE CARE MANAGEMENT

## Corrective Lenses

Visual impairments caused by refractive errors are usually diagnosed as part of a routine eye examination. The person may initiate the diagnostic process in response to chronic headache or an awareness of blurred or failing vision. Eyeglasses and contact lenses are widely used to correct common refractive errors and restore visual acuity. Federal law requires that all prescription glasses be made with impact-resistant lenses. Plastic lenses are lightweight but scratch easily. Hardened and safety lenses have been tempered to make them extremely resistant to breakage.

Contact lenses are made of various types of thin plastic that fit over the cornea. Their popularity is primarily cosmetic, but some people do achieve better vision correction with contact lenses than with glasses.

Contact lenses may be rigid, soft, gas permeable (rigid), extended-wear (soft), or disposable (soft). *Rigid* (hard) lenses are easy to care for, are relatively inexpensive, and correct vision efficiently. However, they are generally uncomfortable and require a prolonged period of adaptation. Wearing time generally does not exceed 12 hours. *Gas-permeable lenses* have the optical quality of hard lenses but are permeable to oxygen and other gases and are generally more comfortable for the wearer.

*Soft* lenses are very flexible and can often be used successfully by persons who cannot tolerate hard lenses. They are higher in cost and require frequent replacement. *Extended-wear* (soft) *contact lenses* can be left in place for as long as a month, but their use is generally limited to 1 week before removal for cleaning and disinfection.

Disposable soft contact lenses are similar to the standard soft contact lenses, but they can be inexpensively manufactured and are discarded after 1 week, thus eliminating cleaning and disinfecting. There is concern that use of any extended-wear contact lens increases the risk of *ulcerative keratitis* (inflammation of the cornea). Extended-wear contact lens users were found to have a 10 to 15 times higher risk of developing ulcerative keratitis than wearers who removed and cleaned their lenses every day.

All contact lenses can cause problems, and careful attention to recommended regimens for cleaning and disinfection are important for the overall success of the wearer.

### Refractive Surgery

Refractive surgery, defined as any operative procedure performed for the purpose of eliminating a refraction error, has become an increasingly viable alternative to glasses and contact lenses for persons with visual impairment related to refraction errors. The *radial keratotomy* is the most common procedure. It is designed to flatten the cornea and decrease myopia by making a series of 3 to 8 radial cuts from the limbus to within 3 mm of the apex of the cornea (Figure 56-4). A more invasive procedure, *incisional keratotomy,* attempts to correct both astigmatism and myopia. *Photorefractive keratotomy* uses an excimer laser to reshape the surface of the cornea and has become increasingly popular. Thin sections of outer cornea can also be removed to correct higher degrees of myopia. All of these procedures are performed in ambulatory surgery centers. Careful preoperative teaching about the goals and limitations of the surgery, as well as the expected postoperative course, is essential. Patients are permitted to gradually resume activities and usually experience a slow improvement of vision over a period of weeks or months. The nurse administers analgesics as needed to keep the patient comfortable and administers antibiotics to decrease the incidence of infection.

### Macular Degeneration

There is no adequate treatment currently available for the non-neovascular form of macular degeneration. Oral zinc may reduce the progression of the disease. A small percentage of patients with neovascular degeneration can benefit from laser therapy to coagulate the abnormal vessels.

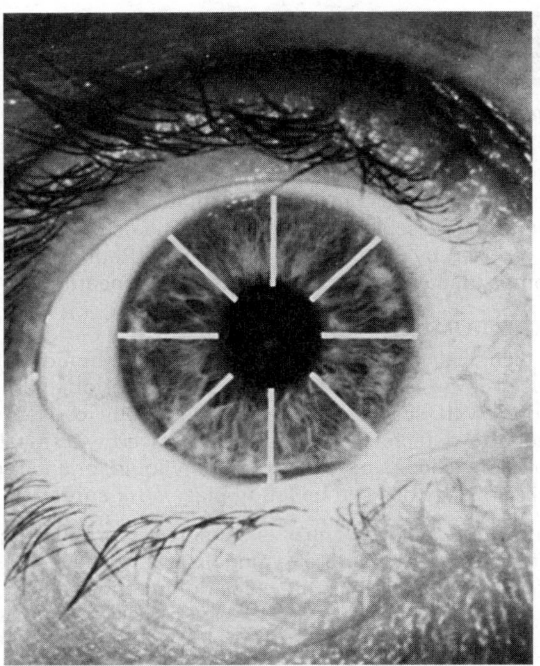

**fig. 56-4** Location of incisions in radial keratotomy.

### Patient/Family Education

Some forms of visual impairment are preventable, and most forms can be slowed or treated with early diagnosis and appropriate therapy. Regular eye examinations by a competent professional are an important health promotion measure throughout life, especially as a person ages. Early identification of eye disorders such as glaucoma is essential to prevent loss of vision. Appropriate intervention for cataracts can restore useful vision, and the rigorous control of systemic diseases such as diabetes and hypertension can minimize the adverse visual consequences.

Multiple opportunities exist for education and intervention with patients and families related to preserving visual function and promoting eye health. The importance of this area is reflected in the *Healthy People 2000* goals. The following objective related to vision is included in that initiative: Reduce visual impairment to no more than 30 cases per 1000 persons from a baseline of 34.5 per 1000. This objective particularly targets people 65 years and older. A target for this group is to reduce the current rate from 87.7 cases per 1000 to 70 cases per 1000.

Maintaining eye health is an important teaching intervention for all patients, not just those experiencing eye problems. The eye is a remarkably resilient organ. It cleans itself through the constant production and excretion of tears and the secretions from the conjunctivae, which also are protective. As a consequence, normal healthy eyes do not need special care or cleaning. Care should be taken not to irritate the eyes or introduce bacteria into the eyes by rubbing them.

Adequate nutrition is as important for eye health as it is for maintaining other body functions. Vitamin deficiencies can cause night blindness (vitamin A), corneal damage (vitamin A), optic neuritis (vitamin B), and other disorders. Although a sufficient vitamin intake is necessary, an excessive amount is wasted and may actually do more harm than good.

It is difficult to predict the course of any progressive visual impairment, and patients rightly fear becoming blind. The nurse ensures that the patient has accurate information about the specific disease, type of vision loss, and prognosis. Opportunities to express fears and frustrations related to declining vision can be helpful to the patient and family. Social support is a key factor in the adjustment of patients to visual impairment. The nurse can also provide referrals for the patient to the numerous community agencies that provide services and support to visually impaired persons as they attempt to incorporate their changing vision status into their daily lives. Integration of declining vision or blindness into one's self-concept can take a long time. A social stigma related to blindness still exists, and patients need ongoing support and understanding.

Visual impairment requires a major life adjustment. Persons need to adjust to both the initial impact of the loss and the subsequent changes that will occur in their life because of the loss of vision. Over time most patients learn new ways or adapt their present ways of doing things to carry out their normal activities. Most recognize that there are some things that they will never be able to do again on their own or that they can do only with help.

The nurse ensures that the patient has any and all visual aids that may be useful to them including magnifying glasses and special reading lights. Patients with progressive macular degeneration need to learn how to optimize their peripheral vision as their central vision deteriorates.

Adjustment is an ongoing process and time is a key variable. Time is needed to grieve for the lost sight and to recognize and come to terms with the implications of the loss. Time is also needed to master many of the difficult tasks and the work associated with adjustment to a visual impairment.

The dependence on others and the necessity to ask for help are two of the most difficult things to which they must adjust. Fluctuating vision leads to frustration and difficulties in planning or implementing tasks.

Figure 56-5 and the following Guidelines for Care Boxes provide useful strategies for assisting the visually impaired person.

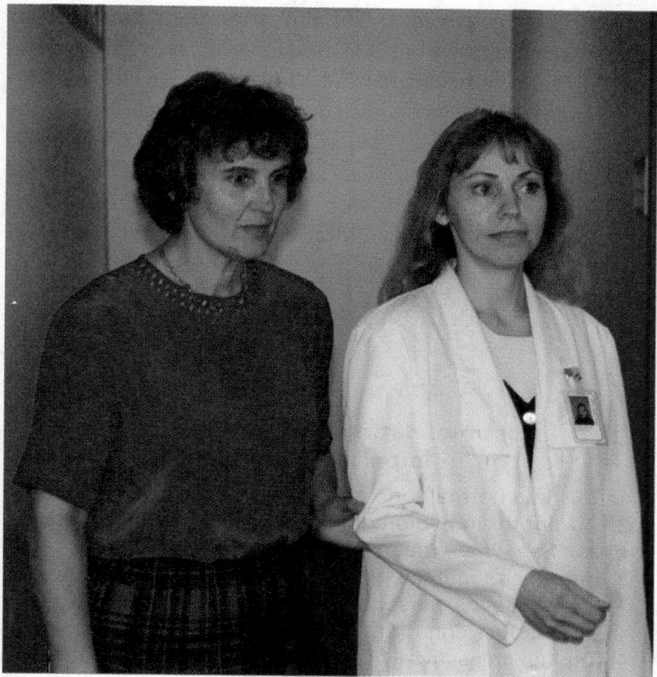

**fig. 56-5** Assisting a visually impaired person to ambulate. Note that woman is holding nurse's arm and is led without being held.

*guidelines for care*

**Facilitating Independence in ADL for Visually Impaired Persons**

1. Place clothing in specific and consistent locations in drawers and closets.
2. Place food and cooking utensils in specific and consistent locations in cupboards and/or refrigerator.
3. Encourage use of cane when walking.
4. Keep furniture and household objects in specific and consistent places.
5. When walking with a blind person, let the person take your arm (Figure 56-5).
6. Provide descriptions of food on the plate using clock placement of food; for example, put the peas at "7 o'clock." Cut food as appropriate.
7. Always permit blind persons to pull out their own chairs and seat themselves.

## INFECTIONS AND INFLAMMATION

Infections and inflammation can occur in any of the eye structures and may be caused by microorganisms, mechanical irritation, or sensitivity to some substance. Inflammation of the eye is the most common acute condition affecting the eye. Conjunctivitis represents about two thirds of the total. Table 56-2 summarizes the common eye infections/inflammations and their management. Conjunctivitis is discussed below. Box 56-2 summarizes ophthalmic drugs used to treat inflammation and infection.

### CONJUNCTIVITIS

#### Etiology/Epidemiology

*Conjunctivitis* (inflammation of the conjunctiva) is a common infection that can occur from a variety of causes. It may result from mechanical trauma such as that caused by sunburn or from infection with organisms such as *staphylococci, streptococci,* or *Haemophilus influenzae.* Two sexually transmitted agents that cause conjunctivitis are *Chlamydia trachomatis* and *Neisseria gonorrhoeae.* Inflammation is often caused by allergic reactions within the body or by external irritants (e.g., poison ivy or cosmetics). Viral agents that cause conjunctivitis include most human adenovirus strains and the herpes simplex viruses.

Acute mucopurulent bacterial conjunctivitis (often called *pinkeye*) is the most common form of conjunctivitis. It is prevalent in school-aged children but can occur at any age. It is highly infectious, especially in crowded environments such as schools and nursing homes. It is usually self-limited and causes no permanent damage.

### Pathophysiology

The symptoms of conjunctivitis vary in severity. Hyperemia and burning are common initial symptoms that progress rapidly to a mucopurulent exudate, which crusts on the base of the eyelashes and is easily transferred to the uninfected eye. Viral infections produce minimal exudate. The conjunctiva are grossly reddened and inflamed. Invasion of the cornea can result in ulceration and even perforation, usually in response to virulent organisms such as *Neisseria gonorrhoeae.* Involvement of the cornea, although rare, is extremely serious and can even result in the loss of the eye. The corneal ulcer is usually identified on slit-lamp examination and may be outlined with the use of sterile fluorescein dye.

### Collaborative Care Management

Treatment of conjunctivitis includes careful cleansing of the eyelids and lashes and the use of topical antibiotics. Warm moist compresses may be used to gently remove firm adherent crusts from the eyes, especially in the morning. The procedure for applying warm compresses is outlined in the following Guidelines for Care Box. Because the drainage material is infectious, it should be disposed of carefully.

**guidelines for care**

**Communicating with the Visually Impaired Person**

1. Talk in a normal tone of voice.
2. Do *not* try to avoid common phrases in speech, such as "See what I mean."
3. Introduce yourself with each contact (unless well known to the person). If in a hospital, knock on the door before entering.
4. Explain any activity occurring in the room or what you will be doing.
5. Announce when you are leaving the room so the person is not put in the position of talking to someone who is no longer there.

**table 56-2** *Eye Infection/Inflammation*

| Disorder | Description | Collaborative Management |
|---|---|---|
| Hordeolum (style) | Common infection of small glands of lid margins, caused by *staphylococcus;* it creates a tender, swollen pustule that gradually resolves or ruptures. | Application of warm compresses 3-4 times per day; antibiotic ointment if severe; incision of pustule if it does not resolve spontaneously |
| Chalazion | Sterile cyst located in the connective tissue in the free edges of the eyelid. Lump is small, hard, and nontender, but may put pressure on the eye and affect vision. | May disappear spontaneously, become infected, or require local excision if impairing vision |
| Trachoma | A chronic infectious form of conjunctivitis believed to be caused by *Chlamydia trachomatis.* Common in Africa and Asia, it is one of the leading causes of blindness worldwide. | Can be effectively treated early in the disease with antibiotics; hard to eradicate once chronic |
| Keratitis | Inflammation of the cornea, it can be superficial or deep, acute or chronic. *Staphylococcus* and *Streptococcus* bacteria and herpes simplex viruses are common causes. Pain, photophobia, and blepharospasm are common. It can result in visual loss. | Steroids to control inflammation, antibiotics, cycloplegics to rest the eye; corneal transplant may be necessary |
| Uveitis | Acute inflammation of the uvea from infection, allergy, toxic agents, and systemic disorders; it causes eye pain, swelling, photophobia, and visual impairment. | May be self-limiting; treatment of underlying cause plus cycloplegics to rest the eye; warm moist compresses to reduce inflammation and increase comfort |
| Blepharitis | Inflammation of the eyelids frequently begins in childhood and recurs causing redness and scaling of the upper and lower lid at the lash borders. | Daily facial cleansing and shampoo to remove scales; local antibiotics may be helpful |
| Corneal ulcer | Infection of the cornea is not common but it can readily lead to ulceration. Ulcers typically cause pain, tearing, and spasms of the eyelid. A greyish white corneal opacity is seen with fluorescein evaluation. | Minor abrasions heal spontaneously and without scarring; comfort measures critical as the pain can be severe; possible need for antibiotics and corticosteroids |

Common ophthalmic antibiotics include polymixin B, bacitracin, and gentamicin in ointment or eye drop form (Box 56-2). Ophthalmic ointments remain in contact with the eye much longer, providing a prolonged effect. There is also less absorption into the lacrimal passages than with eye drops. Eye ointments can however produce a film in front of the eye that may blur vision.

#### Patient/family education

The nurse teaches the patient about the disease and its treatment. The infectiousness of the disorder is emphasized, and the patient is encouraged to avoid crowded environments and to keep the hands away from the face. Frequent hand washing is critical, especially before and after the use of warm compresses or the instillation of eye medications.

**box 56-2 Ophthalmic Drugs Used to Treat Infection/Inflammation**

**ANTIBIOTICS AND ANTIVIRAL DRUGS**

Polymyxin B, bacitracin (Polysporin)
Polymyxin B, neomycin, bacitracin (Neosporin)
Bacitracin
Idoxuridine (IDU)
Gentamicin sulfate (Garamycin)
Chloramphenicol (Chloromycetin, Chloroptic)

**STEROIDS**

Prednisone
Prednisolone acetate
Methylprednisolone (Depo-Medrol)
Triamcinolone (Aristocort)
Dexamethasone (Decadron, Maxidex)
Fluorometholone (FML)

**CYCLOPLEGIC AND MYDRIATIC ACTION**

Atropine sulfate (Atropisol, Isopto Atropine)
Cyclopentolate hydrochloride (Cyclogyl)
Homatropine hydrobromide (Isopto Homatropine)
Scopolamine hydrobromide (Isopto Hyoscine)
Tropicamide (Mydriacyl)

**guidelines for care**

**Applying Warm Moist Compresses**

1. Use sterile technique when infection or ulceration is present; clean technique may be used for allergic reactions.
2. Use separate equipment for bilateral eye infections.
3. Wash hands before treating each eye.
4. Temperature of compress should not exceed 49° C (120° F).
5. Change compresses frequently every 5 minutes as ordered. Always wash hands first.
6. Do not exert pressure on the eyeball.
7. Sterile petrolatum may be used on skin around eyes, if desired, to protect the skin.
8. If sterility is not required, moist heat may be applied by means of a clean face cloth.

The nurse instructs the patient about how to correctly instill the ophthalmic ointment. The procedure is similar to that used for eye drops. The ointment is gently placed directly onto the exposed conjunctiva from the inner to the outer canthus, being careful to avoid the eyelashes or any part of the eye that would contaminate the tip of the tube (Figure 56-6). The nurse warns the patient about the possible blurring of vision. If both eye drops and ointments are to be used, the ointment is applied last. Treatment at bedtime minimizes the adverse effects of blurring of vision.

## EYE TRAUMA AND INJURY

### ETIOLOGY/EPIDEMIOLOGY

Two to 3 million persons each year in the United States sustain an injury to their eyes. Of these, 4000 will have permanent blindness as a result. Most of these injuries are considered to be preventable.

The two major categories of injury are burns and mechanical trauma. Chemical burns can occur in the home, school, and industrial setting and may involve either an acid or an alkali substance. Prompt treatment is essential to prevent permanent eye damage. Ultraviolet burns are also a concern and may occur from excess sun exposure (skiing, outdoor work, or sunbathing) or the use of heat lamps and tanning beds. Thermal burns are less common but may destroy the eyelids and necessitate skin grafting.

Mechanical trauma can include lacerations of the eyelids as well as direct injury to the eye itself. Contusions can cause bleeding into the anterior chamber (*hyphema*). Corneal injuries present unique problems because they are extremely painful and resistance to infection is low. Scarring on the cornea can impair vision. Foreign bodies on the surface of the cornea are estimated to account for about 25% of all eye injuries.[15]

### PATHOPHYSIOLOGY

Although the eye is vulnerable to trauma, its natural protective mechanisms both prevent and minimize minor eye

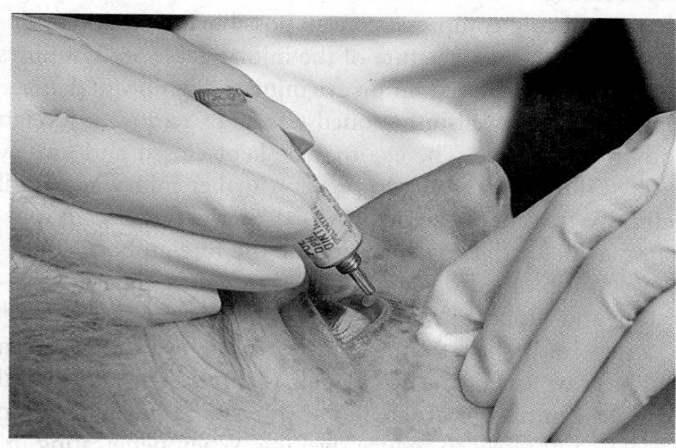

**fig. 56-6** Ophthalmic ointment is squeezed onto conjunctiva of lower lid.

injury. The heavy orbital bone protects the eye from most blunt mechanical injuries. The eye's natural lubricating system is augmented by tears to help flush away chemicals and other foreign bodies, and the blink reflex protects the eye from most low-impact forces.

Acid causes coagulation in the cornea which, although it produces significant local trauma, actually prevents the substance from penetrating and damaging the deeper structures of the eye. Alkaline substances, however, penetrate the corneal epithelium and release proteases and collagenases that can cause corneal necrosis and perforation.

Penetrating injuries or retained foreign bodies can result in *sympathetic ophthalmia,* a serious inflammation of the ciliary body, iris, and choroid that occurs in the uninjured eye. The cause of the acute inflammation is unknown, but it is believed to be some type of autoimmune response. The inflammation can spread rapidly from the uvea to the optic nerve. The uninjured eye becomes inflamed, painful, and photophobic with a decline in visual acuity. Prompt aggressive treatment of eye injuries has decreased the incidence of this rare disorder that can result in the loss of the "good" eye.

## COLLABORATIVE CARE MANAGEMENT

Prompt professional evaluation and care are perhaps the most important aspects of management for eye injuries and may protect the eye from serious visual impairment. First aid measures for eye injury should be widely taught and posted clearly in all settings in which eye injury is a significant risk. Chemical burns are immediately treated with copious flushing of the eye with water (Guidelines for Care Box and Figure 56-7). A litmus paper may be applied to the conjunctiva to determine the pH if the substance is unknown. Irrigation is continued for at least 15 minutes *before* the patient is transferred for further evaluation and treatment. This simple measure may preserve eye function. Further treatment may include topical antibiotics, steroids, and antiglaucoma agents to reduce intraocular pressure. Ultraviolet burns are treated with cool compresses, analgesics, and anesthetics.

Mechanical trauma also requires prompt professional care and evaluation. The risk of infection is accompanied by the risk of losing the eye. Antibiotics, wound suturing, cycloplegic agents, and cold compresses are all possible interventions, depending on the exact nature of the injury. Table 56-3 outlines the basic first aid for common eye injuries. Significant damage can be done by well-intentioned efforts to remove a foreign body from the eye. The eye may be kept closed and loosely covered during transport to prevent further injury and until definitive treatment can be provided. Sterile fluorescein solution may be distilled to help outline the foreign body for removal. Antibiotic drops may be used to reduce the risk of infection and support healing.

Extensive or penetrating injuries to the eye can result in blindness or loss of the eye. Repair is surgically performed if possible. Contusions are treated with rest and the application of cold compresses to reduce swelling. When penetrating injuries occur *no attempt* is made to remove the object or to clean the eye. Professional management is essential.

**guidelines for care**

**Eye Irrigations**

**Purpose**

1. Remove chemical irritants, foreign bodies, and secretions.
2. Cleanse the eye postoperatively (may be done preoperatively).

**Procedure**

1. Prepare solution. Physiological solutions of sodium chloride or lactated Ringer's solution are most commonly used.
2. Position person comfortably toward one side so that fluid cannot flow into the other eye.
3. Use appropriate means (e.g., kidney basin, large towel) to catch irrigating fluid.
4. Use appropriate amounts of solution.
    a. If small amounts are needed (to cleanse eye postoperatively) sterile cotton balls moistened with solution can be used.
    b. If moderate amounts of fluid are needed (removing secretions) a plastic squeeze bottle is used to direct irrigating fluid along the conjunctiva and over the eyeball from inner to outer canthus.
    c. If copious amounts of fluid are needed (that is, for removing chemical irritants), bags of solution such as intravenous bags along with the tubing to direct the flow onto the eye can be used.
5. Avoid directing a forceful stream onto the eye.
6. Avoid touching any eye structures with the irrigating equipment.
7. If there is drainage, wrap a piece of gauze around the index finger to raise the lid and ensure thorough cleansing.

### Patient/Family Education

The nurse may be responsible for community education efforts concerning eye safety and the first aid for eye injuries. The body's natural eye defenses can be appropriately augmented by the use of goggles, shields, and safety lenses for sports and high-risk activities. Children need to be taught about the risks associated with BB guns, slingshots, and even rubber bands. The use of protective sunglasses may also be important, depending on the patient's occupational and leisure time sun exposure. General guidelines for eye safety are summarized in Box 56-3.

# GLAUCOMA

## ETIOLOGY

Glaucoma is an eye disease characterized by progressive optic nerve atrophy and loss of vision. Elevated intraocular pressure (IOP) is the most important risk factor for developing glaucoma. In primary open-angle glaucoma many persons have elevated IOP, but some have normal IOP. Because of this, elevated IOP is no longer a defining characteristic of glaucoma. The term *glaucoma* actually refers to a group of disorders as shown in Table 56-4. The two major forms of glaucoma are *open-angle* and *angle-closure* (formerly called *closed-angle*).

A

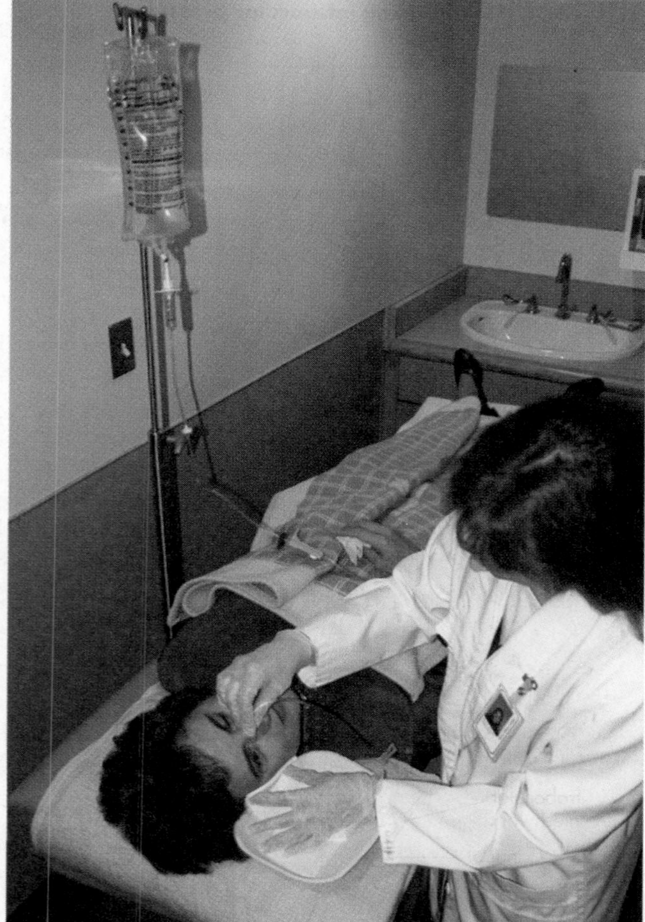

B

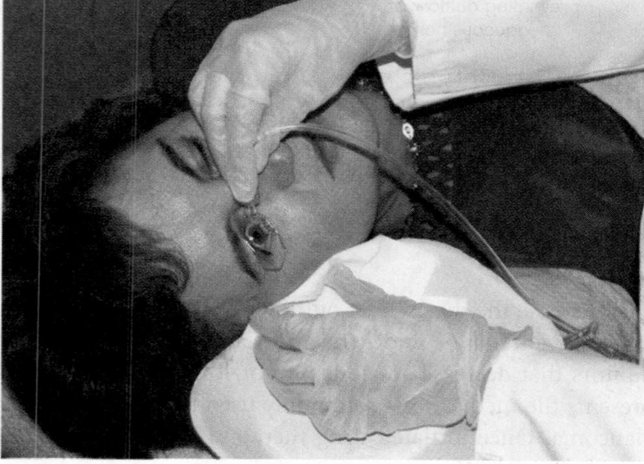

**fig. 56-7 A,** Eye irrigation using an intravenous bag and tubing. **B,** Note lid speculum in place.

The disease is primary when its etiology is unknown, and secondary when it results from another eye disorder such as a forward shift of the iris, pupillary blockage, or contracture of the fibromuscular membrane in the anterior chamber.

## EPIDEMIOLOGY

Glaucoma is the third leading cause of blindness in the general U.S. population and the leading cause among African Americans.[33] The prevalence rate among African Americans is 15 times higher than that of whites, but no explanation currently exists for this wide discrepancy. About 2% of the population older than 40 has glaucoma, and an estimated 1 million additional persons have undiagnosed disease. The incidence is expected to continue to rise as the population ages. Age, race, myopia, and a family history of glaucoma are the only identified risk factors. Angle closure glaucoma is more prevalent in Asian persons. Glaucoma is a major cause of visual impairment and blindness worldwide.

**table 56-3** *First Aid for Eye Injuries*

| Injury | Interventions |
|---|---|
| Burns: chemical, flame | Flush eye immediately for 15 min with cool water or any available nontoxic liquid; seek medical assistance. |
| Loose substance on conjunctiva: dirt, insects | Lift upper lid over lower lid to dislodge substance, produce tearing; irrigate eye with water if necessary; do not rub eye; obtain medical assistance if above interventions fail. |
| Contact injury: contusion, ecchymosis, laceration | Apply cold compresses if no laceration present; cover eye if laceration present; seek medical assistance. |
| Penetrating objects | Do not remove object; place protective shield over eye (for example, paper cup); cover uninjured eye to prevent excess movement of injured eye; seek medical assistance. |

**box 56-3** *Rules of Eye Safety*

1. Spray aerosols away from eyes.
2. Wear protective glasses during active sports such as racquetball.
3. Slowly release steam from ovens, pots, pressure cookers, and microwave popcorn bags.
4. Gaze at solar eclipses only through adequate filters.
5. Wear safety goggles whenever hazardous work is being done or if you are in a workplace area where such hazards exist.
6. Fit all machinery with safeguards.
7. Keep dangerous items and chemicals away from children.
8. Store sharp objects safely.
9. Pick up rocks and stones rather than going over them with a lawn mower.

## PATHOPHYSIOLOGY

The normal balance of production and drainage of aqueous humor allows the IOP to remain relatively constant within the normal range of 10 to 21 mm Hg with a mean pressure of 16 mm Hg. Normal diurnal variations are limited to about 5 mm Hg. Obstruction in any part of the outflow channels for aqueous humor results in a backup of fluid and an increase in IOP (Figure 56-8). A sustained elevation gradually

**table 56-4** *Types of Glaucoma*

| Type | Description |
|---|---|
| Primary open-angle (chronic, simple) | Most common type (90%)<br>Usually caused by obstruction in trabecular meshwork |
| Secondary open-angle | Can occur from an abnormality in the trabecular meshwork or an increase in venous pressure |
| Primary angle-closure (narrow angle, acute) | Outflow impaired as result of narrowing or closing of angle between iris and cornea<br>Intermittent attacks—pressure normal when angle open; if persistent, acute ocular emergency |
| Secondary angle-closure | Can result from ocular inflammation, blood vessel changes, trauma |
| Congenital | Abnormal development of filtration angle; can occur secondary to other systemic eye disorders<br>Rare (0.05%) |

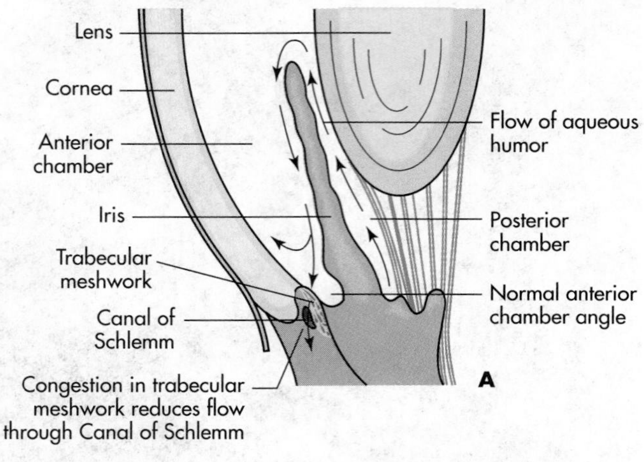


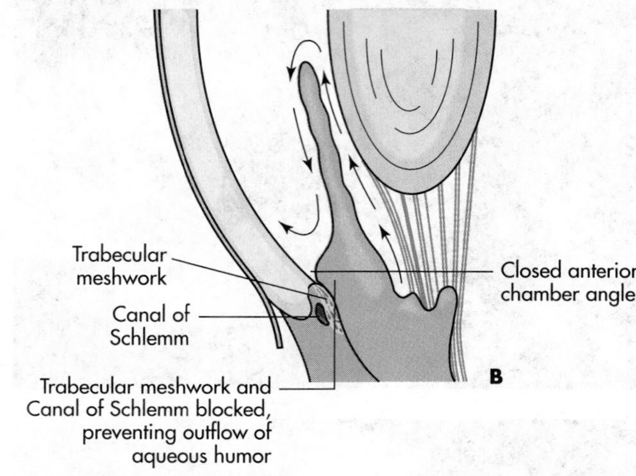


**fig. 56-8** **A,** Chronic open angle glaucoma. Congestion in the trabecular meshwork reduces the outflow of aqueous humor. **B,** Acute angle closure glaucoma. Angle between the iris and the anterior chamber narrows, obstructing the outflow of aqueous humor.

damages the optic nerve and impairs vision. In primary open-angle glaucoma, which represents 90% of all cases, the changes occur slowly, and the damage is insidious. The process can also occur more rapidly in response to injury or infection or as a complication of surgery. Clinical manifestations of glaucoma are summarized in Box 56-4. Figure 56-9 shows the progressive loss of peripheral vision that can occur with glaucoma.

## COLLABORATIVE CARE MANAGEMENT

### Diagnostic Tests

Several diagnostic tests are used to diagnose and monitor glaucoma. These include:

1. Tonometry: measurement of IOP
2. Tonography: estimation of the resistance in the outflow channels by continuously recording the IOP over 2 to 4 minutes[4,6]
3. Ophthalmoscopy: evaluation of the color and configuration of the optic cup
4. Perimetry: measurement of visual function in the central field of vision[6]
5. Gonioscopy: examination of the angle structures of the eye, where the iris, ciliary body, and cornea meet

### Medications

Drug therapy is the foundation of treatment for most forms of glaucoma. The goal of treatment is to lower the individual's IOP and keep it at a level that prevents loss of vision. Drug therapy is administered topically or systemically to lower IOP by either (1) increasing the outflow of aqueous humor or (2) decreasing the production of aqueous humor. Drug options include (1) miotic agents that constrict the pupil and increase the drainage of aqueous humor, (2) prostaglandin agonists that increase the uveoscleral outflow of aqueous humor, and (3) beta adrenergic blockers and carbonic anhydrase inhibitors that decrease aqueous humor formation. Table 56-5 presents the medications commonly used in the treatment of glaucoma. Once initiated drug therapy is continued for the rest of the patient's life.

Angle-closure glaucoma usually requires more aggressive management because it represents an emergency situation with the threat of permanent vision loss if the pressure is not controlled promptly. Intravenous carbonic anhydrase inhibitors may be given in combination with osmotic agents that draw fluid from the intraocular spaces, and topical beta blocker and miotics. Topical steroids may also be given in the attempt to minimize damage to the iris and the trabecular network.

**box 56-4** *clinical manifestations*

***Glaucoma***

**OPEN-ANGLE GLAUCOMA**

Frequently no signs or symptoms in early stages
IOP typically elevated >24 mm Hg
Slow loss of vision
Peripheral vision lost before central (Figure 56-9)
Tunnel vision
Persistent dull eye pain
Difficulty adjusting to darkness
Failure to detect color changes

**ANGLE-CLOSURE GLAUCOMA**

Acute: severe ocular pain, decreased vision, pupil enlarged and fixed, colored halos around lights, eye red, steamy cornea, may cause nausea and vomiting
IOP usually dramatically elevated; may exceed 50 mm Hg
Permanent blindness if marked increase in IOP for 24-48 hours

**CONGENITAL GLAUCOMA**

Enlargement of eye, lacrimation, photophobia, blepharospasm

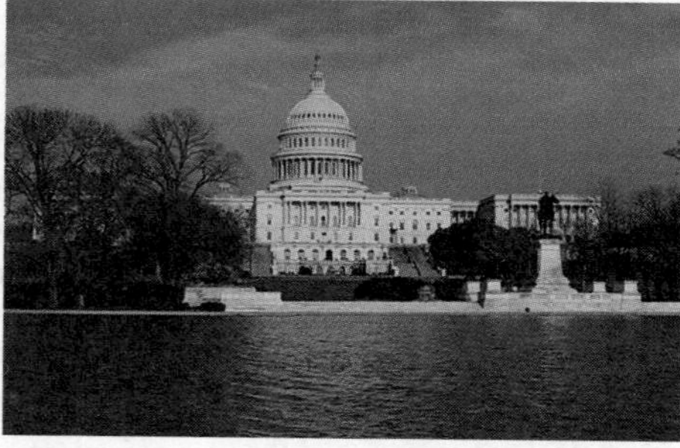
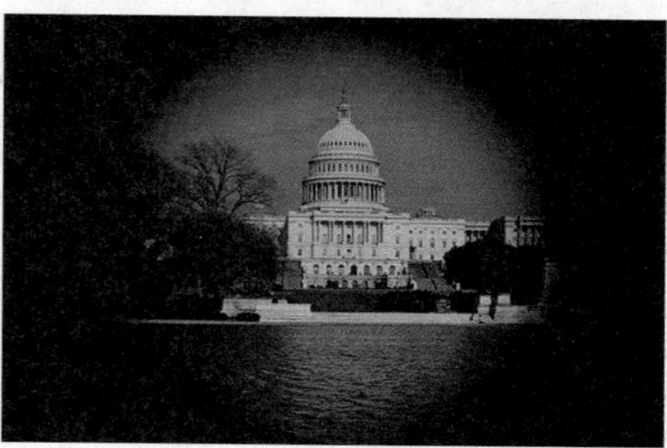
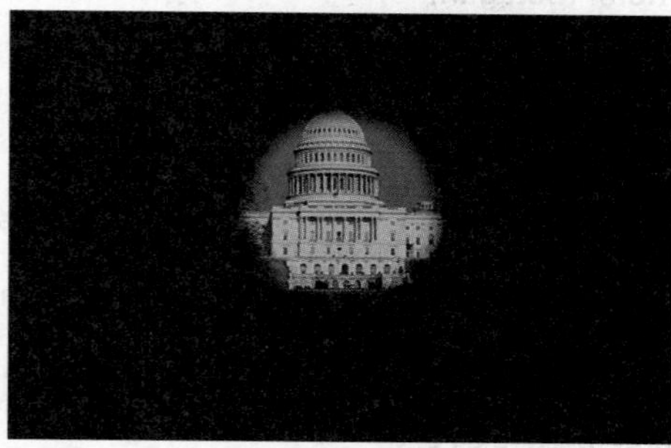

**fig. 56-9** Glaucoma causes a progressive loss of peripheral vision. The changes may be so insidious that extensive irreversible damage occurs before the problem is recognized.

### Treatments

Cyclodestructive procedures such as cyclotherapy and YAG (yttrium, aluminum, and garnet) laser thermal procedures attempt to lower IOP by permanently damaging the ciliary body.[16,48,52] The results of these procedures are unpredictable, and repeat treatment may be necessary to achieve the desired effect. Patients require close follow-up because they have an increased risk of retinal detachment, hemorrhage, and severe inflammation in the treated eye.

### Surgical Management

Surgical intervention is indicated when conservative treatment fails to control the IOP. Two of the common procedures are argon laser trabeculoplasty (ALT) and trabeculectomy. ALT uses a laser beam to produce a non-penetrating thermal burn on the trabecular meshwork that changes the configuration of the meshwork, increases tension in the meshwork, and leads to increased outflow of aqueous humor. Trabeculectomy creates an opening, or fistula, at the limbus under a partial thickness scleral flap. The new opening circumvents the obstruction, and aqueous humor flows into the subconjunctival spaces. Fibrosis can occur at the site of the scleral-flap and interfere with drainage causing the IOP to rise again. Antimetabolites such as 5-fluorouracil and mitomycin C may be given to inhibit fibrosis. Releasable sutures and laser suturelysis can also be used to support drainage at the site.[44] ALT can usually be performed on an outpatient basis whereas trabeculectomy typically requires an overnight hospital stay.

IOP control is achieved in about 85% of all patients, but most (75%) continue to require medications to treat

**table 56-5 Common Medications for Glaucoma**

| Drug | Action | Interventions |
|---|---|---|
| **MIOTICS** | | |
| Cholinergics<br>Pilocarpine HCl (Pilocar, Isopto Carpine)<br>Carbachol (Carbacel) | Contrict the pupil (miosis) by directly stimulating the sphincter muscle.<br>Increase outflow of aqueous humor by ciliary muscle pull on trabecular meshwork. | Evaluate effectiveness.<br>Monitor frequency of use.<br>Inform the patient that blurred vision and poor night vision may occur due to a small pupil. Other side effects include eye, brow, or lid discomfort, or burning sensation with drop instillation. |
| **CHOLINESTERASE INHIBITORS** | | |
| Physostigmine (Eserine)<br>Isoflurophate (Floropryl)<br>Demercarium bromide (Humorsol)<br>Echothiophate iodide (Phospholine Iodide) | Constrict ciliary muscle and iris sphincter; iris is pulled away from anterior chamber angle, allowing drainage of aqueous humor and lowering IOP. | Avoid use of Isoflurophate, Demercarium during pregnancy.<br>Inform patient that blurred vision, watering eyes, browache, and change in vision may occur. |
| **BETA ADRENERGIC ANTAGONISTS** | | |
| Timolol maleate (Timoptic)<br>Betaxolol (Betoptic)<br>Levobunolol (Betagan)<br>Carteolol hydrochloride (Ocupress)<br>Metipranolol (OptiPranolol) | Decrease aqueous humor production and increase the outflow, thereby decreasing IOP. | Evaluate effectiveness.<br>Use caution when administering nonselective beta blockers to patients who have pulmonary or cardiac disease—can cause bronchospasm. |
| **CARBONIC ANHYDRASE INHIBITORS** | | |
| Acetazolamide (Diamox)<br>Ethoxzolamide (Cardrase)<br>Dichlorphenamide (Daranide)<br>Methazolamide (Neptazane)<br>Dorzolamide (Trusopt) | Decrease aqueous humor production by inhibiting carbonic anhydrase in ciliary processes (an enzyme necessary to produce aqueous humor). | Evaluate effectiveness.<br>Monitor for tingling sensation in extremities, tinnitus, gastric upset, or hearing dysfunction.<br>Monitor for signs of hypokalemia. |
| **ADRENERGIC AGENTS** | | |
| Epinephryl borate (Eppy/N, Epinal)<br>Epinephrine hydrochloride (Glaucon)<br>Epinephrine bitartrate (Epitrate)<br>Dipivefrin (Propine)<br>Apraclonidine (Lopidine) | Reduce aqueous humor formation and increase outflow. | Evaluate effectiveness.<br>Monitor for side effects: headache, brow ache, blurred vision, tachycardia, pigment deposits in cornea, conjunctiva, lids. |
| **OSMOTIC AGENTS** | | |
| Glycerin (Osmoglyn)<br>Mannitol (Osmitrol)<br>Isosorbide (Ismotic) | Move water from the intraocular structures, resulting in a marked ocular hypotonic effect, thereby decreasing IOP. | Evaluate effectiveness.<br>Monitor electrolytes for depletion.<br>Monitor glucose levels in patients with type 1 diabetes. Drugs can cause hyperglycemia. |
| **PROSTAGLANDIN AGONISTS** | | |
| Latanoprost (Xalatan) | Increase outflow of aqueous humor. It is used primarily with patients intolerant to or unresponsive to other glaucoma agents. | Monitor renal and hepatic function during treatment.<br>Teach patient about adverse side effects, e.g., burning on administration, blurred vision, itching, and photophobia. |

glaucoma. Nursing care for the person after trabeculectomy is summarized in the Guidelines for Care Box.

*Molteno implants* and other *seton implants,* e.g. Schoket, Krupin, and Ahmed, provide an alternative for patients with glaucoma that is resistant to other forms of surgery.[26,49] In implant surgery, a polymethylmethacrylate plate is implanted against the sclera. A tube is then surgically implanted directly into the anterior chamber. The aqueous humor drains out of the eye through the tube and collects under the plate posteriorly. The plate is designed to block scar tissue formation that could affect aqueous reabsorption or physically block the outflow tube. Overdrainage of aqueous humor is a potential complication that can increase the risk of retinal detachment and choroidal and vitreous hemorrhage.

Acute angle-closure glaucoma is treated with either a laser *peripheral iridotomy* (YAG or argon) or a surgical *peripheral*

**guidelines for care**

**The Person Undergoing Trabeculectomy**

Nursing care for the patient after trabeculectomy includes the following:

1. Routine postanesthesia care
2. Protection of operative eye with patch or shield, positioning patient on back or unoperative side, and safety measures
3. Maintaining comfort in the operative eye
4. Assessment, as appropriate, of the IOP, appearance of the bleb, and anterior chamber depth
5. Administration of medications such as a cycloplegic, a mydriatic, and a combination antibiotic and steroid

*iridectomy,* which penetrates the iris and permanently connects the anterior and posterior chamber of the eye. This prevents the iris from occluding the anterior chamber.

### Diet

Diet does not play a role in the management of glaucoma. Patients experiencing acute angle-closure glaucoma may develop nausea and vomiting from the acute eye pain.

### Activity

Activity does not need to be restricted for the treatment of open-angle glaucoma but the patient is instructed to avoid heavy lifting, isometric exercises, and constipation that would cause straining. The loss of peripheral vision that can result from the disease and the blurred vision and loss of night vision that are common side effects of several of the medications do create safety risks that may need to be addressed through a modification in activity, particularly driving.

### Referrals

Referrals would not be routinely needed in the treatment of glaucoma although patients with acute angle-closure glaucoma will need immediate treatment by an ophthalmic surgeon. Patients with loss of vision may benefit from referrals to the National Federation of the Blind, 1800 Johnson St., Baltimore, MD, 21230, (410) 659-9314; and the National Eye Care Project, toll-free helpline (8 AM to 4 PM Pacific time) (800) 222-3937.

## NURSING MANAGEMENT

## ASSESSMENT

Patients with open-angle glaucoma are typically asymptomatic in the early stages of the disease and may remain asymptomatic if they receive adequate treatment.

Acute angle-closure glaucoma causes an abrupt rise in intraocular pressure and can produce a variety of symptoms. Nausea and vomiting are often so severe in some persons with acute angle-closure glaucoma that an acute abdomen is mistakenly diagnosed. A popular misconception is that symptoms of headache, halos around lights, blurred vision, and eye pain are seen in persons with primary open-angle glaucoma.

### Subjective Data

Data to be collected to assess the patient with glaucoma include:

Sudden-onset severe pain in the eye
Acute blurring of vision
Halos around lights
Possible nausea and vomiting

### Objective Data

Data to be collected to assess the patient with glaucoma include:

Excessive lacrimation
Mild pupil dilation
Hazy, bluish appearance to the cornea
Sharp elevation in IOP (may be >50 mm Hg)
Impaired visual fields (central involvement late in disease process)
Enlarged optic disk cup and disk pallor (by ophthalmoscope)

## NURSING DIAGNOSES

Nursing diagnoses are determined from analysis of patient data. Nursing diagnoses for the patient with open-angle or angle-closure glaucoma may include but are not limited to:

| Diagnostic Title | Possible Etiological Factors |
|---|---|
| Pain | Increased IOP |
| Knowledge deficit: disease process and treatment | Lack of exposure/recall of information or misinterpretation of information |
| Health maintenance, altered | Impairment in vision |

## EXPECTED PATIENT OUTCOMES

Expected patient outcomes for the patient with glaucoma may include but are not limited to:

1. Experiences a decrease in eye pain.
2. Accurately describes the nature of the disease process, components of the treatment plan, and the need for lifelong treatment.
3. Adapts lifestyle and self-care activities to accommodate losses in vision,

## INTERVENTIONS

### Relieving Pain

Aggressive pharmacological intervention is required to control the IOP and reduce the patient's pain. The nurse carefully explains all interventions and assesses the patient's pain level frequently. The nurse administers analgesics as needed to control the pain and carefully evaluates their effectiveness. The nurse modifies the patient's environment by controlling light levels, visitors, and stimulation and offers cool eye compresses to augment comfort. The nurse assists the patient to use relaxation strategies to help control disabling anxiety.

### Patient/Family Education

Glaucoma is a chronic condition, and teaching focuses on the essential knowledge and skills for self-management. The nurse teaches the patient and family about the disease and its treatment and emphasizes that the disease can be controlled through lifelong management but that there is no cure. Vision that has been lost to elevated IOP cannot be restored, but further vision loss can be prevented with careful adherence to the pharmacological regimen and ongoing follow-up. A normal lifestyle is possible with minimal restrictions or modifications.

The nurse instructs the patient about all prescribed medications and their side effects and teaches the patient how to correctly administer topical eye drops. Eye drops are quickly eliminated from the eye and may need to be administered several times a day. Guidelines for administering eye drops are summarized in the Guidelines for Care Box. The nurse recommends that the patient keep a reserve bottle of the medication available if possible in case the drug is lost or spilled. The medication should always be carried in a pocket or purse when traveling and never packed in luggage. A Medic Alert or other information card indicating that the patient has glaucoma and takes a specific medication can be an important safety precaution in case the patient is involved in an accident.

### Supporting Self-Care

The use of miotic drugs causes pupil constriction and may adversely affect the patient's night vision and adaptation to dark places. The nurse assists the patient to plan for any adaptations in home or daily activities to ensure safety. Extra lighting in the home and reducing clutter can be helpful. The nurse cautions the person to carefully evaluate his or her safety for driving at night. The nurse also frankly discusses the adverse side effects of the drugs, including temporary blurred vision after administration and a stinging or burning sensation. Patients need both professional and family support to adhere to the treatment regimen, especially when an absence of disease symptoms makes the disease process seem tenuous, and the treatment can certainly seem worse than the disease. Honesty is an important tool for the nurse to use in all patient education efforts.

**guidelines for care**

**Self-Administration of Eye Drops**

1. Wash the hands thoroughly before administering the medication.
2. Tilt the head back and look up toward the ceiling.
3. Pull the lower lid gently down and out to expose the conjunctiva and create a sac.
4. Bring the dropper from the side and apply the eye drops. Avoid touching the eyelashes, conjunctiva, or surface of the eye with the dropper. Resting the thumb on the forehead can help to stabilize the hand.
5. Close both eyes gently. Do not squeeze them tightly or the medication will be expelled.
6. Apply slight pressure at the inner canthus of the eye to decrease systemic absorption of the medication.
7. If more than 1 drop is to be administered, wait 2-5 minutes before administering the second drop.[21]

### Health promotion/prevention

Early diagnosis and treatment of glaucoma are essential to prevent permanent destruction of fibers on the optic disk. All persons with a family history of glaucoma should have their eyes examined, including measurement of intraocular pressure, every 2 years after the age of 40. Mass screening programs are important for detecting glaucoma in persons who do not have periodic medical eye examinations. because the permanent vision loss it causes is usually preventable.

Once the diagnosis has been made regular medical follow-up is essential to evaluate the effectiveness of treatment. Follow-up every 2 to 3 months may be necessary initially until it is clear the patient's IOP is under control. Adherence to treatment and regular monitoring are the best means available to prevent vision loss from progressive disease activity.

## EVALUATION

To evaluate the effectiveness of nursing interventions, compare patient behaviors with those stated in the expected patient outcomes. Successful achievement of patient outcomes for the patient with glaucoma is indicated by:

1a. Reports no eye pain or headache
b. Has IOP within target range.
2a. Has appointment for follow-up monitoring and care.
b. States commitment to lifelong therapy of the disease.
3. Makes needed alterations in home environment and activities to ensure safety despite impaired night vision or compromised peripheral vision.

## GERONTOLOGICAL CONSIDERATIONS

The incidence of glaucoma increases with aging, and the entire discussion of the disease and its management applies primarily to the older adult. Screening initiatives for glaucoma need to be particularly targeted to this population, because the disease is frequently not diagnosed until irreversible vision loss has already occurred. Adherence issues are particularly challenging in this population. Fixed incomes can make the purchase of any medications difficult. The fact that most patients with glaucoma are asymptomatic can make it difficult for the patient to accept these medication purchases as essential. Compliance with a regimen that does not make you feel better and even compromises your night vision skills can be difficult to achieve. It is also frequently more difficult for patients with any degree of mobility or dexterity impairment, such as with arthritis or other problems, to learn to correctly self-administer eye drops. In addition, most elders are already dealing with some degree of visual impairment, and these impairments frequently have an impact on their ability to drive. Blurred vision and impaired visual acuity for night driving can create significant safety risks for individuals who are already struggling to remain independent. The issues for elders are real and challenging, and the nurse can neither solve nor eliminate them. Honest acknowledgment can be helpful, however, as the nurse attempts to assist the patient to anticipate areas of difficulty and develop strategies for addressing these problems.

## SPECIAL ENVIRONMENTS FOR CARE

### Critical Care Management

Critical care would not be used in the management of glaucoma. Angle-closure glaucoma can represent a real and emergent threat to the patient's vision, but the intense invasive monitoring and supervision inherent in the critical care environment does not add any benefits for management.

### Home Care Management

Glaucoma is a community-based problem. Patients are typically diagnosed in the community and manage their disease process independently in their own homes. Hospitalization is rarely necessary unless the glaucoma does not respond to standard pharmacological treatment, and surgery is indicated. Even in these situations the surgery is typically performed in an ambulatory center or as an overnight procedure. All of the nurse's interventions related to teaching and self-care must be targeted toward the reality of the patient's home situation and the supports available.

## COMPLICATIONS

Vision loss is the primary complication of glaucoma, and preventing vision loss and blindness is the ultimate goal of all therapy. Most patients with glaucoma can be successfully managed with routine pharmacological therapy. Selected patients may require surgical intervention, and in rare instances the disease cannot be successfully controlled, and severe visual impairment or blindness results. Glaucoma-related blindness remains a major international health concern.

# CATARACT

## ETIOLOGY

A *cataract* is a clouding or opacity of the lens that leads to gradual painless blurring and eventual loss of vision (Figure 56-10). Cataracts are generally classified as *senile* (associated with aging), *traumatic* (associated with injury), *congenital* (present at birth), and *secondary* (occurring after other eye diseases).

Senile cataracts are associated with the aging process and are not preventable. There is some evidence that exposure to ultraviolet radiation may significantly contribute to cataract formation, but a cause and effect relationship has not been proven. Speculation exists that antioxidant use, such as the combined intake of vitamins A, C, and E may reduce the risk of senile cataracts, but this is also not proven.

Eye injury is the next most common identifiable cause of cataracts. The transparency of the lens may be destroyed by either a penetrating wound or a contusion. Cataracts may result from the ingestion of injurious substances such as dinitrophenol or naphthalene. Some researchers report that cataracts may result from systemic absorption of hair dyes. The incidence of most traumatic cataracts is preventable through adherence to standard eye safety precautions (see Box 56-3).

Cataracts may also occur secondary to eye diseases, such as uveitis or eye trauma, or with systemic diseases, such as diabetes mellitus, galactosemia, or sarcoidosis.

## EPIDEMIOLOGY

Cataracts are the third leading cause of preventable blindness in the United States, and their incidence increases steadily with age. Visible lens changes are present in 42% of the 52- to 64-year-old population and 5% of this group demonstrate some degree of visual impairment related to the cataract. Sixty to 90% of the population older than 65 years have visible lens changes, and between 25% and 45% of them have some degree of related visual impairment. A higher incidence of cataracts is found among people residing in warm sunny climates. Risk factors for cataract are summarized in the box below.

## PATHOPHYSIOLOGY

Senile cataracts occur because of a decrease in protein, an accumulation of water, and an increase in sodium content that disrupts the normal fibers of the lens. The cause of these pathological changes is unknown. Cataracts usually develop bilaterally, but at different rates.

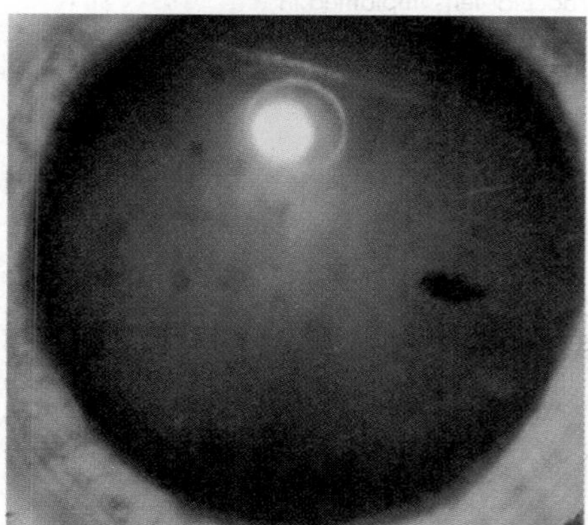

**fig. 56-10** Mature senile cataract viewed through dilated pupil.

**risk factors**

### Cataract

Age: the incidence increases dramatically after age 65
Sex: cataracts are slightly more common in women
Ultraviolet light exposure
- More common in persons living in warm sunny climates
- More common in persons who have worked outdoors extensively

High-dose radiation exposure
Drug effects: use of corticosteroids, phenothiazines, and selected chemotherapeutic agents
Poorly controlled diabetes mellitus: accumulation of sorbitol (by-product of glucose)
Trauma to the eye

The primary symptom of cataracts is a progressive loss of vision. The degree of loss depends on the location and extent of the opacity. Persons with an opacity in the center portion of the lens can generally see better in dim light when the pupil is dilated. The person with *presbyopia* may find that reading without glasses is possible in the early stage of cataract formation because the greater convexity of the lens creates an artificial myopia.

Clinical manifestations of cataract are summarized in Box 56-5.

## COLLABORATIVE CARE MANAGEMENT

### Diagnostic Tests

There are no particular diagnostic tests for cataract. The diagnosis is made with direct inspection of the lens with an ophthalmoscope after pupil dilation. The progression of the cataract is monitored over time. Before surgery A-scan, keratometry, B-scan, endothelial cell counts, and potential acuity meter (PAM) tests may be performed. The A-scan measures the length of the eye and is done to help estimate the power of the intraocular lens (IOL) that will be needed. Keratometry measures the curvature of the cornea and is also used to determine the power of the IOL. A B-scan may be performed to evaluate the health of the retina if a dense cataract obscures visualization through an ophthalmoscope. Endothelial cell counts evaluate the health of the cornea and its ability to withstand surgery.[19] The PAM test enables the surgeon to ensure that cataract surgery will be beneficial in increasing the patient's visual acuity.

### Medications

Medications do not play a role in the management of cataract. Anesthetics, antiinflammatory agents, and antibiotics are all used after surgery to facilitate the healing process and promote patient comfort.

### Treatments

Surgery is the treatment of choice for cataract and can be used with virtually all patients. Various types of lenses are used after surgery to restore the person's vision, but these are discussed under surgical management below.

### Surgical Management

Surgery is the definitive treatment for cataracts, and it can be used safely and effectively with elders of advanced age. The success rate is between 90% and 95%. It was previously believed that a cataract had to "ripen" or mature before it could be successfully removed. Currently, cataracts are removed when the visual impairment interferes with the individual's daily activities. The person's general health is the most important variable.

**box 56-5** *clinical manifestations*

***Cataract***

Gradual, painless blurring and loss of vision
- Peripheral vision may be affected first
- Near vision may initially improve

Glare: at night and in bright light

Halos around lights

Loss of ability to discriminate between hues

Cloudy white opacity on the pupil

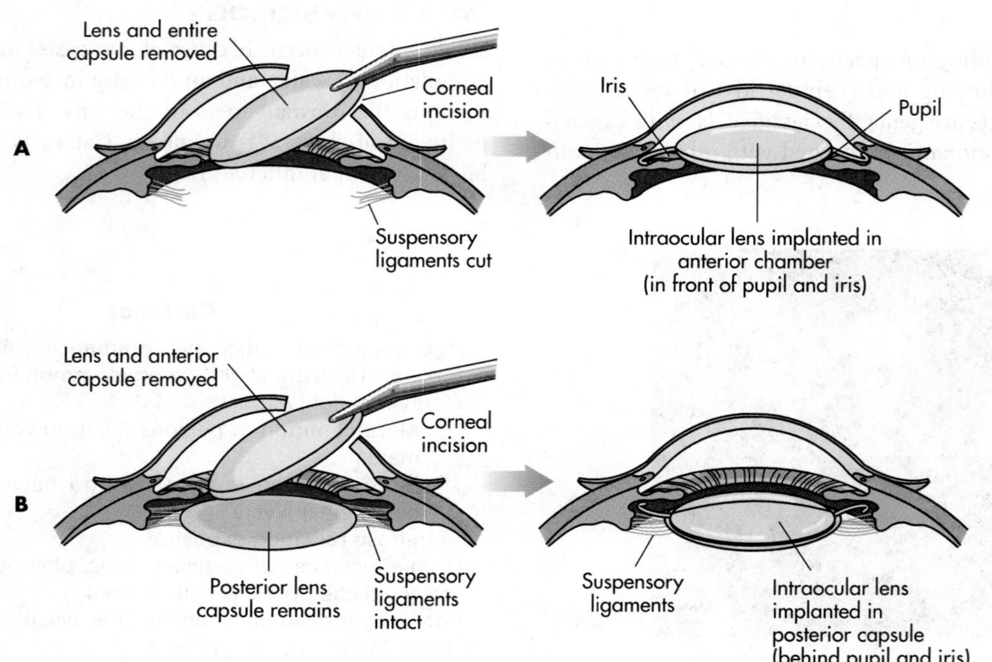


**fig. 56-11 A,** Intracapsular cataract extraction with removal of entire lens and capsule. **B,** Extracapsular cataract extraction leaving the posterior lens capsule intact.

Cataract removal is performed under local anesthesia. The anesthetic is injected behind the eye and in and around the eyelids. The most popular method of cataract removal is the extracapsular cataract extraction (ECCE) (Figure 56-11). In this procedure, only the anterior portion of the lens capsule and the capsule contents are removed, using techniques such as irrigation and aspiration or phacoemulsification (ultrasonic vibration to break up the lens).

Phacoemulsification is performed in about 80% of all cataract patients in North America. This procedure uses a smaller (⅛ inch) incision that promotes healing and decreases postoperative inflammation. Other surgical innovations include making the incision on the sclera rather than the cornea and using a single stitch to close the incision or even no stitch. These innovations are all attempts to facilitate healing and decrease the incidence of postoperative astigmatism.

Extracapsular extraction leaves the posterior lens capsule intact, which avoids disruption of the vitreous humor and facilitates the placement of a lens implant (Figure 56-11). Cataracts can also be removed with intracapsular extraction (ICCE), which involves the removal of the entire lens and its surrounding capsule using a freezing probe that adheres to the surface of the lens. This technique was popular at one time but is rarely used anymore.

Intraocular lens implant (IOC) is the preferred method for replacing the focusing power of the lens. A posterior chamber lens made of polymethylmethacrylate is placed behind the iris at time of surgery and is supported by the posterior portion of the lens capsule that was left in place (Figure 56-11). This type of implant is not dependent on the pupil or iris for support and rarely moves out of position. It is the most frequently used type of lens implant, because it is believed that the lens position most closely approximates the natural lens, and magnification is minimized.

Vision can be restored to near 20/20. The field of implants is rapidly evolving. Currently multifocal, bifocal, and even foldable implants are available. Foldable implants can be folded for insertion into the eye and allow the surgical incision to be even smaller.

If an intraocular lens is not inserted during surgery, the person must wear an external lens. Cataract glasses are the least desirable option but are used if the person cannot tolerate contact lenses. Cataract glasses tend to magnify objects about 25%, making them appear closer than they actually are. The person's field of vision is also narrowed, and a circular blind area (ring scotoma) may occur at the edge of the glasses because the glasses bend the light rays so much that they do not enter the eye. Objects tend to "pop" in and out of the person's visual field as the eyes are moved away from the center of the glasses. An accurate prescription cannot be made for several months until the person's vision stabilizes after surgery.

Contact lenses correct some of the problems encountered with cataract glasses, but not all of them. The extended-wear soft contact lens is commonly used. Interruption of the nerve supply to the cornea from surgery usually facilitates the wearing of a contact lens, but persons with rheumatoid arthritis or any other form of impaired mobility may be unable to insert and maintain contact lenses.

### Diet

Diet does not play a role in the management of cataracts, but it is important that the individual use diet modification and stool softeners or laxatives as necessary after surgery to prevent constipation. Straining during defecation can significantly increase the patient's intraocular pressure.

### Activity

Activity used to be severely curtailed after cataract surgery, but the newer surgical techniques have allowed the restrictions to be significantly eased. Most of the positioning and activity restrictions are focused on preventing increases in the patient's IOP. These are discussed below under Nursing Management.

### Referrals

Referrals are not generally necessary after cataract surgery unless the elder lives alone and is not able to manage self-care safely during the first few days after surgery. A referral for home health supervision or assistance may be appropriate, especially for dressing changes and eye drop administration.

## NURSING MANAGEMENT OF THE PERSON UNDERGOING CATARACT SURGERY

### PREOPERATIVE CARE

Most cataract surgery is performed in ambulatory surgery centers; few patients require hospitalization. Routines for preoperative care vary with the setting and the eye surgeon.

The patient may be asked to perform a face scrub before admission, and the eyelashes may be cut. The pupil of the operative eye is dilated and paralyzed before surgery, and sedation may be initiated. The nurse ensures that the patient has understood all explanations about the surgery and expected postoperative care and restrictions. The nurse also ensures that plans are in place for someone to transport the patient home and hopefully to assist with the patient's care during the first few postoperative days.

### POSTOPERATIVE CARE

Most patients are discharged within a few hours. Immediate care considerations are summarized in the Guidelines for Care Box. Because of the steady advances in surgical technique, patients do not need to restrict their activities in any substantive way, and they are encouraged to resume normal self-care activities as soon as they feel able (Research Box).

#### Protecting the Eye

After any cataract operation, a dressing is applied to the eye and covered with a metal shield to protect the eye from injury. The dressing is usually removed the day of or a day after surgery, but a metal eye shield is worn at night for a few weeks until the eye is healed to avoid accidental bumping of the eye during sleep. The patient is cautioned not to sleep on the operative side for 3 to 4 weeks to prevent pressure on the operated eye. Depending on the technique used to implant the lens, patients may be cautioned not to bend over with the head lower than the waist for about 2 weeks. Other patients have no restrictions on bending. The nurse instructing the patient clarifies with the surgeon what restrictions are necessary, if any.

The use of stool softeners is recommended to prevent constipation and straining. The nurse instructs the patient to avoid rubbing the eye and to continue using the eye shield as instructed.

### Patient/Family Education

The nurse instructs the patient to be careful to prevent soap or water from entering the operative eye during face or hair washing. The nurse also instructs the patient to avoid heavy lifting, active exercise, isometric exercise, or straining during defecation until cleared by the surgeon to prevent abrupt fluctuations in IOP. The nurse reviews plans for follow-up care and ensures that appointments have been made and confirmed.

Most patients receive postoperative medications to relieve inflammation and facilitate healing. Antiinflammatory agents, antibiotics, analgesics, cycloplegics, and mydriatics may all be used. Dilating the pupil alleviates discomfort and prevents the iris from adhering to the lens implant. Pupil dilation necessitates the use of sunglasses as the eye is not able to respond naturally to light. Beta blockers or carbonic anhydrase inhibitors may be administered to reduce aqueous-humor formation and prevent postoperative increases in IOP (Table 56-5).

The nurse ensures that the patient and the caregiver understand the purpose of all prescribed medications and can administer them correctly. Eye drop solutions are commonly prescribed. If the patient is receiving multiple topical solutions or ointments, the nurse reminds the patient to wait 2 to 5 minutes between the administration of each drop and to administer the ointment last (Guidelines for Care Box on p. 1838 and the Research Box, below). The nurse ensures that all discharge instructions are provided to the patient and family in writing for easy reference and that they have a phone number to call if questions or problems arise (Research Boxes, bottoms of columns).

The nurse reviews safety precautions and reminds the patient that depth perception is initially compromised after

**guidelines for care**

**The Person After Cataract Surgery**

1. Position patient on back or unoperated side to prevent pressure on operated eye.
2. Keep side rails up as necessary for protection.
3. Place bedside table on side of unoperated eye (patient then turns toward unoperated side).
4. Place call light within reach.
5. Stress avoidance of actions that increase IOP (for example, sneezing, coughing, vomiting, straining, or sudden bending over with the head below the waist).

**research**

Morlet N, Kelly M: Improving drop administration by patients, *J Ophthal Nurs Technol* 15(2):60-64, 1996.

Twenty-three patients who underwent cataract surgery were observed during eye drop administration to identify problems in their technique. The teaching of the next group of 10 patients was modified to address the problems identified. The performance of this group was then compared with the performance of a group of patients whose drops were administered by a caregiver.

The performance of both groups was found to be equal, and the mean number of drops used was similar in each group. Patients who self-administered drops were found to be most effective when they stabilized the bottle by placing the thumb of their hand against their forehead to administer the drops.

**research**

Reference: McGrory A, Assman S: A study investigating primary nursing, discharge teaching, and patient satisfaction of ambulatory cataract patients, *Insight* 19(2):8-13, 29, 1994.

The purpose of this study was to investigate the impact of the primary nursing model of care on discharge teaching and patient satisfaction of ambulatory cataract patients. Patients were randomly assigned to a primary care group ($N = 36$) and to a control group ($N = 36$).

Patients in the primary care group received pre- and postoperative care from the same nurse as well as a follow-up phone call 24 to 48 hours later. The control group of patients received care from different nurses during each phase of care. Knowledge of self care, normal side effects, and complications was assessed as well as satisfaction with care at the time of discharge. No statistically significant differences were found between the two groups in either measure, although patients in the primary care group scored higher on both measures.

**research**

Reference: Allen M, Oberle K: Follow up of day surgery cataract patients, *J Ophthal Nurs Technol,* 12(5):211-216, 1993.

This telephone survey study explored the informational needs and postoperative course of 33 cataract surgery patients who underwent day surgery. The patients experienced few problems, but expressed uncertainty over the administration of eye drops and the extent of activity restrictions.

The amount, type, and timing of teaching received was inconsistent. No patient received all three kinds of information (procedural, behavioral, and sensory) deemed essential for surgical patients. The majority of patients would have liked more information about how they would feel postoperatively and how they could cope with their various problems and concerns. Much of the teaching was provided in writing, which was inappropriate for many patients after eye surgery.

surgery, and the risk of injury is increased. Special care is taken with any stairs, and driving is prohibited until cleared by the physician.

## GERONTOLOGICAL CONSIDERATIONS

Since cataract is a problem that primarily affects elders, the entire discussion is directed to that population. It is particularly important for the nurse to perform a careful assessment of the patient's support system for care after discharge, physical dexterity to be able to perform dressing changes and medication administration, and understanding of the important components of home care. If a patient needs cataract glasses additional teaching is given for safety precautions to be followed at home. Objects appear larger, and both peripheral vision and depth perception can be seriously compromised after surgery. Extra care must be taken in ambulation, particularly when the patient attempts to go up and down stairs or curbs.

## SPECIAL ENVIRONMENTS FOR CARE

### Critical Care Management

Critical care does not play a role in the treatment of cataract. The surgery is performed in an ambulatory surgery center, and even extremely aged individuals are successfully discharged back to their home environments the same day.

### Home Care Management

The patient is likely to need assistance during the first days after surgery, and if family or friends are not available the nurse ensures that referral for home health supervision is initiated. The acuity of vision in the nonoperative eye may influence the person's ability to perform activities of daily living (ADL) and administer medications safely.

Anticipatory planning can reduce the patient's dependence on others. Items needed for self-care can be temporarily relocated for easy access without bending over at the waist, e.g., slippers and pet supplies. The patient's hair is washed before surgery to delay the need to wash it in the postoperative period. Meals can be prepared ahead and frozen for easy access. Frail elders without strong family or social supports may need a brief admission to an assisted-living facility.

## COMPLICATIONS

Infection, bleeding, and elevated IOP are the major complications of cataract surgery. The patient is instructed to promptly report the incidence of drainage, excessive tearing, bleeding, or a decline in visual acuity. Irritation and discomfort are expected after surgery, but acute pain would indicate a complication and should be reported immediately. When severe pain occurs, it frequently indicates that the position of the iris has been disrupted, causing an acute rise in IOP. This may require surgical correction to preserve the patient's vision.

# RETINAL DETACHMENT

## ETIOLOGY/EPIDEMIOLOGY

Retinal detachment occurs when the outer pigmented layer and the inner sensory layer of the retina separate. Inflammation and bleeding are common contributors to the detachment (Figure 56-12). Myopic degeneration and trauma are the most common causes of detachment, but it is also a frequently complication in eyes that are aphakic (without a lens). In many cases no apparent cause can be found.

## PATHOPHYSIOLOGY

The retina is a smooth, unbroken, multilayered surface. Degenerative holes or tears in the retina can allow vitreous humor to pass through and initiate a detachment *(rhegamatogenous detachment)*. The presence of an inflammatory mass, blood clot, or tumor can also separate the retinal layers *(exudative detachment)*. The vitreous also undergoes some deterioration with aging and can fall forward exerting a traction pull on the inner lining of the retina, causing detachment *(traction detachment)*.

Retinal detachment may occur suddenly or develop slowly. Symptoms include floating spots or opacities before the eyes, flashes of light, and progressive loss of vision in one area. The floating spots are blood and retinal cells that are freed at the time of the tear; they cast shadows on the retina as they drift about the eye. The flashes of light are caused by vitreous traction on the retina. The area of visual loss depends entirely on the location of the detachment.

If the detachment extends to include the macula, blindness results. When the detachment is extensive and occurs quickly, the patient may have the sensation that a curtain has been drawn before the eyes, but there is no pain associated with the detachment.

## COLLABORATIVE CARE MANAGEMENT

The diagnosis of retinal separation is established by ophthalmoscopic examination of the retina to identify the location and extent of the retinal tear. B-scan ultrasonography may be used to improve the accuracy of the diagnosis, particularly if

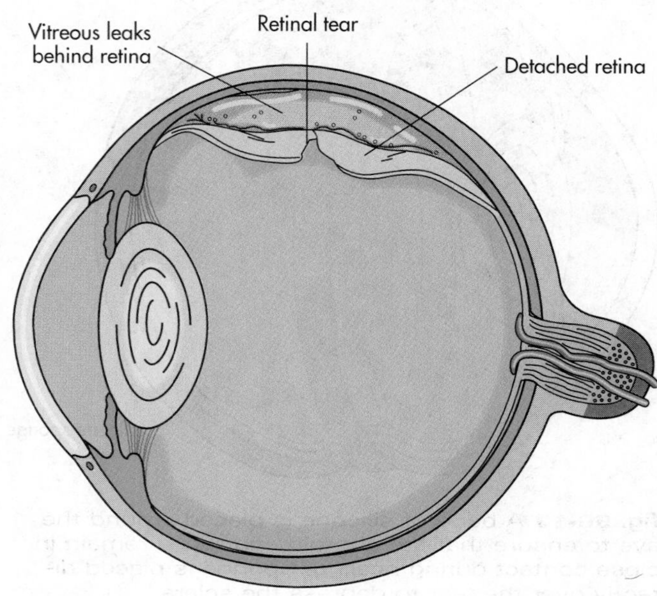


fig. 56-12 Retinal detachment.

the vitreous is opaque. Minor tears and retinal holes are frequently identified as part of a routine eye examination, but if the individual is asymptomatic, no intervention is necessary.

Detachments that compromise vision are repaired surgically if possible. Surgery has a 90% success rate in reattaching the retina. Several different surgical techniques may be used. Fluid is usually first drained from the subretinal space to return the retina to its normal position. The tear is then sealed by producing an inflammatory reaction that causes adhesions to form between the margins of the break and the choroid *(chorioretinitis)*. Diathermy can be used for small tears of recent origin. Needlepoint electrodes are applied to stimulate the inflammatory process. Laser photocoagulation can also provide the energy source to trigger the chorioretinitis. In *cryopexy* or *cryotherapy* subfreezing nitrous oxide or carbon dioxide is applied to the sclera in the area of the tear or hole to produce the inflammatory reaction.

Cryopexy is a commonly used procedure that is frequently combined with a *scleral buckling* procedure in which the sclera and choroid are indented (buckled) toward the break by placing various sizes and shapes of silicone in the region of the break. An encircling band of silicone can also be placed around the eye (Figure 56-13). These procedures ensure that the choroid remains in contact with the tear during healing and reduce the traction pull of any vitreous adhesions. The hole is thereby closed and a water-tight intraretinal space is reestablished.

Pneumatic *retinopexy* may also be used to repair a detachment, particularly small holes on the superior portion of the retina. Cryopexy is performed and followed by the instillation of an expandable gas, such as SF (sulfur hexafluoride) or perfluropane, or oil to tamponade the tear and support healing. The gas or oil is gradually absorbed and replaced with vitreous.

The location and severity of the retinal detachment guide the patient's preoperative care. With small tears the patient may be permitted to continue with normal activities. When the detachment is large, however, or the macula is threatened, the patient needs quiet bedrest and may have both eyes patched to minimize eye movement and prevent extension of the detachment if possible. This is an extremely stressful time for the patient who needs careful teaching about the planned procedure and postoperative care. Patients with eye patches require thoughtful supportive care and frequent monitoring to remain oriented in a strange and frightening environment. The nurse also needs to assist the patient with all routine care.

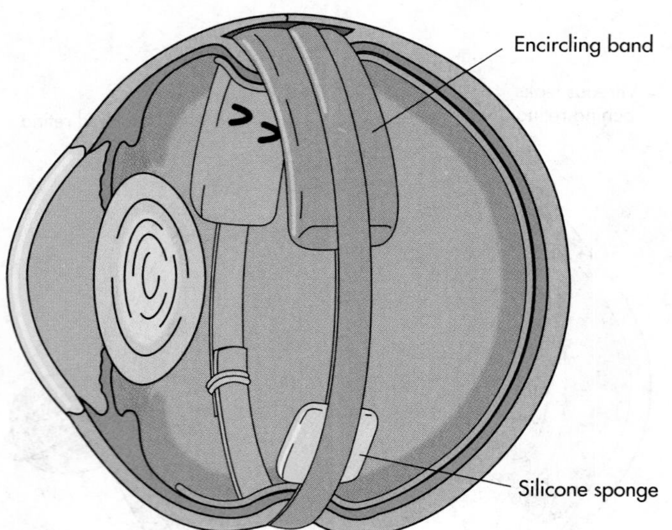


**fig. 56-13** A band of silicone is placed around the eye to ensure that the choroid and retina remain in close contact during healing. Sponge is placed directly over the tear to depress the sclera.

Eye patching may be continued in the postoperative period, depending on the preference of the surgeon. The nurse continues to orient the patient to the environment and ensures patient safety through the use of side rails, assistance with self-care activities, close supervision when the patient is out of bed, and placement of the call bell securely within easy reach. The nurse provides ongoing support and encouragement to the patient and family while the eye patches are in place and while the success of the surgery is in question, reinforcing the >90% success rate. The threat of permanent blindness can be extremely frightening for both patient and family.

The exact location and severity of the detachment also govern the patient's specific activity restrictions in the postoperative period. If a gas or oil bubble has been injected into the eye to reinforce the repair, the patient is positioned so that the gas rises in the eye and presses against the repair. This usually necessitates positioning the patient face down or angled toward the unoperative side. This position can be extremely difficult for patients to maintain, especially elders, and the nurse assists the patient to achieve as much comfort as possible through the use of support pillows and head supports. Positioning restrictions may be in place for as long as 4 to 8 days. The patient is permitted out of bed for brief periods but is encouraged to keep the head parallel with the floor as much as possible. The nurse works to ensure both the patient's safety and relative comfort. The nurse encourages the patient to practice deep breathing every hour to decrease the risk of respiratory infection. Prone positioning significantly compromises respiratory excursion. Coughing is contraindicated because of the risk of elevating IOP.

The nurse attempts to increase the patient's physical and emotional comfort. Eye pain is expected to be moderate, and the nurse administers analgesics as needed and evaluates their effectiveness. Cycloplegic agents may be administered to rest the eye, and corticosteroid drops are given to reduce inflammation. The combined effects of the medications and surgery may cause acute photophobia, and the nurse adjusts the room light to increase the patient's comfort. Vision is initially blurred because accommodation has been paralyzed. Care of the patient after repair of a retinal detachment is presented in the Nursing Care Plan.

### Patient/Family Education

The patient is discharged within a few days. The nurse ensures that the patient or family caregiver can correctly administer all medications and eye drops. The nurse reinforces the need to limit activity, avoid bending over below the level of the waist,

## nursing care plan The Person with Retinal Detachment

**DATA** Mr. A. is a 56-year-old warehouse clerk who complains of decreasing vision in his left eye over the past few days, like "a curtain coming over my eye." He comments that he began to notice spots floating in front of his eye about 2 weeks ago and flashes of light out of the corner of his eye a week ago. He states that he did not get concerned about these, because he thought they were just normal aging changes. He remarks, "I began to get scared when I started to go blind in that eye, and then it didn't take me long to get to my eye doctor." He continues, "I got more scared when the doctor sent me straight to the hospital." Mr. A. states that, except for nearsightedness, he has had no trouble with his eyes. He is generally healthy except for high blood pressure, which is well controlled with medication and diet. Examination of his left eye revealed a superior retinal detachment with inferior visual loss. His visual acuity preoperatively was 20/80. He underwent retinal detachment surgery (scleral buckling) this morning. His left eye is patched, and his orders are for restricted activity.

His admission assessment identified the following:

- He and his wife had little understanding of what has happened to his eye or what the physician is going to do to his eye in the hospital.
- The loss of vision is very frightening to Mr. and Mrs. A. They are also concerned about whether Mr. A. will get any vision back in the eye and whether the visual loss will spread to the other eye.
- Mr. A. has not had any accidents or injuries to his eyes that he can remember.
- Mr. A. is a very active man, swimming and jogging regularly. He comments that he has to do some "good" activity every day so he can feel his best.

**NURSING DIAGNOSIS** *Pain related to inflammation, increased intraocular pressure*

| expected patient outcome | nursing interventions | rationale |
|---|---|---|
| States eye feels comfortable. | Assess the level of discomfort. | Postoperative discomfort is expected, but acute pain suggests increased IOP or hemorrhage. |
| | Apply cool, moist compresses. | Reduces swelling and promotes comfort. |
| | Administer analgesics as required. | Promotes comfort. |
| | Instruct patient to avoid rapid head movements and not to bend head below waist. | Avoids increasing IOP and pain. |

**NURSING DIAGNOSIS** *Anxiety/fear related to surgical procedure and possible loss of vision*

| expected patient outcomes | nursing interventions | rationale |
|---|---|---|
| Shows decreased signs of anxiety. | Give patient and spouse an opportunity to explore concerns about possible loss of vision. | Talking may help decrease anxiety and identify specific fears. |
| Verbalizes fears and feelings of anxiety. | Answer questions honestly. | Information decreases uncertainty and helps person gain control and feel less anxious. |
| | Encourage realistic hope about maintaining vision. | Helps relieve anxiety. |
| | Explore knowledge of disorder and therapy, and correct misunderstandings. | Clarification assists understanding. |

**NURSING DIAGNOSIS** *Risk for injury related to sensory deficit, anxiety, lack of awareness of environmental hazards*

| expected patient outcomes | nursing interventions | rationale |
|---|---|---|
| Experiences no injury. | Orient patient to physical surroundings. | Increase awareness of potential hazards. |
| | Keep bed in lowest position and side rail up on left side. | Ensure safety when patient has eyes patched and is in strange environment. |
| | Assist patient when first getting up after surgery. | Ensure safety. |
| | Instruct patient to avoid sneezing, coughing, and vomiting. Administer cough medicine or antiemetics, if required. | Help avoid increasing IOP. |

*Continued*

## The Person with Retinal Detachment—cont'd

**NURSING DIAGNOSIS** *Risk for injury related to sensory deficit, lack of awareness of environmental hazards—cont'd*

| expected patient outcomes | nursing interventions | rationale |
|---|---|---|
| | Instruct patient to wear eye shield at night or when taking a nap for 2 weeks after surgery. | Prevent accidental bumping of the eye. |
| | Maintain prescribed activity and position restrictions. | Restricted eye movement helps decrease risk of further detachment. |
| | Place bedside table within patient's reach without need to turn head. | Gravity is used to help keep the retina in its proper position. |
| | Assist with ADL as necessary. | Decreased vision and restrictions in activity alter or interfere with familiar ways of doing things. |
| | Orient patient to physical surroundings. | Provides for increased comfort and familiarity. |
| | Place bed so patient is not facing wall and can see others approaching. Approach patient from unaffected side. | Offsets isolation and aids orientation to surrounding environment. |
| | Encourage diversional activities such as radio and conversation. | Provides sensory input and feelings of normalcy. |

**NURSING DIAGNOSIS** *Risk for infection related to surgical repair of detached retina*

| expected patient outcome | nursing interventions | rationale |
|---|---|---|
| Shows no signs or symptoms of infection. | Assess for signs and symptoms of infection. | Allow for early detection. |
| | Use sterile technique when performing eye care and changing dressings. | Decrease possibility of introducing pathogens. |
| | Administer antibiotic drops. | Help prevent infection. |

**NURSING DIAGNOSIS** *Knowledge deficit regarding condition, surgery, postoperative care, and self-care at home related to lack of exposure*

| expected patient outcomes | nursing interventions | rationale |
|---|---|---|
| Patient and his wife can describe retinal detachment and explain the basis for the symptoms experienced. | Teach about the eye and the role of the retina in vision. Explain why flashing lights and spots appear before the eyes and decreased vision occurs. | Increase understanding and promote cooperation with postoperative routine. |
| Patient and wife can verbalize or demonstrate knowledge of surgery, preoperative and postoperative care, and self-care at home. | Teach preoperative routine and surgery. Instruct patient in permitted postoperative activities: | Activities that cause increased IOP may compromise surgery. |
| | 1. Ensure that any prescribed position is maintained. | If a gas bubble is injected to cover the retinal hole, a specific position will be required to ensure that this occurs (usually prone). |
| | 2. Ask physician when a return to work can be made. | |
| | 3. May climb stairs, watch TV, read, and carry out ADL as long as eye is comfortable. | |
| | 4. Avoid driving, heavy house or yard work, or sporting activities before checking with physician. | |
| | 5. May bathe in tub; avoid splashing eyes when washing face. | |
| | 6. Do not bend head below waist: avoid sudden movements. | |
| | Demonstrate ways the patient can make himself comfortable if he must maintain a specific position (e.g., face down). | |

*Continued*

## The Person with Retinal Detachment—cont'd

**NURSING DIAGNOSIS** *Knowledge deficit regarding condition, surgery, postoperative care, and self-care at home related to lack of exposure—cont'd*

| expected patient outcomes | nursing interventions | rationale |
|---|---|---|
| | Demonstrate proper technique of cleaning eye from inner to outer canthus using clean cotton ball for each wipe. Stress hand washing. | Good technique reduces risk of spread of bacteria. |
| | Demonstrate proper technique to administer drops and ointment and apply shield. Stress hand washing. | |
| | Instruct patient and spouse to call doctor if:<br>1. New flashing lights, floaters, or shadows appear.<br>2. Eye pain is severe or persistent.<br>3. Redness of eye or lid increases.<br>4. Quantity of discharge from eye increases or changes to greenish color. | Early intervention can prevent development of complications. |

and to avoid constipation and straining. Activities that require close vision such as reading, needlework, or writing are limited because they require rapid eye movements and accommodation. Watching television and walking are appropriate, although patients with gas bubbles may still have restrictions on positioning their heads. An eyeshield is worn during sleep for about 2 weeks. The nurse instructs the patient to contact the surgeon immediately if acute eye pain develops, eye discharge increases or turns yellow-green, and if symptoms of detachment recur.

## STRABISMUS

### ETIOLOGY/EPIDEMIOLOGY

Strabismus is an ocular misalignment that results from an imbalance in the intraocular muscles. The eyes may be misaligned in any direction, e.g., *esotropia* (turning in), *exotropia* (turning out), *hypertropia* (turning up), or *hypotropia* (turning down). Strabismus is usually associated with childhood, but it can also be a lifelong disorder. Adult strabismus is also associated with brain tumor, head trauma, stroke, and thyroid ophthalmopathy. An estimated 2% to 3% of the general population have some degree of strabismus.

### PATHOPHYSIOLOGY

The ability to move the eyes in all directions and fixate on an object is the function of the six pairs of extraocular muscles (see Chapter 55). Strabismus interferes with the ability to use binocular vision and focus both eyes on an object, often causing double vision. Children with strabismus are frequently able to compensate for the confused images and avoid diplopia. Adults with new-onset strabismus are rarely able to compensate.

### COLLABORATIVE CARE MANAGEMENT

Strabismus is diagnosed through a standard visual fields assessment. A variety of treatment options exist. Glasses with prisms may successfully realign the eyes and restore binocular vision. Eye exercises have been widely prescribed for patients with strabismus to "strengthen" the weak muscles, but there is little evidence of their effectiveness. Surgical correction is the standard treatment. The extraocular muscles are selectively weakened *(recession)*, tightened *(resection)*, or physically shifted *(transposition)* to achieve balanced eye movement. Adjustable sutures can be used to achieve an even more accurate alignment. A slip knot is attached during surgery. Once the anesthetic has worn off the patient's ocular alignment is checked, and minor corrections can be made by tightening or loosening the knot.[29,53]

Drug therapy with *botulinum neurotoxin A* (Botox) may eliminate the need for surgery or be used in conjunction with surgery. Botox is injected into the extraocular muscle and interferes with the release of acetylcholine at the neuromuscular junction. The toxin appears to strengthen the antagonist muscle and weaken the injected muscle over a period of weeks to months.[21,46]

#### Patient/Family Education

Most strabismus surgery is performed on an outpatient basis under either local or general anesthesia. Postoperative care focuses on careful monitoring and preparation of the patient for self-care at home. The eyes may be patched initially for protection, especially if an adjustable suture was used. Patients are instructed to avoid strenuous exercise and heavy lifting until approved by the surgeon. Slight redness, swelling, and irritation are expected, and the nurse instructs the patient to use cold compresses for comfort. Dust and heavy pollen can irritate the eye and should be avoided. The nurse instructs the patient to monitor the eye for healing and to promptly report any sign of infection.

## EYE TUMORS

Both benign and malignant tumors may affect the eye and related structures. They may originate within the eye or metastasize from another primary site. Benign neoplasms include lymphomas, hemangiomas, and mucoceles from the sinuses. Malignant tumors threaten both the patient's vision and life as extension frequently involves vital structures within the brain. The eyelids are vulnerable to any of the standard tumors that affect the skin including nevi and xanthelasma (lipid depositis near the corner of the eye). Positive outcomes frequently require early diagnosis and prompt treatment. Treatment usually involves surgical excision but may also include various forms of radiotherapy.

### MALIGNANT MELANOMA

#### Etiology/Epidemiology

A melanoma involving the eye is rare, but it is the most common form of intraocular tumor in adults. Retinoblastoma is the most common form of eye tumor, but it is congenital and is typically diagnosed in childhood. Melanomas usually occur unilaterally. See Chapter 63 for a more complete discussion of melanoma.

#### Pathophysiology

Malignant melanomas occur in the choroid, ciliary body, and iris. They are slow growing, but they metastasize early due to the vascularity of the choroid. Vision may not be affected until the tumor becomes large or affects the macula (Figure 56-14).

#### Collaborative Care Management

Intraocular malignant melanomas are frequently diagnosed with an ophthalmoscopic examination. Ultrasonography and fundus photography may be useful in documenting the size and placement of the tumor. Fluorescein angiography may be used to document the vascular involvement of the tumor.

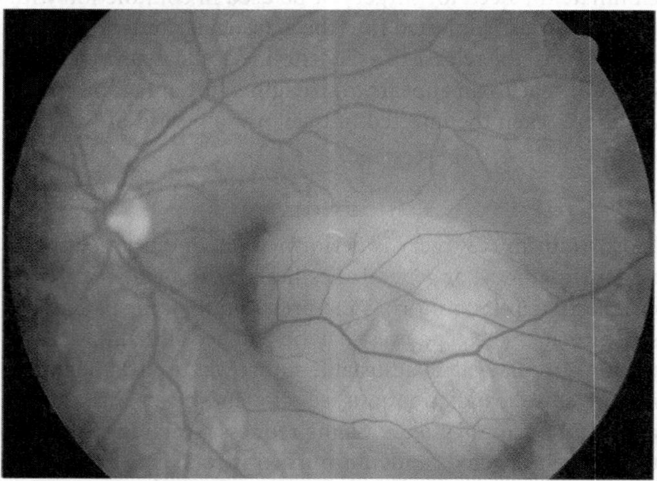

**fig. 56-14** Large choroidal melanoma.

Surgery is the primary treatment for an intraocular melanoma. Treatment is based on the exact size, shape, and location of the tumor. Every effort is made to preserve the patient's vision if possible. Small tumors that involve the iris may be successfully treated with iridectomy, often with removal of the ciliary body as well. Large melanomas of the choroid are usually treated with *enucleation* of the eye, which involves surgical removal of the entire eye including the sclera. *Evisceration* is removal of the contents of the eye with retention of the sclera. *Exenteration* involves removal of the entire eye and all other soft tissues in the bony orbit.

Nonsurgical treatments include radiation therapy, photocoagulation, and brachytherapy, in which radioactive plaques are sutured into the sclera.

If feasible, the eyeball alone is removed, leaving the surrounding layers of fascia (Tenon's capsule) and the muscle attachments. A silicone, plastic, or tantalum implant is inserted into the eye socket, the cut ends of the muscle attachment are overlapped and sutured around it, and the Tenon's capsule and the conjunctiva are closed. This procedure supplies both support and motion for an artificial eye.

A newer implant called *hydroxyapatite,* which has the same consistency as bone, may provide better movement of an ocular prosthesis.[2] The ball-shaped implant is left in place permanently. A plastic conformer is placed in the socket until edema subsides, and an artificial eye (prosthesis) can be inserted because the extraocular muscles strongly anchor to it. This provides superior motion and improved cosmetic appearance.

Pressure dressings are used for 1 or 2 days to help control possible hemorrhage. Headaches or pain on the operative side could indicate a venous thrombosis or the onset of meningitis. Infection is a dangerous complication of eye surgery, and most patients receive prophylactic antibiotics.

A custom-made prosthetic eye can be used as soon as healing is complete and edema has disappeared. Healing is usually

**guidelines for care**

**Care of Prosthetic Eyes**

1. Remove prosthesis: gently depress the lower lid and exert a small amount of pressure under lower edge of prosthesis.
2. Wash prosthesis with soap (for example, Ivory) and water. Soap is less irritating than detergents. Rinse thoroughly.
3. Reinsert prosthesis: place upper portion under upper lid, pull down lower lid and slip lower edge behind lower lid. With finger or thumb, gently pull down on lower lid and slide prosthesis in place.
4. Do not expose the plastic eye to alcohol, ether, or any other solvent; they can damage the eye beyond repair.
5. If rubbing the eye, rub toward the nose. Wiping away from the nose may cause the eye to fall out.
6. Wear a protective patch or goggles when swimming, diving, or water skiing—or remove the eye and store it.
7. If the eye is left out of the socket, store it in water or contact lens solution.

complete 4 to 8 weeks after surgery, although many patients begin to wear a temporary prosthetic eye after only 2 to 3 weeks. Today artificial eyes are made of plastic instead of glass and can be made in shades that closely match the normal eye.

### Patient/family education

The diagnosis of eye malignancy and the need to undergo enucleation creates a crisis situation for the patient and family. The virulence of the malignancy may necessitate immediate surgery with little time to prepare for the loss of the eye either physically or emotionally. The nurse plays an important role in providing support and counseling to the patient during this difficult time. Both the patient and family need to be encouraged to talk about their feelings and concerns and to be helped to adjust their lives when confronted by this serious situation.

When a person has lost one eye, the preservation of sight in the other eye becomes crucial. Wearing impact-resistant glasses provides some protection from injury. Because binocular vision is gone when there is only one functioning eye, depth perception is affected. The nurse teaches the person about the adjustments necessary to carry out normal activities with one eye and about potential safety hazards. Driving a car, for example, is potentially dangerous because of the alteration in depth perception. With patience and practice, however, almost all normal activities are possible.

Care of the prosthetic eye is relatively simple. Frequent removal and cleaning is no longer recommended. Patients are referred for follow-up to an ocularist who will clean and polish the eye to remove salt and protein buildups. This may be done just one to two times per year. Patients who need to care for the eye more frequently for any reason should follow the guidelines outlined in the Guidelines for Care Box on the previous page.

## critical thinking QUESTIONS

1. How would you teach a visually impaired person who is using three different types of eye drops to identify the correct drops?
2. What approaches might you consider for a person with glaucoma who refuses to administer eye drops four times a day as prescribed by the physician?
3. Miss C., 20 years old, has a foreign object floating on the surface of her left eye. The nurse has Miss C. lie on her right side and begins irrigating the left eye with a syringe filled with normal saline. She directs the fluid from the outer to inner canthus. Critique this irrigation procedure.

## chapter SUMMARY

### VISUAL IMPAIRMENT

- Macular degeneration causes loss of central vision and decreased ability to distinguish colors.
- Many systemic diseases have eye manifestations.
- Diabetic retinopathy occurs in about 90% of persons who have had diabetes for 30 years.
- Blindness imposes limitations on mobility, interaction with the environment, and the range of experiences readily available to the sighted person.
- Loss of social supports is a major factor hindering adjustment to a visual impairment.
- Nursing care of the person with a visual impairment includes support and counseling, instruction about the aids and strategies that facilitate living with a visual impairment, and referral to appropriate community agencies.

### INFECTION AND TRAUMA

- Acute bacterial conjunctivitis (pinkeye) is highly contagious.
- After any chemical burn, the eye must be irrigated immediately, before transportation to a physician.

### GLAUCOMA

- In glaucoma, IOP can be increased because of obstruction to the outflow of aqueous humor, causing subsequent optic nerve damage,which may result in decreased visual acuity, visual field defects, and potential blindness. The person with glaucoma may need help to adhere to a lifetime of medication therapy.
- When administering more than one eye drop at a time, wait 2 to 5 minutes between instillations.

### CATARACT

- A cataract is an opacity of the lens. Cataracts most commonly occur as a result of the aging process.
- Cataracts can be successfully removed surgically. Intraocular lens implants restore adequate vision.

### DETACHMENT OF THE RETINA

- Common factors placing the person at risk for a retinal detachment include myopia, trauma, and aphakia.

## References


1. Ai E, Kelly MP: Ophthalmic manifestations of the acquired immunodeficiency syndrome, *J Ophthalmic Nurs Technol* 11(4):148-156, 1992.
2. Albiar E: Hydroxyapatite implants—a new trend in enucleation and orbital reconstructive surgery, *Insight* 17(1):25-28, 1992.
3. Allen MN: Adjusting to visual impairment, *J Ophthalmic Nurs Technol* 9(2):47-51, 1990.
4. Allen MN, Birse E: Stigma and blindness, *J Ophthalmic Nurs Technol* 10(4):147-152, 1991.
5. Beran RF, Stewart C, Doty J: Refractive surgery and the athlete, *J Ophthalmic Nurs Technol* 14(1):11-16, 1995.
6. Best SJ: Visual fields in glaucoma and neuro-ophthalmology, *J Ophthalmic Nurs Technol* 11(2):46-56, 1992.
7. Birt L: Making sense of . . . photorefractive keratectomy, *Nurs Times* 91(44):30-31, 1995.
8. Boyd-Monk H, Steinmentz CG III: *Nursing care of the eye,* Norwalk, Conn, 1987, Appleton & Lange.
9. Bressler SB: *Age-related macular degeneration,* San Francisco, 1995, American Academy of Ophthalmology.
10. Brown RM, Roberts CW: Preoperative and postoperative use of nonsteroidal antiinflammatory drugs in cataract surgery, *Insight* 21(1): 13-16, 1996.
11. Burlew JA: Preventing eye injuries—the nurse's role, *Insight* 16(6): 24-28, 1991.
12. Chialant D et al: Technical and nursing roles in patient care for photorefractive surgery, *J Ophthalmic Nurs Technol* 15(2):52-56, 1996.

13. Eichelbaum JW: Vitamins for cataract and macular degeneration, *J Ophthalmic Nurs Technol* 15(2):65-67, 1996.
14. Elfervig LS: Eye care and AIDS prevention for ophthalmic medical personnel, *J Ophthalmic Nurs Technol* 12(3):117-193, 1993.
15. Fishbaugh J: Lessons on dilation, *Insight* 19(1):30-32, 1994.
16. Fishbaugh J: Overview and new technology in cyclodestructive procedures, *Insight* 19(4):26-29, 1994.
17. Fishbaugh J: Retina: indocyanine green (ICG) angiography, *Insight* 19(3):30-33, 1994.
18. Frederick MC: Care of the patient with AIDS and cytomegalovirus retinitis, *J Ophthalmic Nurs Technol* 13(4):156-160, 1994.
19. Hagan JC, Wyatt B: Preoperative evaluation and workup of the cataract and intraocular lens implant patient, *J Ophthalmic Nurs Technol* 12(3):123-128, 1993.
20. Harkness, BS: Hydroxyapatite eye implant, *Today's Surg Nurse* 18(3): 16-20, 1996.
21. Hill JE, editor: *Ophthalmic procedures—a nursing perspective,* San Francisco, 1994, American Society of Ophthalmic Registered Nurses.
22. Hunt L: Eyeglasses and common complaints, *Insight* 17(3):20-22, 1992.
23. Hunt L: Microwave ovens and eye injuries, *Insight* 17(4):23, 25, 1992.
24. Hunt L: Nutrients and the eye, *Insight* 19(1):25-27, 1994.
25. Kelly JS: Eye examination and vision testing, *Br J Nurs* 5(10):630-634, 1996.
26. Krupin T: Implanted aqueous shunt devices for glaucoma surgery, *J Ophthalmic Nurs Technol* 11(1):23-25, 1992.
27. Levin LA: Ophthalmology, *JAMA* 275(23):1834-1836, 1996.
28. McCoy K: Ophthalmic drug use in the OR, *Insight* 17(4):10-21, 1992.
29. Melhuish JA, Kemp EG: The routine use of adjustable sutures in adult strabismus surgery, *J R Coll Surg Edinburgh* 38:134-137, 1993.
30. National Advisory Eye Council (US): Vision research: a national plan 1983-1987, vol 1, The Report of The National Eye Council, Bethesda, Md, 1983, National Institutes of Health.
31. National Society to Prevent Blindness, Operational Research Department: *Vision problems in the United States: a statistical analysis,* New York, 1980, The Society.
32. New product for seniors, *Futurist,* p 19, July-Aug 1992.
33. Newell FW: *Ophthalmology: principles and concepts,* ed 8, St Louis, 1996, Mosby.
34. Newhourse J: Opening your eyes to intraocular drug administration, *Nursing 94,* p 44-45, June 1994.
35. Parker P: Overview of refractive surgery, *J Ophthalmic Nurs Technol* 13(3):105-109, 1994.
36. Phillips WB: Ocular manifestations of diabetes mellitus, *J Ophthalmic Nurs Technol* 13(6):255-261, 1994.
37. Plona RP, Schremp P: Nursing care of patients with ocular manifestations of human immunodeficiency virus infection, *Nurs Clin North Am* 27(3):793-805, 1992.
38. Rowell M: Eradication of vitamin A deficiency: with five cents and a vegetable garden, *J Ophthalmic Nurs Technol* 12(5):217-224, 1993.
39. Sandler RL: Clinical snapshot: glaucoma, *Am J Nurs* 95(3):34-35, 1995.
40. Servodidio CA: Teaching aids for patients diagnosed with choroidal melanoma, *Insight* 16(6):21-23, 1991.
41. Servodidio CA, Abramson KH: Choroidal melanoma, *Nurs Clin North Am* 27(3):777-790, 1992.
42. Sharp PS: Growth factors in the pathogenesis of diabetic retinopathy, *Diabetes Rev* 3(2):164-172, 1995.
43. Shulman J: Cataract from diagnosis to recovery—the complete guide for patients and families, revised ed, New York, 1993, St. Marten's Griffin.
44. Sivalingam E: Glaucoma: an overview, *J Ophthalmic Nurs Technol* 15(1):15-18, 1996.
45. Smith JF, Eanes MJ: Preventive screening services for diabetic retinopathy, *J Ophthalmic Nurs Technol* 14(3):132-133, 1995.
46. Smith H: The effects of botulinum toxin on ocular tissue, *Nurs Times* 91(4):41-43, 1995.
47. Smith S: Diabetic retinopathy, *Insight* 17(2):20-25, 1992.
48. Spires R: Perfluorcarbon liquid in the management of complex retinal detachments, *J Ophthalmic Nurs Technol* 11(4):157-160, 1992.
49. Sprires R: Contact laser TM transscleral cyclophotocoagulation in the treatment of glaucoma, *J Ophthalmic Nurs Technol* 14(4):154-158, 1995.
50. US Department of Health and Human Services: *Vision research: a national plan 1983-1987—the 1983 report of the National Advisory Eye Council,* NIH Publ No 83-2469, 1983, Washington, DC, The Department.
51. US Department of Health and Human Services, Public Health Service: *Healthy people 2000: midcourse review and 1995 revisions,* Washington, DC, 1995, US Government Printing Office.
52. Vaughan DE, Asbury T, Riordan-Eva P: *General ophthalmology,* ed 14, Norwalk, Conn, 1995, Appleton & Lange.
53. Weston B, Enzenauer RW, Kraft SP, Gayowksy GR: Stability of the postoperative alignment in adjustable strabismus surgery, *J Pediatr Ophthalmol Strabismus* 28(4):206-211, 1991.
54. Woods S: Macular degeneration, *Nurs Clin North Am* 27(3):761-775, 1992.
55. Wu G: *Retina, the fundamentals,* Philadelphia, 1995, WB Saunders.

chapter 57

# ASSESSMENT OF THE Auditory and Vestibular Systems

LINDA T. SCHURING and JANE F. MAREK

## objectives

*After studying this chapter, the learner should be able to:*

1 Describe the basic structure and function of the temporal bone and ear.
2 Use behavioral cues to detect loss of hearing and balance.
3 Describe normal and abnormal physiological changes associated with aging affecting the auditory and vestibular systems.
4 Recognize normal physical assessment features of the ear.
5 Identify specific diagnostic tests for hearing and balance and their associated nursing interventions.

Hearing is one of the five senses, and both hearing and balance are important in activities of daily living. Hearing helps us interact with the environment and adds aesthetic pleasure as well as warning of danger. Hearing is also essential for the normal development and maintenance of speech. The organs of balance are contained within the ear and relay information about the body's position to the brain.

Nurses are involved in every aspect of care of the patient with auditory and vestibular problems, including prevention, detection, and treatment. Auditory problems are common and can interfere with the person's activities of daily living. Auditory problems can occur at any age and may require immediate attention. Every nurse needs to be skillful in examining the outer ear and grossly assessing the patient's hearing and equilibrium. Nurses frequently participate in case findings of persons with hearing and balance disorders. Detection of hearing impairment and/or a balance problem is an important nursing responsibility, and the nurse is frequently the first member of the health care team to be approached by the patient regarding problems with hearing and balance.

## ANATOMY AND PHYSIOLOGY

### THE EAR

The ears are a pair of complex sensory organs located in the middle of both sides of the head at approximately eye level. The position of the ears is important because the use of both ears simultaneously produces binaural hearing, allowing a person to detect the direction of sound and aiding in maintaining equilibrium. A person detects the direction from which a sound comes by the time lag between the sound entry into one ear compared with the sound entry into the other ear and by the intensity of sound in each ears. Each ear is also responsible for sending signals to the brain for the maintenance of equilibrium. Therefore the *two major functions* of the ears are *hearing* and *balance.*

The ears are housed in the "temporal" bones of the skull, which are part of both the base and the lateral wall of the skull. The temporal bones are the hardest bones in the human body and provide adequate protection for the organs of hearing and balance.

Each ear is divided into three parts. The *external ear* includes the pinna or auricle and the external auditory canal and contains a sound collecting tube that terminates at the tympanic membrane (Figure 57-1). The *middle ear* is an air-containing cavity that contains three small bones and a small (eustachian) tube that connects the middle ear to the nasopharynx. The *internal ear* consists of membranous sacs and ducts encased in bony canals. The cochlea, which is specific for hearing, and the vestibular canals, which help to maintain equilibrium, are found in the internal ear.

#### The External Ear

The pinna is primarily composed of cartilage covered by skin and is attached to the side of the head at approximately a 10° angle. The parts of the pinna are illustrated by Figure 57-2. The *concha* is the deepest part and leads to the ear canal.

The ear canal extends from the concha to the eardrum, in an inward, forward, and downward path in an adult. The lumen is irregular and constricts about midway and again near the eardrum. Skin lines the ear canal and furnishes an external covering for the eardrum. The supporting wall of the first half of the ear canal is cartilaginous and the second half is osseous. The skin lining this bony portion of the canal is thin and highly sensitive and contains fine hairs and sebaceous glands.

*Ceruminous glands* (modified sweat glands) produce *cerumen* or *ear wax,* which functions as a protective mechanism. The sticky consistency of wax, along with the fine hairs of the ears, help to cleanse the ear canal of foreign matter.

The funnel shape of the external ear collects sound and channels it toward the eardrum.

#### The Tympanic Membrane

The tympanic membrane protects the middle ear and conducts sound vibrations from the external ear to the ossicles. The eardrum is a thin, semitransparent membrane, obliquely directed

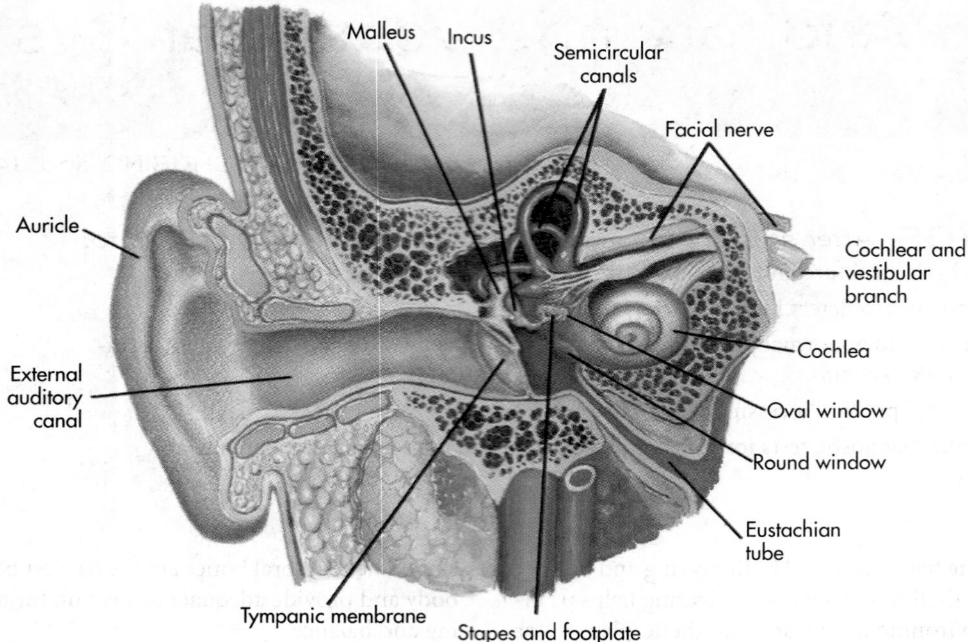


**fig. 57-1** Structures of the ear.

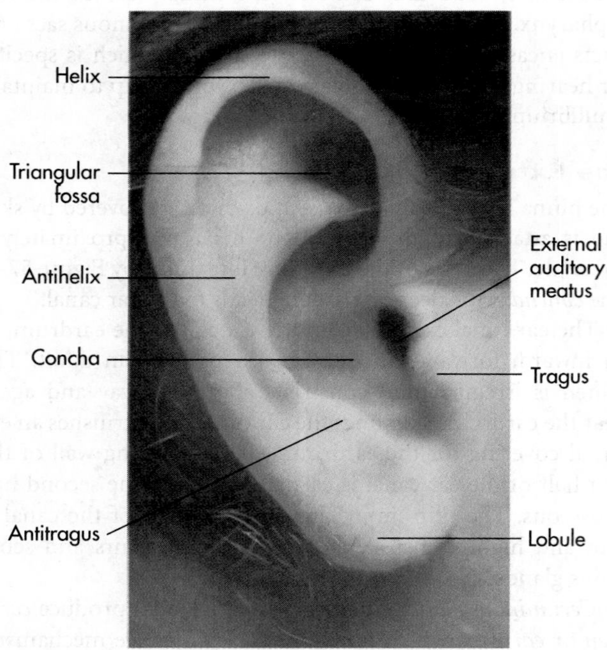


**fig. 57-2** Anatomical structures of the pinna. The helix is the prominent outer rim, whereas the antihelix is the area parallel and anterior to the helix. The concha is the deep cavity containing the auditory canal meatus. The tragus is the protuberance lying anterior to the auditory canal meatus, and the antitragus is the protuberance on the antihelix opposite the tragus. The lobule is the soft lobe on the bottom of the auricle.

downward and inward. Nearly oval in shape, this membrane is approximately 9 mm in diameter and pearly gray in color.

Distinguishing landmarks of the normal eardrum include the *annulus,* which is the thickened border that attaches the eardrum to the temporal bone; the *umbo,* the most depressed point where the first ossicle attaches to the eardrum; the *pars flaccida,* a small triangular area above the short process of the malleus; and the largest portion, the *pars tensa* (Figure 57-3).

The *tympanic membrane* is composed of three layers: an outer skin layer continuous with the skin of the external ear canal, a fibrous middle layer, and an inner mucosal layer continuous with the lining of the middle ear.[1] The pars flaccida is composed of only two layers. The absence of the fibrous middle layer makes the pars flaccida more vulnerable to negative pressure, causing pathological disorders.

### The Middle Ear

The middle ear consists of an air-filled cavity and its contents; the ossicles, the oval and round windows, and the eustachian tube. The middle ear is traversed by a chain of three movable bones that connect the tympanic membrane to the labyrinth (see Figure 57-1).

The ossicles, the *malleus* (hammer), the *incus* (anvil), and the *stapes* (stirrup), are the three smallest bones in the body. The ossicles have been given these common names because of their appearance. The function of the ossicles is to mechanically transmit sound vibrations. They are held in place by muscles, ligaments, and joints and offer protective mechanisms from loud sounds. The ossicles provide an efficient

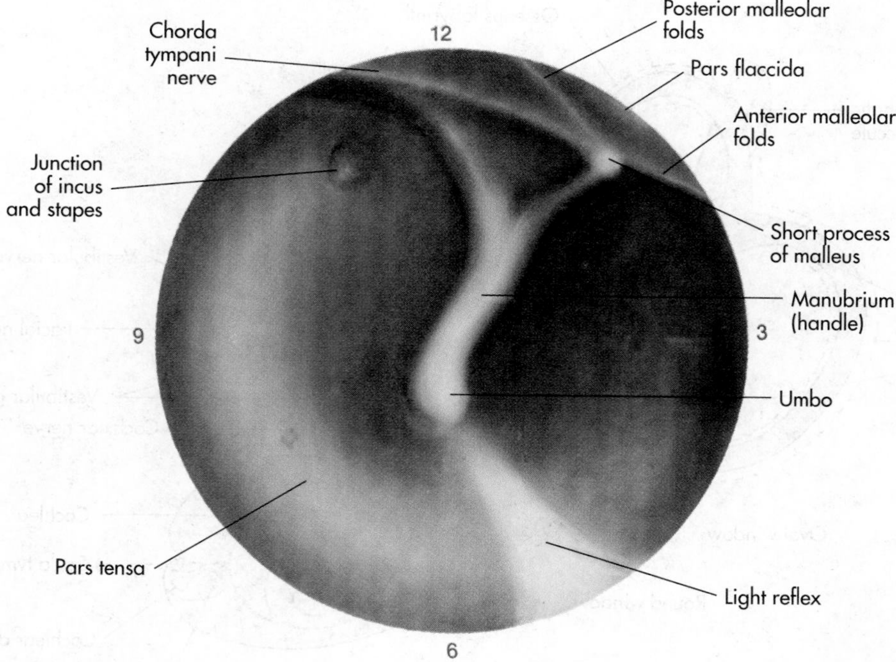


**fig. 57-3** Structural landmarks of the tympanic membrane.

means by which the moving air molecules of sound can be transferred to the fluid molecules that circulate in the inner ear. Liquids offer more resistance than air and need more force to produce movement; the ossicular chain produces this force against the inner ear fluids.[4]

The oval window and the round window are found in the middle ear although the oval window is not a true window, since the footplate of the stapes covers it. The *oval window* is the opening into the inner ear where sound vibrations enter. The *round window* is a true window and provides an exit for sound vibrations from the inner ear.

The *eustachian tube* is a channel approximately 35 mm ($1^1/_2$ in) in length that connects the middle ear with the nasopharynx. The tube is composed of bone, cartilage, and fibrous tissue lined with mucous membrane. The eustachian tube allows air to enter and leave the middle ear and is responsible for both ventilation and pressure regulation, which are necessary for normal hearing.

Only a small segment of the eustachian tube remains open permanently; otherwise the walls are in direct contact with each other. This prevents the sound of normal nasal respiration and one's own voice from passing up the eustachian tube into the middle ear. The tube can be forcibly opened by increasing nasopharyngeal pressure ("popping the ears").

## The Mastoid

The *mastoid* includes the mastoid bone (part of the temporal bone); the mastoid process, which can be felt as a bony protuberance behind the lower portion of the pinna, the mastoid cavity, a large cavity that is continuous with the middle ear; and the mastoid air cells that branch off the mastoid cavity. The cavity and system of air-filled cells contained within the mastoid bone aid the middle ear in adjusting to changes in pressure and lighten the weight of this protective bony structure.

## The Inner Ear

The inner ear is a complex system of intercommunicating chambers and connecting tubes located in the petrous part of the temporal bone. It is the primary organ for hearing and equilibrium. The inner ear is composed of two major structures: the *bony labyrinth* and the *membranous labyrinth,* which lies within but does not completely fill the bony labyrinth.

### Bony labyrinth

The bony labyrinth is the rigid capsule in which the membranous labyrinth lies and consists of the semicircular canals, the vestibule, and the cochlea (Figure 57-4).

There are three semicircular canals: the superior, the lateral (horizontal), and the posterior. These canals provide the sense of balance.

The *vestibule* connects the semicircular canals and the cochlea. The *cochlea* looks like a snail shell and has two compartments. The upper compartment is called the *scala vestibuli* and leads from the oval window to the apex of the cochlea. The lower compartment is called the *scala tympani* and continues from the apex of the cochlea to the round window. This system allows sound vibrations to enter at the oval

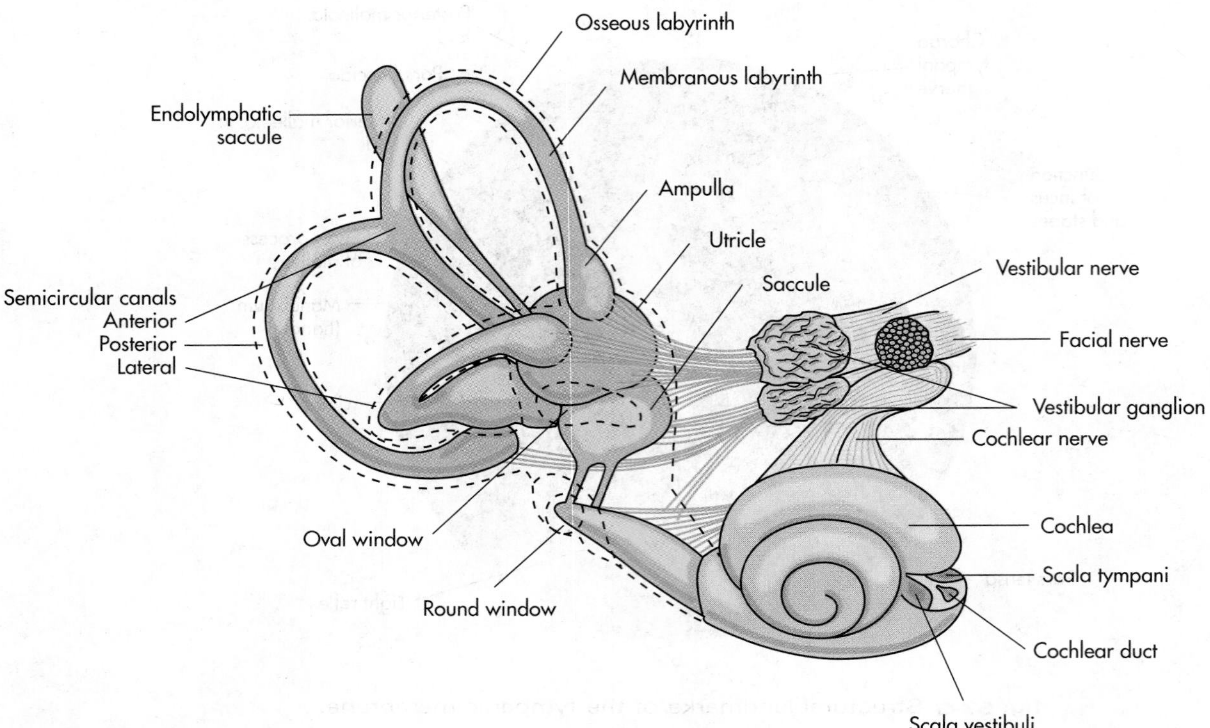


**fig. 57-4** Structures of the inner ear.

window and exit at the round window. The main function of the cochlea is hearing.[8]

### Membranous labyrinth

The membranous labyrinth consists of the utricle, saccule, three semicircular ducts, the cochlear duct, and the organ of Corti. The membranous labyrinth contains a fluid called *endolymph* and is continuously bathed in another fluid, called *perilymph.* The utricle, saccule, and the three semicircular canals are the sense organs responsible for position and balance. The semicircular canals are arranged to sense rotational movement, whereas the utricle and saccule are involved with linear movements. Sound vibrations enter the perilymph at the oval window and travel through the vestibular membrane, enter the cochlear duct, and cause movement of the basilar membrane.

The organ of Corti, the end organ for hearing, is located on the basilar membrane and stretches from the base to the apex of the cochlea.

## SOUND TRANSMISSION

Sound is transmitted from the external ear to the inner ear by two routes, air conduction and bone conduction. *Air conduction* transmits sound vibration through the middle ear, involving the tympanic membrane and the ossicles (Figure 57-5). *Bone conduction* transmits sound vibrations through the skull to the inner ear.

The tympanic membrane conducts sound vibrations to the ossicles. After passage through the ossicles the sound pressure applied to the stapes in the oval window connecting to the inner ear is 22 times greater than the pressure exerted by the sound pressure on the eardrum. The force of the sound vibrations increases after transmission from a larger area to a smaller area.

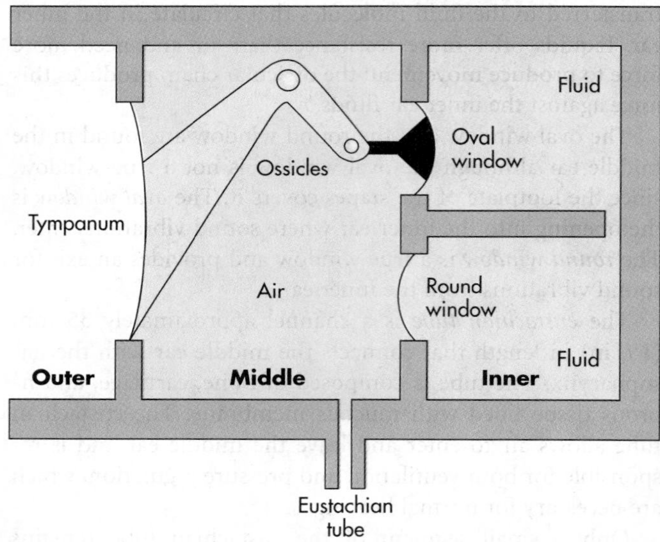


**fig. 57-5** Diagrammatic representation of transmission of sound impulses from outer to inner ear.

Sound energy must be transformed into neural energy for transmission to the brain. The organ of Corti transforms me-

## gerontological assessment

**ASSESSMENT**

External ear
- Enlarged auricle due to continued cartilage formation
- Pendulous earlobes
- Loss of elasticity of pinna

Otoscopic examination
- Eardrum whiter in color, more opaque
- Impacted cerumen due to decreased secretion and increased amounts of keratin, which make cerumen harder and more easily impacted

**COMMON DISORDERS IN ELDERS**
- Presbycusis
- Impacted cerumen
- Tinnitis
- Presbyastasis
- Conductive hearing loss
- Sensorineural hearing loss

### box 57-1 *Behavioral Cues Suggesting Loss of Hearing*

Any adult may exhibit one or more of the following traits:
- Is irritable, hostile, or hypersensitive in interpersonal relations
- Has difficulty hearing upper frequency consonants
- Complains about people mumbling
- Turns up volume on television
- Asks for frequent repetition or misunderstands
- Answers questions inappropriately
- Loses sense of humor; becomes grim
- Leans forward to hear better; face looks serious and strained
- Shuns large- and small-group audience situations
- Appears aloof and "stuck up"
- Complains of ringing in the ears
- Has an unusually soft or loud voice
- Has garbled speech

chanical sound vibrations into neural activity and separates sound into different frequencies. Nerve impulses are transmitted between the ear and the brain by the eighth cranial nerve, the acoustic or vestibulocochlear nerve, which has two branches. The acoustic portion of the ear is innervated by the cochlear branch, and the vestibular portion is innervated by the vestibular branch of the nerve.[2] Electrochemical impulses travel via the acoustic nerve to the temporal cortex of the brain and are interpreted as meaningful sound. In a similar way, the inner ears send impulses to the brain via the vestibular portion of the nerve that are decoded to maintain normal balance.

## PHYSIOLOGICAL CHANGES WITH AGING

As in any other organ system, the ear is affected by changes that occur with normal aging. The cilia that line the ear canal become coarse and stiff with the aging process and thus may decrease hearing acuity. Hair cells in the organ of Corti usually begin to degenerate after age 50. Sclerotic changes occur in the tympanic membrane, which cause it to become more translucent, resulting in conductive hearing loss. Hearing loss may also occur as a result of excess deposition of bone cells in the ossicles, causing fixation of the stapes in the oval window.[2]

Atrophy of the *apocrine glands* causes cerumen to be drier. The cerumen may accumulate and oxidize, decreasing hearing. The most common cause of hearing loss in elderly persons is *presbycusis.* Changes in the delicate labyrinthine structures result in hearing loss, usually in the higher frequencies. The onset of presbycusis typically is in the fifth decade and progresses slowly. The amount of hearing loss is affected by familial differences. Presbycusis is not curable, but some persons benefit from hearing aids.

*Tinnitis* accompanies most types of hearing loss and is a common complaint in the elderly. *Presbyastasis* or *presbyvertigo* is a balance disorder of aging that results from generalized degenerative changes in the labyrinth. Decreased visual acuity and compromised proprioception also contribute to the imbalance. Presbyastasis can be controlled by not cured. Assessment adaptations appropriate to older patients are summarized in the Gerontological Assessment Box.

## ASSESSMENT

### SUBJECTIVE DATA

Before beginning the health history, the nurse attempts to determine if the patient hears well and seeks to validate the patient's functional status with a family member or significant other. Box 57-1 summarizes common behavioral cues that suggest the presence of hearing loss. The individual may also focus on the speaker's face and lips, rather than making eye contact. If the patient has a hearing loss, it is important for the nurse to face the patient directly and speak clearly. If the patient wears a hearing aid, the nurse ensures that it is in use and functioning properly.[6]

The nurse also assesses the patient for any incidence of pain (earache), drainage (otorrhea), tinnitis, or vertigo. An environmental and work history is also obtained. Previous or current occupational exposure to loud noises or living in a noise polluted area may result in hearing loss. Occupational exposure to loud machinery is another potential cause of hearing loss, especially if adequate ear protection is not worn. A history of old trauma, such as a blow to the ears or a foreign body, may result in hearing loss later in life.

The nurse completes a thorough medication history as a variety of drugs are potentially ototoxic. Ototoxic agents directly affect the eighth cranial nerve or the organs of hearing and balance.[3] These drugs cause symptoms such as tinnitus, headache, dizziness, vertigo, nausea, ataxia, nystagmus, or a discernible change in hearing. Table 57-1 summarizes some of the common ototoxic drugs.

The patient is questioned regarding self-care of the ears. Determining the frequency of hearing tests and the method and frequency of cleaning the ears helps the nurse plan appropriate health teaching. Incorrect methods of cleaning the ears, such as the use of cotton-tipped applicators, can lead to impacted cerumen and hearing loss. The nurse asks the patient about any history of ear infections and the method of treatment. A history of chronic ear infections alerts the nurse to the possibility of sequelae.

Dizziness and/or hearing loss can have devastating effects on the patient's quality of life. The nurse carefully explores the extent of disruption of the patient's lifestyle caused by the symptoms and evaluates the patient's emotional response to these disruptions. If the ability to communicate is impaired, the patient may feel socially isolated. The nurse carefully explores the nature and effectiveness of the patient's coping mechanisms. When either balance or hearing is affected, the patient's risk for injury increases, and safety measures are carefully explored.

## OBJECTIVE DATA

### External Ear

The external ear is inspected for size, configuration, and angle of attachment to the head. The configuration of the pinna is observed for gross deformity. Whether the ears protrude and the degree of protrusion, the color of the skin of the ear, and whether any additional skin tags are present are noted. The skin of the ear should be smooth and without breaks or inflammation, especially behind the ear in the crevice. The presence of any lumps or skin lesions is charted by approximate size and location. The nurse also assesses all pierced ear holes for irritation or infection.

The pinna is palpated for the presence of tenderness or nodules. Palpation in the mastoid area may produce pain or discomfort that could indicate inflammation or infection. For direct observation of the ear canal, the adult is asked to tip the head slightly to the opposite side while the nurse pulls the

**table 57-1** *Potentially Ototoxic Drugs*

| Drug | Effect on the Auditory/Vestibular System |
|---|---|
| **AMINOGLYCOSIDES** | Affect auditory and vestibular functions, usually related to persistently high drug levels; elderly patients, persons taking other ototoxic drugs, and persons with preexisting auditory loss most susceptible; damage may be reversible if detected early and drug discontinued; however, may be permanent |
| Gentamicin<br>Tobramycin<br>Streptomycin | Primarily affect vestibular function |
| Amikacin<br>Neomycin<br>Kanamycin | Primarily affect auditory function |
| **VANCOMYCIN** | Elderly and those with hearing loss most susceptible; ototoxicity more common with high serum levels |
| **LOOP DIURETICS**<br>Furosemide<br>Torsemide<br>Bumetanide<br>Ethacrynate sodium<br>Ethacrynate acid | Rapid parenteral administration may cause hearing loss, deafness, or tinnitis |
| **ERYTHROMYCIN** | Hearing loss associated with IV administration of high doses, especially with patients with renal failure |
| **SALICYLATES**<br>Aspirin | Tinnitis, hearing loss, audiometric testing indicated before and/or after long-term therapy; elderly most susceptible; effects generally reversible |
| **NONSTEROIDAL ANTIINFLAMMATORY DRUGS** | Auditory function monitored before and during therapy to prevent ototoxicity; elderly most susceptible |
| **CISPLATIN** | Tinnitis, high-frequency hearing loss |
| **QUININE SULFATE** | Tinnitis, impaired hearing; serum concentrations $\geq$10 mg/ml may confirm toxicity as cause of tinnitis or hearing loss |

pinna up, back, and out. A penlight is used to inspect the ear canal for any abnormalities such as extreme narrowing, excessive wax, redness, scaliness, swelling, drainage, cysts, or foreign objects.

### Tympanic Membrane

Visualization of the tympanic membrane is difficult and requires illumination. The addition of magnification allows a more accurate assessment of the ear. An otoscope consists of a handle, a light source, a magnifying lens, and an attachment for visualizing the ear canal and eardrum (Figure 57-6). Some otoscopes have a pneumatic device for injecting air into the ear canal to test the mobility and integrity of the eardrum.

The diameter of the meatus and the length of the ear canal vary; thus the speculum with the largest diameter that fits comfortably into the ear canal is chosen.

The otoscope is held with the dominant hand, with the hand resting against the patient's head. In this manner, the otoscope is less likely to damage the external canal if the patient moves suddenly. With the nondominant hand, the pinna is pulled up, back, and out, straightening the ear canal. The patient's head is gently tilted away from the nurse, and the speculum inserted slowly and carefully into the ear canal and advanced far enough to create a good seal to facilitate use of the pneumatic bulb.[5] However, the otoscope should not touch the bony walls of the auditory canal as this will be painful. The cartilaginous portion of the canal is normally not tender.

The otoscope is moved in a circular fashion to allow for visualization of the entire ear canal. Any abnormalities such as extreme narrowing of the ear canal, nodules, redness, scaliness, swelling, drainage, cysts, foreign objects, or excessive wax are noted. Color and consistency of cerumen are genetically determined. Dark sticky cerumen is common in whites and African Americans, whereas flaky, dry cerumen that is light brown to grey in color is commonly found in Asian-Americans and Native Americans. Sometimes the ear canal must be cleaned of wax, dead skin, and other debris before the eardrum can be visualized. Hearing remains normal even when 90% to 95% of the ear canal is blocked with cerumen. Total occlusion creates a sudden hearing loss or feeling of fullness in the ear.

The normal eardrum is slightly conical, shiny and smooth, and pearly gray in color. The position of the drumhead is oblique to the ear canal. In the presence of disease, the color of the eardrum changes, and other abnormalities such as retraction, bulging, perforation, or a white plaque in the eardrum may be present. The entire eardrum is carefully inspected, including the border or the annulus. The umbo and the long and short process of the malleus should be easily visible through the eardrum.

The mobility of the eardrum is tested by injecting a small puff of air into the ear canal with the pneumatic device on the otoscope. Gentle movement of the eardrum should occur.

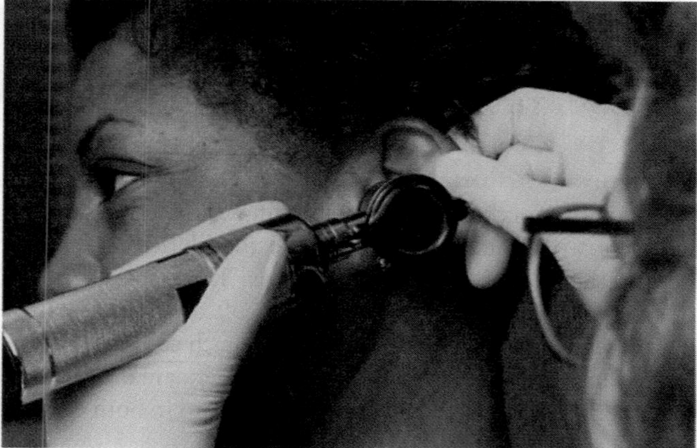

**fig. 57-6** Otoscopic examination. Straighten the external auditory canal by pulling the auricle up and back to examine the ear with the otoscope.

### Middle Ear

Assessment of the middle ear involves evaluating hearing and inspecting the middle ear through the tympanic membrane with the otoscope. Gross assessment of hearing can be accomplished through general conversation and whisper tests that compare one ear to the other. Tuning forks are also used to assess hearing. Typical tuning fork tests are the Weber and Rinne tests (see p. 1859).

### Mastoid

Assessment of the mastoid is performed by palpating the bone behind the pinna. A normal mastoid bone is smooth, hard, and nontender, and the two sides are not always equal in size. This finding is not of pathological significance.

### Inner Ear

The inner ears are not accessible to direct examination. However, some inferences concerning their condition can be made by testing auditory and vestibular function. A gross assessment of the patient's hearing was discussed above. Balance testing assesses the vestibular function of the inner ear.

### Assessment of Balance

Balance and equilibrium depend on four systems being intact: the *vestibular* (the labyrinth or inner ear), the *proprioceptive* (somatosensors of joints and muscles), the *visual* (the eye), and the *cerebellar* (coordination). Sensations transmitted from the muscles and joints and the inner ears are integrated in the brainstem and cerebellum and perceived in the cerebral cortex. Dizziness is most likely to occur when two or more systems are impaired simultaneously or when they transmit sensory information that is contradictory.

Assessment of the inner ear for balance is accomplished by observation of gait, the gaze test for nystagmus, and the Romberg test.

*Gait* is tested by asking the patient to walk away from the nurse and then turn and walk back. Posture, balance, swinging of the arms, and movement of the legs are all observed.

*Nystagmus* is the involuntary, rhythmic oscillation of the eyes and is associated with vestibular dysfunction. The finger of the examiner is placed directly in front of the patient at eye level, and the patient is asked to follow the finger without moving the head. The finger is moved slowly from the midline toward the ear in each direction and the eyes are observed for any jerking movements.

For a *Romberg test,* the patient stands with feet together and the arms at the sides first with the eyes open and then with the eyes closed (Figure 57-7). The ability to maintain an upright posture with eyes closed is assessed. Normally only a minimal amount of swaying occurs. A loss of balance (positive Romberg test) may indicate an inner ear problem (vestibular problem) or cerebellar ataxia. Assessment of gait, nystagmus, and the Romberg test is discussed in more detail in Chapter 51.

## DIAGNOSTIC TESTS

### LABORATORY TESTS

Routine blood and urine tests rarely provide significant information related to disease of the ears. An elevated white blood cell count indicates an infection but is not diagnostic of ear disease.

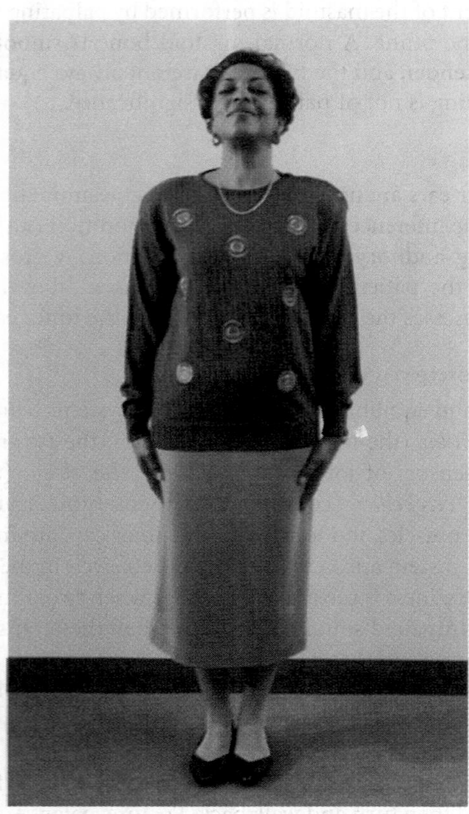

**fig. 57-7** Evaluation of balance with the Romberg test. Person maintains balance with eyes closed.

Drainage from the ear canal can be cultured to identify specific organisms causing infection. Cultures are important for treatment of acute infections, but are less helpful with long-term drainage because gram-negative bacilli cover up the original pathogen.

When clear fluid is found in the ear, it is important to rule out the presence of cerebrospinal fluid. Fistulas, skull fractures, and other head injuries can cause leakage of cerebrospinal fluid with the accompanying risk of meningitis. Cerebrospinal fluid tests positive for glucose on a reagent strip and feels "slippery" to the touch.

### RADIOLOGICAL TESTS

#### Computed Tomography

Computed tomography (CT) scanning can be used to evaluate the temporal bone in thin sections or slices producing more and smaller components than a plain film x-ray. The CT scan can also be done with a contrast medium to improve the imaging of vascular lesions and to increase the clarity of the images. The person is carefully assessed for any allergy to iodine, shellfish, or contrast media, and the nurse prepares the patient for what to expect during the test.

#### Magnetic Resonance Imaging

Magnetic resonance imaging (MRI) uses a large magnet rather than ionizing radiation to emit energy. MRI effectively details soft tissues. Therefore, the membranous organs, nerves, and blood vessels of the temporal bone can be examined. The nurse carefully prepares the patient for the expected sensory experiences associated with MRI, including loud pounding noises and a sense of claustrophobia. Newer MRI machines make less noise, which makes them more comfortable for the patient.

#### Arteriography and Venography

Adjuncts to radiography are arteriography and venography in which contrast medium is injected into blood vessels. These studies are especially useful for diagnosing vascular abnormalities in the temporal bone. Compression of the vessels can be recognized, and tumors of the temporal bone and related structures can be recognized in greater detail.

### SPECIAL TESTS

#### Auditory Acuity Tests

##### *Whispered voice test*

The patient occludes one ear with a finger and the nurse softly whispers two-syllable words toward the unoccluded ear. The patient is then asked to repeat the words. The intensity of the nurse's voice can be increased from a soft, medium, or loud whisper to a soft, medium, or loud voice. Each ear is tested separately, and the patient is asked if hearing is better in one ear than the other. A soft whisper can normally be heard in both ears.

##### *Tuning fork tests*

The tuning fork provides a general estimate of hearing loss. The two major tuning fork tests date from the nineteenth century and are named after their originators: Rinne and Weber.[8]

The tuning fork is set into vibration by striking the tines on the examiner's knuckles or knee, holding only the base of the fork without touching the tines.

**Rinne test.** The Rinne test is performed by placing the vibrating tuning fork against the patient's mastoid process (Figure 57-8, *A*) to assess bone conduction (BC) until the vibrating sound is no longer heard. The still vibrating fork is then placed 1 to 2 cm from the auditory canal to assess air conduction (AC) (Figure 57-8, *B*). The patient is asked to inform the nurse when the sound is no longer heard. The nurse times the intervals the sounds are heard and compares the number of seconds. Normally, air conduction is twice as long as bone conduction. The results are documented as AC > BC. The test is performed on each ear.[9]

The Rinne test is useful in differentiating between conductive and sensorineural hearing losses. When normal conduction pathways are blocked, transmission through the mastoid may be able to bypass the obstruction. Bone conduction therefore lasts longer than air conduction in these situations.

**Weber test.** The vibrating tuning fork is placed on the patient's forehead or teeth (Figure 57-9). Placement on the teeth (even if the patient has false teeth) is generally more reliable. The patient is asked whether the tone is heard equally in both ears or is stronger in the right or left ear. Normally, the sound should be heard equally in both ears.[9] Lateralization, an abnormal finding, indicates the sound is heard better in one ear. The Weber test is useful in identifying patients with unilateral hearing loss. Table 57-2 presents the results of Weber and Rinne tests with normal hearing and with conductive and sensorineural hearing loss.

### Audiometric Hearing Tests

Audiometric hearing tests are conducted in a soundproof booth by an audiologist. Hearing is measured in *decibels,*

**table 57-2** *Tuning Fork Tests for Auditory Acuity*

| Site of Problem | Weber Test | Rinne Test |
|---|---|---|
| **NORMAL HEARING** | | |
| No problem | Tone heard in center of head. | Air conduction lasts twice as long as bone conduction. |
| **CONDUCTIVE LOSS** | | |
| External or middle ear | Tone heard in poorer ear because ear not distracted by room noise. | Bone conduction lasts longer than air conduction. |
| **SENSORINEURAL LOSS** | | |
| Inner ear | Tone heard in better ear because inner ear less able to receive vibrations. | Air conduction lasts longer than bone conduction. |

A

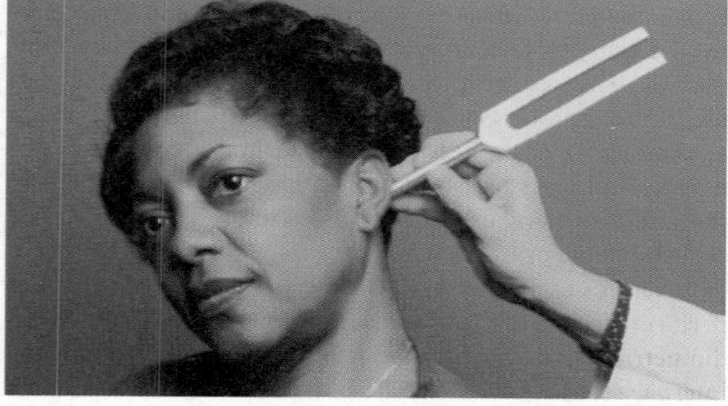

B

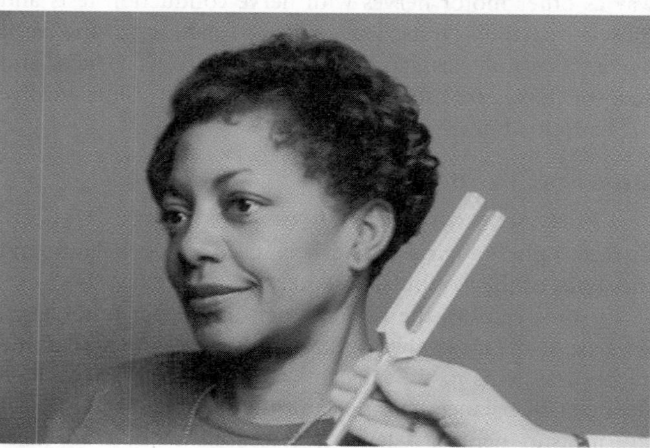

**fig. 57-8** Rinne test. **A,** The vibrating tuning fork is placed on the mastoid bone for bone conduction. **B,** The vibrating tuning fork is placed in front of the ear for air conduction.

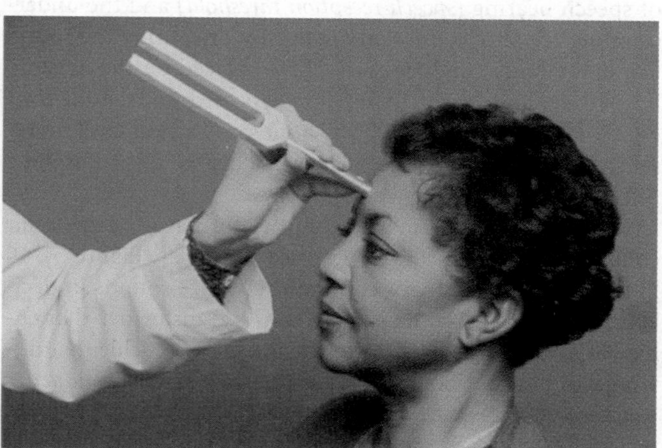

**fig. 57-9** Weber test. The vibrating tuning fork is placed on the midline of the skull.

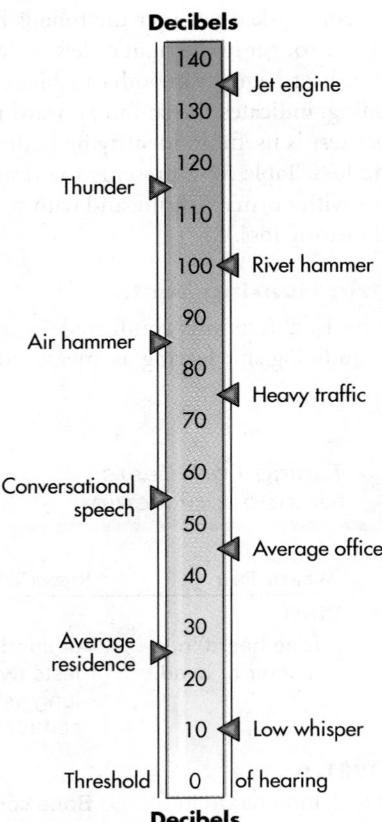


**fig. 57-10** Intensity range of human hearing. Intensity levels of various environmental sounds and situations.

a logarithmic function of sound intensity. The sound is presented through an audiometer, and the patient wears earphones and signals the audiologist when a tone is heard. Responses are plotted on a graph called the *audiogram.* By varying the loudness of the pure tones or speech, a hearing level is established. The earphones are also used to measure the level of speech hearing *(speech reception threshold)* and the understanding of speech *(discrimination).* By presenting the sound through a bone conduction oscillator placed on the mastoid bone, the middle ear structures are bypassed, and a bone conduction level is established. The bone conduction level represents the level at which the cochlea can hear and is commonly referred to as the *nerve hearing level.*

A person with normal hearing would have the same air conduction as bone conduction hearing levels. Figure 57-10 illustrates the intensity of common reference sounds in decibels. Because the middle ear serves as a transformer that enhances and transfers sound to the inner ear (cochlea), a difference in air and bone conduction levels reflects *conductive hearing loss* involving the tympanic membrane, middle ear, or mastoid. Fortunately, most disorders causing conductive hearing loss can be corrected by microsurgery. If air and bone conduction levels are equal but not within the normal range, a *sensorineural nerve hearing loss* is present. Surgery cannot correct most of the problems that cause a sensorineural hearing loss, although a hearing aid can be useful if speech discrimination is adequate. It is quite common for a patient to have both a conductive and sensorineural hearing loss; the combination is called a *mixture hearing loss.*

#### Impedance audiometry

Impedance audiometry or tympanometry can be used for differentiating problems in the middle ear. The test applies pressure to the tympanic membrane and measures the result, creating a distinctive tracing on a graph called a *tympanogram.* Abnormalities of the tympanogram indicate problems of the middle ear, eustachian tube, or the ossicles. Tympanometry can also be used to measure the stapedial muscle reflex and the status of the acoustic nerve. With pathological conditions of the cochlea, acoustic reflexes often occur at less intense stimulation levels. With a retrocochlear lesion, the reflex thresholds are elevated or even absent. With conductive hearing loss, the reflex thresholds may be elevated but usually are absent. The nurse thoroughly explains all aspects of the test before its start.

#### Auditory brainstem response

Brainstem auditory evoked potential testing assesses dysfunction of the auditory nervous system at the level of the eighth cranial nerve (acoustic nerve), pons, or midbrain. Evoked potentials measure and record changes in brain electrical activity that occur in response to auditory sensory stimulation. The test involves placing electrodes on the vertex, mastoid process, or earlobes while the patient is seated in a comfortable chair. Test data are fed into a computer. Abnormal findings suggest dysfunctions at the various levels in the auditory nervous system, for example, a lesion of the acoustic nerve or brainstem.

Seventh cranial nerve (facial nerve) testing may also be performed. Tests of the seventh cranial nerve are related to audiometric tests because the facial and acoustic nerves share the internal acoustic canal. The facial nerve is tested in the same way as other motor nerves with nerve conduction tests and muscle excitability tests. The auxiliary functions of the facial nerve (taste and tearing) can also be measured. The facial and acoustic nerves are usually both involved when lesions involve the temporal bone.

### Balance Testing

#### Electronystagmography

Electrophysiological tests can be used to test balance and the status of the vestibular system.

In some settings the tests are performed by audiologists, because of the close physical proximity of the vestibular and cochlear systems in the labyrinth. Although the physical assessment of balance is important, the most common objective measurement of balance is accomplished by electronystagmography, which measures nystagmus in response to stimulation of the vestibular system. The patient is tested at rest in different positions and with different temperatures in

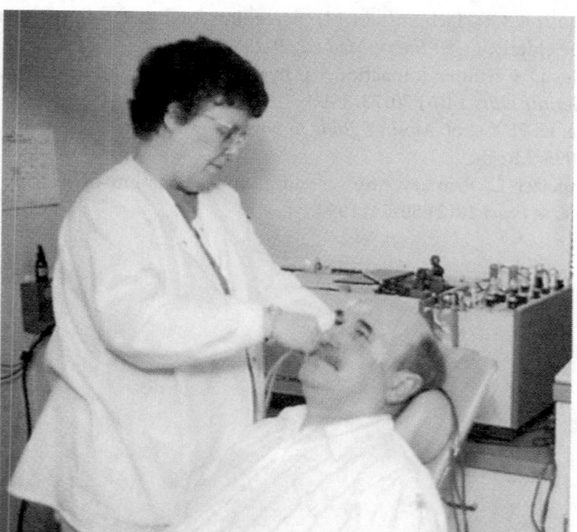

**fig. 57-11** Electrodes are applied to a patient in preparation for electronystagmography.

the ear canals, thus stimulating the semicircular canals. The test results create an *electronystagmogram* that reflects the status of each labyrinth and can point to central nervous system disorders.

The patient is instructed to discontinue any vestibular sedatives or tranquilizers and to avoid alcohol use for at least 24 hours before the test. Patients are also cautioned to avoid a heavy meal before the test because vertigo and nausea may be stimulated. Figure 57-11 shows the application of electrodes for electronystagmography. Because the electrodes are placed with conduction paste, the patient is assisted in washing his or her hair after the procedure.

#### *Platform posturography*

Platform posturography is a computerized test performed while the person is standing (Figure 57-12). This test can separate the balance problem into inner ear, visual, and muscle stretch origins. The platform test helps to identify, quantify, and localize the source of balance disorders. The nurse explains the procedure and the sensations the patient can expect. Although painless, the test can cause vertigo and nausea. Sedatives, tranquilizers and alcohol can alter the test results and should be restricted before the procedure.

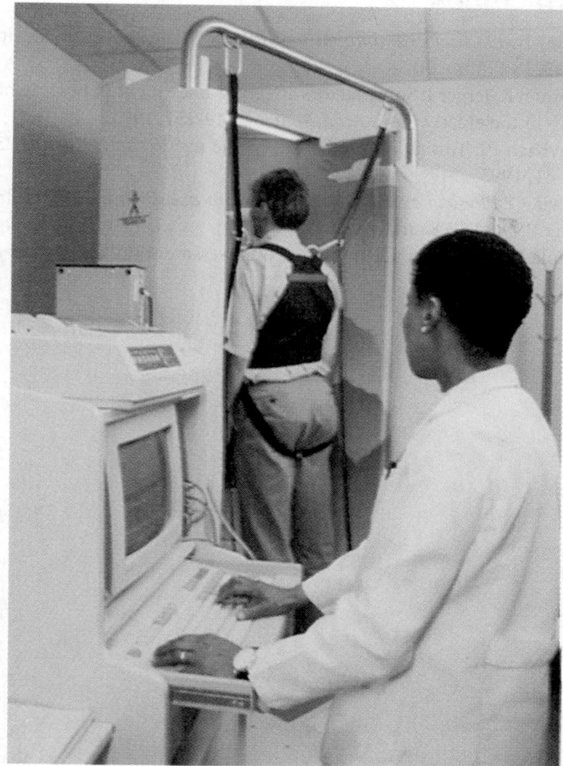

**fig. 57-12** Patient wears a harness during platform posturography examination to protect him from falling.

## chapter SUMMARY

### ANATOMY AND PHYSIOLOGY

- Detection of patients with a hearing impairment or a balance problem is an important nursing responsibility.
- Behavior can alert the nurse to the possibility of hearing impairment.
- The ear is housed in the temporal bone and divided into the external, middle, and inner ear.
- Sound vibrations reach the inner ear by mechanical energy through air conduction and bone conduction.
- The tympanic membrane is a membrane between the external ear canal and the middle ear cleft.
- The otoscope is the most common instrument used to examine the ear.
- The functions of the eustachian tube are ventilation and pressure regulation, both of which are essential for normal hearing.
- The functions of the mastoid bone include helping the middle ear to adjust to pressure changes and decreasing the weight of the skull.
- The inner ear transforms mechanical energy into electrochemical impulses that travel via the acoustic nerve to the temporal cortex of the brain. The brain interprets these impulses as meaningful sound and as balance.
- Nystagmus can be an objective sign of a vestibular problem.

### DIAGNOSTIC TESTS

- Electronystagmography is the test used to measure nystagmus.
- Audiometric tests, usually performed by audiologists, are used to evaluate hearing.

## References

1. Bates B: *Physical examination and history taking,* ed 6, Philadelphia, 1995, JB Lippincott.
2. Chmiel R, Jerger J: Some factors affecting assessment of hearing handicap in the elderly, *J Am Acad Audiol* 4:249-257, 1993.
3. Haybach PJ: Tuning in to ototoxicity: the inside story, *Nursing* 23(6): 34-41, 1993.
4. Jarvis C: *Physical examination and health assessment,* ed 2, Philadelphia, 1996, WB Saunders.
5. Miola E: The otoscope: an update on assessment skills, *J Pediatr Nurs* 9(3):283-286, 1994.
6. Mulrow CD, Lichtenstein MJ: Screening for hearing impairment in the elderly, *J Gen Intern Med* 6:249-258, 1991.
7. Ney D: Cerumen impaction, ear hygiene practices and hearing acuity, *Geriatr Nurs* 14(6):70-73, 1993.
8. Seidel HM et al: *Mosby's guide to physical examination,* ed 3, St Louis, 1995, Mosby.
9. Smelzer C: Primary care screening and evaluation of hearing loss, *Nurse Pract* 18(2):50-54, 1994.

# chapter 58 MANAGEMENT OF PERSONS WITH Problems of the Ear

LINDA T. SCHURING and JUDITH K. SANDS

## objectives After studying this chapter, the learner should be able to:

1 Identify three measures that are important in preventing hearing loss.
2 Compare the etiologies and assessment features of conductive and sensorineural hearing loss.
3 Contrast the pathophysiology and nursing care of patients with external and middle ear infections.
4 Discuss the preoperative and postoperative care of the patient undergoing ear surgery.
5 Relate the signs and symptoms of Ménière's disease to its underlying pathology.
6 Develop strategies for communicating with a hearing-impaired person.

A wide range of disorders can affect the ear including infections, tumors, and trauma, but hearing loss is by far the most common and important ear problem affecting adults. Any problem with the ear threatens the function and acuity of this essential sensory organ and the ability of the individual to interact effectively with the environment. Selected ear problems can also create problems with an individual's sense of balance.

## HEARING LOSS

### ETIOLOGY/EPIDEMIOLOGY

Hearing loss has become the nation's number one disability, affecting 1 of 15 Americans. Millions of people, including 29% of persons age 65 or older have some kind of hearing impairment.[5] Hearing impairment ranges from difficulty in understanding words or hearing certain sounds, to total deafness.

Hearing impairment and dizziness (a major symptom of inner ear problems) can hinder communication with others, limit social activities, and negatively impact employment. Hearing loss diminishes the individual's aesthetic enjoyment of major aspects of daily living and can adversely affect quality of life (see the Research Box).

Hearing loss is a symptom rather than a specific disease or disorder and can be the result of mechanical, sensory, or neural problems. The major types of hearing loss are defined in Box 58-1. Figure 58-1 illustrates the results of problems affecting different structures of the ear. Although some diseases of the ear canal can be helped with medicine or surgery, the vast majority of persons with a hearing impairment cannot be treated effectively. Of all hearing impairments, 80% are caused by nerve deafness for which, at present, there is no known cure.

### PATHOPHYSIOLOGY

*Conductive hearing loss* results from any interference with the conduction of sound impulses through the external auditory canal, the eardrum, or the middle ear. Conductive hearing loss may be caused by anything that blocks the external ear, such as wax, infection, or a foreign body; a thickening, retraction, scarring, or perforation of the tympanic membrane; or any pathophysiological changes in the middle ear affecting or fixing one or more of the ossicles.

**box 58-1** *Types of Hearing Loss*

**Conductive Hearing Loss**
Loss of hearing from a mechanical problem

**Sensorineural Hearing Loss**
Loss of hearing involving the cochlea and auditory nerve; bone and air conduction equal but diminished

**Neural Hearing Loss**
A sensorineural hearing loss originating in the nerve or brainstem

**Fluctuating Hearing Loss**
A sensorineural hearing loss that varies with time

**Sensory Hearing Loss**
A sensorineural hearing loss originating in the cochlea and involving the hair cells and nerve endings

**Sudden Hearing Loss**
A sensorineural hearing loss with a sudden onset

**Central Hearing Loss**
Loss of hearing from damage to the brain's auditory pathways or auditory center

**Functional Hearing Loss**
Loss of hearing for which no organic lesion can be found

**Mixed Hearing Loss**
Elements of both conduction and sensorineural hearing loss

**research**

Reference: Chen HL: Hearing in the elderly: relation of hearing loss, loneliness, and self esteem, *J Gerontol Nurs* 20(6):22-27, 1994.

This descriptive correlational study explored the relationship between hearing handicap and various demographic factors, loneliness, and self-esteem. The sample included 90 individuals older than 65 years of age with perceived hearing loss. They were a volunteer sample drawn from eye, ear, nose, and throat clinics; speech and audiology services; and retirement centers in a large metropolitan area. The participants ranged in age from 65 to 90, were about evenly split between men and women, and tended to be well educated.

Hearing handicap was the focus of study rather than simply hearing loss and was defined as the individual's response to the hearing loss. Various self-report scales were administered to the sample concerning each variable under study. A significant correlation was found between hearing handicap and both loneliness and low self-esteem. The higher the hearing handicap the greater the loneliness and the greater impact on self-esteem. Significant differences were found between the male and female subjects, however. The links between hearing handicap, loneliness, and low self-esteem were much lower among the men who exhibited a much higher correlation with social difficulties associated with hearing loss.

The researchers conclude that the impact of hearing handicap is significant, creating loneliness and negatively affecting self-esteem. In addition, these effects of hearing handicap are much more significant in their effect on women than on men.

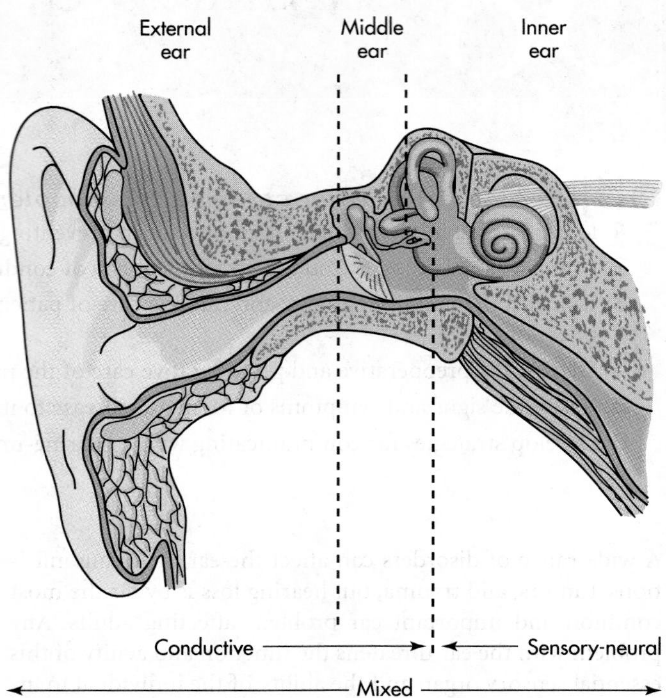


**fig. 58-1** Three types of hearing loss. Conductive loss results from interference with conduction in the external and middle ear; sensorineural loss results from interference with conduction in the inner ear; and mixed hearing loss results from interference with conduction in all three areas.

*Sensorineural hearing loss* results from disease or trauma to the inner ear, neural structures, or nerve pathways leading to the brainstem. Some of the causes of "nerve" deafness are infectious diseases (measles, mumps, and meningitis), arteriosclerosis, ototoxic drugs (Box 58-2), neuromas of cranial nerve VIII, otospongiosis (form of progressive deafness caused by the formation of new abnormal spongy bone in labyrinth), trauma to the head or ear, or degeneration of the organ of Corti occurring most commonly from advancing age *(presbycusis)*.

Central deafness, also known as central auditory dysfunction, results from the inability of the central nervous system to interpret normal auditory stimuli. It is a rare form of sensorineural hearing loss that can result from tumors or a cerebrovascular accident. Hearing ability remains intact, but the patient is deaf.

Noise-induced hearing loss accounts for the major proportion of hearing impairment among people between the ages of 35 and 65.[3] This hearing loss can be traumatic, for example, a sudden loud noise or blast injury. More commonly, a hearing loss occurs over time from repeated injury from noise.

Occupational noise is a primary cause of noise-induced hearing loss in Western society. Other causes of noise-induced hearing loss include the use of firearms and high-intensity music. Noise from rock bands can exceed 120 decibels (dB), and hearing losses have been measured in some members of rock bands. In the United States, the Occupational Safety and Health Administration (OSHA) has established acceptable noise levels for work environments.[5] In general, *exposure to noise levels in excess of 90 dB over an 8-hour day is considered excessive* and should be avoided. Ordinary speech is about 50 dB and heavy traffic about 70 dB; above 80 dB, noise becomes uncomfortable to the human ear. Exposure to levels greater than 85 to 90 dB for months or years can cause cochlear damage. Whatever the cause, noise-induced hearing loss is characterized by a greater loss in the higher frequencies. The sensory cells in the ear are progressively destroyed, and the problem cannot be medically or surgically repaired. The only treatment is to prevent the injury by avoiding noise or by wearing ear protection.

A variety of diseases and disorders affect the ear, and the majority of persons with ear problems experience some degree of hearing loss. Any disease that causes prolonged ear symptoms such as pain, swelling, drainage, a "plugged" feeling, or decreased hearing should be promptly assessed by a health care provider. Many chronic problems such as perforations and necrotic ossicles could be prevented with prompt and adequate medical attention.

Some drugs are potentially toxic to the cochlea, the vestibule of the ear, the labyrinth, or the eighth cranial nerve (Box 58-2). Persons taking ototoxic drugs need to know that symptoms such as dizziness, decreased hearing acuity, and/or

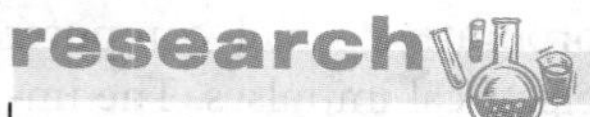

Reference: O'Rourke C et al: Effectiveness of a hearing screening protocol for the elderly, *Geriatr Nurs* 14(2):66-69, 1993.

This study compared the effectiveness of four types of hearing screening tests used to assess hearing in the elderly. The sample of 60 persons was drawn from the pool of individuals aged 56 to 90 years who attended a university-sponsored hearing and speech clinic. Methods to assess hearing included case history, visual inspection, pure-tone screening, and the Hearing Handicap Inventory for the Elderly Screening Version (HHIE-S). The most effective method for hearing screening in the elderly person was found to be the pure-tone screening used in conjunction with the case history and visual inspection. These methods are simple and efficient and could be easily added to the protocols for assessment of older adults, particularly in long-term and extended care facilities.

tinnitus should be promptly reported. Audiometric testing (see Chapter 57) may be indicated.

*Presbycusis* is a hearing loss associated with aging that becomes more common after age 50. Changes in the delicate labyrinthine structures over the decades cause a hearing loss predominantly in the higher frequencies. The incidence of presbycusis increases with age, and the disorder affects almost 50% of persons aged 85 and older.[2] In some persons the amount of hearing loss warrants the use of a hearing aid. Presbycusis cannot be cured.

Hearing loss is frequently accompanied by *tinnitus,* which is defined as a ringing or any other noise in the ear. Tinnitus accompanies most sensorineural hearing losses and is often a warning of impending or worsening hearing loss. Persistent tinnitus is extremely annoying, and the only cure for tinnitus is to correct the underlying condition.

## COLLABORATIVE CARE MANAGEMENT

Hearing loss is often first detected by a family member rather than by the affected person. The earliest sign is not hearing what was once heard. Another common sign is asking for a repetition of what was said. Usually the request is in the form of a question, such as "What did you say?" A hearing loss in one ear is more difficult to detect than bilateral losses. The person may notice the loss only when using a telephone or when having difficulty determining the direction of sounds.

Because the auditory nerve does not regain function, early detection of hearing loss is important. It is essential that routine hearing assessment be incorporated into the annual physical examinations of all persons older than 40 years of age because aging frequently causes degenerative changes in the ear (see the Research Box). Additional testing may be used as indicated (see Chapter 57 for a review of diagnostic tests of auditory function). Box 58-3 presents a sample tool for assessing the hearing-impaired person.

Hearing aids offer assistance to many individuals with hearing impairments. Hearing aids amplify sound in a controlled manner and are used by both hard-of-hearing and deaf persons. Hearing aids make sound louder, but do not improve the ability to hear and the amplication of background noise can be confusing, especially in crowded settings. Therefore persons with decreased discrimination (the ability to understand what is spoken) benefit less from the use of a hearing aid.

**box 58-2** *Ototoxic Drugs*

**AMINOGLYCOSIDE ANTIBIOTICS**
Streptomycin
Neomycin
Kanamycin
Gentamicin
Tobramycin
Netromycin
Amikacin

**OTHER ANTIBIOTICS**
Vancomycin
Viomycin
Polymyxin B (Aerosporin)
Polymyxin E (Colistin/Coly-Mycin)
Erythromycin
Minocycline
Capreomycin

**DIURETICS**
Ethacrynic acid (Edecrin)
Furosemide (Lasix)
Acetazolamide (Diamox)

**OTHER DRUGS**
Quinine
Chloroquine
Nitrogen mustard
Bleomycin
Quinidine
Cisplatin
Salicylates

**box 58-3** *Assessment of the Hearing-Impaired Person*

1. Do you have any problems with your hearing?
2. How long have you had a hearing loss in the:
   right ear?
   left ear?
3. Was anyone in your family hard of hearing before age 50?
4. Are you wearing hearing aids now? How old are they? What type?
5. Have you worked amid loud noise? How long?
6. Do you have head noise or ringing?
7. Is dizziness or unsteadiness a major problem?
8. Have you had previous ear surgery?

Adapted from Sigler BA, Schuring L: *Ear, nose, and throat disorders,* p 275, St Louis, 1993, Mosby.

The evolution in hearing aid development has led to smaller and more effective aids. Hearing aids currently are available that fit into the ear canal, fit within the ear concha, or fit behind the ear. Special hearing aids can transmit sound by radio waves to the opposite ear or by vibration to the inner ear through the skull. In the future, hearing aids will be semiimplantable and ultimately totally implantable within the middle ear and mastoid.

Regardless of the type, the hearing aid consists of the following parts:

1. Microphone to receive sound waves from the air and change sounds into electrical signals
2. Amplifier to increase the strength of the electrical signals
3. Battery to provide the electrical energy needed to operate the hearing aid
4. Receiver (loudspeaker) to change the electrical signals back into sound waves

Figure 58-2 illustrates several common types of hearing aids.

### Implantable Hearing Devices

Three types of implanted hearing devices are either available for use or under development. They are cochlear implants, bone conduction devices, and semiimplantable hearing devices.

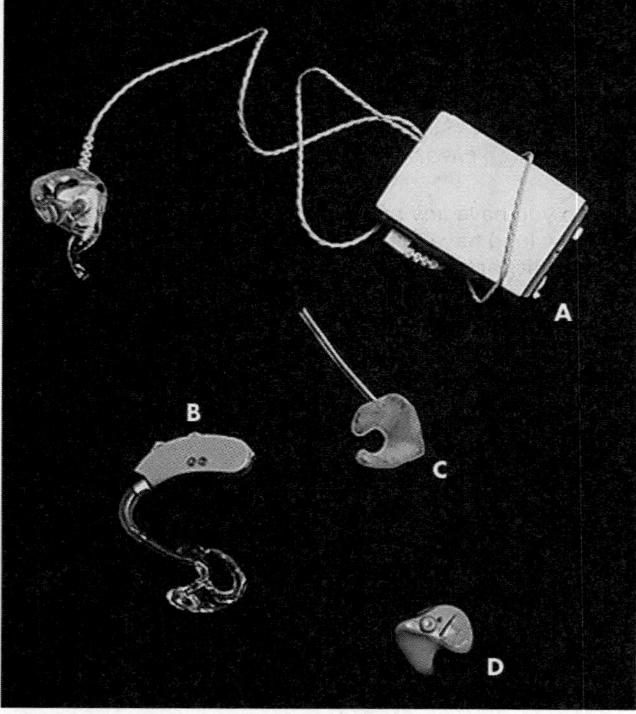


**fig. 58-2** Types of hearing aids. **A,** Older aid with a battery pack worn on the body and a wire connected to the ear mold. **B,** Behind-the-ear battery with ear mold. **C,** Small ear canal mold with battery. **D,** Newer, smaller mold worn in the ear canal.

Cochlear implant devices incorporate a small computer that changes the spoken word to electrical impulses. The impulses are transmitted across the skin to an implanted coil that carries the impulse to the hearing nerve endings in the cochlea by an electrode introduced through the round window. Figure 58-3 shows an externally placed implant, and Figure 58-4 shows an implant placed transmastoid. The best cochlear implants use multiple channels and are able to return about half of the patient's hearing and understanding.

In some cases, sound can be transmitted through the skull to the inner ear by bone conduction devices. Patients with a conductive hearing loss can use a device in which an orthopedic screw is implanted under the skin into the skull. The external device transmits the sound through the skin and is worn above the ear and not in the ear canal. Patients who already use a hearing aid will gain the most from the implantable device.

If hearing loss is irreversible and not amenable to surgical correction or if the person elects not to have surgery, aural rehabilitation may be recommended. Aural rehabilitation includes auditory training, speech reading, and speech training and is designed to maximize the hearing-impaired person's communication skills. Auditory training attempts to increase the hearing-impaired person's listening skills by fine tuning the person's ability to discriminate between similar sounds. Speech reading, formerly called lip reading, is a difficult skill to master but can be an important means of communication. Speech training focuses on the preservation of speech skills (pitch, clarity, and rate) to prevent deterioration as auditory feedback diminishes. Guidelines for communicating with hearing-impaired persons are summarized in the following Guidelines for Care Box.

### Patient/Family Education

Hearing loss is a major health concern in the United States, and nurses play a major preventive role in interactions with all

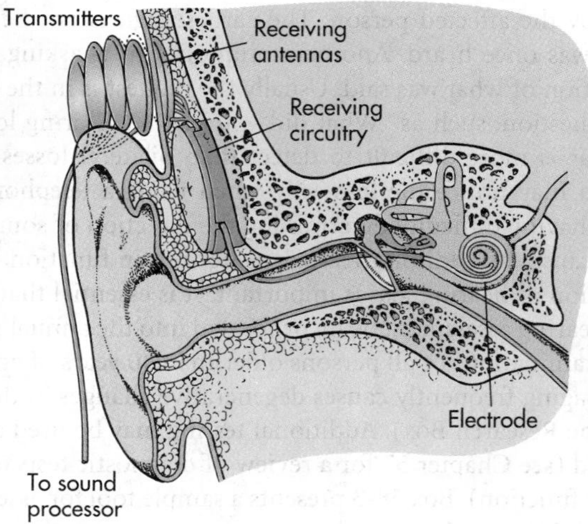


**fig. 58-3** Cochlear implant in place externally.

patients and families. Hearing loss is addressed in the *Healthy People 2000* national health objectives as:

1. Reduce to no more than 15% the proportion of workers exposed to average daily noise levels that exceed 85 dB.
2. Reduce significant hearing impairment to a prevalence of no more than 82 per 1000 people, as measured by self-reported hearing impairment.

Individuals 45 years of age and older are identified as special target populations.

The nurse explores the patient's understanding of the role of noise in hearing loss and encourages moderation of music levels, especially with the use of headphones. The use of protective ear covers in noisy environments is strongly recommended.

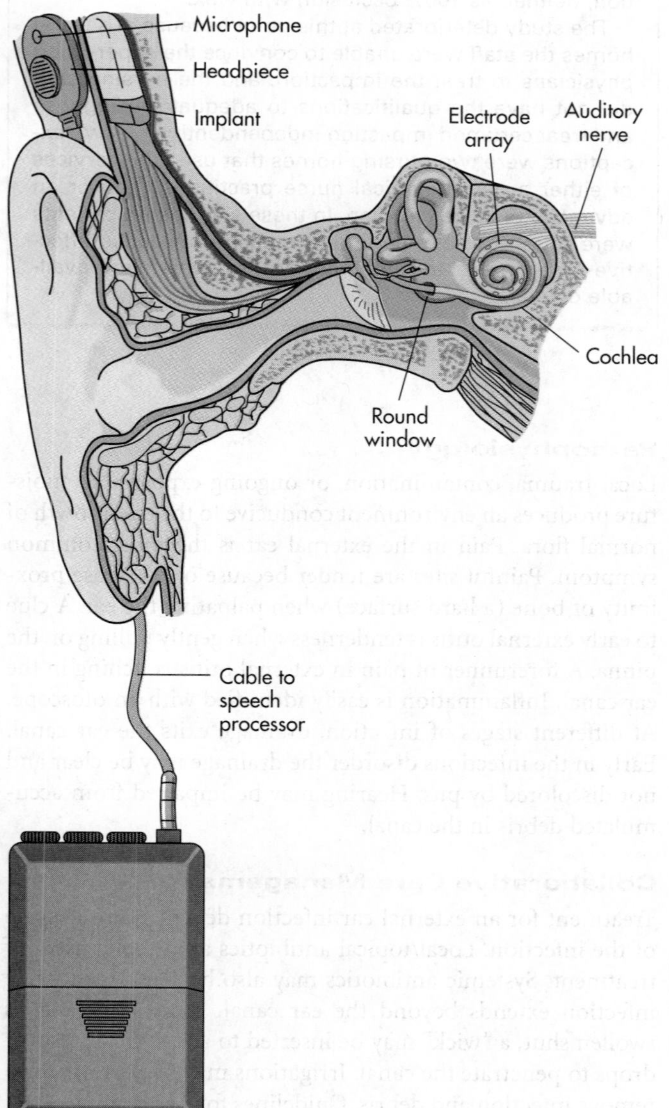


**fig. 58-4** Cochlear implant in place transmastoid through round window into the cochlea.

People should be taught to avoid inserting hard articles into the ear canal, obstructing the ear canal with any object, inserting unclean articles or solutions into the ear, or swimming in polluted water.

The ear canal is generally "self-cleaning." Wax is to the ears what tears are to the eyes; it serves as a protective mechanism. Earwax lubricates the skin and traps foreign material that enters the canal. Therefore wax should not be cleaned out of the ear routinely. The external ear may be washed with soap and water daily while bathing or showering, but the patient is cautioned against routinely using cotton-tipped applicators or other objects to clean the ear. The ear canal and eardrum can easily be damaged, and the applicator may push accumulated wax against the eardrum.

The person with a hearing aid should know how to care for the aid and what to do if the aid does not work. The nurse must also have a basic knowledge of the hearing aid to assist the person who is unable or unwilling to do this when ill. The person is encouraged to use the hearing aid and to store it safely in its case when it is not in use. The Guidelines for Care Boxes on the next page outline hearing aid care and provide trouble-shooting suggestions.

**guidelines for care**

### Communicating with the Hearing-Impaired Person

1. Get the person's attention by touching him or her lightly, flickering the room lights, or raising an arm or hand.
2. Stand facing the patient with the light on your face; this will help the person speech (lip) read.
3. Speak slowly and clearly, but do not overaccentuate words.
4. Speak in a normal tone; do not shout. Shouting overuses normal speaking movements and may cause distortion. If the person has a conductive loss making the voice louder without shouting may be helpful.
5. If the person does not seem to understand what is said, express it differently. Some words are difficult to "see" in speech reading, such as *white* and *red.*
6. Do not smile, chew gum, or cover the mouth when talking to a person with limited hearing.
7. Use phrases to convey meaning rather than one-word answers. Supplement words with body language.
8. Do not show annoyance by careless facial expression. Persons who are hard of hearing depend more on visual clues.
9. Write out proper names or any statement that you are not sure was understood.
10. Encourage the use of a hearing aid if the person has one; allow him or her to adjust it before speaking.
11. Avoid the use of the intercom when communicating with the patient.
12. Do not avoid conversation with a person who has hearing loss.
13. Post a note at the bedside and nurses station alerting personnel that the person is hard of hearing.

**guidelines for care**

**Care of a Hearing Aid**

1. Turn the hearing aid off when not in use.
2. Open the battery compartment at night to avoid accidental drainage of the battery.
3. Keep an extra battery available at all times.
4. Wash the earmold frequently (daily if necessary) with mild soap and warm water and use a pipe cleaner to cleanse the cannula.
5. Do not wear the hearing aid if an ear infection is present.

**guidelines for care**

**What to Do if a Hearing Aid Fails to Work**

1. Check the on-off switch.
2. Inspect the earmold for cleanliness.
3. Examine the battery for correct insertion.
4. Examine the cord plug for correct insertion.
5. Examine the cord for breaks.
6. Replace the battery, cord, or both, if necessary. The life of batteries varies according to amount of use and power requirements of the aid. Batteries last from 2 to 14 days.
7. Check the position of the earmold in the ear. If the hearing aid "whistles," the earmold is probably not inserted properly into the ear canal, or the person needs to have a new earmold made.

**research**

Reference: Mahoney DF: Cerumen impaction: prevalence and detection in nursing homes, *J Gerontol Nurs* 19(4):23-29, 1993.

Cerumen impaction is a common, reversible, and frequently overlooked cause of conductive hearing loss, particularly in the elderly. This study sought to determine the prevalence of impacted cerumen in a population of elderly nursing home residents, evaluate differences in hearing after wax removal, and identify factors impeding detection of the problem.

A sample of 100 stable, cognitively intact elders were selected from among a large pool of residents in a group of nursing homes in a metropolitan area. The participants were screened for the presence of cerumen impaction and hearing loss. Of the participants, 96% were found to be hearing impaired, although few had hearing aids, and 55% were found to have moderate to profound hearing loss. Twenty-five percent had cerumen impaction, defined as 100% occlusion with wax.

The study deteriorated at this point because at several homes the staff were unable to convince the supervising physicians to treat the impaction, and the nursing staff did not have the qualifications to adequately diagnose and treat cerumen impaction independently. The two exceptions were two nursing homes that used the services of either a gerontological nurse practitioner and or an advanced practice clinician. In these settings no patients were found to have cerumen impaction because effective assessment and intervention protocols were available on-site.

## PROBLEMS OF THE EXTERNAL EAR

The external ear may be affected by masses, trauma, wax impaction, and infection (Research Box). External ear infection is by far the most common disorder and is discussed below. The other problems are summarized in Table 58-1.

### EXTERNAL EAR INFECTION (EXTERNAL OTITIS)

#### Etiology/Epidemiology

The most common problems of the external ear are infections, primarily bacterial or fungal. The most frequent infection, called *external otitis,* involves the external ear canal. This infection begins in the skin lining of the ear canal and can occlude the canal. External otitis occurs more frequently in summer than in winter. A localized form of this infection is an *ear canal furuncle* or *abscess.* In the presence of a systemic disease such as diabetes, the external otitis can spread wildly through cartilage and bone and is then termed *malignant external otitis.* The most common form of external otitis is called *swimmer's ear,* because it is prevalent when water remains in the ear canal. In addition, opportunistic fungal infections are common. Occasionally, infection involves only the cartilage of the auricle *(perichondritis),* resulting in necrosis of the cartilage and loss of the distinctive shape of the auricle if not treated quickly.

#### Pathophysiology

Local trauma, contamination, or ongoing exposure to moisture produces an environment conducive to the overgrowth of normal flora. Pain in the external ear is the most common symptom. Painful sites are tender because of the close proximity of bone (a hard surface) when palpating the ear. A clue to early external otitis is tenderness when gently pulling on the pinna. A forerunner of pain in external otitis is itching in the ear canal. Inflammation is easily identified with an otoscope. At different stages of infection, drainage exits the ear canal. Early in the infectious disorder the drainage may be clear and not discolored by pus. Hearing may be impaired from accumulated debris in the canal.

#### Collaborative Care Management

Treatment for an external ear infection depends on the stage of the infection. Local/topical antibiotics are the mainstay of treatment. Systemic antibiotics may also be prescribed if the infection extends beyond the ear canal. If the ear canal is swollen shut, a "wick" may be inserted to allow the antibiotic drops to penetrate the canal. Irrigations may be performed to remove infection and debris. Guidelines for performing an irrigation are summarized in Figure 58-5. Comfort measures are provided to control the symptoms. Abscesses and perichondritis may require excision and drainage.

**table 58-1** *Disorders of the External Ear*

| Disorder | Etiology | Collaborative Management |
|---|---|---|
| Masses<br>Cysts<br>Exostosis (bony protrusions)<br>Infectious polyps<br>Malignant tumors | Most cysts arise from sebaceous glands. Polyps typically arise from the middle ear or tympanic membrane. Malignant tumors are usually basal cell carcinomas on the pinna and squamous cell carcinomas in the canal. | Masses of all types are fairly rare, and if treatment is indicated, surgical excision is performed. Squamous cell carcinomas can invade the underlying tissue and spread throughout the temporal bone. |
| Trauma | Both sharp and blunt force injuries are common. Penetrating injury can damage hearing, but infection and cosmetic appearance are more common concerns. | Supportive care and protection from infection are indicated. Cosmetic surgery may be needed. |
| Foreign bodies | Many options exist. Insects and cotton pieces are the most common. | Remove carefully aided by microscopic visualization. Insects are removed by filling the canal with mineral oil. |
| Pruritis | This frequent complaint in elders results from sebaceous gland atrophy and dry epithelium. Dry cerumen worsens the itching. | Daily application of glycerin or mineral oil drops decreases dryness and softens cerumen. |
| Impacted cerumen | This may result from use of cotton-tipped applicator or other object to clean the ear. Age-related drying of cerumen increases incidence. | Impacted wax is softened and loosened with alternating instillation of glycerine to soften and hydrogen peroxide to loosen the cerumen for removal by warm water irrigation. |

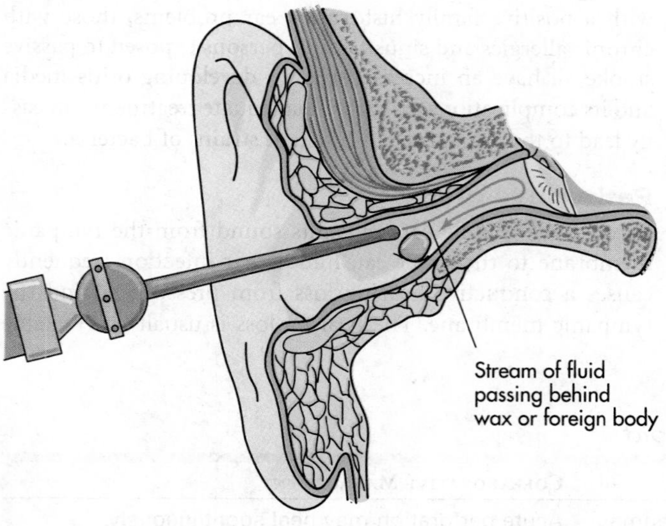


**fig. 58-5** Ear irrigation. **1,** Warm solution to body temperature. **2,** Protect the patient's clothing with a drape and obtain a kidney basin to collect the fluid. **3,** Instruct the patient to tilt the head toward the opposite ear. **4,** Pull the external ear gently upward and backward. **5,** Direct the irrigating fluid toward the upper canal wall so it passes behind the blockage. **6,** Monitor the patient for dizziness or nausea.

### guidelines for care

**Administering Ear Drops**

1. Wash hands before and after the procedure.
2. Warm the ear drops to body temperature before administration. Dizziness may occur from insertion of drops that are too warm or too cold.
3. Instruct the patient to tilt the head so that the ear to be treated is up.
4. Straighten the ear canal by pulling the external ear up and back.
5. Instill prescribed number of drops to run along ear canal.
6. Press gently several times on the tragus of the ear to ensure proper instillation, or hold the head in position for 2 to 3 minutes.
7. Wipe the external ear with a cotton ball or tissue to prevent skin irritation.
8. A cotton ball may be placed in the ear but is not necessary.

#### *Patient/family education*

The nurse instructs the patient/family in the safe administration of ear drops (Guidelines for Care Box). A piece of 1/4-inch-wide gauze may be used to create a wick if necessary. A length of about 1 inch is usually adequate. If an ointment is prescribed to control itching or inflammation, it is applied using a cotton-tipped applicator. The applicator is not inserted any deeper into the ear than the cotton end. A new applicator is used each time.

The nurse instructs the patient to avoid getting water in the ear by using earplugs or cotton with Vaseline. If earplugs are used, thorough cleansing with alcohol or a mild detergent between uses is recommended to prevent reinfection. The patient should not go swimming during this time.

## PROBLEMS OF THE MIDDLE EAR

Infection with its associated complications is the most common disorder of the middle ear, but masses, trauma, and other conditions may occur. The less common disorders of the middle ear are summarized in Table 58-2.

## MIDDLE EAR INFECTION (OTITIS MEDIA)

### Etiology

*Otitis media* is a general term that refers to inflammation of the mucous membranes of the middle ear, eustachian tube, and mastoid. The mucous membranes are continuous with those of the respiratory tract, and infection can easily ascend to the ear. Otitis media is caused by various types of bacteria. Acute otitis media develops suddenly and is usually of short duration.

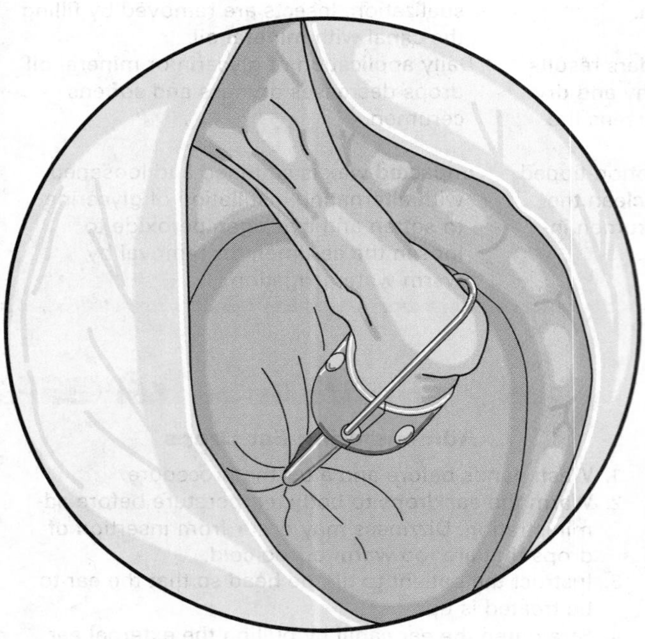

**fig. 58-6** Stapedectomy with Robinson stainless steel prosthesis in place.

Recurrent infection, usually causing drainage and perforation of the tympanic membrane, is called *chronic otitis media*. Between episodes of infection, fluid may collect in the middle ear (*serous otitis media*). Blockage in the eustachian tube creates a vacuum that causes fluid formation. When the inflammation accompanying the infection subsides, the residual fluid may be too thick to drain. Serous otitis media is also found in conjunction with upper respiratory infections or allergies. If fluid is present within the ear for a protracted period of time, the tympanic membrane retracts, and *adhesive otitis media* may develop. Likewise, any long-term blockage of the eustachian tube can also lead to adhesive otitis media and result in hearing loss.

### Epidemiology

Otitis media is classically considered to be a childhood disorder associated with upper respiratory infection. The vast majority of cases occur in children from infancy to school age. The incidence is clearly increased during the colder months in association with the increased incidence of upper respiratory infection. Otitis media may go undiagnosed in the adult population because the symptoms are frequently less dramatic than in the child. Adults are vulnerable to the development of chronic otitis media, particularly if they experienced multiple acute episodes in their youth. Staphylococcus and streptococcus organisms are the predominant causes in adults. Persons with a positive family history for ear problems, those with chronic allergies and sinusitis, and persons exposed to passive smoke all have an increased risk of developing otitis media and its complications as adults. Inadequate treatment can easily lead to the emergence of resistant strains of bacteria.

### Pathophysiology

Because the middle ear transmits sound from the tympanic membrane to the inner ear, middle ear infection frequently causes a conductive hearing loss from pressure behind the tympanic membrane. The hearing loss is usually correctable

**table 58-2** *Disorders of the Middle Ear and Mastoid*

| Disorder | Etiology | Collaborative Management |
|---|---|---|
| Perforated tympanic membrane | Perforations may occur acutely after trauma or as the result of chronic infection. Damage may extend to the ossicles and worsen the hearing loss. | Acute perforation may heal spontaneously. Infection is treated with appropriate local and/or systemic antibiotics. Surgical correction of the perforation may be performed: myringoplasty for the membrane or tympanoplasty if repair includes the middle ear structures. Grafts may be taken from the muscle fascia, a vein, or perichondrium. Success rate is high. |
| Otosclerosis (hardening of the ear) | Problem involves the stapes. Sclerotic bone forms on the stapes limiting its movement and resulting in conductive hearing loss. Underlying cause is unknown. | A hearing aid may be initially prescribed. Advanced disease is treated surgically through stapedectomy in which a prosthesis replaces the otosclerotic footplate. The success rate is high (Figure 58-6). |
| Mastoiditis | Chronic otitis media can result in the extension of the infection into the mastoid cavity. The volume of drainage from the middle ear increases. | Antibiotic therapy is the foundation of care, possibly supplemented by irrigations. Aggressive treatment is appropriate to prevent serious complications. Surgical mastoidectomy may be necessary in rare situations. |

with resolution of the infection. Common additional symptoms include throbbing pain in the affected ear, inflammation, fever, and drainage and bulging of the eardrum with possible perforation. Blood, pus, and other material may be present when perforation occurs. A thick yellow purulent discharge is a common finding with chronic otitis media. *Tympanosclerosis,* a deposit of collagen and calcium within the middle ear, can also result from repeated infection. The deposits can harden around the ossicles and contribute to a worsening of any conductive hearing loss. Because of the anatomy of the temporal bone, middle ear infection can, in rare cases, lead to a life-threatening brain abscess. Box 58-4 summarizes the common symptoms of otitis media.

**box 54-4** *clinical manifestations*

***Otitis Media***

- Throbbing pain in infected ear
- Fever
- Drainage: clear, bloody, or purulent
- Bulging of the eardrum
- Conductive hearing loss, usually reversible with effective treatment

## Collaborative Care Management

### *Diagnostic tests*

The diagnosis of otitis media is usually made based on the patient's symptoms of acute ear pain and fever. Otoscopic examination of the ear canal readily reveals the inflamed bulging tympanic membrane and perforation or drainage if present.

### *Medications*

Antibiotic therapy is the key to treatment of otitis media. Broad-spectrum antibiotics are used unless drainage is present that allows for culture of the organism and sensitivity testing. Chronic infections frequently do not respond to the usual antibiotics and may require local treatment with irrigations and ear drops.[4] Drugs commonly used to treat otitis media are summarized in Table 58-3.

### *Treatments*

An ear wash may be prescribed, particularly if chronic drainage is present that is irritating to the tissue of the ear canal. The most common solution used is boric acid and alcohol, which is obtained by prescription. The solution cleanses the ear of debris and infection and provides a drying agent. When the eustachian tube is chronically obstructed, it may be necessary to remove fluid from the middle ear.

**table 58-3** *Common Medications for* ***Treatment of Otitis Media***

| Drug | Action | Nursing Intervention |
|---|---|---|
| Antibiotics: amoxicillin, trimethoprim sulfamethoxazole, amoxicillin-clavulanate, cefaclor | Inhibits cell wall synthesis, bacteriocidal | 1. Assess for allergies or sensitivities.<br>2. Instruct patient to take medication around the clock, not to miss any doses, and to finish prescription completely.<br>3. Assess for superinfection. |
| Analgesic/antipyretic or narcotic analgesics: acetaminophen with codeine | Central nervous system (CNS) depressant, analgesic, antipyretic, antiinflammatory | 1. Assess vital signs, especially temperature.<br>2. Caution patient not to drive or operate machinery if taking codeine; also not to take other CNS depressants, including alcohol, while taking medication.<br>3. Teach patient to increase fluid and roughage intake to avoid constipation.<br>4. Take medication with meals to decrease possible nausea.<br>5. Do not increase dose; assess effectiveness of pain relief. |
| Antihistamines: chlorpheniramine | H1 receptor antagonist, antiemetic, antitussive, anticholinergic, and local anesthetic actions | 1. Monitor blood pressure (BP) in hypertensive patients.<br>2. Avoid driving a car or operating machinery until drug effects are determined.<br>3. Caution against alcohol use, which may cause an additive effect or drowsiness. |
| Decongestants: pseudoephedrine | Sympathomimetic, acts directly on smooth muscle, produces little congestive rebound that occurs with nasal sprays | 1. Monitor heart rate and BP, especially in patients with cardiac history.<br>2. Teach patient not to take medication before bedtime because of stimulant effect.<br>3. Withhold medication if restlessness or tachycardia occurs.<br>4. Teach patient to avoid other over-the-counter medications, which may contain ephedrine. |

Myringotomies, with or without tubes, are performed to regain normal middle ear and eustachian tube function. *Myringotomy* involves making a tiny incision in the tympanic membrane through which the fluid can be suctioned. To keep the incision open and prevent a reaccumulation of fluid, various types of trans-tympanic tubes can be inserted into the incision (Figure 58-7). These tubes fall out by themselves in 3 to 12 months and rarely have to be removed.

### Surgical management

Surgical intervention may be necessary if attempts to control the infection medically are unsuccessful, and the ossicles become necrotic. Repairing the damage of middle ear infection requires a difficult microsurgical procedure. *Tympano-ossiculoplasty* repairs the necrotic ossicles and creates a new eardrum. The surgical procedure is still being refined, and a variety of middle ear prostheses are available (Figure 58-8). The surgery is often performed in an ambulatory surgery center under local anesthesia and sedation. Tympano-ossiculoplasty is not always successful, but it does restore sound transmission for some patients.

### Diet

Diet does not play a role in the management of otitis media, but patients may wish to modify their diet slightly in response to the fever. Increasing the daily intake of fluids is generally recommended.

### Activity

No particular activity restrictions are included in the management of middle ear infections. Patients who are experiencing significant ear pain and fever may be more comfortable resting and avoiding activity until the antibiotics are able to reduce the severity of the symptoms.

### Referrals

Referrals are not necessary for patients with acute otitis media that responds promptly to treatment with antibiotics.

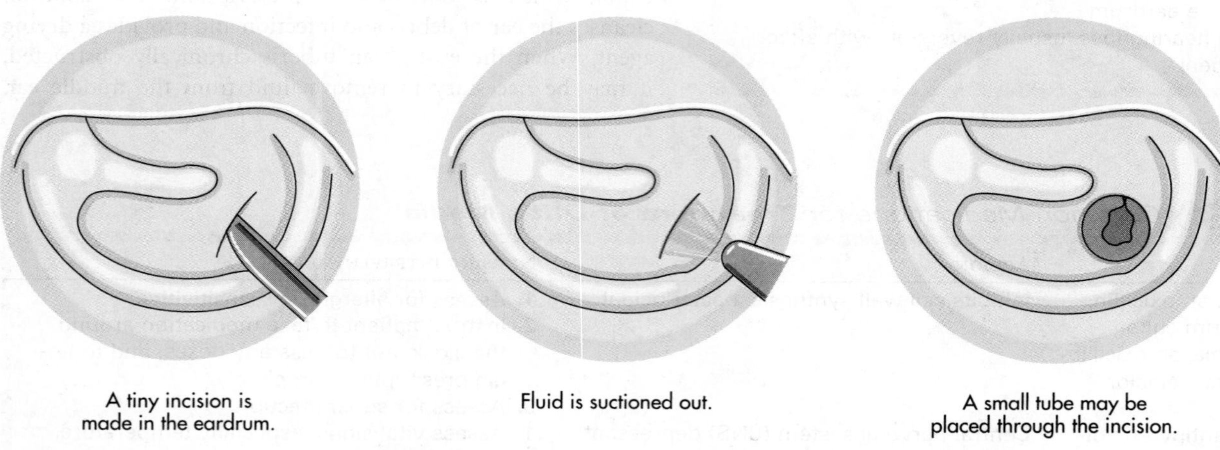

A tiny incision is made in the eardrum.
Fluid is suctioned out.
A small tube may be placed through the incision.


**fig. 58-7** Myringotomy and trans-tympanic tube placement to prevent chronic serous otitis media.

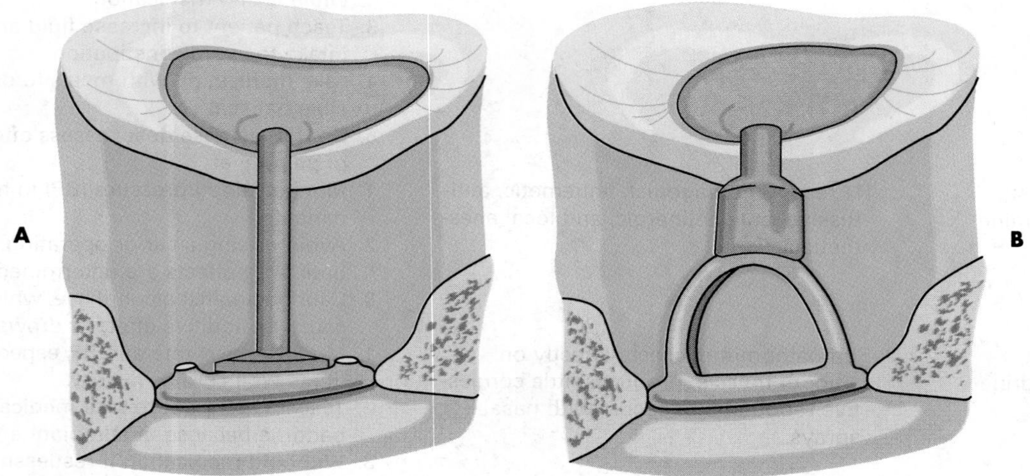


**fig. 58-8** Middle ear prostheses. **A,** Schuring ossicle columnella prosthesis for total ossicular replacement surgery. **B,** Schuring ossicle cup prosthesis for incus replacement surgery.

Patients with chronic otitis media may be referred to a surgeon for correction of complications or to an audiologist if extensive hearing loss occurs.

## NURSING MANAGEMENT

### ASSESSMENT

#### Subjective Data

Data to be collected to assess the patient with a middle ear infection include:

Reports of pain, often severe and throbbing, in the affected ear
Sense of fullness or pressure in the ear
Perceived change in hearing

#### Objective Data

Data to be collected to assess the patient with an ear infection include:

Inflamed, bulging tympanic membrane
Drainage from ear: bloody, serous, or purulent
Perforation of tympanic membrane
Fever

### NURSING DIAGNOSES

Nursing diagnoses are determined from analysis of patient data. Nursing diagnoses for the patient with a middle ear infection may include but are not limited to:

| Diagnostic Title | Possible Etiological Factors |
|---|---|
| Pain | Infection, buildup of fluid in ear spaces, swelling, trauma |
| Knowledge deficit: treatment of otitis, self-care after ear surgery | Lack of exposure to information and skills |

### EXPECTED PATIENT OUTCOMES

Expected patient outcomes for the person with a middle ear infection may include but are not limited to:

1. States that pain is decreased to a manageable level.
2. Performs ear wash correctly; states signs and symptoms to report to health care provider.

### INTERVENTIONS

#### Relieving Pain

Patients with otitis media are rarely admitted to an acute care setting and need to be instructed about self-care. The nurse instructs the patient about the use of all medications (see Table 58-2) and the importance of taking the antibiotic exactly as prescribed for the full course of the prescription. Analgesics may be necessary to successfully control the ear pain until the antibiotic begins to reduce the severity of the inflammation. The nurse encourages the patient to use these medications for comfort and to remain at rest until the antibiotic has demonstrated effectiveness. Reduced physical activity does appear to be helpful in controlling pain.

#### Patient/Family Education

The nurse instructs the patient to avoid getting water in the ear during treatment. This includes showering and shampooing as well as swimming. Commercial ear plugs or other barriers may be used as temporary protection during shampooing. If an ear wash is prescribed, the nurse teaches the patient and a designated family caregiver how to perform this treatment safely at home (Guidelines for Care Box).

Most patients undergoing ear surgery have extremely short hospitalizations. The nurse teaches the patient what to expect after discharge and how to promote healing during the recovery period. The nurse informs the patient that decreased hearing is expected initially from the presence of swelling and packing in the ear. Cracking or popping noises are commonly heard in the affected ear and are expected. Minor earache and discomfort in the cheek and jaw are common, but should be managed effectively with mild analgesics. Dizziness or lightheadedness may also be present initially, and the patient should use caution when getting out of bed and walking. Bleeding and drainage are negligible. A cotton ball frequently provides adequate dressing. Other patient teaching points are summarized in the accompanying Patient/Family Teaching Box.

### EVALUATION

To evaluate the effectiveness of nursing interventions, compare patient behaviors with those stated in the expected patient outcomes. Successful achievement of patient outcomes for the patient with middle ear infection is indicated by:

1a. States that no pain is present in the affected ear
b. Has no ear drainage in the canal and no redness, edema, or itching. The ear canal is clean and healing.

**guidelines for care**

**Performing an Ear Wash**

NOTE: The procedure should be performed by a family member or significant other if possible. It cannot be performed effectively by the patient alone.

1. Wash hands before and after the procedure.
2. Fill a 2 to 3 ounce ear syringe with the solution, warmed to body temperature.
3. Position the patient lying on his or her side with the affected ear up.
4. Place the tip of the syringe gently into the ear canal. Do not be afraid to insert it into the ear.
5. Pump the solution from the syringe back and forth into the ear. Do this vigorously and repeatedly. The fluid must actively move in and out of the ear canal to be effective.
6. Assist the patient to lean over the side and let the solution run out of the ear at the end of the procedure. The patient may experience dizziness with movement.
7. Apply eardrops if instructed.
8. Continue to use the ear wash solution as instructed for about 2 weeks or until the ear is dry and without drainage.

Modified from Sigler BA, Schuring L: *Ear, nose, and throat disorders,* p 261, St Louis, 1993, Mosby.

**patient/family teaching**

**Patient Teaching After Ear Surgery**

1. Sneeze or cough with the mouth open as needed for the first week after surgery.
2. Blow the nose gently as needed, one side at a time.
3. Avoid vigorous activity until approved by the surgeon.
4. Change cotton ball dressing as prescribed.
5. Report any drainage other than a slight amount of bleeding to the surgeon.
6. Keep ear dry for 6 weeks after surgery.
   - Do not shampoo the hair without a barrier.
   - Protect the ear when necessary with two pieces of cotton (outer piece saturated with petrolatum).
7. Avoid loud noisy environments. Do not fly until approved by surgeon.
8. Balance ear pressure as needed by holding nose, closing mouth, and swallowing.

2a. Correctly explains and demonstrates prescribed treatments.
b. Correctly identifies symptoms that need to be reported promptly to a health care provider (otorrhea, decrease in hearing, and return of pain).

## GERONTOLOGICAL CONSIDERATIONS

Middle ear infection can occur at any point in the life span, but it is not a particularly common problem in elders. Early infection may go undiagnosed unless pain is severe because elders frequently experience itching in the ear or blockage with cerumen. All the care and teaching described for the patient with otitis media would also apply to the care of elders with the same diagnosis.

## SPECIAL ENVIRONMENTS FOR CARE

### Critical Care Management

Patients being treated for middle ear infection would never be expected to need critical care management. Otitis media is a community-based infection that the patient can manage effectively at home. Even surgical intervention is at most a 1- to 2-day hospitalization, which would not be expected to need critical care intervention unless catastrophic complications develop.

### Home Care Management

Because middle ear infection is a community-based problem, the entire discussion is appropriate to this setting. Patients need written as well as oral instruction and may require temporary home visiting if no one is available to assist the patient with treatments such as ear washes.

## COMPLICATIONS

The primary complications of middle ear infection are perforation of the eardrum and conductive hearing loss. The hearing loss usually resolves with effective treatment of the infection, but may be permanent if chronic disease is present. Acute perforations also tend to heal spontaneously and without residual problems, but complex situations may require surgical closure of the perforation (see Table 58-2).

*Cholesteatoma* may result from chronic otitis media. In this condition epithelium from the external ear canal enters and extends into the middle ear, usually through a tympanic membrane perforation. The skin forms a sac-like growth that traps debris and puts increasing pressure on the structures of the middle ear. The chronic infection causes cholesterol granules to be deposited within the sac, which gives the growth its name. Surgical excision may become necessary if pressure is causing damage or necrosis to the delicate ear structures. Limited procedures are generally attempted to preserve hearing, but either an open or closed mastoidectomy may be performed.

# PROBLEMS OF THE INNER EAR

Sensorineural hearing loss is the most common inner ear disorder and may occur in conjunction with an identified ear problem or in isolation. The hearing loss is usually incomplete but is frequently progressive. The loss of discrimination (understanding of words) is a characteristic feature of sensorineural hearing loss. The inner ear is so delicate that it does not lend itself to surgical correction or repair. Hearing loss is discussed at the beginning of the chapter.

## ACOUSTIC NEUROMA

### Etiology/Epidemiology

Benign and malignant tumors can involve the inner ear by extension through the temporal bone, but acoustic neuroma is by far the most common lesion. An acoustic neuroma is a benign tumor of the eighth cranial nerve. It is a slow-growing lesion that can occur at any age and usually occurs unilaterally. The tumor typically grows at the point where cranial nerve VIII enters the internal auditory canal, the temporal bone, and may extend into the brainstem. The tumor is more common in women and tends to occur in persons between 30 and 60 years of age.

### Pathophysiology

The tumor arises from the neurilemmal sheath (sheath of Schwann) along the vestibular branch of the nerve and spreads to the cochlear branch. Early diagnosis is important because the tumor can grow and compress the facial nerve and arteries within the ear canal. It is important that the tumor be diagnosed before it becomes intracranial. In rare cases, the pressure of the tumor can become life-threatening. Symptoms include tinnitus, vertigo, and a progressive unilateral loss of ability to hear high-pitched sounds. Disorders of the facial nerve may emerge if the tumor is compressing this structure as well.

### Collaborative Care Management

Acoustic neuromas are treated surgically, usually by a neurosurgeon. Computed tomography scans can show tumors greater than 2 cm in size, but the patient's hearing is usually already compromised by the time the tumor is this large. The technical challenges of the surgery include preservation of both hearing and facial nerve function. Many patient experience some degree of residual hearing loss after treatment.

## MÉNIÈRE'S DISEASE

### Etiology/Epidemiology

Ménière's disease or syndrome, also called idiopathic endolymphatic hydrops, is an uncommon form of vertigo of unknown etiology. A virus is believed to play a role in etiology, but this relationship has not been proven. The disease occurs when the normal fluid and electrolyte balance of the inner ear is disrupted. The diagnosis is based on the presence of a classic triad of symptoms plus a prodromal symptom of fullness or pressure in the involved ear. The triad includes episodic true vertigo, sensorineural hearing loss, and tinnitus. Other disorders can also result in vertigo and balance disturbances. To maintain balance, the brain must integrate data from the vestibular, visual, and proprioceptive systems. Other vestibular disorders are summarized in Table 58-4.

The prevalence of Ménière's disease in the United States is approximately 40 persons per 100,000. Men and women are affected about equally. Peak onset occurs in the fourth decade and the disease is usually diagnosed in persons younger than 60 years of age. The disease usually begins unilaterally but may progress to both ears in 10% to 78% of patients.[1] Family history is significant. Symptoms may be exacerbated during the menstrual cycle in women who experience significant premenstrual fluid retention.

### Pathophysiology

The underlying pathological changes of Ménière's disease include overproduction and defective absorption of endolymph, which increases the volume and pressure within the membranous labyrinth until distention results in rupture and mixing of the endolymph and perilymph fluids. The two fluids have significantly different compositions, and the mixture disrupts the fluid and electrolyte balance within the labyrinth. Classic Ménière's disease attacks last from 2 to 3 weeks, approximately the time required to close the rupture and restore the fluid balance. The symptoms range from mild to incapacitating and include vertigo, tinnitus, and fluctuating sensorineural hearing loss from degeneration of the hair cells. Prodromal symptoms include tinnitus, ear fullness, and hearing loss. Ninety-five percent of patients experience vertigo associated with nausea, vomiting, and ataxia.

Ménière's disease is relatively uncommon, but the symptom of dizziness or vertigo is second only to headache as the most common chronic symptom reported by patients in the United States. *Vertigo,* or *spinning,* is the medical term for dizziness, but dizziness is described in such varied terms that it is almost impossible to accurately define the symptom. Spinning, or vertigo, may be the most common form of dizziness. Other "feelings" include light-headedness, giddiness, imbalance, veering in one direction while walking, unsteadiness, or a vague feeling of uncertainty during changes in body position. Questions that can be used to explore vertigo are presented in Box 58-5. Initially symptoms last less than 2 hours. Altered balance may last up to 2 days. As the disease progresses symptoms last hours to days, and the episodes occur with less warning and are disabling. Because the balance system can compensate, dizziness is usually not present consistently but is episodic. Early in the course of the disease the patient is asymptomatic between episodes, but as the disease progresses, recovery between attacks is incomplete and permanent tinnitus, moderate to severe hearing loss, and chronic unsteadiness may result.

### Collaborative Care Management

The diagnosis of Ménière's disease is established after eliminating other causes of the patient's symptoms. There is no known cure for Ménière's disease, and management is focused on control of symptoms.

A variety of medications may be used in the management of Ménière's disease, primarily in the attempt to control disabling symptoms. Antiemetics and anticholinergics may be

**table 58-4** *Vestibular Disorders*

| Disorder | Definition | Cause (Most Common) | Vertigo | Tinnitus | Hearing Loss |
|---|---|---|---|---|---|
| Vestibular neuronitis | Infection of the vestibular nerve with sudden onset | Virus | First attack most severe, subsequent attacks less severe | | |
| Labyrinthitis | Infection of the labyrinth of the inner ear | Virus, bacteria | Severe vertigo diminishing with time | May or may not be present | Permanent sensorineural loss |
| Benign paroxysmal positional vertigo | Degenerative debris free floating in the endolymph | Idiopathic (many theories) | Positional vertigo with quick head movements or position change | | |
| Presbyastasis (presbyvertigo) | Balance disorder of aging | Degenerative changes of the vestibule | Imbalance when standing/walking, leading to falls and injuries | | |

**box 58-5** *Questions to Assess Vertigo*

When did the dizziness first occur?
Did the dizziness start suddenly or gradually?
Is the dizziness constant, or does it come in "attacks"?
How often do the attacks occur?
How long do the attacks last?
List anything that stops an attack of dizziness or makes it better.
Overall, has the dizziness gotten better or worse since starting?
List anything that brings on an attack of dizziness or makes it worse.
Does the dizziness occur only in certain positions?
Do any other symptoms occur simultaneously with the dizziness such as nausea, vomiting, or ear pressure?
Does stress have any relationship to the dizziness?
Have you ever fallen because of the dizziness?
Do you get dizzy after heavy lifting, straining, exertion, or overwork?
Do you get dizzy if you have not eaten for a long time?
For women: Is your dizziness connected with your menstrual cycle?
How has the dizziness affected the quality of your life?

Adapted from Sigler BA, Schuring L: *Ear, nose, and throat disorders,* pp 276-279, St Louis, 1993, Mosby.

administered during an acute attack to decrease autonomic nervous system activity. Diuretics and vasodilators are helpful to some patients in restoring the proper fluid balance in the inner ear. Other patients may respond to drugs that reduce vestibular impulses and sedatives. Treatment protocols have used more than 50 different medications. Usually a combination of agents can be found that adequately control the patient's symptoms.

The treatment of Ménière's disease is symptom driven, but patients with severe vertigo may profit from vestibular rehabilitation, which teaches labyrinthine compensatory exercises combined with physical therapy. Balance exercises decrease dizziness by helping the brain to compensate for the damaged balance system. Movements that trigger dizziness are repeated rather than avoided. Avoiding dizziness is more comfortable for the patient but does not help the balance system regain its function and compensate for losses. Figure 58-9 illustrates basic balance training exercises.

Surgery may be performed when the patient's symptoms cannot be satisfactorily controlled with medical interventions. The endolymphatic sac procedures include decompression and various forms of shunts. These procedures are designed to reduce the fluid pressure within the labyrinth and control vertigo. A destructive procedure to remove the

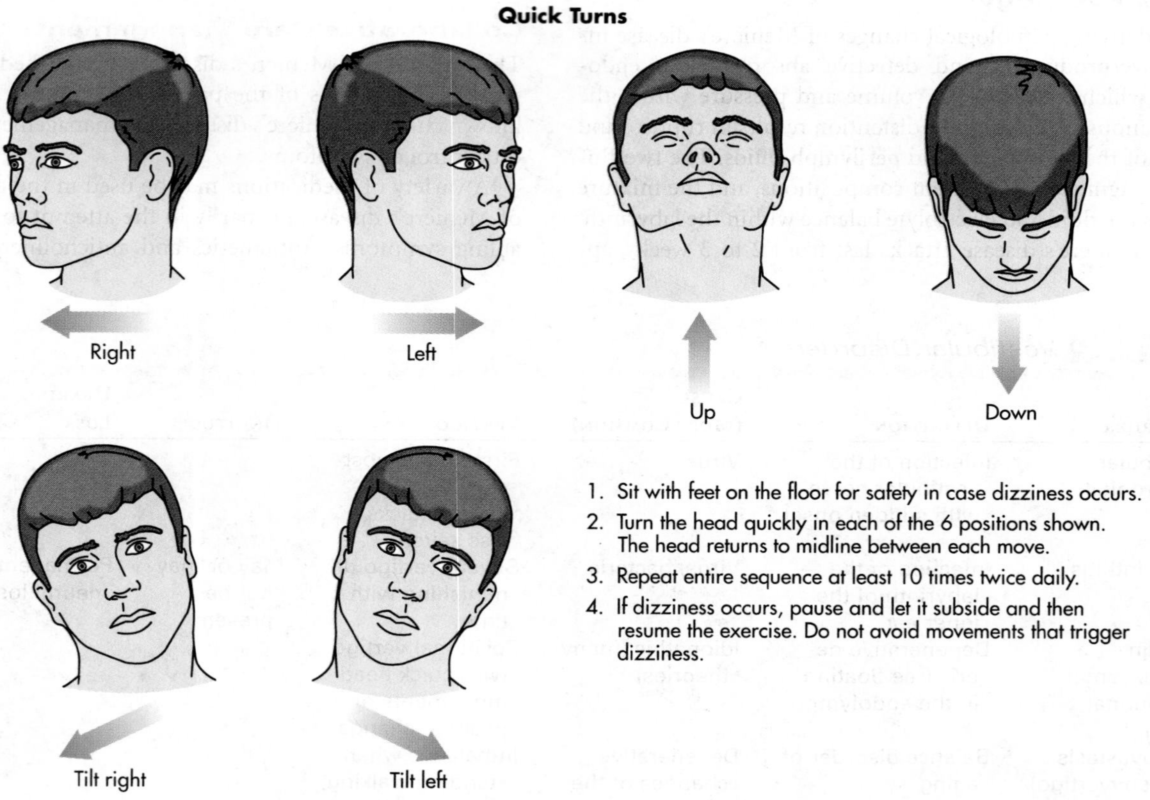

Quick Turns
Right
Left
Up
Down
Tilt right
Tilt left
1. Sit with feet on the floor for safety in case dizziness occurs.
2. Turn the head quickly in each of the 6 positions shown. The head returns to midline between each move.
3. Repeat entire sequence at least 10 times twice daily.
4. If dizziness occurs, pause and let it subside and then resume the exercise. Do not avoid movements that trigger dizziness.


**fig. 58-9** Balance training exercises.

## nursing care plan | The Person with Ménière's Disease

**DATA** Mrs. B. is a 59-year-old schoolteacher. During the past 6 months, she has had three attacks of "whirling in space" or vertigo, fluctuating hearing in the left ear, noise in the left ear or tinnitus, nausea and vomiting, and a sense of fullness or pressure in the left ear. Two attacks have occurred during class, and one attack occurred at home where she lives alone. Embarrassment, fear, anxiety, and uncertainty are some of her feelings. Mrs. B. made an appointment at an otology office where diagnostic tests were performed.

These tests included an audiogram, tympanometry, electronystagmography, auditory brain stem response, a nursing assessment, and physical examination. A diagnosis of Ménière's disease was made. A 1500-mg sodium restricted diet, hydrochlorothiazide 50 mg (HCTZ) PO qd, labyrinthine compensatory exercises, and niacin 100 mg PO tid were prescribed to control the incapacitating attacks of vertigo.

**NURSING DIAGNOSIS** *Anxiety (related to effects of disorder)*

| expected patient outcome | nursing interventions | rationale |
|---|---|---|
| Signs of anxiety are decreased. | Encourage Mrs. B. to explore concerns about decreased hearing and effects of dizziness attacks and to take action in relation to the concerns.<br>Explore Mrs. B.'s knowledge of the disorder and correct misunderstandings.<br>Encourage realistic hope about expected hearing ability as described by physician.<br>Refer Mrs. B. to necessary support services, such as social worker or audiologist. | Expressing concerns and receiving realistic counseling and support reduces helplessness and apprehension. |

**NURSING DIAGNOSIS** *Sensory/perceptual alteration (vestibular, auditory)*

| expected patient outcome | nursing interventions | rationale |
|---|---|---|
| Describes actions to avoid dizziness. | Help Mrs. B. identify avoidable actions that precipitate dizziness attacks. | Understanding cause of dizziness and measures to reduce it may lessen occurrence. |
| Interacts with others accurately. | Encourage Mrs. B. to move slowly and not turn head suddenly when dizziness is present. | |
| | If tinnitus is distressing, increase background noises such as music. | Use of distraction may lessen effects of tinnitus. |
| | If hearing is decreased:<br>**1.** Use measures to facilitate communication with hearing impaired (see the Guidelines for Care Box, p. 1867).<br>**2.** Refer Mrs. B. to an audiologist, if appropriate. | |

**NURSING DIAGNOSIS** *Injury, risk for*

| expected patient outcome | nursing interventions | rationale |
|---|---|---|
| Is not injured from falls. | Explore pattern of dizziness with Mrs. B. | Knowledge of pattern of attacks can be used in planning. |
| | Reinforce need to take prescribed medications. | Therapy may help prevent dizziness, which leads to falls. |
| | Explore home environment to decrease risk for injury. | Knowledge of safety measures reduces possibility of injuries. |

*Continued*

## The Person with Ménière's Disease–cont'd

**NURSING DIAGNOSIS** *Fluid volume deficit, risk for*

| expected patient outcome | nursing interventions | rationale |
|---|---|---|
| Fluid intake is >2500 ml/day.<br>Mucous membranes are moist. | Explain need for fluids, rationale for diuretic.<br>Help Mrs. B. plan ways to maintain a fluid intake >2500 ml/day. | Dehydration may occur from vomiting and from diuretic (HCTZ).<br>Use of a variety of fluids (juices, soups, soft drinks) will increase probability that Mrs. B. will drink >2400 ml/day. |

**NURSING DIAGNOSIS** *Coping, ineffective (individual)*

| expected patient outcome | nursing interventions | rationale |
|---|---|---|
| Identifies coping pattern and resultant effects.<br>Describes alternative coping behaviors. | Make decisions regarding safety of Mrs. B. and others when patient is unable to do so.<br>Assist Mrs. B. to identify usual coping behaviors and the consequences of the behaviors.<br>Assist Mrs. B. to identify personal strengths.<br>Teach Mrs. B. alternative coping behaviors (see Chapter 6). | Support and understanding by caregivers improves coping. Discussing possible coping behaviors assists the patient to choose behaviors that are most functional for her. |

**NURSING DIAGNOSIS** *Knowledge deficit (about pathophysiology of Ménière's disease related to lack of exposure to information)*

| expected patient outcome | nursing interventions | rationale |
|---|---|---|
| Describes nature of disorder, therapy, and safety measures. | Teach Mrs. B. about the disorder, therapy, and need for medical follow-up (see text).<br>Teach Mrs. B. ways to protect herself from injury and to prevent dizziness attacks when possible. | Need for information regarding disease increases learning that assists the patient to care for herself and to live as independently as possible. |

membranous labyrinth, either subtotally through the oval window or totally through the mastoid bone, is called *labyrinthectomy.*

Vestibular nerve surgery destroys the vestibular nerve in the affected ear while attempting to preserve hearing. With any surgery on the vestibular system there is a risk of causing hearing loss and creating chronic vertigo.

### Patient/family education

Diet therapy is frequently quite helpful in controlling the symptoms associated with Ménière's disease. The nurse encourages the patient to follow a low-salt diet and avoid the excess use of caffeine, sugar, monosodium glutamate, and alcohol. The intake of food and fluid is distributed over the course of the day. Some patients are able to achieve significant symptom improvement from diet modification alone.

Patients need clear instructions about how to manage an acute attack of vertigo. The nurse instructs the patient to immediately lie down on a firm surface if possible, loosen the clothing, and close the eyes until the acute vertigo stops. Driving and operating machinery should not be attempted during attacks. Between attacks the patient can resume normal activities but should avoid swimming under water which may cause a loss of orientation.

Loss of balance places the person with vertigo at high risk for falls. The nurse assists the patient to explore ways to increase the safety of the home environment. The nurse reminds the patient of the importance of sitting or lying down at the onset of dizziness to reduce the risk of falls. The nurse advises the patient to avoid ladders, work on roofs or trees, or climbing in high places until the vertigo is controlled. Balance therapy can be extremely helpful in supporting the balance network in the brain, and the nurse reinforces the importance of daily practice with these exercises. Careful adherence to the medication regimen is also discussed.

A Nursing Care Plan for a patient with Ménière's disease can be found on p. 1877 and above.

### critical thinking QUESTIONS

1 Describe how you think you might feel if you were told that you have a significant and permanent hearing loss.

2 Compare and contrast the pathophysiology, clinical manifestations, and assessment parameters for conductive and sensorineural hearing loss.

3 What measures or precautions could you suggest to the patient who has vertigo?

## chapter SUMMARY

### HEARING LOSS

- Disorders that plug the outer ear, add fluid to the middle ear, make the ossicles unmovable, destroy the hair cells of the organ of Corti, or interfere with nerve stimulus transmission over the acoustic nerve can lead to decreased hearing.
- Hearing can be preserved by preventing infection or trauma of the ear, by using ototoxic drugs with caution and seeking medical attention if symptoms occur, and by preventing frequent exposure to loud noises (or using ear protection for constant loud noises).
- Sensorineural hearing loss results from interference with hearing in the inner ear or neural pathways; it may result from a known disorder or may be idiopathic. Presbycusis (hearing loss resulting from aging) is a form of sensorineural hearing loss.
- Cochlear implants are used for patients with no usable hearing at all in either ear.
- Aural rehabilitation includes auditory training, speech reading (lip reading), speech training, (improving speech clarity), and the use of hearing aids.

### PROBLEMS OF THE EXTERNAL EAR

- Ear infections are the most common disorders of the external ear; pain results from pressure from fluid buildup within the enclosed spaces.

### PROBLEMS OF THE MIDDLE EAR

- Otitis media is the most common problem involving the middle ear. It is usually acute and resolves with antibiotics but can also become chronic.
- Serous otitis media develops from a collection of serous fluid in the middle ear when the eustachian tube becomes blocked. Any long-term blockage of the eustachian tube leads to serous otitis media and a hearing loss.
- Ear infections are treated with antibiotics, which are given by ear drops, ear ointments, or systemically. Treatments to remove drainage may include earwash, ear irrigation, or surgery.
- Otosclerosis is the hardening of the ear that involves the stapes bone and causes a conductive hearing loss. Stapedectomy is the surgical procedure that removes and replaces the stapes.

### PROBLEMS OF THE INNER EAR

- Vertigo is the major symptom of disorders (such as labyrinthitis or Ménière's disease) affecting the semicircular canals of the inner ear. Tinnitus (ringing in the ears) often accompanies vertigo.
- Dizziness, like pain, is subject to psychological influences and is second to headache as the most common chronic symptom currently found in the United States.

## References


1. DeLa Cruz A, Robertson DD: Ménière's disease. In Rakel RE, editor: *Conn's current therapy,* ed 2, Philadelphia, 1997, WB Saunders.
2. Leuckenotte AG: *Gerontologic nursing,* St Louis, 1996, Mosby.
3. Nodol JB Jr: Hearing loss, *N Engl J Med* 329(15):1092-1102, 1993.
4. Uphold CR, Graham MV: *Clinical guidelines in adult health,* Gainesville, FL, 1994, Barmarrae Books.
5. US Department of Health and Human Services, Public Health Service: *Healthy people 2000: midcourse review and 1995 revisions,* Washington DC, 1995, US Government Printing Office.

# chapter 59 ASSESSMENT OF THE Musculoskeletal System

JANE F. MAREK

## objectives *After studying this chapter, the learner should be able to:*

1. Contrast the structure and function of the different tissues that compose the musculoskeletal system.
2. Analyze the interrelationship of the tissues of the musculoskeletal system with overall functioning of the system.
3. Discuss the physiological changes that occur in the musculoskeletal system as a result of the aging process.
4. Explain the pathological conditions that can occur within the musculoskeletal system.
5. Relate components of the nursing assessment of the musculoskeletal system, including subjective and objective data.
6. Correlate the diagnostic tests indicated for the person with a musculoskeletal problem, the rationale for each test, and appropriate nursing responsibilities associated with each test.
7. Synthesize a plan of care for a person with a musculoskeletal problem, using relevant subjective and objective data and results of diagnostic tests.

People often take the ability to move about freely in the environment for granted. Activities as simple as making a fist to movements as complex as a ballerina performing a cabriole depend on the structure, function, and integrity of the musculoskeletal system. The musculoskeletal system is one of the body's largest systems and accounts for over 50% of the body's weight. This dynamic system comprises bones, joints, muscles, and supporting structures. All the components of the system work together to produce movement and to supply structure and support. Any disturbance in this well-integrated system results in musculoskeletal dysfunction. Problems can arise as a result of disease affecting the nerves, bones, muscles, or joints or as a result of trauma to these or surrounding structures. Problems arising outside of the musculoskeletal system, such as endocrine or neurological diseases, may also directly affect the system, resulting in some form of disability.

Planning appropriate interventions for individuals with alterations in musculoskeletal functioning requires a careful and thorough assessment, based on the nurse's knowledge and understanding of the anatomy and physiology of the musculoskeletal system. The patient's reaction to the disability and implications of the results of diagnostic studies must also be considered. This chapter discusses the anatomy and physiology of the musculoskeletal system, methods and rationale for obtaining subjective and objective data about patients and their disabilities, and the relevance of selected diagnostic studies.

## ANATOMY AND PHYSIOLOGY

### BONES

The human skeleton is made up of the axial and appendicular skeletons, which consist of 206 bones (Figure 59-1). The axial skeleton consists of 80 bones—the hyoid bone and those of the skull, vertebral column, and thorax. The remaining 126 bones make up the appendicular skeleton, which contains the bones of the upper and lower extremities, pectoral girdle, and pelvic girdle (os coxae). The skeleton makes up 14% of the weight of the adult body.

#### Types

Bones are divided into four types, according to their shape:

1. Long (femur, humerus)
2. Short (carpals): often cuboidal in shape (see Figure 59-1)
3. Flat (skull)
4. Irregular (vertebrae)

Long bones are made up of a diaphysis, a metaphysis, and an epiphysis. The *diaphysis* (midportion) is made of thick cortical bone and contains the medullary cavity, where the marrow is stored. The *diaphyseal* cavity comprises primarily fatty tissues and contains yellow marrow, which is not capable of hematopoiesis. The marrow cavity of the diaphysis connects to the cancellous bone of the *metaphysis,* or broad neck of the long bone. The *epiphysis,* or broad end of the bone, contains the red marrow, which is responsible for hematopoiesis. The *endosteum* lines both yellow and red marrow cavities. The

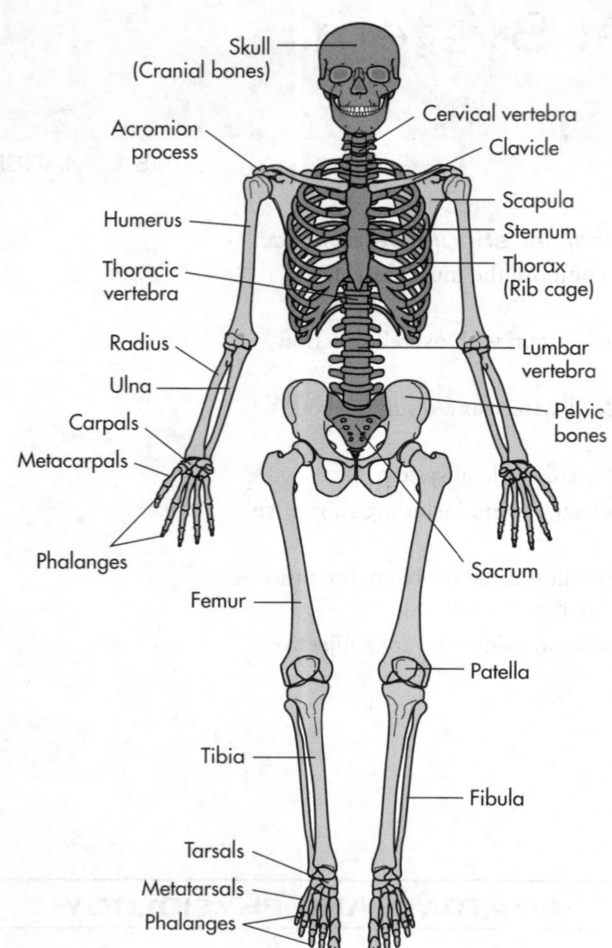


**fig. 59-1** Axial and appendicular skeleton.

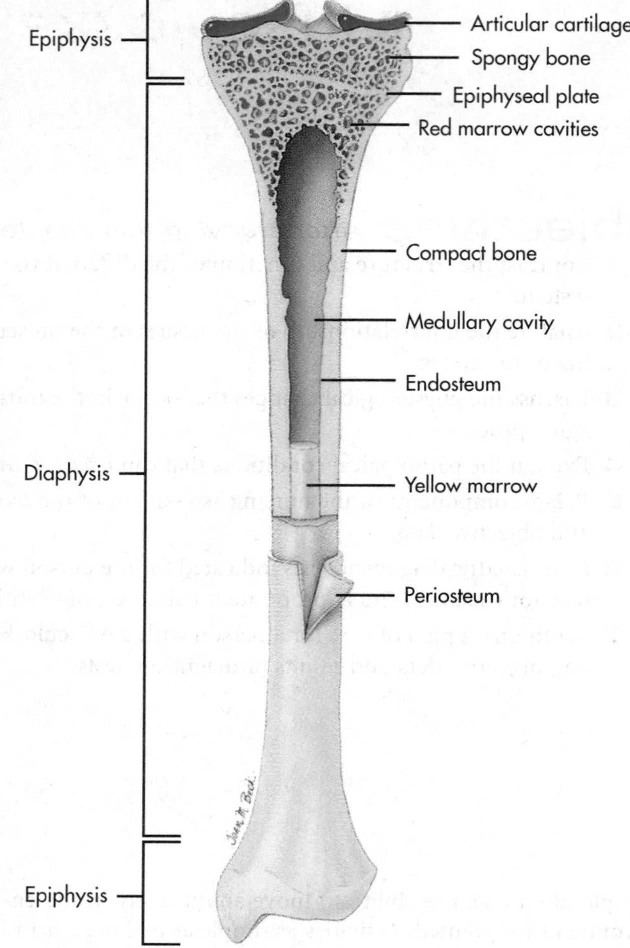


**fig. 59-2** Cross section of a long bone.

epiphysis is made up of spongy bone covered with a thin layer of cortical bone. Its broad end allows weight to be distributed over a greater surface area. A cartilaginous growth plate or *epiphyseal plate* separates the metaphysis from the epiphysis in children. The epiphysis and metaphysis merge after puberty when the epiphyseal plate calcifies. This growth plate, easily seen on x-ray examination in children, is undetectable in adults (Figure 59-2).

Each bone is composed of *cancellous* (spongy) and *cortical* (compact) bone. In the long bones, the cancellous portions are found in the ends of the bones and cortical bone in the shaft (see Figure 59-2). The short and irregular bones have an inner core of cancellous bone with an outer layer of cortical bone. Flat bones have two outer plates of cortical bone with an inner layer of cancellous bone. Cancellous bone is also found in the ends of long bones and in the iliac crests, tibiae, and sternum.

### Structure

Bone, like other connective tissue, is made up of cells, fibers, and ground substance. In addition, unlike other connective tissue, bone contains crystallized minerals, which gives it rigidity (Table 59-1).

Bone is a dynamic substance, continuously synthesizing and resorbing bone tissue. Bone cells allow growth, repair, and remodeling. Bone formation begins in the fetal stage as cartilage formation and continues throughout life. In the mature individual, the first step in bone formation is the initiation of an organic matrix by the bone cells. Next, mineralization takes place as minerals are bound to collagen fibers, providing support and tensile strength to bone.

Three types of bone cells are found in the body. *Osteoblasts,* or bone-forming cells, are responsible for laying down new bone. They produce type I collagen and respond to changing levels of parathyroid hormone (PTH). New bone is formed as the osteoblasts produce osteoid and mineralize the bone matrix. Once this is accomplished, osteoblasts become osteocytes and are trapped in the mineralized bone matrix. *Osteocytes* maintain the mineral content and organic elements of bone. The third type of bone cell, *osteoclasts,* resorb bone during growth and repair. They are able to resorb bone by secreting citric and lactic

**table 59-1** *Structural Elements of Bone*

| STRUCTURAL ELEMENT | FUNCTION |
|---|---|
| **BONE CELLS** | |
| Osteoblasts | Synthesize collagen and proteoglycans; stimulate osteoclast resorptive activity |
| Osteocytes | Maintain bone matrix |
| Osteoclasts | Resorb bone; assist with mineral homeostasis |
| **BONE MATRIX** | |
| Collagen fibers | Lend support and tensile strength |
| Proteoglycans | Control transport of ionized materials through matrix |
| Bone morphogenic proteins | Induce cartilage formation |
| BMP-1 | |
| BMP-2A | |
| BMP-3 | |
| Glycoproteins | |
| Sialoprotein | Promotes calcification |
| Osteocalcin | Inhibits calcium-phosphate precipitation; promotes bone resorption |
| Laminin | Stabilizes basement membranes in bones |
| Osteonectin | Binds calcium in bones |
| Albumin | Transports essential elements to matrix; maintains osmotic pressure of bone fluid |
| α-Glycoprotein | Promotes calcification |
| Minerals (elements) | |
| Calcium | Crystallizes to lend rigidity and compressive strength |
| Phosphate | Regulates vitamin D and thereby promotes mineralization |

From McCance KL, Huether SE: *Pathophysiology: the biologic basis for disease in adults and children,* ed 3, St Louis, 1998, Mosby.

acid and collagenases, which dissolve minerals and break down collagen.

Bone is primarily composed of *organic matrix* and calcium salts. Collagen fibers account for 90% to 95% of the organic matrix; ground substance makes up the remainder. The collagen fibers extend along the lines of tensional force and give bone its great tensile strength.[1] The ground substance functions as a medium for the diffusion of nutrients, oxygen, minerals, and wastes between bone tissue and blood vessels. Ground substance contains extracellular fluid and *proteoglycans,* particularly chondroitin sulfate and hyaluronic acid, which help control the deposition of calcium salts. The *bone morphogenic proteins (BMP),* important substances responsible for inducing cartilage formation, are also found in the bone matrix. The glycoproteins found in the matrix play a role in the calcification, resorption, and metabolism of bone. The minerals contained in the matrix are primarily calcium and phosphate. *Hydroxyapatite (HAT),* the primary bone salt, is formed as a result of the mineralization and crystal formation of calcium and phosphate. Mineralization is the final step in the process of bone formation.

Both cancellous and cortical bone contain the same structural elements, but they differ in the organization of the bone matrix. Concentric layers of bone matrix are called *lamellae.*

The basic unit of cortical bone is the *haversian system* (Figure 59-3, *B*). At the center of this arrangement of concentric rings is the haversian canal, which runs through the long axes of bones. This canal contains blood vessels (capillaries, arterioles, or venules), nerve fibers, and lymphatics. Blood vessels in the canal communicate with blood vessels in the periosteum. Lacunae are small spaces between the rings of the lamellae and contain osteocytes. Canaliculi, very small canals that connect the lacunae and the haversian canal, run parallel to the long axis of the bone. This connection allows the osteocytes access to the nutrient supply. Haversian units (lamellae, haversian canal, lacunae, canaliculi) fit closely together in cortical bone. The hardness and density of cortical bone give it strength and rigidity.

In contrast, *cancellous bone lacks haversian systems.* The lamellae are arranged not in concentric layers but in connecting plates or bars called *trabeculae,* which form an irregular meshwork (Figure 59-3, *A*). The pattern of the trabecular bone depends on the direction of stress in the particular bone. Red marrow fills the spaces between the trabeculae. Lacunae, rich in osteocytes, are distributed among the trabeculae and connected by canaliculi. Capillaries flowing through the marrow provide nutrients to the osteocytes. The fine, thready structure of trabecular bone provides strength to cancellous bone while reducing its weight.

The outer, nonarticulating surfaces of long bones are covered with a white fibrous membrane called the *periosteum.* The outer layer of the periosteum contains blood vessels and nerves that reach the inner bones through Volkmann's canals. Nutrient arteries in the periosteum communicate with the haversian system. Collagenous fibers (Sharpey's fibers) anchor the inner layer of the periosteum to the bone.

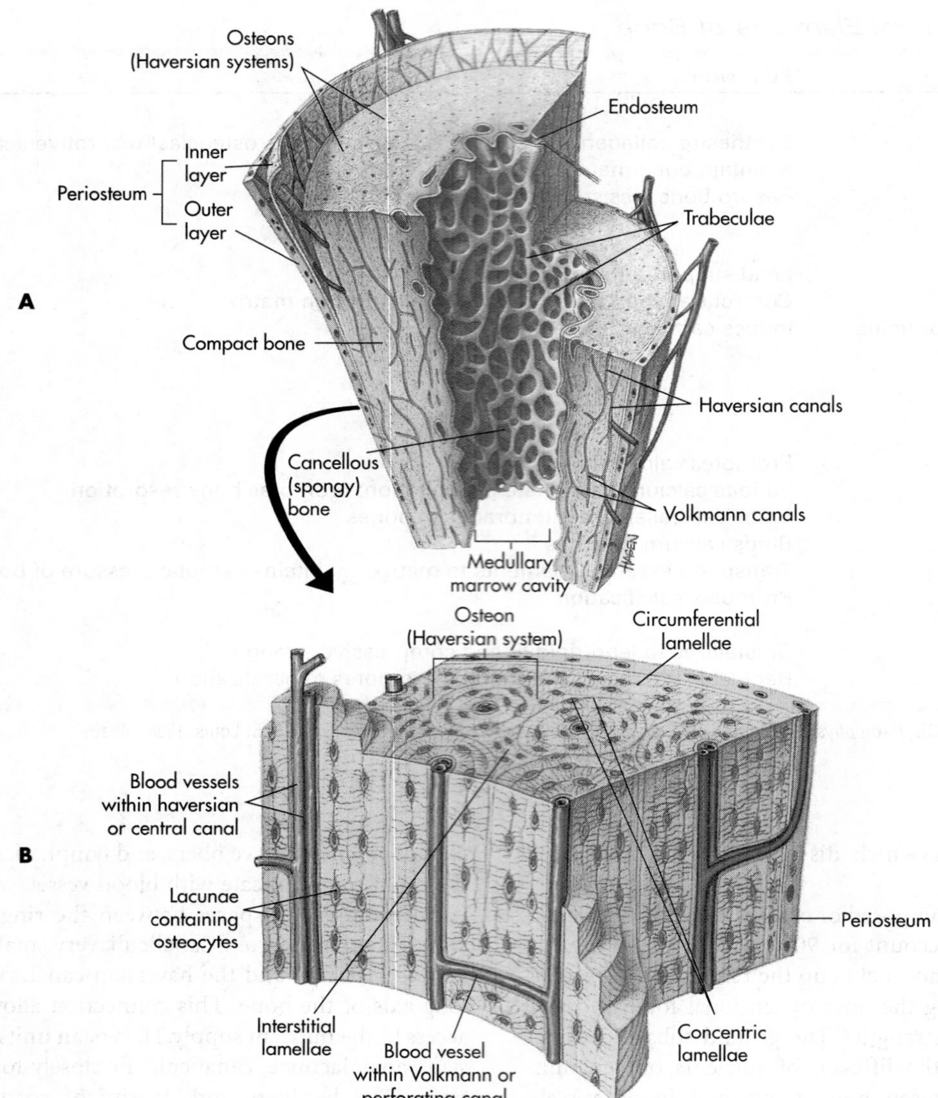


**fig. 59-3** Structure of compact and cancellous bone. **A,** Longitudinal section of a long bone showing both cancellous and compact bone. **B,** A magnified view of compact bone.

Surfaces of bones contain grooves or ridges for nerves and blood vessels, prominences for muscular attachments, and openings for blood vessels and muscles. Articulating surfaces are covered with hyaline cartilage (Figure 59-4).

Blood supply to bone is maintained through the haversian canals, periosteal vasculature, and vessels located in the marrow and ends of bones. Bones are supplied with sensory nerve endings in the periosteum that connect with the central nervous system.

## Function

Bones have five functions:

1. *Support*—of body tissues as provided by the skeletal framework; they also give form and shape to the body.
2. *Protection*—of body organs; for example, the bony casing of the skull protects the brain and the bones of the thorax and pelvis protect the heart, lungs, and reproductive organs.
3. *Movement*—by muscular attachments to bone and by joint movement.
4. *Hematopoiesis*—the marrow of some bones has a hematopoietic function. Normally after birth, red blood cell (RBC) production occurs only in the bone marrow (medullary hematopoiesis). Extramedullary hematopoiesis is usually a sign of disease. In adults, the marrow in the bones of the skull, vertebrae, ribs, sternum, shoulders, and pelvis produces RBCs. The hematopoietic function of bone continues throughout life. Blood cells are produced to replace those lost through disease, bleeding, and cellular aging. An increase in RBC production can be triggered by anemia, hemorrhage, infection, stress, and other disorders that deplete their stores. Medullary hematopoiesis is accomplished by conversion of yellow marrow to red, increased differentiation of daughter cells, and increased growth of stem cells.

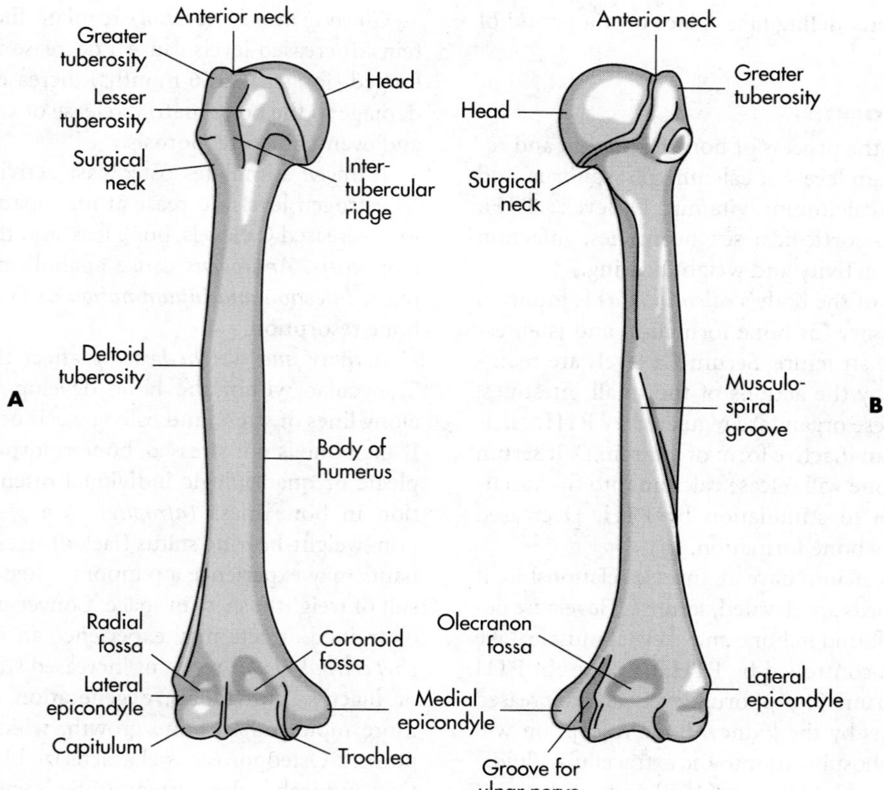


**fig. 59-4** **A,** Anterior view of right humerus. **B,** Posterior view of right humerus. Note groove for ulnar nerve, tuberosities for muscular attachments.

5. *Mineral homeostasis*—bones store calcium, phosphate, carbonate, and magnesium, which are necessary for normal cellular function; approximately 99% of the body's calcium is stored in the skeleton.

## Bone Growth and Remodeling

Longitudinal growth of the long bones emanates from the epiphyseal cartilage, which thickens because of rapid proliferation of the cartilage, and undergoes ossification *(endochondral ossification)*. Growth in the diameter of the bone is accomplished as osteoblasts in the periosteum produce new bone on the outside of the bone *(membranous ossification)*. Bone reaches maturity after puberty.

Bone is continuously being deposited by osteoblasts and continuously being resorbed by active osteoclasts. In the adult, osteoblastic activity occurs on approximately 4% of all surfaces of living bone, resulting in a constant state of bone formation.[1] Osteoclastic activity is present on less than 1% of the bony surfaces of a normal adult.[1]

Except in growing bones, the rate of bone deposition equals the rate of bone destruction until approximately 35 years of age. Thus the total mass of bone remains constant. The value of the equilibrium between bone destruction and formation fulfills some physiologically important functions. Most important, bone responds to the amount of stress to which it is subjected; bone thickens and strengthens itself in response to a heavy load. Secondly, bone can also be reshaped in response to alterations in its mechanical function. These responses are in accordance with Wolff's law (German anatomist 1836-1902): "Every change in form and function of bones or their function alone is followed by definite changes in their external configuration in accordance with mathematical laws." Lastly, in old bone the organic matrix degenerates and the bone becomes weak and brittle; new organic matrix is necessary to maintain the strength and toughness of bone.

*Remodeling* is the process in which existing bone is resorbed and new bone replaces the old. In the first phase (activation), bone cell precursors form osteoclasts in response to a stressor or stimulus. In phase 2 (resorption), masses of osteoclasts form a cutting cone and begin to eat away at the bone for a period of approximately 3 weeks, creating a tunnel or cavity 0.2 to 1 mm in length.[1,3] In cancellous bone this tunnel is parallel to the trabeculae. In cortical bone it follows the longitudinal surface of the haversian system. In phase 3 (formation) the tunnel is then invaded by osteoblasts, and new bone (secondary bone) is laid down in lamellae on the inner surface of the tunnel until it is filled. New bone deposition is complete when the bone begins to encroach on the blood supply of the area. Subsequent lamellae are formed until the tunnel is reduced to a haversian canal around a blood vessel. This process is responsible for the formation of new haversian systems and trabeculae. Areas of new bone are termed *osteons.*

The entire process of remodeling takes place over a period of approximately 4 weeks.

### Influencing Factors

Many factors influence the process of bone formation and resorption, including serum levels of calcium, phosphorus, and alkaline phosphatase; calcitonin; vitamin D levels; PTH; growth hormone; glucocorticoids; sex hormones; infection and inflammation; and activity and weight bearing.

Approximately 99% of the body's *calcium (Ca)* is found in bone. Calcium is necessary for bone formation and is an essential element in bone structure. Serum Ca levels are maintained in homeostasis by the actions of the small intestines, bones, and kidneys. These organs are regulated by PTH, calcitonin, and vitamin $D_1$, an inactive form of vitamin D. If serum Ca levels are low, the bone will release calcium into the vascular system in response to stimulation by PTH. Decreased serum levels of Ca delay bone formation.

*Phosphorus (P)* and calcium have an inverse relationship. If serum levels of phosphorus are elevated, serum Ca levels are decreased. Phosphorus is found in bone and skeletal muscle. Like calcium, phosphorus is controlled by PTH. Increases in PTH cause a decrease in serum phosphorus levels and increased excretion of phosphorus by the kidney. Bone resorption will result in the release of phosphorus into the extracellular fluid.

The enzyme *alkaline phosphatase (ALP)* is found in osteoblasts. It is excreted via the biliary tract and is necessary for the utilization of mineral salts and bone formation. Levels of ALP rise in response to increased osteoblastic activity in the bones (e.g., during fracture healing).

*Calcitonin* is a hormone produced and secreted primarily by the thyroid gland. Calcitonin inhibits bone resorption, inhibits Ca absorption from the gastrointestinal tract, and increases Ca and P excretion from the kidneys.

*Vitamin D* is derived from the action of ultraviolet light on provitamins found in the skin and from vitamin D–enriched foods. Vitamin D is activated in the liver and kidneys through the action of PTH. The activated form, calcitrol, is a hormone necessary for calcium absorption. Activated vitamin D elevates Ca and phosphate levels in the plasma by increasing intestinal absorption of calcium and phosphate and by increasing the release of calcium from bone into the blood. Vitamin D deficiencies can manifest themselves as rickets in children and osteomalacia in adults.

*Parathyroid hormone*, or parathormone, produced by the parathyroid gland, controls serum Ca and phosphorus levels. Decreased serum Ca levels are the stimulus for release of more PTH to keep the serum Ca levels normal. In conjunction with vitamin D, PTH works to stimulate absorption of calcium and phosphorus by the intestinal mucosa. It also causes mobilization of Ca from the bones by promoting osteoclastic activity and bone resorption.

*Growth hormone (GH)* is secreted by the anterior lobe of the pituitary gland and promotes the growth of bone and other tissue. Decreased levels of GH are manifested as dwarfism. Increased levels of GH in children result in gigantism; increased levels of GH in adults result in acromegaly. (See Chapter 34.)

*Glucocorticoids (cortisol)* regulate the metabolism of proteins. Increased levels cause a decrease in protein stores. Prolonged (longer than 6 months) increased levels may result in damage to the bone matrix, release of calcium from the bone, and eventually osteoporosis.

*Estrogen* stimulates osteoblast activity and inhibits PTH. As estrogen levels decrease at menopause, women are at risk for decreased Ca levels, bone loss, and the development of osteoporosis. *Androgens* cause anabolism and increased bone mass. *Infection and inflammation* can cause lysis of bone and bone resorption.

*Activity and weight bearing* affect the structure of bone. Trabeculae within the bone develop and align themselves along lines of stress, and osteogenesis occurs along those lines. If the bone is not stressed, bone resorption occurs. The paraplegic or quadriplegic individual often experiences a reduction in bone mass *(atrophy)* as a result of inactivity and non–weight-bearing status (lack of stress) on the bone. Astronauts may experience a temporary loss of bone mass as a result of weightlessness in space. Conversely, a marathon runner or trained athlete may experience an increase in bony mass *(hypertrophy)* as a result of increased stress on bones. In older or inactive individuals, degeneration and resorption occur more rapidly than bone growth, which may lead to osteoporosis. Osteoporosis is characterized by thin, weakened cortices and trabeculae. Osteoporotic bones are more susceptible to fractures.

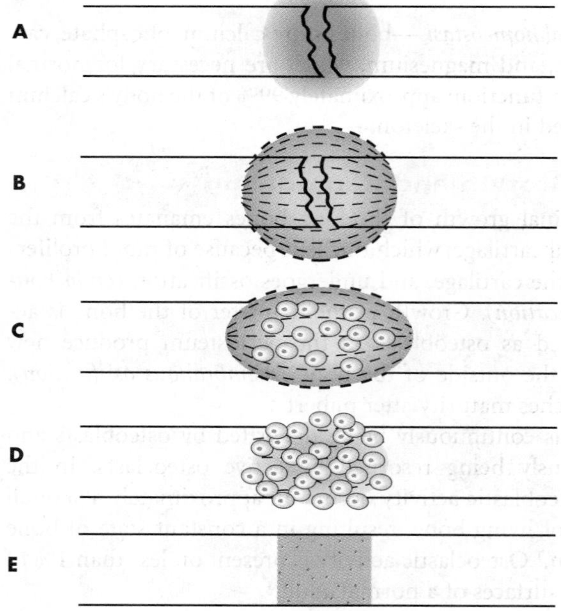


**fig. 59-5** Bone healing (schematic representation). **A,** Bleeding at broken ends of the bone with subsequent hematoma formation. **B,** Organization of hematoma into fibrous network. **C,** Invasion of osteoblasts, lengthening of collagen strands, and deposition of calcium. **D,** Callus formation: new bone is built up as osteoclasts destroy dead bone. **E,** Remodeling is accomplished as excess callus is reabsorbed and trabecular bone is laid down.

### Physiology of Bone Healing

Bone heals by a process termed *callus formation*. Fractures and surgical disruption of bone both heal by the same process. New growth of bone is called a *callus*. Callus formation proceeds in five general stages (Figure 59-5):

1. *Hematoma formation.* Because bone is highly vascular, bleeding occurs at both ends of the fractured bone. Increased capillary permeability permits further extravasation of blood into the injured area. Blood collects in the periosteal sheath or adjacent tissues and fastens the broken ends together.
2. *Fibrin meshwork formation.* Fibroblasts invade the hematoma, forming a fibrin meshwork. White blood cells (WBCs) wall off the area, localizing the inflammation.
3. *Invasion by osteoblasts.* As osteoblasts invade the fibrous union to make it firm, blood vessels develop from capillary buds, thereby establishing a supply for nutrients to build collagen. Granulation tissue, or procallus is formed. Collagen strands become longer and begin to incorporate calcium deposits. Cartilage is formed, and bone morphogenic proteins are present in this stage.
4. *Callus formation.* Osteoblasts form woven bone, known as callus. Osteoblasts continue to lay the network for bone buildup as osteoclasts destroy dead bone and help synthesize new bone. Collagen strengthens and becomes further impregnated with calcium. Calcium and phosphate are deposited as mineral salts. Lamellar or trabecular bone continues to replace the callus.
5. *Remodeling.* Excess callus is reabsorbed, and trabecular bone is laid down along lines of stress in accordance with Wolff's law. Remodeling is an important stage because bone that has not undergone remodeling lacks the mechanical properties necessary for weight bearing.

Factors impeding callus formation are (1) inadequate reduction of the fracture, (2) excessive edema at the fracture site impeding the supply of nutrients to the area, (3) too much bone lost at the time of injury to permit sufficient bridging of the broken ends, (4) inefficient immobilization, (5) infection at the site of injury, (6) bone necrosis, (7) anemia or other systemic conditions, (8) endocrine imbalance, and (9) poor dietary intake. If callus formation does not occur normally and efficiently, the resulting lack of repair is termed *nonunion*, or an *ununited fracture* (See Chapter 60).

## MUSCLES

### Types

Muscles are divided into three major groups:

1. Visceral (smooth, involuntary)
2. Cardiac
3. Skeletal (striated, voluntary, extrafusal)

*Visceral muscle,* such as that in the blood vessels, stomach, and intestines, is innervated by the autonomic nervous system. Therefore visceral muscle is not under voluntary control.

The *cardiac muscle* found in the myocardium has the properties of automaticity, rhythm, and conductivity. The cardiac conduction system and the autonomic nervous system exert control over cardiac muscle.

*Skeletal muscle* accounts for 45% to 50% of an average adult's body weight (Figures 59-6 and 59-7). Muscle is 75% water, 20% protein, and 5% organic and inorganic compounds. Muscle contains 32% of all protein stores necessary for energy and metabolism.[2] Skeletal muscle is innervated by nerve fibers from the cerebrospinal system and can be controlled by will.

The body has approximately 350 skeletal muscles, most in pairs.[2] The function of a muscle determines its shape. Muscle length varies greatly, from 2 to 60 cm. *Fusiform* muscles are elongated and run from one joint to another—for example, the quadriceps, which extends the knee. *Pennate* muscles are broad and flat. Their muscle fibers run obliquely to the muscle's long axis. The deltoid is an example of a pennate muscle.

### Structure

Each skeletal muscle is covered with a layered connective tissue called fascia. The *epimysium,* or outer layer, tapers at each end to form the tendon, which allows joint mobility. The middle layer, or *perimysium,* divides the muscle fibers into fascicles, or bundles of connective tissue. The *endomysium,* or inner layer, is the smallest unit of fibers and surrounds the fascicles[3] (Figure 59-8).

Skeletal muscles are contained within a membrane, the *sarcolemma,* which contains the sarcoplasm or cytoplasm. The sarcolemma can transmit electrical impulses and plays a role in protein synthesis and nutrient supply. Sarcoplasm is similar to cytoplasm and contains proteins and enzymes necessary for the cell's energy production, protein synthesis, and oxygen storage. Small, closely packed fibers (called *myofibrils*) within the sarcoplasm alternate light and dark horizontal stripes and produce the striated appearance that lends this type of muscle its name. The myofibril is the functional unit of muscle contraction. The dark stripes are *A bands,* and the light stripes are *I bands.* Light bands crossing the middle of the dark stripes are called the *H zone,* and dark lines crossing the middle of the light stripes are called *Z lines.* Myofibrils consist of several sections called *sarcomeres* that contain actin and myosin, which are contractile proteins. Each sarcomere is a section that extends from one Z line of a myofibril to the next (Figure 59-9, p. 1890). Bundles of muscle fibers (cells) make up the muscle itself. Glycogen is present in muscle as an energy source.

### Function

Skeletal muscle provides controlled movement and maintains posture. Movement is accomplished by muscle contractions and work production. Muscular contraction is a complex process triggered by nerve impulses arriving at the muscle fiber. Calcium ions, released when the impulse is received, bind to troponin (an inhibitor of the molecular myosin-actin interaction). Once troponin is bound, the myosin-actin interaction takes place, and the sarcomeres of the myofibrils contract. This is known as the *cross-bridge theory,* which replaced the sliding filament theory described by Huxley.[2] The energy for muscle contraction is supplied by the breakdown of adenosine triphosphate (ATP), a substance muscle cells produce by combining adenosine diphosphate (ADP) with

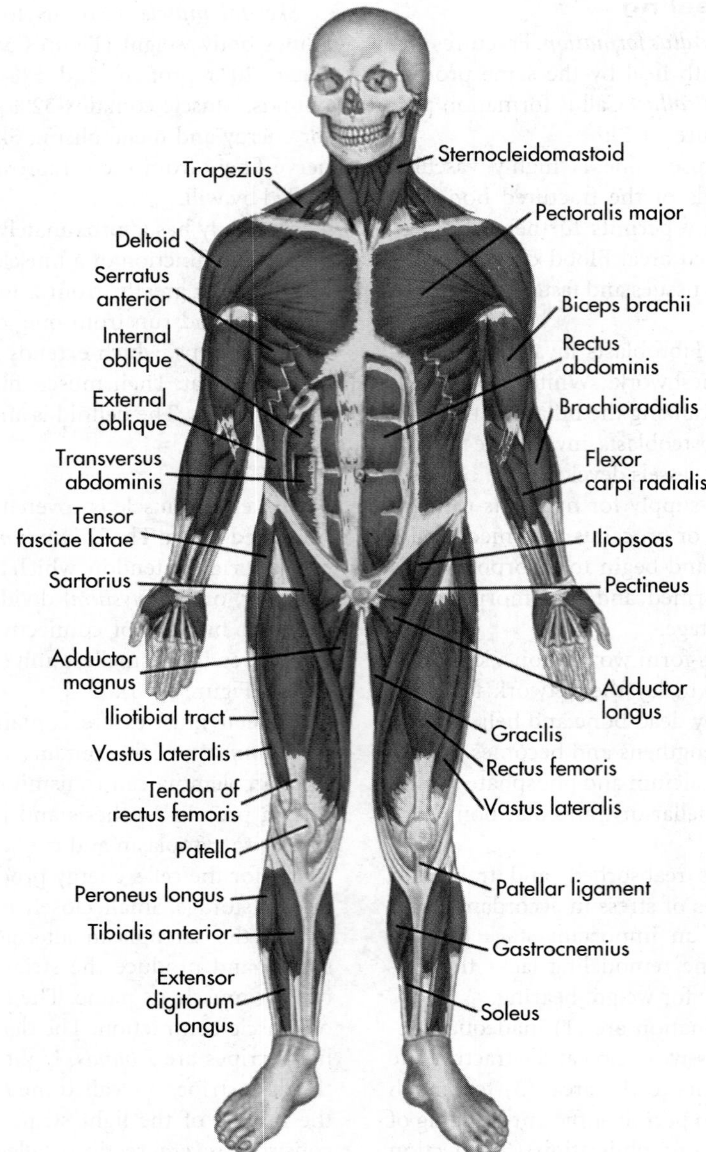


**fig. 59-6** Skeletal muscles of body, anterior view.

creatine phosphate. Relaxation of the muscle occurs when the calcium separates from the troponin[5] (Figure 59-10, p. 1891).

Muscle cells obey the "all or none" law; that is, they contract fully or not at all. This does not mean that the entire muscle contracts fully. Only those individual cells that receive the nerve impulse contract. Adequately oxygenated muscle fibers contract more forcefully than those inadequately oxygenated.

### Types of Contractions

The arrangement of the fibers within the muscle determines the capacity of the forceful contraction of the muscle. Skeletal muscles contract only if they are stimulated. There are many types of contractions:[5]

1. *Tonic:* a continual partial contraction that is vital in maintenance of posture
2. *Isotonic:* a contraction in which tension within the muscle is constant but the length of the muscle changes; can either shorten (concentric contraction) or lengthen (eccentric); examples of concentric contractions: lifting weights or climbing upstairs; eccentric contraction: going down stairs or putting down a weight; eccentric contraction uses less energy and results in pain and stiffness following unaccustomed exercise[2]
3. *Isometric (static or holding):* tension within the muscle increases, but the muscle does not shorten
4. *Twitch:* a jerky reaction to a single stimulus
5. *Tetanic:* a more sustained contraction than the twitch, produced by a series of stimuli in rapid succession
6. *Spasm:* an involuntary contraction caused by stimulation of an entire motor unit
7. *Treppe:* stronger twitch contractions in response to regularly repeated, constant-strength stimuli
8. *Fibrillation:* a synchronous contraction of individual fibers

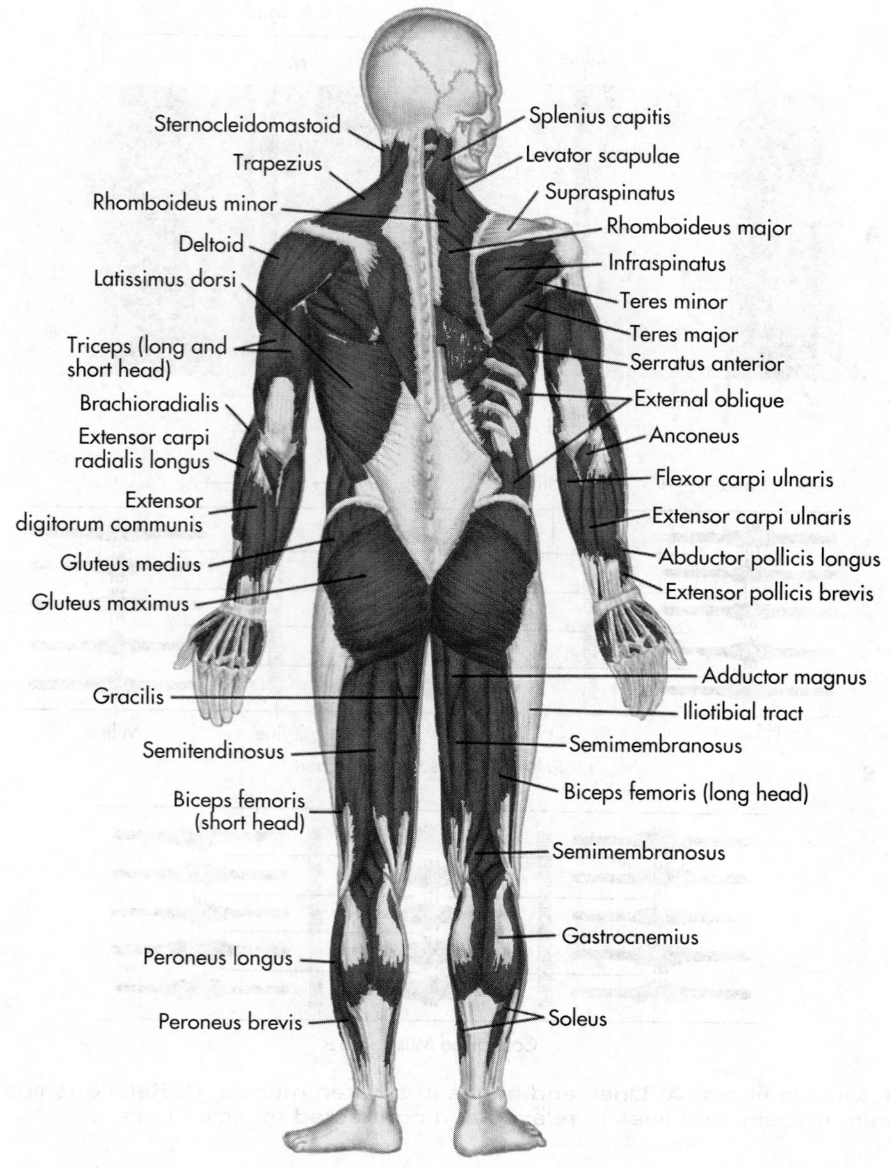


**fig. 59-7** Skeletal muscles of body, posterior view.

9. *Convulsive:* abnormal uncoordinated tetanic contractions occurring in varying groups of muscles

## Mechanism of Muscle Movement

Movements of the body are produced by muscles pulling on bones; the bones serve as levers, and the joints serve as fulcrums for the levers. Most movements depend on several muscles acting in a coordinated manner. To produce movement a muscle acts as a *prime mover,* or *agonist,* as its reciprocal muscle, or *antagonist,* relaxes. *Synergistic* muscles contract at the same time as the prime movers, either to produce the movement or to stabilize a body part so that contraction of the prime movers is more efficient.[5]

## Muscle Metabolism

Energy for a muscle contraction can be generated both aerobically and anaerobically. The two anaerobic processes are called

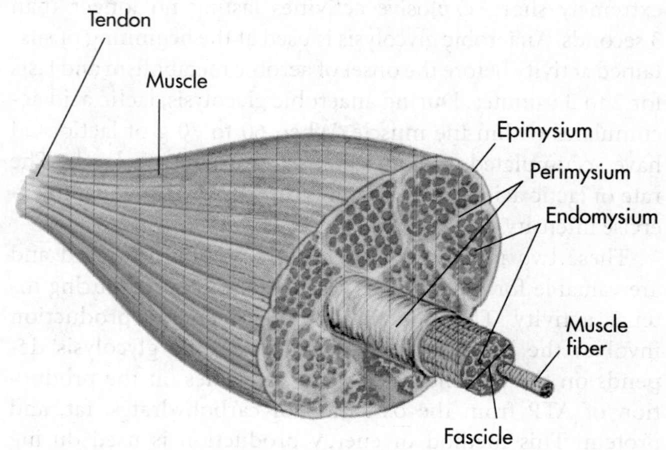


**fig. 59-8** Cross section of skeletal muscle showing muscle fibers and their coverings.

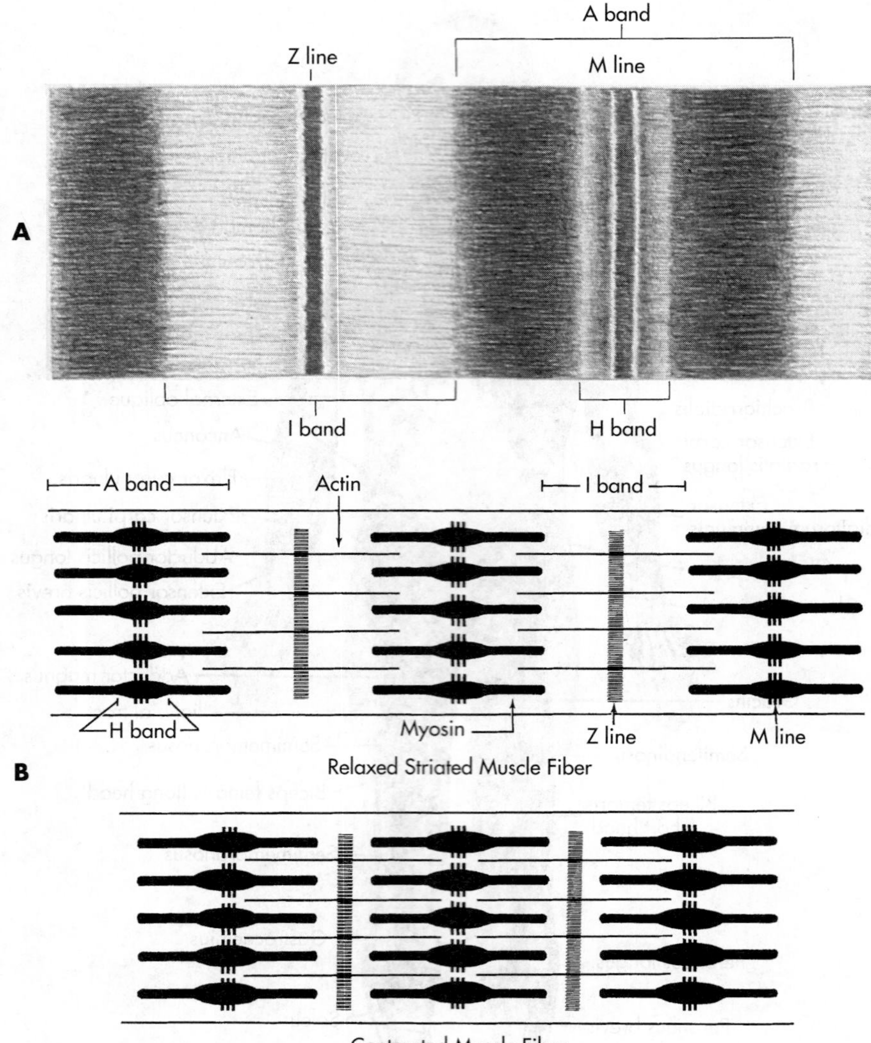


**fig. 59-9** Muscle fibers. **A,** Lines and bands in striated muscle. **B,** Relationships of bands, actin, myosin, and lines in relaxed and contracted muscle fibers.

the ATP-PC (adenosine triphospage-phosphocreatinine) system and anaerobic glycolysis. The ATP-PC system is used for extremely short, explosive activities lasting no longer than 3 seconds. Anaerobic glycolysis is used at the beginning of sustained activity before the onset of aerobic metabolism and lasts for 2 to 3 minutes. During anaerobic glycolysis, lactic acid accumulates within the muscle. When 60 to 70 g of lactic acid have accumulated, the muscle reaches exhaustive levels. The rate of lactic acid accumulation is directly proportional to exercise intensity.

These two methods of energy production are rapid and are valuable for quick bursts of energy to be used during intense activity. The aerobic method of energy production involves the burning of foodstuffs. Aerobic glycolysis depends on the presence of oxygen and relies on the production of ATP from the oxidation of carbohydrates, fat, and protein. This method of energy production is used during prolonged activity.

Efficient muscle contraction depends on an adequate blood supply to and from the muscle fibers. Therefore skeletal muscle is highly vascular. Waste products resulting from the chemical changes that occur during muscle contraction must be transported to the liver to be resynthesized. When waste products are not adequately carried off, muscle fatigue and pain result. Conversely, oxygen must be transported to the muscle fibers to support the work of muscle contraction. Poor muscle work occurs when the oxygen supply is inadequate—for example, in conditions such as anemia, in which the amount of oxygen-carrying hemoglobin is reduced, or trauma, in which circulation to the muscle fibers is interrupted.

## Muscle Innervation

Adequate muscle contraction also depends on effective innervation. The cerebellum is primarily responsible for control of muscle movement (see Chapter 51). Every muscle cell is sup-

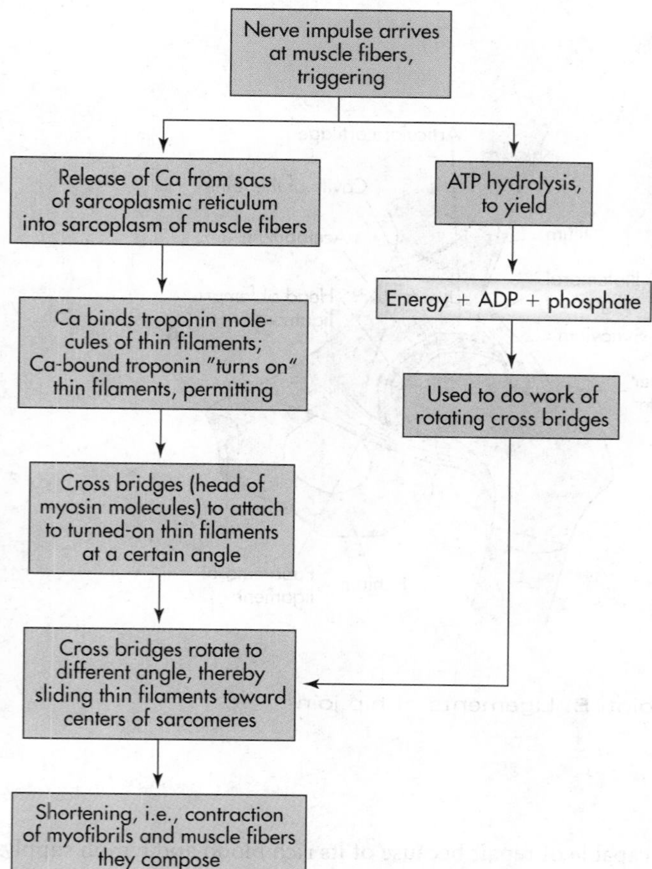


**fig. 59-10** Mechanism of skeletal muscle contraction.

plied with the axon of a nerve cell. Nerve cells that transmit impulses to skeletal muscles are known as somatic motor neurons. The neuron and the muscle cell it activates are called a *motor unit.* The number of motor units per muscle varies significantly. The motor units, made up of lower motor neurons, extend to the skeletal muscle. The axon of one somatic motor neuron may be divided into any number of branches and therefore innervates a like number of muscle cells. The fewer muscle cells innervated, the more precise (or fine) are the resultant movements.

The actual contraction of the muscle is set off by the release of acetylcholine, a chemical contained in small vesicles in the axon terminal. When acetylcholine contracts the sarcolemma, it stimulates the contraction. This reaction takes place across a structure known as the *motor end plate* or *neuromuscular junction,* where the muscle and the nerve are in contact. Damage to the nervous system at the cerebrospinal level or at any point in the nerve's course through the local motor neuron level will result in muscular dysfunction.

## CARTILAGE

Cartilage is composed of fibers embedded in a firm gel. Structurally, cartilage is a strong but flexible material and is avascular. Nutrients reach the cartilage cells by diffusion through the gel from capillaries located in the *perichondrium* (fibrous covering of the cartilage) or, in the case of articular cartilage, through the synovial fluid. Articular cartilage is hyaline cartilage that covers the articulating surface on the ends of bones. The amount or thickness depends on the type of bone and amount of weight and shearing force to which the joint is subjected.

The number of collagenous fibers found in the cartilage determines its type: fibrous, hyaline, or elastic. *Fibrous* cartilage (or fibrocartilage) composes the intervertebral disks. *Hyaline* cartilage is composed of chondrocytes (cartilage cells), type II collagen fibers in the matrix, and protein polysaccharide complexes and water between the matrix and fibers. Its composition gives hyaline cartilage its spongy and elastic qualities, which are crucial to preventing injury to the bone during weight bearing. Articular cartilage reduces friction in the joint and helps distribute weight bearing. Articular cartilage contains 60% to 80% water.[3]

Articular cartilage does not contain any blood vessels, lymph tissue, or nerves. As a result, it is insensitive to pain and does not easily repair itself following injury. Regeneration occurs at the junction of the synovial membrane and cartilage, because of the adjacent blood supply and nutrients supplying the synovial membrane.

Yellow or *elastic* cartilage has the fewest fibers. Elastic cartilage may be found in areas such as the external ear and epiglottis.

## LIGAMENTS

Ligaments are parallel bands of dense fibrous connective tissue that are flexible and tough. They connect the articular ends of bones and provide stability. Ligaments permit movement in some directions but limit movement in others, preventing joint injury. Examples are the medial and lateral collateral ligaments of the knee, which provide mediolateral stability to the knee joint, and the anterior and posterior cruciate ligaments within the joint capsule of the knee, which provide anteroposterior stability (Figure 59-11). Ligaments may also attach to soft tissue to suspend structures, for example, the suspensory ligament of the ovary that passes from the tubal end of the ovary to the peritoneum.

## TENDONS

Tendons are bands of dense fibrous tissue that form the origin and insertion of a muscle to a bone (Figure 59-12). The longitudinal arrangement of fibers gives tendons their tensile strength while preventing tendon damage. The tendon is an extension of the fibrous sheath that envelops each muscle and is continuous with the periosteum at its other end. *Tendon sheaths* are tubular structures of connective tissue that enclose certain tendons, especially in the wrist and ankle. These sheaths are lined with a synovial membrane, which provides lubrication (synovial fluid) for each movement of the tendon. Ligaments and tendons may add extra stability to the capsule. The synovial membrane, or synovium, lines the nonarticulating surfaces of the joint capsule. The synovium is

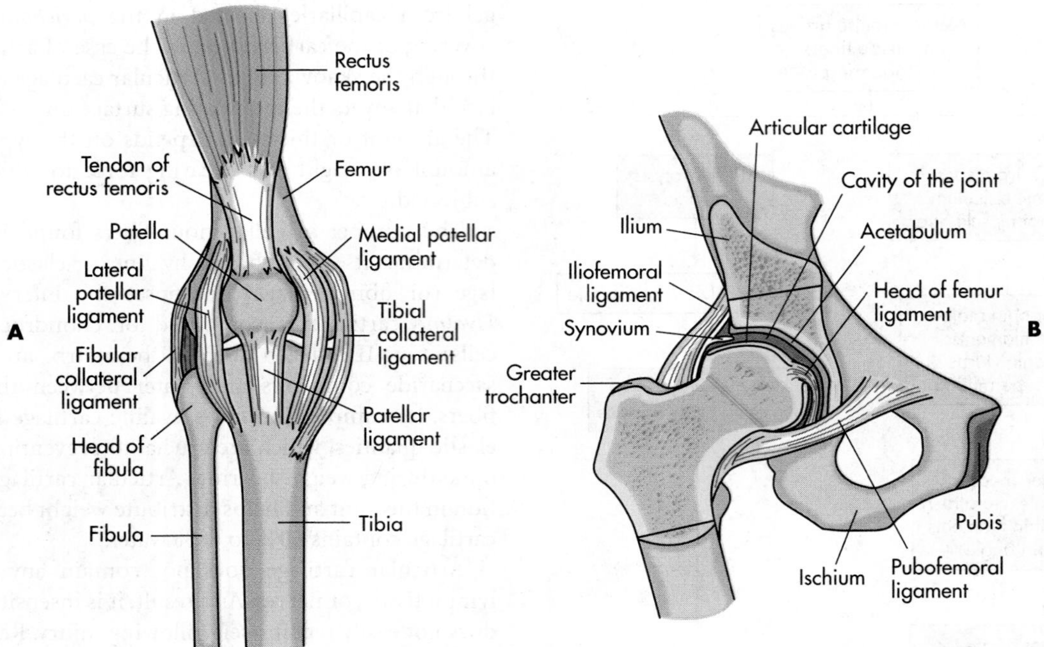


fig. 59-11 A, Ligaments of knee joint. B, Ligaments of hip joint.

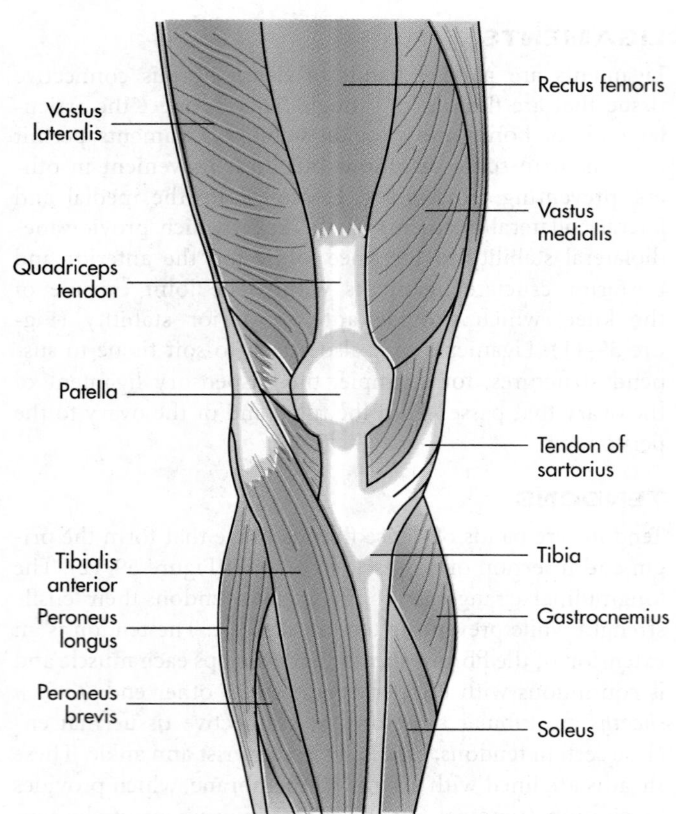


fig. 59-12 Anterior view of tendons around knee joint.

capable of repair because of its rich blood and lymph supply. The synovial membrane secretes synovial fluid into the joint capsule to lubricate the joint (Figure 59-13). Synovial fluid is plasma derived from blood vessels in the synovium. In addition to joint lubrication, *synovial fluid* provides nourishment to articular cartilage and contains leukocytes that have a phagocytic action on bacteria and debris in the joint. A decrease in synovial fluid can lead to destruction of the articular cartilage.

## FASCIA

Fascia is a sheet of loose connective tissue that may be found directly under the skin as superficial fascia or as a sheet of dense, fibrous connective tissue making up the sheath of muscles, nerves, and blood vessels. The latter is known as deep fascia.

## BURSAE

Bursae are small sacs of connective tissue located wherever pressure is exerted over moving parts. They may, for example, occur between skin and bone, between tendons and bone, or between muscles. Bursae are lined with synovial membrane and contain synovial fluid. They serve as cushions between moving parts. One such bursa, the olecranon bursa, is located between the olecranon process and the skin. New bursae can develop as a result of prolonged or increased pressure or friction, often resulting in pain. The shoulder bursa (subacromial) is a common site of bursitis (Figure 59-14).

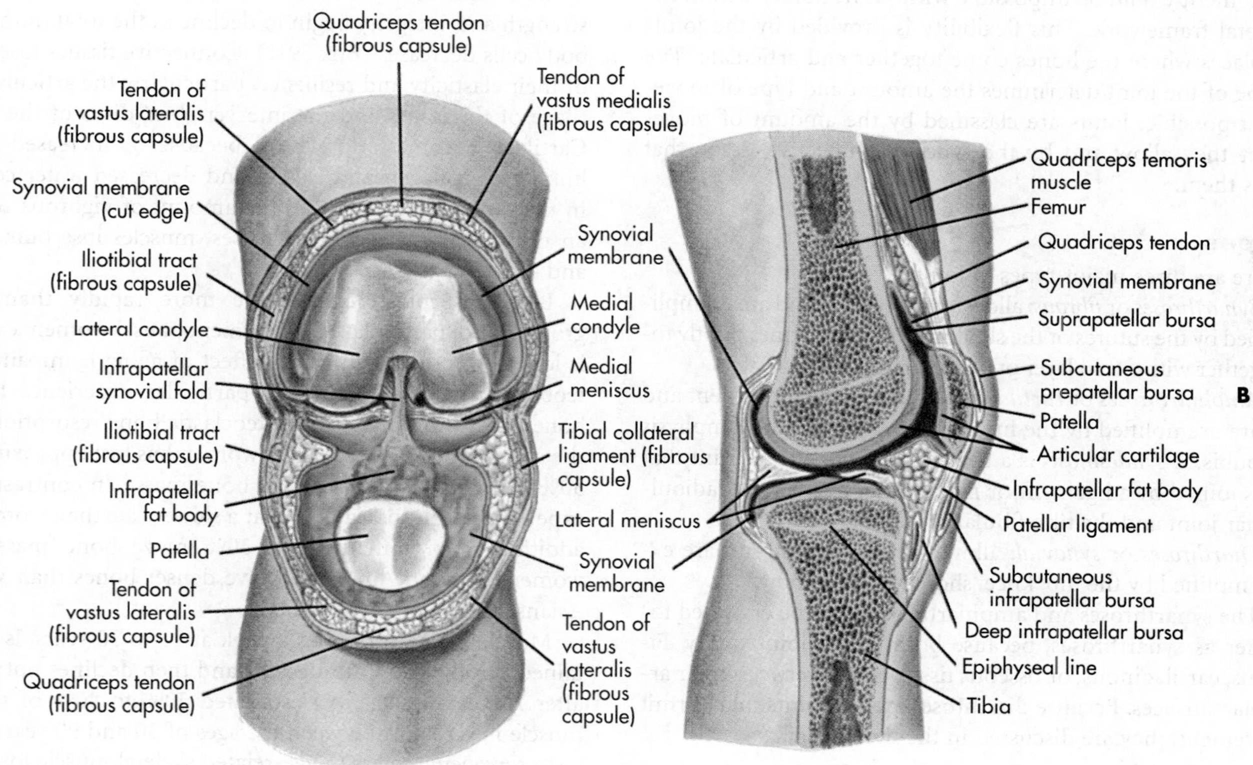
Quadriceps tendon (fibrous capsule)
Tendon of vastus lateralis (fibrous capsule)
Tendon of vastus medialis (fibrous capsule)
Synovial membrane (cut edge)
Synovial membrane
Iliotibial tract (fibrous capsule)
Medial condyle
Lateral condyle
Medial meniscus
Infrapatellar synovial fold
A
Iliotibial tract (fibrous capsule)
Tibial collateral ligament (fibrous capsule)
Infrapatellar fat body
Patella
Synovial membrane
Tendon of vastus lateralis (fibrous capsule)
Tendon of vastus lateralis (fibrous capsule)
Quadriceps tendon (fibrous capsule)
Quadriceps femoris muscle
Femur
Quadriceps tendon
Synovial membrane
Suprapatellar bursa
Subcutaneous prepatellar bursa
B
Patella
Articular cartilage
Infrapatellar fat body
Lateral meniscus
Patellar ligament
Subcutaneous infrapatellar bursa
Deep infrapatellar bursa
Epiphyseal line
Tibia

**fig. 59-13** Knee joint (synovial joint). **A,** Frontal view. **B,** Lateral view.

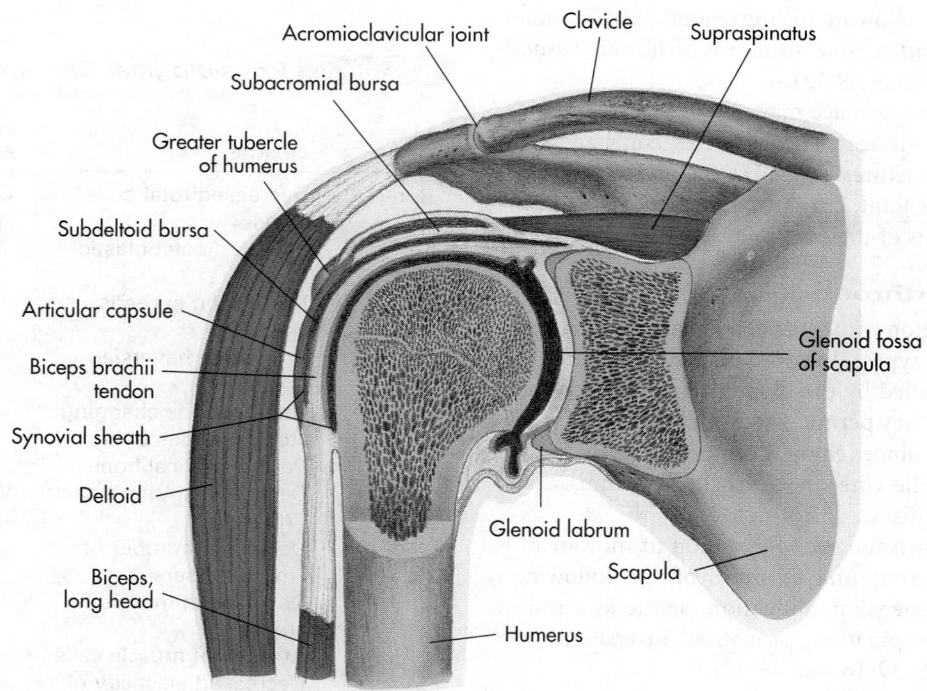
Acromioclavicular joint
Clavicle
Supraspinatus
Subacromial bursa
Greater tubercle of humerus
Subdeltoid bursa
Articular capsule
Biceps brachii tendon
Glenoid fossa of scapula
Synovial sheath
Deltoid
Glenoid labrum
Scapula
Biceps, long head
Humerus

**fig. 59-14** Shoulder joint bursae.

## JOINTS

Movement would be impossible without flexibility within the skeletal framework. This flexibility is provided by the joints or places where the bones come together and articulate. The shape of the joint determines the amount and type of movement possible. Joints are classified by the amount of movement they allow and by the type of connective tissue that joins them.

### Types

There are three major types of joints:

1. *Synarthroses* or *fibrous:* allow no movement and are exemplified by the sutures of the skull. Sutures bind bones tightly together with a thin layer of dense fibrous tissue.
2. *Amphiarthroses* or *cartilaginous:* allow little movement and are exemplified by the intervertebral joints and symphysis pubis. A *syndesmosis* is a type of amphiarthrotic joint that is joined by a ligament or membrane, such as the radioulnar joint and the tibiofibular joint.
3. *Diarthroses* or *synovial*: allow free movement and are exemplified by the hip, knee, shoulder, and elbow.

The synarthroses and amphiarthroses may be classified together as synarthroses, because both lack a joint cavity. Fibrous, cartilaginous, or osseous tissue grows between their articular surfaces. Because diarthroses are the joints that permit movement, they are discussed in the most detail.

#### Structure of Diarthrodial Joints

Each diarthrodial joint contains a small space, or *joint cavity,* between the articulating surfaces of the bones that make up the joint. Articular hyaline cartilage covers the articulating surfaces of both bones, allowing for the smooth, gliding motion of the joint. A *joint capsule,* or sleeve of fibrous tissue, encases the joint (see Figure 59-13).

Small pieces of dense cartilage may also be interposed between the articulating surfaces. These are crescent shaped or half moon–shaped structures *(menisci)* that provide additional cushioning of the joint. Examples are the medial meniscus and lateral meniscus of the knee joint.

#### Function of Diarthrodial Joints

Joints provide the skeleton with both stability and mobility. In addition to the joint types already described, diarthrodial joints are further classified by the shape of their surface and the type of movement they permit. Examples include ball and socket (shoulder, hip), hinge (elbow, knee), pivot (atlas, axis), condyloid (wrist), saddle (first metacarpal, trapezium), and gliding (intervertebral disks).

Each joint has its own range and direction of movement. Diarthrodial joints permit one or more of the following movements: flexion, extension, abduction, adduction, rotation, circumduction, supination, pronation, inversion, and eversion (Figures 59-15, 59-16, and 59-17).

## PHYSIOLOGICAL CHANGES WITH AGING

Physiological changes occur in the musculoskeletal system throughout a person's life span. Childhood and adolescence are a time of rapid growth and development of the structures of the system. However, at maturity and into older age, tissue strength and integrity begin to decline as the total number of body cells decreases (Box 59-1). Connective tissues lose some of their elasticity and resilience, particularly the articular cartilage of the joints and the intervertebral disks of the spine. Cartilage becomes more rigid because of increased cross-linking of collagen and elastin and decreased water content in the ground substance. As the amount of vigorous activity an individual engages in decreases, muscles lose bulk, tone, and strength.

Bone resorption takes place more rapidly than bone growth, and, particularly in postmenopausal women, calcium is lost from bone. A universal effect of aging is impaired osteoblastic activity. Women in particular experience loss of bone density and increased osteoclastic bone resorption with the aging process. By age 70, a woman has lost approximately 50% of her peripheral cortical bone mass.[3] In contrast, men experience bone loss later and at a slower rate than women. In addition, men initially have 30% more bone mass than women.[3] African Americans have denser bones than whites, Asians, and Native Americans.

Muscle strength reaches a peak at 25 to 30 years, is maintained through the fifth decade, and then declines noticeably after 70 years of age. An estimated 30% to 40% of skeletal muscle mass is lost between the ages of 30 and 90 years.[2] The term *sarcopenia* refers to age-related skeletal muscle loss.[3]

Regular exercise (such as walking or swimming) and a nutritionally adequate diet can help reduce the loss of muscle mass and bone density associated with aging. With age the

**box 59-1** *Physiological Changes with Aging*

| TISSUE | CHANGE | POTENTIAL PROBLEM |
|---|---|---|
| Bone | Decreased total bone mass<br>Impaired osteoblastic activity<br>Resorption exceeds growth<br>Erosion of haversian systems<br>Cortical bone changing to cancellous bone<br>Porous cortical bone | Osteoporosis, pathologic fracture, delayed healing |
| Muscles | Decline in strength past 70 years<br>Decline in number of muscle fibers<br>Decrease in muscle mass<br>Atrophy of muscle cells | Weakness, uncoordination, disuse atrophy, slow unsteady gait, poor posture, falls, contractures |
| Joints | Decreased elasticity of cartilage<br>Increased susceptibility to tears in cartilage | Arthritis, decreased range of motion contractures |

shoulders may become stooped and narrower. The knees and hips may be slightly flexed when standing or walking because of pain associated with joint degeneration. Posture becomes stooped as the body attempts to compensate for changes in the center of gravity caused by lower extremity joint flexion and forward thrusting of the head, neck, and shoulders. With these changes, height decreases 6 to 10 cm. Gait may become unsteady because of loss of muscle strength and coordination, and the individual is more susceptible to falls. An estimated one third of persons 65 years and older experience falls annually.[2] Of this number, 2% are hospitalized as a result. Falls are common in nursing homes; an estimated 50% of nursing home residents fall each year. Falls are the number one cause of accidental death in the elderly.[2]

In summary, aging affects the musculoskeletal system (see the Gerontological Assessment Box, p. 1898). Approximately 40% of elderly persons living in the community have arthritis, and 17% report chronic problems of the musculoskeletal system. Independence and the ability to perform activities of daily living (ADL) are commonly affected. Although diseases of the musculoskeletal system are not usually fatal, they do cause chronic pain and disability.[2] However, complications arising as a result of a musculoskeletal problem can be fatal.

Programs of regular exercise (including weight-bearing activities) and resistive muscle strengthening can decrease or prevent some of the age-related changes in the musculoskeletal system.[2] A nutritionally adequate diet is also beneficial.

## SUBJECTIVE DATA

Plans for the care of any person with a musculoskeletal problem are based on a systematic assessment of needs, capabilities, and resources. A thorough assessment includes subjective data gathered from patient and family interviews.

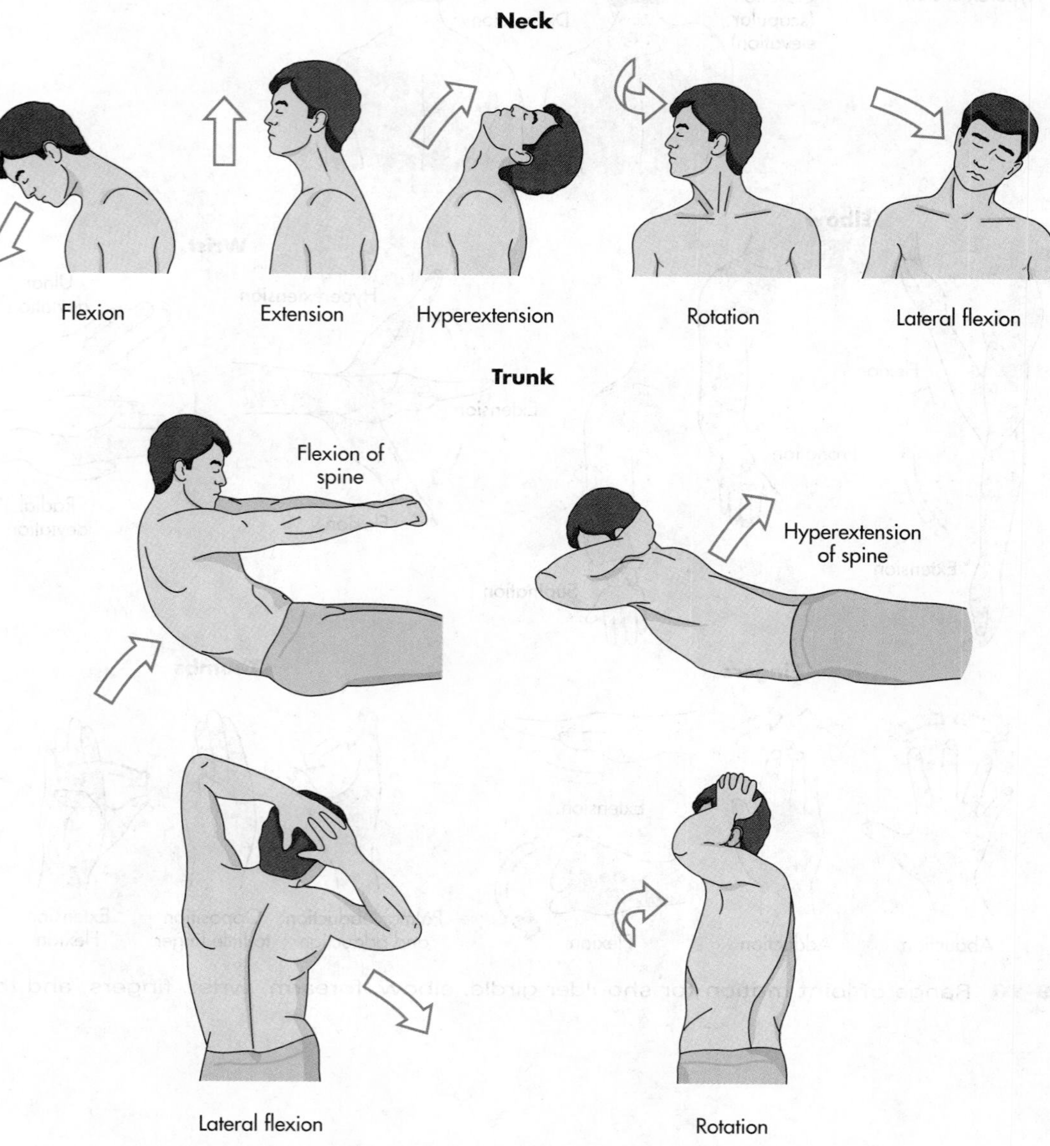


**fig. 59-15** Range of motion for neck and trunk.

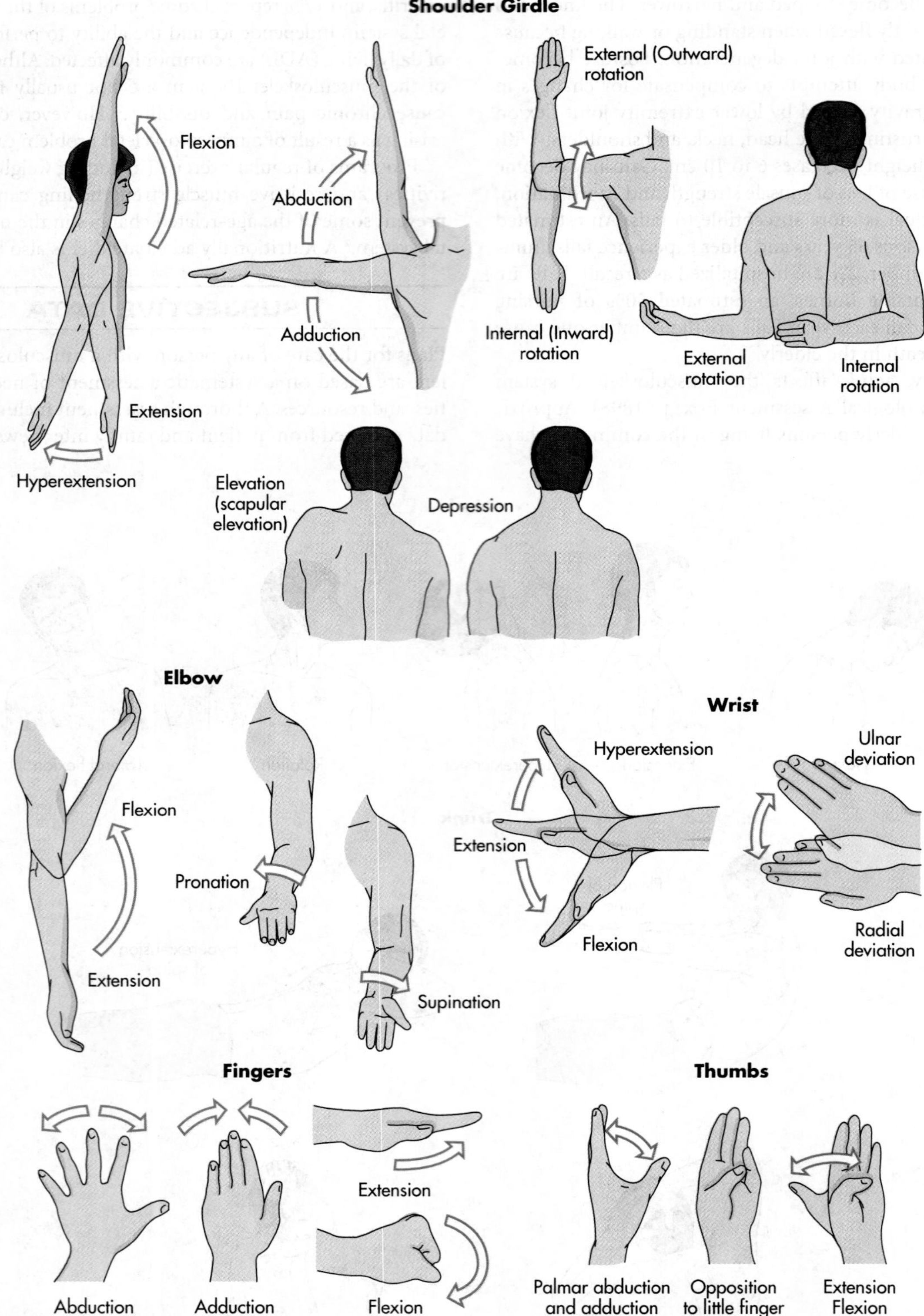


**fig. 59-16** Range of joint motion for shoulder girdle, elbow, forearm, wrist, fingers, and thumbs.

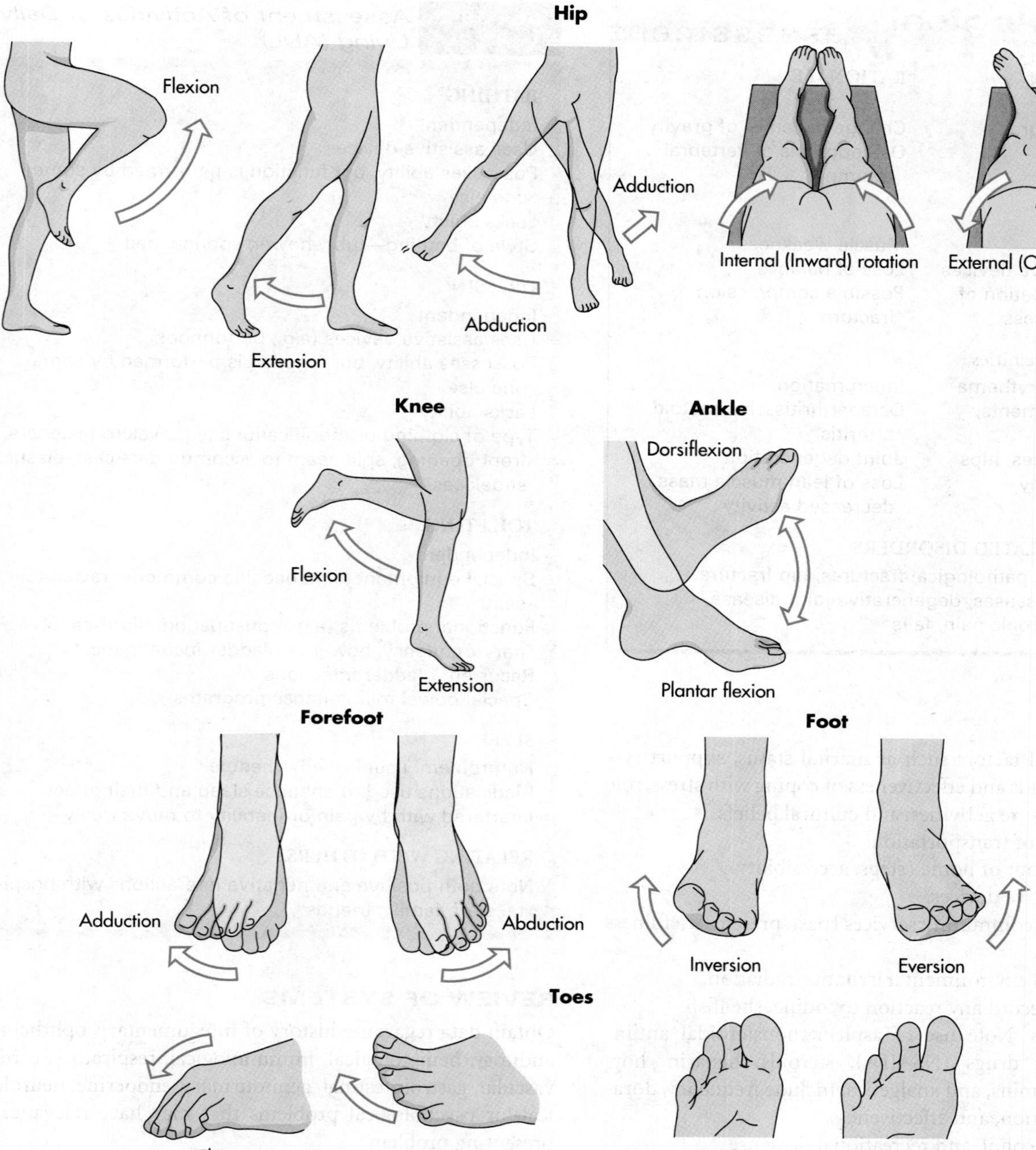


**fig. 59-17** Range of joint motion for hip, knee, ankle, foot, and toes.

## GENERAL HISTORY

Interview the person, gathering the following data:

1. Age. Age can be a predictor of common problems associated with a particular age-group. For example, the elderly are susceptible to falls, older women have an increased risk of osteoporosis, and young men are at a higher risk for trauma.
2. Height and weight. Any changes? If so, were they intentional? What is the person's ideal weight and body mass index? Any loss of height, particularly in the elderly?
3. Nutrition. Dietary intake of calcium, vitamin D, minerals, total calories, fad diets?
4. Occupation (past, present). Sedentary, standing, repetitive movements, safety factors, lifting, ergonomic environment?
5. Exercise regimen. Type, frequency, duration, weight-bearing activity, safety equipment, type of shoes, warm-up, cool-down activities?
6. Ability to perform ADL (Box 59-2), use of adaptive devices.
7. Transfer ability.

## gerontological assessment

| OBSERVATION | RATIONALE |
|---|---|
| **General** | |
| Stooped posture | Change in center of gravity |
| Kyphosis | Osteoporosis of vertebral column |
| **Gait** | |
| Unsteady | Muscle weakness |
| Use of assistive devices | Loss of balance |
| Pain with palpation of spinous process | Possible compression fracture |
| **Joints and Extremities** | |
| Tenderness, erythema | Inflammation |
| Body enlargements, deformities | Osteoarthritis, rheumatoid arthritis |
| Flexion of knees, hips | Joint degeneration |
| Muscle atrophy | Loss of lean muscle mass, decreased activity |

**COMMON RELATED DISORDERS**

Osteoporosis, pathological fractures, hip fracture, rheumatic diseases, degenerative joint disease, kyphosis, chronic pain, falls

8. Psychosocial factors such as marital status, support systems, methods and effectiveness of coping with stress, role changes, leisure activities, and cultural beliefs.
9. Availability of transportation.
10. Physical layout of home (steps, accessibility).
11. Use of assistive devices.
12. Reliance on community services (past, present; usefulness of services).
13. Exposure to environmental irritants, radiation.
14. Allergies. Record any reaction to iodine, shellfish.
15. Medications. Note use of aspirin, nonsteroidal antiinflammatory drugs (NSAIDs), steroids, heparin, hormones, vitamins, and analgesics. Include frequency, duration, indication, and effectiveness.
16. Smoking, alcohol, and recreational drug use.
17. Dominant hand.
18. Childbearing history. Nulliparity is a risk factor for osteoporosis.

## FAMILY HISTORY

1. Genetic disorders, abnormalities
2. Congenital abnormalities
3. Arthritis, scoliosis, ankylosing spondylitis

## MEDICAL AND SURGICAL HISTORY

1. Developmental abnormalities
2. Childhood diseases, illnesses, trauma
3. Chronic illnesses, hospitalizations
4. Past surgeries
5. Age at menopause

### box 59-2 *Assessment of Activities of Daily Living (ADL)*

**BATHING**

Independent
Uses assistive devices
Possesses ability, but function is performed by someone else
Lacks ability
Style of bathing—tub, shower, sponge, bed

**DRESSING**

Independent
Uses assistive devices (e.g., buttonhook)
Possesses ability, but function is performed by someone else
Lacks ability
Type of clothing or modifications (e.g., Velcro fasteners, front opening, split seam to accommodate cast, elastic shoelaces)

**TOILETING**

Independent
Special equipment (e.g., bedside commode, raised toilet seat)
Functional problems (e.g., constipation, diarrhea, urinary frequency, bowel or bladder incontinence)
Recurrent bladder infections
Special bowel maintenance programs

**SLEEP**

No problem, usual sleep schedule
Medications used to enhance sleep and their effect
Interfered with by pain or inability to move freely

**RELATING WITH OTHERS**

Note both positive and negative interactions with hospital staff, family, friends

## REVIEW OF SYSTEMS

Obtain data regarding history of integumentary, ophthalmic, auditory, hematological, immunological, respiratory, cardiovascular, gastrointestinal, genitourinary, endocrine, neurological, or psychological problems that may have relevance to presenting problem.

## HISTORY OF CURRENT PROBLEM

Questions related to the history of the problem should help the patient explain the following:

1. Onset of the problem
2. Circumstances surrounding the onset of the problem: any precipitating or associated events or injuries?
3. Duration of problem
4. Patient's perception of the problem
5. Patient's perception of impact problem has had on lifestyle, ability to carry out ADL
6. Any efforts to treat problem and their effectiveness
7. Adherence to treatment programs
8. Trauma, mechanism of injury, sensations or sounds at time of injury

**table 59-2** *Objective Data (Behavior, Appearance, Skin)*

| Observations | Rationale |
|---|---|
| **BEHAVIOR** | |
| Mental status | Interventions must be based on the person's: |
| Orientation to time, place, person | Ability to relate to reality |
| Ability to understand directions | Ability to act on and retain instruction |
| Capacity to retain information | |
| Attention span | |
| Ability to relate to others | Ability to relate to instruction/intervention in a positive way |
| Is the person's attitude quiet, talkative, tense, guarded, negative, appropriate, inappropriate? | |
| **GENERAL APPEARANCE** | |
| Age, sex | May relate to a specific disorder or attitude toward the disorder |
| Posture | May be characteristic of a specific problem, for example, scoliosis; kyphotic posture in ankylosing spondylitis (see Figure 61-26); guarding of head, neck, and shoulders following whiplash |
| Nutritional status | |
| Overweight | May indicate diminished ability to perform regular exercise or activity. Excess weight causes increased stress on joints |
| Underweight | May indicate inability to secure or prepare nutritional meals or to carry out feeding activities adequately; thin persons, particularly women, may have an increased risk of osteoporosis due to insufficient stress on bones |
| | May relate to specific systemic condition causing anorexia, nausea, vomiting, or malabsorption of food |
| **SKIN** | |
| Turgor (fullness) | Thin papery skin may indicate aging, systemic connective tissue disease, or long-term steroid use; skin is easily broken |
| Texture (feel) | Thick leathery patches over forearms, hands, chest, and face indicate scleroderma; ulcerates easily, especially over joints |
| Integrity | |
| Breaks in skin, ulcerations, reddened areas | Individuals with limited mobility are subject to skin breakdown and pressure ulcers from pressure over skin areas, which interferes with circulation; possibility of shearing forces against sheets, chair surfaces, bedpans, or other surfaces tearing or abrading skin; accurate assessment of potential for skin breakdown is vital in planning for prevention |
| Impaired circulation to extremities | Increased risk of skin breakdown in distal extremities |
| Temperature | Warmth, especially over painful joints, indicative of presence and degree of inflammatory or infectious process within joint |
| Erythema over joints | Indicates inflammation and the need to keep joint at rest |
| | May be present in systemic connective tissue disorders (psoriasis, scleroderma, dermatomyositis); initial observations provide useful baseline to determine effectiveness of treatment |

*Continued*

9. Any history of paresthesias, paralysis, swelling (location and timing), locking, "giving way"
10. Unilateral or bilateral joint involvement
11. Reasons for seeking and expectations of current treatment

## DISCOMFORT ASSOCIATED WITH THE PROBLEM

Because pain or discomfort mark many musculoskeletal problems, questions should elicit the following information about the pain or discomfort:

1. Nature
2. Location
3. Duration
4. Radiating or referred pain
5. Evaluation of pain, using pain rating scale
6. Measures the person has taken to alleviate pain or discomfort
7. Effectiveness of measures taken
8. Effect on daily or leisure activities
9. Associated or precipitating events

## OBJECTIVE DATA

The second area of data collection concerns observations about the person. General observations are made regarding behavior, general appearance, skin, nails, and hair (Table 59-2). In addition, data are collected regarding deformities, strength

**table 59-2** *Objective Data (Behavior, Appearance, Skin)—cont'd*

| OBSERVATIONS | RATIONALE |
|---|---|
| **SKIN—cont'd** | |
| Color change on exposure to cold | Change from *white* (resulting from arteriolar spasm) to *blue* (cyanosis caused by stagnation of blood) to *red* (warming and reactive vasodilation) present in some connective tissue disorders *(Raynaud's phenomenon);* requires specific interventions |
| Bruising | Often present following trauma and consequent to long-term treatment of connective tissue disease with corticosteroids; areas may slough easily and become infected |
| Swelling of extremities or joints | In extremities, may denote prolonged dependent position, lack of activity, circulatory or renal impairment<br>In joints, may indicate presence of *effusion* (serous, purulent, or bloody fluid in the joint capsule); inflamed synovium (feels boggy): indication of need to rest joints involved |
| Bony enlargements | Indicative of disease process, for example, *Heberden's nodes,* in osteoarthritis (hard, irregular swellings over the distal interphalangeal joints of the fingers) or *Bouchard's nodes* (cartilaginous or bony enlargement of the proximal interphalangeal finger joints) (Figure 59-18) |
| Subcutaneous nodules | Indicative of rheumatoid arthritis: hard, mobile swellings commonly found in the subolecranon area |
| Bursal swelling | Indicative of bursal inflammation: palpated as soft swelling over the bursa |
| Synovial cyst | Indicative of hypertrophy of synovial tissue, for example, *Baker's cyst* (swelling in the popliteal area, often extending into the calf) |
| Tophaceous deposits | Indicative of gout: hard translucent swellings over joints or in cartilage such as that of the ear |
| Tenderness | |
| May be elicited by direct pressure, and graded by the amount of pressure required to produce discomfort | Degree of tenderness is usually in direct proportion to severity of inflammation or trauma, for example, in joint inflammation or injured soft tissue or overlying fracture |
| General hygiene | |
| Evidence of uncleanliness of body, clothing | May indicate inability to adequately carry out hygienic requirements (because this may be embarrassing for the individual, plans must be made to introduce self-help devices or to provide assistance in ways that will not be demeaning) |
| **NAILS AND HAIR** | |
| Poorly kept or diseased nails | May indicate lack of strength or inability to reach nails to care for them<br>Change in nail structure may indicate presence of connective tissue disease |
| Poorly kept hair | May indicate inability to lift arms to comb hair |
| Alopecia, scaling of scalp | May indicate connective tissue disease, medications |

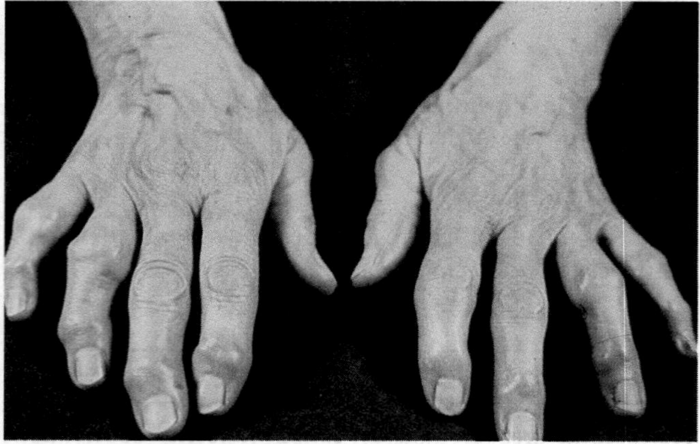

**fig. 59-18** Heberden nodes at the distal interphalangeal joints and Bouchard nodes at the proximal interphalangeal joints.

and range of motion, ability to transfer and ambulate, and ability to perform other ADL.

## INSPECTION

Much information can be gathered even before the physical examination begins. Observe the patient's gait entering the examining room. Note the person's ability to stand, sit, and rise from a chair. If the patient uses assistive devices for ambulation or transferring, observe if the devices are being used properly. While ensuring patient privacy, assess the person's ability to dress and undress. These data will be useful in determining the individual's functional status. Observe the person's posture while standing erect, noting any abnormal curvatures of the spine. A gentle *lordotic* (concave) curve in the lumbar spine is normal, and a gentle *kyphotic* (convex) curve in the thoracic spine is also normal (Figure 59-19). Any exaggeration of these normal curves, such as a lateral curvature or scoliotic curve of the spine, is considered abnormal.

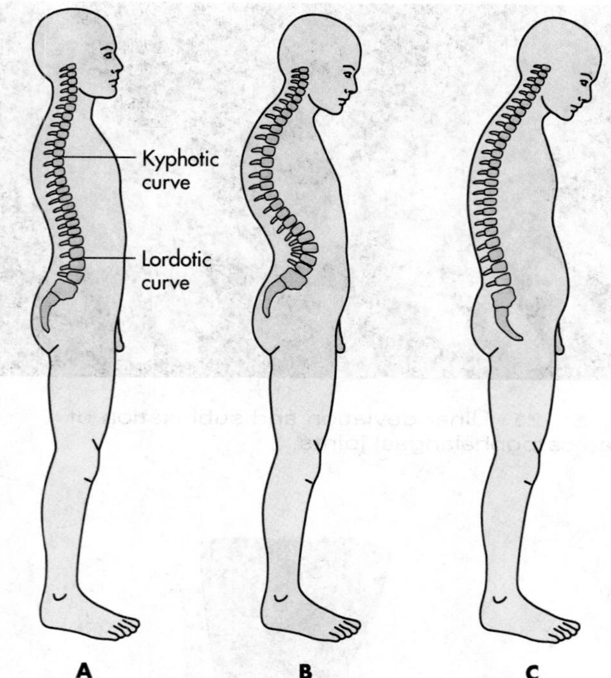


fig. 59-19 A, Curves of spine in good posture. B, Curves of spine in slumping posture. C, Obliteration of spinal curves such as in early spondylitis.

**box 59-3** *Normal Gait Cycle*

| | |
|---|---|
| Stance phase | Begins with heel strike and ends with toe-off |
| Swing phase | Begins with toe-off and continues through heel strike |
| Double support | Brief period when both feet are on ground |

NOTE: Stance phase and swing phase are usually rhythmic and symmetrical. When they are markedly asymmetrical, alteration in gait is called a limp.

Gait (Box 59-3) is the manner or style of walking. An altered gait pattern indicates a pathological process. Have the patient walk 20 to 25 feet. This distance is usually adequate to make an accurate assessment of gait. While observing ambulation, note the presence and type of limp, involved joints, ability to bear weight, balance, and the degree of deformity in the lower extremities. Deformity of the lower extremities (genu varum, talipes varus, and so on) may not be as apparent when the joint is examined at rest as when weight-bearing forces are exerted across the joint. Furthermore, in persons with significant upper extremity involvement, some consideration must be given both to the amount of weight bearing that might be expected from the arms and hands and to the appropriate type of assistive device. For example, the individual with severe rheumatoid involvement of the hands might need a device that permits weight bearing on the forearms.

Other problems, such as cardiovascular disease, respiratory impairment, or anemia, may also affect ambulatory ability and must be considered during the assessment of ambulation. Assessment of transfer and ambulatory ability will help determine a suitable level of activity for the patient. Observe all extremities for overall muscle mass, deformities, asymmetry, and masses. See Box 59-4 for a list of common musculoskeletal deformities.

## PALPATION

In a head-to-toe fashion, palpate all bones, joints, and soft tissue for temperature, swelling, tenderness, pain, or masses. Palpate the spinous processes and intervertebral spaces for tenderness.

## ASSESSMENT OF SENSORY FUNCTION

Assess the person's ability to discern light touch, gentle pressure, pain, and temperature, which will evaluate sensory innervation. Perform each test bilaterally and compare results. Check sensation in the dermatomes, which will show abnormalities in spinal nerve innervation (see Figure 59-24). Also evaluate the person's sense of proprioception (position sense) in the extremities.

## DEEP TENDON REFLEX ACTIVITY

Absent reflexes may indicate neuropathy or a lower motor neuron lesion, whereas brisk reflexes indicate an upper motor neuron lesion. Again, be sure to compare bilateral responses. Figure 59-25 shows the location of tendons and their corresponding spinal level, and Figure 59-26 illustrates the documentation of deep tendon response. The grading of responses is shown in Table 59-3.

## RANGE OF MOTION

*Range of motion* is defined as the normal arc of movement provided for by the structure of a joint. Active range of motion is motion performed independently. Passive range of motion is accomplished with the assistance of someone else or with a mechanical device.

Before testing the muscle strength or range of motion of a joint, some assessment of the position of the person's extremities must be made. Sudden changes from normal may indicate the presence of fractures, dislocations, or ruptures of supporting structures. Typical of this kind of sudden change is the marked external rotation and shortening of the leg following a hip fracture; the inability to extend a "dropped" finger following rupture of an extensor tendon in the hand; or postoperative "dropfoot," a complication that may occur following surgical procedures on the back, hip, or knee because of pressure on or stretching of the sciatic or peroneal nerve.

*Subluxation,* or partial dislocation of a joint, should also be noted. This is often a chronic problem, as in the shoulder of the hemiplegic person or in the wrist of the arthritic person. Its presence is usually accompanied by some loss of function or need for support. Subluxation of the shoulder may be detected by examination: a space can be felt between the head of the humerus and the glenoid cavity of the scapula.

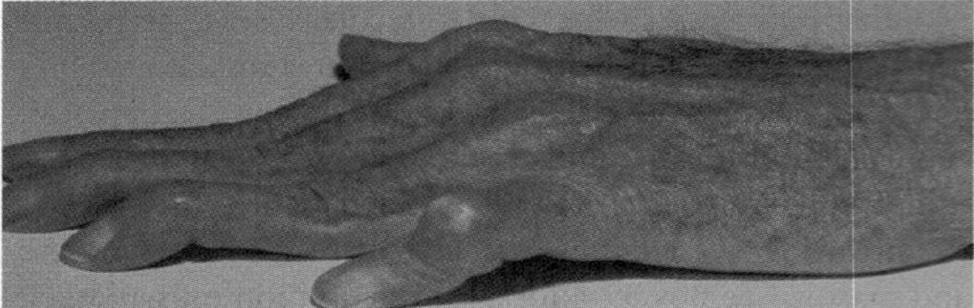

fig. 59-20 Swan neck deformities of fingers in rheumatoid arthritis.

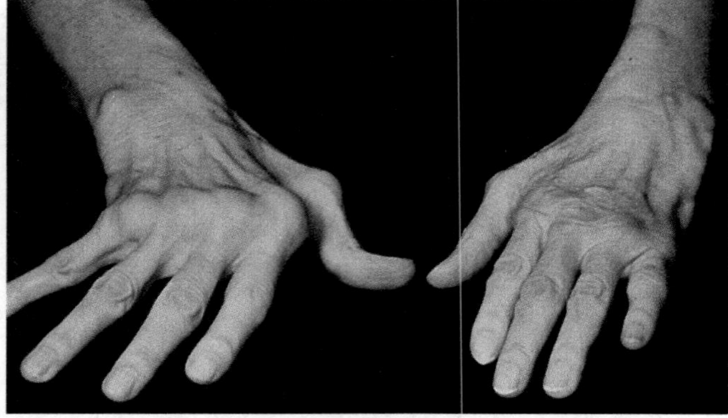

fig. 59-21 Ulnar deviation and subluxation of metacarpophalangeal joints.

**box 59-4** *Common Musculoskeletal Deformities*

**Swan neck deformity**—Flexion contracture of the metacarpophalangeal joint, hyperextension of the proximal interphalangeal joint, and flexion of the distal interphalangeal joints of the fingers (Figure 59-20), found in advanced rheumatoid arthritis

**Ulnar deviation or drift**—Fingers deviate at the metacarpophalangeal joints toward the ulnar aspect of the hand (Figure 59-21)

**Valgus deformities**—Distal arm of the angle of the joint points away from the midline of the body

- **Hallux valgus**—Great toe turns toward the other toes
- **Genu valgum**—"Knock-knees" (Figure 59-22)
- **Talipes valgus**—Eversion of the foot

**Varus deformities**—Distal arm of the angle of the joint points toward the midline of the body

- **Genu varum**—Bowing of the knees (see Figure 61-12)
- **Talipes varus**—Inversion of the foot

**Scoliosis**—Lateral curvature of the spine (see Chapter 61)

**Kyphosis**—Thoracic spinal curvature, the convexity of the curve being posterior

**Atrophy**—Reduction in size of an extremity or body part, for example, wasting of muscles so that they appear to lack the bulk of normal muscle; can result from lack of use or disease process, for example, polymyositis

**Hypertrophy**—Abnormal enlargement of an organ or body part; limitation of function may be associated with enlargement

**Pes planus**—Flat feet (Figure 59-23, *A*)

**Pes cavus**—High instep (Figure 59-23, *B*)

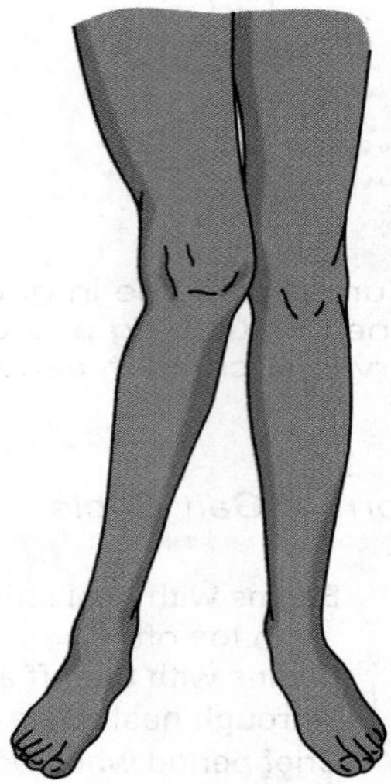

fig. 59-22 Valgus deformity of right knee.

Loss of strength or limitation of joint motion will result in some degree of loss of function. Loss of strength or joint range of motion may be the result of a neurologic, skeletal, muscular, or traumatic disorder.

Range of motion is tested by having the person actively perform the full range of motion of a particular joint (see Figures 59-15, 59-16, and 59-17). In some instances when the person cannot actively move a joint, as with the person who has some form of paralysis, the joint may be passively moved. When passive range of motion is performed, support must be given proximal to the joint being moved (Figure 59-27). Comparing the limitation of movement or instability present in one joint with its contralateral joint is helpful in differentiating normal from abnormal findings.

If a joint cannot be moved beyond a certain point in its normal arc of motion (e.g., a knee that does not extend beyond 130 degrees of flexion), the joint is contracted or a *contracture* is present. Contractures may exist because of soft tissue limitations (following immobilization for treatment of a fracture) or because of bony limitation (Figure 59-28). The location and nature of contractures can significantly limit function. For example, a person who can flex one knee only 15 degrees must climb stairs one at a time.

*Crepitus,* a crunching or grating sensation that is audible or palpable and elicited when the joint is actively or passively moved, is a significant indicator of a pathological condition within the joint. This sensation will also be palpated or heard if the ends of a broken bone move against one another. *In the presence of a possible fracture, no attempt should be made to elicit crepitus.*

A *goniometer* measures degrees of joint movement, comparing findings with expected normal findings. Remember

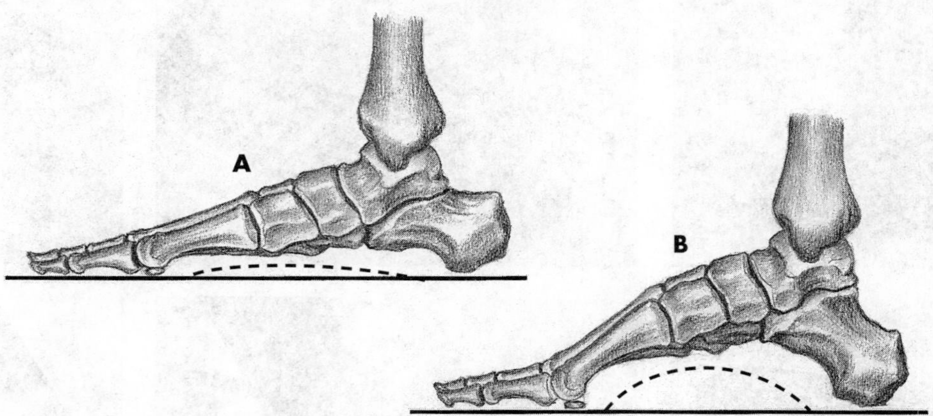


**fig. 59-23** Variations in the longitudinal arch of the foot. **A,** Pes planus (flatfoot). **B,** Pes cavus (high instep).

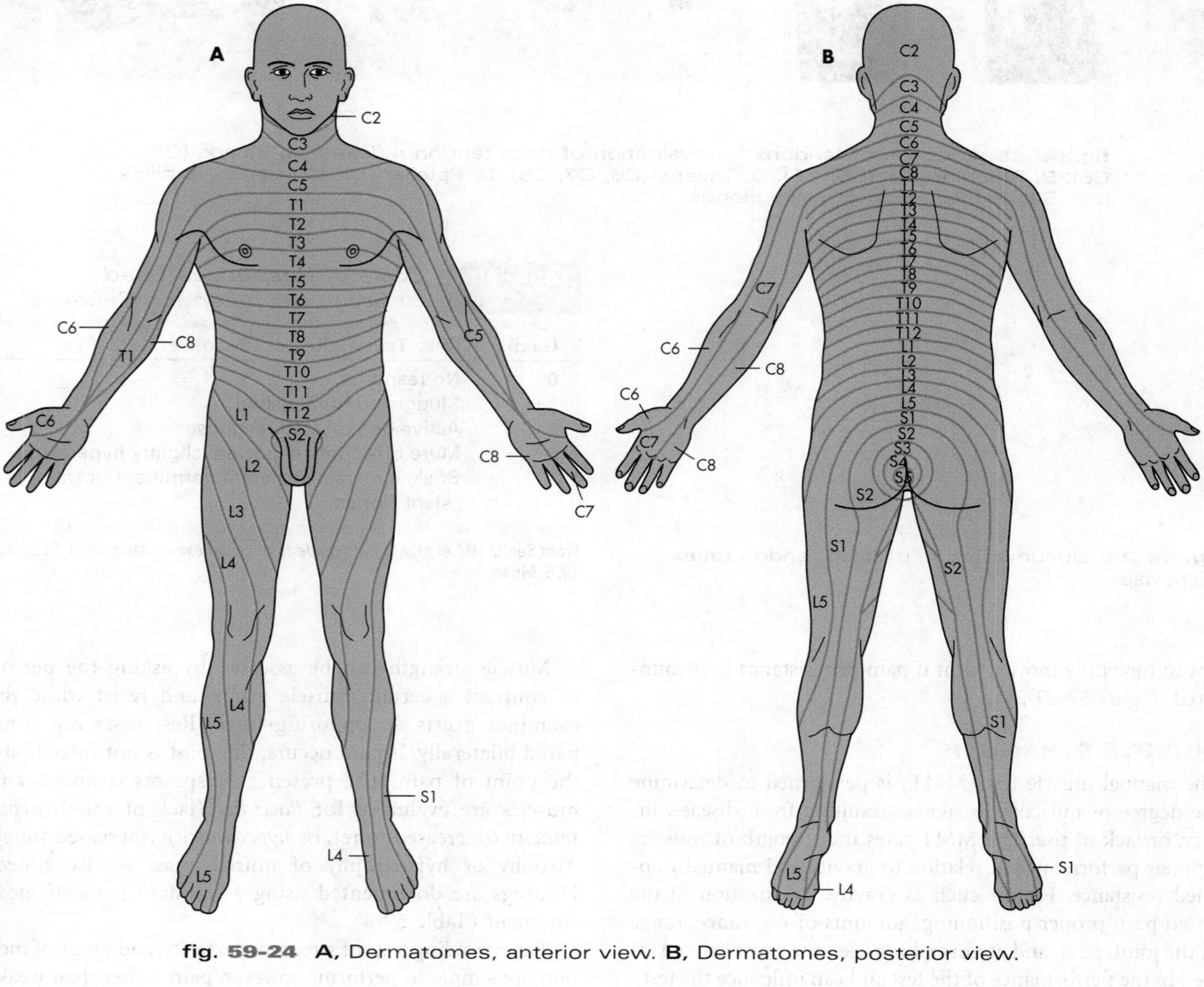

**fig. 59-24** **A,** Dermatomes, anterior view. **B,** Dermatomes, posterior view.

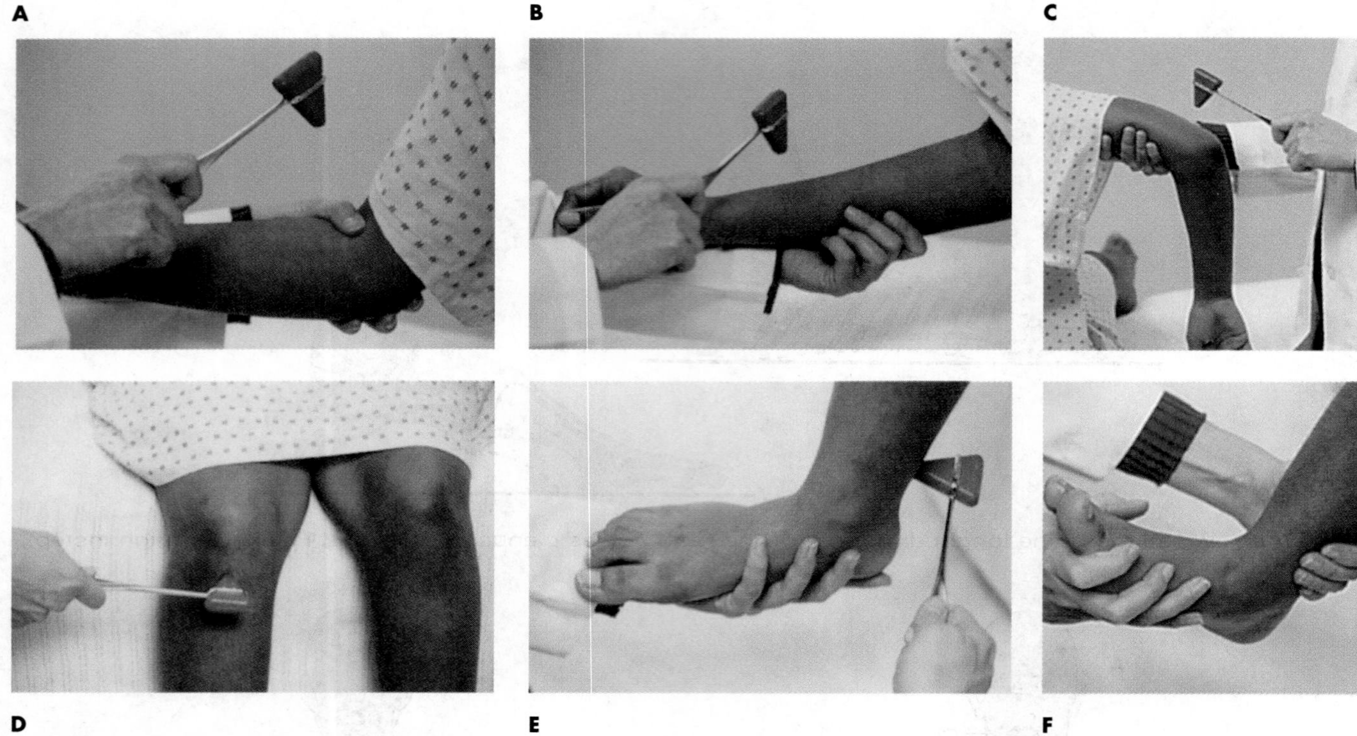


**fig. 59-25** Location of tendons for evaluation of deep tendon reflexes. **A,** Biceps (C5, C6). **B,** Brachioradial (C5, C6). **C,** Triceps (C6, C7, C8). **D,** Patellar (L2, L3, L4). **E,** Achilles (S1, S2). **F,** Evaluation of ankle clonus.

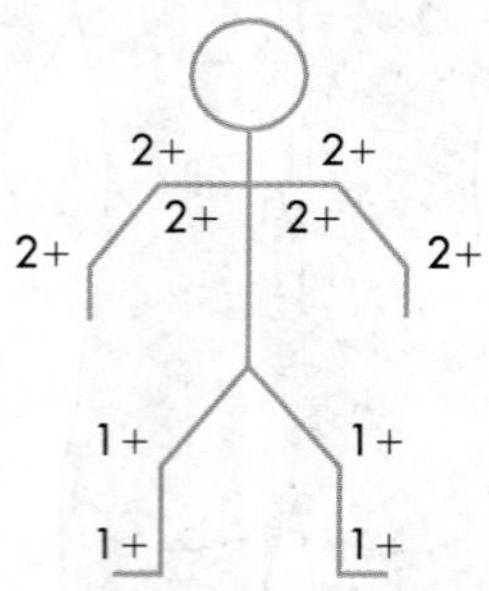


**fig. 59-26** Documentation of deep tendon reflex response.

**table 59-3** *Scale of Responses Used to Score Deep Tendon Reflexes*

| Grade | Deep Tendon Reflex Response |
|---|---|
| 0 | No response |
| 1+ | Sluggish or diminished |
| 2+ | Active or expected response |
| 3+ | More brisk than expected, slightly hyperactive |
| 4+ | Brisk, hyperactive, with intermittent or transient clonus |

From Seidel HM et al: *Mosby's guide to physical examination,* ed 3, St Louis, 1995, Mosby.

not to forcefully move a joint if pain or resistance is encountered (Figure 59-29).

## MUSCLE STRENGTH

The manual muscle test (MMT) is performed to determine the degree of muscular weakness resulting from disease, injury, or lack of use. The MMT rates the strength of muscles by their performance in relation to gravity and manually applied resistance. Factors such as gravity, stabilization of the tested part, proper positioning, amounts of resistance, range of the joint, pain, and abnormal muscle tone must be considered in the performance of the test and can influence the test's objectivity.

Muscle strength can be assessed by asking the person to contract a certain muscle group and resist while the examiner exerts an opposing force. Responses are compared bilaterally. If pain occurs, the joint is not forced past the point of pain. The presence of spasms is noted, and muscles are evaluated for *flaccidity* (lack of tone), *hypotonicity* (decreased tone), or *hypertonicity* (increased tone). Atrophy or hypertrophy of muscle mass is also noted. Findings are documented using a standard scale of measurement (Table 59-4).

The preceding tests of strength, dexterity, and range of motion are simple to perform; however, pain rather than weakness, lack of coordination, or joint limitation may limit the

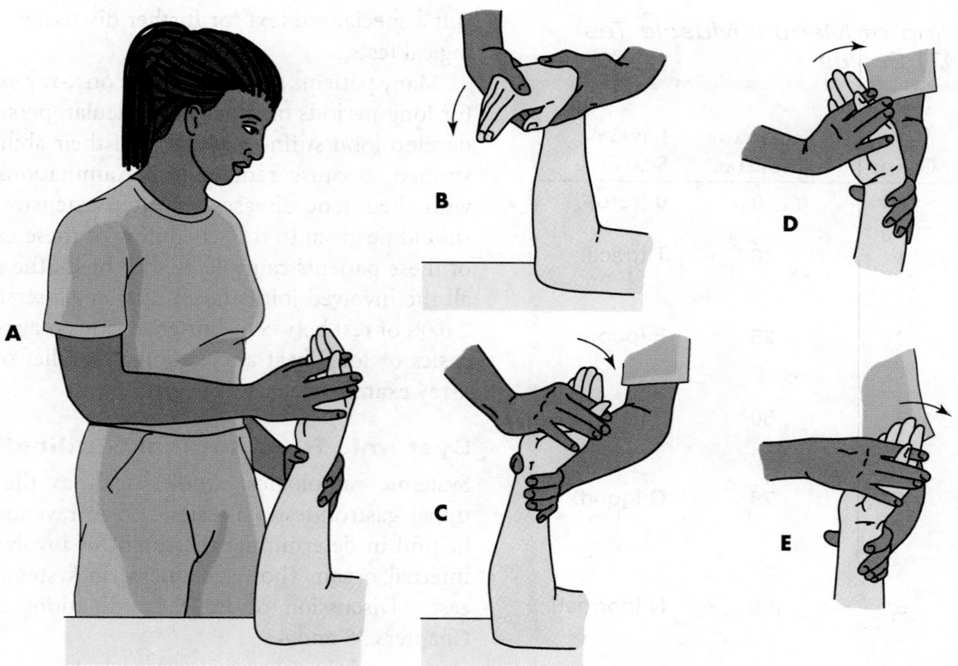


**fig. 59-27** Techniques of passive range of motion. With patient in supine position, upper arm is supported on bed. **A,** Forearm is supported with nurse's hand; hand is supported with nurse's other hand. **B,** Wrist is flexed forward. **C,** Wrist is extended. **D,** Wrist is moved to ulnar side. **E,** Wrist is moved to radial side.

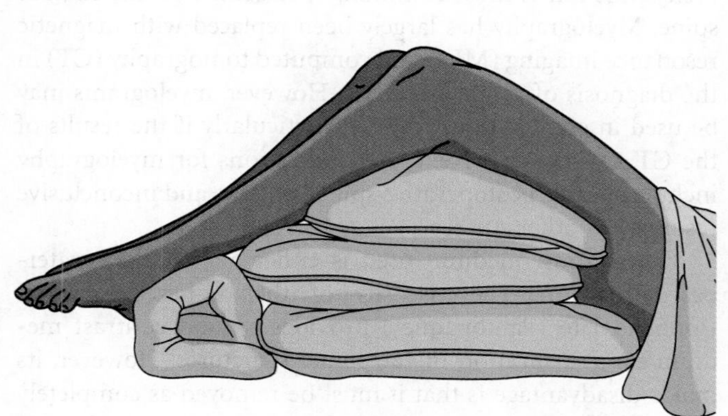

**fig. 59-28** Contractures of hips and knees in patient with rheumatoid arthritis caused by continuous use of pillows to support knees in flexed position.

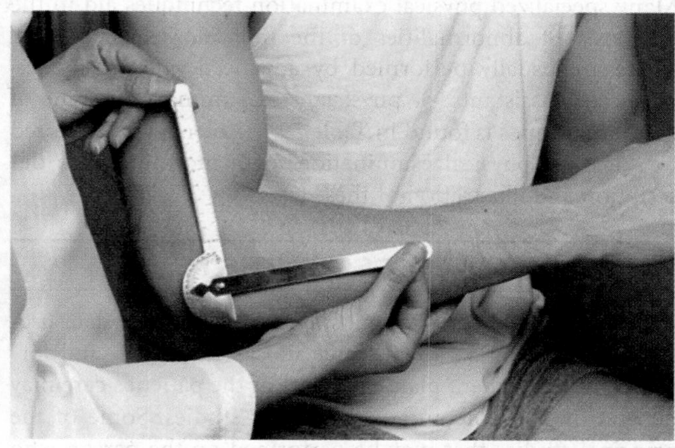

**fig. 59-29** Measurement of joint motion with a goniometer.

person's ability to perform the movement. It is often difficult to differentiate the cause of the deficit. Although quantitatively the same as the effect of the weakness or limitation (i.e., diminished function), pain is qualitatively different because treatment measures will be geared to pain relief rather than to muscle strengthening. The patient may have actual muscle weakness because of chronic pain and consequent lack of use of muscles. It must be remembered that in performing these kinds of tests the person must *not* be moved beyond the point of pain. Pain indicates that something is wrong. Injudicious testing techniques can produce untoward results, for example, the fracture of an osteoporotic bone. The desired result of diagnostic testing is the establishment of a baseline of strength, motion, and dexterity from which interventions to assist the person to gain strength, regain lost motion, and increase functional capacity may be planned and evaluated.

**table 59-4** *Grading of Manual Muscle Test (MMT) Scales*

| Muscle Functional Level | Grade | Percentage of Normal | Lovett Scale |
|---|---|---|---|
| No evidence of contractility | 0 | 0 | 0 (zero) |
| Slight contractility, no movement | 1 | 10 | T (trace) |
| Full range of motion, gravity eliminated* | 2 | 25 | P (poor) |
| Full range of motion with gravity | 3 | 50 | F (fair) |
| Full range of motion against gravity, some resistance | 4 | 75 | G (good) |
| Full range of motion against gravity, full resistance | 5 | 100 | N (normal) |

From Seidel HM et al: *Mosby's guide to physical examination,* ed 3, St Louis, 1995, Mosby.
*Passive movement.

Many specialized physical examination techniques aid in the diagnosis of abnormalities of the musculoskeletal system. These are usually performed by advanced practice nurses, physician's assistants, or physicians. A summary of some of these techniques is found in Table 59-5. The reader is referred to a text on physical examination for a more in-depth description and illustration of these tests.

## DIAGNOSTIC TESTS

As with other illnesses, diagnostic test results offer data useful in diagnosing a patient's musculoskeletal illness and formulating a treatment plan. Elements of the patient's care may depend on the outcome of diagnostic studies. Some of the principal studies that may be performed on the person who has a musculoskeletal problem are described in the following sections.

### LABORATORY TESTS

Laboratory tests consist of two major categories, serological and urinary, as described in Tables 59-6 and 59-7.

### RADIOLOGICAL TESTS

#### Bones and Joints

Radiological tests of bones and joints are imperative for the identification and treatment of fractures. They are also helpful in determining the presence of disease (e.g., rheumatoid arthritis, spondylitis, avascular necrosis, and tumor), as well as the progress and effects of treatment on these disorders. Consult a specialized text for further discussion of specific radiological tests.

Many patients are unable to lie on x-ray examination tables for long periods of time. In particular, persons with arthritis develop joint stiffness and pain if their ability to move is restricted. Because radiological examinations for individuals with rheumatic diseases are often extensive, careful thought should be given to the scheduling of these examinations. Few of these patients can tolerate having all the required views of all the involved joints taken in a single session. Instead, 1 or 2 days of rest between shorter sessions may be required. Analgesics or local heat applications for relief of joint pain after x-ray examinations may be necessary.

#### Systemic Radiological Studies

Systemic radiological studies such as the barium enema, upper gastrointestinal series, and intravenous pyelogram are helpful in determining the extent of involvement of various internal organs (bowel, kidneys) in systemic rheumatic diseases. Discussion of these examinations can be found in Chapters 38 and 43.

#### Myelography

A myelogram is a radiological examination of the spinal canal. A radiopaque solution (or less commonly, air) is injected into the arachnoid space. Myelography is used to identify lesions such as herniated nucleus pulposus, nerve root involvement, spinal stenosis, tumor, or other lesions that may encroach on the spinal canal. It can be performed on the cervical or thoracic spine but is most commonly performed on the lumbar spine. Myelography has largely been replaced with magnetic resonance imaging (MRI) and computed tomography (CT) in the diagnosis of spinal disorders. However, myelograms may be used in conjunction with CT, particularly if the results of the CT are inconclusive. Other indications for myelography include obesity, postoperative spinal surgery, and inconclusive results with other studies.

The contrast medium used is either an oil- or a water-based solution. The viscosity of the oil-based solution (iophendylate [Pantopaque]) provides a good contrast medium for visualization of the spinal structures. However, its major disadvantage is that it must be removed as completely as possible after the examination or it may cause arachnoiditis, encephalopathy, or severe headaches.

These limitations led to the development of the water-soluble, nonionic solutions that are widely used today (metrizamide [Amipaque] and iohexol [Omnipaque]). Water-based dyes are less viscous and fill the canal and narrow spaces easily, allowing good visualization of the structures. They are absorbed into the cerebrospinal fluid and need not be removed after the procedure. Major adverse effects are seizures, nausea, headache, and vomiting after the procedure. Emergency medications and equipment should be immediately available in case of allergic response to the contrast medium. Informed consent is necessary before the procedure.

Patient education is vital before the procedure. A thorough explanation of events before, during, and after the procedure

**table 59-5** *Special Assessment Techniques for the Musculoskeletal System*

| Assessment Technique | Description | Abnormality Detected |
|---|---|---|
| Limb measurement | Measurement in centimeters of extremities from a major landmark | Asymmetrical limb length may indicate pelvic obliquity or hip deformities; discrepancies in circumference may indicate atrophy or paresis of muscle groups; <1 cm discrepancy is normal in most people |
| Ballottement | Compression of the suprapatellar pouch, which is normally snug against the femur | Fluid wave indicates excess fluid in the knee (effusion) |
| Bulge sign | Stroke the medial aspect of the knee, then tap the lateral side of the patella; if fluid is present, a fluid wave or bulge will appear | Effusion, excess fluid in the suprapatellar pouch |
| McMurray's test | External rotation and valgus stress applied to the knee while the leg is held flexed at the knee and hip (patient is lying supine); normally there is no pain or sound | "Click" or pain indicates meniscal tear |
| Drawer test (Anteroposterior and mediolateral) | With the patient supine and the knee flexed, push forward and backward on tibia at the joint line; with the patient supine with knee extended, stabilize the femur and ankle while attempting to abduct and adduct the knee; normally there is little or no movement—assess symmetry of responses | Laxity or movement suggests instability of the anterior or posterior cruciate ligaments or the medial or lateral collateral ligaments of the knee |
| Straight leg raising (LaSegue) test | With the patient supine, raise the leg straight with the knee extended; normally there is no pain | If the maneuver reproduces sciatic pain, it is considered positive and suggests a herniated disk |
| Trendelenburg's test | While the patient stands on one foot and then the other, both iliac crests should appear symmetrical | Asymmetry suggests hip dislocation |
| Thomas test | With the patient lying supine and one leg fully extended and the other flexed on the chest, observe the ability of the patient to keep the extended leg flat on the table | Inability to keep the leg extended suggests a hip flexion contracture in the extended leg that may be masked by increased lumbar lordosis |
| Phalen's test | Flex both wrists together to 90° and hold for 60 seconds; normally this produces no symptoms | Numbness, tingling, or burning in the median nerve distribution suggests carpal tunnel syndrome |
| Tinel's sign | Tap over the median nerve where it passes through the carpal tunnel in the wrist; normally this does not produce any symptoms | Tingling along the median nerve distribution is associated with carpal tunnel syndrome |
| Drop arm test | Raise the affected arm to ~90° of flexion, then have the patient slowly adduct the arm to the side | Inability to lower the arm slowly or smoothly is associated with disruption of the rotator cuff mechanism of the shoulder |
| Scoliosis screening | "Forward bend" test; observe symmetry and height of scapulae, shoulders, iliac crests, rib cage | Asymmetry of scapulae or shoulder height, "winged" iliac crests, demonstrable curve of spine, rib hump indicates scoliosis |

may help allay fears and clarify any misconceptions regarding myelography.

Myelography is an outpatient procedure done in the radiology department by a radiologist with the assistance of a radiology technician. The patient is admitted to the hospital the morning of the procedure. After a clear liquid breakfast, the patient is on NPO status. A careful history should be taken, noting any previous allergic reactions to other contrast agents, iodine, or shellfish. If a water-based solution is being used, the patient may not take amphetamines, phenothiazides, or tricyclic antidepressants for 12 hours before the procedure. These drugs lower the seizure threshold.

If necessary, a sedative may be prescribed before the procedure. In the radiology department, the patient is transferred to the x-ray table. The patient is either placed in the lateral or sitting position for the lumbar puncture. Local anesthetic is injected before the lumbar puncture (see Chapter 51). The myelogram is performed with the patient in the prone position. Approximately 10 ml of cerebrospinal fluid (CSF) is withdrawn and sent to the laboratory for analysis. The contrast medium is then injected, and the x-ray table is moved and tilted, allowing the dye to fill the canal as films are taken. The procedure may take up to 1 hour. Commonly, a CT scan follows the myelography.

**table 59-6** *Serological Tests*

| TEST | RATIONALE FOR PERFORMING TEST |
|---|---|
| Serum muscle enzymes<br>AST (serum aspartate transaminase) (SGOT)<br>Aldolase<br>CPK (creatine phosphokinase) isoenzymes MM, MB | Enzymes can be elevated in the presence of primary myopathic (muscle) diseases. Elevated levels may result from muscle fiber degeneration or from diffusion through a muscle membrane that has increased permeability.<br>Enzyme levels are an index of both progress of the myopathic disorder and effectiveness of treatment. Aldolase levels most commonly used to diagnose and monitor treatment of muscular dystrophy.<br>NURSING PRECAUTION: Intramuscular injections should be avoided when these enzymes are being monitored.<br>*Normal values:* AST = 8-20 U/L<br>Aldolase: 3-8.2 U/dl<br>CPK-MM: 5-70 U/L<br>CPK-MB: 0-7 U/L |
| STS (serological test for syphilis)<br>FTA-ABS (fluorescent treponemal antibody absorption) | False-positive STS results occur in 10-15% of persons with connective tissue diseases, so test may aid diagnosis. FTA-ABS excludes the presence of syphilis. |
| Rheumatoid factor or latex fixation (reaction of rheumatoid factor antibodies with IgG [7S] gamma globulin) | Rheumatoid factor antibodies are found in the sera of individuals with rheumatoid arthritis. Test considered positive if rheumatoid factor is found in titrations of 1:40 or greater. May be positive in persons with systemic lupus erythematosus (SLE).<br>CAUTION: Rheumatoid factor may be found in other conditions, for example, in aging, scleroderma, acute pulmonary tuberculosis, and parenteral narcotic addiction. |
| Antinuclear antibodies (ANA) | Circulating antibodies, which are composed of protein material and called antinuclear antibodies react with cellular nuclei and various individual constituents of cellular nuclei, and can be identified by fluorescent techniques utilizing antihuman gamma globulin labeled with fluorescein. Positive tests are used in diagnosing Sjögren's syndrome, scleroderma, and SLE. Pattern of nuclear staining varies with different diseases. Poor positive predictive value for SLE and other rheumatic diseases.[6] |
| Serum complement | Protein substances that are found in serum and synovial fluid and are associated with immune and inflammatory mechanisms; low levels often occur in SLE and rheumatoid arthritis. |
| Erythrocyte sedimentation rate (ESR) | Increased rate of settling of erythrocytes is an important index of the presence of inflammation.<br>*Normal values:* men, 1-3 mm/hr; women, 4-7 mm/hr |
| Hematocrit | Individuals with systemic connective tissue disease often have normocytic (normal RBCs), normochromic (normal amount of iron carried by RBCs) anemia, in the absence of any abnormal bleeding.<br>Individuals who suffer trauma or undergo major surgery to the musculoskeletal system sustain significant blood loss.<br>Symptoms of anemia (e.g., extreme tiredness, fatigue, weakness) are experienced when hematocrit drops quickly; acute symptoms may be absent if anemia develops gradually or is chronic. Individuals with acute anemia should not be physically stressed.<br>*Normal values:* men, 45-50 vol/dl; women, 40-45 vol/dl |
| Calcium | Immobility and bone demineralization (bone cancers, multiple myeloma) will show increase in serum levels. Rickets, vitamin D deficiency, will show decrease in levels. Malnutrition also results in decreased levels.<br>*Normal value:* 3.9-4.6 mg/dl |
| Alkaline phosphatase | Bone tumor and infections, fractures, Paget's disease, rickets, and other conditions that cause an increase in osteoblastic activity will cause an increase in alkaline phosphatase levels.<br>*Normal value:* 30-85 ImU/ml; elderly, slightly higher<br>In hypophosphatasia (characterized by a defect in bone formation), levels are decreased. |
| Phosphorus | Together with calcium, plays a vital role in bone metabolism. Conditions that cause an increase in calcium levels will cause a decrease in serum phosphates.<br>*Normal values:* 2.5-4.5 mg/dl |
| Anti-DNA antibody | Used in the diagnosis of SLE or to monitor response to treatment. Antibodies to DNA are present in the serum of 60-80% of persons with SLE. |
| C-reactive protein | Used as a nonspecific indicator of infection and inflammation. Commonly used to aid in the diagnosis of rheumatoid arthritis. May also be used to monitor responses to antibiotics or antiinflammatory medication. |
| LE prep | Used in the diagnosis and treatment of SLE. The antinuclear factor in SLE is the LE factor; the LE test detects antinuclear antibodies, but many patients with SLE have negative results. |

**table 59-7** *Urinary Tests*

| Diagnostic Test | Rationale for Test |
|---|---|
| 24-hour urine for creatine-creatinine ratio | In the presence of muscle disease, the ability of muscle to convert creatine is decreased, the amount of creatine excreted by the kidneys increases, and the ratio of urinary creatine to creatinine increases. Periodic studies are helpful in diagnosis and evaluation of progress of treatment of primary myopathies. |
| Urinary uric acid levels (24-hour collection)* | Helpful in diagnosis and decisions regarding treatment modalities for gout. *Normal value:* should not exceed 900-mg uric acid excretion per day |
| Urine for deoxypyridinoline (first or second morning void) routine collection | Deoxypyridinoline (Dpd) cross-links assay provides a quantitative measurement of Dpd, which is excreted unmetabolized in the urine during bone resorption. |

*NOTE: 24-hour urine collections must be accurate to facilitate proper diagnosis and treatment.

After myelography, the patient is returned to his or her room. Fluids are encouraged to replace the removed CSF and to aid in the excretion of the contrast medium. If an oil-based dye was used, the patient is kept flat in bed for approximately 8 hours. If a water-soluble dye was used, bed rest is maintained, with the head of the bed elevated 30 degrees for 24 hours. If air was used, the head of the bed should be kept lower than the trunk for up to 48 hours.

Contrast material has a diuretic effect. Output should be monitored for at least 8 hours after the test. Diet is resumed as tolerated, and fluids are encouraged, regardless of the dye used. The patient should be observed for any reactions to the contrast agent. Headaches, nausea, and vomiting are the most common side effects. Neurological checks are performed hourly. The lumbar puncture site will be covered with a small adhesive strip and should be observed for any bleeding. The patient can be discharged the afternoon of the procedure. Patients should continue with bedrest at home, then gradually resume normal activities. Lifting or strenuous activity should be avoided for 24 hours.

The patient should be taught to check the puncture site for any drainage, swelling, or signs of infection. Anticonvulsants or other medications withheld before the procedure may be resumed in 48 hours. The patient should be instructed to contact the physician if persistent nausea or vomiting develops.

Myelography is contraindicated for persons with multiple sclerosis. Allergy to contrast material or renal impairment affects the choice of contrast medium.

## Bone Densitometry

Bone densitometry measures bone density to aid in the diagnosis of osteoporosis, predict fracture risk, and monitor the effectiveness of treatment protocols. The most widely used method is dual x-ray absorptiometry (DEXA or DXA scan). This noninvasive radiological test measures bone mass and density in the lumbar spine, proximal femur, and wrist. The two types of scanners are the pencil beam fan and fan beam. The fan beam produces images with better resolution in less time. Both emit low-dose radiation, approximately 1 to 3 mrem compared with 20 to 50 mrem for a chest x-ray. The duration of the procedures varies from 30 seconds per site to 4 minutes per site. No special preparation or aftercare for this test is needed. A certified x-ray technologist performs the tests. The patient's results are compared with the bone density expected for someone of the same age, sex, and race and with the peak bone density of a healthy adult of the same age, sex, and race. These scores are known as "young normal" or T-score, and "age-matched" or Z-score. Densities 1 standard deviation below the "normals" represent a reduction in bone mass of about 12% and an increased risk for fracture.

## Arthrography

Arthrography permits visualization of structures within the joint that are not normally seen on routine radiographical films. An arthrogram is usually performed on the knee or shoulder for evaluation of persistent pain or preoperative assessment. Although the knee and shoulder are the most common joints evaluated, the elbow, wrist, hip, and temporomandibular joints may also be visualized.

The joint cavity is injected with radiopaque dye, air, or both. The latter is called a *double-contrast arthrogram.* The dye or air serves as a contrast medium against which the outlines of soft tissue components of the joint may be seen. Tears of the menisci and internal derangement of the joint such as ligament disruption and synovial cysts can be diagnosed with the aid of arthrograms.

Before the examination, the patient should be checked for allergies to iodine or seafood. Patients may experience pain while the joint is expanded by the dye or air, and local anesthetic may be injected before the examination. Analgesics are prescribed after the examination. The patient should be instructed to watch for redness, edema, or unusual pain in the joint after the procedure.

## Radioisotope Bone Scans

Radioisotope bone scans are performed primarily to demonstrate the presence of metastatic disease, tumors, infection (osteomyelitis), and other conditions with increased bone activity. This nuclear scanning test can also be used to diagnose the cause of undetermined bone pain and assess the healing of fractures. Intravenously injected sodium pertechnetate $^{99m}$Tc (technetium) is the isotope most commonly used in this study. The $^{99m}$Tc concentrates in areas of osteoblastic activity involved in the exchange of calcium. Technetium, a bone-seeking radioisotope, is taken up by the bone in areas of adequate blood supply and metabolic activity. *Hot spots* on the scan indicate areas of increased bone turnover, as in the case of fractures, bone healing, and inflammatory responses. *Cold spots*, or areas of decalcified bone, indicate no bone activity, as in lytic lesions. Lesions may be visualized on bone scans as early as 3 to 6 months before the lesions are evident on routine x-ray films. Bone scans are commonly used to rule out bony metastases from the prostate, breast, and lung.

Technetium scans are also of some use in determining the degree of parotid gland involvement in Sjögren's syndrome. The uptake, concentration, and excretion of the isotope by the major salivary glands are measured by a technique called *sequential scintiphotography*.

Persons being prepared for these procedures should know that the procedures are not painful and that the isotopes will not harm them. However, persons may have to remain quietly in one position for 1 hour or more. The radioisotope will be injected intravenously about 2 hours before scanning. The patient is encouraged to drink fluids before the scan and is assessed for iodine or seafood allergies before the examination. Procedures using barium or iodine are not scheduled before the bone scan, because these substances interfere with scanning. The kidneys excrete the radioisotope.

### Computed Tomography

*Tomography* is an x-ray technique by which detailed images of "slices" of tissue are obtained by focusing x-ray beams at predetermined planes or depths of the tissue being studied. Detailed images of the structures at that level are produced, and details of structures surrounding that level are blurred or eliminated. *Computed tomography* (CT scanning) is tomography employing a computer to compose a picture of the tissue being studied. A series of x-ray beams is rotated, 1 degree at a time, around the specific area being examined. With each rotation, a picture is generated that depicts the difference in tissue density. These pictures are extremely clear and detailed. Computed tomography may be used in conjunction with intravenous or oral contrast media to allow better visualization of structures.

The scan picks up disruptions in normal structures. The procedure can be used in diagnosing spinal pathological conditions and tumors and in evaluating the hip before custom joint replacement. The procedure is noninvasive and does not require repositioning of the patient, as does conventional tomography. Disadvantages of CT include poor depiction of intraspinal processes and poor differentiation between disk herniation and postoperative scar tissue.[4] Computed tomography is commonly done after myelography in diagnosing spinal pathological conditions. Patients who are claustrophobic may have difficulty tolerating the procedure, because they must lie in a cylindrical metal scanner for up to 1 hour.

### Magnetic Resonance Imaging

Magnetic resonance imaging (MRI) is a scanning technique that produces tomographical images by using magnetic forces rather than x-ray beams. The patient lies on a nonmagnetic scanning table that slides, head first, into a large cylindrical magnet. The magnet causes the body's atomic protons to line up and spin in the same direction. A radio frequency signal is beamed into the magnetic field, causing the protons to move out of alignment. When the signal stops, the protons move back into alignment and release energy. A receiver coil measures the energy released by the movement of the protons and the time it takes for the protons to return to their aligned position. These measurements provide information regarding the type of tissue in which the protons lie, as well as the condition of the tissue. A computer uses this information to construct an image on a television screen, showing the distribution of protons of hydrogen atoms; the television image may also be recorded on film or magnetic tape. The images produced by MRI are more accurate than CT and myelography.[4]

Patients being prepared for MRI should know that the procedure is painless and requires no special preparation. However, because a magnetic field is used, the patient will be asked to remove any metallic objects, such as jewelry, hairpins, credit cards, and nonpermanent dentures. Patients who have cardiac pacemakers or intracranial vascular aneurysm clips are excluded from MRI. Persons who have metal implants cannot have that area scanned.

As with CT scanning, patients who are claustrophobic may have difficulty being placed in the scanner. Sometimes medication such as diazepam (Valium) is prescribed to help the patient relax. "Open-air" MRI scanners allow the patient to feel less confined but still obtain quality images. These scanners are an option for some patients. During the scan, the patient will hear the hum of the machine, a loud thump when the radio waves are turned on and off, and other machine-like noises. The thumping can be particularly annoying to patients, and many persons are frightened if they are not told what will happen. Scanning time is usually 30 to 90 minutes. Many facilities offer earplugs to reduce outside noise while in the scanner.

Contrast media may be used with MRI to enhance the quality of the images. Gadolinium-DPTA, an intravenous contrast agent often used with MRI to enhance imaging, differentiates recurrent disk herniation from epidural scarring.[4]

### Diskography

A diskogram is a radiological procedure that uses a contrast medium to evaluate the integrity of the intervertebral disks. Diskography is performed on an outpatient basis in the operating room or radiology department with the use of fluoroscopy. The patient is placed in the prone position, and local anesthetic is administered. The patient may require additional sedation, because the procedure can be quite uncomfortable. Needle position is confirmed by fluoroscopy; contrast medium and saline are then injected into the disk space. If a pathological condition is present, injection of the saline reproduces the patient's back or leg pain. Despite the accuracy of myelography, CT, and MRI, the diskogram is still a useful diagnostic tool because the ability to reproduce the patient's symptoms may aid the surgeon in differential diagnosis, especially when several vertebral levels are involved. However, this technique is less specific than myelography.

## SPECIAL TESTS

### Electromyography

Electromyography measures the electrical activity of muscles; an electromyogram (EMG) is a recording of the variations of electrical potentials (voltage) detected by a needle electrode inserted into skeletal muscle. Electromyogram, an electrophysiological test, differentiates between myopathies (muscle diseases) and neuropathies (nerve diseases). The electrical activity can be heard over a loudspeaker and viewed on an oscilloscope and graph at the same time. No electrical activity can be detected in normal muscles at rest, but during volitional movement, action potentials can be detected. In both primary myopathic and neuropathic disorders, specific variations exist in the size of individual motor unit potentials. In neurogenic atrophy, fibrillations may be present in the resting muscle. An EMG provides direct evidence of motor dysfunction and can be used to some extent to detect a dysfunction located in the motor neuron, the neuromuscular junction, or the muscle fibers. Thus it is particularly helpful in the diagnosis of lower motor neuron (LMN) disease, primary muscle disease, and defects in the transmission of electrical impulses at the neuromuscular junction, such as occurs in myasthenia gravis. However, electromyography cannot be used to differentiate specific disease entities in either the myopathic or neuropathic categories.

No special preparation is required for this procedure. The patient may fear that insertion of electrode needles will be painful or that electrical stimulation of the needles will cause severe shock. Although the patient may be reassured that the procedure is not dangerous, some individuals do experience mild to moderate discomfort. Therefore nurses preparing patients for this test should not refer to the test as "painless."

### Biopsy

Biopsies of tissue from a variety of organs are helpful in the diagnosis of disease or disorders affecting the musculoskeletal system. Table 59-8 lists the tissues that may be biopsied, the tests performed, significance of results, and general nursing considerations for patients undergoing biopsy.

**table 59-8** *Types of Biopsies*

| Organ | Test(s) Performed | Positive Results | Nursing Considerations |
|---|---|---|---|
| Skin (punch biopsy) | Immunofluorescent staining—tissue is washed with solution of fluorescein-labeled antihuman gamma globulin antibody | Band of immunofluorescence at epidermal-dermal junction, indicating presence of rheumatic disease (i.e., scleroderma, SLE, psoriatic arthritis) | Biopsy site kept clean and dry with small adhesive bandage until scab develops; hydrogen peroxide (3%) used to cleanse open area prn; only very mild discomfort experienced by patient |
| Muscle (operative procedure) | Histochemical staining | Tissue reveals features of LMN disease, degeneration, inflammatory reaction as in polymyositis, or involvement of specific fibers indicating primary myopathic disease | Patient instructed and prepared for surgery; patient monitored per postanesthesia routine (local or general); mild to moderate pain and stiffness in biopsy area; routine activity encouraged within 24 hours to avoid undue stiffness; dressings changed as necessary |
| Synovium (closed—performed with needle; open—performed in surgery) | Histological examination—synovial fluid obtained at the same time; may be cultured to determine presence of infection | Differentiates various forms of arthritis | Patient instructed about procedure; patient may require postanesthesia monitoring; strict asepsis observed throughout procedure and in caring for the wound; small compression dressing applied to joint, and joint rested for 24 hours to prevent hemorrhage or effusion |
| Buccal mucosa (punch biopsy) | Histological examination of tissue from inside lower lip | Helpful in diagnosing Sjögren's syndrome | Patient instructed about procedure; generally minor discomfort experienced; diet altered to avoid rough and very hot foods (they will irritate the site) |
| Bone (operative procedure) | Microscopic analysis | Can confirm presence of infection or neoplasm | Patient instructed and prepared for surgery; patient monitored per postanesthesia routine; mild to severe discomfort may be experienced; activity restrictions dependent on location and extent of surgical procedure; dressings changed as necessary |

### Joint Aspiration

Joint aspiration *(arthrocentesis)* is performed to obtain a sample of synovial fluid from within the joint cavity. This procedure (performed by introducing a needle into the joint cavity and withdrawing fluid) helps determine the presence of an aseptic inflammatory process such as rheumatoid arthritis or a septic process such as bacterial arthritis. Samples of synovial fluid are cultured and examined both microscopically and chemically.

The synovial fluid is normally straw colored and clear; the viscosity resembles that of clean motor oil. In the presence of inflammation, the fluid becomes turbid and watery. The *mucin clot test* is performed by mixing synovial fluid with glacial acetic acid. Normal synovial fluid forms a white, ropey mucin clot. When inflammation is present, the clot breaks apart easily and becomes flaky (flocculent). The degree of flocculence increases with the degree of inflammation. Also, when inflammation is present, the number of WBCs, the protein content, and the number of polymorphonuclear cells in the synovial fluid are increased, and the glucose content is decreased.

A local anesthetic is usually administered before the procedure. Strict asepsis is observed during the procedure. After the procedure the joint is often wrapped in a small compression (Ace) dressing. The joint may be rested for 8 to 24 hours. Drainage should be managed in accordance with Standard Precautions.

## ENDOSCOPY

### Arthroscopy

*Arthroscopy* (visualization of a joint) is a procedure performed in the operating room, usually in an ambulatory surgical center, under local or regional anesthesia. A specially designed endoscope (arthroscope) is inserted through a small incision into the joint cavity, enabling the physician to visualize the structure and contents of the joint (Figure 59-30). Most arthroscopic procedures are performed on the knee, although the wrist, ankle, hip, shoulder, and temporomandibular joint are also examined and treated with this technique.

The procedure is used to diagnose and treat such conditions as chondromalacia of the knee, ligamentous disruption, meniscal tears, carpal tunnel syndrome, osteoarthritis, rheumatoid arthritis, and impingement syndrome. Endoscopy is also used to perform lumbar and thoracic diskectomy. Analgesics are prescribed postoperatively. The patient is taught to observe the operative site for swelling and signs of infection. The period of time the joint is rested and the use of any immobilizing device is determined by the location and extent of the procedure. The surgeon should be consulted regarding the activity the patient is permitted after the procedure so that damage to the joint may be avoided.

## chapter SUMMARY

### ANATOMY AND PHYSIOLOGY

- Support, protection, and movement are the three mechanical functions of bones. Bones also store calcium and produce RBCs.
- Bone is produced by the process of osteogenesis or endochondral ossification. The bone-building cells are known as osteoblasts; bone cells are osteocytes. Calcium salts in the matrix give bone its characteristic hard quality.
- Bones are classified into four groups based on shape: long, short, flat, and irregular.
- Bone is composed of cancellous (spongy) and compact cortical (dense) bone. Lamellae are concentric cylindrical layers of calcified matrix. The arrangement of lamellae within bone differentiates cancellous and compact bone. The haversian canal is at the center of the lamella.
- Bone reshapes itself in response to alterations of its mechanical function. Osteogenesis occurs along lines of stress. This explains why a person who regularly exercises may have some increase in bone mass, whereas a sedentary person may experience loss of bone substance.
- Circulation of blood to bone is supplied by three routes: through arterioles in the haversian canals, through Volkmann's canals (located in the periosteum), and through vessels in the marrow and the ends of bone.

A

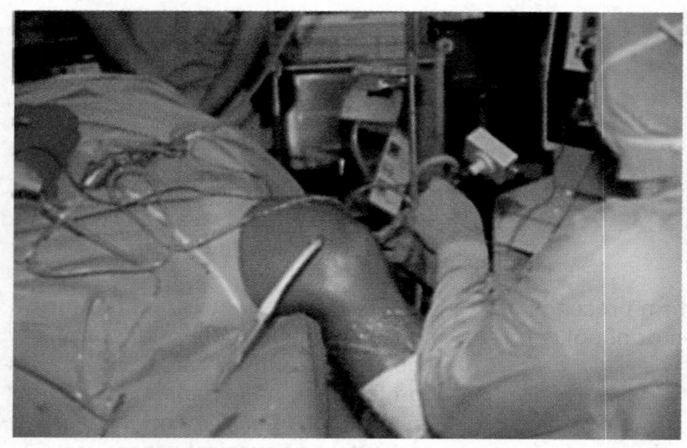

B

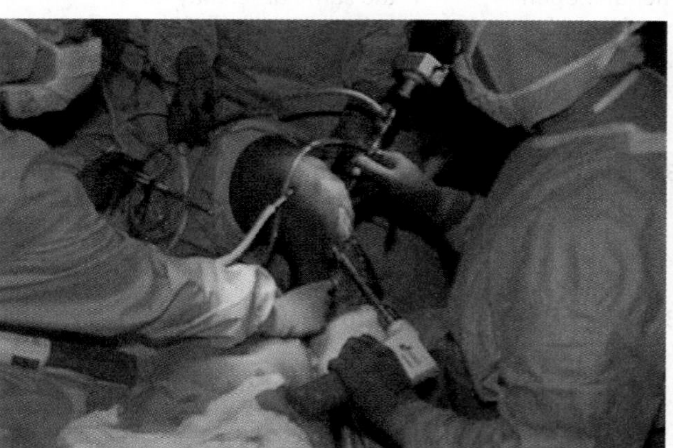

**fig. 59-30** **A,** Arthroscopy of the knee. **B,** Arthroscopically aided reconstruction of anterior cruciate ligament.

Blood supply to the bone can be interrupted by injury to an artery, the periosteum, or the bone itself. Because bones are supplied with sensory nerve endings, pain will result if bone is damaged.

- Callus formation is the process of bone healing and proceeds in five general stages: hematoma formation, fibrin meshwork formation, invasion by osteoblasts, callus formation, and remodeling. Callus formation can be impeded by inadequate reduction of a fracture, excessive edema at a fracture site, extensive bone loss at the time of injury, inefficient immobilization, infection, bone necrosis, anemia or other systemic conditions, endocrine imbalance, and poor dietary intake. Nonunion, or an ununited fracture, results from lack of or inadequate treatment or from abnormal or inefficient callus formation.
- Three major types of muscle are skeletal, visceral, and cardiac.
- The function of muscles is to contract. Body movement is produced by muscles pulling on bones, with bones serving as levers and joints serving as fulcrums for the levers. Muscles act in a coordinated manner, involving prime movers, antagonists, and synergists.
- Cartilage is a material composed of fibers embedded in a firm gel. It is strong, flexible, and avascular. The type of cartilage (fibrous, hyaline, or elastic) is determined by the number of collagenous fibers.
- Ligaments connect the articular ends of bones and provide stability.
- Tendons are dense fibrous tissue bands that form the termination of a muscle and attach it to a bone.
- Small sacs of connective tissue are called bursae. They are located wherever pressure is exerted over moving parts.
- Joints, or the places where bones come together, provide flexibility within the skeletal framework. There are three major classifications of joints: synarthroses, or fibrous joints, provide no movement; amphiarthroses, or cartilaginous joints, allow little movement; and diarthroses, or synovial joints, allow free movement.
- Diarthrodial joints contain a joint cavity between the articulating surfaces of the bones that compose the joint. The articulating surfaces of both bones are covered by articular hyaline cartilage, allowing smooth motion. The joint is encased in a joint capsule, and the capsule is lined with a synovial membrane. Lubrication is provided by synovial fluid secreted by the synovial membrane. Ligaments may be present to provide internal stability to the joint. Menisci (small pieces of dense cartilage) may also be present to provide additional cushioning.
- Physiological changes with aging occur as the total number of body cells decreases, resulting in the decline of tissue strength and integrity. Connective tissues lose elasticity; muscles lose bulk, tone, and strength; bone resorption is more rapid than bone growth; and, particularly in postmenopausal women, calcium is lost from bone, making it softer and more prone to fracture.
- The musculoskeletal, circulatory, and nervous systems are interrelated. Any problem that causes interruption of innervation, contractility, articulation, circulation, or support results in musculoskeletal dysfunction.

### SUBJECTIVE DATA

- Assessment of any person with a musculoskeletal problem includes subjective data elicited from the person and family. This includes a description of the present problem, such as onset and duration, associated pain or discomfort, current medications, effect on performance of ADL, and the patients's and family's perception of the problem.

### OBJECTIVE DATA

- Objective data involve observations of the person. Data also are collected about deformities, strength and range of motion, and the ability to transfer, ambulate, and perform ADL.

### DIAGNOSTIC TESTS

- Some of the principal diagnostic studies performed on a person with a musculoskeletal problem include laboratory examinations (e.g., serological and urinary tests); radiological examinations (e.g., radiographs of bones and joints, systemic radiological studies, and bone density studies; myelography; diskography; arthrography; radioisotope scans; CT scans; MRI); EMG; biopsies; and joint aspiration.
- Arthroscopy is a surgical procedure that provides visualization of a joint via a specially designed endoscope. Biopsy, diagnosis, repair of torn meniscus or ligament, and removal of loose bodies from the joint space can be accomplished with this approach.

## References

1. Guyton AC, Hall JE: *Textbook of medical physiology,* ed 9, Philadelphia, 1996, WB Saunders.
2. Lueckenotte AG: *Gerontologic nursing,* St Louis, 1996, Mosby.
3. McCance KL, Huether SE: *Pathophysiology: the biologic basis for disease in adults and children,* ed 3, St Louis, 1998, Mosby.
4. Patel PR, Lauerman WC: The use of magnetic resonance imaging in the diagnosis of lumbar disc disease, *Orthop Nurs* 16(1):59, 1997.
5. Thibodeau GA, Patton KT: *Anatomy and physiology,* ed 3, St Louis, 1996, Mosby.
6. Slater CA et al: Antinuclear antibody testing: a study of clinical utility, *Arch Intern Med* 8(156):1421, 1996.

chapter 60

# MANAGEMENT OF PERSONS WITH Trauma to the Musculoskeletal System

JANE F. MAREK

## objectives *After studying this chapter, the learner should be able to:*

1. Relate appropriate preventive measures to the causes of bone fractures.
2. Explain various treatment modalities for fracture healing.
3. Correlate complications of fracture with the available treatment regimens.
4. Describe the components of the nursing assessment of the person who has had a fracture.
5. Explain the nursing role in the management of fractures and prevention of complications.
6. Develop a nursing care plan for a person who has undergone surgical repair of a hip fracture.
7. Compare and contrast the nursing care required for a person with a prosthetic implant for hip fracture with that required for a person who has received an internal fixation device.
8. Delineate the special nursing considerations in caring for the patient with a spine fracture.
9. Analyze the various types of soft-tissue trauma and joint injuries.
10. Discuss the nursing care of patients who have sustained soft-tissue trauma and joint injuries.
11. Discuss the special care considerations that a patient who has sustained multiple trauma needs.

The person with musculoskeletal trauma has sustained an interruption in the integrity of one or more components of the system. Musculoskeletal trauma is most commonly manifested as bone fracture, but it may also include injury to soft tissue, muscle, ligament, meniscus, tendon, or joint.

The National Center for Health Statistics estimates that annually an average of 1 of 10 persons suffers acute injury to the musculoskeletal system. The most common injuries are fracture, dislocation, and sprain.

## TRAUMA TO BONE

### FRACTURE

#### Etiology/Epidemiology

Fracture of bone usually occurs as a result of a blow to the body, a fall, or another accident. However, fracture may occur during normal activity or after a minimal injury, if the bone has been weakened by a disease such as primary or metastatic cancer or osteoporosis. This type of fracture is referred to as *pathological* or collapse of the bone. Bone may also fracture when the muscles adjacent are unable to absorb energy as they usually do. This type of fracture is called a *fatigue* or *stress* fracture. *Avulsion* fractures occur when a strong ligamentous or tendinous attachment pulls a fragment of bone away from the rest of the bone.

The highest incidence of fractures is in males 15- to 24-years old and in elderly persons, especially women, aged 65 years and older. Osteoporosis is the most common cause of long bone fractures (see Chapter 61). Neuromuscular instability is an important contributing factor to the risk of falls, which commonly precede a fracture in the elderly population.[13] Wrist, hip, and vertebral fractures are most common in the elderly. Persons in high-risk occupations (e.g., steelworkers and race car drivers) and persons with chronic degenerative or neoplastic diseases are also at higher risk for injury. In this section, fractures in general will be discussed. Later in the chapter, complications of fractures and hip and spine fracture will be discussed.

#### Pathophysiology

##### Types of fractures

A fracture is a complete or partial interruption of osseous tissue. *Complete* fractures penetrate both cortices, producing two bone fragments; only one cortex is broken in *incomplete* fractures. The part of the bone nearest the body is referred to as the *proximal* fragment; the part more distant from the body is called the distal fragment. The proximal fragment is also called the *uncontrollable* fragment, because its location and muscle attachments prevent it from being moved or manipulated when attempting to bring the separate fragments into alignment. The distal fragment is called the *controllable* fragment, because it can usually be moved to bring it into correct relationship to the proximal fragment. Fractures in long bones are designated as being in the proximal, middle, or distal third of the bone.

If the skin over the fracture is intact, the fracture is classified as *simple* or *closed.* A fracture is classified as *compound* or *open* when there is a direct communication between a skin wound and the fracture site. An open or compound fracture has a high risk of contamination, which is an important factor in treatment. Open fractures can be classified into three categories based on the severity of the fracture and the degree of soft-tissue involvement. Type 3 fractures are the most severe and are further subdivided into three subtypes (Box 60-1).[19] When the two bone fragments are in proper alignment with no change from normal position despite the break in continuity of bone, the fracture is referred to as a *nondisplaced* fracture. If the bone fragments have separated at the point of fracture, the fracture is referred to as a *displaced* fracture. The degree of displacement will vary with the type of injury and the condition of the bone and soft tissues. The position of the bone fragments depends on the mechanism of injury. The type, direction, and strength of the force and pull of the attached muscles determine the position of the bone fragments. Bone fragments that slide over each other are termed *overriding.*

The *line of fracture* as revealed by x-ray film or fluoroscopy is usually classified according to type. It may be *greenstick,* with splintering on one side of the bone (this occurs most often in the elderly and in young children); *transverse,* with the break being straight across the bone; *oblique,* with the line of the fracture at an oblique angle to the bone shaft; or *spiral,* with the fracture lines partially encircling the bone. The fracture may be referred to as *telescoped* or *impacted* if the distal fragment is forcibly pushed against and into the proximal fragment. This occurs most often with compression and force applied to the distal fragment. If there are several bone fragments, the fracture is called *comminuted.* (See Figure 60-1 and Box 60-2 for examples of fractures.)

Because bones are more rigid than their surrounding structures, any injury severe enough to cause bone fracture may also cause injury to adjacent muscles, nerves, connective tissue, and blood vessels. The force that causes the fracture is dissipated through the surrounding soft tissue, and small fragments of bone may become embedded in muscle, blood vessels, or nerves.

**box 60-1** *Classifications of Open Fractures*

**TYPE 1**
Length of wound <1 cm
Low-energy injury

**TYPE 2**
Length of wound >1 cm
More energy absorbed during fracture

**TYPE 3**
Length of wound >10 cm
Comminuted fracture with extensive soft-tissue damage
High-energy injury typically from gunshot wounds, motor vehicle accidents, farming accidents

**Type 3A**
Do not require major reconstructive surgery for closure

**Type 3B**
Major soft-tissue defects requiring reconstructive surgery for closure

**Type 3C**
Vascular and neural compromise
Requires major reconstructive procedures

### Healing of fractures

Immobilization of a fractured bone is necessary for healing to take place. Immobilization may be accomplished in any of the following three ways:

1. *Physiological splintage,* a naturally occurring phenomenon related to pain in the affected area that causes guarding, muscle spasm, and avoidance of use; furthermore, there will be a desire to rest the whole body until some repair has occurred
2. *External orthopedic splinting* with devices such as casts, plaster splints, and braces
3. *Internal fixation* with screws, plates, or rods to hold the opposing ends of the fracture in place

Once immobilization is accomplished, the bone heals by the process of callus formation (see Chapter 59).

The clinical manifestations of fracture differ depending on the location and type of fracture and associated soft-tissue in-

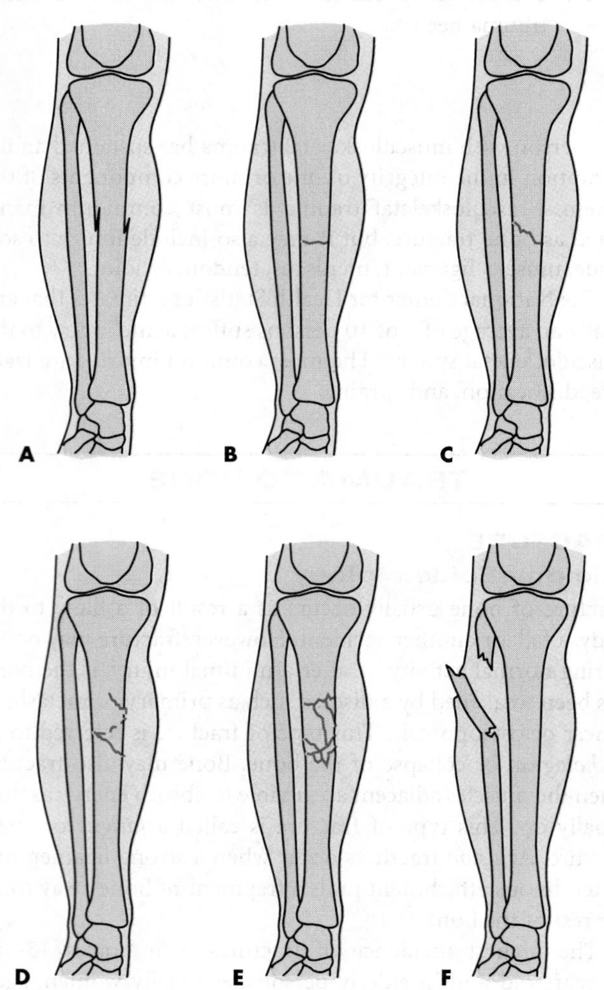


**fig. 60-1** Types of fractures. **A,** Greenstick. **B,** Transverse. **C,** Oblique. **D,** Spiral. **E,** Comminuted. **F,** Open.

juries (Box 60-3). Signs and symptoms characteristic of most fractures include pain, impairment or loss of function, deformity, abnormal or excessive motion, swelling, altered sensation, and radiological evidence of fracture. The immediate pain associated with a fracture is usually severe. Attempts at movement and associated injuries increase the pain. Factors contributing to the pain are associated soft-tissue injuries, muscle spasms, and overriding of fracture fragments. Alterations in sensation are caused by pressure, pinching, or severing of nerves from the trauma or by bone fragments.

Fracture healing begins with hematoma formation 24 to 72 hours after the injury. The healing time required for fractures depends on many factors. The age of the patient and type of bone fractured are important considerations. Adults require a longer healing time than children. Osteoporotic bone, commonly found in the elderly, requires additional healing time. In general, fractures of cancellous bone heal faster than cortical bone fractures because of the rich blood supply. Midshaft fractures of the humerus, ulna, and tibia usually heal slowly because of the poor blood supply. An adequate blood supply enables the bone to bleed with the injury, allowing adequate hematoma formation, which is the first stage of bone healing. A greenstick fracture will take only a few weeks for healing, in contrast to an open, comminuted fracture, which may take up to 2 years for complete healing. Factors conducive to fracture healing include close approximation of fracture fragments, adequate blood supply, surrounding muscular envelope, absence of infection, and adequate immobilization.[19] See Table 60-1 for factors that impede bone healing.

Failure of a fracture to consolidate in the time usually required is called *delayed* union, and failure to form a stable union after 6 months is called *nonunion*.[19] Of the estimated 2 million cases of long bone fractures that occur annually, there will be approximately 100,000 (5%) cases of nonunion.[7] The incidence of nonunion tibial fractures is higher than in other long bones, especially when fracture occurs as a result of a high-energy injury, such as a motor vehicle accident. Certain bones are more likely to result in a nonunion, regardless of proper fracture management. The distal tibia, carpal navicular, and proximal fifth metatarsal have a higher incidence of nonunion.[19] A fracture is considered united when radiographical evidence demonstrates a bony bridge at the fracture site.

Healing with angulation or deformity is called *malunion*. If a fracture is nonunited, there will be excessive mobility at the fracture site, creating a false joint. This is called a *pseudoarthrosis*.

### box 60-2 Types of Fractures

**TYPICAL COMPLETE FRACTURES**

Closed (simple) fracture—Noncommunicating wound between bone and skin
Open (compound) fracture—Communicating wound between bone and skin
Comminuted fracture—Multiple bone fragments
Linear fracture—Fracture line parallel to long axis of bone
Oblique fracture—Fracture line at 45-degree angle to long axis of bone
Spiral fracture—Fracture line encircling bone
Transverse fracture—Fracture line perpendicular to long axis of bone
Impacted—Fracture fragments are pushed into each other
Pathological—Fracture occurs at a point in the bone weakened by disease, for example, by tumor or osteoporosis
Avulsion—A fragment of bone connected to a ligament breaks off from the main bone
Extracapsular—Fracture is close to the joint but remains outside the joint capsule
Intracapsular—Fracture is within the joint capsule

**TYPICAL INCOMPLETE FRACTURES**

Greenstick fracture—Break on one cortex of bone with splintering of inner bone surface
Torus fracture—Buckling of cortex
Bowing fracture—Bending of the bone
Stress fracture—Microfracture
Transchondral fracture—Separation of cartilaginous joint surface (articular cartilage) from main shaft of bone

From McCance KL, Huether SE: *Pathophysiology: the biologic basis for disease in adults and children,* ed 3, St Louis, 1998, Mosby.

## Collaborative Care Management

### Diagnostic tests

Diagnosis is confirmed by x-ray. Other studies may be indicated if multiple injuries have been sustained.

### box 60-3 clinical manifestations

**Fractures**

1. Pain (caused by swelling at the site, muscle spasm, damage to periosteum)
   a. Immediate
   b. Severe
   c. Aggravated by pressure at the site of injury
   d. Aggravated by attempted motion
2. Loss of normal function (the injured part incapable of voluntary movement)
3. Obvious deformity resulting from loss of bone continuity
4. Excessive motion at site (i.e., motion where motion does not usually occur)
5. Crepitus* or grating sound if limb is moved gently
6. Soft-tissue edema in area of injury resulting from extravasation of blood and tissue fluid
7. Warmth over injured area resulting from increased blood flow to the area
8. Ecchymosis of skin surrounding injured area (may not be apparent for several days)
9. Impairment or loss of sensation or paralysis distal to injury resulting from nerve entrapment or damage
10. Signs of shock related to severe tissue injury, blood loss, or intense pain
11. Evidence of fracture on x-ray film

*No attempt should be made to elicit this sign when fracture is suspected, because it may cause further damage and increase pain.

### Medications

1. Analgesics are given as needed to treat pain.
2. Prophylactic antibiotics (initially intravenously, then orally) are given when an open fracture has occurred or surgical intervention is necessary.
3. Tetanus toxoid may be necessary in the case of an open fracture.

### Treatments

Management objectives include the following:

1. Reduce the fracture by realigning the fracture fragments.
2. Maintain the fragments in correct alignment by immobilization.
3. Restore function and prevent excessive loss of joint mobility and muscle tone.

Immediate treatment principles implemented at the time of injury include the following:

1. Maintain airway and assess for signs of shock (see section on multiple trauma).
2. Splint the fracture to prevent movement of the fracture fragments and further injury to the soft tissues by bony fragments. Splinting and immobilization will also decrease pain.
3. Preserve correct body alignment.
4. Elevate the injured body part to decrease edema.
5. Apply cold packs (during the first 24 hours) to reduce hemorrhage, edema, and pain.
6. Observe for changes in color, sensation, circulation, movement, or temperature of injured part.

Secondary management goals include the following:

1. For simple fracture
   a. Optimal reduction (replacing bone fragments in their correct anatomical position)
      (1) Manual manipulation, or *closed reduction* (moving bone fragments into position by applying traction and pressure to distal fragment)
      (2) Traction
      (3) *Open reduction* (surgical intervention that may incorporate use of an internal fixation device)
   b. Immobilization
      (1) External fixation—cast, splint, external fixator device (wires, external frame)
      (2) Traction
      (3) Internal fixation—pins, plates, screws, wires, and prostheses
      (4) Combinations of the above
2. For compound fracture
   a. Surgical debridement and irrigation of wound to remove dirt, foreign material, devitalized tissue, and necrotic bone
   b. Wound culture
   c. Pack the wound
   d. Observe for signs of osteomyelitis, tetanus, and gas gangrene
   e. Wound closure when there is no sign of infection
   f. Reduce fracture
   g. Immobilize fracture
3. Use of bone-growth stimulators that use low-voltage electrical impulses to enhance healing in cases of nonunion

The purpose of immobilization is to hold the broken bone fragments in contact with each other (or in very close approximation) until healing takes place. Immobilization can be accomplished *externally* with external fixation devices (cast, splint, brace, cast brace), traction, or external fixators or *internally* with metal plates, pins, screws, and nails, alone or in combination with bone grafts or prosthetic implants. Both ex-

**table 60-1** *Major Factors That Impede Bone Healing*

| FACTOR | EFFECT ON BONE |
|---|---|
| Excess motion of fracture fragments | Inadequate immobilization, resulting in movement of fragments |
| Poor approximation of fracture fragments | Inaccurate reduction or malalignment of fracture fragments |
| | Excessive bone loss at time of fracture, preventing sufficient bridging of broken ends |
| | Excessive fragmentation of bone, allowing soft tissue to be interposed between bone ends |
| | Inability of patient to comply with restrictions imposed by immobilizing/fixation device(s), resulting in movement of fragments |
| Compromised blood supply | Damage to nutrient vessels |
| | Periosteal or muscular injury |
| | Severe comminution |
| | Avascularity (type of fracture, result of internal fixation device) |
| Excessive edema at fracture site | Tissue swelling impedes supply of nutrients to area of fracture |
| Bone necrosis | Injury to blood vessels impedes supply of nutrients to involved bone |
| Infection at fracture site | Infection disrupts normal callus formation |
| Metabolic disorders or diseases (cancer, diabetes, malnutrition, immunodeficiency, Paget's disease) | Retard osteogenesis |
| Soft-tissue injury | Disruption of blood supply |
| Medication use (e.g., steroids, anticoagulants) | Steroids can cause osteoporosis, avascular necrosis; long-term use of heparin may cause osteoporosis. |

ternal and internal methods can be used, with combinations of the above. The appropriate period of immobilization must be maintained in order to prevent nonunion or malunion.

### Methods of external fixation

**Casts.** The most common external fixation device is the cast. Materials used for casts include plaster of paris, fiberglass, and plastic. All of these materials are available as rolled bandages and are applied over the body part to be immobilized in much the same manner as an Ace bandage. *Plaster,* which has to be moistened before application, dries very slowly, is heavy, and will lose its strength and integrity if it becomes wet after the initial drying. If a plaster cast requires revision, it usually must be removed and a new one applied. However, plaster is less expensive than fiberglass or plastic. *Fiberglass* and *plastic* dry quickly, are lightweight, and may be immersed in water without losing their strength. Plastic casts may be reheated and remolded if revision is necessary. Some types of fiberglass require drying under special ultraviolet lights, and persons wearing fiberglass or plastic casts may suffer maceration of the skin unless they dry the skin thoroughly with a warm air dryer after bathing or showering. Specific advantages or disadvantages of various cast materials are discussed in orthopedic texts.

A cast may incorporate (1) all or a portion of an extremity (Figure 60-2), (2) all or a portion of the trunk and cervical area, or (3) all or a portion of the trunk with all or a portion of one or more extremities. The latter type of cast is called a *spica* cast (Figure 60-3). *Splints* are made from cast material, but they may be thought of as half-casts because they do not encompass a body part. They are applied anteriorly, posteriorly, medially, or laterally and are wrapped in place with bandages, usually Ace bandages. *Cast braces* are made of two separate casts, one applied above a joint and the other below the joint. The two casts are joined by metal or heavy polyethylene hinges that are incorporated into the cast material. Cast braces permit the patient joint mobility below the fracture while still providing immobilization for the fracture fragments.

Casts are applied over skin that has been cleansed and assessed for potential areas of infection or breakdown. Skin lesions are treated with disinfectant before cast application. Before the cast is applied, the skin may be treated with tincture of benzoin and wrapped with cotton padding or stockinette. Bony prominences are padded with sheet wadding or felt to prevent pressure points. For specific techniques of cast application, consult specialized texts.

**Traction.** Traction is the mechanism by which a steady pull is exerted on a part or parts of the body. Traction may be used to accomplish the following:

1. Reduce a fracture
2. Maintain correct alignment of bone fragments during healing
3. Immobilize a limb while soft-tissue healing takes place
4. Overcome muscle spasm
5. Stretch adhesions
6. Correct deformities

*Countertraction* is a force that counteracts the pull of traction. The patient's body may be the countertraction, as with Buck's traction. (In that case the patient's feet should not rest on the foot of the bed.)

*Suspension* is the use of traction equipment, such as frames, splints, ropes, pulleys, and weights, to suspend but not exert a "pull" on a body part. To suspend the part correctly and continuously, the suspension must be balanced by weights. Suspension is often referred to as *balanced suspension.* Balanced suspension is often used in conjunction with traction to allow the patient to move about more freely and easily in bed.

Two types of traction are used: skin traction and skeletal traction. *Skin traction* is achieved by applying wide bands of moleskin, adhesive, or commercially available devices directly to the skin and attaching weights to them. *The pull of the weights is transmitted indirectly to the involved bone or other connective tissue.* Buck's extension and Russell traction are the two most common forms of skin traction for injury to the lower extremities.

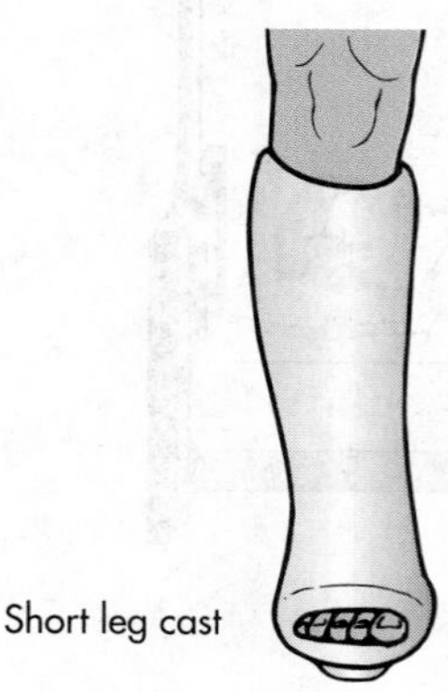


**fig. 60-2** Short leg walking cast.

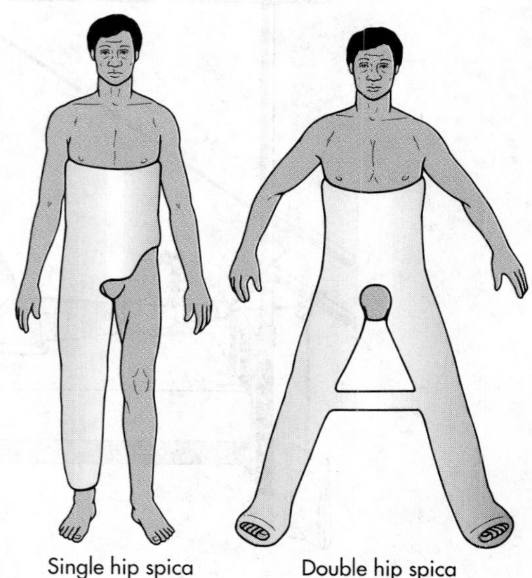


**fig. 60-3** Hip spica casts.

*Buck's extension* is the simplest form of skin traction and provides for straight pull on the affected extremity (Figure 60-4). It is often used to relieve muscle spasm and to immobilize a limb temporarily, for example, to treat a hip fracture before open reduction and internal fixation. If adhesive substances are to be used, the leg is shaved and tincture of benzoin is applied to protect the skin. Adhesive tape or moleskin is then placed on the lateral and medial aspects of the leg and secured with a circular gauze or elastic bandage. The adhesive material should not cover the malleoli, because of the risk of skin breakdown over these bony prominences. The tapes are attached to a spreader bar wide enough to pull the tapes away from the malleoli. Rope is attached to the spreader, passed through a pulley on a crossbar at the foot of the bed, and suspended with weights. The maximum weight that should be applied by skin traction is 2 to 4 kg (5 to 10 lb).[14] Greater amounts of weight can cause skin damage. Commercial foam rubber Buck's extension splints are widely used and are applied with Velcro straps. Contraindications to placing a patient in Buck's extension are stasis dermatitis, arteriosclerosis, allergy to adhesive tape, severe varicosities or varicose ulcers, diabetic gangrene, or marked overriding of bone fragments that would require more than 3.6 kg of weight to reduce the fracture.

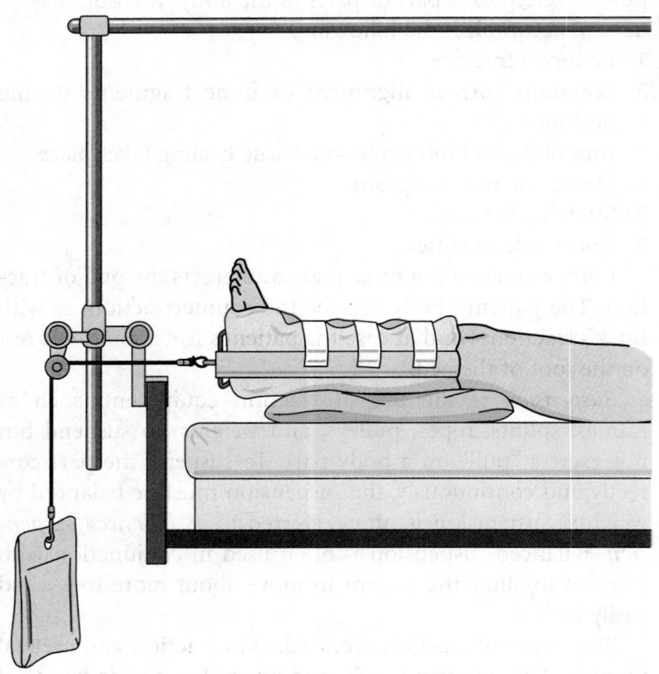

**fig. 60-4** Buck's extension. Heel is supported off bed to prevent pressure on heel; weight hangs free of the bed, and foot is well away from footboard of bed. The limb should lie parallel to the bed unless prevented, as in this case, by a slight knee flexion contracture.

*Russell traction* is sometimes used because it permits the patient to move somewhat freely in the bed and permits flexion of the knee joint (Figure 60-5). It requires an overhead frame attached to the bed and preparation of the leg as for Buck's extension. A foot plate with pulley attachments is used instead of a spreader bar. The knee is suspended in a sling to which a rope is attached. The rope is directed up to a pulley that has been placed on the overhead frame directly above the tibial tubercle of the affected extremity. The rope is then passed down through a pulley on a crossbar at the foot of the bed, back through a pulley on the footplate, back again to another pulley on the crossbar, and then suspended with weights. This arrangement effects a double pull from the crossbar to the footplate, so the traction is approximately double the amount of weight used. Usually the foot of the bed is

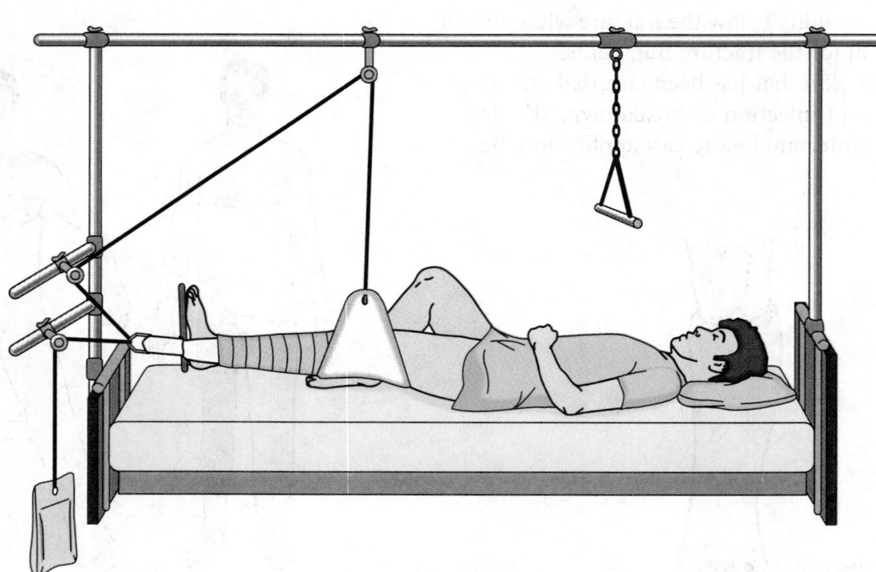

**fig. 60-5** Russell traction. Hip is slightly flexed. Pillows may be used under lower leg to provide support and keep the heel free of the bed.

elevated on blocks (or the bed is put in Trendelenburg's position) to provide countertraction.

Russell traction is used in the treatment of intertrochanteric fracture of the femur when surgery is contraindicated. Either bilateral Russell traction or Buck's extension may be used to treat back pain, because both partially immobilize the patient and reduce muscle spasm.

*Skeletal traction* is traction applied directly to bone. With the patient under local or general anesthesia, a Kirschner wire or Steinmann pin is inserted through bone distal to the fracture; the site of insertion varies with the type of fracture. The pin protrudes through the skin on both sides of the extremity,

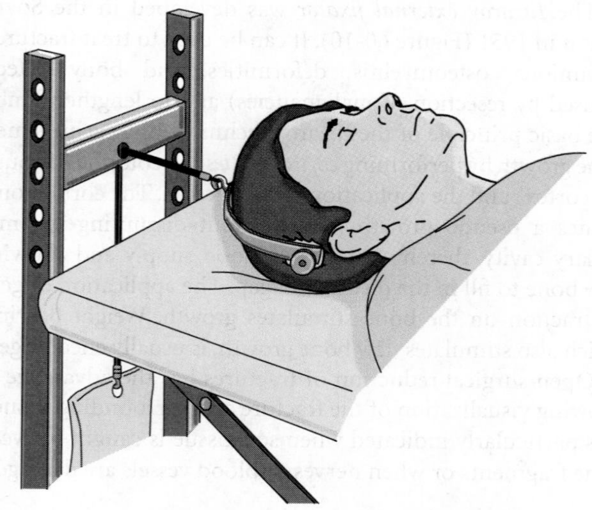

**fig. 60-6** Traction to the cervical spine can be maintained through the use of Crutchfield tongs inserted into the skull.

and the ends of the pin are covered with cork or metal protectors. Small sterile dressings are usually placed over the entry and exit sites of the pin, or pin sites may be left uncovered for easier observation. A U-shaped metal spreader or bow is attached to the pin, and the rope on which the traction weights are hung is tied onto the spreader. Skeletal traction can be used for fractures of the tibia, femur, humerus, and cervical spine. Skeletal traction applied to the cervical spine is achieved through use of tongs applied to the skull (Figure 60-6).

When a balanced suspension apparatus is used in conjunction with skin or skeletal traction, the patient is able to move about in bed more freely without disturbing the line of pull of the traction. The use of a balancing apparatus facilitates nursing measures such as bathing, skin care, and positioning the bedpan. A full- or half-ring Thomas or Hodgen splint is commonly used for suspension of the lower extremity (Figure 60-7). Straps of canvas, muslin, or synthetic lamb's wool are placed over the splint and secured to provide a support for the leg. The areas under the popliteal space and heel are left open to prevent pressure on these parts. If knee flexion or movement of the lower leg is desirable, a Pearson attachment is clamped or fixed to the Thomas splint at the level of the knee.

**Other types of external immobilization.** Other devices for external immobilization of fractures include:

1. Braces made of rigid plastic material
2. Plaster or plastic braces that incorporate metal struts attached to pins inserted into bone, such as a halo brace (Figure 60-8)

### *Surgical management*

A variety of procedures and materials exists for operative fracture fixation. The materials selected and type of procedure performed depend on the individual patient, surgeon, and type of fracture. Materials selected for internal fixation must

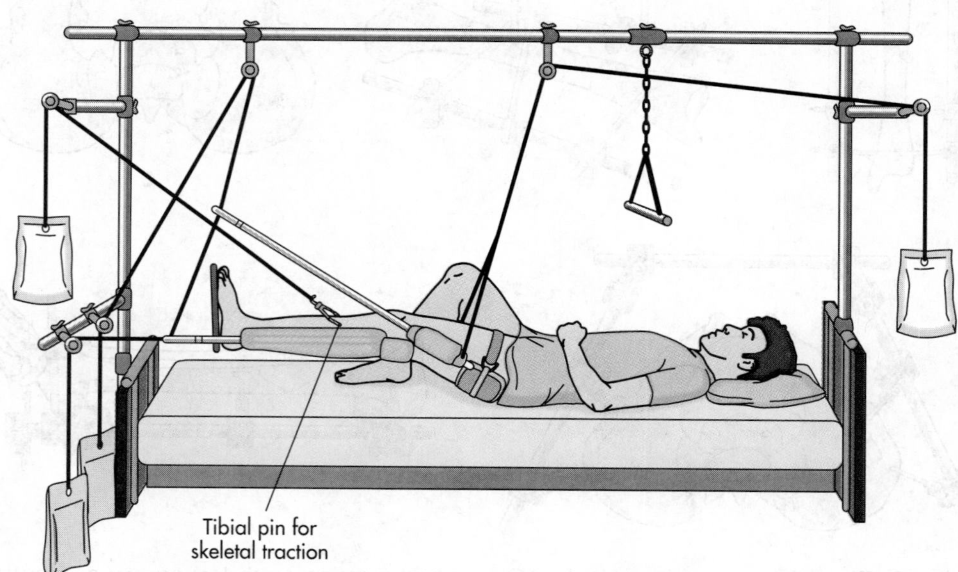


**fig. 60-7** Balanced suspension with Thomas splint and Pearson attachment. This apparatus can be used alone or, as in this case, with skeletal traction.

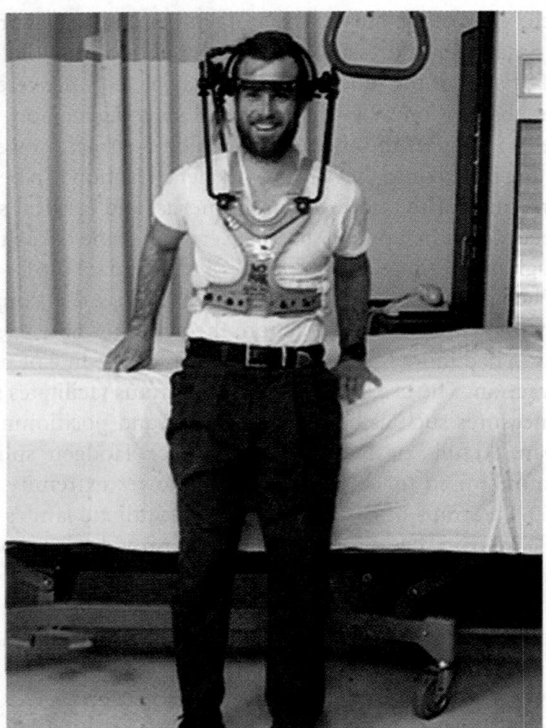

**fig. 60-8** Halo vest. Note the rigid shoulder straps and encompassing vest. Various vest sizes are available prefabricated. The halo ring, superstructure, and vest are magnetic resonance imaging (MRI)-compatible.

be strong and flexible. Two common materials are titanium alloy and stainless steel. Both of these materials provide adequate strength and fatigue resistance to allow healing of the fracture. Both may be contoured to fit irregularities in bone surfaces.

One method of fracture fixation is the external fixation device, which consists of metal struts attached to pins inserted into bone (Figure 60-9). External fixators such as the Hoffman or Synthes devices may be used alone or in conjunction with plaster. All of these devices provide extremely rigid fixation while allowing the patient some degree of mobility. The patient with an external fixator on the lower leg can be out of bed in a wheelchair and can ambulate without bearing weight on the affected leg.

The *Ilizarov external fixator* was developed in the Soviet Union in 1951 (Figure 60-10). It can be used to treat fractures, nonunions, osteomyelitis, deformities, and bony defects (caused by resection of malignancies) and to lengthen limbs. The basic principle of the Ilizarov technique is to achieve new bone growth by performing *corticotomies* (osteotomies through the cortex) and the application of distraction. The corticotomy creates a pseudo–growth plate without disrupting the medullary cavity, thereby preserving blood supply and allowing new bone to fill in the distraction gap. The application of gentle traction on the bone stimulates growth. Weight bearing, which also stimulates new bone growth, is usually encouraged.

Open surgical reduction of fractures has the advantage of allowing visualization of the fracture and surrounding tissues. It is particularly indicated when soft tissue is caught between bone fragments or when nerves or blood vessels are damaged.

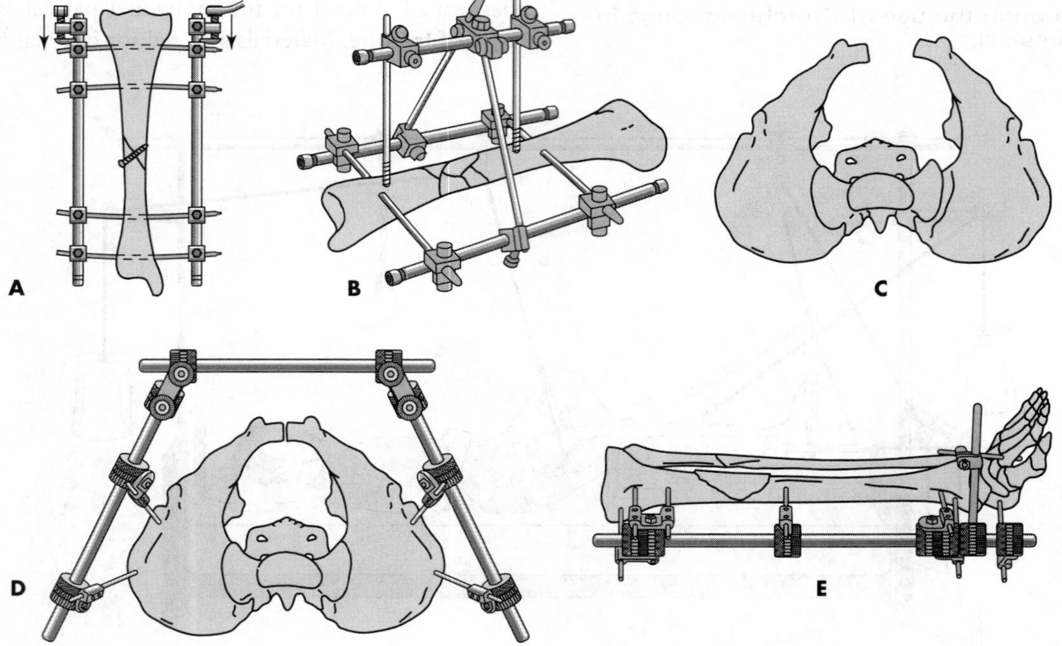


**fig. 60-9** **A,** Tibial fracture with simple AO external fixation with lag screw at fracture site. **B,** AO (Synthes) external fixator with three-dimensional or triangular fixation of comminuted fracture of the tibia. **C,** Pelvic diastasis (dislocation). **D,** Hex-Fix™ external fixator in place, showing reduction of pelvic fracture. **E,** Hex-Fix™ external fixator used to treat tibial fracture. Immobilization of ankle and foot allows soft-tissue healing.

The disadvantages of internal fixation are that it requires anesthesia and carries the risk of infection at the time of surgery. Internal fixation is carried out under the most vigorous aseptic conditions, and patients may receive a course of perioperative prophylactic intravenous antibiotics.

A variety of internal fixation devices are available:

1. Plates and nails (Figure 60-11, *A*)
2. Intramedullary rods (Figure 60-11, *B*)
3. Transfixion screws (Figure 60-12)
4. Prosthetic implants (Figure 60-13, *A* and *B*)—used particularly when survival of the proximal fragment of the fracture is jeopardized, for example, a fracture through or immediately below the femoral head

Rigid internal fixation with hardware is often used in conjunction with bone grafting, particularly when there has been excessive bone loss at the fracture site. *Autogenous* bone grafting (the patient's own bone) from the iliac crest is the gold standard for bone grafting material.[19] However, this procedure has risks, including increased blood loss, potential for infection, and increased pain. Alternatives to this technique include *allograft* (human donor bone) and bone "substitutes." Allograft is bone derived from living or cadaver donors. During total hip arthroplasty (see Chapter 61) the femoral head is removed and may be processed for the bone bank and future grafting. Allograft bone has the risk of transmission of blood and tissue-borne disease, including the human immunodeficiency virus (HIV).

Methods of processing the bone differ. Immunogenicity, sterility, mechanical properties, and bone-stimulation potential depend on the method of collection and processing. Bone that carries the highest risk of viral and bacterial contamination is cadaveric bone collected by sterile technique and used without further processing. However, cadaveric bone also contains the most bone growth factors, and thus it has the greatest potential to stimulate new bone formation.[19] Ethylene oxide, a

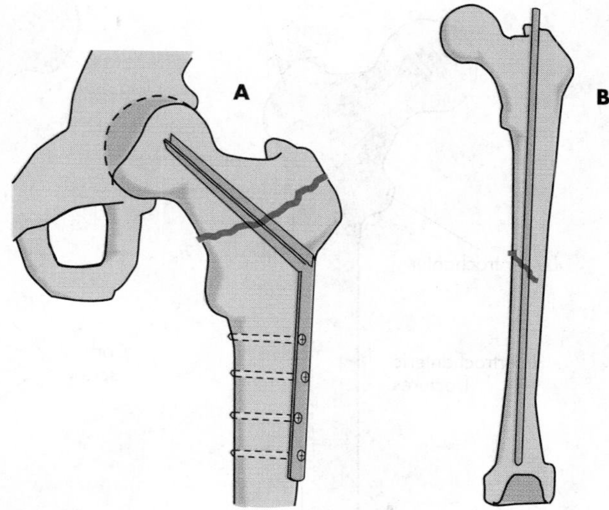


**fig. 60-11** **A**, Neufeld nail and screws, used in repair of intertrochanteric fracture. **B**, Küntscher nail (intramedullary rod) used in repair of midshaft femoral fracture.

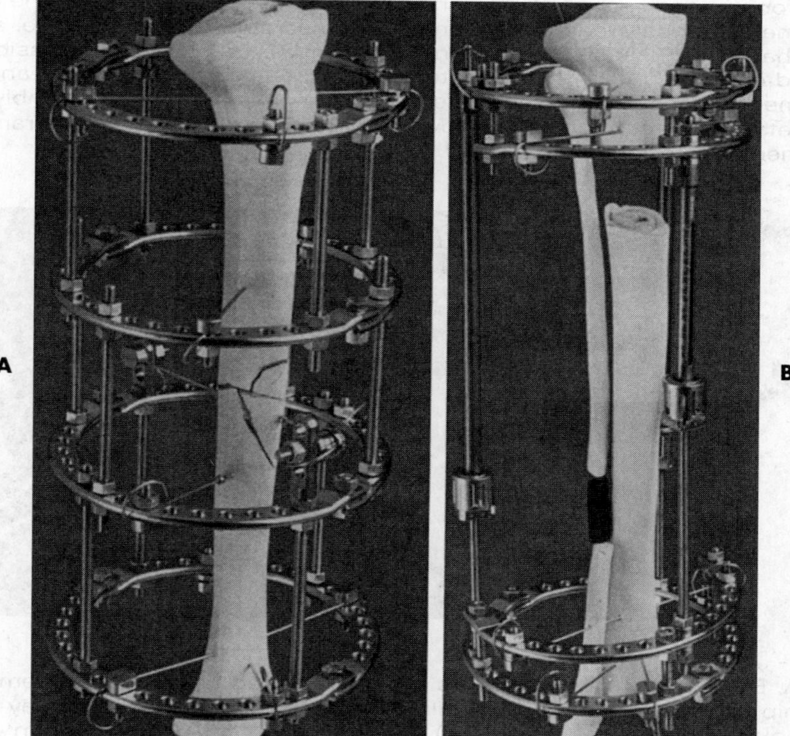


**fig. 60-10** **A**, Ilizarov device in place to treat comminuted fracture. **B**, Ilizarov device assembly for lengthening of tibia.

sterilizing agent, is not able to penetrate large pieces of allograft; therefore large grafts must be secondarily sterilized with gamma radiation. However, even the acceptable dose of gamma radiation may not be sufficient to eliminate HIV.

An alternative to both types of human bone graft materials is *hydroxyapatite* and other similar materials. Hydroxyapatite, a material derived from coral, has been approved by the Food and Drug Administration. This material is useful for filling bone defects, but it does not stimulate bone growth. A similar material, made from collagen and hydroxyapatite, also requires autogenous bone grafting to stimulate bone growth. In addition, it has poor structural properties. These bone

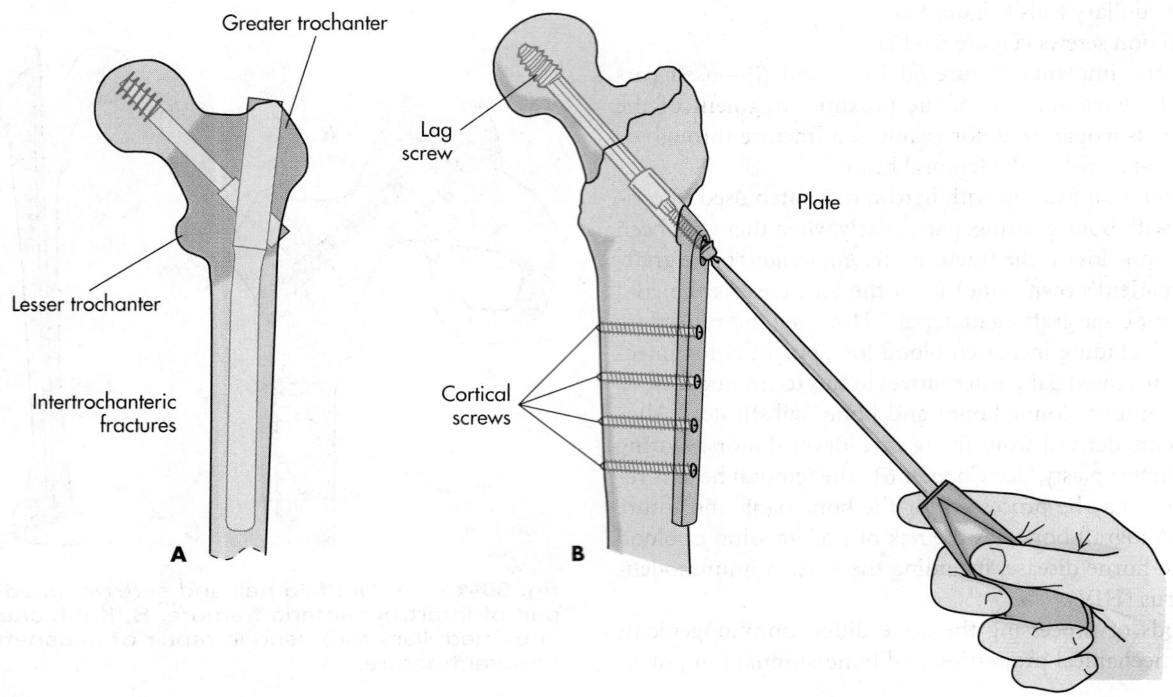


**fig. 60-12 A,** Richards intramedullary hip screw used for proximal femur fractures. Shown here for management of intratrochanteric fracture *(shaded area).* The device consists of intramedullary nail, lag screw, compression screw, centering sleeve, and set screw. **B,** Richards compression screw and plate for hip fracture. Compression screw (shown at end of screwdriver) threads into the distal end of the lag screw and draws the fracture fragments together. The sliding feature of the nail and plate assembly reduces the risk of acetabular penetration and allows weight-bearing forces to be transferred to the bone, rather than to the device.

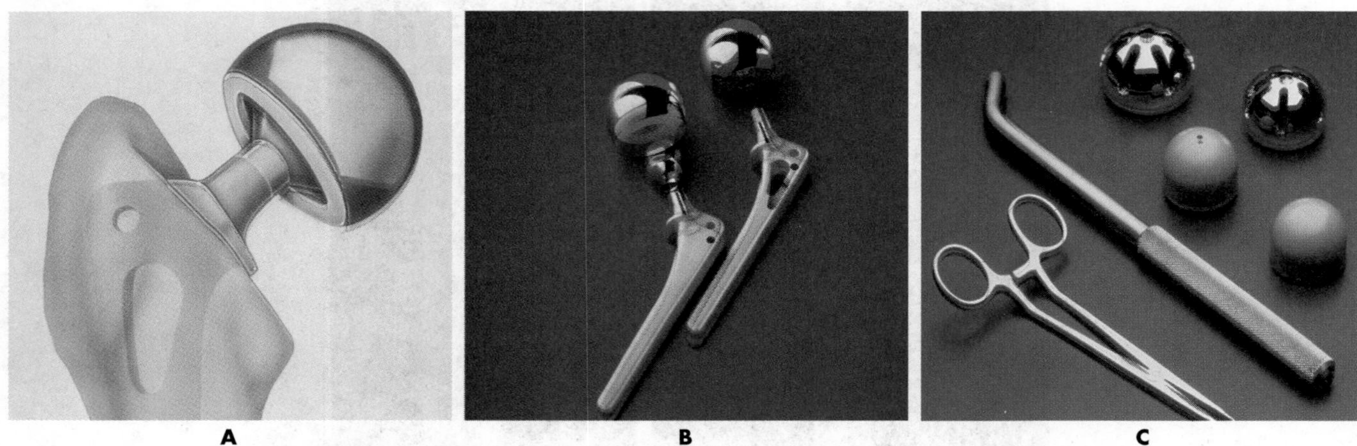


**fig. 60-13 A,** Bipolar modular prosthesis commonly used to replace the femoral head and neck in hip fractures when the vascular supply to the femoral head may be compromised. **B,** Bipolar (left) and unipolar (right) hip prostheses for hip fracture. In unipolar prostheses the femoral head attaches directly to the femoral stem. In bipolar prostheses the femoral head consists of two components. **C,** Instrumentation used for hip prostheses. Trial components used for sizing actual implant.

"pastes" can be injected directly into the fracture site and harden in about 10 minutes. Twelve hours later, they are as strong as normal human bone. Ideally, as with human bone graft, the body eventually resorbs the graft material and transforms it into bone mineral. Fixation with internal devices does not preclude additional fixation with external devices (casts, braces, or traction), particularly in cases of highly complicated fracture or multiple trauma.

In general, the major objective of care is to protect the fixation until healing takes place. Metal, which can fatigue and break, cannot be expected to substitute for intact bone. If the fixation device breaks, healing of the fracture will be disrupted. However, mobilization of patients who have had internal fixation is usually much faster than that for patients who have had external fixation.

Severe open fractures can be treated with antibiotic "beads" placed directly in the wound. Antibiotic-impregnated beads of bone cement (polymethylmethacrylate) are placed temporarily in compound fracture wounds. Tobramycin is commonly used. The wound is then covered with a porous, transparent dressing. This method, first used in total hip arthroplasty, is effective in reducing infection.[9]

#### Diet

A diet high in protein and with sufficient calories is necessary to promote bone and tissue healing. If immobility is prolonged, foods high in calcium (milk, milk products) should be encouraged to prevent hypocalcemia. A negative nitrogen balance may develop if protein intake is insufficient to compensate for catabolism in the immobilized patient. In addition, metabolic needs are increased during healing. Maintenance of ideal body weight is encouraged, to avoid increased stress on the joints. Fluids and fiber should be encouraged to promote bowel and bladder elimination. Vitamin and iron supplements may be prescribed to prevent or treat anemia.

#### Activity

Activity is limited, depending on the individual patient, type and location of fracture, and method of reduction. The physician determines the amount of ambulation, activity, and weight-bearing and prescribes specific exercises. Isometric exercises should be performed while in bed to promote circulation and prevent muscle atrophy.

#### Referrals

Common referrals for persons with fractures include physical therapy and occupational therapy for instructions regarding exercises and proper use of assistive and adaptive devices. Placement in a rehabilitation facility or home care may be necessary for some persons with multiple trauma or complicated fractures.

## NURSING MANAGEMENT

### ASSESSMENT

#### Subjective Data

Subjective data to be collected include the patient's report of:

- Mechanism of injury, events leading up to injury
- Pain
- Loss of sensation or movement of affected part
- Medication history
- Past medical history—as stated earlier, the presence of chronic diseases may affect the healing process.
- Nutritional history—the patient's nutritional status will affect the healing process. Patients with inadequate nutritional intake may require supplements.
- Coping skills, support systems

#### Objective Data

Objective data to be collected include:

- Head-to-toe assessment (see Chapter 59)
- Warmth, edema, or ecchymosis over and surrounding the injured part
- Obvious deformity, changes in normal alignment
- Loss of normal function in the injured part
- Immobilization device(s) applied to the injured part
- Complete neurovascular assessment (Table 60-2)

**table 60-2** *Signs and Symptoms of Neurovascular Impairment*

| Signs and Symptoms | Interpretation |
|---|---|
| Tissue color white (pallor) | Decreased arterial blood supply |
| Tissue color blue (cyanosis) | Venous stasis and poorly oxygenated tissue |
| Prolonged capillary refill | Decreased arterial blood supply |
| Edema | Fluid accumulating in tissues; poor venous return |
| Tissue cold or cool to touch | Decreased arterial blood supply |
| Patient unable to move parts distal to injury or external fixation device; paralysis or paresis | Pressure on nerves innervating parts distal to injury or underlying external fixation device |
| Patient report of extreme pain unrelieved by elevation, analgesic, or repositioning | Pressure on nerves innervating parts distal to injury or underlying external fixation device, ischemia |
| Patient report of heightened or decreased sensation or paresthesia in part distal to injury or underlying external fixation device | Pressure on nerves innervating parts distal to injury or underlying external fixation device |
| Diminished or absent pulses | Arterial injury, vascular compromise secondary to tissue edema |

Comparison of tissue should be made with uninvolved limb to determine the extent of the deviation from normal.

Condition of skin
Indicators of apprehension or fear

## NURSING DIAGNOSES

Nursing diagnoses are determined from analysis of patient data. Various methods of treatment, including surgical repair and immobilization by cast, traction, or external devices, are considered here when discussing nursing diagnoses and interventions. See Chapters 18 and 20 for general preoperative and postoperative care. Nursing diagnoses for the patient with a fracture may include but are not limited to:

| Nursing Diagnoses | Possible Etiological Factors |
|---|---|
| Knowledge deficit: fracture | Lack of experience with fracture, hospitalization, treatment protocols |
| Trauma, risk for | Sensorimotor deficits |
| Mobility, impaired physical | Musculoskeletal impairment, decreased strength and endurance, pain |
| Pain | Injury to bone or soft tissue at fracture site, muscle spasm, edema, surgery, immobility, improper positioning, pressure points |
| Neurovascular dysfunction, risk for peripheral | Pressure, restrictive envelope, mechanical compression, trauma, casts, traction |
| Tissue perfusion, altered, peripheral | Immobility, anesthesia, pressure sites |
| Infection, risk for | Tissue trauma, open fracture, surgical intervention |
| Self-care deficit | Musculoskeletal impairment, pain/discomfort, activity intolerance |
| Home maintenance management, impaired | Surgery, altered mobility, activity restrictions |
| Skin integrity, risk for impaired | Decreased mobility, pressure, shearing forces |
| Nutrition, altered: less than body requirements | Fatigue, pain; increased metabolic needs |
| Powerlessness | Health care environment, decreased mobility |
| Injury, risk for | Systemic complications of fractures |

## EXPECTED PATIENT OUTCOMES

Expected patient outcomes for the patient with a fracture may include but are not limited to:

1. Patient or significant others can explain rationale and course of treatment, including:
   a. Nature of injury and course of treatment that must be followed to prevent injury or infection and to achieve desired result
   b. Preoperative and postoperative routines and treatment protocols if surgical repair of fracture is indicated
   c. Type and duration of weight-bearing and activity restrictions
   d. How to perform or modify activities of daily living (ADL) within prescribed limitations of activity and motion; correct use of adaptive devices
   e. Care for cast, pins, or other immobilization devices, if applicable
   f. Safe use of an ambulatory or other ADL assistive device, if necessary
   g. Safe technique in performing wound care, if necessary
   h. Techniques appropriate to prevent skin breakdown, swelling, and neurovascular impairment
   i. Measures that can be taken for relief of pain or discomfort
   j. Appropriate use of prescribed medications
   k. Plans for follow-up care
   l. Methods to prevent further fracture or injury
2. Patient avoids additional trauma or injury by using adaptive or assistive devices correctly
   a. Patient identifies potential hazards in environment and methods to reduce risk of injury
3. Patient participates in a program of progressive activity
4. Patient states that pain is decreased with a lower rating on a scale of 1 to 10 (1 = no pain, 10 = most severe pain imaginable)
5. Patient maintains intact peripheral neurovascular status in all extremities
6. Patient maintains adequate tissue perfusion
7. Patient does not develop an infection
8. Patient demonstrates ability to do self-care
9. Patient adapts home environment to meet his or her needs
   a. Removes scatter rugs
   b. Positions furniture to provide clear pathway when ambulating with walker or crutches
   c. Places safety devices in bathroom (grab bars, elevated toilet seat, tub rails)
10. Patient maintains skin integrity
11. Patient stabilizes weight at an acceptable level
12. Patient verbalizes sense of power and control of situation
13. Patient is free from additional injury and systemic complications of fractures.

## INTERVENTIONS

### Preventing Trauma and Injury/Promoting Self-Care

As healing progresses and pain diminishes, patients will be more receptive to learning what activities are necessary for a safe return home. The following instructions should be included:

1. How to move comfortably in bed
2. Safe transfer techniques
3. Duration and extent of weight-bearing restrictions
4. Type of activity restrictions
5. Proper use of ambulatory or other ADL assistive devices
6. Use and care of immobilization devices (slings, casts, and pins)
7. Proper positioning of the affected extremity
8. Pain or discomfort relief measures
9. Exercises to maintain strength and enhance circulation

The easiest and most effective way to teach patients self-care is to have them function as independently as possible within their prescribed limitations, using the appropriate assistive devices while they are in the hospital.

### Maintaining Strength and Mobility/Promoting Activity

One objective in the care of the patient who has sustained a fracture is to prevent loss of mobility and muscle tone. This is true for the fractured part, as well as for the rest of the body. The nurse can use the following interventions to assist the patient to maintain mobility, muscle tone, and strength:

1. Allow and encourage the patient to move about to the greatest extent possible within the restrictions of the fracture reduction and the immobilizing devices.
2. Allow and encourage the patient to accomplish as much self-care as possible.
3. Encourage the patient to perform muscle toning (isometric) exercises on a regular basis, for example, quadriceps setting, gluteal setting (see Chapters 18 and 20).
4. Encourage and assist the patient to follow through with exercise programs (including ambulation) prescribed by the physician and taught by the physical therapist and nurse.
5. Encourage and assist patient to resume normal functioning for all ADL (within limits of immobilization or fixation device) as soon as possible, for example, using bedside commode or toilet instead of bedpan.

### Promoting Comfort

The person with a fracture will often have severe pain at the fracture site, pressure from edema in the damaged soft tissues adjacent to the fracture, and spasm of the muscles in the fracture area. Continued pain and muscle spasm can put undue stress on the fracture fragments and retard efforts both to reduce and to maintain reduction of the fracture. Patients who are in severe pain will resist efforts to help them carry out measures designed to prevent complications. If the fracture is repaired by open reduction and internal fixation (ORIF), the patient will have operative pain.

Measures the nurse can take to help reduce pain include the following:

1. During initial stages of treatment, administer prescribed narcotic and nonnarcotic analgesics in appropriate doses at timely intervals.
2. Instruct the patient about principles of pain management and use of patient-controlled analgesia (PCA), if prescribed.
3. Administer prescribed agents such as diazepam (Valium) to reduce muscle spasm.
4. Apply ice compresses, as ordered, to the affected part to reduce swelling and decrease pain.
5. Reposition patient frequently within prescribed position or activity limitations to avoid prolonged pressure over bony prominences and to prevent stiffness.
6. Instruct patient how to use relaxation techniques (deep breathing, imagery) to reduce tension (see Chapters 6 and 20).
7. As pain subsides, negotiate with the patient a reduction in the strength or frequency of analgesic administration.

Positioning is a measure that promotes comfort, provides for adequate ventilation and mobilization of pulmonary secretions, enhances circulation, and relieves pressure on vulnerable skin areas. Before positioning, the nurse should know the following:

1. Location and type of fracture
2. Reduction techniques
3. Special activity or positioning restrictions

The nurse should use the following guidelines for positioning the patient with a fracture:

1. Maintain the alignment of the fracture.
2. Maintain the direction of pull of traction. See the Guidelines for Care Box for the person in traction.
3. Maintain the integrity of the cast. See the Guidelines for Care Box for the person in a cast.
4. Maintain positioning, activity, and weight-bearing restrictions of internal fixation device (if any). See the Guidelines for Care Box for the person with an internal fixation device.

Generally, nurses should avoid changing the position of patients with unreduced, unsplinted fractures. Manipulation of fracture fragments, particularly long bones, may cause release of fat into the vasculature (see the section on fat embolus).

Once the parameters for safe positioning are defined, the nurse should assist the patient to change position at least every 2 hours until the patient can do so independently. Providing an overhead frame with a trapeze helps the patient move in bed.

### Maintaining Intact Neurovascular Status and Tissue Perfusion

Monitoring for neurovascular compromise must be carried out every hour in the initial stages of fracture. Damage to blood vessels or nerves may occur at the time of the fracture or following reduction. Some swelling of a fractured extremity may be expected and is often well controlled by elevating the extremity. However, unrelieved swelling of an extremity that is confined in a cast or compression dressing causes undue pressure on vessels and nerves and can result in circulatory or neurological impairment. Evidence of impaired circulation or sensation must be reported to the physician immediately. Frequency of neurovascular checks can usually be reduced if there is no evidence of compromise within 48 hours of the fracture or reduction (see Table 60-2). Observations of the involved extremity should be compared with observations of the uninvolved extremity to validate deviations from the patient's "normal."

Monitoring neurovascular status of the injured part includes:

1. Palpating for warmth
2. Observing color
3. Assessing length of capillary filling time
4. Questioning patient about pain and paresthesias in injured part
5. Assessing patient's ability to discriminate sensation
6. Observing patient's ability to voluntarily move body part distal to fracture
7. Instituting measures to promote venous blood flow:
   a. Elevate extremities to level slightly above the heart
   b. Apply elastic stockings or intermittent pneumatic compression devices
   c. Use proper positioning techniques
   d. Avoid external compression on pressure sites
   e. Encourage range of motion (ROM) and isometric exercises

**guidelines for care**

### The Person in Traction

1. Patient education
   a. Explain traction in relation to fracture and physician's plan of treatment.
   b. Explain amount of movement permitted and how to achieve it (e.g., how trapeze can be used to assist with movement)
   c. Explain correct body positioning. Maintain proper body alignment.
2. Maintain continuous traction, unless indicated otherwise
   a. Inspect traction apparatus frequently to ensure that ropes are running straight and through the middle of the pulleys; that weights are hanging free; that bedclothes, the bed, or the frame and bars on the bed are not impinging on any part of the traction apparatus.
   b. Check ropes frequently to be sure they are not frayed.
   c. Avoid releasing weights or altering the line of pull of the traction.
   d. Avoid adding weight to the traction.
   e. Check the position of the Thomas splint frequently; if the ring slides away from the groin, readjust the splint to its proper position without releasing traction.
   f. Avoid bumping into or jarring the bed or traction equipment.
   g. Be sure weights are securely fastened to their ropes.
   h. Avoid manipulation of pins.
3. Maintain countertraction
4. Skin care
   a. Encourage the patient to turn slightly from side to side and to lift up on the trapeze to relieve pressure on the skin of the sacrum and scapulae; have the patient lift up for routine skin care to prevent friction and shearing forces.
   b. Avoid padding the ring of the Thomas splint, because this will create dampness next to the skin. Bathe the skin beneath the ring, dry it thoroughly, and powder the skin lightly.
   c. Inspect skin frequently to be sure it is not being rubbed, contused, or macerated by traction equipment; readjust splints or the extremity in the splint to free the skin from pressure.
   d. Keep skin areas around pin sites clean and dry; direct care to pin sites (e.g., cleansing with cotton applicators and hydrogen peroxide, povidone iodine, or alcohol) is controversial. Check with the physician regarding method and frequency of pin care.
5. Toileting
   a. Use a fracture pan with blanket roll or padding as support under the small of the back.
   b. Protect the ring of the Thomas splint with waterproof material when female patients are using the bedpan.

8. Assessing for presence of positive Homans' sign (although not always reliable)
9. Encouraging ambulation if possible
10. Obtaining baseline and ongoing measurements of circumference of both calves for comparison

### Preventing Infection

Interventions to promote wound healing include:

1. Carefully attending to aseptic technique during dressing changes to prevent infection; assessing wound for signs of healing or presence of infection
2. Monitoring drains for correct placement
3. Assessing pin sites regularly; perform pin care as specified to prevent infection
4. Providing and encouraging patient to eat a well-balanced diet to provide the nutritional elements necessary for tissue healing
5. Assessing patient for any systemic signs of infection
6. Monitoring laboratory data (e.g., WBC, C&S, ESR)
7. Assessing patient for therapeutic response to antibiotics if prescribed

### Facilitating Return to Home Environment

Discharge planning should begin at admission. In preparation for the patient's discharge, the following should be determined:

1. Assess probable level of functioning at time of discharge and determine type of assistance and equipment that will be needed.
   a. As necessary, refer to home care team, community health nurse, or other agency that will meet with patient and family to determine what help (aide, homemaker) may be needed. This is especially important for persons who live alone or who will be alone for long periods of time while family members are at work.
   b. Most patients will need a walker or crutches and should be taught to use these before discharge. Remind the patient and family that scatter rugs should be removed so the patient will not trip while walking with an assistive device.
   c. Furniture should be positioned to provide a clear pathway in areas where the patient will be walking, especially between bedroom and bathroom.
   d. Safety devices such as an elevated toilet seat, grab bars, and tub rails should be in place before the patient arrives home. Elevated toilet seats with arms on each side can be rented from a medical supply store or drugstore.
2. Provide guidance about the availability of community resources, such as meals-on-wheels and exercise pools.
3. Assess the patient's support system; encourage family involvement in care.
4. Support the patient's and family's decision-making abilities.
5. Teach and supervise correct use of adaptive devices. In many institutions physical and occupational therapists do much of this teaching. However, the nurse needs to reinforce the teaching and supervise the patient in the correct use of these devices.

guidelines for care

### The Person in a Cast

1. Patient education
   a. Before cast application, explain why and how the cast will be applied.
   b. Advise the patient that the plaster cast will feel warm as it dries.
   c. Explain the extent to which the patient will be immobilized.
   d. Following cast application, explain care of the cast and expectations after discharge.
   e. Instruct patient not to insert sharp objects (coat hangers or pencils) under the cast, because these may abrade the skin and lead to infection.
   f. Cast removal: explain that saw used for removal is noisy; saw will not harm skin.
2. Handling the new cast
   a. Support wet cast with the flat of the hands or on pillows to avoid indentations that will cause pressure on underlying skin.
   b. Place cotton blankets or other absorbent material under the cast to aid the drying process.
   c. Expose the cast to air as much as possible to aid the drying process.
   d. Turn the patient frequently to aid the drying process.
   e. Use a fan to circulate air over the cast.
   f. *Do not apply paint, varnish, or shellac to the cast; plaster is a porous material that allows air to circulate to the skin.*
3. Skin care
   a. Inspect skin at edges of cast and underlying the cast for redness or irritation; apply petal-shaped strips of adhesive tape or moleskin around rough edges of cast.
   b. Remove plaster crumbs from skin with a washcloth moistened with warm water.
   c. Use creams and lotions sparingly, because they may soften the skin and cause the cast to stick to the skin.
   d. Apply waterproof material around perineal area to prevent skin irritation and soiling of and damage to cast.
   e. Attend to patient's report of pain under the cast, particularly over bony prominences, because this may indicate pressure on the skin. If discomfort is not relieved by repositioning, report to physician. Cast pressure may need to be relieved by windowing or bivalving (cutting cast into two halves).
   f. Following cast removal, skin care to remove built-up exudate of secretions and dead skin. Mineral oil and warm water soaks are helpful.
4. Turning
   a. Turning to any position is generally permitted, as long as the integrity of the cast is not compromised and the patient is comfortable.
5. Toileting (for a long leg or hip spica cast)
   a. Use a fracture pan with blanket roll or padding as support under the small of the back
   b. Elevate the head of the bed if permitted, or place the bed in reverse Trendelenburg position.
6. Abdominal discomfort
   a. Spica cast may be "windowed" (cut an opening into cast) to provide relief of abdominal distention or as a port for checking bladder distention.
7. Mobilization
   a. Weight-bearing is at the discretion of the physician, who will prescribe specific limitations.
   b. A cast shoe or a walking heel incorporated into a lower extremity cast will permit weight-bearing without damaging the cast.
8. Prevention of neurovascular problems
   a. Perform neurovascular checks every hour for at least 24 hours after cast application to detect difficulty from swelling or pressure of cast on nerves or vessels. Notify physician of color changes, alterations in sensation, or motion unrelieved by position change; cast may need to be bivalved to relieve pressure.
   b. Elevate affected extremity on pillows until danger of swelling is over (usually 24 to 48 hours).
   c. After mobilization of patient with lower extremity or upper extremity cast, avoid keeping extremity in dependent position for prolonged periods.
   d. After lower extremity cast is removed, encourage patient to wear elastic stocking and elevate affected leg at rest until full mobility is regained.

guidelines for care

### The Person with an Internal Fixation Device

1. Patient education
   a. Prepare the patient for anesthesia.
   b. Explain the surgical procedure and general nursing care after surgery. (See Chapters 18 through 20.)
   c. Postoperatively, explain the limits of motion and weight-bearing to the affected part.
2. Promoting mobility
   a. Determine, in consultation with the physician, the limits of motion and weight-bearing permitted.
   b. Instruct and assist the patient to turn, transfer, and ambulate within the prescribed limits (mobilization may begin as early as the day of surgery).
   c. Instruct and assist the patient to use an appropriate ambulatory aid if the fracture is of a lower extremity.
3. Prevention of neurovascular problems
   a. Perform neurovascular checks every hour for the first 24 to 48 hours; notify the physician of any change from preoperative status, because this may indicate pressure from swelling, constricting bandages, or damage to nerves or vessels at surgery.
   b. Keep affected extremity elevated.
4. Maintenance of immobilization of fracture; considerations for care would be the same as for patients in cast/traction if those devices are used

## Maintaining Skin Integrity

When determining interventions to maintain skin integrity, the nurse must consider ways to prevent skin breakdown, as well as ways to promote wound healing. Measures to prevent skin breakdown include:

1. Identifying skin areas at risk, particularly areas over bony prominences (e.g., heels, sacrum, elbows, scapulae, and ischial tuberosities)
2. Inspecting skin (at least every 8 hours) for signs of pressure (e.g., erythema or induration, nonblanchable areas)
3. Turning (at least every 2 hours) while maintaining fracture immobilization using a turning sheet
4. Moving patient from one surface to another with a pull sheet or roller board
5. Rolling patient onto side or lifting patient to place him or her on a bedpan rather than sliding pan under patient
6. For patient who cannot be fully turned because of traction apparatus or other limiting factors, possibly using one or more of the following pressure-relieving devices:
   a. Sheepskin pads
   b. Flotation pads
   c. Alternating air pressure mattress or alternating air pressure system
   d. Foam mattress
   e. Foam heel or elbow pads
   f. Special bed such as the Clinitron, Mediscus, or Biodyne
   g. Turning frames such as the Foster or Stryker frames
7. Regularly inspecting skin areas in contact with cast edges or traction apparatus and taking appropriate measures to eliminate chafing or rubbing in those areas
8. Assisting patient to keep skin clean and dry, especially under casts, slings, and traction apparatus

## Promoting Nutrition/Stabilizing Weight

The essentials of a nutritious diet, including fruits, vegetables, proteins, and vitamins, are especially important for the individual after a fracture. If mobility is restricted, catabolic activity is accelerated, producing a rapid breakdown of cellular materials, leading to protein deficiency and negative nitrogen balance. Decalcification and demineralization of bone take place during immobility, regardless of the quantity of calcium intake. Therefore increasing dietary calcium above normal requirements is not recommended, because the excess calcium cannot be used. However, a diet high in protein is indicated to overcome protein deficiency and to return the body to a state of positive nitrogen balance. Patients who have had fractures have increased needs for iron, protein, and vitamins if bone repair is to progress normally. Weight gain or loss is to be avoided, especially if the patient is in a cast or molded brace, because it will affect the proper fit of the device.

Interventions the nurse can use to ensure adequate nutrition for the patient include:

1. Encourage the patient to eat regular meals.
2. Allow the patient adequate time to eat.
3. Encourage self-feeding, but help the patient or provide special assistive utensils as necessary.
4. Attend to the patient's need for roughage and fluid as noted and encourage protein intake of 150 to 300 g per day.
5. Position the patient to facilitate comfortable intake of food and fluid.

## Promoting Autonomy and Sense of Control

To promote autonomy, the following interventions may be helpful:

1. Assess and incorporate patient's locus of control (internal or external) into plan of care.
2. Explain course of treatment to patient and family.
3. Provide opportunities for decision making.
4. Incorporate patient preferences into daily plan of care.
5. Allow the patient to manipulate the environment whenever possible.
6. Involve family and significant others in patient's care
7. Assist patient to set realistic goals.

## Preventing Injury from Systemic Complications of Fracture

Complications can arise as a result of the initial trauma, treatment, or the resulting loss of mobility. Systemic complications usually are a result of immobility or surgical intervention and include circulatory, respiratory, gastrointestinal, and urinary complications. See Chapter 20.

### *Preventing circulatory complications*

Individuals who have sustained trauma and are completely or partially immobilized are at risk of developing circulatory complications as a result of the following:

1. Failure of blood vessels in the legs to achieve and maintain a state of vasoconstriction
2. Pooling of venous blood and decreased venous return
3. Decreased cardiac output
4. Increased prothrombin time and platelet adhesiveness

These factors contribute to decreased ability to adapt to an erect posture, increased incidence of deep-vein thrombosis and pulmonary embolus, increased workload on the heart, and decreased tolerance to exercise or activity.

The nurse can use the following interventions to help prevent these complications:

1. Encourage and assist the patient to perform routine active or active-assisted ROM exercises (at least four times per day).
2. Teach and encourage the patient to perform active dorsiplantar flexion and quadriceps setting exercises every 1 to 2 hours.
3. Position the patient so that pressure is not exerted over major vessels.
4. Mobilize the patient slowly and increase activity gradually.
5. Elevate the affected extremity for the first 48 hours; thereafter, elevate the extremity when the patient is at rest.
6. Instruct the patient about the use of antiembolic hose and intermittent pneumatic compression devices.

***Preventing respiratory complications***

Factors that contribute to pooling of secretions in the bronchi and bronchioles are pain on movement or deep breathing, decreased movement, decreased stimulus to cough, and decreased depth of respiration.

Unless interventions are used to facilitate movement and removal of secretions, hypostatic pneumonia can result. Nursing interventions include:

1. Turning patient frequently to mobilize secretions
2. Encouraging patient to perform active or active-assisted ROM exercises to increase depth of respiration
3. Using appropriate pain control measures to improve respiratory effort
4. Teaching and encouraging patient to take maximal sustained inhalations and to cough to mobilize and clear secretions every 2 hours
5. Persons unable to ambulate should be assisted up to a chair at least twice daily. An upright position promotes optimal respiratory function.
6. Encouraging patient to move independently as much as possible to improve respiratory effort

***Preventing gastrointestinal complications***

Individuals who sustain trauma to the spine, pelvis, or extremities commonly experience a slowing or temporary cessation of bowel function. Paralytic ileus is a potential postfracture complication (see Chapter 41). Food and fluids are withheld until bowel sounds are present or the patient passes flatus.

Immobilized persons are at risk for constipation. Contributing factors are changes in normal dietary habits and fluid intake, lack of activity, and use of a bedpan. Interventions the nurse can use to promote gastric motility and prevent constipation include:

1. Turning the patient frequently
2. Elevating the head of the bed (as permitted)
3. Administering stool-softening agents, laxatives, suppositories, or enemas
4. Encouraging the patient to incorporate bulk-building foods such as bran in the diet
5. Encouraging a fluid intake of 2000 to 3000 ml per day
6. Assisting the patient to use a bedside commode or toilet instead of a bedpan when possible

***Preventing urinary complications***

Patients with fractures, particularly if immobilized, are at risk of developing bladder infections and renal stones for the following reasons:

1. Increased serum calcium, because of bone destruction
2. Increased urinary pH (alkaline)
3. Increased citric acid (which precipitates calcium salts)
4. Urinary stasis because of difficulty emptying bladder when using a urinal or bedpan in bed

Nursing interventions to decrease the risk of these problems include:

1. Encouraging a fluid intake of 2000 to 3000 ml per day
2. Encouraging patient to decrease calcium intake
3. Encouraging patient to limit intake of citrus fruits and juices
4. Assisting patient to use a bedside commode or toilet when possible to facilitate emptying the bladder
5. Encouraging male patients to stand to urinate

## Patient/Family Education

Treatment of the acute fracture is usually carried out in the hospital's emergency room or in the operating room before the patient is admitted to the general hospital unit. Patients may have little or no opportunity to become oriented to the hospital or to the care they will be receiving. In addition, they will probably be frightened or overwhelmed by what has happened to them, be experiencing pain, and possibly be groggy from pain medication or anesthesia. Careful and often repeated explanation and direction regarding the following will be necessary:

1. Nature of injury and course of treatment, including follow-up care
2. Positioning
3. Skin care routines
4. Deep breathing and coughing
5. Pain relief measures
6. Exercises to be performed to prevent complications

Direction, explanation, and physical handling must be accomplished gently but efficiently during the initial stages of hospitalization. Patients must be given time to adjust to their situations before they can begin to understand how they can cooperate in their care.

***Health promotion/prevention***

One approach to preventing fracture is to make the home environment safer. Measures that can be taken include:

1. Mounting grab bars on the wall next to a tub or toilet
2. Attaching safety arms around a toilet
3. Removing throw rugs and obstacles from areas used by individuals with neurological or musculoskeletal impairment
4. Ensuring that wheelchairs have adequate locking devices
5. Teaching individuals who must use ambulatory devices and wheelchairs how to use them properly

A second approach is to continue to educate the public regarding the following:

1. The dangers of drinking alcohol and driving
2. Use of seat belts in motor vehicles
3. Attending to safety precautions when climbing ladders and using power tools or heavy equipment
4. Wearing recommended protective clothing (e.g., steel-toed shoes and hard hats for hazardous work at home or on the job)
5. Wearing proper protective clothing while engaging in sports (e.g., protective padding, helmets, and proper fitting running shoes)

A third approach is to continue to educate women about the problem of osteoporosis (see Chapter 61).

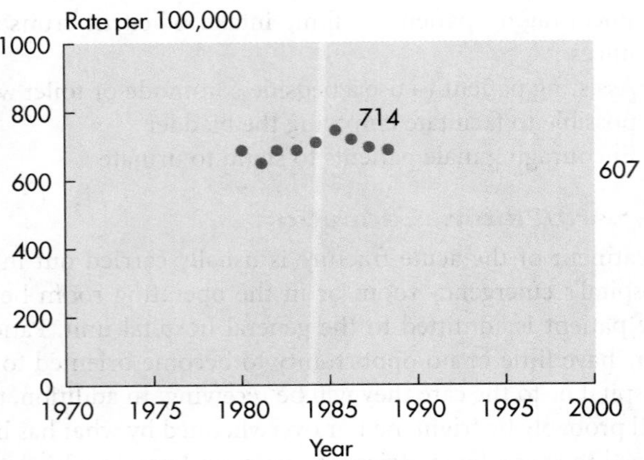


**fig. 60-14** Hip fracture rate among people aged 65 years and older. Note case rate of 714 in 1988 and target goal of 607 cases per 100,000 in the year 2000.

### Healthy People 2000

Goals from *Healthy People 2000* include reducing hospitalizations for hip fracture to 607 per 100,000 (Figure 60-14). White women ages 85 and older were targeted as a special population in 1995. The goal is to reduce hip fractures to 2177 per 100,000 in the year 2000 from a 1988 baseline of 2721 per 100,000.[20] See the section on hip fracture for further discussion.

## EVALUATION

To evaluate the effectiveness of nursing interventions, compare patient behaviors with those stated in the expected patient outcomes. Successful achievement of patient outcomes for the patient with a fracture is indicated by:

1. Correctly describing the nature of the injury and course of treatment, including perioperative routines
   a. Explaining the limitations and duration of motion and activity restrictions
   b. Explaining how to perform ADL using assistive devices
   c. Describing how to care for cast, pins, or other immobilization devices
   d. Demonstrating correct way to walk with cane, walker, or crutches
   e. Explaining how to cleanse wound and apply sterile dressings if applicable
   f. Explaining how to prevent skin breakdown, swelling, and neurovascular impairment
   g. Explaining appropriate use of analgesics
   h. Explaining plans for follow-up care
2. Ambulating safely using a cane, walker, or crutches
3. Participating in a program of progressive exercise
   a. Attends physical therapy sessions as indicated to practice prescribed exercises
   b. Participates in ADL to maximum potential
4. Verbalizing that pain is controlled effectively by:
   a. Rating pain as less than 4 on a scale of 1 to 10
   b. Use of oral analgesics or nonsteroidal antiinflammatory drugs (NSAIDs)
   c. Ice packs for 20 minutes after exercising
5. Maintaining peripheral neurovascular status and adequate tissue perfusion
   a. Pulses present, strong, and symmetrical in both extremities
   b. Limbs warm and pink
   c. Sensation and motor ability intact
   d. Capillary refill less than 3 seconds bilaterally
6. Maintaining infection-free status
   a. Incision appears clean and without excessive swelling, redness, or drainage
   b. Temperature normal
7. Demonstrating ability to do self-care
   a. Does personal care
   b. Dresses self
   c. Walks with cane or other ambulatory aid without assistance; able to ascend, descend stairs safely
8. Preparing home environment to meet safety needs
   a. All scatter rugs removed
   b. Furniture placed conveniently with firm chair with arms in areas frequently used, such as the bedroom and kitchen
   c. Safety bars, elevated toilet seat in bathroom
9. Maintaining skin integrity
   a. Skin clean and well moisturized
   b. Skin intact, free from pressure areas
10. Maintaining weight at acceptable level
   a. Eats varied diet with adequate calories and nutrients to promote healing
   b. Avoids weight gain above ideal weight to prevent placing excess stress on joints
11. Verbalizing feeling in control of situation
12. Demonstrating absence of systemic complications of fracture

## GERONTOLOGICAL CONSIDERATIONS

Older persons who sustain fractures often incur some loss of functional ability. The elderly are prone to fractures for many reasons, including osteoporosis, neoplasm, sensorimotor deficits, and falls. Falls are the most common cause of fracture in the elderly. Bones most commonly fractured are the proximal femur (hip), distal radius (Colles' fracture), vertebrae, and clavicle. Colles' fractures usually occur as a result of placing an outreached hand to break a fall, most commonly in a woman with osteoporosis. Treatment usually consists of closed reduction and immobilization. The majority of clavicular fractures in the elderly are sustained in a manner similar to a Colles' fracture. The fracture usually occurs in the medial third of the clavicle. The patient exhibits swelling, point tenderness, local deformity, and crepitus. Treatment consists of closed reduction and immobilization with a sling or cast. Vertebral fractures are usually pathological and are a result of osteoporosis. The fracture is usually a compression fracture of the vertebral body.

## SPECIAL ENVIRONMENTS FOR CARE

### Critical Care Management

The person who has sustained a fracture does not usually require critical care nursing management. Exceptions include a patient with fat embolism and the victim of multiple trauma.

The patient with a fat embolus is at risk of developing pulmonary edema and adult respiratory distress syndrome (ARDS). Treatment includes oxygen therapy, mechanical ventilation, positive end-expiratory pressure (PEEP), fluid replacement, and administration of steroids (their use is controversial). See Chapter 32 for a full discussion of ARDS.

#### Home care management

The home should be assessed for environmental hazards, including scatter rugs, highly waxed floors, electrical cords, and other potential hazards. Safety equipment such as grab bars, nonskid mats in the bath and tub, secure handrails, elevated toilet seat, elevated chair with arms, and nightlights should be rented or installed in the home if possible.

A home health aide may be required for assistance with ADL. Meals-on-wheels is an excellent resource for those who are unable to purchase or prepare their own meals. If dressing changes or intravenous medications are to be continued at home, a home care agency will be consulted for nursing visits. The patient may be transferred to a rehabilitation facility before going home if extensive therapy is needed.

## COMPLICATIONS OF FRACTURES

Complications of fractures affect the patient's recovery and functional outcome. Early recognition and treatment of complications are extremely important. In this section, fracture blisters, fat embolism syndrome, and compartment syndrome are discussed. Deep vein thrombosis and pulmonary embolus are also complications of fracture and are discussed in Chapters 20, 27, and 32. Impaired fracture healing may result in nonunion, malunion, or pseudoarthrosis. These complications are generally treated with revision of the reduction.

Infection and heterotopic bone formation are also complications of fracture and are discussed here briefly. Infection, which is the leading cause of delayed union and nonunion, occurs primarily in open or compound fractures.[7] Most symptoms of infection occur within 4 weeks of the injury. Pain is the primary symptom, followed by erythema and edema. Infections following open fractures commonly result in osteomyelitis (infection of the bone), which is discussed in Chapter 61.

Heterotopic bone formation occurs as a result of trauma in approximately 10% of cases and may cause pain and restricted joint motion. Evidence of heterotopic ossification is detectable by x-ray as early as 1 to 2 months after injury. Persons with head injuries are more prone to heterotopic bone formation. Treatment consists of surgical resection and, in some cases, low-dose radiation.

### Fracture Blisters

#### Etiology/epidemiology

Fracture blisters are skin bullae and blisters representing areas of epidermal necrosis with separation of the stratified squamous cell layer by edema fluid.[12] They are associated with fractures, twisting types of injuries, and joint trauma. Fracture blisters may also develop as a result of compartment syndrome, as the body attempts to relieve rising tissue pressures. Other factors influence the development of blisters, including the interval between fracture and immobilization. The presence of fracture blisters predisposes the patient to infection, delays in treatment, nonunion, impaired healing, and ultimately a longer hospital stay and increased costs. Research indicates that early surgical reduction results in a lesser incidence of blistering. Patients who underwent ORIF within 24 hours of injury had significantly lower incidence of blistering (2%) than those persons whose surgery was delayed more than 24 hours after injury (8%).[12] The highest incidence of fracture blisters occurs in the ankle, elbow, distal tibia, and foot; anatomical areas with tight skin constraints and little muscle or surrounding fascia, both of which contribute favorably to the formation of fracture blisters. The incidence of fracture blisters is 2.9% of all acute fractures that require hospitalization.[12] In fractures occurring in the areas most likely to develop blistering, the incidence rises to 5.2%.

#### Pathophysiology

After the acute injury, severe tissue edema and swelling develop as a result of damage to bone, ligaments, tendon, and surrounding soft tissues. The vasculature and lymphatic drainage are disrupted, which causes the epidermis to separate from the dermis.[12] Detachment of the epidermis results in disruption of its blood supply, causing necrosis of the epidermal layers. The edema and venous stasis that occur after the injury cause collapse and thrombosis of the affected blood and lymph vessels, which increases circulatory problems. Blisters may result from the local tissue hypoxia. Deep tissue damage may result, necessitating later full-thickness skin grafting. The time period for reepithelialization is an estimated 4 to 21 days.[12]

#### Collaborative care management

Preventive nursing measures include identifying persons at risk and early and frequent assessment of the skin. In addition to fractures associated with a greater incidence of blisters, other risk factors include the presence of diabetes, hypertension, peripheral vascular disease, smoking history, alcohol use, and lymphatic obstruction. Initial treatment measures that may decrease the development of blisters include early immobilization and elevation to limit edema formation, both of which help maintain normal blood and lymphatic circulation. If the patient develops a fracture blister, a dry dressing is recommended for protection. "Popping" the blister is not recommended, because the blister covering provides a biological dressing.[12] A ruptured blister provides an excellent environment for infection; it is moist, provides nutrients (serum), lacks initial phagocytic activity, and has few coexisting microorganisms. If blister rupture occurs, a hydrocolloid dressing is helpful to maintain a moist wound environment. Triple antibiotic ointment and silver sulfadiazine cream have been shown to be beneficial in promoting healing, whereas povidone iodine and hydrogen peroxide may interfere with reepithelialization of the epidermis. Despite treatment, a ruptured blister may result in a full-thickness loss. Intravenous antibiotics are recommended if the wound culture reveals *Staphylococcus aureus.* Anticoagulants such as low-dose heparin or warfarin are prescribed to prevent thrombus formation.

**Patient/family education.** Persons at risk for sustaining high-risk fractures should be taught the etiology of blisters and treatment protocols. This is especially important for patients who are treated in the emergency department or urgent care center and discharged home. The patient and family should be taught the importance of proper wound care, signs and symptoms of infection, dressing techniques, and signs and symptoms of potential complications such as compartment syndrome. Other interventions include teaching the patient and family about the significance of fracture blisters, their effect on healing, and the rationale for delaying fracture fixation if blisters develop. They should be given the name and number of the appropriate person to contact if symptoms develop.

## Fat Embolism Syndrome

### *Etiology/epidemiology*

Fat embolism syndrome (FES) is a potentially fatal complication associated with fractures, multiple crush injuries, total hip arthroplasty, and total knee arthroplasty. Fat embolism syndrome has also been implicated as the cause of death in persons who have been beaten to death.[11] Fat emboli may lead to ARDS, with an associated mortality rate of 50%, especially if the onset is more than 5 days after trauma.

Fat embolism syndrome is most common after fractures of the pelvis, femur, and tibia. Persons with total hip and knee arthroplasties are at risk for FES because of surgical reaming of the intramedullary canal to allow seating of the prosthesis and pressurizing of the medullary canal during sizing of the prosthesis, which may cause fat to enter the venous system. The incidence of FES after long bone fractures is reported to be 0.5% to 4% and up to 10% after multiple fractures or pelvic fracture.[17] An increase in serum glucose and beta-lipoprotein levels may increase the incidence of FES. Fat embolism syndrome usually occurs within 24 hours of injury in 60% of patients and within 48 hours of injury in 85% of patients.

### *Pathophysiology*

On autopsy, fat globules greater than 20 $\mu m$ in diameter have been found in the lungs of 90% of patients with long bone fractures.[11] After fracture, fat globules are released from the bone marrow and local tissue into circulation. The fat molecules enter the venous circulation, travel to the lungs, and embolize the small capillaries and arterioles. Lipase is produced to break down fat molecules into fatty acids. These chemical changes irritate pulmonary tissue and result in deterioration of lung surfactant, increased permeability of the alveolocapillary membrane, interstitial hemorrhage, edema, and atelectasis. Eventually, hypoxemia and ARDS may develop. Fatty acids attract red blood cells (RBCs) and platelets, forming an aggregate, which can lead to disseminated intravascular coagulation (DIC) and emboli to the brain and other vital organs.

Symptoms of FES include hypoxemia, tachypnea, tachycardia, petechiae, fever, lipuria, chest pain, and altered mental status. Alteration in mental status is an important clinical indicator of FES. Approximately 75% of persons with FES develop significant neurological symptoms, which may manifest as restlessness, confusion, lethargy, or coma. Petechiae, considered a "classic" symptom of FES, occur in only 50% to 60% of persons with FES. They usually occur 24 to 48 hours after the injury. They are usually found on the conjunctiva, axilla, chest, and neck and are thought to be caused by capillary occlusion with fat and fibrin. Other causative factors include capillary fragility and platelet defects. The rash does not blanch with pressure but usually disappears within 48 hours of onset. The presence of unexplained fever, especially when accompanied by a change in mental status and petechiae, should alert the caregiver to the possibility of FES. This is a medical emergency, and the physician should be notified immediately.

### *Collaborative care management*

Diagnosis is confirmed by a decrease in arterial $Po_2$, an increase in systemic $Pco_2$ infiltrates on chest x-ray, petechiae, and mental confusion in persons at risk. Pathological examination of the lungs reveals fat globules diffusely distributed throughout the pulmonary vasculature.[19]

Arterial blood gases are obtained to determine the amount of hypoxemia. Fat may be found in the blood and urine. However, lipuria is a normal finding after fracture and therefore is not of clinical significance in the diagnosis of FES. Blood analysis reveals a decreased hemoglobin and platelet count. Chest x-ray films detect changes related to fat embolus in

**table 60-3 Comparison of Fat Embolism and Pulmonary Embolism**

| Fat Embolism | Pulmonary Embolism |
|---|---|
| **PATHOPHYSIOLOGY** | |
| Fat globules released from marrow following fracture(s) enter bloodstream and obstruct pulmonary circulation | Deep vein thrombosis dislodges and obstructs pulmonary circulation |
| **ONSET OF SYMPTOMS** | |
| Usually 1-4 days after injury | Usually 4-10 days after trauma or development of thrombophlebitis but can occur much later |
| **SIGNS AND SYMPTOMS** | |
| Altered mental status | Dyspnea |
| Dyspnea | Chest pain |
| Tachypnea | Apprehension |
| Tachycardia | Anxiety |
| Petechial rash | Cough |
| Fever | Hemoptysis |
| Restlessness | Tachypnea |
| Agitation | Tachycardia |
| | Fever |
| **RISK FACTORS** | |
| Hypovolemia | Venous stasis |
| Shock | Immobility |
| Delayed immobilization of fracture | Obesity |
| Multiple fractures | Trauma |
| | Major surgery |
| | History of heart disease |
| | Age >40 yr |
| | History of deep vein thrombosis, pulmonary embolism |

only one third of patients. If ARDS develops, chest films will show areas of consolidation. A lung scan (VQ scan or ventilation/perfusion scan) may be used to rule out pulmonary embolus (Table 60-3).

The most important nursing interventions are the recognition of patients who are at risk for developing FES and careful monitoring for early detection of clinical indicators of FES. Careful handling of the fractured extremity, especially when turning and positioning the patient, decreases manipulation of the fracture site, thus decreasing the risk of fat emboli.

As stated earlier, medical management is the same as for a person with ARDS. (See Chapter 32.) Adequate hydration and administration of corticosteroids are basic treatment measures. Albumin, a volume expander, has been effective in reducing the incidence of FES.[7,17] Preventive measures include early immobilization (within 24 hours of injury) of patients with long bone fractures. Patients who undergo early stabilization of fractures experience shorter hospital stays and less incidence of respiratory complications than those with late stabilization (more than 48 hours after injury) of fractures.

Early recognition of symptoms, including respiratory insufficiency, decreased oxygenation, mental status changes, unexplained drop in hemoglobin, thrombocytopenia, and the presence of fat in the urine or sputum, should alert the caregiver to the possibility of fat embolus.

**Patient/family education.** The patient and family will require much emotional support and information regarding treatment regimens. Because the onset of FES is abrupt, the patient and family are not prepared to deal with the severity of the situation. Early teaching regarding the risk for developing complications and signs and symptoms may help prepare them if the situation occurs. Early recognition of discrete mental status changes is often best recognized by family or friends. If FES develops, education regarding the rationales for treatment and emotional support while the patient is in the critical care environment are essential.

## Compartment Syndrome

*Compartment syndrome* is a complication of trauma in which increased pressure within a limited anatomical space compromises the circulation, viability, and function of the tissues within that space.[7,18] Compartment syndrome was first recognized more than 100 years ago. In 1881 Volkmann described an upper extremity contracture that he attributed to trauma, swelling, and restrictive dressings. This phenomenon was later termed *compartment syndrome* (Figure 60-15). If unrecognized, compartment syndrome can lead to loss of function, deformity, and possibly amputation. Failure to recognize compartment syndrome has been cited as the most common cause of medical litigation in the United States.[18]

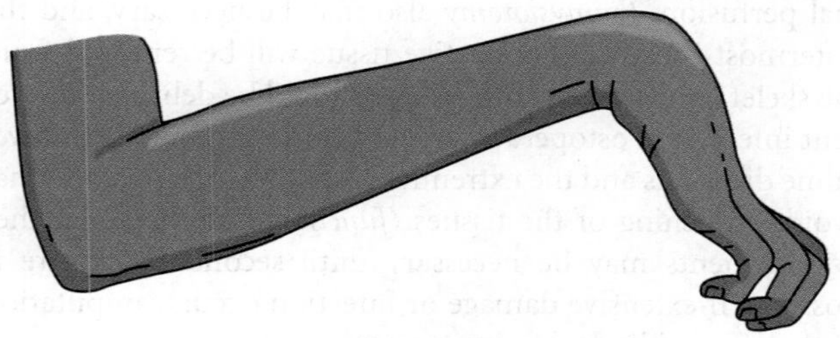

**fig. 60-15** Volkmann's ischemic contracture.

Compartment syndrome can be either acute or chronic. Acute compartment syndrome is usually a complication of trauma. Chronic compartment syndrome commonly occurs in persons who are active in sports such as long-distance running, cycling, dancing, and cross-country skiing. The following section pertains to acute compartment syndrome.

### *Etiology/epidemiology*

For compartment syndrome to occur, there must be a space-limiting sleeve surrounding the tissue and increased tissue pressure. The space-limiting sleeve can be a restrictive dressing, a splint, a cast, fascia, or epimysium. Increased pressure within the compartment results from anything that either increases the contents of the compartment or decreases its size. Compartments consist of muscles, nerves, and blood vessels surrounded by a nonelastic covering. The body contains 46 compartments, 38 of which are in the extremities. These compartments are the most vulnerable to the development of compartment syndrome. The most common sites are the four compartments of the lower leg (deep posterior, superficial posterior, lateral, and anterior) (Figure 60-16), the dorsal and volar compartments of the forearm, and the interosseous compartments of the hand.

Although compartment syndrome usually occurs as a result of trauma, there are several other causes (Box 60-4). Shock can also increase the risk of compartment syndrome.

### *Pathophysiology*

Following trauma, fluid accumulates in the compartment, and fascia cannot expand to accommodate the excess fluid, causing compartment pressure to rise. Increases in tissue and venous pressures result in a decreased arteriovenous gradient. The end result is decreased blood supply and tissue hypoxia. In an attempt to correct the hypoxia, histamine is released, causing vasodilation and increased capillary permeability, which causes compartment pressure to continue to rise. Rising pressures lead to tissue ischemia and eventually necrosis. Peripheral muscle tissue will undergo ischemic changes within 6 hours of injury. Necrotic muscle cannot regenerate and is eventually replaced by dense, fibrous scar tissue. Peripheral neuropathy can develop within 24 hours, and contracture (ischemic paralysis) begins to develop within 4 to 12 hours of ischemia. If extensive ischemic muscle damage occurs, myoglobinuria may occur, leading to systemic complications that include renal failure, metabolic acidosis, hyperkalemia, and sepsis. Normal tissue compartment pressure is 1 to 10 mm Hg. Pressure in excess of 20 mm Hg is abnormal. Sustained pressure readings of 35 to 40 mm Hg usually require prompt treatment with fasciotomy, but this varies with the individual patient.

Early recognition of symptoms and prompt treatment may preserve the function of the limb. Pain is the most common symptom of compartment syndrome. *The patient may report severe, unrelenting pain, unrelieved by analgesia and increased by elevation of the extremity.* The intensity of pain is

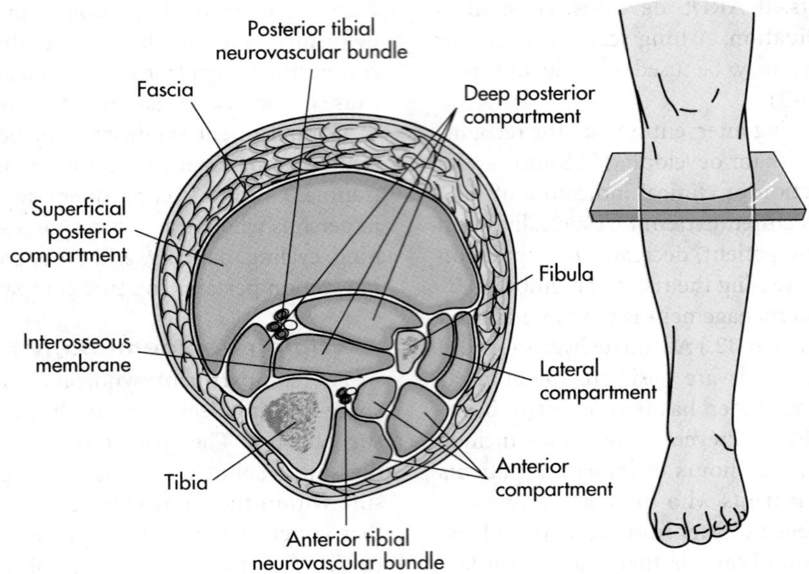


**fig. 60-16** Compartments of lower leg.

**box 60-4** *Causes of Compartment Syndrome*

**BLEEDING**
Vascular injury
Coagulation defect (hemophilia, anticoagulant therapy)

**NEPHROTIC SYNDROME**

**EXCESSIVE MUSCLE USE**
Exercise
Seizures
Tetany
Eclampsia

**TRAUMA**
Fractures
Crush injuries
Hypothermia, frostbite
Burns
Snake or spider bites

**INFILTRATED INFUSIONS**

**SURGERY**

**EXTERNAL PRESSURE**
Positioning (lying on limb)
Surgical tourniquets
Military antishock trousers (MAST)
Circumferential restrictive dressings
Tight cast
Splints

**DECREASED COMPARTMENT SIZE**
Excessive traction
Closure of fascial defects

usually greater than expected for the extent of the injury. As pressures increases, so does the intensity of the pain. Passive movement or stretching of the digits will increase pain. It is important to note that epidural analgesia may mask the onset of compartment syndrome.

Motor and sensory function will also be affected. Hypoesthesia, paresthesia, and muscular weakness or paralysis are common. It may be helpful to remember the five *P's*: *pulselessness, paresthesia, pain, pressure,* and *pallor.* Skin color, temperature, capillary refill, and quality of peripheral pulses are not reliable clinical indicators for the presence of compartment syndrome. If pallor, coolness, slow capillary refill, and diminished or absent pulses are present, extensive and potentially irreversible damage has probably already occurred.

### Collaborative care management

Goals of treatment include (1) decreasing tissue pressure, (2) restoring blood flow, and (3) preserving function of the limb. Removal of external compression devices by splitting dressings or bivalving casts may alleviate early compartment syndrome. If conservative measures fail, surgical intervention may be indicated. *Decompressive fasciotomy* is performed along the complete length of the compartment to open the affected compartments, decrease the pressure, and restore normal perfusion. *Epimysiotomy* also may be necessary, and the outermost sheath of connective tissue will be removed from the skeletal muscle. Necrotic tissue should be debrided to prevent infection. Postoperatively the wound is covered with wet saline dressings and the extremity is splinted in a position that avoids stretching of the tissues *(functional position).* Further debridements may be necessary until secondary closure is possible. If extensive damage or infection occurs, amputation of the affected limb may be necessary.

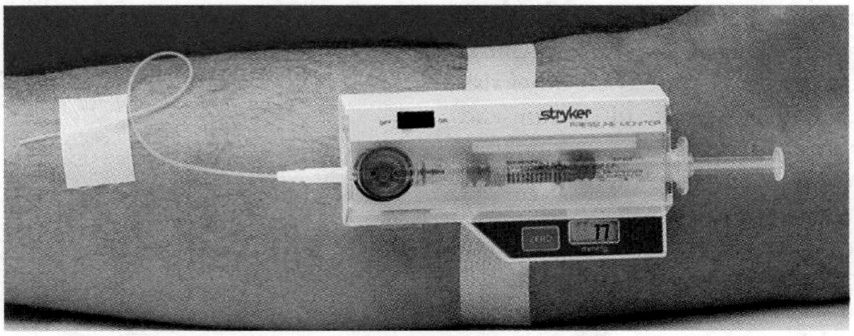

fig. 60-17 Compartment pressure monitor.

Subfascial hyaluronidase, an enzyme that breaks down collagen fibers in fascia and allows fluids to escape from the compromised compartment, is used in some settings. This method has not been demonstrated to be effective. Osmotic diuretics such as mannitol may be given early in compartment syndrome to prevent the need for fasciotomy.[7]

If contractures develop, splints and physical and occupational therapy may be indicated. In some cases, additional surgery such as joint fusion, tenotomy, or tendon transfers may be performed.

As mentioned earlier, recognition of early signs and symptoms may lead to prompt diagnosis and treatment. In an unconscious patient, pain and changes in neurovascular status may be difficult to assess. Therefore, if compartment syndrome is suspected, invasive measurement of compartment pressures can be performed. A variety of systems are available either for one-time use or for continuous monitoring (Figure 60-17). Compartment pressure readings should be evaluated in relation to the clinical picture, because improper use of the device or instrument malfunction may occur.

Segmental limb blood pressures and Doppler-derived ankle-brachial indices are used for evaluation of compartment syndrome. Nerve conduction studies may be performed to evaluate nerve function. Blood tests may show an increase in creatine phosphokinase (CPK), lactate dehydrogenase (LDH), and aspartate aminotransferase (AST), which is indicative of muscle damage. Myoglobinuria indicates muscle cell death and may lead to acute renal failure. Hyperkalemia also indicates muscle damage. Venograms or arteriograms may be ordered to rule out deep vein thrombosis or vascular injury.

Nursing management of the patient with or at risk for developing compartment syndrome includes maintaining neurovascular integrity of the extremities. Careful monitoring of the neurovascular status of the extremities is crucial in the detection and prevention of compartment syndrome. Baseline and ongoing assessments include data regarding both extremities. It is important to compare observations about both extremities. Knowledge of the innervation to the extremities is useful when assessing for deficits. Hourly assessments should be performed and recorded, noting any reports of increased pain, pain that occurs with passive stretching, and alterations in sensory or motor function. The patient with upper extremity involvement should be assessed for the ability to extend, flex, abduct, adduct, and oppose the fingers and thumbs and flex the wrist. If the lower extremities are involved, the ability to extend and flex the toes, perform plantar flexion and dorsiflexion, and invert and evert the foot should be assessed.

If compartment syndrome is suspected, the physician is notified, restrictive dressings are loosened, and the extremity is lowered to the level of the heart. If ice packs are being used, they are removed because the application of cold and elevation of the limb may further impair the circulation.

Dressings, splints, and casts are checked for excessive pressure, and compartment pressures are monitored and recorded. Any significant changes are reported to the physician. Reports of pain are monitored, and the effectiveness of pain relief measures is assessed.

**Patient/family education.** An adequate fluid intake is encouraged. Active ROM to other extremities and ambulation are performed, if possible. Isometric exercises are taught and encouraged. Range-of-motion exercises are continued throughout rehabilitation. The patient may need instructions about crutch use and care of the dressing or splint. The need to elevate and ice the affected extremity should be stressed. The family and patient should be knowledgeable about the symptoms of recurring compartment syndrome and infection. Return to normal activities is gradual and depends on the type of injury.

## HIP FRACTURE

### Etiology/Epidemiology

Hip fractures are a serious problem, especially for elderly persons. The incidence of hip fracture increases with age, doubling every 5 years over 50 years of age; 95% of all hip fractures occur in persons age 50 and older. An estimated one third of the female and one sixth of the male population over 90 years of age will experience a hip fracture. Currently more than 250,000 hip fractures occur annually, and the associated health care costs exceed 7 billion dollars.[5] Repair of a hip fracture is probably the most common surgical procedure for persons over 85 years of age. As the population ages, the number of fractures of the femoral neck is expected to be 500,000.[22]

Risk factors commonly associated with hip fracture include osteoporosis, advanced age, being female and white, decreased estrogen levels (because of postmenopausal changes or bilateral oophorectomy), prior hip fractures, Alzheimer's dementia, institutional residence, and sedentary lifestyle.[5] Other risk factors include an inadequate dietary intake of calcium and vitamin D, excessive dietary protein, caffeine intake, smoking, alcohol use, and use of psychotropic drugs. Although the incidence of hip fracture is most commonly associated with women, the risk of hip fracture in elderly men has increased as well. Black persons over 45 years of age are less likely to experience hip fractures than white persons because of the increased mineral content and increased mass of their bones. Only 1% of black women over 80 years of age experience hip fracture. Among African-American women, thinness, previous cerebrovascular accident, use of assistive devices for walking, and alcohol consumption are associated with an increased risk of hip fracture.[8]

The hospital stay of elderly persons with hip fractures is often complicated and prolonged and may result in chronic disability, transfer to an extended care facility, or death. An estimated 15% of persons hospitalized with a hip fracture die within a short period of time, 30% die within 1 year, and 30% to 50% never return to their prior level of functioning. The older the individual, the lower the chance of regaining prefracture functional status. Factors that negatively influence recovery and increase risk of mortality following hip fracture include being male, preexisting medical problems, cognitive impairment, and the development of postoperative complications.

## Pathophysiology

A hip fracture is a fracture of the proximal femur and may be classified as follows (Figure 60-18)

1. Intracapsular (or femoral neck) fractures—occurring within the hip joint and capsule
   a. Subcapital
   b. Transcervical
   c. Basal neck
2. Extracapsular fractures—occurring outside the hip joint and capsule to an area 5 cm (2 inches) below the lesser trochanter; called intertrochanteric fractures
3. Subtrochanteric fractures—occurring below the lesser trochanter

The location of the fracture is an important consideration in predicting healing. Intracapsular fractures, especially displaced fractures, can disrupt the blood supply to the femoral head (Figure 60-19). They are associated with an increased incidence of nonunion and avascular necrosis of the femoral head.[22] Intertrochanteric fractures occur in the well-nourished vascular metaphyseal region of the hip and do not generally interfere with the blood supply of the proximal femur. Complications associated with intertrochanteric fracture include malunion and shortening of the affected extremity. Intertrochanteric and femoral neck fractures account for approximately 90% of all hip fractures, and subtrochanteric fractures account for approximately 10%.

Signs and symptoms of hip fracture are severe pain at the fracture site, inability to move the leg voluntarily, shortening and external rotation of the leg, and other signs and symptoms consistent with those of any fracture.

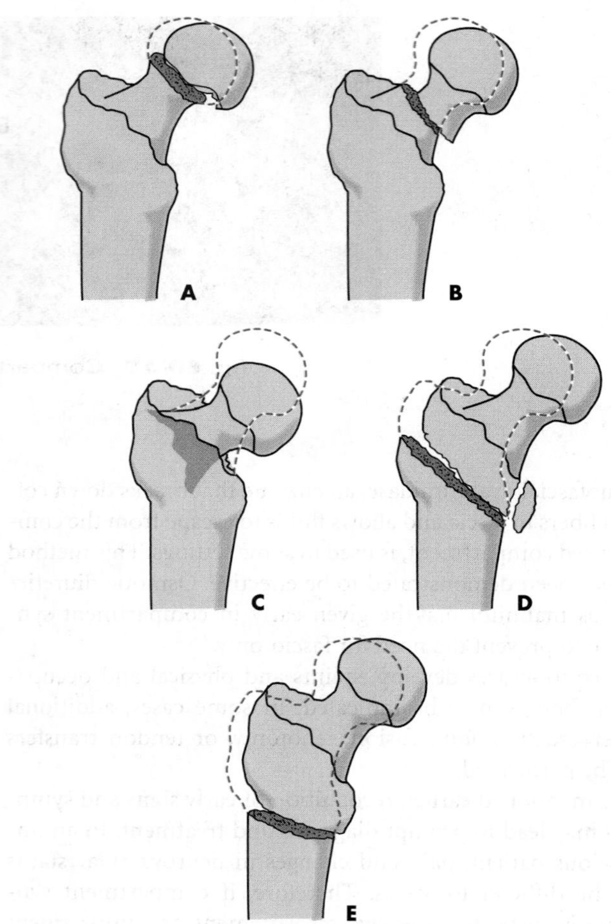


**fig. 60-18** Fractures of the hip. **A,** Subcapital fracture. **B,** Transcervical fracture. **C,** Impacted fracture of base of neck. **D,** Intertrochanteric fracture. **E,** Subtrochanteric fracture.

## Collaborative Care Management

Treatment of hip fracture includes both conservative measures and surgery. Surgical intervention is usually preferred, unless the patient's general medical condition precludes that option. Conservative management involves prolonged immobility with the associated complications but avoids the risks associated with anesthesia. The risks and benefits of both modalities should be discussed by the patient, family, physician, and nurse.

Surgery involves reduction and stabilization of the fracture and insertion of an internal fixation device. A variety of fixation devices are available. The choice of fixation device depends on the location of the fracture, the potential for avascular necrosis of the femoral head, and the personal preference of the surgeon. An impacted intracapsular fracture without displacement may be treated only with bedrest. The following treatments are often chosen for other types of hip fractures:

1. Stable plate and screw fixation; implies non–weight-bearing status for 6 weeks to 3 months
2. Telescoping nail fixation; implies minimal to partial weight-bearing status for 6 weeks to 3 months

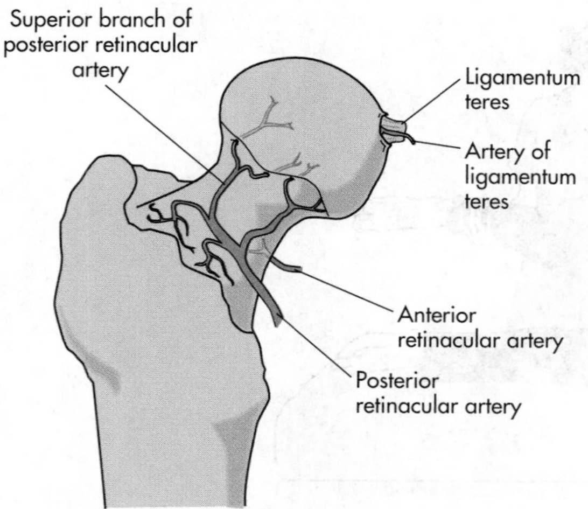


**fig. 60-19** Posterior view of blood supply to head of femur.

3. Prosthetic implant; usually bipolar prosthesis to replace femoral head and neck; implies some position restrictions for 2 weeks to 2 months and partial weight-bearing restrictions for up to 2 months; goals of treatment are to return patient to his or her prefracture level of functioning and prevent further disability

Improving the general medical condition of the elderly patient before surgery, which includes the stabilization of preexisting medical problems and the correction of fluid and electrolyte imbalances, increases the chances for functional recovery. Nursing interventions include those to prevent the most common postoperative complications, such as thromboembolism, pneumonia, alterations in skin integrity, and voiding dysfunction (see Chapter 20). See the accompanying Nursing Care Plan.

Nursing management should include those interventions already noted for general care of patients with fractures, with specific attention to interventions for persons with internal fixation. *Special consideration should be given to persons who have had a prosthetic implant, because there will be specific position restrictions, unless they have external fixation as well.* These include:

1. Avoid hip flexion beyond 60 degrees for up to 10 days.
2. Avoid hip flexion beyond 90 degrees from day 10 to 2 months.
3. Avoid adduction of the affected leg beyond midline for 2 months.
4. Maintain partial weight-bearing status for approximately 2 months.

Suggestions for nursing management include the following:

1. Instruct the patient on the limits of motion to be observed.
2. Avoid positioning the patient on the operative side in bed. This varies by surgeon's preference.
3. Assist the patient to maintain hip abduction (Figures 60-20 and 60-21).
4. Carefully monitor the patient's position during transfer (while the patient is standing and sitting).
5. Provide a chair with armrests and a firm, nonreclining seat; elevate the sitting surface as necessary with pillows or foam cushions to keep the angle of the hip within the prescribed limits when the patient is sitting.

In general, patients who have had *any* kind of internal fixation for fractured hip should avoid elevation of the operated leg when sitting in a chair, because this puts excessive strain on the fixation device.

### Patient/family education

Most patients will be discharged to a rehabilitation facility. The patient and family should be reminded that complete recovery may take as long as 6 months.[1] Recovery is generally measured by the amount of assistance required for ADL (see the Research Box). The patient and family should be assured that the process of healing and recovery is gradual. Home-going instructions include medication instruction, positioning restrictions (see the Nursing Care Plan on p. 1941), weight-bearing restrictions, ambulation techniques with assistive devices, and signs and symptoms suggestive of complications. Adaptive equipment for the home includes elevated toilet seat, grab bars for the bath, long-handled reachers, and an elevated chair with armrests. Many patients are prescribed anticoagulants for as long as 3 months postoperatively. Deep vein thrombosis may occur in as many as 70% of patients after hip fracture.[5] The patient and family should be familiar with medication administration (the patient may be prescribed subcutaneous injections of low-molecular-weight heparin), side effects, and the need for periodic laboratory assessment of coagulation times.

Instructions regarding the prevention of falls, which are the major cause of hip fracture, should also be given. Because osteoporosis is a significant contributing factor to hip fracture, primary prevention should focus on the education of persons at risk for osteoporosis (see Chapter 61). Secondary prevention includes early detection of the disease process and methods to decrease the severity of the disorder. Much emphasis has been placed on women as a high-risk group for hip fracture, but because of the rising incidence of fracture in elderly men, education also needs to be directed toward this previously overlooked group.

## FRACTURE OF THE SPINE

### Etiology/Epidemiology

Spinal or vertebral fractures occur as the result of falls, motor vehicle or diving accidents, or blows to the head or body by heavy objects. With increasing frequency, fractures of the spine are also occurring as the result of osteoporosis and metastatic lesions of the spine. Spinal fracture can occur at any age.

### Pathophysiology

Vertebral fracture may occur with or without displacement. Displaced fracture fragments may place pressure on spinal nerves or injure the spinal cord itself. Such pressure results in partial or complete dysfunction of the body parts innervated by nerves at the level of injury. Depending on the extent of injury to the nervous system, dysfunction may be permanent or temporary.

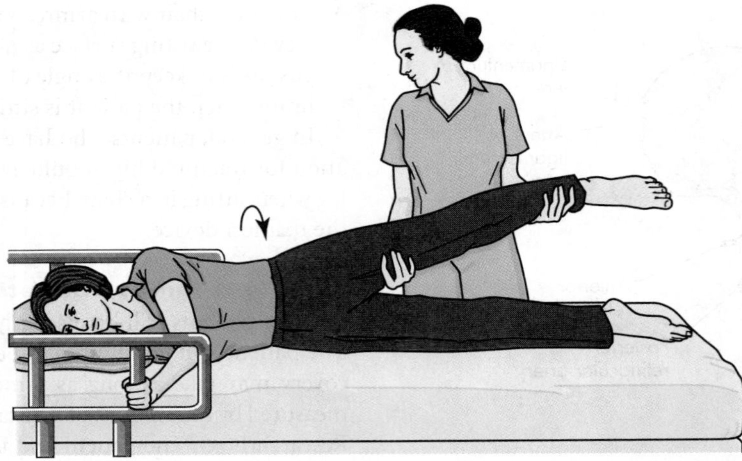

**fig. 60-20** Assisting patient to turn while maintaining abduction of the hip. Leg is supported at the thigh and just above the ankle to avoid putting undue stress on the hip. Abduction pillow may also be used.

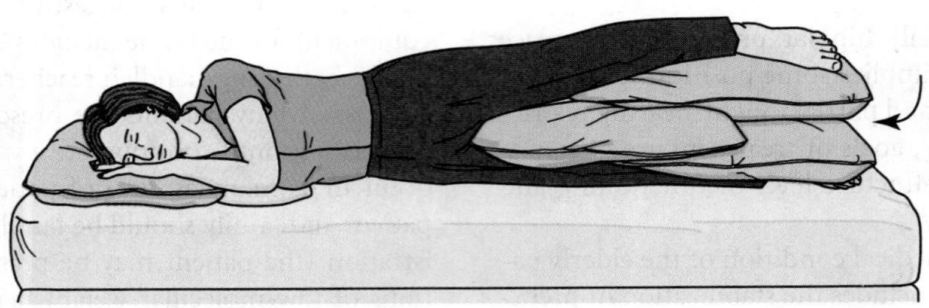

**fig. 60-21** Pillows are staggered in a wedge-shaped arrangement to maintain abduction of the hip.

**research**

Reference: Williams MA, Oberst TM, Bjorklund BC: Posthospital convalescence in older women with hip fracture, *Orthop Nurs* 13(4):55, 1994.

The purpose of the study was to collect data about the recovery of functional abilities and patients' subjective responses during early posthospital convalescence. Patients chosen were relatively healthy prefracture, so recovery and convalescent events would reflect responses to the fracture, rather than responses to preexisting conditions. Specific purposes of the study were to determine "(a) early recovery patterns in function and mood, (b) factors predictive of assistance needed in mobility and perceived mobility compared to prefracture status, (c) problems faced, and (d) advice to others."

Results included the following: (1) The abilities to eat and groom oneself were recovered quickly, whereas independence in bathing, walking, and stair climbing was slow; (2) a rapid gain in mobility was made in the first 7 weeks, with smaller gains thereafter; (3) affective mood distress was low, except in women discharged to nursing homes; (4) somatic mood distress was high, and higher in those discharged to nursing homes; (5) predictors of assistance were factors both susceptible and not susceptible to nursing intervention; (6) problems related to limitations in mobility and difficulty in dressing were identified; and (7) advice to others included the necessity of maintaining a positive outlook, following the advice of health care professionals, and preventing falls.

Data from research regarding patients' perceptions of recovery and identification of common problems can assist nurses in teaching patients about realistic expectations of recovery and regaining mobility.

Fracture can occur at any level of the spine, from occiput through the sacrum. Signs and symptoms of vertebral fracture include pain at the site of injury, partial or complete loss of mobility or sensation below the level of injury, and evidence of fracture or fracture dislocation on routine x-ray examination, myelography, computed tomography (CT) scan, or magnetic resonance imaging (MRI) scan.

### Collaborative Care Management

Long-term goals of treatment are stabilization and reduction of the fracture and decompression (i.e., removal of pressure from spinal nerves or the spinal cord). Immediate management objectives are (1) immobilization of the patient with backboard and cervical collar and (2) immediate transport to a hospital.

*Text continued on p. 1944*

## nursing care plan: Person with an Intracapsular Hip Fracture, Open Reduction, and Internal Fixation with a Prosthetic Implant

**DATA** Mrs. W. is an 81-year-old widowed, Caucasian, retired secretary. This evening she tripped and fell on an icy step when leaving her niece's home. She complained of immediate, severe pain in her left hip and was unable to move her leg. Emergency Medical Services was phoned, and Mrs. W. was accompanied to the hospital by her niece and her niece's husband. In the emergency room it was noted that her left leg was shorter than her right, and it was externally rotated. Her vital signs were stable, and the neurovascular status of the left leg was intact. An x-ray examination revealed an intracapsular femoral neck fracture. Intravenous fluids were initiated. An ECG, a urinalysis, a CBC, and a serum electrolyte study were obtained. She was transferred to the nursing unit with physician's orders for morphine sulfate via PCA pump, bedrest, pneumatic compression devices bilaterally, and diet as tolerated. Five pounds of Buck's traction was applied to the left leg. Informed consent was obtained for surgical repair in the morning. The procedure planned is hemiarthroplasty (prosthetic replacement of the femoral head and neck).

The nursing history identified the following:

- Mrs. W. lives alone in her own apartment in a senior citizen complex.
- Mrs. W. has no children but has nieces and nephews in the area who see her regularly. They assist with shopping and other errands.
- Mrs. W. would like to return to her own apartment after being discharged from the hospital, but she worries that she might need help at home. Her family is considering hiring a home health aide.
- She takes no medications other than aspirin for occasional "stiffness" on awakening.
- She has never been hospitalized and last saw a physician 2 years ago for "the flu."

**NURSING DIAGNOSIS** *Knowledge deficit related to lack of exposure to surgery and treatment protocols*

| expected patient outcomes | nursing interventions | rationale |
|---|---|---|
| Can explain the teaching provided by the nurse about preoperative and general postoperative care.<br>States that she is experiencing less anxiety related to fear of the unknown and misconceptions about surgery and the recovery period. | Assess need for instruction and provide as necessary.<br>Provide written materials pertaining to the surgery, if available in the institution.<br>Review preoperative instruction with patient and family before the surgery; provide examples of prostheses if available.<br>Evaluate patient's understanding of the information taught. | Understanding the surgical procedure and postoperative care should lessen anxiety and promote participation in postoperative routine. |
| | Reinforce information taught. | Reinforcement of information previously taught will improve retention. |
| Will actively participate in plan of care. | Keep patient and family informed of plan of care and rationales for treatment. | Encourage family support and participation in care routines while the patient is hospitalized and after discharge. |
| Will verbalize understanding of need for follow-up care and activity restrictions. | Provide information and rationale for discharge activity restrictions.<br>Collaborative nursing actions include those to identify possible complications of surgery and immobility. Nursing actions include monitoring for the following: | Understanding the rationale for activity restrictions may promote compliance and avoidance of complications. |
| Performs active dorsiflexion, plantar flexion, isometric quadriceps and gluteal setting, and active ROM of unaffected limbs q12h until ambulatory. | Neurovascular compromise: Perform neurovascular checks q2h for the first 24-48 hours. Notify physician of any changes from preoperative status. | Exercising promotes venous return, prevents thrombus formation, and helps maintain muscle tone. |
| Verbalizes understanding of need for postoperative anticoagulation and need for follow-up checkups and laboratory tests. | Administer anticoagulants as ordered. Educate regarding use of anticoagulants and signs and symptoms of bleeding. | Deep vein thrombosis is a common postoperative complication.<br>Bleeding and thrombocytopenia are side effects of some anticoagulants. Coagulation studies are done to monitor drug effectiveness. |
| | Dislocation of the prosthesis: Notify physician if patient complains of sudden onset of increased pain, especially groin pain, particularly if accompanied by deformity or external rotation. | Patient has history of aspirin use. |

Continued

## Person with an Intracapsular Hip Fracture, Open Reduction, and Internal Fixation with a Prosthetic Implant—cont'd

**NURSING DIAGNOSIS** *Knowledge deficit related to lack of exposure to surgery and treatment protocols—cont'd*

| expected patient outcomes | nursing interventions | rationale |
|---|---|---|
| | Impaired skin integrity or impaired wound healing: Monitor pressure areas for signs of redness, monitor temperature, and assess incision for signs or symptoms of infection or excessive drainage. | |
| | Atelectasis/respiratory infection: Monitor breath sounds until patient is ambulatory. Have patient deep breathe and cough every hour until fully ambulatory. Demonstrate and encourage use of incentive spirometer. | If carried out correctly and at appropriate intervals, pulmonary exercises can effectively prevent atelectasis and pneumonia. Frequent monitoring and early detection of complications can speed recovery and increase functional status. |
| | Urinary retention: Assess for urinary retention or stasis. | |
| | Constipation: Assess bowel status each day until patient is able to have a bowel movement. | |
| | Fluid and electrolyte imbalance: Monitor intake and output until patient is taking oral fluids without difficulty, monitor IV fluid rates, and assess patient for fluid volume excess or deficit. | |
| | Monitoring for signs and symptoms of DVT. Application of antiembolic hose and sequential compression devices. Encourage isometric exercises and early ambulation. Perform neurovascular assessment of extremities. Monitor labs for therapeutic effects of anticoagulants. | |
| | By discharge the patient should be instructed in and be able to explain or demonstrate the following: | |
| | Independent ambulation on level surfaces and stairs with appropriate ambulatory aid. | |
| | Activity restrictions to be observed for approximately 2 months or until follow-up with physician, for example, limiting flexion of the affected hip to 90 degrees, avoiding adduction of the affected leg beyond midline, avoiding extreme internal and external rotation of the affected hip, and maintaining partial weight-bearing status with the walker or crutches. | |
| | Independent ADL with assistive devices. | |

**NURSING DIAGNOSIS** *Pain related to surgical procedure*

| expected patient outcomes | nursing interventions | rationale |
|---|---|---|
| Reports decrease or absence of pain after the use of pain relief measures. | Assess patient's pain, and evaluate response comfort measures provided. | Subjective and objective data are important in ascertaining the nature of patient's postoperative pain and determining its management. |

*Continued*

## Person with an Intracapsular Hip Fracture, Open Reduction, and Internal Fixation with a Prosthetic Implant—cont'd

**NURSING DIAGNOSIS** *Pain related to surgical procedure—cont'd*

| expected patient outcomes | nursing interventions | rationale |
|---|---|---|
| Can perform necessary postoperative routine and exercises. | Monitor use and effectiveness of PCA. | PCA avoids peaks and valleys associated with intermittent use of analgesics. |
| | Teach relaxation techniques as appropriate. | Relaxation facilitates rest and may modify the response of pain. |
| | Use other pain-relieving techniques as appropriate, for example, back rubs, repositioning. | A change in type of cutaneous stimulation may result in pain relief. |
| Reports decreasing levels of pain. | As pain decreases, use milder analgesics as prescribed. | Pain may be controlled by less potent analgesics (with fewer untoward side effects) as pain lessens in severity. |
| | Apply ice to operative hip for 48 hours. | Ice reduces swelling at the operative site; swelling contributes to pain. |

**NURSING DIAGNOSIS** *Impaired physical mobility related to alteration in lower limb status after surgical repair of hip fracture*

| expected patient outcomes | nursing interventions | rationale |
|---|---|---|
| Will demonstrate optimal level of mobility with adaptive devices within prescribed limitations of activity by time of discharge. | | |
| Will be free from complications associated with immobility. | Determine from surgeon the limits of motion and weight bearing permitted, keeping in mind the following guidelines:<br>Hip flexion is usually limited to <90 degrees for 2 to 3 months.<br>Adduction beyond midline is prohibited for 2 to 3 months.<br>Extreme internal or external rotation is prohibited for 2 to 3 months.<br>Partial weight bearing on affected body part with the aid of a walker or crutches is usually observed for 2 to 3 months. | Restrictions on positioning are designed to avoid dislocating the prosthesis. |
| | Turn patient from back to unoperated side q2h and prn. Avoid positioning patient on operative side, and observe flexion restrictions when elevating the head of the bed. | Turning and repositioning frequently promote circulation, respiratory effort, and muscle activity. |
| | When turning the patient, hold the operative leg in abduction; use pillows to maintain 30-degree abduction when turning is accomplished. | Prevents adduction of leg. |
| | Assist patient to walk using the appropriate ambulatory aid. Begin walking the first or second postoperative day and increase the frequency and distance of ambulation as tolerated. | Early postoperative activity, including walking, can hasten recovery and prevent postoperative complications. |
| | Begin sitting when patient demonstrates sufficient control of the affected leg to sit within flexion restriction. | Prepares patient for discharge while ensuring that the patient functions safely within prescribed limits on flexion. |
| | Elevate sitting surface with pillows to keep angle of hip within prescribed limits. | Limits hip flexion to 90 degrees. |
| | Reinforce use of assistive devices provided by occupational therapy. | Promotes independence in ADL. Items such as long-handled reachers allow independence, while maintaining positioning restrictions. |

Objectives of surgical management are as follows:

1. Decompression of nerve structures through laminectomy (see Chapter 61) or appropriate reduction of the fracture and removal of fracture fragments
2. Reduction of the fracture through operative procedures or, in some cases, traction (e.g., cervical traction through application of tongs to the skull)
3. Stabilization of the fracture with bone grafting or internal fixation devices such as pedicle screws and plates, Texas Scottish Rite Hospital (TSRH), or Harrington or Luque rods (see Chapter 61)
4. Maintenance of stabilization with external fixation devices such as casts, corsets, or braces as necessary

In the absence of displacement of fracture fragments and pressure on spinal nerves or the spinal cord, compression fractures may be treated with bedrest until the patient's pain subsides. The patient is then gradually mobilized, sometimes with stabilization by a corset or brace.

Many of the nursing interventions required by the patient with spinal fracture are identical to those outlined for the patient with spinal cord injury in Chapter 54. Of special concern are interventions designed for the following:

1. Maintaining the stability of the fracture fixation
   a. Pay strict attention when logrolling the patient for position changes to avoid twisting the spine and placing stress at the fracture site.
   b. Position the patient with pillows between the legs and behind the back when patient is side lying to prevent strain on the back.
   c. Changes of position can be accomplished with the use of special beds that rotate 45 degrees from side to side. Literature indicates that when the spine is unstable, logrolling and the use of turning frames are contraindicated because they can stress the fracture site.
   d. Avoid elevating the head of the bed beyond the prescribed level (usually only 30 degrees and only on the physician's order).
   e. When the patient is to be mobilized, apply prescribed corsets or braces *before* getting the patient out of bed.
2. Preventing neurovascular problems
   a. Perform neurovascular checks every hour for the first 24 to 48 hours postoperatively; report decrease in neuromotor function to the physician, because this may indicate displacement or pressure at the fracture site.
   b. Perform passive ROM to involved extremities at least four times daily to maintain joint motion.
   c. Encourage patient to move noninvolved extremities to the fullest extent possible as frequently as possible to maintain joint motion and promote circulation.
3. Promoting comfort—in addition to usual comfort measures
   a. Reposition the patient frequently.
   b. Wait a few minutes to ascertain the patient's comfort, because small adjustments may be necessary and may not be immediately recognized.
4. Promoting psychological comfort
   a. Recognize that the patient may have feelings of powerlessness, anger, or fear about the situation, particularly if there is sensorimotor deficit.
   b. Encourage the patient to express his or her feelings.
   c. Encourage the patient to take advantage of psychological or social counseling, when available.
   d. If long-term rehabilitation is indicated, prepare the patient for care in a rehabilitation setting.

Other nursing interventions are similar to those for any patient who has a fracture, including interventions for individuals in casts or traction, which are discussed earlier in this chapter.

#### *Patient/family education*

The patient should be taught proper body mechanics and lifting techniques to avoid strain on the spine. If permissible, exercises may be prescribed to strengthen back and abdominal muscles. If a brace or corset is to be worn, instructions are needed regarding skin care and care of the brace.

# TRAUMA TO SOFT TISSUE STRUCTURES

## TRAUMA TO LIGAMENTS AND TENDONS

### Etiology/Epidemiology

Trauma to ligaments and tendons is usually seen in connection with injury to a joint caused by a blow, twisting, or severe stretching. The most common site of ligament damage is the knee, often resulting from a sports injury, because of the anatomy, location, and complex motions of the joint. The Achilles' tendon is susceptible to partial or complete tears, usually caused by a sports injury. Shoulder and ankle injuries are common, particularly sports injuries. Approximately 2 million persons sustain ankle sprains in the United States annually[1] (Table 60-4).

This section contains a general discussion of ligamentous and tendon injuries. A more detailed discussion of anterior cruciate ligament trauma and rotator cuff trauma follows.

### Pathophysiology

The most common ligamentous or tendon injuries are partial or complete tears. Injury to the knee may include damage to the medial, lateral, and posterior ligaments and to the anterior and posterior cruciate ligaments. Injuries may be classified as mild, moderate, or severe:

Mild (class I) injuries—stretching of ligament without obvious tear

Moderate (class II) injuries—several ligament fibers torn with a partial loss of function; partial tear

Severe (class III) injuries—severe or complete disruption of the ligament with resulting instability

Signs and symptoms of class I injuries are mild pain and swelling. Class II injuries are associated with moderate pain and swelling, and persons with class III injuries typically report severe pain, swelling, joint instability, and disability or

**table 60-4** *Common Soft-Tissue Injuries*

| Mechanism of Injury | Symptoms | Treatment |
|---|---|---|
| **MENISCAL** | | |
| Medial and lateral tears usually occur with rotary or extension/flexion injuries of knee | Joint pain<br>Swelling<br>"Locking" | Splint, bracing, or cast<br>Surgical treatment by meniscectomy via arthroscopy or arthrotomy |
| **ANTERIOR CRUCIATE LIGAMENT (ACL)** | | |
| Valgus stress applied to knee while in hyperextension and external rotation<br>Associated with deceleration and changes in direction | Audible "pop" or "snap"<br>Pain<br>Joint effusion<br>Hemarthrosis<br>Joint deformity<br>Joint instability<br>"Giving way" of knee | Treatment depends on age and lifestyle of patient<br>Conservative treatment: quadriceps and hamstring strengthening, bracing, and avoidance of high-risk activities<br>Surgical reconstruction of ACL either open or arthroscopically aided, using autologous or synthetic graft followed by extensive rehabilitation program |
| **ROTATOR CUFF** | | |
| Strain or tear of rotator cuff muscles or tendons of shoulder (supraspinatus, infraspinatus, teres minor, subscapularis)<br>Usually results from falling on an outstretched hand, throwing objects (baseball pitchers), or chronic or excessive use | Severe pain with loss of ability to flex and abduct shoulder | Rest, sling and swath for immobilization, physical therapy, NSAIDs<br>Surgical repair for complete rupture, disability, or chronic pain; followed by physical therapy |
| **ANKLE SPRAIN** | | |
| Approximately 75% of all ankle injuries are sprains; 25% of injuries occur in running and jumping sports<br>Higher incidence in sports—basketball, soccer; also can occur while walking on uneven surfaces; lateral ligaments more susceptible to injury<br>Usually injury results from an inversion and plantar flexion force on ankle (95% as a result of inversion)<br>Position of the foot, type of sport, directional changes, joint laxity, and magnitude of force affect severity of the injury | Swelling<br>Tenderness<br>Reluctance to bear full weight, perform full ROM<br>Deformities<br>Ecchymoses | Rest, ice, elastic compression, elevation for grades I, II sprains<br>Grade II sprains—immobilization by cast or bracing, gradual resumption of activity<br>Aggressive treatment may include primary surgical repair or ankle stabilization procedure |

loss of function. The clinical manifestations of trauma to the knee are listed in Box 60-5.

### Collaborative Care Management

Immediate first aid measures for soft-tissue injuries of the musculoskeletal system can be easily remembered by the mnemonic RICE (rest, ice, compression, elevation):

Rest of the injured part

Ice for at least 48 to 72 hours to decrease bleeding and edema

Compression with elastic bandages, splints, or casts (be sure to monitor for signs of compartment syndrome)

Elevation of the extremity to slightly above the level of the heart to increase venous return and decrease edema

Diagnosis is based on the evaluation of the patient's history and physical examination, including specialized tests to detect ligamentous instability. It is especially important to elicit a complete history of the specific mechanism of injury, which aids in differential diagnosis. X-ray films are used to rule out fracture. Arthrography and arthroscopy may be performed to visualize the extent of the injury.

**box 60-5** ***clinical manifestations***

***Knee Trauma***

- Tenderness
- Swelling, effusion (usually within 2 to 4 hours of injury)
- Pain
- Hematoma
- Disability; "knee gives way"
- Abnormal motion at joint
- Audible pop

#### *Treatment*

1. Mild injuries
   a. Rest
   b. Compression dressing
2. Moderate injuries
   a. Rest
   b. Possible aspiration of excess fluid
   c. Compression dressing to control swelling and further effusion
   d. Support—splint or brace
   e. Strengthening exercises
3. Severe injuries
   a. Surgical repair to prevent disability and instability; possible knee or shoulder surgery performed, through an arthroscope
   b. Modified compression dressing to prevent effusion
   c. Immobilization of the joint for a prescribed time
   d. Remobilization of the joint, sometimes with the aid of a continuous passive motion machine; appropriate strengthening exercises through a program of physical therapy, crutch walking for lower extremity

Postoperative nursing interventions for the patient with a ligamentous or tendon tear include the same considerations as for the partially immobilized patient after fracture reduction and application of an external fixation device.

#### *Patient/family education*

Patient teaching is particularly important. The following information should be included:

1. Information about the nature of the injury and the general nursing care after surgery
2. Use of the brace or cast postoperatively
3. Limitations of motion and weight bearing
4. Use of appropriate ambulatory aids
5. Exercises to perform and frequency of exercising
6. Plans for physician follow-up

Methods to prevent future injury should be stressed. Repetitive injuries may result in posttraumatic degenerative arthritis. Safety equipment, proper footware, and warm-up and cool-down exercises should be a part of any sports activity.

## TRAUMA TO THE ANTERIOR CRUCIATE LIGAMENT

### Etiology/Epidemiology

Trauma to the anterior cruciate ligament (ACL) is the most common ligamentous injury to the knee. It is also the knee injury most often treated surgically. Over 250,000 injuries are diagnosed annually. Ninety percent of all injuries occur in the middle third of the ligament. As mentioned earlier, the anatomy and function of the knee make it vulnerable to injury because of the stresses of motion and load bearing on the joint. Injury usually occurs in instances when the knee is hyperextended and the femur is externally rotated on a fixed tibia. Injuries commonly occur during soccer, football, skiing, and basketball, with the affected leg firmly planted on the ground. The patient usually sustains a twisting type of injury and reports a "pop" as the injury occurs.

### Pathophysiology

The ACL provides support to the knee joint. It is paired with the posterior cruciate ligament to stabilize the knee joint. The ligament originates from the posterior medial aspect of the lateral femoral condyle and crosses (origin of the name cruciate) the knee joint obliquely. The insertion is on the anteromedial aspect of the tibial plateau. The ACL functions primarily to prevent anterior displacement of the tibia, hyperextension, and excessive internal rotation of the knee. Lesser functions include decreasing varus and valgus stresses to the knee while in flexion.

The chief complaint of the patient is usually a report of the knee "giving way" and severe swelling and pain. Effusion usually occurs 2 to 4 hours after the injury. Ruptured blood vessels are the cause of hemarthrosis, which is particularly indicative of ACL injury. Examination of the patient is often difficult because of the pain.

Chronic injury occurs as a result of a missed diagnosis, failure to seek treatment, or unsuccessful nonoperative treatment of an acute injury. The knee will become increasingly unstable anteriorly and "give way" more frequently. Muscle weakness and decreased activity are common.

### Collaborative Care Management

Diagnosis is made by history and physical examination. The drawer test and the Lachman's test are both done to determine the degree of anterior displacement of the tibia and the amount of laxity of the knee. (See Chapter 59.)The pivot shift maneuver also detects anterolateral stability of the knee. It is important to include both knees for comparison. Radiographs and MRI are performed to confirm the diagnosis. X-rays are not useful in diagnosing ACL tears, but they are essential to rule out fractures or avulsion of the ACL from its insertion site.

The patient's age, activity level, type of job and leisure activities, and general medical condition are factors to be considered before determining the type of treatment. If meniscal damage is also present, surgical treatment is highly recommended because the resultant degenerative arthritis is difficult to treat. Options are physical therapy and rehabilitation or surgical intervention and rehabilitation. The goals of treatment are to prevent further damage to the knee (traumatic arthritis and meniscal tears) and allow the patient to return to his or her former level of functioning.

Nonoperative treatment usually consists of NSAIDs; application of ice and heat; electrical stimulation; rest and immobilization for a few days, followed by physical therapy to restore muscle strength; ROM; and weight bearing as quickly as possible. A brace and activity modification to avoid further injury are recommended. If the patient is not willing to modify activity, surgical repair should be considered.

Surgical options include repair with or without augmentation of the ligament and reconstruction using various types of grafts. The procedure is often performed with the aid of arthroscopy, limiting the need to open the joint surgically. A popular reconstructive technique involves the use of a patellar tendon graft with a bone block at both ends; the graft is passed through to the original origin and insertion sites of the ligament. Both autograft and allograft can be used for the patellar tendon, although autograft is preferable.

Controversy surrounds the ideal time between injury and surgical repair. Research indicates that a delay of up to 6 months does not significantly affect outcomes.[15] Patients undergoing reconstruction of a chronic ACL tear may actually attain more joint ROM than those who have had acute injuries repaired. Early reconstruction is indicated for high-performance athletes and those persons who wish to remain active in vigorous sports.

Treatment modalities have dramatically changed the postoperative period following ACL reconstruction. The operative procedure is now performed as an outpatient procedure in many facilities. Previously, a 4- to 5-day hospitalization was required. The degree of pain control is usually the main determinant of length of stay. Newer techniques are aimed at minimizing the amount of postoperative pain control and facilitating early discharge. Bupivacaine is often injected into the knee intraarticularly in the operating room for pain relief of up to 4 hours. Intraarticular morphine also shows promise as an effective method of reducing postoperative knee pain for as long as 3 to 6 hours after injection. Cryotherapy, or the use of cooling pads, is another method of controlling pain, as well as swelling, which contributes to pain.

#### Patient/family education

If surgical repair is performed, patient education centers around postoperative activity restrictions, exercises, weight-bearing limits, brace instruction, crutch walking, and recognition of signs and symptoms of complications. The goals of rehabilitation are to protect the graft, restore ROM, promote early weight bearing, and return to preinjury activity levels.[3] The amount of permissible weight bearing depends on the surgeon's protocols. Generally, touch-down or weight-bearing as tolerated is prescribed postoperatively. Physical therapy sessions usually begin 1 to 4 weeks after surgery. The rehabilitation process can take as long as 1 year. Ankle pumps, quadriceps and hamstring isometrics, and straight-leg raising are taught before discharge. The patient should be cautioned against overdoing exercising too early in the rehabilitation process. The graft often takes up to 12 months to revascularize and up to 24 months to attain preinjury strength.[3] Complications of ACL repair include infection and severe pain. The patient and family should be instructed to call the physician if the patient experiences fever, chills, increased swelling, increased wound drainage, or pain unrelieved by analgesics. The patient and family should also be instructed regarding the appropriate use of prescription pain medication.

## OVERUSE AND TRAUMATIC INJURIES OF THE SHOULDER

### Etiology/Epidemiology

The shoulder is the third most commonly injured joint, after the knee and ankle. Injury commonly occurs during athletic activities. Sports injuries are associated with direct trauma and overuse (as with throwing motions), which causes overloading of the shoulder's supporting structures. Overhead arm motion can stress the soft tissues surrounding the glenohumeral joint, causing injury over a period of time. The large head of the humerus and the comparatively shallow glenoid fossa allow the shoulder to be the most mobile joint in the body. Because of the mobility of the shoulder joint, there are fewer structural restraints to prevent potentially damaging movements. Chronic overuse is insidious in onset and usually results in impingement syndrome. Acute trauma may result in a partial or complete tear of the rotator cuff, dislocation, subluxation, separation, or fracture. Acromioclavicular separation is one of the most common shoulder injuries. Injuries to the rotator cuff usually occur as a result of chronic impingement in persons over the age of 40.

### Pathophysiology

The *rotator cuff* is composed of subscapularis, supraspinatus, infraspinatus, and teres minor muscles and tendons. The rotator cuff functions to stabilize the humeral head in the glenoid while the arm is raised. Primary movements of these muscles are abduction, external rotation, joint stabilization, and, to a lesser extent, internal rotation. *Impingement syndrome* refers to the impingement of the rotator cuff by the acromion, coracoacromial ligament, and acromioclavicular joint. It occurs as the arm is abducted past 90° and the greater tuberosity of the humerus impinges the rotator cuff against the acromion. The impingement causes microtrauma to the cuff, edema, hemorrhage, and cuff shortening. A poor blood supply to the tendons results in decreased potential for healing. Fibrosis, tendinitis, bony changes, rotator cuff tear, or biceps tendon rupture may progressively result. Symptoms of impingement are limited movement, increased pain on external rotation and abduction, weakness on manual muscle testing, muscle atrophy, and point tenderness over the insertion of the rotator cuff. Differentiating the pain occurring from impingement from the pain that occurs as a result of rotator cuff tear is difficult.

### Collaborative Care Management

Treatment is based on the following principles: decrease the inflammatory response by administering NSAIDs or applying ice; alleviate pain; immobilize the joint or provide limitation of motion; and rehabilitate the patient to achieve the maximal functional outcome. Rehabilitation begins with isometrics, passive ROM progressing to active ROM, and exercises to promote strengthening of the rotator cuff and the surrounding muscles. Subacromial cortisone injections, activity modifications to avoid repetitive overhead motions, heat, and electrical stimulation are also prescribed to decrease inflammation and promote healing. The use of cortisone injections should be limited because repeated injections into the cuff may weaken the cuff and predispose the tissues to tearing.

Surgical intervention is indicated if conservative methods fail to improve functioning within 6 months to 1 year. Extremely active persons or athletes may opt for immediate surgical treatment, without a trial of conservative therapy. Most procedures can be performed arthroscopically. Arthroscopic procedures offer the advantage of less discomfort, less chance of infection, and quicker return to overhead activities, usually within 6 to 8 weeks. Laser surgery can also be used for rotator cuff repair and relief of impingement. Rehabilitative exercises are prescribed after surgery, in the same progression as described earlier (Figure 60-22).

### *Patient/family education*

Surgical repair of shoulder injuries is performed on an outpatient basis or requires a short hospitalization. Home-going instructions should include wound care, hygiene methods, medication instruction, signs of infection, and activity restrictions. The patient should be familiar with the proper application of any immobilization devices (slings, splints) and how to inspect the skin for signs of irritation. Passive ROM techniques should be taught, in addition to prescribed exercises. A physical therapist is consulted for initial instruction; the nurse can reinforce teaching. The amount of active ROM and shoulder movement permitted varies, depending on the type of injury and treatment. The patient and family should understand the signs of potential complications, such as decreased sensation in the affected arm, increased pain, unusual swelling, increased drainage from the wound (if applicable), and coolness of the extremity.

## CUMULATIVE TRAUMA DISORDERS

*Cumulative trauma disorder* (CTD) and *repetitive strain injury* (RSI) are relatively new terms for a group of upper extremity soft-tissue musculoskeletal disorders. However, written reports of use-related complaints date back centuries.[21] Less commonly used terms are *work-related upper extremity disorder* and *occupational overuse syndrome.* As these names imply, these disorders are caused by cumulative trauma and overuse of the neck and upper extremities in the workplace. The widespread use of computers in the home and workplace for both recreational and occupational use has been cited as a significant factor in the development of CTD (see the Research Box).

The rising incidence of CTD accounted for over 60% of all new cases of occupational illness in the United States in 1991.[10] The impact of CTD on society is significant. Cumulative trauma disorders reportedly cost 50% more than the average traumatic injury claim and are the basis of a large number of lawsuits filed against employers by data processors, telephone operators, and keyboard operators.[6,10] More time is lost from work because of CTD than from any other musculoskeletal disorder, including lower back pain.[10] The National Institute for Occupational Safety and Health (NIOSH) has named occupational musculoskeletal disorders, including CTD, as one of the top 10 priority work-related conditions.[10] The goal of NIOSH is to promote a better understanding of the incidence, presentation, prevention, treatment, and rehabilitation of these common disorders.[10] The Occupational Safety and Health Administration (OSHA) is in the process of creating ergonomic standards to address work-related disorders.[21] Adoption of such standards would require employers to make efforts to reduce workplace exposure to CTD. How-

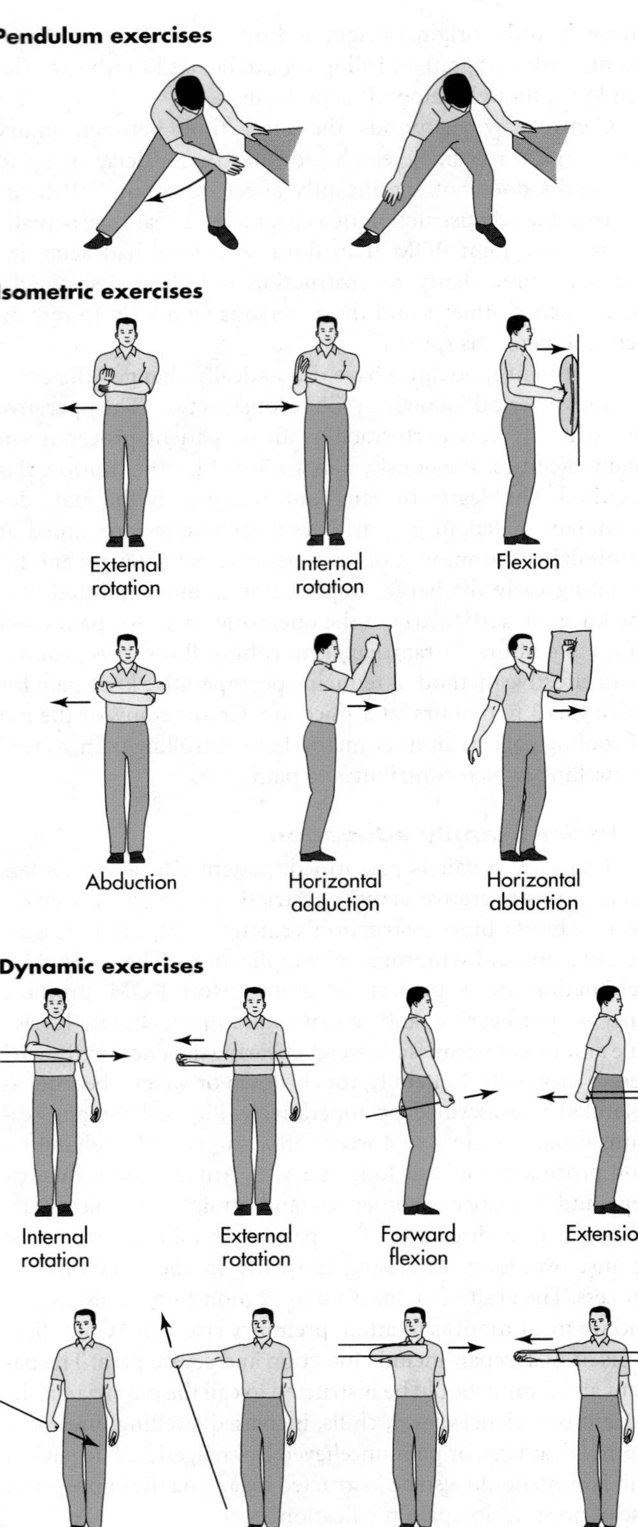


**fig. 60-22** Rehabilitative exercises of the shoulder.

**research**

Reference: Faucett J, Rempel D: Musculoskeletal symptoms related to video display terminal use, *AAOHN J* 44(1):33, 1996.

The increasing incidence of work-related musculoskeletal trauma of the upper extremities, termed *cumulative trauma disorders* (CTD), is of growing concern to health care providers, particularly those in occupational health. Several factors have been associated with the development of CTD, including computer use, repetitive and forceful movements, static posture, and workstation design. Persons at risk include office workers, computer operators, data processors, and newspaper employees.

This study compared video display terminal (VDT) use of newspaper reporters and copy editors in a large metropolitan U.S. city. The purpose was to estimate the average duration of time spent using a VDT, types of job tasks for which a VDT was required, and proportion of time spent per job task. Copy editors reported spending more hours per day using VDTs than the reporters. Copy editors experienced a greater number of musculoskeletal symptoms at a greater number of body sites. Reporters had less VDT use, more flexibility in moving away from their workstation during the day, and more variety of job tasks. Both groups had similar findings on the severity of upper extremity pain and stiffness and the likelihood of meeting the study's criteria for CTD.

More studies producing reliable data defining the amount of time at VDTs and the risk of CTD are needed. Such data can be useful to all nurses as they provide patients with teaching and health promotion guidelines.

ever, the literature reports controversy over whether a definitive causal relationship exists between these upper extremity disorders and the performance of many jobs.[21]

Cumulative trauma disorders can occur in any muscle group that is used repeatedly for long, uninterrupted periods with the body in a relatively fixed posture.[6] Women are affected twice as often as men. Most sources cite repetitive motion as the predominant risk factor for the development of CTD. Other risk factors include obesity; excessive, forceful movements; poor tool design; ergonomic factors in the workplace; vibration exposure; extremes of flexion or extension; and static positioning.[21] The most common CTD include carpal tunnel syndrome, medial and lateral epicondylitis, thoracic outlet syndrome, and de Quervain's tenosynovitis (Table 60-5). Symptoms are primarily those of entrapment neuropathies, including pain and paresthesias. Carpal tunnel syndrome is discussed in detail next.

## Carpal Tunnel Syndrome

### Etiology

Carpal tunnel syndrome (CTS), which was first described in 1854, is caused by pressure exerted on the median nerve of the wrist. The condition occurs most commonly in women 30 to 50 years of age. It usually affects the dominant hand. Many conditions can cause an increase in pressure in the carpal tunnel, thereby producing symptoms of median nerve compression. Symptoms are usually consistent, regardless of etiology. Carpal tunnel syndrome is considered a cumulative trauma disorder because the etiology is often repetitive hand or wrist motions. Because of its association with computer use, CTS has been called the "industrial injury of the information age."[16] It should be stressed that as with all other CTD, the etiology in not always repetitive motion.

### Epidemiology

Inflammatory processes such as rheumatoid arthritis, flexor tenosynovitis, and gout can cause thickening of the flexor synovium, which leads to elevated pressure in the tunnel. Patients receiving long-term hemodialysis for chronic renal failure may be at risk for developing CTS because of synovial edema and amyloid deposits.

Previous trauma may contribute to the development of CTS. Burns, fractures, and dislocations of the wrist can constrict the tunnel by the formation of contractures, scarring, or bony deformities.

Repetitive motion of the wrist may also contribute to the development of CTS. Work-related carpal tunnel syndrome is a CTD caused by job-related tasks that involve certain motions or actions:

1. Forceful grasping or pinching of objects (e.g., tools)
2. Awkward positions
3. Direct pressure over carpal tunnel
4. Repetitive motions
5. Use of vibrating handheld tools

Other conditions that contribute to the development of carpal tunnel syndrome include diabetes, myxedema, pregnancy, abnormalities of the median artery and flexor muscle, ganglions, and lipomas. Alcoholism has also been associated with the development of carpal tunnel syndrome. Certain occupations put workers (typists, computer operators, assembly line workers, and truck drivers) at risk for developing the syndrome.

### Pathophysiology

The median nerve passes through a tunnel bounded by the carpal bones dorsally and the transverse carpal ligament volarly (Figure 60-23). Through this "tunnel" pass nine flexor tendons and the median nerve. The median nerve provides sensation to the radial aspect of the palm and volar surfaces of the thumb, index finger, middle finger, and radial half of the ring finger. The median nerve also innervates the muscles of the anterior forearm and thenar muscles of the thumb, and it supplies sensation to the skin of the thumb, index finger, middle finger, and half of the ring finger. Any narrowing within this canal leads to compression of the medial nerve and CTS.

Initially, pressure on the median nerve causes temporary blockage of the myelinated nerve fibers, which results in numbness and pressure of the hand and fingers. Continued pressure causes ischemia, resulting in axonal death, muscular atrophy, and pain.[2]

**table 60-5** *Common Types of Cumulative Trauma Disorders*

| Disorder | Manifestations | Etiology | Treatment |
|---|---|---|---|
| De Quervain's tenosynovitis | Pain with thumb and wrist movement, pain radiating to forearm, aching over dorsal thumb surface, swelling, decreased pinch-grip strength | Inflammation of the abductor pollicis longus and the extensor pollicis brevis tendons in the first dorsal compartment of the wrist, at the base of the thumb; first described in 1895 as "washerwoman's strain" from wringing clothes; workers at risk include operating room personnel, housekeepers, musicians, and butchers (repetitive pinching and forearm rotation) | Wrist and thumb spica splint, gentle active ROM exercises, joint protection and ergonomically designed workplace and tools; surgical treatment (release of first dorsal compartment) only if conservative measures fail |
| Thoracic outlet syndrome | Pain; paresthesias; swelling; temperature changes; weakness of the forearm, shoulder, arm | Compression of the brachial plexus, subclavian artery, and subclavian vein; mechanical compression; posture of head, neck, shoulders; cervical rib; overhead activities | Physical therapy; patient education about posture, workstation dynamics; ergonomics; physical activity; surgical resection if compression is due to cervical rib |
| Lateral epicondylitis (tennis elbow) | Microscopic tears in the extensor carpi radialis brevis tendon, which originates at the lateral epicondyle of the elbow; repetitive activities | Pain over the lateral epicondyle and extensor muscle mass; increased pain with elbow extension and forceful grip; persons at risk include construction workers, assembly line workers, tennis players (only 5% of identified cases), swimmers, golfers, and carpenters (hammering) | Reduce elbow extension; splinting; cold compresses followed by stretching; electrical stimulation, heat, and ulstrasound; patient education about avoidance of aggravating movements or postures, tool or handle modification; surgical intervention to lengthen and repair the tendon if conservative measures fail |

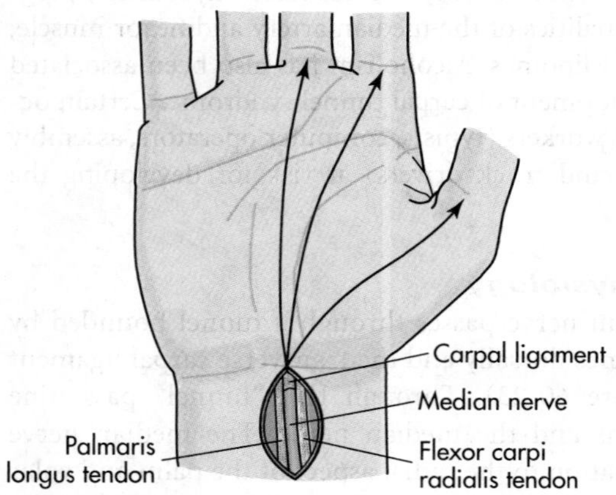


**fig. 60-23** Carpal tunnel syndrome. Volar aspect of wrist retracted to demonstrate position of median nerve. Distribution of median nerve is to thumb and first two fingers.

The severity of symptoms varies. Mild manifestations include intermittent paresthesias, tingling, and pain in the median nerve distribution. The pain may awaken the patient at night; symptoms will persist and increase if not treated. More severe cases of CTS include symptoms of hypoesthesia, awkwardness, and loss of dexterity and pinch strength. The patient may complain of dropping things or changes in handwriting.

Symptoms may be worse at night, perhaps caused by sleeping with the wrists in a flexed position. Complaints usually increase when there has been forced flexion of the wrist for long periods, as with knitting or typing. The patient may describe the hand as "swollen" and may complain of clumsiness. Pain referred to the upper extremity and base of the neck is common.

Long-standing CTS may manifest with pronounced thenar atrophy (the padded area of the palm below the base of the thumb), chronic pain, and major functional impairment secondary to axonal death. The prognosis at this stage is poor, regardless of treatment.[2]

### *Collaborative care management*

Diagnosis is based on patient history, physical examination, and evaluation of diagnostic tests. Other conditions with similar symptoms must be eliminated, including cervical radiculopathy, brachial plexopathy, de Quervain's tenosynovitis, arthritis, and thoracic outlet syndrome. Symptoms can be reproduced by tapping the median nerve at the wrist (positive Tinel's sign). Phalen's test is also used to diagnose carpal tunnel syndrome. The examiner holds the wrists in acute flexion for 60 seconds; if symptoms are reproduced or increased, the test is considered positive. Direct compression of the median nerve at the wrist for 30 seconds will also reproduce or increase symptoms in the presence of carpal tunnel syndrome.

Nerve conduction studies and electromyography are used to evaluate nerve function and muscle abnormalities.

Medical management of the patient with carpal tunnel syndrome includes:

1. Rest
2. Splinting to maintain the wrist in a neutral position—most effective if begun within 3 months of onset of symptoms
3. Local steroid injections
4. Administration of NSAIDs and oral vitamin $B_6$; pyridoxine deficiency has been noted in some persons with CTS
5. Short-term use of diuretics to reduce fluid volume in the carpal tunnel
6. Decompression of the median nerve (an ambulatory procedure)

Surgical intervention is indicated if conservative treatment fails or in the presence of long-standing symptoms. Surgical correction is performed by open or endoscopic release and decompression. Endoscopic release decreases postoperative pain, reduces scarring, and decreases recovery time. Arthroscopic release is contraindicated in patients with rheumatoid arthritis and flexor synovitis.

Nursing management includes the following:

1. Preoperative care
   a. Instruct patient regarding rest, splinting of wrist.
   b. Provide preoperative instruction (see Chapter 18).
   c. Occupational history and job counseling; if occupational factors such as wrist flexing and repetitive tasks contributed to development of the condition, job retraining may be indicated.
   d. Postoperative teaching:
      (1) Instruct patient about follow-up care.
      (2) Lifestyle modification if repetitive motions (workplace or leisure) contributed to disease process.
2. Postoperative care
   a. Promote comfort and circulation:
      (1) Elevate hand and arm for 24 hours; use ice to reduce swelling and pain.
      (2) Encourage active thumb and finger motion within limits imposed by dressing.
      (3) Administer prescribed analgesic as necessary; assess effectiveness.
   b. Prevent complications:
      (1) Check fingers for circulation, sensation, and movement every 1 to 2 hours for 24 hours; instruct patient and family how to recognize symptoms of neurovascular compromise.
   c. Discharge instructions:
      (1) Explain splint care. The splint usually is maintained for 2 to 3 weeks postoperatively.
      (2) Follow up in physician's office within 1 week to assess wound and dressing change.
3. Refer to physical therapist for ROM and strengthening exercises.

**Patient/family education.** Because of the increasing incidence of cumulative trauma–related injuries in the workplace, it is important for nurses to recognize persons at risk and to teach preventive measures. As a result of the number of lawsuits against employers filed by employees, many businesses have initiated programs to decrease the development of CTD. These programs include redesign of the workplace with the focus on ergonomics, stress reduction techniques, and classes to teach proper mechanics and body awareness and reduce computer stress.[2,6] Nurses are in an ideal position to promote wellness and reduce the risks associated with the development of CTS and other CTD.

Depending on the work environment and type of job the patient has, it may be possible to reorganize the work structure to avoid long periods of repetitive motions. The patient should be taught to organize the day in an efficient but diverse schedule. Instruct the patient to take frequent short breaks and to get out of the office chair and move around, exercising the neck, shoulders, and upper extremities. Simple ROM exercises can be performed at the desk, if moving around is not an option. The work space should be redesigned to reduce fatigue and stress, while increasing efficiency.

Instructions regarding body mechanics during computer use are beneficial to both the patient and family. The position of the computer and the person's posture while working are important factors in reducing CTS risk. The patient should be taught to sit erect and lean slightly forward while using the keyboard. The arms should be elevated with the wrists straight to reduce pressure on the nerves, tendons, and muscles of the arms and hands. The forearms and palms should be angled toward each other while typing to reduce fatigue.[2] The keyboard height should be modified to avoid placing the wrists into hyperextension, which stretches the muscles and ligaments. Foam pads on which to rest the wrists while typing are available commercially. When keystroking, the patient should understand that rapid, prolonged movements of the fingers can cause pain. Patients who use the keyboard frequently should be instructed to avoid long fingernails, which cause awkward positioning of the fingers and wrists during keystroke. In addition, general health teaching should be done, including education regarding the benefits of a healthy diet and regular exercise.

## TRAUMA TO JOINTS AND JOINT STRUCTURES

Injuries to joints and joint structures may occur as a *sprain* (tearing of the capsule or ligaments surrounding a joint, including disruption of the synovial membrane), meniscus tear, joint dislocation, or joint subluxation.

Trauma to ligaments and tendons and principles of patient management have been discussed previously. Joint dislocation will be discussed in this section.

The shoulder is susceptible to traumatic dislocation. Closed reduction is the first choice of treatment, followed by rehabilitative exercises. Chronic instability may necessitate surgical stabilization.

### TRAUMATIC HIP DISLOCATION

#### Etiology/Epidemiology

Traumatic hip dislocation usually occurs as a result of a motor vehicle accident, especially if a frontal impact is sustained.

This type of force can drive the victim's knees into the dashboard, forcibly dislocating the hip. Traumatic dislocation of the hip is considered an orthopedic emergency because of the risk of *avascular necrosis (AVN)* of the femoral head. Prompt treatment is critical; reduction within 6 hours of injury decreases the risk of persistent pain, decreased range of motion, and avascular necrosis. Traumatic dislocations occur most commonly in persons under 50 years of age, unless an underlying disease is present, such as a neuromuscular disease or rheumatoid arthritis.

### Pathophysiology

As the hip is forcibly dislocated, the blood supply to the femoral head can be disrupted (see Figure 60-19). Damage to the sciatic nerve is also possible and can result in partial to complete motor and sensory loss in the affected extremity. Sciatic nerve injury is present in 10% to 20% of persons with posterior dislocation. Another potential problem is fracture of the femoral head, acetabulum, or pelvis. The articular surface of the femoral head may be eroded by bone fragments. Clinical manifestations of traumatic hip dislocation can be found in Box 60-6. Most dislocations of the femoral head occur posteriorly with the thigh in flexion. The femoral head cannot be completely displaced from the acetabulum unless the ligamentum teres is torn or ruptured. Anterior dislocation occurs with the hip in extension and external rotation. The femoral head may be palpable anteriorly below the inguinal area. Complications of dislocation include avascular necrosis, infection, malunion, posttraumatic arthritis, and sciatic nerve injury. Avascular necrosis may occur as late as 2 years after the injury.[19] Residual neuropathy occurs in approximately 20% of persons in whom sciatic nerve damage has been sustained.

### Collaborative Care Management

Diagnosis is made on the basis of history, physical examination, and evidence of dislocation on x-ray film.

If possible, the hip is reduced immediately. The patient is given intravenous sedation, and the physician uses manual traction to relocate the hip *(closed reduction)*. If closed reduction is not feasible, or in the presence of acetabular or pelvic fracture, skeletal traction may be used to reduce the hip until surgery is possible. If there is no fracture, *open reduction* is accomplished by opening the hip capsule and relocating the head. For pelvic and acetabular fractures, internal fixative devices are usually used. If avascular necrosis results, prosthetic replacement of the hip is required.

Nursing management of the person with a traumatic hip dislocation is the same as for the patient with a hip fracture. The major emphasis is on keeping the limb in alignment by proper positioning. In addition, some patients will have a brace applied either in surgery (if an orthotist is available) or the next day.

#### *Patient/family education*

The patient is taught active and passive exercises. Teaching also includes prevention of further injury and the use of assistive devices. The use of crutches or a walker is usually required until the patient has progressed to full weight bearing, generally in 4 to 6 weeks.

**box 60-6** *clinical manifestations*

***Traumatic Hip Dislocation***

- Pain
- Deformity
- Decreased range of motion
- Decreased sensation
- Diminished or absent pulses
- Anterior dislocation
  Hip in extension and external rotation; palpable femoral head
- Posterior dislocation
  Hip in flexion and internal rotation; shortening; may be a visible leg length discrepancy when compared with unaffected leg

## MULTIPLE TRAUMA

### ETIOLOGY/EPIDEMIOLOGY

The leading cause of death in the United States for persons under the age of 45 is trauma. Causes of trauma include falls, crush injuries, vehicular (including airplane) accidents, and gunshot wounds. The nature of the injuries sustained in trauma is often extensive, involving multiple organ systems and multiple sites of injury. Approximately 50% of trauma deaths occur at the scene of injury, before medical help can arrive. Death usually results from brainstem trauma, spinal cord injury, hemorrhage, or major organ injuries. The second peak of trauma deaths occurs within 2 hours of injury, as a result of hemorrhage or head, chest, or abdominal injuries. Death during the third peak occurs within days to weeks of the initial injury, usually because of sepsis or multisystem failure.

The fact that many persons with multiple injuries are able to survive and reach treatment facilities is related to treatment improvements at the accident scene, quick methods of transport to hospitals, and advances in the field of emergency medicine and nursing. Regional trauma centers allow transfer of patients to facilities equipped to manage complex care needs of the victim of polytrauma. Personnel in any hospital may be confronted with a multiply injured patient and should be prepared to treat the patient. Often the patient is stabilized and then airlifted to a trauma center.

The most common orthopedic injuries that occur as a result of multiple trauma are pelvic fracture and crush injuries. Approximately 30% of persons involved in multiple trauma sustain a pelvic fracture. Fractures of the pelvis usually occur as a result of motor vehicle accidents, falls, and crush injuries. Depending on the type of fracture and coexisting injuries, closed pelvic fracture has an associated mortality rate of 8% to 15%, and open pelvic fracture has an associated mortality rate of 30% to 50%.[19] Hemorrhage is usually the cause of death. Shearing forces from the impact of trauma cause rupture of blood vessels surrounding the pelvic ring, causing hemorrhage and hypotension. Damage to internal organs, especially urogenital injuries, can occur from shearing forces, bone fragments, and compression. The retroperitoneal space can accommodate up to 4 L of blood before tamponade results. Coagulopathy is a significant problem because of loss of clotting factors and because of continued bleeding at the fracture site. Pelvic fractures are classified by the mechanism of injury and degree of instability.

*Crush injuries* may result from falls, motor vehicle accidents, and blunt trauma, such as being trapped under heavy fallen objects. Multiple fractures and internal bleeding may result, with hemorrhage being the usual cause of death. *Crush syndrome* was first described during World War II. Crush syndrome follows crush injury and is characterized by muscle necrosis, hypovolemia, compartment syndrome, rhabdomyolysis, fluid and electrolyte imbalance, coagulopathy, and renal failure.[4] The development of renal failure increases the mortality rate. Fluid and electrolyte imbalances commonly seen in crush syndrome include hypocalcemia, hyperphosphatemia, hyperkalemia, edema, and third spacing.

## COLLABORATIVE CARE MANAGEMENT

Treatment of victims of multiple trauma is based on the ABCs (**a**irway, **b**reathing, **c**irculation) of airway management with cervical spine control, breathing, and circulation. (See Chapters 21 and 22.) The pelvis and abdomen must be evaluated for fractures and hemorrhage (Box 60-7). Rib and spine fractures may cause life-threatening neurological and cardiovascular injuries.

### box 60-7 Pelvic Fractures

**SIGNS AND SYMPTOMS**

Pain with compression of iliac crests
Asymmetry of iliac crests
Abnormal rotation of femurs
Leg length discrepancy
Lacerations of perineum, vagina, or rectum
Hematuria
Neurological deficits
Hypotension

**DIAGNOSTIC TESTS**

X-ray
CT scan*
Peritoneal lavage to determine presence of intraabdominal bleeding*
Arteriogram: intravenous pyelogram may be done if the patient is stable to determine extent of internal injury

**MANAGEMENT**

Pelvic sling
Skeletal traction
Spica cast
Open reduction and internal fixation
External fixators are the treatment of choice

**ASSOCIATED INJURIES**

Vascular
Genitourinary
Abdominal
Intestinal and rectal

*Controversial.

Obvious fractures are immobilized and splinted, and sterile dressings are applied to open fractures until surgical reduction is feasible. The goals of management are to correct or stabilize any life-threatening problems (e.g., obstructed airway, pneumothorax, bleeding) and then to reestablish the continuity of injured tissues. Musculoskeletal injury may require reduction of fractures and repair of related soft-tissue injury. Because life-threatening problems must be addressed first, musculoskeletal injuries are usually not repaired until the patient has been stabilized. However, sites of fracture or potential fracture must be splinted or otherwise protected until reduction can be effected.

The principles of nursing management are:

1. *Before reduction,* protection of all actual or potential sites of fracture through maintaining splints, traction, or positioning precautions; avoid manipulation of fracture fragments; monitor patient for hemorrhage and other complications.
2. *After reduction,* observation of all the previously discussed principles of nursing management of the patient with a fracture

The challenge for the nurse is to devise a plan of care that takes into account the demands of the variety of fixation techniques, fracture sites, and mobilization or immobilization requirements for that patient. The psychosocial needs and the rehabilitation requirements for individuals who have sustained multiple trauma are often long term and extensive. Consideration of rehabilitation requirements must occur early in the patient's hospital course and be reviewed frequently (see Chapter 7).

### Patient/Family Education

Nurses can play a role in the prevention of multiple trauma by promoting safety awareness among all persons, especially those at risk. Promoting safety in the work environment may prevent industrial or on-the-job accidents. Public awareness of the dangers of driving while intoxicated and the importance of wearing seat belts may help decrease the number of motor vehicle accidents and the injuries sustained in them.

Persons who have sustained multiple trauma may have residual deficits and an extensive rehabilitative process. Teaching focuses on adaptive techniques and measures to prevent further disability (see Chapter 7).

## critical thinking QUESTIONS

**1** Explain how the care of an individual undergoing an open reduction differs from the care of a patient undergoing a closed reduction of a fracture.

**2** Discuss the essential assessment parameters used by the nurse to detect systemic complications of bone fracture.

**3** Develop a health promotion plan for a group of office workers to prevent the development of repetitive motion disorder.

**4** Describe nursing interventions for a 24-year-old man who suffered a pelvic and femoral fracture in a motor vehicle accident. What are potential complications of his injury? What preventive nursing measures are indicated?

**5** What information would be included in the home-going instructions for a person who has undergone an ACL reconstruction in an ambulatory surgery center?

## chapter SUMMARY

### TRAUMA TO BONE

- Musculoskeletal trauma is most commonly manifested as bone fracture but may include injury to other structures of the system.
  1. Fracture of bone is usually the result of a blow to the body, a fall, or an accident, but it may occur during normal activity if the bone is weakened by disease (pathological fracture). A fatigue or stress fracture results when muscles associated with the fractured bone are unable to absorb energy as they usually do.
  2. A bone is fractured when there is a complete or partial (incomplete) interruption of the osseous tissue. Fractures may be further classified as simple (closed) or compound (open), depending on whether the skin over the fracture remains intact. If fracture fragments are moved away from the normal alignment of the bone, the fracture is displaced; if the fragments are not moved out of alignment, the fracture is nondisplaced.
  3. Greenstick, transverse, oblique, spiral, telescoped (impacted), and comminuted are terms that describe the line of the fracture.
  4. Immobilization of fractured bone is necessary for healing to take place. This can be accomplished through physiological splintage, external orthopedic splinting, or internal fixation. Bone heals by the process of callus formation. Complications of bone healing, such as delayed union, nonunion, malunion, and pseudoarthrosis, can occur.
  5. The most pronounced signs and symptoms of fracture usually include pain, loss of normal function, obvious deformity, edema, and ecchymosis.
  6. Medical management of the patient with a fracture focuses on reduction of the fracture, maintenance of correct alignment of the bone fragments, and prevention of excessive loss of joint mobility and muscle tone.
  7. Complications of fracture include fracture blisters, fat embolism syndrome, compartment syndrome, deep vein thrombosis, pulmonary embolus, infection, and heterotopic bone formation.
  8. Nursing interventions emphasize promoting knowledge; controlling pain; maintaining safety; preserving strength and mobility; maintaining skin integrity; preventing systemic complications (circulatory, respiratory, gastrointestinal, and urinary); promoting nutrition; and maintaining immobilization of the reduced fracture.
  9. Internal fixation is carried out with the patient under anesthesia in the operating room. The result is open surgical reduction of the fracture.
- Fractures of the hip are common; they occur more commonly in women than in men.
- Intracapsular fractures occur within the hip joint and capsule. Extracapsular fractures occur outside the hip joint and capsule. Avascular necrosis may result if blood supply to the head of the femur is disrupted as a result of the fracture.
  1. The signs and symptoms of hip fracture include severe pain, inability to move the leg, and shortening and external rotation of the leg.
  2. Medical management of the patient with a hip fracture focuses on reduction and fixation of the fracture.
  3. Nursing management of the patient with a hip fracture includes the same considerations and interventions as for any patient with a fracture. Special considerations relate to specific position restrictions for persons who have had a prosthetic implant.
- Spinal fracture can occur at any age, usually as a result of trauma or, with increasing frequency, as the result of osteoporosis and metastatic lesions.
  1. Fracture can occur at any level of the spine. If fracture fragments are displaced, they may injure the spinal nerves or spinal cord. Dysfunction may be permanent or temporary, depending on the extent of the injury.
  2. The signs and symptoms of vertebral fracture include pain, loss of sensation or mobility below the level of injury, and evidence of fracture or dislocation on x-ray film or other radiological studies.
  3. Immediate medical management of the patient with suspected spinal fracture includes immobilization with backboard and cervical collar and transport to a hospital. The general medical management objectives are stabilization and reduction of the fracture and decompression (i.e., removal of pressure from spinal nerves or the spinal cord).
  4. Nursing management of the patient with spinal fracture may include both interventions required by any patient who has a fracture and those for a patient with a spinal cord injury.

### TRAUMA TO SOFT TISSUE STRUCTURES

- Trauma to ligaments and tendons is usually seen with injury to a joint. The most common site of ligament damage is the knee, followed by the ankle and shoulder. Ligament and tendon injuries may be classified as mild, moderate, or severe, depending on the extent of the tear.
  1. The signs and symptoms of ligament and tendon injury may include tenderness, swelling, pain, effusion, hematoma, disability, and abnormal joint motion. These are not always present and may vary in intensity.
  2. Medical management of persons with trauma to ligaments and tendons is determined by the extent of the damage and may range from rest and immobilization for mild injuries to surgical repair for severe injuries.
  3. Anterior cruciate ligament injury is a common sports-related injury of the knee. Treatment can be conservative or surgical, depending on the individual.
  4. Rotator cuff injuries and impingement syndrome can be a result of trauma to the shoulder. Both conservative and surgical treatments are available.
  5. Soft-tissue injuries are initially managed by rest, ice, compression, and elevation (RICE).

### TRAUMA TO JOINTS AND JOINT STRUCTURES

- Injuries to joints and their structures may occur as sprains, tears of the capsule surrounding the joint, meniscus tears, joint dislocations, or subluxation. Dislocation and subluxation occur as the result of extreme stress applied to the joint, forcing it in an abnormal direction.

1. The signs and symptoms of trauma to the joints and their structures are specific to the type of injury and include pain, swelling, limitation of motion, instability of the joint, and possible impairment of neurovascular status.
2. Joint dislocation and subluxation require reduction and immobilization.
3. Nursing management of the patient with trauma to joints and joint structures is the same as for the person with severe strain, except there will be emphasis on maintaining and improving muscle strength around the injured joint. Patient teaching is a priority and emphasizes performing the prescribed exercises and following through with physical therapy regimens.

## MULTIPLE TRAUMA

- Trauma is the leading cause of death in the United States for persons under 45 years of age.
  1. Causes of trauma include falls, crush injuries, crush syndrome, vehicular accidents, and gunshot wounds. These injuries are often extensive and involve multiple organ systems and multiple sites of injury.
  2. Pelvic fracture and crush injury are the most common injuries resulting from multiple trauma.
  3. The goals of medical management in multiple trauma are to correct or stabilize any life-threatening problems and to repair injured tissues. This would include reduction of fractures and repair of related soft-tissue injury. Because attention to life-threatening problems is the priority of immediate care, musculoskeletal injuries may not be repaired until after the patient has been stabilized. Fracture sites must be splinted until this can be accomplished.
  4. Immediate nursing management of the patient with musculoskeletal trauma focuses on protection of actual and potential sites of injury until they can be repaired.

## References


1. Baumhauer JF et al: A prospective study of ankle injury risk factors, *Am J Sports Med* 23(5):564, 1995.
2. Belmonte K: Carpal tunnel syndrome, *J Am Acad Nurse Pract* 8(11): 511, 1996.
3. Brown FM: Anterior cruciate ligament reconstruction as an outpatient procedure, *Orthop Nurs* 15(1):15, 1996.
4. Cheney P: Early management and physiologic changes in crush syndrome, *Crit Care Nurs Q* 17(2):62, 1994.
5. Cifu DX: Rehabilitation of fractures of the hip, *Phys Med Rehabil* 9(1):125, 1995.
6. Doheny M, Linden P, Sedlak C: Reducing orthopaedic hazards of the computer work environment, *Orthop Nurs* 14(1):7, 1995.
7. Duong TT: Complications of fractures, *Phys Med Rehabil* 9(1):17, 1995.
8. Grisso JA et al: Risk factors for hip fracture: black women, *N Engl J Med* 330(22):1555, 1994.
9. Henry SL, Osterman PA, Seligson D: The antibiotic bead pouch technique in the management of severe compound fractures, *Clin Orthop Related Res* 295:54, 1993.
10. Himmelstein TS et al: Work-related upper-extremity disorders and work disability: clinical and psychosocial presentation, *J Occup Environmental Med* 37(11):1278, 1995.
11. Hiss J, Kahuna T, Kugel C: Beaten to death: why do they die? *J Trauma Injury Infection Crit Care* 40(1):27, 1996.
12. McCann S, Gruen G: Fracture blisters: a review of the literature, *Orthop Nurs* 16(2):17, 1997.
13. Matkovic V, Klisovic D, Ilich JZ: Epidemiology of fractures during growth and aging, *Phys Med Rehabil Clin North Am* 6(3):415, 1995.
14. Mourad LA, Droste MM: *The nursing process in the care of adults with orthopaedic conditions,* ed 3, Albany, NY, 1993, Delmar.
15. Neal LJ: Outpatient ACL surgery: the role of the home health nurse, *Orthop Nurs* 15(4):9, 1996.
16. Norgan GH et al: A program plan addressing carpal tunnel syndrome, *AAOHN J* 43(8):407, 1995.
17. Reed LJ, Keegan MJ: Fat embolism syndrome: a complication of trauma, *Crit Care Nurse* 6:33, 1993.
18. Ross DG: Chronic compartment syndrome, *Orthop Nurs* 15(3):23, 1996.
19. Skinner HB: *Current diagnosis and treatment in orthopedics,* Norwalk, Conn, 1995, Appleton & Lange.
20. US Department of Health and Human Services, Public Health Service: *Healthy people 2000,* Washington, DC, 1995, US Government Printing Office.
21. Vender MI et al: Upper extremity disorders: a literature review to determine work-relatedness, *J Hand Surg* 20A(4):534, 1995.
22. Zuckerman JD: Hip fracture, *N Engl J Med* 334(23):1519, 1996.

# chapter 61 MANAGEMENT OF PERSONS WITH Inflammatory and Degenerative Disorders of the Musculoskeletal System

JANE F. MAREK

## objectives

*After studying this chapter, the learner should be able to:*

1 Compare and contrast the etiology/epidemiology, pathophysiology, and clinical manifestations of rheumatoid arthritis and osteoarthritis.

2 Describe the medical, surgical, and nursing management of persons who have rheumatoid arthritis.

3 Describe the medical, surgical, and nursing management of persons who have degenerative joint disease.

4 Relate the pathophysiology with the collaborative care management for persons with inflammatory and degenerative disorders affecting the joints.

5 Compare the pathophysiology and collaborative care management of the different types of degenerative and inflammatory processes affecting bones.

6 Discuss the incidence, pathophysiology, and clinical manifestations of osteoporosis.

7 Describe the collaborative care management of persons with osteoporosis.

8 Develop a teaching plan for persons at risk for osteoporosis, including preventive measures to reduce the risk of osteoporosis.

9 Relate the pathophysiology and clinical manifestations of degenerative disease of the spine with the medical, surgical, and nursing management of persons who have degenerative disease of the spine.

10 Correlate the pathophysiology and clinical manifestations of scoliosis with medical management of persons with scoliosis and contrast the nursing care required for individuals being treated conservatively with those treated surgically.

11 Relate the etiology, pathophysiology, and treatment for common tumors of the musculoskeletal system.

12 Describe the medical, surgical, and nursing management of the patient with an osteosarcoma.

13 Compare and contrast potential complications after limb salvage surgery and amputation.

14 Discuss the etiology/epidemiology, pathophysiology, and clinical manifestations of disorders affecting the soft tissues of the musculoskeletal system.

15 Explain the medical and nursing interventions used in the care of persons with soft tissue disorders of the musculoskeletal system.

The essence of nursing care for individuals with musculoskeletal problems lies in helping them make the physiological and psychosocial adaptations necessary to cope with a temporary or permanent disability. Inflammatory and degenerative processes can affect all structures in the musculoskeletal system: bones, joint, and soft tissues. This chapter describes common inflammatory and degenerative problems of the musculoskeletal system. Degenerative and inflammatory conditions of the musculoskeletal system are often chronic and disabling. Pain and impaired mobility are major problems that must be considered when planning nursing care. Nursing interventions are focused on assisting the patient to maximize independent functioning and teaching methods of joint protection, energy conservation, and prevention of further disability.

## DISORDERS AFFECTING THE JOINTS

*Arthritis* (inflammation of the joint) is a common disorder of the musculoskeletal system that causes pain and stiffness in the joints. There are more than 100 types of arthritis, and an estimated 40 million persons in the United States have some form of this debilitating disese. Significant health care costs and long-term disability are associated with arthritic conditions. An estimated 50% of persons with arthritis are disabled within 10 years of diagnosis.[55] The number of persons in the United States affected by arthritis continues to increase; it is estimated that 18% of the population will have arthritis by the year 2020.[55]

The following sections will discuss the two main types of arthritis: rheumatoid and osteoarthritis. In addition, other degenerative and inflammatory conditions affecting joints will be discussed.

## RHEUMATOID ARTHRITIS

### Etiology

Rheumatoid arthritis (RA) is a chronic systemic disease affecting primarily the diarthroidial joints and surrounding soft tissues. The disease process is characterized by inflammation of the connective tissues throughout the body. Systemic manifestations include pulmonary, cardiac, vascular, ophthalmological, dermatological, and hematological involvement. Mortality is associated with the extraarticular manifestations of RA and may shorten the individual's life expectancy by 3 to 18 years.

The etiology of rheumatoid arthritis is unknown. However, several theories have been postulated regarding the pathogenesis of RA. Rheumatoid arthritis is thought to be an autoimmune process, specifically the interaction of immunoglobin (Ig) G with rheumatoid factor, which appears to perpetuate the rheumatoid inflammation. A genetic predisposition has also been identified related to certain human leukocyte antigen (HLA) antigens. Another theory postulates that the disease occurs as an altered immune response to an unknown antigen. Possible causative antigens include the Epstein-Barr virus, bacteria, and mycoplasma. Environmental factors have also been thought to trigger the inflammatory response. Prolonged exposure to the antigen causes normal antibodies (Ig) to become autoantibodies and attack host tissues (self-antigen). These autoantibodies, called rheumatoid factors (RF), bind with self-antigens in the blood and synovial membrane to form immune complexes (Figure 61-1).

### Epidemiology

Rheumatoid arthritis is more prevalent in women than men by a ratio of 3:1. It affects 1% to 3% of the population in the United States, with an estimated 200,000 cases diagnosed annually.[45,55] An increased incidence of RA is found in persons older than age 30; RA affects more than 5% of the population older than 70 years of age.[41] The average age of onset is 55 years.[56]

### Pathophysiology

The disease begins in the synovial membrane within the joint. Edema, vascular congestion, fibrin exudate, and cellular infiltrate occur as a result of the inflammatory process. The inflammatory process is triggered by an unknown event that damages or irritates joint tissues. Activated T cells, not present in normal joints, are found in joints affected by rheumatoid arthritis. Macrophages and monocytes are also found in rheumatoid joints and produce cytokines, which affect immune responses and inflammatory reactions. The cytokines, including interleukins, tissue necrosis factor, granulocyte-macrophage colony-stimulating factors, and other growth factors, cause cartilage destruction and increase inflammation.

White blood cells release chemicals (including superoxide radicals and hydrogen peroxide), which destroy both the bacteria and normal cells. Prostaglandins (chemicals that mediate inflammation), leukotrienes (producers of inflammation), and digestive enzymes are released. Particularly damaging to joint tissue is the enzyme collagenase, because it breaks down collagen, the main structural protein of connective tissue. The presence of these substances within the joint attracts more white blood cells, and in rheumatoid arthritis, the process becomes chronic. Continued inflammation leads to thickening of the synovium, particularly where it joins the articular cartilage. At these junctures fibrin develops into a granulation tissue termed *pannus* that covers the surface of the cartilage. The pannus also invades subchondral bone and interferes with the normal nutrition of the articular cartilage, causing necrosis. Pannus formation leads to adhesions between the joint surfaces, and fibrous or bony union *(ankylosis)* develops. Destruction of cartilage and bone, in addition to some weakening of tendons and ligaments, may lead to subluxation or dislocation of joints. Invasion of the subchondral bone may cause eventual regional osteoporosis (Table 61-1).

Pain occurs as a result of cartilage degeneration. Exposed areas of bone due to erosion of cartilage may develop fissures or bone cysts. These cysts, caused by an excessive amount of inflammatory exudate, may develop into draining fistulae, communicating with the skin. Bone spurs and osteophytes (outgrowth of bone) may also occur, decreasing joint mobility and increasing pain.

Constitutional symptoms and a new onset of joint pain are early manifestations of RA. The patient may report lymphadenopathy, malaise, depression, fever, weight loss, fatigue, and generalized aching. Early morning stiffness lasting more than an hour is characteristic. Morning stiffness is thought to occur as a result of synovitis. The person may describe the location of aching and stiffness in general terms as opposed to naming specific joints. This kind of discomfort, commonly referred to as *fibrositis*, is poorly localized. Such discomfort may be the patient's earliest report. These symptoms may be present for some period of time before they are replaced by more specific, or localized, problems (i.e., frank articular inflammation with joint swelling, pain, redness, warmth, and tenderness). In other persons, fibrositis and joint inflammation occur together at the onset (Box 61-1).

The proximal interphalangeal (PIP) and metacarpophalangeal (MCP) joints of the hands and joints are often affected early. As the disease progresses, the fingers develop a characteristic tapering (fusiform) appearance with a classic ulnar deviation of the hand (Figure 61-2). Virtually all joints can become involved, but most common are the joints of the hands, wrists, ankles, elbows, and knees. Shoulder and hip involvement occur later. Joint involvement most often occurs in a

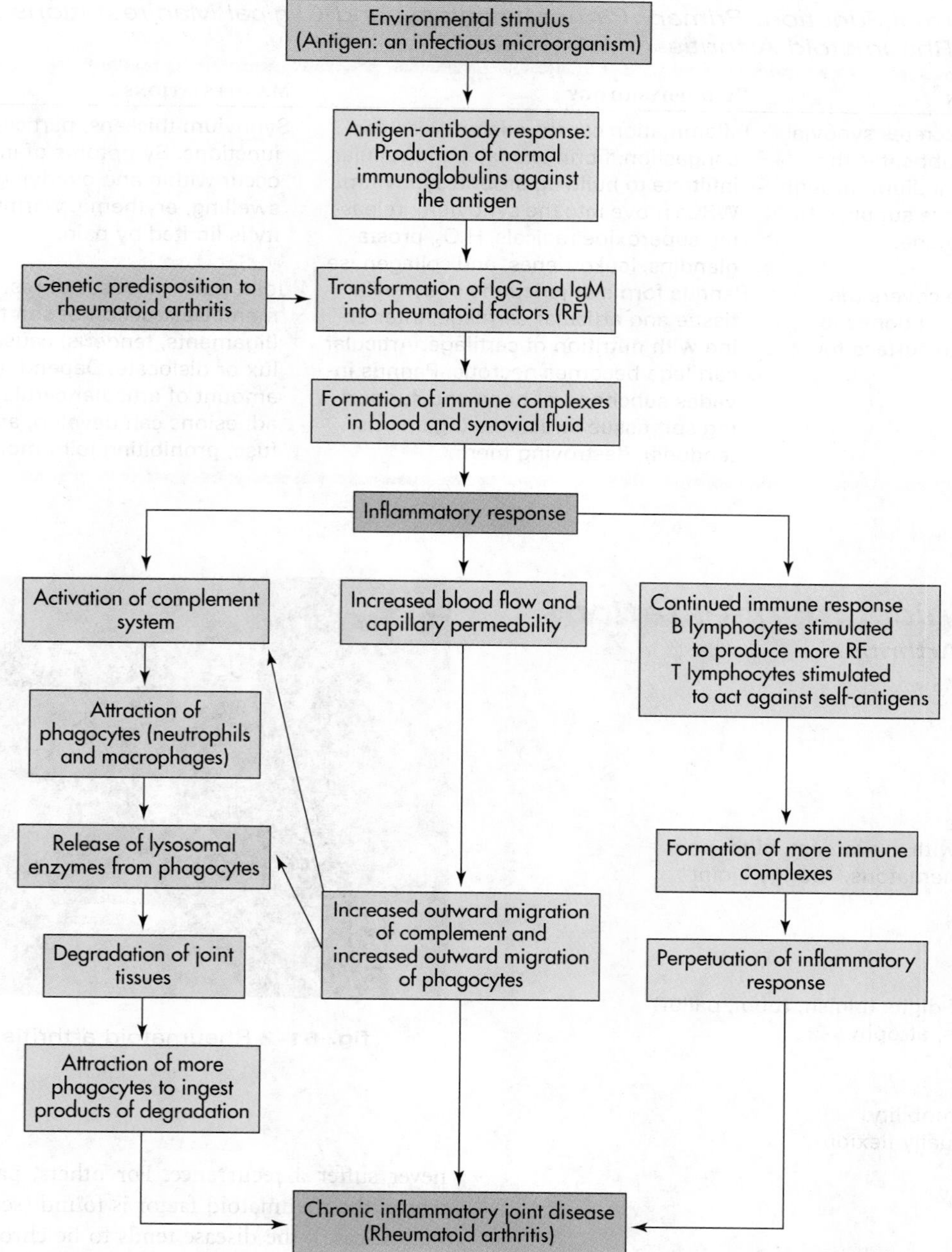


**fig. 61-1** Probable pathogenesis of rheumatoid arthritis.

bilaterally symmetric pattern with involvement of the same joints on both sides of the body.

Joint swelling is caused by inflammation of the synovial membrane, new bone formation, and tissue hyperplasia. The joint feels warm and boggy on palpation and may be erythematous.

Eventually all joints may be affected by RA. Involvement of the temporomandibular joint (TMJ) may limit the person's ability to open the mouth. Spinal involvement is usually limited to the cervical spine, particularly the first and second vertebrae. Subluxation or dislocation of the cervical vertebrae may result in death or paralysis. Both TMJ and cervical spine pathological conditions should be assessed before general anesthesia.

Inflammation of the tendon sheaths, particularly in the wrist, may occur. Muscle spasms contribute to the deformity of involved joints. Muscle atrophy may occur as a result of disuse, secondary to pain. *Rheumatoid nodules* are an aggregate of inflammatory cells around a center of cellular debris and may develop near joints, over body prominences, or along extensor surfaces in the subcutaneous tissues. Twenty percent of persons with RA develop rheumatoid nodules.[41]

**table 61-1** *Normal Function, Primary Pathophysiology, and Clinical Manifestations of Rheumatoid Arthritis*

| Normal Function | Pathophysiology | Manifestations |
|---|---|---|
| Synovial tissue secretes synovial fluid that both lubricates the joint and is the medium through which nutrients are supplied to the articular cartilage. | Inflammation causes edema, vascular congestion, fibrin exudate, and cellular infiltrate to build up around synovium. WBCs move into the synovium, releasing superoxide radicals, $H_2O_2$, prostaglandins, leukotrienes, and collagenase. | Synovium thickens, particularly at articular junctions. Symptoms of inflammation occur within and overlying the joint (pain, swelling, erythema, warmth). Joint mobility is limited by pain. |
| Articular cartilage covers the ends of articulating bones to provide a smooth surface for movement. | Pannus forms at junctions of synovial tissue and articular cartilage, interfering with nutrition of cartilage. Articular cartilage becomes necrotic. Pannus invades subchondral bone and supporting soft tissue structures (ligaments, tendons), destroying them. | Joint pain increases at rest and with movement. Destruction of soft tissue structures (ligaments, tendons) causes joint to sublux or dislocate. Depending on the amount of articular cartilage destroyed, adhesions can develop, and the joints can fuse, prohibiting joint motion. |

**box 61-1** *clinical manifestations*

***Rheumatoid Arthritis***

EARLY SYMPTOMS

Fatigue
Weight loss
Fever
Malaise
Morning stiffness
Pain at rest and with movement, night pain
Edematous, erythematous, "boggy" joint

LATE SYMPTOMS

Pallor
Anemia
Color changes of digits (bluish, rubor, pallor)
Muscle weakness, atrophy
Joint deformities
Paresthesias
Decreased joint mobility
Contractures (usually flexion)
Subluxation
Dislocation
Increasing pain

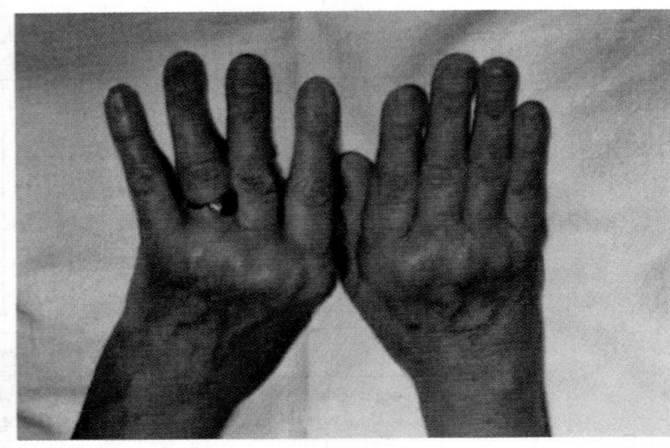

**fig. 61-2** Rheumatoid arthritis of hands.

Rheumatoid arthritis may also affect other body systems, and rheumatoid nodules may form in the heart, lungs, and spleen (Table 61-2). Glaucoma may result from rheumatoid nodule formation on the sclerae. Manifestations of the multisystem involvement of rheumatoid arthritis include pleuritis, pulmonary fibrosis, pericarditis, aortic valve disease, lymphadenopathy, and splenomegaly. Acute necrotizing vasculitis, also common in other autoimmune disorders, may result in a myocardial infarction, cerebrovascular accident, kidney damage, and Raynaud's phenomenon.

The course and severity of the of the RA is unpredictable, marked by periods of exacerbation and remission. Some individuals have been known to recover from a first attack and never suffer a recurrence. For others, particularly those in whom the rheumatoid factor is found (seropositive rheumatoid disease), the disease tends to be chronically progressive. In a small number of individuals the disease may be rapidly progressive, marked by unremitting joint destruction and diffuse vasculitis. This form of the disease is referred to as *malignant rheumatoid disease.* The length of time between exacerbations varies with individuals. Physiological and psychological stress can contribute to exacerbations of the disease.

Patients with an early onset of RA and elevated levels of erythrocyte sedimentation factor (ESR) and rheumatoid factor, and swelling of more than 20 joints tend to have a poorer prognosis.[55] Remission is unlikely after 3 years of sustained disease activity.

If untreated, rheumatoid arthritis tends to relapse and recur in a more severe form. Even with careful management, approximately 10% of patients with rheumatoid arthritis develop a severe crippling form of the disease.

**table 61-2** *Systemic Manifestations of Rheumatoid Arthritis*

| Body System | Clinical Manifestations |
|---|---|
| Cardiovascular | Pericarditis, valvular lesions, myocarditis, vasculitis, Raynaud's phenomenon |
| Pulmonary | Pleurisy; rheumatoid nodules on lungs, pneumoconiosis *(Caplan's syndrome)*; interstitial pneumonitis; pulmonary fibrosis; pulmonary hypertension |
| Neurological | Compression neuropathy, peripheral neuropathy, cervical myelopathy |
| Hematological | Anemia, leukopenia *(Felty's syndrome* when accompanied by hepatosplenomegaly) |
| Renal | Rheumatoid nodules on kidney |
| Dermatological | Rheumatoid nodules, brown lesions on skin due to ischemia, ulcers, draining fistulae |
| Ophthalmological | Scleritis, *sicca syndrome* (keratoconjunctivitis); *Sjögren's syndrome* (keratoconjunctivitis, xerostomia, vaginal dryness); glaucoma; scleromalacia |
| Other | Fever, malaise, weakness |

**box 61-2** *Diagnostic Criteria for Rheumatoid Arthritis*

1. Morning stiffness ≥1 hour and at least 6-week duration
2. Symmetric joint swelling
3. Soft tissue swelling of ≥3 joints for at least 6 weeks
4. Swelling of wrist, MCP, or PIP joints
5. Rheumatoid nodules
6. Positive serum rheumatoid factor test

## Collaborative Care Management

### Diagnostic tests

The American Rheumatism Association has devised a system for the diagnosis of rheumatoid arthritis (Box 61-2). The presence of four of the seven criteria is necessary for the diagnosis of RA.[24,55]

Diagnostic test results usually include the following:

1. An elevated erythrocyte sedimentation rate
2. Positive C-reactive protein test during acute phases
3. Positive antinuclear antibody test
4. Mild leukocytosis
5. Anemia (hypochromic, normocytic)
6. Positive rheumatoid factor or latex fixation test (present in 50% to 90% of patients, depending on disease duration and severity)
7. Narrowing of the joint spaces and erosion of articular surfaces on roentgenographic examination; subluxation, dislocation
8. Inflammatory changes in synovial tissue obtained by biopsy
9. Increased turbidity and decreased viscosity of synovial fluid obtained by arthrocentesis; immune complexes and white blood cells (WBCs) present

### Medications

The purpose of pharmacological therapy is to control inflammation and prevent bone erosion (Table 61-3). The use of nonsteroidal antiinflammatory drugs (NSAIDs) has traditionally been the first line of treatment. Research indicates that the use of disease-modifying antirheumatic drugs (DMARDs) or slow-acting antirheumatic drugs (SAARDS) may be more effective in suppressing symptoms of RA in some persons. The use of DMARDs has been shown to result in less functional disability, less pain, less joint tenderness and swelling, and lower ESR rates than in persons using NSAIDs,[65] although NSAIDs are still considered first-line therapy by some practitioners. Persons with minimal joint involvement and absence of radiological changes are well suited to initial treatment with NSAIDs. NSAIDs, including salicylates, modify the inflammatory process by inhibiting prostaglandin synthetase, but do nothing to prevent bony erosion and alone are usually ineffective in the management of RA. Many agents are available, and patients respond differently to different agents; a 2- to 3-week trial is necessary to judge the effectiveness of therapy.

The American College of Rheumatology recommends that before initiation of therapy with NSAIDs baseline values are obtained for the following: complete blood count (CBC); blood urea nitrogen (BUN), creatinine, liver enzymes, and potassium levels; and urinalysis.[22] Monitoring should be done again in 1 to 3 months, then at 3- to 12-month intervals thereafter. Gastrointestinal side effects can be controlled with the addition of an $H_2$ blocker or sucralfate. Misoprostol has been shown to be effective for reducing the incidence of gastric ulcers and hemorrhage and should be considered in high-risk persons (those with a history of ulcers, the elderly, smokers, and those who are receiving concomitant steroid therapy).[22]

Persons with polyarthritic involvement, persistent inflammation, elevated ESR or positive RF tests, and radiological evidence of bone erosion are usually treated with second-line agents or disease-modifying antirheumatic drugs. Patients frequently receive NSAIDs and DMARDs simultaneously. Therapy with DMARDs is usually begun if a 2- to 3-month trial of NSAIDs is ineffective. DMARDs "modify" the disease by preventing erosions. Formerly used later in the course of RA, these agents are now introduced early in the disease to preserve joint function and improve the overall outcome. The effectiveness of DMARDs may not be evident until after weeks to months of therapy. Disadvantages of DMARD therapy include the high cost, toxic effects, and long onset of action. DMARDs are continued at low doses even after disease control is achieved because of the risk of a rebound effect after drug discontinuation. Careful monitoring is required to prevent the development of toxic effects. Most adverse effects are

table 61-3 Common Medications for **Rheumatoid Arthritis**

| Drug | Action | Intervention |
|---|---|---|
| **NSAIDs, SALICYLATES** | | |
| Diclofenac (Voltaren, Cataflam)<br>Diflunisal (Dolobid)<br>Etodolac (Lodine)<br>Fenoprofen (Nalfon)<br>Ibuprofen (Motrin)<br>Indomethacin (Indocin)<br>Naproxen (Naprosyn)<br>Oxaprozin (Daypro)<br>Piroxicam (Feldene)<br>Sulindac (Clinoril)<br>Tolmetin (Tolectin) | Modify inflammatory process by inhibiting prostaglandin synthetase, analgesic, antipyretic | Monitor patient for dyspepsia, gastritis, hemorrhage, renal and hepatic function, platelet dysfunction, headache, confusion (tinnitis with salicylates). Administer with food (check individual drug, food may interfere with absorption); avoid concomitant use of salicylates and NSAIDs. |
| Diclofenac sodium and misoprostol (Athrotec) | Reduces risk of gastric ulcers | |
| **CORTICOSTEROIDS** | | |
| Prednisone (oral) | Antiinflammatory | Take with food or milk; do not abruptly discontinue medication; monitor patient for fluid and electrolyte balance, glucose levels, hypertension, skin lesions (purpura), decreased healing potential, cataract formation; encourage adequate calcium and vitamin D intake to retard osteoporosis; teach patient to avoid sources of infection. |
| Hydrocortisone (intraarticular) | | Systemic effects are rare with intraarticular use; avoid more than three injections per joint per year. |
| **DMARDs** | | |
| Methotrexate (Rheumatrex), oral or intramuscular | Rapid onset of action inhibits degradation of folic acid, which inhibits DNA synthesis of inflammatory cells | Evaluate renal function before therapy; monitor patient for hepatic and pulmonary toxicity, leukopenia, thrombocytopenia, anemia; explain to patient that nausea, diarrhea, and stomatitis are common; advise patient to use birth control while taking medication; check for drug interactions that may increase toxicity risk. |
| Hydroxychloroquine (Plaquenil) | Mechanism of action unclear; acts on DNA synthesis, antiinflammatory | Inform patient of need for eye examination before therapy and every 6 months thereafter (retinal edema may result in blindness); monitor patient for hematological toxicity, gastrointestinal irritation, and hypertension; evaluate renal function. |
| Sulfasalazine (Azulfidine) | Unknown, antiinflammatory | Monitor patient for neurological and gastrointestinal toxicity, leukopenia, anemia, and Stevens-Johnson syndrome; educate patient about need for CBC and liver function tests throughout therapy. |
| Gold salts (Myochrysine, Ridaura, Solganal), oral and intramuscular | Antiinflammatory mechanism unclear, effect not noted until several months of therapy | Monitor patient for renal and hepatic damage, dermatitis, and mouth ulcerations; inform patient of need for CBC and urinalysis before and at intervals throughout therapy; stress the need for oral hygiene; therapy may cause metallic taste in mouth. Oral gold has fewer side effects. |
| Azathioprine (Imuran) | Unknown, immune suppressant | Monitor patient for blood dyscrasias, hepatitis, and pancreatitis. CBC necessary as baseline and throughout treatment. |
| D-Pencillamine (Depen, Cuprimine) | Unknown | Monitor patient for fever, rash, gastrointestinal upset, blood dyscrasias, and delayed wound healing; assess for penicillin allergy; inform patient of potential for dysgeusia (taste alteration). Food interferes with absorption. Rare side effects include polymyositis and Goodpasture's syndrome. Urinalysis and CBC required before and at intervals during therapy. |
| **ANTINEOPLASTICS** | | |
| Cyclophosphamide (Cytoxan) | Suppresses synovitis; retards bony erosions | Monitor patient for toxic effects including: GI distress, bone marrow supression, alopecia, and hemorrhagic cystitis; inform patient of possible long-term effects including bladder fibrosis and cancer, infections, sterility, and hematological malignancies; inform patient of need for monitoring CBC and urinalysis during therapy; teach patient to increase fluid intake to ensure frequent bladder emptying. |

reversible after the drug is discontinued. Many physicians prescribe two or more DMARDs in combination.

Steroid therapy, oral and intraarticular, is also used in the management of RA. The many side effects associated with steroid use rarely occur with intraarticular injections. More than three injections in the same joint per year is not recommended. The use of low-dose (5 to 7.5 mg) prednisone can significantly reduce the incidence of side effects. This regimen is often effective in controlling inflammation, particularly in elderly persons at risk for NSAID toxicity. Supplemental calcium (1200 to 1500 mg/day) and vitamin D can be prescribed to reduce steroid-induced osteoporosis.

Other pharmacological therapies used to treat RA include cytokines, cytokine agonists, cyclosporine, antibiotics (minocycline), and monoclonal antibodies. These therapies are experimental and are reserved for use in persons who do not respond to conventional therapy.

#### Treatments

The goals of therapy for persons with rheumatoid arthritis are to relieve symptoms, prevent joint destruction, maintain joint function, and promote independence and qualify of life. In addition to pharmacological therapy, occupational and physical therapy are mainstays of treatment to preserve joint mobility and promote independence. An exercise program, designed with the physical therapist, is important for maintaining mobility and preventing muscle atrophy. There is ample evidence to support the fact that exercise can improve the individual's sense of well-being, which is beneficial to an individual trying to cope with a chronic, disabling disease.

Splints and orthoses (braces) are prescribed by the physician and fitted by a physical therapist, occupational therapist, or orthotist. The purposes of splints and braces are as follows:

1. Stabilize or support a joint
2. Protect a joint or body part from external trauma
3. Mechanically correct a dysfunction such as footdrop by supporting the joint in its functional position
4. Assist patients to exercise specific joints

Splints and braces (Table 61-4) are designed to be as lightweight and cosmetically acceptable as possible. Many splints are made of plastic that can be molded to fit the patient (see Figure 61-6). In many instances plastic has replaced metal and leather braces that are often obvious, even though worn under loose-fitting clothing. Shoes may be modified or corrective shoes may be prescribed to provide special support for the feet. Braces can be fitted to the patient's own shoes (Figure 61-3).

Many assistive devices are available for individuals who have impaired upper and/or lower extremity function (Box 61-3). These devices are obtained by referring the patient to an occupational therapist.

Supportive devices or ambulatory aids (walkers, canes, and crutches) are usually recommended for persons who cannot bear weight on one or more joints of the lower extremities. Other indications for use include instability, loss of balance, or pain on weight bearing. The physical therapist evaluates the patient to determine the specific device that will match the patient's needs and abilities. Some considerations regarding choice of device include:

1. Axillary crutches
   a. Require dexterity and a good sense of balance
   b. Permit faster ambulation than walkers
   c. Can be used on stairs
2. Walkers
   a. Provide solid support
   b. Can be used by individuals with loss of balance
   c. Limit speed of ambulation
   d. Are hazardous on stairs or uneven ground
3. Canes
   a. Are less cumbersome than crutches or walkers
   b. Do not permit as effective unloading of weight as a double support

**table 61-4** *Types and Functions of Splints and Braces*

| Type | Function |
|---|---|
| Spring-loaded braces | Oppose the action of unparalyzed muscles and act as partial functional substitutes for paralyzed muscles (Figure 61-3) |
| Resting splints | Maintain a limb or joint in a functional position while permitting the muscles around the joint to relax (Figure 61-4) |
| Functional splints | Maintain the joint or limb in a usable position to enable the body part to be used correctly |
| Dynamic splints | Permit assisted exercise to joints, particularly following surgery to finger joints (Figure 61-5) |

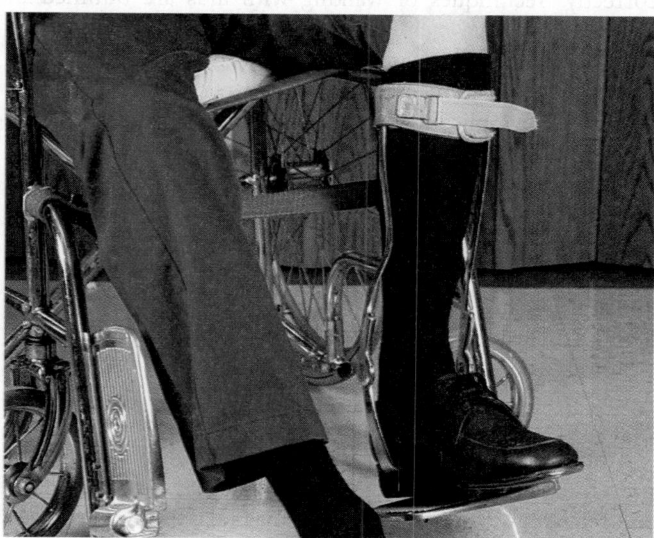

**fig. 61-3** Leg brace.

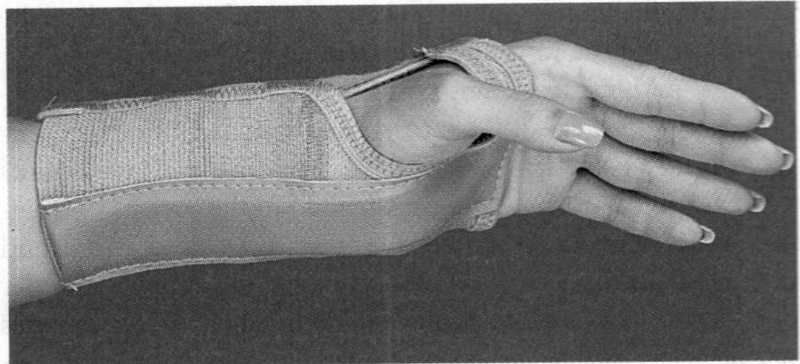

fig. 61-4 Wrist splint.

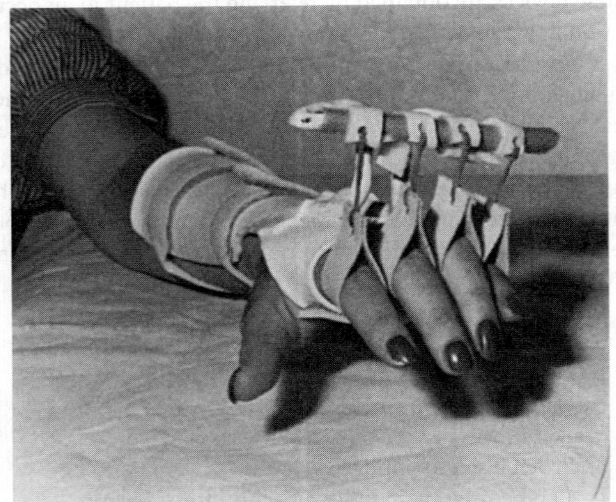

fig. 61-5 Dynamic hand splint.

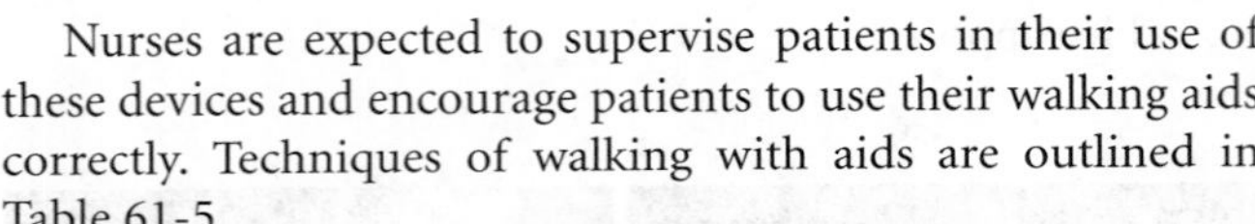

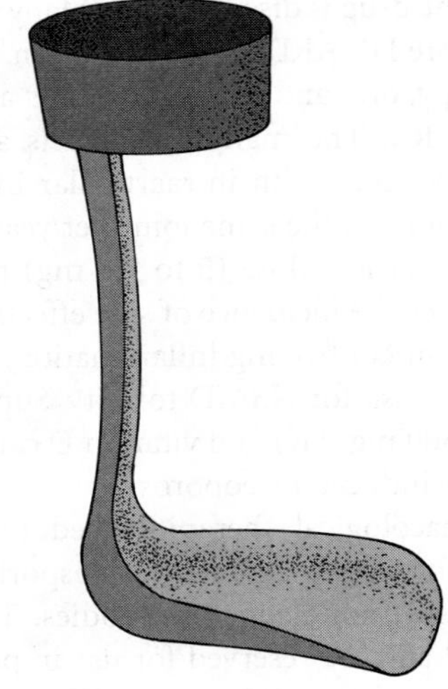

fig. 61-6 Ankle-foot orthosis.

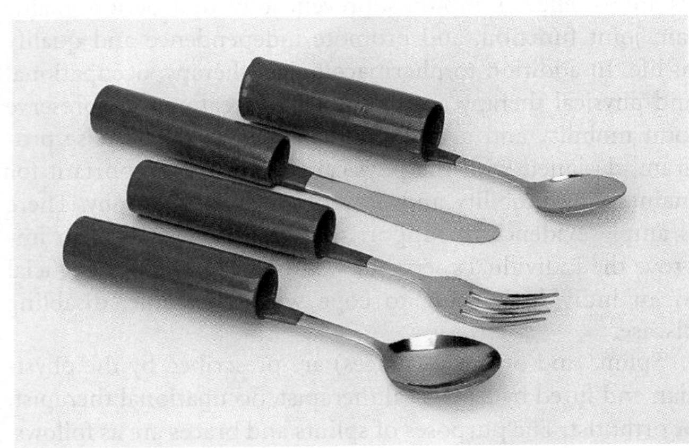

fig. 61-7 Utensils with special handles.

Nurses are expected to supervise patients in their use of these devices and encourage patients to use their walking aids correctly. Techniques of walking with aids are outlined in Table 61-5.

Other treatment modalities for the person with RA include the application of hot and cold packs to the affected joint(s). The application of heat/cold can be achieved by the following:

1. Hydrocollator packs (packs containing chemical filler that expands in water and retains heat; may be heated in pot of water or special machines that maintain a constant temperature of 80° C [174° F])
2. Paraffin baths
3. Electric heating pads that are approved for use with moist towels
4. Electric heating pads that produce moisture
5. Warm soaks, tub soaks, or showers

Application of cold or ice packs is helpful in reducing or preventing swelling (especially after trauma), reducing pain, and relieving stiffness. Cold packs may take the form of plastic bags containing ice, commercially available gel packs that

**box 61-3** *Assistive Devices for Persons with Motor Impairments*

| ASSISTIVE DEVICE | PATIENT LIMITATION |
|---|---|
| Utensil with built-up handle (Figure 61-7) | Cannot adequately close hand |
| Utensil with cuffed handle | Loss of opposition of thumb |
| Combination knife-fork | Loss of only one hand |
| Mug with special handle (Figure 61-8) | Unable to grasp regular cup handle |
| Long-handled shoehorn (Figure 61-9) | Unable to bend to reach feet, hip flexion limitation |
| Long-handled reacher (to reach for or pick up objects) (Figure 61-10) | Unable to stoop or reach, hip flexion limitation |
| Stocking guide (Figure 61-11) | Inability to reach feet, hip flexion limitation |

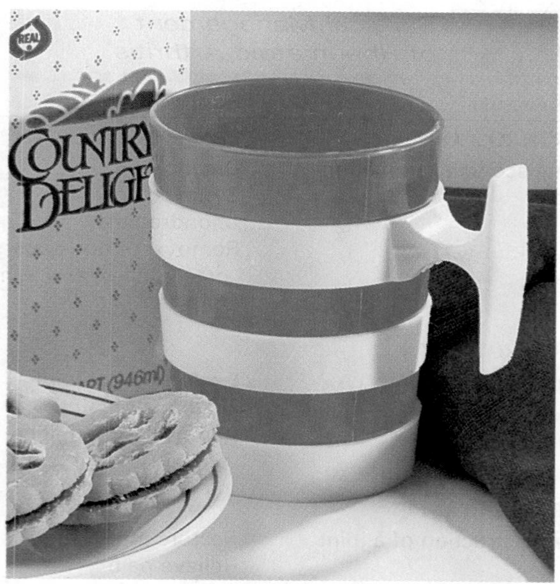
fig. 61-8 Cup with special handle.

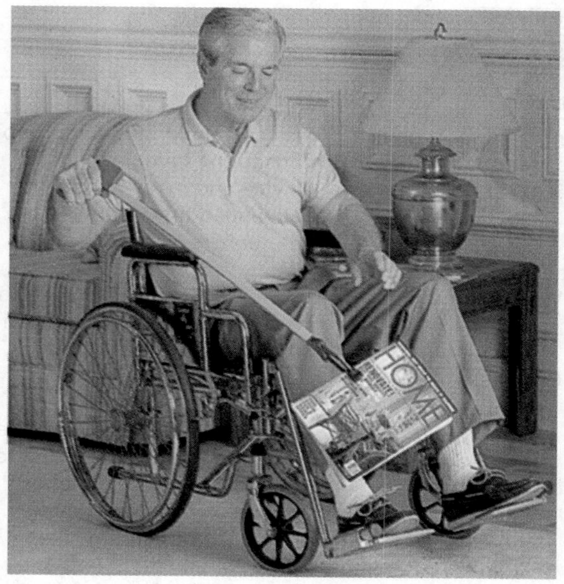
fig. 61-10 Long-handled reachers.

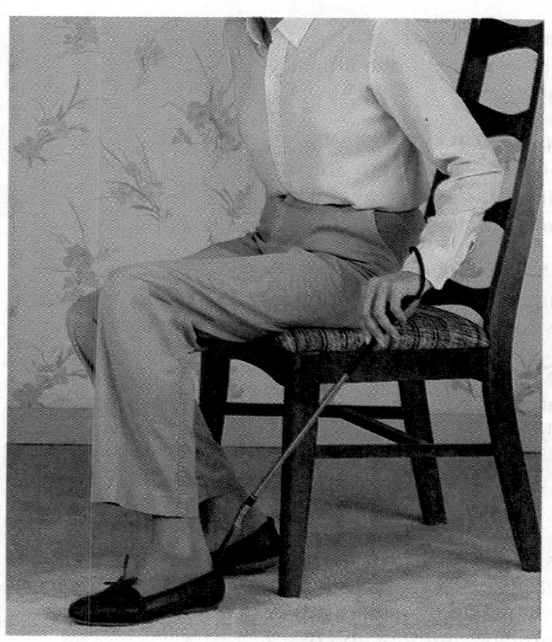
fig. 61-9 Long-handled shoehorn.

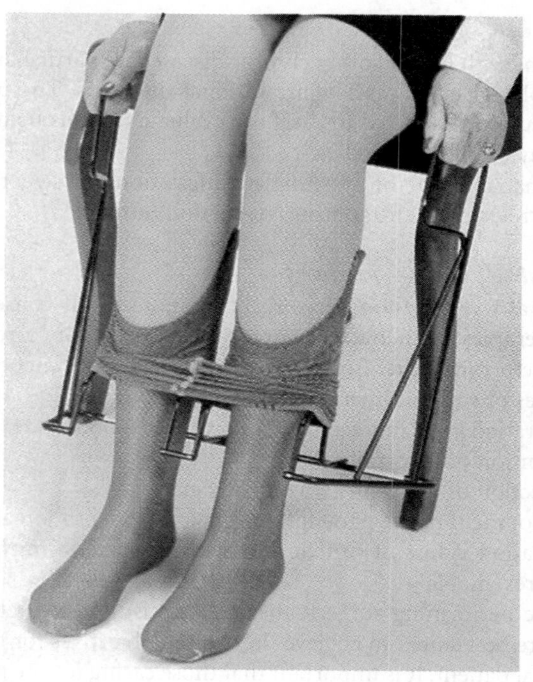
fig. 61-11 Stocking helper.

can be refrozen and reused, or large bags of frozen vegetables (especially for home use).

Heat or cold should be left on for 15 to 20 minutes to achieve maximum effect. Cold packs and moist heat packs should be wrapped in protective towels to prevent burns to the skin, and the skin should be checked 5 minutes after application for any evidence of tissue damage. Heat or cold should be applied with caution to any individual with decreased sensation, because of the risk of injury.

**table 61-5** *Techniques of Walking with Ambulatory Aids**

| Device | Gait |
|---|---|
| Single-support device (cane, quad cane, single crutch) | Device is held in the hand opposite the involved leg<br>Device and involved leg are advanced first, followed by the uninvolved leg |
| Double-support device | |
| Walker | Walker is advanced first, then the involved extremity, then the uninvolved extremity |
| Crutches | 3-point gait—the same as walker gait<br>4-point gait—crutch, opposite leg, opposite crutch, other leg<br>2-point gait—both crutches, both legs (one leg may be non–weight bearing) |

*SPECIAL NOTE: Climbing up stairs is accomplished by moving the uninvolved leg first, then the device and the involved leg; to descend stairs, the involved leg and the device are moved first, then the uninvolved leg. The device and the involved leg always move together.

**table 61-6** *Surgical Management of Rheumatoid Arthritis*

| Procedure | Indication |
|---|---|
| **ARTHROSCOPY** | |
| Endoscopic examination of joint | Diagnosis<br>Synovectomy<br>Chondroplasty<br>Removal of bone spurs, osteophytes, and joint mice |
| **ARTHROTOMY** | |
| Opening of a joint | Exploration of joint<br>Drainage of joint<br>Removal of damaged tissue |
| **ARTHROPLASTY** | |
| Reconstruction of a joint | Restore motion<br>Relieve pain<br>Correct deformity<br>Avascular necrosis |
| **Interposition** | |
| Replacement of part of a joint with a prosthesis or with soft tissue | |
| **Hemiarthroplasty** | |
| Replacement of one articulating surface | |
| **Replacement (Total Joint)** | |
| Replacement of both articulating surfaces of a joint with prosthetic implants | |
| **SYNOVECTOMY** | |
| Removal of part or all of the synovial membrane | Delay the progress of rheumatoid arthritis |
| **OSTEOTOMY** | |
| Cutting a bone to change its alignment | Correct deformity (varus or valgus)<br>Alter the weight-bearing surface of diseased joint to relieve pain |
| **ARTHRODESIS** | |
| Surgical fusion of a joint by removal of articular hyaline cartilage, introduction of bone grafts, and stabilization with internal or external fixation devices | Stabilize a joint<br>Relieve pain |
| **TENDON TRANSPLANTS** | |
| Moving a tendon from its anatomical position | Substitute one tendon for another that is not working<br>Realign tendon function, for example, for stability |

Persons with RA and other chronic diseases are particularly susceptible to "cures" and nontraditional therapies. The patient should be educated to carefully evaluate options before trying any of these "remedies."

For management of systemic manifestations of RA, the reader is referred to the appropriate section of the text.

### *Surgical management*

Referral to an orthopedic surgeon is indicated if conservative therapies are ineffective. Surgery is indicated for correction of deformity, relief from pain, or restoration of function. Objectives of surgical intervention are as follows:

1. Restoration or maintenance of function of a body part
2. Prevention of deformity
3. Correction of deformity if it already exists
4. Development of the patient's powers of compensation and adaptation if loss of function or permanent deformity is not preventable

Before performing surgery, the orthopedist considers the procedure best suited to achieve the desired objectives for the individual patient. It is important that those caring for the patient know and understand what the expected outcomes are so that care may be adapted to achieving them.

A description of commonly performed surgical procedures is found in Table 61-6. Synovectomy is performed early in the disease to decrease pain and retard the degenerative changes in the joint. Osteotomy and joint arthroplasty are performed in advanced disease.

### *Diet*

There is evidence to suggest that ingestion of fish oil (a type of n-3 polyunsaturated fat) as a dietary fat is beneficial to persons with RA. Improvements in terms of the number of swollen joints, duration of morning stiffness, grip strength, NSAID use, and overall evaluation has been seen in several studies.[10] In all cases, fish oil was a supplement to pharmacological therapy. How fish oil produces a therapeutic effect is unknown, but it does suppress inflammatory mediator (prostaglandins, leukotrienes, and cytokines) production. More research is needed to determine the optimal effectiveness of fish oil in the diet.

Persons with RA frequently have anemia. A diet containing iron-rich foods (liver, oysters, clams, organ meat, lean meat, whole grains, legumes, and leafy green vegetables) is recommended to decrease anemia. Calcium and vitamin D supplement can reduce bone resorption.

Fatigue and malaise are common in persons with RA. A diet containing adequate calories and balanced nutrition is necessary to prevent fatigue and increase energy. If the patient is overweight, a weight reduction diet, combined with exercise, is recommended to decrease the strain on weight-bearing joints.

### Activity

Rest is a therapy often used for persons with RA. However, too much rest can at times be as detrimental as too much activity. There are two forms of rest:

1. Absolute rest or no activity
    a. May be required for the whole body or for a specific part of the body
    b. Is accomplished through avoidance of use of the part
    c. Is possibly enhanced by some method of external immobilization (splint, cast, or traction) to ensure inactivity
2. Partial rest or limited activity; some activity permitted, but other activities (e.g., weight bearing, certain movements) are limited

Activity must be balanced with adequate rest. Individuals who have pain and stiffness with or after certain activities must learn to recognize their tolerances and adapt their activities of daily living (ADL) accordingly. This does not mean stopping all activity; it means *modifying* activity.

Exercise is prescribed to accomplish the following:

1. Preserve joint mobility (active and passive range of motion)
2. Maintain muscle tone (active range of motion and isometrics)
3. Strengthen selected muscle groups (resistive exercises performed against resistance provided by another person or by weights)

Exercise may be facilitated by the application of heat or cold or the administration of an analgesic before the exercise period. Exercise is contraindicated in the presence of acute joint or muscle inflammation until the inflammatory process subsides.

Exercise programs should be tailored to the patient's specific needs and capabilities. Nurses need to be aware of the specific exercise program the patient is following and be prepared to provide support and assistance in performing the exercises as needed and reinforcing the purpose, technique, frequency, and duration of the exercises.

### Referrals

Common referrals for persons with rheumatoid arthritis include physical therapy and occupational therapy. A social service consultation may be initiated to assist the patient with discharge needs. The patient and family may benefit from a referral to the Arthritis Foundation. The Arthritis Foundation sponsors support groups, self-help classes, and exercise programs (see the Research Box). The address is: The Arthritis Foundation, 1314 Spring Street NW, Atlanta, GA 30309; (800) 283-7800; (404) 872-7100; Internet address: www.arthritis.org.

## NURSING MANAGEMENT

### ■ ASSESSMENT

#### Subjective Data

Early in the disease, the patient may report chronic fatigue, generalized aching and stiffness in the extremities, and weight loss. As the disease progresses, the patient will report specific joints that are painful, loss of strength, decreased

**research**

Reference: Boutaugh ML, Brady TJ: Quality of life programs of the arthritis foundation, *Orthop Nurs* 15 (5):59-69, 1996.

The Arthritis Foundation is a national nonprofit, voluntary health organization founded to support research for arthritis and improve the quality of life for people with arthritis. The Quality of Life Action Plan outlines the organization's initiatives based on the physical, psychosocial, and economic issues of persons with arthritis. Results of the plan's research on these issues include:

- More than 90% of persons with arthritis report pain; arthritis is the most common cause of physical activity limitations of persons older than 45 years of age, leisure activities are particularly affected; 88% of persons with active arthritis report fatigue; low self-esteem and sexual dissatisfaction can also be present because of the disease.
- The Arthritis Self-Help Course teaches participants about the disease, relaxation techniques, exercises, and coping strategies.
- Similar classes for systemic lupus erythematosus (SLE) and fibromyalgia, and People With Arthritis Can Exercise (PACE) and water exercise classes positively influence participants' levels of depression, pain, helplessness, functioning, quality of life, and ability to manage the disease.
- Patients with chronic pain who perceive family support show a decrease in pain and medication use and an increase in activity.

Nurses can aid patients by educating themselves. Volunteering at the local chapter of the Arthritis Foundation and using video tapes and professional literature will make it easier to refer patients and explain the foundation's services.

mobility, early morning stiffness, and fatigue. Generally, pain will interfere with normal ADL. The patient will also note that affected joints are changing in appearance. Many patients will express fear or despair over loss of function and independence.

### Objective Data

Specific objective data to be gathered by the nurse include:

Inspection and palpation of the same joints on both sides of the body for symmetry, skin color, size, shape, tenderness, heat, and swelling

Limitation of active joint range of motion

Evidence of pain with active range of motion

Evidence of atrophy or loss of tone or tenderness in muscles associated with involved joints

## NURSING DIAGNOSES

Nursing diagnoses are determined from analysis of patient data. Possible nursing diagnoses for the person with rheumatoid arthritis may include but are not limited to:

| Diagnostic Title | Possible Etiological Factors |
|---|---|
| Pain | Inflammation and swelling in joints |
| Self-care deficit (related to bathing/hygiene, dressing/grooming, feeding, toileting) | Pain and musculoskeletal impairment |
| Fatigue | Chronic systemic disease |
| Self-esteem disturbance | Change in body appearance |
| Injury, risk for | Loss of muscle strength and joint motion |
| Sleep disturbance | Chronic systemic disease, pain |
| Knowledge deficit (related to arthritis) | Lack of exposure to information |

## EXPECTED PATIENT OUTCOMES

Expected patient outcomes for the person with rheumatoid arthritis may include but are not limited to:

1. States pain is decreased and verbalizes ways to control pain.
2. Demonstrates improved ability to perform self-care activities and participates in usual activities to fullest extent possible.
3. States factors that lead to fatigue and how fatigue might be avoided.
4. Verbalizes a more positive self-concept.
5. Maintains active joint range of motion within limits of disease to strengthen muscles and prevent injuries.
6. Reports adequate sleep and rest.
7. Explains the disease process, the applicability of treatment measures, and plans for follow-up care.

## INTERVENTIONS

### Promoting Comfort

1. Evaluate the type, amount, and duration of pain.
2. Assess intensity of pain using pain rating scale.
3. Administer medications as ordered.
4. Teach relaxation techniques and alternate methods of pain control.
5. Evaluate effectiveness of pain relief measures.
6. Observe patient for nonverbal signs of pain.
7. Provide heat or cold treatments as appropriate. Nursing responsibilities with heat or cold therapy include:
   a. Helping patient determine which type of application works best
   b. Instructing patient about safety precautions to be observed with that method
   c. Instructing patient about timely application of heat or cold (e.g., before activity or exercise or before going to bed at night) depending on patient's particular needs
   d. Assisting the patient with application
8. Promote frequent changes of position (patients are often more comfortable changing position themselves rather than having someone handle their sore joints).
9. Provide for adequate periods of rest.
10. Encourage use of resting splints.

### Promoting Independence

Most people want to be able to live their lives independently. In the context of this discussion, independence would mean freedom from having to make demands on others for personal and social ADL. However, persons with musculoskeletal problems may be unable to manage one or more activities for themselves. If help from another person is needed to perform a certain function, such as buttoning buttons, the individual is dependent in that area. If an assistive device (e.g., button hook or Velcro closures) can be made available and the use of it can be mastered, the individual can again be independent in that function.

Very few people live truly independent lives; we are interdependent. Families are also structured around interdependent functions. Persons with motor disability may at some time be faced with losing their interdependent role; that is, they may no longer believe they are useful or needed by anyone else.

Nursing interventions to promote maximal independence include:

1. Assess patient's level of functioning and ability to perform self-care activities.
2. Assist with ADL as needed.
3. Provide frequent rest periods to maximize patient participation.
4. Encourage use of supportive and/or assistive devices.

### Reducing Fatigue

1. Encourage patient to discuss factors that cause fatigue.
2. Assess times of greatest fatigue, and structure activities accordingly.
3. Provide for frequent rest periods.
4. Promote comfort by use of medications and other comfort measures.
5. Instruct patient regarding energy conservation techniques (Table 61-7).

**research**

Reference: Neuberger GB, Press AN, Lindsley HB, et al: Effects of exercise on fatigue, aerobic fitness, and disease activity measures in persons with rheumatoid arthritis, *Res Nurs Health* 20:195-204, 1997.

This study evaluated the effects of low-impact aerobic exercise on fatigue, aerobic fitness, and disease activity in 25 adults with RA. The mean age of the sample was 55 years; the range was 30 to 71 years. The mean duration of RA was 9.8 years, with a range of 7 to 30 years. The exercise intervention consisted of participation in a low-impact aerobics class (including warm-up and cool-down) for 1 hour three times weekly for 12 weeks. Participants were separated into different levels of exercise participation: high (31 of 36 classes, $n = 8$); medium (25 to 30 of 36 classes, $n = 9$); and low (24 or fewer of 36 classes, $n = 9$). Fatigue, the Arthritis Impact Measurement Scales (pain measurement, medications, duration of arthritis, and arthritis impact), bicycle ergometer testing, the number of swollen, painful joints (high when RA is active), grip strength, walk time (number of seconds to walk 50 feet), and ESR were measured to determine the effects of exercise on these variables. Subjects were evaluated before beginning the exercise, after 6 weeks of treatment, at termination of treatment, and at 15 weeks post-treatment.

Results indicated that those who exercised more frequently reported less fatigue, while those with less exercise participation reported increased levels of fatigue. All subjects showed increased aerobic fitness, increased grip strength, decreased pain, and decreased walk time. No significant increases in the number of swollen joints or increased ESR levels were found in the subjects. Improvements continued at the 15-week follow-up.

Fatigue is a common finding in persons with RA. Fatigue can be relieved by rest, caused by rest, and lessened by exercise. These data indicate that exercise is an appropriate intervention for lessening fatigue and producing other positive effects, while not contributing to increased symptoms of RA.

6. Assist patient in modifying daily routines to accommodate decreased abilities.
7. Recommend a regular aerobic exercise program to reduce fatigue (see the Research Box).

### Promoting a Positive Self-Concept

A major problem faced by many individuals who have musculoskeletal problems is that the disorder may be disfiguring as well as disabling. Not only must they adapt to functional disability, but they also may have to adapt to "looking different" from other people. Loss or alteration of function or the need to use an assistive device or prosthesis can also cause patients to view themselves as different from others. Depending on the nature and strength of pressures from family, social, or work situations or the individual's degree of self-esteem, the individual may attempt to cover up the disability so as not to lose support, esteem, or a livelihood. If the disability cannot be covered up, some persons may withdraw or limit their contact with others.

**table 61-7** *Joint Protection and Energy Conservation Techniques*

| Technique | Examples |
|---|---|
| Avoid positions of possible joint deformity | Avoid keeping joints in positions of flexion for prolonged periods of time.<br>Avoid twisting motions such as turning a jar lid with small joints. |
| Avoid holding muscles or joints in one position for a long time | When working at a desk, stand up and walk about for a few minutes every half hour. |
| Use the strongest joints for all activities | Use the knees, not the back, when lifting heavy objects.<br>Push a door open with the shoulder, not the wrist.<br>Use a shoulder strap, not a hand-held strap, to carry a heavy purse. |
| Use joints in their best position, maintaining good standing and sitting posture | Avoid reaching or bending when another approach would work as well.<br>Work at a comfortable height. |
| Conserve energy | Avoid trying to accomplish difficult tasks in a single time period.<br>Take breaks during work periods.<br>Slide rather than lift objects.<br>Use a wheeled cart to move objects from one place to another. |

Nursing interventions include:

1. Establish a trusting relationship with the patient.
2. Encourage verbalization of feelings regarding appearance and disease process.
3. Encourage verbalization of positive attributes of self.
4. Support positive coping mechanisms and decision-making abilities.
5. Institute referral to community resources if needed.

### Promoting Mobility and Preventing Injury

Safety devices are items that can be used by the patient to enhance function and prevent accidents when normal function, balance, or dexterity is compromised. Examples of safety devices include safety arms around toilets, grab bars mounted at tubs or showers, elevated toilet seats, adhesive strips on tub or shower floors, hand rails along staircases, and nonskid wax applied to floors. Nurses need to be familiar with the various devices available, help patients learn to use them, and if necessary, advise patients where they may be obtained.

Nursing interventions include:

1. Assess all joints for signs of inflammation and deformity.
2. Assess and record range of motion of all joints.

3. Encourage active range of motion exercises.
4. Provide passive range of motion if needed.
5. Encourage use of splints to rest joint and provide proper alignment.
6. Avoid positions that may produce contractures, for example, pillows under knees when supine or pillows forcing neck into forward flexion.
7. Encourage patient to perform prescribed exercises on a regular basis.
8. Provide appropriate ambulatory devices and supervise patient in their use.
9. Encourage patient to wear shoes, not slippers, for ambulation.

### Patient/Family Education

As for any chronic illness, patient teaching is perhaps the most important aspect of nursing care of patients with rheumatoid arthritis. It is, after all, the patient who will have to recognize response to prescribed therapy, follow the prescribed therapy correctly, and report the effectiveness of therapy to the physician.

It is estimated that hundreds of millions of dollars are spent each year on gadgets, programs, and "medicines" allegedly able to "cure" arthritis. This money is spent by persons with arthritis who often cannot afford the expense. In some instances the disease and associated disability may increase despite all efforts to control the disease process; this is extremely discouraging for the patient, family, and members of the health team. But many more persons are able to live reasonably normal, productive lives while managing their arthritis. Their ability to do so partially depends on their knowledge of the disease and its treatment.

Nurses teaching persons about rheumatoid arthritis (and other rheumatic diseases) may find it helpful to use some of the patient teaching material prepared by the Arthritis Foundation.

Patient teaching should include information about the following:

1. Proper balance of rest and activity; assisting the patient in determining his/her activity tolerance
2. Joint protection and energy conservation techniques
3. Proper use of medications (i.e., names of drugs, dosages, precautions in administration, and side effects or toxic effects)
4. Plans for implementation of the exercise program prescribed by the physician or physical therapist
5. Proper application of heat and/or cold packs
6. Proper use of walking aids and other assistive devices
7. Safety measures to prevent injury
8. Application, appropriate use, and care of splints and braces
   a. Inspect patient's skin after the orthosis has been applied for a short time to be certain it has caused no skin irritation.
   b. Notify the orthotist if adjustments need to be made in the orthosis to make it more comfortable or to relieve chafing.
   c. Instruct patient in the proper application and care of the orthosis.
      (1) Metal braces should be stored upright.
      (2) Leather materials should be treated occasionally with neatsfoot compound or other leather preservative to prevent cracking and drying.
      (3) Orthoses fabricated of molded materials should be stored away from sources of heat.
      (4) If patients fitted with molded orthoses or braces gain or lose weight, the brace may have to be adjusted or replaced.
   d. Assist patient to make the psychological adjustment to wearing the orthosis.
9. Basics of good nutrition and the importance of avoiding weight gain
10. Importance of regular follow-up with the physician
11. Risks of following programs that promise a "cure"
12. Information about local arthritis support groups and programs and services of the Arthritis Foundation

## EVALUATION

To evaluate the effectiveness of nursing interventions, compare the patient's behaviors with those stated in the expected patient outcomes. Successful achievement of patient outcomes for the patient with rheumatoid arthritis is indicated by:

1. Verbalizes pain level is reduced or tolerable; demonstrates effective pain relief measures.
2. Performs own ADL to the fullest extent possible.

3a. Describes plan for balancing rest and exercise and use of cold or heat after exercising.
b. Lists factors that cause fatigue.
c. Describes plans for preventing fatigue, plans for adequate rest periods, and techniques for energy conservation to increase activity level as tolerated.

4. Demonstrates behaviors to promote positive self-esteem; identifies feelings and underlying issues for negative self-perception.
5. Demonstrates active range of motion exercises and strengthening exercises such as straight leg lifts and quadriceps sets; achieves maximum mobility of extremities; is injury free.
6. Demonstrates adequate sleep and rest; sleep is not disturbed by pain.
7. Verbalizes understanding of disease process of RA and rationales for treatment.

### GERONTOLOGICAL CONSIDERATIONS

Early manifestations of rheumatoid arthritis such as fatigue and myalgia are vague and can also be attributed to a number of other conditions. The elderly patient with rheumatic disease probably has at least one other comorbid condition. Fatigue and myalgia can be symptoms of hypothyroidism, a common condition in the elderly population. The onset of RA in the elderly is slightly higher than that at midlife.[37] Care must be taken to be sure that the arthritic symptoms are not a result of a comorbid condition. The elderly patient may not exhibit the typical symptoms associated with RA. In contrast to the usual presentation, the larger joints are usually affected in the elderly, and the onset is usually acute.[37]

An important factor when considering treatment of RA in elderly persons is the choice of drug therapy. It is well known that altered drug metabolism is a physiological event of aging, and the dosage of many drugs needs to be decreased in the elderly. Even with reduced dosages, drug toxicity occurs more frequently and is more serious in the elderly patient.[46] Caution when prescribing dosages is of particular concern with NSAIDs. Research indicates that up to 50% of elderly persons are taking these medications, often at inappropriate dosages.[46] Side effects include gastrointestinal complications and renal toxicity. Renal function may already be impaired in the elderly and drug dosage should depend on age and renal function. The elderly patient with rheumatic arthritis should have baseline values for CBC, chemistry panel, ESR, and thyroid-stimulating hormone level obtained before any pharmacological therapy is initiated. Even medications such as methotrexate and steroids, associated with serious adverse effects, may be safer and more effective than the use of NSAIDs in treating RA in the elderly. Methotrexate, started in doses of 5 to 7.5 mg once weekly, then increased to 15 to 20 mg weekly, is well tolerated in elderly patients. Low-doses of prednisone (5 to 7.5 mg/day) take up to 10 years to produce osteoporosis and may be an alternative therapy for elderly patients, particularly those at risk for developing side effects from NSAIDs. NSAIDs such as aspirin and ibuprofen (dosages up to 400 mg three times daily) have been found to be the best tolerated in persons older than age 65.[46]

Another factor relevant to treatment of RA in elderly persons is the need for modification of the home environment to meet the needs of the individual. Mobility impairments induced by RA, coupled with changes associated with aging (hearing loss, decreased vision, loss of balance, and loss of muscle mass) are potential obstacles to preserving independence and function. Raised toilet seats, support bars in the bathroom, hand railings, avoidance of scatter rugs, and other modifications to prevent injury may allow the person to remain at home and avoid relocation to an extended-care or assisted-living facility. Prevention of falls is an important intervention for the elderly person with RA to avoid fractures and the possible associated complications. Coping with a chronic and potentially disabling condition, in addition to pain and alterations in body image and role performance, may result in depression in the elderly person. Nurses are in an ideal position to provide support and counseling to patients. If depression is suspected, a referral for evaluation is indicated.

## SPECIAL ENVIRONMENTS FOR CARE

### Home Care Management

In addition to the adaptive and assistive devices previously mentioned, adaptations to the home environment may be necessary. Elevated toilet seats and safety equipment for the bathroom can be installed in the home. Doorways should be wide enough to accommodate a walker or wheelchair if necessary. A ramp can be added for access to the front door if there are stairs. Countertops and cupboards can be lowered to accommodate the person who is wheelchair-bound. These modifications may be costly. Patients with severe rheumatoid arthritis are quite disabled and may need the assistance of a family member or friend to complete ADL; if that is not feasible, a home health aide may be needed. The patient should continue in a regular exercise program; eat a nutritious, balanced diet; take medications as prescribed; and participate in follow-up care. Maintenance of social supports and continued participation in social and recreational activities are necessary to prevent social isolation and depression.

## COMPLICATIONS

Complications associated with RA are usually a result of systemic manifestations. Pericarditis occurs in approximately 40% of patients with RA.[23] Pulmonary complications are more frequent than cardiac manifestations and are usually manifested as infiltrates and interstitial pneumonitis. Pulmonary complications may also result from treatment for RA with methotrexate and gold.[23]

Compression neuropathy may develop in the form of carpal and tarsal tunnel syndrome and ulnar nerve palsy. Atlantoaxial subluxation (C1 and C2) is a potentially fatal complication in persons with RA. Cervical subluxation occurs in approximately 15% of persons with RA within 3 years of onset of disease; patients with RA should be carefully screened for cervical subluxation, particularly if they are undergoing general anesthesia.[8] Any patient with a new onset of neck pain or myelopathy should be evaluated for cervical subluxation.

Rheumatoid vasculitis, inflammation and blockage of small blood vessels, is another potentially severe complication of RA. The extremities are most commonly affected, but involvement of the heart, abdominal organs, muscle, and nerves is possible. Treatment for internal organ involvement is usually high-dose corticosteroids (prednisone in doses greater than 60 mg/day) and cyclophosphamide (50 to 200 mg PO daily or 500 to 1000 mg/m$^2$ intravenously).[23] The initial manifestation of vasculitis may be 1- to 3-mm brown spots on the fingers and fingernails, resulting from small areas of skin infarction. Eventually skin ulcers may form, which may be difficult to heal. Concomitant treatment with corticosteroids or other immunosuppressants may compound the problem.

## DEGENERATIVE JOINT DISEASE

### Etiology

*Degenerative joint disease (DJD),* also known as osteoarthritis, hypertrophic arthritis, osteoarthrosis (OA), or senescent arthritis, is an extremely common disease that is probably as old as civilization. Almost everyone older than 40 years of age has hypertrophic changes in the joints. Although symptomatic degenerative joint disease is usually seen in the 50- to 70-year age-group, it has been observed as early as 20 years of age.

### Epidemiology

Women are more severely affected by the disease, although the incidence rates are the same for men and women. Men usually develop symptoms before 45 years of age; women usually do not develop symptoms until after age 55. Women usually develop osteoarthritis in the hands and knees, whereas men typically develop OA in the hips, knees, and spine. Heberden's nodes are 10 times more likely to develop in women than men; there is also a familial tendency noted.[26] An estimated 17 million people in the United States have osteoarthritis serious enough to cause pain. The two forms of osteoarthritis are *primary* (idiopathic) and *secondary.*

Primary joint disease is the most common type of noninflammatory joint disease. Primary degenerative joint disease is distributed throughout the central and peripheral joints of the body, usually affecting the joints of the hand, wrist, neck, lumbar spine, hip, knee, and ankle. The etiology is unknown, but age is an important factor in the development of the disease. The quantity and quality of proteoglycans decrease with the aging process and predispose the cartilage to break down and degenerate. Research suggests a genetic component to the development of osteoarthritis. A mutation of the gene that directs formation of type II collagen has been found in families of persons with osteoarthritis.[26,55]

Osteoarthritis is also common among postmenopausal women. Women taking estrogen replacement therapy appear to have a lower risk of developing the disease, which suggests that estrogen may have a protective effect on cartilage similar to the protective effect it has on bone resorption in osteoporosis.[26]

Secondary joint disease is caused by any condition that damages cartilage, subjects the joints to chronic stress, or causes joint instability. Secondary joint disease is usually limited to the specific joints that were subjected to stress. Causes of secondary disease include trauma and long-term mechanical stressors. Examples of mechanical stressors include obesity, athletics, dancing, or the performance of repetitive tasks; infection; endocrine disorders (acromegaly or hyperparathyrodism); neurological disorders (pain and proprioceptive responses are altered, thereby increasing the risk of abnormal movement or weight bearing); skeletal deformities; and hemophilia (bleeding into the joints). Regular moderate exercise does not appear to cause or increase existing DJD in normal joints.[7,35]

## Pathophysiology

Despite the name *osteoarthritis,* there is not a significant inflammatory component associated with the disorder. A small amount of low-grade inflammation is observed, and mechanical abnormalities in the joints irritate surrounding soft tissues and can cause inflammation. OA is generally termed "noninflammatory" to distinguish it from RA (Table 61-8). Both primary and secondary degenerative joint diseases affect the articular cartilage. Characteristic pathological changes include:

1. Erosion of articular cartilage.
2. Thickening of subchondral bone
3. Formation of osteophytes or bone spurs

Normal articular cartilage is white, translucent, and smooth. When affected by DJD, it becomes yellow and opaque. Areas of cartilage soften, and the surface becomes rough, frayed, and cracked. This process is thought to occur as a result of digestion of the cartilage by enzymes and alteration of the nutrition of the cartilage. Eventually the cartilage is destroyed, and the underlying subchondral bone goes through a remodeling process. *Osteophytes,* or bone spurs, appear at the joint margins and at the sites of attachment of supporting structures. These may break off and appear in the joint cavity as "joint mice."

Persons generally seek medical attention because of pain, usually described as a deep aching in the joint. Weather changes and increased activity tend to increase the pain. Loss of joint motion may be caused by the loss of articular cartilage, muscle spasms, shortening of ligaments, and osteophytes; loss of articular cartilage and subchondral bone can lead to joint subluxation and deformity. As the joint degenerates, the person may report decreased mobility and the sensation of grinding and catching.

Although OA may affect any joint, the joints involved differ with the age and sex of the patient.[7] Arthritis of the hand, more common in women, occurs most often (74%) in persons 65 to 74 years of age (see Figure 61-13). Hip involvement is more common in men; women are more likely to have knee involvement. Arthritic changes in the hip cause an antalgic gait, and pain is usually felt on the outer aspect of the hip, in the groin, buttocks, inner thigh, and knee. Patients with OA of the knee are most likely to report pain with motion, stiffness after inactivity, and decreased flexion. A varus deformity is common (Figure 61-12 and Box 61-4). Osteoarthritis of the spine is the most common cause of low back pain. Patients may report pain, stiffness, and occasionally neurological symptoms. Neurological symptoms can be caused by osteophytes, foraminal stenosis, disc protrusion, or subluxation. Clinical manifestations of DJD are summarized in Box 61-5.

## Collaborative Care Management

Objectives in management include relief of pain, restoration of joint function, and prevention of disability or further progression of the disease.

### *Diagnostic tests*

Diagnosis is made based on evaluation of history and physical assessment and the results of radiological studies. Serological and synovial fluid examinations will be essentially normal. Synovial fluid will be pale yellow or clear with a low leukocyte count, 500 to 2000 cell/$mm^3$. Leukocyte counts in excess of 2000 is indicative of inflammation; a work-up for RA, gout, lupus, and other inflammatory arthropathies should follow. Bloody effusions are usually the result of trauma, fractures of osteophytes or subchondral bone, or synovial or ligamentous tears. Arthroscopy is not necessary for diagnosis of OA, but it is helpful because it allows direct visualization of articular surfaces; early disease may be detected. X-ray films will reveal narrowing of the joint space, osteophyte formation, and eburnation (sclerosis) of subchondral bone. Almost 50% of patients with evidence of OA on x-ray are asymptomatic.

**table 61-8** *Distinguishing Features of Osteoarthritis and Rheumatoid Arthritis*

| | OA | RA |
|---|---|---|
| **ETIOLOGY** | Primary: unknown, genetic component<br>Secondary: mechanical stress, trauma, hormonal | Unknown<br>Theories: overstimulation of inflammatory process; autoimmune, genetic, antigen-antibody reaction, viral |
| **ONSET** | 45 to 55 years<br>Insidious | After age 30<br>Average age 55 years<br>Insidious or acute |
| **PATHOPHYSIOLOGY** | Disease of articular cartilage<br>Biochemical changes leading to deterioration and loss of cartilage<br>Reactive new bone formation<br>Changes in articular surface<br>Areas of exposed bone may occur<br>Formation of osteophytes<br>*No systemic manifestations* | Inflammatory disease of joints, connective tissue with *systemic manifestations*<br>Inflammatory process destroying joint components<br>Formation of pannus<br>Cartilage erosion<br>Soft tissue changes causing joint subluxation and dislocation<br>Formation of rheumatoid nodules |
| **JOINT INVOLVEMENT** | Asymmetrical, monoarticular or polyarticular<br>DIP joints (Heberden's nodes)<br>PIP joints (Bouchard's nodes)<br>First CMC, first MTP<br>Hips, knees, lumbar and cervical spine | Symmetrical, polyarticular<br>PIP joints<br>MCP joints<br>MTP joints<br>Cervical spine<br>Large joints (hip, knee; more common in elderly) |
| **CLINICAL MANIFESTATIONS** | Joint enlargement<br>Crepitus<br>Pain increased with weight bearing, relieved with rest<br>Limitation of joint motion<br>Noninflammatory joint effusion<br>Morning stiffness <1 hour | Fever<br>Weight loss<br>Fatigue<br>Night pain<br>Pain with rest<br>Morning stiffness >1 hour<br>Joint "boggy" with palpation, tender, erythematous<br>Inflammatory joint effusion<br>Subluxation, dislocation<br>Rheumatoid nodules |
| **DIAGNOSTIC DATA** | No laboratory abnormalities<br>Radiographic evidence of joint space narrowing, osteophytes, bony sclerosis | Rheumatoid factor positive in 75-80% of patients; elderly onset positive in 90% of persons[56]<br>Elevated ESR<br>Radiographic evidence of joint space narrowing, bone erosion, osteopenia |

*DIP,* Distal interphalangeal; *PIP,* proximal interphalangeal; *MCP,* metacarpophalangeal; *MTP,* metatarsophalangeal; *CMC,* carpometacarpal.

### Medications

Analgesics, NSAIDs, and intraarticular corticosteroids are the mainstays of pharmacological treatment of OA. The objective of treatment is symptomatic relief of pain; benefits such as improved mobility and functioning have not been established.

Acetaminophen is a first-line agent for treatment. Doses up to 4 g/day may be given in the absence of hepatic or renal disease. Liver function studies must be done at regular intervals while the patient is receiving therapy. Constant pain is best relieved by regular intervals of dosing; intermittent pain may be relieved by as needed dosing. The effectiveness of acetaminophen is similar to that of NSAIDs. Moderate to severe pain can also be managed by propoxyphene, codeine, or tramadol; however, most practitioners try to avoid the use of narcotics in the management of OA.

If acetaminophen is contraindicated (liver or renal disease), NSAIDs are the next choice for therapy. As mentioned earlier, a small degree of inflammation may be present; thus NSAIDs have the advantage of having an antiinflammatory effect. There is no convincing evidence to support the hypothesis that NSAIDs retard articular cartilage degeneration or alter the course of the disease.[7,26,55] In vitro and animal studies differ in the reported effect of NSAIDs on articular cartilage; however there is evidence that indomethacin increases the rate of degeneration in human hip joints.[7]

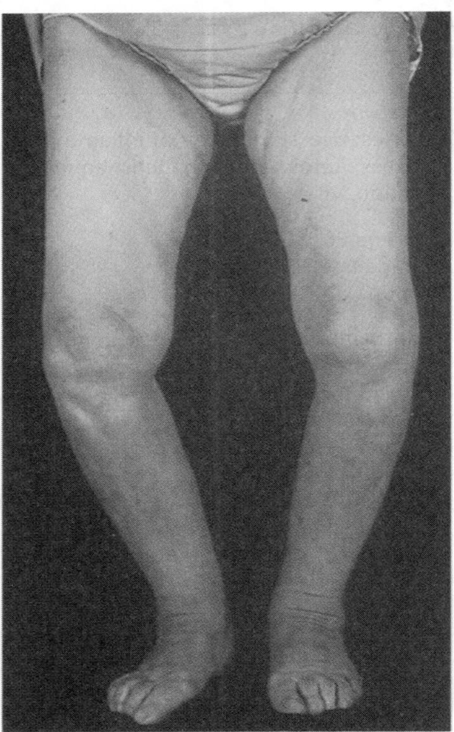

**fig. 61-12** Typical varus deformity of knee osteoarthritis.

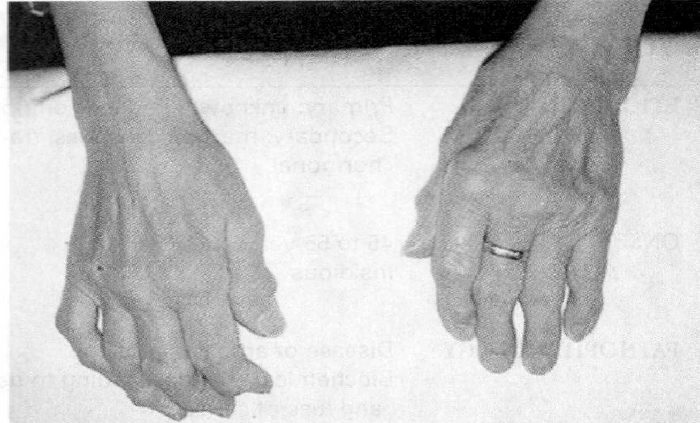

**fig. 61-13** Osteoarthritis.

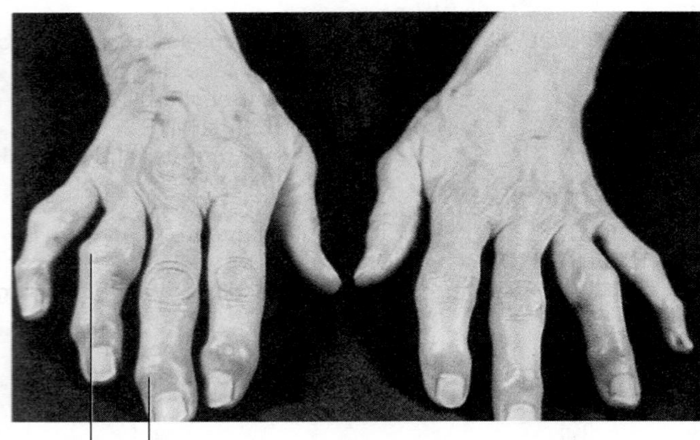


**fig. 61-14** Bouchard's node.

**box 61-4** *Characteristic Changes or Symptoms in Certain Joints*

1. Knee involvement—varus (Figure 61-12), valgus (knocked knees), flexion deformity, crepitus, and limited range of motion
2. Heberden's nodes—bony protuberances occurring on the dorsal surface of the distal interphalangeal joints of the fingers (Figure 61-13)
3. *Bouchard's nodes*—bony protuberances occurring on the proximal interphalangeal joints of the fingers (Figure 61-14)
4. *Coxarthrosis* (degenerative joint disease of the hip)—pain in the hip on weight bearing, with pain progressing to include groin and medial knee pain and limited range of motion

Numerous brands of NSAIDs are on the market. Choice is determined by cost, availability, adverse effects, duration of action, and patient and physician preference; there are no significant differences in effectiveness.[7] Adverse effects with the use of NSAIDs are common and potentially serious. Persons at increased risk include the elderly, those with a history of ulcers, and patients with a history of congestive heart failure, cirrhosis, and diabetes.[55] Elderly patients may benefit from concomitant use of misoprostol to prevent gastrointestinal symptoms. Prescribing an $H_2$ blocker to patients at risk may prevent duodenal ulcers. Arthrotec offers the convenience of both medications in one pill. Renal and hepatic function and blood counts must be monitored regularly while the patient is taking NSAIDs. Certain NSAIDs are available in creme or gel forms (capsaicin creme) for topical application. If capsaicin creme is prescribed, the patient must be instructed to wash the hands thoroughly after application and to avoid contact with mucous membranes because the medication is made from pepper plants.

Intraarticular injection of steroids may be needed if analgesics and NSAIDs are ineffective or as an adjunct to therapy. Unstable or infected joints should never be injected.[55] Steroid injections are effective in controlling pain and improving function. However, repeated injections may actually accelerate joint degeneration. To prevent articular cartilage damage, a joint should not be injected more than three to four times per year. Other complications include infection and cutaneous atrophy.

box 61-5 clinical manifestations

**Degenerative Joint Disease**

| | |
|---|---|
| Pain | Worse with weight bearing, improves with rest, may be accompanied by paresthesias |
| Swelling and joint enlargement | May be from inflammatory exudate or blood entering joint capsule causing an increase in synovial fluid or from fragments of osteophytes entering synovial cavity |
| Decreased range of motion | Depends on amount of destroyed cartilage |
| Muscular atrophy | From disuse, joint instability, and deformity |
| Crepitus | May be present on movement |
| Joint stiffness | Worse in the morning (morning stiffness <1 hour) and after a period of rest or disuse |

*Viscosupplementation,* developed in the 1960s and previously used in Canada and Sweden, is an alternative therapy for OA of the knee. This therapy is based on the fact that synovial fluid in persons with OA is less elastic and viscous than normal synovial fluid. Viscosupplementation is the intraarticular injection of hyaluronan or its derivatives to restore the normal elasticity and viscosity of the synovial fluid and restore the normal balance of hyaluronan within the fluid. Hyaluronan (hyaluronic acid) is a glycosamine polysaccharide and is found in high concentrations in synovial fluid. In persons with OA, the concentration of hyaluronan is decreased, and the amount of synovial fluid is increased. The source of hyaluronan is umbilical cords or rooster combs; available hyaluronan products include Synvisc, Hylan, Hyalgan, and Healon. Injections are given weekly, at least 3 injections are given, and up to 10 injections may be required for efficacy. Relief from pain occurs after the first injection, progresses over a few weeks, and may last 6 months or longer.[48] Complications include infection, pain with injection, headache, gastrointestinal complaints, swelling of the knee, and allergic reaction. Viscosupplementation may be used in combination with other medications for treatment of OA.

### Treatments

Treatment early in the course of DJD can make a significant improvement in the person's quality of life and may alter the course of the disease.[7] Three foci of therapy are relief of pain, joint protection, and physical therapy to stabilize joints and prevent deformity. Joint protection techniques may include weight reduction and the use of canes or splints.

Persons with mild DJD should avoid activities that produce an exacerbation of symptoms, maintain or increase muscle strength and range of motion, and use NSAIDs or mild analgesics as needed. Activities that produce an increase in symptoms are typically load-bearing activities. Maintenance of muscle strength can be attained by engaging in regular exercise. The Arthritis Foundation offers exercise classes at many community centers for persons with arthritis. Exercises to maintain range of motion are indicated and should be performed twice daily, with 10 to 30 repetitions per session.[56] For the patient with decreased function due to DJD, adaptive aids, physical therapy, and pain relief medications can be prescribed. Adaptive devices may be beneficial for completing ADL for persons with DJD of the hands. (See Treatment section for RA for information on assistive and adaptive devices and joint protection techniques, p. 1963-1966.) Persons with advanced DJD, severe pain, or severe limitations in mobility may be candidates for surgical management of their disease.

### Surgical management

Surgical management of the person with osteoarthritis is indicated to relieve pain, improve function, or correct deformity. Surgical procedures include those that preserve or restore articular cartilage and those that realign, fuse, or replace joints. Surgical management usually provides the patient with excellent results; however the patient is at risk for developing surgical complications, including infection, nerve and blood vessel injury, deep venous thrombosis, and pulmonary or fat embolism. Surgery is performed when medications and physical therapy have failed. However, surgery should be performed before severe deformity, joint instability, contracture, or severe muscle atrophy develop, all of which can seriously compromise the outcome and place the patient at a higher risk for developing complications.[7]

Procedures to restore or preserve articular cartilage include joint debridement (via arthroscopy), *abrasion chondroplasty* (abrasion of subchondral bone to stimulate growth of cartilage), and replacement of articular cartilage with grafts. These procedures are not indicated for patients with advanced DJD, because they usually produce only short-term results. An alternative therapy is the transplantation of healthy cartilage cells into the knees of persons with traumatic arthritis or other cartilage defects. Chondrocytes are harvested from a healthy individual, cultured in the laboratory, and injected into patients' knees.[26] Young persons with small areas of damaged cartilage are the ideal candidates for cartilage transplantation.

An *osteotomy* is a surgical incision through a bone. Osteotomy may be thought of as a surgical or intentional fracture. The purpose of osteotomy is to realign a joint or bone or to redistribute the load-bearing surface of a joint to a region that has more articular cartilage (Figure 61-15). Osteotomy is useful for correcting angulation or rotational deformities. The patient is treated similarly to a patient who has suffered a fracture. Persons with stable joints, functional range of motion, adequate musculature, and some remaining articular cartilage benefit the most from osteotomy.

*Arthrodesis* or joint fusion is performed to relieve pain and to restore stability and alignment. Joint fusion, as the term implies, results in lost motion; hence this procedure has limited application. The fusion of one joint increases the load-bearing of adjacent joints, which may accelerate degeneration of those

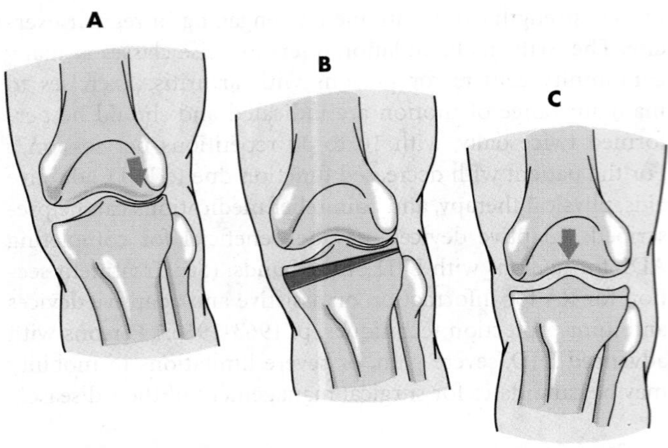


fig. 61-15 Osteotomy of tibia for genu valgum (valgus deformity); anterior view of left knee. **A,** Weight-bearing force is concentrated on one compartment of knee. **B,** Wedge of bone is removed from tibia. Amount of bone removed is determined by how much correction in angulation is necessary. **C,** Distal portion of tibia is swung to proximal portion. Correction of angulation obtained allows weight-bearing forces to be more evenly distributed through both compartments of knee.

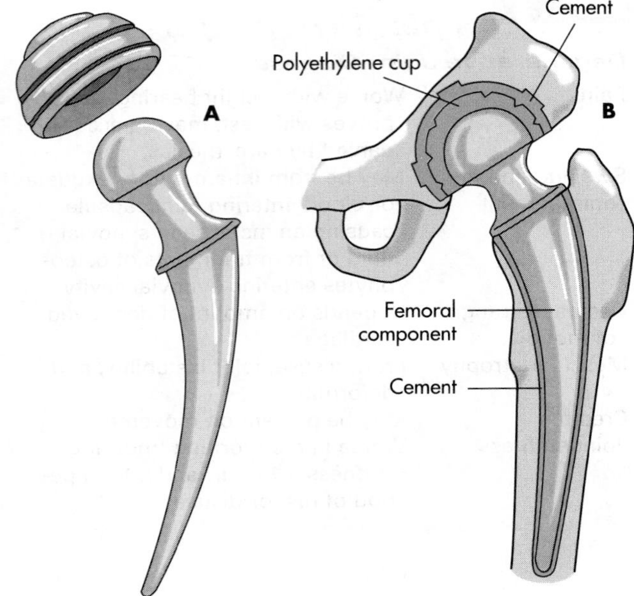


fig. 61-16 **A,** Acetabular and femoral components of total hip prosthesis. **B,** Total hip prosthesis in place.

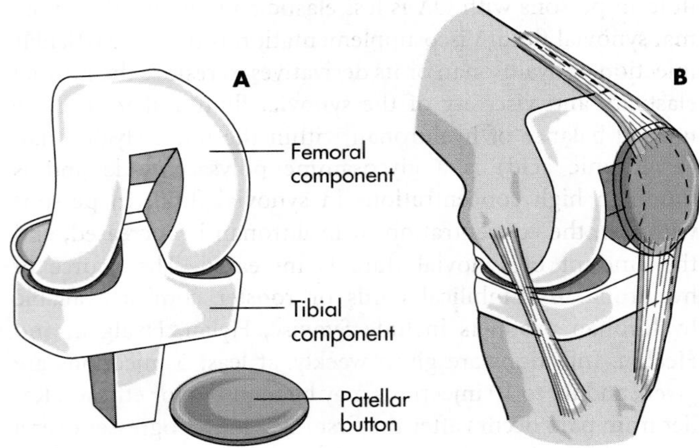


fig. 61-17 **A,** Tibial and femoral components of total knee prosthesis. A patellar button, made of polyethylene, protects the posterior surface of the patella from friction against the femoral component when the knee is moved through flexion and extension. **B,** Total knee prosthesis in place.

joints. Arthrodesis is most commonly performed on the cervical and lumbar spine, interphalangeal joints, first metatarsal joints, and the wrist and ankle.

Joint replacement or *arthroplasty* has been a mainstay of treatment for OA since the 1960s. Sir John Charnley, a pioneer in arthroplasty surgery, first described his success with *hip arthroplasty* in 1961. The hip was the first joint to be successfully replaced and continues to be replaced in many persons with OA. More than 275,000 total hip replacements and an additional 75,000 hip revisions are performed annually in the United States today.[26] Although arthroplasty procedures of the hip and knee are most common, the procedure can also be performed on the shoulder, elbow, ankle, and finger joints (Figures 61-16 and 61-17). Materials for prosthetic implants are metal (titanium or cobalt-chrome alloy), high-density polyethylene, ceramic (low-friction and longer wear), and other synthetic materials (Figure 61-18). Replacement prostheses can be *cemented* to the remaining bone with polymethamethacrylate or uncemented. *Uncemented* prostheses are usually treated with a porous coating that promotes bony ingrowth (Figure 61-18).

The decision whether to implant a cemented or uncemented prosthesis depends upon such factors as the individual patient, bone stock, age, and surgeon preference. Uncemented components are thought to last longer, as the bony growth lessens the likelihood of the prosthesis loosening, which is a consideration with cemented joints. Loosening of the components may lead to implant failure. In addition, uncemented joints are usually easier to replace and revise than cemented joints. An estimated 50% of persons treated with hip arthroplasty will need revision joint surgery within 15 years.[26] The articulating surface of the artificial joint lacks the mechanical properties and durability of normal articular cartilage.

*Total knee arthroplasty* is a technically more difficult procedure than total hip replacement, because of the complex movements of the knee joint. A well-designed firmly implanted knee prosthesis can withstand 20 years' wear in some patients, and 90% to 95% of patients with primary knee replacements are doing well after 15 years. Approximately 20% of patients with total knee replacements undergo revision.[44]

A

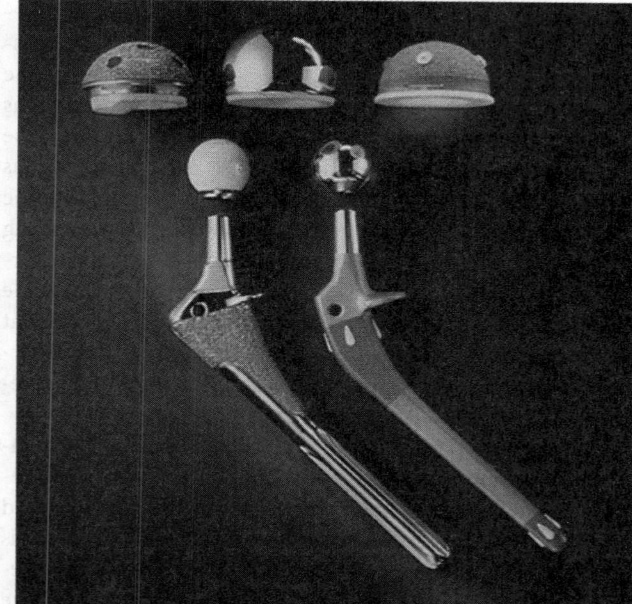

B

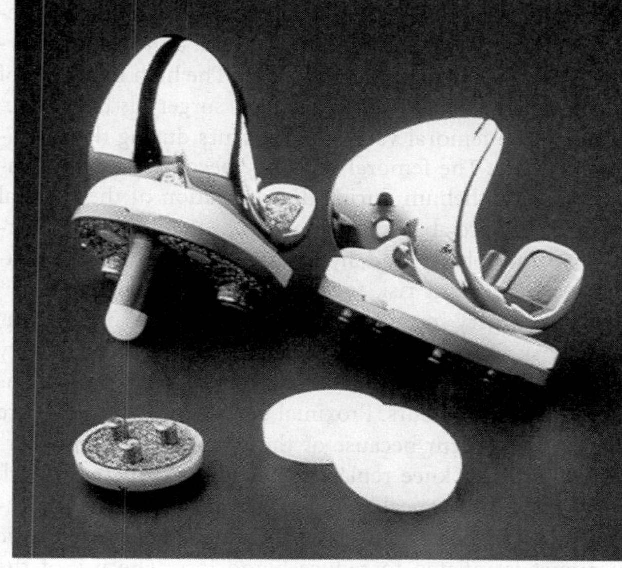

**fig. 61-18** **A,** Hip prostheses. *Left:* porous ingrowth acetabular cup and femoral stem, ceramic femoral head. *Middle:* bipolar head for hemiarthroplasty (component fits on top of femoral head component). Used with either cemented or uncemented femoral stems. *Right:* cemented femoral stem and cemented acetabular cup. **B,** Knee prostheses. *Left:* porous ingrowth femoral and tibial components, porous ingrowth patellar button. *Right:* hybrid: cemented femoral component and patellar button; porous ingrowth tibial component.

The prosthetic implants are subject to fatigue, wear, breakage, and failure. A particular risk associated with total joint arthroplasty is infection, which usually necessitates removal of the prosthesis. Most revisions are done because of component loosening; infection and implant failure are other reasons for revision.

*Total shoulder replacement* was first described in 1893, long before the first hip replacement. Since the 1970s replacement of the shoulder joint has become more common, although less than 5000 replacements were performed in the United States between 1990 and 1992.[69] Long-term results of shoulder replacements are not available, although the short-term (2 and 5 years postimplant) results are encouraging.[69] The surgical procedure is challenging due to the dynamic structure and movements of the joint. The shoulder joint lacks a true socket and depends on soft tissue structures for its stability.

*Total elbow replacements* are primarily performed to relieve the pain and disability associated with rheumatoid arthritis. The patient must have adequate bone stock and ligamentous structures to provide stability to the implanted joint. Both components are usually cemented in place.

Another type of joint replacement is the *interposition arthroplasty,* in which the joint surface on one or both sides is replaced with metal, inert material (polyethylene), fascia, or tendon. Interposition arthroplasty is usually performed on the wrist or metacarpal-phalangeal joints of the finger.

Preventing infection is a priority of care with all joint replacement surgery. Revision surgery carries a higher risk of infection due to the longer operating time. Sources of infection in the operating room include direct contamination of the wound and contamination of the sterile field or personnel. The rate of infection in patients with total hip replacements is approximately 1%, with an estimated 50% to 80% having their origin in the operating room.[1] Measures taken to prevent surgically acquired infection include the use of laminar airflow systems; body exhaust systems for scrubbed and circulating personnel; limited traffic in the operating room and use of an "outside circulating nurse," skin preparation, and strict adherence to sterile technique (Figure 61-19). Preoperative preparation, the use of laminar flow rooms, and prophylactic antibiotics have reduced infection rates for primary total joint replacements to 0.5% to 2%.[35]

### Diet

Appropriate nutritional intake is encouraged to maintain ideal body weight and avoid weight gain. Weight gain places an unnecessary stress on joints, particularly the hips and knees.

### Activity

Emphasis is placed on the following:

1. Unloading the stress on painful weight-bearing joints through the use of canes, walkers, or crutches
2. Range of motion exercises to prevent deformities and contractures; muscle-strengthening exercises to increase or maintain muscle muscle tone and strength

Aerobic exercise should be included in the regimen to increase endurance and increase overall conditioning. Exercise is also beneficial in reducing fatigue, a common complaint in persons with chronic disease. Exercises that maintain joint motion and muscle strength but with minimal joint loading are the best choice for persons with degenerative arthritis.

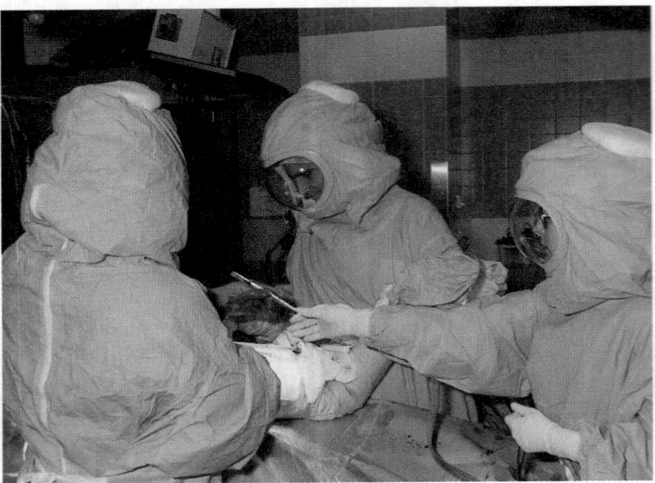

fig. 61-19 Body exhaust system during total joint surgery.

Exercises that include impact loading or tortional loading of joints should be avoided.[7] Water exercises are an excellent choice for the patient with arthritis and as mentioned earlier are offered by the Arthritis Foundation in many locations. In persons with advanced disease, exercise may exacerbate symptoms. Rest relieves most joint pain but should be avoided for prolonged periods, because immobility promotes joint stiffness. Persons with DJD of the lower extremities should also avoid prolonged standing or kneeling.

#### Referrals

In some settings the nurse assumes responsibility for making referrals to other services. Common referrals for persons with degenerative joint disease include physical therapy and occupational therapy.

A Nursing Care Plan for a patient undergoing joint replacement is found on p. 1985.

## NURSING MANAGEMENT OF THE PATIENT WITH JOINT REPLACEMENT SURGERY

### PREOPERATIVE CARE

As described in Chapter 18, preoperative data are usually gathered at a preadmission appointment. Many institutions have brochures, videos, and other teaching aids to enhance preoperative instruction and decrease anxiety. The teaching may also be done in the surgeon's office by an orthopedic nurse specialist. The patient is assessed for risk factors that may influence his or her care intraoperatively or postoperatively (refer to Chapter 18). Major concerns identified by patients with total joint replacements include fear of the unknown, pain, performance, altered body image, dependency, depression, and fatigue.[61] Nursing interventions should focus on providing accurate information on these topics.

The presence of infection is a contraindication to joint replacement surgery. Infection causes loosening of the prosthetic components and may progress to osteomyelitis. The presence of respiratory conditions may delay surgery. Persons with severe chronic obstructive pulmonary disease or those with pneumonia are at particular risk perioperatively, as methylmethacrylate (bone cement) is excreted through the lungs, which may cause pneumonitis or worsen a preexisting respiratory condition. Persons with bleeding or clotting disorders require special care perioperatively. Persons with sickle cell disease or hemophilia often require joint replacement surgery. Measures are taken to control hemorrhage intraoperatively, and prophylactic anticoagulants would not be prescribed for patients with clotting disorders.

The patient and family will require teaching about potential complications and preventive measures after joint replacement surgery. Persons having knee or hip joints replaced are at risk for the development of deep vein thrombosis (DVT) and pulmonary or fat embolism. A history of previous DVT or bilateral knee or hip replacements place the patient at an increased risk. Without prophylactic anticoagulation, the frequency of DVT in persons having hip replacement surgery is as high as 50% to 60% and up to 80% in persons having knee replacement surgery.[5] The high incidence of DVT in patients with hip replacement surgery is due to occlusion of the femoral vein, which occurs during the operative procedure. The femoral vein may become twisted, damaging the endothelium during disarticulation of the femoral head from the acetabulum. These factors, in addition to postoperative immobility and hypercoagulability, place the patient at a significant risk for the development of DVT.[5,51,66] Length of surgery in excess of 30 minutes is the most documented risk factor for DVT.[1] Any joint replacement surgery takes longer than 30 minutes; revision surgery may last as long as 4 or more hours. Proximal deep vein thromboses are more likely to occur because of the surgical technique. Persons having total knee replacement are at an increased risk for DVT due to surgical technique. Intraoperatively, the extremity is wrapped in an elastic bandage and a pneumatic tourniquet is inflated to reduce blood loss. The use of the tourniquet and elastic wrap may damage the endothelial lining of the vein, attracting platelets and causing aggregation and possibly thrombus.[51] In addition, the use of bone cement, which produces release of heat, may cause local venous damage and an increased risk of DVT.[51] The risk of DVT continues into the first 6 weeks postoperatively at an estimated 10%.[5]

Most patients are given a dose of heparin or low-molecular-weight heparin (LMWH) preoperatively, generally 2 to 12 hours before incision time, which is continued postoperatively as prophylaxis.[1,5] Other methods of preoperative prophylaxis for DVT include the placement of a vena cava filter for patients at high risk for DVT.[51] Patients who are taking anticoagulants, steroids, aspirin, and NSAIDs should discontinue these medications before surgery. Steroid therapy needs to be tapered and may take several weeks to discontinue; aspirin and NSAIDs should be discontinued 7 to 10 days preoperatively.[1] Results of coagulation studies should be within the normal range before surgery. Despite the use of prophylaxis, the incidence of DVT in elective orthopedic surgery is estimated to be 20%.[51]

The patient should be informed about autologous donation of blood in sufficient time to allow donation. An iron supplement will be prescribed, if the patient opts for autologous donation. If autologous donation is not planned, the patient's blood will be typed and cross-matched for 2 to 4 units of packed cells. Some surgeons use blood-salvaging techniques intraoperatively to reinfuse blood lost on the surgical field, which decreases the need for postoperative blood transfusions.

A CBC and serum chemistry analysis, coagulation studies (platelets, prothrombin time, activated partial thromboplastin time, and international normalized ratio), urinalysis, chest x-ray, and electrocardiogram will be done at the preadmission appointment, in addition to a complete history and physical examination. The results of the examinations and laboratory testing should be evaluated before the patient's admission to the hospital, in case additional studies are needed, or abnormal results require medical intervention. The serum albumin level is evaluated to identify patients at risk for wound infection. Wound complications are more frequent in persons with serum albumin levels below 3.5 g/dl.[67] Objective data to be gathered regarding the musculoskeletal system include the following: joint range of motion; presence of deformities such as varus, valgus, or flexion; leg length discrepancies; condition of joints, enlargement, erythema, crepitus, and asymmetry; gait; and ability to perform ADL.

The patient is also instructed about the perioperative routine, including respiratory and leg exercises (see Chapter 18). The patient may have a physical therapy evaluation preoperatively and be measured for crutches, a walker, or cane. Persons with arthritis involving the joints of the upper extremity may be fitted with a platform walker, in which most of the upper body weight is distributed on the forearms during ambulation. Platform walkers are particularly beneficial to persons with rheumatoid arthritis, who typically have wrist and finger joint involvement. The patient should be informed about what adaptive equipment will be needed upon discharge. Postoperative pain control is usually achieved with the use of patient-controlled analgesia (PCA) pumps. Both epidural and intravenous pain control are used for patients with joint replacement surgery. The patient should be shown the pump and given instructions regarding its use at the preoperative interview. The patient's pain control is usually managed by the anesthesia staff or the pain management service.

The patient is instructed to be given nothing by mouth after midnight on the day preceding surgery and is admitted to the hospital on the day of surgery. Intravenous antibiotics are begun at least 30 minutes before the incision time to establish a therapeutic level; antibiotics are usually continued for 24 hours postoperatively. The lowest rate of infection occurs when antibiotics are given no more than 2 hours before incision time.[1]

Discharge planning is also begun at the preadmission interview. The length of hospital stay varies with the joint replaced and individual patient's condition. Most patients admitted for hip or knee replacement are discharged after 4 to 6 days. Patients are no longer hospitalized until the are independently ambulatory; hence most patients are discharged to a rehabilitative facility or subacute division for continued therapy. The patient's and family's resources and preferences should be assessed at the preadmission interview to begin planning for transfer after discharge.

## POSTOPERATIVE CARE

### General Considerations

Routine postoperative nursing care for the patient recovering from total joint replacement surgery includes monitoring vital signs and level of consciousness, coughing and deep breathing, monitoring and recording intake and output (including suction drains at operative site), providing adequate nutrition and hydration, managing pain, assessing the surgical site for drainage and signs of infection, maintaining the position of the operative extremity to prevent dislocation of prostheses, performing neurovascular checks, providing skin care, encouraging progressive ambulation, preventing infection, teaching, and monitoring the patient for signs of complications. (See Chapter 20 for general postoperative care.) Priorities of care include interventions to prevent the complications associated with immobility, including constipation, urinary retention, respiratory complications, altered skin integrity, and venous stasis. Nursing interventions specific to the joint replaced are discussed separately following this section.

Deep vein thrombosis is a common complication after both hip and knee replacement. Measures to prevent DVT are the administration of anticoagulants, use of intermittent pneumatic compression devices, antiembolism hose, and leg exercises performed by the patient. As mentioned earlier, the threat of DVT and pulmonary embolism continues 4 to 6 weeks after surgery. Proximal DVT is most often associated with pulmonary embolism. Depending upon the individual patient and surgeon preference, patients are given heparin, low-dose heparin, LMWH (enoxaparin), or warfarin for prophylactic anticoagulation. LMWH has a longer half-life than standard heparin and does not require laboratory testing for twice-daily dosing. LMWH has been shown to be more effective than standard heparin in reducing the incidence of proximal DVT, but showed no difference in preventing distal DVT. LMWH is usually administered subcutaneously twice daily for a period of 7 to 14 days and is highly effective in reducing the incidence of proximal and distal DVT after total hip and knee replacement.[66] Low doses of warfarin can be administered daily based on the patient's daily prothrombin time or INR results. The goal is to maintain a prothrombin time of 15 seconds and a control of 1.5 seconds.[1] Warfarin is continued until there is no risk of embolism.

Studies indicate concomitant use of LMWH and pneumatic compression devices is the most effective means of reducing the incidence of DVT when compared with other measures such as aspirin, dextran, standard heparin, and warfarin.[1] In many institutions, pneumatic compression devices are applied intraoperatively and are continued until the patient is fully ambulatory.

The venous foot pump is an alternative method of decreasing venous stasis and thus the risk of DVT. This device has been shown to be as effective as natural weight bearing in producing adequate pumping action to increase venous return.[1] Nurses should encourage the patient to perform isometric leg exercises every 1 to 2 hours, with 10 repetitions per session. The use of antiembolism hose should be continued until the patient is fully ambulatory. Some institutions include ultrasound or other diagnostic testing to rule out DVT as part of the postoperative protocol.

Early ambulation is the best, safest, and least expensive method of preventing venous stasis.[1] Most patients are assisted out of bed on the first postoperative day, with progressive ambulation and physical therapy (PT) sessions daily to follow. Activity and weight-bearing restrictions vary, depending on the joint replaced, whether or not cement was used, and surgeon protocol. The nurse should assist and encourage the patient to perform active and passive range-of-motion (ROM) exercises, isometrics, and other exercises prescribed by the physical therapist to increase muscle strength and decrease the complications of mobility.

While the patient is receiving anticoagulants, the nurse is responsible for monitoring the patient for signs of bleeding. The stool, urine, and sputum should be monitored for blood; a soft-bristled tooth brush should be used; dental floss should be avoided; electric razors should be used in place of razor blades; and needle punctures should be kept to a minimum. The suction drain and dressing should be assessed for excessive drainage and the patient's coagulation studies and CBC should be monitored daily.

Estimated blood loss during total hip surgery usually ranges from 1000 to 1200 ml and during total knee surgery can be up to 1500 ml.[38,44] Closed wound drainage systems are surgically placed at the time of closing of the incision to prevent hematoma formation and are left in place 24 to 48 hours postoperatively. Studies now indicate that the use of suction drains may be ineffective in preventing hematoma formation and may contribute to increased blood loss and infection.[1,38]

Because of intraoperative blood loss, the patient may require a transfusion postoperatively. Either autologous or homologous blood can be transfused. An alternative is an autotransfusion drain, a closed drainage system that collects and filters the blood, which can then be reinfused intravenously into the patient. These types of drains have not been proven to be cost-effective. Several studies have shown that preoperative autologous donation, intraoperative salvage (see Chapter 19), and postoperative salvage and reinfusion are the most effective means of reducing homologous transfusion in patients receiving total joint replacements.[16]

Used alone, postoperative salvage and reinfusion have been shown to be effective in reducing the amount of autologous blood needed postoperatively. The blood obtained through intraoperative and postoperative salvage methods has several advantages over homologous banked blood. Platelets and clotting factors remain intact in the salvaged blood, the pH of the blood is identical to the patient's, red blood cells are viable, reinfused blood has a greater affinity for oxygen, and the risk of transfusion reaction or transmission of blood-borne diseases is less.[16] Postoperative salvage and reinfusion must be accomplished within 6 hours, according to the American Association of Blood Banks Standards Committee.[16]

In addition to monitoring the drain and dressing site for signs of excessive bleeding, the patient's hemoglobin and hematocrit must be monitored daily. Output from the surgical drain is generally less than 300 ml per shift. Patients are often given an iron supplement postoperatively to prevent anemia.

Preventing infection is a nursing priority for any patient who has had a total joint replacement. A postoperative wound infection can lead to prolonged hospitalization, permanent disability, and removal of the prosthesis with a decreased chance for success in subsequent replacements.[70] More than 50% of infections occur at least 3 months after joint replacement.[70] The cost of treating a patient with a deep wound infection has been estimated to be more than $50,000 with an associated mortality rate of 1% to 4%.[70] Infection rates for persons receiving total hip replacements are 0.1% to 1% and for those receiving knee replacements range from 1% to 4%.[70] Infection rates for persons having elbow replacements are significantly higher (5% to 10%) because of the superficiality of the joint and poor skin coverage for closure.[2]

*Staphylococcus aureus* and *Staphylococcus epidermidis* are the most frequently cultured organisms from hip and knee wounds. The patient's skin has been identified as the major source of infection.[70] Bone and joint infections are particularly difficult to treat because of the multiple channels in bone that may harbor organisms for long periods of time. The use of prophylactic antibiotics in the perioperative period has been effective in reducing the incidence of postoperative infection in patients having hip and knee replacements. Antibiotics should be given as prescribed to maintain therapeutic blood levels.

The patient should be monitored for any signs of infection, including elevated temperature, elevated white blood cell count, and erythema, edema, or drainage from the wound. Dressing changes should be performed using aseptic technique. A report of a dull aching pain or unusual or persistent pain may be an indication of joint infection and should be reported to the physician for further evaluation. The patient and family should be taught to recognize the signs and symptoms of infection.[70] Discharge instructions should include methods of avoiding sources of infection, including the necessity for prophylactic antibiotics when undergoing dental or genitourinary procedures or other invasive procedures and for instances of systemic bacterial infections.

Pain management is an important aspect of nursing care for patients after total joint replacement. Many patients with arthritis have endured years of chronic pain as a result of degenerative changes in the joint. Total joint replacement may offer relief from that pain. However, postoperative pain may be of a different character than that associated with arthritis. The pain after total knee arthroplasty may continue for up to 1 year postoperatively due to reflex sympathetic dystrophy or the components of the total knee.[44] Many institutions use intravenous or epidural PCA as a method of pain control. Morphine and fentanyl are commonly used analgesics. The PCA pump is usually continued for 48 to 72 hours postoperatively; then oral analgesics are ordered as needed. The patient should be monitored for bowel function because of the side effects of the medication and immobility after surgery. Ice is applied to the incision area for the first 48 hours to prevent swelling and to decrease pain. Ice will help decrease pain, particularly after PT sessions. The nurse should consider the patient's PT schedule and make sure the patient is adequately medicated before going to therapy.

### Total Hip Arthroplasty

In addition to general postoperative care, there are some important considerations for care after total hip arthroplasty (see the Guidelines for Care Box). Positioning restrictions protect the prosthesis and depend on the surgical technique and type of prosthesis. After total hip arthroplasty, dislocation of the prosthesis is a serious complication that may require additional surgery or anesthesia to relocate the prosthesis. Signs of possible dislocation include a sudden onset of pain unrelieved by medication, a "popping" sensation associated with movement, loss of movement, leg length discrepancy, and deformity. The affected extremity may be either externally or internally rotated, depending on the direction of the dislocation, and the head of the femoral prosthesis may be palpable.

Extremes of flexion, adduction, or rotation should be avoided, because these motions may cause dislocation (Figure 61-20). Flexion is generally limited to 60° for 6 to 7 days and then to 90° for 2 to 3 months. When the patient is supine or lying on the side, the legs should be kept in abduction; pillows or an abduction splint can be used (Figure 61-21). Positioning the patient on the operative side is usually avoided to prevent adduction of the operative limb. Positioning restrictions are maintained until the hip capsule is well healed and the risk of dislocation has passed. Bone growth around the prosthesis begins in approximately 10 days.[1]

Most patients have some restriction in weight bearing, which limits the distraction force on the prosthesis. Patients with cemented prostheses are usually allowed weight bearing as tolerated. With the help of physical therapists, the goal

**guidelines for care**

#### Postoperative Care of the Person with Total Hip Replacement

1. Positioning
   a. Positioning will depend on the design of the prosthesis and the method of insertion. Restrictions designed to avoid dislocation of the prosthesis usually include the following:
      (1) Flexion is limited to 60° for 6 to 7 days, then 90° for 2 to 3 months.
      (2) No adduction is permitted beyond midline for 2 to 3 months, therefore no side lying on operative side unless ordered by the surgeon. Leg is maintained in abduction when lying supine or on nonoperative side (see Figure 61-21).
      (3) No extreme internal or external rotation is permitted (see Figure 61-20).
2. Wound care
   a. Drains are inserted in wound to prevent formation of hematoma and left in place for 24 to 48 hours.
   b. Maintain constant suction through self-contained suction device.
   c. Note amount and types of drainage.
   d. Use aseptic technique.
   e. Following initial dressing change, change dressing once daily and prn, using aseptic technique. Observe the incision line for signs of infection. The wound may be left open to air if there is no drainage. Staples are removed 7 to 10 days postoperatively.
3. Activity
   a. Observe flexion restrictions when elevating head of bed.
   b. Encourage periodic elevation and lowering of head of bed to provide motion at hip.
   c. Instruct patient in use of overhead trapeze to shift weight and lift for bedpan and change of linen.
   d. Encourage active dorsiplantar flexion exercise of ankles and quadriceps and gluteal setting exercises to promote venous return, prevent thrombus formation, and maintain muscle tone (see Chapter 20).
   e. Patient may be turned to unoperative side with operative leg maintained in abduction and extension.
   f. Begin ambulation as early as the first postoperative day, if tolerated.
      (1) Observe flexion and adduction restrictions.
      (2) Observe weight-bearing restrictions prescribed by surgeon (usually partial weight bearing assisted with walker or crutches).
      (3) Increase amount of walking each day according to patient's tolerance.
   g. Begin sitting when patient demonstrates sufficient control of leg to sit within flexion restrictions (usually requires elevation of sitting surfaces, including use of raised toilet seat).
4. Medications
   a. Prophylactic anticoagulant drugs may be prescribed to decrease risk of thrombus formation.
   b. Initially, control pain with positioning and narcotics, gradually tapered to nonnarcotic analgesics according to patient's tolerance.
5. Discharge instructions
   a. Patient must use ambulatory aid, avoid adduction, and limit hip flexion to 90° for about 2 to 3 months (see Figure 61-20).
   b. A raised toilet seat is to be obtained and used at home until flexion restrictions are removed.
   c. Patient may need a long-handled shoehorn and reacher to facilitate ADL within flexion restriction.
   d. Patient must be made aware of the lifelong need for antibiotic prophylaxis when undergoing invasive procedures or dental work to protect the prosthesis from bacteremic infection.

is for the patient to accomplish safe transfer from bed to chair and toilet, perform prescribed exercises independently, and ambulate with the appropriate weight-bearing restrictions using walker, cane, or crutches. The patient should also be taught to ascend and descend stairs safely. Most patients are able to ambulate without an assistive device by 8 to 12 weeks; muscle strength is restored to 80% of normal by 3 to 6 months postoperatively.[1]

Assistive devices to aid the patient in completing ADL are usually obtained through the occupational therapy department. The patient is given instructions about the use of an elevated toilet seat, which prevents extreme hip flexion; long-

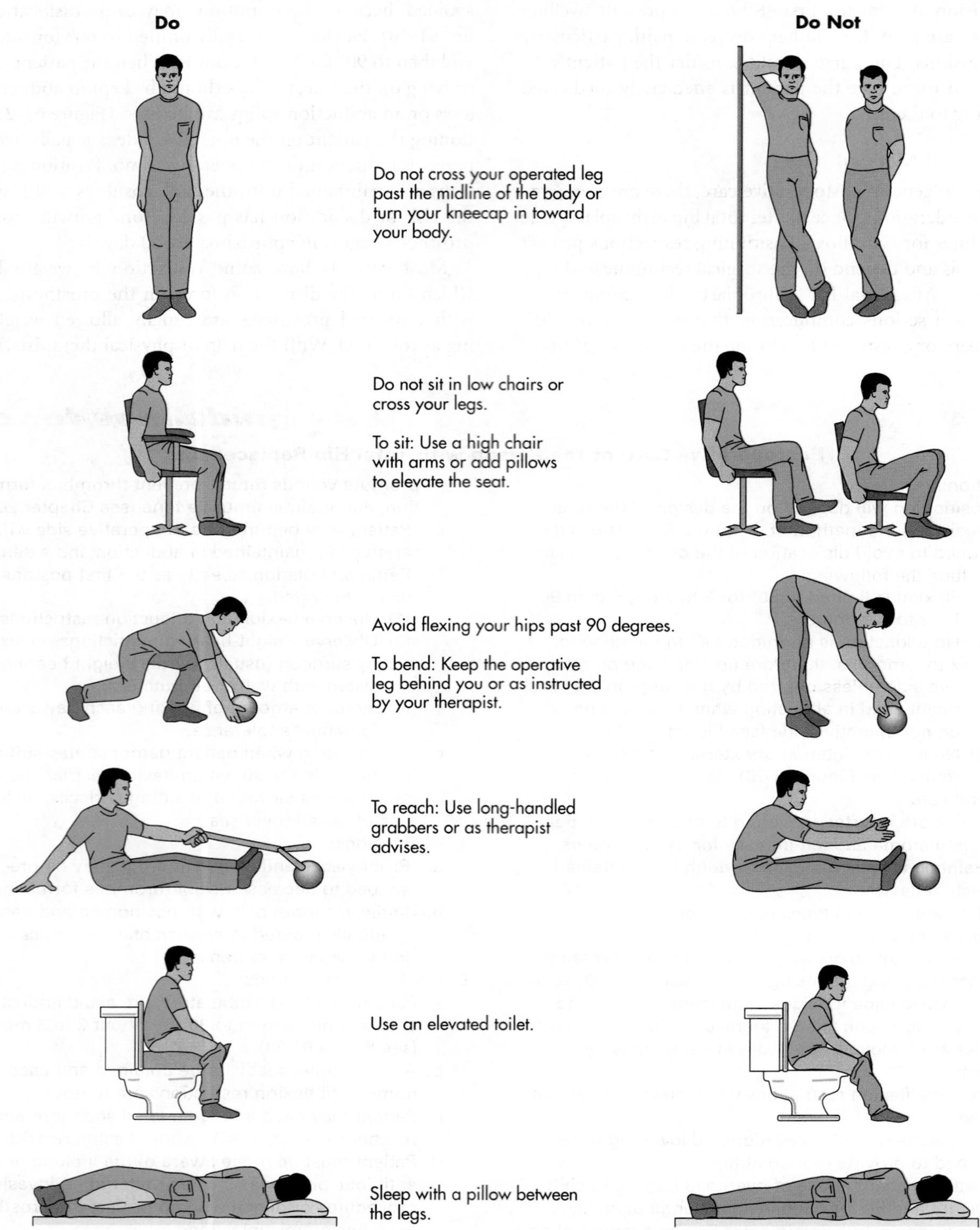
Do
Do Not
Do not cross your operated leg past the midline of the body or turn your kneecap in toward your body.
Do not sit in low chairs or cross your legs.
To sit: Use a high chair with arms or add pillows to elevate the seat.
Avoid flexing your hips past 90 degrees.
To bend: Keep the operative leg behind you or as instructed by your therapist.
To reach: Use long-handled grabbers or as therapist advises.
Use an elevated toilet.
Sleep with a pillow between the legs.

**fig. 61-20** Home-going instructions illustrating *do's* and *do not's* for patients with a total hip replacement. Patients are to avoid extreme flexion (past 90°), adduction, and internal rotation of the operated hip—any of which may cause dislocation of the prosthesis.

handled reachers; and devices that aid in donning shoes and stockings; these items will be used after discharge as well.

### Total Knee Arthroplasty

Postoperative management of persons with total knee replacement may include the use of a continuous passive motion (CPM) machine (Figure 61-22). The CPM machine supports the operative extremity while passively moving it within preset limits of flexion and extension. Use of the CPM machine reduces postoperative swelling, prevents adhesions, decreases pain, and facilitates early mobility. The CPM is usually applied in the operating room or postanesthesia care unit, and patients are encouraged to use the machine while in bed, up to 22 hours per day. Increases in the amount of knee flexion are ordered by the physician. If the CPM is not used, a knee immobilizer is frequently placed over the bulky dressing and is kept in place until the dressing is reduced. Other surgical protocols call for the use of a knee exerciser, which is attached to the overhead frame of the bed and allows the patient to exercise the knee while in bed. The physician will determine when active flexion exercises may begin. There are no real positioning restrictions, although the patient should adhere to the physician's orders regarding the amount weight bearing and knee flexion permitted. Kneeling is usually discouraged. Flexion is increased at intervals. While in bed, the patient is cautioned against having a pillow under the knee, which may cause the knee to remain in a flexed position (see the Guidelines for Care Box).

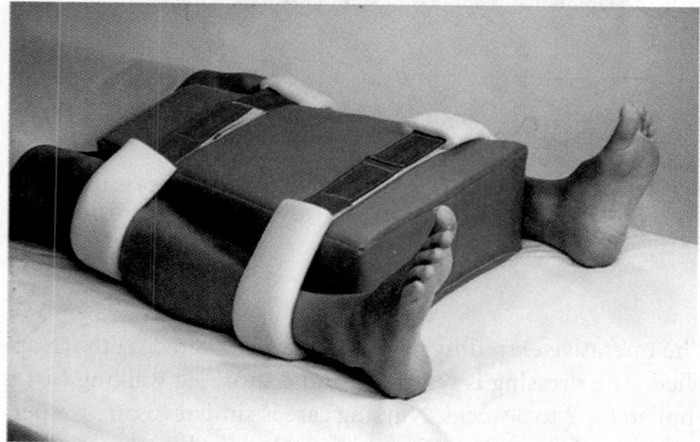

**fig. 61-21** Abduction splint for postoperative hip arthroplasty.

### Total Shoulder Arthroplasty

After total shoulder replacement, the operative extremity is placed in an immobilizer, which is kept in place for 1 to 2 days (Figure 61-23). The sling is then worn at night and for comfort during the day. Passive exercises are initiated immediately after surgery, and pendulum exercises are begun 1 to

**guidelines for care**

**Postoperative Care of the Person with Total Knee Replacement**

1. Positioning
   a. The operative leg(s) is elevated on pillows to enhance venous return for the first 48 hours. Pillows are placed with caution not to flex the knee(s). It is becoming more common for patients to have bilateral total knee replacements at one surgery.
   b. The patient may be turned from side to back to side.
2. Wound care
   a. Care of drains is as for total hip replacement.
   b. Patient is assessed for systemic evidence of loss of blood (hypotension, tachycardia) if bulky compression dressing is used, since it may hold large quantities of drainage before drainage is visible.
   c. Bulky dressings are removed before the patient begins active flexion.
   d. Assess wound for healing and signs of infection. Perform dry sterile dressing change once bulky dressing is discontinued. Leave incision open to air if no drainage.
3. Activity
   a. Passive flexion in a CPM machine within prescribed flexion-extension limits. Patient's leg may remain in machines as much as tolerated (up to 22 hours per day) to facilitate even healing of tissue.
   b. Patient is encouraged to perform active dorsiplantar flexion of the ankles, quadriceps setting, and, after the drain is removed, straight leg-raising exercises.
   c. Patient begins active flexion exercises three to four times per day on about the third postoperative day. The time when active flexion is permitted varies.
   d. Partial weight bearing with an assistive device may be started as early as the first postoperative day and increased as the patient tolerates.
   e. Sitting in a chair with the leg(s) elevated may be started on the first postoperative day.
   f. Patient may be encouraged to wear a resting knee extension splint (immobilizer) on the operative extremity until able to demonstrate quadriceps control (independent straight leg raising).
4. Pain control
   a. Initial control of pain is with narcotics (PCA) and positioning; medication is gradually decreased to nonnarcotic analgesics as patient tolerates.
   b. Ice is usually prescribed to be applied to the knee to reduce swelling and pain.
   c. Patient is encouraged to apply ice to knee(s) for 20 to 30 minutes before and after active flexion exercise.
5. Discharge instructions
   a. Patient must observe partial weight-bearing restriction and use ambulatory aid for approximately 2 months after discharge.
   b. Patient should continue active flexion and straight leg-raising exercises at home.
   c. Patient must be made aware of the lifelong need for antibiotic prophylaxis before invasive procedures or dental work.

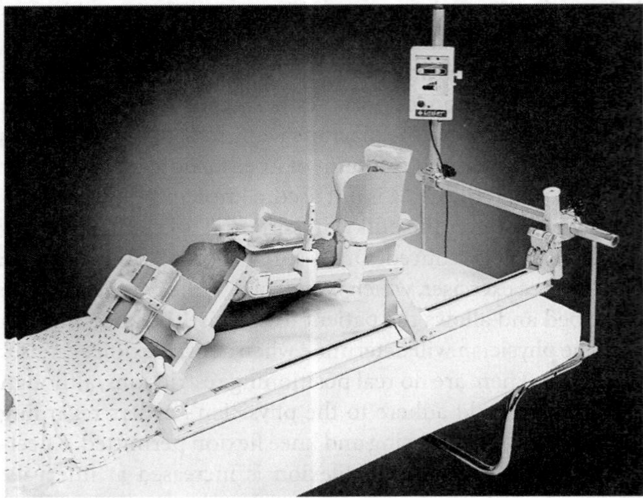

fig. 61-22 Example of CPM machine.

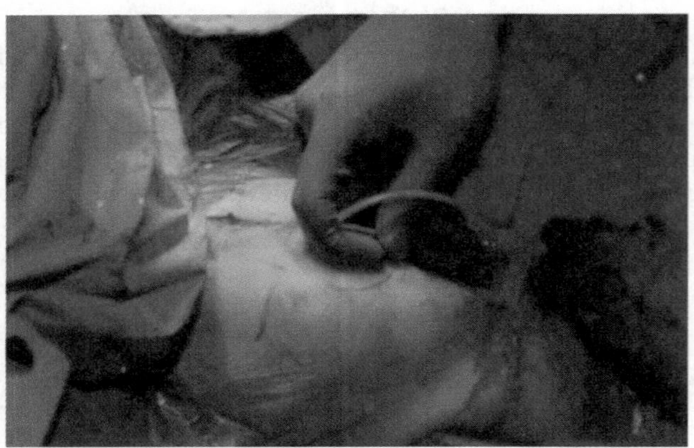

fig. 61-23 Total shoulder arthroplasty with postoperative immobilization. Note Hemovac drain.

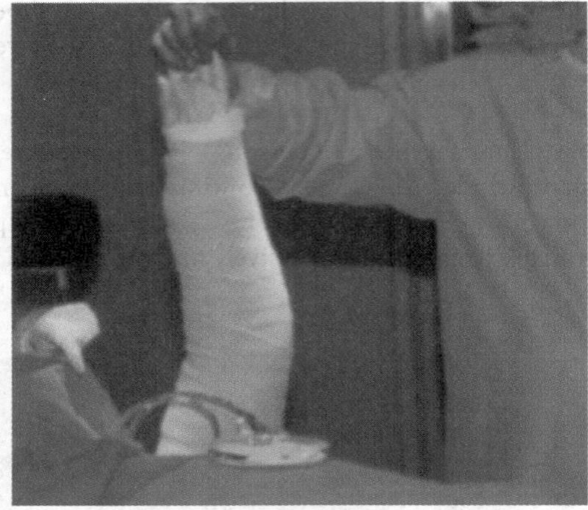

fig. 61-24 Total elbow arthroplasty with postoperative splint and dressing. The elbow is in full extension.

10 days postoperatively (see Chapter 60). Isometric exercises are started the second week. The patient is cautioned to limit the amount of external rotation. Patients having total shoulder replacement may only require overnight hospitalization.

### Total Elbow Arthroplasty

After total elbow replacement, the operative extremity is placed in a plaster splint and bulky dressing (Figure 61-24). The splint may be flexed up to 90°. The arm should be elevated and ice applied. Frequent neurovascular checks are important. The drain is removed within 24 to 36 hours, and the bulky dressing is reduced. Elbow flexion and extension exercises are begun after the dressing is removed. Activity restrictions include limiting lifting to no more than 1 pound for 3 months and less than 5 pounds long term.

### Total Ankle Arthroplasty

Total ankle replacement is performed most frequently for patients with rheumatoid arthritis. Postoperatively, the extremity is placed in a soft compression dressing and plaster splint. The operative extremity should be kept elevated, with ice applied. The dressing is removed, and a short leg walking cast is applied for 2 to 3 weeks. Nursing care is similar to care for person with a fracture (see Chapter 60). Physical therapy and exercises are begun after cast removal.

## GERONTOLOGICAL CONSIDERATIONS

Arthritis is a common problem among the elderly population and may affect their ability to perform ADL and to enjoy usual leisure activities. Osteoarthritis is the most common form of arthritis in the elderly.[46] Over 40% of women older than age 60 have OA. Joint involvement is typically symmetric, and the onset of pain is insidious, progressing to more persistent pain, unrelieved by rest (see the Gerontological Assessment Box, p. 1988.)

Physical therapy is an important treatment for elderly persons with OA. Exercise and PT can improve the quality of life and maintain independence. Resting the affected joint typically provides pain relief, but can contribute significantly to contractures, atrophy of disuse, and osteoporosis.[46] Thus, the elderly patient should be advised to maintain a constant level of physical activity, even in the presence of active arthritis. Passive and active exercises should be performed to maintain range of motion and muscle tone. Swimming and walking are good choices for regular exercise.

Assistive and adaptive devices can improve the quality of life and allow the patient independence in ADL. Orthoses and special shoes for foot problems can help maintain alignment and provide support for diseased joints.

Medications to treat OA should be chosen carefully when elderly patients are treated. The health care provider should be aware of any other medications the patient is taking, which could cause drug interactions. Hepatic and renal function should be evaluated before a pharmacological regimen is prescribed. Acetaminophen in doses up to 4 g is a good choice for elderly patients without renal or hepatic disease. A dose of 4 g of acetaminophen has been shown to be as effective as

*Text continued on p. 1988*

## nursing care plan *The Person with Total Knee Replacement*

**DATA** Mr. K. is a 59-year-old married office manager with osteoarthritis of the right knee. Over the past 8 months, he has had increased pain in his knee with only minimal relief from nonsteroidal antiinflammatory medications prescribed by his nurse practitioner. He reports that he must now ambulate with a cane when his pain is severe. He can no longer participate in many activities he used to enjoy because of his discomfort and limited mobility. After consulting his internist and an orthopedic surgeon, he has decided to undergo elective total knee replacement. Mr. K. is admitted to the nursing division on the morning of the day he is scheduled for surgery. Collaborative nursing actions include those to identify possible complications of the surgery.

The nursing history identified the following:

- Mr. and Mrs. K. reside in a two-story colonial house with the bedroom upstairs.
- Mr. K. plans to return home after this hospitalization and has received a 6 weeks leave of absence from his job.
- He is not taking any medications other than his "arthritis pills" and has no other preexisting medical problems.
- Mr. K. was last hospitalized 18 years ago for a cholecystectomy.
- He attended a total knee replacement class 2 weeks ago as part of his preadmission screening.
- NSAIDs were discontinued 1 week before scheduled surgery date.

Immediate reporting of and treatment of early signs and symptoms may prevent serious complications. Nursing actions to prevent complications include monitoring for the following:

- Atelectasis/respiratory infection: Monitor breath sounds and encourage deep breathing and coughing.
- Neurovascular compromise: Perform vascular checks every 2 hours for the first 24 to 48 hours; notify physician of any changes from preoperative status.
- Assess for bleeding: Monitor VS frequently, check dressing for drainage, measure output from drain; guaiac stool, monitor urine for blood.
- Fluid and electrolyte imbalance: Monitor intake and output until patient is taking oral fluids comfortably; monitor IV fluid intake; measure drain output; assess patient for fluid volume excess or deficit.
- Problems with elimination: Assess for urinary stasis and constipation.
- Impaired skin integrity and/or wound healing: Monitor pressure areas for signs of redness; monitor temperature; assess incision for signs or symptoms of infection or excessive drainage.

**NURSING DIAGNOSIS** *Knowledge deficit related to lack of exposure to total knee replacement surgery*

| expected patient outcomes | nursing interventions | rationale |
|---|---|---|
| States he understands the teaching provided.<br>Will have less anxiety related to fear of the unknown and/or misconceptions regarding the surgery and recovery period. | Preoperatively:<br>**1.** Assess need for further instruction and provide as necessary.<br>**2.** Review preoperative instruction with patient and family before surgery. Use written materials or videos if they are available. Use anatomical model of knee. Show patient examples of knee prostheses.<br>**3.** Evaluate patient's understanding of the information taught. | Understanding the surgical procedure and postoperative recovery should lessen anxiety and promote behaviors that will enhance recovery from surgery. |
| | **4.** Assess if wife is able to assist in care after discharge.<br>**5.** Assess layout of home, number of stairs, proximity of bathroom to bedroom; assess home for potential safety hazards.<br>**6.** If possible, schedule physical therapy (PT) evaluation preoperatively. | Begin planning for discharge before admission.<br>Patient can practice exercises, transfer techniques, ambulation with assistive devices without anxiety of hospitalization, pain, and free from IVs, drains, and catheters.<br>Home may need to be arranged to increase patient's independence and decrease potential for injury postoperatively. |
| | Postoperatively:<br>**1.** Ensure that patient can explain or demonstrate the following:<br>**a.** Independent transfer and ambulation with appropriate ambulatory aid. | |

Continued

## The Person with Total Knee Replacement—cont'd

**NURSING DIAGNOSIS** *Knowledge deficit related to lack of exposure to total knee replacement surgery—cont'd*

| expected patient outcomes | nursing interventions | rationale |
|---|---|---|
| | Postoperatively—*cont'd:*<br>b. Exercises to be performed at home (straight leg raising and active flexion) and with what frequency.<br>c. Activity restrictions, including avoidance of kneeling and jarring activities, that are to be observed for 2 months or until follow-up with the surgeon.<br>2. Evaluate patient's understanding of the need for antibiotic prophylaxis in the future, and reinforce as necessary. | |

**NURSING DIAGNOSIS** *Pain related to knee replacement surgery*

| expected patient outcomes | nursing interventions | rationale |
|---|---|---|
| States he is feeling comfortable. | Assess patient's pain and evaluate response to comfort measures provided. | Subjective and objective data are important to ascertain the nature of the patient's postoperative pain and how to manage it. |
| Is able to perform necessary postoperative routines/exercises because pain is adequately managed. | Patient will have patient-controlled analgesia (PCA) postoperatively.<br>Advise patient to administer dose of PCA before beginning activities, particularly before exercise periods. | It is usually necessary to administer narcotic analgesics the first 48 to 72 hours after surgery. Analgesics have a greater effect if they are administered before pain becomes severe. Self-administered analgesia allows the patient to feel in control of the situation; avoids peaks and valleys of intermittent administration. Patient will perform better in PT if pain is manageable. |
| | Teach relaxation techniques and nonpharmacological methods of pain relief. | Relaxation facilitates rest and may modify the patient's response to pain. |
| | Use other pain-relieving measures as pertinent (e.g., back rubs, repositioning, ice to knee for 30 minutes before and after active flexion exercises). | A change in type of cutaneous stimulation may result in pain relief. Ice is analgesic and reduces swelling. |
| | As pain decreases, use milder analgesics administered orally. | Pain, as it lessens in severity, can be controlled by less potent analgesics that have fewer side effects. |

**NURSING DIAGNOSIS** *Impaired physical mobility related to alterations in lower limb following total knee replacement surgery*

| expected patient outcome | nursing interventions | rationale |
|---|---|---|
| Will demonstrate optimal level of mobility with adaptive devices by time of discharge from hospital. | Turn patient side to back to side every 2 hours and as necessary while bed rest is ordered. | Turning and repositioning frequently provide for better ventilation of the lungs. |
| | Encourage patient to perform active dorsiplantar flexion, isometric quadriceps setting exercises, and, after drain is removed, straight leg raises every 2 hours until fully ambulatory, then 4 times/day. | Exercises of the lower extremities will prevent venous stasis and promote muscle strengthening. |

*Continued*

## The Person with Total Knee Replacement—cont'd

**NURSING DIAGNOSIS** *Impaired physical mobility related to alterations in lower limb following total knee replacement surgery—cont'd*

| expected patient outcome | nursing interventions | rationale |
|---|---|---|
| | Elevate operative leg on pillows in bed and when patient is up in chair for the first 24 to 48 hours. Place pillows so that passive flexion of the knee is avoided. | Elevation of the operative leg on pillows enhances venous return. Flexion contracture is to be avoided. |
| | Assist patient to transfer out of bed on first postoperative day. Weight bearing as tolerated on the operated leg is generally permitted using an assistive device. | The exercise of getting in and out of bed is one means of increasing activity in the early postoperative period. The patient gains numerous physiological benefits from such activity. Weight-bearing restrictions depend upon method of implanting prosthesis. |
| | Assist patient to walk as tolerated, increasing the frequency and the distance walked each day. | Early ambulation is a significant factor in hastening recovery and preventing postoperative complications. |
| | Encourage patient to sit up in a chair as tolerated, especially for meals. | |
| | If continuous passive motion machine is used, patient's leg should be in the machine a minimum of 8 to 12 hours/day and can be in the machine up to 22 hours/day if tolerated. Advance the degrees of flexion according to the surgeon's order. | Passive flexion of the knee may prevent excessive swelling and bruising at the site of the surgery, and it may promote more even healing of the involved joint tissues. |
| | Begin active flexion exercise of the knee on the second postoperative day, and encourage flexion 4 times/day. | Active flexion of the knee is necessary to promote return of function. It is desired that the patient achieve approximately 90° of active flexion before discharge from the hospital. |
| | Encourage use of knee exerciser. | |
| | A knee immobilizer may be worn at night as a night resting splint. | The knee immobilizer splints the resting knee, helping to prevent painful muscle spasm. |

**NURSING DIAGNOSIS** *Impaired home maintenance management related to discharge needs*

| expected patient outcome | nursing interventions | rationale |
|---|---|---|
| Patient and family will express satisfaction with arrangements made to transfer to rehabilitation facility or to manage self-care at home. | Discuss with patient and family any problems they anticipate with management of self-care at home. | Adequate discharge planning will foster safe, successful completion of rehabilitation at home. |
| Knowledgeable about home-going medications. | Determine the type of equipment needed, for example, crutches, walker, or elevated toilet seat; consult PT and OT to obtain supplies. | |
| Is able to administer own anticoagulants (enoxapril subcutaneously or warfarin orally). Patient and family are able to state bleeding precautions and side effects of medication. | Assure that the patient can climb stairs. If not, help the patient to arrange for first floor sleeping arrangements. | |
| Is aware of need for follow-up appointment with surgeon, laboratory appointments to monitor coagulation studies if needed, and physical therapy appointments. If discharged directly home, will need outpatient PT. | | |

## gerontological assessment

**ASSESSMENT**

Assess all elderly persons for muscle strength and tone, gait, sensory deficits, painful joints or muscles, contractures, deformities, and foot problems that may interfere with ambulation and ADL.

Assess availability, condition, and use of assistive aids, such as walkers, canes, or crutches.

Assess environmental factors conducive to falls because elderly persons are at high risk for falls.

**INTERVENTION**

Order assistive aids to foster independence and to increase ambulation, such as walker, cane, lift, and bedside commode.

Encourage an exercise program to maintain baseline muscle and joint function.

Perform active and passive range of motion for elderly persons needing bedrest.

Obtain orders for progressive ambulation as early in hospitalization as possible.

Position extremities in proper body alignment; elderly persons are highly susceptible to flexion contractures.

Teach good foot care and importance of well-fitted shoes.

Request physical therapy for patients with gait or mobility problems.

Request occupational therapy for problems with ADL and fine motor coordination.

Teach elderly persons how to transfer and ambulate safely.

Initiate a fall-prevention program that identifies risk factors and promotes an individualized plan for each patient, depending on ability and tendency to fall.

Use restraints only as a last resort; assess patient every hour while restrained, reevaluate use every 4 to 8 hours; remove them hourly for range of motion.

Be sure environment is free of clutter, bed is kept in lowest position, and night-light illuminates the floor.

2.4 g of ibuprofen in the treatment of OA.[46] Lower doses of NSAIDs are usually indicated for elderly patients to avoid increased toxicity. A CBC, urinalysis, and liver and kidney function tests should be performed before treatment with NSAIDs and at 1- to 3-month intervals thereafter. Increased age has been identified as a significant risk factor for the development of side effects associated with NSAIDs.[46] NSAIDs found to be most toxic to the elderly include indomethacin, tolmetin, and meclofenamate.[46] Sulindac is thought to be a safe choice for the elderly patient with impaired renal function, heart failure, or hypertension.[46] A good choice for the elderly is Arthrotec, a combination of diclofenac sodium (NSAID) and misoprostol (a prostaglandin with antisecretory and mucosal protective properties). The pill is coated with misoprostol (Cytotec); the NSAID medication is at the core. This medication was approved by the Food and Drug Administration (FDA) in 1998.

Many elderly patients with OA require or elect surgical intervention to relieve pain or to improve mobility. Any coexisting disease such as heart disease, hypertension, diabetes, or kidney problems must be stabilized before elective surgery. See Chapters 18 to 20 for perioperative considerations for the elderly patient.

After surgical intervention, the elderly patient may be discharged to a rehabilitative facility to continue with physical therapy and to attain independence in ADL, transfers, and ambulation. If the patient is transferred directly to home, a family member, friend, or home health care referral will be necessary to assist in care.

## SPECIAL ENVIRONMENTS FOR CARE

### Home Care Management

Patients and their families should be informed that the rehabilitative phase after joint replacement lasts at least 1 year. At 1 year, most patients have achieved approximately 90% of functional return. Over the next 2 years, functional ability and muscle strength are increased, reaching a maximum increase at 3 years.[1] Patients and families should be reminded that cooperation in the rehabilitative process is necessary for success. Daily exercise is an important component of the recovery process.

Because of the shortened length of stay (4 to 6 days for total hip replacement), most patients are discharged to a subacute facility or rehabilitative center for physical therapy. Some patients do opt to be discharged directly home. Patients who are discharged to home need a referral for home physical therapy or need to make arrangements for outpatient PT. A home health nurse visit should be scheduled for suture or staple removal.

The follow-up appointment with the orthopedic surgeon is usually at 6 weeks postoperatively. After 6 weeks, patients are allowed a little more flexibility in activity and can usually resume sexual activity. Research indicates that patients want more information regarding sexual activity after total hip replacement, but are hesitant to ask.[1] When it is safe to resume sexual activity is a topic that nurses need to address, preferably at the preoperative visit, but certainly before discharge. Generally 6 to 8 weeks is the recommended time for refraining from sexual intercourse. Persons with joint revisions may need additional time. Other sexual activities (touching or caressing) can be alternatives until intercourse can safely be resumed. Once intercourse is resumed, appropriate positioning of the affected extremity is a key consideration. Persons with hip replacements should continue to observe hip flexion limits of no more than 90°. Extremes of external rotation, adduction, and abduction should be avoided. Persons with joint replacements should assume the passive position during sexual intercourse.[61]

The patient should be cautioned against driving without consulting the surgeon. Patients with total hip replacements generally have sufficient muscle strength to resume driving a car with an automatic transmission at 6 weeks; persons having the right hip replaced may have to wait until 8 weeks.[1]

When the patient has regained maximal strength, he or she may resume low-impact exercise such as walking, swimming, golfing, biking, bowling, and tennis. High-impact activities and exercises that place an increased load on the joints are not recommended as they decrease the longevity of hip prostheses.[1]

Teaching includes information about home-going medications, particularly anticoagulants. The patient and family should be aware of the purpose, side effects, dosage, and method of administration of prescribed medications. The patient and family should be knowledgeable about the signs and symptoms of complications, such as prosthesis dislocation, infection, DVT, fat embolus, and pulmonary embolus.

Temporary rearrangement of the home environment may be necessary, especially if the patient returns directly home. It may be more convenient if the bathroom and bedroom are on the same floor; a bedside commode or urinal can be used temporarily. The bed should be arranged so the patient can exit the bed on the opposite side of the operative leg. The floors and doorways should be free from any obstructions. Throw rugs should be removed. A firm chair with armrests is necessary for persons recovering from total hip or knee surgery. The height of the seat can be raised by adding pillows. The room can be arranged with commonly used items within close reach of the patient. A tote bag can be attached to the patient's walker to carry the phone, reachers, or other necessary items. A raised toilet seat is needed for persons with total knee and hip replacements. For bathing, long-handled sponges allow the patient to wash his or her legs. A walk-in shower is best, and a chair can be added for safety. If the patient has a tub, a sponge bath may be easier for the first few weeks. If the patient has pets, a friend or family member may be needed to help care for them. Small dogs or cats may easily trip a person using a walker, cane, or crutches. The patient should be instructed to wear comfortable, well-fitting, nonskid, walking shoes. Regular follow-up appointments are continued for the first year and as necessary thereafter.

## COMPLICATIONS

Complications associated with total joint replacement include the following: wound infection (superficial or deep), thrombophlebitis or DVT, pulmonary embolus, fat embolus, and dislocation of the prosthesis. Other complications associated with the surgical procedure include urinary tract infection (if an indwelling catheter is used) and pneumonia. It should be stressed that infection is a potentially severe complication after joint replacement. Deep infection may necessitate removal of the prosthesis.

Over 50% of hip infections occur more than 3 months postoperatively. Infections that develop within the first 3 postoperative months are usually superficial or suprafascial infections (Stage I). Deep or subfascial infections are commonly seen within 3 to 24 months postoperatively (Stage II). Infections occurring later than 24 months postoperatively are usually attributed to hematogenous spreading from other locations in the body (Stage III).[70]

Stage II infections are attributed to direct contamination of the wound in the operating room (50% to 80% cases).[2] Symptoms associated with mechanical loosening of the prosthesis resemble those of stage II infections; however loosening rarely occurs in the first year after replacement.[2] A patient's report of a *new* pain in the operative site should be immediately investigated. Conditions such as diverticulitis, cellulitis, abscesses, or seeding resulting from dental procedures, GI procedures, or any surgery can be a source of Stage III infections.

Once an infection occurs, there are several treatment options. The patient's condition and causative organism are major determinants of treatment. Surgical debridement, resection arthroplasty, arthrodesis, amputation, antibiotic therapy, and reimplantation are all options for treating persons with infected total joints. If infection necessitates removal of the prosthesis, first the area is debrided, and then the appropriate antibiotics are administered, based on culture and sensitivity results. Reimplantation of the joint is done between 6 weeks and 1 year, depending upon the causative organism and the condition of the patient. Antibiotics are continued for several weeks. Intraoperatively, antibiotic-treated cement can be used for susceptible organisms during reimplantation. If it is not possible to replace the prosthesis in a patient with a total hip replacement, a *girdlestone* hip results. Fibrous scar tissue replaces the hip joint, but the patient can still ambulate. In the case of a total knee replacement that cannot be replaced, the patient can undergo an arthrodesis, resulting in an immobile knee joint. Patients with severe systemic infection, intractable pain, or extensive bone loss may eventually require an amputation.

Persons with rheumatoid arthritis are more likely to develop major wound complications due to immunosuppressive medications used to treat RA. Patients with diabetes are also at an increased risk for developing infections after total joint replacement.

In addition, DVT, pulmonary embolus, and fat embolus are potentially fatal complications occurring after total knee or hip replacement. An estimated 0.5% to 0.8% of patients develop fat embolus after joint replacement.[44] Pulmonary embolus is fatal in 2% to 3% of patients with total hip replacement and in 1% to 3% of patients with total knee replacement.[44]

Dislocation of the prosthesis is a particular concern for persons with hip replacements. Dislocation can add significant morbidity and possibly an additional surgical procedure. The rate of dislocation in patients with unilateral hip replacement in acute and rehabilitative settings ranges from 1.27% to 2.17%.[32] Half the hip dislocations in the rehabilitation setting occurred during transfers. Safety precautions and education of patients and personnel are necessary during the rehabilitation process and during the acute care phase. See Box 61-6 for other complications of total joint arthroplasty.

## GOUT

### Etiology

*Podagra,* or foot pain, was first described in the fourth century BC. Gout was considered a disease of the wealthy, associated with rich food and wine. *Gout* is a clinical syndrome resulting from the deposition of urate crystals in the synovial fluid, joints, or articular cartilage. Considered a metabolic disorder, gouty arthritis develops as a result of prolonged hyperuricemia (elevated serum uric acid) caused by problems in the synthesis of purines or by poor renal excretion of uric acid.

Gout must be distinguished from *pseudogout,* which occurs as a result of calcium pyrophosphate dihydrate (CPPD) crystals. Pseudogout resembles gout with intraarticular calcium deposits and CPPD crystals in synovial fluid and affects primarily elderly persons. Articular cartilage, menisci, and adjacent tendinous or ligamentous structures are affected by pseudogout. Persons with previous joint trauma or a history

**box 61-6** *Complications of Total Joint Arthroplasty*

**HIP**
- Dislocation
- Infection
- DVT
- Pulmonary embolus
- Fat embolus
- Leg length discrepancy
- Altered gait
- Pneumonia
- Foot drop (secondary to nerve damage)

**KNEE**
- Infection
- DVT
- Pulmonary embolus
- Fat embolus
- Acute compartment syndrome
- Instability
- Loosening of prosthesis
- Patellar fracture
- Poor patellar tracking
- Vascular injury (intraoperative) and hemorrhage
- Reflex sympathetic dystrophy
- Nerve damage

**SHOULDER**
- Infection
- Loosening of the prosthesis
- Glenohumeral instability
- Dislocation, subluxation
- Intraoperative fracture
- Rotator cuff tears
- Deltoid dysfunction
- Nerve damage
- Impingement syndrome
- Pulmonary embolus

**ELBOW**
- Infection
- Dislocation
- DVT
- Pulmonary embolus
- Loosening of prosthesis
- Delayed healing of wound

**ANKLE**
- Infection
- Residual pain
- Impingement
- Loosening of prosthesis

of menisectomy are prone to developing pseudogout. Both disorders resemble rheumatoid arthritis.

## Epidemiology

The prevalence of gout in the United States is between 0.3% and 1%.[27] Gout affects men eight to nine times more frequently than women. It can occur at any age, with the peak age of onset occurring in the fifth decade. Eighty-five percent of all persons with gout have a genetic or familial tendency to develop the disease.

**box 61-7** *Causes of Secondary Gout*

**OVERPRODUCTION OF URIC ACID**
- Paget's disease
- Cancer
- Polycythemia vera
- Multiple myeloma
- Chronic myelocytic and lymphocytic leukemia
- Hemolytic anemias
- Cytotoxic drugs

**UNDEREXCRETION OF URIC ACID**
- Chronic renal insufficiency
- Ketoacidosis
- Lactic acidosis
- Drug ingestion (diuretics, cyclosporine, levodopa, pyrazinamide, low-dose salicylates)

**UNKNOWN ETIOLOGY**
- Hyperparathyroidism
- Hypoparathyroidism
- Hypothyroidism
- Adrenal insufficiency

## Pathophysiology

Hyperuricemia is not necessary for the diagnosis of gout. Uric acid levels are controlled by diet, purine metabolism, and renal clearance. Approximately 25% of persons with chronically elevated uric acid levels will develop gouty arthritis eventually.[27]

Gout is classified as primary or secondary. Underexcretion of uric acid is caused by decreased tubular secretion, increased tubular resorption, or a combination of both. Approximately 75% of patients develop *primary gout* as a result of undersecretion of uric acid. The remaining 25% of persons develop primary gout as a result of overproduction of uric acid. Primary gout is idiopathic; affected persons tend to also have hypertension and obesity.[27]

*Secondary gout* results from an overproduction of uric acid secondary to increased purine catabolism or impaired excretion of uric acid. Secondary gout usually occurs in the acute care setting (Box 61-7).

Urate crystals form in the synovial tissue, causing severe inflammation. The inflammatory process is extremely rapid, occurring over a few hours. Acute symptoms are extreme pain, swelling, and erythema of the involved joints. Typically the first metatarsophalangeal joint of the great toe is involved (50% of patients), but other joints, such as the ankle, heel, knee, or wrist, may also be affected. Pain is so severe that the patient may not tolerate even the weight of a sheet over the joint. Renal damage may occur, especially if recurrent uric acid stones have been present. Between attacks of gout, the patient may be asymptomatic, but repeated attacks can occur with gradually increasing frequency if the disease is untreated. Patients with gouty symptoms may develop *tophi,* or deposits of monosodium urate in their tissues. These consist of a core of monosodium urate with a surrounding inflammatory reaction. Patients with tophaceous deposits (Figure 61-25) tend to have more frequent and more severe episodes of gouty arthritis.

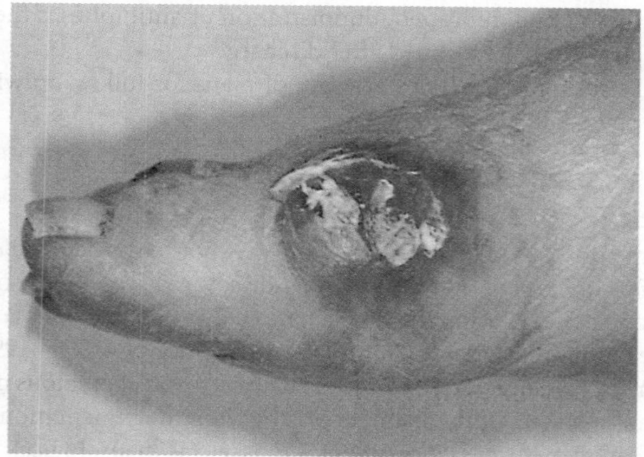

**fig. 61-25** Gouty tophus on right foot.

## Collaborative Care Management

Laboratory studies will indicate an elevated serum uric acid, normal or increased urinary uric acid level over a 24-hour period, and the presence of monosodium urate monohydrate crystals in the synovial fluid and in the tophi. Treatment is focused on control of acute attacks, prevention of recurrent attacks, and long-term uricosuric therapy to prevent formation of tophi.

Colchicine, once considered the mainstay of treatment, is used less frequently for management of acute attacks because of the distressing side effect of diarrhea. The ability to inhibit phagocytosis of urate crystals by neutrophils is the key to colchicine's effectiveness. Colchicine is not effective once an attack has been present for several days. However, in persons who are able to recognize the symptoms of an acute attack, one to two 0.6-mg tablets of colchicine may be taken to thwart the attack. Initially a 1-mg dose is given, followed by 0.5- to 0.6-mg doses every 1 to 2 hours until diarrhea develops (to a maximum of 8 mg). Joint inflammation usually subsides within 48 hours in 75% to 80% of patients.[14] Colchicine may also be given intravenously to avoid gastrointestinal (GI) effects, but it is associated with systemic toxic effects, including bone marrow suppression and liver and kidney damage.

For persons with adequate renal function and no other contraindications, NSAIDs are considered first-line therapy. The maximum dose should be prescribed as early as possible in an acute attack and continued for 5 to 7 days. Although any NSAID may be prescribed, indomethacin has been successful in the treatment of gout.

For persons in whom NSAIDs are contraindicated, the administration of corticosteroids is effective. Intraarticular injections or systemic therapy can be used for treatment of acute attacks.

Future attacks of acute gout can be prevented by the administration of colchicine or NSAIDs. Pharmacological prophylaxis should be initiated before uric acid levels are corrected. Prophylaxis with colchicine decreases the number of acute attacks, regardless of the serum uric acid level. Controversy exists regarding the duration of prophylactic therapy. Treatment for 1 year after the serum uric acid levels return to normal is usually considered adequate.[14] NSAIDs can also be used prophylactically, but are associated with more side effects than colchicine.

Prevention of gouty attacks can be accomplished by identifying and correcting the cause of hyperuricemia. Medications can be given that inhibit the synthesis of urate or increase its secretion. Some causes of hyperuricemia may require lifelong medication to decrease serum levels. Attention should be focused on factors that increase uric acid levels. The factors that contribute to increased urate production are regular alcohol consumption, obesity, and a high purine diet. Alcohol should be avoided because it not only increases production of uric acid but prevents its excretion.

Serum uric acid levels should be lowered to approximately 5 mg/dl, not just to normal range. Uric acid levels less than 5 mg/dl deplete urate stores and prevent tophi and renal damage.[57]

Rest and joint immobilization are recommended until the acute attack subsides. Local application of cold can relieve pain. Application of heat should be avoided, as it will increase the inflammatory process.

### *Patient/family education*

Nursing management includes the following:

1. Patient teaching
   a. Instruct patient in nature of disease.
   b. Instruct patient in proper use of prescribed medications.
   c. Encourage patient to lose weight gradually if overweight.
   d. Encourage lifestyle modifications to control hypertension or adherence to pharmacological regimen.
   e. Encourage patient to take in sufficient fluid to assure daily output of 2000 to 3000 ml.
   f. Advise patient to avoid excessive intake of purines (sweet breads, yeast, heart, herring, herring roe, and sardines and excessive alcohol intake).
   g. Explain to patient that severe dietary purine restriction is not necessary as long as his or her hyperuricemia is well controlled by daily medication therapy.
2. Promoting comfort
   a. Provide absolute rest until the pain of an acute attack subsides.
   b. Avoid touching the joint or moving the affected extremity until the acute pain subsides.

## BACTERIAL OR SEPTIC ARTHRITIS

### Etiology

Bacterial arthritis is the result of invasion of the synovial membrane by microorganisms, most often *Neisseria gonorrhoeae,* meningococci, streptococci, *Staphylococcus aureus,* coliform bacteria, *Salmonella,* and *Haemophilus influenzae.* Bacteria can enter the joint by hematogenous spread, direct inoculation, or extension from an adjacent infection. Hematogenous infection is the most common cause of bacteria arthritis.

Persons with an underlying medical illness are at greatest risk. Immunodeficiency, chronic disease, intravenous drug abuse, local joint surgery or trauma, intraarticular injections, and rheumatoid arthritis also place the person at risk for bacterial arthritis.

### Pathophysiology

Synovial tissues respond to bacterial invasion by becoming inflamed. The joint cavity may become involved, and pus will be present in the synovial membrane and the synovial fluid. If allowed to progress, the infection will cause abscesses in the synovium and subchondral bone, eventually destroying cartilage. Ankylosis of the joint may result. The patient will report pain, swelling, and tenderness of the joint.

### Collaborative Care Management

Joint aspiration is performed to identify the causative organism and determine treatment. Strict aseptic technique must be followed to avoid introducing additional bacteria into the joint. White blood cell counts will be high, and the glucose content of synovial fluid may be reduced. X-ray films taken days to weeks after the onset of infection may reveal loss of joint space and lytic changes in bones.

Treatment should begin immediately. Medical management includes the following:

1. Appropriate antibiotic therapy.
2. Rest or immobilization of the joint
3. Surgical drainage by needle aspiration, arthroscopy, arthrotomy, or a system of irrigation and drainage if infection does not respond to antibiotic therapy or if osteomyelitis is present. Needle aspiration of purulent exudate may be required daily until drainage ceases. Infections of the hip joint must be drained immediately to prevent necrosis of the femoral head.
4. Resumption of active range of motion when infection subsides and motion can be tolerated

Nursing management includes the following:

1. Promoting rest of the affected joint
2. Administering antibiotics on time and as prescribed to maintain blood levels
3. Administering prescribed pain medication as necessary
4. Encouraging the patient to participate in self-care to the extent possible within restrictions of prescribed rest for the joint

#### *Patient/family education*

The results of treatment depend upon the infecting organism, duration of infection before treatment, and host defenses. The patient should be educated about signs and symptoms of bacterial arthritis and about seeking prompt treatment if symptoms recur. Prompt diagnosis and treatment can save the joint from destruction. The immunodeficient patient should be taught how to avoid sources of infection.

Antibiotic therapy may be prescribed for prolonged periods of time; the patient should be encouraged to comply with treatment to ensure eradication of infection. Other teaching includes the following:

1. Instructing in care of cast or other immobilizing device
2. Encouraging active joint motion when motion is permitted
3. Instructing about use of crutches or assistive devices
4. Instructing in proper administration of antibiotics if therapy is to be continued after discharge
5. Ensuring that patient is aware of plans for follow-up with physician

## LYME DISEASE

### Etiology/Epidemiology

Lyme disease (LD) is caused by the tick-borne spirochete *Borrelia burgdorferi.* The disease was discovered in Lyme, Connecticut, in 1976 and declared a nationally notifiable disease by the Centers for Disease Control and Prevention (CDC) in 1991. For surveillance purposes, the presence of an erythematous migrans rash >5 cm in diameter or laboratory documentation of infection with evidence of musculoskeletal, neurological, or cardiovascular disease confirms the diagnosis of Lyme disease.[43] LD is transmitted by ticks, present most commonly on deer, mice, dogs, cats, raccoons, cows, and horses. Deer ticks are responsible for 95% of cases of LD. Birds help spread infected ticks by their migratory flights. The tick bite is usually painless, and the patient may not remember being bitten.

The disease has been reported in most European countries, throughout Asia, and in 45 states and the District of Columbia in the United States. LD is the number one vector-borne disease in the United States. The overall incidence in the United States is 4.4 per 100,000 population (16,461 cases in 1996).[43,59] The disease is prevalent in the northeastern, north-central, and mid-Atlantic regions of the United States. Persons affected have ranged in age from 2 to 88 years, and persons living in endemic areas with outdoor exposure are at risk.[28] The peak months for early clinical manifestations of the disease are June through October. The trend in the United States toward utilization of farmlands and forest increases the contact between humans and vectors and is responsible for the increasing rates of the disease. Humans can be exposed to the ticks in wooded areas and in well-landscaped areas in endemic regions. Transmission of the disease from the tick to humans requires some time. Attachment of the tick for less than 24 hours rarely transmits the disease; attachment for at least 72 hours or more almost certainly transmits the disease.[28] The incubation period from exposure to onset of symptoms is from 3 to 32 days.[28]

### Pathophysiology

LD has been called the "great imitator" because it mimics other disease such as influenza, rheumatoid arthritis, multiple sclerosis, chronic fatigue syndrome, amytrophic lateral sclerosis, fibromyalgia, lupus erythematosus, and Alzheimer's disease.[28,59] Infection with *B. burgdorferi* stimulates inflammatory cytokines and autoimmune mechanisms, which results in Lyme arthritis. Primarily an extracellular organism, *B. burgdorferi* is thought to invade some cells and cross the blood-brain barrier, resulting in the neurological manifestations of LD.

Infection with *B. burgdorferi* can be divided into three stages. Not all patients develop all stages. The early manifestations of the disease are usually self-limiting, and the late manifestations can become chronic (Box 61-8). The arthritis associated with LD is either monoarticular or oligoarticular, affecting the knee and other large joints. Inflammation is a result of immune complex deposition in the synovium.[60] Chronic and recurrent arthritis develops in 10% of persons. If untreated, 50% of persons will develop migratory polyarthritis.[59]

### Collaborative Care Management

The varied signs and symptoms, coupled with the fact that most persons do not remember the tick bite, make diagnosis difficult. Serological tests used to diagnose LD include enzyme-linked immunosorbent assay (ELISA), Western blot, and indirect immunofluorescence assay. Less than 50% of persons with Stage I disease have detectable antibodies; in Stage II disease the percentage rises to 70% to 90%. Both serum and cerebrospinal fluid should be tested to diagnose Lyme disease. Synovial fluid may be sampled if arthritic symptoms are present.

Patients in Stage I disease should be treated with tetracycline or doxycycline to prevent development of further symptoms. During Stages II and III, intravenous therapy is indicated, usually ceftriaxone (crosses the blood-brain barrier), cefotaxime, or penicillin. Administration of ceftriaxone has been associated with biliary problems necessitating cholecystectomy in persons being treated for LD.[28]

The patient should be monitored for development of cardiac and neurological sequelae. Persons with musculoskeletal symptoms resulting in impaired mobility may require PT and occupational therapy (OT), and analgesics to relieve joint pain. Nursing care would be similar to interventions for patients with rheumatoid arthritis (see p. 1968-1970).

#### *Patient/family education*

A vaccine against Lyme disease was approved by the FDA in 1998. One year is required for optimal immunity, and the need for booster shots has not been determined. The vaccine is not for use in children younger than 15 years or in persons with chronic arthritis.

Education is the best prevention against LD (see the Patient/Family Teaching Box). For persons with the disease,

**box 61-8** *clinical manifestations*

***Lyme Disease***

**STAGE I (EARLY LOCALIZED INFECTION)**

Symptoms appear days to 16 weeks after tick bite
Erythema migrans appears in 50% to 70% of patients, resolves spontaneously in a few weeks
Fatigue
Headache
Lethargy
Myalgia, arthralgia
Lymphadenopathy

**STAGE II (EARLY DISSEMINATED INFECTION)**

Symptoms occur weeks to months after tick bite

**Cardiac Symptoms**

Carditis
Dysrhythmias
Heart failure
Pericarditis
Palpitations
Dyspnea

**Neurological Symptoms**

Meningitis
Encephalitis
Cranial and peripheral neuropathy
Myelitis

**Musculoskeletal Symptoms**

Arthralgia, myalgia
Fibromyalgia

**Other Symptoms**

Conjunctivitis, optic neuropathy
Hepatomegaly, hepatitis
Generalized lymphadenopathy

**STAGE III (LATE INFECTION)**

Symptoms occur months to years after tick bite
Monoarticular or oligoarticular arthritis
Chronic arthritis
Acrodermatitis chronica atrophicans (bluish-red, doughy lesions)
Lyme encephalitis, encephalomyelitis
Ataxia
Spastic paresis
Periventricular lesions
Memory loss
Behavioral changes

***patient/family teaching***

**Lyme Disease Prevention**

- Avoid tick-infested areas and sitting directly on the ground. Stay on paths while hiking.
- When outdoors in high-risk areas, wear long sleeves and long pants in light colors (to easily see ticks). Tuck shirt into pants and pants into shoes or socks.
- Wear closed shoes when hiking.
- Use EPA-approved tick repellents on skin and clothing. Wash off repellent thoroughly when returning inside. Avoid spraying repellents directly on skin of small children.
- Check frequently for ticks; pets should be checked also.
- Have pets wear tick collars; do not allow outdoor pets on furniture or bedding,
- If a tick is found, use a fine pointed tweezer to grasp the tick at the point of attachment, gently pull the tick straight out. Place the tick in a sealed jar and have it tested by a local veterinarian or health department. Do not squeeze the tick, doing so may release infected fluids.
- Wash the tick site thoroughly with soap and warm water, apply antiseptic, and disinfect the tweezers. Wash hands. Wash clothes thoroughly.
- Ticks are susceptible to dehydration. Reduce humidity by pruning trees, clearing brush, and mowing the lawn on your property.
- Do not have bird feeders or birdbaths in your yard, these attract animals that may have ticks.
- Keep woodpiles away from the house.
- Keep children's play areas away from wooded areas.
- See a physician or nurse practitioner if flu-like symptoms or a rash develops.

education about the signs and symptoms and complications of later disease is necessary. Patients and families will need to learn about joint protection and energy conservation techniques.

Nurses can provide community education to prevent the disease, especially in areas where the disease is prevalent. Education about the signs and symptoms of the disease is important to ensure early recognition and treatment of persons with LD. If LD is untreated, severe neurological, cardiac, and musculoskeletal manifestations may occur. If the disease is diagnosed, cases should be reported to community health officials. Patients can be referred to: The Lyme Disease Foundation, 1 Financial Plaza, Hartford, CT 06103; (860) 525-2000 or National Hotline (800) 886-LYME; e-mail: lymefnd@aol.com; www.lyme.org.

## SERONEGATIVE ARTHROPATHIES

*Seronegative arthropathies* is a term used to describe a group of diseases characterized by arthritis (arthropathy), in which the rheumatoid factor is *not* present in the serum. Approximately 2 million persons in the United States have seronegative arthropathies. Diseases included in this category are Reiter's syndrome, psoriatic arthritis, enteropathic arthritis, and ankylosing spondylitis (Table 61-9). The majority of persons with ankylosing spondylitis and Reiter's syndrome have a specific gene, HLA-B27, which is found in only 7% of the general population.

These diseases are also known as the *spondyloarthropathies* and have several characteristics (other than a negative rheumatoid factor) in common. These include:

- Frequent bouts of *spondylitis* (inflammation of the vertebrae characterized by stiffness and pain)
- *Enthesitis* (inflammation at tendon attachment sites to bone)
- Presence of the cell marker HLA-B27
- Common extraarticular manifestations (iritis and skin lesions)

Ankylosing spondylitis is discussed in the following section.

**table 61-9** *Seronegative Arthropathies*

| Disorder | Etiology | Signs and Symptoms | Collaborative Management |
|---|---|---|---|
| Reiter's syndrome (Reactive arthritis) | Sexually transmitted organisms or GI bacteria<br>Precipitating event commonly urethritis[25]<br>Common organisms: *Chlamydia, Salmonella, Shigella* | Classic triad: *arthritis, urethritis,* and *conjunctivitis*<br>Acute onset of monoarthropathy or oligoarthropathy<br>Fatigue, fever, generalized aching, joint stiffness, and back pain<br>Arthritis usually affecting the knees, ankles, feet, or wrists<br>Oral or genitourinary lesions; cutaneous lesions on soles and palms | Goals: alleviate pain, maintain joint mobility, and relieve systemic symptoms<br>Medications: antibiotics for underlying infection, NSAIDs, sulfasalazine, methotrexate, ocular or topical steroids[25]<br>PT referral may be indicated; application of heat or cold for comfort<br>Patient education regarding the disease<br>No cure; exacerbations in one third of persons |
| Psoriatic arthritis | Complication of psoriasis<br>Occurs in 7% of persons with psoriasis<br>Possible genetic predisposition<br>May result from abnormal immune response to *Streptococcus* that collects in psoriatic skin lesions | Distal interphalangeal joints of fingers, toes (sausage digits)<br>Spondyloarthropathy similar to ankylosing spondylitis<br>Sacroiliac joint involvement<br>Skin lesions<br>Nail changes (see Chapter 63) | Similar to treatment for rheumatoid arthritis |
| Enteropathic arthritis | Develops in 9-20% of persons with inflammatory bowel disease, specifically ulcerative colitis and Crohn's disease (see Chapter 41)<br>May result from an immune response to intestinal bacteria | Arthritis in multiple joints, particularly the knees, ankles, and wrists<br>Spine, hips, and shoulders also affected<br>Occurs during exacerbations of bowel disease and disappears when bowel symptoms subside<br>In persons with spondylitis, symptoms not correlated with bowel symptoms | Similar to treatment for rheumatoid arthritis |

## Ankylosing Spondylitis

### Etiology

Ankylosing spondylitis is a chronic inflammatory disorder affecting the sacroiliac joints and spine. The etiology is unknown. The course of the disease is marked by remissions and exacerbations.

### Epidemiology

Ankylosing spondylitis affects approximately 300,000 people in the United States, usually between the ages of 20 and 40 years.[26] Men are affected three times more often than women. There is a strong genetic link with the genetic marker HLA-B27, and it is thought that a link between the marker and some form of trigger (perhaps an infection) sets off a reaction in the immune system that leads to the inflammatory process. *Klebsiella* is thought to be the causative organism.[60] African Americans have a lower incidence of the disease, whereas the incidence in Native Americans is 18% to 50%.

### Pathophysiology

Spondylitis means inflammation of the spine. As a result of inflammation, the bones of the spine grow together and ankylose (fuse). The primary site of pathological findings is the *enthesis,* where ligaments, tendons, and joint capsule insert into bone. In ankylosing spondylitis, fibrous ossification and eventually fusion of the joint occur. The joint capsule, articular cartilage, and periosteum are invaded by inflammatory cells that trigger the development of fibrous scar tissue and growth of new bone. The bony growth changes the contour of the vertebrae and forms a new enthesis called a *syndesmophyte* on top of the old one. As the spinal ligaments continue to undergo progressive calcification, the vertebral bodies lose their original contour and appear square, which gives the spine the classic "bamboo" appearance of ankylosing spondylitis. Inflammation usually begins around the sacroiliac joints and progresses up the spine, eventually resulting in fusion of the entire spine. As the inflammatory process involves the costosternal and costovertebral cartilage, it causes chest pain, which is worse on inspiration.

Initial symptoms may include low back pain or aching; pain and swelling of the hips, knees, or shoulders; mild fever; loss of appetite; and fatigue. Low back pain flares and subsides intermittently. Over time, pain subsides and motion of the back becomes restricted. Fusion of the sacroiliac joints and spine up through the cervical vertebrae may occur over a period of 10 to 20 years. As a result of rigidity, fractures may develop at multiple sites. The spine loses its normal lordotic curve and the patient may have either a "poker back" deformity or a kyphosis at the cervicodorsal junction (Figure 61-26). The knees are flexed as the person attempts to move the head upright.

Ankylosing spondylitis is a systemic disease that may affect the eyes, heart, and lungs. One third of persons develop uveitis, which causes tearing, photosensitivity, and ocular pain. Involvement is typically unilateral. Internal organ involvement is rare and occurs in persons with long-standing disease (>20 to 30 years).

### Collaborative care management

Diagnosis is made by history and physical examination and the following findings:

1. X-ray films show the presence of syndesmophytes and "bamboo" spine. Ankylosis of peripheral joints may be seen. Computed tomography (CT) scans and magnetic resonance imaging (MRI) may show changes before they are visible on plain films.
2. Erythrocyte sedimentation rate is elevated.
3. Test for rheumatoid factor is negative.
4. HLA-B27 is present in the serum (test not routinely performed due to expense).

Goals of treatment are to relieve pain, achieve and maintain the best possible alignment of the spine, strengthen the paraspinal muscles, and maintain maximal breathing capacity. Following are the most common interventions:

1. Salicylates
2. NSAIDs (Phenybutazone is effective, but may cause bone marrow toxicity.)
3. Sulfasalazine and systemic steroids are avoided, except for patients with severe eye disease
4. Exercise is an important component of treatment. Swimming in a warm pool is a good choice for exercise. Rest should be discouraged, unless a fracture is present.

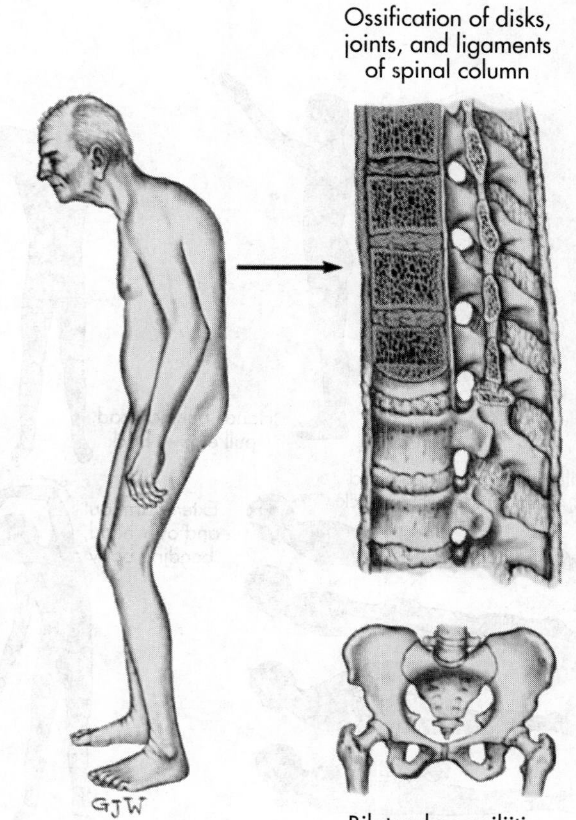


**fig. 61-26** Characteristic posture and sites of ankylosing spondylitis.

5. Physical therapy to maintain mobility and reduce severity of deformity, for example, ROM exercises and lying prone (extension) 3 to 4 times per day for 15 to 30 minutes and deep breathing exercises to promote maximum chest expansion (rib cage mobility is decreased) (Figure 61-27).
6. Heat
7. Use of thoracic lumbar sacral orthosis (TLSO)
8. Cervical head halter traction to decrease muscle spasms and distract the spine
9. Spinal osteotomy and fusion, usually cervical
10. Hip arthroplasty
11. Valve replacement or pacemaker insertion if cardiac involvement present

**Patient/family education.** Patient teaching focuses on the following:

1. Facilitating learning
   a. Nature and course of disease
   b. Prescribed exercises
   c. Appropriate use of prescribed medications
   d. Methods of applying heat to back and hips
2. Promoting maximum mobility and reducing severity of deformity
   a. Maintain proper posture and walk erect.
   b. Provide firm mattress and bed board.
   c. Encourage patient to sleep without pillow under the head to maintain extension of spine; lying prone or supine is recommended; avoid side-lying.

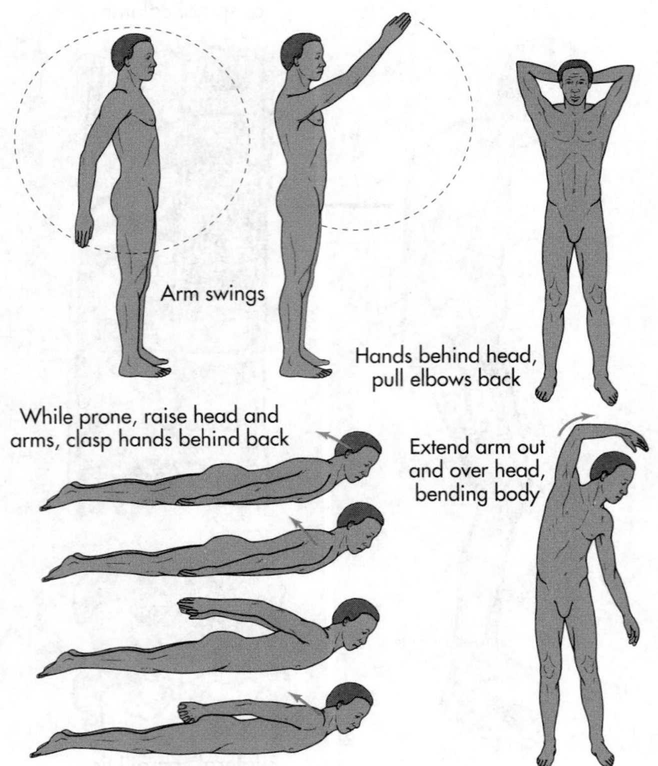
Arm swings
Hands behind head, pull elbows back
While prone, raise head and arms, clasp hands behind back
Extend arm out and over head, bending body

**fig. 61-27** Typical chest-cage stretching and deep chest breathing exercises for ankylosing spondylitis.

   d. Supervise and encourage regular exercises; assist as necessary. Regular deep breathing exercises are important to optimize respiratory function. Persons with ankylosing spondylitis should not smoke.
   e. Encourage participation in ADL and usual activities to the fullest extent possible.
   f. Refer to an occupational therapist for adaptive or supportive devices. Recommend use of long-handled reachers, sponges, and shoe horns for patients with hip involvement.
3. Promoting comfort and relieving pain
   a. Provide heat applications/hydrotherapy, especially before exercises.
   b. Administer prescribed medications on time.
   c. Assess effectiveness of pain relief measures.
4. Promoting acceptance of body image

## AUTOIMMUNE CONNECTIVE TISSUE DISEASES

Several autoimmune disorders affect the joints. These diseases are of unknown etiology and are similar to rheumatoid arthritis, affecting the skin and other organs. These disorders include systemic lupus erythematosus, scleroderma, CREST syndrome (calcinosis cutis, Raynaud's phenomenon, esophageal motility disorder, sclerodactyly, and telangiectasia), and Sjögren's syndrome (Table 61-10). Nursing care for the person with musculoskeletal symptoms are similar to the care for the person with rheumatoid arthritis. Lupus is discussed in the following section.

### SYSTEMIC LUPUS ERYTHEMATOSUS

#### Etiology

Lupus was described as early as the time of Hippocrates. Today, lupus is classified as discoid (see Chapter 63), systemic, and drug induced.[3] Systemic lupus erythematosus (SLE), which means "red wolf" is a chronic inflammatory disease of autoimmune origin that affects primarily the skin, joints, and kidneys, although it may affect virtually every organ of the body. The disease was named after the characteristic rash, the erosive nature of the rash being "likened to the damage wrought by a hungry wolf."[3]

The etiology is unknown. Factors associated with the development of lupus include:

1. Genetic factors may contribute to the development of the disease. Family members of persons with SLE have an increased chance of developing the disease.
2. Environmental factors have been associated with cases of SLE. For example, exposure to ultraviolet light is known to cause exacerbations. Drugs, including procainamide (Pronestyl), isonicotinic acid hydrazide (isoniazid), hydralazine, anticonvulsants, and chlorpromazine, are known to induce lupus-like syndromes. Persons with drug-induced lupus do not develop renal and neurological disease. The symptoms usually resolve after the drug is discontinued. Other areas being considered include a viral origin and disturbances in estrogen metabolism.

3. Alterations in the immune response may cause immune complexes containing antibodies to be deposited in tissue, causing tissue damage.

## Epidemiology

SLE affects women, particularly young and middle-aged adults, 8 to 10 times more often than men. An estimated 500,000 persons in the United States have SLE with 16,000 new cases diagnosed each year.[34] The incidence in African American women is 3 times greater than in white women. Asian and Polynesian persons have an increased incidence over white persons in Hawaii. During the reproductive years the incidence of SLE is 10 times greater in women than in men. Menses and pregnancy can cause an exacerbation of the disease. The risk for developing SLE drops significantly after menopause in women, but remains constant throughout the lifespan in men. Although there is no cure, the course of SLE can usually be controlled. Previously thought to be fatal, 95%

**table 61-10** *Autoimmune Connective Diseases*

| Disorder | Pathophysiology | Clinical Manifestations | Treatment |
|---|---|---|---|
| **Scleroderma (Systemic sclerosis)** | Most common in middle-aged women<br>Causes microvascular damage and fibrous degeneration of tissue in the skin, GI tract, lung, and kidneys | Raynaud's phenomenon<br>GI: dysphagia, gastroesophageal reflux disease (GERD), diarrhea, and malabsorption<br>Renal: hematuria, proteinuria, renal crisis, hypertension<br>Cardiopulmonary: pericarditis, dysrhythmias, pulmonary hypertension, fibrosis<br>Dermatological: hardening, tightening, and thickening of skin; edema, pallor, and deepened pigmentation<br>Musculoskeletal: muscle atrophy, rheumatoid arthritis, tightening of tendons, flexion contractures | Avoidance of cold; protective clothing<br>Skin care for ulcers<br>Thoracic sympathectomy for Raynaud's phenomenon<br>Metoclopramide, cisapride, $H_2$ blockers, and esophageal dilation for GI symptoms<br>Captopril for renal symptoms<br>NSAIDs, calcium channel blockers, prednisone, bronchial lavage for cardiopulmonary symptoms<br>NSAIDs, PT, OT, exercises to maintain joint mobility<br>Splints for contractures and deformities<br>Heat and cold as needed<br>D-Penicillamine and colchicine used to decrease collagen with some success[4] |
| **CREST syndrome (Limited cutaneous scleroderma)** | Variant of scleroderma, classified by the extent of skin thickening<br>More favorable prognosis and less organ involvement | Calcinosis (result of chronic vascular insufficiency)<br>Intracutaneous or subcutaneous calcifications on digital pads, periarticular tissues, extensor surfaces of forearms, olecranon and prepatellar bursae<br>Raynaud's phenomenon<br>Esophageal dysmotility<br>Sclerodactyly<br>Telangiectasia<br>Pulmonary involvement in many patients | As for scleroderma<br>Surgical removal of calcium deposits |
| **Sjögren's syndrome** | Inflammation and dysfunction of the exocrine glands, particularly the lacrimal and salivary glands, which results in dryness of the mouth, eyes, and mucous membranes<br>Lymph nodes, bone marrow, and organ involvement<br>Rheumatoid arthritis in 50% of patients | Xerostomia<br>Dyspareunia<br>Decreased tearing<br>Gritty sensation in eyes<br>Dysphagia<br>Dental caries<br>Cough<br>Enlarged parotid glands<br>Rheumatoid and antinuclear antibody factors positive in most patients<br>Anemia | Artificial tears<br>Vaginal lubrication<br>Surgical punctal occlusion<br>Increased fluid intake, especially with meals<br>Good dental and oral hygiene, especially after meals<br>Avoidance of respiratory infections<br>Increased humidity in home and work environment |

of persons with SLE survive 5 years or longer. Some patients may die as a result of lesions affecting major organs or from secondary infections.

### Pathophysiology

The exact mechanism of pathogenesis is unknown. However, several alterations in the immune system are associated with SLE. Numerous cellular antibodies have been identified in persons with the disorder. Antinuclear antibodies, antibodies to DNA, antihistones, and antibodies to ribonucleoprotein (Smith antigen) are all strongly associated with SLE.

Abnormalities in both B cells and T cells have also been identified in persons with the disease. The appearance of B cells is thought to cause an increase in production of antibodies to self and nonself antigen. These antibodies are responsible for the tissue injury seen in SLE. Most visceral lesions are mediated by type III hypersensitivity, and antibodies against red blood cells are mediated by type II hypersensitivity. An acute necrotizing vasculitis can occur in any tissue. Most lesions are found in the blood vessels, kidney, connective tissues, and skin.

Because of the multisystem involvement and characteristic remissions and exacerbations, the clinical manifestations of SLE can be overwhelming. The American College of Rheumatology has developed criteria for the diagnosis of SLE (Table 61-11). The initial manifestation of SLE is often arthritis, typically a nonerosive synovitis without deformity. Ninety-five percent of persons with SLE develop arthritis. Joint deformity occurs without bony erosion and resembles that of persons with rheumatoid arthritis. Contractures may also develop. In many instances the joint symptoms are transient and respond to treatment. Weakness, fatigue, and weight loss may be present. The patient may report photosensitivity, development of a rash, and at times fever or ar-

**table 61-11** *American College of Rheumatology: Criteria for Classification of Systemic Lupus Erythematosus**

| Criterion | Definition |
|---|---|
| 1. Malar rash | Fixed erythema, flat or raised, over the malar eminences, tending to spare the nasolabial folds |
| 2. Discoid rash | Erythematous raised patches with adherent keratotic scaling and follicular plugging; atrophic scarring may occur in older lesions |
| 3. Photosensitivity | Skin rash as a result of unusual reaction to sunlight, by patient history or physician observation |
| 4. Oral ulcers | Oral or nasopharyngeal ulceration, usually painless, observed by a physician |
| 5. Arthritis | Nonerosive arthritis involving two or more peripheral joints, characterized by tenderness, swelling, or effusion |
| 6. Serositis | (a) Pleuritis—convincing history of pleuritic pain or rub heard by a physician or evidence of pleural effusion, or<br>(b) Pericarditis—documented by electrocardiogram or rub or evidence of pericardial effusion |
| 7. Renal disorder | (a) Persistent proteinuria greater than 0.5 g/dl or greater than 3+ if quantitation not performed, or<br>(b) Cellular casts—may be red blood cell, hemoglobin, granular, tubular, or mixed |
| 8. Neurological disorder | (a) Seizures—in the absence of offending drugs or known metabolic derangements, e.g., uremia, ketoacidosis, or electrolyte imbalance, or<br>(b) Psychosis—in the absence of offending drugs or known metabolic derangements, e.g., uremia, ketoacidosis, or electrolyte imbalance |
| 9. Hematological disorder | (a) Hemolytic anemia—with reticulocytosis, or<br>(b) Leukopenia—less than $4.0 \times 10^9$/L (4000/mm$^3$) total on two or more occasions, or<br>(c) Lymphopenia—less than $1.5 \times 10^9$/L (1500/mm$^3$) on two or more occasions, or<br>(d) Thrombocytopenia—less than $100 \times 10^9$/L ($100 \times 10^3$/mm$^3$) in the absence of offending drugs |
| 10. Immunological disorder | (a) Positive lupus erythematosus cell preparation, or<br>(b) Anti-DNA antibody to native DNA in abnormal titer, or<br>(c) Anti-Sm—presence of antibody to Sm nuclear antigen, or<br>(d) False-positive serological test for syphilis known to be positive for at least 6 months and confirmed by negative *Treponema pallidum* immobilization or fluorescent treponemal antibody absorption test |
| 11. Antinuclear antibody | An abnormal titer of antinuclear antibody by immunofluorescence of an equivalent assay at any point in time and in the absence of drugs known to be associated with drug-induced lupus syndrome |

Data from Tan EM et al: The revised criteria for the classification of systemic lupus erythematosus, *Arthritis Rheum* 25:1271, 1982.

*The classification is based on 11 criteria. For the purpose of identifying patients in clinical studies, a person shall be said to have systemic lupus erythematosus if any 4 or more of the 11 criteria are present, serially or simultaneously, during any interval of observation.

thritis on exposure to sunlight. Erythema, usually in a butterfly pattern, appears over the cheeks and bridge of the nose. The margins of these lesions are bright red, and the lesions may extend beyond the hairline with partial alopecia above the ears. Lesions may also occur on the exposed part of the neck. Lesions spread slowly to the mucous membranes and other tissues of the body, or they may originate there. These lesions do not ulcerate but cause degeneration and atrophy of tissues.

Depending on the organs involved, glomerulonephritis, splenomegaly, hepatomegaly, pleuritis, pericarditis, lymphadenopathy, peritonitis, neuritis, or anemia may be present. Renal and neurological manifestations are among the more serious complications of the disease.

### Collaborative Care Management

Diagnosis is made after evaluation of the history and physical examination and results of laboratory tests. See Table 61-11 for selected laboratory findings.

The immunofluorescence test for antinuclear antibodies (ANAs) is positive in more than 95% of patients with SLE; the higher the titer the more likely the diagnosis of SLE. However, the diagnosis of SLE cannot be made solely upon a positive ANA result, because it is also positive in many other autoimmune disorders, such as systemic sclerosis (both CREST syndrome and diffuse sclerosis), Sjögren's syndrome, and polymyositis. It is also positive in 10% of the normal population. As mentioned earlier, antibodies against double-strand DNA and anti-Smith antigen are positive in 20% to 60% of patients with SLE. The LE cell test is positive in 70% of patients with SLE. The LE cell is any phagocytic leukocyte that has engulfed the nucleus of an injured cell.

The following medications are given for SLE:

1. NSAIDs to control arthritic symptoms; diclofenac, naproxen, and oxaprozin are effective in treating lupus. Renal function must be monitored carefully.
2. Antimalarial drugs, particularly if rash is extensive
3. Corticosteroids for severe neurological and renal involvement or if NSAIDs and antimalarial drugs ineffective
4. Cytotoxic agents if other drugs fail (cyclophosphamide)
5. Ointments or skin creams for rash

Kidney failure is the most common cause of death in persons with lupus. Cyclophosphamide is effective in treating lupus nephritis, but is associated with toxicity. Dialysis or transplant may be indicated for patients with uncontrolled lupus nephritis. Orthopedic surgery may be required for persons with severe arthritic manifestations of SLE.

During exacerbations, persons with SLE are acutely ill. Nursing care will depend upon the symptoms manifested. The patient should be monitored for the effects of medications and the possibility of renal failure. The patient's neurological status must be assessed frequently.

Nursing interventions to maintain musculoskeletal functioning are similar to those for caring for persons with rheumatoid arthritis.

#### Patient/family education

In addition to joint protection and energy conservation techniques, the patient and family will need instruction on ways to resume independence in ADL (see p. 1968).

The patient should be instructed to avoid sun exposure and to apply sunscreen (SPF 15 or higher) liberally when outdoors. Sun exposure exacerbates skin and systemic manifestations. When skin manifestations are present, the patient should be taught to keep the lesions clean and avoid secondary sources of infection. Any cosmetics used on the face should be hypoallergenic. Wigs may be used to mask hair loss.

The patient and family may need help in coping with a chronic systemic disease with an unpredictable course. Compliance may be an issue particularly because strict adherence to the treatment regimen does not necessarily prevent exacerbation.

Because most persons affected with SLE are women in child-bearing years, pregnancy should be addressed. Pregnancy does not induce SLE flares, but pregnancy should be planned in consultation with the patient's physician, usually an obstetrician who treats high-risk patients.

Factors such as fatigue, sun, stress, and infection can exacerbate SLE. The patient and family should be taught measures to deal with stress. Physical changes, such as the rash, alopecia, or joint deformities, may cause problems with body image or social isolation. Nursing interventions can assist the patient in accepting changes and coping with a chronic disease.

## INFLAMMATORY MYOPATHIES

Polymyositis and dermatomyositis are considered to be both rheumatic connective tissue diseases and idiopathic inflammatory myopathies. Both may occur alone or in combination with other rheumatic diseases, most notably scleroderma, SLE, and Sjögren's syndrome.

### Polymyositis/Dermatomyositis

#### Etiology/epidemiology

*Polymyositis* (PM) is a chronic acquired inflammatory disorder of skeletal muscle. When a characteristic skin rash is present, the disorder is called *dermatomyositis* (DM). The etiology of both disorders is unknown, but abnormal reactions of the immune system have been implicated, perhaps triggered by a virus. Autoantibodies are found in the serum of affected individuals. The incidence of both disorders is estimated to be 6 per 1,000,000 population; PM and DM are the most common inflammatory muscle diseases.[41] PM occurs two times more frequently in women than men.

#### Pathophysiology

Both polymyositis and dermatopolymyositis are characterized by inflammation of muscle fibers and connective tissue, resulting in extensive tissue necrosis and destruction of muscle fibers. Both cell-mediated and humoral immune mechanisms are associated with the diseases. Inflammatory cells found at the perimysial and perivascular sites contain B cell and helper T cells in dermatomyositis. Less vascular involvement occurs in polymyositis, and B and T cells are found surrounding the muscle fibers and fascicles.

Results of histological studies of biopsied muscle are variable, but the pathological alterations found, in order of their frequency, are as follows:

1. Primary degeneration of muscle fibers, either focal or extensive
2. Basophilia of some fibers with central migration of the sarcolemmal nuclei
3. Necrosis of parts or entire groups of muscle fibers
4. Inflammation of blood vessels supplying the muscles
5. Interstitial fibrosis varying in severity with the duration and, to some extent, the type of the disease
6. Variation in the cross-sectional diameter of fibers

The initial symptoms of both disorders are similar to those associated with any inflammatory response: fever, swelling, malaise, and fatigue. The diseases, which run a course of exacerbations and remissions, are usually first noted in proximal muscles, in particular the pelvic and shoulder girdles. The weakness is symmetric. Climbing stairs, rising from a chair, and other activities that involve lifting the body become increasingly difficult or impossible. Lifting the arms becomes progressively more difficult, and hair combing may be impossible. Other muscles such as the neck flexors and the muscles of swallowing may also become involved. Muscle pain or tenderness is present in some instances in the early stages.

Clinical manifestations common to both polymyositis and dermatomyositis include dysphagia, dyspnea, decreased esophageal motility, cardiomyopathy, and Raynaud's phenomenon. A dusky red lesion may be found in the periorbital region (*heliotrope*) along with periorbital edema in persons with DM. This dusky red rash may extend over the face, forehead, neck, upper shoulders, chest, and upper back. Scaly lesions on the arms and legs commonly affect the extensor surfaces. Erythema occurs over the metacarpophalangeal and proximal phalangeal joints. Calcinosis can also occur in dermatomyositis.

The weakness of myositis, if it persists, can lead to contractures and atrophy. Individuals with dermatomyositis, particularly if they are older than 50 years of age, have a 40% to 50% greater chance of having evidence of a malignant neoplasm found during the first 5 years of illness than the population at large. Some physicians believe that routine yearly examinations should be performed to define or exclude the presence of neoplasms in these patients during that 5-year period.

### Collaborative care management

Diagnosis is based on the following:

1. History and physical examination including manual muscle test to delineate weakness in specific muscles
2. Electromyogram to delineate a specific pattern of findings to differentiate polymyositis from other types of muscle disease
3. Muscle biopsy to define specific pathological changes in muscle
4. Serum enzyme levels (creatine phosphokinase, lactate dehydrogenase, and aldolase), which are elevated in the presence of active disease
5. 24-hour urine tests to determine abnormal creatine/creatinine ratio

High-dose corticosteroid therapy (prednisone up to 60 mg daily) is used for patients with PM or DM. Serial muscle testing will help document response to treatment. With clinical improvement, steroid dosage should be tapered to 10 to 20 mg daily and continued for 1 year. With exacerbations, high-dose steroid therapy is reinstituted. If steroids are contraindicated or ineffective, an immunosuppressant such as methotrexate is prescribed. Blood counts and liver enzymes should be monitored while the patient is receiving therapy. Cyclosporin has been used effectively in some patients, and hydroxychloroquine may improve the rash in persons with DM.

Nursing responsibilities include the following:

1. Promoting comfort
   a. During acute episodes, assist with frequent changes of position.
   b. Administer prescribed analgesics.
   c. Assist with ADL.
   d. Provide adequate rest.
2. Promoting mobility
   a. Elevate sitting surfaces to facilitate transfer.
   b. Provide appropriate ambulatory device to facilitate comfortable walking.
   c. Provide for frequent changes of position and range of motion to prevent contractures.
   d. Encourage patient to gradually resume independent ADL as symptoms subside.
   e. Refer patient to PT for exercise program to maximize functional ability and maintain mobility. Steroid-induced myopathy may occur with long-term steroid use.
3. Preventing skin breakdown
   a. Reposition patient frequently.
   b. Assess skin for integrity.
   c. Topical steroids may be prescribed for the rash in persons with DM.

**Patient/family education.** Teaching includes the following:

1. Instruct patient and family in nature and course of disease. The patient should be aware of the need for serial laboratory and clinical examinations.
2. Instruct patient in appropriate balance of rest and activity.
3. Instruct patient in use of selected ADL devices to enhance function (e.g., long-handled comb). Home health services may be required during acute phases of illness because of muscle weakness. Family and caregiver support will be needed.
4. Instruct patient in appropriate use of prescribed drugs (how to take them, dosage, side effects, and precautions).

## FIBROMYALGIA SYNDROME

Although fibromyalgia syndrome (FMS) is considered to be a generalized pain syndrome, it is discussed here because of its association with rheumatoid arthritis, SLE, polymyositis, and Sjögren's syndrome. Other generalized pain syndromes affecting the musculoskeletal system include polymyalgia rheumatica, which can be accompanied by a destructive, inflammatory arthritis (Table 61-12). Polymyalgia rheumatica often occurs with giant cell arteritis.

## Etiology/Epidemiology

FMS was established as a diagnosis in 1990,[40] although it has been described for more than 90 years. Fibromyalgia is the cause of more unemployment than rheumatoid arthritis and osteoarthritis combined, resulting in an annual cost in excess of $9.2 billion in the United States. An estimated 5 to 6 million persons in the United States are affected by this disorder, which is characterized by widespread musculoskeletal pain and tenderness to palpation at anatomically defined tender points. A secondary type of fibromyalgia has been identified in persons with rheumatoid arthritis, osteoarthritis, and sleep apnea.

The etiology is unknown, but there is an association between sleep disturbances and fibromyalgia. More than 50% of patients with fibromyalgia have sleep disturbances and symptoms of the disorder occur in unaffected persons when stage 4 non–rapid eye movement (REM) sleep is disrupted.[12] Muscle microtrauma and an imbalance of neurotransmitters have also been implicated as possible causative factors. Trauma or infection may trigger the onset of symptoms.

Symptoms typically occur between the ages of 20 and 40 years, mainly in women (80% to 90%).[41] The prevalence is estimated at 2% and increases with age.

## Pathophysiology

Fibromyalgia may appear with RA or SLE or other pain syndromes and is considered in the differential diagnosis of RA, SLE, polymyalgia rheumatica, myositis, neuropathies, and hypoparathyroidism. The pathophysiology of FMS is not completely understood. Several abnormalities in muscle have been documented in persons with FMS, including lower ATP and ADP levels, higher levels of AMP, and changes in the number of capillaries and fiber area. A general hypothesis is that increased muscle tenderness is the result of generalized pain intolerance, perhaps as a result of central nervous system (CNS) abnormalities (Figure 61-28).

## Collaborative Care Management

The American College of Rheumatology defined diagnostic criteria for FMS in 1990 (Box 61-9 and Figure 61-29). Palpation of the tender points should reproduce pain, not tenderness or pressure. A pressure threshold meter can be used for objectivity. Excessive or inadequate pressure can lead to false-positive or false-negative results. Tender points must be present bilaterally, above and below the waist, and in the midline.

The characteristic symptom of fibromyalgia is a generalized chronic pain, which may be described as "burning or gnawing."[41] Chronic aching, nonrestorative sleep, morning stiffness, and fatigue are commonly reported by patients with FMS. Patients with FMS demonstrate loss of functional abilities similar to patients with RA, yet no radiographic changes in articular structures are found in persons with FMS. An estimated 30% to 40% of persons with FMS also have depression, a finding very similar to the prevalence of depression in persons with RA.[22] Headaches, sensitivity to extreme temperatures, abdominal pain, paresthesias, menstrual irregularities, irritable bowel, and difficulty concentrating may be reported. There are no visible signs of FMS.

There is no cure for FMS. Goals of therapy are to restore sleep and reduce pain. A multidisciplinary approach to managing the person with FMS is most effective. Medications used to treat FMS include tricyclic antidepressants to increase non-REM sleep; amitriptyline, cyclobenzaprine, and imipramine are commonly used.[12,22,40] Fluoxetine, a selected serotonin reuptake inhibitor, can be given in the morning to avoid compounding sleep disturbances. A combination of a tricyclic

**table 61-12** *Polymyalgia Rheumatica*

| Epidemiology | Etiology | Clinical Manifestations | Treatment |
|---|---|---|---|
| Peak incidence: whites older than age 50 years; average age at onset 70 yr<br>Twice as many women as men<br>Incidence in African Americans 15%<br>Affects 54 persons per 100,000 population yearly[62] | Unknown etiology<br>Theories include: trauma to cell-mediated response, immune process; normal aging process; genetic predisposition or environmental influences such as infectious agents, drugs, and toxins[12,40,41] | ESR 50 mm/hr<br>Anemia<br>Elevated C-reactive protein and elevated alkaline phosphatase<br>Creatine kinase normal and rheumatoid factor negative<br>Acute or insidious onset of symptoms<br>Morning stiffness lasting >30 min classic symptom<br>Bilateral aching in the shoulders, neck, and pelvic girdle<br>Knees, elbows, wrists, and metatarsophalangeal joints also affected<br>No radiological evidence of bone erosion<br>Fever, anorexia, night sweats, apathy, depression, weight loss, and malaise | Low-dose steroid therapy, typically prednisone, tapered after 4- to 6-wk course of therapy<br>Possibility of disease recurrence within 18 mo of cessation of prednisone<br>Patient teaching about signs and symptoms of disease and medications<br>Encourage adequate rest and regular exercise |

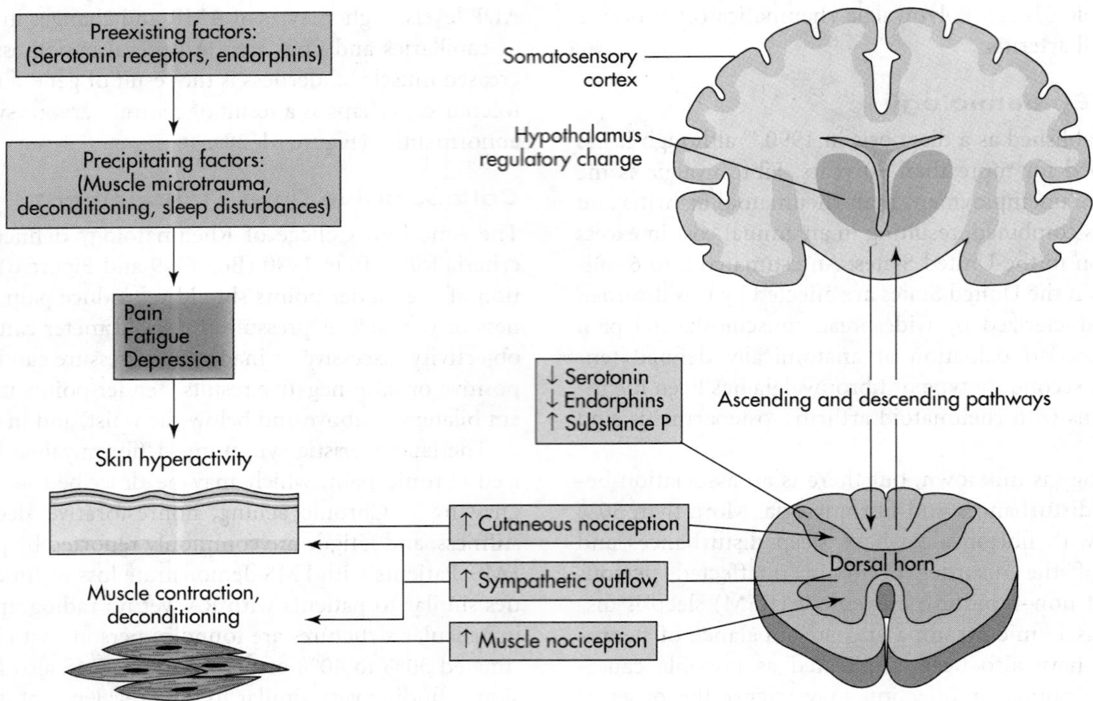


**fig. 61-28** Theoretical pathophysiological model of fibromyalgia.

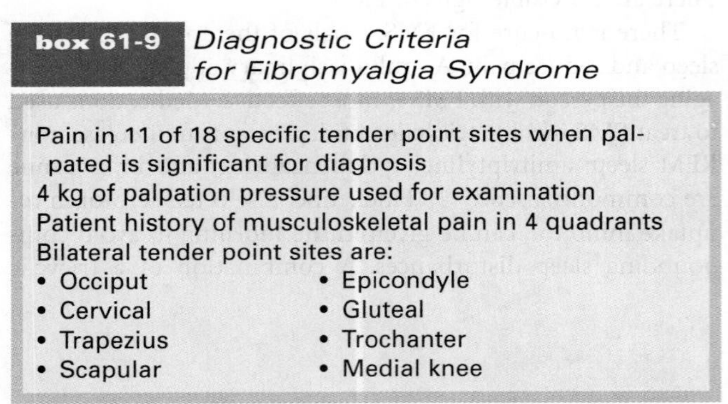

**box 61-9** *Diagnostic Criteria for Fibromyalgia Syndrome*

Pain in 11 of 18 specific tender point sites when palpated is significant for diagnosis
4 kg of palpation pressure used for examination
Patient history of musculoskeletal pain in 4 quadrants
Bilateral tender point sites are:

- Occiput
- Cervical
- Trapezius
- Scapular
- Epicondyle
- Gluteal
- Trochanter
- Medial knee

Data from Golbus J: The locomotor system. In Rakel RE, editor. *Conn's current therapy,* Philadelphia, 1997, WB Saunders.

given at bedtime and an SSRI taken in the morning may be effective in restoring adequate sleep and reducing fatigue. Muscle relaxants can be prescribed to treat muscle spasms; cyclobenzaprine has both antidepressant and muscle relaxant qualities and is a good choice. Tramadol and topical anesthetics have had limited success in controlling pain, but more research is needed. NSAIDs may also be used for pain control.

Exercise is an important treatment modality for persons with FMS. Stretching exercises, PT, and massage can aid in relaxation, reducing fatigue, and improving overall conditioning. Other relaxation techniques such as biofeedback, deep breathing, and meditation can be useful adjuncts to pharmacological therapies. Stress management techniques should be included in treatment. Other treatments that may be effective include heat in the form of whirlpools, moist packs, or hot shower, acupuncture, and acupressure.[40]

### Patient/family education

Support of the patient and family is an important nursing responsibility. FMS affects not only the patient, but the entire family. The patient may have considerable anxiety, especially if diagnosis of the disorder was difficult; the patient may need assurance that she or he is not "crazy." Because of the lack of objective signs of illness, others may doubt the reality of the illness. Psychological counseling may be necessary for some patients. Reassurance and validation of the patient's reports of symptoms are important.

The patient and family should be encouraged to discuss their feelings openly. Stress can cause exacerbations of the disorder, so stress management and reduction techniques are important.

Teaching should include information about the disease and the rationales for treatment. The patient should be taught the relationship between exercise and sleep and other factors that may disturb sleep (alcohol, stress, noise, and pain). Making a lifetime commitment to regular exercise can decrease symptoms and improve well-being.

Nurses can provide support to individuals trying to cope with chronic disease. The principles of therapeutic communication are important when listening to patients' reports of illness and coping strategies. Support groups are available for patients with FMS. The Arthritis Foundation may be helpful as a resource for exercise programs in the community. Another resource is the Fibromyalgia Network. The address is:

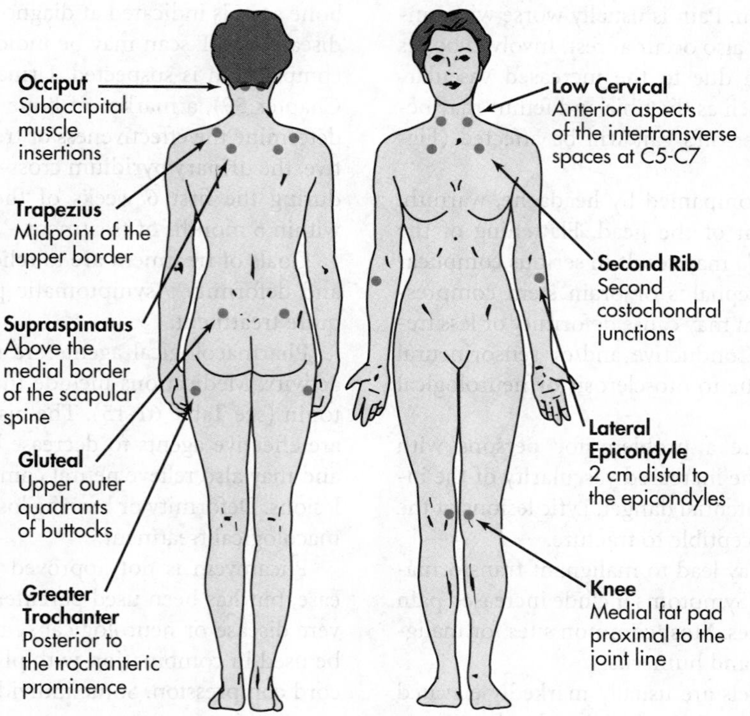

**fig. 61-29** Location of specific tender points for diagnostic classification of fibromyalgia.

5700 Stockdale Highway, Suite 100, Bakersfield, CA 93309; (805) 631-1950.

## DISORDERS AFFECTING THE BONES

### METABOLIC BONE DISEASES

Metabolic bone diseases affect the normal homeostatic functioning of the skeletal system. The etiology of metabolic bone diseases includes hormonal, genetic, and dietary factors. Paget's disease and osteoporosis will be discussed in the following sections.

#### Paget's Disease

##### *Etiology/epidemiology*

Sir James Paget, an English surgeon first described this disorder, also called *osteitis deformans,* in 1876. Characterized by an excess of bone destruction and unorganized bone formation and repair, Paget's disease is the second most common bone disorder in the United States following osteoporosis. The etiology of Paget's disease is unknown, although a genetic predisposition has been identified in 15% to 30% of patients, most probably an autosomal dominant pattern of inheritance.[9] Research suggests that a slow viral infection of the osteoclasts triggers the disease in genetically predisposed individuals. Other causative theories include autoimmune dysfunction, vascular disorders, vitamin D deficiency in childhood, and mechanical stressors to bone.

Paget's disease is a common disorder in Northern Europe, North America, Australia, and New Zealand, but relatively uncommon in other parts of the world. The highest prevalence is in Lancashire, England, where an estimated 6% to 8% of the adult population older than age 55 have radiographic evidence of the disease.[22] An estimated 3% of the United States population older than 55 years of age, mostly of European ancestry, are affected with Paget's disease.[22] The average age at diagnosis is 50 to 60 years of age, and the disease affects slightly more men than women.

The axial skeleton is usually affected by Paget's disease, particularly the vertebrae and skull, although the pelvis, femur, and tibia are other common sites of disease. Most persons are asymptomatic and diagnosis is incidental.

##### *Pathophysiology*

Initial changes in Paget's disease involve an increase in osteoclast-mediated resorption of cancellous bone, in addition to an increase in osteoblast-mediated bone formation. Bone resorption and formation are increased, resulting in a mosaic-like mix of abnormal woven and normal lamellar bone. Mineralization may encroach into the marrow and excessive bone formation usually occurs around partially resorbed trabeculae, causing thickening and hypertrophy. Vascularity is increased at affected portions of the skeleton. Lesions may occur in one or more bones, but the disease does not spread bone to bone.

Deformities and bony enlargement often occur. Bowing of the limbs and spinal curvature may occur in persons with advanced disease. Bone pain is the most common symptom of Paget's disease. Degenerative arthritis may occur at adjacent joints. Microfractures, corticeal swelling, and lytic bone lesions contribute to the pain. Pain is usually worse with ambulation or activity, but may also occur at rest. Involved bones may feel spongy and warm due to the increased vascularity. Weight-bearing bones such as the tibia and femur may become deformed, and the person's gait will be affected (Figure 61-30).

Skull pain is usually accompanied by headache, warmth, tenderness, and enlargement of the head. Flattening of the base of the skull or *platybasia* may result in serious complications of obstructive hydrocephalus or brain stem compression. Facial bone involvement may cause deformity or less frequently, affect the airway. Conductive and/or sensorineural hearing loss may develop due to otosclerosis or neurological abnormalities.

Pathological fractures are a problem for persons with Paget's disease. Because of the increased vascularity of the involved bone, bleeding is a potential danger. Lytic lesions of the long bones are the most susceptible to fracture.

Long-standing disease may lead to malignant transformation, usually osteosarcoma.[9] Symptoms include increased pain and swelling of affected bones. Most common sites for malignancy are the pelvis, femur, and humerus.

Alkaline phosphatase levels are usually markedly elevated as a result of osteoblast activity. Serum calcium levels are usually normal, except with generalized disease or immobilization. The development of kidney stones is a potential complication if immobility is prolonged. Calcium deposits may also occur in the joint spaces. The risk of developing secondary hyperparathyroidism is 15% to 20% in persons with normal serum calcium levels and increased levels of serum alkaline phosphatase.[9] Gout and hyperuricemia (see p. 1989) may develop as a result of increased bone activity, which causes an increase in nucleic acid catabolism. With extensive disease, cardiac involvement may develop as a result of increased vascularity and increased cardiac output.

### Collaborative care management

Radiographs of individuals with Paget's disease will reveal radiolucent areas in the bone, typical of increased bone resorption. Deformities and fractures may also be present. A bone scan is indicated at diagnosis to determine the extent of disease. A CT scan may be indicated if malignancy or neural compression is suspected. Urinary pyridium cross-links (see Chapter 59), a marker of bone turnover, can be followed to determine the effectiveness of treatment. If treatment is effective, the urinary pyridium cross-links should decrease by 50% during the first 6 weeks of therapy and return to normal within 6 months of treatment.

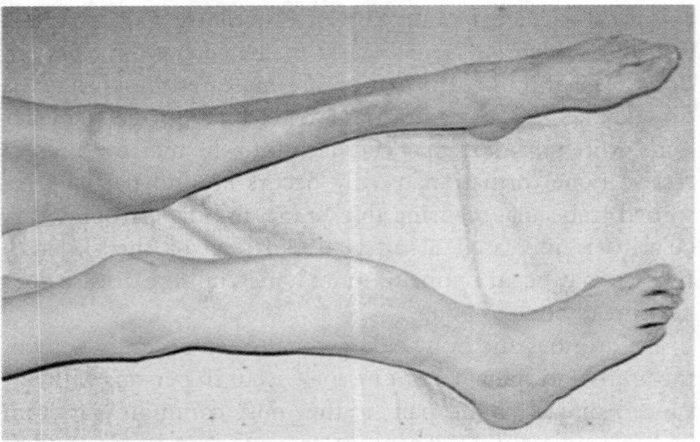

**fig. 61-30** Paget's disease with bilateral tibial deformities.

Goals of treatment are to relieve pain and prevent fracture and deformity. Asymptomatic patients generally do not require treatment.

Pharmacological agents are used to suppress osteoclastic activity. Medications include the bisphosphonates and calcitonin (see Table 61-15). The bisphosphonates and calcitonin are effective agents to decrease bone pain and bone warmth and may also relieve neural compression, joint pain, and lytic lesions. Deformity or hearing loss will not improve with pharmacological treatment.

Plicamycin is not approved for treatment of Paget's disease, but has been used parenterally to treat persons with severe disease or neurological symptoms. Dexamethasone may be used in combination with plicamycin in the case of spinal cord compression. Some individuals may require surgical decompression.

Other treatments include the use of analgesics and NSAIDs. Assistive devices, including canes and walkers, may be needed. A shoe lift may be required for persons with deformities resulting in leg length discrepancy. Deformities may also be corrected by surgical intervention (osteotomy). Open reduction and internal fixation may be necessary for fractures. In some cases, total joint arthroplasty may be indicated for severe degenerative arthritis.

The patient may benefit from a PT referral. Local application of ice or heat may help alleviate pain. However, application of heat may increase the warmth associated with increased vascularity, which some patients find uncomfortable. Massage may be effective in some patients.

**Patient/family education.** The patient and family should receive information regarding the course of disease, complications, and treatments. Instructions for taking medications should be included. The patient should understand the need for follow-up medical care and monitoring for complications.

A regular exercise program should be maintained; walking is best. Patients should avoid extended periods of immobility to avoid hypercalcemia. A nutritionally adequate diet is recommended. Because of the pathological fractures, safety precautions are very important to avoid falls or other injuries. The patient may need assistance in learning to use canes or other ambulatory aids. If deformities are present, the patient may need support in dealing with changes in body image. Referrals to the Arthritis Foundation (see p. 1967) or support groups for Paget's disease are useful resources for patients and their families. The address for The Paget Foundation for Paget's Disease of Bone and Related Disorders is: 200 Varick Street, Suite 1004, New York, NY 10014-4810; (212) 229-1582 or (800) 237-2438; fax: (212) 229-1502; The Paget Foundation, 120 Wall Street, Suite 1602, New York, NY 10005; (212) 509-5335; fax: (212) 509-8492.

## Osteoporosis

### Etiology

Osteoporosis is the most common bone disorder in the Western world and second only to arthritis as a cause of musculoskeletal morbidity in the elderly population. The initial definition of osteoporosis was "too little bone in the bone" by Albright.[47] Although the exact etiology of osteoporosis is unknown, several risk factors have been identified (see the Risk Factors Box). Important risk factors are a low peak bone mass at skeletal maturity, aging, and accelerated postmenopausal bone loss.

Osteoporosis was initially categorized as postmenopausal (women up to age 65 years), senile (any sex over 65 years), and idiopathic. Subsequently it was redefined as Type I and Type II forms of the disease (Table 61-13). In some persons, the two types of osteoporosis overlap.

**risk factors**

**Osteoporosis**

Aging
Female
White race
Nulliparity
Family history
Postmenopause—surgical or natural
Chronic calcium deficiency
Vitamin D deficiency
Sedentary lifestyle
Small frame, low body weight
Chronic smoking
Diet high in protein and fat
Chronic alcohol use
Excessive caffeine intake

**table 61-13** *Types of Osteoporosis*

| | Type I: Postmenopausal | Type II: Senile |
|---|---|---|
| Age | Postmenopausal women (natural or surgically induced)<br>Age of onset 55-75 yr | Women >70 yr<br>Men >80 yr |
| Sex | F:M 6:1 | F:M 2:1 |
| Pathology | Osteoclast mediated<br>Increased resorption | Osteoblast mediated<br>Decreased bone formation |
| Rate of bone loss | Rapid | Slow |
| Type of bone lost | Predominantly trabecular | Cortical and trabecular |
| | Associated with vertebral (compression-type) and distal radial fractures; hip fracture possible | Associated with vertebral (wedge), proximal humerus, tibia, and hip fractures |
| Bone density | >2 SD below normal | Low normal |

Osteoporosis can also be further classified as primary or secondary. *Primary* osteoporosis, the more common form, has no underlying pathological condition. *Secondary* osteoporosis results from another cause or medical condition, such as glucocorticoid-induced osteoporosis (Box 61-10). The focus of treatment of secondary osteoporosis is removal of the underlying cause.

Low bone mass is a critical element in the diagnosis of osteoporosis. The World Health Organization has established the following classifications of bone mass:[21]

- *Normal skeletal status:* Bone mineral density (BMD) of no more than 1 standard deviation below the young adult (30 to 40 years) mean value
- *Osteopenia* (low bone mass): Bone mass values between 1 and 2.5 standard deviations below peak young adult values

**box 61-10** *Causes of Secondary Osteoporosis*

**ENDOCRINE DISORDERS**
Diabetes
Cushing's syndrome
Hyperparathyroidism
Parathyroidism
Hypogonadism
Prolactinoma

**RHEUMATOID ARTHRITIS**

**DRUG-INDUCED**
Glucocorticoids
Heparin
Chronic use of phosphate-binding antacids
Loop diuretics
Anticonvulsants
Barbiturates
Lithium
Chemotherapy

**DISUSE**
Prolonged immobilization (prolonged bedrest, immobilization of limb by casting or splinting)
Paraplegia
Quadriplegia
Lower motor neuron disease

**CHRONIC ILLNESS**
Sarcoidosis
Cirrhosis
Renal tubular acidosis

**CANCER**
Multiple myeloma
Lymphoma
Leukemia

**MALABSORPTION SYNDROME**

**ANOREXIA NERVOSA**

**PROLONGED PARENTERAL NUTRITION**

**ALTERATIONS IN GI AND HEPATOBILIARY FUNCTION**

- *Osteoporosis: Bone mass less than 2.5 standard deviations below the average values measured in young women*
- *Severe osteoporosis:* Low BMD (2.5 or more standard deviations below the mean and a history of one or more pathological (fragility) fractures

The National Osteoporosis Foundation defines osteoporosis as BMD 2 standard deviations or more below the peak adult range.

Decreased bone mass and susceptibility to fracture with little or no trauma are hallmarks of the disease. At age 50, the lifetime risk of spinal, hip, or wrist fracture is 40% in white women and 13% in white men.[21] As bone density decreases by 1 standard deviation, the risk of fracture increases 1.5 to 3 times.[17] Osteoporosis was usually an asymptomatic condition until fracture occurred. With the advent of bone densitometry, the ability to safely and easily measure the amount of bone density allows persons at risk for fracture to be identified before fracture occurs (see Chapter 59). Early intervention can prevent or decrease further bone loss and decrease the risk of fractures.

Bones are constantly undergoing remodeling. The remodeling process is a complex and highly integrated activity that strategically balances the forces of resorption with the process of bone formation. The osteoblastic forces predominate throughout childhood and young adulthood, until peak bone mass is reached at about age 35. After a variable period of relative balance, the resorptive breakdown forces begin to predominate. High rates of bone turnover and progressive loss persist throughout aging. In osteoporosis, the bone is essentially normal, but there is not enough of it to withstand mechanical stresses. Simple bone mass is the major determinant of bone strength and accounts for about 75% to 85% of its variance.

Other factors associated with the development of osteoporosis are related to hormonal balance. The loss of natural estrogen at menopause appears to dramatically increase the process of bony resorption, although the exact mechanism is not well understood. Chronic calcium deficiency is a common problem in the aging population, and adequate calcium is essential to bone production. The mechanism of intestinal absorption of calcium becomes less efficient with advancing age, increasing the demand for calcium. Diets high in fat appear to decrease calcium absorption, and excess protein ingestion—particularly animal protein—increases the excretion of calcium by the kidney. Alcohol may be toxic to osteoblast cells, and chronic use usually results in malnutrition. Alcohol and possibly caffeine also increase calcium excretion. Chronic smoking affects bone remodeling and appears to both lower body estrogen levels and block calcium absorption. Smoking at least one pack of cigarettes per day may result in a 5% to 10% decrease in bone density by the time of menopause.[29]

Lack of exercise is another causative factor. In accordance with Wolff's law (see Chapter 59), bone is a dynamic substance that responds to stressors and weight-bearing forces. Chronic immobility is accompanied by well-documented increases in bone resorption. In normal daily lifestyles, this translates into an increased risk of osteoporosis for individuals with small frames, low body weight, and a sedentary activity pattern.

The use of steroids for treatment of persons with chronic illness is widespread. However successful in controlling conditions such as rheumatoid arthritis or asthma, steroid use is associated with many side effects. Osteoporosis is one of these side effects. Glucocorticoids interfere with calcium metabolism, reduce the synthesis of proteins by osteoblasts in the bone matrix, and may interfere with calcium absorption in the gut and renal tubule.[53] A reduction in serum sex hormone levels has also been noted, particularly in men and postmenopausal women. As a result, up to 30% of trabecular bone is lost within the first few months of steroid treatment. Bone densities of persons receiving long-term steroid therapy are 10% to 20% below normal. Fractures occur in one third of patients after 5 to 10 years of therapy, and the risk of hip fracture is tripled.[53] Persons receiving organ transplants are also at increased risk for fracture. Cyclosporine has also been shown to induce osteopenia, caused by increased bone resorption.[15]

### Epidemiology

Characterized by decreased bone mass and increased susceptibility to fracture, osteoporosis has become a major health problem. Elderly women, frequently affected by osteoporosis, are the fastest growing segment of the United States population. The prolonged longevity of the American population is expected to increase the number of persons affected by osteoporosis. There are 40 million women in the United States older than age 50.[29] More than 50% of those women have radiographic evidence of osteoporosis, and more than 30% of them will suffer fractures as a consequence of osteoporosis.

Twenty million persons in the United States are affected by osteoporosis. More than 1.2 million fractures occur annually as a result of osteoporosis, with more than 300,000 of those being hip fractures.[33] Hip fracture and its sequelae are of major concern. Proximal hip fractures are associated with a significant mortality rate, and most persons never regain their prefracture level of functioning (see Chapter 60). Costs associated with osteoporosis exceed $10 billion annually and are expected reach $62 billion by the year 2020.[30]

The racial distribution of osteoporosis is influenced by differences in bone mass, rather than rates of bone loss. The rate of bone loss among racial groups is constant among persons of the same age.[29] African Americans have approximately 10% greater bone mass than do whites and consequently are at less risk of developing osteoporosis. Persons of northern European or Scandinavian ancestry are at greatest risk of developing osteoporosis.

Considered primarily a women's disease, attention is now being focused on the development of osteoporosis in men. More than 5 million men in the United States have osteoporosis.[21] In 25 years, the incidence of osteoporosis-related hip fracture in men is expected to equal that of women. In men 70 to 80 years of age, the prevalence of osteoporosis is 7%. Interventions to prevent or decrease bone loss in both sexes is well warranted.

### Pathophysiology

In the process of normal bone remodeling, bone formation equals bone resorption. An osteoporotic state develops if bone resorption exceeds bone formation. Age-related bone loss begins in both sexes at approximately age 40 years. Women experience a 35% to 40% loss in trabecular bone and up to 60% of the cancellous bone stores, in contrast; men lose only about two-thirds of that amount throughout life.[41] By the time a person reaches age 75 years, the skeletal mass is reduced 50% from age 30 levels.[47] The skeleton continues to lose bone mass in the hip and appendicular skeleton, even after the age of 80 years.

Two processes of bone loss have been identified: rapid bone loss and gradual bone loss. Rapid bone loss occurs during menopause and is *osteoclast-mediated,* while gradual bone loss is *osteoblast-mediated* and occurs after menopause. The time required to complete one cycle of bone remodeling in a healthy adult is about 4 months; that time is increased to almost 2 years for individuals with osteoporosis.

The remodeling process consists of the following steps: clusters of bone precursor cells respond to a stimulus (drug, hormone, or physical stressor) to activate the remodeling process and form osteoclasts. Osteoclasts form a cutting cone and begin to resorb bone, leaving a resorption cavity. In cortical bone, osteoblasts line the cavity and begin laying down layers (lamellae) of new bone until a haversian canal results (see Chapter 59). Trabeculae are formed in cancellous bone. If this process of remodeling is disrupted, osteoporosis may result. A decrease in the number of bone precursor cells or in the rate of bone formation or an increase in the rate of bone resorption or an increase in the number of stimuli that activate the process can all result in osteoporosis. Osteoporosis will also occur if the whole process is not completed in entirety. Interference in the bone's vascular system will result in a decreased number of bone precursor cells, which may also cause osteoporosis.

Cortical thinning begins at age 40 years, increases with age, and almost ceases late in life. Following menopause, women lose cortical bone at a rate of 2% to 3% per year, returning to normal levels approximately 10 years after menopause.[47] The rate of trabecular bone loss differs. Trabecular bone loss begins earlier in both sexes and is lost in greater amounts. Following menopause, the rate of trabecular bone loss is as high as 8% annually.[29] There are fewer and smaller trabeculae, with large spaces between them, decreasing the bone density. The compressive strength of trabecular bone is related to its density; as the density decreases, so does its compressive force and ability to withstand mechanical stressors. The bones most susceptible to fracture are those rich in trabecular bone, particularly the vertebrae, proximal femur, and distal radius. Cortical bone undergoes osteoporotic changes as well, becoming thin and porous and thus susceptible to fracture. Collapse and deformity may occur as a result of the bone's decreased density.

Osteoporosis has been called the "silent thief" and "the silent disease" because most person affected have no outward manifestations of disease. The disease was not diagnosed unless fracture occurred. Many fractures related to osteoporosis occur without the patient's knowledge, although some are associated with excruciating pain. The earliest manifestation of osteoporosis may be an acute onset of back pain in the mid to low thoracic region as a result of vertebral fracture, occurring at rest or with minimal activity. Vertebral fracture can involve the entire vertebrae (compression) or a portion, usually the anterior section (wedge). Motion of the spine is restricted, especially forward flexion. Anterior compression fractures of the thoracic vertebrae may cause a "dowager's hump" or thoracic kyphosis (Figure 61-31). Loss of height and a protruding abdomen (due to pressure on abdominal viscera) are associated with this condition. Eventually the lower rib cage may rest on the iliac crests. Paravertebral muscle spasm often occurs, but neurological deficits are rare with spontaneous vertebral compression fractures.[29] These postural changes may affect exercise tolerance and food tolerance. The patient will report early satiety and bloatedness. The patient's body image may also be affected as a result of the spinal deformity.

Distal radial fractures (Colles' fractures) usually occur after a fall on a outstretched hand. Fractures of the proximal femur are associated with considerable morbidity and mortality (see Chapter 60). Osteoporotic hip fracture often occurs after little or no trauma. Intracapsular hip fracture is due to bone loss, and intertrochanteric fracture is due to both cortical and trabecular bone loss.

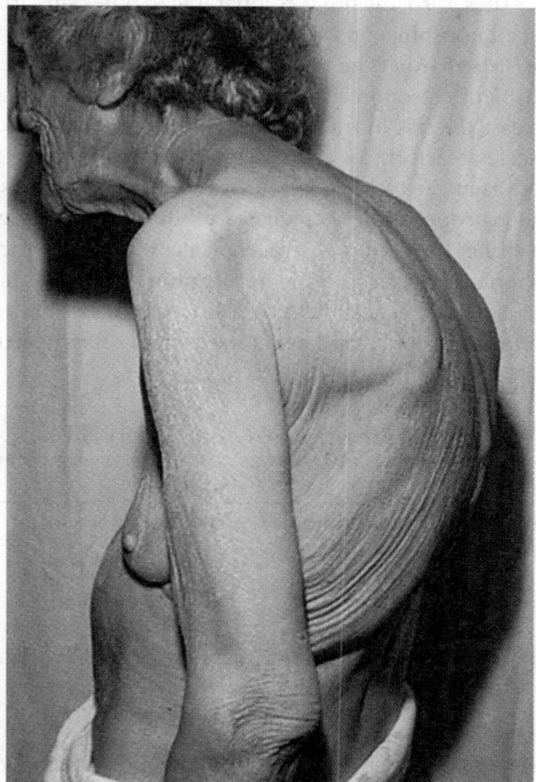

**fig. 61-31** Kyphosis. This elderly woman's condition was caused by a combination of spinal osteoporotic vertebral collapse and chronic degenerative changes in the vertebral column.

### *Collaborative care management*

**Diagnostic tests.** The risk for fracture can be assessed by the patient's risk factors and history and measured precisely with noninvasive diagnostic tools. Measurement of bone mineral density (BMD) and biochemical markers of bone resorption are the basic tools for diagnosis of osteoporosis. Diagnostic techniques can assess extent of disease, effects of treatment, progression of disease, and perhaps most importantly, risk of fracture. Measurement of BMD predicts risk of fracture in both men and women. There are a variety of techniques used to measure bone density at various parts of the skeleton (Table 61-14). Once the diagnosis of osteoporosis is established, BMD studies should be performed every 1 to 2 years to determine response to treatment.

Biochemical markers of bone turnover (urinary deoxypyridine) can be easily assessed by a second-voided morning urine sample (see Chapter 59). Urinary tests can be used alone or in conjunction with BMD studies and are helpful to monitor response to treatment.

The National Osteoporosis Foundation recommends BMD screening for persons with the following risk factors:[21]

Estrogen deficiency
Vertebral abnormalities or osteopenia by x-ray
Primary hyperparathyroidism (asymptomatic)
Long-term glucocorticoid treatment

When elderly women are screened, the hip is the preferred site, because hip fractures are easier to predict than fractures at other sites. Also, the hip is comparable to other sites for predicting all nonspinal and wrist fractures.[21]

**Medications.** The goal of pharmacological therapy for persons with osteoporosis is to prevent further bone loss and to decrease the risk of fracture. Relief of symptoms associated with skeletal deformity and fracture and maximizing functional capacity are other goals of treatment. Medications used to treat osteoporosis either decrease bone resorption or increase bone formation. Estrogen, calcitonin, and the bisphosphonates decrease bone resorption; they also have a greater effect on cancellous bone. Estrogen and alendronate (a bisphosphonate) may have bone formation properties as well. Other drugs that increase bone formation (fluorides, anabolic steroids, calcitrol, testosterone, and parathyroid hormone analogs) are under investigation for use. Medications used to treat osteoporosis are summarized in Table 61-15. Combination therapy using estrogen and bisphosphonates results in a greater increase in BMD than either therapy alone. Mild analgesics are used to relieve pain associated with muscular aches and spasms. Calcitonin has been shown to be effective in relieving pain associated with osteoporotic vertebral fractures.

**Treatments.** Osteoporosis is easier to prevent than to treat. Diet, medications, exercise, and prevention of falls and fractures are the foundations of therapy. There are no specific treatments for persons with osteoporosis. Treatments for persons with fractures are discussed in Chapter 60. Wrist fractures are usually treated by closed reduction and immobilization. Treatment for acute vertebral fractures is bedrest for 1 to 2 days and analgesics. Persons who have sustained a vertebral fracture as a result of osteoporosis may benefit from a corset (fitted by an orthotist) to provide support. Rigid bracing should be avoided as complete immobilization results in bone loss. Pain usually subsides after 6 to 12 weeks as the fracture heals. Activity is essential during the healing period to avoid chronic back symptoms. Calcitonin has been effective in relieving the pain after vertebral fracture. Ultrasound, massage, and local application of heat or cold may alleviate pain and muscle spasms. Assistive or adaptive devices may be needed in the home or work environment. Persons who have had one fracture are at risk for subsequent fractures.

**Surgical management.** Surgical intervention is necessary to repair some fractures. However, vertebral fractures without neurological deficits usually do not require surgical intervention. Wrist fractures may need open reduction for the person to achieve maximum functional results. Almost all hip fractures are managed surgically. Open reduction and internal fixation or prosthetic replacement of the proximal femur (hemiarthroplasty) are procedures for operative treatment of hip fracture. The choice of procedure depends on the location of the fracture and vascular supply to the femoral head. As

**table 61-14** *Methods of Measuring Bone Mineral Density*

| Method | Site | Advantages and Disadvantages |
|---|---|---|
| Radiographic absorptiometry (RA) | Phalanx, metacarpal | Inexpensive, easy to use<br>Lengthy time required for results<br>First technique developed to measure BMD |
| Single-photon and x-ray absorptiometry (SXA, SPA) | Radius, calcaneus | Reasonably precise, inexpensive |
| Dual-photon and dual x-ray absorptiometry (DXA, DPA) | Spine, proximal femur, forearm, whole body | Dual x-ray absorptiometry (DXA) most widely used, allows precise measurement of hip and spine with low radiation exposure<br>Equipment not widely available around country |
| Quantitative CT (QCT) | Spine, radius (both cortical and trabecular) | Rapid results, widely available, able to assess trabecular content of spine<br>Higher exposure to radiation than other methods |
| Quantitative ultrasound (QUS) | Calcaneus, tibia | Inexpensive, portable, no radiation exposure, high sensitivity for predicting fracture risk |

table 61-15 Common Medications for **Osteoporosis**

| Drug | Action | Nursing Intervention |
|---|---|---|
| Calcium | Necessary for bone formation<br>High calcium intake may retard bone loss, insufficient alone to prevent or treat osteoporosis | Daily recommended dose is 1500 mg taken in divided doses of 500 mg/day or 600 mg bid for maximum absorption.<br>Observe for signs of hypercalcemia.<br>Calcium is contraindicated with severe renal disease. |
| Vitamin D: calcitrol, calcifedol | Necessary for bone formation and calcium absorption<br>Improves calcium balance | Effectiveness of therapy depends on adequate calcium intake. Monitor for effects of hypercalcemia. |
| Estrogen replacement therapy (ERT): conjugated estrogen, estropipate, estradiol oral, transdermal patch | Inhibits bone resorption, positive effect on calcium balance, protects against postmenopausal osteoporosis | Inform patients of risks/benefits.<br>Side effects include breast tenderness, vaginal bleeding, hypertension, and DVT.<br>Protective effect shown for coronary artery disease.<br>Prolonged use increases risk of breast cancer by 30%.[33]<br>Use increases risk of endometrial cancer by 1%.[29]<br>Encourage women to have regular gynecological (Papanicolaou smears and uterine biopsy if indicated) and breast examinations during therapy.<br>Usual daily dose is 0.625 mg; half dose is necessary if combined with calcium supplement. |
| Selective estrogen receptor modulators (SERM) anti-estrogens, "designer estrogens": raloxifene (Evista) | Mimics effects of estrogen in some, but not all, tissues.<br>Blocks estrogen's cancer-promoting effects in other tissues.<br>Reduces rate of bone resorption and decreases rate of overall bone turnover.<br>Increases bone density, lowers blood lipids, *does not* increase HDL.<br>Does not adversely affect breast, uterine tissue in clinical trials<br>FDA approved for prevention of osteoporosis in postmenopausal women<br>Inconclusive data regarding decreasing fracture risk | Risk of venous thromboembolic events, similar to risks associated with HRT. Avoid use in women with history of blood clots.<br>Inform patient of side effects, including hot flashes and leg cramps.<br>Smoking should be avoided while taking SERMs.<br>Caution women of childbearing potential to avoid pregnancy. |
| Hormone replacement therapy (HRT): estrogen in combination with progestin | Increases BMD, decreases fracture risk<br>Adding progestin decreases reduces risk of endometrial cancer | Initiation of therapy is recommended early in postmenopausal period.<br>Increases bone mass in women older than age 65 yr. |
| Bisphosphonates: etidronate, pamidronate, alendronate (Fosamax), residronate, taludrinate | Inhibits osteoclast-mediated bone resorption<br>Also used in treatment of Paget's disease<br>Increases bone resorption, increases bone density, and prevents fractures in postmenopausal women with osteoporosis (alendronate)<br>Protects against bone loss during long-term steroid therapy (etidronate) | Administer on an empty stomach (before any food or medications) with full glass of water because of poor absorption.<br>Preferably patient should remain standing or upright for 30 min after administration.<br>Administration with coffee or orange juice decreases bioavailability by 60%.[21]<br>Use is alternative for ERT or HRT.<br>Convenience of once-daily dosing. |
| Calcitonin (human or salmon): intranasal (Miacalcin) | Opposes effect of parathyroid hormone on bone and kidneys<br>Inhibits bone resorption, decreases fracture risk<br>Increases bone mass in persons with steroid-induced osteoporosis<br>Analgesic effect with osteoporotic fractures | Use is limited to parenteral or intranasal administration.<br>Monitor for hypocalcemia.<br>Assess for allergy.<br>Teach importance of reading labels; many over-the-counter products contain calcium.<br>Few systemic effects with intranasal use. |
| Fluoride | Stimulates osteoblasts to form new bone, primarily trabecular<br>Quality of new bone is poor, has decreased tensile strength and elasticity<br>Used only for treatment, not prevention | Patient must have adequate intake of calcium and vitamin D while receiving therapy.<br>Side effects include GI disturbance and ulceration, peripheral edema, and stress microfractures. |

with all types of fractures, the principles of management are to mobilize the patient as quickly as possible to prevent the complications of immobility and to restore the patient to the maximum level of functioning. Surgical fixation of fractures is discussed in Chapter 60 and arthroplasty is discussed on p. 1975-1977.

**Diet.** Adequate nutrition is essential throughout life for a healthy skeleton. Calcium and vitamin D intake should be adequate from childhood through maturity to develop peak bone mass in premenopause, thus protecting against osteoporosis later in life. The importance of adequate calcium intake increases with aging. Vitamin D and calcium absorption is gradually impaired as a result of the aging process. The daily recommended intake of calcium for adults older than 51 years is 1200 mg (Box 61-11). Persons with osteoporosis should have a daily intake of calcium of 1500 mg. If the person is unable to take in adequate calcium in the form of dairy products, supplements are needed. Single doses of calcium should not exceed 600 mg/dose. Calcium-enriched juices and breads, which contain approximately 300 mg of calcium, equal to the calcium content of one glass of milk, are available. Foods rich in calcium include dairy products, green vegetables, and tofu (Table 61-16).

Vitamin D is necessary for calcium absorption and stimulates bone formation. Deficiencies of vitamin D are common in persons with osteoporosis, strict vegetarians, and those living in northern latitudes with restricted sunlight exposure. The recommended daily allowance of vitamin D is 400 IU. Persons with vitamin D deficiencies may require supplements, but persons with sun exposure throughout the year usually do not. Foods rich in vitamin D are milk, fish, and eggs.

Another dietary recommendation for persons with osteoporosis is avoidance of excessive intake of alcohol and caffeine, both risk factors associated with the development of osteoporosis. For persons with fractures, a diet adequate in proteins and vitamin C is necessary to promote wound and tissue healing.

**Activity.** Exercise is a frequently prescribed, but not completely understood, intervention for the prevention and treatment of osteoporosis. Benefits of exercise include increased muscle tone and muscle mass, which may improve balance and flexibility and thus prevent falls. In addition to the benefits of overall well-being and cardiovascular effects, impact-loading exercise seems to be effective in maintaining bone mass.[33] Regular weight bearing or bone stressing (weight training and resistance exercises) is necessary to maintain bone mass in both children and adults. The effects of exercise on peak bone mass are most significant during the years of skeletal growth and have less significance in older adults. Premenopausal women who exercise regularly and have regular menstrual cycles have the greatest bone mass.[33] Amenorrhea leads to bone loss.[33] The ideal amount and type of exercise needed to maintain bone mass have not been determined. Research has shown positive effects of exercise on BMD in postmenopausal women. Weight-bearing or weight-training

**box 61-11 Recommendations for Daily Calcium Intake**

| AGE | DAILY RECOMMENDATION | SERVINGS* |
|---|---|---|
| 1 to 3 years | 500 mg | 2 |
| 4 to 8 years | 800 mg | 3 |
| 9 to 18 years | 1300 mg | 4 |
| 19 to 50 years | 1000 mg | 3 |
| 51+ years | 1200 mg | 4 |

*1 serving is equal to:
1 cup whole, reduced-fat, fat-free or flavored milk
1 cup yogurt
1½ ounces natural cheese
1 cup pudding made with milk

**table 61-16 Major Dietary Sources of Calcium**

| FOOD | QUANTITY | CALCIUM (MG) |
|---|---|---|
| **MILK** | 1 cup (240 ml) | |
| Skim | | 302 |
| 1% | | 300 |
| 2% | | 297 |
| **ICE CREAM** | 1 cup | |
| Hard | | 176 |
| Soft | | 236 |
| **ICE MILK (VANILLA)** | 1 cup | |
| Hard | | 176 |
| Soft | | 274 |
| **CHEESE** | | |
| Cheddar | 1 oz | 204 |
| Swiss | 1 oz | 272 |
| American | 1 oz | 150 |
| Cottage | 1 cup | 155 |
| **BEANS** | | |
| Pinto (cooked) | 1 cup | 86 |
| Soy (cooked) | 1 cup | 131 |
| Navy (cooked) | 1 cup | 95 |
| Green (cooked) | 1 cup | 80 |
| **VEGETABLES** | | |
| Turnip greens (cooked) | 1 cup | 249 |
| Broccoli (cooked) | 1 cup | 90 |
| **TOFU** | 4 oz | 108 |
| **FISH AND SHELLFISH** | | |
| Oysters (raw) | 1 cup | 226 |
| Salmon (canned) | 3 oz | 167 |
| **YOGURT** | | |
| Plain (low fat) | 8 oz | 415 |
| Fruit (low fat) | 8 oz | 343 |
| Frozen (fruit) | 8 oz | 240 |
| Frozen (chocolate) | 8 oz | 160 |

exercise appears to be beneficial in maintaining and, in some cases, increasing BMD.[29] One study demonstrated the effectiveness of a 5-month period of load-bearing exercise in early postmenopausal women. The women were not taking any medications for osteoporosis except calcium supplements. The experimental group had a significant increase in BMD of the radius.[52] These data support other studies indicating that the effects of exercise may be increased by calcium supplementation.[29]

Recommendations for all adults should include a daily (or at least 5 times per week) program of weight-bearing and mild weight-training exercises. Brisk walking or low-impact aerobics are good choices for the older adult. Extension exercises of the spine are beneficial for posture and flexibility, but flexion exercises may contribute to fracture. Jogging may also precipitate vertebral fracture. Walking outdoors has the added benefit of sunlight exposure, essential for vitamin D formation. Swimming or water exercises have no direct effect on bones but are good choices for an aerobic workout.

**Referrals.** Referrals for PT and OT may be necessary for exercise regimens and assistive and adaptive devices. A nutritionist can assist the elderly patient in meal planning to include adequate calcium and vitamin D. National organizations and support groups for patients and family are excellent resources for information about osteoporosis. An example is the Osteoporosis and Related Bone Diseases-National Resource Center, National Osteoporosis Foundation, 1150 17th Street NW, Suite 500, Washington, DC 20036-4603; (202) 223-2226 or (800) 624-BONE; TTY: (202) 466-4315; fax: (202) 223-2237; e-mail: orbdnrc@nof.org.

## NURSING MANAGEMENT OF THE PERSON WITH OSTEOPOROSIS

The nursing management section will pertain to persons with osteoporosis, but *without* fractures. The nursing management of persons with fractures is discussed in Chapter 60.

### ASSESSMENT

#### Subjective Data

The patient should be assessed for the presence of risk factors for osteoporosis. The patient's diet, exercise habits, amount of caffeine and alcohol consumption, and amount and frequency of sunlight exposure are all relevant data. Medications (steroids or heparin) and coexisting medical conditions may be contributing factors to osteoporosis. The medication list should also include over-the-counter preparations. Any family history of osteoporosis should be noted. Female patients should have a gynecological history taken. The regularity of menstrual cycles, pregnancies, time of menopause, and medications are important factors in the development of osteoporosis.

If the patient has an established diagnosis of osteoporosis, what treatments or therapies have been prescribed? In addition, the nurse should question the patient regarding his or her expectations of treatment. A complete assessment of the patient's level of pain should be included in the history. The patient's previous methods of pain control may be beneficial in planning interventions for pain relief.

A history of falls or previous fractures, especially occurring after minimal trauma, is important for planning care. The nurse should assess the patient's home environment for fall hazards and injury potential. Questions that should be asked are the following: Does the patient need to climb stairs? Are the bedroom and bathroom on the same floor? Is the home carpeted?

Psychosocial assessment should include noting any disturbances in self-esteem due to loss of independence or functional ability. Pain or limited mobility may impair the patient's ability to pursue necessary and leisure activities, leading to anxiety, social isolation, and depression. Depression is a common finding in elderly persons. The amount of family support can influence the patient's coping abilities, especially with a chronic degenerative disease.

#### Objective Data

A complete physical examination focusing on the musculoskeletal and neurological system should be performed. The patient's gait, balance, coordination, and sensory ability should be assessed to determine the risk for falls and injury. The patient's baseline level of functioning should be assessed, including the ability to perform ADL.

The physical examination should include an assessment of all joints and extremities. Areas prone to pathological fracture should be thoroughly and carefully assessed. The presence of kyphosis is common in elderly women. When kyphosis is present, a complete respiratory and GI assessment should be performed, as decreased respiratory excursion, respiratory compromise, abdominal distention, ileus, and constipation may occur as a result of the deformity. Tenderness with palpation over the intervertebral disc spaces may indicate a vertebral fracture, so the spine should be palpated gently. Loss of height may be attributed to osteoporosis and vertebral fractures. Loss of motion, particularly flexion, may also occur.

### NURSING DIAGNOSES

Nursing diagnoses are determined from analysis of patient data. Nursing diagnoses for the patient with osteoporosis may include but are not limited to:

| Diagnostic Title | Possible Etiological Factors |
|---|---|
| Injury, risk for | Altered mobility, minimal trauma, falls, advanced age, previous fall |
| Impaired physical mobility | Decreased bone mass, decreased strength, musculoskeletal impairment, pain |
| Self-esteem disturbance | Chronic illness, anxiety, loss of usual role, body changes, limitation in mobility, chronic pain, loss of independence |

## EXPECTED PATIENT OUTCOMES

Expected patient outcomes for the patient with osteoporosis may include but are not limited to:

1. Experiences no injuries, falls, or fractures; relates understanding of factors that contribute to potential injury and steps to correct situation or modify environment.
2. Maintains maximum level of mobility and functioning.
3. Has positive self-esteem and participates in desired activities at fullest level.

## INTERVENTIONS

### Preventing Injury

Pathological fracture can result from minor trauma in the individual with osteoporosis. Falls commonly result in hip fracture, a significant cause of mortality in the elderly person. The environment should be modified to protect the patient from accidental harm or injury.

As stated in the assessment section above, the patient should be assessed for level of consciousness, ability to make judgments, motor strength, coordination, balance, and sensory deficits. Many medications may cause weakness, drowsiness, or dizziness, which pose an additional risk for injury. If adverse effects are occurring, the physician should be consulted for alternatives. Electrolyte imbalances are common in elderly persons and may manifest as mental status changes or weakness. Blood chemistry results should be evaluated for abnormalities.

Instructions should be given about the proper technique for transferring from bed to chair, bending, and lifting. Proper body mechanics can protect the patient from back injuries (Figure 61-32). Excessive flexion of the spine may contribute to compression fracture of the vertebrae. Kyphosis may alter the patient's center of gravity and diminish vision. The patient should be encouraged to maintain an upright posture to improve ambulatory ability and also to enhance respiration. Assistive devices and ambulatory aids may be necessary for some persons. Physical therapy referrals may be needed to teach the patient the proper technique for using a walker or cane. Walkers and canes provide support, decreasing the risk for falls.

The environment should be kept as hazard free as possible while the patient is hospitalized. The bed should be kept in low position, and the need for side rails should be assessed. Confused persons or those receiving sedation should have the side rails elevated. However, careful monitoring of the patient is crucial, as some persons may attempt to climb over the rails and sustain a fall. The call light should be within reach, and the patient should be instructed in its use. Nonskid shoes or slippers can also help prevent falls. Environmental hazards such as equipment, electrical cords, and slippery floors should be eliminated. The home environment should also be assessed for safety hazards (see the Patient/Family Teaching Box, p. 2014).

Exercise is an important intervention for preventing falls. Regular exercise increases energy, muscle tone, strength, flexibility, and coordination, which may help in fall prevention. Range-of-motion exercises should be included in the program to maintain joint mobility. Weight-bearing, regular exercise for 30 minutes, 5 times per week, should be recommended to persons with osteoporosis.

### Promoting Mobility

The patient's ROM and muscle strength should be assessed, and limitations in mobility should be documented. The level of the patient's pain should also be assessed, because unrelieved pain may interfere with mobility. Analgesics should be given as needed, especially before planned activities, such as PT. Active ROM should be encouraged daily; if the patient is unable, passive ROM should be performed by the nurse.

If the patient has a vertebral fracture, a corset may be prescribed to provide support and increase mobility while fracture healing occurs. Encouraging maximum mobility while the fracture heals is recommended to avoid bone loss from immobility. Again, weight-bearing exercises are recommended to maintain bone mass. In addition, strengthening exercises increase circulation to both bone and muscle. PT referrals are an option to teach weight-bearing and resistive exercises. OT can provide the patient with adaptive devices to complete ADL. Participation in ADL should be encouraged to maintain independence, allowing the patient adequate time to complete self-care.

Affected parts of the body can be supported with slings or pillows as needed, especially during periods of rest. Uninterrupted periods of rest should be ensured to increase energy and prevent fatigue throughout the day. Fatigue is common among persons with musculoskeletal impairments. The patient's family and friends should be encouraged to participate in care as they can assist the patient in managing problems associated with immobility.

### Promoting a Positive Self-Image

Osteoporosis, in addition to the effects on musculoskeletal functioning, also significantly affects an individual's social and emotional functioning. Changes in the body and body functioning may cause anxiety. Deformities such as kyphosis, onset of menopause, or decreased mobility as a result of musculoskeletal disease may be difficult changes for the patient to assimilate. Depression is not an uncommon reaction to an altered body image and functional limitations. Kyphosis can result in height loss, spinal deformity, and difficulty wearing one's usual clothing. Dissatisfaction with appearance may cause a patient to avoid going out and pursuing social activities. Patients who experienced previous falls often fear falling again. Explaining the process of aging, menopause, and the effects on bone can help reassure patients that aging and menopause are normal events of life. Knowledge of the treatment and preventive strategies for protecting bone mass can alleviate patients' fears. Nurses can provide support and help patients adapt to change and maintain a positive outlook.

Women with chronic illnesses such as osteoporosis often have to modify their roles as a result of the limitations imposed by disease. These changes often have negative effects, creating feelings of dependency and isolation. Changes in physical appearance may have similar effects.

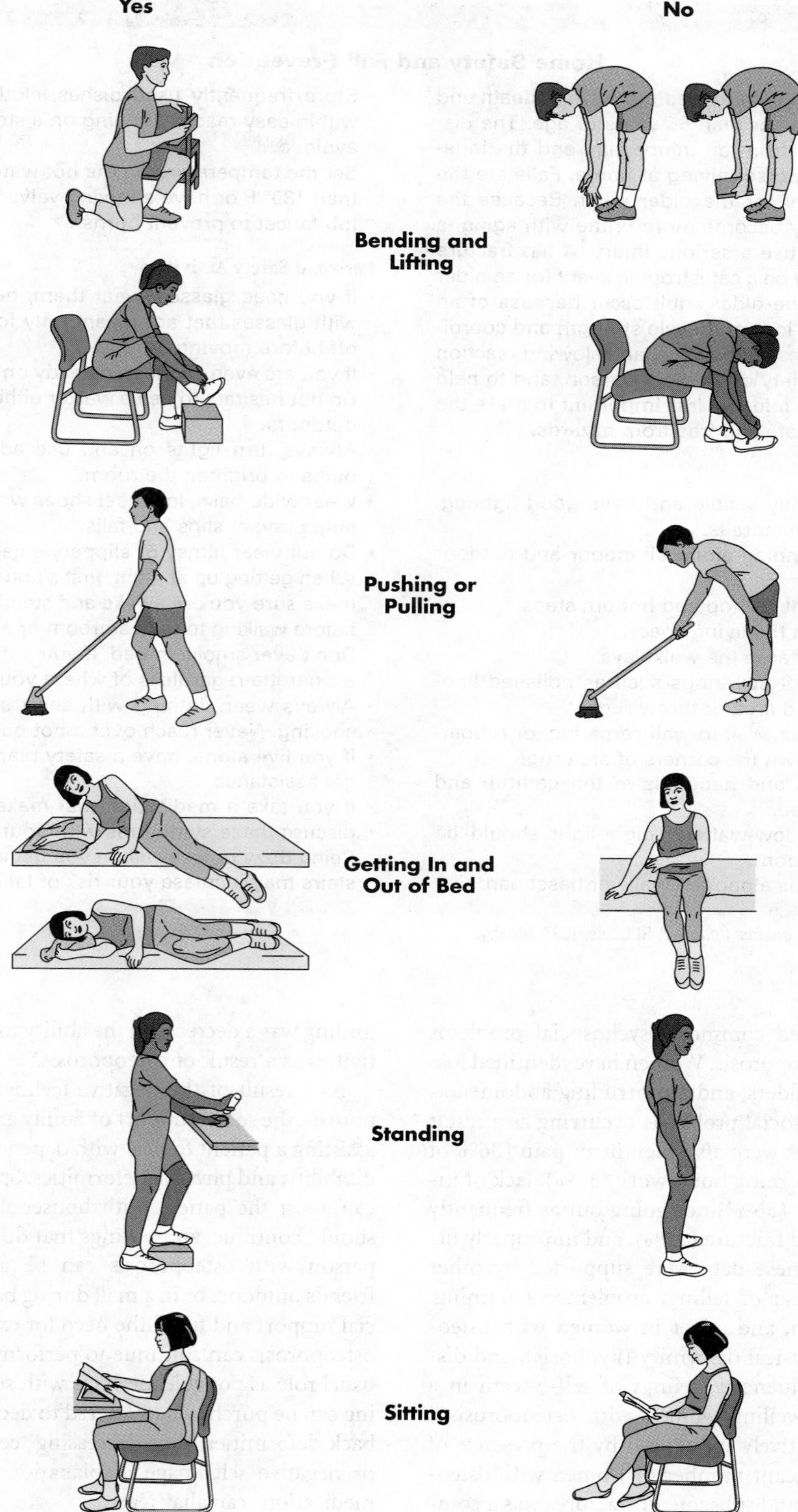


**fig. 61-32** Proper body mechanics.

**patient/family teaching**

### Home Safety and Fall Prevention

Unintentional injury is the third leading cause of death and disability for persons older than 65 years of age. The disability that may result from an injury may end the independence of an older person living at home. Falls are the leading cause of injury for the older adult. Because the bones in the body may become more brittle with aging, a fall may potentially cause a serious injury. A hip fracture secondary to a fall may be a catastrophic event for an older person. Most falls in the older adult occur because of an environmental hazard, loss of muscle strength and coordination, an impaired sense of balance, and slowing reaction time. To ensure the safety of an older person, and to help prevent falls and other injuries, it is important to make the person's living space safe and free from hazards.

**Environmental Safety**

- Steps should be highly visible and have good lighting, nonskid treads, and handrails.
- A strong banister running along all indoor and outdoor steps is essential.
- Clearly mark and light the top and bottom steps.
- Use bright lighting in the living space.
- Remove all floor clutter in the walkways.
- Remove slippery floor coverings such as polished linoleum, small mats, and area or throw rugs.
- Use nonskid floor wax, wall-to-wall carpeting, or rubber-backed rugs. Tack down the corners of area rugs.
- Install nonskid mats and handrails in the bathtub and near the toilet and bed.
- A bedside lamp or low-wattage night-light should be available in the bedroom.
- Secure electrical cords along the walls or baseboards.
- Store frequently used dishes, clothes, and other items within easy reach; climbing on a stool or chair should be avoided.
- Set the temperature on the hot water heater to no hotter than 130° F or have a mixing valve installed on the bathtub faucet to prevent burns.

**Personal Safety Activities**

- If you need glasses, wear them, but never walk around with glasses that are meant only for reading. Take them off before moving around.
- If you are even slightly unsteady on your feet, use a cane. Do not hesitate to use a walker either inside the house or outdoors.
- Always turn lights on and use adequate wattage light bulbs to brighten the room.
- Wear wide-base, low-heel shoes with corrugated soles to help prevent slips and falls.
- Do not wear flimsy or slippery-soled shoes or slippers.
- When getting up at night, first sit on the edge of the bed to make sure you are awake and steady, then turn on a light before walking to the bathroom or around the room.
- Don't ever smoke in bed. If you are sleepy, don't light up a cigarette regardless of where you are sitting.
- Always wear clothing with short sleeves when you are cooking. Never reach over a hot burner on the stove.
- If you live alone, have a safety plan to call for help or to get assistance.
- If you take a medication that makes you dizzy or weak, discuss these symptoms with your health care provider. Being dizzy or weak when you get up to walk or go down stairs may increase your risk of falling.

From *Mosby's patient teaching guides: update 3,* St Louis, 1997, Mosby.

Studies have identified common psychosocial problems arising as a result of osteoporosis. Women have identified loss of height, rounded shoulders, and a protruding abdomen as problematic. Six psychosocial problems occurring as a result of these physical changes were also identified: pain (86% of women), difficulty performing housework (57%), lack of information about disease (36%), not going out as frequently (33%), fear of falling and fracture (22%), and improperly fitting clothes (21%).[71] These data were supported by other studies that identified fear of falling, problems vacuuming, problems traveling, pain, and anger in women with osteoporosis.[71] Back pain, physical deformity (kyphosis), and disability all negatively influenced feelings of self-esteem in a study of community-dwelling women with osteoporosis.[71] Quality of life was negatively influenced by the presence of chronic pain in a significant number of women with osteoporosis.[71] Fear of falling and subsequent fractures was a common finding among women with osteoporosis in several studies.[71] Fear of falling and fracture may limit a person's willingness to go out and pursue necessary or social activities, compounding the problem. Interventions are needed to assist women to adapt to physical changes and to assist them in methods to avoid injury and lessen fears. Another consistent finding was a decrease in the ability to participate in social activities as a result of osteoporosis.

As a result of the negative feelings associated with osteoporosis, the social support of family and friends is essential for assisting a patient to deal with dependency as a result of pain, disability, and physical deformities. Spouses, friends, or family can assist the patient with household tasks. Social contacts should continue, and outings that do not pose hazards to the person with osteoporosis can be arranged. Walking with friends outdoors or in a mall during bad weather can foster social support and fulfill the need for exercise. The woman with osteoporosis can continue to perform as many aspects of her usual role as possible, perhaps with some adaptations. Clothing can be purchased or altered to decrease the prominence of back deformities, thus decreasing feelings of embarrassment or negative self-image. Explanations about treatments and medications can allay fears.

### Patient/Family Education

Teaching the family and patient with osteoporosis should include instructions about the disease process, medications, body mechanics, exercise, and prevention of falls (see the Patient/Family Teaching Box and Figures 61-32 and 61-33).

**patient/family teaching**

### What Is Osteoporosis?

Osteoporosis is the most common metabolic bone disease. It results from the loss of calcium in the bones, causing the bones to become brittle and susceptible to breaking. Osteoporosis, which means "porous bone," is usually not diagnosed until the person suffers a fracture or broken bone.

**Why Are Women Affected More Often?**

One out of four women and half the women older than 65 years of age have osteoporosis to some extent. Most are white women who have gone through menopause. Generally, blacks have greater bone mass than whites, and men have greater bone mass than women. Petite women with small bones and thin bodies have very small bone masses. Thus women are at greater risk of developing osteoporosis if they are white, Asian, or petite.

Osteoporosis is also caused by low estrogen levels that occur in women after menopause. Although the role of estrogen is not clear, it is linked to the processes of bone formation and resorption. Estrogen is thought to reduce bone resorption, to reduce calcium loss through the kidneys, and to increase calcium absorption in the digestive tract. Estrogen protects women who have had an inadequate intake of calcium in their growing years. However, when estrogen levels drop after menopause, bone resorption in women increases greatly.

**What Are the Risk Factors?**

Two major factors for osteoporosis are lack of exercise and inadequate intake of calcium, vitamin D, and protein. Osteoporosis caused by calcium and vitamin D deficiencies affects men and women 70 to 85 years of age. Other risk factors contributing to the disease are these:

1. A family history of osteoporosis
2. Smoking and consuming too much alcohol and caffeine, which interfere with the absorption of calcium
3. Prolonged use of drugs or medications such as steroids, magnesium-based antacids such as Maalox, and heparin
4. Diseases and hormonal disorders such as rheumatoid arthritis, liver disease, certain cancers, and an overactive thyroid gland
5. Poor calcium absorption in the intestines

Although osteoporosis primarily affects middle-aged or older people, it can occur in young adults. Injuries that result in paralysis or long periods of immobility can lead to osteoporosis.

From *Mosby's patient teaching guides: update 3,* St Louis, 1997, Mosby.

The patient and family will also need information about diet, including foods rich in calcium and vitamin D. Patients should be instructed to read the labels of over-the-counter medications, particularly for calcium content.

#### Health promotion/prevention

Teaching should include health promotion techniques, especially for persons at risk of developing osteoporosis. To decrease the risk of osteoporosis in all persons, a diet adequate in calcium and vitamin D and regular weight-bearing exercise should be advocated beginning in childhood to accumulate peak bone mass at skeletal maturity. The elderly, including elderly men, are another at-risk target population. Premenopausal women will benefit from an explanation of the effects of estrogen on bone mass before the need arises. Strategies to prevent osteoporosis should be explained to perimenopausal women (Box 61-12). Screening for BMD should be done for persons at risk of developing osteoporosis or before beginning treatment to determine baseline levels to monitor the effectiveness of treatment.

The National Osteoporosis Foundation is an excellent resource for information about osteoporosis. A newsletter is published quarterly regarding advances in treatments for osteoporosis. *Boning Up on Osteoporosis* is an excellent guide to the treatment and prevention of osteoporosis and is available from the Foundation. National Osteoporosis Week is usually held in May each year.

## EVALUATION

To evaluate the effectiveness of nursing interventions, compare patient behaviors with those stated in the expected outcomes. Successful achievement of patient outcomes for the patient with osteoporosis is indicated by:

1. Is not injured; has had no falls or fractures. Verbalizes knowledge of safety measures, exercises, and preventive strategies to prevent falls, injuries, and fractures
2. Maintains or increases strength and mobility. Demonstrates maximum degree of mobility and functioning.
3. Has positive self-esteem, participates in usual roles to fullest extent, and engages in social activities as desired.

## SPECIAL ENVIRONMENTS FOR CARE

### Home Care Management

Many of the home care considerations for persons with osteoporosis pertain to modification of the home environment to prevent falls or fractures (see the Patient/Family Teaching Box on p. 2014). In addition, a home health care referral may be needed if the patient is unable to complete ADL independently. Homemaking services may also be required. Meals-on-Wheels is an option for patients who are unable to prepare their meals independently. Assistive and adaptive devices may need to be purchased for the home. If the patient does not have the necessary resources, several community agencies may offer assistance. These items may also be rented. If patients are severely disabled or lack family support for care, transfer to an assisted-living or nursing facility may be necessary.

## COMPLICATIONS

Complications of osteoporosis are primarily fractures. Fractures and complications of fracture are discussed in Chapter 60.

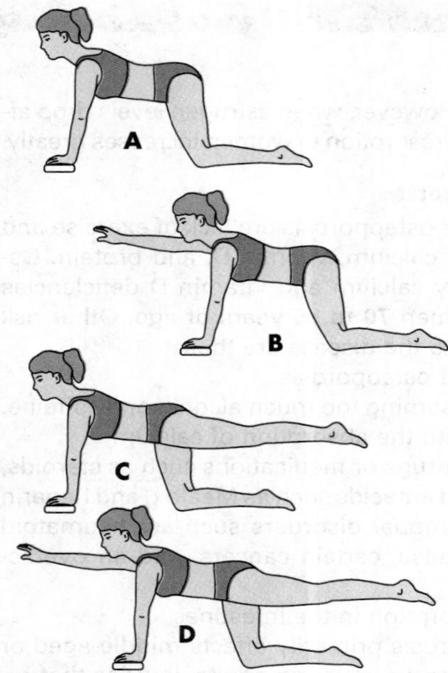


**All Fours Arm/Leg Lifts**
Position yourself on your hands and knees, with your hands directly under your shoulders and your knees directly under your hips (A). Your back should be flat or slightly arched. Lift one arm and hold for 3 seconds (B). Repeat with the other arm. Then lift one leg and hold for 3 seconds (C). Repeat with the other leg. If you can do these exercises comfortably, try lifting your right arm and left leg simultaneously (D), and then your left arm and right leg.

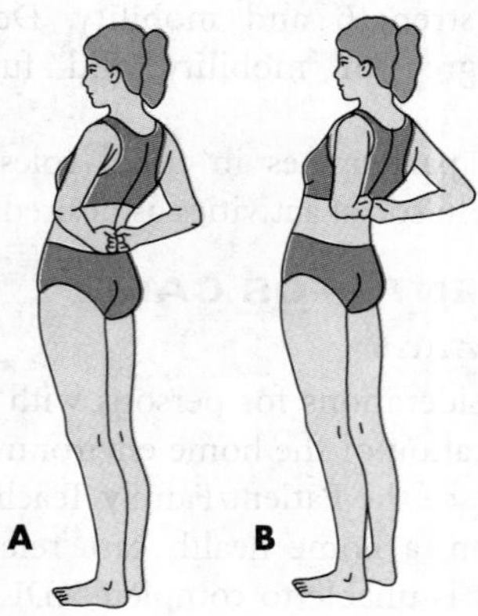


**Standing Back Bend**
Put your fists on your lower back. Arch backwards slowly while taking a deep breath (A). Relax and put your arms down, then repeat, this time with the fists on the middle back (B).

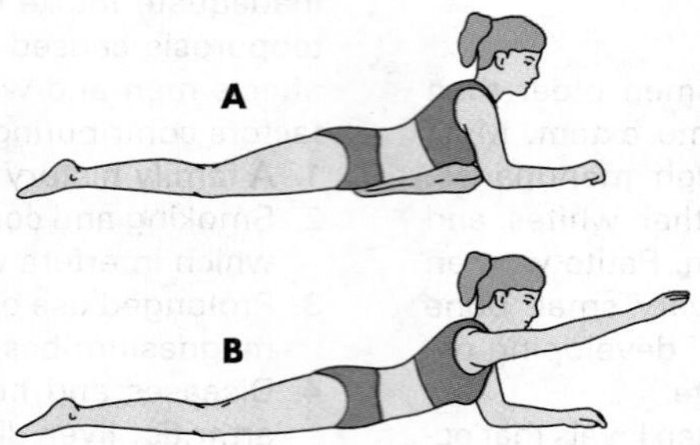


**The Elbow Prop**
Lie on your stomach with your elbows holding the weight of your upper body (A). Stay in this position for 5 minutes the first day; gradually increase the time to half an hour. You may be more comfortable if you put a pillow under your stomach. The elbow prop position helps reverse the effects of bad posture by passively decompressing the vertebrae and disks. To exercise the back as well, reach the right arm forward (B), then the left, and repeat.

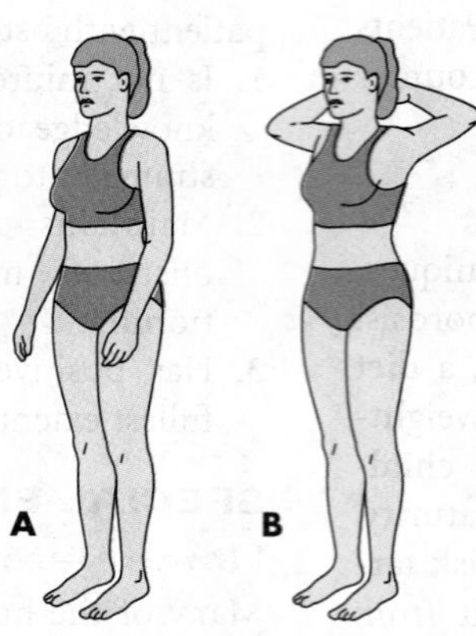


**Isometric Posture Correction**
Stand as tall as you can, with your chin in, not up (A). Place your palms against the back of your head. Simultaneously push your hands against your head while pinching your shoulder blades together (B). Hold for 3 seconds, then relax for 3 seconds. Maintain an erect posture throughout the exercise.

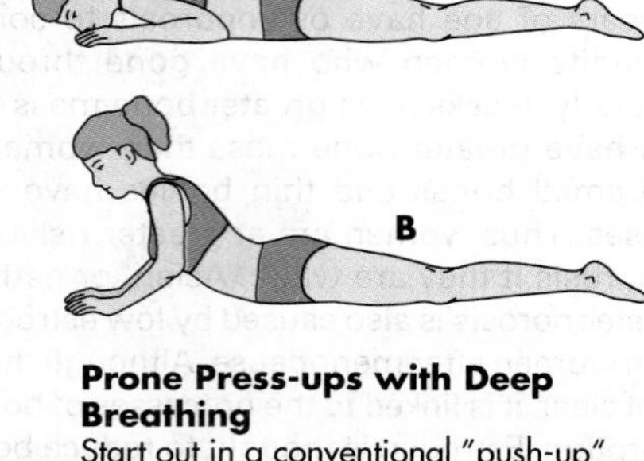


**Prone Press-ups with Deep Breathing**
Start out in a conventional "push-up" position (A). Arch your back, pinching your shoulder blades together (B). As you push up, inhale; as you lie down, exhale. Keep elbows partially bent to protect the back. Make sure you don't lift your pelvis.

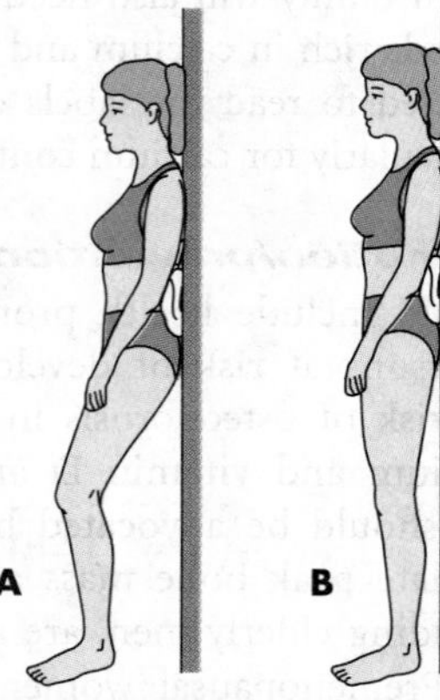


**Standing and Pelvic Tilt**
Stand with your feet about a foot from the wall, with your knees slightly bent and your back straight (A). Use a towel to support your lower back. Slide up and down, keeping the back straight and the stomach muscles contracted. You should be able to plant your feet closer to the wall as you improve.

**fig. 61-33** Exercises for prevention of osteoporosis.

**box 61-12** Healthy People 2000 *Goals—Osteoporosis*

Increase to at least 90% the proportion of perimenopausal women who have been counseled about the benefits and risks of estrogen replacement therapy (combined with progestin when appropriate) for prevention of osteoporosis.

Source: US Department of Health and Human Services, Public Health Service: *Healthy people 2000: midcourse review and 1995 revisions,* Boston, 1996, Jones & Bartlett.

## INFECTIOUS BONE DISEASE

### Osteomyelitis

#### Etiology

Although the development of osteomyelitis is often precipitated by a traumatic event or is a complication of trauma, it is included with the degenerative disorders because of its chronic and debilitating aspects. Osteomyelitis is an infection of the bone. It is most commonly caused by bacteria but can also be caused by fungi, parasites, and viruses.

#### Epidemiology

The two types of osteomyelitis are classified by the mode of entry of the pathogen. *Exogenous osteomyelitis,* or as described by the Waldvogel system as secondary to a contiguous source of infection,[35,39] is caused by a pathogen from outside the body. Examples include pathogens from an open fracture or surgical procedure, particularly joint replacements or procedures involving instrumentation. The infection can also be caused by human and animal bites and fist blows to the mouth. The most common organism found in human bites is *Staphylococcus aureus* and in animal bites is *Pasteurella multocida.* The infection spreads from the soft tissues to the bone. Risk factors for developing exogenous osteomyelitis are chronic illness or diabetes, alcohol or drug abuse, and immunosuppression. In persons with diabetes or vascular disease, osteomyelitis occurs most frequently in the feet. Pain may be absent due to neuropathy. The onset is insidious: initially cellulitis progressing to the underlying bone.

*Hematogenous osteomyelitis* is caused by blood-borne pathogens originating from infectious sites within the body. Examples include sinus, ear, dental, respiratory, and genitourinary infections. In hematogenous osteomyelitis the infection spreads from the bone to the soft tissues and can eventually break through the skin, becoming a draining fistula. This type of osteomyelitis is more common in infants, children, and elderly persons. In elderly persons, men are more commonly affected. *S. aureus* is the most common causative organism. Other responsible organisms include *streptococcus B, Haemophilus influenzae, Salmonella,* and gram-negative bacteria. *Salmonella* is linked with sickle cell anemia, and gram-negative organisms are associated with infections occurring in elderly and immunocompromised individuals. *Pseudomonas aeruginosa* is common in persons with a history of IV or IM drug abuse.[35]

**box 61-13** *Classification of Long-Bone Osteomyelitis by Cierny-Mader System*

**Stage 1: Medullary**
Necrosis limited to medullary canal and endosteal surfaces

**Stage 2: Superficial**
Bone necrosis only at exposed surface

**Stage 3: Localized**
Bone stable; sequestrum through one cortex, well-marginated infection

**Stage 4: Diffuse**
Unstable bone, infection all around bone, through both cortices

Acute osteomyelitis, left untreated or unresolved after 10 days is termed *chronic osteomyelitis.* Osteomyelitis of long bones can also be categorized by the stages of infection (Box 61-13).[39]

#### Pathophysiology

Necrotic bone is the distinguishing feature of chronic osteomyelitis. In hematogenous osteomyelitis the organisms reach the bone through the circulatory and lymphatic systems. The bacteria lodge in the small vessels of the bone, triggering an inflammatory response. Blockage of the vessel causes thrombosis, ischemia, and necrosis of the bone. The femur, tibia, humerus, and radius are commonly affected. Infections of the pelvic organs frequently spread to the pelvis and vertebrae. The pathophysiology of osteomyelitis is similar to that of infectious processes in any other body tissue.

Bone inflammation is marked by edema, increased vasculature, and leukocyte activity. Exudate seals the bone's canaliculi, extends into the metaphysis and marrow cavity, and finally reaches the cortex. New bone, laid down over the infected bone by osteoblasts, is termed *involucrum.* Openings in the involucrum allow infected material to escape into soft tissues. The infectious process weakens the cortex, thereby increasing the risk of pathological fracture. *Brodie's abscesses* are characteristic of chronic osteomyelitis. These are isolated, encapsulated pockets of microorganisms surrounded by bone matrix, usually found in long bones. These pockets of virulent organisms are capable of reinfection at any time. The microscopic channels found in bone allow bacteria to proliferate without being affected by the body's defenses.[41]

In patients with exogenous osteomyelitis the infection begins in the soft tissues, disrupting muscle and connective tissues, and eventually forming abscesses. Signs and symptoms associated with soft tissue infection are most common.

Chronic osteomyelitis is difficult to treat. Recurrent infection, areas of dead bone (*sequestrum*), and scar tissue are contributing factors to its resistance to treatment. Complications of chronic osteomyelitis include sepsis, nonunion, draining fistulae, shortening of the affected extremity, and eventual amputation.[35]

The clinical manifestations of osteomyelitis vary with the individual, type of responsible organism, precipitating event, and type of infection (acute or chronic). The patient may report fever, malaise, anorexia, and headache. The affected body part may be erythematous, tender, and edematous. There may be a fistula draining purulent material.

### Collaborative care management

Blood tests reveal an increase in WBCs, erythrocyte sedimentation rate, and C-reactive protein levels. A culture and sensitivity test of the drainage will reveal the causative organisms and identify appropriate antibiotic therapy. Blood cultures will determine the presence or absence of septicemia. MRI and a radionuclide bone scan may be performed. Pathological changes are visible after the infection is present for 7 to 10 days. If an open debridement is necessary, pathological examination of the tissues will confirm the diagnosis of osteomyelitis.

Treatment is difficult and costly. The goals of treatment are as follows:

1. Complete removal of dead bone and affected soft tissue
2. Control of infection
3. Elimination of dead space (after removal of necrotic bone)

Many modes of treatment are available. Which treatment modality is used depends on the area of bone involved, causative organism, ability to maintain a functional limb, duration of treatment, and expected outcomes. Treatment options include the following:

1. Antibiotic therapy: Intravenous antibiotics may be prescribed for up to 6 weeks, and oral antibiotic therapy may continue for up to 6 months.
2. Irrigation and drainage system: This involves a surgical procedure in which holes are drilled into the cortex of the bone, allowing continuous infusion of antibiotic solution and drainage of inflammatory exudate. Drains are usually removed after a few days to prevent secondary infection.[60]
3. Analgesics and antipyretics as necessary.

When conservative modalities fail to control the infection, surgical intervention is indicated. Many types of surgery are possible, from simple debridement to amputation. Debridement involves removal of sequestrum and surrounding granulation tissue. Temporary placement of polymethylmethacrylate antibiotic beads in the wound is done after debridement.[35,60] Antibiotics continue to be released into the wound for up to 30 days (see Chapter 60). With placement of antibiotic beads, antibiotic levels at the infection site are higher than after systemic administration.[31] The wound is closed and covered; 2 to 4 weeks later, the beads are removed, and reconstruction is performed. Other options include the use of allograft bone, the Ilizarov technique (see Chapter 60), and the *Papineau bone graft.* The Papineau technique was introduced in the 1970s as a means to treat osteomyelitis occurring in the diaphysis of long bones. It consists of removal of infected and necrotic bone, immobilization (usually achieved by an external fixator [see Chapter 60]), delayed cancellous bone grafts, and finally soft tissue closure. This technique has been shown to be highly successful in the treatment of chronic osteomyelitis.

Revascularization procedures including local pedicle flaps and myocutaneous flaps are commonly performed for recurrent osteomyelitis.[35,60] Hyperbaric oxygen treatments have been used for gas gangrene and chronic osteomyelitis. In addition, patients are also treated with antibiotics and surgical debridement.

Nursing management of the patient with osteomyelitis includes the following:

1. Using aseptic technique during dressing changes
2. Observing the patient for signs and symptoms of systemic infection
3. Encouraging range-of-motion exercises to prevent contractures and flexion deformities
4. Administering antibiotics on time and as prescribed
5. Administering analgesics and/or antipyretics as prescribed; monitoring patient for effectiveness
6. Promoting rest of affected joint or limb. The affected extremity should be handled carefully to avoid pathological fracture. Splints are often used for immobilization.
7. Encouraging participation in ADL to fullest extent
8. Instructing the patient in correct use of assistive devices as needed

**Patient/family education.** If home-going therapy is prescribed, the proper administration of antibiotics should be taught. A discussion of drug side effects should be included. Long-term antibiotic therapy can be performed at home with the help of a home health nurse. The patient and family can also administer antibiotics with periodic visits by the nurse. Dressing changes may also be performed at home. The patient and family can be taught an aseptic technique.

Persons with total joint implants need instruction regarding the signs and symptoms of infection and avoiding sources of infection. The patient with an acute infection should be instructed to avoid the use of heat and exercise, which increase circulation and may spread infection. Information regarding follow-up care should be provided.

If surgery is performed, perioperative instructions are necessary (see Chapter 18). Persons with radical resections, flaps, external fixators, or amputations will need emotional support in accepting body image changes and decreased mobility and independence. The patient and family will need much support in coping with a chronic illness. Depression may occur in response to a chronic illness. The patient and family may need support and referrals for financial assistance, particularly if they lack insurance or they have insufficient coverage.

## DISORDERS AFFECTING THE SPINE

### LOW BACK PAIN

#### Etiology/Epidemiology

Low back pain (LBP) is one the most common conditions a nurse will encounter in any practice setting. Although a common disorder, LBP is also a challenge to health care professionals. Worldwide, it is estimated that up to 80% of the population experience LBP at some time during the life span.[36] Second only to respiratory problems in the number of primary care office visits and time lost from work, LBP is also a major cause of permanent work disability.[68] In the United States, medical costs from LBP alone exceed $24 billion annually.[11] Each year more than 7 million people in the United States are treated for LBP, 2 million of those are new patients.[68] LBP is a challenge to the health care professional because it is a *symptom,* not usually attributable to a specific cause or disease. Eighty percent of cases of LBP are idiopathic. Indeed, in approximately 80% of persons with LBP without neurological symptoms the pain will resolve within 4 to 6 weeks without specific treatment.[22,68] Some patients will develop chronic pain conditions, and approximately 15% have LBP attributable to specific causes, including herniated disk, spinal stenosis, compression fracture, systemic disease related to the spine, and systemic disease unrelated to the spine.[22] The most common systemic conditions related to LBP are malignancy and infection.[68] Persons in whom a systemic cause of LBP should be suspected include those younger than 20 years or older than 50 years and those with a history of cancer, symptoms of fever or chills, and unexplained weight loss. Other symptoms that require immediate attention include severe pain, significant neurological deficit, sensory loss in the saddle area, abdominal pain, and trauma.[22]

Approximately 2% of Americans have had back surgery, and many patients in back pain clinics have had two or more spine procedures.[68] The United States has the highest rate for back surgery among industrialized countries. The emerging opinion is that many of these procedures are unnecessary and are often associated with poor results in terms of relieving pain.[68] Surgery is necessary in an estimated 1% of persons with LBP.[58]

Low back pain affects the area below the ribs and gluteal muscles, often radiating to the thighs. An acute low back problem as defined by the Agency for Health Care Policy and Research is "an activity intolerance due to low back or back-related symptoms of less than 3 months duration."[68] Chronic pain persists longer than 12 weeks. The most common cause is a lumbar strain after lifting or twisting. Men and women are affected equally, but women report more symptoms after age 60. Risk factors associated with LBP include occupational hazards (repetitive motions, prolonged exposure to vibrations, and forward bending and twisting motions of the spine), smoking, osteoporosis, and hyperthyroidism.

## Pathophysiology

The pathophysiology of common causes of back pain including herniated disc, spinal stenosis, and spondylolisthesis is discussed on p. 2021-2022. If disk herniation is the cause of back pain, the pain comes from the irritated dura and spinal nerves, as the nucleus pulposus lacks intrinsic innervation. Pain can arise from the joint capsule, ligaments, or muscles in the lumbar spine. The ligamentous structures of the lumbar spine are richly supplied with pain receptors and are susceptible to tears, sprains, and fracture. Muscle sprains and strains are also common causes of back pain. See Chapter 12 for a discussion of the theories of pain.

## Collaborative Care Management

A detailed history and complete physical examination are required for accurate diagnosis and treatment of the person with LBP. The patient should be asked about any associated symptoms, any neurological deficits, and any loss of bowel or bladder control. The presence of bowel or bladder symptoms should alert the health care provider to the possibility of *cauda equina syndrome,* which needs emergency surgical intervention. Cauda equina syndrome is compression of the caudal sac by herniated disk material. The presence of abdominal pain may suggest the presence of abdominal aortic aneurysm.

The physical examination should include neurological assessment, ROM, and muscle testing. Limits in forward flexion are commonly found, with localized pain in the lumbosacral area. Screening for malignancy should also be done. Specialized tests including straight leg raising (see Chapter 59) and crossed leg raising should be incorporated into the examination. A complete assessment of the pain should be done. The patient's descriptors of the pain are important in determining the effect the pain has had on the person's lifestyle.

Routine laboratory examinations are not indicated. Controversy exists regarding the appropriateness of ordering x-rays at the first visit. Federal guidelines recommend a conservative approach, but research indicates that for more than 50% of patients seen for LBP, lumbar films are ordered at the first visit.[68] Plain films are recommended only for persons older than age 50, those with symptoms suspicious of systemic disease, and persons with radiculopathy.[68] CT scan and MRI are used only for persons in whom surgery is indicated.

Most persons with LBP respond well to conservative therapy. A multidisciplinary approach is necessary. Patients benefit from an early return to work and physical activity. Prolonged bedrest and missed work are actually harmful, reinforcing the concept of illness and disability.[68] Bedrest is limited to 2 to 3 days for patients with radiculopathy. For those without neurological symptoms bedrest is not recommended or at most for 1 to 2 days.[58,68] Inactivity results in loss of strength and endurance, promotes dysfunction, and increases the risk of microtrauma.[58] Back exercises to strengthen lumbar musculature are indicated for treatment of LBP. Stretching and extension exercises have shown positive results, whereas flexion exercises have been of little benefit.[58,68] A PT referral is beneficial to instruct patients in the proper method to perform exercises. Lumbar and pelvic traction have not been effective in relieving pain and are not recommended.[68] The application of heat or cold applied within 48 hours of onset of symptoms, or heat for symptoms persisting over 48 hours is effective in reducing pain. Massage therapy has provided some patients with temporary relief. Previously recommended, transcutaneous electrical stimulation has little objective effect in increasing functional status, although the placebo effect is high.[68] Other treatments include trigger-point therapy and spinal manipulation. See Chapter 12 for other nonpharmacological methods of pain control.

Pharmacological treatments include NSAIDs, analgesics, and muscle relaxants. Medications should not be used for longer than 12 weeks, because of the risk of side effects.[58] Tricyclic antidepressants have been used in treating chronic pain, although the results are not conclusive.[68] Steroid injections have also been used with some success.

Interventions addressing psychosocial needs are important in the management of persons with LBP. Depression and substance abuse are common in persons with LBP.[11] Secondary gain may be a motive in some persons, making treatment difficult. Persons whose pain has persisted for longer than 3 months may need a psychological referral.

### *Patient/family education*

The patient and family will need education about the pathogenesis of back pain, particularly if no specific cause is found. Reassurance that most persons with back pain respond favorably to conservative treatment and are able to return to work and leisure activities can help decrease anxiety about long-term effects of the pain on lifestyle. If appropriate, information about lifestyle changes such as cessation of smoking, weight loss, and institution of a regular exercise program should be given. Body weight should be maintained within 10% of the ideal body weight. If environmental conditions such as occupational hazards are contributing to the LBP, perhaps a modification in the work environment can be made. In some cases, employment retraining may be indicated.

Persons with depression or substance abusers should be referred to a psychologist or counselor for additional therapy. Cognitive coping strategies have been used effectively in helping patients cope with chronic pain. Patients' positive perceptions of their self-efficacy may assist them in implementing strategies to relieve pain and cope with a chronic pain condition. Self-efficacy theory states that a person's perceived ability to carry out a behavior necessary for a desired outcome positively influences the probability the person will perform the behavior.[36] Nurses can assist patients in learning these behaviors.

Providing information about proper body mechanics and methods to avoid back injury are very important. The proper ways to sit, stand, bend, and lift objects should be demonstrated to all patients with LBP (see Figure 61-32). When seated, feet should rest flat on the floor or stool. Knees should be higher than the hip with the arms supported. When lifting, bend the knees, not the back and do not lift objects higher than the level of the elbows. While sleeping supine, place a pillow under the knees. A firm mattress or bed board is beneficial for adequate support. Giving the patient information to prevent further episodes of back pain allows the patient responsibility for management of the condition and some sense of control. Many back pain clinics have a "Back School" where patients are referred and taught principles of body mechanics, posture, and exercises. Regular aerobic exercise in addition to back-strengthening exercise should be done for at least 30 minutes 5 times per week (Figure 61-34). Walking and swimming are good choices for persons with LBP. Some persons may believe that exercise will do further harm to the back; they will need reassurance and encouragement to participate in a regular exercise program.

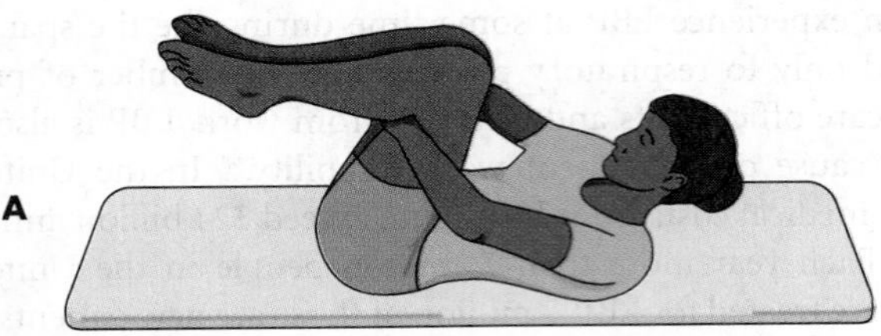


**Back Roll**

The back roll stretches your back, buttocks, and neck muscles. Lie on your back on the floor, relax, and bring your knees to your chest. Clasp your hands behind your knee and rock back and forth, from your buttocks to your neck. Slowly return to the starting position. Repeat 5 to 10 times.

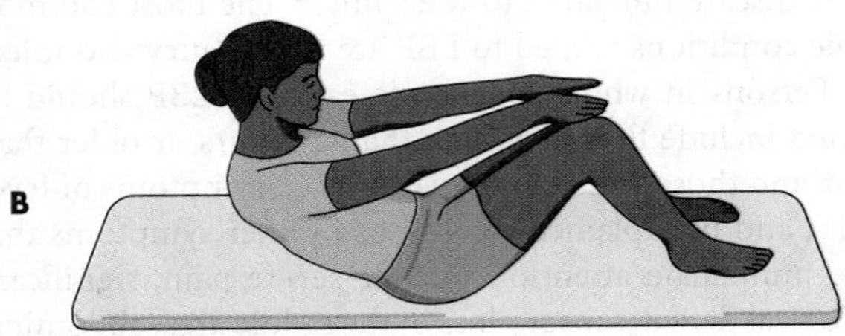


**Partial Sit-ups**

Partial sit-ups strengthen your abdominal muscles. Lie flat on your back on the floor with your knees bent and feet flat on the floor. Tuck in your chin and tighten your abdomen. Slowly raise your head and neck while reaching out with your hands to touch your knees. Hold your knees for a count of five and slowly return to the starting position. Repeat 5 to 10 times.

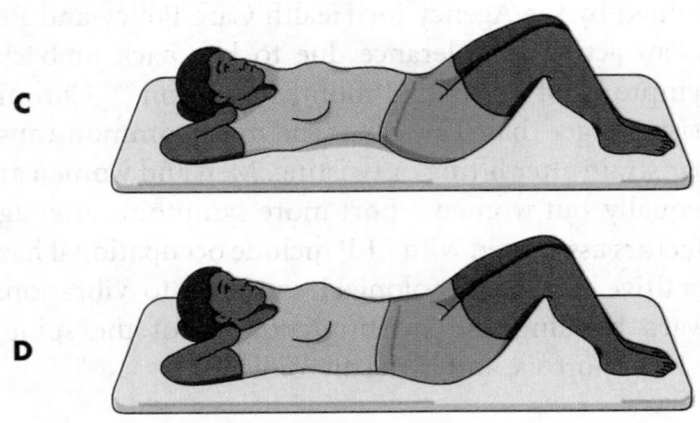


**Pelvic Tilt**

The pelvic tilt strengthens your abdominal and back muscles. Lie flat on your back on the floor with your knees bent and feet flat on the floor. Join your hands behind your head. Firmly tighten your buttock and abdominal muscles, pressing your lower back flat against the floor. Hold for a count of five and relax muscles. Repeat 5 to 10 times.

**fig. 61-34** Exercises for lower back pain. **A,** Back roll; **B,** partial sit-ups; **C** and **D,** pelvic tilt.

Support groups may help the individual with LBP. Exercising at community centers may provide the person with companionship. For persons with chronic pain, a referral to a pain support group may be indicated. Information can be obtained at the following address:

The American Pain Society, 4700 West Lake Avenue, Glenview, IL 60025; (847) 375-4715; Internet address: info@ampainsoc.org.

## DEGENERATIVE DISORDERS OF THE SPINE

A number of degenerative disorders that affect the cervical, thoracic, and lumbar portions of the spine are treated by surgical intervention. The collaborative care and nursing management sections will pertain to persons with any of the these disorders.

### Etiology

Degenerative disease of the spine is a common but difficult problem. The spine has 23 intervertebral disk joints and 46 posterior facet joints (Figure 61-35), all of which are subjected to stresses and strains in holding the human body upright and moving it about. The vertebrae in the spinal column are articulated in a series of "couplets" that are able to move through an intervertebral disk joint and two posterior facet joints. The intervertebral disks are composed of an outer layer of cartilage called the *anulus fibrosus* and an inner layer of cartilage called the *nucleus pulposus.* Several common problems arise with these structures in degenerative disease of the spine. These include degenerative disc disease, herniated intervertebral disk, spinal stenosis, spondylolisthesis, and spondylosis.

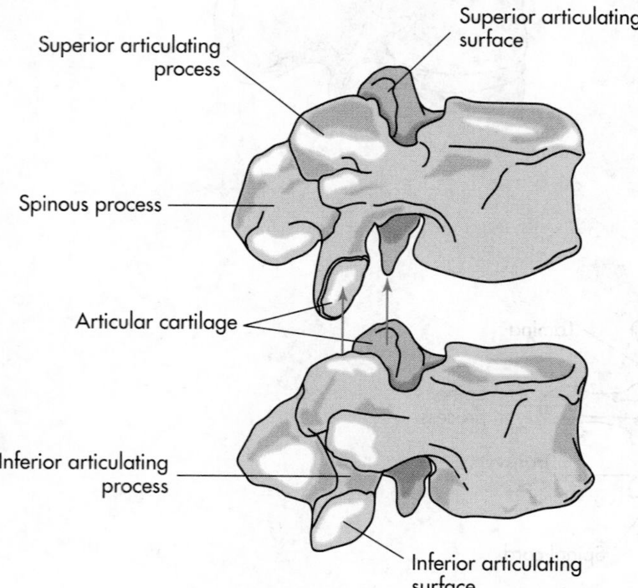


**fig. 61-35** Posterior facet joints of lumbar vertebrae. Each vertebra has four surfaces by which it articulates with its adjacent vertebrae: two on its superior aspect and two on the inferior. Superior articulating surfaces are medially located; inferior articulating surfaces are laterally located. These joints are diarthrotic, having a joint capsule with a synovial lining.

Degenerative disc disease (DDD) develops as a result of biochemical and biomechanical changes in the intervertebral discs. The gelatinous mucoid material of the nucleus pulposus is replaced with fibrocartilage as a result of aging. The water content of the disc changes from 90% during childhood to 70% by 60 years of age.[60]

Spinal stenosis occurs as result of aging, degenerative disk disease, spondylosis, osteophyte formation, or a congenital condition. The disc space is narrowed, losing its resiliency, and may be unstable at the affected levels. Smoking is a risk factor for the development of disc degeneration and herniation. Other identified risk factors include sedentary lifestyle and extensive motor vehicle driving.

Heredity plays a role in spondylolysis, occurring more frequently in conjunction with other congenital spine defects.

### Epidemiology

Degenerative disorders of the spine develop most commonly in persons older than age 50. Cervical spondylosis is found in 90% of men older than age 50 and in 90% of women older than age 60.[60] Disc herniation is seen in persons of all ages, but the peak incidence is between 35 to 45 years of age. The rate for surgical treatment of disk herniation in the United States is three times as high as that in Sweden.[60]

### Pathophysiology

Pathophysiological changes associated with degenerative disc disease include spinal stenosis (narrowing of the spinal canal), spondylosis (degeneration and stiffness of the vertebral joints), subluxation, and vertebral degeneration. Initial disc changes are followed by facet arthropathy, osteophyte formation, and ligamentous instability. Myelopathy and radiculopathy (disease involving a spinal nerve root) may follow. The degenerative process usually involves synovitis, which causes cartilage erosion, leading to the formation of osteophytes.

*Herniated intervertebral disk* is a protrusion of the nucleus pulposus through a tear or rupture in the anulus. Herniation can occur anteriorly, posteriorly, or laterally. Extrusion of the disk material may impinge on a nerve root or on the spinal cord (Figure 61-36). Herniation may occur as a result of trauma, a sharp or sudden movement, or degeneration. In the cervical spine, herniation usually occurs at the more mobile segments, C5-6, C6-7, and C4-5.[60] Ninety percent of lumbar herniations occur at the L5-S1 and L4-5 levels (Box 61-14).[60] Herniation of thoracic disks is rare. Symptoms may develop immediately or take years to manifest themselves. The location and size of the herniation will determine the signs and symptoms associated with the herniation. Pain associated with disk herniation may be caused by direct pressure of disc fragments on the nerve root, by breakdown products from a degenerated nucleus pulposus, or by an autoimmune reaction. The nurse's knowledge of dermatomes and spinal nerve innervation will aid in the assessment of a patient with a herniated intervertebral disk (Table 61-17). Another consideration is the size of the patient's spinal canal. A slight herniation may cause significant symptoms in an individual with a congenitally narrow canal.

*Spinal stenosis* is a narrowing of the spinal canal or intervertebral foramina at any level, creating pressure on the involved nerve root(s), resulting in neurological symptoms. Spinal stenosis results from enlargement of the ligamentum flavum, laminae, and facet joints. Osteophyte formation may cause neuroforaminal stenosis. Joint instability and subluxation may result. The most commonly involved segments are L4-5 and then L3-4.[6]

*Spondylolisthesis* is a forward slipping of one vertebra on another. Spondylolisthesis can be a congenital abnormality or be caused by degenerative changes, trauma, or bone disease. Spondylolysis is often the cause. *Spondylolysis* refers to a structural defect of the lamina, usually in the lumbar spine. The pars interarticularis (between the superior and inferior articular facets) is usually the site of the defect. The degree of spondylolisthesis is graded on a scale of 1 to 4, depending on the percentage of slip that is shown on x-ray films of the spine. Grades 3 and 4 are usually treated surgically. Spondylolisthesis usually occurs at L5-S1 but can also occur at the L4-5 and L3-4 levels.[60] The forward slip of the vertebra can cause nerve impingement, manifested by motor and sensory deficits at the level(s) involved, such as pain, weakness, and/or bowel and bladder involvement. The slip may be detected when the spinous processes are palpated.

## Collaborative Care Management

### Diagnostic tests

Diagnostic tests to determine defects in the spine include x-ray films, myelography, CT scanning, and MRI. See Chapter 59 for more information.

### Medications

Conservative management of degenerative problems of the spine includes the use of antiinflammatory agents (usually NSAIDs). Concomitant use of alcohol or aspirin may increase

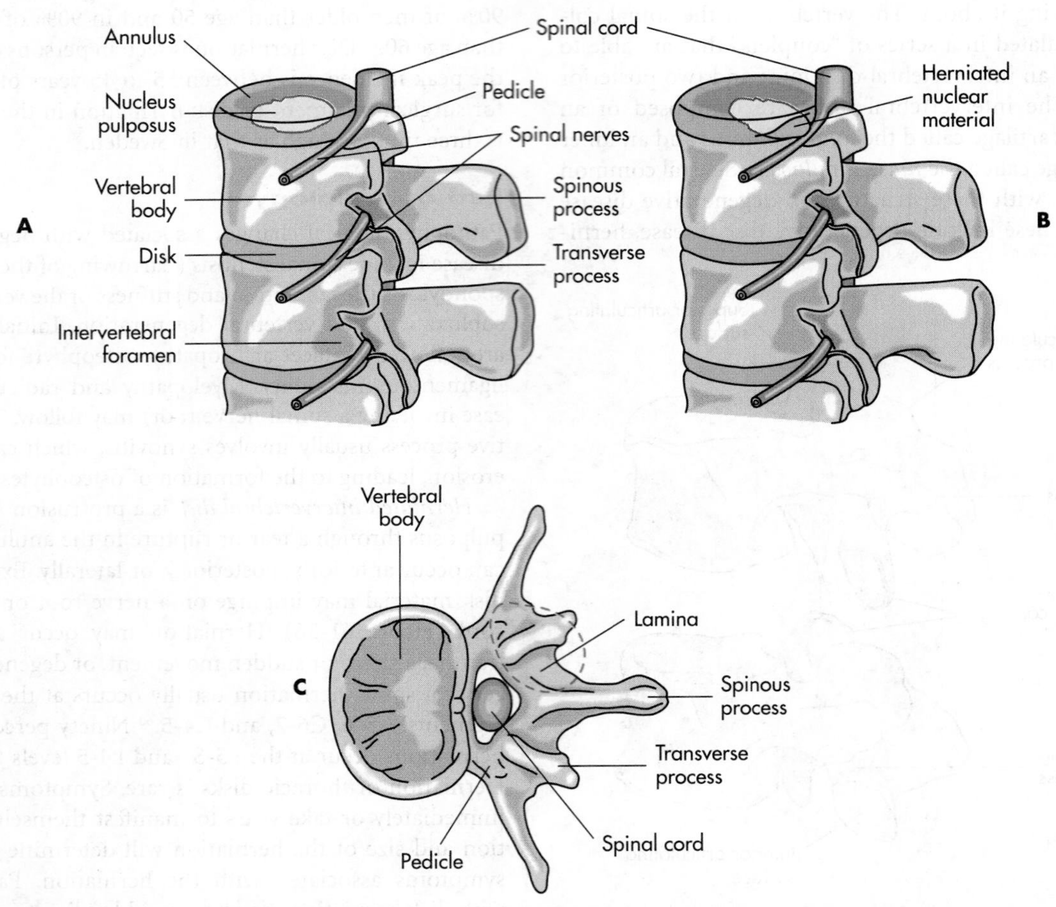


**fig. 61-36** Compression of spinal cord and nerve root. **A,** Disks, composed of a cartilaginous outer layer (anulus fibrosus) and a gel-like inner layer (nucleus pulposus), lie between vertebral bodies. Spinal nerves exit the spinal cord laterally just above the pedicle. **B,** Laminae compose posterior portions of vertebrae. Each pedicle joins with a lamina *(dotted line)*; the transverse and spinous processes project from laminae. **C,** When nucleus pulposus herniates posteriorly through its fibrous covering and the posterior longitudinal ligament, it may compress the spinal cord and trap the nerve root. The surgical approach to relieve this compression is through lamina, posterior to the transverse process.

gastrointestinal irritation and bleeding tendencies and therefore should be avoided. Pain relief is usually noted after 1 week of therapy.

The use of narcotic analgesics is usually avoided, especially over a prolonged period of time, because of the risks of dependency and tolerance. However, short-term use of opiates is appropriate in some cases. Oral corticosteroids are useful for treating pain for short periods of time; long-term use is not recommended.

Skeletal muscle relaxants may also be prescribed. The patient should be cautioned against driving or engaging in potentially hazardous activities because of drowsiness, a frequent side effect of muscle relaxants. The patient should be informed that the use of alcohol or other CNS depressants will enhance the effect of the muscle relaxant. Muscle relaxants frequently cause dry mouth, and the nurse can instruct the patient in measures to counteract this side effect.

**box 61-14** *Possible Signs and Symptoms of Herniated Intervertebral Disk*

CERVICAL

- Decreased range of motion of cervical spine
- Paresthesias of upper extremities, depending on nerve root involved
- Weakness or atrophy of upper extremity musculature, depending on level involved
- Pain in affected nerve root distribution
- Abdominal reflex activity
- May have motor or sensory disturbances in lower extremities

LUMBAR

- Sciatica in 40% of persons
- Tenderness or pain with palpation of disk spaces and sciatic notch
- Painful and/or decreased range of motion of lumbar spine
- Motor and sensory impairment in affected nerve root distribution (may note discrepancies in calf circumference, weakness in lower extremity muscle groups, pain and numbness in dermatomal distribution)
- Decreased or absent reflexes
- Bowel or bladder impairment
- Positive straight leg raising (Lasegue's test): straight leg raising with opposite leg flat will produce leg pain or radicular symptoms
- Pain radiating down leg in dermatomal distribution
- Pain relieved by lying down

Antiinflammatory medications or local anesthetics may be injected directly into the affected joint or structure (epidural space to relieve nerve root pain). The use of steroid injections should be limited because of adverse effects on tissue healing and the risk of osteoporosis. Epidural steroids have a 50% success rate in short-term treatment of spinal stenosis.[60]

### Treatments

Conservative treatment is implemented initially. Pain control and return to functioning are the goals of treatment. Conservative management is given a trial before surgical intervention is considered, unless neurological deficits are present.

Bedrest is indicated for 1 or 2 days at most, followed by a physical therapy regimen. Ultrasound, application of heat and cold, massage, pelvic traction to relieve muscle spasms, and physical therapy referrals for back-strengthening exercises are common treatment modalities. Spinal manipulation, joint immobilization, and deep massage are also indicated, usually by a physical therapist, chiropractor, or physician. Spinal manipulation is contraindicated for patients with documented disk herniation, because of the risk of neurological deficits. Exercises should be taught by a physical therapist initially, then can be performed independently by the patient. Two to three sessions per week for a 6- to 8-week period are recommended for strengthening exercises. Isometrics, dynamic exercises, and exercise machines are all used. Exercises can be performed at home, or at the health club or gym and should be performed regularly to maintain progress.

Passive decompression for disk herniation (forcing the protruded disc material out) can be used for younger patients with neurological deficits. Disadvantages include breaking off of the fragment and migration caudally or cephalad. *Chemonucleolysis,* or injection of enzyme, has been used to dissolve disk material (chymopapain injections). Chymopapain, an enzyme extracted from papaya plant, hydrolyzes the proteoglycans and is injected directly into the disc to degrade the nucleus pulposus. Adverse effects include allergic reaction (possibly fatal) and neurological deficits. Risks associated with chymopapain injection are lower than those associated with surgical intervention. However, this procedure is not performed frequently in the United States because of potential adverse effects. The risk of life-threatening anaphylaxis can be decreased by using lower doses of chymopapain. Blood tests, performed before chemonucleolysis, can determine whether or not the patient is allergic to the chymopapain. The patient should also be questioned regarding allergy to meat tenderizers, which are similar in composition to chymopapain.

**table 61-17** *Lumbar Disk Herniation*

| Level of Herniation | Nerve Root | Reflex | Sensation | Muscle Testing |
|---|---|---|---|---|
| L3-4 | L4 | Patellar | Medial aspects of leg and foot | Inversion of foot (tibialis anterior) |
| L4-5 | L5 | — | Lateral aspect of leg and dorsal surface of foot | Extension of toes (extensor hallucis longus) |
| L5-S1 | S1 | Achilles | Lateral aspect of foot | Eversion of foot (peroneus longus, brevis) |

Corsets or braces are sometimes prescribed to provide external support to the spine, especially during physical activity. Braces and corsets are fitted by an orthotist.

The injection of *sclerosants* (or proliferants) into a specific incompetent structure stimulates local inflammatory repair processes. Injections are painful, and repeated injections may be necessary to achieve results.[42]

### Surgical management

Most spinal disorders are treated conservatively. Surgery is indicated when conservative modalities fail or for the following reasons: neurological deficits, such as loss of bowel or bladder control or loss of motor function; severe, intractable pain; bony instability; and progressive deformity with resultant loss of function.

Spinal surgery is also performed for fractures (see Chapter 60) and tumors. A variety of procedures are performed on the cervical, thoracic, and lumbar spine. Surgical approaches to the spine include anterior, as for a cervical discectomy; transthoracic or retroperitoneal, for anterior spinal fusion; and posterior, as for a lumbar laminectomy. Box 61-15 gives examples of commonly performed types of spine surgery.

Spinal surgery may involve the use of instrumentation. A number of different implants are on the market today. Instrumentation is used to maintain correction of deformity, stabilize the spine, prevent neurological damage, enhance bony fusion, avoid external immobilization, and allow for early mobilization, thereby facilitating rehabilitation. The type of instrumentation used depends on the pathological condition, individual patient, and surgeon preference. Table 61-18 gives examples of spinal instrumentation.

Some types of spinal surgery involve the use of bone grafts. Bone grafts function as a form of scaffolding into which osteogenic cells grow and/or as a means of mechanical support. In addition to their use in spinal fusions, they are also used for patients with fractures, tumors, and joint replacements. Three types of bone grafts are autograft, xenograft, and allograft. *Autograft,* using the patient's own bone or that of an identical twin, has the best result. *Xenograft* is a graft taken from a different species, for example, bovine bone. Xenografts are rarely used in the United States. *Allograft* is human bone harvested from either a cadaver or living donor. In addition, bone substitute may be used for bone graft (see Chapter 60). The success of the bone graft depends partially on the type of fixation of the graft and the site and condition of the host recipient.

Both cortical and cancellous bone can serve as graft material. Allogeneic and autogenic cortical grafts both initially act as weight-bearing struts to provide support until the host bone has incorporated and remodeled the graft and is able to bear weight. Freshly implanted autografts are capable of osteogenesis, the process of bone synthesis by graft or host cells. Cancellous bone, because of its larger surface area, has greater potential for osteogenesis than does cortical bone. Host bone is produced by *osteoconduction,* a process in which mesenchymal cells of the host differentiate into osteoblasts.

Initially, all types of bone graft are partially resorbed. Incorporation of the bone graft takes place in overlapping stages. It begins by *creeping substitution* (gradual resorption of the graft, and finally replacement of the graft by new bone). Both autografts and allografts produce an acute inflammatory response within the first week, followed by the formation of fibrous granulation tissue and an increase in osteoclastic activity. This is followed by osteoinduction, which is probably regulated by bone morphogenic protein, which promotes new bone production by the host. Bone morphogenic protein is present in fresh autografts and in modified allografts, but autoclaving for sterilization destroys bone morphogenic protein. Osteoinduction is followed by osteoconduction, characterized by capillary growth and infiltration of the graft by perivascular tissue and osteoprogenitor cells of the host. This process may last for several months in cancellous autografts and for years in cortical autografts or allografts. Cancellous grafts are eventually completely replaced, whereas cortical grafts remain a mixture of necrotic graft bone and viable host bone. As remodeling takes place, the graft is resorbed and replaced by living bone, subject to Wolff's law (see Chapter 59).

Advantages of autografts are tissue compatibility and low cost. Disadvantages include a limited supply of bone, weakened donor site with a potential for fracture, and an added surgical site that can cause considerable pain for 2 to 3 years. The most common sites for graft harvesting are the iliac crests and the fibulae.

Advantages of allograft are fewer surgical sites, and thus less pain. Allografts also come in a variety of sizes and shapes. Disadvantages include a limited and costly supply and a high graft failure rate. Allografts trigger local and systemic immune responses that may affect their failure rate. Freezing and freeze-drying implants have decreased rejection, but frozen implants still have a 25% failure rate. There is also a danger of transmitting diseases such as acquired immunodeficiency syndrome (AIDS) and hepatitis B with allograft bone.

Surgical techniques have evolved to replace the traditional open approach to spinal surgery and instrumentation. *Microdiscectomy* involves a surgical incision, but much smaller than that with the open approach. The use of MRI and other imaging techniques allows direct access to the disc through a very small incision. Decompression and disc removal can be accomplished with less exposure and thus less pain and a shorter hospital stay. The surgeon must have considerable experience to

**box 61-15** *Types of Spinal Surgery*

**Laminectomy**—Removal of a portion of the lamina, the posterior arch of the vertebra, to gain access to the disk and spinal canal

**Discectomy**—Removal of all or part of a herniated intervertebral disk

**Foraminotomy**—Widening of the intervertebral foramen to allow free passage of the spinal nerve

**Spinal fusion**—Stabilization of two or more vertebrae by insertion of bone grafts with or without the addition of hardware (rods, plates, screws, or cages) to achieve vertebral stability

**Decompression**—Release of pressure or impingement on spinal nerve roots by removal of osteophytes, bone, or soft tissues

**table 61-18** *Common Types of Spinal Instrumentation*

| Indications | Approach | Components | Advantages and Disadvantages |
|---|---|---|---|
| **COTREL-DUBOUSSET (CD) (HORIZON)** | | | |
| Idiopathic scoliosis, kyphosis, trauma | Posterior | Parallel rods<br>Hooks<br>Screws<br>C-rings<br>Cross-link plate | *Advantages:* ability to correct rib hump deformity; early mobilization; bracing not necessary<br>*Disadvantages:* time-consuming, difficult technique, difficult to revise; hook shift; expensive |
| **HARRINGTON** | | | |
| Thoracolumbar fracture scoliosis | Posterior | Rods<br>Hooks<br>Screws | *Disadvantages:* increased immobility postoperatively; instrument failure, breakage; loss of correction; inability to control rod; loss of lumbar lordosis; need to fuse above and below level of pathological condition, resulting in immobile spine; requires bracing<br>*Advantages:* rigid fixation, uncomplicated technique |
| **KANEDA** | | | |
| Thoracolumbar fracture<br>Kyphosis<br>Compromised spinal canal | Anterior (transthoracic retroperitoneal) | Threaded rods<br>Staples<br>Vertebral body screws<br>Nuts | *Advantages:* rigid fixation<br>*Disadvantages:* possible damage to vascular structures |
| **LUQUE** | | | |
| Scoliosis<br>Kyphosis<br>Thoracolumbar fracture | Posterior | L-shaped rods<br>Sublaminar wires | *Advantages:* rigid stabilization; ability to contour rod<br>*Disadvantages:* risk of neural damage associated with sublaminar wiring |
| **PEDICLE SCREW AND PLATE SYSTEMS (ROY CAMILLE, AO, STEFFEE, DANEK)** | | | |
| Spinal instability<br>Spinal stenosis<br>Thoracolumbar fracture<br>Pseudoarthrosis<br>Failed instrumentation<br>Tumor<br>Spondylosis<br>Spondylolithesis | Posterior | Screws<br>Plates<br>Rods<br>Cables | *Advantages:* reduces deformity, restores alignment, and achieves stability while fusing fewer levels; rigid fixation; early, less painful mobility postoperatively<br>*Disadvantages:* screw breakage, failure; pseudoarthrosis; loosening of hardware; lengthy procedure; proximity of pin, screw to neural elements |
| **TSRH (TEXAS SCOTTISH RITE HOSPITAL) (PEDICLE SCREW AND PLATE)** | | | |
| Scoliosis<br>Spinal fracture<br>Tumor<br>Kyphosis | Anterior or posterior | Parallel rods<br>Cross-link plates<br>Hooks | *Advantages:* easily revised; can be adapted for anterior use; easily contoured rods; early ambulation<br>*Disadvantages:* pseudoarthrosis; hardware failure |
| **UNIT** | | | |
| Neuromuscular scoliosis | Posterior | Precontoured, continuous rod<br>Sublaminar wiring | *Advantages:* ends of rods able to be implanted in pelvis; stability: little rod migration; good correction of rotational deformities; correction of pelvic obliquity<br>*Disadvantage:* risk to neural elements associated with sublaminar wiring |
| **FUSION CAGES (MOSS, BAK)** | | | |
| Spinal stenosis<br>Tumor<br>Interbody fusion<br>Spinal instability | Anterior<br>Posterior<br>Endoscopic | Metal cage<br>Screws with bone graft or bone substitute | *Advantages:* immediate stabilization; allows bony ingrowth from superior and inferior vertebral bodies into matrix of bone graft; can be used in a variety of approaches, particularly endoscopic; uncomplicated technique; high success rate<br>*Disadvantages:* long-term results unknown |
| **Z PLATE** | | | |
| Instability<br>Corpectomy<br>Fusion | Anterior | Z-shaped plates and screws | *Advantages:* rigid stabilization<br>*Disadvantages:* hardware failure; pseudoarthrosis |

perform the procedure with limited exposure. The success rates for open discectomy and microdiscectomy are equal.

An alternative to microsurgery is another less invasive method of accessing the spinal structures. *Endoscopic* approaches to the spine allow the surgeon to perform discectomy, decompression, and fusion through endoscopic portals.[18] These procedures can be performed at the cervical, thoracic, and lumbar levels. Procedures performed without fusion can usually be performed as an outpatient procedure. Patients having endoscopic fusions can expect a 2- to 4-day hospital stay. Not all patients are candidates for less invasive techniques. Persons with multilevel disease or previous spine surgery may not be candidates for these techniques.

#### Diet

Although a special diet is not indicated for the treatment of degenerative disorders of the spine, weight reduction may be advised in the case of an overweight individual. Every effort should be made to attain or maintain ideal body weight to decrease the mechanical stressors on the back, as well as other joints.

#### Activity

Emphasis should be placed on the following:

1. Encouraging rest (complete or modified, depending on the severity of symptoms)
2. Promoting comfort
    a. Encourage slight elevation of head of bed and flexion of the knees when supine.
    b. Roll patient onto bedpan rather than lifting onto bedpan.
    c. Use fracture bedpan or small bedpan.
    d. Instruct patient in logrolling technique.
    e. Instruct patient in proper body mechanics.
3. Promoting circulation
    a. Encourage patient to perform active dorsiplantar flexion of the ankles at regular intervals.
4. Referring for physical therapy

The physical therapist will instruct the patient in a program to strengthen the muscles of the back and abdomen, which will increase support of the vertebral column. Exercises to increase flexibility, which will enable the person to bend and move with less chance of injury are also prescribed. Aerobic exercises, such as swimming, may be prescribed to improve overall conditioning and to maintain or reduce weight, without placing stress on the back. The patient should be taught to avoid lifting heavy objects (generally over 10 lb), participating in contact sports, and extreme twisting or bending of the spine.

#### Referrals

A referral to a back school or occupational therapist may be initiated to assist the patient and family to function effectively within the confines of the patient's disability. Emphasis is placed on body mechanics and modifications of daily routines to decrease the possibility of further injury. Job retraining may be indicated. Sometimes a referral to a pain management center is initiated, especially in the case of an individual having difficulty coping with chronic pain. If back or leg pain persists longer than 6 weeks or if a psychological component of pain is suspected, a psychological referral may be indicated.

## NURSING MANAGEMENT OF THE PATIENT WITH SPINE SURGERY

### PREOPERATIVE CARE

Preoperative nursing care that is relevant to persons undergoing all types of spinal surgery will be discussed. Persons having elective spinal surgery are admitted on the morning of their surgery. Preoperative teaching and testing are completed and evaluated before admission. Preoperative evaluation may include the following: complete history and physical examination; laboratory work including complete blood count, urinalysis, SMA/18, prothrombin time, partial thromboplastin time, type and screen or crossmatch of blood; chest x-ray; electrocardiogram; and diagnostic tests related to the spine, such as x-ray films, myelography, CT scans, and MRI.

Some patients may elect to participate in an autologous or donor-directed blood program. The optimal period for autologous donation is 4 to 6 weeks before the scheduled surgery date. The last donation must be completed at least 72 hours before surgery. The patient must have a hemoglobin (Hb) of at least 11 g/dl and a hematocrit (Hct) of 33% to be eligible for autologous donation. Iron replacement therapy is prescribed for autologous donors. These are recommendations of the National Blood Resource Group, and institutional policies may vary. If unable to participate in an autologous donor program, some patients may opt to obtain their own donors (designated or directed donors) in an effort to reduce chances of transmissible diseases. Some agencies recommend that designated (directed) donor blood be irradiated to reduce graft versus host reaction. The number of units requested will depend on the type of surgery planned. Bony fusion of multiple levels usually results in a greater blood loss because of muscle stripping required for exposure and the decortication of the host bed.

If postoperative bracing is required, the patient will be fitted for the brace and given instructions for its use preoperatively. An orthotist measures and fabricates the brace. Many types of braces are available, depending on the type of procedure performed. Some examples are cervical four-poster braces, thoracic lumbar sacral orthosis (TLSO), and soft corsets.

General preoperative teaching should be given to the patient and family (see Chapter 18). Many patients are curious about the types of implants to be used. If a sample of the instrumentation is available, it may be helpful to show it to the patient. The patient should also be informed about the location and extent of the surgical incision(s). If a spinal fusion with autologous graft is planned, an explanation of donor site location and degree of postoperative pain is beneficial. The patient should also be informed if allograft bone is to be used.

The patient should be given instructions in performing logrolling technique, isometric exercises, incentive spirometry, and coughing and deep breathing. Instructions are also given regarding general postoperative care, such as postanesthesia care, care of IV lines and catheters, vital sign routines, and pain management.

## POSTOPERATIVE CARE

Postoperative care of the patient recovering from spinal surgery includes interventions to prevent or minimize respiratory, elimination, and circulatory complications. The use of elastic stockings and pneumatic sleeves applied in the operating room is continued postoperatively. Patients are instructed to perform isometric exercises hourly while awake. Anticoagulants are prescribed postoperatively as prophylaxis against deep vein thrombosis and pulmonary embolism. The patient is evaluated daily for signs of vein thrombosis.

Monitoring of hemoglobin and hematocrit levels is important, especially if the patient has experienced an extensive blood loss during surgery. The surgical site and dressing should be assessed for signs of infection and hemorrhage. Clear drainage may indicate leakage of cerebrospinal fluid and should be reported to the surgeon.

With any spinal procedure, careful monitoring of neurological function is critical. Knowledge of the patient's baseline functioning is vital when monitoring for changes postoperatively. Neurovascular checks to the extremities are performed hourly in the immediate postoperative period and less frequently thereafter. The patient's ability to detect touch and discern sharp from dull is tested. Motor strength in the extremities is evaluated, and any changes are reported to the surgeon. Neurological changes can occur up to 72 hours after surgery. Drainage from surgical drains should be assessed and measured. Drains are usually removed after 24 to 36 hours. If a fusion has been done, the donor site should be assessed for hemorrhage.

Urinary retention is common after spinal surgery. If the patient does not have an indwelling catheter, he or she should be assessed for the ability to void. Lying flat in bed can make voiding difficult, particularly for male patients. Patients without fusion are usually allowed out of bed the evening of surgery, which may facilitate the ability to void. The physician may order that the patient be catheterized if unable to void after 8 hours.

Correct positioning of the patient after spinal surgery is important. When turning, patients should be logrolled to keep the spinal column straight. If bracing is required postoperatively, the patient may be in bed without the brace, but it must be worn while ambulating. A straight-backed chair should be used for sitting to avoid twisting the back.

Discharge planning focuses on teaching and performing ADL. Assistive devices such as long-handled brushes, shoehorns, and grabbers may be necessary to avoid extreme bending or reaching. If bracing is used, the patient and family should be able to demonstrate the proper technique when applying and removing the brace. The patient should be taught to assess the skin for evidence of pressure or breakdown, and the patient or family member should be instructed how to inspect the wound for any signs of infection.

### Lumbar Spine Surgery

The length of stay for persons having lumbar spine surgery varies. Patients having endoscope disc removal may go home the same day; persons with fusions may be hospitalized for up to 4 days (see the Guidelines for Care Box). Note the differ-

**guidelines for care**

**Postoperative Care of the Person with Lumbar Spinal Surgery**

1. Positioning
   a. Head of bed is kept flat.
   b. Patient is encouraged to logroll to change position from side to back to side.
   c. Use of a turning sheet is advised until patient can assist with turning.
2. Neurological checks to assess motor and sensory function
3. Wound care (drains placed in wound to prevent hematoma formation, if necessary)
   a. Maintain constant suction through drain as required.
   b. Maintain drain free of contamination.
   c. Monitor for excessive output from drains. Output ranges from 20 to 250 ml/8 hr for the first 24 hours, tapers for 12 hours postoperatively, and usually is removed 24 to 36 hours postoperatively. Drains that allow reinfusion of serous drainage may be used.
   d. Inspect surgical area frequently for evidence of excess drainage or formation of hematoma (bulging of tissues surrounding surgical site).
   e. If a spinal fusion has been done, inspect donor sites (usually iliac crest) for drainage, hematoma.
4. Promoting comfort
   a. Reposition patient frequently.
   b. Administer narcotic medications as needed; gradually reduce to nonnarcotic analgesics as patient tolerates.
   c. Monitor use and effectiveness of PCA pump, if ordered.
   d. Use fracture bedpan.
5. Promoting mobility
   a. Activity out of bed varies. Patients with fusion may need bedrest for 1 to 2 days.
   b. Transfer patient out of bed with as little time spent in the sitting position as possible.
      (1) Start transfer with patient in a side-lying position at the edge of the bed.
      (2) Have the patient push off the bed with the uppermost hand and the lowermost elbow.
      (3) One person assists by guiding the patient's trunk and another assists the patient's legs over the side of the bed.
      (4) Reverse process for return to bed.
   c. The patient may be permitted to walk as much as tolerated, with an assistive aid if necessary.
   d. Braces or corsets, if prescribed, are applied *before* the patient gets out of bed.
   e. Encourage patient to participate in ADL within prescribed limits of mobility.
6. Discharge instructions
   a. Do not lift or carry anything heavier than 2.25 kg (5 lb).
   b. Do not drive a car until permitted by surgeon.
   c. Avoid twisting motions of the trunk.

ences in care for patients undergoing lumbar spine surgery with and without fusion in the Clinical Pathway on p. 2029 and 2031.

### Cervical Spine Surgery

Persons undergoing cervical spinal surgery may require tongs or halo traction (see Chapter 60) or a halo brace. The person will have edema of the throat in the early postoperative period, requiring careful assessment of the airway and ability to swallow (see the Guidelines for Care Box). The estimated length of stay for persons undergoing procedures on the cervical spine is 3 days. A Clinical Pathway for a person undergoing cervical fusion is found on p. 2035.

### Thoracic Spine Surgery

Anterior approaches to the thoracic spine may involve entering the chest cavity, and if so, nursing care will include postoperative measures required following thoracotomy (see Chapter 32). Mobility restrictions are more prolonged than with lumbar surgery, because the thoracic spine is more mobile; consequently, there is greater risk of dislodging grafts through improper motion (see the Guidelines for Care Box on p. 2033).

## GERONTOLOGICAL CONSIDERATIONS

As stated earlier, degenerative changes occur as the skeleton ages. Degenerative disc disease and spinal stenosis primarily affect the elderly population.

Disc degeneration causes the facet joints and posterior ligamentum flavum to hypertrophy in an attempt to stabilize the posterior elements of the spine. These anatomic changes result in a narrowed spinal canal. Consequently, nerve roots may not receive an adequate blood supply and nutrition, depending upon the diameter of the person's spinal canal. The onset of spinal stenosis is usually insidious and physical symptoms may take years to manifest. Care must be taken to differentiate spinal stenosis from peripheral vascular disease, as the claudication (leg pain and weakness after walking) symptoms are similar. In persons with spinal stenosis, the pain in the legs is reproduced by walking and relieved by resting. Back pain often accompanies the leg pain, probably as a result of facet arthritis and degenerative disc disease.

Neurological deficits are rare in persons with spinal stenosis, presumably because the insidious nature of the disease allows the nerve roots time to accommodate to changes in canal dimensions.[6] Surgical intervention is done not because of neurological deficits but to increase the patient's ability to

*Text continued on p. 2033*

**guidelines for care**

### Postoperative Care of the Person with Cervical Spinal Surgery

1. Positioning
   a. Keep head of bed elevated 30 to 45°, particularly if anterior surgical approach was used, to decrease swelling in throat and facilitate respiration.
   b. If patient is in cervical brace, position is not restricted except by patient's tolerance.
   c. If patient is in cervical traction, patient may be turned side to back to side to patient's tolerance.
2. Promoting safety
   a. Assess airway and respiratory function frequently. Airway may be compromised by swelling.
   b. Provide suction equipment and tracheotomy set in patient's room until swelling in throat subsides and patient is swallowing and breathing normally.
   c. Check adjustment screws and straps frequently to ensure there is no loosening of the brace.
   d. Advise physician or orthotist of loosening of brace consequent to decrease in edema so brace can be readjusted.
3. Wound care
   a. Inspect surgical area, including iliac crest donor site, frequently for evidence of excess drainage or formation of hematoma. Use ice bag to donor site for comfort.
   b. If *tong or halo traction* is being used, pin care may be required (see Chapter 60).
4. Promoting comfort and relieving pain
   a. Provide ice chips to soothe sore throat.
   b. Make progressive diet changes slowly; patient will have difficulty swallowing and will be afraid of choking. Full liquids or semi-solids (ice cream, custards, jello, nectars) are often better tolerated than clear juice or broth; however, milk products may increase mucous production.
   c. Administer analgesics as for any patient having spine surgery. Donor sites often cause more discomfort than does neck incision.
   d. Patient may require aerosol treatments or humidification of air to loosen mucous secretions or make breathing more comfortable.
5. Promoting mobility
   a. If patient is in traction, encourage patient to perform ankle dorsiplantar flexion exercises and quadriceps setting on a regular basis to promote circulation and maintain leg strength.
   b. If patient is in a brace, out-of-bed activity, including walking, may begin as soon as patient tolerates.
   c. Provide for temporary use of walker if donor site pain restricts mobility.
   d. Encourage patient to participate in ADL to greatest extent possible.
6. Discharge instructions
   a. Wear brace at all times.
   b. Report any difficulty with brace to physician immediately.
   c. Do not drive a car during period that brace must be worn.
   d. Report symptoms of graft dislodgement (dysphagia and a feeling of "fullness" in the throat).

## clinical pathway Lumbar Discectomy

**Directions:**
1. Review CCT approximately every 8°
2. Appropriate and completed interventions need no additional documentation.
3. Cross through any interventions that are not applicable.
4. Circle any intervention not completed.
5. The plan of care—nursing interventions and outcome evaluation statements—may be added to the CCT as necessary.

DRG 215 Expected LOS 2
Physician(s) ______
Admit Date ______
Discharge Date ______
Surgery/Procedure ______
Date of Surgery/Procedure ______

Comorbid Conditions:
☐ CHF
☐ IDDM
☐ Angina
☐ COPD ☐ UTI
☐ Malignant HTN
☐ Dehydration

Imprint/Label

Complications during this admission:
☐ DVT
☐ PE
☐ Infection
☐ Continued wound drainage
☐ Urinary retention
☐ Ileus
☐ Stroke
☐ Mental status change
☐ Cardiac (dysrhythmia)
Other

Title: **Lumbar Discectomy**

Risk Factors: ☐ Obesity ☐ ETOH/Substance Abuse ☐ Smoking ☐

| DATE | PROBLEM LIST | DISCHARGE CRITERIA | DATE INITIALLY MET | MET ON DISCHARGE | |
|---|---|---|---|---|---|
| | | | | YES | NO |
| | 1. Knowledge deficit<br>2. Pain<br>3. Impaired mobility<br>4. Impaired skin (potential)<br>5. Impaired gas exchange (potential)<br>6. Altered tissue perfusion (potential)<br>7. Constipation (potential) | 1. Vital signs baseline.<br>2. Pain controlled by PO pain meds.<br>3. Incision well approximated/no signs of infection.<br>4. Patient ambulates independently.<br>5. Patient/caregiver has knowledge, resources, and ability to safely provide care outside the hospital environment.<br>Explain any discharge criteria not met: | | | |

| PLAN | TEAM MEMBERS | | HOMEGOING EQUIPMENT/SUPPLIES | NEEDED | ORDERED | PATIENT EDUCATION |
|---|---|---|---|---|---|---|
| Patient to be discharged on:<br>Date: ______<br>To: ☐ Home ☐ SNF<br>☐ Rehab ☐ Other<br>☐ Intermediate care<br>Gold Form Must Be Completed ☐<br>Gold Form completed ______ (date/initials) | Case Manager: ______<br>Social Worker: ______<br>Alternate Site Coordinator(s): ______ | Physical Therapy: <br>Occupational Therapy: ______<br>Pastoral Care: ______<br>Nutrition Service: ______ | Wheelchair<br>Bedside Commode<br>Walker<br>Crutches<br>Oxygen<br>Hospital Bed<br>Other: | | | ☐ Medication<br>☐ Discharge needs<br>☐<br>☐ |

Notes:

Courtesy of The Cleveland Clinic Foundation, Department of Advance Practice Nursing, Cleveland, OH.

*CCT,* Coordinated care track; *CHF,* congestive heart failure; *COPD,* chronic obstructive pulmonary disease; *UTI,* urinary tract infection; *HTN,* hypertension; *DVT,* deep vein thrombosis; *PE,* pulmonary embolism; *ETOH,* alcohol; *SNF,* skilled nursing facility; *POD,* postoperative day; *ASC,* alternate site coordinator; *SS,* social services; *IS,* incentive spirometer; *PT,* physical therapy; *PAS,* pneumatic antiembolic stocking; *LE,* lower extremity; *CL,* clear liquid; *N/C,* nasal cannula.

*Continued*

## *Lumbar Discectomy—cont'd*

| TIME/FRAME LOCATION | HOSPITAL DAY POD DAY OF SURGERY DATE UNIT | HOSPITAL DAY POD #1 DATE UNIT | HOSPITAL DAY POD #2 DATE UNIT | HOSPITAL DAY POD DATE UNIT |
|---|---|---|---|---|
| **Discharge Planning** | Identify primary caregiver ______<br>If Pt lives alone consult ASC (44663) for home care<br>Consult SS (46552) as needed | Visit from nurse clinician and ASC for home care | | |
| **Patient Education** | Orient to room<br>Review IS, PCA<br>Review importance of logrolling | Transfer techniques<br>No sitting >30 min<br>Importance of logrolling<br>"Do's & Don'ts" (nurse clinician)<br>Anticipate D/C in AM | D/C instruction:<br>Review transfer technique<br>"Do's & Don'ts", pain control<br>S/S infection<br>Review dressing; change if needed | |
| **Tests/Procedures/ Consults** | | Assess need for PT/consult<br>Consult PT if pt requires assistance with ambulating | | |
| **Allied Health Interventions** | | PT gait training prn | PT gait training prn | |
| **Nursing/Medical Interventions** | PCA pump assess pain level q4h<br>Bed rest logroll q2h<br>Assess dressing/skin—protect heels<br>IS as ordered; $O_2$ via N/C prn<br>Lung sounds qs<br>IVF as ordered; monitor I/O<br>PAS stockings bilateral LEs<br>Neuro/vascular checks qs<br>Monitor voiding patterns<br>CL liquid/regular diet | DC pump by PM (dinner time)<br>Begin PO pain meds-assess 4 hrs<br>OOB to chair; no sitting >30 min<br>No bed pans; ambulate to BR by PM<br>Assess dressing; skin-protect heels<br>IS as ordered; $O_2$ via N/C prn<br>Lung sounds qs<br>DC IV by PM; continue to monitor I/O<br>PAS stockings bilat LE's<br>Neuro checks qs<br>Select diet | PO pain meds<br>Continue independent ambulation<br>Dressing change<br>Select diet<br>DC $O_2$ if $O_2$ >92% room air<br>Monitor voiding patterns<br>Assess Neuro status | |
| **Outcome Criteria** | Moves arms/legs freely with full sensation<br>Orientation × 3<br>VS stable, lungs clear<br>UO >240 ml/shift<br>Pain controlled with analgesics<br>Pt compliant with logrolling<br>Incision/dressing with scant drainage | Ambulates with assistance in room<br>Pain controlled on PO meds by PM<br>Tolerates diet<br>Baseline bladder<br>Pt understands "Do's & Don'ts" | Verbalizes understanding of D/C instructions<br>Meets D/C criteria<br>Ambulates independently in room<br>Pain controlled with PO meds<br>Verbalizes understanding of limitations/precautions/"Do's & Don'ts"<br>Patient states S/S of infection<br>Pt/SO performs dressing change if needed | |

## clinical pathway Lumbar Fusion

| | PREADMISSION | DAY OF SURGERY DAY 1 | POD #1 DAY 2 | POD #2 DAY 3 | POD #3 DAY 4 | POD #4 DAY 5 |
|---|---|---|---|---|---|---|
| **Outcomes: Medical/Health Status** | Potential problems identified | 1. Surgery completed<br>2. Medically stable<br>3. Neurologically intact<br>4. Acceptable level of pain | 1. Medically stable<br>2. Neurologically intact<br>3. Incision dry or minimal drainage<br>4. Acceptable level of pain | 1. Medically stable<br>2. Neurologically intact<br>3. Incision healing with minimal drainage<br>4. Acceptable level of pain | 1. Medically stable<br>2. Neurologically intact<br>3. Incision healing<br>4. Acceptable level of pain | 1. Neurologically intact<br>2. Medically stable<br>3. Incision(s) clean and dry<br>4. Acceptable level of pain |
| **Tests** | PAT protocol | Hct/Hb (PACU)<br>Labs pertinent to patient's condition | Hct + Hb | Hct only if indicated | Hct<br>X-ray-standing: AP & lateral lumbar spine | |
| **Treatment** | | I/O × 48 hr<br>NV q2h × 24 hr<br>VS q4h × 24 hr<br>Foley → CD<br>Hemovac → self-suction<br>IS q1h W/A<br>TEDs/SCDs<br>Inspect Incision(s) q shift<br>Turning schedule, logroll q2h | I/O q shift<br>NV q8h<br>VS q4h → q8h<br>Foley → CD<br>Hemovac → self-suction<br>IS q2h W/A<br>TEDs/SCDs<br>Inspect incision(s) q shift<br>Ambulate today/up chair with corset | I/O q shift; D/C if PO >400 ml q shift<br>NV q8h<br>Teds<br>D/C SCDs<br>D/C Hemovac per MD<br>IS q2-4h W/A<br>Dressing change PM<br>Inspect incision(s) q shift<br>Continue ambulation with corset | TEDs<br>IS q2-4 h W/A<br>Dressing change PM<br>Inspect incision(s) q shift<br>Continue ambulation with corset | TEDs<br>Ambulate with corset<br>Inspect incision(s) |
| **Medications/ IV Fluids** | Assess for use of NSAIDS + Discontinue | PCA: morphine or Demerol or IM analgesics or PO analgesics<br>Intraoperative antibiotics<br>Postoperative antibiotics<br>IV fluids | Maintain PCA + begin weaning<br>IV fluids<br>Continue postoperative antibiotics | D/C PCA; convert to oral pain management<br>D/C IV fluids; convert to IIP if need to finish IV antibiotics | D/C IIP if applicable | Outplacement prescriptions:<br>PO analgesics<br>Colace<br>$FeSO_4$<br>Muscle relaxant<br>Other medications |
| **Nutrition** | | NPO, few ice chips | NPO, few ice chips | CL diet if passing flatus, and (+) bowel sounds.<br>Advance as tolerated | Regular diet | Regular diet |

Courtesy MetroHealth Medical Center, Cleveland, OH.

Continued

*PAT,* preadmission testing; *AP,* anteroposterior; *VS,* vital signs; *CD,* continuous drainage; *SCDs,* sequential compression devices; *PCA,* patient-controlled anesthesia; *IIP,* intermittent infusion plug; *PST,* physical therapy; *IS/C,* incentive spirometer/cough.

## Lumbar Fusion—cont'd

| | PREADMISSION | DAY OF SURGERY DAY 1 | POD #1 DAY 2 | POD #2 DAY 3 | POD #3 DAY 4 | POD #4 DAY 5 |
|---|---|---|---|---|---|---|
| **Consults** | Initial nursing evaluation<br>PST<br>Care Management<br>Orthotic Specialties | | Orthotic Specialties<br>Occupational therapy/physical therapy if indicated | | | |
| **Outcomes: Functional Status** | Fitted for corset | BR, logroll q2h<br>Ankle pumps q2h W/A and with VS at night | Progressive ambulation with corset<br>Up chair<br>Assist ADL | Continue ambulation with corset<br>Up chair<br>Assist ADL | Continue ambulation with corset<br>Up chair<br>Assist ADL | Ambulates with/without assistive device<br>Transfers independently<br>Stairs with/without assistance<br>Independent with ADL |
| **Outcomes: Educational** | Patient verbalizes understanding of surgical routine, exercises, precautions, equipment<br>Review pathway<br>Lumbar fusion home care booklet given | Education complete<br>IS/C and DB<br>Logrolling/BR<br>PCA/IV meds | OT initiated on use of adaptive equipment<br>PT instruct on use of walker/cane if needed | Teaching completed | Teaching completed | Verify lumbar fusion homecare booklet given |
| **Outcomes: Community Re-entry** | Discharge plans completed | Discharge plans verified after surgery | Verify equipment ordered<br>Adjustments made on corset | | Verify equipment ordered | Discharge plans implemented |
| **Discharge Targets** | 1. Incision(s) clean and dry, healing well<br>2. Neurologically intact<br>3. Medically stable<br>4. Independent with ambulation/ADL<br>5. Patient to be discharged before hospital day 5 (POD #4)<br>6. Acceptable level of pain<br>7. Spinal alignment appropriate<br>8. Spinal implants intact<br>9. Nutrition—ileus resolved and taking PO satisfactorily | | | | | |

**guidelines for care**

### Postoperative Care of the Person with Thoracic Spinal Surgery

Same as for lumbar surgery with the following additions and exceptions:

1. Positioning
   a. Head of bed may often be elevated to 30°.
2. Wound care
   a. If pleural cavity is entered, a chest tube will be inserted and must be managed postoperatively (see Chapter 32).
3. Promoting comfort
   a. Assist patient to splint chest while coughing.
4. Promoting mobility
   a. Encourage and assist patient in vigorous pulmonary hygiene measures.
   b. Assist patient to maintain bed rest for 1 to 2 days with strict attention to avoidance of twisting or bending motions to prevent dislodging grafts.
   c. Discourage patient from vigorous pulling or pushing with the arms because weight bearing through the arms poses a threat to the integrity of the graft.
   d. Brace is routinely prescribed and must be applied before patient is allowed out of bed.
   e. Permit patient to perform whatever activities are comfortable within the limitations of the brace.
   f. Encourage patient to participate in ADL within prescribed limits of mobility.
5. Discharge instructions
   a. Apply and remove the brace before getting out of bed.
   b. Wear the brace whenever out of bed; assess skin under brace.

walk longer distances and function independently. Performing the surgery in elderly nonambulatory patients is not recommended. A complete medical evaluation of the patient is recommended preoperatively. A healthy patient will benefit both subjectively and objectively from the surgical procedure.[6]

## SPECIAL ENVIRONMENTS FOR CARE

### Home Care Management

Because of shortened lengths of stay, considerable recovery from spinal surgery takes place at home. The patient and family should understand the indications for the prescribed medications. If narcotic analgesics are prescribed, the patient should understand the precautions associated with administration.

A follow-up appointment with the surgeon usually 6 weeks after surgery is necessary to evaluate progress. Before that, a home care nurse may visit to remove sutures or staples if used for skin closure. The patient or family member should evaluate the incision for signs of infection and healing. Dressing changes should be done daily or as needed until the wound is free of drainage; then the incision may remain open to air. Any excessive or purulent drainage should be reported to the physician. A nutritionally adequate diet should be recommended to promote wound healing. The patient may require some assistance with meal preparation, until energy reserves are restored. Cigarette smoking is not recommended and actually delays bone healing.

Depending upon the degree of mobility restrictions, the patient may require assistance with ADL. Clothing should be loose fitting, especially if worn under a brace. The patient may benefit from long-handled reachers and sponges if back flexion is limited. The occupational therapist can supply these and other assistive devices before discharge. An elevated toilet seat should be obtained. Bathing may be easier if a shower chair is used. If the patient does not have a shower, a sponge bath is best until activity restrictions are lifted. Special attention should be given to the skin if a brace is worn. A cotton T-shirt should be worn under the brace. Sensible low-heeled walking shoes with a nonskid sole are a good choice for footwear.

An exercise program should be recommended once healing is progressing. Walking is a safe and effective exercise for patients recovering from back surgery. Activities should be resumed gradually, allowing adequate time for rest and sleep. Driving is usually not permitted until cleared by the surgeon at the 6-week appointment. If a cervical collar is needed, the patient may not drive until the collar is removed. Driving with a halo vest is illegal in most states. When riding in a car as a passenger, the patient should be encouraged to comply with safety belt laws. To avoid injury, proper body mechanics are required for getting in and out of an automobile. The patient should be encouraged to comply with recommendations for activity and mobility restrictions to prevent dislodgment of the graft if a fusion was performed. Physical activities that involve bending, twisting, and lifting should be avoided until cleared by the surgeon. Lifting is generally restricted to objects lighter than 10 lb. For reference, a gallon of milk weighs about 9 lb. Parents with small children may require assistance with child care in the early postoperative period.

Symptoms to report immediately to the surgeon include increased temperature, new onset of neurological deficit, bleeding from the incision(s), or new onset of pain. The patient should be reminded that numbness and tingling present before surgery do not always abate immediately after surgery. Months or years may be needed for resolution of symptoms, and occasionally symptoms never completely resolve.

Most persons can return to work after 6 weeks. The work environment should be modified to include proper body mechanics and ergonomic design. The patient should avoid staying in one position for prolonged periods of time. Frequent breaks to get up and move about should be taken if possible. If the patient's job involves heavy manual labor, vocational retraining may be an option.

Modification of the home environment should be considered if potential hazards exist. Safety is a key concern for the patient recovering from spinal surgery. Falls and injury can cause neurological injury or graft displacement.

## COMPLICATIONS

Complications associated with general anesthesia are important considerations after surgery. These include complications such as atelectasis, paralytic ileus, and urinary retention,

Infection is a complication associated with the operative procedure. When instrumentation is used, the risk for infection increases. There is also a risk for hardware failure.

Posterior approaches to the spine are performed with the patient in the prone position, using a variety of frames and positioning devices. Complications can arise from positioning techniques and lengthy procedures. Potential complications include pooling of blood in the lower extremities; pressure areas on the knees, forehead, chest, and other bony prominences; and neuropathies as a result of local ischemia caused by prolonged pressure.

Complications of the procedure and the postoperative period include dural tear and cerebrospinal fluid leakage, blood loss, hypovolemia and decreased cardiac output, hematoma formation, infection, instrumentation or graft failure, pseudoarthrosis, loss of correction of deformity, persistence of pain and/or deficits, neurological impairment or loss, deep vein thrombosis, pulmonary embolism, fluid volume overload, and fat embolism.[60] Monitoring of *sensory evoked potentials* is frequently used as a method of reducing injury to the neural elements intraoperatively. Before surgery begins, electrodes are placed on the patient's scalp and extremities. Baseline data are collected, and impulse transmissions through the posterior columns of the spinal cord are monitored throughout the procedure. Any changes indicate possible injury, and the patient is given a "wake-up test." The level of anesthesia is lightened sufficiently to allow the patient to follow commands to move the extremities. Inability to do these tasks is considered indicative of neurological impairment. This monitoring technique allows the surgeon an opportunity to explore, ascertain, and possibly correct the cause of neurological loss before closing the incision.

A complication frequently occurring in the postoperative period of spinal fusion patients is inappropriate antidiuretic hormone secretion (SIADH).[13] Contributing factors include decreased blood volume, the use of anesthetic agents and analgesics, and physical and emotional stressors (see Chapters 15 and 34). Postoperative monitoring of spinal fusion patients should include accurate measurement of intake and output. Be suspicious of SIADH if the patient exhibits decreased Hb and Hct (which should be normal 2 to 4 days postoperatively), and the blood pressure and pulse remain within the patient's normal range.

Complications associated with approaches to the cervical spine include vascular injury and injury to the laryngeal nerve because of the proximity of these structures to the surgical site. Complications associated with surgical correction of thoracic spine disorders also include those associated with thoracic surgery (see Chapter 32), because the thoracic cavity is entered in an anterior approach to the thoracic spine.

When fusions are performed, complications include graft failure, infection, and pseudoarthrosis. The use of hardware is associated with potential complications including hardware failure or loosening, infection, damage to neurovascular structures, and adverse reactions to implant materials.[18]

Endoscopic procedures, although less invasive, are also associated with complications. Complications include visceral injury; instrument breakage or failure; $O_2$ retention in abdomen, chest, or vasculature; hypoxia to local tissues; infection; $CO_2$ absorption; and scar tissue formation.[18]

## SCOLIOSIS

### Etiology/Epidemiology

Scoliosis can be classified as nonstructural or structural. Nonstructural scoliosis is also termed *postural* or *functional* and is caused by posture, pain, leg length inequality, and other factors. This form of scoliosis is usually easily corrected, either by exercise or by removing the underlying cause. An important distinction is the absence of vertebral rotation. However, untreated nonstructural scoliosis can progress to structural scoliosis.

*Structural scoliosis* involves a rotational deformity of the vertebrae. It is further divided into three major categories:

1. *Congenital scoliosis* (present at birth) occurs as a result of vertebral malformations in fetal life and accounts for 15% of structural scoliosis cases.
2. *Neuromuscular scoliosis* results as a consequence of several diseases and represents approximately 15% of cases. Curves generally appear early and progress rapidly.
3. *Idiopathic scoliosis* has an unknown cause, but genetic factors have been linked to the development of disease. It accounts for approximately 65% to 80% of cases and affects 1% to 4% of all children.[41,60] Idiopathic scoliosis is further divided into three groups, depending on the age of onset (Box 61-16). Girls account for 90% of persons affected with idiopathic scoliosis and also more frequently have curves of the spine greater than 20°.

### Pathophysiology

Scoliosis may develop in localized areas of the spinal column or involve the whole spinal column. Curvatures may be S shaped or C shaped (Figure 61-37).

The earliest pathological changes begin in the soft tissues. Muscles and ligaments shorten on the concave side of the curve, progressing to deformities of the vertebrae and ribs. In skeletally immature persons vertebral formation occurs as asymetrical forces are applied to the epiphysis by the shortened

*Text continued on p. 2037*

**box 61-16** *Classification of Scoliosis*

**CONGENITAL**

**NEUROMUSCULAR CAUSES**

Cerebral palsy
Charcot-Marie-Tooth disease
Syringomyelia
Spinal cord injury
Poliomyelitis
Myelomeningocele
Muscular dystrophy
Neurofibromatosis
Marfan's syndrome

**IDIOPATHIC**

Infantile: 0 to 3 years of age
Juvenile: 3 to 10 years of age
Adolescent: older than 10 years of age

## clinical pathway *Cervical Fusion*

| | PREADMISSION | DAY OF SURGERY<br>DAY 1 | POD #1<br>DAY 2 | POD #2<br>DAY 3 | POD #3<br>DAY 4 |
|---|---|---|---|---|---|
| **Outcomes: Medical/Health Status** | Potential problems identified | 1. Surgery completed<br>2. Medically stable<br>3. Neurologically intact<br>4. Acceptable level of pain | 1. Medically stable<br>2. Neurologically intact<br>3. Incision(s) healing well with minimal drainage<br>4. Acceptable level of pain | 1. Medically stable<br>2. Neurologically intact<br>3. Bone graft position satisfactory<br>4. Incision(s) healing well with minimal drainage<br>5. Acceptable level of pain | 1. Medically stable<br>2. Neurologically intact<br>3. Incision(s) clean & dry<br>4. Acceptable level of pain |
| **Tests** | PAT protocol | Hct | Hct | Hct<br>AP and lateral x-ray of neck | |
| **Treatment** | | I/O × 48 hr<br>NV q2h × 24 h<br>VS q4h × 24 h<br>Foley → CD<br>IS q1h W/A<br>TEDs/SCDs<br>Tonsil suction set up at bedside<br>Trach set at bedside<br>Maintain 2-poster brace<br>Inspect incision(s) q shift<br>Check scalp pressure points q shift<br>Check brace pressure points q shift<br>Phili Collar at bedside | I/O q shift<br>NV q8h<br>VS q4h → q8h<br>Foley → CD<br>IS q2h W/A<br>TEDs/SCDs<br>Tonsil suction set up at bedside<br>Maintain 2-poster brace<br>Inspect incision(s) q shift<br>Check scalp pressure points q shift<br>Check brace pressure points q shift<br>Initial dressing change done per MD<br>Phili Collar at bedside | VS q8h<br>I/O q shift D/C if po >400 ml q shift<br>IS q2-4h W/A<br>NV q8h<br>TEDs<br>D/C SCDs<br>D/C Foley<br>Tonsil suction and trach set at bedside<br>Maintain 2-poster brace<br>Inspect incision(s) q shift<br>Dressing change prn<br>Check scalp pressure points q shift<br>Check brace pressure points q shift<br>Phili Collar at bedside | TEDs<br>Maintain 2-poster brace<br>Inspect incision(s) |
| **Medications/ IV Fluids** | Assess for use of NSAIDS + Discontinue | PCA: morphine/Demerol<br>IM analgesics<br>PO analgesics<br>Intraoperative antibiotics<br>Postoperative antibiotics<br>IV fluids | Maintain PCA or change to PO after assessing pain status<br>IV fluids<br>Continue postoperative antibiotics<br>IV fluids | D/C PCA; convert to oral pain medications<br>IIP if need to finish IV antibiotics | D/C IIP if applicable<br>Outplacement prescriptions:<br>PO analgesics<br>Colace<br>$FeSO_4$<br>Muscle relaxants |
| **Nutrition** | | NPO, few ice chips | Progress diet as tolerated | | Regular diet |

Courtesy of MetroHealth Medical Center, Cleveland, OH.
For abbreviations see Clinical Pathway for Lumbar Fusion.

## Cervical Fusion—cont'd

| | PREADMISSION | DAY OF SURGERY DAY 1 | POD #1 DAY 2 | POD #2 DAY 3 | POD #3 DAY 4 |
|---|---|---|---|---|---|
| **Consults** | Initial nursing evaluation<br>PST<br>Care Management<br>Orthotic Specialties | | Physical therapy<br>Occupational therapy if indicated<br>Orthotic Specialties for brace adjustments | | |
| **Outcomes: Functional Status** | Fitted for 2-poster brace. | Dangle at bedside postoperative night<br>Head of bed ↑ 20–30°<br>Ankle pumps q2h W/A and with VS at night | Progressive ambulation<br>Up chair<br>ADL | Continue ambulation<br>Up chair<br>ADL | Ambulates with/without assistive device<br>Transfers independently<br>Stairs with/without assistance<br>Independent with ADL |
| **Outcomes: Educational** | Patient verbalizes understanding of surgical routine, exercises, precautions, equipment<br>Review pathway<br>Cervical fusion home care booklet given | Education complete re:<br>IS/C and DB<br>Activity level<br>PCA/PO meds<br>Tonsil suction<br>IV therapy | Teach patient how to wash hair, apply clothes<br>Show patient/family cervical fusion book<br>Instruction given on walker/cane if needed.<br>OT: instruction initiated on use of adaptive equipment if needed | Teaching completed | Verify cervical fusion homebook given<br>Teaching completed |
| **Outcomes: Community Re-entry** | Discharge plans completed | Discharge plans verified after surgery | Verify equipment ordered<br>Adjustments made on brace if necessary | | Discharge plans implemented |
| **Discharge Targets** | 1. Incision(s) clean and dry, healing well<br>2. Neurologically intact<br>3. Medically stable<br>4. Independent with ambulation/ADL<br>5. Patient to be discharged before hospital day 4 (POD #3)<br>6. Acceptable level of pain | | | | |

and tight soft tissue structures on the concave side of the curve.

The Scoliosis Research Society has devised a method of classifying curves. Deformities are classified by magnitude, direction, location, and etiology. Curve direction is designated by the convex side of the curve.

The degree of rotation of the curve is important, because it determines the amount of impingement on the rib cage. The amount of vertebral compression and twisting depends on the position of the vertebrae in the curve. The forces of compression are greatest on the apical vertebrae, which become the most deformed. Deformity progresses quickly during skeletal growth and slows later in life, but the greatest increase in curvature may occur in adult life. Gravity and an increase in upper body weight may increase the deformity in adulthood. With curves greater than 35° to 40°, especially lumbar curves that lack rib support, the curve may continue to progress at the rate of 1°/year. Curves greater than 60° have a significant effect on pulmonary function. Curves of 40° to 50° should be followed for progression, usually with x-ray films every 2 to 5 years.[60]

The individual can initially have slight, mild, or severe deformity. Early deformity may not be obvious except on specific examination. In the early stages, individuals may note that clothing does not fit correctly or hang evenly, because the height of the shoulders is uneven. Pain is not usually an accompanying factor.

Persons affected with structural scoliosis may exhibit asymmetry of hip height; pelvic obliquity (tilting of the pelvis from the normal horizontal position); inequalities of shoulder height; scapular prominence; rib prominence; and rib humps, which are posterior, unilateral humpings of the rib cage visible on forward bending. In severe cases, cardiopulmonary and digestive function may be affected because of compression or displacement of internal organs. Total lung capacity, vital capacity, and maximum voluntary ventilation are decreased in persons with scoliosis. Cardiac output may also be compromised. Significant deviations in balance of the curve may also affect gait patterns.

Right thoracic, right thoracic and left lumbar, and right thoracolumbar curves are most common in idiopathic scoliosis. A *compensatory curve* may develop, allowing the head to be centered over the pelvis. In general, compensatory curves are of a lesser degree, more flexible, and less rotated.

## Collaborative Care Management

A complete radiological examination of the spine is performed. Curve angles, flexibility, and degree of vertebral rotation are calculated. Radiographs may also be done to determine skeletal maturity. In patients with severe thoracic scoliosis, pulmonary function studies may be completed to evaluate the degree of restrictive lung disease.

Treatment depends on the individual patient and the degree of lateral curvature.

1. Early or postural scoliosis may be amenable to postural exercise or exercise combined with traction. Cotrel's traction, which is a combination of a cervical head halter with 5 to 7 lb and pelvic traction with 10 to 20 lb, may be used.
2. When the curve is flexible (less than 40°) and the patient is cooperative, bracing, in combination with exercise, may be sufficient to correct the deformity (e.g., Milwaukee brace, Risser cast, or halofemoral or helopelvic traction [Figure 61-38]). Maintaining ideal weight is a consideration in reducing the stress on the spine. The patient should be advised against weight gain, especially if bracing is prescribed, because the brace is specifically fitted and contoured to the individual. The brace can usually accommodate a 10 lb gain or loss.
3. Transcutaneous electrical muscle stimulation may be used to stimulate the muscles on the convex side of the curve. Repeated stimulation strengthens the muscles and pulls the spine into alignment. The patient usually uses the stimulator at night.

Surgery is indicated for patients when conservative management has failed to halt curve progression, for those with severe, progressing curves, intractable pain, or compromised pulmonary function, or for cosmesis. Many individuals with neuromuscular scoliosis are unable to walk. Surgical correction is sometimes performed in these patients to facilitate the ability to transfer or to increase sitting ability or tolerance. Surgical correction is usually performed when curves are greater than 45° (Figure 61-39).[31]

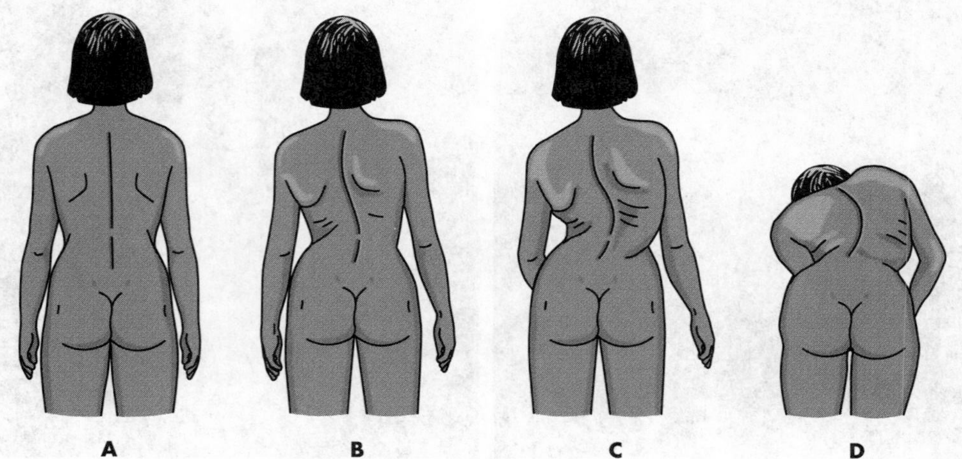


**fig. 61-37** Normal spinal alignment and abnormal spinal curvatures associated with scoliosis. **A,** Normal; **B,** mild; **C,** severe; **D,** rotation and curvature of scoliosis.

Surgical correction usually involves a posterior approach to the spine with instrumentation and bony fusion. Patients with severe, rigid curves and pelvic obliquity frequently require a staged procedure. A transthoracic or retroperitoneal approach to the spine is performed first, followed by a posterior procedure in 1 to 2 weeks. Many types and combinations of types of instrumentation are available. The type used is based on the individual patient and surgeon preference. Refer to Table 61-18 for examples of commonly used implants and see also Figure 61-39.

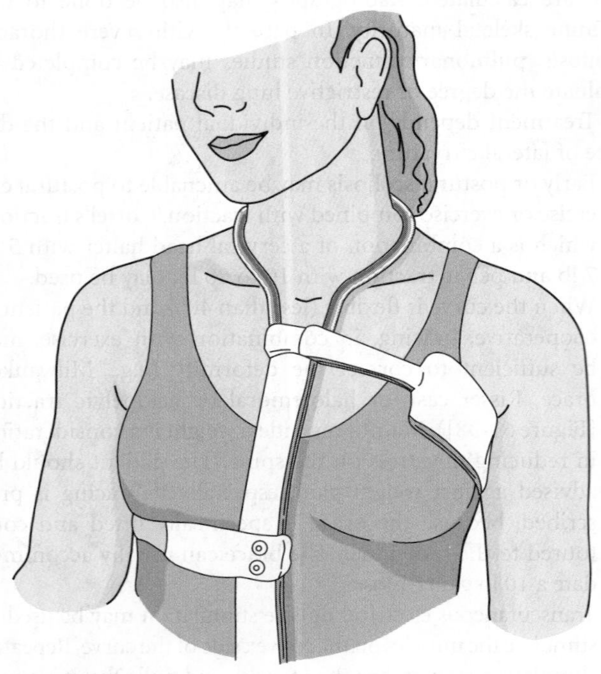

**fig. 61-38** Milwaukee brace.

Complications of scoliosis fusion are similar to those described in the spinal surgery section above. The incidence of paralysis, both temporary and permanent, has been estimated to be 4% by the Scoliosis Research Society.[60]

Nursing management of the patient with surgery of the spine was discussed in the previous section. This nursing care is also applicable to the patient with a scoliosis fusion. Particular attention should be paid to assessment of respiratory function, management of pain, and acceptance of changes in body image.

### *Patient/family education*

For individuals for whom conservative interventions are being used, patient instruction is most important for achieving the desired outcomes. Points to be stressed in teaching are as follows:

1. Instruct patient regarding the disease process and rationales for treatment.
2. Explain and discuss the patient's and family's expectations of treatment.
3. Instruct and supervise patient in performance of prescribed exercises and use of traction equipment.
4. Advise patient that wearing brace need not restrict normal or desired activities.
5. Instruct patient how to apply, remove, and care for brace.
6. Instruct and supervise patient in method of inspecting the skin.

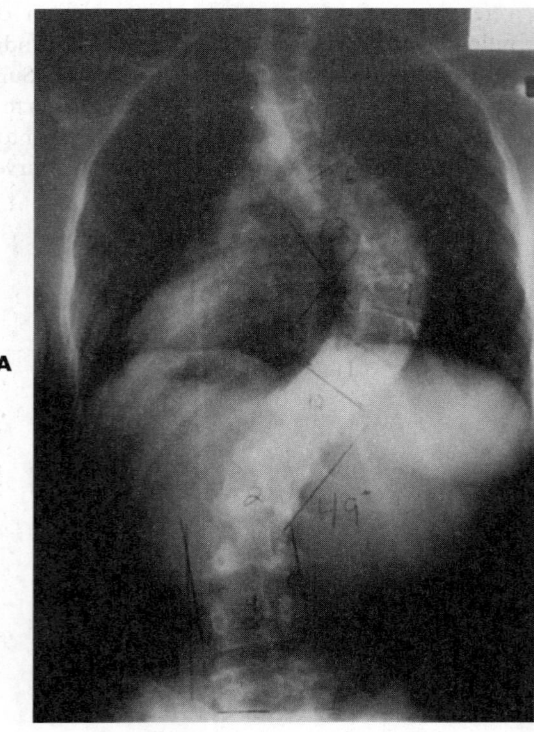

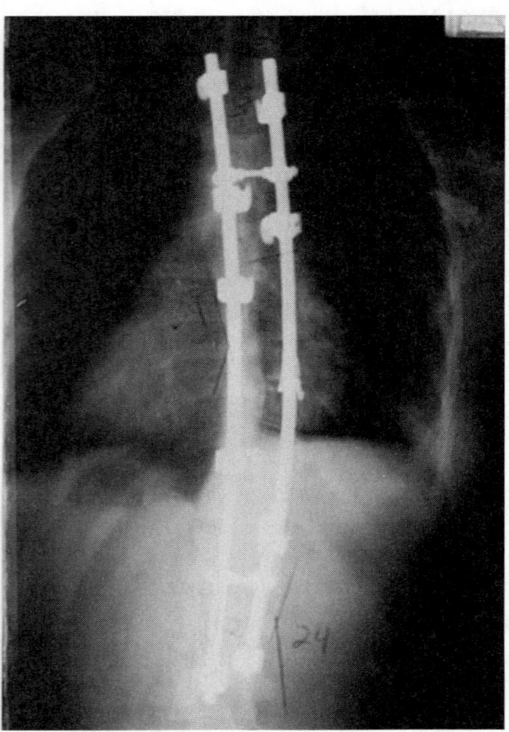

**fig. 61-39 A,** Preoperative radiograph of adult with idiopathic scoliosis. **B,** Postoperative film showing correction of curve with Cotrel-Dubousset instrumentation in place.

7. Advise patient regarding the selection of loose-fitting but attractive clothing that conceals the brace (particularly important for women and adolescents).
8. Inform patient and family of support groups.

Persons who have undergone spinal fusion will need teaching as described in the spinal surgery section above. In addition, the patient and family must be knowledgeable regarding brace care and application (Figure 61-40).

There are no specific measures to prevent scoliosis. However, attention to proper posture may be effective in preventing some types of nonstructural scoliosis in both children and adults.

The Scoliosis Research Society recommends annual screening of all children aged 10 to 14 years. Scoliosis screening is mandated by law in some states; others have voluntary screening programs.[64] The U.S. Preventive Services Task Force has insufficient evidence to recommend either for or against routine screening of asymptomatic adolescents.

Interested patients and families can be referred to support groups: Scoliosis Association Incorporated, PO Box 811705, Boca Raton, FL 33481-1705; (800) 800-0669; National Scoliosis Foundation, 72 Mount Auburn Street, Watertown, MA 02172; (617) 926-0397.

## DISORDERS AFFECTING THE HANDS AND FEET

### DUPUYTREN'S CONTRACTURE

#### Etiology

Dupuytren's contracture, first described in the early 1800s by a French surgeon, is a progressive condition marked by hypertrophic hyperplasia of the palmar fascia that results in a flexion deformity of the distal palm and fingers (Figure 61-41). The cause of Dupuytren's contracture is unknown. A familial tendency has been noted.

#### Epidemiology

Dupuytren's contracture appears most commonly in persons of Northern European ancestry, between 40 and 60 years of age. White men, middle aged or older, are affected by a ratio of 7:1. When affected, women seem to experience only mild deformity. Dupuytren's deformity is associated with diabetes, epilepsy, alcoholism, penile lesions (Peyronie's disease), and hyperplasia of the plantar fascia (Lederhose's disease). Although occupation does not contribute to the development of the disease, repetitive occupational trauma may increase the severity of preexisting disease.[60] The most deforming cases of

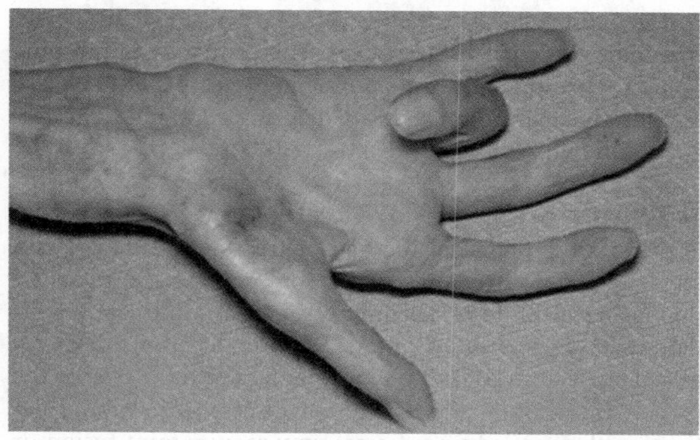

**fig. 61-41** Dupuytren's contracture.

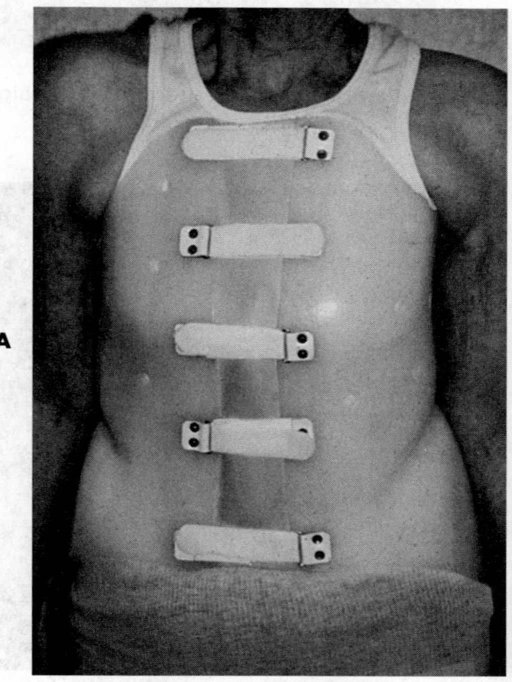

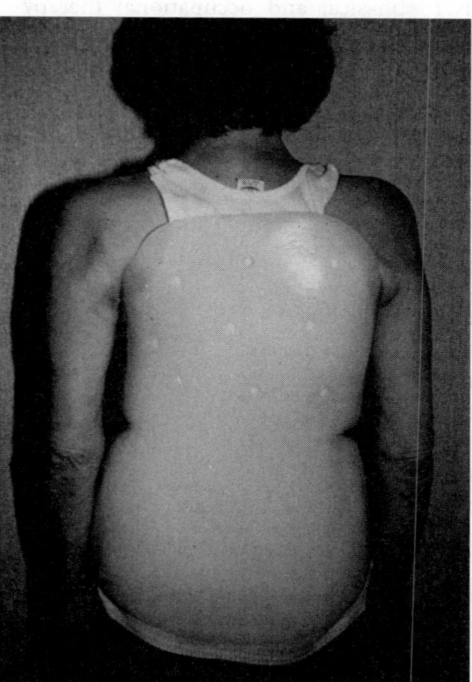

**fig. 61-40** **A,** Anterior view of thoracolumbar sacral orthosis (TLSO). **B,** Posterior view of TLSO. Note cotton shirt worn under brace.

Dupuytren's seem to occur in persons with a family history and an onset of disease before age 40.

### Pathophysiology

Deformity results from changes mediated by the myofibroblasts, which is not completely understood. The anatomy of the palmar fascia is distorted.

Dupuytren's contracture may take up to 20 years to reach maximum deformity. It often occurs bilaterally and symmetrically. Hyperplasia and progressive fibrosis of the palmar fascia on the ulnar side of the band cause progressive shortening of the pretendinous bands of the ring and small fingers. The bands shorten and the metacarpophalangeal joints are drawn into flexion contractures. Web space contractures and scissoring of the fingers develop from ligamentous contracture. The proximal interphalangeal joint may also be involved. The skin of the palm is drawn down, forming tight puckers and nodules.

Depending on the severity of the deformity and hand dominance, the patient may experience difficulty in grasping objects. Burning pain may accompany attempts at grasping. Usually, the main complaints are deformity and mild interference with hand function.

### Collaborative Care Management

Surgery is the preferred method of treatment. Persons with fixed flexion contractures of 30° or more at the metacarpophalangeal or proximal interphalangeal joints are candidates for surgical intervention. Surgical repair involves regional fasciectomy or subtotal palmar fasciectomy to allow the patient full motion. Recurrence of disease is common. Patients with more advanced cases may require joint fusion or amputation if neurovascular structures are involved. Splints worn at night may decrease residual flexion contractures of the digits. Referrals to physical and occupational therapy are necessary postoperatively for exercises to regain ROM and splinting. Some patients may develop sympathetic dystrophy postoperatively and require hospitalization for elevation of the hand and administration of sympathetic blockers and steroids.[60]

Surgical repair is performed as an outpatient procedure. The most common postoperative complications are hematoma and inadequate skin closure. Nursing management focuses on postoperative care:

1. Elevating hand to control swelling.
2. Checking fingers for circulation, sensation, and movement every 1 to 2 hours
3. Administering prescribed analgesics as necessary to maintain comfort
4. Encouraging active extension of fingers
5. Encouraging patient to begin using hand in self-care activities after 2 to 3 days

#### *Patient/family education*

The patient and family will need instruction about care of the dressing and splint. The hand should be elevated for comfort and to decrease swelling. A sling may be worn. The patient should be instructed to contact the surgeon if the fingers become cool, pale, or painful, or if paresthesias, increased pain, or decreased movement is experienced. The splint should be maintained until the follow-up visit. Analgesics will be prescribed as needed. If the patient's dominant hand is affected, assistance in ADL may be needed. The patient can generally return to work in a few days. A PT referral is indicated for postoperative ROM exercises. The patient and family should understand the signs and symptoms of recurrent disease.

## HALLUX VALGUS

### Etiology/Epidemiology

More than 80 million persons in the United States have foot problems that cause pain, deformity, and disability. *Hallux valgus* is the lateral angulation of the proximal phalanx on the metatarsal head of the great toe. This common foot problem is often bilateral (Figure 61-42). Depending upon the degree of angulation, prominence of the medial eminence may occur, resulting in the bunion deformity (Figure 61-43).

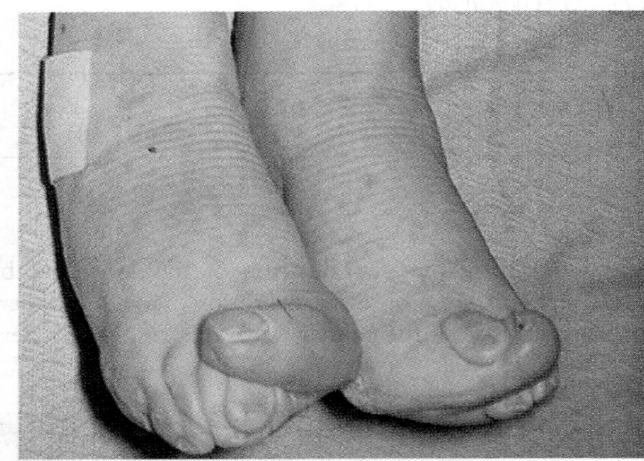

**fig. 61-42** Bilateral hallux valgus.

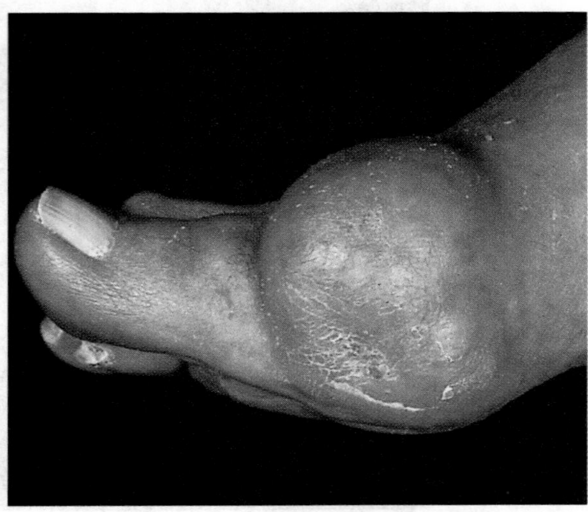

**fig. 61-43** Bunion.

Women develop hallux valgus deformity 10 to 15 times more frequently than do men.[13,60] In women, the deformity is most common in the sixth decade. There is also a familial tendency: 68% of patients have a family history of hallux valgus.[13] Persons who wear shoes have a higher incidence than those who do not.[13,60] The prevalence of hallux valgus in Japan increased significantly after World War II when the traditional clog-type shoe was replaced by Western style footwear.[13] The type of shoes worn also contributes to the development of the deformity; pointed toe shoes that cause crowding and angulation of the toes are associated with development of hallux valgus and bunion. Other associated factors include pes planus (flat foot), chronic tightening of the Achilles tendon, spasticity, and rheumatoid arthritis.

## Pathophysiology

Lateral deviation of the proximal phalanx causes pressure on the medial metatarsal head and attenuation and contracture of the joint capsule. The adjacent sesamoid bones, anchored by the adductor tendon and transverse metatarsal ligament, become subluxed. The flexor and extensor hallicus longus, which insert at the base of the distal phalanx, also deviate laterally, contributing more to the deformity. The medial eminence of the metatarsal head becomes prominent and a protective bursa forms as it rubs against shoes. The great toe may cause crowding and deformity of the seond toe.

## Collaborative Care Management

Diagnosis is made by history and physical examination. The type of shoes worn, occupation, and amount of exercise are important points to include in the history. The gait and neurovascular status of the feet are important points of the objective examination. Corns and callus may also be present, and the patient may have flat feet. Radiographs will confirm the diagnosis and define the severity of the deformity.

Conservative treatment includes encouraging the patient to wear proper-fitting shoes of the correct size and shape to allow room for the toes; this alone may alleviate the problem. Shoes should be wide enough to accommodate the medial eminence. A protective pad can be taped under the metatarsal head to change the weight-bearing pressure. Insoles can be purchased to cushion the foot in shoes. A pad can be placed over the corn or bunion to decrease pain and pressure. Medications such as NSAIDs or acetaminophen can be prescribed for pain relief.

If conservative treatment fails or the patient is reluctant to change footwear, surgical intervention may be indicated. There are more than 130 procedures to correct hallux valgus and bunions.[60] Keller bunionectomy, Chevron osteotomy, Stone procedure, Mitchell osteotomy, and Mayo arthroplasty are just a few of the many procedures. Surgical management of bunion and hallux valgus includes the following principles (Figure 61-44):[13,60]

- Correction of metatarsal deformity by osteotomy
- Resection of bone or arthroplasty using a Silastic implant (gap arthroplasty)
- Arthrodesis of the first metatarsophalangeal joint
- Revision of soft tissue structures

Before consenting to surgery, the patient should be completely informed of the risks and benefits of the procedure. After bunion surgery, it is not always possible to wear whatever type of shoes are desired.[60] The surgical procedure is not indicated for cosmesis, but to correct a structural deformity.[60]

Postoperatively the foot is wrapped in a soft, bulky dressing, and in some patients a splint or cast is applied. The patient will wear a postoperative cast shoe and ambulate with crutches or a walker until full weight-bearing is permitted.

### Patient/family education

Bunion surgery is usually performed as an outpatient procedure, and the patient and family will need discharge instructions. The cast shoe is worn for approximately 2 weeks or until the splint or cast is removed. Activity and weight bearing should be limited during that time. Two to 4 weeks postoperatively, round-toed, lacing shoes or sandals can be worn and a bunion splint is worn at night for approximately 6 weeks. At 6 weeks, full activity can be resumed. The patient will need teaching about wearing proper fitting shoes and avoiding pointed-toe shoes. High-heeled shoes, which alter the weight-bearing pressure on the feet, should be avoided. A PT referral may be required for some patients. A podiatry consult for custom shoes may be required for patients with severe deformity. Teaching should be done regarding proper foot care (see the Patient/Family Teaching Box).

The patient may need support in accepting body image changes associated with the appearance of the feet. Because bunions often occur bilaterally, the patient should be taught to assess the other foot for signs of beginning deformity. Finally, the patient should be educated about the signs and symptoms of infection and any medications that may be prescribed.

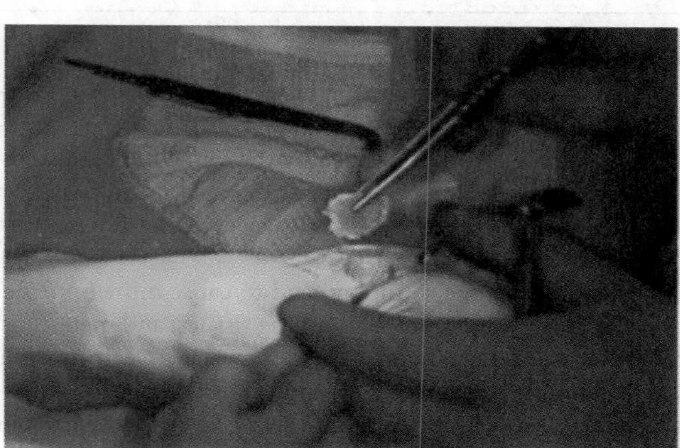

**fig. 61-44** Surgical correction of bunion and hallux valgus. Medial eminence is removed.

**patient/family teaching**

**Good Foot Care**

**How to Prevent Feet Problems**

In addition to recognizing common problems, there are many things that you can do to promote healthy feet and prevent problems. Follow these guidelines:

- Walk regularly. This will improve circulation, increase flexibility, and encourage bone and muscle development. Walking is very important for maintaining overall foot health.
- Always wear comfortable shoes that provide proper support. The shoes should be sufficiently wide and have low enough heels so that you feel no leg fatigue, leg or foot cramps, or pain.
- Massage your feet to improve circulation and promote relaxation of the feet at least daily.
- If you have bunions, wear shoes that are extra long or wide. This will help ease pressure on your toes. In addition, use donut-shaped bunion cushions or mole-skin to take pressure off of the joints.
- Wear heel pads or cushions in the bottom of your shoes to protect your heels if you walk on hard surfaces for long times.
- Wash your feet every day in warm water. Dry them by blotting with a towel, rather than rubbing.
- If your feet perspire a lot, dust your feet with talc or a hygienic foot powder. You may also sprinkle some powder into your shoes. Do not use cornstarch powder because it may lead to a fungal infection.
- Trim your nails shortly after you have taken a bath or shower, while they are soft. Cut the nails straight across with a toenail clipper.
- Do not go barefoot outdoors, especially if you are in an area that is not your own yard. A foreign body may cut or puncture your foot.
- Inspect your feet every day for cuts, blisters, and scratches. Provide care as needed and observe for proper healing.

From *Mosby's patient teaching guides: update 3,* St Louis, 1997, Mosby.

## TUMORS OF THE MUSCULOSKELETAL SYSTEM

### ETIOLOGY

Tumors may arise from any of the structures of the musculoskeletal system (Tables 61-19 and 61-20). The type of tumor is determined and classified by the tissue of origin (Figure 61-45). Tumors can be benign or malignant and can affect both adults and children. Musculoskeletal tumors comprise 3% of all malignant tumors.

Generally, malignant tumors tend to cause more bone destruction, invasion of the surrounding tissues, and metastasis. Benign bone tumors tend to be less destructive to normal bone, do not invade soft tissues, and are not capable of metastasis. Common tumors of the musculoskeletal system, their characteristics, and treatment are described in Table 61-21.

The cause of bone tumors is unknown. A tumor can be defined as a new growth or hyperplasia of cells. This growth may be in response to inflammation or trauma. Others are a result of a spontaneous, rapid, poorly differentiated proliferation of cells.

**table 61-19** *Common Tumors of the Musculoskeletal System*

| Benign | Malignant |
|---|---|
| **BONE** | |
| Osteoma | Osteosarcoma |
| **CARTILAGE** | |
| Osteochondroma | Chondrosarcoma |
| Enchondroma | |
| Periosteal | |
| Chondroblastoma | |
| **FIBROUS** | |
| Fibroma | Fibrosarcoma |
| **BONE MARROW** | |
| Giant cell | Ewing's sarcoma |
| | Myeloma |
| **UNCERTAIN CELL** | |
| Unicameral bone cyst | |
| Aneurysmal bone cyst | |

See also Table 61-20.

### EPIDEMIOLOGY

The incidence of bone tumors varies with age. Adults 30 to 35 years of age have a low incidence of bone tumor. The incidence increases slowly after age 35. Adolescents and adults older than the age of 60 years have the highest incidence of bone tumor, related to metastatic tumors.[41]

Approximately 6000 primary bone and soft tissue tumors are diagnosed annually in the United States.[50] Osteosarcoma is the most common type of primary bone tumor, representing 20% of all cases.[41]

Other factors are associated with the development of bone tumors. A history of Paget's disease or radiation therapy increases the risk of development of a bone tumor. Bone tumors can also occur as a result of metastases from other primary sites of neoplasias. Cancers of the breast, prostate, kidney, thyroid, and lungs frequently metastasize to bone. One half of the million cancers diagnosed annually in the United States metastasize to bone.[50] Common sites for metastases include the spine, ribs, pelvis, hip, and proximal long bones.[50] Bony metastases are common in persons older than age 40. Survival rates for those with metastatic disease depend on the primary tumor site and range from 6 months to 4 years.[50]

### PATHOPHYSIOLOGY

The pathophysiology of neoplasms is found in Chapter 11. Bone tumors commonly cause bone destruction and erosion of the cortex. Benign bone tumors have a controlled growth

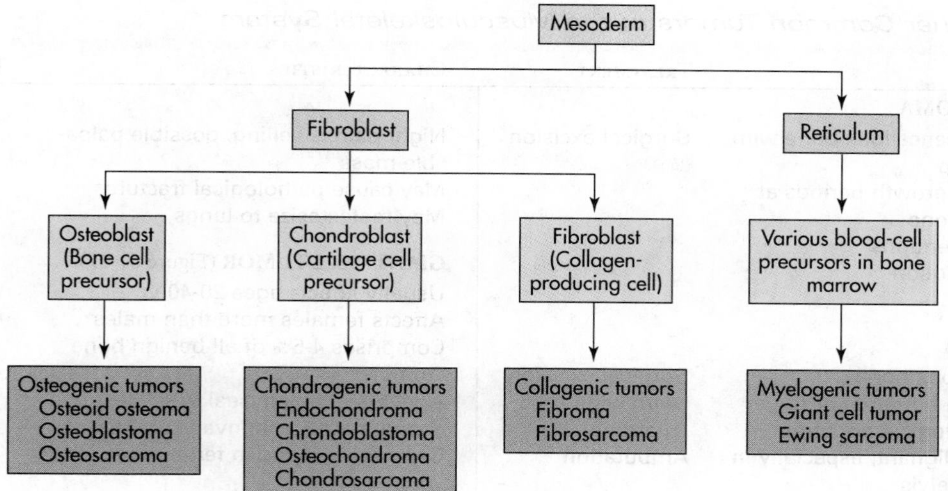


**fig. 61-45** Derivation of bone tumors.

**table 61-20** *Muscle Tumors*

| CHARACTERISTICS | TREATMENT |
|---|---|
| **LEIOMYOMA** | |
| Affects smooth muscle, usually uterus | Surgical excision |
| Palpable mass | |
| Tenderness | |
| **RHABDOMYOMA** | |
| Affects striated muscle | Surgical excision |
| Rare | |
| Tenderness | |
| **LEIOMYOSARCOMA** | |
| Affects smooth muscle, usually uterus, stomach, or small bowel | Surgical excision with wide margins |
| | Radiation |
| Radical growth | Chemotherapy |
| **RHABDOMYOSARCOMA** | |
| Affects striated muscle, usually in inguinal, popliteal, or gluteal areas | Radiation |
| | Surgical excision |
| | Chemotherapy |
| Slow-growing mass | |
| Tenderness | |

rate, normally compressing and displacing rather than invading normal bone tissue. This eventually leads to weakening of the normal bone. Other types of tumors destroy normal bone either by resorption or disruption of the blood supply to the bone. Three patterns of bone destruction have been identified:[41]

1. *Geographical:* Characterized by slow-growing tumors; there is an identifiable margin between the normal and abnormal bone.
2. *Moth-eaten:* The margins are less defined; this type of destruction characterizes rapidly proliferating tumors and malignancies.
3. *Permeative:* Tumor and normal bone are meshed with no perceivable margins.

A staging system has been developed for bone tumors.[25] Malignancies are classified according to their growth patterns and sites of metastases (Table 61-22).

The rest of this section refers only to osteosarcoma.

## OSTEOSARCOMA

Osteosarcoma exhibits a moth-eaten pattern of bone destruction with poorly defined margins (Figure 61-46). Osteoid and callus produced by the tumor invade and resorb normal cortical bone. The tumor erodes through the cortex and periosteum and eventually invades soft tissues. Metastasis to the lungs is common.

Ninety percent of osteosarcomas occur in the metaphyses of long bones, especially the distal femur and proximal tibia.[41] Pain and swelling are frequently reported. The initial complaint of pain is often described as dull, aching, and intermittent, but the pain rapidly increases in intensity and duration. Night pain is common. Other frequent complaints include generalized malaise, anorexia, and weight loss.

Two types of lesions are seen with metastatic tumors. Bone destruction exceeds bone formation in *lytic* lesions, commonly seen in lung metastases. Tumors in which bone formation exceeds bone destruction are termed *blastic* lesions, as seen in prostate metastases. Bone lysis generally occurs with metastatic disease and hypercalcemia may occur in 10% to 20% of persons[50] (see Chapter 15). Another potential problem of persons with metastatic disease is pathological fracture. An estimated 9% of persons with metastatic disease incur pathological fractures. Pathological fractures can occur with any activity and pose a significant risk to persons with metastatic bone lesions.

**table 61-21** *Other Common Tumors of the Musculoskeletal System*

| Characteristics | Treatment |
|---|---|
| **OSTEOCHONDROMA** | |
| Compromise of cancellous bone with cartilaginous cap<br>Develops during growth periods at metaphysis of bone<br>Also appears in tendons<br>May limit joint motion<br>May recur | Surgical excision |
| **ENCHONDROMA** | |
| Destroys cancellous bone<br>Usually occurs in humerus or finger<br>Can cause pathological fractures<br>May become malignant, especially in long bones or pelvis | Surgical excision with wide margins<br>Amputation |
| **CHONDROSARCOMA** | |
| Usually affects persons 50-70 yr old<br>Comprises 20% of all bone tumors<br>Affects males more than females<br>Slow growing, insidious onset<br>Most common in humerus, femur, pelvis<br>Local pain, swelling<br>May have palpable mass<br>Severe, persistent pain<br>May infiltrate joint space and soft tissue<br>May metastasize to lung tissue<br>May recur | Surgical excision<br>Amputation |
| **FIBROSARCOMA** | |
| Usually affects persons 30-50 yr old<br>Affects females more than males<br>Occurs in bony fibrous tissue of femur and tibia<br>Comprises 4% of primary malignant bone tumors<br>May result from radiation therapy, Paget's disease, or chronic osteomyelitis<br>Night pain, swelling, possible palpable mass<br>May cause pathological fractures<br>May metastasize to lungs | Wide surgical excision<br>Amputation |
| **GIANT CELL TUMOR** (Figure 61-47) | |
| Usually affects ages 20-40 yr<br>Affects females more than males<br>Comprises 4-5% of all benign bone tumors<br>Appears in epiphyseal area, destroys bone matrix, can invade soft tissues<br>Commonly found in femur, tibia, or humerus<br>Dull, aching night pain<br>Limitation of motion<br>Swelling<br>High incidence of recurrence | Wide excision<br>May require bone graft<br>Amputation |
| **MYELOMA, MULTIPLE MYELOMA (MULTIFOCAL)** | |
| Poor prognosis<br>Common in persons >40 yr<br>Affects males more than females<br>Comprises 27% of bone tumors<br>Higher incidence in African Americans<br>Neoplastic proliferation of plasma cells<br>Causes cortical and medullary bone lysis and infiltrates bone marrow<br>Aching, intermittent pain in spine, pelvis, ribs, or sternum<br>Pain increased with weight bearing<br>May complain of weight loss, malaise, or anorexia<br>Causes pathological fractures | Palliative treatment<br>Radiation<br>Chemotherapy |
| **OSTEOMA** | |
| Usually affects persons 10-20 yr old<br>Comprises 20% of benign bone tumors<br>Slow growth | Treatment only if symptomatic, then excision |

**table 61-22** *Surgical Staging System for Bone Tumors*

| Stage | Grade | Site (T) | Metastasis (M) |
|---|---|---|---|
| IA | Low ($G_1$) | Intracompartmental ($T_1$) | None ($M_0$) |
| IB | Low ($G_1$) | Extracompartmental ($T_2$) | None ($M_0$) |
| IIA | High ($G_2$) | Intracompartmental ($T_1$) | None ($M_0$) |
| IIB | High ($G_2$) | Extracompartmental ($T_2$) | None ($M_0$) |
| IIIA | Low ($G_1$) | Intracompartmental or extracompartmental ($T_1$ or $T_2$) | Regional or distant ($M_1$) |
| IIIB | High ($G_2$) | Intracompartmental or extracompartmental ($T_1$ or $T_2$) | Regional or distant ($M_1$) |

Data from Simon SR, editor: *Orthopaedic basic science*, Chicago, 1994, American Academy of Orthopaedic Surgeons.

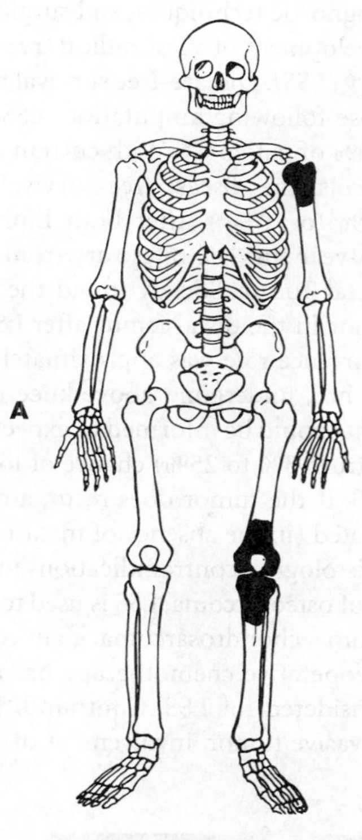


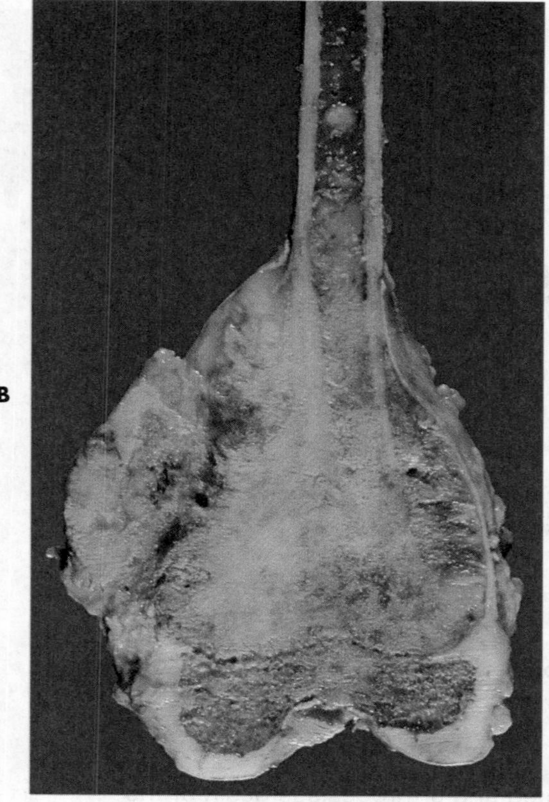


**fig. 61-46** Osteosarcoma. **A,** Common locations of osteosarcoma. **B,** Femur has a large mass involving the metaphysis of the bone; the tumor has destroyed the cortex, forming a soft-tissue component.

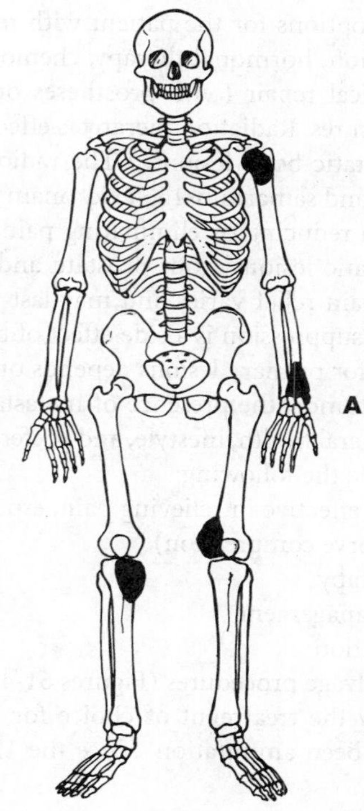


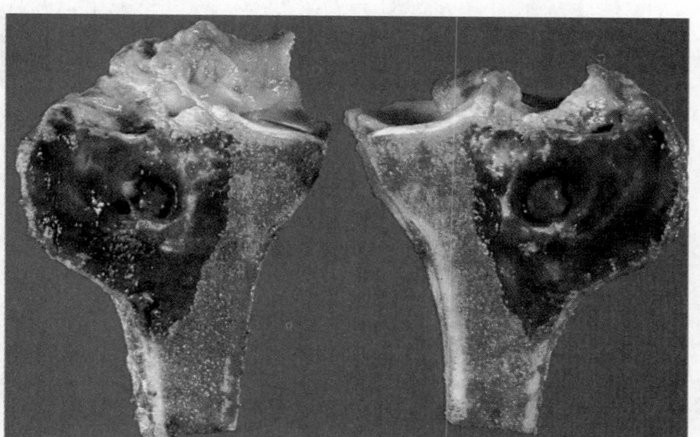


**fig. 61-47** Giant cell tumor. **A,** Common skeletal locations. **B,** Gross picture of cell tumor on bone (epimetaphysis).

## Collaborative Care Management

Bone biopsy is used to confirm the diagnosis. Because of the rapid growth rate of osteosarcomas, the prognosis is poor. Death, usually from pulmonary complications as a result of metastases, may occur within 2 years of diagnosis if the tumor is left untreated.

X-ray films, CT scan, MRI, and bone scans will show tumor location and size. X ray films have limited use as 50% of trabecular bone must be destroyed before lesions are visible. Blood tests will reveal an elevated serum alkaline phosphatase level. Chest x-ray film will confirm the presence of metastases.

Treatment options for the patient with metastatic disease include radiation, hormonal therapy, chemotherapy, surgical excision, surgical repair (with prostheses or hardware) and palliative measures. Radiation therapy is effective in palliating 70% of metastatic bone lesions.[54] The radiopharmaceuticals strontium-89 and samarium-153 exidronam have shown limited success in reducing or eliminating pain in persons with blastic metastatic lesions from prostate and breast cancer.[54] Duration of pain relief varies and may last up to 6 months. Bone marrow suppression is a side effect of both drugs.

Treatment for primary lesions depends on the size and location of the tumor; the presence of metastases; and the patient's age, general health, lifestyle, and preferences. Treatment options include the following:

1. Radiation (effective in relieving pain, especially from fracture and nerve compression)
2. Chemotherapy
3. Surgical management
   a. Amputation
   b. Limb salvage procedures (Figures 61-48 and 61-49)

Historically the treatment of choice for high-grade bone sarcomas has been amputation. Since the 1980s advances in chemotherapy, diagnostic techniques, and surgical techniques have led to the development of a less radical treatment option: *limb salvage surgery (LSS)*. Disease-free survival rates after LSS are similar to those following amputation. LSS may be successful in up to 80% of patients.[41] With current adjuvant chemotherapy protocols, the disease-free survival rate for osteosarcoma is 40% to 70%.[19] After both limb salvage and amputation, the 5-year survival rates vary from 40% to 70%. The Musculoskeletal Tumor Society found the rate for local recurrence of tumor in the distal femur after LSS to be 10%. The reported recurrence rate was approximately the same as for patients who had undergone above-knee amputation.[14] Generally, a patient should be informed to expect a 5% to 10% (reported ranges from 3% to 25%) chance of local tumor recurrence after LSS. If the tumor does recur, amputation will probably be indicated (in the absence of metastases).

There are no histological contraindications to LSS. In addition to treatment of osteosarcoma, LSS is used to treat patients with Ewing's sarcoma, chondrosarcoma, giant cell tumor, and other tumors. Preoperative chemotherapy has allowed more persons to be considered for LSS. Contraindications to LLS include a large invasive tumor, involvement of the neurovas-

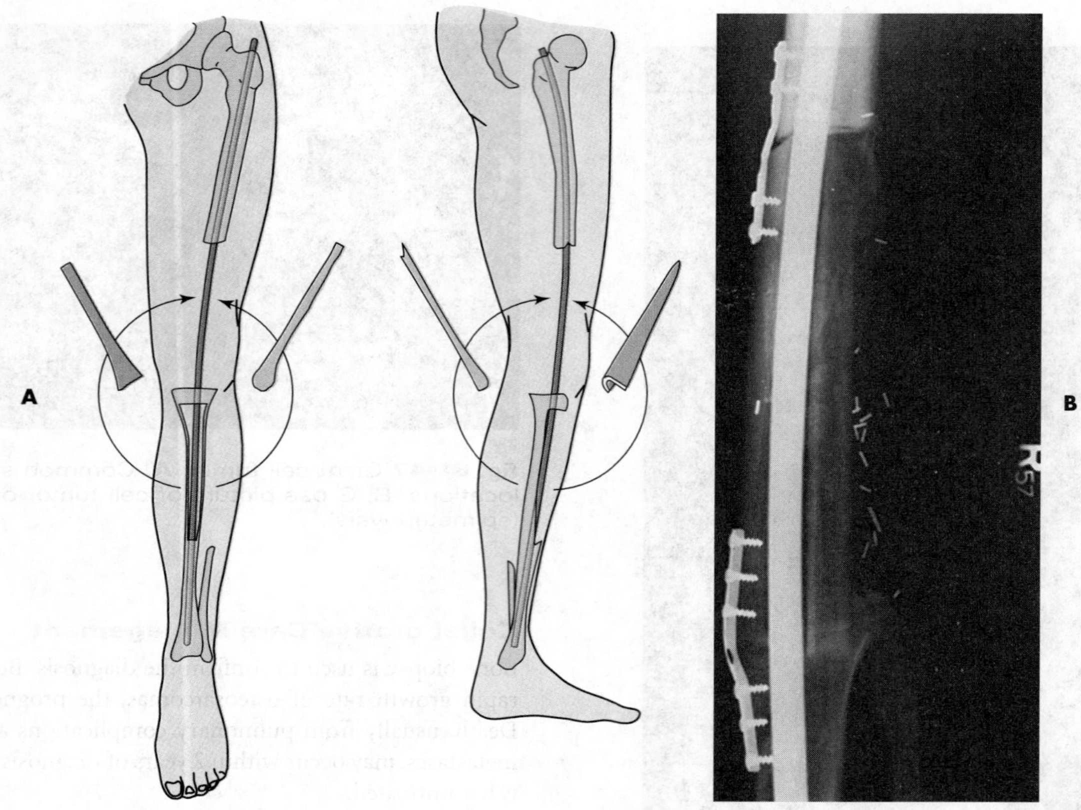


**fig. 61-48 A,** When the distal femur has been resected and arthrodesis is desired, the anterior one third of the tibia and proximal fibula may be used to span the defect. The extremity is stabilized with a long fluted intramedullary rod. When the proximal tibia is resected, the anterior one third of distal femur and a segment of fibula are used to span defect. An iliac bone graft is added to improve strength of reconstruction. Allograft segments also have proven successful in filling defects. **B,** Postoperative radiograph of patient who had resection arthrodesis for stage IIB tumor in distal femur. He uses no external aids and is fully active.

cular bundle, inability to achieve tumor-free margins, or a technically difficult surgical approach, such as a tumor in the distal tibia. However, LSS results in more complications than amputation (Box 61-17).

In addition to LSS and amputation, other surgical techniques are available to the patient with a bone malignancy. As mentioned earlier, which modality is used depends on many factors. Other surgical procedures are as follows:

1. Pelvic resection, including hemipelvectomy
2. Hip disarticulation
3. Rotationplasty (for skeletally immature individuals)

*Rotationplasty* involves an intercalary amputation with a 180° distal limb rotation. When used for a distal femur lesion, the tumor area including the knee joint is resected. The end result includes the foot pointing toward the buttock and the ankle becoming the knee joint. This procedure provides knee flexion and extension potential with the use of a prosthesis and also accommodates limb growth in children. It provides more function than a high level above-knee amputation or hip disarticulation. Patients may experience a disturbance of body image. Research is needed to determine whether patients prefer LSS to amputation as a treatment option. Data indicate that psychological adjustment is better after lower extremity amputation than following upper extremity amputation and that patients prefer a surgical technique that allows them knee motion.

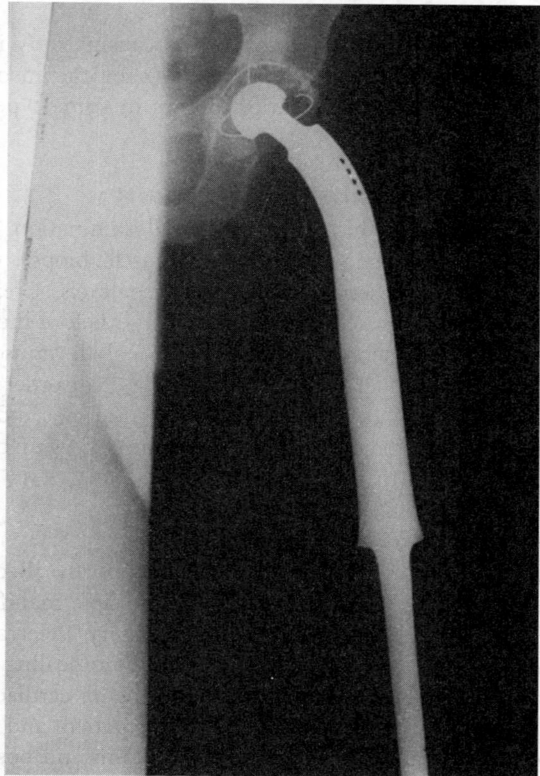

**fig. 61-49** This custom-made total hip was used to replace the proximal femur and hip joint of a 50-year-old woman with a chondrosarcoma. She has had no recurrence of tumor and walks with a modest limp while using a cane, but has no active abduction of the hip.

### Patient/family education

Nursing care for the patient with cancer is discussed in Chapter 11. Nursing care for the patient undergoing LSS is challenging. The patient and family, who may still be trying to cope with the diagnosis of cancer, are now faced with difficult decisions regarding treatment options. Nursing interventions focus on education and support. Nursing interventions include but are not limited to the following:

1. Discussion of diagnosis, prognosis, and treatment options
2. Exploration of the patient's understanding of the risks, benefits, and expected outcomes of treatments available
3. Preoperative preparation regarding perioperative experience, including use of allograft, hardware, and possible need for transfusion
4. Explanation of potential complications
5. Exploration of the patient's expected functional abilities (Patients should understand that a "normal" limb is not a reasonable expectation after LSS and that there will be some degree of residual disability.)
6. Instruction on and supervision of correct use of supportive devices
7. Support of decision-making abilities of the patient and family
8. Referral to support groups or community services
9. Promotion of independence within capabilities
10. Encouragement of effective coping strategies
11. Promotion of mobility
12. Promotion of acceptance of body image
13. Prevention of complications

**box 61-17** *Complications of Limb Salvage Surgery and Amputation*

**LIMB SALVAGE SURGERY**

Local recurrence of tumor
Wound and skin necrosis: the procedure may necessitate extensive soft tissue flaps
Deep infection (incidence of 6-13%; may be increased by the immunosuppressant action of chemotherapy)
Neurovascular complications
Deep vein thrombosis
Nonunion
Hemorrhage
Implant and/or graft failure
Arthritis (long-term)

**AMPUTATION**

Infection
Wound necrosis
Phantom limb pain
Contractures
Skin breakdown

**table 61-23** *Common Types of Muscular Dystrophy*

| DYSTROPHY | GENETICS | ONSET | PROGRESSION | MUSCULAR DISTRIBUTION |
|---|---|---|---|---|
| Duchenne | X-linked recessive<br>Only males affected | 18 months to 3 years | Rapid, death from cardiac or respiratory failure by third decade | Symmetrical shoulder and hip involvement<br>Cardiac involvement and mental retardation common |
| Becker | X-linked recessive<br>Only males affected | 5-25 years | Gradual, normal life span, inability to walk ~25 years after onset of disease | Pelvic and shoulder muscle atrophy |
| Limb-girdle | Autosomal dominant or recessive<br>Either sex affected | Variable, second or third decade | Variable, shortened life span, severe disability by 15-20 years after onset of disease | Pelvic and shoulder girdle, neck muscles |
| Facioscapulohumeral (Landouzy-Dejerine) | X-linked autosomal dominant<br>Either sex affected | Usually second decade | Moderate, normal life span | Facial, neck, shoulder girdle, and pelvic muscles |
| Myotonic (Steinert) | Autosomal dominant<br>Either sex affected | Birth to fourth decade | Gradual, if adult onset | Muscle atrophy<br>Delayed muscle relaxation, eyelids, facial, neck muscles<br>Cataract development<br>Dysphagia<br>Hypersomnolence |

## DISORDERS AFFECTING THE MUSCLES

### MUSCULAR DYSTROPHY

#### Etiology/Epidemiology

The muscular dystrophies are a group of familial disorders characterized by varying degrees of skeletal muscle weakness and degeneration, leading to disability and deformity. Classification has traditionally been by phenotype, mode of inheritance, rate of progression, and distribution of involvement. At least 10 types of muscular dystrophy have been identified; of these, 5 types are commonly seen in adults (Table 61-23).

Duchenne muscular dystrophy (MD), discovered in 1868, is the most common, affecting 1 in 3500 male births.[44] Becker's dystrophy is also an X-linked recessive disease, but is less common than Duchenne's. Other types of MD seen in adults can occur in either sex. Children with MD rarely live past 25 years of age.

The mechanism of the genetic defects is unknown. Theories include defects in muscle cell membranes and biochemical abnormality.

#### Pathophysiology

The genetic abnormality in MD causes a defect in the intracellular metabolism of the muscle fibers. Defects in creatine metabolism and intracellular enzymes in the glycolytic system have been identified.[41] Muscle cells exhibit phagocytosis and necrosis, with dissolution of myofilaments. The striation of the fibers is altered, and the fibers are either hypertrophied or atrophied. Eventually, muscle fibers are replaced with fat and connective tissue, causing fatty infiltration and fibrosis. There is no pattern of the involved muscle fibers. Mental retardation occurs in some types of muscular dystrophy.

#### Collaborative Care Management

Diagnosis is made by history and physical examination. Laboratory and diagnostic data include muscle biopsy, electromyography, and serum muscle enzyme levels. Creatine kinase levels are elevated during infancy and before the onset of weakness. There is no cure for any of the muscular dystrophies. Treatment varies with the type of disorder (Table 61-24). Genetic counseling is important. Steroids and immunosuppressants have been used with some success in treating persons with MD.

##### *Patient/family education*

Nursing care of the person with MD is supportive. Because of the severity of the disability and the multiple manifestations, a multidisciplinary approach is necessary. Referrals to PT and OT can assist the patient and family in dealing with ADL and problems with mobility. Monitoring for cardiac and other system involvement is important. The patient and family should be aware of the signs and symptoms and possible complications of MD. Prevention of the complications associated with immobility is vital. Medication teaching is necessary if the patient is receiving steroids or immunosuppressants. Emotional support is vital, especially for parents of children with MD. The family may need help dealing with feelings such as grief and guilt about disease transmission. Genetic counsel-

**table 61-24** *Treatment for Common Types of Muscular Dystrophy*

| TYPE | TREATMENT |
|---|---|
| Duchenne | Function of unaffected muscles maintained; muscle fiber breakdown hastened by strenuous exercise<br>PT for ROM<br>Orthoses, braces, use of wheelchair<br>Surgical release of contractures<br>Spinal fusion<br>Respiratory exercises |
| Becker | Surgical release of contractures, tenotomies<br>Ambulation maintained as long as possible<br>Monitor for cardiac complications |
| Limb-girdle | PT for ROM, contracture development rare; patient usually ambulatory up to 20 years after diagnosis |
| Facioscapulohumeral | PT for exercises<br>Orthoses<br>Preserve ambulation<br>Wheelchair for distance<br>Surgical stabilization to prevent winged scapulae<br>Arthrodesis of scapulae to ribs |
| Myotonic | Monitor for cardiac and endocrine disorders<br>Aspiration precautions for dysphagia<br>Decreased esophageal motility, feeding tube may be necessary<br>Cataract surgery<br>Pemoline or methylphenidate for somnolence |

ing should be offered to appropriate individuals. Encouraging ambulation and mobility to the fullest extent should be balanced with ensuring adequate rest and sleep to prevent fatigue. Family members will need instruction about transfer techniques for wheelchair-bound patients. A lift may be necessary if the family members are unable to assist with transfers. The Muscular Dystrophy Association is a good resource for patients and families of persons with MD. All states have local chapters.

## critical thinking QUESTIONS

1 What are the similar features of the spondyloarthropathies? How do they differ?

2 A patient is admitted to the hospital with systemic manifestations of rheumatoid arthritis. The patient remarks, "I thought I just had arthritis. How did this happen?" Develop a teaching plan for this patient.

3 Mr. B., a 70-year-old patient, is admitted 6 months after a right knee replacement, with right knee pain, an elevated temperature, and general malaise. What are probable causes for his symptoms? What treatment might you expect? Develop a discharge teaching plan for Mr. B.

4 You are asked to speak to a group of perimenopausal women at a local community center. The topic is "Healthy Bones." Describe essential components of your presentation.

5 How might the diagnosis of idiopathic scoliosis affect the body image of an adolescent female? What nursing interventions would be appropriate?

6 Mrs. X. is a 73-year-old woman admitted for a left hip revision arthroplasty. She has a history of dislocation. Devise a teaching plan for her to prevent further dislocations of the prosthesis.

## chapter SUMMARY

### DISORDERS AFFECTING THE JOINTS

- Rheumatoid arthritis is an idiopathic, chronic, systemic disease most prominently manifested as an inflammation in the synovium of the diarthrodial joints.
- The disease process begins as an inflammation of the synovium. The process becomes chronic and leads to thickening of the synovium and formation of granulation tissue. The cartilage becomes necrotic. Destruction of cartilage and bone may lead to dislocation of the joints.
- Early manifestations of the disease may include complaints of fever, weight loss, fatigue, generalized discomfort that is poorly localized (fibrositis), and morning stiffness. These symptoms may later be replaced by more specific (localized) pain and articular inflammation with swelling, redness, warmth, and tenderness.
- The joints of the hands and the feet are often affected early. The joints of the hands, wrists, feet, ankles, elbows, and knees are most commonly involved, usually in a bilaterally symmetric pattern. Shoulder involvement and hip involvement are later phenomena.
- The course of rheumatoid arthritis varies greatly from patient to patient and is marked by periods of exacerbation and remission.
- Diagnostic findings usually indicative of rheumatoid arthritis include an elevated erythrocyte sedimentation rate, mild leukocytosis, positive rheumatoid factor, narrowing of the joint spaces and erosion of articular surfaces on x-ray films, inflammatory changes in synovial tissue (biopsy), and increased turbidity and decreased viscosity of synovial fluid (needle aspiration).
- The goals of therapy are preservation of joint function, prevention and correction of deformity, and improvement in quality of life.
- Nursing management consists of measures to promote comfort, promote mobility, encourage good nutrition, and promote improved self-esteem. Patient teaching is stressed.
- Surgical intervention may be warranted when rheumatoid arthritis has caused severe joint destruction. Common procedures are synovectomy, arthrotomy, arthrodesis, and arthroplasty.

- Degenerative joint disease (or osteoarthritis) is the result of degeneration of the articular cartilage of the synovial joints. Unlike rheumatoid arthritis, it is not systemic. It is an extremely common disease. Symptomatic degenerative joint disease is usually noted in the 50- to 70-year-old age-group, although most persons older than 40 years have hypertrophic changes of the joints.
- Two forms of osteoarthritis exist: primary, for which the cause is unknown; and secondary, which can be the result of trauma, infection, fracture, another type of arthritis, stress on weight-bearing joints from obesity, unusual wear and tear on joints associated with certain occupations, or a genetic disposition.
- The target organ of degenerative joint disease is the articular cartilage. This normally white, translucent, smooth cartilage becomes yellow and opaque with softened areas and a rough or frayed surface. The cartilage is digested by enzymes and is eventually destroyed. The underlying bone develops osteophytes (spurs of new bone) that may break off into the joint cavity.
- Persons with degenerative joint disease have pain, stiffness, and limited range of motion, particularly in the large weight-bearing joints and in the joints of the hand. Inflammation is usually not present, and tenderness is mild. The joints may become enlarged (deformed). Crepitation and changes in the alignment of the extremity may be present.
- Medical management objectives include relief of pain, restoration of joint function, and prevention of disability or further disease progression. Surgery may be indicated. Common surgical procedures include arthroscopic surgery for debridement, osteotomy for realignment, arthrodesis, and replacement arthroplasty.
- Nursing management of persons with degenerative joint disease focuses on teaching persons about the disease process and measures to exert control over their situation. Patients who undergo surgery require special postoperative care. Of particular importance are the mobility restrictions after total hip replacement, the exercise program after total knee replacement, and prevention of infection after any total joint replacement.
- Gout is a metabolic disorder that results from prolonged hyperuricemia. Urates are deposited in and around joints, usually in the knee or foot. Bacterial arthritis is a result of infection in which the synovial membrane is invaded by microorganisms.
- Lyme disease is caused by the tick-borne spirochete *Borrelia burgdorferi*. Characterized by an erythematous rash, the disease has musculoskeletal, neurological, and cardiovascular manifestations. Prevention is the best treatment. Tetracycline or doxycycline is given to infected persons. Nursing interventions are similar to those for patients with arthritis.
- A number of diseases resemble each other, characterized by arthritis, a negative rheumatoid factor test, spondylitis, enthesitis, extraarticular symptoms, and the presence of HLA-B27.
- Known as the seronegative arthropathies, ankylosing spondylitis is the prototype disease. Others include Reiter's syndrome, psoriatic arthritis, and enteropathic arthritis. Care is similar to care for persons with RA.
- Ankylosing spondylitis is an idiopathic, chronic, progressive disorder affecting the joints of the hips and spine.
- As a result of the inflammatory process within the spine, the bones of the spine fuse (ankylose). Inflammation usually begins at the sacroiliac joints and progresses up the spine, resulting in fusion of the entire spine.
- Early symptoms may include low back pain and pain and swelling of the hips, knees, or shoulders. Mild fever, anorexia, and fatigue may also be present. Symptoms flare and subside. Eventually pain may decrease and motion of the back becomes restricted. Fusion of the sacroiliac joints and spine may occur, resulting in a kyphosis at the cervicodorsal junction.
- Medical management consists of exercise, rest, heat, and antiinflammatory analgesics. Spinal osteotomy or hip arthroplasty may be necessary for persons with severe symptoms.
- Nursing management centers on patient teaching, promotion of comfort and correct posture, and prevention of complications.
- Systemic lupus erythematosus (SLE) is a chronic inflammatory disease of unknown cause. It affects women more often than men. Its course can be controlled by corticosteroids, but some patients do die as a result of lesions affecting major organs or from secondary infections.
- Pathological manifestations of SLE include synovial involvement, severe vasculitis, renal involvement, and lesions of the nervous system.
- The initial manifestation of SLE is often arthritis, but the joint symptoms may be transient. The patient may complain of sensitivity to the sun. Erythema, usually in a butterfly pattern, can appear over the cheeks and bridge of the nose. The patient may also have findings of glomerulonephritis, pleuritis, pericarditis, peritonitis, neuritis, or anemia. Laboratory findings are specific to the organs involved.
- Medical management begins conservatively with rest, exercise, and medications. Kidney dialysis or transplant may be necessary for uncontrolled lupus nephritis, or total hip replacement may be necessary for avascular necrosis resulting from high-dose steroid therapy.
- Nursing management centers on patient teaching and promoting comfort and ADL.
- Polymyositis and dermatomyositis are idiopathic inflammatory diseases of striated (voluntary) muscle.
- Diagnostic tests for polymyositis include manual muscle test, electromyogram, muscle biopsy, serum enzyme measurements, and 24-hour urine tests.
- Medical management consists of rest and treatment with corticosteroids, and nursing management addresses teaching, prevention of skin breakdown, and promotion of comfort and mobility.

## DISORDERS AFFECTING BONE

- Paget's disease is a metabolic bone disease of unknown etiology characterized by excessive bone destruction and unorganized bone formation and repair. There is a high incidence in persons of Northern European ancestry, especially in persons older than 55 years of age.
- The axial skeleton is affected most, although the pelvis, femur, and tibia are also affected.
- Bony enlargement and deformity are common manifestations. Pain is common and neurological deficits may occur as a result of bony compression.
- Pathological fractures may occur. Persons with long-standing disease should be monitored for osteosarcoma.
- Treatment goals are to relieve pain and prevent deformity and fracture. Bisphosphonates and calcitonin may be prescribed.
- Osteoporosis is the most common musculoskeletal disorder in older adults.

- Osteoporosis is a degenerative disorder of bone metabolism that is caused by a greater rate of bone resorption than bone formation. It occurs more frequently in white, postmenopausal women. The loss in bone mass predisposes the individual to pathological fractures, especially of the vertebrae and hips.
- Type I osteoporosis involves rapid bone loss and is caused primarily by estrogen depletion, resulting in increased osteoclast activity.
- Type II osteoporosis is related to general aging and is primarily associated with decreased osteoblast activity. It affects men and women about equally.
- Estrogen replacement therapy with progestins minimizes the associated risks of breast and uterine cancer.
- A diet adequate in calcium and active weight-bearing exercise are essential throughout life to minimize bone loss from osteoporosis.
- Medical management includes exercise, dietary supplements of calcium and vitamin D, and estrogen therapy. The goal of treatment is to slow bone loss. Nursing management focuses on education and identification of risk factors. Other interventions include promoting comfort, mobility, and safety to maximize independence and reduce potential for injury.
- Osteomyelitis is a bone infection caused by either exogenous or internal pathogens. The most common causative organism for both types is *Staphylococcus aureus.* It is treated with oral and intravenous antibiotic therapy, suction irrigation systems, and surgical debridement of infected bone.

## DISORDERS AFFECTING THE SPINE

- Low back pain is a common cause of disability and time lost from work. Frequently the etiology is not known.
- Treatment is usually conservative. Exercise, proper body mechanics, and pain management are important interventions.
- Degenerative disease of the spine is a common but difficult problem. The intervertebral disks and facet joints of the spine are subjected to a great deal of stress in maintaining upright posture and providing mobility. Herniated nucleus pulposus, osteophyte formation, spondylolisthesis, and spinal stenosis are several conditions that result from degenerative changes in the spine.
- Degenerative diseases of the spine are clinically manifested as low back pain, sciatic pain radiating down the leg (e.g., with herniated nucleus pulposus), and neurological signs and symptoms (e.g., with herniated nucleus pulposus, stenosis, and osteophyte formation). Conservative medical management consists of rest, heat, medications, and traction to relieve muscle spasm. Surgical interventions are carried out to decompress nerve roots and to stabilize the spine. Spinal surgery procedures include laminectomy, discectomy, foraminotomy, and spinal fusion.
- Conservative nursing management consists of patient teaching, promoting comfort, and promoting lower extremity circulation.
- Nursing care after spinal surgery focuses on positioning (logrolling) and mobility, wound care, and patient comfort. Postoperative nursing interventions will differ depending on the level at which the spinal surgery was performed (e.g., lumbar, thoracic, or cervical).
- Scoliosis is a lateral deviation of the spine from the midline. Scoliosis may develop in localized areas of the spine or involve the whole spinal column. The amount of impingement on the rib cage is determined by the degree of rotation of the curve. Stability of the spine and mobility of the trunk are affected by the balance of the curve.
- Scoliosis deformity can be slight, mild, or severe. Early deformity may not be easily detected but will increase with growth and age. The cardiopulmonary system can be impaired in advanced scoliosis. Medical management for early scoliosis includes exercise with or without traction, bracing in combination with exercise for curves less than 40°, and corrective surgery if the curve exceeds 40° and other measures have failed.
- Nursing management of persons with scoliosis consists of patient instruction for persons who are being treated conservatively. Patients who undergo surgery require special postoperative care. The risk for pulmonary, gastrointestinal, and fluid balance complications after spinal fusion for scoliosis is high. Preventing such problems is a primary objective of the nurse.

## DISORDERS AFFECTING THE HANDS AND FEET

- Hallux valgus, a lateral deviation of the great toe toward the midline, is a common foot problem.
- Bunion deformity frequently accompanies hallux valgus. A bunion develops as the medial eminence of the metatarsal head becomes prominent and a protective bursa forms as it rubs against shoes. Narrow-toed, high-heeled shoes crowd the toes.
- Conservative treatment consists of changing shoe styles, using protective pads or insoles, and NSAIDs.
- If conservative treatment fails, surgical correction may be indicated.
- A soft dressing and special shoe are worn after surgery. Crutches or a walker may be necessary.
- Dupuytren's contracture is a deformity of the palmar fascia that causes the ring and sometimes the little finger to flex into the palm and lose the capacity to be extended. Surgical removal of the involved palmar fascia may be required if conservative measures to relieve symptoms are ineffective. Nursing management then addresses postoperative care.

## TUMORS OF THE MUSCULOSKELETAL SYSTEM

- Benign and malignant tumors of the musculoskeletal system include those arising from muscle, bone, cartilage, fibrous tissue, and bone marrow.
- Some examples of benign tumors include osteoma, osteochondroma, leiomyoma, and giant cell tumor. Treatment methods include surgical excision and amputation.
- The most common primary bone tumor is osteosarcoma. It is a rapidly growing neoplasm that causes a moth-eaten pattern of bone destruction. Metastasis to the lungs is common.
- Treatment of osteosarcoma includes chemotherapy and surgical excision, either by amputation or limb salvage techniques.
- Limb salvage procedures have many potential complications but offer an alternative to amputation. The patient must be fully informed about both procedures and their risks, benefits, and expected outcomes.
- Nursing interventions for patients with bone tumors focus on teaching, support, promotion of independence, and acceptance of body image.

## DISORDERS AFFECTING THE MUSCLES

- The muscular dystrophies are a group of familial disorders characterized by varying degrees of skeletal muscle

weakness and degeneration, leading to disability and deformity. Mental retardation occurs in some types.
- At least 10 types have been identified; 5 are commonly seen in adults.
- Classification is done by phenotype, mode of inheritance, rate of progression, and muscular involvement.
- The etiology is unknown. Muscle cell membrane defects and biochemical abnormalities have been identified. Muscle fibers are eventually replaced with fat and connective tissue.
- Treatment is supportive, as there is no cure.
- Treatment is focused on preserving function and mobility. Physical therapy, assistive and adaptive devices, surgical release of contractures, steroids, and immunosuppressants are examples of treatments for persons with MD.
- Nursing management is also supportive. Monitoring for complications of immobility is important. Referrals for genetic counseling may be indicated.

## References


1. Altizer L: Total hip arthroplasty, *Orthop Nurs* 14(4):7-18, 1995.
2. Anderson LP, Dale KG: Infections in total joint replacements, *Orthop Nurs* 17(1):7-11, 1998.
3. Bertino LS, Lu LC: The bite of a wolf: systemic lupus erythematosus, *Rehab Nurs* 18(3):173-178, 1993.
4. Bertsch C: CREST syndrome: a variant of systemic sclerosis, *Orthop Nurs* 14(2):53-60, 1995.
5. Bregqvist D, et al: Low molecular-weight heparin (enoxaparin) as prophylaxis against venous thromboembolism after total hip replacement, *N Engl J Med* 335(10) 696-700, 1996.
6. Bridwell KN: Lumbar spinal stenosis: diagnosis, management, and treatment, *Clin Geriatr Med* 10(4):677-701, 1994.
7. Buckwatter JA, Martin J: Degenerative joint disease, *Clin Symp* 47(2): 1-32, 1995.
8. Casey ATH, Crockard HA, Bland JM, et al: Surgery on the rheumatoid cervical spine for the non-ambulant myelopathic patient—too much, too late? *Lancet* 347:1004-1007, 1996.
9. Clarke BL: Paget's disease of bone. In Rakel RE, editor: *Conn's current therapy,* Philadelphia, 1997, WB Saunders.
10. Cleland LG, Hill CL, James MJ: Diet and arthritis, *Baillière's Clin Rheumatol* 9(4):771-785, 1995.
11. Connelly C: Patients with lowback pain: how to identify the few who need extra attention, *Postgrad Med* 100(6):143-156, 1996.
12. Cunningham ME: Becoming familiar with fibromyalgia, *Orthop Nurs* 15(2):33-36, 1996.
13. Donley BG, et al: Diagnosing and treating hallux valgus: a conservative approach for a common problem, *Cleve Clin J Med* 64(9):469-474, 1997.
14. Emmerson BT: Drug therapy the management of gout, *N Engl J Med* 334(7):445-451, 1996.
15. Epstein S: Post-transplantation bone disease: the role of immunosuppressive agents and the skeleton, *J Bone Miner Res* 11(1):1-7, 1996.
16. Evans RL, Rubash HE, Albrecht SA: The efficacy of postoperative autotransfusion in total joint arthroplasty, *Orthop Nurs* 12(3):11-18, 1993.
17. Favus MJ: Diagnosis and treatment of osteoporosis in the elderly, *Nurs Home Med* 5(suppl B):1B-9B, 1997.
18. Forsythe LL: Laparoscopic fusion procedures, *AORN* 66(4):637-643, 1997.
19. Gebhardt MC, et al: The use of bone allografts for limb salvage in high-grade extremity osteosarcoma, *Clin Orthop Relat Res* 270:181-194, 1990.
20. Geier K: Perioperative blood management, *Orthop Nurs* Jan/Feb suppl, pp 9-10, 1998.
21. Genant HK, et al: Osteoporosis: a treatment approach to long-term care patients, *Nurs Home Med* 5(suppl G):1G-24G, 1997.
22. Golbus J: The locomotor system. In Rakel RE, editor: *Conn's current therapy,* Philadelphia, 1997, WB Saunders.
23. Halverson PB: The spondyloarthropathies, *Orthop Nurs* 16(4):21-27, 1997.
24. Halverson PB: Extraarticular manifestations of rheumatoid arthritis, *Orthop Nurs* 14(4):47-50, 1995.
25. Harootunian AM: Is it Reiter's syndrome? *J Am Acad Nurse Practitioners* 9(9):427-430, 1997.
26. Harvard Medical School Health Publication Group: *Arthritis, a Harvard Health Letter special report,* Boston, Mass, 1995, the Group.
27. Holland NW, Agudelo CA: Hyperuricemia and gout. In Rakel RE, editor: *Conn's current therapy,* Philadelphia, 1997, WB Saunders.
28. Ismeurt RL, Wilson LW, Long CO: Lyme disease, *Home Health Care Nurse* 13(3):28-33, 1995.
29. Kaplan FS: Prevention and management of osteoporosis, *Clin Symp* 47(1):1-32, 1995.
30. Kessenich CR, Rosen CJ: Vitamin D and bone status in elderly women, *Orthop Nurs* 15(3):67-71, 1996.
31. Klem, KW: Antibiotic bead chains, *Clin Orthop Relat Res* 295:63-76, 1993.
32. Krotenberg R, et al: Incidence of dislocation following hip arthroplasty for patients in the rehabilitation setting, *Am J Phys Med Rehabil* 74(6):444-447, 1995.
33. Lane JM, et al: Osteoporosis: diagnosis and treatment, *J Bone Joint Surg* 78-A(4):618-632, 1996.
34. Lash AA: Why so many women? SLE, *Dermatol Nurs* 6(2):92-96, 1994.
35. Lew DP, Waldvogel FA: Osteomyelitis, *N Engl J Med* 336(14):999-1007, 1997.
36. Lin CC, Ward SE: Perceived self-efficacy and outcome expectancies in coping with chronic low back pain, *Res Nurs Health* 19:299-310, 1996.
37. Luekenotte AG: *Gerontologic Nursing,* St Louis, 1996, Mosby.
38. Mac HL, Reynolds MA, Treston-Aurand J, Henke JA: Comparison of autoreinfusion and standard drainage systems in total joint arthroplasty patients, *Orthop Nurs* 12(3):19-25, 1993.
39. Mader JT, Calhoun J: Long-bone osteomyelitis: diagnosis and treatment, *Hosp Pract* October 15, pp 73-86, 1994.
40. Maurizio SJ, Rogers JL: Recognizing and treating fibromyalgia, *Nurse Practitioner* 22(12):18-28, 1997.
41. McCance KL, Huether SE: *Pathophysiology: the biologic basis of disease in adults and children,* ed 3, St Louis, 1998, Mosby.
42. Mooney V, Saal JA, Saal JS: Evaluation and treatment of low back pain, *Clin Symp* 48(4):1-32, 1996.
43. Massachusetts Medical Society: Lyme disease US, 1995, *MMWR* 45(23), 1996.
44. Mourad LA: Musculoskeletal system. In Thompson JM, et al, editors: *Mosby's clinical nursing,* ed 4, St Louis, 1997, Mosby.
45. Mourad LA, Droste MM: *The nursing process in the care of adults with orthopaedic conditions,* ed 3, Albany, NY, 1993, Delmar Publishers.
46. Nesher G, Moore TL: Clinical presentation and treatment of arthritis in the aged, *Clin Geriatr Med* 10(4):659-672, 1994.
47. Nordin BEC and others: The definition, diagnosis, and classification of osteoporosis, *Phys Med Rehabil Clin North Am* 6(3):395-410, 1995.
48. Peyron JG: Intraarticular hyaluronan injections in the treatment of OA: state-of-the-art-review, *J Rheumatol* 20(39):10-16, 1993.
49. Pfister HW, Wilske B, Weber K: Lyme boreliosis: basic science and clinical aspects, *Lancet* 343:1013-1016, 1994.

50. Piasecki PA: Nursing care of the patient with metastatic bone disease, *Orthop Nurs* 15(4):25-34, 1996.
51. Proctor MC, Greenfield LJ, Marsh EE: Prophylaxis for thromboembolism in elective orthopaedic surgery, *Orthop Nurs* 16(5):51-56, 1997.
52. Pruitt LA, Taaffe DR, Marcus R: Effects of a one-year high-intensity versus low-intensity resistance training on bone mineral density in older women, *J Bone Miner Res* 10(11):1788-1795, 1995.
53. Reid IA: Preventing glucocorticoid-induced osteoporosis, *N Engl J Med* 337(6):420-421, 1997.
54. Robinson RG, et al: Strontium 89 therapy for the palliation of pain due to osseous metastases, *JAMA* 274(5):420-424, 1995.
55. Ross C: A comparison of osteoarthritis and rheumatoid arthritis: diagnosis and treatment, *Nurse Practitioner* 22(9):20-41, 1997.
56. Sanders RD: Aching and inflamed joints, *Fam Pract Audio Digest* 44(13):1996.
57. Schumacher HR: Crystal-induced arthritis: an overview, *Am J Med* 100(2A):2A-46S-2A-51S, 1996.
58. Shiple BJ: Treating low back pain, *Physician Sports Med* 25(8):51-66, 1997.
59. Sigal LN: Myths and facts about Lyme disease, *Cleve Clin J Med* 64(4):203-209, 1997.
60. Skinner HB: *Current diagnosis and treatment in orthopaedics,* Norwalk, Conn, 1995, Appleton & Lange.
61. Spica MM, Schwab MD: Sexual expression after total joint replacement, *Orthop Nurs* 15(5):41-44, 1996.
62. Terrazas D: Managing polymyalgia rheumatica and giant cell arteritis in the primary care setting, *J Am Acad Nurse Practitioners* 9(6):289-292, 1997.
63. US Department of Health and Human Services, Public Health Service: *Healthy People 2000: midcourse review and 1995 revisions,* Boston, 1996, Jones & Bartlett.
64. US Preventive Services Task Force: Screening for adolescent idiopathic scoliosis, *Nurse Practitioner* 19(9):39-45, 1994.
65. van der Heide A, et al: The effectiveness of early treatment with "second-line" anti-rheumatic drugs: a randomized, controlled trial, *Ann Intern Med* 15(124):699-707, 1966.
66. Warwick D, et al: Perioperative low-molecular-weight heparins, *Br J Bone Joint Surg* 77-B(5):715-719, 1995.
67. Wilde AH: Management of infected knee and hip prostheses, *Curr Opin Rheumatol* 5:317-32, 1993.
68. Wipt JE, Chaquette DL: Low back pain: selective evaluation and management, *Fed Practitioner* 14(8):8-24, 1997.
69. Wirth MA, Rockwood CA: Current concepts review: complications of total shoulder replacement arthroplasty, *J Bone Joint Surg* 78-A (4):603-616, 1996.
70. Yandrich TJ: Preventing infection in total joint replacement surgery, *Orthop Nurs* 14(2):15-19, 1996.
71. Zimmerman SI, Fox KM, Magaziner J: Psychosocial aspects of osteoporosis, *Phys Med Rehabil Clin North Am* 6(3):441-451, 1995.

# chapter 62 ASSESSMENT OF THE Skin

VICKIE WEAVER

## objectives

*After studying this chapter, the learner should be able to:*

1. Relate the structures of the skin to their functions.
2. Explain physiological skin changes in elderly persons.
3. Describe guidelines and parameters for assessment of the skin and accessory structures.
4. Differentiate among various skin lesions.

## ANATOMY AND PHYSIOLOGY OF THE SKIN

The integument, or skin, is the largest organ of the body. It is exposed to the external environment and provides the first line of defense of the body; yet at the same time it is affected by changes in the internal environment. (See Chapter 10 for a review of biological defense mechanisms.) Assessment of the integument provides data about how the person is affected by and is coping with both external and internal environments. Data obtained in the assessment provide the basis for identification of actual or potential nursing problems related to the skin, infection, fluid and electrolyte imbalances, nutritional imbalances, or inadequate oxygenation of tissues. Baseline observations are useful for identifying changes that may occur.

### STRUCTURE OF THE SKIN

The skin is composed of three major layers: the epidermis, the dermis, and subcutaneous tissue (Figure 62-1). The epidermis consists of five layers. The outermost layer is a thin layer of closely packed, dead squamous cells that contain keratin, a fibrous protein, that gives skin its color. This dead cell layer is called the stratum corneum. The innermost layer, stratum basale or basement membrane, is also called the stratum germinativum. The stratum germinativum gives rise to new cells to renew the outermost layer which lacks blood vessels and is constantly being shed. Between these two layers are three other layers: the stratum lucidum, stratum granulosum, and stratum spinosum, identified in Figure 62-1. These three layers are involved in keratin formation.

The second main layer, the dermis, or corium, is connected to the epidermis by the stratum basale. The dermis is composed of bundles of collagen fibers that act to support the epidermis. It is well supplied with nerves and blood vessels and contains appendages such as the sweat glands, sebaceous glands, and hair follicles.

The third layer of skin is subcutaneous tissue, composed of loose connective tissue filled with fat cells. Fat conducts heat only one fourth as rapidly as do other tissues and thus serves as the heat insulator of the body. It also serves as a cushion and is a storage site for energy. The subcutaneous layer also anchors the other two layers to supportive structures (e.g., muscle, tendon, and bone).

Thickness of the skin varies over different areas of the body. Exposed areas such as hands and face usually have thicker skin that contains more keratin in the epidermis. The skin on the inner aspect of the arms is thinner and therefore more sensitive to heat.

Sweat glands excrete directly to the surface of the skin and are under the control of the sympathetic nervous system. The two types of sweat glands are eccrine and apocrine. The eccrine glands are distributed throughout the body and are more abundant in the forehead, palms, and soles of the feet. Eccrine glands assist in the heat-regulating mechanisms of the body. The apocrine glands are found mainly in the axillary and genital regions. Some of the protoplasm of these secretory cells is secreted with the fluid, and it is bacterial decomposition of the sweat from these glands that is responsible for body odor. Sweat glands of the axilla, palms, and soles are mostly under control of the stress response.

Sebaceous glands secrete an oily, odorless fluid (sebum) into the hair follicles. Earwax is sebum from glands in the external ear canal. Sebum protects the hair follicle from infection and lubricates the skin.

### FUNCTIONS OF THE SKIN

#### Protection

The outermost layer of the epidermis, the stratum corneum, is a relatively impermeable layer of tightly packed flat cells that protects the underlying tissue from the outer environment. A normal amount of nonpathogenic bacteria is present on the outer surface of the skin, but the dryness of the surface keeps

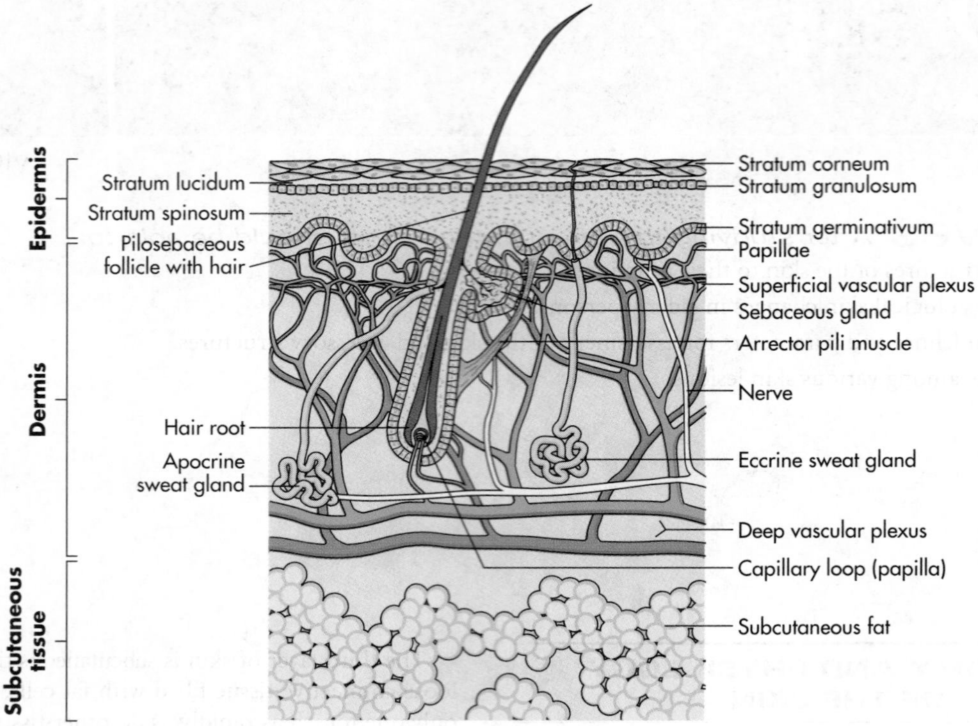

**fig. 62-1** Anatomy of skin and skin layers.

the number small because microorganisms require moisture for growth. Bacteria that penetrate hair follicles usually are removed by the sebum. Fat-soluble substances such as emollient lotion can penetrate the skin by passing through the hair follicles and sebaceous glands.

An intact skin is the first line of defense against bacterial and foreign-substance invasion, slight physical trauma, heat, or ultraviolet rays. When the skin is exposed to environmental factors such as pressure, friction, and internal shearing forces, the epidermis is compressed to the depth of the supporting structures (i.e., bone). With prolonged exposure the capillary bed within the dermis and the greater vessels within the subcutaneous tissue become occluded, causing tissue ischemia to the area. If the ischemia is not reversed by removing the source of pressure, cellular death is imminent and the skin's defensive line is jeopardized.

Scraping or stripping the surface of the skin (e.g., removal of tape or the use of razors without shaving cream) can weaken the epidermis. Once the barrier has weakened, permeability to bacteria, drugs, and other foreign substances is increased. Large amounts of drugs can be absorbed by extensive denuded skin areas. Epidermis that becomes extremely dry may crack, which leads to breaks in the surface. If it remains wet for long periods of time, it becomes macerated, and the moisture provides a medium for bacterial growth.

Mucous membranes, although continuous with the stratum corneum, are somewhat protected from the external environment. Fluids and other substances such as certain drugs can be absorbed through the mucous membranes.

### Heat Regulation

Body temperature is controlled by *radiation* of heat from the surface of the skin, conduction of heat from skin to other objects or air, removal of heat by air currents on the skin *(convection),* or evaporation of water from skin surfaces. Insensible water evaporation from the skin and lungs occurs at a rate of 600 to 1000 ml/day. On a hot day the only way the body can lose heat is by evaporation, and anything that restricts evaporation under these conditions will increase body temperature. The blood vessels of the skin help control body temperature by constricting in cold environments to promote conservation of heat and dilating in warm environments to promote loss of heat by radiation. These mechanisms help maintain a constant internal body temperature.

### Sensory Perception

The skin contains receptor endings of nerves responsible for sensing pain, touch, heat, and cold. Through the stimulation of these nerve endings, a person is able to communicate with the immediate external environment. Distribution of the sensory endings is generalized; however, certain areas of the body have more than other areas. The hands, for example, have a higher concentration than the forearms.

### Excretion

Water lost through the skin is a factor in maintaining water balance in the body. Salt is lost through excessive sweating in addition to water loss. A person can become acclimatized to a

**table 62-1** *Changes in Skin, Hair, and Nails as a Result of Aging*

| Parameter | Observable Changes | Cause |
|---|---|---|
| **SKIN** | | |
| Color | Paleness in white skin | Decreased vascularity of dermis; loss of melanocytes |
| | Liver or brown spots (senile lentigines) | Hyperpigmentation, clusters of melanocytes |
| | Purple patches (senile purpura) | Blood leaking from poorly supported fragile capillaries |
| Types | Keratoses | Overgrowth and thickening of the cornified epithelium |
| | Seborrheic | Benign; raised; tan to black in color; greasy |
| | Actinic or senile | Slow-growing; localized thickening of outer skin layers caused by chronic, prolonged skin exposure; premalignant lesion that may develop into squamous cell carcinoma |
| Moisture | Dry skin (xerosis), decreased perspiration | Decreased sebaceous and sweat gland activity |
| Elasticity, turgor | Loose folds and wrinkles | Loss of collagen and elastic fibers |
| | Decreased turgor, tenting | Decreased elasticity |
| Texture | Some rough areas | Environmental effects over time and less moisture |
| | Thin, more transparent skin | Thinning of epidermis from decreased vascularity of dermis; loss of underlying tissue |
| | Skin tags (acrochordons) | Overgrowth of normal skin |
| **HAIR** | | |
| Color | Grayness | Decreased number of melanocytes in follicle |
| Consistency | Thinner on head and body | Decreased density and rate of hair growth |
| | Coarser in nose of men | Increased density of nasal hair |
| Distribution | Loss of hair on head and body | Decreased rate of hair growth; decreased hormones; decreased peripheral circulation |
| | Increased hair on face of women | Higher androgen to estrogen ratio |
| **NAILS** | More brittle<br>Longitudinal ridges<br>Thickening and yellowing of toenails | Slowing of nail growth; decreased peripheral circulation |

continually hot environment, however, and the amount of salt lost decreases over time.

### Vitamin D Production

Synthesis of vitamin D takes place in the skin by the effect of sunlight (ultraviolet rays). Vitamin D is necessary in the metabolism of calcium and phosphorus.

### Expression

Because the skin is the part of the body that is visible to others, it is a means of communicating feelings. Also, because of its visibility, skin is largely involved in a person's body image. Individuals become concerned when there is fear of or presence of disfigurement.

## PHYSIOLOGICAL CHANGES WITH AGING

Many skin changes may be observed as the person ages (Table 62-1). These changes result primarily from loss of subcutaneous tissue, degeneration of collagen and elastic fibers, loss of melanocytes, increased capillary fragility, decreased secretion of sweat glands, hormonal changes, and overexposure to environmental elements.

The skin loses its elasticity and becomes loose and wrinkled. Exposed areas may be thickened, but in general the skin becomes thinner, drier, and more fragile. There are fewer hair follicles; therefore absorbency of fat-soluble substances is less. Lesions appear, the most common of which are senile lentigines (brown spots, Figure 62-2) or senile purpura (red to purple ecchymoses seen on exposed areas). Seborrheic keratoses (see Chapter 63) are more common than actinic keratoses. Changes in the appearance of the hair and nails also occur.

The elderly person is also more likely to have one or more chronic diseases and to be taking medications that can cause skin changes. Dry skin may cause itching and if scratched, can lead to skin breakdown. Stasis dermatitis may occur with a marked decrease in circulation to the legs. Skin infections occur more readily because of increased epidermal permeability.

Some general principles related to assessment and health teaching and a listing of common disorders in the elderly are listed in the Gerontological Assessment Box.

## SUBJECTIVE DATA

The patient history is an important part of the health assessment and is included with the physical examination. If during a general history, the patient describes a skin problem or skin discomfort (itching or superficial pain), then further data are obtained, including the following information.[5]

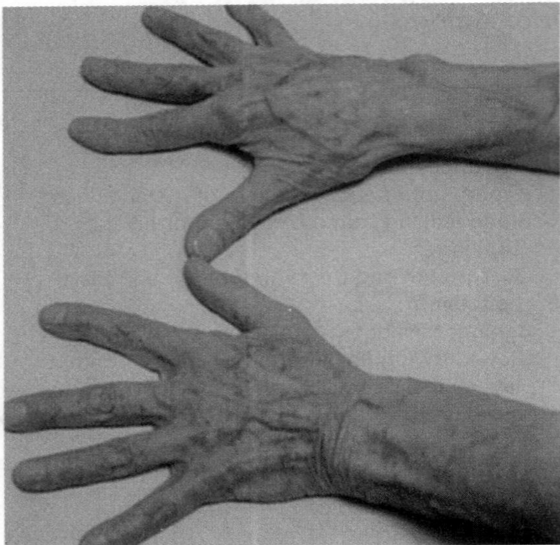

**fig. 62-2** Hands of older adult. Note prominent veins and thin appearance of skin.

1. Usual skin condition: usual appearance, color, moisture, texture, or integrity
2. Onset of the problem: initial sites—when changes were first noticed; skin appearance at onset; any other symptoms noted at time of onset, such as pain or itching
3. Changes since onset: changes in location of lesions; changes in appearance; increase in size; new symptoms such as pain or itching
4. Specific known cause: for example, contact with poison ivy, exposure to a known allergen, or stress
5. If cause is unknown:
   a. Recent exposure to sensitizing substances, such as metals, chemicals, detergents, or poisonous plants
   b. Prescriptions for a new drug such as penicillin
   c. Occupation that may cause contact with potential skin irritants or hands constantly in water
   d. Recreational activities, for example, painting, camping, or gardening
   e. Exposure to sun (burn, photosensitivity, or skin cancer) or cold (frostbite)
6. Alleviating factors: physician-prescribed or self-prescribed
7. Psychological reaction to skin changes: withdrawal from social activities; cosmetics for coverup; feelings about the problem (body image)

Latex allergies are becoming increasingly common among health care workers and patients since the initiation of the use of Universal Precautions in 1987.[2] Populations most at risk for a latex sensitivity or true allergic reaction include children and adults with spina bifida, children who have had multiple surgeries before the age of 5, persons with congenital urological anomalies, employees of the rubber industry, and health care workers. Sensitivity reactions may be immediate or delayed and range from symptoms of contact dermatitis to systemic anaphylactic reactions. While performing a physical assessment on an individual within one of the high-risk categories, the nurse should question the person about previous signs of sensitivity such as itchy, watery eyes when in contact with latex balloons, condoms, and catheters or after previous contact with a health care worker wearing latex gloves. (See Chapter 19 for further discussion of latex allergy.)

**gerontological assessment**

**ASSESSMENT**

Assess for presence of dryness and intactness of skin, skin infections, and lesions.

Identify medications currently taken by patient, and assess potential for photosensitivity (see Table 63-4). Thiazides and phenothiazides are medications commonly taken by elders.

**INTERVENTION**

Teach patient to avoid frequent baths, especially hot baths, that cause additional skin dryness. Tell patient to apply lotion to skin immediately after bathing.

Teach patient to report early signs of skin infection to physician. The elderly person's decreased immune response may delay healing. The elderly person with herpes zoster needs protection from secondary infection such as pneumonia.

Teach patient to perform self-skin assessment routinely.

Teach patient to differentiate benign skin lesions commonly seen with aging (brown spots and bruises) from potentially malignant lesions and to report the latter to physician.

**COMMON DISORDERS IN ELDERS**

Benign skin tumors
Skin cancers
Dermatitis medicamentosa
Skin infections, especially herpes zoster
Stasis dermatitis of legs

## OBJECTIVE DATA

### METHODS OF ASSESSMENT

The skin is an organ that can be examined by direct inspection and observation with no tools but a good light. Palpation also is used in gathering data about certain types of lesions. See principles related to skin assessment in the Guidelines for Care Box.[5]

Data that can be obtained from physical assessment of the skin include not only dermatological problems but also information about the person's overall health status. A systematic head-to-toe skin assessment usually is conducted while other significant data in the initial interview and physical assessment of the person are gathered. Specific areas of the skin are reassessed as potential or existing problems are identified.

### PARAMETERS OF GENERAL SKIN ASSESSMENT

The objective data to be collected when examining the skin for general health status include skin color, temperature, moisture, elasticity, turgor, texture, thickness, and odor.

**guidelines for care**

**Skin Assessment Techniques**

1. Be prepared: Have a good light available and well-controlled room temperature. If the lighting is inadequate, lesions may be missed or described inaccurately. If the room temperature is not well controlled, vasoconstriction, vasodilation, and papillary erections occur, giving false data.
2. Be systematic: If only some parts of the skin are inspected, an important parameter may be omitted or a lesion missed.
3. Be thorough: Look at all areas carefully. If the person is lying down, be sure to examine the back, especially the sacral area. Lift folds of tissue, such as under the breasts or gluteal folds. The examiner's embarrassment or anticipated embarrassment of the examinee may result in inadequate data. Do not forget to assess the mucous membranes as well.
4. Be specific: When lesions are identified, describe the lesions using metric system and established parameters (e.g., color, size, and shape).
5. Compare right side with left side: When observing changes in skin color or tissue shape, always compare one side of the body with the other to differentiate structural from pathological changes as well as symmetry of manifestation.
6. Record the data: Unrecorded data are lost data. Baseline observations indicating normality or abnormality are needed for comparison with subsequent findings. Changes need to be recorded to determine progress toward achieving desired outcomes.
7. Use appropriate technique: Palpation is used during physical assessment of the skin. Lesions are palpated for density, induration, and tenderness. Standard Precautions (see Chapter 10) need to be observed during palpation, and the examiner should determine whether it is appropriate to use gloves.

## Color

Changes in skin color are best observed in the lips, mucous membranes of the mouth, earlobes, fingernails and toenails, and the extremities. The lips show rapid color changes. Color of the skin varies with the amount of melanin in the cells and with the blood supply (Table 62-2). Skin color may be masked by cosmetics or tanning. Inaccurate assessment of skin color may be attributed to factors such as conducting the examination in a poorly lit room, room temperature extremes, the presence of edema, poor hygiene, or positioning.

## Pigmentation

Melanin formation requires the amino acid tyrosine, the enzyme tyrosinase, and molecular oxygen. Variations of general pigmentation are seen within one individual; an increase in pigmentation usually is seen on exposed surfaces and in the areola of the nipples. Conversely, decreased pigmentation is seen on unexposed surfaces and on the palms and soles of dark-skinned persons.

Hyperpigmentation occurs normally in some persons as a genetic factor (dark skin). Pigmentary changes are more common in African Americans than in whites because of the greater amount of melanin in dark skin. Light-skinned persons may have increased pigmentation from the effects of sunlight (tanning). Melanin is formed in the basal cells of the stratum basale and then gradually moves to the surface, where it is cast off and the tan fades. Elderly light-skinned persons may normally develop irregular brown patches. Hyperpigmentation may occur with x-ray therapy as a result of activation of tyrosinase. This type of hyperpigmentation fades slowly but may be long-lasting. Hydroquinone with salicylic acid or with retinoic acid inhibits the tyrosinase reaction. Hyperpigmentation also occurs with inflammations, acne vulgaris, drug eruptions, neurodermatitis, and pityriasis rosea.

Hypopigmentation occurs normally in some persons as a genetic factor (light skin). Albinos have a congenital inability to produce melanin. Severe trauma can destroy melanin-producing cells and result in hypopigmentation (scar tissue). Some healthy persons develop a condition called vitiligo, in which there is a failure of melanin formation in certain areas, primarily around orifices and hairy areas, producing sharply demarcated white patches. Vitiligo also can occur with hyperthyroidism, pernicious anemia, and adrenocortical insufficiency. One treatment for small patches of vitiligo is methoxypsoralen administered orally plus exposure to sunlight or long-wave ultraviolet light. Other causes of hypopigmentation include atopic dermatitis, tinea, and pityriasis alba.

## Dark Skin

Assessment of dark-skinned persons is more difficult than that of light-skinned persons because color changes are less obvious. Often other signs and symptoms must be used to reach a conclusion. For example, when a skin area is inflamed, the erythema may not be noticeable, and the involved area must be palpated for warmth and edema. Rashes may not be visible and must be determined by palpation if the rash is papular or by patient reports of pruritus. Suggestions for assessment of dark skin are presented in Box 62-1.

Melanin, which gives skin its general color, is produced by melanocytes. The skin of darkly pigmented persons does not contain more melanocytes, but the melanocytes are larger and produce more melanin.[4] Pigmented skin offers more protection from ultraviolet radiation; hence dark skin reacts less to sunlight and skin cancers occur less frequently.

Skin color changes will be seen best in areas of lesser pigmentation, which include the lips, areas around the mouth, mucous membranes, conjunctivae, earlobes, nail beds, palms, and soles. The sclerae of many dark-skinned persons contain fatty deposits with carotene, giving the sclerae a yellowish tinge.[4] In these persons, jaundice will have to be determined by other signs, such as bile in the urine or feces.

Loss of redness provided by the blood produces grayish or dull tones rather than pallor. This sign may be difficult to observe by the untrained eye. Grayish or dull tones can be visualized best in the lips, mucous membranes, conjunctivae, and nail beds. Cyanosis also gives the skin a grayish or dull tone because of loss of redness. Areas of lesser pigmentation,

**table 62-2** *Skin Color Changes*

| Physiology | Conditions |
|---|---|
| **REDNESS (ERYTHEMA)** | |
| Vasodilation: more rapid blood flow, more oxygenated blood giving a reddish hue | Blushing, heat, inflammation, fever, alcohol ingestion, extreme cold (below 15° C), hot flushes, polycythemia |
| **WHITENESS (PALLOR)** | |
| Vasoconstriction: slower blood flow, less blood in capillaries | Cold, fear, shock |
| Partially obstructed blood flow: less blood in capillaries | Vasospasm, thrombus, narrowed vessels, arterial insufficiency |
| Fluid between blood vessels and skin surface | Edema |
| Decreased oxygenation of blood from decreased hemoglobin | Anemia |
| Loss of melanin | Vitiligo |
| **BLUISH (CYANOSIS)** | |
| Deoxygenated hemoglobin seen in earlobes, lips, mucous membranes of mouth, nail beds | Heart or lung disease, inadequate respiration, peripheral blood vessel obstruction, venous disease, cold, anxiety |
| **YELLOW (JAUNDICE)** | |
| Increased bile pigment in blood eventually distributed to skin and mucous membranes and to sclera of eye | Liver disease, obstruction of bile ducts, chronic uremia, rapid hemolysis |
| **BROWN** | |
| Increased melanin deposits: normal in brown-black races | Aging, sunburn; anterior pituitary, adrenal cortex, or liver disease |
| **DULLNESS** | |
| Vasoconstriction in dark skin | Cold, fear, shock |
| Partially obstructed blood flow in dark skin | Vasospasm, thrombus, narrowed vessels, arterial insufficiency |
| Fluid between blood vessels and skin surface in dark skin | Edema |

**box 62-1** *Tips for Assessing Dark Skin*

1. Skin color should be observed in the sclerae, conjunctivae, buccal mucosa, tongue, lips, nail beds, palms, and soles.
2. Inspection should be accompanied by palpation, especially if inflammation or edema is suspected.
3. Findings should always be correlated with the patient's history to arrive at a nursing diagnosis.
4. Pallor in brown-skinned patients may present as a yellowish brown tinge to the skin. In a black-skinned patient the skin will appear "ashen-gray." It can be difficult to determine. Pallor in dark-skinned individuals is characterized by absence of the underlying red tones in the skin.
5. Jaundice may be observed in the sclera but should not be confused with the normal yellow pigmentation of the dark-skinned black patient. The best place to inspect is in that portion of the sclera that is observable when the eye is open. If jaundice is suspected, the posterior portion of the hard palate should also be observed for a yellowish cast. This is most effective when done in bright daylight.
6. The oral mucosa of dark-skinned individuals may have a normal freckling of pigmentation that may also be evident in the gums, the borders of the tongue, and the lining of the cheeks.
7. The gingivae normally may have a dark blue color that may appear blotchy or be evenly distributed.
8. Petechiae are best observed over areas of lighter pigmentation—the abdomen, gluteal areas, and volar aspect of the forearm. They may also be seen in the palpebral conjunctiva and buccal mucosa.
9. To differentiate petechiae and ecchymosis from erythema, remember that pressure over the area will cause erythema to blanch but will not affect either petechiae or ecchymosis.
10. Erythema usually is associated with increased skin temperature, so palpation should also be used if an inflammatory condition is suspected.
11. Edema may reduce the intensity of the color of an area of skin because of the increased distance between the external epithelium and the pigmented layers. Therefore, darker skin would appear lighter. On palpation the skin may feel "tight."
12. Cyanosis can often be difficult to determine in dark-skinned individuals. Familiarity with the precyanotic color is often helpful. However, if this is not possible, close inspection of the nail beds, lips, palpebral conjunctiva, palms, and soles should show evidence of cyanosis.
13. Skin rashes may be assessed by palpating for changes in skin texture.

including the earlobes, palms, and soles, are assessed for signs of cyanosis.

### Blood Supply

The degree of blood supplied to the skin produces color changes. The rate of blood flow through the skin is highly variable because of its function in heat control. The blood vessels are innervated by the sympathetic nervous system; thus vasoconstriction occurs with the neuroendocrine response to stressors. With vasoconstriction, smaller amounts of blood pass through the vessels, producing decreased redness; a dark skin becomes dull and gray and a light skin whiter (pallor). Vasodilation increases the amount of oxygenated blood flow, and the skin acquires a reddish color (erythema). Vascular flush areas of the body are the "butterfly" band from cheek to cheek across the nose, the neck, upper portion of the chest, flexor surfaces of the extremities, and genital areas.

Changes in blood composition also can alter skin color. Excess deoxygenated hemoglobin gives a bluish tint (cyanosis) to the skin and mucous membranes. An excess of bile pigment results in a yellowish tint to the skin and sclerae of the eyes, although the sclerae of dark-pigmented persons may always have a yellowish tint.

### Temperature

The temperature of the skin is regulated by vasoconstriction or vasodilation. If an excess amount of heat is being produced within the body, such as with fever or exercise, or if heat from the external environment increases, the sympathetic centers in the hypothalamus are inhibited and vasodilation occurs. An increase in the amount of blood flow creates a sensation of warmth on the skin. This also occurs with hyperthyroidism. A local inflammation of the skin or underlying tissue also produces vasodilation; this is part of the inflammatory response. Cold skin is caused by vasoconstriction as a result of sympathetic stimulation. Diseases such as hypothyroidism also can contribute to skin coolness. To assess the temperature of the skin use the backs of the fingers, which are more sensitive than the finger tips.

### Moisture

Skin is assessed as being dry, moist, or oily. Dry skin is frequently seen in the elderly person because of decreased activity of the sebaceous glands. Dry skin and mucous membranes also are seen in persons who are dehydrated as water moves from the cells into the intravascular compartments. Persons with hypothyroidism have thick, dry, leathery skin.

Moist skin is caused by the presence of water or sweat on the surface. Overheating produces sweating. Persons with hyperthyroidism have moist, smooth skin. Some persons have more effective sweat mechanisms than others. Stressors, shock, or any situation that stimulates the sympathetic nervous system will cause increased fluid loss through the sweat glands (diaphoresis). Inasmuch as vasoconstriction occurs simultaneously with stimulation of the sympathetic nervous system, the skin is cold and wet (clammy).

Oily skin frequently is seen in the adolescent. Excess sebum formation by the sebaceous glands may lead to blocking of the follicular orifices, resulting in blackheads (comedo), acne, or sebaceous cysts.

### Elasticity, Mobility, and Turgor

The skin is highly elastic and moves freely over most areas. It loses its mobility when it becomes stretched; this occurs with edema, when the interstitial spaces become filled with fluid. Skin becomes rigid in the person with scleroderma, a collagen disease, as a result of collagenous fibrosis of the tissue. Turgor is tissue tension and is measured by the speed of the skin's return to normal position of fullness after it has been stretched. It should be noted that decreased skin turgor is a normal assessment finding in the elderly. Decreased turgor indicates dehydration of the tissue or extreme weight loss. To assess elasticity and turgor, a portion of skin over the sternum is picked up (elasticity) and the speed of return to normal is assessed (turgor). To assess hydration status of an elderly patient, the nurse should examine the mucous membranes. Skin that has decreased turgor will remain for a few seconds in a fold ("tenting") before returning slowly to normal (Figure 62-3).

### Texture

Roughness may occur normally on exposed areas, especially elbows and the soles of the feet. The skin of an infant is usually soft and smooth, whereas that of an elderly person may be rough and lack underlying tissue substance (atrophy). Roughness also may occur with hypothyroidism. Hypertrophic scarring, also known as keloid formation, can contribute to roughness of skin.

### Thickness

Normal skin is uniformly thin over most of the body except over the palms and soles. A callus, or painless overgrowth of

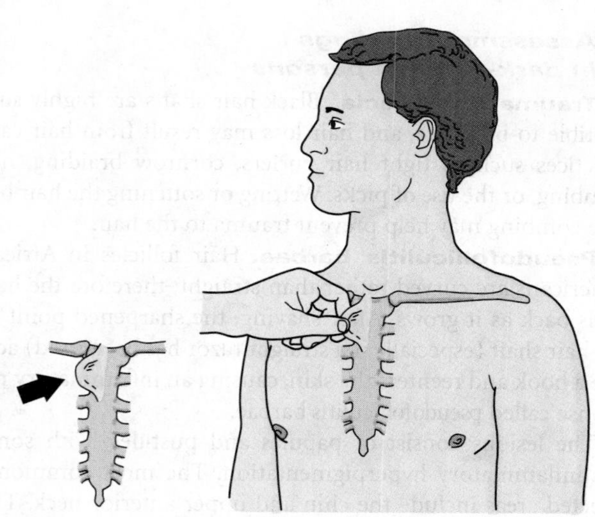

**fig. 62-3** Examination of skin turgor. Tenting of the skin over the sternum occurs with decreased skin turgor.

epidermis, may develop over these areas as a result of pressure or friction.

### Odor

Normal clean skin usually is free of odor except for areas that contain apocrine sweat glands. Odor occurs because of bacterial composition of protein matter. Some draining skin lesions may produce an odor.

## ACCESSORY STRUCTURES

### Hair

If the patient is wearing a wig or other hairpiece, this should be removed temporarily for inspection of any remaining hair and the scalp. It is easy to miss lesions on the scalp, and the patient can assist by indicating areas of itching, pain, or roughness.

Hair growth, pattern, and distribution are indicators of the person's general state of health.[3] Excessive hair growth (hypertrichosis) usually is related to heredity or hormonal changes. Hair loss (alopecia) occurs normally with age, especially in some men. Abnormal hair loss may be caused by hormonal imbalance, general ill health, infections of the scalp, typhoid fever, chronic liver disease, stressors, or drugs (antimetabolites or heparin). Changes in hair distribution of the body may be caused by hormonal changes. Hair loss on the dorsum of the toes may indicate decreased arterial circulation. Common misconceptions about hair growth include the following: shaving promotes the growth of dark, coarse hairs; singeing alters growth; brushing and massaging increase hair growth; and hair "turns gray overnight." None of these is true. The hair shaft is an inert structure, and changes occur over time as a result of hormonal activity and the availability of nutrients to the bulb at the base of the hair root.

Hair should be free of lice or nits. Nits are the eggs of the lice and are found embedded on hair strands. They are observed as small, glistening, grayish specks along the hair shaft near the scalp.

#### *Assessment findings in dark-skinned persons*

**Traumatic alopecia.** Black hair shafts are highly susceptible to breakage, and hair loss may result from hair care practices such as tight hair curlers, cornrow braiding, hot combing, or the use of picks. Wetting or softening the hair before combing may help prevent trauma to the hair.

**Pseudofolliculitis barbae.** Hair follicles in African Americans are curved rather than straight; therefore the hair curls back as it grows. After shaving, the sharpened point of the hair shaft (especially if a straight razor has been used) acts like a hook and reenters the skin, causing an inflammatory response called pseudofolliculitis barbae.

The lesions consist of papules and pustules, with some postinflammatory hyperpigmentation. The most commonly affected areas include the chin and upper anterior neck. The legs and axilla may also develop pseudofolliculitis from shaving. Treatment consists of letting the hair grow. As the beard is growing, a brush or rough wash-cloth may be used to dislodge ingrowing hairs. If shaving is done, a foil-guarded shaver is recommended. A mild depilatory may be used in place of shaving. Lesions may be treated with topical steroids or antibiotics.

### Nails

The appearance of the nails changes with age and with ill health. Changes in hardness, brittleness, roughness, or shape may indicate some metabolic diseases, nutritional imbalances including vitamin deficiencies, or digestive disturbances. Pale nail beds and poor capillary return (slow return to normal color after the nail is pinched) may indicate hypoxia or anemia. Capillary refill is normally less than 3 seconds. *Clubbing* of the nails refers to the elimination of the small concave portion at the base of the nail by soft tissue growth. Normally, the angle between the nail base and the fingernail is approximately 160°. Early clubbing is present when the angle increases to 180° or more. The mechanism of clubbing is not understood, but occurs with certain diseases associated with chronic hypoxia (Figure 62-4).

The epithelial lining of the nail bed is usually inert. The nail is affixed to the nail bed, and both move outward as the nail grows. The epithelial lining of the nail bed loses its inert quality in the presence of inflammatory lesions such as those that occur with psoriasis or ringworm, and the nail bed begins to keratinize. Horny masses collect under the nail, resulting in a thickening deformity of the nail and possible separation from the nail bed.[6]

Paronychia, an infection of the tissue surrounding the nail, is characterized by red, shiny skin and painful swelling. The

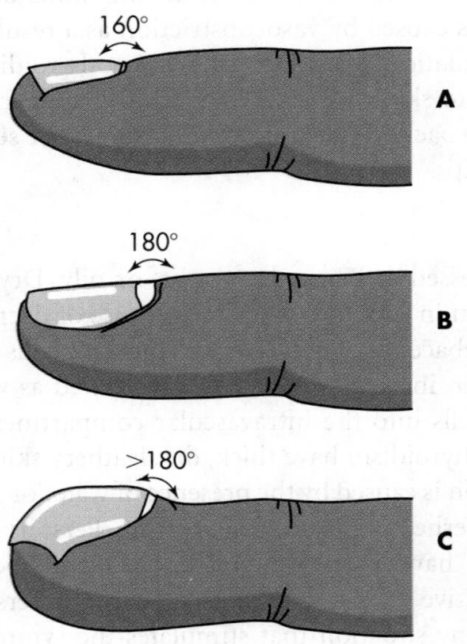


**fig. 62-4** Clubbing. **A,** Normal nail; nail base angle 160°. **B,** Early clubbing; nail base angle 180°. **C,** Late clubbing.

infection may result from trauma or from certain diseases such as psoriasis or dermatitis. If the nail is lost, it usually will grow back unless the nail bed has been injured.

## LESIONS

When lesions are observed, the following parameters are used for description: type, color, size, shape and configuration, texture, effect of pressure, arrangement, distribution, and variety.

### Type

Use of medical terminology facilitates communication (Table 62-3). For example, use of the term vesicle immediately establishes the lesion as a clear, fluid-filled lesion smaller than 1 cm. Figure 62-5 presents common appearance along with descriptions for macule, plaque, nodule, scale, papule, wheal, and crust.

### Color

Color of lesions varies among pale, brown, red, and normal pigmentation. Color helps to identify whether the lesion is part of normal aging, an inflammatory process, or an infection. For example, café au lait spots (French for coffee with milk) are pale tan macules. They are usually normal but also associated with neurofibromatosis.

### Size

The metric system is used for measurement. If a metric ruler is not available, the size of a lesion can be estimated by measuring a portion of one's finger to use as a gauge.

### Shape and Configuration

Shape describes the contour of a lesion and includes round, oval, and asymmetrical. Configuration refers to the sharpness

**table 62-3** *Types of Skin Lesions*

| Observed Skin Changes | Differentiation | Term | Example |
|---|---|---|---|
| **CHANGE IN COLOR OR TEXTURE** | | | |
| Spot | Circumscribed; flat; color change | Macule | Freckle |
| Discoloration (reddish purple) | Bleeding beneath the surface; injury to tissue | Contusion | Bruise |
| Soft whitening | Caused by repeated wetting of skin | Maceration | Between toes after soaking |
| Flake | Dry cells of surface | Scale | Dandruff; psoriasis |
| Roughness from dried fluid | Dry exudate over lesions | Crust ("scab") | Eczema, impetigo |
| Roughness from cells | Leathery thickening of outer skin layer | Lichenification | Callus on foot |
| **CHANGE IN SHAPE** | | | |
| Fluid-filled lesions | Less than 1 cm; clear fluid | Vesicle | Blister; chickenpox |
| | Greater than 1 cm; clear fluid | Bulla | Large blister, pemphigus |
| | Small, thick yellowish fluid (pus) | Pustule | Acne |
| Solid mass, cellular growth | Less than 1 cm | Papule | Small mole; raised rash |
| | 1 to 2 cm | Nodule | Enlarged lymph node |
| | Greater than 2 cm | Tumor | Benign or malignant tumor |
| | Excess connective tissue over scar | Keloid | Overgrown scar |
| Swelling of tissue | Generalized swelling; fluid between cells | Edema | Inflammation; swelling of feet |
| | Circumscribed surface edema; transient; some itching | Wheal ("hive") | Allergic reaction |
| **BREAKS IN SKIN SURFACES** | | | |
| Oozing, scraped surface | Loss of superficial structure of skin | Abrasion | "Floor burn"; scrape |
| Scooped-out depression | Loss of deeper layers of skin | Ulcer | Pressure or stasis ulcer |
| Superficial linear skin breaks | Scratch marks, frequently by fingernails | Excoriations | Scratching |
| Linear cracks or cleft | Slit or splitting of skin layers | Fissure | Athlete's foot |
| Jagged cut | Tearing of skin surface | Laceration | Accidental cut by blunt object |
| Linear cut, edges approximated | Cutting by sharp instrument | Incision | Knife cut |
| **VASCULAR LESIONS** | | | |
| Small, flat, round, purplish, red spot | Intradermal or submucous hemorrhage | Petechia | Bleeding tendency, decreased platelets; vitamin C deficiency |
| Spider-like, red, small | Dilation of capillaries, arterioles, or venules | Telangiectasis | Liver disease, vitamin B deficiency |
| Discoloration, reddish purple | Escape of blood into tissue | Ecchymosis | Trauma to blood vessels |

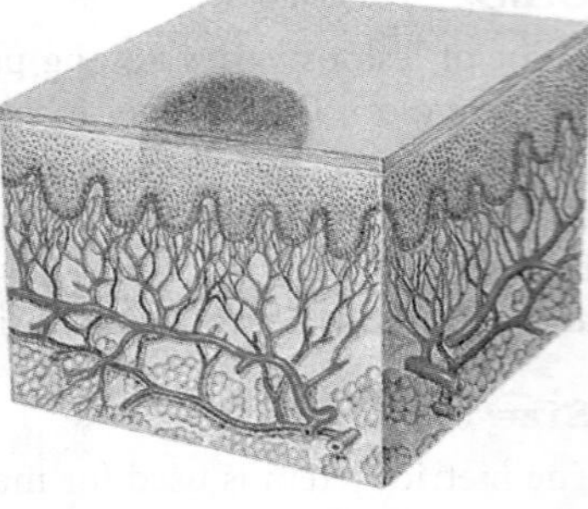

Macule—flat; nonpalpable; circumscribed; less than 1 cm in diameter; brown, red, purple, white, or tan
Examples: Freckles; flat moles; rubella; rubeola


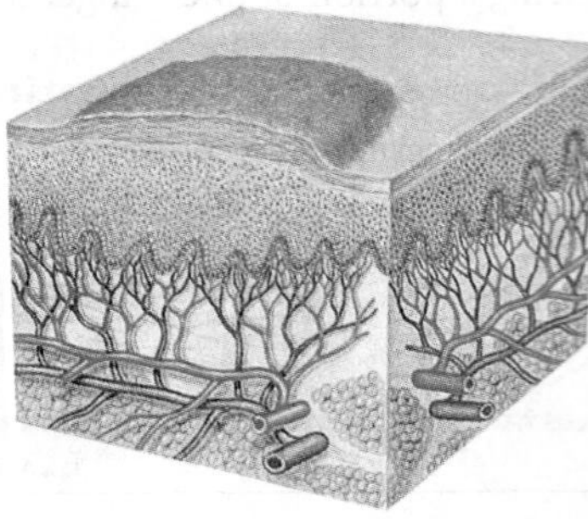

Plaque—elevated; flat topped; firm; rough; superficial papule greater than 1 cm in diameter; may be coalesced papules
Examples: Psoriasis; seborrheic and actinic keratoses


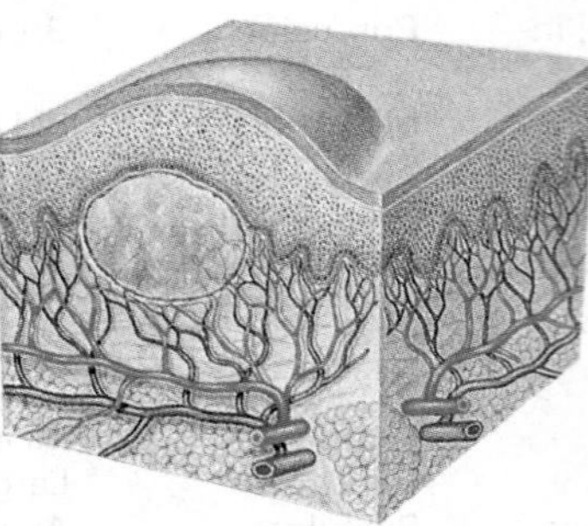

Nodule—elevated; firm; circumscribed; palpable; deeper in dermis than papule; 1 to 2 cm in diameter
Examples: Erythema nodosum; lipomas


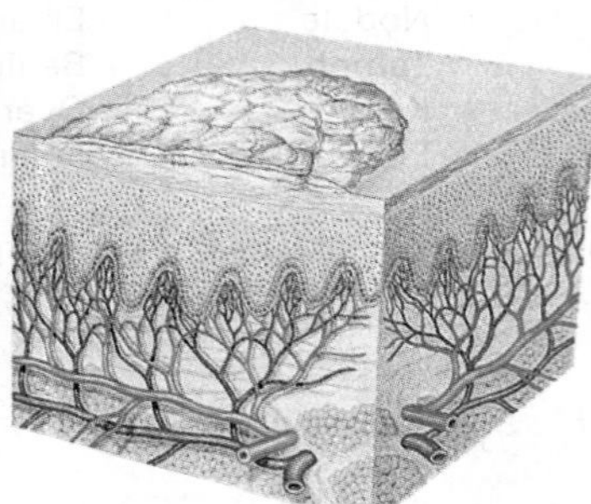

Scale—heaped-up keratinized cells; flaky exfoliation; irregular; thick or thin; dry or oily; varied size; silver, white, or tan
Examples: Psoriasis, exfoliative dermatitis


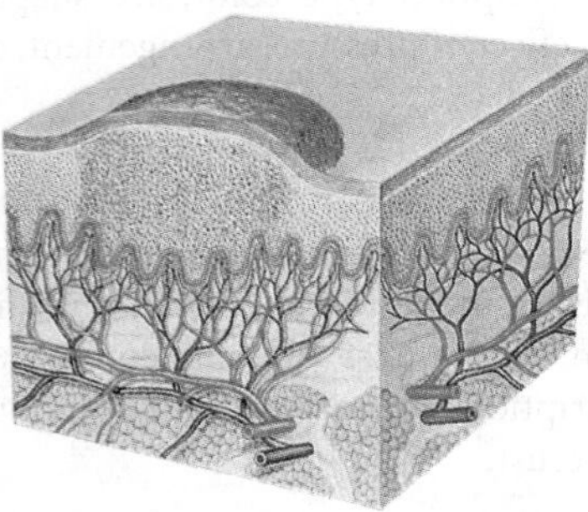

Papule—elevated; palpable; firm; circumscribed; less than 1 cm in diameter; brown, red, pink, tan, or bluish red
Examples: Warts; drug-related eruptions; pigmented nevi


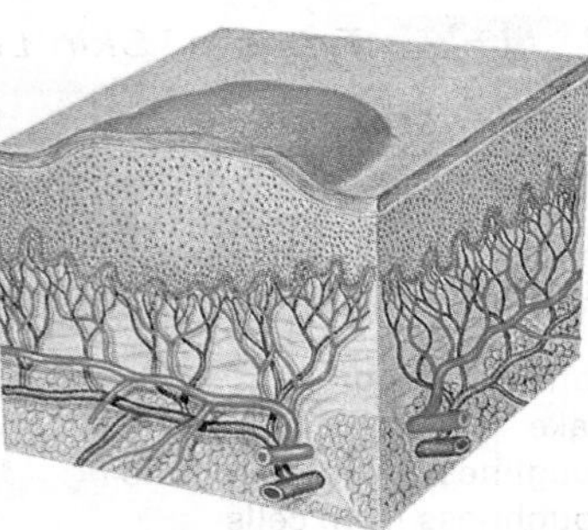

Wheal—elevated; irregular-shaped area of cutaneous edema; solid, transient, changing; variable diameter; pale pink with lighter center
Examples: Urticaria; insect bites


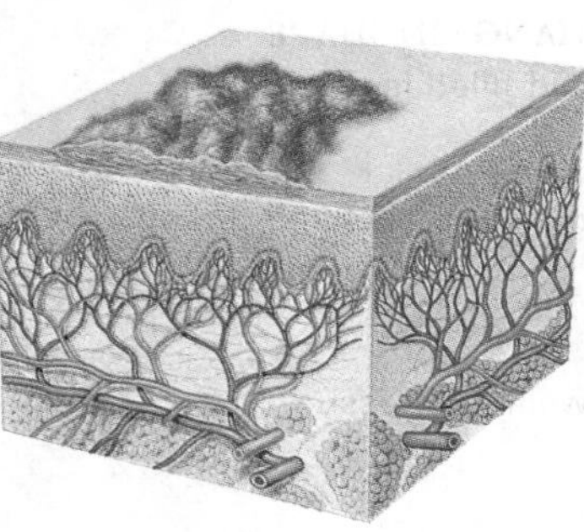

Crust—dried serum, blood, or purulent exudate; slightly elevated; size varies; brown, red, black, tan, or straw
Examples: Scab on abrasion; eczema


**fig. 62-5** Common skin lesions.

of demarcation of the lesion, that is, whether it is discrete or diffuse.

### Texture

The lesion is described as being rough or smooth, dry or moist, and on the surface or deeply penetrating into the tissue. Alterations in texture may occur as a result of scarring. Keloids are hard, raised, shiny growths of collagen tissue that usually originate from a scar and then grow beyond the wound, often with claw-like projections. Keloids usually flatten and become less obvious with time. The patient may elect to have the keloid excised, although treatment can result in formation of a new keloid. To decrease the potential for recurrence, surgery is usually followed by intralesional steroids, radiation, electron beam therapy, or pressure garments.

Although keloids are seen in all races, they are much more prevalent in African Americans than in whites. Keloids occur most often in young women. Highly susceptible areas for keloid growth include the sternum, mandible, ear, and neck.

### Blanching Test

Some vascular lesions blanch when pressure is applied and then return to their original color. Other lesions remain the same with pressure. The blanching test is performed by applying pressure to the lesion, and if circulation is normal, color will return to normal in about 5 seconds.

### Arrangement

Some lesions occur in patches, whereas others occur diffusely over the body. This is an important parameter when describing rashes.

### Distribution

Some lesions occur in certain parts of the body, such as on exposed areas as with contact dermatitis or on main body areas as in chickenpox. The lesions may follow the area of distribution of one of the spinal nerves as in herpes zoster.

### Variety

In some diseases, such as smallpox, the lesions may all occur at the same time. In chickenpox the lesions occur in crops so that there may be lesions at different stages of development at the same time.

## DIAGNOSTIC TESTS

Diagnostic tests usually are performed to confirm diagnoses of certain skin disorders. However, most skin disorders are diagnosed by physical assessment.

### LABORATORY TESTS

#### Tzanck Smear

Vesicular disorders can be differentiated by a Tzanck smear. The top of the vesicle is cut, and a smear is taken from the base of the vesicle. Examination of the smear can reveal a virus (herpes simplex or zoster) or acantholytic cells (pemphigus). The test shows a negative reaction for vesicles from burns, erythema multiforme, or dermatitis herpetiforme.

#### Potassium Hydroxide Test

If the causative factor is believed to be a fungus, a potassium hydroxide (KOH) examination may be carried out. The lesion is scraped with a knife blade, and the scraping is placed on a slide, which is set in a KOH solution for microscopic study.

#### Culture

If the primary lesion is a pustule, a culture specimen of the pustule contents may be obtained to identify the causative organism. Streptococci and staphylococci are commonly seen.

### SPECIAL TESTS

#### Skin Biopsy

Specimens of skin lesions may be obtained either by incision and suturing or by punch biopsy, which does not require suturing. A punch biopsy has a sharp edge that cuts through previously anesthetized skin and removes a core from the lesion for analysis. Bleeding can be stopped by direct pressure or by electrodesiccation.

#### Patch Testing

If allergic dermatitis is suspected, patch testing is performed to determine the source of the allergen. Standard concentration samples of suspected allergens are applied to the skin. Minute quantities of the products are held next to the skin by hypoallergenic tape, usually on the forearm and upper portion of the back. The patches are removed 48 hours after application, and the sites are assessed after 20 minutes for swelling or vesicle formation. Because delayed reactions are possible, sites should be reevaluated in 1 week.[1]

#### Diascopy

Diascopy is used to differentiate between types of pigmented lesions. Diascopy consists of pressing a transparent object such as a glass side over a pigmented lesion. The lesion caused by dilated blood vessels will whiten with pressure as the blood is pushed to the periphery. Other lesions caused by melanin changes or increased blood in dilated vessels (e.g., erythema, spider angiomas, telangiectasis) will not change color.

#### Wood's Light

To assist in the diagnoses of fungal infections of the hair and skin (tinea), the hair is illuminated by a special filter (Wood's filter) attached to an ultraviolet lamp. The infected hairs fluoresce brilliant green or appear luminous under the light.

## chapter SUMMARY

### ANATOMY AND PHYSIOLOGY OF THE SKIN

- Functions of the skin include protection, heat regulation, sensory perception, excretion, vitamin D production, and expression.
- Skin changes in elderly persons include hypopigmented and hyperpigmented areas, dry skin, decreased perspiration, decreased elasticity and turgor, wrinkles and loose folds, and thinner skin with some roughened areas.
- Skin color changes result from changes in melanin production, vascular dilation or constriction, changes in hemoglobin and red blood cells, and increased bile pigment.
- Skin temperature changes result from vascular dilation or constriction; some causes include fever, exercise, skin inflammations, and sympathetic inhibition or stimulation.
- Elasticity of the skin is the ability of the skin to stretch; turgor is tissue tension and is measured by the ability of the skin to return to normal after being stretched.
- Hair loss results normally from aging; hair also may be lost with decreased oxygenation, general ill health, stressors, drugs, or chronic liver disease.
- Nail changes may occur from aging, metabolic diseases, nutritional deficiencies, or decreased oxygenation.

### SUBJECTIVE DATA

- In-depth subjective data are obtained if a problem is identified during a general assessment.
- Subjective data include usual skin condition, onset of problem, any changes, possible causes, alleviating factors, and psychological responses to changes in the skin.

### OBJECTIVE DATA

- Solid tissue growths, according to size, include papules, nodules, and tumors. Fluid-filled lesions by size include vesicles and bullae; if the fluid is pus, it forms a pustule.
- Breaks in skin surfaces include abrasions, ulcers, excoriations, fissures, lacerations, and incisions.
- Vascular lesions include petechiae (intradermal or submucous bleeding), telangiectasis (dilated capillaries), or ecchymosis (bruise).

### DIAGNOSTIC TESTS

- Skin diseases are primarily diagnosed by direct observation; diagnostic tests include the Tzanck smear, potassium hydroxide test, culture of a pustule, diascopy, Wood's light test, patch testing, and skin biopsy.

## References

1. Anderson KN, Anderson LE, Glanze WD, editors: Mosby's medical, nursing, and allied health dictionary, ed 5, St Louis, 1998, Mosby
2. Blaylock B: Latex allergies: overview, prevention and implications for nursing care, Ostomy/Wound Manage 41(5):10-12, 1995.
3. Guyton AC, Hall JE: Textbook of medical physiology, ed 9, Philadelphia, 1996, WB Saunders.
4. Irwin MJ: Assessing color changes for dark skinned patients, Adv Clin Care 6(6):8-10, 1991.
5. Malasanos L, Barkauskas V, Stoltenberg-Allen K, editors: Health assessment, ed 4, St Louis, 1990, Mosby.
6. Moschella SL, Hurley HP: Dermatology, ed 3, Philadelphia, 1991, WB Saunders.

# chapter 63 MANAGEMENT OF PERSONS WITH Problems of the Skin

VICKIE WEAVER and JANE F. MAREK

## objectives *After studying this chapter, the learner should be able to:*

1. Relate the psychological effects of dermatological problems.
2. Describe general nursing interventions for patients with dermatological problems.
3. Explain the etiology, pathophysiology, and interventions for parasitic infestations, fungal and bacterial infections, and viral diseases of the skin.
4. Describe the collaborative care management for secretory disorders of the skin.
5. Compare preventive measures and interventions for different types of dermatitis.
6. Identify different skin reactions that may result from systemic factors.
7. Describe the nature and management of psoriasis.
8. Contrast the different benign and malignant skin tumors and their management.
9. Correlate preventive and early intervention measures for pressure ulcers.
10. Develop an individualized nursing care plan for the patient with a pressure ulcer.

Prevention of dermatological conditions relieves the patient of discomfort and is cost effective, because many skin conditions are chronic. This chapter discusses specific dermatological problems, including their etiology and epidemiology, pathophysiology, and collaborative care management.

A discussion of care of persons undergoing dermatological surgery, care of healthy skin, methods of prevention and treatment follows. A discussion of pressure ulcers concludes the chapter.

## COMMON SKIN PROBLEMS

Skin problems may result from various causes, such as parasitic infestations; fungal, bacterial, or viral infections; reactions to substances encountered externally or taken internally; and new growths. A major skin problem is pressure ulcers. Many skin manifestations have no known cause; others are hereditary. Specific information relevant to each problem is presented next.

### PARASITIC INFESTATIONS

The major parasitic infestations are pediculosis and scabies.

#### Pediculosis

##### *Etiology/epidemiology*

*Pediculosis* (lice infestation) occurs mostly among children. Many children get head lice from their classmates or from people on crowded buses. Control and treatment of pediculosis in middle- and upper-income populations can be hampered by refusal of parents to admit that their children have pediculosis.

Pediculi (lice) are most often found among people who live in overcrowded dwellings with inadequate hygiene facilities. Pediculosis occurs less commonly in African Americans than in other races.

##### *Pathophysiology*

Lice obtain their nutrition by sucking blood from the skin. They leave their eggs or nits on the skin surface attached to hair shafts, and this results in the transfer from person to person.

Three types of lice infest humans: the head louse, the body louse, and the pubic louse. The head louse *(Pediculus humanus capitis)* attaches itself to the hair shaft, laying about eight eggs a day. The eggs are firmly attached to the hair or threads of clothing; ova hatch in 1 week. They may be viewed with a hand lens or flashlight and appear as grayish, glistening oval bodies. The head louse is usually confined to the scalp and beard. Transmission of head lice may also occur through use of infected persons' hats, brushes, or combs.

The body louse *(Pediculus humanus corporis)* resides chiefly in the seams of clothing around the neck, waist, and thighs. The bite causes minute hemorrhagic points and severe itching. Transmission is by direct contact or by way of clothing, bedding, and towels.

The pubic louse *(Phthirus pubis)* differs slightly from the head and body louse. It resembles a tiny crab, having claw-like pincers that attach firmly to the pubic hair. Nits are visible in the pubic hair. *Phthirus pubis* is transmitted by sexual contact, bed clothing, towels, and occasionally toilet seats.

Diagnosis is made by physical examination of the appropriate body part. A magnifying glass may be helpful. Other symptoms include pinpoint erythema, raised macules, and pruritus. The bite of the insect—with contamination from saliva, head parts, and feces—causes intense itching. Scratching may lead to further trauma, with the possibility of secondary infection and enlarged cervical lymph nodes.

#### Collaborative care management

Treatment of pediculosis consists of topical application of a pediculicide, such as lindane (Kwell, Scabene), permethrin (Nix), pyrethrin (RID, A-200 Pyrinate), or malathion 0.5% (Prioderm). When pyrethrin products or lindane are used, a second application in 7 to 10 days may be necessary.[10] Directions for application differ according to the product and body location. Pediculicides are not used on eyebrows or eyelashes because of potential eye irritation or sensitization. If eyelashes are infested, nits are removed and petrolatum jelly is applied to smother the lice.

**Patient/family education.** Patients are usually able to carry out their own treatment. The focus of nursing care is to identify infected persons and teach them about the nature of pediculosis and prevention of its spread.

Contacts should be evaluated for infestation and treated if necessary. Persons with head lice should be instructed to soak combs, brushes, and hair utensils in hot water and pediculicide shampoo for 15 minutes. Clothing and bedding should be laundered in hot water and dried on high heat or dry-cleaned.

### Scabies

#### Etiology/epidemiology

Scabies is caused by the female itch mite *(Sarcoptes scabiei)*. Scabies is prevalent during periods of overcrowding. The incidence of scabies has increased worldwide since the 1960s. The reason for the increase is unknown and is thought to be multifactorial, including sexual promiscuity, increased worldwide travel, and ecological changes.[7]

Scabies occurs among persons in all age-groups and socioeconomic levels. Scabies is also common in nursing homes as a result of crowded conditions and debilitated patients with weakened immune systems.[10] Scabies is usually transmitted by prolonged contact; therefore it is commonly observed among several members of a family.

#### Pathophysiology

The female itch mite penetrates the stratum corneum and burrows into the skin. Within several hours of skin penetration, the itch mite lays a large number of eggs and deposits fecal pellets. The larvae mature in 10 to 14 days and move to the skin surface, where the females are impregnated; the cycle then repeats itself. The incubation period varies, but often a long period elapses before symptoms are noted. Delayed hypersensitivity is thought to be a major factor in the lapse between infestation and symptoms. The incubation period in persons with no previous exposure is 4 to 6 weeks.[10]

The classic symptoms of scabies are intense itching and lesions that resemble wavy, brownish, threadlike lines occurring most commonly on the hands (especially the interdigital webs), flexor surface of the wrists, posterior inner surface of the elbows, anterior axillary folds, nipples in the female, belt line, gluteal creases, and male genitalia (Figures 63-1 and 63-2). The head and neck are rarely involved. Pruritus may be severe, especially at night. Pruritus is thought to be a result of a hypersensitivity reaction.[10] Secondary infections with excoriations and pustules may result from scratching. Scratching destroys the burrows. Vesicles are filled with serous fluid and may contain mites.

Diagnosis is made by identifying the itch mite. The mite is removed from the end of a burrow with a pointed scalpel blade, or the entire burrow is sliced off, placed on a slide with glycerol or mineral oil, and examined under a microscope. If the burrows are not yet visible, mineral oil may be applied to the skin to aid in identification of the burrows.

#### Collaborative care management

The goal of therapy is elimination of the itch mite and treatment of complications.

1. Scabies treatment (patient, all family members)
   a. Lindane (Kwell, Scabene)
      (1) Apply at bedtime in a thin layer over the *entire* body from *neck down.*
      (2) Wash off in 8 to 12 hours.
      (3) Give a second treatment in 24 hours if prescribed.
   b. Crotamiton 10% (Eurax)
      (1) Crotamiton 10% is less effective than lindane.
      (2) Bathe before initial application and after each treatment.
      (3) Repeat treatment as prescribed.
   c. Benzyl benzoate
      (1) Give two overnight treatments 1 week apart as prescribed.
      (2) Not widely available; apply as directed by physician.
2. Treatment for complications from scabies
   a. Postscabies dermatitis with pruritus: topical or oral corticosteroids

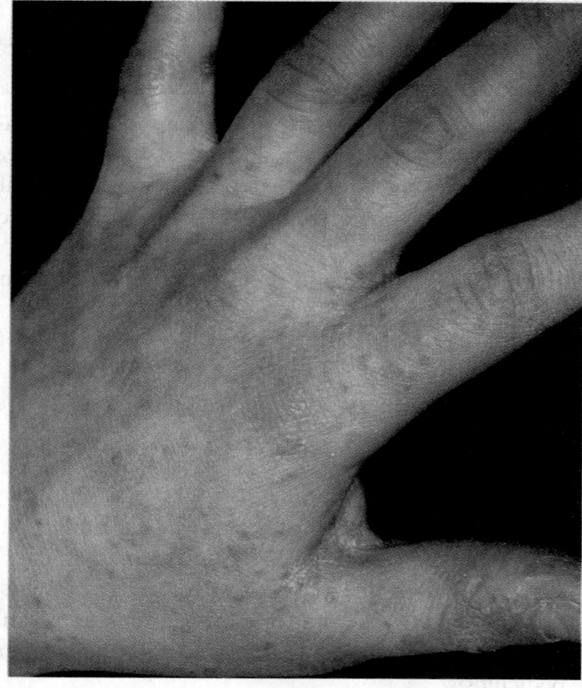

**fig. 63-1** Scabies. Tiny vesicles and papules in the finger webs and back of the hand.

b. Secondary infections: systemic antibiotics
c. Postscabies papules or nodules: coal tar gels

**Patient/family education.** As with pediculosis, patient education is the primary intervention. Because scabies spreads within families, the patient and family members need to know the nature of the disease and the need for all family members to receive treatment, even if they are asymptomatic. Some patients experience shame and guilt when they learn the diagnosis; a nonjudgmental attitude with explanations of methods of control may help these patients cope with their feelings.

Teaching the patient with scabies includes the following:

1. All family members should be treated simultaneously, whether or not symptoms are present.
2. Be sure that *all* external body areas below the neck are covered by the prescribed scabicide.
3. Wash underclothing and bed and bath linens in hot water on the day of treatment; dry in dryer or iron after dry; clothing and bedding that cannot be laundered should be placed in plastic bags for at least 1 week. Parasites cannot survive longer than 4 days off of human skin.
4. Signs and symptoms may not disappear until 1 or 2 weeks after treatment; pruritus of hands and feet may persist for up to 3 months.[8]

## FUNGAL INFECTIONS

Fungi are larger and more complex than bacteria. They may be unicellular, such as yeasts, or multicellular, such as molds. Many types are pathogenic to humans, causing common skin disorders or serious systemic diseases, such as blastomycosis. Certain types of fungi cause few symptoms, whereas others produce inflammatory or hypersensitivity reactions.

### Candidiasis

#### Etiology/epidemiology

*Candida albicans*, a yeastlike fungus, normally inhabits the gastrointestinal tract, mouth, and vagina, but not usually the skin. Candidiasis (moniliasis), the inflammation associated with the organism's overgrowth on the skin, is caused by the toxins that are released. Some predisposing factors causing an overgrowth of *C. albicans* are pregnancy, use of birth control pills, poor nutrition, antibiotic therapy, diabetes mellitus, other endocrine diseases, inhalational corticosteroids, and immunosuppressed conditions. Yeast thrives in a warm, moist environment, such as the perineum and intertriginous areas. The epidemiology of candidiasis is unknown.

#### Pathophysiology

Overgrowth of *C. albicans* causes candidiasis. Candidiasis of the mucous membrane is thrush. The lesions are white spots that look like milk curd on the buccal mucosa and may extend down the esophagus. Vaginal thrush causes intense itching with a thick, white vaginal discharge. Candidiasis of the skin appears as pruritic, eroded, moist, inflamed areas with vesicles and pustules, and it occurs mostly in body folds, such as beneath the breasts, in the intergluteal fold, or in the groin. The classic clinical sign of candidiasis is the presence of satellite lesions on the periphery of the general inflammation

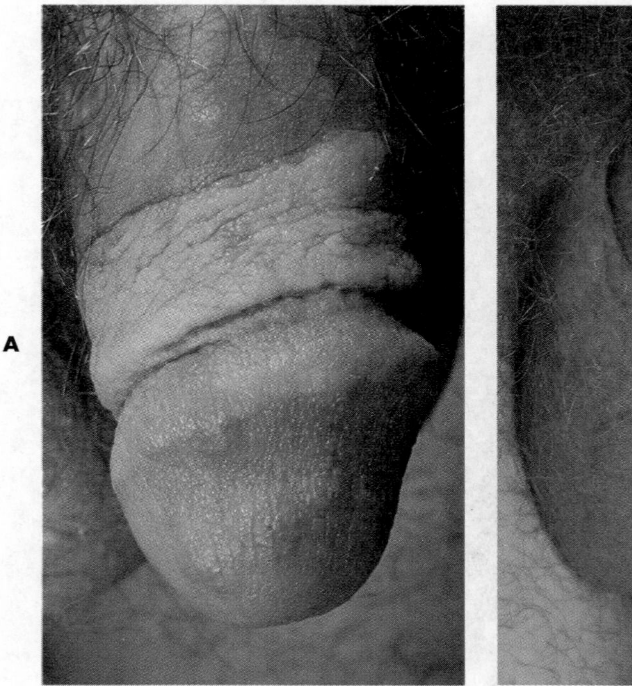


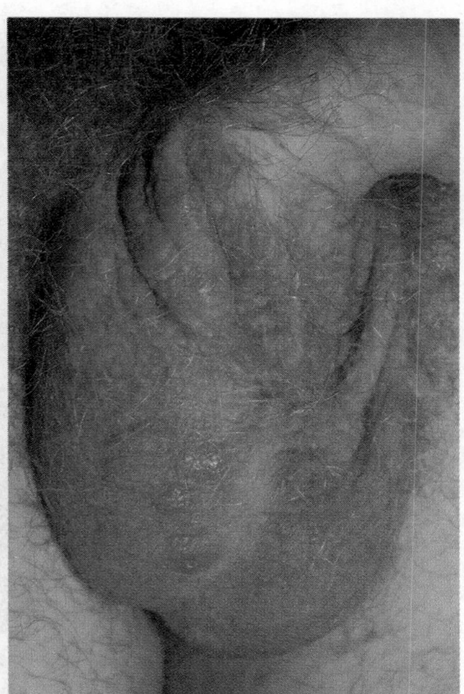


**fig. 63-2 A,** Eroded papules on the glans is a highly characteristic sign of scabies. **B,** An established infestation of the penis and scrotum. Large papules may remain after appropriate therapy and sometimes require treatment with intralesional steroids.

(Figures 63-3 and 63-4). Diagnosis of candidiasis at any site is made by clinical appearance and microscopic examination.

### Collaborative care management

Treatment is aimed at elimination of the precipitating factors. Other measures include keeping the skin dry to avoid maceration; wearing loose, absorbent clothing; and using topical medications, such as powders, that help keep the skin dry. Nystatin (Mycostatin), an antifungal available in tablets, powder, or vaginal suppositories; amphotericin; clotrimazole (Mycelex); ciclopirox (Loprox); and ketoconazole (Nixoral) are effective against yeast infections.

**Patient/family education.** The primary focus is prevention by teaching persons at high risk for the development of candidiasis and eliminating such factors as a warm, moist environment. A second focus is early detection by teaching careful assessment of mucous membranes and skin folds. This should be done daily and all early lesions reported immediately. Many patients, such as persons with immunosuppression, will be receiving preventive therapy. They need to be taught about the therapy, encouraged to comply, and taught self-assessment measures.

## Dermatophytoses

There are several different types of dermatophytoses (tinea) or superficial fungal infections of the skin and its appendages. The most common types are tinea capitis, tinea corporis, tinea cruris, and tinea pedis.

### Tinea capitis

**Etiology/epidemiology.** Tinea capitis, inappropriately called ringworm of the scalp, can be caused either by a species of *Microsporum* or by *Trichophyton* fungi. The most common causative agent in the United States is *Microsporum audouinii.* The infection is transmitted readily, especially in crowded conditions where poor hygiene exists, although many children show a high resistance. Minor scalp trauma facilitates implantation of the spores; therefore the infection can be spread by contaminated barbers' instruments, combs, or sharp brushes. Tinea capitis has a worldwide distribution, primarily among prepubertal children.

**Pathophysiology.** The characteristic lesion is round, with erythema, a slight scaling, and some pustules appearing at the edge of the lesion (Figure 63-5, *A*). Hair loss occurs, with the hair shaft broken off at skin level. The hair loss is only temporary, because the lesions usually heal without scarring. Although tinea capitis is usually noninflammatory, a painful inflammatory condition called a *kerion* may develop. Infected hairs placed under a Wood's light will fluoresce a blue-green color.

**Collaborative care management.** Griseofulvin is an antifungal agent effective in the treatment of all the dermatophytoses. The adult dose for tinea capitis is 500 mg orally, and absorption is enhanced when the medication is administered after a high-fat meal. The infection usually resolves within 4 to 6 weeks. A mild antifungal agent, such as tolnaftate (1%) or haloprogin, may be applied twice daily.

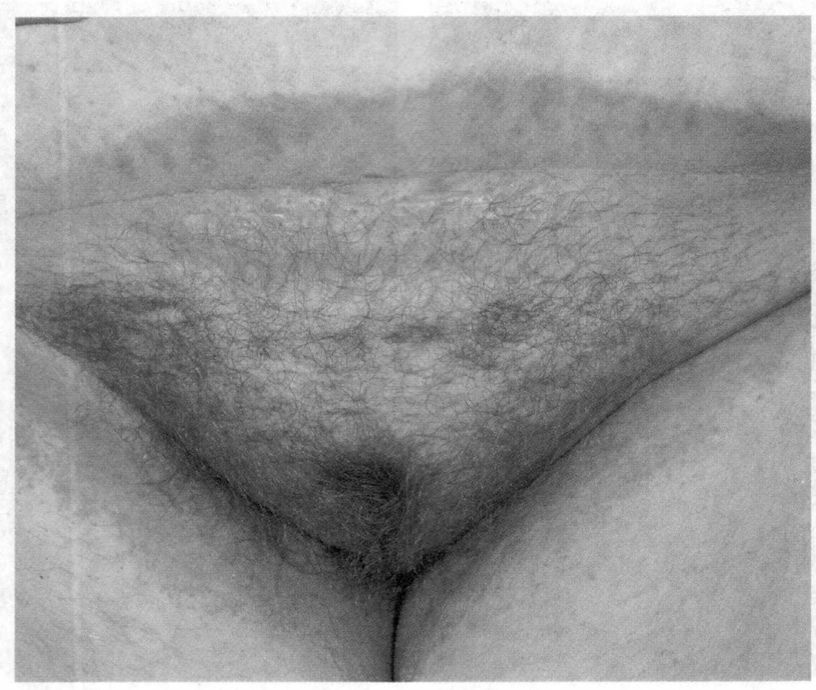

**fig. 63-3** Candida intertrigo. The overhanging abdominal fold and groin area are infected in this obese patient.

***Patient/family education.*** Patient teaching focuses on helping the patient understand the rationale for the treatment regimen. The scalp should be shampooed at least twice a week. Cutting the hair short facilitates shampooing but may cause psychological trauma for some children; therefore the hair is best left at an acceptable length. If inflammation occurs, the scalp is shampooed daily.

### *Tinea corporis and tinea cruris*

**Etiology/epidemiology.** Tinea corporis and tinea cruris are dermatophytic infections. Tinea corporis occurs in children living in hot, humid climates. Tinea cruris, commonly referred to as "jock itch," occurs most commonly in men, especially those who have tinea pedis and those who frequently wear athletic supporters or tight shorts. It also occurs in women who wear tight pantyhose or slacks.

**Pathophysiology.** The lesions of tinea corporis occur on nonhairy parts of the body and are flat with an erythematous scaling border and clearing center (Figure 63-5, *B*). The lesions of tinea cruris occur in the warm, moist, intertriginous areas of the groin. The lesions are bilateral and extend outward from the groin along the inner thigh. The color ranges from brown to red, scaling is absent, and pruritus is usually present.

**Collaborative care management.** Mild infections are treated with topical fungicides. Oral griseofulvin is given for severe infections.

***Patient/family education.*** Because the dermatophytes thrive in moist, warm environments, the affected areas should be kept clean and dry, and overbathing should be avoided. A bland dusting powder can be used to promote dryness. Loose underclothing should be worn.

### *Tinea pedis*

**Etiology/epidemiology.** The most common dermatophytosis is tinea pedis, or athlete's foot. There are several forms of tinea pedis. Tinea pedis is rarely seen in children or women but is widespread among young men, especially those wearing shoes in hot climates. Walking barefoot in gymnasiums or around swimming pools will not necessarily lead to a tinea infection; however, susceptible persons will acquire it regardless of their activities.

**Pathophysiology.** The most common form of tinea pedis is the intertriginous form. The fungal involvement usually begins in the toe webs, especially in the fourth interspace, and may extend to the undersurface of the toes or onto the plantar surface. The person may be asymptomatic or may experience itching and burning in the affected area. The nails may become discolored, thickened, or distorted *(onychomycosis).* Tinea pedis is often confused with other foot eruptions, such as simple intertrigo (chronic bacterial infection of the intertriginous areas of the toes), contact dermatitis, or psoriasis.

**Collaborative care management.** Treatment depends on the stage of infection. Most persons have a chronic low-grade infection that is controllable with topical antifungal

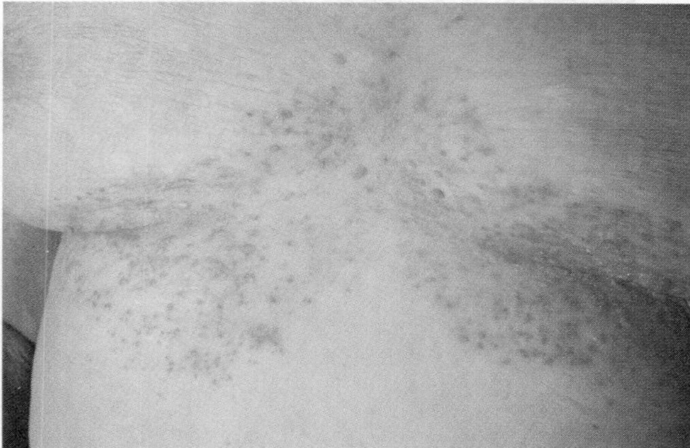

**fig. 63-4** Candidiasis under the breast. There are several moist, red papules with a fringe of white scale.

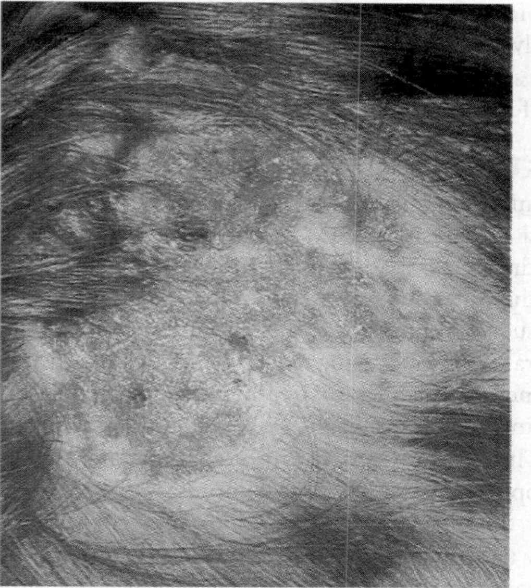

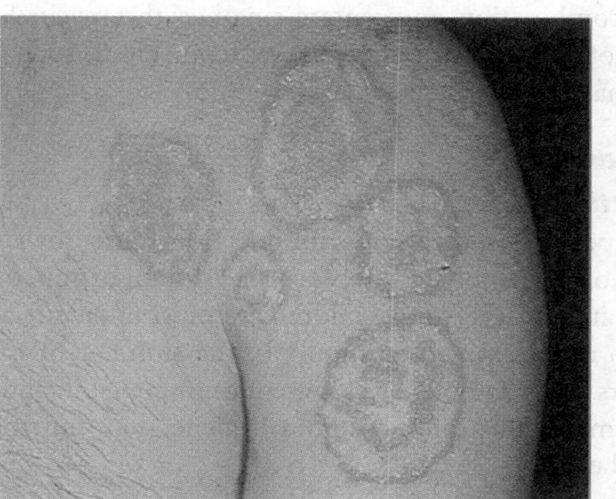

**fig. 63-5 A,** Tinea capitis. **B,** Tinea corporis.

drugs. When thick, chronic, scaling lesions are present, the topical antifungal drugs cannot penetrate the lesion; therefore a strong peeling ointment, such as Whitfield's ointment, can be applied thinly to the lesions at bedtime, followed by an antifungal cream in the morning. If the lesions become acutely inflamed, they are treated with foot soaks with a bland solution, such as Burow's solution, followed by a topical antimicrobial agent. A systemic antibacterial agent, such as penicillin or erythromycin, may be prescribed. Oral griseofulvin is prescribed only for severe infections that do not respond to local treatment.[8]

***Patient/family education.*** The person with tinea pedis needs to be taught meticulous foot hygiene. After the toes are dried thoroughly, a light dusting of antifungal powder is applied to promote dryness. Caking of the powder should be avoided. Socks should be of an absorbent material, such as cotton, and may need to be changed more than once daily to promote dryness. Wearing white socks does not affect the course of the infection. A major focus of nursing is to initiate activities that lessen infection, such as wearing sandals, going barefoot (to decrease tissue moisture), and using good foot hygiene, which includes washing the feet frequently and drying well between the toes. Preventive actions, such as prophylactic footbaths in public places, are not effective.

## BACTERIAL INFECTIONS

Skin infections may result from loss of skin integrity or from altered host resistance. Most bacteria that normally inhabit the skin are nonpathogenic. Pathogenic bacteria that penetrate the outer skin layer may cause a superficial skin infection, such as impetigo or superficial folliculitis, or they may penetrate deeper, causing a deep folliculitis or a furuncle.

General principles of treatment for bacterial skin infections include cleansing the skin well and applying an antibiotic. The skin is cleansed with soap and water or with hexachlorophene. Water or saline compresses or heat may be used to dry the horny layer of the skin. Topical antibiotics commonly used include the hydroxyquinilones, such as Vioform; neomycin, bacitracin, or polymyxin (Polysporin), either alone or in combination; and gentamicin or erythromycin. Systemic antibiotics are used only when systemic signs, such as fever and malaise, are present.

### Impetigo

#### *Etiology/epidemiology*

Impetigo is a common skin infection caused by staphylococci or $\beta$-hemolytic streptococci. Although impetigo may occur in any age-group, children are most often affected. Impetigo occurs more commonly in the summer or early fall. Factors that promote development of impetigo include tropical climates, uncleanliness, poor hygiene, poor nutrition, and poor health.

#### *Pathophysiology*

Impetigo begins as a small, thin-walled vesicle that ruptures easily and leaves a weeping denuded spot. It becomes pustular and dries to form a honey-colored crust that appears stuck on the skin (Figure 63-6). The process, which is superficial, may extend below the crust. Impetigo is usually confined to the face but may occur elsewhere. If untreated, impetigo may last for several weeks with new lesions forming.

#### *Collaborative care management*

Treatment consists of maintaining cleanliness and applying topical antibiotics. The crusts must be removed and the lesions washed gently two or three times daily to prevent further crust formation. Warm soaks or saline compresses may be necessary to soften crusts that adhere firmly. Topical antibiotics are applied at least three times daily. Systemic antibiotics may be prescribed.

**Patient/family education.** Nursing care focuses on helping the patient understand and carry out the regimen. Teaching focuses on prevention of spread of infection. Family members and the patient should wash their hands thoroughly with a bacteriostatic soap after contact. Patients should use personal towels. Linens should be laundered after the first day of treatment.

### Folliculitis

#### *Etiology/epidemiology*

Folliculitis is usually caused by *Staphylococcus aureus,* but occasionally it is caused by other bacteria, both gram-negative and gram-positive organisms. The infection may be caused by drainage from other infected lesions. Predisposing factors include uncleanliness, maceration, infection, chemical irritation, and injury. *Pseudofolliculitis,* seen most commonly in African American men, occurs in the beard area. Stiff hairs emerge from the follicle, curve, and reenter the skin, causing a chronic low-grade irritation.

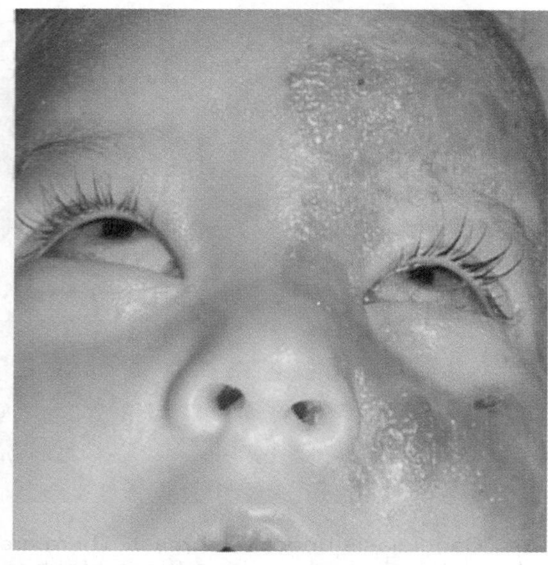

**fig. 63-6** Impetigo. Note characteristic crusting.

#### Pathophysiology

Bacterial infections of the hair follicle may be superficial in the epidermis around the hair follicle or deep in the tissue surrounding both the lower and upper portions of the hair follicle. Deep folliculitis produces a more severe inflammatory response. *Sycosis barbae* (barber's itch) is a deep folliculitis of the beard. The hairs do not fall out or break, such as occurs with tinea barbae. *Hordeolum* (stye) is a deep folliculitis of the cilia of the eyelids (see Chapter 56). There is usually swelling of the surrounding eyelid, with crusting along the edge of the eyelid.

#### Collaborative care management

Treatment of superficial folliculitis includes cleansing with soap and water and applying topical antibiotics. Warm compresses are applied to encourage resolution of deep folliculitis. Topical antibiotics, such as Neosporin, hasten healing.

**Patient/family education.** Nursing management focuses on teaching patients about the prescribed therapy and about avoiding predisposing factors.

### Furuncles and Carbuncles

#### Etiology/epidemiology

Furuncles (boils) are a deep folliculitis that originates either from a superficial folliculitis or as a deep nodule around the hair follicle. *Furunculosis* is the appearance of several furuncles. An infection that involves several surrounding hair follicles is termed a *carbuncle.* The causative organism is usually *Staphylococcus,* but occasionally furuncles can be caused by other bacteria. Both furuncles and carbuncles occur most often in obese, poorly nourished, fatigued, or otherwise susceptible persons whose hygiene may be poor; in debilitated elderly people; and in persons with poorly controlled diabetes mellitus.

#### Pathophysiology

Local swelling and redness occur, together with severe local pain, which is decreased by moving the involved part as little as possible. Within 3 to 5 days the lesion becomes elevated or "points up," the surrounding skin becomes shiny, and the center or "core" turns yellow. A carbuncle has several cores. The boil will usually rupture spontaneously, but it may be surgically incised and drained. As drainage occurs, the pain is immediately relieved. The drainage soon changes from a yellow purulent material to a serosanguineous discharge. All drainage usually subsides within a few hours to a few days; the redness and swelling subside gradually. Furuncles are likely to occur on the face, neck, forearms, groin, and legs, whereas carbuncles are usually limited to the nape of the neck and the back.

#### Collaborative care management

Hot, wet dressings are used to help bring the boil to a head, but these dressings are discontinued as soon as drainage occurs to prevent skin maceration and spread of infection. As the boil drains, care must be taken to keep the infected discharge off the surrounding skin, because organisms may be harbored in hair follicles and furunculosis may recur. Systemic antibiotics may be prescribed. Strict adherance to Standard Precautions is essential in the care of persons with boils or carbuncles.

Furuncles and carbuncles tend to recur in susceptible individuals. Staphylococci causing them are often resistant to local treatment and to antibiotics.

**Patient/family education.** Nursing care focuses on preventing the spread of the infection. Patients are cautioned to keep their hands away from the discharge to prevent spread of infection.

### Erysipelas

#### Etiology/epidemiology

Erysipelas is a type of cellulitis usually caused by a hemolytic streptococcus and *S. aureus* (Figure 63-7). Elderly people with poor resistance are most often affected. Erysipelas may follow a puncture wound, ulcer, or chronic dermatitis.

#### Pathophysiology

Erysipelas was a serious disease before the advent of antibiotics. It is characterized by localized inflammation and swelling of the skin and subcutaneous tissues, usually of the face, scalp, hands, and genitalia. A bright, sharp line separates the diseased skin from the normal skin. The lesions are hot and red. The infection spreads via the lymphatic system and bloodstream.

#### Collaborative care management

Gram stain and culture and sensitivity will determine the appropriate antibiotic treatment. Local lesions should be immobilized and elevated to decrease local edema. Wet-to-dry dressings may decrease pain and dry up bullous lesions. Moist heat may also be used. If abscess formation occurs, incision and drainage may be indicated.

**Patient/family education.** Nursing care focuses on helping patients assume responsibility for treatment and completing the treatment. It is imperative that the patient complete the course of prescribed antibiotic therapy.

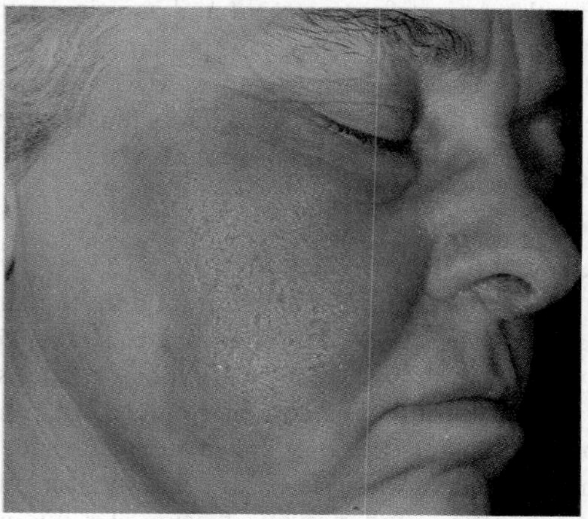

**fig. 63-7** Cellulitis. Acute phase with intense erythema.

# VIRAL DISEASES

## Warts

### Etiology/epidemiology

Warts develop from hypertrophy of epidermal cells as a result of a viral infection. The infection is not highly contagious but does spread along the dermis through autoinfection. It is seen most commonly in older children and young adults.

### Pathophysiology

Warts are benign skin growths that grow in a variety of shapes. The common wart is a small, circumscribed, painless, hyperkeratotic papule usually seen on the extremities, especially the hands. *Filiform warts* are slender fingerlike projections occurring mostly on the face and neck. *Plantar warts* grow inward from the pressure on the soles of the feet and may be painful. They are differentiated from calluses by lack of skin lines over the surface. Warts that develop in the anogenital region have a lighter-colored surface and a cauliflower-like appearance, and they may cause itching. Anogenital warts may be spread either by sexual activity or by other means. Some genital warts in women may predispose the woman to cancer of the cervix.

### Collaborative care management

There are numerous treatments for warts, but no one method is effective. If only a few painless warts are present, no treatment is necessary, and the wart will probably disappear in time.

The most commonly used therapeutic measures for common warts are electrodesiccation and cryosurgery. In electrodesiccation, the top of the wart is seared gently to soften the keratinized surface and then curetted off and the bleeding points cauterized. This method is not used for plantar warts. Cryosurgery consists of freezing the lesion with a substance such as liquid nitrogen. Cauterant chemicals—such as formalin, phenol, nitric acid, cantharidin, salicylic acid, or podophyllum—may be used. Recalcitrant warts may respond to radiation therapy. Surgical excision is seldom used, because painful scarring may result.

**Patient/family education.** Nursing care focuses on preparing the patient for treatment and assisting with treatment. Warts sometimes disappear spontaneously or under psychological suggestion, thus creating a basis for numerous folktales on how to get rid of warts. Nurses must help patients avoid potentially dangerous home remedies.

## Herpes Simplex

### Etiology/epidemiology

One of the most common viruses found in humans is the herpes simplex virus (HSV). It occurs as two similar yet serologically different strains, type 1 and type 2. Herpes simplex virus has a DNA-containing core surrounded by a phospholipid covering. Factors that may precipitate recurrence of herpes simplex lesions include fever, upper respiratory tract infection, exhaustion, and nervous tension. Lesions also are more common during the menses and after direct exposure to the sun's rays.

### Pathophysiology

The type 1 virus is found primarily in lesions of the face and mouth (fever blister, cold sore), eye (keratitis), and brain (encephalitis). Type 2 is associated with a lesion of the genitalia that can be transmitted by sexual contact (see Chapter 50).

There are two phases to HSV infection. Primary infection is acquired by direct exposure to the virus, usually through mucocutaneous contact with an infected individual. After the initial infection, the virus travels to a sensory nerve ganglion and becomes latent. Reactivation of the virus causes disease recurrence. Most persons experience the initial contact with HSV (type 1) as young children. The HSV remains in the cells of the sensory nerves that supply the affected areas and causes recurrent lesions when the person is subjected to stress. The appearance of vesicles is preceded by several hours by a sensation of burning or itching. A cluster of vesicles on an erythematous base appears at the mucocutaneous junctions of the lips or nose or as an inflammation of the cornea of one eye with photophobia and tearing. The type 2 virus lesions occur in the vagina or cervix of the woman or on the penile skin of the man. The lesions are painful and may crack open. A crust gradually forms, and the lesions heal in about 10 days. Herpes simplex virus can be identified by a Tzanck smear (see Chapter 62).

### Collaborative care management

The development of antiviral compounds has helped in the treatment of HSV. Topical use of acyclovir, idoxuridine, or vidarabine has been effective in preventing corneal ulceration and visual impairment in herpetic keratitis. Acyclovir is effective systemically in treating primary genital herpes simplex and preventing recurrent episodes if suppressive dosages are maintained. However, if the drug is stopped, the frequency of recurrence is not altered.

The antivirals have been found to reduce the mortality in herpes simplex encephalitis and disseminated herpetic infection of the newborn, but they do not prevent all the complications. Herpes simplex viral infections resistant to acyclovir have been found in persons with acquired immunodeficiency syndrome (AIDS).[7] These have been treated effectively with foscarnet.[7] Zidovudine in combination with acyclovir may be used for treatment of chronic HSV infection in HIV-positive persons.

Patients with frequent recurrence may benefit from subcutaneous interferon-alfa. Although not FDA approved for this use, topical interferon alfa and interferon-beta ointments have been shown to reduce recurrence and duration of labial and genital herpes.[3]

**Patient/family education.** Patient education is the primary nursing intervention needed for patients with herpes. Information should be given about the etiology, treatment methodology, and measures to prevent secondary infection.

## Herpes Zoster

### Etiology/epidemiology

Herpes zoster, or shingles, is caused by the same virus (varicella-zoster) that causes varicella (chickenpox). Varicella is believed to be the primary infection in a nonimmune host, whereas herpes zoster is thought to be the response in a partially immune host. Although herpes zoster is far less communicable than is chickenpox, persons who have not had chickenpox may develop it after exposure to the vesicular lesions of persons with herpes zoster. For this reason, susceptible persons should not care for patients with herpes zoster. It is one of the most persistent and exasperating conditions in elderly patients and leads to discouragement and demoralization. Herpes zoster may recur in rare circumstances. Herpes zoster often occurs in persons with AIDS and Hodgkin's disease and in individuals with lymphoid and some bone cancers because of reduced cell-mediated immunity.

### Pathophysiology

In herpes zoster, clusters of small vesicles usually form in a line. They follow the course of the peripheral sensory nerves and often are unilateral (Figure 63-8). Because they follow nerve pathways, the lesions never cross the midline of the body. However, nerves on both sides of the body can be involved. Two thirds of persons with herpes zoster develop lesions over thoracic dermatomes, and the remainder show involvement of the trigeminal nerve with lesions on the face, eye, and scalp. The rash develops first as macules but progresses rapidly to vesicles. The fluid becomes turbid, and crusts develop and drop off in about 10 days.

Malaise, fever, itching, and pain over the involved area may precede the eruption of the lesions. If vesicles develop within 1 to 2 days after the initial pain symptoms, the lesions usually clear in 2 to 3 weeks, but if the vesicles develop over a period of 1 week, a prolonged course can be expected.

Discomfort from pain and itching is the major problem with herpes zoster. The pain may vary from a light burning sensation to a deep visceral-type pain, and it may be intermittent or constant. It usually persists for up to 4 weeks. In approximately 50% of persons over age 60, the pain may last for months or years.[3] Enlargement of the lymph nodes may also occur with the rash.

### Collaborative care management

For many patients, no treatment is prescribed for herpes zoster. However, for persons with immunosuppression, treatment is given. Acyclovir (Zovirax) accelerates healing and reduces acute pain and is given orally in high doses (400 mg to 800 mg, every 4 hours, five times a day for 5 to 6 days). In severe infections, acyclovir may be given intravenously; lower doses are effective intravenously. Because acyclovir may precipitate in renal tubules, drinking fluids should be encouraged. Although acyclovir does not prevent postherpetic neuralgia, it may reduce its severity. Treatment must be initiated within 48 to 72 hours of the appearance of vesicles. Vidarabine is also effective in treating people with herpes zoster, but it has the potential for more side effects than acyclovir; it is also indicated for treatment of patients with resistance to acyclovir. Dosing for both drugs must be adjusted for patients with impaired renal function. Famciclovir, similar to acyclovir, is used for uncomplicated cases of acute herpes zoster in patients who are immunocompromised. As with acyclovir, famciclovir has been shown to reduce the duration of postherpetic neuralgia (PHN).[3]

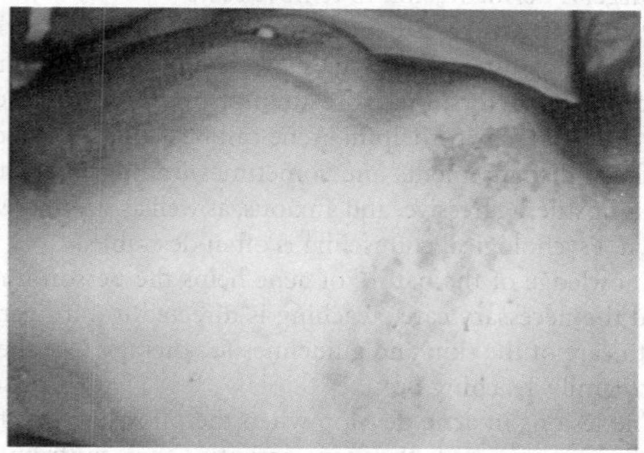

**fig. 63-8** Herpes zoster.

Analgesics are prescribed for pain relief. Aspirin, with or without codeine, is often effective; meperidine (Demerol) may be needed for severe pain. Nonsteroidal antiinflammatory drugs (NSAIDs) are usually ineffective. Systemic steroids, such as prednisone, may decrease the incidence of postherpetic neuralgia and decrease herpetic pain. However, steroid therapy should not be used in immunocompromised persons. Sedatives may also be helpful, especially at bedtime. Local discomfort may be relieved by calamine lotion or by application of a vinegar solution (one-fourth cup white vinegar in 2 quarts lukewarm water). Burow's solution (5% aluminum acetate) applied as a cool compress may provide local relief and quicken drying of the vesicles.[3] Loose clothing helps minimize contact with the affected area. Patients should avoid exposure to highly susceptible persons (those who have not had chickenpox or who are immunocompromised).

Postherpetic neuralgia occurs in about 10% of persons after herpes zoster infection, mostly in elderly persons. The pain usually lasts less than 1 year but may persist for many years. The pain is always present with superimposed sharp pain episodes. Because the pain results from nervous system damage, it does not respond well to usual pain therapies, and thus a multimodal approach is more effective. Local application of capsaicin cream may provide some pain relief. A tricyclic antidepressant is commonly prescribed. Combining nortriptyline, a tricyclic antidepressant, with an anticonvulsant has been used successfully in some cases. Transcutaneous electrical nerve stimulation (TENS) may be tried initially, although it usually is not effective on a long-term basis. Narcotics are avoided because of the persistence of the pain and potential for addiction. Neurosurgical procedures are usually ineffective. Because the pain can become an all-consuming part of the patient's life, ongoing evaluation of the impact on the patient functionally and socially and ongoing supportive counseling are helpful.

**Patient/family education.** Patient and family education to prevent spread of infection is important. Patients should be educated regarding the course of the disease and possible complications. Patients and family should receive information regarding treatments and medications. Nursing care focuses on helping patients deal with the postherpetic neuralgia. (For a complete discussion of chronic pain, see Chapter 12.)

## ACNE

### Acne Vulgaris

#### Etiology/epidemiology

Acne vulgaris, a common skin disease, is seen in 80% of adolescents, but may also occur in adults. The cause of acne is thought to be multifactorial. Some of the common causes that have been postulated are free fatty acids, endocrine effects, stressors, diet, heredity, and infection. Diet has been essentially ruled out as a causative factor, but none of the other factors have been demonstrated conclusively. Acne occurs at puberty, when the sebaceous glands are stimulated by androgens, and is often found to be common within families. Acne is more quiescent in summer months.

#### Pathophysiology

At puberty, sebaceous glands undergo enlargement from androgen stimulation. Sebum is released, passed through the follicular canal, and combined with sebaceous gland cell fragments, epidermal cells (keratin), and bacteria. At this time the triglycerides in the sebum are hydrolyzed to glycerol and free fatty acids. The sebum and debris may become plugged in the hair follicle to form an *open comedo* (blackhead) if it is at the surface or a *closed comedo* (whitehead) if it is below the surface (Figure 63-9). The dark color of the blackhead is melanin, not dirt, and results from passage of melanin from the adjoining epidermal cells.

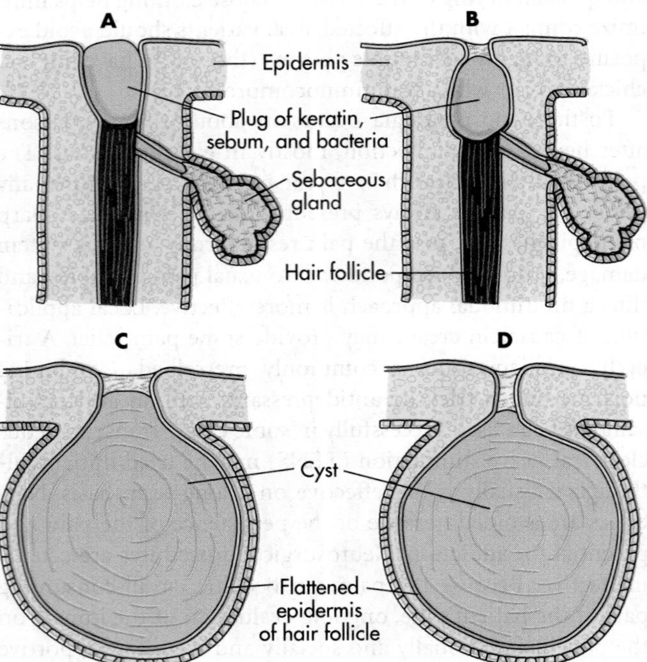


**fig. 63-9** Formation of lesions in acne vulgaris. **A,** Open comedo (blackhead), early stage. **B,** Closed comedo (whitehead), early stage. **C,** Cyst formation in open comedo, advanced stage. **D,** Cyst formation in closed comedo, advanced stage.

Inflammatory lesions apparently develop from the escape of sebum into the dermis, which then serves as an irritant, causing an inflammatory reaction. Free fatty acids may also be an irritant in the follicle itself.

Acne occurs mostly on the face and neck, upper chest, and back, although the upper arms, buttocks, and thighs may also be involved. Comedones are the first visible signs, and the skin is characteristically oily. The inflammatory lesions include papules, pustules, nodules, and cysts. Superficial lesions may resolve in 5 to 10 days without scarring, but large lesions last for several weeks and often result in scarring. The typical scar resembles an old volcano (ice-pick scar); however, many other sizes and shapes may result, depending on the depth and extent of the inflammatory lesions.

The extent of the lesions varies greatly. Some persons have only a few small lesions. Many adolescents have several lesions that peak at ages 16 to 18 years of age and then slowly resolve. A few persons develop severe nodular acne that may not resolve for 10 to 15 years.

#### Collaborative care management

Treatment of acne may be topical, systemic, intralesional, or surgical and includes the following:

1. Topical therapy
   a. Basic method of therapy
   b. Agents: benzoyl peroxide, vitamin A acid (tretinoin), antibiotics (topical erythromycin), sulfur-zinc lotion
2. Removal of comedones with a comedo extractor
3. Systemic therapy
   a. Used with topical therapy for severe nodular or cystic acne
   b. Isoretinoic acid (Accutane)
      (1) A vitamin A acid analog
      (2) Side effects: dry lips and conjunctiva, brittle hair, tenderness of fingertips and toetips, hypertriglyceridemia, birth defects
   c. Systemic antibiotics
   d. Estrogens for female patients who have not responded to other therapies
4. Intralesional corticosteroid therapy for cysts of severe acne
5. Surgery: dermabrasion to remove scars

**Patient/family education.** Counseling and teaching are the major nursing strategies. Stress appears to be one of the causative factors; therefore attempts to identify and cope with stressors may be helpful. Acne can be a stressor, producing facial disfigurements and sometimes leading to behavior that is hostile, aggressive, and anxious, as well as shy and withdrawn. Psychological counseling is often desirable.

Knowledge of the nature of acne helps the person understand the necessary care. Teaching is directed toward general health care of the skin and guidelines for therapy (see the Patient/Family Teaching Box).

The lesions in acne develop when the pilosebaceous follicles become plugged; therefore activities that contribute to occlusion of the follicles are to be avoided. Hair and hands should be kept away from the face. Loose clothing prevents pressure over the follicles, and tight collars should not be worn. The skin should be kept clean. Greasy, oil-based cosmetics may be occlusive and plug up the follicles. Any food that appears to cause acne flare-ups in a given individual is best avoided.

### Acne Rosacea

#### Etiology/epidemiology

Acne rosacea is a skin condition that usually affects persons over 25 years of age. The cause is unknown. Over the years many causative factors have been suggested, including bacteria, vitamin deficiency, hormonal imbalance, alcohol, caffeine, psychological factors, and heredity.

#### Pathophysiology

Acne rosacea begins with redness over the cheeks and nose, followed by papules, pustules, and enlargement of superficial blood vessels. Years of acne rosacea lead to an irregular, bulbous thickening of the skin of the distal part of the nose *(rhinophyma)*, with a red-purple discoloration and dilated follicles.

#### Collaborative care management

There is no specific treatment for acne rosacea. Some persons respond to tetracycline and topical peeling agents, but there is no specific treatment for the vascular component. Rhinophyma may be treated by plastic surgery.

**Patient/family education.** Teaching about the disease and possible treatment is necessary. Avoiding stimuli that cause vasodilation is usually appropriate.

## DERMATITIS

Dermatitis, a superficial inflammation of the skin, refers to several different conditions resulting in the same type of lesions. Dermatitis is often classified arbitrarily according to specific features, such as cause, pattern, age, or type of treatment required. Some common types of dermatitis are listed in Table 63-1 and are discussed in more detail in succeeding paragraphs. The term *eczema* is often used synonymously with dermatitis but usually refers to the chronic type.

Regardless of the cause, the lesions in any dermatitis follow a characteristic pattern. Initially, erythema and local edema are followed by vesicle formation with oozing and then crusting and scaling. If the dermatitis persists, there will be evidence of excoriation from scratching and thickening of the skin, and the color becomes more brownish. Secondary infection may result.

### Contact Dermatitis

#### Etiology/epidemiology

Contact dermatitis is caused by external agents and may affect various parts of the body (Table 63-2). The two types of contact dermatitis are irritant and allergic. *Irritant contact dermatitis* can occur in any person on contact with a sufficient concentration of an irritant. Mechanical irritation may result

**patient/family teaching**

**The Person with Acne**

1. Preventive measures
   a. Keep hands and hair away from the face.
   b. Avoid constricting clothing over lesions.
   c. Shampoo hair and scalp frequently.
   d. Avoid exposure to oils and greases.
   e. Eat a well-balanced diet and avoid any foods that appear to cause skin flare-ups.
2. General skin care
   a. Keep skin clean; wash face 2 to 3 times daily.
   b. Use a medicated soap or agent prescribed by physician.
   c. Avoid vigorous rubbing of the skin.
   d. Use cosmetics that are water-based, rather than cream-based, and avoid those that contain wax esters (myristates, palmitates, stearates).
   e. Never leave cosmetics on face at night.
3. During therapy
   a. Follow the prescribed therapy even when immediate improvement is not noted for 2 to 3 weeks.
   b. Expect skin desquamation during therapy.
   c. Avoid using self-remedies during therapy.
   d. Remove cosmetics before applying topical medications.
   e. Avoid exposure to direct sunlight if using tretinoin or taking tetracycline (photosensitivity).
   f. Avoid pregnancy if taking Accutane (possibility of birth defects).

**table 63-1** *Types of Dermatitis*

| TYPE | CAUSE | CHARACTERISTICS |
|---|---|---|
| Contact (Fig. 63-10) | External agents | Site and pattern of lesions depend on exposure pattern (linear, angular, etc.)<br>Itching a major symptom |
| Atopic | Hypersensitivity reaction, hereditary | Itching a major symptom<br>Lesions caused by scratching |
| Lichen simplex chronicus | Stasis, irritants, psychological factors | Itching a major symptom<br>Lesions caused by scratching |
| Seborrheic (Fig. 63-11) | Unknown | Erythematous, scaly (e.g., dandruff) |
| Nummular | Unknown | Coin-shaped lesions<br>Severe itching |
| Stasis | Decreased circulation | Erythema, edema<br>Lesions may develop from trauma<br>Itching may be severe |

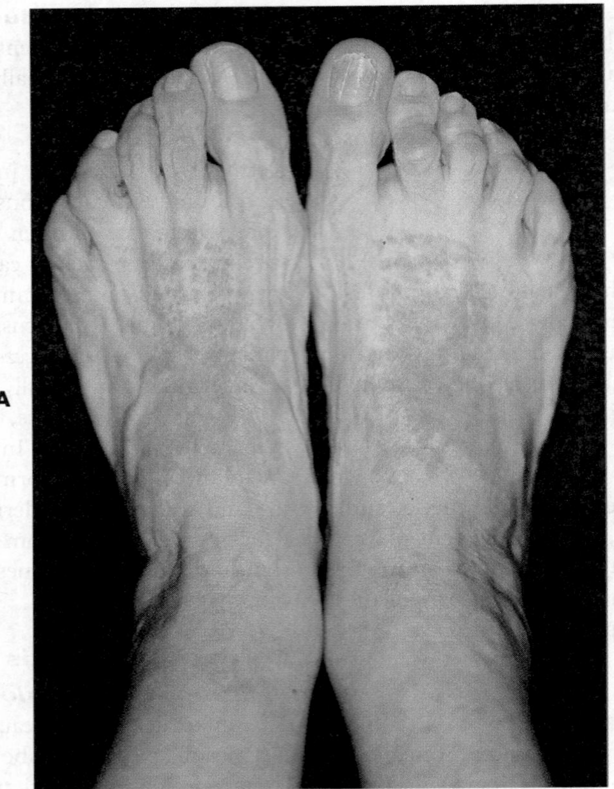


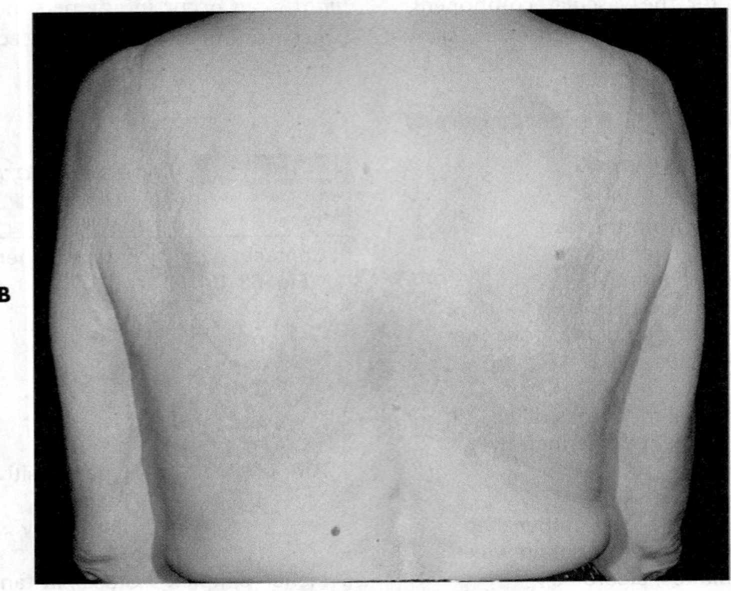


**fig. 63-10, A,** Shoe contact dermatitis. Sharply defined plaques formed under a shoe lining impregnated with rubber cement. **B,** Allergic contact dermatitis to spandex rubber in a bra.

from wool or glass fibers. Chemical irritants include acids, alkalies, solvents, detergents, and oils commonly found in cleaning compounds, insecticides, and industrial compounds. Biological irritants include urine, feces, and toxins from insects or aquatic plants. People whose hands and feet are constantly wet often develop irritant contact dermatitis.

*Allergic contact dermatitis* is a cell-mediated hypersensitivity immune reaction from contact with a specific antigen (see Figure 63-10, *B*). Many compounds can cause sensitization under specified conditions. Typical antigens include poison ivy, synthetics, industrial chemicals, drugs (for example, sulfanilamide or penicillin), and metals (especially nickel and

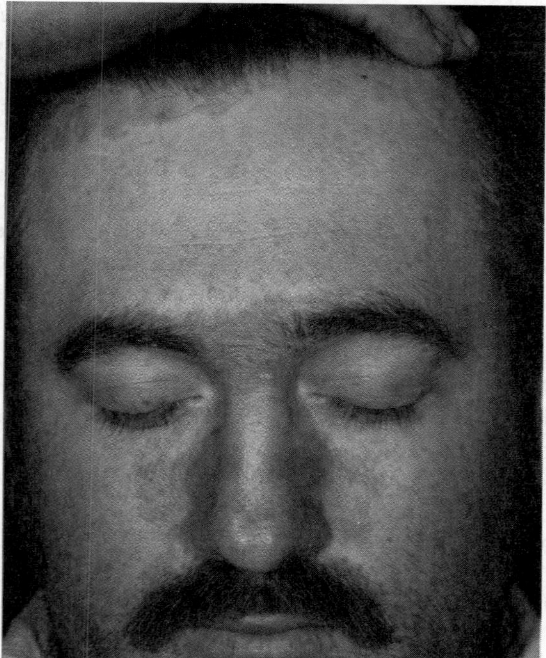

**fig. 63-11** Seborrheic dermatitis in an adult with extensive involvement in all of the characteristic sites.

chromate). Once the skin has been sensitized, further contact with the sensitizing substance will produce an eczematous reaction. The sensitizing allergen may reach the site by direct contact; by indirect contact, such as transmission by animals, from one part of the body to the other by the hands, or on clothing; or by the air, as in smoke.

### Pathophysiology

Characteristic dermatitis lesions appear sooner in irritant contact dermatitis than in the allergic type; however, the onset and appearance vary, depending on the type and concentration of the irritant. The lesions develop on the exposed areas, particularly the more sensitive areas, such as the dorsal rather than the palmar surface of the hands. If the irritant can be spread by the hands, as in poison ivy, lesions may involve other nonexposed areas. When contact dermatitis is suspected but the agent is unknown, patch testing (see Chapter 62) may be carried out, or the environment may be manipulated to exclude suspected agents.

### Collaborative care management

Weeping uninfected lesions respond rapidly to wet dressings with water or Burow's solution for 20 minutes four times daily. Crusts and scales are not removed but are allowed to drop off naturally as the skin heals. Topical corticosteroids are applied to dry lesions. Systemic corticosteroids may be given in acute extensive exacerbations but are not used to treat a mild contact dermatitis. Systemic antibiotics are prescribed when infection is present. Severe pruritus may be eased by antihistamines; plain calamine lotion may be applied for pruritus from poison ivy.

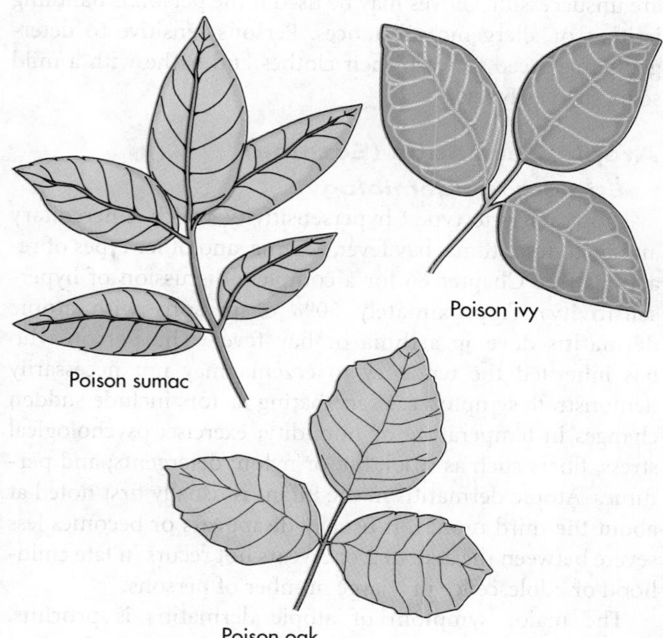


**fig. 63-12** Typical leaves of poison sumac, poison ivy, and poison oak.

**table 63-2** *Common Causes of Contact Dermatitis of Different Areas*

| AREA | CAUSE |
|---|---|
| Face/scalp/ears | Cosmetics, hair care products, jewelry, cleansers, sunscreen, contact lens solution, metals (especially nickel), glasses |
| Neck | Perfumes, clothing (especially wool) |
| Trunk, axillae | Deodorants, clothing, perfumes, laundry products |
| Arms/hands | Poison ivy, oak, and sumac; jewelry; nickel, etc., in watchbands<br>Detergents and other cleansers, gloves |
| Legs/feet | Medication for "athlete's foot," shoes |

**Patient/family education.** The primary focus of nursing care is prevention. Contact dermatitis may be prevented by avoiding the irritating or sensitizing substance whenever possible. All persons should know how to recognize the leaves of poisonous plants—such as poison ivy, poison oak, or poison sumac—that grow where they live (Figure 63-12). Persons walking in areas where poison ivy grows need to protect the skin by wearing appropriate clothing. If contact with poison ivy is suspected, symptoms may be averted by immediately rinsing the skin for 15 minutes with running water to remove the resin before skin penetration occurs.

The person who develops a sensitivity to material encountered in the living or working environment may need to consider a permanent change of environment if other measures are unsuccessful. Gloves may be used if the person is handling irritant or allergenic substances. Persons sensitive to detergents may need to wash their clothes and bathe with a mild soap, such as Ivory.

## Atopic Dermatitis (Eczema)

### *Etiology/epidemiology*

Atopy refers to type I hypersensitivity, which is hereditary and includes asthma, hay fever, eczema, and other types of reactions (see Chapter 66 for a complete discussion of hypersensitivity). Approximately 50% of persons with atopic dermatitis develop asthma or hay fever. The person who has inherited the tendency to eczema may not necessarily demonstrate symptoms. Exacerbating factors include sudden changes in temperature or humidity; exercise; psychological stress; fibers such as wool, fur, or nylon; detergents; and perfumes. Atopic dermatitis in the infant is usually first noted at about the third month. It usually disappears or becomes less severe between the ages of 2 or 3 years but recurs in late childhood or adolescence in a large number of persons.

The major symptom of atopic dermatitis is pruritus. Chronic scratching leads to eczematous lesions and subsequent lichenification. Healing usually occurs without scarring, but hypopigmentation or hyperpigmentation may result.

### *Pathophysiology*

Persons with atopic dermatitis have dry, highly sensitive skin with a lowered threshold to pruritus, so that minor stimuli cause intense itching. There is a marked tendency toward vasoconstriction of superficial blood vessels, and the skin blanches readily. Cold and low humidity are poorly tolerated because of drying effects. Heat and high humidity are also poorly tolerated because vasodilation increases the inflammatory reaction, thus aggravating the dermatitis and causing increased itching and discomfort. Lesions become localized to the flexor surfaces of the neck (Figure 63-13), to the eyelids, behind the ears, in the antecubital and popliteal areas, and at the wrists. The erythema is dusky, and excoriations may become secondarily infected. By the late twenties or early thirties the lesions usually disappear, but they may recur at a later date as chronic hand or foot eczema.

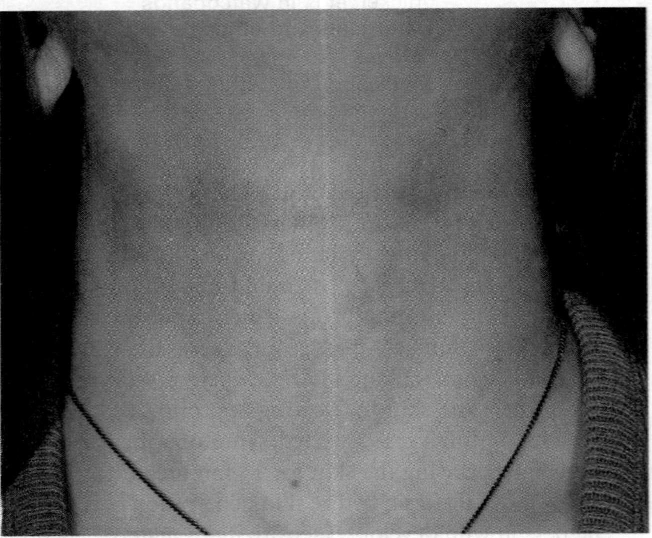

**fig. 63-13** Atopic dermatitis. Classic appearance of erythema and diffuse scaling about the neck.

Persons with atopic dermatitis are highly susceptible to viral infections, especially herpes, and to bacterial infections, such as those caused by staphylococci or $\beta$-hemolytic streptococci. There is also an increased incidence of fungal infections, such as tinea. Lymph nodes draining affected areas may be enlarged.

### *Collaborative care management*

There is no cure for atopic dermatitis, but symptoms can be controlled. The focus of therapy is relief of pruritus to break the itch-scratch cycle that leads to lesions. The major form of topical therapy consists of corticosteroid cream or ointment. Fluorinated corticosteroids may be used for localized lesions in adults but are used less often in children and *never on the face.* An occlusion wrap over the steroid in adults may enhance the steroid effect but may lead to folliculitis. Topical antibiotics are rarely used. Cool compresses with water or Burow's solution are helpful for acute phases when weeping lesions are present.

Systemic therapy includes antihistamines, especially at night when itching is more intense. Antibiotics, such as penicillin or erythromycin, may be given systemically to treat bacterial infections. Systemic corticosteroids may be given for a limited period to those with severe atopic eczema.

**Patient/family education.** Patient education is the major focus of care and should stress prevention of hypersensitivity and control of signs and symptoms. Patients should keep the skin hydrated and avoid temperature extremes and irritating substances (see the Patient/Family Teaching Box).

## Other Types of Dermatitis

### *Lichen simplex chronicus*

Lichen simplex chronicus (LSC) is a chronic skin condition that results from repeated scratching. Psychological factors are thought to be involved. Although more common in females and Asians, LSC may occur in both genders and all races. Itching initiates the condition in normal skin and may occur as a result of stasis or an irritant, or it may occur without any known cause. Lichen simplex chronicus is more commonly found on the hands, perineum, legs, and occipital region of the scalp.

Once itching starts, the itch-scratch cycle is initiated and scratching becomes a habit. The skin becomes excoriated, and lichenified plaques result. Lesions disappear if scratching ceases, but it is difficult for the person to stop scratching. Itching is often worse at night. Topical corticosteroids are the treatment of choice. In hairless areas, corticosteroid tape (Cordran tape) is effective if the medicated tape covers the area, so that further excoriation is reduced.

### *Seborrheic dermatitis*

Seborrheic dermatitis may occur primarily in areas of increased sebaceous gland activity on the face, ears, scalp, chest, and back. The cause is unknown. Mild seborrheic dermatitis is often seen in the scalp in the form of erythema and dandruff and can be controlled easily by shampooing with selenium sulfide (Selsun Blue) shampoo. More extensive seborrheic dermatitis leads to red scaly plaques and is treated with topical hydrocortisone.

#### Nummular dermatitis

Nummular dermatitis is a chronic condition of uncertain cause occurring most commonly in middle-aged or older men. The lesions of nummular dermatitis are coin shaped and are found on the dorsum of the hand, the extensor surfaces of the extremities, and the buttocks. Itching is often severe. The skin is usually dry; therefore frequent bathing is inadvisable. Exposure to sunlight may be helpful. Treatment consists of topical corticosteroids and antibiotic therapy if bacteria are isolated by culture.

#### Stasis dermatitis

Stasis dermatitis is a common skin condition of the lower extremities in older persons. It is usually preceded by varicosities and poor circulation. With the reduction in venous return from the legs, substances normally carried away by the circulation remain in the tissues causing irritation. The skin is often reddened and edematous. Pruritus may be severe. Scratching causes breaks in the skin, which become infected via hands, clothing, and other sources.

The most important treatment for stasis dermatitis is prevention with careful attention to the treatment of peripheral vascular conditions and preventing constriction of the circulation to the extremities (see Chapter 27). Acute weeping lesions are treated with wet compresses and elevation of the legs.

## SKIN REACTIONS FROM SYSTEMIC FACTORS

### Dermatitis Medicamentosa

#### Etiology/epidemiology

*Dermatitis medicamentosa,* or drug rash, can be caused by almost any drug. The rash occurs as a result of gradual accumulation of the drug or because of antibodies that develop in response to a component of the medication. Skin manifestations from drugs may have a nonallergic or an allergic basis. Commonly seen skin reactions include erythematous rashes, purpura, vesicles, bullae, ulcers, and urticaria (Table 63-3). The reactions can appear at any time, but the onset is usually sudden.

#### Pathophysiology

Most skin reactions are caused by hypersensitivity reactions to drugs. Type I anaphylactic (urticaria, angioedema), type II cytotoxic (cellular injury), type III immune complex (serum sickness), or type IV cell-mediated (allergic contact dermatitis, allergic photosensitivity) reactions may occur. Some drugs may have combined reactions; for example, penicillin may produce both type I and type III reactions. Allergic contact dermatitis is commonly seen with drugs used topically. The rash is often bright red, semiconfluent, macular and papular, generalized, and bilateral. Hypersensitivity occurs early when previous sensitization has taken place.

*Photosensitivity* may occur with certain drugs and may take one of two forms, phototoxicity or photoallergy (Table 63-4). *Phototoxicity* may occur in any person taking a photosensitive drug and results from the reaction of the drug (chemical) with radiant energy, particularly ultraviolet light. Sunscreens are not effective in preventing photosensitivity reactions. Photoallergic reactions are cell-mediated (type IV) hypersensitivity reactions; therefore they affect only a small group of persons after several sensitizing exposures of drug and sunlight.

**patient/family teaching**

**The Person with Atopic Dermatitis**

1. Avoid soap over lesions (soap is an irritant); use soap minimally over nonaffected areas.
2. Soak affected areas for 15 to 20 minutes in warm water for hydration; pat skin dry, then *immediately* apply recommended lotion or cream to seal in moisture.
3. Wet wraps may be used in place of soaking; wraps permit evaporation, which cools the skin, thus decreasing pruritus.
4. Apply corticosteroids in a thin layer and rub in well; do not use fluorinated corticosteroid on the face.
5. Avoid wool, fur, or rough fibers against the skin; they act as irritants and cause itching.
6. Avoid overheating that increases sweating, leading to itching. Wear loose, light clothing in hot weather. Air conditioning promotes comfort. Sunlight is beneficial to the skin.
7. Avoid excessive cold that dries the skin.
8. Avoid anything that aggravates the eczema.
9. Rinse all garments and bed linens twice to avoid residue of cleansing agents.
10. Consult dermatologist for appropriate laundry agents to prevent irritations from clothing.
11. Seek medical care if eczema becomes worse.

**table 63-3** *Skin Reactions to Common Medications*

| REACTION | MEDICATION |
|---|---|
| Erythematous rash | Antibiotics, sulfonamides, thiazide diuretics, barbiturates, phenylbutazone |
| Purpura (ecchymosis, petechiae) | Thiazides, sulfonamides, barbiturates, anticoagulants |
| Mucocutaneous lesions (vesicles, bullae, ulcers) | Sulfonamides, penicillins, barbiturates, phenylbutazone |
| Urticaria | Penicillins, streptomycin, tetracycline, insulin, aspirin, dyes, ACTH, antiserum |

#### Collaborative care management

Treatment of dermatitis medicamentosa consists of stopping the drug and treating the symptoms with cool, moist compresses; antihistamines (for pruritus); and topical and systemic corticosteroids. Photosensitivity can be prevented by avoiding direct sunlight on the skin when taking a drug with photosensitivity effects.

**Patient/family education.** Patient and family education focuses on prevention by making sure people are aware of drugs to which they are allergic. The patient or family member should know the specific drug name and type of reaction. A Medic Alert bracelet may be beneficial. Allergy information should be documented on the patient's record. Nursing care also focuses on helping the patient comply with treatment.

### Exfoliative Dermatitis

#### Etiology/epidemiology

Exfoliative dermatitis is a rare, generalized dermatitis. In most cases, the cause is unknown, but the disease may be associated with other types of dermatitis or with a lymphoma, or it may be the result of a drug reaction.

#### Pathophysiology

The onset of exfoliative dermatitis may be rapid or insidious and consists of an elevated temperature and a generalized erythema, followed by extensive scaling (exfoliation). Pruritus may be present, and the lesions often become infected. Loss of large amounts of water and protein from the skin leads to hypoproteinemia, weight loss, and difficulty with temperature control. Heart failure may occur in elderly patients. Death may result from overwhelming infection or circulatory collapse.

#### Collaborative care management

Therapy consists of maintaining fluid balance and preventing infection. Methods used to prevent infection in patients with burns are applicable (see Chapter 64). All drugs are discontinued as potential causative factors, although antibiotics may be started after culture and sensitivity tests of infected lesions. Oral corticosteroids are given for severe cases. Daily baths followed by application of petrolatum to the skin promote comfort.

**Patient/family education.** Patient and family are educated regarding the course of the disease and rationales for treatment. Nursing care focuses on promotion of comfort and management of signs and symptoms.

**table 63-4** *Drug Photosensitivity*

| Reaction | Symptoms | Drugs |
|---|---|---|
| Phototoxicity | Resembles sunburn (erythema, edema, vesicles) | Coal tar derivatives<br>Psoralens<br>Tetracycline<br>Nalidixic acid<br>Sulfanilamide<br>Declomycin<br>Chlorpromazine<br>Certain dyes |
| Photoallergy | Resembles eczema (exudative papules and vesicles, urticaria, lichenification) | Diuretics (thiazides)<br>Phenothiazines<br>Oral hypoglycemics<br>Griseofulvin |

### Erythema Multiforme

#### Etiology/epidemiology

Erythema multiforme (EM) is a self-limiting inflammation of the skin and mucous membranes in genetically susceptible persons. Episodes of the disease may be single, recurrent, or, rarely, continuous. Although it is usually mild, EM may progress to a toxic epidermal necrolysis type of illness. Erythema multiforme is classified as major or minor. The major type is also described as the severe bullous form or *Stevens-Johnson syndrome.* Both forms are thought to be a cell-mediated immune response to relevant antigens. The responsible agent usually can be identified. Medications that can trigger erythema multiforme include phenytoin, carbamazepine, sulfonamides, NSAIDs, allopurinol, and certain antibiotics (particularly cephalosporins). Drugs, not infection, are thought to be responsible for the severe bullous form of the disorder.

Infections that cause EM include mycoplasmal pneumonia, chickenpox, hepatitis B, infectious mononucleosis, and herpes simplex, which is the most common. Herpes simplex triggers 60% to 70% of cases of recurrent EM.[3] More unusual causes of EM include systemic lupus erythematosus, lymphoma, leukemia, radiation therapy, and reactions to vaccinations, particularly hepatitis B.

#### Pathophysiology

Erythema multiforme may affect the skin and mucous membranes or solely the skin. Episodes of the disease usually last for 1 to 3 weeks. The clinical lesions are characteristically erythematous papules acrally distributed. The rash is painful and itchy, and it may progress to the bullous variety. The rash occurs on the dorsa of the hands, palms, knees, feet, and elbows. The oral cavity may be affected by blisters progressing to erosion of the entire oral mucosa and lips. Conjunctivitis may occur, progressing to corneal opacity. If the genital mucosa become involved, adhesions may result as a long-term complication. The skin eruptions may be preceded by fever, chest pain, and arthralgia. Severe cases may be confused with toxic epidermal necrolysis. If the triggering agent is herpes simplex, EM usually occurs 7 to 10 days after the onset of the herpes infection. It is not possible to culture HSV from an EM lesion, but DNA studies have shown the presence of the virus within cutaneous lesions.[3]

#### Collaborative care management

A single attack of EM does not usually require treatment. Any suspected triggering agent is discontinued and symptoms treated. Topical steroids may be prescribed to relieve itching and burning. Systemic steroids seem to prolong episodes of the disease. A sedating antihistamine such as hydroxyzine may be of use. Even if HSV has been determined to be the cause of

EM, acyclovir is not useful once the rash has appeared. Oral care is an important aspect of care. Antiseptic mouthwashes are advised. Oral lesions have improved with the use of fluocinonide and clobetasol propionate.[3] Persons with eye and oral involvement, as well as those with the severe bullous type (Stevens-Johnson syndrome), need to be treated as inpatients. A skin biopsy may be needed to rule out other possible causes. Individuals with extensive blistering should be treated as burn patients and admitted to an intensive care unit (see Chapter 64).

Intravenous or enteral feeding may be indicated for persons with extensive oral involvement. Protective dressings should be applied to prevent secondary infection. Caution must used when choosing the appropriate antibiotic therapy, because Stevens-Johnson syndrome is triggered by drugs. Systemic steroids are indicated for the treatment of patients with severe cases of EM. Steroids are effective in reducing fever and aiding symptomatic relief but do not significantly affect morbidity or mortality rate. Skin lesions may take weeks to heal, and systemic steroids may delay the healing process. The risk-benefit ratio should be considered, particularly in elderly patients, before prescribing systemic steroids. Cyclosporine has been shown to be of use in treating patients with severe cases of EM. Patients with recurrent EM that is disabling may be treated with a short course of oral acyclovir. Treatment should be initiated at the earliest sign of EM. For persistent or frequently recurring cases, acyclovir 400 mg orally twice a day for 6 to 12 months should induce remission. If the patient fails to respond to acyclovir, dapsone and antimalarial drugs have been shown to be effective. If all other treatments fail, azathioprine is an option for suppressing attacks, although this use is not currently approved by the Food and Drug Administration (FDA).

**Patient/family education.** The patient with any type of EM needs support and education throughout diagnosis and treatment. Initially, other disorders causing blistering must be considered, and the patient will require support during this time. Education is needed regarding the medications prescribed, including administration, dosing, and side effects. Nursing care is supportive and includes baths, soaks, oral care, and dressings. Thorough explanations should accompany treatments. Patients and family will require teaching regarding the course of the disease, complications, possible triggers, and recurrences. The relationship between herpes simplex and episodes of erythema multiforme should be explained.

## INFECTIOUS DISEASES

Communicable diseases, such as measles, chickenpox, smallpox, scarlet fever, and typhoid fever, produce skin reactions (Table 63-5). Nodes and hemorrhagic spots in the skin also accompany severe acute rheumatic fever.

## LUPUS ERYTHEMATOSUS

One of the more common tissue diseases that may result in skin conditions is lupus erythematosus (LE). There are two forms, systemic lupus erythematosus (SLE) (see Chapter 61) and discoid lupus erythematosus (DLE).

### Etiology/Epidemiology

Discoid lupus erythematosus is a chronic, relatively benign skin condition that has worldwide distribution among all races, occurring most often in the fourth decade of life. It rarely occurs in children or elderly persons. Precipitating factors include physical trauma and stress.

### Pathophysiology

The lesions of DLE are well demarcated and erythematous, have a characteristic scaly border with an atrophied center, and vary in size. The most common sites are the cheeks (butterfly pattern), nose, ears, scalp, and chest, although other parts of the body—including mucous membranes—may also be involved. Discoid lupus erythematosus occurs in the absence of other signs, symptoms, and serological abnormalities of SLE. About 15% to 20% of persons with SLE will have DLE, and 5% to 10% of persons who initially have DLE will develop SLE.[7]

### Collaborative Care Management

There is no cure for DLE. Palliative measures include topical steroid therapy under occlusive wraps, intralesional steroid

**table 63-5** *Skin Reactions of Some Communicable Diseases*

| Disease | Cause | Incubation Period (Days) | Place of Rash Origin | Skin Lesions |
|---|---|---|---|---|
| Measles (rubeola) | Rubeola virus | 11 (8-14) | Face | Pink macular-papular rash; lesions coalesce |
| German measles; 3-day measles (rubella) | Rubella virus | 14-21 | Face | Pink macular-papular rash; lesions usually discrete; may coalesce |
| Scarlet fever (scarlatina) | Hemolytic streptococcus | 1-3 | Neck, chest | Bright red (scarlet) macules (pinpoint) |
| Chickenpox (varicella) | Varicella-zoster virus | 14-21 | Back, chest | Macule, papule, vesicle, crust; lesions at different stages |
| Smallpox (variola) | Variola virus | 12 (7-21) | Face | Macule, papule, vesicle, crust; lesions all at same stage |
| Typhoid fever | *Salmonella typhosa* | 14 (7-21) | Abdomen | Macular rash |

therapy, antimalarial therapy with chloroquine (Aralen), hydroxychloroquine sulfate (Plaquenil), or quinacrine hydrochloride (Atabrine).

#### Patient/family education

Nursing care is focused on assisting patients and their families to live with a chronic, incurable disease. Education is necessary regarding palliative and preventive care. Preventive measures include avoiding physical trauma, using sunscreen to prevent sunburn, and wearing warm clothing to protect against cold and wind. If stress is a precipitating factor, measures to reduce stress can be instituted (see Chapter 6). Patients with DLE are not usually hospitalized. Education regarding the course of the disease, treatment, and possible complications should enable the patient to cope effectively with a chronic illness.

## PAPULOSQUAMOUS DISEASES

Papulosquamous diseases are characterized by papular, scaly lesions. Common disorders are psoriasis, pityriasis rosea, and lichen planus.

### Psoriasis

#### *Etiology/epidemiology*

Psoriasis is a genetically determined, chronic, epidermal proliferative disease. The etiology is unknown. There are no specific precipitating factors for the majority of persons; however, some people may develop exacerbations after climatic changes, stressors, trauma, infections, or drugs (propranolol, lithium). Pregnant women often experience a remission of symptoms. Approximately 1% to 2% of the population of North America and Western Europe has psoriasis, and 3% to 5%[9] of this group has associated inflammatory arthritis.[9] There is a higher incidence of psoriasis among whites and a lower incidence among the Japanese, Native Americans, and people of West African origin. Men and women are equally affected. Psoriasis occurs in all ages but is less common among children and elderly persons. Approximately one third of cases of psoriasis occur in persons younger than 20 years of age.

#### *Pathophysiology*

The turnover time for normal skin is 28 days. After the basal cell divides, it normally takes 14 days to reach the stratum corneum and an additional 14 days for this cell to be sloughed off. In psoriasis the time is accelerated to 3 to 4 days.[8]

The lesions of psoriasis are elevated, erythematous, and sharply circumscribed, with a silvery-white scale (Figure 63-14). Removal of the scale usually results in a characteristic pinpoint bleeding called the *Auspitz phenomenon.* The primary lesion is a papule; these papules then join to form plaques. In the African American person, the plaques may appear purple. Lesions may occur over the entire body but are found more commonly on the scalp, elbows, shins, intergluteal cleft, and trunk. Beefy red lesions may be observed in an acute flare-up. Nail changes occur in 10% to 50% of patients with psoriasis. The nails of persons with psoriasis have characteristic involvement; there may be pitting of the nails, yellowish discoloration, oil drop or salmon patches, leukonychia (whitening of the nail), splinter hemorrhage, and onycholysis (separation of the nail from the nailbed).

The four types of psoriasis are psoriasis vulgaris, generalized pustular psoriasis, localized pustular psoriasis, and erythrodermic psoriasis. An outbreak of psoriasis vulgaris may follow streptococcal pharyngitis. Generalized psoriasis usually requires the patient to be admitted to the hospital. Most patients have a history of a plaque-type of psoriasis developing to pustules on an erythematous base, which eventually develop into pools of pustules. Other symptoms include fever, chills, arthralgia, hypocalcemia, and leukocytosis. Flare-ups of the disease may be triggered by discontinuing systemic steroids for a plaque-type of psoriasis. Erythrodermic psoriasis, as the name implies, produces a red coloration of the skin with a desquamative scale over most of the body. It is associated with problems in temperature regulation, hypoalbuminemia, pedal edema, and high-output cardiac failure caused by inflammatory vasodilation.

Psoriatic arthritis occurs in approximately 3% to 4% of persons with psoriasis, occurring with the lesions, preceding the lesions, or occurring in the absence of skin lesions. Presentation of the arthritis varies; it may manifest as an asymmetrical oligoarthropathy, it may affect mainly the distal interphalangeal joints, or it may cause a severely debilitating type of joint disease (see Chapter 61).

#### *Collaborative care management*

Because of the overproduction of skin in psoriasis, treatment is based on slowing mitotic activity. Initially the lesions may be treated with topical keratolytic agents or topical

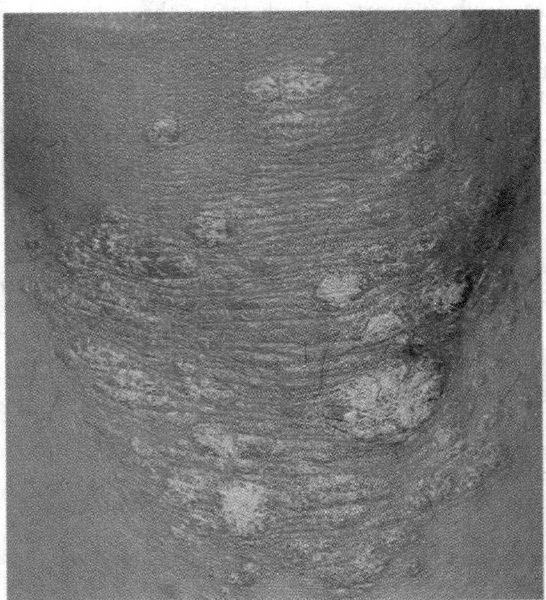

**fig. 63-14** Psoriasis. Note characteristic silvery scaling.

steroids with occlusive wraps and wet dressings to decrease inflammation (Table 63-6).

The application of emollients is important in the treatment of patients with any type of psoriasis. The emollient decreases the amount of scale on the psoriatic plaques and the thickness of the plaque. White petrolatum or a hydrated ointment, applied several times a day, is effective. If the psoriasis becomes resistant to these treatments, coal tar or anthralin therapy is used.

Both coal tar and anthralin therapy are messy and can stain clothing. Calcipotriene (or Dovenex), a vitamin $D_3$ derivative, is effective in inhibiting the proliferation of keratinocytes. Calcium levels must be monitored during therapy, because calcipotriene is systemically absorbed. The use of calcipotriene is not indicated for the treatment of widespread psoriasis because of the large body surface area involved and the risk of systemic absorption.

Ultraviolet (UV) light inhibits DNA synthesis, thus slowing the rapid skin cell growth. Ultraviolet light is divided into different waves: UVC (long), UVB (middle), and UVA (short). UVC is a potent carcinogen and can cause severe burns, so it is not used in treatment of psoriasis. Exposure to sunlamps or blacklight lamps without other therapy may benefit patients with psoriasis. The combination of tar and ultraviolet (UVB) light, known as the *Goeckerman regimen,* is a widely used form of therapy for patients with psoriasis.

Photochemotherapy (Psoralen with ultraviolet [UVA] light [PUVA]) is used for severe psoriasis when other therapies have not been effective. Etretinate (Tegison), a vitamin A derivative, and methoxsalen (Psoralen) are photosensitizing agents that react with the ultraviolet energy. The drugs are taken 2 hours before exposure to the ultraviolet light; dose is based on body weight. Moderate flare-up of

**table 63-6** *Psoriasis Therapy*

| TYPE | ACTION | COMMENTS |
|---|---|---|
| Bland emollients (petrolatum, mineral oil) | Hydration of skin | Use for mild lesions<br>Facilitate scale removal |
| Keratolytics (salicylic acid, ammoniated mercury) | Hydration and softening of skin<br>Antimitotic | Avoid using on face<br>Cover with occlusive wraps<br>May cause skin maceration and folliculitis<br>Not applied to irritated skin |
| Corticosteroids | Antimitotic<br>Antiinflammatory | Topical use for most lesions; cover with occlusive wraps; may cause folliculitis<br>Intralesional use for plaques<br>Rarely given systemically<br>May produce rebound psoriasis when withdrawn |
| Coal tar preparations | Action unknown<br>Have keratolytic, antipruritic, and photosensitizing effects | May cause folliculitis with long-term use<br>Avoid direct sunlight for 24 hours after use<br>Avoid use on face<br>Stain skin, hair, and clothing<br>Available as cream, lotion, gel, solution, and shampoo<br>May be used with ultraviolet light therapy (Goeckerman regimen) |
| Anthralin products | Antimitotic<br>Inhibition of enzyme metabolism | May cause skin irritation<br>Not applied to open skin areas<br>Petrolatum is used to protect normal skin during therapy<br>Wear gloves during application; stains skin, hair, and clothing<br>Avoid using on face |
| Photochemotherapy with ultraviolet light | Inhibition of DNA synthesis | May cause pruritus, erythema, vesicles, flare-up of lesions, transient nausea<br>May be carcinogenic for light-skinned persons or those previously exposed to x-ray therapy<br>Avoid direct sunlight for 12 to 24 hours after ingestion of Psoralen |
| Methotrexate | Antimitotic<br>Inhibition of DNA synthesis | For severe lesions not amenable to other treatment<br>Given orally unless nausea is present<br>Requires close monitoring of hematological, renal, and liver functioning |
| Synthetic retinoids | Correction of abnormal cell differentiation | Experimental therapy<br>Side effects: pruritus, lip edema, sore mouth, thirst, fragile skin, peeling of palms and soles<br>May be used with anthralin or ultraviolet therapies |

psoriasis *(Koebner's phenomenon)* may occur after treatment. Methotrexate is reserved for persons with severe psoriasis that is recalcitrant to other treatments.

Generalized pustular psoriasis is a potentially life-threatening disorder. The person is usually hospitalized, and renal function and calcium metabolism are carefully monitored. Most other types of psoriasis can be managed effectively on an outpatient basis.

**Patient/family education.** Most patients with psoriasis are treated on an ambulatory basis. A new approach to therapy has been the establishment of psoriasis day care centers where patients come daily for treatments, rest, and counseling. Because the lesions are commonly found in visible skin areas, persons with psoriasis face a socially disabling disease. They may need help in identifying and coping with their feelings and with changes that may occur in their lifestyle.

The disease is not curable and may wax and wane continuously. Lesions may fade with treatment, only to recur in the same area or elsewhere. Patients who are unaware of this characteristic of the disease may lose confidence in the physician and seek a quick cure elsewhere. Because psoriasis is so common and so resistant to treatment, manufacturers of patent remedies find a lucrative field for their products among persons with the disease. Teaching for individuals who have psoriasis is summarized in the Guidelines for Care Box.

### Pityriasis Rosea

#### Etiology/epidemiology

Pityriasis rosea is a noncontagious skin condition. The etiology is thought to be viral. Common, with worldwide distribution, the disease affects all races and occurs most commonly in women, adolescents, and young adults. Seventy-five percent of cases occur in persons 10 to 35 years of age.[10] The incidence is higher in the winter months.

#### Pathophysiology

The initial symptom is usually a 2 to 10 cm, single oval lesion *(herald patch)* with a thin, scaly border and yellowish center, appearing most often on the trunk, upper arm, or thigh. The herald patch usually precedes other lesions by 1 to 30 days. A generalized eruption of multiple erythematous macules follows the herald patch, followed by papules. A fine scale is usually present. The distribution of lesions is often in long axes running parallel to each other and on the trunk, which creates a "Christmas tree" distribution.[10] The skin usually clears in 6 to 8 weeks, and the condition does not recur.

Treatment options consists of topical steroids and colloid baths. Ultraviolet therapy may be used. Exposure to sunlight (to the point of minimal erythema) will speed disappearance of the lesions and relieve itching.[10] The patient should be cautioned against sunburn.

**Patient/family education.** Nursing care is essentially symptomatic and includes assisting patients with topical steroids and colloid baths if itching is present. Nurses will be helping patients primarily by educating them.

**guidelines for care**

**Teaching the Person with Psoriasis**

1. Nature of psoriasis: noncurable, recurrence of symptoms.
2. Reduce episodes of rapid-spreading psoriasis (flare-ups) by avoiding skin trauma (injuries, sunburn, infections), extremes of temperature, and stress.
3. Shampoo hair frequently to remove scales. If scalp has plaques, use a tar shampoo (Polytar, Sebutone) for 10 minutes before rinsing. Presoften thick plaques with mineral oil the night before a morning shampoo; use a fine-toothed comb to remove loose scales.[9]
4. Avoid self-medication, particularly when receiving prescribed therapy.
5. Apply topical medications in a thin layer for most lesions; use a thick layer over plaques.
6. Monitor for side effects of medications (see Table 63-6).
7. Seek medical follow-up during periods of exacerbation.

## BULLOUS DISEASES

### Pemphigus Vulgaris

#### Etiology/epidemiology

The cause of pemphigus vulgaris is thought to have an autoimmune basis. Rare, but worldwide, pemphigus vulgaris occurs primarily in persons between the ages of 40 and 60, with a higher incidence among Jewish persons.

#### Pathophysiology

Pemphigus vulgaris is characterized by enormous bullae that appear all over the body and on the mucous membranes. Tissue injury results from circulating autoantibodies that bind to the structural proteins within the epidermis. Blister formation occurs above the stratum basalis. Healing is commonly associated with the development of postinflammatory hyperpigmentation, rather than scarring. The lesions break and are followed by crusts and scarring. The disease is characterized by *acantholysis* (cells slip past one another and fluid accumulates between the cells). By placing the thumb firmly on the skin and exerting lateral sliding pressure, the upper epidermis can be dislodged, resulting in erosion or blister *(Nikolsky's sign)*. A Tzanck test will identify acantholytic cells. Infection of the crust produces a foul odor, and toxemia may result. If the disease is untreated, death usually ensues in about 1 year, secondary to sepsis.

#### Collaborative care management

Hospitalization is usually required for skin care and monitoring of drug effects. The treatment of choice for severe pemphigus is systemic corticosteroids in large doses; the dose is gradually reduced as improvement is noted. Immunosuppressants—such as methotrexate, cyclophosphamide, and azathioprine—may be given to reduce the corticosteroid dose. Gold therapy (gold sodium thiomalate) may be given alone or in combination with corticosteroids for chronic therapy.

Nursing care of the person with severe pemphigus can be a challenge. Stryker frames may be used to help the person change position painlessly and to prevent weight bearing on raw surfaces. Air mattress or flotation systems may be used to reduce surface pressure on skin and promote comfort. Dakin's solution compresses may be applied to oozing lesions to help control odor and infection. Infection is a major concern because of the immunosuppressive effects of drug therapy. Special mouth care is required for mouth lesions, and bland diets are more easily tolerated.

**Patient/family education.** Emotional support and encouragement of both patient and family are extremely important. Patients may fear rejection because of their appearance, and they need evidence of continued family and staff interest and attention. The risk for altered body image and social isolation is high.

Patients and family should be taught general skin lesion care. The patient should be given information regarding medication use and side effects.

## TUMORS OF THE SKIN

Skin cell growths may develop from the epidermis, from sebaceous or sweat glands, from the melanocyte system, or from mesodermal tissue (for example, connective or vascular tissue). Most skin tumors are benign, and even those that are malignant—with the exception of such tumors as malignant melanoma—are often less serious than tumors elsewhere in the body.

### Keratosis (Benign Lesion)

The term *keratosis* refers to any cornification or growth of the horny layer of the skin. Different types of keratosis include corns and calluses, warts, and seborrheic and actinic (senile) keratosis (Table 63-7).

### Premalignant Lesions

Skin lesions that may lead to malignancy include actinic keratosis (as previously described), leukoplakia, Bowen's disease, and pigmented moles. The term *premalignant* does not imply that all of the lesions will become malignant but that the tendency to become malignant exists (Table 63-8).

### Malignant Lesions

Malignant lesions of the skin include squamous cell carcinoma, keratoanthoma, basal cell epitheliomas, and malignant melanoma (Table 63-9). See Chapter 67 for a discussion of AIDS-related Kaposi's sarcoma.

#### *Malignant melanoma*

**Etiology.** Malignant melanoma usually develops from a pigmented nevi, although it may arise from healthy skin. Three lesions are considered precursors of melanoma: *dysplastic nevi, congenital nevi,* and *lentigo maligna.* Chronic exposure is associated with its development. There is a genetic predisposition to melanoma; 10% of persons with melanoma have an affected parent or sibling.

**Epidemiology.** Malignant melanoma is increasing more rapidly than any other malignancy, with 34,100 new cases expected annually.[2] If in situ melanoma are included in this estimate, the number increases to 80,000 annually. Alarmingly, the death rate is also increasing and is second only to lung cancer. If current trends continue, in the year 2000, 1 in 90 Caucasian persons in the United States will develop melanoma. This increase may be due in part to increased sun exposure and a thinning of the ozone layer, in addition to other unknown and uncontrollable factors. Melanoma is more common in light-skinned persons. The lifetime risk of a Caucasian developing a melanoma is currently 1:150. Persons at risk include those with a previous melanoma, fair-skinned

**table 63-7** *Keratoses: Etiology, Appearance, and Treatment*

| Type of Lesion | Etiology | Appearance | Treatment |
|---|---|---|---|
| Corns | Pressure, ill-fitting shoes | Center core that thickens inwardly, pain with pressure, usually occur on toes | Felt pad with center hole to relieve pressure, properly fitting shoes; corn will recur if pressure not relieved |
| Callus | Constant pressure on plantar surface of foot; can also occur on palmar surface of hands | Thickening of horny layer of skin | Relief of pressure, regular massage with softening lotion or creams |
| Seborrheic keratoses (Figure 63-15, *A*) | Normal aging process, rarely develop into malignancy; must distinguish from actinic keratoses, which have malignancy potential | Large, darkened, greasy warts usually on trunk, less often on scalp, face, and proximal extremities; sudden increase in number and size may indicate a gastrointestinal malignancy | No treatment except for cosmetic reasons or constant irritation; may be removed by curettage, electrodesiccation, or liquid nitrogen |
| Dermatosis papulosa nigra | Seborrheic keratoses in African American persons | Small, pedunculated, heavily pigmented | Same as for seborrheic keratoses |
| Actinic keratoses (Figure 63-15, *B*) (senile, solar) | Chronic exposure to solar irradiation; occur on exposed areas of skin; light-skinned persons most vulnerable<br>Approximately 25% evolve to squamous cell carcinoma (evidenced by a rapid increase in size of lesion) | Round or irregular, red-brown to gray in color with dry, scaly appearance<br>Surrounding skin usually dry and wrinkled from overexposure to sun | Protective clothing, sunscreens; removal by curettage, liquid nitrogen therapy, dermabrasion, electrodesiccation, large lesions by excision; multiple lesions may be treated with topical application of 1-5% 5-fluorouracil cream |

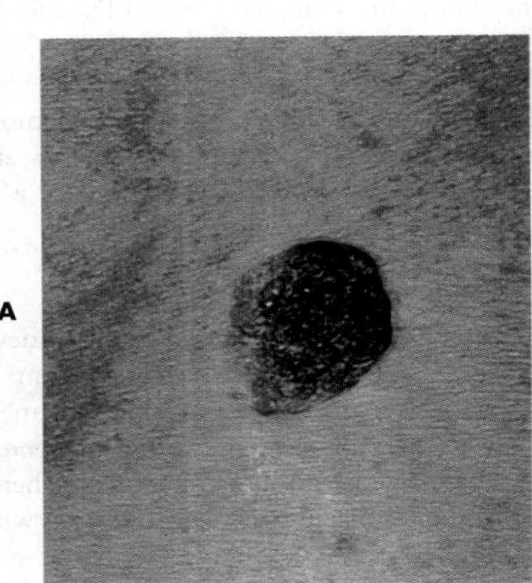


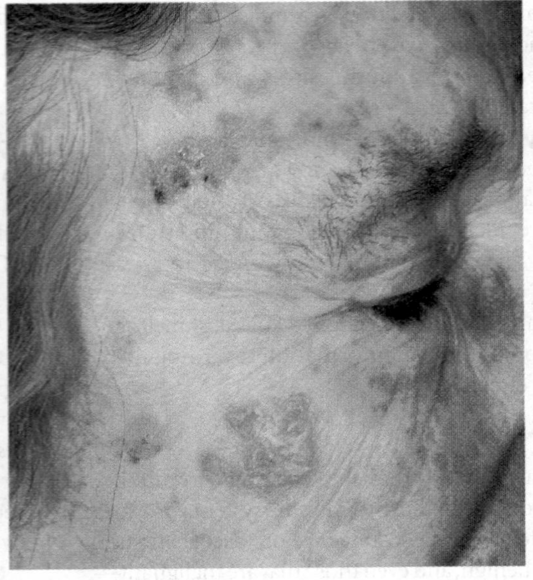


fig. 63-15 A, Seborrheic keratosis. B, Actinic (senile) keratosis.

**table 63-8** *Premalignant Lesions: Etiology, Appearance, and Treatment*

| Lesion | Etiology | Appearance | Treatment |
|---|---|---|---|
| Leukoplakia | Unknown causes and external irritants such as poor-fitting dentures, cheek biting, and pipe and cigarette smoking. Chronic maceration, friction, and senile atrophy may lead to vaginal leukoplakia. | Mucous membranes develop thickened, white patches of keratinized cells, which may eventually lead to squamous cell carcinoma.<br>Erythroplakia (red or red and white patches) of the mouth has a higher malignancy potential than leukoplakia. | Prevention by removal of causative factors; inspection of mouth, mucous membranes; dental care for rough teeth, proper-fitting dentures. Large lesions are usually surgically excised, and a biopsy is performed. Benign lesions may be removed by electrodesiccation. |
| Bowen's disease | Chemical carcinogens; occurs on older, light-skinned men.<br>Also called squamous cell carcinoma in situ.<br>Persons affected are at higher risk of developing other malignancies. | Widely distributed, sharply demarcated brown plaques, although a single lesion may exist. | Surgical excision, cryotherapy, curettage and electrodesiccation, carbon dioxide laser therapy, 5-fluorouracil cream or solution. |
| Pigmented nevi (moles) | Most are harmless, but others may be dysplastic, precancerous, or cancerous.<br>Changes in a mole that require immediate attention:<br>Development of a ring of new pigment around the base<br>Development of uneven pigmentation<br>Sudden growth<br>Loss of hair<br>Bleeding | Present on most persons regardless of skin color; may be flat, raised, prominent, or hairy. Color ranges from tan to black.<br>Dysplastic moles usually occur on the upper back in males and on the legs in females. (Refer to malignant melanoma section for further discussion.) | Biopsy and excision of suspicious lesions. To help remember the characteristics of malignant moles, the American Cancer Society has developed the mnemonic **ABCD**:<br>**A**symmetry of borders<br>**B**order irregularity<br>**C**olor blue-black or variegated<br>**D**iameter >6 mm |

persons, persons who tend to burn rather than tan, red- or blonde-haired persons, and persons with multiple nevi. The mean age of diagnosis is 40 years of age.

**Pathophysiology.** Major classifications of melanoma include lentigo maligna melanoma, superficial spreading melanoma, nodular melanoma, and acral-lentiginous melanoma. The most common is the superficial spreading type, which accounts for 70% of all melanomas.

Nodular melanoma carries the worst prognosis. Survival rates for primary localized melanomas after excision are 90% to 98%. The survival rate for other stages ranges from 5% to 80%.[2] Staging is based on tumor size, affected lymph nodes,

**table 63-9** *Malignant Lesions: Etiology, Appearance, and Treatment*

| Lesion | Etiology | Appearance | Treatment |
|---|---|---|---|
| Squamous cell carcinoma (Fig. 63-16) | Unknown; may arise from actinic keratoses, Bowen's disease, or leukoplakia | If precursor was premalignant lesion, the lesion will be indurated and surrounded by an inflammatory base. New lesions appear as a firm keratotic nodule with an indurated base. Lip or ear lesions may metastasize to regional lymph nodes. Lesions on hair-bearing areas rarely metastasize. | Prevention and early detection. Removal by excision, curettage with electrodesiccation, irradiation, or chemosurgery (for treatment of tumors without well-defined borders). A dressing is applied with a fixative paste such as zinc chloride; removal of the dressing removes malignant tissue. Reapplication is usually necessary. |
| Keratoanthoma | Occurs on normal skin areas exposed to sun, tar, oils; noninvasive and does not metastasize | Microscopically similar to squamous cell carcinoma. Grows rapidly to 1-2 cm, remains quiescent for 2-8 weeks, then regresses spontaneously. Dome-shaped, shiny, pink lesion contains a keratinous plug, which is expelled as the nodule shrinks. | Excision and biopsy. |
| Basal cell epithelioma | Unknown; most common malignant tumor affecting light-skinned persons over age 40; primarily occurs over hairy areas that contain pilosebaceous follicles | Translucent appearance, color from flesh to pale pink with a few telangiectatic vessels across the surface. Rarely metastatic if treated. | If untreated, tumors become locally invasive with severe tissue destruction, infection, and hemorrhage. If untreated, metastasizes to bone, lung, and brain. Treatment depends on site and extent of tumor: curettage with electrodesiccation, excision, irradiation, and chemosurgery. |
| Kaposi's sarcoma | Unknown; theories include viral causes, immunosuppression, and sexually transmitted agents. Categorized by groups affected:<br>Elderly men of Jewish and Mediterranean ancestry<br>Endemic in black Africans<br>Renal transplant recipients<br>AIDS related | Slowly progressing red, purple, or brown plaques or nodules scattered widely over the body on the skin or mucous membranes, especially the mouth. Lesions have been found in lymph nodes, gastrointestinal tract, and lungs. Lesions do not blanch with pressure and are painless. | Diagnosis by punch biopsy. Treatment options: surgery, radiation, and chemotherapy. Patients at high risk should be taught self-assessment for early detection of lesions. |

and metastases. The tumor arises from melanocytes. Responsible for the biosynthesis and transport of melanin, these cells are most commonly found in the basal layer of the epidermis and eye, but are also found in the meninges, alimentary and respiratory tracts, and lymph nodes. Contained in each melanocyte is a *melanosome,* an organelle that synthesizes the pigment. In melanoma, the melanosome is abnormal or absent. Atypical melanocytes proliferate along the basal layer of the epidermis; when the melanocytes invade the dermis, the lesion is considered malignant. There is a radical growth phase in each type of melanoma; the length of time of this phase varies. Melanoma is staged, as are other cancers, depending on the extent of tumor and metastases.

Tumors occur most commonly on the head, neck, and lower extremities. The lesions vary considerably in appearance, some with deep pigmentation, irregular borders, and

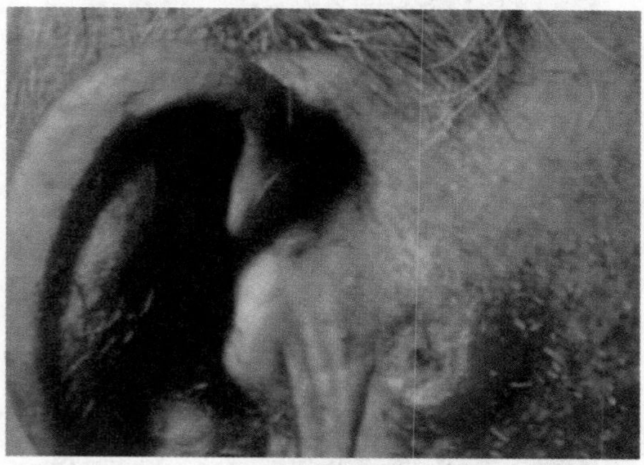

**fig. 63-16** Squamous cell carcinoma in infratemporal area, one of the most common sites for this tumor.

surrounding erythema, and others with irregular pigmentation (yellow, blue, black) and irregular surfaces (Figure 63-17). The rate of growth varies. Late changes include bleeding and ulceration. The incidence of metastasis from malignant melanoma is high and depends on the depth of invasion. Metastasis occurs first to the regional lymph nodes and then by hematogenous spread to the lungs, liver, and other areas.

#### Collaborative care management

***Diagnostic tests.*** As in all malignancies, confirmation of diagnosis is by biopsy. Suspicious pigmented lesions should be biopsied with sufficient margins to determine the depth of invasion and provide staging information. Electrocoagulation, curettage, shaving, and burning should not be used on a suspicious mole.

***Medications.*** Metastatic malignant melanoma is resistant to currently available systemic chemotherapeutic agents. The drug used most successfully is dacarbazine (DTIC), with an overall response rate of 10% to 28%, depending on disease site.[2] Indicated as treatment for surgically unresectable advanced metastatic melanoma, DTIC can be administered on an outpatient basis. Other chemotherapeutic agents with similar response rates but more toxicity include the nitrosureas and cisplatin. Some combinations of agents useful in treating metastatic disease include dacarbazine (DTIC), carmustine (BCNU), cisplatin, and tamoxifen; bleomycin, vindesine, lomustine (CCNU ), and dacarbazine (DTIC); and cisplatin and vincristine. Responses to these combinations are reportedly as high as 40% to 50% in persons with lung or soft tissue metastases.[2]

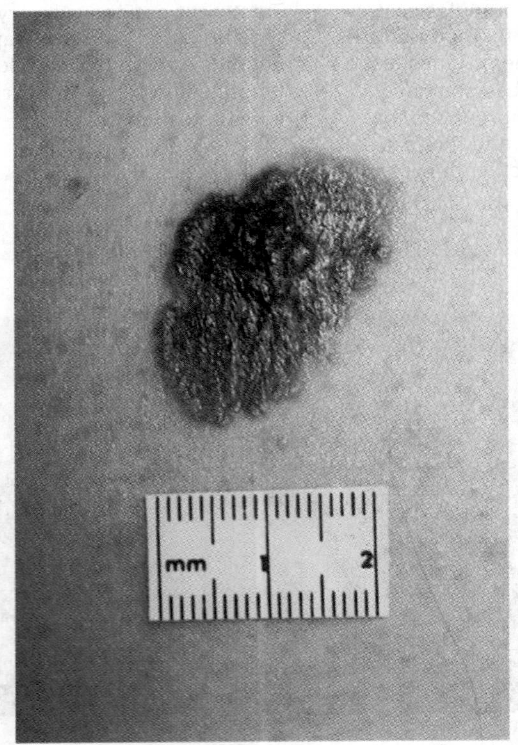


**fig. 63-17** Malignant melanoma. Note asymmetry of borders, size >6 mm, and color.

An expensive, investigational, and controversial treatment of advanced melanoma is isolated limb perfusion. Hyperthermia, in addition to vascular perfusion of chemotherapy through an isolated region, allows high concentrations of chemotherapeutic agents to be administered to the extremity with minimal systemic toxicity. The drug most commonly used in this technique is melphalan. Other drugs include thiotepa, cisplatin, and doxorubicin.

Patients with recurrent and in-transit metastases can also be treated with injection therapy with dinitrochlorobenzene (DNCB), and $CO_2$ laser vaporization. High-dose interferon has recently been shown to result in a small but significant improvement in both disease-free and overall survival rates. Interferon treatment is both costly and potentially toxic. Lower-dose interferon therapy results in less toxicity but does not result in a survival benefit. Radiation has not been clinically proven to be beneficial.

***Surgical management.*** Once the diagnosis of malignant melanoma is made, a wide excision is indicated. Removing an appropriate margin of tissue surrounding the lesion decreases the chance of local recurrence. Surgical margins for primary cutaneous melanoma are determined by the thickness of the lesion. Patients with intermediate-thickness melanoma may elect to undergo lymph node dissection, but long-term outcomes have not been improved by elective lymph node dissection. Therapeutic lymph node dissection is indicated for persons with clinically enlarged regional nodes, after cytological confirmation of metastatic disease. Fine-needle aspiration biopsy is the preferred method of biopsy because of the minimally invasive nature of the procedure. If needle biopsy is not possible, excisional biopsy is recommended before lymphadenectomy. Regional lymphadenectomy may be indicated for palliative purposes as well.

Many other types of surgical treatment of skin lesions are usually performed by dermatologists either in the office, ambulatory unit, or surgical suite. The following section discusses different types of dermatological surgery.

***Dermatological surgery.*** Treatment of skin lesions by dermatologists sometimes includes removal of skin lesions. Superficial skin lesions involving only the epidermis can be removed easily by various means; deep lesions involving the dermis, such as with some cancers, are removed with full-thickness skin excision.

*Tangential surgery.* Superficial lesions can be removed by slicing off the lesion with a sharp blade. It is especially useful for removal of flat lesions. The entire lesion may be removed for diagnosis. Hemostasis is obtained with pressure or gelatin foam.

*Curettage.* Curettage is the scraping or scooping out of a superficial lesion with a curette, a spoon-shaped, sharp-edged instrument. A local anesthetic is usually injected around the lesion before curettage (Figure 63-18). Hemostasis is accomplished with a chemical styptic, such as ferric chloride or Monsel's solution; with gelatin foam; or by electrocoagulation. Lesions that may be removed by curettage include seborrheic keratosis, actinic keratosis, basal cell epitheliomas, leukoplakia, warts, and nevi.

*Punch biopsy.* After the patient receives a local anesthetic, a punch is used to remove deep lesions up to 10 mm in diameter. The tissue is then sent for biopsy. Small punch biopsies may be closed with a suture. Larger biopsies may be partially closed; they then heal by secondary intention. Hemostasis can be obtained with gelatin foam packing. Punch biopsies are used for identification of basal cell carcinomas and for removal of small, deep, round lesions.

*Cryosurgery.* Tissue can be destroyed by rapid freezing with substances such as liquid oxygen, carbon dioxide snow or gas, liquid nitrogen, dichlorodifluoromethane (Freon), or nitrous oxide. Carbon dioxide snow and liquid nitrogen are most commonly used. The rapid freezing causes formation of intracellular ice, which destroys the cell membranes and produces cell dehydration. Cryosurgery is commonly used for removing skin tumors (benign and malignant), warts, and keloids.

Although the procedure usually is not painful, a tingling pain occurs when the freezing substance is applied and may be uncomfortable for some persons, particularly if multiple lesions are treated. Therefore a local anesthetic may be necessary. Analgesics may promote patient comfort during thawing.

Tissue necrosis may not be evident until 24 hours after cryosurgery. A clear or hemorrhagic bulla forms during the first day, but inflammatory reactions and bleeding are usually absent. A serous exudate occurs during the first week, followed by eschar or crust formation. The crust drops off in 3 to 4 weeks as the underlying tissue heals. Scarring usually results. Hypopigmentation may occur, because melanocytes are highly vulnerable to freezing.

*Electrosurgery.* Electric current may be used in dermatological surgery to remove tissue and to control bleeding. *Electrodesiccation* is the drying of tissue by means of a monopolar current through the needle electrode. *Electrofulguration* is a form of electrodesiccation in which the needle electrode is held close to, rather than inserted into, the tissue, thus spraying the area with sparks. Bipolar current is used for *electrocoagulation,* which coagulates the tissue, curtailing capillary bleeding, and for electrosection, which cuts the tissue. Delayed bleeding may occur, especially from electrocoagulation, and may alarm the unprepared patient. The bleeding can be easily controlled by direct pressure.

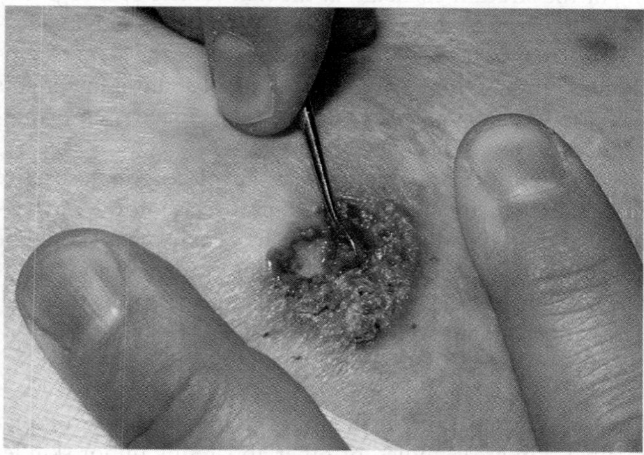

**fig. 63-18** Curettage of inflamed seborrheic keratosis.

Electrosurgery is usually performed after the patient has received a local anesthetic. Sedation is rarely necessary. After most uses of electrosurgery, the wound is left exposed for air drying. Dressings may be used if the area is subject to frequent trauma or rubbing or if oozing is present. The wound may be wiped with 70% alcohol to hasten drying. A hemostatic nonocclusive dressing may be made by covering the wound with Gelfoam powder and tape.

**Diet.** No special diet is prescribed for persons undergoing dermatological surgery. The patient should, however, be encouraged to have a nutritionally balanced diet both preoperatively and postoperatively to enhance healing of tissues.

**Referrals.** If the lesion removed was malignant, the patient may benefit from a referral to a support group, the American Cancer Society, or a hospice. If the patient's family is involved as primary caregivers, they may need periodic relief from their responsibilities. Referrals to social services may be indicated depending on the individual patient and family situation.

## NURSING MANAGEMENT OF THE PATIENT UNDERGOING DERMATOLOGICAL SURGERY

### PREOPERATIVE CARE

Regardless of the type and extent of the surgery, the patient and family need preoperative teaching. This may be done in a variety of settings, depending on the type of procedure planned. Teaching should include specifics regarding the location and extent of incision, any postoperative activity limitations, and any special postoperative care needs. Information should be included regarding the anesthetic options available. See Chapter 18 for further discussion of preoperative preparation of the patient.

### POSTOPERATIVE CARE

After surgery, the patient will require care and monitoring as described in Chapter 20. If a malignant lesion was removed, the patient is followed closely, checked at 3-month intervals for the subsequent 2 years, and then checked annually.

If metastasis occurs, the nursing care focuses on helping the patient understand the treatment and its side effects. The patient is confronted with many physical problems, as well as psychoemotional problems such as fear of cancer, loss of health, and fear of dying (see Chapters 8 and 11).

After superficial skin surgery, the patient is instructed not to remove the crust (scab), which acts as a protection (healing occurs under the crust). The crust should be kept as dry as possible; if it gets wet, it should be patted dry. Alcohol may be applied and allowed to evaporate. Makeup may be used over the crust. The crust may be left uncovered or may be covered with an adhesive bandage. Signs of redness, edema, or pain should be reported to the surgeon.

After deep skin surgery, the wound is usually bandaged and the patient is given specific instructions for care by the surgeon. Aspirin should be avoided for 7 days before and after surgery because of its anticoagulant properties, which may lead to postoperative bleeding.

The patient and family will require an explanation about the treatments that may be performed postoperatively or prescribed for home care. They will also require teaching regarding the care of healthy skin and steps to prevent further damage to the skin. A discussion of such topics follows.

### Avoiding Causative Agents

The first step in preventing dermatological conditions is avoiding the causative agent, which may be a specific antigen, a contact irritant, a microorganism, trauma, direct sunlight, or an insect. Instructing the person to avoid a known causative agent is preventive medicine; however, it may not be that simple. Many dermatological diseases have no known cause or are hereditary. Unfortunately, once the mechanism of the disease is known, it is not always possible to remove the triggering factors. Occasionally, symptoms may persist long after the agent is removed. Therefore major responsibilities of the nurse include education of the patient about measures that promote rest, methods that decrease emotional stress, the need for good nutrition, and the need to closely observe sites to determine changes in skin conditions.

### Cleansing

Bathing is an essential element of skin care. The frequency of skin cleansing is individualized according to need and patient preference. The outer layer of skin cells and the perspiration are acidic, and their presence inhibits the life and growth of harmful bacteria. However, a normal flora of bacteria grow in acidity and act as the skin's protection. Strong soaps that are alkaline in reaction may neutralize this protective acid condition of the skin. They may also remove the oily secretion of the sebaceous glands, which lubricates the outer skin layers and contributes to their health. Removal of excess oil and scale or debris is sometimes necessary to facilitate the absorption of medication, promote healing, and enhance the appearance of the skin. In psoriasis, for example, removal of scale by mechanical means and slowing of skin metabolism are prime objectives.

Normal skin should be washed often enough to remove excess oils and excretions and to prevent odor. Care must be taken not to cause drying or irritation. After showering, the skin can be patted dry and lotion applied to prevent drying. Maintaining a proper degree of hydration in the skin prevents dryness and itching, which may lead to scratching, excoriation, and further trauma. Hydrating the stratum corneum, or outer layer of skin, may be accomplished by soaking in a tub of water for 20 to 30 minutes and then immediately applying a lubricating lotion or cream. This application of a cream prevents the rapid loss of water from the skin surface.

### Sunlight

Sunlight, particularly UV light, is damaging to the skin. Ultraviolet light is termed *actinic,* meaning photochemically active radiation. UVA light contributes to aging and carcinogenesis of the skin.[6] UVB light leads to burning and activation of melanin, which produces tanning. Suntans eventually lead to permanent roughening and wrinkling of the skin; therefore there is no such thing as a "safe tan." Tanning parlors should be avoided because they use UV light to produce the tan. Long-term sun exposure is the major cause of skin cancer.

The way to protect against UV rays is to block the rays. The rays may be blocked by opaque clothing, umbrellas, hats, or other screening aids; by avoiding sun exposure between 10 AM and 3 PM; or by selected sunscreens. The best sunscreens have a sun protection factor (SPF) of 15 or more. Sunscreens are removed easily with water and must be reapplied after swimming or heavy sweating. Lips must be protected with sunscreens or dark lipstick. Ultraviolet light has stronger effects at high altitudes (where there is less atmosphere to absorb the rays) and at the equator (where the sun is closer to the earth); therefore additional protection is required in these places. Persons who have been diagnosed as having a skin condition that is aggravated by UV light or who are taking photosensitive drugs should avoid the sun, if possible, or ensure adequate protection. Lesions caused by photosensitivity resulting from certain medications appear abruptly and are widespread, symmetrical, and bright red. Medications that enhance photosensitivity include penicillin, antihypertensives, diuretics, oral hypoglycemics, and NSAIDs.

### Nutrition

Balanced nutrition plays an important role in preventing the occurrence of skin lesions. The nutrients considered essential to the maintenance of healthy skin include protein, vitamin C, iron, and zinc. Some skin lesions may be directly associated with dietary intake. Excessive dryness of the skin and thickening of the stratum corneum at the hair follicle openings may be caused by nutritional deficiencies. Elevated blood lipid levels caused by hyperlipoproteinemia may take the form of xanthomas on the skin surface. Restriction of sodium in patients who are receiving glucocorticoid steroids may lessen or prevent edema as a side effect.

Hypersensitive individuals may be placed on restrictive diets to exclude intake of known causative agents or as a diagnostic tool to identify causative agents. Food labels should be read carefully to determine whether the product or food additive contains the agent the hypersensitive person is to avoid. The patient should know the type of diet to be followed.

### Observations of Changes

Care of normal skin includes regular observation of pigmented skin areas, moles, or other apparently minor skin lesions. Any change in size, color, or general appearance should be reported to a physician at once because a change in moles or new skin growths is one of the danger signals of cancer. The patient should be taught the warning signs of skin lesions (see Chapter 62).

### Dangers of Self-Treatment

People should be urged to seek medical help when skin conditions develop. Although skin diseases rarely cause death, they may be reflections of serious systemic illness and can account for much discomfort and for serious interruption of work and other activities. Many persons are inclined to rely on the advice of friends or the local druggist or on medications they may have on hand. Each individual's skin reacts differently to treatment, and the skin that is already irritated or diseased may respond violently to inexpert treatment. Because of changes in the skin, medications prescribed previously for a similar skin ailment in the same patient may not produce a favorable response. Medications may deteriorate, and for this reason old medications are not safe. Medications without expiration dates should be discarded. The person may be spared much discomfort and expense by consulting a specialist when symptoms first develop and before a mild skin condition becomes a serious problem.

### Psychological Care

A certain degree of "beauty orientation" exists in Western culture. Beauty pageants are popular, and advertisements in the media use beautiful models to attract the reader. Beauty is culturally defined. Cosmetics to enhance good looks are extensively used by women, as well as men. Therefore skin diseases or physical defects that detract from "good looks" often produce psychological reactions.

A person's emotional reaction to a deformity or defect must not be underestimated. Pride in oneself and the ability to think well of oneself and to regard oneself favorably in comparison with others are essential to the development and maintenance of a well-integrated personality. Every person who has a defect or is physically challenged, particularly if the defect is conspicuous to others, suffers from some threat to emotional security. The extent of the emotional reaction and the amount of maladjustment that follows depend on the individual's personality and ability to cope with emotional insults. Disfigurements almost invariably lead to disturbing experiences. The child who has webbed fingers may be ridiculed at school; the adolescent girl who has acne scars may be self-conscious and avoid social situations; and the young man with a posttraumatic scar on his face may be refused a sales job. Under any of these circumstances, the individual may withdraw from a society that is unkind. The defect may be used to justify failure, avoid responsibility, or justify striking out against an unkind society.

Skin diseases that produce marked disfigurement of visible body surfaces can alter the person's body image. Feelings of decreased worth by persons with large, draining lesions or with severe disfigurement are reinforced during interactions with others. Some people are repelled when viewing persons with severe skin diseases, or they may experience a threat to their own body integrity and physically withdraw to avoid interaction. Persons may also experience nonverbal messages of disgust when others view them for the first time. This can be even more disturbing when those nonverbal messages are sent by significant others or by health professionals. In working with the person with severe skin disease, the nurse first examines his or her own feelings that could be expressed nonverbally in a negative manner.

### Relief of Pruritus

*Pruritus,* or itching, is a cutaneous symptom that provokes the desire to scratch and is caused by repetitive low-frequency stimulation of C fibers. These C fibers are similar to but different from the C fibers that transmit pain stimuli. Itching can be produced by mechanical stimulation of the skin or by chemical mediators, primarily the kinins. Itching occurs only in the skin, certain mucous membranes, and the eyes. The areas most sensitive to itching are the nostrils, mucocutaneous junctions, external ear canals, and perineum.

Pruritus can be caused by any irritating substance that interrupts the stratum corneum layer of the skin, or it can be a result of certain systemic diseases (Box 63-1). Not all infectious diseases that produce rashes cause itching. One of the most common causes is dry skin, sometimes occurring as a result of excessive bathing, particularly with "bubble bath," which has a drying effect. Factors that can intensify itching include vasodilation, tissue anoxia, and circulatory stasis. Whatever the cause, pruritus ranges from an annoyance to a severe, distressing, or exhausting problem.

Pruritus leads to the motor response of scratching. Persons with intense itching may severely excoriate the skin by digging deeply into the skin with their fingernails when trying to alleviate the itch. Persons with generalized itching may be observed to be in almost constant motion—twisting, rubbing, and scratching.

A major step in treating patients with pruritus is to attempt to remove the itch stimuli and break the itch-scratch cycle. Cold causes vasoconstriction and will provide some relief. Hydration in a tepid bath followed by the application of an emollient lotion is helpful. Cornstarch or oatmeal preparations may be added to the bath. Topical corticosteroids decrease inflammation leading to vasoconstriction. In some persons, antihistamines, such as diphenhydramine, or tranquilizers are of value.

**box 63-1** *Common Causes of Pruritus*

- Dry skin
- Skin irritants: plastic or glass fibers, wool, plant products, insects
- Drug reactions
- Psychogenic reactions
- Infectious diseases
- Infestation: hookworm
- Systemic diseases: obstructive biliary disease, uremia, diabetes mellitus
- Neoplasia: Hodgkin's disease, leukemia, lymphoma

**table 63-10** *Preparations Commonly Used for Baths or Soaks*

| Substance | Effect | Suggested Actions |
|---|---|---|
| Colloids: oatmeal, cornstarch, soybean powder | Antipruritic, drying | Tub surfaces become very slippery; support person to prevent falls. |
| Potassium permanganate $KMNO_4$ | Antifungal, drying, deodorizing | Strain pulverized tablet through cheesecloth to prevent irritation; stains surfaces and linens. |
| Burow's solution (aluminum acetate) | Antibacterial, drying | Commonly used for soaks. |
| Sulfur bath suspension | Antibacterial | Rinse body with tepid water after bath to remove residual sulfur particles. |
| Tar preparations: Balnetar, Zetar, Alma-Tar, Polytar | Antipruritic, moisturizing | Do not use soap with tar baths. |
| Bath oils: Alpha-Keri, Jeri-Bath, Domol | Antipruritic, moisturizing | Tub surfaces may become slippery. |

The awareness of pruritus may be more acute during the night because of a decrease in diverting stimuli. Cool, light, nonrestrictive bed clothing may help allay itching. Excessive drying of the skin caused by high room temperature and low humidity can also increase pruritus. Pruritus occurs readily in an elderly person who already has dry skin. Usually a room temperature of 20° C (68° to 70° F) and humidity of 30% to 40% are best for the person with pruritus.

### Temperature Control

Temperature control is an important need in persons with dermatological problems. The individual who has a generalized flush, or erythema, and the one who has an extensive exfoliative dermatitis may be losing body heat at an abnormally increased rate and may need a room temperature of 32.2° C (90° F) or more to maintain normal body temperature. Care must be taken to avoid chilling, particularly after baths, when compresses are used, or when parts of the body are exposed. The person with pruritus benefits from a cool environment.

### Therapeutic Baths and Soaks

Baths or soaks may be prescribed to remove exudates from an affected extremity, to moisturize or dry the skin, to relieve pruritus, or to provide antibacterial or antifungal therapy (Table 63-10). Frequent baths or soaks tend to dry the skin; the application of lotion or cream immediately after a bath or soak will moisturize the skin.

Hard crusts or thickened exudates from skin disorders are often soaked with physiological saline solution, peroxide, or mild soap in warm water. These crusts or exudates are removed only when prescribed by the physician.

Tub baths may be given to cleanse the skin before therapy (such as for psoriasis), to relieve general body pruritus, or to provide therapy (for example, potassium permanganate, sulfur, or tar baths). During cleansing baths, special attention is given to intertriginous areas, where creams and topical medications may collect. Persons with arthropathic psoriasis may find it difficult to use a tub because of limited mobility. A lift may be used with the hospitalized patient; if a lift is not available, sitting on a chair under a gentle shower is the next best alternative to a cleansing bath. Guidelines for therapeutic baths and soaks are described in the Guidelines for Care Box.

**guidelines for care**

**Baths and Soaks**

1. The water temperature should be of comfort to patient (usually 32° to 38° C, or 90° to 100° F).
2. Medication should be completely dissolved while tub is filling.
3. The soak should last 20 to 30 minutes.
4. To prevent patient falls when oils or colloids are added to the water, persons are assisted in and out of the water.
5. A rubber mat will help prevent slipping.
6. The skin is *patted,* not rubbed, dry to avoid skin irritation.
7. Creams or ointments are applied *immediately* after the bath to retain skin moisture.
8. After a medicated bath, cleanse tub as follows:
   a. Pour 1 cup of bleach into used tub water.
   b. Let bleach stand in water for 5 minutes.
   c. Wipe sides and bottom of tub.
   d. Drain tub and clean as usual.

### Topical Medications

Applications of medications to the skin surface may take many forms. Wet dressings, creams, pastes, ointments, and lotion can be used. The nurse should know the purpose for which a local application is ordered, the drugs contained in the preparation, and any toxic signs that may occur from the preparation's use.

#### *Types of topical medications*

Many different topical medications are used for persons with dermatological problems. Antibacterial or antifungal topical medications (Table 63-11) are used for bacterial or fungal infections.

Corticosteroids are among the most commonly used drugs because of their antiinflammatory, vasoconstrictive, and antipruritic effects. Topical corticosteroids differ in their antiinflammatory effects, ranging from low to very high potency. Hydrocortisone is of low potency. Some corticosteroids, such as triamcinolone acetonide (Aristocort, Kenalog), vary in potency depending on the dose. Greasy ointments are usually more potent and have a greater lubricating effect than creams. Fluorinated corticosteroids are powerful agents and may

**table 63-11** *Common Topical Antibiotic and Antifungal Medications*

| Generic Name | Trade Name | Vehicle | Comments |
|---|---|---|---|
| **ANTIBACTERIAL** | | | |
| Bacitracin | Baciguent | Ointment | Effective against gram-positive organisms (nonprescription) |
| Neomycin, bacitracin, and polymyxin B | Neosporin | Cream, ointment | Broad-spectrum antibiotic effect |
| Bacitracin and polymyxin B | Polysporin | Ointment | Same as Neosporin |
| Gentamicin | Garamycin | Cream, ointment | Broad-spectrum antibiotic |
| Chloramphenicol | Chloromycetin | Cream | Broad-spectrum antibiotic |
| Clioquinol | Vioform | Lotion, cream, ointment | Has both antibacterial and antifungal effects; useful for eczema and tinea |
| Nitrofurazone | Furacin | Solution, cream, ointment | Broad-spectrum antibiotic |
| Povidone-iodine | Betadine | Solution | Kills gram-negative and gram-positive organisms, fungi, viruses, protozoa, yeasts |
| Mafenide | Sulfamylon | Cream | Effective against both gram-positive and gram-negative bacteria; used for burns |
| Silver sulfadiazine | Silvadene | Cream | Effective against bacteria and yeast; used for burns |
| **ANTIFUNGAL** | | | |
| Tolnaftate | Tinactin Pitrex | Powder, cream, solution | Useful for tinea |
| Nystatin | Mycostatin Nilstat | Powder, cream, ointment | Useful against wide variety of yeasts, especially *Candida* |
| Amphotericin B | Fungizone | Lotion, cream, ointment | Effective against *Candida* |
| Clotrimazole | Lotrimin | Cream, solution, lotion | Broad-spectrum antifungal |
| Haloprogin | Halotex | Cream, solution | Synthetic agent useful for superficial fungal infections |
| Miconazole nitrate | Micatin | Cream, lotion, powder | Synthetic agent useful for tinea |

cause epidermal, dermal, and subcutaneous atrophy, leading to development of petechiae and ecchymoses, as well as to irritation and burning. The fluorinated corticosteroids are not used on the face, where they may cause a rosacea-like dermatitis. Systemic effects are unlikely with the less potent topical corticosteroids but may occur with drugs of high potency.

Occlusive dressings potentiate the effect of topical corticosteroids and other medications. An airtight plastic film is applied over medicated skin, producing moisture retention, skin maceration, and decreased evaporation, which enhances the effects of the medication. Occlusion is primarily for (1) dermatoses of palms and soles, (2) psoriatic lesions on smooth bare skin, (3) localized patches of lichenified dermatitis, and (4) extensive, severe, steroid-responsive dermatitis. The affected area should be occluded only when prescribed by the physician. Plastic wrap is good for occluding small areas. Plastic gloves may be used on hands and plastic bags on feet. Plastic garment bags or large trash bags may be used for the trunk, with holes cut for head and arms. Plastic suits are available for total body occlusion. Lesions are usually occluded at night, usually not for more than 8 hours at a time. Plastic suits are usually worn during the day for 4 hours. The patient should be monitored for potential complications, including candidal infections, sweat retention, and folliculitis.

### Vehicles for topical medications

Topical medications can be prepared in a variety of bases (Table 63-12). Powders are effective in reducing friction and moisture in intertriginous areas. Lotions must be shaken well, because the insoluble powder may settle. The addition of alcohol increases the cooling effect of a lotion. Ointments do not usually leave an oily residue on the skin unless they have a petrolatum base. A nonporous covering, such as plastic, should not be used over an ointment unless so prescribed,

**table 63-12** *Comparison of Vehicles for Topical Medications*

| Base | Effect |
|---|---|
| **POWDER** | |
| Dry | Drying by absorbing moisture; cooling by evaporating moisture |
| **LOTION** | |
| Powder suspended in water or oil | Protective, cleansing, cooling, antipruritic effect depending on drug and base used |
| **CREAMS AND OINTMENTS** | |
| Emulsions of oil and water | Covering the skin to prolong contact of medication with skin—good skin penetration; warming effect |
| **PASTE** | |
| 50% or more powder in ointment base | Holds medication for long period with slower skin penetration |

because the heat retention may increase percutaneous absorption of the medication.

### Application of topical medications

Gloves are worn for protection when applying topical medications. Powders should first be sprinkled into the gloved hand and then applied to the skin to avoid getting excess powder into the air and thus causing irritation to the mucous membrane. Powders should be used sparingly to prevent caking and should not be used on wet surfaces, because this leads to caking. Cornstarch is *not* suggested because it encourages growth of yeast, bacteria, and fungi.

Lotions with a water or alcohol base are applied by patting gently. A gauze pledget should be used for applying extremely thin lotions. Lotions with an oily base are applied thinly and evenly with the palm of the gloved hand. A small area of skin is often tested to determine whether the person will tolerate the cream or lotion over the entire body. The topical medication is applied to a small (silver-dollar size) area on the person's forearm. The time and the exact location of the trial are recorded, and the skin response to the trial medication is read 24 hours later. Crude coal tar is commonly tested in this manner.

Ointments may be applied with gloved hands. If a dressing is to be applied, the ointment may be spread on the dressing with a tongue blade before application to the skin. Anthralin may be caustic to normal skin, so gloves should always be worn. Crude coal tar is always applied in firm, long, downward strokes to prevent folliculitis, because tar is an irritant. Creams, as opposed to ointments, may be rubbed in.

Some topical medications, such as crude coal tar, are often removed before other treatments. Crude coal tar must be removed in the morning before ultraviolet light therapy by applying corn oil in long, downward strokes over the skin surface and then wiping with gauze pledgets, leaving a thin film of tar. A general rule is to remove only the excess ointment or ointments having a consistency of cold cream before a bath or wet dressing. Cottonseed oil or a gauze pledget may be used to remove caked, oil-based lotions.

## Medicated Dressings

### Open wet dressings

Wet dressings are used over various skin lesions for cooling, drying, antipruritic, vasoconstricting, or debriding effects. Plain tap water or physiological saline may be used, or medications may be added. An astringent effect may be obtained through the use of Burow's solution (Domeboro, Buro-Sol, Bluboro), 1:20 or 1:40 dilution. Potassium permanganate ($KMnO_4$), one 300 mg tablet in 1500 ml (1:5000) or one 300 mg tablet in 3000 ml (1:10,000), has an antimicrobial and drying effect. All tablet crystals must be thoroughly dissolved to prevent chemical burning of the skin. Potassium permanganate should not be used on the face. Silver nitrate ($AgNO_3$), 0.5%, is also an antimicrobial and is often used in the treatment of burns. Both $KMnO_3$ and $AgNO_3$ stain skin and cloth.

The type of dressing material used for a wet dressing should be one without cotton filling, because cotton leaves particles and a residue on the skin, which may cause irritation. Several layers of fine-mesh gauze are ideal, and roller gauze or Kerlix may be used for extremities. A mask for the face may be designed by cutting out openings for the eyes, nose, and mouth from several thicknesses of gauze. At home the person can use lint-free, muslin-type cotton material such as old clean sheets, handkerchiefs, cloth diapers, or muslin dish towels. These materials need not be sterilized but should be washed or discarded every 24 hours.

The best effects of wet dressings are obtained by several treatment periods spaced across the person's waking hours. The solution is applied at room temperature to prevent the marked vasoconstriction with subsequent vasolidation that occurs with cold solutions (see the Guidelines for Care Box). Although the dressings can be kept wet by adding solution with the dressings in place, this practice usually leads to excessive dripping. Dressings *must* be removed, soaked, and reapplied when $KMnO_4$ or $AgNO_3$ is used, because evaporation can increase the solute on the dressings, increasing the dose and causing a chemical burn or irritation. Occlusive plastic wraps should be avoided unless specifically ordered by the physician.

### Closed wet dressings

Wet dressings can be covered with a nonpermeable material, such as plastic wrap, specifically to retain heat, if an early abscess is present, to soften excessive keratinized tissue, or to enhance penetration of a topical medication. This method is not commonly used, because interference with evaporation contributes to skin maceration.

### Wet-to-dry dressings

Wet-to-dry dressings are used to debride wounds or ulcerations. A fine-mesh gauze is moistened with the prescribed solution, placed over the lesion, and allowed to dry. The crust and debris are removed as the dressing is pulled off dry. This process is usually repeated every 4 to 8 hours. Normal saline

**guidelines for care**

**Applying Open Wet Dressings**

1. Prepare solution to be applied at room temperature. Sterility is not required.
2. Soak dressing thoroughly in solution.
3. Protect bed or clothing with towels, bath blanket, flannel squares, etc.
4. Wring out dressings—they should be wet but not dripping.
5. Apply dressings in smooth layers (two to four layers) to involved areas. Wrap fingers and toes separately, and wrap joints so that they can bend.
6. Remove, soak, and reapply dressings *before* they dry (that is, every 3 to 5 minutes).
7. Continue treatment for 20 to 30 minutes.
8. Pat skin dry.

solution is the most common solution used; however, half-strength Dakin's solution is also used for this purpose.

## GERONTOLOGICAL CONSIDERATIONS

In general, the elderly adult is at higher risk for alterations in integumentary function because of a variety of factors, including the normal aging process, with its associated changes in the skin, and the environment, particularly the sun. In one study, 75% of persons over 64 years of age were found to have cherry angiomas.[5] Although these are benign lesions, the patient may need education and reassurance regarding the nature of the lesion. Types of melanoma common in the elderly include lentigo melanoma and acral-lentiginous melanoma, which have a mean age at diagnosis of 60 years.

An elderly patient undergoing dermatologic surgery is at increased risk simply because of age. Many elderly persons have multiple coexisting chronic diseases, which adds to the morbidity and mortality rate. For further discussion of the needs of the elderly postoperative patient, see Chapter 20.

## SPECIAL ENVIRONMENTS FOR CARE

### Home Care

Many persons with dermatological disorders are not hospitalized; therefore patient teaching is an important component of nursing care. Key points of discussion for patient teaching are described in the Guidelines for Care Box. It is best to *write out* instructions specifically, because verbal instructions are easily forgotten. Preprinted teaching protocols provide an effective adjunct to adult learning. Patients often apply medications in excess amounts or with vigorous rubbing; these procedures may counteract all benefits or make the condition worse.

***guidelines for care***

**Teaching the Person with a Dermatological Disorder**

1. Nature of the disorder (cause, preventive measures, acuity or chronicity, symptoms requiring medical follow-up)
2. Treatment modalities to be carried out at home (soaks, baths, medicated dressings)
3. Special precautions to be observed during treatment, such as the following:
   a. Avoiding nonporous coverings over dressings, unless ordered
   b. Completely dissolve tablets or crystals in baths or soaks
   c. Avoiding excessive rubbing of medication over lesions
   d. Applying thin layers of lotions or powders
4. Prescribed medication regimens: route of administration, vehicle to be used, dose, frequency, duration of topical application, side effects, where supplies can be obtained.
5. Ways to promote socialization with others when disfiguring dermatological lesions are present

Dressing procedures are sometimes costly and complex. These patients will benefit from a home health referral to assist with teaching, as well as community financial resources.

# PRESSURE ULCERS

## ETIOLOGY

*Pressure ulcers* are defined by the National Pressure Ulcer Advisory Panel (NPUAP) as lesions caused by unrelieved pressure against soft tissue, usually over bony prominences. For many years, pressure ulcers were incorrectly termed *decubitus ulcers.* The Latin definition of the term *decubitus* implies lying flat, and *decubitus* was therefore correctly changed to *pressure* after it was ascertained that one could develop a pressure ulcer while assuming any body position, in any body location, and from any source of pressure (internal, as well as external). Risk factors for pressure ulcers include moisture, nutritional deficits, shear stress, alterations in mobility and perception, and abnormal serum albumin and hemoglobin levels.

## EPIDEMIOLOGY

Pressure ulcers are nonselective; that is, they can occur among those in any age-group or any ethnic population and regardless of socioeconomic status. Attempts have been made to estimate the financial burden of the pressure ulcer problem; however, research has been limited and inconsistent. Some studies estimate that $11.5 billion is expended annually on products for pressure ulcer management. Attempts to estimate the cost of an individual pressure ulcer also have been unsuccessful. Conservative estimates of the cost of treatment for one pressure ulcer range from $5000 to $30,000.

The NPUAP reviewed over 800 available manuscripts in an attempt to define the scope of the problem and has concluded that the incidence and prevalence of pressure ulcers in various health care settings are high enough to warrant concern. Clinical Practice Guidelines,[1] nationally accepted standards of care, were established and reviewed for validity based on that manuscript review.

Estimates of the prevalence of pressure ulcers in skilled care facilities are approximately 23%; in acute care facilities, 9%; and much greater in certain high-risk populations, such as patients with a spinal cord injury. An estimated 60,000 people die annually because of complications from pressure ulcers.

## PATHOPHYSIOLOGY

Unrelieved pressure causes cellular necrosis. The cellular necrosis occurs from vascular insufficiency and causes tissue destruction. The pathophysiology of pressure ulcers is outlined in Table 63-13. Box 63-2 presents the stages of pressure ulcers.

## COLLABORATIVE CARE MANAGEMENT

Pressure ulcers have been identified as primarily a nursing problem, but they require collaboration with the entire health

**table 63-13** *Normal Function, Pathophysiology, and Clinical Manifestations of Pressure Ulcers*

| Normal Function | Pathophysiology | Clinical Manifestations |
|---|---|---|
| Microvasculature: capillaries supply tissue needs of oxygenated blood and nutrients | Pressure applied to soft tissue compresses capillaries, distorting structure and occluding blood flow | Ischemia at first, followed by reactive hyperemia |
| Sympathetic response | Compensation by increased shunting of capillary circulation to area under pressure; capillaries increase permeability and leak fluid into tissues | Tissue edema and inflammation |
| Capillary walls lined with endothelial cells; platelets flow smoothly through microvessels | Endothelial cells disrupted, platelets aggregate, and thrombi form in capillaries and lead to cellular death | Erythema that may or may not resolve once pressure source is removed |
| Intact skin as the body's protective mechanism | Cellular death leads to tissue necrosis | Pressure ulcer with visible tissue damage, described by stages (Box 63-2) |

**box 63-2** *Stages of Pressure Ulcers*

STAGE 1

Nonblanchable erythema, redness that remains present over an area under pressure 30 minutes after pressure source is removed. Epidermis remains intact.

STAGE 2

Epidermis is broken, superficial lesion, no measurable depth. Partial-thickness skin loss.

STAGE 3

Full-thickness skin loss down through the dermis, may include subcutaneous tissue, may undermine adjacent skin.

STAGE 4

Full-thickness skin loss extending into supportive structures, such as muscle, tendon, and bone; may undermine and have various sinus tracts.

NOTE: If eschar (dead leathery tissue) is present, pressure ulcers cannot be accurately staged.

care team for effective resolution. Management includes interventions designed to control chronic disease symptomatology that affects healthy integument, such as medication regulation to keep glucose levels within normal limits and measures to promote optimal tissue perfusion and oxygenation. The correct product for treatment of pressure ulcers must be ordered. Products chosen inappropriately for wound management could cause more tissue damage or delay healing. A discussion of common treatment modalities for management of pressure ulcers follows.

### Diagnostic Tests

No specific laboratory tests assist with diagnosis of pressure ulcers. Related laboratory examinations pertinent to risk factors may be used. Open, draining ulcers may require culture and sensitivity to identify pathogens and determine appropriate antibiotics.

### Medications

There are no particular medications for pressure ulcers. Antibiotics are used if an infection is present.

### Treatment

More than 100 products exist as purported treatment measures for pressure ulcers. These are discussed in Table 63-14.

### Surgical Management

Some patients with wounds qualify for surgical intervention. Surgeons perform myocutaneous flaps and skin grafts of various levels, depending on the patient's physical condition, compliance level, and type of wound. Surgical interventions are discussed in Chapter 64.

### Diet

Patients with wounds require additional protein and calorie intake to assist with tissue regeneration on a cellular level. A well-balanced diet is sufficient to maintain healthy skin; however, most patients with any identified risk factors are not eating a well-balanced diet. Protein supplementation in balanced amounts is helpful. Only a registered dietitian can accurately determine a balance of demand and replacement that will be therapeutic for the patient. Research also suggests that supplemental vitamin C and zinc, as well as a multiple vitamin with iron, help stimulate wound healing on a cellular level.

### Activity

As discussed earlier, the more independently active the patient is, the lower the risk of pressure ulcer formation and the greater the chances of wound healing. The key factor related to wound healing is the removal of the causative agent(s). Regardless of the treatment prescribed for wound care, if the pressure is not relieved by the patient or the nurse, wound healing will not occur.

### Referrals

Many disciplines have become involved with wound-healing modalities. Physical therapists receive some education about

**table 63-14** *Products Used to Treat Pressure Ulcers*

| CATEGORY | EXAMPLE |
|---|---|
| **EXUDATE ABSORPTION** | |
| Dextronomer beads | Debrisan |
| Copolymer starch dressings | Absorption dressing<br>Duoderm granules |
| Calcium alginates (absorb exudate, as well as release calcium on a cellular level—stimulates angiogenesis) | Kaltostat<br>Sorbsan<br>Algosteril |
| **DEBRIDEMENT** | |
| Enzymatic | Elase ointment<br>Travase<br>Santyl<br>Panafil<br>Biozyme C |
| Wet-to-dry dressings* | Gauze in many forms (4 × 4, kerlex) |
| **WOUND PROTECTION, INSULATION, AND MILD ABSORPTION** | |
| Hydrocolloids (waxy pectin adhesive dressings that provide an optimal wound environment) | Duoderm<br>Restore<br>Tegasorb<br>Ultec |
| Transparent dressings (thin, adhesive dressings that support the microenvironment for cellular regeneration) | Tegaderm<br>Bioclusive<br>OpSite<br>Acu-Derm<br>Polyskin |
| Polyurethane foam dressings (nonadhesive; some assist with odor control) | Allevyn<br>Lyofoam<br>EpiLock |
| Hydrogel dressings (nonadherent; have a topical soothing effect; varied in thickness) | Elasto-Gel<br>Vigilon<br>Second Skin |

NOTE: Research suggests that wounds heal most effectively in a moist, natural environment, with a clean, debris- and necrotic-free wound area. Dressings and interventions are all designed with these principles in mind. Several have other added benefits that are discussed separately within each category.

*Solutions used vary according to preference of physician; most common solution is normal saline.

wound healing. Nurses and physicians receive minimal education about products and principles of wound healing. A nursing specialty has evolved over the past 30 years called enterostomal therapy (ET) nursing. Enterostomal therapy nurses are nationally recognized as leaders in the wound care arena and are an active part of the NPUAP. If your institution does not have an ET nurse on staff, the Wound, Ostomy and Continence Nurses Society in California can refer you to the closest person; contact this organization by calling 714-476-0268, or through the Internet by www.wocn.org.

## NURSING MANAGEMENT

A holistic approach to nursing management of the patient with a pressure ulcer contains four components: (1) controlling the contributing factors by reduction or elimination, (2) supporting the host, (3) optimizing the microenvironment based on principles of wound healing, and (4) providing education for patients and caregivers.

**research**

Reference: Tourtual DM, Reisenberg LA, Korutz CJ, et al: Predictors of hospital-acquired heel pressure ulcers, *Ostomy Wound Manage* 43(9):24, 1997.

Pressure ulcers are a serious and expensive health care problem. An estimated 1 million persons in the United States suffer from pressure ulcers. The cost to heal an ulcer is estimated at $2000 to $3000, and over 6.4 million dollars are spent annually on the treatment of ulcers.

Heel ulcers prolong a patient's hospital stay, delay recovery, and increase rehabilitation time. The National Pressure Ulcer Prevalence Survey indicates that the prevalence of heel ulcers has increased to 30% in 1993 from 19% in 1989, while the prevalence of ulcers in other locations remained the same.

The purpose of this prospective, descriptive study was to evaluate predictors of hospital-acquired heel ulcers. The sample consisted of 291 patients. Assessment consisted of demographics, Braden scale, and daily heel assessment. The subjects' heels were assessed after being elevated off the bed for 20 minutes. The staging system defined by the National Pressure Ulcer Advisory Consensus Development Conference was used (stages I through IV). In this study, the sensitivity of the Braden scale was found to be 100% and the specificity from 64% to 90%.

Twenty-six percent of patients developed heel ulcers, mostly stage I (94.6%); the remaining were stage II. Ulcers occurred more frequently in white female patients. Other variables statistically significant between the ulcer and nonulcer group included age; length of stay; incontinence; limb weakness; preventive moisture applied to heels; decreased appetite, albumin, and protein levels; and Braden scale results. Incontinence and moisture (on Braden scale) as variables associated with the development of heel ulcers were unexpected findings. Results also indicated that no new scoring tool has improved sensitivity or specificity over the total Braden scale. The Braden scale may be the best predictive tool for heel ulcer development.

## ASSESSMENT

Most pressure ulcers can be prevented if the nurse is diligent about assessment and appropriate interventions. Not all interventions are within the scope of nursing practice; therefore a multidisciplinary leadership approach as recommended by the NPUAP is important. Prevention can be accomplished only when the nurse has identified those patients at high risk for development of pressure ulcer. Many "assessment tools" are available (see the Research Box). Currently only two tools are cited in the Clinical Practice Guidelines[1] as valid and research based; these are the Norton and Braden scales. Most institutions incorporate information from one or both of these tools while developing their own tool.

Assessment tools consider both extrinsic and intrinsic factors that contribute to alterations in skin integrity. The Norton scale (Figure 63-19) examines the patient's general health and mental status and levels of mobility, activity, and continence. Simple to use, this tool leaves much room for nursing judgment within the specific areas. These areas are scored from 1 to 4, and a total is calculated. The lower the total number of points, the greater the risk the patient has for skin breakdown. The Braden scale is more specific, providing explanations for each score the patient is given (Figure 63-20). The areas scored in this tool include the patient's levels of sensory perception, mobility, nutrition, and activity, as well as the presence or absence of moisture, friction, and shear. Once again, a number is assigned for each parameter, the total is calculated, and the lower the score, the greater the risk factor.

Nursing assessment of wounds is discussed in the next section. Once a wound has developed, the nurse is responsible for periodic assessments to determine whether the plan of care continues to be effective. Institutional policies differ on the frequency of assessments, so the term *periodic* has been adopted by the NPUAP to offer general guidelines while allowing flexibility for individual care settings.

## Subjective Data

Pressure ulcers generally do not cause subjective symptomatology, except for pain if the patient has sensation at the level of the wound. Pain management before dressing changes is a nursing consideration, as is providing restful periods for the patient to promote the optimal environment for wound healing. Cellular regeneration is slowed when the body is under stress, such as pain or fever. Management of pain is discussed in detail in Chapter 12.

## Objective Data

A staging classification system, as detailed in Box 63-2, is helpful for the nurse in determining the appropriate interventions for a particular wound; however, it is not an all-inclusive tool. Important wound characteristics—such as appearance of the wound bed, drainage, odor, and size—are not obtained using staging alone. In most cases, staging allows the nurse to determine only the depths of tissue involvement. However, if the wound is covered with necrotic tissue, the depth of tissue damage cannot be ascertained. To appropriately evaluate and document pressure ulcers, the nurse also must assess the size, color, and presence of exudate.

### Size

The nurse should measure circumference of wound, diameter or length, and width if irregular shape exists. The depth of the wound can be measured by inserting a sterile applicator and comparing depth with measurements on a wound measuring guide. Sizing the wound not only assists with staging, but can help determine the size and type of dressing(s) required. Accurate sizing of the wound is required by Medicare for reimbursement of home care dressing supplies.

### Color

The color of wounds gives the examiner information about vascular supply, infection, healthy versus necrotic tissue, and nutritional status. "Healthy" wounds have a beefy-red, granu-

**Norton Scale**

| A<br>*Physical condition* | B<br>*Mental state* | C<br>*Activity* | D<br>*Mobility* | E<br>*Incontinence* | *Total Score* |
|---|---|---|---|---|---|
| 4 Good | 4 Alert | 4 Ambulant | 4 Full | 4 Not | |
| 3 Fair | 3 Apathetic | 3 Walks with help | 3 Slightly limited | 3 Occasional | |
| 2 Poor | 2 Confused | 2 Chairbound | 2 Very limited | 2 Usually urine | |
| 1 Bad | 1 Stupor | 1 Bedrest | 1 Immobile | 1 Double incontinence | |

**Norton Plus Scale**
(For determining high risk for pressure sores)

| *Check ONLY if YES* | *YES* |
|---|---|
| Diagnosis of diabetes | ____ |
| Diagnosis of hypertension | ____ |
| Hematocrit (M) <41% | ____ |
| (F) <36% | ____ |
| Hemoglobin (M) <14 g/dl | ____ |
| (F) <12 g/dl | ____ |
| Albumin level <3.3 g/dl | ____ |
| Febrile >99.6°F | ____ |
| 5 or more medications | ____ |
| Changes in mental status to confused, lethargic within 24 hours | ____ |
| ***TOTAL Number of Checkmarks*** | |
| Norton Scale Score | ____ |
| Minus total from above | ____ |
| Norton Plus Score | ____ |

**fig. 63-19** Norton Scale and Norton Plus Scale.

lar appearance. If the wound bed is pale, check the hemoglobin level. Necrotic tissue is white, yellow, gray, or black. Certain infections will change the color of a wound bed (*Pseudomonas* can produce greenish drainage on the wound bed).

### Exudate

Wound drainage should be assessed for amount, color, and consistency. Odor is also an indicator for assessment. Infected wounds generally produce large amounts of odorous drainage. Be as objective as possible while documenting. Terms such as *small, moderate,* and *large* are subjective. Be as descriptive as possible, such as "drainage of serosanguineous liquid, nonodorous, quarter sized on 4 × 4." Other general parameters to assess include presence of undermining or sinus tracts in wound, condition of surrounding skin, and foreign bodies in wound (e.g., sutures, orthopedic hardware).

## NURSING DIAGNOSES

Nursing diagnoses are determined from analysis of patient data. Nursing diagnoses for the patient with a pressure ulcer may include but are not limited to:

| Diagnostic Title | Possible Etiological Factors |
|---|---|
| Skin integrity, risk for impaired | Nutritional deficit, prolonged immobility, decreased hemoglobin and advanced age, serum albumin levels |
| Infection, risk for | Lack of knowledge, decreased nutrition, decreased immune response, loss of skin integrity |
| Mobility, impaired physical | Intolerance to activity, decreased strength/endurance, pain/discomfort, perceptual/cognitive impairment, neuromuscular impairment, musculoskeletal impairment, depression, severe anxiety |
| Tissue perfusion, altered (skin) | Decreased blood flow, immobility, pressure |
| Self-care deficit: wound treatments | Location of wound, impaired mobility |

See the accompanying Nursing Care Plan.

## EXPECTED PATIENT OUTCOMES

Expected patient outcomes for the patient with a pressure ulcer may include but are not limited to:

1. Patient is discharged with intact skin.
2. At discharge there is active wound healing, as evidenced by a clean, granular wound bed, minimal serosanguineous drainage, and no necrotic tissue present.
   a. No clinical signs or symptoms of infection are present (pain, tenderness, fever, induration, surrounding erythema, increased drainage).
3. Patient shows evidence of achievement or return to maximal level of functioning.
4. No evidence of nonblanchable erythema is present.
5. Patient or caregiver states the following aspects of a continued care program: measures to reduce or relieve pressure to skin, importance of well-balanced diet, ways to manage incontinence/moisture, and treatment measures as indicated.

## INTERVENTIONS

### Preventing

1. Reduce or relieve pressure by instituting a schedule of turning the patient a minimum of every 2 hours and using available pressure relief devices for bed and chair.
2. Inspect the skin at regular intervals for signs of early breakdown.
3. Maintain skin in soft, elastic state through use of lotions; avoid massage.
4. Control incontinence and moisture next to skin.
5. Reduce or eliminate shear and friction.
6. Provide optimal nutrition; consult with dietitian.

A summary of preventive interventions can be found in the Guidelines for Care Box on p. 2106.

### Protecting

1. Use aseptic technique and Standard Precautions for the prevention of infection.
2. Monitor for clinical signs and symptoms of infection every shift and report as appropriate.

### Restoring

1. Involve patient in activity schedule as much as possible. Increasing activity levels assists with restoration to an optimal level of functioning.
2. Increase nutritional intake with adequate calorie, protein, and vitamins and minerals; work with dietitian.

### Patient/Family Education

1. Teach patient and caregiver about the need for continued interventions to prevent recurrence.
2. Instruct on dressing and intervention techniques.

Many of the preventive measures described in the Guidelines for Care Box can be taught to the patient and his or her family.

## EVALUATION

To evaluate the effectiveness of nursing interventions, compare patient behaviors with those stated in the expected patient outcomes. Emphasis is placed throughout this discussion on early interventions for prevention of pressure ulcers. It remains the nurse's individual responsibility to be knowledgeable about preventive strategies and interventions in harmony with the Clinical Practice Guidelines. Adherence to national standards affords the nurse increased professional power, as well as autonomy, thus promoting feelings of professional satisfaction while maintaining high-quality patient care. If the nurse functions at the level established by the national standards, the patient will exhibit:

1. Intact skin or at least a decrease in the size of the pressure ulcer
2. A wound with no signs and symptoms of infection (e.g., the sore is clean, drainage is clear, temperature is normal)
3. Maximal functioning
4. Minimal and blanchable erythema
5. Implementation of pressure-reducing measures and measures to control moisture and incontinence

| **Patient's name** | | **Evaluator's name** |
|---|---|---|
| **Sensory perception**<br>Ability to respond meaningfully to pressure-related discomfort | **1. Completely limited:**<br>Unresponsive (does not moan, flinch, or grasp) to painful stimuli, due to diminished level of consciousness or sedation,<br>**OR**<br>limited ability to feel pain over most of body surface. | **2. Very limited:**<br>Responds only to painful stimuli. Cannot communicate discomfort except by moaning or restlessness,<br>**OR**<br>has a sensory impairment that limits the ability to feel pain or discomfort over ½ of body. |
| **Moisture**<br>Degree to which skin is exposed to moisture | **1. Constantly moist:**<br>Skin is kept moist almost constantly by perspiration, urine, etc. Dampness is detected every time patient is moved or turned. | **2. Moist:**<br>Skin is often but not always moist; linen must be changed at least once a shift. |
| **Activity**<br>Degree of physical activity | **1. Bedfast:**<br>Confined to bed. | **2. Chairfast:**<br>Ability to walk severely limited or nonexistent. Cannot bear own weight and/or must be assisted into chair or wheelchair. |
| **Mobility**<br>Ability to change and control body position | **1. Completely immobile:**<br>Does not make even slight changes in body or extremity position without assistance. | **2. Very limited:**<br>Makes occasional slight changes in body or extremity position but unable to make frequent or significant changes independently. |
| **Nutrition**<br>Usual food intake pattern | **1. Very poor:**<br>Never eats a complete meal. Rarely eats more than ⅓ of any food offered. Eats 2 servings or less of protein (meat or dairy products) per day. Takes fluids poorly. Does not take a liquid dietary supplement,<br>**OR**<br>is NPO and/or maintained on clear liquids or IV for more than 5 days. | **2. Probably inadequate:**<br>Rarely eats a complete meal and generally eats only about ½ of any food offered. Protein intake includes only 3 servings of meat or dairy products per day. Occasionally will take a dietary supplement,<br>**OR**<br>receives less than optimum amount of liquid diet or tube feeding. |
| **Friction and shear** | **1. Problem:**<br>Requires moderate to maximum assistance in moving. Complete lifting without sliding against sheets is impossible. Frequently slides down in bed or chair, requiring frequent repositioning with maximum assistance. Spasticity, contractures, or agitation leads to almost constant friction. | **2. Potential problem:**<br>Moves feebly or requires minimum assitance. During a move, skin probably slides to some extent against sheets, chair, restraints, or other devices. Maintains relatively good position in chair or bed most of the time but occasionally slides down. |

**fig. 63-20** Braden Scale for predicting pressure ulcer risk.

## GERONTOLOGICAL CONSIDERATIONS

Many of the changes in the skin associated with aging predispose the elderly person to the development of pressure ulcers. The thinning of the epidermis makes the skin more prone to injury. Adhesion of the epidermis to the dermis is decreased and accompanied by a decrease in skin elasticity; allowing the skin to be easily stretched and deformed. The skin is a less effective barrier against infection, bruising, and water loss. In addition, thermal regulation and the ability to perceive touch and pain are decreased in the elderly person. Excessive pressure may not be well perceived in the elderly patient. Any coexisting neurological deficits may compound the problem.

With the application of shearing forces, the epidermal-dermal attachment may weaken and allow the skin layers to separate. A blister forms and eventually ruptures, leaving a flap of skin with uneven edges, called a *skin tear* (see the Research Box, p. 2107). Persons who require assistance with moving in bed or transfers are at risk for the development of skin tears caused by shearing forces. Frequent bathing with drying soaps can dry elderly patients' skin. The use of emollient soaps and moisturizers is recommended; moisturizing the skin is best performed during and after bathing.

Because of the numerous predisposing factors present in the elderly, they are at greater risk for pressure ulcers. Predisposing factors include: (1) anemia; (2) poor nutrition; (3) de-

| | | Dates of assessment | | | |
|---|---|---|---|---|---|
| **3. Slightly limited:** Responds to verbal commands but cannot always communicate discomfort or need to be turned, **OR** has some sensory impairment that limits ability to feel pain or discomfort in 1 or 2 extremities. | **4. No impairment:** Responds to verbal commands. Has no sensory deficit which would limit ability to feel or voice pain or discomfort. | | | | |
| **3. Occasionally moist:** Skin is occasionally most, requiring an extra linen change approximately once a day. | **4. Rarely moist:** Skin is usually dry; linen requires changing only at routine intervals. | | | | |
| **3. Walks occasionally:** Walks occasionally during day but for very short distances, with or without assistance. Spends majority of each shift in bed or chair. | **4. Walks frequently:** Walks outside the room at least twice a day and inside room at least once every 2 hours during waking hours. | | | | |
| **3. Slightly limited:** Makes frequent though slight changes in body or extremity position independently. | **4. No limitations:** Makes major and frequent changes in position without assistance. | | | | |
| **3. Adequate:** Eats over ½ of most meals. Eats a total of 4 servings of protein (meat, diary products) each day. Occasionally will refuse a meal, but will usually take a supplement if offered, **OR** is on a tube feeding or TPN regimen, which probably meets most of nutritional needs. | **4. Excellent:** Eats most of every meal. Never refuses a meal. Usually eats a total of 4 or more servings of meat and dairy products. Occasionally eats between meals. Does not require supplementation. | | | | |
| **3. No apparent problem:** Moves in bed and in chair independently and has sufficient muscle strength to lift up completely during move. Maintains good position in bed or chair at all times. | | | | | |
| | **Total score** | | | | |

**fig. 63-20, cont'd** Braden Scale for predicting pressure ulcer risk.

creased albumin; (4) decreased mobility; (5) thinning of skin and loss of subcutaneous cushion; (6) drug therapy, such as glucocorticoids; (7) incontinence; (8) comorbid conditions or use of sedatives that interfere with sensory perception, natural shifting of body position, or turning in bed; and (9) use of restraints.

Pressure ulcers can develop not only in those confined to bed but also in those confined to a sitting position. The ulcers occur whenever pressure is allowed to be maintained. Ulcers can occur on the head, shoulders, or lower back if a recumbent position is maintained. If a side-lying position is maintained, ulcers can develop on hips, ankles, and the pinna of the ear. Sitting promotes ulcers on the buttocks. The underside of the scrotum can be injured with shearing and pressure.

Measures to prevent and treat pressure ulcers are the same for the elderly as for any person. The only difference is that tissue, because of the predisposing factors, is damaged more quickly, so more frequent position changes and inspections need to be implemented. Many hospitalized elders require dietary measures to improve nutrition to prevent pressure ulcers. Also, many elderly persons require use

*Text continued on p. 2107*

## nursing care plan *Person with a Pressure Ulcer*

**DATA** Mrs. M. is a 79-year-old widow. She has a history of hypertension, congestive heart failure (CHF), obesity, and degenerative joint disease (DJD). She is right-hand dominant. She lives alone in her own home; an adult daughter lives nearby. Mrs. M. is active and attends a local senior center for social activities. Mrs. M. is admitted for a left cerebrovascular accident (CVA) with right hemiparesis.

**NURSING ASSESSMENT**

A&O × 3, seems depressed
Dysphagia
Incontinent of urine and stool
Right hemiparesis
+2 pitting edema of the lower extremities
Bruise on the sacrum from a previous fall
Generalized dry skin
Height 65 inches
Weight 180 pounds
Braden scale 12

**VITAL SIGNS**

Temperature 36.9° C
Pulse 92
Respirations 18
Blood pressure 142/88

**MEDICATIONS**

Lisinopril 10 mg bid
Furosemide 40 mg qd
Digoxin 0.125 mg qd
Heparin 5000 U q12h subcutaneously
Motrin 800 mg tid

Collaborative management is focused on preventing any further neurological events or deficits, promoting nutrition, preventing aspiration, controlling hypertension, preventing any worsening CHF, promoting mobility and independence, preventing injury, and psychological support. A skin tear is present on the sacrum, stage II pressure ulcer. Mrs. M. is transferred to a subacute division for physical and occupational therapy. The heparin has been discontinued, and the patient is on a mechanical soft diet and transfers with the assistance of one person.

**NURSING DIAGNOSIS** *Impaired skin integrity related to immobility and mechanical forces*

| expected patient outcome | nursing interventions | rationale |
|---|---|---|
| Displays healing of pressure ulcer without complications.<br>Participates in prevention measures and treatment program. | Assess skin every shift and prn. Assess areas of redness for ability to blanch. Document Braden scale results weekly. | Frequent assessment allows for early recognition of skin changes, effectiveness of treatment, and preventive measures. Areas of nonblanchable erythema indicate increased pressure, which can easily progress to ulcers. The Braden scale is a reliable tool for predicting pressure ulcer risk; the patient's initial score of 12 places her at risk for pressure ulcer development. |
| | Turn patient every 2 hours, and post the turning schedule. Pad bony prominences. Elevate the heels off the mattress. | Rotation of body position promotes adequate blood flow and avoids prolonged pressure on any one part. Padding reduces pressure on skin over bony prominences, which are prone to breakdown because of tissue necrosis. The heels are susceptible to breakdown, and elevation avoids pressure. |
| | Avoid massaging reddened areas. | Massage of areas under pressure may lead to further tissue injury. |
| | Use emollient soap, moisturize skin after bathing, and keep perianal area clean and dry. Provide bowel and bladder training; avoid use of diapers and plastic pads. | Emollient soaps prevent drying of the skin and may be an effective preventive measure for heel ulcer formation. Contamination of the perianal area with feces or urine may speed skin breakdown and cause infection. Continence of urine and stool decreases the patient's risk of skin ulcer development. Increased moisture and decreased ventilation increase the risk of pressure ulcer development. |
| | Assess patient's caloric needs; promote nutritionally adequate diet and adequate fluid intake. | Adequate nutrition is necessary for tissue healing. Fluid intake less than 800 ml/day increases the risk of pressure ulcer development. |

*Continued*

## Person with a Pressure Ulcer—cont'd

**NURSING DIAGNOSIS** *Impaired skin integrity related to immobility and mechanical forces—cont'd*

| expected patient outcome | nursing interventions | rationale |
|---|---|---|
| | Monitor the patient's serum albumin, protein, and CBC results. | Assesses the patient's protein stores (necessary for healing and tissue integrity). Albumin less than 3.0 is a risk factor in the development of pressure ulcers. Protein needs are increased to maintain a positive nitrogen balance to aid in healing and general health. CBC results may indicate infection or anemia. |
| | Obtain nutritional consult. | The patient is overweight and would benefit from a weight reduction diet, but needs adequate nutrients for tissue healing. The patient's history of dysphagia must be considered when making food choices. |
| | Avoid shearing forces (e.g., use of turning sheet, pull sheet, appropriate transfer and position change techniques). | Shearing forces predispose the skin to injury and breakdown. Adequate personnel prevent injury from shearing forces or friction. The patient has a history of DJD, which decreases the mobility of involved joints. |
| | Employ safety precautions and fall prevention measures. | The patient is elderly, has neurological deficits, and has a history of previous falls, all of which predispose the patient to another fall or dermal injury. |
| | Use egg crate mattress on bed and seat cushion on wheelchair. | Provides padding, decreases pressure. |
| | Perform passive range of motion on affected extremities. Teach patient and daughter techniques. Promote active range of motion of unaffected extremities. Promote ambulation and a regular exercise program. | Promotes circulation, prevents complications associated with immobility. Patient and family involvement in the treatment program increases success in attaining goals. The patient has a history of DJD, which may decrease motion of involved joints. A regular exercise program enhances circulation, promotes general health, decreases stress, and aids in weight reduction. |
| | Encourage maximal participation in activities of daily living (ADL). | Allows patient some sense of control and independence. Patient is right-handed with right-sided paresis, so she may need additional assistance in ADL. Occupational therapy consult can provide patient with assistive and adaptive devices to increase independence. |
| | When sitting, encourage elevation of legs. | Promotes venous return, reduces edema formation. Patient has history of CHF, edema. |
| | Use appropriate barrier dressings and topical agents on sacral wound. | Protocols are determined by physician or skin care specialist nurse. Proper medication and treatment are necessary for ulcer healing. |
| | Keep sheets clean and dry; avoid wrinkling. | Moisture increases risk of breakdown, and wrinkled areas may cause increased pressure. |
| | Assess and record wound and surrounding tissue with each dressing change. Document size and depth. | Monitor progress of healing, and detect any complications or infection. Some institutions may take color |

Continued

## Person with a Pressure Ulcer—cont'd

**NURSING DIAGNOSIS** *Impaired skin integrity related to immobility and mechanical forces—cont'd*

| expected patient outcome | nursing interventions | rationale |
|---|---|---|
| | Assess patient's need for analgesia before dressing change. Explain all procedures to patient and family. | photographs to monitor ulcer progress. The patient will tolerate dressing changes if pain is controlled. Knowledge of treatment will decrease anxiety. |
| | Provide psychological support, encourage patient to express feelings, and assess support systems. | The patient has a history of chronic disease, which may contribute to feelings of powerlessness and depression. Further loss of independence or ability to perform usual role may cause depression and anxiety. Ventilation of feelings is important in adapting to changes, and support can make lifestyle changes easier. Use of previously effective coping skills may be useful in other stressful situations. |
| | Teach patient and daughter skin assessment techniques, measures to promote healthy skin, and measures to prevent future skin breakdown. | Identification of risk factors and use of preventive measures are the best methods of preventing pressure ulcers. Discharge is planned to daughter's home. |

## guidelines for care

### Interventions to Prevent Pressure Ulcers

**Incontinence**
- Cleanse skin after each episode of incontinence. Check incontinent patients frequently.
- Assess causative factors of incontinence.
- Contain urine and feces in absorbent products that control moisture and exposure to skin; plastic-lined products can contribute to the problem.
- Minimize moisture next to skin from any source.

**Nutritional deficits**
- Collaborate with dietitian to assess for optimal nutritional support.
- Assess for symptoms of nutritional compromise (decreased appetite and subsequently less oral intake; serum albumin level of less than 3-3.5 gm/dl; Hgb level of less than 10 gm/dl; signs and symptoms of dehydration, including thirst, poor skin turgor, and dry mucous membranes; elevated hematocrit and serum sodium levels).

**Skin care and early treatment measures**
- Inspect skin at regular intervals, at least daily, frequency determined by institutional policy (e.g., every shift instead of daily) and patient degree of risk. A head-to-toe inspection should be conducted, with attention to intertriginous areas and bony prominences.
- Bathing schedule should be developed according to patient preference, institutional policy, and general skin condition. Use a mild cleansing agent, and avoid water temperature extremes.
- Assess environmental factors, such as temperature and humidity, for contribution to skin condition.
- Lubricate skin with emollient lotions. Avoid lotion with scents or high alcohol contents.
- Avoid vigorous massage.

**Alterations in mobility/activity**
- Reposition patient at least every 2 hours.
- Use position pillows or foam wedges to separate skin areas in contact with each other or to assist with maintaining positions. Use cautiously because these devices can become an additional source of pressure if not properly placed.
- Heels should be elevated off of bed surfaces with supportive pillows. Heel protectors help reduce friction.
- Avoid positioning directly onto trochanter. Place patient more appropriately into 30 degree side-lying position.
- Elevating the head of the bed centers all body weight directly over the pelvic triangle. It is best to keep the degree of elevation to less than 45 degrees, if possible.
- To reduce friction and shear, use lifting devices to raise patient in bed, rather than dragging patient across the surface of the bed.
- A pressure reduction or relief device should be used for all patients at risk of pressure ulcer formation.
- Patients in wheelchairs and other chairs should be taught to shift weight and have pressure-reducing surfaces on which to sit.

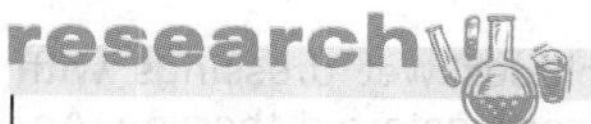

Reference: Mason SR: Type of soap and the incidence of skin tears among residents of a long-term care facility, *Ostomy Wound Manage* 43(8):26, 1997.

A *skin tear* is defined as the separation of the dermis from the epidermis, usually as a result of shearing. When subjected to shearing, the elderly person's skin may separate, causing bleeding and blistering, which can lead to a skin tear. Daily bathing and the use of pure soaps and deodorant soaps are drying to elderly patients' skin.

This study evaluated the effectiveness of emollient antibacterial soap compared with non-emollient soap in improving skin quality and reducing the incidence of skin tears in residents of a long-term care facility. The sample consisted of 43 patients ranging in age from 59 to 102 years (mean 85.5 years). There were 39 women and 4 men in the sample. Residents were ambulatory, bed-bound, or chair-bound, and all required at least moderate assistance with bathing. Subjects were bathed three times per week, using plain, non-emollient antibacterial soap or an emollient antibacterial soap. The total rate of skin tears over the 4-month period for the non-emollient soap was 28.5% compared with 18.3% for the emollient soap. The non-emollient soap was used exclusively during the first and third months and the emollient soap exclusively during the second and fourth months of the study. Results indicated that the incidence of skin tears decreased (37%) during the months the emollient soap was used and increased (43%) during the third month, when the non-emollient soap was reintroduced. There was an overall improvement in the residents' skin and the skin of the nursing personnel who bathed the residents. These results support the effectiveness of emollient soaps as a method of decreasing the incidence of skin tears in the elderly.

of special beds and padding for chairs, if immobilization is required.

## SPECIAL ENVIRONMENTS FOR CARE

### Home Care Management

Many persons at high risk for pressure ulcerations are sent home with these same risk factors. Thus the family or other caregiver must know all the interventions, including proper positioning techniques, use of protective devices, and proper nutrition.

If a pressure ulcer has developed, the caregiver may have to continue treatment measures after discharge. The caregiver must know how to do the treatment, the frequency of the treatment, safety precautions for self, how to dispose of used dressings, and what type of inspection to implement with each treatment. The caregiver must also know what changes need to be reported immediately.

Most patients sent home with pressure ulcers should have a referral to a home health care agency. The home care nurse can help the caregiver establish routines at home, obtain supplies most economically, and store supplies appropriately. The home care nurse can help the caregiver gain confidence in doing treatments. Additionally, the home care nurse can make sure that the patient's nutritional needs are met and an appropriate frequency and technique for change in position is maintained.

Most persons at home with pressure ulcers have many other physiological or psychosocial needs. The home health nurse can help the caregiver develop routines to meet these other needs and also obtain assistance to provide some respite.

## COMPLICATIONS

Most complications associated with pressure ulcers are the sequelae of infection. In addition, if the patient has undergone surgical intervention, the complications associated with anesthesia and surgery are potential problems. See Chapter 20 for a discussion of postoperative care and complications. If the pressure ulcer becomes infected, the infection may spread to the bloodstream, and sepsis may result. Osteomyelitis is another potential complication, requiring possible surgical intervention and long-term intravenous antibiotics (see Chapter 61). In a patient with alterations in mobility, extensive pressure ulcers may result in further immobility. For example, a person with spinal cord injury with a pressure ulcer on the buttocks or sacral area may have to spend an extended period of time lying prone, with all pressure off the affected area. In such instances, the patient is not allowed to sit in his or her wheelchair.

If contamination of the pressure ulcer with bowel contents is a problem, some surgeons will perform a temporary colostomy to prevent potential contamination of the wound. The colostomy is reversible after healing has occurred.

To prevent infection, the nurse must carefully monitor the wound for size, both depth and dimension; the type of drainage; and the presence of granulation tissue. The patient must be monitored for signs and symptoms of systemic infection.

Psychological support for both the patient and family is important because of the length of time required for treatment and healing. Depression and social isolation, particularly in the elderly patient, may be a sequela of treatment for pressure ulcers.

## critical thinking QUESTIONS

1 Discuss how a disease such as scabies as opposed to an ankle ulcer may affect the person emotionally.

2 Explain the major psychosocial needs of persons with psoriasis.

3 What nursing interventions would be appropriate for a patient experiencing a disturbance in body image as a result of a dermatological condition?

4 What are the risk factors for pressure ulcers? What nursing approaches would you prescribe for an obese 60-year-old patient with diabetes mellitus who has neuropathy and is wheelchair-bound?

## chapter SUMMARY

### COMMON SKIN PROBLEMS

- Some dermatological disorders may be prevented by removal of known causative agents, protecting the skin against ultraviolet rays, keeping the skin clean and hydrated, eating a balanced diet, monitoring for early signs of skin changes, and seeking medical help when skin conditions develop.
- Skin lesions can create changes in body image. Social interactions may be altered when there is considerable disfigurement.
- Pruritus leads to skin excoriation from scratching; it may be relieved by cold applications, hydration in a tepid oatmeal bath followed by application of emollient lotion, and maintaining room temperature at a moderate temperature with increased humidity.
- Medications used for therapeutic baths or soaks include colloids, potassium permanganate, Burow's solution, sulfur, tar preparations, and oils. These baths or soaks are given for antipruritic, antifungal, antibacterial, and moisturizing or drying effects.
- The most commonly used topical medications are corticosteroids; the types vary in potency. Occlusion over the corticosteroid increases absorption and should be used only by prescription. Topical antibiotic and antifungal medications may also be prescribed.
- Vehicles for topical medications include powders, lotions, creams, ointments, and pastes.
- Wet dressings are commonly used over skin lesions for cooling, drying, antipruritic, or vasoconstricting effects.
- Parasitic infestations include pediculosis and scabies; treatment includes applications of pediculicides and scabicides.
- Fungal skin infections include candidiasis and the dermatophytoses (tinea). Treatment includes applying topical fungicides, keeping the skin dry, and wearing loose clothing or shoes, as appropriate.
- Bacterial skin infections include impetigo, folliculitis, furuncles and carbuncles, and erysipelas. Management includes cleansing the skin well and applying topical antibiotics; soaks are used to remove crusts. Heat is applied to furuncles until drainage occurs; incision and drainage may be necessary. Care must be taken to prevent spread of infection to other skin areas or to other persons.
- Viral skin infections include warts, herpes simplex (fever blister), and herpes zoster (shingles). Acyclovir may be prescribed for herpes infections. Pain is a problem with herpes infections and may persist after the lesions have healed.
- Acne results from multiple factors and is seen mostly in adolescents. The lesions result from blockage of hair follicles by sebum, leading to inflammations. Treatment may be with topical drying agents, removal of comedones, and systemic therapy with isoretinoic acid, antibiotics, estrogens, or intralesional corticosteroids for severe acne.
- Types of dermatitis include contact (from external agents), atopic (hypersensitivity reaction), seborrheic, nummular, stasis dermatitis, and lichen simplex chronicus. Typical lesions include erythema, followed by vesicle formation with oozing, followed by crusting and scaling; itching is common. Treatment commonly includes wet dressings with water or Burow's solution and corticosteroid therapy. Antibiotics are given for superimposed infections.
- Skin reactions from systemic factors include dermatitis medicamentosa (drugs), exfoliative dermatitis, erythema multiforme, lesions of communicable diseases, and lupus erythematosus.
- Psoriasis is a genetically determined, papulosquamous disease; no cure exists. The lesions are scaling plaques. Treatment consists of bland emollients and keratolytics to hydrate and soften the skin, corticosteroids, coal tar preparations, anthralin products (antimitotic), and photochemotherapy.
- Benign skin growths are keratoses (corns, calluses, seborrheic, actinic); premalignant growths include leukoplakia, Bowen's disease, and pigmented nevi.
- Benign nevi (moles) are symmetrical, with even borders and uniform color, and are usually smaller than 6 mm; malignant melanomas are asymmetrical, with uneven borders and multiple colors, and are usually larger than 6 mm.
- A major contributing factor to the incidence of some skin growths (actinic keratoses, squamous cell carcinomas, keratocanthomas, malignant melanomas) is unprotected exposure to the sun. Most skin cancers, *except* malignant melanomas and some squamous cell carcinomas (on lips or ears), do not metastasize.
- Types of dermatological surgeries for superficial lesions include tangential surgery, curettage, cryosurgery, and electrosurgery. Deep lesions are removed by punch biopsy or by excision.

### PRESSURE ULCERS

- National Clinical Practice Guidelines were established to guide practitioners with high-quality preventive and management interventions.
- Nurses' primary responsibility lies with prevention of and early intervention in those with pressure ulcers.

## References


1. Clinical Practice Guidelines: *Pressure ulcers in adults: prediction and prevention,* Washington, DC, 1992, US Department of Health and Human Services.
2. Coit DG: Malignant melanoma. In Rakel RE: *Conn's current therapy,* Philadelphia, 1997, WB Saunders.
3. Donohue FC, Spieluogel RL: Viral diseases of the skin. In Rakel RE: *Conn's current therapy,* Philadelphia, 1997, WB Saunders.
4. Guyton AC, Hall JE: *Textbook of medical physiology,* ed 9, Philadelphia, 1996, WB Saunders.
5. Loescher LJ: Skin cancer prevention and detection update, *Semin Oncol Nurs* 9(3):184, 1993.
6. Morris-Hicks LE, Lewis DJ: Management of chronic resistive scabies: a case study, *Geriatr Nurs* 16(5):230, 1995.
7. Price SA, Wilson LM, editors: *Pathophysiology: clinical concepts of disease processes,* ed 5, St Louis, 1997, Mosby.
8. Stein JH et al: *Internal medicine,* ed 4, St Louis, 1994, Mosby.
9. Teirney L et al: *Current medical diagnosis and treatment,* ed 33, Norwalk, Conn, 1994, Appleton & Lange.
10. Uphold CR, Graham MV: *Clinical guidelines in adult health,* Gainesville, Fla, 1994, Barmarrae Books.

chapter 64

# MANAGEMENT OF PERSONS WITH Burns

DIANE E. FRITSCH and LYNNE C. YURKO

## objectives

*After studying this chapter, the learner should be able to:*

1. Describe the assessment of the burn patient including extent, location, and etiology of the burn.
2. Differentiate among the three periods of a major burn.
3. Describe emergency care for a major burn.
4. Compare interventions for replacing body fluids, preventing infection, promoting nutrition and mobility, and providing emotional support during the three periods of burn care.
5. Identify learning needs of the patient with burns.
6. Discuss preventive measures for populations at risk for burn injury.

## ETIOLOGY

Burns are caused by flame, scald, direct contact, chemicals, electrical current, and radiation. Burn injuries are in many respects the worst of all tragedies an individual can experience. An intensive burn is accompanied by an overwhelming insult to the patient physically and psychologically and is catastrophic in cost and suffering to the family involved.

## EPIDEMIOLOGY

Approximately 2.5 million people suffer a thermal injury each year in the United States. Of these victims, 60,000 are admitted to hospitals and more than 7000 die as a result of burn injury. Injury is frequently a result of the victim's own action. This is particularly true for elderly persons, whose burns frequently are caused by the ignition of clothing when cooking or smoking. Scald injuries are the most frequent type of injury, but flame injury is more serious. The direct cost of treating burn injuries is more than $1 billion a year. Indirect costs (pain, suffering, and disability) amount to several billion dollars more per year.[14]

Recent statistics indicate that burns and fires occur at a U.S. national rate of 2.1 per 100,000 population. (It is believed to be higher, but most states do not require official reporting.) Rural areas and lower income sections of large cities have the highest death rates.[14]

## PATHOPHYSIOLOGY

Traditionally, burns have been classified as first, second, or third degree. The terms *first, second,* and *third degree* are not descriptive of the injury because they are based only on the visual characteristics of the burn wound. The injury of a burn extends beyond what can be seen. More accurate terms are *partial thickness* and *full thickness,* which graphically describe the burn and indicate depth and severity of the tissue injury (Figure 64-1).

Partial-thickness burns are characterized by destruction in varying depths from the epidermis (outer layer of skin) to the dermis (middle layer of skin). Partial-thickness burns of the skin involve a "part" of the epidermis and dermis. The depth of tissue injury is described further as *superficial* partial thickness, involving only the epidermis, or *deep* partial thickness, involving the entire epidermis and part of the dermis. Partial-thickness burns are likely to be painful because nerve endings have been injured and exposed, but they have the ability to heal because a portion of the epithelial cells are not destroyed. The presence of blisters often indicates deep partial-thickness injury. They may increase in size as the result of continuous exudation and collection of tissue fluid. During the healing phase, dryness and itching are common and are caused by increased vascularization of sebaceous glands, reduction of secretions, and decreased perspiration.

Full-thickness burns include destruction of the epidermis and the entire dermis, as well as possible damage to the subcutaneous layer, muscle, and bone. Nerve endings are destroyed, resulting in a painless wound. *Eschar,* a leathery covering composed of denatured protein, may form as the result of surface dehydration. Black networks of coagulated capillaries may be seen. Full-thickness burns require skin grafting because the destroyed tissue is unable to epithelialize. Often a deep partial-thickness burn may convert to a full-thickness burn due to infection, trauma, or decreased blood supply.

As a result of burns, normal skin function is diminished, resulting in physiological alterations. These include (1) loss of protective barriers, (2) escape of body fluids, (3) lack of temperature control, (4) destroyed sweat and sebaceous glands, and (5) a diminished number of sensory receptors. The severity of these alterations depends on the extent of the burn and the depth of the damage.

A major burn injury is one of the most serious forms of trauma an individual can experience. Virtually every organ system is affected. A shock state, known as *burn shock,* develops that is both a hypovolemic and a cellular shock. Two stages occur after severe burns: the immediate hypovolemic

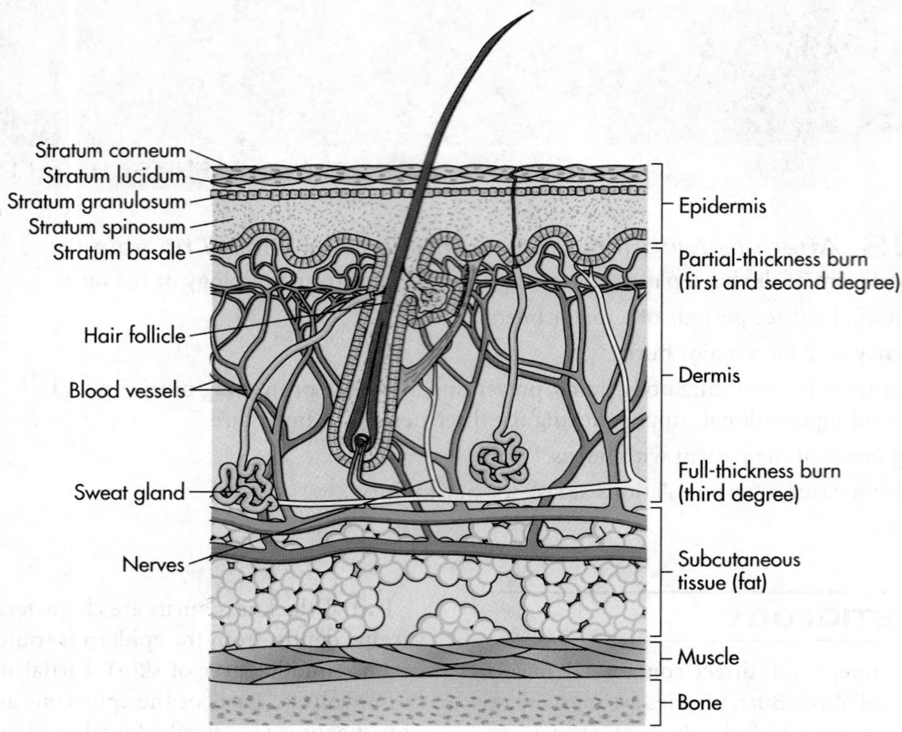


**fig. 64-1** Levels of human skin involved in burns.

stage and the diuretic stage. Figure 64-2 presents an overview of the pathophysiological changes seen with a severe burn.

## HYPOVOLEMIC STAGE

The hypovolemic stage begins at the time of burn injury and lasts for the first 48 to 72 hours. It is characterized by a rapid shift of fluid from the vascular compartments into the interstitial spaces. When tissues are burned, vasodilation, increased capillary permeability, and changes in the permeability of tissue cells in and around the burn area occur. As a result, abnormally large amounts of extracellular fluid (ECF), sodium chloride, and protein pass through the burned area to cause blister formation and local edema or escape through the open wound.

Visible fluid loss makes up only a small part of the fluid lost from the circulating blood and other essential fluid compartments. Most of the fluid loss occurs deep in the wound where the fluid extravasates into the deeper tissues. Burns occurring in highly vascular areas such as muscle tissue or the face are believed to cause a greater fluid shift than comparable burns of other parts of the body. One half of the ECF of the body can shift from its normal distribution to the site of a severe burn. Patients with large surface area burns experience edema throughout the body that can impair peripheral circulation by compressing the circulatory vessels in an extremity. This can lead to a decrease in peripheral pulses or complete absence of circulation to the extremity. The ECF constitutes about 20% of the body weight. Three fourths of it surrounds the cells, and one fourth is found in blood plasma (Table 64-1). For a person weighing 68 kg (150 lb), this means that from

**table 64-1** *Approximate Division of Total Body Fluid into Compartments**

| Body Fluid Compartments | Liters of Fluid: Lean Adult Weighing 45 kg | Liters of Fluid: Lean Adult Weighing 68 kg |
|---|---|---|
| Intravascular (plasma) | 2.8 | 4.2 |
| Interstitial | 8.4 | 12.5 |
| Intracellular | 22.3 | 33.3 |
| TOTAL | 33.5 | 50.0 |

*Note that the smaller the individual, the less fluid he or she has in each compartment, and that plasma is reduced most markedly with decrease in size. The normal size and body type of the individual are considered when fluid replacement is ordered.

4.5 to 6.5 kg or from 5 to 7.5 L of fluids may be removed from the interstitial spaces and bloodstream.

The body can partially compensate for this fluid shift with intense peripheral vasoconstriction for approximately 1 to 2 hours after the burn injury. During this compensatory period, blood pressure may be normal to slightly elevated, pulse rapid (greater than 100 beats/min), and the patient oliguric. As the compensatory mechanisms fail, the classic picture of *hypovolemic shock*—hypotension, tachycardia, oliguria, acidosis, and hypoxia—is seen. These changes are summarized in Figure 64-3.

As a result of these fluid shifts, *dehydration* of nondamaged tissue cells may occur. More fluids and sodium than protein are lost initially from the capillaries. This increases the

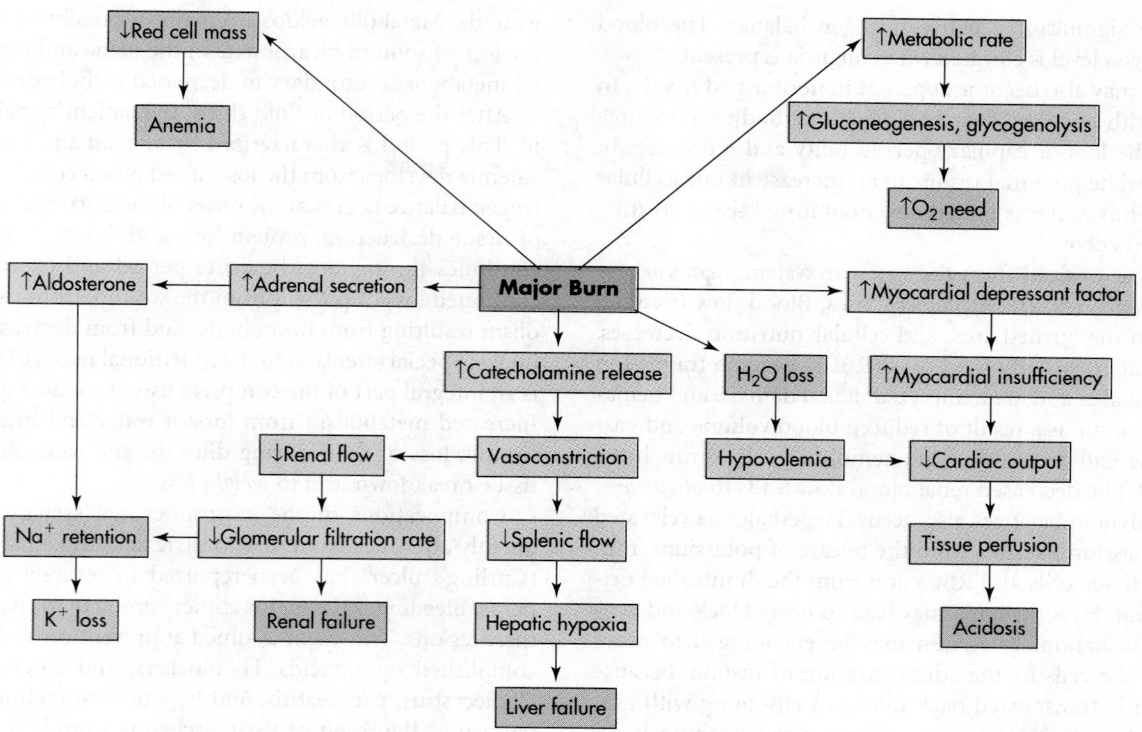


**fig. 64-2** Overview of pathophysiology of a major burn.

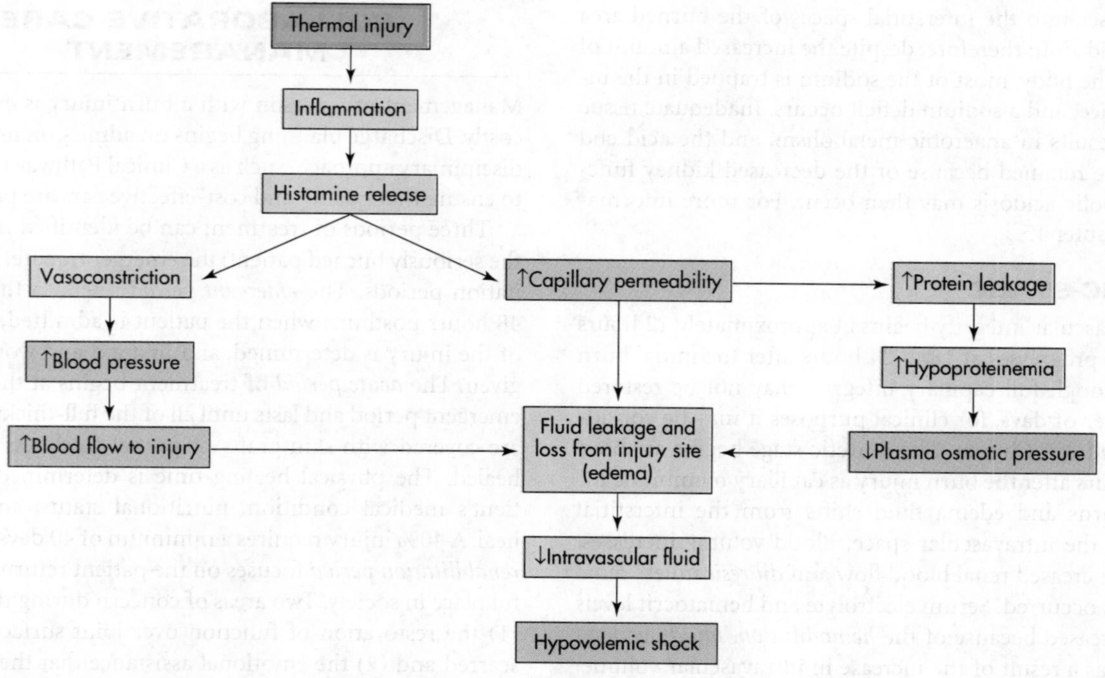


**fig. 64-3** Flow diagram of fluid shifts resulting in hypovolemic shock.

capillary osmotic pressure, leading to dehydration with pronounced *edema* in the burned area.

As protein continues to be lost into the burned area because of the increased capillary permeability, *hypoproteinemia* results. The increased amount of protein in the tissue spaces is a further contributing factor to edema formation. Proteins may be lost through the open wounds. The lymphatic system, which normally functions to remove increased tissue fluid, becomes overloaded and inefficient, contributing to edema formation. Nitrogen is lost through the kidney from catabolism, leading to significant negative nitrogen balance. The blood urea nitrogen level is elevated when oliguria is present.

Edema may also become apparent in nonburned tissues. In patients with burns greater than 30% total body surface area (TBSA), the loss of capillary permeability and a decrease in cell membrane potential results in an increase in intracellular sodium. Thus, water is pulled into nonburned tissue creating generalized edema.[22]

With loss of fluid from the vascular system, *hemoconcentration* occurs, and the *hematocrit* rises. Blood flow becomes sluggish in the burned area, and cellular nutrition decreases. Large numbers of red blood cells (RBCs) become trapped in the burned area and are hemolyzed. Renal damage and hematuria may occur as a result of reduced blood volume and passage of the end products of the hemolyzed cells through the glomeruli. The decreased renal blood flow leads to *oliguria*.

Electrolyte imbalances also occur. Hyperkalemia (elevated serum potassium) results from the release of potassium from damaged tissue cells and RBCs and from the diminished urinary output. Hyperkalemia may lead to heart block and ventricular fibrillation. Potassium may be encouraged to move back into the cells by the administration of insulin, because potassium is transported back into the cells along with glucose (see Chapter 15 for more information). Sodium is retained by the body as a result of the endocrine response to stress. Aldosterone secretion is increased, leading to increased sodium reabsorption by the kidney. This sodium, however, quickly passes into the interstitial spaces of the burned area with the fluid shift; therefore, despite the increased amount of sodium in the body, most of the sodium is trapped in the interstitial space, and a sodium deficit occurs. Inadequate tissue perfusion results in anaerobic metabolism, and the acid end products are retained because of the decreased kidney function. Metabolic acidosis may then occur. For more information see Chapter 15.

## DIURETIC STAGE

Return of vascular integrity begins at approximately 12 hours and rapidly progresses at 18 to 24 hours after the initial burn injury. Although full capillary integrity may not be restored for a number of days, for clinical purposes it may be considered restored at 24 hours. The diuretic stage begins at about 48 to 72 hours after the burn injury as capillary membrane integrity returns and edema fluid shifts from the interstitial spaces into the intravascular space. Blood volume increases, leading to increased renal blood flow and *diuresis* unless renal damage has occurred. Serum electrolyte and hematocrit levels will be decreased because of the *hemodilution*. *Fluid overload* may occur as a result of the increase in intravascular volume. The patient's vital signs, breath sounds, and urinary output are used to determine the amount of intravenous fluid replacement. Dehydration may occur if rapid urinary fluid losses deplete the intravascular reserve. Sodium deficit continues because of the loss of sodium through the burn wound and through the increase in urine output. Hypokalemia results from potassium moving back into the cells or being excreted in the urine. Protein continues to be lost from the wounds. Metabolic acidosis remains a possibility because of the loss of sodium bicarbonate in the urine and the increased fat metabolism secondary to decreased carbohydrate intake.

After the period of fluid shifts, the patient remains acutely ill. This period is characterized by *anemia* and *malnutrition*. Anemia develops from the loss of red blood cells. Negative nitrogen balance begins at the onset of the burn and is the result of tissue destruction, protein loss, and the stress response. It continues throughout the acute period and is secondary to continued loss of protein from the wound, from tissue catabolism resulting from immobility, and from decreased protein intake. Special attention to the nutritional needs of the patient is an integral part of the comprehensive care during this time. Increased metabolism from loss of water and heat from the wound, loss of fluid during diuresis, and catabolism during tissue breakdown lead to *weight loss*.

Complications of the gastrointestinal system occur frequently after thermal injury. Gastric and duodenal ulceration (Curling's ulcer) has been reported in severely burned patients. Bleeding is the major clinical problem for patients with these lesions. Treatment is aimed at prevention and is best accomplished by antacids, $H_2$ blockers, and enteral feedings. Cholecystitis, pancreatitis, and hepatic dysfunction may also be seen as the result of tissue ischemia from hypoperfusion. The differences in changes between the hypovolemic and diuretic stages are summarized in Table 64-2.

# COLLABORATIVE CARE MANAGEMENT

Management of a person with a burn injury is extensive and costly. Discharge planning begins on admission using a multidisciplinary approach, such as a Clinical Pathway (see p. 2114), to ensure that quality and cost-effective care are provided.

Three periods of treatment can be identified in the care of the seriously burned patient: the emergent, acute, and rehabilitation periods. The *emergent period* refers to the first 24 to 48 hours postburn when the patient is admitted, the severity of the injury is determined, and first aid and wound care are given. The *acute period* of treatment begins at the end of the emergent period and lasts until all of the full-thickness wounds are covered with skin grafts or partial-thickness wounds are healed. The physical healing time is determined by the patient's medical condition, nutritional status, and ability to heal. A 40% injury requires a minimum of 40 days to heal. The *rehabilitation period* focuses on the patient returning to a useful place in society. Two areas of concern during this phase are (1) the restoration of function over joint surfaces that were scarred and (2) the emotional assistance that the patient and family will need. The rehabilitation of the patient actually begins during early hospitalization and is addressed throughout the hospital stay. After the initial discharge, the patient may require emotional assistance and counseling, and many readmissions may be necessary for reconstructive procedures. Emotional and social healing depends on each patient's ability to cope with a new body image and society's acceptance of the change in the patient's physical appearance.

**table 64-2** *Physiological Changes with Burns*

| Hypovolemic Stage | | Diuretic Stage | |
|---|---|---|---|
| **Mechanism** | **Result** | **Mechanism** | **Result** |
| **EXTRACELLULAR FLUID SHIFT** | | | |
| Vascular to interstitial | Hemoconcentration<br>Edema at burn site | Interstitial to vascular | Hemodilution |
| **RENAL FUNCTION** | | | |
| Decreased renal blood flow from decreased blood pressure and decreased cardiac output | Oliguria | Increased renal blood flow from increased blood volume | Diuresis |
| **SODIUM LEVEL** | | | |
| $Na^+$ reabsorbed by kidneys *but* $Na^+$ lost in exudate and trapped in edema fluid | Sodium deficit | $Na^+$ loss with diuresis (becomes normal in 1 week) | Sodium deficit |
| **POTASSIUM LEVEL** | | | |
| $K^+$ released as result of tissue and red blood cell injury; decreased $K^+$ excretion from decreased renal function | Hyperkalemia | $K^+$ moves back into cells; $K^+$ lost by diuresis (begins 4-5 days after the burn) | Hypokalemia |
| **PROTEIN LEVEL** | | | |
| Protein lost into tissues by increased capillary permeability | Hypoproteinemia | Loss of protein during continued catabolism | Hypoproteinemia |
| **NITROGEN BALANCE** | | | |
| Tissue catabolism; protein loss in tissues; more nitrogen lost than taken in | Negative nitrogen balance | Tissue catabolism, protein loss, immobility | Negative nitrogen balance |
| **ACID BASE BALANCE** | | | |
| Anaerobic metabolism from decreased tissue perfusion; increased acid end products; decreased renal function (causing retention of acid end-products); loss of serum bicarbonate | Metabolic acidosis | Sodium bicarbonate lost in diuresis; hypermetabolism with increased metabolic end products | Metabolic acidosis |
| **STRESS RESPONSE** | | | |
| Occurs because of trauma | Decreased renal blood flow | Occurs because of prolonged nature of injury and psychological threat to self | Stress ulcers |

Each of the three periods and the management required is discussed below.

## EMERGENT PERIOD

The goals of management during the emergent period, the first 24 to 48 hours after a burn, are to (1) secure the airway, (2) support circulation by fluid replacement, (3) keep the patient comfortable with analgesics, (4) prevent infection through careful wound care, (5) maintain body temperature, and (6) provide emotional support. The nurse and physician work collaboratively to achieve these goals. The specific details of treatment are discussed below under Nursing Management.

### Prehospital Care and First Aid

At the scene of a burn injury, the first action should be to remove the victim from the hazardous environment. Length of exposure to the causative agent is directly related to the severity of the injury (Guidelines for Care Box).

**guidelines for care**

**Prehospital Care of Major Burns**

1. Remove victim from source of burn.
2. Douse with water and remove nonadherent smoldering clothing to stop the burning process.
3. If chemical burn, carefully remove clothing and flush wound with large amounts of water.
4. If electrical burn and victim is still in contact with electrical source, do *not* touch victim. Remove electrical source with dry nonconductive object.
5. Establish patent airway and assess for inhalation injury. Give oxygen if available.
6. Check peripheral pulses to assess circulatory status.
7. Assess and initiate treatment for injuries requiring immediate attention.
8. Remove tight-fitting jewelry or clothing.
9. Cover burn with moist sterile or clean cover.
10. Cover victim with warm, dry cover to prevent heat loss.
11. Transport victim to nearest medical facility.

## clinical pathway *Extensive Burns Without (Prior to) Surgery and After Surgery (Post Op Day 6)*

DRG: ______
EXPECTED LOS: ______
ADMIT DATE: ______
ACTUAL LOS: ______
DISCHARGE DATE: ______

(page 1 of 2)

ATTENDING PHYSICIAN: ______

**CONSULTS:**
SOCIAL WORK OT/PT CHILD LIFE PHARMACY
NUTRITION CARE MANAGEMENT PASTORAL CARE
(Initial when complete in shaded box) ☐

Authors:
R. Fratianne, M.D.
C. Brandt, M.D.
Lynne Yurko, R.N.
Burn Team

Metro Health Medical Center
Cleveland, Ohio

| | (EMERGENT PHASE) | | (ACUTE PHASE Day 3) | | (REHABILITATION PHASE 1 Week Prior to Discharge) |
|---|---|---|---|---|---|
| **ELEMENTS** | **DAY 1** | **DAY 2** | | **DISCHARGE** | **OUTCOMES** |
| **Diagnostic Testing** | ☐ Chem 7&11 —— daily ——→<br>☐ EKG<br>☐ Cultures (Wound)<br>☐ Tox Screen<br>☐ Sickle Cell<br>☐ CBC/Diff<br>☐ Platelets<br>☐ PT/PTT<br>☐ Type & screen<br>☐ Pre-albumin q Mon & Thur<br>☐ 24 hr. Urine q Sun & Wed<br>☐ UA<br>☐ Chest X-Ray<br>☐ Refer to DVT Protocol<br>☐ Testing for premorbid condition<br>☐ ABG with Respiratory Symptoms —— ABGs with ventilator or O2 therapy changes | ☐ CBC ——→<br>☐ Chest X-Ray<br>☐ Repeat abnormal Lab findings<br>☐ Evaluation for Chest X-ray | Reassess Lab needs according to results daily<br>☐ Cultures (wound) —— ☐ q Mon & Wed ——→<br>Reassess Lab needs according to results daily<br>☐ SW assessment (within 5 working days) | | 1. Patient will maintain a balanced metabolic state.<br>2. Patient with/without acute respiratory insult will maintain optimal airway/ pulmonary function. |
| **Medications/ IV Therapy** | ☐ Vitamins<br>☐ Minerals<br>☐ Stool Softener (when on bedrest)<br>☐ Fluid/colloid resus.<br>**Peds: 2-4cc/kg/% TBSA Burned plus 1/2 maintenance: Monitor Urine Output for .5-1 cc/hr<br>**Adult: 4cc/kg/% TBSA Burned (Monitor Urine output 30-50 cc/hr)<br>☐ IV Catheter sites rethread day 3 and changed day 6<br>☐ Routine IV Protocols: Adult and Peds.<br>☐ Pain Management/Assessment —— Pain Scale Daily<br>☐ $H_2$ Blockers<br>☐ Tetanus Proph.<br>☐ Immunization status/Peds | | ☐ Antibiotics per culture or wound assessment ——→<br>☐ IV: fluids or IIP ——→ | | 1. Patient maintains optimal cardiac and circulatory status.<br>2. Patient will attain a self-identified acceptable level of pain relief.<br>3. Absence of clinical signs of IV infiltration, site infection, line occlussion or thrombophlebitis. |
| **Treatments** | ☐ Wound care protocol ——→ ☐ assists with wound care ——→ ☐ performs wound care ——→ until discharge<br>☐ Routine care protocol until discharge<br>☐ Isolation<br>☐ Weight | ☐ Weight ☐ Weight | ☐ Weight daily ☐ Weight ☐ Weight | ☐ Weight daily | 1. Patient will remain free from wound infection/wound related sepsis.<br>2. Burns heal without complications. |

| | (EMERGENT PHASE) | | | (ACUTE PHASE Day 3) | | (REHABILITATION PHASE 1 Week Prior to Discharge) |
|---|---|---|---|---|---|---|
| **ELEMENTS** | **DAY 1** | **DAY 2** | | | **DISCHARGE** | **OUTCOMES** |
| **Treatments (cont'd)** | Grid pediatric < 12 yrs.<br>Splinting →<br>Positioning →<br>Evaluate for pressure relief (Low air loss bed)<br>P/T & O/T ROM | | | Reassess —<br>Reassess —<br>ADL When appropriate | Plan Discharge Needs<br>Plan Discharge Needs | 3. Unburned skin integrity will be maintained.<br>4. Patient will maintain or attain optimal level of function.<br>5. Patient will have daily periods of rest/sleep. |
| **Nutrition** | Tube Feeding per Protocol<br>Nutrition Screen → | Nasojejunal Tube placement in 24 hours | | Advance Diet According to needs | | Patient will maintain or achieve optimal nutrition status. |
| **Activity** | May be bedrest or up to chair with activity as tolerated<br>P/T & O/T ROM Exercise<br>Child Life planning → | | | Increase activity to ambulating independently<br>Gym Program — | Independent with exercise program | Patient will maintain/attain an optimal level of functioning. |
| **Assessment and Monitoring** | Standard Medical H+P<br>I+O →<br>Standard Nursing Assessment on admit and q8 hours<br>S.W. Consultation for patient and family →<br>Photo Permit Signed<br>Photos on admit and weekly →<br>Pastoral Care Assessment within 3 days<br>Cardiac Monitor/Pulse Ox — | | | Assess I&O monitoring needs<br>DC Monitors when non-critical | | 1. Patient will maintain a balanced metabolic state. (For age and stage of recovery)<br>2. Stable Cardiac Rhythm<br>3. Identify needed spiritual/religion support.<br>4. Identify patient's faith group/religion denomination to determine spiritual response. |
| **Patient/Family Education** | Emergent Care Teaching →<br>Orient to:<br>1. Unit<br>2. Burn Injury<br>3. Infection Control<br>Initiate Learning Pathway →<br>Patients/Families told clergy can be contacted<br>Pastoral Care consultation for patient & family. | | Evaluate Home and resources available for discharge<br>Educate Pt./Family on Burn Recovery Process →<br>Follow through to home care<br>Gym Program introduced<br>Educate Nutritional Requirements | Acute Care Teaching → | Rehab Teaching | 1. Patient/Caregiver response/interactions are appropriate for phase of injury.<br>2. Patient/caregiver will participate in the total management of care.<br>3. Patient/caregiver response & intervention demonstrates adaptation to injury. |
| **Discharge Planning** | Diet<br>Visitor Booklet<br>Education Pack | | Videos<br>Discharge Class<br>Diet<br>Adult Support Group | OT/PT recommendations (for Discharge) | Wound Care Instruction Complete<br>Outpatient Plans complete<br>Follow-up Appointments Made<br>OT/PT teaching complete<br>Diet Instructions complete as appropriate. | 1. Patient/Caregiver will verbalize/demonstrate an understanding of post-hospital care and follow-up requirements.<br>2. Patient reenters society at preburn status/or makes adjustments.<br>3. Appropriate sacramental/religious rites will be offered. |


IIP, intermittent infusion plug.

The most common causative agents for burn injury are fire, scalding fluids, chemicals, and electricity. Other types of injuries result from contact with hot surfaces. Regardless of the cause, the burning process must be stopped.

Flame and flash injuries are the second most common types of burn injury and are commonly associated with an inhalation injury if the burn has occurred in a closed space. These injuries may occur from house fires (caused by smoking in bed or children playing with matches) or ignited gasoline or propane. Injuries may be combined partial- and full-thickness burns. The amount and duration of the flame will determine the depth of the injury. In the case of fire, flames should be extinguished, flammable or hot material removed from the victim, and the victim and rescuer removed from the unventilated or hazardous surroundings. If clothing is on fire, the victim's first reaction is to run, which only fans the flames. The best intervention is to stop the person, wrap him or her in a blanket, coat, sheet, or towel, and roll him or her on the ground to exclude oxygen and thereby put out the fire. The rule is *stop, drop,* and *roll.* The victim should never stand because this will cause the flames and smoke to engulf the facial area, possibly igniting the hair and causing an inhalation injury. Any water source can be used to extinguish flames, cool the burn, or dilute the chemical unless the victim is still in contact with an electrical source. Once all flame is extinguished, clothing (excepting clothing that adheres to the burned area), jewelry, and debris are carefully removed. Any clothing removed should be saved for possible analysis of flammability.

*Contact burns* occur from direct contact with a hot substance, such as hot metal, stoves, hot tar, or irons. The area of burn is usually confined to the area where the substance came into contact with the skin. The treatment goal is to stop the burning process.

*Scald burns* are the most common burn injury, particularly in children. Scald injury may be caused by steam or hot fluids and may affect a widespread area (Figure 64-4). Scald injury is related to the temperature of the liquid and length of exposure. Initial care consists of cooling the skin with cool water. First aid follows the same treatment plan as for a flame burn, that is, stop the burning process.

*Chemical burns* are usually the result of accidents in homes or industry but may be the result of a deliberate assault on an individual. Household chemical burns may be caused by drain cleaners, disinfectants, and other chemicals used in the home. Industrial chemicals such as strong acids (hydrochloric), alkali, and organic compounds such as phenol and petroleum products (gasoline) are common causes of chemical burns. Thousands of chemicals are in use today and exposure to them may cause thermal injury. The severity of the injury is related to the chemical involved, its concentration, length of exposure, and the immediate treatment. Treatment should include irrigation of the area with copious amounts of water or saline.[23] Serious burns to the eyes may occur whenever a chemical splashes onto the face. Treatment includes careful irrigation of the eye with water. Adequacy of the irrigation is determined by testing a sample of the irrigated fluid with litmus paper to test for the presence of acid or alkali. Ingestion of noxious chemicals may burn the upper gastrointestinal tract. These burns are difficult to treat and frequently cause complications.

*Electrical burns* pose a special hazard to the victim because the total body surface area of the burn is not always apparent and is often internal. Dysrhythmias and neurological dysfunction are common.[23] Extreme care must be taken when removing the victim from the electrical source to prevent a similar injury to the rescuer.

Initial management follows the completion of the primary assessment of a head to toe evaluation and ongoing management of the ABCs: airway, breathing, and circulation. A secondary assessment is performed as long as the patient has no life-endangering injuries. The secondary assessment includes the mechanism of injury and medical history including

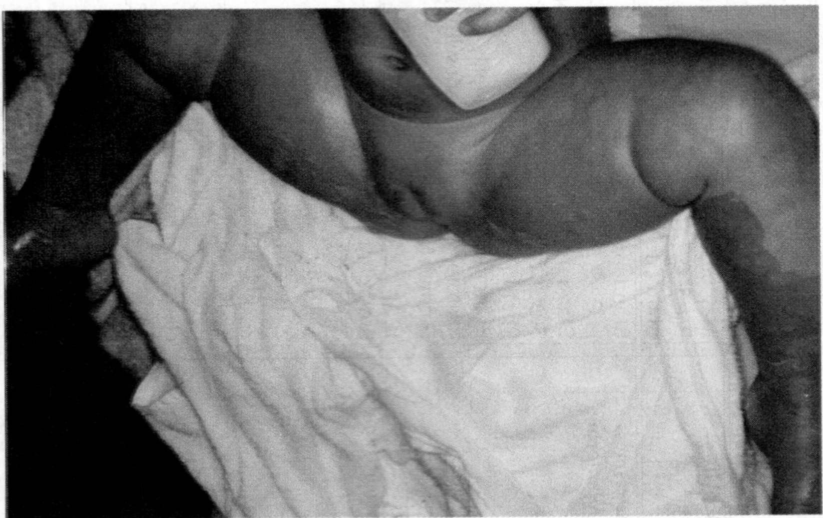

**fig. 64-4** Child with scald burns on lower extremities and perineum.

allergies and medications the patient is taking. During this assessment the burn wound is evaluated and treated. Life-threatening conditions are cared for before the burn wound.

Burn wounds are covered with dressings dampened with normal saline or water, which eases the pain, reduces edema, and prevents evaporation of body water. The patient's entire body is wrapped in a dry cover to prevent heat loss. Ice should never be used because sudden vasoconstriction causes severe shifting of body fluids and may increase the depth of injury. Although sterile dressings are preferred, clean dressings may be used because all dressings will be removed when the patient arrives at the medical facility. Oils, salves, and ointments should never be used on burns.

Standard Precautions should be followed whenever there is a possibility of exposure to blood or other body fluids. This includes the wearing of gown, gloves, mask, and eye protection. Initial care of the person with a major burn in the emergency department is summarized in the Guidelines for Care Box.

### Pain Relief

In the prehospital period, pain in extensive burns is best controlled by gentle and minimal handling and by application of dressings to exclude air from burned surfaces. The degree of pain is usually inversely proportional to the depth of the burn injury. As mentioned earlier, full-thickness burns are usually painless because nerve endings have been destroyed.

In small partial-thickness burns, cool (not cold) compresses applied to the burn may provide some relief as long as the victim is kept warm. Ice packs are contraindicated because they may cause further skin injury and hypothermia.

### Transporting the Burn Victim

Burns are often more severe than they first appear to be; therefore, even patients with burns that appear to be superficial should be seen by a physician. The hospital or burn center should be notified before a burn victim is transported so that they have time to prepare for the patient's arrival.

Transfer of the patient should not be delayed because of difficulty in establishing an intravenous line. The American Burn Association teaches that an IV line is not necessary if the patient is less than 60 minutes from the hospital. When an IV line is established the recommended solution is Ringer's lactate infused at 500 ml/hr for an adult and 250 ml/hr for a child age 5 years or older. No IV lines are recommended for children younger than age 5.[18]

For obviously small burns fluids may be given by mouth with caution. Large burns cause decreased peristalsis, and nothing should be given by mouth. Patients with large burns or who have inhaled smoke may vomit, and attention is given to preventing them from aspirating vomitus.

Patients with major burns should be transported to a regional burn center. The American Burn Association's 1996-1997 report of burn centers in North America lists 135 hospitals in the United States that have burn care centers. These burn units are located throughout the country, and most are found in major medical centers in urban areas. Canada has 12 burn care centers.[5]

**guidelines for care**

**Initial Treatment of Major Burns in Emergency Department**

1. Establish airway.
2. Initiate fluid therapy by intravenous catheters.
3. Insert indwelling catheter for hourly urine measurement.
4. Insert nasogastric tube to remove stomach contents and prevent gastric distention.
5. Insert central intravenous catheter, if appropriate.
6. Manage pain by intravenous narcotics in small frequent doses.
7. Provide tetanus prophylaxis.

## EMERGENCY ROOM MANAGEMENT

Rapid and efficient care is essential in the emergency room management of the victim with a major burn (see the Guidelines for Care Box). If any respiratory distress is present, an airway is established. Prophylactic intubation is initiated if any heat or smoke has been inhaled, or if the head, neck, or face is involved. Inhalation injuries are best managed with controlled ventilation because swelling of the upper airway can progress to obstruction (Figure 64-5). Endotracheal intubation is preferred over a tracheostomy. Edema of the respiratory passages frequently subsides within a few days after the initial injury; therefore surgery of the airway should be avoided. Depending

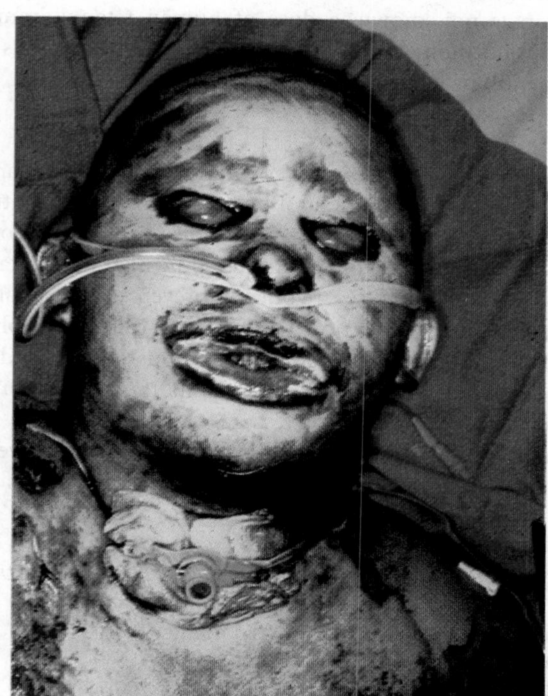

**fig. 64-5** Patient with massive upper airway edema requiring a tracheotomy to prevent airway obstruction.

on the severity of symptoms, emergency treatment may include oxygen, suctioning, and postural drainage.

After an airway has been established, circulatory support is addressed. Fluid is best replaced through two large-caliber peripheral intravenous catheters. Placement of these catheters is through an unburned site to prevent the introduction of infection. An indwelling urinary catheter is inserted to adequately monitor urine output. Hourly urine output measurements are used as a guide to the adequacy of fluid (plasma volume) replacement.

Almost every patient whose burn involves more than 15% of total body surface area (TBSA) develops thirst and an ileus. Oral fluids will not pass beyond the stomach (therefore, they will not relieve thirst), and they create a threat of regurgitation and aspiration. A nasogastric tube is inserted and attached to suction to prevent gastric distention.

### Medications

Morphine sulfate is the drug of choice for pain relief and is given intravenously in small increments (2 to 4 mg). A morphine drip can be used and titrated to the patient's pain. *No medication of any kind should be given intramuscularly or subcutaneously because it may pool and be absorbed later when cardiac output and blood pressure improve.* Large doses of sedatives and analgesics are avoided because of the danger of respiratory depression and the potential for masking other symptoms.

Tetanus prophylaxis is given in the emergency room. Tetanus toxoid is administered if the patient has been previously immunized but has not received tetanus toxoid in the preceding 5 years. If information about prior tetanus immunization is not known, a dose of human tetanus-immune globulin hormone is administered, and an active tetanus immunization program is begun.

### Treatments

Replacing fluids and electrolytes (fluid resuscitation) is an essential part of the treatment of burn victims and is instituted as soon as the severity of the burn and the patient's condition are known (Box 64-1). Ideally, fluid therapy is started within an hour after a severe burn to prevent the onset of hypovolemic shock. Insertion of two large-caliber peripheral catheters or one large-caliber central venous catheter and one large-caliber peripheral catheter permits the rapid administration of fluids and electrolytes.

Fluids administered during the first 48 hours are given to maintain circulating blood volume. Additional fluids and electrolytes are added to replace losses from vomiting or from nasogastric drainage. Two types of fluids are considered when calculating the needs of the patient: crystalloids and colloids.

*Crystalloids* may be isotonic or hypertonic. Isotonic solutions, such as lactated Ringer's or physiological (0.9%) sodium chloride, do not generate a difference in osmotic pressure between the intravascular and interstitial spaces. Thus large amounts of fluids are required to restore and maintain the intravascular volume. Hypertonic salt solutions have a milliosmolar content of 400 to 600 (280 to 300 mosm is isotonic), thus creating an osmotic pull of fluid from the interstitial space back to the depleted intravascular space. The use of hypertonic solutions decreases the amount of fluid a patient needs during resuscitation,[15] which helps decrease burn tissue edema and minimizes cardiopulmonary complications (pulmonary edema and congestive heart failure).

The most common formula used to calculate fluid requirements is the Parkland formula which follows. In the first three 8-hour periods (24 hours) lactated Ringer's solution (RL) is administered according to this formula:

$$4 \text{ ml RL} \times \text{weight (kg)} \times \text{\% BSA burned} = \text{ml RL for the first 24 hours}$$

Because blood volume falls most rapidly and edema increases most rapidly in the first 8 hours, intravenous replacement is accomplished at a rapid rate. One half of the total amount calculated is given in the first 8 hours after the injury. *The time is calculated from the time of injury,* not from the time emergency care was initiated. In the second 8-hour period, one fourth of the total amount of calculated lactated Ringer's solution is given and in the third 8-hour period, the remaining one fourth is given. For example, if a patient weighing 75 kg has a 70% TBSA burn, the fluid requirements are:

1. 4 ml lactated Ringer's × 75 kg × 70% = 21,000 ml needed over the first 24 hours
2. one half is needed in the first 8 hours
   $\frac{1}{2} \times 21{,}000 = 10{,}500$ ml in 8 hours, or 1312 ml/hr
3. one fourth is needed in each of the next two 8-hour periods
   $\frac{1}{4} \times 21{,}000 = 5250$ ml in 8 hours, or 656 ml/hr

*Colloids* may also be used to replace body fluids.[8] Traditionally, the use of colloids in the first 24 hours was avoided because of the leak of protein through the capillaries into the interstitial space. The capillary permeability caused by the burn injury begins to close at 12 hours. At this time patients may receive colloids such as fresh-frozen plasma, albumin, or dextran. The oncotic pressure generated by the colloids also helps pull fluid back into the intravascular space. In addition, fresh-frozen plasma is beneficial in restoring lost clotting factors. Red blood cells are used only if the patient has had a significant loss or destruction of red cells.

During the second 24 hours postburn, one half to two thirds of the initial 24-hour volume is required. Also during this second 24-hour period colloid solutions are used to replace intravascular volume once capillary permeability significantly decreases.

After the first 48 to 72 hours, the patient enters the diuretic stage or phase as edema reabsorption occurs. The urinary out-

**box 64-1** *Indications for Fluid Resuscitation*

Burns greater than 20% TBSA in adults
Burns greater than 10% TBSA in children
Patient older than 65 or younger than 2 years of age
Patient with preexisting disease that would reduce normal compensatory responses to minor hypovolemia (i.e., cardiac or pulmonary disease or diabetes)

put increases dramatically and is no longer a reliable guide to fluid needs, and fluid needs are assessed by measuring serum and urine electrolyte levels. Fluid replacement, using 5% dextrose and water, is based on patient assessment. If dehydration occurs from diuresis, fluid replacement therapy is continued until blood volume is stabilized. Potassium may be added to the intravenous fluid because of potassium losses in the urine. The patient is monitored closely for signs of *water intoxication* or *pulmonary edema*.

## NURSING MANAGEMENT

### ASSESSMENT

Assessment of the person who has sustained a severe burn depends on the severity of the burn injury.

#### Subjective Data

Knowledge of circumstances surrounding the burn injury is extremely valuable in the management of a burn victim. This information can be obtained from either the burn victim or witnesses to the event. Data should include:

- How the burn injury occurred
- When the burn injury occurred
- Duration of contact with the burning agent
- Location (enclosed area suggests possibility of smoke inhalation and/or carbon monoxide poisoning)
- Presence of an explosion (suggests possibility of other injuries)

The burn victim's age and general health may modify treatment. Elderly patients and very young patients have a higher mortality rate than a young adult with the same percentage of burn. Preexisting endocrine, pulmonary, cardiovascular, or renal disease or a history of drug abuse will decrease a victim's ability to cope with severe burns. Because most burn patients will require topical and systemic therapy with a number of drugs, allergies and drug sensitivities must be determined and documented.

#### Objective Data

Burns may be categorized as major, moderate, or minor on the basis of the size of the burn and the presence of complicating factors (Box 64-2).

##### *Assessing the severity of the burn injury*

**Medical history.** Identification of known and unknown disorders may prevent fatal complications in the burn victim. A prior illness, such as diabetes or renal failure, may become acute during the postburn phase. The physiological stress seen with the burn may exacerbate a latent disease process or worsen an already active process and thus increase mortality. Diabetes and chronic obstructive pulmonary disease may be aggravated, or patients with arteriosclerotic heart disease may develop a myocardial infarction.

**Size and depth of burn.** For adults, the "rule of nines" is used to determine the size of the burn. The percentage of TBSA burned is estimated with the use of charts that depict anterior and posterior drawings of the body. In adults, the body is divided into areas equal to multiples of 9% (Figure 64-6). In clinical practice, the burned area is shaded in on the drawings, and the amount of body surface burned is calculated from the shaded areas. Calculations are modified

**box 64-2** *Classification of Severity of Burns*

**MAJOR BURN INJURIES**

- Partial-thickness injury greater than 25% TBSA (greater than 20% in children less than 10 years and adults more than 40 years)
- Greater than 10% TBSA, full-thickness (children and adults)
- Involvement of face, eyes, ears, hands, feet, or perineum
- Electrical burns
- Burns complicated by inhalation injury or major trauma
- Burns in patients with preexisting disease (diabetes, congestive heart failure, or chronic renal failure)

**MODERATE BURN INJURIES**

- 15-25% TBSA in adults, partial-thickness (10-20% TBSA in children less than 10 years and adults more than 40 years)
- 2-10% TBSA full-thickness
- Burns with no concurrent injury
- Burns in patients with no preexisting disease

**MINOR BURN INJURIES**

- Less than 15% TBSA in adults (10% in children or elderly persons)
- Less than 2% TBSA full-thickness injury
- Burns in patients with no preexisting disease

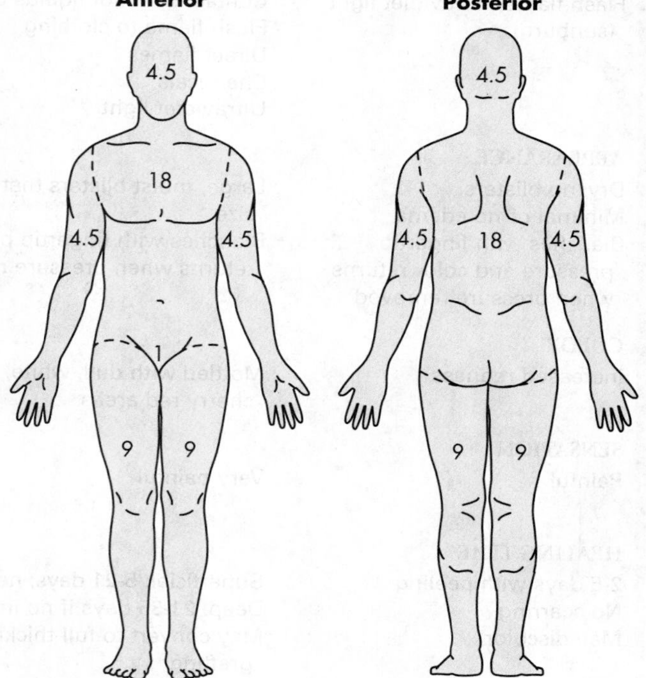


**fig. 64-6** Rule of nines.

for infants and children younger than 10 years of age because of their relatively larger head and smaller body (consult a pediatric textbook for these figures). The depth of the burn injury is evaluated on the basis of appearance, color, and sensation (Table 64-3).

**Age of victim.** The severity of a burn also depends on the age of the victim. Infants younger than 2 years of age and adults older than 60 years have a higher mortality rate than persons in other age-groups with a similar size injury. The infant has a weak antibody response to infection, and in older victims the serious burn may aggravate the degenerative processes or exacerbate a preexisting health problem.

**Body part involved.** The body part involved is an important factor in evaluating the severity of a burn. The part of the body burned must be considered when the severity of the burn is estimated: a 3% burn of the anterior surface of the thigh is not as serious as a 3% burn to the neck, face, or perineal area. Injuries that involve cosmetic and functional areas of the body require a long period of recovery because of both physical and emotional reactions to the burn injury. A burn of the face, hands, and feet requires extensive, meticulous care, and extensive physical and occupational therapy. A burn of the head, neck, and chest may also involve injury to the respiratory tract and result in severe respiratory distress. Burns of the perineum are difficult to manage because of the potential for contamination and infection. The circumferential, or encircling burn, of a limb, the neck, or the chest has serious consequences. This type of burn will cause constrictive contraction of the skin and produce a tourniquet effect that may impair breathing and/or circulation.

**Mechanism of injury.** Identifying the causative agent is of prime importance because the nature of the agent has a direct effect on prognosis and treatment. As mentioned earlier, mechanisms of burn injury are flame and flash, contact, scald, chemical, and electric. The factors determining the severity of burns are summarized in Box 64-3.

## NURSING DIAGNOSES

Nursing diagnoses are determined from analyses of patient data. Nursing diagnoses for the person with burns during the emergent period may include but are not limited to:

**table 64-3** *Characteristics of Depth of Burn Injury*

| Superficial Partial-Thickness (First-Degree) | Deep Partial-Thickness (Second-Degree) | Full-Thickness (Third-Degree) |
|---|---|---|
| **SKIN DEPTH** | | |
| Epidermis | Entire epidermis, partial dermis<br>Sweat glands, hair follicles intact | Epidermis, dermis<br>Extends to subcutaneous tissue, possibly muscle and bone |
| **CAUSE** | | |
| Flash flame, ultraviolet light (sunburn) | Contact with hot liquids or solids<br>Flash flame to clothing<br>Direct flames<br>Chemicals<br>Ultraviolet light | Contact with hot liquids or solids<br>Flame<br>Chemicals<br>Electrical contact |
| **APPEARANCE** | | |
| Dry, no blisters<br>Minimal or no edema<br>Blanches with fingertip pressure and color returns when pressure removed | Large, moist blisters that will increase in size<br>Blanches with fingertip pressure and color returns when pressure removed | Dry with leathery eschar<br>Charred vessels visible under eschar<br>Blisters rare but thin-walled blisters that do not increase in size may be present<br>No blanching with pressure |
| **COLOR** | | |
| Increased redness | Mottled with dull, white, tan, pink, or cherry red areas | White, charred, dark tan, black, red |
| **SENSATION** | | |
| Painful | Very painful | No pain<br>Nerve endings dead |
| **HEALING TIME** | | |
| 2-5 days with peeling<br>No scarring<br>May discolor | Superficial: 5-21 days; no grafting<br>Deep: 21-35 days if no infection<br>May convert to full-thickness and require grafting | No healing potential<br>Requires excision and grafting<br>Healing of grafts may take months |

| Diagnostic Title | Etiological Factors |
|---|---|
| Airway clearance, ineffective | Tracheobronchial edema, obstruction, secretions |
| Fluid volume deficit (hypovolemic stage) | Abnormal fluid loss: movement of fluid from intravascular to interstitial space; evaporation |
| Fluid volume excess (diuretic stage) | Movement of fluid from interstitial to intravascular space |
| Hypothermia | Impaired temperature regulatory mechanisms; wound exposure to environment |
| Infection, risk for | Break in skin integrity |
| Skin integrity, impaired | Burn injury, impaired perfusion |
| Pain, acute | Trauma, exposure of nerve endings |
| Anxiety | Threat of death, situational crisis |

## EXPECTED PATIENT OUTCOMES

Expected patient outcomes for the burn-injured patient during the emergent phase include:

1. Maintains a patent airway, adequate oxygenation, and ventilation.
2. Exhibits no signs of fluid deficit.
3. Exhibits no signs of fluid excess.
4. Has a body temperature greater than 37° C.
5. Does not develop an infection.
6. Has no further tissue loss.
7. Achieves an acceptable level of pain
8. Verbalizes concerns and does not appear to be anxious.

## INTERVENTIONS

### Maintaining a Patent Airway

Persons who are burned on the face and neck or those who have inhaled flame, steam, or smoke are observed closely for signs of laryngeal edema and airway obstruction. Data indicating potential or existing inhalation injury are outlined in Box 64-4.

Adequate ventilation and oxygenation may be possible with the victim breathing room air; however, when any inhalation injury has occurred, it is best to give oxygen. When smoke is inhaled, carbon monoxide binds with hemoglobin, displacing oxygen. High carboxyhemoglobin levels impair tissue oxygenation resulting in tissue asphyxia. Providing the victim with 100% oxygen by mask will reverse this condition. If the victim is in respiratory distress or has a suspected inhalation injury endotracheal intubation may be necessary.[4a]

**box 64-3** *Factors Determining Severity of Burns*

- Size of burn
- Depth of burn
- Age of victim
- Body part involved
- Mechanism of injury
- History of cardiac, pulmonary, renal, or hepatic disease
- Injuries sustained at time of burn

### Maintaining Fluid Volume

During fluid resuscitation, adequate volume is assessed by monitoring mental status, vital signs, peripheral perfusion, body weight, and urine output. A 15% to 20% weight gain in the first 72 hours of resuscitation is anticipated. Significant laboratory measurements include serum and urine electrolytes, serum and urine osmolality, and hematocrit. Hourly urine output is the most accessible and generally a reliable index of adequate fluid replacement. Fluid should be titrated to ensure an output of 30 to 50 ml/hr. The most common reasons for a urine output below 30 ml/hr, indicating insufficient fluid replacement, are that the calculated fluid replacement is behind schedule and the severity of the burn has been underestimated. The urine is observed for color and analyzed for the presence of blood. The physician is notified if hematuria or a positive Hemastix reaction is present.

Other clinical criteria that indicate adequate resuscitation are pulse rate of 120 beats/min or less, central venous pressure in the low to normal range, pulmonary artery end-diastolic pressure in the low to normal range, and mental lucidity (Box 64-5).

Decreasing blood pH is an indication that fluids have not been given in sufficient quantities to maximize tissue perfusion. Anaerobic metabolism ensues when the metabolic tissue requirements are not met during resuscitation.

After the first 48 to 72 hours, the patient enters the diuretic stage or phase as edema reabsorption occurs. The urinary output increases dramatically and is no longer a reliable guide

**box 64-4** *Factors Determining Inhalation Injury and/or Potential Airway Obstruction*

- Burns to face and neck
- Singed hairs, nasal hair, beard, eyelids or eyelashes
- Intraoral charcoal, especially on teeth and gums
- Brassy cough
- Hoarseness
- Copious sputum production
- Carbonaceous sputum
- Burn injury that has occurred in a closed space
- Smell of smoke on victim's clothes or on victim
- Respiratory distress

**box 64-5** *Signs of Adequate Fluid Resuscitation*

- Clear sensorium
- Pulse <120 beats/min
- Urine output: 30 to 50 ml/hr (adult)
- Systolic blood pressure: 100 mm Hg
- Central venous pressure: 5 to 10 mm Hg
- Pulmonary capillary wedge pressure (PCWP): 5 to 15 mm Hg
- Blood pH normal range: 7.35 to 7.45

to fluid needs. Fluid needs are assessed by measuring serum and urine electrolyte levels. Fluid replacement, using 5% dextrose and water, is based on individual patient assessment. If dehydration occurs from diuresis, fluid replacement therapy is continued until blood volume is stabilized. Potassium may be added to the intravenous fluid because of potassium losses in the urine. The patient is monitored closely for signs of water intoxication or pulmonary edema.

Patients may complain of moderate to severe thirst during this period. Aggressive oral hygiene may alleviate patient discomfort. If oral fluids are permitted, accurate recording of ingested fluids is important. Unlimited oral intake and failure to measure it may provide too much fluid in the circulating blood, resulting in water intoxication.

### Maintaining Body Temperature

Maintenance of body temperature is a critical factor for the severely burned patient because of the loss of some of the ability to regulate body temperature. The environment must be heat controlled and kept warmer than usual. Drafts must be eliminated. A heat lamp or warming lights should be available. Prolonged exposure to air is avoided. Exposed areas of the body are covered with sterile sheets and blankets to decrease the loss of body heat through the open wounds while other areas of the burn are being cleansed.

### Providing Initial Wound Care

Care of the burn wound can be delayed until all first aid measures have been initiated. Wound care should be carried out carefully and with as little discomfort to the patient as possible. One of the most important factors to be considered in wound care is that the patient has lost the ability to withstand infection in the area where the skin is damaged or destroyed. The goals of the initial wound care are as follows:

1. Cleanse the wound to eliminate or decrease the dead tissue and debris that serve as the media for bacterial growth.
2. Prevent further destruction of viable skin.
3. Provide for patient comfort.

During the admission procedure, the burn wound and the entire body are washed to remove dirt and debris as well as loose dead tissue on the burned areas. Detergents or antiseptic preparations are effective cleansing agents. Gentle cleansing with gauze is effective in removing dead tissue without causing further tissue damage.

All hair in and around the burn wound is shaved and wiped off the skin because hair attracts and shelters bacteria. Singed hair is clipped short to avoid bacterial contamination of the wound.

Firm, intact blisters can remain undisturbed because they are a natural protective and pain-free dressing. If the blisters are broken and the epidermis is separated, loose tissue must be debrided.

After the wound is cleaned and before a dressing is applied, cultures of the wound are obtained. Baseline cultures provide information about organisms present in the wounds at the time of admission. Prophylactic antibiotics are usually not indicated.

Photographs are taken on admission and at intervals during the patient's hospitalization. These pictures provide a record of the appearance of the burn wound on admission, before the application of topical therapy, and during the healing process.

The constricting effect of nonviable tissue (eschar) from a full-thickness injury to the chest, neck, or extremities is an early complication. Edema forming rapidly under the constricting eschar will produce a tourniquet effect that causes occlusion of venous and arterial circulation and may result in *ischemic necrosis,* especially with unburned areas distal to the constrictive eschar. Frequent monitoring of distal pulses is part of an ongoing assessment to ensure uninterrupted vascular flow to all extremities. Extremities should be monitored for signs and symptoms of circulatory compromise, including diminished peripheral pulses, decreased capillary refill, paleness or cyanosis, temperature decrease, and increase in pain or paresthesia. It may be necessary to monitor circulation every 15 minutes.

Circumferential burns of the neck and chest can lead to constriction of chest wall expansion and airway compromise resulting in respiratory distress.[11] Monitoring chest excursions, respiratory rate, and ventilator settings, if the person is intubated, for high pressures and low tidal volume is part of the respiratory assessment.

Treatment of the constricting effects of the eschar is an *escharotomy,* which is performed on the burn unit. An escharotomy is a linear surgical incision through the burn eschar that releases the constriction caused by the full-thickness injury (Figure 64-7). Escharotomies are painless procedures because the nerve endings have been damaged by the burn.

### Providing Comfort

The patient is kept as comfortable as possible by gentle handling of the burn areas and by keeping the wounds covered so that air does not reach them. Small doses of morphine are given intravenously.

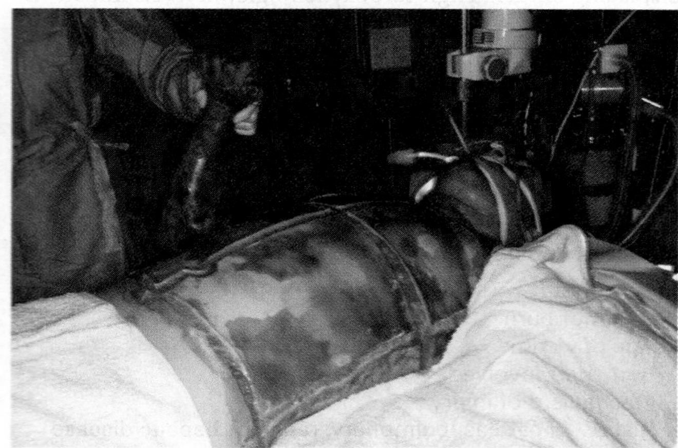

**fig. 64-7** Linear escharotomy used to alleviate circulatory and pulmonary constriction.

### Providing Emotional Support

Patients with significant burn injury receive a profound insult to their body and self-image. They are aware that they may not survive, which causes fear and helplessness. The shock and pain of the accident, the chaos and rush to the hospital, and the unknown surroundings and people all intensify the emotional stress.

The nurse spends the most time with the patient and has a considerable influence on the patient's psychological adjustment. Interventions that can be used to reassure the patient and alleviate anxiety include the following:

1. Identify self to patient.
2. Orient patient to the surroundings.
3. Describe basis of physical symptoms (skin loss, pain, and cold).
4. Explain the equipment and procedures to be used in treatment.

### Patient/Family Education

#### Health promotion/prevention

Nurses can help prevent accidental burns by participating in health education programs that stress fire prevention and the consequences of fires such as burns, deformities, and death. Nurses also can promote legislation that would control hazardous practices and make working and living environments safer. Community health nurses are in an unusually advantageous position to recognize unsafe practices in the home and to help families develop safe habits of living. Nurses can raise the awareness of patients and the community to the burn problem with education and burn awareness campaigns (Figure 64-8).

Prevention programs can be developed to highlight seasonal activities that result in burn injuries (Box 64-6). Approximately 80% of all accidental burns occur in the home and are caused primarily by ignorance, carelessness, and the curiosity of children. More than 35% of all fire and burn injuries involve children playing with matches and cigarette lighters. Prevention focuses on teaching parents and others caring for children to keep matches and cigarette lighters out of the reach of children.

Although about 80% of all homes now have smoke detectors, 30% of these units are nonfunctioning either because of no batteries or faulty electrical connections. Prevention includes teaching the following. (1) All homes should have working smoke detectors on each level of the home and in the hallway outside of the bedrooms. (2) Batteries should be tested periodically and changed twice yearly in the spring and the fall. In states and countries with time changes such as the change between Eastern Standard and Daylight Savings times in the United States, battery changes can be timed to coordinate with these time changes. Batteries should never be removed for the reason that they go off during cooking as it is easy to forget to replace them. (3) In most cities in the United States, the fire department will install smoke detectors free of charge to the elderly and others unable to do so for themselves. Fire departments in many communities have free smoke detectors for those unable to afford them.

Burn injuries to adults are most often related to accidents while they are cooking, using microwave ovens, or smoking or otherwise using matches. Burns commonly occur when a person is distracted while cooking or falls asleep while smoking. Prevention centers on teaching persons of all ages to be especially careful of scald burns when using microwave ovens. Scald burns occur when the power of the microwave is underestimated, and all users need to be educated about the safe use of these ovens. Smokers need to be reminded to never smoke in bed, to be particularly careful about falling asleep while smoking and sitting in overstuffed furniture, and to be sure that cigarettes are completely extinguished, especially before going to bed.

Although sunburn may not be thought of as a burn, even a relatively mild burn over a large portion of the body

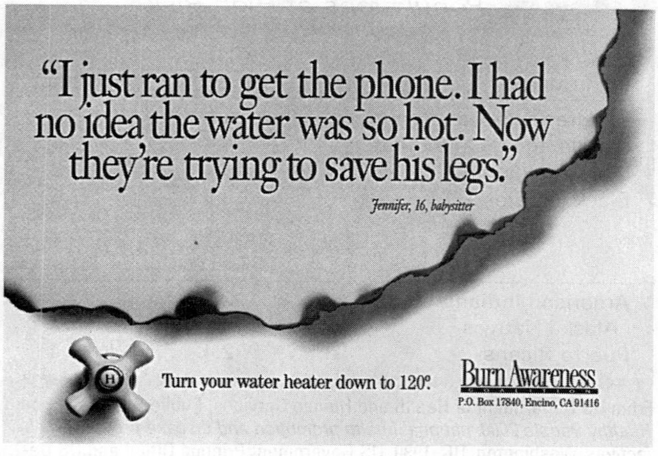

fig. 64-8 Sample burn prevention poster.

**box 64-6** *Seasonal Causes of Burn Injuries*

|  |  |
|---|---|
| Spring | Barbecuing<br>Burning leaves<br>Overheated radiators<br>Gasoline (lawnmowers) |
| Summer | Sun exposure<br>Fireworks<br>Beach activity<br>Sun-heated surfaces (tar, asphalt, sand) |
| Fall | Hot liquids<br>Yard clean-up<br>Candles<br>Halloween activities |
| Winter | Holiday activities<br>Fireplaces<br>Hot liquids<br>Woodburning stoves/space heaters<br>Electrical wires |

From Lillico S: *Burn awareness kit,* Encino, Calif, 1996, Burn Awareness Coalition.

can cause changes in fluid distribution and kidney damage. Camp nurses should keep this in mind when they present educational programs for camp counselors and campers. Emphasis is on the proper use of sunscreen products, the need to use a sunscreen with at least a skin protector factor (SPF) of 15, and the need to limit the time spent in the sun.

Each year there is an increased demand for careful inspection and regulation of places housing the ill and infirm. The elderly are frequently housed in old and nonfireproof structures from which they may not be able to escape if a fire occurs. Nurses can be involved to exert necessary pressure to ensure that adequate measures are taken to bring structures up to the fire code and to ensure that there is a fire evacuation plan. Basic fire prevention programs in all health care facilities should include one mock evacuation drill yearly.

Another facet of fire prevention programs focuses on places where large numbers of persons congregate such as schools, theaters, and sports arenas. Laws regulating public buildings require hinged doors that swing outward, draperies and decorations that are fireproof, and stairways with special fire doors in new apartment buildings and hotels. Smoke detectors and sprinkler systems are required in new buildings and residential health care facilities.

In fire prevention programs, emphasis should be placed on the special needs of the disabled. They are at higher risk for burn injury because of their inability to rapidly evacuate from unsafe situations (Box 64-7).

The government's role in fire prevention centers around laws designed to protect the public. For example, rigid enforcement of laws requiring that industrial products be labeled when they are known to be flammable and that new products be tested carefully for their flammable qualities before being placed on the market is further evidence of government efforts to protect the public from accident by fire.

**box 64-7** *Safety Measures to Be Observed by the Disabled*

Set hot water heater thermostat at 120° F or less with installation of valves in bathrooms that regulate water temperature.

Develop a fire escape plan. Keep exit routes free of clutter and have two escape routes. Do not include windows with bars in the escape plan. All windows with bars should have a quick release feature for easy removal.

Turn handles of pans to back of stove when cooking. Do not wear clothing with loose sleeves when cooking. Double check that stoves are turned off after cooking.

Keep whistle by bed to alert rescuers where you are or to warn others of a fire. The fire department will place a placard in your bedroom window to assist fire fighters in locating you should a fire occur.

Keep eyeglasses, dentures, keys, and flashlight near your bedside in case of an emergency.

Smokers should use large, deep ashtrays and never smoke in bed.

Industry can be made safer by constant vigilance of management in cooperation with fire safety officers and health care professionals to identify hazards and implement a safety program. All chemicals should be labeled, and antidotes should be identified and available. A core group of every workforce should be versed in emergency treatment of all types of burns for the protection of every employee.

The Surgeon General's report on goals to be achieved by 2000 included goals for a reduction in fire deaths for children younger than age 4, adults 65 and older, black males, and black females. When these objectives were reviewed in 1995, goals were set for two additional groups: American Indian/Alaska natives and Puerto Ricans. The goals for all groups are summarized in Table 64-4.

## EVALUATION

To evaluate effectiveness of nursing interventions compare patient's behaviors with those stated in the expected outcomes. Indications of successful achievement of patient outcomes for the patient with burns follow.

### Emergent Phase

1. Maintains patent airway, adequate ventilation, and oxygenation.
   a. Has absence of stridor and adventitious breath sounds.
   b. Has $Po_2 > 80$ and $Pco_2 < 45$.
   c. Has carboxyhemoglobin level <10%.
2. Overcomes fluid deficit and maintains optimal fluid and electrolyte balance.
   a. Has urinary output of 30 to 50 ml/hr in adults or 1 to 2 ml/kg/hr in children.
   b. Has electrolytes within normal limits.
   c. Has normal sensorium.
   d. Has systolic blood pressure >100 mm Hg.
   e. Has heart rate <120 beats/min.
   f. Has pH between 7.35 and 7.45.

**table 64-4** *Goals per 100,000 People for Reduction in Fire Deaths Among Populations at High Risk*

| Populations | 1987 Baseline | 2000 Target |
|---|---|---|
| Children age 4 and younger | 4.4 | 3.3 |
| People age 65 and older | 4.4 | 3.3 |
| Black males | 5.7 | 4.3 |
| Black females | 3.4 | 2.6 |
| | 1990 Baseline | 2000 Target |
| American Indians/ Alaska Natives | 2.1 | 1.4 |
| Puerto Ricans | 2.4 | 2.0 |

From US Department of Health and Human Services, Public Health Service: *Healthy People 2000: national health promotion and disease prevention objectives,* Washington, DC, 1990, US Government Printing Office and US Department of Health and Human Services, Public Health Service: *Healthy People 2000: midcourse review and 1995 revisions,* Washington, DC, 1995, US Government Printing Office.

3. Exhibits no signs of fluid excess.
   a. Limited tissue edema.
   b. Minimal fluid weight gain.
   c. No signs of pulmonary edema.
   d. Urinary output 30-50 ml/hr.
4. Maintains normal body temperature.
   a. Has body temperature between 37° and 38.5° C.
5. Shows no evidence of a wound infection.
   a. Wound appears clean.
   b. Has temperature <38.5° C.
   c. Routine wound cultures are obtained on admission and are scheduled for every 3 days.
   d. There is documentation of Standard Precautions or protective gowns, sterile gloves, hats, and masks being worn when caring for the open burn wounds.
6. Burn wound shows no evidence of further tissue loss.
7. Controls pain.
   a. Sleeps between treatments.
   b. Does not have elevated vital signs.
   c. Appears relaxed and indicates pain is reduced after receiving morphine.
8. Does not appear to be anxious.
   a. Listens to explanations from staff.
   b. Begins to verbalize concerns about the accident and asks questions about future.

## SPECIAL ENVIRONMENTS FOR CARE

### Critical Care Management

Patients who suffer burn injuries require specialized care, which is best obtained in a burn unit. A multidisciplinary team including surgeons, nurses, physical and occupational therapists, social workers, microbiologists, clergy, child life workers, psychologists, volunteers, and other disciplines is involved in the approach to care. Nurses working in the burn unit need to provide critical care for patients of all age-groups. They must understand wound care, infection control, and rehabilitation requirements of burn patients. Nurses also need to understand the different types of dressings including BioBrane, porcine, and artificial skin such as Integra, AlloDerm, and cultured epithelium.

Patient support services need to be available through rehabilitative and outpatient services. With patients being discharged earlier, education about their care requirements and wound care is generally completed after discharge. Treatment plans and teaching for all patients start at the onset of injury and continue throughout their course of healing whether they are in the hospital or are being treated in an outpatient setting. All team members are available, and resources are provided to patients and families at the different levels of healing. Support groups are available to assist patients with resocialization and coping with their burn injury for many years after their discharge.

# COLLABORATIVE CARE MANAGEMENT

## ACUTE PERIOD

The acute period of treatment begins at the end of the emergent period and lasts until the burn wound is healed. The length of this period varies. If the burn is a partial-thickness injury, the acute period extends for 10 to 20 days; if the burn is a full-thickness injury over a large percentage of the body requiring surgery for skin grafting, the acute period may last for months.

During the acute period the two main principles of management are (1) treatment of the burn wound and (2) avoidance, detection, and treatment of complications. The most common complications are infection (septicemia and pneumonia), renal disease, and heart failure.

### Diagnostic Tests

Laboratory testing during the acute period focuses on monitoring the patient's fluid and electrolyte balance. Chemistry profiles may be obtained once or twice daily during the patient's critical phase while fluid resuscitation is in progress. Complete blood counts are monitored to assess the patient's white blood cell count and hemoglobin and hematocrit. Wound cultures are obtained once or twice weekly to track the bacterial colonization of the wounds. Ongoing surveillance of wound cultures is essential for early treatment of infection. Evaluation of nutritional status is monitored through prealbumin levels and urine urea nitrogen (see Diet, p. 2128). Patients who are intubated or have inhalation injuries require periodic chest x-rays. In addition, bronchoscopy is performed on patients with inhalation injuries to assess the degree of injury to the lungs.

### Medications

Administration of medications for the burn patient is supportive in nature. Analgesia is essential for pain control. The most commonly used agents are opioids such as morphine sulfate, meperidine, and codeine (see Promoting Comfort, p. 2132). Patients with major burns may require agents to prevent stress ulcers, e.g., ranitidine, cimetidine, or sulcrulfate. Systemic antimicrobial agents are used only when evidence of infection is present. Topical antimicrobial agents are applied to the burn wounds based on depth of injury and wound culture results (Table 64-5). In addition, many burn patients have preexisting illnesses and require ongoing medication management of their current health problems.

### Treatments

For the burn patient, wound care is a major treatment. Depending on the depth and location of the wound, dressing changes are performed once, twice, or three times daily (see Promoting Skin Integrity, p. 2130).

#### *Skin grafts*

Skin grafts are applied to cover the burn wound and speed healing, to prevent contractures, and to shorten convalescence. Successful grafting reduces the patient's vulnerability to infection and prevents the loss of body heat and water vapor from the open wound. Grafting may be performed for cosmetic or functional purposes during the rehabilitative period. Most skin grafts are applied between the third and twenty-first days after the initial injury, depending on the depth and extent of the burn and the condition of the base.

**table 64-5** *Topical Medications and Wound Coverings Used in Burn Therapy*

| Drug/Wound Covering | Action | Interventions |
|---|---|---|
| Mafenide acetate (Sulfamylon®) | Bacteriostatic against gram-negative and gram-positive organisms<br>Penetrates thick eschar<br>Effective against *Pseudomonas* organisms<br>Causes pain on application<br>Inhibits epithelial tissue development | Monitor for metabolic acidosis especially when applied to 40% TBSA or more (inhibits carbonic anhydrase activity).<br>Apply ¼-inch layer directly to wound or impregnate into gauze dressing 2-3 times daily.<br>Monitor for allergic rash.<br>Discontinue when wound is clean and eschar has separated. |
| Silver sulfadiazine (Silvadene®) | Broad-spectrum activity against gram-negative, gram-positive, and *Candida* organisms<br>Does not cause electrolyte imbalances<br>Is painless and somewhat soothing<br>May cause skin rash<br>May cause transient decrease in white blood cell count for 24-48 hr after initiation<br>Inhibits epithelial tissue development and should be discontinued when eschar is no longer present | Apply ¼-inch layer applied directly to wound or impregnated into gauze dressing 2-3 times daily.<br>Repeated application may develop slimy, grayish appearance, simulating an infection despite negative cultures. |
| Silver nitrate | Bacteriostatic against gram-positive and gram-negative bacteria<br>Poorly penetrates eschar<br>Stains clothing and linen<br>Causes pain on application<br>Colors tissue black | Staining of tissue black makes wound assessment more difficult. |
| Aluminum salts: Burow's solution | Astringent providing a strong antimicrobial effect by creating an environment unconducive to bacteria (particularly gram-negative)<br>Retards epithelialization and should be discontinued when infection subsides | Monitor for resolution of infection.<br>Apply with a gauze dressing. |
| Hypochlorites: Dakin's solution | Effective against gram-negative bacteria and spores<br>May be used as an antimicrobial after skin grafting | Monitor for tissue irritation. It should have a strong odor of chlorine. |
| Bacitracin | Prevents drying of wound<br>Weak antimicrobial effects<br>May be used in conjunction with gauze dressing, xeroform, and scarlet red | Maintain a complete covering of the wound, particularly if used in an open technique (e.g., on the face). |
| Collagenase | Enzyme that digests collagen in necrotic tissue<br>Does not harm healthy tissue | Apply to deep partial- and full-thickness burns where eschar exists.<br>Monitor for separation of eschar and discontinue use. |
| BioBrane® | No antimicrobial properties<br>Semisynthetic wound covering composed of nylon, Silastic, and collagen membrane that binds with the wound fibrin forming a skin substitute, allowing for healing<br>Remains adherent to wound until healing occurs | Apply to a clean, partial thickness wound immediately after injury or as a covering for donor sites. |
| Scarlet red | No antimicrobial properties<br>Fine mesh gauze impregnated with lanolin, olive oil, and petrolatum with a red dye. Promotes epithelial tissue development and protects wound | Monitor for signs of infection.<br>Monitor for and maintain adherence to wound.<br>Maintain a smooth, single layer. |
| Xeroform | Provides a protective skin substitute to allow for epithelial tissue development<br>Minimal antimicrobial properties | Apply to clean partial-thickness wounds.<br>Monitor for and maintain adherence to wound.<br>Monitor for signs of infection.<br>Maintain a smooth, single layer. |
| Calcium alginate | Dressing composed of nonwoven fabric pad composed of calcium alginate<br>Calcium alginate ions exchanged with sodium ions on the wound to form protective, fibrous gel<br>Provides protective barrier, promoting healing and promoting exudate absorption | Remove calcium alginate dressing for wound care, monitoring for wound healing and infection. |

**table 64-6** *Types of Grafts*

| GRAFT | SOURCE | COVERAGE |
|---|---|---|
| Autograft | Patient's own nonburned skin removed and applied to burn | Permanent |
| Cultured skin | Patient's skin removed in small squares and grown in Petri dishes to large sizes and then grafted | Permanent |
| Homograft | Another of the same species (e.g., cadaver skin obtained 6-24 hr after death) and applied within 5 days | Temporary |
| Heterograft | Another species (e.g., pig skin) | Temporary |
| Synthetic substitute | Man-made substitute that has properties similar to skin | Temporary |
| Integra® (artificial skin) | Two-layer man-made membrane used to replace dermis and covered with autograft forming functional dermis and epidermis | Permanent |
| AlloDerm® | Man-made collagen matrix used to provide dermal layer covered with autograft | Permanent |

Grafts are obtained from various sources (Table 64-6). An autograft is a graft of skin obtained from the patient's own body. A *homograft* is a graft of skin obtained from a cadaver 6 to 24 hours after death. A *heterograft* is a graft of skin obtained from another species, such as a pig.

Synthetic substitutes for skin are currently being developed and used in burn units throughout the United States. Integra, AlloDerm, and cultured epithelium are new products currently available. All of them are expensive. The products alone may cost $20,000 per patient. Cost effectiveness is still being evaluated.

Homografts, heterografts, and synthetic substitutes are intended to provide temporary coverage while the burn wound heals. As the wound heals, these temporary coverings are gradually rejected and are easily removed from the newly healed skin.

The advantage of a temporary graft is to reduce water, electrolyte, and protein losses at the burn surface. The covered wound is less painful and allows the patient freedom of movement. Temporary grafts may be used until the patient is ready for autografts. Often, autografting is delayed as a result of complications such as pneumonia or gastric hemorrhage.

*Split-thickness skin grafts* are used most frequently in the early stages of wound treatment (Figure 64-9). The grafts include two upper layers of skin (epidermis) and part of the middle layer (dermis) but are not taken so deep to prevent regeneration of the skin at the site from which they are taken (donor site). The grafts are removed with a dermatome blade from almost any unburned part of the body. The sizes of these grafts are determined by the sites available and the area to be covered. Grafts may be placed on the recipient bed by two

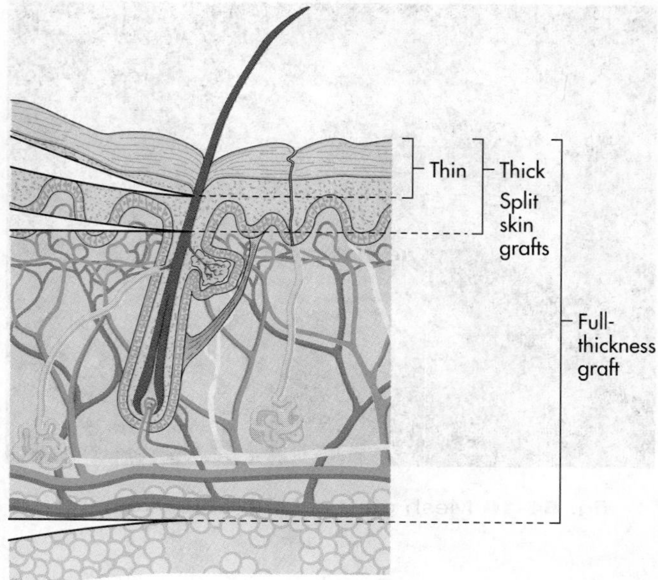


**fig. 64-9** Levels of the skin involved in thin- and thick-split skin grafts and full-thickness grafts.

methods: stamping and meshing. Stamping uses "postage stamp"-sized grafts of donor skin applied over the recipient bed. This technique is generally used with a wound that is unclean because it allows drainage of excess debris. Meshing involves taking the sheet of skin after it is removed from the donor and feeding it into a meshing instrument that perforates the sheet with tiny slits. The meshing of the graft makes it more distensible so that it can be stretched to cover wider areas of the body surface (Figure 64-10).

*Full-thickness grafts* are composed of layers of skin down to the subcutaneous tissue. They give a better cosmetic appearance than split-thickness grafts when healed and are used early in wound management and if there is a well-defined area of full-thickness burn. Areas that benefit from full-thickness grafts are the hands, neck, and face. Full-thickness grafts can also be used in rehabilitative stages to restore body function and to repair areas of released skin contractures.

Tangential excision and grafting is a surgical procedure in which the necrotic tissue or eschar is excised down to viable tissue or fascia and immediately covered without autograft or skin substitute. The procedure is best performed between the second and fifth burn day. This technique is used with a well-defined partial-thickness injury in which deep epidermal cells remain intact for primary healing. Advantages of tangential excision and grafting are outlined in Box 64-8.

Graft sites require skilled nursing management. Autografts are delicate and should not be dislodged. The grafted area may be covered with a large, occlusive, bulky dressing to hold new skin securely in place. Splints may be applied in the operating room to provide immobilization and maintain position.

The dressing remains intact for 48 to 72 hours unless there is purulent drainage with a strong odor. The dressing is removed slowly and carefully to not disturb the graft.

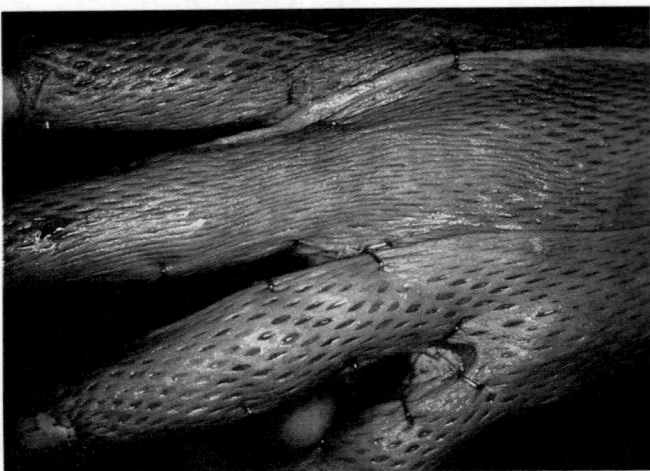

fig. 64-10 Mesh graft covering burn to hand.

**box 64-8 Advantages of Tangential Excision and Grafting**

- Decreases hospitalization
- Prevents potential conversion of burn to full thickness by removing necrotic tissue before infection occurs
- Diminishes anxiety and lessens trauma to multiple graftings
- Allows early grafting and early restoration of function
- Reduces scar formation because of use of full-thickness graft

After grafting the donor site represents a wound similar to that of a partial-thickness injury. Care of the donor site is as important as care of the graft itself, because donor sites that fail to heal result in a net enlargement of the patient's open wound surface. Donor sites may be treated by a variety of methods. One method is covering the exposed surface with fine mesh gauze, Xeroform, or a synthetic dressing and leaving it exposed to the air. Exposing the donor site to a heat lamp also promotes healing, because, as the drainage from the wound dries, it serves as a protective covering. The site usually heals within 2 weeks. Another method is to cover the site with sterile gauze and a pressure dressing.

Many patients complain of severe pain in the donor site, and the nurse should not hesitate to give medications for pain. The pain should subside in 24 to 48 hours as the wound dries. The wound is inspected daily for any signs of infection (erythema, purulent drainage, or foul odor). If infection develops, antibiotics may be administered, and the wound may be treated with wet dressings.

### Diet

Metabolism is increased after moderate to severe burns because of stress, fluid loss, hypercatabolism, and immobility, and energy requirements may be as much as 100% to 300% more than the patient's preburn status.[16] Shivering and elevated levels of catecholamines, cortisol, and glucagon present after thermal injury increase oxygen consumption and heat production and deplete liver and muscle glycogen and fat deposits resulting in negative nitrogen balance and weight loss. Protein is broken down to provide amino acids for gluconeogenesis, preventing amino acids from incorporating into protein. This decreased rate of protein production prolongs wound healing and increases the patient's susceptibility to infection.

A burn patient remains catabolic until caloric intake exceeds caloric expenditure. This *catabolic* state may last for days or months depending on the severity of the burn. The patient's energy and protein requirements become those needed for normal homeostasis plus those required to offset the catabolic state and repair the burn injury.

#### Nuritional assessment

Maintenance of a nutritional support program is critical to survival and is initiated on admission. The goals of the nutritional support program are to establish oral intake as soon as possible and to maintain sufficient caloric and protein intake to restore tissue loss. A team approach provides comprehensive input and integrates the efforts of the patient, physician, nurse, pharmacist, dietitian, and occupational and physical therapists.

A nutritional assessment is made during the first days of the burn injury and includes anthropometric measurements (to determine actual weight loss compared with ideal weight), laboratory studies (electrolytes, liver function tests, and urine), and skin testing (if indicated to determine immune response) (see Chapter 66).

The admission assessment provides a baseline against which progress can be evaluated. Twenty-four-hour urine specimens and urea nitrogen tests may be obtained two to three times a week to evaluate the patient's nitrogen balance. Evaluation of albumin and protein levels is also necessary. The current trend is to follow *prealbumin levels (PAB)*. Urinary nitrogen and serum albumin levels can be affected by insensible protein loss and hydration status. Albumin's half-life of 20 days makes day-to-day evaluation of albumin difficult to interpret. On the other hand, prealbumin, which has a short half-life of 20 to 25 hours, provides a sensitive indicator of nutritional status and the patient's response to feeding.[13]

Nutritional requirements for the burn patient are highly variable, depending on the extent and depth of injury and the patient's age, gender, preburn nutritional status, and preexisting diseases. Total caloric needs may be as high as 3500 to 5000 calories per day. Calories are provided to the patient as 20% protein, 50% carbohydrate, and 30% fat. Dietitians in burn centers most commonly use the Curreri formula and variations of the Harris-Benedict equation. These formulae are used as a guide to begin nutritional support. Ongoing nutritional assessment is essential to modify the diet to provide the patient with appropriate support.[7,13]

Protein is essential to replace nitrogen loss through the wound and in urine and to promote tissue repair and healing. Protein needs in the adult increase from a normal of 0.8 g/kg of body weight to 1.5 to 3.0 g/kg. Protein calories must be dedicated to the wound and not used for energy needs. This is accomplished by providing the patient with sufficient carbohydrate and fat for energy use.

Increased carbohydrate and fat intake is provided to avoid protein catabolism and meet the patient's energy needs. Approximately 5 mg/kg/min of glucose is provided. Excessive carbohydrate administration is avoided to prevent increased carbon dioxide production and hyperglycemia.[13] In addition to calories, fat provides fat-soluble vitamins and essential fatty acids. Calories provided by fat are limited to 30% because of the adverse effect that high-fat levels have on the immune system.[2,7]

Vitamin and mineral supplements are essential for optimal wound healing. Vitamins C and A, zinc, and iron are provided at doses higher than the recommended daily allowances. Vitamins A and C have roles as cellular antioxidants and are required for collagen synthesis. Patients may receive as much as 1000 mg of vitamin C and 5,000 to 10,000 IU of vitamin A per day. Zinc levels decrease because of increased nitrogen excretion in the urine during the acute phase. Zinc is essential for wound healing and has a key role in immune function. Patients receive supplementation of up to 25 mg/day.[6] Iron may be supplied to treat anemia caused from blood loss after skin grafting.

#### *Feeding methods*

Enteral feeding (oral or tube feeding) is the preferred method for the burn patient. A paralytic ileus or gastric dilation is frequently seen in the severely burned patient due to shock, stress, or sepsis. This may limit the patient's ability to tolerate gastric feedings for the first few weeks. Commonly, small-bore feeding tubes are inserted into the duodenum or endoscopically into the jejunum so that feedings may be initiated within the first 24 hours of injury. Early feeding decreases hypermetabolism, improves nitrogen balance, minimizes bacterial translocation from the gut secondary to muscle atrophy, and decreases diarrhea and hospital length of stay.[7] Total parenteral nutrition is generally reserved for patients who are unable to tolerate enteral feeding.

Oral feeding is encouraged whenever possible. However, it is difficult for the patient to consume the number of calories needed from food alone because of pain and decreased gastric motility. Therefore, a combination of food by mouth with supplements, such as milk shakes or Ensure, and tube feedings may be necessary to meet the patient's nutritional requirements.

### Activity

Physical and occupational therapy are necessary for the burn patient and begin on admission. Collaboration between nurses and the therapists is essential. The patient is encouraged to move about and to ambulate as much as possible. Patients with major burns or those who require mechanical ventilation may only tolerate bedrest and range of motion exercises. As soon as hemodynamic and pulmonary stability is achieved, the patient may sit in a chair and then ambulate. The patient is encouraged to assist with self-care as much as possible.

### Referrals

Referrals to other services are determined by the needs of the patient. For example, patients with other conditions such as diabetes may require consultation from an expert to assist in managing the diabetes during the acute period of their burn. Consultation with a psychiatrist may be indicated for patients whose burns were self-inflicted or for those who are having difficulty adjusting to their postburn appearance.

## NURSING MANAGEMENT

### ASSESSMENT

#### Subjective Data

Burn patients are often frightened and anxious about their injury and the associated treatments. These responses can be compounded by the intensive care unit environment.

Burn patients experience both physical and psychological pain. Physical pain is usually focused on specific activities such as wound cleansing and debridement, dressing changes, and physical therapy. The nurse must assess the patient's reaction to pain and intervene appropriately.

#### Objective Data

The nurse must perform a thorough head-to-toe assessment of the burn patient every 8 hours. Data should include mental status; vital signs; breath sounds; bowel sounds; dietary intake; motor ability; intake and output; weight pattern; circulatory assessment; and observation of burn wounds, grafts, and donor site. Purulent drainage, abnormal color, foul odor, redness or swelling in surrounding normal skin, or presence of healing should be noted. Changes in these parameters from shift to shift or from day to day make further investigation necessary.

### NURSING DIAGNOSES

Nursing diagnoses are determined from analysis of patient data. Possible nursing diagnoses for the person with burns during the acute phase may include but are not limited to:

| Diagnostic Title | Etiological Title |
|---|---|
| Skin integrity, impaired | Burn injury, nutritional deficit |
| Infection, risk for | Break in skin integrity; impaired immune response |
| Altered nutrition: less than body requirements | Increased metabolic needs, protein losses through wounds, decreased appetite |
| Pain, acute | Exposed nerve endings, immobility |
| Fluid volume deficit | Increased fluid loss via evaporation through the burn wound |
| Mobility, impaired | Splinting after a graft procedure, activity intolerance, depression, decreased strength and endurance |
| Anxiety | Changes in health status/role functioning; situational crisis |

| | |
|---|---|
| Coping, ineffective individual | Situational crisis, personal vulnerability, ineffective support systems |
| Coping, ineffective family, compromised | Inadequate or incorrect information, temporary family disorganization, role changes |
| Body image disturbance | Loss/change of body parts, function |
| Knowledge deficit | Unfamiliarity with burn injury and treatment |
| Self-care deficit | Intolerance to activity, pain, musculoskeletal impairment |
| Hypothermia | Exposure of wounds to environment |

## ■ EXPECTED PATIENT OUTCOMES

Expected patient outcomes for the burn injured patient during the acute phase include but are not limited to:

1. Burn wound clean and exhibits healing.
2. Is free of pathogenic organisms and signs and symptoms of infection.
3. Has a positive nitrogen balance and wound healing.
4. Reports a decreasing and acceptable level of pain.
5. Exhibits signs of adequate fluid balance.
6. Maintains full range of motion.
7. Exhibits reduced anxiety.
8. Exhibits functional coping mechanisms.
9. The family exhibits functional coping mechanisms.
10. Begins to develop a realistic body image.
11. Explains his or her treatment regimen.
12. Demonstrates increased ability to perform self-care activities.
13. Has body temperature greater than 37° C.

## ■ INTERVENTIONS

### Promoting Skin Integrity

Expert assessment skills are required to monitor wounds during healing and to detect any signs of infection. The wound eschar that forms after burn injury is conducive to bacterial growth because it contains dead tissue and is moist and warm. Daily cleansing and mechanical debridement help remove the eschar. Washing and friction remove the debris and support healthy tissue regeneration. Hydrotherapy using tubs or shower carts facilitates the removal of medications and loosens debris, sloughing eschar, and exudate. It is a comfortable method for removal of dressings and facilitates range-of-motion exercise with minimal energy expenditure and discomfort. The solution used in a tub may be plain water, normal saline, or an electrolytically balanced solution. To minimize the chance of infection, sterile technique is used during dressing care and a clean environment is maintained. The use of gowns, masks, gloves, aprons, goggles, and a plastic disposable tub liner will decrease the chance of contamination between patients. Tubbing is usually performed once or twice daily and should not exceed 30 minutes to prevent exposure and chilling. Tubbing is initiated after the patient's vital signs and fluid balance have stabilized.

If the patient has a wound infection, tubbing is avoided to prevent spread of bacteria through the water to other parts of the body. Hydrotherapy is also contraindicated if the patient experiences any sudden changes in temperature, heart rate, blood pressure, or respiratory rate.

The current trend in wound cleansing is to use a shower cart with the same isolation measures as with tubbing. The patient is placed on a special stretcher, which allows for drainage and has a hose system that allows for the control of water temperature and flow, thus maintaining patient comfort.

#### *Methods of treatment*

Different methods of treating the burned area may be used, depending on the location of the burn, its size and depth, the facilities available, and the patient's response to therapy. One method may be replaced with another during the course of treatment. Those commonly used today include the open or exposure method, the semiopen method, and the closed or occlusive method.

**Open or exposure method.** The exposure of treatment was accidentally discovered to be effective in 1888 when, during a serious steamboat fire on the Mississippi River, those in attendance ran out of bandages and later observed that the neglected persons fared better than those who received more intensive treatment. Today the exposure method is used most often in the treatment of burns involving the face, neck, perineum, and broad areas of the trunk. The burned area is cleansed and exposed to air (Figure 64-11). The exudate of a partial-thickness burn dries in 48 to 72 hours and forms a hard crust that protects the wound. Epithelialization occurs beneath this crust and may be complete in 14 to 21 days. The crust then falls off spontaneously, leaving a healed, unscarred surface. The dead skin of a full-thickness burn is dehydrated and converted to black, leathery eschar in 48 to 72 hours. Loose eschar may be gradually removed through hydrotherapy and/or debridement. Uninfected eschar acts as a protective covering. The danger of infection exists as bacteria proliferate beneath the eschar. Spontaneous separation, produced by bacterial action, occurs unless surgical debridement is performed first.

Isolation technique is essential when the exposure method is used. The nurse caring for the patient should wear a sterile gown, mask, apron, and goggles; sterile linen may be used on

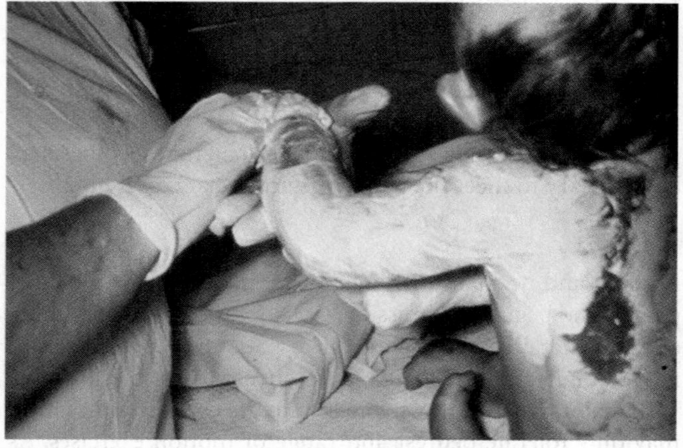

**fig. 64-11** Full-thickness burn being treated with silver sulfadiazane.

the bed. A cradle may be used on the bed because no clothing or bed clothes are allowed directly over burned areas. If the burn is extensive, a CircOlectric bed draped with a sheet is an ideal way to care for the patient. The patient can be kept from embarrassing exposure by wearing a halter and loin cloth. Lights or heat lamps may be used with caution to provide warmth. Advantages of the open method are that the wound is easily inspected, and the patient has maximal freedom to perform exercises for the prevention of contracture and the improvement of circulation.

Patients having exposure treatment complain of pain and chilling. Pain may be controlled by administering morphine sulfate, meperidine hydrochloride (Demerol), or salicylates as ordered. Discomfort can be decreased if drafts are avoided, and the temperature of the room is kept at 24.4° C (85° F). Patients lose more heat from burned surfaces than from normal skin surfaces, because the vascular bed that normally contracts and retains heat in the body is lost. The humidity of the room also should be controlled. Humidity of 40% to 50% is usually considered satisfactory. Portable electric humidifiers and dehumidifiers can be used to achieve and maintain this level.

**Semiopen method.** The semiopen wound care method consists of covering the wound with topical antimicrobial agents and a thin layer of gauze to help keep the agent in contact with the wound. This method permits the passage of wound exudate through the dressing without the loss of antimicrobial cream. The success of semiopen care depends on cleaning the wound once or twice a day, either at the bedside, in the hydrotherapy tank, or on the spray table. Meticulous semiopen wound care speeds debridement, enhances the development of granulation tissue, and makes earlier grafting possible.

**Closed or occlusive method.** In the closed or occlusive method of burn treatment, the wounds are washed, and dressings are changed at least once a day, or in some instances once each shift. Commonly, the dressing consists of gauze impregnated with topical ointments with a gauze wrap. Counterpressure wrappings (elastic bandages) may be applied. When a dressing is in place, nursing observation includes monitoring for signs of impaired circulation (numbness, pain, and tingling) and for signs of infection (odor on dressings, elevated temperature, and elevated pulse rate).

#### Topical agents

The application of topical agents to the burn wound can help decrease infection and hasten healing. These agents are effective because damage to the blood vessels in the burn area prevents systemic antibiotics from reaching the burn wound. Antibiotics may be given prophylactically or may be withheld until an infection occurs. Table 64-5 summarizes some of the commonly used topical wound agents.

#### Dressings

Large bulky dressings are rarely used for large burns except in select instances because infection control is more difficult and partial-thickness burns may develop into full-thickness wounds. The purposes of applying some light covering include prevention of infection from exogenous sources, facilitation of debridement, maximal contact by topical agents, and prevention of fluid evaporation with loss of body heat. The type of dressing that is usually applied consists of a single layer of fine-mesh gauze impregnated with a topical medication and held in place by a wrapping of a coarse gauze.

The dressing change is usually a painful procedure requiring analgesics. Analgesics should be given 30 minutes before the procedure for maximal effectiveness. Most dressing changes are performed after hydrotherapy, which loosens the dressing making it easier to remove and lessens pain. Additional debridement of eschar and dead tissue may be performed before the new dressing is applied.

Wet dressings may be used with silver nitrate or normal saline applications. Normal saline is applied to clean granulation tissue or to new grafts to maintain moisture or is used with fine-mesh gauze to provide for slight debridement. A single layer of fine-mesh gauze is usually placed over the wound, covered with thick gauze pads to maintain moisture, and held in place with a gauze wrapping. The dressings must be kept wet.

### Preventing Infection

The burn patient is at tremendous risk for infection.[9] Measures to prevent infection begin at the time the patient is admitted to the hospital and continue until healing is complete. The break in skin integrity destroys the body's first line of defense. In addition, changes in the immune system occur as a result of the burn injury, creating a state of immunosuppression postburn. Damaged tissue triggers the release of the inflammatory cytokine cascade. The release of these cytokines (tumor necrosing factor and interleukins) impairs the function of lymphocytes, macrophages, and neutrophils, increasing the risk of infection. The nutritional deficit that occurs also decreases the burn patient's ability to fight infection.

Sources of infection may be *endogenous* or *exogenous*. Bacteria that survive in the hair follicles and glands are a source of endogenous infection. In addition, after burn injury, bacteria that normally live in the intestinal tract migrate or translocate across the intestinal wall and spread to the general circulation by way of the lymphatic system. Local and systemic infections *(septicemia)* are the most common complications of burns and are the major cause of death, particularly in burns covering more than 25% of the body.

Organisms commonly causing burn wound infection include *Pseudomonas aeruginosa, Acinetobacter,* enterococci, and *Staphylococcus aureus.* These organisms are normally found on the skin or in the intestine and become a source of infection. Treatment of antimicrobial resistant organisms, such as methicillin-resistant *S. aureus* and vancomycin-resistant enterococci, is an increasingly difficult problem in burn centers.

Fungal infections have an increased incidence in burn patients because of the use of broad-spectrum antibiotics. *Candida albicans,* which normally is found in the gastrointestinal tract, accounts for the majority of the fungal infections. Cultures of the patient's wound may be taken on admission and at biweekly intervals to determine the presence of bacteria and their sensitivity to antibiotics.

Infection is usually the cause of any deterioration in the condition of a burn patient. Signs of infection include erythema and edema at the wound edges, increasing pain, odor, drainage, and decreasing function. The wound may show changes in color from red to violet, dark brown, or black. Tissue necrosis may occur.

Signs of sepsis in the burn patient are the following:

1. Change in sensorium
2. Fever
3. Tachypnea
4. Tachycardia
5. Paralytic ileus (decreased tolerance of feedings)
6. Abdominal distention
7. Oliguria

To prevent the introduction of exogenous organisms into the wound, strict adherence to Standard Precautions is essential. Persons with upper respiratory infections should not be permitted near the patient. Thorough wound cleansing is necessary to remove the debris that acts as a media for bacterial growth. Placing the severely burned patient in a special burn unit can decrease the possibility of infection because the unit environment is specifically equipped for infection control. If the patient is cared for in a general hospital unit, a private room is essential, and all equipment needed by the patient remains in the room.

### Providing Nutrition

Planning, collaboration, and ingenuity are required to ensure that the patient receives adequate nutritional support. An oral diet is encouraged whenever possible. The patient's food preferences are determined, and the family is encouraged to bring favorite foods from home. Care is coordinated so that meal times are relaxed and not associated with other procedures, such as wound care. A social situation can be created by having burn patients eat together or with family members. Pain medication is provided so that the patient is comfortable. Coordination with occupational therapy staff is essential if the patient needs assistive devices to hold utensils and cups.

Patients unable to consume sufficient calories orally require tube feedings. Continuous feedings are provided when requirements are high. As the patient begins to eat orally, tube feedings may be provided overnight, allowing the patient to eat during the day. Calorie counts are essential to monitor the patient's progress.

Monitoring the patient's nutritional status is an ongoing process. Weight loss and gain are monitored daily during the critical phase and biweekly as the wounds heal. Initially, weight gain occurs because of fluid retention. As diuresis occurs, the patient's weight decreases due to fluid loss. Significant weight loss reflects protein loss and loss of fat reserves and muscle mass. Prealbumin, urine urea nitrogen balance, and cholesterol levels are obtained.

The patient's tolerance of feeding is monitored by evaluating bowel function. Diarrhea may be a problem for patients receiving antibiotics or tube feedings. Commonly, burn patients have difficulties with constipation due to administration of opioids and decreased activity. Stool softeners, laxatives, and increased fluid intake may be provided.

Weight loss and gain are monitored for evaluation of nutritional status. Weight gain occurs initially because of fluid retention; however, after diuresis there is a marked loss of weight. Severe weight loss is closely related to protein loss resulting in negative nitrogen balance or the loss of body cell mass and the enormous amount of body fluid lost through the burn wound itself. As with other metabolic responses, weight loss depends on the extent of injury: the greater the burn, the greater the weight loss.

### Promoting Comfort

Pain control is a major part of the burn patient's care. Uncontrolled pain affects all aspects of recovery, including tolerance of wound care, ability to eat, mobility, wound healing, and psychological adjustment. Acute pain is most successfully managed with narcotics. The methods and routes of administration are carefully evaluated on an individual basis. Attention is paid to pain management needs during dressing changes and other daily activities. During dressing changes, parenteral narcotics are given to achieve rapid onset of action. The use of anesthetic agents such as ketamine, fentanyl, and self-administered nitrous oxide may be beneficial for some patients. (The Guidelines for Care Box outlines nursing interventions during dressing change.)

An around-the-clock approach to pain management is essential for the burn patient. Undermedication may occur if the patient fears becoming addicted and fails to report pain or if the nurse fails to adequately evaluate the degree of pain. The use of a numerical analog scale in which the patient rates the pain helps determine whether the pain is being adequately controlled. Providing medication at frequent intervals helps to maintain ongoing comfort. Time-released morphine and patient-controlled analgesia are also viable options.

Physiological pain may be induced or aggravated by loneliness and depression. The patient's complaint of pain may be an indication of unmet emotional needs that can be addressed with the use of presence, touch, or diversional activities. Anxiety about anticipated procedures and sleep deprivation may increase the amount of pain experienced by the patient. Patients experiencing posttraumatic stress disorder report higher levels of pain.[6] Interventions may include the use of antianxiety medication and nonpharmacological methods such as meditation or relaxation exercises. (See Chapter 12 for further discussion of pain management.)

### Maintaining Fluid Balance

To prevent fluid volume deficit the patient is weighed daily on the same scale, in the same amount of clothing, at the same time of day. A careful record is kept of the weights. Electrolytes

#### guidelines for care

**Minimizing Pain During Dressing Changes**

Provide analgesic medications before dressing change.
Provide clear explanation to gain patient's cooperation.
Handle burned areas gently.
Use sterile technique (infection causes increased pain).
Encourage patient to participate in treatment whenever possible.
Use distraction (for example, radio or conversation) and relaxation techniques when appropriate.

are monitored by frequent blood chemistry analyses. Fluid intake is planned in conjunction with the daily diet, which is high in protein and potassium. Fluids are offered on a regular basis, and a careful record is kept of all intake and output.

Patients are taught the importance of maintaining fluid and electrolyte balance after discharge and the need to notify their health care provider immediately if they experience weight loss accompanied by headache, lightheadedness, fatigue, decreased urinary output, irritability, or rapid pulse, which are signs of fluid deficit or an increase in fatigue, abdominal distention, anorexia, vomiting, constipation, muscle cramps, paresthesia, or confusion, which are signs of electrolyte imbalance. They are also taught to eat potassium-rich foods such as oranges, bananas, and potatoes daily.[12]

### Promoting Range of Motion

As the patient's wounds heal and pain is controlled, the patient is encouraged to do range-of-motion exercises on a regular schedule. The nurse provides assistance and support as needed with the goal of the patient being able to perform them independently. The patient and family are taught the importance of range-of-motion exercises in preventing or minimizing contractures. Physical and occupational therapists are involved in helping the patient improve range of motion.

### Relieving Anxiety

A burn injury is a sudden, unexpected event. Its impact on psychological well-being is enormous, and promoting mental health is a major area of the burn patient's care. The psychological responses in the emergent period are related to the threat of survival. During the acute period, a variety of behaviors may be seen. (See Table 64-7 for a summary of psychological responses.) As the patient becomes aware of the extent of the injury and begins to evaluate its implications on his or her life, many problems may occur that affect the ability of both the patient and family to cope with the situation.

**table 64-7** *Psychological Reactions to Severe Burns*

| Definition | Behavior Exhibited | Nursing Approach |
|---|---|---|
| **CONSERVATION, WITHDRAWAL** | | |
| Decreased interaction with environment as an immediate response to serious injury<br>Occurs immediately after injury and may last for first 1-2 weeks<br>Protective value to self (may be mistaken for depression) | Decreased interaction with environment, staff, family<br>Keeps eyes closed frequently, sleeps, remains immobile | Avoid forcing patient to deal with situation<br>Supportive environment<br>Provide ongoing information on status and care |
| **DENIAL** | | |
| Protective, unconscious defense mechanism<br>Helps relieve anxiety due to threat to life, limb, self | Patient denies extent of injury, loss of limb, loss of others in accident<br>May acknowledge the loss but not the impact | Support patient<br>Avoid forcing patient to deal with fears<br>Answer questions honestly<br>Provide information in small doses over time |
| **REGRESSION** | | |
| Patient returns to earlier ways of coping with stress<br>May exhibit childlike behaviors | Assertive, demanding, temper tantrums<br>Tearful, cling to dependent relationships | Avoid attacking and responding negatively to behavior exhibited<br>Acknowledge patient's difficulty in coping<br>Encourage and reward positive behaviors and independence |
| **ANGER AND HOSTILITY** | | |
| Angry, agitated behavior in response to a perceived wrong, loss of control<br>Grieving response | Angry, agitated, hostile to staff and family | Encourage verbalization of frustration<br>Avoid responding directly to anger<br>Provide choices and control<br>Assist patient to search for meaning to injury |
| **DEPRESSION** | | |
| The extent of injury becomes distorted and impacts the patient's sense of worthiness and self-esteem | Degrading comments about self<br>Sleep disturbances, decreased appetite, generalized slowing, poor motivation | Acknowledge the loss<br>Focus patient on realistic expectations |
| **ANXIETY** | | |
| Fear and threat to self as a result of injury | Restlessness, agitation, difficulty in following instructions, poor memory, easily startled | Support patient<br>Acknowledge fears<br>Provide information in small frequent doses |

Nurses play a major role in maintaining and restoring the patient's mental health. Pain plays a significant role in the patient's level of anxiety and is commonly identified by patients as the worst part of their hospital stay. Controlling pain assists in decreasing anxiety,[16] (see Promoting Comfort, p. 2132).

Ongoing education is imperative to assist the patient to understand the care given and to make realistic plans for the future. It is important for the patient to maintain a sense of hope for the future so that he or she can resume a normal life. Without hope, the patient will have less ability to cope, a sense of failure, and less gratifying interpersonal relationships (Research Box).[3]

Those individuals who adjust well after a burn injury have characteristics in common. Those who had positive experiences before the injury are better able to deal with the consequences of a burn injury. In addition, they have family and other social supports available to them. They can engage others in their care and are able to revise their self-image in a realistic and positive manner.

Emotional recovery from a burn injury is slower than physical recovery. Two thirds of those with major burns have some degree of psychological disability for as long as 6 months after discharge from the hospital (Table 64-7).[6,16]

Burn-injured persons are also at risk for the development of posttraumatic stress disorder (PTSD). In this condition symptoms occur after a psychologically traumatic event that would be considered outside the range of normal human experience.[1] Symptoms of PTSD include the following:

1. Reexperiencing the trauma in dreams or intrusive recollections
2. A numbed response to the environment, such as decreased interest or detachment
3. An exaggerated startle response
4. Sleep disturbance
5. Guilt about having survived the event, especially if others did not
6. Avoidance of activities that arouse recollections of the event

### research

Reference: Anderson FD, Maloney JP, Redland AR: Study of hope in patients with critical burn injuries, *J Burn Care Rehabil* 14:207-214, 1993.

Previous research suggests the importance of hope in the recovery of a critically ill patient. The authors identify hope as a dynamic process with past, present, and future dimensions. The purpose of this study was to examine the factors that affect the critically ill burn patient to determine nursing interventions that influence the patients' perceptions of hope. A convenience sample of nine white men (aged 18 through 58 with burn sizes ranging from 23% to 70% TBSA) was used. Semistructured interviews were conducted using open-ended questions to determine the patients' perception of hope related to their burn experience. The results indicated the importance of the present dimension of hope as determined by the patient's interpretation of present circumstances. Caregivers, e.g., nurses, played a significant role in the patient's perception of hope. Eight categories were identified that had an impact on the patient's perception: (1) nurturance of the patient by the caregiver (more personal contact and nurturing increased hope); (2) validation of personal worth; (3) feelings of powerlessness (limited control, decreased hope); (4) trust in the caregiver or significant other (confidence in the competence of the caregiver, increased hope); (5) support of other patients with burns; (6) reality surveillance (reflection of the reality of progress by the caregiver increased levels of hope); (7) treatment affiliations (pain associated with treatments negatively affected hope); and (8) sick role responsibility. The study supported the role of nurses in promoting hope in critically ill burn patients. Interventions can be focused based on the patient's physiological and psychological stages of recovery.

### Promoting Effective Coping of Patient and Family

The nurse should explore with the patient how she or he coped with stressful events in the past. It is important to remember that some patients (especially males) were raised to be stoic when in pain or distress. Other patients were encouraged to express their feelings openly. Nurses should support the patient's coping style unless the patient indicates that he or she would be interested in exploring new methods of coping.

Relaxation exercises, meditation, and soothing audio tapes may be useful in helping the patient cope with pain and other stressors. In some situations, hypnosis may be used with the goal of having the patient develop the ability to induce self-hypnosis during dressing changes and other stressful events.

Patients are usually helped to cope if they are kept fully informed about what is planned for their care and what will be expected of them during various treatments. Then they are not forced to cope with unexpected events that can be very upsetting, especially when they have had to give up most of their independence.

Families, like patients, cope best when they are kept fully informed and have a realistic understanding of what lies ahead for the patient. The family can be deeply disrupted by a serious burn to a family member. Initially, they are concerned about the patient's survival and need careful explanations of what is being done for the patient and why. The explanations may need to be repeated more than once because the family may be too distressed to comprehend what they are being told.

Social workers are helpful in exploring the family's concerns about role disruptions, plans for child care, financial concerns, and their own feelings of distress. Often the family requires considerable support from health professionals to work through their own feelings before they can be supportive to the patient. The burn team members meet to decide who will provide what support to the family.

The family can best provide realistic support to the patient when they have accurate knowledge about what the patient will experience at each step in the recovery process. The family also needs information about community resources available to them and the patient.

### Promoting a Positive Body Image and Self-Concept

A burn wound, especially a large one, presents a serious challenge to the patient's self-concept. As the patient's condition improves, he or she may express a desire to view the burned area. The burn team assesses the readiness of the patient to view the burned area and decides which members of the burn team will be present when the viewing occurs. If the patient desires, a family member or another support person may be present.

The patient is encouraged to express how he or she feels about the changed appearance. Individual counseling may be necessary for some patients as they integrate the change in their appearance into their self-concept. Other patients will benefit from being referred to a patient support group where they meet other patients in various stages of recovery. The group may be led by a nurse, social worker, psychologist, or other health professional experienced in working with burn patients. Knowledge about the patient's coping style can help determine whether individual or group therapy or both will be recommended to the patient.

### Encouraging Self-Care Activities

The patient is encouraged to participate as much as possible in his or her own care. Independence in activities of daily living (ADL) is supported. Some patients will require more encouragement than others in assisting with tasks such as wound care. It is important that the patient be involved in developing a daily plan of care including meal selection, time of treatments, rest periods, therapy, and socialization.

### Preventing Hypothermia

Room temperature is maintained at 83° to 85° F with 40% to 50% humidity. Care is taken to limit wound exposure time during dressing changes.

## EVALUATION

To evaluate the effectiveness of nursing interventions compare patient behaviors with those stated in the expected outcomes. Successful achievement of patient outcomes for the patient with burns during the acute phase is indicated by:

1. Skin integrity is reestablished
   a. Shows wound healing
   b. Shows hypertrophic scarring
   c. Is able to perform skin care
2. Absence of wound or systemic infection
   a. Shows no pathogenic organisms from wound culture
   b. Has no signs of systemic infection
      (1) Fever
      (2) Tachypnea
      (3) Tachycardia
      (4) Paralytic ileus
      (5) Oliguria
3. Has optimal nutritional status
   a. Has protein and caloric intake adequate to meet calculated needs
   b. Has positive nitrogen balance indicated by normal prealbumin and albumin levels
   c. Maintains preburn weight
   d. Has no diarrhea or constipation
4. Adequate pain control
   a. Rates pain control as acceptable
   b. Has no physical signs of pain, e.g., tachycardia, diaphoresis, splinting of body parts, or protective movement
   c. States is able to sleep
   d. Is able to perform self-care
5. Adequate fluid balance
   a. Has stable weight as measured by daily weighing
   b. Has blood levels of $Na^+$ and $K^+$ within normal limits
   c. Has balance of intake and output
   d. Has good skin turgor
6. Exhibits full range of motion
   a. Moves arms and legs through range of motion several times daily
   b. Is able to perform ADL with no or minimal assistance
7. Exhibits reduced anxiety
   a. Appears relaxed and calm
   b. Has normal vital signs
   c. Listens quietly to explanations from staff and asks appropriate questions about future
8. Effective coping of patient
   a. Uses relaxation and meditation techniques during dressing changes and other stressful events
   b. Verbalizes a realistic appraisal of life situation
   c. Discusses resources available to assist with changes in lifestyle
9. Effective coping of family or significant other(s)
   a. Is realistically supportive of patient
   b. Uses counseling and other services in adjusting to changes in family
10. Develops realistic body image and self-concept
   a. Is able to look at and touch burned areas
   b. Verbalizes feelings about change in appearance and grieving for former self
   c. Verbalizes ways appearance could be improved (makeup, etc.)
11. Understands treatment regimen
   a. Is able to explain daily routine after discharge
   b. Discusses resources available after discharge
   c. States name of person to call in case of an emergency
   d. States date and time of follow-up visit
12. Performs self-care with minimal assistance
   a. Feeds self
   b. Dresses self
   c. Maintains hygiene and grooming
   d. Changes dressing with assistance of significant other
13. Maintains normothermia
   a. Understands importance of avoiding chilling
   b. Takes temperature daily

## GERONTOLOGICAL CONSIDERATIONS

Gerontological considerations are summarized in the box at right.

# COLLABORATIVE CARE MANAGEMENT

## REHABILITATION PERIOD

Rehabilitation begins at the time of admission.[19] However, rehabilitation as the third stage of treatment begins when the patient's burn is reduced to less than 20% TBSA, and the patient is capable of assuming some self-care activity. The principles of management are to return the patient to a productive place in society and to accomplish functional and cosmetic reconstruction. Rehabilitation does not end when the patient is discharged. It may take from 2 to 5 years after discharge for the patient to reach a maximal level of emotional and physical adjustment.

### Diagnostic Tests

Specific diagnostic testing during the rehabilitation period depends on the patient's condition and progress toward goals. Overall, limited testing is required. Evaluation of nutritional status (prealbumin and urine urea nitrogen measurements) and the presence of infection (complete blood counts and wound and/or blood cultures) may be necessary.

### Medications

The number of medications prescribed decreases as the patient progresses through the rehabilitation period. As wounds heal, less analgesia is required, and antimicrobial agents are prescribed only for documented infections.

### Treatments

As burn wounds continue to heal only minimal wound care is necessary. This may be performed by the patient in an outpatient clinic or in the home. When reconstructive procedures are performed, more extensive wound care will be necessary.

### Surgical Management

Initial skin grafting is completed during the acute period. However, the patient may require reconstructive surgery to improve function and plastic surgery to reform ears, noses, or eyelids during the rehabilitation period. Scar tissue and contractures commonly occur 1 to 2 years postburn and may require additional skin grafting.

### Diet

Nutritional requirements continue to decrease, and vitamin supplements are no longer necessary. A well-balanced diet with adequate fluid intake is encouraged.

### Activity

Optimal function is the goal of rehabilitation. Physical and occupational therapy are provided in inpatient rehabilitation settings, in outpatient settings, or in the home.

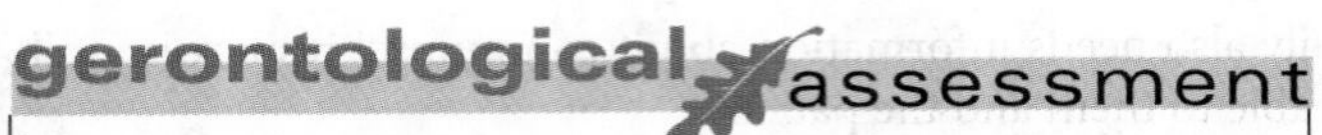


**EPIDEMIOLOGY**

Incidence of burn injury in the home is disproportionately higher than for younger adults.
One third of all those who die in residential fires are elderly persons.
Elderly persons are at a higher risk for burn injury because of:
Thinner skin, which is less resistant to heat
Decreased mobility and reaction time
Visual and hearing impairments that decrease ability to evaluate danger
Living in older homes, which may have faulty wiring, poor heating systems, or no smoke detectors
Flame injury is the most common type of burn injury.
Inhalation injury occurs more often in elderly persons than in younger persons because of their inability to escape the fire.

**AGING CHANGES THAT AFFECT RECOVERY FROM BURN INJURY**

Overall mortality is higher than in younger adults.
Reserve capacity of organ systems is diminished.
Cardiovascular system:
- Cardiac response to burn shock is impaired because of
- Lower cardiac output
- Coronary atherosclerosis
- Decreased baroreceptor response to volume changes
- All of these put elderly persons at risk for cardiac failure.

Pulmonary:
- Decreased elasticity of thoracic cage and decreased number and efficiency of alveoli make elderly persons more prone to hypoxia, hypoventilation, and atelectasis.

Immunological:
- Elderly persons have diminished host resistance and impaired cell-mediated and humoral immunity.
- Elderly persons are more prone to infection and sepsis and have decreased ability to combat infection.

Wound healing:
- Diminished inflammatory response
- Increased healing time
- Decreased tolerance of wound excision and grafting

**MANAGEMENT CONSIDERATIONS**

Carefully assess cardiac status during burn resuscitation.
Monitor response to fluid volume administration:
- Hypotension
- Monitor breath sounds for onset of pulmonary edema
- May require the use of pulmonary artery catheter to adequately evaluate
- Urinary output

Monitor for early signs of respiratory failure.
- Mobilize patient as soon as possible.
- Provide pulmonary hygiene.

Prevent infection.
- Monitor for early signs of complications such as mental status changes, ileus, wound drainage, and temperature changes (especially hypothermia).

Promote nutritional intake.
Provide thorough wound care.

### Referrals

In promoting the patient's return to full function, referrals may be made to agencies that can facilitate reintegration into society. Patients requiring a change in vocation will be referred to a vocational counselor and those who continue to have difficulty adjusting to their injuries will be referred for psychological care.

## NURSING MANAGEMENT

## ■ ASSESSMENT

### Subjective Data

The patient must be helped to maintain range of joint motion to prevent scars from healing in positions that will result in deformity. Complaints of pain and pressure should not be overlooked because damage may occur from an improperly applied splint or poor positioning. It is important that patients understand why ambulation or motion is necessary even though it may be painful.

The emotional impact of a severe burn is enormous. The psychological scars last forever and affect the victim and family for the rest of their lives. The extent to which the family unit adapts affects how the patient reacts to his or her new body image and feelings of self-worth.

The hospital environment and hospital personnel influence the adaptation process. In the immediate postburn period, the nurse is primarily concerned with physiological survival of the patient. At the same time, the nurse must be able to identify psychological problems and coping mechanisms of the patient and family.

### Objective Data

The nurse is responsible for assessing the patient's response to positioning, splinting, and exercise and the ability of the patient and family to perform daily wound care after discharge. Correct positioning must be maintained to avoid the development of contractures. The splinted limb is assessed for adequate circulation, cyanosis, and temperature and the presence of pulses. Exercise, ADL, and ambulation must be continuously assessed for patient tolerance, both physically and emotionally. Complete and comprehensive instructions of wound and dressing care followed by return demonstrations are necessary before discharge.

## ■ NURSING DIAGNOSES

Nursing diagnoses are determined from analysis of patient data during the rehabilitative period. Nursing diagnoses for the person with burns may include but are not limited to:

| Diagnostic Title | Etiological Factors |
|---|---|
| Mobility, impaired physical | Pain, decreased strength and endurance, contractures |
| Self-care deficit | Intolerance to activity, musculoskeletal impairment |
| Body image disturbance | Loss/change of body parts and/or function |
| Skin integrity, impaired, risk for | Nutritional deficit, fragile new tissue |
| Pain, chronic | Joint, tissue contractures |
| Coping, ineffective individual | Situational crisis, ineffective support systems |
| Coping, ineffective family, compromised | Inadequate or incorrect information; temporary family disorganization, role changes |
| Knowledge deficit | Unfamiliarity with burn injury |

## ■ EXPECTED PATIENT OUTCOMES

Expected patient outcomes for the burn-injured patient during the rehabilitation phase include but are not limited to:

1. Achieves full range of motion and physical activity consistent with desired levels.
2. Performs ADL.
3. Develops a realistic image of self and makes alterations needed in daily activities.
4. Has healed tissue remain intact.
5. Reports decreased pain.
6. Demonstrates effective coping mechanisms and develops a realistic plan for the future.
7. The family demonstrates effective coping mechanisms.
8. Verbalizes understanding of treatments and demonstrates wound care and exercises.

## ■ INTERVENTIONS

### Promoting Mobility

As the survival rate of patients with large and deeper burns increases, so does the challenge to maintain optimal functioning and cosmetic results. The percentage of patients with joint limitations increases as the degree and extent of burns increases. Although these patients may be critically ill, their rehabilitative needs must be addressed immediately. A comprehensive program of positioning, splinting, exercise, ambulation, and activities of daily living must begin on the first or second day postburn and be carried through until after discharge. Any delays in initiating treatment will be detrimental to the patient's ultimate functional outcome. Contractures are among the most serious long-term complications of burns today. They result from muscle and joint stiffening, skin grafting, and prolonged bedrest (Research Box). Although occupational and physical therapists are primarily responsible for addressing the patient's rehabilitation needs during all phases of the patient's recovery, the nurse is responsible for assuring that all their recommendations are followed.

#### *Therapeutic positioning*

Therapeutic positioning—placing body parts in antideformity positions—is vital to the prevention of burn contractures. The patient must be repositioned in bed (side-lying, supine, or prone) frequently and regularly around the clock. Correct positioning varies, depending on the area of the body burned (Table 64-8). Positioning can be enhanced by placing patients on a Stryker frame, a Foster bed, a CircOlectric bed, or one of the many different types of low-air-loss beds or mattresses currently available. These beds facilitate the use of the

**table 64-8** *Therapeutic Positioning for the Burn Patient*

| Area Burned | Description of Position |
|---|---|
| Neck | No pillow |
| | Towel roll under cervical spine |
| | Neck splint |
| Shoulder | 90° abduction, neutral rotation |
| | Elbow splint may be used to aid in maintaining position |
| Axilla | Abduction with 10° to 15° forward flexion and external rotation |
| | Support abducted arm with suspension from IV pole or bedside table |
| | Axilla splint |
| Elbow | Extension |
| | Support extended arm on bedside table, foam trough |
| | Elbow splint |
| Hand | Hand splint |
| Dorsal surface | Flexion |
| Palmar surface | Hyperextension |
| Hip | Extension with neutral rotation |
| | Supine with lower extremity extended |
| | Prone-lying (if medically appropriate) |
| | Trochanter roll |
| | Foam wedge along lateral aspect of thigh |
| | Knee or long leg splint |
| Knee | Extension |
| | Prone-lying (if medically appropriate) |
| | Patient out of bed with lower extremities extended and elevated |
| | Knee splint |
| Ankle | Dorsiflexion |
| | Padded footboard with heels free of pressure |
| | Ankle splint |

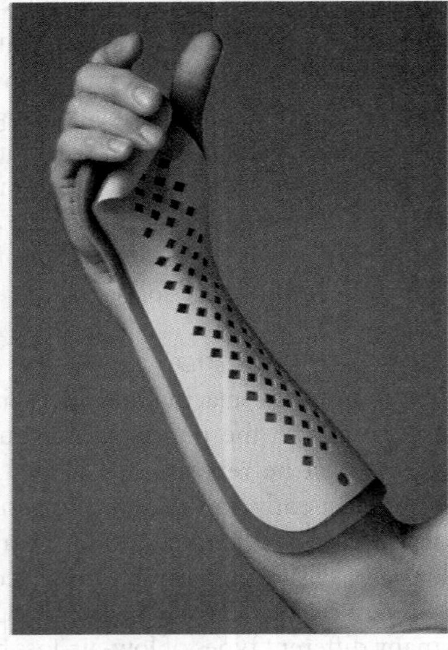

**fig. 64-12** Orthoplast hand splint.

**research**

Reference: Baker RAU et al: Degree of burn, location of burn, and length of hospital stay as predictors of psychosocial status and physical functioning, *J Burn Care Rehabil* 17:327-333, 1996.

Using the Burn-Specific Health Scale, the authors investigated the relationship between degree of burn, location of burn, length of hospital stay, and psychosocial and physical status. The tool, which assesses dysfunction and distress in the physical, mental, social, and general areas of health, was administered to a convenience sample of 31 patients admitted to a burn center at the first-alert stage (stable, alert, and oriented) and predischarge. Overall, the patients had a higher level of social and mental functioning than physical functioning at both first-alert and predischarge stages. In addition, patients reported a lower level of functioning in each of the four areas of health (except mobility and role activities) predischarge than at the first-alert stage. Results indicated that patients with first-degree burns reported lower functioning in the physical domain only in the first-alert stage. By discharge, patients with first-degree burns reported lower functioning in all psychological and physiological areas. The location of the burn predicted functioning, e.g., patients with hand burns reported lower physical function than patients with head burns. In general, patients who stayed longer in the hospital reported lower physical functioning, particularly in mobility and hand function. This study dispels the myth that the more serious the burn, the more serious the physical and psychological impact. Patients with minor burns may suffer significant physical and emotional effects.

bedpan and urinal, permit change of position with a minimum of handling, and permit larger skin surfaces to remain freer from body pressure than is possible when the patient lies on a regular mattress. These special beds are particularly useful when both the back and front of the trunk, thighs, and legs have been burned. These beds allow turning of the patient with minimal handling and thus help decrease pain.

Prolonged rest in a semi-Fowler's position or with the pillow pushing the head forward must be avoided, even though many patients like this position because it enables them to see about the room better. The bed can often be turned so that the patient can look about without having to assume positions that may lead to the formation of contractures. The bedside table may be changed from one side of the bed to the other at intervals to stimulate other body positions.

**Splints.** Splints prevent or correct contractures and immobilize joints after grafting. They are custom-made and often molded directly on the patient to assure optimal conformity (Figure 64-12). It is the responsibility of the nurse to apply the splint properly and according to an established schedule. An improperly applied splint can promote contractures and lead to additional complications. The nurse assesses the splinted limb for adequate circulation, cyanosis, temperature, and the presence of pulses. Complaints of pain and pressure should be assessed because damage may occur with an improperly applied splint. Some physicians prefer to use the open method of treatment and use frequent exercise instead of splinting to prevent contractures.

**Exercises and ambulation.** Exercises for prevention and correction of contractures are begun as soon as the patient is stable. Active exercises are preferred, although active assistance and gentle pressure exercises may be more realistic. Supervision by a physical or occupational therapist is desirable. Exercises may be performed more easily in water and may be done concurrently with dressing changes if the patient is able to tolerate the activity (Figure 64-13). Continuous passive pressure motion devices may be used to prevent contractures of affected joints. When burns are completely covered (by healing or by graft), exercises may be performed more easily in an occupational therapy or physical therapy department where the patient may benefit from a change in environment.

Ambulation decreases the risk of thromboemboli and renal calculi, promotes optimal ventilation, helps maintain range of motion and strength in the lower extremities; orients the patient to the environment, and provides a sense of functional independence. Patients who have large burns have less ability to tolerate activity and will require a progressive approach to mobilization. Initially the patient may need to be transferred with maximal assistance onto a stretcher chair and progress to a sitting position. Gradually, the patient may progress to a standing pivot transfer into a nearby chair and eventually ambulate with minimal assistance. Before getting out of bed, an elastic bandage support must be applied to the lower extremities to prevent venous stasis, edema, and orthostatic hypotension.

### Promoting Self-Care

One of the ultimate goals in the rehabilitation of the burned patient is to maintain or restore the patient's independence in performing ADL. The occupational therapist aids in this process by selecting activities appropriate to the patient's medical, physical, and mental status. Activities that the nurse can encourage are self-feeding, telephoning, reading mail, and assisting with grooming or burn wound management. The nurse supports the information taught by the physical and occupational therapists so that progress can be continued on the nursing unit, in the clinic, or in the home.

After the wounds are healed, the long recuperative process begins, accompanied by the realization of endless implications for the future. Burns on the face make adjustments particularly difficult. Different kinds of fears include death, pain, disfigurement, prolonged hospitalization, loss of job security, disruption of lifestyle, and reaction of family and friends.

### Promoting a Positive Body Image

Regardless of its size, a burn injury represents a change in the individual's perception of self. As the burn heals, the patient must deal with a new appearance. The patient must have the opportunity to talk about concerns or fears. Some patients may be unable to discuss these with their family or significant others. The nurse must be prepared to listen actively and help the patient accept changes in appearance. The patient must be allowed to grieve for the loss of the former self. However, the patient should be encouraged to focus on the positive aspects of self.

To the adolescent, the thought of being different or conspicuous may be unbearable. If possible, the patient should see facial burns only after being prepared for the experience. The patient will need support and understanding to cope with his or her image in the mirror. The patient will exhibit readiness by asking to look in the mirror. Interaction with other burn patients who are further along in the healing process may help the patient feel that recovery is possible. In some cases, the recovery is very good, and although differences in skin pigmentation remain, the redness that accompanies healed burn wounds often fades considerably within a few months. Pigmentation problems are more acute for persons with brown or black skin. Their healed skin may be a different shade, freckled, or whitish. Commercial makeup products that help blend skin tones are available.

### Promoting Skin Integrity

#### *Preventing scarring*

Whenever a wound of connective tissue heals, hypertrophic scarring will occur unless the skin adheres to the underlying structure. Hypertrophic scarring results from the

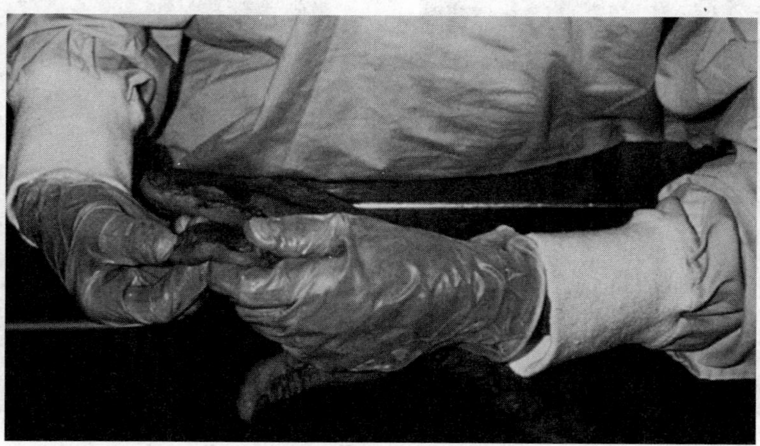

**fig. 64-13** Passive range-of-motion exercise during hydrotherapy.

overgrowth and overproduction of tissue. This occurs especially in areas of stress and movement such as the hands, legs, and chest (Figure 64-14). The thickened rigid scar that results may later cause contractures. The application of controlled constant pressure to the surface of an immature scar will reduce the scar and leave a smooth pliable tissue. If this pressure is applied to new healthy tissue, hypertrophic scarring can be prevented (Figure 64-15). The pressure garment, a specially designed elastic woven material, provides tridimensional control. It is fitted to each patient individually and then custom made. Until the garment is completed, bandages can be used for a pressure dressing.

Even though pressure garments help decrease the formation of thick, disfiguring scars, patient acceptance is a problem. The garments are uncomfortable and make the patient warm, especially during hot weather. They must be tight enough to produce the 24 mm Hg of pressure required to exceed capillary pressure to be effective in reducing edema and scar formation. The patient must wear the garments 23 hours a day for 6 months to a year.

A plan for exercise and splinting must be established before discharge. To prevent scar contracture, daily therapy sessions may be necessary for several weeks or months. The occupational therapist can develop aids to help with the activities of daily living.

### Promoting Comfort

Although less severe, pain remains a problem during the rehabilitation phase. Small areas of skin may remain open and continue to require dressing changes. In addition, newly healed skin is sensitive. Physical and occupational therapy and increasing activity may result in discomfort. Interventions are focused on administration of analgesics, diversional activities, relaxation techniques, and providing information about what the patient can expect. Daily hydrotherapy helps the patient relax tense muscles.

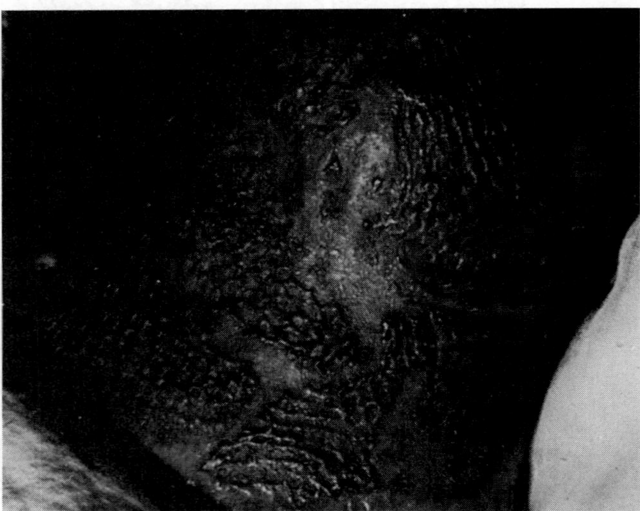

**fig. 64-14** Hypertrophic scarring over chest and abdomen.

### Facilitating Individual and Family Coping

After discharge, the patient continues to adjust to temporary or permanent function loss, cosmetic disfigurement, and the reactions of others. The ability to manage depends on coping mechanisms before the burn, the severity and site of the burn, and the reaction of others. The patient's adaptation to these changes can be evaluated during outpatient visits when the burn team and appropriate personnel are available.[15]

Follow-up care may not take place at the institution where the patient was hospitalized. The burn team members may need to contact their counterparts in the community to plan follow-up care. If possible, a member of the follow-up team should visit the patient in the hospital before discharge.

Job retraining may be necessary if the burn injury caused loss of joint function or other physical limitations that prevent the patient from returning to former employment. The local office of the State Labor and Industry Board can assign a vocational counselor to help the patient return to the workforce. Even if retraining cannot begin for several months, the contact with the vocational counselor and anticipation of retraining may help the patient look beyond immediate problems and think of the future.

### Facilitating Learning

#### *Discharge teaching*

Before discharge, burned patients and their families have a great need for education so that they may take increasing responsibilities for their own care. Discharge teaching involves the entire burn team, who work together to prepare the patient and family for discharge.

Early discharge planning accomplishes two goals. First, it helps solve problems early. For example, if the patient's

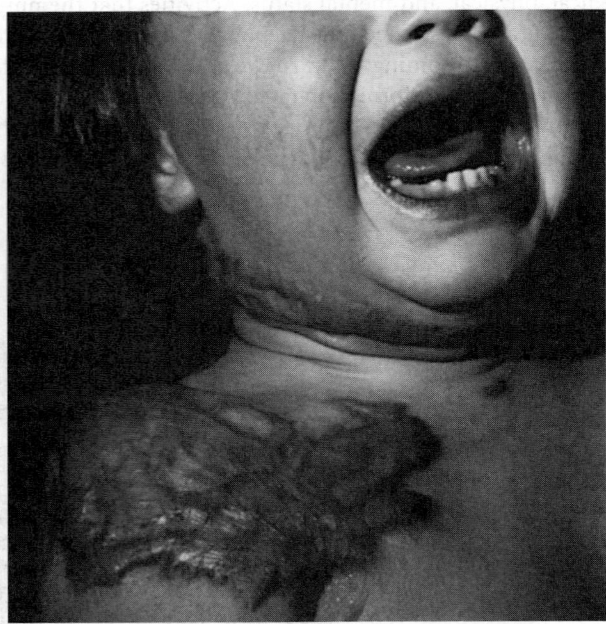

**fig. 64-15** Scar formation occurring from lack of pressure dressing application.

house burned and needs to be repaired, the family may need to relocate. This could be done before discharge, thus preventing the added stress of moving after discharge. Second, early discharge planning emphasizes the future. If discharge is discussed, the patient and his or her family may realize more quickly that recovery and return to home are possible.

Complete and comprehensive instructions followed by return demonstrations contribute to learning the necessary skills to be independent in self-care activities after discharge. Patients with a major burn should not be discharged from the hospital until they can care for themselves physically, with assistance if necessary, and are prepared to meet the stresses involved in returning to their former living patterns. Teaching priorities are summarized in the Guidelines for Care Box below.

A major goal in discharge teaching is to prevent excessive scar formation by exercising, splinting, and applying pressure dressings. If these methods are not effective, reconstructive surgery may be necessary. A patient recovering from a major burn may need 12 to 18 months to achieve complete wound healing.

Instructions should include how to care for the healed graft and nongrafted areas. Signs and symptoms of complications, including areas that may blister and break down, and signs of infection are also addressed.

An example of written discharge instructions is provided in the Guidelines for Care Box on the next page, and a Nursing Care Plan is presented on p. 2143-2144. Written instructions should include the name and phone number of a physician or nurse who the patient may call with questions or problems concerning follow-up care. A referral may be made to the Visiting Nurse Association or another home health agency that may be of assistance in dressing the patient's wounds at home.

## EVALUATION

To evaluate the effectiveness of nursing interventions, compare patient behaviors with those stated in the expected outcomes. Successful achievement of patient outcomes for the patient with burns is indicated by:

1. Has full range of motion and mobility.
   a. Demonstrates exercise program for the prevention and control of contractures.
   b. Is able to perform ADL.
2. Performs self-care.
   a. Cares for own burn scars and applies dressings as necessary.
   b. Performs daily routines without assistance.
3. Has realistic body image.
   a. Speaks openly about change in appearance.
   b. Participates in activities with nonburned persons.
   c. Presents self positively.

**guidelines for care**

### Teaching the Person with a Burn

- Patient/significant other verbalizes understanding of:
  - Pathophysiology of burn process
  - Depth and percentage of injury
  - Functions of the skin
  - Need for fluid replacement
- Knowledge of healing process:
  - Nutritional requirements
  - Infection control measures
  - Rationale for wound management
    - Hydrotherapy and debridement
    - Topical agents
    - Grafting
  - Scar formation
    - Stages of development
    - Use of Ace bandage or pressure garments
    - Use of cosmetics and prosthetics
  - Purpose of occupational and physical therapy toward improved mobility
    - Level of activity
    - Prescribed exercises
- Pain management
  - Relation of pain to depth of injury
  - Pain control options
    - Analgesics
    - Diversional activities
    - Meditation
    - Relaxation exercises
- Discharge needs:
  - Skin care for healed areas
    - Protection from sun
    - Avoidance of chemical irritants
    - Increased sensitivity
    - Blister formation
  - Skin care for open areas
    - Prescribed dressing
    - Application
    - Abnormal conditions
  - Application and care of pressure garments
  - Home care needs
    - Care of clothing
    - Cleanliness of dressing change area, that is, shower/bathtub
    - Adaptation of home environment, that is, handicap rails in bathtub or shower area
  - Nutritional needs
    - Basic four food groups
    - Relationship of dietary intake to healing process
  - Emotional readjustment
    - To new body image
    - Emotional reactions that may develop at home
      - Nightmares/flashbacks
      - Grief
      - Isolation
      - Depression
  - Dealing with reactions of others
  - Options for increasing social activity

**guidelines for care**

## Discharge Instructions for the Person with a Burn

We on the burn team are happy to see that you are able to go home. To ensure you the speediest possible recovery, it is important that you are able to care for yourself and recognize problems that may interfere with your complete recovery.

If any of the following occur, please call the hospital and ask for the Burn Clinic. The nurse will be able to assist you.

1. Healed area breaking open: cover with clean dressing.
2. Formation of blisters
3. Signs of infection:
   a. Fever, temperature over 38° C (100.4° F)
   b. Redness, pain, swelling, hardness, or warmth in or around wound or any other part of body
   c. Increased or foul-smelling drainage from wound
4. Problems with your Ace bandages or Jobst garment such as improper fit, formation of blisters, or opening of healed area underneath

Your first clinic appointment will be on ______.

### Bathing

Bathing or showering daily in your usual manner cleans the wounds, especially the ones that are still open.

1. Check the water and be sure to adjust the temperature to a warm and comfortable level. Your skin is more sensitive to extra heat or cold and can be easily injured.
2. Wash gently with a clean, soft washcloth, using a mild detergent soap such as Dial or Ivory. Be careful not to rub too hard so as not to disturb the grafted areas. Avoid harsh or deodorant soaps.
3. Rinse skin thoroughly after washing.
4. Dry thoroughly.
5. Apply specific dressing as instructed.

### Care for Burn Wound

These are your guidelines for the care of your burn wound. During this time, look at the involved areas and note any changes that need to be reported.

1. Wash hands.
2. Remove dressing and dispose of in paper bag or wrap in newspaper.
3. Wash hands.
4. Wash open area with a clean soft washcloth and Dial or Ivory soap and water. Use a clean towel and washcloth with each dressing change.
5. Rinse skin well with plain water.
6. Wash hands.
7. Apply dressing as described below.
8. Wear gloves. Wash basin or bathtub with a disinfectant such as Lysol.
9. Wash hands.

### Care of Clothing

When you are discharged, you may find that healed burn areas are sensitive to harsh detergents, fabric softeners, and clothing dyes. If you are sensitive, we suggest the following:

1. Launder new clothing before use by machine or hand with a detergent free of additives.
2. Rinse clothes twice.
3. Do not use fabric softeners.
4. If you have open burns or a healed area that opens, wash all clothes separately from those of other family members.
5. Scarlet red ointment will permanently stain clothing.
6. If dyes used in clothing cause irritation, wear white articles.
7. Wear loose-fitting clothing.

### Ace Bandages

You have been taught to put on your own Ace bandages while in the hospital, but if you do have a problem with this, please notify the Burn Clinic. It is also important that you know how to care for them and understand problems that occur.

1. If they are too loose, they will be ineffective and must be rewrapped.
2. If they are too tight, they will cause discomfort, numbness, tingling, and puffiness and must be rewrapped.
3. They must be worn for a long period of time, probably 6-12 months to be effective, so please do not stop wearing them until your doctor tells you.
4. To care for your Ace bandages:
   a. Hand wash with a mild detergent in cold water.
   b. Towel dry.
   c. Lay flat to dry.

### Pressure Garment

You have been taught to put on your Jobst garment while in the hospital, but if you have a problem with this, please notify the Burn Clinic. It is also important that you know how to care for it and understand problems that can occur.

1. If it is too loose, it will be ineffective and you will require a new garment.
2. If it is too tight, it will cause discomfort, numbness, and tingling. Do not wear it if this occurs, but notify the Burn Clinic as soon as possible.
3. To care for your pressure garment:
   a. Hand wash with a mild detergent in cold water.
   b. Towel dry.
   c. Lay flat to dry.

### Diet

A well-balanced diet is important as your burn wound continues to heal. Be sure to include meat, milk products, breads and cereals, and fruits and vegetables in your diet.

### Your Emotions

It is not uncommon to feel blue or let down after you go home. The Burn Support Group meets every Thursday to help you.

Courtesy Comprehensive Burn Center, MetroHealth Medical Center, Cleveland.

## nursing care plan The Person with a Burn

**DATA** Mr. W. is a 63-year-old retired man with a history of adult onset diabetes, diabetic neuropathy, peripheral vascular disease, and hypertension. The evening before admission to the hospital, he had filled his bathtub at home to soak his feet. Without checking the water temperature with his hands, he placed his feet and lower legs in the tub to soak for approximately 20 minutes. Because of decreased sensation in his feet and legs, he was unaware of the hot water temperature. On removing his feet from the tub, he noticed that his legs were bright red. The next morning he noticed that his skin remained bright red and was blistering and weeping. After evaluation in the emergency department, he was admitted to the burn center.

In the burn center, Mr. W.'s wounds are cleansed with water and a mild soap. Nonadherent skin is removed. An initial wound culture is obtained. The wounds are assessed and are dark red with poor capillary refill. His burn is determined to be a 10% TBSA, deep partial-thickness burn, circumferential from the toes to midcalf bilaterally. A wound culture and admission photographs are obtained.

The nursing history also identified the following:

- Mr. W. states he controls his diabetes by "watching what I eat" and takes an oral hypoglycemic. He does not monitor his blood glucose level.
- He lives alone in a two-story home. His daughter lives in the same city, but they have limited contact.

Objective data included the following:

- Blood pressure of 158/90
- Peripheral pulses present by Doppler only
- Diminished sensation in his lower extremities but identifies a burning, throbbing pain
- Blood glucose of 204 mg/dl

**NURSING DIAGNOSIS** *Impaired skin integrity related to thermal injury*

| expected patient outcome | nursing interventions | rationale |
|---|---|---|
| Burn wounds will heal without complications. | Perform wound care (hydrotherapy and debridement) as prescribed using strict asepsis. | Meticulous wound care is essential to remove nonviable tissue, protect viable tissue, prevent infection, and promote healing. |
| | Assess wounds with each dressing change for evidence of healing or infection. | Topical wound agents may change daily, depending on the condition of the wound. Early detection of wound infection is essential to prevent deterioration of the wound and the development of systemic infection. |
| | Limit patient ambulation. Maintain leg elevation when in chair or bed. | Leg dependence in a patient with leg burns promotes edema. Increased edema at the burn site results in decreased tissue perfusion. |
| | Administer vitamins and minerals (vitamin A, ascorbic acid, and zinc) as ordered. | Vitamin A, zinc, and ascorbic acid are required for wound healing. |
| | Monitor blood glucose levels before meals and at bedtime. | Poorly controlled diabetes impairs wound healing and promotes infection. Burn injury affects diabetes control due to stress of the illness and hypermetabolism (for major burns). |

**NURSING DIAGNOSIS** *Risk for infection related to loss of skin integrity and diabetes*

| expected patient outcome | nursing interventions | rationale |
|---|---|---|
| Has no wound infection. | Monitor for signs and symptoms of infection (temperature elevation, altered sensorium, and elevated white blood cell count). | Early detection of infection will allow for the appropriate selection of systemic or topical antimicrobial agents. |
| | Assess the wound during each dressing change for signs of local infection. | Infection of the burn wound may be reflected by erythema at the wound edges; pale, mottled, dry appearance of the wound; and purulent, foul-smelling drainage. The presence of a wound infection will effect the type of topical agent selected. |

Continued

## The Person with a Burn—cont'd

**NURSING DIAGNOSIS** *Risk for infection related to loss of skin integrity and diabetes—cont'd*

| expected patient outcome | nursing interventions | rationale |
|---|---|---|
| | Obtain a wound sample for culture twice weekly, as ordered. | Tracking bacterial colonization of the wound allows for early detection of pathogens. |
| | Maintain aseptic wound technique and thorough cleansing of equipment and hydrotherapy tubs/tables. | This prevents cross-contamination of bacteria between patients that may cause infection. |

**NURSING DIAGNOSIS** *Pain related to tissue injury*

| expected patient outcome | nursing interventions | rationale |
|---|---|---|
| States pain is controlled. | Assess pain level using a 1 to 10 pain rating scale every 4 hours during wound care and during physical therapy. | Determination of patient's perception of pain assists in the appropriate analgesic agent and dose. |
| | Administer analgesia around the clock. | Burn pain is constant. |
| | Provide analgesia before hydrotherapy and wound care and therapy. | Pain will increase during wound care and physical therapy. Pain control allows for more active participation by the patient. |
| | Maintain elevation of legs while in bed and in the chair. | Pain increases in dependent leg positions related to venous pooling and edema formation. |
| | Instruct patient in nonpharmacological methods of pain control, e.g., imagery or distraction. | Nonpharmacological methods of pain control are effective *adjuvant* therapies along with opioids. |

**NURSING DIAGNOSIS** *Altered health maintenance related to lack of knowledge of burn process, treatment regimen, signs and symptoms of complications, and burn injury prevention*

| expected patient outcome | nursing interventions | rationale |
|---|---|---|
| Verbalizes understanding of wound care needs. Performs wound care. | Assess patient's physical and cognitive ability to perform wound care. | Patient's ability to perform wound care will help to determine discharge needs, i.e., home health care versus performing by self. |
| Identifies skin care for healed areas. | Instruct patient to: Apply lotion 2-3 times a day. | Lotion helps to maintain moisture of newly healed tissue and prevent tissue breakdown. Newly healed skin is prone to itching, flaking, and dryness. |
| | Wear clean socks and well-fitting shoes. | Tight shoes will predispose healed areas of the feet to tissue breakdown. |
| Identifies actions that predispose to burn injury. | Avoid exposure of healed wounds to chemicals or extremes in temperature. | Tissue is fragile initially and will easily reinjure. |
| | Provide patient with a bath thermometer to assess the temperature of the water before bathing. | Decreased sensation of feet from diabetic neuropathy limits ability to determine temperature of the water. Water temperature should be 100-105° F. |
| | Instruct patient to turn the temperature of his home hot water tank down to 130° F. | Water temperatures of 150° F (a common hot water tank setting) will result in a full-thickness burn in approximately 1 second. At 130° F 30 seconds are required, decreasing the possibility of burn injury. |

4. Maintains skin integrity.
   a. Identifies techniques to prevent breakdown of healed areas, e.g., protection from sun, exposure to harsh chemicals, use of lubricating lotions, and proper use of pressure garments.
5. Controls pain.
   a. Rates pain control as acceptable.
   b. States is able to sleep.
   c. Is able to perform daily routines without increasing pain.
6. Exhibits positive coping behaviors
   a. Identifies alterations in personal situation and identifies strategies to improve it.
   b. Develops positive body image.
   c. Reintegrates into the community.
7. Family exhibits positive coping behavior.
   a. Family identifies alterations in patient's and family situation and identifies strategies to improve it.
8. Understands treatment regimen.
   a. Is able to explain daily routine and the reasons for it.
   b. Discusses hospital and community resources available for assistance.
   c. States date and time of next medical follow-up.
   d. States name of health care provider to call in an emergency.

## COMPLICATIONS

Complications may occur at any period in burn managment. The most common complications are wound infections, contractures, and psychological problems with some persons developing posttraumatic stress syndrome. Each of these conditions is discussed within the chapter.

## critical thinking QUESTIONS

1 Two 30-year-old men are brought to the emergency room after burns from a house fire. One man has a partial-thickness burn, and the other has a full-thickness burn. What subjective data would help differentiate these two types of burns?

2 Incorporating general principles of psychological care, develop one nursing approach for each of the following patient responses to a severe burn: withdrawal; regression; anger/hostility; and depression.

3 What factors would you consider in determining how aggressively to care for a healthy 80-year-old woman who suffers a 60% TBSA deep-partial and full-thickness burn?

4 Discuss the differences in priorities of care during the emergent and rehabilitative phases of burn injury.

## chapter SUMMARY

### ETIOLOGY/EPIDEMIOLOGY

- The severity of a burn injury depends on the age of the victim, the body part involved, the burning agent, the size and depth of the burn wound, and the victim's medical history.

### NURSING MANAGEMENT

- The initial care for a burn includes removing the victim from the source of the burn and dousing the burn with water.
- The initial systemic response to a burn is the shift of fluid from the intravascular to the interstitial space, creating hypovolemia. This is treated with a calculated dose of lactated Ringer's solution. After 48 to 72 hours, the fluid shifts from the interstitial to the intravascular space and hypervolemia occurs.
- Emotional support to the victim and the victim's family is an important role for nurses.
- Burn wounds must be assessed on a daily basis.
- Correct splinting and positioning are the best methods for preventing contractures.
- There is no way to predict the appearance of a burn wound after healing.

## References


1. American Psychiatric Association: *Diagnostic and statistical manual of mental disorders,* ed 4, Washington, DC, 1994, American Psychiatric Association.
2. Bagley SM: Nutritional needs of the acutely ill with acute wounds, *Crit Care Nurs Clin North Am* 8:150-167, 1996.
3. Bernstein NR, O'Connell K, Chedekel D: Patterns of burn adjustment, *J Burn Care Rehabil* 13:4-12, 1992.
4. Blumenfeld M, Schoeps MM: Psychological reactions. In Blumenfeld M, Schoeps MM, editors: *Psychological care of the burn and trauma patient,* Baltimore, 1993, Williams & Wilkins.

4a. Carrougher GJ: *Burn care and therapy,* St Louis, 1998, Mosby.

5. Committee on the Organization and Delivery of Burn Care: *Burn care resources in North America* 1996-1997, New York, 1996, American Burn Association.
6. Davis ST, Sheely-Adolphson P: Psychosocial interventions: pharmacologic and psychologic modalities, *Nurs Clin North Am* 32(2):331-342, June 1997.
7. Gamiel Z, DeBiasse MA, Demling RH: Essential microminerals and their response to burn injury, *J Burn Care Rehabil* 17:264-272, 1996.
8. Gordon M, Goodwin CW: Initial assessment, management, and stabilization, *Nurs Clin North Am* 32(2):237-249, 1997.
9. Greenfield E, McManus AT: Infectious complications: prevention and strategies for their control, *Nurs Clin North Am* 32(2):297-310, June 1997.
10. Hildreth M, Gottschlich M: Nutritional support in the burned patient. In Herndon DN, editor: *Total burn care,* London, 1996, WB Saunders.
11. Jordan BS, Harrington DT: Management of the burn wound, *Nurs Clin North Am* 32(2):252-274, 1997.
12. Kim MJ, Mc Farland GK, McLane AM: *Pocket guide to nursing diagnoses,* ed 7, St Louis, 1997, Mosby.
13. Klein DG, Fritsch DE, Amin SG: Wound infection following trauma and burn injuries, *Crit Care Nurs Clin North Am* 7:627-641, 1995.
14. Lillico S: *Burn awareness kit,* Encino, Calif, 1996, Burn Awareness Coalition.
15. Mertens DM, Jenkins ME, Warden GD: Outpatient burn management, *Nurs Clin North Am* 32(2):343-364, June 1997.
16. Molter NC: When is the burn injury healed? Psychosocial implications of care, *AACN Clin Issues Crit Care Nurs* 4:424-432, 1993.
17. Munster AM: The immunological response and strategies for intervention. In Herndon DN, editor: *Total burn care,* London, 1996, WB Saunders.
18. Nebraska Burn Institute: *Advanced burn life support,* Lincoln, Nebr, 1994, The Institute.
19. Pessina MA, Ellis SM: Rehabilitation, *Nurs Clin North Am* 32(2):365-374, June 1997.

20. Rodriguez DJ: Nutrition in patients with severe burns: state of the art, *J Burn Care Rehabil* 17:62-70, 1996.
21. US Department of Health and Human Services: *Healthy People 2000: national health promotion and disease prevention objectives*, Washington, DC, 1990, US Government Printing Office.
22. Warden GD: Fluid resuscitation and early management. In Herndon DN, editor: *Total burn care*, London, 1996, WB Saunders.
23. Winifree J, Barillo DJ: Nonthermal injuries, *Nurs Clin North Am* 32(2):275-296, June 1997.
24. Wolfe RR: Metabolic responses to burn injury, nutritional implications. In Herndon DN, editor: *Total burn care*, London, 1996, WB Saunders.

# chapter 65 ASSESSMENT OF THE Immune System

CAROL GREEN-NIGRO

**objectives** *After studying this chapter, the learner should be able to:*

1. Review the structure and function of the immune system.
2. Differentiate between natural and acquired immunity.
3. Discuss changes that occur within the immune system with normal aging.
4. Identify subjective and objective data relative to actual or potential alterations in immune functioning.
5. Describe common diagnostic tests used to identify immune alterations.
6. Explore nursing implications for immune-related diagnostic tests.

This chapter provides a brief overview of the structure and function of the immune system, essential components of natural and acquired immunity, related assessment data, and diagnostic tests of immune function. Immune alterations are presented in Chapters 66 and 67.

## ANATOMY AND PHYSIOLOGY

### REVIEW OF THE IMMUNE RESPONSE

The human organism exists in a world of potential biological insults. Fortunately, the body's immune system protects the body from biological insults by distinguishing "self" cells from "nonself" cells and destroying those substances that are not self. Nonself cells such as microorganisms, pollens, and foods are generally known as *antigens*. The unique network of specialized immune cells provides protection from antigens, disposes of cellular debris, destroys malignant cells, and neutralizes foreign substances. A unique property of the immune system is its ability to remember the identity of antigens so that when a second encounter occurs a swifter, more effective defense is evoked.

The immune system has two levels of defense: natural or nonspecific immunity and specific or acquired immunity. These basic responses are meshed together to give individuals their own unique immunological reaction to antigens. This variation in immunological response occurs because each person has a different genetic background, is exposed to different environmental conditions, and responds differently to antigen stimulation.[14]

The properties that make the immune system unique also make immune disorders difficult to diagnose and treat. How a person will respond to any new substance cannot be predicted, and the medical treatment itself may place the individual at risk for pathogenic invasion. It is important for nurses to understand the functions of the immune system and its relationship to health and disease to support appropriate immune responses, or intervene when the immune response is excessive.

The immune system is composed of specialized cells and organs located throughout the body. Primary immune organs, also known as *primary lymphoid organs,* include the bone marrow and thymus. Lymphocytes migrate to these organs where they mature. Lymphocytes that migrate to the thymus gland are called *T lymphocytes.* Those that migrate to the bone marrow are called *B lymphocytes.*

The lymph nodes, spleen, tonsils, appendix, and patches of specialized lymphoid tissues that lie beneath the mucous membrane layer of the respiratory, gastrointestinal, and genitourinary tracts are the *secondary lymphoid organs.* Lymph nodes are small, bean-shaped structures that occur along lymphatic vessels. Lymph nodes not only filter foreign substances from lymph, but also store macrophages and B cells that, when stimulated, can rapidly proliferate and differentiate into immunoglobulin producing cells (Figure 65-1).

The spleen lies inferiorly and posteriorly to the stomach in the upper left quadrant of the abdomen. The spleen is also a major storage depot for macrophages and lymphocytes, both of which can launch an immune response when stimulated by blood-borne antigens. The spleen is composed of two types of tissues: white pulp and red pulp. White pulp primarily contains B lymphocytes, which support immune surveillance and lymphocyte proliferation.

*Mucosa-associated lymphoid tissues* are patches of specialized cells similar to those found in the spleen. They block submucosal entry of antigens into the area where they are located, e.g., the respiratory, gastrointestinal, and gentiourinary tracts and skin. The tonsils, Peyer's patches, and appendix are known as *gut-associated lymphoid tissues.* The tonsils filter out air-borne and ingested antigens. The appendix and Peyer's patches specifically protect against alimentary antigens. Collectively, the lymphoid cells and organs act in concert to protect skin surfaces, mucous membranes, blood, lymph, and internal organs from foreign invasion.[15]

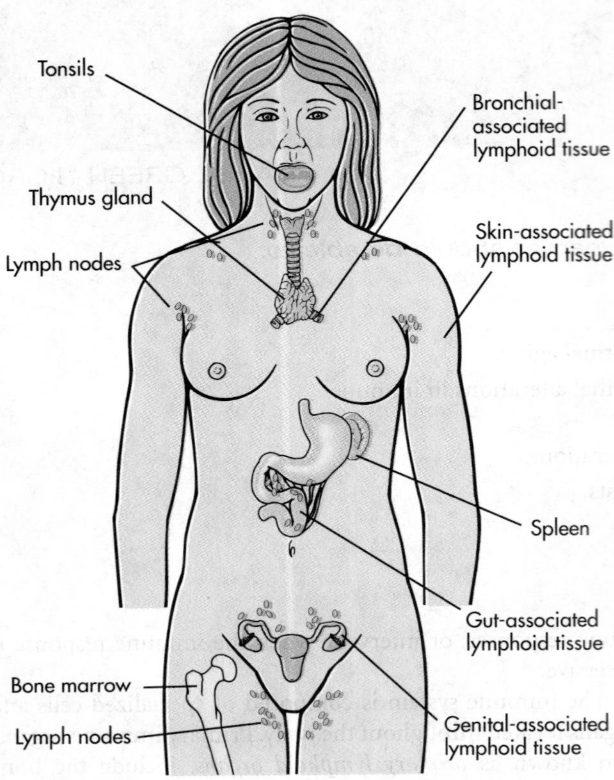


**fig. 65-1** Structures of the immune system.

## NATURAL AND ACQUIRED IMMUNITY

*Natural immunity* is nonspecific immunity, meaning that the reaction is always the same. Only the degree of response varies. Natural immunity is composed of anatomic and chemical barriers that nonspecifically recognize and respond to damaged self cells or foreign antigens. *Acquired immunity* begins after birth as the result of the immune system's response to repeated antigenic stimulation.

### Natural Immunity

The skin, mucous membranes, protective secretions, enzymes, phagocytic cells, and protective proteins provide the body with natural immunity. When intact, body surfaces such as the skin and mucous membranes provide the first line of defense from antigenic attack. Organs are structured to provide physical barriers against foreign invasion, and their surfaces have chemical barriers that prevent microbial growth. If antigens are successful in penetrating these barriers, a host of chemical substances within the body further impede their progress. Gastric acid and lysosomes (enzymes found in secretions throughout the body) are examples of chemical substances that attack foreign, or nonself, antigens.

Phagocytic cells, such as granulocytic white blood cells and macrophages, play a key role in natural immunity. In response to tissue injury or the presence of infectious microorganisms, chemotactic substances are carried via the blood to the bone marrow where phagocytic cells are formed and stored until they are needed. When signaled for release, the cells are drawn by chemotactic substances to the site of injury. They leave the blood vessels and move into the tissues where they engulf and destroy foreign, nonself materials.

A variety of proteins also play a role in natural immunity. They are released early in infection and help mediate the immune response. *Interferon*, a protein substance produced when cells are damaged by viruses, protects surrounding cells from invasion by the same virus. Interferon also increases the phagocytic ability of macrophages, which facilitates removal of the antigen. *Acute phase proteins* are another group of proteins that multiply during acute infections and promote initiation of the complement cascade (Figure 65-2).

### Acquired Immunity

Specific, acquired immunity recognizes and acts against very specific foreign antigens. An *antigenic determinant* is the part of an antigen molecule that can be recognized and bound by immune cells. Antigenic determinants elicit the formation and proliferation of reactive proteins (antibodies) and cells (cytoxic lymphocytes) that bind to the antigenic determinant to activate or destroy the antigen. Acquired immunity possesses memory, which allows the system to remember prior contact with antigenic material and respond faster and more efficiently to subsequent encounters with the same antigen. Acquired immunity consists of two functional components: a cell-mediated system that provides cytotoxic lymphocytes and a humoral-mediated system that provides circulating antibodies.

#### Cell-mediated acquired immunity

Some antigens, such as viruses and mycobacteria, are incapable of activating B lymphocytes to produce antibodies. It is therefore the responsibility of the T lymphocytes to provide protection against such antigens. T cell lymphocytes, responsible for cell-mediated or cellular immunity, make two important contributions to immune defense. They are vital to the coordination of cellular and humoral immunity and they directly attack antigens. T lymphocytes are produced in the bone marrow and mature in the thymus gland. From the thymus gland they migrate to regional lymph nodes and the spleen where they populate the medullary regions. Each mature immunosensitive T cell lymphocyte is capable of responding to a specific antigen. Upon exposure to its specific antigen, the T cell proliferates. Cells are shed into the circulation where they are transported throughout the body.

Several T cell lymphocyte subsets act to regulate T cell function and augment production of antibodies by B cells. *Helper/inducer T cells* ($T_H$ or $T_4$) are essential for activating other T lymphocyte cells, B lymphocyte cells, natural killer cells, and macrophages. Without the helper T cell, B cells are unable to make sufficient antibody against most invading antigens. *Cytotoxic T cells* ($T_c$) attack and destroy antigen or antigenically labeled cells on site. Specifically, they kill virus-infected cells, tumor cells, and foreign graft cells.[10] T cells known as *suppressor T cells* ($T_s$ or $T_8$) operate to prevent or

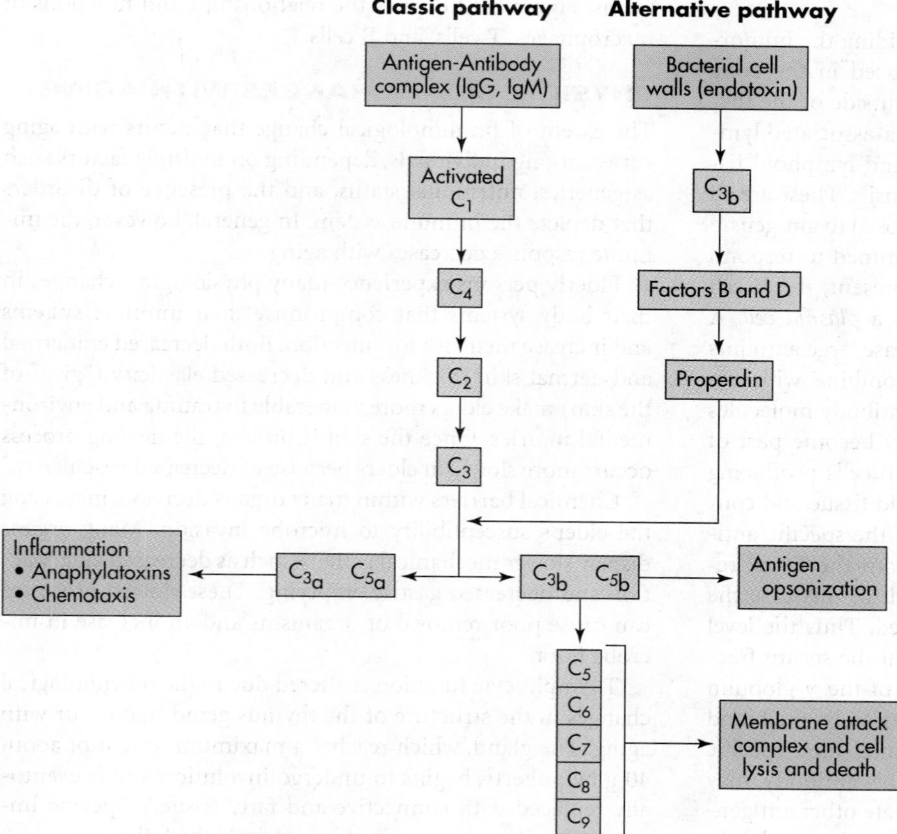


**fig. 65-2** Pathways of activation of the complement cascade. Complement components are cleaved into fragments (denoted by *lowercase letters*) during activation. Many of the fragments are biochemical mediators of inflammation. The classic pathway usually is activated by antigen-antibody complexes through component C1, whereas the alternative pathway is activated by many agents, such as bacterial polysaccharides, through component C3b.

modify the functions of the two systems. It is thought that they may turn off the specific immune reaction when it is no longer needed. *Delayed cells* ($T_d$) are involved in delayed hypersensitivity involving fungi and mycobacteria allergic responses.[15] The last subset of T lymphocytes is the *memory T cell* ($T_M$). They are named for their ability to remember contact with specific antigens and immediately respond upon subsequent exposure.

T lymphocyte cells work primarily by secreting potent chemical messengers known as *cytokines*, or specifically *lymphokines.* Lymphokines are soluble substances that recruit and activate nonspecifically reactive phagocytes, including components of the inflammatory response and lymphokine-activated killer cells.[10] T helper cells produce a lymphokine known as *interleukin-2 (IL-2)*, which stimulates the production of *natural killer (NK)* cells that target tumor cells and virally infected cells. NK cells are similar to the cytotoxic T cell subset, but do not need to recognize a specific antigen to attack. Once activated by IL-2, NK cells release potent chemicals that kill on contact.[11] Table 65-1 summarizes the functions of the various T lymphocytes.

**table 65-1** *Functions of Various T Lymphocytes*

| T Lymphocyte | Function(s) |
|---|---|
| T helper cell ($T_4$, $T_H$) | Release lymphokines that: Regulate antibody production by B cells; Activate other T cells; Activate macrophages; Activate natural killer cells |
| T suppressor cell ($T_8$, $T_S$) | Prevent or modify the functions of T cells and B cells; May suppress the immune reaction when no longer needed |
| Cytotoxic ($T_c$) cell | Kill virus infected cells, tumor cells, and foreign graft cells |
| Delayed ($T_d$) cell | Delayed hypersensitivity; Inflammatory response |
| T memory cell ($T_M$) | Induce secondary immune response |

### Humorally mediated immunity

*B cell lymphocytes,* the lymphocytes providing the humorally mediated immune response, are produced in the bone marrow and undergo maturation at a site outside of the thymus, such as in the bone marrow or mucosa-associated lymphoid tissues. They migrate to the spleen and lymphoid tissues located along the gut, bronchus, and tonsils. These are all strategic locations that are continuously exposed to antigens.[15]

The immunosensitive B cells are programmed to respond to a single antigen. When the antigen is present, the B cell begins to proliferate and differentiate into a *plasma cell.* A plasma cell is designed to synthesize and release large amounts of *immunoglobulin* (antibody) that will combine with the antigen that caused its production. These antibody molecules are released into the circulation where they become part of the γ-globulin fraction of the serum. The B cells producing the immunoglobulin remain in the lymphoid tissue and continue to synthesize additional molecules of the specific antibody. Note that this process is different from the T cell response where cytotoxic T cells are released; in this case the B cells remain, and their product is released. Thus the level of active specific antibodies begins to rise in the serum fraction *(antibody titer),* as well as in the level of the γ-globulin fraction in general. These antibodies are carried by the blood and other body fluids to where they encounter their specific antigen and bind to it. Upon binding, the antibody may inactivate the antigen, precipitate it, or activate other antigen-damaging processes (such as the complement cascade) to remove it.

The immunoglobulins are subdivided into different classes on the basis of molecular structure and function. The generic symbol for immunoglobulins is Ig, and each of the classes is designated by a letter of the alphabet: IgG, IgM, IgA, IgE, and IgD. The predominant immunoglobulin is IgG. Table 65-2 summarizes the characteristics of immunoglobulins.

The B cell system is similar to the T cell system in that it is controlled by helper and suppressor T cells, forms memory ($B_M$) cells, and is rendered self-tolerant by the same mechanisms. Figure 65-3 depicts the relationships and functions of macrophages, T cells, and B cells.

## PHYSIOLOGICAL CHANGES WITH AGING

The extent of immunological change that occurs with aging varies among individuals, depending on multiple factors such as genetics, nutritional status, and the presence of disorders that deplete the immune system. In general, however, the immune response decreases with aging.

Elderly persons experience many physiological changes in their body systems that compromise their immune systems and increase their risk for infection. Both decreased epidermal and dermal skin thickness and decreased elasticity ("give" of the skin) make elders more vulnerable to trauma and environmental injuries. Once the skin is broken, the healing process occurs more slowly in elders because of decreased vascularity.[2]

Chemical barriers within many organs decrease, increasing the elder's susceptibility to microbe invasion. Many organs display slower mechanical activity such as decreased ciliary action and decreased gastric emptying. These slowed processes can cause poor removal of organisms and an increase in microbe flora.

T lymphocyte function is altered due to the morphological changes in the structure of the thymus gland that occur with aging. The gland, which reaches a maximum weight of about 40 g by puberty, begins to undergo involution and is eventually replaced with connective and fatty tissue.[15] Specific immune response changes in elders include the following.

1. Decreased relative proportions of $CD_4$ and $CD_8$, which affect immune system regulation. This may explain why autoantibodies are increased in this age group.
2. Low rate of T lymphocyte proliferation in response to a stimulus, without an overall decrease in the number of T cells. This tends to cause elders to respond more slowly to allergic stimulants.
3. Cytotoxic (killer) T cells decrease in number; therefore the normal antigen specific cytotoxicity is diminished. This produces a reduced response to foreign material.

**table 65-2** *Characteristics of Immunoglobulins*

| Class | Relative Serum Concentration (%) | Location | Characteristics |
|---|---|---|---|
| IgG | 76 | Plasma, interstitial fluid | Is only immunoglobulin that crosses placenta<br>Fixes complement<br>Is responsible for secondary immune response |
| IgA | 15 | Body secretions, including tears, saliva, breast milk, colostrum | Lines mucous membranes and protects body surfaces |
| IgM | 8 | Plasma | Fixes complement<br>Is responsible for primary immune response<br>Provides specific antitoxin action when combined with IgG<br>Forms antibodies to ABO blood antigens |
| IgD | 1 | Plasma | Is present on lymphocyte surface<br>Assists in the differentiation of B lymphocytes |
| IgE | 0.002 | Plasma, interstitial fluids, exocrine secretions | Causes symptoms of allergic reactions<br>Fixes to mast cells and basophils<br>Assists in defense against parasitic infections |

From Lewis SM, Collier IC, Heitkemper MM: *Medical-surgical nursing: assessment and management of clinical problems,* ed 4, St Louis, 1996, Mosby.

4. Production of IL-2 by T helper cells is reduced. This further decreases the stimulation of the T lymphocytes and NK cells.
5. T cell function is reduced in response to certain viral antigens, allografts (transplants from other persons), and tumor cells.

B cell responsiveness also decreases, but is thought to be the result of a decline in helper T cell function.[15] Elders experience an increased frequency of bacterial infections possibly due to a defect in antibody function. The total immunoglobulin concentration is not changed with age, but there is an increase in the level of IgA and IgG antibodies.[15]

Elders experience multiple chronic illnesses, are hospitalized more frequently than younger persons, and undergo treatments that put them at risk for infection. Chronic illness may cause elders to be less mobile, and immobility, coupled with altered immune responses, increases the risk of complications such as pneumonia and skin breakdown.[18] Gerontological patient considerations for assessment are summarized in the accompanying box.

The end result of immune system changes in the elderly is an increased incidence of infections, increased number of tumors, and an increased incidence of autoimmune disorders.[18] Common infections tend to be more severe, with slower recovery and less probability of developing effective immunity after an infection.[17]

## SUBJECTIVE DATA

Persons at increased risk for infection (children, elderly, immunosuppressed, or immunodeficient) need to be identified so that preventive measures can be taken and early treatment

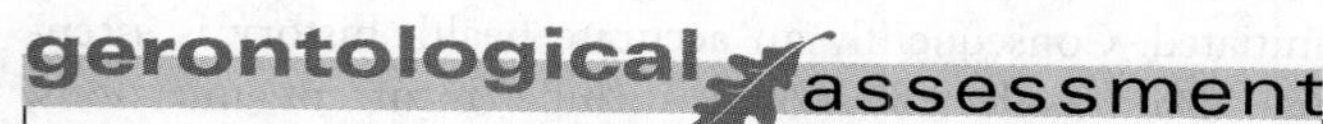

**gerontological assessment**

**ASSESSMENT**

Skin

Assessment for intact skin is very important. Decreased thickness, elasticity, and neurosensory function along with decreased awareness of injury makes aging skin more vulnerable to trauma. Torn skin provides an opening for microorganism invasion.

Respiratory

Elders are at high risk for respiratory infection due to decreased ciliary action, reduced respiratory muscle strength, and decreased gag and cough reflexes, which reduce their ability to expel inhaled organisms.

Cardiovascular

Cardiac output is decreased while peripheral resistance is increased in elders. These changes result in decreased circulation to the tissues, delay inflammation, and increase their risk for ischemic injury.

Gastrointestinal

Elders experience decreased gastric emptying and decreased secretion of HCl and selected dietary enzymes, resulting in less efficient digestion and decreased production of serum proteins.

Immune

Elders are at increased risk for infections because of the decreased number and size of lymph nodes.

**COMMON DISORDERS IN THE ELDERLY**

Infections, especially bacterial pneumonia, urinary tract infection, tetanus, herpes zoster
Malignancies
Autoimmune disorders
Malnutrition
Skin breakdown

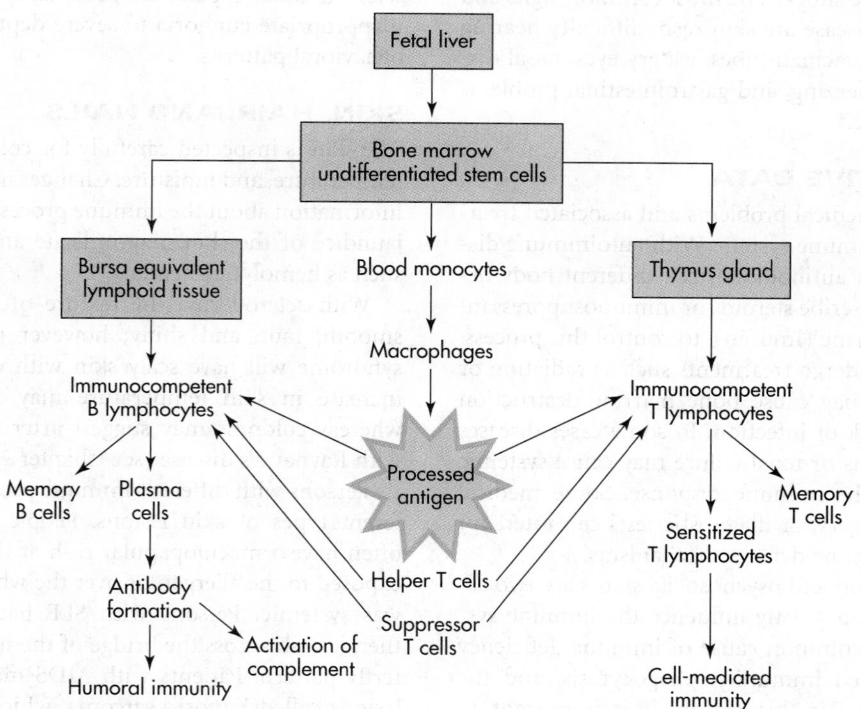


**fig. 65-3** Relationships and functions of macrophages, B lymphocytes, and T lymphocytes in an immune response.

initiated. Consequently an accurate health history is essential. Data collected should include recurrent infections, known allergies, history of autoimmune disorders, diet, and any therapy or environmental factors that may affect the immune system.

## INFECTION HISTORY

Recurrent infections can be a good indication that the immune system is compromised. Ask the patient what infections have occurred and when they occurred. Also investigate whether the patient has any insight into what might be causing these infections; this information provides data for future teaching, as well as assessment.

Fevers may occur with the inflammatory response, with an impaired immune system, or from rapid proliferation of white blood cells (WBCs).[12] The pattern of the fever can provide clues to the type of infective process involved. Data are collected about the fever onset, range and duration, and the presence of night sweats and chills. High fevers of 39° to 40° C may indicate serum sickness, whereas low-grade fevers may indicate allergies.[12] Fever may also be a sign of transplant rejection.

Enlarged lymph nodes usually accompany inflammation but may also be seen with Hodgkin's disease or non-Hodgkin's lymphoma, or they may be a sign of transplant rejection. Location of the enlarged nodes provides data about the source of the inflammation.

## ALLERGY HISTORY

Allergic symptoms are triggered by a variety of allergens; therefore data are collected regarding allergens such as food, contrast media, medications, or other substances. The reactions to particular allergens can vary from a slight rash to life-threatening anaphylactic shock. The most common signs and symptoms of allergic disease are skin rash, difficulty hearing from obstruction of eustachian tubes, watery eyes, nasal discharge, coughing or wheezing, and gastrointestinal problems such as diarrhea or colic.[4]

## OTHER SUBJECTIVE DATA

The patient's current medical problems and associated treatments can affect the immune system. With autoimmune diseases, the patient's own antibodies attack different body organs and physicians prescribe steroids or immunosuppressant drugs, such as azathioprine (Imuran), to control this process. Patients with cancer undergo treatments such as radiation or chemotherapy, which may cause bone marrow destruction leading to increased risk of infection. In some cases diseases such as diabetes mellitus or renal failure may cause systemic changes that depress the immune response. Some medical treatments, such as surgery, or diagnostic tests can interrupt the integrity of the immune defense mechanisms.

The patient's nutrition and psychosocial status are two aspects of lifestyle that can greatly influence the immune system. Malnutrition is a common cause of immune deficiency (defects in cell-mediated immunity, phagocytosis, and the complement system).[15] For this reason, it is important to collect data about nutritional habits. Explore with patients their usual eating habits and present appetite. Stress can compromise immune functioning by increased release of cortisol. If the patient has experienced recent stressors, it is important to investigate this more completely. How has the patient coped with this stressor and how has it changed relationships with others? Does the person possess any of the risk factors for human immunodeficiency virus (HIV) infection (history of blood transfusions, illicit drug use, high-risk occupations such as nursing and medical technology, homosexuality, unprotected sexual intercourse, or multiple sexual partners)?

An environmental assessment can help identify factors in the patient's environment that might be causing allergies. Common allergens include animal dander, house dust, mold, and mites located in homes and chemicals or items used in the home, work, or with hobbies. Data about potential allergens will help to identify sources that may be controlled.

# OBJECTIVE DATA

Disorders of the immune system are more difficult to assess objectively because of less obvious physical markers. However, observations can be made about the person's general behavior, as well as about the skin, lymph nodes, lungs, ears, eyes, nose, throat, and other body systems, that may suggest immune dysfunction.

## PATIENT BEHAVIOR

The inflammation and cellular destruction that can occur with many immune disorders can cause problems in cognition, which in some diseases, such as acquired immunodeficiency syndrome (AIDS) and systemic lupus erythematosus (SLE), may develop into dementia. Patients with multiple sclerosis often experience personality changes, varying from inappropriate euphoria to severe depression, which can alter behavioral patterns.

## SKIN, HAIR, AND NAILS

The skin is inspected carefully for color, skin turgor, texture, temperature, and moisture. Changes in skin color can provide information about the immune process involved; for example, jaundice of the skin may indicate an autoimmune disorder such as hemolytic anemia.

With scleroderma the texture of the skin is very thick, smooth, taut, and shiny; however patients with Sjögren's syndrome will have scaly skin with decreased sweating. An increase in skin temperature may indicate inflammation, whereas coldness may suggest arterial insufficiency as seen with Raynaud's disease (see Chapter 27).

Persons with different immune problems demonstrate different types of skin lesions. People with allergic reactions often have a maculopapular rash at the site where they were exposed to the allergen or over the whole body if the allergen was systemic. Persons with SLE have a characteristic erythemic rash across the bridge of the nose and cheek in a butterfly pattern. Patients with AIDS may have malignant skin lesions called Kaposi's sarcoma, which are typically maculopapular and range in color from pink to bluish-purple (see

Chapter 67). Patients with rheumatoid arthritis experience bony spurs located primarily over the knuckles and finger joints (see Chapter 61).

Some autoimmune processes will cause notable patches of alopecia or dry, brittle. and broken hair. The nails show changes in color, configuration, or brittleness.

## EARS, EYES, NOSE, AND THROAT

The physical assessment of the ears of patients with allergies may reveal serous otitis media with retracted tympanic membranes, indicating obstruction of the eustachian tubes and fluid collection within the ear. The patient may be noted to repeat questions many times because of difficulty with hearing.

Periorbital edema may be seen in certain autoimmune disorders or hypersensitivity reactions. Dark circles, referred to as "allergic shiner," may be noted under the eyes of allergy patients because of chronic nasal obstruction resulting in venous stasis.[4] Changes in the conjunctiva, such as discoloration and vascular hemorrhage, can be caused by certain autoimmune disorders.

Nasal obstruction may cause the patient to breathe through the mouth, and the voice will have a nasal tone. Examination of the mouth and throat will identify any lesions in the mucous membrane or changes in mucosal color. Many autoimmune disorders cause oral lesions, and immunosuppressed patients may experience thrush, a white exudate that occurs over the tongue and mucous membranes.

## LYMPH NODES

Assessment of the lymph nodes includes inspection, as well as palpation, beginning at the neck and extending to the entire body. The location, size, surface characteristics, consistency, symmetry, mobility, and discomfort with palpation of the lymph nodes are documented. Inflamed, tender, or fixed nodes indicate the need for further investigation, and their location will help to identify the possible source of infection by the pattern of node involvement and usual drainage route (Figures 65-4 and 65-5).

## RESPIRATORY SYSTEM

Because persons with allergies typically show respiratory symptoms and immunosuppressed patients are particularly prone to pneumonias, it is critical that a complete respiratory assessment be made. Special attention is made to cough pattern, sputum color, skin color, the work of breathing, and lung sounds. Patients with pneumonia will display tachypnea and thick yellow or green sputum and use accessory muscles

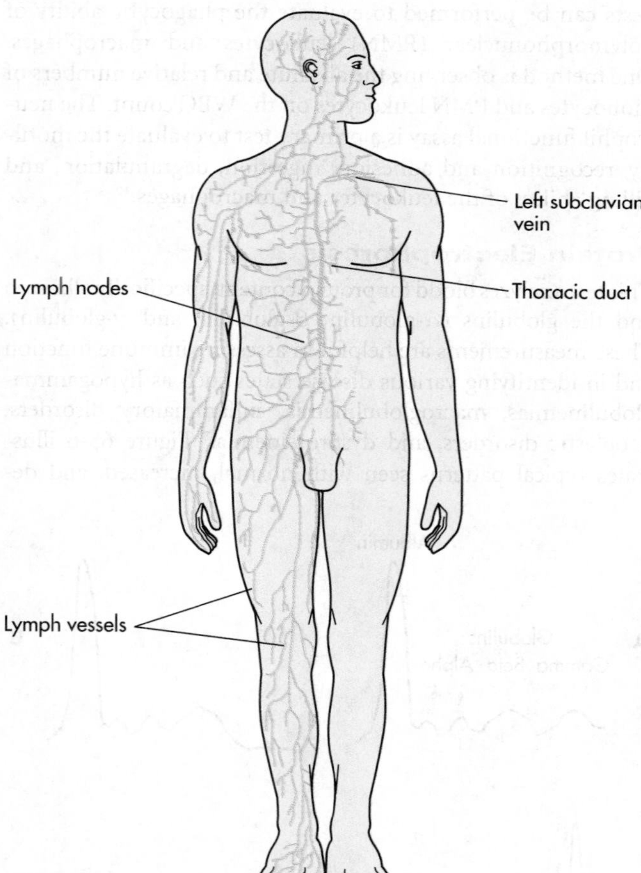


**fig. 65-4** The lymphatic system. Lymph nodes are found at junctures of lymphatic vessels and form a complete network, draining and filtering lymph derived from the tissue spaces. They are either superficial or visceral, draining the skin or deep tissues and internal organs of the body. The lymph eventually reaches the thoracic duct, which drains into the left subclavian vein and thus back into the circulation.

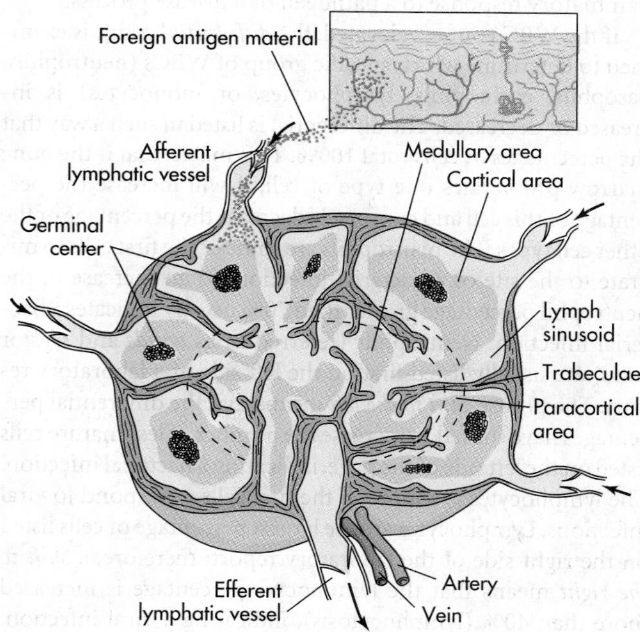


**fig. 65-5** Structure of a lymph node. Lymph nodes are organized into three main areas: the outer cortex, where B cells proliferate and mature; the deeper paracortex, populated mainly by macrophages and T cells; and the inner medulla, containing both B cells and T cells. Macrophages, B cells, and T cells interact with each other, often in the presence of antigen percolating through the node, resulting in the inductive phase of the immune response.

to breathe. Allergic patients will typically wheeze and cough, but experience little or no dyspnea. An allergic cough characteristically is hacking and nonproductive.

## DIAGNOSTIC TESTS

Laboratory tests, skin tests, and biopsies are the main sources of diagnostic evaluation of the immune system.

### LABORATORY TESTS

Laboratory tests are used to assess the patient's immune status, identify the offending antigen, and monitor the effectiveness of treatment. The white blood cell count with differential, erythrocyte sedimentation rate, C-reactive protein, total complement activity test, and phagocytic cell function tests measure the natural, nonspecific inflammatory response and phagocytosis. Protein electrophoresis, immunoelectrophoresis, autoantibody tests, and antigen tests measure specific, acquired immune processes.

#### White Blood Cell Count with Differential

The WBC count with differential provides information about the type of infection and the body's response to it. Normally a healthy adult will have a WBC count between 5,000 and 10,000/cm$^3$; the healthy elder range is typically 3,000 to 9,000/cm$^3$. *Leukopenia,* a WBC count less than 5,000, often signifies a compromised inflammatory response or a viral infection. *Leukocytosis,* a WBC count greater than 10,000, indicates an inflammatory response to a pathogen or a disease process.[3]

If the WBC count is elevated, the *differential* count is examined to determine which specific group of WBCs (neutrophils, basophils, eosinophils, lymphocytes, or monocytes) is increased or decreased. The differential is listed in such a way that the percentages of cells total 100%. This means that if the bone marrow proliferates one type of cell, it will increase the percentage of this cell and conversely decrease the percentage of the other cell types. The neutrophils are some of the first cells to migrate to the site of a bacterial infection, so an increase in the neutrophil percentage greater than 70% usually indicates a bacterial infection. Neutrophils (referred to as *bands* and *segs* or *stabs*) are usually listed first on the left side of a laboratory report. The phrase *shift to the left* means that the differential percentages have shifted to increase the number of less mature cells listed on the left side of the page, indicating a bacterial infection. The lymphocytes are some of the first cells to respond to viral infections. Lymphocytes are the largest percentage of cells listed on the right side of the laboratory report; therefore, a *shift to the right* means that the lymphocyte percentage is increased more than 40% (lymphocytosis), indicating a viral infection. An increase in eosinophils is associated with allergic disorders.[13]

#### Erythrocyte Sedimentation Rate (ESR)

The ESR or sed rate is the rate at which red blood cells (RBCs) settle and is expressed in millimeters/hour. An increased ESR indicates that there are increased globulins, fibrinogen, or other substances in the blood, which make it clump faster than normal, usually because of infection, malignancy, or collagen vascular disease.[3] The ESR is frequently higher in healthy elders.[1]

#### C-Reactive Protein (CRP)

CRP measures an abnormal protein found 18 to 24 hours after certain inflammatory processes. It is commonly used to distinguish inflammatory from noninflammatory diseases, such as osteoarthritis from rheumatoid arthritis. It is also used to monitor treatment effects of inflammatory diseases.[7]

#### Total Complement Activity ($CH_{50}$)

The $CH_{50}$ is a screening tool for the complement cascade. In healthy adults it ranges from 75 to 100 mg/dl. A positive test for CRP or an elevated $CH_{50}$ indicates the presence of inflammation, but does not identify the source. Healthy elders typically show higher values for these protein tests than younger adults.[1] Low values on the complement activity test indicate complement deficiency.

#### Phagocytic Cell Function Tests

Tests can be performed to evaluate the phagocytic ability of polymorphonuclear (PMN) leukocytes and macrophages. One method is observing the absolute and relative numbers of monocytes and PMN leukocytes on the WBC count. The neutrophil functional assay is a primary test to evaluate the motility, recognition and adhesion, ingestion, degranulation, and killing ability of the leukocytes and macrophages.[12]

#### Protein Electrophoresis

This test analyzes blood for protein content, specifically albumin and the globulins ($\alpha$-globulin, $\beta$-globulin, and $\gamma$-globulin). These measurements are helpful in assessing immune function and in identifying various disease states such as hypogammaglobulinemias, macroglobulinemia, inflammatory disorders, neoplastic disorders, and dysproteinemia.[3] Figure 65-6 illustrates typical patterns seen with normal, increased, and de-

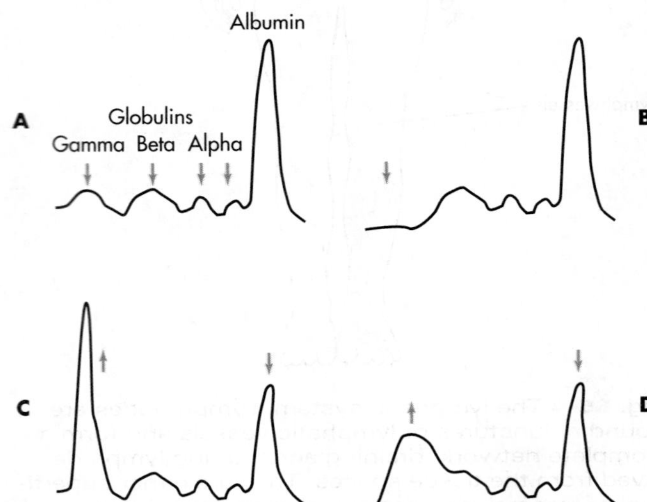


**fig. 65-6** Electrophoretic patterns. **A,** Normal. **B,** Hypogammaglobulinemia. **C,** Monoclonal gammopathy. **D,** Polyclonal gammopathy.

creased immunoglobulin levels. Immunoglobulins can be either increased or decreased when immune disorders are present.

### Immunoelectrophoresis

Immunoelectrophoresis separates serum electrophoretically and then tests for reaction with IgG, IgA, or IgM antisera. It is used to help differentiate between various immunological disorders. The test shows relative but imprecise quantities of immunoglobulins. IgG, IgA, and IgM can be measured quantitatively via an agar plate impregnated with antisera specific to the immunoglobulin. The immunoglobulin, placed in the center of the agar plate, diffuses rapidly forming a visible precipitate ring. The smaller the precipitate ring, the smaller the concentration of immunoglobulin. The ring diameter is compared to a standard measure to determine the immunoglobulin level. Normal adult IgG levels are 600 to 1800 mg/dl; IgA levels are 100 to 400 mg/dl; and IgM levels are 60 to 150 mg/dl. Nephelometry is another rapid yet accurate quantitative measurement of IgG, IgM, and IgA. The specific antibody is introduced into a fluid containing the specific antigen. The interaction of the antigen and antibody makes the fluid turbid; the degree of turbidity is measured by a photometric instrument. IgD and IgE immunoglobulins are generally present in amounts too small to measure. Table 65-3 presents a summary of the clinical significance of altered levels of immunoglobulins.

### Radioallergosorbent Test (RAST)

This test is a quantitative evaluation of IgE. Studies have shown that results of the RAST correlate well with skin testing for allergies. This form of testing is very expensive, but it is useful in patients taking antihistamines that suppress skin reaction or in patients with skin diseases.[7]

### Antibody Screening Tests

Numerous tests are available to detect antibodies formed against specific bacteria, viruses, fungi, or parasites. The *enzyme-linked immunosorbent assay* (ELISA) is used to detect antibodies to HIV. Because the ELISA can give false-positive results, a positive test is followed by a Western blot test. The Western blot identifies specific antibodies toward various fragments of the HIV and definitely confirms the presence of the virus. Antibody screening tests confirm the presence of antibodies toward a particular antigenic source but do *not* necessarily mean that the person has the disease. Test results can be influenced by medications, infections, or chronic diseases.

### Autoantibody Tests

Abnormal antibodies that the body produces against itself are termed *autoantibodies*. Autoantibodies injure self tissues and produce the symptoms associated with autoimmune conditions. Several tests are useful in confirming the presence of autoantibodies. *Rheumatoid factor (RF)* is an abnormal protein consisting of IgM antibodies found in the serum of persons with rheumatoid arthritis and other autoimmune diseases. *Antinuclear antibodies (ANAs)* or anti-DNA antibodies are γ-globulins formed against properties of the cell nucleus. Tests for ANAs are positive in a large number of patients with autoimmune disorders such as SLE. Healthy elders have increased antibodies (ANAs and RF), but the clinical relevance of these increases is unclear.[1,14]

**table 65-3** *Summary of the Clinical Significance of Altered Levels of Immunoglobulin*

| Class of Immunoglobulin | Increased Level | Decreased Level |
|---|---|---|
| IgG | IgG myeloma bacterial infections, hepatitis A, glomerulonephritis, rheumatoid arthritis, SLE, AIDS | Agammaglobulinemia, IgA myeloma, IgA deficiency, chronic lymphocytic leukemia, type I dysgammaglobulinemia, lymphoid aplasia, combined immunodeficiency, common variable immunodeficiency, X-linked hypogammaglobulinemia |
| IgM | Hepatitis A and B, Waldenström's macroglobulinemia, trypanosomiasis, chronic infections, type I dysgammaglobulinemia, hepatitis, SLE, rheumatoid arthritis, Sjögren's syndrome, AIDS | Lymphoid aplasia, hypogammaglobulinemia, chronic lymphocytic leukemia, IgG myeloma, IgA myeloma, agammaglobulinemia |
| IgA | SLE, rheumatoid arthritis, IgA myeloma, glomerulonephritis, chronic liver disease | Ataxia, telangiectasia, hypogammaglobulinemia, acute and chronic lymphocytic leukemia, IgA deficiency, combined immunodeficiency, common variable immunodeficiency, X-linked hypogammaglobulinemia, agammaglobulinemia, IgG myeloma, chronic infections (especially upper respiratory type) |
| IgE | Atopic disorders: allergic rhinitis, allergic asthma, atopic dermatitis, Wiskott-Aldrich syndrome with eczema, parasitic infestation, hyperimmunoglobulin E | Associated with IgA deficiency, intrinsic (nonallergic) asthma |
| IgD | Eczema, skin disorders | Unknown |

From Mudge-Grout CL: *Immunologic disorders,* St Louis, 1993, Mosby.

### Antigen Tests

Laboratory tests are used to isolate specific serum antigens. Some tests recognize the presence of invading antigens. For example, a positive result for $HB_SAG$ indicates the presence of the hepatitis B surface antigen, a specific antigenic determinant of the hepatitis B virus. Other tests isolate the antigenic properties of the antibodies toward RBCs. The indirect Coomb's test indicates serum antibodies to RBCs, which are not connected to the cell. It can be used to identify the patient's Rh factor. ABO and Rh typing are used to help determine blood type compatibility, and thereby reduce the possibility of transfusion reactions. The direct Coomb's test detects antibodies coating the RBCs that are not detected by ABO typing. A positive test facilitates diagnosing hemolytic disease and autoimmune disorders.[12]

The LE cell test is used to help confirm the diagnosis of systemic lupus erythematosus, a classic autoimmune disorder. LE cells are neutrophils that contain large groups of abnormal DNA in their cytoplasms and are seen in 70% to 80% of SLE patients. *Cryoglobulins* are abnormal serum proteins that precipitate at low temperatures, subsequently causing the affected person to experience increased sensitivity to cold. The presence of these proteins in the serum is associated with immune system disorders.[12]

Certain subsets of T lymphocyte cells called *clusters of differentiation* (CD) provide the clinician with information about the extent of immunodeficiency present in patients with AIDS. When the $CD_4$ levels fall below certain parameters, immunorestorative therapy is initiated. Infection and autoimmune disorders can also result in reduced $CD_4$ levels. Other T cell subsets are used to detect T cell leukemias, T cell lymphoma, or B cell tumors.[12]

## SPECIAL TESTS

### Biopsy

A lymph node biopsy may be performed in patients with lymphadenopathy to determine whether inflammation or malignancy is present. A synovial biopsy may be performed to obtain synovial fluid from a joint to differentiate among various types of arthritis or bone malignancies.

The nurse's role in a biopsy includes teaching the patient about the procedure and assisting the physician during the procedure. Most biopsies are completed under local anesthetic in an ambulatory setting. After anesthesia is effective, the patient should perceive only a pressure sensation; pain generally indicates insufficient anesthesia. After biopsy, the area is covered with a bandage, and the patient is instructed to monitor for bleeding and infection. Postbiopsy discomfort can be relieved by analgesics.

### Skin Tests

Skin tests are a simple, relatively painless, and inexpensive means to diagnose particular IgE-mediated allergies. The suspected allergen can be delivered by intradermal injection, or a scratch, prick, or puncture of the skin. Skin tests are influenced by skin reactivity to the allergen, amount of allergen administered, and degree of host mast cell sensitivity. Elderly persons tend to have a poorer response to skin testing due to changes in their mast cell reactivity.[10] Although intradermal skin tests are the most sensitive, they can also produce a systemic reaction, anaphylaxis, or a false-positive reaction. The scratch test is difficult to standardize and has the highest probability of producing a systemic reaction, anaphylaxis, or a false-positive reaction. The prick test enables more substances to be tested at one time than other methods, but bleeding can cause false-positive results. Closely placed sites can also interfere with accurate interpretation of results. The puncture method is used more than the other skin testing methods because of greater reliability, safer administration, and easier use with children.

### Anergy Tests

Skin testing may also be used to screen patients for T cell immunodeficiency. Specific antigens, including purified protein derivative, *Candida,* mumps antigen, streptokinase-streptodornase, coccidiodin, histoplasmin, and trichophyton, are injected intradermally. Reactions are read at 24-, 48-, and 72-hour intervals. The reactions determine *hypersensitivity,* not the presence of disease. More than 90% of healthy persons will show a response to one of these antigens within 48 hours.[12] Areas of induration are carefully measured with a ruler. Indurations of 5 mm or greater are recorded as positive. A person who does not react to any of these antigens is said to be anergic. Anergy is associated with immunodeficiency disorders.

Nurses frequently administer skin tests. The correct amount of allergen must be administered by the correct method to ensure patient safety and test reliability. Emergency equipment should be available before skin tests are administered because of the risk of anaphylaxis, and the patient should be monitored for at least 30 minutes after allergen administration.

## NURSING IMPLICATIONS FOR LABORATORY TESTING

Many of the tests presented in this chapter require little nursing intervention to prepare the patient for the test. Additionally, they require little or no observation after the test. Even so, a clear understanding of the various tests will allow the nurse to conduct routine teaching and answer patient questions accurately.

## chapter SUMMARY

### ANATOMY AND PHYSIOLOGY

- The protective mechanisms of the body may be natural, nonspecific (anatomic and chemical barriers, complement, phagocytes, or acute phase proteins) or acquired, specific (T cell or B cell lymphocytes).
- Immunological responses generally decrease with aging, leading to increased incidence of infection. The elderly are also admitted to the hospital for longer time periods and undergo more invasive procedures than younger persons.

### SUBJECTIVE DATA

- Nursing assessment includes comprehensive subjective data obtained from a thorough history of infections, allergies, and current health problems.

### OBJECTIVE DATA

- Objective data are not as obvious in immunological disorders but include general behavior, skin, ears, eye, nose and throat, and lymph node assessment.

### DIAGNOSTIC TESTS

- Laboratory tests, skin tests, and biopsies provide important data to identify the type of immune process or immune dysfunction.
- Laboratory tests include those that test the natural, nonspecific immune functioning (WBC count with differential, ESR, CRP, $CH_{50}$, and phagocytic cell functioning) and acquired immune functioning (qualitative and quantitative evaluation of immunoglobulins and antibody and antigen tests).
- Skin testing can aid in recognition of anergic and allergic persons.
- Nurses perform many skin tests.
- Lymph node biopsies are performed to diagnose inflammation and malignancy.

## References


1. Cavalieri TA, Chopra A, Bryman P: When outside the norm is normal: interpreting lab data in the aged, *Geriatrics* 45(5):66-70, 1992.
2. Fenske NA, Lober CW: Skin changes of aging: pathological implications, *Geriatrics* 45(3):27-35, 1990.
3. Fischbach F: *Common laboratory and diagnostic tests,* Philadelphia, 1995, JB Lippincott.
4. Gibbs L: Assessment and management of allergic patients, *ORL-Head Neck Nurs* 10(3):10-16, 1992.
5. Huether SE, McCance KL: *Understanding pathophysiology,* St Louis, 1996, Mosby.
6. Korenblat PE, Wedner HJ: *Allergy theory and practice,* ed 2, Philadelphia, 1991, WB Saunders.
7. Kushner I: C-reactive protein and the acute-phase response, *Hosp Pract* 25(3H):13-28, 1990.
8. Lewis SM, Collier IC, Heitkemper MM: *Medical-surgical nursing: assessment and management of clinical problems,* ed 4, St Louis, 1996, Mosby.
9. Lockey RF: Future trends in allergy and immunology, *JAMA* 268(20):2991-2992, 1992.
10. McCance KL, Huether SE: *Pathophysiology: the biologic basis for disease in adults and children,* ed 3, St Louis, 1998, Mosby.
11. McKenry LM, Salerno E: *Mosby's pharmacology in nursing,* ed 20, St Louis, 1998, Mosby.
12. Mudge-Grout CL: *Immunologic disorders,* St Louis, 1993, Mosby.
13. Pagana KD, Pagana TJ: *Diagnostic and laboratory test reference,* St Louis, 1997, Mosby.
14. Patterson R et al: *Allergic diseases,* Philadelphia, 1993, JB Lippincott.
15. Price S, Wilson L: *Pathophysiology,* ed 5, St Louis, 1997, Mosby.
16. Roitt IM, Brostoff J, Male DK: *Immunology,* ed 4, St Louis, 1996, Mosby.
17. Stanley M, Beare P: *Gerontological nursing,* Philadelphia, 1995, FA Davis.
18. US Department of Health and Human Services: *Health: United States 1991 and prevention profile,* Pub No (PHS) 92-1232, US Department of Health and Human Services, 1991, Hyattsville, Md.

# chapter 66 MANAGEMENT OF PERSONS WITH Problems of the Immune System

CAROL GREEN-NIGRO

## objectives

*After studying this chapter, the learner should be able to:*

1. Compare primary and secondary immunodeficiency disorders.
2. Develop a nursing care plan for the patient with an immunodeficiency disorder, addressing physical, psychosocial, and educational needs.
3. Describe the pathophysiological changes that occur in a patient with monoclonal and polyclonal gammopathies.
4. Discuss nursing problems and interventions necessary for a patient experiencing multiple myeloma.
5. Examine the differences in immunological reactions that occur between the four classifications of hypersensitivity disorders.
6. Delineate the nursing interventions that are imperative to prevent a hypersensitivity reaction.
7. Formulate a nursing care plan that includes discharge teaching for a patient with a type I hypersensitivity disorder.
8. Explain the pathophysiological factors involved in immunological blood reactions.
9. Depict the role of the nurse caring for patients with serum sickness.
10. List three examples of type IV hypersensitivity reactions.
11. Outline the possible etiologies of autoimmune disease.
12. Describe nursing management for the person with chronic fatigue syndrome.

In the normal healthy individual the immune response is a protective one. That protection, however, depends on an intact immune system. Four primary aberrations in immunity can lead to disease: (1) Deficiency of one or more immune components results in immunodeficiency; (2) an abnormal production of antibodies is known as gammopathy; (3) an exaggerated or inappropriate immune response manifests as hypersensitivity; and (4) an immunological attack on host cells is known as autoimmunity. These four immune disorders serve as the basis of organization for this chapter.

## IMMUNODEFICIENCIES

The four components of the immune system—antibody-mediated (B cell) immunity, cell-mediated (T cell) immunity, phagocytosis, and complement—act together and independently to protect the individual from infection and disease. Immunodeficiency, whether primary (congenital) or secondary (acquired), produces chronic or recurrent infections that can lead to death.

### ETIOLOGY/EPIDEMIOLOGY

Primary immunodeficiencies are rare congenital disorders that occur naturally from defects of the immune system. They are seen mostly in infants and young children. For instance, agammaglobulinemia occurs in 1:50,000 people, and severe combined immunodeficiency disorders occur in 1:100,000 to 1:500,000 live births. Chromosomal abnormalities have been noted in some primary immunodeficiency disorders, but despite modern medical advances in understanding the immune system, the biological errors of most primary immunodeficiencies remain unknown.[4]

The most common immunodeficiencies are secondary or acquired. Any factor that interferes with the normal growth or expression of the immune system can lead to a secondary immunodeficiency. Major contributing factors include age, nutrition, environmental chemicals, drugs that induce immunosuppression, and pathogens. Human immunodeficiency virus (HIV) causes a serious secondary immunodeficiency, acquired immunodeficiency syndrome (AIDS) (discussed in detail in Chapter 67). Specific conditions that can suppress immunity are presented in Table 66-1.

Many chemicals have immunosuppressive effects in exposed humans. T lymphocytes seem to be affected more severely than other immune cells. Examples of potentially damaging environmental chemicals are asbestos, dioxin, insecticides, and heavy metals.[5] Much is unknown in this area, including the effect of chemical exposure when coupled with the aging process.

Generalized immunosuppression can be artificially induced to decrease unwanted immune reactions, such as those related to hypersensitivity reactions, autoimmune diseases, neoplasia, or organ rejection.[8] Specific antigens can be administered to a hypersensitive person in small amounts over time. The antigenic stimulation forms circulating antibodies (immunoglobulins [Ig]) of the IgG class that combine with

**table 66-1** *Conditions That Can Suppress Immunity*

| CONDITION | EFFECT ON IMMUNE SYSTEM |
|---|---|
| Nephrotic syndrome<br>Burns<br>Protein-losing enteropathy | Loss of serum protein |
| Severe liver disease | Decreased protein synthesis |
| Cancer<br>Alcoholism<br>Malabsorption | Severe malnutrition; decreased protein synthesis |
| Uremia<br>Diabetes mellitus<br>Infections (especially viral)<br>Autoimmune disorders | Decreased T cell function |
| Lymphomas<br>Leukemias | Alterations in B cell and T cell numbers and function |

the antigen to block contact with immunocompetent cells or IgE-coated mast cells, thus suppressing the immune response. An adaptation of this method is used by allergists to desensitize persons allergic to specific antigens such as pollens.

A slightly different method involves administration of a specific antibody, which then combines with the antigen to block contact with the immunocompetent cell. This method has been used successfully in obstetrics to prevent the sensitive Rh-negative mother from responding to the Rh-positive fetus during pregnancy.

Antilymphocytic globulin (ALG) and antithymocytic globulin (ATG) are antisera prepared by isolating the active globulin fraction from the serum of horses, goats, or rabbits that have been immunized with human lymphocytes or thymocytes.[8] These antisera decrease all lymphocytes, although T cells are more affected than B cells. Because these globulins are xenogeneic (from another species), serum sickness may occur, and this limits their use to short-term therapy.

Monoclonal antibodies (MoAbs) also produce immunosuppression. They are derived from single cells and directed toward specific subpopulations of lymphocytes, such as helper T cells (muromonab-CD3).[8] Monoclonal antibodies are useful for cancer immunotherapy (see Chapter 11) and for reversing renal allograft rejection (see Chapter 68).

Irradiation is another method by which immune suppression can be achieved. Irradiation suppresses both primary and secondary immune responses, although primary suppression is more effective (see Chapter 11). Irradiation destroys lymphocytes, either directly or through depletion of precursor stem cells.

Drugs that are commonly employed for immunosuppression are described in Table 66-2 and in more detail in Chapter 68. Corticosteroids have both antiinflammatory and immunosuppressive effects. Therefore persons receiving corticosteroid therapy are highly susceptible to superimposed infections. If infections are present, their severity may increase despite the minimizing of symptoms caused by the antiinflammatory effects. Cyclosporine is a primary immunosuppressant used for organ transplantation. It acts by inhibiting helper T cells and facilitating development of suppressor T cells.

Cytotoxic drugs (such as alkylating agents, antifolates, and antimetabolites) have the potential to destroy any cell that is replicating; therefore immunosuppression occurs through the destruction of rapidly dividing, immunologically stimulated cells. Cytotoxic drugs act by interfering with the basic metabolic processes. B cell reduction is greater than T cell reduction.

## PATHOPHYSIOLOGY

Primary immunodeficiency disorders are characterized by a blockage of immunological cell development or function that results in B cell, T cell, complement, or phagocytic cell deficiency (Figure 66-1). Recurrent infections or infection treatment failures generally prompt the clinician to suspect the presence of immunodeficiency. Without treatment, most individuals suffering from these deficiencies will die of overwhelming infections early in life.[4]

Persons with B cell deficiencies have reduced circulating immunoglobulins, referred to as hypogammaglobulinemia. Severe disease produces agammaglobulinemia, totally or nearly absent immunoglobulins.[14] Individuals with B cell deficiencies are particularly susceptible to infections from pyrogenic bacteria, such as streptococci, staphylococci, *Pseudomonas,* and *Haemophilus influenzae,* and infections that affect the eyes, sinuses, ears, nose, and lungs.[18]

T cell deficiencies produce lymphopenia with greatly reduced T cell numbers and function. Patients are at increased risk for malignancies, viral infections (cytomegalovirus and herpes), fungal infections *(Candida),* protozoan infections *(Pneumocystis),* and mycobacterial infections.[10]

Patients who are both T cell and B cell deficient are at high risk for developing nearly every type of infection. Individuals with phagocytic disorders are at risk for developing mild to severe bacterial infections, whereas those with complement deficits have problems that range from recurrent infections to autoimmune diseases. Signs and symptoms depend on the site of infection and type of infecting organism. Table 66-3 presents a summary of primary immunodeficiencies.

## COLLABORATIVE CARE MANAGEMENT

The primary goals of collaborative management for patients with suspected immunodeficiency disorders are to (1) identify those at risk for the disorder, (2) prevent infection or effectively treat existing infections, and (3) replace missing humoral or cellular immunological factors.

Diagnostic tests for immunodeficiencies include complete blood count (CBC) with differential, erythrocyte sedimentation rate (ESR), antibody titers, absolute neutrophil counts, and $CH_{50}$. Fetoscopy and chromosome analysis have aided in the early detection of some of the primary immunodeficiencies. See Chapter 65 for a more detailed discussion of diagnostic tests for primary and secondary immunodeficiency states.

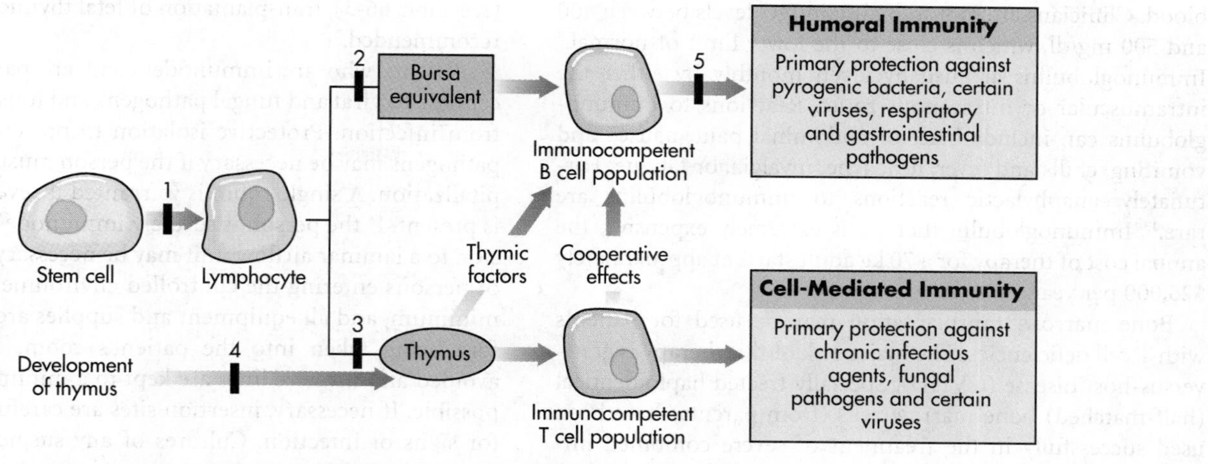

**fig. 66-1** Causes of immunodeficiencies. Abnormalities at *1* result in combined humoral and cell-mediated immunodeficiency. Blockage at *2* produces agammaglobulinemia. Blockage at *3* or *4* results in drastic reduction in T cell-mediated function and, because of cooperative effects on B cell system, some reduction in humoral response. Abnormalities in synthesis of specific immunoglobulin classes are reflected by blockage at *5*. Some blockages result in complete deficiency; others show up as reduction in response.

**table 66-2** *Major Immunosuppressive Drug Categories*

| Immunological Action | Indications for Use |
|---|---|
| **CORTICOSTEROIDS (e.g., Prednisone)** | |
| Inhibit T cell proliferation<br>Decrease interleukin-2 production<br>Decrease macrophage and neutrophil function<br>Inhibit T helper and T suppressor cell activity | Disease in which immune disorder is unknown<br>Autoimmune diseases (e.g., systemic lupus erythematosus)<br>Allergic disorders (e.g., asthma)<br>Transplant rejection (e.g., kidney transplant) |
| **CYTOTOXIC DRUGS** | |
| **Alkylating Agents (e.g., Cyclophosphamide)** | |
| Interfere with DNA, RNA, and protein synthesis<br>Lymphocytolytic<br>Depress B cell, macrophage, and monocyte function | Autoimmune diseases (e.g., systemic sclerosis)<br>Lymphomas<br>Leukemias<br>Granulomatous diseases (e.g., thyroiditis) |
| **Antimetabolites (e.g., Azathioprine)** | |
| Interfere with RNA, DNA, and protein synthesis<br>Depress bone marrow and antibody production<br>Depress T cell function | Autoimmune disease (e.g., multiple sclerosis, systemic lupus erythematosus)<br>Organ transplantation<br>Pemphigus (e.g., skin disease)<br>Neoplasia (e.g., cancers) |
| **Antifolates (e.g., Methotrexate)** | |
| Cause deficiency of folate coenzymes preventing synthesis of thymine and purines | Autoimmune disease (e.g., rheumatoid arthritis)<br>Neoplasia (e.g., cancers) |
| **TRANSPLANT IMMUNOSUPPRESSANTS (e.g., Cyclosporine, Sandimmune)** | |
| Inhibits helper T cell, lymphokine, and interleukin-2 production<br>Facilitates suppressor T cell development | Allograft rejection<br>Graft-versus-host disease |

Medications, either antibiotics or replacement of immunological factors, are the primary approach to treatment of all types of immunodeficiencies. Patients who already have infections are prescribed antibiotics and fungicides to treat the infecting organisms.

For patients with antibody deficiencies (hypogammaglobulinemia), immunoglobulin replacement therapy, which contains primarily IgG with small amounts of other antibodies, is a common form of treatment. The optimal dose of IgG is maintained by monitoring the trough levels of IgG in the blood. Clinicians attempt to maintain IgG levels between 400 and 500 mg/dl, which is close to the lower limit of normal.[5] Immunoglobulins are usually given monthly by either the intramuscular or intravenous route. Reactions to immunoglobulins can include back or abdominal pain, nausea and vomiting, chills and fever, headache, myalgia, or fatigue. Fortunately, anaphylactic reactions to immunoglobulins are rare.[13] Immunoglobulin therapy is extremely expensive; the annual cost of therapy for a 70 kg adult starts at approximately $25,000 per year.

Bone marrow transplantation may be used for patients with T cell deficiencies. The major risk of this therapy is graft-versus-host disease (GVHD). Specially treated haploidentical (half-matched) bone marrow cells (from parents) have been used successfully in the treatment of severe combined immunodeficiency disorder. In the case of DiGeorge syndrome (see Table 66-3), transplantation of fetal thymic tissue may be recommended.[2]

Patients who are immunodeficient are particularly susceptible to viral and fungal pathogens and must be protected from infection. Protective isolation to prevent exposure to pathogens may be necessary if the person must undergo hospitalization. A single room is warranted if severe leukopenia is present. If the person is severely immunodeficient, admission to a laminar airflow unit may be necessary. The number of persons entering the controlled environment is kept to a minimum, and all equipment and supplies are sterilized before being taken into the patient's room. Injections are avoided and invasive lines are kept to a minimum whenever possible. If necessary, insertion sites are carefully monitored for signs of infection. Cultures of any suspicious drainage are obtained.

**table 66-3** *Selected Primary Immunodeficiencies*

| Disorder | Basis of Deficiency |
|---|---|
| **B CELL DEFICIENCIES** | |
| Bruton's agammaglobulinemia | Sex-linked depression of all immunoglobulin classes. Failure of prelymphocytes to mature into B lymphocytes. All serum immunoglobulins are decreased. |
| Common variable immunodeficiency (CVID) | Variable degree of ability to synthesize primarily IgA or IgM in adults. High concentrations of autoantibodies and abnormal immunoglobulins. |
| Selective IgA deficiency | Total absence or severe deficiency of IgA. The B lymphocytes that normally produce IgA are unable to convert to IgA-producing plasma cells. |
| **T CELL DEFICIENCIES** | |
| DiGeorge syndrome (thymic hypoplasia) | Nongenetic failure of thymic development related to abnormal embryonic development of head and neck tissues and cells. Normal or increased serum immunoglobulins; decreased T cells. |
| **MIXED T CELL AND B CELL DEFICIENCIES** | |
| Severe combined immunodeficiency disease (SCID) | Defect in stem cell differentiation and maturation of T and B cells. T and B cells are decreased or absent. |
| Wiskott-Aldrich syndrome | Sex-linked IgM and T cell deficiency in males. Tendency toward bleeding because of low numbers of platelets. |
| Ataxia-telangiectasia | Autosomally recessive deficit in IgA and IgE. Decreased or normal T cells. |
| Nezelof syndrome | Congenital failure of embryonic thymic development. Normal or increased serum immunoglobulins. Lymphopenia. |
| **PHAGOCYTIC CELL DEFICIENCIES** | |
| Chronic granulomatous disease | Sex-linked genetic disease in males that results in failure to destroy phagocytized organisms and particles. |
| Chédiak-Higashi syndrome | Autosomal recessive disorder with abnormal granule formation, neutrophil chemotactic response, and intracellular killing of microorganisms. |
| **COMPLEMENT DEFICIENCIES** | |
| C1, C3, and C4 | Develop bacterial infections. More prone to autoimmune processes (systemic lupus erythematosus, glomerulonephritis, Sjögren's syndrome). |
| Hereditary angioedema | Autosomal dominant disorder associated with C1 inhibitor deficiency. Results in large amount of vasoactive peptides and increased vascular permeability. |

## PATIENT/FAMILY EDUCATION

Immunodeficient or immunosuppressed patients and their families need to know the nature of the immunodeficiency and how to avoid infection. Many patients do not require hospitalization, but they do need to be taught about infection control measures to follow at home. The nurse educates significant others about signs and symptoms of infection and what symptoms need to be reported to the clinician. People who have infections such as colds or chickenpox should be requested not to visit. The nurse teaches about the use of protective strategies such as hand washing, dietary precautions (e.g., thorough cooking of meat products), and washing of fruits and vegetables. Careful attention should be given to elders because they are already at a higher risk for infection from a decline in T cell function and overall decrease in immune response efficiency.[19] (See the accompanying Patient/Family Teaching Box.)

A balanced, nutritious diet is an important part of treatment for persons with immunodeficiency diseases. The diet should include all food groups, with adequate calories and protein to support tissue building. There are no specific activity restrictions; however, the nurse cautions patients about becoming overly tired. Patients with immunodeficiency disorders need to understand the importance of ongoing follow-up care. Referrals to community or home health nurses for continued assessment and treatment of infections may be necessary. Hospice care may be appropriate for patients with terminal primary or secondary immunodeficiency disorders.

**patient/family teaching**

**The Person with Immunodeficiency**

1. Nature of immunodeficiency (the inability of the body to adequately fight infection)
2. Measures to prevent infection
   a. Avoid persons with infections (especially colds)
   b. Avoid bumping or breaking the skin
   c. Inspect skin daily for lesions
   d. Eat a well-balanced diet with sufficient calories to maintain ideal weight
   e. Drink at least six glasses of fluid daily
   f. Avoid becoming overly fatigued
   g. Get a sufficient amount of sleep every night
   h. Avoid letting water stand unchanged around the house, such as in vases, to prevent bacterial growth
   i. Keep indoor pets clean
   j. Avoid placing fresh flowers or plants in bedroom
   k. Avoid using cold-mist humidifiers, to prevent infections from gram-negative bacteria
   l. Do not take routine immunizations or have immediate family take them
   m. Take prophylactic antibiotics before any manipulative or invasive procedure, such as dental work, biopsies, endoscopies, arteriograms
   n. Keep scheduled follow-up appointments with health care provider
3. Report signs of infection to health care provider immediately, including increased temperature, redness, or swelling of skin or mucous membranes; change in color of sputum; coughing; unusual drainage; diarrhea

# GAMMOPATHIES

Gammopathies, also termed *hypergammaglobulinemias,* are elevated levels of gamma globulin in serum resulting from its overproduction. The normal synthesis of an immunoglobulin is the result of the proliferation and plasma cell differentiation of a single clone of B cells in response to an antigenic signal. In gammopathies, a single clone or multiple clones of plasma cells begin to overproduce immunoglobulins.

Monoclonal gammopathies involve a single B cell clone with an electrophoretic pattern that is characterized by a single sharp peak in the gamma globulin region. Monoclonal gammopathies are commonly referred to as plasma cell dyscrasias. Multiple myeloma and macroglobulinemia are plasma cell dyscrasias that have distinctive clinical patterns. Multiple myeloma is discussed in the following section.

Polyclonal gammopathies involve the overproduction of virtually all classes of immunoglobulins in response to inappropriate antigenic stimulation. The electrophoretic pattern of polyclonal gammopathies is characterized by a diffuse increase in the gamma globulin curve. Polyclonal gammopathies are summarized in Table 66-4.

## MULTIPLE MYELOMA

### Etiology/Epidemiology

Multiple myeloma is the most serious and prevalent of the plasma cell dyscrasias. It affects approximately 28 of every 100,000 Americans each year.[1] The median age of onset is 60 years, and African Americans are affected twice as often as whites. The origin is unknown, but studies have shown associations with agricultural occupations and radiation or benzene exposure.[3]

**table 66-4** *Polyclonal Gammopathies (Hypergammaglobulinemia)*

| ETIOLOGIES | CHARACTERISTICS |
|---|---|
| Infectious diseases<br>Chronic bacterial infections (lung abscess and osteomyelitis) | Diffuse increase in antibody synthesis as a result of inappropriate antigen stimulation<br>IgG and IgM most commonly involved immunoglobulins |
| Connective tissue disease<br>Systemic lupus erythematosus<br>Rheumatoid arthritis<br>Chronic active liver disease | The immunoglobulin levels reflect the severity of disease<br>High levels of dysfunctional immunoglobulins depress the synthesis of normal immunoglobulins, leaving the person susceptible to infection |

## Pathophysiology

Multiple myeloma is a B cell cancer that originates in the bone marrow and moves out into the hard bone tissue, causing bone erosion. The disease is characterized by numerous malignant tumor masses located throughout the skeletal system, occasionally invading soft tissues.[12] The onset is slow and insidious, so symptoms may not develop until late in the disease. By the time of diagnosis, bone lesions are typically present in the skull, spine, and pelvis.

Diagnosis is based on computed tomography (CT) scans and radiography that show a "punched-out" type of bone lesion or generalized osteoporosis of the axial skeleton. Laboratory values may show increased serum calcium from bone demineralization and increased serum uric acid from protein breakdown. The CBC with differential shows anemia, leukopenia, and thrombocytopenia, depending on the amount of bone marrow involvement. The levels of normal immunoglobulins are decreased. The $B_2$ microglobulin test provides an estimate of tumor burden. Less than 0.6 trillion cells per square meter indicates low burden; greater than 1.2 trillion cells per square meter indicates high burden and advanced disease.[4] Twenty percent of patients have impaired renal function as a result of hypercalcemia and hyperuricemia. Box 66-1 summarizes the clinical manifestations of multiple myeloma.

## Collaborative Care Management

Glucocorticoids and calcitonin are used to reduce the lytic bone destruction and hypercalcemia. Oral melphalan combined with prednisone is the treatment of choice to reduce tumor load. Other chemotherapy agents such as vincristine sulfate and doxorubicin are used for patients with resistant tumors. The use of interferon-α between chemotherapy treatments has been shown to be of some value in prolonging remissions. Intensive chemotherapy supported with bone marrow transplant has resulted in remission for approximately 50% of patients with advanced disease.[1,2]

Bone plasmocytomas respond well to local radiation treatments. If the bone damage to the spine is extensive, orthopedic fixation devices may be used for stabilization and to prevent cord compression. If the patient has renal failure, dialysis may be necessary to correct the severe azotemia, hypercalcemia, and fluid overload.

**box 66-1** *clinical manifestations*

***Multiple Myeloma***

Frequent recurrent infections (especially respiratory)
Anemia, leukopenia, thrombocytopenia; abnormal immunoglobulin formation, depressed normal immunoglobulin formation
Skull, spine, and pelvis fractures
Spinal cord compression—paraplegia, quadraplegia
Hypercalcemia, hyperuricemia, renal insufficiency, renal failure

## Patient/Family Education

The major problems encountered by the patient with multiple myeloma are pathological fractures, fluid overload caused by kidney failure, and infection. Nursing interventions, therefore, are focused around three areas: safety during mobility, fluid balance, and infection prevention.

Patients with multiple myeloma have extremely fragile bones because of bone destruction by the plasmacytomas. Ambulation is encouraged to prevent further bone demineralization associated with immobility. Safety is of vital importance because of the risk of fractures; a fall could be disastrous. Skeletal pain may be a deterrent to ambulation; therefore a lightweight spinal brace, analgesics, and local radiotherapy are used to control the pain. The nurse encourages the family to remove throw rugs from the home to eliminate a potential source of falls. If the patient is completely immobile, careful turning is important. In late stages, even a tug on the arm or a turn toward the bed rail could cause a fracture. A lift sheet and the assistance of several people are necessary to facilitate moving the patient gently and safely.

Patients and families are taught that adequate hydration is necessary to prevent renal complications from the increased amounts of urates and calcium being excreted in the urine. Fluid intake needs to be sufficient to ensure a urinary output of a minimum of 1500 ml per 24 hours. If the patient is unable to maintain adequate fluid intake orally or requires nothing-by-mouth (NPO) status for diagnostic or surgical procedures, intravenous fluids are administered. The patient is weighed daily to assess for fluid retention. The nurse monitors the patient's blood urea nitrogen (BUN) and serum creatinine levels frequently to evaluate renal function.

The nurse instructs the patient and family about measures to prevent infection, including avoiding persons with infections. The patient is reminded to seek medical attention for any signs of impending infection. Frequent turning and deep breathing exercises are encouraged to prevent atelectasis and pneumonia. A Nursing Care Plan for a patient with multiple myeloma is found on p. 2165.

# HYPERSENSITIVITIES

The immune system is always ready to respond to foreign substances. Under certain circumstances, however, this response may harm as well as protect. Occasionally, re-exposure of a previously sensitized person to a specific antigen results in an exaggerated or inappropriate immune response that produces injury to local tissues or a dramatic systemic effect that can cause death. Such reactions are called hypersensitivity reactions, or allergies. The antigen producing the hypersensitivity reaction is referred to as an allergen. Whether an allergic response occurs and to what degree depends on a combination of interrelated factors that are summarized in Box 66-2, p. 2167.

Hypersensitivities can be divided broadly into two categories based on the components of the immune system involved in mediating the hypersensitivity reaction: humoral

## nursing care plan Person with Multiple Myeloma

**DATA** Mr. T. is a married, 66-year-old African-American farmer admitted for primary treatment of multiple myeloma. Mr. T. has worked on his family farm his entire adult life. He has been in excellent health until 2 years ago, when he began experiencing a series of bacterial infections. The multiple myeloma was diagnosed during a recent episode of pneumonia. He was immediately started on high-dose corticosteroid treatment, but his disease is believed to be fairly advanced and he has consented to aggressive treatment with chemotherapy plus radiotherapy to reduce the mass of the multiple bone tumors.

His nursing history also revealed the following:

- His wife is in failing health, and with no children in the area the couple is extremely concerned about losing the farm.
- Mr. T. has been experiencing severe fatigue over the last 9 months but has been reluctant to discuss this symptom with anyone. When directly asked, he admits to chronic bone pain in his lower back and pelvis.
- Mr. T. neither smokes nor drinks alcohol, and he and his wife have a strong religious faith, believing that "nothing happens for no reason."
- Mr. T. believes himself to be a strong person and is confident that he can regain his health and strength after treatment.

Admission diagnostic data include the following:

- CBC—Hgb 9.6 g; Hct 28%; WBC 6000
- Chemistry—serum calcium 12.1 mg/dl; creatinine 2.1 mg/dl; uric acid 10.0 mg/dl
- CT scan and x-rays show presence of multiple bone tumors and "punched-out" lesions, plus evidence of widespread osteoporosis

**NURSING DIAGNOSIS** *Chronic pain related to presence of bony tumors and osteoporosis*

| expected patient outcome | nursing interventions | rationale |
|---|---|---|
| States pain is controlled at manageable levels with pharmacological and nonpharmacological interventions. | **1.** Complete a thorough pain history, including the following:<br>**a.** Rating of severity, duration, frequency<br>**b.** Factors that exacerbate and relieve pain<br>**c.** Pain control strategies in use at home<br>**d.** Effects of pain on daily activities, appetite, sleep, mood, general coping<br>**e.** Knowledge of physiological basis for pain | **1.** Chronic pain is a complex challenge and usually requires a multifocal management plan. It is essential to fully understand the patient's situation before planning any interventions. |
| | **2.** Initiate referral to the pain management team. | **2.** Chronic pain is best managed by a multidisciplinary team of specialists who can explore the entire scope of management options for the patient. |
| | **3.** Administer NSAIDs as ordered, and encourage patient to use the medication on a consistent basis. | **3.** Chronic pain management is best achieved with constant blood levels of analgesics rather than peaks and valleys. |
| | **4.** Explore patient's preferences in terms of nonpharmacological pain management strategies, and encourage him to begin incorporating these strategies into his daily routines. | **4.** Nonpharmacological strategies work most effectively when patients are receptive to them. These strategies often require practice before they are fully effective. |
| | **5.** Explore effectiveness of heat/cold for pain relief. | **5.** Heat and cold are usually effective in reducing musculoskeletal types of pain. |

**NURSING DIAGNOSIS** *Risk for injury related to bone dimineralization*

| expected patient outcome | nursing interventions | rationale |
|---|---|---|
| Identifies injury risks in home environment and modifications that can be made to reduce these risks. | **1.** Ensure safety in hospital environment.<br>**a.** Ensure adequate lighting, and keep floor free of clutter.<br>**b.** Encourage patient to change positions slowly and avoid sudden, jarring movements.<br>**c.** Equip bed with firm mattress. | **1.** Hospital environment contains new surroundings that increase risk of falls and injury. Pathological fracture can occur from sudden movements when bone matrix is fragile. Firm mattress supports the skeleton and maintains vertebrae and joints in optimal position. |

*Continued*

## Person with Multiple Myeloma–cont'd

**NURSING DIAGNOSIS** *Risk for injury related to bone dimineralization—cont'd*

| expected patient outcome | nursing interventions | rationale |
|---|---|---|
| Accurately states the physiological nature of his disease-related risk for injury. | **2.** Explore home safety concerns with patient and wife, including equipment, rugs, polished floors. | **2.** Most falls and injuries occur at home. Most homes contain numerous hazards that can be prevented or lessened with minor adaptations. |
| | **3.** Explore use of light braces or other assistive devices. Consider adding nonslip pads and hand grips, particularly in the bathroom. | **3.** The use of supports can allow the patient to remain active yet reduce the risk of injury. |
| Maintains a high daily fluid intake to prevent kidney stone formation from excess calcium. | **4.** Encourage a daily fluid intake sufficient to ensure at least 1500 ml of urine output daily. Fluid intake of approximately 3000 ml per day is recommended. | **4.** Bone demineralization creates severe hypercalcemia. Adequate fluids are the best strategy for preventing the development of kidney stones. |

**NURSING DIAGNOSIS** *Fatigue related to inadequate tissue oxygenation*

| expected patient outcome | nursing interventions | rationale |
|---|---|---|
| Establishes priorities for daily activities; balances activity and rest effectively to complete desired daily activities | **1.** Discuss the severity of the fatigue and patient's understanding of the physiological cause. | **1.** Fatigue has been denied by the patient. Patients often consider fatigue to be a sign of weakness; physical basis for symptoms may not be clearly understood. |
| | **2.** Encourage patient to prioritize daily activities and "let go" of unessential tasks. | **2.** Fatigue compromises ability to participate in daily activities. It is important that the patient's available energy be used to complete priority activities. |
| | **3.** Explore strategies to:<br>**a.** Modify existing activities, conserving energy where possible<br>**b.** Seek assistance or delegate activities<br>**c.** Pace activities throughout the day to allow for periods of rest | **3.** Many daily activities can be modified to consume less energy, but this requires being willing to think about routine activities in different ways. Accepting the reality of fatigue may allow the patient to consider ways of seeking assistance or delegating activities that would not usually be considered acceptable. |

**NURSING DIAGNOSIS** *Risk for infection related to inadequate internal defenses*

| expected patient outcome | nursing interventions | rationale |
|---|---|---|
| Demonstrates knowledge of risk factors for infection in daily life; practices appropriate precautions to prevent infection. | **1.** Teach the importance of thorough, frequent hand washing. | **1.** Hand washing remains one of the most effective strategies to prevent infection. |
| | **2.** Limit visitors if needed; avoid contact with any person with active infection. | **2.** Patient may require assistance explaining the need to limit visitors to avoid infections. |
| | **3.** Monitor vital signs, and encourage patient to report the development of any signs of infection. | **3.** Overt symptoms of infection may be missing in immunocompromised individuals. |
| | **4.** Encourage frequent deep breathing, position changes, and routine hygiene. | **4.** Immobility in the hospitalized patient can quickly progress to respiratory infection. |
| | **5.** Encourage patient to limit contact with fresh plants and soil and to wash fresh fruits and vegetables thoroughly. Explore implications for home routines on the farm. | **5.** Normal pathogens in soil and on foods can be sources of infection in the immunocompromised patients. Farmers are at particular risk. |

**box 66-2** *Factors That Determine an Allergic Response*

1. *Responsiveness of the host to the allergen.* If the host is highly sensitive to the antigen, a greater than normal chance exists that a tissue-damaging reaction will occur.
2. *Amount of allergen.* Generally, the greater the amount of allergen contacted, the more severe the reaction.
3. *Nature of the allergen.* Any foreign protein or protein-containing component can serve as an allergen when coupled with a normal tissue protein carrier. Examples include pollens, foods, animal dander, house dust, and feathers.
4. *Route of entrance of the allergen.* Allergens may gain host entry via the respiratory tract, through epidermal or mucosal surfaces, by injection, or through the digestive tract.
5. *Timing of exposure to the allergen.* If the host's contacts with the allergen are widely separated by time, the immunological mediators may be so dilute that there is little response. Conversely, if frequent contact is made with the allergen, reactions are more likely to occur.
6. *Site of the allergen–immune mediator reaction.* A reaction can occur in the tissues with little consequence; however, the same reaction occurring in the bloodstream can lead to a severe reaction.
7. *Host's threshold of reactivity.* The host's immune system can be changed by factors such as stress, fatigue, or infection, all of which can decrease the responsiveness of the immune system to potential allergens.

response (B cell mediated) or cellular response (T cell mediated). This basic division corresponds with the older clinical symptom division of immediate and delayed, which described the timing of the appearance of clinical symptoms and the speed of skin test reactions when a host was challenged with various allergens.

Hypersensitivity reactions are generally classified into four types, as shown in Table 66-5. Type I, type II, and type III reactions are mediated by the humoral system, whereas type IV reactions are those of the cell-mediated system. Because type I, type II, and type III hypersensitivities are the result of interactions involving circulating antibodies, they can be transferred from a sensitized host to a nonsensitized host by serum transfer. Type IV sensitivities can be transferred by lymphocyte exchange only.

## TYPE I HYPERSENSITIVITIES

Type I hypersensitivity (anaphylactic) reactions include a wide variety of conditions. All of these diseases are characterized by a rapid and exaggerated response directed by IgE antibodies toward some external substance.

### Etiology

The tendency to become hypersensitive and produce IgE antibodies in response to an antigen is inherited as a dominant trait. This tendency is referred to as atopy. If both parents are atopic, there is a high probability that the children will be atopic. What an individual becomes hypersensitive to, however, is determined by the allergens to which that individual is exposed. A person does not inherit a specific allergy; the allergy manifests itself in response to the allergens to which the person is exposed. Allergic rhinitis, hay fever, asthma, atopic eczema (atopic dermatitis), venom hyperreactivity, and food allergy are examples of atopic diseases, which are often divided into two categories: seasonal and perennial. Seasonal allergens include pollens from trees, grasses, and weeds. Symptoms are produced when the person reacts to a brief tree season, followed by the grass and then weed season. Perennial allergens such as house dust, mites, molds, food, venom, and animal dander are present throughout the year, and the individual can experience symptoms at any time.

There are nonatopic disorders that are also mediated by IgE (e.g., urticaria/angioedema and systemic anaphylaxis). These disorders lack the genetic link or specific organ hyperresponsiveness displayed by atopic disease. The allergic form of urticaria is usually caused by foods, especially eggs, fish, and nuts, or by drugs such as penicillins, sulfonamides, cephalosporins, aspirin, and other nonsteroidal antiinflammatory drugs (NSAIDs). Angioedema is a form of urticaria, but it involves the subcutaneous tissue rather than the skin.

A more severe form of nonatopic reaction in humans is systemic anaphylaxis. Anaphylaxis is most often associated with drugs such as penicillin, streptokinase, and amphotericin B; insect or snake venoms; or foods, although almost any antigen to which the individual is hypersensitive has the potential for producing anaphylaxis.

### Epidemiology

Allergic disease can begin at any age, but the most common onset is from 2 to 15 years. Of the immediate hypersensitivity reactions, atopic disorders are most common. More than 15% of the population reacts to antigens that are not antigenic for the remainder of the population. Allergic diseases are estimated to account for approximately 10% of all patient visits to the primary care provider's office.[18] The occurrence of anaphylaxis (life-threatening hypersensitivity) is rare, occurring in approximately 0.4 cases per million a year in the general population. No association has been found between gender, race, or geographic area and an increased risk of developing anaphylaxis.

### Pathophysiology

Type I hypersensitivities are mediated by the IgE class of immunoglobulins. For type I reactions to occur, the individual must initially come into contact with the allergen that sensitizes the B lymphocytes to produce IgE antibodies. This primary contact is known as a sensitizing dose. The IgE antibodies, once produced, have a tendency to attach to the

**table 66-5** *Summary of Hypersensitivity Reactions*

| | Immune System Mediators | Allergens | Response to Intradermal Skin Test | Pathophysiological Effects | Examples |
|---|---|---|---|---|---|
| **HUMORAL (IMMEDIATE)** | | | | | |
| I—Anaphylactic | IgE bound to mast cells | Exogenous antigens | Wheal and flare within 30 min, edema | Release of histamines, kinins, chemotactic factors, and active products of arachidonic acid metabolism (leukotrienes, prostaglandins, and thromboxanes) from mast cells, which affect smooth muscle, mucous glands | Systemic anaphylaxis, atopic allergies, hay-fever, insect sting reactions |
| II—Cytotoxic | IgG or IgM (plus complement) | Foreign cells or alteration of cell surface antigens | Not done | Direct cytotoxic destruction of cells | Hemolytic disease of the newborn (Rh), transfusion reactions |
| III—Immune complex | IgG or IgM (plus complement) | Soluble antigens | Erythema and edema within 3-8 hr | Acute inflammatory reaction; primarily polymorphonuclear neutrophil leukocytes | Serum sickness, Arthus reaction, glomerulonephritis |
| **CELLULAR (DELAYED)** | | | | | |
| IV—Cell mediated | T cells, macrophages | Infectious agent, contact allergens, foreign tissues, cancer cells | Erythema and induration within 24-48 hr | Tissue destruction, primarily lymphocytes and macrophages | Tuberculin reaction, skin graft rejection, poison ivy |

surface of mast cells and basophils. On subsequent contact with the allergen (termed the *shocking dose* or *challenging dose*), the individual exhibits the symptoms of type I hypersensitivity.

Mast cells are found in virtually all tissues of the body and are often in close proximity to blood vessels, whereas basophils circulate in the blood. Mast cells are particularly abundant in the skin, nasal region, and lungs. Both mast cells and basophils have numerous, membrane-bound vacuoles containing potent, pharmacologically active substances (histamine, kinins, chemotactic factors, and active products of arachidonic acid metabolism [leukotrienes, prostaglandins, and thromboxanes]).[21] When IgE immunoglobulins bind to the surface of these cells by the Fc portion of the immunoglobulin molecule, the antigen-binding site of the molecule is left exposed to bind the allergen at the surface of the cell (Figure 66-2).

On second exposure to the allergen, the allergen becomes bound to the IgE, causing mast cell degranulation, which releases the internal agents of the cell into the environment. These mediators cause vasodilation, smooth muscle contraction, increased vascular permeability, and increased mucous gland secretion. Repeated cycles of exposure to allergens and type I responses can lead to chronic diseases.

The clinical manifestations of type I hypersensitivity reactions reflect changes in a wide variety of organs, because the reactions do not occur at the site of the antigen-antibody reaction. Rather, they occur in the organs where the pharmacologically active mediators exert their actions. If the mediators remain confined to a local area, the tissue reactions remain localized. This is known as local anaphylaxis. If the mediators become released systemically, the response is known as systemic anaphylaxis (Figure 66-3).

Atopic diseases are rarely life threatening, but the symptoms can be uncomfortable and may cause the individual to miss school or work. The local hypersensitivity that most people demonstrate in response to a mosquito bite is a classic example of this type of reaction; the intradermal injection of the mosquito anticoagulants produces a wheal-flare type of reaction within a matter of minutes. Box 66-3 lists the clinical manifestations associated with type I atopic hypersensitivity.

Nonatopic diseases can range from a local reaction such as hives or angioedema to a systemic reaction such as anaphy-

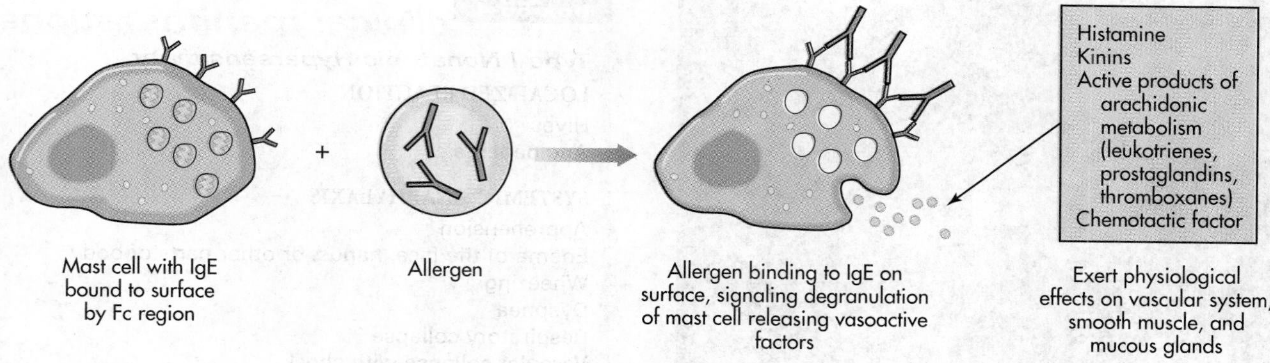

Mast cell with IgE bound to surface by Fc region

Allergen

Allergen binding to IgE on surface, signaling degranulation of mast cell releasing vasoactive factors

Histamine
Kinins
Active products of arachidonic metabolism (leukotrienes, prostaglandins, thromboxanes)
Chemotactic factor

Exert physiological effects on vascular system, smooth muscle, and mucous glands

**fig. 66-2** Mediators of type I hypersensitivity.

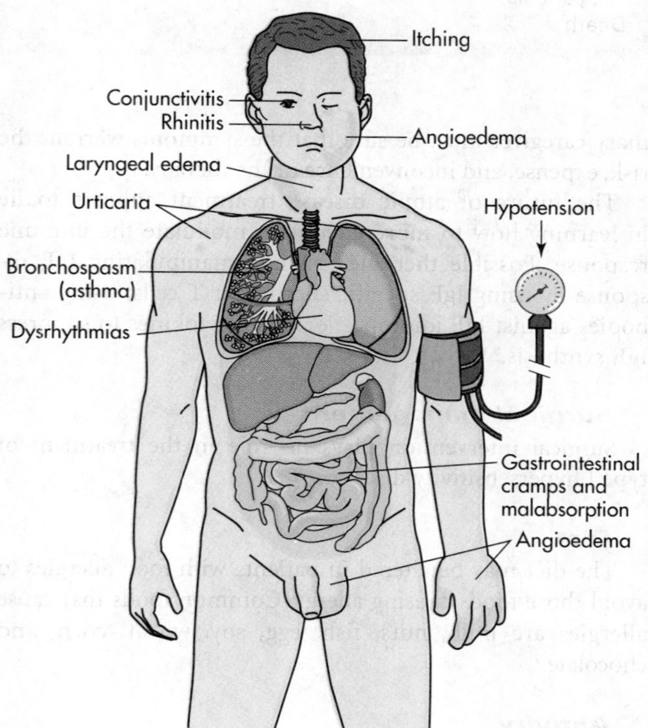


**fig. 66-3** Clinical manifestations of type I hypersensitivity reactions.

lactic shock. Hives (urticaria) are pruritic lesions characterized by a pale pink elevated edge (wheal) on an erythematous background (Figure 66-4). Urticaria are generally transient and may reappear in different body areas. A chronic form of urticaria is produced by factors other than IgE-mediated hypersensitivity in response to heat, cold, or various light waves. Cholinergic urticaria, yet another form, occurs as a response to stress or physical exertion. Angioedema is a form of urticaria that involves the subcutaneous tissue rather than the skin. It can involve an entire anatomical part, such as the eyelid, thumb, or lip; swelling is present, but not pruritus.

**box 66-3** ***clinical manifestations***

***Type I Atopic Hypersensitivity***

**RESPIRATORY**
- Rhinorrhea
- Watery, itching eyes
- Obstruction of eustachian tubes
- Sneezing
- Sinusitis
- Headache
- Facial pain
- Bronchospasm
- Dyspnea
- Stridor
- Tachypnea
- Wheezing
- Cyanosis
- Use of accessory muscles for breathing
- Flaring of nares

**DERMAL**
- Hives
- Rash
- Angioedema

**ABDOMINAL**
- Nausea
- Vomiting
- Cramping
- Diarrhea

**GENERAL**
- Fever
- Diaphoresis
- Malaise
- Joint pain
- Hematopoietic suppression
- Anxiety
- Anaphylaxis

The initial symptoms of systemic anaphylaxis are apprehension and sneezing. Edema and itching occur at the site when injected drugs or venoms are the allergens. These mild reactions are rapidly followed (sometimes in a matter of seconds or minutes) by severe manifestations that lead to vascular collapse and shock. Death may ensue unless rapid action is taken. Box 66-4 lists the clinical manifestations associated with type I nonatopic hypersensitivity.

## Collaborative Care Management

### *Diagnostic tests*

A health history, including an environmental assessment, is one of the most valuable diagnostic tools for the practitioner evaluating the patient with type I hypersensitivities. With atopic patients, skin tests and the radioallergosorbent test (RAST) may be helpful in determining therapy. The results of skin tests or the RAST must be correlated with the patient's history, however, to accurately identify the cause of the allergic reaction (see Chapter 65).

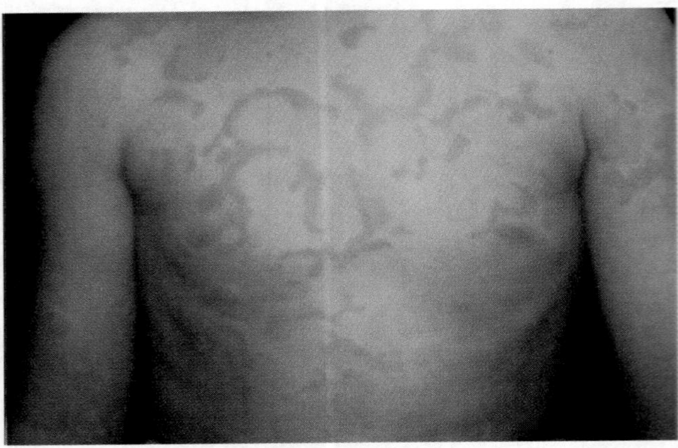

fig. 66-4 Urticaria.

box 66-4 **clinical manifestations**

***Type I Nonatopic Hypersensitivity***

LOCALIZED REACTION
Hives
Angioedema

SYSTEMIC ANAPHYLAXIS
Apprehension
Edema of the face, hands, or other parts of body
Wheezing
Dyspnea
Respiratory collapse
Vascular collapse with shock
- Rapid, weak pulse
- Falling blood pressure
- Cyanosis

Death

#### *Medications*

Drug therapy for atopic allergies is primarily for symptom relief. Urticaria and angioedema are usually self-limiting; therefore treatment is often not required. Anaphylaxis is treated with epinephrine to shorten its duration and prevent relapse (Table 66-6).

#### *Treatments*

Avoidance therapy, in which the patient is taught to reduce exposure to triggering antigens, is the most effective treatment to decrease allergic attacks. This therapy appears to be more effective with food, drug, and allergens such as animal dander, but it can also be useful to treat seasonal allergies. For instance, limiting outdoor activities and staying in air-conditioned settings when the pollen counts are high decrease seasonal allergy symptoms.

Immunotherapy is about 80% effective in diminishing symptoms of allergic rhinitis in patients with atopic IgE-mediated disease, particularly allergies from pollens and house dusts. Hyposensitization appears to affect the immune system by two mechanisms: stimulation of suppressor T cells specific to depression of IgE responses, and stimulation of IgG production specific to the allergen.[5] Increasing amounts of allergen are injected at weekly intervals, starting with a dose to which the person has been found sensitive by skin testing. If large local reactions occur during therapy, the dose is repeated or lowered until better tolerated (Box 66-5).

Systemic reactions, although uncommon, may occur within 30 minutes of injection. Treatment includes placing the person in a supine position and administering epinephrine.[21] If signs and symptoms of systemic anaphylactic shock are noted, oxygen is administered and intravenous fluids are infused rapidly to support blood pressure. (See Chapter 17 for treatment of shock.)

Although immunotherapy is widely used, controversy over this 75-year-old therapy still exists because of its potential for anaphylaxis and death. Consequently, before immunotherapy is chosen as a viable treatment option, the patient and primary caregiver must be sure that the symptoms warrant the risk, expense, and inconvenience of the therapy.

The future of atopic disease treatment appears to lie in learning how to more effectively modulate the immune response. Possible therapies include manipulating IgE response by using IgE-specific suppressor T cells; using antibodies against IgE idiotopes; or using cytokines to suppress IgE synthesis.[8,11]

#### *Surgical management*

Surgical intervention plays no role in the treatment of type I hypersensitivity disease.

#### *Diet*

The diet may be altered in patients with food allergies to avoid those foods causing allergy. Common foods that cause allergies are milk, nuts, fish, egg, soy, wheat, corn, and chocolate.[7]

#### *Activity*

The activity of the patient is not restricted. Atopic patients are encouraged to avoid activities when certain allergens or pollutants are high. Pollen counts are usually the highest between the hours of 12 midnight and 8 AM and on dry, windy days.

#### *Referrals*

Atopic individuals who have not achieved control of their symptoms with avoidance therapy and symptom-treating drugs may be referred to allergists for testing and immunotherapy.

## NURSING MANAGEMENT

### ■ ASSESSMENT

Nursing interventions are based on the patient's knowledge about the disorder and on the source or form of allergy present. This information is obtained by taking a history.

**table 66-6** *Common Medications for **Type I Hypersensitivities***

| Drug | Action | Nursing Implications |
|---|---|---|
| **ANTIHISTAMINES** | | |
| Diphenhydramine (Benadryl)<br>Chlorpheniramine (Chlor-Trimeton)<br>Brompheniramine (Dimetane)<br>Terfenadine (Seldane)<br>Astemizole (Hismanal)<br>Loratadine (Claritin) | Antihistamine; compete with histamine for effector cell $H_1$ receptor sites, thus preventing the action of histamine | May produce significant drowsiness (Benadryl) or central nervous system stimulation (Chlor-Trimeton); causes dry mouth; may produce blurred vision<br>Contraindicated in hypersensitivity, narrow-angle glaucoma, pregnancy, breast feeding, lower respiratory tract disease, acute asthma attacks, or within 14 days of taking monoamine oxidase inhibitors<br>Advise to take 1 hour before or 1 hour after meals to facilitate drug absorption |
| **DECONGESTANTS** | | |
| Phenylephrine (Neo-Synephrine)<br>Pseudoephedrine (Sudafed) | Stimulate alpha-adrenergic receptors to shrink respiratory mucous membranes | May produce nausea, vomiting, headache, anxiety, tremors, dizziness, seizures, tachycardia, hypertension, dysrhythmias, mucous membrane irritation, or dry mouth<br>Monitor blood pressure and pulse; give several hours before bedtime if drug produces sleeplessness<br>Contraindicated in patients with hypertension<br>Teach patient to stop drug if tremors or restlessness occur |
| **MAST CELL DEGRANULATOR INHIBITOR** | | |
| Cromolyn sodium inhaler (Intal)<br>Cromolyn sodium nasal spray (Nasalcrom) | Inhibit mast cell release of histamine and slow-reacting substance of anaphylaxis, thus preventing an allergic response | For prophylactic use only<br>May produce nasal irritation and burning, sneezing, cough, or throat irritation; dry mouth; nausea and vomiting; angioedema or bronchospasm<br>Do not give in hypersensitivity, acute asthma, or to patients with a history of coronary artery disease or dysrhythmias<br>Teach effective use of inhaler for accurate dosing |
| **CORTICOSTEROIDS** | | |
| Prednisone<br>Methylprednisone<br>Decadron phosphate<br>Vancenase<br>Beconase<br>Nasalide | Suppress migration of polymorphonuclear leukocytes and fibroblasts, thereby reducing inflammation | Contraindicated in patients with hypersensitivity, psychoses, fungal infections, AIDS, tuberculosis<br>Monitor for thrombocytopenia, increased intraocular pressure, poor wound healing, nausea, diarrhea, headache, and mood changes<br>Monitor daily weight, serum potassium levels, blood glucose levels, blood pressure, signs of infection, mood changes<br>Give with food or milk to decrease GI irritation<br>Caution patient not to stop taking drug abruptly and to notify health care provider if infection develops |
| **ADRENALIN** | | |
| Epinephrine | Opposes the action of histamine through vasoconstriction to raise blood pressure; promotes bronchiole relaxation to facilitate breathing; stimulates both alpha and beta receptors to reproduce effects of sympathetic nervous system | Temporary relief from anaphylaxis, hypersensitivity reactions, bronchospasm, and acute asthma attacks<br>Contraindicated in hypersensitivity, narrow-angle glaucoma, dysrhythmias<br>Monitor for anxiety, tremors, palpitations, tachydysrhythmias, hypertension, pulmonary edema |
| **AMINOPHYLLINE** | | |
| Theophylline (Theo-Dur) | Xanthine blocks phosphodiesterase, thus increasing cyclic AMP, which alters intracellular calcium and ion movement; produces respiratory tract relaxation and bronchodilation and increases pulmonary blood flow | Monitor for central nervous system stimulation, dizziness, anxiety, restlessness, seizures, tachycardia, dysrhythmias, nausea, vomiting, insomnia<br>Contraindicated in hypersensitivity to xanthine and in patients with history of tachydysrhythmias<br>Avoid intake of stimulant foods such as coffee, tea, and colas<br>Monitor theophylline blood levels<br>Avoid smoking because it interferes with absorption |

**box 66-5** *clinical manifestations*

***Immunotherapy Reactions***

| LOCAL | SYSTEMIC |
|---|---|
| Redness | Nasal stuffiness |
| Edema | Sneezing |
| Pruritus | Reddening of conjunctiva |
| Tenderness | Chest tightness |
| | Wheezing |
| | Fainting |
| | Apprehension |
| | Anaphylactic shock |

### Subjective Data

Subjective data to be obtained include:

- History of allergic reactions in the past (e.g., type, frequency, or perceived causes)
- Familial history of allergies
- Recent exposure to sensitizing substances
- Changes in living, working, or environmental conditions
- Characteristics of present environment (house, clothing, plants, trees, or animals)
- Increased stress in recent past (aggravates asthmatic response—see the Research Box)
- Types of symptoms: respiratory, dermal, gastrointestinal, or general
- Alleviating factors, either prescribed by physician or self-prescribed

All patients should be questioned about allergies and sensitivities to drugs before any drug therapy is initiated. If there is a positive history, the physician is consulted before a new drug is given; when a new drug is given, the patient is monitored closely for allergic responses.

### Objective Data

Objective data to be obtained include:

- Rashes (location, color)
- Mouth breathing
- Difficulty hearing (plugged eustachian tubes)
- Nasal obstruction
- Flaring nares
- Pale bluish turbinates that are edematous with clear secretions
- Tearing
- Dark areas under eyes (venous dilation of skin)
- Scleral or conjunctival infections
- Increased respiratory rate
- Audible wheezing
- Use of accessory muscles for breathing
- Anxious expression

**research**

Reference: Kang DH, Coe CL, McCarthy DO, Ershler WB: Immune responses to final exams in healthy and asthmatic adolescents, *Nurs Res* 46(1):12, 1997.

This study explored the responses of the immune system to the stress of final exams in healthy adolescents and adolescents with asthma. The sample consisted of 87 students who were divided into three groups—healthy, mild asthma not requiring regular medication, and severe asthma requiring daily medication. The students completed a 2-week health diary and had blood drawn for immunological analysis at midsemester, during final exams, and after final exams.

The stress of final exams altered the immune response of all three groups of students, and no significant differences were found between the three groups related to their health status. During exam week the levels of natural killer cells was significantly lower, while lymphocyte proliferation and neutrophil superoxide release were significantly higher. The first two changes returned to baseline within 2 weeks after exams, while the neutrophil reactivity continued to rise. The study offers further evidence of the links between life stress and immune system function.

## ■ NURSING DIAGNOSES

### Atopy

| Diagnostic Title | Possible Etiological Factors |
|---|---|
| Health maintenance, altered | Effects of allergy on preferred lifestyle |
| Knowledge deficit: environmental and life-style modifications to control allergies | Lack of exposure, inadequate information about allergy treatment |

### Anaphylaxis

| Diagnostic Title | Possible Etiological Factors |
|---|---|
| Airway clearance, ineffective | Excess secretion production, bronchoconstriction |
| Cardiac output, decreased | Inadequate venous return to heart, peripheral vasodilation |

## ■ EXPECTED PATIENT OUTCOMES

Expected outcomes for the person with a type I hypersensitivity may include but are not limited to:

### Atopy

1. Maintains health status by verbalizing:
   a. Understanding of disease process
   b. Understanding of the substances that are allergenic and approaches for avoidance
   c. Plans to alter habits or environment to reduce exposure to allergens
2. Demonstrates knowledge of treatments by verbalizing:
   a. Rationale for immunotherapy (if applicable)
   b. The need for constant availability of an anaphylaxis emergency kit for self-treatment (if anaphylaxis is a possibility)
   c. Understanding of drug therapy prescribed to relieve symptoms

### Anaphylaxis

1. Maintains patent airway
2. Shows no clinical manifestations of shock

## ■ INTERVENTIONS

### Promoting Effective Disease Management

The major nursing responsibility in the care of the person with an atopic allergy is teaching the patient and family about the nature of the disorder and the methods that can be used to avoid the allergen. Results of allergy testing, assessment findings, and patient history are reviewed with the patient and family so they understand which allergens need to be controlled or avoided. Patients are taught the importance of controlling their living and working environments to reduce the risk of reactions. For example, air conditioning is desirable to reduce pollens in hot weather. If animal dander is a source of allergy and the removal of a family pet is unacceptable to the family, the nurse can suggest that the pet be kept outdoors (see the Patient/Family Teaching Box).

### Teaching about Immunotherapy and Anaphylaxis

Anaphylaxis can occur following exposure to offending antigens or from immunotherapy. The patient and family need to be taught about such reactions and how to deal with them. The nurse instructs both the patient and family about signs and symptoms that need to be reported, potential reactions that can result in the need for emergency measures, and use of emergency care kits. If immunotherapy is elected as a treatment choice, the risks and benefits, schedules, and costs of such therapy are discussed. The patient is informed that immunotherapy can be reinstituted if symptoms recur. The nurse explains all prescribed medications, including desired actions, dosage schedules, and potential side effects. The importance of maintaining drug schedules for prophylactic drugs, such as cromolyn, is stressed, and the patient and family are reminded that these drugs are of no value during an acute allergic attack.

### Promoting Effective Airway Clearance

Death from anaphylaxis occurs from asphyxiation because of upper airway edema and congestion, irreversible shock, or a combination of these factors (see the section on clinical manifestations of type I nonatopic anaphylaxis).[12] The primary concern of the nurse is making certain that the patient has a patent airway. The patient is positioned in high Fowler's position to maximize ventilation; an oral airway is inserted if necessary, and secretions are removed by suction or by encouraging the patient to cough. Oxygen therapy may be given according to doctor's orders or facility protocols. The nurse encourages slow, deep breathing. The administration of epinephrine or bronchodilators such as aminophylline may be necessary to decrease bronchospasm. In severe cases, tracheostomy may be necessary to maintain a patent airway. The patient is monitored closely both during and after anaphylaxis.

**patient/family teaching**

**The Person with Atopic Allergy**

The nurse instructs the patient to:

1. Avoid allergen, if possible.
   a. Animal dander
      (1) Avoid fur-bearing pets, if possible, or keep pets outdoors.
      (2) Avoid furniture stuffed with horsehair or feathers.
   b. Pollen spores
      (1) Use air conditioning if possible; keep windows closed at night; if using air conditioner in car, start car, roll down windows, and allow air conditioner to run for 10-15 minutes before entering car.
      (2) Limit time outdoors between sunset and sunrise, especially when windy.
      (3) Do not hang wash outside to dry. (Pollen and molds stick to wet wash.)
      (4) Avoid gardening, raking leaves, mowing lawn, or being near freshly cut grass.
      (5) Keep car windows closed when driving.
      (6) Minimize number of indoor plants.
      (7) Vacation in selected geographical areas, such as beach or sea, that are free of specific allergen during seasonal height, if possible.
   c. House dust
      (1) Use synthetic materials; avoid wool and cotton.
      (2) Use a minimum of lint-producing articles.
      (3) Put away articles that are difficult to dust.
      (4) Dust with damp cloth daily.
      (5) Use air conditioner, if possible.
      (6) Change furnace filter every month when in use.
2. Use all medications as prescribed and report the incidence of side effects.

### Supporting Effective Cardiac Output

Respiratory compromise quickly leads to decreased cardiac output that can produce death within a matter of minutes. The nurse is alert for clinical manifestations that indicate anaphylactic shock and is prepared to address the problem should it occur. At the first sign of anaphylaxis, the patient is given epinephrine 1:1000 solution 0.3 to 0.5 ml subcutaneously or intramuscularly. If shock continues, albuterol (Ventolin) or epinephrine administered through aerosol treatments may be administered. Vasopressors such as dopamine or metaraminol bitartrate (Aramine) may be prescribed for severe shock to assist in increasing the blood pressure and increasing cardiac output. (See Chapter 17 for treatment of shock.)

### Patient/Family Education

Allergic individuals are advised to alert health care workers of their allergies when animal sera, allergenic extracts, or contrast media containing iodide need to be given for any reason, so that epinephrine can be readily available. The patient is then monitored for at least 30 minutes after administration of such substances. Any reaction that occurs within a few minutes forewarns of an impending emergency.

Because persons with a history of allergies are more likely to develop anaphylactic reactions to drugs than those without such a history, all patients are questioned about allergies and drug sensitivities before drug therapy is initiated. High-risk persons are instructed to wear an identification bracelet or tag at all times that indicates the known allergy. Such tags may be obtained from Medic Alert or other commercial sources.

## EVALUATION

Successful achievement of patient outcomes for the patient who is atopic is indicated by:

### Atopy

1a. Verbalizes understanding of the allergens to which she or he is sensitive
b. Verbalizes changes in environment or habits that will decrease exposure to allergens
c. Modifies lifestyle and environment to reduce exposure to allergens
2. Shows no tachycardia, dyspnea, use of accessory muscles for breathing, stridor, cyanosis, or nasal flaring and maintains a systolic blood pressure greater than 100
2a. Verbalizes the purpose and expected outcomes of immunotherapy
b. Verbalizes the need for an easily accessible anaphylaxis kit
c. Verbalizes knowledge of medications, drugs prescribed, actions, side effects, and demonstrates correct use of medications in anaphylaxis kit

### Anaphylaxis

1. Maintains patent airway
2. Shows no tachycardia, dyspnea, use of accessory muscles for breathing, stridor, cyanosis, or nasal flaring, and maintains a systolic blood pressure greater than 100

## GERONTOLOGICAL CONSIDERATIONS

Older adults have a decreased ability to respond to immunological events and undergo changes in their patterns of immunological response. These changes may lead to decreased responsiveness to allergens. However, studies indicate that between 27% and 38% of adults with a history of childhood allergic asthma have a recurrence of the disease in later life. Because there are no conclusive data to support that older adults have fewer hypersensitivities than younger adults, they are assessed for allergies and taught the same emergency interventions as younger adults. If elders are unable to care for themselves, it is particularly important that the nurse instruct the family or caregiver how to deal with potential and actual hypersensitivities.[6]

## SPECIAL ENVIRONMENTS FOR CARE

### Critical Care Management

Critical care management plays no role in the routine management of atopic allergy but may be essential to monitor a patient in anaphylactic shock. Persons experiencing anaphylaxis and anaphylactic shock will require hospitalization until they are free of respiratory distress. Tracheostomy may be required when airway compromise is severe. Anaphylaxis has a propensity to recur as emergency medications are excreted from the body. Therefore patients are likely to remain hospitalized until the likelihood of recurrence has passed. (See Chapter 17 for treatment of shock.)

### Home Care Management

Except in the case of anaphylaxis, people with atopic hypersensitivities will be cared for at home and seen as necessary in the primary caregiver's office or outpatient clinic. The home environment should be altered to decrease the risk of exposure to allergens (see earlier discussion regarding home maintenance).

Persons with type I hypersensitivities should be aware of situations in which the allergens to which they are sensitive may be found. Persons who are sensitive to insect stings should learn the emergency care to take after a sting. Sting emergency medical kits are available commercially and should be readily available. Both the person and family are taught how to use the self-injecting syringe to administer the 1:1000 epinephrine HCl. If the patient is unable to use the syringe or give the injection, an inhalation high-dose epinephrine taken from a metered-dose aerosol (found in some emergency kits) may be used (see the Patient/Family Teaching Box).

## COMPLICATIONS

The primary complication of type I hypersensitivities is anaphylactic shock, which can lead to death within minutes without emergency treatment. This complication was previously discussed, and a detailed discussion of shock can be found in Chapter 17.

## TYPE II HYPERSENSITIVITIES

Type II hypersensitivity is classically illustrated by the reactions that occur in mismatched blood transfusion reactions. The underlying mechanism of type II (cytotoxic) hypersensitivities involves the direct binding of IgG or IgM immunoglobulins

**patient/family teaching**

**The Person with Type I Hypersensitivity: Sting**

The nurse instructs the patient and family concerning the following:

1. Emergency care for the specific allergy
2. Availability and use of commercially prepared emergency kit
3. Concentration and route of emergency use epinephrine (1:1000 epinephrine injection)
4. Use of self-injecting syringe of epinephrine supplied with kit (spring loaded; can be given through clothing)
5. Emergency procedure if sting occurs
   a. Immediately swallow the uncoated antihistamine tablet
   b. Inject the epinephrine
   c. If unable to self-inject, inhale high-dose epinephrine from metered-dose aerosol* (if included in kit)

*Epinephrine is rapidly absorbed through respiratory tract and will help relieve bronchoconstriction and bronchospasms; not recommended as primary treatment because it does not correct hypotension.

to an antigen on the surface of a cell. This antibody labeling then triggers the destruction of the cell by phagocytic attack, nonspecific lymphocytic attack, or lysis of the cell through the operation of the full complement cascade (see Chapter 10). Figure 66-5 illustrates the mechanism of type II hypersensitivity reactions.

## Blood Transfusion Reactions

Blood replacement therapy is used when there has been excessive blood loss (whole blood or blood components) or in the treatment of diseases of the hematopoietic system.

Although whole blood may be administered, specific blood components are increasingly used. Blood can be fractionated into red blood cells (RBCs), platelets, and plasma (Table 66-7), either by centrifuge or by automated cell separators. Blood can also be withdrawn from a donor, a portion separated from the blood, and the remainder returned to the donor (apheresis). Using blood components rather than whole blood is a more efficient use of an increasingly scarce commodity (blood) for an increased number of recipients, prevents fluid overload, and gives the recipient only the blood components required, thus decreasing the incidence of side effects.

### *Etiology/epidemiology*

There are many antigens on the surface of RBCs, but two major systems are significant clinically in terms of potential immunological reactions: the ABO system and the Rh system.

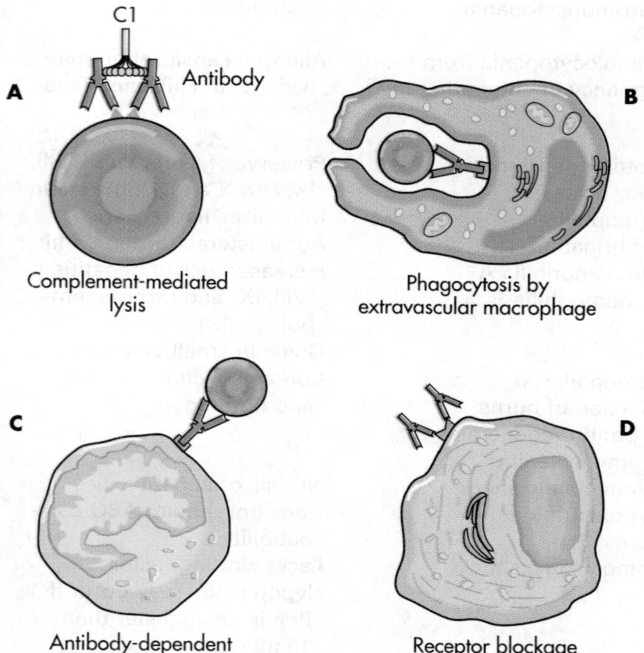


**fig. 66-5** Mechanisms of type II, tissue-specific reactions. Antigens on the target cell bind with antibody and are destroyed or prevented from functioning by **A,** complement-mediated lysis; **B,** clearance by macrophages in tissues; **C,** antibody-dependent cell-mediated cytotoxicity (ADCC); or **D,** the modulation or blockage of receptors on the target cell.

The human leukocyte antigen (HLA) system relates to leukocytes and platelets.

**ABO system.** Four major blood groups are found in humans: A, B, AB, and O (Table 66-8). Erythrocyte antigens inherited from our parents give us our blood types.[16] Within 3 months of birth the individual has formed antibodies against the other types of major erythrocyte antigens. The exact cause of this antibody formation is not clear, but it is suspected that something antigenically similar to the antibodies are found in the environment and these stimulate antibody formation.[20] For example, a person with type A blood will possess anti-B antibodies within the serum. These antibodies, called isohemagglutinins, are usually of the IgM class. Antibodies formed in this way are capable of cross-reacting with the A or B antigens on the surface of the "foreign" ABO types. Because type AB blood contains both antigens, persons with type AB may receive blood from any other blood type (Figure 66-6). Persons with type O may donate blood to other types, but because both antigens are absent in type O, they may not receive another type without experiencing a reaction.

These antibodies are naturally present in the serum; therefore mismatched blood cells from a transfusion will be immediately coated by the isohemagglutinins, causing the agglutination of the introduced cells and the rapid lysis of the cells by complement. The products released by the lysed cells are then dumped into the bloodstream.

**Rh system.** The Rh system is more complex, because there are at least 27 different antigens in this system. The D antigen is the most significant clinically, because it is more immunogenic than any other Rh antigen, and it is usually the antigen involved in hemolytic disease of the newborn. When the term *Rh positive* is used, the presence of antigen Rh-D is implied; the term *Rh negative* indicates the absence of antigen D. Approximately 85% of the population has Rh-positive blood.

When the Rh-negative person is first exposed to Rh-positive blood, Rh antibodies are formed. On subsequent exposures to Rh-positive blood, the Rh antibody binds to its corresponding antigen on the surface of the RBCs containing the Rh antigen. The Rh antibodies do not usually fix complement; therefore there is no immediate hemolysis as occurs in the ABO system. Instead, the Rh-antigen RBCs are rapidly broken down by macrophages in the spleen, with conversion of hemoglobin to bilirubin, resulting in jaundice.

**Other erythrocyte antigens.** Other groups of erythrocyte antigens that can form antibodies are grouped into the Kidd, Duffy, Kell, and MNS systems.[20] The antibodies can cause hemolytic reactions if antigen-positive blood is transfused into a sensitized recipient. These antibodies cause more problems in patients who are chronically transfused.[9]

**HLA system.** Another system that has clinical significance in blood transfusion is the HLA system. Human leukocyte antigens are found on many types of tissue cells and on blood leukocytes and platelets. The system is more complex than the RBC antigen systems, and thousands of combinations of antigens may occur. Sensitization may occur through pregnancy or through exposure to platelets

**table 66-7** *Types of Blood Components*

| Blood Component | Description | Usage | Comments |
|---|---|---|---|
| **RED BLOOD CELLS (RBCs)** | | | |
| Packed RBC (PRBCs) | RBCs separated from plasma and platelets | Anemia<br>Moderate blood loss | Decreased risk of fluid overload as compared with whole blood |
| Autologous PRBCs | Same as packed RBC | Elective surgery for which blood replacement is expected | Units may be stored for up to 35 days |
| Washed RBCs | RBCs washed with sterile isotonic saline before transfusion | Previous allergic reactions to transfusions | Increased removal of immunoglobulins and protein |
| Frozen RBCs | RBCs frozen in a glycerol solution; cells washed after thawing to remove the glycerol | Storage of rare type blood<br>Storage of autologous blood for future use | Relatively free of leukocytes and microemboli<br>Expensive |
| Leukocyte-poor RBCs | RBCs from which most leukocytes have been removed | Previous sensitivity to leukocyte antigens from prior transfusions or from pregnancy | Fewer RBC than packed RBC; washed leukocyte-poor RBC units have more RBC than nonwashed |
| Neocytes | RBC units with high number of reticulocytes (young RBCs) | Transfusion-dependent anemias | Fewer problems with iron overload<br>Expensive |
| **OTHER CELLULAR COMPONENTS** | | | |
| Platelets | | | |
| Random donor packs | Platelets separated from RBCs by centrifuge; given in 50 ml of plasma | Thrombocytopenia<br>Disseminated intravascular coagulation (DIC) | Plasma base is rich in coagulation factors<br>Platelet preparations can also be packed, washed, or made leukocyte poor |
| Pheresis packs | Platelets from an HLA-matched donor, separated by apheresis | Allosensitized persons with thrombocytopenia | Requires specialized techniques |
| Granulocytes | Granular leukocytes separated by apheresis | Granulocytopenia from malignancy or chemotherapy | Allergen sensitization may occur with chills and fever |
| **PLASMA COMPONENTS** | | | |
| Fresh frozen plasma (FFP) | Freezing of plasma within 4 hr of collection | Clotting deficiencies<br>Liver disease<br>Hemophilia<br>Defibrination | Preserves factors V, VII, VIII, IX, and X and prothrombin<br>Minimizes hepatitis risk<br>Administered through a filter |
| Factor concentrates VIII and IX | Prepared from large donor pools<br>Heated to inactivate HIV | VIII: hemophilia A<br>IX: hemophilia B | Increased risk of hepatitis (VIII, IX) and thromboembolism (IX)<br>Given in small volumes |
| Cryoprecipitate | Precipitated material obtained from FFP when thawed | Hemophilia A<br>Infection of burns<br>Hypofibrinogenemia<br>Uremic bleeding | Contains factors VIII, XIII, and fibrinogen |
| Serum albumin<br>Normal serum albumin (NSA)<br>Plasma protein fraction (PPF) | Albumin chemically processed from pooled plasma | Hypovolemic shock<br>Hypoalbuminemia<br>Burns<br>Hemorrhagic shock | No risk of hepatitis<br>Does not require ABO compatibility<br>Lacks clotting factors<br>Hypotension may occur if PPF is given faster than 10 ml/min |
| Immune serum globulin | Obtained from plasma of preselected donors with specific antibodies | Hypogammaglobulinemia<br>Prophylaxis for hepatitis A, tetanus | Given intramuscularly |

**table 66-8** *ABO Blood Groups*

A—antigen A is present on cell; anti-B antibodies in serum
B—antigen B is present on cell; anti-A antibodies in serum
AB—antigens A and B are present on cell; no antibodies in serum
O—neither antigen A nor B is present on cell; anti-A and anti-B antibodies in serum

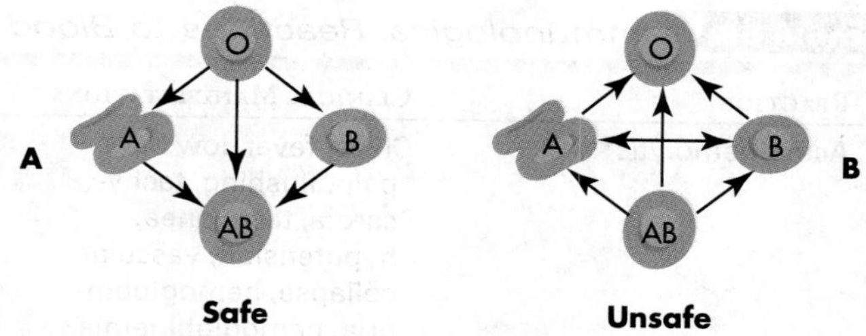


**fig. 66-6** Blood groups and their donor/recipient relationships. **A,** Safe. **B,** Unsafe.

and white blood cells (WBCs) during transfusions. Repeated transfusions of blood cells may lead to transfusion reactions.

Although there are numerous types of adverse reactions to blood transfusions, they occur in only approximately 2% to 5% of all transfusions.[9] The incidence of each type of reaction is included in the following discussion of pathophysiology.

### Pathophysiology

Transfusion reactions can be broadly grouped into immunological and nonimmunological types. Table 66-9 presents an overview of each of the major types of immunological transfusion reactions along with their associated clinical manifestations and management.

**Immunological transfusion reactions.** *Acute hemolytic transfusion reaction* is the most serious adverse reaction to blood transfusion. It occurs within the first 30 minutes of blood administration. Hemolytic reactions are responsible for about 90% of all transfusion-related deaths but fortunately account for only 0.5% to 1% of all reactions. Studies of hemolytic reactions have shown that mistakes in specimen collection and labeling and inadequate patient identification are the primary errors that lead to hemolytic reactions.[17] Acute hemolytic reactions are caused by antigen-antibody complexes on the erythrocyte membrane. These complexes activate the Hageman factor (coagulation factor XII) and the complement cascade. The Hageman factor initiates the kinin system, causing increased capillary permeability, arteriole vasodilation, and hypotension.[20] The activated complement system initiates intravascular hemolysis, as well as histamine and serotonin release from the mast cells. Hageman factor and free incompatible erythrocyte stroma (covering) activate the intrinsic clotting cascade causing disseminated intravascular coagulation (DIC).[15]

*Febrile nonhemolytic reactions* are one of the most common transfusion reactions. They occur because the recipient becomes sensitized to the donor's WBCs, platelets, or plasma. Symptoms usually begin 30 minutes after the start of the infusion. Although this reaction is not usually serious, it is uncomfortable for the patient. Patients with a history of febrile nonhemolytic reaction may be premedicated with Tylenol and Benadryl or receive leukocyte-poor RBCs to prevent recurrence.

Another common transfusion reaction is the *allergic transfusion reaction.* It is caused by sensitivity of the recipient to foreign plasma proteins. Common symptoms include hives, rash, and urticaria. If the symptoms are mild, the patient is treated with antihistamines and the transfusion is restarted slowly. A more severe allergic reaction (anaphylaxis) can occur rarely.[12] The patient will show symptoms of bronchospasm, respiratory distress, and shock.

*Delayed hemolytic reactions* occur 7 to 14 days after the transfusion and are thought to be the result of sensitization of the recipient's immune system to the transfused erythrocyte antigens. The recipient may also have been previously sensitized but have antibody titers that are undetectable at the time of the transfusion.

*Posttransfusion graft-versus-host disease (PT-GVHD)* is relatively rare but has recently been reported more frequently because of increased use of purposeful immunosuppression in certain treatments (e.g., bone marrow transplantation). The donor lymphocytes begin to reject the patient's host cells 4 to 30 days after the infusion of blood.

*Noncardiac pulmonary edema* is thought to be caused by a high titer of leukocyte antibodies in either the donor or recipient plasma. These antibody-to-granulocyte reactions cause granulocyte aggregates that are filtered out by the lung. The antibodies attached to the granulocytes initiate the complement cascade and promote histamine release, causing an influx of inflammatory cells into the lung.

**Nonimmunological transfusion reactions.** Blood transfusion can result in reactions that are not immunological in nature. These include circulatory overload, sepsis, and transmission of disease. These reactions are summarized in Box 66-6. Clinical manifestations associated with nonimmunological transfusion reactions are presented in Box 66-7.

### Collaborative care management

Prevention is the key to management of transfusion reactions. Accurate prescreening of potential donors, meticulous laboratory testing, and close patient monitoring are all essential components of care. Blood received from volunteer donors through the American Red Cross Blood Service or hospital blood banks is preferred to that of paid donors, because paid donors may be less likely to report past or present diseases that may be transmitted to the recipient. Common screening guidelines for blood donation are outlined in Box 66-8.

**table 66-9** *Immunological Reactions to Blood Transfusion*

| Reaction | Clinical Manifestations | Management | Prevention |
|---|---|---|---|
| Acute hemolytic* | Chills, fever, low back pain, flushing, tachycardia, tachypnea, hypotension, vascular collapse, hemoglobinuria, hemoglobinemia, bleeding, acute renal failure, shock, cardiac arrest, death | Treat shock.<br>Draw blood samples for serological testing. To avoid hemolysis from the procedure, use a new venipuncture (not an existing central line) and avoid small-gauge needles. Send urine specimen to the laboratory.<br>Maintain BP with IV colloid solutions. Give diuretics as prescribed to maintain urine flow.<br>Insert indwelling catheter or measure voided amounts to monitor hourly urine output. Dialysis may be required if renal failure occurs.<br>Do not transfuse additional red blood cell–containing components until the transfusion service has provided newly crossmatched units. | Meticulously verify and document patient identification from sample collection to component infusion.<br>Transfuse blood slowly for first 15-20 minutes with nurse at patient's side. |
| Febrile, nonhemolytic (most common)* | Sudden chills and fever (rise in temperature of greater than 1° C [2° F]), headache, flushing, anxiety, muscle pain | Give antipyretics as prescribed. Do not give aspirin to thrombocytopenic patients.<br>*Do not restart transfusion.* | Consider leukocyte-poor blood products (filtered, washed, or frozen). |
| Mild allergic* | Flushing, itching, urticaria (hives) | Give antihistamines as directed.<br>If symptoms are mild and transient, restart transfusion slowly.<br>Do not restart transfusion if fever or pulmonary symptoms develop. | Treat prophylactically with glucocorticosteroids or antihistamines (Decadron, Benadryl) given 30-60 min before transfusion. |
| Anaphylactic* | Anxiety, urticaria, wheezing, tightness and pain in chest, difficulty swallowing, progressing to cyanosis, shock, and possible cardiac arrest | Initiate CPR if indicated.<br>Have epinephrine ready for injection (0.4 ml of a 1:1000 solution subcutaneously or 0.1 ml of 1:1000 solution diluted to 10 ml with saline for IV use).<br>*Do not restart transfusion.* | Transfuse extensively washed red blood cell products from which all plasma has been removed. Alternatively, use blood from IgA-deficient donor. |
| Delayed hemolytic | Fever, chills, back pain, jaundice, anemia, hemoglobinuria | Monitor adequacy of urinary output and degree of anemia.<br>Treat fever with Tylenol.<br>May need further blood transfusion. | Do more specific type and crossmatch when giving patient blood. |
| Posttransfusion graft-versus-host disease | Anorexia, nausea, diarrhea, high fever, rash, stomatitis, liver dysfunction | No effective treatment.<br>Administer steroids. | Give irradiated blood products. |
| Noncardiac pulmonary edema | Fever, chills, hypotension, cough, orthopnea, cyanosis, shock | Stop transfusion.<br>Continue IV saline.<br>Give oxygen prn.<br>Administer steroids as directed.<br>Give furosemide (Lasix) and epinephrine as ordered. | |

*Modified from *National blood resource education program's transfusion therapy guidelines for nurses,* NIH Pub No 90-2668, 1990.

**box 66-6** *Major Nonimmunological Transfusion Reactions*

**CIRCULATORY OVERLOAD**

Can occur when blood is given too rapidly or in large quantities. The elderly are particularly vulnerable. Patients develop signs of fluid overload and pulmonary congestion. The transfusion is stopped and oxygen and diuretics may be administered.

**SEPSIS**

Bacterial contamination may occur at any time during the collection or handling of blood. Signs of sepsis begin almost immediately. The transfusion is stopped, and the patient receives antibiotics and treatment for shock if it occurs.

**DISEASE TRANSMISSION**

Hepatitis, CMV, and HIV are the most common diseases transmitted by blood transfusions. Hepatitis A and B are effectively identified with current screening capabilities, but hepatitis C is still readily transmissible.

**box 66-7** *clinical manifestations*

***Nonimmunological Transfusion Reactions***

| CIRCULATORY OVERLOAD | SEPSIS |
|---|---|
| Dyspnea | Fever >40° C |
| Chest tightness | Abdominal cramps |
| Headache | Nausea |
| Hypertension | Vomiting |
| Tachypnea | Diarrhea |
| Cough | Septic shock |
| Cyanosis | |
| Peripheral edema | |
| Jugular vein distention | |
| Rales | |
| Abnormal heart sounds | |
| Hypertension | |

One method of preventing immunological blood transfusion reactions and disease transmission is by using the person's own blood for replacement. In planned autologous transfusion, blood is collected at regular intervals before anticipated use, such as forthcoming surgery. The blood is then stored or frozen until needed. This method is especially useful for persons with rare blood types, for those whose religious beliefs preclude receiving donor blood, or when several units of blood are expected to be necessary during surgery (e.g., selected heart surgeries or joint replacements).

Autotransfusion, which consists of collecting, filtering, and immediately reinfusing the person's own blood, may be performed in the emergency department, the operating room suite during surgery, or in the critical care unit. The blood is suctioned into a bag and passes through a filter to remove microaggregates. When the bag is full, it is disconnected from the

**box 66-8** *Screening Guidelines for Blood Donors*

Persons with any of the following are not permitted to donate blood:

1. History of infectious diseases such as hepatitis, HIV infection and AIDS, tuberculosis, syphilis, or malaria
2. Malignant diseases
3. Allergies or asthma
4. Polycythemia vera
5. Abnormal bleeding tendencies
6. Hypotension (current)
7. Anemia (current)
8. Recent pregnancy or major surgery
9. Men with at least one homosexual or bisexual contact since 1975 (concern for AIDS)
10. International travel to malarial areas or high-risk countries (concern for AIDS)
11. Blood transfusion during last 6 months
12. History of jaundice
13. Diseases of the heart, lung, or liver
14. Immunizations or vaccinations with attenuated viral vaccine rubella or rabies vaccine
15. Hgb level below 13.5 g/dl for men or 12.4 g/dl for women
16. Abnormalities in vital signs, particularly fever

system and the blood is infused into the patient with an administration set, using a standard or microembolic filter.

Most of the serious reactions that occur during transfusions are the result of human error. Type, screen, and crossmatching of blood in the laboratory must be accurate. Typing is confirmed by testing the recipient's serum against commercial A and B cells to detect isoagglutinins. The recipient's serum is then screened for alloantibodies that were not found in the typing. A crossmatch tests the compatibility between donor and recipient directly. The blood from each is mixed and observed for hemolysis. More complete antibody identification is performed in patients who have been sensitized to the less important antigenic systems (Kell, Kidd, Duffy, and MNS systems).[16]

Blood transfusions are carefully monitored and follow strict institutional protocols. Guidelines for care of the person receiving a blood transfusion are outlined in the box on the next page. If a patient reports any of the symptoms associated with transfusion reaction, the nurse immediately stops the transfusion and keeps the vein patent by administering normal saline. The primary care provider is notified immediately. Patients who exhibit any sign of anaphylaxis or hemolytic reaction receive frequent vital sign monitoring and are assessed for signs of impending shock, renal failure, or DIC. The blood and tubing are returned to the laboratory for analysis, and a first-voided urine specimen is collected to analyze for signs of hemolysis. The patient's hemoglobin and hematocrit levels are carefully monitored to determine the extent of the reaction. Patients who experience mild allergic reactions to blood may receive premedication with an antihistamine if they should need transfusion in the future. A Clinical Pathway for a patient receiving a blood transfusion can be found on p. 2181.

**Patient/family education.** Informed consent is necessary before the administration of blood; therefore the patient and family are queried about their understanding of the procedure, and permission for the transfusion is secured. The nurse answers questions and clarifies misunderstandings about blood transfusions. The prospect of receiving blood is frightening to many individuals because of concerns about contracting AIDS. The nurse reassures patients and families that blood is carefully screened and tested for disease before being prepared for transfusion.

Teaching also includes information about how the blood will be administered, approximately how long the transfusion will take, and signs and symptoms associated with transfusion reactions. Patients are encouraged to promptly report any unusual sensations experienced during the transfusion. They are also informed that their vital signs will be frequently monitored throughout the procedure, and that this is normal protocol and does not mean that a reaction is actually occurring.

## TYPE III HYPERSENSITIVITIES

Type III hypersensitivities result in injury to tissues from the deposit of immune complexes in various tissues, where they may trigger complement activation. Serum sickness is the type III hypersensitivity of clinical importance.

### guidelines for care

#### The Patient Receiving a Blood Transfusion

1. Carefully check all of the following:
   a. Identity of patient to receive transfusion
   b. The label of the unit of blood for the name of the person for whom it is intended; make certain that it matches the patient's wristband before administering the blood
   c. Expiration date of the blood
   d. Color and consistency of blood (if the bag appears to have clots, gas, or a dark purple color, it could be contaminated and should not be infused)
2. Obtain baseline vital signs and check again at frequent intervals throughout the procedure.
3. Administer all blood products through micron mesh filters.
4. Assess patient for any unusual sensations felt throughout the transfusion. (This information may help with early identification of any reactions that occur.)
5. Infuse blood within 4 hours after it is taken from the blood bank (to prevent bacterial growth).
6. If blood cannot be infused within 4 hours, return it to the blood bank for proper refrigeration.
7. Follow facility guidelines for proper disposal of empty blood bag and tubing.
8. Record patient's response to the infusion.
9. Report any adverse effect to the primary care provider immediately.
10. Return the blood bag and tubing to the laboratory for testing if a reaction occurs.

### Serum Sickness

#### *Etiology/epidemiology*

Serum sickness can develop from 1 to 3 weeks after the administration of foreign serum. This type of serum (horse or rabbit antilymphocyte antibodies) is used in the prevention and treatment of transplant rejection. Serum sickness reactions may also occur with the administration of certain drugs (e.g., antimicrobials such as penicillin and sulfonamides).

#### *Pathophysiology*

The pathogenesis of serum sickness lies in the union of soluble antigens (foreign serum proteins) and immunoglobulins of the IgM and IgG classes. The complexes formed in these interactions are not properly cleared by the reticuloendothelial system (RES) because of their small size, which tends to defy phagocytosis. The complexes can then bind complement, initiating the complement cascade and resulting in chemotaxis, vasodilation, and cell lysis.

The chemotactic factors released by the complement cascade lead to an influx of phagocytes, which tend to intensify the inflammatory response. Complement also aids in phagocytosis by depositing complement protein fragments onto the immune complexes. Large complexes are then successfully removed by the RES (Figure 66-7).

The antigen-antibody reactions of serum sickness occur in many organs, but the kidneys, choroid plexus, joints, skin, and lungs are primarily affected. Itching and discomfort at the injection site are usually the first symptoms noted. These are followed by lymphadenopathy, fever, uritcaria or erythematous rash, angioedema of the face, and joint pain. Splenomegaly, abdominal pain, headache, nausea, and vomiting may also occur.

People with complement deficiencies have an increased risk of developing chronic type III disease. Intermediate-sized complexes remain in circulation and are large enough to activate complement.[17]

#### *Collaborative care management*

Serum sickness is a self-limiting disease. Mild symptoms respond well to antihistamines and salicylates. More severe symptoms are treated with steroids such as prednisone, and relief of symptoms is often obtained within hours. Epinephrine is given if an anaphylactic reaction occurs.

**Patient/family education.** Patients who develop serum sickness are concerned about the cause of this unusual disorder and how it is treated. They are taught that serum sickness is a reaction to foreign protein, that symptoms can be controlled, and that it is a self-limiting condition. Patients placed on steroids are taught about the actions and potential side effects of the drug and cautioned against abruptly discontinuing the medication. Persons who develop serum sickness are encouraged to inform future health care providers of their tendency toward hypersensitivity.

## TYPE IV HYPERSENSITIVITIES

Cell-mediated immune mechanisms function in host defense against chronic bacterial and fungal infections, rejection of

**clinical pathway** *Blood Transfusion*

COLLABORATIVE CARE PATH

| ADDRESSOGRAPH | COLLABORATIVE CARE PATH<br>Case Type: Blood Transfusion<br>DRG# Expected LOS<br>Key: Nurse's initials = Met; U = Unmet → continued | | | | |
|---|---|---|---|---|---|
| **PROBLEM LIST AND OUTCOMES** | **DATE UNIT #1** | **DATE UNIT #2** | **DATE UNIT #3** | **DATE UNIT #4** | **DATE UNIT #5** |
| Knowledge deficit R/T need for transfusion | Verbalizes understanding of procedure and symptoms to report to nurse | → | → | → | → |
| Potential for adverse physical effects R/T administration of blood component therapy | Demonstrates no adverse physical effects (see symptoms of reaction) | → | → | → | → |
| TESTS | H&H postinfusion as ordered | → | → | → | → |
| TREATMENTS | Check Nsg H&P for previous transfusion history | → | → | → | → |
| | Establish adequate IV access | → | → | → | → |
| | VS: prior to getting unit from bloodbank, 15min & 1hr after start of infusion | → | | | |
| | Temperature elevation prior to starting blood is reported to physician for pre-treatment | → | → | → | → |
| | Blood started within 15 minutes of pickup | → | → | → | → |
| | Infuse unit in 4 hours or less as ordered | → | → | → | → |
| | Check VS immediately & 1 hr after infusion is complete | → | → | → | → |
| | Transfusion form completed and returned to blood bank within 8 hours. | → | → | → | → |
| | **If symptoms occur:**<br>Stop infusion, notify MD & Blood Bank, KVO IV w/ normal saline, assist pt. to collect specimens, send bag, tubing, & saline to lab, complete suspected transfusion reaction form. | → | → | → | → |
| | **Benign urticaria (hives with no other symptoms):**<br>Notify physician, treat symptoms, no workup required | | | | |
| TEACHING | Instruct pt. & family on rationale, procedure symptoms to report of reaction | Reinforce teaching | → | → | → |
| SYMPTOMS OF REACTION:<br><br>Reviewed blood/tissue 1/21/97<br>BLDTRANS.WK1 1/14/97 | Fever (1.5° F rise), Chills, Shock, Excessive bleeding, BP change, Chest pain, Back pain, Flushing, Oliguria, Dyspnea, Hemoglobinuria, Urticaria (Hives) with other symptoms, Jaundice, Itching, Rash | | | | |

*H&H*, Hgb & Hct; *KVO*, keep vein open.

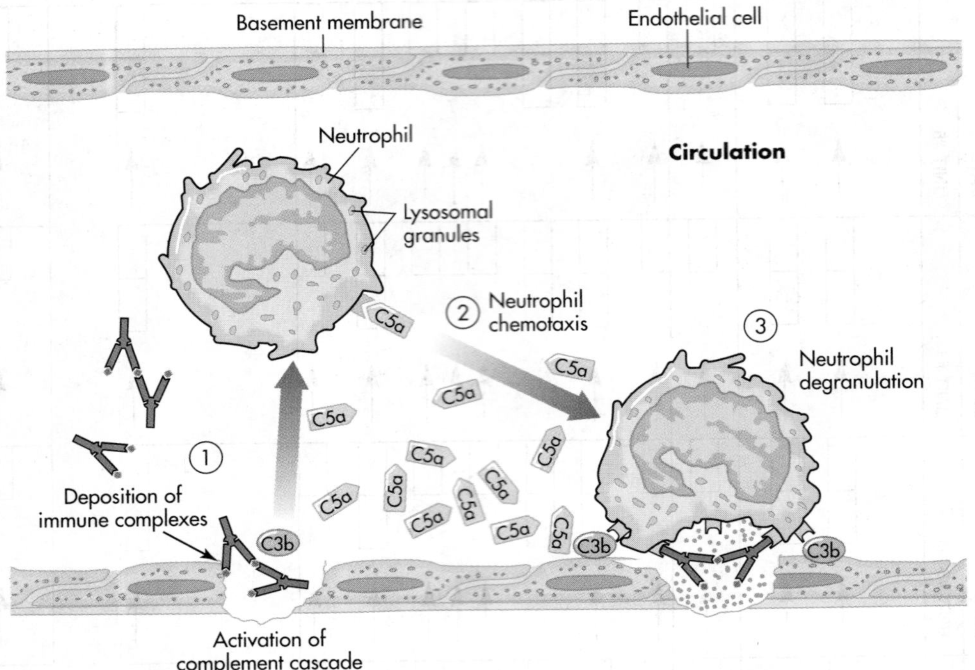


**fig. 66-7** Mechanism of type III, immune complex-mediated reactions. Immune complexes are deposited in the vessels or other healthy tissue, where they activate the complement cascade and generate complement fragments including C5a *(1)*. C5a is chemotactic for neutrophils, which migrate into the inflamed area *(2)* and attach to the IgG and C3b in the immune complexes. The neutrophils degranulate a variety of degradative enzymes that destroy healthy tissues *(3)*.

foreign tissue cells, and surveillance for cancer cells. However, they can also produce adverse effects in the form of delayed-type hypersensitivity. Three major areas of concern are hypersensitivity reactions in response to infection, contact dermatitis, and tissue transplant rejection.

## Etiology/Epidemiology

Type IV hypersensitivity reactions are elicited by environmental antigens that are not usually immunogenic but become so after binding with carrier proteins in the host. Once bound, they evoke a cell-mediated immune response. Industrial chemicals, detergents, cosmetics, foods, metals, clothing, and topical medications are common causes of type IV hypersensitivity.[12]

## Pathophysiology

Type IV hypersensitivities are cell mediated (delayed type), involving T cells. Macrophages pick up antigens identified as "foreign" to the body. These macrophages take pieces of the antigen and present them to the T lymphocytes, which become sensitized for this type of antigen. The next time the person comes in contact with this particular antigen, the sensitized lymphocyte can form cytotoxic T cells or activate nonspecific phagocytic cells. The cytotoxic T lymphocyte can destroy the antigen directly by breaking down the cell membrane, causing lysis and cell death. This direct approach also appears to be the major factor in acute allograft rejection. The sensitized T lymphocyte can also activate nonspecific phagocytic cells (macrophages and polymorphonuclear leukocytes) through release of lymphokines.

Allergic contact dermatitis is one of the most commonly encountered types of allergic disease. Usually, both the route of sensitization and the clinical manifestations are produced by direct dermal contact. The allergen attaches to skin proteins, which function as haptens to stimulate the proliferation of a T cell population sensitized to the allergen. After sensitization, subsequent contact with the contact allergen leads to the formation of an erythematous, vesiculated (blistered) lesion. The inflamed area itches, burns, or stings.

The body's reaction to the tubercle bacillus *(Mycobacterium tuberculosis)* is another classic example of a type IV hypersensitivity. The organism itself is not directly toxic to human cells or tissues. As a result, the tubercle bacillus may invade the tissues of a nonsensitized host and establish residence in the host tissues, causing virtually no damage. However, in the course of time, as the organism sheds antigenic material, the cell-mediated immune response is triggered. The sensitized lymphocytes and the activated macrophages attack not only the organism, but also the tissues surrounding the organism. This process is aimed at destroying the foreign organism; however, in the course of the attack, tissue destruction may result. The lesions associated with tuberculosis (such as caseation necrosis cavitation) and general toxemia are results of the hypersensitivity.

After the initial sensitization with the infectious organism, subsequent contact with the tuberculosis organism or even an extract of a purified protein from the organism will elicit a hypersensitivity reaction. This is the basis of the Mantoux tuberculin skin test. The skin rashes of smallpox and measles and the lesions of herpes simplex virus are all examples of an infectious type IV hypersensitivity.

The transfer of healthy tissues and organs from one individual to replace damaged or diseased tissues of another has been surgically possible for many years. The early attempts at transplant failed because of the rejection process resulting from type IV hypersensitivity. The foreign tissue or organ serves as the allergen against which the cell-mediated response is directed. Cytotoxic T lymphocytes attack and destroy the tissues directly, resulting in destruction of transplanted tissues.[12] A discussion of organ transplantation can be found in Chapter 68.

### Collaborative Care Management

Treatment for contact dermatitis includes elimination of known allergens, decreased exposure, or both. Topical antiinflammatory agents such as corticosteroid creams may be useful in reducing the discomfort associated with itching and decreasing healing time. For severe reactions, systemic corticosteroids and antihistamines may be necessary. There is no specific treatment, other than treatment of the underlying infection, for hypersensitivity reactions to infective agents. If secondary infection develops as a result of the patient scratching the area, antibiotics may be prescribed. Immunosuppression therapy is used to control transplant rejection.

#### *Patient/family education*

The nurse provides the patient and family with information about the hypersensitivity reaction and how it manifests. Specific antigens are identified and strategies are planned to reduce exposure. Patients with contact dermatitis are cautioned to avoid scratching lesions, because scratching may further spread the lesion or infect the site. Patients are also taught how to use topical corticosteroids. Patients on systemic corticosteroids are cautioned to never abruptly stop taking their medication. (For care of the person with contact dermatitis, see Chapter 63.)

## AUTOIMMUNE DISEASES

### ETIOLOGY/EPIDEMIOLOGY

Autoimmunity is influenced by genetic, hormonal, viral, and environmental factors. Autoimmune disorders run in families but are not passed on by simple mendelian inheritance. Human leukocyte antigens and non-HLA antigens have a well-documented association with certain autoimmune diseases. Many individuals with these same gene markings, however, do not have the disease, so there is not a direct relationship between the genetic predisposition and the disease.

The role of sex hormones is not clearly understood, but autoimmune diseases are far more common in females than in males. Interactions of the host with certain environmental agents such as bacteria, viruses, drugs, and toxins have been shown to initiate autoimmune disease.

### PATHOPHYSIOLOGY

Autoimmunity, the formation of antibodies against self-tissues, is a natural phenomenon. Certain responses such as autorecognition and autoimmunity are necessary for removal of dead cells and cell components and response to viral and microbial infections.[14] However, when autoimmunity causes injury to host cells it is described as pathological. A self-attack is referred to as autoimmune disease or autohypersensitivity. These self-reactions are not usually immunologically initiated; the etiological (causative) agent lies outside the immune system, but the immune response serves as the pathogenic mechanism.

The meaning of the presence of autoantibodies and autosensitive T cell clones is not clear. These self-reactive immunoglobulins are often associated with pathological states in the body but can also be isolated from the serum of "normal" individuals, especially older persons.

The process of autoimmunity is theorized to include the following:

1. *Release of sequestered antigens.* If an antigen does not come into contact with the immune system during fetal development when the tolerance to self normally develops, it is not registered as a self-antigen, and clones of immunoresponsive cells to that antigen remain reactive. As a result of trauma or infection, these antigens may be exposed to the immune system. If this occurs, they elicit an immune response.
2. *Activation of suppressed clones.* If one of the functions of the suppressor T cell is to suppress the activation of certain clones of potentially self-reactive T cells or B cells, it is possible through some loss of suppressor function that these "forbidden" clones are allowed to proliferate.
3. *Synthesis of cross-reactive antibodies.* Antibodies synthesized in response to certain foreign antigens may have cross-reactivity with similar antigenic components within human tissues. Contact with antigens called heterophile antigens may trigger the production of autoantibodies. This process is theorized to account for the damage of rheumatic heart disease.
4. *Alteration of self-antigens.* Normal body proteins may be altered by chemicals, infectious organisms, or therapeutic drugs and present new antigenically active groups to the immune system. Autoimmune hemolytic anemia may result from alteration of the Rh antigens of the RBC, rendering it antigenic. Certain antibiotics can have a similar effect.

Autoimmune disorders are grouped into categories according to the part of the body involved. Autoimmune diseases that are organ specific produce chronic inflammatory changes in a specific organ. Non–organ-specific autoimmune disorders are characterized by chronic inflammatory changes in many different organs and tissues throughout the body. Box 66-9 presents a listing of selected autoimmune disorders.

**box 66-9** *Classification of Autoimmune Disorders*

**ORGAN SPECIFIC**

**Blood**
Autoimmune hemolytic anemia
Idiopathic thrombocytopenic purpura

**Heart**
Rheumatic fever

**Central Nervous System**
Multiple sclerosis
Guillain-Barré syndrome

**Muscles**
Myasthenia gravis

**Endocrine System**
Addison's disease
Autoimmune thyroiditis (Hashimoto's disease)
Graves' disease
Hypothyroidism

**Eye**
Uveitis

**Gastrointestinal System**
Pernicious anemia
Ulcerative colitis

**Kidneys**
Glomerulonephritis
Goodpasture's syndrome

**Skin**
Pemphigus vulgaris

**NON–ORGAN SPECIFIC**
Systemic lupus erythematosus
Rheumatoid arthritis
Progressive systemic sclerosis

## COLLABORATIVE CARE MANAGEMENT

The treatment for many autoimmune disorders is suppression of cell-mediated immunity and control of clinical manifestations. This is primarily achieved through treatment with systemic corticosteroid therapy. Initial doses of 60 mg of oral prednisone often bring about a noticeable decrease in symptoms. Once symptoms are controlled, dosages are slowly decreased and then discontinued until the next exacerbation occurs. Cytotoxic drugs, such as cyclosphosphamide, azathioprine, and methotrexate, are sometimes prescribed for patients with severe or persistent manifestations. The treatment of specific autoimmune disorders is discussed in other chapters of this textbook.

### Patient/Family Education

Emotional support and patient teaching are important aspects of care for the person with an autoimmune disorder. Patients are taught about their illness, symptoms that warn of exacerbation, and any measures that may reduce the chances for exacerbation. Teaching includes manifestations that need to be reported immediately versus those that can be managed at home.

The nurse encourages patients to eat a well-balanced diet, maintain daily exercise patterns that do not result in fatigue, and get plenty of rest and sleep. The nurse also explains the anticipated benefit of prescribed medications, dosage schedules, and adverse effects, especially when the patient is taking corticosteroids or other immunosuppressive drugs. The patient is cautioned against abruptly withdrawing steroid medications, because abrupt cessation can result in adrenal insufficiency or crisis. The nurse stresses the importance of close follow-up care. The patient and family are referred to available local support groups.

# CHRONIC FATIGUE SYNDROME

Chronic fatigue syndrome (CFS), also known as chronic fatigue immune dysfunction syndrome (CFIDS) or myalgic encephalomyelitis, is a condition in which the person experiences extreme fatigue that appears suddenly and that eventually becomes debilitating. Accompanying manifestations, such as muscle aches, headache, weakness, joint discomfort, and tender lymph nodes, may go unnoticed because they are similar to the flu. Unlike the flu, however, the fatigue and other symptoms remain or reappear frequently.

## ETIOLOGY/EPIDEMIOLOGY

The exact cause of CFS is unknown. At one time, the Epstein-Barr virus (EBV) was thought to be the causative agent because elevated levels of the antibodies were noted in individuals with CFS. The disease also occurs, however, in people who lack EBV antibodies. The human herpesvirus-6, enteroviruses, and retroviruses are being investigated as possible etiologies.[15]

Chronic fatigue syndrome is diagnosed in females two to four times more often than in males, which may be due to biological, psychological, or social factors (see the Research Box). Mislabeled as "yuppie flu" because it was mainly reported by well-educated, affluent women in their thirties and forties, CFS is now recognized in people of all ages, races, and socioeconomic classes.[15]

## PATHOPHYSIOLOGY

Chronic fatigue syndrome often begins after an infection such as gastroenteritis, bronchitis, or a cold. In other cases, no specific triggering event can be identified, or its occurrence may be associated with a period of severe stress. Because the symptoms of CFS are also associated with many other conditions, it is difficult to diagnose. The Centers for Disease Control and Prevention (CDC) published the first case definition of CFS and a set of diagnostic criteria in 1988. A revised set of diagnostic criteria is presented in Box 66-10. The primary clinical manifestation of CFS is prolonged, debilitating fatigue that is accompanied by any or all of the symptoms listed in Box 66-10.

## COLLABORATIVE CARE MANAGEMENT

Treatments for CFS have included antiviral agents, antidepressants, and immunomodulators, but these treatments have

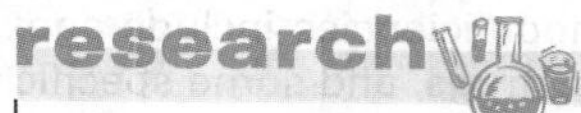

Reference: Jason LA et al: Prevalence of chronic fatigue syndrome related symptoms among nurses, *Eval Health Prof* 16(4):385, 1993.

This study attempted to determine the prevalence of CFS-related symptoms in a sample of nurses. Chronic fatigue syndrome has not been acknowledged by many physicians, and data about its incidence and prevalence have been highly variable when physician diagnosing and reporting has been the sole method of data collection.

Mailed questionnaires were sent to a sample of 3400 nurses drawn from the roster of the Illinois Nurses Association (INA) and American Holistic Nurses Association (AHNA). A 43% response rate was obtained with 1474 completed questionnaires. The participants were asked to respond to the presence of the diagnostic symptoms, major and minor, established to support a diagnosis of CFS. Two hundred participants met these criteria by self-report. The respondents exhibited a prevalence rate significantly higher than those reported in previous studies. Members of AHNA had rates almost twice as high as members of the INA. The researchers suggest that this may reflect a natural gravitation of persons with chronic illness to the holistic group or a greater willingness to acknowledge the legitimacy of fatigue-related symptoms. It is also possible that nurses are exposed in their work to more viruses and have a naturally higher prevalence rate than the general population. Further validation and replication of these findings are indicated.

not been proven effective. Other treatments are aimed at controlling symptoms. Nonsteroidal antiinflammatory drugs may be beneficial in reducing body aches or fever, and nonsedating antihistamines have been useful for relieving allergic symptoms. There is no cure for this disease.[15]

## Patient/Family Education

Education for the patient with CFS should focus on how to manage fatigue to improve functioning and quality of life. The nurse carefully assesses the extent of the patient's symptoms and physical limitations. The nurse helps the patient identify potential triggers of fatigue and avoid situations or activities that adversely affect energy levels. Periods of activity are scheduled at times when the patient feels better and are alternated with rest periods. Exercise may seem contradictory in the presence of fatigue, but exercise improves conditioning and energy utilization and can restore energy. The patient is assisted to develop an individualized exercise program that incorporates a gradual increase in intensity and duration. The nurse helps the patient incorporate exercise in a manner that does not exacerbate fatigue, yet promotes regular participation.

A well-balanced diet is essential to promote adequate energy stores and is therefore another important part of patient/family education. Nighttime sleep should be as free of interruption as possible, and daytime naps are avoided if they interfere with nighttime rest. The patient may also benefit from relaxation, meditation, massage, imagery, touch, music, or biofeedback. See Chapter 6 for these and other measures to help reduce stress.

### box 66-10 Diagnostic Criteria for Chronic Fatigue Syndrome

**MAJOR CRITERIA**

- New, debilitating, persistent, or relapsing fatigue that does not improve with rest and that has impaired daily activities by 50% over 6 months or longer
- Absence of other conditions that produce similar symptoms (autoimmune diseases, cardiac disease, cancer, HIV, AIDS, gastrointestinal dysfunction, hepatic problems, endocrine dysfunction, neuromuscular complaints, psychiatric problems, etc.)

**MINOR CRITERIA**

- Four or more of the 11 symptoms must be present

**SYMPTOMS**

Symptoms must have started after fatigue onset and persisted or recurred for 6 months or longer.

- Low-grade fever
- Sore throat
- Cervical or axillary adenopathy
- Generalized muscular weakness
- Myalgia
- Prolonged fatigue (≥24 hours) after exercise that was previously tolerated
- New onset of generalized headache
- Noninflammatory arthritis
- Complaints of one or more of the following: photophobia, transient visual scotomata, forgetfulness, excessive irritability, confusion, difficulty thinking, inability to concentrate, or depression
- Insomnia or hypersomnia
- Onset of symptoms over a few hours to a few days

**SIGNS**

Must be documented by a physician on two occasions at least 1 month apart.

- Low-grade fever
- Nonexudative pharyngitis
- Palpable/tender cervical or axillary lymph nodes of 2 cm or less

Modified from Holmes GP et al: *Ann Intern Med* 108(3):387, 1998.

Chronic fatigue syndrome is a disease with overwhelming subjective symptoms, and patients experiencing persistent debilitating fatigue are commonly treated with overt skepticism if not direct accusations of malingering by health care providers. The symptoms of CFS may be attributed to life stress, unhappiness, or "female problems," or simply labeled as psychosomatic. The nurse plays an important role in reassuring the patient about both the validity and severity of the symptoms. The nurse also includes the family in all discussions and teaching sessions about disease etiology and management. Family support is critical to the patient because many occupational and family roles may have to be reduced or eliminated in the face of overwhelming fatigue (see the Research Box). The nurse also encourages the patient and family to contact local or national CFS support groups to establish a network of information and support for dealing with this debilitating chronic disease.

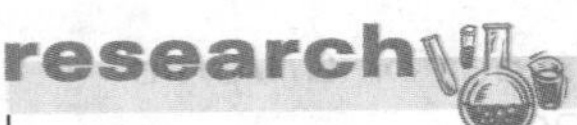

Reference: Goodwin SS: The marital relationship and health in women with chronic fatigue and immune dysfunction syndrome: views of wives and husbands, *Nurs Res* 46(3):138, 1997.

The purpose of this study was to describe the association between the marital relationship and the health of the wife with CFS. A convenience sample of 130 couples was recruited from CFS support groups and advertisements in disease-related publications. This resulted in a fairly affluent and well-educated sample. Seventy-seven percent of the women had worked full time before their illness; only 3% currently worked full time.

Instruments were administered that measured marital adjustment, marital empathy, marital support, and symptom presence and severity. The analysis showed no significant differences in the husbands' and wives' reported marital relationship variables. Significant differences were found between the wives' and husbands' descriptions of symptoms. Wives reported significantly more symptoms. Small but significant associations were found between scores for marital adjustment, conflict and support, and CFS symptoms. Higher education and longer marriages were associated with fewer problems and symptoms, but the relationship between these findings remains elusive.

## critical thinking QUESTIONS

1 You are caring for two patients, Tim and Ralph. Tim has a primary immune deficiency disease, and Ralph has a secondary immune deficiency. How will the care of these two patients be similar? How will it be different?

2 Mary resided in a warm and dry climate for 30 years. After moving to another climate, Mary developed an upper respiratory infection for which her physician gave her an injection of penicillin. Mary stated that she had never been given penicillin, but that she had no known allergies. Within 20 minutes after receiving the penicillin, Mary developed symptoms of anaphylaxis. What explanation can be given for Mary's reaction?

3 Mrs. M. was recently diagnosed with seasonal allergies to pollens and grasses. She cleans houses 3 days each week, and she lives in a house near a large open field. What additional data, if any, do you need to collect from Mrs. M., and what do you need to include in her teaching plan?

4 Compare and contrast the four mechanisms of autoimmune disease. Name several diseases that may result from each of these mechanisms. What aspect of care is similar for any patient with autoimmune disease, regardless of cause?

## chapter SUMMARY

### IMMUNODEFICIENCIES

- Primary immunodeficiencies are congenital. Secondary immunodeficiencies are acquired. Major factors in the development of secondary immunodeficiencies include age, nutrition, exposure to chemicals, drugs, and some specific disorders.
- Immunosuppression may be induced by antigen or antibody administration, immunological methods, irradiation, or immunosuppressive drugs.
- Screening tests for immune deficiencies include ESR, absolute lymphocyte or neutrophil counts, $CH_{50}$, antibody titers, and skin tests.
- Collaborative care management of primary immunodeficiencies consists of identification of those at risk, prevention of or effective treatment of infection, and replacement of missing humoral or cellular immunological factors.
- Nursing management of the immunodeficient person involves prevention of infection, maintaining optimal nutrition and hydration, and educating the patient and family.

### GAMMOPATHIES

- Gammopathies are excessive production of immunoglobulins, the most common of which is multiple myeloma.
- Multiple myeloma is characterized by proliferation of plasma cells causing lytic bone disease, bone marrow infiltration, and proliferation of monoclonal proteins.
- Collaborative care management of patients with multiple myeloma is aimed at decreasing tumor bulk, preventing kidney failure, and preventing further bone demineralization.
- Nursing management of patients with multiple myeloma includes preventing pathological fractures, fluid volume overload, and infection.

### HYPERSENSITIVITIES

- Hypersensitivity reactions are exaggerated or inappropriate responses to specific antigens (allergens).
- Hypersensitivities depend on the responsiveness of the host to the allergen; the amount, nature, route of entrance, and timing of exposure of the allergen; site of the allergen–immune mediator reaction; and the host's threshold of reactivity.
- Type I hypersensitivities are mediated by IgE immunoglobulins attached to mast cells and basophils. When the allergen binds to the IgE, histamine, kinins, chemotactic factors, and active products of arachidonic metabolism are released, producing a systemic reaction (anaphylaxis) or a local allergic reaction.
- Hypersensitivity can occur only in a previously sensitized host.
- Anaphylaxis is the most severe form of type I hypersensitivity.
- Drug therapy for anaphylaxis consists of epinephrine, antihistamines, and corticosteroids.
- Nursing management of the patient in anaphylaxis includes maintaining a patent airway and adequate cardiac output.
- Atopic illnesses are typically initiated by seasonal or perennial allergens. Symptoms are usually not life threatening but are uncomfortable.
- Collaborative care management of atopic illnesses includes use of antihistamines, decongestants, steroids, and cromolyn sodium; avoidance of exposure to allergens; and immunotherapy (hyposensitization).
- Nursing management of patients with atopic allergy includes education about hyposensitization, side effects of medications, and recognition and treatment of anaphylaxis.

- Type II hypersensitivities are cytotoxic reactions from the direct binding of IgG or IgM immunoglobulins to the surface of foreign cells to trigger cell lysis; an example is blood transfusion reactions.
- The major antigens of RBCs are AB antigens, Rh antigens, and HLA antigens.
- Rh-positive reactions indicate presence of antigen Rh-D; Rh-negative indicates absence of antigen Rh-D.
- Immunological reactions to blood transfusions include acute hemolytic, febrile nonhemolytic, mild allergic, anaphylactic, delayed hemolytic, graft-versus-host diseases, and noncardiac pulmonary edema.
- Nonimmunological complications of blood transfusions include circulatory overload, sepsis, and transmission of diseases.
- Type III hypersensitivities are characterized by immune complexes formed by the union of IgM or IgG with soluble antigens.
- Type IV hypersensitivities are cell mediated (T cell reactions).

### AUTOIMMUNE DISEASES

- Autoimmune diseases are the result of an immune response to one's own antigens, usually because of an agent from outside the immune system.
- Immune intolerance may be the result of sequestered antigens, activation of suppressed clones, synthesis of cross-reactive antibodies, or alteration of self-antigens.

### CHRONIC FATIGUE SYNDROME

- The exact cause of chronic fatigue syndrome is unknown.
- The person with CFS experiences unrelenting fatigue, which may become debilitating.
- Nursing management of CFS includes educating the patient and family about the syndrome, methods to conserve energy, and measures to reduce fatigue.

## References


1. Alexanian R, Dimopoulos M: The treatment of multiple myeloma, *N Engl J Med* 330(7):484, 1994.
2. Attal M, Harousseau JL, Stoppa AM, et al: A prospective, randomized trial of autologous bone marrow transplantation and chemotherapy in multiple myeloma, *N Engl J Med* 335(2):91, 1996.
3. Barlogie B, Alexanian R, Jagannath S: Plasma cell dyscrasias, *JAMA* 268(20):2946, 1992.
4. Buckley RH: *Immunological disorders,* St Louis, 1993, Mosby.
5. Buckley RH, Schiff RI: The use of intravenous immune globulin in immunodeficiency diseases, *N Engl J Med* 324(2):110, 1991.
6. Burke MM, Walsh MB: *Gerontologic nursing,* St Louis, 1997, Mosby.
7. Gibbs L: Assessment and management of the allergic patient, *ORL Head Neck Nurs* 10(3):10, 1992.
8. Hadden JW, Smith DL: Immunopharmacology, immunomodulation, and immunotherapy, *JAMA* 268(20):2964, 1992.
9. Huston CJ: Emergency! Hemolytic transfusion reaction, *Am J Nurs* 96(3):47, 1996.
10. Immune Deficiency Foundation: *IDF patient/family handbook for primary immune deficiency diseases,* Towson, Md, 1993.
11. Lockey RF: Future trends in allergy and immunology, *JAMA* 268(20):2991, 1992.
12. McCance K, Huether S: *Pathophysiology,* ed 2, St Louis, 1997, Mosby.
13. Mudge-Grout CL: *Immunologic disorders,* St Louis, 1993, Mosby.
14. Nakamura MC, Nakamura RM: Contemporary concepts of autoimmunity and autoimmune diseases, *J Clin Lab Anal* 6(5):275, 1992.
15. Office of Communications, National Institute of Allergy and Infectious Diseases, and National Institutes of Health, Fact Sheet: *Chronic fatigue syndrome,* 1995, Public Health Service, US Department of Health and Human Services.
16. Pavel J: Red cell transfusions for anemia, *Semin Oncol Nurs* 6(2):117, 1990.
17. Roitt I: *Essential immunology,* ed 8, London, 1994, Blackwell.
18. Rosen FS, Cooper MD, Wedgewood RJ: Medical progress: the primary immunodeficiencies, *N Engl J Med* 333(7):431, 1995.
19. Smeltzer SC, Bare BG: *Textbook of medical-surgical nursing,* ed 8, Philadelphia, 1996, JB Lippincott.
20. Stites DP, Terr AL, editors: *Basic and clinical immunology,* Norwalk, Conn, 1991, Appleton & Lange.
21. Wener M: Basic clinical immunology, *Hosp Med* 28(1):69, 1992.

# chapter 67 MANAGEMENT OF PERSONS WITH HIV Infection and AIDS

CAROL GREEN-NIGRO

## objectives

*After studying this chapter, the learner should be able to:*

1 Describe the epidemiology of human immunodeficiency virus (HIV) infection.
2 Identify the causative agent of HIV infection.
3 Discuss the infection and replication process of the human immunodeficiency virus.
4 Distinguish among primary, secondary, and tertiary prevention measures for HIV infection.
5 Describe the continuum of HIV infection.
6 Differentiate among the various opportunistic infections that can occur with AIDS in regard to symptomatology and collaborative care management.
7 Compare and contrast nursing care for the person with HIV infection and acquired immunodeficiency syndrome.
8 Discuss the role of the nurse in addressing psychosocial, legal, and ethical issues related to the HIV epidemic.

One of the most dreaded communicable diseases is infection with the human immunodeficiency virus (HIV). Individuals infected with this virus have, thus far, eventually developed acquired immunodeficiency syndrome (AIDS). AIDS severely compromises the body's ability to fight various infections and some forms of cancer. The incidence of HIV infection and AIDS continues to increase steadily in the United States and worldwide. Therefore nurses must understand the critical concepts related to this problem. AIDS was considered to be universally fatal until quite recently. Advances in drug treatment, however, are delaying the onset of AIDS for selected persons infected with HIV and are providing new hope to thousands of infected individuals.

## ETIOLOGY

AIDS is an acquired viral disease. The virus integrates itself into CD4 (T4 helper) cells, causing immune dysfunction and rendering the infected person unusually susceptible to life-threatening infections and malignancies.

The origin of HIV is still largely unknown. Evidence appears to support the hypothesis of an African origin, because an AIDS-like illness was reported in the early 1960s in central Africa. It is further hypothesized that the most likely source of human infection was from nonhuman primates.

The causative agent of AIDS is infection with HIV, a human retrovirus that belongs to the lentivirus subfamily. Several human retroviruses have been identified. Two of them, HIV-1 and HIV-2, have been associated with T4 helper cell depletion, resulting in loss of cellular immunity characterized by AIDS. HIV-1 is the predominant cause of AIDS in the United States, accounting for greater than 95% of AIDS cases. HIV-2 seems to be limited in geographical distribution and is most prevalent in West Africa.[16] Although there has been scientific and clinical progress and development of new treatments and comprehensive models of care, HIV disease remains an incurable disease, spreading rapidly throughout the United States and worldwide.

## EPIDEMIOLOGY

AIDS was first identified in the United States in 1981 following an investigation of five Los Angeles men who developed unusual opportunistic infections. By late 1982 at least 100 cases had been reported, and the Centers for Disease Control and Prevention (CDC) issued its first definition of AIDS. In 1985 HIV was identified as the causative agent of AIDS. Since then, the CDC has revised its definition of AIDS twice, in an effort to more accurately reflect an evolving understanding of the infection process. To date, at least 270,000 Americans have died of AIDS.[6]

Throughout the pandemic, the numbers of those infected have steadily increased each year. Early in the U.S. epidemic, more than 80% of those infected were homosexual men. Currently, less than 50% of infections occur in this group. Those persons now at greatest risk for acquiring HIV infection in the United States include heterosexual women and their children and intravenous (IV) drug users. African Americans and Hispanic Americans are at greater risk than white Americans.[8]

AIDS is the number one killer of persons between the ages of 25 and 44 years.[25] In 1994 the World Health Organization estimated that worldwide there were 17 million people infected with HIV, over 6 million people had died of AIDS, 5 million children had been orphaned, and approximately 8500 people are becoming infected daily, in spite of vigorous educational efforts.[29] In South Africa 15% of women of childbearing age are infected with HIV. By the year 2010, the life expectancy in Zambia is expected to fall from 66 to 33 years; in Zimbabwe, from 70 to 40 years; and in Uganda, from 59 to 31 years. Statistics show that HIV infection rates are rapidly increasing in India, Southeast Asia, Latin America, and the Caribbean, because most of the new pharmacological treatments are beyond the financial reach of these populations.[29]

Before the introduction of the newer drug therapies the mortality rate in the United States approached 80% within 3 years of an AIDS diagnosis. It may be even higher in developing countries where treatment is virtually nonexistent[18] (Figure 67-1).

The routes for transmission of HIV are well documented: (1) directly from person to person by sexual contact; (2) direct inoculation with contaminated blood products, needles, or syringes; and (3) from infected mother to her fetus or newborn. HIV has been cultured from a variety of body fluids, including blood, semen, vaginal secretions, cerebrospinal fluid (CSF), saliva, tears, and breast milk. However, blood, semen, and vaginal secretions are the primary routes of infection. Epidemiological studies indicate that transmission through body fluids such as saliva, tears, and breast milk is inefficient and unlikely to produce infection.

HIV is a blood-borne sexually transmitted disease (STD). Sexual practices, including vaginal or anal penetration without a condom and possibly oral sexual practices, are associated with a high risk for infection. The use of contaminated needles for subcutaneous (SC), intramuscular (IM), or IV injection represents another serious risk for HIV infection. Women who are HIV infected may pass the virus on to their newborns via three potential routes: during gestation, during delivery, and rarely via breast milk.[19] HIV is not transmitted by casual contact, including sneezing, coughing, spitting, handshakes, contact with potential secretions on toilet seats, bathtubs, showers, swimming pools, utensils, dishes, or linens used by infected persons. Mosquito bites are not a source of infection.

Blood transfusions are not a significant source of HIV infection today. In the United States each unit of donated blood is tested for HIV infection, as well as several other blood-borne infections, such as hepatitis B. HIV screening of blood products has been conducted since 1985; only recipients of transfusions before that time were at risk for infection via the blood supply. It is possible, however, for a contaminated unit of blood to test negative for HIV if the donor has not yet formed antibodies to the virus at the time of donation. Nevertheless, the risk of exposure to HIV via the U.S. blood supply is estimated to be 1 in 400,000 units of blood.[8]

Risk factors for HIV infection are summarized in the following Risk Factors Box. The risk of HIV transmission to health care workers prompted the development and imple-

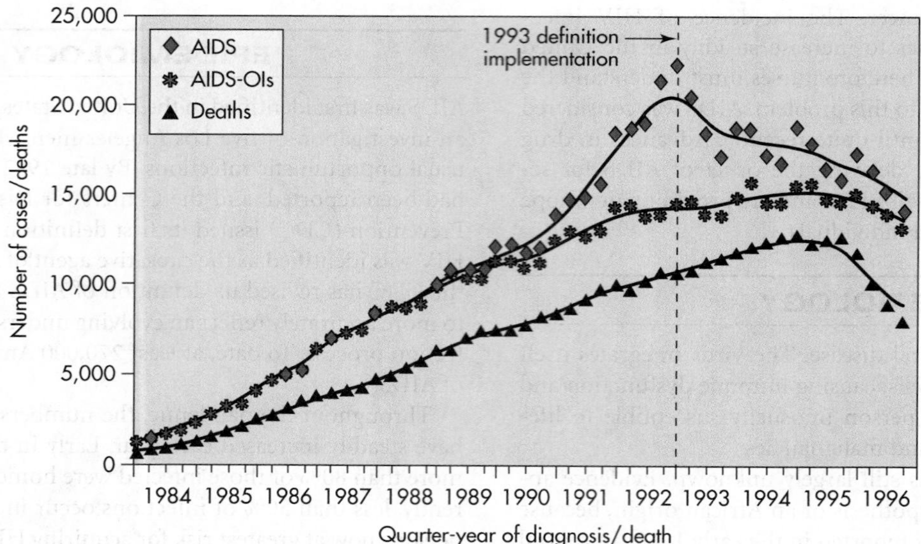


Estimated incidence of AIDS includes persons diagnosed using the 1993 expanded surveillance case definition, including persons whose AIDS diagnosis is based on evidence of severe immunosuppression (HIV-infected persons with $CD4^+$ T-lymphocyte counts of less than 200 cells/μL or a $CD4^+$ percentage of less than 14). Estimated AIDS-OI incidence is the sum of the observed AIDS-OI incidence and the incidence based on estimated dates of AIDS-OI diagnosis for persons reported with AIDS based only on severe immunosuppression. Points on the figure represent quarterly incidence; lines represent smoothed incidence. Estimated incidence of AIDS, estimated AIDS-OIs, and deaths are all adjusted for delays in reporting. Estimates are not adjusted for incomplete reporting of cases.

**fig. 67-1** Estimated incidence of AIDS, AIDS-opportunistic illness (AIDS-OI), and deaths in persons with AIDS, adjusted for delays in reporting, by quarter-year of diagnosis/death, United States, 1984-1996.

mentation of Standard Precautions by the Centers for Disease Control and Prevention. These principles, which are summarized in Box 67-1, are to be used in the care of all patients at all times.

## PATHOPHYSIOLOGY

The natural history of HIV infection is associated with an unpredictable course of disease progression. Many patients undergo a prolonged period of clinically silent infection, often lasting more than 10 years.[16,17] Although the virus is consistently detectable throughout this time, patients typically have only subtle immunological alterations. Once the patient becomes symptomatic, however, decreases in the number of T4 helper cells can be detected and viral replication increases.

The life cycle of HIV is similar to that of the other retroviruses. Mature virions interact with specific host receptors and then use the host cell for viral replication. HIV interacts with the CD4 glycoprotein, which occurs on the membrane of specific cells, primarily the CD4+ (T4) helper lymphocytes. The CD4 protein may also be found on the surface of several other cells as well, including some monocytes, macrophages, glial cells, and gastrointestinal (GI) cells. Presence of the CD4 glycoprotein allows the virus to fuse to the host cell. The viral core is subsequently injected into the cell cytoplasm, where the viral ribonucleic acid (RNA) genome is translated into deoxyribonucleic acid (DNA) by a retroviral enzyme called reverse transcriptase. Infection and subsequent viral replication eventually deplete the host's T4 helper cells, resulting in a dramatic loss of the protective immune response against invading microorganisms (Figure 67-2).

Several potential cofactors may be associated with HIV disease progression. These cofactors, which may be viral, host, or environmental, are thought to directly influence the replication of HIV or the severity of its pathogenic effects. Viral cofactors that may influence the progression of the disease include herpes simplex virus, cytomegalovirus (CMV), and Epstein-Barr virus (EBV). Host cofactors may include a variety of cytokines and intracellular mediators. Environmental cofactors may include repeated exposure to HIV, which may induce hyperactivation of the immune system, resulting in an expansion of the pool of HIV-replicating cells. As viral replication increases, depleting the body of T4 lymphocytes, the body's defense mechanisms are progressively weakened. Infections that were once disarmed by the healthy immune system are eventually able to cause serious and potentially life-threatening disease. The spectrum of HIV infection ranges from asymptomatic infection to potentially life-threatening opportunistic infection. In the past, clinicians used an informal staging system categorizing patients as (1) HIV positive, (2) having AIDS-related complex (ARC), and (3) having AIDS. In this staging system, HIV positive referred to those patients who were completely asymptomatic but HIV positive. Those patients classified as having ARC exhibited constitutional symptoms, including persistent generalized lymphadenopathy, persistent fevers, involuntary weight loss, or diarrhea. Any patient who had experienced an opportunistic infection was classified as having AIDS.

**risk factors**

**HIV**

Sexual practices*
- Unprotected sex
- Multiple sexual partners
- Anal or oral sexual activity
- Improper condom use or condom breakage
- Open sore, lesions, or irritation in the genital area

Contaminated blood

Contaminated needles

Occupational exposure
- All health care workers—acute care, long-term care, and home care
- Dental workers
- Corrections officers and law enforcement personnel

Perinatal exposure (during pregnancy, birth, or breast feeding)

NOTE: Approximately 25% of children of HIV-positive mothers are infected with the virus.

*NOTE: An individual's sexual *practices* create the HIV risk, not sexual preferences. The only true "safe sex" involves two seronegative partners in a monogamous relationship.

**box 67-1 Centers for Disease Control and Prevention Standard Precautions**

NOTE: Standard Precautions are to be used in the care of all patients and apply to blood, all body fluids, secretions, excretions (except sweat), and nonintact skin and mucous membranes.

1. Hands must be washed between patient contacts and after contact with blood or body fluids, or articles contaminated by them. Hands are also to be washed after gloves are removed.
2. Gloves are worn for any patient contact involving blood, body fluids, secretions, excretions, nonintact skin, mucous membranes, or contact with contaminated items.
3. Gowns should be worn if soiling with blood or body fluid is likely to occur.
4. Masks, eye protection, or face shields should be worn if splashes or sprays of blood or body fluids are likely during care activities.
5. All sharp instruments and needles should be discarded in a puncture-resistant container. Needles should be disposed of uncapped.
6. Contaminated linen should be placed in leak-proof bags for disposal.

NOTE: Additional precautions may be necessary to decrease the risk of infection with specific organisms. These precautions are instituted on a per patient basis and include airborne precautions, droplet precautions, and contact precautions. They are not needed for care of the HIV-positive patient unless a specific opportunistic infection such as tuberculosis is also present.

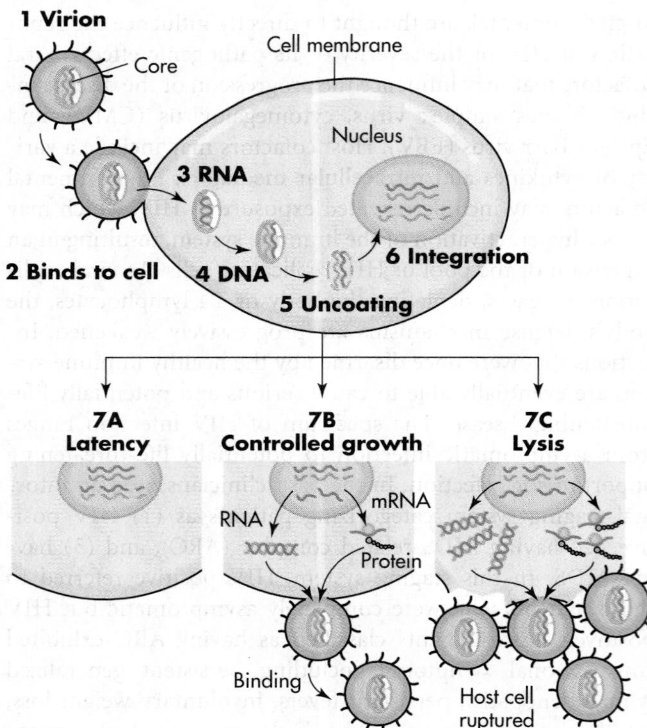


**fig. 67-2** Infection and cellular outcomes of HIV. HIV infection begins *(1)* when a virion, or virus particle, *(2)* binds to the outside of a susceptible cell and fuses with it, *(3)* injecting the core proteins and two strands of viral RNA. Uncoating occurs, during which the core proteins are removed and the viral RNA is released into the infected cell's cytoplasm. *(4)* The double-stranded DNA (provirus) migrates to the nucleus, *(5)* uncoats itself, and *(6)* is integrated into the cell's own DNA. The provirus then can either: *(7A)* remain latent or *(7B)* activate cellular mechanisms to copy its genes into RNA, some of which are translated into viral proteins or ribosomes. The proteins and additional RNA then are assembled into new virions that bud from the cell. The process can take place slowly, sparing the host cell *(7B)*, or so rapidly that the cell is lysed or ruptured *(7C)*.

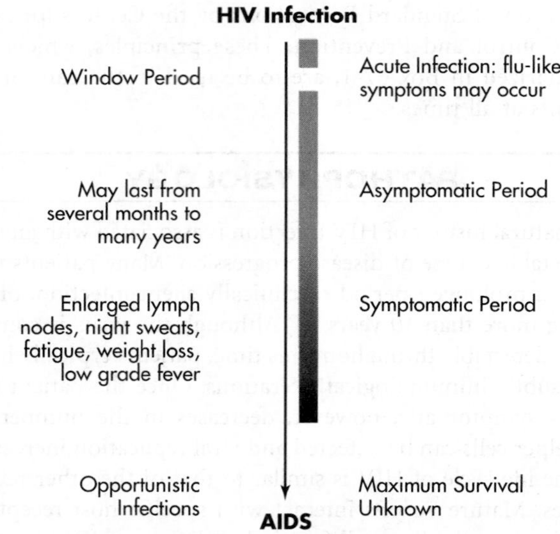


**fig. 67-3** Spectrum of HIV infection. The initial phase of infection may be followed by a period of latency that may last from several months to several years. During this time the person may be completely asymptomatic or experience only mild symptoms. AIDS is said to exist when opportunistic infections are present and CD4 cell counts drop.

Today, clinicians have become much more sophisticated about the staging of HIV disease. Although we usually refer to end-stage HIV disease as AIDS, most clinicians use the CDC Classification System for HIV Infection in Adults, which has evolved over time and incorporates both laboratory and clinical stages[8] (Box 67-2).

The early phase of infection with HIV varies from person to person. Some individuals experience symptoms similar to the flu or mononucleosis, consisting of fever, fatigue, nausea, vomiting, headache, rash, or lymphadenopathy. Symptoms may be mild or serious enough to warrant hospitalization. It is during this time that the viral load (amount of HIV virus present) is very high, CD4 helper cells drop dramatically, and the person converts to seropositive HIV status.[24]

The initial phase of infection may be followed by a period of latency that may last from several months to 10 years or more. During this time the person may be completely asymptomatic or experience only mild symptoms such as fatigue. As the immune system becomes further compromised, the symptoms of AIDS develop. Figure 67-3 depicts the spectrum of HIV infection. Clinical manifestations associated with AIDS are primarily those of opportunistic infections. Common symptoms are summarized in Box 67-3. Symptoms of specific opportunistic infections are presented later in this chapter. Figure 67-4 illustrates the scope of HIV infection in the body and the range of organs and tissues that can be affected.

## PULMONARY SYSTEM

Pulmonary infection from a variety of organisms is a constant threat to the person with HIV and is often the first manifestation of HIV infection. Pulmonary infections can very rapidly lead to severe hypoxemia. Compromised respiratory function can also result from pulmonary infiltration by a lymphoma.

## GASTROINTESTINAL SYSTEM

Numerous GI problems associated with opportunistic infections or chemotherapy may plague the person with HIV infection. Common problems include granulomatous hepatitis, drug toxicity hepatitis, or coinfection with a hepatitis virus; masses or lesions from lymphomas and Kaposi's sarcoma; cholangitis or cholestasis; and pancreatic lesions. Patients may have difficulty eating or swallowing or may experience dyspepsia, diarrhea, and weight loss. Loss of lean muscle mass is common.

## box 67-2 1993 Revised Human Immunodeficiency Virus Classification for Adolescents and Adults

The revised Centers for Disease Control and Prevention (CDC) classification system for human immunodeficiency virus (HIV)–infected adolescents and adults emphasizes the importance of CD4+ lymphocyte testing in the clinical management of HIV-infected clients. The classification system is divided into laboratory and clinical categories as follows.

**LABORATORY CATEGORIES**

Category 1: greater than or equal to 500 CD4+ cells
Category 2: 200 to 499 CD4+ cells
Category 3: less than 200 CD4+ cells

**CLINICAL CATEGORIES**

Category A: One or more of the following conditions occurring in an adolescent or adult with documented HIV infection. Conditions listed in categories B and C must not have occurred.

- Asymptomatic HIV infection
- Persistent generalized lymphadenopathy
- Acute (primary) HIV infection with accompanying illness or history of acute HIV infection

Category B: Symptomatic conditions occurring in an HIV-infected adolescent or adult that are not included among conditions listed in clinical category C and that meet at least one of the following criteria:

- The conditions are attributed to HIV infection or are indicative of a defect in cell-mediated immunity.
- The conditions are considered by physicians to have a clinical course or management that is complicated by HIV infection.

Examples of conditions in clinical category B include but are not limited to:

- Bacterial endocarditis, meningitis, pneumonia, or sepsis
- Candidiasis, vulvovaginal; persistent for more than 1 month, or poorly responsive to therapy
- Candidiasis, oropharyngeal (thrush)
- Cervical dysplasia, severe; or carcinoma
- Constitutional symptoms, such as fever (>38.5° C) or diarrhea lasting more than 1 month
- Hairy leukoplakia, oral
- Herpes zoster (shingles), involving at least two distinct episodes or more than one dermatome
- Idiopathic thrombocytopenic purpura
- Listeriosis
- *Mycobacterium tuberculosis* infection, pulmonary
- Nocardiosis
- Pelvic inflammatory disease
- Peripheral neuropathy

Category C: Any condition listed in the 1987 surveillance case definition for AIDS and affecting an adolescent or an adult. For classification purposes, once a category C condition has occurred, the person will remain in category C.

- The conditions in clinical category C are strongly associated with severe immunodeficiency, occur frequently in HIV-infected patients, and cause serious morbidity or mortality.
- According to the proposed classification system, HIV-infected patients would be classified on the basis of both:
  - The lowest accurate (not necessarily the most recent) CD4+ lymphocyte determination
  - The most severe clinical condition diagnosed regardless of the patient's current clinical condition

From CDC: Revised classification system for HIV infection and expanded surveillance case definition for AIDS among adolescents and adults, *MMWR* 41(51):961, 1992.

### NERVOUS SYSTEM

HIV is able to cross the blood-brain and blood-CSF barriers and infect microglia and possibly other cells, resulting in encephalopathy. This process results in loss of cognitive and motor function. Many of the opportunistic infections can affect the central nervous system. Peripheral neuropathy with loss of motor function often occurs.

### INTEGUMENT

The initial infection with HIV may cause macular roseola eruptions. Later, seborrheic dermatitis, psoriasis, and Kaposi's sarcoma lesions can occur, along with cutaneous infections.

### OPHTHALMIC

HIV makes the eye vulnerable to invasion by CMV, which can result in blurring of vision and decreased acuity. The lesions are progressive unless treated early and aggressively.

### HEMATOLOGICAL SYSTEM

Thrombocytopenia, anemia, and neutropenia may be present with HIV. The causes of these problems are not known, but HIV may decrease production, and drug side effects include both impaired production and increased destruction of blood cells.

### CARDIOVASCULAR SYSTEM

Opportunistic infections can result in pericarditis or myocarditis. Severe pulmonary hypertension associated with multiple episodes of *Pneumocystis carinii* pneumonia can cause right ventricular failure.

### ENDOCRINE

Although not as common as other system dysfunctions, all endocrine glands can be infiltrated with HIV. The adrenal gland is most commonly affected. Adrenal insufficiency may result from invasion by infective organisms, invasion by a tumor, or drug therapy.

### MUSCULOSKELETAL

Rheumatological manifestations of HIV are common and vary from mild to severe. Arthralgia is seen with acute infection and may also result from drug therapy. Myalgia,

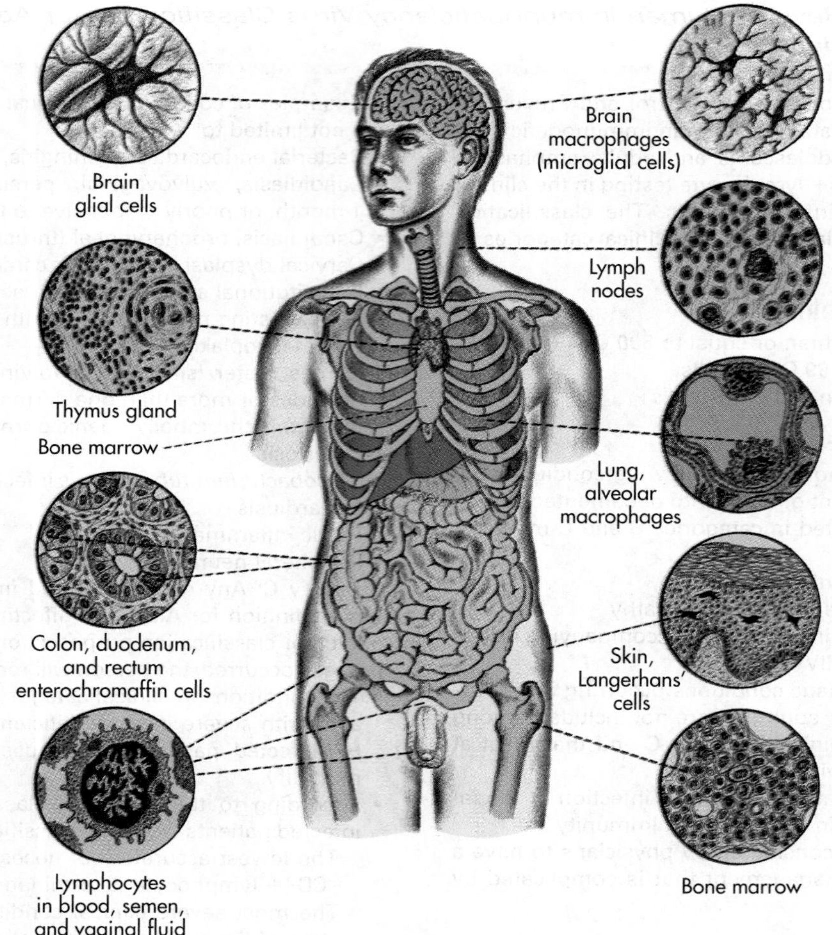


**fig. 67-4** Distribution of tissues that can be infected by human immunodeficiency virus (HIV). Infection is closely linked to the presence of CD4 receptors on host tissue, with the possible exceptions of glial cells in the brain and chromaffin cells in the colon, duodenum, and rectum.

**box 67-3** ***clinical manifestations***

***HIV/AIDS***

| | |
|---|---|
| Chills and fever | Malaise |
| Night sweats | Fatigue |
| Dry productive cough | Oral lesions |
| Dyspnea | Skin rash |
| Lethargy | Abdominal discomfort |
| Confusion | Diarrhea |
| Stiff neck | Weight loss |
| Seizures | Lymphadenopathy |
| Headache | Progressive generalized edema |

weakness, and wasting may also occur. The cause of these rheumatological manifestations is unknown.

### FLUID AND ELECTROLYTE BALANCE

Fluid and electrolyte imbalance and acid-base imbalance from a variety of causes, including renal, GI, endocrine, or drugs, can occur. Prerenal or acute renal failure caused by hypovolemia, interstitial nephritis caused by invasion of renal tissue by tumors or infective organisms, and glomerulosclerosis from HIV-associated nephropathy are common causes of renal dysfunction in HIV.

## COLLABORATIVE CARE MANAGEMENT

### DIAGNOSTIC TESTS

The most commonly used test is the enzyme-linked immunosorbent assay (ELISA), a highly specific test for HIV antibodies that has a sensitivity of 93.4% to 99.6%. A positive ELISA must be confirmed by the Western blot technique. Both the ELISA and the Western blot depend on antibody formation. Approximately 90% of the population will form antibodies in response to HIV exposure within 6 weeks to 3 months after exposure, although this period may be as long as 6 months. A negative antibody test may occur in the "window phase" between the dates of actual exposure leading to infection and development of detectable serum antibodies. Because newborns maintain maternal antibodies for as long as 18 months, antibody testing is unreliable until the infant is 18 months of age.

Plasma HIV RNA levels measure the amount of virus in the person's serum, which is a reflection of active viral replication, or viral load. The steeper the rate of increase in plasma HIV RNA, the greater the risk of disease progression. A plasma HIV RNA level of less than 10,000 copies/ml is considered low risk for development of AIDS. Levels between 10,000 and 100,000 copies/ml double the risk for developing AIDS, and greater than 100,000 copies/ml indicates a high risk for developing AIDS.[4]

HIV RNA levels are measured periodically to determine the risk for disease progression and to monitor the effectiveness of antiretroviral therapy. Therapy is aimed at reducing plasma HIV RNA levels to below the limit of detection by the sensitive assay. For accuracy, two HIV RNA assays are completed within 1 to 2 weeks of one another, and both values are used to establish a baseline for the infected person. It is important for nurses to understand that suppression of HIV RNA levels to below the limits of detection does not mean that HIV infection has been eliminated or that virus replication has been halted completely. It simply means that HIV levels have been reduced to such a degree that they cannot be measured by present methods.[28] New tests that can detect viral loads of between 20 and 100 copies/ml are being developed, which will improve the practitioner's ability to predict HIV disease progression.

CD4+ T cell counts are used to measure the extent of immune damage that has occurred as a result of HIV infection and its complications and to monitor the immunological benefit of antiretroviral therapy. CD4 refers to the particular protein expressed on the surface of the T4 helper lymphocyte. CD4+ T cell counts should be obtained on all newly diagnosed persons, and once every 6 months as long as the counts are above 500 cells/ml. When the counts decrease to less than 500 cells/ml, the assessments should occur every 3 months. Should the cell count fall below 200, more frequent monitoring is advisable.[2] Figure 67-5 illustrates the relationship among HIV viral load, CD4 lymphocyte counts, and HIV antibody levels at various points along the HIV continuum.

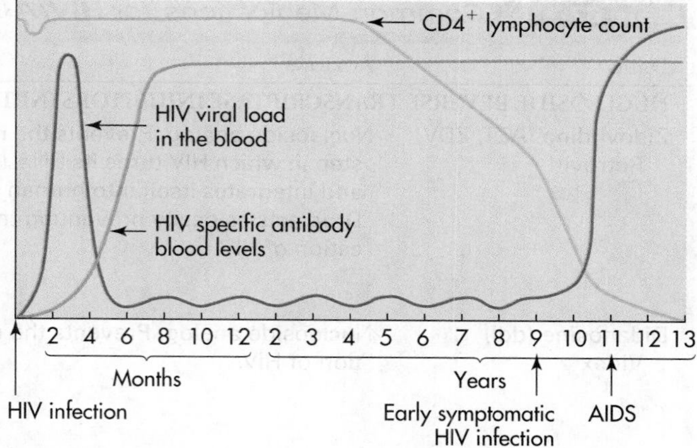


**fig. 67-5** Viral load in the blood and CD4+ lymphocyte counts over the spectrum of human immunodeficiency virus (HIV) infection.

## MEDICATIONS

Recent drug developments have significantly improved the outlook for many HIV-infected persons. Three classes of antiretroviral agents have been approved for use in the United States for the management of HIV. Antiviral agents such as AZT, ddl, d4T, 3TC, and ddC are known as nucleoside reverse transcriptase inhibitors (NRTIs). They act by being incorporated into the growing DNA chains by viral reverse transcriptase, thereby interfering with viral replication.[27] Protease inhibitors (PIs) such as Indinavir, Ritonavir, Saquinavir, and Nelfinavir prevent HIV from making the long protein molecules necessary to create new viruses, thus halting replication of infectious virus. Viruses continue to be produced, but they are noninfectious and unable to attack and destroy immune cells. Nevirapine and Delavirudine are nonnucleoside reverse transcriptase inhibitors (NNRTIs, or nucleoside analogs), the newest group of drugs that block HIV replication by protecting non–HIV infected cells.[12]

Protease inhibitors have stimulated much interest among practitioners recently because they produce greater viral suppression than NRTIs alone. When used in combination with NRTIs, they produce viral suppression and immune recovery to a far greater degree than earlier treatment protocols.[12] Table 67-1 summarizes the medications commonly used to treat AIDS. New drugs are undergoing constant development and clinical trials.

Studies are being undertaken to determine the risk versus benefit of placing newly infected persons on antiretroviral agents such as the protease inhibitors. Many clinicians used to take a conservative approach to treatment and simply monitor asymptomatic patients, but it is currently believed to be essential to initiate aggressive drug therapy before significant immunodepletion occurs. Box 67-4 presents a summary of risk versus benefit of early therapy for HIV.

All patients with advanced HIV disease, and those with symptomatic HIV infection without AIDS, should be treated with PI and NRTI combinations regardless of plasma viral levels.[24] The goal of treatment with combination therapy is to suppress plasma HIV RNA levels to below detectable levels on assay and elevate CD4+ T cell counts for as long as possible.[23]

There are disadvantages to antiretroviral therapy, and the decision to initiate therapy must be a joint decision between the patient and practitioner. Patients are likely to experience drug toxicity and numerous side effects, must be compliant with large pill burdens and tightly prescribed administration regimens, be able to financially withstand the cost of therapy, and be prepared to accept that drug resistance can develop, which may limit future therapy options. Drug resistance can develop if viral replication is not sufficiently suppressed or the person is already infected with a resistant strain of HIV.[10,25] See Table 67-2 for indications for initiation of antiretroviral therapy.

**table 67-1** *Common Medications for **HIV/AIDS***

| Drug | Actions | Interventions |
|---|---|---|
| **NUCLEOSIDE REVERSE TRANSCRIPTASE INHIBITORS (NRTIs)** | | |
| Zidovudine (AZT, ZDV) Retrovir | Nucleoside analog. Prevents the initial step in which HIV turns its RNA into DNA and integrates itself into human genes. Drug acts as decoy preventing the replication of HIV. | Monitor for bone marrow suppression: anemia or neutropenia.<br>Monitor for GI intolerance, headache, insomnia, asthenia.<br>Monitor for drug effectiveness.<br>Teach patient/significant other regarding drug dose, schedule, and possible adverse effects. |
| Didanosine (ddl) Videx | Nucleoside analog. Prevents the replication of HIV. | Monitor for drug-associated pancreatitis, peripheral neuropathy, nausea, diarrhea.<br>Monitor CD4+ cell counts for drug effectiveness.<br>Teach patient/significant other regarding drug dose, schedule, and possible adverse effects. |
| Zalcitabine (ddC) Hivid | Nucleoside analog. Prevents replication of HIV. | Monitor for peripheral neuropathy, stomatitis.<br>Monitor for drug effectiveness.<br>Teach patient/significant other regarding drug dose, schedule, and possible adverse effects. |
| Stavudine (d4T) Zerit | Nucleoside analog. Prevents replication of HIV. | Monitor for peripheral neuropathy.<br>Monitor for drug effectiveness.<br>Teach patient/significant other regarding drug dose, schedule, and possible adverse effects. |
| Lamivudine (3TC) Epivir | Nucleoside analog. Prevents replication of HIV. | Minimal toxicity noted.<br>Monitor for drug effectiveness.<br>Teach patient/significant other regarding drug dose, schedule and possible adverse effects. |
| **NONNUCLEOSIDE REVERSE TRANSCRIPTASE INHIBITORS (NNRTIs)** | | |
| Nevirapine Viramune | Blocks HIV replication by protecting non–HIV infected cells. | Monitor for rash.<br>Monitor drug effectiveness.<br>Drug interactions: rifampin, rifabutin, oral contraceptives, protease inhibitors. |
| Delavirudine Rescriptor | Blocks HIV replication. | Monitor for rash.<br>Do not administer within 1 hour of antacids.<br>Drug interactions: terfenadine, astemizole, alprazolam, midazolam, cisapride, rifabutin, rifampin.<br>Drugs that decrease drug effectiveness: phenytoin, carbamazepine, phenobarbital.<br>Increases drug levels of clarithromycin, dapsone, rifabutin, ergot alkaloids, dihydropyrides, quinidine, warfarin, indinavir, saquinavir. |

Adapted from Guidelines for the use of antiretroviral agents in HIV-infected adults and adolescents, Panel on Clinical Practices for Treatment of HIV Infection, Department of Health and Human Services and the Henry J. Kaiser Foundation, 1997.

*Continued*

Recommendations for antiretroviral treatment of established HIV infection include one highly active protease inhibitor combined with two NRTIs. The most effective combination is believed to be ZDV, ddl, and Nevirapine. An alternative protocol that is less likely to produce sustained viral suppression is Saquinavir with ZDV and ddl. The use of two NRTIs without a protease inhibitor has shown some nonsustained viral suppression but is not generally recommended therapy. Monotherapies (NRTIs used alone) are no longer prescribed because they do not produce adequate viral suppression. There is one exception, however. ZDV may be used prophylactically for pregnant women who have low HIV RNA and high CD4+ T cell counts to prevent perinatal transmission of HIV.[24]

## TREATMENTS

There are no special treatments in the early stages of HIV infection. Respiratory treatments may become necessary as the patient's disease progresses. Standard Precautions are necessary when the patient is hospitalized or being treated at home. Treatments associated with maintenance and improvement of nutritional status also usually become necessary. Specific treatments related to opportunistic infections are discussed later in this chapter.

## SURGICAL MANAGEMENT

Surgery does not play a role in the standard management of HIV. Patients may undergo surgical biopsy of skin lesions,

**table 67-1** *Common Medications for* ***HIV/AIDS*** *—cont'd*

| Drug | Actions | Interventions |
|---|---|---|
| **PROTEASE INHIBITORS** | | |
| Indinavir<br>Crixivan | Protease inhibitors interfere with the step of HIV replication in which the virus makes the long protein chains necessary to reproduce itself from DNA. The long protein chains must be cut by a protease enzyme in order to turn the proteins into the correct length to create HIV. Protease inhibitors interfere with this step of the process, rendering the virus noninfectious. The defective viruses are not able to infect or destroy immune cells. | Monitor CD4+ cells and viral load for drug effectiveness.<br>Teach patient/significant other about drug dose, schedule, and potential side effects.<br>Monitor for nephrolithiasis, GI intolerance, headache, asthenia, blurred vision, dizziness, rash, metallic taste, thrombocytopenia.<br>Drug interactions: rifampin, terfenadine, astemizole, cisapride, triazolam, ergot alkaloids, ketoconazole, rifabutin, midazolam. |
| Ritonavir<br>Norvir | Protease inhibitor. | Monitor CD4+ cells and viral load for drug effectiveness.<br>Teach patient/significant other about drug dose, schedule, and potential side effects.<br>Monitor for GI intolerance, nausea, vomiting, diarrhea.<br>Must be kept refrigerated.<br>Drug interactions: meperidine, piroxicam, flecainide, quinidine, rifampin, bepridil, terfenadine, cisapride, bupropion, clozapine, diazepam, alprazolam, dihydroergotamine, ergotamine. |
| Saquinavir<br>Invirase | Protease inhibitor. | Monitor CD4+ cells and viral load for drug effectiveness.<br>Teach patient/significant other about drug dose, schedule, and potential side effects.<br>Monitor for GI intolerance, nausea, diarrhea, headache, elevated transaminase enzymes.<br>Drug interactions: rifampin, rifabutin, astemizole, terfenadine, cisapride. |
| Nelfinavir<br>Viracept | Protease inhibitor. | Monitor for diarrhea.<br>Monitor CD4+ cells and viral load for drug effectiveness.<br>Teach patient/significant other about drug dose, schedule, and potential side effects.<br>Drug interactions: rifampin, astemizole, terfenadine, cisapride, midazolam, triazolam. |

treatment of internal Kaposi's sarcoma lesions that do not respond to chemotherapy, or drainage of abscesses or other sites of infection. These all represent management of AIDS complications, however, and are not primary therapies for HIV disease.

## DIET

No special diet is indicated for persons with HIV, even though nutritional deficits commonly develop from both the disease itself and the opportunistic infections associated with the disease. Anorexia, nausea, and diarrhea are commonly associated with antiretroviral therapy, further contributing to nutritional alterations. Many persons with AIDS develop wasting syndrome, especially toward the later stages of the disease. Wasting syndrome is defined as nonvoluntary weight loss in excess of 10% to 15% of normal baseline weight. The exact etiology of this problem is unknown but is thought to be related to chronic diarrhea, fatigue, and weakness.[15]

Each patient must be carefully monitored to evaluate the adequacy of intake, any food intolerances, and ways to promote a high-calorie, high-protein diet. In the later stages of disease when infections and muscle wasting prevent adequate food intake, intravenous nutritional support may be necessary.

## ACTIVITY

There are no activity restrictions for the person with HIV infection. A pattern of rest and activity should be encouraged to help maintain lean body mass and prevent deconditioning. More frequent rest periods are necessary for individuals with AIDS because fatigue is a common complaint. During acute infections, activity may need to be restricted. Increasing the

**box 67-4** *Risks and Benefits of Early Antiretroviral Therapy for the Asymptomatic HIV-Infected Person*

**POTENTIAL BENEFITS**
Potential reduction of viral load
Control of viral replication and mutation
Prevention of progressive immunodeficiency
Delayed progression from HIV infection to AIDS
Decreased risk of resistance
Decreased risk of drug toxicity

**POTENTIAL RISKS**
Reduction in quality of life from side effects of drug therapy
Earlier development of drug resistance
Limited choice of antiretroviral agents for future use
Risk of dissemination of drug-resistant virus
Unknown long-term toxicity
Unknown duration of drug effectiveness

Adapted from: Guidelines for use of antiretrovial agents in HIV-infected adults and adolescents, Panel on Clinical Practices for Treatment of HIV Infection, US Department of Health and Human Services, *Federal Register* 1997.

**table 67-2** *Indications for Initiation of Antiretroviral Therapy*

| Clinical Category | CD4+ T Cell Count HIV RNA Count | Recommendation |
|---|---|---|
| Asymptomatic | CD4+ T cells >500/mm³ **AND** HIV RNA <10,000 (bDNA) | Some clinicians treat; others delay therapy and monitor. |
| Asymptomatic | CD4+ T cells <500/mm³ **OR** HIV RNA >10,000 (bDNA) | Treatment should be offered. |
| Symptomatic (opportunistic infection) | Any value | Treat. |

From Guidelines for use of antiretrovial agents in HIV-infected adults and adolescents. Panel on Clinical Practices for Treatment of HIV Infection. US Department of Health and Human Services, *Federal Register* 1997.

amount of sleep and reducing sleep interruptions may be effective in increasing the adequacy of sleep and combating fatigue.

## REFERRALS

Most HIV-infected individuals are managed on an outpatient basis. The goal of such management is for the person to receive needed services so that hospitalizations can be minimized. Consequently, a thorough assessment of the HIV-infected person should be undertaken to determine whether referrals need to be made. In some settings the nurse assumes responsibility for making referrals. In other settings, a multidisciplinary approach is taken and referrals are made by various health care professionals.

Social services should always be consulted, whether the HIV-infected person is being cared for at home or hospitalized. This department can ensure that the individual is covered by insurance or has completed the application process for Medicare/Medicaid and associated programs. Social services can also facilitate contact with a variety of services, including food pantries, housing assistance, community AIDS services, and support groups. For hospitalized persons, social services can assist with discharge planning and facilitating home care.

Referrals are commonly made to physical and occupational therapists. Some HIV-infected individuals have difficulty with exercise tolerance related to acute infections, fever, fatigue, and nutritional deficits. Physical and occupational therapy may assist HIV-infected persons to return to their usual state of activity and improve their ability to perform activities of daily living (ADL).

Psychiatry, counseling, or spiritual referrals may be desired or requested by HIV-infected individuals. The nurse must assess each individual and family for need and interest in such referrals.

# NURSING MANAGEMENT

## ASSESSMENT

Health assessment of all patients should include an appraisal of potential risk factors for HIV infection. Obtaining a complete, accurate sexual history, including past and present sexual activities, requires skillful interviewing techniques and a professional relationship based on trust. Nurses need to be able to explain the need for information on intimate sexual activities and phrase questions in appropriate but comprehensive terms. The sexual history, in addition to identifying individuals at risk for possible HIV infection, may also be an opportunity for health education concerning risk reduction and disease prevention. A discussion on taking a sexual history can be found in Chapter 46.

Some HIV-infected individuals are asymptomatic; others report nonspecific flulike symptoms. The clinical diversity of HIV infection can make identification and assessment of infected persons difficult.

### Subjective Data

Subjective data to be collected include:
- History of clinical manifestations
- Complaints of weakness, fatigue, headache
- Factors that exacerbate or relieve symptoms
- Ability to perform ADL
- Current drug therapy
- Risk factors (unprotected sex, exposure to blood or blood products, needle exposure, use of mood-altering drugs)
- Other medical problems
- Surgical history

### Objective Data

Objective data to be collected include:
- Nutritional status, height, weight
- Vital signs

Skin and mucous membranes (turgor, temperature, integrity, lesions)
Respiratory status (cough, dyspnea, crackles, wheezing)
Gastrointestinal status (presence of diarrhea)
Urinary status (urine color, quality, and quantity)
Mental status (alertness, orientation)

## NURSING DIAGNOSES

Nursing diagnoses are determined from analysis of subjective and objective data. Nursing diagnoses for the person with HIV disease may include but are not limited to:

| Diagnostic Title | Possible Etiological Factors |
|---|---|
| Infection, risk for | Compromised host defenses |
| Fatigue | Chronic inflammatory process and side effects of drug therapy |
| Nutrition, altered: less than body requirements | Anorexia, drug side effects, and chronic diarrhea |
| Home maintenance management, impaired | Compromised functional abilities and inadequate support mechanisms |
| Individual coping, ineffective | Chronic worry and uncertainty about the future |

## EXPECTED OUTCOMES

Expected outcomes for the person with HIV disease may include but are not limited to:

1. Reports absence of infection, or infections diagnosed early in disease process
2a. Engages in routine daily activities with fatigue controlled
b. Maintains independence in self-care ADL
c. Demonstrates usual strength and activity tolerance
3a. Maintains present weight or weight returns to within 0.5 kg of preillness weight
b. Verbalizes need to increase caloric intake; increases intake to 3000 calories per day as tolerated
4. Verbalizes and demonstrates adequate knowledge of disease, communicability, treatment, and lifestyle changes as applicable
5. Engages in communication that leads to sharing of feelings, decision making, and problem resolution as pertinent

## INTERVENTIONS

The HIV epidemic in the United States has brought not only a dismal prognosis, but also severe social stigmatization, public fear, and a growing number of legal and ethical concerns. Nurses providing care in a variety of settings face many of these issues, which may jeopardize the quality of patient care. In addition, nurses caring for patients face many personal stresses, including fear of personal contamination and disease transmission to family members, and burnout related to caring for terminally ill patients. The professional commitment needed by nurses who provide care to HIV-infected patients requires clarification of personal values and renewed dedication to service (Research Box).

**research**

Reference: Sherman DW: Nurses' willingness to care for AIDS patients and spirituality, social support, and death anxiety, *Image J Nurs Sch* 28(3):205, 1996.

The purpose of this study was to examine relationships among spirituality, perceived social support, death anxiety, and nurses' willingness to care for AIDS patients. Willingness to care was found to positively correlate with spirituality and perceived social support and negatively correlate with death anxiety. The study supported the theoretical proposition that the fear of death paralyzes action and limits one's ability to make responsible choices and to relate lovingly and freely with others. The study findings suggest that social support at work from administrators and colleagues, as well as the support of patients themselves, is important to nurses and should be fostered.

### Preventing Infection

Infection is a major complication of HIV disease. The already compromised AIDS patient, in particular, should be protected from further infectious insults. The nurse assesses vital signs, skin integrity, mucous membranes, respiratory status, GI function, and mental status routinely for signs of possible infection. Laboratory data are monitored when signs of infection are present. A low-microbial diet is recommended for patients with absolute neutrophil counts less than 500 cells/cm$^3$. Meticulous asepsis is essential. The nurse educates significant others about signs and symptoms of infection and when to report them to the clinician. Visitors can be requested to wear a mask during their visit to the home if the patient's condition warrants it. People who have infections such as colds or chickenpox should be requested not to visit until they are well. The nurse reinforces the importance of protective strategies, including hand washing, scrupulous personal hygiene, dietary precautions such as thorough cooking of meat products and washing of fruits and vegetables, removing fresh plants and flowers from the patient's bedroom, and keeping inside pets clean.[4]

The need for control of infections does not mean that the person with HIV disease should be socially isolated. It is important that patients maintain their usual social relationships to prevent feelings of social isolation. Many communities have support groups with volunteers who are willing to make routine visits or become the patient's "buddy" or "ally." This can be of particular benefit to those who have no nearby relatives or significant others.

### Controlling Fatigue

Fatigue is a primary complaint of persons with HIV infection or disease; therefore energy management is important. The nurse assesses the person's ability to perform ADL, including weakness, gait, endurance, strength, and motor and sensory deficits. The importance of balancing activities with rest periods in order to maintain normal or near-normal activity levels is stressed. The nurse encourages the person to respect the signs and symptoms of fatigue that require activity reduction. The use of assistive devices, such as wheelchairs, canes, or walkers, can help conserve energy.

The nurse and patient may have to be creative in finding ways to help the person conserve energy in a home environment that may be less than optimal, because the majority of persons are cared for at home. The environment is arranged so that items of necessity are within easy reach. Items used on a daily basis need to be conveniently located and readily accessible. Attention is also given to conditions that may jeopardize patient safety, such as stairs, use of small scatter rugs, or lack of handrails on bathtubs. The support of family members or significant others can be solicited to assist with home maintenance tasks to prevent or relieve the patient's fatigue.

Environmental stimuli can be adjusted so that a restful night's sleep can be achieved. At least 6 to 8 hours of sleep per night are recommended. Visits from a home health aide or community support group can be arranged to assist the patient with physical care when necessary.

### Promoting Nutrition

The nutritional status of patients with HIV disease may range from normal to extreme cachexia during the later stages of illness. Therefore the nurse assesses the nutritional status of all patients and promotes food intake necessary to maintain maximal health and functioning. Current dietary intake, likes and dislikes, dietary restrictions, food tolerances and intolerances, and height and weight are all assessed. The nurse also assesses the patient for signs of altered nutrition or factors that may alter nutritional status, such as decreased weight, decreased muscle strength and tone, decreased energy levels, anorexia, nausea, stomatitis, impaired swallowing, or self-care deficits. Teaching includes the side effects of drug therapy that may affect nutritional status. Eating toast or dry crackers and drinking beverages 30 minutes before meals may be effective in reducing nausea. Antiemetics may be necessary for severe nausea and vomiting. Oral analgesics and topical anesthetics can often aid in reducing mouth pain. The nurse encourages the patient to perform mouth care before meals, sit in a chair to eat, eat with others, and take meals in pleasant surroundings. These measures can be successful in promoting an adequate oral intake.

A high-calorie, high-protein diet divided into six small meals per day is recommended. Specific food likes and dislikes are incorporated into meal planning to enhance intake. If the patient is losing weight, the nurse keeps a calorie and protein count or food diary for 1 week to determine the presence of deficits. Teaching includes normal nutrient requirements, calories required to maintain or gain weight, and the distribution of nutrients and calories in food. The nurse assists the patient with feeding and encourages the use of adaptive equipment if needed. Impaired swallowing is reported promptly to the physician. Family members, friends, or community agencies can be an important source of support and can be contacted to provide meals, visit during mealtimes, or assist with feeding.

### Promoting Effective Home Management

Caring for the person with HIV disease at home places heavy physical, psychological, and financial burdens on both the patient and caregiver. The nurse assesses the patient for functional abilities, disabilities, and extent of illness, as well as the caregiver's ability and willingness to perform needed care. The patient is encouraged to maintain self-care to the extent possible, without incurring injury. Not only is the activity provided during self-care physiologically important, it also provides a sense of control for the individual. It is important for the nurse to educate the person in safety measures and the importance of calling for assistance when needed. Diet, activities, self-monitoring needs, prevention of infection, stress reduction (see Chapter 6), and follow-up are all discussed. The nurse reviews treatment protocols, particularly drug regimens, and teaches the patient about drug dosages, administration schedules, and side effects. The nurse encourages the patient to anticipate unpleasant drug side effects and plan strategies for addressing them, such as napping or using a cool cloth to the head to relieve nausea.

The nurse assists the patient to consider the consequences of disease progression and the potential for further physical and mental deterioration. The patient-caregiver relationship is assessed, and the nurse attempts to anticipate how the stressors of disease progression may affect that relationship. A therapeutic nursing relationship built with empathy, acceptance, and support is essential. HIV-infected people often feel stigmatized by their disease. An empathetic nurse can do much to support individuals simply by taking time to talk to them at times other than when providing physical care. The nurse encourages the patient and caregiver to explore and express their feelings and fears and helps them identify past and current coping strategies, as well as effective and ineffective components of their relationship. The use of effective coping strategies is reinforced.

The early success of the protease inhibitor drug protocols has added new uncertainties to the lives of persons with HIV. Dramatic successes have been widely reported, with some patients experiencing a drop in their viral load to undetectable levels. It is often difficult for patients to know how to use this newfound well-being, especially if their lives have been fully consumed with disease management. Returning to work is rarely an option because of ongoing fatigue and financial concerns, but the person may no longer be overtly sick. This creates new and unexpected challenges for patients and caregivers, who must both find new ways to relate and effectively use this gift of time. The persistent threat of disease recurrence is also always present and can easily create a state of chronic anxiety in which the present is difficult to enjoy because of pervasive worries over how long the respite will last.

A wide range of knowledge, skills, and resources may be needed to provide care at home during various stages of HIV and AIDS, and the nurse needs to carefully explore the availability and adequacy of those resources. Family members, friends, clergy, and community support groups available to assist the patient and caregiver are thoroughly explored. The services of such resources can be enlisted to provide rest periods or time away from home for the caregiver. Referrals to home health agencies, social workers, AIDS support groups, respite care, spiritual counselors, and other community resources are initiated as available.

Some individuals with AIDS may be able to continue to work as their disease progresses, whereas others find it necessary to quit because they can no longer meet the physical requirements of their job. Inadequate health insurance coverage forces some patients to stop working prematurely and seek disability to qualify for medical assistance to cover the costs of drug therapy. This step makes it nearly impossible for patients to then return to work at some point in the future even if their health status allows it. Loss of work generally means loss of income and eventual loss of independence. The impact of lost income and the psychological impact of inability to work both need to be explored. Information about how and where to apply for financial assistance and medical care should be provided before it becomes a crisis, to reduce the burden on both patient and caregiver. The nurse needs to use all available multidisciplinary resources, including social services, clergy, public and private mental health resources, and special funding initiatives such as the Ryan White Fund, to assist patients in their efforts to self-manage AIDS in their home environment.

### Supporting Individual Coping

HIV-infected persons have many fears and concerns, including fear of losing their jobs and independence, fear of becoming debilitated, fear of bodily changes, and fear of death. Fear produces anxiety, which can result in ineffective coping patterns. The recognition of fear is often the first step in alleviating it. The nurse assesses the patient's psychological response to the situation and availability of support systems and helps the patient identify additional sources of financial and physical support. Patients are encouraged to talk about their concerns and assisted to identify ways of dealing with those concerns. The nurse encourages patients to maintain social and community activities with persons who have common interests and goals and use available support groups because they offer a safe place for individuals to express themselves.[20] Uncontrolled fear may interfere with care. In this case a counseling referral should be considered (Research Box).

**research**

Reference: Barroso J: Self-care activities of long-term survivors of acquired immunodeficiency syndrome, *Holistic Nurs Pract* 10(1):44, 1995.

The purpose of this study was to identify self-care activities of persons who had survived acquired immunodeficiency syndrome (AIDS) for at least 3 years. Twenty subjects reported behavioral changes needed to restructure their lives toward normalcy and taking care of themselves: (1) discontinuing negative habits; (2) improving their nutrition, rest, and exercise habits; (3) accepting responsibility for their own health; and (4) decreasing their level of stress.

A Nursing Care Plan for a person with HIV/AIDS can be found on p. 2203.

### Patient/Family Education

#### Health promotion/prevention

Because HIV is a multifaceted national and international problem, the first priority of care is to halt the spread of infection. To achieve this goal, the U.S. Department of Health and Human Services, Public Health Service, has developed *Healthy People 2000* objectives related to HIV infection (Box 67-5).[34] Prevention efforts must include accurate, reliable, and clear information about risk factors for HIV disease and ways to decrease these risks by limiting exposure to infected blood, semen, or vaginal secretions.

Persons identified with HIV infection have numerous knowledge needs, including but not limited to prevention of transmission, treatment options, legal and medical rights, and community resource availability. The nurse begins by assessing the patient's current knowledge base and includes the patient's significant other in teaching. The importance of collaborative planning for future care is stressed. Depending on the extent of the patient's knowledge, teaching involves all aspects of the disease and its treatment.

The patient and caregiver are assisted to organize information so that it is readily available and easy to understand. Emergency phone numbers and phone numbers for community resources need to be readily accessible. The nurse reviews the patient's plan of care and current treatment protocols and answers questions as needed to clarify information. The importance of physician visits and follow-up care is stressed.[13] During the later stages of disease, education may shift from providing specific information about the disease to keeping patients informed and discussing their wishes in regard to their own care.

## ■ EVALUATION

To evaluate the effectiveness of nursing interventions, compare client behaviors with those stated in the expected client outcomes. Successful achievement of outcomes for the person with HIV disease may include but are not limited to:

1. Is free of secondary infections; has normal temperature, clear lungs, intact skin

2a. Accomplishes desired tasks with fatigue controlled

b. Maintains self-care in feeding, bathing, hygiene, dressing, grooming, toileting

3. Regains weight with maintenance of desired body weight

4a. Interacts with family in a supportive manner, allowing family to help patient accomplish own goals

b. Maintains prescribed medical treatments and medications, returns for follow-up care, reports changes in health status as necessary

5a. Maintains social interaction and participation in activities

b. Freely verbalizes fears and concerns

## GERONTOLOGICAL CONSIDERATIONS

Even though most cases of HIV in the elderly have been traced to blood transfusions, the issues surrounding HIV infection

**box 67-5** Healthy People 2000 *Objectives Related to HIV/AIDS*

- Confine the prevalence of HIV infection to no more than 400 per 100,000 people.
- Confine annual incidence of diagnosed AIDS cases to no more than 43 per 100,000 population.
- Increase to at least 80% the proportion of HIV-infected people who know their serostatus.
- Increase to at least 75% the proportion of primary care and mental health care providers who provide appropriate counseling on the prevention of HIV and other sexually transmitted diseases.
- Reduce to no more than 1 per 250,000 units of blood and blood components the risk of transfusion-transmitted HIV infection.
- Extend to all facilities where workers are at risk for occupational transmission of HIV regulations to protect workers from exposure to blood-borne infections, including HIV infection.
- Increase to at least 50% the proportion of large businesses and to 10% the proportion of small businesses that implement a comprehensive HIV/AIDS workplace program.
- Increase to at least 95% the proportion of schools that provide appropriate HIV and other STD education curricula for students in 4th to 12th grade, preferably as part of comprehensive school health education program, based on scientific information that includes the way HIV and other STDs are prevented and transmitted.
- Increase to at least 90% the proportion of students who received HIV and other STD information, education, or counseling on their college or university campus.
- Increase to at least 90% the proportion of cities with populations over 100,000 that have outreach programs to contact drug users (particularly injecting drug users) to deliver HIV risk reduction messages.
- Increase to at least 50% the proportion of family planning clinics, maternal and child health clinics, sexually transmitted disease clinics, tuberculosis clinics, drug treatment centers, and primary care clinics that provide on-site primary prevention and provide or refer for secondary prevention services for HIV infection and bacterial sexually transmitted diseases (gonorrhea, syphilis, and chlamydia) to high-risk individuals and their sex or needle-sharing partners.

From US Department of Health and Human Services, Public Health Service: *Healthy people 2000: midcourse review and 1995 revisions,* Washington, DC, 1995, US Government Printing Office.

in this population have not been adequately addressed. Approximately 10% of AIDS cases in the United States involve people who are 50 years or older,[5] and the incidence is projected to rise steadily.

Recognition of HIV infection in elderly persons may be difficult for several reasons. A diagnosis of AIDS may be missed in elderly persons, who commonly experience symptoms such as pneumonia, dementia, shortness of breath, weakness, fatigue, poor nutritional intake, and weight loss. In addition, caregivers may fail to evaluate thoroughly such risk factors as IV drug use and unprotected sex in this age-group.

Care and counseling of the older adult with HIV infection or HIV disease will be similar to that of the younger adult, except that age-related changes will need to be incorporated into the plan of care. Elderly persons with compromised immune functions or chronic illnesses often have little reserve to resist or fight the multiple infections that accompany the HIV infection. In general, this age-group exhibits more side effects from aggressive antibiotic therapy used to fight infections of any kind. They will consequently be at greater risk for the development of adverse effects associated with aggressive HIV drug therapy.

Because older adults are not generally targeted as an at-risk group for HIV infection, they are often neglected when it comes to AIDS outreach and teaching.[32] Nurses must keep in mind that the elderly are sexually active and be prepared to provide health teaching about HIV infection and transmission when appropriate (Research Box).[5]

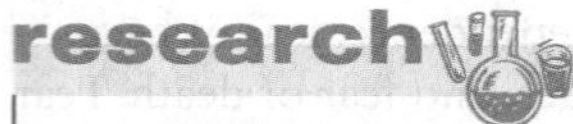

Reference: Rose MA: Knowledge of human immunodeficiency virus and acquired immunodeficiency syndrome, perception of risk, and behaviors among older adults, *Holistic Nurs Pract* 10(1):10, 1995.

The purpose of this study was to assess the knowledge of older adults about HIV and AIDS. The author queried 458 older adults at senior citizen meal sites about their general knowledge of AIDS, their perceptions of susceptibility and seriousness of the disease, and risk behaviors associated with HIV transmission. The majority of subjects responded correctly to all but two questions: nearly 73% thought that the cause of AIDS was unknown, and more than half thought it was possible to get AIDS by donating blood. Most subjects (80%) had no sex partners during the previous year; of those who engaged in sex, many had never used condoms.

## SPECIAL ENVIRONMENTS FOR CARE

### Critical Care Management

The majority of individuals with HIV disease are cared for at home and are followed on an outpatient basis. The occasion may arise, however, when it is necessary to hospitalize the person for induction therapy or to treat severe physical compromise related to opportunistic infections. Critical care management of overwhelming infections may include aggressive intravenous antibiotic therapy or respiratory support. All medical and nursing efforts are directed at controlling or eliminating symptoms.

## nursing care plan | Person with HIV/AIDS

**DATA** Trudy is a 51-year-old Cauasian hair stylist who lives with her 76-year-old mother, her primary caregiver. Eight years ago she was diagnosed as being HIV positive, 3 years after receiving several blood transfusions following an automobile accident. Trudy has been divorced for 14 years and has one adult son who lives in another state. Trudy has been able to work full time until recently. Since her diagnosis, Trudy has been undergoing drug therapy with AZT and more recently with combination antiretroviral drugs. Trudy has been under close outpatient supervision for the past 3 months because of increasing fatigue and a 10-pound weight loss. She is being admitted to the hospital today for complaints of fever, night sweats, myalgia, malaise, chest discomfort, dry nonproductive cough, abdominal discomfort, and diarrhea.

**PHYSICAL EXAMINATION** Bilaterally diminished lung sounds with coarse rales, respiratory rate 28 and mildly labored; axillary adenopathy, oral temperature 101.8° F, heart rate 92 and regular; clear sensorium, abdomen firm and tender with the presence of hyperactive bowel sounds.

**PHYSICIAN ORDERS** Oxygen by nasal cannula, 4 L/min; bed rest with bathroom privileges; diet as tolerated; lactated Ringer's solution at 125 ml/hr. Prepare for diagnostic bronchoscopy, stool specimen to laboratory. Diagnosis: suspected *Pneumocystis carinii* pneumonia and *Cryptosporidium.*

The nursing history also identified the following:

- Trudy is concerned about her condition and fears the inability to return to full-time work.
- Trudy is concerned about the health of her mother, who has diabetes mellitus and arthritis.
- Trudy has not told her son that she is HIV positive.
- Trudy does not date and is not sexually active, a choice she made following her HIV-positive diagnosis.

Collaborative nursing actions include monitoring for the following:

- Temperature
- Lung sounds, sputum production, chest discomfort, pulse oximetry
- Intake and output, number and consistency of stools
- Ability to sleep, appetite, food and fluid intake, weight
- Fatigue, ability to perform activities of daily living (ADL)
- Side effects of antiretroviral drugs
- Ability to discuss concerns, indications of anxiety
- Laboratory results of CD4 cell counts, HIV RNA levels, serum electrolytes

**NURSING DIAGNOSIS** *Altered nutrition, less than body requirements, related to diarrhea*

| expected patient outcome | nursing interventions | rationale |
|---|---|---|
| Describes a meal plan with adequate calories and fluid; ceases to lose weight; serum albumin, serum electrolytes remain within normal limits. | Fluid management: | |
| | Maintain accurate intake and output. | To determine if fluid output is excessive when compared with intake. |
| | Monitor hydration status. | To determine adequacy of fluid intake. |
| | Administer IV therapy as ordered. | To prevent fluid volume deficits and cellular dehydration. |
| | Nutrition management: | |
| | Weigh daily and monitor trends. | Weight is a clinical indicator of adequate nutrition. |
| | Encourage six small meals, excluding dairy products and raw fruits and vegetables. | Small meals prevent gastric distention and nausea; lactose in dairy products may enhance diarrhea; raw foods contain naturally occurring microorganisms that may increase infection in compromised hosts. |

**NURSING DIAGNOSIS** *Skin integrity, risk for impaired secondary to diarrhea*

| expected patient outcome | nursing interventions | rationale |
|---|---|---|
| Skin breakdown will not occur. | Skin surveillance: | |
| | Inspect skin and mucous membranes. | To detect skin deterioration. |
| | Monitor for redness, breakdown. | Redness denotes skin irritation and precedes skin breakdown. |
| | Skin care: topical treatments. | |
| | Keep rectal area clean and dry. | Prevents secondary infections and spread of existing infections. |
| | Apply protective cream to reddened areas. | Protects the skin from caustic effects of diarrhea. |

*Continued*

## Person with HIV/AIDS–cont'd

**NURSING DIAGNOSIS** *Infection, risk for related to immunodeficiency secondary to HIV infection*

| expected patient outcome | nursing interventions | rationale |
|---|---|---|
| Will remain free of new opportunistic infections; will identify ways to avoid new infections. | Infection protection: | |
| | Monitor for signs and symptoms of infection. | To identify new infections so treatment can be instituted early. |
| | Monitor hematology studies. | To detect signs of infection. |
| | Screen all visitors for communicable disease. | To protect the immunocompromised person from sources of new infections. |
| | Infection control: | |
| | Use Standard Precautions. | To prevent spread of infection. |
| | Ensure aseptic handling of all IV lines. | To prevent secondary infection from contaminated equipment. |
| | Wash hands before and after rendering care. | To prevent nosocomial infection. |

**NURSING DIAGNOSIS** *Breathing pattern, ineffective related to respiratory infection* (Pneumocystis carinii)

| expected patient outcome | nursing interventions | rationale |
|---|---|---|
| Reports increased comfort with breathing; uses effective cough technique. | Respiratory monitoring: | |
| | Monitor rate, rhythm, effort of respirations. | To detect respiratory complications and monitor effectiveness of treatment. |
| | Auscultate lung sounds. | |
| | Airway management: | |
| | Encourage slow, deep breathing. | To alleviate dyspnea. |
| | Instruct how to cough effectively. | To prevent stasis of secretions. |
| | Increase fluid intake. | To promote liquefaction of secretions for easy expectoration. |
| | Oxygen therapy: | |
| | Administer supplemental oxygen as ordered. | To enhance oxygenation and prevent hypoxia. |

**NURSING DIAGNOSIS** *Activity intolerance related to decreased oxygen transport and reduced energy reserves*

| expected patient outcome | nursing interventions | rationale |
|---|---|---|
| Is free of dyspnea with activity; reports feeling rested. | Energy management: | |
| | Monitor nutritional intake. | To ensure adequate energy reserves. |
| | Monitor sleep pattern. | To ensure adequate nighttime rest to enhance daytime energy. |
| | Organize daily activities. | To conserve energy. |

**NURSING DIAGNOSIS** *Fear related to change in health status; threatened loss of independence, job, and income*

| expected patient outcome | nursing interventions | rationale |
|---|---|---|
| Identifies previous coping strategies for stress; verbalizes sources of fear; verbalizes decreased anxiety/fear | Anxiety reduction: | |
| | Explain all procedures. | Decreases anxiety that often occurs when unfamiliar procedures are scheduled. |
| | Encourage verbalization of fears, concerns. | Venting of feelings often decreases anxiety. |
| | Discourage decision making while under extreme stress. | Stress inhibits one's ability to problem solve and approach decisions in a rational manner. |
| | Coping enhancement: | |
| | Explore past effective coping strategies. | Patterns of past successful coping are indicators of present resources and strengths. |

The decision to treat infections aggressively depends on the patient's and family's wishes and the extent of physical deterioration present. It is important for the nurse to understand and support the patient's wishes in this regard. Persons with early HIV disease are likely to request aggressive treatment, whereas persons who have experienced repeated infections and HIV wasting syndrome may not desire aggressive therapy.

### Home Care Management

There was a time when HIV-infected patients were cared for primarily in hospitals. In recent years a shift has occurred from hospital-based care to home care. Diagnostic testing and monitoring are performed in the outpatient setting. With improvements in antiretroviral therapy and treatments for opportunistic infections, continuing therapy can now be accomplished at home (Research Box).

A vital resource for the person with HIV disease is the assistance and support of a competent and dependable caregiver. That person may be a spouse, companion, friend, or relative. During the early stages of disease, the patient may rely on the caregiver to help diminish mood fluctuations, provide encouragement, foster motivation, and assist with some aspects of daily care. As the condition of the person with HIV deteriorates, however, the caregiver's role is significantly increased to include physical, psychological, and financial support.[22] Consequently, caregiver burden has become an important issue. It is important to assist caregivers to find suitable outlets for their own emotions. They should be encouraged to maintain adequate rest and nutrition so that they will have the physical stamina to meet the demands placed on them. Use of community resources, family members, or friends should be encouraged to provide time periods away from the physically ill individual for the purpose of shopping, work, or recreation.[31]

Persons with HIV disease who do not have a dependable support system are at a considerable disadvantage. Not only will they require earlier referrals for home care and other community services, but they will not have the day-to-day comfort and encouragement offered by a close personal companion. In many cases, it is the nurse who will have to fill part of the void by being a compassionate listener, offering encouragement, and fostering hope.

**research**

Reference: Baigis-Smith J, Gordon D, McGuire DB, Nanda J: Health-care needs of HIV-infected persons in hospital, outpatient, home, and long term care settings, J Assoc Nurses AIDS Care 6(6):21, 1995.

This study was undertaken to describe the health care needs of persons with HIV or AIDS in various health care settings. The sample consisted of 386 HIV-positive or AIDS patients and 40 nurses. Needs of HIV patients related to decreased physical endurance, decreased physical mobility, and sensory deficits. The most urgent needs reported by patients in all settings were financially related. Patients in hospital and outpatient facilities reported more needs that those in other settings; those in long-term care reported more needs than those in home care.

## COMPLICATIONS

The complications of HIV disease present a complex picture of opportunistic infections, neoplasms, or conditions related to immunodeficiency. When CD4 cell counts fall below 500/mm$^3$, signs and symptoms of immune deficiency are likely to be noted; when counts fall below 200/mm$^3$, opportunistic infections and neoplasms are encountered.[24] Bacterial, fungal, protozoal, and viral infections are the four categories of opportunistic infections seen in immunodeficient individuals. Kaposi's sarcoma is the most commonly seen neoplasm associated with HIV disease, but non-Hodgkin's lymphoma and cervical cancers also occur.

The infections associated with HIV disease are called opportunistic because the organisms producing the infection do not ordinarily produce disease. Such organisms are found throughout the environment but are rendered harmless by the intact immune system and do not cause disease. In patients with HIV infection, however, the organisms multiply, thrive, and produce disease because the immune regulators are severely compromised. Opportunistic infections are not limited to persons with HIV disease, but may affect any person who is immunodeficient or immunosuppressed as a result of chronic illness or chemotherapy.

Persons with HIV disease may experience one or more infections at the same time, producing numerous problems that present a challenge for both the physician and the nurse. The patient may be on several antibiotics for extended periods of time, causing an increased incidence of side effects and the potential for the development of drug resistance. It is not uncommon for opportunistic infections to return when antibiotics are reduced or discontinued. Recommendations have been developed to prophylactically treat some of the opportunistic infections commonly associated with severe immune compromise. The goal of treatment is to prevent infection or reduce its incidence and severity. Prophylactic interventions are summarized in Table 67-3. This section reviews common opportunistic infections and other complications associated with HIV disease.

## AIDS-RELATED OPPORTUNISTIC INFECTIONS

### Bacterial Infections

#### *Mycobacterium avium complex*

**Etiology/epidemiology.** *Mycobacterium avium* and *Mycobacterium intracellulare* are closely related nontuberculous or atypical mycobacteria that are usually grouped together as *M. avium* complex (MAC). These organisms are widespread in the environment, with high concentrations found in water, soil, unpasteurized dairy products, and aerosol droplets. There is a low incidence of clinical disease in the normal host because of the low pathogenicity of the organism, but MAC is the most common bacterial infection in AIDS, occurring in up to 50% of patients late in the course of HIV infection.

**table 67-3** *Prophylactic Treatment of Common Opportunistic Infections*

| INFECTION | PROPHYLACTIC INTERVENTIONS | COMMENTS |
|---|---|---|
| Pneumococcal pneumonia | Pneumococcal vaccine. | Provide as soon as possible during course of infection; antibody response is optimal when CD4+ cells are >350/μl. |
| Hepatitis B virus (HBV) | Hepatitis B vaccine series; screen and vaccinate those who show no evidence of previous HBV infection. | Provide as soon as possible during course of infection; encourage vaccine in injecting drug users, sexually active gay men, and sex partners or household contacts of HBV-infected individuals. |
| Herpes simplex virus (HSV) 1 and 2 | Low-dose acyclovir therapy may be initiated if prompt treatment of outbreaks is not sufficient for control. | Provide ongoing assessment and intervention. |
| Pulmonary tuberculosis | Treat if PPD is >5 mm reactive or if patient is anergic or at risk. INH for 12 mo. Consider directly observed therapy. (Clinical disease requires treatment with four or more drugs.) | Rule out active or extrapulmonary disease, which requires multidrug therapy; remember that a negative PPD in the presence of HIV does not exclude a diagnosis of tuberculosis; provide ongoing assessment and intervention. |
| *Pneumocystis carinii* pneumonia (PCP) | Trimethoprim-sulfamethoxazole (TMP-SMX) (drug of choice) or dapsone or pentamidine per inhalation. | Initiate when CD4+ cells go below 200/μl; offer TMP-SMX to any patient with a history of PCP, regardless of CD4+ cell count; oral drugs that provide systemic effect are preferred. |
| *Mycobacterium avium* complex (MAC) | Rifabutin. | Initiate when CD4+ cells go below 100/μl; rifabutin has caused dose-related uveitis (above 600 mg/day), which is reversible with drug withdrawal or dose reduction. |
| Toxoplasmosis | Trimethoprim-sulfamethoxazole (TMP-SMX) or dapsone with pyrimethamine and folinic acid. | Initiate when CD4+ cells go below 100/μl. |

From Lewis et al: *Medical-surgical nursing*, ed 4, St Louis, 1996, Mosby.

**Pathophysiology.** *Mycobacterium avium* complex is generally manifested as a tuberculosis-like pulmonary process. The majority of people who are colonized with MAC but who do not have HIV infection are asymptomatic. It is unusual to find an HIV-infected person with MAC who is asymptomatic. Many HIV patients have symptoms that can be attributed either to MAC or to profound immunodeficiency. Persistent fevers as high as 104° F (40° C) are the most common symptom. Weight loss and diarrhea are other commonly occurring symptoms.

*Mycobacterium avium* complex is most often disseminated and may be found in every organ. Physical examination may reveal lymphadenopathy or hepatosplenomegaly. Other clinical manifestations of MAC include fatigue, anorexia, night sweats, and weakness. It is thought to be a major contributing factor to the development of wasting syndrome.[4]

**Collaborative care management.** Most people with MAC have high-grade bacteremia; consequently, a single blood culture is usually sufficient for diagnosis. Diagnosis can also be confirmed by culture of MAC from other normally sterile body sites such as the liver, bone, or lymph nodes.[11]

The most common laboratory abnormality associated with MAC is anemia. A sudden fall in hematocrit or the need for repeat transfusions may be associated with disseminated MAC. An elevated alkaline phosphatase level may indicate direct liver involvement.

Use of combination therapy for the treatment of MAC has the best success. Table 67-4 lists drugs that are likely to have activity against MAC and are most widely used in various drug combinations. Because disseminated MAC is associated with significant morbidity and mortality, it is rational to attempt to prevent MAC in patients at risk.

Patients at highest risk for first occurrence of MAC are those with less than 100 CD4 cells/μl. Persons with HIV infection should receive prophylactic chemotherapy if their CD4+ T lymphocyte counts are less than 50 cells/μl. Prophylactic drug therapy is still in clinical trials, but clarithromycin, azithromycin, and rifabutin are commonly used. Use of these drugs is particularly advantageous because they also confer protection against other respiratory bacterial infections. Persons who have been diagnosed with MAC infection should be continued on full therapeutic doses of antimycobacterial agents for life.[35]

**Patient/family education.** Teaching for the person with MAC is similar to teaching for HIV disease in general. No special diet is required; however, weight loss is a common problem, and oral, enteral, or parenteral supplementation may be necessary. There are no specific activities or activity restrictions. Fatigue is usually present and may be a limiting factor in activity levels. Patients are encouraged to stay as active as possible. Supplemental oxygen may be necessary to prevent hypoxia, in which case the patient and family are instructed

**table 67-4** Common Medications for *Mycobacterium avium* Complex

| Drug | Actions | Interventions |
|---|---|---|
| Rifampin (Rifadin) | Bacteriostatic and bactericidal; inhibits DNA-dependent polymerase activity, thereby decreasing replication | Monitor for rash, hepatotoxicity, neutropenia<br>Assess skin integrity<br>Monitor liver function studies, CBC<br>Institute neutropenic precautions if necessary<br>May turn urine orange |
| Clarithromycin (Biaxcin) | Inhibits protein synthesis by binding to the 50S ribosomal subunit of susceptible bacteria | Monitor for nausea, abdominal pain, diarrhea, hepatotoxicity<br>Assess nutritional status<br>Monitor intake and output<br>Monitor liver function studies |
| Azithromycin (Zithromax) | Same as clarithromycin | Monitor for nausea, abdominal pain, diarrhea, hepatotoxicity<br>Same as clarithromycin |
| Amikacin (Amikin) | Bactericidal; inhibits protein synthesis in susceptible organisms | Monitor for ototoxicity, nephrotoxicity<br>Obtain peak and trough as ordered<br>Monitor renal studies |
| Streptomycin (Streptomycin) | Bactericidal; interferes with bacterial protein synthesis | Monitor for ototoxicity, nephrotoxicity<br>Same as amikacin |
| Ciprofloxacin (Cipro) | Bactericidal; Interferes with conversion of intermediate DNA into high-molecular DNA | Monitor for nausea, abdominal pain, diarrhea, rash<br>Monitor nutritional status<br>Assess hydration status<br>Assess skin integrity |
| Ethambutol (Myambutol) | Inhibits RNA synthesis, decreasing organism replication | Monitor for nausea, abdominal pain, changes in visual acuity<br>Monitor nutritional status<br>Assess visual acuity and monitor for changes |
| Clofazime | Binds to mycobacterial DNA, inhibiting growth of organism | Monitor for nausea, abdominal pain<br>Assess and monitor nutritional status<br>Educate patient that drug may cause hyperpigmentation |

about how and when to use oxygen. The nurse educates patients and families about drug therapy and side effects, symptoms that should be reported to the physician, and the need for drug therapy for the remainder of their lives.

Because most persons with MAC are likely to have end-stage HIV disease with significant immune compromise, the patient and family should be informed about the availability of community resources. In particular, a respiratory therapist may be able to provide valuable insights into managing respiratory difficulties.

### *Mycobacterium tuberculosis*

**Etiology/epidemiology.** *Mycobacterium tuberculosis* is affecting increasing numbers of immunodeficient or immunosuppressed individuals. HIV is thought to be one of the most important factors responsible for the increased incidence of *M. tuberculosis* in the United States. In fact, the CDC recommends that all HIV-positive persons be skin tested annually for tuberculosis, and those with positive results should be placed on prophylactic isoniazid for a full year.[35] This respiratory disease represents a complex community health illness that is discussed in detail in Chapter 32.

**Pathophysiology.** *Mycobacterium tuberculosis* is a bacterial infection that most commonly affects the lungs, but it can also affect the kidneys, intestines, lymph nodes, liver, spleen, joints, or central nervous system. It is characterized by inflammation, the formation of organ tubercles, caseation, necrosis, fibrosis, and calcification. Persons who have been exposed to *M. tuberculosis* and have calcified tubercles may later develop active disease in the presence of immune deficiency. Common clinical manifestations include fever, chills, night sweats, fatigue, cough, hemoptysis, dyspnea, chest pain, fatigue, and lymphadenopathy.

**Collaborative care management.** All HIV-infected persons who have a positive tuberculin skin test (TST) (≥5 mm induration) should be suspected of having active tuberculosis and should undergo diagnostic evaluation. HIV-infected persons who are symptomatic should undergo diagnosis even if their TST is negative.[35] Definitive diagnosis of tuberculosis is made when acid-fast *M. tuberculosis* bacilli are identified in sputum or tissue samples.

Five primary drugs are used to treat tuberculosis: isoniazid, rifampin, pyrazinamide, streptomycin, and ethambutol. HIV-infected persons who have a positive TST but who are asymptomatic should undergo prophylaxis for tuberculosis with isoniazid (INH) for a full year. HIV-infected persons with active tuberculosis are placed on a multi-drug treatment plan and kept on respiratory isolation while chemotherapy is initiated and until sputum specimens are free of the bacillus. Chronic suppressive therapy for the HIV-infected person who has completed chemotherapy for active tuberculosis is not necessary or recommended.[35]

Drug resistance has become a serious problem in recent years, and multidrug-resistant strains of *M. tuberculosis* are now recognized. Drug-resistant strains can develop when drug therapy is inadequate or the patient fails to take the prescribed medication for the length of time necessary to eradicate the tuberculosis bacillus.

**Patient/family education.** Care of the person with *M. tuberculosis* is primarily based on clinical manifestations and the need for early infection control measures. Respiratory treatments, supplemental oxygen, or both may be necessary to enhance oxygenation, and total parenteral nutrition may be necessary to prevent further weight loss. There are no activity restrictions; however, patients often restrict their own activities because of fatigue. Patients are encouraged to alternate activities with rest periods to conserve energy and reduce dyspnea. Fatigue and dyspnea, along with drug therapy, often result in anorexia and weight loss; consequently, the patient is instructed about ways to maintain adequate caloric and fluid intake.

It is essential that the patient and family be taught the importance of compliance with treatment regimens in order to prevent drug resistance and recurrent active tuberculosis. It may be necessary to monitor the patient's medication use to ensure compliance. Teaching includes drug dosages, schedules, and anticipated side effects.

Signs and symptoms of recurrent disease are reviewed, and the nurse encourages the patient to maintain close follow-up care. *Mycobacterium tuberculosis* is a reportable disease, and the patient and family need to be informed that local health authorities will be contacting them and monitoring treatment.

## Fungal Infections

Fungal infections are a common problem among HIV-infected patients. The three most commonly encountered diseases—candidiasis, cryptococcosis, and histoplasmosis—will be addressed.

### Candidiasis

**Etiology/epidemiology.** Thrush (candidiasis), caused by *Candida albicans,* may be one of the earliest signs of HIV infection. It is normally found in the mouth, GI tract (throat, esophagus, stomach, or bowel), vagina, and skin. Not usually pathogenic, *Candida* can become pathogenic when the immune system is altered by disease, diabetes, cancer, or immune-suppressing drugs. In HIV-infected people, mucocutaneous *Candida* infections of the mouth are most common, followed by infections of the esophagus, skin, rectum, and vagina. Although annoying, oral or vaginal candidiasis presents no significant risk of mortality. Disseminated infections, however, although rare, can be associated with significant morbidity and mortality. There are no known measures to reduce exposure to this fungus.[35]

**Pathophysiology.** *Candida albicans* is characterized by the formation of white, curdlike patches, erythema, and ulcers on mucous membranes. The patches are painful and often bleed when disturbed or removed. Oral lesions occur as thrush. Esophageal lesions produce irritation and dysphagia. Vaginal infections are associated with itching, irritation, and discharge (often described as thick and cheesy). Rectal lesions also produce itching and irritation. Disseminated infections are characterized by high fever, chills, and hypotension.

A *Candida* infection is usually diagnosed by its characteristic appearance of glistening white patches on the tongue or oral mucosal surfaces or creamy white vaginal discharge. Scrapings of the lesions and examination under a microscope allow identification of the yeast organism. Candidal infections can progress to other mucocutaneous sites as well. Oral infections, when left untreated, can progress into the esophagus. Diagnostic scraping of these lesions may then require an endoscopic procedure to obtain the sample and assess the extent of infection.

**Collaborative care management.** The current recommended treatment and maintenance therapy for mouth and esophageal candidiasis is oral fluconazole or ketoconazole. However, fluconazole-resistant strains of *C. albicans* are emerging. Alternative treatments include ketoconazole, itraconazole, clotrimazole, and nystatin.[35] Vaginal yeast infections may be treated with nystatin cream, ointments, or suppositories. For persistent or systemic infections, amphotericin may be required. Table 67-5 presents an overview of these drugs.

Although candidiasis is a common complication of HIV infection, primary prophylactic drug therapy is not recommended because the mortality rate is low and therapy for acute infections is highly effective. Persons with repeated episodes of esophageal candidiasis, however, are considered candidates for chronic suppression therapy with fluconazole.[35]

**Patient/family education.** There are no dietary restrictions, and patients may eat whatever they can tolerate. Oral candidal lesions make it difficult, however, for patients to tolerate temperature extremes and spicy foods. Soft foods may be better tolerated. Use of a soft-bristled toothbrush for oral hygiene will decrease the risk of pain and bleeding. Referral to a dietitian may be necessary for patients having difficulty maintaining their nutrition because of pain from oral lesions.

Patients with disseminated disease require amphotericin therapy and are likely to be acutely ill. Many patients receiving this drug experience fatigue, which may greatly reduce activity tolerance. Patients may need assistance in establishing an activity regimen they can tolerate. A gynecological referral is initiated for patients who have recurrent vaginal yeast infections. A dermatologist may be consulted regarding lesions that do not resolve.

### Cryptococcosis

**Etiology/epidemiology.** *Cryptococcus neoformans* is a yeastlike fungus that is ubiquitous and occurs worldwide. The organism is found in pigeon droppings and can be retrieved in nesting places, soil, fruit, and fruit juices. *Cryptococcus neoformans* can remain viable for up to 2 years even in desiccated pigeon feces. Neither person-to-person nor animal-to-person transmission has been documented. The disease is naturally acquired from the environment, where the organism is aerosolized and inhaled. In patients with prolonged, severe immunodeficiency caused by HIV, the immune system may no

**table 67-5** *Common Medications for* **Candida** ***Infections***

| Drug | Actions | Interventions |
|---|---|---|
| Fluconazole (Diflucan) | Fungistatic; fungicidal; inhibits ergosterol biosynthesis, producing damage to fungal cell wall | Monitor for headache, nausea, vomiting, hepatotoxicity, gynecomastia<br>Monitor liver function studies, CBC<br>Monitor nutritional status |
| Ketoconazole (Nizoral) | Fungistatic; fungicidal; inhibits fungal enzymes; alters cell membrane; prevents fungal metabolism | Same as fluconazole |
| Clotrimazole (Mycelex) | Fungistatic; fungicidal; changes integrity of cell membrane, allowing leakage of cell nutrients and halting fungal replication | Monitor for nausea and vomiting<br>Monitor liver function studies<br>Monitor nutritional status |
| Nystatin (Mycostatin) | Fungistatic; fungicidal; same as clotrimazole | Monitor for nausea, vomiting, epigastric pain, diarrhea<br>Assess nutritional status<br>Educate patient about swish-and-swallow procedure |
| Amphotericin (Fungizone) | Fungistatic; increases cell membrane permeability, thus inhibiting replication; decreases potassium, sodium, and nutrients in fungal cell | Monitor for fever with shaking chills, headache, anorexia, malaise, generalized pain<br>Treat symptoms of discomfort during therapy |

longer be competent against *C. neoformans,* and cryptococcosis can develop. Cryptococcal infection usually manifests as meningitis in HIV-infected patients.

**Pathophysiology.** *Cryptococcus* primarily affects the central nervous system and lungs, but it can also affect the skin, mouth, bones, liver, and kidneys. Pulmonary cryptococcal infection is generally asymptomatic, but in some patients it causes dyspnea, cough, and chest discomfort. Central nervous system findings include low-grade fever, headache, blurred vision, dizziness, memory changes, irritability, nausea or vomiting, lassitude, fatigue, and convulsions. If untreated, coma and death can occur as a result of cerebral edema or hydrocephalus. Cryptococcal skin lesions are painless, red papules that may be similar in appearance to Kaposi's sarcoma.

**Collaborative care management.** Diagnosis of *Cryptococcus* is achieved by identification of the fungus in the CSF. The organism may also be detected by antigen testing in urine or serum. Cryptococcal antigen titers and cultures of blood or CSF are the most reliable diagnostic measures. Computed tomography (CT) of the head may be performed to rule out hydrocephalus and to look for focal lesions. Chest radiographs are helpful if cryptococcal pneumonia is suspected.

Central nervous system infection can be fatal if appropriate therapy is not instituted in a timely manner. The primary drug used to treat an initial cryptococcal infection is amphotericin B; however, studies have shown that fluconazole and itraconazole can also reduce the frequency of cryptococcal infections in HIV-infected persons. HIV-infected persons with CD4+ T lymphocyte counts less than 50 cells/$\mu$l may be considered for prophylactic treatment with fluconazole. Patients who have had an episode of *Cryptococcus* infection are generally placed on lifelong suppressive therapy.[35] In addition to the usual IV infusion of amphotericin B, intrathecal administration has been used in patients failing to respond to IV infusion.

Other medications used include flucytosine and fluconazole. Flucytosine is an oral agent and is given in combination with amphotericin B. Fluconazole is less toxic than amphotericin and is better tolerated but may not be as efficacious in certain patients. The side effects and nursing implications of drug therapies for cryptococcosis are discussed in Table 67-6.

As with many of the opportunistic infections associated with HIV disease, the successful treatment of the initial acute infection does not cure the patient. Long-term suppressive therapy is necessary to prevent recurrence. Primary prophylaxis (instituted before the patient ever develops an initial infection) and long-term suppressive therapy may be accomplished with oral fluconazole therapy.

**Patient/family education.** There are no special dietary considerations for this infection. Patients need to be encouraged to maintain a healthy and well-balanced diet. Activity restrictions are as needed. For example, patients with meningitis may experience somnolence or confusion; consequently, activity restrictions may be necessary to protect the patient from injury. Patients and families should be educated and counseled about the modes of transmission of *Cryptococcus* and cautioned about contact with infected animals, human or animal feces, soil, and sexual practices that may result in oral exposure to feces.

As with other serious opportunistic infections that occur in late-stage disease, patients with cryptococcal infections may require multiple referrals. Social services, home nursing services, physical or occupational therapy, and psychiatry or counseling may be appropriate.

### Histoplasmosis

**Etiology/epidemiology.** *Histoplasma capsulatum* causes a common, usually benign fungal infection, histoplasmosis, that occurs primarily in the lungs. *Histoplasma capsulatum* is present in the soil where bird and bat excrement collect. The most likely sources of soil contamination in endemic areas

**table 67-6** *Common Medications for* ***Cryptococcosis***

| DRUG | ACTIONS | INTERVENTIONS |
|---|---|---|
| Flucytosine | Antiinfective; antibiotic; antifungal; converted to fluorouracil within fungal cell, inhibiting fungal cell metabolism | Monitor for anemia, jaundice, skin rash, itching, sore throat, fever, unusual bleeding/bruising, confusion, diarrhea, nausea, vomiting, headache, light-headedness, drowsiness<br>Assess for signs of unusual bleeding<br>Monitor nutritional status |
| Fluconazole (Diflucan) | Fungistatic; fungicidal; inhibits ergosterol biosynthesis, producing damage to fungal cell wall | Monitor for headache, nausea, vomiting, hepatotoxicity, gynecomastia<br>Monitor liver function studies, CBC<br>Monitor nutritional status |
| Amphotericin (Fungizone) | Fungistatic; increases cell membrane permeability, thus inhibiting replication; decreases potassium, sodium, and nutrients in fungal cell | Monitor for fever with shaking chills, headache, anorexia, malaise, generalized pain<br>Treat symptoms of discomfort during therapy |

are blackbird roosts, pigeon roosts, chicken houses, chicken manure, fertilizer, and sites frequented by bats such as caves, attics, old buildings, and hollow trees. The major endemic areas in the United States are the middle, central, and south central states. Although many individuals in endemic areas have been infected with *H. capsulatum,* the organism usually does not cause significant pulmonary disease. In immunocompromised patients, however, acute and life-threatening illness may develop.

**Pathophysiology.** Histoplasmosis in HIV-infected persons may manifest as acute pulmonary infection or disseminated disease. Acute pulmonary disease produces lung cavitations similar to those seen in *M. tuberculosis.* Symptoms often resemble the symptoms of influenza, including fever, cough, chest pain, fatigue, myalgias, anorexia, and headache. Disseminated disease produces generalized lymphadenopathy, hepatosplenomegaly, anemia, and thrombocytopenia. Progressive, disseminated disease is fatal in about 90% of cases.

**Collaborative care management.** Chest radiographs are unreliable and are normal in up to 30% of individuals with disseminated histoplasmosis. Because histoplasmosis most often manifests as disseminated disease in HIV-positive patients, bone marrow biopsy and cultures, examination and culture of pulmonary tissue and secretions, and blood cultures are the most common means of establishing a diagnosis.

Disseminated histoplasmosis in AIDS is invariably fatal if not treated aggressively with antifungal therapy. Amphotericin B and fluconazole are the drugs of choice in induction therapy for acute infection. These agents are discussed in Table 67-6. Patients who have been diagnosed with histoplasmosis will require lifelong suppressive treatment with itraconazole. HIV-infected individuals with CD4+ T lymphocyte counts less than 100 cells/$\mu$l may be considered for prophylactic therapy with itraconazole; however, concerns over drug toxicities, interactions, drug resistance, and cost may delay prophylactic treatment.[35]

**Patient/family education.** No standard protocols for diet or activity exist for histoplasmosis. Dietary teaching is aimed at maintenance of a healthful and well-balanced diet. Activities will depend on the patient's symptoms and activity tolerance. Fatigue may significantly limit physical activity; therefore frequent rest periods are encouraged. Amphotericin B can cause fever, chills, and nausea, and antiemetics and antipyretics may be necessary to enhance comfort during therapy.

Patients placed on prophylactic therapy are taught the signs and symptoms of drug toxicity and informed about potential drug interactions. As with other serious opportunistic infections that occur in late-stage disease, patients with histoplasmosis may require multiple referrals. Dietary services, social services, home nursing services, physical or occupational therapy, and psychiatry or counseling may be appropriate.

## Protozoal Infections

Protozoal infections are caused by a variety of organisms, many of which are parasitic. The organisms that most commonly cause protozoal opportunistic infections are *Cryptosporidium, Pneumocystis carinii,* and *Toxoplasma gondii.*

### *Cryptosporidium*

**Etiology/epidemiology.** *Cryptosporidium* is a parasite present in a variety of animal species, including birds, reptiles, fish, cattle, sheep, and humans. It is a well-recognized pathogen in both immunologically intact individuals and immunocompromised hosts, such as persons with HIV disease. In addition to animal-to-human transmission, person-to-person transmission has also been documented among daycare centers, household contacts, hospital patients, and health care workers. Water-borne transmission has also been documented. Chlorination of water does not kill *Cryptosporidium.*

**Pathophysiology.** The most common site of *Cryptosporidium* infection is the small intestine. It is a self-limiting disease in immune-competent individuals; however, it is extremely pathogenic in immunocompromised persons. It can affect the entire GI tract, producing fever, nausea, vomiting, abdominal pain and cramping, and severe watery diarrhea. Death from profound malabsorption, electrolyte imbalances, malnutrition, and dehydration may occur.

**Collaborative care management.** Diagnosis is made by identifying *Cryptosporidium* oocytes in fresh or formalin-preserved stool specimens. No effective anticryptosporidial therapy currently exists for either treatment or prevention.[26] Nearly 100 drugs have been tried without success. The National Institutes of Health are conducting clinical trials with the drug nitazoxanide (NTZ), originally developed to treat worms in dogs, as a potential treatment. Octreotide may be used to reduce the volume of stool. Otherwise therapy is aimed at controlling pain and decreasing peristalsis.

**Patient/family education.** Education of the HIV-infected person should emphasize modes of transmission and ways to avoid contact with the organism. Patients and families should be advised to avoid contact with infected animals, contaminated drinking water, lake water, diaper-age infants and children, and human and animal feces.

Patients with *Cryptosporidium* require IV therapy for fluid replacement and may require total parenteral nutrition (TPN) to replace fluids, calories, and nutrients lost through the massive volumes of diarrhea. Some patients find that reducing the bulk in their diet reduces the volume of their stools. Some form of nutritional supplementation is usually necessary to maintain adequate nutritional status. If octreotide is prescribed, patient education about the drug is essential. Side effects may include hyperglycemia, hypoglycemia, abdominal pain, nausea, vomiting, pain at the injection site, headache, fatigue, dizziness, edema, facial flushing, and hepatic dysfunction. The patient is taught how to self-monitor stool volume to assess the drug's effectiveness.

Frequent perineal care is essential for the person experiencing *Cryptosporidium* diarrhea. The patient is instructed to use nondrying soaps and to keep the skin clean and dry. Protective topical creams or lotions are applied to prevent skin cracking and breakdown.

### *Pneumocystis carinii*

**Etiology/epidemiology.** *Pneumocystis carinii* pneumonia (PCP) is the most common severe opportunistic infection associated with HIV infection. *Pneumocystis carinii* is a ubiquitous organism with worldwide distribution. It can be found in the air, on food, and in water, although most transmission appears to be via airborne routes. Most healthy children have acquired *P. carinii* infection by 4 years of age. It is not highly virulent, and infection in a normal host is usually asymptomatic. In the immunocompromised host, however, *P. carinii* can cause fulminant disease. *Pneumocystis* occurs in 90% of HIV-infected persons in the United States and is the leading cause of death.[3]

**Pathophysiology.** *Pneumocystis carinii* is generally confined to the lungs, although extrapulmonary *Pneumocystis* can occur. The infection causes increased permeability of alveolar capillary membranes, degenerative lung cell changes, and diffuse alveolar injury, resulting in impaired gas exchange and altered lung compliance. Without treatment, the infection leads to respiratory insufficiency and death.[1] Clinical manifestations include dyspnea, nonproductive cough, intermittent fever, fatigue, anorexia, weight loss, and tachypnea. Persons with advanced disease may also exhibit crackles, decreased breath sounds, and cyanosis.

**Collaborative care management.** Bronchoalveolar and transbronchial biopsies are usually performed to identify *P. carinii* in patients with pneumonia. If unsuccessful, an open lung biopsy via thoracotomy may be performed as a last resort. Chest radiograph may reveal pneumonia, although 5% to 10% of chest radiographs in AIDS patients with PCP appear normal. Pulmonary function studies usually reveal decreased vital capacity, decreased total lung capacity, and decreased single-breath diffusing capacity of carbon monoxide. Arterial blood gas studies may reveal hypoxemia, hypocarbia, and an increase in the alveolar-arterial oxygen gradient, particularly with exercise.

Presumptive diagnosis of PCP may be made according to the following CDC guidelines: (1) history of dyspnea on exertion or nonproductive cough of recent onset; (2) chest radiographical evidence of diffuse bilateral interstitial infiltrates or gallium scan evidence of diffuse bilateral pulmonary disease; (3) arterial blood gas analysis showing an arterial oxygen tension of less than 70 mm Hg, a low respiratory diffusing capacity, or an increase in the alveolar-arterial oxygen tension gradient; and (4) no evidence of bacterial pneumonia.

The most effective treatments for PCP are IV pentamidine isethionate or either IV or oral cotrimoxazole (trimethoprim and sulfamethoxazole). Cotrimoxazole is the preferred therapy because it is better tolerated. Many patients, however, are sensitive to sulfa drugs such as cotrimoxazole, which may limit the medication options. Other therapies that may be used include aerosolized pentamidine, trimetrexate, clindamycin, primaquine, or atovaquone. Table 67-7 summarizes information about pentamidine and co-trimoxazole.

Significant progress has been made in controlling PCP. Primary prophylaxis with cotrimoxazole is recommended for patients who have not yet developed PCP but have CD4 T lymphocyte counts less than 200 cells/$\mu$l, exhibit unexplained fever for 2 weeks or longer, or have a history of oropharyngeal candidiasis. For patients who cannot tolerate co-trimoxazole, dapsone, dapsone with pyrimethamine and leucovorin, and inhaled pentamidine are recommended. An advantage of dapsone is that it is also protective against toxoplasmosis. Secondary prophylaxis is recommended after the first episode of PCP.[35] The use of prophylactic therapy has significantly reduced the number of PCP recurrences, ultimately reducing the mortality rate.

**Patient/family education.** Drug therapy for PCP may produce severe adverse effects in immunodeficient individuals, including bone marrow suppression, fever, nausea, vomiting, and hepatotoxicity. Patients are encouraged to seek follow-up care and report signs of adverse or toxic drug effects. The nurse assesses the patient's drug administration technique to ensure that inhaled drugs reach the lung bases. Supplemental oxygen may be necessary to enhance oxygenation when dyspnea is severe. Mechanical ventilation may improve the chance of survival for persons with advanced disease who develop respiratory failure.

There are no special diet or activity recommendations for the person with PCP. A well-balanced, nutritional diet with

**table 67-7** Common Medications for **Pneumocystis carinii *Pneumonia***

| Drug | Actions | Interventions |
|---|---|---|
| Pentamidine isethionate (Pentam 300) | Interferes with protozoan DNA and RNA synthesis, thus interfering with parasite reproduction | |
| Intravenous | | Monitor for blood dyscrasias, rapid irregular pulse, hyperglycemia, hypoglycemia, diabetes mellitus, skin rash, hypotension, pain at injection site<br>Monitor blood and renal studies<br>Rotate injection sites |
| Inhalation | | Implement respiratory therapy precautions<br>Administer bronchodilators as indicated<br>Monitor for chest pain, congestion, cough, dyspnea, pharyngitis, wheezing, skin rash, metallic taste, pneumothorax |
| Co-trimoxazole (Bactrin, Septra) (sulfamethoxazole and trimethoprim) | Trimethoprim: antiinfective and folic acid antagonist; interferes with bacterial cell growth<br>Sulfamethoxazole bacteriostatic sulfonamide; halts the multiplication of bacteria | Monitor for hemolytic, megaloblastic, or aplastic anemia; agranulocytosis, skin rash, Stevens-Johnson syndrome, dysphagia, nausea, vomiting, stomatitis, headache, convulsions<br>Contraindicated in hypersensitivity to sulfa agents<br>Give oral preparation with full glass of water<br>Monitor intake and output |

adequate fluid intake is encouraged. Activity will depend on the person's degree of illness. Dyspnea often results in fatigue; therefore activities should be alternated with rest periods. As with other serious opportunistic infections, the person with *Pneumocystis* infection may require multiple referrals. A respiratory therapy referral for airway management is essential. A sample Clinical Pathway for a patient with pneumocystis carinii pneumonia is presented on p. 2213.

### *Toxoplasma gondii*

**Etiology/epidemiology.** *Toxoplasma gondii* is a protozoan that occurs worldwide and infects both humans and domestic animals. The definitive hosts are members of the cat family, although not all cats are infected, and toxoplasmosis has been documented in locales without cats. Transmission of *Toxoplasma* in humans is primarily through ingestion of meats and vegetables containing oocysts. The prevalence of *Toxoplasma* tissue cysts in meat consumed by humans may be as high as 25%. Cockroaches, earthworms, snails, and slugs may serve as transport hosts for the oocysts. Approximately 50% of American adults have been infected with *Toxoplasma.* Human-to-human transmission is from mother to fetus, by blood transfusion, or by organ transplantation.

**Pathophysiology.** Toxoplasmosis infection does not generally cause significant illness in healthy hosts. It is, however, a major cause of encephalitis in persons with AIDS. Toxoplasmosis produces localized and disseminated infections. Localized infections may be mild and are manifested by symptoms similar to mononucleosis. Disseminated infections are serious and include signs and symptoms such as headache, confusion or delirium, fever, encephalitis, vomiting, hemiparesis, seizures, and loss of vision.

**Collaborative care management.** Persons newly diagnosed with HIV infection should be tested for *Toxoplasma* antibodies to detect latent toxoplasmosis infection.[35]

Because *Toxoplasma* usually causes encephalitis, definitive diagnosis generally requires brain biopsy. Presumptive diagnosis is most often accomplished by (1) brain-imaging evidence of a lesion with a mass effect, (2) recent onset of focal neurological abnormality, (3) serum antibody to toxoplasmosis, or (4) successful response to therapy for toxoplasmosis.

HIV-infected persons who are seropositive for toxoplasmosis and who have CD4+ counts of less than 100/$\mu$l are started on prophylactic drug therapy with co-trimoxazole. If they cannot tolerate co-trimoxazole, dapsone with pyrimethamine can be used as alternative therapy. It is recommended that persons who have been diagnosed with toxoplasmosis be placed on suppressive drug therapy for the remainder of their lives.[35] The primary therapy for toxoplasmosis in persons with AIDS is a combination of sulfadiazine and pyrimethamine (Table 67-8 on p. 2216). Adjunctive therapy include dexamethasone (Decadron) for cerebral inflammation associated with abscesses and phenytoin (Dilantin) for seizures induced by infection. Approximately 40% to 60% of patients may have severe adverse reactions during the initial treatment phase, and alternative regimens, including cessation of sulfadiazine or addition of clindamycin, may be required.[35]

**Patient/family education.** The nurse warns HIV-infected persons against eating raw or undercooked meat; advises them to wash their hands after contact with raw meat or contact with soil and to wash raw fruit and vegetables before eating them; and recommends that they avoid changing cat litter if they own a cat.

There are no specific dietary or activity restrictions for the person with toxoplasmosis. Patients with mental status changes or seizures may require safety precautions. Because drug therapy can cause blood dyscrasias, teaching includes signs and symptoms of drug toxicity and the importance of follow-up monitoring. As with other opportunistic infections, patients with toxoplasmosis may require multiple referrals.

*Text continued on p. 2216*

## clinical pathway Pneumonia with Immunocompromise

Expected LOS: 5 days
Developed by Team

| | DAY/HOUR/VISIT | | | |
|---|---|---|---|---|
| | ADMISSION | 1 | 2 | 3 |
| **Consults** | Dietician | | | |
| **Tests** | Chem 18 with LDH<br>CBC<br>CXR<br>Blood cultures × 2, AFB × 1, Fungal × 1<br>RC: ABG<br>RC: Sputum C&S & GM stain<br>Silver Stain (order on misc. requisition) | Lab as Ordered<br><br>Monitor reports<br>Alert MD to any microscopic evidence of organisms<br>Sputum results called | →<br><br>Consider line placement (PICC, Midline) if antibiotics to be prolonged<br>→ | →<br><br>→ |
| **Medication** | Antibiotics IV<br>*Antibiotics started within 1 hr of admission<br>PO meds as ordered | Continue until DC'd<br><br>→ | →<br><br>→ | →<br><br>→ |
| **Treatment** | IV Fluids<br>RC: treatments as ordered<br>$O_2$: titrate $O_2$ to 95% & notify MD<br>NSG: Advanced Directive in chart<br>Report abnormal labs<br>Nsg Assessment q shift<br>resp rate & rhythm, lung aeration, abnorm. gas exchange<br>Functional level assessed based on Karnofsky scale (see page 2) | Continue until DC'd<br>→<br>Continue until DC'd<br><br>→ | →<br>RC TX or MDI<br>→<br><br>→<br>Reassess functional level based on Karnofsky scale (see page 2)<br>Reassess appropriateness of Advanced Directive | S.L.<br>→<br>→<br><br>→ |
| **Diet** | Advera/Ensure supplement TID | Food intake recorded<br>24 hr Calorie Count<br>NPO p MN if bronch in AM<br>Advera/Ensure supplement TID | NPO p MN if bronch in AM<br>Advera/Ensure supplement TID | Advera/Ensure supplement TID |
| **Activity** | As ordered, encourage activity<br>Assist to chg position q2h from sitting to lying as tolerated<br>NSG: If ADL rating 3-4, order for PT/OT/TR assessment obtained | Chair (for meals)<br>→ | Chair (for meals)<br>(× 3 for _____ min)<br>Ambulate with assist<br>Reassess for need for PT/OT evaluation | →<br>(3 × for _____ min.)<br>Ambulate ad lib |
| **Teaching** | Orient to room and routines<br>Review intended effect of therapy and CCP & goals<br>RC: Instruct on treatment plans and $O_2$ safety (if applicable) | Reinforce teaching<br>Discuss changes in diet, activity, medications if appropriate | Reinforce teaching<br>Discuss possibility of move to SNU or home with Home Health if appropriate | → |
| **Discharge Planning** | Assess for barriers to discharge<br>NSG: If from LTC facility, VNA, home $O_2$, financial issues, notify Social Services | NSG: Notify Resource Nurse of any changes in discharge plans | SS/NSG: Discuss with physician if pt is candidate for move to SNU ie., IV therapy, IM injection, rehabilitative nsg procedures, or PT/OT needed | If candidate for SNU prepare for discharge<br>RC: If going home on $O_2$, make home arrangements |

Columbia Overland Park Regional Medical Center, Overland Park, KS.

## Pneumonia with Immunocompromise—cont'd

Expected LOS: 5 days
Developed by Team

| | DAY/HOUR/VISIT | | | |
|---|---|---|---|---|
| | ADMISSION | 1 | 2 | 3 |
| Team Problem Identification | | Intermediate Goals | | |
| Anxiety R/T hospitalization | NSG: Pt. /family verbalizes concerns | → | → | → |
| Knowledge deficit R/T tests/ procedures disease process | NSG: Verbalizes understanding of tests/procedures | → | → | → |
| | NSG: Verbalizes understanding of information on the teaching pathway & goals/CCP | | | |
| | NSG: Pt/family verbalize agreement with Advance Directive/Living Will status | | | |
| | RC: Verbalizes understanding of $O_2$ therapy and aerosol TX | → | RC: Verbalizes understanding of correct method to use MDI | RC: Demonstrates independence in use of MDI |
| Home maintenance management impaired R/T disease process | NSG: Verbalize beginning knowledge of home care needs | → | Verbalizes agreement with current discharge plans | |
| Potential for injury R/T unfamiliar environment | NSG: Verbalizes understanding of safety measures | Demonstrates compliance with safety measures | No injury | → |
| | RC: Verbalize understanding of safety R/T oxygen therapy | | | |
| Ineffective breathing pattern R/T disease process | NSG: Demonstrates comfortable breathing pattern | → | → | → |
| | RC: Adequate ventilation/respiration per ABG results. $PaO_2 > 60$ ($PaO_2$ = to pre disease with or without $O_2$, and $SpO_2 > 90$.) | RC: Verbalizes a sense of improvement from respiratory treatments | → | → |
| Potential alteration in nutrition R/T disease process | NSG: Verbalizes understanding of need for adequate nutritional intake | NSG: Demonstrates tolerance of nutritional regimen | → | → |
| Potential alteration in self care R/T disease process | NSG: Demonstrates tolerance of activity levels without respiratory distress | NSG: Demonstrates able to sit up in the chair for 30 min | → | NSG: Demonstrates returning to pre-illness care abilities |

| Signatures: NSG | 7-3 | 7-3 | 7-3 | 7-3 |
|---|---|---|---|---|
| | 3-11 | 3-11 | 3-11 | 3-11 |
| RC (Respiratory Care) | 11-7 | 11-7 | 11-7 | 11-7 |
| | 7-3 | 7-3 | 7-3 | 7-3 |
| | 3-11 | 3-11 | 3-11 | 3-11 |
| | 11-7 | 11-7 | 11-7 | 11-7 |
| SS | | | | |
| Baseline Data: | | | | |

| DISCHARGE DAY*********** 4 | |
|---|---|
| Nursing Diagnosis | |
| Anxiety R/T hospitalization | NSG: Pt./family demonstrate appropriate coping mechanisms |
| Knowledge deficit R/T tests/procedures disease process | NSG: Verbalizes understanding of tests/procedures |
| Home maintenance management impaired R/T disease process | NSG: Verbalize understanding of discharge plans/instructions |
| Potential for injury R/T unfamiliar environment | NSG: No injury |
| Ineffective breathing pattern R/T disease process | NSG: Demonstrates optimal ventilation with measures taken<br>RC: Verbalizes a sense of improvement from resp. treatments |
| Potential alteration in nutrition R/T disease process | NSG: Demonstrates tolerance of nutritional regimen |
| Potential alteration in self care R/T disease process | NSG: Demonstrates pre-illness self care abilities |
| Signatures: NSG | |
| | 7-3 |
| | 3-11 |
| RC | 11-7 |
| | 7-3 |
| | 3-11 |
| SS | 11-7 |

**table 67-8** *Common Medications for* ***Toxoplasmosis***

| Drug | Actions | Interventions |
|---|---|---|
| Sulfadiazine PO | Bacteriostatic sulfonamide; halts the multiplication of bacteria but does not fully kill the mature microorganism | Maintain fluid intake of 1500 ml/day.<br>Educate patient about the importance of maintaining drug dosage and schedules<br>Monitor for fever, blood dyscrasias<br>Monitor liver and renal studies |
| Pyrimethamine PO | Inhibits folic acid metabolism in organism; stops growth of fertilized gametes to inhibit parasitic transmission | Contraindicated if hypersensitivity exists<br>Monitor for CNS stimulation, convulsions, tremors, fatigue, nausea, vomiting, anorexia, diarrhea, gastritis, thrombocytopenia, leukopenia, megaloblastic anemia, agranulocytosis<br>Monitor liver and renal studies |
| Clindamycin PO, (Cleocin) IM, IV | Antibacterial agent that suppresses protein synthesis; binds to 50S subunit of bacterial ribosomes | Monitor for rash, urticaria, nausea, vomiting, diarrhea, pseudomembraneous colitis, vaginitis, leukopenia, eosinophilia, agranulocytosis<br>Monitor liver studies<br>Contraindicated if hypersensitivity exists<br>Competes with chloramphenicol and erythromycin |

## Viral Infections

### Etiology/epidemiology

Cytomegalovirus and herpes simplex virus (HSV) types 1 and 2 are widespread in the general population. Cytomegalovirus infection is caused by *Cytomegalovirus,* a virus belonging to the herpesvirus family. Seroprevalence of CMV ranges from 30% to 100% in the United States.[33] It is found in breast milk, saliva, cervical secretions, semen, feces, urine, and blood.

Herpes simplex virus is caused by *Herpesvirus hominis.* Type 1 HSV is transmitted via oral and respiratory secretions. Type 2 HSV is transmitted by sexual contact. Both CMV and HSV remain dormant in tissues after initial infection and are reactivated in the presence of HIV and immunodeficiency.

### Pathophysiology

Cytomegalovirus is thought to spread throughout the body via lymphocytes or mononuclear cells. Cytomegalovirus is usually asymptomatic in the immune-competent host and can exist as a latent or chronic infection. In the immune-compromised host, CMV is pathogenic and produces symptoms. Disseminated infection can produce inflammatory reactions in the lungs, GI tract, liver, central nervous system, and eyes, leading to chorioretinitis, pneumonitis, encephalitis, adrenalitis, colitis, esophagitis, cholangitis, and hepatitis. Cytomegalovirus is a significant cause of blindness in persons with HIV disease.[33]

Herpes simplex virus type 1 affects the skin and mucous membranes, producing painful vesicular lesions. Similar lesions are produced by HSV type 2, but they occur in the genital or perianal region. Disseminated herpes infections affect the brain, liver, and lungs, producing blindness, seizures, deafness, and death.

### Collaborative care management

Cytomegalovirus and HSV types 1 and 2 are diagnosed by identification of antibodies in the serum. Parenteral or oral gancyclovir, parenteral foscarnet, and parenteral cidofovir are the drugs of choice for both treatment and prophylaxis of CMV infections. Prophylaxis is not always recommended, however, because of costs, limited effectiveness, and side effects. Chronic suppressive therapy or maintenance therapy is recommended for persons with recurrent disease.[25]

Herpes simplex virus is treated effectively with acyclovir. Prophylaxis is not generally recommended because acyclovir is an effective treatment for acute episodes. Persons who tend to have chronic herpes lesions are candidates for daily suppressive therapy with acyclovir. Intravenous foscarnet and cidofovir are alternative drugs that can be used when acyclovir is not effective.[25]

### Patient/family education

HIV-infected persons should be advised that CMV is shed in saliva, semen, and cervical secretions and that HSV is spread by oral and sexual contact. Latex condoms must be used during sexual contact to reduce the risk of viral transmission. Use of good hygienic practices, such as hand washing, can significantly reduce the risk of infection.

There are no specific dietary or activity restrictions for the person with CMV or HSV. Teaching regarding antiviral therapy should include signs and symptoms of drug toxicity and the importance of follow-up monitoring. All HIV-positive individuals are provided with home screening tools for identifying early CMV-related visual changes and are encouraged to have regular professional eye screening. Cytomegalovirus retinitis rapidly progresses toward blindness. As with other opportunistic infections, patients with viral infections may require multiple referrals.

## HIV-Related Cancer

### Etiology/epidemiology

Kaposi's sarcoma is by far the most common neoplasm found in patients with HIV infection. Kaposi's sarcoma is a rare cancer that may occur in elderly non–HIV infected persons. It has commonly been associated with HIV but may affect any person who is immunosuppressed or immunodeficient. The incidence of unexplained cases of Kaposi's sarcoma was one of the initial manifestations of the onset of HIV infection in this country.

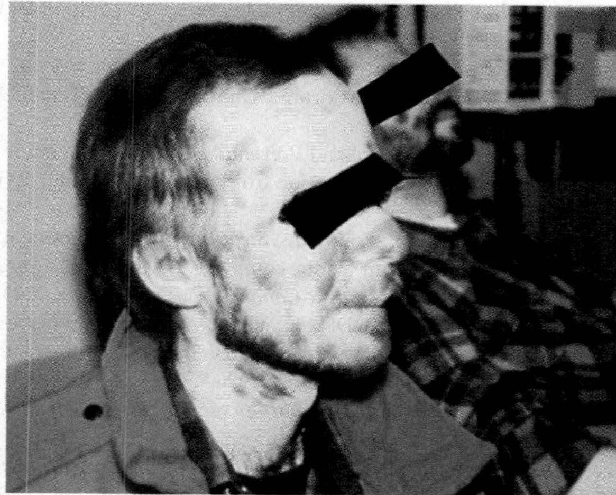

**fig. 67-6** Kaposi's sarcoma lesions on the face and neck.

### Pathophysiology

The exact cause of Kaposi's sarcoma is unknown. Kaposi's sarcoma lesions may appear on the skin, mucous membranes, mouth, tongue, tonsils, sclera, or conjunctiva and may also affect the internal organs. Lesions extend from the mid dermis upward into the epidermis and appear as dark blue, purple, or red papules (Figure 67-6). They may ulcerate and are associated with pain and itching. Systemic manifestations include lymphatic obstruction with resulting edema, dyspnea or respiratory distress when the lungs are affected, and digestive problems when the GI tract is involved.

### Collaborative care management

Kaposi's sarcoma is diagnosed by skin biopsy, but high suspicion exists when persons with lesions are immunocompromised. Local lesions can be surgically removed, but systemic lesions are treated with radiation or chemotherapy.[28] Doxorubicin, vinblastine, vincristine, and etoposide are agents of choice for treatment of Kaposi's sarcoma. Kaposi's sarcoma is not a major cause of death in persons with HIV disease; however, systemic disease can result in the need for medical or surgical intervention. A more complete discussion of Kaposi's sarcoma can be found in Chapter 63.

### Patient/family education

There are no known measures to prevent Kaposi's sarcoma; consequently, patients need information regarding what to expect and how to care for lesions. The nurse explains infection prevention methods such as keeping draining lesions covered, avoiding scratching or picking at lesions, and keeping lesions clean and dry. Skin care protocols are implemented for ulcerated areas. Patients are encouraged to express their feelings about the changes in appearance produced by Kaposi's sarcoma. If chemotherapy is elected, education must include an explanation of medications, potential side effects, drug interactions, and signs and symptoms that need to be reported to the physician.

## critical thinking QUESTIONS

1. Jill engaged in unprotected sex 2 weeks ago. Concerned, she decided to have her blood drawn to determine her HIV status. Four days later Jill learns that her ELISA was negative. What conclusions can be drawn about Jill's ELISA findings?
2. How is the care of the person with AIDS similar to and different from the care of a person with a primary immunodeficiency or someone who is receiving immunosuppressive drugs?
3. Ted and Joe both have AIDS. Ted has *Mycobacterium avium* complex and Joe has *Pneumocystis carinii* pneumonia. What elements of care will be the same for both of these patients?
4. You have been asked to talk to a group of high school freshmen about AIDS. What information do you think will be most relevant to this group? What information is irrelevant or not appropriate for their age-group?
5. Your co-worker confides in you that he thinks his assigned patient, who has AIDS, deserves the disease because he is gay. Discuss the ramifications of your co-worker's attitude toward his AIDS patient. Should this patient be assigned to another nurse? Why or why not?
6. Mr. R is a 69-year-old man who contracted AIDS 5 years ago after receiving massive blood transfusions following an automobile accident in the early 1980s. Given Mr. R's age, how will his care differ from that of a 25- or 30-year-old?
7. Your AIDS patient has several opportunistic infections, one of which is Kaposi's sarcoma. No treatment has been ordered for the problem. Given your understanding of Kaposi's sarcoma, explain why the disease is not being medically treated.

## chapter SUMMARY

### ETIOLOGY

- The human immunodeficiency virus (HIV), a retrovirus, is the cause of acquired immunodeficiency syndrome (AIDS).

### EPIDEMIOLOGY

- The routes of HIV transmission are (1) intimate sexual contact; (2) parenteral exposure to blood, blood-containing body fluids, and blood products; and (3) from mother to child during the perinatal period.

### PATHOPHYSIOLOGY

- HIV targets primarily the T4 helper lymphocytes, producing immune system dysfunction.

### PREVENTION

- Testing for HIV is accomplished through the use of an antibody test; most individuals produce antibodies within 6 weeks to 3 months of exposure.
- Most HIV-positive individuals remain relatively asymptomatic as their T4 helper cell counts decrease to about 500 cells/$\mu$l.
- Zidovudine (AZT) therapy is usually initiated in asymptomatic patients with CD4 counts less than 500 cells/$\mu$l.

- As CD4 counts decrease below 500 cells/μl, the risk for opportunistic infections, cancers, and HIV encephalopathy increases.

## COLLABORATIVE CARE MANAGEMENT

- Currently, no known cure exists for HIV infection. Survival rates have been extended with early-intervention antiretroviral therapy and appropriate primary and secondary prophylaxis against opportunistic infections.

## NURSING MANAGEMENT

- Nursing care in early stages focuses on preventing infection, maintaining adequate nutrition, helping the patient cope, promoting home maintenance management, decreasing fatigue, maintaining self-care, preventing social isolation, and controlling fear.
- Most nursing care is delivered in the outpatient setting.
- Teaching is a major intervention.
- Prevention of infections and treatment of active infections are major goals of care.

## COMPLICATIONS

- Opportunistic organisms are ubiquitous and are often widespread in the general population, although they typically do not cause disease in persons with a competent immune system.
- Bacterial infections include *Mycobacterium avium* complex, which causes fever, diarrhea, and profound wasting.
- Fungal infections include (1) candidiasis, which often causes thrush or a vaginal infection; (2) cryptococcosis, which causes meningitis; and (3) histoplasmosis, which causes disseminated infection with fever and weight loss.
- Protozoal infections include (1) cryptosporidiosis, which causes fulminant diarrhea and has no known therapy; (2) *Pneumocystis carinii* infection, which usually manifests as pneumonia and may progress to acute respiratory failure; or (3) toxoplasmosis, which usually causes encephalitis.
- Viral infections include cytomegalovirus infection, which most often causes retinitis; if not treated, this leads to permanent blindness.
- Most opportunistic infections are not eliminated from the body and require secondary prophylaxis to prevent recurrence.
- HIV can cross the blood-brain barrier, attach to microglial cells, and cause encephalopathy or neuropathy and motor dysfunction.
- Non-Hodgkin's lymphomas, Kaposi's sarcoma, and cervical cancer occur because of the depletion of T4 lymphocytes.

## References


1. Ad Hoc Subpanel on Opportunistic Infections Research Subgroups Report: *NIH and AIDS research program,* 1997.
2. Agency for Health Care Policy and Research: *Evaluation and management of early HIV infection,* Rockville, Md, 1994, US Department of Health and Human Services.
3. Bartlett JB: *The Johns Hopkins hospital guide to medical care of patients with HIV infection,* ed 4, Baltimore, 1994, Williams & Wilkins.
4. Black JM, Matassarin-Jacobs E: *Medical-surgical nursing,* ed 5, Philadelphia, 1997, WB Saunders.
5. Burke MM, Walsh MB: *Gerontologic nursing: wholistic care of the older adult,* ed 2, St Louis, 1997, Mosby.
6. Centers for Disease Control and Prevention (CDC): *HIV/AIDS surveillance report,* Atlanta, 1997, Department of Health and Human Services.
7. Centers for Disease Control and Prevention (CDC): 1993 revised classification system for HIV infection and expanded surveillance case definition for AIDS among adolescents and adults, *MMWR* 41(17):1, 1992.
8. Centers for Disease Control and Prevention (CDC): Update: acquired immunodeficiency syndrome: United States, *MMWR* 42(28): 517, 1993.
9. Centers for Disease Control and Prevention (CDC): Zidovudine for the prevention of HIV transmission from mother to infant, *MMWR* 43(16):285, 1994.
10. Ferreira T: Current HIV treatments, *Step Perspective* 8(1):8, 1994.
11. Gordin F: Mycobacterium avium complex (MAC): natural history and clinical issues, *Opportunistic Complications HIV* 2(1):1, 1993.
12. HIV/AIDS Bureau and AIDS Surveillance Program: Protease inhibitors: a new class of antiviral for HIV infection, *Massachusetts HIV/AIDS Quarterly Review* 3(2):14, 1996.
13. Jaffe MS, Skidmore-Roth L: *Home health nursing: assessment and care planning,* ed 3, St Louis, 1997, Mosby.
14. Lewis SM, Collier IC, Heitkemper MM: *Medical surgical nursing: assessment and management of clinical problems,* ed 4, St Louis, 1996, Mosby.
15. LeMone P, Burke K: *Medical-surgical nursing,* Menlo Park, Calif, 1996, Addison-Wesley.
16. Lucey D: The first decade of human retroviruses: a nomenclature for the clinician, *Mil Med* 156(10):555, 1991.
17. Lusso P, Gallo R: Pathogenesis of AIDS, *J Pharm Pharmacol* 44(suppl 1):160, 1992.
18. Mann J: Global AIDS: further evolution of the pandemic and the response, *HIV Advisor* 7(3):3, 1993.
19. McCance K, Huether S: *Pathophysiology: the biologic basis for disease in adults and children,* ed 3, St Louis, 1998, Mosby.
20. McClusky JC, Bulechek GM: *Nursing interventions classification (NIC),* St Louis, 1997, Mosby.
21. Mellors J et al: Prognosis in HIV-1 infection predicted by quantity of virus in plasma, *Science* 272:1167, 1997.
22. Miller JF: *Coping with chronic illness,* ed 2, Philadelphia, 1992, FA Davis.
23. O'Brien WA et al: Changes in plasma HIV-1 RNA and CD4+ lymphocyte counts and the risk of progression of AIDS, *N Engl J Med* 334(7):426, 1996.
24. Panel on Clinical Practices for Treatment of HIV Infection: *Guidelines for the use of antiretroviral agents in HIV-infected adults and adolescents,* 1997, US Department of Health and Human Services and the Henry J Kaiser Family Foundation, Rockville, Md.
25. Panther L: 10th international conference on AIDS: a review, *Step Perspective* 6(3):1, 1994.
26. Polaski AL, Tatro SE: *Luckmann's core principles and practice of medical-surgical nursing,* Philadelphia, 1996, WB Saunders.
27. Price SA, Wilson LM: *Pathophysiology,* ed 5, St Louis, 1997, Mosby.
28. *Report of the NIH panel to define principles of therapy of HIV infection,* Washington, DC, 1997, Office of AIDS Research of the National Institutes of Health, US Government Printing Office.
29. Schouten J: 11th international conference on AIDS: a review, *Step Perspective* 8(2):1, 1996.
30. Sherman DW: Nurses' willingness to care for AIDS patients and spirituality, social support, and death anxiety, *Image J Nurs Sch* 28(3): 205, 1996.
31. Stanhope M, Lancaster J: *Community health nursing: promoting health of aggregates, families, and individuals,* ed 4, St Louis, 1996, Mosby.
32. Stanley M, Beare P: *Gerontology nursing,* Philadelphia, 1995, FA Davis.
33. Torres G, Link D: Opportunistic infections update, *Treatment Issues* 8(1):12, 1994.
34. US Department of Health and Human Services, Public Health Service: *Healthy people 2000: midcourse review and 1994 revisions,* Washington, DC, 1995, US Government Printing Office.
35. USPHS/IDSA guidelines for the prevention of opportunistic infections in persons infected with human immunodeficiency virus, *MMWR* 46(16):RR-12, 1997.

chapter 68

# MANAGEMENT OF PERSONS WITH Organ/Tissue Transplants

MARILYN ROSSMAN BARTUCCI

## objectives *After studying this chapter, the learner should be able to:*

1. Describe the criteria used to select candidates for transplantation.
2. List the general organ and tissue donor criteria and the steps of the donor evaluation process.
3. Examine the influences of current and past legislative initiatives on organ donation and transplantation.
4. Construct a plan of care for the organ donor family.
5. Differentiate among hyperacute, acute, and chronic rejection.
6. Discuss the histocompatibility testing and matching required for transplantation.
7. Compare mode of action, indications for use, dosage, administration, side effects, and nursing interventions for the commonly used immunosuppressive agents.
8. Describe the major infections for which the immunosuppressed transplant recipient is at high risk.
9. Describe the general nursing diagnoses and care needs of the transplant recipient before and after transplantation.
10. Design care plans that address the common needs and interventions for persons with corneal, kidney, liver, pancreas, heart, lung, or bone marrow transplants.

## OVERVIEW OF TRANSPLANTATION

Organ transplantation has evolved from being a medical experiment to a major therapeutic intervention for selected patients. Advances in organ procurement and preservation, surgical technique, tissue typing and matching, management of the immune system, and the prevention and treatment of rejection have dramatically increased the demand for organs and tissues for transplantation.

In 1996, 34,688 cornea,[19] 12,080 kidney, 4064 liver, 2344 heart, 1022 pancreas, 800 lung, and 39 heart-lung transplants were performed in the United States.[36] Approximately 550,000 patients benefitted from bone allografts, 5000 from heart valve allografts, more than 1000 from arterial and venous allografts, and 15,000 from tendon and cartilage allografts.[2] Transplantation offers new life to individuals dying of liver, heart, and lung failure, and it restores lost body function and improves quality of life for individuals with kidney failure, diabetes, blindness, heart disease, and bone disease.

Conservative medical management of patients with end-stage kidney, liver, heart, or lung disease is costly. Although transplant procedures are expensive, the current success rates have made transplantation a cost-effective treatment option compared with traditional medical management. For example, a patient undergoing chronic hemodialysis costs the federal government, through Medicare, about $40,000 per year just for dialysis. The cost of a kidney transplant is approximately $50,000 for the initial hospitalization and approximately $20,000 per year for follow-up care and immunosuppressive medications. Because greater than 75% of transplants function for 5 years, the cost for transplant is $130,000, as opposed to $200,000 for 5 years of chronic hemodialysis. Likewise, patients with end-stage liver, heart, or lung disease have multiple costly hospital admissions for conservative management of their disease before death occurs. Table 68-1 shows the estimated cost of hospitalization for each transplant procedure and the current success rates.[35,36]

Other financial factors that increase the cost-effectiveness of transplantation include the potential earning power of the transplant recipient and the discontinuation of existing disability benefits. Transplantation can restore dignity and quality to the lives of patients and families dealing with end-stage organ disease and allow patients to once again become productive members of society.

Although many types of organ/tissue transplants are performed, this chapter focuses on allograft transplantation (transplantation of organs/tissues from one member of a species to another member of the same species) of solid organs (kidney, liver, heart, pancreas, and lung), corneas, and bone marrow.

### SHORTAGE OF DONOR ORGANS

Every year, the number of patients awaiting organs for transplantation increases. On the last day of 1996, there were over 50,000 people awaiting solid organs in the United States, a 14% increase from 1995 and a 212% increase from 1988.[36] Every day, approximately 12 people die because of the large gap between the small available supply and the great demand for

**table 68-1** *Organ Transplant Success Rates and Average Costs for Transplant Hospitalization*

| Organ | Graft Survival Rate (%) | Patient Survival Rate (%) | Average Cost ($) |
|---|---|---|---|
| Kidney | | | |
| Cadaver | 84.2 | 94.2 | 50,000 |
| Live donor | 92.7 | 97.7 | 40,000 |
| Heart | 84.2 | 85.1 | 80,000 |
| Heart and lung | 72.4 | 72.4 | 150,000 |
| Lung | 74.1 | 75.7 | 150,000 |
| Liver | 75.2 | 83.7 | 80,000 |
| Pancreas | 68.3 | 82.5 | 50,000 |
| Kidney and pancreas | 85.1 | 91.6 | 70,000 |

NOTE: Success rates are reported by the percentage of functioning grafts after 1 year because the greatest number of organs fail within the first year from rejection, technical problems, or other complications.

Data from UNOS: *UNOS Update* July-August 1996, Richmond, Va, 1996.

organs. The shortage reflects both organ accessibility and availability. Only an estimated 40% of organs from people who die meeting donor eligibility criteria are actually donated each year.[18] Despite extensive public awareness campaigns and the existence of laws mandating that all families be given the opportunity to donate the organs of a loved one who dies, the ratio of potential to actual donors has not been affected.

Some of the difficulties of the organ procurement process relate to the definition and declaration of death. Both the medical profession and lay public agree that the absence of a heartbeat and respirations are acceptable criteria for a declaration of death. However, advances in life-support technology enable health care professionals to maintain respiration and circulation in individuals whose brain function is minimal or absent and have created uncertainty about what constitutes death. Although the 1981 Uniform Definition of Death Act includes the cessation of all functions of the brain as a criterion for death, many health care professionals feel uncertainty over implementing this criterion.[29] People are strongly conditioned to view a breathing body with a beating heart as alive even when those functions result only from life-support systems.

## ORGAN SOURCES

Because of the disparity between the supply and demand for organs, there is ongoing interest in increasing the potential organ donor pool with the use of living donors, non–heart-beating donors (NHBDs), marginal donors, and animals.

### Living Donors

Living donors have been used in kidney transplantation since 1954. In the past, donors were restricted to blood relatives (i.e., parents, children, siblings). More recently, unrelated donors have been added to the donor pool. These donors are not blood relatives, but have an emotional relationship with the potential recipient (e.g., spouse, stepparent, stepchild, friend). The advantages of a live donor include (1) improved patient and graft survival rates; (2) immediate availability of an organ; (3) the ability to schedule the surgery when the recipient is in the best possible medical condition; and (4) immediate functioning of the organ because there is minimal preservation time. In 1996, 3511 live donor kidney transplants were performed in the United States, accounting for 29% of the total.[36]

More recently, living donors have also become sources for livers, pancreata, lungs, and hearts. The concept of living donor liver transplantation grew out of the need for appropriately sized livers for the smallest patients, those weighing less than 15 kg. The initial work with reduced-size and split-liver transplants established the feasibility of using a portion of an adult liver in a pediatric patient. Live donors have also been used in pancreas transplantation. The donor gives up a portion of the tail of the pancreas but is left with enough islet cells to produce adequate amounts of insulin to remain non-diabetic. Living donor lung transplantation was first performed in 1990 when a 12-year-old received a right upper lobe from her mother.[22] Living heart donors donate their healthy hearts when they become heart-lung recipients. This is called a domino transplant but is rarely performed anymore because of the increased success of lung transplant alone.

Ethical concerns that arise when people donate organs or portions of organs include (1) the risk of surgical complications for the healthy donor, (2) loss of income if the donor is a primary wage earner, (3) uncertain outcomes for the recipient, and (4) guilt experienced by the donor if the recipient dies.[14] These concerns for the donor must be weighed against the future that organ donation offers to people with end-stage liver, lung, or heart disease who may otherwise die waiting for a cadaver donor with the right match. Respect for autonomy supports the right of the donor to assume these risks if the donor's decision is informed, free from coercion, and truly autonomous.

Patients who have been declared dead by traditional cardiopulmonary criteria rather than brain death criteria are another source of transplantable organs. These are NHBDs because organ procurement takes place after the heart has stopped beating. Before the institution of brain death criteria these donors were the major source of transplantable kidneys, but problems with extended ischemia time leading to cell and tissue damage limited their usefulness. Recently, two different methods for procuring organs from NHBDs have been developed to address this problem: (1) in situ organ preservation immediately after cardiopulmonary arrest, and (2) procurement from patients who die after choosing to forego life-sustaining treatment.[37]

In situ organ preservation involves the infusion of cooled preservation solution through a catheter inserted into the abdominal aorta immediately after death has been declared. This process must be instituted immediately after asystole. Unfortunately, obtaining family consent for the procedure is difficult, because the family does not have time to adjust to the news of their loved one's death before having to make a decision about organ donation.

The alternative method, allowing patients and families the option of donating organs after they have decided to forego life-sustaining treatment, has two advantages. First, because the decision for organ donation is made by the patient and family before death, there is time for them to discuss, reflect, and give informed consent before the initiation of any invasive procedure. Second, the time and place of death are controlled to minimize warm ischemia time. The patient is taken to the operating room, where a surgical team begins organ removal and preservation within minutes of the declaration of death. No reliable data exist about the number of these patients, but it is estimated that the use of NHBDs could increase the potential donor pool by 20% to 25%.[10]

### Cadaver Donors

The criteria for cadaver donors have been liberalized to include increasing age (up to 70 years), diabetes, hypertension, some infections, high-risk social history but negative human immunodeficiency virus (HIV) test, some hemodynamic instability, some chemical imbalances, and increased organ preservation time. These expanded criteria could add 25% to 39% to the cadaver donor supply.[1] A careful evaluation, including histological assessment of the recovered organs, is made before transplantation, and careful, long-term follow-up is provided to ensure that patient and graft survival rates are comparable to those obtained with traditional cadaver donors. The decision to transplant a marginal donor organ requires not only a thorough anatomical and physiological evaluation of the organ, but also a similar evaluation of the recipient, including age, comorbid conditions, and immunological compatibility.[1,12]

### Xenografts

Xenografting, the transplantation of animal organs into humans, has become an attractive option. Although significant advances have been made in our understanding of xenotransplantation, a clinically useful procedure has not yet been developed. The major obstacle to success is hyperacute rejection, which occurs when the human recipient produces xenoreactive antibodies that destroy the organ. The transmission of viral diseases from animal to human is another concern. Potential advantages of xenografting include a readily available organ supply, fewer patient deaths on the waiting list, lower organ procurement costs, a more elective surgical procedure, and size matching for donor and recipient. Research in this area is ongoing.

## ROLE OF NURSING IN THE DONATION PROCESS

Nurses are commonly the first health care professionals to identify a potential organ donor and make the appropriate referral to the local organ procurement organization (OPO). Nurses are in the best position to provide compassionate support to families and are well prepared both educationally and through experience to help the family through this crisis. Studies indicate that 87% of the general public is knowledgeable about transplantation and willing to donate organs at the time of death.[20] However, in an emergency situation the family cannot be expected to initiate the idea of donation. The nurse provides both sufficient factual information and the emotional support needed for the next of kin to arrive at a decision about organ/tissue donation.

A common concern that arises in the minds of caregivers relates to whether organ donation and transplantation are supported by their religious group. Although the specific standards and positions about transplantation vary both within and among various faiths and denominations, the major religious groups in the United States all support donation and transplantation. Many groups (e.g., Roman Catholics, Amish, Moslems, and Jews) view donation as an act of charity, fraternal love, and self-sacrifice. Hindus, Jehovah's Witnesses, and various Protestant groups express the belief that donation is a matter of individual conscience.

Requests for organ/tissue donation must be carefully timed and sensitive to the needs of the family. The donation process is initiated only after the physician has communicated to the family the hopelessness of the clinical situation and the family has had time to assimilate this information. Once the next of kin have been informed of their family member's death, the physician, nurse, procurement coordinator, or hospital designee can offer the family the opportunity to donate organs/tissues. The discussion takes place in a comfortable, private area, conducive to the family's expression of grief. The success of the request usually reflects the attitude exhibited by the caregivers during this sensitive period. The request for donation is handled as part of the natural support provided to a family at the time of a loved one's death. It is the death that is the most important event, not the donation. The family is approached, not to acquire organs, but to show compassion and offer assistance and support during their bereavement (see the Guidelines for Care Box on p. 2222). The discussion begins with an expression of sympathy and allows the family time to express their feelings. It is important that the caregivers verify the family's understanding of the loved one's condition, and reexplain, if necessary, why the patient is considered to be dead.

It has been shown that initiating a request for organ/tissue donation before the family has had time to assimilate the news of their loved one's death results in a high rate of denied consent. Separating the explanation of the certainty of death of a loved one and the request for donation allows for a period of acceptance and results in a statistically significant improvement in the consent rate (60% versus 18%).[21]

The organ procurement team responds to commonly expressed family concerns such as pain experienced by the donor, payment, disfigurement of the body, funeral delays, and confidentiality. A brief reexplanation of brain death can allay fears related to pain during the organ/tissue procurement surgery. The team informs the family that the procurement agency pays all costs associated with the procurement of the organ/tissue and care of the donor, including laboratory tests, operating room costs, surgeon fees, and intravenous fluids and medications. The family remains financially responsible for all health care costs incurred up to the pronouncement of death. Families are often concerned about

**guidelines for care**

### Talking with Families About Organ and Tissue Donation

1. Make sure that death has been declared and discussed with the family and the family has been given time to assimilate this information.
2. Contact the local organ procurement organization (OPO) to make referral and to determine medical suitability for organ/tissue donation.
3. Try to determine the beliefs of the potential donor; that is, has a donor card been signed?
4. Identify the legal next of kin and any other family members or significant others who should be included in the discussion.
5. Provide a comfortable, private place for discussion between the health team members and the family.
6. Ascertain what the family understands about brain death and the hope of recovery.
7. Speak slowly, be sensitive, refer to the potential donor by name, and do not be afraid to refer to the potential donor as dead.
8. Provide adequate, accurate information on the options available to the family related to discontinuing life support.
9. Provide adequate, accurate information on organ/tissue donation, including informed consent, evaluation required, and that there is no cost to the family.
10. Ensure that the family understands that organ/tissue donation will not interfere with the timing of the funeral service or with an open casket service.
11. Provide time for the family to discuss the request and make the decision.
12. Request written consent only after the family has had time to make the decision and has given an affirmative response.

whether donation interferes with an open-casket funeral. Assurance can be given that the donor will appear normal, and donation does not preclude use of an open casket. Funeral delays usually are not necessary unless procurement teams are coming from various parts of the country. After procurement, the body is released to the funeral home. Gifts of organs or tissues are confidential. No one who receives a transplant is told the identity of the donor, and donor families are told only the age and sex of the various recipients and how they are doing after transplantation.

Health care professionals often fear that asking grieving families for organ/tissue donation adds to the family's grief. Studies have consistently shown, however, that the strongest advocates of donation are donor families, who view donation as the highest form of charity, giving the ultimate gift, life, to another person.[11]

## ORGAN DONATION AND ALLOCATION

Organ procurement organizations are responsible for organ recovery in the United States. These organizations have offices in major cities and provide services on a local, state, and regional basis. Organ procurement organizations provide 24-hour assistance to evaluate potential donors, discuss donation with the next of kin, and assist with physical assessment and hemodynamic monitoring to maintain organ function until surgical removal. They also implement organ recovery and placement through the United Network for Organ Sharing (UNOS) allocation policies. In addition, they provide follow-up bereavement support for donor families and information regarding the outcome of the donation. They also provide feedback to the donor hospital regarding the transplant outcomes.

The UNOS operates under the auspices of the U.S. Department of Health and Human Services. Organ procurement organizations and transplant centers are members of UNOS, and UNOS maintains the national waiting list of persons needing transplants and uses a system that computer matches potential recipients with donor organs. The present criteria for allocating extrarenal transplants are (1) blood type compatibility, (2) organ size, (3) medical urgency, (4) geographic location, and (5) time on waiting list. Kidneys are transplanted locally based on blood type compatibility and a point system, unless there is a potential recipient with a perfect human leukocyte antigen (HLA) match somewhere else in the country. Each waiting list patient in the local area is assigned points based on the quality of the HLA match, waiting time, and the presence of preformed antibodies.

Traditionally, one of the biggest obstacles to organ/tissue donation has been the failure to identify potential donors early in the process. Nurses must be knowledgeable about donor eligibility criteria and know how to activate the organ procurement process. Organ donors are previously healthy individuals who have suffered an irreversible brain injury. The most common causes of injury are cerebral trauma from motor vehicle accidents or gunshot wounds, intracerebral or subarachnoid hemorrhage, and anoxic brain damage resulting from a drug overdose or cardiac arrest. The brain-dead donor must have effective cardiovascular function and must be supported on a ventilator to preserve organ function. The age range for most suitable donors is newborn to 70 years of age. The age of the donor is generally less important than the quality of organ function. The donor must be free of malignancy, sepsis, and communicable diseases, including HIV, hepatitis B and C, syphilis, and tuberculosis, and have no history of intravenous drug abuse.

Unlike organ donors, tissue donors (donors of eyes, bone, skin, heart valves, etc.) do not need to have a beating heart. Death is pronounced, and tissue may be recovered hours after the heart has stopped beating. Care of the organ donor is presented in the Nursing Care Plan.

## RECIPIENT SELECTION

Because the supply of organs/tissues is limited, appropriate recipient selection is important for both a successful outcome and the best use of this scarce resource. Candidacy is determined by a wide variety of medical and psychosocial

## nursing care plan *Organ Donor*

**DATA** Mr. G. is a 31-year-old married man who is the father of three young children. He was involved in a serious accident while riding his motorcycle. He was struck directly by a car at moderate speed and, although he was wearing a helmet, he sustained multiple trauma, including a severe head injury.

Despite aggressive initial management Mr. G. did not respond to treatment and has since met the criteria for brain death. His wife has been informed of his status and has been approached about organ donation. Despite her shock and grief Mrs. G. is clear that donation is something her husband would have wanted, and she has just signed permission. The organ procurement process has been initiated.

Collaborative care interventions for Mr. G. include the following:

- Frequent monitoring of vital signs, intake and output, central venous pressure, PWP, electrocardiogram
- Vasopressor administration to support blood pressure within established parameters
- Mechanical ventilation
- Use of heating/cooling blankets to maintain normothermia

**NURSING DIAGNOSIS** *Decreased cardiac output related to central nervous system dysfunction (loss of vasomotor control), hypovolemia*

| expected patient outcome | nursing interventions | rationale |
|---|---|---|
| Normal cardiac output as evidenced by systolic blood pressure greater than 100 mm Hg, heart rate within normal limits, and central venous pressure greater than 10 cm $H_2O$ or 7 mm Hg. | 1. Monitor hourly heart rate and blood pressure.<br>2. Maintain continuous electrocardiographic monitoring.<br>3. Monitor hourly central venous or pulmonary artery pressures.<br>4. Monitor hourly fluid intake and output.<br>5. Administer intravenous fluids as ordered.<br>6. Administer vasopressors as ordered and monitor for untoward effects.<br>7. Obtain serum cardiac enzymes as ordered. | Patient's regulatory mechanisms are partially or severely compromised. An adequate output is essential for maintaining an adequate level of perfusion to the tissues. Vital signs and hemodynamic parameters are basic measures of cardiac output. |

**NURSING DIAGNOSIS** *Impaired tissue perfusion related to central nervous system dysfunction, hypovolemia*

| expected patient outcome | nursing interventions | rationale |
|---|---|---|
| Adequate tissue perfusion as evidenced by systolic blood pressure greater than 100 mm Hg, central venous pressure greater than 10 cm $H_2O$ or 7 mm Hg, urine output greater than 2 to 3 ml/kg per hour, good quality peripheral pulses, absence of cyanosis, and normal blood pH, urea nitrogen, and creatinine. | 1. Monitor hourly heart rate, blood pressure, central venous pressure, or pulmonary artery pressure.<br>2. Monitor quality of peripheral pulses.<br>3. Monitor skin temperature and color.<br>4. Check capillary refilling in fingertips.<br>5. Observe nailbeds and lips for cyanosis.<br>6. Obtain arterial blood gases as indicated.<br>7. Obtain serum electrolytes, blood urea nitrogen, and creatinine.<br>8. Administer vasopressors as ordered, and document changes in blood pressure and urine output after administration. | Sustaining organ and tissue perfusion is the primary challenge before organ harvest.<br>Critical monitoring of basic physical assessment parameters provides insight into status of peripheral perfusion. |

*Continued*

## Organ Donor–cont'd

**NURSING DIAGNOSIS** *Impaired gas exchange related to central nervous system dysfunction (loss of respiratory mechanics), neurogenic pulmonary edema, aspiration pneumonia*

| expected patient outcomes | nursing interventions | rationale |
|---|---|---|
| Adequate gas exchange as evidenced by $Pa_{O_2}$ between 80 and 120 mm Hg, oxyhemoglobin saturation above 90%, $Pa_{CO_2}$ between 35 and 45 mm Hg, IMV rate between 8 and 14 breaths per minute, tidal volume 12 to 15 ml/kg, pH 7.35 to 7.45, hemoglobin 12% to 18% to maximize content of oxygen in arterial blood.<br>Adequate ventilation as evidenced by normal breath sounds bilaterally on auscultation and equal bilateral chest wall movement with respiration. | 1. Monitor mechanical ventilation.<br>2. Auscultate breath sounds bilaterally.<br>3. Obtain arterial blood gases every 4 to 6 hours and after ventilator changes.<br>4. Observe tracheobronchial secretions for amount, color, consistency, and odor.<br>5. Maintain patent airway with sterile suctioning to remove tracheobronchial secretions.<br>6. Turn every 2 hours and administer chest physiotherapy. | Brain-dead patients lack any ventilatory drive and must be mechanically ventilated.<br>Physical assessment and blood gases provide insight into the adequacy of gas exchange.<br>Turning, suctioning, and chest physiotherapy help mobilize secretions to avoid stasis. |

**NURSING DIAGNOSIS** *Risk for fluid volume deficit related to diabetes insipidus*

| expected patient outcome | nursing interventions | rationale |
|---|---|---|
| Adequate fluid and electrolyte balance as evidenced by stable vital signs, appropriate urine output, stable weight, and normal serum and urine electrolytes. | 1. Monitor hourly intake and output.<br>2. Daily weights.<br>3. Monitor urine specific gravity every 2 hours.<br>4. Monitor serum and urine electrolytes and osmolality.<br>5. Administer intravenous maintenance and replacement fluids.<br>6. Administer aqueous vasopressin as ordered and document changes in urine output after administration. | Brain-dead patients commonly develop an imbalance of pituitary secretion of antidiuretic hormone.<br>Monitoring intake and output, urine specific gravity, and urine and serum osmolality best assess the patient's fluid status.<br>Daily weights reveal subtle and dramatic shifts in body fluid.<br>IV fluids need to be administered to replace heavy fluid losses in urine.<br>Vasopressin replaces antidiuretic hormone effect and reduces fluid losses. |

**NURSING DIAGNOSIS** *Impaired thermoregulation related to central nervous system dysfunction (damage to hypothalamus)*

| expected patient outcome | nursing interventions | rationale |
|---|---|---|
| Adequate temperature control as evidenced by normal body temperature, 97° to 100° F. | 1. Monitor body temperature for hyperthermia or hypothermia.<br>2. Restore normal body temperature with the use of heating/cooling blankets as indicated.<br>3. Warm intravenous fluids before administration if hypothermia is present. | Without adequate central regulation the patientís temperature can fluctuate out of control.<br>Frequent monitoring is essential. Cooling or rewarming may be necessary. |

*Continued*

factors that vary among transplant centers. These factors include disease status, therapeutic benefits of transplantation, age, functional ability, and presence of family support. A careful evaluation is completed before transplant to attempt to identify and minimize potential complications after transplant. Contraindications for transplantation include disseminated malignancies, chronic infections (except hepatitis B and C), and ongoing psychosocial problems such as noncompliance with medical regimens and chemical dependency (see the Research Box).

### PAYMENT FOR TRANSPLANTATION

Reimbursement for transplantation occurs through private insurance, self-payment, Medicare, and Medicaid. Private insurance and managed care companies currently reimburse at a fixed rate, and reimbursement may not equal the actual charges. The recipient may be responsible for the difference.

Medicare is the primary payer for kidney transplant and certain heart, liver, and bone marrow transplants, but restrictions for coverage include the length and extent of the patient's disability, age of the recipient, underlying disease

*Text continued on p. 2226*

## Organ Donor–cont'd

**NURSING DIAGNOSIS** *Risk for infection related to presence of indwelling catheters and an endotracheal tube*

| expected patient outcome | nursing interventions | rationale |
|---|---|---|
| Absence of infection as evidenced by clear urine, WBC count within normal limits, absence of fever, and absence of purulent secretions and purulent wound drainage. | 1. Careful hand washing.<br>2. Obtain complete blood count with differential.<br>3. Maintain aseptic care of indwelling Foley catheter, observing urine for cloudiness, sediment, and odor.<br>4. Monitor wounds, incisions, and puncture sites for erythema and drainage.<br>5. Culture secretions, urine, and blood as indicated.<br>6. Administer antibiotics as ordered. | General asepsis is the best preventive measure.<br>Presence of infection is monitored through blood work, results of cultures, and status of all wounds, incisions, and drainage sites.<br>Prophylactic antibiotics may be administered to prevent sepsis. |

**NURSING DIAGNOSIS** *Grieving related to imminent death or death of a loved one*

| expected patient outcome | nursing interventions | rationale |
|---|---|---|
| Completion of the first task of grieving as evidenced by the family's ability to discuss feelings about loss of a loved one.<br>Knowledge and understanding of the normal grief process as evidenced by the family's ability to identify thoughts, feelings, behaviors, and physical sensations they experience as a result of their loss.<br>Support system(s) in place as evidenced by the presence of other family members, friends, clergy, or counselor to help the family begin to work through their grief. | 1. Assess and evaluate accuracy of family's perceptions of loved one's condition.<br>2. Listen attentively and with empathy to accounts of circumstances leading up to trauma.<br>3. Encourage family to talk about loved one.<br>4. Allow family to visit any time and participate in care if they so desire.<br>5. Explain variety of thoughts, feelings, behaviors, and physical sensations family may experience as normal part of healthy grieving.<br>6. Evaluate support systems (e.g., other family members, friends, clergy).<br>7. Refer for bereavement therapy if appropriate.<br>8. Reinforce altruism and benefit of the gift of organ donation. | Brain death is a difficult concept because patient's heart still beats.<br>Coping with traumatic losses is fostered by allowing wife to relive and process the circumstances. This includes talking about the patient's life and qualities.<br>Quiet time at the bedside can facilitate movement through the grief process.<br>Brief discussion of grief can help the wife understand the nature of her physical and emotional responses.<br>Support systems are an essential coping resource, and bereavement therapy may help the wife to cope with this traumatic loss.<br>Organ donation is a gift of life from sudden death. This is a comfort to many survivors. |

## research

Reference: Douglas S, Blixen D, Bartucci MR: Relationship between pretransplant noncompliance and posttransplant outcomes in renal transplant recipients, *Journal of Transplant Coordination* 6:53, 1996.

Kidney transplant is a successful treatment for end-stage renal disease. Posttransplant graft survival in part depends on patients' compliance with the treatment regimen. An estimated 5% to 18% of kidney transplant recipients are noncompliant with their posttransplant medical treatment, including taking prescribed medications, coming to office visits, and obtaining regular laboratory tests. From 60% to 90% of these patients lose their graft or die.

This study examined the relationship between pretransplant noncompliance and posttransplant outcomes. Using a longitudinal retrospective chart audit, pretransplant and post-transplant data were collected for 126 kidney transplant recipients over a 3-year period. Patients were identified as noncompliant before transplant if there was written documentation of consistently missed medications, dialysis treatments, or office visits. Patients were identified as noncompliant after transplant if there was written documentation of consistently missed medications, laboratory tests, or office visits. Of the 23 patients (18.3%) identified as noncompliant before transplant, 61% lost their graft or died after transplant. Statistically significant correlations between pretransplant noncompliance and graft loss and between pretransplant and posttransplant noncompliance were found.

requiring transplantation, and the transplant center that will perform the procedure. Medicare not only covers the transplant procedure and hospitalization, but 80% of the cost of immunosuppressive medications for 36 months from the day of hospital discharge. After 3 years, the recipient either pays out of pocket or purchases a supplemental insurance policy that covers the medications.

## IMMUNOLOGY AND TRANSPLANTATION

Successful transplantation of allografts requires manipulation of the recipient's immune system. All cells and tissues in the body have markers or antigens on the cell membrane surface. These antigens allow cells to be recognized by other cells as either "self" or "nonself." (See Chapter 65.) The antigens distributed on the surface of the cells of any one person are unique for that person, except for identical twins, and are controlled by the genes. These cell markers are important in protecting the body from invasion by foreign substances. Because foreign substances have different markers, they can be recognized as nonself by the immune system.

The B and T lymphocytes of the immune system are the surveillance cells that can recognize the cell membrane markers as foreign (nonself) or nonforeign (self). When the markers on cell membranes are recognized as foreign (nonself), the B and T lymphocytes are activated; they then differentiate, proliferate, and clone to be able to attack and destroy the foreign substance.

The ability of immune cells to recognize foreign substances is the result of genetic factors on chromosome 6. This region of the chromosome is called the major histocompatibility complex and codes for human leukocyte antigens (HLA), which initiate the process of rejection and serve as the targets for immunological attack against the transplanted organ. Although these antigens are called human leukocyte antigens, the HLA genetic complex encodes cell membrane markers or antigens on almost all cells in the body. The HLA antigenic complex is classified into two groups. Class I HLAs are encoded by three loci on chromosome 6—loci A, B, and C. Class II HLAs are encoded at four loci—referred to as D, DR, DQ, and DP. Class I HLAs are expressed by almost all cells, including leukocytes, platelets, and cells of most solid organs. Class II HLAs are expressed on fewer cells; however, these antigens are found on many of the immune system cells, including B and some T lymphocytes, macrophages, monocytes, and vascular endothelium.[30,31]

One hundred antigens have been identified in the HLA system. Because of the millions of combinations of antigens that are possible, the chance of two unrelated persons having an identical combination of histocompatibility genes is less than 1 in 20 million. Any cell surface protein configuration that is different from a person's own is an antigen capable of provoking the immunological defense response.[8]

Each person has two number 6 chromosomes, and each chromosome will encode for seven specific HLAs, one for each specific locus. Each person inherits one number 6 chromosome and thus one set of seven HLAs, or one haplotype, from each parent (Figure 68-1). Therefore, using mendelian inheritance principles, two siblings have a 25% possibility of sharing both haplotypes, a 25% possibility of sharing neither haplotype, and a 50% possibility of sharing one haplotype.

A second antigen system important to the acceptance of transplant tissue is the ABO blood typing system. The ABO antigens are on red blood cells (RBCs) and other tissues. Some minor RBC antigens, particularly the Lewis system, are important to transplantation rejection or acceptance and are assessed in recipients and donors. The RHO antigen system is not thought to have a role in the survival or rejection of transplanted tissue or organs.

### TISSUE TYPING AND MATCHING PROCEDURES

In preparation for transplant, some tissue typing and leukocyte crossmatching may be performed. See Box 68-1 for a description of the major tests that may be used to establish compatibility between the donor and recipient.

The number and types of tests vary among transplant centers and by the organ being transplanted. Several reasons exist for this variability. All the antigens play some role in allowing self cells to be differentiated from nonself cells and are found on at least some of the immune system cells. However, the individual locations of the HLA and RBC antigens are not equally important in activating the immune system to attack the nonself transplant tissue. The purpose of histocompatibility testing is to identify the antigens at each locus. The immunogenicity of transplanted organs also varies from most allogeneic to least allogeneic as follows: bone marrow, skin, islets of Langerhans, heart, kidney, and liver. In addition, the

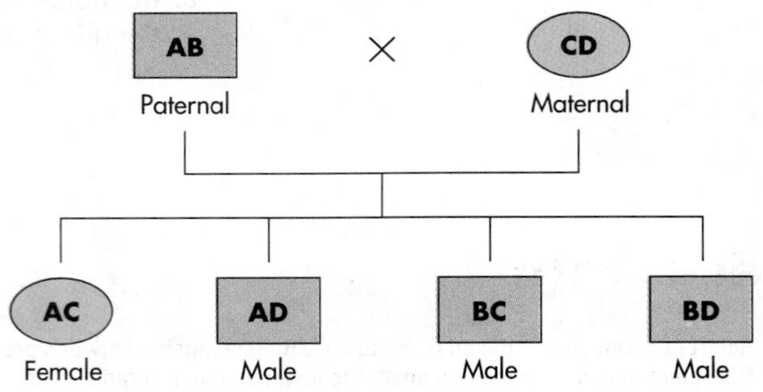


**fig. 68-1** Inheritance of HLA haplotyes. A haplotype is the combination of alleles at each locus on a single chromosome and is almost always inherited as a unit. Haplotype designations are given by A, B, C, and D. Paternal haplotypes are A and B, and maternal haplotypes are C and D. Offspring of this mating inherit one haplotype from each parent and will have one of four possible combinations of haplotypes: AC, AD, BC, and BD. Statistically, 25% of the offspring will be HLA identical (e.g., AC and AC), 25% will be totally HLA nonidentical (e.g., AC and BD), and 50% will be HLA haploidentical (e.g., AC and AD).

preservation time of many organs is too short to allow all these various tests to be completed before transplant.

### Histocompatibility Testing for Different Types of Transplants

Transplantation of organs from live donors is associated with maximal histocompatibility testing. Transplantation of a kidney from a live donor, for example, requires the establishment of ABO compatibility, HLA matching by means of microlymphocytotoxicity testing, and mixed leukocyte (or lymphocyte) culture (MLC). White blood cell (WBC) crossmatch and mixed lymphocyte crossmatch are also conducted.

Because of the very short preservation times of the heart, liver, lung, and pancreas, only minimal histocompatibility testing is possible. With a heart transplant, ABO compatibility is established and a mixed lymphocyte crossmatch is carried out. In liver transplants, the ideal transplant comes from an identical ABO donor. However, incompatible matches are acceptable in emergency situations. Human leukocyte antigen typing and matching and MLC testing are not thought to be as clinically important in liver transplantation as in other types of transplants.

Successful allograft bone marrow transplantation requires maximal compatibility between donor and recipient. This compatibility is identified by microlymphocytotoxicity testing for class I HLAs and by MLC testing for class II HLAs. However, ABO and RH compatibility is not necessary. If a transplant with ABO-incompatible bone marrow is planned, the recipient must undergo plasma exchange to eliminate antibodies against the ABO group of the donor.[34]

Histocompatibility testing, although possible for corneal transplants, is controversial. Sight is restored without HLA matching 95% of the time, and ABO compatibility has not been shown to increase the success of the transplant. However, class I HLA matching may be beneficial for patients who are at high risk for allograft rejection resulting from corneal vascularization.[26]

Research is ongoing to improve histocompatibility testing and identify the most important antigen matching for various transplants. As new information and technology accumulate, tissue-matching procedures for transplants may change.

## DRUG THERAPY TO PREVENT REJECTION

The goal of immunosuppressive drug therapy is to adequately suppress the immune response to prevent rejection of the transplanted organ while maintaining sufficient immunity to prevent overwhelming infection. Many of the medications used have adverse effects. By using a combination of medications that each work in a different phase of the immune response, effective immunosuppression can be achieved with lower doses of each drug while minimizing side effects (Figure 68-2). Immunosuppressive protocols are highly variable among transplant centers, with different combinations of medications used. The major groups of immunosuppressive

**box 68-1** *Tests Used for Tissue Typing and Matching*

**ABO COMPATIBILITY**

Tests surface antigens on RBCs and other tissues; compatibility is same as for blood transfusions; recipient would have antibodies to any ABO antigens present on donor cells and not on recipient cells.

**MINOR RBC ANTIGEN TESTING**

Tests surface antigens on RBCs; transplant recipients who have had multiple transfusions may have antibodies to known minor RBC antigens.

**MICROLYMPHOCYTOTOXICITY TESTING**

Detects class I HLA antigens (A, B, C) and matches these antigens between recipient and donor.

**MIXED LEUKOCYTE CULTURE OR MIXED LYMPHOCYTE CULTURE (MLC)**

Lymphocytes of the potential donor are treated to prevent them from responding. In this way an estimate of the response of a potential recipient (living cells) to a potential donor (treated cells) can be made. The MLC is primarily the result of HLA-D differences between donor and recipient. A low response of the recipient's cells to the donor's cells is predictive of a successful transplant. This test is helpful in live donor transplants. Because the test takes approximately 7 days to complete, it cannot be used for cadaver transplants.

**T CELL CROSSMATCH**

A positive crossmatch occurs when the recipient has demonstrable circulating antibodies against the donor's T cell antigens. These circulating cytotoxic antibodies are detected by incubating donor lymphoid cells in recipient serum in the presence of complement. After a period of incubation, a marker of cell death is added to the suspension, and the proportion of dead cells is counted. The presence of significant numbers of dead cells indicates a positive crossmatch and predicts a poor outcome after transplantation (i.e., hyperacute rejection).

**PANEL REACTIVE ANTIBODY (PRA)**

A blood test using lymphocytotoxic antibodies to determine the presence of preformed antibodies to HLA antigens. The results range from 0% to 100% and reflect the percentage of antigens on the test panel against which the potential recipient has preformed antibodies. If a potential recipient is found to have antibodies against specific HLA antigens, an organ donor carrying those antigens would not be suitable for that recipient because of the increased risk of rejection. A high PRA means that a potential transplant recipient has antibodies against many HLA antigens, and finding a suitable donor will be more difficult.

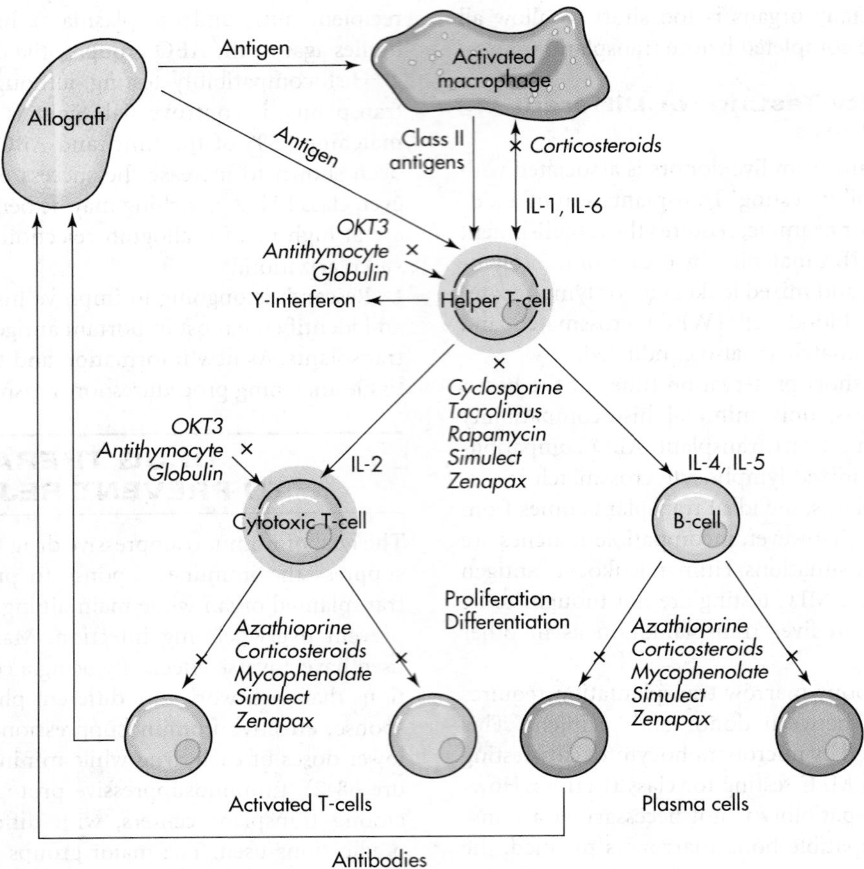


**fig. 68-2** Sites of action for immunosuppressive agents.

agents are (1) mycophenolate mofetil (CellCept), azathioprine (Imuran), or cyclophosphamide (Cytoxan); (2) corticosteroids; (3) cyclosporine (Neoral), tacrolimus (Prograf), or sirolimus (Rapamycin); and (4) antilymphocyte globulin, antithymocyte globulin, or OKT3. These medications plus their mechanism of action and nursing interventions can be found in Table 68-2.

Mycophenolate mofetil is a lymphocyte-specific inhibitor of purine synthesis with antiproliferative effects on both T and B lymphocytes.[33] This drug appears to be most effective when used in combination with the macrolide immunosuppressive agents cyclosporine, tacrolimus, or sirolimus. Its effects are additive because it acts later in the lymphocyte activation pathway by an entirely different mechanism. Mycophenolate mofetil has replaced azathioprine as a first-line agent in the immunosuppressive regimen because of its greater lymphocyte-specific effects.

Cyclosporine is used in most transplant centers in the United States. This fungus extract prevents the production and release of interleukin-2 (IL-2) from T-helper lymphocytes. Because the proliferation and maturation of T-cytotoxic lymphocytes are mediated by IL-2, cyclosporine alters the cell-mediated attack against the transplanted organ. This drug does not cause bone marrow suppression or alter the normal inflammatory response. Cyclosporine is used in conjunction with steroids and mycophenolate mofetil. Many of the side effects of cyclosporine are dose related. Cyclosporine is nephrotoxic. For this reason, drug levels are followed closely to prevent toxicity.

Like cyclosporine, tacrolimus inhibits cytokine production (including IL-2), inhibits expression of IL-2 receptors, and blocks cell division. It is 100 times more potent than cyclosporine but is never used in combination with cyclosporine because of the nephrotoxicity of both drugs. Tacrolimus does not cause hirsutism or gingival hyperplasia and is often selected over cyclosporine for women and adolescents to prevent these distressing side effects.

Sirolimus is a new immunosuppressive agent with structural similarities to tacrolimus. The ability of this drug to prevent chronic rejection and to halt preexisting graft vascular disease makes it unique. Sirolimus suppresses lymphocyte proliferation, but it mediates its effects without directly affecting nucleotide or cytokine synthesis.[25] It also inhibits unpurified B cells from synthesizing antibody. In relatively low doses it has a synergistic effect with cyclosporine or corticosteroids.

Antilymphocyte globulin (ALG) and antithymocyte globulin (ATG) are also used to suppress the immune response in many transplant centers. These agents are prepared by

*Text continued on p. 2232*

table 68-2 Common Medications for **Prevention of Rejection After Organ Transplantation**

| DRUG | ACTION | NURSING INTERVENTION |
|---|---|---|
| Azathioprine (Imuran) | An antimetabolite that suppresses proliferation of rapidly dividing cells, including sensitized T and B cells | • Institute infection control measures<br>• Monitor hematocrit, white blood cell count, and platelet count<br>• Assess for signs and symptoms of infection or bleeding<br>• Administer oral antifungal agent as ordered<br>• Decrease dose as ordered<br>• Assess for jaundice<br>• Monitor serum transaminases, alkaline phosphatase, bilirubin, and coagulation factors<br>• Assess for nausea, vomiting, and abdominal pain<br>• Monitor serum amylase and lipase<br>• Inspect oral mucous membranes<br>• Assess for hair loss<br>• Maintain good oral hygiene |
| Mycophenolate mofetil (CellCept) | Inhibits purine synthesis, which suppresses proliferation of T and B cells | • Decrease dose as ordered<br>• Monitor GI status (nausea, vomiting, diarrhea, abdominal cramps, dyspepsia)<br>• Monitor daily weight<br>• Monitor intake and output<br>• Administer antiemetics as ordered<br>• Administer antidiarrheal agents as ordered<br>• Institute infection control measures<br>• Monitor white blood cell count |
| Corticosteroids (prednisone) | Suppresses inflammatory response, prevents proliferation of T-cytotoxic lymphocytes | • Instruct patient about all potential side effects<br>• Administer low-sodium diet<br>• Monitor daily weights<br>• Administer low-fat, low-cholesterol diet if cholesterol elevated<br>• Consult dietitian<br>• Instruct patient to watch calorie intake carefully and eat low-calorie snacks between meals<br>• Administer oral corticosteroids with food to minimize GI upset<br>• Administer antacids, $H_2$ receptor blockers as ordered<br>• Perform guaiac tests on stool and emesis<br>• Observe for abdominal pain and rebound tenderness<br>• Report complaints of acid indigestion, esophageal or gastric burning<br>• Monitor blood glucose<br>• Administer insulin as ordered<br>• Instruct patient regarding diabetes, if newly acquired<br>• Inspect skin<br>• Avoid skin trauma and use of adhesive tape<br>• Inspect oral mucous membranes<br>• Maintain good oral hygiene<br>• Administer oral antifungal agents<br>• Monitor wound healing<br>• Assess and report complaints of bone or joint pain<br>• Consult physical therapy<br>• Administer calcium or vitamin D as ordered<br>• Monitor changes in muscle strength<br>• Instruct patient to exercise regularly to counteract muscle weakness |

From Bartucci MR: Nursing care of the immunosuppressed patient. In Chabalewski F, editor: *Donation and transplantation: nursing curriculum,* Richmond, Va, 1996, UNOS.

*Continued*

**table 68-2** *Common Medications for* ***Prevention of Rejection After Organ Transplantation—cont'd***

| Drug | Action | Nursing Intervention |
|---|---|---|
| Corticosteroids (prednisone)—*cont'd* | | • Assess presence of psychosis, euphoria, depression, irritability<br>• Consult psychiatrist if necessary<br>• Assess for peripheral edema<br>• Monitor blood pressure<br>• Administer antihypertensive medication as ordered<br>• Administer diuretics as ordered |
| Cyclophosphamide (Cytoxan) | An alkylating agent that interferes with DNA, RNA, and protein synthesis | • Institute infection control measures<br>• Monitor hematocrit, white blood cell count, and platelet count<br>• Assess for signs and symptoms of infection<br>• Assess for hematuria<br>• Encourage increased water intake with each dose<br>• Assess for hair loss<br>• Reduce dose as ordered |
| Cyclosporine (Neoral, Sandimmune) | Prevents production and release of interleukin-2, inhibits maturation of T-cytotoxic lymphocyte precursors | • Instruct patient about all side effects<br>• Obtain true trough cyclosporine levels<br>• Decrease dose as ordered<br>• Monitor serum creatinine, blood urea nitrogen, potassium, serum transaminases, alkaline phosphatase bilirubin, and coagulation factors<br>• Review medication list for drugs that increase or decrease cyclosporine metabolism<br>• Assess patient for peripheral edema and high blood pressure<br>• Administer diuretics as ordered<br>• Administer antihypertensive medications as ordered<br>• Monitor neurological status (tremors, paresthesias) and assure patient that these side effects are dose related<br>• Assess for jaundice<br>• Instruct patient in use of depilatories if hirsutism occurs<br>• Instruct patient to see dentist for teeth cleaning every 6 months or more often if gingival hyperplasia is present<br>• Instruct patient in proper oral hygiene, including flossing |
| Tacrolimus (Prograf) | Prevents production and release of interleukin-2, inhibits maturation of T-cytotoxic lymphocyte precursors; 100 times more potent than cyclosporine | • Instruct patient about all side effects<br>• Obtain true trough levels<br>• Decrease dose as ordered<br>• Monitor serum creatinine, blood urea nitrogen, and potassium<br>• Monitor neurological status (headache, confusion, seizures). Assure patient that these side effects are dose related<br>• Monitor GI status (anorexia, nausea, vomiting, diarrhea, weight loss)<br>• Monitor daily weights<br>• Monitor intake and output<br>• Monitor blood glucose<br>• Administer insulin or oral hypoglycemic agents as ordered<br>• Educate patient regarding diabetes, if newly acquired |

*Continued*

**table 68-2** Common Medications for **Prevention of Rejection After Organ Transplantation—cont'd**

| Drug | Action | Nursing Intervention |
|---|---|---|
| Muromonab-CD3 (OKT3, Orthoclone) | A monoclonal antibody that removes circulating T lymphocytes | • Administer prescribed acetaminophen, diphenhydramine, and hydrocortisone at time of IV infusion<br>• Administer IV push over 30-60 seconds<br>• Treat symptomatically and provide for patient comfort<br>• Weigh daily (patient should be within 3% of his or her dry weight)<br>• Prepare patient for chest radiograph to assess congestion<br>• Assess for peripheral edema<br>• Auscultate lungs before the first dose is administered for baseline comparison<br>• Administer prescribed diuretics<br>• Monitor GI status (nausea, vomiting, diarrhea)<br>• Administer antiemetics as ordered<br>• Administer antidiarrheal agents as ordered<br>• Monitor intake and output<br>• Administer IV fluids as ordered<br>• Monitor temperature<br>• Administer acetaminophen as ordered<br>• Report complaints of headache<br>• Administer analgesics as ordered<br>• Report complaints of photophobia and keep room darkened<br>• Arrange for outpatient administration to complete course |
| Antilymphocyte globulin (ALG)<br>Antithymocyte globulin (ATG) | A polyclonal antibody directed against lymphocytes; reduces circulating lymphocytes, decreases lymphocyte proliferation | • Monitor temperature<br>• Administer acetaminophen/diphenhydramine, as ordered<br>• Monitor platelet count<br>• Decrease dose as ordered if platelets <100,000<br>• Administer through central line over 4-6 hr |
| Sirolimus (Rapamycin, Rapamune) | Suppresses lymphocyte proliferation, inhibits B cells from synthesizing antibody | • Monitor gastrointestinal status for nausea, vomiting, diarrhea<br>• Monitor daily weight<br>• Monitor intake and output<br>• Administer antiemetics as ordered<br>• Administer antidiarrheal agents as ordered<br>• Monitor cholesterol and triglyceride levels<br>• Decrease dose as ordered<br>• Monitor surgical wound for infection and delayed healing |
| Chimeric anti–IL-2 Receptor Antibody (Simulect)<br>Daclizumab (Humanized anti-TAC, Zenapax) | Monoclonal antibody against IL-2 receptor; blocks T cell activation and proliferation | • Administer by IV infusion over 15-30 min through peripheral vein<br>• Arrange for outpatient infusion to complete course of therapy after discharge |

immunizing horses, goats, or rabbits with human lymphocytes (for ALG) or thymocytes (for ATG). The antibody made against human lymphocytes or thymocytes is then purified and administered intravenously. Their mechanism of action is not known. Both ALG and ATG are used for induction to prevent rejection immediately after transplantation or less commonly to treat an acute rejection episode.

Allergic reactions to the foreign proteins contained in the immunosuppressive agents are common but usually are not severe enough to preclude use. Fever, arthralgias, and tachycardia commonly occur. These reactions can be attenuated by administering the preparation slowly, over 4 to 6 hours, and premedicating patients with acetaminophen (Tylenol) and diphenhydramine hydrochloride (Benadryl). Patients may develop antibodies against the antisera that limit the drugs' effectiveness during subsequent courses of treatment. The main toxicities of these antisera are lymphopenia and thrombocytopenia caused by antibody contaminants that are not completely removed during preparation of the antisera.

Monoclonal antibodies are usually used for treating acute rejection episodes, but they may also be used for induction to prevent acute rejection after transplantation. OKT3 was the first of these monoclonal antibodies to be used. OKT3 is a mouse monoclonal antibody that reacts with the T3 antigen found on the surface of human thymocytes and mature T cells. Thus OKT3 is an anti–antigen receptor antibody that interferes with the function of the T lymphocyte, the pivotal cell in the response to graft rejection. This agent reverses 95% of acute rejection episodes.

A flulike syndrome that lasts through the first few days of treatment is caused by vasoactive substances released from the T3 cells during treatment. All patients receive Tylenol, Benadryl, and corticosteroids at the time of intravenous infusion to reduce the severity of the symptoms. Severe pulmonary reactions manifested by dyspnea, wheezing, or acute respiratory failure have occurred in some patients.

The side effects associated with OKT3 virtually mandate hospital admission during treatment. However, all of the side effects tend to subside within 3 to 5 days, making a switch to outpatient administration feasible (see the Research Box).

**research**

Reference: Hricik DE et al: Outpatient use of OKT3 for the treatment of acute allograft rejection, *Clin Transplant* 4:19, 1990.

All patients receiving OKT3 experience side effects for the first 3 to 5 days, mandating hospital admission. Outpatient administration is feasible once side effects subside. A retrospective chart review of 79 consecutive renal transplant patients who received OKT3 over a 3-year period was done to (1) determine the percentage of patients able to receive outpatient therapy; (2) compare clinical variables in patients receiving outpatient therapy versus those hospitalized; and (3) identify conditions precluding outpatient therapy. Forty-seven percent of patients received one to six outpatient doses; 136 of 856 total doses (16%) were administered as outpatient therapy. There were no significant differences in patient age, previous rejection episodes, or number of diabetic persons in the inpatient and outpatient groups. The decision to use outpatient therapy did not depend on ultimate rejection reversal after OKT3 administration. Peak serum creatinine levels during treatment were higher in the inpatient group. All patients exhibited fever for at least 1 day, but inpatients were febrile for more days. Of the 46 patients remaining hospitalized, 17 had difficulty with transportation or concern about compliance with daily office visits. In conclusion, almost half the patients had decreased length of stay because of outpatient therapy. Persistent fever and renal dysfunction were the main factors precluding outpatient therapy.

## KIDNEY TRANSPLANT

### ETIOLOGY

Kidney transplant is primarily used to treat patients experiencing end-stage renal disease resulting from diabetes, hypertension, and glomerulonephritis. The advantages of kidney transplantation include the reversal of many of the pathophysiological changes associated with renal failure as normal kidney function is restored. It also eliminates the patient's dependence on dialysis and its accompanying dietary restrictions, provides the opportunity to return to normal life activities (including employment), and is less expensive than dialysis after the first year. Some patients who are approaching end-stage renal disease may be transplanted before they require dialysis if a kidney becomes available. This approach is most advantageous for children, whose physical and mental development is significantly impaired by renal failure, and for patients with diabetes, who have a much higher mortality rate on dialysis than nondiabetics.

### EPIDEMIOLOGY

Kidney transplant is the oldest and most common type of transplant procedure. The first kidney transplant was performed in the early 1950s, and the procedure is now well established as a viable and desirable alternative to dialysis as a treatment for end-stage renal disease. Currently, over 100,000 persons in the United States have received kidney transplants, and about 11,000 new transplants are performed each year. However, more than 160,000 people are being maintained on dialysis, and the lack of available organs is significant. More than 20,000 people are currently on the transplant list waiting for an available organ.

### COLLABORATIVE CARE MANAGEMENT

#### Diagnostic Tests

The diagnostic testing for transplant is discussed on p. 2226. Kidney transplant is associated with maximal histocompatibility testing, especially in situations involving a live donor. ABO compatibility, HLA matching, WBC crossmatch, and mixed lymphocyte crossmatch are all performed.

### Medications

Patients undergoing kidney transplant will be started and maintained on the full battery of immunosuppressive therapy that is outlined on p. 2227-2232. Immunosuppressive therapy is maintained for life to preserve the transplanted kidney.

### Treatments

Patients awaiting kidney transplant continue on their regular schedule of dialysis right up to the time of transplant. Dialysis is conducted as close to the surgery as possible to ensure that the patient is in the best possible metabolic condition to withstand the rigors of surgery. Living donor kidneys usually begin to function immediately after surgery. Cadaver kidneys may experience a delay in functioning, and the patient might need to have dialysis resumed after surgery to maintain physiological homeostasis.

### Surgical Management

The donor kidney is carefully dissected free with its renal artery and vein intact. The ureter is also dissected with great care to preserve the periureteral vascular supply. The kidney is removed, flushed with a chilled, sterile electrolyte solution, and prepared for transplant into the recipient. The procedure takes about 2 hours.

The transplanted kidney is placed extraperitoneally, in the iliac fossa (Figure 68-3). Generally the peritoneal cavity is not entered. The patient's own kidneys are not removed unless they are infected or are the cause of significant hypertension. The patient's kidneys are left intact to maintain erythropoietin production, blood pressure control, and prostaglandin synthesis and metabolism.[23] Efficient revascularization is critical to prevent ischemic injury to the kidney.

The donor ureter is used to the extent possible. If long enough, the donor ureter is tunneled through the bladder submucosa and sutured in place. This allows the bladder to clamp down on the ureter as it contracts for micturition, thereby preventing reflux of urine up the ureter into the transplanted kidney. The entire transplant surgery takes about 3 hours.

### Diet

Before surgery the patient with end-stage renal disease continues on the renal failure diet that has been prescribed. One of the major benefits of successful kidney transplantation is the ability to eat a more normal diet without the extensive restrictions of protein, fluid, sodium, and potassium that are characteristic of the management of end-stage renal disease. However, the patient will need to continue to control the sodium and calorie content of the diet after transplant to manage the side effects of high-dose steroid administration as part of the overall plan for immunosuppression.

### Activity

Activity restrictions are not necessary after successful kidney transplantation. The patient typically experiences a significant improvement in energy level and mood and is able to gradually resume a more active role in family and social activities. The ultimate goal is to support the patient's return to gainful employment.

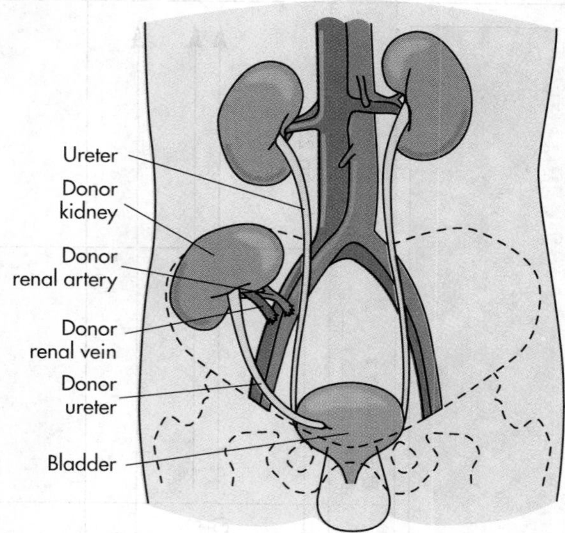


**fig. 68-3** Location of a transplanted kidney showing the anastomosis of the renal artery, renal vein, and ureter.

### Referrals

Various referrals may be needed for patients undergoing kidney transplantation. The patient requires long-term follow-up by a transplant service. The services of a dietitian may be helpful as the patient attempts to understand the differences in diet restrictions that are in place after transplant. The patient may need assistance understanding and managing the complex medication regimen and usually profits from involvement with a support group. The psychological and emotional responses to transplantation are highly unpredictable, but they can be profound, especially when a kidney has been donated by a family member.

A Clinical Pathway that outlines the care for a patient undergoing kidney transplant is found on p. 2234.

## NURSING MANAGEMENT OF THE PERSON UNDERGOING KIDNEY TRANSPLANT

### PREOPERATIVE CARE

Nursing care of the patient in the preoperative phase includes emotional and physical preparation for surgery. Because the patient and family may have been waiting 2 to 3 years for the transplant, a review of the operative procedure and what can be expected in the immediate postoperative recovery period is important. The nurse informs the patient that there is a 20% chance the kidney will not function immediately and dialysis may be required for the first few

*Text continued on p. 2239*

## clinical pathway *Kidney Transplant*

**UNIVERSITY HOSPITALS**
of Cleveland

CARE PATH NAME: KIDNEY TRANSPLANT
DRG: ELOS: 7 days
Expected Disposition: Home
Surgery Date: ___/___/___
Pre-op Dry Weight: ___ Kg

Collaborative Problem List
1. Impaired Home Maintenance Management
2. Potential for Infection
3. Knowledge Deficit
4. Fluid and Electrolyte Imbalance
5. Pain Management
6.
7.

| FOCUS | PRE-OP<br>DATE: ___/___/___ | DAY OF SURGERY<br>DATE: ___/___/___ | POST-OP DAY 1<br>DATE: ___/___/___ | POST-OP DAY 2<br>DATE: ___/___/___ | POST-OP DAY 3<br>DATE: ___/___/___ | POST-OP DAY 4<br>DATE: ___/___/___ |
|---|---|---|---|---|---|---|
| **Laboratory/ Tests/ Procedures** | • Chem 23<br>• CBC + Diff<br>• PT/PTT<br>• Urine C&S<br>• T&C 2 U PRBC<br>• Check CMV status<br>• Chemstick if diabetic<br>• CMV IgG quantitative | • Immediately Post-op: Chem 7, CBC<br>• 8 hours post-op: Chem 7, CBC<br>• CXR on arrival to PACU | • CBC + Diff<br>• Chem 23<br>• CD3 level if on OKT3<br>• CXR<br>• Ultrasound as indicated per protocol | • Chem 7 →<br>• Urine for bacteria/ fungus<br>• CBC (Diff if on OKT3) →<br>• CD3 level if on OKT3 →<br>• CYA level starting day 2 of therapy → | → | • Chem 23 |
| **Consults/ Referrals** | | | • Consider PT Consult<br>• Dietary screen and evaluation | | | |
| **Physical Assessment** | • VS q4h<br>• Weight<br>• Baseline skin assessment<br>• Renal assessment regarding need for dialysis | • BP, AP, Rq 1/2 h until stable then q2h-q4h then q4h prn<br>• Temp. immediately and q2h × 16 h then q4h<br>• CVP q2-4 × 16 h then q 4 h<br>• Pulse ox baseline and prn →<br>• Urine output q1h × 24 h then q4h × 24 then qs | • VS q4h with CVP<br>• Urine output q4h weight<br>• Bowel sounds | • VS q4h<br>• I&O q shift →<br>• Weight →<br>• Pulse ox × 2 | • VS q shift → | → |
| **Activity** | • Up ad lib | • Bed rest | • Out of bed → chair | | | |
| **Treatments** | • Fleet enemas × 2<br>• Hibiclens shower<br>• SCDs with patient to OR<br>• Apply Teds pre-op | • $O_2$ per order, wean as tolerated<br>• CVP dressing<br>• JP dressing →<br>• Incision dressing<br>• Incentive spirometry q1h W/A →<br>• Foley care →<br>• Guaiac stools →<br>• SCDs and Teds → | • D/C $O_2$ if RA pulse ox > 92%<br>• Incision care | • Up with assistance<br>• CVP dressing<br>• D/C JP if output <30 cc →<br>• Remove incision dressing | • Out of bed ad lib →<br>• Incentive spirometry q2h W/A → | • CVP dressing<br>• D/C Foley |

| FOCUS | PRE-OP DATE: ___/___/___ | DAY OF SURGERY DATE: ___/___/___ | POST-OP DAY 1 DATE: ___/___/___ | POST-OP DAY 2 DATE: ___/___/___ | POST-OP DAY 3 DATE: ___/___/___ | POST-OP DAY 4 DATE: ___/___/___ |
|---|---|---|---|---|---|---|
| **Diet** | • NPO | • NPO, ice chips<br>• Advance as tolerated | • Diabetic/or any other diet restrictions as indicated → | → | → | → |
| **Medications** | • On call to OR: Antibiotic, Solumedrol 250 mg IV, Imuran 5 mg/kg IV maximum dose—500 mg<br>• Induction Options: OKT3, ATG, Cyclosporine, MMF, Neoral | • Solumedrol 60 mg q6h IV →<br>• Antibiotic<br>• Fluid replacements | → (Solumedrol 60 mg q6h IV)<br>• Imuran or Mycophenolate<br>• OKT3, ATG, Cyclosporine, Neoral<br>• Gancyclovir 2.5 mg/kg qd if CMV (+) or CMV (−) receiving (+) organ<br>• MSO4 prn | • Solumedrol 60 mg IV q8h<br>• OKT3, ATG, Cyclosporine, Neoral →<br>• Gancyclovir →<br>• Bactrim ss or Trimethoprim qd →<br>• Colace →<br>• Clotrimazole →<br>• Acyclovir →<br>• Zantac → | • Solumedrol 60 mg IV q12h<br>• Tylenol #3<br>• Cytogam if donor CMV (+) and recipient (−) | → (Imuran or Mycophenolate; OKT3, ATG, Cyclosporine, Neoral; Gancyclovir; Bactrim ss or Trimethoprim qd; Colace; Clotrimazole; Acyclovir; Zantac)<br>• Prednisone 1 mg/kg/day<br>• OKT3, CYA or ATG<br>• Tylenol or Darvon |
| **Patient/ Family Teaching** | • View pre-op transplant video<br>• Orient to Tower 9 | | • Give teaching materials to patient<br>• Renal transplant booklet<br>• Preprinted cards<br>• I&O sheet<br>• Outcome criteria form | • Review of meds and teaching material with patient/family → | → | • Continued review and if ready, take test |
| **Discharge Planning** | | • Social Worker review notes from information appointments | • Review chart, interview RN and patient →<br>• Collect psychosocial data (insurance, financial issues, discharge needs) → | →<br>→<br>• Psychosocial assessment, support and education/ information → | →<br>→<br>→<br>• Initial note in chart<br>• Discuss prescription plan | • Arrange financial applications<br>• Begin arranging prescription plans<br>• Meet/talk with family prn<br>→<br>• Consult/refer to other disciplines prn<br>• For patients using mail order program, arrange forms with physicians |

University Hospitals' carepaths have been developed to assist clinicians in patient management and clinical decision-making. The carepaths are intended to meet the needs of patients in most circumstances. They are not intended to replace a clinician's judgment or establish a protocol for all patients with this diagnosis.

*SCDs*, Sequential compression devices; *AP*, apical pulse; *JP*, Jackson-Pratt.

SP-9601 (01/05/96)

*Continued*

## Kidney Transplant—cont'd

| FOCUS | PRE-OP<br>DATE: ___/___/___ | DAY OF SURGERY<br>DATE: ___/___/___ | POST-OP DAY 1<br>DATE: ___/___/___ | POST-OP DAY 2<br>DATE: ___/___/___ | POST-OP DAY 3<br>DATE: ___/___/___ | POST-OP DAY 4<br>DATE: ___/___/___ |
|---|---|---|---|---|---|---|
| **Intermediate Outcomes** | 1. Viewed video<br>2. Negative cross-match | 1. Hemodynamically stable<br>2. CVP 10-12<br>3. Euvolemic with fluid replacements<br>4. Vital signs returned to baseline<br>5. K + <6.0<br>6. Equal and clear breath sounds<br>7. Pain controlled | 1. Hemodynamically stable<br>2. CVP 10-12<br>3. Euvolemic with or without fluid replacements<br>4. Vital signs at baseline<br>5. Decrease in BUN and Cr from pre-op<br>6. Equal and clear breath sounds<br>7. Pain controlled<br>8. Teaching material given to patient/family<br>9. Immunosuppression dosages adjusted | 1. Hemodynamically stable<br>2. Euvolemic without fluid replacements<br>3. Decrease in BUN and Cr<br>4. Electrolytes WNL<br>5. Equal and clear breath sounds<br>6. Pain controlled<br>7. Ambulating<br>8. Tolerating oral meds and diet<br>9. Teaching begun<br>10. JP removed if drainage is <30 cc for 24 h<br>11. Immunosuppression dosages adjusted<br>12. Wound dry and approximated | 1. Hemodynamically stable<br>2. Euvolemic<br>3. Decrease in BUN and Cr<br>4. Electrolytes WNL<br>5. Equal and clear breath sounds<br>6. Pain controlled<br>7. Actively participates in ADLs<br>8. Ambulates at baseline<br>9. Has bowel movement<br>10. Initial Social Worker note in chart<br>11. Teaching continues<br>12. JP removed if drainage is <30 cc for 24 h<br>13. Immunosuppression dosages adjusted<br>14. Wound dry and approximated | 1. Hemodynamically stable<br>2. Euvolemic<br>3. Decrease in BUN and Cr<br>4. Electrolytes WNL<br>5. Equal and clear breath sounds<br>6. Actively participates in ADL<br>7. Pain controlled<br>8. Ambulates at baseline<br>9. Has bowel movement<br>10. Teaching continues<br>11. Foley discontinued<br>12. JP removed if drainage is <30 cc for 24 h<br>13. Immunosuppression dosages adjusted<br>14. Wound dry and approximated<br>15. Financial and prescription arrangements made |
| **Intermediate Outcomes RN Signature Days** | ☐ Met<br>☐ Not Met (see notes)<br>#s not met ______<br>Signature ______ | ☐ Met<br>☐ Not Met (see notes)<br>#s not met ______<br>Signature ______ | ☐ Met<br>☐ Not Met (see notes)<br>#s not met ______<br>Signature ______ | ☐ Met<br>☐ Not Met (see notes)<br>#s not met ______<br>Signature ______ | ☐ Met<br>☐ Not Met (see notes)<br>#s not met ______<br>Signature ______ | ☐ Met<br>☐ Not Met (see notes)<br>#s not met ______<br>Signature ______ |
| **Intermediate Outcomes RN Signature Evenings** | ☐ Met<br>☐ Not Met (see notes)<br>#s not met ______<br>Signature ______ | ☐ Met<br>☐ Not Met (see notes)<br>#s not met ______<br>Signature ______ | ☐ Met<br>☐ Not Met (see notes)<br>#s not met ______<br>Signature ______ | ☐ Met<br>☐ Not Met (see notes)<br>#s not met ______<br>Signature ______ | ☐ Met<br>☐ Not Met (see notes)<br>#s not met ______<br>Signature ______ | ☐ Met<br>☐ Not Met (see notes)<br>#s not met ______<br>Signature ______ |
| **Intermediate Outcomes RN Signature Nights** | ☐ Met<br>☐ Not Met (see notes)<br>#s not met ______<br>Signature ______ | ☐ Met<br>☐ Not Met (see notes)<br>#s not met ______<br>Signature ______ | ☐ Met<br>☐ Not Met (see notes)<br>#s not met ______<br>Signature ______ | ☐ Met<br>☐ Not Met (see notes)<br>#s not met ______<br>Signature ______ | ☐ Met<br>☐ Not Met (see notes)<br>#s not met ______<br>Signature ______ | ☐ Met<br>☐ Not Met (see notes)<br>#s not met ______<br>Signature ______ |

| FOCUS | POST-OP DAY 5<br>DATE: ___/___/___ | POST-OP DAY 6<br>DATE: ___/___/___ | POST-OP DAY 7<br>DATE: ___/___/___ |
|---|---|---|---|
| **Laboratory/ Tests/ Procedures** | • CBC (Diff if on OKT3)<br>• Chem 7<br>• CD 3 level if on OKT3<br>• CYA level | →<br>→<br>→<br>→ | →<br>→<br>→<br>→ |
| **Consults/ Referrals** | • Consider Home Team referral | | |
| **Physical Assessment** | • VS qs<br>• I&O qs<br>• Weight | →<br>→<br>→ | →<br>→<br>→ |
| **Activity** | • OOB ad lib | → | → |
| **Treatments** | • Guaiac stools<br>• Incentive spirometry q2h W/A | →<br>• CVP dressing | →<br>• D/C central line |
| **Diet** | • Diabetic or any other diet restriction as indicated | → | → |
| **Medications** | • Prednisone—taper as indicated<br>• Imuran or Mycophenolate<br>• OKT3, ATG, Neoral or Cyclosporine<br>• Gancyclovir<br>• Bactrim<br>• Colace<br>• Clotrimazole<br>• Acyclovir<br>• T3 or Darvon<br>• Zantac | →<br>→<br>→<br>→<br>→<br>→<br>→<br>→<br>→<br>→ | • D/C Gancylovir<br>• Acyclovir<br><br>**SrCr** / **Dosage**<br><1.4 / 800 mg PO q6h<br>1.5-2.5 / 800 mg PO q8h<br>2.6-4.5 / 800 mg PO q12h<br>>4.5 / 800 mg PO q24h<br>HD / 800 mg PO q48h |

*Continued*

## Kidney Transplant—cont'd

| FOCUS | POST-OP DAY 5<br>DATE: __/__/__ | POST-OP DAY 6<br>DATE: __/__/__ | POST-OP DAY 7<br>DATE: __/__/__ |
|---|---|---|---|
| **Patient/ Family Teaching** | • Take test<br>• Diet teaching prn | • Review material as needed and retake test if needed | • Review homegoing med dosages, clinic and lab test follow-up appointments |
| **Discharge Planning** | • Arrange financial applications<br>• Arrange prescription plans<br>• Meet/talk with family prn<br>• Other D/C plans<br>• Psychosocial assessment, support, and education/information | • Transportation arrangements prn →<br>• Other D/C plans carried out prn →<br>• Final note in chart with D/C plan<br>Psychosocial assessment, support, and education/information → | |
| **Homegoing Medications** | • Mail order prescription forms completed and faxed by 2:00 PM. (If weekend/holiday D/C anticipated must do this by 2:00 PM, Friday). | • Delivery of medications prn → | |
| **Intermediate Outcomes** | 1. Hemodynamically stable →<br>2. Euvolemic →<br>3. Electrolytes WNL →<br>4. Independent in ADL and ambulation →<br>5. Has bowel movement →<br>6. Test taken and passed with 90% or continue med review<br>7. Scale and thermometer arranged for home<br>8. JP removed if drainage is <30 cc for 24 hr<br>9. Immunosuppression dosage assessed →<br>10. Financial and prescription plans arranged<br>11. Cyclosporine levels assessed and adjusted | | 1. D/C to home with written instructions<br>2. Medications available to take at home<br>3. Refer to discharge order form |
| **Intermediate Outcomes RN Signature Days** | ☐ Met<br>☐ Not Met (see notes)<br>#s not met ______<br>Signature ______ | ☐ Met<br>☐ Not Met (see notes)<br>#s not met ______<br>Signature ______ | ☐ Met<br>☐ Not Met (see notes)<br>#s not met ______<br>Signature ______ |
| **Intermediate Outcomes RN Signature Nights** | ☐ Met<br>☐ Not Met (see notes)<br>#s not met ______<br>Signature ______ | ☐ Met<br>☐ Not Met (see notes)<br>#s not met ______<br>Signature ______ | ☐ Met<br>☐ Not Met (see notes)<br>#s not met ______<br>Signature ______ |

weeks. In addition, the rationale for the immunosuppressive therapy and the importance of preventing infection after surgery are stressed.

To ensure that the patient is in optimal physical condition for surgery, an electrocardiogram (ECG), chest x-ray, and laboratory studies are performed. Dialysis is often required to achieve optimal fluid, electrolyte, and acid-base balance, as well as to remove excess nitrogenous wastes. Because dialysis may be required after transplant, the patency of the vascular access must be maintained. The extremity containing the vascular access is wrapped in Kerlix and labeled "dialysis access." This identification reminds all caregivers to avoid using the affected extremity for blood pressure measurement, phlebotomy, or intravenous infusions.

## POSTOPERATIVE CARE

### Care of the Donor

The postoperative care of a live donor is similar to that provided after a nephrectomy (see Chapter 44). The donor can easily become a forgotten person in the transplant process because most of the attention is focused on the recipient. The pain of a nephrectomy is significant, and adequate analgesia is essential to ensure comfort, promote ambulation, and prevent atelectasis and possible pulmonary complications. Most donors are discharged within 3 to 5 days and can usually return to work in 1 month.

The majority of kidney donors feel good about the donation because of the improved health of their family member or significant other. Nurses caring for live donors need to acknowledge the precious gift they have given.

Care of the cadaver donor is outlined in the Nursing Care Plan on p. 2223.

### Care of the Recipient

#### Maintaining fluid and electrolyte balance

The first priority of care for the recipient is maintenance of fluid and electrolyte balance. Kidney transplant recipients often spend the first 24 hours after surgery in the intensive care unit because of the close monitoring required. Rapid diuresis may take place soon after the blood supply to the kidney is reestablished, especially in live donor transplants. This diuresis is due to (1) the kidney's ability to filter blood urea nitrogen (BUN), which acts as an osmotic diuretic; (2) the abundance of fluids administered intravenously during the operation; and (3) the renal tubular dysfunction, which inhibits the kidney from concentrating urine normally. Urine output during this phase may be as high as 1 L per hour, slowing down as the BUN and serum creatinine levels return toward normal. The patient's urine output is measured and replaced with intravenous fluids hourly for the first 12 to 24 hours. Central venous pressure readings are essential for monitoring the patient's postoperative fluid status. Dehydration is avoided to prevent renal hypoperfusion and further tubular damage. The patient's electrolyte levels are closely monitored to assess for hypokalemia, which is often associated with rapid diuresis. Hyponatremia can also result from the kidney tubules' inability to concentrate. Delayed graft function occurs in 20% of patients receiving cadaver kidneys that have been preserved for longer than 24 hours. The ischemic damage from prolonged preservation results in acute tubular necrosis (ATN), which can last anywhere from several days to weeks, followed by gradually improving kidney function. These patients may need to be discharged from the hospital on dialysis. Dialysis is discontinued when the patient's urine output increases and serum creatinine and BUN levels normalize. Some patients develop high-output ATN—that is, they are able to excrete fluid but unable to excrete metabolic wastes or regulate electrolytes. Other patients experience oliguric or anuric ATN. These patients are at risk for fluid overload in the immediate postoperative period.

A sudden decrease in urine output in the early postoperative period may be caused by dehydration, rejection, a technical complication such as vascular thrombosis, or an obstruction that impedes urine flow. Any decrease in output is thoroughly investigated. A blood clot in the Foley catheter is a common cause of early obstruction. Because the catheter remains in the bladder for 3 to 5 days after surgery to allow the bladder anastomosis to heal, its patency must be ensured. The physician may order careful sterile catheter irrigation to dislodge the occluding clots.

Most patients undergo ultrasonography within 24 hours of transplantation to assess the kidney's vascular supply and look for any fluid collections, such as hematoma, lymphocele, or urine leak. The presence of hydronephrosis, with or without a dilated ureter, may indicate obstruction.

Once the patient has sufficiently recovered from the operative procedure, nursing care involves ongoing assessment, diagnosis, intervention, and evaluation of the patient's response to the transplant. This includes the prevention or treatment of allograft rejection, prevention of and monitoring for infection, and monitoring for the complications of surgery and immunosuppression. Some institutions still use protective isolation, but scrupulous patient hygiene and thorough staff hand washing are two of the most effective interventions to prevent infection. The nurse carefully assesses all insertion sites for invasive lines and devices. People with active infections should not visit or care for the patient. Environmental cleanliness is carefully assessed and ensured.

#### Patient/family education

Patient/family education is an integral part of a smooth transition from hospital to home. The first priority for discharge preparation is medication teaching. Patients and their families must be able to explain the action, dosage, and potential adverse effects of all medications. A written list of discharge medications with the administration schedule is supplied for the patient to use as a home resource.

Patients should be able to describe the signs and symptoms of rejection and infection and when and how to contact the transplant office if symptoms are present (Box 68-2). A follow-up appointment is scheduled, along with instructions for any routine laboratory testing. Careful timing of cyclosporine and tacrolimus administration is essential if 12-hour trough level testing is scheduled.

**box 68-2** *Signs and Symptoms of Acute Rejection in the Renal Transplant Patient*

Decrease in urine output
Fever greater than 37.7° C (100° F); may be masked by steroid therapy
Pain or tenderness over grafted kidney
Edema
Sudden weight gain: 2 to 3 pounds in a 24-hour period
Hypertension
General malaise
Increase in serum creatinine and BUN
Decrease in creatinine clearance
Evidence of rejection on ultrasound or biopsy

The nurse also discusses postdischarge activity limitations, sexuality issues, and dietary recommendations. Most patients can return to work in 6 to 12 weeks. Heavy lifting (more than 20 pounds) is avoided for the first 6 weeks, until the incision completely heals. Regular exercise is encouraged to counteract the proximal muscle weakness associated with steroid administration.

Patients can resume sexual intercourse after 4 to 6 weeks. Women of childbearing age are encouraged to postpone pregnancy for at least 1 year after transplant to ensure stable renal function and allow for lower doses of immunosuppressives. Barrier contraceptive methods such as condoms, diaphragms, and foam are recommended. Oral contraceptives and intrauterine devices are not recommended because of the risks of thrombophlebitis and infection. Some women prefer to use contraceptive injections because they are easier and are more reliable in protecting against pregnancy.

The dietitian is an excellent resource for educating patients and families about good eating habits. Steroids commonly stimulate appetite, and the dietitian can offer suggestions for low-calorie snacks to minimize weight gain. The dietitian also provides teaching about cholesterol restriction because of the risk of hyperlipidemia associated with the use of steroids and cyclosporine. Although most renal patients are accustomed to following a low-sodium diet, a review of foods to avoid and hidden sources of sodium in fast food and convenience foods may help the patient minimize the salt- and water-retaining effects of steroids.

## GERONTOLOGICAL CONSIDERATIONS

The incidence of end-stage renal disease is increasing most rapidly in the elderly population, which makes issues related to kidney transplantation particularly relevant for this group. Almost one third of all new cases of end-stage renal disease are diagnosed in persons over 65 years of age. Age itself is not an absolute contraindication for kidney transplant, and transplants are successfully performed in healthy elders. However, a higher incidence of concurrent health problems and systemic disorders may contraindicate transplant for any particular person. Arteriosclerosis and atherosclerosis are also more common in this population and may be a factor in the transplant decision.

Elders typically experience a decline in immune system function, and the immunosuppressive regimen may leave the individual extremely vulnerable to infection. The accelerated incidence of malignancy related to immunosuppression is also a concern, because cancer is already much more common among the elderly. Many elders undergoing transplant also have type II diabetes mellitus, and the need for high-dose corticosteroid therapy may seriously compromise the regimen for glucose control and impair wound healing.

## SPECIAL ENVIRONMENTS FOR CARE

### Critical Care Management

Patients undergoing solid organ transplant are typically cared for in a critical care unit during the early postoperative period. Meticulous monitoring of all cardiovascular and fluid and electrolyte parameters is critical, and hemodynamic monitoring necessitates critical care placement. If the patient stabilizes promptly, the stay in the critical care unit is usually brief.

### Home Care Management

Hospitalization for successful kidney transplant is typically brief, and patients are rapidly discharged to their home environments. Discharge teaching is initiated as soon as the patient is able to focus and attend to it, and all teaching is supplemented by written materials prepared at an appropriate reading level for the patient's understanding.

Preventing infection and adhering to the immunosuppressive regimen are two major areas of emphasis. The nurse stresses the importance of meticulous personal hygiene, frequent mouth care, and a liberal intake of fluids to prevent urinary stasis. Infections, besides occurring more frequently, also tend to generalize more rapidly in patients after transplant and can quickly result in sepsis.

Adherence to a complex immunosuppressive drug regimen is difficult and cannot be assumed. The nurse lays the groundwork for successful regimen management and ensures that all necessary appointments have been made to initiate appropriate follow-up. Patients with ongoing needs for wound care management are referred for home health supervision.

# COMPLICATIONS

## REJECTION

The major reason for transplant failure is rejection. There are three types of rejection: hyperacute, acute, and chronic. A special type of rejection that occurs in recipients of allogeneic bone marrow transplants is graft-versus-host disease (GVHD).

### Hyperacute Rejection

Hyperacute rejection occurs at the time of transplantation or within 48 hours after the transplant. It is mediated by the humoral immune system. Preformed circulating cytotoxic antibodies to incompatible ABO blood group antigens, antigens on the vascular endothelium, or histocompability antigens are responsible for the hyperacute rejection. The combination of the preformed antibody with the antigen causes activation of complement, entrapment of formed blood elements and clotting factors, massive intravascular coagulation, and necrosis of the graft from decreased perfusion. The degranulation of phagocytic cells causes the release of hydrolytic enzymes that also cause tissue destruction.

To date, hyperacute rejection has occurred only in kidney transplants.[30] The liver seems to be particularly protected from hyperacute rejection, possibly because of the type of blood flow and the large cell mass of the liver. Hyperacute rejection is prevented by ensuring ABO blood group compatibility and avoiding transplantation if positive lymphocyte crossmatches occur (WBC crossmatch).[30] A special type of hyperacute rejection is accelerated rejection. This type of rejection occurs over 3 to 5 days and may be reversed if caught early.

### Acute Rejection

Acute rejection usually occurs from 1 week to 3 months after the transplantation. Acute rejection episodes may recur at any time. Acute rejection is mediated by both the humoral and the cellular immune systems. In acute rejection, foreign antigens are trapped by macrophages. This macrophage-antigen interaction can stimulate differentiation and maturation of various B cell and T cell lines. The activated B and T cells cause destruction of the transplanted tissue directly or indirectly through activation of other immune cells. Acute rejection is treated by pharmacological interventions consisting of increased doses of steroids, the use of monoclonal antibodies (e.g., OKT3), or polyclonal antibodies such as ATG or ALG.

### Chronic Rejection

Chronic rejection occurs 3 months or longer after transplantation. It is mediated by both the cellular and the humoral immune systems and results in slow, progressive loss of graft function. Chronic rejection remains the major unresolved problem in transplantation, because it is less responsive to current immunosuppressive therapies. Mycophenolate mofetil has been shown to slow or halt the progression of chronic rejection. Sirolimus may have a similar action, although human trials are still in progress.[25,33]

## HYPERTENSION

Hypertension is a well-known complication of kidney failure that is rarely cured by kidney transplant. In fact, hypertension occurs in approximately 70% of kidney transplant recipients and up to 90% of patients transplanted with other solid organs such as hearts, livers, lungs, and pancreata. Hypertension has been attributed to the effects of antirejection drugs such as prednisone, cyclosporine, and tacrolimus.

## INFECTION

Infection remains a major cause of morbidity and mortality after transplantation. The transplant recipient is at risk for infection resulting from alteration of the body's normal defense mechanisms by surgery, immunosuppressive medications, and the effects of end-stage organ disease. Advancing age plus the presence of other illnesses such as diabetes mellitus, lupus, and malnutrition further impair the immune response. The signs and symptoms of infection can be subtle, and prompt diagnosis and treatment are important.

The most common infections observed in the first month after transplantation are similar to those acquired by any postoperative patient, including wound and intravenous line infections, pneumonia, and urinary tract infections. Viral infections, especially cytomegalovirus (CMV), Epstein-Barr virus (EBV), herpes simplex virus (HSV), and varicella-zoster virus (VZV), may occur as primary or reactivated infections. Reactivation occurs when a virus is dormant in a patient and becomes reactivated after transplantation because of pharmacological immunosuppression. Primary infections that occur after transplantation can often be traced to an exogenous source such as the donated organ or blood transfusion. Matching the CMV status of the donor and recipient is not considered to be practical because of the shortage of donor organs and the high incidence (70%) of previous exposure to CMV in the normal population. The risk of acquiring CMV disease from the donor has been significantly reduced by the use of prophylaxis with anti-CMV hyperimmune globulin in high-risk patients.

## MALIGNANCIES

The incidence of malignancies is approximately 5% in transplant recipients, a rate 100 times greater than that in the general population. The increased incidence is related to an altered immune system caused by the chronic immunosuppressive therapy. Common malignancies include cancer of the skin, lips, cervix, and lymphomas.

# HEART TRANSPLANT

## ETIOLOGY/EPIDEMIOLOGY

The first heart transplant was performed in 1967. The procedure has evolved into a viable treatment option for patients with terminal cardiac disease. End-stage cardiomyopathy is the pathology in more than 50% of the patients needing transplant; inoperable coronary artery disease (CAD) is the next most common cause.

Donor availability is a serious problem with cardiac transplantation, and the waiting period may be prolonged. As the patient's condition deteriorates, extended hospitalization may be required until a suitable donor can be found. These patients are usually physiologically unstable and may require intensive treatment in a critical care setting because of the need for complex drug therapy, intraaortic balloon pump therapy, or the placement of a ventricular assist device.

Potential candidates for heart transplant are usually less than 60 years of age and are free of systemic illnesses or diseases in other organ systems that would limit their chances for long-term survival. Donor matching includes ABO blood group compatibility, negative lymphocyte crossmatch, and avoidance of a CMV-positive donor if the recipient is CMV negative. Human leukocyte antigen screening is not usually performed and has no proven benefit in light of the scarcity of donors.

## COLLABORATIVE CARE MANAGEMENT

Heart transplant surgery consists of the removal of the diseased heart (leaving the posterior walls of the recipient's atria to spare the sinoatrial node), followed by anastomosis of the atria, aorta, and pulmonary arteries.[13,22] Figure 68-4 shows the recipient's atrial cuffs and great vessels after cardiectomy, at the beginning of the left atrial suture line, and after the completed cardiac transplant.

The patient who undergoes heart transplant receives care similar to that of any patient having open heart surgery (see Chapter 26). A clinical pathway may be used to specifically guide the patient's postoperative care (see the Research Box). A healthy donor heart usually functions well and the patient's cardiac output stabilizes. Dysrhythmias are common in the initial postoperative period, and hypervolemia can result from fluid replacement and high-dose corticosteroid therapy.

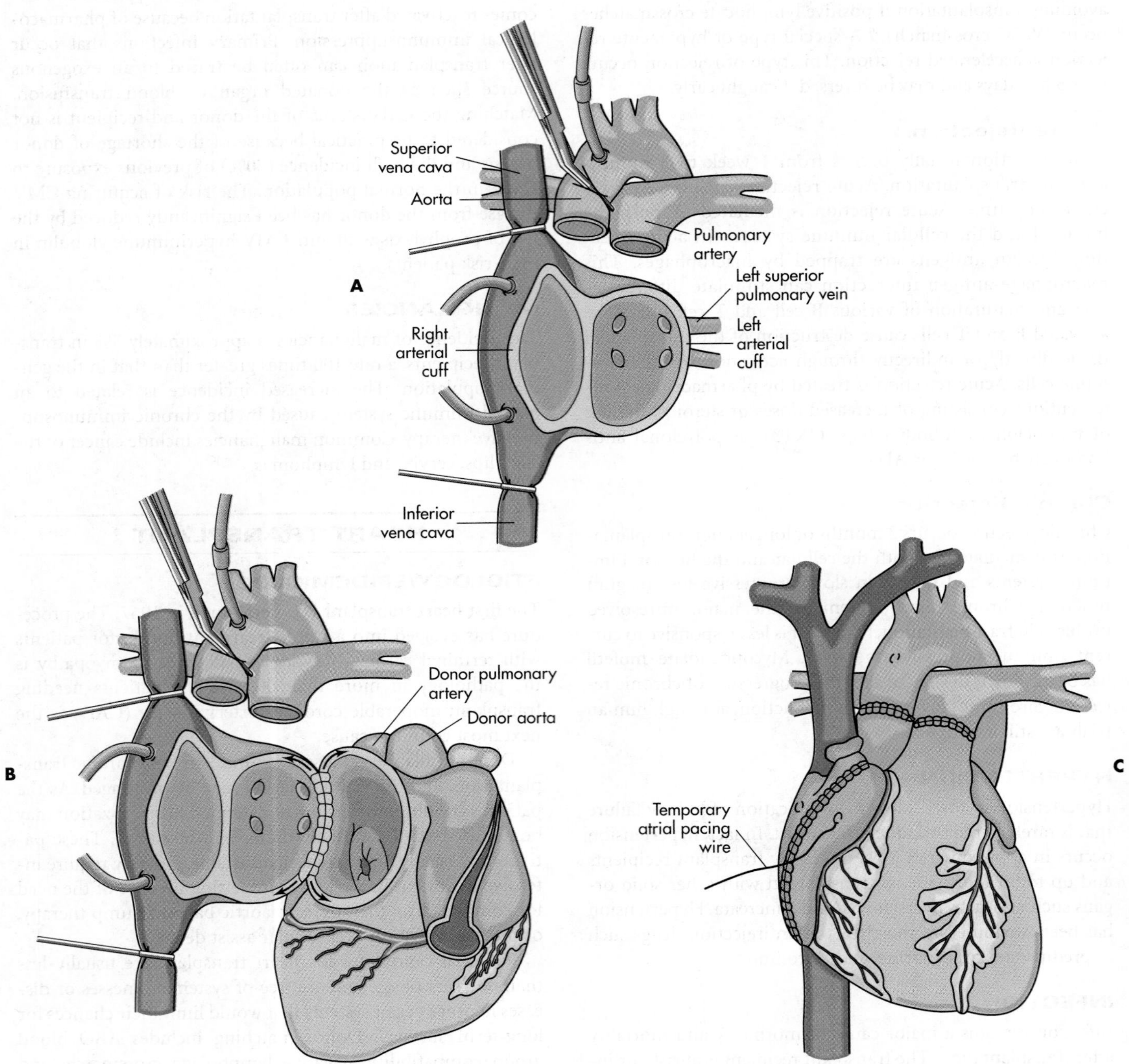


**fig. 68-4 A,** Recipient atrial cuffs and great vessels after cardiectomy. **B,** Beginning of left atrial suture line. Arrows indicate direction of suture line. **C,** Completed cardiac transplant.

These complications are managed with the same treatments used for other cardiac patients. Critical care placement is usually maintained until the patient's condition stabilizes.

Either acute or chronic rejection of the transplanted heart can occur. Endometrial biopsy is performed to confirm the presence of rejection. Biopsies are used routinely to monitor the patient's progress because the classic signs of rejection may or may not be present. Potential symptoms are presented in Box 68-3.

The patient showing signs of rejection may be treated with increasing doses of immunosuppressive agents. Additionally, methylprednisolone boluses, lymphocytic immune globulin, or OKT3 may be given. The patient needs considerable support during rejection episodes because of the potentially life-threatening nature of rejection and the anxiety associated with the threat of losing the new heart.

Chronic rejection is insidious and is characterized by graft atherosclerosis, which can result in myocardial ischemia, myocardial infarction, or cardiac failure. The ischemia and infarction may not be associated with pain because the transplanted heart is denervated. No effective treatment exists to stop the chronic rejection process or the associated atherosclerosis. Treatment focuses on interventions to improve cardiac function until another heart becomes available.

### Patient/Family Education

Preparation for discharge involves the same teaching as discussed for the kidney transplant recipient. Health care measures to improve cardiac fitness, particularly exercise, are reviewed. Patients who have had long waits for donor hearts may have become virtually immobilized before surgery, and they need to very gradually increase their activity and fitness. The patient and family must understand the plan for repeat cardiac catheterization with biopsies and the timing intervals for these monitoring tests.

**research**

Reference: Noedel NR et al: Critical pathways as an effective tool to reduce cardiac transplantation hospitalization and charges, *Journal of Transplant Coordination* 6(1):14, 1996.

Cardiac transplantation is a well-established treatment for end-stage cardiac disease, but it is costly in terms of charges and resources. Managed care organizations attempt to control costs by dictating shorter lengths of stay and eliminating tests and treatments that they believe may be unnecessary.

This retrospective review of 74 cardiac transplants evaluated the influence of critical pathways on the clinical management, length of hospitalization, and hospital charges. Transplant patients were divided into two groups. One group received standard primary care nursing and the other received care guided by a critical pathway. The number of intensive care unit days was significantly smaller for patients treated by critical pathway, as were the length of hospitalization and cost of hospital care. No statistically significant differences were found between the two groups with regard to complications, readmissions, or number of home care services used. The critical pathway provided for systematic delivery of care and decreased length of hospitalization and costs without compromising safety or quality.

## LIVER TRANSPLANT

### ETIOLOGY/EPIDEMIOLOGY

The first liver transplant was performed in 1963, and the procedure has since become a therapeutic option for both adults and children with liver failure. Liver transplant is used to treat biliary atresia, fulminant hepatic failure, cirrhosis, hepatitis, metabolic disorders, and primary hepatic malignancy. Cirrhosis of the liver is the major pathology in adult patients seeking transplant, and the importance of abstinence from alcohol creates unique dilemmas in the selection procedures for liver transplant recipients. The use of transplant to treat liver cancer is also controversial because of the high rate of recurrence, even when there is no evidence of disseminated disease.

Bilirubin concentrations greater than 10 mg/dl, a serum albumin concentration less than 2.5 mg/dl, and a prothrombin time greater than 5 seconds beyond the control value are clinical features predictive of the need for liver transplant. Other criteria include incapacitating encephalopathy, recurrent variceal bleeding not controlled by sclerotherapy, intractable ascites that does not respond to diuretic therapy or paracentesis, and recurrent spontaneous bacterial peritonitis.[15]

### COLLABORATIVE CARE MANAGEMENT

A liver transplant takes 8 to 12 hours and involves the removal of the recipient's diseased liver followed by implantation of the donor liver allograft. The diseased liver is removed en bloc. A venovenous bypass system may be used to allow normal hemodynamic values to be maintained while the recipient is without a liver. This bypass system helps prevent venous hypertension, circulatory instability, and excessive bleeding. The

**box 68-3** *Signs and Symptoms of Acute Rejection in the Heart Transplant Patient*

**SIGNS**

Fluid retention, peripheral edema, crackles, jugular venous distention (JVD), $S_3$ gallop
Pericardial friction rub
ECG changes: dysrhythmias and decreased voltage
Decreased cardiac output
Hypotension
Cardiac enlargement

**SYMPTOMS**

Fatigue, lethargy
Dyspnea
Decreased tolerance for exercise

liver transplant procedure is the most technically complex of the solid organs because of the intricate vascular and biliary anastomoses that are required (Figures 68-5 and 68-6).

The major postoperative complications include rejection, infection, and occlusion of vessels. The liver is less susceptible to acute rejection than the kidneys, but adequate immunosuppressive therapy is still a priority concern. The extensive nature of the surgery and the patient's preoperative liver failure combine to significantly increase the risk of postoperative complications.

Postoperatively, the patient is admitted to an intensive care unit because the initial care is both challenging and complex. Constant monitoring of the patient's hemodynamic status and liver function is critical. Bedrest is maintained for several days. The patient's liver function tests, including serum transaminases, bilirubin, albumin, and clotting factors, often show improvement within 24 hours if a complication does not occur. Immunosuppressive therapy is started before surgery and continued on a regular schedule after the procedure. Worsening liver function, fever, swelling, and tenderness of the liver are all warning signs of a complication. Infection is a crucial concern and can be bacterial, viral, or fungal in nature. The risk of infection is greatest during the first 3 months after surgery. Common organisms responsible for infection in transplant recipients are presented in Box 68-4.

### Patient/Family Education

Preparation for discharge involves the same teaching discussed for the kidney transplant recipient. In addition, the patient with alcoholic cirrhosis is counseled that the ongoing involvement with a chemical dependency program is an essential strategy to prevent relapse.

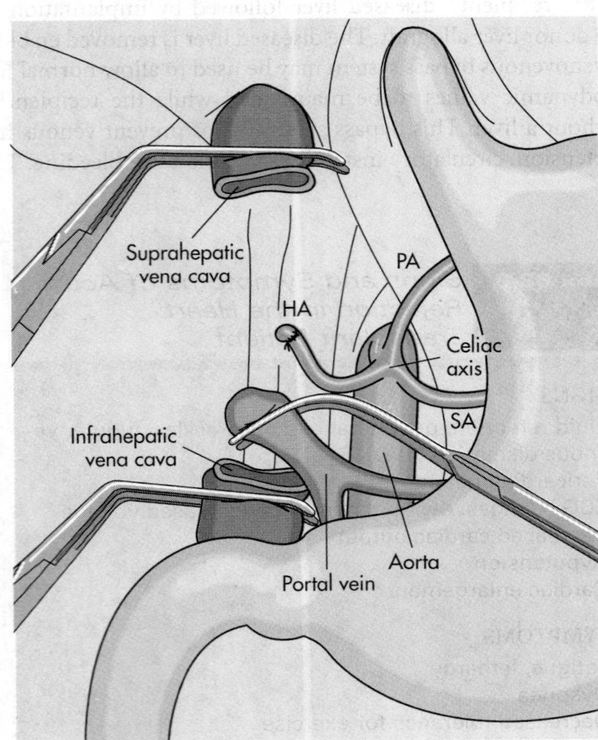


**fig. 68-5** Vascular anastomoses of liver transplant.

## LUNG TRANSPLANT

### ETIOLOGY/EPIDEMIOLOGY

Successful transplantation of the lungs did not become a reality until the 1980s. Advances in surgical technique and immunosuppressive therapy have raised the 1- and 2-year survival rates for lung transplants to about 75%. The procedure is used with patients under 60 years of age who are not active smokers and who suffer from advanced pulmonary diseases such as pulmonary hypertension, emphysema, cystic fibrosis, and sarcoidosis. Single and double lung transplants may be used, as well as a combined heart-lung transplant.

Single lung transplantation has been used for restrictive lung disease, because the decreased compliance and increased

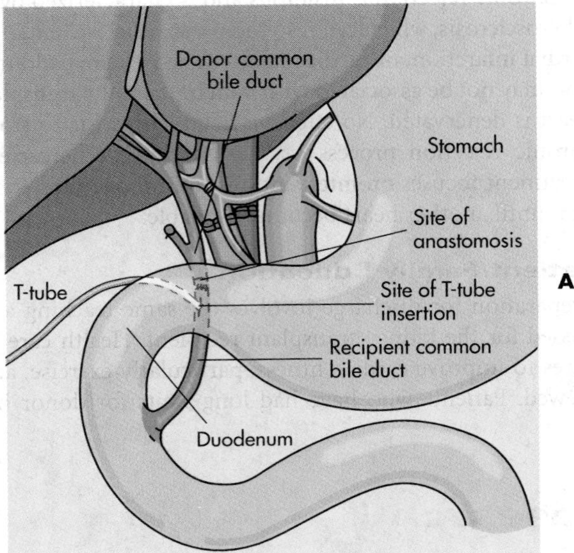


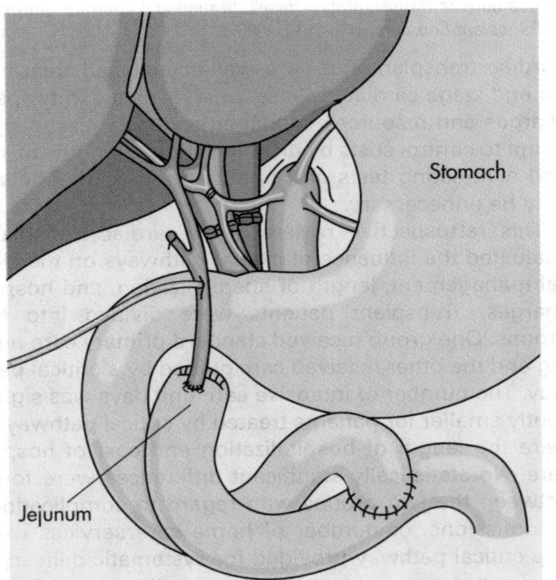


**fig. 68-6** Biliary anastomoses of liver transplant. **A,** choledochocholedochostomy **B,** choledochojejunostomy.

pulmonary resistance of the recipient's remaining lung result in preferential ventilation and perfusion of the transplanted lung. Double lung transplants are typically used in persons with emphysema or cystic fibrosis.

## COLLABORATIVE CARE MANAGEMENT

Single lung transplants are performed through an anterolateral thoracotomy (Figure 68-7). Some patients require cardiopulmonary bypass, especially those patients with primary pulmonary hypertension. The double lung transplant procedure has been modified to a bilateral single lung transplant procedure with individual bronchial anastomoses (see Figure 68-7). Cardiopulmonary bypass is required in the double lung procedure.

When heart-lung procedures are performed with the use of cardiopulmonary bypass the recipient's heart is first removed and the phrenic nerves are isolated. Enough left atrium is removed to allow the donor's right lung to fit into the right pleural space. The lungs are then removed individually by dividing the inferior pulmonary ligaments and transecting the pulmonary hilar structures. The donor's heart-lung bloc is placed into the recipient's chest, and the tracheal anastomosis is completed (Figure 68-8).

The patient is placed in an intensive care unit after surgery. The most important aspects of care are promoting adequate airway clearance and gas exchange and instituting care to prevent the major complications associated with lung transplantation. Poor gas exchange is a common complication and may be caused by reperfusion edema of the lung, impaired cough, infection, or rejection. Appropriate immunosuppressive therapy is initiated, and the patient is monitored closely for rejection.

**box 68-4** *Organisms Responsible for Infections in Transplant Recipients*

**BACTERIAL INFECTIONS**

Gram-negative organisms, including *Pseudomonas aeruginosa, Serratia marcescens, Proteus rettgeri, Enterobacter cloacae, Legionella pneumophila,* and various *Nocardia* species

**VIRAL INFECTIONS**

Herpesviruses, including herpes simplex viruses 1 and 2, varicella-zoster virus, cytomegalovirus, and Epstein-Barr virus

**FUNGAL INFECTIONS**

Candidal species (most often *C. albicans*) and other fungi, including *Aspergillus fumigatus, Cryptococcus neoformans, Coccidioides immitis,* and *Histoplasma capsulatum*

**PARASITIC INFECTIONS**

Include *Pneumocystis carinii* and *Toxoplasma gondii*

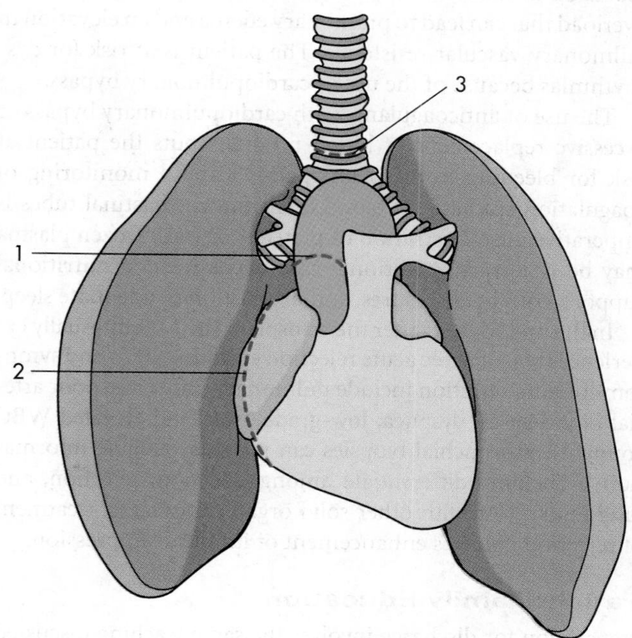


**fig. 68-8** Anastomotic sites in heart-lung transplantation. *1,* Aorta; *2,* right atria; and *3,* trachea.

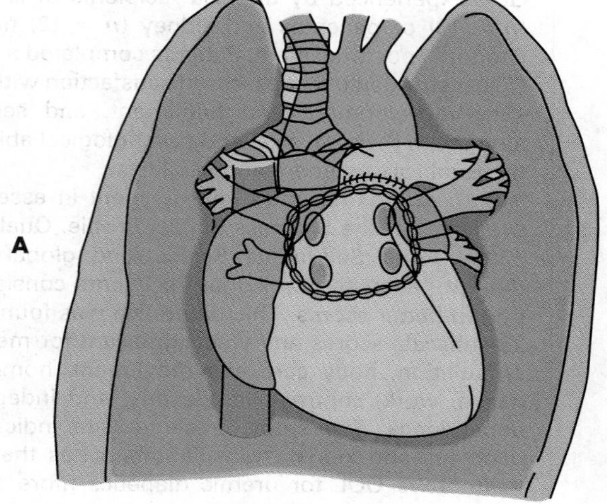


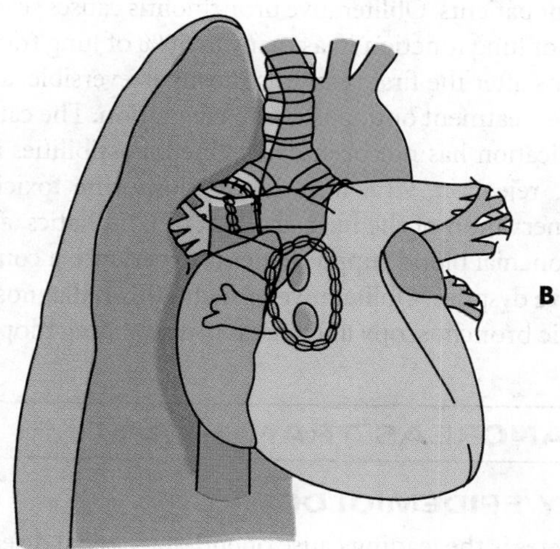


**fig. 68-7** Anastomoses for **A,** double-lung and **B,** single-lung transplantation.

One difference in the immunosuppressive regimen for lung transplants is that corticosteroids are not used for the first 7 to 14 days after the transplant. Corticosteroids jeopardize the healing of the tracheal and bronchial anastomoses; therefore OKT3 is used instead. Once healing has occurred, immunosuppressive therapy with corticosteroids is initiated.

Aggressive respiratory care is critical. It is difficult for the patient to clear the airway because the transplanted lung (or lungs) is denervated below the level of the trachea and mucociliary clearance is decreased. Care includes frequent position changes and deep breathing along with postural drainage and coughing. Supplemental oxygen is necessary. The patient with a lung transplant is prone to cardiovascular complications from hypervolemia or hypovolemia, myocardial irritability, or decreased contractility. Hemodynamic status is carefully managed to maintain adequate cardiac output without fluid overload that can lead to pulmonary edema and an elevation in pulmonary vascular resistance. The patient is at risk for dysrhythmias because of the use of cardiopulmonary bypass.

The use of anticoagulants with cardiopulmonary bypass or excessive replacement of blood products puts the patient at risk for bleeding from coagulopathy. Careful monitoring of coagulation studies and blood loss from mediastinal tubes is imperative. Administration of platelets or fresh frozen plasma may be necessary. Additional care needs include nutritional support, comfort measures, and promotion of adequate sleep.

In the first 6 weeks after the transplant the patient usually experiences two or three acute rejection episodes. Signs and symptoms of lung rejection include pulmonary infiltrates, poor arterial blood gases, dyspnea, low-grade fever, and elevated WBC count. Transbronchial biopsies can provide valuable information by helping differentiate among infection, rejection, and lung injury.[28] As with other solid organ transplants, treatment of rejection involves enhancement of immunosuppression.

### Patient/Family Education

Preparation for discharge involves the same teaching discussed for the kidney transplant recipient. The importance of adherence to the regimen and regular follow-up is stressed. Infection is a risk for any transplant patient but is of particular concern for lung transplant patients. Obliterative bronchiolitis causes severe deterioration of lung function in as many as 50% of lung transplant recipients after the first year. It is mostly irreversible, and the only viable treatment option is retransplantation. The cause of this complication has not been determined. Possibilities include chronic rejection, viral infection, cyclosporine toxicity, long-term denervation of the lung, the lack of lymphatics, and the loss of bronchial blood supply. Patients experience a cough and progressive dyspnea. Obliterative bronchiolitis is diagnosed with fiberoptic bronchoscopy and transbronchial lung biopsy.

## PANCREAS TRANSPLANT

### ETIOLOGY/EPIDEMIOLOGY

Because diabetes is the leading cause of end-stage renal disease in the United States, pancreas transplants are being performed with increasing frequency and a marked improvement in overall outcomes. Simultaneous transplantation of both the kidney and pancreas (KP) from the same donor into a patient with type I diabetes mellitus and end-stage renal disease accounts for 85% of all pancreas transplants.[4,36] Kidney and pancreas transplantation has resulted in significantly better 1-year pancreas graft survival, exceeding 80%, than pancreas transplant alone.

The goals of pancreas transplantation are to eliminate the need for exogenous insulin and dietary restrictions and to prevent or stabilize the microvascular and neuropathic complications of the diabetes. The recipient eligibility criteria for KP transplantation are similar to those for kidney transplantation except that the age range is more restricted at 18 to 45 years, and cardiovascular clearance must be obtained from a cardiologist.[7] Some centers do not consider diabetics with secondary complications such as blindness or severe peripheral vascular disease to be acceptable candidates for KP transplantation. It is generally agreed that pancreas transplantation should be offered to a select group of patients who are at low to moderate cardiac risk, highly motivated, and well informed about the benefits and risk associated with the procedure. The risks include greater morbidity, an increased rate of acute rejection, and an increased risk of cardiac death.[17] The accompanying Research Box presents the results of a study on quality of life in patients receiving KP transplants.

### COLLABORATIVE CARE MANAGEMENT

In the combined KP transplant the recipient's own pancreas is left in place and continues to perform its exocrine function

**research**

Reference: Hathaway DK et al: A prospective study of changes in quality of life reported by diabetic recipients of kidney-only and pancreas-kidney allografts, *Journal of Transplant Coordination* 4(1):12, 1994.

The purpose of this study was to explore whether pancreas transplantation improves the patient's quality of life (QOL) to the extent that the additional risks associated with the procedure and long-term care are warranted. This prospective study examined changes in QOL experienced by diabetic recipients of kidney only ($n$ = 13) or pancreas and kidney ($n$ = 12) transplants 6 months posttransplant. Patients completed a battery of QOL instruments that assessed satisfaction with life, personal development and fulfillment, and self-esteem, along with their physical and psychological ability to fulfill usual role-related responsibilities.

Both groups reported improvement in essentially all subscales of the Sickness Impact Profile, Quality of Life Index, Adult Self-Image Scales, and global QOL, although pancreas and kidney recipients consistently reported better scores. This difference was found in 22 of 23 subscale scores and was significant for measures of ambulation, body care and movement, home maintenance, work, control over destiny, and independence-dependence. The study presents data indicating that pancreas and kidney transplantation has the potential to improve QOL for uremic diabetics more than does kidney-only transplantation.

while the transplanted pancreas provides endocrine function. The donor pancreas is placed intraperitoneally in the pubic area. Most centers use a bladder drainage technique to handle the exocrine juices from the donor pancreas. The head of the donor pancreas is anastomosed to the dome of the recipient's bladder with a segment of the donor's duodenum. The donor kidney is placed in the iliac fossa as described earlier (Figure 68-9).

The KP transplant recipient has nursing care needs similar to those of any patient after extensive abdominal surgery. Blood glucose levels are monitored closely in the immediate postoperative period as an indicator of graft perfusion. Increasing glucose levels during this time may indicate graft dysfunction as a result of thrombosis. Metabolic acidosis may also occur from the loss of bicarbonate in the exocrine pancreatic juices that are eliminated in the urine. Supplemental sodium bicarbonate may be added to the patient's intravenous infusions or may be administered orally.

The extra digestive juices and fluids that are excreted in the urine account for an additional 1000 to 1500 ml of fluid output daily. Consequently, fluid replacement must be adjusted to compensate for these additional losses. The KP recipient may need to drink more than 5 L of fluid daily to prevent fluid deficits.

The diagnosis of pancreas rejection is difficult because specific parameters are late indicators of rejection. Hyperglycemia becomes apparent only after 90% of the pancreas is damaged. A major advantage of urinary drainage is the ability to monitor amylase and bicarbonate levels in the urine and detect a rejection episode before hyperglycemia occurs. The exocrine pancreas typically malfunctions approximately 3 days before the endocrine pancreas; therefore decreases in urine amylase and urine pH can be early indicators of pancreatic rejection. Changes in kidney function also precede signs of pancreas rejection, and an increase in serum creatinine is an important warning sign. Reversal of rejection in the kidney nearly always is associated with preservation of pancreas graft function as well.

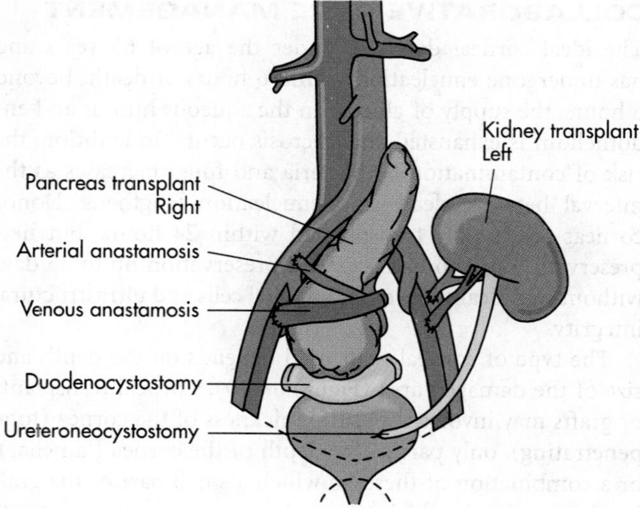


**fig. 68-9** Diagram of the combined kidney-pancreas transplant.

### Patient/Family Education

Many patients find it difficult to maintain an adequate oral fluid intake because they are so accustomed to the fluid restrictions of dialysis, and they do not have a normal response to thirst. Some patients are discharged from the hospital with a venous access device in place for home intravenous fluid administration. One to two liters of fluid can be administered at night to ensure an adequate fluid balance. In most patients, the exocrine juices produced by the pancreas and excreted in the urine significantly decrease after the first 2 months. The patient can then discontinue intravenous supplementation and maintain fluid balance with oral intake alone. Before discharge, it is critical that KP transplant recipients be instructed in the signs and symptoms of dehydration, including a decrease in weight, dizziness (especially with position changes), increased pulse rate, and generalized weakness. All KP transplant recipients must also be alert to signs and symptoms of metabolic acidosis, including weakness, anorexia, nausea, and vomiting.

If a bladder drainage procedure is used, the patient is also instructed to monitor the urine pH with a dipstick to detect early signs of pancreas rejection. If the patient's vision is impaired, a family member or significant other is taught how to perform the test.

## BONE MARROW TRANSPLANT

### ETIOLOGY/EPIDEMIOLOGY

Bone marrow transplant (BMT) is used to treat a wide variety of malignant and nonmalignant disorders. The malignant diseases amenable to BMT are the leukemias, lymphoma, and selected solid tumors. Five-year disease-free survival rates average 50%. The nonmalignant diseases requiring BMT include immunological deficiency disease, aplastic anemia, and thalassemia. Five-year disease-free survival rates for these conditions average 80%.[32]

There are three types of bone marrow donors: allogeneic, the use of marrow from an HLA-matched donor, most often a sibling; syngeneic, from an identical twin; or autologous bone marrow transplantation (ABMT), in which patients serve as their own donors. With the hope of making BMT more accessible to patients who lack an HLA-matched sibling, many centers are exploring the use of partially matched or unrelated donors. Advances in histocompatibility testing have enabled researchers to more clearly define disparity between the recipient and the donor. In general, as the disparity between the donor and recipient increases, the incidence and severity of graft-versus-host disease and the risk of graft failure increase, and the survival rate decreases. Donor registries have been established in the United States and abroad to assist in the search for HLA-matched unrelated donors. The National Marrow Donor Program has a registry of more than 200,000 donors.

The type and extent of disease are the primary determinants of a patient's eligibility for BMT. The risk of relapse after transplantation is reduced if BMT is performed in patients whose disease is in complete remission or those who have minimal residual disease at the time of transplantation. Additional eligibility criteria include age, the lack of preexisting organ toxicity or comorbid conditions, and the availability of a suitable marrow donor.

## COLLABORATIVE CARE MANAGEMENT

In preparation for BMT, the recipient undergoes intensive chemoradiotherapy to eradicate residual disease, make space in the recipient's marrow for donor cell engraftment, and establish immunosuppression to prevent the rejection of donor marrow in allogeneic transplants.

Bone marrow stem cells capable of engraftment can be obtained from peripheral blood, fetal liver tissue, fetal umbilical cord blood, cadavers, or the sternum or pelvis of a live donor. Most autologous or allogeneic bone marrow is obtained by multiple needle aspirations from the posterior iliac crests with the donor under general or spinal anesthesia. The amount of marrow extracted ranges from 600 to 2500 ml. Complications of bone marrow donation include bruising, bleeding, pain at aspiration sites, infection, transient neuropathies, and hypotension secondary to volume loss.

After processing, the marrow is given to the recipient intravenously, frozen at −140° C, or cryopreserved at −196° C and kept for 3 years or more. The bone marrow reinfusion process is technically similar to blood transfusion and takes 2 to 4 hours. The recipient is hydrated with intravenous fluids containing sodium bicarbonate before and after marrow infusion. This ensures adequate renal perfusion and urine alkalinization if red cell hemolysis occurs as a result of incompatibility or trauma. All BMT recipients can expect a red tinge to their urine for up to 12 hours after marrow infusion because of mild intravascular red cell lysis.

The recipient is closely monitored during reinfusion. Many of the common problems seen after transplantation result from the conditioning regimen of radiation and chemotherapy required before transplant. Gastrointestinal complications are the most common problems and include anorexia, nausea, vomiting, diarrhea, stomatitis, and mucositis. Bone marrow suppression can also result in bleeding and infection.

### Graft-versus-Host Disease

Persons who receive allogeneic bone marrow are at risk for graft-versus-host disease (GVHD), depending on the degree to which the donor and recipient are HLA incompatible. Irradiation and chemotherapy are used before allogeneic transplant to destroy the recipient's immunocompetent cells. The donor's immunocompetent cells, once they engraft in the recipient, recognize other cells of the recipient as foreign and attack them. The tissue and organs most often affected are the skin, liver, and gastrointestinal tract.[32] Graft-versus-host disease can occur as an acute or a chronic process. Histocompatibility testing and effective immune suppression are used to prevent or minimize GVHD.

### Patient/Family Education

Patients can be discharged after BMT when they are afebrile, are able to maintain an adequate oral intake, and have met or exceeded specific blood count criteria, including a platelet count greater than 15,000, a granulocyte count greater than 500, and a hematocrit above 30%. Important components of discharge teaching are similar to those discussed for the kidney transplant recipient. Preventing infection is a priority concern. In addition, BMT recipients must be knowledgeable about bleeding precautions and the signs and symptoms of GVHD.

# CORNEA TRANSPLANT

## ETIOLOGY/EPIDEMIOLOGY

Although cornea transplantation is not a lifesaving procedure, it has great potential for enhancing quality of life. The importance of this technology is underscored by the number of Americans, young and old, with impaired vision resulting from corneal damage. Defective corneas cause blindness in more than 40,000 Americans each year. The leading causes of corneal damage requiring transplant are keratoconus, Fuchs' dystrophy, herpes simplex keratitis, pseudophakic bullous keratopathy, and chemical burns.[26] Corneal transplants are successful in 95% of patients, but the degree of visual acuity restored can be highly variable. It is not unusual for patients to require eyeglasses or contact lenses to correct refractive error.

Patients considering cornea transplant must be evaluated for other ocular conditions that can affect visual acuity after transplant. These conditions include strabismus, amblyopia, retinal disease, glaucoma, and previous cataract surgery. A complete examination of all ocular structures is performed to determine existing conditions that can affect graft survival. The eye is carefully assessed for infection, because corneal transplantation cannot be performed in the presence of infection.

## COLLABORATIVE CARE MANAGEMENT

The ideal corneal donor is under the age of 65 years and has undergone enucleation within 6 hours of death. Beyond 6 hours, the supply of glucose in the aqueous humor and endothelium is exhausted and necrosis occurs. In addition, the risk of contamination by bacteria and fungi increases as the interval between death and enucleation lengthens. Donor corneas are usually transplanted within 24 hours, but new preservation methods can extend preservation up to 35 days without significant loss of endothelial cells and ultrastructural integrity.

The type of corneal graft used depends on the depth and size of the damaged area (Figure 68-10). Corneal transplants or grafts may involve the entire thickness of the cornea (total penetrating), only part of the depth of the cornea (lamellar), or a combination of these, in which a small part of the graft involves the entire thickness of the cornea (partial penetrating). The penetrating graft establishes least well and the surgeon seldom uses a donor eye that is more than 48 hours old.

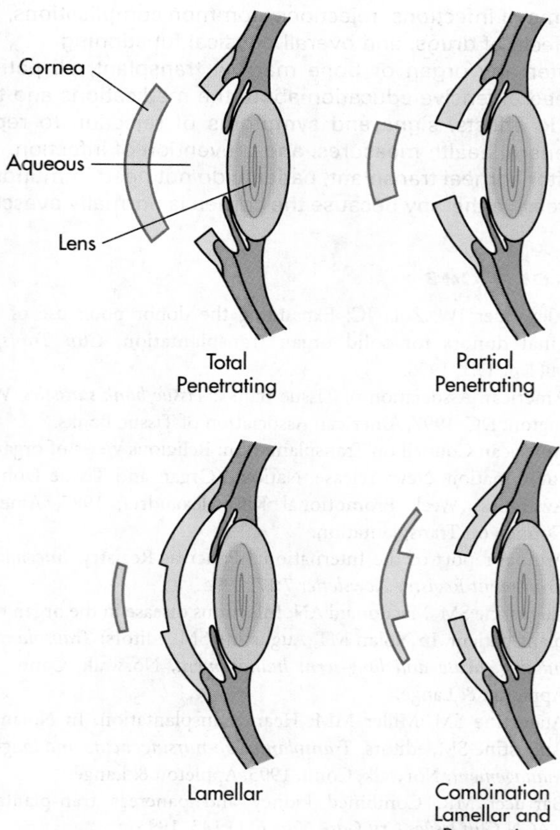


**fig. 68-10** Types of corneal grafts currently in use. Note that the lamellar graft defect does not penetrate the entire thickness of cornea.

The patient is permitted out of bed after recovery from the anesthetic. Discharge takes place within 2 to 4 days. The eye is covered with a sterile eye pad, and a metal or plastic shield is placed over the pad for extra protection. The patient continues to wear the shield at night for several weeks. Cornea grafts heal very slowly because of the lack of blood vessels in the cornea and require 3 to 6 months for complete healing.[26]

### Patient/Family Education

Patient teaching includes instruction about medications and assessment for graft rejection. Patients are usually discharged on cycloplegic, steroid, and sulfa eye drops.

Because the cornea is normally avascular, the recipient's immune cells are not exposed to the cornea, and thus immunosuppressive therapy is not required. However, patients are instructed to check for graft rejection daily for the rest of their lives. The eye is checked at the same time each day for redness; an increase in redness, irritation, or discomfort; or a decrease in vision. Any symptoms that persist or increase in severity in a 24-hour period should be reported to the surgeon.

Many persons expect to have their vision restored immediately after the graft. Vision, however, is sometimes poor while the sutures remain in place. Once the sutures are removed, vision usually improves remarkably. The sutures may remain in place for at least 1 year, and the patient is evaluated monthly during that time.

## critical thinking QUESTIONS

**1** The following patients are all awaiting liver transplant:

a Harry, a 46-year-old patient with alcoholic cirrhosis and liver failure. Harry first entered an alcohol treatment program when he was placed on the transplant list 2 months ago. His condition is deteriorating rapidly, but he is not hospitalized.

b Millie, a 22-year-old woman who is in liver failure related to an acetaminophen overdose. She has just been placed on the list but is in full liver failure.

c Stanley, a 65-year-old man with idiopathic cirrhosis who is hospitalized and fading in and out of hepatic coma. He has been on the transplant list for 3 years.

A liver has just become available in Millie's home state. The liver is an excellent ABO and HLA match for Harry, who lives halfway across the country. Who should get the transplant? What criteria did you use to make your decision?

**2** Kidney and pancreas transplant may allow a patient with type I diabetes mellitus to stop taking insulin and relax his diet restrictions. Given the cost of the procedure and its associated rejection and complication rates, should health insurance plans be required to cover it for anyone seeking it? Why or why not?

**3** Compatible Asian/Pacific Islander bone marrow donors are in extremely short supply nationwide. You live in an urban area with a dense population of this ethnic group. Design a community outreach program targeted at getting Asian/Pacific Islander ethnic group members typed as potential bone marrow donors.

**4** John Gray is a 32-year-old father of three who has been pronounced brain dead after a motorcycle accident. Outline a plan for approaching his young wife about organ donation.

## chapter SUMMARY

### TRANSPLANTATION CRITERIA

- Transplantation of organs/tissues is a major therapeutic intervention for selected patients.
- Legislation has been passed to increase the supply of organs and the fair allocation of donated organs; the family or guardians of all potential donors must be approached about donating organs.
- Organ donors must be brain dead and have no preexisting disease of the organ(s) being recovered, no transmissible diseases or sepsis, no history of intravenous drug abuse, no malignancies, and no death of unknown etiology.
- The potential donor must have been maintained hemodynamically until the organs are recovered.
- To decrease the potential transmission of HIV, criteria for the exclusion of high-risk persons have been identified even if the HIV test is negative.

- The patient selection criteria for transplant are the presence of end-stage disease that is unresponsive to conventional therapy or worsening despite aggressive medical management, ability to achieve improvement in quality and quantity of life, and financial means to cover the cost of the procedure and the immunosuppressive medications required to prevent rejection of the allograft.
- Medicare covers the cost of kidney, liver, and heart transplants; some transplants are covered by state programs; and third party payers cover some transplants.

### IMMUNOLOGY AND TRANSPLANTATION

- Successful allogeneic transplantation requires manipulation of the recipient's immune system with drugs to prevent rejection.
- Three types of rejection occur: hyperacute, acute, and chronic.
- Rejection results from activation of humoral or cellular immune responses to mismatched class I and II HLAs, ABO antigens, and minor red blood cell antigens.
- Acute rejection is an immune response that occurs from approximately 7 days after the transplant to 3 months after the transplant. Immunosuppressive therapy is used to prevent and treat acute rejections.
- Chronic rejection is a slow, progressive process that occurs 3 months or more after the transplant and leads to loss of function of the transplant.
- Azathioprine or CellCept, corticosteroids, and cyclosporine or tacrolimus are the immunosuppressive agents used in all types of transplants to prevent acute rejections.
- Bolus doses of corticosteroids, OKT3, and lymphocyte immune globulin are used to treat acute rejection episodes.

### COLLABORATIVE MANAGEMENT OF TRANSPLANT PATIENTS

- A major focus of nursing care is the prevention or early detection of infections, which the transplant patient is at risk for because of immunosuppression.
- Once the patient decides to undergo transplant and is accepted, nursing care needs to focus on helping the patient and family deal with the waiting period, helping the patient manage the end-stage failure carefully, and helping the patient implement appropriate preventive health practices to maintain as healthy a state as possible.
- After transplantation, all patients must be monitored carefully for rejection and infection. Rejection signs and symptoms are unique for each type of transplant but include a decrease in function of the transplanted organ.
- Other major complications after renal transplant include acute tubular necrosis, fluid and electrolyte imbalance, hemorrhage, and occlusion of the renal artery or vein.
- Heart transplants are associated with the following additional major complications: hemorrhage, cardiac tamponade, and hemodynamic instability.
- Lung transplant patients are at risk for reperfusion edema of the lung, hemodynamic instability, coagulopathy, and pulmonary infections.
- Pancreatic transplant patients are at risk for peritonitis and multiple respiratory complications.
- Patients who undergo allogeneic bone marrow transplants are at risk for acute and chronic complications resulting from the conditioning radiation therapy or chemotherapy and acute and chronic graft-versus-host disease.
- After any organ or bone marrow transplant, all patients need consistent, detailed monitoring for signs and symptoms of infections, rejections, common complications, side effects of drugs, and overall physical functioning.
- After any organ or bone marrow transplant, all patients need extensive education about the medications and their side effects, signs and symptoms of rejection to report, general health measures, and prevention of infection.
- After corneal transplant, patients do not need immunosuppressive therapy because the cornea is normally avascular.

## References


1. Alexander JW, Zola JC: Expanding the donor pool: use of marginal donors for solid organ transplantation, *Clin Transplant* 10(1 pt 1):1, 1996.
2. American Association of Tissue Banks: *Tissue bank statistics,* Washington, DC, 1997, American Association of Tissue Banks.
3. American Council on Transplantation: Religious views of organ/tissue donation. News release, National Organ and Tissue Donation Awareness Week Promotional Kit, Alexandria, 1987, American Council on Transplantation.
4. Annual report of the International Pancreas Registry, *International Transplant Registry Newsletter* 7:17, 1994.
5. Augustine SM, Macdonald AN: Infectious disease in the organ transplant patient. In Nolan MT, Augustine SM, editors: *Transplantation nursing, acute and long-term management,* Norwalk, Conn, 1995, Appleton & Lange.
6. Augustine SM, Miller MM: Heart transplantation. In Nolan MT, Augustine SM, editors: *Transplantation nursing, acute and long-term management,* Norwalk, Conn, 1995, Appleton & Lange.
7. Bartucci MR: Combined kidney and pancreas transplantation, *AACN Clin Issues Crit Care Nurs* 6(1):143, 1995.
8. Bartucci MR: Nursing care of the immunosuppressed patient. In Chabalewski F, editor: *Donation and transplantation: nursing curriculum,* Richmond, 1996, UNOS.
9. Bartucci MR: Organ donation. In Clochesy JM et al, editors: *Critical care nursing,* Philadelphia, 1993, WB Saunders.
10. Bartucci MR: Organ donation. In Clochesy JM et al, editors: *Critical care nursing,* ed 2, Philadelphia, 1996, WB Saunders.
11. Bartucci MR: Organ donation: a study of the donor family perspective, *J Neurosci Nurs* 19(6):305, 1987.
12. Briceno J, Lopez-Cillero P, Ruflan S, et al: Impact of marginal quality donors on the outcome of liver transplantation, *Transplant Proc* 29(1-2):477, 1997.
13. Cupples SA: Stress and coping among transplant patients and their families. In Nolan MT, Augustine SM, editors: *Transplantation nursing, acute and long-term management,* Norwalk, Conn, 1995, Appleton & Lange.
14. Caplan A: Must I be my brother's keeper? Ethical issues in the use of living donors as sources of livers and other solid organs, *Transplant Proc* 25(2):1997, 1993.
15. Coleman J, Wise BV, Mendoza M, Kaczmarek CA: A nursing perspective on adult and pediatric liver transplantation. In Nolan MT, Augustine SM, editors: *Transplantation nursing, acute and long-term management,* Norwalk, Conn, 1995, Appleton & Lange.
16. Douglas S, Blixen C, Bartucci MR: Relationship between pretransplant noncompliance and posttransplant outcomes in renal transplant recipients, *Journal of Transplant Coordination* 6(2):53, 1996.
17. Douzdjian V, Abecassis M, Corry R, Hunsicker L: Simultaneous pancreas-kidney versus kidney-alone transplants in diabetics: increased risk of early cardiac death and acute rejection following pancreas transplants, *Clin Transplant* 8(3 Pt 1):246, 1994.
18. Evans R, Orians C, Ascher N: The potential supply of organ donors: an assessment of the efficiency of organ procurement efforts in the United States, *JAMA* 267(2):239, 1992.

19. Eye Bank Association of America: *1996 eye bank statistics,* Washington, DC, 1997, Eye Bank Association of America.
20. Gaedeke MK: Overview of organ and tissue donation. In Chabalewski F, editor: *Donation and transplantation: nursing curriculum,* Richmond, 1996, UNOS.
21. Garrison RN, Bentley FR, Raque GH: There is an answer to the shortage of organ donors, *Surg Gynecol Obstet* 173(5):391, 1991.
22. Goldsmith MF: Mother to child: first living donor lung transplant, *JAMA* 264(21):2724, 1990.
23. Hathaway DK, Hartwig MS, Milstead J, et al: A prospective study of changes in quality of life reported by diabetic recipients of kidney-only and pancreas-kidney allografts, *Journal of Transplant Coordination* 4(1):12, 1994.
24. Hricik DE, Bartucci MR, Seller MC, Schulak JA: Outpatient use of OKT3 for the treatment of acute allograft rejection, *Clin Transplant* 4(3):19, 1990.
25. Kaufman D, Jones J, Matas A: New immunosuppressive agents: FK506, rapamycin, RS-61443, 15-deoxyspergualin, *Journal of Transplant Coordination* 2(3):20, 1992.
26. Navarro VB, Tolley FM: Corneal transplantation. In Nolan MT, Augustine SM, editors: *Transplantation nursing, acute and long-term management,* Norwalk, Conn, 1995, Appleton & Lange.
27. Noedel NR, Osterloh JF, Brannan JA, et al: Critical pathways as an effective tool to reduce cardiac transplantation hospitalization and charges, *Journal of Transplant Coordination* 6(1):14, 1996.
28. Owens SG, Wallop JM: Heart-lung and lung transplantation. In Nolan MT, Augustine SM, editors: *Transplantation nursing, acute and long-term management,* Norwalk, Conn, 1995, Appleton & Lange.
29. President's Commission for the Study of Ethical Problems in Medicine and Biomedical and Behavioral Research: *Defining death: medical, legal, and ethical issues in the determination of death,* Washington, DC, 1981, US Government Printing Office.
30. Rohrer KS: Transplantation immunology. In Nolan MT, Augustine SM, editors: *Transplantation nursing, acute and long-term management,* Norwalk, Conn, 1995, Appleton & Lange.
31. Roitt IM, Brostoff J, Male D: *Immunology,* ed 3, St Louis, 1994, Mosby.
32. Shivnan JC, Ohly KV, Hanson JL: Bone marrow transplantation. In Nolan MT, Augustine SM, editors: *Transplantation nursing, acute and long-term management,* Norwalk, Conn, 1995, Appleton & Lange.
33. Siconolfi L: Mycophenolate mofetil: immunosuppression on the cutting edge, *AACN Clin Issues* 7(3):390, 1996.
34. Workman ML, Ellorhorst-Ryan J, Hargrave-Koertge V: *Nursing care of the immunocompromised patient,* Philadelphia, 1993, WB Saunders.
35. United Network for Organ Sharing: *Financing transplantation, what every patient needs to know,* ed 3, Richmond, 1996, UNOS.
36. United Network for Organ Sharing: *1996 transplant statistics,* Richmond, 1997, UNOS.
37. Youngner S, Arnold R: Ethical, psychosocial, and public policy implications of procuring organs from non–heart-beating cadaver donors, *JAMA* 269(21):2769, 1993.

# Selected Bibliography

## Chapter 1
## Issues Affecting Adult Health Care


### General

Center for Studying Health System Change: The trajectory of managed care, *Issue Brief* 9:1-4, 1997.

Harris IB: New expectations for professional competence. In Curry L, Wergin JF, editors: *Educating professionals: responding to new expectations for competence and accountability,* San Francisco, 1993, Jossey-Bass.

Mortality patterns—United States, 1993, *MMWR* 45(8):161-164, 1996.

Pew Health Professions Commissions: *Critical challenges: revitalizing the health professions for the twentyfirst century,* San Francisco, 1995, The Commissions.

Young M: Professions face technology-based practice, *Center Licensing Eval Accred Regul* 8(5), 1996.

### Case Management

Bower KA: *Case management by nurses,* Washington, DC, 1992, American Nurses Publishing.

Clafin N: Interdisciplinary patient and family education, *J Hosp Qual* 18(2): 16-21, 1996.

Cronin CJ, Maklebust J: Case-management care: capitalizing on the CNS, *Nurs Manage* 40(3):38-47, 1989.

Day C: The evolution of case management: one organization's experience, *Nurs Case Manage* 1(2):54-58, 1996.

Dunstron J: How managed care can work for you, *Nursing '90* 20(10):56-59, 1990.

Etheredge MLS: *Collaborative care: nursing case management,* Chicago, 1989, American Publishing.

Ethridge P, Lamb GS: Professional nursing case management improves quality, access and cost, *Nurs Manage* 20(3):30-35, 1989.

Newman M, Lamb GS, Michaels C: Nurse case management the coming together of theory and practice, *Nurs Health Care* 12(8):404-408, 1991.

Perez C: The next frontier in clinical pathways: the journey to outcomes management, *Nurs Case Manage* 1(2):75-78, 1996.

Robinson JA, Robinson KJ, Lewis DJ: Balancing quality of care and cost effectiveness through case management, *Am Nephrol Nurs Assoc J* 19(2):182-188, 1992.

Sobkowski DH, Maquera V: Critical path case management: the headache clinic, *Best Pract Benchmarking Healthcare* 1(4):198-202, 1996.

Tahan HA: A ten-step process to develop case management plans, *Nurs Case Manage* 1(3):112-121, 1996.

Zander K: Nursing case management: strategic management of cost and quality outcomes, *J Nurs Adm* 18(5):23-30, 1988.

### Health Care Cost and Reform

Adams TP: Case mix index: nursing's new management tool, *Nurs Manage* 27(9):31-32, 1996.

Caplan A: Do ethics and money mix? The moral implications of the corporation of medical care. In Baer EB, Fagan CM, Gordon S, editors: *Abandonment of the patient,* New York, 1996, Springer.

Handley T: Need for reform is in the numbers, *Kansas City Health Care Times* 2(7):5, 1993.

Jaret P: Nurses—the final guardians, *Newsweek* 104:16, 1984.

Kennedy EM: Congress and the national health policy, Rosenhause lecture, *Am J Public Health* 68:241-244, 1978.

Kerr CE: The case for managed care. In Baer EB, Fagan CM, Gordon S, editors: *Abandonment of the patient,* New York, 1996, Springer.

Olendski MC: *Cautionary tales,* Wakefield, Mass, 1973, Contemporary Publications.

Packard NJ: The price of choice: managed care in America, *Nurs Adm Q* 17(3):8-15, 1993.

Rakich JS, Longest BB, Darr K: *Managing health services organizations,* ed 2, Philadelphia, 1985, WB Saunders.

Schondelmeyer B: Home health care is a growing business, *Kansas City Health Care Times* 2(2):4, 1993.

Sobkowski DH, Maquera V: Critical path case management: the headache clinic, *Best Pract Benchmarking Healthcare* 1(4):198-202, 1996.

Tahan HA: A ten-step process to develop case management plans, *Nurs Case Manage* 1(3):112-121.

Weissenstein E: Medicare, Medicaid are next targets for reform, *Mod Healthcare* 26(33):26, 1996.

Young QD: The case against profit-driven managed care. In Baer EB, Fagan CM, Gordon S, editors: *Abandonment of the patient,* New York, 1996, Springer.

### Quality Care and Improvement

Bergman R: Hitting the mark, *Hosp Health Networks* 68(8):48-51, 1994.

Cesta TG: The link between continuous quality improvement and case management, *J Nurs Adm* 23(6):55-61, 1993.

Czarmeclo MT: Benchmarking: a data-oriented look at improving health care performance, *J Nurs Care Qual* 10(3):1-6, 1996.

Dienemann J: *Continuous quality improvement,* Washington, DC, 1992, American Nurses Publishing.

Frommer AG: Benchmarking, monitoring and moving through the continuum of the clinical pathway system, *Best Pract Benchmarking Healthcare* 1(3):157-160, 1996.

Juran JM: *Juran on quality leadership: how to go from here to there,* Wilton, Conn, 1987, Juran Institute.

Juran JM: *Juran on planning for quality,* New York, 1988, Free Press.

McKeon T: Benchmarks and performance indicators: two tools for evaluating organizations results and continuous quality improvement efforts, *J Nurs Care Qual* 10(3):12-17, 1996.

Saldon R, Tanner FW: Quality management program boosts financial performance, *Provider* 18(10):56-57, 1992.

### Role of Nursing

Doddato T: Advanced practice education for the twenty-first century, *N&HC Perspect Community* 16(5):266-269, 1995.

Dropplemann PG, Thomas SP: Anger in nurses: don't lose it, use it, *Am J Nurs* 96(4):26-31, 1996.

Glaister JA, Sapp AJ, Esparza D: Nurses practicing nursing independently, *N&HC Perspect Community* 17(3):128-132, 1996.

Huston CL: Unlicensed assistive personnel: a solution to dwindling health care resources or the precursor to the apocalypse of registered nursing? *Nurs Outlook* 44(2):67-73, 1996.

Koerner J: Differentiated practice: the evolution of professional nursing, *J Prof Nurs* 8:335-341, 1992.

Kotthoff E: Current trends and issues in nursing in the U.S.: the primary health care nurse practitioner, *Int Nurs Rev* 28:24-28, 1981.

Lavin J, Enright B: Charting with managed care in mind, *RN* 47-48, August 1996.

Levick ML, Jones CB: The nursing practice environment, staff retention, and quality of care, *Res Nurs Health* 19:331-343, 1996.

Manthey M et al: Primary nursing—a return to the concept "my nurse" and "my patient," *Nurs Forum* 9:65-83, 1970.

McCloskey JC: Recognizing the management role of all nurses, *N&HC Perspect Community Health* 16(6):307-308, 1995 (guest editorial).

Mundinger MO: Advanced nursing practice is the answer what is the question? *N&HC Perspect Community Health* 16(5):254-259, 1995.

Mosher C, Rademacher K, Day G, Fanelli D: Documenting for patient-focused care, *Nurs Econ* 14(4):218-223, 1996.

Neisser-Frankson C: Positioning the CNS in a changing market, *Clin Nurse Specialist* 8(6):319, 329, 1994.

O'Flynn AI: The preparation of advanced practice nurses: current issues, *Nurs Clin North Am* 31(3):429-438, 1996.

O'Koren ML: Reflections on facilitating collaboration between nursing services and nursing education, *J Prof Nurs* 2:72-74, 1986 (editorial).

Papenhausen JL: Case management: a model of advanced practice? *Clin Nurse Specialist* 1:47-52, 1990.

Paulen A: A time for reassessment, *Cancer Nurs* 9:2, 1986 (editorial).

Soehren PM, Schumann LL: Enhanced role opportunities available to the CNS/nurse practitioner, *Clin Nurse Specialist* 8(3):123-127, 1994.

Trey B: Managing interdependence on the unit, *Health Care Manage Rev* 21(3):72-82, 1996.

## Chapter 2 Cultural Care Nursing

### Cultural Care

Boyle JS: The practice of transcultural nursing, *Transcultural Nurs Soc Newslett* 7:2, 1987.

Giger JN, Davidhizar RE: *Transcultural nursing assessment and intervention,* ed 2, St Louis, 1995, Mosby.

Go GV: Changing populations and health. In Edelman CL, Mandle C, editors: *Health promotion through the life-span,* ed 3, St Louis, 1994, Mosby.

Lipson J: Culturally competent nursing care. In Lipson J, Dibble S, Minarik P, editors: *Culture and nursing care: a pocket guide,* San Francisco, 1996, University of San Francisco Press.

McGee P: Culturally sensitive and culturally comprehensive care, *Br J Nurs* 3(15):789-792, 1996.

Spector R: *Cultural diversity in health and illness,* ed 4, Norwalk, Conn, 1996, Appleton & Lange.

Spector R: *Guide to heritage assessment and health traditions,* Norwalk, Conn, 1996, Appleton & Lange.

### Traditional and Alternative Therapies

Budge EAW: *Amulets and superstitions,* New York, 1978, Dover Publications (originally published in London, 1930, Oxford University Press).

Buehler J: Traditional Crow Indian health beliefs and practices, *J Holistic Nurs* 10(1):18-33, 1992.

Eisenberg DM et al: Unconventional medicine in the United States: prevalence, costs, and patterns of use. *N Engl J Med* 328:251, 1993.

Fadiman A: *The spirit catches you and you fall down,* New York, 1997, Farrar, Straus, Giroux.

Fejos P: Man, magic, and medicine. In Goldstone I, editor: *Medicine and anthropology,* New York, 1959, International Universities Press.

Maloney C, editor: *The evil eye,* New York, 1976, Columbia University Press.

Weil A: *Health and healing,* Boston, 1983, Houghton Mifflin.

## Chapter 3 Promoting Healthy Lifestyles

### Prevention and Health Promotion

Bigbee JL, Jansa N: Strategies for promoting health protection. *Nurs Clin North Am* 26:895-913, 1991.

Caserta MS: Health promotion and the older population: expanding our theoretical horizons. *J Community Health* 20(3):283-292, 1995.

Frauman AC, Nettle-Carlson B: Predictors of a health promoting life style among well adult clients in a nursing practice, *J Am Acad Nurse Pract* 3(4): 174-178, 1991.

Koplan JP, Livengood JR: The influence of changing demographic patterns on our health promotion priorities, *Am J Prev Med* 10(suppl 3):42-44, 1994.

Landis BJ, Brykczynski KA: Employing prevention in practice, *Am J Nurs* 97(8):40-46, 1997.

Palank CL: Determinants of health-promotive lifestyle, *Nurs Clin North Am* 26:815-832, 1991.

Pencak M: Workplace health promotion programs, *Nurs Clin North Am* 26(1):233-239, 1991.

Pruitt RH: Effectiveness and cost efficiency of interventions in health promotion, *J Adv Nurs* 17:926-932, 1992.

Turjanica MA: Prevention: what is the cost? *MedSurg Nurs* 4(6):474-478, 1995.

### Nutrition and Weight Management

American Institute for Cancer Research: 50 top nutrition tips, *Nursing* 26(7): 55-56, 1996.

Herron DG: Strategies for promoting a healthy dietary intake. *Nurs Clin North Am* 26:875-884, 1991.

Keithley JK, Keller A, Vazquez MG: Promoting good nutrition: using the food guide pyramid in clinical practice, *MedSurg Nurs* 5(6):397-403, 1996.

Manson JE, Faich GA: Pharmacotherapy for obesity—do the benefits outweigh the risks? *N Engl J Med* 335(9):659-660, 1996.

Moore SA: Educating the family and the patient about nutrition, *Primary Care* 21(1):69-83, 1994.

Navia JM: A new perspective for nutrition: the health connection, *Am J Clin Nutr* 61(suppl):407S-409S, 1995.

Popkin BM, Siega-Riz AM, Haines PS: A comparison of dietary trends among racial and socioeconomic groups in the United States, *N Engl J Med* 335(10):716-720, 1996.

Russell RM: Nutrition, *JAMA* 273(21):1699-1700, 1995.

Shafer L, Gillespie A, Wilkins L, Borra ST: Position of the American Dietetic Association: nutrition education for the public, *J Am Diet Assoc* 96(11): 1183-1187, 1996.

### Exercise

Anonymous: Physical activity: counseling adults and older adults, *Nurse Pract* 22(4):159-171, 1997.

Evans WJ, Cyr-Campbell D: Nutrition, exercise, and healthy aging, *J Am Diet Assoc* 97(6):632-638, 1997.

Levine GN, Balady GJ: The benefits and risks of exercise training, *Adv Intern Med* 38:57-79, 1993.

Shephard RJ: Exercise and relaxation in health promotion, *Sports Med* 23(4):211-217, 1997.

Smith F, Iliffe S: Exercise prescription in primary care, *Br J Gen Pract* 47:272-273, 1997.

### Regimen Adherence

Nichols J: Changing public behavior for better health: is education enough? *Am J Prev Med* 10(suppl 3):19-21, 1994.

Redland AR, Stuitbergen AK: Strategies for maintenance of health-promoting behaviors, *Nurs Clin North Am* 28(2):427-442, 1993.

Simons MR: Interventions related to compliance, *Nurs Clin North Am* 27(2): 477-484, 1992.

### Smoking Cessation

Daughton DM et al: Confronting cigarette addiction: a guide to efficient clinical intervention, *Intern Med* 15(9):68-71, 1994.

Lewis SF, Fiore MC: Smoking cessation: what works? What doesn't? *J Respir Dis* 16(5):497-501, 1995.

Nett LM: How you and your team can help smokers quit, *J Respir Dis* 14(suppl 10):S26, 1993.

## Chapter 4
## Nursing Practice with Elders

### Assessment of Elders


Ebersole P, Hess P: *Toward healthy aging: human needs and nursing response,* ed 5, St Louis, 1998, Mosby.

Lenihan AA: Identification of self-care behaviors in the elderly: a nursing assessment tool, *J Prof Nurs* 4(4):285-288, 1988.


### Functional Assessment in Elders


Clinical guidelines: adult screening for cognitive and functional impairments, *Nurs Pract* 21(4):112-115, 1996.

Cress ME et al: Relationship between physical performance and self-perceived physical function, *J Am Geriatr Soc* 43:93-101, 1995.

Finch M, Kane RL, Philp I: Developing a new metric for ADLs, *J Am Geriatr Soc* 43:877-884, 1995.

Hungelmann J et al: Development of the JAREL spiritual well-being scale. In Caroll-Johnson RM, editor: *Classification of nursing diagnoses, Proceedings of the Eighth Conference, North American Diagnosis Association,* Philadelphia, 1989, JB Lippincott.

Miller C: Identify adverse medication effect when assessing function, *Geriatr Nurs* 17:295-296, 1996.

Stabler SP: Screening the older population for cobalamin (vitamin B12) deficiency, *J Am Geriatr Soc* 43:1290-1297, 1995.


## Chapter 5
## Ethical Decision Making in Nursing

### General


Arras JD, Steinbock B, editors: *Ethical issues in modern medicine,* ed 4, Mountain View, Calif, 1995, Mayfield.

Bayles MD: *Professional ethics,* Belmont, Calif, 1981, Wadsworth.

Bowle NE: *Making ethical decisions,* New York, 1986, McGraw-Hill.

Benjamin M, Curtis J: *Ethics in nursing,* ed 3, New York, 1992, Oxford University Press.

Daly BJ: Ethics in critical care. In Clochesy JM et al, editors: *Critical care nursing,* Philadelphia, 1993, WB Saunders.

Davis GC: Nursing values and health care policy, *Nurs Outlook* 36:289-292, 1988.

Iserson KV, Mahowald MB: Acute care research: is it ethical? *Crit Care Med* 20:1032-1037, 1992.

SUPPORT Principal Investigators: A controlled trial to improve care for seriously ill hospitalized patients: the Study to Understand Prognoses and Preferences for Outcomes and Risks of Treatment (SUPPORT), *JAMA* 274:1591-1598, 1995.

Veatch RM, Fry ST: *Case studies in nursing ethics,* Philadelphia, 1987, JB Lippincott.

Wright RA: *Human values in health care,* New York, 1987, McGraw-Hill.


### Moral Agency


American Nurses Association: *Code for nurses,* Washington, DC, 1985, The Association.

American Nurses Association: *Ethics in nursing,* Washington, DC, 1988, The Association.

Bandman EL, Bandman B: *Nursing ethics through the life span,* ed 2, Norwalk, Conn, 1992, Appleton & Lange.

Barnett TJ: Are there employment risks to ethical decisions? *Nurs Forum* 28(1):17-21, 1993.

Benner P, Tanner CA, Chesla CA: *Expertise in nursing practice: caring, clinical judgment, and ethics,* New York, 1996, Springer.

Caskey CT: Medical genetics, *JAMA* 277(23):1869-1870, 1997.

Hedin BA: Nursing, education, and sterile ethical fields, *Adv Nurs Sci* 11(3):43-52, 1989.

Mohr WK: Ethics, nursing, and health care in the age of "reform," *Nurs Health Care* 17(1):16-21, 1996.

Purtillo R: *Ethical dimensions in the health professions,* ed 2, Philadelphia, 1993, WB Saunders.

Silva MC: The American Nurses Association's code for nurses: purposes, content, and enforceability, *Health Matrix* 11(2):55-63, 1989.

Solomon MZ et al: Decisions near the end of life: professional views on life-sustaining treatments, *Am J Public Health* 83(1):14-22, 1993.


### Common Ethical Issues in Acute Care


Abrams FR: Advance directives: when the patient cannot communicate. In Monagle JF, Thomasma DC, editors: *Medical ethics,* Rockville, Md, 1988, Aspen.

Asch DA: The role of critical care nurses in euthanasia and assisted suicide, *N Engl J Med* 334:1374-1379, 1996.

Badzek LA: What you need to know about advance directives, *Nursing '92* (6):58-59, 1992.

Bosek MSD: Disregarding a physician's order: insurrection or comparison? *MedSurg Nurs* 4(5):396-400, 1995.

Brock D: Death and dying. In Veatch RM, editor: *Medical ethics,* Boston, 1989, Jones & Bartlett.

Brock D: Voluntary active euthanasia, *Hastings Cent Rep* 23(2):10-22, 1992.

Brody H: Assisted death—a compassionate response to a medical failure, *N Engl J Med* 327:1384-1388, 1992.

Burt RA: The Supreme Court speaks—not assisted suicide but a constitutional right to palliative care, *N Engl J Med* 337(17):1234-1236, 1997.

Caralis PV, Davis B, Wright K, Marcial E: The influence of ethnicity and race on attitudes toward advance directives, life-prolonging treatments, and euthanasia, *J Clin Ethics* 4(2):155-165, 1993.

Cohen ED, Davis M, editors: *AIDS: crisis in professional ethics,* Philadelphia, 1994, Temple University Press.

Collins E, Mozdzierz G: Ethical considerations in treating oncology patients in the intensive care unit, *Crit Care Nurs Q* 18(4):44-53, 1996.

Daly BJ: Withdrawal of food and fluid, *AACN Clin Iss Crit Care Nurse* 1(1):187-195, 1990.

Drane JF, Coulehan JL: The best-interest standard: surrogate decision making and quality of life, *J Clin Ethics* 6(1):20-29, 1995.

Emanuel L: Advance directives: what have we learned so far? *J Clin Ethics* 4:8-16, 1993.

Evans D: An ethical dilemma: the dishonest doctor, *Nurs Forum* 30(3):5-11, 1995.

Ferrell BR, Rivera LM: Ethical decision making in oncology, *Cancer Pract* 3(2):94-99, 1995.

Foley KM: Competent care for the dying instead of physician-assisted suicide, *N Engl J Med* 336(1):54-58, 1997.

Howe EG: The vagaries of patients' and families' discussing advance directives, *J Clin Ethics* 4(1):3-7, 1993.

Idemoto B et al: Implementing the Patient Self-Determination Act, *Am J Nurs* 93:21-25, 1993.

Jennings B: Active euthanasia and foregoing life-sustaining treatment: can we hold the line? *J Pain Sympt Manage* 6:312-316, 1991.

Lo B: The clinical use of advance directives. In Monagle JF, Thomasma DC, editors: *Medical ethics,* Rockville, Md, 1988, Aspen.

Marsden C: "Do Not Resuscitate" orders and end-of-life care planning, *Am J Crit Care* 2:177-179, 1993.

Meisel A: The legal consensus about foregoing life-sustaining treatment: its status and prospects, *Kennedy Inst Ethics J* 2:309-346, 1992.

Meyer C: End-of-life care: patients' choices, nurses' challenges, *Am J Nurs* 93(2):40-47, 1993.

Mezcy M, Latimer B: The Patient Self-Determination Act, *Hastings Cent Rep* 23(1):16-20, 1993.

O'Brien LA: Nursing home residents preferences for life-sustaining treatments, *JAMA* 274:1775-1779, 1995.

Oddi LF: Disclosure of human immunodeficiency virus status in healthcare settings, *J Intraven Nurs* 17(2):93-101, 1994.

President's Commission for the Study of Ethical Problems in Medicine and Biomedical and Behavioral Research: *Deciding to forego life-sustaining treatment: ethical, medical, and legal issues in treatment decisions,* Washington, DC, 1983, US Government Printing Office.

Rachels J: Euthanasia. In Regan T, editor: *Matters of life and death,* New York, 1986, Random House.

Scanlon C: Euthanasia and nursing practice—right question, wrong answer, *N Engl J Med* 334:1401-1402, 1996.

Schwarz JK: Living wills and health care proxies, *Nurs Health Care* 13(2):92-96, 1992.

Silverman HJ, Fry ST, Armistead N: Nurses' perspectives on implementation of the patient self-determination act, *J Clin Ethics* 5(1):30-37, 1994.

Stolman C et al: Evaluation of patient, physician, nurse, and family attitudes toward Do Not Resuscitate orders, *Arch Intern Med* 150:653-658, 1990.

Veatch RM: Foregoing life-sustaining treatment: limits to the consensus, *Kennedy Inst Ethics J* 3:1-20, 1993.

Vergara M, Lynn-McHale DJ: Withdrawing life support: who decides? *Am J Nurs* 95(11):47-49, 1995.

### Resources for Ethical Decision Making

Blake DC: The hospital ethics committee, *Hastings Cent Rep* 22(1):6-11, 1992.

Brennan TA: Ethics committees and decisions to limit care, *JAMA* 260:803-807, 1988.

Edwards BS: When the physician won't give up, *Am J Nurs* 93(9):34-37, 1993.

Lo B: Behind closed doors: promises and pitfalls of ethics committees, *N Engl J Med* 317:46-50, 1987.

Simpson KH: The development of a clinical ethics consultation service in a community hospital, *J Clin Ethics* 3:124-130, 1992.

Slome LR et al: Physician-assisted suicide and patients with human immunodeficiency virus disease, *N Engl J Med* 336(6):417-421, 1997.

Talone P: Ethics and managed care: beyond helplessness, *MedSurg Nurs* 5(3):212-214, 1996.

Viens DC: A history of nursing's code of ethics, *Nurs Outlook* 37(1):45-49, 1989.

Winslow GR: From loyalty to advocacy: a new metaphor for nursing, *Hastings Cent Rep* 14(3):32-39, 1984.

### Ethical Theories and Principles

Beauchamp TL, Childress JF: *Principles of biomedical ethics,* ed 3, New York, 1989, Oxford University Press.

Chell B: Competency: what it is and what it isn't. In Monagle JF, Thomasma DC, editors: *Medical ethics,* Rockville, Md, 1988, Aspen.

Committee on Ways and Means, US House of Representatives: *Health care resources book,* Washington, DC, 1991, US Government Printing Office.

Gorovitz S: Informed consent and patient autonomy. In Callahan JC, editor: *Ethical issues in professional life,* New York, 1988, Oxford University Press.

Pinch WJE: Feminism and bioethics, *MedSurg Nurs* 5(1):53-56, 1996.

Rikowski E: *Equal justice,* Oxford, 1991, Clarendon.

Veatch RM: Models for ethical medicine in a revolutionary age, *Hastings Cent Rep* 2(3):5-7, 1972.

Wiens AG: Patient autonomy in care: a theoretical framework for nursing, *J Prof Nurs* 9(2):93-103, 1993.

### Resolving Ethical Dilemmas

Haggarty MC: Ethics: nurse patron or nurse advocate? *Nurs Manage* 16(5): 34o-34u, 1985.

Halloran MC: Rational ethical judgments utilizing a decision-making tool, *Heart Lung* 11:566-570, 1982.

Hastings Center: *Guidelines on the termination of life-sustaining treatment and the care of the dying,* Indianapolis, 1987, Indiana University Press.

Holly CM: The ethical quandaries of acute care nursing practice, *J Prof Nurs* 9:110-115, 1993.

Levine-Artif J: Preventive ethics: the development of policies to guide decision-making, *AACN Clin Iss Crit Care Nurse* 1(1):169-177, 1990.

Novak J: An ethical decision-making model for the neonatal intensive care unit, *J Perinat Nurs* 1(3):57-67, 1988.

## Chapter 6 Stress, Stressors, and Stress Management

### General

Aguilera DC: *Crisis intervention: therapy and methodology,* ed 7, St Louis, 1994, Mosby.

Ashmore R: Post-traumatic stress disorder: symptoms, treatment, prevention, *Ment Health Nurs* 16(2):18-21, 1996.

Blair DT, Ramones VA: Understanding vicarious traumatization, *J Psychosoc Nurs* 34(11):24-30, 1996.

Clark CC: Post traumatic stress disorder: how to support, *Am J Nurs* 97(8), 26-32, 1997.

Fester C, Anderson RM: Empowerment: from philosophy to practice, *Patient Educ Couns* 26(1-3):139-144, 1995.

Figley CR: *Compassion fatigue: Coping with secondary traumatic stress disorder in those who treat the traumatized,* New York, 1995, Brunner/Mazel.

Humphrey JH: *Stress among older adults: understanding and coping,* Springfield, Ill, 1992, Charles C Thomas.

Kennedy P, Grey N: High pressure areas, *Nurs Times* 93(29):26-31, 1997.

McCain NL et al: The influence of stress management training on HIV disease, *Nurs Res* 45(4):246-252, 1996.

Siegrist J: Self, social structure, and health promoting behavior in hypertensive patients, *Patient Educ Couns* 26(1-3):215-218, 1995.

## Chapter 7 Chronic Illness and Rehabilitation

### General

Diamond M, Jones SI: *Chronic illness across the life span,* Norwalk, Conn, 1983, Appleton-Century Crofts.

Granger CV: Health accounting-functional assessment of the long term patient. In Kottke FJ, Stillwell GK, Lehmann JF, editors: *Krusen's handbook of physical medicine and rehabilitation,* Philadelphia, 1982, WB Saunders.

Henry WF: Chronic care needs to be a higher priority, *Hospitals* 68, February 20, 1991.

Hines Martin VP: A research review: family caregivers of chronically ill African American elderly, *J Gerontol Nurs* 28(2):25-29, 1992.

Institute of Medicine: *The second fifty years promoting health and preventing disability,* Washington, DC, 1990, National Academy Press.

Kahn KL et al: Comparing outcomes of care before and after implementation of the DRG-based prospective payment system, *JAMA* 264(15):1984-1988, 1990.

Kane RL: Improving the quality of long-term care, *JAMA* 273(17):1376-1383, 1995.

Lasker RD, Lee PR: Improving health through health system reform, *JAMA* 272(16):1292-1298, 1994 (editorial).

Lubkin JM: *Chronic illness: impact and interventions,* Boston, 1986, Jones & Bartlett.

Mackenbach JP, Louman CWN, van der Meder JBW: Differences in the misreporting of chronic conditions, by level of education, the effect of inequalities in prevalence rates, *Am J Public Health* 86(5):706-711, 1996.

McGinnis JM, Lee PR: Healthy people 2000 at mid decade, *JAMA* 273(14):1123-1124, 1995.

Murphy JF, Hepworth JT: Age and gender differences in health services utilization, *Res Nurs Health* 19:323-329, 1996.

Older Americans present a double challenge preventing disability and providing care, *Am J Public Health* 82(3):287-288, 1991 (editorial).

Olson PV, editor: The hazards of immobility, *Am J Nurs* 67:780-797, 1969.

Papazian R: What is enough, *Harvard Health Lett* 20(11):6, 1995.

Shepherdson N: Free from falling, *Arthritis Today* 24-26, September/October 1996.

Sorensen K, Armis DB: Understanding the world of the chronically ill, *Am J Nurs* 67:811-817, 1967.

Stewart AJ et al: Functional status and well-being of patients with chronic conditions, *JAMA* 262(7):907-913, 1989.

Verbrugge LM, Patrick DL: Seven chronic conditions: their impact on US adults' activity levels and use of medical services, *Am J Public Health* 85(2):173-182, 1995.

Watson PG: The Americans with Disabilities Act: more rights for people with disabilities, *Rehabil Nurs* 15(6):325-328, 1990.

Woog P, editor: *The chronic illness trajectory framework—the Corbin and Strauss nursing model,* New York, 1992, Springer.

### Ethnicity and Health

Council on Ethical and Judicial Affairs: Black white disparities in health care, *JAMA* 263(17):2344-2346, 1990.

Gornick ME, Eggers PW, Reilly TW et al: Effects of race and income on mortality and use of services among Medicare beneficiaries, *N Engl J Med* 335(11):791-799, 1996.

Schwartz E et al: Black/white comparisons of deaths preventable by medical interventions: United States and the District of Columbia 1980-1986, *Int J Epidemiol* 19(3):591-598, 1990.

Van Horne WA, Tonnoson TV, editors: *Ethnicity and health,* Madison, 1988, University of Wisconsin System Institute on Race and Ethnicity.

## Home Care/Nursing Home Care

Braden CJ: A test of self help model, learned response to chronic illness experience, *Nurs Res* 39(1):42-47, 1990.

Closson BL, Mattingly LJ, Finne KM, Larson JA: Telephone evaluation: application of Orem's self-care model, *Rehabil Nurs* 19(5):287-292, 1994.

Heidrich SM: Mechanisms related to psychological well-being in older women with chronic illnesses, age and disease comparisons, *Res Nurs Health* 19:225-235, 1996.

Katz JN, Larson MG, Phillips CB et al: Comparative measurement of short and longer health status instruments, *MedCare* 30(10):917-925, 1992.

Kahn KL et al: Comparing outcomes of care before and after implementation of the DRG based prospective payment system, *JAMA* 264(15):1984-1988, 1990.

Kemper P, Murdaugh CM: Lifetime use of nursing home care, *N Engl J Med* 324(9):595-600, 1991.

Metzler DJ, Harr J: Positioning your patient properly, *Am J Nurs* 96(3):33-37, 1996.

Papazian R: A call for help, *Harvard Health Lett* 20(6):1-4, 1995.

Patrick DL, Erickson P: *Health status and health policy, quality of life in health care evaluation and resource allocation,* New York, 1993, Oxford University Press.

Robertson JF, Cummings CC: What makes long-term care nursing attractive? *Am J Nurs* 91(11):41-46, 1991.

Rowe MA, The impact of internal and external resources on functional outcomes in chronic illness, *Res Nurs Health* 19:485-497, 1996.

Shamansky SI, editor: Home health care, *Nurs Clin North* Am 23(2):305-455, 1988.

Shaughnessy PW, Kramer AM: The increased needs of patients in nursing homes and patients receiving home health care, *N Engl J Med* 322(1):21-27, 1990.

Testa MA, Simonson DC: Assessment of quality of life outcomes, *N Engl J Med* 334(13):835-840, 1996.

Welch HG, Wennberg DE, Welch WP: The use of Medicare home health care services, *N Engl J Med* 335(5):324-329, 1996.

## Family—Family Care Givers

Black J: Can performance appraisals ensure that family members are prepared to provide adequate care? *Plast Surg Nurs* 16(2):70, 1996.

Bock DJ: A case manager's practical tips for family caregivers, *J Case Manage* 4(4):128-131, 1955.

Burton LM: Age norms, the timing of family role transitions, and intergenerational caregiving among aging African American women, *Gerontologist* 36(2):199-208, 1996.

Ell K: Social networks, social support and coping with serious illness: the family connection, *Soc Sci Med* 42(2):173-183, 1996.

England M, Roberts BL: Theoretical and psychometric analysis of caregiver strain, *Res Nurs Health* 19:499-510, 1996.

Mahoney DF, Shippee-Rice R: Training family caregivers of older adults: a program model for community nurses, *J Community Health Nurs* 11(2):71-78, 1994.

Nolan M, Keady J, Grant G: Developing a typology of family care: implications for nurses and other service providers, *J Adv Nurs* 21(2):256-265, 1995.

Norum J: Cancer patients dying at home—care providers' experience, *J Cancer Care* 4(4):157-160, 1995.

Quinn J: Family caregivers: a crucial element in our long-term care system, *J Case Manage* 4(4):119, 1995.

Richter JM, Roberts KA, Bottenberg DJ: Communicating with persons with Alzheimer's disease: experiences of family and formal caregivers, *Arch Psychiatry Nurs* 9(5):279-285, 1995.

Ruppert RA: Caring for the lay caregiver, *Am J Nurs* 96(3 Nurs Pract Extra Ed):40-46, 1996.

Smith CE: Quality of life in long-term total parenteral nutrition patients and their family caregivers, *JPEN: J Parenter Enteral Nutr* 7(6):501-506, 1993.

Smith CE: Quality of life and caregiving in technological home care, *Annu Rev Nurs Res* 14:95-118, 1996.

Toseland RW: *Group work with the elderly and family caregivers,* New York, 1995, Springer.

Weeks SK, O'Connor PC: Taking on the family caregiver role: nurses' sensitivity to the needs of prospective family caregivers, *Rehabil Nurs Res* 5(1):16-22, 1996.

## Psychosocial

Burchardt CS et al: Quality of life of adults with chronic illness: a psychometric study, *Res Nurs Health* 12:347-354, 1989.

Foxall MJ, Edberg JY: Loneliness of chronically ill adults and their spouses, *Iss Ment Health Nurs* 10(2):149-167, 1989.

Leidy NK: A structural model of stress, psychosocial resources, and symptomatic experiences in chronic physical illness, *Nurs Outlook* 34(4):230-236, 1990.

Pollock G: The mourning liberation process in health and disease, *Psychiatr Clin North Am* 10(3):345-354, 1987.

Pollock SE: Human responses to chronic illness: physiologic and psychosocial adaptation, *Nurs Res* 36:90-95, 1986.

Primomo J, Yates BC, Woods NF: Social support for women during chronic illness: the relationship among sources and types top adjustment, *Res Nurs Health* 13:153-161, 1990.

## Rehabilitation—General

Brandstater ME: Physical medicine and rehabilitation, *JAMA* 273(21):1710-1712, 1995.

Evans RL, Connis RT, Hendricks RD, Haselkom JK: Multidisciplinary rehabilitation versus medical care: a meta-analysis, *Soc Sci Med* 40(12):1699-1706, 1995.

Fuhrer MJ, editor: *Rehabilitation outcomes, analysis and measurement,* Baltimore, 1987, Paul H Brookes.

Heinemann AW, Linacre JM, Wright BJ et al: Prediction of rehabilitation outcomes with disability measures, *Arch Phys Med Rehabil* 75:133-143, 1994.

Kochersberger G, Hjelema F, Westlund R: Rehabilitation in the nursing home: how much, why, and with what results, *Public Health Rep* 109(3):372-376, 1994.

May BJ, Dennis JK: Caregivers. In *Home health and rehabilitation: concepts of care,* Philadelphia, 1993, FA Davis.

Rader MC, Vaughen JL: Management of the frail deconditioned patient, *South Med J* 87(5):561-565, 1994.

Tate DG, Forchheimer M, Daugherty J, Maynard F: Determining differences in post discharge outcomes among catastrophically and noncatastrophically sponsored outpatients with spinal cord injury, *Am J Phys Med Rehabil* 73(2):89-97, 1994.

Velozo CA, Magalhaes MS, Pan AW, Leiter P: Functional scale discrimination at admission and discharge: Rasch analysis of the level of rehabilitation scale—III, *Arch Phys Med Rehabil* 76:706-712, 1995.

Wahlquist G: The family in rehabilitation, *Rehabil Nurs* 12:62, 1987.

Weber DC, Fleming KC, Evans JM: Rehabilitation of geriatric patients, *Mayo Clin Proc* 70:1198-1204, 1995.

Wright B: *Physical disability: a psychological approach,* ed 2, New York, 1983, Harper & Row.

Wright BA: Value-laden beliefs and principles for rehabilitation, *Rehabil Lit* 12:266-269, 1981.

## Rehabilitation Nursing

Buchanan LC: A rehabilitation clinical nurse specialist: evaluation of the role in a home health care setting, *Holistic Nurs Pract* 6(2):42-50, 1992.

Carpenter C: The experience of spinal cord injury: the individual's perspective—implications for nursing practice, *Phys Ther* 74(7):614-628, 1994.

Derstine JB: The rehabilitation clinical nurse specialist of the 1990s: roles assumed by recent graduates, *Rehabil Nurs* 17(3):139-140, 1992.

Doyle DL, Stern PN: Negotiating self care in rehabilitation nursing, *Rehabil Nurs* 17(6):319-322, 326, 1992.

Habel M, Garland G: Rehabilitation nursing novices: changing the acute care mind set, *Rehabil Nurs* 15(2):73-76, 1990.

Hoeman SP: *Rehabilitation nursing, process and application,* ed 2, St Louis, 1996, Mosby.

Ross B: The impact of reimbursement issues on rehabilitation nursing practice and patient care, *Rehabil Nurs* 17(5):236-238, 1992.

Safran DG, Graham JD, Osberg JS: Social supports as a determinant of community based care utilization among rehabilitation patients, *HSR: Health Serv Res* 28(6):729-750, 1994.

Sawin KJ, Heard L: Nursing diagnoses used most frequently in rehabilitation nursing practice, *Rehabil Nurs* 17(5):256-262, 1992.

## Chapter 8 Loss, Grief, and Dying

### Change and Transition

Birney M: Psychoneuroimmunology: a holistic framework for the study of stress and illness, *Holistic Nurs Pract* 5(4):32-38, 1991.

Brammer L: *How to cope with life transitions: the challenge of personal change,* Bristol, Penna, 1990, Hemisphere.

Holmes T, Rahe R: Social readjustment rating scale, *J Psychosom Res* 11:213-218, 1967.

Kobasa S: Stressful life events, personality, and health, *J Pers Soc Psychol* 37:1-11, 1979.

Levenson J, Bemis C: The role of psychosocial factors in cancer onset and progression, *Psychosomatics* 32:124-132, 1991.

Streff M: Examining family growth and development, *Adv Nurs Sci* 3(4):61-69, 1981.

### Loss and Grief

Benoliel J: Loss and terminal illness, *Nurs Clin North Am* 20(2):439-448, 1985.

Brice C: Mourning throughout the life cycle, *Am J Psychoanal* 42(4):315-325, 1982.

Carroll R: Mourning: a concern for medical-surgical nurses, *MedSurg Nurs* 2(4):301-303, 1993.

Cousins N: *Anatomy of an illness,* New York, 1979, WW Norton.

Cowles K, Rodgers B: The concept of grief: a foundation for nursing research and practice, *Res Nurs Health* 14(2):119-127, 1991.

Martocchio B: Grief and bereavement: healing through hurt, *Nurs Clin North Am* 20(2):327-334, 1985.

Pollock S: Human responses to chronic illness: physiologic and psychologic adaptation, *Nurs Res* 35:90-95, 1986.

### Influencing Factors

Callahan D: Frustrated mastery: the cultural context of death in America. In *Caring for patients at the end of life* (Special Issue), *West J Med* 163:226-230, 1997.

Cobb S: Social support as a moderator of life stress, *Psychosomatics* 38(5):300-315, 1976.

Cutcliff J: How do nurses inspire and instill hope in terminally ill HIV patients? *J Adv Nurs* 22(5):888-895, 1995.

Dufault K, Martocchio B: Hope: its spheres and dimensions, *Nurs Clin North Am* 20:379-391, 1980.

Flach F: *Resilience: Discovering a new strength at times of stress,* New York, 1988, Fawcett Columbine.

Frankl V: Self-transcendence as a human phenomenon, *J Humanistic Psychol* 6:97-106, 1966.

Gamlin R: Using hope to cope with loss and grief, *Nurs Standard* 9(48):33-35, 1995.

Grey R: The psychospiritual care matrix: a new paradigm for hospice care givers, *Am J Hospice Palliat Care* 13(4):19-25, 1996.

Hickey S: Enabling hope, *Cancer Nurs* 9:133-137, 1986.

Highfield M: Spiritual health of oncology patients, *Cancer Nurs* 15(1):1-8, 1992.

Lambert C, Lambert V: Hardiness: its development and relevance to nursing, *Image* 19(2):92-95, 1987.

Leininger MM, editor: *Cultural care, diversity and universality: a theory of nursing,* New York, 1991, National League for Nursing.

Martocchio B: Family coping: helping families help themselves, *Semin Oncol Nurs* 1(4):292-297.

McGoldrick M: *Living beyond loss: death in the family,* New York, 1991, WW Norton.

Miller J: Hope-inspiring strategies of the critically ill, *Appl Nurs Res* 2:23-29, 1989.

Nishimoto P: Venturing into the unknown: cultural beliefs about death and dying, *Oncol Nurs Forum* 23(6):889-894, 1996.

Osterman P, Schwartz-Barcott D: Presence: four ways of being there, *Nurs Forum* 31(2):23-29, 1996.

Rustoen T: Hope and quality of life: two central issues for cancer patients—a theoretical analysis, *Cancer Nurs* 18(5):355-361, 1995.

Norbeck J: Social support, *Adv Nurs Sci* 3(4):43-54, 1981.

Scanlon C: Creating a vision of hope: the challenge of palliative care, *Oncol Nurs Forum* 7:491-496, 1989.

### Death and Dying

Brabant J, Forsyth C, Melancon C: Grieving men: thoughts, feelings, and behaviors following deaths of wives, *Hospice J* 8(4):33-47, 1992.

Bryan E: The death of a twin, *Palliat Med* 9(3):187-192, 1995.

Carse J: *Death and existence:* A *conceptual history of human mortality,* New York, 1980, John Wiley & Sons.

Curry L, Stone J: The grief process: a preparation for death, *Clin Nurs Specialist* 5(1):17-22, 1991.

Durham E, Weiss L: How patients die, *Am J Nurs* 97(12):41-47, 1997.

Galloway S: Young adults: reactions to the death of a parent, *Oncol Nurs Forum* 17(6):899-904, 1990.

Harper G: *Living with dying: finding meaning in chronic illness,* Grand Rapids, Mich, 1992, William B Eardmans.

Kastenbaum R, Aisenberg R: *The psychology of death,* New York, 1976, Springer.

Levine S: *Healing into life and death,* Garden City, NY, 1987, Anchor.

Long M: Death and dying and recognizing approaching death, *Clin Geriatr Med* 12(2):359-368, 1996.

Schneidman E: *Voices of death,* New York, 1980, Harper & Row.

Sowell R: The lived experience of survival and bereavement following the death of a lover from AIDS, *Image* 23(2):89-94, 1991.

Waltman R: When a spouse dies, *Nursing '92* 22(7):48-51, 1992.

### Quality of Dying

Brody R: Assisted death—a compassionate response to a medical failure, *N Engl J Med* 327:1384-1388, 1992.

Byock I: Consciously walking the fine line: thoughts on a hospice response to assisted suicide and euthanasia, *J Palliat Care* 9(3):25-28, 1993.

Coyle N: The euthanasia and physician-assisted suicide debate: issues for nursing, *Oncol Nurs Forum* 19(7):41-46, 1992.

Mech A: Assisted suicide: a patient's right? *Nurs Policy Forum* 2(4):5, 1996.

Meyer C: 'End-of-life' care: patient choices, nurses' challenges *Am J Nurs* 2:40-47, 1993.

Zerwekh J: Do dying patients really need IV fluids? *Am J Nurs* 97(3):26-31, 1997.

### Grief Support

Carmack B: Balancing engagement/detachment in AIDS-related multiple losses, *Image* 4(1):9-14, 1992.

Carnevali D, Reiner A: *The cancer experience: nursing diagnosis and management,* Philadelphia, 1990, JB Lippincott.

Hall M: Letting go, *Nursing '96* 11:54-56, 1996.

Hammer M, Nichols D: A ritual of remembrance . . . grief suffered by nurses themselves, *Maternal Child Nurs* 17(6):310-313, 1992.

Heiney S, Wells S: Strategies for organizing and maintaining successful support groups, *Oncol Nurs Forum* 16(6):803-812, 1989.

Hittle J: Dealing with grief: grieving together, *Am J Nurs* 95(7):55-57, 1995.

Karl G: Survival skills for psychic trauma, *J Psychosoc Nurs* 27(4):15-19, 1989.

Lane PS: Critical incident stress de-briefing for healthcare workers, *Omega* 28(4):301-315, 1993-94.

LeShan L: *Counseling the dying,* New York, 1964, Thomas Nelson.

Longman A: Effectiveness of a hospice community bereavement program, *Omega* 27(2):165-175, 1993.

Mian P: Sudden bereavement: nursing interventions in the ED, *Crit Care Nurse* 10:30-40, 1990.

Morse J, Bottorff J, Anderson G et al: Expanding expressions of caring, *J Adv Nurs* 17(6):809-821, 1992.

Moseley J: Developing a bereavement program in a university hospital setting, *Oncol Nurs Forum* 15:151-155, 1988.

Pheifer W, Houseman C: Bereavement and AIDS: a framework for intervention, *J Psychosoc Nurs* 26:21-26, 1988.

Puckett P, Hinds P, Milligan M: Who supports you when your patient dies? *RN* 59(10):48-50, 1996.

Quill T: *A midwife through the dying process,* Baltimore, 1996, John Hopkins Press.

Raphael B: Preventive interventions with the recently bereaved, *Arch Gen Psychiatry* 34(12):1450-1454, 1977.

Rickel L: Making mountains manageable: maximizing quality of life through crisis intervention, *Oncol Nurs Forum* 14(4):29-34, 1987.

Rubin J: Critical incident stress debriefing: helping the helpers, *J Emerg Nurs* 16:255-258, 1990.

Spencer L: How do nurses deal with their own grief when a patient dies on an intensive care unit, and what help can be given to enable them to overcome their grief effectively? *J Adv Nurs* 19(6):1141-1150, 1994.

### Grief Resolution

Curry L, Stone J: Moving on: recovery after the death of a spouse, *Clin Nurse Specialist* 6(4):80-90, 1992.

Kallenberg K, Soderfeld B: Three years later: grief, view of life, and personal crises after death of a family member, *J Palliat Care* 8(4):13-19, 1992.

Kaprio J: Mortality after bereavement: a prospective study of 95,647 widowed persons, *Am J Public Health* 77:283-287, 1987.

Merrill E: Never too late to grieve, *Nursing '95* 25(4):75, 1995.

Murphy S: An explanatory model of recovery from disaster loss, *Res Nurs Health* 12:67-76, 1989.

Weinberg N: Self-blame, other blame, and desire for revenge: factors in recovery from bereavement, *Death Studies* 18(6):583-593, 1994.

Wolfelt A: Toward an understanding of complicated grief: a comprehensive overview, *Am J Hospice Palliat Care* 8(2):28-30, 1991.

Wortman C, Silver R: The myths of coping with loss, *J Consult Clin Psychol* 57:349-357, 1989.

## Chapter 9
## Impact of Illness on Mentation

### Confusion

Bliwise DL: What is sundowning? *J Am Geriatr Soc* 42(9):1009-1011, 1994.

Evans C et al: Caring for the confused geriatric surgical patient, *Geriatr Nurs* 14(5):237-241, 1993.

Foreman MD, Zane D: Nursing strategies for acute confusion in elders, *Am J Nurs* 96(4):44-51, 1996.

Hall GR, Wakefield B: Acute confusion in the elderly, *Nursing* 26(7):32-37, 1996.

Holt J: How to help confused patients, *Am J Nurs* 93(8):32-36, 1993.

Innouye SK: The dilemma of delirium, *Am J Med* 97(9):278-288, 1994.

Ludwick R, O'Toole AW: The confused patient—nurses knowledge and interventions, *J Gerontol Nurs* 22(1):44-49, 1996.

Matthiesen V et al: Acute confusion: nursing intervention in older patients, *Orthopaed Nurs* 13(2):21-29, 1994.

Miller J: A clinical project to reduce confusion in hospitalized older adults, *MedSurg Nurs* 5(2):436-444, 1996.

Morency CR et al: Research considerations: delirium in hospitalized elders, *J Gerontol Nurs* 20(8):24-30, 1994.

Shedd PP, Kobokovich LJ, Slattery MJ: Confused patients in the acute care setting: prevalence, intervention and outcomes, *J Gerontol Nurs* 21(4):5-12, 1995.

Valente SM: Recognizing depression in elderly patients, *Am J Nurs* 94(12):18-24, 1994.

Wallace M: The sundown syndrome, *Geriatr Nurs* 15(3):164-166, 1994.

Williams-Russo P et al: Postoperative delirium: predictors and prognosis in elderly orthopedic patients, *J Am Geriatr Soc* 40(2):759-767, 1992.

Yeaw EM, Abbate JH: Identification of confusion among the elderly in an acute care setting, *Clin Nurse Specialist* 7(4):192-197, 1993.

### Restraints

Blakeslee JA, Goldman BD, Papougenis D, Torell CA: Making the transition to restraint free care, *J Gerontol Nurs* 17(2):4-8, 1991.

Cohen C et al: Old problem, different approach: alternatives to physical restraints, *J Gerontol Nurs* 22(2):23-29, 1996.

Ejaz F et al: Restraint reduction: can it be achieved? *Gerontologist* 34(5):694-699, 1994.

Janelli LM, Kanski GW, Neary MA: Physical restraints: has OBRA made a difference? *J Gerontol Nurs* 20(6):17-21, 1994.

Leger-Krall S: When restraints become abusive, *Nursing* 24(3):54-56, 1994.

Neufeld R: Alarm devices instead of restraints? *J Am Geriatr Soc* 40(2):191-193, 1992.

Quinn CA: Nurses' perceptions about physical restraints, *West J Nurs Res* 15(2):148-162, 1993.

Scherer YK et al: Restrained patients: an important issue for critical care nursing, *Heart Lung* 2(4):77-83, 1993.

Stolley J: Freeing your patient from restraints, *Am J Nurs* 95(2):27-31, 1995.

Weick MD: Physical restraints: an FDA update, *Am J Nurs* 92(11):74-76, 78, 80, 1992.

Werner D et al: Reducing restraints—impact on staff attitudes, *J Gerontol Nurs* 20(12):19-23, 1994.

## Chapter 10
## Inflammation and Infection

### General

APIC: *APIC infection control and applied epidemiology: principles and practice,* St Louis, 1996, Mosby.

Beaumont E: Technology scorecard: focus on infection control, *Am J Nurs* 97(12):51-54, 1997.

Benenson AS, editor: *Control of communicable disease manual,* Washington, DC, 1995, American Public Health Association.

Centers for Disease Control and Prevention: Addressing emerging infectious disease threats: A prevention strategy for the United States, *MMWR* 43(RR-5):1-18, 1994.

Centers for Disease Control and Prevention: Update: provisional Public Health Service recommendations for chemoprophylaxis after occupational exposure to HIV, *MMWR* 45(22):468-472, 1996.

Cohen FL, Larson E: Emerging infectious diseases: nursing responses, *Nurs Outlook* 44(4):164-168, 1996.

Crow S, Penn R: Controlling nosocomial infection in the intensive care unit, *J Crit Illness* 11(6):380-391, 1996.

Diekema DJ, Bradley ND: Employee health and infection control, *Infect Control Hosp Epidemiol* 16:292-301, 1995.

Gardner P et al: Adult immunizations, *Ann Intern Med* 12(1 part 1):35-40, 1996.

Gerberding JL: Prophylaxis for occupational exposure to HIV, *Ann Intern Med* 125(6):497-501, 1996.

Holtzclaw BJ: The febrile response in critical care: state of the science, *Heart Lung* 21(5):482-501, 1992.

Osguthorpe NC, Morgan EP: An immunization update for primary health care providers, *Nurse Pract* 20(6):52-65, 1995.

Reiss PJ: Battling super bugs, *RN* 59(3):36-41, 1996.

Tablan OC et al: Guideline for prevention of nosocomial pneumonia, *Infect Control Hosp Epidemiol* 15:587-627, 1994.

Wood JJ, Gold HS, Moellering RC: Drug therapy: antimicrobial-drug resistance, *N Engl J Med* 335(19):1445-1453, 1996.

## Chapter 11
## Cancer

### General

Barraclough J: *Cancer and emotion: a practical guide to psycho-oncology,* ed 2, New York, 1994, John Wiley & Sons.

Bonan-Crawford D, Orlick M: Helping patients with cancer achieve their work potential, *Clin Perspect Oncol Nurs* 1(1):1-11, 1994.

Clark JC, McGee RF: *Core curriculum for oncology nursing,* ed 2, Philadelphia, 1992, WB Saunders.

Dow KH, editor: *Nursing care in radiation oncology,* Philadelphia, 1992, WB Saunders.

Fox BH: The role of psychological factors in cancer incidence and prognosis, *Oncology* 9(3):245-253, 1995.

Greenspan D: Xerostoma: diagnosis and management, *Oncology* 10(suppl 3): 7-11, 1996.

Haskell CM, editor: *Cancer treatment,* ed 4, Philadelphia, 1995, WB Saunders.

Lewis CE, O'Sullivan C, Barraclaugh J, editors: *The psychoimmunology of cancer: mind and body in the fight for survival,* Oxford, 1994, Oxford University Press.

Loescher LJ: Genetics in cancer prediction, screening, and counseling. Part II: the nurse's role in genetic counseling, *Oncol Nurs Forum* 22(suppl 2):16-19, 1995.

Mahon SM, Casperson DS: Hereditary cancer syndrome. Part 2: psychosocial issues, concerns, and screening—results of a qualitative study, *Oncol Nurs Forum* 22(2):775-782, 1995.

McCorkle R et al, editors: *Cancer nursing: a comprehensive textbook,* ed 2, Philadelphia, 1996, WB Saunders.

Ottery FD: Cancer cachexia, *Cancer Pract* 2(2):123-130, 1994.

Peckham M, Pinedo HM, Veronesi U, editors: *Oxford textbook of oncology,* Oxford, 1995, Oxford University Press.

Perry MC, editor: *The chemotherapy source book,* Baltimore, 1992, Williams & Wilkins.

Powe BD: Cancer fatalism among African-Americans: a review of the literature, *Nurs Outlook* 44(1):18-21, 1996.

Schweid L, Etheredge CS, Werner-McCullough M: Will you recognize these oncological crises? *RN* 9:23-28, 1994.

Watson RR, Mufti SI, editors: *Nutrition and cancer prevention,* Boca Raton, Fla, 1996, CRC Press.

Williams JK: Principles of genetics and cancer, *Semin Oncol Nurs* 13(2):68-73, 1997.

### Patient and Family Education

Freeman HP, Muth BJ, Kerner JF: Expanding access to cancer screening and clinical follow-up among the medically underserved, *Cancer Pract* 3(1):19-30, 1995.

Gyauch TM: Implementing a cancer education program for family and friend caregivers, *J Oncol Manage* 18-22, November/December 1995.

Nichols BS, Misra R, Alexy B: Cancer detection: how effective is public education? *Cancer Nurs* 19(2):98-103, 1996.

Reding DJ, Krauska ML, Lappe KA, Fischer VV: Cancer education interventions for rural populations, *Cancer Pract* 2(5):353-359, 1994.

### Chemotherapy

Almedrones L, Campana P, Dantis EC: Arterial, peritoneal, and intravascular access devices, *Semin Oncol Nurs* 11(3):194-202, 1995.

Bociek RG, Armitage JO: Hematopoietic growth factors, *CA Cancer J Clin* 46(3):165-184, 1996.

Dodd MJ, Onishi K, Dibble SL, Larson PJ: Differences in nausea, vomiting, and retching between younger and older outpatients receiving cancer chemotherapy, *Cancer Nurs* 19(3):155-161, 1996.

Hadaway LC: Comparison of vascular access devices, *Semin Oncol Nurs* 11(3):154-166, 1995.

Mishaw KB: Chemoprevention, *Nurs Interventions Oncol* 8(3):3-6, 1996.

Prescott LM: New polytherapy approaches for cancer treatment, *COPE* 12(3):26-27, 1996.

Spivak JL: Cancer-related anemia: its causes and characteristics, *Semin Oncol Nurs* 21(suppl 3):3-8, 1994.

### Radiation Therapy

Campbell MK, Pruitt JJ: Radiation therapy: protecting your patient's skin, *RN* 46-47, January 1996.

Dunne-Daly CF: Skin and wound care in radiation oncology, *Cancer Nurs* 18(2):144-162, 1995.

Fieler VK: Side effects and quality of life in patients receiving high-dose rate brachytherapy, *Oncol Nurs Forum* 24(3):545-553, 1997.

Iwamato RR: A nursing perspective on radiation-induced xerostomia, *Oncology* 10(suppl 3):12-15, 1996.

Johnson JE, Fieler VK, Wlasowicz G et al: The effects of nursing care guided by self-regulation theory on coping with radiation therapy, *Oncol Nurs Forum* 24(6):1041-1050, 1997.

Kirkbride P: The role of radiation therapy in palliative care, *J Palliat Care* 11(1):19-26, 1995.

Sitton E: Early and late radiation-induced skin alterations. Part I: mechanisms of skin changes, *Oncol Nurs Forum* 19(5):801-807, 1992.

### Biotherapy

Karius D, Marriott MA: Immunologic advances in monoclonal antibody therapy: implications for oncology nursing, *Oncol Nurs Forum* 24(3):483-494, 1997.

Payne JY: Will gene therapy revolutionize medicine? *Nurs Interventions Oncol* 8:9-12, 1996.

Post-White J: The immune system, *Semin Oncol Nurs* 12(2):89-96, 1996.

Rieger PT: Future projection in biotherapy, *Semin Oncol Nurs* 12(2):163-171, 1996.

### The Elderly

Dubin S: Geriatric assessment, *Am J Nurs* 96(5):49-50, 1996.

Dwyer J: Nutritional problems of elderly minorities, *Nutr Rev* 52(8):S24-S27, 1994.

Knobf T, Fulmer TT, Mion LC: Geriatric perspective for oncology nursing practice, *Curr Iss Cancer Nurs Pract* 2(3):1-14, 1993.

Lee M: Drugs and the elderly: do you know the risks? *Am J Nurs* 96(6):24-31, 1996.

### Cancer Pain

Brant JM: The use of access devices in cancer pain control, *Semin Oncol Nurs* 11(3):203-212, 1995.

Brown RI, Sullivan E: Helping families of chronic pain cancer patients to cope, *Am J Nurs* 6(suppl):22-28, 1996.

Ferrell BR, Rhiner M, Rivera LM: Empowering patients to control pain, *Curr Iss Cancer Nursing Pract Updates* 2(4):1-9, 1993.

McCaffery M, Ferrell BR, Turner M: Ethical issues in the use of placebos in cancer pain management, *Oncol Nurs Forum* 23(10):1587-1593, 1996.

Skobel S: Epidural narcotic administration: what nurses should know, *Oncol Nurs Forum* 23(10):1555-1560, 1996.

Zech DF, Grond S, Lynch J et al: Validation of World Health Organization guidelines for cancer pain relief: a 10-year prospective study, *Pain* 63(1):65-76, 1995.

### Nutrition

Grendel CG, Costello MC: Nutrition screening: an essential assessment parameter, *MedSurg Nurs* 5(3):145-154, 1996.

Grendel CG, Whitmer K, Barsevick A: Quality of life and nutritional support in patients with cancer, *Cancer Pract* 4(2):81-87, 199.

Hallwell B: Antioxidants: sense or speculation? *Nutr Today* 29(6):15-19, 1994.

### Home Management

Blesch KS: Rehabilitation of the cancer patient at home, *Semin Oncol Nurs* 12(3):219-225, 1996.

McEnroe LE: Role of the oncology nurse in home care: family-centered practice, *Semin Oncol Nurs* 12(3):188-192, 1996.

McNally JC, Bohnet NL, Lindquist ME: Hospice nursing, *Semin Oncol Nurs* 12(3):238-243, 1996.

Salvaggio RJ: Meeting the challenge of home therapy for the patient with cancer, *Clin Perspect Oncol Nurs* 1(3):1-12, 1995.

Yost LS: Cancer patients and home care, *Cancer Pract* 3(2):83-87, 1995.

## Chapter 12 Pain and Pain Control

### General

Alspach G: Pain management: dispelling some myths, *Crit Care Nurse* 14(5):13-15, 1994.

Bostrom J, Batina M: Managing pain in a diverse medical-surgical patient population, *MedSurg Nurs* 3(6):469-474, 486, 1994.

Bowman JM: Perceptions of surgical pain by nurses and patients, *Clin Nurs Res* 3(1):69-76, 1994.

Closs SJ: Pain in elderly patients: a neglected phenomenon? *J Adv Nurs* 19(6):1072-1081, 1994.

Ferrell BR: Controlling pain: switching to a longer acting opioid, *Nursing* 24(2):22-24, 1994.

Ferrell B et al: The Pain Resource Nurse Training Program: a unique approach to pain management, *J Pain Sympt Manage* 8:549-556, 1994.

Ferrell B, Whedon M, Rollins B: Pain and quality assessment/improvement, *J Nurs Care Qual* 9:69-85, 1995.

Gordon DB, Ward SE: Correcting misconceptions about pain, *Am J Nurs* 95(7):43-45, 1995.

Hitchcock LS, Ferrell BR, McCaffery M: The experience of chronic nonmalignant pain, *J Pain Sympt Manage* 9(5):312-318.

Lindaman C: Talking to physicians about pain control, *Am J Nurs* 95(1):36-37, 1995.

McCaffery M: Analgesics—mapping out pain relief, *Nursing* 26(1):41-46, 1996.

McCaffery M: Ensuring pain relief, *Nursing* 24(9):81-82, 1994.

McCaffery M, Ferrell BR: Does the gender gap affect pain control decisions? *Nursing* 22(8):48-51, 1992.

McCaffery M, Ferrell BR, O'Neill-Page E: Does life-style affect your pain-control decisions? *Nursing* 22(4):58-61, 1992.

McGuire L: The nurse's role in pain relief, *MedSurg Nurs* 3(2):94-98, 1994.

Miakowski C: Current concepts in the assessment and management of acute pain, *MedSurg Nurs* 2(1):28-32, 40, 1993.

Pasero CL: Help for chronic pain sufferers, *Am J Nurs* 94(10):17, 1994.

Pasero CL, McCaffery M: Avoiding opioid induced respiratory depression, *Am J Nurs* 94(4):25-30, 1994.

Pasero CL et al: Pain control: antidepressants for pain relief, *Am J Nurs* 95(2):22-24, 1995.

### Pain Assessment

Arathuzik D: Preliminary assessment: the Pain Inventory and the Pain Coping Tool, *Am J Hospice Palliat Care* 11(5):25-29, 1994.

Briggs M: Principles of acute pain assessment, *Nurs Standards* 9(19):23-27, 1995.

Kohr J: Measuring your patient's pain, *RN* 58(4):39-40, 1995.

McCaffery M: How reliable is your patient's pain assessment? *Nursing* 24(1):19-20, 1994.

McCaffery M, Ferrell BR: Nurses' assessment of pain intensity and choice of analgesic dose, *Contemp Nurse* 3(2):68-74, 1994.

### Nonpharmacologic Pain Relief Strategies

Altsberger DB: Relaxation therapy: its potential as an intervention for acute postoperative pain, *J Post Anesth Nurs* 10(1):2-8, 1005.

Borneman T: Controlling pain: using nondrug interventions to relieve pain, *Nursing* 25(2):21-22, 1995.

Funk B: Controlling pain: using cognitive interventions, *Nursing* 25(3):30, 1995.

Kurz JM: Therapeutic touch for postop pain? *Am J Nurs* 94(9):48D, 1994.

### Epidural Pain Control

Hambleton NE: Dealing with complications of epidural analgesia, *Nursing* 24(10):55-57, 1994.

Lawrence S et al: Epidural analgesia for effective pain control, *Critical Care Nurse* 15(1):20-21, 1995.

Naber L, Jones G, Halm M: Epidural analgesia for pain control, *Crit Care Nurse* 14(5):69-72, 77-85, 1994.

Wild L, Coyne C: The basics and beyond: epidural analgesia, *Am J Nurs* 92(4):26-34, 1992.

### Issues in Pain Control

Bates MS, Edward WT, Anderson KO: Ethnocultural influences on variation in chronic pain experience, *Pain* 52:101-112, 1993.

Bates MS, Rankin-Hill L: Control, culture and chronic pain, *Soc Sci Med* 39(5):629-645, 1993.

Cain JM, Hammes BJ: Ethics and pain management: respecting the patient's wishes, *J Pain Sympt Manage* 8(7):474-482, 1994.

Dahlberg N, Pendle S: Developing an acute pain service in a multicultural setting, *J Post Anesth Nurs* 9(2):96-100, 1994.

Faucett J, Gordon N, Levine J: Differences in post operative pain severity among four ethnic groups, *J Pain Sympt Manage* 9(6):383-389, 1994.

Ferrell BR: Using placebos ethically: controlling pain, *Nursing* 24(3):28, 1994.

Fox AE: Confronting the use of placebos for pain, *Am J Nurs* 94(9):42-46, 1994.

Henkleman WJ: Inadequate pain management: ethical considerations, *Nurs Manage* 25(1):48A-B, 48D, 1994.

Kumasaka L: My pain is God's will, *Am J Nurs* 96(6):45-47, 1996.

Scholz MJ: Pain clinic: assessing safety of opioids for chronic pain, *RN* 58(4):71, 1995.

Ufema J: Pacebos: sugar coated pain, *Nursing* 24(9):31, 1994.

Walsh SA et al: A place for placebos? *Am J Nurs* 95(2):18, 1995.

Wenger AF: The cultural meaning of symptoms, *Holistic Nurs Pract* 7(2):22-35, 1993.

## Chapter 13 Sleep Disorders

### General

Hobson JH: *Sleep,* New York, 1995, WH Freeman.

Kryger MH, Roth R, Dement WB: *Principles and practice of sleep medicine,* ed 2, Philadelphia, 1993, WB Saunders.

### Physiology of Sleep

Dunlap J, Loros J, editors: *Biological clocks,* Oxford, 1997, Oxford University Press.

Kandel ER, Schwartz JH, Jessell TM: *Principles of neural science,* New York, 1991, Elsevier Science.

Moore-Ede MC, Sultzman FM, Fuller CE: *The clocks that time us: physiology of the circadian timing system,* Cambridge, Mass, 1982, Harvard University Press.

### Parasomnias

Ferber R, Kryger M: *Principles and practice of sleep disorders in the child,* Philadelphia, 1995, WB Saunders.

Schaeffer CE: *Clinical handbook of sleep disorders in children,* Arcade, NY, 1995, Aronson.

### Insomnia

"Insomnia," *Sleep* 19(suppl 3):S1-S41, 1996.

Mendelson WB: Insomnia and related sleep disorders, *Psychiatr Clin North Am* 16(4):841-851, 1993.

Vafi H, Vafi P: *How to get a great night's sleep: step by step practical advice,* Holbrook, Mass, 1994, Adams Publishing.

### Sleep Apnea

Hoffstein V: Is snoring dangerous to your health? *Sleep* 19(6):506-516, 1996.

Johnson TS, Halberstadt J: *Phantom of the night: overcome sleep apnea and snoring,* Cambridge, Mass, 1994, New Technology.

Noureddine SN: Sleep apnea: a challenge in critical care, *Heart Lung* 25(1):37-42, 1996.

Saunders NA, Saunders CE: Sleep and breathing, *Lung biology in health and disease,* ed 2, New York, 1993, Marcel Dekker.

Strollo PJ, Rogers RM: Obstructive sleep apnea, *N Engl J Med* 334(2):99-104, 1996.

Young T et al: The occurrence of sleep-disordered breathing among middle-aged adults, *N Engl J Med* 328(17):1230-1235, 1993.

### Narcolepsy

Aldrich MS: Sleep-related spells associated with parasomnias and narcolepsy, *Semin Neurol* 15(2):194-202, 1995.

Rogers AE, Aldrich MS: The effect of regularly scheduled naps on sleep attacks and excessive daytime sleepiness associated with narcolepsy, *Nurs Res* 42(2):111-117, 1993.

### Sleep in the Elderly

Bliwise DL: Sleep in normal aging and dementia, *Sleep* 16(1):40-81, 1993.

Foreman MD, Wykle M: Nursing standard of care protocol: sleep disturbance in the elderly, *Geriatr Nurs* 16(5):238-243, 1995.

Gall K et al: Night life: nocturnal behavior patterns among hospitalized elderly, *J Gerontol Nurs* 16(10):31-37, 1990.

### Sleep and Shift Work

Alward RR, Monk TH: A 'round the clock profession: coping with the effects of shift work, *Am Nurse* 27(5):18-19, 1995.

Chadwick DJ, Ackrill K, editors: *Circadian clocks and their adjustment,* New York, 1995, Wiley & Sons.

Deacon S, Arendt J: Adapting to phase shifts, *Physiol Behav* 59(4-5):665-673, 1995.

Eastman C et al: Light treatment for sleep disorders: consensus report VI, shift work, *J Biol Rhythms* 10(2):157-164, 1995.

Wetterberg L: Light and biological rhythms, *J Intern Med* 235(1):5-19, 1994.

## Chapter 14 Substance Abuse

### General

Abadinsky H: *Drug abuse: an introduction,* Chicago, 1993, Nelson-Hall.

American Medical Association: AMA reports hidden epidemic of elderly alcoholism, *Am Med News* 38(7):11, 1995.

Brust JC: *Neurological aspects of substance abuse,* Boston, 1993, Butterworth-Heinemann.

Burns E et al: *An addictions curriculum for nurses and other helping professionals. Level A: basic knowledge and practice.* Columbus, 1991, The Ohio State University College of Nursing.

Burns E et al: *An addictions curriculum for nurses and other helping professionals. Level B: advanced knowledge and practice,* Columbus, 1991, The Ohio State University College of Nursing.

Carr LA: The pharmacology of mood-altering drugs of abuse, *Primary Care Clinicians Office Pract* 20(1):51-70, 1993.

Centers for Disease Control and Prevention: Update: alcohol-related traffic crashes and fatalities among youth, United States, 1982-94, *JAMA* 274:1904-1905, 1995.

Cohen JB: Smokers' knowledge and understanding of advertised tar numbers: health policy implications, *Am J Public Health* 86:18-24, 1996.

Corrigan JD, Rust E, Lamb-Hart GL: The nature and extent of substance abuse problems in persons with traumatic brain injury, *J Head Trauma Rehabil* 10(3):29-46, 1995.

Day M: Agony and ecstasy. . . . substance abuse is not going to go away: and nurses will have to deal with it, *Nurs Times* 91(44):102, 1995.

Galanter M, Kleber HD: *Textbook of substance abuse treatment,* Washington, DC, 1994, American Psychiatric Press.

Gigliotti E, Naegle MA, D'Arcangelo JS: Fetal effects of maternal alcohol and drug use. In Naegle MA, editor: *Substance abuse education in nursing,* New York, 1992, National League for Nursing.

Hartwell TD et al: Aiding troubled employees: the prevalence, cost, and characteristics of employee assistance programs in the United States, *Am J Public Health* 86:804-8, 1996.

*Mosby's medical, nursing, and allied health dictionary,* ed 4, St Louis, 1994, Mosby.

Naegle MA: *Substance abuse education in nursing,* vol 2, New York, 1992, National League for Nursing.

Naegle MA: The need for alcohol abuse-related education in nursing curricula, *Alc Health Res World* 18(2):154, 1994.

Pierce JP, Gilpin E: How long will today's new adolescent be addicted to cigarettes? *Am J Public Health* 86(2):253-256, 1996.

Riley JA: Dual diagnosis: commodal substance abuse or dependency and mental illness, *Nurs Clin North Am* 29(1):29-34, 1994.

Schonberg KS, editor: *Substance abuse: a guide for health professionals,* Elk Grove, Ill, 1996, American Academy of Pediatrics.

Sullivan EJ: *Nursing care of clients with substance abuse,* St Louis, 1995, Mosby.

Turnball JM, Roszell DK: Dual diagnosis, *Primary Care Clin Office Pract* 20(1):181-190, 1993.

Wilson MD, Joffe A: Adolescent medicine, *JAMA* 273:1657-1660, 1995.

### Prevention

Carnegie Corporation: Making America drug free: a new vision of what works, *Carnegie Q* 37(3):1-7, 1992.

Perry CL et al: Project Northland: outcomes of a communitywide alcohol use prevention program during early adolescence, *Am J Public Health* 86(6): 956-965, 1996.

### Alcoholism

Buchsbaum DG: Quick, effective screening for alcohol abuse, *Patient Care* 29:56-62, 1995.

Chiang PP: Perioperative management of the alcohol-dependent patient, *Am Fam Physician* 52:2267-2274, 1995.

Flandermeyer A et al: Nursing care of women who abuse alcohol, *MedSurg Nurs Q* 1(1):122-139, 1992.

Hyman SE: A man with alcoholism and HIV infection, *JAMA* 274(10):837-843, 1995.

Mirand AL, Welte JW: Alcohol consumption among the elderly in a general population, *Am J Public Health* 86:978-984, 1996.

National Highway Traffic Safety Administration: The cost of alcohol related traffic crash injuries, Washington DC, 1994, The Administration.

Sobell LC, Cunningham JA, Sobell MA: Recovery from alcohol problems with and without treatment: prevalence in two population surveys, *Am J Public Health* 86:966-792, 1996.

Tweed SH, Ryff CD: Family climate and parent-child relationships: recollections from a nonclinical sample of adult children of alcoholic fathers, *Res Nurs Health* 19:311-321, 1996.

Urbano-Marquez A et al: The greater risk of alcoholic cardiomyopathy in women compared with men, *JAMA* 274:149-155, 1995.

WHO Brief Intervention Study Group: A cross-national trial of brief interventions with heavy drinkers, *Am J Public Health* 86(6):948-955, 1996.

### Substance Abuse

Bell K: Identifying the substance abuser in clinical practice, *Orthop Nurs* 11(2):29, 1992.

Chen K, Kandal DB: The natural history of drug use from adolescence to the mid-thirties in a general population sample, *Am J Public Health* 85(1):41-47, 1995.

Cummings KH et al: Trends in smoking initiation among adolescents and young adults, *MMWR* 44(28):521-525, 1996.

Dubiel S: Action stat! Cocaine overdose, *Nursing '90* 20(3):33, 1990.

McCusker J et al: The effectiveness of alternative planned durations of residential drug abuse treatment, *Am J Public Health* 85(10):1426-1429, 1995.

Paul S, York D: Cocaine abuse: an expanding healthcare problem for the 1990s, *Am J Crit Care* 1(1):109-113, 1992.

Ross TM: Gammahydroxybutyrate overdose: two cases illustrate the unique aspects of this dangerous recreational drug, *J Emerg Nurs* 21(5):374-376, 1995.

Wadler GI: Drug use update, *Med Clin North Am* 78(2):439-455, 1995.

### Codependency

Cullen A: Burnout: why do we blame the nurse, *Am J Nurs* 95(11):23-27, 1995.

Herrick C: Codependency characteristics: risks, progression, and strategies for healing, *Nurs Forum* 27(3):12-19, 1992.

Klebanoff N: *Caring and nursing: exploration in feminist perspectives. Codependency: caring or suicide for nurses and nursing,* NLN Pub No 14-2369, 1991.

### Impaired Nurse

Bugle L: A study of drug and alcohol use among Missouri RNs, *J Psychosoc Nurs* 34(7):41-44, 1996.

Committee on Chemical Dependency Issues: *Model guidelines: a nondisciplinary alternative program for chemically impaired nurses,* Chicago, Ill, 1994, Council of State Boards of Nursing.

Green P: The chemically dependent nurse, *Nurs Clin North Am* 24(1):81-94, 1989.

Hughes TL: Chief nurse executives' responses to chemically dependent nurses, *Nurs Manage* 26(3):37-40, 1995.

Lippman H: Addicted nurses: tolerated, tormented, or treated? *RN* 55(4):36, 1992.

Miller H: Addiction in a coworker: getting past the denial, *Am J Nurs* 90(5):72, 1990.

## Chapter 15 Fluid and Electrolyte Imbalance

### Maintenance of Fluid and Electrolyte Imbalance

Metheny NM: *Fluid and electrolyte balance nursing considerations,* ed 3, Philadelphia, 1996, Lippincott.

McDougal JE: Bringing electrolytes to life: an imagery game, *Nurse Educator* 17(6):8-10, 1992.

Terry J: The major electrolytes: sodium, potassium, and chloride, *J Intrav Nurs* 17(5):240-247, 1995.

### Fluid Imbalance

Convertino VA et al: American College of Sports Medicine position standards: exercise and fluid replacement, *Med Sci Sports Exerc* 28(1):1-vii, 1996.

Cosgray R, Davidhizar R, Giger JN, Kreisal R: A program for water-intoxicated patients at a state hospital, *Clin Nurse Specialist* 7(2):55-61, 1993.

Sims J: Making sense of tonicity and IV therapy, *Nurs Times* 92:42-43, 1996.

### Electrolyte Imbalance

Maughan RJ, Leiper JB, Shirreffs SM: Factors influencing the restoration of fluid and electrolyte balance after exercising in the heat, *Br J Sports Med* 31(3):175-182, 1997.

Rose BD: *Clinical physiology of acid-base and electrolyte disorders,* ed 4, New York, 1994, McGraw-Hill.

## Chapter 16 Acid-Base Imbalance

### General

Burrell LO, Gerlach MJ, Pless BS: *Foundations of contemporary nursing practice,* ed 2, Stamford, Conn, 1997, Appleton & Lange.

Chulay M, Guzzetta C, Dossey B: *AACN handbook of critical care nursing,* Stamford, Conn, 1997, Appleton & Lange.

Kidd PS, Wagner KD: *High acuity nursing,* ed 2, Stamford, Conn, 1997, Appleton & Lange.

## Chapter 17 Shock

### General

Abello PA, Buchman TG, Bukley GB: Shock and multiple organ failure. In Armstrong P, editor: *Free radicals in diagnostic medicine,* New York, 1994, Plenum Press.

Marino PA: *The ICU book,* Philadelphia, 1991, Lea & Febiger.

Rice V: Shock, a clinical syndrome: an update. Part 3: therapeutic management, *Crit Care Nurse* 11(6):34-39, 1991.

### Etiology

Hazinski MF: Mediator-specific therapies for the systemic inflammatory response syndrome, sepsis, severe sepsis and septic shock: present and future approaches, *Crit Care Nurs Clin North Am* 6(2):309-319, 1994.

Shelton BK: Disorders of homeostasis in sepsis, *Crit Care Nurs Clin North Am* 6(2):373-388, 1994.

West MA, Wilson W: Hypoxia alterations in cellular signal transduction in shock and sepsis, *New Horz* 4(2):168-178, 1996

### Physiology

Higgins TL, Chernow B: Receptor physiology and pharmacology in circulatory shock. In Silvak E et al, editors: *The high risk patient: management of the critically ill,* Baltimore, 1995, William & Wilkins.

Shoemaker WC et al: Hemodynamic and oxygen transport monitoring to titrate therapy in shock, *Crit Care Med New Horz* 1(1):145-157, 1993.

Suhl J: Patients with septic shock. In Clochsey J et al, editors: *Critical Care Nursing,* Philadelphia, 1993, WB Saunders.

Tortora JG, Grabowski SR: The cardiovascular system: blood vessels and hemodynamics. In Tortora JG, Grabowski SR, editors: *Principals of anatomy and physiology,* New York, 1993, Harper Collins College Press.

### Pathophysiology

Crowley SR: The pathogenesis of septic shock, *Heart Lung* 25(2):124-134, 1996.

Hinshaw LB: Sepsis/septic shock: participation of the microcirculation, *Crit Care Med* 24(6):1072-1078, 1996.

Huston MC: Pathophysiology of shock, *Crit Care Clin North Am* 2(2):143-149, 1990.

Littleton MT: Prostaglandin's and leukotrienes as mediators of shock and trauma, *Crit Care Nurs Q* 11(2):11-20, 1988.

Shoemaker WC: Pathophysiology, monitoring and therapy of acute circulatory problems, *Crit Care Nurs North Am* 6(2):295-307, 1994.

Vollman KM: Adult respiratory distress syndrome: mediators on the run, *Crit Care Nurs Clin North Am* 6(2):341-358, 1994.

### Clinical Manifestations

Alverdy JC, Levine ES: Principles of blood replacement. In Sivak DE et al, editors: *The high risk patient: management of the critically ill,* Baltimore, 1995, Williams & Wilkins.

Baron BJ, Scalea TM: Acute blood loss, *Emerg Med Clin North Am* 14(1):35-55, 1996.

Rady MY: Triage of critically ill patients, *Emerg Med Clin North Am* 14(1):13-33, 1996.

Ramamoorthy S: Current understanding and treatment of sepsis, *Infect Med* 12(6):261-268, 274 1995.

Rogers GR: Cardiovascular shock, *Med Clin North Am* 13(4):794-809, 1995.

Von Ruden KT: Sequelae of massive fluid resuscitation in trauma patients, *Crit Care Nurs Clin North Am* 6(3) 463-472, 1994.

### Nursing Management

Mancinelli-Van Atta J, Beck SL: Preventing hypoxemia and hemodynamic compromise related to endotracheal suctioning, *Am J Crit Care* 1(3):62-79, 1996.

Phipps WJ: The patient with pulmonary problems. In Long BC, Phipps WJ, Cassmeyer VL, editors: *Medical surgical nursing: a nursing approach,* ed 3, St Louis, 1993, Mosby.

Rice V: Shock, a clinical syndrome: an update. Part 4: nursing care of the shock patient, *Crit Care Nurse* 11(7):28-32, 35-40, 42-43, 1991.

Shoemaker WC: Pathophysiology, monitoring and therapy of acute circulatory problems: the expanded role of the physiologically oriented critical care nurse, *Am J Crit Care* 1(1):38-53, 1992.

Wiessner WH et al: Treatment of sepsis and septic shock, *Heart Lung* 24(5):380-392, 1995.

Wilson EW et al: Effects of backrest position on hemodynamic and right ventricular measurements in critically ill adults, *Am J Crit Care* 5(4):264-270, 1996.

Yared JP: Pitfalls in hemodynamic and respiratory monitoring. In Sivak DE et al, editors: *The high risk patient: management of the critically ill,* Baltimore, 1995, Williams & Wilkins.

### Planning

Ackerman MH: The systematic inflammatory response, sepsis and multiple organ dysfunction: new definitions for an old problem, *Crit Care Nurs Clin North Am* (2):243-250, 1994.

American Society of Anesthesiologists, Inc: Practice guidelines for blood component therapy: a report by the American Society of Anesthesiologist Task Force on blood component therapy, *Anesthesiology,* 84:732-747, 1996.

American Society of Anesthelogists, Inc: Practice guidelines for pulmonary artery catheterization: a report by the American Society of Anesthesiologists Task Force on pulmonary artery catheterization, *Anesthesiology* 78:380-394, 1993.

Barone JE: Treatment strategies in shock: use of oxygen transport measurements, *Heart Lung* 20(1):81-86, 1991.

Bone RC: A critical evaluation of new agents for treatment of sepsis, *JAMA* 266(12):168-1691, 1991.

Cadwell AC: Intra-aortic balloon counterpulsation timing, *Am J Crit Care* 5(4):254-261, 1996.

Calandra T et al: Treatment of gram-negative septic shock with human IgG antibody to *Escherichia coli* j5: a prospective double blind, randomized trial, *J Infect Dis* 158(2):312-319, 1988.

Cone A: The use of colloids in clinical practice, *Br J Hosp Med* S4(4):156-159, 1995.

Cronin L et al: Corticosteroids treatment for sepsis: a critical appraisal and meta-analysis of the literature, *Crit Care Med* 23(8):1430-1439, 1995.

Gannon DM et al: An evaluation of the efficacy of postoperative blood salvage after total joint arthroplasty, *J Arthroplasty* 1(2):109-114, 1991.

Gorelick K et al: Randomized placebo-controlled study of *E5 monoclonal* antitoxin antibody. In Larrick J, Borrebaeck C, editors: *Therapeutic monoclonal antibodies,* New York, 1990, Stockton Press.

Krausz MM: Controversies in shock research: hypertonic resuscitation: pros and cons, *Shock* 3(1):69-72, 1995.

Lefering R, Neugebauer EAM: Steroid controversy in sepsis and septic shock: a meta-analysis, *Crit Care Med* 23(7):1294-1303, 1995.

McCarthy S et al: Cytokine production and its manipulation by vasoactive drugs, *New Horz* 4(2):252-264, 1966.

McSwain NE: Pneumatic anti-shock garment: state of the art 1988, *Ann Emerg Med* 17(5):506-526, 1988.

Overlie PA: Emergency cardiopulmonary support with circulatory support devises, *Cardiology* 84:231-237, 1994.

Owings JT, Holcraft JW: Fluid resuscitation of the critically ill patient. In Sivak DE et al, editors: *The high risk patient: management of the critically ill,* Baltimore, 1995, Williams & Wilkins.

Shoemaker WC et al: Resuscitation from severe hemorrhage, *Crit Care Med* 24(2):S12-S23, 1966.

Wampler RK, Baker BA, Wright WM: Circulatory support of cardiac interventional procedures with the Hemopump(TM) Cardiac Assist Systems, *Cardiology* 84:194-201, 1994.

## Chapter 18 Preoperative Nursing

### Surgical Procedures

DeFazio-Quinn DM: Ambulatory surgery: an evolution, *Nurs Clin North Am* 32(2):377-386, 1997.

Moran S, Kent G: Quality indicators for patient information in short-stay units, *Nurs Times* 91(4):37-40, 1995.

### Informed Consent

Brazell NE: The significance and application of informed consent, *AORN J* 65(2):377-386, 1997.

Brick J: Informed consent and perioperative nursing, *AORN J* 63(1):258-261, 1996.

Chiarella M: The consent form: perils and possibilities, *ACORN J* 8(4):21-22, 1995.

Chiarella M: The consent form: perils and possibilities. Part 2, *ACORN J* 9(1):29-30, 1996.

Erlen JA: When the patient lacks decision-making capacity, *Orthop Nurs* 14(4):51-54, 1995.

Golanowski M: Do not resuscitate: informed consent in the operating room and postanesthesia care unit, *J Post Anesth Nurs* 10(1):9-11, 1995.

Pape T: Legal and ethical considerations of informed consent, *AORN J* 65(6): 1122-1127, 1997.

### Assessment

Lancaster KA: Patient teaching in ambulatory surgery, *Nurs Clin North Am* 32(2):417-427, 1997.

Litwack K: Care of the special needs patient, *Nurs Clin North Am* 32(2):457-467, 1997.

William GD: Preoperative assessment and health history interview, *Nurs Clin North Am* 32(2):395-415, 1997.

### Nursing Interventions

Burden N: Patient and family education in the ambulatory surgery setting, *Semin Perioperative Nurs* 3(3):145-152, 1994.

Edmondson M: Day surgery: handling patients' complaints, *Nurs Standard* 9(47):25-28, 1995.

Estey A, Kemp M, Allison S, Lamb C: Evaluation of a patient information booklet, *J Nurs Staff Dev* 9(6):278-282, 1993.

Hunt AH: Humor as a nursing intervention, *Cancer Nurs* 16(1):34-39, 1993.

Jones LA: Patient information issues in the ambulatory surgery setting, *Today's OR Nurse* 9-12, March/April 1995.

Maksud DP, Anderson RC: Psychological dimensions of aesthetic surgery: essentials for nurses, *Plast Surg Nurs* 15(3):137-178, 1995.

Meeker BJ: Preoperative patient education: evaluating postoperative patient outcomes, *Patient Educ Counsel* 23:41-47, 1994.

Mick DJ: The patient on display, *Crit Care Nurse* 16(2):148, 1996.

Newton V: Care in pre-admission clinics, *Nurs Times* 92(1):27-28, 1996.

Oetker-Black SL, Kauth C: Evaluating a revised self-efficacy scale for preoperative patients, *AORN J* 62(2):244-250, 1995.

Recker D: Patient perception of preoperative cardiac surgical teaching done pre- and postadmission, *Crit Care Nurse* 14(1):52-58, 1994.

Tusek D, Church JM, Fazio VW: Guided imagery as a coping strategy for perioperative patients, *AORN J* 66(4):644-649, 1997.

Winter MJ, Paskin S, Baker T: Music reduces stress and anxiety of patients in the surgical holding area, *J Post Anesth Nurs* 9(6):340-343, 1994.

Wolford ET: Timing of perioperative antibiotic administration, *AORN J* 65(1):109-115, 1997.

## Chapter 19 Intraoperative Nursing

### General

Dougherty J: Same-day surgery: the nurse's role, *Orthop Nurs* 15(4):15-18, 1996.

Hankela S, Kiikkala I: Intraoperative nursing care as experienced by surgical patients, *AORN J* 63(2):435-442, 1996.

### Intraoperative Patient Care Team

Hylka SC, Beschle JC: The role of advanced practice nurses in surgical services, *AORN J* 66(3):481-485, 1997.

### The Surgical Environment

AORN recommended practices for use and selection of barrier materials for surgical gowns and drapes, *AORN J* 63(3):650-654, 1996.

Kurz A, Sessler DI, Lenhardt R: Perioperative normothermia to reduce the incidence of surgical-wound Infection and shorten hospitalization, *N Engl J Med* 334(19):1209-1215, 1996.

Wheelock SM, Lookkinland S: Effect of surgical hand scrub time on subsequent bacterial growth, *AORN J* 65(6):1087-1097, 1997.

### Anesthesia

Kurpiers E, Scharine J, Lovell SL: Cost-effective anesthesia: desflurane versus propofol in outpatient surgery, *J Am Assoc Nurses Anesth* 64(1):69-75, 1996.

Haines MM: AANA journal course: update for nurse anesthetist—pulmonary aspiration revisited. Changing attitudes toward preoperative fasting, *J Am Assoc Nurse Anesth* 63(5):389-396, 1995.

McLaughlin ME: The intraoperative administration of ketorolac tromethamine in evaluating length of stay in a same day surgery unit, *J Am Assoc Nurse Anesth* 62(5):433-436, 1994.

Stein RH: The perioperative nurse's role in anesthesia management, *AORN J* 63(5):794-801, 1995.

### Malignant Hyperthermia

Beck CF: Malignant hyperthermia: are you prepared? *AORN J* 59(2):367-378, 1994.

Dunn D: Malignant hyperthermia, *AORN J* 65(4):728-754, 1997.

Golinski M: Malignant hyperthermia: a review, *Plast Surg Nurs* 15(1):30-33, 1995.

### Nursing Management

Leske JS: Anxiety of elective surgical patients' family members, *AORN J* 57(5): 1091-1101, 1993.

Leske JS: Intraoperative progress reports decrease family members' anxiety, *AORN J* 64(3):424-436, 1996.

## Chapter 20
## Postoperative Nursing

### General

Ledwith SP: Therapeutic touch and mastectomy: a case study, *RN* 51-53, July 1995.

### Special Care Considerations

Badgwell MJ: The postanesthesia care unit: a high-risk environment for bloodborne and infectious respiratory pathogens, *J Post Anesth Nurs* 11(2): 66-70, 1996.

Brooks-Brunn JA: Protecting the lungs, *Reflections,* 1st quarter 1997.

Dennison RD: Nurse's guide to common postoperative complications, *Nursing '97* 56-59, November 1997.

Einhorn GW, Chang P: Postanesthesia care unit dilemmas: prompt assessment and treatment, *J Post Anesth Nurs* 9(1):28-33, 1994.

Krenzischek DA, Frank SM, Kelly S: Forced-air warming versus routine thermal care and core temperature measurement sites, *J Post Anesth Nurs* 10(2):69-77, 1995.

Sanford MM: Rewarming cardiac surgical patients: warm water versus warm air, *Am J Crit Care* 6(1):39, 1997.

Wall MP: Postoperative respiratory complications, *Perspect Respir Nurs* 6(4): 1-4, 1995.

### Gerontological Considerations

Demaagd G: High-risk drugs in the elderly population, *Geriatr Nurs* 16:198-207, 1995.

### Nursing Management

Atsberger DB: Relaxation therapy: its potential as an intervention for acute postoperative pain, *J Post Anesth Nurs* 10(1):2-8, 1995.

Beck VP: On the lookout for impaired wound healing, *Nursing '98* 28(1):32hn1-32hn4, 1998.

Hiser RM, Chiles K, Fudge M, Gray SE: The use of music during the immediate postoperative recovery period, *AORN J* 65(4):777-785, 1997.

Marley RA, Moline BM: Patient discharge from the ambulatory setting, *J Post Anesth Nurs* 11(1):39-49, 1996.

Morris J: Monitoring post-operative effects in day-surgery patients, *Nurs Times* 91(10):32-34, 1995.

Strimike CL, Wojcik JM, Stark BA: Incision care that really cuts it, *RN* 60(7): 22-26, 1997.

## Chapter 21
## Emergency Care Environment

### General

Cole F, Ramirez E: The emergency nurse practitioner: an educational model, *J Emerg Nurs* 23(2):112-115, 1997.

Gordon S: The tapestry of care, *J Emerg Nurs* 23(2):148-152, 1997.

Harvey C, Dixon M, Padberg N: Support group for families of trauma patients: a unique approach, *Crit Care Nurse* 15(4):59-63, 1995.

Mayer T, Cates R, Royalty D: Customer service and triage, *Top Emerg Med* 19(2):28-39, 1997.

Rhee K, Bird J: Perceptions and satisfaction with emergency department care, *J Emerg Med* 14(6):679-683, 1996.

Sheehy S: *Emergency nursing principles and practice,* ed 3, St Louis, 1992, Mosby.

Wolcott B, Bell W: Demand management: the future of triage in emergency medicine, *Top Emerg Med* 19(2):64-62, 1997.

Zimmerman P: Delegating to assistive personnel, *J Emerg Nurs* 22(3):206-212, 1996.

## Chapter 22
## Critical Care Environment

### General

Atkinson B: The current state of critical care, *Intens Care Nurs* 7(2):73-79, 1991.

Baker C: Discomfort to environment noise: heart rate responses of sick patients, *Crit Care Nurs Q* 15(2):75-90, 1992.

Carnevale F: High technology and humanity in intensive care: finding a balance, *Intens Care Nurse* 7(1):23-27, 1991.

Chesla CA, Stannard D: Breakdown in the nursing care of families in the ICU, *Am J Crit Care* 6(1):64-71, 1997.

Henneman B: Building the model ICU, *Crit Care Nurs Q* 12(8):112-114, 1992.

Hickey MI, Leske JS: Needs of families of critically ill patients: state of the science and future directions, *Crit Care Clin North Am* 4(4):645-649, 1992.

Lazure LLA, Baun MM: Increasing patient control of family visiting in the coronary care unit, *Am J Crit Care* 4(3):157-164, 1995.

Lewis DJ, Robinson JA: ICU nurses coping measures and response to work related stressors, *Crit Care Nurse* 12(2):18-26, 1992.

McConnell EA: Medical devices and medical futility: when is enough enough? *Nursing* 27(8):32hn1-32hn4, 1997.

Porte-Gendron RW et al: Baccalaureate nurse educators' and critical care nurse managers' perceptions of clinical competencies necessary for new graduate baccalaureate critical care nurses, *Am J Crit Care* 6(2):147-158, 1997.

## Chapter 23
## Home Care Environment

### Trends and Issues in Home Care

Allen SA: Medicare case management, *Home Healthc Nurse* 12(3):21-27, 1994.

Brent N: Healthcare reform: implications for home health care nursing and agencies, *Home Healthc Nurse* 12(1):10-11, 1994.

Dee-Kelly PA, Heller S, Sibley M: Managed care: an opportunity for home care agencies, *Nurs Clin North Am* 29(3):471-481, 1994.

Grossman D: Cultural dimensions in home health nursing, *Am J Nurs* 96(7):33-36, 1996.

Knollmueller R: The role of prevention in home health care nursing practice, *Home Healthc Nurse* 11(1):21-23, 1993.

Martin KS: Past, present, and future, *Home Health Focus* 1(12):1-2, 1995.

Smith CE et al: Financial and technological costs of high technology home care, *Nurs Econ* 10(5):369-373, 1992.

Stulginsky MM: Nurses' home health experience. Part I: the practice setting, *Nurs Health Care* 14(8):402-407, 1993.

Stulginsky MM: Nurses' home health experience. Part II: the unique demands of home visits, *Nurs Health Care* 14(9):476-485, 1993.

Zang SA, Bailey NC: *Home care manual: making the transition,* Philadelphia, 1997, JB Lippincott.

### Discharge Planning

Hester LE: Coordinating a successful discharge plan, *Am J Nurs* 96(6):35-37, 1996.

Zarle ND: Continuity of care: balancing care of elders between health care settings, *Nurs Clin North Am* 24:697-706, 1989.

### Patient Teaching

Carr P: Needs to know, wants to know, ought to know, *Home Healthc Nurse* 8(4):34-36, 1990.

Chachkes E, Christ G: Cross cultural issues in patient education, *Patient Educ Couns* 27:13-21, 1996.

Chang BL, Hirsch M: Video intervention: producing videotapes for use in nursing practice and education, *J Contin Educ Nurs* 25(6):263-267, 1994.

Dollahite J, Thompson C, McNew R: Readability of printed sources of diet and health information, *Patient Educ Couns* 27:123-134, 1996.

Grieco AJ: The importance of the family in patient education and care, *Patient Educ Couns* 27:1-3, 1996 (editorial).

Hellwig K: Health teaching: the crux of home care nursing, *Home Healthc Nurse* 8(4):35-37, 1990.

Matthis E: Family caregivers want education for their caregiving roles, *Home Health Care* 10(4):19-22, 1991.

Mayo AM: Teaching family/significant other nursing, *J Contin Educ Nurs* 24(1):7-31, 1993.

Rakel BA: Intervention related to patient teaching, *Nurs Clin North Am* 27(2):397-405, 1992.

Redman BK: Patient education at 25 years: where we have been and where we are going, *J Adv Nurs* 18:725-730, 1993.

Rohret L, Ferguson KJ: Effective use of patient education illustrations, *Patient Educ Couns* 1:73-75, 1990.

### Documentation

Anderson K: Deceptive documentation in home healthcare nursing, *Home Healthc Nurse* 10(6):31-35, 1992.

Ellenbecker CA, Shea K: Documenting in home health care practice: evidence of quality care, *Nurs Clin North Am* 29(3):495-506, 1994.

Magliozzi H: Home care: charting that makes it through the Medicare maze, *RN* 53(6):75-77, 1990.

## Chapter 24 Assessment of the Cardiovascular System

### General

Barbiere CC: A new device for control of bleeding after transfemoral catheterization, *Crit Care Nurse* 15(5):51-53, 1995.

Bean LC: Cardiac imaging after acute myocardial infarction: identification of patients at continual risk, *Postgrad Med* 92(8):93-100, 1992.

Beattie S et al: The use of cardiac catheterization data to design nursing care plans, *Crit Care Nurse* 10(6):43-51, 1990.

Beattie S, Meinhardt L: Transesophageal echocardiograph: advanced technology for the cardiac patient, *Crit Care Nurse* 12(3):42-48, 1992.

Darovic GO: *Hemodynamic monitoring: invasive and noninvasive clinical applications,* ed 2, Philadelphia, 1993, WB Saunders.

Feinstein SB: Myocardial perfusion: contrast echocardiography perspectives, *Am J Cardiol* 69(20):36H-41H, 1992.

Frizzel J: Transesophageal echocardiography, *Am J Nurs* 97(9):17-18, 1997.

Jain DJ, Zaret BL: Assessment of right ventricular function: role of nuclear imaging techniques, *Cardiol Clin* 10(1):23-39, 1992.

Jarvis C: *Physical examination and health assessment,* ed 2, Philadelphia, 1996, WB Saunders.

Perez A: Cardiac monitoring—mastering the essentials, *RN* 59(8):32-38, 1996.

Tilkien A, Conover M: *Understanding heart sounds and murmurs,* ed 3, Philadelphia, 1993, WB Saunders.

Veram MS: Thallium-201 single photon emission computed tomography (SPECT) in the assessment of coronary artery disease, *Am J Cardiol* 70(14):3E-9E, 1992.

Verdeber A et al: Preparation for cardiac catheterization, *J Cardiovasc Nurs* 7(1):75-77, 1992.

US Public Health Service: Put prevention into practice: blood pressure, *J Am Acad Nurse Pract* 9(1):27-32, 1997.

## Chapter 25 Management of Persons with Coronary Artery Disease and Dysrhythmias

### Coronary Artery Disease

Albert NM: High risk unstable angina: keeping pace with current research findings, *AACN Clin Iss* 6(1):110-120, 1995.

Arubi-Norris N: Sexual concerns after an MI, *Am J Nurs* 97(8):48-49, 1997.

Arnold SE: What you should know about cardiac stress testing: your patient has questions—here's how to answer them, *Nursing* 27(1):58-61, 1997.

Brown C et al: Pearls for practice—coronary restenosis, *J Am Acad Nurse Pract* 8(6):283-287, 1996.

Ellerbeck EF et al: Quality of care for Medicare patients with acute myocardial infarction, *JAMA* 273(19):1509-1543, 1995.

Fair JM, Berra K: Life-style changes and coronary heart disease: the influence of nonpharmacologic interventions, *J Cardiovasc Nurs* 9(2):12-24, 1995.

Franklin BA: Diagnostic and functional exercise testing: test selection and interpretation, *J Cardiovasc Nurs* 10(1):8-29, 1995.

Futterman LG, Lemberg L: Endothelium: the key to medical management of coronary artery disease, *Am J Crit Care* 6(2):159-167, 1997.

Gillum RF: The epidemiology of cardiovascular disease in black Americans, *N Engl J Med* 335(21):1597-1599, 1996 (editorial).

Grodstein F et al: Postmenopausal estrogen and progestin use and the risk of cardiovascular disease, *N Engl J Med* 335(7):453-461, 1996.

Gulanick M et al: Patients' responses to the angioplasty experience—a qualitative study, *Am J Crit Care* 6(1):24-30, 1997.

Hayes DD: Understanding coronary atherectomy, *Am J Nurs* 96(12):38-45, 1996.

Ide B: Bedside electrocardiographic assessment, *J Cardiovasc Nurs* 9(4):10-23, 1995.

Juran NB et al: Survey of current practice patterns for percutaneous transluminal coronary angioplasty, *Am J Crit Care* 5(6):442-448, 1996.

Kendler BS: Recent nutritional approaches to the prevention and therapy of cardiovascular disease, *Progr Cardiovasc Nurs* 12(3):3-23, 1997.

Mangan B: Structuring cardiology services for the 21st century, *Am J Crit Care* 5(6):406-411, 1996.

Miller LA et al: Care of the elective intracoronary stent patient, *Crit Care Nurs Q* 18(4):77-91, 1996.

Montes P: Managing outpatient cardiac catheterization, *Am J Nurs* 97(8):34-37, 1997.

Mueller IW: Common questions about sex and sexuality in elders, *Am J Nurs* 97(7):61-64, 1997.

O'Donnell L: Complications of MI—beyond the acute stage, *Am J Nurs* 96(9):25-31, 1996.

Scherck KA: Recognizing a heart attack: the process of determining illness, *Am J Crit Care* 6(4):267-273, 1997.

Schickel S et al: Removal of femoral sheaths by registered nurses: issues and outcomes, *Crit Care Nurse* 16(2):32-36, 1996.

Thompson EJ, Nelson CM: Dobutamine stress echocardiography: a new, non-invasive method for detecting ischemic heart disease, *Heart Lung* 25(2):87-97, 1996.

Turner DM: Right ventricular myocardial infarction: detection, treatment, and nursing implications, *Crit Care Nurse* 15(1):22-27, 1995.

Tyler DO: Activity progression in acute cardiac patients, *J Cardiovasc Nurs* 12(1):16-32, 1997.

Warner CD: Triaging and interpreting chest pain, *J Cardiovasc Nurs* 12(1):84-92, 1997.

Wood AJJ: Adjunctive drug therapy of acute myocardial infarction—evidence from clinical trials, *N Engl J Med* 335(22):1660-1667, 1996.

Zell KA: Syndrome X: a discussion of angina and normal coronary arteries, *Am J Crit Care* 5(2):99-101, 1996.

### Dysrhythmias

Banerji S, Kayser SR: Pharmacology news—antiarrhythmic drug therapy. Part IV: ventricular arrhythmias, *Progr Cardiovasc Nurs* 12(3):32-36, 1997.

Dunbar SB, Summerville JG: Cognitive therapy for ventricular dysrhythmia patients, *J Cardiovasc Nurs* 12(1):33-44, 1997.

Futterman LG, Lemberg L: Amiodarone: a late comer, *Am J Crit Care* 6(3):232-239, 1997.

Ghosh RJ: Clinical notebook: introducing the cardiac rhythm interpretation tree, *J Emerg Nurs* 21(3):226-227, 1995.

Hayes D: Bradycardia—keeping the current flowing, *Nursing* 27(6):50-55, 1997.

Karnes N: Critical care educator: adenosine—a quick fix for PSVT, *Nursing* 25(7):55-56, 1995.

Kusumoto FM, Goldschlager N: Medical progress—review articles, *Cardiac Pacing* 334(2):89-98, 1996.

Lenhart RC: Pacemaker assessment and care plans in long-term care, *Geriatr Nurs* 16(6):276-280, 1995.

Lewandowski D, Jacobson C: AV blocks: are you up to date? *Am J Nurs* 95(12):27-33, 1995.

Perez A: Cardiac monitoring—mastering the essentials, *RN* 59(8):32-38, 1996.

Ruffy R: The automatic implantable defibrillator: it can be done, but should it? *J Cardiovasc Electrophysiol* 6(8):649-651, 1995.

Sauve MJ: Long-term physical functioning and psychosocial adjustment in survivors of sudden cardiac death, *Heart Lung* 24(2):133-144, 1995.

Scrima DA: Clinical care—foundations of arrhythmia interpretation, *MedSurg Nurs* 6(4):193-202, 1997.

Severson A, Baldwin L, DeLoughery TG: International normalized ratio in anticoagulant therapy: understanding the issues, *Am J Crit Care* 6(2):88-92, 1997.

Snowberger P: Arrhythmia review—torsades de pointes, *RN* 58(8):34-35, 1995.

Sopher SM, Camm JA: Atrial fibrillation: maintenance of sinus rhythm versus rate control, *Am J Cardiol* 77:24A-37A, 1996.

Stahl L: How to manage common arrhythmias in medical patients, *Am J Nurs* 95(3):36-41, 1995.

Symanski BJ, Marriott HJL: Ventricular tachycardia, diagnosis and misdiagnosis: a case report, *Heart Lung* 24(2):121-123, 1995.

Yacone-Morton LA: Cardiovascular drugs—antiarrhythmics, *RN* 58(4):26-35, 1995.

## Chapter 26 Management of Persons with Inflammatory Heart Disease, Heart Failure, and Persons Undergoing Cardiac Surgery

### Endocarditis

Bansal RC: Infective endocarditis, *Med Clin North Am* 79(5):1205-1240, 1995.

### Heart Failure

Ahrens SG: Managing heart failure: a blueprint for success, *Nursing* 25(12): 27-31, 1995.

Beattie S, Pike C: Left ventricular diastolic dysfunction: a case report, *Crit Care Nurse* 16(2):37-50, 1996.

Bove LA: Now! Surgery for heart failure, *RN* 58(5):26-30, 1995.

Brown KK: Surgical therapy of chronic heart failure and severe ventricular dysfunction, *Crit Care Nurs Q* 18(1):45-55, 1995.

Dracup K: Heart failure secondary to left ventricular systolic dysfunction: therapeutic advances and treatment recommendations, *Nurse Pract* 21(9): 56-68, 1996.

English MA, Mastrean MB: Congestive heart failure: public and private burden, *Crit Care Nurs Q* 18(1):1-6, 1995.

Grady KL: When to transplant: recipient selection for heart transplantation, *J Cardiovasc Nurs* 10(2):58-70, 1996.

Janowski MJ: Managing heart failure, *RN* 59(2):34-39, 1996.

Meyer MS: Congestive heart failure: meet the challenge, *MedSurg Nurs* 4(5):341-349, 1995.

Miller MM: Current trends in the primary care management of chronic congestive heart failure, *Nurse Pract* 19(5):64-70, 1994.

Moser DK: Maximizing therapy in the advanced heart failure patient, *J Cardiovasc Nurs* 10(2):29-46, 1996.

Moyer JA: Factors related to length of ICU stay for CABG patients, *Dimensions Crit Care Nurs* 13(4), 1994.

Parenti C: Pulmonary embolism after coronary artery bypass surgery, *Crit Care Nurs Q* 17(3):48-50, 1994.

Reiley P, Howard E: Predicting hospital length of stay in elderly patients with congestive heart failure, *Nurs Econ* 13(4):210-216, 1995.

Sherman A: Critical care management of the heart failure patient in the home, *Crit Care Nurs Q* 18(1):77-87, 1995.

Venner GH, Seelbinder JS: Team management of congestive heart failure across the continuum, *J Cardiovasc Nurs* 10(2):71-84, 1996.

Wright JM: Pharmacologic management of congestive heart failure, *Crit Care Nurs Q* 18(1):32-44, 1995.

Yacone-Morton LA: First line therapy for CHF, *RN* 58(2):38-44, 1995.

### Cardiac Surgery

Alvarez MG, O'Brien M: Right gastroepiploic artery conduit use in myocardial revascularization, *AORN J* (60)5:763-777, 1994.

Earp JK: The gastroepiploic arteries as alternative coronary artery bypass conduits, *Crit Care Nurse* 14(1):24-30, 1994.

LeNoble E: Clinical rounds: cardiac pre-admission teaching program, *CJCN* 4(3-4):16-24, 1993.

Loos F: Understanding mediastinitis: nursing's role in prevention and treatment, *CJCN* 4(1):11-15, 1993.

Moyer JA: Factors related to length of ICU stay for CABG patients, *Dimensions Crit Care Nurs* 13(4), 1994.

Parenti C: Pulmonary embolism after coronary artery bypass surgery. *Crit Care Nurs Q* 17(3):48-50, 1994.

Quaal SJ: Ask the experts, *Crit Care Nurse* 17(3):100-101, 1997.

Quaal SJ: Caring for the intra-aortic balloon pump patient: most frequently asked questions, *Crit Care Nurs Clin North Am* 8(4):471-476, 1996.

Schaefer KM: Sleep disturbances post coronary artery bypass surgery, *Progr Cardiovasc Nurs* 11(1):5-14, 1996.

## Chapter 27 Management of Persons with Vascular Problems

### Hypertension

Alderman M, Elliott W, Oparil S, Wood A: Addressing multiple risks in hypertensive therapy, *Patient Care* 28(14):64-76, 1994.

Anonymous: New drugs—losartan (Cozaar)—an antihypertensive in a class by itself, *Am J Nurs* 95(12):56-57, 1995.

Chase S: Antihypertensives, *RN* 59(6):33-39, 1996.

Cuddy R: Hypertension: keeping dangerous blood pressure down, *Nursing* 25(8):35-41, 1995.

Haefele L, Dumas MA: Controlling hypertension in the elderly, *Am J Nurs* 96(11):2-7, 1996.

Hutchins L: Drug therapy for hypertension and hyperlipidemia, *J Cardiovasc Nurs* 9(2):37-53, 1995.

Johannsen JM: Update: guidelines for treating hypertension, *Am J Nurs* 93(3):42-49, 1993.

Kuncl H, Nelson KM: Antihypertensive drugs, *Nursing* 27(8):46-49, 1997.

Noel H: Essential hypertension: evaluation and treatment, *J Am Acad Nurse Pract* 6(9):421-438, 1994.

Solomon J: Hypertension—new drug therapies, *RN* 57(1):26-33, 1994.

Uber L, Uber W: Hypertensive crisis in the 1990's, *Crit Care Nurs Q* 16(2):27-34, 1993.

### Chronic Arterial Occlusive Disease

Blank CA, Irwin GH: Peripheral vascular disorders, *Nurs Clin North Am* 25(4):777-794, 1990.

Bright LD, Georgi S: Peripheral vascular disease. Is it arterial or venous? *Am J Nurs* 92(9):34-43, 1992.

Cameron J: Arterial leg ulcers, *Nurs Standard* 10(26):51-56, 1996.

Cantwell-Gab K: Identifying chronic peripheral arterial disease, *Am J Nurs* 96(7):40-46, 1996.

Harris AH, Brown-Etris M, Troyer-Caudle J: Managing vascular leg ulcers. Part 1: assessment, *Am J Nurs* 96(1):38-44, 1996.

Harris AH, Brown-Etris M, Troyer-Caudle J: Managing vascular leg ulcers. Part 2: treatment, *Am J Nurs* 96(1):40-47, 1996.

Hodges H: Raynaud's disease: pathophysiology, diagnosis, and treatment, *J Am Acad Nurse Pract* 7(4):159-164, 1995.

Husband LL: The management of the client with a leg ulcer, *J Adv Nurs* 24(3): 53-59, 1996.

### Acute Arterial Disease

Appleton DL, LaQuaglia JD: Vascular disease and postoperative nursing management, *Crit Care Nurse* 5(5):34-42,1985.

Beal K, Danzig B: Lasers in vascular surgery, *Nurs Clin North Am* 25(3):711-719, 1990.

Coen SD, Silverman E: Peripheral intra-arterial thrombolytic therapy for acute arterial occlusion, *Crit Care Nurse* 16(10):23-29, 1994.

Hall LT: Endovascular surgery: an overview, *Progr Cardiovasc Nurs* 5(2):43-49, 1990.

Hatswell EM: Abdominal aortic aneurysm surgery. Part II: major complications and nursing implications, *Heart Lung* 23(4):337-343, 1994.

### Venous Disease

Blondin MM, Titler MG: Deep vein thrombosis and pulmonary embolism prevention: what role do nurses play? *Med Surg Nurs* 5(3):205-208, 1996.

Bright LD: Deep vein thrombosis, *Am J Nurs* 95(6):48-49, 1995.

Bright LD, Georgi S: How to protect your patient from DVT, *Am J Nurs* 94(12):28-32, 1994.

Gibbar-Clements T, Shirrell D, Free C: PT and APTT—seeing beyond the numbers, *Nursing* 27(7):49-51, 1997.

Handerhan B: Recognizing pulmonary embolism, *Nursing* 21(4):92-93, 1991.

Hickey A: Catching deep vein thrombosis in time, *Nursing* 24(10):34-41, 1994.

Hull RD, Pineo GF: Low molecular weight heparin treatment of venous thromboembolism, *Progr Cardiovasc Dis* 37(2):71-78, 1994.

Kayser SR: Management of venous thromboembolic (VTE) disease. Part I: prevention, *Progr Cardiovasc Nurs* 10(4):31-36, 1995.

Kayser SR: Management of venous thromboembolic (VTE) disease. Part II: treatment, *Progr Cardiovasc Nurs* 11(1):36-40, 46, 1996.

Keep NB: Identifying pulmonary embolism, *Am J Nurs* 95(4):42-45, 1995.

Lancaster R, Dinwiddie JR: Filters that trap emboli, *RN* 54(9):56-59, 1991.

Lilly LL, Guanci R: A cautious look at heparin, *Am J Nurs* 96(5):14-16, 1996.

Majoros KA, Moccia JM: Pulmonary embolism: targeting an elusive enemy, *Nursing* 26(4):26-31, 1996.

Nunnelee JD: Minimize the risk of DVT, *RN* 58(12):28-31, 1995.

Raimer F, Thomas M: Clot stoppers—using anticoagulant safely and effectively, *Nursing* 25(3):35-43, 1995.

Sparks KS: Are you up to date on weight-based heparin dosing? *Am J Nurs* 96(4):33-37, 1996.

White VM: T-PA for pulmonary embolism, *Am J Nurs* 96(9):34, 1996.

## Chapter 28 Assessment of the Hematologic System

### General

Baer DM: Schilling test, *Med Lab Observer* 26(1):10, 1994.

Beutler E et al: *Williams hematology,* ed 5, New York, 1995, McGraw-Hill.

Evalt BL et al: *Diagnostic hematology: anemia,* US Department of Health and Human Services, 1992, World Health Organization.

Hoffman R: *Hematology basic principles and practice,* New York, 1995, Churchill Livingstone.

Spivak JL, Eichner ER: *The fundamentals of clinical hematology,* ed 3, Baltimore, 1993, John Hopkins University Press.

## Chapter 29 Management of Persons with Hematologic Problems

### Anemia

Erickson JM: Anemia, *Semin Oncol Nurs* 12(1):2-14, 1996

Hawley K: Clinical snapshot: pernicious anemia, *Am J Nurs* 96(11):52-53, 1996.

Tinkle M: Folic acid and food fortification: implications for the primary care practitioner, *Nurse Pract* 22(3):105-114, 1997.

### Hemoglobinopathy

Anionwu EN: Sickle cell and thalassemia: some priorities for nursing research, *J Adv Nurs* 23(5):853-856, 1996.

Anionwu EN: Haemoglobinopathies, *Pract Nurse* 13(7):374-379, 1997.

Bailey G: Educating young adults about sickle cell and thalassemia, *Health Visitor* 69(12):499-500, 1996.

Bunn HF: Pathogenesis and treatment of sickle cell disease, *N Engl J Med* 337(11):762-769, 1997.

Buswell C: Beta thalassemia, *Prof Nurse* 12(2):145-147, 1996.

Embury SH, Hebbel RP, Mohandas N: *Sickle cell disease: basic principles and clinical practice,* Boston, 1994, Raven.

Nash KB: *Psychosocial aspects of sickle cell disease: past, present, and future directions of research,* 1994, Haworth Press.

### Leukemia

Bertero C, Eriksson D, Ek A: Explaining different profiles in quality of life experiences in acute and chronic leukemia, *Cancer Nurs* 20(2):100-104, 1997.

Collins PM: Diagnosis and treatment of chronic leukemia, *Semin Oncol Nurs* 6(1):31-43, 1990.

Greco MG, Balbi M, Saracino L, Milanesi M: Improvement of supportive nursing care in cancer patients autografted with bone marrow and mobilized peripheral haematopoietic progenitors, *Eur J Cancer Care* 5(1):21-25, 1996.

Pitler LR: Hematopoietic growth factors in clinical practice, *Semin Oncol Nurs* 12(2):115-129, 1996.

### Lymphoma

Cambell K: Lymphomas: aetiology, classification and treatment, *Nurs Times* 92(9):44-45, 1996.

Gale D: *Oncology nursing care plans,* El Paso, Tex, 1995, Skidmore-Roth.

Glass AG, Karnell LH, Menck HR: The national cancer data base report on non-Hodgkin's lymphoma, *Cancer* 80(12):2311-2320, 1997.

Gruenwald SL et al: *Cancer nursing principles and practice,* ed 3, Boston, 1993, Bartlett & Jones.

Johnson MH, Moroney CE, Gay CF: Relieving nausea and vomiting in patients with cancer: a treatment algorithm, *Oncol Nurs Forum* 24(1):51-57, 1997.

Lundquist DM, Stewart FM: An update on non-Hodgkin's lymphomas, *Nurse Pract* 19(10):41-50, 1994.

Warmkessel JH: Caring for patients with non-Hodgkin's lymphoma, *Nursing* 27(6):48-49, 1997.

## Chapter 30 Assessment of the Respiratory System

### General

Beare PG, Myers JL: *Adult health nursing,* St Louis, 1994, Mosby.

Copstead LC: *Perspectives on pathophysiology,* Philadelphia, 1995, WB Saunders.

Ignatavicius DD, Workman ML, Mishler MA: *Medical-surgical nursing,* Philadelphia, 1995, WB Saunders.

Monahan FD, Drake T, Neighbors M: *Nursing care of adults,* Philadelphia, 1994, WB Saunders.

Preusser BA et al: Quantifying the minimum discard required for accurate arterial blood gases, *Nurs Res* 38(5):276-279, 1989.

Smeltzer SC, Bare BG: *Medical-surgical nursing,* Philadelphia, 1996, Lippincott.

Szaflarski NL: Preanalytic error associated with blood gas/pH measurement, *Crit Care Nurse* 16(3):89-100, 1996.

Thelan LA, Davie JK, Urden LD, Lough ME: *Critical care nursing,* St Louis, 1994, Mosby.

Weilitz PB, Lueckenotte A: Respiratory assessment of older adults: part I, *Perspect Respir Nurs* 6(1):4, 1995.

Wilkins MA, Dexter JR, Murphy RLH, DelBono EA: Lung sound nomenclature survey, *Chest* 98(4):886-889, 1990.

## Chapter 31 Management of Persons with Problems of the Upper Airway


### General

Glass C et al: Nurses' ability to achieve hyperinflation and hyperoxygenation with a manual resuscitation bag during endotracheal suctioning, *Heart Lung* 22:158-165, 1993.

Groothius JR: Viral respiratory infections. In Rakel RE, editor: *Conn's current therapy 1993,* Philadelphia, 1993, WB Saunders.

Pichichero MB: Streptococcal pharyngitis. In Rakel RE, editor: *Conn's current therapy 1993,* Philadelphia, 1993, WB Saunders.

Scher RI, Richtsmeiler SJ: Otolaryngology: head and neck surgery. In Sabiston DC, Lyerly KH, editors: *Sabiston essentials of surgery,* ed 2, Philadelphia, 1994, WB Saunders.

Warshawsky MF et al: Endotracheal intubation—induced upper airway obstruction, *Heart Lung* 25:69-71, 1996.

### Sinus Conditions

Leach JL, Schaeffer S: Sinusitis. In Rakel RE, editor: *Conn's current therapy 1993,* Philadelphia, 1993, WB Saunders.

Miller WE: The role of the outpatient nurse in endoscopic sinus surgery, *ORL Head Neck Nurs* 10(3):20-24, 1992.

Newman LJ et al: Chronic sinusitis: relationship of computed tomographic findings to allergy, asthma and eosinophilia, *JAMA* 271:363-367, 1994.

Williams JW, Simel DL: Does this patient have sinusitis? Diagnosing acute sinusitis by history and physical examination, *JAMA* 270:1242-1246, 1993.

### Allergies

Gibbs L: Assessment and management of the allergic patient, *ORL Head Neck Nurs* 10(3):10-16, 1992.

Howard BA: Guiding allergy sufferers through the medication maze, *RN* 57(4):26-31, 1994.

Mabry CS, Mabry RL: Making the diagnosis of allergy, *ORL Head Neck Nurs* 14(1):13-14, 1996.

McConnell EA: How to instill nose drops, *Nursing '93* 24(7):18, 1993.

Nurse's guide to O.T.C. allergy products, *Nursing '93* 24(9):67-70, 1993.

Patten BC, Holt JA: When your patient is allergic, *Am J Nurs* 92(9):58-61, 1992.

Pope AM: Indoor allergens—assessing and controlling adverse health effects, *JAMA* 269:2721, 1993.

Rodman MJ: OTC interactions: cough, cold, and allergy preparations, *RN* 56(2):38-42, 1993.

Simons FE, Simons KJ: The pharmacology and use of $H_1$-receptor-antagonist drugs, *N Engl J Med* 330:1663-1670, 1994.

Tips for taking O.T.C. allergy products(patient teaching aid), *Nursing '93* 24(9):71-72, 1993.

### Head and Neck Cancer

Droughton ML, Krech RL: Head and neck cancer resection and reconstruction: from past to present, *Today's OR Nurs* 14(9):25-34, 1992.

Eliachar MD, Oringher SF: Performance and management of long-term tracheostomy, *Operative Techn Otolaryngol Head Neck Surg* 1(1)56-63, 1990.

Hatfield BO: Cost effective trach teaching, *RN* 60(3):48-49, 1997.

Johns ME, Niparko JK: Otolaryngology—head and neck surgery, *JAMA* 270:243-245, 1993.

Logemann JA: Rehabilitation of the head and neck cancer patient, *Semin Oncol* 21:359-365, 1994.

Mancinelli-Van Atta J, Bech SL: Preventing hypoxemia and hemodynamic compromise related to endotracheal suctioning, *Am J Crit Care* 1:62-79, 1992.

Martin JW et al: Postoperative care of the maxillectomy patient, *ORL Head Neck Nurs* 12(3):15-20, 1994.

Merlano M et al: Treatment of advanced squamous-cell carcinoma of the head and neck with alternating chemotherapy and radiotherapy, *N Engl J Med* 327:1115-1121, 1992.

Roberts NK: The selective approach to successful stomal management at home, *ORL Head Neck Nurs* 13(14):12, 1995.

Strohl RA: The etiology and management of acute and late sequelae of radiation therapy, *ORL Head Neck Nurs* 13(4):23, 1995.

Trudeau MD, Schuller DE: Mechanisms for vocal communication following total laryngectomy, *Cancer Treat Res* 52:117-131, 1990.


## Chapter 32 Management of Persons with Problems of the Lower Airway


### General

Carroll P: Tradition or science? Splitting the difference in respiratory care, *RN* 26-29, May 1996.

Hsia CC: Mechanisms of the disease: respiratory function of hemoglobin, *N Engl J Med* 3348(4):239-247, 1998.

Huston CJ: Carbon monoxide poisoning, *Am J Nurs* 96(1):48, 1996.

Manning HL, Schwartzstein RM: Physiology of dyspnea, *N Engl J Med* 333(23):1547-1553, 1995.

### Acute Respiratory Distress Syndrome

Amato BP et al: Effect of protective ventilation strategies on mortality in the acute respiratory distress syndrome, *N Engl J Med* 338(6):347-354, 1998.

Angelucci P: A new weapon against ARDS, *RN* 22-24, November 1996.

Anzueto A et al: Aerosolized surfactant in adults with sepsis-induced acute respiratory distress syndrome, *N Engl J Med* 334(22):1471-1521, 1996.

Brandstatter RD et al: Adult respiratory distress syndrome: a disorder in need of improved outcome, *Heart Lung* 26(1):3-14, 1997.

Hudson LD: Protective ventilation for patients with acute respiratory distress syndrome, *N Engl J Med* 338(6):385-386, 1998 (editorial).

Kollef MH, Schuster DP: The acute respiratory distress syndrome, *N Engl J Med* 332(1):27-37, 1995.

Moss M et al: The role of chronic alcohol abuse in the development of acute respiratory distress syndrome in adults, *JAMA* 275:50-54, 1996.

O'Hanlon-Nichols T: Clinical snapshot: adult respiratory distress syndrome, *Am J Nurs* 95:42, 1995.

Weg JG et al: The relation of pneumothorax and other air leaks in mortality in acute respiratory distress syndrome, *N Engl J Med* 338(1):341-346, 1998.

### Asthma

Barnes PJ: Inhaled glucocorticoids for asthma, *N Engl J Med* 332(13):868-875, 1995.

Centers for Disease Control and Prevention: Asthma surveillance programs in public health departments—United States, *MMWR* 45(37):802-804, 1996.

Centers for Disease Control and Prevention: Surveillance for asthma—United States, 1960-1995, *MMWR* 47(no. SS-1):1-27, 1998.

Chiocca E, Russo L: Action stat: acute asthmatic attack, *Nursing '97* 28:43, 1997.

Drazen JM et al: Comparison of regularly scheduled with as-needed use of albuterol in mild asthma, *N Engl J Med* 335(12):841-847, 1996.

Devine EC: Meta-analysis of the effects of psychoeducational care in adults with asthma, *Res Nurs Health* 19:367-376, 1996.

Eisenbeis C: Full partner in care, *Nursing '96* 27(1):48-51, 1996.

Mathews PJ: Using a pek flow meter, *Nursing '97* 28:57-59, 1997.

Middelton AD: Managing asthma: it takes teamwork, *Am J Nurs* 97(1):39-43, 1997.

Nelson HS: $\beta$-Adrenergic bronchodilators, *N Engl J Med* 333(8):499-506, 1995.

Postma DS et al: Genetic susceptibility to asthma-bronchial hyperresponsiveness coinherited with a major gene for atopy, *N Engl J Med* 333(14):894-900, 1995.

Tarlo SM et al: A worker's compensation claim population for occupational asthma: comparison of sub-groups, *Chest* 107:634-641, 1995.

### Blastomycosis

Booker KJ: Blastomycosis-induced respiratory failure: the successful application of continuous positive airway pressure, *Heart Lung* 25(5):384-387, 1996.

### Cancer of the Lung

Held JL: Caring for a patient with lung cancer, *Nursing '95* 26(10):34-43, 1995.

Sarna L, Brecht ML: Dimensions of symptoms distress in women with advanced lung cancer: a factor analysis, *Heart Lung* 26(1):23-30, 1997.

### Closed Suctioning

Galvin WF, Cusano AL: Making a clean sweep using a closed tracheal system, *Nursing '98* 28(6):50, 1998.

Kite-Powell DM et al: Optimizing outcomes in ventilator-dependent patients: challenging critical care practice, *Crit Care Nurs Q* 19(3):77-90, 1996.

Tasota FJ, Hoffman LA: Terminal weaning from mechanical ventilation: planning and process, *Crit Care Nurs Q* 19(3):36-51, 1996.

### Chronic Obstructive Pulmonary Disease (COPD)

Anderson KL: The effect of chronic obstructive pulmonary disease on quality of life, *Res Nurs Health* 18:547-556, 1995.

Bauldoff GS et al: Home-based upper arm exercise training for patients with chronic obstructive pulmonary disease, *Heart Lung* 25(4):288-294, 1996.

Breslin EH: Respiratory muscle function in patients with chronic obstructive pulmonary disease, *Heart Lung* 25(4):271-285, 1996.

Lareau SC, Breslin EH, Meek PM: Functional status instruments: outcome measures in the evaluation of patients with chronic obstructive pulmonary disease, *Heart Lung* 25(3):212-224, 1996.

Leidy NK, Traver GA: Psychophysiologic factors contributing to functional performance in people with COPD: are there gender differences? *Res Nurs Health* 18:535-546, 1995.

Whittemore AS, Perlin SA, DiCiccio Y: Chronic obstructive pulmonary disease in lifelong nonsmokers: results from NHANES, *Am J Public Health* 85(5):702-706, 1995.

### Cystic Fibrosis

Konston MW et al: Effect of high-dose ibuprofen in patients with cystic fibrosis, *N Engl J Med* 332(13):848-854, 1995.

Ramsey BW: Management of pulmonary disease in patients with cystic fibrosis, *N Engl J Med* 335(3):179-188, 1996.

### Mechanical Ventilation

Brody H et al: Sounding board: withdrawing intensive life-sustaining treatment—recommendations for compassionate clinical management, *N Engl J Med* 336(9):652-657, 1997.

Dickens MD: Pharmacology of neuromuscular blockade: interactions and implications for concurrent drug therapies, *Crit Care Nurs Q* 18(2):1-12, 1995.

Ely EW et al: Effect on the duration of mechanical ventilation on identifying patients capable of breathing spontaneously, *N Engl J Med* 335(25):1864-1869, 1996.

Hillberg RE, Johnson DC: Noninvasive ventilation, *N Engl J Med* 337(24):1746-1752, 1997.

Knebel A et al: A guide to noninvasive intermittent ventilatory support, *Heart Lung* 26(4):307-316, 1997.

Logan J, Jenny J: Qualitative analysis of patient's work during mechanical ventilation and weaning, *Heart Lung* 26(2):140-147, 1997.

Noll ML, Byers JF: Weaning from mechanical ventilation, *Heart Lung* 24(3):220-227, 1995.

Swigart V et al: Letting go: family willingness to forgo life support, *Heart Lung* 25(6):483-494, 1996.

### Oxygen Therapy

Caliano C, Clifford DW, Titano K: Oxygen therapy: giving your patient breathing room, *Nursing '95* 26:33-38, 1995.

Carroll P: Pulse oximetry at your fingertips, *RN* 60(2):22-26, 1997.

Carroll P: When you want humidity, *RN* 60(5):31-35, 1997.

Goodfellow LM: Application of pulse oximetry and the oxyhemoglobin dissociation curve, *Crit Care Nurs Q* 20(2):22-27, 1997.

Lewis P et al: The effect of turning and backrub on mixed venous oxygen saturation in critically ill patients, *Am J Crit Care* 6(2):132, 1994.

Mathews PJ: Safely delivering a breath of fresh air, *Nursing '95* 26(5):66-69.

### Pneumonia

Bartlett JG, Mundy LM: Community-acquired pneumonia, *N Engl J Med* 333(24):1618-1624, 1995.

Bregeon F et al: Relationship of microbiologic diagnostic criteria to morbidity and mortality in patients with ventilator-associated pneumonia, *JAMA* 277(8):655-662, 1997.

Brooks-Brunn JA: Postoperative atelectasis and pneumonia, *Heart Lung* 24(2):94-115, 1995.

Carroll P: Preventing nosocomial pneumonia, *RN* 61(6):44-48, 1998.

Centers for Disease Control and Prevention: Guidelines for the prevention of nosocomial pneumonia, *MMWR* 46(no. RR-1):1-79, 1997.

Centers for Disease Control and Prevention: Outbreaks of pneumococcal pneumonia among unvaccinated residents in chronic care facilities—Massachusetts, October 1995, Oklahoma, February 1996, and Maryland, May-June 1996, *MMWR* 46(3):60-62, 1997.

Centers for Disease Control and Prevention: Recommendations of the Advisory Committee on Immunization Practices (ACIP), *MMWR* 46(no. RR-8):1-24, 1997.

Centers for Disease Control and Prevention: Surveillance for penicillin-nonsusceptible *Streptococcus pneumoniae*—New York City, 1995, *MMWR* 46(14):297-299, 1997.

Crowe HM: Nosocomial pneumonia: problems and progress, *Heart Lung* 25(5):418-421, 1996.

Doern GV, Brueggeann A, Holley HP, Rauch AM: Antimicrobial resistance of *Streptococcus pneumoniae* recovered from outpatients in the United States during winter months of 1994 to 1995: results of a 30-center national surveillance study, *Antimicrob Agents Chemother* 40:1208-1213, 1996.

Gleason PP et al: Medical outcomes and antimicrobial costs with use of American Thoracic Society guidelines for outpatients with community-acquired pneumonia, *JAMA* 278(1):32-39, 1997.

Howland WA: Defending your patient against nosocomial pneumonia, *Nursing '95* 25(8):62-63, 1995.

Tuomanes EL, Austrian R, Masure HR: Pathogenesis of pneumococcal infection, *N Engl J Med* 332(19):1280-1284, 1995.

### Pneumothorax

Hayden C: Spontaneous pneumothorax: a mother's perspective, *Am J Nurs* 98(4):16 BB-EE, 1998.

### Pulmonary Embolism

Decousis H et al: A clinical trial of venal caval filters in the prevention of pulmonary embolism in patients with proximal deep-vein thrombosis, *N Engl J Med* 338(7):409-415, 1998.

Keep NB: Identifying pulmonary embolism, *Am J Nurs* 95(4):52, 1995.

Majoras KA, Moccia JM: Pulmonary embolism, *Nursing '96* 27(4):26-30, 1996.

White VM: Nursing rounds t-PA for pulmonary embolism, *Am J Nurs* 96(9):34, 1996.

### Sarcoidosis

Newman LS, Rose CS, Maier LA: Sarcoidosis, *N Engl J Med* 336(17):1224-1234, 1997.

Zitkus BS: Clinical snapshot: sarcoidosis, *Am J Nurs* 97(10):40-41, 1997.

### Smoking

Barendregt MA, Bonneux L, van der Maas: The health costs of smoking, *N Engl J Med* 337(15):1052-1057, 1997.

Celermajer DS et al: Passive smoking and impaired endothelium-dependent arterial dilatation in healthy young adults, *N Engl J Med* 334(3):150-154, 1996.

Conrad KM et al: The worksite environment as a cue to smoking reduction, *Res Nurs Health* 19:21-31, 1996.

Centers for Disease Control and Prevention: State-specific prevalence of cigarette smoking—United States, 1995, *MMWR* 45(44):962-966, 1996.

Centers for Disease Control and Prevention: Tobacco use among high school students—United States, 1997, *MMWR* 47(12):229-233, 1998.

Centers for Disease Control and Prevention: Selected cigarette smoking initiation and quitting behaviors among high school students—United States, 1997, *MMWR* 47(19):386-389, 1998.

Centers for Disease Control and Prevention: Cigarette smoking before and after an excise tax increase and a anti-smoking campaign—Massachusetts, 1990-1996, *MMWR* 45(44):966-970, 1996.

Escobedo LG, Peddicord JP: Smoking prevalence in US birth cohorts: the influence of gender and education, *Am J Public Health* 86(2):231-236, 1996.

Franzgote M et al: Screening for adolescent smoking among primary care physicians in California, *Am J Public Health* 87(8):1341-1345, 1997.

Gold DR et al: Effects of cigarette smoking on lung function in adolescent boys and girls, *N Engl J Med* 335(13):931-937, 1996.

Greenlund KJ et al: Cigarette smoking attitudes and first use among third-through sixth-grade students: the Bogalusa heart study, *Am J Public Health* 87(8):1345-1348, 1997.

Meirer KJ, Licard MJ: The effect of cigarette taxes on cigarette consumption 1955-1994, *Am J Public Health* 87(7):1126-1130, 1997.

Parmet WE, Daynard RA, Gottlieb MA: The physician's role in helping smoke-sensitive patients to use the Americans with Disabilities Act to secure smoke-free workplaces and public spaces, *JAMA* 276(11):909-913, 1996.

Rigotti NA et al: The effect of enforcing tobacco sales laws and adolescents' access to tobacco and smoking behavior, *N Engl J Med* 337(15):1044-1051, 1997.

Schoenbaum M: Do smokers understand the mortality effects of smoking? Evidence from the health and retirement study, *Am J Public Health* 87(5):755-759, 1997.

Taylor CB et al: A nurse-managed smoking cessation program for hospitalized smokers, *Am J Public Health* 86(11):1557-1560, 1996.

Thun MJ et al: Excess mortality among cigarette smokers: changes in a 20-year interval, *Am J Public Health* 85(9):1223-1230, 1995.

Walsh RA et al: A smoking cessation program at a public antenatal clinic, *Am J Public Health* 87(7):1201-1204, 1997.

### Thoracic Surgery

Carroll P: Chest tubes made easy, *RN* 58(12):46-55, 1995.

Carroll P: Salvaging blood from the chest: chest drainage autologous transfusion or autotransfusion (ATS), *RN* 59(9):33-39, 1996.

Colizza DF: Action stat: dislodged chest tubes, *Nursing '95* 26(9):33, 1995.

Colt HG: Thoracoscopy: a prospective study of safety and outcome, *Chest* 108:324-329, 1995.

Dickey DM: Bilateral lung volume reduction surgery for treatment of emphysema, *AORN J* 63(2):355-372, 1996.

Lazzara D: Why is the Heimlich chest drain valve making a comeback? *Nursing '96* 27(12):50-53, 1996.

McGraw LR: Lung volume reduction surgery: an overview, *Heart Lung* 26(2):131-137, 1997.

Miracle V, Miller D: Lung volume reduction surgery, *Nursing '97* 28(9):65-66, 68, 1997.

Rogers RM, Sciurba FC, Keenan RJ: Lung reduction surgery in chronic obstructive lung disease, *Med Clin North Am* 80(3):623-644, 1996.

Sciurba FC et al: Improvement in pulmonary function and elastic recoil after lung reduction surgery for diffuse emphysema, *N Engl J Med* 334(17):1095-1099, 1996.

Waldhausen JA, Pierce WS, Campbell DB: *Surgery of the chest,* ed 6, St Louis, 1996, Mosby.

### Trauma

Collins PM, Benedict JL: Pleural effusion, *Am J Nurs* 96(7):38-39, 1996.

Gaedeke MK, Cross J: Action stat: blunt chest trauma, *Nursing '96* 27(2):33, 1996.

Laskowski-Jones L: Meeting the challenge of chest trauma, *Am J Nurs* 95(9):23-29, 1995.

Rutter KM: Action stat: tension pneumothorax, *Nursing '95* 26(4):33, 1995.

### Tuberculosis

Agerton T et al: Transmission of a highly drug resistant strain (strain W1) of *Mycobacterium tuberculosis, JAMA* 278(13):1073-1077, 1977.

Buchanan RJ: Compliance with tuberculosis drug regimens: incentives and enablers offered by public health departments, *Am J Public Health* 87(2):2014-2017, 1997.

Centers for Disease Control and Prevention: Nucleic acid amplification tests for tuberculosis, *MMWR* 45(43):950-951, 1997.

Centers for Disease Control and Prevention: Clinical update: impact of HIV protease inhibitors in the treatment of HIV-infected tuberculosis patients with rifampin, *MMWR* 45(42):921-925, 1996.

DeCock K et al: Research issues involving HIV-associated tuberculosis in resource-poor countries, *JAMA* 276(18):1502-1507, 1996.

Field KW, Vezeau TM: Nursing interventions for MDR-TB, *Am J Nurs* 98(6):16E, 16H, 16J, 1998.

Frieden TR et al: A multi-institutional outbreak of highly-drug resistant tuberculosis epidemiology and clinical outcomes, *JAMA* 276(15):1229-1235, 1996.

Gold HS, Moellering RC: Antimicrobial-drug resistance, *N Engl J Med* 335(19):1445-1453, 1996.

Grimes DE, Grimes RM: Tuberculosis: what nurses need to know to help control the epidemic, *Nurs Outlook* 43(4):164-173, 1995.

McCombs SB et al: Tuberculosis surveillance in the United States: case definitions used by state health departments, *Am J Public Health* 86(5):728-731, 1996.

McKenna MT, McCray E, Onorato I: The epidemiology of tuberculosis among foreign-born persons in the United States, 1986-1993, *N Engl J Med* 332(16):1071-1076, 1995.

Michele TM et al: Transmission of *Mycobacterium tuberculosis* by fiberoptic bronchoscope, identification by DNA fingerprinting, *JAMA* 278(13):1093-1095, 1997.

Moore M et al: Trends in drug-resistant tuberculosis in the United States, 1993-1996, *JAMA* 278(10):833-837, 1997.

Pablos-Mendez A et al: Global surveillance for antituberculosis-drug-resistance, 1994-1997, *N Engl J Med* 338(23):1641-1649, 1998.

Pablos-Mendez A, Sterling ER, Frieden TR: The relationship between delayed or incomplete treatment and all-cause mortality in patients with tuberculosis, *JAMA* 275(15):1223-1228, 1996.

Pablos-Mendez A, Blustein J, Knirsch CA: The role of diabetes mellitus in the higher prevalence of tuberculosis among Hispanics, *Am J Public Health* 87(4):574-579, 1997.

Small P: Tuberculosis research balancing the portfolio, *JAMA* 276(18):1512-1513, 1996.

Snider DE, Castro KG: The global threat of drug resistant tuberculosis, *N Engl J Med* 338(23):1689-1690, 1998 (editorial).

Tuberculosis in New York City—focal transmission of an often fatal disease, *JAMA* 276(15):1259-1260, 1996 (editorial).

Zuber LF et al: Long-term risk of tuberculosis among foreign-born persons in the United States, *JAMA* 278(4):304-307, 1997.

## Chapter 33 Assessment of the Endocrine System

### General

Agana-Defensor R, Proch M: Pheochromocytoma: a clinical review, *AACN Clin Iss Crit Care Nurs* 3:309-318, 1992.

Aron DC, Tyrell JB, Wilson CB: Current concepts in diagnosis and management of pituitary tumors, *West J Med* 162:340, 1995.

Bilezikian JP et al: *The parathyroids,* Boston, 1994, Raven Press.

Giefer CK, Cassmeyer VL: The syndrome of primary aldosteronism: a case study, *MedSurg Nurs* 3:277-284, 1994.

Goldsmith C: Hypothyroidism: easy to treat, but often overlooked, *Nurseweek* 11(22):12-13, 1997.

Greenspan FS, editor: Thyroid diseases, *Med Clin North Am* 75:1, 1991.

Ladenson PW et al: Comparison of administration of recombinant human thyrotropin with withdrawal of thyroid hormone for radioactive iodine scanning in patients with thyroid carcinoma, *N Engl J Med* 337(13):888-896, 1997.

Melmed S, editor: Acromegaly, *Endocrinol Metab Clin North Am* 21:483, 1992.

Melmed S, editor: *The pituitary,* Cambridge, Mass, 1995, Blackwell.

Molitch ME: Neuroendocrinology. In Felig P, Baxter JD, Frohman LA, editors: *Endocrinology and metabolism,* ed 3, New York, 1995, McGraw-Hill.

Singer PA et al: Treatment guidelines for patients with hyperthyroidism and hypothyroidism, *JAMA* 273:808, 1995.

Strewler GJ: Mineral metabolism and metabolic bone disease. In Greenspan FS, editor: *Basic and clinical endocrinology,* ed 5, Norwalk, Conn, 1997, Appleton & Lange.

Utinger RD: Follow-up of patients with thyroid carcinoma, *N Engl J Med* 337(13):928-930, 1997.

Wartofsky LM, editor: The thyroid gland. In Becker KL, editor: *Principles and practice of endocrinology and metabolism,* ed 2, Philadelphia, 1995, JB Lippincott.

## Chapter 34 Management of Persons with Problems of the Pituitary, Thyroid, Parathyroid, and Adrenal Glands

### Thyroid

Goldsmith C: Hypothyroidism: easy to treat, but often overlooked, *Nurseweek* 11(22):12-13, 1997.

Greenspan FS, editor: Thyroid diseases, *Med Clin North Am* 75:1, 1991.

Ladenson PW et al: Comparison of administration of recombinant human thyrotropin with withdrawal of thyroid hormone for radioactive iodine scanning in patients with thyroid carcinoma, *N Engl J Med* 337(13):888-896, 1997.

Singer PA et al: Treatment guidelines for patients with hyperthyroidism and hypothyroidism, *JAMA* 273:808, 1995.

Utinger RD: Follow-up of patients with thyroid carcinoma, *N Engl J Med* 337(13):928-930, 1997.

Wartofsky LM, editor: The thyroid gland. In Becker KL, editor: *Principles and practice of endocrinology and metabolism,* ed 2, Philadelphia, 1995, JB Lippincott.

### Parathyroid

Bilezikian JP et al: *The parathyroids,* Boston, 1994, Raven Press.

Strewler GJ: Mineral metabolism and metabolic bone disease. In Greenspan FS, editor: *Basic and clinical endocrinology,* ed 5, Norwalk, Conn, 1997, Appleton & Lange.

### Hypothalamus and Pituitary

Aron DC, Tyrell JB, Wilson CB: Current concepts in diagnosis and management of pituitary tumors, *West J Med* 162:340, 1995.

Melmed S, editor: Acromegaly, *Endocrinol Metab Clin North Am* 21:483, 1992.

Melmed S, editor: *The pituitary,* Cambridge, Mass, 1995, Blackwell.

Molitch ME: Neuroendocrinology. In Felig P, Baxter JD, Frohman LA, editors: *Endocrinology and metabolism,* ed 3, New York, 1995, McGraw-Hill.

### Adrenals

Agana-Defensor R, Proch M: Pheochromocytoma: a clinical review, *AACN Clin Iss Crit Care Nurs* 3:309-318, 1992.

Giefer CK, Cassmeyer VL: The syndrome of primary aldosteronism: a case study, *MedSurg Nurs* 3:277-284, 1994.

## Chapter 35 Management of Persons with Diabetes Mellitus and Hypoglycemia

### General

Boitard C, Caillat-Zucman S, Timsit J: Insulin-dependent diabetes and human leucocyte antigens, *Diabetes Metab* 23(suppl 2):22-28, 1997.

Campbell RK, Campbell LK, White JR: Insulin lispro: its role in the treatment of diabetes mellitus, *Ann Pharmacother* 30(11):1263-1271, 1996.

Carel JC, Lotton C, Bourgneres P: Prediction and prevention of type 1 diabetes: what can be expected from genetics? *Diabetes Metab* 23(suppl 2):29-33, 1997.

Colwell JA: Intensive insulin therapy in type II diabetes: rationale and collaborative clinical trial results, *Diabetes* 45(suppl 3):S87-S90, 1996.

DeFronzo R: Lilly Lecture 1987. The triumvirate: b-cell, muscle, liver: a collusion responsible for NIDDM, *Diabetes* 37:667-687, 1987.

DeGroot LJ, editor: *Endocrinology,* Philadelphia, 1995, WB Saunders.

Diabetes Control and Complications Trial Research Group: Effects of intensive diabetes therapy on neuropsychological function in adults in the Diabetes Control and Complications Trial, *Ann Intern Med* 124(4):379-388, 1996.

Edelstein SI, Knowler WC, Bain RP et al: Predictors of progression from impaired glucose tolerance to NIDDM: an analysis of six prospective studies, *Diabetes* 46(4):701-710, 1997.

Fonseca V, Wall J: Diet and diabetes in the elderly, *Clin Geriatr Med* 11(4):613-624, 1995.

Forbes GB: The abdomen:hip ratio: normative data and observations on selected patients, *Int J Obes* 14:149-157, 1990.

Froguel P: Tracking down genes to cure diabetes: An achievable task for the 21st century? *Diabetes Metab* 23(suppl 2):8-13, 1997.

Garcia-Palmieri MR, Perea-Lopez RM: Coronary disease in women, *P R Health Sci* 15(4):283-288, 1996.

Grossman E, Messerli FH: Diabetic and hypertensive heart disease, *Ann Intern Med* 125(4):304-310, 1996.

Hellman R, Regan J, Rosen H: Effect of intensive treatment of diabetes on the risk of death or renal failure in NIDDM and IDDM, *Diabetes Care* 20(3):258-264, 1997.

Henry RR: Glucose control and insulin resistance in non-insulin-dependent diabetes mellitus, *Ann Intern Med* 124(1 part 2):97-103, 1996.

Hinson J, Riordan K, Hemphill D et al: Hypertension education: an important and neglected part of the diabetes education curriculum? *Diabetes Educ* 23(2):166-170, 1997.

Ido Y, Kilo C, Williamson JR: Interactions between the sorbitol pathway, non-enzymatic glycation, and diabetic vascular dysfunction, *Nephrol Dial Transplant* 11(suppl 5):72-75, 1996.

Kozak GP, editor: *Clinical diabetes mellitus,* Philadelphia, 1982, WB Saunders.

Peterson CM, Jovanovic-Peterson L: Randomized crossover study of 40% vs. 55% carbohydrate weight loss strategies in women with previous gestational diabetes mellitus and non-diabetic women of 130-200% ideal body weight, *J Am Coll Nutr* 14(4):369-375, 1995.

Pozzilli P: Prevention of insulin-dependent diabetes: where are we now? *Diabetes Metab Rev* 12(2):127-135, 1996.

Sheard NF: The diabetic diet: evidence for a new approach, *Nutr Rev* 53(1):16-28, 1995.

Stern Z, Levy R: Analysis of direct cost of standard compared with intensive insulin treatment of insulin-dependent diabetes mellitus and cost of complications, *Acta Diabetol* 33(1):48-52, 1996.

Wilson PW: Established risk factors and coronary artery disease: the Framingham Study, *Am J Hypertens* 7(7 part 2):7S-12S, 1994.

## Chapter 36 Assessment of the Hepatic System

### General

Jones A, Aggeler B: Structure of the liver. In Haubrich WS, Schaffner F, Berk E, editors: *Gastroenterology,* ed 5, vol 3, Philadelphia, 1995, WB Saunders.

Zucker S, Gollan J: Physiology of the liver. In Haubrich WS, Schaffner F, Berk E, editors: *Gastroenterology,* ed 5, vol 3, Philadelphia, 1995, WB Saunders.

## Chapter 37 Management of Persons with Problems of the Hepatic System

### General

Crab D, Lumeng L: Alcoholic liver disease. In Haubrich WS, Schaffner F, Berk E, editors: *Gastroenterology,* ed 5, vol 3, Philadelphia, 1995, WB Saunders.

Kowdley KV: Update on therapy for hepatobiliary diseases, *Nurse Pract* 21(7):78-88, 1996.

Okuda K, Kondo Y: Primary carcinoma of the liver. In Haubrich WS, Schaffner F, Berk E, editors: *Gastroenterology,* ed 5, vol 3, Philadelphia 1995, WB Saunders.

### Hepatitis

Alter HJ et al: The incidence of transfusion-associated hepatitis G virus infection and its relation to liver disease, *N Engl J Med* 336(11):747-754, 1997.

Alter MJ et al: Acute non-A-E hepatitis in the US and the role of hepatitis G virus infection, *N Engl J Med* 336(11):741-746, 1997.

Breese JS et al: Hepatitis C virus infection associated with administration of intravenous immune globin, *JAMA* 276(19):1563-1567, 1996.

Clinical Guidelines: Hepatitis B immunization/prophylaxis: recommendations for adults/older adults, *Nurse Pract* 21(12):64-70, 1996.

Davis G, Lau J: Hepatitis C. In Haubrich WS, Schaffner F, Berk E, editors: *Gastroenterology,* ed 5, vol 3, Philadelphia 1995, WB Saunders.

Gutch D et al: Assessment of hepatitis C viremia using molecular amplification technologies: correlations and clinical implications, *Ann Intern Med* 123:321-329, 1995.

Hoofnagle J: Hepatitis B. In Haubrich WS, Schaffner F, Berk E, editors: *Gastroenterology,* ed 5, vol 3, Philadelphia 1995, WB Saunders.

Jeffers L et al: Hepatitis C virus infection in patients with acute and chronic liver disease of unknown etiology, *Hepatology* 22(4 part 2):182A, 1996.

Krawczynski D: Hepatitis E. In Haubrich WS, Schaffner F, Berk E, editors: *Gastroenterology,* ed 5, vol 3, Philadelphia 1995, WB Saunders.

Kuhns MC: Viral hepatitis. Part 2: treatment, prevention and special precautions, *Lab Med* 26(7):186-792, 1995.

Lemon SM, Thomas DL: Vaccines to prevent viral hepatitis, *N Engl J Med* 336(3):196-204, 1997.

Linnen J et al: Molecular cloning and disease association of hepatitis G virus: a transfusion-transmissible agent, *Science* 271:505-508, 1996.

McMahon B et al: Hepatitis A. In Haubrich WS, Schaffner F, Berk E, editors: *Gastroenterology,* ed 5, vol 3, Philadelphia 1995, WB Saunders.

Moradpour D: Understanding hepatitis B virus infection, *N Engl J Med* 332(4):1092-1093, 1995.

Rizzetto M et al: Hepatitis D (delta). In Haubrich WS, Schaffner F, Berk E, editors: *Gastroenterology,* ed 5, vol 3, Philadelphia 1995, WB Saunders.

Schaffner F: Introduction to viral hepatitis. In Haubrich WS, Schaffner F, Berk E, editors: *Gastroenterology,* ed 5, vol 3, Philadelphia 1995, WB Saunders.

Shetty K, Carey W: Fever, abdominal pain, and jaundice in a 43-year-old woman, *Cleve Clin J Med* 64(4):216-219, 1997.


### Biliary Cirrhosis


Coy D, Blei A: Portal hypertension. In Haubrich WS, Schaffner F, Berk E, editors: *Gastroenterology,* ed 5, vol 3, Philadelphia 1995, WB Saunders.

Ferenci P: Hepatic encephalopathy. In Haubrich WS, Schaffner F, Berk E, editors: *Gastroenterology,* ed 5, vol 3, Philadelphia 1995, WB Saunders.

Kaplan M et al: Sustained biochemical and histologic remission of primary biliary cirrhosis in response to medical treatment, *Ann Intern Med* 126:682-688, 1997.

Lindor K: Primary biliary cirrhosis: questions and promise, *Ann Intern Med* 126:733-735, 1997.


### Liver Failure


Runyon B: Ascites in liver disease. In Haubrich WS, Schaffner F, Berk E, editors: *Gastroenterology,* ed 5, vol 3, Philadelphia 1995, WB Saunders.


## Chapter 38 Assessment of the Gastrointestinal, Biliary, and Exocrine Pancreatic Systems

### General


Barker LR, Burton JR, Zieve PD: *Principles of ambulatory medicine,* Baltimore, 1995, Williams & Wilkins.

*Illustrated guide to diagnostic tests,* Springhouse, Penna, 1994, Springhouse.

Jarvis C: *Physical examination and health assessment,* ed 2, Philadelphia, 1996, WB Saunders.

Pagana KD, Pagana TJ: *Mosby's diagnostic and laboratory test reference,* ed 2, St Louis, 1997, Mosby.

Stone R: Acute abdominal pain, *Nurse Pract* 21(12):19-30, 35-39, 1996.

Thibodeau GA, Patton KT: *Anatomy and physiology,* ed 2, St Louis, 1996, Mosby.

Thompson JM, Wilson SF: *Health assessment for nursing practice,* St Louis, 1996, Mosby.


## Chapter 39 Management of Persons with Problems of the Mouth and Esophagus

### Problems of the Mouth


Baker C: A functional status scale for measuring quality of life outcomes in head and neck cancer patients, *Cancer Nurs* 18(6):452-457, 1996.

Mah MA, Johnston C: Concerns of families in which one member has head and neck cancer, *Cancer Nurs* 16(5):382-387, 1993.

Languis A, Bjorvell H, Lind MG: Oral and pharyngeal cancer patients perceived symptoms and health, *Cancer Nurs* 16(3):214-221, 1993.

Vigneswaran N, Tilashalski K, Rodu B, Cole P: Tobacco use and cancer, *Oral Surg Oral Med Oral Pathol* 80(2):178-181, 1995.

Whitney RG: Vincent's angina, periodontitis, and stomatitis, *Nursing* 25(4): 32-33, 1995.

Winn DM: Diet and nutrition in the etiology of oral cancer, *J Clin Nutr* 61(suppl):437s-455s, 1995.

Wright JM: Oral precancerous lesions and conditions, *Semin Dermatol* 13(2): 125-131, 1994.


### Esophageal Reflux Disease


Castell DO, Richter JE, Spechler SJ: Achieving better outcomes for patients with GERD, *Patient Care* 30(8):20-42, 1996.

Fennerty MB, Sampliner RE: Gastroesophageal reflux disease, *Hosp Med* 29(4):28, 32-34, 37-40, 1993.

Grainger SL, Klass HJ, Rake MO, Williams JG: Prevalence of dyspepsia: the epidemiology of overlapping symptoms, *Postgrad Med* 70(821):154-161, 1994.

Long K, Long R: Treating gastroesophageal reflux disease, *Nurse Pract Forum* 5(2):63-64, 1994.

Marshall JB: Severe gastroesophageal reflux disease, *Postgrad Med* 97(5):98, 100-106, 1995.

Miller CA: Alleviating the discomfort of gastroesophageal reflux disease, *Geriatr Nurs* 15(3):171-172, 1993.

Morton LS, Fromkes JJ: Gastroesophageal reflux disease: diagnosis and medical therapy, *Geriatrics* 48(3):60-66, 1993.

Pope CE: Acid-reflux disorders, *N Engl J Med* 331(10):656-660, 1994.

Robinson M: Gastroesophageal reflux disease, *Postgrad Med* 95(2):88, 90, 93-94, 99-102, 1994.

Spiro HM: Hiatus hernia and reflux esophagitis, *Hosp Pract* 29(1):51-54, 61, 65-66, 1994.


### Esophageal Surgery


Alpers DA: Laparoscopic Nissen fundoplication, *Semin Periop Nurs* 4(3):162-167, 1995.

Campbell AD, Ferrara BE: Toupet partial fundoplication, *AORN J* 57(3):671-673, 675-676, 678-679, 1993.

Lee NL, Broome A, Pappas TN: Laparoscopic fundoplication: an alternate approach in the surgical treatment of esophageal reflux, *Today's OR Nurse* 16(3):44-45, 1994.

Stengel JM, Dirado R: Laparoscopic Nissen fundoplication to treat gastroesophageal reflux, *AORN J* 61(3):483-484, 486-489, 1995.

Weant CA: Easing the pain of esophageal surgery, *RN* 58(8):26-30, 1995.


### Esophageal Cancer


Blot WJ: Esophageal cancer trends and risk factors, *Semin Oncol* 21(3):403-407, 1994.

Daniel BT, Shuey KM: Role of the nurse in managing the patient with esophageal cancer, *Nurs Interventions Oncol* 5(2):14-22, 1993.

Franceschi S: Role of nutrition in the etiology of oesophageal cancer in developed countries, *Endoscopy* 25(suppl):613-616, 1993.

Munoz N: Epidemiologic aspects of esophageal cancer, *Endoscopy* 25(suppl): 609-612, 1993.

Nabeya K, Hanaoka SL, Nymura T: What is the ideal treatment for early esophageal cancer? *Endoscopy* 25(suppl):670-671, 1993.

Reed PI, Johnston BJ: The changing incidence of esophageal cancer, *Endoscopy* 25(suppl):606-608, 1993.

Sideranko S: Esophagogastrectomy, *Crit Care Nurs Clin North Am* 5(1):177-183, 1993.

### Achalasia

Aliberti L: Managing esophageal achalasia: medical and nursing implications, *Gastroenterol Nurs* 16(3):126-130, 1994.

Saunderlin G: Esophageal achalasia, *Gastroenterol Nurs* 15(5):191-193, 1993.

## Chapter 40 Management of Persons with Problems of the Stomach and Duodenum

### Peptic Ulcer Disease

Anderson ML: *Helicobacter pylori* infection, *Postgrad Med* 96(6):40-50, 1994.

Anonymous: The management of NSAID ulcers, *Emerg Med* 25(13):41-42, 1993.

Anonymous: Aspirin and ulcer bleeding, *Nurses Drug Alert* 19(7):51, 1995.

Anonymous: Antibacterial therapy for gastric ulcers, *Nurses Drug Alert* 19(5):40, 1995.

Anonymous: Ranitidine prophylaxis for recurrent bleeding ulcers, *Nurses Drug Alert* 18(5):36-37, 1994.

Anonymous: Nizatidine for NSAID ulcer prevention, *Nurses Drug Alert* 18(1):4-5, 1994.

Anonymous: Preventing NSAID induced ulcers, *Nurses Drug Alert* 17(10):79, 1993.

Brozenec SA: Ulcer therapy update, *RN* 59(9):48-53, 1996.

Cerda JJ, Go MF, Loeb D, Westblom U: A revolution in peptic ulcer disease, *Patient Care* 28(9):19-33, 1994.

Conwell CF, Lyell R, MacMillan RW: Prevalence of *Helicobacter pylori* in family practice patients with refractory dyspepsia: a comparison of tests available in the office, *J Fam Pract* 41(3):245-252, 1995.

Fay M, Jaffe P: Diagnostic and treatment guidelines for *Helicobacter pylori, Nurse Pract* 21(7):28-34, 1996.

Fedotin MS: *Helicobacter pylori* and peptic ulcer disease, *Postgrad Med* 94(3):38-45, 1993.

Fennerty MB et al: *Helicobacter pylori: the new factor in management of ulcer disease,* Bethesda, Md, 1994, American Gastroenterological Association Foundation.

Heigh RI: Use of NSAIDs, *Postgrad Med* 96(6):63-69, 1994.

Heslin JM: Peptic ulcer disease, *Nursing* 27(1):34-39, 1997.

Hixson LJ, Kelley CL, Jones WN, Tuohy CD: Current trends in the pharmacotherapy for peptic ulcer disease, *Arch Intern Med* 152:726-731, 1992.

Holt S: Over the counter histamine $H_2$ receptor antagonists, *Drugs* 47(1):1-11, 1994.

Lilley LL, Guanci R: Adverse effects of NSAIDS, *Am J Nurs* 95(8):17, 1995.

Monmaney T: Marshall's hunch, *The New Yorker* 64-72, September 20, 1993.

Netchvolodoff CV: Refractory peptic lesions, *Postgrad Med* 93(4):143-154, 163, 1993.

Parent K: Acid reduction in peptic ulcer disease, *Postgrad Med* 96(6):53-59, 1994.

Sonnenberg A, Everhart JE: The prevalence of self reported peptic ulcer in the United States, *Am J Public Health* 86(2):200-205, 1996.

Sung JJY et al: Antibacterial treatment of gastric ulcers associated with *Helicobacter pylori, N Engl J Med* 332(3):139-142, 1995.

Walsh JH, Peterson WL: The treatment of *Helicobacter pylori* infection in the management of peptic ulcer disease, *N Engl J Med* 333(15):984-991, 1995.

Ziller SA, Netchvolodoff CV: Uncomplicated peptic ulcer disease, *Postgrad Med* 93(4):126-140, 1993.

### GI Bleeding

Anonymous: Gastric hemorrhage prophylaxis, *Nurses Drug Alert* 18(12):91, 1994.

Anonymous: Prevention of upper GI bleeding, *Nurses Drug Alert* 18(5):37, 1994.

Cook DJ et al: Risk factors for gastrointestinal bleeding in critically ill patients, *N Engl J Med* 330(6):377-381, 1994.

Gardner SS, Messner RL: Gastrointestinal bleeding, *RN* 55(12):43-46, 1992.

Kankaria AG, Fleischer DE: The critical care management of nonvariceal upper gastrointestinal bleeding, *Crit Care Clin* 11(2):347-366, 1995.

Qureshi WA, Netchvolodoff CV: Acute bleeding from peptic ulcers, *Postgrad Med* 93(4):167-178, 1993.

Rush C: Gastrointestinal bleeding, *Nursing* 26(8):33, 1995.

### Stress Ulcers

Anonymous: Stress ulcer prophylaxis and nosocomial pneumonia, *Nurses Drug Alert* 18(5):38, 1994.

Anonymous: Do $H_2$ blockers lead to nosocomial pneumonia? *Emerg Med* 25(12):63, 1993.

Anonymous: When to use stress ulcer prophylaxis, *Emerg Med* 25(7):57, 1993.

Bezarro ER: Changing perspectives of the $H_2$ antagonists for stress ulcer prophylaxis, *Crit Care Nurs Clin North Am* 5(2):325-331, 1993.

DePriest JL: Stress ulcer prophylaxis, *Postgrad Med* 98(4):159-168, 1995.

Fisher RL, Pipkin GA, Wood JR: Stress related mucosal disease, *Crit Care Clin* 11(2):323-343, 1995.

Neill KM, Rice KT, Ahern HL: Comparison of two methods of measuring gastric pH, *Heart Lung* 22(4):349-355, 1993.

Prevost SS, Oberle A: Stress ulceration in the critically ill patient, *Crit Care Nurs Clin North Am* 75(4):853-863, 1993.

### Gastric Cancer

Barkin JS et al: What's new in stomach cancer? *Patient Care* 26:22-59, 1992.

Fuchs CS, Mayer RJ: Gastric carcinoma, *N Engl J Med* 333(1):32-41, 1995.

Hansson LE, Nyren O, Hsing AW et al: The risk of stomach cancer in patients with gastric or duodenal ulcer disease, *N Engl J Med* 335:242-249, 1996.

Hendlisz A, Bleiberg H: Diagnosis and treatment of gastric cancer, *Drugs* 49(5):711-720, 1995.

Onishi K, Miaskowski C: Mechanisms and management of gastric cancer, *Cancer Nurs* 19(3):187-196, 1996.

### Surgery for Obesity

Benotti PN, Forse A: The role of gastric surgery in the multidisciplinary management of severe obesity, *Am J Surg* 169:351-367, 1995.

Calloway CW et al: Obesity: a quartet of approaches, *Patient Care* 26:157-199, 1992.

Consensus Development Conference Panel: Gastrointestinal surgery for severe obesity, *Ann Intern Med* 115(12):956-961, 1991.

Grace DM: Gastric restriction procedures for treating severe obesity, *Am J Clin Nutr* 55(suppl 2):556S-559S, 1992.

Kral JF: Overview of surgical techniques for treating obesity, *Am J Clin Nutr* 55(suppl 2):552S-555S, 1992.

Sugarman HJ et al: Gastric bypass for treating severe obesity, *Am J Clin Nutr* 55(suppl 2):560S-566S, 1992.

## Chapter 41 Management of Persons with Problems of the Intestines

### Inflammatory Bowel Disease

Bateson MC: Gastroenterology. II: small and large bowel, pancreas and biliary system, *Postgrad Med J* 70:620-624, 1994.

Belluzzi A, Brignola C, Campieri M et al: Effect of an enteric coated fish oil preparation on relapses in Crohn's disease, *N Engl J Med* 334(24):1557-1560, 1996.

Bitton A, Peppercorn MA: Emergencies in inflammatory bowel disease, *Crit Care Clin* 11(2):513-527, 1995.

Cox J: Inflammatory bowel disease: implications for the medical-surgical nurse, *MedSurg Nurs* 4(6):427-437, 1995.

Drossman DA, Thompson WG, Whitehead WE: Approaching IBS with confidence, *Patient Care* 26:175-210, 1992.

Giese LA, Terrell L: Sexual health issues in inflammatory bowel disease, *Gastroenterol Nurs* 19(1):12-17, 1996.

Hanauer SB: Inflammatory bowel disease, *N Engl J Med* 334(13):841-846, 1996.

Kinash RG, Fischer DG, Lukie BE, Carr TL: Coping patterns and related characteristics in patients with IBD, *Gastroenterol Nurs* 15:9-16, 1993.

Scott-Conner CEH: Current surgical management of inflammatory bowel disease, *South Med J* 87(12):1232-1241, 1994.

Thomas GAO, Rhodes J, Mani V et al: Transdermal nicotine as maintenance therapy for ulcerative colitis, *N Engl J Med* 332(15):988-992, 1995.

Tooson JD, Varilek GW: Inflammatory diseases of the colon, *Postgrad Med* 98(5):46-74, 1995.

## Constipation and Diarrhea

Anand A et al: Epidemiology, clinical manifestations, and outcome of *Clostridium difficile*-associated diarrhea, *Am J Gastroenterol* 89(4):519-523, 1994.

Bennett RG, Greenough WB: Approach to acute diarrhea in the elderly, *Gastroenterol Clin North Am* 22(3):517-533, 1993.

Eckler JAL: Defending against diarrhea, *Nursing* 26(3):22-23, 1996.

Hall GR et al: Managing constipation using a research based protocol, *MedSurg Nurs* 4(1):11-18, 1995.

Roberts MI: Diarrhea: a symptom, *Holistic Nurs Pract* 7(2):73-80, 1993.

Spollett GR: Nutritional management of common gastrointestinal problems, *Nurse Pract Forum* 5(1):24-27, 1994.

van der Horst ML, Sykula J, Lingley K: The constipation quandary, *Can Nurse* 90(1):25-30, 1994.

## Bowel Surgery

Bosley CL: Applying perianal pouches with confidence, *Nursing* 25(6):58-61, 1995.

Carr CS et al: Randomised trial of safety and efficacy of immediate post operative enteral feeding in patients undergoing gastrointestinal resection, *BMJ* 312(4):869-871, 1996.

Deziel DJ, Swanstrom L, Turec K: Laparoscopy's changing state of the art, *Patient Care* 30(10):42-54, 1996.

Fazio VW: Surgery of the colon and rectum, *Am J Gastroenterol* 89(8):S106-S115, 1994.

Galloway SC, Graydon JE: Uncertainty, symptom distress and information needs after surgery for cancer of the colon, *Cancer Nurs* 19(2):112-117, 1996.

Hampton BG, Bryant RA: *Ostomies and continent diversions: nursing management*, St Louis, 1992, Mosby.

Minard G, Kudsk KA: Is early feeding beneficial? How early is early? *New Horiz* 2(2):156-163, 1994.

Novak LT: Accelerated recovery technique: a new approach to abdominal surgery, *RN* 56(3):19-23, 1993.

Penney C: Innovations in gastrointestinal diseases, *Practitioner*, 238(10):694-699, 1994.

Provenzale D et al: Health related quality of life after ileoanal pull through, *Gastroenterology* 113(1):7-14, 1997.

## Tube Feeding

Belcaster A: Helping your patients avoid refeeding syndrome, *Nursing* 27(9):32hn8, 1997.

Bockus S: When your patient needs tube feedings, *Nursing* 23(7):34-42, 1993.

Davis AE, Arrington K, Fields-Ryan S, Pruitt JO: Preventing feeding associated aspiration, *MedSurg Nurs* 4(2):111-120, 1995.

Eisenberg PG: Causes of diarrhea in tube-fed patients: a comprehensive approach to diagnosis and management, *Nutr Clin Pract* 8(3):119-123, 1993.

Eisenberg PG: Feeding formulas, *RN* 57(12):46-52, 1994.

Eisenberg PG: Gastrostomy and jejunostomy tubes: a nurse's guide to tube feeding. Part 2, *RN* 57(11):54-60, 1994.

Estoup M: Approaches and limitations of medication delivery in patients with enteral feeding tubes, *Crit Care Nurse* 14(1):80-81, 1994.

Fater KH: Determining nasoenteral feeding tube placement, *MedSurg Nurs* 4(1):27-31, 1995.

Forloines-Lynn S: How to smooth the way for cyclic tube feedings, *Nursing* 26(3):57-60, 1996.

Forloines-Lynn S: Knowing how to manage the complications of tube feeding, *Nursing* 26(3):32m-32p, 1996.

Heavner B: Tube feeding choices: more than a game of chance, *Nursing* 26(10):32a-32d, 1996.

Heximer B: Spontaneous balloon rupture, *RN* 59(7):22-27, 1996.

Klang MG: Medicating tube fed patients, *Nursing* 26(1):18, 1996.

Matarese LE: Rationale and efficacy of specialized enteral nutrition, *Nutr Clin Pract* 9(2):58-64, 1994.

Mateo MA: Nursing management of enteral tube feedings, *Heart Lung* 25(4):318-323, 1996.

Metheny N, Reed L, Berglund G, Wehrle MA: Visual characteristics of aspirates from feeding tubes as a method for predicting tube location, *Nurs Res* 43(5):282-287, 1994.

Metheny N, Reed L, Worshek M, Clark J: How to aspirate fluid from small bore feeding tubes, *Am J Nurs* 93(5):86-88, 1993.

Miller D, Miller HW: Giving meds through the tube, *RN* 58(1):44-47, 1995.

Ouellette F: Pulmonary aspiration of enteral feedings: a model for prevention, *J Home Health Care Pract* 7(2):45-55, 1995.

Pratt JC, Tolbert CG: Tube feeding aspiration, *Am J Nurs* 96(5):37, 1996.

Ricciardi E, Brown D: Managing PEG tubes, *Am J Nurs* 94(10):29-31, 1994.

Saunderlin G: Mechanical bowel preparation in review, *MedSurg Nurs* 4(4):267-278, 1995.

Scanlan M, Frisch S: Nasoduodenal feeding tubes: prevention of occlusion, *J Neurosci Nurs* 24(5):256-259, 1992.

Shuster MH, Mancino JM: Ensuring successful home tube feeding in the geriatric population, *Geriatr Nurs* 15(2):67-81, 1994.

Sweed MR, Guenter P, Jones S: Nursing implications for the adult patient receiving nutritional support, *Med Surg Nurs* 4(2):99-110, 1995.

Viall CD: Location, location, location, *Nursing* 26(9):43-45, 1996.

Wurzback ME: Long term care nurses' ethical convictions about tube feeding, *West J Nurs Res* 18(1):63-76, 1996.

Young CK, White S: Preparing patients for tube feeding at home, *Am J Nurs* 92(4):46-53, 1992.

## Total Parenteral Nutrition

Anonymous: Correcting common problems with parenteral nutrition, *Nursing* 26(4):24p-24r, 1996.

Gianino S, Seltzer R, Eisenberg P: The ABC's of TPN, *RN* 59(2):42-47, 1996.

Masoorli S: Home IV therapy comes of age, *RN* 59(10):22-25, 1996.

Viall C: Taking the mystery out of TPN, *Nursing '95* 25(4):34-41, 1995.

## Bowel Obstruction

Anonymous: Bowel obstruction, *Am J Nurs* 93(5):51, 1993.

Barnie DC, Currier J: What's that GI tube being used for? *RN* 58(8):45-48, 1995.

McConnell EA: Loosening the grip of intestinal obstruction, *Nursing* 24(3):34-41, 1994.

McConnell EA: Managing a nasoenteric decompression tube, *Nursing* 24(3):18, 1994.

Peterson KJ, Solie CJ: Caring for the patient with intestinal obstruction, *Am J Nurs* 94(10):48A-48B, 1994.

Roberts MK: Assessing and treating volvulus, *Nursing* 22(2):56-57, 1992.

## Bowel Cancer

Ahlquist DA et al: Accuracy of fecal occult blood screening for colorectal neoplasia, *JAMA* 269(10):1262-1267, 1993.

Allison JE, Tekewa IS, Ransom LJ, Adrain AL: A comparison of fecal occult blood tests for colorectal cancer screening, *N Engl J Med* 334(3):155-159, 1996.

Bond JH, Volk EE, Wexner SD: Colorectal cancer: effective treatment, diligent follow-up, *Patient Care* 30(10):20-41, 1996.

Burris J, McGovern P: Mass colorectal cancer screening, *AAOHN J* 41(4):186-191, 1993.

Catalano MF, Grace ND: Getting to the cause of rectal bleeding, *Patient Care* 30(19):32-59, 1996.

Dammel T: Fecal occult blood testing, *Nursing* 27(7):44-45, 1997.

Dominitz JA, McCormick LH, Rex DK: Colorectal cancer: latest approaches to prevention and screening, *Patient Care* 30(7):124-149, 1996.

Ellis DJ, Reinus JF: Lower intestinal hemorrhage, *Crit Care Clin* 11(2):369-387, 1995.

Giovannucci E et al: Aspirin and the risk of colorectal cancer in women, *N Engl J Med* 333(10):609-614, 1995.

Giovannucci E, Willett WC: Dietary factors and the risk of colon cancer, *Ann Med* 26(6):443-452, 1994.

Launoy G, Herbert C, Gignoux M: Screening for colorectal cancer: the role of the general practitioner, *Am J Public Health* 84(10):1693-1694, 1994.

Mandel JS et al: Reducing mortality from colorectal cancer by screening for fecal occult blood, *N Engl J Med* 328(19):1365-1371, 1993.

Mayer RJ, Thomas P: Colon cancer: knowledge is power, *Harvard Health Lett* 20(12):4-6, 1995.

Meissner JE: Caring for patients with colorectal cancer, *Nursing* 26(11):60-61, 1996.

O'Connell MJ, Rich TA, Steele GD: Low rectal Ca: sphincter-sparing strategies, *Patient Care* 22:32-48, 1992.

Ransohoff DF, Lang CA: Sigmoidoscopic screening in the 1990's, *JAMA* 269(10):1278-1281, 1993.

Reddy BS: Dietary fat, calories, and fiber in colon cancer, *Prev Med* 22:738-749, 1993.

Toribara NW, Sleisenger MH: Screening for colorectal cancer, *N Engl J Med* 332(13):861-867, 1995.

Truszkowski JA, Summers RW: Colorectal neoplasms, *Postgrad Med* 98(5):97-112, 1995.

Winawer SJ et al: Risk of colorectal cancer in the families of patients with adenomatous polyps, *N Engl J Med* 334(2):82-87, 1996.

Witt ME: Current management of adults with colorectal cancer, *MedSurg Nurs* 2(2):105-111, 1993.


### Ostomies


Blaylock B: Enhancing self care of the elderly client: practical teaching tips for ostomy care, *J ET Nurs* 18(4):118-121, 1991.

Hampton B, Bryant R: *Ostomies and continent diversions: nursing management,* St Louis, 1992, Mosby.

Krasner D: Six steps to successful stoma care, *RN* 56(7):32-38, 1993.

Long LV: Ileostomy care—overcoming the obstacles, *Nursing '91* 21(10):73-75, 1991.

Paulford-Lecher N: Teaching your patient stoma care, *Nursing '93* 23(9):47-49, 1993.


### Anorectal Disorders


Metcalf A: Anorectal disorders, *Postgrad Med* 98(5):81-94, 1995.

Rao SSC: Functional colonic and anorectal disorders, *Postgrad Med* 98(5):115-126, 1995.

Shoji BT, Becker JM: Colorectal disease in the elderly patient, *Surg Clin North Am* 74(2):293-316, 1995.


## Chapter 42 Management of Persons with Problems of the Gallbladder and Exocrine Pancreas

### Gallbladder Disease


Babb RR: Managing gallbladder disease with prostaglandin inhibitors, *Postgrad Med* 94(1):127-128, 130, 203-205, 1993.

Diehl AK: Laparoscopic cholecystectomy: too much of a good thing? *JAMA* 270(12):1469-1470, 1993.

Everhart JE: Contributions of obesity and weight loss to gallstone disease, *Ann Intern Med* 119(10):1029-1035, 1993.

Fenster LF, Lonborg R, Thirlby RC, Traverso LW: What symptoms does cholecystectomy cure? *Am J Surg* 169(5):533-538, 1995.

Gauwitz DF: Endoscopic cholecystectomy: the patient friendly alternative, *Nursing* 20(12):58-59, 1992.

Ghiloni BW: Cholelithiasis: current treatment options, *Am Fam Physician* 48(5):762-768, 1993.

Giurgiu DI, Roslyn JJ: Treatment of gallstones in the 1990's, *Prim Care Clinicians Office Pract* 23(3):497-513, 1996.

Legorreta AP et al: Increased cholecystectomy rate after the introduction of laparoscopic cholecystectomy, *JAMA* 270(12):1429-1432, 1993.

Moscati RM: Cholelithiasis, cholecystitis, and pancreatitis, *Emerg Med Clin North Am* 14(4):19-37, 1996.

National Institutes of Health: National Institutes of Health Consensus Development Conference Statement on Gallstones and Laparoscopic Cholecystectomy, *Am J Surg* 165(4):390-398, 1993.

Ondrusek RS: Cholecystectomy: an update, *RN* 56(1):28-31, 1993.

Pinto KM: Acalculous cholecystitis: a case report, *Nurse Pract* 21(10):120-122, 1996.

Price P, Hartranft TH: New trends in the treatment of calculus disease of the biliary tract, *J Am Board Fam Pract* 8(1):22-28, 1995.

Schweisinger WH, Diehl AK: Changing indications for laparoscopic cholecystectomy, *Surg Clin North Am* 76(3):493-504, 1996.

Shaw B: Primary care for women: management and treatment of gastrointestinal disorders, *J Nurse Midwifery* 41(2):75-79, 1996.

Stillman A: Laparoscopic cholecystectomy, *AORN J* 57(2):429-436, 1993.

Vanek VW, Rhodes R, Dallis DJ: Results of laparoscopic versus open cholecystectomy in a community hospital, *South Med J* 88(5):555-566, 1995.


### Pancreatitis


Ambrose MS, Dreher HM: Pancreatitis—managing a flareup, *Nursing* 26(4):33-39, 1996.

Baker CC, Huynh T: Acute pancreatitis—surgical management, *Crit Care Clin* 11 (2):311-322, 1995.

Domingues-Munoz JE, Malfertheiner P: Management of severe acute pancreatitis, *Gastroenterologist* 4:248-253, 1993.

Evans JD et al: Outcome of surgery for chronic pancreatitis, *Br J Surg* 84(5):624-629, 1997.

Forsmark CE, Toskes PP: Acute pancreatitis-medical management, *Crit Care Clin* 11(2):295-306, 1995.

Gupta PK, Al-Kawas FH: Acute pancreatitis: diagnosis and management, *Am Fam Physician* 52(2):435-443, 1995.

Haber P et al: Individual susceptibility to alcoholic pancreatitis: still an enigma, *J Lab Clin Med* 125(3):305-312, 1995.

Haber PS, Pirola RC, Wilson JS: Clinical update: management of acute pancreatitis, *J Gastroenterol Hepatol* 12(3):189-197, 1997.

Huber D, Hemstrom M: GI nursing: the community health aspect, *Gastroenterol Nurs* 16(2):219-222, 1994.

Kohn CL, Brozenec S, Foster PF: Nutritional support for the patient with pancreatobiliary disease, *Crit Care Nurs Clin North Am* 5(1):37-45, 1993.

Krumberger JM: Acute pancreatitis, *Crit Care Nurs Clin North Am* 5(1):185-201, 1993.

Marshall JB: Acute pancreatitis: a review with an emphasis on new developments, *Arch Intern Med* 153(6):1185-1193, 1993.

Marulendra S, Kirby DF: Nutrition support in pancreatitis, *Nutr Clin Pract* 10(2):45-53, 1995.

McClave SA, Greene LM, Snider HL: Comparison of the safety of early enteral vs. parenteral nutrition in mild acute pancreatitis, *JPEN J Parenter Enteral Nutr* 21(1):14-20, 1997.

McConnell E, Lewis LW: Managing the patient with pancreatitis, *Nursing* 21(11):98-102, 1991.

Meier PB: Who gets and what causes pancreatitis? *J Lab Clin Med* 125(3):298-300, 1995.

Murr MM et al: Pancreatic cancer, *CA Cancer J Clin* 44(2):304-314, 1994.

Noone J: Acute pancreatitis: an Orem approach to nursing assessment and care, *Crit Care Nurse* 15(4):27-37, 1995.

Peterson KJ, Solie CJ: Interpreting lab values in pancreatitis, *Am J Nurs* 94(11):45A-45B, 56F, 1994.

Sidhu SS, Tandon RK: The pathogenesis of chronic pancreatitis, *Postgrad Med* 71(2):67-70, 1995.

Smith A: When the pancreas fails, *Am J Nurs* 91(9):38-48, 1991.

Thompson C: Managing acute pancreatitis, *RN* 55(3):52-54, 1992.

Vaona B et al: Food intake of patients with chronic pancreatitis after onset of the disease, *Am J Clin Nutr* 65(3):851-854, 1997.


### Pancreatic Cancer


Greifzo S, Dest V: When the diagnosis is pancreatic cancer, *RN* 54(3):38-41, 1991.

Price TF, Payne RL, Oberleitner MG: Familial pancreatic cancer in South Louisiana, *Cancer Nurs* 19(4):272-282, 1996.

## Chapter 43 Assessment of the Renal System


### Pyelonephritis

McMurray B, Wrenn K, Wright S: Usefulness of blood cultures in pyelonephritis, *Am J Emerg Med* 15(2):137-140, 1997.

### Renal Artery Stenosis

Pickering T, Mann S: Is there a role for non-invasive screening tests in diagnosing renal artery stenosis? *J Hypertens* 14(11):1265-1266, 1996.


## Chapter 44 Management of Persons with Problems of the Kidney and Urinary Tract


### Polycystic Kidney Disease

McCarthy S, McMullen M: Autosomal dominant polycystic kidney disease, *ANNA J* 24(1):45-53, 1997.

### Urinary Tract Infection

Holmes H, editor: *Mastering geriatric care,* Springhouse, Penna, 1997, Springhouse.

Marchiondo K: A new look at urinary tract infection, *Am J Nurs* 98(3):34-39, 1998.

### Pyelonephritis

Johnson J: Recognizing and treating acute pyelonephritis, *Emerg Med* 24(3): 24-26, 29-30, 33, 1992.

Millar L: Pyelonephritis, *Hosp Pract* 28(suppl 2):31-35, 1993.

### Renal Tuberculosis

Wiseman K: Tb: an old disease with a new face, *ANNA J* 22(6):541-556, 1995.

### Nephrotic Syndrome

Adhikari M: Comparison of noninvasive methods for distinguishing steroid sensitive nephrotic syndrome from focal glomerulosclerosis, *J Lab Clin Med* 129(1):47-52, 1997.

### Renal Artery Stenosis

Grafe D, Hanson S: Sonographic detection of renal artery stenosis, *J Diagn Med Sonogr* 11(2):67-75, 1995.

Ram C, Fierro G: Secondary hypertension: when to suspect and how to diagnose renal artery stenosis, *Consultant* 35(10):1454-1458, 1995.

Rimmer J: The consequences of renal artery stenosis, *Hosp Pract* 29(3):29-30, 32, 35, 1994.

### Renal Calculi

Beare P, Myers J: *Principles and practice of adult health nursing,* St Louis, 1994, Mosby.

Ruth-Shad L: Renal calculi, *Am J Nurs* 95(11):50, 1995.

Shellenbarger T, Krouse A: Treating and preventing kidney stones, *MedSurg Nurs* 3(5):389-394, 1994.

### Renal Trauma

Sheehy S, Jimmerson C: *Manual of clinical trauma,* St Louis, 1996, Mosby.

### Renal/Urinary Malignancies

Hald D, Aehring T, Razor B: The pathogenesis and management of urethelial malignancies, *J Wound Ostomy Continence Nurs* 23(3):144-149, 1996.

Klein E: Options in the surgical treatment of bladder cancer, *J ET Nurs* 19(4):122-125, 1992.

Letzig M, Conway A: Interleukin 2 therapy for renal cell carcinoma: indications, effects, and nursing implications, *Crit Care Nurse* 16(5):20-22, 26, 1996.

### Urinary Diversions

Golden T, Ratliff C: Development and implementation of a clinical pathway for radical cystectomy and urinary system reconstruction, *J Wound Ostomy Continence Nurs* 24(2):3, 1997.

Raleigh E, Berry M, Montie J: A comparison of adjustments to urinary diversions: a pilot study, *J Wound Ostomy Continence Nurs* 22(1):58-63, 1995.

Walsh B: Urostomy and urinary pH, *ET Nurs* 9(4):110-113, 1992.

### Urinary Retention

Duffy L et al: Clean intermittent catheterization: safe, cost effective bladder management for male residents of VA nursing homes, *J Am Geriatr Soc* 43(8):865-870, 1995.

Jolley S: Intermittent catheterization for post-operative urine retention, *Nurs Times* 93(33):46-47, 1997.

Jolley S, Tuneycliff L: No holding back—post operative urinary retention, *Nurs Times* 92(41):80, 82, 1996.

Kirton C: Assessing for bladder distention, *Nursing* 27(4):64, 1997.

Kurdtz M, VanZandt K, Burns J: Comparison study of home catheter cleaning methods, *Rehabil Nurs* 20(4):212-214, 1995.

Moore D, Edwards K: Using a portable bladder scan to reduce the incidence of nosocomial UTI, *MedSurg Nurs* 6(1):39-43, 1997.

Newman D, Smith D, Goetz G: Neurogenic bladder dysfunction causing urinary retention, *J Home Health Care Pract* 4(4):45-60, 1992.

Williams M, Wallhage M, Dowling G: Urinary retention in hospitalized elderly women, *J Gerontol Nurs* 19(2):7-14, 1993.

Wren K, Wren T: Postsurgical urinary retention, *Urol Nurs* 16(2):45-49, 1996.

### Urinary Incontinence

Catanzaro J: Managing incontinence: an update, *RN* 59(10):39-45, 1996.

Cliner J: A nursing management protocol for incontinence, *Rehabil Nurs* 19(3):141-144, 1994.

Connor P, Kooker B: Nurse's knowledge, attitudes, and practices in managing urinary incontinence in the acute care setting, *MedSurg Nurs* 5(2):87-92, 1996.

Johnson V, Gary M: Urinary incontinence: a review, *J Wound Ostomy Continence Nurs* 22(1):8-15, 1995.

Ouslander J et al: Predictors of successful prompted voiding among incontinent nursing home residents, *JAMA* 273(17):1366-1370, 1995.

Resnick B, Slocum D, Ra L, Moffett P: Geriatric rehab: nursing interventions and outcomes focusing on urinary function and knowledge of medicine, *Rehabil Nurs* 21(3):142-147, 1995.

Resnick N: Urinary incontinence in older adults, *Hosp Pract* 27(10):139-142, 1992.

Resnick N, Gillyatt P: Staying dry, *Harvard Health Lett* 21(2):3-5, 1995.

### Diuretics

Holcomb S: Understanding the ins and outs of diuretic therapy, *Nursing* 24(2):34-40, 1997.


## Chapter 45 Management of Persons with Renal Failure


### Renal Diets

Rigalleau V et al: Low protein diet in uremia: effects of glucose metabolism and energy production rate, *Kidney Int* 5(9):1222-1227, 1997.

Varella L, Utermoklen V: Nutritional support for the patient with renal failure, *Crit Care Nurs Clin North Am* 5(1):79-96, 1993.

### Dialysis

Dirkes S: A dialysis alternative more nurses can run, *RN* 60(5):20-26, 1997.

Dunetz P: Coordinating care for dialysis patients, *Nursing* 24(9):32hn1-32hn4, 1997.

Naylor M, Roe B: A study of the efficacy of dressings in preventing infections of CAPD catheter exit sites, *J Clin Nurs* 6(1):17-24, 1997.

Newman L, Hanslik T, Tessman M: Cost effective automated peritoneal dialysis for patients with average to low transport . . . an 8-10 mL mixed APD/CAPD regimen, *ANNA J* 21(5):271-273, 1994.

Ponferrada et al: Home visit effectiveness for peritoneal dialysis patients, *ANNA J* 20(3):333-336, 1993.

Stark J: Dialysis choices: turning the tide in acute renal failure, *Nursing* 22(2):41-46, 1997.

### Acute Renal Failure

Algren R et al: Anartide in acute renal failure, *N Engl J Med* 336(12):828-834, 1997.

Catts L: Renal disorders and their management. In Urden LD, Lough ME, Stacy KM, editors: *Priorities in critical care nursing,* ed 2, St Louis, 1996, Mosby.

Humes H: Acute renal failure: the promise of new therapies, *N Engl J Med* 336(12):870-871, 1997.

King B: Detecting acute renal failure, *RN* 57(3):34-39, 1994.

King B: Preserving renal function, *RN* 60(8):34-40, 1997.

Olivero J: Post surgical acute renal failure: which patients are at greatest risk, *J Crit Illness* 9(7):679-685, 1994.

Pesola G, Akhaven I, Carion G: Urinary creatinine excretion in the ICU: low excretion does not mean inadequate collection, *Am J Crit Care* 12(6):462-466, 1993.

Wood J, Bosely C: Acute post renal failure: reversing the problem: here's how to recognize and respond to this potentially fatal renal condition, *Nursing* 25(3):48-50, 1995.

### Chronic Renal Failure/End Stage Renal Disease

Blanford N: Renal transplantation: a case study of the ideal, *Crit Care Nurse* 13(1):46-55, 1993.

Goodnough L, Monk T, Andriole T: Erythropoietin therapy, *N Engl J Med* 336(13):933-938, 1997.

Guerrero S, Gomez N: Dealing with end stage renal disease, *Am J Nurs* 97(10):44-51, 1997.

Harries F: Psychosocial care in end stage renal failure, *Prof Nurse* 12(2):124-126, 1996.

Price C: Issues related to care of the critically ill patient with end stage renal disease, *AACN Clin Iss Crit Care Nurse* 3(3):585-595, 1992.

Rowe M: The impact of internal and external resources on functional outcomes in chronic illness, *Res Nurs Health* 19(6):485-497, 1996.

## Chapter 46 Assessment of the Reproductive System and Sexuality

### General

Berek JS, Adashi EY, Hillard PA: *Novak's gynecology,* ed 12, Baltimore, 1996, William & Wilkins.

Ernster V: Mammography screening for woman aged 40-49—a guidelines saga and a clarion call for informed decision making, *Am J Public Health* 87:1103-1106, 1997.

Ferreira N: Sexually transmitted *Chlamydia trachomatis, Nurse Pract Forum* 8:70-76, 1997.

Isacson C, Kurman RJ: The Bethesda system: a new classification for managing Pap smears, *Contemp OB/GYN* 6:67-74, 1995.

Lee KR, Ashfaq R, Birdsong GG et al: Comparison of conventional Papanicolaou smears and a fluid-based, thin-layer system for cervical cancer screening, *Obstet Gynecol* 90:278-284, 1997.

Mouton J, Roel V, van der Meijden W et al: Detection of *Chlamydia trachomatis* in males and female urine specimens by using the amplified *Chlamydia trachomatis* test, *J Clin Microbiol* 35(6):1369-1372, 1997.

Paukku M, Puolakkainen M, Apter D et al: First void urine testing for *Chlamydia trachomatis* by polymerase chain reaction in asymptomatic women, *Sex Transm Dis* 24(6):343-346, 1997.

Peterson E: Laboratory detection of *Chlamydia trachomatis, West J Med* 167(1):36, 1997.

Wertlake PT, Francus K, Newkirk GR: Effectiveness of the Papanicolaou smear and speculoscopy as compared with the Pap smear alone: a community based clinical trial, *Obstet Gynecol* 90:421-427, 1997.

Worthington S, Rubin M: Nurse-midwifery evaluation and management of cervical pathology and the colposcopic examination, *J Nurse Midwifery* 38(suppl 2):36S-41S, 1993.

Younkin EQ, Davis MS: *Women's health, a primary care clinical guide,* Norwalk, Conn, 1994, Appleton & Lange.

## Chapter 47 Management of Women with Reproductive Problems

### Infections/Inflammations

Acuzzio J, Joegsberg B: PID: hard to find but essential to treat, *Contemp OB/GYN-NP* 1(2):6-11, 1993.

Kottman LM: Pelvic inflammatory disease—clinical overview, *J Obstet Gynecol Neonatal Nurs* 24(8):759-761, 1995.

Overman B: The vagina as an ecologic system, *J Nurse Midwifery* 38(3):146-151, 1993.

Reed BD, Eyler A: Vaginal infections—diagnosis and management, *Am Fam Physician* 47(8):1805-1818, 1993.

Thomason J, Scaglione N: Basics of managing bacterial vaginosis, *Contemp OB/GYN-NP* 1(3):15-17, 1993.

### Menstrual Disorders

Clark-Coller T: Dysfunctional uterine bleeding and amenorrhea: differential diagnosis and management, *J Nurse Midwifery* 36(1):49-62, 1991.

Colbry S: A review of toxic shock syndrome: the need for education still exists, *Nurse Pract* 17(9):39-46, 1992.

Creehan PA: Toxic shock syndrome: an opportunity for nursing intervention, *J Obstet Gynecol Neonatal Nurs* 24(6):557-561, 1995.

Endicott J et al: PMS: new treatment that really works, *Patient Care* 30(7):88-96, 1996.

Garner C: Endometriosis: what you need to know, *RN* 60(1):27-31, 1997.

Garner C: Uses of GnRH agonists, *J Obstet Gynecol Neonatal Nurs* 23(7):563-570, 1994.

Hanrahan SN: Historical review of menstrual shock syndrome, *Women's Health* 21(2-3):141-165, 1994.

Lewis LL: One year in the life of a woman with premenstrual syndrome, *Nurs Res* 44(2):11-115, 1995.

Pepping PB: Endometriosis—a nursing perspective, *Innovations Women's Health Nurs* 1(1):2-5, 1994.

### Structural Problems/Hysterectomy

Bernhard LA: Understanding fibroids, *Innovations Women's Health Nurs* 1(2):21-14, 1994.

Ravkinar V, Chen E: Hysterectomies: what are the indications? *Obstet Gynecol Clin North Am* 21(9):405-411, 1994.

Wood N: The use of vaginal pessaries for uterine prolapse, *Nurse Pract* 17(7):31-38, 1992.

### Cancer of the Female Reproductive System

Barber H, Creasman W, Knapp R: A rational approach to ovarian masses, *Patient Care* 27(1):50-72, 1993.

Blesch K, Prohaska T: Cervical cancer screening in older women: issues and interventions, *Cancer Nurs* 14(3):141-147, 1991.

Brucks JA: Ovarian cancer—the most lethal gynecologic malignancy, *Nurs Clin North Am* 27(4):835-845, 1992.

Colodny CS: Colposcopy and cervical biopsy, *Patient Care* 29(11):66-71, 1995.

Dillon P: Ovarian cancer: confronting the "silent killer," *Nursing* 24(5):66-69, 1994.

Dumas MAS: What it's like to belong to the cancer club, *Am J Nurs* 96(4):40-42, 1996.

Fox S, Haney LT: Taxol: new hope for cancer patients, *RN* 57(11):33-36, 1994.

Held JL: Cancer care—preventing cervical cancer, *Nursing* 25(2):24-26, 1995.

Ivey C: When your patient has ovarian cancer, *RN* 57(11):26-32, 1994.

Lilly L, Scott H: What you need to know about taxol, *Am J Nurs* 93(12):46-50, 1993.

Lowdermilk DL: Home care of the patient with gynecologic cancer, *J Obstet Gynecol Neonatal Nurs* 24(2):157-160, 1995.

McMullin M: Holistic care of the patient with cervical cancer, *Nurs Clin North Am* 27(4):847-858, 1992.

Moore D: New therapies for ovarian cancer, *Female Patient* 18(9):29-32, 1993.

Shurpin KM: Ovarian cancer, *Am J Nurs* 97(4):34-35, 1997.

Thompson SD, Szukiewicz-Nugent JM, Walczak JR: When ovarian cancer strikes, *Nursing* 26(10):33-38, 1996.

Wender R: Cancer screening in primary care, *Female Patient* 18(6):33-39, 1993.

### Infertility

Hirsch AM, Hirsch SM: The long term psychosocial effects of infertility, *J Obstet Gynecol Neonatal Nurs* 24(6):517-520, 1995.

## Chapter 48 Management of Persons with Problems of the Breast

### General

Bilimoria MM, Morrow M: The woman at increased risk for breast cancer: evaluation and management strategies, *CA Cancer J Clin* 45(5):263-278, 1995.

Boyle DM, Engelking C, Blesch KS et al: Oncology Nursing Society Position Paper on Cancer and Aging: the mandate for oncology nursing, *Oncol Nurs Forum* 19(6):913-933, 1992.

Clark JC, Mc Gee RF: *Core curriculum for oncology nursing*, ed 2, Philadelphia, 1992, WB Saunders.

Eddleman J, Warren C: Cancer resource center, *Cancer Pract* 2(5):371-378, 1994.

Galassi A: Long-term sequelae of primary breast cancer, *Innovations Oncol Nurs* 10(3):54-57, 1994.

Gale D, Charette J: *Oncology nursing care plans,* El Paso, Tex, 1994, Skidmore-Roth.

Groenwald SL, HansenFrogge M, Goodman M, Yarbro C: *Cancer symptom management,* Boston, 1996, Jones & Bartlett.

Hetelekidis S, Schnitt SJ, Morrow M, Harris JR: Management of ductal carcinoma in-situ, *CA Cancer J Clin* 45(4):244-253, 1995.

Langer AS, Dow KH: The breast cancer advocacy movement and nursing, *Oncol Nurs* 1(3):1-12, 1994.

Markman M: An update on breast cancer: evolving treatments and persistent questions, *Cleve Clin J Med* 63(1):48-56, 1996.

McCorkle R, Grant M, Frank-Stromborg M, Baird S, editors: *Cancer nursing,* ed 2, Philadelphia, 1996, WB Saunders.

Miaskowski C, Dibble SL: Prevalence and morbidity of pain in women with breast cancer, *Innovations Breast Cancer Care* 1(1):6-8, 1995.

Otto S, editor: *Oncology nursing,* ed 3, St Louis, 1997, Mosby.

Tokarsky JM, McLaughlin MA: Advantages of using clinical pathways for breast cancer patients, *Innovations Breast Cancer Care* 1(2):26-29, 1995.

### Adjuvant Therapy

Bilezikian JP: Major issues regarding estrogen replacement therapy in postmenopausal women, *J Women's Health* 3(4):273-281, 1994.

Bonadonna G, Valagussa P, Zucali R, Salvadori B: Primary chemotherapy in surgically resectable breast cancer, *CA Cancer J Clin* 45(4):227-243, 1995.

Boothe VA, Pommier RF, Vetto JT: Tamoxifen in the treatment and chemoprevention of breast cancer, *Cancer Pract* 2(5):335-342, 1994.

Esparza-Guerra LT: Docetaxel: advancing the treatment of metastatic breast cancer, *COPE* 16-18, May/June 1996.

Faulkenberry JE, Mante MP: Taxol: nursing interventions, *Nurs Interventions Oncol* 6:3-8, 1994.

Jacobson JA et al: Ten year results of conservation with mastectomy in the treatment of stage I and II breast cancer, *N Engl J Med* 332(17):907-911, 1995.

Osborne CK, Elledge RM, Fuqua AW: Estrogen receptors in breast cancer therapy, *Sci Am Sci Med* 32-41, January/February 1996.

Perry MC, editor: *The chemotherapy source book,* Baltimore, 1992, Williams & Wilkins.

Veronesi U et al: Radiotherapy after breast-preserving surgery in women with localized cancer of the breast, *N Engl J Med* 328(22):1587-1591, 1993.

### Genetics

Bove CM, Fry ST, MacDonald DJ: Presymptomatic and predisposition genetic testing: ethical and social considerations, *Semin Oncol Nurs* 13(2):135-140, 1997.

Biesecker BB: Psychological issues in cancer genetics, *Semin Oncol Nurs* 13(2):129-134, 1997.

Jenkins J: Educational issues related to cancer genetics, *Semin Oncol Nurs* 13(2):141-144, 1997.

Lerman C, Croyle RT: Emotional and behavioral responses to genetic testing for susceptibility to cancer, *Oncology* 10(2):191-195, 1996.

Mahon SM, Casperson DS: Hereditary cancer syndrome. Part II: psychosocial issues, concerns, and screening—results of a qualitative study, *Oncol Nurs Forum* 22(5):775-782, 1995.

Weber BL: Genetic testing for breast cancer, *Sci Am SCI MED* 12-21, January/February 1996.

Williams JK: Principles of genetics and cancer, *Semin Oncol Nurs* 13(2):68-73, 1997.

### Lymphedema

Carter BJ: Women's experiences of lymphedema, *Oncol Nurs Forum* 24(5):875-882, 1997.

Farncombe M, Daniels G, Cross L: Lymphedema: the seemingly forgotten complication, *J Pain Sympt Manage* 9(4):269-276, 1994.

Granda C: Nursing management of patients with lymphedema associated with breast cancer therapy, *Cancer Nurs* 17(3):229-235, 1994.

Mitchell HS: Breast cancer and arm lymphoedema—what can be done? *J Cancer Care* 4(2):61-67, 1995.

Newman ML, Brennan M, Passik S: Palliative care rounds: lymphedema complicated by pain and psychological distress; a case with complex treatment needs, *J Pain Sympt Manage* 12(6):376-379, 1996.

### Prevention/Screening

Douglass M, Bartolucci A, Waterbor J, Sirles A: Breast cancer early detection: differences between African American and white women's health beliefs and detection practices, *Oncol Nurs Forum* 22(5):835-837, 1995.

Grier S: Breast cancer: prevention and detection, *Oncol Patient Care* 3(3):5-6, 13, 1993.

Loescher LJ: Strategies for preventing breast cancer, *Innovations Oncol Nurs* 9(1):15-19, 1993.

McCance KL, Mooney KH, Field R, Smith KR: Influence of others in motivating women to obtain breast cancer screening, *Cancer Pract* 4(3):141-146, 1996.

Mettlin C, Smart CR: Breast cancer detection guidelines for women aged 40-49 years: rationale for the ACS reaffirmation of recommendations *CA Cancer J Clin* 44(4):248-255, 1994.

Salazar MK: Hispanic women's beliefs about breast cancer and mammography, *Cancer Nurs* 19(6):437-446, 1996.

Schildkraut JM, Lerman C, Lustbader E, Rimer BK: Adherence to mammography among subgroups of women at high risk for breast cancer, *J Women's Health* 4(6):645-654, 1995.

### Psychoemotional Issues

Deane KA, Degner LF: Determining the information needs of women after breast biopsy procedures, *AORN J* 65(4):767-768, 775-776, 1997.

DeGrasse CE, Hugo K: Supportive care needs of women undergoing breast diagnosis and their families: a focus for nursing interventions, *Can Oncol Nurs J* 6(4):185-190, 1996.

Hilton BA: Getting back to normal: the family experience during early stage breast cancer, *Oncol Nurs Forum* 23(4):605-614, 1996.

Northhouse LL, Tocco KM, West P: Coping with a breast biopsy: how healthcare professionals can help women and their husbands, *Oncol Nurs Forum* 24(3):473-470, 1997.

### Quality of Life

Ferrell BR: Overview of breast cancer: quality of life, *Oncol Patient Care* 3(3):7-9, 1993.

Hilton BA: Getting back to normal: the family experience during early stage breast cancer, *Oncol Nurs Forum* 23(4):605-614, 1996.

Limoges M, Thompson CH: Peer counseling: enhancing women's adjustments to breast cancer, *Innovations Oncol Nurs* 10(4):1-19, 1993.

### Sexuality and Body Image

Anderson MS, Johnson J: Restoration of body image and self-esteem for women after cancer treatment, *Cancer Pract* 2(5):345-349, 1994.

Horwood KV, O'Conner AP: Sexuality and breast cancer: overview of issues, *Innovations Oncol Nurs* 10(2):30-33, 51, 1994.

### The Elderly

Blustein J: Medicare coverage, supplemental insurance and the use of mammography by older women, *N Engl J Med* 332(17):1138-1143, 1995.

Byrne A, Carney DN: Cancer in the elderly, *Curr Probl Cancer* 17(3):145-220, 1993.

Ludwick R, Rushing B, Biordi DL: Breast cancer and the older woman: information and images, *Health Care Women Int* 15:235-242, 1994.

Masetti R et al: Breast cancer in women 70 years of age or older, *J Am Geriatr Soc* 44(4):390-393, 1996.

Silliman RA et al: Breast cancer care in old age: what we know, don't know, and do, *J Natl Cancer Inst* 85(3):190-197, 1993.

## Chapter 49 Management of Men with Reproductive Problems

### Benign Prostatic Hyperplasia (BPH)

*Benign prostatic hyperplasia: diagnosis and treatment,* Clinical Practice Guidelines No 8, Rockville, Md, 1994, Agency for Health Care Policy and Research, Public Health Service, US Department of Health and Human Services.

Bruskewitz R, Cassel C: Benign prostatic hyperplasia: intervene or wait? *Hosp Pract* 27(8):99-115, 1992.

Hicks RJ, Cook JB: Managing patients with benign prostatic hyperplasia, *Am Fam Physician* 52(1):135-142, 1995.

McConnell JD: Benign prostatic hyperplasia: hormonal treatment, *Urol Clin North Am* 22(2):387-399, 1995.

Miller CA: New medication for the treatment of benign prostatic hyperplasia, *Geriatr Nurs* 14(2):111-112, 1993.

Roehrborn CG: The Agency for Health Care Policy and Research: clinical guidelines for the diagnosis and treatment of benign prostatic hyperplasia, *Urol Clin North Am* 22(2):445-453, 1995.

### Prostate Cancer

Brenner ZR, Krenzer ME: Update on cryosurgical ablation for prostate cancer, *Am J Nurs* 95(4):44-48, 1995.

D'Elia FL, Yomella LG: Prostate cancer update, *Compr Ther* 21(1):35-40, 1995.

Greifzu S, Tiedemann D: Prostate cancer: the pros and cons of treatment, *RN* 58(6):22-26, 1995.

Held JL, Osborne DM, Volpe H, Waldman A: Cancer of the prostate: treatment and nursing implications, *Oncol Nurs Forum* 21(9):1517-1529, 1994.

Keetch DW, Moore S, Shea L: Cryosurgical ablation of the prostate, *AORN J* 61(5):807-820, 1995.

Moore S et al: Nerve sparing prostatectomy, *Am J Nurs* 92(4):59-64, 1992.

Pobursky J: Prostate cancer: detection, treatment options, *Today's OR Nurse* 17(3):5-9, 1995.

### Impotence

Bryant R, Boarini J: Treatment options for men with sexual dysfunction, *J ET Nurs* 19(4):131-142, 1992.

Kuritzky L: Solutions for patients with erectile dysfunction, *Hosp Pract* 30(12):24G-24K, 1995.

Montorsi F, Guazzoni G, Rigatti P et al: Pharmacological management of erectile dysfunction, *Drugs* 50(3):465-479, 1995.

O'Keefe M, Hunt DK: Assessment on treatment of impotence, *Med Clin North Am* 79(2):415-433, 1995.

### Miscellaneous

Donovan DA, Nicholas PK: Prostatitis: diagnosis and treatment in primary care, *Nurse Pract* 22(4):144-156, 1997.

Gordon SI, Brenden MA, Wyble JS et al: When the Dx is penile cancer, *RN* 60(3):41-44, 1997.

Hans JM, Butta PG, Giruin S: A comprehensive and efficient process for counseling patients desiring sterilization, *Nurse Pract* 22(6):52-66, 1997.

Higgs D: The patient with testicular cancer: nursing management of chemotherapy, *Oncol Nurs Forum* 17:243-249, 1990.

Kaler S: Epididymitis in the young adult male, *Nurse Pract* 15(5):10-16, 1990.

Lasater S: Testicular cancer, a perioperative challenge, *AORN J* 51(2):513-526, 1990.

Tonetti J, Tonetti J: Testicular torsion or acute epididymitis? Diagnosis and treatment, *J Emerg Nurs* 16(2):96-98, 1990.

## Chapter 50 Management of Persons with Sexually Transmitted Diseases

### General

Bonny AE, Biro FM: Recognizing and treating STDS in the adolescent, *Contemp OB/GYN* 37-57, November 1997.

Centers for Disease Control and Prevention: Sexual behaviors that contribute to unintended pregnancy and STDs, including HIV infection, *MMWR* 45(SS-4):16-19, 1996.

Lande RE: Controlling sexually transmitted diseases, *Popul Rep Ser L* No 9, 1993.

### Bacterial Vaginosis

Ahmed-Jushuf IH, Shahmanesh M, Arya OP: The treatment of bacterial vaginosis with a 3 day course of 2% clindamycin cream: results of a multicentre, double blind, placebo controlled trial, *Genitourin Med* 71:254-256, 1995.

Fischbach F et al: Efficacy of clindamycin vaginal cream versus oral metronidazole in the treatment of bacterial vaginosis, *Obstet Gynecol* 82(3):405-411, 1993.

Hill GB, Livengood CH: Bacterial vaginosis-associated microflora and effect of topical intravaginal clindamycin, *Am J Obstet Gynecol* 171(5):1198-1204, 1994.

Hillier SL et al: Association between bacterial vaginosis and preterm delivery of a low-birth-weight infant, *N Engl J Med* 333(26):1737-1742, 1995.

Meis PJ et al: The preterm prediction study: significance of vaginal infections, *Am J Obstet Gynecol* 173(4):1231-1235, 1995.

### Chlamydia

Alexander LL et al: A national survey of nurse practitioner chlamydia knowledge and treatment practices of female patients, *Nurse Pract Am J Prim Health Care* 21(5):48-53, 1996.

Bell TA: *Chlamydia trachomatis* infections in adolescents, *Med Clin North Am* 74(5):1225-1233, 1990.

Ferreira N: Sexually transmitted *Chlamydia trachomatis, Nurse Pract Forum* 8(2):70-76, 1997.

Hillis SD, Wasserheit JN: Screening for chlamydia—a key to the prevention of pelvic inflammatory disease, *N Engl J Med* 334(21):1399-1400, 1996.

Kent ALJ: *Chlamydia trachomatis*: prevalence and risk factors in a family planning setting, *Nurse Pract Am J Prim Health Care* 19(8):30-34, 1994.

Magid D et al: Doxycycline compared with azithromycin for treating women with genital *Chlamydia trachomatis* infections: an incremental cost-effectiveness analysis, *Ann Intern Med* 124(4):389-399, 1996.

Rodgers K: CDC recommends aggressive treatment of chlamydia, *Drug Top* 13(23):51, 1995.

### Human Papilloma Virus

Adimora A, Quinlivan E: Human papillomavirus infection: recent findings on progression to cervical cancer, *Postgrad Med* 98(3):109-120, 1995.

Brodell R, Miller D: Human papillomavirus infection: treatment options for warts, *Am Fam Physician,* 53(1):135-143, 148-150, 1996.

Ghim S et al: Human papillomaviruses: their clinical significance in the management of cervical carcinoma, *Oncology* 9(4):279-285, 1995.

Schiffman M, Vittorio C: Epidemiology of human papillomaviruses, *Dermatol Clin* 13:561-574, 1995.

Stone K: Human papillomavirus infection and genital warts: update on epidemiology and treatment, *Clin Infect Dis* 1(suppl 20):91-97, 1995.

Stegbauer CC: College health providers' knowledge, attitudes, and management practices of genital HPV infection, *Nurse Pract* 21:122-128, 1996.

### Syphilis

Rolfs RT, Nakashima AK: Epidemiology of primary and secondary syphilis in the United States, 1981 through 1988, *JAMA* 264(11):1432-1437, 1990.

Thomas JC, Kulik AL, Schoenbach V: Syphilis in the south: rural rates surpass urban rates in North Carolina, *Am J Public Health* 85(8):1119-1122, 1995.

Tillman J: Syphilis: an old disease, a contemporary perinatal problem, *J Obstet Gynecol Neonatal Nurs* 21:209-213, 1992.

### Trichomonas

Hamed KA, Studemeister AE: Successful response of metronidazole-resistant trichomonal vaginitis to tinidazole, *Sex Transm Dis* 19(6):339-340, 1992.

Nyirjesy P et al: Paromomycin for nitroimidazole-resistant trichomoniasis, *Lancet* 346(8982):1110, 1995.

Paisarntantiwong R et al: The relationship of vaginal trichomoniasis and pelvic inflammatory disease among women colonized with *Chlamydia trachomatis, Sex Transm Dis* 22(6):344-347, 1995.

Tidwell BH et al: A double-blind placebo-controlled trial of single-dose intravaginal versus single-does oral metronidazole in the treatment of trichomonal vaginitis, *J Infect Dis* 170(1):242-246, 1994.

Weinberger MW, Harger JH: Accuracy of the Papanicolaou smear in the diagnosis of asymptomatic infection with trichomonas vaginalis, *Obstet Gynecol* 82(3):425-429, 1993.

## Chapter 51 Assessment of the Nervous System

### General

Ackerman L: Interventions related to neurologic care, *Nurs Clin North Am* 27(2):325-335, 1992.

Barker E: Eleven neuro myths to retire now, *RN* 60(6):26-29, 1997.

Cochran I et al: Stroke care: piecing together the long term picture, *Nursing* 24(6):34-41, 1994.

Glick OJ: Normal thought processes: an overview, *Nurs Clin North Am* 28(4):715-727, 1993.

Hickey J: *Neurological and neurosurgical nursing,* ed 4, Philadelphia, 1995, JB Lippincott.

Jarvis C: *Physical examination and health assessment,* ed 2, Philadelphia, 1996, WB Saunders.

Johnson CC: After a brain injury: clearing up the confusion, *Nursing* 25(11):39-45, 1995.

Morgan S: A passage through paralysis, *Am J Nurs* 92(4):54-58, 1992.

Olson E et al: The hazards of immobility, *Am J Nurs* 90(3):43-48, 1990.

Rankin J: The nursing diagnosis: swallowing, impaired and bedside assessment of swallowing in neurologically involved cases, *J Neurosci Nurs* 24:117-118, 1992.

Snyder M, editor: *A guide to neurological and neurosurgical nursing,* ed 2, New York, 1991, Delmar.

St George CL: Spasticity: mechanisms and nursing care, *Nurs Clin North Am* 28(4):819-827, 1993.

Thibodeau GA, Patton KT: *Anatomy and physiology,* ed 3, St Louis, 1996, Mosby.

US Department of Health and Human Services, Public Health Service: *Healthy people 2000: national health promotion and disease prevention objectives,* Washington, DC, 1990, US Government Printing Office.

Wilson LD: Sensory perceptual alteration: diagnosis, prediction, and intervention in the hospitalized adult, *Nurs Clin North Am* 28(4):747-765, 1993.

Zasler N: Sexuality in neurologic disability: an overview, *Sex Disabil* 9(1):11-27, 1991.

## Chapter 52 Management of Persons with Traumatic, Neoplastic, and Related Problems of the Brain

### Altered Level of Consciousness

Foreman M: Complexities of acute confusion, *Geriatr Nurs* 11(3):136-139, 1990.

Potter PA, Perry AG: *Basic nursing theory and practice,* ed 3, St Louis, 1995, Mosby.

Strittmatter WJ: Altered mental status and coma. In Civetta JM et al, editors: *Critical care,* ed 3, Philadelphia, 1997, JB Lippincott.

### Intracranial Pressure

Bader MK, Littlejohns L, Palmer S: Ventriculostomy and intracranial pressure monitoring: in search of a 0% infection rate, *Heart Lung* 24(2):166-172, 1995.

Barker E: *Neuroscience nursing,* St Louis, 1994, Mosby.

Fraser C: This dementia patient can be helped, *RN* 59(1):38-44, 1996.

Hickey JV: *The clinical practice of neurological and neurosurgical nursing,* ed 3, Philadelphia, 1992, JB Lippincott.

Morrison CA: Brain herniation syndromes, *Crit Care Nurse* 7(5):34-38, 1987.

Reichenbach SL: Neuromuscular blockade: when paralysis is intentional, *RN* 58(6):42-48, 1995.

Specht DM: Cerebral edema, *Nursing* 25(11):34-38, 1995.

### Headache

Bartelink M, van Weel C: Migraine in female patients in family practice, *Headache Q Curr Treat Res* 6:204-207, 1995.

Nussbaum E: Migraines, *Am J Nurs* 96(10):36-37, 1996.

Silberstein SD: Differential diagnosis of headache, *Hosp Med* 30:49-73, 1994.

Sheftell F: Beating migraines: how to use the new medications and behavioral techniques to stop your pain, *Health Confidential* 19(4):13-14, 1996.

### Epilepsy

Dilorio C, Henry M: Self-management in persons with epilepsy, *J Neurosci Nurs* 27:338-343, 1995.

Fowler S: Horizons: epilepsy education, *J Neurosci Nurs* 27:375-376, 1995.

Kelly M: Status epilepticus, *Am J Nurs* 95(8):50, 1995.

Russell A: Epilepsy, *Emerg Nurse* 4:9-15, 1996.

### Tumors

Arbour RB: Stereotactic localization and resection of intracranial tumors, *J Neurosci Nurs* 25:14-21, 1993.

Borozny M, Gray E, Ratel M: Nursing concerns associated with radical skull base surgery: a case study, *J Neurosci Nurs* 25:45-51, 1993.

Foote AW, Holcombe J: Acoustic neuroma: suggestions for helping the patient adapt after translabyrinthine surgery, *J Neurosci Nurs* 26:162-165, 1994.

O'Hanlon-Nichols T: Intracranial tumors, *Am J Nurs* 96(4):38-39, 1996.

### Craniocerebral Trauma

Brucia J, Rudy E: The effect of suction catheter insertion and tracheal stimulation in adults with severe brain injury, *Heart Lung* 25(4):295-303, 1996.

Hillier SL, Metzer J: Awareness and perceptions of outcomes after traumatic brain injury, *Brain Inj* 11(7):525-536, 1997.

Johnson CA: After a brain injury: clearing up the confusion, *Nursing* 25(11):39-45, 1995.

Kirby MY, Long CJ: Minor head injury: attempts at clarifying the confusion, *Brain Inj* 10(3):159-186, 1996.

Rowland J et al: Motorcycle helmet use and injury—outcome and hospitalization costs from crashes in Washington state, *Am J Public Health* 86(1):41-45, 1996.

Sosin DM et al: Trends in death associated with traumatic brain injury, 1979-1992, *JAMA* 273(22):1778-1780, 1995.

### Meningitis

Chiocca EM: Meningococcal meningitis, *Am J Nurs* 95(12):25, 1995.

Jackson LA et al: Serogroup C meningococcal outbreaks in the United States, *JAMA* 273(5):383-389, 1995.

Meissner JE: Caring for patients with meningitis, *Nursing* 25(7):50-51, 1995.

## Chapter 53 Management of Persons with Vascular, Degenerative, and Autoimmune Problems of the Brain

### Cerebral Vascular Disease

Anonymous: What's new in drugs: better use of warfarin means fewer CVAs, *RN* 59(1):71, 1996.

Anonymous: Horizons: new stroke treatment, *J Neurosci Nurs* 27(4):260, 1995.

Bronstein KS, Chadwick LR: Ticlopidine hydrochloride: its current use in cerebrovascular disease, *Rehabil Nurs* 19(1):17-20, 58, 1994.

Camp YG, Davis TM, Salter JP, Pierce LL: Stop and look: two approaches to manage stroke patients, *J Neurosci Nurs* 27(1):24-28, 1995.

Dancer S: Redesigning care for the nonhemorrhagic stroke patient, *J Neurosci Nurs* 28(3):183-189, 1996.

Gauwitz DF: How to protect the dysphagic stroke patient, *Am J Nurs* 95(8):3408, 1995.

Hafsteinsdottir TB: Neurodevelopmental treatment: application to nursing and effects on the hemiplegic stroke patient, *J Neurosci Nurs* 28(1):36-47, 1996.

Hayn MA, Fisher TR: Stroke rehab, *Nursing* 27(3):40-46, 1997.

Hydo B: Designing an effective clinical pathway for stroke, *Am J Nurs* 95(3):44-51, 1995.

Janowski MJ: A road map for stroke recovery, *RN* 59(3):26-30, 1996.

Lugger KE: Dysphagia in the elderly stroke patient, *J Neurosci Nurs* 26(2):78-84, 1994.

Macabasco AC, Hickman JL: Thrombolytic therapy for brain attack, *J Neurosci Nurs* 27(3):138-151, 1995.

Moore K, Trifiletti E: Stroke: the first critical days, *RN* 57(2):22-28, 1994.

Moore K: Stroke: the long road back, *RN* 57(3):50-55, 1994.

Mower DM: Brain attack—treating acute ischemic CVA, *Nursing* 27(3):35-39, 1997.

Murphy KB: Depression and stroke patients: the key to successful adaptation, *MedSurg Nurs* 4(3):225-228, 235, 1995.

Pierce L, Rodrigues-Fisher L, Buettner M et al: Frequently selected nursing diagnoses for the rehabilitation client with stroke, *Rehabil Nurs* 20(3):138-143, 186, 1995.

Tyson JM: Janforum: on being a "stroke" patient, *J Advanced Nursing* 21(2): 412-414, 1995.

Weber CE: Stroke: brain attack, time to react, *AACN Clin Issues* 6(4):562-575, 1995.

### Multiple Sclerosis

Anonymous: MS: What it is, what it does, what works against it, *RN* 58(7):49, 1995.

Anonymous: Cladribine aims at the source of MS . . . multiple sclerosis, *Am J Nurs* 94(9):50, 1994.

Clark C: Nursing care for multiple sclerosis, *Orthop Nurs* 10(1):21-33, 1991.

Coffey K: Multiple sclerosis: the inner world, *Home Healthc Nurse* 5(5):33-36, 1995.

Halper J, Holland N: *Comprehensive nursing care in multiple sclerosis,* New York, 1996, Demos Vermande.

Keating MM, Ostby PL: Education and self-management of interferon beta 1-b therapy for multiple sclerosis, *J Neurosci Nurs* 28(6):350-358, 1996.

Kelley C: The role of interferons in the treatment of multiple sclerosis, *J Neurosci Nurs* 27(4):114-120, 1995.

Mascarella J, Hudson D: Dysimmune neurologic disorders, *AACN Clin Issues Crit Care Nurse* 14(2):675-683, 1994.

Meissner JE: Caring for patients with multiple sclerosis, *Nursing* 24(8):60-61, 1994.

Miller CM, Hens M: Multiple sclerosis: a literature review, *J Neurosci Nurs* 25(3):174-179, 1993.

Radice B: Nursing and peer support: a winning combination, *RN* 58(7):47-49, 1995.

Ross AP: Nursing interventions for persons receiving immunosuppressive therapies for demyelinating pathology, *Nurs Clin North Am* 28(4):832-838, 1993.

Stewart-Amidei C: New treatment options for MS, *J Neurosci Nurs* 27(2):132-133, 1995.

Wilson BA: Nursing pharmacology: interferon beta for treatment of multiple sclerosis, *MedSurg Nurs* 4(2):151-153, 1995.

### Parkinson's Disease

Biziere KE, Kurth MC: *Living with Parkinson's disease,* New York, 1996, Demos Vermande.

Cerrato PL: Diet therapy helps this drug work better, *RN* 54(2):71-72, 74, 1991.

Cochran JW, Kessler ES, Wittenborn R: Neurologic disease: 5 scenarios to manage, *Patient Care* 32-51, 1994.

Fitzsimmons B, Bunting LK: Parkinson's disease: quality of life issues, *Nurs Clin North Am* 28(4):807-818, 1993.

Habermann-Little B: An analysis of the prevalence and etiology of depression in Parkinson's disease, *J Neurosci Nurs* 23(3):165-169, 1991.

Marr J: The experience of living with Parkinson's disease, *J Neurosci Nurs* 23(5):325-330, 1991.

Parr-Day K: Postanesthesia care of the pallidotomy patient, *J Post Anesth Nurs* 9(5):274-247, 1994.

Rawlins K: One RN's view of using fetal tissue in procedures . . . now there's more proof that fetal tissue helps against Parkinson's, *RN* 59(1):10, 1996.

Taira F: Facilitating self-care in clients with Parkinson's disease, *Home Healthc Nurse* 10(4):23-27, 1991.

Toledo LW: The postanesthesia patient with Parkinson's disease, *J Post Anesth Nurs* 7(1):32-37, 1992.

Vernon GM, Jenkins M: Health maintenance behaviors in advanced Parkinson's disease, *J Neurosci Nurs* 27(4):229-235, 1995.

Weekly NJ: Parkinsonism: an overview, *Geriatr Nurs Am J Care Aging* 16(4): 169-171, 1995.

Whitehouse C: A new source of support: the nurse practitioner role in Parkinson's disease and dystonia, *Prof Nurse* 9(7):448, 450-451, 1994.

### Myasthenia Gravis

Hardy EM, Rittenberry K: Myasthenia gravis: an overview, *Orthop Nurs* 13(6): 37-42, 1994.

Hickey JV: Myasthenic crisis—your assessment counts, *RN* 5:54-58, 1991.

Lohi E, Lindberg C, Andersen O: Physical training effects in myasthenia gravis, *Arch Phys Med Rehabil* 74(11):1178-1180, 1993.

Lopate G, Pestronk A: Autoimmune myasthenia gravis, *Hosp Pract* 28(1):109-112, 115-117, 121-122, 1993.

Mascarella JJ, Hudson DC: Dysimmune neurologic disorders, *Crit Care Nurse* 2(4):675-684, 1991 (AACN clinical issues).

### Amyotrophic Lateral Sclerosis

Anonymous: Horizons: gene therapy for ALS, *J Neurosci Nurs* 27(4):260, 1995.

Burwinkel K: Diligent nursing for these patients may mean hospice . . . ALS demands diligent nursing care, *RN* 58(7):9-10, 1995.

Mitsumoto H, Norris FH: *Amyotrophic lateral sclerosis: a comprehensive guide to management,* New York, 1994, Demos Vermande.

Shellenbarger T, Stover J: ALS demands diligent nursing care . . . amyotrophic lateral sclerosis, *RN* 58(3):30-32, 34-36, 1995.

Thomas S: Motor neurone disease: a progressive disease requiring a coordinated approach, *Prof Nurse* 8(9):583-585, 1993.

### Guillain-Barré Syndrome

Anderson SB: Guillain-Barré syndrome; giving the patient control, *J Neurosci Nurs* 24(3):158-162, 1992.

Barall-Inman RA: Question and answer: Guillain-Barré syndrome, *J Am Acad Nurse Pract* 7(4):165-169, 1995.

Hund EF, Borel CO, Cornblath DR et al: Intensive management and treatment of severe Guillain-Barré syndrome, *Crit Care Med* 21(3):433-446, 1993.

Morgan SP: A passage through paralysis . . . Guillain-Barré syndrome, *Am J Nurs* 91(10):70-74, 1991.

Murray DP: Impaired mobility: Guillain-Barré syndrome, *J Neurosci Nurs* 25(2):100-104, 1993.

Penrose NJ: Guillain-Barré syndrome: a case study, *Rehabil Nurs* 18(2):88-90, 94, 1993.

Ross AP: Nursing interventions for persons receiving immunosuppressive therapies for demyelinating pathology, *Nurs Clin North Am* 28(4):829-838, 1993.


## Chapter 54 Management of Persons with Problems of the Spinal Cord and Peripheral Nerves

### Spinal Cord Injury


American Association of Spinal Cord Injury Nurses: Standards of spinal cord injury nursing practice, *SCI Nurs* 11(1):33-37, 1994.

Bach CA, McDaniel RW: Quality of life in quadriplegic adults: a focus group study, *Rehabil Nurs* 18(6):364-367, 1993.

Chiles BW, Cooper PR: Acute spinal injury, *N Engl J Med* 334(8):514-520, 1996.

Curry K, Casady L: The relationships between extended periods of immobility and decubiti formation in the acutely spinal cord-injured individual, *J Neurosurg Nurs*, 24(4):185-189, 1992.

Gilbert M, Counsell CM: Coordinated care for the SCI patient, *SCI Nurs* 12(3):87-89, 1995.

Huston CJ, Boelman R: Autonomic dysreflexia, *Am J Nurs* 95(6):55, 1995.

Laskowski-Jones L: Acute SCI: how to minimize the damage, *Am J Nurs* 93(12):22-31, 1993.

Lehman CA: Risk factors for pressure ulcers in the spinal cord injured in the community, *SCI Nurs* 12(4):110-114, 1995.

Nolan S: Current trends in the management of acute spinal cord injury, *Crit Care Nurs Q* 17(1):64-78, 1994.

Richmond TS: Spinal cord injury, *Nurs Clin North Am* 25(1):57-69, 1990.

Rose DD et al: Cervical spine injury, *AORN J* 57(4):830-850, 1993.

Spoltore TA, O'Brien AM: Rehabilitation of the spinal cord injured patient, *Orthop Nurs* 14(3):7-16, 1995.

Thomason SS: Preventing and detecting unique complications in the spinal cord injured, *Home Healthc Nurse* 8(5):16-21, 1990.


### Cranial Nerve Disorders


Dyck PJ, Haase G, May M: When you suspect Bell's palsy, *Patient Care* 26(1):151-168, 1992.

Geary S: Nursing management of cranial nerve dysfunction, *J Neurosci Nurs* 27(2):102-108, 1996.

Levins TT: Bell's palsy versus trigeminal neuralgia questioned, *J Emerg Nurs* 20(2):86-87, 1994.

McConaghy DJ: Trigeminal neuralgia: a personal review and nursing implications, *J Neurosci Nurs* 26(2):85-90, 1994.

Weir AM, Pentland B, Crosswaite A et al: Bell's palsy: the effect on self-image, mood state and social activity, *Clin Rehabil* 9(2):121-125, 1995.

Wollenberg SP: Primary care diagnosis and management of Bell's palsy, *Nurse Pract* 18(12):15-19, 1994.


## Chapter 55 Assessment of the Visual System

### General


Follmer BA, Smith SC: Electrophysiology testing and the ophthalmic registered nurse, *Insight* 19(14):12-18, 1994.

Hunt L: Aging and the visual system, *Insight* 18(3):6-7, 18, 1993.

Hunt L: Ophthalmic nursing assessment, *Insight* 17(3):9-11, 1992.

Kelly JS: Visual impairment among older people, *Br J Nurs* 2(2):110-116, 1993.


## Chapter 56 Management of Persons with Problems of the Eye

### Visual Impairment


Allen MN: Adjusting to visual impairment, *J Ophthalmic Nurs Technol* 9(2):47-51, 1990.

Birt L: Making sense of . . . photorefractive keratectomy, *Nurs Times* 91(44): 30-31, 1995.

Eichenbaum JW: Vitamins for cataract and macular degeneration, *J Ophthalmic Nurs Technol* 15(2):65-67, 1996.

Hunt L: Nutrients and the eye, *Insight* 12(1):25-27, 1994.

Parker P: Overview of refractive surgery, *J Ophthalmic Nurs Technol* 13(3): 105-109, 1994.

Rowell M: Eradication of vitamin A deficiency: with five cents and a vegetable garden, *J Ophthalmic Nurs Technol* 12(5):217-224, 1993.

Woods S: Macular degeneration, *Nurs Clin North Am* 27(3):761-775, 1992.


### Eye Manifestations of Systemic Disease


Ai E, Kelly MP: Ophthalmic manifestations of the acquired immunodeficiency syndrome, *J Ophthalmic Nurs Technol* 11(4):148-156, 1992.

Frederick MC: Care of the patient with AIDS and cytomegalovirus retinitis, *J Ophthalmic Nurs Technol* 13(4):156-160, 1994.

Phillips WB: Ocular manifestations of diabetes mellitus, *J Ophthalmic Nurs Technol* 13(6):255-261, 1994.

Plona RP, Schremp P: Nursing care of patients with ocular manifestations of human immunodeficiency virus infection, *Nurs Clin North Am* 27(3):793-805, 1992.

Smith S: Diabetic retinopathy, *Insight* 17(2):20-25, 1992.


### Glaucoma and Cataract


Hagan JC, Wyatt B: Preoperative evaluation and workup of the cataract and intraocular lens implant patient, *J Ophthalmic Nurs Technol* 12(3):123-128, 1993.

Newhouse J: Opening your eyes to intraocular drug administration, *Nursing* 24(6):44-45, 1994.

Sandler RL: Clinical snapshot: glaucoma, *Am J Nurs* 95(3):34-35, 1995.

Sivalingam E: Glaucoma: an overview, *J Ophthalmic Nurs Technol* 15(1):15-18, 1996.


## Chapter 57 Assessment of the Auditory and Vestibular Systems

### General


Chmiel R, Jerger J: Some factors affecting assessment of hearing handicap in the elderly, *J Am Acad Audiol* 4:249-257, 1993.

Haybach PJ: Tuning in to ototoxicity: the inside story, *Nursing* 23(6):34-41, 1993.

Miola E: The otoscope: an update on assessment skills, *J Pediatr Nurs* 9(3):283-286, 1994.

Mulrow CD, Lichtenstein MJ: Screening for hearing impairment in the elderly, *J Gen Intern Med* 6:249-258, 1991.

Ney D: Cerumen impaction, ear hygiene practices and hearing acuity, *Geriatr Nurs* 14(6):70-73, 1993.

Smelzer C: Primary care screening and evaluation of hearing loss, *Nurse Pract* 18(2):50-54, 1994.


## Chapter 58 Management of Persons with Problems of the Ear

### General


Chen HL: Hearing in the elderly: relation of hearing loss, loneliness and self esteem, *J Gerontol Nurs* 20(6):22-27, 1994.

Ekstrom I: Communicating with the deaf patient, *Plast Surg Nurs* 14(1):31-33, 1994.

Foote A, Holcombe J: Acoustic neuroma: suggestions for helping the patient adapt after translabyrinthine surgery, *J Neurosci Nurs* 26(3):162-165, 1994.

Goldenberg R, Brown M, Cunninghem S: Laser stapedectomy, *AORN J* 59(6):411-415, 1992.

Mahoney DF: Cerumen impaction: prevalence and detection in nursing homes, *J Gerontol Nurs* 19(4):23-29, 1993.

O"Rourke CM et al: Effectiveness of a hearing screening protocol for the elderly, *Geriatr Nurs* 14(2):66-69, 1993.

Shelp SG: Your patient is deaf, now what? *RN* 60(2):37-40, 1997.

Smith LE: Communicating with patients who are deaf, *J Am Acad Physician Assist* 5(1):37-39, 1992.

Walbrecker J: Knowing the signs, *RN* 60(2):40-41, 1997.

Webber-Jones J: Doomed to deafness? *Am J Nurs* 92(11):37-39, 1992.

## Chapter 59 Assessment of the Musculoskeletal System

### General

Hoppenfeld S: *Physical examination of the spine and extremities*, Norwalk, Conn, 1976, Mosby.

Long JS: Shoulder arthroscopy, *Orthop Nurs* 15(2):21, 1996.

Maldonado A, Barger M: Primary care for women: comprehensive assessment of common musculoskeletal disorders, *J Nurse Midwifery* 40(2):202, 1995.

## Chapter 60 Management of Persons with Trauma to the Musculoskeletal System

### Trauma

Childre F, Winzeler A: Cumulative trauma disorder: a primary care provider's guide to upper extremity diagnosis and treatment, *Nurse Pract Forum* 6(2): 106, 1995.

Childs SA: Musculoskeletal trauma, *Crit Care Clin North Am* 6(3):483, 1994.

Cunningham ME: Bursitis and tendinitis, *Orthop Nurs* 13(5):13, 1994.

Hager CA, Brncick N: Fat embolism syndrome: a complication of trauma, *Orthop Nurs* 17(2):41, 1998.

Kuwada GT: Current concepts in the treatment of ankle sprains, *Clin Podiatr Med Surg* 12(4):653, 1995.

Paletta JH: Nursing care of sports-related injuries, *Orthop Nurs* 16(6):43, 1997.

Reid DC: *Sports injury assessment and rehabilitation,* New York, 1992, Churchill Livingstone.

### Hip Fracture

Birge SJ, Morrow-Howell N, Proctor, EK: Hip fracture, *Clin Geriatr Med* 10(4):589, 1994.

Cifu DX: Rehabilitation of fractures of the hip, *Phys Med Rehabil* 9(1):125, 1995.

Cralk RL: Disability following hip fracture, *Phys Ther* 74(5):387, 1994.

Cummings SR et al: Risk factors for hip fracture in white women, *N Engl J Med* 332(12):767, 1995.

Dargent-Molina P et al: Fall-related factors and the risk of hip fracture: the EPIDOS prospective study, *Lancet* 348:145, 1996.

Eldar R, Tamir A: Determinants of rehabilitation following fracture of the hip in elderly patients, *Clin Rehabil* 9:184, 1995.

Garnero P et al: Markers of bone resorption predict hip fracture in elderly women: the EPIDOS prospective study, *J Bone Miner Res* 11(10):1531, 1996.

Greenspan SL et al: Fall severity and bone mineral density as risk factors for hip fracture in ambulatory elderly, *JAMA* 271(2):128, 1994.

Grisso JA et al: Risk factors for hip fracture in black women, *N Engl J Med* 330(22):1555, 1994.

Koval KJ et al: Ambulatory ability after hip fracture, *Clin Orthop Relat Res* 310:150, 1995.

Lamb KV, Waszkiewicz M, Davis-Kipnis N: Dual disabilities: when a stroke patient fractures a hip, *Orthop Nurs* 15(5):13, 1996.

McCracken AL, Gilster SD: Outcomes of people with a fractured hip and dementia who reside in a specialized nursing home, *Top Geriatr Rehabil* 11(1):20, 1995.

Michelson JD et al: Epidemiology of hip fractures among the elderly, *Clin Orthop Relat Res* 311:129, 1995.

Pellino TA: How to manage hip fractures, *Am J Nurs* 94(4):46, 1994.

Perry CR: Intracapsular fractures of the proximal femur, *Clin in Geriatr Med* 10(4):647, 1994.

Santry J: Hip fractures: can nursing make the difference? *Br J Nurs* 3(7):335, 1994.

Williams MA, Oberst MT, Bjorklund BC: Posthospital convalescence in older women with hip fracture, *Orthop Nurs* 13(4):55, 1994.

Wolinsky FD, Fitzgerald JF, Stump TE: The effect of hip fracture on mortality, hospitalization, and functional status: a prospective study, *Am J Public Health* 87(3):398, 1997.

Zinsmeister D: The diagnosis and treatment of hip fractures, *J Am Acad Physician Assist* 6(8):542, 1993.

## Chapter 61 Management of Persons with Inflammatory and Degenerative Disorders of the Musculoskeletal System

### General

Gerber DE, McGuire SL: Community resources for clients with mobility problems, *Orthop Nurs* 15(6):35, 1996

Pellino TA: Relationships between patient attitudes, subjective norms, perceived control, and analgesic use following elective orthopedic surgery, *Res Nurs Health* 20:97, 1997.

Proctor MC, Greenfield LJ, Marsh EE: Prophylaxis for thromboembolism in elective orthopaedic surgery, *Orthop Nurs* 16(5):51, 1997.

Wynd CA, Wallace M, Smith KM: Factors influencing postoperative urinary retention following orthopaedic surgical procedures, *Orthop Nurs* 15(1):43, 1996.

### Arthritis

American College of Rheumatology Ad Hoc Committee on Clinical Guidelines: Guidelines for monitoring drug therapy in rheumatoid arthritis, *Arthritis Rheum* 39(5):723, 1996.

Brown S, Williams A: Women's experiences of rheumatoid arthritis, *J Adv Nurs* 21:695, 1995.

Hochberg MC et al: Guidelines for the medical management of osteoarthritis, *Arthritis Rheum* 38(11):1541, 1995.

Kantor TG: Current nonsteroidal antiinflammatory drug applications for rheumatic diseases, *Prim Care* 20(4):955, 1993.

Krug B: Rheumatoid arthritis and osteoarthritis: a basic comparison, *Orthop Nurs* 16(5):73, 1997.

Mazanec DJ: Pharmacology of corticosteroids in synovial joints, *Phys Med Rehabil Clin North Am* 6(4):815, 1995.

Nesher G, Moores TL: Clinical presentation and treatment of arthritis in the aged, *Clin Geriatr Med* 10(4):659, 1994.

Pigg JS: Case management of the patient with arthritis, *Orthop Nurs* 16(suppl 2):33, 1997.

Rankin JA: Pathophysiology of the rheumatoid joint, *Orthop Nurs* 14(4):39, 1995.

Schilke JM et al: Effects of muscle-strength training on the functional status of patients with osteoarthritis of the knee joint, *Nurs Res* 45(2):68, 1996.

Wetherbee LL: Caring for clients with arthritis, *Home Healthc Nurse* 12(1):13, 1994.

### Rheumatic and Inflammatory Disorders

Brander VA et al: Rehabilitation in joint and connective tissue diseases, *Arch Phys Med Rehabil* 76:47, 1995.

Bynum DT: Clinical snapshot: gout, *Am J Nurs* 97(7):36, 1997.

Carpenter DR, Hudacek S: Polymyalgia rheumatica: a comprehensive review of this debilitating disease, *Nurse Pract* 19(6):50, 1994.

Dattwyler RJ et al: Ceftriaxone compared with doxycycline for the treatment of acute disseminated Lyme disease, *N Engl J Med* 337(5):289, 1997.

Leondike MR, Shattuck MA: Intravenous cyclophosphamide in lupus nephritis, *J Intravenous Nurs* 16(1):23, 1993.

McCauliffe DP, Sontheimer RD: Dermatologic manifestations of rheumatic disorders, *Prim Care* 20(4):925, 1993.

Oddis CV, Medsger TA: Inflammatory myopathies, *Balliere's Clin Rheumatol* 9(3):497, 1995.

Reinhard JD, Calkins E: Geriatric issues in the diagnosis and management of patients with rheumatic disorders, *Prim Care* 20(4):911, 1993.

Ulek LJ: Special nursing considerations for SLE patients, *MedSurg Nurs* 4(2): 146, 1995.

### Total Joint Arthroplasty

Blaylock B et al: Tape injury in the patient with total hip replacement, *Orthop Nurs* 14(3):25, 1995.

Cohen MS, Whitman K: Calcium phosphate bone cement—the Norian skeletal repair system in orthopaedic surgery, *AORN J* 65(5):958, 1997.

Crutchfield J et al: Preoperative and postoperative pain in total knee replacement patients, *Orthop Nurs* 15(2):65, 1996.

Henry SL, Hood GA, Seligson D: Long-term implantation of gentamycin-polymethylmethacrylate antibiotic bead, *Clin Orthop Relat Res* 295:47, 1993.

Lin PC, Lin LC, Lin JJ: Comparing the effectiveness of different educational programs for patients with total knee arthroplasties, *Orthop Nurs* 16(5):43, 1997.

Ljung P, Bornmyr S, Svensson H: Wound healing after total elbow replacement in rheumatoid arthritis, *Acta Orthop Scand* 66(1):59, 1995.

Muntz JE: Perioperative DVT and pulmonary embolism: diagnosis, management, and treatment, *Orthop Nurs* 16(suppl 2):25, 1997.

Owens R: Total shoulder arthroplasty, *AORN J* 65(5):927, 1997.

Schmalzried TP, Noordin S, Amstutz HC: Update on nerve palsy associated with total hip replacement, *Clin Orthop Relat Res* 344:188, 1997.

### Spine Disorders

Krause TM: Case management through a multidisciplinary spinal evaluation, *Orthop Nurs* 16 (suppl 2):46, 1997.

### Metabolic Bone Diseases

Adachi JD et al: Intermittent etidronate therapy to prevent corticosteroid-induced osteoporosis, *N Engl J Med* 337(6):382, 1997.

Chestnut CH: Medical treatment of osteoporosis, *Phys Med Rehabil Clin North Am* 6(3):639, 1995.

Delmas PD, Meunier PJ: The management of Paget's disease of bone, *N Engl J Med* 336(8):558, 1997.

Edelson GW, Kleerekoper M: Bone mass, bone loss, and fractures, *Phys Med Rehabil Clin North Am* 6(3):455, 1995.

Galsworthy TD, Wilson PL: Osteoporosis it steals more than bone, *Am J Nurs* 96(6):27, 1996.

Gunby MC, Morley JE: Epidemiology of bone loss with aging, *Clin Geriatr Med* 10(4):557, 1994.

Hangartner TN: Osteoporosis due to disuse, *Phys Med Rehabil Clin North Am* 6(3):579, 1995.

Herzenberg MA: Osteoporosis independent study, *Orthop Nurs* 17(2):63, 1998.

Hunt AH: The relationship between height changes and bone mineral density, *Orthop Nurs* 15(3):57, 1996.

Kessenich CR, Rosen CJ: Vitamin D and bone status in elderly women, *Orthop Nurs* 15(3):67, 1996.

Lindsay R: Secondary prevention of osteoporosis, *Phys Med Rehabil Clin North Am* 6(3):629, 1995.

Marguiles JY et al: The relationship between degenerative changes and osteoporosis in the lumbar spine, *Clin Orthop Relat Res* 324:145, 1996.

Matkovic V et al: Primary prevention of osteoporosis, *Phys Med Rehabil Clin North Am* 6(3):595, 1995.

Mazess RB: Dual-energy x-ray absorptiometry for the management of bone disease, *Phys Med Rehabil Clin North Am* 6(3):507, 1995.

Nordins BEC et al: The definition, diagnosis, and classification of osteoporosis, *Phys Med Rehabil Clin North Am* 6(3):395, 1995.

Paier GS: Specter of the crone: the experience of vertebral fracture, *Adv Nurs Sci* 18(3):27, 1996.

Zimmerman SI, Fox KM, Magaziner J: Psychosocial aspects of osteoporosis, *Phys Med Rehabil Clin North Am* 6(3):441, 1995.

## Chapter 62 Assessment of the Skin

### Age Related Skin Changes

Young E: *Geriatric dermatology*, Philadelphia, 1993, Lea & Febiger.

### Pathophysiology

Ganong WF: *Review of medical physiology*, ed 16, East Norwalk, Conn, 1993, Appleton & Lange.

McCance K, Huether S: *Pathophysiology*, ed 3, St Louis, 1998, Mosby.

### Physical Assessment

Barakauskas V et al: *Health and physical assessment*, St Louis, 1994, Mosby.

## Chapter 63 Management of Persons with Problems of the Skin

### General

Habif TP: *Clinical dermatology: a color guide to diagnosis and therapy*, St Louis, 1996, Mosby.

Hess CT: Fundamental strategies for skin care, *Ostomy Wound Manage* 43(8):32-40, 1997.

Hill M, Labik M, Vanderbilt D: Managing skin care with the care map system, *J Wound Ostomy Continence Nurs* 24(1) 26-37, 1997.

Miller L: Maintaining skin integrity: setting the standard in a rehabilitation facility, *Rehab Nurs* 20(5):273-277, 1995.

Milne CT, Corbett LQ: The skin care workshop: an innovative training program to implement clinical guidelines, *J Gerontol Nurs* 23(1):49-52, 1997.

### Age Related Skin Changes

Jeter KF, Lutz JB: Skin care in the frail, elderly, dependent, incontinent patient, *Adv Wound Care* 9(1):29-34, 1996.

### Photosensitivity

Miller CA, Summer skin precautions to protect against adverse medication effects, *Geriatr Nurs* 17(4):193-194, 1996.

### Bacterial, Viral, and Fungal Diseases

Gentry LO: Dermatologic manifestations of infectious diseases in cardiac transplant patients, *Infect Dis Clin North Am* 8(3):523-532, 1994.

Kemmerly SA: Dermatologic manifestations of infections in diabetics, *Infect Dis Clin North Am* 8(3):637-654, 1994.

Le Fort SM: Herpes zoster and postherpetic neuralgia: the need for early intervention in the elderly, *Nurse Pract* 14(3):30-41, 1989.

### Infestations

Morris-Hicks-LE, Lewis-DJ: Management of chronic resistive scabies: a case study, *Geriatr Nurs* 16(5):230-236, 1995.

### Pressure Ulcers

Bostrom J, Mechanic J, Lazar N et al: Preventing skin breakdown: nursing practices, costs, outcomes, *Appl Nurs Res* 9(4):184-188, 1996.

Declair V: The usefulness of topical application of essential fatty acids (EFA) to prevent pressure ulcers, *Ostomy Wound Manage* 43(5):48-52, 54, 1997.

Goode PS, Thomas DR: Pressure ulcers: local wound care, *Clin Geriatr Med* 13(3):543-552, 1997.

Hunter SM, Langemo DK, Olson B et al: The effectiveness of skin care protocols for pressure ulcers, *Rehabil Nurs* 20(5):250-255, 1995.

Maklebust J: *Pressure ulcers: guidelines for prevention and nursing management*, Springhouse, Penna, 1996, Springhouse.

Pieper B, Weiland M: Pressure ulcer prevention within 72 hours of admission in a rehabilitation setting, *Ostomy Wound Manage* 43(8):14-25, 1997.

Sprung P, Zizheng H, Ladin DA: Hydrogels and hydrocolloids: an objective product comparison, *Ostomy Wound Manage* 44(1):36-51, 1998.

Vogelpohl T: What do nursing students learn about pressure ulcers? A survey of content on pressure ulcers in nursing school textbooks, *Decubitus* 6(2):48-50, 52, 1993.

Wells JA, Karr D: Interface pressure, wound healing, and satisfaction in the evaluation of a non-powered fluid mattress, *Ostomy Wound Manage* 44(2): 38-54, 1998.

Zahid BMN, Salzberg CA: Surgical management of pressure ulcers, *Ostomy Wound Manage* 43(8):44-51, 1997.

Zernike W: Preventing heel pressure sores: a comparison of heel pressure relieving devices, *J Clin Nurs* 3:375-380, 1994.

## Chapter 64 Management of Persons with Burns

### General

Byers JF, Flynn MB: Acute burn injury: a trauma case report, *Crit Care Nurse* 16:55-66, 1996.

Faldmo L, Kravitz M: Management of acute burns and burn shock resuscitation, *AACN Clin Iss Crit Care Nurs* 4:351-366, 1993.

Herndon DN, editor: *Total burn care,* Philadelphia, 1996, WB Saunders.

Marvin J: Thermal injuries. In Cardona VD et al, editors: *Trauma Nursing: from resuscitation through rehabilitation,* ed 2, Philadelphia, 1994, WB Saunders.

Trofino RB: *Nursing care of the burn-injured patient,* Philadelphia, 1991, FA Davis.

US Department of Health and Human Services: *Healthy people 2000: midcourse review and 1995 revisions,* Washington, DC, 1995, US Government Printing Office.

### Etiology, Prevention, and Health Education

Brigham PA, McLoughlin E: Burn incidence and medical care use in the United States: estimates, trends, and data sources, *J Burn Care Rehabil* 17: 95-107, 1996.

Clark DE, Katz MX, Campbell SM: Decreasing mortality and morbidity rates after the institution of a statewide burn program, *J Burn Care Rehabil* 13: 261-270, 1992.

### Classification

Trofino RB, Orr PM: Types of burns, In Trofino RB: *Nursing care of the burn-injured patient,* Philadelphia, 1991, FA Davis.

### Pathophysiology of Severe Burns

Caine RM: Patients with burns. In Clochesy JM et al, editors: *Critical Care Nursing,* ed 2, Philadelphia, 1996, WB Saunders.

Kramer GC, Nguyen TT: Pathophysiology of burn shock and burn edema. In Herndon DN, editor: *Total burn care,* Philadelphia, 1996, WB Saunders.

Morehouse JD et al: Resuscitation of the thermally injured patient, *Crit Care Clin* 8:355-365, 1992.

Robins EV: Burn shock, *Crit Care Nurs Clin North Am* 2:299-307, 1990.

### Periods of Treatment

Bolinger B: Burn care in the home, *J Wound Ostomy Continence Nurs* 22:122-127, 1995.

Boyce ST et al: Comparative assessment of cultured skin substitutes and native skin autograft for treatment of full-thickness burns, *Ann Surg* 222:743-752, 1995.

Bridigare CM, Brown KR: Role of the burn nurse: emergent care, *Top Emerg Med* 17:61-69, 1995.

Chang A et al: Rehabilitation after burn injury, *Trauma Q* 11:180-187, 1994.

Chang P et al: Prospective, randomized study of the efficacy of pressure garment therapy in patients with burns, *J Burn Care Rehabil* 16:473-475, 1995.

Deitch EA: Infection and sepsis in burn patients, *Trauma Q* 11:157-165, 1995.

Demling RH: Fluid replacement in burned patients, *Surg Clin North Am* 67:15-30, 1987.

Faldmo L, Kravitz M: Management of acute burns and burn shock resuscitation, *AACN Clin Issues Crit Care Nurs* 4:351-366, 1993.

Fratianne RB et al: When is enough enough? Ethical dilemmas on the burn unit, *J Burn Care Rehabil* 13:600-604, 1992.

Greenfield E, Jordan B: Advances in burn wound care, *Crit Care Nurs Clin North Am* 8:203-215, 1996.

Helvig EI et al: Development of burn outcomes and quality indicators: a project of the ABA Committee on Organization and Delivery of Burn Care, *J Burn Care Rehabil* 16:208-211, 1995.

Ireton-Jones CS, Gottschlich MM: The evolution of nutrition support in burns, *J Burn Care Rehabil* 14(suppl):272-280, 1993.

Kravitz M: Immune consequences of burn injury, *AACN Clin Iss* 4:399-413, 1993.

Kravitz M: Outpatient wound care, *Crit Care Nurs Clin North Am* 8:217-223, 1996.

Miller SF: Surgery in the burned patient, *Top Emerg Med* 17:35-39, 1995.

Molter NC: Pain in the burn patient. In Puntillo KA, editor: *Pain in the critically ill,* Gaithersburg, Md, 1991, Aspen.

Nguyen TT et al: Current treatment of severely burned patients, *Ann Surg* 223:14-25, 1996.

Peate WF: Outpatient management of burns, *Am Fam Physician* 45:1321-1332, 1992.

Robins EV: Immunosuppression of the burned patient, *Crit Care Nurs Clin North Am* 2:767-774, 1989.

Smith DJ et al: Burn wounds: infection and healing, *Am J Surg* 167:46S-48S, 1994.

Tomkins RG, Burke JF: Alternative wound coverings. In Herndon DN, editor: *Total burn care,* Philadelphia, 1996, WB Saunders.

Trofino RB, editor: *Nursing care of the burn-injured patient,* Philadelphia, 1991, FA Davis.

Waltman M: Assessing the severity of the burn injury, *Top Emerg Med* 17:17-24, 1995.

Ward RS: Pressure therapy for the control of hypertonic scar formation after burn injury: a history and review, *J Burn Care Rehabil* 12:257-262, 1991.

Wong L, Munster AM: New techniques in burn wound management, *Surg Clin North Am* 73:363-371, 1993.

Weber JM, Tompkins DM: Improving survival: infection control and burns, *AACN Clin Iss Crit Care Nurs* 4:414-423, 1993.

## Chapter 65 Assessment of the Immune System

### General

Adair MN, Nygard NK, Maddox RW, Adair JB: New behavioral strategies for enhancing immune function, *AIDS Patient Care* 5(6):297-300, 1991.

Blaylock B: The aging immune system and common infections in elderly patients, *J ET Nurs* 20(2):63-67, 1993.

Ershler WB: The influence of an aging immune system on cancer incidence and progression, *J Gerontol* 48(1):83-87, 1993.

Krenitsky J: Nutrition and the immune system, *AACN Adv Pract Acute Crit Care* 7(3):359-369, 1996.

Kubena KS, McMurray DN: Nutrition and the immune system: a review of nutrient-nutrient interactions, *J Am Diet Assoc* 96(11):1156-1164, 1996.

Meliska CJ et al: Immune function in cigarette smokers who quit smoking for 31 days, *J Allergy Clin Immunol* 95(4):901-910, 1995.

O'Brien JM, Reilly NJ: Comparison of tape products on skin integrity, *Adv Wound Care* 8(6):26-39, 1995.

Phillips MC, Olson LR: The immunologic role of the gastrointestinal tract, *Crit Care Clin North Am* 5(1):107-120, 1993.

Post-White J: The immune system, *Semin Oncol Nurs* 12(2):89-96, 1996.

Workman ML: Essential concepts of inflammation and immunity, *Crit Care Clin North Am* 7(4):601-615, 1995.

## Chapter 66 Management of Persons with Problems of the Immune System

### General

Bancroft B: Immunology simplified, *Semin Perioper Nurs* 3(2):70-78, 1994.

Bauer CL: Commentary on differences in immunosuppressant agents, *AACN Nurs Scan Crit Care* 3(4):14, 1993.

Blaylock B: The aging immune system and common infections in elderly patients, *J Enteros Ther Nurs* 20(2):63-67, 1993.

Gibbs L: Assessment and management of the allergic patient, *ORL Head Neck Nurs* 10(3):10-16, 1992.

Gritter M: Latex hypersensitivity, *Nursing* 25(5):33, 1995.

Hadden JW, Smith DL: Immunopharmacology, immunomodulation, and immunotherapy, *JAMA* 268(20):2964-2969, 1992.

Immune Deficiency Foundation: *IDF patient/family handbook for primary immune deficiency diseases,* Towson, Md, 1993, The Foundation.

Johnson CCS: Knowledge of immunology is essential to plan effective nursing care for immunocompromised patients, *Intens Crit Care Nurs* 10(2): 121-126, 1994.

Lockey RF: Future trends in allergy and immunology, *JAMA* 268(20):2991-2992, 1992.

Nakamura MC, Nakamura RM: Contemporary concepts of autoimmunity and autoimmune diseases, *J Clin Lab Anal* 6(5):275-289, 1992.

Rosen FS, Cooper MD, Wedgewood RJ: Medical progress: the primary immunodeficiencies, *N Engl J Med* 333(7):431-430, 1995.

Shronts EP: Basic concepts of immunology and its application to clinical nutrition, *Nutr Clin Pract* 8(4):177-183, 1993.

Thompson G, Ruane-Morris M, Lawton S: Lines of defense—hypersensitivity, *Nurs Times* 90(4):48-51, 1994.

Workman ML: Essential concepts of inflammation and immunity, *Crit Care Nurs Clin North Am* 7(4):601-615, 1995.

Workman ML: The immune system: your defensive partner and offensive foe, *AACN Clin Iss Crit Care Nurs* 4(3):453-470, 1993.

### Blood Transfusions

Fitzpatrick L, Fitzpatrick T: Blood transfusion: keeping your patient safe, *Nursing* 27(8):34-42, 1997.

Harovas J, Anthony HH: Managing transfusion reactions, *RN* 56(12):32-36, 1993.

Harovas J, Anthony HH: Your guide to trouble free transfusions, *RN* 56(11): 26-34, 1993.

Huston CJ: Emergency! Hemolytic transfusion reaction, *Am J Nurs* 96(3):47-49, 1996.

Pavel J: Red cell transfusions for anemia, *Semin Oncol Nurs* 6(2):117-122, 1990.

## Chapter 67 Management of Persons with HIV Infection and AIDS

### General

Abercrombie PD: Women living with HIV infection, *Nurs Clin North Am* 31(1):97-106, 1996.

Aiken LH et al: Nurse practitioner managed care for persons with HIV infection, *Image* 25(3):172-177, 1993.

Anastasi JK, Sun V: Controlling diarrhea in the HIV patient, *Am J Nurs* 96(8):35-41, 1996.

Anonymous: A new class of anti-HIV drugs debuts, *Am J Nurs* 96(7):59-60, 62-63, 1996.

Bechtel-Boenning C: State of the art: antiviral treatment of HIV infection, *Nurs Clin North Am* 31(1):1-13, 1996.

Breault AJ, Polifroni EC: Caring for people with AIDS: nurses' attitudes and feelings, *J Adv Nurs* 17:21-27, 1992.

Cerrato PL: HIV report: always a death sentence? *RN* 59(8):22, 24-27, 1996.

Fegan C: Cryptosporidial disease in the adult HIV infected patient, *J Assoc Nurses AIDS Care* 3:17-20, 1996.

Flaskerud JH, Ungvarski PJ: *HIV/AIDS: a guide to nursing care,* ed 3, Philadelphia, 1995, WB Saunders.

Gloersen B et al: The phenomena of doing well in people with AIDS, *West J Nurs Res* 15(1):44-47, 1993.

Gray J: HIV report: meeting psychosocial needs, *RN* 59(8):23-27, 1996.

Grayce-Barnes KB: Nutrition, immunity and HIV disease, *Physician Assist* 19(8):57-58, 60, 62-65, 1995.

Hurley PM, Ungvarski PJ: Home health care needs of adults living with HIV disease/AIDS in New York City, *J Assoc Nurses AIDS Care* 5(2):33-40, 1994.

Kelly PJ, Holman S: The new face of AIDS, *Am J Nurs* 93(3):26-34, 1993.

Kenny P: HIV infection, *Nursing* 26(8):27-35, 1996.

Lisanti P, Zwolski K: Understanding the devastation of AIDS, *Am J Nurs* 97(7):26-34, 1997.

Merrill A: AIDS and malnutrition: dual assaults on the body, *Home Healthc Nurse* 13(1):56-63, 1995.

Roccograndi JF, Clements KS: Managing AIDS-related meningitis, *RN* 56(11):36-39, 1993.

Rose MA: Concerns of women with HIV/AIDS, *J Assoc Nurses AIDS Care* 4(3):40, 44, 1993.

Rose MA, Clark-Alexander B: Quality of living and coping styles of HIV-positive women with children, *J Assoc Nurses AIDS Care* 7(2):28-30, 1996.

Sax P: Viral load testing, *AIDS Clin Care* 8(4):31-32, 1996.

Schmidt J, Crespo-Fierro M: Who says there's nothing we can do? *RN* 58(10):30-35, 1995.

Ungvarski PJ: Adults and HIV/AIDS: clinical considerations for care management, *J Care Manage* 1(3):40-42, 45-46, 49, 51-63, 1995.

Ungvarski PJ: Meeting the challenge of HIV/AIDS, *Imprint* 42(4):51-54, 1995.

Ungvarski PJ: Waging war on HIV wasting, *RN* 59(2):26-33, 1996.

Whipple B, Scura KW: The overlooked epidemic: HIV in older adults, *Am J Nurs* 96(2):22-28, 1996.

## Chapter 68 Management of Persons with Organ/Tissue Transplant

### General

Corley MC, Sneed G: Criteria in the selection of organ transplant recipients, *Heart Lung* 23(6):446-457, 1994.

Duffy M, Uber L: Immunosuppressive medications, *Dialysis Transplant* 23(6):303-305, 1994.

Hussar DA: Immunosuppressant: tacrolimus, *Nursing* 24(2):54, 1994.

Jahanansouz F, Kriett JM: Transplantation: a review of immunosuppressive agents, *Crit Care Nurs Q* 15(4):13-22, 1993.

Lancaster L: Immunogenetic basis of tissue and organ transplantation and rejection, *Crit Care Nurs Clin* 4(1):1-24, 1992.

Lange S: Psychosocial, legal, ethical and cultural aspects of organ donation and transplantation, *Crit Care Nurs Clin* 4(1):25-42, 1992.

Martinelli AML: Organ donation: barriers, religious aspects, *AORN J* 58(2): 236-252, 1993.

Olbrisch ME, Levenson JL: Psychosocial assessment of organ transplant candidates, *Psychosomatics* 36(3):236-243, 1995.

Peterson R: An emerging cancer risk: organ transplantation, *Cancer Nurs* 16(6):468-472, 1993.

Smith SL: The cutting edge in organ transplantation, *Crit Care Nurse* 4(suppl):10-11, 26, 1993.

### Specific Organ Transplants

Bartucci MR: Combined kidney and pancreas transplantation, *AACN Clin Iss Crit Care Nurs* 6(1):143-153, 1995.

Benning CR, Smith A: Psychosocial needs of family members of liver transplant patients, *Clin Nurse Specialist* 8(5):28-288, 1994.

Blanford NL: Renal transplantation: a case study of the ideal, *Crit Care Nurse* 3(3):570-584, 1992.

Bratton LB, Griffin LW: A kidney donor's dilemma: the sibling who can donate—but doesn't, *Soc Work Health Care* 20(2):75-96, 1994.

Bronsther O et al: Prioritization and organ distribution for liver transplantation, *JAMA* 271(2):140-143, 1994.

Corley MC et al: Patient and nurse criteria for heart transplant candidacy, *MedSurg Nurs* 4(3):211-215, 1995.

Douglas S, Blixen C, Bartucci MR: Relationship between pretransplant noncompliance posttransplant outcomes in renal transplant recipients, *J Transplant Coord* 6:53-58, 1996.

Fallon L, Lerner L: Renal transplantation, *MedSurg Nur Q* 1(3):27-37, 1993.

Gholson CF, McDonald J, McMillan R: Liver transplantation: when is it indicated and what can be expected afterwards? *Postgrad Med* 97(2):101-104, 107-109, 113-114, 1995.

Grady KL et al: Symptom distress in cardiac transplant patients, *Heart Lung* 21:490-494, 1992.

Hilton BA, Starzomski RD: Family decision making about living related kidney donation, *ANNA J* 21(6):346-355, 1994.

Juneau B: Psychologic and psychosocial aspects of renal transplantation, *Crit Care Nurs Q* 17(4):62-66, 1995.

Smith SL, Ciferni M: Liver transplantation for acute hepatic failure: a review of clinical experience and management, *Am J Crit Care* 2(2):137-144, 1993.

Vargo RL: Bridging to transplant: mechanical support for heart failure, *Crit Care Nurs Clin North Am* 5(4):649-659, 1993.

Wood RP et al: Liver transplantation: the last 10 years, *Surg Clin North Am* 74(5):1133-1154, 1994.

# Illustration Credits

**Chapter 1** 1-2, Source National League for Nursing: *Prism—the NLN Research and Policy Quarterly* 1(1):1, 1993.

**Chapter 2** 2-1, 2-3, From Potter PA, Perry AG: *Fundamentals of nursing: concepts, process, and practice*, ed 4, St Louis, 1997, Mosby; 2-4, From Spector RE: *Cultural diversity in health and illness*, Stamford, Conn, 1996, Appleton & Lange.

**Chapter 3** 3-1, 3-3, 3-4, Source US Dept of Agriculture; 3-2, redrawn from Pender NJ: *Health promotion in nursing practice*, ed 2, East Norwalk, Conn, 1987, Appleton & Lange; 3-5, Report of the Dietary Guidelines Advisory Committee on the Dietary Guidelines for Americans, 1995.

**Chapter 4** 4-1, Source US Bureau of the Census; 4-2, Redrawn from Ebersole P, Hess P: *Toward healthy aging: human needs and nursing response*, ed 5, St Louis, 1998, Mosby; 4-3, Redrawn from Sbrocco T, Weisberg RB, Barlow DH: Sexual dysfunction in older adults: assessment of psychosocial factors, *Sexuality and Disability* 13(3):201, 1995.

**Chapter 6** 6-5, Redrawn from Aguilera DC: *Crisis intervention: theory and methodology*, ed 7, St Louis, 1994, Mosby.

**Chapter 7** 7-6, From Potter PA, Perry AG: *Basic nursing: theory and practice*, ed 3, St Louis, 1995, Mosby; 7-7, Courtesy CLG Photographics, St Louis; 7-8, From Elkin MK, Perry AG, Potter PA: *Nursing interventions and clinical skills*, St Louis, 1996, Mosby; 7-9, From Dittmar SS: *Rehabilitation nursing: process and application*, St Louis, 1989, Mosby.

**Chapter 8** 8-1, Modified from Aguilera DC: *Crisis intervention: theory and methodology*, ed 7, St Louis, 1994, Mosby.

**Chapter 9** 9-1, From Thibodeau GA, Patton KT: *Anatomy and physiology*, ed 3, St Louis, 1996, Mosby; 9-2, from Golstein MF, Rovner BW: Mini mental state examination in clinical practice, *Hospital Practice* 22, 1A:99, 1987; 9-3, From Pfeiffer E: SPMSQ for the assessment of organic brain deficit in elderly patients, *Journal of the American Geriatrics Society* 23:433, 1975.

**Chapter 11** 11-1, From Szarka C, Generosa G, Engstrom P: *Curr Probl Cancer* 15:6, 1994; 11-2, 11-14, Modified from Goodman M: *Cancer: chemotherapy and care*, Part I, Syracuse, NY, Bristol Laboratories; 11-3, Modified from *CA* Jan/Feb 1997; 11-5, 11-11, From Lewis SM, Collier IC, Heitkemper MM: *Medical- surgical nursing: assessment and management of clinical problems*, ed 4, St Louis, 1996, Mosby; 11-12, Adapted from Krakoff IH: *CA* 46(3):134, 1996; 11-13, Modified from Makwell MB, Maher KE: *Semin Oncol Nurs* 8(2):117, 1992; 11-16, courtesy Arrow International, Reading, Penn; 11-17, 11-18, Redrawn from LaRocca JC, Otto SE: *Pocket guide to intravenous therapy*, ed 3, St Louis, 1997, Mosby; 11-19, Courtesy Infusaid Corp, Norwood, Mass.

**Chapter 12** 12-6, Redrawn from Watt-Watson JH, Donovan MI: *Pain management: nursing prospective*, St Louis, 1992, Mosby; 12-7, Adapted from McCaffery M, Beebe A: *Pain: clinical manual for nursing practice*, St Louis, 1989, Mosby.

**Chapter 17** 17-3, 17-7, From Daily EK, Schroeder J: *Techniques in bedside hemodynamic monitoring*, ed 5, St Louis, 1994, Mosby; 17-6, Redrawn from Asheervath I, Blevins D: *Handbook of clinical nursing practice*, Norwalk, Conn, 1986, Appleton & Lange; 17-8, Courtesy The Jobst Institute, Toledo, Ohio.

**Chapter 18** 18-1, 18-2, 18-3, Courtesy University Hospitals of Cleveland, Cleveland, Ohio; 18-4, Courtesy Mt. Sinai Medical Center, Cleveland, Ohio.

**Chapter 19** 19-9, 19-10, From Elkin MK, Perry AG, Potter PA: *Nursing interventions and clinical skills*, St Louis, 1996, Mosby.

**Chapter 20** 20-1 Redrawn from Litwack K: *Post anesthesia care nursing*, ed 2, St Louis, 1995, Mosby; 20-3, Courtesy MetroHealth System, Cleveland, Ohio; 20-4B, redrawn from Canobbio MM: *Cardiovascular disorders*, St Louis, 1990, Mosby.

**Chapter 21** 21-1, Courtesy University of Virginia Medical Center, Charlottesville, Va.

**Chapter 22** 22-1, Redrawn from *Waiting room survival guide*, ed 2, Washington, DC, Foundation for Critical Care, 1993.

**Chapter 23** 23-1, Source National Association for Home Care; 23-2, Source Health Care Financing Administration.

**Chapter 24** 24-5, Redrawn from Thompson JM, Wilson SF: *Health assessment for nursing practice*, St Louis, 1996, Mosby; 24-8, 24-24, 24-25, 24-26, Redrawn from Conover MB: *Understanding electrocardiography: arrhythmias and the 12-lead ECG*, ed 6, St Louis, 1992, Mosby; 24-12, 24-13, From Thibodeau GA, Patton KT: *Anatomy and physiology*, ed 3, St Louis, 1996, Mosby; 24-18, 24-19, 24-20, 24-22, Redrawn from Kinney MR et al: *Comprehensive cardiac care*, ed 7, St Louis, 1991, Mosby; 24-29, Redrawn from Daily EK, Schroeder JS: *Techniques in bedside hemodynamic monitoring*, ed 5, St Louis, 1994, Mosby.

**Chapter 25** 25-2, From Huether SE, McCance KL: *Understanding pathophysiology*, St Louis, 1996, Mosby.

**Chapter 26** 26-1, From Anderson WAD, Scotti TM: *Synopsis of pathology*, ed 10, St Louis, 1980, Mosby; 26-2, From Kissane JM: *Anderson's pathology*, ed 9, St Louis, 1990, Mosby; 26-5, Redrawn from Konstam M et al: *Heart failure: evaluation and care of patients with left ventricular systolic dysfunction*. Clinical Practice Guideline No. 11. AHCPR Publication No. 94-0612. Rockville, MD: Agency for Health Care Policy and Research, Public Health Service, US Dept. of Health and Human Services, June 1994; 26-6, Redrawn from Kissane IM: *Anderson's pathology*, ed 9, St Louis, 1990, Mosby; 26-8, 26-9, 26-10, 26-11, 26-12, 26-13, 26-16, from Beare PG, Myers JL: *Adult health nursing*, ed 3,

St Louis, 1998, Mosby; 26-24B, Courtesy Medtronic, Minneapolis, Minn; 26-14C, Courtesy St Jude Medical, Inc, St Paul, Minn.

**Chapter 27** 27-3, 27-6, 27-7, 27-12, From Lewis SM, Collier IC, Heitkemper MM: *Medical-surgical nursing: assessment and management of clinical problems*, ed 4, St Louis, 1996, Mosby; 27-4, 27-10, From Kamal A, Brockelhurst IC: *Color atlas of geriatric medicine*, ed 2, St Louis, 1991, Mosby; 27-5, Courtesy LoGerfo FW, Boston; 27-11, Redrawn from *AJN*, December 1994; 27-13, From Lofgren KA: *Varicose veins*. In Haimovici H, editor: *Vascular surgery: principles and techniques*, Oxford, 1976, Blackwell Science, Ltd; 27-14, From Belch JJF et al: *Color atlas of peripheral vascular diseases*, ed 2, 1996, Mosby-Wolfe.

**Chapter 28** 28-2, From McCance KL, Huether SE: *Pathophysiology: the biologic basis for disease in adults and children*, ed 3, St Louis, 1998, Mosby; 28-4, 28-5, Redrawn from Yasko J: *Guidelines for cancer care: symptom management*, Reston, Va, 1983, Reston Publishing.

**Chapter 29** 29-6, Redrawn from Yasko J: *Guidelines for cancer care: symptom management*, Reston, Va, 1983, Reston Publishing; Redrawn from Rosenberg SA, Kaplan HS: *Calif Med* 113:23, 1970.

**Chapter 30** 30-2, 30-6, From Beare PG, Myers IL: *Adult health nursing*, ed 3, St Louis, 1998, Mosby; 30-5, From Lewis SM, Collier IC, Heitkemper MM: *Medical-surgical nursing: assessment and management of clinical problems*, ed 4, St Louis, 1996, Mosby; 30-8, Redrawn from Price SA, Wilson LM: *Pathophysiology: clinical concepts of disease processes*, ed 5, St Louis, 1997, Mosby; 30-11, Modified from Talbot L, Meyers-Marquardt M: *Pocket guide to critical care assessment*, ed 3, St Louis, 1997, Mosby; 30-15, Redrawn from Seidel HM et al: *Mosby's guide to physical examination*, ed 3, St Louis, 1995, Mosby; 30-16, Redrawn from Stillwell S, Randall E: *Pocket guide to cardiovascular care*, ed 2, St Louis, 1994, Mosby; 30-18, From Talbot L, Meyers-Marquardt M: *Pocket guide to critical care assessment*, ed 3, St Louis, 1997, Mosby; 30-20, Redrawn from Spearman CB, Sheldon RL, Egan DF: *Egan's fundamentals of respiratory therapy*, ed 5, St Louis, 1990, Mosby.

**Chapter 31** 31-1, 31-2, 31-4, 31-5, 31-7, 31-8, 31-11, 31-14, 31-15, 31-16, 31-17, 31-19, Redrawn from Schuller DE, Schleuning AJ: *Otolaryngology: head and neck surgery*, ed 8, St Louis, 1994, Mosby; 31-9, From Gruber RP, Peck GC: *Rhinoplasty: state of the art*, St Louis, 1993, Mosby; 12-10, From Beare PG, Myers JL: *Adult health nursing*, ed 3, St Louis, 1998, Mosby; 31-23, Courtesy CLG Photographics, St Louis; 31-25, 31-29, From Lewis SM, Collier IC, Heitkemper MM: *Medical-surgical nursing: assessment and management of clinical problems*, ed 4, St Louis, 1998, Mosby; 31-27, 31-28, Redrawn from Kaplow R, Bookbinder M: *Heart Lung* 23(1):59, 1994; 31-30, 31-31, Source The Cleveland Clinic Foundation, Cleveland, Ohio, 1996.

**Chapter 32** 32-2, 32-3, 32-38, 32-32, From Potter PA, Perry AG: *Fundamentals of nursing: concepts, process, and practice*, ed 4, St Louis, 1997, Mosby; 32-4, 32-5, 32-7, Source Centers for Disease Control and Prevention; 32-6, 32-18, 32-19, 32-20, 32-22, 32-23, 32-29, From McCance KL, Huether SE: *Pathophysiology: the biologic basis for disease in adults and children*, ed 3, St Louis, 1998, Mosby; 32-8, From Des Jardins T, Burton GG: *Clinical manifestations and assessment of respiratory disease*, ed 3, St Louis, 1995, Mosby; 32-33, Courtesy DePaul Health Center, St Louis; 32-34, From Sorrentino SA: *Mosby's assisting with patient care*, St Louis, 1998, Mosby; 32-35, Courtesy Ballard Medical Products, Draper, Utah.

**Chapter 33** 33-2, 33-3, 33-5, 33-6, 33-13, Redrawn from McCance KL, Huether SE: *Pathophysiology: the biologic basis for disease in adults and children*, ed 3, St Louis, 1998, Mosby; 33-7, 33-8, Redrawn from Thibodeau GA, Patton KT: *Anatomy and physiology*, ed 3, St Louis, 1996, Mosby.

**Chapter 34** 34-1, From Shapiro LM, Buchalter MB: *Color atlas of hypertension*, London, 1992, Wolfe; 34-4, From Bergman LV and Associates, Cold Spring, NY; 34-5, Courtesy Dr. Jeffrey Hurwitz. From Bingham BJ et al: *Atlas of clinical otolaryngology*, St Louis, 1992, Mosby; 34-6, From Hall R, Evered DC: *Color atlas of endocrinology*, ed 2, St Louis, 1990, Year Book Medical Publishers; 34-8, From Lewis SM, Collier IC, Heitkemper MM: *Medical-surgical nursing: assessment and management of clinical problems*, ed 4, St Louis, 1996, Mosby.

**Chapter 35** 35-1, Data from National Institute of Diabetes and Digestive and Kidney Diseases, National Information Clearinghouse, National Institutes of Health: Diabetes Statistics, NIH Publication No. 96-3926, 1995; 35-10, US Dept of Agriculture; 35-12, 35-13, From Lewis SM, Collier IC, Heitkemper MM: *Medical-surgical nursing: assessment and management of clinical problems*, ed 4, St Louis, 1996, Mosby.

**Chapter 36** 36-1, 36-2, From Thibodeau GA, Patton KT: *Anatomy and physiology*, ed 3, St Louis, 1996, Mosby; 36-3, 36-4, Redrawn from McCance KL, Huether SE: *Pathophysiology:* the biologic basis for disease in adults and children, ed 3, St Louis, 1998, Mosby.

**Chapter 37** 37-1, Courtesy Invacare Corp, Elyria, Ohio; 37-3B, From Lewis SM, Collier IC, Heitkemper MM: *Medical-surgical nursing: assessment and management of clinical problems*, ed 4, St Louis, 1996, Mosby; 37-4, 37-5, 37-7, From Beare PG, Myers JL: *Adult health nursing*, ed 3, St Louis, 1998, Mosby; 37-6, Courtesy Davol Rubber Company, Providence, RI.

**Chapter 38** 38-3, 38-4, From Thibodeau GA, Patton KT: *Anatomy and physiology*, ed 3, St Louis, 1996, Mosby; 38-12, Courtesy Olympus America, Inc, Mehlville, NY.

**Chapter 39** 39-1, 39-4, From Lewis SM, Collier IC, Heitkemper MM: *Medical-surgical nursing: assessment and management of clinical problems*, ed 4, St Louis, 1996, Mosby.

**Chapter 40** 40-12, From Beare PG, Myers JL: *Adult health nursing*, ed 3, St Louis, 1998, Mosby.

**Chapter 41** 41-22, From Elkin MK, Perry AG, Potter PA: *Nursing interventions and clinical skills*, St Louis, 1996, Mosby.

**Chapter 42** 42-3, From Apstein MD, Carey MC: Biliary tract stones and associated diseases. In Stein JH, editor: *Internal medicine*, ed 4, St Louis, 1994, Mosby.

**Chapter 43** 43-4, From Thibodeau GA, Patton KT: *Anatomy and physiology*, ed 3, St Louis, 1996, Mosby; 43-5, Redrawn from Thibodeau GA, Patton KT: *Anatomy and physiology*, ed 3, St Louis, 1996, Mosby.

**Chapter 44** 44-2, From Brundage DJ: *Renal disorders*, St Louis, 1992, Mosby; 44-3, From Kissane JM, editor: *Anderson's pathology*, ed 9, St Louis, 1990, Mosby; 44-7, From Beare PG, Myers JL: *Adult health nursing*, ed 3, St Louis, 1998, Mosby; 44-8, Redrawn from Thompson JM et al: *Mosby's clinical nursing*, ed 4, St Louis, 1997, Mosby.

**Chapter 45** 45-1, Redrawn from McCance KL, Huether SE: *Pathophysiology: the biologic basis for disease in adults and children*, ed 3, St Louis, 1998, Mosby; 45-2, Redrawn from Urden LD et al: *Priorities in critical care nursing*, ed 2, St Louis, 1996, Mosby; 45-7, From Lewis SM, Collier IC, Heitkemper MM: *Medical-surgical nursing: assessment and management of clinical problems*, ed 4, St Louis, 1996, Mosby.

**Chapter 46** 46-1, 46-2, 46-3, 46-5, 46-13, 46-17, From Lowdermilk DL, Perry SE, Bobak IM: *Maternity & women's health care*, ed 6, St Louis, 1997, Mosby; 46-4, 46-6, 46-9, 46-10, 46-11, From Seidel HM et al: *Mosby's guide to physical examination*, ed 3, St Louis, 1995, Mosby; 46-8, 46-12, 46-20, Redrawn from Gillenwater JY et al: *Adult and pediatric urology*, ed 3, St Louis, 1996, Mosby; 46-14, Redrawn and modified from the Nursing Research Consortium on Violence and Abuse, 1991.

**Chapter 47** 47-1, 47-5, From Lewis SM, Collier IC, Heitkemper MM: *Medical-surgical nursing: assessment and management of clinical problems*, ed 4, St Louis, 1996, Mosby; 47-2, 47-16, Redrawn from Herbst A et al: *Comprehensive gynecology*, ed 2, St Louis, 1992, Mosby; 47-3, 47-14, From Beare PG, Myers JL: *Adult health nursing*, ed 3, St Louis, 1998, Mosby; 47-4, Redrawn from Wong DL, Perry SE: *Maternal child nursing care*, St Louis, 1998, Mosby; 47-15, From Seidel HM et al: *Mosby's guide to physical examination*, ed 3, St Louis, 1995, Mosby.

**Chapter 48** 48-1, From Parker SL et al: Cancer statistics, *CA* 46(1):5, 1996; 48-2, Source National Center for Health Statistics; 48-3, 48-4, From Seidel HM et al: *Mosby's guide to physical examination*, ed 3, St Louis, 1995, Mosby; 48-6, From Powell DE, Stelling CB: *The diagnosis and detection of breast disease*, St Louis, 1994, Mosby; 48-10, Courtesy Active, Inc, Kalamazoo, Mich; 48-11, Redrawn from *Reach to recovery exercises after breast surgery*, No. 4668-PS, Atlanta, 1996, American Cancer Society.

**Chapter 49** 49-1, 49-2, 49-4, From Seidel HM et al: *Mosby's guide to physical examination*, ed 3, St Louis, 1995, Mosby; 49-8, From Lowdermilk DL, Perry SE, Bobak IM: *Maternity and women's health care*, ed 6, St Louis, 1997, Mosby; 49-10, From Beare PG, Myers JL: *Adult health nursing*, ed 3, St Louis, 1998, Mosby.

**Chapter 50** 50-1, 50-2, 50-3, 50-4, 50-5, 50-6, Source Centers for Disease Control and Prevention.

**Chapter 51** 51-2, 51-3, 51-4, 51-5, 51-9, 51-10, 51-12, 51-13, 51-14, From Thibodeau GA, Patton KT: *Anatomy and physiology*, ed 3, St Louis, 1996, Mosby; 51-11, From Beare PG, Myers JL: *Adult health nursing*, ed 3, St Louis, 1998, Mosby; 51-16, Scott Bodell.

**Chapter 52** 52-2, Redrawn from Thelan LA et al: *Critical care nursing*, ed 2, St Louis, 1994, Mosby; 52-7, 52-8, 52-10, 52-11, 52-14, Redrawn from Barker E: *Neuroscience nursing*, St Louis, 1994, Mosby.

**Chapter 53** 53-5, 53-10B, 53-12, From Lewis SM, Collier K, Heitkemper MM: *Medical-surgical nursing*, ed 4, St Louis, 1996, Mosby; 53-7, 53-10A, Redrawn from *Recovering from a stroke*, Dallas, 1994, American Heart Association; 53-9, Redrawn from *The One Handed Way*, Dallas, 1994, American Heart Association; 53-15, Redrawn from Rudy E: *Advanced neurologic and neurosurgical nursing*, St Louis, 1984, Mosby; 53-17, From Perkin GD, Hochberg FH, Miller DC: *Atlas of clinical neurology*, ed 2, London, 1993, Gower Medical Publishing.

**Chapter 54** 54-11, Courtesy Zimmer, Inc, Warsaw, Ind; 57-8, From Lewis SM, Collier IC, Heitkemper MM: *Medical-surgical nursing: assessment and management of clinical problems*, ed 4, St Louis, 1996, Mosby; 54-13, Courtesy Acromed Corporation, Cleveland, Ohio; 54-14, Courtesy Kinetic Concepts, San Antonio, Tex; 54-16, Courtesy Sammons Preston, A Bissell Healthcare Company, Bolingbrook, Ill; 54-20, Redrawn from Chipps E, Clanin N, Campbell V: *Neurologic disorders*, St Louis, 1992, Mosby.

**Chapter 55** 55-2, 55-3, Redrawn from Stein HA, Slatt BJ, Stein RM: *Ophthalmic terminology: speller and vocabulary builder*, ed 3, St Louis, 1992, Mosby; 55-4, 55-8, Redrawn from Newell FW: *Ophthalmology: principles and concepts*, ed 8, St Louis, 1996, Mosby; 55-6, From Elkin MK, Perry AG, Potter PA: *Nursing interventions and clinical skills*, St Louis, 1996, Mosby; 55-7, 55-11, From Thompson JM, Wilson SF: *Health assessment for nursing practice*, St Louis, 1996, Mosby; 55-12, From Seidel HM et al: *Mosby's guide to physical examination*, ed 3, St Louis, 1995, Mosby; 55-13, From Ragling EM, Roper-Hall MJ: *Eye injuries*, London, 1986, Gower Medical Publishing; 55-15, From Lewis SM, Collier IC, Heitkemper MM: *Medical-surgical nursing: assessment and management of clinical problems*, ed 4, St Louis, 1996, Mosby.

**Chapter 56** 56-3 Redrawn from Stein HA, Slatt BJ, Stein RM: *The ophthalmic assistant: fundamentals in clinical practice*, St Louis, 1988, Mosby; 56-9, From Sorrentino SA: *Mosby's textbook for nursing assistants*, ed 4, St Louis, 1995, Mosby.

**Chapter 57** 57-1, 57-2, From Seidel HM et al: *Mosby's guide to physical examination*, ed 3, St Louis, 1995, Mosby; 57-3, From Wong DL: *Whaley and Wong's nursing care of infants and children*, ed 5, St Louis, 1995, Mosby; 57-6, 57-7, 57-8, 57-9, 57-11, 57-12, From Sigler BA, Schuring LT: *Ear, nose, and throat disorders*, St Louis, 1994, Mosby.

**Chapter 58** 58-2, Courtesy CLG Photographics, St Louis; 58-6, 58-7, 58-9, Redrawn from Sigler BA, Schuring LT: *Ear, nose, and throat disorders*, St Louis, 1994, Mosby.

**Chapter 59** 59-1, 59-4, 59-9, 59-11, 59-12, Redrawn from Thompson JM et al: *Mosby's clinical nursing*, ed 4, St Louis, 1997, Mosby; 59-2, 59-3, 59-8, From Thibodeau GA, Patton KT: *Anatomy and physiology*, ed 3, St Louis, 1996, Mosby; 59-6, 59-7, From McCance KL, Huether SE: *Pathophysiology: the biologic basis for disease in adults and children*, ed 3, St Louis, 1998, Mosby; 59-13, From Thompson JM et al: *Mosby's clinical nursing*, ed 4, St Louis, 1997, Mosby; 59-14, 59-19, 59-21, 59-22, 59-26, 59-28, From Seidel HM et al: *Mosby's guide to physical examination*, ed 3, St Louis, 1995, Mosby; 59-27, Redrawn from Seidel HM et al: *Mosby's guide to physical examination*, ed 3, St Louis, 1995, Mosby; 59-32, From Mourad LA: *Orthopedic disorders*, St Louis, 1991, Mosby; 59-33, From Gregory B: *Perioperative nursing series: orthopaedic surgery*, St Louis, 1994, Mosby.

**Chapter 60** 60-1, 60-22, Courtesy Rocky Shepheard, New London, Ohio; 60-2, 60-3, From Lewis SM, Collier IC, Heitkemper MM: *Medical-surgical nursing: assessment and management of clinical problems*, ed 4, St Louis, 1996, Mosby; 60-8, Courtesy Acromed Corporation, Cleveland, Ohio; 60-10, Courtesy Smith & Nephew; 60-13, Courtesy Zimmer, Inc, Warsaw, Ind, 60-17, Courtesy Stryker Instruments, Kalamazoo, Mich.

**Chapter 61** 61-1, 61-28, 61-29, 61-45, From McCance KL, Huether SE: *Pathophysiology: the biologic basis for disease in adults and children*, ed 3, St Louis, 1998, Mosby; 61-2, 61-13, 61-15, 61-30, 61-31, 61-41, 61-42, 61-43, From Kamal A, Brockelhurst JC: *Color atlas of geriatric medicine*, ed 2, St Louis, 1991, Mosby; 61-3, From Sorrentino SA: *Assisting with patient care*, St Louis, 1999, Mosby; 61-4, 61-7, 61-8, 61-9, 61-10, 61-11, Courtesy Sammons Preston, A Bissell Healthcare Corp, Bolingbrook, Ill; 61-12, From Doherty M: *Color atlas and text of osteoarthritis*, London, 1994, Wolfe; 61-18, 61-21, Courtesy Zimmer, Inc, Warsaw, Ind; 61-19, Courtesy Depuy Orthopaedics, Inc, Warsaw, Ind; 61-22, Courtesy OrthoLogic Corp, Phoenix, Ariz; 61-23, 61-24, 61-44, From Gregory B: *Perioperative nursing series: orthopaedic surgery*, St Louis, 1994, Mosby; 61-25, From Dieppe P et al: *Arthritis and rheumatism in practice*, London, 1991, Gower; 61-26, Redrawn from Mourad L: *Orthopedic disorders*, St Louis, 1991, Mosby; 61-27, From Lewis SM, Collier IC, Heitkemper MM: *Medical-surgical nursing: assessment and management of clinical problems*, ed 4, St Louis, 1996, Mosby; 61-32, Redrawn from The National Osteoporosis Foundation: *Osteoporosis Report* 13(1):8, Spring 1997, Washington, DC; 61-34, From Beare PG, Myers JL: *Adult health nursing*, ed 3, St Louis, 1998, Mosby; 61-46, 61-47, From Damjanov I, Linder J, editors: *Anderson's pathology*, ed 10, St Louis, 1996, Mosby; 61-48, 61-49, From American Academy of Orthopaedic Surgeons: *Instructional Course Lectures*, vol 33, St Louis, 1984, Mosby.

**Chapter 62** 62-1, Redrawn from Thompson JM et al: *Mosby's clinical nursing*, ed 4, St Louis, 1997, Mosby; 62-2, 62-5, From Seidel HM et al: *Mosby's guide to physical examination*, ed 3, St Louis, 1995, Mosby.

**Chapter 63** 63-1, 63-2, 63-3, 63-4, 63-5, 63-7, 63-10, 63-11, 63-13, 63-14, 63-15, 63-18, From Habif TP: *Clinical dermatology*, ed 3, St Louis, 1996, Mosby; 63-6, Courtesy Antoinette Hood, MD, Dept of Dermatology, University of Indiana School of Medicine, Indianapolis, Ind; 63-8, Courtesy Wellcome Foundation, Ltd; 63-16, Courtesy Gary Monheit, MD, University of Alabama at Birmingham School of Medicine, Birmingham, Ala; 63-17, From Mackie RM: *Skin cancer*, ed 2, St Louis, 1996, Year Book Medical Publishers; 63-19, From Norton D, McLaren R, Exton-Smith AN: *An investigation of geriatric nursing problems in hospital*, Edinburgh, 1975, Churchill-Livingstone; 63-20, Copyright Braden B and Bergstrom N, 1988. Reprinted with permission.

**Chapter 64** 64-4, From Zitelli BJ, Davis HW: *Atlas of pediatric physical diagnosis*, ed 3, St Louis, 1997, Mosby; 64-5, From Lewis SM, Collier IC, Heitkemper MM: *Medical-surgical nursing: assessment and management of clinical problems*, ed 4, St Louis, 1996, Mosby; 64-7, 64-11, 64-13, 64-14, 64-15, Courtesy Burn Center, MetroHealth Medical Center, Cleveland, Ohio; 64-8, Courtesy Burn Awareness Coalition, Encino, Calif; 64-10, From Wong DL: *Whaley and Wong's nursing care of infants and children*, ed 5, St Louis, 1995, Mosby; 64-12, Courtesy Zimmer Inc, Warsaw, Ind.

**Chapter 65** 65-1, 65-3, From Lewis SM, Collier IC, Heitkemper MM: *Medical-surgical nursing: assessment and management of clinical problems*, ed 4, St Louis, 1996, Mosby; 65-2, Redrawn from Huether SE, McCance KL: *Understanding pathophysiology*, St Louis, 1996, Mosby.

**Chapter 66** 66-3, 66-5, 66-7, Redrawn from McCance KL, Huether SE: *Pathophysiology: the biologic basis for disease in adults and children*, ed 3, 1998, Mosby; 66-4, From McCance KL, Huether SE: *Pathophysiology: the biologic basis for disease in adults and children*, ed 3, 1998, Mosby.

**Chapter 67** 67-1, Source Centers for Disease Control and Prevention; 67-2, 67-4, Redrawn from McCance KL, Huether SE: *Pathophysiology: the biologic basis for disease in adults and children*, ed 3, St Louis, 1998, Mosby; 67-5, From Lewis SM, Collier IC, Heitkemper MM: *Medical-surgical nursing: assessment and management of clinical problems*, ed 4, St Louis, 1996, Mosby; 67-6, From Grimes DE, Grimes RM: *AIDS and HIV infection*, St Louis, 1994, Mosby.

**Chapter 68** 68-1, 68-2, Redrawn from Chabalewski FL: Donation and transplantation, *Nursing Curriculum*, 1996; 68-4, 68-5, 68-6, 68-7, 68-8, Redrawn from Smith SL: *Tissue and organ transplantation: implications for professional nursing practice*, St Louis, 1990, Mosby.

# Index

## C

## D

## E

## G

## I

## N

## S

## NURSING CARE PLAN



## CLINICAL PATHWAY



## PATIENT/FAMILY TEACHING

## PATIENT/FAMILY TEACHING—cont'd



## GUIDELINES FOR CARE